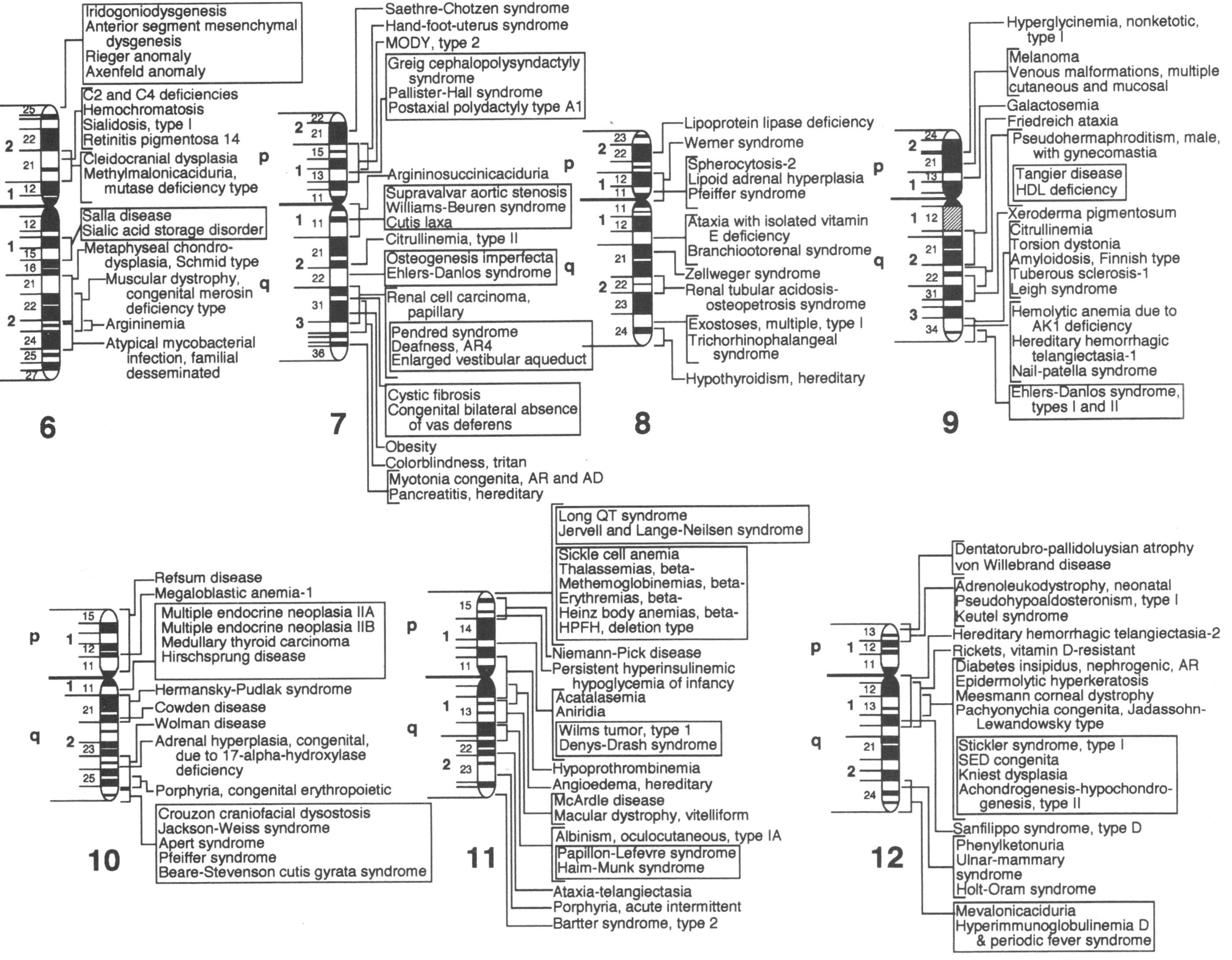

Iridogoniodysgenesis
Anterior segment mesenchymal dysgenesis
Rieger anomaly
Axenfeld anomaly
C2 and C4 deficiencies
Hemochromatosis
Sialidosis, type I
Retinitis pigmentosa 14
Cleidocranial dysplasia
Methylmalonicaciduria, mutase deficiency type
Salla disease
Sialic acid storage disorder
Metaphyseal chondrodysplasia, Schmid type
Muscular dystrophy, congenital merosin deficiency type
Argininemia
Atypical mycobacterial infection, familial desseminated
6
Saethre-Chotzen syndrome
Hand-foot-uterus syndrome
MODY, type 2
Greig cephalopolysyndactyly syndrome
Pallister-Hall syndrome
Postaxial polydactyly type A1
Argininosuccinicaciduria
Supravalvar aortic stenosis
Williams-Beuren syndrome
Cutis laxa
Citrullinemia, type II
Osteogenesis imperfecta
Ehlers-Danlos syndrome
Renal cell carcinoma, papillary
Pendred syndrome
Deafness, AR4
Enlarged vestibular aqueduct
Cystic fibrosis
Congenital bilateral absence of vas deferens
Obesity
Colorblindness, tritan
Myotonia congenita, AR and AD
Pancreatitis, hereditary
7
Lipoprotein lipase deficiency
Werner syndrome
Spherocytosis-2
Lipoid adrenal hyperplasia
Pfeiffer syndrome
Ataxia with isolated vitamin E deficiency
Branchiootorenal syndrome
Zellweger syndrome
Renal tubular acidosis-osteopetrosis syndrome
Exostoses, multiple, type I
Trichorhinophalangeal syndrome
Hypothyroidism, hereditary
8
Hyperglycinemia, nonketotic, type I
Melanoma
Venous malformations, multiple cutaneous and mucosal
Galactosemia
Friedreich ataxia
Pseudohermaphroditism, male, with gynecomastia
Tangier disease
HDL deficiency
Xeroderma pigmentosum
Citrullinemia
Torsion dystonia
Amyloidosis, Finnish type
Tuberous sclerosis-1
Leigh syndrome
Hemolytic anemia due to AK1 deficiency
Hereditary hemorrhagic telangiectasia-1
Nail-patella syndrome
Ehlers-Danlos syndrome, types I and II
9
Refsum disease
Megaloblastic anemia-1
Multiple endocrine neoplasia IIA
Multiple endocrine neoplasia IIB
Medullary thyroid carcinoma
Hirschsprung disease
Hermansky-Pudlak syndrome
Cowden disease
Wolman disease
Adrenal hyperplasia, congenital, due to 17-alpha-hydroxylase deficiency
Porphyria, congenital erythropoietic
Crouzon craniofacial dysostosis
Jackson-Weiss syndrome
Apert syndrome
Pfeiffer syndrome
Beare-Stevenson cutis gyrata syndrome
10
Long QT syndrome
Jervell and Lange-Neilsen syndrome
Sickle cell anemia
Thalassemias, beta-
Methemoglobinemias, beta-
Erythremias, beta-
Heinz body anemias, beta-
HPFH, deletion type
Niemann-Pick disease
Persistent hyperinsulinemic hypoglycemia of infancy
Acatalasemia
Aniridia
Wilms tumor, type 1
Denys-Drash syndrome
Hypoprothrombinemia
Angioedema, hereditary
McArdle disease
Macular dystrophy, vitelliform
Albinism, oculocutaneous, type IA
Papillon-Lefevre syndrome
Haim-Munk syndrome
Ataxia-telangiectasia
Porphyria, acute intermittent
Bartter syndrome, type 2
11
Dentatorubro-pallidoluysian atrophy
von Willebrand disease
Adrenoleukodystrophy, neonatal
Pseudohypoaldosteronism, type I
Keutel syndrome
Hereditary hemorrhagic telangiectasia-2
Rickets, vitamin D-resistant
Diabetes insipidus, nephrogenic, AR
Epidermolytic hyperkeratosis
Meesmann corneal dystrophy
Pachyonychia congenita, Jadassohn-Lewandowsky type
Stickler syndrome, type I
SED congenita
Kniest dysplasia
Achondrogenesis-hypochondrogenesis, type II
Sanfilippo syndrome, type D
Phenylketonuria
Ulnar-mammary syndrome
Holt-Oram syndrome
Mevalonicaciduria
Hyperimmunoglobulinemia D & periodic fever syndrome
12

The Metabolic & Molecular Bases of Inherited Disease

eighth edition

EDITORS

Charles R. Scriver, M.D.C.M.
Alva Professor of Human Genetics, Professor of Pediatrics, Faculty of Medicine, Professor of Biology, Faculty of Science, McGill University; Director (retired), deBelle Laboratory of Biochemical Genetics and Biochemical Genetics Clinical Unit, McGill University–Montreal Children's Hospital Research Institute, McGill University Health Centre, Montreal, Quebec, Canada

Arthur L. Beaudet, M.D.
Henry and Emma Meyer Professor and Chair, Department of Molecular and Human Genetics, Professor, Departments of Pediatrics and Molecular and Cellular Biology, Baylor College of Medicine, Houston, Texas

William S. Sly, M.D.
Alice A. Doisy Professor of Biochemistry and Molecular Biology, Chair, Edward A. Doisy Department of Biochemistry and Molecular Biology, Professor of Pediatrics, St. Louis University School of Medicine, St. Louis, Missouri

David Valle, M.D.
Professor of Pediatrics and Molecular Biology, Howard Hughes Medical Institute, McKusick-Nathans Institute of Genetic Medicine. The Johns Hopkins University School of Medicine, Baltimore, Maryland

ASSOCIATE EDITORS

Barton Childs, M.D.
Emeritus Professor of Pediatrics, The Johns Hopkins University School of Medicine, Baltimore, Maryland

Kenneth W. Kinzler, Ph.D.
Professor of Oncology, The Johns Hopkins University School of Medicine, Baltimore, Maryland

Bert Vogelstein, M.D.
Investigator, Howard Hughes Medical Institute, Clayton Professor of Oncology and Pathology, The Johns Hopkins University School of Medicine, Baltimore, Maryland

The Metabolic & Molecular Bases of Inherited Disease

eighth edition

VOLUME II

EDITORS

Charles R. Scriver, M.D.C.M.
Arthur L. Beaudet, M.D.
William S. Sly, M.D.
David Valle, M.D.

ASSOCIATE EDITORS

Barton Childs, M.D.
Kenneth W. Kinzler, Ph.D.
Bert Vogelstein, M.D.

McGraw-Hill
Medical Publishing Division

New York St. Louis San Francisco Auckland Bogotá Caracas Lisbon London Madrid Mexico City Milan Montreal New Delhi San Juan Singapore Sydney Tokyo Toronto

McGraw-Hill
A Division of The **McGraw-Hill** *Companies*

The Metabolic and Molecular Bases of Inherited Disease, 8th Edition

1234567890 KGPKGP 09876543210

ISBNs
0-07-913035-6
0-07-136319-X (vol. 1)
0-07-136320-3 (vol. 2)
0-07-136321-1 (vol. 3)
0-07-136322-X (vol. 4)
This book was set in Times Roman by Progressive Information Technologies, Inc.
The editors were Martin J. Wonsiewicz, Susan R. Noujaim, and Peter J. Boyle;
the production supervisor was Richard Ruzycka; the text designer was José R. Fonfrias;
the cover designer was Elizabeth Schmitz; Barbara Littlewood prepared the index.
Quebecor Printing/Kingsport was printer and binder.
This book is printed on acid-free paper.

Library of Congress Cataloging-in-Publication Data

The metabolic and molecular bases of inherited disease / editors,
Charles R. Scriver . . . [et al.].–8th ed.
p.; cm.
Includes bibliographical references and index.
ISBN 0-07-913035-6 (set)
1. Metabolism, Inborn errors of 2. Medical genetics. 3. Pathology, Molecular. I. Scriver, Charles R.
[DNLM: 1. Hereditary Diseases. 2. Metabolic Diseases. 3. Metabolism, Inborn Errors.
WD 200 M5865 2001]
RC627.8 . M47 2001
616′.042–dc21

00-060957

INTERNATIONAL EDITION
ISBNs 0-07-116336-0
0-07-118833-9 (vol. 1)
0-07-118834-7 (vol. 2)
0-07-118835-5 (vol. 3)
0-07-118836-3 (vol. 4)

Notice

CONTENTS

VOLUME I

PART 1
INTRODUCTION

PART 2
PERSPECTIVES

PART 5
CHROMOSOMES

PART 6
DIAGNOSTIC APPROACHES

PART 7
CARBOHYDRATES

VOLUME II

PART 8

AMINO ACIDS

PART 9
ORGANIC ACIDS

PART 10
DISORDERS OF MITOCHONDRIAL FUNCTION

PART 11
PURINES AND PYRIMIDINES

PART 12
LIPIDS

PART 17
VITAMINS

PART 18
HORMONES

PART 19
BLOOD

PART 20
IMMUNE AND DEFENSE SYSTEMS

PART 21
MEMBRANE TRANSPORT DISORDERS

VOLUME IV

PART 22
CONNECTIVE TISSUE

PART 23
CARDIOVASCULAR SYSTEM

PART 24
KIDNEY

PART 25
MUSCLE

PART 26
LUNG

PART 27
SKIN

PART 28
NEUROGENETICS

PART 29
EYE

PART 30
MULTISYSTEM INBORN ERRORS OF DEVELOPMENT

CONTRIBUTORS

Lauri A. Aaltonen, M.D. [34]*
Senior Fellow, Academy of Finland, Dept. of Medical Genetics, Haartman Institute, Finland
Lauri.aaltonen@helsinki.fi

Frank Accurso, M.D. [201]
Dept. of Pediatrics, University of Colorado School of Medicine; Director, The Mike McMorris Cystic Fibrosis Center, The Children's Hospital, Denver, Colorado
accurso.frank@tchden.org

Milton B. Adesnik, Ph.D. [16]
Professor of Cell Biology, Dept. of Cell Biology, New York University School of Medicine, New York, New York
Adesnm01@popmail.med.nyu.edu

Björn A. Afzelius, M.D. [187]
Professor Emeritus, Wenner-Gren Institute, Stockholm University, Arrhenius Laboratories, Stockholm, Sweden
Bjorn.Afzelius@zub.su.se

Naji Al-Dosari, M.D. [57]
Duke University, Durham, North Carolina
naji@acpub.duke

Rando L. Allikmets, Ph.D. [243]
Dept. of Ophthalmology, Columbia University, New York, New York
rla22@columbia.edu

Robert J. Alpern, M.D. [195]
Dean, Southwestern Medical School, Ruth W. and Milton P. Levy, Sr., Chair in Molecular Nephrology, Atticus James Gill Chair in Medical Science, Div. of Nephrology, UT Southwestern Medical Center at Dallas, Dallas, Texas
Robert.alpern@email.swmed.edu

Wallace L.M. Alward, M.D. [242]
Dept. of Opthalmology and Visual Sciences, University of Iowa College of Medicine, Iowa City, Iowa
wallace-alward@uiowa.edu

Joanna S. Amberger, M.D. [1]
McKusick-Nathans Institute of Genetic Medicine, Johns Hopkins University School of Medicine, Baltimore, Maryland
joanna@peas.welch.jhu.edu

Donald C. Anderson, M.D. [188]
Professor, Dept. of Pediatrics, Baylor College of Medicine, Vice President and Chief Scientific Officer, Pharmacia & Upjohn, Kalamazoo, Michigan
donald.c.anderson@pnu.com

Karl E. Anderson, M.D. [124]
Professor of Preventive Medicine and Community Health, Internal Medicine, and Pharmacology and Toxicology, Dept. of Preventive Medicine and Community Health, University of Texas Medical Branch, Galveston, Texas
karl.anderson@utmb.edu

Mary E. Anderson, Ph.D. [96]
Assistant Professor, Dept. of Microbiology and Molecular Cell Sciences, University of Memphis, Memphis, Tennessee
Mary@mmcs.memphis.edu

Generoso Andria, M.D. [152]
Professor of Pediatrics, Department of Pediatrics, Federico II University, Naples, Italy

Stylianos E. Antonarakis, M.D., D.Sc. [13, 172]
Professor and Director of Medical Genetics, Div. of Medical Genetics, University of Geneva Medical School, Geneva, Switzerland
stylianos.antonarakis@medicine.unige.ch

Irwin M. Arias, M.D. [125]
Professor and Chairman, Dept. of Physiology, Tufts University, Boston, Massachusetts
irwin.arias@tufts.edu

Gerd Assmann, M.D., F.R.C.P [118, 122, 142]
Professor of Medicine, Director, Institute for Clinical Chemistry and Lab Medicine, Director, Institute for Arteriosclerosis Research, Westfälische Wilhelms-University, Münster, Germany
assmann@uni-muenster.de

Arleen D. Auerbach, Ph.D. [31]
Associate Professor, Laboratory of Human Genetics and Hematology, The Rockefeller University, New York, New York
auerbac@rockvax.rockefeller.edu

Perti Aula, M.D. [141, 200]
Professor of Medical Genetics, Medical Genetics Dept., University of Helsinko, Haartman Institute, Haartmaninkatu, Finland
Perti.aula@helsinki.fi

Salvatore Auricchio, M.D. [75]
Professor, Dept. di Pediatria, Università Federico II Napoli, Italy

Andrea Ballabio, M.D. [149, 166, 225]
Professor of Medical Genetics, Second University of Naples, Director, Telethon Institute of Genetics and Medicine (TIGEM), Naples, Italy
ballabio@tigem.it

Peter G. Barth [130]
Professor of Pediatric Neurology, University of Amsterdam Academic Medical Centre, Emma Children's Hospital and Clinical Chemistry, Amsterdam, The Netherlands
p.g.barth@amc.uva.nl

Stephen B. Baylin, M.D. [58]
Professor of Oncology and Medicine, Associate Director for Research, The Johns Hopkins Oncology Center, Baltimore, Maryland
sbaylin@jhmi.edu

Philip A. Beachy, M.D. [205]
Professor of Molecular Biology and Genetics, Howard Hughes Medical Institute, The Johns Hopkins University School of Medicine, Baltimore, Maryland
pbeachy@jhmi.edu

Arthur L. Beaudet, M.D. [1, 229]
Henry and Emma Meyer Professor and Chair, Dept. of Molecular and Human Genetics, Professor, Depts. of Pediatrics and Molecular and Cellular Biology, Baylor College of Medicine, Houston, Texas
abeaudet@bcm.tmc.edu

Michael A. Becker, M.D. [106]
Professor of Medicine
Dept. of Medicine University of Chicago School of Medicine, Chicago, Illinois
mbecker@medicine.bsd.uchicago.edu

*The numbers in brackets following each contributor's name refer to chapters written or co-written by that contributor.

David M.O. Becroft, M.D. [113]
Dept. of Obstetrics and Gynecology, University of Auckland School of Medicine, Auckland, New Zealand
David.Genevieve.Becroft@extra.co.nz

Lenore K. Beitel, Ph.D. [161]
Research Scientist, Lady Davis Institute for Medical Research, Sir M.B. Davis–Jewish General Hospital, Montreal, Quebec, Canada
mdtm001@musica.mcgill.ca

John W. Belmont, M.D., Ph.D. [185]
Dept. of Molecular and Human Genetics, Baylor College of Medicine, Houston, Texas
jbelmont@bcm.tmc.edu

Merrill D. Benson, M.D. [209]
Professor of Medicine, Pathology and Medical Genetics, Dept. of Medical and Molecular Genetics, Indiana University School of Medicine, Indianapolis, Indiana
mdbenson@iupui.edu

Wolfgang Berger, M.D. [239]
Max-Planck-Institute for Molecular Genetics, Berlin, Germany
berger@molgen@mpg.de

Michel Bergeron, M.D. [196]
Professor of Physiology, Dept. of Physiology, Université de Montréal, Montreal, Quebec, Canada
Bergermi@ere.umontreal.ca

Sten Erik Bergstrom, M.D. [187]
Dept. of Pediatrics, Huddinge University Hospital, Stockholm, Sweden

Ernest Beutler, M.D. [127, 146, 182]
Chairman, Dept. of Molecular and Experimental Medicine, Scripps Clinic and Research Foundation, La Jolla, California
beutler@scripps.edu

Daniel G. Bichet, M.D. [163]
Professor of Medicine, University of Montreal, Director, Clinical Research Unit, Hopital du Sacre-Coeur de Montreal, Montreal, Quebec, Canada
D-Binette@crhsc.umontreal.ca

Sandra H. Bigner, M.D. [57]
Professor of Pathology, Dept. of Pathology, Duke University Medical Center, Durham, North Carolina
Bigne002@mc.duke.edu

David F. Bishop, Ph.D. [124]
Professor of Human Genetics, Dept. of Human Genetics, Mount Sinai School of Medicine, New York, New York
David.bishop@mssm.edu

Ingemar Björkhem, M.D., Ph.D. [123]
Professor and Head Physician, Dept. of Medical Laboratory Sciences and Technology, Division of Clinical Chemistry, Karolinska Institutet, Huddinge University Hospital, Huddinge, Sweden
Ingemar.Bjorkhem@chemlab.hs.sll.se

E. Joan Blanchette-Mackie, M.D. [145]
Chief, Sect. of Lipid Cell Biology, Laboratory of Cell Biochemistry and Biology, National Institute of Diabetes and Digestive and Kidney Diseases, Bethesda, Maryland
eb78u@nih.gov

Nenad Blau, M.D., Ph.D. [78]
Associate Professor, Div. of Clinical Chemistry and Biochemistry, Dept. of Pediatrics, University Children's Hospital, Zurich, Switzerland
blau@access.unizh.ch

Kirsten Muri Boberg, M.D., Ph.D. [123]
Dept. of Clinical Chemistry, Rikshospitalet, Oslo, Norway
kirsten.boberg@online.no

Sir Walter F. Bodmer, M.D., Ph.D., F.R.C.Path, F.R.S. [11]
Imperial Cancer Research Fund Laboratories, University of Oxford, Institute of Molecular Medicine, John Radcliffe Hospital, Oxford, United Kingdom
walter.bodmer@hertford.ox.ac.uk

C. Richard Boland, M.D. [32]
Professor of Medicine; Chief, Gastroenterology, University of California, San Diego, La Jolla, California
CRBOLAND@UCSD.EDU

Dirk Bootsma, M.D. [28]
Dept. of Cell Biology and Genetics, Erasmus University, Rotterdam, The Netherlands
Bootsma@gen.fgg.eur.nl

Thomas H. Bothwell, M.D., D.Sc. [127]
Emeritus Professor of Medicine, Honorary Professorial Research Fellow, Faculty of Medicine, University of Witwatersrand, Medical School, Johannesburg, South Africa
014jozo@chiron.wits.ac.za

G. Steven Bova, M.D. [56]
Assistant Professor, Depts. of Pathology, Urology and Oncology, Johns Hopkins Hospital, Pelican Laboratory, Baltimore, Maryland
gbov@jhmi.edu

Bernard Brais, M.D., MPhil, Ph.D. [216]
Direction de L'IREP, Centre de recherche du CHUM, Hopital Notre-Dame, Montreal, Quebec, Canada

David S. Bredt, M.D., Ph.D. [168]
Associate Professor of Physiology, Dept. of Physiology, University of California, San Francisco
bredt@phy.ucsf.edu

Jan L. Breslow, M.D. [121]
Frederick Henry Leonhardt Professor, Director, Laboratory of Biochemical Genetics and Metabolism, The Rockefeller University, New York, New York
breslow@rockvax.rockefeller.edu

Martijn H. Breuning, M.D. [248]
Dept. of Clinical Genetics, Centre for Human and Clinical Genetics, Leiden University Medical Centre, Leiden, The Netherlands M.H.Breuning@kgc.azl.nl

H. Bryan Brewer, Jr., M.D. [118, 122]
Chief, Molecular Disease Branch, National Heart, Lung, and Blood Institute, Bethesda, Maryland
bryan@mdb.nhlbi.nih.gov

Garrett M. Brodeur, M.D. [21, 60]
Div. of Oncology, Children's Hospital of Philadelphia, Philadelphia, Pennsylvania
brodeur@email.chop.edu

Dieter Brömme, Ph.D. [137]
Associate Professor of Human Genetics, Mount Sinai School of Medicine, New York, New York
brommd01@doc.mssm.edu

Michael D. Brown [105]
Assistant Professor, The Center for Molecular Medicine, Emory University School of Medicine, Atlanta, Georgia
mdbrown@gen.emory.edu

Michael S. Brown, M.D. [120]
Regental Professor, Johnson Center for Molecular Genetics, University of Texas Southwestern Medical Center, Dallas, Texas
mike.brown@utsouthwestern.edu

George J. Broze, Jr., M.D. [175]
Professor of Medicine, Cell Biology and Physiology, Washington University School of Medicine, Barnes-Jewish Hospital at Washington University, St. Louis, Missouri
gbroze@im.wustl.edu

John D. Brunzell, M.D. [117]
Professor of Medicine, Program Director, General Clinical Research Center, Dept. of Medicine, University of Washington School of Medicine, Seattle, Washington
brunzell@u.washington.edu

Saul W. Brusilow, M.D. [85]
Professor of Pediatrics Emeritus, The Johns Hopkins Hospital, Baltimore, Maryland
sbru@jhmi.edu

Manuel Buchwald, O.C., Ph.D., F.R.S.C. [31]
Professor, Molecular and Medical Genetics, University of Toronto, Chief of Research and Director, Research Institute, Hospital for Sick Children, Toronto, Ontario, Canada
Manuel.Buchwald@sickkids.on.ca

Peter H. Byers, M.D. [205]
Professor, Dept. of Pathology and Medicine, Dept. of Pathology, University of Washington, Seattle, Washington
pbyers@u.washington.edu

Daniel P Cahill, M.D., Ph.D. [22]
Dept. of Oncology, The Johns Hopkins University School of Medicine, Baltimore, Maryland

Paul Cairns, M.D. [54]
Fox Chase Cancer Center, Philadelphia, Pennsylvania 19111

Giovanna Camerino, Ph.D. [62]
Professor Biologia Generale E Genetica Medica, Universitá Di Pavia, Pavia, Italy
camerino@unipv.it

Hubert Carchon, Ph.D. [74]
Assistant Professor, University of Leuven, Centre for Metabolic Disease, Leuven, Belgium
hubert.carchon@med.kuleuven.ac.be

Eugene D. Carstea, M.D. [145]
Director, Saccomanno Research Institute, St. Mary's Hospital and Medical Center, Grand Junction, Colorado
gcarstea@stmarygj.com

Webster K. Cavenee, M.D. [36]
Director, Ludwig Institute for Cancer Research, University of California, San Diego, La Jolla, California

Aravinda Chakravarti, Ph.D. [251]
Henry J. Knott Professor and Director, McKusick-Nathans Institute of Genetic Medicine, Johns Hopkins University School of Medicine, Baltimore, Maryland
aravinda@jhmi.edu

Arlene B. Chapman, M.D. [215]
Associate Professor of Medicine, Director, Hypertension and Renal Disease Research Center, Emory University School of Medicine, Atlanta, Georgia
arlene_chapman@emory.org

Robert W. Charlton, M.D. [127]
Emeritus Professor, University of Witwatersrand Medical School, Johannesburg, South Africa
014jozo@chiron.wits.ac.za

Christiane Charpentier, Ph.D. [66]
Biologist, INSERM-Paris France, Metabolic/Diabetes Unit-Dept. of Pediatrics, Hopital Necker Enfants Malades, Paris, France
Elisabeth.saudubray@nck.ap_hop_paris.fr

Yuan-Tsong Chen, M.D., Ph.D. [71]
Professor of Pediatrics and Genetics, Chief, Div. of Medical Genetics, Duke University Medical Center, Durham, North Carolina
chen0010@mc.duke.edu

Russell W. Chesney, M.D. [194]
Le Bonheur Professor and Chair, Dept. of Pediatrics, Le Bonheur Children's Medical Center, University of Tennessee, Memphis, Tennessee
rchesney@utmem.edu

Barton Childs, M.D. [2, 3, 4]
Emeritus Professor of Pediatrics, The Johns Hopkins University School of Medicine, Baltimore, Maryland

Kathleen R. Cho, M.D. [53]
Associate Professor, Depts. of Pathology and Internal Medicine, University of Michigan Medical School, Ann Arbor, Michigan
kathcho@umich.edu

Streamson C. Chua, Jr. [157]
Dept. of Medicine, Columbia University College of Physicians and Surgeons, New York, New York

David T. Chuang, Ph.D. [87]
Associate Professor, Dept. of Biochemistry, University of Texas Southwestern Medical Center, Dallas, Texas
david.chuang@utsouthwestern.edu

Dominic W. Chung, Ph.D. [171]
Dept. of Biochemistry School of Medicine, University of Washington, Seattle, Washington
chung@u.washington.edu

Carmen Cifuentes-Diaz, Ph.D. [231]
Laboratoire de Neurogénétique Molécularie, INSERM, GENOPOLE, Evry, France
c.diaz@genopole.inserm.fr

James E. Cleaver, M.D. [28]
Dept. of Dermatology, University of California at San Francisco Cancer Center, San Francisco, California
jcleaver@cc.ucsf.edu

J.B. Clegg [181]
Institute of Molecular Medicine, John Radcliffe Hospital, Oxford, United Kingdom

Bruce E. Clurman, M.D. [23]
Assistant Professor, Fred Hutchinson Cancer Research Center, Seattle, Washington
bclurman@fhcrc.org

Anne-Marie Codori, Ph.D. [49]
Dept. of Psychiatry and Behavioral Sciences, The Johns Hopkins University School of Medicine, Baltimore, Maryland

Joy D. Cogan, M.D. [162]
Research Assistant Professor of Pediatric Genetics, Div. of Genetics, Vanderbilt University School of Medicine, Nashville, Tennessee
joy.cogan@mcmail.vanderbilt.edu

Francis S. Collins, M.D., Ph.D. [39]
National Human Genome Research Institute, Bethesda, Maryland
Fc23@nih.gov

Mary Ellen Conley, M.D. [184]
St. Jude Children's Research Hospital, University of Tennessee School of Medicine, Memphis, Tennessee
maryellen.conley@stjude.org

David N. Cooper, Ph.D. [13]
Professor of Human Molecular Genetics, Institute of Medical Genetics, University of Wales College of Medicine, Cardiff, Wales, United Kingdom
cooperdn@cardiff.ac.uk

Valerie Cormier-Daire, M.D., Ph.D. [99]
Dept. of Medical Genetics, Hopital Necker Enfants Malades, Paris, France
cormier@necker.fr

Richard G.H. Cotton, Ph.D., D.Sc. [1, 78]
Professor, Mutation Research Centre, Director, Mutation Research Centre, St. Vincent's Hospital, Fitzroy, Victoria, Australia
cotton@ariel.ucs.unimelb.edu.au

Fergus J. Couch, M.D. [47]
Assistant Professor, Dept. of Laboratory Medicine and Pathology, Mayo Foundation and Clinic, Rochester, Minnesota
Couch.Fergus@mayo.edu

Diane Wilson Cox, M.D., Ph.D. [219]
Professor and Chair, Dept. of Medical Genetics, Genetics Sect. Head, Child Health, Capital Health Authority, Dept. of Medical Genetics, University of Alberta, Edmonton, Alberta, Canada
diane.cox@ualberta.ca

Rody P. Cox, M.D., Ph.D. [86]
Professor of Internal Medicine, Dept. of Internal Medicine, University of Texas, Southwestern Medical Center, Attending Physician, Parkland Memorial Hospital and St. Paul University Hospital, Dallas, Texas
rcox@mednet.swmed.edu

William J. Craigen, M.D., Ph.D. [14]
Dept. of Molecular and Human Genetics, Baylor College of Medicine, Houston, Texas
wcraigen@bcm.tmc.edu

Donnell J. Creel, Ph.D. [220]
Research Professor, Moran Eye Center, University of Utah School of Medicine, Salt Lake City, Utah
Donnell.creel@hsc.utah.edu

Frans P.M. Cremers, Ph.D. [236]
Associate Professor, Dept. of Human Genetics University Medical Center Nymegen, Nymegen, The Netherlands
F.Cremers@Antrg.azn.nl

Valeria Cizewski Culotta, Ph.D. [126]
Associate Professor, Dept. of Environmental Health Sciences, Johns Hopkins University, School of Hygiene and Public Health, Baltimore, Maryland
vculotta@JHSPH.edu

Garry R. Cutting, M.D. [201]
Professor of Pediatrics and Medicine, McKusick-Nathan Institute of Genetic Medicine, The Johns Hopkins University, Baltimore, Maryland
gcutting@jhmi.edu

Christopher J. Danpure, Ph.D. [133]
Professor of Molecular Cell Biology, MRC Laboratory for Molecular Cell Biology, University College London, London, United Kingdom
c.danpure@ucl.ac.uk

Earl W. Davie, Ph.D. [169]
Dept. of Biochemistry School of Medicine, University of Washington, Seattle, Washington

Alessandra d'Azzo, Ph.D. [152]
Professor, Member, Dept. of Genetics, St. Jude Children's Research Hospital, Memphis, Tennessee
sandra.dazzo@stjude.org

Samir S. Deeb, Ph.D. [117, 238]
Research Professor of Medicine and Genetics, Dept. of Genetics, University of Washington School of Medicine, Seattle, Washington
deeb@genetics.washington.edu

Robert J. Desnick, Ph.D., M.D. [124, 137, 139, 144, 150]
Professor and Chairman, Human Genetics, Professor of Pediatrics; Attending Physician, Dept. of Human Genetics, Mount Sinai School of Medicine, New York, New York
rjdesnick@mcvax.mssm.edu

Harry C. Dietz, M.D. [206]
Associate Investigator, Howard Hughes Medical Institute, Professor, Dept. of Pediatrics, Medicine and Molecular Biology and Genetics, McKusick-Nathan Institute of Genetic Medicine, Johns Hopkins University School of Medicine, Baltimore, Maryland
hdietz@jhmi.edu

Mary C. Dinauer, M.D., Ph.D. [189]
Novz Letzter Professor of Pediatrics and Medical and Molecular Genetics, Riley Hospital for Children, Indiana University School of Medicine, Director, Herman B. Wells Center for Pediatric Research, Indianapolis, Indiana
mdinauer@iupui.edu

Jiahuan Ding, M.D., Ph.D. [101]
Director, Molecular Diagnostics, Senior Scientist, Associate Professor, Baylor University, Waco, Texas, Institute of Metabolic Disease, Baylor University Medical Center, Dallas, Texas
j.ding@baylordallas.edu

Michael J. Dixon, M.D. [246]
Professor of Dental Genetics, School of Biological Sciences, Dept. of Dental Medicine and Surgery, University of Manchester, Manchester, United Kingdom
mdixon@fs1.scg.man.ac.uk

Patricia A. Donohoue, M.D. [159]
Associate Professor, Dept. of Pediatrics, Div. of Endocrinology, University of Iowa Hospitals, Dept. of Pediatrics, The Children's Hospital of Iowa, Iowa City, Iowa
patricia-donohoue@uiowa.edu

Thaddeus P. Dryja, M.D. [235]
Professor of Ophthalmology, Harvard Medical School, Dept. of Ophthalmology, Massachusetts Eye and Ear Infirmary, Boston, Massachusetts
dryja@helix.mgh.harvard.edu

Louis Dubeau, M.D., Ph.D. [51]
Professor, Dept. of Pathology, USC/Norris Comprehensive Cancer Center, Keck School of Medicine of USC, Los Angeles, California
ldubeau@hsc.usc.edu

Thomas D. DuBose, Jr., M.D. [195]
Peter T. Bohan Professor and Chair, Dept. of Internal Medicine, Professor of Molecular and Integrative Physiology, University of Kansas School of Medicine, Kansas City, Kansas
tdubose@kumc.edu

Jacques E. Dumont, M.D., Ph.D. [158]
Professor of Biochemistry, Head, Institut de Recherche interdisciplinaire, Faculté de Medecine, Université Libre de Bruxelles, Brussels, Belgium
jedumont@ulb.ac.be

Marinus Duran, M.D. [128]
Academic Medical Center, Laboratory Genetic Metabolic Diseases, University of Amsterdam, Amsterdam, The Netherlands
m.duram@amc.uva.nl

Michael J. Econs, M.D. [197]
Associate Professor of Medicine and Medical and Molecular Genetics, Indiana University School of Medicine, Indianapolis, Indiana
mecons@iupui.edu

Lora Hedrick Ellenson, M.D. [52]
Associate Professor and Director, Div. of Gynecologic Pathology, Weill Medical College of Cornell University, New York, New York
lhellens@med.cornell.edu

Nathan A. Ellis, M.D. [59]
Associate Member, Dept. of Human Genetics, Memorial Sloan-Kettering Cancer Center, New York, New York
n-ellis@ski.mskcc.org

Lynne W. Elmore, Ph.D. [59]
Research Associate, Dept. of Pathology, School of Medicine, Virginia Commonwealth University, Richmond, Virginia
LWElmore@hsc.vcu.edu

Charis Eng, M.D., Ph.D. [45]
Assoc. Professor of Medicine and Human Cancer Genetics, The Ohio State University; Hon. Fellow, CRC, Human Cancer Genetics Research Group, Univ. of Cambridge, United Kingdom; Director, Clinical Cancer Genetics Program, Ohio State University, Columbus, Ohio
Eng-1@medctr.osu.edu

Christine M. Eng, M.D. [150]
Associate Professor, Dept. of Molecular and Human Genetics, Baylor College of Medicine, Houston, Texas
ceng@bcm.tmc.edu

Charles J. Epstein, M.D. [63]
Professor of Pediatrics, Co-Director, Program of Human Genetics, Chief, Div. of Medical Genetics, Dept. of Pediatrics, University of California at San Francisco, California
cepst@itsa.ucsf.edu

Charles T. Esmon, Ph.D. [170]
Head, Cardiovascular Biology Research Program, Oklahoma Medical Research Foundation, Investigator, Howard Hughes Medical Institute, Oklahoma Medical Research Foundation, Oklahoma City, Oklahoma
charles-esmon@omrf.ouhsc.edu

Lindsay A. Farrer, Ph.D. [234]
Genetics Program, Boston University School of Medicine, Boston, Massachusetts
farrer@neugen.bu.edu

Eric R. Fearon, M.D. [26]
Div. of Molecular Medicine and Genetics, University of Michigan Medical Center, Ann Arbor, Michigan
fearon@umich.edu

Andrew P. Feinberg, M.D., M.P.H. [18]
King Fahd Professor of Medicine, Oncology and Molecular Biology and Genetics, Johns Hopkins Medical School, Baltimore, Maryland
afeinberg@jhu.edu

Anthony H. Fensom, Ph.D. [143]
Prince Philip Laboratory, Guy's Hospital, London, United Kingdom

Wayne A. Fenton, Ph.D. [94, 155]
Dept. of Genetics, Yale University School of Medicine, New Haven, Connecticut
wayne.fenton@yale.edu

Malcolm A. Ferguson-Smith, F.R.S. [62]
Professor, Dept. of Clinical Veterinary Medicine, University of Cambridge, Centre for Veterinary Science, Cambridge, United Kingdom

Clair A. Francomano, M.D. [210]
National Center for Human Genome Research, National Institutes of Health, Bethesda, Maryland
clairf@nhgri.nih.giv

Deborah L. French, Ph.D. [177]
Assistant Professor of Medicine and Immunobiology, Div. of Hematology, Mount Sinai School of Medicine, New York, New York
dfrench@mssm.edu

Frank E. Frerman, Ph.D. [95, 103]
Professor of Pediatrics, Dept. of Pediatrics, University of Colorado Health Science Center, Denver, Colorado
Frank.frerman@uchsc.edu

Carol Freund, Ph.D. [240]
Dept. of Clinical Bioethics, National Institutes of Health, Bethesda, Maryland
cfreund@nih.gov

Theodore Friedmann, M.D. [107]
Dept. of Pediatric/Molecular Genetics, University of California, San Diego, Center for Molecular Genetics, La Jolla, California
tfriedmann@ucsd.edu

Tony Frugier, MSc [231]
Laboratoire de Neurogénétique Moléculaire, INSERM, GENOPOLE, Evry, France
t.frugier@genopole.inserm.fr

Elaine Fuchs, Ph.D. [221]
Amgen Professor of Basic Sciences, HHMI, Dept. of Molecular Genetics and Cell Biology, University of Chicago, Chicago, Illinois
lain@midway.uchicago.edu

Lars Fugger, M.D., Ph.D. [12]
Professor, Dept. of Clinical Immunology, Aarhus University Hospital, Aarhus, Denmark
fugger@inet.uni2.dk

T. Mary Fujiwara, MSc [163]
Assistant Professor, Depts. of Human Genetics and Medicine, McGill University, Div. of Medical Genetics, Montreal General Hospital, Montreal, Quebec, Canada
fujiwara@bagel.epi.mcgill.ca

Toshiyuki Fukao, M.D., Ph.D. [102]
Department of Pediatrics, Gifu University School of Medecine, Gifu, Japan
toshi-gif@umin.ac.jp

William A. Gahl, M.D., Ph.D. [199, 200]
Head, Sect. on Human Biochemical Genetics, Heritable Disorders Branch, National Institute of Child Health and Human Development, Bethesda, Maryland
bgahl@helix.nih.gov

David Gailani, M.D. [175]
Assistant Professor of Pathology and Medicine, Director, Clinical Coagulation Laboratory, Vanderbilt Hospital, Hematology/ Oncology Div., Vanderbilt University, Nashville, Tennessee
dave.gailani@mcmail.vanderbilt.edu

Hans Galjaard, M.D., Ph.D. [152]
Professor of Clinical Genetics, Dept. of Clinical Genetics, Erasmus University Medical Faculty, Rotterdam, The Netherlands
galjaard@algm.azr.nl

Carlos A. Garcia, M.D. [227]
Professor, Dept. of Psychiatry and Neurology, Tulane University Health Sciences Center, New Orleans, Louisiana
cgarcia2@tulane.edu

Paolo Gasparini, M.D. [191]
Medical Genetics Service, IRCCS-Ospedale CSS, San Giovanni Rotondo, Foggia, Italy
genetcss@fg.nettuno.it

Richard A. Gatti, M.D. [29]
Professor, Dept. of Pathology, School of Medicine, University of California, Los Angeles, Los Angeles, California
rgatti@mednet.ucla.edu

Bruce D. Gelb, M.D. [137]
Associate Professor of Pediatrics and Human Genetics, Mount Sinai School of Medicine, New York, New York
gelbb01@doc.mssm.edu

James L. German, III, M.D. [30]
Professor, Dept. of Pediatrics, Weill Medical College of Cornell University, New York, New York
jlg2003@mail.med.cornell.edu

Gregory G. Germino, M.D. [215]
Associate Professor of Medicine, Div. of Nephrology, Johns Hopkins University School of Medicine, Baltimore, Maryland
ggermino@welch.jhu.edu

Ali Gharavi, M.D. [211]
Assistant Professor of Medicine, Mount Sinai School of Medicine, New York, New York; Visiting Assistant Professor, Dept. of Genetics, Yale University School of Medicine, New Haven, Connecticut
ali.gharavi@yale.edu

K. Michael Gibson, Ph.D. [91]
Director, Biochemical Genetics Laboratory, Associate Professor, Dept. of Molecular and Medical Genetics, Biochemical Genetics Lab, Oregon University Health Sciences, Portland, Oregon
gibsonm@ohsu.edu

Volkmar Gieselmann, M.D. [148]
Professor and Director, Biochemisches Institut, Christian-Albrechts-Universitat Zu Kiel, Kiel, Germany
office@biochem.uni-kiel.de

Rachel H. Giles, Ph.D. [248]
Dept. of Immunology, University Medical Center Utrecht, Utrecht, The Netherlands
R.Giles@lab.azu.nl

David Ginsburg, M.D. [178]
Warner-Lambert/Parke-Davis Professor of Medicine and Human Genetics, Investigator, Howard Hughes Medical Institute, The University of Michigan Medical Center, Ann Arbor, Michigan
ginsburg@umich.edu

Jonathan David Gitlin, M.D. [126]
Helene B. Roberson Professor of Pediatrics, Professor of Pathology and Immunology, Director, Division of Pediatric Immunology and Rheumatology, Washington University School of Medicine, St. Louis Children's Hospital, St. Louis, Missouri
gitlin@kidsal.wustl.edu

Richard Gitzelmann, M.D. [70]
Professor Emeritus, Div. of Metabolic and Molecular Pediatrics, University Children's Hospital, University of Zurich, Zurich, Switzerland

M. Goedert, M.D., Ph.D. [234]
MRC Laboratory of Molecular Biology, Cambridge, England, United Kingdom
mg@mrc-lmb.cam.ac.uk

Joseph L. Goldstein, M.D. [120]
Paul J. Thomas, Professor of Genetics and Chair, Dept. of Molecular Genetics, University of Texas Southwestern Medical Center, Dallas, Texas
joseph.goldstein@utsouthwestern.edu

Peter N. Goodfellow, B.Sc., D.Phil. [62]
Senior Vice President, Discovery Biopharmaceutical Research and Development, SmithKline Beecham, Harlow, Essex, United Kingdom
peter_n_goodfellow@sbphrd.com

Stephen I. Goodman, M.D. [95, 103]
Chief, Sect. of Genetics, Metabolism, and Birth Defects, Professor of Pediatrics, Dept. of Pediatrics, School of Medicine, University of Colorado Health Science Center, Denver, Colorado
stephen.goodman@uchsc.edu

Paul Goodyer, M.D. [191]
Professor of Pediatrics, McGill University, Montreal Children's Hospital, Nephrology Dept., Montreal, Quebec, Canada
paul.goodyer@muhc.mcgill.ca

Jerome L. Gorski, M.D. [247]
Professor of Pediatrics and Human Genetics, Director, Div. of Pediatric Genetics, Div. of Clinical Genetics, Dept. of Pediatrics, University of Michigan, Ann Arbor, Michigan
jlgorski@umich.edu

André Gougoux, M.D. [196]
Professor of Medicine, CHUM (Pavillon Notre Dame), Université de Montréal, Montreal, Quebec, Canada

Stephen J. Gould, Ph.D. [129]
Associate Professor, Dept. of Biological Chemistry, The Johns Hopkins University School of Medicine, Baltimore, Maryland
sgould@jhmi.edu

Gregory A. Grabowski, M.D. [146]
Director, Div. and Program in Human Genetics, Children's Hospital Research Foundation, Cincinnati, Ohio
grabg0@chmcc.org

Denis M. Grant, Ph.D. [9]
Genetics and Genomic Biology Programme, Research Institute, Hospital for Sick Children, Toronto, Ontario, Canada
grant@sickkids.on.ca

Roy A. Gravel, Ph.D. [94, 153]
Professor, Cell Biology and Anatomy, University of Calgary, Calgary, Alberta, Canada
rgravel@ucalgary.ca

Eric D. Green, M.D., Ph.D [10]
Chief, Genome Technology Branch, Director, NIH, Intramural Sequencing Center, National Human Genome Research Institute, Bethesda, Maryland
egreen@nhgri.nih.gov

Daniel L. Greenberg, M.D. [169]
Dept. of Medicine, University of Washington Medical Center, Division of Hematology, Seattle, Washington
robin@u.washington.edu

James E. Griffin, M.D. [160]
Professor of Internal Medicine, Diana and Richard C. Strauss Professor in Biomedical Research, University of Texas Southwestern Medical Center, Dallas, Texas
jgrif2@mednet.swmed.edu

Markus Grompe, M.D. [79]
Dept. of Molecular/Medical Genetics and Dept. of Pediatrics, Oregon Health Sciences University, Portland, Oregon
grompem@ohsu.edu

James Gusella, M.D. [40]
Molecular Neurogenetics Unit, Massachusetts General Hospital, Charlestown, Massachusetts

David H. Gutmann, M.D., Ph.D. [39]
Associate Professor, Director, Neurofibromatosis Program, St. Louis Children's Hospital, Dept. of Neurology, Washington University, St. Louis, Missouri
gutmannd@neuro.wustl.edu

Daniel A. Haber, M.D., Ph.D. [38]
Associate Professor of Medicine, Harvard Medical School, Director, Center for Cancer Risk Analysis, Massachusetts General Hospital Cancer Center, Lab of Molecular Genetics, Charlestown, Massachusetts
haber@helix.mgh.harvard.edu

Theodora Hadjistilianou, M.D. [36]
Associate Professor, Dept. of Ophthalmology, University of Siena School of Medicine, Siena, Tuscany, Italy

Judith G. Hall, M.D. [15]
Dept. of Pediatrics, British Columbia Children's Hospital, Vancouver, British Columbia, Canada
judyhall@interchange.ubc.ca

Ada Hamosh, M.D., M.P.H. [1, 90]
Associate Professor of Pediatric, McKusick-Nathans Institute of Genetic Medicine, The Johns Hopkins University School of Medicine, Johns Hopkins Hospital, Baltimore, Maryland
ahamosh@jhmi.edu

Folker Hanefeld, M.D. [84]
Professor of Pediatrics and Child Neurology, Georg-August-Universitat, Zentrum Kinderheilkunde, Abt. Padiatrie, Schwerpunkt Neuropadiatrie, Germany

Isabel Hanson, M.D. [240]
Molecular Medicine Center, Western General Hospital, Edinburgh, United Kingdom
isabel.hanson@ed.ac.uk

Jean-Pierre Hardelin [254]
Unite de Genetique des Deficits Sensoriels, Institut Pasteur, Paris, France

Peter S. Harper, M.D. [217]
Professor and Consultant in Medical Genetics, University of Wales College of Medicine, Heath Park Institute of Medical Genetics, Cardiff, United Kingdom
harperps@cardiff.ac.uk

Curtis C. Harris, M.D. [59]
Chief, Laboratory of Human Carcinogenesis, National Cancer Institute, Bethesda, Maryland
Curtis_Harris@NIH.GOV

Klaus Harzer, M.D. [134]
Professor, Neurochemical Laboratory, University of Tübingen, Institut für Hirnforschung, Tübingen, Germany
hirnforschung@uni-tuebingen.de

Richard J. Havel, M.D. [114, 115]
Professor Emeritus, Cardiovascular Research Institute, University of California School of Medicine, San Francisco, California
dargank@curi.ucsf.edu

J. Ross Hawkins, Ph.D. [62]
Principal Scientist of Development Incyte Genomics, Ltd. Cambridge, United Kingdom
Ross.Hawkins@incyte.com

Michael R. Hayden, M.D., ChB, Ph.D., FRCP(C), FRSC [223]
Professor of Medical Genetics, Centre for Molecular Medicine and Therapeutics, University of British Columbia, Vancouver, British Columbia, Canada
mrh@cmmt.ubc.ca

Vincent J. Hearing, M.D. [220]
Laboratory of Cell Biology, National Institutes of Health, Bethesda, Maryland

Jacqueline T. Hecht, Ph.D. [210]
Dept. of Pediatrics, University of Texas Medical School, Houston, Texas
jhecht@ped1.med.uth.tmc.edu

Peter Hechtman, Ph.D. [82]
Associate Professor of Biology, Human Genetics, and Pediatrics, McGill University, Dept. of Biochemical Genetics, Montreal Children's Hospital, Montreal, Quebec, Canada
Peter@uww.debelle.mcgill.ca

James F. Hejtmancik, M.D., Ph.D. [241]
National Eye Institute, National Institutes of Health, Bethesda, Maryland
f3h@helix.nih.gov

Raoul C. M. Hennekam, Ph.D., M.D. [248, 249]
Pediatrician and Clinical Geneticist, Dept. of Pediatrics and Institute for Human Genetics, Academic Medical Center, University of Amsterdam, Amsterdam, The Netherlands
r.c.hennekam@amc.uva.nl

Meenhard Herlyn, Ph.D. [44]
Professor, The Wistar Institute, Philadelphia, Pennsylvania
herlynm@wistar.upenn.edu

Michael S. Hershfield, M.D. [109]
Dept. of Medicine and Biochemistry, Duke University Medical Center, Durham, North Carolina
msh@biochem.duke.edu

Hugo S.A. Heymans [130]
Professor of Pediatrics, Director and Chairman. Emma Children's Hospital and Clinical Chemistry, University of Amsterdam Academic Medical Centre, Amsterdam, The Netherlands
h.s.heymans@amc.uva.nl

Howard H. Hiatt, M.D. [73]
Professor of Medicine, Harvard Medical School, Senior Physician, Div. of General Medicine, Dept. of Medicine, Brigham and Women's Hospital, Boston, Massachusetts
hhiatt@partners.org

D.R. Higgs [181]
Institute of Molecular Medicine, John Radcliffe Hospital, Oxford, United Kingdom
drhiggs@molbiol.ox.ac.uk

Katherine A. High, M.D. [173]
William H. Bennett Professor of Pediatrics, UPENN School of Medicine, Director of Research, Hematology Div., Director, Hematology and Coagulation Laboratories, Children's Hospital of Philadelphia, Philadelphia, Pennsylvania
high@email.chop.edu

Adrian V. S. Hill, D.Phil., D.M. [7]
Professor of Human Genetics, Wellcome Trust Centre for Human Genetics, Headington, Oxford, United Kingdom
adrian.hill@imm.ox.ac.uk

Akira Hirono, M.D., Ph.D. [182]
Research Associate, Okinaka Memorial Institute for Medical Research, Tokyo, Japan
Ncc01353@nifty.nc.jp

Rochelle Hirschhorn, M.D. [135]
Professor of Medicine and Cell Biology, Chief, Div. of Medical Genetics, Dept. of Medicine, New York University School of Medicine, New York, New York
hirscr01@mcrcr0.med.nyu.edu

Helen H. Hobbs, M.D. [120]
Professor, Depts. of Internal Medicine and Molecular Genetics, The University of Texas Southwestern Medical Center at Dallas, Dallas, Texas
helen.hobbs@utsouthwestern.edu

Jan H.J. Hoeijmakers, M.D. [28]
Dept. of Cell Biology and Genetics, Erasmus University, Rotterdam, The Netherlands
hoeijmakers@gen.fgg.eur.nl

Sandra L. Hofmann, M.D., Ph.D. [154]
Associate Professor of Internal Medicine, Hamon Center for Therapeutic Oncology Research, University of Texas Southwestern Medical Center, Dallas, Texas
hofmann@simmons.swmed.edu

Jeffrey M. Hoeg, M.D. [118]
Chief, Section on Molecular Biology, Molecular Disease Branch, National Institutes of Health, Bethesda, Maryland
Deceased 7/21/98.

Michael D. Hogarty, M.D. [21]
Div. of Oncology, The Children's Hospital of Philadelphia, Philadelphia, Pennsylvania
hogartym@email.chop.edu

Edward J. Hollox, Ph.D. [76]
Institute of Genetics, University of Nottingham, Queens Medical Centre Nottingham, United Kingdom
Ed.Hollox@Nottingham.ac.uk

Edward W. Holmes, M.D. [110]
Vice Chancellor and Dean, School of Medicine, University of California, San Diego, California

John B. Holton, Ph.D. [72]
Emeritus Consultant Clinical Scientist, Clinical Biochemistry, Southmean Hospital, Bristol, United Kingdom

John J. Hopwood, Ph.D. [149]
Professor & Head, Lysosomal Diseases Research Unit, Dept. of Chemical Pathology, Women's and Children's Hospital, North Adelaide, South Australia
john.hopwood@adelaide.edu.au

Ourania Horaitis, B.Sc. [1]
Co-ordinator, HUGO Mutation Database Initiative, Mutation Research Centre, St. Vincent's Hospital, Fitzroy, Melbourne, Victoria, Australia
horaitis@ariel.ucs.unimelb.edu.au

D. Jonathan Horsford, B.Sc. [240]
Program in Developmental Biology, Hospital for Sick Children, Toronto, Ontario, Canada
djhors@sickkids.on.ca

Arthur L. Horwich, M.D. [85]
Professor of Genetics and Pediatrics, Investigator, HHMI, Yale School of Medicine/HHMI, New Haven, Connecticut
horwich@csb.yale.edu

James R. Howe, M.D. [35]
Assistant Professor, Dept. of Surgery, University of Iowa College of Medicine, Iowa City, Iowa
James_howe@uiowa.edu

Ralph H. Hruban, M.D. [50]
Professor of Pathology and Oncology, The Johns Hopkins University, School of Medicine, Dept. of Oncology and Pathology, Baltimore, Maryland
rhruban@jhmi.edu

Chien-an A. Hu, Ph.D. [81]
Research Associate, McKusick-Nathans Institute of Genetic Medicine, Johns Hopkins University School of Medicine, Baltimore, Maryland
cahu@welch.jhu.edu

Lynn D. Hudson, Ph.D. [228]
Acting Chief, Lab of Developmental Neurogenetics, National Institute of Neurologic Disorders and Stroke, National Institutes of Health, Bethesda, Maryland
hudsonl@ninds.nih.gov

Donald E. Hultquist [180]
Associate Chair, Dept. of Biological Chemistry, University of Michigan Medical School, Ann Arbor, Michigan
hultquis@umich.edu

Keith Hyland, Ph.D. [78]
Associate Professor, Baylor University, Associate Professor, University of Texas Southwestern Medical Center, Senior Research Scientist, Baylor University Medical Center, Institute of Metabolic Diseases, Dallas, Texas
k.hyland@baylordallas.edu

Akitada Ichinose, M.D., Ph.D. [171]
Professor and Chairman, Dept. of Molecular Pathological Biochemistry, Yamagata University School of Medicine, Yamagata, Japan
aichinos@med.id.yamagata-u.ac.jp

Yiannis A. Ioannou, Ph.D. [150]
Associate Professor, Dept. of Human Genetics, Mount Sinai School of Medicine, New York, New York
yiannis.ioannou@mssm.edu

William B. Isaacs, Ph.D. [56]
Professor of Urology and of Oncology, Dept. of Urology, The Johns Hopkins University School of Medicine, Baltimore, Maryland
wisaacs@mail.jhmi.edu

Dirk Isbrandt, M.D. [84]
Research Scientist, Universitat Hamburg, Zentrum fur Molekulare Neurobiologie Hamburg, Institut fur Neurale Signalverarbeitung, Hamburg, Germany
isbrandt@uni-hamburg.de

Jaak Jaeken, M.D., Ph.D. [74, 112, 148]
Professor of Pediatrics, University of Leuven; Director, Center for Metabolic Disease, University Hospital Gasthuisberg, Leuven, Belgium
Jaak.jacken@uz.kuleuven.ac.be

Ernst R. Jaffe, M.D. [180]
Distinguished University Professor of Medicine Emeritus, Albert Einstein College of Medicine, Bronx, New York
(Deceased)

Cornelis Jakobs, Ph.D. [91, 132]
Associate Professor, Head Metabolic Unit, Dept. of Clinical Chemistry, Vrije Universiteit Medical Centre, Amsterdam, The Netherlands
C.Jakobs@AZVU.nl

Anu Jalanko, Ph.D. [141]
Senior Scientist, Dept. of Human Molecular Genetics, National Public Health Institute, Helsinki, Finland
Anu.jalanko@ktl.fi

Joanna C. Jen, M.D. [204]
Assistant Professor, Dept. of Neurology, UCLA School of Medicine, Los Angeles, California
jjen@ucla.edu

Gerardo Jimenez-Sanchez, M.D., Ph.D. [3,4]
McKusick-Nathans Institute of Genetic Medicine, Johns Hopkins University School of Medicine, Baltimore, Maryland
gjimenez@jhmi.edu

H.A. Jinnah, M.D., Ph.D. [107]
Assistant Professor, Dept. of Neurology, Johns Hopkins Hospital, Baltimore, Maryland
hjinnah@welch.jhu.edu

Hans Joenje, Ph.D. [31]
Senior Scientist, Dept. Clinical and Human Genetics, Free University Medical Center, Amsterdam, The Netherlands
H.Joenje.HumGen@med.vu.nl

Jean L. Johnson, M.D. [128]
Assistant Research Professor, Dept. of Biochemistry, Duke University Medical Center, Durham, North Carolina
jean_johnson@biochem.duke.edu

Keith J. Johnson, Ph.D. [217]
Professor of Genetics, Head, Div. of Molecular Genetics, Institute of Biomedical and Life Sciences, University of Glasgow, Glasgow, United Kingdom
K.Johnson@bio.gla.ac.uk

Michael V. Johnston, M.D. [90]
Professor of Neurology and Pediatrics, The Johns Hopkins University School of Medicine, Kennedy Krieger Institute, Baltimore, Maryland
johnston@kennedykrieger.org

Michael M. Kaback, M.D. [153]
Professor, Depts. of Pediatrics and Reproductive Medicine, University of California, San Diego, Children's Hospital and Health Center, San Diego, California
mkaback@ucsd.edu

Steven E. Kahn, M.B., Ch.B. [67]
Associate Professor of Medicine, University of Washington, Staff Physician, VA Puget Sound Health Care System, Seattle, Washington
skahn@u.washington.edu

Muriel I. Kaiser-Kupfer, M.D. [241]
Chief, Ophthalmic Genetics, National Eye Institute, Bethesda, Maryland
kaiserm@box-k.nih.gov

Anne Kallioniemi, M.D. [20]
Cancer Genetics Branch, National Human Genome Research Institute, Bethesda, Maryland

Werner Kalow, M.D. [9]
Professor Emeritus, Dept. of Pharmacology, University of Toronto, Toronto, Ontario, Canada
w.kalow@utoronto.ca

Naoyuki Kamatani, M.D. [108]
Professor and Director, Institute of Rheumatology, Tokyo Women's Medical University, Tokyo, Japan
kamatani@ior.twmu.ac.jp

Alexander Kamb, Ph.D. [44]
Chief Scientific Officer, Arcaris, Inc., Salt Lake City, Utah
kamb@arcaris.com

John P. Kane, M.D., Ph.D. [114, 115]
University of California, San Francisco, California
Kane@itsa.ucsf.edu

Hitoshi Kanno, M.D., Ph.D. [182]
Assistant Professor, Dept. of Biochemistry, Nihon University School of Medicine, Tokyo, Japan
hikanno@med.nihon-u.ac.jp

Josseline Kaplan [237]
Unite de Recherches sur les Handicaps, Genetiques de L'Enfant, INSERM, Hôpital des Enfants Malades, Paris, Cedex, France

George Karpati, M.D., FRCP(C), FRS(C) [216]
Director, Neuromuscular Research, Dept. Neurology/Neurosurgery, Montreal Neurological Institute, McGill University, Montreal, Quebec, Canada
mcgk@musica.mcgill.ca

Seymour Kaufman, Ph.D. [77]
Emeritus Chief, Laboratory of Neurochemistry, National Institute of Mental Health, National Institutes of Health, Bethesda, Maryland
kaufman@codon.nih.gov

Haig H. Kazazian, Jr., M.D. [172]
Chairman, Dept. of Genetics, University of Pennsylvania School of Medicine, Philadelphia, Pennsylvania
kazazian@mail.med.upenn.edu

Mark T. Keating, M.D. [203]
Professor of Medicine and Human Genetics, Eccles Institute of Human Genetics, University of Utah/Howard Hughes Medical Institute, Eccles Institute of Human Genetics, Salt Lake City, Utah
mark@howard.genetics.utah.edu

Richard I. Kelley, M.D., Ph.D. [249]
Associate Professor of Pediatrics, Johns Hopkins University, Director of Metabolism, Kennedy Krieger Institute, Baltimore, Maryland
kelle_ri@jhuvms.hcf.jhu.edu

Scott E. Kern, M.D. [50]
Associate Professor of Oncology, Johns Hopkins University School of Medicine, Baltimore, Maryland
sk@jhmi.edu

Keith Kerstann, M.A. [105]
The Center for Molecular Medicine, Emory University School of Medicine, Atlanta, Georgia
kkersta@gen.emory.edu

Richard A. King, M.D. [220]
Professor, University of Minnesota, Minneapolis, Minnesota
kingx002@tc.umn.edu

Kenneth W. Kinzler, Ph.D. [17, 27, 48]
Professor of Oncology, The Johns Hopkins University School of Medicine, Baltimore, Maryland
kinzlke@jhmi.edu

D. Richard Klausner, M.D. [41]
Director, National Cancer Institute, Bethesda, Maryland
Klausner@helix.nih.gov

Michael Koenig, M.D. [232]
Professor of Medical Genetics, University of Louis Pasteur, Strasbourg; Adjunct Director of the Genetics Diagnosis Laboratory, Institute de Genetique et de Biologie Moleculaire et Cellulaire, CNRS-INSERM-ULP, Illkirch, Strasbourg, France
mkoenig@igbmc.u-strasbg.fr

Thomas Kolter, Ph.D. [134]
Kekule-Institut für Organische Chemie und Biochemie, der Reinnischen Friedrich-Wilhelms Universität Bonn, Bonn, Germany
kolter@snchemie1.chemie.uni-bonn.de

Stuart Kornfeld, M.D. [138]
Professor of Medicine, Div. of Hematology-Oncology, Dept. of Medicine, Washington University School of Medicine, St. Louis, Missouri
skornfel@im.wustl.edu

Kenneth H. Kraemer, M.D. [28]
Research Scientist, Basic Research Laboratory, National Cancer Institute, Bethesda, Maryland
kraemerk@nih.gov

Jan P. Kraus, Ph.D. [88]
Professor of Pediatrics and Cellular/Structural Biology, Dept. of Pediatrics, University of Colorado School of Medicine, Denver, Colorado
jan.kraus@uchsc.edu

Michael Krawczak, M.D. [13]
Professor, Institute of Medical Genetics, University of Wales College of Medicine, Cardiff, Wales, United Kingdom
krawczak@cardiff.ac.uk

Berry Kremer, M.D., Ph.D. [223]
Professor, Dept. of Neurology, University Medical Center Nijmegen, The Netherlands
h.kremer@czzoneu.azn.nl

Anjli Kukreja, Ph.D. [69]
Research Associate, Weill College of Medicine, Cornell University, New York
anjlik@hotmail.com

Bert N. La Du, Jr., M.D., Ph.D. [92]
Emeritus Professor of Pharmacology, Dept. of Pharmacology, University of Michigan Medical School, Ann Arbor, Michigan
bladu@umich.edu

Marie Lambert, M.D. [79]
Service de genetique medicale, Centre de recherche, Ste-Justine Hospital, Montreal, Quebec, Canada
lamberma@medclin.umontreal.ca

Risto Lappatto, M.D., Ph.D. [111]
Consultant Pediatrician, University of Helsinki, Helsinki, Finland
Risto.Lapatto@helsinki.fi

Agne Larsson, M.D., Ph.D. [96]
Professor of Pediatrics, Chairman, Dept. of Pediatrics, Children's Hospital, Karolinska Institutet, Huddinge University Hospital, Stockholm Sweden
agne.larsson@klinvet.ki.se

David H. Ledbetter, Ph.D. [65]
Professor and Chair, Dept. of Human Genetics, The University of Chicago, Chicago, Illinois
dhl@genetics.uchicago.edu

Rudolph L. Leibel, M.D. [157]
Chief, Division of Molecular Genetics, Co-Director, Naomi Berrie Diabetes Center, Professor of Pediatrics and Medicine, Columbia University College of Physicians & Surgeons, New York, New York
RL232@columbia.edu

Eran Leitersdorf, M.D. [123]
Professor of Medicine, Dorothy and Maurice Bucksbaum Chair in Molecular Genetics, Head, Center for Research, Prevention, and Treatment of Atherosclerosis, Dept. of Medicine, Hadassah University Hospital, Jerusalem, Israel
eran1@hadassah.org.il

Christoph Lengauer, M.D. [22]
The Johns Hopkins Oncology Center, Baltimore, Maryland
lengauer@jhmi.edu

Thierry Levade, Ph.D. [143]
Laboratoire de Biochemie, Maladies Metaboliques, CJF INSERM, Institut Louis Bugnard, Toulouse, France

Jacqueline Levilliers [254]
Unite de Genetique des Deficits Sensoriels, Institut Pasteur, Paris, France

Harvey L. Levy, M.D. [80, 88, 193]
Associate Professor of Pediatrics, Harvard Medical School, Senior Associate in Medicine and Genetics, Children's Hospital, Boston, Massachusetts
levy_h@al.tch.harvard.edu

Richard Alan Lewis, M.D. [243]
Professor, Dept. of Ophthalmology, Medicine, Pediatrics and Molecular Human Genetics, Baylor College of Medicine, Houston, Texas
rlewis@bcm.tmc.edu

Roland Libau, M.D. [12]
Postdoctoral Fellow, Dept. of Microbiology and Immunology, Stanford University School of Medicine, Stanford, California

Uri A. Liberman, M.D., Ph.D. [165]
Professor of Physiology and Medicine, Head, Dept. of Endocrinology and Metabolism, Rabin Medical Center, Beilinson Campus, Sackler School of Medicine, Tel-Aviv University, Petach-Tikvah, Israel
uliberman@clalit.org.il

Richard P. Lifton, M.D. [211]
Associate Investigator, Howard Hughes Medical Institute, Chair, Dept. of Genetics, Professor of Genetics, Internal Medicine & Molecular Biophysics, Yale University School of Medicine, New Haven, Connecticut
richard.lifton@yale.edu

W. Marston Linehan, M.D. [41]
Chief, Urologic Oncology Branch, National Cancer Institute, Bethesda, Maryland
Wml@nih.gov

Thomas Linke, M.D. [143]
Institute fur Organisch Chemie, Bonn, Germany

A. Thomas Look, M.D. [19]
Dept. of Experimental Oncology, St. Jude Children's Research Hospital, Memphis, Tennessee
Thomas.look@stjude.org

Marie T. Lott, M.A. [105]
Research Specialist, Supervisor, Center for Molecular Medicine, Emory University School of Medicine, Atlanta, Georgia
mtlott@gen.emory.edu

James R. Lupski, M.D., Ph.D. [65, 227, 243]
Cullen Professor of Molecular and Human Genetics and Professor of Medicine, Dept. of Molecular and Human Genetics, Baylor College of Medicine, Houston, Texas
jlupski@bcm.tmc.edu

Andreas Lux, Ph.D. [212]
Research Associate, Dept. of Genetics, Duke University Medical Center, Durham, North Carolina

Samuel E. Lux, IV, M.D. [183]
Robert A. Stranahan Professor of Pediatrics, Harvard Medical School Chief, Div. of Hematology/Oncology, Children's Hospital, Boston, Massachusetts
lux@genetics.med.harvard.edu

Lucio Luzatto, M.D., Ph.D. [179]
Scientific Director, Instituo Nazionale per la Ricerca sul Cancro, Genova, Italy
luzzatto@hp380.ist.unige.it

Stanislas Lyonnet, M.D., Ph.D. [251]
Professor of Genetics, University of Paris, Dept. de Genetique et Unite, INSERM, Hospital Necker-Enfants Malades, Paris, France
lyonnet@necker.fr

Mack Mabry, M.D. [58]
Div. of Radiology, The Johns Hopkins Hospital, Baltimore, Maryland

Mia MacCollin, M.D. [40]
Assistant Professor of Neurology, Massachusetts General Hospital, Charlestown, Massachusetts
maccollin@helix.mgh.harvard.edu

Noel Keith Maclaren, M.D. [69]
Professor of Pediatrics, Director, Juvenile Diabetes, Weill College of Medicine, Cornell University, New York
NKMaclaren@aol.com

Edward R. B. McCabe, M.D., Ph.D [97, 167]
Professor and Executive Chair, Dept. of Pediatrics UCLA School of Medicine; Physician-in-Chief, Mattel Children's Hospital at UCLA, Los Angeles, California
emccabe@pediatrics.medsch.ucla.edu

Hugh O. McDevitt, M.D. [12]
Professor of Microbiology and Immunology, Stanford University School of Medicine, Stanford, California
hughmcd@stanford.edu

Roderick R. McInnes, M.D., Ph.D. [80, 240]
University of Toronto Tanenbaum Chair in Molecular Medicine, Professor of Pediatrics and Molecular Genetics, University of Toronto, Head, Program in Developmental Biology, Research Institute, Hospital for Sick Children, Toronto, Ontario, Canada
mcinnes@sickkids.on.ca

Victor A. McKusick, M.D. [1]
Professor , McKusick-Nathans Institute of Genetic Medicine, Johns Hopkins University School of Medicine, Baltimore, Maryland
McKusick@peas.welch.jhu.edu

Roger E. McLendon, M.D. [57]
Associate Professor; Director of Anatomic Pathology Services; Chief, Sect. of Neuropathology, Duke University Medical Center, Durham, North Carolina
roger.mclendon@duke.edu

Michael J. McPhaul, M.D. [160]
Professor, Dept. of Internal Medicine, Div. of Endocrinology and Metabolism, University of Texas Southwestern Medical Center, Dallas, Texas
mcphaul@pop3.utsw.swmed.edu

Robert W. Mahley, M.D., Ph.D. [119]
Director, Gladstone Institute of Cardiovascular Disease, Professor of Pathology and Medicine, University of California, San Francisco
rmahley@gladstone.ucsf.edu

David Malkin, M.D. [37]
Associate Professor of Pediatrics, University of Toronto, Program in Cancer and Blood Research, Research Institute, Hospital for Sick Children, Toronto, Ontario, Canada
David.malkin@sickkids.on.ca

Ned Mantei, Ph.D. [75]
Professor, Swiss Federal Institute of Technology, Institute for Cell Biology, Zurich, Switzerland
mantei@cell.biol.ethz.ch

Douglas A. Marchuk, Ph.D. [212]
Assistant Professor, Dept. of Genetics, Duke University Medical Center, Durham, North Carolina
march004@mc.duke.edu

Sandrine Marlin [254]
Unite de Genetique des Deficits Sensoriels, Institut Pasteur, Paris, France

Karen L. Marsh, Ph.D. [246]
University of Manchester, School of Biological Sciences, Manchester, United Kingdom

George M. Martin, M.D. [8]
Professor of Pathology, Adjunct Professor of Genetics, Director, Alzheimer's Disease Research Center, Attending Pathologist, Medical Center, University of Washington School of Medicine, Seattle, Washington
gmmartin@u.washington.edu

Martín G. Martín, M.D. [190]
Dept. of Pediatrics, Gastroenterology, UCLA School of Medicine, Los Angeles, California
mmartin@mednet.ucla.edu

Paula Martin, Ph.D. [214]
Dept. of Biochemistry, University of Oulu, Finland
paula.martin@oula.fi

Stephen J. Marx, M.D. [43, 165]
Chief, Genetics and Endocrinology Sect., National Institutes of Health, Bethesda, Maryland
stephenm@intra.niddk.nih.gov

Gert Matthijs, Ph.D. [74]
Assistant Professor, Center for Human Genetics, University Hospital of Leuven, Centre for Human Genetics, Leuven, Belgium
gert.matthijs@med.kuleuven.ac.be

Atul Mehta, M.D. [179]
Consultant Hematologist, Dept. of Hematology, Royal Free Hospital, London, United Kingdom
atul.mehta@rfh.nthames.nhs.uk

Judith Melki, M.D., Ph.D. [231]
Neurogénétique Moléculaire, INSERM, GENOPOLE, Evry, France
j.melki@genopole.inserm.fr

Paul S. Meltzer, M.D., Ph.D. [20]
Sect. of Molecular Cytogenetics, Lab of Cancer Genetics, National Institutes of Health, Bethesda, Maryland

Claude J. Migeon, M.D. [159]
Professor of Pediatrics, Div. of Pediatric Endocrinology, The Johns Hopkins University School of Medicine, Baltimore, Maryland
cmigeon@welchlink.welch.jhu.edu

Tetsuro Miki, Ph.D. [33]
Geriatric Research Education and Clinical Center, University of Washington, Seattle, Washington

Beverly S. Mitchell [109]
Wellcome Professor of Cancer Research, University of North Carolina, Lineberger Comprehensive Cancer Center, Chapel Hill, North Carolina

Grant A. Mitchell, M.D. [79, 102]
Div. of Medical Genetics, Hopital Ste-Justine, Montreal, Quebec, Canada
mitchell@justine.umontreal.ca

Shiro Miwa, M.D. [182]
Director, Okinaka Memorial Institute for Medical Research, Tokyo, Japan

Maria Judit Molnar, M.D., Ph.D. [216]
Dept. of Neurology, Medical University of Debrecen, National Institute of Psychiatry and Neurology, Budapest, Hungary
molnarm@jaguar.dote.hu

Jill A. Morris, Ph.D. [145]
Senior Research Biologist, Dept. of Pharmacology, Merck Research Laboratories, West Point, Pennsylvania
jill_morris@merck.com

Ann B. Moser, BA [131]
Kennedy Krieger Institute, Baltimore, Maryland
mosera@kennedykrieger.org

Hugo W. Moser, M.D. [131, 143]
Professor of Neurology and Pediatrics, Johns Hopkins University, Director of Neurogenetics, Kennedy Krieger Institute, Baltimore, Maryland
moser@kennedykrieger.org

Björn Mossberg, M.D., Ph.D. [187]
Chief Physician, Dept. of Respiratory Medicine and Allerology, Huddinge University Hospital Stockholm, Sweden
bjorn.mossberg@lungall.hs.sll.se

Arno G. Motulsky, M.D., D.Sc. [127, 238]
Professor Emeritus Active of Medicine and Genetics, Attending Physician, University of Washington Hospital, Div. of Medical Genetics, Dept. of Medicine, University of Washington, Seattle, Washington
agmot@u.washington.edu

S. Harvey Mudd, M.D. [88]
Guest Scientist, Laboratory of Molecular Biology, National Institute of Mental Health, National Institutes of Health, Bethesda, Maryland
sbm@codon.nih.gov

Maximilian Muenke, M.D. [245, 250]
Chief, Medical Genetics Branch, National Human Genome Research Institute, National Institutes of Health, Bethesda, Maryland
muenke@nih.gov

Joseph Muenzer, M.D., Ph.D. [136]
Associate Professor of Pediatrics, Dept. of Pediatrics, University of North Carolina at Chapel Hill, North Carolina
muenzer@css.unc.edu

Arnold Munnich, M.D., Ph.D. [99, 237]
Professor, Dept. of Pediatrics, INSERM, Hopital des Enfants Malades, Hopital Necker, Paris, France
munnich@necker.fr

Jun Nakura, M.D., Ph.D. [33]
Department of Geriatric Medicine, School of Medicine, Ehime University, Ehime, Japan
nakura@ m.ehime-u.ac.jp

Eiji Nanba, M.D. [151]
Associate Professor, Gene Research Center, Tottori University, Yonago, Japan
enanba@grape.med.tottori-u.ac.jp

William M. Nauseef, M.D. [189]
Professor, Inflammation Program and Dept. of Medicine, University of Iowa, Iowa City, Iowa
william-nauseef@uiowa.ed

Barry D. Nelkin, Ph.D. [58]
Associate Professor of Oncology, Johns Hopkins University School of Medicine, Baltimore, Maryland
bnelkin@jhmi.edu

Edward B. Neufeld, Ph.D. [145]
National Heart, Lung, and Blood Institute, Bethesda, Maryland
neufelde@mail.nih.gov

Elizabeth F. Neufeld, Ph.D. [136]
Professor and Chair Biological Chemistry, Dept. of Biological Chemistry, UCLA School of Medicine, Los Angeles, California
eneufeld@mednet.ucla.edu

Peter E. Newburger, M.D. [189]
Professor of Pediatrics and Molecular, Genetics/Microbiology; Director, Pediatric Hematology/Oncology, University of Massachusetts Medical School, Worcester, Massachusetts
peter.newburger@ummed.edu

Peter J. Newman, Ph.D. [177]
Senior Investigator, Vice President and Assoc. Director for Research, The Blood Center, Milwaukee, Wisconsin
pjnewman@bcsew.edu

Irene F. Newsham, Ph.D. [36]
Dept. of Anatomy and Pathology, Medical College of Virginia, Richmond, Virginia
inewsham@hsc.vcu.edu

Jeffrey L. Noebels, M.D., Ph.D. [230]
Professor of Neurology, Neuroscience, and Molecular and Human Genetics, Dept. of Neurology, Baylor College of Medicine, Houston, Texas
jnoebels@bcm.tmc.edu

Josette Noël, M.D. [196]
Assistant Professor, Dept. of Physiology, Université de Montréal, Montreal, Quebec, Canada
josette.noel@umontreal.ca

Lawrence M. Nogee, M.D. [218]
Associate Professor, Dept. of Pediatrics, Div. of Neonatology, Johns Hopkins University School of Medicine, Baltimore, Maryland
lnogee@welch.jhu.edu

Virginia Nunes, Ph.D. [191]
Medical and Molecular Genetics Center, L'Hospitalet de Llobregat, Barcelona, Catalunya, Spain
vnunes@iro.es

Robert L. Nussbaum, M.D. [252]
Chief, Genetic Diseases Research Branch, National Human Genome Research Institute, Bethesda, Maryland
rlnuss@nhgri.nih.gov

William S. Oetting, M.D. [220]
Assistant Professor, University of Minnesota, Minneapolis, Minnesota
bill@lenti.med.umn.edu

Harry T. Orr, M.D. [226]
University of Minnesota, Institute of Human Genetics, Minneapolis, Minnesota
harry@lenti.med.umn.edu

Akihiro Oshima, M.D. [151]
Visiting Investigator, Dept. of Veterinary Science, National Institute of Infectious Diseases, Tokyo, Japan
oshima@nih.go.jp

Manuel Palacín, M.D. [191]
Professor, Biochemistry and Molecular Biology, Faculty of Biology, Dept. of Biochemistry and Physiology, University of Barcelona, Barcelona, Spain
mnpalacin@porthos.bio.ub.es

Cristina Panozzo, Ph.D. [231]
Laboratoire de Neurogénétique Moléculaire, INSERM, GENOPOLE, Evry, France
c.panozzo@genopole.inserm.fr

Lucie Parent, M.D. [196]
Associate Professor, Dept. of Physiology, Université de Montréal, Montreal, Quebec, Canada
lucie.parent@umontreal.ca

Peter Parham, Ph.D. [12]
Professor of Structural Biology and of Microbiology and Immunology, Stanford University, Stanford, California
Peropa@leland.stanford.edu

Morag Park, M.D. [25]
Molecular Oncology Group, Royal Victoria Hospital, Montreal, Quebec, Canada
morag@lan1.molonc.mcgill.ca

Keith L. Parker, M.D., Ph.D. [159]
Professor of Internal Medicine and Pharmacology, Dept. of Internal Medicine, UT Southwestern Medical Center, Dallas, Texas
kparke@mednet.swmed.edu

Ramon Parsons, M.D., Ph.D. [45]
Assistant Professor, Columbia Institute of Cancer Genetics, Columbia University, New York, New York
rep15@columbia.edu

Marc C. Patterson, M.D. [145]
Consultant, Div. of Child and Adolescent Neurology, Mayo Clinic, Rochester, Minnesota
mpatterson@mayo.edu

Leena Peltonen, M.D., Ph.D. [141, 154]
Professor and Chair of Human Genetics, Dept. of Human Genetics, UCLA School of Medicine, Los Angeles, California
lpeltonen@mednet.ucla.edu

Peter G. Pentchev, Ph.D. [145]
Chief, Sect. of Cellular and Molecular Pathophysiology, Developmental and Metabolic Neurology Branch, National Institutes of Neurological Disorders and Stroke, Bethesda, Maryland
peter.pentchev@xtra.co.nz

Isabelle Perrault, M.D. [237]
Unite de Recherches sur les Handicaps, Genetiques de L'Enfant, INSERM, Hôpital des Enfants Malades, Paris, France

Gloria M. Petersen, Ph.D. [49]
Professor of Clinical Epidemiology, Consultant, Mayo Foundation, Mayo Clinic, Rochester, New York
peterg@mayo.edu

Christine Petit [254]
Unite de Genetique des Deficits Sensoriels, Institut Pasteur, Paris, France
cpetit@pasteur.fr

Fred Petrij, M.D. [248]
Clinical Genetics Registrar, Dept. of Clinical Genetics, Erasmus University, Rotterdam, The Netherlands
petrij@kgen.azr.nl

James M. Phang, M.D. [81]
Chief, Metabolism and Cancer Susceptibility Sect., Basic Research Laboratory, Div. of Basic Sciences, National Cancer Institute, Frederick, Maryland
phang@mail.ncifcrf.gov

John A. Phillips, III, M.D. [162]
Professor of Pediatrics and Biochemistry, Div. of Medical Genetics, Vanderbilt University School of Medicine, Nashville, Tennessee
john.phillips@mcmail.vanderbilt.edu

Joram Piatigorsky, Ph.D. [241]
Chief, Laboratory of Molecular and Developmental Biology, National Eye Institute, Bethesda, Maryland
joramp@intra.nei.nih.gov

Leonard Pinsky, M.D. [161]
Professor, Depts. of Medicine, Human Genetics, Biology and Pediatrics, McGill University, Lady Davis Institute for Medical Research, Sir M.B. Davis–Jewish General Hospital, Montreal, Quebec, Canada
rrosenzw@ldi.jgh.mcgill.ca

Eleanor S. Pollak, M.D. [173]
Assistant Professor of Pathology and Laboratory Medicine, Hospital of the University of Pennsylvania, Associate Director, Clinical Coagulation Laboratory, The Children's Hospital of Philadelphia, Philadelphia, Pennsylvania
pollak@mail.med.upenn.edu

Bruce A.J. Ponder, Ph.D., F.R.C.P. [42]
CRC Professor of Oncology, University of Cambridge, Cambridge Institute for Medical Research, Cambridge, United Kingdom
bajp@mole.bio.cam.ac.uk

Mortimer Poncz, M.D. [177]
Professor of Pediatrics, University of Pennsylvania Medical Center, Philadelphia, Pennsylvania

Daniel Porte, Jr., M.D. [67]
Professor of Medicine, University of California San Diego; Staff Physician, VA San Diego Health Care System, San Diego, California
dporte@ucsd.edu
poncz@email.chop.edu

Steven M. Powell, M.D. [55]
Assistant Professor of Medicine, Div. of Gastroenterology, University of Virginia Health Systems, Charlottesville, Virginia
SMP8N@virginia.edu

James M. Powers, M.D. [131]
Dept. of Pathology, University of Rochester Medical Center, Rochester, New York

Richard L. Proia, Ph.D. [153]
Chief, Genetics of Development and Disease Branch, National Institute of Diabetes and Digestive and Kidney Diseases, National Institutes of Health, Bethesda, Maryland
proia@nih.gov

Kathleen P. Pratt, Ph.D. [171]
Instructor, Department of Biochemistry, University of Washington, Seattle
kpratt@u.washington.edu

Stanley B. Prusiner, M.D. [224]
Director, Institute for Neurodegenerative Diseases, Professor of Neurology and Biochemistry, Dept. of Neurology, University of California, San Francisco, California

Louis J. Ptáček, M.D. [204]
Associate Professor, Associate Investigator, Dept. of Neurology Human Genetics, Howard Hughes Medical Institute, University of Utah, Salt Lake City, Utah
ptacek@genetics.utah.edu

Jennifer M. Puck, M.D. [185]
Head Chief, Immunologic Genetics Sect., National Human Genome Research Institute, Genetics and Molecular Biology Branch, Bethesda, Maryland
jpuck@nhgri.nih.gov

Leena Pulkkinen, Ph.D. [222]
Jefferson Institute of Molecular Medicine, Dept. of Dermatology and Cutaneous Biology, Jefferson Medical College, Thomas Jefferson University, Philadelphia, Pennsylvania
leena.pulkkinen@mail.tju.edu

Reed E. Pyeritz, M.D., Ph.D. [206]
Professor of Human Genetics, MCP Hahnemann School of Medicine, Philadelphia, Pennsylvania
pyeritz@yahoo.com

Kari O. Raivio, M.D. [111]
Professor of Perinatal Medicine, School of Medicine, University of Helsinki, Helsinki, Finland
kari.raivio@helsinki.fi

Stanley C. Rall, Jr., Ph.D. [119]
Investigator, Gladstone Institute of Cardiovascular Disease, San Francisco, California

Bonnie W. Ramsey, M.D. [201]
Dept. of Pediatrics, University of Washington School of Medicine, Children's Hospital Regional Medical Center, Seattle, Washington
bramsey@u.washington.edu

Ahmed Rasheed [57]
Research Assistant Professor, Duke University Medical Center, Durham, North Carolina
a.rasheed@duke.edu

Gerald V. Raymond, M.D. [129]
Assistant Professor, Neurology, Kennedy Krieger Institute, Johns Hopkins University School of Medicine, Baltimore, Maryland
raymond@kennedykrieger.org

Andrew P. Read, MA, Ph.D., FRC Path, FmedSci [244]
Professor of Human Genetics, Dept. of Medical Genetics, St. Mary's Hospital, University of Manchester, Manchester, United Kingdom
andrew.read@man.ac.uk

Jonathan J. Rees, MBBS, FRCP [46]
Professor and Chairman, Dept. of Dermatology, The University of Edinburgh, Edinburgh, Scotland, United Kingdom
Jonathan.rees@ed.ac.uk

Samuel Refetoff, M.D. [158]
Professor of Medicine and Pediatrics, Director, Endocrinology Laboratory, Depts. of Medicine and Pediatrics and the J.P. Kennedy Jr. Mental Retardation Research Center, The University of Chicago, Chicago, Illinois
refetoff@medicine.bsd.uchicago.edu

Arnold J.J. Reuser, Ph.D. [135]
Associate Professor of Cell Biology, Erasmus University Rotterdam, Dept. of Clinical Genetics, Rotterdam, The Netherlands
reuser@ikg.fgg.eur.nl

William B. Rizzo, M.D. [98]
Professor of Pediatrics, Human Genetics, Biochemistry, and Molecular Biophysics, Dept. of Pediatrics, Medical College of Virginia, Virginia Commonwealth University, Richmond, Virginia
wrizzo@hsc.vcu.edu

James M. Roberts, M.D. [23]
Div. of Basic Sciences, Fred Hutchinson Cancer Research Center, Seattle, Washington 98104

Brian H. Robinson, Ph.D. [100]
Professor, Depts. of Biochemistry and Pediatrics, Program Head, Metabolism, Senior Scientist, Genetics and Genomic Biology, Hospital for Sick Children, Toronto, Ontario, Canada
bhr@sickkids.on.ca

Charles R. Roe, M.D. [101]
Institute of Metabolic Disease, Baylor University Medical Center, Dallas, Texas
cr.roe@baylordallas.edu

Hans-Hilger Ropers, M.D., Ph.D. [236, 239]
Professor, Dept. of Human Genetics, Max-Planck-Institute fuer Molekulare Genetik, Berlin, Germany
Ropers@molgen.mpg.de

Michael Rosenbaum, M.D. [157]
Associate Professor of Clinical Pediatrics and Clinical Medicine, Div. of Molecular Genetics, Russ Berrie Research Center, Columbia University College of Physicians and Surgeons, New York, New York
mr475@columbia.edu

David S. Rosenblatt, M.D. [94, 155]
Professor of Human Genetics, Medicine, Pediatrics, and Biology, Director, Div. of Medical Genetics, McGill University Health Centre, Royal Victoria Hospital, Montreal, Quebec, Canada
mc74@musica.mcgill.ca

Agnes Rötig, Ph.D. [99]
Dept. of Genetics, INSERM, Hopital Necker, Paris, France
roetig@necker.fr

Jayanta Roy Chowdhury, M.D., M.R.C.P. [125]
Professor of Medicine and Molecular Genetics, Dept. of Medicine and Molecular Genetics, Albert Einstein College of Medicine at Yeshiva University, Bronx, New York
chowdhur@aecom.yu.edu

Namita Roy Chowdhury, Ph.D. [125]
Professor of Medicine and Molecular Genetics, Albert Einstein College of Medicine, Bronx, New York

Jean-Michel Rozet, M.D. [237]
Unite de Recherches sur les Handicaps, Genetiques de L'Enfant, INSERM, Hôpital des Enfants Malades, Paris, France

Edward M. Rubin, M.D., Ph.D. [121]
Head, Genome Sciences Dept., Lawrence, Berkeley Laboratory, University of California at Berkeley, Berkeley, California
emrubin@lbl.gov

Charles M. Rudin, M.D. [24]
Assistant Professor of Medicine, University of Chicago Medical Center, Chicago, Illinois
crudin@medicine.bsd.uchicago.edu

Elena I. Rugarli, M.D. [225]
Researcher, Telethon Institute of Genetics and Medicine (TIGEM), Milan, Italy
rugarli@tigem.it

David W. Russell, Ph.D. [160]
Eugene McDermott Distinguished Professor of Molecular Genetics, University of Texas Southwestern Medical Center Dallas, Texas
russell@utsw.swmed.edu

Pierre Rustin, Ph.D. [99]
Dept. of Genetics, INSERM, Hopital Des Enfants-Malades, Paris, France
rustin@necker.fr

David D. Sabatini, M.D., Ph.D. [16]
Frederick L. Ehrman Professor and Chairman, Dept. of Cell Biology, New York University School of Medicine, New York, New York
Sabatd01@popmail.med.nyu.edu

Richard L. Sabina, Ph.D. [110]
Associate Professor of Biochemistry, Dept. of Biochemistry, Medical College of Wisconsin, Milwaukee, Wisconsin
sabinar@mcw.edu

J. Evan Sadler, M.D., Ph.D. [174]
Professor, Depts. Of Medicine, Biochemistry and Molecular Biophysics; Investigator, Howard Hughes Medical Institute, Washington University School of Medicine, St. Louis, Missouri
esadler@im.wustl.edu

Amrik S. Sahota, Ph.D., F.A.C.M.G. [108]
Dept. of Genetics, Nelson Biological Laboratories, Rutgers University, Piscataway, New Jersey
sahota@nel-exchange.vutgers.edu

Mika Saksela, M.D. [111]
Research Associate, Children's Hospital, University of Helsinki, Helsinki, Finland
Mika.Saksela@Helsinki.fi

Julian R. Sampson, M.D. [233]
Professor of Medical Genetics Institute of Medical Genetics, University of Wales, College of Medicine, Cardiff, United Kingdom
wmgjrs@cardiff.ac.uk

Konrad Sandhoff, Ph.D. [134, 143, 153]
Director and Professor of Biochemistry, Kekule-Institut fur Organische Chemie und Biochemie, Universitat Bonn, Bonn, Germany
sandhoff@uni-bonn.de

Michael C. Sanguinetti, Ph.D. [203]
University of Utah, Eccles Institute of Human Genetics, Salt Lake City, Utah
mike.sanguinetti@hci.utah.edu

Silvia Santamarina-Fojo, M.D, Ph.D. [118]
Chief, Section on Cell Biology, Molecular Disease Branch, National Institutes of Health, Bethesda, Maryland
silvia@mdb.nhlbi.nih.gov

Carmen Sapienza, Ph.D. [15]
Professor of Pathology and Laboratory Medicine, Associate Director, Fels Institute for Cancer Research, Temple University School of Medicine, Philadelphia, Pennsylvania
sapienza@unix.temple.edu

Shigeru Sassa, M.D., Ph.D. [124]
Emeritus Head, Laboratory of Biochemical Hematology, The Rockefeller University, New York, New York
sassa@rockvax.rockefeller.edu

Jean-Marie Saudubray, M.D. [66]
Director of the Metabolic/Diabetes Unit, Professor, Dept. of Pediatrics, Hopital Necker Enfants Malades, Paris, France
Elisabeth.saudubray@nck.ap_hop_paris.fr

Alan J. Schafer, Ph.D. [253]
Vice President Genetics, Incyte Genomics, Cambridge, United Kingdom
alan.schafer@incyte.com

Gerard Schellenberg, Ph.D. [33]
Veterans Affairs Medical Center, Seattle, Washington
zachdad@u.washington.edu

Detlev Schindler, M.D. [139]
Director, Cell Culture, Biochemistry and Flowcytometry Div.; Associate Professor of Human Genetics, Dept. of Human Genetics, University of Wuerzburg, Wuerzburg, Germany
schindler@biozentrum.uni-wuerzburg.de

Jerry A. Schneider, M.D. [199]
Professor of Pediatrics; Benard L. Maas Chair in Inherited Metabolic Disease, Dean for Academic Affairs, Office of the Dean, School of Medicine, University of California, San Diego School of Medicine, La Jolla, California
jschneider@ucsd.edu

Edward H. Schuchman, Ph.D. [144]
Professor of Human Genetics, Dept. of Human Genetics, Mount Sinai School of Medicine, Member, Institute for Gene Therapy and Molecular Medicine, New York, New York
schuchman@msvax.mssm.edu

C. Ronald Scott, M.D. [89]
Professor, Dept. of Pediatrics, University of Washington School of Medicine, Seattle, Washington
crscott@u.washington.edu

Charles R. Scriver, M.D.C.M. [1, 5, 77]
Alva Professor of Human Genetics, Professor of Pediatrics, Faculty of Medicine, Professor of Biology, Faculty of Science, McGill University; McGill University-Montreal Children's Hospital Research Institute, McGill University Health Centre, Montreal, Quebec, Canada
mc77@musica.mcgill.ca

Udo Seedorf, M.D. [142]
Institut fur Klinische Chemie and Laboratoriumsmedizin, Zentrallaboratorium Westfalische Wilhelms-Universitat, Munster, Germany
seedorfu@uni-muenster.de

Christine E. Seidman, M.D. [213]
Investigator, Howard Hughes Medical Institute
Professor Medicine and Genetics, Director, Cardiovascular Genetics Center, Dept. of Medicine, Brigham and Women's Hospital, Harvard Medical School, Boston, Massachusetts
cseidman@rascal.med.harvard.edu

Jonathan G. Seidman, Ph.D. [213]
Henrietta B. and Frederick H. Bugher Professor of Cardiovascular Genetics, Investigator, Howard Hughes Medical Institute, Harvard Medical School, Boston, Massachusetts

Giorgio Semenza, M.D. [75]
Professor, Dept. of Biochemistry, Swiss Institute of Technology, Laboratorium fur Biochemie, Zurich, Switzerland; Professor, Dept. of Chemistry and Medical Biochemistry, University of Milan, Milan, Italy
giorgio.semenza@unimi.it
semenza@bc.biol.ethz.ch

Gul N. Shah, Ph.D. [208]
Assistant Research Professor, Edward A. Doisy Dept. of Biochemistry and Molecular Biology, Saint Louis University School of Medicine, St. Louis, Missouri
shahgn@slu.edu

Lisa G. Shaffer, Ph.D. [65]
Associate Professor, Dept. of Molecular and Human Genetics, Baylor College of Medicine, Houston, Texas
lshaffer@bcm.tmc.edu

Larry J. Shapiro, M.D. [166]
W.H. and Marie Wattis Distinguished Professor, Chairman, Dept. of Pediatrics, University of California Medical Center, San Francisco, California
Lshapiro@peds.ucsf.edu

Val C. Sheffield, M.D., Ph.D. [242]
Professor of Pediatrics, Associate Investigator, Howard Hughes Medical Institute, Dept. of Pediatrics, Div. of Medical Genetics, University of Iowa Hospital and Clinic, Iowa City, Iowa
Val-sheffield@uiowa.edu

Stephanie L. Sherman, Ph.D. [64]
Dept. of Genetics Emory University School of Medicine, Atlanta, Georgia
ssherman@genetics.emory.edu

Vivian E. Shih, M.D. [87]
Professor of Neurology, Harvard Medical School, Director, Amino Acid Disorder Laboratory/Metabolic Disorders Unit, Massachusetts General Hospital, Charlestown, Massachusetts
vshih@partners.org

John M. Shoffner, M.D. [104]
Director, Molecular Medicine, Molecular Medicine Laboratory, Children's Healthcare of Atlanta, Atlanta, Georgia
john.shoffner@choa.org

David Sidransky, M.D. [54]
Dept. of Otolaryngology-HNS, The Johns Hopkins University School of Medicine, Baltimore, Maryland
dsidrans@jhmi.edu

Olli Simell, M.D. [83, 192]
Professor of Pediatrics, Dept. of Pediatrics, University of Turku, Turku, Finland
Olli.simell@utu.fi

H. Anne Simmonds, Ph.D. [108]
Purine Research Unit, Guy's Hospital, London Bridge, London, United Kingdom
anne.simmonds@kcl.ac.uk

Ola H. Skjeldal, M.D., Ph.D. [132]
Div. of Pediatrics, Ullevaal University Hospital, Oslo, Norway
ola.skjeldal@klinmed.uio.no

William S. Sly, M.D. [1, 138, 208]
Alice A. Doisy Professor of Biochemistry and Molecular Biology, Chair, Edward A. Doisy Dept. of Biochemistry and Molecular Biology, Professor of Pediatrics, St. Louis University School of Medicine, St. Louis, Missouri
slyws@slu.edu

C. Wayne Smith, M.D. [188]
Head, Sect. of Leukocyte Biology; Professor, Depts. of Pediatrics, Microbiology and Immunology, Sect. of Leukocyte Biology, Children's Nutrition Research Center, Baylor College of Medicine Houston, Texas
cwsmith@bcm.tmc.edu

Kirby D. Smith, Ph.D. [131]
Professor of Pediatrics, Kennedy Krieger Institute, McKusick-Nathans Institute of Genetic Medicine, The Johns Hopkins University School of Medicine, Baltimore, Maryland
smithk@mail.jhmi.edu

Oded Sperling, Ph.D. [198]
Professor and Chairman of Clinical Biochemistry, Dept. of Clinical Biochemistry, Rabin Medical Center, Petah-Tikva, Israel
odeds@post.tau.ac.il

Allen M. Spiegel, M.D. [164]
Director, National Institute of Diabetes and Digestive and Kidney Diseases, Bethesda, Maryland
allens@amb.niddk.nih.gov

Peter H. St. George-Hyslop, M.D. [234]
Professor, Dept. of Medicine, Center for Research in Neurodegenerative Diseases, University of Toronto, Toronto, Ontario, Canada
p.hyslop@utoronto.ca

Beat Steinmann, M.D. [70]
Professor, Div. of Metabolism and Molecular Pediatrics, University Children's Hospital, Zurich, Switzerland
beat.steinmann@kispi.unizh.ch

Sylvia Stöckler-Ipsiroglu, M.D. [84]
Dept. of Pediatrics, University Hospital Vienna, Laboratory for Inherited Metabolic Diseases, Wahringergurtel, Vienna, Austria

Edwin M. Stone, M.D., Ph.D. [242]
Dept. of Ophthalmology and Visual Sciences, University of Iowa College of Medicine, Iowa City, Iowa
edwin-stone@viowa.edu

Pietro Strisciuglio, M.D. [152]
Associate Professor of Pediatrics, Dept. of Pediatrics, "Magna Graecia", Catanzaro, Italy
strisciuglio_unicz@libero.it

Sharon F. Suchy, Ph.D. [252]
Staff Scientist, Genetic Disease Research Branch, National Human Genome Research Instit, Bethesda, Maryland
suchy@nhgri.nih.gov

Kathleen E. Sullivan, M.D., Ph.D. [186]
Assistant Professor of Pediatrics, Children's Hospital of Philadelphia, Philadelphia, Pennsylvania

Andrea Superti-Furga, M.D. [202]
Div. of Metabolism and Molecular Pediatrics, University of Zurich, Universitaets-Kinderklinik, Zurich, Switzerland
asuperti@access.unizh.ch

Kinuko Suzuki, M.D. [145, 147, 153]
Professor of Pathology and Lab Medicine, Dept. of Pathology and Lab Medicine, School of Medicine, University of North Carolina at Chapel Hill
kis@med.unc.edu

Kunihiko Suzuki, M.D. [147, 153]
Director Emeritus, Neuroscience Center, Professor of Neurology and Psychiatry, School of Medicine, University of North Carolina at Chapel Hill, North Corolina
Kuni.Suzuki@attglobal.net

Yoshiyuki Suzuki, M.D. [147, 151]
Professor and Director, Nasu Institute for Developmental Disabilities, Clinical Research Center, International University of Health and Welfare, Otawara, Japan
suzukiy@iuhw.ac.jp

Dallas M. Swallow, Ph.D. [76]
Professor of Human Genetics, The Galton Laboratory, Dept. of Biology, University College London, London, United Kingdom
dswallow@hgmp.mrc.ac.uk

Lawrence Sweetman, Ph.D. [93]
Professor, Institute of Biomedical Studies, Baylor University; Director, Mass Spectrometry Lab, Institute of Metabolic Disease, Baylor University Medical Center, Dallas, Texas
l.sweetman@baylordallas.edu

Alan Richard Tall, M.D. [121]
Tilden Weger Bieler Professor of Medicine, Dept. of Medicine, Div. of Molecular Medicine, Columbia University College of Physicians and Surgeons, New York, New York
art1@columbia.edu

Robert M. Tanguay, Ph.D. [79]
Laboratoire de genetique cellulaire et developpementale, Pavillon Charles-Eugene Marchand, Université Laval, Ste-Foy, Quebec, Canada
robert.tanguay@rsvs.ulaval.ca

Robin G. Taylor, Ph.D. [80]
Dept. of Genetics, The Hospital for Sick Children Research Institute, Toronto, Canada
rgtaylor@alumni.haas.org

Simeon I. Taylor, M.D., Ph.D. [68]
Lilly Research Fellow, Lilly Research Laboratories, Indianapolis, Indiana

Harriet S. Tenenhouse, Ph.D. [197]
Professor of Pediatrics and Human Genetics, Auxiliary Professor of Biology, Div. of Medical Genetics, McGill University, Montreal Children's Hospital Research Institute, Montreal, Quebec, Canada
mdht@www.debelle.mcgill.ca

Jess G. Thoene, M.D. [199]
Karen Gore Professor; Director, Hayward Genetics Center, Human Genetics Program, Tulane University School of Medicine, New Orleans, Louisiana
jthoene@mailhost.tcs.tulane.edu

George H. Thomas, Ph.D. [140]
Professor of Pediatrics, Pathology and Medicine, The Johns Hopkins University School of Medicine, Director of Kennedy Krieger Institute Genetics Laboratory Baltimore, Maryland
thomasg@kennedykrieger.org

Craig B. Thompson, M.D. [24]
Abramson Family Cancer Research Institute, University of Pennsylvania, Philadelphia, Pennsylvania
drt@mail.med.upenn.edu

Beat Thöny, Ph.D. [78]
Associate Professor, Division of Clinical Chemistry & Biochemistry, Div. of Chemistry and Biochemistry, University of Zurich, Zurich, Switzerland
bthony@kispi.unizh.ch

Roland Tisch, Ph.D. [12]
Postdoctoral Fellow, Dept. of Microbiology and Immunology, Stanford University School of Medicine, Stanford, California

Jay A. Tischfield, Ph.D. [108]
MacMillan Professor and Chair, Dept. of Genetics, Rutgers University, Professor of Pediatrics and Psychiatry, Robert Wood Johnson Medical School, Piscataway, New Jersey

John A. Todd, M.D. [6]
Professor, Dept. of Medical Genetics, Cambridge University; Institute for Medical Research, Addenbrooke's Hospital, Cambridge, United Kingdom
john.todd@cimr.cam.ac.uk

Douglas M. Tollefsen, M.D., Ph.D. [176]
Professor of Medicine, Hematology Div., Washington University Medical School, St. Louis, Missouri
tollefsen@im.wustl.edu

Eileen P. Treacy, M.D. [5]
Associate Professor of Human Genetics and Pediatrics; Director, Biochemical Genetics Unit, Div. of Medical Genetics, Dept. of Biochemical Genetics, Montreal Children's Hospital, Montreal, Quebec, Canada
mcet@musica.mcgill.ca

Jeffrey M. Trent, M.D., Ph.D. [20]
Chief, Lab of Cancer Genetics, National Human Genome Research Institute, Bethesda, Maryland
jtrent@nih.gov

Mark A. Trifiro, Ph.D. [161]
Associate Professor, Dept. of Medicine, McGill University; Associate Physician, Dept. of Medicine, Lady Davis Institute for Medical Research, Sir Mortimer B. Davis Jewish General Hospital, Montreal, Canada, Quebec
mdtm@musica.mcgill.ca

Karl Tryggvason, M.D. [214]
Div. Matrix Biology, Dept. of Medical Biochemistry and Biophysics, Karolinska Institut, Stockholm, Sweden
karl.tryggvason@mbb.ki.se

William T. Tse, M.D., Ph.D. [183]
Children's Hospital/Dana-Farber Cancer Institute, Div. of Hematology/Oncology, Boston, Massachusetts
William_tse@dfci.harvard.edu

Edward G.D. Tuddenham, M.D. [172]
Professor, MRC/CSC, Hammersmith Hospital, London, United Kingdom
etuddenh@rpms.ac.uk

Eric Turk, Ph.D. [190]
Dept. of Physiology, UCLA School of Medicine, Los Angeles, California
eturk@mednet.ucla.edu

Linda A. Tyfield, M.D. [72]
Consultant Clinical Scientist, Hon. Sr. Research Fellow, Dept. of Child Health, University of Bristol, Molecular Genetics Unit, The Lewis Laboratories, Southmead Hospital, Bristol, United Kingdom
linda.tyfield@bristol.ac.uk

Jouni Uitto, M.D., Ph.D. [222]
Jefferson Institute of Molecular Medicine, Dept. of Dermatology and Cutaneous Biology, Jefferson Medical College, Philadelphia, Pennsylvania
jouni.uitto@mail.tju.edu

Gerd M. Utermann, M.D. [116]
Professor and Chair, Institute for Medical Biology and Human Genetics, Leopold-Franzens University of Innsbruck, Innsbruck, Austria
Gerd.Utermann@uibk.ac.at

David Valle, M.D. [1, 3, 4, 5, 81, 83, 129]
Professor of Pediatrics Genetics and Molecular Biology, Investigator Howard Hughes Medical Institute, McKusick-Nathans Institute of Genetic Medicine, The Johns Hopkins University, Baltimore, Maryland
dvalle@jhmi.edu

Georges Van den Berghe, M.D. [70, 112]
Professor, Dept. of Biochemistry and Cellular Biology, University of Louvain Medical School, Director of Research, Laboratory of Physiological Chemistry, Christian de Duve Institute of Cellular Pathology, Brussels, Belgium
vandenberghe@bchm.ucl.ac.be

Peter van Endert, M.D. [12]
Postdoctoral Fellow, Dept. of Microbiology and Immunology, Stanford University School of Medicine, Stanford, California

Albert H. van Gennip, M.D. [113]
Laboratory Genetic Metabole Diseases, Academic Medical Center, University of Amsterdam, Amsterdam, The Netherlands

Veronica van Heyningen, D.Phil., F.R.S.E. [240]
Head of Cell and Molecular Genetics Sect., MRC Human Genetics Unit, Western General Hospital, Edinburgh, Scotland, United Kingdom
v.vanheyningen@hgu.mrc.ac.uk

Marie T. Vanier, M.D., Ph.D. [145]
Directeur de Recherche INSERM, Lyon-Sud Medical School, Oullins, France
vanier@univ-lyonl.fr

André B.P. Van Kuilenburg, M.D. [113]
Laboratory Genetic Metabole Diseases, Academic Medical Center, University of Amsterdam, Amsterdam, The Netherlands

Emile Van Schaftingen, M.D., Ph.D. [74]
Professor of Biochemistry, Laboratory of Physiological Chemistry, ICP, Universite Catholique de Louvain, Brussels, Belgium
vanschaftingen@bchm.ucl.ac.be

Gilbert Vassart, M.D., Ph.D. [158]
Head, Dept. of Medical Genetics, Institut de Recherche Interdisciplinaire, Universite Libre de Bruxelles, Brussels, Belgium
gvassart@ulb.ac.be

Bert Vogelstein, M.D. [17, 27, 48]
Investigator, Howard Hughes Medical Institute, Clayton Professor of Oncology and Pathology, The Johns Hopkins University School of Medicine, Baltimore, Maryland
vogelbe@welch.jhu.edu

Arnold von Eckardstein, M.D. [122]
Institut für Klinische Chemie und Laboratoriumsmedizin, Zentrallaboratorium, Westfälische Wilhelms-Universität Münster, Münster, Germany
vonecka@uni-muenster.de

Kurt von Figura, Ph.D. [84, 148]
Director and Professor, Institute of Biochemistry II Zentrum Biochemie und Molekulare Zellbiologie Georg-August-Universitat Gottingen, Gottingen, Germany
kfigura@gwdg.de

Tom Vulliamy, Ph.D. [179]
Clinical Scientist, Honorary Lecturer, Dept. of Hematology, Imperial College of School of Medicine, Hammersmith Hospital, London, United Kingdom
t.vulliamy@ic.ac.uk

Douglas C. Wallace, Ph.D. [105]
Robert W. Woodruff, Professor of Molecular Genetics, Professor and Director, Center for Molecular Medicine, Emory University School of Medicine, Atlanta, Georgia
dwallace@gen.emory.edu

John H. Walter, M.D. [72]
Consultant Pediatrician, Willink Biochemical Genetics Unit, Royal Manchester Children's Hospital, Pendlebury, Manchester, United Kingdom
john@jhwalter.demon.co.uk

Ronald J.A. Wanders, Ph.D. [130, 132]
Professor of Clinical Enzymology and Inherited Diseases, University of Amsterdam Academic Medical Centre, Emma Children's Hospital and Clinical Chemistry, Amsterdam, The Netherlands
wanders@amc.uva.nl

Stephen T. Warren, Ph.D. [64]
Rollins Research Center, Emory University School of Medicine, Atlanta, Georgia
swarren@bimcore.emory.edu

Paul A. Watkins, M.D., Ph.D. [131]
Associate Professor, Neurology, Dept. of Neurogenetics, Kennedy Krieger Institute, Johns Hopkins University, Baltimore, Maryland
watkins@kennedykrieger.org

Sir David J. Weatherall, M.D., FRS [181]
Regius Professor of Medicine, Institute of Molecular Medicine, John Radcliffe Hospital, Headington, Oxford, United Kingdom
janet.watt@imm.ox.ac.uk

Barbara L. Weber, M.D. [47]
Professor of Medicine and Genetics; Director, Breast Cancer Program; Assoc. Director, Cancer, Control and Population Science, University of Pennsylvania Cancer Center, Philadelphia, Pennsylvania
weberb@mail.med.upenn.edu

Dianne R. Webster, Ph.D [113]
National Testing Center, Lab Plus Auckland Hospital, Auckland, New Zealand

Lee S. Weinstein, M.D. [164]
Investigator, Metabolic Disease Branch, National Institute of Diabetes and Digestive Kidney Diseases, Bethesda, Maryland

Michael J. Welsh, M.D. [201]
Investigator, Howard Hughes Medical Institute, Dept. of Internal Medicine, University of Iowa College of Medicine, Iowa City, Iowa
mjwelsh@blue.weeg.uiowa.edu

David A. Wenger, Ph.D. [147]
Professor of Neurology and Biochemistry and Molecular Pharmacology, Jefferson Medical College, Philadelphia, Pennsylvania
David.wenger@mail.tju.edu

Jeffrey A. Whitsett, M.D. [218]
Div. of Pulmonary Biology, Children's Hospital Medical Center, Cincinnati, Ohio
jeff.whitsett@chmcc.org

Michael P. Whyte, M.D. [207]
Professor of Medicine, Pediatrics, and Genetics, Div. of Bone and Mineral Diseases, Washington University School of Medicine, Barnes-Jewish Hospital, Medical Scientific Director, Center for Metabolic Bone Disease and Molecular Research, Shriners Hospital for Children, St. Louis, Missouri
mwhyte@shrinenet.org

Andrew O.M. Wilkie, M.D., F.R.C.P. [245]
Senior Research Fellow in Clinical Science, Wellcome Trust, Institute of Molecular Medicine, John Radcliffe Hospital, Headington, Oxford, United Kingdom
awilkie@worf.molbiol.ox.ac.uk

Douglas Wilkin, Ph.D. [210]
Medical Genetics Branch, National Human Genome Research Institute, Bethesda, Maryland

Huntington F. Willard, Ph.D. [61]
Henry Wilson Payne Professor and Chairman of Genetics, Director, Center for Human Genetics, Case Western Reserve University School of Medicine, Cleveland, Ohio
hfw@po.cwru.edu

Julian C. Williams, M.D., Ph.D. [93]
Associate Professor of Pediatrics, USC School of Medicine, Head, Div. Of Med. Genetics, Children's Hospital LA, Med. Dir., Dept. of Pathology and Laboratory Medicine Genetics Laboratories, Los Angeles, California
jwilliams@chlais.usc.edu

Jean D. Wilson, M.D. [160]
Charles Cameron Sprague Distinguished Chair in Biomedical Science, Clinical Professor of Internal Medicine, Dept. of Internal Medicine, University of Texas Southwestern Medical Center, Dallas, Texas
jwils1@mednet.swmed.edu

Jerry A. Winkelstein, M.D. [186]
Dept. of Pediatrics, Johns Hopkins University School of Medicine, Baltimore, Maryland
jwinkels@welchlink.welch.jhu.edu

Barry Wolf, M.D., Ph.D. [156]
Associate Chair for Research, Head, Div. of Pediatric Research, Professor, Div. of Human Genetics, University of Connecticut School of Medicine, Director of Pediatric Research, Connecticut Children's Medical Center, Hartford, Connecticut
bwolf@hsc.vcu.edu

Allan W. Wolkoff, M.D. [125]
Professor, Albert Einstein College of Medicine, Liver Research Center Bronx, New York
wolkoff@aecom.yu.edu

W.G. Wood [181]
Institute of Molecular Medicine, John Radcliffe Hospital, Oxford, United Kingdom

Ronald G. Worton, C.M., Ph.D., F.R.S.C. [216]
CEO and Scientific Director, Ottawa General Hospital Research Institute, University of Ottawa, Ottawa, Ontario, Canada
rworton@ogh.on.ca

Ernest M. Wright, D.Sc. [190]
Professor and Chair, Dept. of Physiology, UCLA School of Medicine, Los Angeles, California
ewright@mednet.ucla.edu

Charles John Yeo, M.D. [50]
Professor and Attending Surgeon, Dept. of Surgery and Oncology, The Johns Hopkins Hospital, Baltimore, Maryland
cyeo@jhmi.edu

Chang-En Yu, M.D., Ph.D. [33]
Veterans Affairs Puget Sound Health Care System, Seattle Div. and the Dept. of Medicine, University of Washington, Seattle, Washington
changeyu@u.washington.edu

Berton Zbar, M.D. [41]
Chief, Laboratory of Immunology, National Cancer Institute-Frederick Cancer, Research Facility, Frederick, Maryland
zbar@mail.ncifcrf.gov

Huda Y. Zoghbi, M.D. [226, 255]
Professor, Dept. of Pediatrics and Molecular and Human Genetics; Investigator Howard Hughes Medical Institute, Baylor College of Medicine, Houston, Texas
hzoghbi@bcm.tmc.edu

PREFACE TO THE EIGHTH EDITION

Following "the new synthesis" of Mendelism and Darwinism, Theodosins Dobzhansky stated that biology makes sense only in the light of evolution.[1] A corollary to that opinion would say that medicine without biology does not make sense. This book, now in its eighth edition, presents evidence that biology, as we come to know it in the era of genomics, is helping to make better sense of medicine.

In its first edition,[2] this book, then known as *The Metabolic Basis of Inherited Disease* (MBID), focused almost exclusively on the Mendelian diseases falling into the category known as "inborn errors of metabolism." For the next five editions, MBID served as a medical companion to human biochemical genetics which had its own seminal text.[3] Then, to acknowledge the increasing relevance of molecular biology and molecular genetics, for the seventh edition we changed its title to: *The Metabolic and Molecular Bases of Inherited Disease* (*MMBID*). There were further changes in the seventh edition: complex genetic traits were increasingly recognized, cancer being a notable new section of the book, and even more so in the CD-ROM update of the print edition. Chromosomal disorders had appeared in the sixth edition and they increased their presence in the seventh, along with a chapter dedicated to imprinting.

The eighth edition of MMBID, now appearing in the first year of the twenty-first century, contains new chapters on the history of the inborn errors of metabolism (Chapter 3), their impact on health (Chapter 4) and their response to treatment (Chapter 5). This edition further reveals how genetics is contributing to the understanding of complex traits and birth defects as well as the Mendelian diseases with nominal pathways of metabolism or development. It is not surprising then that MMBID-8 should have chapters on aging and hypertension or on Hirschsprung disease, for example. In brief, this book is becoming a "textbook of medicine," as predicted by one reviewer of an earlier edition.[4]

Five questions formulated as such by Victor McKusick among others have been of abiding interest in medicine since at least the time of Osler: (1) What is the problem? (2) How did it happen? (3) What is the cause? (4) What can be done? (5) Will it happen again? The questions address the corresponding issues of diagnosis, pathogenesis, ultimate and proximal cause, treatment and prevention, and inherited risks of recurrence. As for cause, the theme of special interest shared by every entity discussed in this book is *mutation*: mutation that modifies phenotype, contributes to pathogenesis of the disease and, in various ways, identifies a key component in a "pathway" or "network" responsible for homeostasis and functional integrity.

MMBID-8 is being published as genome projects, both human and nonhuman, yield information and knowledge about the organization and nucleotide sequences of genomes. The allied field of research, now called genomics, has been called "a journey to the center of biology."[5] Comparative genomics reveals that homeostasis of energy metabolism and many aspects of intermediary metabolism are encoded in genes with a very long evolutionary history (see Chapter 4). Moreover, a number of the human disorders can be analyzed functionally in yeast in a manner some will call "biochemical genomics"[6] and there is a corresponding database cross-referencing human and yeast phenotypes.[7] Accordingly, Dobzhansky's angle of vision is increasingly validated.

At the same time, the genomes of *C. elegans* and *Drosophila* are telling us that development of multicellular organisms is controlled by the major portion of the corresponding genomes and each organism has particular programs for particular body plans. New sections and chapters in MMBID-8 are devoted to various disorders of development in *H. sapiens*.

It follows that biology is indeed a shared language for medicine.[8] However, shared language does not preclude particular language to deal with variant phenotypes (the diseases), their clinical consequences, and the specialization in clinical expertise required to address them. In recognition of this, the book contains material in the particular languages of counseling, testing and screening, and treatment; indeed, in a language increasingly accessed on Web sites by patients who want to know. The particular language extends beyond phenotype, counseling, and so on; it reaches the patient. Every patient who has one of the so-called "single-gene" diseases described in this book has an "orphan" disease; furthermore, because of biological individuality, each patient has his or her own private (orphan) form of unhealth. In other words, this book is an ultimate guidebook for *individualized medicine*.

MMBID-8 will contribute to an instauration of the clinician-investigator, a colleague who has been much marginalized by successes in the basic science and molecular and cellular biology and the corresponding contributions to medical science. The original editions of MBID were written largely by clinician-investigators; or by basic scientists who still retained a familiarity with patients or did research that was patient-oriented and disease-oriented.[9] However, in the more recent editions of MMBID, the chapters themselves and the majority of the references cited in them were more often than not authored by persons doing basic research, sometimes rather remote from the patient's primary problem. But, as the "genome project" moves from its structural to a functional phase and into biochemical- and pharmacogenomics, the editors of MMBID recognize a need for the return of the clinician-investigator. The latter must share equal status with the basic scientist so that science can be translated quickly into benefits for patients. That is why some chapters in MMBID-8 (e.g., 66 and 99) are devoted to clinical algorithms.

The prefaces to MBID-6 and MMBID-7 described how the editors chose material for Chapters and Parts of these editions. In the seventh edition, we said: "If there is an identifiable molecular explanation for the disease — and it affects a dynamic phenotype, metabolic or otherwise — then it is a candidate for inclusion .... The expansion of topics here is selective and obviously not inclusive of all possibilities." Although MMBID-8 has not changed its title, it has changed in many other ways. It has three new associate editors (Barton Childs, Kenneth Kinzler, and Bert Vogelstein), new chapters have appeared (the total is now 255) and the number of authors now exceeds 500. That the printed and bound book exceeds 7000 pages is not really a surprise, but it is an abiding reason to have portable and online versions of the book.

A survey undertaken by some of the editors, by some of our readers and owners of the seventh edition showed that 70% used the book at least once per week. Half those persons believed the book should grow beyond its original domain; that content of MMBID-7 was appropriate; and over 90% of the readers welcomed the prospect of a Web version.

The editors intend to keep MMBID-8 "user friendly;" and also to keep it up to date. We hope a portable version of MMBID-8 will be available for those who wish to have something they can carry home; there will be a Web version. In this latter format, MMBID will become a "continuous book," able to update all material and to incorporate new topics as they become pertinent to our stated mission. Accordingly, as more and more scientific print literature goes "on line" in one format or another, MMBID will do likewise;

the web version will allow MMBID to reincarnate itself through a long and healthy life.

So much seems to change between editions of MMBID; for example, a new team — Susan Noujaim, Peter Boyle, Marty Wonsiewicz, and others at McGraw-Hill — have translated formidable stacks of typescript into a book agreeable to the publisher. On the other hand, stability can still be found in the life of this book; the editors are still working with the same colleagues: Lynne Prevost and Huguette Rizziero (CRS), Grace Watson (AB), Elizabeth Torno (WS), Sandy Muscelli (DV); while Kathy Helwig helped the new editors (BC, KK, and BV). The process of reading manuscripts and proofs was yet again lightened by the tolerant support of our families and by colleagues at the places of business.

REFERENCES

1. Dobzhansky TH: "Nothing in biology makes sense except in the light of evolution." *Am Biol Teach* **35**:125, 1973.
2. Stanbury JB, Wyngaarden JB, Fredrickson DS (eds.): *The Metabolic Basis of Inherited Disease*. McGraw-Hill Book Co., New York. 1960.
3. Harris H: The principles of human biochemical genetics. *Frontiers of Biology* (Neuberger A, Tatum EL (eds.), Vol. 19. North Holland Pub. Co., London, 1970. North-Holland Research Monographs.
4. Childs B: Book Review. *The Metabolic Basis of Inherited Disease*. 6th ed. 2 volumes. Scriver CR, Beaudet AL, Sly WS, Valle D (eds.). *Am J Hum Genet* **46**:848, 1990.
5. Lander ES, Weinberg RA: Genomics: Journey to the center of biology. *Science* **287**:1777, 2000.
6. Carlson M: The awesome power of yeast biochemical genomics. *Trends Genet* **16**:49, 2000.
7. Bassett DE Jr., Boguski MS, Spencer F, Reeves R, Kim SH, Weaver T, Hieter P: Genome cross-referencing and XREFdb: Implications for the identification and analysis of genes mutated in human disease. *Nat Genet* **15**:339, 1997.
8. Scriver CR: American Pediatric Society Presidential Address 1995. Disease, war and biology: Language for medicine — and pediatrics. *Pediatric Res* **38**:819, 1995.
9. Goldstein JL, Brown MS: The clinical investigator: Bewitched, bothered, and bewildered — but still beloved. Editorial. *J Clin Invest* **99**:2803, 1997.

PREFACE TO THE SEVENTH EDITION

The sixth edition of *The Metabolic Basis of Inherited Disease* experienced "transition, transformation, and challenge." Transition continues in the seventh edition with the arrival of many new authors. Challenge remains, like the mountain whose peak is never in view while the climb proceeds. And there is transformation again, not least with the title: *The Metabolic and* Molecular *Bases of Inherited Disease*. The new word is significant.

A reviewer of the sixth edition reminds us of the original plan for the book: to present "the pertinent clinical, biochemical, and genetic information concerning those metabolic anomalies grouped under Garrod's engaging term 'inborn errors of metabolism.' "[1] The term *molecular* is a belated but natural homecoming for Garrod. During his lifetime, Garrod's views grew to encompass inherited susceptibility to any disease originating in our chemical individuality. These ideas emerged fully developed, for their time, in Garrod's second book. *The Inborn Factors in Disease*. That we have been slow to perceive the reach of his thinking is a theme of his recent biographer.[2] To accept it and put it to use requires the means to test its validity. Molecular analysis of the genetic variation causing or predisposing to disease provides the opportunity. The inborn errors of metabolism are simply our most obvious illustrations of the genetic variation that affects health and the molecular underpinnings of that variation. A corresponding analysis of multifactorial diseases is the obvious next step in the understanding of disease.[3] Need we say that MMBID-7 is nothing less than a textbook of molecular medicine, encompassing the diseases about which we know most? We predict that the "classic" textbooks of medicine in the future will look more and more like MMBID.

Change in the title of MBID did something else: it solved a problem the editors created for themselves in MBID-6, again commented on by the above-mentioned reviewer.[1] When we included topics not overtly "metabolic" in the sixth edition, for example, Down and fragile X syndromes, primary ciliary dyskinesia, collagen disorders and the muscular dystrophies, we moved well beyond the canonical theme of inborn errors of *metabolism*. The nonmetabolic topics are further expanded in this edition because they conform to a *logic of disease*, as it is called by Barton Childs in Chapter 2. The manifestations of any "genetic" disease are explained by a process (pathogenesis) that originates in part or in full form an intrinsic cause (mutation); and, since genotype is one of the determinants of the phenotype (disease), it follows that diagnosis, treatment, and counseling should be motivated form the genetic point of view because the disease involves both the patient and his or her family.

If there is an identifiable molecular explanation for the disease—and it affects a dynamic phenotype, metabolic or otherwise—then it is a candidate for inclusion in the seventh edition. The expansion of topics here is selective and obviously not inclusive of all possibilities. If this were the case, the table of contents would resemble the McKusick catalog, *Mendelian Inheritance in Man*! Nevertheless, yet a further 32 chapters are new to this edition of MBID while 31 others were introduced in the sixth edition; new ideas appear again and again in virtually all "old" chapters. Will it be three volumes—or more—for the eighth edition? (A CD-ROM format is under serious consideration for the next edition.) The Summary Table, immediately preceding Chapter 1, surveys the information in MMBID-7.

In the first section of the book, the following major new themes appear:

- A logic of disease based on genetic and evolutionary concepts that challenges conventional medical thinking (Chapter 2).
- Mutational mechanisms, including dynamic mutations (elastic or unstable DNA) (Chapter 3) and the methods to detect them (Chapter 1).
- Pharmacogenetics (Chapter 4) as a classical illustration of multifactorial disease (with ultimate and proximate causes) and of the "idiosyncratic reaction to drugs"—to recall Garrod's felicitous phrase.
- Diagnostic algorithms for the patient with an inborn error of metabolism (Chapter 5).
- Mapping of genes (genomics) (Chapter 6), along with an increased awareness that mutant gene expression may involve more than conventional Mendelian inheritance: for example, imprinting and mosaicism (Chapter 7).
- How cellular organelles, protein targeting and posttranslational modification, and the HLA complex affect expression of "genetic" disease (the subjects of Chapters 8 and 9, respectively).
- Cancer appears as a major theme for the first time in this edition (Chapters 10 to 15). Cancers are products of genetic damage. Modified events in pathways release cells from the normal controls of replication and growth. The cascades of events controlled by proto-oncogenes are counterparts of Garrod's pathways of metabolism. Because cancers can involve constitutional mutations, somatic mutations, or both, they further expand the conceptual boundaries of the book.
- Processes of inactivation harbored on the X chromosome (Chapter 16) and knowledge about the testis-determining factor and primary sex reversal (Chapter 17) are topics new to the section on chromosomes, itself an innovation of the sixth edition.

An awesome expansion of information continues in old and new chapters. The new chapters include, for example, insulin gene defects (Chapter 22); a completely new look at nonketotic hyperglycinemia (Chapter 37); diseases of the mitochondrial genome (Chapter 46); the apolipoprotein (a) molecule and its association with heart disease (Chapter 58); oxalosis as a peroxisomal disorder (Chapter 75); lysosomal enzyme activator proteins (Chapter 76); Pompe disease as a disease of lysosome function (Chapter 77) rather than a disease of carbohydrate metabolism; Lowe syndrome, separated from the Fanconi syndrome, following positional cloning of the gene (Chapter 123); Marfan syndrome, a disease of fibrillin dysfunction (Chapter 135); the muscular dystrophies (Chapters 140 and 141), and hypertrophic cardiomyopathy (Chapter 142). All is not new; in recognition of tradition, the spelling of *alcaptonuria* has reverted to *alkaptonuria* (Chapter 39).

A new section on disease of the eye (Chapters 143 to 146) includes retinitis pigmentosis, choroideremia, and disorders of color vision and crystallins. Discussions of epidermolysis bullosa (Chapter 149). Huntington disease (Chapter 152), and prion-related diseases (Chapter 153) reflect emerging molecular information on diseases of skin and brain. Chapter 154, the last in the book, catches recent developments involving half a dozen diseases.

The authors of chapters about particular diseases were asked to remember the needs of physicians and families, and they provide up-to-date information on diagnosis, treatment, and counseling. (These aspects are dealt with an even greater depth in a book that functions as our companion—the excellent *Inborn Metabolic*

Diseases: Diagnosis and Treatment, edited by J. Fernandes, J-M. Saudubray, and K. Tada.)

Some 200 authors wrote for MBID-6; 302 have written for MMBID-7; they have achieved the continuing transformation of this text. While so much seems to change overnight in molecular biology and genetics, stability can be found in the life of this book. Gail Gavert, Mariapaz Ramos-Englis, J. Dereck Jeffers, Peter McCurdy, and their colleagues have translated formidable stacks of typescript into a book agreeable to the publisher. The editors are still working with the same colleagues: Lynne Prevost and Huguette Rizziero (CRS), Grace Watson (AB), Elizabeth Torno (WS), and Sandy Muscelli (DV), Loy Denis was again our editorial coordinator until the last stages of this edition; her successor is Catherine Watson. The process of reading manuscripts and proofs was lightened by the tolerant support of our families and by colleagues at the place of business.

As this edition went to press, Harry Harris died. A giant in our field, his imprint is apparent everywhere in the book.

REFERENCES

1. Childs B: Book Review: *The Metabolic Basis of Inherited Disease*, 6th ed. *Am J Hum Genet* **66**:848, 1990.
2. Bearn AG: *Archibald Garrod and the Individuality of Man*. New York, Oxford University Press, 1993, 227 pp.
3. King RA, Rutter JI, Motulsky AG: *The Genetic Basis of Common Diseases*. New York, Oxford University Press, 1993, 978 pp.

PREFACE TO THE SIXTH EDITION

This edition of *The Metabolic Basis of Inherited Disease* marks a transition, a changing of the guard, as it were, among the editors. The sixth edition also reflects a transformation in the field of endeavor it encompasses; and there is a challenge too — for future editions. Transitions can be difficult and transformations sometimes produce unhappy results; neither need be the case here. Challenges can invigorate.

THE TRANSITION

Stanbury-Wyngaarden-'n-Fredrickson, collectively, were one famous "author" known to everyone in the field. This extraordinary editorial organism piloted the novel and timely book they had introduced and then edited through four successful editions. By a remarkable fision — or was it fusion? — the fifth edition was placed under the care of Stanbury-Wyngaarden-'n-Fredrickson, Goldstein 'n Brown. Now that giant has stepped aside, handing the challenge to a new team. The new editors have discovered how great the former ones were — if they hadn't known it before. Very large shoes had to be filled!

THE TRANSFORMATION

The sixth edition has many new features, notably the evidence of molecular genetics in one chapter after another. If *The Metabolic Basis of Inherited Disease* has had an abiding rationale, it was that the cause of all diseases listed in it was Mendelian and the diseases (so-called inborn errors of metabolism) were exceptions to be treasured for their illumination of human biology and for the insight they gave into pathogenesis of disease. But always there was a feeling that one did not understand cause as well as one should because not much was known about the genes. That situation is changing. There are new data about loci and structures of numerous normal genes and about the mutations affecting the phenotype encoded by them.

With 31 new chapters, the book is approximately one-third larger than it was. Accordingly, this edition appears for the first time in a two-volume format. It is a change undertaken with reluctance, but size of type, weight of paper, and the like had been adapted to the limit in the previous edition to accommodate the mass of information presented there. We elected to revise and print all chapters instead of using a précis of some, as in the last edition. Authors were encouraged to focus on up-to-date material and to use previous editions as archives of older material. But the wealth of new information neutralized contraction of the old. Hence the option taken here; to divide the book into two volumes, between separate covers.

New topics in the sixth edition include the following: There is a formal discussion of gene mapping and the medical use of genome markers (Chapter 6). Down syndrome (Chapter 7) and fragile X syndrome (Chapter 8) illustrate how any genetic disorder can eventually accommodate to our views of molecular genetics. They are the thin edge of the wedge toward understanding a great deal about human genetic disease and the editors introduce these chapters with some trepidation, realizing they could well be the very thin edge of a very big wedge — one of our challenges for future editions. One new chapter (122) covers the lactose deficiency polymorphism. This disorder does not fit the paradigm of a rare inborn error because it is so common; on the other hand, it does represent a Mendelian disadaptive phenotype for some individuals. There is a whole new section on peroxisomal diseases (Chapters 57–60) and Chapter 3 covers organelle biogenesis. Contiguous gene syndromes appear in this edition for the first time. The retinoblastoma story (Chapter 9) began as a contiguous gene syndrome; the new chapter encompasses this and analogous phenomena. Chapter 5 on oncogenes is new. The genes for retinoblastoma, chronic granulomatosus disease, and Duchenne muscular dystrophy are now known through techniques of "reverse" or "indirect" genetics. They are harbingers of what is to come in other diseases and they are topics developed at some length in this edition. Two appendices to Chapter 1, experiments in this edition, list: (1) the Mendelian disorders that can be diagnosed at the DNA level through oligonucleotide probes or by tightly linked markers that associate with alleles encoding mutant gene products; useful probes and their sources are catalogued in this appendix; (2) the mapped loci and their chromosomal assignments in the most current version of Victor McKusick's famous catalog available as we went to press. Perhaps a future edition will also catalog what we know about the mutant alleles at the loci encoding disease. Meanwhile the summary table grows in Chapter 1. It was introduced for the first time in the fifth edition and it is continued here for two reasons: first to show, in a simple manner, the growth of subject material between the last and present editions; second, to show how the white spaces in the fifth edition table are being filled in.

THE CHALLENGE

The future holds the potential for a separate chapter delineating the biochemical basis of each variant listed in McKusick's *Mendelian Inheritance in Man*. If this is the case, there will be many hundred chapters in subsequent editions of MBID. In addition, most monogenic disorders are not monogenic but modified through other loci by definable biochemical mechanisms; and most diseases are caused by polygenic and multifactorial mechanisms which also have a biochemical basis. Cytogenetic disorders have a biochemical basis as well, and in some instances the phenotypes may be determined by one or a few loci. These all represent effects of the constitutional genotypes on the phenotype, but there is also the role of somatic mutation in the pathogenesis of malignancies whether inherited or sporadic. With the explosion of information virtually assured, the challenge of how to focus and mold future editions is a daunting one.

This book has not grown unattended. In addition to the herculean efforts of some 200 authors and their assistants, others assured a safe passage during the development of the book, notably Dereck Jeffers and Gail Gavert at McGraw-Hill; Loy Denis, who served as coordinator for the editors and authors; and our own assistants: Lynne Prevost and Huguette Rizziéro (CRS), Grace Watson (AB), Elizabeth Torno (WS), and Sandy Muscelli (DV). But especially we thank our extraordinary predecessors for their nurture and care of a book many of us have come to admire and need. If this edition meets with the approval of its former editors, we will have partially done the job we acquired; the readers will ultimately decide whether it was done satisfactorily.

Last, an acknowledgment to our families; they know more about this book than they bargained for . . .!

Charles R. Scriver
Arthur L. Beaudet
William S. Sly
David Valle

The Metabolic & Molecular Bases of Inherited Disease

eighth edition

AMINO ACIDS

PART 8

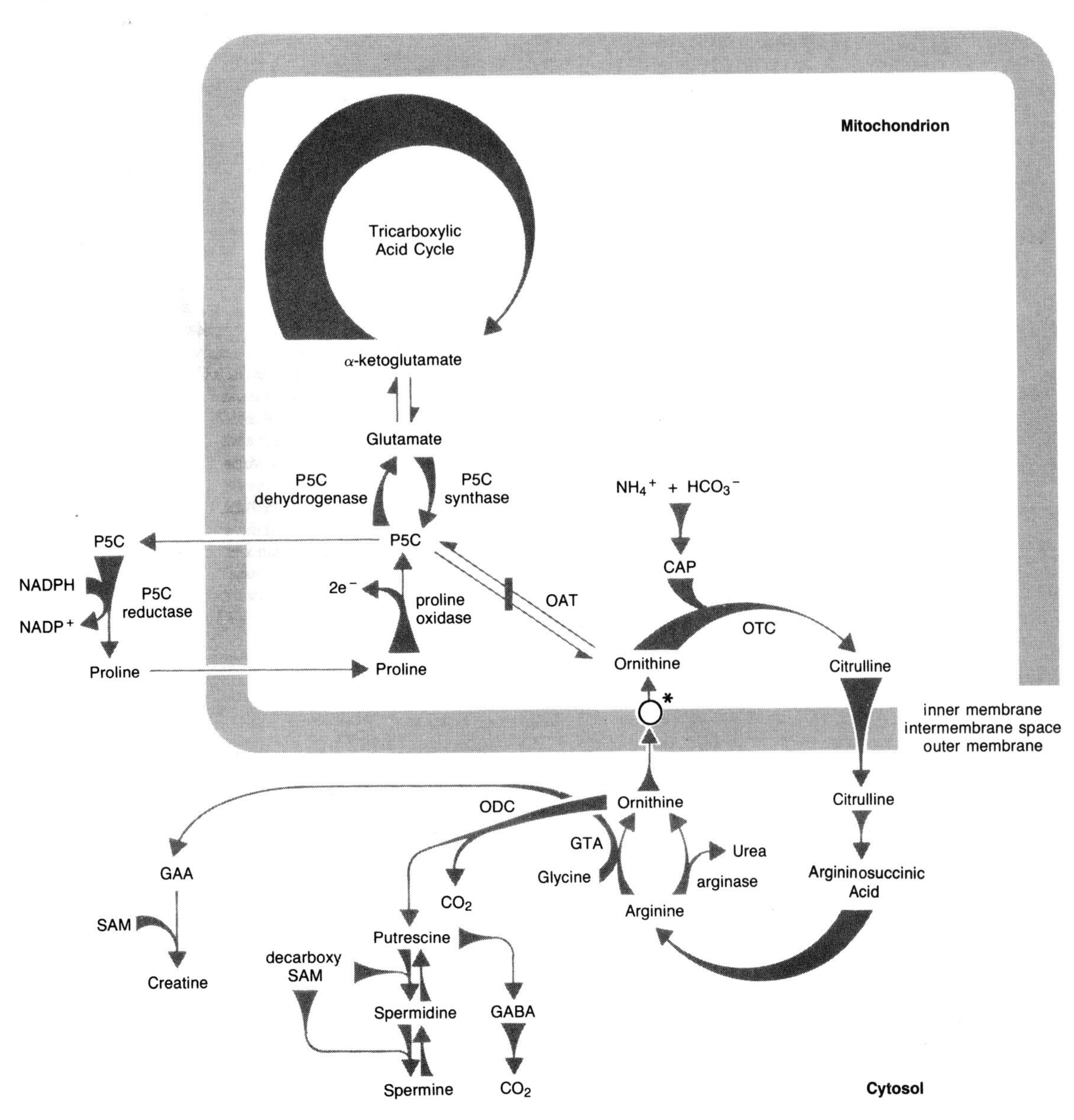

CHAPTER 77

Hyperphenylalaninemia: Phenylalanine Hydroxylase Deficiency

Charles R. Scriver ▪ Seymour Kaufman

1. **Hyperphenylalaninemia [phenylketonuria (PKU) and non-PKU hyperphenylalaninemia (HPA) are the clinical forms discussed here] is an autosomal recessive (*Mendelian*) trait (OMIM 261600) with *multifactorial cause*: mutation in the human phenylalanine hydroxylase (symbol *PAH*) gene and exposure to dietary phenylalanine are both necessary and sufficient conditions. The proximal phenotype (phenylalanine hydroxylation dysfunction) is under the control of multiple loci encoding phenylalanine hydroxylase protein and several enzymes necessary for synthesis and recycling of its tetrahydrobiopterin cofactor; *locus heterogeneity* thus enters the diagnosis of *hyperphenylalaninemia*. The intermediate (metabolic) and distal (cognitive) phenotypes of PKU disease both behave as *complex traits* that elude consistent interindividual genotype/phenotype correlations. The phenylalanine hydroxylase gene harbors great *allelic diversity*: several hundred disease-causing mutations are recorded in *PAHdb*, a public on-line locus-specific mutation database (http://www.mcgill.ca/pahdb).**
2. **The HPAs are disorders of phenylalanine hydroxylation. The minimum requirements for the normal reaction, which occurs mainly in liver in human subjects, are *phenylalanine hydroxylase enzyme*, a monooxygenase (EC 1.14.16.1), oxygen, L-phenylalanine substrate, and tetrahydrobiopterin (BH_4) cofactor. For the pterin cofactor to function as a catalyst, BH_4 must be regenerated from the carbinolamine byproduct (4α-hydroxytetrahydropterin) of the hydroxylation reaction. This is achieved by a recycling pathway in which *4α-carbinolamine dehydratase* (formerly known as phenylalanine hydroxylase-stimulating protein) converts the carbinolamine to the quinonoid dihydropterin, which, as the substrate for *dihydropteridine reductase* in the presence of reduced pyridine nucleotide, is converted back to BH_4. A pathway exists for biosynthesis of this obligatory cofactor involving *guanosine triphosphate cyclohydrolase*, *6-pyruvoyltetrahydropterin synthase*, and *sepiapterin reductase*. The recycling and synthesis pathways, enzymes, genes for, and diseases of BH_4 homeostasis are discussed in Chap. 78.**
3. ***Hyperphenylalaninemia* is defined as a plasma phenylalanine value of more than 120 μM (more than 2 mg/dl). Whether forms of HPA due to altered integrity of phenylalanine hydroxylase enzyme (PAH) should be subdivided into different forms — notably *phenylketonuria* (plasma phenylalanine >1000 μM, diet phenylalanine tolerance <500 mg/day) and *non-PKU* forms (plasma phenylalanine <1000 μM, diet tolerance >500 mg/day) — is a moot point if all degrees of persistent HPA are harmful to cognitive development (a hypothesis still awaiting rigorous confirmation). For purposes of diagnosis, counseling, and treatment the non-PAH enzyme deficiencies affecting BH_4 homeostasis must be ruled out.**
4. **The human *PAH* gene covers 100 kb of genomic DNA on chromosome 12, band region q22–q24.1. It has 13 exons and a complex 5′ untranslated region containing *cis*-acting, *trans*-activated regulatory elements. The nucleotide sequence for a full-length cDNA is known (GenBank U49897). The gene is rich in intragenic polymorphic markers, including biallelic restriction fragment length polymorphism (RFLP) and single-nucleotide polymorphism (SNP) alleles, a tetranucleotide short tandem repeat (STR) acting as a fast molecular clock in intron 3, and a variable number of tandem repeats (VNTR, 30-bp-long cassettes) in the 3′ untranslated region (UTR). The polymorphic sites are in linkage disequilibrium and describe a large series of extended and minihaplotypes. The *PAH* gene also harbors several hundred disease-causing alleles associated with HPA, among which only a half-dozen account for the majority of mutant chromosomes in Europeans and Orientals; the remainder are rare, even private, alleles.**
5. **The human *PAH* gene has developmental- and tissue-specific transcription/translation. Its hepatic and renal translation product is a 452-amino-acid polypeptide homologous in several domains with the subunits of tyrosine and tryptophan hydroxylases. The crystal structure of the catalytic domain of human PAH polypeptide has been resolved at 2 Å for residues 117 to 427. The enzyme is homooligomeric and functions in alternating activated and deactivated states, in dimeric and tetrameric conformations. The effect of mutant alleles can now be studied by molecular modeling *in silico*.**
6. **The effects of disease-causing PAH mutations on a patient can be measured at three levels: proximal (enzymic),**

A list of standard abbreviations is located immediately preceding the index in each volume. Additional abbreviations used in this chapter include: BH_4 = tetrahydropterin [(*6R*)-L-*erythro*-5,6,7,8-tetrahydrobiopterin]; DHPR = dihydropteridine reductase; $DMPH_4$ = 6,7-dimethyltetrahydropterin; GTP-CH = guanosine triphosphate cyclohydrolase; HPA = hyperphenylalaninemia; $6MPH_4$ = 6-methyltetrahydropterin; PAH = phenylalanine hydroxylase enzyme (phenylalanine 4-monooxygenase); *PAH* = phenylalanine hydroxylase gene (human), and symbol in mouse is *Pah*; *Pah* = phenylalanine hydroxylase gene (mouse); PAL = phenylalanine ammonia lyase; PKU = phenylketonuria; 6-PTS = 6-pyruvoyltetrahydropterin synthase; qBH_2 = quinonoid form of dihydrobiopterin; RFLP = restriction fragment length polymorphism; SNP = single nucleotide polymorphism; STR = short tandem repeat; VNTR = variable number of tandem repeats.

intermediate (metabolic), and distal (cognitive function). Enzyme dysfunction can be measured *in vitro* directly by hepatic biopsy or indirectly by expression analysis when the mutation is expressed in a plasmid construct in mammalian or bacterial cell systems or in a cell-free transcription/translation system. *In vitro* expression analysis enables *in vivo* hepatic PAH activity to be predicted with considerable accuracy. *In vivo* flux rates for phenylalanine hydroxylation/oxidation can be measured by two different isotopic methods. All studies of genotype-phenotype correlations reveal reasonable correlations at the proximal (enzyme) level; but, at intermediate (metabolic) and distal (cognitive) levels, phenotypes have emergent properties and behave as complex traits in which the effects of *PAH*, the major locus, is modulated by "modifiers."

7. **Pathogenic *PAH* alleles produce their effects on PAH enzyme by various mechanisms and behave in broad terms: as *null* alleles (no activity), V_{max} alleles (reduced activity), *kinetic* alleles (altered affinity for substrate or cofactor), and *unstable* alleles (increased turnover and loss of PAH protein). Findings have occasionally been taken to signify negative allelic complementation as a mechanism of mutant genotype expression.**
8. **Newborn screening for PKU occurs in many societies and is a potent resource for ascertainment and sampling of mutant *PAH* genes. Incidence data for HPA (5 to 350 cases/million live births) and mutation analysis together reveal nonuniform distribution of cases and alleles in populations. Human genetic diversity at the *PAH* locus complements data from analysis of mitochondrial DNA, the Y chromosome, and classical polymorphisms. The distribution and types of *PAH* alleles indicate how migration, genetic drift, natural selection (perhaps), recurrent mutation, and intragenic recombination over the past 100,000 years might account for the present-day incidence of PKU, the observed mutation-haplotype associations, and the nonuniform distribution of cases and major alleles in modern populations.**
9. **Pathogenesis of the most important disease phenotype (impaired cognitive development and neurophysiological functions) in HPA is undoubtedly complex in nature, but there is an emerging consensus that phenylalanine itself, at elevated concentrations, is the harmful molecule. Several strains of mice mutagenized by the alkylating agent *N*-ethyl-*N*-nitrosourea, with documented mouse phenylalanine hydroxylase (*Pah*) gene mutations and deficient hepatic enzyme activity, are new orthologous resources to study pathogenesis and treatment to control the phenotypic effects of the mutant genotype.**
10. **Newborn screening with measurement of blood phenylalanine is the most reliable method for early detection of HPA. Classification of phenotype into severe and less severe forms, and exclusion of BH_4-deficient probands, require measurements of phenylalanine, pterins, and neurotransmitter derivatives in urine, plasma, and cerebrospinal fluid (CSF), along with various assays of enzyme activity (see Chap. 78). If it is requested, prenatal diagnosis for PKU is feasible by DNA analysis of mutations and haplotypes.**
11. **Treatment of HPA requires restoration of blood phenylalanine to values as near normal as possible, as early as possible, for as long as possible, perhaps for a lifetime. At present, it seems that any deviation from this policy may incur a cost in structure and function of brain in classical PKU patients; whether this will also occur in non-PKU HPA is still unclear, but opinion favors a prudent (protreatment) position, contrary to an earlier policy of no treatment. Among the modalities of treatment, the low-phenylalanine diet is still paramount but needs to be improved in organoleptic properties and nutrient composition, notably of the essential fatty acids and the relative ratios of amino acids. Alternative modalities include enzyme substitution with phenylalanine ammonia lyase (promising) and gene therapy (in a holding pattern).**
12. **Maternal HPA, a toxic embryopathy/fetopathy, causes congenital malformations, microcephaly, and permanently impaired cognitive development. It is a consequence of intrauterine phenylalanine excess in the fetal compartment and derived from a positive transplacental gradient. All females of reproductive age with HPA should receive reproductive counseling, social support, and continued or renewed treatment to restore euphenylalaninemia before conception and throughout pregnancy. Meticulous treatment of maternal HPA is compatible with a normal outcome for the fetus.**
13. **Virtually all the major themes and issues now considered to be important in PKU were recognized by Penrose over half a century ago. The fundamental questions are the same then and now; only the tools and opportunities to address them have changed.**

PREFACE

This chapter cannot aspire to be a total overview of hyperphenylalaninemia (HPA) and its principal disease type,† even though it touches most aspects of the topic. Rather, it is a close analysis of the enzyme involved, phenylalanine hydroxylase (PAH), the corresponding human gene (*PAH*) with its alleles, their disease-causing effects, and how the latter occur and can be prevented.

In 1994, a symposium‡ was held to celebrate the 60th anniversary of Asbørn Følling's German-language report[3] on a new inborn error of metabolism; another in 1995 celebrated the 40th anniversary of effective therapy of this genetic disease. The disease, renamed *phenylketonuria* in 1935 by Penrose,[4] had been called *Imbecilitas phenylpyrouvica* by Følling to recognize its effect on cognitive development.§ Eleven years later, for his inaugural address as Galton Professor at University College London,[6] Penrose chose phenylketonuria (PKU) as his topic. Among the many themes running through his remarkable analysis of this now classic genetic disease, Penrose observed that PKU was the first to exhibit a chemical explanation for mental retardation.

With the hindsight of 6 decades, major milestones on this journey of discovery about PKU can be recognized: (1) In the 1930s, it is shown that both the disease (mental retardation) and the major metabolic abnormality (hyperphenylalaninemia) are accounted for by autosomal recessive inheritance‡ of a deleterious gene;[3,4] the OMIM entry is 261600. (2) In the 1950s, PKU patients are shown to have deficient activity of hepatic phenylalanine hydroxylase (symbol PAH; EC 1.14.16.1), the key enzyme controlling L-phenylalanine catabolism.[7] (3) In the same decade, a

†This chapter is an overview of both recent developments and well-established themes in the Mendelian hyperphenylalaninemias. A *Medline* search identified over 400 new entities (since MMBID-7e) on hyperphenylalaninemia and phenylketonuria. All of these could not be cited.

‡The symposium was published [*Acta Paediatr Scand* 83(suppl 407), 1994]. It opens with an elegant essay, written by his son Ivar, about Asbjørn Følling and his discovery of PKU.[1] Another symposium, opened by Horst Bickel, the "father of PKU therapy," covering this and other topics was published thereafter [*Eur J Pediatr* 155(suppl 1), 1996].

§Asbjørn Følling later renamed "his" disease, preferring to call it *oligophrenia phenylpyrouvica*,[2] a name more compatible with the wide range of mental deficiency he had discovered in patients with PKU. The same article extends the evidence in his Norwegian cases for autosomal recessive inheritance of the disease, adding support to similar claims made early by himself,[3] Penrose,[4] and Jervis.[5]

diet restricting intake of phenylalanine, an essential amino acid for humans, is proposed[8] and shown to ameliorate the HPA of PKU, thus offering the potential to prevent mental retardation.[8a] (4) In the 1960s, a simple test for population screening is developed[9] that provides the opportunity for early diagnosis, treatment, and prevention of PKU disease. (5) In the 1960s and 1970s, treatment of this particular genetic disease is seen as a prototype for the treatment of other genetic diseases,[10] and it is shown to be truly effective in preventing mental retardation in PKU.[11] (6) In the 1980s, mapping and cloning of the phenylalanine hydroxylase gene comes first in rodent[12] and then in *Homo sapiens sapiens*[13] (human gene symbol, *PAH*; GenBank cDNA sequence, U49897.1), followed in the 1990s by worldwide mutation analysis and recognition that extensive mutant allelic heterogeneity accounts for PKU and related HPA.[14] (7) In the 1970s, there is recognition[15,16] that locus heterogeneity must exist to account for all components of phenylalanine hydroxylation *in vivo* and to account for a mysterious subset of patients with "malignant" HPA. (The present chapter no longer covers details of the diseases caused by mutations in the genes controlling synthesis and recycling of tetrahydrobiopterin (BH_4), cofactor for phenylalanine hydroxylase, wherein lies the explanation for once-called malignant HPA; those diseases are now described in Chap. 78).

In the 1990s, it becomes evident that PKU and the HPAs are more than Mendelian traits; they also have the features of multifactorial, multilocus, and complex traits. Therefore, they serve as prototypes for thinking more broadly on the nature of so-called Mendelian disease.

Since the last edition of this chapter (published in 1995), two advances are particular highlights. First, the catalytic core of human phenylalanine hydroxylase[17,18] and the regulatory domain (N-terminus) of rat enzyme[18a] have been crystallized and its structure at 2 Å resolution can now be visualized so that (virtual) molecular modeling *in silico* of mutation effects can begin. Second, the vast allelic diversity, both disease-causing and neutral polymorphic in type, at the *PAH* locus is being recorded in an electronic database (http://www.mcgill.ca/pahdb).[14] But whatever one might like to call "progress," it is chastening to realize, by rereading his article,[6] that Penrose anticipated much of our present knowledge; the difference between then and now is simply the evidence, obtained with tools not available in Penrose's own lifetime, and the evidence shows that he was a very foresighted geneticist—as were so many of his colleagues.

INTRODUCTION

The generic term for a phenotype distinguished by phenylalanine concentrations persistently elevated above the distribution of its plasma values in healthy controls is *hyperphenylalaninemia*. This disturbance in metabolic homeostasis can have clinical consequences depending on its pathogenesis and its degree. The major associated clinical manifestation is impaired cognitive development and function resulting from neurochemical imbalance: postnatally in affected cases and prenatally in the fetus of an affected pregnant woman. The genetic causes of HPA include mutations (alleles) in the gene (symbol *PAH*) encoding L-phenylalanine hydroxylase enzyme (PAH); at loci for at least two enzymes in the pathway for synthesis of tetrahydrobiopterin, also known as BH_4 [(*6R*)-L-*erythro*-5,6,7,8-tetrahydrobiopterin], the cofactor for the hydroxylation reaction; and at the loci for 4αcarbinolamine dehydratase and dihydropteridine reductase (DHPR), enzymes that regenerate BH_4 from the oxidized biopterin by-product of the hydroxylation reaction. Most mutations at the *PAH* locus cause PKU: some cause a lesser degree of HPA (so-called non-PKU HPA), where the associated risk of mental retardation is less than it is in classical PKU.

BH_4 homeostasis serves two additional hydroxylation reactions involving L-tryptophan and L-tyrosine, notably in brain. The hydroxylated derivatives of these substrates, 5-hydroxytryptophan and L-dopa, respectively, are precursors of serotonin and catecholamines which, as neurotransmitters, influence brain development and function. Accordingly, diagnosis of BH_4-deficient variants of HPA is relevant for prognosis and treatment. Less than 2 percent of newborn infants with persistent HPA have a disorder of BH_4 homeostasis (see Chap. 78 and the relevant Web site: www.bh4.org).

Nomenclature. This chapter deals with the HPAs associated with primary deficiency of PAH function caused by variant disease-causing alleles in the *PAH* gene. If all degrees of HPA are a risk factor for impaired cognitive development, then it may not matter whether we classify the trait into its more consistently severe (PKU) or usually milder (non-PKU HPA) forms; we will worry about prognosis in either form. One could thus argue for the use of a single name—*phenylketonuria*; indeed, Smith recommends acceptance of the term phenylketonuria (PKU) "as a scientifically sound, collective noun for the family and disorders due to PAH deficiency."[19] We concur, yet there is the issue of common practice. The literature is now well populated with papers naming the severe and mild forms of HPA as "PKU HPA" and "non-PKU HPA," respectively; we use both these terms here knowing each implicates some degree of harm to the central nervous system.

Whereas the clinical distinction between PKU and non-PKU HPA may be arbitrary, it currently rests on recognition of higher plasma phenylalanine values in PKU (more than 1000 μM; more than 16.5 mg/dl) in the untreated state, and on lower tolerance for dietary phenylalanine in PKU (less than 500 mg/day).[20] Others have suggested similar but quantitatively different criteria for classification of PAH enzyme-deficient HPA,[21] but the intention is similar: higher ambient blood phenylalanine levels and lower dietary tolerance are associated with a more PKU-like phenotype and thus greater hazard of impaired cognitive development.

Hyperphenylalaninemia (HPA): A Framework for Understanding Why This "Simple" Phenotype Has "Complex" Explanations

Whereas PKU is a classic Mendelian disease, its metabolic phenotype (HPA) and the associated disease (mental retardation) are the result of more than the effect of a single mutant allele. To be aware of this is to have a framework for understanding HPA and its attendant diseases; and so-called Mendelian disease in general.

HPA Is a Mendelian Inborn Error of Metabolism. PKU is listed under entry 261600 in the McKusick *Catalogs of Mendelian Inheritance in Man* (OMIM). When Følling found an increased frequency of consanguinity among the parents of his patients, he recognized evidence for autosomal recessive inheritance; he also found an aberrant metabolic state in the propositi he investigated.[1,3] Lionel Penrose almost immediately recognized the disorder as a new *inborn error of metabolism*[4] and as the first form of mental retardation to have an overt chemical feature;[6] he communicated accordingly with Garrod.[22] Since then, all human mutations causing primary impairment of PAH enzyme integrity have been shown to map to the *PAH* locus at chromosome 12q22-q24.1[23] in keeping with the involvement of a major gene in PKU and related forms of HPA. *Incidence* of the autosomal recessive metabolic phenotype and its disease, when due to primary deficiency of phenylalanine hydroxylase function, is on average 1 in 10,000 live births in Europeans; *prevalence* of persons affected by and coping with the implications of persistent HPA will be the same. But in a source population of 100 million people, the subset following contemporary recommendations for treatment of HPA would generate 500,000 patient treatment years in half a century.

HPA in PKU Is Multifactorial. Dietary intake of L-phenylalanine, an essential nutrient for *Homo sapiens sapiens*, is required to produce HPA in the mutant phenotype. Dietary experience and mutant genotype are thus both necessary components of cause. Accordingly, the metabolic phenotype is multifactorial and therein lies the original opportunity for treatment through restriction of dietary phenylalanine.

HPA Is Genetically Heterogeneous. PKU indeed manifests HPA, but not all HPA is necessarily PKU. The phenylalanine hydroxylating reaction requires tetrahydrobiopterin (BH_4) cofactor. Mutation in a gene controlling any one of the several stages of synthesis or recycling of BH_4 can cause HPA. Recognition of this fact is a necessary part of the diagnosis, workup, counseling, and treatment of every patient with persistent HPA (see Chap. 78 and Web site, www.bh4.org).

PKU Disease and the Attendant Metabolic Phenotype Are Complex Traits. Analysis of genotype-phenotype correlations in untreated PKU patients shows no consistent relationship, either interfamilial or intrafamilial, between predicted severity of the *PAH* mutation effect and cognitive development (IQ or DQ scores).[24] Long ago, Penrose had noticed discrepancies in IQ values within PKU sibships[6] and further recognized that whereas phenylalanine values in normal and PKU populations behaved as a discontinuous metrical trait, IQ values resembled a *quasi-discontinuous* trait. Since intelligence itself is a complex trait, the failure to correlate IQ with the *PAH* mutation effect is not surprising. However, even blood phenylalanine values themselves, more proximate than cognitive function to the primary mutant gene effect on enzyme function, do not correlate consistently with predicted effect of the mutant *PAH* genotype. For example, the same mutant genotype can be associated with both severe (PKU) and mild (non-PKU) forms of HPA,[25] and whereas *in vivo* measures of L-phenylalanine oxidation rates show the gene dosage expected for a Mendelian trait, the corresponding plasma phenylalanine values do not.[26,27] This evidence implies that whereas the oxidative step has a high sensitivity coefficient for phenylalanine homeostasis,[28] PAH enzyme function is not the only determinant of phenylalanine homeostasis. Phenylalanine homeostasis is apparently under the control of a set of *quantitative trait loci*.

Multiple *PAH* Alleles. Even half a century after Følling's description of PKU, it was customary to refer to *the* PKU mutation, and to record it by the single symbol *a* (for a recessive allele). In the molecular era of PKU studies, though, it is apparent that the mutant human *PAH* locus harbors hundreds of disease-causing alleles ($a_1 + a_2 + a_3 \ldots a_n$); a few are prevalent, most are rare, even *private*.[14] PKU fits an emerging view of *Mendelian* disease in general: the majority of disease-causing alleles at the relevant locus will be rare; only a few will be prevalent.[29]

PHENYLALANINE HOMEOSTASIS

Claude Bernard recognized that constancy of the internal milieu was a necessary condition of life;[30] Walter B. Cannon called it *homeostasis*.[31] The phenylalanine content of blood, or of any other body fluid, is a metrical trait that observes a central tendency (homeostasis). HPA is recognized when the value for non-peptide-bound (free) phenylalanine is greater than the normal frequency distribution; the normal range of values represents one steady state and the range of deviant values in HPA reflects a different steady state, which may or may not have consequences for health.

The metabolic steady state is a dynamic one in which the concentrations of metabolites in the system remain fixed in the face of fluxes through it.[32] Any persistent change in a flux will eventually change the steady state value. Regulatory mechanisms control homeostatic systems so that steady state values experience only minor, transitory changes within certain limits under usual circumstances.[33] The dispersion of plasma phenylalanine values around the central tendency (the mean or *homing* value) fits this model (Fig. 77-1) and shows that the plasma phenylalanine value is a quantitative (complex) trait. It reflects both intraindividual or interindividual biologic variation (V_G) and the range of experience

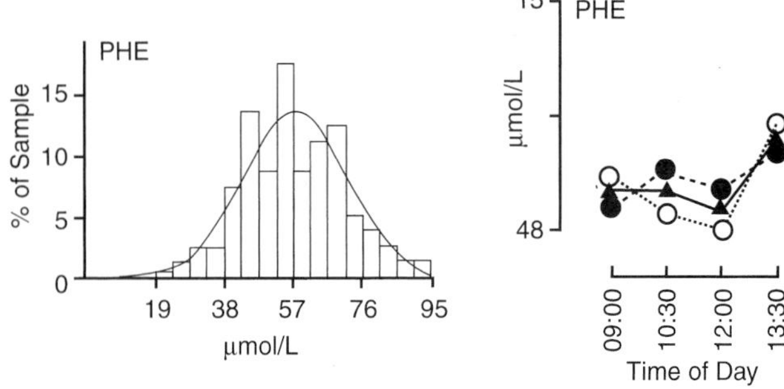

Fig. 77-1 A: The frequency distribution of plasma phenylalanine values (*n* = 80) in adult human subjects (*n* = 10) studied twice (fasting and fed) at four different times of the day. B: Mean values (▲) for infradiem variation in plasma phenylalanine in fasted (•) and fed (○) subjects. (*Both figures adapted from Scriver et al.*[34] *Used by permission.*)

encountered by the individual (V_E).[34] The normal value for plasma phenylalanine *within* an individual shows infradiem oscillation[34] which is not greater than about half of the nadir value (Fig. 77-1). The broad similarity in values *between* individuals implies that their homeostatic mechanisms are similar and have descended through shared human evolution; the outlier values are of greatest interest since they reflect unusual biologic diversity or experience. Evidence for heritability (h^2), which in the broad sense is $V_G/V_G + V_E$, is found in twin studies;[35] plasma phenylalanine values are more similar within monozygotic twin pairs than they are between non-twin subjects. Accordingly, an individual has a *private* plasma amino acid phenotype, with values distributed over a range narrower than the *public* distribution of values for a population of unrelated individuals.[34] Thus, the blood phenylalanine value should indeed be viewed as a quantitative trait in which the biologic factors controlling it are the *quantitative trait loci*.[34,36]

Normal Plasma Values

The normal plasma free phenylalanine value is not significantly different in young and adult subjects.[34,37] The normal adult value under physiological conditions is 58 ± 15 μM (mean and standard deviation); the corresponding values in children (mean age, 8 years) and adolescents (mean age, 16 years) are 62 ± 18 μM and 60 ± 13 μM, respectively. Gender affects the value only in adolescents (male values are higher).[37] Values in newborns and older infants are similar to those in older subjects.[35]

Determinants of the Steady State

Fluid compartments in the body [e.g., plasma and cerebrospinal fluid (CSF)] may have quite different concentrations of free phenylalanine but, at the steady state, the compartments are in a state of equilibrium, albeit at far from chemical equilibrium.[32] (This fundamental feature will lie behind the proposal to use enzyme substitution therapy with oral phenylalanine ammonia lyase to treat PKU; see the section "Treatment of PKU.") The flux of free phenylalanine through pools in the human body comprises inputs and runouts (Fig. 77-2), and there are ways to measure net flux rates *in vivo*.[38] Input of phenylalanine has two major sources: *exogenous* from dietary phenylalanine, and *endogenous* from bound (polypeptide) and free amino acid stores, the latter located largely in muscle.[35] Runout involves incorporation into bound pools, oxidation to tyrosine, and conversion to minor metabolites; net runout by oxidation can be measured in vivo by measurement of labeled CO_2 in expired air derived from a tracer-dose of labeled L-phenylalanine.[26,39]

Input. L-Phenylalanine is an essential amino acid in humans, and a (dietary) source is necessary both to maintain phenylalanine homeostasis and to meet requirements for endogenous protein synthesis.[40,41] The nutritional requirement for L-phenylalanine is

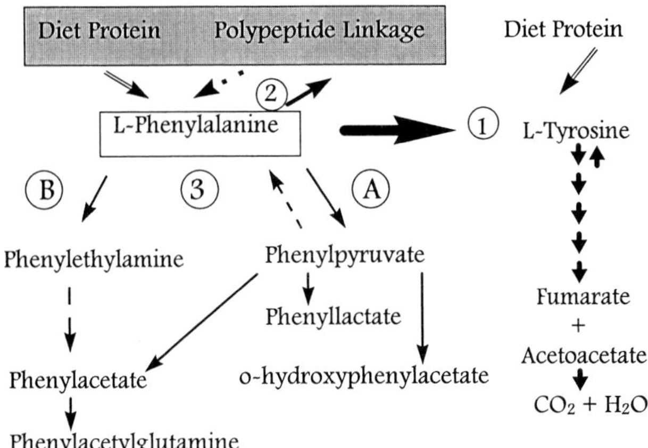

Fig. 77-2 Major inputs (⇒) and runouts (→) of free L-phenylalanine in human metabolism. Inputs of this essential amino acid to the pool of freely diffusible solute are from dietary protein [hence the minimal dietary requirement (Table 77-1)] and turnover of endogenous (bound, polypeptide) pools. Runout is by (1) hydroxylation to tyrosine (reaction 1 catalyzed by phenylalanine hydroxylase, followed by oxidation); (2) incorporation into bound (polypeptide) pools (reaction 2); and (3) by transamination (A) and decarboxylation (B). The approximate proportional importance of the three runouts is 3:1:trace at normal steady state (see the discussion in Scriver et al[435]).

difficult to estimate in normal subjects because catabolic runout perturbs the estimate of the anabolic requirement. Accordingly, the blocked catabolic state (as in a person with totally deficient PAH enzyme activity) is useful to estimate the actual human requirement. Empirical estimates in treated PKU patients indicate that the minimum requirement to support protein synthesis is on the order of 200 to 500 mg/day in infants and young children (depending in part on the mutant *PAH* genotype) and probably not more than 1.5 times greater in older children. The requirement for phenylalanine is greater in the absence of tyrosine in subjects with intact phenylalanine hydroxylation.[40–42] Thus, the range of phenylalanine requirement in PKU patients and in normal subjects probably reflects interindividual differences in the biologic determinants of homeostasis, as well as allelic differences at the *PAH* locus in the PKU subjects. Estimates of the requirement in adults (Table 77-1) are probably lower than the true value,[40] and values obtained by kinetic analysis with isotope-labeled amino acid in adults resemble those for young children when expressed per unit of total protein requirement (Table 77-1). This revisionist view may influence treatment of HPA in affected pregnant women.

Turnover of endogenous peptide-bound pools contributes input to the plasma phenylalanine pool value.[42–44] When nutrition is inadequate, protein catabolism occurs and free L-phenylalanine is released; as a consequence, plasma phenylalanine values will initially rise in PKU patients in early negative nitrogen balance. Failure to recognize this phenomenon can confound treatment of PKU patients during intercurrent illness.

Runout. Input of phenylalanine will expand the plasma phenylalanine pool unless there is compensating runout. Incorporation into protein, oxidation, and conversion of phenylalanine to other metabolites (Fig. 77-2) provide runout on a background of interorgan amino acid flow and cellular uptake. The relative contributions of these components to phenylalanine homeostasis have theoretical interest and practical relevance.

In a series of important theoretical studies,[28,45,46] it was reasoned that each component in a network of steady-state determinants has a value, called the *sensitivity coefficient*, proportional to its importance in setting the summation property (value = 1) of the steady state maintained by the network. Relative quantitative values for the components of phenylalanine runout have been measured.[47,48] At physiological concentrations, incorporation into protein and hydroxylation to tyrosine account for about one-quarter and three-quarters of total free phenylalanine runout, respectively; conversion to phenylpyruvic acid is of minor significance and occurs only at elevated plasma concentrations of phenylalanine;[47] conversion to phenylethylamine is a trivial part of the whole. Whereas stress, feeding, and fasting modulate phenylalanine oxidation,[42,44] on average about half the control of runout is accounted for by a first step, which is uptake of phenylalanine by cells, notably hepatocytes;[48] the remainder occurs by events after this step (hydroxylation, protein incorporation, and metabolite formation). Direct measures in human subjects confirm that hepatic uptake and oxidation of phenylalanine are almost equally important determinants of the steady state value for plasma phenylalanine in mammals[43] and, from the PKU phenotype, we see that the *PAH* gene behaves as the *major* locus in the genetic make up of this complex trait. On the other hand, since the sensitivity coefficient of the hydroxylation component in the system is considerably less than 1.0 (because the system maintaining phenylalanine homeostasis has many components), it follows that HPA is not a dominant phenotype and must be recessive and, furthermore, that the heterozygote, under usual conditions, will not show significant HPA, in keeping with theory.[28]

Alternative Phenylalanine Conversion Pathways. Conversion to tyrosine is the major metabolic pathway for phenylalanine runout[47] (Fig. 77-2). Conversion of phenylalanine to nontyrosine derivatives constitutes only a minor alternative under normal conditions; more details of the latter reactions are given in previous editions of this text[49–51] and elsewhere.[52]

The initial reaction in the most significant alternative pathway is transamination of L-phenylalanine to form phenylpyruvate; this and the subsequent metabolic transformations in the transamination pathway (Fig. 77-2) are restricted to the alanine side chain of the molecule. Only when the major catabolic pathway is blocked and phenylalanine concentration is much increased does the transamination pathway become functionally significant. The reaction is induced by substrate and is not fully operative in immature newborns or in the early phase of HPA.[52] Rates of phenylalanine disposal by the alternative pathways do influence the mutant metabolic phenotype in PKU, and siblings with identical mutant *PAH* genotypes can have different rates for disposal of minor metabolites.[53]

Decarboxylation of phenylalanine to phenylethylamine (Fig. 77-2) is not an important route for disposal of excess phenylalanine in humans at any time. Monoamine oxidase inhibitors, which block further metabolism of phenylethylamine, do little to alter its level in human subjects.[54]

A controversial finding, originating in low-dose continuous *in vivo* infusions of isotopically labeled L-phenylalanine in PKU subjects,[53,55,56] implied that pathways other than the one mediated by PAH enzyme, may be more significant for disposal of

Table 77-1 Estimates of Phenylalanine Requirement in Humans*[40,41]

	$g \cdot day^{-1}$	$mg \cdot kg^{-1} \cdot day^{-1}$	$mg \cdot g^{-1}$ Protein
Infant		25–90	
Preschool child	200–500†[41]	69	63
Older child	200–500	22	22
Young adult	14	19	
Young male adult	39‡		

*Estimates made in normal subjects with normal phenylalanine hydroxylase enzyme (PAH) activity and receiving tyrosine in the diet.

†Estimates made in patients with severe deficiency of PAH activity (classical phenylketonuria).

‡Estimated by oral tracer studies in subjects receiving various phenylalanine intakes without added tyrosine.[42]

phenylalanine in humans than credited heretofore. The findings introduced a logical inconsistency and a vexing question: If patients with *de facto* HPA have "normal" hydroxylating activity by whatever means, why do they have HPA?[27] New findings,[26,39,57] where rates of phenylalanine hydroxylation have been measured *in vivo* in various ways, both in patients and in control subjects, show that phenylalanine hydroxylation *is* impaired as predicted, in the PKU and non-PKU HPA types of phenylalaninemia. A satisfactory explanation for the earlier and contrary findings[53,55,56] has now emerged.¶

Interorgan Phenylalanine Flow and Uptake. PAH enzyme is active in hepatocytes in humans (and in kidney) (see below and Lichter-Konecki et al[77a,77b]), but phenylalanine is incorporated into protein in all tissues, and metabolic conversion of phenylalanine to various metabolites also occurs in tissues other than liver. Accordingly, interorgan fluxes are an integral part of runout for this amino acid;[58] and there must be phenylalanine transport across plasma membranes before it can enter its intracellular pathways. L-Phenylalanine uptake by mammalian cells is mediated by carriers that are coupled to the inward-oriented Na^+ gradient in apical membranes of renal[59,60] and intestinal epithelia,[61] and by Na^+-independent carriers in other plasma membranes (cited in Christensen[58,62,63]). The nephron, which contains both high affinity and low affinity carriers for phenylalanine,[59] achieves near-total reabsorption of the amino acid from filtrate under physiological conditions. The systems do not saturate even at high phenylalanine concentrations in filtrate,[35,64] which means the transporters continue to function in the homeostatic network and contribute to the HPA of PKU.

Phenylalanine enters parenchymal cells from plasma and extracellular fluid on a Na^+-independent, weakly concentrative carrier, which accepts both branched chain and aromatic amino acids; it exits from cells on a system shared by neutral-charge amino acids.[62,63] Hepatic uptake of phenylalanine is a significant component in the runout flux.[48] Interactions between amino acids on the carriers can perturb these fluxes[65–67] and may play a role in the pathogenesis of the brain phenotype in PKU.

Kaufman[67a] proposes a quantitative model for metabolism of phenylalanine at steady state in fasted human subjects that takes into account disposal by the hydroxylation and transamination reaction (decarboxylation being a negligible reaction in this context) and input from net protein degradation. From available empirical data, Kaufman assigned values: K_m (mM) for hydroxylase and transaminase, 0.54 and 1.37 respectively; the corresponding V_{max} (μmol/ml per hour), 0.9 and 0.063 respectively; phenylalanine release from protein degradation, 0.012 μmol/ml per hour. Assuming that blood levels reflect tissue levels, Kaufman then tested the validity of his model against data for normal subjects, heterozygotes, and mutant homozygotes with PKU. The model was satisfactory and sufficiently robust to show that HPA could not be explained by putative transaminase deficiency and that alternative pathways for significant phenylalanine disposal (e.g., on tyrosine hydroxylase) do not exist.

THE PHENYLALANINE HYDROXYLATING SYSTEM

The most important single determinant of phenylalanine homeostasis in humans is the hydroxylation reaction. To understand the mutant phenotypes associated with HPA, the normal components of the hydroxylation should be known.

General Characteristics

The phenylalanine hydroxylation reaction is an obligatory and rate-limiting step in the catabolic pathway that leads to the complete oxidation of phenylalanine to CO_2 and water.[68] The ketogenic (e.g., acetoacetate) and gluconeogenic (e.g., fumarate) products of phenylalanine catabolism (Fig. 77-2) contribute to the organism's pool of two-carbon metabolites and glucose. In view of the brain's partial dependence on a peripheral supply of glucose, the ability of phenylalanine to provide gluconeogenic substrates, in this context, plays a role in normal brain development and function. Hydroxylation of phenylalanine plays another role in mammalian metabolism: it provides the organism with an endogenous supply of the nonessential amino acid—tyrosine. When hydroxylation is deficient, tyrosine becomes an *essential* amino acid. The formal name for PAH enzyme is L-phenylalanine-4-monooxygenase (EC 1.14.16.1), a mixed-function oxidoreductase.

Tissue Distribution of Hydroxylating Activity

It was thought, at one time, that PAH is not present in nonhepatic mammalian tissues.[69] However, subsequent studies demonstrated appreciable activity in mouse kidney and pancreas[70] and in rat and guinea pig kidney.[71] The putative presence of hydroxylase activity in pancreas has not been confirmed.[72] Rat kidney PAH is in an unusual state of activation relative to the rat liver enzyme[72] and, at the resting blood phenylalanine concentration, kidney enzyme might account for as much as 20 to 30 percent of the total phenylalanine hydroxylase activity in rats.[72] The status of the kidney hydroxylase in humans was unclear. Ayling and her coworkers reported hydroxylase activity in kidney,[73,74] whereas others found none in either human or nonhuman primate kidney.[75] In support of the latter evidence, rat phenylalanine hydroxylase cDNA hybridizes with rat kidney mRNA but not with baboon kidney mRNA.[76] Further studies[77] did not find any hydroxylase activity in various human nonhepatic tissues and cells. However, new evidence based on analysis of mRNA, immunohistochemistry, and assay of enzymic activity indicates that human kidney expresses significant phenylalanine hydroxylase protein and enzyme activity.[77a,77b]

PAH is not present in brain,[78] contrary to an earlier claim;[79] the finding has bearing on pathogenesis of the brain phenotype in PKU. Brain does contain another enzyme, tyrosine hydroxylase, which catalyzes the conversion of phenylalanine to tyrosine at a rate comparable to its ability to hydroxylate tyrosine.[80] Perhaps tyrosine hydroxylase, acting on phenylalanine, provides the developing brain with a significant fraction of the tyrosine it needs for protein synthesis;[81] whether it might in PKU is not known.

Evidence has been reported that PAH and 4α-carbinolamine dehydratase are present together in human melanocytes and keratinocytes, where they are postulated to play a role in melanin formation.[82] In the proposed scenario, hydroxylation of phenylalanine provides the tyrosine essential for melanin synthesis; further, the depigmentation disorder vitiligo, constitutes a lack of the dehydratase with accumulation of 7-biopterin, which inhibits phenylalanine hydroxylase,[83] leading to disruption of the supply of tyrosine and consequent impairment of melanin synthesis.

Although the presence of 4α-carbinolamine dehydratase in normal human epidermal keratinocytes has been unequivocally demonstrated, the conclusion that phenylalanine hydroxylase is also present[82] is not strongly supported. The enzyme that hydroxylates phenylalanine in both melanocytes and keratinocytes could be tyrosine hydroxylase. Indeed, if as postulated, phenylalanine hydroxylase were essential for melanin synthesis, PKU patients would be expected to show irreversible signs of this defect. PKU patients do tend to have fair skin, but this defect in

¶The discrepancy between the earlier and recent findings was mentioned in an editorial[57a] accompanying the article by Van Spronsen et al;[57] this elicited a response from Scott C. Denne (personal communication, September 11, 1998), who explained how a technical issue involving mass spectrometry and stable isotope ratios could account for the problem. Thompson and Halliday[56] used d_2 tyrosine to measure tyrosine Ra, whereas Van Spronsen et al[57] used [^{13}C]tyrosine, with consequences for the magnitude of the background shift effect. The larger magnitude of the background shift effect would account for essentially all of the phenylalanine hydroxylation measured in the earlier study; thus, the significant hydroxylation flux report in that study was apparently an artifact.

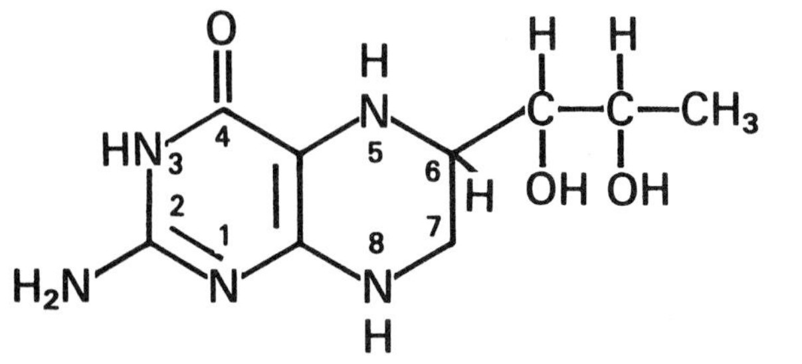

Fig. 77-3 Structure of tetrahydrobiopterin [2-amino-4-hydroxy-6(L-*erythro*-1′,2′-dihydroxypropyl)-tetrahydropteridine], of BH_4, the natural coenzyme (cofactor) for phenylalanine hydroxylase.

pigmentation is reversed when the plasma phenylalanine level is reduced, a finding consistent with the evidence that excess phenylalanine inhibits tyrosinase-mediated melanin synthesis.[84]

Vitiligo patients could have HPA due to their deficiency of dehydratase and putative impairment of phenylalanine hydroxylation. The patients do not have ambient HPA. Following an oral load of phenylalanine, phenylalanine clearance from plasma in about half of the patients was apparently slower than in a group of healthy controls.[85] The evidence is tenuous, and the rate constants, calculated from the kinetics of the decrease of phenylalanine in patients and controls, appear to be indistinguishable.

The phenomenon of *illegitimate transcription* is relevant to a discussion of the tissue distribution of phenylalanine hydroxylase. The term was coined to describe the low level of transcription of tissue-specific genes in nonspecific cells.[85] Gene transcripts of phenylalanine hydroxylase (as well as tyrosine hydroxylase) have been detected in white blood cells, erythroleukemic cells, and chorionic villus cells.[86] To date, the levels of transcripts detected are too low to know whether their occurrence is of any functional significance. The phenomenon has, however, proved to be of value in the identification of PKU-associated mutations in phenylalanine hydroxylase in circulating lymphocytes.[87,88]

The Hydroxylating System

The hepatic phenylalanine hydroxylating system consists of three essential components: PAH, DHPR, and the unconjugated pterin tetrahydrobiopterin (2-amino-4-hydroxy-6-[L-*erythro*-1′,2′-dihydroxypropyl]tetrahydropteridine),[15,89] in addition to a stimulating protein,[90] isolated in pure form from rat liver,[91] which, although not essential, can markedly stimulate the hydroxylation reaction *in vivo*. Originally called phenylalanine hydroxylase stimulator (PHS),[90] this protein was later shown to be the aforementioned dehydratase.[92,93]

The structure of BH_4 is shown in Fig. 77-3. Like all other naturally occurring compounds of this type, BH_4 is a 2-amino-4-hydroxypteridine (trivial name, *pterin*); it is classified as an unconjugated pterin to distinguish it from its relatives, the folates. The latter compounds are called *conjugated pterins* because their pterin rings are conjugated with a *para*-aminobenzoyl-glutamate(s) substituent at position 6 of the pteridine ring. Unlike the folates, BH_4 is not a vitamin for mammals, since they can synthesize it. Several synthetic tetrahydropterins with simple alkyl substituents at position 6, such as 6-methyltetrahydropterin ($6MPH_4$) and 6,7-dimethyltetrahydropterin ($DMPH_4$), are even more active than BH_4 in the phenylalanine hydroxylating system.[94]

The reactions catalyzed by PAH, DHPR, and PHS (the dehydratase) in the presence of the pterin appear in Fig. 77-4. PAH catalyzes a coupled reaction in which phenylalanine is oxidized to tyrosine and the tetrahydropterin is oxidized to the corresponding 4a-hydroxytetrahydropterin (also called 4α-carbinolamine). The conversion of carbinolamine to quinonoid dihydropterin and water is catalyzed by 4α-carbinolamine dehydratase,[92,93] formerly known as PAH-stimulating protein. The oxygen in the *para* position of the benzene ring of the tyrosine product is derived from molecular oxygen rather than from water;[95] accordingly, the hydroxylase is an oxygenase. During the hydroxylation reaction, the second atom of oxygen in the oxygen molecule is normally reduced to the level of water.

The minimum requirements for phenylalanine hydroxylation are the hydroxylase, oxygen, L-phenylalanine, and BH_4, but under these conditions BH_4 can function only stoichiometrically (i.e., the amount of tyrosine formed cannot exceed the amount of BH_4 present). For the pterin coenzyme to function catalytically, there must be another component of the system: it is DHPR (along with a reduced pyridine nucleotide). Although the reductase is active with both NADH and NADPH, NADH is the better substrate *in vitro*.[96–98] It is not known whether NADH or NADPH, or both, function with the reductase *in vivo*. In addition to the NADH-dependent DHPR-catalyzed regeneration of BH_4 from quinonoid

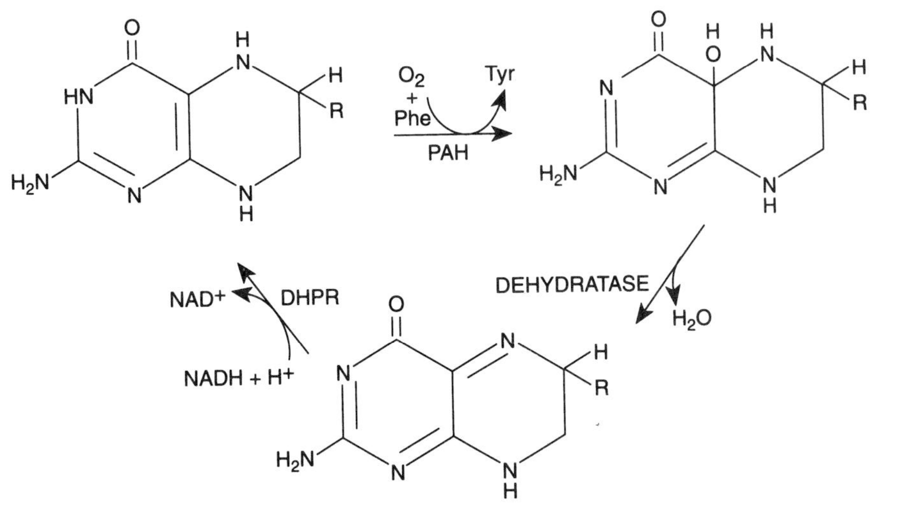

Fig. 77-4 The conversion of phenylalanine to tyrosine is catalyzed by the phenylalanine hydroxylation system. The overall reaction is the sum of three reactions, each catalyzed by a separate enzyme. In the presence of an *active tetrahydropterin* cofactor like the naturally occurring substance, BH_4 (R = $-CHOH-CHOH-CH_3$), phenylalanine hydroxylase (PAH) catalyzes a coupled reaction in which phenylalanine is converted to tyrosine and BH_4 to a carbinolamine, the corresponding *4α-hydroxytetrahydropterin*. The carbinolamine is then converted to the *quininoid dihydropterin* by a dehydratase (4α-carbinolamine dehydratase). The cycle is completed by the action of dihydropteridine reductase (DHPR), which catalyzes the NADH-mediated reduction of the quinonoid dihydropterin back to the tetrahydropterin. (The pterin substrates for the three reactions are indicated in *italics*.)

dihydrobiopterin (qBH_2), reduction of the latter compound to BH_4 can also proceed nonenzymatically in the presence of millimolar concentrations of reducing agents such as mercaptans and ascorbate.[99] Attempts to demonstrate ascorbate-mediated regeneration of BH_4 in humans have not been successful.

The complete absence of phenylalanine hydroxylase, DHPR, or BH_4 leads to persistent HPA. By contrast, because the reaction catalyzed by the dehydratase can occur quite rapidly by nonenzymatic routes,[92] it was predicted that the complete absence of this enzyme would cause only mild or transient HPA.[100] This prediction was validated in a patient with the mild phenotype who excretes 7-BH_4 and harbors two mutations in the gene for the dehydratase, one inherited from the mother (C82R) and the other from the father (E87X).[101] The results of *in vitro* studies of the activity of these two engineered alleles were also coherent with this prediction. The C82R mutant had about 40 percent of the activity of the wild-type dehydratase enzyme,[102,103] whereas the E87X allele was devoid of activity, in part because of its instability.[102] The predicted effects of these two mutations, combined *in vivo*, would much reduce the dehydratase activity.[102]

In addition to its catalytic function in the regeneration of BH_4 (see Fig. 77-4), the dehydratase also plays a completely unrelated role in regulating gene transcription, a striking example of a phenomenon dubbed *molecular opportunism*.[104] Upon cloning and sequencing the dehydratase, it was found that this protein is identical to DCoH, the dimerization cofactor of hepatocyte nuclear factor (HNF1).[105,106] The dimeric form of the latter protein regulates transcription of a large number of genes in the liver, intestine, and kidney, including those coding for albumin, α_1-antitrypsin, and fibrinogen. DCoH enhances this transcriptional activity by combining with HNF1 dimers and stabilizing them (for a review, see Mendel and Crabtree[107]). Involvement of the dehydratase in a gene transcription system raised questions about whether mutations that affect dehydratase activity also affect its transcription-enhancing activity. A detailed analysis of the effect of some mutations on both of these activities showed that those decreasing dehydratase activity to less than 1 percent of wild type decrease transcriptional activity only modestly (by about 10 percent) and have no effect on binding DCoH to HNF1, a clear indication that dehydratase activity is not essential for the binding.[108] The same conclusion was reached from a study that focused on the binding of allelic dehydratase (C82R) to HNF1.[109] These findings may explain why dehydratase-deficient patients do not appear to suffer from the global metabolic consequences that would be expected from disruption of the activity of the DCoH/HNF1 transcription system.

Although the DNA and amino acid sequences of mouse, rat, and human phenylalanine hydroxylases are strikingly similar,[110] there are noteworthy physiological differences between the human enzyme and the rodent enzyme.[111] In primates phenylalanine hydroxylase is present mainly or only in liver, whereas in rodents it is also present in kidney, albeit at a lower level. Moreover, the developmental pattern is different with activity in humans being detected during the second trimester, whereas in rats it is not present until just before birth. In addition, fetal development of phenylalanine hydroxylase in rats is regulated by glucocorticoids and cyclic AMP (cAMP).[111]

Structural and functional studies of the 5′ flanking region of the phenylalanine hydroxylase gene have defined some of the features that are essential for the regulation of the phenylalanine hydroxylase gene and have identified some of the characteristics that may account for these differences[112] (see the section "The *PAH* Gene" and Fig. 77-6). As shown in transgenic mice, a 9-kb DNA fragment upstream of the human gene contains all of the *cis*-acting elements needed to direct tissue-specific and developmental stage-specific expression of phenylalanine hydroxylase *in vivo*.[113] Like other typical housekeeping genes, human *PAH* gene utilizes multiple transcriptional initiation sites.[114] The promoter regions of the mouse and human phenylalanine hydroxylase genes are similar in their lack of a TATA-like sequence.[115] Expression of the mouse phenylalanine hydroxylase gene depends on a hormone-responsive and tissue-specific enhancer located 3.5 kb upstream as well as on the presence of cAMP and steroid hormones such as dexamethasone. Furthermore, activity of this enhancer has been shown to require the hepatocyte-enriched transcription factors HNF1 and C/EBP.[115]

Experiments carried out on HNF1 knockout mice complement the *in vitro* studies and show that phenylalanine hydroxylase belongs to the group of proteins whose genes are indeed regulated by HNF1;[116] the gene coding for phenylalanine hydroxylase is completely silent in the knockout. These animals, however, are not true models for PKU, because they also have a severe Fanconi syndrome caused by proximal renal tubule dysfunction; they die around the time of weaning.[116]

Any attempt to relate the results obtained with the HNF1 knockout mice to PKU in humans has been hampered, until recently, by the lack of evidence that HNF1 regulates the expression of human phenylalanine hydroxylase. That gap was at least partially closed with the demonstration that the 9-kb human phenylalanine hydroxylase 5′ flanking fragment[114] contains two HNF1-binding sites located at 0.5 kb upstream.[117] Cotransfection experiments showed that HNF1 markedly transactivated the 9-kb DNA fragment (linked to a reporter gene) in Chinese hamster ovary cells. Moreover, although DCoH, by itself, lacked this ability, it could enhance the HNF1-mediated transactivation of the 9-kb fragment. These effects of HNF1 and DCoH were observed in the absence of added hormones, in contrast to the hormonal dependence of the effect of HNF1 on the expression of the mouse *Pah* gene,[115] an indication that regulation of expression of human phenylalanine hydroxylase by hormones, if it occurs, does not follow the same pattern as that for the mouse enzyme.

Further studies of the promoter region in the mouse *Pah* gene[116] reveal multiple DNase-hypersensitive sites in the normal animal, reflecting an open chromatin structure and low degree of methylation, both characteristic of transcriptionally active genes. By contrast, the corresponding region of the gene in the HNF1-knockout mouse has a relatively closed chromatin structure and the hypermethylation pattern of a silent gene. These results suggest that HNF1 is essential for chromatin remodeling and DNA methylation that accompany transcriptional activation.

Dihydrofolate reductase (DHFR) (EC 1.6.99.7) may also play a role in hydroxylation of phenylalanine *in vivo*. This enzyme has a well-established role in one-carbon metabolism catalyzing the reduction of 7,8-dihydrofolate:

$$\text{NADPH} + \text{7,8-dihydrofolate} \rightarrow \text{NADP}^+ + \text{tetrahydrofolate} \qquad \text{(Eq. 77-1)}$$

The enzyme can also catalyze the analogous reaction with 7,8-dihydrobiotperin:[118]

$$\text{NADPH} + \text{H}^+ + \text{7,8-dihydrobiopterin} \rightarrow \text{NADP}^+ + \text{tetrahydrobiopterin} \qquad \text{(Eq. 77-2)}$$

The second reaction assumes importance for phenylalanine hydroxylation when the rate of the DHPR-catalyzed reduction of qBH_2 lags behind the rate of the PAH-catalyzed formation of the quinonoid derivative (Fig. 77-4). Under such conditions, the extremely unstable qBH_2 will undergo a rearrangement to the corresponding 7,8-dihydrobiopterin;[118] the latter is not a substrate for DHPR. Therefore, when DHPR limits the rate of phenylalanine hydroxylation, DHFR could salvage some of the biopterin diverted to the 7,8-dihydro derivative and thereby potentially support some phenylalanine hydroxylation. However, since the near-total absence of DHPR leads to HPA (see Chap. 78), it is evident that neither DHFR, nor any other enzyme, is as effective as DHPR at sustaining normal rates of phenylalanine hydroxylation.

The reactions depicted in Fig. 77-4 were the first to establish a metabolic role for an unconjugated pterin and to reveal the coenzyme role of BH_4. It was shown subsequently that BH_4 and

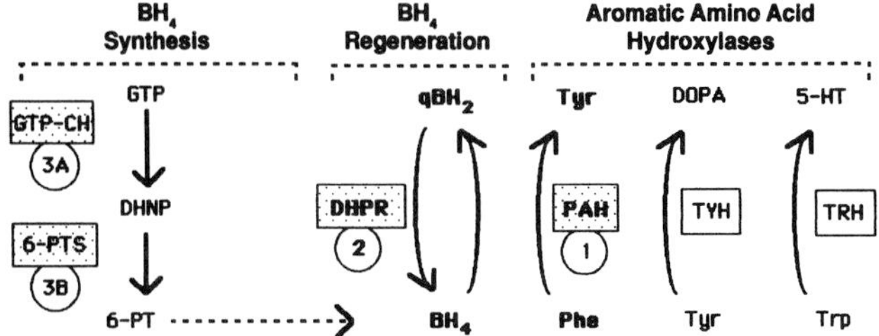

Fig. 77-5 Scheme to show the hydroxylation reactions for phenylalanine, tyrosine, and tryptophan, each requiring BH_4 cofactor and therefore dependent on synthesis and maintenance of BH_4. The pathway for BH_4 synthesis is only sketched (see Chap. 78 for details). Maintenance of BH_4 requires regeneration from dihydropteridine reductase (DHPR) in the presence of dehydratase (not shown here; see Fig. 77-4) and DHPR. Enzymes involved in the Mendelian hyperphenylalaninemias (*shaded jammed*) are disorders of (1) primary hydroxylase activity (this chapter), (2) maintenance of BH_4 (Chap. 78), and (3) BH_4 synthesis (Chap. 78). GTP-CH, GTP cyclohydrolase; 6PTS, 6-pyruvoyl tetrahydropterin synthase; PAH, TYH, and TRH, phenylalanine hydroxylase, tyrosine hydroxylase, and tryptophan hydroxylase, respectively; DHNP, dihydroneopterin. (*Reproduced from Scriver et al.*[831] *Used by permission.*)

DHPR play precisely the same roles in the hydroxylating systems for phenylalanine, tyrosine, and tryptophan[119–121] (Fig. 77-5). Accordingly, BH_4 and DHPR are essential for the biosynthesis of the neurotransmitters dopamine, norepinephrine, and serotonin. A fuller realization of the *in situ* role of BH_4 and DHPR in these other hydroxylating systems became clear with the discovery of variant forms of PKU caused by defects in BH_4 regeneration and synthesis (see Chap. 78).

Phenylalanine Hydroxylase

Physical Properties. Many of the properties of PAH were first determined with enzyme purified from rat liver extracts.[122] The properties of the human liver enzyme are similar to those of the rat enzyme, with the exceptions mentioned below.

Rat Enzyme. Essentially pure rat liver PAH appeared initially to be a mixture of two different polymeric forms.[122] Based on a determination of their Stokes radii and sedimentation constants, molecular weights of 210,000 and 100,000 were calculated for the major and minor species, respectively. Since the molecular weight of the subunit(s) is about 49,000 to 51,000,[122] the two forms are putative tetramers and dimers, respectively. A more detailed study of the oligomeric composition of the pure rat liver enzyme isolated by high-performance gel-permeation chromatography showed that the mixture consists of 75 to 80 percent tetramer and 20 to 25 percent dimer at 25°C.[123] When assayed with the synthetic pterin cofactor, $6MPH_4$, both species had identical specific activities; when assayed with BH_4, the specific activity of the tetramer was five times that of the dimer.[123]

Existence of the rat enzyme in solution as a mixture of tetramers and dimers[123] has been disputed, with some reports claiming that rat PAH exists solely as tetramers,[124] with others[125] detecting only dimers. Most studies, however, have confirmed the original finding[122] of a mixture of tetramers and dimers.[126–129] Variables that account for some of these inconsistent findings have been delineated:[128] (1) Dimers are detected when the protein concentration is less than 5 μg/ml, whereas at relatively high concentrations of protein (more than 20 μg/ml), the distribution shifts in the direction of tetramers.[128] (2) In phosphate buffer, an increase in pH from 6.0 to 8.0 shifts the distribution from tetramers to dimers.[128] (3) Preincubation of the hydroxylase with phenylalanine increases conversion of dimers to tetramers.[123,125,126]

Human Enzyme. Until recently, there were questions about whether the physical and regulatory properties of human phenylalanine hydroxylase are identical with those of the well-studied rat liver enzyme.[20] With the cloning, expression, and successful purification of human phenylalanine hydroxylase, most of these questions have been answered.

At pH 7.0, the oligomeric composition of recombinant human phenylalanine hydroxylase isolated from *Escherichia coli* as a maltose-binding fusion protein is a mixture of inactive aggregated forms and catalytically active hexamers, tetramers, and dimers with the relative proportion of the active species being 14, 70, and 16 percent, respectively; the subunit size is about 50 kDa.[130] When expressed in *E. coli* cells, with a system that does not involve the use of a maltose-binding fusion protein, the oligomeric composition of human phenylalanine hydroxylase at pH 6.8 is a mixture of tetramers, and dimers (80:20 parts), of subunit size of about 52 kDa, and with no evidence of higher aggregates.[131] This composition is not significantly different from that found for rat liver phenylalanine hydroxylase.[123,132]

As with the rat liver enzyme, the proportion of dimeric human enzyme is augmented by increasing the pH to alkaline values (pH 8 to 9).[128] Preincubation of human phenylalanine hydroxylase with L-phenylalanine shifts the equilibrium in the direction of the tetrameric form,[130] as seen with rat[123,125,132] and bovine hepatic enzymes.[126]

The ability to determine distinctive catalytic properties of the two species and their ready separation during gel-permeation chromatography indicate that the dimer and tetramer are not in rapid equilibrium even under assay conditions.

Human phenylalanine hydroxylase resembles rat liver phenylalanine hydroxylase in being phosphorylated by cAMP-dependent protein kinase, phosphorylation resulting in activation.[100] Recombinant human phenylalanine hydroxylase incorporates between 0.6 mol[131] and 0.97 mol[130] of phosphate per phenylalanine hydroxylase subunit, resulting in 1.5-fold and 1.2-fold activation, respectively, of the BH_4-dependent activity. This modest degree of human enzyme activation is less than the two- to fourfold activation observed with either rat liver[133,134] or recombinant rat enzyme.[135]

An even more striking difference in regulatory properties between recombinant human phenylalanine hydroxylase and its rat counterpart has been observed with other known activators of the latter enzyme. Whereas preincubation with phenylalanine or lysolecithin activates the BH_4-dependent activity of the rat enzyme 8-fold and 25-fold, respectively, the human hydroxylase is activated only 2.2-fold by either of these treatments.[131] Similar results were reported for the uncleaved fusion products of human phenylalanine hydroxylase with the maltose-binding protein.[136]

The K_m for phenylalanine (measured with BH_4 as the cofactor) of recombinant human phenylalanine hydroxylase is 50 μM,[131] a value close to the normal level of phenylalanine in human plasma and notably lower than the K_m value (280 μM) for the recombinant rat liver enzyme.[135] The corresponding values for the human fusion protein and its cleavage products are closer to those of the recombinant rat hydroxylase.[130] Most of the other catalytic properties of human phenylalanine hydroxylase are similar to those of the rat enzyme.[130,131,136]

Just as was found with rat liver phenylalanine hydroxylase,[83,137] 7-tetrahydrobiopterin ($7\text{-}BH_4$) has cofactor activity with human recombinant phenylalanine hydroxylase.[131] Significantly, this pterin is also a potent inhibitor of the human enzyme when tested against the likely hepatic concentration of BH_4. Moreover, the inhibition shows the same peculiar pattern as the one that was originally reported for rat liver phenylalanine hydroxylase, i.e., greater inhibition at higher phenylalanine concentrations[83] with 50 percent inhibition by 5 μM $7\text{-}BH_4$ occurring at 100 μM phenylalanine.[131] Based on the inhibition of rat phenylalanine hydroxylase by $7\text{-}BH_4$, it was proposed that this inhibition could account for the mild HPA observed in patients with suspected deficiency of 4α-carbinolamine dehydratase who excrete $7\text{-}BH_4$.[83,138] The demonstration that HPA patients who excrete $7\text{-}BH_4$ are indeed deficient in the dehydratase,[101] together with the evidence that this pterin is a potent inhibitor of human phenylalanine hydroxylase,[131] strongly support the proposed mechanism for the HPA seen in dehydratase-deficient patients.

Human phenylalanine hydroxylase is only moderately stimulated by the several agents (e.g., phenylalanine and lysolecithin) that markedly activate rat hydroxylase; the finding suggests that the human enzyme is in a relatively activated state.[131] If these unusual *in vitro* properties of the human enzyme accurately reflect the enzyme's state of activation *in vivo*, it would mean that some earlier notions about phenylalanine homeostasis in humans that were derived from properties of rat liver phenylalanine hydroxylase would have to be modified.[131] At resting blood and hepatic levels of phenylalanine, the rat enzyme has very low activity, but it is poised to be massively activated in response to a physiological demand, such as that resulting from eating a protein-rich meal or, to a lesser extent, from glucagon-stimulated phosphorylation activation. By contrast, the properties of recombinant human phenylalanine hydroxylase indicate that its basal activity is relatively high even without phenylalanine- or glucagon-mediated activation. This higher basal activity of human enzyme may explain why the mean normal plasma phenylalanine concentration in adult human subjects is 58 μM[34] and in the rat is 96 μM.[139] The structural basis for the relatively activated state of human phenylalanine hydroxylase is unknown.

The human phenylalanine hydroxylase subunit comprises 452 amino acids.[140] Structure of the catalytic domain of human enzyme has now been determined by x-ray crystallography of residues 117 to 424 at 2-Å resolution.[18] The findings are providing unique insights into the way the enzyme functions and how various mutations affect integrity and function. The properties of the truncated species of the crystallized enzyme differ from those of the intact protein in several important respects. First, as originally shown for the rat liver enzyme,[141,142] proteolytic removal of 11 kDa (about 100 amino acid residues) from the N-terminus stimulates by approximately 30-fold the BH_4-dependent activity of the protease-resistant catalytic domain that is located toward the central portion of the molecule. As a result, the isolated remaining species can no longer be activated by preincubation with L-phenylalanine. Recent results with the catalytic domain of human phenylalanine hydroxylase are in accord with these results.[136] Second, results of limited proteolysis of rat hydroxylase[142] show that removal of a 5-kDa portion (about 45 amino acid residues) from the C-terminus does not lead to activation, destroys the enzyme's ability to form tetramers, eliminates the cooperative binding of phenylalanine, and implicates the carboxy-terminus in the formation of tetramers from two dimers.[142] The properties of the engineered truncated species of human phenylalanine hydroxylase used in the crystallization studies are coherent with these earlier results of studies of the rat liver enzyme. The truncated human enzyme occurs almost exclusively as dimers and does not show positive cooperativity of binding of phenylalanine;[136] the stretch of amino acids that determines these two properties has been narrowed to 25 residues at the C-terminus.[136] If rat enzyme is an appropriate model for human PAH structure, both N-terminal and C-terminal portions of the complete polypeptide are required for multimerization.

The approximate dimensions of the monomers and dimers are 50 × 45 × 45 Å and 85 × 45 × 45 Å, respectively. The essential Fe^{+3} atom sits in a crevice 10 Å below the surface of the protein on the floor of the active center. It is coordinated to residues H285 and H290 and one oxygen atom in residue F330. Through the use of site-directed mutagenesis, the two equivalent histidine residues in rat phenylalanine hydroxylase had previously been shown necessary for iron binding.[143] The side chain of residue Y325, highly conserved in the aromatic amino acid hydroxylases, is in close proximity to the iron atoms, raising the possibility that it may have a role in catalysis.[18]

A motif of 27 amino acids (H263 → H289), which is also highly conserved, has been proposed previously to be responsible for BH_4 binding.[144,145] Ten of these residues are located in the active site.

Dimerization of phenylalanine hydroxylase monomers is mediated by the interaction of two symmetry-related loops (residues 414 to 420), located close to the C-terminus of the crystallized truncated species.

To date, no mutations known to cause PKU have been found in any of the amino acid residues involved in binding of the iron atom. On the other hand, 22 (of over 250) missense *PAH* mutations affect residues lining the active site crevice; five (F263, C265, T278, E280, and P281) are in the pterin-binding motif.[18]

Two mutations together account for almost 50 percent of PKU patients in the Northern European population; they are both in the C-terminal end of the catalytic domain. The splice defect allele (IV12nt1g → a) deletes exon 12[146] and interferes with tetramer formation; when expressed in COS cells, the allele is a null, mainly due to instability of the protein.[146,147] The other common mutation, R408W, is located at the start of the tetramerization helix; replacement of the arginine by the larger tryptophan residue could interfere with the proper folding of the tetramer. When expressed in COS cells, it has less than 1 percent of wild-type activity,[147,148] the level of immunoreactive phenylalanine hydroxylase is comparably low, and the low activity results from protein instability, at least when expressed in COS cells.[147,149] Since the crystallized truncated species lacks the N-terminal regulatory domain, we do not yet know how this domain exerts its characteristic negative control over the catalytic domain.

Human phenylalanine hydroxylase may degrade in part in the nonlysosomal, ATP-dependent, ubiquitin-mediated proteolytic pathway[150] (this study was done in a nonhepatic cell system). If the finding applies to liver cells, some unstable mutant forms of phenylalanine hydroxylase (e.g., R408W) could be degraded by the ubiquinating system more rapidly than the normal enzyme; this is probably not the case, however, for some of the unstable mutant human PAH polypeptides, and further investigation is necessary (P.J. Waters, M. Parniak, and C.R. Scriver, unpublished data).

Rat liver phenylalanine hydroxylase contains one atom of iron per subunit. The iron is essential for catalytic activity,[151,152] although its role has not been elucidated. The claim that the enzyme contains one atom of copper and a bound molecule of FAD[153] has not been confirmed.

Regulation of Phenylalanine Hydroxylase

Human liver PAH and rat liver PAH have some significant differences in their regulated properties, and the following should be read with that in mind.

Since PAH catalyzes the rate-limiting step in the major pathway by which phenylalanine is catabolized to CO_2 and water, and thus has the highest sensitivity coefficient.[28] for metabolic runout of phenylalanine (Fig. 77-2), it is a likely site for regulation of phenylalanine homeostasis.[68] The enzyme can play this role because its catalytic activity is exquisitely sensitive to changes in concentrations of its substrate, phenylalanine. This sensitivity assures that exposure of tissues to high levels of phenylalanine will be kept to a minimum, while it also assures that the hydroxylase-catalyzed conversion of phenylalanine to tyrosine will not lead to depletion of phenylalanine to the point where normal protein synthesis is compromised.

This delicate balance is accomplished by a synergistic interaction between two types of regulating mechanisms: activation by phenylalanine and activation/deactivation by phosphorylation/dephosphorylation. Together, they accommodate short-term regulation of PAH activity. These mechanisms enable a more responsive coupling between hydroxylase activity and tissue levels of phenylalanine than could be achieved by an enzyme having simple Michaelis-Menten kinetics. The Michaelis-Menten relationship describes a rectangular hyperbolic response in the initial velocity to variation in substrate concentration; it shows that activity of the enzyme is geared to availability of substrate. While it may constitute an adequate regulatory mechanism at substrate concentrations at or below K_m values, it is a relatively insensitive coupling device at higher substrate concentrations.

Regulation by Substrate and Cofactor. The first evidence for short-term regulation of rat liver PAH was the 20- to 30-fold increase in the BH_4-dependent activity upon brief exposure to a phospholipid such as lysolecithin;[141,154] by contrast, activity of the enzyme in the presence of $DMPH_4$, a synthetic pterin cofactor, was only slightly increased by lysolecithin treatment.[154] The sigmoid relationship between initial velocity and phenylalanine concentration in the presence of BH_4 changed to hyperbolic with lysolecithin.[141,154] Diverse treatments of PAH such as limited proteolysis[141] and alkylation of a single sulfhydryl group[155] also markedly increased the BH_4-dependent hydroxylase activity. In the presence of BH_4 PAH is predominantly in a low-activity form, expressing only 3 to 5 percent of its potential activity.

Although there is no evidence to indicate that any of the aforementioned modes of activation are of physiological significance, they delineate some of the characteristics of the activated hydroxylase. Activation by substrate is probably involved in acute physiological regulation of PAH. It was a process independently discovered by Nielson,[97] who used $6MPH_4$ to assay the enzyme, and by Kaufman,[90] who used BH_4, the natural cofactor. The activation process was later reported by several groups.[125,156–158] The results of these studies can be accommodated by a single model that depicts PAH in equilibrium between a low-activity conformation, E, and an active conformation, E′.[158]

$$\text{Phe} \rightarrow \overset{E'}{\underset{E}{\uparrow\downarrow}} \leftarrow BH_4 \qquad \text{(Eq. 77-3)}$$

According to this formulation, the E′ conformation of PAH can be stabilized by the binding of phenylalanine to a regulatory site, whereas the E conformation can be stabilized by the binding of BH_4 in the absence of, or prior to, phenylalanine binding. In contrast to the natural coenzyme BH_4, synthetic analogues such as $DMPH_4$ are not effective in pushing the equilibrium in the direction of E; hence, more of the enzyme would exist as E′.

Studies of the inactivation of rat liver phenylalanine hydroxylase by bombarding it with high-energy electrons have provided additional structural details about how the pterin cofactor and phenylalanine interact to regulate the activity of the enzyme. From the loss of activity as a function of radiation dose, it was shown that the target size or minimum mass necessary for the $6MPH_4$-dependent activity is the dimer, with radiation causing physical destruction of one monomer at a time. By contrast, low doses of irradiation actually increase the BH_4-dependent activity; this phase is followed by a decrease in activity at higher doses, with the target size again corresponding to a dimer. The results with BH_4 support the important conclusion that this pterin inhibits or inactivates tetramers but not dimers and that a radiation hit in any part of the tetramer relieves the inhibition, resulting in activation at low doses of radiation.[159]

Parallel studies of the radiation-induced loss of the phenylalanine-activated hydroxylase indicate that phenylalanine increases the interactions between the subunits in a dimer and weakens the interactions between dimers in a tetramer. Furthermore, pretreatment of the enzyme with phenylalanine prevents the increase in BH_4-dependent activity seen at low doses of radiation, which appears to require a tetrameric structure. Phenylalanine activation, therefore, appears to be due in part to its ability to remove the BH_4-mediated inhibition of the activity of tetramers.[160]

The pterin-binding site on PAH is being mapped by photoaffinity labeling[161] and with a monoclonal anti-idiotype antibody.[162,163] These procedures have identified different pterin-binding sites. The divergent results are not necessarily incompatible but definitive identification of the pterin-binding site(s) is likely to come with x-ray diffraction analysis of PAH crystals. At the present stage of crystal analysis,[18] one can try to confirm whether the motif of 27 residues (H263 → H289), which includes 10 residues in the active site,[18] also contains a postulated BH_4-binding region.[145,163] Photoaffinity labeling identified residue C236 in rat enzyme as the reactive sulfhydryl associated with activation of PAH;[161] C237 is the corresponding residue in human enzyme, and site-directed mutagenesis (C237D) increases the activation state.[164]

The model (Eq. 77-3) assumes that there is a second site distinct from the catalytic site that binds phenylalanine which, when occupied, leads to activation. Phenylalanine increases the binding of PAH to a hydrophobic matrix,[124] and it changes the fluorescence of the enzyme.[165] These observations support the model, since they imply that phenylalanine changes the conformation of the enzyme. The notion that activation by phenylalanine might involve binding of phenylalanine to a second site with a regulatory role was first postulated by Tourian.[125] The amount of phenylalanine bound by rat liver PAH hydroxylase is 1.5 mol phenylalanine per 1 mol PAH subunit;[155] this finding provides direct experimental support for the existence of a second phenylalanine-binding site. Regulatory or activator sites for phenylalanine are absent in the dimeric species of the rat enzyme; they are formed or become functional only when two dimers interact to form tetramers,[123] a process favored by preincubation of the enzyme with phenylalanine.[123,125]

Regulation by Phosphorylation/Dephosphorylation of Subunits. Activity of the hydroxylase is increased severalfold by phosphorylation, a reaction catalyzed by cAMP-dependent kinase.[133] Activation by phosphorylation is fully expressed when the enzyme is assayed in the presence of BH_4 but not in the presence of $DMPH_4$ or $6MPH_4$.[133] Activation is accompanied by the incorporation of about 0.70 mol inorganic phosphate per subunit $M_r = 50{,}000$.[133] Because less than stoichiometric amounts of phosphate are incorporated into the pure hydroxylase *in vitro*, it seems likely that PAH isolated from rat liver is already partially phosphorylated, and, indeed, five different preparations[122] of the native enzyme had an average of 0.31 mol (range, 0.23 to 0.42) phosphate per 1 mol of subunit $M_r = 50{,}000$.[133]

The phosphorylated form of human hepatic PAH is recognized by a monoclonal antibody, and this reagent was used to show that binding of antibody correlates closely with the phosphorylation state of PAH in crude cell extracts from rat liver.[166] It was also shown that dibutyryl cAMP stimulates phosphorylation of PAH in isolated rat kidney tubules.[166]

The amino acid sequence at the serine [^{32}P]phosphorylation site of rat liver phenylalanine hydroxylase is SRK[^{32}P]-SNFGQQ.[167] The amount of this peptide is at least twice that calculated from the radioactivity of the sample, implying that it contains a substantial amount of endogenous phosphate.[167] The finding provides independent evidence that hepatic PAH, in untreated rats, is a mixture of phosphorylated and nonphosphorylated forms. It also provides an explanation for an earlier claim that rat PAH exists as three isozymes (designated *Pi*, *Kappa*, and *Upsilon* for PKU).[168] Chemical analysis showed that the preparation contained different amounts of protein-bound phosphate, with the predominant form corresponding to the monophosphorylated tetramer ($M_r = 200{,}000$), the second most prevalent form corresponding to the diphosphorylated tetramer.[169] The catalytic properties of the two forms of PAH were fully consistent with their states of phosphorylation: relative PAH activity (in the presence of BH_4) was higher for the diphosphorylated tetrameric form than for the monophosphorylated species.[169] These results indicate that the major, if not the sole, structural determinant for elution time of different forms of PAH on a calcium phosphate column (the method used for isolating *isozymes*[168]) is the amount of protein-bound phosphate in PAH.

A phosphatase has been purified from rat liver extracts that catalyzes dephosphorylation of PAH.[170] Its properties include relative lack of sensitivity to protein phosphatase inhibitors (types 1 and 2); activity in the absence of added cations; and ability to catalyze the dephosphorylation of a variety of phosphorylated proteins, including glycogen synthase and phosphorylase *a*.[171]

Accordingly, on this evidence, and from studies with antibodies,[172,173] this PAH phosphatase would be classified as a type-2A phosphatase.[174]

Activation of rat liver PAH by phosphorylation has physiological significance. Glucagon causes fourfold activation of rat hepatic PAH *in vivo*[175] and *in vitro*.[176] The effect is rapid and transient, it involves phosphorylation,[175,177,178] and it can be elicited by repeat injections, implying that decay of the activated state is not due to proteolytic degradation of the hydroxylase. The effect of glucagon is detectable when PAH is assayed in the presence of BH_4 but not in the presence of synthetic cofactor analogues such as $DMPH_4$.

Glucagon and insulin have broadly opposing metabolic effects *in vivo*. Insulin depletion increases *in situ* phenylalanine hydroxylation activity in rats.[179] Addition of glucagon to hepatocytes from diabetic rats further stimulates this elevated activity.[177] These results were confirmed in studies of PAH activity in liver extracts from rats 3 days after the onset of diabetes.[180] Although the state of phosphorylation of the enzyme was not measured, PAH appeared to be more highly phosphorylated in diabetic livers. The diabetic state increases not only the BH_4-dependent PAH activity but also the $DMPH_4$- (and $6MPH_4$)-dependent activities,[171,180] suggesting that the increased PAH activity seen in diabetic rats may be due not only to an increased degree of phosphorylation but perhaps also to an increased amount of hydroxylase protein.

Effect of Ligands on PAH. Phenylalanine and BH_4 have opposite effects on the rate of phosphorylation and activation of purified rat liver PAH. Significant concentrations of the naturally occurring 6-*R* diastereoisomer of BH_4 (6 to 8 mM) inhibit phosphorylation and activation by 80 percent, whereas 200 μM L-phenylalanine stimulates both processes to a modest extent; phenylalanine can completely overcome the inhibition caused by BH_4.[158] Inhibition of phosphorylation is quite specific for the 6-*R* diastereoisomer of BH_4; relatively large concentrations of $6MPH_4$ or $DMPH_4$ do not inhibit it.[158,181] The phosphorylated PAH requires less phenylalanine to be activated than does the nonphosphorylated form:[181,182] 29 and 51 μM phenylalanine were required to obtain half-maximal activation of the phosphorylated and nonphosphorylated forms, respectively. These findings are again consistent with the notion that the enzyme exists as an equilibrium mixture of high (E′)-activity and low (E)-activity conformations (Eq. 77-3). Inhibition of phosphorylation in the presence of BH_4 and stimulation in the presence of phenylalanine imply that the active form of PAH (E′) is a better substrate for phosphorylation than the low-activity form (E).

It seems likely that the opposing effects of BH_4 and phenylalanine on direct activation of the enzyme and on kinase-mediated activation is a dominant feature of the physiological regulation of hepatic PAH. In the case of the kinase reaction, the effect of BH_4 could be to limit the extent of phosphorylation, and thus activation, when the levels of hepatic phenylalanine are very low and high hydroxylase activity is not required. This would be true under basal conditions. Higher concentrations of phenylalanine would then be able to overcome the inhibitory effect of BH_4, allowing an increase in the extent of phosphorylation and activation of the hydroxylase when the organism needs higher hydroxylase activity to catabolize excess phenylalanine. This inhibitory effect of BH_4 would then serve to protect against depletion of the organism's pool of phenylalanine below essential levels.

Activation of PAH by phosphorylation and phenylalanine are probably synergistic modes of regulation. Phosphorylation (and activation) by cAMP-dependent protein kinase is stimulated by phenylalanine,[158,181] whereas phosphorylation sensitizes the enzyme to activation by phenylalanine.[177,181,183] A useful adaptive consequence of these interlocking control mechanisms is enhanced responsiveness of PAH activity to altered levels of phenylalanine.

This regulatory process in rats would be triggered by the ingestion of a protein-containing meal.[171] Pancreatic glucagon secretion is stimulated by protein feeding.[184] Blood glucagon increases in association with the postprandial rise in blood amino acids, and amino acids are potent stimulators of pancreatic glucagon release.[185,186] Since glucagon activates hepatic adenylate cyclase with an increase in hepatic cAMP levels, it follows that activation of cAMP-dependent protein kinase and phosphorylation-mediated activation of PAH will attend protein feeding. A consequence of this regulatory response to a postprandial rise of blood phenylalanine is accelerated catabolism of the amino acid to maintain homeostasis.

Since phenylalanine is also a glycogenic amino acid (Fig. 77-2), activation of phenylalanine hydroxylase may also be geared to increased gluconeogenesis.[171] This limb of the regulatory process would be coupled to the blood glucose level. A fall in blood glucose would increase glucagon release and suppress insulin release, resulting in phosphorylation-mediated activation of PAH with a resultant gluconeogenic effect.

Is Human Liver PAH Regulated by Phosphorylation/Dephosphorylation? There is evidence both for[187] and against[188] phosphorylation of human PAH. Any failure to detect phosphorylation-mediated activation of the human enzyme in earlier studies[188] is best explained[171] by assuming the preparation of human enzyme was already highly phosphorylated. Crude human liver PAH is not activated by exposure to cAMP-dependent protein kinase, and the same is true of crude guinea pig and monkey liver PAH.[171] By comparison, rat liver enzyme appears to be unusually responsive to activation by phosphorylation.

Long-Term Regulation of Hepatic Phenylalanine Hydroxylase. (*This section is an unreferenced précis of the corresponding text in Chap. 15 of MMBID, 6th edition.*) The possibility that phenylalanine hydroxylase activity in rat liver is under the control of steroid hormones has been intensively investigated during the last 25 years. Modest stimulatory effects of glucocorticoids on PAH *in vivo* were reported in some studies but not in others. The way the results were expressed apparently affected interpretation, since the response is greater per whole liver weight than per gram wet liver weight or per milligram liver protein. There is general agreement that the modest steroid-induced increase in hepatic PAH activity involves new protein synthesis since the response is blocked by inhibitors of protein synthesis.

Rat kidney PAH is unaffected by cortisol treatment, another indication that kidney and liver enzymes are different in rat species. Adrenalectomy modestly decreases rat hepatic PAH activity, and glucocorticoids restore it to the level found in steroid-treated controls.

PAH regulation by glucocorticoids in cultured hepatoma cells resembles that in the whole animal. Hydrocortisone and dexamethasone stimulate PAH activity to levels seen in adult rat liver. Cell density, serum, cAMP analogue, and insulin each increase enzyme activity. (*End of précis.*)

Control of PAH Activity and Synthesis in Tissue Culture. An active serum factor that stimulates PAH in cultured hepatocytes has not yet been identified. It is nondialyzable, precipitates with 50% saturated ammonium sulfate, and is altered by heat,[189,190] implying it is a protein. Serum-mediated stimulation of PAH in cultured hepatocytes is additive to the effects of insulin[189,190] and hydrocortisone,[189] indicating that the stimulation cannot be explained solely by the presence of these two hormones.

Stimulatory effects were found with serum and dexamethasone but not with insulin in a hepatoma cell line adapted to grow in serum-free medium.[191] Insulin actually inhibited the induction of PAH by serum or dexamethasone,[191] a finding concordant with in situ observations (see above).

Studies in cultured cells elucidate further the multiple forms of PAH. Normal adult rat liver contains different forms of PAH in different states of phosphorylation,[134,175] with different isoelectric points.[192] The form corresponding to half-phosphorylated tetramers (containing 0.05 mol Pi per 1 mol of hydroxylase subunit), designated form III,[134,169] has an isoelectric point of 5.60; form II is the most and form I the least prevalent. H_4 hepatoma cells contain a single form of the hydroxylase,[193,194] which is similar in its behavior to the half-phosphorylated tetramers. By immunochemical criteria, the single species of PAH in hepatoma cells is distinct from the three forms present in normal adult rat liver and the single form in rat kidney.[192,193] Treatment of hepatoma cells with hydrocortisone selectively "induces" the expression of the two forms that are present in adult liver but missing in hepatoma cells,[194] i.e., the pattern after hydrocortisone treatment of cultured cells is similar to that in rat liver. The notion that hydrocortisone induced the expression of different hydroxylase isozymes is not relevant, since the so-called isozymes[168] differ only in their states of phosphorylation.[169] The hydrocortisone effect is a complex one involving some kind of posttranslational modification of the enzyme, in addition to its effect on the amount of the enzyme in the cells.

Fetal Development of Phenylalanine Hydroxylase. Early reports that fetal and newborn mammals have PAH activity far below mature levels[195,196] are not correct.[197,198] PAH activity is detectable in human liver as early as week 8 of fetal life and reaches adult levels by the second trimester;[198–201] mutant forms of human PAH are expressed by midtrimester.[202] Catalytic properties of the human fetal liver PAH appear to be the same as those of the adult enzyme.[198,201]

Dihydropteridine Reductase

(*This enzyme and its role in BH_4 metabolism are discussed in more detail in Chap. 78.*) DHPR, an essential dimeric enzyme in the hydroxylating systems for phenylalanine, tyrosine, and tryptophan (Fig. 77-5), is widely distributed in animal tissues.[96] Whereas its occurrence in brain and adrenal medulla[96] is not surprising in view of its role in the tyrosine hydroxylation system in these tissues, and in the tryptophan hydroxylation system in brain, why DHPR should be found in tissues such as heart and lung, which have little or no aromatic amino acid hydroxylating activity, is obscure. Its wide tissue distribution, together with BH_4, hints at undiscovered roles for both BH_4 and DHPR. For example, BH_4 is the cofactor for nitric oxide synthase,[203,204] an important enzyme active in lung, and recycling of BH_4 may be required there (see Chap. 168). In addition to its role in regenerating BH_4, it has been proposed that DHPR plays an ancillary role (together with dihydrofolate reductase) in brain to keep folate in the tetrahydro form.[205] DHPR activity has been detected in cultured fibroblasts,[206] amniocytes,[207] lymphocytes,[208] leukocytes,[209] erythrocytes,[210] and platelets.[211,212] DHPR deficiency is a cause of human HPA, so it should be considered in the diagnostic investigation (see below) and treatment adapted accordingly (see Chap. 78).

Biosynthesis of BH_4

(*This topic and its relevance to HPA are described in further detail in Chap. 78.*) The cofactor function of BH_4 in the hydroxylation reaction with aromatic amino acids is related to its ability to reduce molecular oxygen; BH_4 provides electrons and in turn it is oxidized to qBH_2.[15,213] The consumption of BH_4 is stoichiometric during hydroxylation of substrate. Whereas the DHPR-catalyzed reaction regenerates (recycles) BH_4 from qBH_2 moment by moment, so that cofactor functions catalytically, the steady state of BH_4 is ultimately dependent on biosynthesis from precursors. Its fundamental role in cellular biochemistry and pathogenesis of disease is a large topic;[111,214] its specific relevance to the human HPAs is the subject of Chap. 78.

As outlined in Eq. 77-3, a dominant theme in the acute regulation of phenylalanine hydroxylase is the balance between the activating effect of phenylalanine and the deactivating effect of BH_4. A variation of this theme also operates to regulate the mammalian biosynthesis of BH_4 and explains how phenylalanine itself controls the synthesis of BH_4 through a regulatory protein that interacts with GTP-cyclohydrolase. All three genes involved in the *de novo* biosynthesis pathway yielding BH_4 have been cloned, sequenced, and mapped to chromosomes. There is evidence that elevated amounts of the end products of hydroxylase-dependent tryptophan and tyrosine pathway down-regulate BH_4 synthesis.

THE *PAH* GENE: RELATIONSHIPS BETWEEN GENOTYPE AND PHENOTYPE

Comment. Over 98 percent of mutations associated with human HPA occur at the *PAH* locus, and the remainder at the loci dedicated to synthesis and regeneration of tetrahydrobiopterin (Chap. 78) The *PAH* gene has a structure and regulatory elements typical of many housekeeping genes: it harbors several hundred alleles, some of which are polymorphic and neutral in their effect on PAH enzyme activity, but most are a cause of HPA. The on-line locus-specific mutation database (www.mcgill.ca/pahdb) is a prototype in the human mutation database initiative taking place at the interface between human genomics and genetics. After mutation analysis, what to do with the information? Hence the interest in correlations between genotype and phenotype; the *PAH* locus shows that all that is phenotype in the disease (PKU) is not always explained by allelic variation at the *PAH* locus. *PAH* alleles have also been part of human history apparently since the "out of Africa" radiation and in their polymorphic forms from before that event.

The *PAH* Gene

Isolation of a human *PAH* cDNA began with synthesis and authentication of a rat cDNA from liver mRNA purified by polysome immunoprecipiation.[12,215] A human liver cDNA library probed with the rat clone produced a full-length cDNA clone (*h PAH* 247) about 2.4 kb in length; it encodes a polypeptide of 452 amino acids, predicted molecular weight 51,862 daltons[140] and sequence nearly identical to that proposed for the human protein.[157,216] Meanwhile, others obtained cDNA clones in the rat,[217] mouse,[110] and human[218] genomes. Rodent and human sequences, both DNA and protein, are similar, with 92 percent overall polypeptide homology and 96 percent similarity at the C-terminal end.[140,215,217] *In vitro* expression of the human or rat *PAH* cDNA is sufficient to assemble a homopolymeric protein with phenylalanine hydroxylating activity in the presence of pterin cofactor.[219,220] The human *PAH* locus, mapped by *in situ* hybridization, is on chromosome 12, band region q22-q24.1.[23]

The full genomic sequence for *PAH* spanning more than 90 kb has not yet been reported. The cDNA sequence[112,140,221] (GenBank U49897) contains 13 exons comprising less than 3 percent of the genomic length; with the exception of exon 13 (more than 892 bps), none exceeds 197 bps in size. The intronic splice site nucleotide sequences are all conventional. Exon border types vary; most are type 3 (beginning after the third nucleotide of a codon); codons 118 and 236 introduce type-1 borders spanning introns 3 and 6 respectively; codons 170, 281, and 400 introduce type-2 borders spanning introns 5, 7, and 11 respectively. The structure of the gene is represented to scale in Fig. 77-6.

PAH has a rich repertoire of restriction fragment length polymorphism (RFLP) sites and polymorphic markers (Fig. 77-6) for analysis of the gene[140] from which a large number of informative haplotypes are derived[221] [see Fig. 77-6 and the section "The *PAH* Gene: Allelic Variation (Mutations)"].

The 5′ untranslated region of the gene (Fig. 77-6), now well characterized,[112] has five potential cap sites upstream from the actual methionine translation initiation codon in exon 1; multiple cap sites are a feature of many housekeeping genes. The *PAH* gene lacks a proximal TATA box but has several elements (Fig. 77-6), which include four GC-rich domains as putative Sp1-binding sites (another housekeeping feature), a CCAAT sequence (a target for

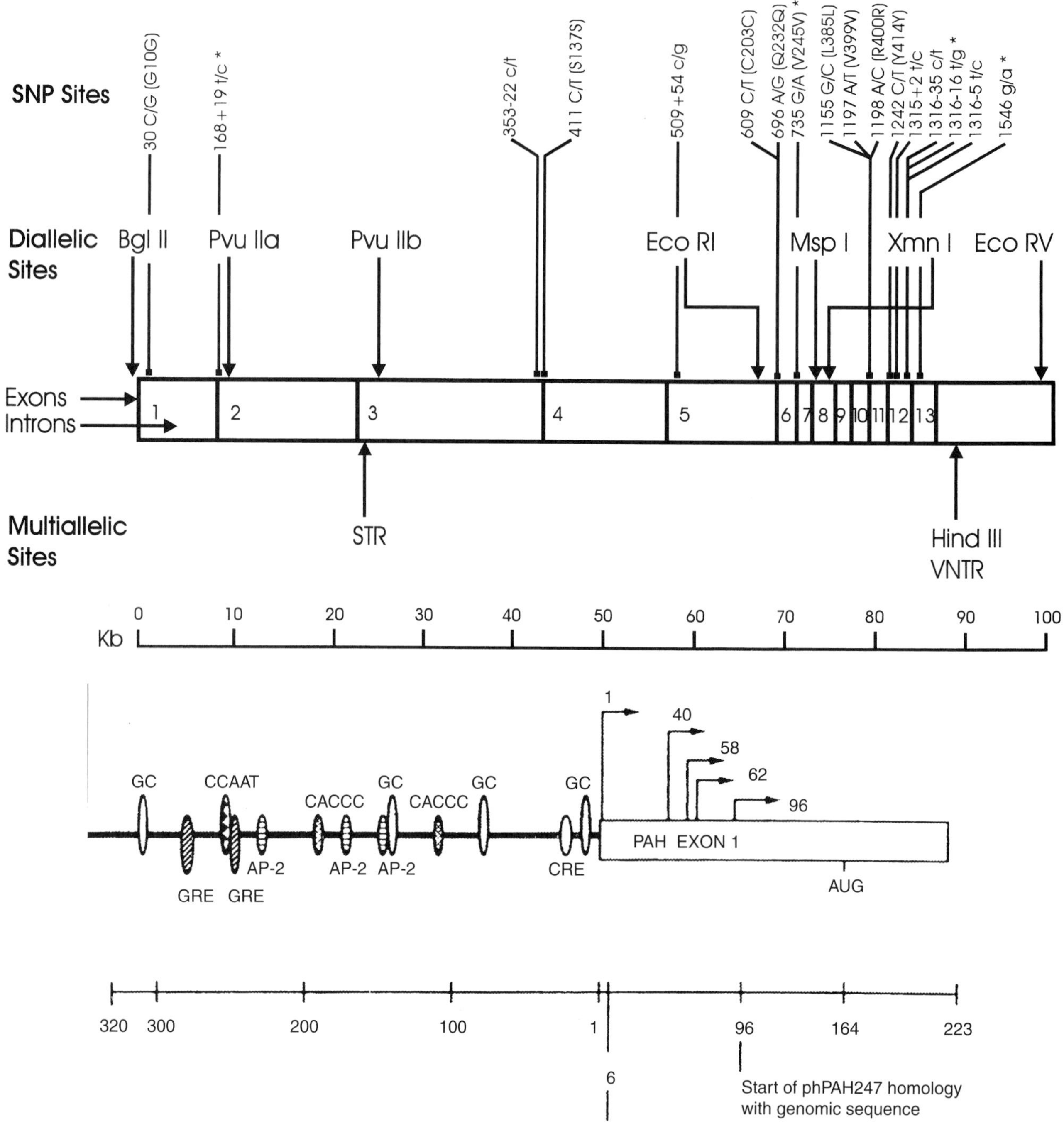

Fig. 77-6 Basic structure of the human phenylalanine hydroxylase (*PAH*) gene. The locus covers approximately 100 kb of genomic DNA on chromosome 12p. The cDNA sequence is deposited at GenBank (NCBI) under U49897. The top shows to scale the relative sizes and positions of exons and introns in *PAH* genomic sequence, and positions of polymorphic sites (multiallelic sites are shown below the gene). Biallelic restriction fragment length polymorphism sites and single-nucleotide polymorphic (SNP) sites are placed above it. SNPs are identified by their systematic (nucleotide) names, as recommended.[234] See the text for discussion of *PAH* polymorphisms. The bottom depicts the 5′ end of the gene as described by Konecki et al.[112] (*Reproduced from reference 112 with permission of the American Chemical Society.*)

factors regulation efficiency of transcription), GRE and CACCC sites (elements involved in regulation mediated by glucocorticoids), several activator protein 2 (Ap-2)-binding sites, and one partial cAMP response element (CRE). The 5′ region of human *PAH*, 3.5 kb upstream and beyond the 0.5-kb region described above, contains a sequence very similar to the mouse liver-specific hormone-inducible *PAH* gene enhancer; this region binds HNF1;[117] dose-dependent HNF1-mediated transactivation of *PAH* gene expression is further potentiated by DCoH. Thus, DCoH, which is identical to phenylalanine hydroxylase simulator (PHS), and is also a 4α-carbinolaminase dehydratase, participates both in regeneration of tetrahydrobiopterin cofactor and in *PAH* gene expression. A 5′ *PAH* construct fused to a *CAT* reporter gene and expressed in transgenic mice showed that expression of the human *PAH* gene is specific both for tissue and for stage of development.[113] The 5′ flanking regions of rat[222,223] and mouse[115] genes encoding phenylalanine hydroxylase have features and elements very similar to those of the human gene.

Evolutionary Aspects. *PAH* is in a gene family[224] of aromatic L-amino hydroxylases that includes L-tyrosine 3-monooxygenase (gene symbol *TYH*; EC 1.14.16.2)[18,225] and L-tryptophan 5-monoozygenase (gene symbol *TPH*; EC 1.14.16.4);[226] the latter are tetrahydrobiopterin-requiring apoenzymes catalyzing rate-limiting steps in pathways leading to synthesis of neurotransmitters. Primary structures of the polypeptide products have remained similar throughout evolution within and between species,[18,217,226] and intron/exon boundaries in the genes are conserved.[227] *PAH*, *TPH*, and *TYH* are likely to have evolved over 75 million years from a common ancestral entity by duplication and divergence,[226,228] *PAH* and *TPH* being more closely related to each other than to *TYH*.

The three hydroxylases share features of their domain structures;[18,217,226] C-terminal regions are more conserved, and N-terminal regions are more divergent. The former region contains the determinants for hydroxylating activity[142] and BH_4 binding,[162,163] whereas the latter contains the determinants for substrate specificity[142] and phosphorylation-mediated activation.[229,230] The genes have significant differences: genomic *TYH* (smaller than 10 kb)[231] is small relative to *PAH*; *TPH* is probably of intermediate size if one extrapolates from the corresponding mouse data.[227] Human *TYH* transcribes several species of mRNA[232] but not so with *PAH* and *TPH*.

The *PAH* Mutation Database (*PAHdb*)

Discovery of variant alleles in the *PAH* gene has outpaced the ability to record them in the print literature; a response on behalf of the *PAH* Mutation Analysis Consortium (90 investigators in 28 countries) is *PAHdb*, a relatively large, curated (edited and maintained), public (on-line) relational locus-specific mutation database (http://www.mcgill.ca/pahdb),[14] with links to the PKU entry (261600) in OMIM (http://www.ncbi.nlm.nih.gov/omim) and the reference nucleotide sequence (U49897) in GenBank at the U.S. National Center for Biotechnology Information (http://www.ncbi.nlm.nih.gov/); *PAHdb* is listed in the genomic databases at the EBI (European Bioinformatics Institute) (http://www2.ebi.ac.uk/mutation) and at the Human Genome Mutation Database (http://www.cf.ac.uk/uwcm/mg/hgmd0.html). The PAH polypeptide amino acid sequence is recorded in the SWISS-PROT database (entry P00439). *PAHdb* is part of the HUGO Mutation Database Initiative,[233] an international project with an integrated approach to the documentation of mutations in genomes.

PAH alleles are systematically named by nucleotide affected; the latter are numbered from the A, of the ATG translation initiation (codon 1), located at nt473 from the 5′ end of the cDNA (GenBank U49897); nucleotides 5′ to this nucleotide are given negative numbers in *PAHdb*. The GenBank sequence numbers nucleotides from the first 5′ base; there is software to find the ATG codon and adjust numbering of nucleotides when naming mutations.

PAHdb contains entities (real-world concepts such as *mutation*) and attributes (such as the *name* of the mutation). The former are distributed into conceptual modules containing attributes and descriptors of the corresponding entities.[14]

PAH alleles are given both systematic and trivial names, in a context according to current guidelines.[234] For example, the codon-1 mutation that disrupts translation initiation in the human *PAH* gene[235] can be named HSAP:PAH:U49897:c.1A→G (M1V), where the terms indicate species, gene, reference sequence, systematic name of the mutation (centered on the nucleotide change in cDNA sequence), and its trivial name (amino acid change, methionine to valine, at position 1 in the PAH polypeptide sequence).

PAHdb maintains an edited off-line copy recording hundreds of alleles (both disease-causing mutations and neutral polymorphisms), dozens of polymorphic haplotypes, in thousands of records (associations), distributed into more than 60 data tables; dated mirror copies are deposited on the website, where they can be interrogated with a search engine on a dedicated server (http://www.debelle.ca/pahdb).

The several hundred PAH mutations, each different by state, have been ascertained in patients with HPA and are assumed to be disease-causing, whereas the associated polymorphic alleles and haplotypes are assumed to be neutral in effect. However, possible modifying influences of the latter on *PAH* gene function have not yet been systematically investigated. Meantime, each allele different by state from all others receives a unique identifier (UID) in *PAHdb*. In addition to relationships of data, the database provides a clinical page for public use (http://www.mcgill.ca/pahdb/handout/handout.htm), and a page that describes mutagenized (enu) mouse strains, useful counterparts of human PAH enzyme deficiency[236] (see the section "Animal Models").

There is an on-line database for mutations in the genes encoding enzymes for BH_4 synthesis and regeneration (http://www.bh4.org), and another for the corresponding diseases and patients (http://www.unizh.ch/~blau.biodef1.html). Further details appear in Chap. 78.

The *PAH* Gene: Allelic Variation (Mutations)

The word *mutation* is used here to mean allelic variation in the nucleotide sequence of the *PAH* gene.[237] *PAH* mutations are most frequently, but not exclusively, ascertained in persons with persistent postnatal HPA attributable to phenylalanine hydroxylase dysfunction; this constitutes a bias of ascertainment. The mutations are of two types: (1) polymorphic and neutral in their effect on phenotype, or (2) pathogenic through impairment of PAH enzyme function. Alleles are called polymorphic when their frequency is 0.01 or greater in the population; whether every polymorphic allele is truly neutral and without a phenotypic effect cannot be stated with certainty. Alleles are considered likely to be disease-causing (pathogenic)[238] when they segregate in affected persons, are inherited codominantly, are unambiguously null (e.g., frameshift, protein truncation, splice defective, large deletion), or are missense and affect a conserved residue[226,239,240] (over half of missense *PAH* alleles do so[224]), or the mutation is known to impair PAH enzyme function in an *in vitro* expression system.[147]

Polymorphic Alleles. The *PAH* cDNA sequence contains a large number of recognized polymorphisms (Fig. 77-6), with the likelihood of more yet to be recognized in the introns when the full genome sequence for *PAH* is known. Polymorphisms occur in three forms: (1) *Biallelic restriction fragment length polymorphisms*,[221,241] named from the corresponding restriction enzyme (*Bgl*II, *Pvu*IIa, *Pvu*IIb, *Eco*RI, *Msp*I, *Xmn*I, and *Eco*RV). With the exception of the *Eco*R sites, which require analysis by Southern blotting, *PAH* RFLPs can be analyzed by methods based on polymerase chain reaction (PCR) amplification [*Bgl*II,[242] *Pvu*IIa,[243] *Pvu*IIb (R.C. Eisensmith, unpublished), *Msp*I,[244] and *Xmn*I[245]]. (2) *Multiallelic polymorphisms*, which include an hypervariable sequence (variable number of tandem repeats or VNTR) of 30-bp cassettes harboring at least 10 alleles (differing by number of repeats) in a *Hin*dIII fragment 3 kb downstream from the last exon in *PAH*;[246,247] and a series of short tandem [tetranucleotide $(TCTA)_n$] repeats (STRs) harboring at least 9 alleles in the third intron of *PAH*.[248–250] (3) *Single-nucleotide polymorphisms* (SNPs), which are silent (non-RFLP) alleles, for example: c.1546g/a which occurs at about 0.20 frequency in the 3′UTR of *PAH* on both mutant and normal chromosomes;[251] and a silent c.696A/G polymorphism ($q = 0.08$–0.63) in codon 232 (Q232Q).[252]

Polymorphic Haplotypes. RFLP, STR, and VNTR alleles can be combined to generate extended *PAH*-locus haplotypes. A *mini-haplotype* comprising only the STR, *Xmn*I, and VNTR alleles is an alternative because it is informative, accessible to PCR-based analysis,[253] and easy to obtain. The extended (*full*) *PAH* haplotypes are named with Arabic numbers[254] and at least 87 are known (see *PAHdb*). A matrix (Fig. 77-7) summarizes

Haplotype	BglII	PvuIIa	STR 228	STR 232	STR 236	STR 240	STR 244	STR 248	STR 252	STR 256	PvuIIb	EcoRI	MspI	XmnI	VNTR 3	VNTR 7	VNTR 8	VNTR 9	VNTR 11	VNTR 12	VNTR 13	EcoRV	N
10	−	+				o					−	+	+	−			o					−	2
1, 24, 25	−	+		o	o	o	o	o	o		−	−	+	−	o	o	o		o	o		−	63
2, 12, 27	−	+		o	o	o	o	o			−	−	+	−	o	o	o		o	o	o	+	28
8, 41	−	+				o	o	o	o		−	+	+	−	o	o		o				+	5
3, 31	−	+		o		o					−	+	−	+	o	o	o					−	8
4, 19	−	+		o	o	o	o				−	+	−	+	o		o					+	30
28	−	+		o	o	o	o				−	−	−	+	o							+	6
16	−	+			o	o	o				−	+	−	−	o							+	4
36	+	−				o	o				+	−	+	−		o		o				−	2
novel	+	−						o	o		+	−	+	−	o					o		+	3
5, 21	+	−				o	o	o	o	o	+	+	+	−				o	o			+	17
18	+	−			o						+	+	−	+	o							+	1
7	+	−	o	o	o	o					−	+	−	+			o					−	13
40	+	−	o	o							−	−	−	+			o					−	4
30	+	+	o								−	−	−	+			o					−	1
9	+	+					o				−	+	+	−			o					+	1
11, 69	+	−				o	o			o	−	+	+	−	o		o	o				+	4
34	+	−				o					−	+	+	−			o					−	1
32	+	−	o					o			−	−	+	−			o					−	3
26	+	+									−	−	+	−			o					−	1

Fig. 77-7 Extended polymorphic haplotypes in the human phenylalanine hydroxylase (*PAH*) gene are derived from seven biallelic restriction fragment length polymorphisms and two multiallelic sites (STR, short tandem repeat; and VNTR, variable number of tandem repeats) (see Fig. 77-6 for their relative positions in the gene). Most, but not all, known haplotypes are summarized in this matrix. Fragment sizes (in basepairs) of the STR alleles are those as identified by Zschocke et al;[832] they are 2 bp shorter than as described in the original report by Goltsov et al.[246] The numbers in *right-hand column* illustrate a typical frequency distribution of haplotypes in a human population (in this case, French Canadians from Eastern Quebec[262]). (Figure designed by Mary Fujiwara.)

extended *PAH* haplotype configurations derived from seven biallelic and two multiallelic sites in a population of European descent; the variety of configurations would be vastly increased if SNPs were included. Whereas several thousand different extended polymorphic *PAH* haplotypes could be generated from combinations of RFLP, STR, and VNTR alleles,[224] far fewer have actually been observed on human chromosomes. Figure 77-7 includes an observed frequency distribution of haplotypes on a set of normal chromosomes from a defined population: only a few haplotypes are prevalent and most are uncommon, and this is typical of all human populations analyzed up to now. The apparent shortage of *PAH* haplotypes is explained by linkage disequilibrium across the 100-kb region of the extended haplotype.[255–257,257a] *PAH* haplotype heterogeneity is much greater on mutant and normal chromosomes in Europeans[258] than it is on chromosomes in Asians.[259] It is predicted that *PAH* haplotype diversity will be found to be greater in African populations than in Europeans, assuming the latter are descendant of a small founding group emerging out of Africa some 100,000 years ago (see reference 257a).

Particular *PAH* haplotypes tend to harbor the prevalent disease-causing mutations in European populations;[224] for example, haplotype 7 is usually associated with the prevalent PKU-causing mutation G272X in Norway, haplotype 2 with R408W in Eastern Europe, haplotype 1 with R408W on the northwestern fringes of Europe, haplotype 3 with IVS12nt1 in Northern Europe, haplotype 9 with I65T in Western Europe and the Iberian Peninsula, and haplotype 6 with IVS10nt-11 in Anatolia, Southeastern Europe, and the Mediterranean. Codominant segregation of polymorphic *PAH* haplotypes, in association with the known mutant genotype, when the latter has been ascertained from a propositus, is compatible with carrier detection and prenatal diagnosis, without recourse to mutation analysis itself.[13,253,260]

Polymorphic haplotypes at the *PAH* locus can be used to study human evolution and the histories of human populations without reliance on disease-causing alleles.[257a] Although the latter can be particularly informative in this regard,[224,261] they are much rarer and therefore may not be available for this type of analysis, for example, in Africa (see the section "Population Genetics of PKU and Pathogenic *PAH* Alleles"). Divergence between African, European, and Asiatic populations, with support for the "out of Africa" hypothesis,[257a] has been documented by *PAH* polymorphic haplotype analysis:[257] the ancestral haplotypes on which some modern configurations arose can be postulated;[252] the origins, by geographic region and population, of a particular allele can be surmised;[251] and the particular genetic structure (at the *PAH* locus) of a population can be described by its haplotype configuration and used to unravel demographic histories;[262] and haplotypes can serve as migration traces over large geographic regions and time frames[263] (see the section "Population Genetics").

Pathogenic Alleles. *PAHdb* assigns unique identifiers to each new *PAH* mutation[14] when the allele is distinct by state from all others. When this chapter was prepared, 417 different alleles were documented in the *PAH* gene (Fig. 77-8). The vast majority are known (or presumed to be) causes of PKU or non-PKU HPA, having been ascertained through patients. The disease-causing mutations are 94 percent of all *PAH* alleles and fall into five classes: missense, 62 percent of all alleles; small deletions (less than 22 bp), 13 percent; modifiers of mRNA splicing, 12 percent; termination nonsense alleles, 6 percent; and small insertions, 1 percent; large deletions are rare in this gene.[264] Two patterns of mutation frequency distribution, now being seen at many human loci harboring pathogenetic alleles,[29] are clearly apparent at the *PAH* locus[261] (see the section "Population Genetics"). First, only a few alleles, five in the case of *PAH*, account for the majority of all mutant chromosomes in the human population while the remainder are rare. Second, the distributions, both geographic and by population, are nonrandom so that the history of a particular allele often corresponds to the history of the population in which it is found.

Phenotypic Effects of PAH Mutations

Comment. A *PAH* disease-causing mutation has an effect at three phenotype levels: (1) on enzyme integrity and function (a proximate level); (2) on phenylalanine homeostasis and thus on its concentration in body fluids (the intermediate level); and (3) on the brain, its function, and on cognitive development (a distal level). The likelihood that categorical genotype-phenotype correlations can be found at all phenotype levels of this autosomal recessive trait is confounded by the extent of allelic heterogeneity, the complexity of phenylalanine homeostasis, and the fact that the

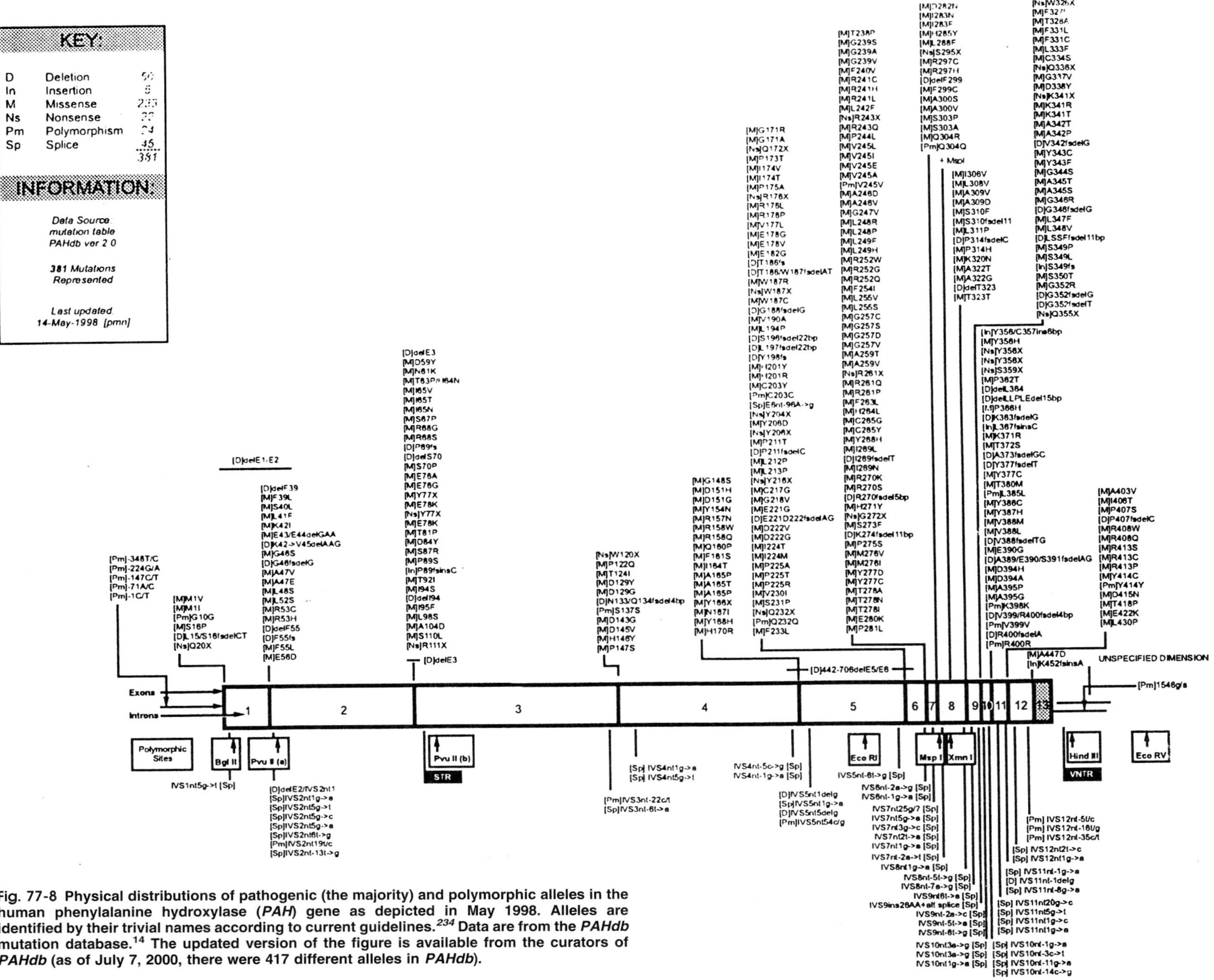

Fig. 77-8 Physical distributions of pathogenic (the majority) and polymorphic alleles in the human phenylalanine hydroxylase (*PAH*) gene as depicted in May 1998. Alleles are identified by their trivial names according to current guidelines.[234] Data are from the *PAHdb* mutation database.[14] The updated version of the figure is available from the curators of *PAHdb* (as of July 7, 2000, there were 417 different alleles in *PAHdb*).

distal phenotype (IQ) is a classic complex trait.[264a] We discuss the relationships: first at the most proximal level (PAH enzyme), then at the most distal level (brain), and last at the intermediate level, because phenylalanine appears to be the mediator between a mutant *PAH* genotype and its association with hazard to cognitive development and function.

Effect of Mutation on Enzymic (Hydroxylating) Function. Nonhepatic human tissues, notably kidney, show evidence of harboring significant phenylalanine hydroxylating activity.[77a,77b] The effect of *PAH* mutations can be assessed either directly or indirectly by three quite different approaches: (1) by enzyme assay, on a tissue biopsy sample, *in vitro*; (2) by an isotopic method *in vivo*; or (3) by *in vitro* gene expression analysis. The first two methods measure the effect of mutant genotype (as homoallelic or heteroallelic forms of homozygosity, or in the heterozygote) on enzymatic function in patients, whereas the third measures the effect of a particular allele, placed in a recombinant gene construct, on homopolymeric *PAH* (enzyme) activity, unless a variant of the yeast two-hybrid expression system is used.

Hepatic Enzyme Activity in Biopsy Samples. Several early studies, using the relatively crude assay of the day, identified deficient enzymatic activity by direct assay on liver samples from PKU patients.[7,265–267] Corroboration with more refined assays followed.[268–270] These and other studies identified CRM^+ and CRM^- hepatic enzyme phenotypes in PKU,[271–274] and very low enzyme activity with apparently normal affinity for substrate was observed in several patients.[275,276] The largest single study of hepatic PAH enzyme activity[277] used a reliable assay on liver biopsy material obtained from a group of very well monitored patients with HPA; patients with typical PKU had less than 1 percent normal activity whereas those with non-PKU HPA had more enzymatic activity, usually more than 5 percent normal (Fig. 77-9). This particular study also showed that impaired hydroxylating activity and primary deficiency of PAH enzyme integrity are not synonymous: some patients, who had HPA *in vivo*, yet had "intact" phenylalanine hydroxylating activity *in vitro*, actually had a primary disorder of BH_4 cofactor metabolism.[277]

Interindividual variation in hepatic enzyme activity in PKU patients[277] has been attributed to allelic heterogeneity.[278] The issue of *PAH* allelism and possible allelic interaction, usually of negative type, at the polypeptide level, came to prominence in several studies. For example, propositi with non-PKU HPA had hepatic enzyme activity about 5 percent of normal and their parents had activity about 13 percent of normal (mean of six subjects), which in the latter is a level much lower than the expected half-normal value for heterozygotes.[279] Some obligate heterozygotes for the PKU phenotype again had enzyme activity well below expectation (14 to 44 percent of normal).[273,280,281] The deviant *in vitro* gene dose effects seen in these subjects imply negative cooperativity at the subunit level of PAH enzyme (a dominant negative mutation effect); whether this unusual dose effect also occurs *in vivo* is not yet known. Meanwhile, one must question why heterozygotes with low *in vitro* activity would not have HPA, and why patients with considerable *in vitro* activity nonetheless have HPA.

***Isotopic Studies* In Vivo.** Phenylalanine hydroxylating activity can be estimated by an indirect assay *in vivo* following intravenous infusion of substrate: the rate at which labeled phenylalanine is converted to tyrosine is measured in plasma (Fig. 77-9).[57,68,282–289] With only one exception,[53,55,56] phenylalanine hydroxylating activities measured in this way were shown to be deficient in patients with the PKU phenotype; in some patients, the *in vivo* findings were also corroborated by direct *in vitro* measurements of hepatic enzyme activity in biopsy material.[284] The method itself is validated by evidence that regulated adaptation of PAH enzyme activity under physiological conditions is observed.[286] The logical inconsistency in any evidence for a normal conversion rate of phenylalanine to tyrosine in PKU patients, as in reports from one group,[53,55,56] and the discrepancy between those unexpected findings and all other observations, particularly in a set of experiments replicating the conditions of the anomalous studies,[57] has since been explained (see footnote ¶).

Phenylalanine hydroxylating activity (more precisely, the *oxidation rate*) can also be assayed *in vivo*, as a flux through the whole pathway, with a noninvasive approach where labeled L-phenylalanine — [1-^{14}C] or [1-^{13}C] — is ingested and labeled CO_2 in expired air is measured subsequently.[26,39] This approach has the virtue of simplicity. It shows the predicted gene dose effect (Fig. 77-9), confirms by an independent approach that *in vivo hydroxylating* activity is deficient in PKU patients, and is sensitive enough to distinguish between the two phenotype classes (PKU and non-PKU HPA phenotype).[26] It is not sufficiently sensitive to correlate a particular mutant genotype with phenotype within the class.[26]

***Nonisotopic Studies* In Vivo.** A simple, nonisotopic method (which involves several blood samples over 72 h) has been devised to assess *PAH activity in vivo*.[290] An oral load of L-phenylalanine (0.6 mmol/kg body weight) is given after an overnight fast, and blood samples are drawn at 0, 1, 2, 3, 4, 24, 48, and 72 h. Patients with genotypes predicted to harbor severe, intermediate, or mild *PAH* alleles manifest the corresponding PKU, variant PKU, and non-PKU HPA phenotypes apparent in the rates at which they clear the load from plasma. The observed rates were concordant with the clinical classification based on pretreatment plasma phenylalanine values and daily diet phenylalanine tolerance.[21,290] The method, of course, measures all parameters of phenylalanine runout and not PAH activity alone.

In Vitro *Expression Analysis.* This is yet another way to demonstrate the effect of a *PAH* allele on the corresponding hydroxylating activity. Expression analysis was used early in the study of PKU alleles to analyze the effect of a natural human R408W allele.[148] An expression vector [p91023(B)] containing the mutant *PAH* cDNA, created by site-directed mutagenesis, and a plasmid construct containing normal cDNA sequence are separately transfected into cultured mammalian (COS) cells; PAH enzyme activity is then assayed with synthetic cofactor ($6MPH_4$). When related to wild-type activity, the R408W expression levels for enzyme activity and for PAH immunoreactive protein are less than 1 percent and for mRNA are 100 percent. When the R408W allele is reanalyzed in another expression system with natural cofactor (BH_4), the original findings are corroborated.[291]

The molecular basis of phenotype heterogeneity in PAH-deficient HPA was then analyzed for several alleles by *in vitro* expression analysis in a landmark study,[149] its major findings being corroborated by additional reports.[292,293] The results show that *PAH* mutations, such as R408W, with a "severe" effect on enzyme function *in vitro* are associated with a severe PKU phenotype *in vivo*, whereas mutations with a "mild" effect in vitro are associated with a corresponding phenotype *in vivo* (Fig. 77-10).

At least 45 natural human *PAH* alleles have now been analyzed by *in vitro* expression[147] (search also on *PAHdb*). While their major effects are described in the original publications and in a review,[147] it has been suggested they can be grouped under four broad headings[294] as (1) *knockout* (null) alleles (undetectable activity), (2) V_{max} alleles (reduced activity), (3) *kinetic* alleles that alter affinity (K_m) for substrate (or cofactor), and (4) *unstable* alleles that increase turnover (loss) of PAH subunit.

Expression analysis of *PAH* alleles is informative in various ways and sometimes offers a surprise; for example, the Y204C "missense" allele has normal expression activity *in vitro* yet behaves as a severe allele *in vivo*: it is in fact a splice mutation (c.611A → g, E6nt-96A → g) masquerading as a missense allele.[295] Substitution of S231 by proline (S231P) in exon 6 causes complete loss of enzymatic activity,[296] as does S349P, a missense allele in exon 10,[297] and F299C in exon 8.[147,294] Each of

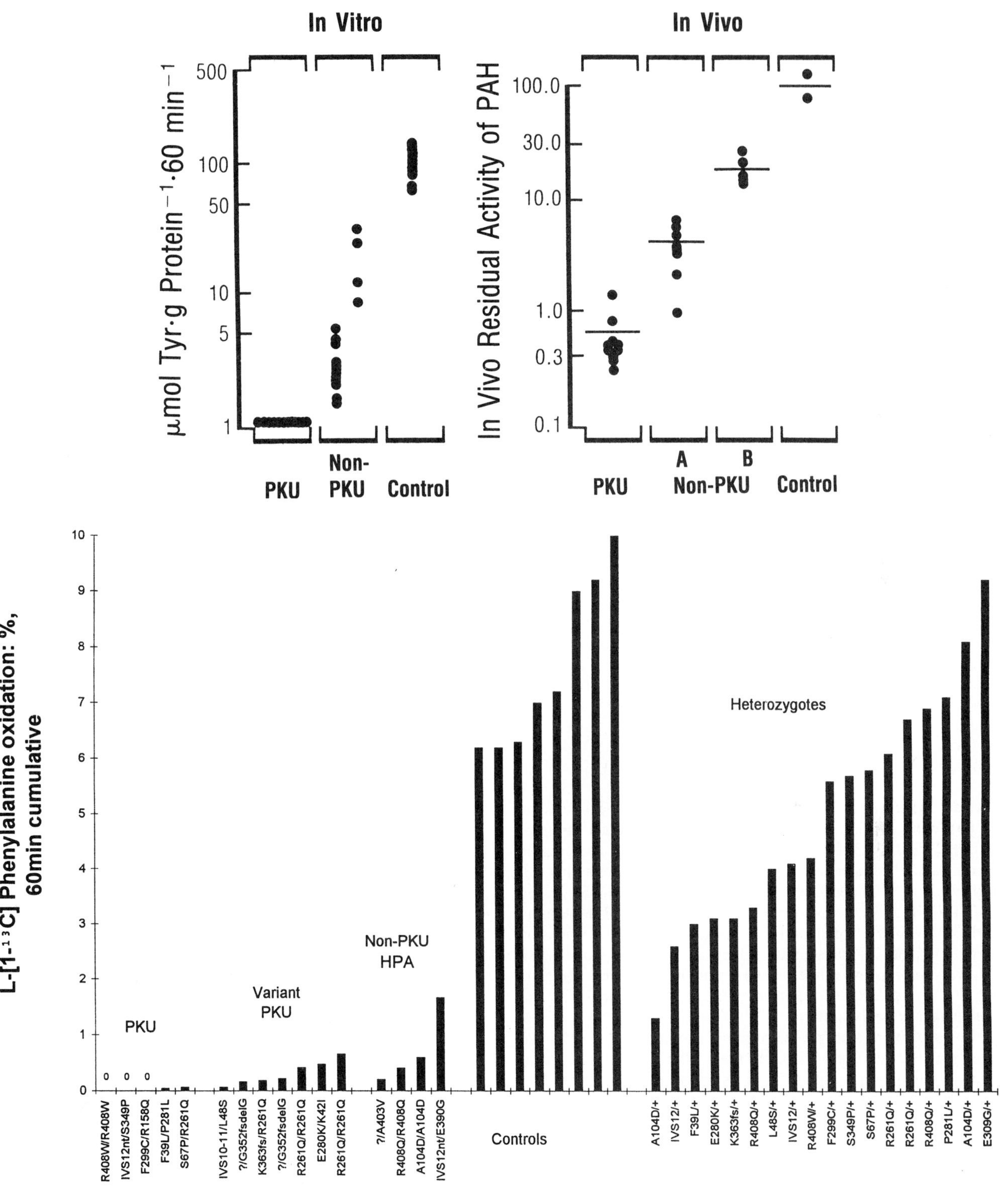

Fig. 77-9 Measured activity of phenylalanine hydroxylase enzyme. Top: *In vitro* on hepatic needle-biopsy material (left), *in vivo* by isotope infusion (right). Bottom: Measured *in vivo* by ingestion of isotope and analysis of expired $^{13}CO_2$. The *in vivo* data (top) were obtained by infusion of heptadeuterated phenylalanine followed by measurement of the rate of tyrosine labelling at steady state. The *in vivo* assay in the bottom figure measures cumulative expired $^{13}CO_2$ for 80 min after ingestion of a tracer dose of L-[1-^{13}C]phenylalanine; propositi in this study were persons with phenylketonuria, variant PKU, and non-PKU HPA and the corresponding heterozygotes of known genotype (indicated on abscissa). The figure is a composite of data from Bartholomé et al,[277] Trefz et al,[284] and Treacy et al.[26]

these alleles behaves as a functional null being associated with undetectable activity both in a bacterial (*E. coli*) expression system and in mammalian COS cells where their expression involves loss of protein along with catalytic activity.[147] The bacterial system affords the greater scope for detailed kinetic analysis of missense mutations affecting the V_{max} value, with or without an effect on the K_m value (e.g., R252Q/G and L255V).[147,294] A K_m mutant (D143G) has been investigated in three different expression

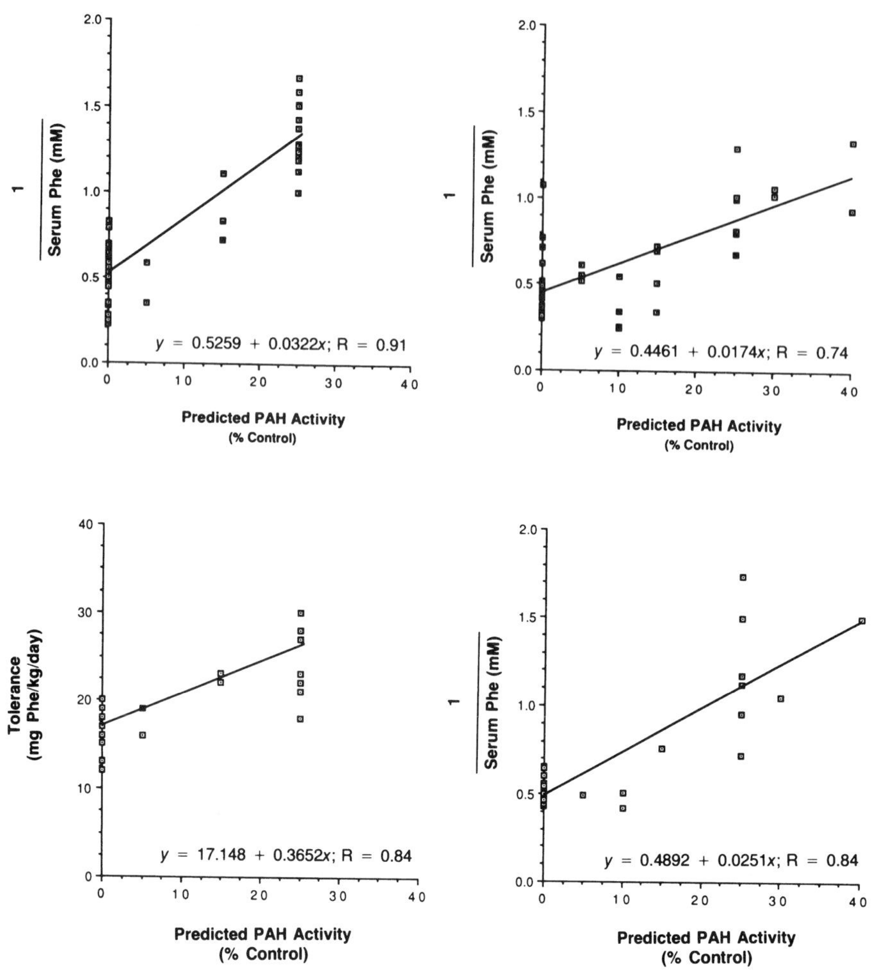

Fig. 77-10 Relationships between predicted phenylalanine hydroxylase activity (by in vitro expression analysis) and biochemical phenotypes in hyperphenylalaninemia patients. Least-squares analysis was used to calculate regressions, for which equations and correlation coefficients are shown. (Top left) Relationship between predicted phenylalanine hydroxylase activity and 1/pretreatment serum phenylalanine levels in Danish phenylketonuria (PKU) patients (n = 51). (Top right) Relationship between predicted phenylalanine hydroxylase activity and 1/pretreatment serum phenylalanine levels in German PKU patients (n = 44). (Bottom left) Relationship between predicted phenylalanine hydroxylase activity and phenylalanine tolerance at age 5 years in Danish PKU patients (n = 48). (Bottom right) Relationship between predicted phenylalanine hydroxylase activity and 1/serum phenylalanine 72 h after an oral protein load at age 6 months in German PKU patients (n = 23). (*From Okano et al.*[149] *Used by permission.*)

systems (human kidney cells, *E. coli*, and cell-free reticulocyte lysate) with consistent results.[298] Five other mutant proteins (R158Q, P244L, A322G, V388M, and R408Q) all show decreased specific activity and behave as stable mutants in a mammalian cell expression system. Missense mutations such as G46S,[299] and A104D or R157N,[300] cause primary instability of the PAH subunit, with or without aggregation, in several different expression systems. There is substantial evidence now from expression analysis that many missense *PAH* mutations impair enzyme activity by defective oligomerization, reduced stability, and accelerated proteolytic turnover.[264a,299,300,300a,300b,300c]

In vitro expression provides some insight on the predicted effects of *PAH* alleles *in vivo*, but the limitations of the different assay systems and the differences between them must be recognized.[147] The latter include considerations of the particular host expression system (mammalian, bacterial, and cell-free systems), design of the vector (e.g., fusion or nonfusion protein products), assay method for catalytic activity (e.g., which pterin cofactor is used, with or without enzyme activation), and how the results are normalized (e.g., to transfection efficiency and mRNA expression level). All of these factors are taken into account when translating *in vitro* data into predictions and interpretations of *in vivo* phenotype. The predicted residual activity of PAH enzyme in a patient is taken to be the average of the *in vitro* activities for each allele in the mutant genotype.[149,224] Since correlations between predicted PAH activity and the observed phenotype are generally good, it is assumed that events such as allelic complementation are unusual in PKU. Thus, it seems that data from *in vitro* expression of homopolymeric mutant PAH in mammalian cells are quite robust and useful to predict and counsel for the corresponding metabolic phenotypes in patients.[224,301] But there are limitations to this comforting agreement.[147]

Estimates from *in vitro* expression analysis of mutation severity do not translate categorically into estimates of *in vivo* hepatic activities,[291] because enzymatic activities in the mammalian cell systems are, in general, higher than those measured in the latter,[277,279] and higher than the corresponding *in vivo* estimates, when allelic effects can be compared directly both *in vitro* and *in vivo*.[26] The major cause of the discrepancy appears to lie in transient overexpression of the *PAH* gene in these expression systems. Steady state levels of hepatic enzyme *in vivo* reflect the balance between synthesis and degradation. Synthesis from an unintegrated and unstable cDNA in the host cell differs from synthesis off the genomic *PAH* gene with its regulatory elements and physiological controls all intact, and the latter may differ in hepatic and cultured expression cells. In this regard, it seems wiser to use human cell lines for expression, such as the human embryonal kidney cell line A293 in place of monkey kidney (COS) cells. Other systems have specific advantages for particular applications: bacterial cells do not normally express PAH, but expression of the gene in a bacterial system enables production of larger amounts of PAH (and other proteins)[302] than is feasible in mammalian cell culture systems. Cell-free systems, such as the rabbit reticulocyte lysate system,[299] containing lysate, the cDNA vector, and T7 polymerase, allow selective and rapid synthesis of radiolabeled PAH protein at reasonable levels in a controlled environment. The enzyme produced in this system is functional and is produced as a mixture of tetramers and dimers with only minor amounts of aggregates.

In vitro expression analysis has also been used to study the effect of six *artificial* human *PAH* alleles (none has been found *in vivo*) on structure-function relationships of the enzyme[164,303] (search also on *PAHdb*). They are informative about conformational changes associated with the processes of PAH enzyme activation. Artificial W120F/I and W187F alleles decrease protein stability and increase aggregation. The K_m for phenylalanine in the presence of BH4 cofactor is increased by the W187F and W326F alleles but decreased by the W120I, W120F, C237S, and C237D alleles. Mutation of C237 leads to an increased activation state of the enzyme and some perturbation of its structure.[164]

At least 22 artificial alleles in the homologous rat gene have been used to analyze structure-function relationships in this, the best studied, species of mammalian PAH enzyme. Among the findings (search on *PAHdb* for details) was replacement of S16, normally a phosphorylation site for PAH, by anionic residues (E16 or D16); this constitutively activates the enzyme.[304] The P281L allele greatly increases the K_m value for substrate,[305] while various E286 alleles identify this residue as critical for pterin function.[306] Removal of the C-terminal domain of rat PAH reduces enzymic activity.[129] The artificial L448A mutation, which could disrupt a leucine zipper/coiled-coil domain, affects assembly of tetramers from dimers.[129] [Note: A human mutation in residue 447 (A447D) is disease-causing.[307]]

***"Virtual" Molecular Modeling* (In Silico).** A fourth approach to study the effects of *PAH* alleles on the protein product is now feasible and is referred to in the foregoing section on PAH enzyme. The crystal structures of the catalytic domain of human PAH enzyme (residues 118 to 424) and regulatory domain (N-terminal region) have been resolved at 2.0 Å and provide the first structural view of how mutations occurring in exons of the gene could affect protein integrity.[18,308–309b] PAH crystal structure shows that the enzyme crystallizes as a homotetramer with each monomer consisting of a catalytic domain and a tetramerization domain.[308] The latter functions as a domain-swapping arm that interacts with the other monomers to form an anti-parallel coiled-coil. At least 12 PKU-causing mutations affect the interface of catalytic and tetramerization domains. R408W, the most prevalent of all PKU-causing alleles, affects the highly conserved arginine position on the hinge loop connecting the tetramerization arm to the core of the monomer; R408 forms a hydrogen bond with the main chain carbamyl of L308, A309, and L311;[308] mutations affecting these residues all cause PKU.[14] Replacement of arginine 408 by tryptophan presumably disrupts alignment of the arms severely; replacement by glutamine would be less disruptive and the R408Q allele is indeed associated with milder forms of HPA in patients[25] and with considerable enzyme activity by *in vitro* expression analysis.[147]

Amino acid residues affected by missense *PAH* alleles can be mapped according to their distance from the essential iron atom, coordinating with H285, H290, and E330 residues.[18] [The human H285Y mutation causes PKU (J. Zschocke, personal communication, 1997; see *PAHdb*).] Modeling shows residues involved in pterin binding[309b] and mutations that modify the shape of the active site (e.g., P281L);[18] a salt bridge and an H-bond network are disrupted by the E280K mutation, which also affects ionic interaction with R158. Mutations (e.g., S349P and S349L) can be identified that alter chain folding near the active site or disrupt hydrogen bonding with the H285 residue and coordination with the Fe^{+3} ion. The A322T and A322G alleles produce non-PKU HPA by altering contacts between A322 in helix α9, and residue S251 in helix α6; residue L255 helps to define the shape of the active site and allele L255S produces the PKU phenotype. L255V, which only alters separation of helices α6 and α9, is associated with a milder phenotype *in vivo*. Although modeling of *PAH* mutants is still in its early stages, these developments should yield better understanding about mutation effects on protein structure, subunit interaction, and catalytic activity of PAH and analogous aromatic amino acid hydroxylases.[308–309a]

Effects of Mutation on Nonenzymic Phenotypes. Despite limitations in translating data from *in vitro* analysis of *PAH* alleles into the clinical equivalent, the overall correlations are reasonable between putative PAH enzyme activity *in vivo* and either the metabolic phenotype (plasma phenylalanine level, clearance after loading, and dietary tolerance)[67,149,224,290,310,311] or the IQ score attained in a patient.[24,312–314] Yet problematic and interesting deviations have been noted[36] in the observed phenotype, from that predicted, in untreated PKU patients.

Discordant correlations between genotype and (clinical) phenotype should not be a surprise, since they are everywhere apparent in patients with monogenic diseases.[315] Summers[316] illustrates this theme with examples from cystic fibrosis and the hemoglobinopathies, to which could be added examples from the corresponding chapters in this book, diseases such as Gaucher (Chap. 146), Marfan (Chap. 206), Hartnup (Chap. 193), low-density lipoprotein receptor deficiency (Chap. 120), and androgen receptor dysfunction (Chaps. 160 and 161). PKU is another example.

One can ask either of two questions and expect to be baffled by evidence: Can I predict phenotype from genotype? Can I predict genotype from phenotype? Interpretations of discrepancies tend to focus on possible modifiers of phenotype in single gene disorders; the modifiers include stochastic or environmental variation, and genetic factors. Among the latter may be allelic variation (in the same gene, so-called malleable genotypes) and postzygotic mutation. Modifier genes may produce their effects by direct interaction with the major gene, by modulating alternative pathways or parallel systems, or by more distant effects, all of which tend to shift our view from the simple Mendelian trait to the biologic reality that most phenotypes are in fact *complex traits*.[264a,316] In brief, no genetic disease is uninfluenced by other genes.[317] A careful study of phenotypes in PKU and non-PKU HPA will show that the same mutant genotype is not necessarily associated with an identical phenotype in different individuals.

Effect on IQ and Brain Function. Penrose[6] knew that untreated siblings with PKU could attain quite different levels of cognitive development. Discrepancy between a particular *PAH* genotype and a differential effect on the IQ score in different untreated PKU patients was "rediscovered" many years later and observed both within and between families[24,36,312–314,318] (Fig. 77-11). Since IQ must be one of the most complex of complex human traits, it is perhaps surprising that any correlation, even a weak one, between IQ score and genotype at the solitary *PAH* locus should be found.

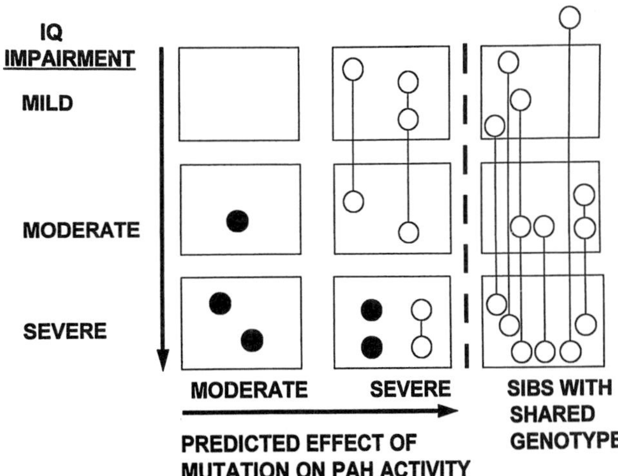

Fig. 77-11 IQ impairment classified as severe, moderate, or mild from IQ scores in untreated phenylketonuria (PKU) adults correlated with mutant human phenylalanine hydroxylase (*PAH*) genotypes predicted to have moderate or severe effect on hepatic *PAH* enzyme activity from the in vitro expression data. *Filled circles* are data for singletons. *Open circles with joining lines* are siblings. Mutation data for "sibs with shared genotype" are incomplete, and enzymic activity could not be predicted; these untreated PKU sibs with the same (unknown) genotype can have different cognitive phenotypes. (*Adapted from data by Ramus et al.*[24])

Yet there *is* broad concordance: *PAH* alleles with a "severe effect *in vitro*" are likely to cause PKU with low IQ scores in the untreated state, whereas mild *PAH* alleles are likely to cause non-PKU HPA with higher IQ scores. A correlation is also seen between predicted severity of an allele, the metabolic phenotype, and magnetic resonance imaging (MRI) findings in brain.[319] All this we know, and it implies that one mediator of the genotypic effect on cognitive development and brain function is likely to be the phenylalanine level itself in body fluids:[24] the level is higher in PKU than in non-PKU HPA. But more than the *PAH* genotype and its effect on the metabolic (phenylalanine) phenotype has to be taken into account.

Weglage et al[320] used *in vivo* nuclear magnetic resonance (NMR) spectroscopy to measure free phenylalanine concentrations in brain in four untreated adult patients with classical PKU (genotypes unknown), all with similar plasma phenylalanine values (1200 to 1500 μM). Two patients were retarded and had severe brain myelin (MRI) abnormalities, whereas two patients had normal IQ scores and minimal myelin abnormalities. The former (low IQ) pair had high brain phenylalanine levels (650 and 670 μM), whereas the latter (normal IQ) pair had brain phenylalanine levels below detectability. In a second study[321] using similar analytic techniques, the same group evaluated two siblings with the homoallelic R408W genotype, poor treatment compliance, similar high blood phenylalanine levels (yet different WAIS-R IQ scores (90 and 77)), and different degrees of brain white matter change (detected by MRI). The sib with the higher IQ and less severe MRI signs accumulated less phenylalanine in brain and cleared it faster over 40 h after a standard load test than did the sib with the more severe phenotype. A third study[321a] in 11 typical PKU patients and three untreated adult PKU patients with normal intelligence corroborated the findings under both static and kinetic conditions, and these important observations are further corroborated by independent observations.[321b] The findings imply that interindividual variation in brain phenylalanine transport is another factor to explain interindividual differences in IQ scores in PKU.[320] Phenylalanine transport from blood to brain is a mediated and complex process (see the section "Pathogenesis: Metabolic Phenotypes and Neurotoxicity"). A transport component from blood across the hepatic cell plasma membrane has elsewhere been shown to be a significant component in whole-body phenylalanine homeostasis.[48] Transporter genes, like enzyme genes, are subject to allelic variation. Perhaps (polymorphic) allelic variation in a brain phenylalanine transporter is a modifier of PKU-causing *PAH* genotypes. The in vivo NMR observations[320–321b] are preliminary, but their importance is obvious and they must be confirmed.

Effect on Phenylalanine Homeostasis. One of the early analyses of correlations between mental and biochemical phenotypes in untreated PKU[36] suggested that *modifiers* must be involved to explain a discordant genotype-phenotype relationship. Treacy et al[53] have since been able to demonstrate by isotope tracer analysis in two siblings with PKU of known mutant *PAH* genotype [R408W + I65T] that significant differences in metabolic runout of phenylalanine, to form the minor metabolites (pathway 3B, Fig. 77-2), could account for consistent and significant differences in dietary phenylalanine tolerances.

Treacy et al then analyzed phenylalanine hydroxylation rates in vivo in patients with different clinical forms of HPA.[26] They showed broad correlations between mutant genotypes of predicted severe, intermediate, or mild effect and the corresponding metabolic phenotype, but again there was discordance in the correlations among some individuals. This led to the conclusion that whereas phenylalanine oxidation *in vivo* is largely under the control of the *PAH* locus, this being evident in the gene dose effect on phenylalanine oxidation in controls, obligate heterozygotes, and propositi, and oxidation by the hydroxylase pathway is the major component in phenylalanine homeostasis, yet the homeostasis value cannot be explained solely by hepatic hydroxylating activity. Accordingly, as expected of an important biochemical and physiological process, whole-body phenylalanine homeostasis has features of a complex quantitative trait,[26] with the feature known as an *emergent property*.[322]

Discordance between predicted PAH activity and oxidation rates *in vivo* may also reflect interactions between different species of mutant PAH subunits. Until data are available from a yeast two-hybrid system for *in vitro* expression, present results all reflect the effect of only one mutant allele on PAH activity, because the mutant enzyme in current expression systems[147] is always *homoallelic*. Most PKU patients in outbred populations are not homoallelic in mutant genotype: about three-quarters of PKU propositi are heteroallelic as shown in many different studies,[307,323–325] and the corresponding values (*j*) for homozygosity are low in a wide range of human populations harboring PKU-causing alleles (see the section "Population Genetics of PKU and *PAH* Alleles"). It follows that phenotypes need to be correlated with genotypes in the patients themselves rather than by prediction from *in vitro* expression analysis.

Interindividual phenotypic variation within a family is sometimes explained by an unusual degree of allelic variation within the family. There are families in which three different *PAH* alleles, instead of two, segregate to cause different forms of HPA within the family.[326–329] Another way in which an extended range of allelic variation at the *PAH* locus could modulate expression of the major disease-causing allele would be through interaction between polymorphic and disease-causing alleles. No examples of such interactions are known so far. Yet another mechanism of phenotype modulation exists when a second allele in *cis* alters expression of the first. A classic example exists in galactosemia (see Chap. 72 transferase-deficient type) where the E203K allele in *cis* neutralizes expression of the Duarte allele (N314D).[329a] Several examples are now known of two alleles occurring in *cis* on a PAH *gene* (C. Aulehla-Scholtz, personal communication, 1998; see also *PAHdb*), but their effect on the HPA has not been examined in detail yet.

Genotype-Based Prediction of Phenotype: Large Studies. A meta-analysis of 31 reports on 365 patients expressing 73 different PAH mutations (44 missense and 29 null) in 161 different mutant genotypes has revealed a number of examples of discordant relationships.[25] To avoid any difficulty in classifying a *PAH* allele as severe, intermediate, or mild, when the genotype is heteroallelic for two different missense alleles, the authors restricted their analysis to individuals in whom the genotype was either homoallelic or *functionally hemizygous*, a term suggested for a *PAH* genotype comprising a missense allele paired with a null;[290,324] 109 homoallelic patients (29 different genotypes) and 181 patients with functionally hemizygous genotypes harboring 34 different missense alleles were analyzed. The majority (37 of 48) of the classifiable genotypes conferred a consistent *in vivo* phenotype classifiable by conventional criteria[20,21] as severe (PKU), intermediate (variant PKU), or mild (non-PKU HPA). However, 11 *PAH* alleles conferred inconsistent phenotypes in two or more patients: G46S, L48S, R158Q, R261Q, and V388M were associated with both PKU and variant PKU; E390G, A403V, and R408Q were associated with variant PKU and non-PKU HPA; the A300S allele was associated with both of the outlier classes (PKU and non-PKU HPA); and I65T and Y414C were found in all three phenotype classes.

A second large study of genotype-phenotype relationships[330] supports, in broad terms, the findings in the first. The second study was based on data from seven European centers and 686 patients, and capitalized on 297 functionally hemizygous genotypes. The authors classified the PAH enzyme-dependent metabolic phenotype into four categories (Kayaalp et al[25] settled for three)—classical PKU, moderate PKU, mild PKU, and non-PKU HPA—using dietary phenylalanine tolerance at 2 to 5 years of age and pretreatment blood phenylalanine levels to classify 105 different *PAH* alleles and found full concordance between the predicted and

Table 77-2 Inconsistent Genotype-Phenotype Correlations in Patients with Homoallelic and Functionally Hemizygous Genotypes

Allele	Genotype State	Number of Patients Clasified as*		
		PKU	Variant PKU	Non-PKU HPA
165T	Homoallelic	1	1	1
	FH	4	3	1
R261Q	Homoallelic	3	8	
	FH	6	3	
Y414C	Homoallelic	—	4	4
	FH	6	4	6

*Clinical classification by conventional criteria.[20,21]

ABBREVIATIONS: FH, functionally hemizygous; HPA, hyperphenylalaninemia; PKU, phenylketonuria.

Adapted from Kayaalp et al.[25]

observed phenotype in 184 patients who were not functionally hemizygous but were homoallelic or heteroallelic for mutations with an assigned severity of effect. Inconsistencies between the predicted phenotype and the observed phenotype were observed in 88 patients at rates varying from 4 to 25 percent between the seven centers; rather than attribute this to *modifier genetic effects*, the authors reasonably suggest that intercenter discrepancies in phenotype classification are a more likely source. Nonetheless, several alleles (notably L48S, I65T, R158Q, R261Q, and Y414C), whose effects were not explained by genotypic or phenotypic misclassification, were associated with more than one phenotype in the European multicenter study, and all five alleles were included by Kayaalp et al in their set of alleles with ambiguous expression.[25] Details for three of these alleles are shown in Table 77-2.

The two studies covering over 1000 patients both support similar conclusions: (1) *PAH* genotype classification is broadly predictive of metabolic (and clinical) phenotype and therefore useful for counseling and treatment, and (2) a small subset of ambiguities highlight the fact that HPA due to PAH enzyme deficiency involves more than simple predictable *PAH* allele expression (i.e., a *single gene* effect).

Mutation Effects in Heterozygotes: Significance for Classification

Identification of a heterozygote carrying a disease-causing *PAH* allele has long been a challenge (see the section "Diagnosis of Heterozygotes"). This is the case because the phenotypic effect of a single mutant *PAH* allele on phenylalanine homeostasis is recessive, as predicted[28] and observed (Fig. 77-12). Nonetheless, to discern whether predicted severity of a *PAH* allele is reflected in a corresponding metabolic phenotype continues to attract attention. A subject, identified by newborn screening, had persistent non-PKU HPA (less than 325 μM); studies later in life revealed euphenylalaninemia and identified "heterozygosity" by DNA analysis (IVS9nt6t → /+); another allele was not recognized, and the unusual circumstance of heterozygosity with neonatal hyperphenylalaninemia was declared.[331]

Several studies have examined the metabolic phenotype in obligate heterozygotes, attempting to find a genotype-phenotype correlation. Overnight fasting followed by an oral phenylalanine load (100 mg/kg) segregated heterozygotes as a group with varying degrees of efficiency[332] according to the fasting plasma phenylalanine value, the postload plasma clearance of phenylalanine, and the postload rise in tyrosine, but there was no correlation in any of the metrical parameters with the predicted severity of the *PAH* allele.[332]

In an earlier study, a discriminate function of plasma amino values for phenylalanine and tyrosine (the dependent variable), related to in vitro expression activity of the *PAH* allele (the independent variable), did yield a significant correlation ($r = 0.40$, $n = 140$, $p < 0.001$).[333] In another study,[26] a measure of *in vivo* hydroxylating activity, using $^{13}CO_2$ excretion after ingestion of labeled phenylalanine, revealed a gene dose effect in heterozygotes as a group (Figs. 77-9 and 77-12); however, considerable interindividual variation was found among different heterozygotes expressing the same mutant allele (Fig. 77-9). The latter finding makes it no easier than it was to classify a heterozygote by this new measure of phenotype. Heterozygosity is still classified just as well by a simple plasma amino acid algorithm[26] and best by DNA analysis.

POPULATION GENETICS OF PHENYLKETONURIA AND PATHOGENIC *PAH* ALLELES

Comment. Universal newborn screening for PKU finds individuals with HPA, and a reliable incidence for the screened population can thus be calculated. Because screening covers many different human societies worldwide, it enables wide sampling of human genetic variation at the *PAH* locus. The corresponding variation in nucleotide composition can be detected by several methods of DNA analysis.

Character of the *PAH* Locus

The locus is rich in allelic variation, both polymorphic in its biallelic and multiallelic forms (Figs. 77-6 and 77-7) and in a large number of less prevalent disease-causing alleles (Fig. 77-8). This autosomal locus behaves as a single 100-kb block of DNA in *Homo sapiens sapiens* and, having been sampled many thousand times, its information complements that gained from the analysis of haploid mitochondrial and Y-chromosomal DNA[334] and from classical protein polymorphisms.[335,336] From the classical studies, a mosaic human genetic geography has emerged that reflects demic expansion and human evolution during the past 100,000 years.[335,337,338] *PAH* alleles can be viewed as a unique set of biologic memories connecting individuals, families, and communities who share the contingent histories that are echoes of the past. The historical and social accidents of migration, genetic drift, gene flow, assortative mating (endogamy, inbreeding), and recurrent mutation, alone or together, with or without selection by heterozygote advantage, have contributed to the frequencies and distributions of *PAH* alleles seen in modern human populations.[261]

Polymorphic *PAH* haplotypes are used to analyze human evolution.[252,257,257a] They also show particular associations between the haplotype and a pathogenic allele[224] (see polymorphisms in

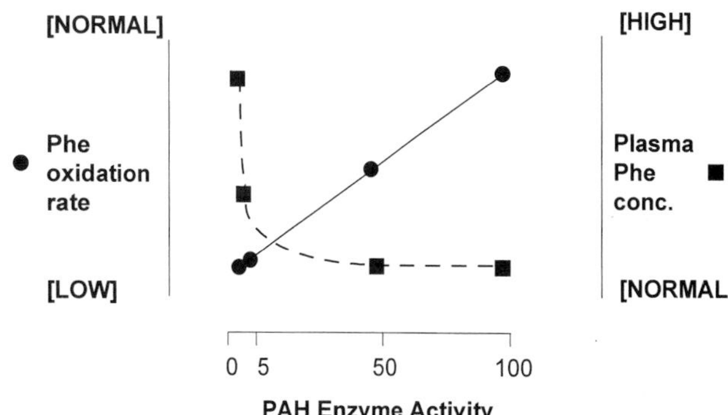

Fig. 77-12 A stylized summary of evidence for (1) the recessive nature of the plasma amino acid phenotype in the phenylalanine hydroxylase (PAH)-deficient hyperphenylalaninemias (plasma phenylalanine values, *right ordinate*), and (2) gene-dosage effect on the rate of hydroxylase-dependent oxidation of phenylalanine in vivo from $^{13}CO_2$ in expired air (*left ordinate*). Original data in Rosenblatt and Scriver[421] and Treacy et al[26] (*From Scriver.[27] Used by permission of the American Society for Clinical Investigation.*)

the section "The *PAH* Gene"). The following text focuses on the rare pathogenic alleles as causes of HPA and what they offer to human population genetics.

Hyperphenylalaninemia: A Special Opportunity in Human Population Genetics

The HPAs offer both advantages and limitations for the study of mechanisms by which pathogenic alleles achieve their particular frequencies and distributions in human populations.

Advantages. (1) Frequencies and classifications of HPA are being systematically documented through newborn-screening programs (Table 77-3). (2) The molecular basis of *PAH* allelic diversity is being determined by DNA analysis[339–341] notably by a very efficient use of PCR amplification, denaturing gradient gel electrophoresis, and direct sequence analysis.[342,343] (3) Associations between prevalent disease-causing mutations and polymorphic haplotype backgrounds are being recognized. (4) Alleles and their associations with haplotypes, populations, and phenotypes are being documented systematically in a relational mutation database (*PAHdb*).[14]

Limitations. (1) Alleles are identified mainly through affected propositi, rarely otherwise, thus introducing a bias of sampling. (2) Populations are sampled mainly through screening programs that are not operative in all human societies and populations; again there is a bias of sampling. (3) Mutation characterization is feasible in only about 3 percent of the whole *PAH* gene. (4) Analysis of population-specific mutant chromosomes is rarely 100 percent efficient (although it often exceeds 95 percent): allele frequencies are relative, rarely absolute, for the selected sample, and they are not true estimates of population frequencies. (5) Parental alleles are not uniformly analyzed (and reported) and *de novo* mutations are likely to be underestimated.

Implications in Nonuniform Incidence Rates

Penrose speculated on the apparently elevated frequency of this harmful autosomal recessive disease in Europeans:[6] he offered several explanations, including consanguinity, hypermutability, and selective advantage of heterozygotes. Nor did the nonuniform distribution of PKU cases in European populations escape his notice. It was never a dry season in Penrose's fertile mind.

Newborn screening provides data to corroborate Penrose's view of incidence and allelic frequency. Assuming Hardy-Weinberg equilibrium, incidence rates reveal an aggregate frequency for pathogenic alleles (both PKU and non-PKU HPA) in the *polymorphic* range in certain populations; having been collected from many different populations, incidence rates also show nonuniform distribution of PKU, more so than for non-PKU HPA (Table 77-3).

Table 77-3 Incidence of Hyperphenylalaninemia Phenotypes by Population: Examples

Phenotype	Association	Incidence (cases/million births)	References*
Phenylketonuria (PKU)	In "Oriental" populations		
	China	60	834, 835, 836
	Japan	8	837, 838
	In "European" populations		
	Turkey	385	344
	Yemenite Jews (in Israel)	190	371
	Scotland	190	
	Czechoslovakia	150	
	Hungary	90	
	Denmark	85	
	France	75	
	Norway	70	
	United Kingdom	70	
	Italy	60	
	Canada	45‡	605
	Finland	5	
	In "Arabic" populations	Up to 165§	334
Non-PKU hyperphenylalaninemia	In "Oriental" populations		
	Japan	4	357, 838
	In "Europeans" (except Finland)	15–75	562, 605, 839
	In "Arabic" populations	"Low"	334

*Newborn screening is the direct source for incidence data.[562,605,835,839,840] Incidence has also been estimated indirectly from consanguinity rates in Norway[348] and in Italy.[349]
†Data were also taken from Woolf and Lentner.[840a]
‡Data are the average of eight provincial screening programs in Canada with an annual cohort of approximately 400,000 births. [605]
§Reviewed in Teebi and Farag,[334] covering Arabic populations (including Bedouins) in Eqypt, Jordan, Iraq, Kuwait, Lebanon, the Maghreb (North Africa), and Palestine/Israel and Sudan. (The data also cover Jewish populations in Arab nations, including Morocco, Tunisia, and Yemen.)

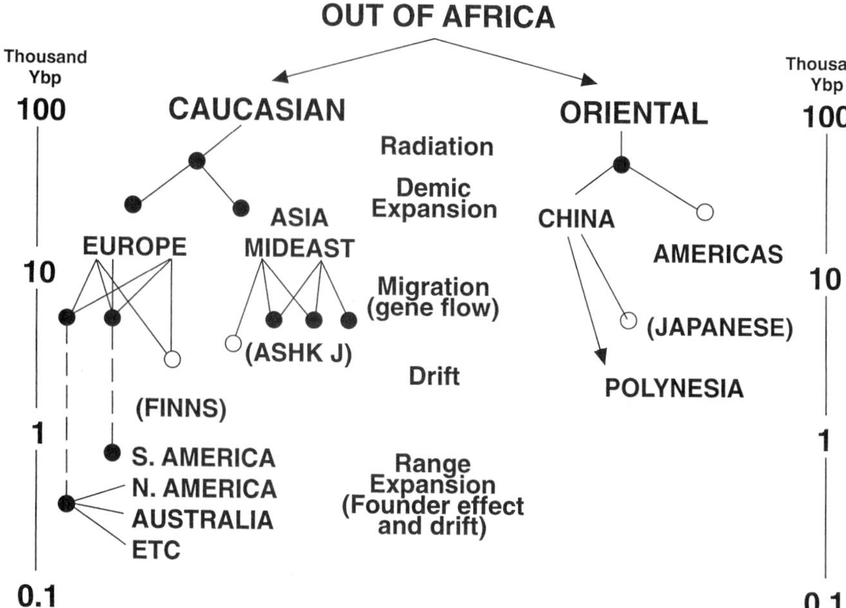

Fig. 77-13 Human history hypothesized from the viewpoint of allelic diversity at the human phenylalanine hydroxylase (*PAH*) gene locus. Following an "out of Africa" migration and divergence, different sets of phenylketonuria (PKU)-causing alleles arose in Europeans (Caucasians) and Asian Orientals and were acted on by genetic drift. Founder effect is the likely explanation for relative rarity of PKU alleles in American aboriginals, Japanese, Ashkenazi, and Finnish populations (also in Polynesians). Demic expansion, migrations, and gene flow disrupt "trees of descent" in pre- and post-Neolithic eras (10,000 ybp). Range expansion and creation of neo-European populations overseas (from 1000 ybp) explain the "overseas" distributions from European sources of certain *PAH* alleles.

The possibility that inbreeding could explain the high incidence of PKU is likely in Turkey[344–346] and has been confirmed by formal analysis in the Pakistani community in the West Midlands of the United Kingdom[347] and in Arabic countries for PKU,[334] but it is not a satisfactory explanation for the (lesser) incidence of PKU in either Norway[348] or Italy.[349] The Italian study showed further, even before the human *PAH* gene had been cloned, that PKU is the result of mutation at only one locus and locus heterogeneity need not be taken into account to explain the elevated incidence of such a severe disease as untreated PKU, an interpretation that has proved to be realistic, since only about 2 percent of propositi with HPA are not explained by mutations at the *PAH* locus (see Chap. 78).

Implications in Nonuniform Allelic Distributions

The *PAH* locus of *Homo sapiens sapiens* has accumulated an impressive array of alleles, each different by state and identity (Figs. 77-6 and 77-8), during demic expansion over the past 100,000 years (see also Fig. 77-13). Among the disease-causing *PAH* mutations, only a few (between four and six in most populations) make up a majority of the total (Table 77-4), and this pattern is emerging as the norm for most pathogenic alleles in human genes.[29]

Distribution of disease-causing *PAH* mutations by race is not uniform. Such alleles are almost invisible in Africans (see Beighton, p. 90, of Scriver et al[261]), and there are different sets of the prevalent alleles in Europeans (Caucasians) and Orientals (Table 77-4). Although sampling of PKU alleles in Africans, in Africa, has only been very modest and almost incidental, the findings in African descendants living in the United States[307,350] and the United Kingdom,[351] where screening occurs, show a dearth of "African" *PAH* mutations, implying that the disease-causing mutations might not have originated in Africa (an hypothesis).

Table 77-4 Relative Frequency Distributions (%) of the Most Prevalent Disease-Causing *PAH* Alleles in Europeans and Orientals

Rank Order	European (n = 3630)*	%	Oriental (n = 210)*	%
1	R408W	31	R243Q	13
2	IVS12nt1	11	R413P	13
3	IVS10nt-11	10	E6nt-96 (Y204C)	13
4	I65T	5	IVS4nt-1	7
5	Y414C	5	R111X	7
6	R261Q	4	Y356X	5
7	Others	38	Others	44

*n is the denominator of all independent chromosomes analyzed.

SOURCE: Adapted from Eisensmith and Woo,[224] and original data from *PAHdb* (reference 14).

Sampling has not been as extensive in Orientals as in Europeans, but the Oriental data are sufficient[352–358] to show, first, that incidence of PKU is similar among Orientals (in mainland Asia) and in Europeans (Table 77-3), but much lower in the Japanese;[353,357] second, that the alleles among Orientals as a group are quite different from those in Europeans, and different again between Japanese and other Orientals[353,357,359,360] (Table 77-5). The Japanese data are compatible with genetic drift in the founding of this island population. The differences in *PAH* allelic distribution among Europeans and Orientals overall, and the deficiency of "African" alleles, suggest that *PAH* mutations entered the human genome after migration out of Africa and persisted following divergence (radiation) to form Caucasian and Oriental populations (as suggested in Fig. 77-13).

At one time, PKU was said to be rare in Arabic populations but, when searched for, it has been found widely,[334,361] and the mutations are often particular to Arabic chromosomes.[362–365] In Kuwait, incidence is 1 in 6500 for PKU and 1 in 20,000 for non-PKU HPA.[366] Likewise, the supposedly low incidence of PKU in Pakistan and India may reflect bias of ascertainment more than absence of alleles: PKU does occur there; unusual alleles, both deletion[264] and missense,[367] are found in propositi from the Asian subcontinent; and when a Pakistani population is accessed by newborn screening, the incidence of PKU is 1 in 14,500 (equivalent to the corresponding European cohort in the United Kingdom), but, because of consanguinity in the Pakistani community, the *PKU gene frequency* is lower (1 in 713) compared with the European cohort (1 in 112).[347]

Extensive allelic diversity in the *PAH* gene implies something else. In the majority of contemporary populations where PKU is found, random mating appears to be the norm. Therefore, homoallelic mutant *PAH* genotypes should be in the minority, a hypothesis that can be tested in two ways: first, by enumeration of homoallelic mutant genotypes and, second, by the use of pathogenic *PAH* alleles to measure homozygosity (j) at the

Table 77-5 Expected Homozygosity at the *PAH* Locus in Patients with Phenylketonuria (a Measure of Allelic Heterogeneity in Human Populations and Geographic Regions)

Population/Region	*J**	*N*†	Mutation Detection Rate (%)	References
Yemenite Jews	1.0	44	100	371
Southern Poland	0.44	80	91.3	679
Iceland	0.26	34	100	386
Tataria	0.19	27	100	375
Denmark	0.17	378	98.4	301, 376¶
Northern Ireland	0.14	242	99.6	323
Australia (Victoria)	0.11	83	97.6	387
Norway	0.10	236	99.6	841, 842
Netherlands	0.08	68	92.6	383
Germany	0.06	90	95.6	384¶
Quebec	0.06‡	142	96.5	325¶
United States	0.06§	294	94.9	307
Sicily	0.06	106	98.1	377

*$j = \Sigma x_i^2$ where x_i is relative frequency of each allele different by state and identity; when analysis of state was not 100%, the uncharacterized alleles are given the aggregate frequency 1/N.
†*N* number of chromosomes available.
‡Variation in *j* by population and geographic subregion in Quebec was 0.05 to 0.08.[325]
§Variation in *j* by region in the United States was 0.05 to 0.10.[307]
¶Includes unpublished data from source.

PAH locus. The enumeration is possible by use of the locus-specific mutation database (*PAHdb*): it contains data on 493 Europeans with HPA genotypes; only 28 percent of the propositi are homoallelic *PAH* mutants. *PAH* homozygosity has been measured directly in a wide range of political and ethnic groups (Table 77-5): only one (Yemenite Jews) shows high homozygosity for pathogenic alleles (due to a major founder effect), whereas the majority show low homozygosity. Where consanguineous mating is a convention, as in Muslim populations,[334] one anticipates evidence of higher homozygosity for pathogenic *PAH* alleles.

Centers of Diffusion and Gene Flow

Demic expansion and migration, in both Europe and Asia[335] (as implied in Fig. 77-13), are likely ways that *PAH* alleles spread through human populations. Distinctive geographic distributions with interpopulation variation for the most prevalent *PAH* mutations (Table 77-6) imply they had origins in multiple centers of diffusion in Europeans[368] and Orientals.[369,370] Assuming that relative frequencies of pathogenic alleles will shed light on their *absolute frequencies* where newborn screening is the norm and that frequency clines can be implied, the corresponding maps have been created indicating centers of diffusion for several *PAH* alleles.[224] The data further imply genetic drift in comparative isolation at the time the centers of diffusion developed, an hypothesis compatible with other measures of human genetic diversity.[337]

Table 77-6 Major Geographic Distributions of Prevalent (Phenylketonuria) Pathogenic *PAH* Mutations

In Europe		In the Orient	
Region	**Allele [haplotype]***	**Region**	**Allele**
Northwest	R408W [H1]	North China	R243Q
North	IVS12nt1[H3]	South China	IVS4nt-1
Northeast and east	R408W [H2]	South Korea	IVS4nt-1 E6nt-96 (Y204C)
Southeast	IVS10nt–11 [H6]		
Southwest and west	I65T [H9]	Japan	R413P

*Haplotypes are named according to Eisensmith and Woo.[843]
Data taken from *PAHdb*[14] and Eisensmith and Woo.[224]

Genetic Drift. The pathogenic *PAH* alleles are useful records of the "dance to the music of time" that molds human societies. The extent of their variation ranges between extremes: at one end of the spectrum are strong effects of drift on *PAH* alleles, as illustrated by one unique (deletion) allele in Yemenite Jews living in Israel,[371] and the less extreme example of two solitary alleles in European Gypsies (IVS10nt-11 on haplotype 34 and R252W haplotype unspecified).[372–374] At the other end is a loss of rare alleles by negative founder effect illustrated by Finns, Ashkenazi Jews, and Japanese, among whom PKU is a very rare disorder, in contrast to its higher frequency in geographic neighbors and parent populations (Table 77-3). In between these extremes, there is the allelic turbulence one expects to find when long-established populations have intermingled.

Migration. The allelic composition of the *PAH* gene among PKU patients in the non-Slavic population of Tataria,[375] a region in the former USSR, reveals mutations that could have been introduced by conquest and movement along trade routes: from Eastern Europe (the R408W mutation on haplotype 2), from Turkic populations (the IVS10nt-11 mutation on haplotype 6), and from Scandinavia (IVS12nt1 and a particular frameshift allele, the latter otherwise found only in Scandinavians). No Oriental mutations are found in Tatarian PKU patients. Together the findings at the *PAH* locus imply that this population was formed mainly by people from Caucasian rather than Oriental background, a hypothesis yet to be tested by analysis of other nuclear genes and mitochondrial DNA.

The different patterns of allelic diversity among HPA patients in Denmark[301,376] and in Sicily[377] reflect the different political and linguistic histories of the regions. Denmark and Sicily are physically distant from each other, and any historical mingling of gametes would likely be the result of extraordinary events in the formation of those populations. Within Italy itself, there is a significant difference in the composition of *PAH* alleles in PKU patients from the northern and southern regions of the country:[378,379] the distribution of alleles in Italy apparently reflects the different demographic and cultural histories of the northern and southern regions.

Examples compatible with the effects of migration are seen in outlier regions, such as the British Isles[351,380] and the Iberian Peninsula.[381] Alleles identified in these two regions have the attributes of having arrived there in people who came from elsewhere in Europe.

Complex "untree-like" allelic diversity, represented by both prevalent and rare *PAH* alleles, is seen in Denmark,[376] France,[382] the Netherlands,[383] and Germany,[384] for example, and it complements evidence derived from analysis of classical polymorphisms.[336] Most European populations have not evolved according to simple "trees" of descent but are "networks" of lineages reflecting historical migration and intermingling. (For more information on allelic profiles in different political and geographic regions, readers are encouraged to search the *PAH* mutation database.)

Range Expansion

PAH mutations make particularly evocative records of range expansion by neo-Europeans[385] from countries of origin to island populations, the Americas, and Australasia, for example (Fig. 77-13). The evidence lies in studies from Iceland,[386]

Australia (Victoria State),[387] the United States,[307] Quebec Province in Canada,[325] Mexico,[388] Costa Rica,[389] and parts of South America.[390,391] Range expansions over the past half-millennium were usually initiated by small numbers of individuals and, when colonization was successful, demic expansion by natural increase would follow, with or without new immigration. These are the conditions under which recent founder effects could still be manifest, and the *PAH* locus again offers examples: (1) The M1V allele, prevalent in Quebec[325] and rare in France,[382] has narrow time and space clusters for its origin in France and entry into New France;[392] its distribution in Quebec today clearly reflects the history of its French Canadians.[325] (2) The Y377fsdelT mutation in Iceland accounts for 40 percent of mutant *PAH* alleles there.[386] The mutation is associated with RFLP haplotype 4, VNTR 3, and STR234. Genealogical reconstruction for five generations in families harboring the mutation identifies ancestors from an isolated part of Southern Iceland, and the mutation has not been seen on any European chromosomes outside Iceland. Since the tetranucleotide STR locus is a "fast" molecular clock,[393] the presence of only one STR allele in the *PAH* haplotype bearing Y377fsdelT is compatible with a "recent" origin for the pathogenic mutation, but other considerations may refute that hypothesis.[394] Other *PAH* mutations occur in Iceland, notably several Scandinavian alleles, including F299C, none of which incidentally is prevalent in either Ireland or Scotland. Along with historical and linguistic evidence, genetic evidence indicates that the Icelandic population is predominantly of Scandinavian origin, with little contribution from the British Isles (as once proposed). (3) Mariners from the Iberian Peninsula discovered South America, and colonization by their followers apparently introduced two *PAH* alleles (IVS10nt-11 and V388M), both prevalent in the Iberian Peninsula[381,395] and now accounting for 5 to 30 percent of *PAH* mutations in South American populations.[390,391,396]

Range expansion did not necessarily result in greater homozygosity for the rare pathogenic alleles in the descendant populations (Table 77-5), and Quebec is an illuminating example in this respect.[325] *PAH* homozygosity (pathogenic alleles) in Quebec overall is low ($j = 0.06$) and is not significantly higher in the linguistic and cultural subsets of the population in Eastern and Western Quebec and in Montreal. Groups of settlers from France before 1759, from the British Isles and Ireland after 1759, and from Eastern Europe and Mediterranean nations after 1945 have each introduced different and identifiable *PAH* alleles into the population,[325] of which the geographic and demographic distributions in the province reflect the histories of the different communities that make up Quebec today.

Molecular Mechanisms Introducing Novel *PAH* Alleles and Haplotype Associations

Penrose suggested *recurrent mutation* as a possible explanation for the frequency of PKU in European populations.[6] The hypothesis might be rephrased to ask: Is the PAH gene *hypermutable*?

***De Novo* Mutations.** At least one *de novo PAH* allele (M1I) has been reported[397] on over 12,000 independent mutant PAH chromosomes. The sampling of biologic parents of PKU propositi is incomplete, however, and the true rate of *de novo PAH* mutation is not known. Whatever the case, $\mu = Sq^2$ must be a small value for pathogenic *PAH* mutations.

Recurrent Mutation. A predicted mutability profile exists for the cDNA sequence of *PAH* (Fig. 77-14). The majority of the *predicted hypermutable* regions coincide with the 24 CpG dinucleotide sites in the gene.[398] CpG sites are 40 times more mutable than any other dinucleotide sequences,[237,399] and they can experience C → T or G → A transition mutations during deamination of 5′ methylcytosine (see Chap. 13). For this to occur, it is assumed that cytosine in the dinucleotide was methylated, a hypothesis tested and confirmed by analysis of a CpG-type mutation in the *PAH* gene, (Singh S. and Scriver CR, unpublished data, 2000) Among the pathogenic *PAH* mutations, CR at least 23 are known to be CpG-type alleles;[398] another 8 occur at CpG sites but are not C → T or G → A transitions, and seven regions containing CpG sites have no reported mutations in the *PAH* gene (Fig. 77-14).

The following illustrates putative recurrent mutation in the *PAH* gene. Ramus et al[400] identified two different mutations in codon 408 of the gene: R408W (c.1222C → T) and R408Q (c.1223G → A). They proposed that codon 408 is a mutational "hotspot." Their observation followed upon an earlier report[401] stating that the identical R408W mutation (c.1222C → T) occurred on two different RFLP haplotypes in the Quebec population: one allele was on "conventional" haplotype 2, and the other was on "novel" haplotype 1; recurrence, gene conversion, or a single intragenic recombination were all compatible with this event.[401] Genealogical reconstructions in the families in which R408W was segregating on haplotype 1 in the Quebec population repeatedly included Celtic ancestors from Scotland and Ireland.[402] It was proposed that a search for this particular allele in European populations would find a center of diffusion in Northwest Europe, different from the center of diffusion for the R408W on haplotype 2 and compatible with a recurrent mutational event.[402] The hypothesis was tested by haplotype analysis of over 1200 European chromosomes harboring the R408W mutation.[403] Those carrying haplotype 1 were most prevalent and clustered on the northwest fringes of Europe, whereas those carrying haplotype 2 clustered in Eastern Europe.[403] By analyzing the flanking 5′ STR alleles and by sequencing the 3′ VNTR markers of normal and mutant chromosomes, Byck et al[404] had already produced the molecular evidence compatible with recurrence as the likely mechanism for appearance of the CpG-type R408W mutation on two different haplotypes in two different European populations.

The human R408W mutation is actually found on seven different haplotype backgrounds. Although the mechanism of recurrence has been supported by molecular evidence in only the one study,[404] from analysis of the associated haplotype configurations, it seems likely that recurrent mutation is the source of R408W on haplotype 5 in Europeans (references 405–408 and L. Kozak to *PAHdb*) and on haplotype 44 in Orientals[409] (Fig. 77-15). On the other hand, the R408W mutation on haplotype 41 in Europeans[410] and Orientals,[411] on haplotype 34 in Portuguese patients,[412] and on haplotype 27 in a Belgian patient (L. Michiels to *PAHdb*) can be explained, in each case, either by mutation (or gene conversion) at a single RFLP site or by an intragenic recombination, in which case the R408W mutation is identical by descent (Fig. 77-15).

The E280K allele occurs on haplotypes 1 and 2, a finding compatible with recurrence.[413] The molecular evidence to support this hypothesis, obtained by analyzing nucleotide sequences flanking the CpG-type c.838G → A (E280K) allele, supports a recurrent mutational process.[398]

Intragenic Recombination. *PAH* alleles are useful markers in evidence of a classic mechanism by which evolution has generated genomic diversity: genetic recombination.[414] R408W mutations are not the only ones that appear to have changed haplotype by intragenic recombination. S76P alleles on haplotypes 1 and 4, G218W on haplotypes 2 and 1, and V245A on haplotypes 7 and 3 have all been identified on chromosomes in Europeans and in their descendants abroad; in each case, a single recombination within the *PAH* gene can explain the association of one mutation with two haplotypes.[325] An IVS12nt1 allele, found almost exclusively on haplotype 3, has been found once on a foreign haplotype; this event is explained by a double intragenic recombination.[325]

Multiple associations between a pathogenic *PAH* allele at a non-CpG site and a polymorphic haplotype have been identified in the case of the prevalent (and ancient) IVS10nt-11 splice allele.

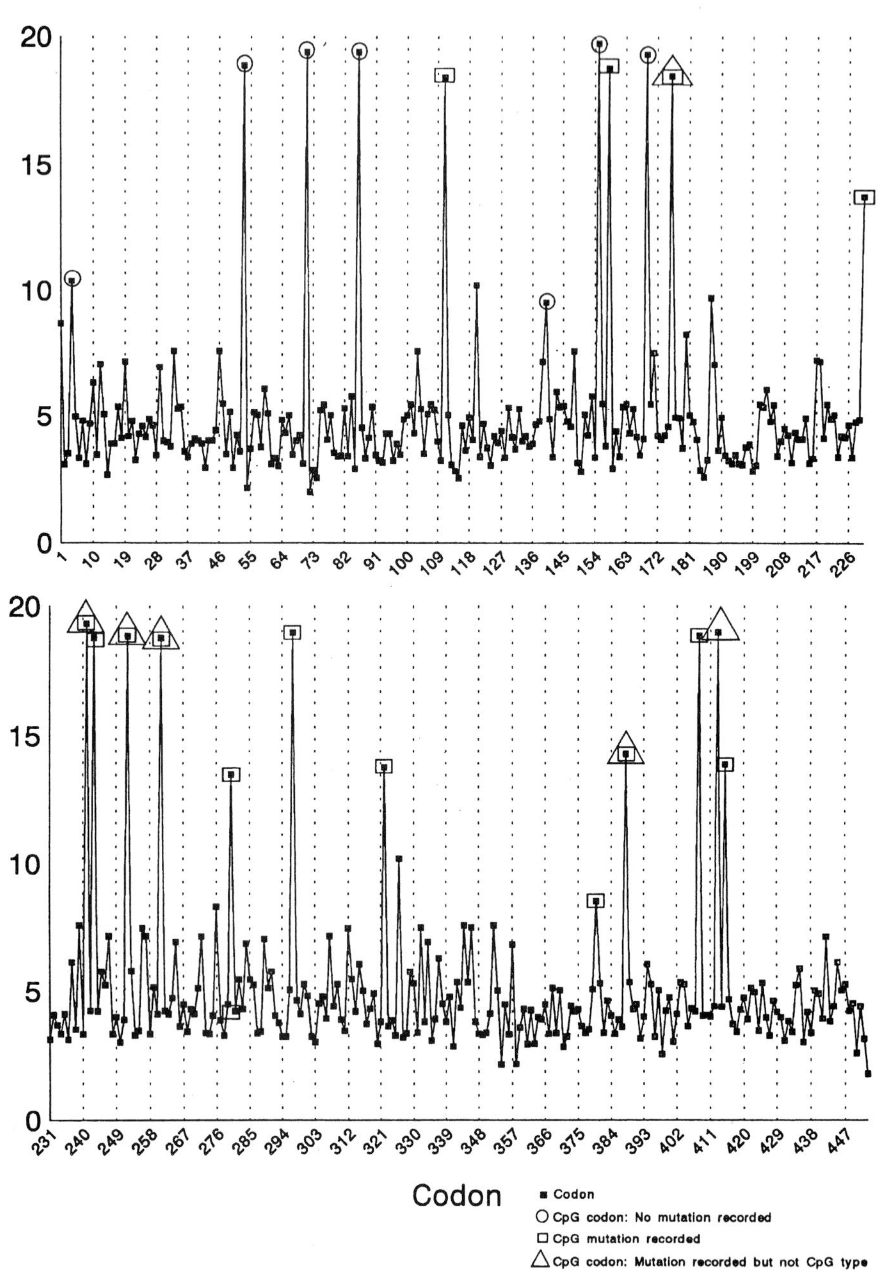

Fig. 77-14 The mutability profile for the human phenylalanine hydroxylase (*PAH*) gene and cDNA sequence *predicted* by the MUTPRED software.[237] Three classes of hypermutable CpG sites occur in the *PAH* gene: ○, sites with no reported alleles; □, sites with CpG-type (C → T or G → A) mutations; △, sites at which the mutation is *not* CpG type. (*From Byck et al.*[398] *Used by permission of Wiley-Liss Inc.*)

Recombination could explain the majority of the associations (Fig. 77-16).

Selective Advantage: Is It a Mechanism?

Are any of the foregoing mechanisms, by themselves, sufficient to explain the incidence of PKU in temperate-zone populations? Consider the evidence once more.

- Involvement of *multiple loci* that could accumulate larger numbers of mutational hits to cause HPA can be discounted, since more than 98 percent of cases are the consequence of phenotypic homozygosity for mutations at the *PAH* locus alone.
- Although some pathogenic *PAH* alleles are the result of *recurrent mutation*, an overall higher rate of disease-causing mutational events at the *PAH* locus can be dismissed, since the majority of patients in the population carry only a few prevalent alleles with their particular haplotype associations.
- *Inbreeding* is a likely contributor only in some populations and, even there, it is a modest one.[346]
- *Founder effect* is only an occasional mechanism to account for the high relative frequency of an occasional allele in a particular population.
- The presence of many different prevalent alleles in different populations is compatible with *genetic drift* (see W. Bodmer in Scriver et al[261]), but can genetic drift be responsible for the high global incidence of PKU in temperate-zone populations today? And would it act on a wide variety of alleles independently? The answer is a tentative "yes," because the set of deleterious *PAH* alleles is still small relative to the whole population size, and thus particularly susceptible to random genetic drift (see D. Hartl, p. 93, in Scriver et al[261]).

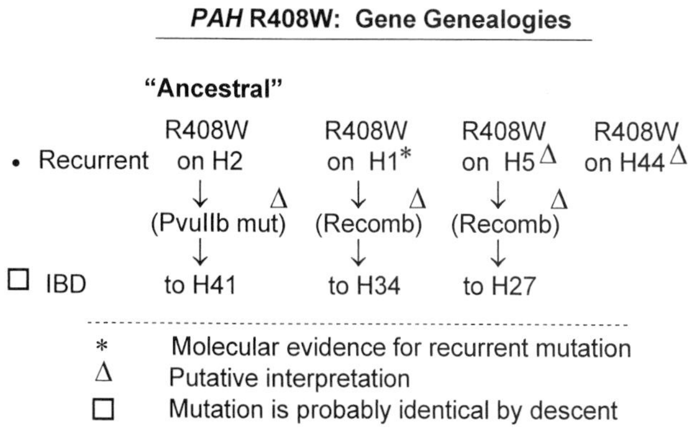

***PAH* R408W: Gene Genealogies**

"Ancestral"

• Recurrent	R408W on H2	R408W on H1*	R408W on H5Δ	R408W on H44Δ
	↓ Δ	↓ Δ	↓ Δ	
	(PvuIIb mut)	(Recomb)	(Recomb)	
	↓	↓	↓	
□ IBD	to H41	to H34	to H27	

* Molecular evidence for recurrent mutation
Δ Putative interpretation
□ Mutation is probably identical by descent

Fig. 77-15 A "gene genealogy" for the phenylketonuria-causing R408W allele. The mutation, always identical by state (c.1222 C → T) is found on seven different extended haplotypes [H]. Sequence analysis by Byck et al[404] of normal and mutant [H1] and [H2] chromosomes reveals the likelihood that one of these versions of R408W in Europeans is a recurrent mutation at a CpG site. Inspection of the other haplotype associations with R408W point to a total of four recurrent alleles and three that are identical by descent on intragenic recombinant copies of the human phenylalanine hydroxylase (*PAH*) gene.

The weight of evidence would seem to favor random genetic drift. Meanwhile, the debate continues (see the "Discussion," p. 95, in Scriver et al[261]), and it includes *selective advantage*.

When only a few in a large set of disease-causing recessive alleles account for the major fraction of the aggregate frequency distribution, selective advantage is a mechanism to consider.[415] Selection of *PAH* alleles (the objects) will occur if the process acts on a phenotype that confers an advantage and is encoded by the corresponding gene. Selection can act indirectly or directly: in the former case, through "hitchhiking" at a closely linked locus and, in the latter, on the primary locus. For example, the γ-interferon locus in region 12q24.1 is physically linked to *PAH*, but there is no evidence that it is involved in the selection of *PAH* alleles. Selection is more likely to have occurred if it could act on a phenotype encoded directly by the *PAH* locus in heterozygotes carrying disease-causing *PAH* alleles. Conventional wisdom sees a

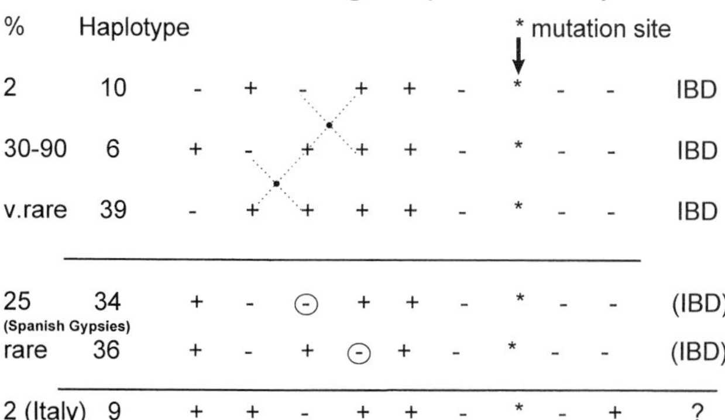

Fig. 77-16 The human phenylalanine hydroxylase (*PAH*) gene mutation c.1066nt-11g → a (IVS10nt-11) is prevalent in populations of Southeastern Europe and the Mediterranean. The allele occurs on six different haplotypes at the relative frequencies (%) shown.[430] Its occurrence on different haplotypes is compatible with identity by descent (IBD) assuming (1) intragenic recombination between haplotypes 6, 10, and 39; or (2) mutation/gene conversion at a restriction fragment length polymorphism (RFLP) site. The origin of the IVS10 mutation on haplotype 9 is unclear. The RFLP sites not named here are shown in Fig. 77-6. The physical site of the IVS10nt-11 mutation in the gene is shown here.

disadaptive or, at best, a neutral effect of a mutant allele in the PKU heterozygote,[416] but if a disadaptive effect is acting in contemporary populations, its effect must be small.[417] Regardless of its magnitude, a disadaptive effect will not increase the frequency of mutant *PAH* alleles.

Increase can occur only through a process that confers an advantage in fitness. In the case of PKU, a simple calculation shows that heterozygote advantage, in terms of surviving offspring, can only be 1 percent (or less) greater than for normal homozygotes, so the advantage is marginal. Selective advantage was advocated[418] when the first PKU-causing alleles were characterized and reported,[148,419] but that hypothesis has since been rejected by its initial advocate (see K.K. Kidd, p. 94, in Scriver et al[261]). Since the selection process must act on a phenotype[420] before it can influence frequency of the allele (the object), plasma phenylalanine levels in heterozyzgotes[421,422] might be the designated phenotype on which the process acts. The actual influence of heterozygosity on this recessive metrical phenotype is very small, however, and it is difficult to imagine how the experience at work in selection would discern it. If selection acts at a more proximal level (e.g., on PAH enzyme itself), it will have been acting not only on *null* phenotypes caused by prevalent alleles such as IVS12nt1, IVS10nt-11, and R408W but also on the V_{max} phenotype caused by the prevalent I65T allele. How this would occur is unknown.

Selective advantage is ultimately expressed in gametic selection, better survival to reproductive age, or higher rates of reproduction among heterozygotes. There is evidence for[346,423,424] and against[425,426] these alternatives in the case of PKU. Such conflicting evidence may reflect bias in the original studies because the families sampled were ascertained through PKU probands. Corrections have since been made for such bias,[427,428] but the ambiguities remain.

It may never be possible to identify the agent of selection. Ochratoxin A, a mycotoxin in grains and lentils, has been proposed as a candidate[428] without supporting evidence. It may never be possible to quantify the effects of the putative selective process for several reasons. First, such effects may have existed only in the past and are no longer acting. Second, since PKU is much less frequent than other genetic disorders where this mechanism has been invoked,[415] the effects of heterozygote selection may be too small to detect reliably. If magnitude of the selective effect on *PAH* alleles is indeed small, yet still stronger than the magnitude of genetic drift, then it must have acted on a large number of individuals or a particular demographic strata to produce the observed incidence of mutant *PAH* alleles and of PKU disease. Furthermore, this selective advantage must have existed in several temperate regions of the world where populations were exposed to different climates, cultures, diets, and infective agents. Despite the persistent fascination with the possibility of positive selection, on theoretical grounds[429] there is no need to invoke it to explain the very variable frequencies of these pathogenic recessive *PAH* alleles; genetic drift will do as an explanation.

The IVS10nt-11 *PAH* Allele: A Paradigm

This *PAH* mutation, a splice allele, with systematic name c.1066-11g → a, also known by the trivial names IVS10nt-11 and IVS10nt546, illustrates many of the themes presented in this section on population genetics.

- IVS10nt-11 in the homoallelic genotype unambiguously confers a PKU phenotype *in vivo*.[25,373]
- Its geographic distribution is nonuniform and is most prevalent in Southern and Southeastern Europe, particularly in the Anatolian region of modern-day Turkey, where it appears to have originated.[430] From observed frequencies in various Mediterranean populations, and the corresponding incidence of PKU, the highest relative frequency of the allele (0.32) is found in Turkey,[345] where the estimated absolute (population) frequency is 0.003456.[346,430] Endogamy and consanguinity

contribute to the high prevalence of this mutant genotype in this particular region.[346]

- IVS10nt-11 is embedded in what has been called an "ancestral" haplotype [RFLP haplotype 6, STR 252 (Goltsov length), VNTR 7], but this particular association is not exclusive. IVS10nt11 is also found on several RFLP haplotypes and, in most cases, this finding is compatible with intragenic recombination or point mutation at an RFLP site (see Fig. 77-16). Since the allele does not involve a CpG site, it is unlikely to be recurrent, and the majority of its mutation-haplotype associations are compatible with identity by descent. Haplotype data indicate a time horizon (origin) for the mutation at least 5000 to 10,000 years ago.[430]
- Associations between IVS10nt-11, and haplotypes on chromosomes from patients in Turkey, Israel and Italy,[430] Greece,[431] and the Iberian Peninsula,[381,395,430,432] indicate a post-Neolithic *demic expansion and diffusion* (gene flow) from the eastern regions westward across the Mediterranean basin. These data, derived from DNA analysis at the *PAH* locus, are concordant with the gradients of several classical (non-DNA) polymorphic markers in the same region.[336,338]
- The IVS10nt-11 allele on haplotype 6 is a tracer for *migration* (gene flow) overland to Tataria;[375] and of range expansion overseas to North America,[307,325] South America,[391] and Australia.[387]
- The IVS10nt-11 mutation is found on a unique haplotype [RFLP 34, STR 230 (Zschocke length), VNTR 7] in Spanish Gypsies,[373] where it is a marker for *founder effect* with drift in relative genetic isolation. There is no need to invoke selective advantage to explain the incidence of this allele, or of PKU, in this population.

PATHOGENESIS: METABOLIC PHENOTYPES AND NEUROTOXICITY

Comment. Whereas the enzyme deficiency is a hepatic phenotype, the major clinical effect of HPA in the PKU phenotype is on brain development and function. It follows that the variant metabolic phenotype must be at least a necessary, if perhaps not a sufficient, explanation for neurotoxicity. (Chapter 78 describes how disorders of tetrahydrobiopterin synthesis and maintenance have both indirect effects, through abnormal phenylalanine homeostasis, and direct effects, by impairment of tryptophan and tyrosine hydroxylations, on brain development and function.) Here, we discuss metabolic phenotypes associated with mutation at the *PAH* locus affecting integrity of PAH enzyme and how these alleles, through their subsequent effect on the metabolic phenotype, may ultimately affect the brain.

Is There a Threshold Value of Plasma Phenylalanine for Neurotoxicity?

There are no abnormal metabolites in PKU—only normal metabolites in abnormal amounts.[51] Phenylalanine itself is probably the chief villain in neurotoxicity.[47] Derivatives of phenylalanine (Fig. 77-2) are not present at sufficient concentration to be toxic in PKU,[433] their concentrations, in CSF for example,[434] bear no relation to those used to show toxic effects *in vitro* and in animal experiments (see Scriver et al[435] for an overview), and a recent study in the mutant mouse ortholog of PKU[433a] denies the relevance of metabolites other than phenylalanine itself.

Induction of temporary HPA in treated PKU patients provokes acute measurable impairment of higher integrative brain functions[436] and abnormal electroencephalographic tracings.[437,438] Under these conditions, urine dopamine excretion[436] and plasma L-dopa levels[437] correlate inversely with plasma phenylalanine and directly with measures of brain dysfunction. These effects on brain function appear when plasma phenylalanine exceeds 1300 μM,[436] a significant value that correlates with concentrations that alter transport and distribution of phenylalanine in brain (see below). Whereas such measurements say little about the profile of brain metabolites, direct,[433a] and indirect evidence from NMR studies[439] in animal models and in PKU patients (see below), from analysis of CSF metabolites,[434,440,441] and from miscellaneous studies[442,443] indicates that high plasma phenylalanine levels do indeed affect brain chemistry and thus brain function.

The threshold value for plasma phenylalanine for its acute neurotoxic effect (1300 μM) does not necessarily correspond to the value associated with chronic neurotoxicity in PKU. Evidence for a lower value in the latter case is apparent, first, in brain white matter where the changes visible by MRI can be found in *treated* patients with much lower levels of chronic HPA (less than 600 μM[444]) and, second, in *treated* PKU patients where IQ scores are distributed below the normal range despite long-term maintenance of plasma phenylalanine values below 300 μM.[445] On the other hand, in *untreated* non-PKU HPA where plasma phenylalanine levels are below 600 μM, there may be no significant abnormalities.[446]

These findings have implications for treatment because they suggest that the putative threshold value for plasma phenylalanine is different for acute and chronic effects on brain. They also imply that any degree of persistent HPA could be harmful to brain particularly during early life and further hint that something in the dietary mode of treatment may have a mildly detrimental effect on outcome. If there is recurrence of HPA in later life, for whatever reason, a reversible acute neurotoxicity will certainly appear first; if the HPA persists, irreversible chronic neurotoxicity could be a consequence.

How Might Deviant Phenylalanine Metabolism Be Neurotoxic?

Pathogenesis can be considered from three viewpoints: (1) a putative deficiency of tyrosine in brain, (2) the effect of phenylalanine on transport and distribution of metabolites in brain, and (3) an effect on neurochemical processes. No single process by itself seems sufficient to explain the PKU brain phenotype, but however complex the process, the ultimate effect will be a disturbance of normal chemical homeostasis in brain.

Tyrosine Deficiency? Complete deficiency of PAH enzyme activity promotes tyrosine to the status of an essential dietary amino acid, from which a line of reasoning called the *justification hypothesis*[447] proposes jeopardy first for the PKU fetus, and then in postnatal life, for two reasons: (1) The affected fetus/newborn cannot obtain tyrosine from its own supply of phenylalanine, and (2) the maternal supply of tyrosine to the fetus is compromised by maternal heterozygosity. However, the hypothesis is not supported by at least five different lines of evidence: (1) Postnatal tyrosine supplementation alone without reduction of phenylalanine intake does not prevent mental retardation in PKU.[448] (2) Postnatal phenylalanine restriction by itself should not be beneficial according to the hypothesis, yet it is, and it appears to prevent neurotoxicity (see the section "Treatment of PKU"). (3) There is no consistent or pathologic reduction in plasma tyrosine content in untreated PKU patients.[449] (4) There is no evidence of significant tyrosine deficiency in cord blood samples obtained from newborns with PKU or with non-PKU HPA.[450] (5) Tyrosine supplements during treatment of PKU sufficient to increase plasma tyrosine levels do not improve neurophysiological parameters or neuropsychological functions.[451,452]

Although the findings pertain only to extracellular tyrosine, the corresponding intracellular values are probably higher than the extracellular values in PKU, since the mechanisms by which tyrosine is depleted from plasma in the disease lead to intracellular accumulation;[62,63] and because intracellular tyrosine is increased in persons homozygous or heterozygous for *PAH* mutations.[453,454] However, these particular findings pertain only to parenchymal cells; brain itself has not been studied.

Effect on Transport Processes and Metabolic Distribution in Brain. The transmembrane fluxes of phenylalanine in somatic cells, mediated by the system L carrier,[58] achieve net intracellular accumulation of phenylalanine.[453,454] During HPA, intracellular phenylalanine concentration is further increased.[455] Several neutral amino acids interact with membrane transport systems other than system L to achieve concentrative uptake into parenchymal cells; phenylalanine does not interfere with this process.[58] These same amino acids, however, leave parenchymal cells on system L, and this flux is blocked when intracellular phenylalanine is elevated. Accordingly, amino acids sharing the carrier are likely to be sequestered in parenchymal tissues in the presence of HPA.[62,63,456] The corresponding transport relationships are different in brain: here, an excess of phenylalanine impedes cellular influx rather than efflux of these amino acids (see below). Thus, the presumed net effect of HPA on interorgan traffic of amino acids, such as the essential branched-chain group, tryptophan and tyrosine, will be to deprive brain and to sequester them in parenchymal tissues.[456]

Transport of phenylalanine across the blood-brain barrier has been measured *in vitro* in a human brain capillary preparation.[457,458] A high-affinity system ($K_m \sim 20$ μM) operates on the blood side of the capillary endothelium, while a very high affinity system ($K_m \sim 0.25$ to 0.30 μM) operates at its brain surface. This arrangement keeps phenylalanine concentration in the interstitial fluid low and stable during the diurnal fluctuations in its plasma level.[34,459] Under normal conditions, it will operate to deliver phenylalanine more efficiently to brain cells than to parenchymal cells, where system L has less affinity for this substrate.

Amino acid uptake on system L across the blood-brain barrier can be measured noninvasively *in vivo* by positron emission tomography using a labeled [^{11}C] inert substrate (aminocyclohexane carboxylate).[460] These, and other studies *in vivo*,[461] show that affinity for phenylalanine uptake (K_m value) is the same both *in vivo* and *in vitro*.[457] The *in vivo* studies[461] also show competition between large neutral amino acids, such as branched chain amino acids, tyrosine, and tryptophan, and phenylalanine on the blood-brain barrier transport system. Phenylalanine has the highest affinity for the system. Accordingly, elevated concentrations of phenylalanine could impair uptake of branched chain amino acids, tyrosine, and tryptophan into brain, and the availability of amino acids from blood for brain is predicted to be impaired by modest supraphysiological concentrations of phenylalanine in the range of 200 to 500 μM.[462] Inhibition has been demonstrated *in vivo* in PKU patients and fits prediction closely.[460]

Brain uptake and content of phenylalanine *in vivo* in human PKU has also been measured by other methods. The intravenous double-indicator technique estimates *in vivo* transport of phenylalanine and other amino acids across the blood-brain barrier:[463,464] the relevant carrier shows saturation in the hyperphenylalaninemic state with inhibition of leucine transport.[465] NMR spectroscopy measures free phenylalanine content and distribution in brain:[466–469] PKU subjects have elevated brain phenylalanine levels and show saturation of the separate transport processes from plasma to interstitial fluid and from extracellular space into brain cells.[466]

Interindividual variation in these *in vivo* studies was substantial and is probably not an artifact; it may explain the interindividual variation in cognitive development, as observed in untreated PKU sibs and patients with similar mutant *PAH* genotypes.[24] At plasma concentrations below 1300 μM, the brain/plasma phenylalanine ratio is about 0.25 (range, 0.15 to 0.50); the transport process at the blood-brain barrier saturates at 1300 μM.[468,469]

The important studies using NMR spectroscopy to measure brain free-phenylalanine content[320,321a,462] (referred to above in this section on "Effect [of *PAH* Alleles] on IQ and Brain Function") imply that interindividual variation exists in the transport of phenylalanine into brain cells and that concentrations of free phenylalanine in brain tissue are one of the ultimate determinants of brain phenotype in PKU. There is NMR evidence[469a] in a crossover study that large neutral amino acids will compete with phenylalanine at the blood-brain barrier and, whereas the adverse effect of excess phenylalanine on the other amino acids may be pathogenic in PKU, diet supplements of large neutral amino acids, if harmless themselves, could block the potentially harmful flux of phenylalanine.

Competition for uptake between amino acids occurs on carriers in other membranes in brain. Phenylalanine inhibits transport of tyrosine[470] and tryptophan[471] in synaptosomal plasma membrane vesicles. Hence, the combined effects of tyrosine sequestration cells in tissues and inhibition of uptake in brain might reduce tyrosine availability for synthesis of neurotransmitters in the brain in the hyperphenylalaninemic state.[472]

Although metabolite levels in CSF do not necessarily reflect the corresponding levels in synaptosomal, interstitial, and intracellular spaces (in brain), CSF tyrosine is significantly increased relative to its plasma level in PKU patients,[434,473] and CSF phenylalanine values are also elevated.[434,473] These findings suggest that phenylalanine and tyrosine compete for a carrier that serves their exit from both brain and CSF into blood. The putative interactions between aromatic amino acids during transport may also affect availability of 5-hydroxytryptophan for serotonin synthesis.[474]

Whereas some argue that competitive interactions on membrane transporters in brain are not sufficient to explain neurotoxicity,[475,476] others[111] have raised questions about validity of the data supporting this argument, while yet others[47,477–479] suggest that the interactions between amino acids during transport in brain might be used to advantage in the treatment of PKU. Dietary supplements of branched chain amino acids, sufficient to double their own plasma values, will reduce phenylalanine levels in plasma and CSF in PKU patients[477] and improve psychological test performance.[478] Corresponding studies in rats show that lysine infusion reduces the harmful effects of HPA on brain development in suckling animals,[479] but the mechanism of the lysine effect is not clear.

[Renal handling of phenylalanine and derivatives has intrinsic interest but has only marginal influence on neurotoxicity and is not discussed here (see Scriver et al[435] for details).]

Effects on Neurochemistry and Metabolism. Phenylalanine has a bulky apolar side chain that could perturb water structure, but at the typical concentrations found in body water of PKU patients it does not perturb water structure *in vitro*[480] (the study was done to discover whether phenylalanine might have anesthetic-like properties).

Studies relating function with neurochemistry in a rat model of induced HPA show impaired performance of a cognitive task dependent on frontal cortex,[481,482] which experiences the greatest reduction in homovanillic acid (HVA) content.[482] Only modest degrees of HPA are required to produce the effect. However, the studies were done in an induced rat model that has significant limitations (see the section "Animal Models").

The cause of defective brain myelination in PKU has long been a focus of interest. There are many explanations for this abnormality,[483–489] but none is comprehensive. Additional evidence from MRI[490,491] indicates that the process of dysmyelination[492] is more prevalent than had been suspected, even in well-treated PKU patients[491] and in non-PKU HPA.

The myelination problem has been studied in the enu2 mouse, a counterpart of human PKU (see the section "Animal Models"). MRI and histologic studies do not reveal a dysmyelination,[493] or abnormalities in cytoarchitecture or histomorphometry. However, more recent histologic and biochemical studies of enu2 mouse brain, and on *in vitro* cultured oligodendrocytes from brain of wild-type control mice (BRBR strain) exposed to abnormal concentrations of L-phenylalanine in the medium (up to 3500 μM), suggest that myelinating oligodendrocytes adopt a nonmyelinating phenotype and overexpress a glial fibrillary acid protein (GFAP).[494] Increased turnover of myelin as a component of brain dysfunction[495,496] is associated with loss of neurotransmitter (muscarinic acetylcholine) receptor density in the enu2 mouse model.[497,498] Related studies in a rat model (made hyperphenylalaninemic by phenylalanine loading with PAH enzyme inhibition by DL-α-methylphenylalanine) that used measurements of neural cell adhesion molecule (NCAM), GFAP, and hyaluronate-binding activity found these parameters were grossly altered in brain exposed to HPA.[499] A similar model demonstrated deficits in myelin basic protein neurofilament staining and maturation of myelin and axons; early onset HPA produced permanent deficits in axon myelination in outer cortical layers.[500]

Brain protein synthesis is perturbed by excessive phenylalanine. It has been monitored by positron emission tomography in PKU patients and shown to be impaired by HPA,[501] an effect that is attributed to polysome disaggregation[502] and inhibition of translation initiation.[503] Although inhibition of brain protein synthesis is an intracellular event, it is directly proportional to the degree of HPA *in vivo et situ* in rats.[504] The adverse effect of phenylalanine on brain protein synthesis can be offset by augmenting the pool of large neutral amino acids.[505] [These findings may be relevant to treatment (see below).]

Polysome disaggregation also occurs in heart and brain of fetal rats exposed to maternal HPA,[506] a finding that could bear on the embryopathy/fetopathy associated with maternal HPA in mice[507] and humans.[508] Excessive protein degradation is not a factor in the "cytotoxic" effects of HPA.[509]

Brain histology and cellular development are altered in human PKU,[510] the corresponding "artificial" animal models,[500,510–515] and the enu2 mouse.[494] The number and spread of dendritic basilar processes of large pyramidal cells are reduced by HPA in rat pups;[511] high levels of phenylalanine and its metabolites, both in culture[512] and *in vivo*,[513,514] decrease proliferation and increase loss of neurons. DNA content is decreased in the affected brain cells,[514] and its synthesis is impaired.[515] The net effect is impaired brain growth.[500] Long exposure to the deviant metabolic phenotype impairs development of brain architecture in untreated PKU patients, with abnormalities in myelination, width of the cortical plate, cell density and organization, dendritic arborization, and number of synaptic spines.[510]

To summarize, phenylalanine itself is probably the neurotoxic agent in PKU. Metabolites of phenylalanine are not found in the human (or mouse) disease at sufficiently high concentrations to disturb metabolic and chemical relationships in brain. Whatever their mechanism, the neurotoxic consequences of PKU are either acute and reversible, or chronic and irreversible; they both affect neuropsychological function.

Is Phenylalanine the Sole Factor in the Neurotoxicity of Phenylketonuria?

Outcome with dietary treatment is not optimal for many PKU patients (see the section "Treatment of PKU"). The cause has generally been assumed to be imperfect compliance with the treatment protocol, leading to attendant HPA. But could this "failure of treatment" be a function of the treatment modality itself—the low-phenylalanine diet—rather than persistence of HPA, no matter how mild? Perhaps toxicity or important deficiency in the diet modality is the problem.

Cockburn notes,[516] "Much of the increase in grey matter weight [of human brain] is due to the development of the complex arborisations and synaptosome formation which subserve neuronal function and the learning processes. Myelination proceeds rapidly after birth and in this process neuroglial cells envelop the axons of cortical neurones.... 60% of the total energy intake of the infant during the first year is utilized by the brain and much of the energy used to construct neuronal membranes and deposit myelin comes from fat in human milk and infant formulas. Fat, however, is not simply a source of hydrocarbon for energy production but is comprised of a series of complex hydrocarbon structures [fatty acids] necessary for the creation of membranes." Cockburn and his colleagues and others[517,518] have built a case for the importance of long chain polyunsaturated fatty acids, notably decosahexaenoic acid [C 22:6 (n-3)] (DHA), in the diet of human infants. This fatty acid is present in human milk but at much lower concentrations in the infant formulas currently in use. The DHA content of cerebral cortex is significantly higher in breast-fed infants when compared with that of formula-fed infants.[519] The "requirement" for DHA could be met by a dietary supplement of 30 mg/day (about 0.2 g/100 g fatty acid) in the diet of formula-fed infants.[520] The requirement is related to the inability of liver to synthesize DHA from α-linolenic acid [C 18:3 (n-3)] in the first months of life.[521] Cockburn[516] cites evidence "that preterm infants fed human milk have a higher developmental status at 18 months and a higher intelligence quotient in later childhood than those fed infant formulas." This outcome is thought not to be explained by the social environment.[522] Are the findings relevant to PKU?

Patients with PKU can have a very low dietary intake of DHA (and arachidonic acid[518]) when low-phenylalanine diet products replace cow or human milk feedings. The majority of PKU diets in infancy also provide only a low intake of α-linolenic acid, which might replace DHA when hepatic synthesis of DHA matures later in infancy.[523] Diet-treated PKU children have erythrocyte membranes that are poorly populated with DHA molecules,[517,523] a deficit likely to be reflected in membranes of the nervous system. Breast feeding, in the 20- to 40-day postnatal interval before low-phenylalanine diet treatment usually begins, is linked to higher IQ scores among PKU patients.[524] Accordingly, disappointments in the outcome of treatment in the PKU patient population might be as much related to deficiency of DHA in early infancy as to some degree of chronic HPA. The hypothesis deserves further investigation, careful review of the treatment diet compositions, and possible supplementation with DHA, particularly during infancy, in the treated PKU patient. The findings also heighten the relevance in seeking possible alternatives to the dietary mode of treatment (see the section "Treatment of PKU").

ANIMAL MODELS

Animal models have long served to study pathogenesis of the disease phenotype in PKU. Now certain of them also enable studies on new ways to treat HPA.

Artificial Models

Hyperphenylalaninemic animal models are not homologues of human PKU when they are achieved by the use of exogenous phenylalanine loads and chemical agents to block the phenylalanine hydroxylation reaction.[47] Such studies, done mainly in rats, were a major source of data about the putative effects of HPA on brain metabolites and chemistry.[525,526] However, the phenylalanine load used to produce HPA in the animals produced an additional burden of tyrosine when PAH enzyme activity was left intact. Accordingly, it was necessary to inhibit the enzyme to obtain the requisite HPA without hypertyrosinemia. Unfortunately, the agents used for this purpose (*p*-chlorophenylalanine and α-methylphenylalanine, for example) had additional effects, notably inhibition of tetrahydrobiopterin-requiring hydroxylating reactions in brain[527] with secondary consequences for neurochemistry.

A Natural Model

Better opportunities to obtain a mammalian counterpart of human PKU now exist in mice.[236,528] The mouse gene has been cloned and characterized, it controls expression of hepatic PAH enzyme activity, and there are strong homologies between mouse and human phenylalanine hydroxylase genes and enzymes.[110] The mouse *Pah* locus is in a linkage group on chromosome 10,[529] homologous to the region on human chromosome 12, where *PAH* is located. Mutations at the mouse *Pah* locus have been produced by chemical mutagenesis with *N*-ethyl-*N*-nitrosourea.[530] The first strain with evidence of mutant phenylalanine hydroxylation to be produced by this method had a defect in GTP-cyclohydrolase 1.[531–534] Other mutant strains were subsequently identified, with mutation at the *Pah* locus affecting phenylalanine hydroxylase function.[236,535] These strains are orthologues of human PKU and non-PKU HPA. The mutations have been characterized:[536] the enu1 mouse, a counterpart of non-PKU HPA, is homozygous for the mutation c.364T → C in exon 3 (V106A); and the enu2 mouse, a counterpart for human PKU, is homozygous for a mutation in exon 7 [c.835T → C (F263S)]. The enu1 mouse has normal plasma phenylalanine and normal behavior on the mouse breeder diet (Teklad number 8626), whereas the enu2 mouse has a 10- to 20-fold elevation of plasma phenylalanine, excretes phenylketones in the urine when fed the breeder diet, and has changes in behavior and in coat color. A hybrid strain heteroallelic for the exon-3 and exon-7 mutations has been produced[537] that offers advantages for the manipulation of blood phenylalanine levels. These animals are described in more detail at the *PAHdb* website (http://www.mcgill.pahdb/mouse/Sarkissian.htm).

The orthologous enu mouse strains are being used to study, for example, pathogenesis of brain disease,[493,498] the effect of maternal HPA on fetal cardiac organogenesis,[507] and the efficacy of enzyme substitution therapy with phenylalanine ammonia lyase.[537–539]

UNUSUAL HUMAN CLINICAL FEATURES

This brief section reminds readers that PKU is still a disease in which the phenotype may encompass more than the effects of allelic variation at the *PAH* locus, and all that is phenylketonuric or HPA is not always what we think it to be. The important disorders of tetrahydrobiopterin homeostasis as causes of HPA are described in Chap. 78.

Oddities of Clinical Phenotype in Phenylketonuria

Early diagnosis and treatment has made the classical PKU phenotype a matter of historical rather than current interest,[11] and for 20 years there were no new articles on the natural history of PKU. Thus, the "oddity" here is a report, in 1991, on progress of 51 never-treated PKU patients during 22 years.[540] One-quarter of the patients had developed epilepsy, half were profoundly retarded (IQ < 35), half were moderately impaired (IQ 36 to 67), and about 5 percent had IQ values above 68. The average serum phenylalanine value for the group had fallen from 1694 to 1180 μM, under apparently similar dietary conditions, during the two decades. The findings indicate the relevance of early diagnosis and treatment for PKU and again beg better understanding of pathogenesis in the brain component of PKU disease.

Reports of novel clinical manifestations affecting skin, teeth, eyes, postnatal growth, and behavior in PKU patients continue to appear (see Scriver et al[435]), as do reports (see Scriver et al[435]) on the chance coexistence of PKU with another Mendelian phenotype (cystinuria, Fahr disease, Duchenne muscular dystrophy, neonatal myotonic dystrophy, galactosemia, hypo-β-lipoproteinemia, or pyruvate kinase deficiency) and now with cystic fibrosis.[541] None of these cases has provided evidence for chromosomal microdeletion syndromes involving the *PAH* locus. The occurrence of schizophrenia in a PKU patient adds fuel to the biogenic amine theory in psychiatric disorders.[542] Abnormalities in the metaphyseal end plate of long bones, once considered to be a postnatal effect in untreated PKU, are now being attributed to intrauterine metabolic imbalance;[543] the findings are not exclusive to PKU. There is decreased bone mineral density, particularly of trabecular bone, in adolescent- and adult-age treated PKU patients,[544,545] and the frequency of fractures in the adolescent group is elevated.[546] Scleroderma-like changes,[547] perhaps related to secondary abnormalities of tryptophan metabolism, occur in PKU patients.[548] There is a possible link between peptic ulcer and untreated PKU in adolescents and young adults.[549] Insofar as the number of cases with any of these "unusual" findings is usually small, relative to all PKU cases, it is unwise to claim cause-and-effect relationships between them and PKU. To illustrate: A link between untreated classical PKU and cataract had been proposed;[550] the observation occurred in two affected sibs and a third unrelated case. A later study,[551] which included a review of the "cataract literature" in PKU, and direct observations of 46 untreated adult PKU cases, showed that the prevalence of cataracts in PKU (6.5 percent) was similar to that in a control sample of intellectually disabled (non-PKU) adults, and in age-matched controls in the general population.

How might one counsel a family in which there is a PKU child affected with congenital heart disease: chance association or cause and effect? A study in the Netherlands[552] found the association of congenital heart disease with PKU to be at least 3.7 times the expected national rate for all cases and 4.1 times the European rate. A putative effect of the maternal phenotype as a possible cause of the association has not been ruled out here.

Agoraphobia, depression, and anxiety are seen following termination of treatment in young adult PKU patients,[553] and symptoms subside when treatment is reinstated. Agoraphobia is now recognized to be a prevalent symptom in untreated PKU patients.[553]

Another significant (clinical) finding is the evidence obtained by MRI for dysmyelination in the brain of PKU patients who are either inadequately treated or in whom treatment is prematurely terminated.[444,490,491,554–557] Such changes are reversible, by restoring euphenylalaninemia, if they are of recent onset;[541,556,557] they probably reflect increased turnover in the fast component of myelin.[495] In the context of recent concepts of cognitive development and brain function,[496] such changes in myelin structure and function might alter patterns of neuronal connectivity and diminish permanent synaptic connection in hyperphenylalaninemic patients.[489] Whatever the pathogenesis and true significance of the abnormal MRI findings, they influence our view of treatment for PKU.[558]

Miscellaneous Forms of Hyperphenylalaninemia/Phenylketonuria

A patient with confirmed severe deficiency of hepatic PAH activity had a normal urine pattern of phenylalanine derivatives, no phenylpyruvic aciduria, plasma phenylalanine values above 1000 μM, and low tolerance for dietary phenylalanine (about 350 mg/day[559]). By definition, this patient had "non-phenylketonuric PKU with PAH deficiency"—an apparent contradiction in terms. Was transamination of phenylalanine (runout 3B, Fig. 77-2) attenuated in this person? Cases without phenylketones in the presence of HPA, in which PAH activity was not measured, were said to have a deficiency of phenylalanine transamination.[560,561] However, transaminase deficiency alone will not cause HPA when PAH activity is normal.[47] Perhaps these "transaminase deficient" patients were truly deficient in hydroxylating activity with relative transaminase deficiency. HPA was persistent in these patients, making them different from persons with 4α-carbinolamine dehydratase deficiency in whom postnatal HPA is transient.[102]

The normal postnatal attenuation of transaminase activity in neonates, particularly preterm infants, can be a cause of missed cases if detection of phenylpyruvic acid in urine (by the ferric chloride test) is the basis of the screening test.[52,562,563] This test for PKU is no longer recommended in the newborn (see the section "Screening").

Persistent phenylketone excretion without HPA was reported in two sisters.[564] The condition is benign and its mechanism obscure. A mutant transaminase with increased affinity for phenylalanine is one (imaginative) explanation.

A puzzling case[565] had apparent PAH deficiency, intact DHPR activity, and no evidence of a defect in biopterin metabolism. The clinical course was "malignant" at birth, death occurring at 46 days. The authors proposed two disorders: PKU and a neurodegenerative disease. Since the report contains no details about the enzyme assays and no quantitative data for hepatic PAH and DHPR activities, the possibility that this patient had DHPR deficiency cannot be excluded.

SCREENING AND DIAGNOSIS

Comment. Guthrie and Susi published their landmark description of a simple phenylalanine method for detecting phenylketonuria in large populations of newborn infants in 1963,[9,566] and many years later it is apparent that applications of the method, and its derivatives, have "gone around the world, changed the natural history of a disease (phenylketonuria) and, through genetic screening, [have] introduced new concepts and approaches to the practice of medicine and health care"[566a] This section describes the principles and practices that made screening for PKU a prototype for genetic screening.

Principles

The rationale for population screening of newborns is *early* medical intervention.[567] The goal in diagnosis of *HPA* is *correct* medical intervention. These objectives require different processes and resources.

A *medical* screening test identifies individuals who probably have a disease from those who probably do not.[568] A *genetic* screening test finds persons who apparently are at risk of incipient or established disease, in themselves or their relatives, because of genotype.[567] On the order of 10 million newborn infants are screened annually worldwide for HPA, and relatives of affected probands are now interested in knowing their genotype and they seek testing. Accordingly, PKU screening and testing have become one of the most widely applied "genetic" tests in health care,[569] the procedure is now seen as the gold standard against which screening for other inborn errors of metabolism can be judged,[569a] and it soon may be enhanced by the use of tandem mass spectrometry.[569b]

Screening

The screening tests in greatest use identify the level of phenylalanine in blood. An alternative phenotype, such as urine phenylpyruvic acid that can be identified by the ferric chloride test, is an unreliable way to detect PKU.[570] Screening at the level of the *PAH* genotype, by DNA (mutation) analysis,[341] will not replace a reliable phenotype test for HPA because of vast allelic heterogeneity and the fact of locus heterogeneity in HPA.

The most reliable newborn-screening tests employ microbiologic, enzymatic, chromatographic, or fluorometric methods to measure the phenylalanine content of dried capillary (not cord) blood samples collected on filter paper. Phenylalanine in blood spots on properly stored filter paper is stable for years,[571,572] and accurate retrospective measurements are feasible. How the blood sample is taken from the newborn, its effect on the baby, and the efficiency of the procedure have been analyzed.[573] A Microlance needle for venipuncture on the dorsum of the hand (compared with two sizes of lancets for sampling by heel prick) has proved to be less painful, more successful on the first attempt, and faster. The microbiologic[9] and chromatographic[574,575] methods are both semiquantitative, with limitations on accuracy at low phenylalanine concentrations. Enzymic[576–579] and fluorometric[580] methods are fully quantitative down to the lowest plasma phenylalanine levels and have the added advantage of a low coefficient of variation.[572,581] The technical issues are relevant. A crucial attribute of a screening test is its sensitivity; which is its ability to minimize the frequency of false-negative results. An enzymic test based on an NADH-detecting biosensor has special promise for this purpose.[582] Because PKU screening is best done soon after birth, and because blood phenylalanine begins to rise in the affected infant only after separation from the placenta, capillary blood phenylalanine values in affected cases will be lower the closer the day of testing is to the day of birth (Fig. 77-17). Therefore, the sensitivity of the test is impaired when it is done

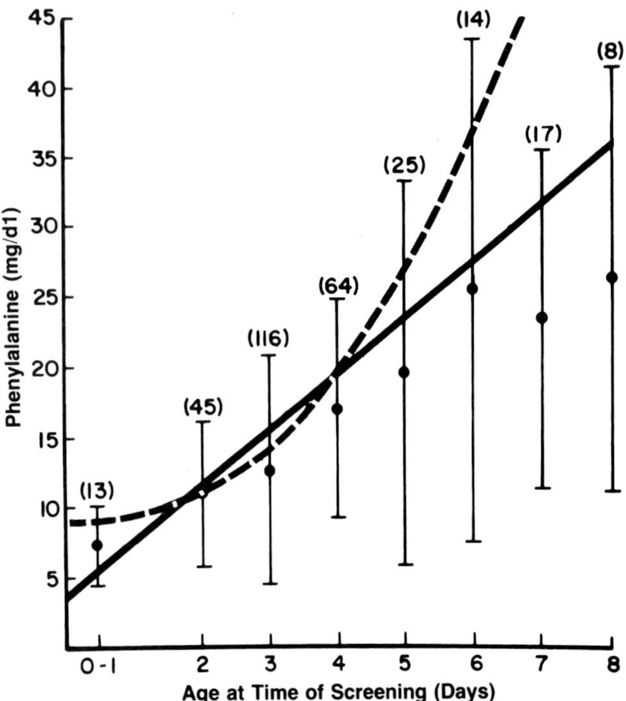

Fig. 77-17 Retrospective analysis of blood phenylalanine values (mean ± 2 SD), related to age, in neonates with confirmed persistent hyperphenylalaninemia and a diagnosis of phenylketonuria. Regressions are for male infants (*solid line*) and female infants (*broken line*). Original data are from Holtzman et al.[603,833] (*From Scriver.[604] Used by permission.*)

early (e.g., on day 1 or 2 of life).[583,584] Accordingly, it would be desirable to use a fully quantitative test on the early samples to separate abnormal from normal values as accurately as possible; the issue is particularly relevant when an infant has non-PKU HPA.[585] A review of neonatal screening for HPA in Britain[562] found that all false-negative tests in that program were associated with tests done by the semiquantitative microbiologic inhibition assay and that none was associated with the fully quantitative fluorometric assay.

The sacrifice of sensitivity in PKU screening, a vexing issue, originates in new obstetric practices. Infants are more likely now to be discharged from birthing units very soon after birth; for example, a quarter of term newborns in the United States are discharged by 24 h.[586] Because the obstetric practice is unlikely to change in the culture of cost saving, the search for a better screening practice has to focus elsewhere.[562,581,583,584,587–589] Routine follow-up (repeat) testing of infants to capture those with false-negative first tests is deemed to be inefficient and expensive,[587,590,591] but nonetheless is being recommended in parts of the United States.[586,592] To convert the test from semiquantitative to fully quantitative status has technical merits[562,581,589] but would require a massive retooling of most screening programs. A compromise would be to use a modified fluorometric method[593] or one of the enzymic methods;[576–579,582] another would be to lower the cutoff level for the microbial inhibition assay.[584] Any (quantitative) method applied to filter-paper blood samples should compensate for the effect of climate and season on the phenylalanine value.[594,595] The threshold (cutoff) value signifying HPA can be lowered to improve sensitivity but at some loss in specificity and predictive value:[596,597] a value of 150 μM (2 mg/dl) should detect all neonatal cases of PKU, unless there is a biologic reason[585] for a normal value in an affected infant at the time of the test.

Whereas a screening program will not detect every case of persistent HPA, the error rate is low (two studies found that only about 1 in 70 cases of PKU is missed[570,598]) and can be lower still.[585] The principal causes for missed cases are noncompliance with the process and errors of procedure,[570,598,599] but biologic causes are also important.[585,600–602] The very existence of the latter ought to cool legal ardor for compensation on the assumption that all missed cases are errors of process. Reanalysis of the original filter-paper blood sample obtained from several "missed" PKU cases has revealed normal blood phenylalanine values at the time of the original screening test.[562,583,585,600–602] The phenomenon is rare in the typical PKU phenotype but occurs more frequently in non-PKU HPA and seems more likely to affect female infants[585,603–605] (Fig. 77-17). Accordingly, some females with HPA probably escape detection and will be ignorant of the risk to offspring in their maternal HPA later in life.

False results, either positive or negative, arise also from artifacts: they include ampicillin contamination of the sample,[606–608] total parental nutrition with some proprietary amino acid solutions,[609] and even lot-to-lot variability in the filter paper affecting absorbency and metabolite recovery.[610]

As experience with neonatal screening for PKU and allied disorders continues to grow, the need to improve education and follow-up increases.[562,611] Meanwhile, society will accept a modest rate of false-positive tests[612] as a "cost" for maximizing the sensitivity of screening. In overall economic terms, screening for PKU is cost-effective.[591,613,614]

Diagnosis and Differential Diagnosis

A positive screening test identifies a newborn with HPA. The diagnostic test identifies the cause of the phenotype in the particular infant.

Some infants with positive first tests have only transient HPA of no further clinical significance. Rarely the cause will be 4α-carbinolamine dehydratase deficiency (see Chap. 78) where the metabolic trait may persist for days or weeks; or it could be an effect of maternal HPA[615] but only for the first day or two of life. Among the infants with persistent HPA, the major cause (over 98 percent of cases) is mutation at the *PAH* locus. Some *PAH* alleles cause the PKU phenotype in which the plasma phenylalanine concentration exceeds 1000 μM (16.5 mg/dl) on a normal diet. Other alleles cause non-PKU HPA in which the phenylalanine value is consistently below 1000 μM on a normal diet. The distinction is relevant because harm to cognitive development is more likely to occur at the higher levels of phenylalanine in *PAH* deficiency.

Some infants (less than 2 percent) with persistent HPA have impaired synthesis or recycling of tetrahydrobiopterin (BH_4) (see Chap. 78), for which there is an international register[616] (see http://www.bh4.org), and these patients require specific treatment to offset the deficiency of BH_4. Since the plasma phenylalanine value alone does not distinguish between BH_4-impaired and BH_4-sufficient forms of HPA, every case of persistent HPA must be investigated further to rule out the disorders of BH_4 metabolism.

Differential Diagnosis. A detailed discussion of diagnostic tests and procedures, is given in the 6th edition of this text; a précis, which includes Table 77-7, is given here.

Table 77-7 Diagnostic Tests for Follow-up of Neonatal Hyperphenylalaninemia

Test Procedure	Approximate Normal Values or Response in Affected Case
1. Plasma (or blood) phenylalanine and tyrosine (μM) with normal protein intake	Phenylalanine 40–130 Tyrosine 50–140
2. Phenylalanine load (100 mg/kg orally), measurements at 0, 1, 2, 4, and 6 h when baseline phenylalanine <180 μM	Excessive rise (>5× baseline) of phenylalanine and deficient rise (<3× baseline) of tyrosine with deficient PAH hydroxylation. Deficient rise (<5× baseline) in defects of BH_4 synthesis.
3. Urine total biopterin and neopterin concentrations (mmol/mol creatinine); neonates have the higher neopterin values	Biopterin 0.4–2.5 Neopterin 0.1–5.0 % Biopterin 20–80
4. BH_4 load (7.5 mg/kg orally), plasma phenylalanine and tyrosine at 0, 1, 2, 4, 6, and 24 h (0 h phenylalanine should be >200 μM)	Fall in phenylalanine indicates BH_4 synthesis is deficient
5. Plasma (or dried blood spot) total biopterin (ng/ml; *Crithidia fasciculata* assay)	Plasma biopterin 1.4–3 BH_4 synthesis is deficient 2.4–6
6. CSF concentrations of HVA and 5-H1AA (nmol/ml; neonates have the higher values)	HVA 400–1000 5-H1AA 200–400
7. CSF total biopterin and neopterin (nmol/ml; neonates have the higher values)	Biopterin 12–40 Neopterin 10–30
8. Percentage of total biopterin as BH_4 in urine and CSF	Urine 60–80 CSF 90–98
9. Total folate (ng/ml; *Lactobacillus caseii*) in serum, red cells, and CSF	Serum 3–12 RBC 150–500 CSF 25–50

ABBREVIATIONS: CSF, cerebrospinal fluid; HVA, homovanillic acid; 5-H1AA, 5-hydroxyindoleacetic acid; RBC, red blood cells.

SOURCE: Adapted from Smith.[844]

Tests at the Metabolite Level

For Phenylalanine (Whole Blood or Plasma). The normal value is less than 150 μM in neonates and less than 120 μM in older subjects.[34,35,37]

For Phenylalanine Metabolites. There are no reliable alternatives to measurement of phenylalanine itself for diagnosis (or screening). Measurement of phenylpyruvic and/or related metabolites (see Fig. 77-2) is not recommended, because formation of phenylpyruvate, the "classical" urine metabolite, depends on transaminase activity,[197] and it may be attenuated in the neonate. Moreover, there is almost fourfold interindividual variation in the substrate (phenylalanine) concentration in plasma at which the keto acid is produced in PKU patients.[563]

By a Phenylalanine Loading Test. A loading test is not recommended in newborns. Three days of protein feeding at normal levels of intake has been used in older subjects to classify the variant phenotype.[21]

By the Plasma Phenylalanine Response to BH_4. The BH_4 dose (see Table 77-7) can be given orally, but intravenous infusion is more reliable. The phenylalanine level must be elevated when the test is done; a fall in the level after BH_4 loading indicates BH_4 deficiency. The test could be misinterpreted when BH_4 cannot function as a catalytic component of the hydroxylating reaction, as in DHPR deficiency.[617] (Note: BH_4 is available for clinical use from B. Schircks, Jona, Switzerland CH8645.)

For Pterin Metabolites. Measurements are done reliably only in laboratories with expertise. Pterin metabolite patterns are abnormal in plasma, CSF, and urine in generalized disorders of BH_4 homeostasis (see Chap. 78). The so-called peripheral form of 6-pyruvoyltetrahydropterin synthase (6-PTS) deficiency may be present when initial pterin levels in CSF are not abnormal. Biopterin can be measured in dried blood spots on filter paper. BH_4 levels are high in untreated cases with ambient HPA and intact BH_4 synthesis[618] and low in disorders of BH_4 homeostasis.

Pterin metabolites (total biopterin and neopterin) can be measured in urine by several methods; relative amounts and normal values are age dependent. PAH enzyme deficiency confers elevated pterin levels with normal neopterin/biopterin ratios, DHPR deficiency produces elevated total pterin levels and low BH_4 levels, 6-PTS deficiency elevates neopterin levels and neopterin/biopterin ratios, and guanosine triphosphate cyclohydrolase (GTP-CH) deficiency produces low pterin values and normal ratios.

For Neurotransmitter Metabolites. Levels of homovanillic acid and 5-hydroxyindoleacetic acid, derivatives of tyrosine and tryptophan, respectively, are usually depressed in disorders of BH_4 synthesis and recycling but not equivalently in PKU.

Tests at the Enzyme Level

For PAH Enzyme. Direct measurement of PAH enzyme activity requires liver biopsy. Indirect *in vivo* assays are feasible by stable isotope infusions[619] and by ingestion of ^{14}C-labeled [39] or ^{13}C-labeled phenylalanine;[26] they show high intraindividual correlation, they correlate with *in vitro* assays of PAH activity, and they will demonstrate deficient phenylalanine hydroxylating activity in vivo. (For the four tests listed next, see Chap. 78 for full discussion.)

For DHPR. Activity is measured in many tissues, including liver biopsy material, cultured skin fibroblasts and amniocytes, erythrocytes, leukocytes, platelets, and in dried blood spots on filter paper. An automated assay of DHPR activity in eluates from dried blood spots on filter paper has been developed.[620]

For 4α-Carbinolamine Dehydratase. Activity can be measured in blood lymphocytes and scalp hair-root cells.[621]

For GTP-CH. Activity is measured in liver biopsy material and phytohemagglutinin-stimulated mononuclear leukocytes. GTP-CH activity is normally low in unstimulated white blood cells and should not be mistaken for an inherited deficiency.

For 6-PTS. Activity is measured in liver biopsy material and erythrocytes.

Diagnosis by DNA Analysis

The *PAH* locus can be analyzed both for the disease-causing mutation and for associated polymorphic haplotype. Venous blood, dried blood spots, buccal cells (obtained by saline mouthwash), cultured skin fibroblasts, and other cells are convenient sources of DNA or mRNA transcripts. Analytic methods include Southern blotting (for large deletions), heteroduplex analysis, single-strand conformational polymorphism, denaturing gradient gel electrophoresis, chemical cleavage of mismatch, restriction enzyme digestion, allele-specific oligonucleotide hybridization,[339–341] and analysis of "illegitimate" (mRNA) transcripts generated by reverse-transcript PCR.[86,622] Detection of a mutation requires *proof of causation*[238] to rule out an artifact or the possibility that it is a neutral polymorphic variant. Nor does a negative finding by any one method exclude a mutation of clinical significance, since no single method can detect all *PAH* alleles. Diagnosis of the mutant *PAH* genotype has some clinical relevance, since it is often possible to predict a severe or a mild effect on enzyme function[149,290,301] and to counsel accordingly.

Prenatal Diagnosis

Indications for prenatal diagnosis exist in the HPAs.[202,623] Treatment under some conditions may be difficult to obtain or administer, and prognosis for a fully normal outcome can still be uncertain.[624,625] Accordingly, there may be an interest in avoidance of recurrent disease. Where the option is permitted, families at risk should know that prenatal diagnosis is feasible.[626]

Fetal diagnosis for PAH deficiency is feasible by DNA analysis.[627] Unless the mutant alleles in the proband are known, polymorphic markers (RFLPs), in gametic association with the PKU alleles, are the mainstay of fetal diagnosis. The approach requires analysis of parental haplotypes and of the association between haplotype and *PAH* mutation. Three-quarters of affected cases are likely to be genetic compounds for PKU alleles, and this has implications for prenatal diagnosis by either haplotype or mutation analysis. Amniocytes and chorion villus samples can be sources of DNA for analysis; maternal contamination of the chorionic villus sample is a hazard.

Diagnosis of Heterozygotes (*PAH* Locus)

Identification of *PAH* heterozygosity is sometimes required. Two relatively simple approaches are available. One involves the use of isotopes.[26,39,628] The tests are done with small substrate loads and measurements are made under quasi-steady state conditions, circumstances that maximize the sensitivity coefficient of PAH enzyme activity in vivo. Large loads of unlabeled phenylalanine lose this advantage but nonetheless have been widely used since first described so many years ago.[629] The results obtained with high-dose loads, followed by measurement of the plasma clearance rate, are influenced by route of administration (oral or intravenous load), pregnancy, contraceptive medication, sex, age, and body weight;[630] allelic heterogeneity further complicates matters.[631,632]

Carrier classification without the use of substrate loads or isotopic tracers can be achieved by taking a single semifasting, noontime blood sample in which phenylalanine and tyrosine are measured quantitatively;[421,633,634] the effect of circadian variation should be taken into account if another time is chosen.[34] A quadratic discriminant function incorporating the prior probability of heterozygosity,[635,636] and linear discriminant functions that do not,[637–640] are about equally efficient for purposes of carrier classification. Measurement of labeled CO_2 following administration of isotope-labeled phenylalanine offers no particular advantage over the discriminant-function approach applied to ambient plasma phenylalanine levels.[26,39]

The advantages and disadvantages of genetic testing by DNA analysis are those already described. On the other hand, it is a very reliable method if the alleles have been identified in an affected family member.

TREATMENT OF PHENYLKETONURIA

Comment. In 1965, the Third International Congress of Human Genetics addressed the topic of treatment in medical genetics. In the discussion, reference was made to "treatment undertaken to modify the environment in which the [person] lives. The otherwise... potentially deleterious mutation is thus offset, and the individual prospers. The principles of therapy in this realm are generally clear. In most instances, they are immediately applicable to [*Homo sapiens*], and many examples of practical success can be documented."[10] Treatment of PKU is one of the classic examples of euphenic therapy (Lederberg's term) where a normal (or near normal) phenotype is restored without modification of the mutant genotype. Because recognized approaches to treatment have been in use for sufficient time to assess the degree of success,[641] and its big success is prevention of mental retardation,[11] PKU is one of those diseases in which process and outcome variables deserve ongoing analysis. In the meantime, more stringent treatment of HPA is being recommended.[19,642,643] Forty years of PKU treatment were reviewed at a recent international symposium [see *Eur J Pediatr* **155**(suppl 1), 1996]‡ where the major good news was again reiterated along with evidence that refinement of treatment protocols is indicated. The PKU story, in both good and less good parts, reveals how difficult it is for *Homo modificans* (a descendant of *H. sapiens sapiens*) to act as a substitute for the normal *PAH* genotype.

Treatment by Low-Phenylalanine Diet

The mainstay of treatment for PKU is the low-phenylalanine diet,[8,8a] and treatment by diet has been feasible since the mid 1950s.[644–646] When started in the neonatal period, it modifies the metabolic phenotype and prevents the neuropsychological consequences of HPA. Optimal treatment of PKU requires (1) early onset of treatment (within 1 month of birth); (2) continuous treatment throughout childhood and adolescence, perhaps for life, and certainly through conception and pregnancy in the affected female (to benefit the fetus); and (3) severe restriction of phenylalanine intake to the small amounts sufficient to hold plasma phenylalanine values as close as possible to the normal range yet sufficient to support protein synthesis (excessive restriction will impair growth and development). The precise tolerance for phenylalanine (200 to 500 mg/day) varies among patients with PKU, even among those with the same mutant *PAH* genotype.

Response to Early Treatment. A prospective controlled trial of treatment by selective restriction of phenylalanine intake, beginning early in postnatal life, was never attempted. However, some of the alternatives to a proper trial have proved to be unpromising: (1) A single case treated purposefully from early infancy only by means of a tyrosine supplement, and with no restriction of phenylalanine intake, nonetheless expressed the PKU phenotype.[448] (2) L-Dopa therapy alone, in adult PKU patients off treatment since 10 years of age, does not improve frontal lobe and other brain functions.[647] (3) Never-treated contemporary PKU patients continue to manifest the classical PKU phenotype;[36,540] by contrast, patients treated continuously and carefully, following neonatal diagnosis, avoid severe impairment of cognitive development and function (see Fig. 15-11 in Scriver et al[435]).

An early study of 28 PKU sib pairs[648] matched the index case, who presented with a late diagnosis and mental retardation, with the sib who had been diagnosed and treated for PKU from the neonatal period. The difference in intellectual development between the early-treated sib (IQ values all above 80) and late-diagnosed sib (mean IQ, 45; range, 30 to 81) was significant. In another historical study,[649] when 36 early-treated PKU cases and their unaffected siblings were compared, the mean IQ values were 94 and 99, respectively.

A large ongoing collaborative study is still evaluating the outcome of early-treated PKU cases.[650] IQ scores measured in 111 PKU children at 4 years of age, whose treatment began between 3 and 92 days after birth,[651] yielded a mean score of 93 (Stanford Binet Intelligence Scale) for the whole group, and cases treated from the first month had a higher mean score (IQ, 95) than those first treated between 31 and 65 days of age (IQ, 85). Evaluation of 132 PKU children at 6 years of age[652] found a mean IQ score of 98; regression analysis showed that scores at 6 years were related to maternal intelligence, age at onset of treatment, and average lifetime plasma phenylalanine values during treatment. Evaluation of outcome in 55 patients at 8 years of age[653] found early treatment compatible with attainment of a "normal" IQ score (WISC Full Scale IQ score, 100). However, the PKU probands, as a group, had a small IQ deficit relative to their normal sibs, whose mean IQ score was 107 ($p = 0.001$), and patients who terminated treatment early scored lower than those who continued it longer.[653]

Among 95 patients treated since the neonatal period and evaluated at 12 years of age,[654] 23 had maintained blood phenylalanine levels below 900 μM for the full 12 years, whereas the remainder had not been able to maintain this degree of control. IQ scores correlated positively with age reached at loss of dietary control and with the midparental IQ score, and negatively with age at which treatment began and with mean blood phenylalanine value during treatment. The best test scores were obtained by the patients treated longest and with blood phenylalanine values kept consistently below 900 μM.

Independent corroborating evidence exists for the efficacy of treatment.[620,655–657] For example, outcomes are known for 808 PKU patients born between 1964 and 1971 in the United Kingdom and followed prospectively; in this study, IQ scores were adjusted to account for the rise in normal scores (+ 0.3 IQ points per year) since standardization of the test in 1932.[657,658] PKU patients showed a 4-point deficit (1) for each month's delay after birth until onset of treatment, (2) for each rise of 300 μmol/L in average blood phenylalanine level with insufficient treatment, and (3) for each 5-month period during infancy when blood phenylalanine values remain below 120 μM due to excessive treatment.[657]

More recent studies from the United Kingdom[659] and in the United States[660] confirm that dietary treatment achieving mean blood phenylalanine levels below 360 μmol/L in early childhood is compatible with normal executive function (higher goal-directed mental activity, organized in nature and dependent of good control of attention):[659] the longer and better the control of phenylalanine levels, the better the cognitive and motor function, behavioral temperament, and executive function.[660–660b] These new studies uphold the recent recommendations for more stringent treatment.[643]

Many early-treated PKU patients were found to have subtle performance deficits in conceptual, visual spatial, and language-related tasks;[442,661–664] in reading and arithmetic skills;[653,654] and in motor coordination, attention span, response time, and problem-solving ability.[653,661,662,664–670] Despite these selective deficits, well-treated PKU patients have satisfactory lives:[671] they meet their genetic potential for height,[672,673] although they tend to be overweight,[674,675] have normal pubertal development[676] and gainful employment.[318]

Whereas social class can have an effect on outcome,[657] and parental skills influence compliance with it,[677] treatment of PKU need not disrupt the family,[678] a fact of some relevance when counseling a family about recurrence risks and the burden of PKU (see Scriver and Clow,[623] Riess et al,[624] and Barwell and Pollitt[625] for views of "burden" by PKU families).

To summarize,[642] (1) the benefits of early treatment in ameliorating the clinical impact of PKU are well established: (2) early-treated children have mean IQ scores approximately half a standard deviation lower than scores for their unaffected sibs and the corresponding population norm; (3) a high proportion of early-treated subjects, not just a minority of poorly treated cases, exhibit some degree of intellectual impairment attributable to events in early childhood; and (4) while subtle neuropsychological impairments are cause for concern, most early-treated PKU children function within the broad normal range of ability and can attend ordinary schools.

Subtle Deficits in Outcome. PKU is no longer associated with mental retardation and severe neurophysiological dysfunction, and early treatment is the explanation. However, to repeat, outcomes for the majority of well-treated patients are not completely normal. New measures of problem solving, abstract reasoning, and executive functions show impairments;[679,680,680a,680b] behavior may be more extrovert along with negative task orientation;[681] the frequency of neurotic and emotional disorder[682] and hyperkinetic behavior can be twice normal.[683] Disordered function in the prefrontal cortex is thought to be at the source of these problems.[482,684]

Response to Termination of Treatment. There has long been a concern that premature termination of treatment in mid childhood might impair later intellectual and neuropsychological performance.[685–687] As a result, quite early in the history of PKU

Table 77-8 Effect of Treatment Termination on IQ scores of Patients with Phenylketonuria

Design	*n*	IQ Points (Change)	Significance	Tested at Age (year)	Months Off Diet (Mean)	Reference
Controlled trial	14	−3.8	NS	6	24	688
Longitudinal	17	−6.3	Yes*	8	41	685
Longitudinal	6	−7.8	Yes*	3.6	12	686
Longitudinal	6	−14.2	Yes*	6.6	48	686
Longitudinal	16	−8.3	<0.001†	11	34	687
Longitudinal	7	−9.1	<0.05†	13	44	687
Longitudinal	30	−0.8	NS	6	24	689a
Controlled trial	55	−5	<0.01	6	24	689b
Controlled trial	115	+18‡	NS	8	24	689c
Longitudinal	14	−14	<0.005	11	6	691

*Stated to be significant.
†Significance applies to treatment-terminated patients only; those who continued treatment on a relaxed regimen had less change in IQ scores.[687]
‡The diet-termination group showed significant deterioration on school achievement data (WRAT scores) relative to the treatment continuation group.

treatment, there was a small controlled trial of continued versus terminated treatment.[688,689] Only a small deficit in IQ (4 points) was found in 6-year-olds, 2 years after termination of treatment. Thus, it seemed that to terminate treatment at this early age would not be cause for concern; nonetheless, the authors of the report recommended a longer period of observation in a larger number of subjects.[688] Conditions for that larger study were fulfilled,[685–687,689a,689b,689c] which provided unambiguous evidence that IQ scores in PKU patients are usually compromised by premature termination of their treatment (Table 77-8). The phenomenon has been called *late onset phenylalanine* intoxication,[690] whose initial features are like those that follow any induced increase in blood phenylalanine levels of the PKU subject.[436–438] A significant fall in the IQ score (by 5 to 30 points) is observed when treatment is terminated in midchildhood;[639,686,687] the fall is less when treatment is relaxed rather than terminated.[687] It is now generally agreed that premature termination of treatment is followed by deficits in performance in most patients.[318,442,691–694] One controlled prospective study of early- and well-treated PKU patients, however, found no deterioration in cognitive ability following termination of low-phenylalanine diets over the next 10 years.[695]

Termination of treatment affects more than the IQ score. There are abnormal neurologic features in later life,[696] deviant electroencephalographic findings,[691,692] and decreased levels of neurotransmitter metabolites in body fluids.[693,697] The latter are analogous to the findings produced by purposeful phenylalanine intoxication.[437,438] Impaired vigilance and reaction times,[693] deficits in social quotients measured on the Vineland scale[694] and behavioral problems[442,682] are also seen.

Termination of treatment is associated with abnormal brain white matter visualized by MRI.[444,490,491,554,556,696] The clinical relevance of this finding is unclear, since it occurs even in well-treated patients still on treatment.[491] Nonetheless, there is some evidence, not all of it consistent,[444,490,555] that the MRI changes are more severe in patients with a history of higher levels of phenylalanine.[490,491] For example, two adolescent patients with non-PKU HPA, both untreated, had no MRI findings; their phenylalanine levels had apparently never exceeded 600 μM.[444] The MRI findings, if of a shorter duration in treated PKU patients, disappear when treatment reduces blood phenylalanine levels,[556,557,698] implying that the abnormality in this circumstance is one of dysmyelination rather than demyelination.[698] Although the changes in white matter are more common than overt neurologic changes,[642] and perhaps more prevalent than measurable neuropsychological deficits, their association with long-term HPA of some degree seems undeniable.

Stringency of Treatment: The Threshold Argument. Is there a tolerable degree of HPA in the PKU treated patient and in the untreated patient with so-called non-PKU HPA? There is no clear answer to this question, so far. Until all causes of cognitive dysfunction, MRI abnormalities and the like, including the diet itself,[523,524] have been ferreted out, we are left to assume that the phenylalanine molecule is the primary troublemaker at every stage of life in patients with HPA. While keeping in mind that persons with untreated non-PKU HPA achieve normal cognitive function in the presence of persistent but modest HPA (less than 600 μM), the extensive studies in this cohort of *untreated* persons with well-documented non-PKU HPA found no significant abnormalities in 28 persons at mean age 21.8 years.[446,699,700] The latter findings require us to question whether the low-phenylalanine diet modality has some undesirable consequences that were avoided in the untreated HPA patients (see the section "Pathogenesis: Metabolic Phenotypes and Neurotoxicity").

In reality, there may be no threshold value for blood phenylalanine, in *treated* PKU patients, at which the brain will escape an effect of persistent HPA.[642] The results in one study[445] imply that even very modest HPA (less than 300 μM in the treated case) may incur cognitive dysfunction, but again, this finding could implicate something harmful in the process or modality of treatment itself. Evidence for the argument against safety in an arbitrary threshold value has come mainly from treated patients with classical PKU[445,656–658] but has also been advanced from other observations:[684,701] in all treated patients, outcome correlates with the quality of treatment and the ambient blood phenylalanine value. Meanwhile, the prudent position remains the one proposed in recent guidelines: treat PKU as early, as well, and as long as possible.[642,643]

Stringency of Treatment: Prolongation. Although some patients were advised long ago that treatment would be for life,[702] most received different advice at the time of diagnosis. In the United States, for example, there was no standard policy for continuation or termination of treatment until the late 1970s.[703] When the evidence began to emerge that early termination of treatment might have undesirable consequences, the majority of American clinics changed policy and began to recommend treatment for the duration.[704] Unfortunately for patients who had already discontinued treatment, it was difficult to reinstate it successfully.[705,706] With hindsight, it seems illogical that treatment would have been terminated in patients with classical PKU, but patients, families, and advisors all had their reasons to do so; among them, the adverse social conditions of the treatment (a restriction and a drastic change of lifestyle), the inadequate organoleptic properties of the low-phenylalanine diet products (poor flavor and offensive smell), and the awkward nutritional considerations (how to keep the intake of phenylalanine far below normal when the intake of other nutrients must be increasing while the patient is growing). Considerations such as these are among the reasons to consider alternative forms of therapy (see below).

Risk of brain dysfunction due to HPA persists throughout life, although risk in adulthood is apparently less than in childhood during development of brain functions, and short-term (3 month) HPA does not affect intellectual performance, memory, and behavior in previously well-treated adolescents.[707] Nonetheless, guidelines recommend that treatment should continue beyond childhood, through adolescence and into adulthood, certainly during conception and pregnancy, and perhaps for the lifetime of all patients.[642,643] To comply can be beneficial,[707a] is clearly difficult to achieve,[797b] and will require better support programs[708] and better resources than are presently in place for treatment during late adolescence and into later life.[696,709] As long as the dietary mode of treatment has the imperfections familiar to anyone who has experienced it, compliance will be a problem beyond childhood. Adolescent patients, well treated in the first decade, can tolerate 3 months of HPA (at levels of 1000 to 1300 μM) without evidence of neurotoxicity,[707,710] but whether their executive functions are immune to harm, or whether a longer period of HPA can be tolerated, has yet to be analyzed. Abnormal neurologic features can occur in adult patients after termination of treatment with rise of blood phenylalanine to the aforementioned levels.[696]

The Modalities for Dietary Treatment: Implications. Protein intake by itself cannot be reduced sufficiently to prevent HPA in PKU without causing deficiencies of other essential amino acids. PKU patients are "consumers with special needs,"[711] and they need selective restriction of phenylalanine intake. Tolerance for dietary phenylalanine (from 200 to 500 mg/day[712]) to maintain plasma phenylalanine levels at "nontoxic" levels in young PKU patients is far below the normal intake. Tolerance increases significantly only during the latter half of a pregnancy.[713]

A semisynthetic diet, selectively low in phenylalanine content and presumed to be adequate in other nutrients, is used to treat PKU. Several commercial products (modified protein hydrolysates or mixtures of free amino acids) provide the other essential amino acids in adequate amounts.[41] Although these products have nutrient compositions and proportions vastly different from human milk,[714] some have been formulated to resemble human milk in most aspects,[715] and efforts are being made to improve their composition and organoleptic properties.[711,716] However, they are still unlike human milk in their content of essential fatty acids.[516,518,520,523,524] Whereas PKU and normal subjects have similar nitrogen requirements,[717–719] classical PKU patients provide evidence that the recommendations for protein requirements in humans can be refined.[720,721] The artificial diets used to treat PKU alter body composition. They incur low levels of trace minerals (zinc, selenium, iron, copper, and chromium) and cholesterol.[435,722] Absence of preformed arachidonic acid and the C22:6(n-3) fatty acid (docosahexaenoic acid) in PKU treatment diets[517,518] distorts the fatty-acid composition of plasma and erythrocytes in patients and perhaps also in brain.[517,523,723]

Treatment of PKU can be made more physiological and plasma phenylalanine homeostasis can be improved[724] by distributing protein intake throughout the day[725] and by increasing the nonphenylalanine protein intake to a least 3 g/100 kcal.[726] These measures may also avoid the growth retardation seen in some treated patients[727,728] and, when combined with more appealing treatment products, may prevent feeding problems.[729]

The dietary mode of treatment has many pitfalls. First, there can be long-term hypophenylalaninemia from excessive treatment[657,730] or persistent HPA with undertreatment, and both will affect outcome adversely. Second, the poor organoleptic properties (taste and smell) of most low-phenylalanine products affect compliance adversely. Third, in the absence of full understanding of pathogenesis, and without assurance that phenylalanine levels in brain can be normalized by dietary means alone in PKU, it is still unclear whether supplements of certain free L-amino acids (leucine, isoleucine, valine, tyrosine, tryptophan, and lysine) are helpful, necessary, or advisable[47,475–479] (see the section "Pathogenesis: Metabolic Phenotypes and Neurotoxicity" and Pietz et al[469a]). A supplement of L-tyrosine (100 mg/kg body weight daily) increased plasma tyrosine but produced no change in neuropsychological performance according to double-blind crossover studies with measurements of three neurophysiological parameters.[451,452] Others claim some benefit from tyrosine supplements at a higher dose (180 mg/kg per day).[731] Supplements of breast milk are considered beneficial in young PKU infants on diet treatment,[732] and the supply of docosahexaenoic acid in breast milk may contribute to higher IQ scores in PKU patients treated early with breast-milk supplements.[524]

The Special Problem of Aspartame. L-Aspartyl-L-phenylalanine methyl ester (trivial name, Aspartame) is an artificial sweetener; upon hydrolysis, it releases free L-phenylalanine, L-aspartic acid, and methanol. Aspartame is widely marketed and has replaced over 12 percent of the total sweeteners consumed annually in America, for example. Its wide availability makes it a potential hazard in the dietary management of PKU (e.g., a quart of Koolaid contains 280 mg phenylalanine, more than half the daily allowance of the amino acid for a PKU patient). Accordingly, those dealing with HPA must know about Aspartame, read product labels, and adjust daily diets accordingly.

Is Aspartame a hazard for PKU heterozygotes, notably pregnant heterozygotes? Studies in normal subjects and heterozygotes, done at 90th and 99th centiles of projected Aspartame intakes with single-bolus ingestion (the worst-case scenario), found no significant disturbance of blood phenylalanine, tyrosine, and large neutral amino acid levels in response to the load,[733] and those findings have been corroborated.[734]

Positron-emission tomography showed a nonsignificant decrease in brain amino acid transport[735] measured with an inert marker following ingestion of Aspartame. Aspartame loading does not change behavior in rats[736] and has no effect on photically induced myoclonus in baboons.[737] Notwithstanding such esoteric studies, PKU heterozygotes will find reassurance that a meal of hamburger and a milk shake can safely replace a craving for Aspartame-flavored sustenance.[738]

In summary, the overall advantages of treating HPA with the low-phenylalanine diet are clear: (1) reversal of key biochemical abnormalities, (2) improved neuropsychological performance, and (3) prevention of neurologic deterioration. The disadvantages are also clear: (1) difficulty in obtaining full compliance with the treatment process, (2) the need for complex social support, (3) risks of nutrient imbalance and deficiency, and (4) persisting uncertainty that dietary treatment in its present formulations and by itself can achieve all that is desired.[19,523,524]

Enzyme Therapy

If enzymatic activity were restored in PKU patients, to deal with the primary problem (enzyme deficiency) there would be no need for the low-phenylalanine diet. Two approaches to *enzyme therapy* have been considered.

Enzyme Replacement. Heterologous partial transplantation of normal liver (or implantation of normal hepatocytes) could replace some of the lost enzyme activity in PKU patients and would constitute somatic *multigene* therapy. No initiatives in this direction have been reported. In theory, only a small replacement of enzyme activity would be needed to convert this autosomal recessive phenotype from homozygous mutant to heterozygous.[28]

Enzyme Substitution. Phenylalanine ammonia lyase (PAL) (EC 4.3.1.5) is a robust autocatalytic protein that does not require a cofactor[739] and will convert L-phenylalanine stoichiometrically to a nontoxic derivative (*trans*-cinnamic acid).[740] PAL is similar to histidine ammonia lyase (see Chap. 80), and the catalytically competent form of PAL requires posttranslational conversion of a serine residue to dehydroalanine; the conversion is autocatalytic.[739] In a chemically induced rat model of HPA, microencapsulated native PAL placed in the intestinal lumen lowered intestinal, plasma, and tissue phenylalanine more effectively than did a low-phenylalanine diet.[741–743] The ability of a recombinant PAL to treat HPA[537–539] in phenylalanine hydroxylase-deficient mice[236] has provided proof of both the pharmacologic and the physiological principle for this form of enzyme-substitution therapy.[538] PAL has been administered to PKU patients in a reactor placed in extracorporeal circulation,[744,745] and in enteric-coated capsules given orally;[740,746] in both cases, the trial was sufficient to observe a modest fall in blood phenylalanine but too brief to be meaningful otherwise. The very high cost of the native enzyme has been overcome by using a recombinant gene from *Rhodosporidium toruloides*[747] expressed in nonpathogenic *E. coli* and purified by column chromatography.[537]

Gene Therapy

The limitations of conventional dietary therapy and the dearth of initiatives in enzyme therapy give gene therapy for PKU a profile it might not otherwise have. The promise lies in putting a normal *PAH* gene in place of, or in addition to, the mutant gene in somatic cells in a patient. Although germ-line therapy would constitute a potential "cure" for the next and successive generations of PKU individuals, it is presently a remote possibility for technical and ethical reasons. On the other hand, the requirements for somatic gene therapy are at hand: a cloned *PAH* cDNA is available, an efficient way to deliver the incoming gene to the target cell exists in a recombinant adenoviral vector, integration of the gene into the nuclear genome of the target cell is feasible, there is reasonable assurance that it will be expressed and transmitted to daughter cells, and an orthologous (PKU) mouse model is available to evaluate somatic gene therapy.[748–750]

A human *PAH* cDNA has already been expressed in a variety of cultured mammalian cells. Expression is transient when integration of the cDNA is not stable, but, when a recombinant retrovirus is used as a vector to infect cells, integration is stable and the *PAH* gene is transmitted to subsequent generations. A functional *PAH* gene has been introduced successfully into NIH 3T3 mouse fibroblasts,[751] Hepal-a mouse hepatoma cells,[751] and normal mouse hepatocytes in primary culture.[752]

Cultures of primary hepatocytes from phenylalanine hydroxylase-deficient mouse[535] have been transfected with a wild-type mouse *Pah* cDNA,[753] using a variant of the LNCX retrovirus;[754] and with an asialooromucoid-poly(L-lysine) DNA complex.[755] Transduced cells express high levels of mouse *Pah*-specific mRNA enzyme activity, and immunoreactive protein.[753,755] Phenylalanine hydroxylase-deficient mice have also been treated *in vivo et situ* with a recombinant adenoviral vector containing a human *PAH* cDNA;[756] the HPA phenotype was normalized in 1 week, but the effect did not persist.

A novel form of gene therapy with a human *PAH* cDNA has been examined in the *Pah*^{enu2} mouse model.[757] The gene was placed in a construct with promoter elements from mouse muscle creatine kinase; this transgene expressed PAH enzyme activity in cardiac and skeletal muscle but not in liver or in kidney. The heterologous PAH enzyme expression *in vivo* required repeated large doses (1.0 μmol/g body weight) of BH_4 to produce an effect on the HPA characteristic of nontransgenic *Pah*^{enu2} mice. These are the first data to suggest that the locus-specific PAH enzyme (and gene), when expressed in heterologous tissue and supplied with abundant cofactor, can restore euphenylalaninemia.

If hepatocyte transplantation becomes feasible in humans (it has been done in rabbits and dogs[758,759]), the patient's own hepatocytes could be obtained, transduced *ex vivo* in primary culture with the normal gene, and then reimplanted. Transduction of hepatocytes *in vivo* with recombinant retroviruses or other hepatotropic viruses, or by delivery of DNA into target organs through receptor-mediated endocytosis,[760,761] has been tried for other diseases and is under consideration in PKU.[755,756] Any real progress in human gene therapy is likely to reflect a perceived failure of all other forms of treatment and will depend on better methods for gene transfer and better gene expression *in vivo*.[762] Meanwhile, it is reported[762a] that T cells from PKU patients, which contain in situ BH_4 cofactor, transfected with recombinant retrovirus will produce significant levels of PAH enzyme activity. This interesting observation merits corroboration.

MATERNAL HYPERPHENYLALANINEMIA

Comment. Inborn errors of metabolism interact with the process of reproduction.[763] The effects include infertility, the effect of pregnancy on maternal metabolic control, the effect of a metabolic defect in the fetus itself on morphogenesis and development, and the effect of the maternal metabolic phenotype on fetal development. Maternal HPA is in the latter category. It is harmful to embryo and fetus because it is a form of metabolic teratogenesis[508] and, as such, it resembles the fetal alcohol syndrome and the effects of maternal diabetes mellitus. The problem has long been recognized,[764,765] as has the potential for intrapartum treatment to prevent harm to the fetus.[766] However, achievements still fall short of expectations because we have yet to learn how to identify, counsel, and treat every mother with HPA and the fetus at risk.[10,767,768] Should we fail, the incidence of HPA-associated disease could rebound to levels experienced before newborn screening came into practice.[10,769]

A Metabolic Embryopathy

Maternal HPA is unquestionably a cause of embryopathy and fetopathy.[10,508,769–771] Its consequences include microcephaly, impaired cognitive development, congenital heart disease, esophageal atresia, dysmorphic facial features, and intrauterine growth retardation.[508] Fetal ultrasonography, in the second trimester, will detect some of these anomalies but not microcephaly; in the first trimester, it will date gestational age and determine whether the pregnancy is viable, facts relevant to counseling and treatment.[772] Maternal HPA can cause hypoplasia of the corpus callosum in the fetus, but the changes in white matter seen in postnatal PKU are absent.[772] Paternal HPA does no harm to the product of conception.[773,774]

Whereas there is no doubt that unmodified maternal HPA is a hazard for the fetus, there is controversy[508] about whether its effect is felt at every level of maternal HPA[775] or has a threshold for the effect.[776,777] Based on the evidence, there seems to be a dose-dependent relationship between the maternal phenylalanine level and its impact on fetal outcome, with the possibility of a threshold effect on cognitive development at the 400 μM maternal phenylalanine level.[763,778] The prudent interpretation thus views all degrees of maternal HPA as a hazard to the fetus but with lower risk when the maternal phenotype is the milder non-PKU form of HPA.[778,779]

Pathogenesis

The normal transplacental gradient for phenylalanine favors the fetus from early pregnancy.[780] The fetal/maternal ratio is 1.5 on average when there is maternal HPA,[780–782] but there is interindividual variation with higher values in early pregnancy. Values overall range from 1.1 to 2.9.[782,783] It follows that one cannot predict the phenylalanine pool size in a particular fetus from the corresponding maternal level other than to say that it will be the same as or greater than the maternal value. From this, it follows that the aim of treatment is to keep the maternal plasma phenylalanine value as near to normal as early as possible in the pregnancy.

An excess of phenylalanine is harmful to the embryo[784,785] probably through the same mechanisms that make it harmful to the central nervous system of the postnatal human infant.[508,780] The phenotypic effect is divorced from whatever the *PAH* genotype may be in the fetus,[786] nor does the effect require accumulation of metabolites derived from phenylalanine itself;[787] since they are apparently harmless to the fetus.[788] Among the likely mechanisms for the effect are competition between phenylalanine and other amino acids for uptake by fetal tissues, and perhaps by the placenta.[780,781,789–791]

Several experimental models exist to study the problem,[792–796] but many of these have used pharmacologic manipulations where inhibitors of phenylalanine hydroxylation are combined with a phenylalanine load to produce HPA in the maternal compartment. Should the inhibitor reach the fetus, its own effect cannot be dissociated from the effect of phenylalanine alone. Accordingly, the preferred model is one such as a PAH-deficient mouse strain[236] in which the effect of the maternal phenylalanine level could be manipulated purposefully and is the result of mutation affecting phenylalanine hydroxylating activity in the maternal compartment.[797]

One further idea about pathogenesis of the effect of maternal HPA on the fetus should be mentioned. The *justification hypothesis* indicts tyrosine deprivation rather than phenylalanine excess as the important pathogenic event in PKU.[447] A formal test of the hypothesis, made by measuring phenylalanine and tyrosine in cord-blood samples from infants with PKU or non-PKU HPA, and from matched controls, found no deficiency of tyrosine in offspring with HPA born to mothers heterozygous for a mutant *PAH* allele.[450] Nonetheless, the hypothesis persists as an echo[798] to a new study[799] that found midpregnancy plasma tyrosine values lower in women being treated for maternal HPA than in controls (untreated pregnant non-HPA women). Because the plasma tyrosine levels of the HPA women could be increased by a dietary supplement of tyrosine, these findings might be seen to validate the justification hypothesis.[798] In a response from Levy,[800] and with a careful reading of the primary paper,[799] however, one finds no support for the idea that the harmful effects of maternal HPA are anything but a result of phenylalanine excess. Whether one supplements maternal tyrosine intake or not, the primary goal in the management of the HPA pregnancy remains reduction of the maternal phenylalanine pool size to safe levels.

Preventing the Fetal Effects of Maternal Hyperphenylalaninemia

Prevention requires broad awareness of the problem, recognition and identification of women with HPA in the reproductive age group, and a planned pregnancy so that the maternal plasma phenylalanine level will be normal or at least below 400 μM from conception to delivery.[508,643,780]

Better awareness of the hazard in maternal HPA requires better education of all those involved in maternal health, obstetrics, and prenatal care; even well-established programs do not track all women at risk.[801] Better detection of the woman with HPA in the reproductive age group will come with a combination of initiatives:[801] First, by tracking women already known to regional treatment programs,[802] perhaps through patient registers,[803,804] while recognizing that tracking and follow-up of cases will be better for persons whose HPA was treated in childhood and adolescence and less so for the forms not treated.[802] Second, by realizing that the cohort of women now at or over 30 years of age (in the late 1990s) were, in general, not screened in the newborn period and thus among them will be women with unsuspected HPA.[801] They can be detected by measuring their blood phenylalanine, and a case for doing so systematically as a health care policy has been proposed.[767,768,801] The third method, by all accounts the least desirable, is through the birth of a microcephalic infant signaling unsuspected maternal HPA.[801,805–808]

A woman with HPA is counseled about the merits of treatment and the need to normalize her phenylalanine levels before conception or as early as possible in the first month of pregnancy. Whereas the early evidence that such treatment made a difference was rather modest,[809] data from the international studies are now quite convincing.[508,778,810–813] Treatment is recommended when maternal phenylalanine levels clearly exceed 400 μM,[763,778] and it should begin before conception. Under these circumstances, risk to the fetus, excepting that for impaired cognitive development, will be no greater than for the general population.[508] But whether any delay in treatment, once conception has occurred, is not without any risk is still uncertain. Accordingly, counseling should be cautious, and the family should know that the delay in onset of treatment is seen by some as reason to consider termination of pregnancy when the option is allowed.[780]

The prospective studies will eventually provide observations on outcomes of several hundred pregnancies. As it happens, some fetal outcomes, even in the carefully designed prospective studies, have been cause for concern. In some trials, maternal blood phenylalanine values were not restored uniformly to the normal range in the critical first trimester—not even below 600 μM on average in one study.[807] Dysmorphic facial features may occur in offspring, and the frequency of these abnormalities correlates positively with the maternal phenylalanine values.[802,814] Head circumference, body length, and body weight can be below normal,[807,815] and, in general, these occurrences correlate with the intrapartum maternal plasma phenylalanine values.[775,807,816–818] Thus, better ascertainment of women at risk, more effective counseling, and more rigorous treatment of maternal HPA, maintaining maternal phenylalanine values below 400 μM, are all indicated.[814,816]

Outcome in cognitive development is of particular interest, and the fetal age at which control of maternal metabolism is attained is an important factor in determining the outcome. A variety of tests in multiple studies[813,819] show that the best outcomes are achieved with the earliest, most adequate, and persistent treatment of the mother under the best social conditions.

Now that the efficacy of rigorous preconception-intrapartum treatment of maternal HPA is no longer in doubt, many studies[713,775,780,800a,808,809,817,820] are showing how difficult the means can be to achieve the desired effect. It is clear that social support, awareness, and education are important for compliance with treatment.[708,800a,802,821–824] The ultimate goal is clear: to restore maternal plasma phenylalanine to a level where it is harmless to the product of conception. What is involved to achieve that goal is well illustrated by one report.[713] A 27-year-old patient with classical PKU reinstated her dietary treatment 10 weeks before conception and continued it until delivery of a normal infant at term. Weekly plasma phenylalanine values were maintained in the range 50 to 150 μM, with rare exception. Dietary phenylalanine tolerance rose from 6 mg/kg per day (about 300 mg/day) to 30 mg/kg per day at term; at the same time, her intake of tyrosine increased to meet requirements for protein synthesis. The diet was supplemented with a mixture of nonphenylalanine amino acids in a proprietary formula. The striking increase in dietary phenylalanine tolerance experienced during the second and third trimesters is a feature of pregnancy in affected women,[780,817,818,825] representing both enhanced protein synthesis in the fetal-maternal unit and new capacity for phenylalanine metabolism gained from the heterozygous fetus.

The willingness of a woman to return to (or continue) treatment before and during a pregnancy is likely to be influenced not only by the nutritional content[826] but also by the qualitative (organoleptic) features of the therapeutic diet. Some products are more suitable than others for the particular task,[713,827,828] and their use is associated with satisfactory fetal outcomes.[713,775] A new inoffensive amino acid mix is compatible with good compliance,[716] as is the use of gelatin encapsulation to mask offensive features of dietary products.[829] Whether supplements of branched chain amino acids[791] are an essential part of dietary treatment is still unclear,[790] and they were not needed to achieve satisfactory results in the "ideal case" just referred to.[713] Tyrosine supplementation will improve maternal levels, if indicated,[799] but excessive tyrosine supplementation is undesirable because it could impair cellular uptake of other amino acids.[780]

The breast milk of a mother with HPA will contain levels of phenylalanine some two- to threefold higher than those in her plasma, and higher still in colostrum.[830] This would be taken into account if she elects to breast feed her heterozygous infant, who would be monitored accordingly.

Thus, maternal HPA continues to be an important challenge[508,643,807,809,816] despite more than 40 years of awareness that it would become such in the global management of PKU.[10,764,765,769] It is a problem that must be resolved; otherwise, all achievements in the prevention of mental retardation associated with PKU and related forms of HPA will have been gained at the cost of a terrible Faustian bargain.

ACKNOWLEDGMENTS

The authors acknowledge invaluable contributions from members of the PAH Mutation Analysis Consortium and from the following colleagues (in alphabetic order): Louis Baumier, Susan Byck, Annie Capua, Kevin Carter, Randy Eisensmith, Mary Fujiwara, Debby Lambert, Harvey Levy, Ken Morgan, Piotr Nowacki, Michael Parniak Lynne Prevost, Christineh Sarkissian, Ray Stevens, Eileen Treacy, Linda Tyfield, and Paula Waters. There would be much less to report without the generosity of Savio Woo and colleagues who shared the hPAH 247 probe and PCR primers so generously, and without the commitment of Per Guldberg and Flemming Güttler to develop a powerful DGGE method for mutation analysis. The authors' own efforts were supported by the National Institutes of Health and by the Medical Research Council (Canada), the Network of Centers of Excellence (Canadian Genetic Diseases Network), and Le Fonds de la Recherche en santé du Quebéc (for the Quebec Network of Applied/Molecular genetics). Nothing appearing in this chapter would have been possible without the *in silico* manipulations of Lynne Prevost, Huguette Rizziero, and Marge Schnackenberg.

REFERENCES

1. Folling I: The discovery of phenylketonuria. *Acta Paediatr Suppl* **407**:4, 1994.
2. Folling A, Mohr OL, Ruud L: Oligophrenia phenylpyrouvica: A recessive syndrome in man. *Skr Nor Vitensk Akad Oslo i Mat Naturvidensk Kl* **1**, 1945.
3. Folling A: Uber Ausscheidung von Phenylbrenztraubensäure in den Harn als Stoffwechselanomalie in Verbindung mit Imbezillitat. *Hoppe-Seylers Z Physiol Chem* **277**:169, 1934.
4. Penrose LS: Inheritance of phenylpyruvic amentia (phenylketonuria). *Lancet* **2**:192, 1935.
5. Jervis GA: The genetics of phenylpyruvic oligophrenia. *J Ment Sci* **85**:719, 1939.
6. Penrose LS: Phenylketonuria: A problem in eugenics. *Lancet* **1**:949, 1946. (Republished *Ann Hum Genet* **62**:193, 1998).
7. Jervis GA: Phenylpyruvic oligophrenia: Deficiency of phenylalanine oxidizing system. *Proc Soc Exp Biol Med* **82**:514, 1953.
8. Woolf LI, Vulliamy DG: Phenylketonuria with a study of the effect upon it of glutamic acid. *Arch Dis Child* **25**:487, 1951.

8a. Bickel H, Gerrard J, Hickmans EM: Influence of phenylalanine intake on phenylketonuria. *Lancet* **2**:812, 1953.

9. Guthrie R, Susi A: A simple phenylalanine method for detecting phenylketonuria in large populations of newborn infants. *Pediatrics* **32**:318, 1963.
10. Scriver CR: Treatment in medical genetics, in Crow JF, Neel JV (eds): *Proceedings of the Third International Congress of Human Genetics*. Baltimore, Johns Hopkins Press, 1967, p 45.
11. MacCready RA: Admissions of phenylketonuric patients to residential institutions before and after screening programs of the newborn infant. *J Pediatr* **85**:383, 1974.
12. Robson KJH, Chandra T, MacGillivray RTA, et al: Polysome immunoprecipitation of phenylalanine hydroxylase mRNA from rat liver and cloning of its cDNA. *Proc Natl Acad Sci USA* **79**:4701, 1982.
13. Woo SLC, Lidsky AS, Güttler F, et al: Cloned human phenylalanine hydroxylase gene allows prenatal diagnosis and carrier detection of classical phenylketonuria. *Nature* **306**:151, 1983.
14. Scriver CR, Waters PJ, Sarkissian C, et al: *PAHdb*: A locus specific knowledge base. *Hum Mutat* **15**:99, 2000.
15. Kaufman S: The phenylalanine hydroxylating system from mammalian liver. *Adv Enzymol* **35**:245, 1971.
16. Danks DM, Bartholomé K, Clayton BE, et al: Malignant hyperphenylalaninemia: Current status. *J Inherited Metab Dis* **1**:49, 1978.
17. Erlandsen H, Martinez A, Knappskog PM, et al: Crystallization and preliminary diffraction analysis of a truncated homodimer of human phenylalanine hydroxylase. *FEBS Lett* **406**:171, 1997.
18. Erlandsen H, Fusetti F, Martinez A, et al: Crystal structure of the catalytic domain of human phenylalanine hydroxylase reveals the structural basis for phenylketonuria. *Nature Struct Biol* **4**:995, 1997.

18a. Kobe B, Jennings IG, House CM, et al: Structural basis of autoregulation of phenylalanine hydroxylase. *Nature Struct Biol* **6**:442, 1999.

19. Smith I: Treatment of phenylalanine hydroxylase deficiency. *Acta Paediatr Scand Suppl* **407**:60, 1994.
20. Scriver CR, Kaufman S, Eisensmith E, et al: The hyperphenylalaninemias, in Scriver CR, Beaudet AL, Sly WS, Valle D (eds): *The Metabolic and Molecular Bases of Inherited Disease*. New York, McGraw-Hill, 1995, p 1015.
21. Guttler F: Hyperphenylalaninemia: Diagnosis and classification of the various types of phenylalanine hydroxylase deficiency in childhood. *Acta Paediatr Scand* **280**:1, 1980.
22. Bearn AG: *Archibald Garrod and the Individuality of Man*. Oxford, Clarendon, 1993, p 145.
23. Lidsky AS, Law ML, Morse HG, et al: Regional mapping of the phenylalanine hydroxylase gene and the phenylketonuria locus in the human genome. *Proc Natl Acad Sci USA* **82**:6221, 1985.
24. Ramus SJ, Forrest SM, Pitt DB, et al: Comparison of genotype and intellectual phenotype in untreated PKU patients. *J Med Genet* **30**:401, 1993.
25. Kayaalp E, Treacy E, Waters PJ, et al: Human phenylalanine hydroxylase mutations and hyperphenylalaninemia phenotypes: A metanalysis of genotype-phenotype correlations. *Am J Hum Genet* **61**:1309, 1997.
26. Treacy EP, Delente JJ, Elkas G, et al: Analysis of phenylalanine hydroxylase genotypes and hyperphenylalaninemia phenotypes using L-[1-^{13}C]phenylalanine oxidation rates in vivo: A pilot study. *Pediatr Res* **42**:430, 1997.
27. Scriver CR: An ongoing debate over phenylalanine hydroxylase deficiency in phenylketonuria. *J Clin Invest* **101**:1, 1998.
28. Kacser H, Burns JA: The molecular basis of dominance. *Genetics* **97**:639, 1981.
29. Weiss KM: Is there a paradigm shift in genetics? Lessons from the study of human diseases. *Mol Phylogenet Evol* **5**:259, 1996.
30. Bernard C: *Les Phenomenes de la Vie*. Paris, Libraire J-B Bailliere et Fils, 1878.
31. Cannon WB: Organization for physiological homeostasis. *Physiol Rev* **9**:399, 1929.
32. Cohn RM, Palmieri MJ, McNamara PD: Non equilibrium thermodynamics, noncovalent forces, and water, in Herman RH, Cohn RM, McNamara PD (eds): *Principles of Metabolic Control in Mammalian Species*. New York, Plenum, 1980, p 63.
33. Murphy EA, Pyeritz RE: Homeostasis VII: A conspectus. *Am J Med Genet* **24**:735, 1986.
34. Scriver CR, Gregory DM, Sovetts D, et al: Normal plasma free amino acid values in adults: The influence of some common physiological variables. *Metabolism* **34**:868, 1985.
35. Scriver CR, Rosenberg LE: *Amino Acid Metabolism and Its Disorders*. Philadelphia, WB Saunders, 1973, p 40.
36. Langenbeck U, Lukas HD, Mench-Hoinowski A, et al: Correlative study of mental and biochemical phenotypes in never treated patients with classic phenylketonuria. *Brain Dysfunct* **1**:103, 1988.
37. Gregory DM, Sovetts D, Clow CL, et al: Plasma free amino acid values in normal children and adolescents. *Metabolism* **35**:967, 1986.
38. Krempf M, Hoerr RA, Marks L, et al: Phenylalanine flux in adult men: Estimates with different tracers and route of administration. *Metabolism* **39**:560, 1990.
39. Lehmann WD, Fischer R, Heinrich HC, et al: Metabolic conversion of L-[U-^{14}C] phenylalanine to respiratory $^{14}CO_2$ in healthy subjects, phenylketonuria heterozygotes and classic phenylketonurics. *Clin Chim Acta* **157**:253, 1986.
40. Young VR, Pellett PL: Protein intake and requirements with reference to diet and health. *Am J Clin Nutr* **45**:1323, 1987.
41. American Academy of Pediatrics Committee on Nutrition: Special diets for infants with inborn errors of metabolism. *Pediatrics* **57**:783, 1976.

42. Basile-Filho A, El-Khoury AE, Beaumier L, et al: Continuous 24-h L-[1-^{13}C]phenylalanine and L-[3,3-$^{2}H_2$]tyrosine oral-tracer studies at an intermediate phenylalanine intake to estimate requirements in adults. *Am J Clin Nutr* **65**:473, 1997.
43. Sanchez M, El Khory AE, Castillo L, et al: Twenty-four hour intravenous and oral tracer studies with L-[1-^{13}C]phenylalanine and L-[3,3-$^{2}H_2$]tyrosine at a tyrosine-free generous phenylalanine intake in adults. *Am J Clin Nutr* **63**:532, 1996.
44. Berke EM, Gardner AW, Goran MI, et al: Resting metabolic rate and the influence of the pretesting environment. *Am J Clin Nutr* **55**:626, 1992.
45. Kacser H, Burns JA: The control of flux. *Symp Soc Exp Biol* **27**:65, 1973.
46. Kacser H, Porteous JW: Control of metabolism: What do we have to measure? *Trends Biochem Sci* **12**:5, 1987.
47. Kaufman S: Phenylketonuria: Biochemical mechanisms. *Adv Neurochem* **2**:1, 1976.
48. Salter M, Knowles RG, Pogson CI: Quantification of the importance of individual steps in the control of aromatic amino acid metabolism. *Biochem J* **234**:635, 1986.
49. Knox WE: Phenylketonuria, in Stanbury JB, Wyngaarden JB, Fredrickson DS (eds): *The Metabolic Basis of Inherited Disease*. New York, McGraw-Hill, 1960, p 321.
50. Knox WE: Phenylketonuria, in Stanbury JB, Wyngaarden JB, Fredrickson DS (eds): *The Metabolic Basis of Inherited Disease*. New York, McGraw-Hill, 1966, p 258.
51. Knox WE: Phenylketonuria, in Stanbury JB, Wyngaarden JB, Fredrickson DS (eds): *The Metabolic Basis of Inherited Disease*. New York, McGraw-Hill, 1972, p 266.
52. Scriver CR, Rosenberg LE: *Amino Acid Metabolism and Its Disorders*. Philadelphia, WB Saunders, 1973, p 298.
53. Treacy E, Pitt JJ, Seller J, et al: In vivo disposal of phenylalanine in phenylketonuria: A study of two siblings. *J Inherit Metab Dis* **19**:595, 1996.
54. Rampini S, Vollman JA, Bosshard HR, et al: Aromatic acids in urine of healthy infants, persistent hyperphenylalaninemia, and phenylketonuria, before and after phenylalanine load. *Pediatr Res* **8**:704, 1974.
55. Thompson GN, Walter JH, Halliday D: In vivo enzyme activity in inborn errors of metabolism. *Metabolism* **799**:807, 1990.
56. Thompson GN, Halliday D: Significant phenylalanine hydroxylation in vivo in patients with classical phenylketonuria. *J Clin Invest* **86**:317, 1990.
57. Van Spronsen FJ, Reijngoud D-J, Smit GPA, et al: Phenylketonuria (PKU): The in vivo hydroxylation rate of phenylalanine into tyrosine is decreased. *J Clin Invest* **101**:2875, 1998.
57a. Scriver CR: An ongoing debate over phenylalanine hydroxylase deficiency in phenylketonuria. *J Clin Invest* **101**:2613, 1998.
58. Christensen HN: Interorgan amino acid nutrition. *Physiol Rev* **62**:1193, 1982.
59. Kragh-Hansen U, Rigaard-Petersen H, Jacobsen C, et al: Renal transport of neutral amino acids: Tubular localization of Na^+-dependent phenylalanine and glucose-transport systems. *Biochemistry* **220**:15, 1984.
60. Samarzija I, Fromter E: Electrophysiological analysis of rat renal sugar and amino acid transport: III. Neutral amino acids. *Pflugers Arch* **393**:199, 1982.
61. Berteloot A, Khan AH, Ramaswamy K: K^+ and Na^+-gradient-dependent transport of L-phenylalanine by mouse intestinal brush border membrane vesicles. *Biochim Biophys Acta* **691**:321, 1982.
62. Christensen HN: Where do the depleted plasma amino acids go in phenylketonuria? *Biochem J* **236**:929, 1986.
63. Christensen HN: Hypothesis: Where the depleted plasma amino acids go in phenylketonuria, and why. *Perspect Biol Med* **30**:186, 1987.
64. Owens CWI: Effects of phenylalanine analogues on renal tubular reabsorption of amino acids in the rat. *Clin Sci Mol Med* **53**:355, 1977.
65. Pardridge WM: Phenylalanine transport at the human blood-brain barrier, in Kaufman S (ed): *Amino Acids in Health and Disease: New Perspectives*. New York, AR Liss, 1987, p 43.
66. Smith QR: Kinetic analysis of neutral amino acid transport across the blood-brain barrier, in Kaufman S (ed): *Amino acids in Health and Disease: New Perspectives*. New York, AR Liss, 1987, p 65.
67. Shershen H, Debler EA, Lajtha A: Alterations of cerebral amino acid transport processes, in Kaufman S (ed): *Amino Acids in Health and Disease: New Perspectives*. New York, AR Liss, 1987, p 87.
67a. Kaufman S: A model of human phenylalanine metabolism in normal subjects and in phenylketonuric patients. *Proc Natl Acad Sci USA* **96**:3160, 1999.
68. Milstien S, Kaufman S: Studies on the phenylalanine hydroxylase system in vivo: An in vivo assay based on the liberation of deuterium or tritium into the body water from ring-labelled L-phenylalanine. *J Biol Chem* **250**:4782, 1975.
69. Udenfriend S, Cooper JR: The enzymatic conversion of phenylalanine to tyrosine. *J Biol Chem* **194**:503, 1952.
70. Tourian A, Goddard J, Puck TT: Phenylalanine hydroxylase activity in mammalian cells. *J Cell Physiol* **73**:159, 1969.
71. Berry HK, Cripps R, Nicholls K, et al: Development of phenylalanine hydroxylase activity in guinea pig liver. *Biochim Biophys Acta* **261**:315, 1972.
72. Rao DN, Kaufman S: Purification and state of activation of rat liver phenylalanine hydroxylase. *J Biol Chem* **261**:8866, 1986.
73. Ayling JE, Pirson WD, At-Janabi JM, et al: Kidney phenylalanine hydroxylase from man and rat: Comparison with the liver enzyme. *Biochemistry* **13**:78, 1974.
74. Ayling JE, Helfand GD, Pirson WD: Kidney phenylalanine hydroxylase from man and rat: Comparison with the liver enzyme. *Enzyme* **20**:6, 1975.
75. Murthy LI, Berry HK: Phenylalanine hydroxylase activity in liver from humans and subhuman primates: Its probable absence in kidney. *Biochem Med* **12**:392, 1975.
76. Robson KJ, Chandra T, MacGillivray RT, et al: Polysome immunoprecipitation of phenylalanine hydroxylase mRNA from rat liver and cloning of its cDNA. *Proc Natl Acad Sci USA* **79**:4701, 1982.
77. Crawfurd MD, Gibbs DA, Sheppard DM: Studies on human phenylalanine mono-oxygenase: I. Restricted expression. *J Inherit Metab Dis* **4**:191, 1981.
77a. Lichter-Konecki U, Hipke CM, Konecki DS: Human phenylalanine hydroxylase gene expression in kidney and other non-hepatic tissues. *Mol Genet Metab* **67**:308, 1999.
77b. Tessari P, Deferrari G, Robaudo R: Phenylalanine hydroxylase across the kidney. *Kidney Int* **56**:2168, 1999.
78. Abita JP, Dorche C, Kaufman S: Further studies on the nature of phenylalanine hydroxylation in brain. *Pediatr Res* **8**:714, 1974.
79. Wapnir RA, Hawkins RL, Stevenson JH: Ontogenesis of phenylalanine and tryptophan hydroxylation in rat brain and liver. *Biol Neonate* **118**:85, 1971.
80. Katz I, Lloyd T, Kaufman S: Studies on the phenylalanine and tyrosine hydroxylation by rat brain tyrosine hydroxylase. *Biochim Biophys Acta* **445**:567, 1976.
81. Kaufman S: Aromatic amino acid hydroxylases, in Krebs E (ed): *The Enzymes: Phosphorylation Control*. 3rd ed. New York, Academic, 1987.
82. Schallreuter KU, Wood JM, Ziegler I, et al: Defective tetrahydrobiopterin and catecholamine biosynthesis in the depigmentation disorder vitiligo. *Biochim Biophys Acta* **1226**:181, 1994.
83. Davis MD, Ribeiro P, Tipper J, et al: 7-Tetrahydrobiopterin, a naturally occurring analogue of tetrahydrobiopterin, is a cofactor for and a potential inhibitor of the aromatic amino acid hydroxylases. *Proc Natl Acad Sci USA* **89**:10,109, 1992.
84. Miyamoto M, Fitzpatrick TB: Competitive inhibition of mammalian tyrosinase by phenylalanine and its relationship to hair pigmentation in phenylketonuria. *Nature* **179**:199, 1957.
85. Schallreuter KU, Zschiesche M, Moore J, et al: In vivo evidence for compromised phenylalanine metabolism in vitiligo. *Biochem Biophys Res Commun* **243**:395, 1998.
86. Sarkar G, Sommer SS: Access to a messenger RNA sequence on its protein product is not limited by tissue or species specificity. *Science* **244**:331, 1989.
87. Ramus SJ, Forrest SM, Cotton RG: Illegitimate transcription of phenylalanine hydroxylase for detection of mutations in patients with phenylketonuria. *Hum Mutat* **1**:154, 1992.
88. Abadie V, Jaruzelska J, Lyonnet S, et al: Illegitimate transcription of the phenylalanine hydroxylase gene in lymphocytes for identification of mutations in phenylketonuria. *Hum Mol Genet* **2**:31, 1993.
89. Kaufman S: The structure of phenylalanine hydroxylation cofactor. *Proc Natl Acad Sci USA* **50**:1085, 1963.
90. Kaufman S: A protein that stimulates rat liver phenylalanine hydroxylase. *J Biol Chem* **245**:4751, 1970.
91. Huang CY, Max EE, Kaufman S: Purification and characterization of phenylalanine hydroxylase-stimulating protein from rat liver. *J Biol Chem* **248**:2435, 1973.

92. Kaufman S: Studies on the mechanism of phenylalanine hydroxylase: Detection of an intermediate, in Pfleiderer W (ed): *Chemistry and Biology of Pteridines*. New York, Walter de Gruyter, 1975, p 291.
93. Lazarus RA, Benkovic SJ, Kaufman S: Phenylalanine hydroxylase stimulator protein is a 4α-carbinolamine dehydratase. *J Biol Chem* **258**:10,960, 1983.
94. Kaufman S, Levenberg B: Further studies on the phenylalanine hydroxylation cofactor. *J Biol Chem* **234**:2683, 1959.
95. Kaufman S, Bridgers WF, Eisenberg G, et al: The source of oxygen in the phenylalanine hydroxylase and the dopamine–β-hydroxylase catalyzed reaction. *Biochim Biophys Res Acta* **9**:497, 1962.
96. Craine JE, Hall ES, Kaufman S: The isolation and characterization of dihydropteridine reductase from sheep liver. *J Biol Chem* **247**:6082, 1972.
97. Neilsen KH: Rat liver phenylalanine hydroxylase: A method for the measurement of activity, with particular reference to the distinctive features of the enzyme and the pteridine cofactor. *Eur J Biochem* **7**:360, 1969.
98. Scrimgeour KG, Cheema S: Quininoid dihydropterin reductase. *Ann NY Acad Sci* **186**:115, 1971.
99. Kaufman S: Studies on the mechanism of the enzymatic conversion of phenylalanine to tyrosine. *J Biol Chem* **234**:2677, 1959.
100. Kaufman S: Phenylketonuria and its variants. *Adv Hum Genet* **13**:217, 1983.
101. Citron BA, Kaufman S, Milstien S, et al: Mutation in the 4α-carbinolamine dehydratase gene leads to mild hyperphenylalaninemia with defective cofactor metabolism. *Am J Hum Genet* **53**:768, 1993.
102. Johnen G, Kowlessur D, Citron BA, et al: Characterization of the wild-type of 4a-carbinolamine dehydratase and two naturally occurring mutants associated with hyperphenylalaninemia. *Proc Natl Acad Sci USA* **92**:12,384, 1995.
103. Koster S, Thöny B, Macheroux P, et al: Human pterin-4 alpha-carbinolamine dehydratase/dimerization cofactor of hepatocyte nuclear factor-1 alpha: Characterization and kinetic analysis of wild-type and mutant enzymes. *Eur J Biochem* **231**:414, 1995.
104. Doolittle RF: More molecular opportunism. *Nature* **336**:18, 1988.
105. Citron BA, Davis MD, Milstien S, et al: Identity of 4α-carbinolamine dehydratase, a component of the phenylalanine hydroxylation system, and DCoH, a transregulator of homeodomain proteins. *Proc Natl Acad Sci USA* **89**:11,891, 1992.
106. Hauer CR, Rebrin I, Thony B, et al: Phenylalanine hydroxylase-stimulating protein/pterin-4α-carbinolamine dehydratase from rat and human liver. *J Biol Chem* **268**:4828, 1993.
107. Mendel DB, Crabtree GR: HNF-1, a member of a novel class of dimerizing homeodomain proteins. *J Biol Chem* **266**:677, 1991.
108. Johnen G, Kaufman S: Studies on the enzymatic and transcriptional activity of the dimerization cofactor for hepatocyte nuclear factor 1. *Proc Natl Acad Sci USA* **94**:491, 1997.
109. Sourdive DJD, Transy C, Garbay S, et al: The bifunctional DCoH protein binds to HNF1 independently of its 4α-carbinolamine dehydratase activity. *Nucleic Acids Res* **25**:1476, 1982.
110. Ledley FD, Grenett HE, Dunbar BS, et al: Mouse phenylalanine hydroxylase. Homology and divergence from human phenylalanine hydroxylase. *Biochem J* **267**:399, 1990.
111. Kaufman S: *Tetrahydropterin: Basic Biochemistry and Role in Human Disease*. Baltimore, Johns Hopkins University Press, 1997.
112. Konecki DS, Wang Y, Trefz FK, et al: Structural characterization of the 5′ region of the human phenylalanine hydroxylase gene. *Biochemistry* **31**:8363, 1992.
113. Wang Y, Demayo JL, Hahn TM, et al: Tissue- and development-specific expression of the human phenylalanine hydroxylase/chloramphenicol acetyltransferase fusion gene in transgenic mice. *J Biol Chem* **267**:15,105, 1992.
114. Wang Y, Hahn TM, Tsai SY, et al: Functional characterization of a unique liver gene promoter. *J Biol Chem* **269**:9137, 1994.
115. Faust DM, Catherin AM, Barbaux S, et al: The activity of the highly inducible mouse phenylalanine hydroxylase gene promoter is dependent upon a tissue-specific, hormone-inducible enhancer. *Mol Cell Biol* **16**:3125, 1996.
116. Pontoglio M, Barra J, Hadchouel M, et al: Hepatocyte nuclear factor 1 inactivation results in hepatic dysfunction, phenylketonuria, and renal Fanconi syndrome. *Cell* **84**:575, 1996.
117. Lei X, Kaufman S: Identification of hepatic nuclear factor 1 binding sites in the 5′ flanking region of the human phenylalanine hydroxylase gene: Implication of a dual function of phenylalanine hydroxylase stimulator in the phenylalanine hydroxylation system. *Proc Natl Acad Sci USA* **95**:1500, 1998.
118. Kaufman S: Metabolism of phenylalanine hydroxylation cofactor. *J Biol Chem* **242**:3934, 1967.
119. Brenneman AR, Kaufman S: The role of tetrahydropteridine in the enzymatic conversion of tyrosine to 3,4-dihydroxyphenylalanine. *Biochem Biophys Res Commun* **17**:177, 1964.
120. Shiman R, Akino M, Kaufman S: Solubilization and partial purification of tyrosine hydroxylase from bovine adrenal medulla. *J Biol Chem* **246**:1330, 1971.
121. Friedman PA, Kappelman AH, Kaufman S: Partial purification and characterization of tryptophan hydroxylase from rabbit hindbrain. *J Biol Chem* **247**:4165, 1972.
122. Kaufman S, Fisher DB: Purification and some physical properties of phenylalanine hydroxylase from rat liver. *J Biol Chem* **245**:4745, 1970.
123. Parniak MA, Kaufman S: Catalytically active oligomeric species of phenylalanine hydroxylases. *Biochemistry* **24**:3379, 1985.
124. Shiman R, Gray DW, Pater A: A simple purification of phenylalanine hydroxylase using a novel pteridine matrix. *J Biol Chem* **254**:11,300, 1979.
125. Tourian A: Activation of phenylalanine hydroxylase by phenylalanine. *Biochim Biophys Acta* **242**:345, 1971.
126. Doskeland AL, Ljones T, Skotland T, et al: Phenylalanine-4-monooxygenase from bovine and rat liver: Some physical and chemical properties. *Neurochem Res* **7**:407, 1982.
127. Webber S, Harzer G, Whiteley JM: Isolation of rat liver phenylalanine hydroxylase using a novel pteridine matrix. *Anal Biochem* **106**:63, 1980.
128. Kappock JT, Harkins PC, Friedenberg S, et al: Spectroscopic and kinetic properties of unphosphorylated rat hepatic phenylalanine hydroxylase expressed in *Escherichia coli*: Comparison of resting and activated states. *J Biol Chem* **270**:30,532, 1995.
129. Hufton SE, Jennings IG, Cotton RG: Structure/function analysis of the domains required for the multimerisation of phenylalanine hydroxylase. *Biochim Biophys Acta* **1382**:295, 1998.
130. Martinez A, Knappskog PM, Olafsdottir S, et al: Expression of recombinant human phenylalanine hydroxylase as fusion protein in *Escherichia coli* circumvents proteolytic degradation by host cell proteases. *Biochem J* **306**:589, 1995.
131. Kowlessur D, Citron BA, Kaufman S: Recombinant human phenylalanine hydroxylase: Novel regulatory and structural properties. *Arch Biochem Biophys* **333**:85, 1996.
132. Parniak MA: Organization of the catalytic and regulatory sites of rat liver phenylalanine hydroxylase, in Curtius H-C, Blau N (eds): *Unconjugated Pterins and Related Biogenic Amines*. Berlin, Walter de Gruyter, 1987, p 327.
133. Abita J, Milstien S, Chang N, et al: In vitro activation of rat liver phenylalanine hydroxylase by phosphorylation. *J Biol Chem* **251**:5310, 1976.
134. Donlon J, Kaufman S: Modification of the multiple forms of rat hepatic phenylalanine hydroxylase by in vitro phosphorylation. *Biochem Biophys Res Commun* **78**:1011, 1977.
135. Citron BA, Davis MD, Kaufman S: Purification and biochemical characterization of recombinant rat liver phenylalanine hydroxylase produced in *Escherichia coli. Protein Exp Purif* **3**:93, 1992.
136. Knappskog PM, Flatmark T, Aarden JM, et al: Structure/function relationships in human phenylalanine hydroxylase: Effect of terminal deletions on the oligomerization, activation and cooperativity of substrate binding to the enzyme. *Eur J Biochem* **242**:813, 1996.
137. Curtius H, Matasovic A, Schoedon G, et al: 7-Substituted pterins. *J Biol Chem* **265**:3932, 1990.
138. Alder C, Ghisla S, Rebrin I, et al: Suspected pterin-4α-carbinolamine dehydratase deficiency: Hyperphenylalaninemia due to inhibition of phenylalanine hydroxylase by tetrahydro-7-biopterin. *J Inherited Metab Dis* **15**:405, 1992.
139. Delvalle JA, Greengard O: The regulation of phenylalanine hydroxylase in rat tissues in vivo: The maintenance of high plasma phenylalanine concentrations in sucking rats — A model for phenylketonuria. *Biochem J* **154**:613, 1976.
140. Kwok SCM, Ledley FD, Dilella AG, et al: Nucleotide sequence of a full-length complementary DNA clone and amino acid sequence of human phenylalanine hydroxylase. *Biochemistry* **24**:556, 1985.
141. Fisher DB, Kaufman S: The stimulation of rat liver phenylalanine hydroxylase by lysolecithin and alpha-chymotrypsin. *J Biol Chem* **248**:4345, 1973.
142. Iwaki M, Phillips RS, Kaufman S: Proteolytic modification of the amino-terminal and carboxyl-terminal regions of rat hepatic phenylalanine hydroxylase. *J Biol Chem* **261**:2051, 1986.

143. Gibbs BS, Wojchowski D, Benkovic SJ: Expression of rat liver phenylalanine hydroxylase in insect cells and site-directed mutagenesis of putative non-heme iron-binding sites. *J Biol Chem* **268**:8046, 1993.
144. Stoll J, Kozak CA, Goldman D: Characterization and chromosomal mapping of a cDNA encoding tryptophan hydroxylase from a mouse mastocytoma cell line. *Genomics* **7**:88, 1990.
145. Hufton SE, Jennings IG, Cotton GH: Structure and function on the aromatic amino acid hydroxylases. *Biochem J* **311**:353, 1995.
146. Marvit J, Dilella AG, Brayton K, et al: GT to AT transition at a splice donor site causes skipping of the preceding exon in phenylketonuria. *Nucleic Acids Res* **15**:5613, 1987.
147. Waters PJ, Parniak MA, Nowacki P, et al: In vitro expression analysis of mutations in phenylalanine hydroxylase: Linking genotype to phenotype and structure to function. *Hum Mutat* **11**:14, 1998.
148. Dilella AG, Marvit J, Brayton K, et al: An amino-acid substitution involved in phenylketonuria is in linkage disequilibrium with DNA haplotype 2. *Nature* **327**:333, 1987.
149. Okano Y, Eisensmith RC, Guttler F, et al: Molecular basis of phenotypic heterogeneity in phenylketonuria. *N Engl J Med* **324**:1232, 1991.
150. Doskeland AP, Flatmark T: Recombinant human phenylalanine hydroxylase is a substrate for the ubiquitin-conjugating enzyme system. *Biochem J* **319**:941, 1996.
151. Fisher DB, Kirkwood R, Kaufman S: Rat liver phenylalanine hydroxylase, an iron enzyme. *J Biol Chem* **247**:5161, 1972.
152. Gottschall DW, Dietrich RF, Benkovic SJ, et al: Phenylalanine hydroxylase. Correlation of the iron content with activity and the preparation and reconstitution of the apoenzyme. *J Biol Chem* **257**:845, 1982.
153. Gillam SS, Woo SLC, Woolf LI: The isolation and properties of phenylalanine hydroxylase from rat liver. *Biochem J* **139**:731, 1974.
154. Fisher DB, Kaufman S: The stimulation of rat liver phenylalanine hydroxylase by phospholipids. *J Biol Chem* **247**:2250, 1972.
155. Parniak MA, Kaufman S: Rat liver phenylalanine hydroxylase: Activation by sulfhydryl modification. *J Biol Chem* **256**:6876, 1981.
156. Ayling JE, Helfand GD: Effect of pteridine cofactor structure on regulation of phenylalanine hydroxylase activity, in Pfleiderer W (ed): *Chemistry and Biology of Pteridines*. New York, Walter de Gruyter, 1975, p 304.
157. Shiman R, Gray DW: Substrate activation of phenylalanine hydroxylase: A kinetic characterization. *J Biol Chem* **255**:4793, 1980.
158. Phillips RS, Kaufman S: Ligand effects on the phosphorylation states of hepatic phenylalanine hydroxylase. *J Biol Chem* **259**:2474, 1984.
159. Davis MD, Parniak MA, Kaufman S, et al: Structure-function relationships of phenylalanine hydroxylase revealed by radiation target analysis. *Arch Biochem Biophys* **325**:235, 1996.
160. Davis MD, Parniak MA, Kaufman S, et al: The role of phenylalanine in structure-function relationships of phenylalanine hydroxylase revealed by radiation target analysis. *Proc Natl Acad Sci USA* **94**:491, 1997.
161. Gibbs BS, Benkovic SJ: Affinity labeling of the active site and the reactive sulfhydryl associated with activation of rat liver phenylalanine hydroxylase. *Biochemistry* **30**:6795, 1991.
162. Jennings I, Cotton R: Structural similarities among enzyme pterin binding sites as demonstrated by a monoclonal anti-idiotypic antibody. *J Biol Chem* **265**:1885, 1990.
163. Jennings IG, Kemp BE, Cotton RGH: Localization of cofactor binding sites with monoclonal anti-idiotype antibodies: Phenylalanine hydroxylase. *Proc Natl Acad Sci USA* **88**:5734, 1991.
164. Knappskog PM, Martinez A: Effect of mutations at Cys237 on the activation stage and activity of human phenylalanine hydroxylase. *FEBS Lett* **409**:7, 1997.
165. Phillips RS, Parniak MA, Kaufman S: Spectroscopic investigation of ligand interaction of hepatic phenylalanine hydroxylase: Evidence for a conformational change. *Biochemistry* **23**:3836, 1984.
166. Green AK, Cotton RGH, Jennings I, et al: Experimental determination of the phosphorylation state of phenylalanine hydroxylase. *Biochem J* **265**:563, 1990.
167. Wretborn M, Humble E, Ragnarsson U, et al: Amino acid sequence at the phosphorylation site of rat liver phenylalanine hydroxylase and phosphorylation of a corresponding peptide. *Biochem Biophys Res Commun* **93**:403, 1980.
168. Barranger JA, Geiger PJ, Nuzino A, et al: Isozymes of phenylalanine hydroxylase. *Science* **175**:903, 1972.
169. Donlon J, Kaufman S: Relationship between the multiple forms of rat hepatic phenylalanine hydroxylase and degree of phosphorylation. *J Biol Chem* **255**:2146, 1980.
170. Jedlicki E, Kaufman S, Milstien S: Partial purification and characterization of rat liver phenylalanine hydroxylase phosphatase. *J Biol Chem* **252**:7711, 1977.
171. Kaufman S: Regulation of the activity of hepatic phenylalanine hydroxylase. *Adv Enzyme Regul* **25**:37, 1986.
172. Alemany S, Tung HYL, Shenolkar S, et al: The protein phosphatases involved in cellular regulation: Antibody to protein phosphatase-2A as a probe of phosphatase structure and function. *Eur J Biochem* **145**:51, 1984.
173. Pelech S, Cohen P, Fisher MJ, et al: The protein phosphatases involved in cellular regulation: Glycolysis, gluconeogenesis and aromatic amino acid breakdown in rat liver. *Eur J Biochem* **145**:39, 1984.
174. Ingebritsen TA, Cohen P: Protein phosphatases: Properties and role in cellular regulation. *Science* **221**:331, 1983.
175. Donlon J, Kaufman S: Glucagon stimulation of rat hepatic phenylalanine hydroxylase through phosphorylation in vivo. *J Biol Chem* **253**:6657, 1978.
176. Abita J, Chamras H, Rosselin G, et al: Hormonal control of phenylalanine hydroxylase activity in isolated rat hepatocytes. *Biochem Biophys Res Commun* **92**:912, 1980.
177. Carr FPA, Pogson CI: Phenylalanine metabolism in isolated liver cells: Effects of glucagon and diabetes. *Biochem J* **198**:655, 1981.
178. Garrison JC, Wagner JD: Glucagon and the Ca^{2+}-linked hormones angiotensin II, norepinephrine, and vasopressin stimulate the phosphorylation of distinct substrates in intact hepatocytes. *J Biol Chem* **257**:13,155, 1982.
179. Santana MA, Fisher MJ, Baie AJ, et al: The effect of experimental diabetes on phenylalanine metabolism in isolated liver cells. *Biochem J* **227**:169, 1985.
180. Donlon J, Beirne D: Modifications of rat hepatic phenylalanine hydroxylase due to diabetes or high protein diet. *Biochem Biophys Res Commun* **108**:746, 1982.
181. Doskeland P, Doskeland SO, Ogreid D, et al: The effect of ligands of phenylalanine 4-monooxygenase on the cAMP-dependent phosphorylation of the enzyme. *J Biol Chem* **257**:11,242, 1984.
182. Shiman R, Mortimore GE, Schworer CM, et al: Regulation of phenylalanine hydroxylase activity by phenylalanine in vivo, in vitro and in perfused rat liver. *J Biol Chem* **257**:11,213, 1982.
183. Shiman R: Relationship between the substrate activation site and catalytic site of phenylalanine hydroxylase. *J Biol Chem* **225**:10,029, 1980.
184. Muller WA, Faloona GR, Aquilar-Parada F, et al: Abnormal α-cell function in diabetes. *N Engl J Med* **283**:109, 1970.
185. Rocha DM, Faloona GR, Unger RH: Glucagon-stimulating activity of 20 amino acids in dogs. *Clin J Invest* **51**:2346, 1972.
186. Guttler F, Kuhl C, Pedersen L, et al: Effects of oral phenylalanine load on plasma glucagon, insulin, amino acid and glucose concentrations in man. *Scand J Clin Lab Invest* **38**:255, 1978.
187. Smith SC, Kemp BE, McAdam WJ, et al: Two apparent molecular weight forms of human and monkey phenylalanine hydroxylase are due to phosphorylation. *J Biol Chem* **259**:11,284, 1984.
188. Abita J, Blandin-Savoja F, Rey F: Phenylalanine hydroxylase: Evidence that the enzyme from human liver might not be a phosphoprotein. *Biochem Int* **7**:727, 1983.
189. McClure D, Miller M, Shiman R: Correlation of phenylalanine hydroxylase activity with cell density in cultured hepatoma cells. *Exp Cell Res* **90**:31, 1975.
190. Tourian A: Control of phenylalanine hydroxylase synthesis in tissue culture by serum and insulin. *J Cell Physiol* **87**:15, 1976.
191. Sorimachi K, Niwa A, Yasumura Y: Hormonal regulation of tyrosine aminotransferase and phenylalanine hydroxylase in rat hepatoma cells continuously cultured in a serum-free medium: Effect of serum, dexamethasone and insulin. *Cell Struct Funct* **6**:61, 1981.
192. Tourian A, Treiman L, Abe K: Three immunologically distinct isozymes of phenylalanine hydroxylase. *Biochemistry* **14**:4055, 1975.
193. Tourian A: A unique identity of rat hepatoma phenylalanine hydroxylase. *Biochem Biophys Res Commun* **68**:51, 1976.
194. Miller MR, Shiman R: Hydrocortisone induction of phenylalanine hydroxylase isozymes in cultured hepatoma cells. *Biochem Biophys Res Commun* **68**:740, 1976.
195. Reem GH, Kretchmer N: Development of phenylalanine hydroxylase in liver of the rat. *Proc Soc Exp Biol Med* **96**:458, 1957.

196. Kenny FT, Kretchmer N: Hepatic metabolism of phenylalanine during development. *J Clin Invest* **38**:2189, 1959.
197. Brenneman AR, Kaufman S: Characteristics of the phenylalanine-hydroxylating system in newborn rats. *J Biol Chem* **240**:3617, 1965.
198. Friedman PA, Kaufman S: A study of the development of phenylalanine hydroxylase in fetuses of several mammalian species. *Arch Biochem Biophys* **146**:321, 1971.
199. Ryan WL, Orr W: Phenylalanine conversion to tyrosine by the human fetal liver. *Arch Biochem Biophys* **113**:684, 1986.
200. Jakubovic A: Phenylalanine-hydroxylating system in the human fetus at different development ages. *Biochim Biophys Acta* **237**:469, 1971.
201. Raiha NCR: Phenylalanine hydroxylase in human liver during development. *Pediatr Res* **7**:1, 1973.
202. Ledley FD, Koch R, Jew K, et al: Phenylalanine hydroxylase expression in liver of a fetus with phenylketonuria. *Pediatrics* **113**:463, 1988.
203. Tayeh MA, Marletta MA: Macrophage oxidation of L-arginine to nitric oxide, nitrite, and nitrate: Tetrahydrobiopterin is required as a cofactor. *J Biol Chem* **264**:19,654, 1989.
204. Kaufman S: The phenylalanine hydroxylating system. *Adv Enzymol Relat Areas Mol Biol* **67**:77, 1994.
205. Pollock RJ, Kaufman S: Dihydropteridine reductase may function in tetrahydrofolate metabolism. *J Neurochem* **31**:115, 1978.
206. Kaufman S, Holtzman NA, Milstien S, et al: Phenylketonuria due to a deficiency of dihydropteridine reductase. *N Engl J Med* **293**:785, 1975.
207. Milstien S, Holtzman NA, O'Flynn ME, et al: Hyperphenylalaninemia due to dihydropteridine reductase deficiency. *J Pediatr* **89**:763, 1976.
208. Firgaira FA, Cotton RGH, Danks DM: Dihydropteridine reductase deficiency diagnosis by assays on peripheral blood-cells. *Lancet* **2**:1260, 1979.
209. Narisawa K, Arai N, Ishizawa S, et al: Dihydropteridine reductase deficiency: Diagnosis by leukocyte enzyme assay. *Clin Chim Acta* **105**:335, 1980.
210. Narisawa K, Arai N, Hayakawa H, et al: Diagnosis of dihydropteridine reductase deficiency by erythrocyte assay. *Pediatrics* **68**:591, 1981.
211. Abelson HT, Gorka C, Beardsley GP: Identification of dihydropteridine reductase in human platelets. *Blood* **53**:116, 1979.
212. Shen R, Abell CW: Purification of dihydropteridine reductase from human platelets. *J Neurosci Res* **6**:193, 1981.
213. Rembold S, Gyure WL: Biochemistry of the pteridines. *Angew Chem* **11**:1061, 1972.
214. Duch DS, Smith GK: Biosynthesis and function of tetrahydrobiopterin. *J Nutr Biochem* **2**:411, 1991.
215. Robson KJH, Beattie W, James RJ, et al: Sequence comparison of rat liver phenylalanine hydroxylase and its cDNA clones. *Biochemistry* **23**:5671, 1984.
216. Friedman PA, Kaufman S: Some characteristics of partially purified human liver phenylalanine hydroxylase. *Biochim Biophys Acta* **293**:56, 1973.
217. Dahl H-H, Mercer JFB: Isolation and sequence of a cDNA clone which contains the complete coding region of rat phenylalanine hydroxylase: Structural homology with tyrosine hydroxylase, glucocorticoid regulation, and use of alternate polyadenylation sites. *J Biol Chem* **261**:4148, 1986.
218. Speer A, Dahl H-H, Riess O, et al: Typing of families with classical phenylketonuria using three alleles of the Hind III linked restriction fragment polymorphism, detectable with a phenylalanine hydroxylase cDNA probe. *Clin Genet* **29**:491, 1986.
219. Ledley FD, Grenett HE, Dilella AG, et al: Gene transfer and gene expression of human phenylalanine hydroxylase. *Science* **228**:77, 1985.
220. Choo KH, Filby RG, Jennings IG, et al: Vectors for expression and amplification of cDNA in mammalian cells: Expression of rat phenylalanine hydroxylase. *DNA* **5**:529, 1986.
221. Dilella AG, Kwok SCM, Ledley FD, et al: Molecular structure and polymorphic map of human phenylalanine hydroxylase gene. *Biochemistry* **25**:743, 1986.
222. McDowell IL, Fisher MJ: The immediate 5′-flanking region of the rat phenylalanine hydroxylase-encoding gene. *Gene* **153**:289, 1995.
223. McDowell IL, Fisher MJ: Analysis of the 5′-flanking region of the rat phenylalanine hydroxylase gene. *Biochem Soc Trans* **24**:424S, 1996.
224. Eisensmith RC, Woo SLC: Molecular genetics of phenylketonuria: From molecular anthropology to gene therapy, in Hall JC, Dunlap JC (eds): Advances in Genetics. **32**:199, 1995.
225. Fauquet M, Grima B, Lamaroux A, et al: Cloning of quail tyrosine hydroxylase: Amino acid homology with other hydroxylases discloses functional domains. *J Neurochem* **50**:142, 1988.
226. Grenett HE, Ledley FD, Reed LL, et al: Full-length cDNA for rabbit tryptophan hydroxylase: Functional domains and evolution of aromatic amino acid hydroxylases. *Proc Natl Acad Sci USA* **84**:5530, 1987.
227. Stoll J, Goldman D: Isolation and structural characterization of the murine tryptophan hydroxylase gene. *J Neurosci Res* **28**:457, 1991.
228. Neckameyer WS, White K: A single locus encodes both phenylalanine hydroxylase and tryptophan hydroxylase activities in *Drosophila*. *J Biol Chem* **267**:4199, 1992.
229. Campbell DG, Hardie DG, Vulliet PR: Identification of four phosphorylation sites in the N-terminal region of tyrosine hydroxylase. *J Biol Chem* **261**:10,489, 1986.
230. Pigeon D, Ferrara P, Gros F, et al: Rat pheochromocytoma tyrosine hydroxylase is phosphorylated on serine 40 by an associated protein kinase. *J Biol Chem* **262**:6155, 1987.
231. Kobayashi K, Kaneda N, Ichinose H, et al: Structure of the human tyrosine hydroxylase gene: Alternative splicing from a single gene accounts for generation of four mRNA types. *J Biochem* **103**:907, 1988.
232. Nagatsu T: Genes for human catecholamine-synthesizing enzymes. *Neurosci Res* **12**:315, 1991.
233. Cotton RGH, McKusick V, Scriver CR: The HUGO Mutation Database Initiative. *Science* **279**:11, 1998.
234. Antonarakis SE and the Nomenclature Working Group: Recommendations for a nomenclature system for human gene mutations. *Hum Mutat* **11**:1, 1998.
235. John SWM, Rozen R, Laframboise R, et al: Novel PKU mutation on haplotype 2 in French-Canadians. *Am J Hum Genet* **45**:905, 1989.
236. Shedlovsky A, McDonald JD, Smyula D, et al: Mouse models of human phenylketonuria. *Genetics* **134**:1205, 1993.
237. Cooper DN, Krawczak M: *Human Gene Mutation*. Oxford, UK, Bios Scientific, 1993.
238. Cotton RGH, Scriver CR: Proof of "disease-causing" mutation. *Hum Mutat* **12**:1, 1998.
239. Morales G, Requena GM, Jimenez-Ruiz A, et al: Sequence and expression of the *Drosophila* phenylalanine hydroxylase mRNA. *Gene* **93**:213, 1990.
240. Onishi A, Liotta LJ, Benkovic SJ: Cloning and expression of *Chromobacterium violaceum* phenylalanine hydroxylase in *Escherichia coli* and comparison of amino acid sequence with mammalian aromatic amino acid hydroxylases. *J Biol Chem* **266**:18,454, 1991.
241. Lidsky AS, Ledley FD, Dilella AG, et al: Extensive restriction site polymorphism at the human phenylalanine hydroxylase locus and application in prenatal diagnosis of phenylketonuria. *Am J Hum Genet* **37**:619, 1985.
242. Dworniczak B, Wedemeyer N, Horst J: PCR detection of the BglII RFLP at the human phenylalanine hydroxylase (PAH) locus. *Nucleic Acids Res* **19**:1958, 1991.
243. Dworniczak B, Wedemeyer N, Eigel A, et al: PCR detection of the PvuII (Ea) RFLP at the human phenylalanine hydroxylase (PAH) locus. *Nucleic Acids Res* **19**:1958, 1991.
244. Wedemeyer N, Dworniczak B, Horst J: PCR detection of the MspI (Aa) RFLP at the human phenylalanine hydroxylase (PAH) locus. *Nucleic Acids Res* **19**:1959, 1991.
245. Goltsov AA, Eisensmith RC, Woo SLC: Detection of the XmnI RFLP at the human phenylalanine hydroxylase locus by PCR. *Nucleic Acids Res* **20**:927, 1992.
246. Goltsov AA, Eisensmith RC, Konecki DS, et al: Associations between mutations and a VNTR in the human phenylalanine hydroxylase gene. *Am J Hum Genet* **51**:627, 1992.
247. Latorra D, Stern CM, Schanfield MS: Characterization of human AFLP systems apolipoprotein B, phenylalanine hydroxylase, and D1S80. *PCR Methods Applications* **3**:351, 1994.
248. Goltsov AA, Eisensmith RC, Naughton ER, et al: A single polymorphic STR system in the human phenylalanine hydroxylase gene permits rapid prenatal diagnosis and carrier screening for phenylketonuria. *Hum Mol Genet* **2**:577, 1993.
249. Zschocke J, Graham CA, McKnight JJ, et al: The STR system in the human phenylalanine hydroxylase gene: True fragment length obtained with fluorescent labelled PCR primers. *Acta Paediatr Scand Suppl* **407**:41, 1994.
250. Giannattasio S, Lattanzio P, Bobba A, et al: Detection of microsatellites by ethidium bromide staining: The analysis of an STR system in the human phenylalanine hydroxylase gene. *Mol Cell Probes* **11**:81, 1997.

251. Ramus SJ, Cotton RGH: Polymorphism in the 3′ untranslated region of the phenylalanine hydroxylase gene detected by enzyme mismatch cleavage: Evolution of haplotypes. *Hum Genet* **96**:741, 1995.
252. Lichter-Konecki U, Schlotter M, Konecki DS: DNA sequence polymorphisms in exonic and intronic regions of the human phenylalanine hydroxylase gene aid in the identification of alleles. *Hum Genet* **94**:307, 1994.
253. Eisensmith RC, Goltsov AA, Woo SL: A simple, rapid, and highly informative PCR-based procedure for prenatal diagnosis and carrier screening of phenylketonuria. *Prenat Diagn* **14**:1113, 1994.
254. Eisensmith RC, Woo SLC: Updated listing of haplotypes at the human phenylalanine hydroxylase (PAH) locus [Letters to the editor]. *Am J Hum Genet* **51**:1445, 1992.
255. Chakraborty R, Lidsky AS, Daiger SP, et al: Polymorphic DNA haplotypes at the human phenylalanine hydroxylase locus and their relationship with phenylketonuria. *Hum Genet* **76**:40, 1987.
256. Feingold J, Guilloud-Bataille M, Feingold N, et al: Linkage disequilibrium in the human phenylalanine hydroxylase. *Dev Brain Dysfunct* **6**:26, 1993.
257. Degioanni A, Darlu P: Analysis of the molecular variance at the phenylalanine hydroxylase (PAH) locus. *Eur J Hum Genet* **2**:166, 1994.
257a. Kidd JR, Pakstis AJ, Zhao H, et al: Haplotypes and linkage disequilibrium at the phenylalanine hydroxylase locus, *PA*, in a global representation of populations. *Am J Hum Genet* **66**:1882, 2000.
258. Daiger SP, Chakraborty R, Reed L, et al: Polymorphic DNA haplotypes at the phenylalanine hydroxylase (PAH) locus in European families with phenylketonuria (PKU). *Am J Hum Genet* **45**:310, 1989.
259. Daiger SP, Reed L, Huang S-H, et al: Polymorphic DNA haplotypes at the phenylalanine hydroxylase (PAH) locus in Asian families with phenylketonuria (PKU). *Am J Hum Genet* **45**:319, 1989.
260. Romano V, Dianzani I, Ponzone A, et al: Prenatal diagnosis by minisatellite analysis in Italian families with phenylketonuria. *Prenat Diagn* **14**:959, 1994.
261. Scriver CR, Byck S, Prevost L, et al: The phenylalanine hydroxylase locus: A marker for the history of phenylketonuria and human genetic diversity. *Ciba Found Symp* **197**:73, 1996.
262. Byck S, Morgan K, Blanc L, et al: The *PAH* locus and population genetic variation: The Quebec example [abstr]. *Am J Hum Genet* **59**:A33, 1996.
263. Bender C, Buchler A, Schmidt-Mader B, et al: Haplotype analysis and a new Msp1-polymorphism at the phenylalanine hydroxylase gene in the Arabian population. *Eur J Pediatr* **153**:392, 1994.
264. Guldberg P, Henriksen KF, Mammen KC, et al: Large deletions in the phenylalanine hydroxylase gene as a cause of phenylketonuria in India. *J Inherited Metab Dis* **29**:845, 1997.
264a. Scriver CR, Waters PJ: Monogenic traits are not simple: Lessons from phenylketonuria. *Trends Genet* **15**:267, 1999.
265. Udenfriend S, Bessman S: The hydroxylation of phenylalanine and antipyrene in phenylpyruvic oligophrenia. *J Biol Chem* **203**:961, 1953.
266. Wallace HW, Moldave K, Meisier A: Studies on conversion of phenylalanine to tyrosine in phenylpyruvic oligophrenia. *Proc Soc Exp Biol Med* **94**:632, 1957.
267. Mitoma C, Auld RM, Udenfriend S: On the nature of enzymatic defect in phenylpyruvic oligophrenia. *Proc Soc Exp Biol Med* **94**:634, 1957.
268. Kaufman S: Phenylalanine hydroxylation cofactor in phenylketonuria. *Science* **128**:1506, 1958.
269. Cotton RGH: The primary molecular defects in phenylketonuria and its variants. *Int J Biochem* **8**:333, 1977.
270. Choo KH, Cotton RG, Danks DM, et al: Genetics of the mammalian phenylalanine hydroxylase system: Studies of human liver phenylalanine hydroxylase subunit structure and of mutations in phenylketonuria. *Biochem J* **181**:285, 1979.
271. Choo KH, Cotton RGH, Danks DM, et al: Genetics of the mammalian phenylalanine hydroxylase system: Studies of human liver phenylalanine hydroxylase subunit structure and of mutations in phenylketonuria. *Biochem J* **181**:285, 1979.
272. Choo KH, Cotton RGH, Jennings IG, et al: Observations indicating the nature of the mutation in phenylketonuria. *J Inherit Metab Dis* **2**:79, 1980.
273. Bartholomé K, Dresel A: Studies on the molecular defect in phenylketonuria and hyperphenylalaninemia using antibodies against phenylalanine hydroxylase. *J Inherit Metab Dis* **5**:7, 1982.
274. Yamashita M, Minato S, Arai M, et al: Purification of phenylalanine hydroxylase from human adult and foetal livers with a monoclonal antibody. *Biochem Biophys Res Commun* **133**:202, 1985.
275. Friedman PA, Fisher DB, Kang ES, et al: Detection of hepatic phenylalanine 4-hydroxylase in classical phenylketonuria. *Proc Natl Acad Sci USA* **70**:552, 1973.
276. Friedman PA, Kaufman S, Kang-Song E: Nature of the molecular defect in phenylketonuria and hyperphenylalaninemia. *Nature* **240**:157, 1972.
277. Bartholomé K, Lutz P, Bickel H: Determination of phenylalanine hydroxylase activity in patients with phenylketonuria and hyperphenylalaninemia. *Pediatr Res* **9**:899, 1975.
278. Bartholomé K, Olek K, Trefz F: Compound heterozygotes in hyperphenylalaninemia. *Hum Genet* **65**:405, 1984.
279. Kaufman S, Max EE, Kang ES: Phenylalanine hydroxylase activity in liver biopsies from hyperphenylalaninemia heterozygotes: Deviation from proportionality with gene dosage. *Pediatr Res* **9**:632, 1975.
280. Grimm U, Knapp A, Schlenza K, et al: Phenylalaninhydroxylase-Aktivität beiketerozygoten Analgeträgen für das Phenylketerurie-Gen. *Acta Biol Med Germ* **36**:1179, 1977.
281. Bartholomé K: Genetics and biochemistry of the phenylketonuria: Present state. *Hum Genet* **51**:241, 1979.
282. Curtius HC, Völlmin JA, Baerlocher K: The use of deuterated phenylalanine for the elucidation of the phenylalanine-tyrosine metabolism. *Clin Chim Acta* **37**:277, 1972.
283. Trefz FK, Erlenmaier T, Hunneman DH, et al: Sensitive in vivo assay of the phenylalanine hydroxylating system with a small intravenous dose of heptadeutero-L-phenylalanine using high pressure liquid chromatography and capillary gas chromatography/mass fragmentography. *Clin Chim Acta* **99**:211, 1979.
284. Trefz FK, Bartholomé K, Bickel H, et al: In vivo residual activities of the phenylalanine hydroxylating system in phenylketonuria and variants. *J Inherited Metab Dis* **4**:101, 1981.
285. Trefz FK, Byrd DJ, Blaskovics ME, et al: Determination of deuterium labelled phenylalanine and tyrosine in human plasma with high pressure liquid chromatography and mass spectrometry. *Clin Chim Acta* **73**:431, 1976.
286. Clarke JTR, Bier DM: The conversion of phenylalanine to tyrosine in man: Direct measurement by continuous intravenous tracer infusions of L-(ring-$^2H_5$) phenylalanine and L-(1-^{13}C) tyrosine in the postabsorptive state. *Metabolism* **31**:999, 1982.
287. Matalon R, Matthews DE, Michals K, et al: The use of deuterated phenylalanine for the in vivo assay of phenylalanine hydroxylase activity in children. *J Inherit Metab Dis* **5**:17, 1982.
288. Lehmann WD, Theobald N, Fisher R, et al: Stereospecificity of phenylalanine plasma kinetics and hydroxylation in man following oral application of a stable isotope-labelled pseudo-racemic mixture of L- and D-phenylalanine. *Clin Chim Acta* **128**:181, 1983.
289. Lehmann WD, Heinrich HC: Oral versus intravenous L-phenylalanine loading compared by simultaneous application of L-(^2H_5N) phenylalanine. *Clin Chim Acta* **147**:261, 1985.
290. Guldberg P, Mikkelsen I, Henriksen KF, et al: In vivo assessment of mutations in the phenylalanine hydroxylase gene by phenylalanine loading: Characterization of seven common mutations. *Eur J Pediatr* **154**:551, 1995.
291. Svensson E, Eisensmith RC, Dworniczak B, et al: Two missense mutations causing mild hyperphenylalaninemia associated with DNA haplotype 12. *Hum Mutat* **1**:129, 1992.
292. Okano Y, Hase Y, Lee D-H, et al: Molecular and population genetics of phenylketonuria in Orientals: Correlation between phenotype and genotype. *J Inherited Metab Dis* **17**:156, 1994.
293. Svensson E, Von Dobeln U, Eisensmith RC, et al: Relation between genotype and phenotype in Swedish phenylketonuria and hyperphenylalaninemia patients. *Eur J Pediatr* **152**:132, 1993.
294. Flatmark T, Knappskog PM, Bjorgo E, Martinez A: Molecular characterization of disease related mutant forms of human phenylalanine hydroxylase and tyrosine hydroxylase [abstr] *Chemistry & Biology of Pteridines & Folates* 1997, Pfliederer W, Rokos H (eds.): Blackwell Science, Berlin, 1997, p. 503
295. Ellingsen S, Knappskog PM, Eiken HG: Phenylketonuria splice mutation (EXON6nt-96A $\rightarrow$ g) masquerading as missense mutation (Y204C). *Hum Mutat* **9**:88, 1997.
296. Dianzani I, Knappskog PM, De Sanctis L, et al: Novel missense mutation in the phenylalanine hydroxylase gene leading to complete loss of enzymatic activity. *Hum Mutat* **6**:247, 1995.
297. Knappskog PM, Eiken HG, Martinez A, et al: The PKU mutation S349P causes complete loss of catalytic activity in the recombinant phenylalanine hydroxylase enzyme. *Hum Genet* **95**:171, 1995.
298. Knappskog PM, Eiken HG, Martinez A, et al: PKU mutation (D143G) associated with an apparent high residual enzyme activity:

Expression of a kinetic variant form of phenylalanine hydroxylase in three different systems. *Hum Mutat* **8**:236, 1996.
299. Eiken HG, Knappskog PM, Apold J, et al: PKU mutation G46S associated with increased aggregation and degradation of the phenylalanine hydroxylase enzyme. *Hum Mutat* **7**:228, 1996.
300. Waters PJ, Parniak MA, Hewson AS, et al: Alterations in protein aggregation and degradation due to mild and severe missense mutations (A104D, R157N) in the human phenylalanine hydroxylase gene (*PAH*). *Hum Mutat* **12**:344,1998.
300a. Waters PJ, Parniak MA, Akerman BR, et al: Missense mutations in the phenylalanine hydroxylase gene (*PAH*) can cause accelerated proteolytic turnover of PAH enzyme: A mechanism underlying phenylketonuria. *J Inherit Metab Dis* **22**:208, 1999.
300b. Bjorgo E, Knappskog PM, Martinez A, et al: Partial characterization and three-dimensional-structural localization of eight mutations in exon 7 of the human phenylalanine hydroxylase gene associated with phenylketonuria. *Eur J Biochem* **257**:1, 1998.
300c. Waters PJ, Parnick M, Akerman BR, et al: Characterisation of phenylketonuria missense substitution, distant from the phenylalanine active site, illustrates a paradigm to mechanise a potential reduction of phenotype. *Mol Genet Metab* **69**:101, 2000.
301. Guldberg P, Henriksen FF, Thöny B, et al: Molecular heterogeneity of nonphenylketonuria hyperphenylalaninemia in 25 Danish patients. *Genomics* **21**:453, 1994.
302. Das A: Overproduction of proteins in *E. coli*: Vectors, hosts and strategies. *Methods Enzymol* **182**:93, 1990.
303. Knappskog PM, Haavik J: Tryptophan fluorescence of human phenylalanine hydroxylase produced in *Escherichia coli*. *Biochemistry* **34**:11,790, 1995.
304. Kowlessur D, Yang X, Kaufman S: Further studies of the role of Ser-16 in the regulation of the activity of phenylalanine hydroxylase. *Proc Natl Acad Sci USA* **92**:4743, 1995.
305. Quinsey NS, Lenaghan CM, Dickson PW: Identification of Gln^{313} and Pro^{327} as residues critical for substrate inhibition in tyrosine hydroxylase. *J Neurochem* **66**:908, 1996.
306. Dickson PW, Jennings IG, Cotton RGH: Delineation of the catalytic core of phenylalanine hydroxylase and identification of glutamate 286 as a critical residue for pterin function. *J Biol Chem* **269**:20,369, 1994.
307. Guldberg P, Levy HL, Hanley WB, et al: Phenylalanine hydroxylase gene mutations in the United States: Report from the Maternal PKU Collaborative Study. *Am J Hum Genet* **59**:84, 1996.
308. Fusetti F, Erlandsen H, Flatmark T, et al: Structure of tetrameric human phenylalanine hydroxylase and its implications for phenylketonuria. *J Biol Chem* **273**:16,962, 1998.
309. Flatmark T, Stevens RC: Structural insight into the aromatic amino acid hydroxylases and their disease-related mutant forms. *Chem Res* **99**:2137, 1999.
309a. Erlandsen H, Stevens RC: The structural basis of phenylketonuria. *Mol Genet Metab* **68**:103, 1999.
309b. Erlandsen H, Bjorgo E, Flatmark T, Stevens RC: Crystal structure and site-specific mutagenesis of pterin-bond human phenylalanine hydroxylase. *Biochemistry* **39**:2208, 2000.
310. Svensson E, Von Döbeln U, Eisensmith RC, et al: Relation between genotype and phenotype in Swedish phenylketonuria and hyperphenylalaninemia patients. *Eur J Pediatr* **152**:132, 1993.
311. Eiken HG, Knappskog PM, Motzfeldt K, et al: Phenylketonuria genotypes correlated to metabolic phenotype groups in Norway. *Eur J Pediatr* **155**:544, 1996.
312. Di Silvestre D, Koch R, Groffen J: Different clinical manifestations in three siblings with identical phenylalanine hydroxylase genes. *Am J Hum Genet* **48**:1014, 1991.
313. Güttler F, Guldberg P, Henriksen KF: Mutation genotype of mentally retarded patients with phenylketonuria. *Dev Brain Dysfunct* **6**:92, 1993.
314. Trefz FK, Burgard P, König T, et al: Genotype-phenotype correlations in phenylketonuria. *Clin Chim Acta* **217**:15, 1993.
315. Romeo G, McKusick VA: Phenotypic diversity, allelic series and modifier genes. *Nature Genet* **7**:451, 1994.
316. Summers KM: Relationship between genotype and phenotype in monogenic diseases: Relevance to polygenic diseases. *Hum Mutat* **7**:283, 1996.
317. Lander ES, Schork NJ: Genetic dissection of complex traits. *Science* **265**:2037, 1994.
318. Koch R, Fishler K, Azen C, et al: The relationship of genotype to phenotype in phenylalanine hydroxylase deficiency. *Biochem Mol Med* **60**:92, 1997.
319. Walter JH, Tyfield LA, Holton JB, et al: Biochemical control, genetic analysis and magnetic resonance imaging in patients with phenylketonuria. *Eur J Pediatr* **152**:822, 1993.
320. Weglage J, Moller HE, Wiedermann D, et al: In vivo NMR spectroscopy in patients with phenylketonuria: Clinical significance of interindividual differences in brain phenylalanine concentrations. *J Inherit Metab Dis* **21**:81, 1998.
321. Weglage J, Wiedermann D, Moller H, et al: Pathogenesis of different clinical outcomes in spite of identical genotypes and comparable blood phenylalanine concentration in phenylketonuria. *J Inherit Metab Dis* **21**:181, 1998.
321a. Moller HE, Weglage J, Wiedermann D, Ullrich K: Blood-brain barrier phenylalanine transport and individual vulnerability in phenylketonuria. *J Cereb Blood Flow Metab* **18**:1184, 1998.
321b. Moats RA, Scadeng M, Nelson MD Jr: MR imaging and spectroscopy in PKU. *Ment Retard Dev Disabil Res Rev* **5**:132, 1999.
322. Mayr E: *The Growth of Biological Thought: Diversity, Evolution and Inheritance*. Cambridge, Belknap Press of Harvard University Press, 1982.
323. Zschocke J, Graham CA, Carson DJ, et al: Phenylketonuria mutation analysis in Northern Ireland: A rapid stepwise approach. *Am J Hum Genet* **57**:1311, 1995.
324. Romano V, Guldberg P, Guttler F, et al: PAH deficiency in Italy: Correlations of genotype to phenotype in the Sicilian population. *J Inherit Metab Dis* **19**:15, 1996.
325. Carter KC, Byck S, Waters PJ, et al: Mutation at the phenylalanine hydroxylase gene (*PAH*) and its use to document population genetic variation: The Quebec experience. *Eur J Hum Genet* **6**:61, 1998.
326. Avigad S, Kleiman S, Weinstein M, et al: Compound heterozygosity in nonphenylketonuria hyperphenylalaninemia: The contribution of mutations for classical phenylketonuria. *Am J Hum Genet* **49**:393, 1991.
327. Ledley FD, Levy HL, Woo SLC: Molecular analysis of the inheritance of phenylketonuria and mild hyperphenylalaninemia in families with both disorders. *N Engl J Med* **314**:1276, 1986.
328. Tyfield LA, Meredith AL, Osborn MJ, et al: Genetic analysis of treated and untreated phenylketonuria in one family. *J Med Genet* **27**:564, 1990.
329. Guldberg P, Levy HL, Koch R, et al: Mutation analysis in families with discordant phenotypes of phenylalanine hydroxylase deficiency: Inheritance and expression of the hyperphenylalaninaemias. *J Inherit Metab Dis* **17**:645, 1994.
329a. Lai K, Langley SD, Dembure PP, et al: Duarte allele impairs biostability of human galactose-1-phosphate uridyltransferase in human lymphoblasts. *Hum Mutat* **11**:28, 1998.
330. Guldberg P, Rey F, Zschocke J, et al: A European minicenter study of phenylalanine hydroxylase deficiency: Classification of 105 mutations and a general system for genotype-based prediction of metabolic phenotype. *Am J Hum Genet* **63**:71, 1998.
331. Roch R, Guttler F, Guldberg P, et al: Mild hyperphenylalaninemia and heterozygosity of the phenylalanine hydroxylase gene. *Mol Genet Metab* **63**:148, 1998.
332. Spada M, Dianzani I, Bonetti G, et al: Phenylalanine and tyrosine metabolism in phenylketonuria heterozygotes: Influence of different phenylalanine hydroxylase mutations. *J Inherit Metab Dis* **21**:236, 1998.
333. Svensson E, Iselius L, Hagenfeldt L: Severity of mutation in the phenylalanine hydroxylase gene influences phenylalanine metabolism in phenylketonuria and hyperphenylalaninemia heterozygotes. *J Inherit Metab Dis* **17**:215, 1994.
334. Teebi AS, Farag T: *Genetic Disorders Among Arab Populations*. New York, Oxford University Press, 1997.
335. Cavalli-Sforza LL, Menozzi P, Piazza A: Demic expansions and human evolution. *Science* **259**:639, 1993.
336. Cavalli-Sforza LL, Piazza A: Human genomic diversity in Europe: A summary of recent research and prospects for the future. *Eur J Hum Genet* **1**:3, 1993.
337. Mountain JL, Cavalli-Sforza LL: Multilocus genotypes, a tree of individuals, and human evolutionary history. *Am J Hum Genet* **61**:705, 1997.
338. Cavalli-Sforza LL, Menozzi P, Piazza A: *The History and Geography of Human Genes*. Princeton, Princeton University Press, 1994.
339. Cotton RGH: Current methods of mutation detection. *Mutat Res* **285**:125, 1993.
340. Grompe M: The rapid detection of unknown mutations in nucleic acids. *Nature Genet* **5**:111, 1993.
341. Cotton RGH: *Mutation Detection*. New York, Oxford University Press, 1997.

342. Guldberg P, Güttler F: "Broad-range" DGGE for single-step mutation screening of entire genes: Application to human phenylalanine hydroxylase gene. *Nucleic Acids Res* **22**:880, 1993.
343. Guldberg P, Güttler F: Mutations in the phenylalanine hydroxylase gene: Methods for their characterization. *Acta Paediatr Scand* **407**:27, 1994.
344. Ozalp I, Coskun T, Ceyhan M, et al: Incidence of phenylketonuria and hyperphenylalaninemia in a sample of the newborn population. *J Inherit Metab Dis* **9**(suppl 2):237, 1986.
345. Ozgüç M, Özalp I, Coskun T, et al: Mutation analysis in Turkish phenylketonuria patients. *J Med Genet* **30**:129, 1993.
346. Woolf LI: Phenylketonuria in Turkey, Ireland and West Scotland. *J Inherit Metab Dis* **17**:246, 1994.
347. Hutchesson AC, Bundey S, Preece MA, et al: A comparison of disease and gene frequencies of inborn errors of metabolism among different ethnic groups in the West Midlands, U.K. *J Med Genet* **35**:366, 1998.
348. Saugstad LF: Frequency of phenylketonuria in Norway. *Clin Genet* **7**:40, 1975.
349. Romeo G, Menozzi P, Ferlini A, et al: Incidence of classic PKU in Italy estimated from consanguineous marriages and from neonatal screening. *Clin Genet* **24**:339, 1983.
350. Eisensmith RC, Martinez DR, Kuzman AI, et al: Molecular basis of phenylketonuria and a correlation between genotype and phenotype in a heterogeneous Southeastern US population. *Pediatrics* **97**:512, 1996.
351. Tyfield LA, Stephenson A, Cockburn F, et al: Sequence variation at the phenylalanine hydroxylase gene in the British Isles [abstr]. *Am J Hum Genet* **60**:388, 1997.
352. Wang T, Okano Y, Eisensmith R, et al: Molecular genetics of phenylketonuria in Orientals: Linkage disequilibrium between a termination mutation and haplotype 4 of the phenylalanine hydroxylase gene. *Am J Hum Genet* **45**:675, 1989.
353. Okano Y, Hase Y, Lee D, et al: Frequency and distribution of phenylketonuric mutations in Orientals. *Hum Mutat* **1**:216, 1992.
354. Wang Y, Okano Y, Eisensmith RC, et al: Identification of three novel PKU mutations among Chinese: Evidence for recombination or recurrent mutation at the PAH locus. *Genomics* **10**:449, 1992.
355. Li J, Eisensmith RC, Wang T, et al: Phenylketonuria in China: Identification and characterization of three novel nucleotide substitutions in the human phenylalanine hydroxylase gene. *Hum Mutat* **3**:312, 1994.
356. Gu XF, Zhang M, Chen RG: Phenylketonuria mutations in southern Chinese detected by denaturing gradient gel electrophoresis in exon 7 of *PAH* gene. *J Inherit Metab Dis* **18**:753, 1995.
357. Okano Y, Isshiki G: Newborn mass screening and molecular genetics of phenylketonuria in East Asia. *Southeast Asian J Trop Med Public Health* **26**:123, 1995.
358. Sun G, Jiang L, Zhang X, et al: Novel mutations identified in exon 7 of phenylalanine hydroxylase gene in Chinese. *I Chuan Hsueh Pao* **24**:492, 1997.
359. Goebel-Schreiner B, Schreiner R: Identification of a new missense mutation in Japanese phenylketonuric patients. *J Inherit Metab Dis* **16**:950, 1993.
360. Okano Y, Hase Y, Shintaku H, et al: Molecular characterization of phenylketonuric mutations in Japanese by analysis of phenylalanine hydroxylase mRNA from lymphoblasts. *Hum Mol Genet* **3**:659, 1994.
361. Teebi AS, Al-Awadi SA, Farag TI, et al: Phenylketonuria in Kuwait and Arab countries. *Eur J Pediatr* **146**:78, 1987.
362. Kleiman S, Schwartz G, Woo SLC, et al: A 22-bp deletion in the phenylalanine hydroxylase gene causing phenylketonuria in an Arab family. *Hum Mutat* **1**:344, 1992.
363. Kleiman S, Bernstein J, Schwartz G, et al: A defective splice site at the phenylalanine hydroxylase gene in phenylketonuria and benign hyperphenylalaninemia among Palestinian Arabs. *Hum Mutat* **1**:340, 1992.
364. Kleiman S, Li J, Schwartz G, et al: Inactivation of phenylalanine hydroxylase by a missense mutation, R270S, in a Palestinian kinship with phenylketonuria. *Hum Mol Genet* **2**:605, 1993.
365. Hashem N, Bosco P, Chiavetta V, et al: Preliminary studies on the molecular basis of hyperphenylalaninemia in Egypt. *Hum Genet* **98**:3, 1996.
366. Teebi AS, Al-Awadi SA, Al-Awqati MA, et al: Neonatal screening of phenylketonuria and congenital hypothyroidism in Kuwait: A preliminary report [abstr]. *Proc. 6th Nat. Neonatal Screening Symposium 1988*, p 150.
367. Guldberg P, Lou HC, Henriksen KF, et al: A novel missense mutation in the phenylalanine hydroxylase gene of a homozygous Pakistani patient with non-PKU hyperphenylalaninemia. *Hum Mol Genet* **2**:1061, 1993.
368. Eisensmith RC, Okano Y, Dasovich M, et al: Multiple origins for phenylketonuria in Europe. *Am J Hum Genet* **51**:1355, 1992.
369. Wang T, Okano Y, Eisensmith RC, et al: Founder effect of a prevalent PKU mutation in the Oriental population. *Proc Natl Acad Sci USA* **88**:2146, 1991.
370. Wang T, Okano Y, Eisensmith RC, et al: Identification of a novel phenylketonuria (PKU) mutation in the Chinese: Further evidence for multiple origins of PKU in Asia. *Am J Hum Genet* **48**:628, 1991.
371. Avigad S, Cohen BE, Bauer S, et al: A single origin of phenylketonuria in Yemenite Jews. *Nature* **334**:168, 1990.
372. Kalanin J, Takarada Y, Kagawa S, et al: Gypsy phenylketonuria: A point mutation of the phenylalanine hydroxylase gene in Gypsy families from Slovakia. *Am J Med Genet* **49**:235, 1994.
373. Desviat LR, Pérez B, Ugarte M: Phenylketonuria in Spanish Gypsies: Prevalence of the IVS10nt546 mutation on haplotype 34. *Hum Mutat* **9**:66, 1997.
374. Tyfield LA, Meredith AL, Osborn MJ, et al: Identification of the haplotype pattern associated with the mutant PKU allele in the Gypsy population of Wales. *J Med Genet* **26**:499, 1989.
375. Kuzman AI, Eisensmith RC, Goltsov AA, et al: Complete spectrum of PAH mutations in Tataria: Presence of Slavic, Turkic and Scandinavian mutations. *Eur J Hum Genet* **3**:246, 1995.
376. Guldberg P, Henriksen KF, Güttler F: Molecular analysis of phenylketonuria in Denmark: 99% of the mutations detected by denaturing gradient gel electrophoresis. *Genomics* **17**:141, 1993.
377. Guldberg P, Romano V, Ceratto N, et al: Mutational spectrum of phenylalanine hydroxylase deficiency in Sicily: Implications for diagnosis of hyperphenylalaninemia in Southern Europe. *Hum Mol Genet* **2**:1703, 1993.
378. Dianzani I, Giannattasio S, De Sanctis L, et al: Genetic history of phenylketonuria mutations in Italy. *Am J Hum Genet* **55**:851, 1994.
379. Dianzani I, Giannattasio G, De Sanctis L, et al: Characterization of phenylketonuria alleles in the Italian population. *Eur J Hum Genet* **3**:294, 1995.
380. Zschocke J, Mallory JP, Eiken HS, et al: Phenylketonuria and the peoples of Northern Ireland. *Hum Genet* **100**:189, 1997.
381. Pérez B, Desviat LR, Ugarte M: Analysis of the phenylalanine hydroxylase gene in the Spanish population: Mutation profile and association with intragenic polymorphic markers. *Am J Hum Genet* **60**:95, 1997.
382. Abadie V, Lyonnet S, Melle D, et al: Molecular basis of phenylketonuria in France. *Dev Brain Dysfunct* **6**:120, 1993.
383. Van der Sijs-Bos CJM, Diepstraten CM, Juyn JA, et al: Phenylketonuria in the Netherlands: 93% of the mutations are detected by single-strand conformation analysis. *Hum Hered* **46**:185, 1996.
384. Guldberg P, Mallmann R, Henriksen KF, et al: Phenylalanine hydroxylase deficiency in a population in Germany: Mutational profile and nine novel mutations. *Hum Mutat* **8**:276, 1996.
385. Crosby AW: *Ecological Imperialism: The Biological Expansion of Europe 900–1900*. Cambridge, UK, Cambridge University Press. 1986.
386. Guldberg P, Zschocke J, Dagbjartsson A, et al: A molecular survey of phenylketonuria in Iceland: Identification of a founding mutation and evidence of predominant Norse settlement. *Eur J Hum Genet* **5**:376, 1997.
387. Ramus SJ, Treacy EP, Cotton RGH: Characterization of phenylalanine hydroxylase alleles in untreated phenylketonuria patients from Victoria, Australia: Origin of alleles and haplotypes. *Am J Hum Genet* **56**:1034, 1995.
388. Nicolini H, Cruz C, Camarena B, et al: Molecular analysis of the phenylalanine hydroxylase gene in Mexican phenylketonuric patients. *Arch Med Res* **26**:53, 1995.
389. Santos M, Kuzmin AI, Eisensmith RC, et al: Phenylketonuria in Costa Rica: Preliminary spectrum of PAH mutations and their associations with highly polymorphic haplotypes. *Hum Hered* **46**:128, 1996.
390. Perez B, Desviat LR, Die M, et al: Presence of the Mediterranean PKU mutation IVS10 in Latin America. *Hum Mol Genet* **2**:1289, 1993.
391. Perez B, Desviat LR, De Lucca M, et al: Mutation analysis of phenylketonuria in South Brazil. *Hum Mutat* **8**:262, 1996.
392. Lyonnet S, Melle D, Debrakeleer M, et al: Time and space clusters of the French-Canadian M1V phenylketonuria mutation in France. *Am J Hum Genet* **51**:191, 1992.

393. Weber JL, Wong C: Mutation of human short tandem repeats. *Hum Mol Genet* **2**:1123, 1993.
394. Rannala B, Slatkin M: Likelihood analysis of disequilibrium mapping, and related problems. *Am J Hum Genet* **62**:459, 1998.
395. Rivera I, Leandro P, Lichter-Konecki U, et al: Relative frequency of IVS10nt546 mutation in a Portuguese phenylketonuric population. *Hum Mutat* **9**:272, 1997.
396. Desviat LR, Pérez B, De Lucca M, et al: Evidence in Latin America of recurrence of V388M, a phenylketonuria mutation with high in vitro residual activity. *Am J Hum Genet* **57**:337, 1995.
397. Eiken HG, Knappskog PM, Apold J, et al: A de novo phenylketonuria mutation: ATG (Met) to ATA (Ile) in the start codon of the phenylalanine hydroxylase gene. *Hum Mutat* **1**:388, 1992.
398. Byck S, Tyfield L, Carter K, et al: Prediction of multiple hypermutable codons in the human PAH gene: Codon 280 contains recurrent mutations in Quebec and other populations. *Hum Mutat* **9**:316, 1997.
399. Cooper DN, Youssoufian H: The CpG dinucleotide and human genetic disease. *Hum Genet* **78**:151, 1988.
400. Ramus S, Forrest SM, Saleeba JA, et al: CpG hotspot causes second mutation in codon 408 of the phenylalanine hydroxylase gene. *Hum Genet* **90**:147, 1992.
401. John SWM, Rozen R, Scriver CR, et al: Recurrent mutation, gene conversion, or recombination at the human phenylalanine hydroxylase locus: Evidence in French-Canadians and a catalog of mutations. *Am J Hum Genet* **46**:970, 1990.
402. Treacy E, Byck S, Clow C, et al: "Celtic" phenylketonuria chromosomes found? Evidence in two regions of Quebec province. *Eur J Hum Genet* **1**:220, 1993.
403. Eisensmith RC, Goltsov AA, O'Neill C, et al: Recurrence of the R408W mutation in the phenylalanine hydroxylase locus in Europeans. *Am J Hum Genet* **56**:278, 1995.
404. Byck S, Morgan K, Tyfield L, et al: Evidence for origin, by recurrent mutation, of the phenylalanine hydroxylase R408W mutation on two haplotypes in European and Quebec populations. *Hum Mol Genet* **3**:1675, 1994.
405. Zygulska M, Eigel A, Dworniczak B, et al: Molecular analysis of phenylketonuria in the population of Southern Poland. *Dev Brain Dysfunct* **6**:129, 1993.
406. Zschocke J, Graham CA, Stewart FJ, et al: Automated sequencing detects all mutations in Northern Irish patients with phenylketonuria and mild hyperphenylalaninemia. *Acta Paediatric* **(Suppl 407)**:37, 1994.
407. Kalaydjieva L, Dworniczak B, Aulehla-Scholz C, et al: Classical phenylketonuria in Bulgaria: RFLP haplotypes and frequency of the major mutations. *J Med Genet* **27**:742, 1990.
408. Kozak L, Kuhrova V, Blazkova M, et al: Phenylketonuria mutations and their relation to RFLP haplotypes at the PAH locus in Czech PKU families. *Hum Genet* **96**:472, 1995.
409. Tsai TF, Hsiao KJ, Su TS: Phenylketonuria mutation in Chinese haplotype 44 identical with haplotype 2 mutation in northern-European Caucasians. *Hum Genet* **84**:409, 1990.
410. Kadasi L, Polakova H, Ferakova E, et al: PKU in Slovakia: Mutation screening and haplotype analysis. *Hum Genet* **95**:112, 1995.
411. Lin C-H, Hsiao K-J, Tsai T-F, et al: Identification of a missense phenylketonuria mutation at codon 408 in Chinese. *Hum Genet* **89**:593, 1992.
412. Caillaud C, Vilarinho L, Vilarinho A, et al: Linkage disequilibrium between phenylketonuria and RFLP haplotype-1 at the phenylalanine hydroxylase locus in Portugal. *Hum Genet* **89**:69, 1992.
413. Okano Y, Wang T, Eisensmith RC, et al: Recurrent mutation in the human phenylalanine hydroxylase gene. *Am J Hum Genet* **46**:919, 1990.
414. Weber JL: Know thy genome. *Nat Genet* **7**:343, 1994.
415. Flint J, Harding RM, Clegg JB, et al: Why are some genetic disease common? Distinguishing selection from other processes by molecular analysis of globin gene variants. *Hum Genet* **91**:91, 1993.
416. Yao Y, Matsubara Y, Narisawa K: Rapid detection of phenylketonuria mutations by non-radioactive single-strand conformation polymorphism analysis. *Acta Pediatr Jpn* **36**:231, 1994.
417. Vogel F: Phenotypic deviations in heterozygotes of phenylketonuria (PKU). *Prog Clin Biol Res* **177**:337, 1985.
418. Kidd KK: Phenylketonuria. Population genetics of a disease. *Nature* **327**:282, 1987.
419. Dilella AG, Marvit J, Lidsky AS, et al: Tight linkage between a splicing mutation and a specific DNA haplotype in phenylketonuria. *Nature* **322**:799, 1986.
420. Sober E: *The Nature of Selection: Evolutionary Theory in Philosophical Focus*. Cambridge, MIT Press, 1984.
421. Rosenblatt D, Scriver CR: Heterogeneity in genetic control of phenylalanine metabolism in man. *Nature* **218**:677, 1968.
422. Gold RJM, Maag UR, Neal JL, et al: The use of biochemical data in screening for mutant alleles and in genetic counseling. *Ann Hum Genet* **37**:315, 1974.
423. Woolf LI, McBea MS, Woolf FM, et al: Phenylketonuria as a balanced polymorphism: The nature of the heterozygote advantage. *Ann Hum Genet* **38**:461, 1975.
424. Saugstad LF: Heterozygote advantage for the phenylketonuria allele. *J Med Genet* **14**:20, 1977.
425. Saugstad LF: Increased "reproductive casualty" in heterozygotes for phenylketonuria. *Clin Genet* **4**:105, 1973.
426. Paul TD, Greco JJ, Brandt TK, et al: Is there a heterozygote advantage in the birthweight and number of children born to PKU heterozygotes? [Abstract]. *Am J Hum Genet* **31**(suppl):A104, 1979.
427. Ten Kate LP: On estimating the actual rate of foetal loss in families with an autosomal recessive disorder and Woolf's data on PKU. *Ann Hum Genet* **41**:463, 1978.
428. Woolf LI: The heterozygote advantage of phenylketonuria. *Am J Hum Genet* **38**:773, 1986.
429. Thompson EA, Neel JV: Allelic distribution and allele frequency distribution as a function of social demographic history. *Am J Hum Genet* **60**:197, 1997.
430. Cali F, Dianzani I, Desviat LR, et al: The STR252-IVS10nt546-VNTR7 phenylalanine hydroxylase mini-haplotype in five Mediterranean samples. *Hum Genet* **100**:350, 1997.
431. Traeger-Synodinos J, Kanavakis E, Kalogerakou M, et al: Preliminary mutation analysis in the phenylalanine hydroxylase gene in Greek PKU and HPA patients. *Hum Genet* **94**:573, 1994.
432. Rivera I, Leandro P, Lichter-Konecki U, et al: Population genetics of hyperphenylalaninemia resulting from phenylalanine hydroxylase deficiency in Portugal. *J Med Genet* **35**:301, 1998.
433. Kaufman S: An evaluation of the possible neurotoxicity of metabolites of phenylalanine. *J Pediatr* **114**:895, 1989.
433a. Sarkissian CN, Scriver CR, Mamer OA: Measurement of phenyllactate, phenylacetate, and phenylpyruvate by negative ion chemical ionization–gas chromatography/mass spectrometry in brain of mouse genetic models of phenylketonuria and non-phenylketonuria hyperphenylalaninemia. *Anal Biochem* **280**:242, 2000.
434. Antoshechkin AG, Chentsova TV, Tatur VY, et al: Content of phenylalanine, tyrosine and their metabolites in CSF in phenylketonuria. *J Inherit Metab Dis* **14**:749, 1991.
435. Scriver CR, Kaufman S, Woo SLC: The hyperphenylalaninemias, in Scriver CR, Beaudet AL, Sly WS, Valle D (eds): *The Metabolic Basis of Inherit Disease*. New York, McGraw-Hill, 1989, p 495.
436. Krause W, Halminski M, McDonald L, et al: Biochemical and neuropsychological effects of elevated plasma phenylalanine in patients with treated phenylketonuria. *J Clin Invest* **75**:40, 1985.
437. Krause W, Epstein C, Averbrook A, et al: Phenylalanine alters the mean power frequency of electroencephalograms and plasma L-DOPA in treated patients with phenylketonuria. *Pediatr Res* **20**:1112, 1986.
438. Epstein CM, Trotter JF, Averbrook A, et al: EEG mean frequencies are sensitive indices of phenylalanine effects on normal brain. *Neurophysiology* **72**:133, 1989.
439. Avison MJ, Herschkowitz N, Novotny EJ, et al: Proton NMR observation of phenylalanine and an aromatic metabolite in the rabbit brain in vivo. *Pediatr Res* **27**:5660, 1990.
440. Lukkelund C, Nielson JB, Lou HC, et al: Increased neurotransmitter biosynthesis in phenylketonuria induced by phenylalanine restriction of by supplementation of unrestricted diet with large amounts of tyrosine. *Eur J Pediatr* **148**:238, 1988.
441. Bach FW, Nielsen JB, Buchholt J, et al: Correlation between cerebrospinal fluid phenylalanine and β-endorphin in patients with phenylketonuria. *Neurosci Lett* **129**:131, 1991.
442. Smith I: The hyperphenylalaninemias, in Lloyd JK, Scriver CR (eds): *Genetic and Metabolic Disease in Pediatrics*. London, Butterworths, 1985, p 166.
443. Lou HC, Lykkelund C, Gerdes AM, et al: Increased vigilance and dopamine synthesis by large doses of tyrosine or phenylalanine restriction in phenylketonuria. *Acta Paediatr Scand* **76**:560, 1987.
444. Bick U, Fahrendorf G, Ludoph AC, et al: Disturbed myelination in patients with treated hyperphenylalaninemia: Evaluation with magnetic resonance imaging. *Eur J Pediatr* **150**:185, 1991.

445. Michel U, Schmidt E, Batzler U: Results of psychological testing of patients aged 3–6 years. *Eur J Pediatr* **149**(suppl 1):34, 1990.
446. Weglage J, Ullrich K, Pietsch M, et al: Untreated non-phenylketonuric-hyperphenylalaninemia: Intellectual and neurological outcome. *Eur J Pediatr* **155(suppl1)**:S26, 1996.
447. Bessman SP, Williamson ML, Koch R: Diet, genetics, and mental retardation: Interaction between phenylketonuric heterozygous mother and fetus to produce non-specific diminution of IQ—Evidence in support of the justification hypothesis. *Proc Natl Acad Sci USA* **75**:1562, 1978.
448. Batshaw ML, Valle D, Bessman SP: Unsuccessful treatment of phenylketonuria with tyrosine. *J Pediatr* **99**:159, 1981.
449. Koepp P, Held KR: Serum-tyrosine in patients with hyperphenylalaninaemia. *Lancet* **2**:92, 1977.
450. Scriver CR, Cole DEC, Houghton SA, et al: Cord-blood tyrosine levels in the full-term phenylketonuric fetus and the "justification hypothesis." *Proc Natl Acad Sci USA* **77**:6175, 1980.
451. Smith ML, Hanley WB, Clarke JTR, et al: Randomised controlled trial of tyrosine supplementation on neuropsychological performance in phenylketonuria. *Arch Dis Child* **78**:116, 1998.
452. Pietz J, Landwehr R, Kutscha A, et al: Effect of high-dose tyrosine supplementation on brain function in adults with phenylketonuria. *J Pediatr* **127**:936, 1995.
453. Thalhammer O, Pollak A, Lubec G, et al: Intracellular concentrations of phenylalanine, tyrosine and α-aminobutyric acid in 13 homozygotes and 19 heterozygotes for PKU compared with 26 normals. *Hum Genet* **54**:213, 1980.
454. Thalhammer O, Lubec G, Konigshofer H, et al: Intracellular phenylalanine and tyrosine concentration in homozygotes and heterozygotes for phenylketonuria (PKU) and hyperphenylalaninemia compared with normals. *Hum Genet* **60**:320, 1982.
455. Andrews TM, McKeran RO, Watts RWE, et al: Relationship between the granulocyte content and the degree of disability in phenylketonuria. *Q J Med New Ser* **XLII**:805, 1973.
456. De Cespedes C, Thoene JG, Lowler K, et al: Evidence for inhibition of exodus of small neutral amino acids from non-brain tissues in hyperphenylalaninaemic rats. *J Inherit Metab Dis* **12**:166, 1989.
457. Choi TB, Pardridge WM: Phenylalanine transport at the human blood-brain barrier. *J Biol Chem* **261**:6536, 1986.
458. Hargreaves KM, Pardridge WM: Neutral amino acid transport at the human blood-brain barrier. *J Biol Chem* **263**:19,392, 1988.
459. Maher TJ, Glaeser BS, Wurtman RJ: Diurnal variations in plasma concentrations of basic and neutral amino acids and in reduced concentrations of aspartate and glutamate: Effects of dietary protein intake. *Am J Clin Nutr* **39**:722, 1984.
460. Koeppe RA, Mangner T, Betz AL, et al: Use of [^{11}C]aminocyclohexane carboxylate for the measurement of amino acid uptake and distribution volume in human brain. *J Cereb Blood Flow Metab* **10**:727, 1990.
461. Momma S, Aoyagi M, Rapoport SI, et al: Phenylalanine transport across the blood-brain barrier as studied with the in situ brain perfusion technique. *J Neurochem* **48**:1291, 1987.
462. Pardridge WW: Blood-brain barrier carrier-mediated transport and brain metabolism of amino acids. *Neurochem Res* **23**:635, 1998.
463. Knudsen GM: Application of the double-indicator technique for measurement of blood-brain barrier permeability in humans. *Cerebrovasc Brain Metab Rev* **6**:1, 1994.
464. Knudsen GM, Pettigrew KD, Patlak CS, et al: Blood-brain barrier permeability measurements by double-indicator method intravenous injection. *Am J Physiol* **266**:H987, 1994.
465. Knudsen GM, Hasselbalch S, Toft PB, et al: Blood-brain barrier transport of amino acids in healthy controls and in patients with phenylketonuria. *J Inherited Metab Dis* **18**:653, 1995.
466. Moller HE, Weglage J, Wiedermann D, et al: Kinetics of phenylalanine transport at the human blood-brain barrier investigated in vivo. *Brain Res* **778**:329, 1997.
467. Novotny EJ Jr, Avison MJ, Herschkowitz N, et al: In vivo measurement of phenylalanine in human brain by proton nuclear magnetic resonance spectroscopy. *Pediatr Res* **37**:244, 1995.
468. Moller HE, Vermathen P, Ullrich K, et al: In vivo NMR spectroscopy in patients with phenylketonuria: Changes of cerebral phenylalanine levels under dietary treatment. *Neuropediatrics* **26**:199, 1995.
469. Pietz J, Kreis R, Boesch C, et al: The dynamics of brain concentrations of phenylalanine and its clinical significance in patients with phenylketonuria determined by in vivo ^{1}H magnetic resonance spectroscopy. *Pediatr Res* **38**:657, 1995.
469a. Pietz J, Kreis R, Rupp A, et al: Large neutral amino acids block phenylalanine transport into brain tissue in patients with phenylketonuria. *J Clin Invest* **103**:1169, 1999.
470. Aragon MC, Gimenez C, Valdiveso F: Inhibition by L-phenylalanine of tyrosine transport by synaptosomal plasma membrane vesicles: Implications in the pathogenesis of phenylketonuria. *J Neurochem* **39**:1185, 1982.
471. Herrero E, Aragon MC, Gimenez C, et al: Inhibition by L-phenylalanine of tryptophan transport by synaptosomal plasma membrane vesicles: Implications in the pathogenesis of phenylketonuria. *J Inherit Metab Dis* **6**:32, 1983.
472. Peterson NA, Shah SN, Raghupathy E, et al: Presynaptic tyrosine availability in the phenylketonuric brain: A hypothetical evaluation. *Brain Res* **272**:189, 1983.
473. Ratzmann GW, Grimm U, Jahrig K, et al: On the brain barrier system function and changes of cerebrospinal fluid concentrations of phenylalanine and tyrosine in human phenylketonuria. *Biomed Biochim Acta* **43**:197, 1984.
474. Piel N, Lane JD, Huther G, et al: Impaired permeability of the blood-cerebrospinal fluid barrier in hyperphenylalaninemia. *Neuropediatrics* **13**:88, 1982.
475. Hommes FA: The role of the blood-brain barrier in the aetiology of permanent brain dysfunction in hyperphenylalaninemia. *J Inherit Metab Dis* **12**:41, 1989.
476. Hommes FA, Lee JS: The effect of plasma valine, isoleucine and leucine on the control of the flux through tyrosine- and tryptophan-hydroxylase in the brain. *J Inherited Metab Dis* **13**:151, 1990.
477. Berry HK, Bofinger MK, Hunt MM, et al: Reduction of cerebrospinal fluid concentrations of phenylalanine, after oral administration of valine, isoleucine, and leucine. *Pediatr Res* **16**:751, 1982.
478. Jordan MK, Brunner RL, Hunt MM, et al: Preliminary support for the oral administration of valine, iosleucine and leucine for phenylketonuria. *Dev Med Child Neurol* **27**:33, 1985.
479. Heuther G, Kaus R, Neuhoff V: Amino acid depletion in the blood and brain tissue of hyperphenylalaninemic rats is abolished by the administration of additional lysine: A contribution to the understanding of the metabolic defects in phenylketonuria. *Biochem Med* **33**:334, 1985.
480. Neal JL, Scriver CR: Abnormally high concentrations of hydrophobic-side-chain amino acids do not affect cell function by modifying water structure in phenylketonuria and branched-chain aminoaciduria. *IRCS* **2**:1700, 1974.
481. Welsh MC: A prefrontal dysfunction model of early-treated phenylketonuria. *Eur J Pediatr* **155**:S87, 1996.
482. Diamond A, Ciaramitaro V, Donner E, et al: An animal model of early-treated PKU. *J Neurosci* **14**:3072, 1994.
483. Shah SN: Fatty acid composition of lipids of human brain myelin and synaptosomes: Changes in phenylketonuria and Down's syndrome [Minireview]. *Int J Biochem* **10**:477, 1979.
484. Johnson RC, Shah SM: Effects of α-methylphenylalanine plus phenylalanine treatment during development of myelin in rat brain. *Neurochem Res* **5**:709, 1980.
485. Dwivedy AK, Shah SN: Effect of hyperphenylalaninemia on polyphosphoinositides content of rat brain. *Experientia* **38**:1458, 1982.
486. Heuther G, Kaus R, Neuhoff V: Brain development in experimental hyperphenylalaninemia: Myelination. *Neuropediatrics* **13**:177, 1982.
487. Matsuo K, Hommes F: Regional distribution of the phenylalanine-sensitive ATP-sulphurylase in brain. *J Inherited Metab Dis* **10**:62, 1987.
488. Baba H, Sato S, Inuzuka T, et al: Developmental changes of myelin-associated glycoprotein in rat brain: Study on experimental hyperphenylalaninemia. *Neurochem Res* **12**:459, 1987.
489. Hommes AF: On the mechanism of permanent brain dysfunction in hyperphenylalaninemia. *Biochem Med Metab Biol* **46**:277, 1991.
490. Shaw DWW, Maravilla KR, Weinberger E, et al: MR imaging of phenylketonuria. *Am J Nutr Res* **12**:403, 1991.
491. Thompson AJ, Smith I, Kendall BE, et al: MRI changes in early treated patients with phenylketonuria. *Lancet* **2**:1224, 1991.
492. Ullrich K, Möller H, Weglage J, et al: White matter abnormalities in phenylketonuria: Results of magnetic resonance measurements. *Acta Paediatr* **407(Suppl)**:78, 1994.
493. Kornguth S, Anderson M, Markley MJ, et al: Near-microscopic magnetic resonance imaging of the brains of phenylalanine hydroxylase-deficient mice, normal littermates, and of normal BALB/c mice at 9.4 Tesla. *Neuroimage* **1**:220, 1994.

494. Dyer CA, Kendler A, Philibotte T, et al: Evidence for central nervous system glial cell plasticity in phenylketonuria. *J Neuropathol Exp Neurol* **55**:795, 1996.
495. Hommes FA, Moss L: Myelin turnover in hyperphenylalaninaemia: A re-evaluation with the HPH-5 mouse. *J Inherited Metab Dis* **15**:243, 1992.
496. Changeux JP, Danchin A: Selective stabilization of developing synapses as a mechanism for the specification of neuronal networks. *Nature* **264**:705, 1976.
497. Hommes FA: The effect of hyperphenylalaninaemia on the muscarinic acetylcholine receptor in the HPH-5 mouse brain. *J Inherited Metab Dis* **16**:962, 1993.
498. Hommes FA: Loss of neurotransmitter receptors by hyperphenylalaninemia in the HPH-5 mouse brain. *Acta Paediatr Scand Suppl* **407**:120, 1994.
499. Ushakova GA, Gubkina HA, Kachur VA, et al: Effect of experimental hyperphenylalaninemia on the postnatal rat brain. *Int J Dev Neurosci* **15**:29, 1997.
500. Reynolds R, Burri R, Herschkowitz N: Retarded development of neurons and oligodendroglia in rat forebrain produced by hyperphenylalaninemia results in permanent deficits in myelin despite long recovery periods. *Exp Neurol* **124**:357, 1993.
501. Paans AMJ, Pruim J, Smit GPA, et al: Neurotransmitter positron emission tomographic-studies in adults with phenylketonuria: A pilot study. *Eur J Pediatr* **155**:S78, 1996.
502. Binek PA, Johnston TC, Kelly CJ: Effect of α-methylphenylalanine and phenylalanine on brain polyribosomes and protein synthesis. *J Neurochem* **36**:1476, 1981.
503. Esliger M-A, Theriault GR, Gauthier D: In vitro localization of the protein synthesis defect associated with experimental phenylketonuria. *Neurochem Res* **14**:81, 1989.
504. Wall KM, Pardridge WM: Decreases in brain protein synthesis elicited by moderate increases in plasma phenylalanine. *Biochim Biophys Res Acta* **168**:1177, 1990.
505. Binek-Singer P, Johnston TC: The effects of chronic hyperphenylalaninemia on mouse brain protein synthesis can be prevented by other amino acids. *Biochem J* **206**:407, 1982.
506. Okano Y, Chow IZ, Isshiki G, et al: Effects of phenylalanine loading on protein synthesis in the fetal heart and brain of rat: An experimental approach to maternal phenylketonuria. *J Inherit Metab Dis* **9**:15, 1986.
507. McDonald JD, Dyer CA, Gailis L, et al: Cardiovascular defects among the progeny of mouse phenylketonuria females. *Pediatr Res* **42**:103, 1997.
508. Levy H, Ghavami M: Maternal phenylketonuria: A metabolic teratogen. *Teratology* **53**:176, 1996.
509. Schöoter J, Schott KJ, Purtill MA, et al: Lyosomal protein degradation in experimental hyperphenylalaninemia. *J Inherit Metab Dis* **273**:273, 1986.
510. Bauman ML, Kemper TL: Morphologic and histoanatomic observations of the brain in untreated human phenylketonuria. *Acta Neuropathol* **58**:55, 1982.
511. Cordero ME, Trejo M, Colombo M, et al: Histological maturation of the neocortex in phenylketonuric rats. *Early Hum Dev* **8**:157, 1983.
512. Swaiman KK, Wu SR: Phenylalanine and phenylacetate adversely affect developing mammalian brain neurons. *Neurology* **34**:1246, 1984.
513. Huether G, Neuhoff V: Use of α-methylphenylalanine for studies of brain development in experimental phenylketonuria. *J Inherit Metab Dis* **4**:67, 1981.
514. Heuther G, Neuhoff V, Kaus R: Brain development in experimental hyperphenylalaninemia: Disturbed proliferation and reduced cell numbers in the cerebellum. *Neuropediatrics* **14**:12, 1983.
515. Johnson RC, Shah SN: Effect of hyperphenylalaninemia induced during suckling on brain DNA metabolism in rat pups. *Neurochem Res* **9**:517, 1984.
516. Cockburn F: Neonatal brain and dietary lipids. *Arch Dis Child* **70**:F1, 1994.
517. Giovannini M, Agostoni C, Biasucci G, et al: Fatty acid metabolism in phenylketonuria. *Eur J Pediatr* **155**:S132, 1966.
518. Agostini C, Riva E, Galli C, et al: Plasma arachidonic acid and serum thromboxane B_2 concentrations in phenylketonuric children are correlated with dietary compliance. *Z Ernahrungswiss* **37**:122, 1998.
519. Farquharson J, Jamieson EC, Abbasi KA, et al: Effect of diet on the fatty acid composition of the major phospholipids of infant cerebral cortex. *Arch Dis Child* **72**:198, 1995.
520. Farquharson J, Cockburn F, Patrick WA, et al: Effect of diet on infant subcutaneous tissue triglyceride fatty acids. *Arch Dis Child* **69**:589, 1993.
521. Farquharson J, Jamieson EC, Logan EW, et al: Age- and dietary-related distributions of hepatic arachidonic and docosahexaenoic acid in early infancy. *Pediatr Res* **38**:361, 1995.
522. Farquharson J, Cockburn F, Patrick WA, et al: Breastfeeding, dummy use, and adult intelligence. *Lancet* **347**:1764, 1996.
523. Cockburn F, Clark BJ, Caine EA, et al: Fatty acids in the stability of neuronal membrane: Relevance to PKU. *Int Pediatr* **11**:56, 1996.
524. Riva E, Agostoni C, Biasucci G, et al: Early breastfeeding is linked to higher intelligence quotient scores in dietary treated phenylketonuric children. *Acta Paediatr Scand* **85**:56, 1996.
525. Lane JD, Neuhoff V: Phenylketonuria: Clinical and experimental considerations revealed by the use of animal models. *Naturwissenschaften* **67**:227, 1980.
526. Vorhees CV, Butcher RE, Berry HK: Progress in experimental phenylketonuria: A critical review. *Neurosci Biobehav Rev* **5**:177, 1981.
527. Hoshiga M, Hatakeyama K, Watanabe M, et al: Autoradiographic distribution of [^{14}C]tetrahydrobiopterin and its developmental change in mice. *J Pharmacol Exp Ther* **267**:971, 1993.
528. McDonald JD: The PKU mouse project: Its history, potential and implications. *Acta Paediatr Scand Suppl* **407**:122, 1994.
529. Ledley FD, Ledbetter SA, Ledbetter DH, et al: Localization of mouse phenylalanine hydroxylase locus on chromosome 10. *Cytogenet Cell Genet* **47**:125, 1988.
530. McDonald JD, Bode VC, Dove WF, et al: The use of *N*-ethyl-*N*-nitrosourea to produce mouse models for human phenylketonuria and hyperphenylalaninemia. *Prog Clin Biol Res* **340C**:407, 1990.
531. Bode V, McDonald J, Guenet J, et al: *hph*-1: A mouse mutant with hereditary hyperphenylalaninemia induced by ethylnitrosourea mutagenesis. *Genetics* **118**:299, 1988.
532. McDonald JD, Bode V: Hyperphenylalaninemia in the *hyp*-1 mouse mutant. *Pediatr Res* **23**:63, 1988.
533. McDonald JD, Cotton R, Jennings I, et al: Biochemical defect of the *hph*-1 mouse mutant is a deficiency of GTP-cyclohydrolase activity. *J Neurochem* **50**:655, 1988.
534. Hyland K, Gunasekera RS, Engle T, et al: Tetrahydrobiopterin and biogenic amine metabolism in the hph-1 mouse. *J Neurochem* **67**:752, 1996.
535. McDonald JD, Bode V, Dove W, et al: $Pah^{hph\text{-}5}$: A mouse mutant deficient in phenylalanine hydroxylase. *Proc Natl Acad Sci USA* **87**:1965, 1990.
536. McDonald JD, Charlton CK: Characterization of mutations at the mouse phenylalanine hydroxylase locus. *Genomics* **39**:402, 1997.
537. Sarkissian CN, Boulais DM, McDonald JD, et al: A heteroallelic mutant mouse model: A new orthologue to human hyperphenylalaninemia. *Mol Genet Metab* **69**:88, 2000.
538. Sarkissian C, Shao Z, Blain F, et al: A different approach to treatment of phenylketonuria: Phenylalanine degradation with recombinant phenylalanine ammonia lyase. *Proc Natl Acad Sci* USA **96**:2339, 1999.
539. Safos S, Chang TM: Enzyme replacement therapy in ENU2 phenylketonuric mice using oral microencapsulated phenylalanine ammonia-lyase: A preliminary report. *Artif Cells Blood Substitutes Immobilization Biotechnol* **23**:681, 1995.
540. Pitt DB, Danks DM: The natural history of untreated phenylketonuria. *J Pediatr Child Health* **27**:189, 1991.
541. Greeves LG, McCarthy HL, Redmond A, et al: Coexistence of cystic fibrosis and phenylketonuria. *Ulster Med J* **66**:59, 1997.
542. Swiwach RS, Sheikha S: Delusional disorder in a boy with phenylketonuria and amine metabolites in the cerebrospinal fluid after treatment with neuroleptics. *J Adolesc Health Care* **22**:244, 1998.
543. Fisch RO, Feinberg SB, Weisberg S, et al: Bony changes of PKU neonates unrelated to phenylalanine levels. *J Inherit Metab Dis* **14**:890, 1991.
544. Hillman L, Schlotzhauer C, Lee D, et al: Decreased bone mineralization in children with phenylketonuria under treatment. *Eur J Pediatr* **155**:S148, 1996.
545. Schwahn B, Mokov E, Scheidhauer B, et al: Decreased trabecular bone mineral density in patients with phenylketonuria measured by peripheral quantitative computed tomography. *Acta Paediatr Scand* **87**:61, 1998.
546. Greeves LG, Carson DJ, Magee A, et al: Fractures and phenylketonuria. *Acta Paediatr Scand* **86**:242, 1997.

547. Haktan M, Aydin A, Bahat H, et al: Progressive systemic scleroderma in an infant with partial phenylketonuria. *J Inherit Metab Dis* **12**:486, 1989.
548. Nova MP, Kaufman M, Halperin A: Scleroderma-like indurations in a child with phenylketonuria: A clinicopathologic correction and review of the literature. *J Am Acad Dermatol* **26**:329, 1992.
549. Greeves LG, Carson DJ, Dodge JA: Peptic ulceration and phenylketonuria: A possible link? *Gut* **29**:691, 1988.
550. Kawashima H, Kawano M, Masaki A, et al: Three cases of untreated classical PKU: A report on cataracts and brain calcification. *Am J Med Genet* **29**:89, 1988.
551. Pitt DB, O'Day J: Phenylketonuria does not cause cataracts. *Eur J Pediatr* **150**:661, 1991.
552. Verkerk PH, Van Spronsen FJ, Smith GPA, et al: Prevalence of congenital heart disease in patients with phenylketonuria. *J Pediatr* **119**:282, 1991.
553. Waisbren SE, Levy HL: Agoraphobia in phenylketonuria. *J Inherit Metab Dis* **14**:755, 1991.
554. Villasana D, Butler IJ, Williams JC, et al: Neurological deterioration in adult phenylketonuria. *J Inherit Metab Dis* **12**:451, 1989.
555. Pearsen KD, Gean-Marton A, Levy HL, et al: Phenylketonuria: MR imaging of the brain with clinical correlation. *Radiology* **177**:437, 1990.
556. Thompson AJ, Smith I, Brenton D, et al: Neurological deterioration in young adults with phenylketonuria. *Lancet* **336**:602, 1990.
557. Battistini S, De Stefano N, Parlanti S, et al: Unexpected white matter changes in an early treated PKU case and improvement after dietary treatment. *Funct Neurol* **6**:177, 1991.
558. Naidu S, Moser HW: Value of neuroimaging in metabolic diseases affecting the CNS. *Am J Nutr Res* **12**:413, 1991.
559. Yudkoff M, Segal S: Absent phenylalanine hydroxylase activity without phenylketonuria. *Eur J Pediatr* **134**:85, 1980.
560. Auerbach VH, DiGeorge AM, Carpenter GG: Phenylalaninemia: A study of the diversity of disorders which produce elevation of blood concentration of phenylalanine, in Nyhan W (ed): *Amino Acid Metabolism and Genetic Variation*. New York, McGraw-Hill, 1967, p 11.
561. Blau K, Levitt GA, Harvey DR: Hyperphenylalaninemia with defective transamination. *Clin Chim Acta* **132**:43, 1983.
562. Smith I, Cook B, Beasley M: Review of neonatal screening programme for phenylketonuria. *BMJ* **303**:333, 1991.
563. Knox WE: Retrospective study of phenylketonuria: Relation of phenyl-pyruvate excretion to plasma phenylalanine. *PKU Newslett no. 2*, 1970.
564. Wadman SK, Ketting D, De Bree PK, et al: Permanent chemical phenylketonuria and a normal phenylalanine tolerance in two sisters with a normal mental development. *Clin Chim Acta* **65**:197, 1975.
565. Westwood A, Barr DG: Phenylketonuria with a progressive neurological disorder not responsive to tetrahydrobiopterin. *Acta Paediatr Scand* **71**:859, 1982.
566. Guthrie R: The introduction of newborn screening for phenylketonuria. *Eur J Pediatr* **155**:S4, 1996.
566a. Scriver CR: Commentary: "A simple phenylalanine method for detecting phenylketonuria in large populations of newborn infants; by R, Guthrie and A Susi, Pediatrics 1963. **32**:318–343.". *Pediatrics* **102(Suppl)**:236, 1998.
567. National Academy of Sciences: *Genetic Screening: Programs, Principles and Research*. Washington, DC, National Research Council, 1975.
568. Wilson JMG, Jungner G: *Principles and Practice of Screening for Disease. Public Health Papers No. 34*. Geneva, World Health Organizationy, 1968.
569. American Academy of Pediatrics Committee on Genetics: Newborn screening fact sheets. *Pediatrics* **83**:449, 1989.
569a. Seymour CA, Thomason MJ, Chalmers RA, et al: Newborn screening for inborn errors of metabolism: A systematic review. *Health Technol Assessment* **1**(11):i-iv, 1-95, 1997.
569b. Pollitt RJ, McCabe CJ, Booth A, et al: Neonatal screening for inborn errors of metabolism: Cost, yield and outcome. *Health Technol Assessment* **1**(7):i-iv, 1-202, 1997.
570. Medical Research Council Steering Committee for the MRC/DHSS Phenylketonuria Register. Routine neonatal screening for phenylketonuria in the United Kingdom 1964–78. *BMJ* **1**:1680, 1981.
571. Levy HL, Simmons JR, MacCready RA: Stability of amino acids and galactose in the newborn screening filter paper blood specimen. *J Pediatr* **107**:757, 1985.
572. Spierto FW, Hearn TL, Gardner FH, et al: Phenylalanine analyses of blood-spot control materials: Preparation of samples and evaluation of interlaboratory performance. *Clin Chem* **31**:235, 1985.
573. Larsson BA, Tannfeldt G, Lagercrantz H, et al: Venipuncture is more effective and less painful than heel lancing for blood tests in neonates. *Pediatrics* **101**:882, 1998.
574. Scriver CR, Davies E, Cullen AM: Application of a simple method to the screening of plasma for a variety of aminoacidopathies. *Lancet* **2**:230, 1964.
575. Efron ML, Young D, Moser HW, et al: A simple chromatographic screening test for the detection of disorders of amino acid metabolism: A technique using white blood or urine collected on filter paper. *N Engl J Med* **270**:1378, 1994.
576. Keffler S, Denmeade R, Green A: Neonatal screening for phenylketonuria: Evaluation of an automated enzymatic method. *Ann Clin Biochem* **31**:134, 1994.
577. Campbell RS, Hollifield RD, Varsani H, et al: Development of an enzyme-mediated assay for phenylalanine in blood spots. *Ann Clin Biochem* **31**:140, 1994.
578. Wendel U, Hummel W, Langenback U: Monitoring of phenylketonuria: A colorimetric method for the determination of plasma phenylalanine using L-phenylalanine dehydrogenase. *Anal Biochem* **180**:91, 1989.
579. Wendel U, Koppelkamm M, Hummel W, et al: A new approach to the newborn screening for hyperphenylalaninemias: Use of L-phenylalanine dehydrogenase and microtiter plates. *Clin Chim Acta* **192**:P165, 1990.
580. McCaman MW, Robins E: Fluorometric method for the determination of phenylalanine in serum. *J Lab Clin Med* **59**:885, 1992.
581. Kirkman HN, Carroll CL, Moore EG, et al: Fifteen-year experience with screening for phenylketonuria with an automated fluorometric method. *Am J Hum Genet* **34**:743, 1982.
582. Huang T, Warsinke A, Kuwana T, et al: Determination of L-phenylalanine based on an NADH-detecting biosensor. *Anal Chem* **70**:997, 1998.
583. American Academy of Pediatrics Committee on Genetics: New issues in newborn screening for phenylketonuria and congenital hypothyroidism. *Pediatrics* **69**:104, 1982.
584. McCabe ERB, McCabe L, Mosher GA, et al: Newborn screening for phenylketonuria: Predictive validity as a function of age. *Pediatrics* **72**:390, 1983.
585. Hanley WB, Demshar H, Preston MA, et al: Newborn phenylketonuria (PKU) Guthrie (BIA) screening and early hospital discharge. *Early Hum Dev* **47**:87, 1997.
586. Sinai LN, Kim SC, Casey R, et al: Phenylketonuria screening: Effect of early newborn discharge. *Pediatrics* **96**:605, 1995.
587. Schoen EJ, Cunningham GC, Koch R: More on newborn screening for phenylketonuria: Recommendations of the Committee on Genetics. *Pediatrics* **72**:139, 1983.
588. Levy HL, Mitchell ML, Ridley SE: Newborn screening. *Pediatrics* **73**:417, 1984.
589. Scriver CR: More on newborn screening for phenylketonuria: In reply. *Pediatrics* **72**:141, 1983.
590. Sepe SJ, Levy HL, Mount FW: An evaluation of routine follow-up blood screening of infants for phenylketonuria. *N Engl J Med* **300**:606, 1979.
591. US Congress: Healthy children: Investing in the future, in Anonymous (ed): *Newborn Screening for Congenital Disorders*. Washington, DC, US Office of Technology Assessments, 1988, p 93.
592. American Academy of Pediatrics Committee on Genetics: Issues in newborn screening. *Pediatrics* **89**:345, 1992.
593. Gerasimova NS, Steklova IV, Tuuminen T: Fluorometric method for phenylalanine microplate assay adapted for phenylketonuria screening. *Clin Chem* **35**:2112, 1989.
594. Hill JB: A climatological factor influencing the determination of phenylalanine in blood of newborn infants in North Carolina. *Biochem Med* **2**:261, 1969.
595. Lambert DM: The genetic epidemiology of hyperphenylalaninemia in Quebec [abstr]. Thesis submitted to the Faculty of Graduate Studies and Research, McGill University, Montreal, 1994.
596. Clemens PC, Neumann SJ, Wulke AP, et al: Newborn screening for hyperphenylalaninemia on day 5: Is 240 μmol/liter the most appropriate cut-off level? *Prev Med* **19**:54, 1990.
597. Doherty LB, Roh RFJ, Levy HL: Detection of phenylketonuria in the very early newborn blood specimen. *Pediatrics* **87**:240, 1991.

598. Holtzman C, Slazyk WE, Cordero JF, et al: Descriptive epidemiology of missed cases of phenylketonuria and congenital hypothyroidism. *Pediatrics* **78**:553, 1986.
599. McCabe ERB, McCabe L: Screening for PKU in sick or premature neonates. *J Pediatr* **103**:502, 1983.
600. Binder J, Johnson CF, Saboe B, et al: Delayed elevation of serum phenylalanine level in a breast-fed child. *Pediatrics* **63**:334, 1979.
601. Morris AF, Holton JB, Burman D, et al: Phenylalanine and tyrosine levels in newborn screening blood samples. *Arch Dis Child* **58**:271, 1983.
602. Walker V, Clayton BE, Ersser RS, et al: Hyperphenylalaninemia of various types among three-quarters of a million neonates tested in a screening programme. *Arch Dis Child* **56**:759, 1981.
603. Holtzman NA, Meek AG, Mellits ED, et al: Neonatal screening for phenylketonuria: III. Altered sex ratio; extent and possible causes. *J Pediatr* **85**:175, 1974.
604. Scriver CR: Screening for medical intervention: The PKU experience in human genetics. *Prog Clin Biol Res* **103B**:437, 1982.
605. Laberge C, Ferreira P, Grenier A, et al: Hyperphenylalaninémies: Expérience canadienne et québecoise. *Arch Fr Pediatr* **44**:643, 1987.
606. Mabry CC, Reid MC, Kuhn RJ: A source of error in phenylketonuria in phenylketonuria testing. *Am J Clin Pathol* **90**:279, 1988.
607. Wilcken B, Brown ARD, Liu A, et al: Correspondence and corrections: Eliminating some possible errors in phenylketonuria screening. *Am J Clin Pathol* **92**:396, 1989.
608. Kremensky I, Kalalydjieva L: Avoiding sources of error in PKU screening. *Am J Clin Pathol* **921**:396, 1989.
609. Mitton SG, Burston D, Brueton MJ: Hyperphenylalaninemia in parenterally fed newborn infants. *Lancet* **2**:8626, 1988.
610. Slazyk WE, Phillips DL, Therrell BL Jr, et al: Effect of lot-to-lot variability in filter paper on the quantification of thyroxin, thyrotopin, and phenylalanine in dried-blood specimens. *Clin Chem* **34**:53, 1988.
611. Meaney FJ: Computerized tracking for newborn screening and follow-up: A review. *J Med Syst* **12**:69, 1988.
612. Sorensen JR, Levy HL, Mangione TW, et al: Parental response to repeat testing of infants with "false-positive" results in a newborn screening program. *Pediatrics* **73**:183, 1984.
613. Bush JW, Chen MM, Patrick DL: Health status index in cost effectiveness: Analysis of PKU program, in Berg RL (ed): *Health Status Indexes Hospital Research and Educational Trust.* London, Health Status Indexes Hospital Research and Educational Trust, 1973, p 172.
614. Dagenais DL, Courville L, Dagenais MG: A cost-benefit analysis of the Quebec Network of Genetic Medicine. *Soc Sci Med* **20**:601, 1985.
615. Levy HL, Lobbregt D: Postnatal clearance of maternally derived phenylalanine in offspring of maternal phenylketonuria: Implications for newborn screening. *Screening* **4**:79, 1995.
616. Blau N, Barnes I, Dhondt JL: International database of tetrahydrobiopterin deficiencies. *J Inherited Metab Dis* **19**:8, 1996.
617. Kaufman S: Unsolved problems in diagnosis and therapy of hyperphenylalaninemia caused by defects in tetrahydropterin metabolism. *J Pediatr* **109**:572, 1986.
618. Leeming RJ, Blair JA, Green A, et al: Biopterin derivatives in normal and phenylketonuric patients after oral loads of L-phenylalanine, L-tyrosine, and L-tryptophan. *Arch Dis Child* **51**:771, 1976.
619. Trefz FK, Bartholomé K, Bickel H, et al: In vivo determination of phenylalanine hydroxylase activity using heptadeutero-phenylalanine and comparison to the in vitro assay values. *Monogr Hum Genet* **9**:108, 1978.
620. Surplice IM, Griffiths PD, Green A, et al: Dihydropteridine reductase activity in eluates from dried blood spots: Automation of an assay for a national screening service. *J Inherit Metab Dis* **13**:169, 1990.
621. Lei XD, Kaufman S: Human white blood cells and hair follicles are good sources of mRNA for the pterin carbinolamine dehydratase/dimerization cofactor of HNF1 for mutation detection. *Biochem Biophys Res Commun* **248**:432, 1998.
622. Chelly J, Concordet JP, Kaplan JC, et al: Illegitimate transcription: Transcription of any gene in any cell type. *Proc Natl Acad Sci USA* **86**:2617, 1989.
623. Scriver CR, Clow CL: Avoiding phenylketonuria: Why parents seek prenatal diagnosis. *J Pediatr* **113**:495, 1988.
624. Riess O, Michel A, Speer A, et al: Introduction of genomic diagnosis of classical phenylketonuria to the health care system of the German Democratic Republic. *Clin Genet* **32**:209, 1987.
625. Barwell BE, Pollitt RJ: Attitude des parents vis-à-vis du diagnostic prénatal de la phenylcétonurie. *Arch Fr Pediatr* **44**:665, 1987.
626. Cleary MA, Wraith JE: Antenatal diagnosis of inborn errors of metabolism. *Arch Dis Child* **66**:816, 1991.
627. Woo SLC: Prenatal diagnosis and carrier detection of classic phenylketonuria by gene analysis. *Pediatrics* **74**:412, 1984.
628. Lehmann WD, Theobald N, Heinrich HC, et al: Detection of heterozygous carriers for phenylketonuria by a L-($^2H_5$)phenylalanine stable isotope loading test. *Clin Chim Acta* **138**:59, 1984.
629. Hsai D, Driscoll KW, Troll W, et al: Detection of phenylalanine tolerance tests of heterozygous carriers of phenylketonuria. *Nature* **178**:1239, 1956.
630. Blitzer MG, Bailey-Wilson JE, Shapira E: Discrimination of heterozygotes for phenylketonuria, persistent hyperphenylalaninemia and controls by phenylalanine loading. *Clin Chim Acta* **161**:347, 1986.
631. Woolf LI, Cranston WI, Goodwin BL: Genetics of phenylketonuria. *Nature* **213**:882, 1967.
632. Woolf LI, Goodwin BL, Cranston WI, et al: A third allele at the phenylalanine-hydroxylase locus in mild phenylketonuria (hyperphenylalaninemia). *Lancet* **1**:114, 1968.
633. Hilton MA, Sharpe JN, Hicks LG, et al: A simple method for detection of heterozygous carriers of the gene for classic phenylketonuria. *J Pediatr* **109**:601, 1986.
634. Guneral F, Ozalp I, Tatlidil H: Heterozygous carriers of classical phenylketonuria in a sample of the Turkish population: Detection by a spectrofluorimetric method. *J Inherited Metab Dis* **14**:741, 1991.
635. Gold RJM, Maag UR, Neal JL, et al: The use of biochemical data in screening for mutant alleles and in genetic counselling. *Ann Hum Genet* **37**:315, 1974.
636. Westwood A, Raine DN: Heterozygote detection in phenylketonuria. *J Med Genet* **12**:327, 1975.
637. Freehauf CL, Lezotte D, Goodman SI, et al: Carrier screening for phenylketonuria: Comparison of two discriminant analysis procedures. *Am J Hum Genet* **36**:1180, 1984.
638. Paul TD, Brandt IK, Elsas LJ, et al: Phenylketonuria heterozygote detection in families with affected children. *Am J Hum Genet* **30**:293, 1978.
639. Wenger SL, Vieira PW, Breck JM, et al: Relative reliability of three different discriminant analysis methods for detecting PKU gene carriers. *Clin Genet* **30**:38, 1986.
640. Sartorio R, Greco L, Carrozzo R, et al: A simplified test to detect PKU heterozygotes by discriminant analysis in mentally retarded children and their mothers. *Clin Genet* **33**:241, 1988.
641. Holton JB: Long-term results of treatment of some inherited metabolic diseases. *Pediatr Rev Commun* **8**:139, 1995.
642. Medical Research Council Working Party on Phenylketonuria: Phenylketonuria due to phenylalanine hydroxylase deficiency: An unfolding story. *BMJ* **306**:115, 1993.
643. Cockburn F, Barwell BE, Brenton DP, et al: Recommendations on the dietary management of phenylketonuria. *Arch Dis Child* **68**:426, 1993.
644. Bickel H, Gerrard J, Hickmans EM: Influence of phenylalanine intake on the chemistry and behaviour of a phenylketonuric child. *Acta Paediatr Scand* **43**:64, 1954.
645. Woolf LI, Griffiths R, Moncrieff A: Treatment of phenylketonuria with a diet low in phenylalanine. *BMJ* **1**:57, 1955.
646. Armstrong MD, Tyler FH: Studies on phenylketonuria: I. Restriction phenylalanine intake in phenylketonuria. *J Clin Invest* **34**:565, 1955.
647. Ullrich K, Weglage J, Oberwittler C, et al: Effect of L-dopa on visual evoked potentials and neuropsychological tests in adult phenylketonuria patients. *Eur J Pediatr* **155**:S74, 1996.
648. Smith I, Wolff OH: Natural history of phenylketonuria and influence of early treatment. *Lancet* **2**:540, 1974.
649. Dobson JC, Kushida E, Williamson M, et al: Intellectual performance of 36 phenylketonuria patients and their nonaffected siblings. *Pediatrics* **58**:53, 1976.
650. Williamson M, Dobson C, Koch R: Collaborative study of children treated for phenylketonuria: Study design. *Pediatrics* **60**:815, 1977.
651. Dobson JC, Williamson ML, Azen C, et al: Intellectual assessment of 111 four-year-old children with phenylketonuria. *Pediatrics* **60**:822, 1977.
652. Williamson ML, Koch R, Azen C, et al: Correlates of intelligence test results in treated phenylketonuric children. *Pediatrics* **68**:161, 1981.
653. Koch R, Azen C, Friedman EG, et al: Paired comparisons between early treated PKU children and their matched sibling controls on intelligence and school achievement test results at eight years of age. *J Inherit Metab Dis* **7**:86, 1984.

654. Azen CG, Koch R, Friedman EG, et al: Intellectual development in 12-year old children treated for phenylketonuria. *Am J Dis Child* **145**:35, 1991.
655. Smith I, Beasley M: Intelligence and behaviour in children with early treated phenylketonuria. *Eur J Clin Nutr* **43**:1, 1988.
656. Smith I, Beasley MG, Wolff OH, et al: Behaviour disturbance in the 8-year-old children with early-treated phenylketonuria. *J Pediatr* **112**:403, 1988.
657. Smith I, Beasley MG, Ades AE: Intelligence and quality of dietary treatment in phenylketonuria. *Arch Dis Child* **65**:472, 1990.
658. Flynn JR: The mean IQ of Americans: Massive gains 1932–1978. *Physiol Bull* **95**:29, 1984.
659. Griffiths P, Campbell R, Robinson P: Executive function in treated phenylketonuria as measured by the one-back and two-back versions of the continuous performance test. *J Inherit Metab Dis* **21**:125, 1998.
660. Arnold GL, Kramer BM, Kirby RS, et al: Factors affecting cognitive, motor, behavioural and executive functioning in children with phenylketonuria. *Acta Paediatr Scand* **87**:565, 1998.
661. Holtzman NA, Kronmal RA, Van Doorninck W, et al: Effect of age at loss of dietary control on intellectual performance and behaviour of children with phenylketonuria. *N Engl J Med* **314**:593, 1986.
662. Pennington BF, Van Doorninck W, Azen C, et al: Effect of age at loss of dietary control on intellectual performance and behaviour of children with phenylketonuria. *Am J Ment Defic* **89**:467, 1985.
663. Rapoport D, Saudubray JM, Ogier H, et al: Psychological prospects and scholastic performance of 33 children with early diagnosis of hyperphenylalaninemia. *Arch Fr Pediatr* **273**:1983, 1983.
664. Melnick CR, Michals KK, Matalon R: Linguistic development of children with phenylketonuria and normal intelligence. *J Pediatr* **98**:269, 1981.
665. Berry HD, O'Grady DJ, Perlmutter LJ, et al: Intellectual development and academic achievement of children treated early for phenylketonuria. *Dev Med Child Neurol* **21**:311, 1979.
666. Faust D, Libon D, Pueschel S: Neuropsychological functioning in treated phenylketonuria. *Int J Psychiatr Med* **16**:169, 1986.
667. Netley C, Hanley WB, Rudier HL: Phenylketonuria and its variants: Observations on intellectual functioning. *Can Med Assoc J* **131**:751, 1984.
668. Fischer K, Azen C, Henderson R, et al: Psychoeducational findings among children treated for phenylketonuria. *Am J Ment Defic* **92**:65, 1987.
669. Welsh MC, Pennington BF, Ozonoff S, et al: Neuropsychology of early-treated phenylketonuria: Specific executive function deficits. *Child Dev* **61**:1697, 1990.
670. Desonneville LHJ, Schmidt E, Michel U, et al: Preliminary neuropsychological test results. *Eur J Pediatr* **5**(suppl 1):39, 1990.
671. Koch R, Yusin M, Fishler K: Successful adjustment to society by adults with phenylketonuria. *J Inherit Metab Dis* **8**:209, 1985.
672. Holm VA, Kronmal RA, Williamson M, et al: Physical growth in phenylketonuria: II. Growth of treated children in the PKU collaborative study from birth to 4 years of age. *Pediatrics* **63**:700, 1979.
673. Lyonnet S, Caillaud C, Rey F, et al: Molecular genetics of phenylketonuria in Mediterranean countries: A mutation associated with partial phenylalanine hydroxylase deficiency. *Am J Hum Genet* **44**:511, 1989.
674. White JE, Kronmal RA, Acosta PB: Excess weight among children with phenylketonuria. *J Am Coll Nutr* **1**:293, 1982.
675. McBurnie MA, Kronmal RA, Schuett VE, et al: Physical growth of children treated for phenylketonuria. *Ann Hum Biol* **18**:357, 1991.
676. Scaglioni S, Virdis R, Zucotti G, et al: Pubertal maturation and classical phenylketonuria. *J Inherit Metab Dis* **9**:285, 1986.
677. Fehrenbach AMB, Petersen L: Parental problem-solving skills, stress, and dietary compliance in phenylketonuria. *J Consult Clin Psychol* **57**:237, 1989.
678. Kazak AE, Reber M, Snitzer L: Childhood chronic disease and family functioning: A study of phenylketonuria. *Pediatrics* **81**:224, 1988.
679. Zygulska M, Eigel A, Pietrzyk JJ, et al: Phenylketonuria in Southern Poland: A new splice mutation in intron 9 at the PAH locus. *Hum Mutat* **4**:297, 1994.
680. Griffiths P, Tarrini M, Robinson P: Executive function and psychosocial adjustment in children with early treated phenylketonuria: Correlation with historical and concurrent phenylalanine levels. *J Intellect Disabil Res* **41**:317, 1997.
680a. Diamond A, Prevor MB, Callender G, Druin D: Prefrontal cortex cognitive deficits in children treated early and continuously for PKU. *Monogr Soc Res Child Dev* **62**:1, 1997.
680b. Welsh MC, Pennington BF, Ozonoff S, et al: Neuropsychology of early-treated phenylketonuria: Specific executive function deficits. *Child Dev* **61**:1697, 1990.
681. Kalverboer AF, Van der Schot LWA, Hendrikx MMH, et al: Social behaviour and task orientation in early-treated PKU. *Acta Paediatr Scand Suppl* **407**:104, 1994.
682. Ris MD, Weber AM, Hunt MM, et al: Adult psychosocial outcome in early-treated phenylketonuria. *J Inherit Metab Dis* **20**:499, 1997.
683. Burgard P, Armbruster M, Schmidt E, et al: Psychopathology of patients treated for phenylketonuria: Results of the German collaborative study of phenylketonuria. *Acta Paediatr Scand Suppl* **407**:108, 1994.
684. Diamond A: Phenylalanine levels of 6–10 mg/dl may not be as benign as once thought. *Acta Paediatr Scand Suppl* **407**:89, 1994.
685. Smith I, Lobascher M, Stevenson J, et al: Effect of stopping the low phenylalanine diet on the intellectual progress of children with phenylketonuria. *Ann Clin Biochem* **14**:134, 1977.
686. Cabalska B, Duczynska N, Borzymowska J, et al: Termination of dietary treatment in phenylketonuria. *Eur J Pediatr* **126**:253, 1977.
687. Smith I, Lobascher ME, Stevenson JE, et al: Effect of stopping low-phenylalanine diet on intellectual progress of children with phenylketonuria. *BMJ* **2**:723, 1978.
688. Holtzman NA, Welcher DW, Mellits ED: Termination of restricted diet in children with phenylketonuria: A randomized controlled study. *N Engl J Med* **293**:1121, 1975.
689. Holtzman NA: Anatomy of a trial. *Pediatrics* **60**:932, 1977.
689a. Koff E, Kammerer B, Boyle P, et al: Intelligence and phenylketonuria: Effects of diet termination. *J Pediatr* **94**:534, 1979.
689b. Williamson M, Koch R, Berlow L: Diet discontinuation in phenylketonuria. *Pediatrics* **63**:823, 1979.
689c. Koch R, Azen CG, Friedman EG, et al: Preliminary report on the effects of diet discontinuation in PKU. *J Pediatr* **100**:870, 1982.
690. Woolf IL: Late onset phenylalanine intoxication. *J Inherit Metab Dis* **2**:19, 1979.
691. Seashore MR, Friedman E, Novelly RA, et al: Loss of intellectual function in children with phenylketonuria after relaxation of dietary phenylalanine restriction. *Pediatrics* **75**:226, 1985.
692. Behbehari AW: Termination of strict diet therapy in phenylketonuria: A study on EEG sleep patterns and computer spectral analysis. *Neuropediatrics* **16**:92, 1985.
693. Lou HC, Güttler F, Lykkelund C, et al: Decreased vigilance and neurotransmitter synthesis after discontinuation of dietary treatment for phenylketonuria in adolescents. *Eur J Pediatr* **144**:17, 1985.
694. Matthews WS, Barabas G, Cusack E, et al: Social quotients of children with phenylketonuria before and after discontinuation of dietary treatment. *Am J Ment Defic* **91**:92, 1986.
695. Rey F, Abadie V, Plainguet F, et al: Long-term follow up of patients with classical phenylketonuria after diet relaxation at 5 years of age: The Paris study. *Eur J Pediatr* **155**:S39, 1996.
696. McDonnell GV, Esmonde TF, Hadden DR, et al: A neurological evaluation of adult phenylketonuria in Northern Ireland. *Eur Neurol* **39**:38, 1998.
697. Neilsen JB, Lou HC, Guttler F: Effects of diet discontinuation and dietary tryptophan supplementation on neurotransmitter metabolism in phenylketonuria. *Brain Dysfunct* **1**:51, 1988.
698. Walter JH, White F, Wraith JE, et al: Complete reversal of moderate/severe brain MRI abnormalities in a patient with classical phenylketonuria. *J Inherit Metab Dis* **20**:367, 1997.
699. Weglage J, Schmidt E, Funders B, et al: Sustained attention in untreated non-PKU-hyperphenylalaninemia. *J Clin Exp Neuropsychol* **18**:343, 1996.
700. Weglage J, Ullrich K, Pietsch M, et al: Intellectual, neurologic, and neuropsychologic outcome in untreated subjects with nonphenylketonuria hyperphenylalaninemia. *Pediatr Res* **42**:378, 1997.
701. Smith I, Beasley MG, Ades AE: Effect of intelligence of relaxing the low phenylalanine diet in phenylketonuria. *Arch Dis Child* **66**:311, 1991.
702. Naughten ER: Continuation vs discontinuation of diet on phenylketonuria. *Eur J Clin Nutr* **43**:7, 1989.
703. Schuett VE, Gurda RG, Brown ES: Diet discontinuation policies and practices of PKU clinics in the United States. *Am J Public Health* **70**:498, 1980.
704. Schuett VE, Brown ES: Diet policies of PKU clinics in the United States. *Am J Public Health* **74**:501, 1984.

705. Schuett VE, Brown ES, Michals K: Reinstitution of diet therapy in PKU patients from twenty-two US clinics. *Am J Public Health* **75**:39, 1985.
706. Hogan SE, Gates RD, Macdonald GW, et al: Experience with adolescents with phenylketonuria returned to phenylalanine-restricted diets. *J Am Diet Assoc* **86**:1203, 1986.
707. Griffiths P, Smith C, Harvie C: Transitory hyperphenylalaninemia in children with continuously treated phenylketonuria. *Am J Ment Retard* **102**:27, 1997.
707a. Koch R, Moseley K, Ning J, et al: Long-term beneficial effects of the phenylalanine-restricted diet in late-diagnosed individuals with phenylketonuria. *Mol Genet Metab* **67**:148, 1999.
707b. Walter JH, White FJ: Biochemical control in phenylalanine: What is achievable? [abstr A22]. *J Inherit Metab Dis* **22**(suppl 1):63, 1999.
708. Levy HL, Waisbren SE: PKU in adolescents: Rationale and psychosocial factors in diet continuation. *Acta Pediatr Scand Suppl* **407**:92, 1994.
709. Fisch RO, Matalon R, Weisberg S, et al: Phenylketonuria: Current dietary treatment practices in the United States and Canada. *J Am Coll Nutr* **16**:147, 1997.
710. Griffiths P, Ward N, Harvie A, et al: Neuropsychological outcome of experimental manipulation of phenylalanine intake in treated phenylketonuria. *J Inherit Metab Dis* **21**:39, 1998.
711. Scriver CR: Mutants: Consumers with special needs. *Nutr Rev* **29**:155, 1971.
712. Acosta PB, Trahms C, Wellman NS, et al: Phenylalanine intakes of 1- to 6-year old children with phenylketonuria undergoing therapy. *Am J Clin Nutr* **38**:694, 1983.
713. Thompson GN, Francis DEM, Kirby DM, et al: Pregnancy in phenylketonuria: Dietary treatment aimed at normalizing maternal plasma phenylalanine concentration. *Arch Dis Child* **66**:1346, 1991.
714. Nayman R, Thomson E, Scriver CR, et al: Observations on the composition of milk-substitute products for treatment of inborn errors of amino acid metabolism: Comparisons with human milk. *Am J Clin Nutr* **32**:1279, 1979.
715. Link RM, Wachtel U: Clinical experiences with an amino acid preparation in children with phenylketonuria. *Rev Med Liege* **39**:429, 1984.
716. Buist NRM, Prince AP, Huntington KL, et al: A new amino acid mixture permits new approaches to the treatment of phenylketonuria. *Acta Paediatr Suppl* **407**:75, 1994.
717. Acosta PB, Wenz E, Williamson M: Nutrient intake of untreated infants with phenylketonuria. *Am J Clin Nutr* **30**:198, 1977.
718. Kindt E, Halvorsen S: The need of essential amino acids in children: An evaluation on the intake of phenylalanine, tyrosine, leucine, isoleucine, and valine in children with phenylketonuria, tyrosine amino transferase defect and maple syrup urine disease. *Am J Clin Nutr* **33**:279, 1980.
719. Kindt E, Motzfeldt K, Halvorsen S, et al: Protein measurements in infants and children: A longitudinal study of children treated for phenylketonuria. *Am J Clin Nutr* **37**:778, 1983.
720. Kindt E, Motzfeldt K, Halvorsen S, et al: Is phenylalanine requirement in infants and children related to protein intake? *Br J Nutr* **51**:435, 1984.
721. Kindt E, Lunde HA, Gjessing LR, et al: Fasting plasma amino acid concentrations in PKU children on two different levels of protein intake. *Acta Paediatr* **77**:60, 1988.
722. Gropper SS, Acosta PB, Clarke-Sheehan N, et al: Trace element status of children with PKU and normal children. *J Am Diet Assoc* **88**:459, 1988.
723. Galli C, Agostoni C, Mosconi C, et al: Reduced plasma C-20 and C-22 polyunsaturated fatty acids in children with phenylketonuria during dietary intervention. *J Pediatr* **119**:562, 1991.
724. Macdonald A, Rylance GW, Asplin D, et al: Does a single plasma phenylalanine predict quality of control in phenylketonuria? *Arch Dis Child* **78**:122, 1998.
725. Cockburn F, Clark BJ: Recommendations for protein and amino acid intake in phenylketonuric patients. *Eur J Pediatr* **155**:S125, 1996.
726. Acosta PB, Yannicelli S: Protein intake affects phenylalanine requirements and growth of infants with phenylketonuria. *Acta Paediatr Suppl* **407**:66, 1994.
727. Van der Schot LW, Doesburg WH, Sengers RCA: The phenylalanine response curve in relation to growth and mental development in the first years of life. *Acta Paediatr Suppl* **407**:68, 1994.
728. Van Spronsen FJ, Verkerk PH, Van Houten M, et al: Does impaired growth of PKU patients correlate with the strictness of dietary treatment? *Acta Paediatr* **86**:816, 1997.
729. Macdonald A, Rylance GW, Asplin DA, et al: Feeding problems in young PKU children. *Acta Paediatr Suppl* **407**:73, 1994.
730. Hanley WB, Linsao L, Davidson W, et al: Malnutrition with early treatment of phenylketonuria. *Pediatr Res* **4**:318, 1970.
731. Lou HC: Dopamine precursors and brain function in phenylalanine hydroxylase deficiency. *Acta Pediatr Suppl* **407**:86, 1994.
732. McCabe L, Ernest AE, Neifert MR, et al: The management of breast feeding among infants with phenylketonuria. *J Inherited Metab Dis* **12**:467, 1989.
733. Filer LJ Jr, Stegink LD: Aspartame metabolism in normal adults, phenylketonuric heterozygotes, and diabetic subjects. *Diabetes Care* **12**:67, 1989.
734. Curtius H, Wolf E, Blau N: Effect of high-protein meal plus aspartame ingestion on plasma phenylalanine concentrations in obligate heterozygotes for phenylketonuria. *Metabolism* **43**:413, 1994.
735. Koeppe RA, Shulkin BL, Rosenspire KC, et al: Effect of aspartame-derived phenylalanine on neutral amino acid uptake in a human brain: A positron emission tomography study. *J Neurochem* **56**:1526, 1991.
736. Mullenix PJ, Tassinari MS, Schunior A, et al: No change in spontaneous behaviour of rats after acute oral doses of aspartame, phenylalanine, and tyrosine. *Fund Appl Toxicol* **16**:495, 1991.
737. Meldrum BS, Nanji N, Cornell RG: Lack of effect of aspartame of L-phenylalanine on photically induced myoclonus in the baboon, *Papio papio*. *Epilepsy Res* **4**:1, 1989.
738. Stegink LD, Filer LJ Jr, Brummel MC, et al: Plasma amino acid concentrations and amino acid ratios in normal adults and adults heterozygous for phenylketonuria ingesting a hamburger and milk shake meal. *Am J Clin Nutr* **53**:670, 1991.
739. Hodgins D: Yeast phenylalanine ammonia lyase: Purification, properties, and the identification of catalytically essential dehydroalanine. *J Biol Chem* **246**:2977, 1971.
740. Hoskins JA, Holliday SB, Greenway AM: The metabolism of cinnamic acid by healthy and phenylketonuric adults: A kinetic study. *Biomed Mass Spectrom* **11**:296, 1984.
741. Bourget L, Chang TM: Phenylalanine ammonia-lyase immobilized in semipermeable microcapsules for enzyme replacement in phenylketonuria. *FEBS Lett* **180**:5, 1985.
742. Bourget L, Chang TMS: Phenylalanine ammonia-lyase immobilized in microcapsules for the depletion of phenylalanine in plasma in phenylketonuric rat model. *Biochim Biophys Acta* **883**:432, 1986.
743. Bourget L, Chang TMS: Effects of oral administration of artificial cells immobilized phenylalanine ammonia-lyase on intestinal amino acids in phenylketonuric rats. *Biomater Artif Cells Artif Organs* **17**:161, 1989.
744. Ambrus CM, Anthone S, Norvath C, et al: Extracorporeal enzyme reactors for depletion of phenylalanine in phenylketonuria. *Ann Intern Med* **106**:531, 1987.
745. Larue C, Munnich A, Charpentier C, et al: An extracorporeal hollow fibre reactor for phenylketonuria using immobilized phenylalanine ammonia lyase. *Dev Pharmacol Ther* **9**:73, 1986.
746. Hoskins JA, Jack G, Wade HE, et al: Enzymatic control of phenylalanine intake in phenylketonuria. *Lancet* **1**:392, 1980.
747. Gilbert HJ, Clarke IN, Gibson RK, et al: Molecular cloning of the phenylalanine ammonia lyase gene from *Rhodosporidium toruloides*. *J Bacteriol* **161**:314, 1985.
748. Eisensmith RC, Woo SLC: Gene therapy for phenylketonuria. *Acta Paediatr Scand Suppl* **407**:124, 1994.
749. Fang B, Eisensmith RC, Woo SLC: Phenylketonuria: A model for hepatic gene therapy. *Ment Retard Dev Disabil Res Rev* **1**:56, 1995.
750. Eisensmith RC, Woo SLC: Gene therapy for phenylketonuria. *Eur J Pediatr* **155**:S16, 1996.
751. Ledley FD, Grenett H, McGinnis-Shelnutt M, et al: Retroviral-mediated gene transfer of human phenylalanine hydroxylase into NIH 3T3 and hepatoma cells. *Proc Natl Acad Sci USA* **83**:409, 1986.
752. Peng H, Armentano D, MacKenzie-Graham L, et al: Retroviral-mediated gene transfer and expression of human phenylalanine hydroxylase in primary mouse hepatocytes. *Proc Natl Acad Sci USA* **85**:8146, 1988.
753. Liu T-J, Kay MA, Darlington GJ, et al: Reconstitution of enzymatic activity in hepatocytes of phenylalanine hydroxylase-deficient mice. *Somat Cell Mol Genet* **18**:89, 1992.
754. Miller AD, Rosman GJ: Improved retroviral vectors for gene transfer and expression. *BioTechniques* **7**:980, 1989.

755. Cristiano RJ, Smith LC, Woo SLC: Hepatic gene therapy: Adenovirus enhancement of receptor-mediated gene delivery and expression in primary hepatocytes. *Proc Natl Acad Sci USA* **90**:2122, 1993.
756. Fang B, Eisensmith RC, Li XHC, et al: Gene therapy for phenylketonuria: Phenotypic correction in a genetically deficient mouse model by adenovirus-mediated hepatic gene transfer. *Gene Ther* **1**:247, 1994.
757. Harding CO, Wild K, Chang D, et al: Metabolic engineering as therapy for inborn errors of metabolism: Development of mice with phenylalanine hydroxylase expression in muscle. *Gene Ther* **5**:683, 1998.
758. Murthy LI, Berry HK: Phenylalanine hydroxylase activity in liver from humans and subhuman primates: Its probable absence in kidney. *Biochem Med* **12**:392, 1975.
759. Kay MA, Baley P, Rothenberg S, et al: Expression of human α_1-antitrypsin in dogs after autologous transplantation of retroviral transduced hepatocytes. *Proc Natl Acad Sci USA* **89**:89, 1992.
760. Wilson JM, Grossman M, Wu CH, et al: Hepatocyte-directed gene transfer in vivo leads to transient improvement in hypercholesterolemia in low density lipoprotein receptor-deficient rabbits. *J Biol Chem* **267**:963, 1992.
761. Wu GY, Wilson JM, Shalaby F, et al: Receptor-mediated gene delivery in vivo. *J Biol Chem* **266**:14,338, 1991.
762. Whittle N: Gene therapy: The gutless approach pays off. *Trends Genet* **14**:136, 1998.
762a. Lin CM, Tan Y, Lee YM, et al: Expression of human phenylalanine hydroxylase activity in T lymphocytes of classical phenylketonuria children by retroviral-mediated gene transfer. *J Inherit Metab Dis* **20**:742, 1997.
763. Levy HL: Reproductive effects of inborn errors of metabolism, in Farriaux J, Dhondt J (eds): *New Horizons in Neonatal Screening*. Amsterdam, Excerpta Medica, 1994, p 61.
764. Dent CE: Relation of biochemical abnormality to development of mental defect in phenylketonuria: Discussion to paper by Armstrong, M.D, in Ross Labs (ed): *Report of 23rd Ross Pediatric Research Conference: Etiological Factors in Mental Retardation*. Columbus, OH, Ross Labs, 1957, p 32.
765. Mabry CC, Dennison JC, Nelson TL, et al: Maternal phenylketonuria: A cause of mental retardation in children without the metabolic defect. *N Engl J Med* **269**:1404, 1963.
766. Allan JD, Brown JK: Maternal phenylketonuria and foetal brain damage: An attempt at prevention by dietary control, in Holt KS, Coffey VP (eds): *Some Recent Advances in Inborn Errors of Metabolism*. Edinburgh, Livingstone, 1968, p 14.
767. Hanley WB: Prenatal testing for maternal phenylketonuria (MPKU). *Int Pediatr* **9**:33, 1994.
768. Hanley WB, Platt LD, Bachman RP, et al: Undiagnosed maternal phenylketonuria: The need for prenatal selective screening or case finding. *Am J Obstet Gynecol* **180**:986, 1999.
769. Kirkman HN: Projections of a rebound in frequency of mental retardation from phenylketonuria. *Appl Res Ment Retard* **3**:319, 1992.
770. Lenke RR, Levy HL: Maternal phenylketonuria and hyperphenylalaninemia: An international survey of untreated and treated pregnancies. *N Engl J Med* **303**:1202, 1980.
771. Lipson A, Beuhler B, Bartley J, et al: Maternal hyperphenylalaninemia fetal effects. *J Pediatr* **104**:216, 1984.
772. Levy HL, Lobbregt D, Platt LD, et al: Fetal ultrasonography in maternal PKU. *Prenat Diagn* **16**:599, 1996.
773. Fisch Ro, Matalon R, Weisberg S, et al: Children of fathers with phenylketonuria: An international survey. *J Pediatr* **118**:739, 1991.
774. Levy HL, Lobbregt S, Koch R, et al: Paternal phenylketonuria. *J Pediatr* **118**:741, 1991.
775. Drogari E, Smith I, Beasley M, et al: Timing of strict diet in relation to fetal damage in maternal phenylketonuria: An international collaborative study by the MCR/DHSS Phenylketonuria Register. *Lancet* **2**:927, 1987.
776. Levy HL, Waisbren SE: Effects of untreated maternal phenylketonuria and hyperphenylalaninemia on the fetus. *N Engl J Med* **309**:1269, 1983.
777. Waisbren SE, Levy HL: Effects of untreated maternal hyperphenylalaninemia on the fetus: Further study of families identified by routine cord blood screening. *J Pediatr* **116**:926, 1990.
778. Levy HL, Waisbren SE, Lobbregt D, et al: Maternal mild hyperphenylalaninemia: An international survey of offspring outcome. *Lancet* **344**:1589, 1994.
779. Levy HL, Waisbren SE, Lobbregt D, et al: Maternal non-phenylketonuric mild hyperphenylketonuric mild hyperphenylalaninemia. *Eur J Pediatr* **155**:S20, 1996.
780. Brenton DP, Haseler ME: Maternal phenylketonuria, in Fernandes J, Saudubray J, Tada K (eds): *Inborn Metabolic Diseases: Diagnosis and Treatment*. Berlin, Springer-Verlag, 1990, p 175.
781. Brenton DP: Maternal phenylketonuria. *Eur J Clin Nutr* **43**:13, 1988.
782. Hanley WB, Clarke JTR, Schoonkey TW: Maternal phenylketonuria (PKU): A review. *Clin Biochem* **20**:149, 1987.
783. Schoonheyt WE, Clarke JTR, Hanley WB, et al: Feto-maternal plasma phenylalanine concentration gradient from 19 weeks gestation to term. *Clin Chim Acta* **225**:165, 1994.
784. Roux C, Rey F, Lyonnet S, et al: An animal model for maternal phenylketonuria. *J Med Genet* **28**:718, 1992.
785. Denno KM, Sadler TW: Phenylalanine and its metabolites induce embryopathies in mouse embryos in culture. *Teratology* **42**:565, 1990.
786. Levy HL, Lenke RR, Koch R: Lack of fetal effect on blood phenylalanine concentration in maternal phenylketonuria. *J Pediatr* **104**:245, 1984.
787. Levy HL, Naylor EW, Mamunes P: Tissue amino acids and organic acids in the maternal phenylketonuria (MPKU) fetus: Implications for the pathogenesis of fetal damage in MPKU [abstr]. *Am J Hum Genet* **49**:43, 1988.
788. Dorland L, Poll-The BT, Duran M, et al: Phenylpyruvate, fetal damage, and maternal phenylketonuria syndrome. *Lancet* **341**:1351, 1993.
789. Kudo Y, Boyd CAR: Transport of amino acids by the human placenta: Predicted effects thereon of maternal hyperphenylketonuria. *J Inherited Metab Dis* **13**:617, 1990.
790. Gardiner RM: Transport of amino acids across the blood-brain barrier: Implications for treatment of maternal phenylketonuria. *J Inherit Metab Dis* **13**:627, 1990.
791. Vorhees CV, Berry HK: Branched chain amino acids improve complex maze learning in rat offspring prenatally exposed to hyperphenylalaninemia: Implications for maternal phenylketonuria. *Pediatr Res* **25**:568, 1989.
792. Brass CA, Isaacs CE, McChesney R, et al: The effects of hyperphenylalaninemia on fetal development: A new animal model of maternal phenylketonuria. *Pediatr Res* **16**:388, 1982.
793. Loo YH, Potempska A, Wang P, et al: Experimental maternal phenylketonuria: An examination of two animal models. *Dev Neurosci* **6**:227, 1983.
794. Sato T, Imura E, Murata A, et al: Effects of maternal phenylalanine or tyrosine hydroxylase inhibition on postnatal maturation of catecholamine and amino acid metabolism in rats. *Acta Pediatr Jpn* **30**:56, 1988.
795. Sadova D, Sutcliffe D: The effects of maternal hyperphenylalaninemia on learning in mature rats. *Life Sci* **43**:1119, 1988.
796. Kirby ML, Miyagawa ST: The effects of high phenylalanine concentration on chick embryonic development. *J Inherit Metab Dis* **13**:634, 1990.
797. Dyer CA, Philibotte T, Levy H, et al: Mechanisms of hypomyelination and gliosis in a genetic mouse model for phenylketonuria [abstr]. *J Neurochem* **64**:S111, 1995.
798. Bessman SP: Historical perspective: Tyrosine and maternal phenylketonuria, welcome news. *Am J Clin Nutr* **67**:357, 1998.
799. Rohr FJ, Lobbregt D, Levy HL: Tyrosine supplementation in the treatment of maternal phenylketonuria. *Am J Clin Nutr* **67**:473, 1998.
800. Levy HL: Reply to SP Bessman. *Am J Clin Nutr* **67**:488, 1998.
801. Mowat DR, Hayden MC, Thompson SM, Wilcken B: Maternal phenylketonuria: A continuing problem. *Med J Aust* **170**:592, 1999.
802. Waisbren SE, Doherty LB, Bailey IV, et al: The New England maternal PKU project: Identification of at-risk women. *Am J Public Health* **78**:789, 1988.
803. Smith I, Wolff OH: MRC/DHSS Phenylketonuria Register. *Newsletter no. 5*:2, 1978.
804. Cartier L, Clow CL, Lippman-Hand A, et al: Prevention of mental retardation in offspring of hyperphenylalaninemic mothers. *Am J Public Health* **72**:1386, 1982.
805. Gungor N, Tokath A, Coskun T, et al: Microcephaly in a hyperphenylalaninemic infant leading to the diagnosis of maternal hyperphenylalaninemia. *Eur J Pediatr* **155**:257, 1996.
806. Superti-Furga A, Steinmann B, Duc G, et al: Maternal phenylketonuria syndrome in cousins caused by mild, unrecognized phenylketonuria in their mothers homozygous for the phenylalanine hydroxylase Arg-261-Gln mutation. *Eur J Pediatr* **150**:493, 1991.

807. Koch R, Hanley W, Levy H, et al: A preliminary report of the collaborative study of maternal phenylketonuria in the United States and Canada. *J Inherit Metab Dis* **13**:641, 1990.
808. Naughten E, Saul IP: Maternal phenylketonuria: The Irish experience. *J Inherited Metab Dis* **13**:658, 1990.
809. Güttler F, Lou H, Andresen J, et al: Cognitive development in offspring of untreated and preconceptionally treated maternal phenylketonuria. *J Inherited Metab Dis* **13**:665, 1990.
810. Koch R, Levy HL, Matalon R, et al: The international collaborative study of maternal phenylketonuria: Status report 1994. *Acta Paediatr Scand Suppl* **407**:111, 1994.
811. Koch R, Levy HL, Matalon E, et al: The international collaborative study of maternal phenylketonuria: 1994 status report, in Platt LD, Koch R, De la Cruz F (eds): *Genetic Disorders and Pregnancy Outcome*. New York, Parthenon, 1997, p 41.
812. Friedman EG, Koch R, Azen C, et al: The International collaborative study on maternal phenylketonuria: Organization, study design and description of the sample. *Eur J Pediatr* **155**:S158, 1996.
813. Hanley WB, Koch R, Levy HL, et al: The North American maternal phenylketonuria collaborative study: Developmental assessment of the offspring—Preliminary report. *Eur J Pediatr* **155**:S169, 1996.
814. Rousse B, Azen C, Roch R, et al: Maternal Phenylketonuria Collaborative Study (MPKUCS) offspring: Facial anomalies, malformations, and early neurological sequelae. *Am J Med Genet* **69**:89, 1997.
815. Rohr FJ, Doherty L, Waisbren JE, et al: New England Maternal PKU Project: Prospective study of untreated and treated pregnancies and their outcomes. *J Pediatr* **110**:391, 1987.
816. Smith I, Glossop J, Beasley M: Fetal damage due to maternal phenylketonuria: Effects of dietary treatment and maternal phenylalanine concentrations around the time of conception. *J Inherited Metab Dis* **13**:651, 1990.
817. Clark BJ, Cockburn F: Management of inborn errors of metabolism during pregnancy. *Acta Paediatr Scand Suppl* **373**:43, 1991.
818. Matalon R, Michals K, Azen C, et al: Maternal PKU collaborative study: The effect of nutrient intake on pregnancy outcome. *J Inherit Metab Dis* **14**:371, 1991.
819. Waisbren SE, Chang P, Levy HL, et al: Neonatal neurological assessment of offspring in maternal PKU. *J Inherit Metab Dis* **21**:39, 1998.
820. Platt LD, Koch R, Azen C, et al: Maternal phenylketonuria collaborative study, obstetric aspects and outcome: The first 6 years. *Am J Obstet Gynecol* **166**:1150, 1992.
821. Cohen BE, Weiss R, Hadar R, et al: Group work with adolescent PKU girls and their mothers. *J Inherit Metab Dis* **11**:199, 1988.
822. Waisbren SE, Rokni H, Bailey I, et al: Social factors and the meaning of food in adherence to medical diets: Results of a maternal phenylketonuria summer camp. *J Inherit Metab Dis* **20**:21, 1997.
823. Waisbren SE, Shiloh S, St. James P, et al: Psychosocial factors in maternal phenylketonuria: Prevention of unplanned pregnancies. *Am J Public Health* **81**:299, 1991.
824. Waisbren SE, Hamilton BD, St. James PJ, et al: Psychosocial factors in maternal phenylketonuria: Women's adherence to medical recommendations. *Am J Public Health* **85**:1636, 1995.
825. Hyanek J, Viletova H, Soukup J, et al: Changes in phenylalanine tolerance while monitoring the dietetic treatment of pregnant women suffering from hyperphenylalaninemia. *J Inherit Metab Dis* **11**:427, 1988.
826. Acosta PB: Nutrition support of maternal phenylketonuria. *Semin Perinatol* **19**:182, 1995.
827. Wardley BL, Taitz LS: Clinical trial of a concentrated amino acid formula for older patients with phenylketonuria. *Eur J Clin Nutr* **42**:81, 1988.
828. Owada M, Abe M, Ono M, et al: Successful treatment of maternal phenylketonuria with a formula consisting of low phenylketonuria peptide as a protein source. *J Inherit Metab Dis* **11**:341, 1988.
829. Kecskemethy HH, Lobregt D, Levy HL: The use of gelatin capsules for ingestion of formula in dietary treatment of maternal phenylketonuria. *J Inherit Metab Dis* **16**:111, 1993.
830. Fox-Bacon C, McCamman S, Therou L, et al: Maternal PKU and breastfeeding: Case report of identical twin mothers. *Clin Pediatr* **36**:539, 1997.
831. Scriver CR, Kaufman S, Woo SLC: Mendelian hyperphenylalaninemia. *Annu Rev Genet* **22**:301, 1988.
832. Zschocke J, Graham CA, McKnight JJ, et al: The STR system in the human phenylalanine hydroxylase gene: True fragment length obtained with fluorescent labelled PCR primers. *Acta Paediatr* **407**:41, 1994.
833. Holtzman NA, Mellits ED, Kallman CH: Neonatal screening for phenylketonuria: II. Age dependence of initial phenylalanine in infants with PKU. *Pediatrics* **53**:353, 1974.
834. Wang T, Okano Y, Eisensmith RC, et al: Founder effect of a prevalent phenylketonuria mutation in the Oriental population. *Proc Natl Acad Sci USA* **88**:2146, 1991.
835. Liu SR, Zuo QH: Newborn screening for phenylketonuria in eleven districts. *Chin Med J [Engl]* **99**:113, 1986.
836. Chen RG, Pan XS, Qian DL: Twenty-one cases of phenylketonuria out of 348,767 newborns in Shanghai, China. *J Inherited Metab Dis* **12**:485, 1989.
837. Aoki K, Wada Y: Outcome of the patients detected by newborn screening in Japan. *Acta Paediatr Scand* **30**:429, 1988.
838. Aoki K: Follow-up study of the patients detected by newborn screening in Japan. *Jpn J Pediatr Med* **23**:1887, 1991.
839. Thalhammer OE: A collaborative study: Frequency of inborn errors of metabolism especially PKU, in some representative newborn screening centres around the world. *Humangenetik* **30**:273, 1975.
840. Szabo L, Somogyi C, Mâté M: Experience based on 800,000 newborn screening tests of the Budapest phenylketonuria centre. *Acta Paediatr Hung* **26**:113, 1985.
840a. Woolf LI, Lentner C: *Geigy Scientific Tables*, vol 4, 8th ed. Basel, 1986, p 231.
841. Eiken HG, Knappskog PM, Boman H, et al: Relative frequency, heterogeneity and geographic clustering of PKU mutations in Norway. *Eur J Hum Genet* **4**:205, 1996.
842. Eiken HG, Knappskog PM, Guldberg P, et al: DGGE analysis as supplement to SSCP analysis of the phenylalanine hydroxylase gene: Detection of eight (one de novo, seven inherited) of nine remaining Norwegian PKU mutations. *Hum Mutat* **8**:19, 1996.
843. Eisensmith RC, Woo SLC: Updated listing of haplotypes at the human phenylalanine hydroxylase (PAH) locus. *Am J Hum Genet* **51**:1445, 1992.
844. Smith I: Disorders of tetrahydrobiopterin metabolism, in Fernandes J, Saudubray J, Tada K (eds): *Inborn Metabolism Diseases: Diagnosis and Treatment*. Berlin, Springer-Verlag, 1991, p 183.

CHAPTER 78

Disorders of Tetrahydrobiopterin and Related Biogenic Amines

Nenad Blau ■ Beat Thöny
Richard G. H. Cotton ■ Keith Hyland

1. Tetrahydrobiopterin (BH_4) deficiencies are disorders affecting phenylalanine homeostasis, and catecholamine and serotonin biosynthesis. The minimum requirements for the normal reaction(s) are the apoenzymes, phenylalanine-4-hydroxylase (PAH), tyrosine-3-hydroxylase (TH), or tryptophan-5-hydroxylase (TPH), oxygen, the corresponding aromatic amino acids, phenylalanine, tyrosine, or tryptophan, and BH_4. The complete hydroxylating system, in each case, consists of the two additional BH_4-regenerating enzymes: pterin-4α-carbinolamine dehydratase (PCD) and dihydropteridine reductase (DHPR). BH_4 is synthesized from guanosine triphosphate (GTP) catalyzed sequentially by GTP cyclohydrolase I (GTPCH), 6-pyruvoyl-tetrahydropterin synthase (PTPS), and sepiapterin reductase (SR). The first two steps are clinically relevant.

2. BH_4 deficiency comprises a heterogeneous group of disorders caused by mutations at one of the genes encoding enzymes involved in the biosynthesis (GTPCH or PTPS) or regeneration (PCD or DHPR) of BH_4. Phenotypically, it presents mostly with hyperphenylalaninemia (HPA) and deficiency of the neurotransmitter precursors, L-dopa and 5-hydroxytryptophan, and thus may be detected through neonatal phenylketonuria (PKU)-screening programs. However, some mutant variants may present without HPA and some with normal neurotransmitter homeostasis: Brain nitric oxide synthase (NOS) may also be affected by a deficit of the essential cofactor BH_4.

3. The genes of the corresponding enzymes are located and characterized in normal and mutant genomes. GTPCH (six exons) is on chromosome 14 (region 14q22.1-q22.2) and harbors 42 mutations, most of them associated with non-HPA dopa-responsive dystonia (DRD). PTPS (six exons) maps to human chromosome 11 (region 11q22.3-q23.3) and harbors over 28 mutations associated with HPA, some having a mild peripheral phenotype. PCD (four exons) is on chromosome 10 (region 10q22), with seven mutations described and associated with benign transient HPA. DHPR (seven exons) maps to chromosome 4 (region 4p15.3) and harbors 21 mutations, all associated with HPA and neurotransmitter deficiency.

4. Mutations of a single allele of the GTPCH gene or of two alleles of the tyrosine hydroxylase (TH) gene can lead to DRD. The spectrum of clinical symptoms in these disorders is wide and does not always include dystonia. Therapy with low-dose L-dopa normally alleviates most symptoms. Detection and differentiation of dominantly inherited GTPCH deficiency from recessively inherited TH deficiency requires measurement of pterins (neopterin and biopterin), and neurotransmitter metabolites in cerebrospinal fluid (CSF). Confirmation of a diagnosis requires enzymatic and molecular analysis in the case of dominantly inherited GTPCH deficiency and molecular analysis for TH deficiency as no suitable tissue is available for TH enzyme assay.

5. Treatment of BH_4 deficiencies requires restoration of normal blood phenylalanine concentration by BH_4 supplementation (2 to 10 mg/kg per day) or diet and replacement therapy with the neurotransmitter precursors L-dopa (+ carbidopa) and 5-hydroxytryptophan, and supplements of folinic acid in DHPR deficiency. Treatment should be initiated as early as possible (and perhaps continued for a lifetime).

6. Detection and differentiation of BH_4 deficiencies among HPAs require measurement of pterins (neopterin and biopterin) in urine, DHPR activity in blood from a Guthrie card, and neurotransmitter metabolites in CSF. If requested, prenatal diagnosis is possible by enzyme assay, measurement of metabolites in amniotic fluid, or DNA analysis in all forms of BH_4 deficiency.

7. The catecholamines [dopamine (DA), norepinephrine (NE), and epinephrine (E)], together with serotonin (5-hydroxytryptamine or 5HT), are major neurotransmitters that are involved with the control of brain homeostasis, behavior, and movement. The initial synthesis steps require hydroxylation of tyrosine to L-dopa, via the action of TH, for the catecholamines, and hydroxylation of

A list of standard abbreviations is located immediately preceding the index in each volume. Additional abbreviations used in this chapter include: 5HT = 5-hydroxytryptamine (serotonin); 5HTP =5-hydroxytryptophan; AADC = aromatic L-amino acid decarboxylase; AR = aldose reductase; BH_4 = tetrahydrobiopterin [(6R)-L-*erythro*-5,6,7,8-tetrahydrobiopterin]; COMT = catechol *O*-methyltransferase; CR = carbonyl reductase; CRM = cross-reactive material; DA = dopamine; DAHP = 2,4-diamino-6-hydroxypyrimidine; DCoH = dimerization cofactor for the hepatocyte nuclear factor 1α; DHFR = dihydrofolate reductase; DHPR = dihydropteridine reductase; DRD = dopa-responsive dystonia; DβH = dopamine β-hydroxylase; E = epinephrine; GTPCH = GTP cyclohydrolase I; HNF-1α = hepatocyte nuclear factor 1α; HPA = hyperphenylalaninemia; HVA = homovanillic acid; IFN-γ = interferon-γ; MAO = monoamine oxidase; MHPG = 3-methoxy-4-hydroxyphenylglycol; NE = norepinephrine; NOS = nitric oxide synthase; PAH = phenylalanine-4-hydroxylase; PCD = pterin-4α-carbinolamine dehydratase; PET = positron-emission tomography; PTPS = 6-pyruvoyl-tetrahydropterin synthase; RT-PCR = reverse transcriptase-polymerase chain reaction; SR = sepiapterin reductase; TH = tyrosine-3-hydroxylase; TPH = tryptophan-5-hydroxylase.

tryptophan to 5-hydroxytryptophan (5HTP), via the action of tryptophan hydroxylase (TPH), for 5HT. L-Dopa and 5HTP are then decarboxylated by aromatic L-amino acid decarboxylase (AADC) to yield DA and 5HT, respectively. DA can then be further hydroxylated in a reaction catalyzed by dopamine *β*-hydroxylase (D*β*H) to form NE, which in turn can be methylated by phenylethanolamine *N*-methyltransferase to form E. Catabolism of the active neurotransmitters is completed by catechol *O*-methyltransferase (COMT), and monoamine oxidase A (MAO-A) and monoamine oxidase B (MAO-B).

8. **Inherited disorders affecting catecholamine and 5HT metabolism have been described at the level of TH, AADC, D*β*H, and MAO-A. Although there is some overlap of clinical features, the main phenotypic features of each disease are different. Characteristic features are occulogyric crises, temperature instability and ptosis in AADC deficiency, parkinsonian features in early cases or dystonia in later-onset cases of TH deficiency, orthostatic hypotension in adolescence in D*β*H deficiency, and signs of violent, often sexual aggression, in males with MAO-A deficiency.**
9. **The genes for TH, AADC, D*β*H, and MAO-A are located and characterized in normal and mutant genomes. TH (14 exons) is on chromosome 11 (region 11p15.5) and harbors three mutations. AADC (15 exons) maps to chromosome 7 (region 7p12.1-p12.3) and harbors six point mutations causing single amino acid substitutions. D*β*H (12 exons) is on chromosome 9 (region 9q34.3). No mutations on this gene have been described. MAO-A (15 exons) maps to the X chromosome (region Xp11.4-p11.3). A single mutation creating a termination codon has been described.**
10. **Treatment of the neurotransmitter defects attempts restoration of normal central neurotransmitter levels. This is achieved by administration of L-dopa (+ carbidopa) in TH deficiency, or MAO inhibitors and DA agonists in AADC deficiency. Trials with vitamin B_6 should also always be attempted. Dihydroxyphenylserine restores NE levels in D*β*H deficiency. Treatment is not available in MAO-A deficiency, but avoidance of amine-containing foods may help prevent aggressive episodes. Detection and differentiation of the defects of catecholamine and serotonin metabolism require the measurement of catecholamines, 5HT, and their metabolites in either CSF, plasma, or urine. Prenatal diagnosis is possible by fetal liver enzyme assay in AADC deficiency, and by DNA analysis where mutations in previous siblings have been described.**

Primary and secondary disorders of serotonin (5-hydroxytryptamine or 5HT) and catecholamine metabolism with special attention to tetrahydrobiopterin (BH_4) deficiencies are the subject of this chapter. The combined deficiencies of biogenic amine neurotransmitters are due to BH_4 being the essential cofactor of both tyrosine and tryptophan hydroxylase (TPH), the rate-limiting enzymes in the biosynthesis of dopamine (DA) and 5HT. In general, these defects are also known as *atypical* or *malignant* phenylketonuria (PKU), although some of them may also present without hyperphenylalaninemia (HPA) (see also Chap. 77). Accordingly, this chapter is divided into three parts dealing with disorders with or without HPA, as well as with primary disorders of catecholamine and serotonin metabolism.

This chapter has adapted material from previous editions of this text and, in addition to the updates, the present chapter contains considerable new material.

TETRAHYDROBIOPTERIN

Pteridines constitute a large and structurally varied group of natural compounds involved in the biosynthetic pathways of cofactors and vitamins. The base structure of these heterocyclic compounds is a pteridine moiety (Fig. 78-1). Derivatives with the structure 2-amino-4-oxo are designated by the term *pterins.* Pterins can be divided into two groups. Those derived from folic acid, containing a *p*-aminobenzoate group plus glutamate, are designated as conjugated pterins (not shown). Unconjugated pterins contain neither of these two groups; instead, a substitution occurs mainly at the 6-position of the ring nucleus. Pterins are present in physiological fluids and tissues in reduced and oxidized

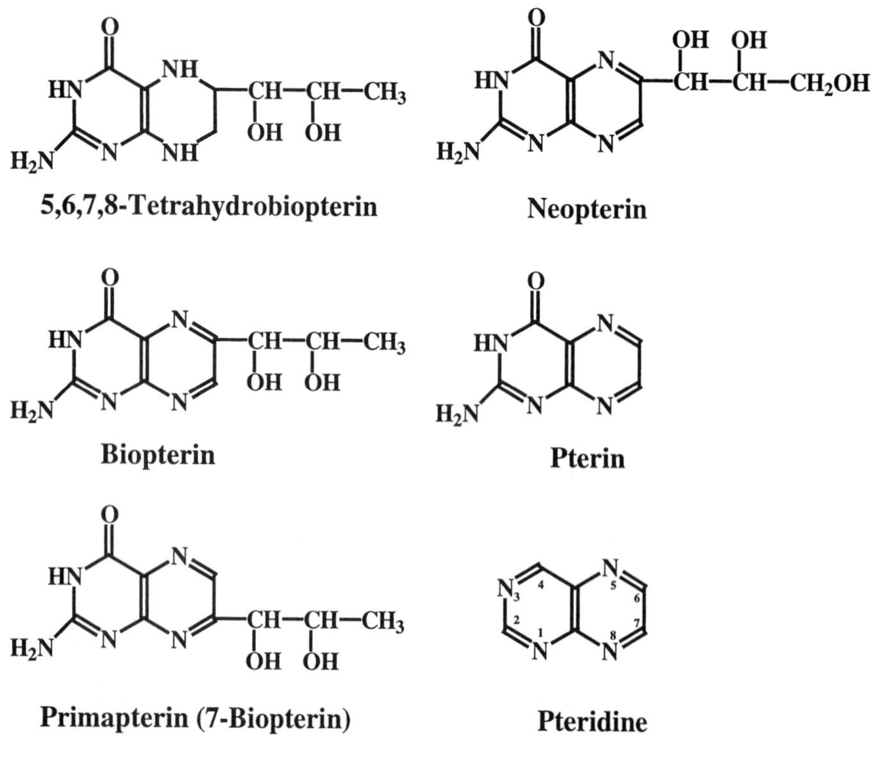

Fig. 78-1 Chemical structure of naturally occurring pterins and their different oxidation stages.

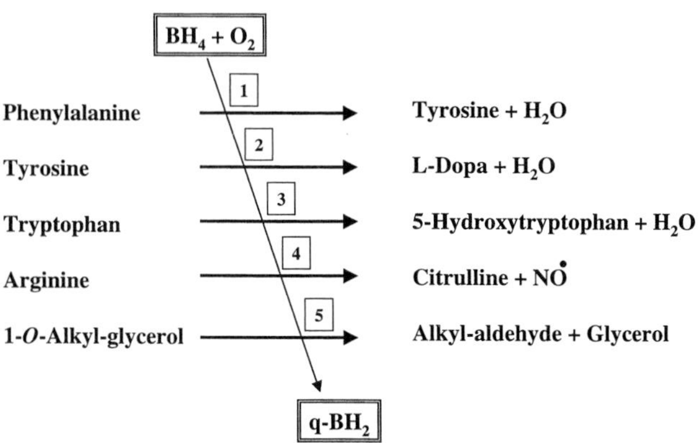

Fig. 78-2 Tetrahydrobiopterin-dependent enzymatic reactions: (1) phenylalanine-4-hydroxylase; (2) tyrosine-3-hydroxylase; (3) tryptophan-5-hydroxylase; (4) nitric oxide synthase; (5) glyceryl-ether monooxygenase. BH_4, tetrahydrobiopterin; q-BH_2, quinonoid dihydrobiopterin.

forms (Fig. 78-1), but only the 5,6,7,8-tetrahydro form is biologically active.

The best established function of BH_4 in humans is that of the natural cofactor for phenylalanine-4-hydroxylase (PAH; EC 1.14.16.1), tyrosine-3-hydroxylase (TH; EC 1.14.16.2), and tryptophan-5-hydroxylase (TPH; EC 1.14.16.4); the latter two are key enzymes in the biosynthesis of biogenic amines. In addition to the hydroxylation of aromatic amino acids, BH_4 serves as the cofactor for nitric oxide synthase (NOS; EC 1.14.23) and glyceryl-ether monooxygenase (EC 1.14.16.5) (Fig. 78-2).

Because the allowed number of references and the space to discuss all relevant aspects of BH_4-dependent reactions are limited, readers are asked to refer to the recent book by Kaufman[1] for further information.

Phenylalanine Hydroxylating System

For a more extensive discussion on the phenylalanine hydroxylating system, readers are referred to Chap. 77.

The phenylalanine hydroxylating system[2,3] comprises numerous components, such as (1) the phenylalanine hydroxylase peptide with a subunit molecular mass of 51672, which can exist as a homotetramer or a homodimer; (2) iron, which is complexed in the phenylalanine hydroxylase protein; (3) BH_4 substrate, which is recycled after oxidation and is synthesized in humans; (4) phenylalanine substrate mainly from diet; and (5) oxygen, which provides the oxygen atom for the tyrosine product. Further components are coupled to this system that allow normal function: (6) pterin-4α-carbinolamine dehydratase (PCD), which eliminates water from the oxidized pterin; and (7) dihydropteridine reductase (DHPR), which regenerates BH_4 by using NADH (Fig. 78-3).

Phenylalanine hydroxylase is activated by phenylalanine in what is thought to be a conformational change. Phosphorylation at serine 16 in rat enzyme has also been shown to activate phenylalanine hydroxylase. Several effectors have been demonstrated in vitro, but it is not sure whether these are relevant in vivo.

Defects in BH_4 synthesis, its recycling, and in phenylalanine hydroxylase can give rise to HPA.

Phenylalanine hydroxylase is present in the liver due to its function of metabolizing dietary phenylalanine. The human organism is thought not to have measurable PAH activity in kidney.

Biosynthesis of the Tetrahydrobiopterin Cofactor

Although the location of BH_4 biosynthetic enzymes has not been studied extensively at the cellular level, it is generally believed that they are present in all organs and many tissues of the human body.[4] At least the BH_4 cofactor itself is present in all tissues and body fluids that have been examined. Cells generate BH_4 by two distinct pathways: by the *de novo* biosynthetic pathway that uses guanosine triphosphate (GTP) as a precursor (Fig. 78-4) and by the *salvage* pathway that depends on preexisting dihydropterins (Fig. 78-5).[5,6] The de novo biosynthesis, which is discussed in detail below, turns out to be essential for viability, as genetic defects in two biosynthetic genes are associated with life-threatening conditions if not treated with an external supply of synthetic BH_4 (see below). Although it is not known to what extent the salvage pathway plays a role in vivo, several cell-culture and animal studies have shown that exogenous dihydropterins are converted to BH_4, most probably by dihydrofolate reductase (DHFR; EC 1.5.1.3) (see also the section "Sepiapterin Reductase and Alternative Reductases").[5]

In the following, genetic and biochemical aspects of the biosynthesis from GTP to BH_4 are presented (see also Table 78-1 and Fig. 78-4). The three enzymes — GTP cyclohydrolase I (GTPCH), 6-pyruvoyl-tetrahydropterin synthase (PTPS), and sepiapterin reductase (SR) — are the required (and sufficient) enzymes to produce BH_4 under in vivo and in vitro conditions.[6–8]

GTP Cyclohydrolase I. GTPCH is the first enzyme of BH_4 biosynthesis. It has been purified and/or extensively studied in diverse organisms such as bacteria, fungi, slime molds, phytoflagellates, plants, fly, chicken, rodents, and humans.[9–14] GTPCH is considered to be the rate-limiting enzyme in rodents but not in humans. The enzyme catalyzes the complex conversion from the purine nucleotide GTP to dihydroneopterin triphosphate, involving imidazole ring opening, formate release, and an Amadori rearrangement of the ribose moiety[15] (Fig. 78-4). The human enzyme is, as purified enzyme but also in tissue extracts, rather unstable and has a calculated molecular weight of 279,000. The

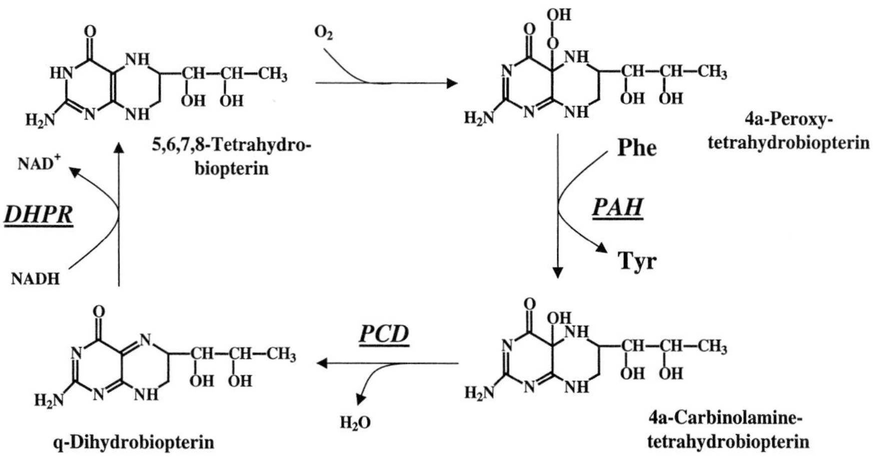

5,6,7,8-Tetrahydrobiopterin; 4a-Peroxy-tetrahydrobiopterin; 4a-Carbinolamine-tetrahydrobiopterin; q-Dihydrobiopterin; O_2; Phe; PAH; Tyr; PCD; H_2O; DHPR; NAD^+; NADH

Fig. 78-3 Regeneration of tetrahydrobiopterin. DHPR, dihydropteridine reductase; PAH, phenylalanine-4-hydroxylase; PCD, pterin-4α-carbinolamine dehydratase; Phe, phenylalanine; Tyr, tyrosine.

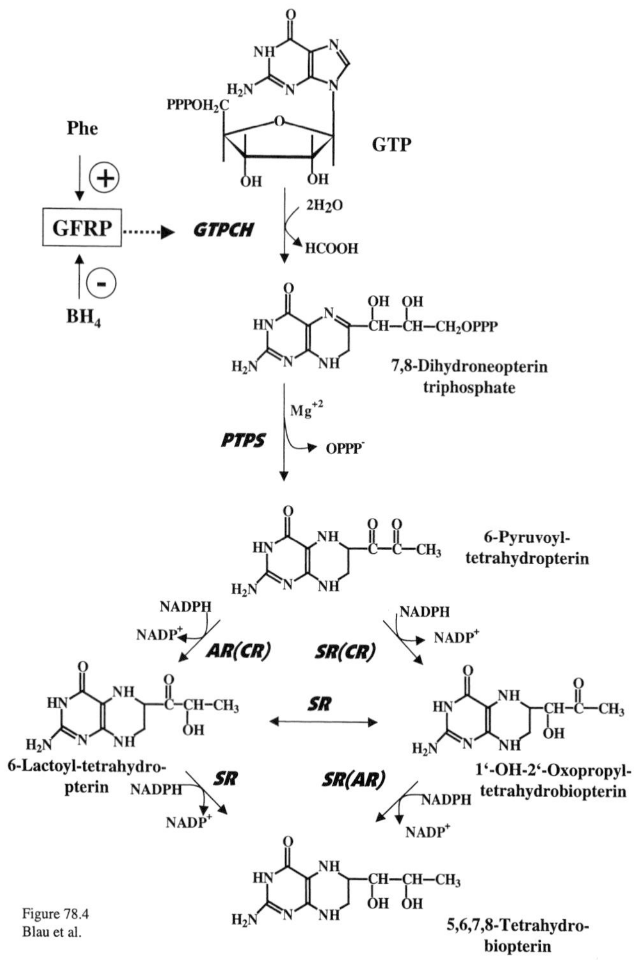

Figure 78.4
Blau et al.

Fig. 78-4 Biosynthesis of tetrahydrobiopterin. GTPCH, GTP cyclohydrolase I; PTPS, 6-pyruvoyl tetrahydropterin synthase; AR, aldose reductase; SR, sepiapterin reductase; CR, carbonyl reductase; GFRP, GTPCH feedback regulatory protein.

latter is based on the 250 codons from the complete open reading frame of the cDNA,[16] and on the assumption that the active enzyme is homodecameric like the *Escherichia coli* GTPCH.[17] From the latter, the crystal structure was solved and turned out to be a barrel-like complex consisting of a dimer of pentamers with 10 equivalent active sites.[18,19] The K_m value of approximately 30 μM for the rat and human GTPCH is in the range of the physiological GTP substrate concentration.[14,20,21] Recombinant expression of the active mammalian enzyme in bacterial cells or eukaryotic cell background enabled the wild-type enzyme as well as mutant forms to be investigated in kinetic analyses.[22] Furthermore, modifications such as phosphorylation[23,24] and/or protein–protein-complex formation(s)[25] will be important in future studies for the characterization and understanding of the active enzyme.

GTPCH is encoded by a single-copy gene, *GCH1*, located to chromosome 14q22.1-q22.2 and composed of six exons (Fig. 78-6), spanning about 30 kb.[22,26,27] It appears that from this gene three types of alternatively spliced cDNAs, types 1, 2, and 3, with different 3′ ends are expressed in human liver, whereas only the *full-length* type-1 cDNA is present in a pheochromocytoma cDNA library.[16,28] Type-1 cDNA containing an open reading frame coding for 250 amino acids exhibits the greatest similarity to that reported for mice and rats. Furthermore, the 250 codons from type-1 cDNA, but not from the shorter forms of type-2 and type-3 cDNAs, gave rise to a catalytically active enzyme when expressed individually in bacterial cells.[29] Nevertheless, alternative subunit complexes of GTPCH multimers other than homopolymers from the 250-amino-acid monomer of type-1 cDNA may assemble into active in vivo complexes.

The level of expression and enzyme activity of GTPCH are highly regulated in various tissues and cells by multiple and cell-specific signaling mechanisms (see also the section "Regulation of Tetrahydrobiopterin Homeostasis"). In situ hybridization with GTPCH-mRNA and immunologic detection with GTPCH antibodies in rodents documented the presence of GTPCH in cell groups synthesizing monoaminergic neurotransmitters, adrenal gland, and liver.[50–53] In other cell types such as macrophages, lymphocytes, or fibroblasts, GTPCH expression appears not to be constitutive but can be induced by cytokines such as interferon-γ and tumor necrosis factor α.[54,55] In superior cervical ganglia (sympathetic neurons), GTPCH expression is modulated by various factors: cytokines such as leukemia inhibitory factor and ciliary neurotrophic factor were found to decrease GTPCH expression, whereas nerve growth factor enhanced GTPCH expression.[56] On the posttranslational level, GTPCH activity in liver is modulated by the GTPCH feedback regulatory protein (GFRP) (see the section "Regulation of Tetrahydrobiopterin Homeostasis").

The inhibitor used for GTPCH is 2,4-diamino-6-hydroxypyrimidine (DAHP).[57] A median effective concentration of DAHP against rat GTPCH is 0.7 mM and, in cell-culture experiment, it has been used at concentrations of 1 to 20 mM.[58]

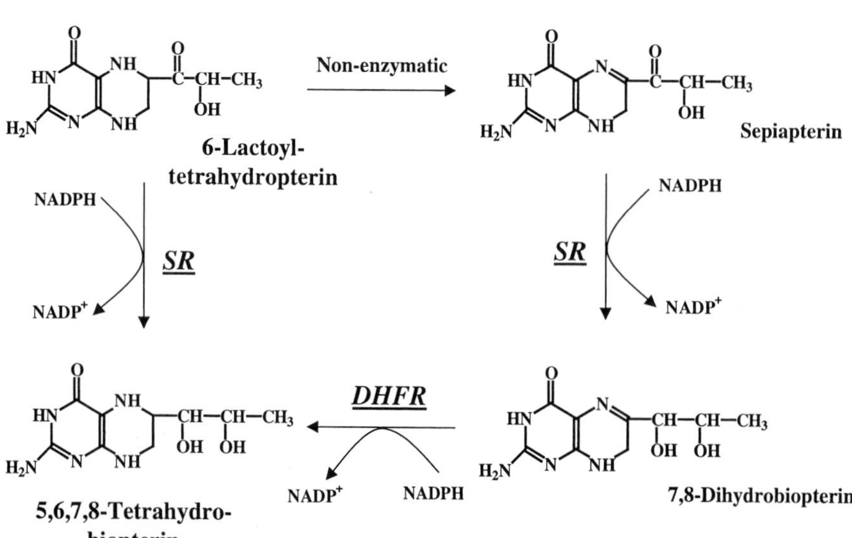

Fig. 78-5 Salvage pathway of tetrahydrobiopterin via sepiapterin. SR, sepiapterin reductase; DHFR, dihydrofolate reductase.

Table 78-1 Metabolic Enzymes and Corresponding Genes from Humans

Enzyme	EC No.*	Molecular Mass	Amino Acids Per Subunit	Gene Symbol	Chromosome Location	No. of Exons	Accession Numbers* cDNA	Genomic DNA
GTPCH	3.5.4.16	279-kDa homodecamer	250	*GCH1*	14q22.1-q22.2	6	U19523	D38602 D38603 U19256 to U19259
PTPS	4.6.1.10	97.5-kDa homohexamer	145	*PTS*	11q22.3-q23.3	6	M97655	L76259
				PTS-P1¶	9p12-p13¶		—	L76260¶
SR	1.1.1.153	56-kDa homodimer	261	*SPR*	2p14-p12	3	M76231	ABO17547, ABO17528
PCD	4.2.1.96	47.6-kDa homotetramer	103†	*PCBD*	10q22	4	L41559	L41560
DHPR	1.6.99.7	51.5-kDa homodimer	244	*QDPR*	4p15.3	7	X04882	—
PAH	1.14.16.1	51.7-kDa homotetramer	452	*PAH*	12q22-q24.2	13	U49897	—
TH	1.14.16.2	55.9- to 59.2-kDa homotetramer	497	*TH1*‡	11p15.5	14	X05290	D00269 to D00292
			501	*TH2*‡				
			524	*TH3*‡			Y00414	M23597
			528	*TH4*‡			M17589	
TPH	1.14.16.4	51-kDa homotetramer	444	*TPH*	11p15.1	11	L29306	X83212 X83213
AADC	4.1.1.28	53.9-kDa homodimer	480	*DDC*	7p12.1-p12.3	15	M76180	M77828 M84588 to M84601 M88070
MAO-A	1.4.3.4	59.7-kDa homodimer	527	*MAO-A*	Xp11.4-p11.3	15	M69226 M68857	M68843 to M68857
DβH	1.14.17.1	64.9-kDa homotetramer	603	*DBH*	9q34.3	12	Y00096	X13255 to X13268

*EC number and symbols are approved by the nomenclature committees.
†Without the starting methionine.
‡Alternately spliced products.
§EMBL/GenBank.
¶Retro-pseudogene.
ABBREVIATIONS: GTPCH = GTP cyclohydrolase I; PTPS = 6-pyruvoyl-tetrahydropterin synthase; SR = sepiapterin reductase; PCD = pterin-4α-carbinolamine dehydratase; DHPR = dihydropteridine reductase; PAH = phenylalanine-4-hydrolase; TH = tyrosine-3-hydrolase; TPH = tryptophan-5-hydrolase; AADC = aromatic L-amino acid decarboxylase; MAO-A = monoamine oxidase A; DβH = dopamine β-hydroxylase.

6-Pyruvoyl-tetrahydropterin Synthase. PTPS was purified and characterized from several species and various tissues and appears to be a highly conserved protein.[59–61] PTPS converts dihydroneopterin triphosphate to 6-pyruvoyl tetrahydropterin by a two-step reaction involving internal redox transfer and triphosphate elimination[5,59,62,62a] (see Fig. 78-4). The K_m value for the dihydroneopterin triphosphate substrate is around 10 μM, and the reaction is strictly Mg^{2+} dependent.[63] The human and rat PTPS, which are the best-characterized enzymes, are homohexameric, heat-stable, Zn^{2+}-containing metalloproteins of

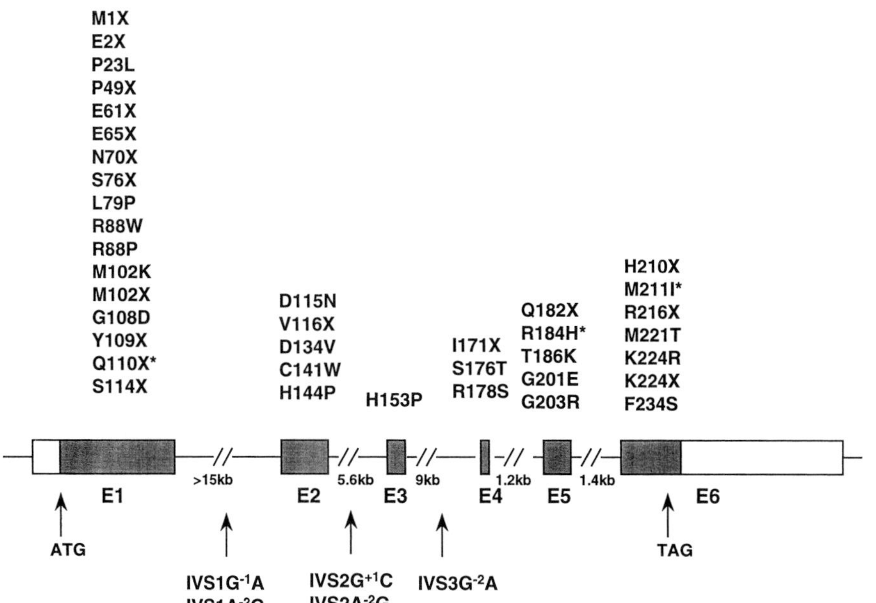

Fig. 78-6 Genomic structure and location of mutations in human *GCH1* gene. Mutations are listed in the BIOMDB database.[231] For original data, see the References.[22,26,30–49] HPA-causing mutations are marked with *asterisk*.

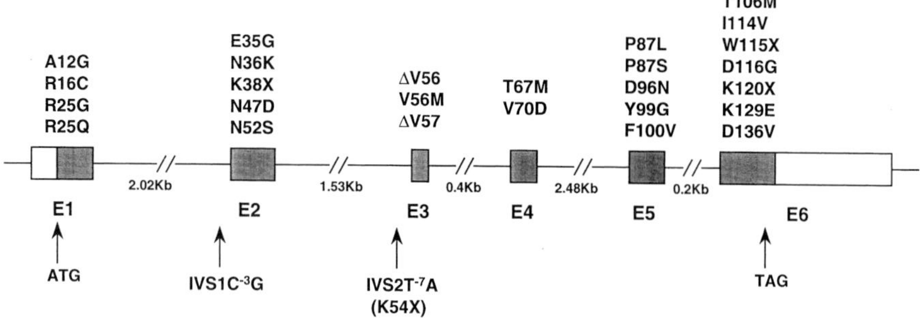

Fig. 78-7 Genomic structure and location of mutations in human *PTS* gene. Mutations are listed in the BIOMDB database.[231] For original data, see the References 65, 70, 73–78.

97.5 kDa.[62–65] Crystal-structure analysis revealed that the hexameric enzyme is formed by face-to-face association of two trimers with an overall barrel-like shape enclosing a hydrophilic pore. The six catalytic sites, each containing a binding site for Zn^{2+} ion, are located at the trimer interface. Furthermore, crystallographic analysis showed that PTPS and GTPCH share a common subunit fold and oligomerization mode.[8,62,66] Investigations on the recombinant human wild-type and mutant enzymes (see also below) indicated a requirement for posttranslational modification for in vivo activity. Correspondingly, a phosphoserine modification by a cyclic-GMP-dependent protein kinase at the single site (serine 19) was identified to be critical for normal activity.[65,6767a]

The PTPS cDNA, which was isolated from human brain and peripheral organs, contains an open reading frame for a polypeptide with 145 amino acids and predicts a molecular weight of 16,387.[68,69] Its corresponding gene *PTS* was localized to chromosome 11q22.3-22.3 and consists of six exons with variable length (Fig. 78-7).[70] One splicing polymorphism was repeatedly observed in several human cells that results in skipping of the 23-bp exon 3. As a consequence, the open reading frame is interrupted and a truncated, nonfunctional PTPS is synthesized. The concurrent observation of low PTPS activity with normal levels of mRNA but deleted for exon 3 indicates that alternative splicing may have a regulatory function.[71,72] Such an exon-3 deletion is also "conserved" in the nonfunctional retro-pseudogene *PTPS-P1*, which has a high similarity to the 3′ portion of the PTPS cDNA and is located on chromosome 9p12-p13.[70] Although PTPS is considered to be constitutively expressed and active, the enzyme is not present at least in many subregions of the rat brain (A. Résibois and B. Thöny, unpublished observation). The presence of PTPS activity in dermal fibroblasts, erythrocytes, and lymphocytes is of diagnostic value.

Sepiapterin Reductase and Alternative Reductases. The last step in cofactor biogenesis involves the SR, which converts 6-pyruvoyl tetrahydropterin to BH_4 in an NADPH-dependent manner.[6] A two-step reduction is necessary to convert both side-chain keto groups into hydroxy functions with proper stereochemistry (Fig. 78-4). The enzyme was purified from different sources, and corresponding cDNAs are available.[79–81] The human SR and the murine SR, which are highly homologous, are dimeric enzymes with a predicted molecular mass of 56 kDa. From the recombinant mouse liver SR, the crystal structure of a ternary complex with recombinant protein and the substrates NADP and sepiapterin or the product BH_4 are available.[82] The human cDNA encoding the 261 amino acids for the SR monomer was isolated, and its gene *SPR* was mapped to chromosome 2p14-12.[27] The genomic organization of the mouse and human *SPR* genes encoding SR is very similar.[82a,b] They both span a region of 4–5 kb and the reading frames are split into three exons. No alternative splice variants have been observed. Only the mouse harbors a genomic pseudogene (*Sprp*), which contains exons 1 and 2 plus the intervening and partial flanking sequences for these two exons, with an overall similarity to the functional *SPR* gene of 82%. Transcriptional start sites have been determined for the *SPR* genes from both species.

Under in vitro conditions with purified enzymes, the Ca^{2+}/calmodulin-dependent protein kinase II and protein kinase C phosphorylated SR and thereby modified the kinetic properties of the enzyme.[83] In vivo data for the significance of SR phosphorylation are not available. Feedback inhibition of SR activity in rat brain by catecholamine and an indoleamine was reported.[84] The most effective compound is *N*-acetylserotonin, with K_i of 0.2 μM for the rat enzyme. The effect of *N*-acetylserotonin on BH_4 levels varies according to the cell type.[58] Crystallographic analysis of indoleamine bound to SR confirmed the inhibition of the reductase activity for pterins.[82]

Although SR is sufficient to complete BH_4 biosynthesis, alternative carbonyl reductases (CRs) and/or aldose reductases (ARs) may participate in the diketo reduction of the carbonyl side chain in vivo.[85,86] AR (or CR) can convert 6-pyruvoyl tetrahydropterin to 6-lactoyl-tetrahydropterin, or 1′-OH-2′oxopropyl-tetrahydropterin to BH_4 in NADPH-dependent reactions. On the other hand, CR converts 6-pyruvoyl-tetrahydropterin to 1′-OH-2′oxopropyl-tetrahydropterin. Furthermore, 6-lactoyl-tetrahydropterin and 1′-OH-2′oxopropyl-tetrahydropterin are isomerized by SR (Fig. 78-4). This is of special interest in the context of inborn errors of pterin metabolism that have not been observed for SR. If alternative reductases can compensate for potential defects in SR activity, AR and CR in a concerted action may be responsible for such an effect. Support for this pathway is in part found in the presence of detectable 6-lactoyl-tetrahydropterin as a biosynthetic intermediate, at least in some tissues such as brain. As shown in Fig. 78-4, only AR or CR can synthesize 6-lactoyl-tetrahydropterin that is converted to BH_4 by SR.[6]

In the *salvage* pathway in Fig. 78-5, SR converts non-enzymatically generated sepiapterin to dihydrobiopterin. DHFR then completes BH_4 biosynthesis by a second NADPH-dependent reduction step.[5] The salvage pathway was demonstrated in cell culture and in vivo to be a methotrexate-sensitive route (i.e., DHFR dependent).[87]

Regeneration of the Tetrahydrobiopterin Cofactor

Enzymatic defects in both BH_4-regenerating enzymes, PCD and DHPR, were described. As de novo biosynthesis of BH_4 is not sufficient for controlling hepatic phenylalanine and brain monoamine neurotransmitter homeostasis, regeneration of the cofactor is essential. A reaction scheme with PAH and the enzymes catalyzing recycling of the pterin cofactor is shown in Fig. 78-3.

Pterin-4α-Carbinolamine Dehydratase. PCD was purified from human and rat liver, but the enzyme was also found to be present in kidney, brain, skin, and hair follicles.[88–93] PCD catalyzes the dehydration of 4α-hydroxy-tetrahydrobiopterin to quinonoid dihydrobiopterin (Fig. 78-3). Catalytic activity of PCD in fetal liver is detectable as early as 6.7 weeks and increases linearly with time, reaching 31 percent of adult value by 17.3 weeks of gestational age.[94] The mature human and rat liver proteins are identical in amino acid sequence, with 103 residues and a

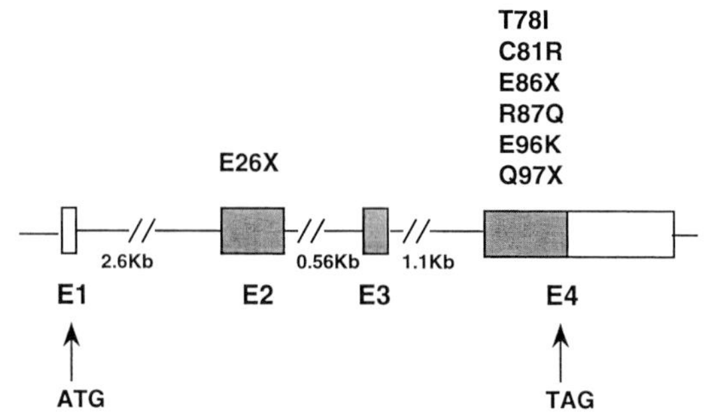

Fig. 78-8 Genomic structure and location of mutations in human *PCDB* gene. Mutations are listed in the BIOMDB database.[231] For original data, see the References 99, 102, 103.

Table 78-2 Properties of Human Dihydropteridine Reductase[117]

Molecular weight	
Sedimentation equilibrium	50,000
Gel filtration	47,500
Gradient gel electrophoresis	54,000
Subunit	26,000
Cross-linked dimer	58,000
Isoelectric point	7.0 ± 1.0
K_m (NADH 37°C, pH 7.2)	29 μM
K_m (NADPH 37°C, pH 7.2)	770 μM
K_m BH_4	17 μM

ABBREVIATION: BH_4 = tetrahydrobiopterin.

molecular weight of 11,909 for the monomer. Furthermore, no protein modification other than cotranslational cleavage of the starting methionine and acetylation of the N-terminal alanine was found for the liver enzyme.[89] PCD is a homotetrameric protein of 47.6 kDa, and its crystal structure and location of the active site have been determined.[95–98]

The corresponding gene, *PCBD*, was located on human chromosome 10q22 and is expressed from a single, four-exon-containing gene (Fig. 78-8), from which the 103-amino-acid active PCD is encoded by exons 2 to 4 only.[99–101]

A second, regulatory function of PCD is the binding and enhancing of transcriptional activity of the hepatic nuclear factor (HNF) 1α. For this second role, PCD is also termed DCoH for dimerization cofactor for HNF-α.[104] DCoH forms a heterotetrameric complex with N-terminal dimerization domains of the HNF-1α dimer. The physiological role of the nuclear DCoH dimer is still unclear.[105,106] PhhA from *Pseudomonas aeruginosa* is encoded by a gene organized within an apparent operon including homologous mammalian PCD/DCoH and aromatic aminotransferase.[107]

Dihydropteridine Reductase. DHPR is an essential enzyme in the hydroxylating systems for phenylalanine, tyrosine, and tryptophan (see Fig. 78-3) and is widely distributed in animal tissues.[108] Its occurrence in brain and adrenal medulla[108] is not surprising in view of its role in the tyrosine hydroxylation system in these tissues and in the tryptophan hydroxylation system in brain. Why DHPR should be found in such tissues as heart and lung, however, which have little or no aromatic amino acid hydroxylating activity, is obscure. Its wide tissue distribution, together with BH_4, hints at undiscovered roles for both BH_4 and DHPR. In addition to its role in regenerating BH_4, it has been proposed that DHPR plays an ancillary role (together with DHFR) in brain to maintain folate in the tetrahydro form.[109] DHPR activity has been detected in cultured fibroblasts,[110] amniocytes,[111] lymphocytes,[112] leukocytes,[113] erythrocytes,[114] and platelets.[115,116]

The human enzyme was purified from liver.[117] The molecular weight was determined to be 50,000 daltons (sedimentation equilibrium) and 47,500 daltons (gel filtration). On sodium dodecyl sulfate gel electrophoresis, a single subunit was shown to be 26,000 daltons. Other properties are listed in Table 78-2. A complex of NADH and DHPR has been demonstrated that is stable to gel electrophoresis. The two subunits are identical.

Detailed studies by immunoprecipitation and two-dimensional electrophoresis have shown that DHPR from liver, Epstein-Barr virus-transformed lymphocytes, and fibroblasts are identical.[118] Antigenic determinants were also shown to be identical.[113,118] Two species were seen in some two-dimensional gels, and indirect evidence indicates that one is derived from the other by posttranslational modification, as similar proteolytic fingerprints are derived from both species. It is concluded, therefore, that the DHPR proteins in these three tissues are derived from the same structural gene. This is supported by the fact that DHPR deficiency has occurred in all tissues so far examined in patients with DHPR deficiency.[112,119]

Studies on the crystal structure of rat and human DHPR[120,121] show that the dimer is formed by the hydrophobic interaction of a pair of helices from each subunit. The two active sites are 30 Å apart. These studies have shown that DHPR is distinct from another pteridine reductase, DHFR, differing in mechanism and active site. In fact, DHPR has been categorized as a member of the so-called Tyr-$(Xaa)_3$-Lys-containing family of reductases and dehydrogenases due to the presence of this active site motif.

Asp37 (rat sequence numbering) also belongs to this family and was earlier designated as required for cofactor (NADH) binding.[122] Modeling experiments have suggested that Trp86, Asn186, and the Tyr and Lys of the motif (146 and 150, respectively) are in the active site.

A more detailed study[123] by crystallization of mutant rat DHPR showed that residues 37, 150, and 186 are involved in cofactor binding and, when any of these residues are mutated, a partially active enzyme results. Tyr146 was also shown to be essential. These equate to amino acids 41, 90, 190, 150, and 154 in the human protein, respectively.

Human cDNA[124] contains an open reading frame of 732 nucleotide pairs, encoding a protein of 244 amino acids. The molecular weight of 25,744 predicted from the cDNA sequence was similar to the values reported for human liver[117,118] and platelet[116] DHPR. Rat DHPR (720 bp and 240 amino acids) differs from the human protein at 10 residues.

The predicted amino acid sequence of human DHPR has no apparent similarity with any other protein of known sequence. This result was somewhat surprising, since two other enzymes, DHFR[125] and methylene tetrahydrofolate reductase,[126] also act on substituted pterin substrates and utilize a pyridine nucleotide cofactor. Furthermore, methylene tetrahydrofolate reductase catalyzes the reduction of quinonoid dihydrobiopterin to BH_4[126] and, in tissues like brain that have low dihydrofolate activities, DHPR probably functions together with DHFR to maintain folate in the tetrahydro form.

The only similarities in the corresponding sequence of DHPR and DHFR are in regions known to contain the binding sites for methotrexate and the pyridine nucleotide cofactors. These results suggest that the analogous activities of DHPR and DHFR represent vestigial homologies at loci that have diverged in evolution to the point at which sequence similarity can no longer be demonstrated by statistical means.

The gene comprises seven exons ranging in size from 83 to 562 bp, with the corresponding introns flanked by canonical splice junctions. Primers are available for the analysis of these exons for mutation analysis. The introns vary in size from 1.7 to 10 kb.[127] The gene has been localized to band p15.3 on chromosome 4.[128]

Regulation of Tetrahydrobiopterin Homeostasis

BH_4 controls its own biosynthesis by a feedback regulatory circuit through the action of the GFRP.[129–131] The mature form of the rat liver GFRP is a homopentamer of 52 kDa, consisting of subunits with 83 amino acid residues and a calculated subunit mass of 9.5 kDa. GFRP is able to form specific complexes with GTPCH and to modulate the activity of the latter. The regulatory protein mediates end-product feedback inhibition of GTPCH by BH_4, which is reversed by phenylalanine (Fig. 78-4). In HPA patients with PAH deficiency, the action of GFRP is thus thought to be responsible for high plasma BH_4. Based on mRNA expression studies from rat tissue, GFRP is found not only in liver and kidney, but also in testis, heart, brain, and lung. It was suggested that GFRP may thus play a role in BH_4-dependent systems other than phenylalanine metabolism.[130]

At least in one report, age-related changes in BH_4 levels were documented from rat studies with decreased biosynthesis in several brain regions and increased production in adrenal glands with aging.[132]

Other Functions of Tetrahydrobiopterin

Besides the requirement of BH_4 for the aromatic amino acid hydroxylases and the NOS enzymes, at least one more enzyme, the glyceryl-ether monooxygenase (EC 1.14.16.5), was described to be dependent on the reduced pteridine cofactor[133] (Fig. 78-2). In addition, the dopamine β-hydroxylase (DβH; EC 1.14.17.1) in the pathway from DA to noradrenaline was recently reported to depend also on the BH_4 cofactor.[134] Besides the direct requirement of BH_4 as a cofactor for enzymatic reactions, various additional but less defined roles have been attributed to the cofactor.[135] This includes the requirement of BH_4 for cell proliferation and mitosis,[136–139] neurotransmitter-releasing factor,[140–142] cell-mediated immunity and inflammation,[143] antioxidative activity,[144] and melanogenesis.[139,145]

Pterin Metabolism and Immune Response

Stimulation of cellular immune response results in enhanced GTPCH gene expression mainly in monocytes and macrophages from peripheral blood.[54,55,146,147] Stimulatory agents are endotoxins (lipopolysaccharide) or release of growth-promoting cytokines (interferon-γ and interleukins) and tumor necrosis factor α by activated T lymphocytes following immune-stimulating diseases like AIDS, autoimmune and inflammatory responses, and malignant diseases.[148] Since human macrophages lack PTPS activity, stimulated GTPCH expression leads not only to enhanced dihydroneopterin triphosphate biosynthesis, but also to the accumulation of dephosphorylated and oxidized plasma neopterin and thus elevated urinary excretion of neopterin. Moderate stimulation of PTPS activity in various cells correlating with higher cellular BH_4 levels was reported by several authors in response to cytokine and cyclic-AMP (cAMP) treatment.[55,149–152] Although neopterin serves as a marker for the stimulated human immune system, the biologic significance of the cytokine-induced pteridine biosynthesis is not known.

TETRAHYDROBIOPTERIN-DEPENDENT HYPERPHENYLALANINEMIAS

The first patients with BH_4-dependent HPA were identified in 1969 by Tada et al.[153] Two siblings with mild HPA were at that time described as "a genetic variant of phenylketonuria" (PKU) but later characterized as DHPR deficient.[154] In 1974, Smith,[155] in London, described three children with "PKU" who had an unusual clinical course. Despite early diagnosis and treatment with a low-phenylalanine diet, these patients developed progressive neurologic symptoms and died at an early age. Independently, Bartholomé,[156] in Heidelberg, reported a similar case of "atypical" HPA unresponsive to dietary treatment. The atypical course, high tolerance for phenylalanine, and normal PAH activity in liver biopsy specimen in Bartholomé's patient, led to the speculation that this syndrome was a new form of HPA, probably due to a defect in the metabolism of BH_4. Smith[155] reasoned that a defect in the metabolism of BH_4 in brain tissue would also result in a defective turnover of the neurotransmitters L-dopa, noradrenaline, adrenaline, and serotonin. In the following years, a number of cases of BH_4 deficiency were described, and it was suggested that all of these patients suffered from a defect in BH_4 metabolism.[110,157–164] Because all untreated patients show severe cerebral deterioration and most of them die at an early age, it was suggested that this clinical syndrome should be called "malignant" HPA.[119,165]

Based on the speculation that pterins might be used in the treatment of PKU, Smith et al[157] proposed that patients with BH_4 deficiency might benefit from substitution with reduced pterins. Indeed, Danks et al[162] showed that intravenous administration of synthetic BH_4 decreases the serum phenylalanine levels and, therefore, can function as a cofactor substituting for hepatic PAH in vivo. Meanwhile, therapy with L-dopa, carbidopa, and 5-hydroxytryptophan (5HTP), alone or in combination with BH_4, was shown to be of benefit for patients with various forms of BH_4 deficiency.[166–173]

Because BH_4 deficiency may cause a severe but treatable disease, it became necessary to develop selective screening tests for detection early in infancy. Every newborn with even slight but persistent HPA should be tested for BH_4 deficiency. Such tests have been introduced in many developed countries, but even today older children are invariably detected because of the appearance of clinical symptoms, such as hypotonia of the trunk, hypertonia of the extremities, and often myoclonic seizures, unresponsive to a low-phenylalanine diet. Although according to the literature the frequency of BH_4 deficiency was estimated to be 1 to 2 percent among cases with HPA (see the section "Population Genetics"), in some countries, like Turkey and Saudi Arabia, because of consanguinity the incidence is even higher.

Nomenclature of Tetrahydrobiopterin Deficiencies

The BH_4 deficiencies are a very heterogeneous group of diseases, and different clinical and biochemical criteria define and characterize the variants. The primary enzyme defect, its severity, outcome of the BH_4 challenge, reactivity with the antibodies against the protein, type of mutation, and responses to therapy are some of the criteria used to define a specific defect. The terms *severe/general* or *mild/peripheral/partial* should be used according to the actual need for treatment with neurotransmitter precursors.[174] Accordingly, the nomenclature given in Table 78-3 applies. Use of older terms such as "atypical PKU" (non-PKU HPA) or "malignant PKU" should be avoided because, in most cases, a BH_4 deficiency is no longer lethal.

There are, in addition, a number of genetic disorders related to BH_4 deficiency without HPA, e.g., 6,10-methylenetetrahydrofolate reductase deficiency and the skin depigmentation disorder vitiligo or dopa-responsive dystonia (DRD) (see the section "Non-Hyperphenylalaninemia Tetrahydrobiopterin Defects").

Table 78-3 Classification and Nomenclature of the Tetrahydrobiopterin (BH_4) Deficiencies

Enzyme Defect	Phenotype	Treatment
GTPCH deficiency	Severe	NT + BH_4
PTPS deficiency	Severe	NT + BH_4
	Mild	BH_4
	Transient	BH_4*
DHPR deficiency	Severe	NT + diet† Folinic acid
	Mild	Diet†
PCD deficiency	Transient	BH_4*

*Treatment with BH_4 in the first months of life.
†Low phenylalanine.
ABBREVIATIONS: GTPCH = GTP cyclohydrolase I; PTPS = 6-pyruvoyl-tetrahydropterin synthase; DHPR = dihydropteridine reductase; PCD = pterin-4α-carbinolamine dehydratase; NT = neurotransmitter precursors L dopa and 5-hydroxytryptophan.

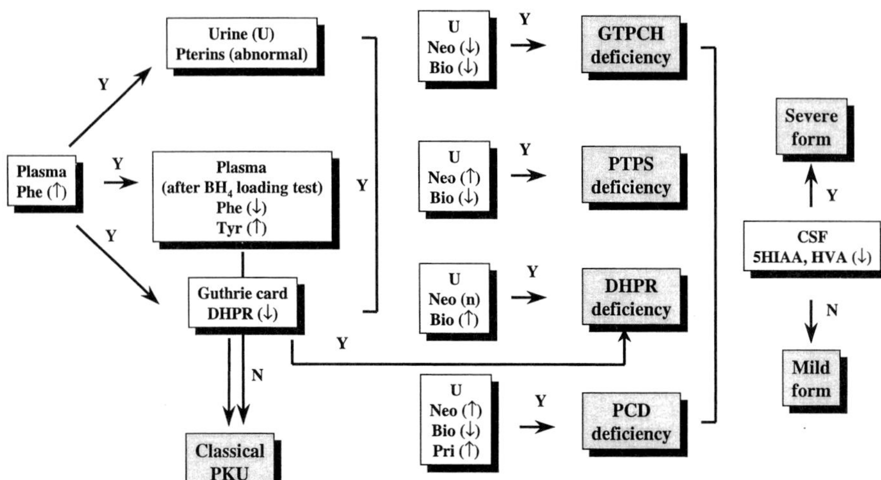

Fig. 78-9 Diagnostic flowchart for differentiation of hyperphenylalaninemia (HPA) variants. Abnormal urinary pterin profile, positive tetrahydrobiopterin (BH_4)-loading test, and decreased dihydropteridine reductase (DHPR) activity suggest BH_4 deficiency. Generally, increased urinary pterins but normal BH_4-loading test and normal DHPR activity are typical in patients with phenylketonuria (PKU). Cerebrospinal fluid (CSF) neurotransmitter metabolites discriminate between severe and mild forms of BH_4 deficiency.

Clinical Observations

Symptoms can become manifest during the first weeks of life but usually are noted at about 4 months of age. When information about the neonatal period is provided, however, a careful review indicates that abnormal signs (poor sucking, decreased spontaneous movements, and "floppy baby") can be noticed even during the neonatal period. Birth is generally uneventful, except that there is a higher incidence of prematurity and lower birth weights in typical (severe) PTPS deficiency.[175]

Severe Forms. The clinical course of the illness is similar in untreated patients with typical (severe) forms of GTPCH, PTPS, and DHPR deficiencies.[176,177] The variable but common symptoms are mental retardation, convulsions (grand mal or myoclonic attacks), disturbance of tone and posture, drowsiness, irritability, abnormal movements, recurrent hyperthermia without infections, hypersalivation, and swallowing difficulties. Diurnal fluctuation of alertness and neurologic symptoms are also reported.[178] There is very limited data about microcephaly in GTPCH-deficient patients; however, microcephaly is frequently observed in PTPS deficiency (52 percent) and in DHPR deficiency (33 percent). In a number of DHPR-deficient patients where there were serial head measurements, progressive microcephaly was noted with increasing age, whether patients were treated or not.

Mild (Peripheral or Partial) Forms. The absence of clinical signs, theoretically, defines phenotypically atypical forms. In some infants with a PTPS deficiency, however, neonatal hypotonia or acute but transient behavioral abnormalities, neurovegetative signs, and sleeping difficulties were noted. In two patients with a DHPR deficiency investigated, there were no signs of neurologic symptoms until 2 years of age. However, one patient later developed deceleration in head growth velocity, whereas psychomotor development continued to be normal for age.[179] In patients with PCD deficiency, slight upper limb tremors after stimulation and a moderate tendency to hypertonia were noticed in one child,[180] and transient hypotonia and motor delay in another.[181] With control of blood phenylalanine levels, symptoms receded.

Screening and Diagnosis

Biochemical data obtained from the International Database of BH_4 Deficiencies (BIODEF)[178] are summarized in Table 78-4. Because BH_4 deficiencies are a group of diseases that can be detected but not identified through neonatal mass screening for HPA, selective screening for a BH_4 deficiency is essential in every newborn with even slightly elevated phenylalanine levels.[182,183] Screening for a BH_4 deficiency should be done in all newborns with plasma phenylalanine levels higher than 120 μM, as well as in older children with neurologic signs and symptoms. The following tests are recommended:

1. Analysis of pterins in urine
2. Measurement of DHPR activity in blood from Guthrie card
3. Loading test with BH_4
4. Analysis of pterins, folates, and neurotransmitter metabolites in cerebrospinal fluid (CSF)
5. Enzyme activity measurement

The first two tests are essential and enables all BH_4 defects to be differentiated. With some limitations, the BH_4-loading test is an additional, useful diagnostic tool for the rapid differentiation between classic PKU and BH_4 variants. Analysis of neopterin, biopterin, 5-methyltetrahydrofolic acid, and the neurotransmitter metabolites, 5-hydroxyindoleacetic acid (5HIAA) and homovanillic acid (HVA), enables differentiation between severe and mild forms of BH_4 deficiencies. A diagnostic flowchart is shown in Fig. 78-9.

The degree of HPA can vary from very mild to plasma phenylalanine concentrations as high as 2500 μM (Table 78-4). There are at least two reports on patients with GTPCH deficiency missed in the newborn screening for PKU because of the initially normal blood phenylalanine levels.[33,184] Therefore, testing for BH_4 deficiency should also be considered in older patients without HPA and with neurologic symptoms of "unknown origin."

Pterins in Urine. Commonly occurring pterins used for differential diagnosis are listed in Table 78-5. Oxidized pterins are highly fluorescent and can be detected with specificity and sensitivity after high-performance liquid chromatography (HPLC) in urine, blood, CSF, and amniotic fluid.[185–188] The method of Niederwieser et al[189] utilizes an automatic HPLC system with the capability for column switching. This method involves minimal pretreatment of the biologic sample (i.e., oxidation with MnO_2), separates complex mixtures of pterins in a short time, and uses fluorometric detection. Coulometric or amperometric detection is used to quantify the reduced pterins in urine and CSF.[190] Reduced pterins and catecholamines can be separated and detected simultaneously by dual-electrode amperometry and ultraviolet absorption.[191,192] Either native urine[186] or urine dried on filter paper[193,194] may be used for selective screening. The use of ascorbic acid protects the reduced pterins from oxidation; however, this may yield poor results when oxidized with MnO_2. Drying an unoxidized urine sample on filter paper is also not recommended. In instances of long shipping times or extreme temperatures, the reduced pterins must be stabilized by oxidation for BH_4 deficiency to be differentiated from classic PKU. Using differential oxidation with iodine at acidic and alkaline conditions,

Table 78-4 Biochemical Data Collected from the BIODEF Database

	GTPCH Deficiency	PTPS Deficiency	DHPR Deficiency	PCD Deficiency	PKU Patients	Controls* (1 mo to 2 yr)
Plasma (μM)						
Phenylalanine	90–1200	240–2500	180–2500	180–1200	> 800	< 120
Urine (mmol/mol creatinine)†						
Neopterin	0.14 (0.09–0.20)	21.86 (4.95–51.16)	6.22 (0.48–23.23)	15.38 (4.07–22.48)	4.60 (1.11–16.94)	0.3–4.0
Biopterin	0.09 (0.04–0.18)	0.14 (0–0.45)	10.19 (3.78–25.56)	1.11 (0.67–1.47)	3.00 (1.21–8.14)	0.5–3.0
Primapterin	ND	ND	Traces	0.76 (0.44–0.93)	Traces	Traces
% Biopterin	36.9 (24.1–54.5)	1.0 (0–5.0)	66.5 (25.3–93.5)	12.4 (3.2–26.6)	32.3 (12.8–75.2)	44–77
CSF (nM)†						
Neopterin	1.0 (0.05–3.0)	173 (11–449)	19 (11–70)	50 (43–117)	37 (6–118)	9–40
Biopterin	4.8 (1.5–7.5)	10 (0.8–42)	51 (25–117)	44 (16–96)	75 (15–143)	10–50
% Biopterin	87 (65–99)	3 (1–9)	74 (46–86)	49 (22–78)	68 (25–88)	32–87
Homovanillic acid	34 (15–48)	152 (11–368)	90 (19–204)	384 (170–602)	378 (47–1174)	100–900
5-Hydroxyindoleacetic acid	112 (61–183)	57 (5–154)	24 (4–75)	205 (135–300)	188 (14–471)	120–500
Residual enzyme activity (%)	< 1‡	< 30§; < 1¶	< 5§; <1 ¶	< 30**	< 1‡	
Loading test with BH_4						
20 mg/kg body weight	+	+	+	+	–	
7.5 mg/kg body weight	+	+	±	+	–	

*Range.
†Mean (range).
‡Liver.
§Erythrocytes.
¶Fibroblasts.
**Small intestine (mucosa); one patient.
+Indicates a reduction in plasma phenylalanine concentration following oral BH_4-loading test.

ABBREVIATIONS: GTPCH = GTP cyclohydrolase I; PTPS = 6-pyruvoyl-tetrahydropterin synthase; DHPR = dihydropteridine reductase; PCD = pterin-4α-carbinolamine dehydratase; PKU = phenylketonuria; BH_4 = tetrahydrobiopterin; ND = not detectable.
SOURCE: From Blau et al[177] (with modifications). Used by permission.

tetrahydrobiopterin, dihydrobiopterin, and fully oxidized biopterin can be measured.[185] At acidic conditions, all three oxidation states of biopterin are transformed to biopterin. BH_4 and quinonoid dihydrobiopterin are unstable under alkaline conditions and are converted to pterin following side-chain cleavage. The difference between biopterin concentration after acidic and alkaline oxidation represents, therefore, the concentration of BH_4.

Blood spots on Guthrie cards can also be used for screening of inherited BH_4 deficiency,[195] but this method may show some limitations in patients with the mild/peripheral phenotype and is not informative if phenylalanine concentrations are normal. The biopterin bioassay with the protozoon *Crithidia fasciculata* used in this method provides a measure of the combined activity of BH_4, dihydrobiopterin, biopterin, and sepiapterin but cannot include another important metabolite, neopterin[196].

Urinary pterins should be analyzed at elevated plasma phenylalanine levels and not during treatment with a low-phenylalanine diet. Healthy newborns excrete relatively higher levels of pterins than children or adults.[189,197]

Patients with classic PKU excrete generally more neopterin and biopterin in urine than normal controls.[198,199] This is due to the activation of GTPCH by phenylalanine via GFRP (see the section "Regulation of Tetrahydrobiopterin Homeostasis"). At serum phenylalanine concentrations ranging from 43 to 1004 μM, a good correlation was found with serum biopterin and neopterin levels.[200] Following oral loading with phenylalanine (100 mg/kg body weight), serum and red blood cell biopterin concentrations increased in patients with classic PKU, as well as in patients with a DHPR deficiency, but not in those with PTPS deficiency. The kinetics of the biopterin response to simple phenylalanine loading was characterized by its early increase in serum, followed by its increase in erythrocytes. Similar information, consistent with biopterin transfer from serum into erythrocytes, was obtained by performing a combined phenylalanine and BH_4-loading test.[200] In view of the relative stability of blood biopterin concentrations and their direct correlation with serum phenylalanine levels, serum and

Table 78-5 Pterins Used in the Differential Diagnosis of Tetrahydrobiopterin (BH_4) Deficiencies

Metabolite	Precursor	Metabolic Route*
Neopterin	Dihydroneopterin Triphosphate	1. Phosphatases 2. Nonenzymatic oxidation
Monapterin	Dihydroneopterin Triphosphate	1. Epimerase 2. Phosphatases 3. Nonenzymatic oxidation
Isoxanthopterin	Pterin	1. Xanthine oxidase
Biopterin	q-Dihydrobiopterin	1. Tautomerization 2. Nonenzymatic oxidation
Primapterin	Carbinolamine-4α-BH_4	1. Nonenzymatic isomerization
Pterin	q-Dihydrobiopterin, BH_4	1. Nonenzymatic side-chain cleavage

*Enzymatic and nonenzymatic steps in the breakdown of precursor.

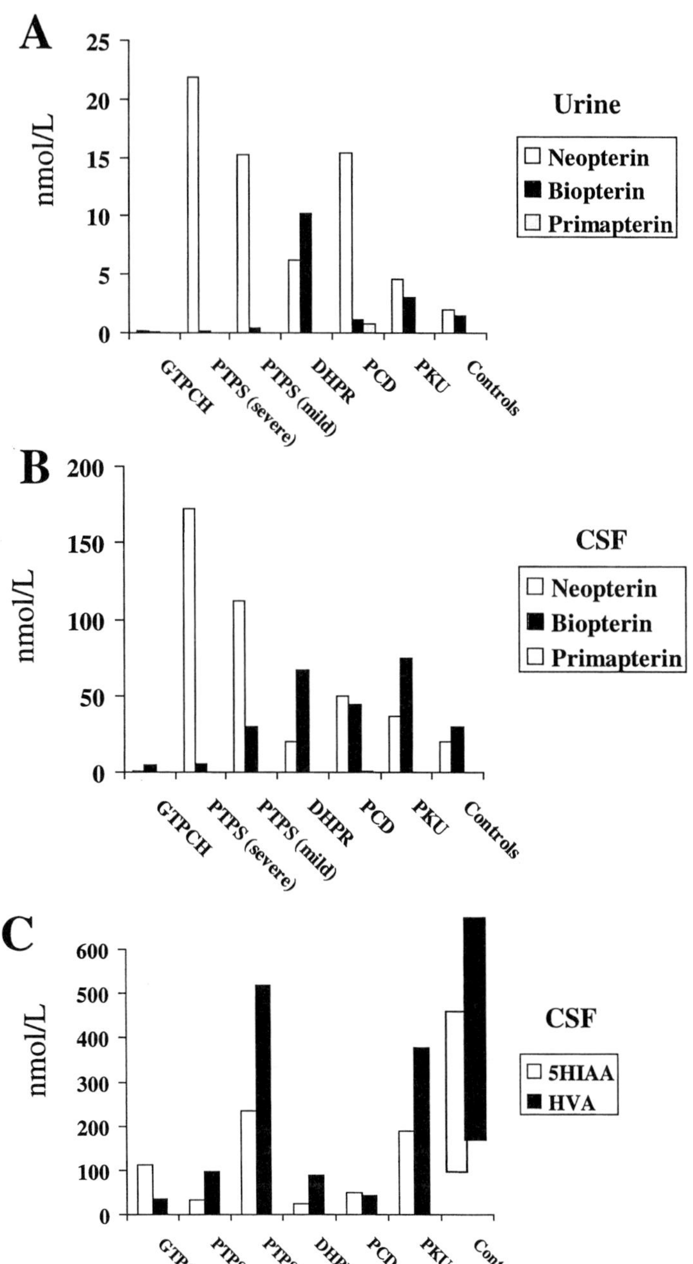

Fig. 78-10 Typical mean values of (A) urinary and (B) cerebrospinal fluid (CSF) pterins and (C) neurotransmitter metabolites 5-hydroxyindoleacetic acid (5HIAA) and homovanillic acid (HVA) in patients with different forms of hyperphenylalaninemia (HPA). Data from the BIODEF database.[178]

urine biopterin measurements should be corrected, taking into account the actual plasma phenylalanine level.

Typical urinary pterin profiles are as follows: neopterin and biopterin are very low in GTPCH deficiency; neopterin and monapterin (isomer of neopterin) are very high in PTPS deficiency and there are only traces of biopterin; neopterin is normal or slightly increased and biopterin is very high in DHPR deficiency; and neopterin is initially high, biopterin is in the subnormal range, and primapterin (7-substituted biopterin) is present in PCD deficiency (Fig. 78-10*A*). By two-dimensional plotting of total urinary biopterin versus percentage of biopterin, of the sum of neopterin plus biopterin, variants of HPA can be differentiated (Fig. 78-11).

Dihydropteridine Reductase Activity in Blood. Measurement of DHPR activity in dry blood spots of Guthrie cards is a widely used and routine method for the diagnosis of DHPR deficiency. The method of Arai et al[201] uses the reduction of BH_4 to quinonoid dihydropterin in the presence of ferricytochrome C. In the presence of NADH, quinonoid dihydropterin is reduced back to BH_4 by DHPR. The formation of ferrocytochrome C is monitored spectrophotometrically. Only 5 μl of blood is required for the assay in erythrocytes. An automated assay of DHPR activity in eluates from dried blood spots on filter paper has been developed.[202]

Tetrahydrobiopterin-Loading Tests. Two types of loading tests have been used in the differential diagnosis of BH_4 deficiencies:

1. Simple oral BH_4 loading
2. Combined phenylalanine and BH_4 loading

Historically, the first method tried,[162] and predicted as the most convenient to selectively screen among HPAs, exploited the

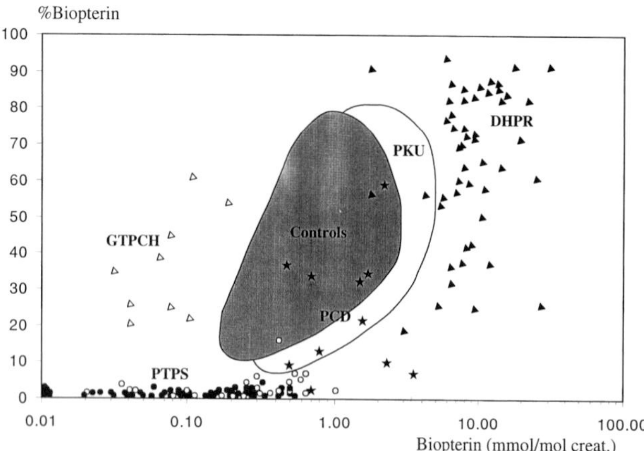

Fig. 78-11 Differentiation of BH_4 deficiency variants by two-dimensional semilogarithmic plotting of urinary biopterin/creatinine ratio versus percentage of biopterin [100*biopterin/(biopterin + neopterin)]. Data obtained from the BIODEF database.[178] △, GTP cyclohydrolase I (GTPCH) deficiency; •, 6-pyruvoyl-tetrahydropterin synthase (PTPS) deficiency (severe form); ○, PTPS deficiency (mild form); ▲, DHPR deficiency; ★, PCD deficiency.

lowering of plasma phenylalanine in BH_4-deficient patients after administration of exogenous BH_4. Intravenous loading with 2 mg/kg BH_4 was originally proposed by Danks et al.[163] With the increased purity and availability of this synthesized cofactor (BH_4), an oral loading test (2.5 mg/kg body weight) was introduced by Niederwieser et al[203] and standardized at a dose of 7.5 mg/kg by the same group.[172] This very simple test discriminated between patients with PAH and BH_4 deficiencies. It soon became obvious, however, that some DHPR-deficient patients could be misdiagnosed, in as much as their serum phenylalanine levels were not lowered by BH_4,[204] thus introducing an unacceptable limitation if this was the sole test performed (Fig. 78-12*A*). The observation that BH_4 nonresponsiveness in DHPR deficiency correlates with the presence of a mutant enzyme,[205] and that this can be overcome by increasing the dose (20 mg/kg body weight) of the administered synthetic cofactor,[206] led to a new standard protocol for the BH_4-loading test. The foregoing observations do not clarify the paradox of why in DHPR deficiency BH_4 does not function in a stoichiometric way but catalytically.[207]

Theoretically, BH_4 should barely lower the plasma phenylalanine levels in these cases if there is a stoichiometric conversion of phenylalanine to tyrosine. By analyzing the time course and changes of plasma phenylalanine concentrations in patients with PKU and a DHPR deficiency, alternately loaded with only phenylalanine (100 mg/kg body weight) and with BH_4 (7.5 or 20 mg/kg body weight) in addition to phenylalanine, it was demonstrated that 6 to 10 times more phenylalanine is hydroxylated per mole of administered BH_4 in DHPR-deficient patients than is expected from the equimolar ratio.[208,209] This corresponds to a daily intake of 8 to 20 mg/kg BH_4. Obviously, some BH_4 recycling occurs in patients with DHPR deficiency, and initial plasma phenylalanine levels may be critical for the outcome of a loading test. Furthermore, it should be stressed that at least one DHPR-deficient patient has been described who did not respond to the ingestion of a higher concentration of BH_4 (20 mg/kg body weight).[210] The lack of response in these patients might be explained by a specific mutation causing unresponsiveness, the coexistence of DHPR deficiency and PKU, or defective BH_4 absorption. Therefore, every loading test regardless of outcome, i.e., positive or negative, has to be confirmed by an enzymatic analysis.

In patients with PCD deficiency, BH_4 loading increases urinary primapterin excretion.[211]

***The Simple BH₄*-Loading** Test. The simple BH_4-loading test (7.5 to 20 mg/kg body weight) has been used in more than 120 patients with different forms of BH_4 deficiencies (Fig. 78-12). Figure 78-12*B* shows marked differences between the slopes obtained in patients with GTPCH or PTPS deficiency and those with DHPR deficiency, but the basal phenylalanine values have to be taken into account. The blood phenylalanine level needs to be elevated (more than 400 μM) for this test to be interpretable. It is customary for a PKU diet to be stopped 2 days before a loading test. A BH_4 test kit is now available and distributed by Dr. Schircks Laboratories (Jona, Switzerland) and should be used at the recommended dosage of 20 mg/kg body weight about 30 min before a regular meal.

In premature newborns with HPA, tyrosine tolerance is markedly reduced, and administration of relatively high doses of BH_4 seems to be warranted. Two preterm newborns with HPA developed transient tyrosinemia after a challenge with BH_4 (20 mg/kg).[212] Simultaneously with plasma phenylalanine decrease, tyrosine rose in almost equimolar concentrations. A lower dose of BH_4 (5 mg/kg per day) restored plasma tyrosine and phenylalanine to normal levels in both infants.

***The Combined Phenylalanine–BH₄*-Loading** Test. Phenylalanine (100 mg/kg body weight) plus BH_4 (20 mg/kg body weight) given orally enables selective screening of all BH_4 deficiencies when pterin analysis is not available or when a clear diagnosis has not previously been made.[208] In its simplest form, this test can be interpreted using only four blood spots from a Guthrie card. In preliminary experiments, the ingestion interval of phenylalanine and BH_4 was 1 h.[213] Three patients with classic PKU, three patients with DHPR deficiency, and two patients with PTPS deficiency were loaded with phenylalanine (100 mg/kg body weight) and 1 h later with BH_4 (20 mg/kg body weight). Plasma phenylalanine levels were measured before and 1, 3, 5, 9, 13, and 25 h after the phenylalanine administration. Although all patients with BH_4 deficiencies responded to BH_4 loading, phenylalanine levels normalized after 9 h in PTPS-deficient patients and after 13 h in DHPR-deficient patients. There was no response in PKU

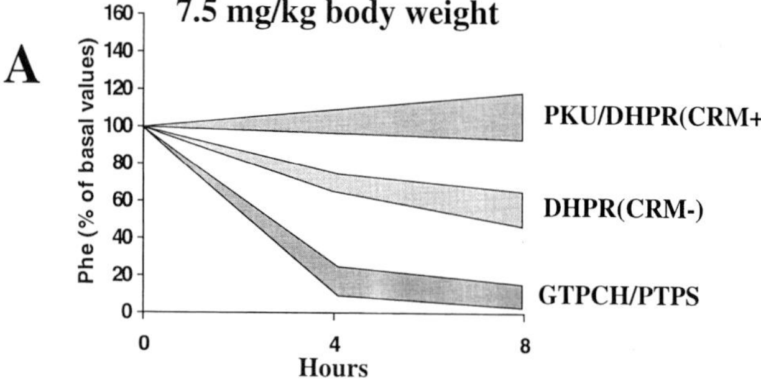

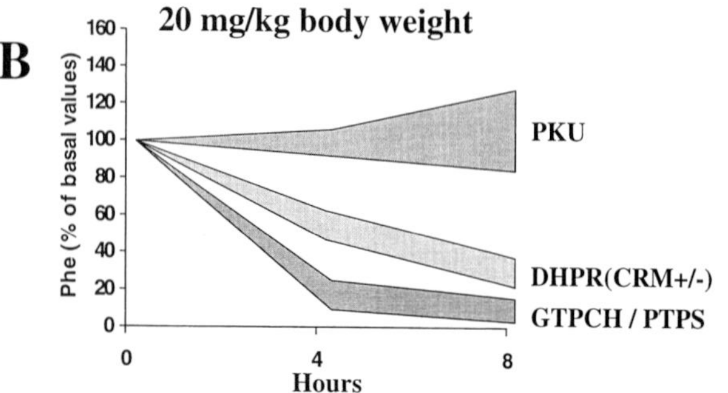

Fig. 78-12 Typical results of a simple loading test with (A) 7.5 mg tetrahydrobiopterin (BH_4)/kg and with (B) 20 mg BH_4/kg in patients with HPA.

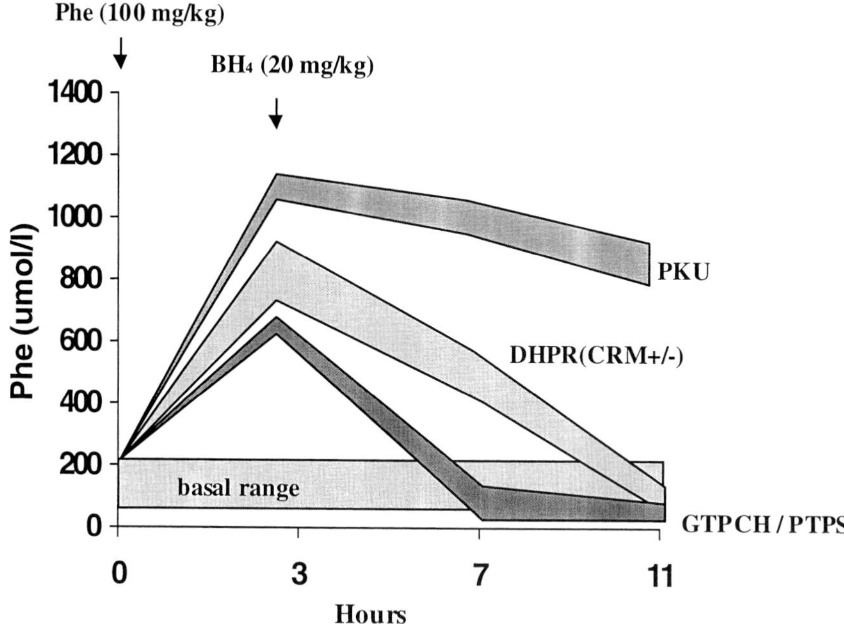

Fig. 78-13 Combined phenylalanine (100 mg/kg) and tetrahydrobiopterin (20 mg/kg) loading test in patients with hyperphenylalaninemia (HPA).

patients. Plasma phenylalanine levels peaked 1 h after phenylalanine administration in PTPS-deficient patients and 3 to 5 h in a DHPR-deficient patient. Because individual differences in phenylalanine and BH_4 gut absorption velocity could interfere with the outcome, the test was modified to its present form. Now, BH_4 is administered 3 h after a standard dose of 100 mg/kg body weight of phenylalanine. This amount of phenylalanine matches the mean daily intake in infants on a "free" diet. The amino acid must be administered when the plasma phenylalanine level is normal, thus producing a safe degree of HPA, sufficient for the interpretation of the test. Due to cofactor recycling, a normal function, PTPS-deficient patients responded maximally within 4 h to the combined loading test, regardless of the administered dose of BH_4 (7.5 or 20 mg/kg body weight). DHPR-deficient patients took 8 h to respond clearly to the 20 mg/kg body weight ingestion of BH_4. There was virtually no response to BH_4 ingestion in PKU patients, and plasma phenylalanine levels peaked in all cases 3 h after phenylalanine administration (Fig. 78-13).

As expected, the response in one case of a GTPCH deficiency was quite similar to that observed in PTPS deficiency.[214] Comparison of the outcomes of the simple phenylalanine and combined loading tests confirmed that cofactor administration is totally ineffective in altering the time course of serum phenylalanine concentrations. Thus, the differential lowering of plasma phenylalanine after the combined test with 20 mg/kg body weight BH_4 allows a clear distinction of BH_4 deficiencies from PKU and also of defects in BH_4 synthesis versus those due to defects in BH_4 regeneration.

Pterins, Folates, and Neurotransmitter Metabolites in Cerebrospinal Fluid. To distinguish between the different variants of BH_4 deficiency, i.e., severe and mild (peripheral, partial) forms, quantification of neopterin, biopterin, and the neurotransmitter metabolites, 5HIAA and HVA, in CSF is essential.[215] In patients with DHPR deficiency, measurement of 5-methyltetrahydrofolic acid is important due to its connection with folate metabolism.

5HIAA and HVA are easily quantified by using HPLC with electrochemical detection, which is discussed in more detail in the section "Catecholamines and Serotonin Neurotransmitters." Except for the mild (peripheral, partial) forms of GTPCH, PTPS, and PCD deficiencies, 5HIAA and HVA are dramatically decreased in the CSF of patients with the severe form of BH_4 deficiency (Table 78-4).[216–218] The ratio of HVA/5HIAA is much lower in patients with GTPCH deficiency (0.3) than in those with PTPS deficiency (2.6) or DHPR deficiency (3.8).[177] In controls, this ratio is between 1.5 and 3.5 (see the section "Catecholamines and Serotonin Neurotransmitters"). The levels of both metabolites decrease with age in all BH_4 deficiencies, and a similar correlation was found in control children.[219] In the mild forms of a DHPR deficiency, 5HIAA is usually decreased, while HVA levels are normal.[179]

Concentrations of neopterin and biopterin in CSF are also found to be age related.[220–222] Particularly in neonatal samples, biopterin concentration is much higher in the first days of life than at the age of 1 month (H. Shintaku, personal communication). Generally, in patients with BH_4 deficiencies, the pterin pattern is similar to that found in urine except that, in GTPCH deficiency, biopterin is always slightly higher than neopterin (Fig. 78-10*B*).[177]

Two enzymes are thought to be involved in the regeneration of BH_4 through salvage pathways. DHFR can synthesize BH_4 from oxidized forms such as 7,8-dihydrobiopterin, and 5,10-methylenetetrahydrofolate reductase can regenerate BH_4 from quinonoid dihydrobiopterin through 5-methyltetrahydrofolic acid.[223] The following reaction catalyzed by 5,10-methylenetetrahydrofolate reductase may have an important implication for folate metabolism:

$$\text{q-dihydrobiopterin} + \text{5-}CH_3\text{-THF} \rightarrow BH_4 + \text{5,10-}CH_2\text{-THF}$$

Supportive evidence for folate deficiency in the central nervous system (CNS) includes low CSF levels of 5-methyltetrahydrofolic acid and frequent occurrence of basal ganglia calcifications similar to those found in congenital folate malabsorption.[224,225] Measurement of 5-methyltetrahydrofolic acid in CSF with HPLC and electrochemical detection[226] is, therefore, important in the differential diagnosis of DHPR deficiency.

GTP Cyclohydrolase I Deficiency (OMIM 233910)

GTPCH deficiency is a rare form of HPA with 16 cases listed in the International BIODEF Database.[178] The clinical course of illness is similar in all untreated patients and associated with those found in the severe forms of PTPS and DHPR deficiencies.[227–230] Most of the patients were screened for HPA at 4 to 11 days of age and had plasma phenylalanine levels of 300 to 1200 μM. At least three patients with GTPCH deficiency passed the newborn PKU-screening program because of initially normal blood phenylalanine values.[33,184]

Genotype. Cloning of the human GTPCH cDNA and structural analysis of the corresponding *GCH1* gene enabled detection of two missense mutations (R184H and M211I)[22,33] and one nonsense mutation (Q110X),[72] causing BH_4-deficient HPA (Fig. 78-6). Mutations are listed in the International BIOMDB Database.[231] One female and one male patient with HPA were both found to be homozygotes (R184H and M211I), and one male was a compound heterozygote (Q110X) with one allele not yet defined. Functional characterization of the amino acid changes was done for the R184H and M211I mutant proteins by recombinant expression in *E. coli.* The analysis revealed that the GTPCH activity was completely abolished, as compared with wild-type protein.[41]

Enzyme Phenotype. GTPCH activity is measurable in liver[232] and in cytokine-stimulated mononuclear cells[233] or fibroblasts.[234,235] It is low both in liver and in phytohemagglutinin-stimulated blood lymphocytes (below 4 percent of normal).[227,228] Two obligate heterozygotes had 30 and 46 percent of normal activity in stimulated lymphocytes.[233] An alternative indirect approach to determine the GTPCH activity is measurement of intracellular neopterin and biopterin concentrations in the patient's primary fibroblasts after stimulation with interferon-γ (IFN-γ)/ tumor necrosis factor α.[235] In two patients with GTPCH deficiency, neopterin (8 and 10 pmol/mg protein) and biopterin (22 and 83 pmol/mg protein) production were markedly reduced when compared with controls (neopterin = 20 to 70 pmol/mg protein; biopterin = 160 to 350 pmol/mg protein), indicating low residual GTPCH activity (N. Blau, personal communication).

Metabolic Phenotype. In GTPCH deficiency, biosynthesis of pterins is blocked at a very early stage and almost no pterins can be formed. The urinary excretion of neopterin, biopterin, isoxanthopterin, and pterin is very low, although the relative proportion of pterins is normal[227–230a] (Table 78-4). In CSF, neopterin and biopterin as well as the neurotransmitter metabolites, 5HIAA and HVA, were also very low (Table 78-4 and Fig. 78-10*C*). The biopterin content was always slightly higher. In one patient,[236] serotonin turnover was normal despite a severe reduction in DA synthesis. The authors suggested that in this patient GTPCH activity was normal in serotonin-producing cells within the CNS but reduced in dopaminergic neurons and hepatocytes. This could be due to the fact that different forms of GTPCH are specific for various cell types.

Clinical Phenotype. Untreated patients with typical BH_4 deficiency show a virtually similar picture of progressive neurologic deterioration, regardless of the different enzyme defects.[176] The clinical manifestation of GTPCH deficiency is variable, but common symptoms are mental retardation, convulsions, disturbance of tone and posture, abnormal movements, hypersalivation, and swallowing difficulties (Table 78-6).[222]

It has been claimed that neopterin may play an active role in the cell-mediated immune response; however, cell proliferation and differentiation, and all humoral and cellular functions tested in one of these patients, were found to be normal.[237]

6-Pyruvoyl-tetrahydropterin Synthase Deficiency (OMIM 261640)

PTPS is the most prevalent and most heterogeneous form of HPA not attributed to PAH deficiency. So far, 208 cases (57 percent of all cases of BH_4 deficiencies) are listed in the International BIODEF Database;[178] of these, 168 patients have the typical severe form, 35 an atypical mild peripheral/partial form, and two were described as having a transient form (see the previous edition of this book for citations of older articles).

Genotype. Since the cloning of the human PTPS cDNA was published,[68] 28 different disease-causing mutations have been reported from 42 PTPS-deficient patients and are summarized in Fig. 78-7.[231] Originally, all mutation detection was based on PTPS-cDNA screening by reverse transcriptase-polymerase chain reaction (RT-PCR) product sequencing mostly from skin fibroblasts, in some instances from lymphoblasts, as an mRNA source. However, the clarification of the genomic structure of the corresponding *PTS* gene, enabled on the one hand, either the confirmation of mutations at the genomic DNA level or the detection of the two splice-site mutations,[70,76] and, on the other hand, new mutations were identified by screening exonic DNA.[72,72a] The mutations described so far are distributed throughout all six exons in the *PTS* gene (Fig. 78-7), even though there seems to be a proportionally high number of mutations in exons 2 and 5 among the Chinese and Korean mutant alleles studied (alleles N52S and P87S).[75,78,238,239] A 14-bp deletion detected in exon 6 from one patient (allele K120X/361del14bp) was found to overlap with a 7-bp direct repeat, which might have been involved in generating such a mutation during DNA replication processes.[77,240]

There is at least one splicing allele, observed in normal fibroblasts, hepatoma cell lines, and in neuronal cells, that results in skipping of exon 3 (deletion of bp T_{164} to G_{168} in the cDNA).[69,241] Remarkably, the exon-3 deletion is "conserved" in the human retro-pseudogene *PTS-PI*, which has 74 percent similarity to the 3′ portion of the PTPS cDNA and is located on chromosome 9p12-p13.[70] The 23-bp exon-3 deletion leads to a frameshift and premature stop codon in the normal PTPS cDNA. Such a potential truncated PTPS peptide, if expressed at all in vivo, was shown to be completely inactive (expressed as a K54X allele).[65] Whether the exon-3 deleted splice variant is a spontaneous polymorphism or has some regulatory function cannot be answered at this time.

So far, two splice-site mutations have been described in PTPS-deficient patients. In one case, a mutation responsible for a four codon deletion was identified as a genomic $c^{-3} \rightarrow g$ transversion at the 3′-acceptor splice site of intron 1 that results in a cryptic splice-site usage within exon 2 [allele Δ(K23-S32)].[76] A second splice-site mutation was identified as being caused by a 3′-acceptor splice-site alteration, a $t^{-7} \rightarrow a$ transversion in intron 2, which leads to skipping of exon 3, thus giving rise to the PTPS-deficient allele K54X.[70]

Individual mutant PTPS have been studied to various degrees, including in vitro studies of purified, recombinant proteins, transient expression in transfected COS-1 cells, and examination of cross-reactive material in primary skin fibroblasts. For some mutants, no experimental information on stability or activity is available.

As expected, all mutations that cause protein truncations such as a premature stop codon or internal amino acid deletions, alleles Δ(K29-532), K54X, ΔV57, and K120X/361del14bp, lead to unstable and enzymatically completely inactive mutant PTPS. Furthermore, most of the point mutations causing single amino acid exchanges were shown to be unstable and/or to be significantly reduced in their activity when transfected into COS-1 cells (alleles T76M, P87S, P87L, D96N, and D136V). An exception to this behavior of anticipated inactivity or instability were the mutant alleles Rl6C, R25Q, and K129E. Whereas the R25Q mutant was found to be degraded in primary fibroblasts from the respective patient, the Rl6C and K129E mutants appeared to be stable in the patient's fibroblasts, although no enzymatic activity was observed. All three mutants exhibited significant in vitro PTPS activity when assayed as purified, recombinant proteins.[65] However, whereas enzyme activities of Rl6C and R25Q were reduced to almost background when expressed in mammalian COS-1 cells, the K129E mutant was three times more active than the wild-type protein when tested in the COS-1 or the hepatoma cells Hep G2, which is in contrast to its inactivity in fibroblasts. This behavior of enzymatic activity that depends on cellular background as opposed to the in vitro activity of purified enzymes suggests the occurrence of posttranslational modification(s) as a requirement for maximal PTPS activity. In the case of the R25Q and K129E alleles, the effect of the single amino acid exchanges is still unclear and awaits further characterization. A critical role for such a postulated modification, however, was demonstrated by investigating the Rl6C mutant that appeared not to be phosphorylated and is active in vivo, whereas the wild-type enzyme was found to be phosphorylated, thus suggesting an essential role of phosphorylation for normal in vivo activity of PTPS.[65,67a]

In general, it is expected that recurrent mutations must have similar treatment protocols and disease outcome. Such a comparative follow-up must be acknowledged especially in the case of the relatively high frequency of the "Asian PTPS alleles" N52S and P87S. A central question concerns, e.g., the correlation of certain mutations with a given clinical subtype of PTPS deficiency. It appears to be unlikely that alternative exons with tissue specificity play an important role, since it was shown that only a single *PTS* gene is present in the human genome that expresses the identical functional mRNA in peripheral tissues, such as blood or liver, and in neuronal tissues.[69,70] So far, four patients with the mild form of PTPS deficiency were investigated on the molecular level (alleles R16C, K38X, N47D, D116G, K120X/361del14bp, and K129E);[77] almost all other mutations are from the central type of deficiency. In a recent report, a homozygous mutation (I114V) was found to be associated with mild HPA in a patient with generalized dystonia and diurnal fluctuation of symptoms.[242] A dominant negative allele (N47D) in a compound heterozygote (N47D/D116G) patient was shown to cause a transient hyperphenylalaninemia.[77a] In contrast the isolated central form seems to be associated with hemizygosity on chromosome 11 q and a mutant allele (Y99C).[77b]

Enzyme Phenotype. Several enzyme assays have been developed for the measurement of enzymes converting dihydroneopterin triphosphate to BH_4.[243–246] PTPS (originally called *phosphate-eliminating enzyme*) activity was severely deficient in liver biopsy samples from patients with clinical and metabolic phenotypes indicative of impaired BH_4 synthesis.[247] The HPLC method is based on the measurement of BH_4 derived from the substrate dihydroneopterin triphosphate in the presence of NADPH, magnesium, DHPR, and SR. The same assay was used to measure PTPS activity in erythrocytes[248] and cultured skin fibroblasts.[249] Erythrocytes, which normally contain PTPS activity, expressed the mutant phenotype (less than 5 percent of normal activity) in these patients.[250] Some patients with PTPS deficiency have mild clinical features (peripheral/partial form).[251–253] They have a partial deficiency of erythrocyte PTPS activity (5 to 23 percent of normal activity).[254,255]

Terms such as "typical," "peripheral," or "partial" relating to patients with BH_4 deficiency have been used to describe different clinical and metabolic phenotypes. However, the corresponding erythrocyte PTPS activities have not been predictive of the clinical phenotype or its apparent prognosis. "Typical" patients can have erythrocyte PTPS activities as high as 20 percent of normal,[254,256] yet patients with the "peripheral" variant can have activity as low as 5 percent of normal.[77,255,257] Erythrocyte PTPS activity remained unchanged in a patient with a disease progression from "peripheral" to "central" phenotype.[258] Despite the low PTPS activity (less than 5 percent of normal controls), this patient has normal plasma phenylalanine levels without any treatment.

The enzyme activities encompass what seem to be homozygous, compound heterozygous, and obligate heterozygous phenotypes.[254,255] The heterozygote can be clinically symptomatic in the neonatal period[254,255] and have an expressed metabolic phenotype in adult life.[251,252,255] One explanation for severe loss of PTPS activity in erythrocytes of homozygotes is a dominant negative mutation effect[255] originating in a heteropolymeric PTPS enzyme; the normal enzyme is a hexamer of identical subunits.[66] In seven of eight obligate heterozygotes, erythrocyte PTPS activity was 19 to 23 percent of normal instead of half of normal.[255] Investigation of 37 obligate heterozygotes revealed median erythrocyte PTPS activity of 22 percent (range, 10 to 37 percent) (N. Blau, unpublished observation).

PTPS activity in patients' cultured skin fibroblasts is below 1 percent of the wild-type control, which is at detection level of the assay.[76,259] One patient with the mild "peripheral" form exhibited an activity equivalent to 1 percent of normal controls.[77] Unfortunately, these results did not distinguish between the observed severe "typical" and mild "peripheral" type of PTPS deficiency, as reflected by the different serum phenylalanine concentrations and neurotransmitter levels in CSF. Fibroblasts from a child with PTPS deficiency are not able to synthesize biopterin upon stimulation with cytokines.[235]

Metabolic Phenotype. Dihydroneopterin triphosphate cannot be converted to 6-pyruvoyl-tetrahydropterin (Fig. 78-4), resulting in an accumulation of dihydroneopterin triphosphate in the tissue of patients with this defect. 6-Pyruvoyl-tetrahydropterin is readily dephosphorylated by pyrophosphatase and excreted as dihydroneopterin and its oxidation product, neopterin. High concentrations of neopterin, monapterin (an isomer of neopterin), and 3′-hydroxysepiapterin, and only traces of biopterin, are found in the urine of patients with PTPS deficiency (Table 78-4). These patients present with the highest urinary neopterin levels, and the ratio of neopterin to biopterin is the highest among BH_4 deficiencies. With regard to HPA, phenylalanine concentrations in plasma are generally around 1200 μM.

In the severe (typical) form of PTPS deficiency, the neurotransmitter status is similar to that in patients with GTPCH deficiency (Table 78-4). In mild (peripheral/partial) forms of PTPS deficiency, neopterin levels are almost as high as in the typical form, both in urine and in CSF, and the biopterin level is slightly higher but still just under the lower normal range (Fig. 78-10*B*). However, the overlap of the urinary biopterin values plotted against the percentage of biopterin [%biopterin = biopterin × 100/(neopterin + biopterin)] does not allow clear discrimination between these two groups on a case-to-case basis (Fig. 78-11). It appears that the degree of HPA is also significantly lower, with a median concentration of around 500 μM. Some infants have been recognized because of a reinvestigation of their mild HPA.

The most striking biochemical difference between the atypical and typical forms of PTPS deficiency is that in the atypical form normal levels of neurotransmitter metabolites can be detected in CSF (Fig. 78-10*C*).

An intermediate PTPS deficiency with urinary pterins consistent with the severe form and normal CSF neurotransmitter metabolites was described by Endres et al.[260] The classification of this patient as an "intermediate" type is based on the appearance of clinical signs and symptoms and a decrease in 5HIAA after withdrawal of BH_4 therapy.

Clinical Phenotype. About 80 percent of all patients with PTPS deficiency are referred to as having severe "typical" forms, presenting with characteristic truncal hypotonia and increased limb tone with pronated hand posture.[261] A decrease in activity or loss of head control may herald the onset of a progressive neurologic degenerative disease.[256] Ultimately, these patients become hypertonic especially in the lower extremities.[168] There may be bradykinesia, episodic "lead pipe" rigidity or "cogwheel" rigidity.[256,262] One patient was reported to present with "stiff-baby syndrome" with cervical torticollis and progressive axial and appendicular rigidity without seizures.[263] Another PTPS-deficient patient presented with unusual episodes of coarse "rubral-like" tremor in arms and legs and orofacial dyskinesia, suggesting a secondary DA deficiency.[264] Symptoms of generalized dystonia with marked diurnal fluctuations were reported in two adult patients.[242,265]

Difficulty in swallowing, oculogyric spasms, somnolence, irritability, hyperthermia, seizures, and impaired neurophysiological development are all part of the clinical picture, depending on the stage of the disease (Table 78-6).[222]

Table 78-6 Clinical and Demographic Data Collected from the BIODEF Database

Signs and Symptoms	GTPCH Deficiency	PTPS Deficiency	DHPR Deficiency	PCD Deficiency
Progressive mental and physical retardation despite treatment for phenylketonuria	+	+	+	
Variable tone with marked hypotonia to opistotonus and spasticity	+	+	+	(+)
Temperature instability	+	+	+	
Seizures—myoclonic or tonic clonic	+	+	+	
Microcephaly	(+)	+	+	
Hypersalivation	+	+	+	
Lethargy and irritability	+	+	+	
Chorea/athetosis		+	+	
Rash—eczema		+	+	
Pneumonia		+	+	
Sudden death		+	+	
Demographic data*				
Number of patients (% of total)†	16 (4)	208 (58)	113 (31)	19 (5)
Caucasians (total)	14	143	89	15
Turkish	1	12	31	
Arab	3	32	21	2
Chinese	1	24	3	
Japanese		113	4	
African	1	1	5	
Mixed		2	2	2
Indonesian, Indian, Mongolian, Pakistani, Vietnamese		9		
Unknown		13	6	

*Updated 1998.
†Nine patients unclassified.
ABBREVIATIONS: GTPCH = GTP cyclohydrolase I; PTPS = 6-pyruvoyl-tetrahydropterin synthase; DHPR = dihydropteridine reductase; PCD = pterin-4α-carbinolamine dehydratase.
SOURCE: From Blau et al.[177] Used by permission.

Patients with the atypical forms of PTPS deficiency may have phenotypic changes with increasing age and should be reevaluated after infancy. At least two cases have been well documented,[258,266] and more are listed in the BIODEF database,[178] in which the CSF neurotransmitters were found to be normal in the first months of life, but one of the infants became progressively neurologically abnormal between 1 and 2 years of age, with very low CSF neurotransmitter levels.

Pterin-4α-Carbinolamine Dehydratase Deficiency (OMIM 264070 and 126090)

PCD deficiency ("primapterinuria") was first recognized by Dhondt et al[180] in a patient with HPA, whose urine contained a very high neopterin level, a low biopterin level, and an unknown compound "X." The same pterin pattern was found in another patient, and it was hypothesized to be a new variant of BH_4 deficiency.[181] CSF pterin and neurotransmitter metabolite levels were normal in both cases. Intensive laboratory investigation revealed that the unknown compound X was a 7-isomer of biopterin (primapterin) (Fig. 78-1), and that these patients exhibited substantial excretion of additional 7-substituted pterins (anapterin and 7-neopterin) in urine.[267] The observation that oral administration of BH_4 increases the excretion of biopterin and primapterin while the ratio remains constant (at about 1), suggested that the 7-substituted biopterin derivative was formed endogenously from BH_4.[268] This hypothesis was confirmed by additional tests, including loading experiments using dihydrobiopterin and sepiapterin[211,269] and deuterated BH_4.[270] The formation of primapterin from BH_4 was shown to proceed nonenzymatically in vitro via a "spiro" intermediate, and this could be prevented by addition of PCD.[271,272] It was subsequently proposed that "primapterinuria" was caused by a deficiency of PCD, the first enzyme in recycling of BH_4 (Fig. 78-3).

So far, 19 patients with PCD deficiency are registered in the BIODEF database.[178]

Genotype. Surprisingly, PCD is a bifunctional protein, with a second function as a dimerization cofactor (DCoH) for HNF-1α. Thus, DCoH was proposed to have a general transcriptional function by binding to HNF-1α and stimulating transcriptional activity.[89,104,273,274] The corresponding gene *PCBD* is characterized by a protein-coding region divided into four exons over 5 kb (Fig. 78-8).[101]

A patient with compound heterozygous mutations (E86X and C81R) in the *PCBD* gene, encoding the corresponding mutant PCD protein with reduced dehydratase activity, was described.[99,275,276] Analysis of DNA from 10 patients identified the following mutations (Fig. 78-8): three patients homozygous for the missense mutations E96K and T87I and five homozygous for the nonsense mutations E86X and Q97X, one compound heterozygote with the mutations E96K and Q97X, and one patient with two different homozygous mutations: E26X in exon 2 and R87Q in exon 4.[102,103] In two families, parents were investigated and found to be obligate heterozygotes for particular mutations. One sibling was found to be unaffected. Recombinant expression in *E. coli* revealed that the mutant proteins, T78I, E86X, and Q97X, are almost entirely in the insoluble fraction, in contrast to the wild type, which is expressed as a soluble protein. These data support the proposal that HPA in combination with urinary primapterin may be due to autosomal recessive inheritance of mutations in the *PCBD* gene, specifically affecting the dehydratase activity. Six of seven mutations are located in exon 4, with the mutant allele Q97X the most common (32 percent of all mutant alleles).[231]

Enzyme Phenotype. PCD was originally detected as a contaminant in a preparation of rat PAH as a consequence of its ability to stimulate the BH_4-dependent hydroxylation of phenylalanine.[277] This stimulating protein (PCD) was subsequently purified from rat liver, and its activity was shown to be due to the catalysis of dehydration of the 4α-carbinolamine intermediate. PCD catalyzes a reaction (Fig. 78-3) that can also occur nonenzymatically.[278] PCD activity was also shown to be present in human liver, and its absence is concomitant with the formation of 7-substituted pterins.[271] The only two tissues that express relatively high PCD activity are liver and kidney, which are also the only two tissues that express PAH activity.[90] PCD activity, as a rule, is low in those tissues that contain high levels of tyrosine and TPH activity, except for the pineal gland. Catalytic activity of PCD is detectable as early as 6.7 weeks and increases linearly with time, reaching 31 percent of the adult value at 17.3 weeks of gestational age.[94]

In one patient with PCD deficiency, enzyme activity in jejunal biopsy was reduced to 29 percent of normal (J.E. Ayling and N. Blau, in preparation).

Metabolic Phenotype. Most patients with PCD deficiency were initially diagnosed as having the mild forms of PTPS deficiency. In the newborn period, they present with variably elevated phenylalanine levels. The levels may rise transiently to the 1200- to 2000-μM range (Table 78-4). Excretion of neopterin in urine is increased, the biopterin level is in the subnormal range (Fig. 78-10*A*), and CSF pterin and neurotransmitter metabolite levels are normal in two cases.[180,279] The most striking finding is the occurrence of primapterin (7-biopterin) in the urine of these patients. The mean concentration of primapterin in urine of these patients was 0.76 mmol/mol creatinine (range, 0.37 to 1.86).[178] Although the percentage of urinary biopterin is rather low in the early neonatal period (5 to 15 percent of the sum of neopterin and biopterin), excretion of primapterin parallels that of biopterin regardless of age. About 30 to 50 percent of total biopterins are excreted in urine as primapterin. Previously, it was shown that both endogenous and exogenous BH_4 as well as sepiapterin and dihydrobiopterin induce production of primapterin in patients with primapterinuria.[211,280] On the other hand, introduction of a phenylalanine-restricted diet reduces excretion of all pterins, due to the negative feedback effect on GTPCH via the feedback regulatory protein.[130] Thus, actual primapterin concentration in urine depends on plasma phenylalanine levels and liver concentrations of tetrahydrobiopterin.

Although generally high plasma phenylalanine concentrations correlate well with plasma and red blood cell neopterin and biopterin,[200] it is not clear why these patients excrete extremely high levels of neopterin and why HPA is a transient condition. One possible explanation is that PCD is not fully active in the early newborn period. The low activity in fetal liver was proposed to be responsible for the high ratio of primapterin to biopterin observed in amniotic fluid of normal pregnancies.[281] This was confirmed by the findings that PCD activity in fetal liver increases with gestational age.[94]

Clinical Phenotype. In the early neonatal period, some of these patients present with clinical manifestations of neurologic impairment, like transient abnormality on electroencephalogram and progressive hypotonia with delay in motor development[181] or slight upper limb tremors after stimulation.[180] In one of the patients, there was a report of eczema probably unrelated to the disease (C.L. Green, personal communication). Generally, these patients show no significant clinical abnormalities other than transient alterations in tone.[222]

Dihydropteridine Reductase Deficiency (OMIM 261630)

The first confirmed reports of DHPR deficiency[110,282] described a 14-month-old boy in whom seizures and progressive neurologic deterioration had developed despite good treatment of his "PKU" beginning in week 3 of life. DHPR activity was absent in a liver biopsy sample, and specific antibodies failed to detect DHPR protein in the sample.[110] Hepatic PAH activity and the BH_4 level were adequate. This latter point is unexplained. Since this first report, investigators have cloned the human DHPR cDNA and gene, characterized mutations causing DHPR enzyme deficiency, identified heterogeneity at levels of genotype and phenotype, and initiated effective treatment. A total of 113 cases of DHPR deficiency are listed in the BIODEF Database of Tetrahydrobiopterin Deficiencies[178] (1998 version): 109 with the severe form, two with the atypical mild form, and two with the central non-HPA form (see also the section "Dihydropteridine Reductase Deficiency Without Hyperphenylalaninemia"). The condition is autosomal recessive.

Genotype. The mutations in DHPR deficiency were reviewed in 1995,[283] and a current listing is presented in Fig. 78-14. The recent completion of the intron/exon structure of the *QDPR* gene[127] has enabled a wider range of mutations to be examined, with not only coding mutations accessible through cDNA but also mutation resulting in RNA-splicing defects amenable to investigation.

Examination of the mutations in this gene reveals little other than random mutation. Thus, the 19 mutations and two polymorphisms are spread evenly along the coding sequence (Fig. 78-14). This number of mutations has been restricted perhaps by the lack of intron/exon structure and sequence, which makes searching for mutations easier in the case of individual patients. This information has recently become available.[127] The mutations are mainly missense, with three splicing mutations and four insertions/deletions.

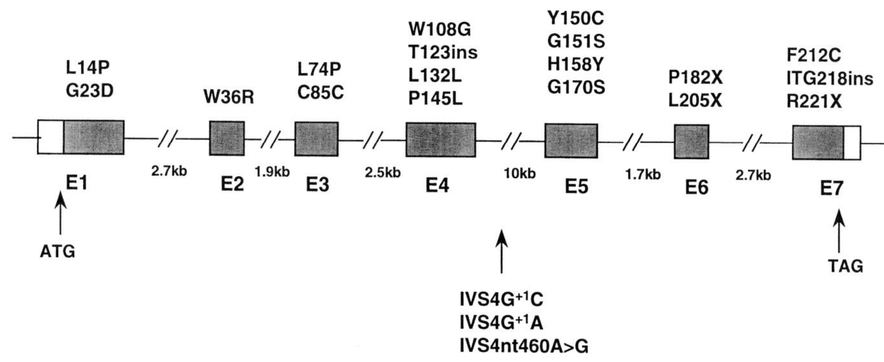

Fig. 78-14 Genomic structure and location of mutations in human *QDPR* gene. Mutations are listed in the BIOMDB database.[231] For original data, see the References 127, 179, 283–290.

There does appear to be a preponderance of mutations described in the Southern Europe/Mediterranean populations, but this still might be due to a sampling bias, which indicates that about half of the patients are from this area.[178,178a] In vitro expression of mutations has been performed only in a minority of cases and, in some cases, this activity is surprisingly high (e.g., W108G and G151S), without an obvious explanation.

Computer modeling on the crystal structure of DHPR[291] provided logical reasons for the diminished activities. Only one human mutation has been found in the five codons identified by structural studies as essential (see above): this is codon 150. However, other mutations are in the vicinity of these residues and thus likely influence enzyme activity.

There is very little recurrence of mutations in unrelated individuals and, where it has occurred, could be because CpG nucleotides are involved rather than being due to founder effect or any other phenomenon.[231]

Enzyme Phenotype. Most affected patients have complete or nearly complete deficiency of DHPR activity.[178,292] Molecular heterogeneity was recognized early[293] to include cross-reactive material (CRM)-positive and CRM-negative forms.[294] Among the former, some have low specific activity (uncommon), whereas others have loss of activity proportional to the loss of DHPR protein (apparent protein stability mutants) (P. Smooker and R.G.H. Cotton, personal communication). For reasons not yet well understood, patients completely lacking DHPR enzyme activity and immunoreactive DHPR protein ($DHPR^-/CRM^-$) can have a less severe form of HPA than patients expressing mutant DHPR proteins devoid of catalytic activity but with nearly normal levels of immunoreactive protein ($DHPR^-/CRM^+$).[205,295] It has been proposed that CRM-positive DHPR binds BH_4, making it unavailable. The CRM-positive form of DHPR deficiency, which seems to be prevalent in the Italian population,[295] has a poor prognosis and is less responsive to therapy.[205]

DHPR activity has been measured in obligate heterozygotes. The expectation is that the phenotype value (DHPR activity) will be about half of normal in heterozygotes. Most heterozygotes fulfill this expectation, but this was not the case in two unrelated obligate heterozygotes whose DHPR activities were 11 and 26 percent of normal.[111] Patients with the atypical mild form of DHPR deficiency show 4 to 10 percent residual activity in cultured fibroblasts.[179] DHPR is a homodimeric enzyme, and the finding in the two heterozygotes is suggestive of negative allelic complementation or a dominant negative mutation effect. Such an effect might account for unusual cases of so-called partial DHPR deficiency.[296–298]

Metabolic Phenotype. Quinonoid dihydrobiopterin, formed from BH_4 through a hydroxylation reaction, is an extremely unstable compound and tautomerizes readily to 7,8-dihydrobiopterin. Since 7,8-dihydrobiopterin is not a substrate for DHPR, patients with DHPR deficiency excrete very high amounts of total biopterin. In most cases, the percentage of biopterin is greater than 80 percent[186,299](Table 78-4 and Fig. 78-10*A*). In addition, owing to the lack of BH_4 in these patients, there is no feedback inhibition of GTPCH and, therefore, pterin biosynthesis is generally activated. Normal to slightly increased concentrations of neopterin can be found in the urine of these patients, and there is an overlapping in the percentage of biopterin with PKU patients (Fig. 78-11).

Although most DHPR-deficient patients were detected by screening the urinary pterins,[300–305] some newborns can be missed if the urine is collected during treatment with a low-phenylalanine diet.[183,292] Some patients might not be detected, even with normal diets.

The pterin pattern in the CSF is similar to that in the urine, and distribution of the neurotransmitter metabolites is similar to that observed in PTPS deficiency (Table 78-4 and Fig. 78-10*B*). The decrease of 5HIAA is more pronounced than that of HVA (Fig. 78-10*C*).[178] CSF levels of 7,8-dihydrobiopterin and dihydroxanthopterin are elevated in DHPR deficiency,[306] and it is likely that these act as inhibitors of aromatic amino acid hydroxylases.[307,308] There is no excessive accumulation of quinonoid dihydrobiopterin in CSF from patients with DHPR deficiency, and the percentage of total BH_4 (BH_4 + quinonoid dihydrobiopterin) is the same as that found in controls.[219]

Defective folate metabolism is a consequence of DHPR deficiency[224,309] because the normal enzyme helps to maintain folate in the active tetrahydro form.[109,223]

Clinical Phenotype. The clinical course of illness is similar to that seen in severe forms of GTPCH and PTPS deficiencies (Table 78-6). In addition, extensive neuronal loss, calcification, and abnormal vascular proliferation were noted in the central cortex, white matter, basal ganglia, and thalamus.[225,310–314]

Treatment

The prognosis of severity of BH_4 deficiency is closely related to the degree of HPA and to impaired biogenic amine production. Therefore, a combination of therapies to correct this metabolic clutter must be promptly applied after diagnosis. The goals of treatment of a BH_4 deficiency are (1) control of HPA and (2) correction of neurotransmitter deficiencies. In infants with DHPR deficiency, in addition, tetrahydrofolate homeostasis has to be restored.

Control of Blood Phenylalanine Levels. Although BH_4-deficient infants exhibit a higher dietary phenylalanine tolerance (300 to 700 mg/day) than patients with classic PKU, a limiting factor in the response to neurotransmitter therapy may be a fluctuating plasma phenylalanine level. The diet can be calculated following the lines used in PKU, also supplementing tyrosine. High plasma phenylalanine levels alter the dose-affected relationship of neurotransmitter precursors by interfering with their membrane transport or by competitive inhibition of tyrosine and TPH.[315] Therefore, the blood phenylalanine concentrations have to be more rigidly controlled than in PAH deficiency. Some patients on neurotransmitter treatment have had neurologic problems when phenylalanine concentrations were above 360 μM.

In patients with GTPCH and PTPS deficiency, administration of BH_4 appears to be the most efficient therapy in controlling blood phenylalanine levels. A single, small daily dose (2 to 5 mg/kg) is sufficient in synthesis defects, whereas larger and fractionated daily doses (20 mg/kg, given in three to four doses) are necessary in some DHPR-deficient patients.[209] However, the required dose of BH_4 to reduce neopterin and increase urine biopterin is 5 to 10 mg/kg per day.[316] In some exceptional cases, when the parents and/or the child will not accept dietary treatment, a combination of a low-protein diet and BH_4 (3 to 6 mg/kg per day) may be therapeutic.[218] BH_4 is available from two sources only (Schircks Laboratories, Jona, Switzerland; and Suntory, Tokyo, Japan), and is expensive (about $200/g). Thus, for a 20-kg child on 10 mg BH_4/kg per day, estimated yearly costs are around $15,000 and increase with age. Two different forms are produced, (6R,S)-BH_4 and (6R)-BH_4, but only the (6R)-BH_4 form is biologically active. The (6R,S)-BH_4 form contains about 30 percent of the 6S isomer, and thus the dosage used is about one-third higher than that for the (6R)-BH_4 form.

Neurotransmitter Replacement. L-Dopa and 5HTP administration in combination represents a common therapeutic approach to all BH_4 deficiency variants.[317] Carbidopa, an inhibitor of peripheral aromatic amino acid decarboxylase, reduces the therapeutic requirements of L-dopa.[166] Two different preparations of L-dopa are commercially available, with 10% or 25% of carbidopa. Use of L-dopa/25% carbidopa, as slow-release preparation (Sinemet Depot), seems to be beneficial in patients with the severe form of BH_4 deficiency.[318] Analysis of neurotransmitter metabolites represents a crucial point and the only way to monitor the efficacy of the therapy. In practice, the

Table 78-7 Therapy of Tetrahydrobiopterin (BH_4) Deficiencies

Therapy	Age	Doses/ Day	PTPS/GTPCH Deficiency	DHPR Deficiency
Combined therapy				
Phenylalanine-low diet	Initially	—	No	Yes
or				
BH_4 (mg/kg per day)	Initially	1–2	2–5	No
L-Dopa (mg/kg per day) + 10% carbidopa	Initially	3–4	1–3	1–3
	<2 years	3–4	<7	<7
	>2 years	3–4	8–10	8–10
5-Hydroxytryptophan (mg/kg per day)	Initially	3–4	1–2	1–2
	<2 years	3–4	<5	<5
	>2 years	3–4	6–8	6–8
Folinic acid (mg/day)	Initially	1	No	10–20
BH_4 monotherapy				
BH_4 (mg/kg per day)	Initially	1–2	5–20	No

ABBREVIATIONS: PTPS = 6-pyruvoyl-tetrahydropterin synthase; GTPCH = GTP cyclohydrolase I; DHPR = dihydropteridine reductase.

optimal dosage of each component can be determined only on a clinical basis and should be adjusted to the requirements of each patient while looking for adverse effects.[171,319] Diurnal fluctuations are also often observed and may require changes in the schedule of drug administration. Daily doses and the number of administrations have to be individually adjusted according to a patient's age and requirements (Table 78-7). When higher doses of neurotransmitter precursors are necessary, patients may show prominent overdose effects or on-off phenomena.[319] Adverse symptoms due to overtreatment are often similar to those seen before introduction of therapy. Adverse symptoms more specific to 5HTP administration have been reported (tachycardia, diarrhea, and anorexia).[176] Good results have recently been obtained in similar cases with the concurrent administration of L-deprenyl, a selective monoamine oxidase (MAO) B inhibitor, allowing dosage reduction of the administered precursors by curtailing their catabolism.[320–322] Although this therapy has been widely used,[323–326] its potential risk during neonatal brain development is not known. Data on long-term treatment are still scarce, and it is not known whether neurotransmitter precursors or carbidopa might have significant side effects.

Although administration of BH_4 to these patients might also appear to offer a reasonable therapy, reports that this pterin does not readily enter the brain from the periphery[327] makes it seem unlikely that this treatment would prevent the neurologic damage that is characteristic for these patients. Kapatos and Kaufman[328] and others[329] have shown that substantial amounts of peripherally administered BH_4 do enter the brain when larger doses (5 to 20 mg/kg per day) are given. Despite substantial amounts of peripherally administered BH_4 found in CSF,[170] only a few patients respond at the central level to BH_4 monotherapy by normalizing their neurotransmitter production.[168,169,178,330] The successful treatment of one patient with 6-methyl-BH_4 could not be replicated with two other patients.[330] Trials with 6-hydroxymethyl-BH_4, a BH_4 analogue that showed three- to sixfold better penetration into the rat brain and good cofactor activity for PAH, also failed in one patient.[331]

In patients with a mild form of BH_4 deficiency, BH_4 monotherapy (5 to 10 mg/kg per day) seems to be efficient.[178]

Folinic Acid Supplementation. Administration of folinic acid (10 to 20 mg/day) is recommended to restore normal CSF folate levels in patients with DHPR deficiency. This therapy may reverse both the demyelinating processes and the calcification of the basal ganglia in patients with DHPR deficiency. Several DHPR-deficient patients were treated with folinic acid (5-formyltetrahydrofolic acid) and many showed some improvement.[224,225,332]

Follow-up. Treatment monitoring can be implemented either clinically, by evaluating the minimal dose effective in relieving carential symptoms, or biochemically, by periodically measuring the CSF concentration of HVA and 5-HIAA.[178] In cases where lumbar puncture is not possible, monitoring by serum prolactin is a useful alternative approach.[333] Since DA is the essential inhibitory factor of prolactin secretion, its plasma concentrations may reflect the actual DA synthesis and serve as an extremely sensitive marker for the hypothalamic DA content under different therapeutic regimens. Immense prolactinemia was documented in several BH_4-deficient patients.[178,263,318] Quantification of CSF 5-methyltetrahydrofolate should be done in patients with DHPR deficiency.[309]

Gene Therapeutic Approaches. For PTPS and DHPR deficiencies, successful gene delivery into primary patients' fibroblasts with the respective genetic defects were reported. The latter experiment involved the lipofection reagent for cDNA transfection to restore DHPR enzyme activity in deficient cells from one patient.[334] For PTPS deficiency, primary skin fibroblasts from various patients were reported for successful, retrovirus-mediated gene delivery.[335] In subsequent approaches, either double transduction with a GTPCH and a PTPS expressing retroviral vector, or a single transduction with vectors containing the two genes, demonstrated that the BH_4-biosynthetic pathway can be restored and cofactor is secreted.[336,337] Implantations of autologous cells that are genetically modified in vitro for continuous secretion of BH_4 cofactor may open new strategies for treatment of PTPS deficiency.

Drug Interference. Some drugs have been reported to be strong inhibitors of DHPR and thus may cause adverse effects in patients with BH_4 deficiency. Particularly, trimethoprim-sulfamethoxazole, a widely used antibiotic for bacterial sinusitis, urinary tract infections, and otitis media, interferes with pterins and folate metabolism. This drug was shown to induce adverse effects in a patient with DHPR deficiency.[338] Methotrexate, another DHFR inhibitor, is also an important medication for therapy of neoplasia in the pediatric population. In patients with acute lymphoblastic leukemia (ALL), methotrexate therapy caused impaired cerebral and biogenic amine metabolism.[339] Some patients with ALL receiving chemotherapy with methotrexate, PEG-asparaginase, cyclophosphamide, doxorubicin, daunorubicin, cytarabine, thioguanine, vincristine, and vepresid, developed HPA with plasma phenylalanine concentrations between 150 and 1400 μM.[340] In contrast to inherited DHPR deficiency, PAH activity can be restored in these patients by BH_4 supplementation.

Generally, any drug intervention in patients with BH_4 deficiency may interfere with pterin metabolism and therefore requires careful follow-up.

Prenatal Diagnosis

Although only 1 to 2 percent of newborns with HPA are deficient in the BH_4 cofactor, there is virtue in performing a prenatal diagnosis of a potential BH_4 deficiency in families at risk so that options may be exercised.[341] Analysis of pterins (neopterin and biopterin) in amniotic fluid is commonly used for the prenatal diagnosis of BH_4 deficiencies.[281]

In a GTPCH deficiency, levels of neopterin and biopterin in amniotic fluid are very low.[342] High levels of neopterin and very low levels of biopterin are characteristic of a PTPS deficiency.[250] The heterozygous fetuses excrete increased levels of neopterin and relatively low concentrations of biopterin.[281] This also has been documented by an increased ratio of neopterin to biopterin (6.7 to 11.0; controls, 2.7 to 3.7).[343] In a fetus suffering from a DHPR deficiency, a characteristic finding is increased biopterin and normal to slightly elevated neopterin excretion in amniotic fluid.[281] The enzyme activity determined in cultured amniocytes, fetal erythrocytes, and chorionic villi is complementary to the analysis of pterins. Table 78-8 summarizes the sample sources that can be used for analyses.

Prenatal diagnoses have been performed in 31 families at risk for BH_4 deficiencies[281,344] (N. Blau, personal communication). In 12 families with a child already affected with a DHPR deficiency, four fetuses were diagnosed as homozygotes and six as heterozygotes for the defect, whereas two were normal. In 18 families with a child affected with a PTPS deficiency, six fetuses were homozygous, eight were heterozygous, and four were normal. One fetus has been diagnosed to be heterozygote for GTPCH deficiency. Most diagnoses were performed by measuring pterins in amniotic fluid (see above) and enzyme activity in fetal erythrocytes for PTPS deficiency[250] or DHPR deficiency,[345] or amniocytes for DHPR deficiency[344] or PTPS deficiency (N. Blau, personal communication), or by molecular analysis using chorionic villi as a source of genomic DNA for DHPR deficiency[288] or PTPS deficiency (N. Blau, personal communication).[75] So far, a single prenatal diagnosis of a DHPR deficiency has been performed using an RFLP analysis.[346] A single polymorphic marker (IVS2 + 14T/C) was reported in the human PTPS gene.[241]

Table 78-8 Material Used for the Prenatal Diagnosis of Tetrahydrobiopterin Deficiencies

Fetal sample (Reference Method)	GTPCH Deficiency	PTPS Deficiency	DHPR Deficiency
Amniotic fluid (Neo/Bio)	+	+	+
627			
Erythrocytes	−	+	+
248			
Stimulated lymphocytes	+	−	+
233			
Cultured amniocytes	−	+	+
249			
281			
628			
Stimulated amniocytes	−	+	+
235			
N. Blau, unpublished			
Chorionic villi	−	+	+
628			
Liver tissue	+	+	+
232			
250			
DNA	+	+	+
288			
75			
N. Blau, unpublished			

ABBREVIATIONS: GTPCH = GTP cyclohydrolase I; PTPS = 6-pyruvoyl-tetrahydropterin synthase; DHPR = dihydropteridine reductase; Neo, neopterin; Bio, biopterin.

These investigations also advanced our knowledge of BH_4 metabolism during fetal development. All key enzymes of the metabolic pathway for BH_4 synthesis and regeneration are expressed early in fetal tissues, with the possible exception of PCD activity. This allows the fetus to be autotropous for its cofactor requirements. In normal fetuses and those heterozygous for a DHPR deficiency, primapterin (7-biopterin) is increased relatively to 6-biopterin (see also the section "Pterin-4α-Carbinolamine Dehydratase Deficiency"). This indicates that PCD activity may be expressed differently during life.

Population Genetics

All variants of BH_4 deficiencies have an autosomal recessive trait. Affected patients are homozygotes or compound heterozygotes, although there is evidence for symptomatic heterozygosity in patients with a PTPS deficiency.[255] The frequency of all BH_4 deficiencies is uncertain, but, assuming they represent altogether about 1 to 2 percent of PKU patients, the combined frequency of BH_4 deficiencies is approximately $1{:}10^{-6}$ live births. Data from newborn and selective screening programs reveal regional (demographic) variations in the frequency of BH_4 deficiencies. In the Piemonte region and the southern parts of Italy, 10 percent of all patients with HPA are accounted for by BH_4 deficiencies. In Turkey, the incidence is even higher (15 percent).[347] It is 19 percent in Taiwan[348] and 20 percent in Brazil.[349] Saudi Arabia has the highest incidence (68 percent).[256] Marriage customs in Saudi Arabia are largely dictated by tribal traditions, and the majority of patients with BH_4 deficiencies are children of first-cousin marriages within tribal boundaries and belong to distantly related families. One particular tribe, for example, that may have more than 100,000 members could be conceptualized as a family possessing a highly conserved genetic constitution.[256]

BIODEF Database. An international database of BH_4 deficiencies (BIODEF) was initiated in 1992 as a joint venture of J.L. Dhondt (France) and N. Blau.[178] A cumulative experience in diagnosis and treatment of BH_4-deficient patients appeared necessary to obtain an overview of the management and outcome of the disease. In this database, the most common findings from the compilation of data on more than 360 patients have been tabulated. Some of the preliminary cumulative data have been published.[177,292,350,351] The two databases BIODEF (patient database) and BIOMDB (mutation database)[231] are established as an information resource and retrieval system on the Internet that includes clinical, biochemical, and molecular information on variants of BH_4 deficiency. The BIOMDB database includes additional mutation information on patients with the dominant form of GTPCH deficiency (see the section "Non-Hyperphenylalaninemia Tetrahydrobiopterin Defects"). Both databases are accessible from the BH_4 home page (http:/www.unizh.ch/~blau/bh4.html). Data were collected from over 60 pediatric departments, biochemistry departments, and screening laboratories, worldwide, over the last 20 years. Some of the data were obtained from the literature. The following information was provided by the clinic on a questionnaire:

1. Patient's identification data, including birth date, ethnic origin, consanguinity, and parents' and siblings' other information

2. Birth information, including data on weight, height, head circumference, and clinical status
3. Screening data on HPA: age when screened, initial blood phenylalanine level, loading test, diet tolerance, etc.
4. Screening data about pterins in urine, plasma, and CSF, and loading test with BH_4
5. Initial concentrations of neurotransmitters and folates in CSF
6. Measurements of related enzyme activities in tissue and blood cells
7. Clinical symptoms before and after initiation of treatment, including electroencephalogram (EEG), computed tomography (CT), and magnetic resonance imaging (MRI) data
8. Treatment and follow-up of therapy, including therapy protocols, clinical examinations, and neurochemical investigations in the CSF
9. Literature references
10. DNA analysis data, including amino acid and nucleotide aberrations, type of mutation, location in gene, number of alleles found, phenotype information, biochemical characterization of mutant proteins, and references (BIOMDB Database)

A total of 365 patients with BH_4 deficiency have been diagnosed as a result of selective screening carried out during the last 20 years. Of these 365 patients, 208 had PTPS deficiency, 113 had DHPR deficiency, 19 had PCD deficiency, 16 had GTPCH deficiency, and 9 are still unclassified (Table 78-6). Of the 208 patients with PTPS deficiency, 35 are defined as atypical variants requiring no neurotransmitters substitution. Since the introduction of a routine screening program for BH_4 deficiency in 1979, an average of 14 patients per year have been detected worldwide.

BIODEF data reveal that the mortality rate is higher among patients with a DHPR deficiency than among those with a PTPS deficiency; however, some DHPR-deficient patients who died were born in the 1970s (data not shown). They were diagnosed late and probably not treated adequately.

Symptoms can manifest during the first weeks of life but usually are noted at about 4 months of age. The variable but common symptoms listed in the BIODEF database are shown in Table 78-7. Preliminary information from the database documents that approximately 68 percent of the patients with BH_4 deficiencies are Caucasians, 9 percent are Chinese, and 6 percent Japanese. There is no demographic information available for approximately 12 percent of the registered patients. In the Turkish population, there is an equal distribution of PTPS and DHPR deficiencies (Table 78-6).

NON-HYPERPHENYLALANINEMIA TETRAHYDROBIOPTERIN DEFECTS

Historically, defects of BH_4 metabolism have been identified during follow-up studies designed to establish the cause of HPA found either during newborn screening or at a later date in a child with neurologic signs of unclear origin. It is now apparent that HPA is not a prerequisite for onset of clinical symptoms where there is defective BH_4 metabolism. Autosomal dominantly inherited and compound heterozygote forms of GTPCH deficiency, together with an apparent CNS-localized form of DHPR deficiency, have recently been recognized, none of which have been associated with HPA in infancy.

Dominantly Inherited GTP Cyclohydrolase I Deficiency (Segawa Disease, Hereditary Progressive Dystonia, Dopa-Responsive Dystonia)

The first reports of a dystonia with marked diurnal variation that was responsive to L-dopa were described in Japanese patients in the 1970s.[352,353] Since then, many other similar cases have been described but the underlying etiology was not elucidated until 1994, when the condition was associated with mutations on a single allele of the gene for GTPCH.[26] Many mutations have since been characterized, and it is clear that the disorder is transmitted as an autosomal dominant trait with sex-influenced reduced penetrance. Penetrance estimates are 15 percent in men and 45 percent in women.[354] There does not appear to be a difference in the penetrance between maternally and paternally transmitted offspring; hence, sex-related penetrance in the disorder is probably not due to genomic imprinting.[36] Dominantly inherited GTPCH deficiency has a worldwide distribution, there is no evidence for an increased prevalence in any ethnic group, and prevalence is estimated at 0.5 per million.[355]

Clinical Phenotype. Dominantly inherited GTPCH deficiency classically presents as a dystonic gait disorder in childhood, with symptom onset at an average age of 5 to 6 years.[353,354] Early motor development is generally normal, but there are some descriptions of cases with delay in attainment of early motor milestones.[354] The first symptom is generally a dystonic posture of the foot, with muscle dystonia spreading to the other extremities within several years. Occasionally, onset has been with torticollis, retrocollis, arm dystonia, poor coordination, or slowness in dressing before the development of leg signs.[354] The symptoms often, but not always, show a marked diurnal variation, being worse in the evening and being alleviated in the morning after sleep. There is concurrent or subsequent development of Parkinson signs and a dramatic response to low-dose L-dopa therapy.[356]

Half of the patients have no family history of dystonia.[357] In older children, the occurrence of hyperactive reflexes and apparent extensor plantar responses and the presence of spastic diplegia have led to the misdiagnosis of cerebral palsy.[358,359] Severity of symptoms seems to correlate with the age at onset, and appearance of the symptoms is not limited to the childhood years, there being cases of early-adult, as well as late-adult, presentation.[357]

The clinical phenotype is undoubtedly not yet totally clear, as mutations in the GTPCH gene have been described in patients with apparent primary torsion dystonia who were highly responsive to anticholinergic drugs.[45]

Enzyme Phenotype. Details of the tissues and cells in which GTPCH activity can be measured are described in the section "GTP Cyclohydrolase I." Activity in phytohemagglutinin-stimulated mononuclear blood cells varied from 0.3 to 3.6 pmol/h/mg prot. in seven patients with dominantly inherited GTPCH deficiency and from 9.0 to 46.1 pmol/h/mg prot. in controls.[26] A more recent report suggests that some normal cells may not be activated by phytohemagglutinin, making false-positive results likely.[31] An alternative indirect approach to measure the GTPCH activity is the measurement of intracellular neopterin in unstimulated transformed lymphoblasts.[31]

Metabolic Phenotype. Dominantly inherited GTPCH deficiency leads to a decreased synthesis of BH_4 within the CNS, as manifested by reduced levels of BH_4 and neopterin in CSF.[358,360] The BH_4 deficiency is not as severe as that seen in the autosomal recessive form of GTPCH deficiency, but it is apparently sufficient to decrease the activity of tyrosine hydroxylase (TH) and reduce DA turnover, as CSF levels of HVA are generally reduced.[357,360] BH_4 is also required for the activity of TPH, but the reduction in BH_4 concentration seems to have less of an effect on this enzyme, and hence serotonin concentration, as levels of CSF 5HIAA have been reported as either low, unchanged, or elevated.[357]

Peripherally, BH_4 is also required for the activity of PAH in the liver. HPA has not been described in dominantly inherited GTPCH deficiency, but the presence of a reduced liver concentration of BH_4 can be exposed by stressing the system with a phenylalanine load. Phenylalanine conversion to tyrosine is slow, resulting in prolonged high ratios of phenylalanine to tyrosine. Low levels of plasma biopterin and an inappropriate rise in plasma biopterin level after the phenylalanine load provide further evidence for compromised peripheral biopterin synthesis.[361]

Genotype. Defects have been characterized at the molecular level in many cases[26,42,362,363] (Fig. 78-6). There is great allelic heterogeneity, and there is evidence to suggest a relatively high spontaneous mutation rate of the GTPCH gene.[36] Changes at the DNA level have involved missense mutations,[26] deletions,[26] base transition at the splice acceptor site of intron 1,[362] base transition at the conserved consensus sequence GT at the 5′ end of intron 2 which led to skipping of the entire exon 2 in the mature mRNA,[38] and nonsense mutations.[26,42,362] There have also been cases where mutations have not been found in either the coding exons or the exon/intron boundaries, and it is assumed that a mutation exists in the untranslated or regulatory portion of the gene.[26,30,42] In two families where no mutation was found, there was evidence for genetic linkage between the family and the GTPCH locus,[26,30] and, in one family, GTPCH activity was greatly reduced in phytohemagglutinin-stimulated mononuclear blood cells from two affected family members.[26] A C-to-A transversion in exon 5 was described that predicted a missense mutation (Thr186Lys); instead, the base change led to the production of a novel transcript lacking exon 5 and part of exon 6.[40]

It is suggested that the defect in the GTPCH gene is essential but not sufficient for the onset of clinical phenotype and that some regulatory gene/process may be involved in the lowered expression of GTPCH in affected patients.[39,362,364] In the first patients described, GTPCH activity in phytohemagglutinin-stimulated lymphoblasts was less than 20 percent of that of controls. Mutations in the GTPCH gene on a single allele necessitates the formation of a chimeric protein composed of wild-type and mutant subunits, assuming that transcription and translation function normally. Dominant negative effects between wild-type and mutant subunits were excluded in one patient with a frameshift mutation that led to the production of a mutant subunit that was not able to interact with the wild-type protein.[26] The relative levels of mutant mRNA encoding GTPCH might contribute to enzymatic and clinical variations.[38,39] Togari et al[16] reported three species of human GTPCH cDNA in a human liver cDNA library. Type 1 encodes the normal full-length subunit, whereas types 2 and 3 encode truncated inactive subunits. It is speculated that the ratio of type 1 to type 2 regulates the GTPCH gene expression under physiological conditions, since both are generated by naturally occurring splicing events.[40]

Pathophysiology. Mutations in the GTPCH gene and a reduced rate of synthesis of BH_4 can explain many of the findings in dominantly inherited GTPCH deficiency. The low CSF BH_4 levels in patients and the improvement of symptoms following administration of BH_4 or L-dopa point to BH_4 deficiency and an abnormality in monoamine metabolism as the mechanism underlying the dystonic symptoms. The intracellular concentration of BH_4 is thought to be close to the K_m for TH; hence, under normal conditions, changes in BH_4 concentration can regulate TH activity.[365] Reduced levels of BH_4 due to decreased synthesis would compromise TH activity and lead to decreased DA turnover in the dopaminergic neurons of the nigrostriatal system. Microdialysis studies have shown that BH_4 stimulates DA release;[366] BH_4 deficiency may therefore also prevent the normal release of DA into the synapse.

The diurnal fluctuation in symptoms in most patients points to a possible metabolic recuperation during periods of inactivity. The requirement for DHPR for the maintenance of monoamine biosynthesis would suggest that turnover of BH_4 is slow relative to that of the monoamine neurotransmitters. Experiments in cultured neurons have shown the half-life of BH_4 to be relatively short (4.5 h),[367] and it has been postulated[26] that, even in the presence of a low activity of GTPCH, BH_4 levels can rise at night during the period of dopaminergic quiescence to concentrations sufficient to maintain DA metabolism at a level that ameliorates dystonic symptoms but that the synthesis rate is not sufficient to maintain BH_4 levels during the day when DA turnover is higher.

The exquisite sensitivity to L-dopa in patients with dominantly inherited GTPCH deficiency shows that the dopaminergic deficit is likely marginal and that steps after the production of L-dopa can function correctly following normalization of DA synthesis. Studies with positron-emission tomography (PET) support this concept, as they have generally shown normal striatal 6-[^{18}F]fluoro-L-dopa uptake, implying a normal number of presynaptic nigrostriatal dopaminergic neurons and adequate activity of dopa decarboxylase.[368,369] One single neuropathologic, neurochemical study has been performed.[370] The number of neurons, TH immunoreactivity, and enzyme activity in the substantia nigra were normal, implying intact nigrostriatal DA neuron cell bodies. In the striatum, TH protein, TH activity, and DA content were reduced, but GBR 12935 binding to the DA transporter was normal, indicating a normal number of cells containing reduced levels of TH.[370] The mechanism for the reduction in TH protein concentration remains obscure but may involve a role for BH_4 in the regulation of TH gene expression or TH protein stability.[371]

Although heterozygote carriers of a mutation in the GTPCH gene can get clinical symptoms, the reduced penetrance and the greater prevalence of the clinical phenotype in women compared with men suggest that factors additional to genetic mutations in GTPCH must also be involved in phenotypic expression. CNS BH_4 concentrations do not appear to be relevant, as asymptomatic gene carriers have reduced CSF BH_4 levels that are indistinguishable from their symptomatic relatives.[360] DA D_2 receptor upregulation is also not likely to be a major determinant for defining clinical state, since penetrance as striatal, DA D_2 receptor binding is increased in both asymptomatic and symptomatic gene carriers, as shown by [^{11}C]raclopride PET.[372]

Treatment and Prognosis. Treatment with low-dose L-dopa together with a peripheral dopa-decarboxylase inhibitor is generally extremely effective. The required dose of L-dopa has varied from 50 to 2000 mg/day, depending on the patient and the presence of the peripheral decarboxylase inhibitor. In individual patients, treatment should be started at lower doses and the optimal therapeutic level established by titration. Chorea may appear as a side effect early in treatment but should respond to dose adjustment.[357]

The long-term partial deficit of DA does not appear to be detrimental, as complete recoveries have been made in symptomatic patients even after 58 years without treatment, and response to treatment appears to be stable for at least 20 years.[373]

Diagnosis. Until 1994, a presumed diagnosis of DRD was generally achieved by careful examination of the clinical phenotype followed by a trial of L-dopa. Confirmation of the diagnosis in a patient responding to L-dopa requires, however, follow-up tests, as TH deficiency[374,375] and PTPS deficiency[265,376] can have similar clinical phenotypes, and there are many types of dystonia and other movement disorders that can respond in some degree to L-dopa. Concentrations of BH_4 and neopterin in CSF are low in dominantly inherited GTPCH deficiency,[360,376] and generally there is a reduced level of HVA.[354,360] Definitive diagnosis is achieved by detection of mutations in the GTPCH gene; however, there is no common mutation, making this a tedious process. Measurement of GTPCH activity in phytohemagglutinin-stimulated lymphocytes can demonstrate decreased GTPCH activity,[26] but some normal cells are not activated by this process, making for a high likelihood of a false-positive result.[31] Neopterin measurement in transformed lymphoblasts may provide a more reliable test, as a small study[31] showed all known carriers of a GTPCH mutation to have lower values than controls. More studies in a greater number of patients are required before it will be clear whether this test will provide a definitive diagnosis.

An oral phenylalanine-loading test (100 mg/kg) has also been developed to aid in diagnosis.[361] The test exposes the partial deficiency of BH_4 in the liver, which manifests as an inability to

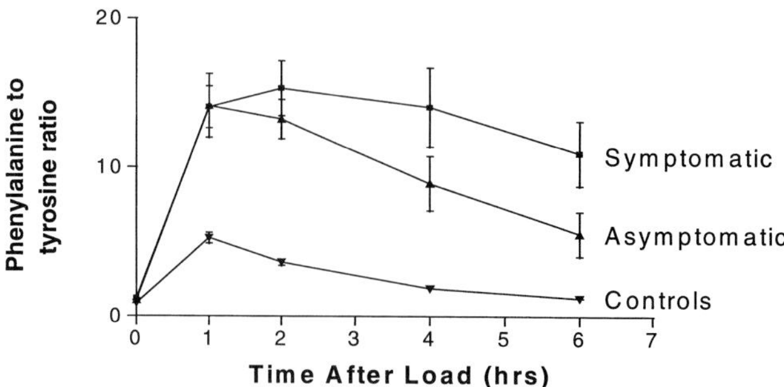

Fig. 78-15 Plasma phenylalanine-to-tyrosine ratios following an oral phenylalanine load in patients with dominantly inherited GTP cyclohydrolase I (GTPCH) deficiency. Patients (11 symptomatic and 9 asymptomatic) and controls (20) received 100 mg/kg L-phenylalanine orally. Blood samples were taken prior to, and 1, 2, 4 and 6 h after the load, and plasma was separated and analyzed for phenylalanine and tyrosine. Values show the mean ± SEM. There is no overlap between control and patient data sets at 1, 2, or 4 h after the load.

convert phenylalanine to tyrosine at a normal rate, leading to elevated phenylalanine-to-tyrosine ratios in plasma for a period of at least 6 h following the load (Fig. 78-15). Abnormal phenylalanine/tyrosine profiles can also be seen in other conditions. PKU heterozygotes, in whom there is a primary defect in phenylalanine hydroxylase, also have delayed clearance of phenylalanine and decreased production of tyrosine following a phenylalanine load.[377,378] These heterozygotes do not have HPA without a phenylalanine load but may have a slightly raised fasting phenylalanine-to-tyrosine ratio. Distinction can be made between a GTPCH deficiency and a PKU heterozygote by inclusion of plasma biopterin measurement. Phenylalanine levels control BH_4 synthesis,[129] and phenylalanine loading leads to a rapid rise in plasma biopterin in humans with and without PKU.[379] In patients with dominantly inherited GTPCH deficiency, biopterin levels do not rise appropriately in response to an increase in plasma phenylalanine,[361] whereas, in PKU heterozygotes, the plasma biopterin rise is the same or greater than that seen in controls.[380] Further proof of the defect in BH_4 metabolism can be demonstrated by preloading the patient with BH_4 prior to repeating the phenylalanine-loading test. The phenylalanine/tyrosine profiles are normalized in GTPCH deficiency but remain abnormal in PKU heterozygotes.[119]

Compound Heterozygotes of GTP Cyclohydrolase I Deficiency

Two patients have been described with generalized dystonia responsive to L-dopa and severe developmental delay.[381] Neither had overt HPA in infancy. The first, a girl, was a child from a family with three previous generations affected with autosomal dominantly inherited GTPCH deficiency. She presented at an age of 6 months with symptoms suggestive of autosomal recessively inherited GTPCH deficiency. Dystonia of the legs was also present, which by 1 year had become generalized.

Diagnosis of GTPCH deficiency was inferred from a finding of low levels of HVA, 5HIAA, BH_4, and neopterin in CSF.[37] Treatment at the age of 3 years with L-dopa (8 mg/day, as Sinemet, increased to 20 mg qid over the next 2 years) led to marked improvement in dystonic symptoms and development. Sudden deterioration of motor function at age 5 years was associated with an elevated plasma phenylalanine concentration (968 μM). Treatment with BH_4 (2 mg/kg per day increasing over 4 months to 10 mg/kg per day) led to complete resolution of the HPA and rapid improvement in neurologic function. Mutation analysis showed a 1-bp deletion in exon 2 on one allele, which shifts the translational reading frame and predicts a premature stop codon in exon 2. The other allele contained a T-to-C transition in exon 6, resulting in a substitution of a methionine residue with a threonine residue at codon 221.[37]

The second patient, a boy, had a clinical course more typical of dominantly inherited GTPCH deficiency.[37] Between the ages of 4 and 6 years, he lost motor and speech function and developed generalized dystonia and symmetric hyperreflexia with bilateral extensor plantar responses. Intellect remained intact. At age 14 years, diagnosis of GTPCH deficiency was inferred from a finding of low levels of HVA, 5HIAA, BH_4, and neopterin in CSF.[37] Initiation of L-dopa (10 mg/day as Sinemet, slowly increased to 80 mg/day) greatly improved motor function.

Mutation analysis showed a G-to-A transition in exon 1 on one allele, causing a glycine-to-aspartic acid substitution at codon 108. The other allele showed an A-to-G transition in exon 6, predicting an amino acid substitution of lysine with arginine at codon 224.[37,361]

Although persistent HPA was not present in either of these children, the oral phenylalanine-loading test clearly demonstrated compromised liver phenylalanine metabolism and virtually no increase in plasma biopterin.[361]

Dihydropteridine Reductase Deficiency Without Hyperphenylalaninemia

There is one single report of a child with a presumed CNS-localized form of DHPR deficiency that does not lead to HPA.[382] The child had psychomotor retardation, spasticity, dystonia, microcephaly, growth retardation, and a severe deficiency of DA and serotonin within the CNS, as shown by greatly decreased levels of HVA and 5HIAA in CSF. Plasma phenylalanine, urinary and plasma total neopterin and biopterin, and red cell DHPR activity were all in the normal range; the CSF profile of pterins was typical for DHPR deficiency,[383] however, with normal levels of BH_4 but increased levels of 7,8-dihydrobiopterin and oxidized biopterin. Sequencing of all coding exons of the DHPR gene failed to detect any mutations. Abnormal conversion of phenylalanine to tyrosine following oral phenylalanine loading demonstrated decreased phenylalanine hydroxylase activity in the liver. Low-dose therapy with L-dopa, carbidopa, and selegiline (L-deprenyl) resulted in significant improvement in neurologic status and development. It is possible that a molecular defect lies in the 5′-regulatory region of the DHPR gene and that it only affects expression of a central form of the DHPR protein.

Most cases of BH_4 deficiency are detected at newborn screening because of the presence of HPA. With current practice, it is unlikely that a working diagnosis of GTPCH deficiency or DHPR deficiency will be pursued if plasma phenylalanine concentration is found to be normal. The two compound heterozygotes for GTPCH deficiency and the patient with presumed CNS-localized DHPR deficiency demonstrate that forms of these conditions exist that are isolated to the CNS and that the absence of HPA should not be used to exclude the possibility of BH_4 deficiency. Careful examination of clinical symptoms and investigation of CSF neurotransmitter metabolites and pterins are therefore essential for diagnosis.

Catecholamine and Serotonin Neurotransmitters

The catecholamines [DA, norepinephrine (NE), and epinephrine (E)] and serotonin (5HT) are important neurotransmitters within the central and peripheral nervous systems. Within the CNS, they are the primary modulators of psychomotor function, with roles, among others, in the regulation of motor coordination, arousal, emotional stability, processing of sensory input, reward-driven learning, memory, appetite, mood, sleep, vomiting, and the secretion of anterior pituitary and other hormones.[384–394] Peripherally, they are involved in thermoregulation, modulation of peripheral pain mechanisms, and regulation of vascular tone and blood flow.[395,396]

The pathways for the synthesis and catabolism of the catecholamines and 5HT are shown in Fig. 78-16. The amines are formed from tryptophan and tyrosine in reactions catalyzed by TPH and TH. These two enzymes are rate limiting for the synthesis of their respective neurotransmitters, and both require

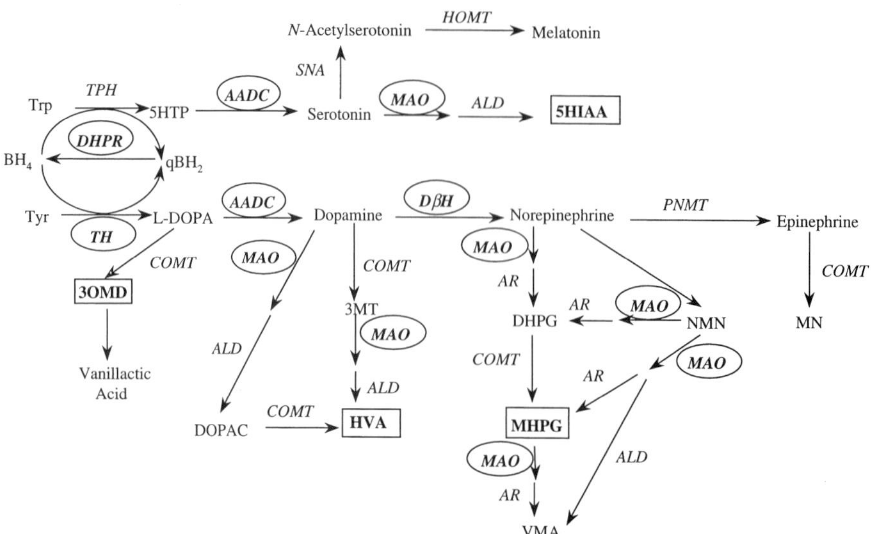

Fig. 78-16 Synthesis and catabolism of serotonin and the catecholamines. Trp, tryptophan; 5HTP, 5-hydroxytryptophan; 5HIAA, 5-hydroxyindoleacetic acid; BH_4, tetrahydrobiopterin; qBH_2, quinonoid dihydrobiopterin; Tyr, tyrosine; 3OMD, 3-*O*-methyldopa; DOPAC, dihydroxyphenylacetic acid; 3MT, 3-methoxytyramine; HVA, homovanillic acid; DHPG, dihydroxyphenylglycol; MHPG, 3-methoxy-4-hydroxyphenylglycol; VMA, vanillylmandelic acid; NMN, normetanephrine; MN, metanephrine; DHPR, dihydropteridine reductase; TPH, tryptophan hydroxylase; TH, tyrosine hydroxylase; AADC, aromatic L-amino acid decarboxylase; COMT, catechol-*O*-methyltransferase; MAO, monoamine oxidase; SNA, serotonin *N*-acetylase; HOMT, hydroxyindole-*O*-methyltransferase; ALD, aldehyde dehydrogenase; DβH, dopamine β-hydroxylase; AR, aldehyde reductase; PNMT, phenylethanolamine-*N*-methyltransferase. The major cerebrospinal fluid (CSF) markers used to diagnose defects are *boxed*. Enzymes with known inherited defects are *circled*.

BH_4 and molecular oxygen for their activity.[397] Hydroxylation of tyrosine and tryptophan leads to the formation of 3,4-dihydroxy-L-phenylalanine (L-dopa) and 5HTP, which are then decarboxylated by pyridoxine-dependent aromatic L-amino acid decarboxylase (AADC) to form the active neurotransmitters. Within the noradrenergic system, DA can be further hydroxylated in a reaction catalyzed by DβH to form NE, which in turn can be methylated to form E, via the action of phenylethanolamine *N*-methyltransferase, which uses *S*-adenosylmethionine as the methyl group donor. Within the pineal gland, 5HT is first acetylated using 5HT *N*-acetylase and then methylated using *S*-adenosylmethionine to form melatonin in a reaction catalyzed by 5-hydroxyindole *O*-methyltransferase.

A schematic representation of the synthesis, storage, release, and reuptake of DA is provided in Fig. 78-17. The catecholamines and 5HT are synthesized in the cytoplasm, and specific vesicles are used to store the active neurotransmitters prior to release into the synaptic cleft. Transport of DA and 5HT into synaptic vesicles within the brain occurs using the vesicle monoamine transporter 2 (VMT2),[398] which uses a transvesicular electrochemical proton gradient to drive the uptake process.[399] The VMT2 transporter has been cloned.[400] Inside the vesicle, catecholamines are complexed with adenosine triphosphate (ATP) and acidic proteins, whereas 5HT is stored in the absence of ATP. Generation of an action potential leads to Ca^{2+} influx, fusion of the vesicle with the neuronal membrane, and release of the vesicle contents into the synaptic cleft.

Five (D_1 to D_5) DA receptors have been cloned;[401,402] they fall into two classes, the D_1-like (D_1 and D_5) and the D_2-like (D_2, D_3, and D_4) receptors. These classes are differentiated according to their positive (D_1-like) or negative (D_2-like) coupling to cAMP. All are G-protein linked and belong to the 7-domain transmembrane superfamily. NE receptors are also members of the 7-transmembrane, G-protein-linked superfamily, and there are three classes, α_1, α_2, and β, all of which have subdivisions. The α_1 receptors act via phospholipase C and the phosphoinositide pathway and open calcium channels. The α_2 receptors inhibit adenylate cyclase, whereas the β receptors stimulate adenylate cyclase.[403] Serotonin receptors are classified into seven major classes ($5HT_1$ to $5HT_7$), each of which contains several subclasses.[404] All members of the $5HT_1$ class are 7-transmembrane, G-protein-coupled receptors thought to be negatively linked to adenylate cyclase. The $5HT_2$ receptors couple via the phosphoinositol hydrolysis signal transduction system, and classes $5HT_{4-7}$ activate adenylate cyclase. Unlike the other 5HT receptors, $5HT_3$ receptor subunits form a pentameric ligand-gated cation channel that is selectively permeable to Na^{2+}, K^+, and Ca^{2+} ions.[404]

Following receptor interaction and depolarization of postsynaptic membranes, termination of the signal involves either enzymatic degradation, diffusion out of the synapse, or removal from the synapse by the Na^+/Cl^--dependent neurotransmitter transporters. Specific high-affinity reuptake transporter systems for DA, NE, and 5HT are present within the presynaptic membrane,[405] and the human DA,[406] NE,[407] and 5HT[408] transporters have been cloned. These transporter systems are the primary targets for a wide variety of clinically important antihypertensives, stimulants, antidepressants, and stimulant drugs of abuse.[409] Enzymatic catecholamine inactivation occurs either by methylation of the catechol moiety via the action of catechol *O*-methyltransferase (COMT) or by the formation of acidic metabolites using either MAO, aldehyde dehydrogenase, or aldehyde reductase. Inactivation of 5HT occurs via the action of MAO and aldehyde dehydrogenase.

Inborn errors that directly affect catecholamine and 5HT metabolism have been described at the level of TH, AADC, DβH, and MAO-A. The presence of the multiple types of receptors and transporters, together with the other enzymes involved with synthesis and catabolism of these neurotransmitters, implies that many more defects have yet to be discovered. Indeed, putative defects affecting the DA D_2 receptor[410] and the DA transporter[411] have already been described.

Tyrosine and Tryptophan Hydroxylases

TH[412,413] and TPH,[413,414] though mechanistically and structurally closely related to PAH,[413] perform very different functions in that they are key enzymes in the synthesis of neurotransmitters derived from the products L-dopa and 5HTP, respectively, whereas phenylalanine hydroxylase is involved with the metabolism of dietary phenylalanine. This has different regulatory features.

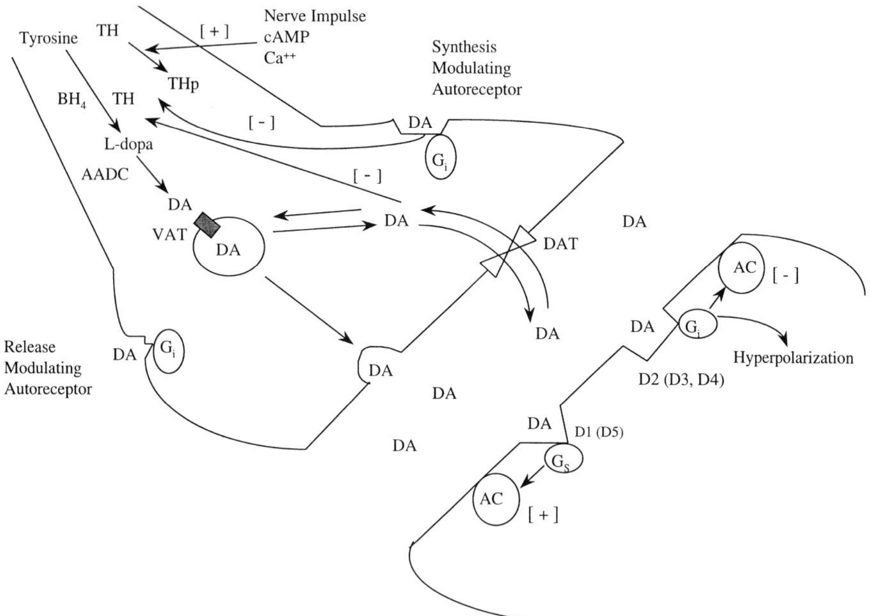

Fig. 78-17 Schematic of a dopamine (DA) nerve terminal. Generation of a nerve impulse leads to Ca^{2+} influx, fusion of the vesicle with the neuronal membrane, and release of the contents of the vesicle into the synaptic cleft. This process is terminated by the action of the release-modulating autoreceptors. The nerve impulse also activates tyrosine hydroxylase (TH) by phosphorylation, resulting in increased affinity for tetrahydrobiopterin (BH_4) and decreased affinity for DA, which acts as a feedback inhibitor. Reversal of the process occurs by activation of the synthesis-modulating autoreceptors by DA and by end-product inhibition by intraneuronal DA. The autoreceptors have a high affinity for DA (nM) and appear to act via a G_i regulatory protein. The vesicular amine transporter (VAT) facilitates the uptake of cytoplasmic DA into the synaptic vesicles, preventing its catabolism. The postsynaptic DA receptors have a low affinity for DA (μM) and are coupled positively (D_1) or negatively (D_2) with adenylate cyclase either via a G_s protein (D_1) or via a G_i protein (D_2). Stimulation of the latter leads to hyperpolarization. It is currently not clear whether D_1 and D_2 receptor types are located on the same neuron. The plasma membrane DA transporter (DAT) acts to remove DA from the synaptic cleft. TH_p, phosphorylated TH; AADC, aromatic L-amino acid decarboxylase; AC, adenylate cyclase.

The three hydroxylases have many features[3,413] in common:

1. Substrates are identical except for the three different aromatic amino acids specific to each of them. The similarity is such that each of these specific hydroxylases can use the other two amino acids as substrates.
2. Each is an iron-containing enzyme.
3. All are homotetramers.
4. All have subunit molecular masses between 51,000 and 59,000.
5. The K_m for BH_4 lies between 13 and 30 μM.
6. Each has a catalytic core that is extremely conserved, with up to 87 percent conservation, between tyrosine and phenylalanine hydroxylase, for example. Key residues are absolutely conserved. This has led to suggestions that all three genes evolved from a primordial locus.[413]
7. Conservation of the intron/exon boundaries in relation to PAH (12 introns) is identical, except for one extra in a different position in each case at the 5′ end, one in TH with an extra central intron, and one extra in PAH at the 3′ end. One intron contained by the other two is missing two-thirds of the way along the coding sequence of TPH.
8. A motif at the C-terminus resembling a leucine zipper allows subunit binding.
9. Each enzyme can be regulated by phosphorylation.

The following are the main differences:

1. The favored substrate.
2. The N-terminal regulatory sequence is specific for each enzyme.
3. Amino acid substrate K_m with that for PAH (200 to 300 μM) being more appropriate for a liver-metabolizing function than the other two being 6 to 11 μM for TH and 12.5 to 32 μM for TPH, these latter being more appropriate for a synthetic pathway. Because of the considerable conservation in the catalytic fragment, it is thought that the reaction mechanisms are the same or similar for all three enzymes.

Tyrosine Hydroxylase. TH (EC 1.14.16.2) is a mixed-function monooxygenase found in adrenal medulla and catecholaminergic neurons of the peripheral and central nervous systems. The enzyme catalyzes the oxidation of tyrosine to L-dopa in a reaction requiring molecular oxygen, ferrous iron, and BH_4 (Fig. 78-2). The enzyme may act through a sequential mechanism in which all substrates bind to the protein before the hydroxylation reaction occurs.[415] Mutagenesis studies first identified His331 and His336 as the coordinating amino acid residues.[416] Later, crystallization of the portion of TH responsible for catalytic activity and for tetramerization showed the iron in a deep active site pocket coordinated by the two histidines together with Glu376. This structure is expected to be similar to the catalytic domains of PAH and TPH.

TH was initially purified from bovine adrenal medulla and rat pheochromocytoma cells and shown to have a molecular weight of 60,000 daltons.[417,418] The native holoenzyme exists as a tetramer and, in most species, is present as a homotetramer. Tetramer formation occurs via sequences in the C-terminal catalytic domain, with the C-terminal leucine zippers being important determinants.[419,420]

The gene for TH has been isolated from several species both as cDNA clones[421–425] and genomic clones.[426–429] The human gene for TH[430] is localized to chromosome 11p15.5[431] (see Table 78-1 for a summary). It should be noted that TH and TPH are close to each other on the same chromosome, indicating that they are likely to have arisen from a precursor by gene duplication.

Four different forms of TH mRNA and protein (h TH1, 2, 3, and 4) are found in various human tissues.[430,432] The variants arise following differential splicing of a single gene copy using two splice donor sites in the first exon and inclusion or exclusion of the second exon.[427,428] The possible in vivo forms of the TH enzymes are, therefore, extremely complex and are differentiated by 12 and 81 nucleotide inserts in the N-terminal regulatory region that cause changes in the four[430] potential phosphorylation sites and subtly alter the kinetic characteristics of the final enzyme product.[412,433–435] One of the four TH isoforms, hTH3, escapes activity regulation by phosphorylation and is always more active than phosphorylated hTH1, a property that might be relevant in disease.[436]

The regulation of TH has been reviewed in detail.[412] Because of its importance, there is extensive literature. The eight regulatory mechanisms that have been found or proposed are

1. Reversible feedback inhibition by catecholamines.
2. TH can be irreversibly inhibited by bound catecholamines in an iron complex.[437] This inhibition can be reversed by phosphorylation at Ser40.[438]
3. Allosteric regulation in the case of polyanions which increase activity, but the only one relevant in vivo may be phospholipid, which occurs in membranes.
4. Protein phosphorylation and activation of the N-terminal regulatory portions (codons 1 to 165). Four possible serine residues (8, 19, 31, and 40) can be phosphorylated and have been shown to be phosphorylated by up to eight different kinases.[412] Only Ser40 has been shown to have a dramatic effect on activity, with the other three being less dramatic, and their in vivo significance is not proven.
5. Enzyme stability has been shown to be decreased by phosphorylation,[439] but its in vivo significance is unclear.
6. Transcriptional regulation has been shown to occur by changes in the physiological state of the animal. For example, cold stress induced TH activity in the chromaffin cells of the adrenal medulla.[440] Current work is involved in defining the promoter and enhancer sequences and the proteins involved.[441]
7. Alternate splicing may have a role, as four different forms of TH mRNA have been found in human tissues.[436] All four protein forms have been identified in human brain,[432] but a functional role is yet to be established.
8. RNA stability may be regulated posttranscriptionally, as conditions stimulating gene transcription also increase the half-life of the mRNA.[442]
9. Translational regulation may be important in vivo, as it has been found[443] that, in pheochromocytoma cells, enzyme activity, but not mRNA, increased with glucocorticoid and cAMP. With these multiple points of regulation, it is assumed that these permit different cells serving different functions to control catecholamine synthesis in response to their unique needs.

Using linkage analysis or polymorphic sites within the human TH gene, several investigators have studied whether changes in the TH gene might be associated with various neurologic diseases. Changes in the TH gene do not seem to be involved in the pathogenesis of affective disorder,[444–449] autosomal dominant parkinsonism,[450] Tourette syndrome,[451] or autism.[451,452] The frequency of a rare variant of a common microsatellite tetrarepeat allele in the TH gene has, however, been associated with schizophrenia,[453] suicide attempt;[454] alcohol-withdrawal delirium,[455] and lower plasma levels of HVA and 3-methoxy-4-hydroxyphenylglycol (MHPG).[456,457] This tetrarepeat appears to be involved in the regulation of TH gene expression.[453]

Tryptophan Hydroxylase. TPH is found in the serotoninergic neurons of the CNS. This enzyme was initially purified from a variety of tissues, but the recovery has been low.[458–460] The cloning of this gene from humans[461] will enable easier study, and the gene has been localized to 11p15.1[462,463] (see Table 78-1 for a summary). The sequence[461] indicates that Ser58 (in the regulatory domain), 260, and 443 are candidates for phosphorylation and, hence, regulation.

TPH activity can also be regulated via a variety of mechanisms, but this has not been so extensively studied:

1. The phospholipid polyanion increases the activity two- to fourfold, but in vivo significance is not proven.
2. Protein phosphorylation at Ser58 in the putative regulatory domain (codons 1 to 92), but in vivo significance is not established.[464]
3. Transcriptional regulation has not been proven even though the promoter has been characterized, with no glucocorticoid or cAMP response elements being identified.[465]

Using linkage analysis or polymorphic sites within the TPH gene, several investigators have studied whether changes in this gene might be associated with various neurologic diseases. TPH genotype has been associated with suicidal behavior in several studies,[466,467] but in other studies the TPH gene was not a susceptibility factor.[468,469] The TPH gene may also be involved in susceptibility to manic-depressive illness.[470]

Aromatic L-Amino Acid Decarboxylase. AADC (EC 4.1.1.28) is a single enzyme that catalyzes the decarboxylation of L-dopa to DA and 5HTP to 5HT. AADC will also decarboxylate histidine, tyrosine, phenylalanine, and tryptophan.[471,472] The enzyme is expressed in neuronal cells, where it is involved in the synthesis of neurotransmitters, and in nonneuronal cells, such as kidney, liver, lung, endothelial cells, and spleen, where its function remains unclear. The enzyme has been highly purified from human pheochromocytoma, and pig and rat kidney, it requires pyridoxal phosphate as cofactor and is thought to be a homodimer composed of identical subunits with an approximate M_r of 50 kDa.[473] Each subunit binds one molecule of pyridoxal phosphate via the *S*-amino group of a lysine residue.[474] The K_m values for L-dopa (70 to 90 μM) and 5HTP (100 to 200 μM) as substrates are similar in both recombinant expressed and purified native enzymes from both human and bovine sources, and all forms of the enzyme have maximum activity in the presence of 10^{-5} to 10^{-4} M pyridoxal phosphate.[475–477] The calculated K_m for each substrate greatly exceeds the endogenous substrate concentration, suggesting AADC is not saturated in vivo.

There is a high degree of homology in amino acid sequence between AADC from the different mammalian species, and many subsets of amino acids are even more highly conserved.[478] These include the pyridoxal phosphate-binding site encompassing human residues 267 to 317,[479] a proposed active site cysteine at residue 111,[480] and extended regions of amino acids from residues 64 to 155, 182 to 204, and 271 to 317.[478]

Human AADC is encoded by a single gene copy[481] that was mapped to chromosome band 7p12.1-p12.3 by in situ hybridization.[482,483] The gene is over 85 kbp in length and is composed of 15 exons[482] (see Table 78-1 for a summary). Full-length cDNAs for human AADC from pheochromocytoma[479] and liver[484] have been cloned and characterized. There are two forms of human AADC mRNA that differ only in their 5′ untranslated regions. These encode an identical amino acid sequence of 480 amino acid residues, with a molecular mass of 53.9 kDa. The different 5′ untranslated regions are encoded by two distinct exons, exon N1 being designated the neuronal type and exon L1 the nonneuronal type; the two forms of mRNA are produced by alternative usage of these two first exons. Distinct promoters directing neuronal and nonneuronal expression of AADC were found in rats,[485,486] humans,[484] and pigs.[487] The transcriptional starting site of human AADC mRNA was located around G of position −111 relative to the first ATG. There was no typical TATA box or CAAT box within 540 bp of the transcriptional starting point, but an AT-rich motif (5′-CATAAAT) at −29 was implicated as the possible alternate TATA box.[482,486,488] Other potential regulatory elements, including ERE, Pit/GHF-1, POU/Oct 1,2, E4TF1, HSE, MRE, NFY, NF-B, AP-3, and C2, have also been described.[482] The nonneuronal promoter is probably regulated by HNF-1.[487]

Alternative splicing also exists in the coding region of the human AADC mRNA. Differential splicing in this area leads to the formation of a short-version transcript that lacks exon 3.[477,489] These data provide evidence that two different protein products could be derived from the single *DDC* gene. Enzymatic analysis of the recombinant expression product of the transcript lacking exon 3 demonstrated that the protein formed had no activity with either L-dopa or 5HTP as substrate; it is therefore unclear whether this protein has any physiological significance.[477]

Several factors appear to regulate AADC levels. Physiological stimuli and pharmacologic agents that affect DA receptors change AADC activity. In rat retina, DA D_1 receptor agonists and α_2-adrenoreceptor agonists prevent the rise in AADC activity seen in response to light,[490] and haloperidol up-regulates activity.[474] Similar up-regulation is seen in striatum following activation of DA D_1 and D_2 receptors.[491] Direct phosphorylation of AADC via a Ca^{2+}, AMP-dependent protein kinase may play an important role in the short-term regulation of AADC,[150] and long-term regulation may involve altered gene expression, as AADC mRNA levels can be regulated by several agents. Reserpine,[492] MAO-B inhibitors,[493] AADC inhibitors,[494] interleukin 1β, prostaglandin E_2,[495] and DA receptor antagonists[496] all increase AADC mRNA concentration.

An SspI polymorphism[497] and a GAGA deletion polymorphism in the untranslated exon 1 of the human *DDC* gene[498] have been described.

Dopamine β-Hydroxylase. DβH (EC 1.14.17.1) catalyzes the hydroxylation of DA to form NE. It is a glycoprotein consisting of a 290-kDa homotetramer containing 75-kDa subunits with 2 atoms of copper per subunit. The enzyme also requires molecular oxygen and ascorbic acid for activity, and the K_m for DA is around 5×10^{-3} M.[499] DβH is localized in synaptic vesicles in NE- and E-containing neurons in brain and retina, in NE-containing neurons of the peripheral ganglia and nerves, and in chromaffin granules in NE- and E-containing adrenomedullary cells. DβH is found both tightly bound to the vesicular membrane and as a soluble form that is secreted together with NE or E following appropriate stimulation.

Human DβH is encoded by a single gene copy[500] that was mapped to chromosome 9q34 by in situ hybridization.[501] The gene is approximately 23 kbp long and is composed of 12 exons[500,502] (see Table 78-1 for a summary). cDNAs of DβH from bovine adrenal glands,[473,503] rat pheochromocytoma,[504] and human pheochromocytoma[500] have been cloned. Alternative use of two polyadenylation sites in exon 12 generates two different mRNA types designated type A (2.7 kb) and type B (2.4 kb), which differ only in the 3′ untranslated region. Type A contains a 3′ extension of 300 bp at the end of type B. Both mRNAs encode the same amino acid sequence of 603 amino acid residues, with a molecular mass of 64.9 kDa.

The region upstream of exon 1 of the human DβH gene was first characterized by Kobayashi and coworkers. The transcription initiation site is located 52 bp from the initiation codon. Several transcriptional regulatory elements were found near the transcription initiation site. These included TATA, CCAAT, CACCC, and GC boxes, and sequences homologous to glucocorticoid and cAMP response factors.[500] Transcription induction by either cAMP or glucocorticoids and the presence of many putative elements that may be involved in cAMP and glucocorticoid regulation of the DβH gene expression have since been demonstrated in many systems.[505–508] The cAMP-inducible transcription appears to act via cAMP-dependent protein kinase,[509] and the presence of Ca^{2+} may act as a negative modulator of this activation process.[510] Other factors said to regulate expression of the DβH gene include transcription factor AP-2,[511] insulin-like growth factor I,[512] pituitary adenylate cyclase-activating polypeptide,[513] and prostaglandin E_2.[514] The 4-kb 5′ flanking region is essential for tissue-specific expression. This region, at position −181 to −174 bp from the transcription start site of the human gene, contains a cAMP-response element that acts as a positive genetic element which interacts with a cell-specific silencer.[508,515,516] This silencer shows sequence homology with the neural-restrictive silencer element and is conserved in both human and rat DβH genes.[517] Potential *cis*-regulatory motifs, AP1 and YY1, occur proximal to and overlap with the cAMP-response element, and this area interacts with multiple nuclear proteins, including cAMP-binding protein and transcription factor YY1 in a cell-specific manner. It therefore appears that multiple proteins bind to the 5′-proximal area in a cell-specific manner and coordinately regulate the cell type-specific transcriptional activation of the DβH gene.[518]

Several studies have investigated whether polymorphic sites within the human DβH gene are associated with differences in human plasma DβH activity or are linked to various neurologic diseases. During the early studies to characterize the human DβH gene, seven clones were identified by screening of a pheochromocytoma cDNA library.[500] The clones differed from each other at six nucleotides located in various portions of the cDNA. The difference at nucleotide 910 (G to T) caused an amino acid change between Ala and Ser. Expression of the two cDNAs in COS cells showed that the presence of the serine decreased DβH activity, and it was speculated that the genetic variations in human serum DβH activity may depend on the presence or absence of the allele containing T at position 910.[519] It is important to check for population stratification when testing for associations between the serine variant and clinical phenotypes, as there is significant heterogeneity in allele frequency across different population samples.[520] Typing of allelic fragments utilizing the polymorphic $(GT)_n$ repeat[521] indicates that the human DβH gene is likely controlled via a codominant mechanism associated with the repeat.[522] This polymorphic microsatellite repeat,[523] together with a MspI polymorphic site in intron 9 and a TaqI polymorphic site,[524] have been associated with biochemical variability of the catecholamine pathway in schizophrenia. In contrast, an earlier linkage and association study had concluded that the DβH gene seemed to make no strong contribution to the etiology of schizophrenia.[525]

Monoamine Oxidase. MAO (monoamine O_2 oxidoreductase; EC1.4.3.4.) catalyzes the oxidative deamination of biogenic and dietary amines.[526] The two forms of the enzyme are classified as monoamine oxidase A (MAO-A) and monoamine oxidase B (MAO-B) on the basis of their differential sensitivity to inhibitors and preferential affinity for substrates. MAO-A preferentially oxidizes 5HT and NE, whereas MAO-B preferentially oxidizes β-phenylethylamine. Both oxidize DA. The two forms are expressed in most tissues and are located in the outer membrane of the mitochondria.

The two MAO proteins are encoded by separate genes that share approximately 70 percent overall homology in amino acid sequence;[527] both have been mapped to the X chromosome in the p11.23-11.4 region[528,529] (see Table 78-1 for a summary). It is likely that the two closely linked forms in humans represent the products of a duplication event that occurred more than 500 million years ago.[527] cDNAs that encode human MAO-A and MAO-B have been cloned. The deduced amino acid sequences showed the A and B forms to have subunit molecular weights of 59.7 and 58.8 kDa, respectively,[530] very similar to those found in rats (59.6[531] and 58.4 kDa).[532]

Comparisons of MAO-A and MAO-B from human, bovine, and rat species show great similarity (85 to 88 percent) in the amino acid sequences of each enzyme.[533] The human protein consists of a FAD-containing homodimer. Both MAO-A and MAO-B contain a redox-active disulfide at the catalytic center.[534] The N-terminal region of the two isoenzymes is not involved in determining the different substrate specificities of MAO-A and MAO-B.[535] Rather, aromatic and aliphatic residues seem to determine the substrate selectivity of MAO-A and MAO-B, respectively, as a single mutation in which Phe208 in MAO-A was substituted by the corresponding residue of Ile in MAO-B was sufficient to convert the MAO-A substrate specificity to that of the MAO-B specificity.[536]

In human, rat, and bovine MAO-A and MAO-B, the covalent binding site for FAD is near the C-terminal region, and there are features characteristic of an adenosine diphosphate-binding fold in the N-terminal region, suggesting that this region is also involved in the binding of FAD.[533,537]

The human MAO-A gene extends over 80 kb and is composed of 15 exons.[527,538] MAO-B also is comprised of 15 exons,[538] and exons 11, 12, and 13 are centered around the FAD-covalent binding site, which is in exon 12, and are highly conserved between the two human MAO-A and MAO-B genes. The human MAO-A and MAO-B genes are arranged tail to tail and are separated by 40 to 45 kb.[527] There are two species of MAO-A mRNA: 2.1 kb and 4.3 kb. The longer message has an extension of 2.2 kb in the 3′ noncoding region that is contained entirely within exon 15. The two messages probably arise from alternative use of two polyadenylation sites present in the same exon.[527]

There is some controversy over the exact site of the promotor for the human MAO-A gene. Initially, it was suggested that the core promotor region of human MAO-A was comprised of two 90-bp repeats, each of which contained two Sp1 elements and lacked a TATA box.[539] Later, the primary transcription initiation site was said to occur at a putative initiator (Inr) element located between −30 and −40 (5′ to the ATG initiation codon).[540] When the Inr-like sequence was added to the core promotor described above, however, the promotor activity decreased, suggesting that the Inr-like sequence acts as a negative *cis* element instead of a transcription initiator.[541]

The MAO-B core promotor region contains two sets of overlapping Sp1 sites that flank a CACCC element all upstream of a TATA box.[539]

Several studies have investigated whether polymorphic sites within the human MAO-A or MAO-B genes are linked to neurologic disease. No clear-cut association has been found with Parkinson disease,[542–544] Tourette syndrome,[545] drug abuse,[545] schizophrenia,[546–548] or bipolar disorder.[549,550]

Screening and Diagnosis

The defects affecting catecholamine and 5HT metabolism cannot be diagnosed by simple basal metabolite analysis in peripheral fluids. Dominantly inherited GTPCH deficiency can be suspected on clinical grounds when presentation is a dystonic gait disorder in childhood. Mildly affected individuals and the early-onset forms can, however, present a confusing clinical picture. Similarly, the early clinical features of TH and AADC deficiency are nonspecific and, as yet, the early clinical features in DβH deficiency and MAO-A or MAO-B deficiency, or the yet to be described deficiencies of TPH, COMT, or phenylethanolamine *N*-methyltransferase, remain uncertain.

Evidence for all of these conditions can be obtained by examination of neurotransmitter metabolites (5HIAA, HVA, 3-*O*-methyldopa, and MHPG), and BH_4 and neopterin profiles in CSF by using HPLC with electrochemical and fluorescence detection.[551] Follow-up tests are then performed as appropriate to confirm a diagnosis (Fig. 78-18). Neurotransmitter metabolite and pterin values must be compared with age-related reference ranges, as there is a near logarithmic drop in concentration of these metabolites in the first year of life, with values then plateauing

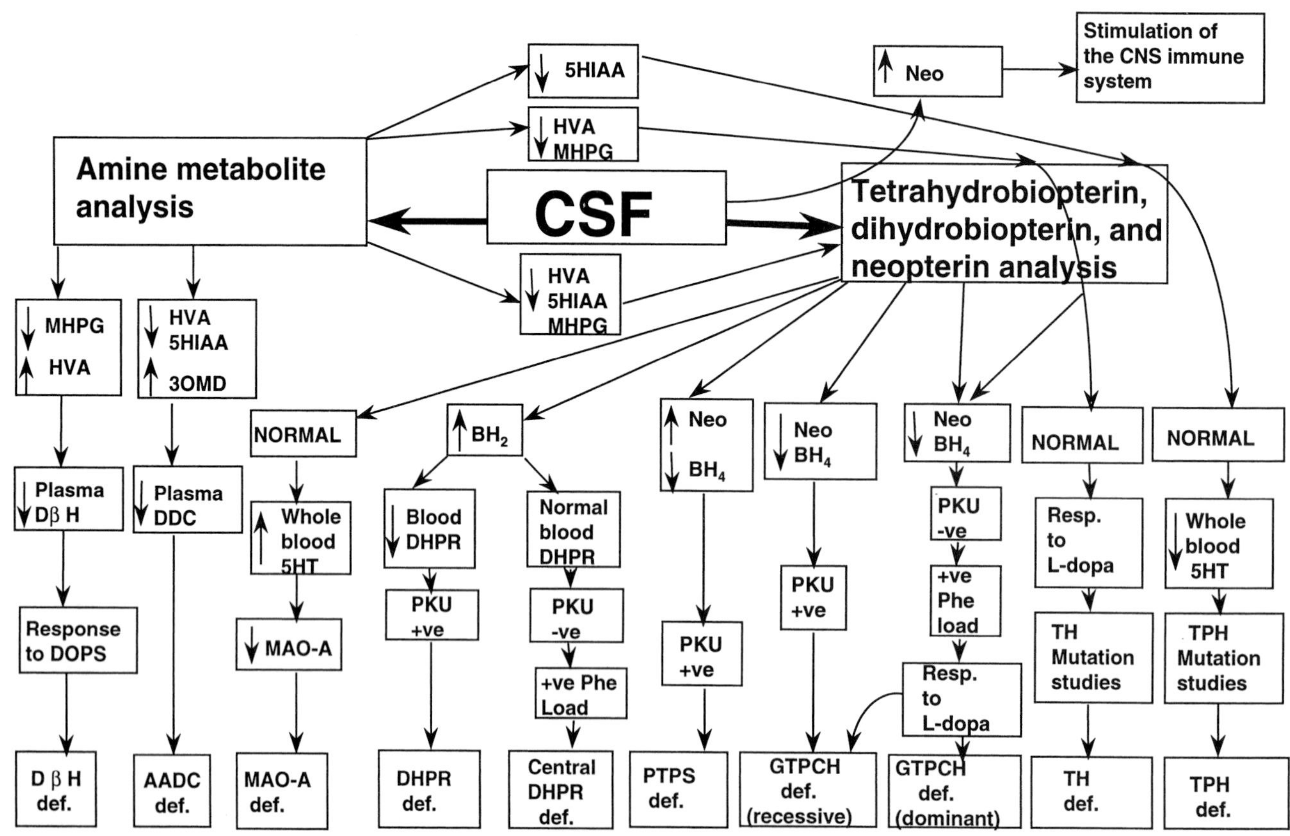

Fig. 78-18 Cerebrospinal fluid (CSF) investigations: diagnostic flowchart. Each CSF sample is analyzed for neurotransmitter metabolites, tetrahydrobiopterin and neopterin. MHPG, 3-methoxy-4-hydroxyphenylglycol; HVA, homovanillic acid; 5HIAA, 5-hydroxyindoleacetic acid; 3OMD, 3-*O*-methyldopa; BH_4, tetrahydrobiopterin; BH_2, 7,8-dihydrobiopterin; Neo, neopterin; DOPS, dihydroxyphenylserine; Phe, phenylalanine; 5HT, serotonin; DβH, dopamine β-hydroxylase; AADC, aromatic L-amino acid decarboxylase; DHPR, dihydropteridine reductase; PTPS, 6-pyruvoyl-tetrahydropterin synthase; PKU, phenylketonuria; GTPCH, GTP cyclohydrolase; TH, tyrosine hydroxylase; TPH, tryptophan hydroxylase; MAO-A, monoamine oxidase A; DDC, L-dopa decarboxylase.

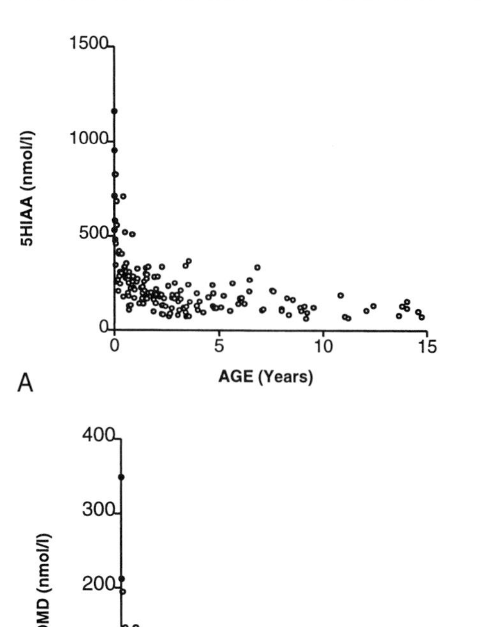

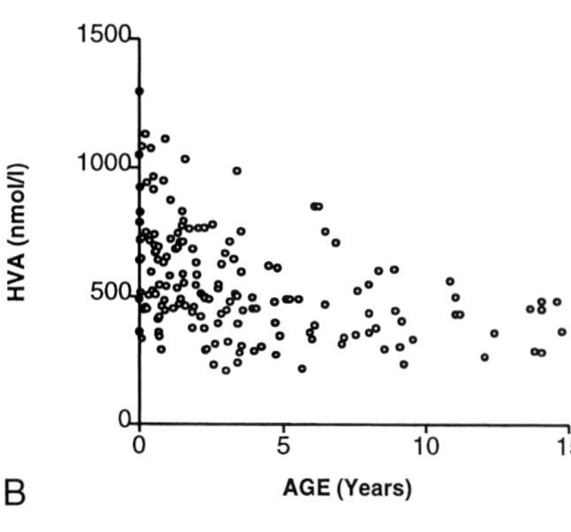

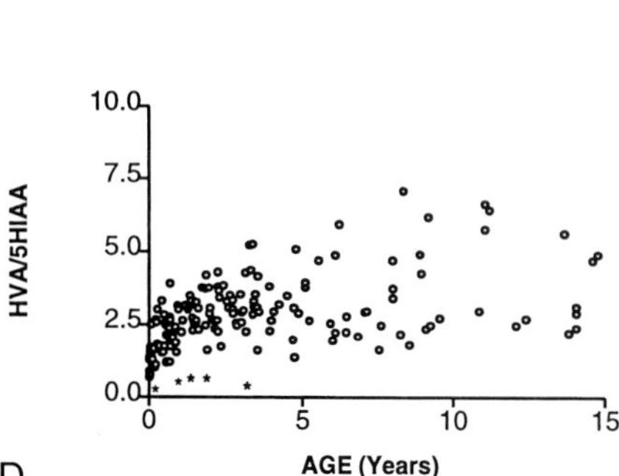

Fig. 78-19 The relationship between age and cerebrospinal fluid (CSF) concentration of (*A*) 5-hydroxyindoleacetic acid, (*B*) homovanillic acid, (*C*) 3-*O*-methyldopa, and (*D*) the ratio of homovanillic acid to 5-hydroxyindole acetic acid. The *asterisk* represents data from patients with tyrosine hydroxylase deficiency or dominantly inherited GTP cyclohydrolase (GTPCH) deficiency. 5HIAA, 5-hydroxyindoleacetic acid; HVA, homovanillic acid; 3OMD, 3-*O*-methyldopa.

gently to the lower levels found in adults (Fig. 78-19 and Table 78-9).[551] CSF must be collected in the same manner as that used to establish reference ranges, as there is a rostrocaudal gradient of neurotransmitter metabolites in CSF.[552] Handling of specimens is also critical, as the neurotransmitter metabolites and the pterins are labile. CSF for analysis of pterins should be collected into a separate tube containing antioxidants,[553] and all samples should be frozen immediately following collection and stored below −70°C at all times prior to analysis.

There is a very close linear relationship between HVA and 5HIAA concentrations in CSF, so a plot of HVA against 5HIAA can be used to indicate an abnormality.[551] Except for the early neonatal period, the ratio of HVA/5HIAA is always greater than 1 (Fig. 78-19), so a plot of this ratio against age can also aid in diagnosis.

Analysis of CSF pterins in children with undiagnosed neurologic disease has an additional benefit outside of its use in the diagnosis of monoamine defects. Neopterin is released from macrophages following stimulation by interferon-γ.[554] An elevation of this pterin in CSF therefore acts as nonspecific marker indicating that the immune system has been stimulated within the CNS. As such, measurement of CSF neopterin can provide information as to whether neurologic symptoms may be related to an infectious process or some other condition that affects the CNS immune system status.

Diagnosis of Tyrosine Hydroxylase Deficiency. A summary of metabolite levels in TH deficiency is presented in Table 78-10. The concentration of HVA and MHPG in CSF from patients with TH deficiency is consistently low, whereas 5HIAA concentrations are normal.[374,375,555,556] BH_4 and neopterin levels are normal, allowing a distinction to be made between a putative case of TH deficiency and cases of dominantly or recessively inherited GTPCH deficiency where pterin levels are low.[178,354] Indirect evidence for a central DA deficiency can also be obtained by a finding of elevated serum prolactin, as the release of this hormone from the anterior pituitary gland is regulated by the tuberoinfundibular DA system.[557] A positive response to low-dose L-dopa also

Table 78-9 Reference Values in Cerebrospinal fluid for Tetrahydrobiopterin (BH_4), 7,8-Dihydrobiopterin (BH_2), Total Neopterin (Neo), and the Metabolites of Serotonin, Dopamine, and Norepinephrine

Age (years)	BH_4	BH_2	Neo	5HIAA	HVA	MHPG	3OMD
<0.5	24.9–127	<0.4–14	4.7–78	179–1159	324–1299	98–168	<350
0.5–1	24.7–60.4	<0.4–14	5.2–44.5	108–520	294–1115	51–112	<100
1–2	17.5–53	<0.4–14	5.3–55.7	101–338	300–1036	47–81	<100
2–5	19.1–60.2	<0.4–14	5.0–54.4	74–370	212–989	39–73	<100
5–10	19.1–54.1	<0.4–14	5.4–33.8	66–338	218–852	39–73	<100
1–16	19.0–44.3	<0.4–14	6.2–25.5	68–190	148–563	28–60	<100
Adult	12–30	<0.4–14	6.0–50	55–130	98–376	28–60	<100

ABBREVIATIONS: 5HIAA = 5-hydroxyindoleacetic acid; HVA = homovanillic acid; MHPG = 3-methoxy-4-hydroxyphenylglycol; 3OMD = 3-*O*-methyldopa.
NOTE: All values are nM.

Table 78-10 Biochemical Data from Patients with Tyrosine Hydroxylase Deficiency[555,585]

Sample	HVA	5HIAA	MHPG	VMA	NE	E	DA
Cerebrospinal fluid (nM)	18–117 (384–1142)	151–268 (110–1028)	2–13 (35–277)				
Urine	1.3–5.3 (2–15) (μmol/mmol creatinine)	3.4–10 (1–12) (μmol/mmol creatinine)		1.0–1.2 (2–15) (μmol/mmol creatinine)	3.8–13.5 (7–100) (nmol/mmol creatinine)	4.5–50.9 (1–30 (nmol/mmol creatinine)	14–293 (50–975) (nmol/mmol creatinine)

NOTE: Reference ranges are in parentheses and are for children less than 5 years of age.
ABBREVIATIONS: HVA = homovanillic acid; 5HIAA = 5-hydroxyindolacetic acid; MHPG = 3-methoxy-4-hydroxyphenylglycol; VMA = vanilmandelic acid; NE = norepinephrine; E = epinephrine; DA = dopamine.

provides good indirect evidence for TH deficiency if pterin metabolism has been shown to be normal. Currently, identification of mutations in the gene for TH is the only way to confirm the diagnosis, as there is no easily accessible source of this enzyme that can be used for kinetic studies.

Diagnosis of Aromatic L-Amino Acid Decarboxylase Deficiency. A summary of metabolite levels in AADC deficiency is presented in Table 78-11. Diagnosis is made by finding reduced levels of 5HIAA and HVA in CSF in conjunction with elevated levels of 3-*O*-methyldopa, L-dopa, and 5HTP in CSF, plasma, and urine.[215,558,559] Vanillactic acid accumulates following transamination of 3-*O*-methyldopa;[560] the elevations are not marked, however, and urine organic acid profiles must be carefully studied if this compound is to be recognized. Definitive diagnosis may be attained by the measurement of AADC activity (L-dopa as substrate) in plasma where activities have ranged from 0 to 8 percent of control values.[559,561,562] The activity of L-dopa decarboxylase in the plasma of parents has varied between 16 and 58 percent of that found in controls.

AADC activity is not present in amniocytes or chorionic villi, and the only prenatal diagnosis has been made following a fetal liver biopsy with biochemical assay of enzymatic activity. The assay predicted a carrier and was confirmed following the birth of a clinically normal girl.[558]

Diagnosis of Dopamine β-Hydroxylase Deficiency. A summary of metabolite levels in DβH deficiency is presented in Table 78-12. DβH deficiency is a primary autonomic neuropathy and must be distinguished from other conditions that lead to chronic failure of the autonomic nervous system. These include the Riley-Day syndrome, a familial dysautonomia;[563] Bradbury-Eggleston syndrome, a peripheral autonomic failure;[564] and the Shy-Drager syndrome, multiple-system atrophy causing central autonomic failure.[565]

DβH deficiency should be considered in any adult with chronic orthostatic hypotension. Measurement of plasma DβH activity in isolation cannot be used to make a definitive diagnosis, as 3 to 4 percent of the normal adult population have near zero levels.[566] The NE/DA ratio in plasma is normally around 10, but in patients with DβH deficiency it is below 0.1, and such a finding is probably pathognomonic for the disease.[567] Additional information can be obtained by demonstration of reduced or absent levels of NE and its metabolites (normetanephrine and vanillylmandelic acid in urine, and MHPG in CSF) combined with elevated levels of L-dopa, DA, and its metabolites (HVA, 3-methoxytyramine, and/or 3,4-dihydroxyphenylacetic acid).

An increase in blood pressure and correction of the orthostatic hypotension in response to dihydroxyphenylserine is also diagnostic. This compound is decarboxylated by AADC to yield NE, and its administration leads to elevation of plasma and urine NE concentrations to near normal levels.[568,569]

DβH deficiency can be distinguished from other forms of autonomic failure where both sympathetic and parasympathetic systems are involved. Physiological autonomic tests specific to DβH deficiency include a lack of pressure response to mental arithmetic, isometric handgrip, or cold pressure testing.[570] Tyramine fails to increase plasma NE levels and leads to a decrease in blood pressure.[571] The Valsalva maneuver causes a drop in blood pressure and increased heart rate reflecting parasympathetic withdrawal, and there is no pressure overshoot in phase IV of the maneuver, demonstrating disruption of the integrity of the baroreflex arc.[572,573] Sympathetic failure can be further confirmed by the absence of a hemodynamic response to α- and β-adrenoceptor antagonists.[573] A normal sweating response demonstrating integrity of the sympathetic cholinergic innervation of eccrine sweat glands together with preservation of parasympathetic function as shown by a normal sinus arrhythmia also help distinguish DβH deficiency from other forms of autonomic failure where there is both sympathetic and parasympathetic involvement. In the eye, pupil size does not change following conjunctival instillation of methacholine, homatropine, or hydroxyamphetamine, showing intact parasympathetic and deficient sympathetic innervation.[569,574]

A diagnosis of DβH deficiency has not been made in infancy but should be considered if there is a history of previous in utero or infant death, unexplained hypotension, hypoglycemia, hypothermia, or ptosis of the eyelids. Profiles of DA, NE, and their metabolites will likely reflect those seen in adults; hence, diagnosis can probably be made by measurement of catechols in plasma, CSF, and urine. A patient with Menkes disease or occipital horn syndrome might have a similar neurochemical pattern, and these diseases should be excluded.[575]

Diagnosis of Monoamine Oxidase-A and -B Deficiencies. A summary of metabolite levels in MAO-A deficiency is presented in Table 78-13. MAO-A deficiency should be considered in males who show prominent behavioral disturbance, especially if there is a family history and linkage to proximal Xp.[576] MAO-A deficiency leads to raised urinary levels of MAO substrates (5HT, normetanephrine, 3-methoxytyramine, and tyramine) and a reduction in the level of their metabolites (5HIAA, vanillylmandelic acid, HVA, and MHPG).[576,577] The urinary concentrations of individual metabolites can be within the normal range, but the substrate-to-product ratios of 3-methoxytyramine/HVA and normetanephrine/vanillylmandelic acid are discriminative for the defect.[577] In the one family where measurements were performed, these ratios were used to distinguish between affected males, carrier females, and normal controls.[576,577] Either 24-h or spot urines can be used for testing.[578] Measurement of MAO-A activity in dexamethasone-stimulated fibroblasts is used to confirm diagnosis.[576] This cannot be used to detect carrier females, as their activities fall within the control range. It is likely that CSF levels of HVA and 5HIAA are also reduced in MAO-A deficiency, but CSF has not been analyzed.

MAO-B deficiency has been described only in association with Norrie disease[579,580] where there was an increase in phenylethylamine in urine. Targeted inactivation of MAO-B in

Table 78-11 Biochemical Data from Patients with Aromatic L-Amino Acid Decarboxylase (AADC) Deficiency[559,561,562]

Sample	HVA	5HIAA	3OMD	L-Dopa	5HTP	5HT	NE	E	VLA	AADC (pmol/min/ml)
Cerebrospinal fluid (nM)	4.1–60 (154–1098)	0–27 (89–608)	308–1650 (<300)	44–311 (<10)	58–139 (<10)					
Plasma (nM)			9100–10,580 (<80)	535–1306 (<25)	186–250 (<20)		<1 (0.5–3.1)	<0.1 (0.1–1.1)		<1–5.3 (36–129)
Whole blood (nM)						66–218 (551–1740)				
Urine (nmol/mmol creatinine)			12,280–14,270 (100–604)	1540–2080 (<50)	1490–2087 (<50)				650–5070 (<100)	

NOTE: Reference ranges are in parentheses and are for children less than 5 years of age.
ABBREVIATIONS: HVA = homovanillic acid; 5HIAA = 5-hydroxyindolacetic acid; 3OMD = 3-*O*-methyldopa; 5HTP = 5-hydroxytryptophan; 5HT = serotonin; NE = norepinephrine; E = epinephrine; VLA = vanillactic acid.

Table 78-12 Biochemical Data from Patients with Dopamine β-Hydroxylase Deficiency[568,569]

Sample	NE	E	DA	HVA	MHPG	L-Dopa	DHPG	DOPAC	3MT	NM	VMA
Cerebrospinal fluid (nM)	<0.03 (0.25–2)	<0.03 (0.03–0.15)	0.5–1.8 (0–0.15)	580 (40–450)	16 (36–70)	16 (4–7)					
Plasma (nM)	ND (0.2–7.2)	ND (0.03–1.0)	3.4 (0–1.0)			19.25 (6.8–11.3)	<0.05 (4.8–8.2)	55 (7.2–19.1)			
Urine (μmol/mol/ creatinine)	<0.5 (10–52)	<0.5 (2–11)	310 (60–220)	5600 (850–2800)	<20 (600–1500)				280 (60–140)	<5 (50–200)	<5 (800–2200)

NOTE: Reference ranges are in parentheses.

ABBREVIATIONS: NE = norepinephrine; E = epinephrine; DA = dopamine; HVA = homovanillic acid; MHPG = 3,methoxy-4-hydroxyphenylglycol; DHPG = 3,4-dihydroxyphenylglycol; DOPAC = 3,4-dihydroxyphenylacetic acid; 3MT = 3-methoxytyramine; NM = normetanephrine; VMA = vanilmandelic acid; ND = not detected.

Table 78-13 Biochemical Data from Patients with Monoamine Oxidase-A Deficiency[576]

Sample	NM (T)	3MT (T)	5HT (F)	TA (T)	VMA (F)	HVA (F)	MHPG (T)	5HIAA (F)
Urine (nmol/mmol creatinine)	52–78 (1–18)	14–34 (13–29)	124–233 (11–68)	1329–4554 <560	200–400 (500–7600)	400–500 (1000–5000)	100–200 (100–2100)	800–1400 (300–5100)

NOTE: Values are reported as total (T, following deconjugation) or free (F). Reference ranges are in parentheses.

ABBREVIATIONS: NM = normetanephrine; 3MT = 3-methoxytyramine; 5HT = serotonin; TA = tyramine; VMA = vanilmandelic acid; HVA = homovanillic acid; MHPG = 3-methoxy-4-hydroxyphenylglycol; 5HIAA = 5-hydroxyindoleacetic acid.

mice also increased levels of phenylethylamine and did not affect 5HT, NE, or DA metabolism, demonstrating the primary role of MAO-B in the metabolism phenylethylamine.[581] A deficiency is confirmed by measurement of the MAO-B activity in platelets.[579]

It is important that patients not eat amine-rich foods such as bananas or dates in the period prior to testing.

Cerebrospinal Fluid Metabolite Profiles Expected to Be Found in the Deficiencies of Tryptophan Hydroxylase and Catechol-*O*-Methyltransferase. A decrease in the concentration of 5HIAA in CSF in the presence of normal levels of HVA, MHPG, BH_4, and neopterin would suggest an isolated deficiency of TPH. Such a defect that affects only 5HT metabolism has yet to be described. A secondary TPH deficiency occurs in the defects of BH_4 metabolism, suggesting that primary mutations affecting TPH would not be lethal.

Similarly, central and peripheral inhibitors of COMT are well tolerated in humans, so it is highly likely that cases of inherited COMT deficiency already exist. The expected pattern of neurotransmitter metabolites in CSF and peripheral fluids in COMT deficiency would be elevations of dihydroxyphenylacetic acid and DA, and decreased levels of HVA and 3-methoxytyramine. It is likely that isolated defects affecting both of these enzymes already exist, but we are unaware of the clinical symptoms that would be associated with the diseases.

Tyrosine Hydroxylase Deficiency (OMIM 191290)

Patients with primary defects in TH were positively identified in the mid-1990s following the identification of point mutations in the TH gene and subsequent demonstration of decreased activity in the recombinant expressed mutant proteins. The mutations were inherited in an autosomal recessive manner, and patients were designated as having autosomal recessively inherited DRD following dramatic response to low-dose L-dopa therapy.[374,375,556]

Genotype. Three mutations in the TH gene have been reported to lead to clinical symptoms (Table 78-14 and Fig. 78-20). The first described was a point mutation in exon 11 resulting in an amino acid exchange of Gln381 to Lys381.[375] Kinetic examination of the recombinant mutant protein showed the enzyme to have a reduced affinity for tyrosine, with a residual activity of about 15 percent of that of the wild-type protein.[374] The second mutation was a 614T > C transition in exon 5 resulting in an amino acid exchange of Leu205 to Pro205. Activity of the recombinant mutant protein was between 0.3 and 16 percent of that of the wild-type protein, depending on the expression system used.[555] Three unrelated Dutch patients had a point mutation in exon 6 (698G>A) resulting in the substitution of Arg233 by His.[556] In addition, a frequent sequence variant in the human TH gene has been reported.[582]

Enzyme Phenotype. TH activity is currently not measurable in any easily accessible tissues or body fluids. Evidence for a defect in the enzyme has to be obtained by indirect means by measurement of DA and NE metabolites in CSF and urine. Activity of enzymes involved in catecholamine metabolism has been reported in human skin keratinocytes,[583] and the mRNA of TH is also present in these cells.[584] Cultured keratinocytes may therefore provide a system in which TH activity can be measured directly.

Metabolic Phenotype. Metabolite profiles in TH deficiency are summarized in Table 78-14. TH deficiency leads to lowered levels of L-dopa and lowered CNS concentrations of catecholamines as demonstrated by the low concentrations of HVA and MHPG in CSF. As expected, 5HT metabolism appears unaffected, as CSF 5HIAA levels are normal.[374,375,555,556] A detailed investigation of

Table 78-14 Mutations Identified in the *TH*, *DDC*, and *MAOA* Genes

Gene	Mutant Designation	Mutant Subtype	Nucleotide Aberration	Amino Acid Aberration	Location in Gene	Reference
TH	L205P	Substitution	614T > C	Leu > Pro at 205	Exon 5	555
	R233H	Substitution	698G > A	Arg > His at 233	Exon 6	556
	Q381K	Substitution	1141C > A	Gln > Lys at 381	Exon 11	375
DDC		Polymorphism	GAGA deletion −61∼ −57		Exon 1	498
	A91V	Substitution	1400C > T	Ala > Val at 91	Exon 3	498
	G102S	Substitution	1432G > A	Gly > Ser at 102	Exon 3	498
	S147R	Substitution	2249A > C	Ser > Arg at 147	Exon 5	498
	S250F	Substitution	3471C > T	Ser > Phe at 250	Exon 7	498
	A275T	Substitution	4028G > A	Ala > Thr at 275	Exon 8	498
	F309L	Substitution	4529T > C	Phe > Leu at 309	Exon 9	498
MAOA	Q296X	Substitution, truncation	936C > T	Gln > Stop at 296	Exon 8	576

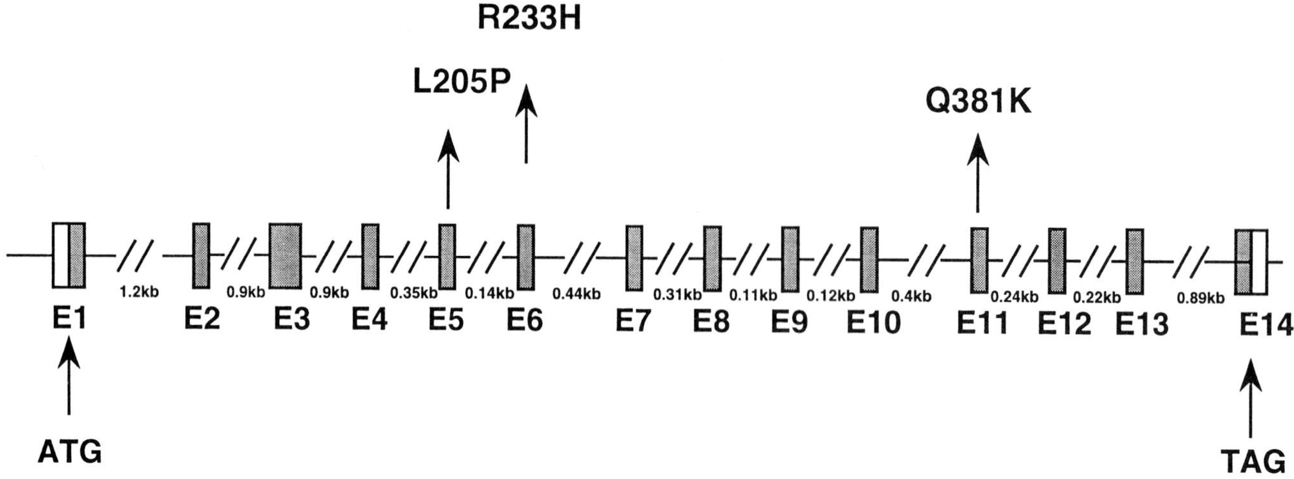

Fig. 78-20 Genomic structure and location of mutations in human *TH* gene.

four Dutch patients showed that urinary catecholamines and metabolites were often in the normal range, and in one patient there was an unexplained elevation of urinary E.[585] Studies have not been performed to determine whether plasma catecholamines are affected in TH deficiency.

Clinical Phenotype. Clinical features in TH deficiency are summarized in Table 78-15. Descriptions of clinical phenotype in the cases of TH deficiency are limited. No details are available from the first cases described, although they are reported to have DRD.[374,375]

One infant had symptoms of jerky movements of upper and lower limbs at 3 months and went on to develop generalized rigidity with little spontaneous movements. An EEG showed nonspecific generalized dysrhythmia, with normal findings on brain CT and MRI scans as well as routine biochemical tests. By 6 months of age, there was an expressionless face, ptosis, drooling, tremulous tongue movements, severe head lag, and truncal hypotonia. There was marked constant tremor in the upper limbs and occasional myoclonic jerks, and tone in the limbs was variable and of cogwheel type. Deep tendon reflexes were reduced, and there were persistent asymmetric tonic neck and Moro reflexes. No diurnal variation in symptoms was noted.[555]

In three other patients, psychomotor retardation, hypertonic tetraparesis, hypokinesia, and axial hypotonia developed within the first few months of life. There was no diurnal variation in the symptoms. EEG showed a monomorph background pattern, and the results of brain MRI and CT scans were normal.[556]

Table 78-15 Signs and Symptoms in the Deficiencies of Tyrosine-3-Hydroxylase (TH), Aromatic L-Amino Acid Decarboxylase (AADC) Dopamine β-Hydroxylase (DβH); and Monoamine Oxidase A (MAO-A)

Signs and Symptoms	TH Deficiency	AADC Deficiency	DβH Deficiency	MAO-A Deficiency
Oculogyric crises	+	+		
Dystonia with diurnal variations	±	±		
Parkinsonian symptoms	+	+		
Tremor	+	+		
Hypokinesia	+	+		
Truncal hypotonia	+	+		
Variable tone with marked hypotonia to opistotonus and spasticity	+	+		
Bilateral ptosis	+	+	±	
Drooling	+			
Sweating		+		
Temperature instability		+		
Chorea/athetosis	+	+		
Miosis	+	+		
Irritability	+	+		
Mental retardation/ development al delay	±	+		±
Hypothermia			±	
Hypoglycemia			±	
Orthostatic hypotension			+	
Aggressive/violent behavior				+
Stereotyped hand movements				±

Table 78-16 Therapy for the Deficiencies of Tyrosine-3-Hydroxylase (TH), Aromatic L-Amino Acid Decarboxylase (AADC), Dopramine β-Hydroxylase (DβH), and Monoamine Oxidase A (MAO-A).

Daily Therapy	Doses/ Day	TH Deficiency	AADC Deficiency	DβH Deficiency	MAO-A Deficiency
L-Dopa (mg/kg) + 10% carbidopa	3–5	2–3	*	No	No
Tranylcypromine (mg)	2	No	4	No	No
Bromocriptine (mg)	2	No	2.5	No	No
Pergolide (mg)	2	No	0.05–2	No	No
Vitamin B_6 (mg)	2	No	†Up to 800	No	No
Dihydroxyphenylserine (mg)	2–3	No	No	250–500	No

*A trial of L-dopa should be attempted.
†A trial with vitamin B_6 should be attempted.

Animal Model. Gene targeting was used to produce mice lacking in TH. Initial studies concluded that TH deficiency led to death in utero via a mechanism probably involving cardiovascular failure.[586] It was unclear whether the pathology was a result of DA deficiency or NE deficiency. Restoration of TH expression specifically in noradrenergic neurons in these animals was achieved by targeting the TH coding sequence to the noradrenergic-specific DβH promotor by homologous recombination in embryonic stem cells.[587] The resulting mice were therefore able to produce NE but still unable to produce DA in the dopaminergic cells. In these animals, pups were born at the expected frequency but within a few weeks became hypoactive and stopped feeding. Administration of L-dopa corrected these abnormal behaviors. It was concluded that DA is essential for movement and feeding but not for the development of the neuronal circuits that control these behaviors, as the nigrostriatal DA system appeared intact.

Treatment. A summary of treatment used in TH deficiency is presented in Table 78-16. Treatment with low-dose L-dopa has been extremely effective. Initiation of L-dopa (2 mg/kg, five times daily) resulted in an optimal sustained clinical response in one child. When reviewed at the age of 4 years, there were no abnormal neurologic signs, and her development was appropriate for her age.[555,588] Treatment with L-dopa and carbidopa, 3 and 0.75 mg/kg, three times daily, respectively, led to rapid clinical improvement in the other cases where details of treatment were given.[556,589]

Aromatic L-Amino Acid Decarboxylase Deficiency (OMIM 107930)

The first case of AADC deficiency was identified in 1990,[590] and a full description was published in 1992.[561] Since then, the present author (Hyland) is aware of nine other cases of which details in three cases have been published.[559,562,591] There appears to be no ethnic trend for the disease. Monozygotic twins and an isolated case were of Middle Eastern origin.[559,561,590] Two were of strictly German origin (unpublished data). Two were Americans: one had Irish, Scottish, French, and English heritage on the maternal side, and Italian heritage on the paternal side; the other had Portuguese and Irish heritage on the maternal side, and English, Welsh, and Irish heritage on the paternal side (unpublished data). The ethnic origin of the other case was not described.[591]

Genotype. Direct genomic sequencing of the AADC gene in six patients with AADC deficiency revealed six point mutations causing single amino acid substitutions (Table 78-14 and Fig. 78-21). Four patients were homozygotes, and one was a compound heterozygote. A single point mutation on one allele in one patient was discovered, but the mutation on the other allele was not located. A 4-bp GAGA deletion was found in the untranslated exon 1 in two patients. Sequencing of 38 control samples revealed that 11 were wild type, 15 were heterozygous, and 12 were homozygous for the deletion, suggesting that the GAGA deletion is a common polymorphism that may be useful for linkage analysis in the future.[498]

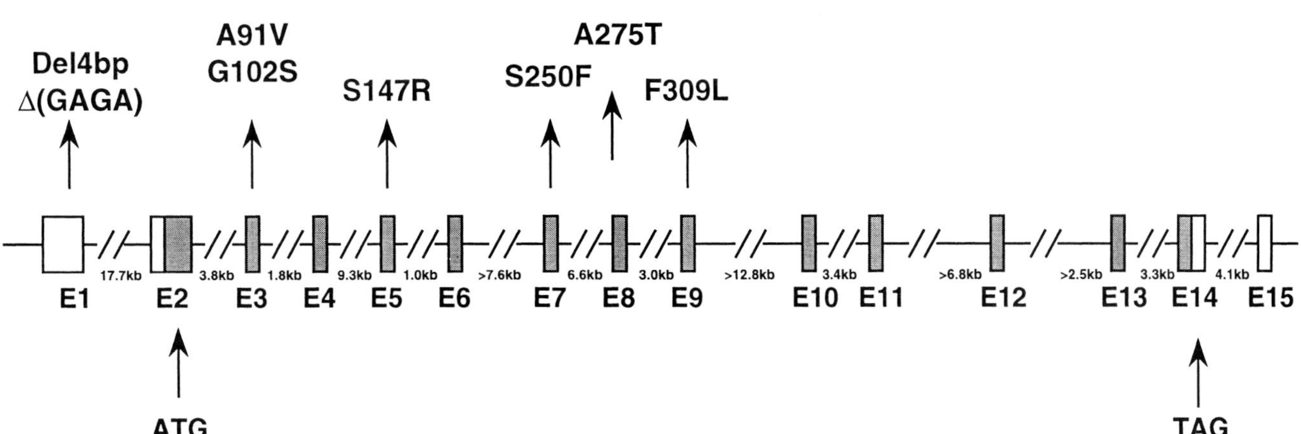

Fig. 78-21 Genomic structure and location of mutations in human *AADC* gene.

One of the patients investigated showed an L-dopa-responsive movement disorder, suggesting the possibility of a mutation affecting the substrate-binding site. Sequencing revealed a homozygous G-to-A substitution converting glycine to serine at position 102 (G102S) in exon 3. Kinetic characterization of the recombinant mutant and wild-type proteins yielded an apparent K_m of 11.6 mM (L-dopa) for the wild-type protein, with that of the G102S mutation being at least 50-fold greater. Glycine 102 lies within a region (residues 61 to 126)[478] that is identical in all mammalian species examined to date. This, together with the aforementioned data and a report describing zero AADC activity in a splicing variant that lacks the amino acids coded by exon 3,[477] suggest that the region around amino acid 102 is critical for L-dopa binding.

Enzyme Phenotype. AADC activity (with L-dopa as substrate) is measurable in plasma and liver.[592] In patients, plasma enzyme activity has ranged from 8 percent to less than 1 percent of that of controls, with heterozygotes generally having approximately 50 percent activity of adult controls.[558,559,562,591] In the index cases, there was a distinct reduction in enzyme activity with age, and adults have lower values than infants and children.[558] Reference to age-related values is therefore important. AADC activity is not measurable in chorionic villi, cultured fibroblasts, or amniocytes, and the only prenatal diagnosis performed utilized a fetal liver biopsy sample taken at 21 weeks of gestation.[558]

Metabolic Phenotype. Metabolite profiles in AADC deficiency are summarized in Table 78-11. AADC deficiency leads to a central and peripheral deficiency of the catecholamines and of 5HT.[559,561,562,591] Low levels of the catecholamine metabolites (HVA and MHPG) and the 5HT metabolite (5HIAA) are found in CSF. Concentrations of whole blood 5HT, plasma catecholamines, and urine metabolites are also very low, showing that AADC deficiency is global.[559,561] The AADC substrates L-dopa and 5HTP also accumulate. L-Dopa is rapidly methylated to 3-*O*-methyldopa, and concentrations of this product are greatly elevated, as its half-life in plasma and CSF is about 18 h.[561] The methylation reaction uses *S*-adenosylmethionine as the methyl group donor, and the demand for this is such that concentrations decrease, as shown by low levels of *S*-adenosylmethionine in CSF.[561,593] Whether there are any pathologic consequences of *S*-adenosylmethionine deficiency remains unclear. Vanillactic acid accumulates in urine following transamination of 3-*O*-methyldopa.[560] Abeling and coworkers described a case in whom there was an unexplained normal concentration of HVA in urine.[591]

Clinical Phenotype. A summary of clinical features is presented in Table 78-15. As in most other recessively inherited diseases, the clinical phenotype of AADC deficiency is heterogeneous, although there appear to be some cardinal features. Overall, the symptoms, if untreated, are very similar to those seen in the defects of BH_4 metabolism. Gestational and neonatal problems include fetal sinus bradycardia, mild-to-severe temperature instability, lethargy, poor feeding, ptosis, and miosis. More major symptoms develop around 2 months of age, with the appearance of generalized hypotonia together with paroxysmal movements consisting of arm and leg extension, rolling eyes, cyanosis, extreme irritability, a tendency to be easily startled, continuing temperature instability, and developmental delay. Sleep disturbance is typical. Other abnormal movements have included sudden myoclonic jerks, flexor spasms, head drops, orofacial dystonia, tongue thrusting, and right torticollis (K. Swoboda, personal communication).[559,561,562] A very characteristic clinical phenotype eventually develops consisting of an extrapyramidal movement disorder, often preceded by oculogyric crises accompanied by convergence spasm. Symptoms typically deteriorate throughout the day and are partially ameliorated following a nap or after nighttime sleep.

Autonomic features are variable, with symptoms including ptosis, miosis, a reverse Argyll Robertson pupil, chronic or paroxysmal nasal congestion, paroxysmal sweating, temperature instability, gastrointestinal reflux, and constipation. In the first described cases, postural drop in blood pressure was not present at 9 months but was noted at 1 year of age.[561]

In most cases, brain MRI scans were normal (K. Swoboda, personal communication);[559,562] however, mild cerebral atrophy was demonstrated in the initial cases at the age of 9 months.[561] Similarly, EEG patterns are mostly normal, although one case had significant background EEG abnormalities, with frequent spike or polyspike and wave bursts (K. Swoboda, personal communication).

Endocrine abnormalities may arise as a result of the peripheral and central catecholamine deficiency. Korenke et al observed significant hypoglycemia following patients' failure to awake after sedation for an MRI scan,[562] and elevated prolactin may be present due to disinhibition of prolactin release in the absence of normal central levels of DA (K. Swoboda, personal communication). Linear growth was delayed in all patients, and delayed bone age has been reported.[562]

A mild form of AADC deficiency was briefly described, with the child presenting with minor motor retardation at the age of 1 year.[591]

In general, all parents have been asymptomatic,[559,561] though minor autonomic symptoms may be present (K. Swoboda, personal communication).

Treatment. A summary of the treatment used in AADC deficiency is presented in Table 78-16. Treatment in AADC deficiency is aimed at correcting the peripheral and central deficiency of 5HT and the catecholamines. In most cases, the defect can not be corrected by neurotransmitter precursor therapy; therefore, treatment has relied on stimulation of the dopaminergic system with DA agonists and the use of MAO inhibitors to prevent the breakdown of the small amounts of 5HT and the catecholamines that are formed. Administration of tranylcypromine, a nonspecific MAO inhibitor, raised plasma NE and whole blood 5HT levels, reduced sweating, and improved spontaneous movement, tone, and color[559,561] and bromocriptine and pergolide, DA agonists, abolished the oculogyric crises and slightly increased spontaneous movement. Pyridoxine (up to 400 mg daily) had no clinical effect on most of the patients[559,561] but did augment the effects seen following L-dopa administration to the three siblings who were L-dopa responsive (G. Hoffmann, personal communication). A trial with pyridoxine is therefore recommended. In the original cases reported, optimum treatment resulted from tranylcypromine (4 mg twice daily), bromocriptine (2.5 mg twice daily), and pyridoxine (100 mg twice daily) in combination.[561] At 8 years of age, substitution of pergolide, a more potent DA agonist (gradually increased from 0.05 mg twice daily to 2 mg twice daily), for bromocriptine resulted in a reduction in the severity of the symptoms that appeared during the day. A similar effect has been noted in another case (unpublished data). In one patient, administration of oxymetazoline hydrochloride (Afrin) led to immediate reversal of nasal congestion, whereas pseudoephedrin, phenylpropanolamine hydrochloride, chlorpheniramine, brompheniramine, and ephedrin had no benefit (K. Swoboda, personal communication).

Short-term, continuous intravenous DA infusion was attempted in two infants with AADC deficiency. This led to reversal of ptosis and nasal congestion, a decrease in blood pressure lability, improvement in mean blood pressure, and improved levels of alertness and attentiveness. A long-term trial in one patient had to be abandoned because of recurrent line sepsis, progressive failure to thrive, and continued failure to show motor progress. Introduction of midodrine hydrochloride, a direct α-adrenergic agonist, following discontinuation of DA, helped to decrease blood pressure lability and to maintain a mean blood pressure within the normal range (K. Swoboda, personal communication).

Worsening of symptoms during the first months of life and improvement of motor symptoms upon institution of treatment in all patients suggests that early diagnosis and treatment of AADC deficiency probably improve prognosis. The twins reported by Hyland et al,[561] who were diagnosed at the age of 10 months, were able to walk without support by the age of 8 years, speak a few words in two languages, and had good comprehension (K. Hyland, unpublished observation). In contrast, the patients reported by Maller et al and Korenke et al, in whom treatment was instituted much later, showed only some minor motor amelioration.[559,562] Response to therapy also appears to depend on the severity of the enzyme defect, as a child with virtually absent plasma AADC activity, diagnosed and treated from 5 months of age, has made little developmental progress, although treatment significantly ameliorated many of her motor symptoms (K. Swoboda and K. Hyland, unpublished observations).

Dopamine β-Hydroxylase Deficiency (OMIM 223360)

In 1986 and 1987, a syndrome of autonomic failure characterized by severe orthostatic hypotension, noradrenergic failure, and ptosis of the eyelids, with maintenance of normal parasympathetic and sympathetic cholinergic function, was reported.[569,572] DβH deficiency was implicated after the demonstration of low or absent NE, E, and their metabolites, elevated DA levels, and absence of DβH activity in plasma. Fewer than 10 cases have been reported so far, and the mode of inheritance is assumed to be autosomal recessive, but as yet the molecular mechanism to explain the deficiency has not been defined.

Genotype. Studies in CSF, plasma, and tissue have shown a lack of immunoreactive protein,[594] but a specific defect at the DNA or mRNA level that explains the absence of DβH activity has yet to be found.

Enzyme Phenotype. DβH activity is measurable in plasma, and in all cases of DβH deficiency the activity has been undetectable. DβH activity measurement in plasma is, however, not suitable as a key diagnostic tool, as very low activity can be found in 3 to 4 percent of the normal population.[567] Diagnosis is therefore achieved by measurement of plasma catecholamines, by testing of autonomic function, and by a finding of a therapeutic response to dihydroxyphenylserine.

Metabolic Phenotype. Metabolite profiles in DβH deficiency are summarized in Table 78-12. Deficiency of DβH leads to a lack of NE and E, and accumulation of DA and L-dopa in plasma, urine, and CSF. The metabolites of these reflect the changes in the neurotransmitters. In urine, the DA metabolites HVA and 3-methoxytyramine are elevated, whereas the levels of NE metabolites vanillylmandelic acid and normetanephrine are decreased. Similar changes are seen in CSF, where the levels of MHPG are decreased and the levels of HVA are elevated.[567]

Clinical Phenotype. A summary of clinical features is presented in Table 78-15. DβH deficiency has been diagnosed only in adulthood following the onset of severe orthostatic hypotension and noradrenergic failure. There is no evidence of other neurologic defects. Retrospective case histories have described delay in opening of eyes, ptosis of the eyelids, hypotension, hypothermia, and hypoglycemia in the newborn period,[567] and there are reports of spontaneous abortions and stillbirths in mothers of affected patients.[567,569] This, together with a high mortality rate in homozygous embryos from "knockout" DβH-deficient mice,[595] suggest that human adults diagnosed with DβH deficiency may have a mild form of the disease and that a more severe form may exist that leads to death in early infancy or in utero.

Symptoms worsen with age. Children develop postural hypotension and syncope on exercising.[596] In adolescence and early adulthood, there is profound orthostatic hypotension, systolic blood pressure of less than 80 mmHg, and low to normal values in the supine position.[567] Other symptoms include nasal stuffiness, reduced exercise tolerance, prolonged or retrograde ejaculation, continuing ptosis of the eyelids, hypoprolactinemia, hyperextensible or hyperflexible joints, nocturia, high palate, hypomagnesemia, seizures following hypotension, mild behavioral changes, hypotonic skeletal muscles, brachydactyly, sluggish deep tendon reflexes, weak facial musculature, raised blood urea nitrogen, atrial fibrillation, and T-wave abnormalities (ECG).[567,597] Sleep duration is normal, but the duration of rapid eye movement (REM) sleep is decreased.[598]

Animal Model. Gene targeting was used to produce mice lacking in DβH. The major feature was death of most of the homozygous embryos in utero via a mechanism probably involving cardiovascular failure.[595] Rescue was achieved by administration of dihydroxyphenylserine. Most of the heterozygous pups born to homozygous females died within a few days of birth, due to a deficit in maternal nurturing, suggesting that NE is responsible for long-lasting changes that promote maternal behavior during development and parturition in mice.[599] As E and NE are thought to control adiposity and energy balance, the animals were investigated as a potential model for obesity. The animals had an increased food intake, were cold intolerant because of impaired vasoconstriction, and were unable to induce thermogenesis in brown tissue via the uncoupling protein. In spite of this, they did not become obese because of an underlying increased basal metabolic rate. The mechanism for this increased rate was not determined.[600] Study of older homozygote animals has provided evidence for a role of NE in motor function, learning, and memory.[601] Ptosis and reductions in male fertility, hind-limb extension, post-decapitation convulsions, and uncoupling protein expression were all reversed by dihydroxyphenylserine administration.[602]

Pathophysiology. NE and E are the main determinants of peripheral vascular tone and hence of arterial pressure. The major symptom of orthostatic hypotension seen in DβH deficiency is therefore mainly caused by the lack of a pressor effect from these catecholamines. Sympathetic nerves remain intact,[603] but firing rates in muscle are accelerated.[604] DA is stored in sympathetic noradrenergic terminals instead of NE. Release of DA contributes to the drop in blood pressure either by means of a diuretic effect in the kidney or via a vasodepressor effect that occurs through direct vasodilation.[605,606] The circadian rhythm in blood pressure is also reversed, and a higher blood pressure at night causes pressure natriuresis[598] that, with the diuretic effect from the high DA concentration, probably explains the nocturia. The ptosis of the eyelids reflects failed noradrenergic control of levator function.[572] The elevated DA levels may contribute to hypothermia, and hypoglycemia reported in infancy may result from the lack of a calorigenic effect in the absence of E.[567]

Treatment. A summary of the treatment used in DβH deficiency is presented in Table 78-16. In adults, 250 to 500 mg of dihydroxyphenylserine, two to three times daily, improved blood pressure and ameliorated or totally prevented the orthostatic hypotension.[568,569,596,607]

Monoamine Oxidase Deficiency (OMIM 309850)

MAO deficiency has been described as a defect affecting only MAO-A,[608] as a combined deficiency of both MAO-A and MAO-B in association with Norrie disease,[579,609] an X-linked syndrome characterized by congenital blindness, hearing loss, and variable mental retardation,[610,611] and as an isolated deficiency of MAO-B in conjunction with Norrie disease.[579]

Genotype. In the single family reported with MAO-A deficiency, the initial molecular evidence for MAO deficiency was obtained from a finding of a maximum multipoint Lod score of 3.69 using a CA-repeat polymorphism in the structural gene for MAO-A.[576,608]

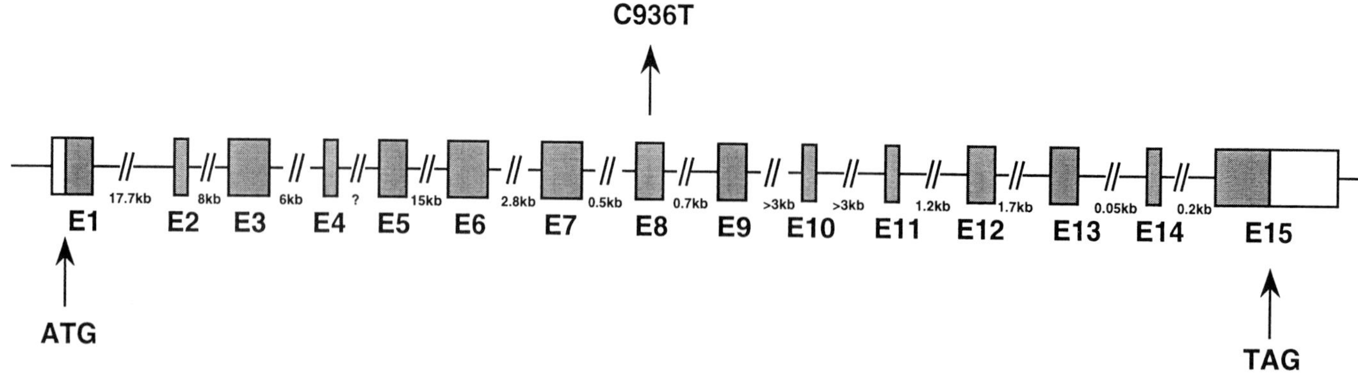

Fig. 78-22 Genomic structure and location of mutations in human *MAO-A* gene.

The diagnosis was confirmed by finding zero activity of this enzyme in dexamethasone-stimulated fibroblasts,[576] and by location of a nonconservative C-to-T mutation at position 936 that changed a glutamine (CAG) codon to a termination (TAG) codon at position 296 of the deduced amino acid sequence (Table 78-14 and Fig. 78-22).[576]

MAO-B deficiency, described in two brothers, was caused by a microdeletion in the X chromosome. The distal deletion breakpoint lay in intron 5 of the MAO-B gene, with the deletion extending proximally into the Norrie gene.[579]

Enzyme Phenotype. MAO-A activity can be measured in dexamethasone-stimulated fibroblasts[576] and MAO-B activity in platelets.[579] MAO-A activity was negligible in three affected males, and low-to-moderate activity was found in two carrier females and one noncarrier female from the same family.[576] Likewise, MAO-B activity was negligible in the patient with Norrie disease in whom the deletion included part of the MAO-B gene.[579]

Metabolic Phenotype. Metabolite profiles in MAO-A deficiency are summarized in Table 78-13. In MAO-A deficiency, the catabolism of DA, NE, and 5HT is impaired. Levels of the MAO-A substrates (normetanephrine, 3-methoxytyramine, and tyramine) are therefore elevated, and there are reduced amounts of the MAO-A oxidation products (VMA, HVA, MHPG, and 5HIAA).[577,579,608]

The neurochemical and behavioral abnormalities seen in MAO-A deficiency were not found in two brothers who had MAO-B deficiency associated with Norrie disease.[579] The only biochemical abnormality detected in these two patients was an elevation of phenylethylamine in their urine. Similar elevations of phenylethylamine have been found in MAO-B-deficient mice.[581]

Clinical Phenotype

Isolated Monoamine Oxidase-A Deficiency. A summary of clinical features is presented in Table 78-15. A single large Dutch family with MAO-A deficiency has been investigated.[608] The condition is X linked, and detailed information was available from 8 of a total of 14 affected males. Early case histories were not available. The main symptoms were mild mental retardation (IQ score, around 85) and behavioral abnormalities. No consistent congenital abnormalities were noted. One patient had clubfoot. There were no specific dysmorphic signs. All had a tendency toward stereotyped hand movements (plucking or fiddling, hand wringing), and all had behavioral problems, with repeated occurrences of excessive, sometimes violent, aggression often triggered by anger. The incidents included attempted rape and other forced sexual activity, stabbing, and fighting. Other abnormal behavior included arson, exhibitionism, and voyeurism. The aggressive behavior tended to occur during periods of 1 to 3 days and was associated with reduced sleep and night terrors. Cardiovascular difficulty was also described.[612] Unaffected males and obligate female carriers within the family functioned normally. Transgenic mice lacking the MAO-A gene also show violent behavior, providing confirmatory evidence for the link between abnormal behavior and MAO-A deficiency.[613]

Monoamine Oxidase Deficiency Associated with Norrie Disease. Patients with X-chromosome deletions, including MAO-A and MAO-B, as well as the Norrie disease gene, had severe mental retardation, abnormal peripheral autonomic function, autistic-like behavior, and atonic seizures.[579,609] Two brothers with a complex deletion involving the Norrie disease gene and a part of the MAO-B structural gene, but with an intact MAO-A gene, had no psychiatric symptoms or mental retardation.[579] The clinical features that might be found in an isolated case of MAO-B deficiency are unknown; however, cataplexy and abnormal REM sleep might be features.[580] The involvement of deletions of the X chromosome in areas other than the structural genes for MAO-A and MAO-B makes further interpretation of the clinical data in these patients difficult. More information on Norrie disease can be found in Chap. 240.

Pathophysiology. Aggressive behavior in animals and humans has been associated with central and peripheral changes in monoamine metabolism.[613–618] MAO-A knockout mice also exhibit aggressive behavior;[613] it is likely, therefore, that the imbalance in central monoamine metabolism underlies the aggressive behavior seen in patients with MAO-A deficiency. However, since MAO-A deficiency raises 5HT levels, it provides an interesting exception to the low-serotonin paradigm of impulsive aggression.[619] REM sleep deprivation may also be involved in the development of aggressive behavior, as MAO-A inhibitors suppress REM sleep,[620] and REM sleep deprivation produces shock-induced fighting.[621]

The activities of MAO-A and MAO-B vary widely in humans, and these variations may contribute to a predisposition to various diseases, including schizophrenia, alcoholism, and affective disorders.[622,623] In the case of MAO-A, the variation in enzyme activity does not appear to be related to altered gene structure, as there is a high conservation of coding sequence in the human MAO-A gene.[624]

Animal Model. A line of transgenic mice was isolated in which transgene integration caused a deletion in the gene encoding MAO-A. 5HT and NE levels were elevated in brain. The elevation of 5HT during critical periods of development of the somatosensory cortex caused a lack of the characteristic barrel-like clustering of layer-IV neurons,[625] and adult mice had abnormal behavior, including enhanced aggression by males[613] and alterations in emotion.[626]

Treatment. Specific treatment for MAO deficiency has not been described. The TPH inhibitor, parachlorophenylalanine, might be beneficial, as this agent corrected behavioral alterations in the transgenic mouse model of MAO-A deficiency.[613] Dietary intervention by avoiding foods rich in amines may also help.

REFERENCES

1. Kaufman S: *Tetrahydrobiopterin: Basic Biochemistry and Role in Human Disease*. Baltimore, Johns Hopkins University Press, 1997.
2. Kaufman S: The phenylalanine hydroxylating system from mammalian liver. *Adv Enzymol* **35**:245, 1971.
3. Hufton SE, Jennings IG, Cotton RGH: Structure and function of the aromatic amino acid hydroxylases. *Biochem J* **311**:353, 1995.
4. Katoh S, Akino M: Biosynthesis of tetrahydrobiopterin in animals. *Zool Sci* **3**:745, 1986.
5. Thöny B, Auerbach G, Blau N: Tetrahydrobiopterin biosynthesis, regeneration and functions. *Biochem J* **347**:1, 2000.
6. Duch DS, Smith GK: Biosynthesis and function of tetrahydrobiopterin. *J Nutr Biochem* **2**:411, 1991.
7. Hatakeyama K, Hoshiga M, Suzuki S, Kagamiyama H: Enzymatic synthesis of 6R-(U-^{14}C)tetrahydrobiopterin from (U-^{14}C)GTP. *Anal Biochem* **209**:1, 1993.
8. Auerbach G, Nar H: The pathway from GTP to tetrahydrobiopterin: Three-dimensional structures of GTP cyclohydrolase I and 6-pyruvoyl-tetrahydropterin synthase. *Biol Chem* **378**:185, 1997.
9. Blau N, Niederwieser A: GTP cyclohydrolases: A review. *J Clin Chem Clin Biochem* **23**:169, 1985.
10. Sohta Y, Ohta T, Masada M: Purification and some properties of GTP cyclohydrolase I from spinach leaves. *Biosci Biotech Biochem* **61**:1081, 1997.
11. Shen RS, Alam A, Zhang YX: Human liver GTP cyclohydrolase I: Purification and some properties. *Biochimie* **71**:343, 1989.
12. De Saizieu A, Vankan P, Van Loon AP: Enzymic characterization of *Bacillus subtilis* GTP cyclohydrolase I: Evidence for a chemical dephosphorylation of dihydroneopterin triphosphate. *Biochem J* **306**(pt 2):371, 1995.
13. Cha KW, Jacobson KB, Yim JJ: Isolation and characterization of GTP cyclohydrolase I from mouse liver: Comparison of normal and the *Hph-1* mutant. *J Biol Chem* **266**:12,294, 1991.
14. Hatakeyama K, Harada T, Suzuki S, Watanabe Y, Kagamiyama H: Purification and characterization of rat liver GTP cyclohydrolase I: Cooperative binding of GTP to the enzyme. *J Biol Chem* **264**:21,660, 1989.
15. Nar H, Huber R, Meining W, Bacher A, Fischer M, Hosl M, Ritz H, et al: Structure and mechanism of GTP cyclohydrolase I of *Escherichia coli*. *Biochem Soc Trans* **24**:S37, 1996.
16. Togari A, Ichinose H, Matsumoto S, Fujita K, Nagatsu T: Multiple mRNA forms of human GTP cyclohydrolase I. *Biochem Biophys Res Commun* **187**:359, 1992.
17. Steinmetz MO, Plüss C, Christen U, Wolpensinger B, Lustig A, Werner ER, Wachter H, et al: Rat GTP cyclohydrolase I is a homodecameric protein complex containing high-affinity calcium-binding sites. *J Mol Biol* **279**:189, 1998.
18. Nar H, Huber R, Meining W, Schmid C, Weinkauf S, Bacher A: Atomic structure of GTP cyclohydrolase I. *Structure* **3**:459, 1995.
19. Nar H, Huber R, Auerbach G, Fischer M, Hösl C, Ritz H, Bacher A, et al: Active site topology and reaction mechanism of GTP cyclohydrolase I. *Proc Natl Acad Sci USA* **92**:12,120, 1995.
20. Blau N, Niederwieser A: The application of 8-aminoguanosine triphosphate, a new inhibitor of GTP cyclohydrolase I, to the purification of the enzyme from human liver. *Biochim Biophys Acta* **880**:26, 1986.
21. Hatakeyama K, Harada T, Kagamiyama H: IMP dehydrogenase inhibitors reduce intracellular tetrahydrobiopterin levels through reduction of intracellular GTP levels: Indications of the regulation of GTP cyclohydrolase I activity by restriction of GTP availability in the cells. *J Biol Chem* **267**:20,734, 1992.
22. Ichinose H, Ohye T, Matsuda Y, Hori T, Blau N, Burlina A, Rouse B, et al: Characterization of mouse and human GTP cyclohydrolase I genes: Mutations in patients with GTP cyclohydrolase I deficiency. *J Biol Chem* **270**:10,062, 1995.
23. Imazumi K, Sasaki T, Takahashi K, Takai Y: Identification of a Rabphilin-3A-interacting protein as GTP cyclohydrolase I in PC12 cells. *Biochem Biophys Res Commun* **205**:1409, 1994.
24. Hesslinger C, Ziegler I, Kremmer E, Hülter L: IgE-mediated signal transduction regulates tetrahydrobiopterin synthesis in mast cells: A model system for posttranslational modulation of GTP cyclohydrolase I, in Pfleiderer W, Rokos H (eds): *Chemistry and Biology of Pteridines and Folates*. Berlin, Blackwell Science, 1997, p 559.
25. Sakamoto H, Fujita K, Ikegame M, Teradaira R, Kuzuya H: Different complex forms of human liver GTP cyclohydrolase I. *Biog Amines* **12**:55, 1996.
26. Ichinose H, Ohye T, Takahashi E, Seki N, Hori T, Segawa M, Nomura Y, et al: Hereditary progressive dystonia with marked diurnal fluctuation caused by mutation in the GTP cyclohydrolase I gene. *Nature Genet* **8**:236, 1994.
27. Thöny B, Heizmann CW, Mattei MG: Human GTP cyclohydrolase I gene and sepiapterin reductase gene map to region 14q21-q22 and 2p14-p12, respectively, by in situ hybridization. *Genomics* **26**:168, 1995.
28. Nomura T, Ichinose H, Sumi-Ichinose C, Nomura H, Hagino Y, Fujita K, Nagatsu T: Cloning and sequencing of cDNA encoding mouse GTP cyclohydrolase I. *Biochem Biophys Res Commun* **191**:523, 1993.
29. Gütlich M, Jaeger E, Rucknagel KP, Werner T, Rodl W, Ziegler I, Bacher A: Human GTP cyclohydrolase I: Only one out of three cDNA isoforms gives rise to the active enzyme. *Biochem J* **302**:215, 1994.
30. Bandmann O, Nygaard TG, Surtees R, Marsden CD, Wood NW, Harding AE: Dopa-responsive dystonia in British patients: New mutations of the GTP cyclohydrolase I gene and evidence for genetic heterogeneity. *Hum Mol Genet* **5**:403, 1996.
31. Bezin L, Nygaard TG, Neville JD, Shen H, Levine RA: Reduced lymphoblast neopterin detects GTP cyclohydrolase dysfunction in dopa-responsive dystonia. *Neurology* **50**:1021, 1998.
32. Beye K, Lao-Villadoniga JI, Vecino-Bilbao B, Cacabelos R, De la Fuente-Fernandez R: A novel point mutation in the GTP cyclohydrolase I gene in a Spanish family with hereditary progressive and dopa responsive dystonia. *J Neurol Neurosurg Psychiatry* **62**:420, 1997.
33. Blau N, Ichinose H, Nagatsu T, Heizmann CW, Zacchello F, Burlina AB: A missense mutation in a patient with guanosine triphosphate cyclohydrolase I deficiency missed in the newborn screening program. *J Pediatr* **126**:401, 1995.
34. De la Fuente-Fernandez R: Mutations in GTP-cyclohydrolase I gene and vitiligo. *Lancet* **350**:640, 1997.
35. Furukawa Y: GTP cyclohydrolase I gene mutations in hereditary progressive and dopa-responsive dystonia. *Ann Neurol* **40**:134, 1996.
36. Furukawa Y, Lang AE, Trugman JM, Bird TD, Hunter A, Sadeh M, Tagawa T, et al: Gender-related penetrance and de novo GTP cyclohydrolase I gene mutations in dopa-responsive dystonia. *Neurology* **50**:1015, 1998.
37. Furukawa Y, Kish SJ, Bebin EM, Jacobson RD, Fryburg JS, Wilson WG, Shimadzu M, et al: Dystonia with motor delay in compound heterozygotes for GTP cyclohydrolase I gene mutations. *Ann Neurol* **44**:10, 1998.
38. Hirano M, Tamaru Y, Nagai Y, Ito H, Imai T, Ueno S: Exon skipping caused by a base substitution at a splice site in the GTP cyclohydrolase I gene in a Japanese family with hereditary progressive dystonia/ dopa-responsive dystonia. *Biochem Biophys Res Commun* **213**:645, 1995.
39. Hirano M, Tamaru Y, Ito H, Matsumoto S, Imai T, Ueno S: Mutant GTP cyclohydrolase I mRNA levels contribute to dopa-responsive dystonia onset. *Ann Neurol* **40**:796, 1996.
40. Hirano M, Imaiso Y, Ueno S: Differential splicing of the GTP cyclohydrolase I RNA in Dopa-responsive dystonia. *Biochem Biophys Res Commun* **234**:316, 1997.
41. Ichinose H, Blau N, Matalon R, Nagatsu T: Genomic organization of mouse and human GTP cyclohydrolase I genes and mutations found in human gene. *Pteridines* **6**:104, 1995.
42. Ichinose H, Ohye T, Segawa M, Nomura Y, Endo K, Tanaka H, Tsuji S, et al: GTP cyclohydrolase I gene in hereditary progressive dystonia with marked diurnal fluctuation. *Neurosci Lett* **196**:5, 1995.
43. Illarioshkin SN, Markova ED, Slominsky PA, Miklina NI, Popova SN, Limborska SA, Tsuji S, et al: The GTP cyclohydrolase I gene in Russian families with dopa-responsive dystonia. *Arch Neurol* **55**:789, 1998.
44. Imaiso Y, Taniwaki T, Yamada T, Yoshimura T, Hirano M, Ueno S, Kaneda N, et al: A novel mutation of the GTP-cyclohydrolase I gene in a patient with hereditary progressive dystonia/dopa-responsive dystonia. *Neurology* **50**:517, 1998.
45. Jarman PR, Bandmann O, Marsden CD, Wood NW: GTP cyclohydrolase I mutations in patients with dystonia responsive to anticholinergic drugs. *J Neurol Neurosurg Psychiatry* **63**:304, 1997.

46. Nitschke M, Steinberger D, Heberlein I, Otto V, Müller U, Vieregge P: Dopa responsive dystonia with Turner's syndrome: Clinical, genetic, and neurophysiological studies in a family with a new mutation in the GTP cyclohydrolase I gene. *J Neurol Neurosurg Psychiatry* **64**:806, 1998.
47. Steinberger D, Weber Y, Korinthenberger R, Deuschl G, Benecke R, Martinius J, Müller U: High penetrance and pronounced variation in expressivity of GCH1 mutations in five families with Dopa-responsive dystonia. *Ann Neurol* **43**:634, 1998.
48. Tamaru Y, Hirano M, Ito H, Kawamura J, Matsumoto S, Imai T, Ueno S: Clinical similarities of hereditary progressive/dopa responsive dystonia caused by different types of mutations in the GTP cyclohydrolase I gene. *J Neurol Neurosurg Psychiatry* **64**:469, 1998.
49. Weber Y, Steinberger D, Deuschl G, Benecke R, Müller U: Two previously unrecognized splicing mutations of GCH1 in Dopa-responsive dystonia: Exon skipping and one base insertion. *Neurogenetics* **1**:125, 1997.
50. Nagatsu I, Ichinose H, Sakai M, Titani K, Suzuki M, Nagatsu T: Immunocytochemical localization of GTP cyclohydrolase I in the brain, adrenal gland, and liver of mice. *J Neural Transm* **102**:175, 1995.
51. Lentz SI, Kapatos G: Tetrahydrobiopterin biosynthesis in the rat brain: Heterogeneity of GTP cyclohydrolase I mRNA expression in monoamine-containing neurons. *Neurochem Int* **28**:569, 1996.
52. Dassesse D, Hemmens B, Cuvelier L, Resibois A: GTP cyclohydrolase I-like immunoreactivity in rat brain. *Brain Res* **777**:187, 1997.
53. Hwang O, Baker H, Gross S, Joh TH: Localization of GTP cyclohydrolase in monoaminergic but not nitric oxide-producing cells. *Synapse* **28**:140, 1998.
54. Werner ER, Werner-Felmayer G, Fuchs D, Hausen A, Reibnegger G, Yim JJ, Pfleiderer W, et al: Tetrahydrobiopterin biosynthetic activities in human macrophages, fibroblasts, THP-1, and T 24 cells: GTP-cyclohydrolase I is stimulated by interferon-gamma, and 6-pyruvoyl tetrahydropterin synthase and sepiapterin reductase are constitutively present. *J Biol Chem* **265**:3189, 1990.
55. Ziegler I, Schott K, Lubbert M, Herrmann F, Schwulera U, Bacher A: Control of tetrahydrobiopterin synthesis in T lymphocytes by synergistic action of interferon-gamma and interleukin-2. *J Biol Chem* **265**:17,026, 1990.
56. Stegenga SL, Hirayama K, Kapatos G: Regulation of GTP cyclohydrolase I gene expression and tetrahydrobiopterin content in cultured sympathetic neurons by leukemia inhibitory factor and ciliary neurotrophic factor. *J Neurochem* **66**:2541, 1996.
57. Gal EM, Nelson JM, Sherman AD: Biopterin III: Purification and characterization of enzymes involved in the cerebral synthesis of 7, 8-dihydrobiopterin. *Neurochem Res* **3**:69, 1978.
58. Hatakeyama K: Measurement of biopterin and the use of inhibitors of biopterin biosynthesis, in Michael A (ed): *Methods in Molecular Biology: Nitric Oxide Protocols*. Totowa, NJ: Humana, 1998 .
59. Takikawa S, Curtius HC, Redweik U, Ghisla S: Purification of 6-pyruvoyl-tetrahydropterin synthase from human liver. *Biochem Biophys Res Commun* **134**:646, 1986.
60. Hasler T, Curtius HC: Purification and characterization of 6-pyruvoyl tetrahydropterin synthase from salmon liver. *Eur J Biochem* **180**:205, 1989.
61. Park YS, Kim JH, Jacobson KB, Yim JJ: Purification and characterization of 6-pyruvoyl-tetrahydropterin synthase from *Drosophila melanogaster*. *Biochim Biophys Acta* **1038**:186, 1990.
62. Bürgisser D, Thöny B, Redweik U, Hess D, Heizmann CW, Huber R, Nar H: 6-Pyruvoyl tetrahydropterin synthase, an enzyme with a novel type of active site involving both zinc binding and an intersubunit catalytic triad motif: Site-directed mutagenesis of the proposed active center, characterization of the metal binding site and modeling of substrate binding. *J Mol Biol* **253**:358, 1995.
62a. Ploom T, Thöny B, Yin J, Lee S, Nar H, Leimbacher W, Richardson J, Huber R, Auerbach G: Crystallographic and Kinetic Investigations on the Mechanism of 6-Pyruvoyl Tetrahydropterin Synthase. *J Mol Biol* **206**:851 1999.
63. Bürgisser DM, Thöny B, Redweik U, Hunziker P, Heizmann CW, Blau N: Expression and characterization of recombinant human and rat liver 6-pyruvoyl tetrahydropterin synthase: Modified cysteine residues inhibit the enzyme activity. *Eur J Biochem* **219**:497, 1994.
64. Inoue Y, Kawasaki Y, Harada T, Hatakeyama K, Kagamiyama H: Purification and cDNA cloning of rat 6-pyruvoyl-tetrahydropterin synthase. *J Biol Chem* **266**:20791, 1991.
65. Oppliger T, Thöny B, Nar H, Bürgisser D, Huber R, Heizmann CW, Blau N: Structural and functional consequences of mutations in 6-pyruvoyltetrahydropterin synthase causing hyperphenylalaninemia in humans: Phosphorylation is a requirement for in vivo activity. *J Biol Chem* **270**:29,498, 1995.
66. Nar H, Huber R, Heizmann CW, Thöny B, Bürgisser D: Three-dimensional structure of 6-pyruvoyl-tetrahydropterin synthase, an enzyme involved in tetrahydrobiopterin synthesis. *EMBO J* **13**:1255, 1994.
67. Thöny B, Leimbacher W, Scherer-Oppliger T, Heizmann CW, Blau N: Molecular analysis of tetrahydrobiopterin deficiency due to 6-pyruvoyl-tetrahydropterin synthase mutations: 2-D gel analysis of the in vivo phosphorylation state, in Pfleiderer W, Rokos H (eds): *Chemistry and Biology of Pteridines and Folates*. Berlin, Blackwell Science, 1997, p 713.
67a. Scherer-Oppliger T, Leimbacher W, Blau N, Thöny B: Serine 19 of Human 6-Pyruvoyltetrahydropterin Synthase Is Phosphorylated by cGMP Protein Kinase II. **274**:31341 1999.
68. Thöny B, Leimbacher W, Bürgisser D, Heizmann CW: Human 6-pyruvoyltetrahydropterin synthase: cDNA cloning and heterologous expression of the recombinant enzyme. *Biochem Biophys Res Commun* **189**:1437, 1992.
69. Kluge C, Leimbacher W, Heizmann CW, Blau N, Thöny B: Isolation of 6-pyruvoyl-tetrahydropterin synthase cDNAs from human brain. *Pteridines* **7**:91, 1996.
70. Kluge C, Brecevic L, Heizmann CW, Blau N, Thöny B: Chromosomal localization, genomic structure and characterization of a single human gene (PTS) and retropseudogene for 6-pyruvoyltetrahydropterin synthase. *Eur J Biochem* **240**:477, 1996.
71. Meyer M, Werner-Felmayer G, Werner ER, Heufler-Tiefenthaler C, Thöny B, Leimbacher W: Characterization of 6-pyruvoyl-tetrahydropterin synthase messenger RNA from human myelomonocytic THP-1 cells, in Pfleiderer W, Rokos H (eds): *Chemistry and Biology of Pteridines and Folates*. Berlin, Blackwell Science, 1997, p 623.
72. Thöny B, Blau N: Mutations in the GTP cyclohydrolase I and 6-pyruvoyl-tetrahydropterin synthase genes. *Hum Mutat* **10**:11, 1997.
72a. Romstad A, Guldberg P, Levy HL, Blau N, Güttler F: Single-step mutation scanning of the 6-pyruvoyl-tetrahydropterin synthase gene in patients with hyperphenylalaninemia. *Clin Chem* **45**:2102 1999.
73. Ashida A, Owada M, Hatakeyama K: A missense mutation (A to G) of 6-pyruvoyltetrahydropterin synthase in tetrahydrobiopterin-deficient form of hyperphenylalaninemia. *Genomics* **24**:408, 1994.
74. Imamura T, Okano Y, Shintaku H, Hase Y, Oura T, Isshiki G: Molecular characterization of 6-pyruvoyl-tetrahydropterin synthase (PTPS) deficiency in Japanese. *Am J Hum Genet* **57**(4 suppl):A180, 1995.
75. Liu TT, Hsiao KJ, Lu SF, Wu SJ, Wu KF, Chiang SH, Liu XQ, et al: Mutation analysis of the 6-pyruvoyl-tetrahydropterin synthase gene in Chinese hyperphenylalaninemia caused by tetrahydrobiopterin synthesis deficiency. *Hum Mutat* **10**:76, 1998.
76. Oppliger T, Thöny B, Kluge C, Matasovic A, Heizmann CW, Ponzone A, Spada M, et al: Identification of mutations causing 6-pyruvoyl-tetrahydropterin synthase deficiency in four Italian families. *Hum Mutat* **10**:25, 1997.
77. Thöny B, Leimbacher W, Blau N, Harvie A, Heizmann CW: Hyperphenylalaninemia due to defects in tetrahydrobiopterin metabolism: Molecular characterization of mutations in 6-pyruvoyl-tetrahydropterin synthase. *Am J Hum Genet* **54**:782, 1994.
77a. Scherer-Oppliger T, Matasovic A, Laufs S, Levy HL, Quackenbush EJ, Blau N, Thony B: Dominant negative allele (N47D) in a compound heterozygote for a variant of 6-pyruvoyltetrahydropterin synthase deficiency causing transient hyperphenylalaninemia. *Human Mutation* **13**:286 1999.
77b. Blau N, Scherer-Oppliger T, Baumer A, Riegel M, Matasovic A, Schinzel A, Jaeken J, et al: Isolated central form of tetrahydrobiopterin deficiency associated with hemizygosity on chromosome 11q and a mutant allele of PTPS. *Human Mutat* 16:54, 2000.
78. Yoo HW, Kim GH: Identification of mutations in Korean patients with atypical PKU caused by 6-pyruvoyl-tetrahydropterin synthase deficiency. *Am J Hum Genet* **61**(suppl):A397, 1997.
79. Citron BA, Milstien S, Gutierrez JC, Levine RA, Yanak BL, Kaufman S: Isolation and expression of rat liver sepiapterin reductase cDNA. *Proc Natl Acad Sci USA* **87**:6436, 1990.
80. Oyama R, Katoh S, Sueoka T, Suzuki M, Ichinose H, Nagatsu T, Titani K: The complete amino acid sequence of the mature form of rat sepiapterin reductase. *Biochem Biophys Res Commun* **173**:627, 1990.

81. Ichinose H, Katoh S, Sueoka T, Titani K, Fujita K, Nagatsu T: Cloning and sequencing of cDNA encoding human sepiapterin reductase: An enzyme involved in tetrahydrobiopterin biosynthesis. *Biochem Biophys Res Commun* **179**:183, 1991.
82. Auerbach G, Herrmann A, Gütlich M, Fischer M, Jacob U, Bacher A, Huber R: The 1.25 A crystal structure of sepiapterin reductase reveals its binding mode to pterins and brain neurotransmitters. *EMBO J* **16**:7219, 1997.
82a. Lee SW, Park IY, Hahn Y, Lee JE, Seong CS, Chung JH, Park YS: Cloning of mouse sepiapterin reductase gene and characterization of its promoter region. *Biochim Biophys Acta* **1445**:165 1999.
82b. Ohye T, Hori T, Katoh S, Nagatsu T, Ichinose H: Genomic Organization and Chromosomal Localization of the Human Sepipterin Reductase Gene. *Biochem Biophys Res. Comm.* **251**:597 1988.
83. Katoh S, Sueoka T, Yamamoto Y, Takahashi SY: Phosphorylation by Ca^{2+}/calmodulin-dependent protein kinase-II and protein kinase-C of sepiapterin reductase, the terminal enzyme in the biosynthetic pathway of tetrahydrobiopterin. *FEBS Lett* **341**:227, 1994.
84. Katoh S, Sueoka T, Yamada S: Direct inhibition of brain sepiapterin reductase by a catecholamine and an indoleamine. *Biochem Biophys Res Commun* **105**:75, 1982.
85. Milstien S, Kaufman S: The biosynthesis of tetrahydrobiopterin in rat brain. Purification and characterization of 6-pyruvoyl tetrahydropterin (2′-oxo)reductase. *J Biol Chem* **264**:8066, 1989.
86. Park YS, Heizmann CW, Wermuth B, Levine RA, Steinerstauch P, Guzman J, Blau N: Human carbonyl and aldose reductases: New catalytic functions in tetrahydrobiopterin biosynthesis. *Biochem Biophys Res Commun* **175**:738, 1991.
87. Nichol CA, Lee CL, Edelstein MP, Chao JY, Duch DS: Biosynthesis of tetrahydrobiopterin by de novo and salvage pathways in adrenal medulla extracts, mammalian cell cultures, and rat brain in vivo. *Proc Natl Acad Sci USA* **80**:1546, 1983.
88. Huang CY, Max EE, Kaufman S: Purification and characterization of phenylalanine hydroxylase-stimulating protein from rat liver. *J Biol Chem* **248**:4235, 1973.
89. Hauer CR, Rebrin I, Thony B, Neuheiser F, Curtius HC, Hunziker P, Blau N, et al: Phenylalanine hydroxylase-stimulating protein/pterin-4 α-carbinolamine dehydratase from rat and human liver: Purification, characterization, and complete amino acid sequence. *J Biol Chem* **268**:4828, 1993.
90. Davis MD, Kaufman S, Milstien S: Distribution of 4α-hydroxytetrahydropterin dehydratase in rat tissues: Comparison with the aromatic amino acid hydroxylases. *FEBS Lett* **302**:73, 1992.
91. Schallreuter KU, Wood JM, Ziegler I, Lemke KR, Pittelkow MR, Lindsey NJ, Gutlich M: Defective tetrahydrobiopterin and catecholamine biosynthesis in the depigmentation disorder vitiligo. *Biochim Biophys Acta* **1226**:181, 1994.
92. Lei XD, Woodworth CD, Johnen G, Kaufman S: Expression of 4alpha-carbinolamine dehydratase in human epidermal keratinocytes. *Biochem Biophys Res Commun* **238**:556, 1997.
93. Lei XD, Kaufman S: Human white blood cells and hair follicles are good sources of mRNA for the pterin carbinolamine dehydratase/dimerization cofactor of HNF1 for mutation detection. *Biochem Biophys Res Commun* **248**:432, 1998.
94. Rebrin I, Bailey SW, Ayling JE: Activity of the bifunctional protein 4α-hydroxy-tetrahydropterin dehydratase/DCoH during human fetal development: Correlation with dihydropteridine reductase activity and tetrahydrobiopterin levels. *Biochem Biophys Res Commun* **217**:958, 1995.
95. Ficner R, Sauer UH, Stier G, Suck D: Three-dimensional structure of the bifunctional protein PCD/DCoH, a cytoplasmic enzyme interacting with transcription factor HNF1. *EMBO J* **14**:2034, 1995.
96. Endrizzi JA, Cronk JD, Wang WD, Crabtree GR, Alber T: Crystal structure of DCoH, a bifunctional, protein-binding transcriptional coactivator. *Science* **268**:556, 1995.
97. Cronk JD, Endrizzi JA, Alber T: High-resolution structures of the bifunctional enzyme and transcriptional coactivator DCoH and its complex with a product analogue. *Protein Sci* **5**:1963, 1996.
98. Köster S, Stier G, Ficner R, Hölzer M, Curtius H-C, Suck D, Ghisla S: Location of the active site and proposed catalytic mechanism of pterin-4α-carbinolamine dehydratase. *Eur J Biochem* **241**:858, 1996.
99. Citron BA, Kaufman S, Milstien S, Naylor EW, Greene CL, Davis MD: Mutation in the 4α-carbinolamine dehydratase gene leads to mild hyperphenylalaninemia with defective cofactor metabolism. *Am J Hum Genet* **53**:768, 1993.
100. Thöny B, Heizmann CW, Mattei MG: Chromosomal location of two human genes encoding tetrahydrobiopterin-metabolizing enzymes: 6-pyruvoyl-tetrahydropterin synthase maps to 11q22.3-q23.3, and pterin-4α-carbinolamine dehydratase maps to 10q22. *Genomics* **19**:365, 1994.
101. Thöny B, Neuheiser F, Blau N, Heizmann CW: Characterization of the human PCBD gene encoding the bifunctional protein pterin-4α-carbinolamine dehydratase/dimerization cofactor for the transcription factor HNF-1 alpha. *Biochem Biophys Res Commun* **210**:966, 1995.
102. Thöny B, Neuheiser F, Kierat L, Blaskovics M, Arn AH, Ferreira P, Rebrin I, et al: Hyperphenylalaninemia with high levels of 7-biopterin is associated with mutations in the PCBD gene encoding the bifunctional protein pterin-4α-carbinolamine dehydratase (PCD) and transcriptional coactivator (DCoH). *Am J Hum Genet* **62**:1302, 1998.
103. Thöny B, Neuheiser F, Kierat L, Rolland MO, Guibaud P, Schlüter T, Germann R, et al: Mutations in the pterin-4α-carbinolamine dehydratase gene cause a benign form of hyperphenylalaninemia. *Hum Genet* **103**:162, 1998.
104. Mendel DB, Khavari PA, Conley PB, Graves MK, Hansen LP, Admon A, Crabtree GR: Characterisation of a cofactor that regulates dimerization of mammalian homeodomain protein. *Science* **254**:1762, 1991.
105. Hansen LP, Crabtree GR: Regulation of the HNF-1 homeodomain proteins by DCOH. *Curr Opin Genet Dev* **3**:246, 1993.
106. Suck D, Ficner R: Structure and function of PCD/DCoH, an enzyme with regulatory properties. *FEBS Letters* **389**:35, 1996.
107. Zhao G, Xia T, Song J, Jensen RA: *Pseudomonas aeruginosa* possesses homologues of mammalian phenylalanine hydroxylase and 4α-carbinolamine dehydratase/DCoH as part of a three-component gene cluster. *Proc Natl Acad Sci USA* **91**:1366, 1994.
108. Craine JE, Hall ES, Kaufman S: The isolation and characterisation of dihydropteridine reductase from sheep liver. *J Biol Chem* **247**:6082, 1972.
109. Pollock RJ, Kaufman S: Dihydropteridine reductase may function in tetrahydrofolate metabolism. *J Neurochem* **31**:115, 1978.
110. Kaufman S, Holtzman NA, Milstien S, Butler LJ, Krumholz A: Phenylketonuria due to a deficiency of dihydropteridine reductase. *N Engl J Med* **293**:785, 1975.
111. Milstien S, Holtzman NA, O'Flynn ME, Thomas GH, Butler IJ, Kaufman S: Hyperphenylalaninemia due to dihydropteridine reductase deficiency: Assay of the enzyme in fibroblasts from affected infants, heterozygotes, and in normal amniotic fluid cells. *J Pediatr* **89**:763, 1976.
112. Firgaira FA, Cotton RG, Danks DM: Dihydropteridine reductase deficiency diagnosis by assays on peripheral blood-cells. *Lancet* **2**:1260, 1979.
113. Narisawa K, Arai N, Ishizawa S, Ogasawara Y, Onuma A, Iinuma K, Tada K: Dihydropteridine reductase deficiency: Diagnosis by leukocyte enzyme assay. *Clin Chim Acta* **105**:335, 1980.
114. Narisawa K, Arai N, Hayakawa H, Tada K: Diagnosis of dihydropteridine reductase deficiency by erythrocyte enzyme assay. *Pediatrics* **68**:591, 1981.
115. Abelson HT, Gorka C, Beardsley GP: Identification of dihydropteridine reductase in human platelets. *Blood* **53**:116, 1979.
116. Shen RS, Abell CW: Purification of dihydropteridine reductase from human platelets. *J Neurosci Res* **6**:193, 1981.
117. Firgaira FA, Cotton RGH, Danks DM: Isolation and characterisation of dihydropteridine reductase from human liver. *Biochem J* **197**:31, 1981.
118. Firgaira FA, Choo KH, Cotton RGH, Danks DM: Molecular and immunological comparison of human dihydropteridine reductase in liver, cultured fibroblasts, and continuous lymphoid cells. *Biochem J* **197**:45, 1981.
119. Danks DM, Schlesinger P, Firgaira F, Cotton RG, Watson BM, Rembold H, Hennings G: Malignant hyperphenylalaninemia: Clinical features, biochemical findings, and experience with administration of biopterins. *Pediatr Res* **13**:1150, 1979.
120. Varughese KI, Skinner MM, Whiteley JM, Matthews DA, Xuong NH: Crystal structure of rat liver dihydropteridine reductase. *Proc Natl Acad Sci USA* **89**:6080, 1992.
121. Varughese KI, Xuong NH, Kiefer PM, Matthews DA, Whiteley JM: Structural and mechanistic characteristics of dihydropteridine reductase: A member of the Tyr-(Xaa)(3)-Lys-containing family of reductases and dehydrogenases. *Proc Natl Acad Sci USA* **91**:5582, 1994.

122. Grimshaw CE, Matthews DA, Varughese KI, Skinner M, Xuong NH, Bray T, Hoch J, et al: Characterisation and nucleotide binding properties of a mutant dihydropteridine reductase containing an aspartate 37-isoleucine replacement. *J Biol Chem* **267**:15,334, 1992.
123. Kiefer PM, Varughese KI, Su Y, Xuong NH, Chang CF, Gupta P, Bray T, et al: Altered structural and mechanistic properties of mutant dihydropteridine reductases. *J Biol Chem* **271**:3437, 1996.
124. Dahl HH, Hutchison W, McAdam W, Wake S, Morgan FJ, Cotton RG: Human dihydropteridine reductase: Characterisation of a cDNA clone and its use in analysis of patients with dihydropteridine reductase deficiency. *Nucleic Acids Res* **15**:1921, 1987.
125. Blakeley RL: Eukariotic dihydrofolate reductase. *Adv Enzymol* **70**:23, 1995.
126. Matthews RG, Kaufman S: Characterisation of the dihydropteridine reductase activity of pig liver methylenetetrahdrofolate reductase. *J Biol Chem* **255**:6014, 1980.
127. Dianzani I, De Santis L, Smooker PM, Gough TJ, Alliaudi C, Brusco A, Spada M, et al: Dihydropteridine reductase deficiency: Physical structure of the QDPR gene, identification of two new mutations and genotype-phenotype correlations. *Hum Mutat* **12**:267, 1998.
128. Brown RM, Dahl HH: Localization of the human dihydropteridine reductase gene to band p15.3 of chromosome 4 by in situ hybridization. *Genomics* **1**:67, 1987.
129. Harada T, Kagamiyama H, Hatakeyama K: Feedback regulation mechanisms for the control of GTP cyclohydrolase I activity. *Science* **260**:1507, 1993.
130. Milstien S, Jaffe H, Kowlessur D, Bonner TI: Purification and cloning of the GTP cyclohydrolase I feedback regulatory protein, GFRP. *J Biol Chem* **271**:19743, 1996.
131. Yoneyama T, Brewer JM, Hatakeyama K: GTP cyclohydrolase I feedback regulatory protein is a pentamer of identical subunits: Purification, cDNA cloning, and bacterial expression. *J Biol Chem* **272**:9690, 1997.
132. Hossain MA, Masserano JM, Weiner N: Age-related changes in tetrahydrobiopterin and GTP cyclohydrolase activity in the brain and adrenal gland of rats. *Neurobiol Aging* **16**:627, 1995.
133. Taguchi H, Armarego WLF: Glyceryl-ether monooxygenase [EC 1.14.16.5]: A microsomal enzyme of ether lipid metabolism. *Med Res Rev* **18**:43, 1998.
134. Dashman T, Samuels S, Leshinsky Silver E, Kolodny E, Axelrod F: Tetrahydrobiopterin (BH_4): Cofactor for dopamine beta hydroxylase (D-beta-H). *FASEB J* **11**:A1311, 1997.
135. Kaufman S: New tetrahydrobiopterin-dependent systems. *Annu Rev Nutr* **13**:261, 1993.
136. Smith GK, Duch DS, Edelstein MP, Bigham EC: New inhibitors of sepiapterin reductase: Lack of an effect of intracellular tetrahydrobiopterin depletion upon in vitro proliferation of two human cell lines. *J Biol Chem* **267**:5599, 1992.
137. Anastasiadis PZ, States JC, Imerman BA, Louie MC, Kuhn DM, Levine RA: Mitogenic effects of tetrahydrobiopterin in PC12 cells. *Mol Pharmacol* **49**:149, 1996.
138. Anastasiadis PZ, Bezin L, Imerman BA, Kuhn DM, Louie MC, Levine RA: Tetrahydrobiopterin as a mediator of PC12 cell proliferation induced by EGF and NGF. *Eur J Neurosci* **9**:1831, 1997.
139. Schallreuter KU, Wood JM, Korner C, Harle KM, Schulz-Douglas V, Werner ER: 6-Tetrahydrobiopterin functions as a UVB-light switch for de novo melanogenesis. *Biochim Biophys Acta* **1382**:339, 1998.
140. Koshimura K, Miwa S, Watanabe Y: Dopamine-releasing action of 6R-L-erythro-tetrahydrobiopterin: Analysis of its action site using sepiapterin. *J Neurochem* **63**:649, 1994.
141. Tani Y, Ishihara T, Kanai T, Ohno T, Andersson J, Lilja A, Antoni G, et al: Effects of 6r-L-erythro-5,6,7,8-tetrahydrobiopterin on the dopaminergic and cholinergic receptors as evaluated by positron emission tomography in the rhesus monkey. *J Neural Transm* **102**:189, 1995.
142. Shiraki T, Koshimura K, Kobayashi S, Miwa S, Masaki T, Watanabe Y, Murakami Y, et al: Stimulating effect of 6R-tetrahydrobiopterin on Ca^{2+} channels in neurons of rat dorsal motor nucleus of the vagus. *Biochem Biophys Res Commun* **221**:181, 1996.
143. Perez-Sala D, Diaz-Cazorla M, Ros J, Jimenez W, Lamas S: Tetrahydrobiopterin modulates cyclooxygenase-2 expression in human mesangial cells. *Biochem Biophys Res Commun* **241**:7, 1997.
144. Kojima S, Ona S, Iizuka I, Arai T, Mori H, Kubota K: Antioxidative activity of 5,6,7,8-tetrahydrobiopterin and its inhibitory effect on paraquat-induced cell toxicity in cultured rat hepatocytes. *Free Radic Res* **23**:419, 1995.
145. Schallreuter KU, Zschiesche M, Moore J, Panske A, Hibberts NA, Herrmann FH, Metelmann HR, et al: In vivo evidence for compromised phenylalanine metabolism in vitiligo. *Biochem Biophys Res Commun* **243**:395, 1998.
146. Schoedon G, Troppmair J, Fontana A, Huber C, Curtius HC, Niederwieser A: Biosynthesis and metabolism of pterins in peripheral blood mononuclear cells and leukemia lines of man and mouse. *Eur J Biochem* **166**:303, 1987.
147. Ziegler I, Hultner L, Egger D, Kempkes B, Mailhammer R, Gillis S, Rodl W: In a concerted action kit ligand and interleukin 3 control the synthesis of serotonin in murine bone marrow-derived mast cells: Up-regulation of GTP cyclohydrolase I and tryptophan 5-monooxygenase activity by the kit ligand. *J Biol Chem* **268**:12,544, 1993.
148. Wachter H, Fuchs D, Hausen A, Reibnegger G, Weiss G, Werner ER, Werner-Felmayer G: *Neopterin: Biochemistry, Methods, Clinical Application.* Berlin, Walter de Gruyter, 1992.
149. Schott K, Yodoi J, Schwulera U, Ziegler I: Control of pteridine biosynthesis in the natural killer-like cell line YT. *Biochem Biophys Res Commun* **176**:1430, 1991.
150. Zhu M, Hirayama K, Kapatos G: Regulation of tetrahydrobiopterin biosynthesis in cultured dopamine neurons by depolarization and cAMP. *J Biol Chem* **269**:11,825, 1994.
151. Hirayama K, Kapatos G: Expression and regulation of rat 6-pyruvoyltetrahydropterin synthase mRNA. *Neurochem Int* **26**:601, 1995.
152. Linschied P, Schaffner A, Blau N, Schoedon G: Regulation of 6-pyruvoyl-tetrahydropterin synthase activity and messenger RNA abundance in human vascular endothelial cells. *Circulation* **98**:1703, 1998.
153. Tada K, Yoshida T, Mochizuku K, Konno T, Nakagawa H, Yokoyama Y, Takada G, et al: Two siblings with hyperphenylalaninemia: Suggestion to a genetic variant of phenylketonuria. *Tohoku J Exp Med* **100**:249, 1969.
154. Tada K, Narisawa K, Arai N, Ogasawara Y, Ishizawa S: A sibling case of hyperphenylalaninemia due to a deficiency of dihydropteridine reductase: Biochemical and pathological findings. *Tohoku J Exp Med* **132**:123, 1980.
155. Smith I: Atypical phenylketonuria accompanied by a severe progressive neurological illness unresponsive to dietary treatment. *Arch Dis Child* **49**:245, 1974.
156. Bartholomé K: A new molecular defect in phenylketonuria. *Lancet* **2**:1580, 1974.
157. Smith I, Clayton BE, Wolff OH: New variant of phenylketonuria with progressive neurological illness unresponsive to phenylalanine restriction. *Lancet* **1**:1108, 1975.
158. Bartholomé K, Lutz P, Bickel H: Determination of phenylalanine hydroxylase activity in patients with phenylketonuria and hyperphenylalaninemia. *Pediatr Res* **9**:899, 1975.
159. Bartholomé K, Byrd DJ, Kaufman S, Milstien S: Atypical phenylketonuria with normal phenylalanine hydroxylase and dihydropteridine reductase activity in vitro. *Pediatrics* **59**:757, 1977.
160. Brewster TG, Abroms IF, Kaufman S, Breslow JL, Moskowitz MA, Villee DB, Snodgrass RS: Atypical PKU, seizures, and developmental delay with dihydropteridine reductase deficiency. *Pediatr Res* **10**:446, 1976.
161. Butler IJ, Holtzman NA, Kaufman S, Koslow SH, Krumholz A: Phenylketonuria due to deficiency of dihydropteridine reductase. *Pediatr Res* **9**:349, 1975.
162. Danks DM, Cotton RG, Schlesinger P: Tetrahydrobiopterin treatment of variant form of phenylketonuria. *Lancet* **2**:1043, 1975.
163. Danks DM, Cotton RG, Schlesinger P: Variant forms of phenylketonuria. *Lancet* **1**:1236, 1976.
164. Rey F, Blandin Savoja F, Rey J: Atypical phenylketonuria with normal dihydropteridine reductase activity. *N Engl J Med* **295**:1138, 1976.
165. Danks DM: Pteridines and phenylketonuria: Report of a workshop— Introductory comments. *J Inherited Metab Dis* **1**:47, 1987.
166. Bartholomé K, Byrd DJ: L-Dopa and 5-hydroxytryptophan therapy in phenylketonuria with normal phenylalanine-hydroxylase activity. *Lancet* **2**:1042, 1975.
167. Butler IJ, O'Flynn ME, Seifert W Jr, Howell RR: Neurotransmitter defects and treatment of disorders of hyperphenylalaninemia. *J Pediatr* **98**:729, 1981.

168. Endres W, Niederwieser A, Curtius HC, Wang M, Ohrt B, Schaub J: Atypical phenylketonuria due to biopterin deficiency: Early treatment with tetrahydrobiopterin and neurotransmitter precursors, trials of monotherapy. *Helv Paediatr Acta* **37**:489, 1982.
169. Endres W, Niederwieser A, Curtius HC, Ohrt B, Schaub J: Dihydrobiopterin deficiency: Monotherapy with tetrahydrobiopterin (BH_4) and diacetyl BH_4. *Pediatr Res* **16**:694, 1982.
170. Kaufman S, Kapatos G, McInnes RR, Schulman JD, Rizzo WB: Use of tetrahydropterins in the treatment of hyperphenylalaninemia due to defective synthesis of tetrahydrobiopterin: Evidence that peripherally administered tetrahydropterins enter the brain. *Pediatrics* **70**:376, 1982.
171. McInnes RR, Kaufman S, Warsh JJ, Van Loon GR, Milstien S, Kapatos G, Soldin S, et al: Biopterin synthesis defect: Treatment with L-dopa and 5-hydroxytryptophan compared with therapy with a tetrahydropterin. *J Clin Invest* **73**:458, 1984.
172. Niederwieser A, Curtius HC, Wang M, Leupold D: Atypical phenylketonuria with defective biopterin metabolism: Monotherapy with tetrahydrobiopterin or sepiapterin, screening and study of biosynthesis in man. *Eur J Pediatr* **138**:110, 1982.
173. Schaub J, Daumling S, Curtius HC, Niederwieser A, Bartholome K, Viscontini M, Schircks B, et al: Tetrahydrobiopterin therapy of atypical phenylketonuria due to defective dihydrobiopterin biosynthesis. *Arch Dis Child* **53**:674, 1978.
174. Blau N, Thöny B, Heizmann CW, Dhondt JL: Tetrahydrobiopterin deficiency: From phenotype to genotype. *Pteridines* **4**:1, 1993.
175. Smith I, Dhondt JL: Birthweight in patients with defective biopterin metabolism. *Lancet* **1**:818, 1985.
176. Dhondt JL: Tetrahydrobiopterin deficiencies: Lessons from the compilation of 200 patients. *Dev Brain Disfunct* **6**:139, 1993.
177. Blau N, Barnes I, Dhondt JL: International database of tetrahydrobiopterin deficiencies. *J Inherited Metab Dis* **19**:8, 1996.
178. Blau N, Dhondt JL: BIODEF: International Database of Tetrahydrobiopterin Deficiencies. http://www.bh4.org/biodef1.html, 1998.
178a. De Sanctis L, Alliaudi C, Spada M, Farrugia R, Cerone R, Bisucci G, Meli C, Zammarchi E, Coskun T, Blau N, Ponzone A, Dianzani I: Genotype-phenotype correlation in dihydropteridine reductase deficiency. *J Inher Metab Dis* **23**:333 2000.
179. Blau N, Heizmann CW, Sperl W, Korenke GC, Hoffmann GF, Smooker PM, Cotton RGH: Atypical (mild) forms of dihydropteridine reductase deficiency: Neurochemical evaluation and mutation detection. *Pediatr Res* **32**:726, 1992.
180. Dhondt JL, Guibaud P, Rolland MO, Dorché C, André S, Forzy G, Hayte JM: Neonatal hyperphenylalaninaemia presumably caused by a new variant of biopterin synthetase deficiency. *Eur J Pediatr* **147**:153, 1988.
181. Blaskovics M, Giudici TA: A new variant of biopterin deficiency. *N Engl J Med* **319**:1611, 1988.
182. Dhondt JL: Strategy for the screening of tetrahydrobiopterin deficiency among hyperphenylalaninaemic patients: 15-years experience. *J Inherited Metab Dis* **14**:117, 1991.
183. Blau N, Thöny B, Spada M, Ponzone A: Tetrahydrobiopterin and inherited hyperphenylalaninemias. *Turk J Pediatr* **38**:19, 1996.
184. Michelson D, Page SW, Casey R, Trucksess MW, Love LA, Milstien S, Wilson C, et al: An eosinophilia-myalgia syndrome related disorder associated with exposure to L-5-hydroxytryptophan. *J Rheumatol* **21**:2261, 1994.
185. Fukushima T, Nixon JC: Analysis of reduced forms of biopterin in biological tissues and fluids. *Anal Biochem* **102**:176, 1980.
186. Dhondt JL, Largilliere C, Ardouin P, Farriaux JP, Dautrevaux M: Diagnosis of variants of hyperphenylalaninemia by determination of pterins in urine. *Clin Chim Acta* **110**:205, 1981.
187. Hyland K, Howells DW: Analysis and clinical significance of pterins. *J Chromatogr* **429**:95, 1988.
188. Curtius HC, Blau N, Kuster T: Pterins, in Hommes FA (ed): *Techniques in Diagnostic Human Biochemical Genetics*. New York, Wiley-Liss, 1991, p 377.
189. Niederwieser A, Curtius HC, Gitzelmann R, Otten A, Baerlocher K, Blehova B, Berlow S, et al: Excretion of pterins in phenylketonuria and phenylketonuria variants. *Helv Paediatr Acta* **35**:335, 1980.
190. Howells DW, Smith I, Hyland K: Estimation of tetrahydrobiopterin and other pterins in cerebrospinal fluid using reversed-phase high-performance liquid chromatography with electrochemical and fluorescence detection. *J Chromatogr* **381**:285, 1986.
191. Tani Y, Ishihara T: Simultaneous measurement of tetrahdrobiopterin (THBP) and biogenic amines by liquid chromatography with electrochemical detection. *Life Sci* **46**:373, 1990.
192. Xie FM, Kissinger PT, Niwa O: Determination of tetrahydrobiopterin and its analogues in biological samples by microbore liquid chromatography. *J Liquid Chromatogr Related*[AU90] *Technol* **20**:825, 1997.
193. Narisawa K, Hayakawa H, Arai N, Matsuo N, Tanaka T, Naritomi K, Tada K: Diagnosis of variant forms of hyperphenylalaninemia using filter paper spots of urine. *J Pediatr* **103**:577, 1983.
194. Blau N, Kierat L, Heizmann CW, Endres W, Giudici T, Wang M: Screening for tetrahydrobiopterin deficiency in newborns using dried urine on filter paper. *J Inherited Metab Dis* **15**:402, 1992.
195. Leeming RJ, Barford PA, Blair JA, Smith I: Blood spots on Guthrie cards can be used for inherited tetrahydrobiopterin deficiency screening in hyperphenylalaninaemic infants. *Arch Dis Child* **59**:58, 1984.
196. Leeming RJ, Hall SK, Friday H, Hurley P, Green A: A microtitre plate method for measuring biopterin with cryopreserved *Crithidia fasciculata*, in Ayling JE, Nair MG, Baugh CM (eds): *Chemistry and Biology of Pteridines and Folates*. New York, Plenum, 1993, p 267.
197. Dhondt JL, Farriaux JP, Largilliere C, Dautrevaux M, Ardouin P: Pterin metabolism in normal subjects and hyperphenylalaninaemic patients. *J Inherited Metab Dis* **4**:47, 1981.
198. Dhondt JL, Ardouin P, Hayte JM, Farriaux JP: Developmental aspects of pteridine metabolism and relationships with phenylalanine metabolism. *Clin Chim Acta* **116**:143, 1981.
199. Leeming RJ, Hall SK, Surplice IM, Green A: Relationship between plasma and red cell biopterins in acute and chronic hyperphenylalaninaemia. *J Inherited Metab Dis* **13**:883, 1990.
200. Ponzone A, Guardamagna O, Spada M, Ponzone R, Sartore M, Kierat L, Heizmann CW, et al: Hyperphenylalaninemia and pterin metabolism in serum and erythrocytes. *Clin Chim Acta* **216**:63, 1993.
201. Arai N, Narisawa K, Hayakawa H, Tada K: Hyperphenylalaninemia due to dihydropteridine reductase deficiency: Diagnosis by enzyme assays on dried blood spots. *Pediatrics* **70**:426, 1982.
202. Surplice IM, Griffiths PD, Green A, Leeming RJ: Dihydropteridine reductase activity in eluates from dried blood spots: Automation of an assay for a national screening service. *J Inherited Metab Dis* **13**:169, 1990.
203. Niederwieser A, Curtius HC, Viscontini M, Schaub J, Schmidt H: Phenylketonuria variants. *Lancet* **1**:550, 1979.
204. Lipson A, Yu J, O'Halloran M, Potter M, Wilken B: Dihydropteridine reductase deficiency: Non-response to oral tetrahydrobiopterin load test. *J Inherited Metab Dis* **7**:69, 1984.
205. Cotton RGH, Jennings I, Bracco G, Ponzone A, Guardamagna O: Tetrahydrobiopterin non-responsiveness in dihydropteridine reductase deficiency is associated with the presence of mutant protein. *J Inherited Metab Dis* **9**:239, 1986.
206. Ponzone A, Guardamagna O, Ferraris S, Bracco G, Cotton RG: Screening for malignant phenylketonuria. *Lancet* **1**:512, 1987.
207. Kaufman S: Phenylketonuria and its variants. *Adv Hum Genet* **13**:217, 1983.
208. Ponzone A, Guardamagna O, Spada M, Ferraris S, Ponzone R, Kierat L, Blau N: Differential diagnosis of hyperphenylalaninemia by a combined phenylalanine-tetrahydrobiopterin loading test. *Eur J Pediatr* **152**:655, 1993.
209. Ponzone A, Guardamagna O, Dianzani I, Ponzone R, Ferrero GB, Spada M, Cotton RGH: Catalytic activity of tetrahydrobiopterin in dihydropteridine reductase deficiency and indications for treatment. *Pediatr Res* **33**:125, 1993.
210. Endres W, Ibel H, Kierat L, Blau N, Curtius HC: Tetrahydrobiopterin and "non-responsive" dihydropteridine reductase deficiency. *Lancet* **2**:223, 1987.
211. Blau N, Kierat L, Curtius HC, Blaskovics M, Giudici T: Hyperphenylalaninaemia presumably due to carbinolamine dehydratase deficiency: Loading tests with pterin derivatives. *J Inherited Metab Dis* **15**:409, 1992.
212. Blau N, Beck M, Matern D: Tetrahydrobiopterin induced neonatal tyrosinaemia. *Eur J Pediatr* **155**:832, 1996.
213. Ponzone A, Guardamagna O, Ferraris S, Ferrero GB, Blau N, Curtius HC, Kierat L, et al: Heterogeneity of tetrahydrobiopterin deficiency: Combined phenylalanine-tetrahydrobiopterin loading test, in Curtius HC, Ghisla S, Blau N (eds): *Chemistry and Biology of Pteridines 1989*. Berlin, Walter de Gruyter, 1990, p 414.
214. Ponzone A, Ferraris S, Spada M, Blau N, Piovan S, Burlina AB: Combined phenylalanine-tetrahydrobiopterin loading test in GTP cyclohydrolase I deficiency. *Eur J Pediatr* **153**:616, 1994.

215. Blau N, Hoffmann GF: Differential diagnosis of disorders of biogenic amines metabolism. *Eur J Pediatr Neurol* **2**:219, 1998.
216. Koslow SH, Butler IJ: Biogenic amine synthesis defect in dihydropteridine reductase deficiency. *Science* **198**:522, 1977.
217. Butler IJ, Koslow SH, Krumholz A, Holtzman NA, Kaufman S: A disorder of biogenic amines in dihydropteridine reductase deficiency. *Ann Neurol* **3**:224, 1978.
218. Smith I, Hyland K, Kendall B: Clinical role of pteridine therapy in tetrahydrobiopterin deficiency. *J Inherited Metab Dis* **8**:39, 1985.
219. Hyland K, Heales SJR: Tetrahydrobiopterin and quinonoid dihydrobiopterin concentrations in CSF from patients with dihydropteridine reductase deficiency. *J Inherited Metab Dis* **16**:608, 1993.
220. Sawada Y, Shintaku H, Isshiki G: Pteridine values in cerebrospinal fluid in sick children, in Wachter H, Curtius HC, Pfleiderer W (eds): *Biochemical and Clinical Aspects of Pteridines*. Berlin, Walter de Gruyter, 1985, p 635.
221. Hyland K, Surtees RAH, Heales SJR, Bowron A, Howells DW, Smith I: Cerebrospinal fluid concentrations of pterins and metabolites of serotonin and dopamine in a pediatric reference population. *Pediatr Res* **34**:10, 1993.
222. Blau N, Blaskovics M: Hyperphenylalaninemia, in Blau N, Duran M, Blaskovics M (eds): *Physician's Guide to the Laboratory Diagnosis of Metabolic Diseases*. London, Chapman and Hall, 1996, p 65.
223. Kaufman S: Some metabolic relationships between biopterin and folate: Implications for the "methyl trap hypothesis." *Neurochem Res* **16**:1031, 1991.
224. Irons M, Levy HL, O'Flynn ME, Stack CV, Langlais PJ, Butler IJ, Milstien S, et al: Folinic acid therapy in treatment of dihydropteridine reductase deficiency. *J Pediatr* **110**:61, 1987.
225. Woody RC, Brewster MA, Glasier C: Progressive intracranial calcification in dihydropteridine reductase deficiency prior to folinic acid therapy. *Neurology* **39**:673, 1989.
226. Hyland K, Surtees R: Measurement of 5-methyltetrahydrofolate in cerebrospinal fluid using HPLC with coulometric electrochemical detection. *Pteridines* **3**:149, 1992.
227. Niederwieser A, Blau N, Wang M, Joller P, Atares M, Cardesa-Garcia J: GTP cyclohydrolase I deficiency, a new enzyme defect causing hyperphenylalaninemia with neopterin, biopterin, dopamine, and serotonin deficiencies and muscular hypotonia. *Eur J Pediatr* **141**:208, 1984.
228. Naylor EW, Ennis D, Davidson AG, Wong LT, Applegarth DA, Niederwieser A: Guanosine triphosphate cyclohydrolase I deficiency: Early diagnosis by routine urine pteridine screening. *Pediatrics* **79**:374, 1987.
229. Dhondt JL, Farriaux JP, Boudha A, Largilliere C, Ringel J, Roger MM, Leeming RJ: Neonatal hyperphenylalaninemia presumably caused by guanosine triphosphate-cyclohydrolase deficiency. *J Pediatr* **106**:954, 1985.
230. Matalon R, Michals K, Blau N, Rouse B: Hyperphenylalaninemia due to inherited deficiencies of tetrahydrobiopterin. *Adv Pediatr* **36**:67, 1989.
230a. Coskun T, Karagöz T, Kalkanoglu S, Tokatli A, Özalp I, Thöny B,Blau N: Guanosine triphosphate cyclohydrolase I deficiency. A rare cause of hyperphenylalainemia. *Tur J Pediatr* **41**:231, 1999.
231. Blau N, Thöny B, Dianzani I: BIOMDB: Database of Mutations Causing Tetrahydrobiopterin Deficiency. http://www.bh4.org.
232. Blau N, Niederwieser A: Guanosine triphosphate cyclohydrolase I assay in human and rat liver using high-performance liquid chromatography of neopterin phosphates and guanine nucleotides. *Anal Biochem* **128**:446, 1983.
233. Blau N, Joller P, Atares M, Cardesa-Garcia J, Niederwieser A: Increase of GTP cyclohydrolase I activity in mononuclear blood cells by stimulation: Detection of heterozygotes of GTP cyclohydrolase I deficiency. *Clin Chim Acta* **148**:47, 1985.
234. Werner ER, Werner-Felmayer G, Fuchs D, Hausen A, Reibnegger G, Wachter H: Parallel induction of tetrahydrobiopterin biosynthesis and indoleamine 2,3-dioxygenase activity in human cells and cell lines by interferon-gamma. *Biochem J* **262**:861, 1989.
235. Milstien S, Kaufman S, Sakai N: Tetrahydrobiopterin biosynthesis defects examined in cytokine-stimulated fibroblasts. *J Inherited Metab Dis* **16**:975, 1993.
236. Walter JH, Brand M, Bridge C, Heales S: Normal serotonin in a patient with deficient tetrahydrobiopterin synthesis, in *SSIEM Meeting Abstracts Book* 20, 1993.
237. Joller PW, Blau N, Atares M, Niederwieser A: Guanosine-triphosphate cyclohydrolase deficiency: Analysis of the influence on immune parameters in a girl, in Curtius HC, Pfleiderer W, Wachter H (eds): *Biochemical and Clinical Aspects of Pteridines*. Berlin, Walter de Gruyter, 1983, p 167.
238. Hsiao KJ, Liu TT, Wu SJ, Wu KF, Chiang SH: The mutations found in 6-pyruvoyl-tetrahydropterin synthase deficient phenylketonuria, in *Third ISNS Meeting Abstracts*. Boston, 1996, p 63.
239. Liu TT, Hsiao KJ: Identification of a common 6-pyruvoyl-tetrahydropterin synthase mutation at codon 87 in Chinese phenylketonuria caused by tetrahydrobiopterin synthesis deficiency. *Hum Genet* **98**:313, 1996.
240. Krawczak M, Cooper DN: Gene deletions causing human genetic disease: Mechanisms of mutagenesis and the role of the local DNA sequence environment. *Hum Genet* **86**:425, 1991.
241. Liu TT, Lu SF, Hsiao KJ: Genomic structure of 6-pyruvoyl-tetrahydropterin synthase gene and a T/C polymorphism detected in Chinese. *J Biomed Lab Sci* **10**:39, 1998.
242. Hanihara T, Inoue K, Kawanishi C, Sugiyama N, Miyakawa T, Onishi H, Yamada Y, et al: 6-Pyruvoyl-tetrahydropterin synthase deficiency with generalized dystonia and diurnal fluctuation of symptoms: A clinical and molecular study. *Mov Disord* **12**:408, 1997.
243. Yoshioka S, Masada M, Yoshida T, Mizokami T, Akino M, Matsuo N: Atypical phenylketonuria due to biopterin deficiency: Diagnosis by assay of an enzyme involved in the synthesis of sepiapterin from dihydroneopterin triphosphate. *Zool Sci* **1**:74, 1984.
244. Dhondt JL, Cotton RGH, Danks DM: Liver enzyme activities in hyperphenylalaninemia due to a defective synthesis of tetrahydrobiopterin. *J Inherited Metab Dis* **8**:47, 1985.
245. Kerler F, Schwarzkopf B, Katzenmaier G, Le Van Q, Schmid C, Ziegler I, Bacher A: Biosynthesis of tetrahydrobiopterin: A sensitive assay of 6-pyruvoyltetrahydropterin synthase using ($2'$-^{3}H) dihydroneopterin $3'$- triphosphate as substrate. *Biochim Biophys Acta* **990**:15, 1989.
246. Werner ER, Werner-Felmayer G, Fuchs D, Hausen A, Reibnegger G, Wels G, Yim JJ, et al: 6-Pyruvoyl tetrahydropterin synthase assay in extracts of cultured human cells using high-performance liquid chromatography with fluorescence detection of biopterin. *J Chromatogr* **570**:43, 1991.
247. Niederwieser A, Leimbacher W, Curtius HC, Ponzone A, Rey F, Leupold D: Atypical phenylketonuria with "dihydrobiopterin synthetase" deficiency: Absence of phosphate-eliminating enzyme activity demonstrated in liver. *Eur J Pediatr* **144**:13, 1985.
248. Shintaku H, Niederwieser A, Leimbacher W, Curtius HC: Tetrahydrobiopterin deficiency: Assay for 6-pyruvoyl-tetrahydropterin synthase activity in erythrocytes, and detection of patients and heterozygous carriers. *Eur J Pediatr* **147**:15, 1988.
249. Guzman J, Blau N: 6-Pyruvoyl tetrahydropterin synthase in human tissues and cell lines. *Pteridines* **3**:43, 1992.
250. Niederwieser A, Shintaku H, Hasler T, Curtius HC, Lehmann H, Guardamagna O, Schmidt H: Prenatal diagnosis of "dihydrobiopterin synthetase" deficiency, a variant form of phenylketonuria. *Eur J Pediatr* **145**:176, 1986.
251. Hreidasson S, Valle D, Holtzman N, Coyle J, Singer H, Kapatos G, Kaufman S: A peripheral defect in biopterin synthesis: A new mutant? *Pediatr Res* **16**:192a, 1982.
252. Hoganson G, Berlow S, Kaufman S, Milstien S, Schuett V, Matalon R, Naylor E, et al: Biopterin synthesis defects: Problems in diagnosis. *Pediatrics* **74**:1004, 1984.
253. Dhondt JL, Meyer M, Malpuech G: Problems in the diagnosis of tetrahydrobiopterin deficiency. *Eur J Pediatr* **147**:332, 1988.
254. Niederwieser A, Shintaku H, Leimbacher W, Curtius HC, Hyanek J, Zeman J, Endres W: "Peripheral" tetrahydrobiopterin deficiency with hyperphenylalaninaemia due to incomplete 6-pyruvoyl tetrahydropterin synthase deficiency or heterozygosity. *Eur J Pediatr* **146**:228, 1987.
255. Scriver CR, Clow CL, Kaplan P, Niederwieser A: Hyperphenylalaninemia due to deficiency of 6-pyruvoyl tetrahydropterin synthase: Unusual gene dosage effect in heterozygotes. *Hum Genet* **77**:168, 1987.
256. Al-Aqeel A, Ozand PT, Gascon G, Nester M, Al Nasser M, Brismar J, Blau N, et al: Biopterin-dependent hyperphenylalaninemia due to deficiency of 6-pyruvoyl tetrahydropterin synthase. *Neurology* **41**:730, 1991.
257. Allanson J, McInnes R, Bradley L, Tarby T, Naylor E, Nardella M: Combined transient and peripheral defects in tetrahydrobiopterin synthesis. *J Pediatr* **118**:261, 1991.
258. Ponzone A, Blau N, Guardamagna O, Ferrero GB, Dianzani I, Endres W: Progression of 6-pyruvoyl-tetrahydropterin synthase deficiency

from a peripheral into a central phenotype. *J Inherited Metab Dis* **13**:298, 1990.

259. Oppliger T, Thöny B, Leimbacher W, Scheibenreiter S, Brandt NJ, Heizmann CW, Blau N: Mutation analysis in patients with 6-pyruvoyl-tetrahydropterin synthase deficiency. *Pteridines* **6**:141, 1995.
260. Endres W, Niederwieser A, Leimbacher W, Curtius HC: Heterogeneity of tetrahydrobiopterin deficiency due to 6-pyruvoyl tetrahydropterin synthase deficiency, in Nicola P, Ponzone A, Cerutti F (eds): *Juvenile Diabetes, Hyperammonemias, Hyperphenylalaninemias*. Milan, Masson, 1988, p 269.
261. Ozand PT: Hyperphenylalaninemia and defective metabolism of tetrahydrobiopterin, in Nyhan WL, Ozand PT (eds): *Atlas of Metabolic Disease*. London, Chapman and Hall Medical, 1998, p 117.
262. Kaufman S, Berlow S, Summer GK, Milstien S, Schulman JD, Orloff S, Spielberg S, et al: Hyperphenylalaninemia due to a deficiency of biopterin: A variant form of phenylketonuria. *N Engl J Med* **299**:673, 1978.
263. Allen RJ, Young W, Bonacci J, Persico S, Andruszewski K, Schaefer AM: Neonatal dystonic parkinsonism, a "stiff baby syndrome," in biopterin deficiency with hyperprolactinemia detected by newborn screening for hyperphenylalaninemia, and responsiveness to treatment. *Ann Neurol* **28**:434, 1990.
264. Factor SA, Coni RJ, Cowger M, Rosenblum EL: Paroxysmal tremor and orofacial dyskinesia secondary to a biopterin synthesis defect. *Neurology* **41**:930, 1991.
265. Tanaka K, Yoneda M, Nakajima T, Miyatake T, Owada M: Dihydrobiopterin synthesis defect: An adult with diurnal fluctuation of symptoms. *Neurology* **37**:519, 1987.
266. Schulpis KH, Covanis A, Loumakou M, Frantzis N, Papandreou O, Divolli A, Missiou Tsagaraki S, et al: A case of 6-pyruvoyl-tetrahydropterin synthase deficiency after screening 1,500,000 newborns in Greece. *J Inherited Metab Dis* **14**:845, 1991.
267. Curtius HC, Kuster T, Matasovic A, Blau N, Dhondt JL: Primapterin, anapterin, and 6-oxo-primapterin, three new 7-substituted pterins identified in a patient with hyperphenylalaninemia. *Biochem Biophys Res Commun* **153**:715, 1988.
268. Blau N, Curtius HC, Kuster T, Matasovic A, Schoedon G, Dhondt JL, Guibaud P, et al: Primapterinuria: A new variant of atypical phenylketonuria. *J Inherited Metab Dis* **12**:335, 1989.
269. Curtius HC, Matasovic A, Schoedon G, Kuster T, Guibaud P, Giudici T, Blau N: 7-Substituted pterins: A new class of mammalian pteridines. *J Biol Chem* **265**:3923, 1990.
270. Adler C, Curtius HC, Wetzel E, Viscontini M, Giudici TA, Blaskovics M, Rolland MO, et al: Loading experiments with 6R,S-tetrahydro-L-(3′-$^2H_1$)biopterin. *Helv Chim Acta* **75**:1237, 1992.
271. Curtius HC, Adler C, Rebrin I, Heizmann C, Ghisla S: 7-Substituted pterins: Formation during phenylalanine hydroxylation in the absenceof dehydratase. *Biochem Biophys Res Commun* **172**:1060, 1990.
272. Davis MD, Kaufman S, Milstien S: Conversion of 6-substituted tetrahydropterins to 7-isomers via phenylalanine hydroxylase-generated intermediates. *Proc Natl Acad Sci USA* **88**:385, 1991.
273. Citron BA, Davis MD, Milstien S, Gutierrez J, Mendel DB, Crabtree GR, Kaufman S: Identity of 4α-carbinolamine dehydratase, a component of the phenylalanine hydroxylation system, and DCoH, a transregulator of homeodomain proteins. *Proc Natl Acad Sci USA* **89**:11,891, 1992.
274. Thöny B, Neuheiser F, Hauer CR, Heizmann CW: Molecular cloning and recombinant expression of the human liver phenylalanine hydroxylase stimulating factor revealed structural and functional identity to the dimerization cofactor for the nuclear transcription factor HNF-1α. *Adv Exp Med* **338**:103, 1993.
275. Johnen G, Kowlessur D, Citron BA, Kaufman S: Characterization of the wild-type form of 4α-carbinolamine dehydratase and two naturally occurring mutants associated with hyperphenylalaninemia. *Proc Natl Acad Sci USA* **92**:12,384, 1995.
276. Köster S, Thöny B, Macheroux P, Curtius HC, Heizmann CW, Ghisla S: Characterization of human pterin-4α-carbinolamine dehydratase/dimerization cofactor of hepatocyte factor-1α, and of the Cys81-mutant involved in hyperphenylalaninemia. *Pteridines* **6**:123, 1995.
277. Kaufman S: A protein that stimulates rat liver phenylalanine hydroxylase. *J Biol Chem* **254**:4751, 1970.
278. Lazarus RA, Benkovic SJ, Kaufman S: Phenylalanine hydroxylase stimulator protein is a 4α-carbinolamine dehydratase. *J Biol Chem* **258**:10,960, 1983.
279. Blaskovics M, Giudici TA, Blau N: Primapterinuria: A clinical update. *Pteridines* **3**:33, 1992.
280. Adler C, Ghisla S, Rebrin I, Haavik J, Heizmann CW, Blau N, Kuster T, et al: 7-substituted pterins in humans with suspected pterin-4α-carbinolamine dehydratase deficiency: Mechanism of formation via non-enzymatic transformation from 6-substituted pterins. *Eur J Biochem* **208**:139, 1992.
281. Blau N, Kierat L, Matasovic A, Leimbacher W, Heizmann CW, Guardamagna O, Ponzone A: Antenatal diagnosis of tetrahydrobiopterin deficiency by quantification of pterins in amniotic fluid and enzyme activity in fetal and extrafetal tissue. *Clin Chim Acta* **226**:159, 1994.
282. Kaufman S, Milstien S, Bartholome K: New forms of phenylketonuria. *Lancet* **2**:708, 1975.
283. Smooker PM, Cotton RGH: Molecular basis of dihydropteridine reductase deficiency. *Hum Mutat* **5**:279, 1995.
284. Dianzani I, Howells DW, Ponzone A, Saleeba JA, Smooker PM, Cotton RGH: Two novel mutations in the dihydropteridine reductase gene in patients with tetrahydrobiopterin deficiency. *J Med Genet* **30**:465, 1993.
285. Howells DW, Forrest SM, Dahl HH, Cotton RG: Insertion of an extra codon for threonine is a cause of dihydropteridine reductase deficiency. *Am J Hum Genet* **47**:279, 1990.
286. Ikeda H, Matsubara Y, Mikami H, Kure S, Owada M, Gough T, Smooker PM, et al: Molecular analysis of dihydropteridine reductase deficiency: Identification of two novel mutations in Japanese patients. *Hum Genet* **100**:637, 1997.
287. Smooker PM, Howells DW, Cotton RGH: Identification and in vitro expression of mutations causing dihydropteridine reductase deficiency. *Biochemistry* **32**:6443, 1993.
288. Smooker PM, Cotton RGH, Lipson A: Prenatal diagnosis of DHPR deficiency by direct detection of mutation. *Prenat Diagn* **13**:881, 1993.
289. Smooker PM, Christodoulou J, McInnes RR, Cotton RGH: A mutation causing DHPR deficiency results in a frameshift and a secondary splicing defect. *J Med Genet* **32**:220, 1995.
290. Zhang HP, Yang N, Armarego W: In vitro mutagenesis of human dihydropteridine reductase at the active site and at sites found in reductase deficient children. *Pteridines* **7**:126, 1996.
291. Varughese KI, Xuong NH, Whiteley JM: Structural and mechanistic implications of incorporating naturally occurring aberrant mutations of human dihydropteridine reductase into a rat model. *Int J Pept Protein Res* **44**:278, 1994.
292. Dhondt JL: Tetrahydrobiopterin deficiencies: Preliminary analysis from an international survey. *J Pediatr* **104**:501, 1984.
293. Firgaira FA, Choo KH, Cotton RG, Danks DM: Heterogeneity of the molecular defect in human dihydropteridine reductase deficiency. *Biochem J* **198**:677, 1981.
294. Firgaira FA, Cotton RGH, Danks DM: Human dihydropteridine reductase deficiency: Demonstration of $DHPR^-CRM^+$, and $DHPR^-CRM^-$ mutants, in Blair JA (ed): *Chemistry and Biology of Pteridines*. Berlin, Walter de Gruyter, 1983, p 771.
295. Ponzone A, Guardamagna O, Ferraris S, Bracco G, Niederwieser A, Cotton RG: Two mutations of dihydropteridine reductase deficiency. *Arch Dis Child* **63**:154, 1988.
296. Nakabayashi H, Owada M, Kitagawa T: A mild case of dihydropteridine reductase deficiency with residual activity in erythrocytes. *J Inherited Metab Dis* **7**:135, 1984.
297. Grobe H, Bartholome K, Milstien S, Kaufman S: Hyperphenylalaninaemia due to dihydropteridine reductase deficiency. *Eur J Pediatr* **129**:93, 1978.
298. Sahota A, Leeming RJ, Blair JA, Armstrong RA, Green A, Cohen BE: Partial dihydropteridine reductase deficiency and mental retardation. *J Inherited Metab Dis* **9**:247, 1986.
299. Niederwieser A, Ponzone A, Curtius HC: Differential diagnosis of tetrahydrobiopterin deficiency. *J Inherited Metab Dis* **8**(suppl 1):34, 1985.
300. Hyland K, Smith I, Leonard JV: Biopterins in arginase, dihydropteridine reductase and phenylalanine hydroxylase deficiency. *J Neurol Neurosurg Psychiatry* **50**:242, 1987.
301. Hayakawa H, Narisawa K, Arai N, Tada K, Matsuo N, Tanaka T, Naritomi K: Differential diagnosis of variant forms of hyperphenylalaninemia by urinary pterins. *J Inherited Metab Dis* **6**:123, 1983.
302. Milstien S, Kaufman S, Summer GK: Hyperphenylalaninemia due to dihydropteridine reductase deficiency: Diagnosis by measurement of oxidized and reduced pterins in urine. *Pediatrics* **65**:806, 1980.

303. Young JH, Walker V, Tippett PA, Clayton BE: Dihydropteridine reductase deficiency in an 18-year-old boy. *J Inherited Metab Dis* **6**:111, 1983.
304. De Almeida IT, Leandro PP, Portel R, Cabral A, Eusebio F, Tasso T, Matasovic A, et al: Tetrahydrobiopterin deficiency in Portugal: Results of the screening for hyperphenylalaninemia, in Ayling JE, Nair MG, Baugh CM (eds): *Chemistry and Biology of Pteridines and Folates*. New York, Plenum, 1993, p 263.
305. Pogson D: Issues for consideration in dihydropteridine reductase (DHPR) deficiency: A variant form of hyperphenylalaninaemia. *J Intellect Disab Res* **41**(pt 3):208, 1997.
306. Hyland K, Howells DW, Collins JE, Smith I: Methotrexate, and deficiencies of dihydropteridine reductase and phenylalanine hydroxylase: Effects on CSF biopterins in children, in Levine RA, Milstien S, Kuhn DM, Curtius HC (eds): *Pterins and Biogenic Amines in Neuropsychiatry, Pediatrics and Immunology*. Grosse Pointe, MI, Lakeshore, 1989, p 335.
307. Heales SJR, Hyland K: Inhibition of phenylalanine hydroxylase by dihydropterins: A mechanism for impaired aromatic amino acid hydroxylation in dihydropteridine reductase deficiency. *Pteridines* **2**:116, 1990.
308. Nagatsu T, Mitzutani K, Nagatsu I, Matsuura S, Sugimoto T: Pteridines as cofactor or inhibitor of tyrosine hydroxylase. *Biochem Pharmacol* **21**:45, 1972.
309. Goldstein DS, Hahn SH, Holmes C, Tifft C, Harvey-White J, Milstien S, Kaufman S: Monoaminergic effects of folinic acid, L-DOPA, and 5-hydroxytryptophan in dihydropteridine reductase deficiency. *J Neurochem* **64**:2810, 1995.
310. Longhi R, Valsasina R, Butte C, Paccanelli S, Riva E, Giovannini M: Cranial computerized tomography in dihydropteridine reductase deficiency. *J Inherited Metab Dis* **8**:109, 1985.
311. Schmidt H, Ullrich K, Korinthenberg R, Peters PE: Basal ganglion calcification in hyperphenylalaninemia due to deficiency of dihydropteridine reductase. *Pediatr Radiol* **19**:54, 1988.
312. Coskun T, Besim A, Özalp I, Erylimaz M: Intracranial calcifications in dihydropteridine reductase deficiency. *Turk J Pediatr* 32:259, 1990.
313. Takashima S, Chan F, Becker LE: Cortical dysgenesis in a variant of phenylketonuria (dihydropteridine reductase deficiency). *Pediatr Pathol* **11**:771, 1991.
314. Gudinchet F, Maeder P, Meuli RA, Deonna T, Mathieu JM: Cranial CT and MRI in malignant phenylketonuria. *Pediatr Radiol* **22**:223, 1992.
315. Ponzone A, Guardamagna O, Ferraris S, Biasetti S, Bracco G, Niederwieser A: Neurotransmitter therapy and diet in malignant phenylketonuria. *Eur J Pediatr* **146**:93, 1987.
316. Al-Aqeel A, Ozand PT, Gascon G, Hughes H, Reynolds CT, Subramanyan SB: Response of 6-pyruvoyl-tetrahydropterin synthase deficiency to tetrahydrobiopterin. *J Child Neurol* **7**:26, 1992.
317. Kaufman S, Kapatos G, Rizzo WB, Schulman JD, Tamarkin L, Van Loon GR: Tetrahydropterin therapy for hyperphenylalaninemia caused by defective synthesis of tetrahydrobiopterin. *Ann Neurol* **14**:308, 1983.
318. Birnbacher R, Scheibenreiter S, Blau N, Bieglmayer C, Frisch H, Waldhauser F: Hyperprolactinemia: A tool in treatment control of tetrahydrobiopterin deficiency—Endocrine studies in an affected girl. *Pediatr Res* **43**:472, 1998.
319. Tanaka Y, Matsuo N, Tsuzaki S, Araki K, Tsuchiya Y, Niederwieser A: On-off phenomenon in a child with tetrahydrobiopterin deficiency due to 6-pyruvoyl tetrahydropterin synthase deficiency (BH_4 deficiency). *Eur J Pediatr* **148**:450, 1989.
320. Schuler A, Blau N, Ponzone A: Monoamine oxidase inhibitors in tetrahydrobiopterin deficiency. *Eur J Pediatr* **154**:997, 1995.
321. Spada M, Schuler A, Blau N, Ferraris S, Lanza C, Ponzone A: Deprenyl in 6-pyruvoyl tetrahydropterin synthase deficiency. *Pteridines* **5**:144, 1995.
322. Spada M, Blau N, Meli C, Ferrero GB, De Sanctis L, Ferraris S, Ponzone A: Different strategies in the treatment of dihydropteridine reductase deficiency. *Pteridines* **7**:107, 1996.
323. Giugliani R, Da-Costa JC, Dutra-Filho CS, Dutra JC, Pereira MLS, Niederwieser A: Successful therapy of hyperphenylalaninemia due to defective tetrahydrobiopterin metabolism in two siblings. *Rev Bras Genet* **9**:685, 1986.
324. Snyderman SE, Sansaricq C, Pulmones MT: Successful long term therapy of biopterin deficiency. *J Inherited Metab Dis* **10**:260, 1987.
325. Endres W, Blau N, Curtius HC: Differential diagnosis and treatment of tetrahydrobiopterin deficient hyperphenylalaninemia, in Levine RA, Milstien S, Kuhn DM, Curtius HC (eds): *Pterins and Biogenic Amines in Neuropsychiatry, Pediatrics and Immunology*. Grosse Pointe, MI, Lakeshore, 1989, p 317.
326. Al-Aqeel A, Gascon G, Nester M, Ozand P: The treatment of biopterin-dependent PKU by combined use of tetrahydrobiopterin (BH_4) and neurotransmitter precursors. *Neurology* **40**:356, 1990.
327. Hoshiga M, Hatakeyama K, Watanabe M, Shimada M, Kagamiyama H: Autoradiographic distribution of [^{14}C]tetrahydrobiopterin and its developmental change in mice. *J Pharmacol Exp Ther* **267**:971, 1993.
328. Kapatos G, Kaufman S: Peripherally administered reduced pterins do enter the brain. *Science* **212**:955, 1981.
329. Ponzone A, Biasetti S, Ferraris S, Guardamagna O, Curtius HC, Kierat L, Blau N: Differential entrance of tetrahydrobiopterin into the brain of patients with 6-pyruvoyl tetrahydropterin synthase deficiency, in Levine RA, Milstien S, Kuhn DM, Curtius HC (eds): *Pterins and Biogenic Amines in Neuropsychiatry, Pediatrics and Immunology*. Grosse Pointe, MI, Lakeshore, 1989, p 325.
330. Leupold D: Tetrahydrobiopterin monotherapy in two siblings with dihydrobiopterin deficiency, in Wachter H, Curtius HC, Pfleiderer W (eds): *Biochemical and Clinical Aspects of Pteridines*. Berlin, Walter de Gruyter, 1982, p 307.
331. Leupold D, Lehmann H, Curtius HC, Niederwieser A: 6-Pyruvoyl-tetrahydropterin synthase deficiency: Therapeutic trial with two different synthetic pterin analogues in three patients, in Curtius HC, W. Pflciderer, H. Wachter (eds): *Unconjugated Pterins and Related Biogenic Amines*. Berlin, Walter de Gruyter, 1987, p 293.
332. Lipson AH, Earl JW, Wilcken B, Yu JS, O'Halloran M, Cotton RG: Successful treatment of dihydropteridine reductase deficiency, with an interesting effect of 5-hydroxytryptophan deficiency on sleep patterns. *J Inherited Metab Dis* **14**:49, 1991.
333. Spada M, Ferraris S, Ferrero GB, Sartore M, Lanza C, Perfetto F, De Sanctis L, et al: Monitoring treatment in tetrahydrobiopterin deficiency by serum prolactin. *J Inherited Metab Dis* **19**:231, 1996.
334. Mikami H, Matsubara Y, Hayasaka K, Narisawa K, Obinata M, Watanabe A, Haginoya K, et al: Molecular analysis of dihydropteridine reductase deficiency and restoration of the enzyme activity by gene transfer. *J Inherited Metab Dis* **13**:787, 1990.
335. Thöny B, Leimbacher W, Stuhlmann H, Heizmann CW, Blau N: Retrovirus-mediated gene transfer of 6-pyruvoyl-tetrahydropterin synthase corrects tetrahydrobiopterin deficiency in fibroblasts from hyperphenylalaninemic patients. *Hum Gene Ther* **7**:1591, 1996.
336. Laufs S, Blau N, Thöny B: Retrovirus-mediated double transduction of the GTPCH and PTPS genes allows 6-pyruvoyl-tetrahydropterin synthase deficient human fibroblasts to synthesize and release tetrahydrobiopterin. *J Neurochem* **71**:33, 1998.
337. Laufs S, Kim SH, Kim S, Blau N, Thöny B: Reconstitution of a metabolic pathway with triple-cistronic IRES-containing retroviral vectors for correction of tetrahydrobiopterin deficiency. *J Gene Med* **2**:22, 2000.
338. Woody RC, Brewster MA: Adverse effects of trimethoprim-sulfamethoxazole in a child with dihydropteridine reductase deficiency. *Dev Med Child Neurol* **32**:639, 1990.
339. Millot F, Dhondt JL, Mazingue F, Mechinaud F, Ingrand P, Guilhot F: Changes of cerebral biopterin and biogenic amine metabolism in leukemic children receiving 5 g/m^2 intravenous methotrexate. *Pediatr Res* **37**:151, 1995.
340. Blau N, Curtius AC, Kierat L, Leupold D, Kohne E: Hyperphenylalaninemia caused by dihydropteridine reductase deficiency in children receiving chemotherapy for acute lymphoblastic leukemia. *J Pediatr* **115**:661, 1989.
341. Blau N, Niederwieser A, Curtius HC, Kierat L, Leimbacher W, Matasovic A, Binkert F, et al: Prenatal diagnosis of atypical phenylketonuria. *J Inherited Metab Dis* **12**(suppl 2):295, 1989.
342. Dhondt JL, Tilmont P, Ringel J, Farriaux JP: Pterins[AU108] analysis in amniotic fluid for the prenatal diagnosis of GTP cyclohydrolase deficiency. *J Inherited Metab Dis* **13**:879, 1990.
343. Shintaku H, Hsiao KJ, Liu TT, Imamura T, Hase Y, Chen RG, Isshiki G, et al: Prenatal diagnosis of 6-pyruvoyl tetrahydropterin synthase deficiency in seven subjects. *J Inherited Metab Dis* **17**:163, 1994.
344. Guardamagna O, Spada M, Ponzone A, Viora E, Ponzone R, Binkert F, Matasovic A, et al: Prenatal diagnosis of dihydropteridine reductase deficiency in a twin pregnancy. *Pteridines* **3**:19, 1992.
345. Bracco G, Iavarone A, Pagliardini S, Levis F, Guardamagna O, Ferraris S, Ponzone A: Dihydropteridine reductase activity in fetal tissues, in Curtius HC, Blau N, Levine RA (eds): *Unconjugated Pterins and Related Biogenic Amines*. Berlin, Walter de Gruyter, 1987, p 265.

346. Dahl HH, Wake S, Cotton RG, Danks DM: The use of restriction fragment length polymorphisms in prenatal diagnosis of dihydropteridine reductase deficiency. *J Med Genet* **25**:25, 1988.
347. Coskun T, Özalp I, Tokatli A, Blau N, Niederwieser A: Hyperphenylalaninemia due to tetrahydrobiopterin deficiency: A report of 16 cases. *J Inherited Metab Dis* **16**:605, 1993.
348. Hsiao KJ, Chiang SH, Liu TT, Chiu PC, Wuu KT: Tetrahydrobiopterin deficient phenylketonuria detected by neonatal screening in Taiwan, in Curtius HC, Ghisla S, Blau N (eds): *Chemistry and Biology of Pteridines 1989*. Berlin, Walter de Gruyter, 1990, p 402.
349. Jardim LB, Giugliani R, Coelho JC, Dutra CS, Blau N: Possible high frequency of tetrahydrobiopterin deficiency in south Brazil. *J Inherited Metab Dis* **17**:223, 1994.
350. Dhondt JL: *Register of Tetrahydrobiopterin Deficiencies*. Lille, France, Milupa, 1991.
351. Blau N, Dhondt JL, Dianzani I, Thöny B: BIODEF and BIOMDB international databases of tetrahydrobiopterin deficiencies, in Pfleiderer W, Rokos H (eds): *Chemistry and Biology of Pteridines and Folates*. Berlin, Blackwell Scientific, 1997, p 719.
352. Segawa M, Ohmi K, Itoh S, Aoyama M, Hayakawa H: Childhood basal ganglia disease with remarkable response to L-DOPA, hereditary basal ganglia disease with marked diurnal fluctuation. *Shinryo (Tokyo)* **24**:667, 1971.
353. Segawa M, Hosaka A, Miyagawa F, Nomura Y, Imai H: Hereditary progressive dystonia with marked diurnal fluctuation, in Eldridge R, Fahn S (eds): *Advances in Neurology*. New York, Raven, 1976, p 215.
354. Nygaard TG, Snow BJ, Fahn S, Calne DB: Dopa-responsive dystonia: Clinical characteristics and definition, in Segawa M (ed): *Hereditary Progressive Dystonia with Marked Diurnal Fluctuation*. Lancester, UK, Parthenon, 1993, p 3.
355. Nygaard TG: Dopa-responsive dystonia, in Tsui JKC, Calone DB (eds): *Neurological Disease and Therapy: Handbook of Dystonia*. New York, Marcel Dekker, 1995, p 213.
356. Nygaard TG, Wooten GF: Dopa-responsive dystonia: Some pieces of the puzzle are still missing. *Neurology* **50**:853, 1998.
357. Nygaard TG: Dopa-responsive dystonia: Delineation of the clinical syndrome and clues to pathogenesis. *Adv Neurol* **60**:577, 1993.
358. Fink JK, Filling-Katz MR, Barton NW, Macrae PR, Hallett M, Cohen WE: Treatable dystonia presenting as spastic cerebral palsy. *Pediatrics* **82**:137, 1988.
359. Boyd K, Patterson V: Dopa responsive dystonia: A treatable condition misdiagnosed as cerebral palsy. *BMJ* **298**:1019, 1989.
360. Takahashi H, Levine RA, Galloway MP, Snow BJ, Calne DB, Nygaard TG: Biochemical and fluorodopa positron emission tomographic finding in an asymptomatic carrier of the gene for dopa-responsive dystonia. *Ann Neurol* **35**:354, 1994.
361. Hyland K, Fryburg JS, Wilson WG, Bebin EM, Arnold LA, Gunasekera RS, Jacobson RD, et al: Oral phenylalanine loading in Dopa-responsive dystonia: A possible diagnostic test. *Neurology* **48**:1290, 1997.
362. Furukawa Y, Shimadzu M, Rajput AH, Shimizu Y, Tagawa T, Mori H, Yokochi M, et al: GTP cyclohydrolase I gene mutations in hereditary progressive and dopa-responsive dystonia. *Ann Neurol* **39**:609, 1996.
363. Ichinose H, Nagatsu T: Molecular genetics of hereditary dystonia: Mutations in the GTP cyclohydrolase I gene. *Brain Res Bull* **43**:35, 1997.
364. Nagatsu T, Ichinose H: GTP cyclohydrolase I gene, tetrahydrobiopterin, and tyrosine hydroxylase gene: Their relations to dystonia and parkinsonism. *Neurochem Res* **21**:245, 1996.
365. Levine RA, Miller L, Lovenberg W: BH_4 in striatum: Localization in dopamine nerve terminals and role in catecholamine synthesis. *Science* **214**:919, 1981.
366. Koshimura K, Miwa S, Lee K, Fujiwara M, Watanabe Y: Enhancement of dopamine release in vivo from the rat striatum by dialytic perfusion of 6R-L-erythro-5,6,7,8-tetrahydrobiopterin. *J Neurochem* **54**:1391, 1990.
367. Kapatos G: Tetrahydrobiopterin synthesis rate and turnover time in neuronal cultures from embryonic rat mesencephalon and hypothalamus. *J Neurochem* **55**:129, 1990.
368. Sawle GV, Leenders KL, Brooks DJ, Harwood G, Lees AJ, Frackowiak RS, Marsden CD: Dopa-responsive dystonia: [^{18}F]Dopa positron emission tomography. *Ann Neurol* **30**:24, 1991.
369. Okada A, Nakamura K, Snow BJ, Bhatt MH, Nomoto M, Osame M, Calne DB: PET scan study on the dopaminergic system in a Japanese patient with hereditary progressive dystonia (Segawa's disease): Case report. *Adv Neurol* **60**:591, 1993.
370. Rajput AH, Gibb WR, Zhong XH, Shannak KS, Kish S, Chang LG, Hornykiewicz O: Dopa-responsive dystonia: Pathological and biochemical observations in a case. *Ann Neurol* **35**:396, 1994.
371. Hyland K, Gunasekera RS, Engle T, Arnold LA: Tetrahydrobiopterin and biogenic amine metabolism in the Hph-1 mouse. *J Neurochem* **67**:752, 1996.
372. Kishore A, Nygaard TG, Delafuentefernandez R, Naini AB, Schulzer M, Mak E, Ruth TJ, et al: Striatal D_2 receptors in symptomatic and asymptomatic carriers of Dopa-responsive dystonia measured with [C-^{11}]-raclopride and positron-emission tomography. *Neurology* **50**:1028, 1998.
373. Nygaard TG, Marsden CD, Fahn S: Dopa-responsive dystonia: Long term treatment response and prognosis. *Neurology* **41**:174, 1991.
374. Knappskog PM, Flatmark T, Mallet J, Lüdecke B, Bartholomé K: Recessively inherited L-DOPA-responsive dystonia caused by a point mutation (Q381K) in the tyrosine hydroxylase gene. *Hum Mol Genet* **4**:1209, 1995.
375. Lüdecke B, Dworniczak B, Bartholomé K: A point mutation in the tyrosine hydroxylase gene associated with Segawa's syndrome. *Hum Genet* **93**:123, 1995.
376. Fink JK, Barton N, Cohen W, Lovenberg W, Burns RS, Hallett M: Dystonia with marked diurnal variation associated with biopterin deficiency. *Neurology* **38**:707, 1988.
377. Westwood A, Raine DN: Heterozygote detection in phenylketonuria: Measurement of discriminatory ability and interpretation of the phenylalanine loading test by determination of the heterozygote likelihood ratio. *J Med Genet* **12**:327, 1975.
378. Saraiva JM, Seakins JWT, Smith I: Plasma phenylalanine and tyrosine levels revisited in heterozygotes for hyperphenylalaninemia. *J Inherited Metab Dis* **16**:105, 1993.
379. Leeming RJ, Blair A, Green A, Raine DN: Biopterin derivatives in normal and phenylketonuric patients after oral load of L-phenylalanine, L-tyrosine, and L-tryptophan. *Arch Dis Child* **51**:771, 1976.
380. Alös T, Bel Y, Cabello ML, Catala JL, Dalmau J, Ferre J, Garcia AM, et al: Improved identification of heterozygotes for phenylketonuria using blood neopterin and biopterin. *J Inherited Metab Dis* **16**:457, 1993.
381. Bebin EM, Fryburg JS, Trugman JM: Dopa-responsive dystonia (DRD) presenting in the first year of life. *Neurology* **45**(suppl 4):A184, 1995.
382. Blau N, Thöny B, Renneberg A, Arnold LA, Hyland K: Dihydropteridine reductase deficiency localized to the central nervous system. *J Inherited Metab Dis* **21**:433, 1998.
383. Howells D, Smith I, Leonard J, Hyland K: Tetrahydrobiopterin in dihydropteridine reductase deficiency. *N Engl J Med* **314**:520, 1986.
384. Le Moal M, Simon H: Mesocorticolimbic dopaminergic network: Functional and regulatory roles. *Physiol Rev* **71**:155, 1991.
385. Vande Kar LD: Neuroendocrine pharmacology of serotionergic (5HT) neurons. *Annu Rev Pharmacol Toxicol* **31**:289, 1991.
386. Koob GF: Drugs of abuse: Anatomy, pharmacology and function of reward pathways. *Trends Pharmacol Sci* **13**:177, 1992.
387. Jackson DM, Westlind-Danielsson A: Dopamine receptors: Molecular biology, biochemistry and behavioural aspects. *Pharmacol Ther* **64**:291, 1994.
388. Caine SB, Koob GF: Modulation of cocaine self-administration in the rat through D-3 dopamine receptors. *Science* **260**:1814, 1993.
389. Jacobs BL, Fornal CA: Serotonin and motor activity. *Curr Opin Neurobiol* **7**:820, 1997.
390. Pani L, Gessa GL: Evolution of the dopaminergic system and its relationships with the psychopathology of pleasure. *Int J Clin Pharmacol Res* **17**:55, 1997.
391. Goldman-Rakic PS: The cortical dopamine system: Role in memory and cognition. *Adv Pharmacol* **42**:707, 1998.
392. Grace AA, Gerfen CR, Aston-Jones G: Catecholamines in the central nervous system: Overview. *Adv Pharmacol* **42**:655, 1998.
393. Haller J, Makara GB, Kruk MR: Catecholaminergic involvement in the control of aggression: Hormones, the peripheral sympathetic, and central noradrenergic systems. *Neurosci Biobehav Rev* **22**:85, 1998.
394. Stockmeier CA: Neurobiology of serotonin in depression and suicide. *Ann NY Acad Sci* **836**:220, 1997.
395. Goldstein DS: Catecholamines in the periphery: Overview. *Adv Pharmacol* **42**:529, 1998.
396. Yildiz O, Smith JR, Purdy RE: Serotonin and vasoconstrictor synergism. *Life Sci* **62**:1723, 1998.
397. Kaufman S: Regulatory properties of pterin dependent hydroxylases: Variation on a theme, in Usdin E, Weiner N, Youdim MBH (eds):

Function and Regulation of Monoamine Enzymes. New York, Macmillan, 1981, p 165.
398. Scherman D: Dihydrotetrabenazine binding and monoamine uptake in mouse brain regions. *J Neurochem* **47**:331, 1986.
399. Schuldiner S, Shirvan A, Linial M: Vesicular neurotransmitter transporters: From bacteria to humans. *Physiol Rev* **75**:369, 1995.
400. Liu Y, Peter D, Roghani A, Schuldiner S, Prive GG, Eisenberg D, Brecha N, et al: A cDNA that suppresses MPP+ toxicity encodes a vesicular amine transporter. *Cell* **70**:539, 1992.
401. Gingrich JA, Caron MG: Recent advances in the molecular biology of dopamine receptors. *Annu Rev Neurosci* **16**:299, 1993.
402. Civelli O, Bunzow JR, Grandy DK: Molecular diversity of the dopamine receptors. *Annu Rev Pharmacol Toxicol* **32**:281, 1993.
403. Goldstein DS: Catecholamine receptors and signal transduction: Overview. *Adv Pharmacol* **42**:379, 1998.
404. Hoyer D, Clarke DE, Fozard JR, Hartig PR, Martin GR, Mylecharane EJ, Saxena PR, et al: International Union of Pharmacology classification of receptors for 5-hydroxytryptamine (Serotonin). *Pharmacol Rev* **46**:157, 1994.
405. Amara SG, Kuhar MJ: Neurotransmitter transporters: Recent progress. *Annu Rev Neurosci* **16**:73, 1993.
406. Giros B, El Mestikawey S, Godinot N, Zheng K, Han H, Yang-Feng T, Caron MG: Cloning, pharmacological characterization, and chromosomal assignment of the human dopamine transporter. *Mol Pharmacol* **42**:383, 1992.
407. Porzgen P, Bonisch H, Bruss M: Molecular cloning and organization of the coding region of the human norepinephrine transporter gene. *Biochem Biophys Res Commun* **227**:642, 1996.
408. Ramamoorthy S, Bauman AL, Moore KR, Han H, Yang-Feng T, Chang AS, Ganapathy V, et al: Antidepressant- and cocaine-sensitive human serotonin transporter: Molecular cloning, expression, and chromosomal localization. *Proc Natl Acad Sci USA* **90**:2542, 1993.
409. Amara SG: Monoamine transporters: Basic biology with clinical implications. *Neuroscientist* **1**:259, 1995.
410. Zschocke K, Hoffmann GF, Assmann B, Brautigam C, Hoffken H, Wevers RA: Disturbance of dopaminergic neurotransmission in infantile parkinsonism and neonatal epileptic encephalopathy. *J Inherited Metab Dis* **20**(suppl 1):2, 1997.
411. Hyland K, Chang YT, Arnold LA, Ford B, De Vito DC: Ballistic movement disorder associated with low cerebrospinal fluid ratio of homovanillic acid to 5-hydroxyindoleacetic acid: A defect in the dopamine transporter? *J Inherited Metab Dis* **21**(suppl. 2):7, 1998.
412. Kumer SC, Vrana KE: Intricate regulation of tyrosine hydroxylase activity and gene expression. *J Neurochem* **67**:443, 1996.
413. Grenett HE, Ledley FD, Reed LL, Woo SL: Full-length cDNA for rabbit tryptophan hydroxylase: Functional domains and evolution of aromatic amino acid hydroxylases. *Proc Natl Acad Sci USA* **84**:5530, 1987.
414. Boadle-Biber MC: Regulation of serotonin synthesis. *Prog Biophys Mol Biol* **60**:1, 1993.
415. Fitzpatrick PF: Mechanistic studies of tyrosine hydroxylase. *Adv Exp Med Biol* **338**:81, 1993.
416. Ramsey AJ, Daubner SC, Ehrlich JI, Fitzpatrick PF: Identification of iron ligands in tyrosine hydroxylase by mutagenesis of conserved histidinyl residues. *Protein Sci* **4**:2082, 1995.
417. Haavik J, Andersson KK, Petersson L, Flatmark T: Soluble tyrosine hydroxylase (tyrosine 3-monooxygenase) from bovine adrenal medulla: Large-scale purification and physicochemical properties. *Biochim Biophys Acta* **953**:142, 1988.
418. Andersson KK, Vassort C, Brennan BA, Que LJ, Haavik J, Flatmark T, Gros F, et al: Purification and characterization of the blue-green rat phaeochromocytoma (PC12) tyrosine hydroxylase with a dopamine-Fe(III) complex: Reversal of the endogenous feedback inhibition by phosphorylation of serine-40. *Biochem J* **284**(Pt 3):687, 1992.
419. Lohse DL, Fitzpatrick PF: Identification of the intersubunit binding region in rat tyrosine hydroxylase. *Biochem Biophys Res Commun* **197**:1543, 1993.
420. Vrana KE, Walker SJ, Rucker P, Liu X: A carboxyl terminal leucine zipper is required for tyrosine hydroxylase tetramer formation. *J Neurochem* **63**:2014, 1994.
421. Grima B, Lamouroux A, Blanot F, Biguet NF, Mallet J: Complete coding sequence of rat tyrosine hydroxylase mRNA. *Proc Natl Acad Sci USA* **82**:617, 1985.
422. D'Mello SR, Weisberg EP, Stachowiak MK, Turzai LM, Gioio AE, Kaplan BB: Isolation and nucleotide sequence of a cDNA clone encoding bovine adrenal tyrosine hydroxylase: Comparative analysis of tyrosine hydroxylase gene products. *J Neurosci Res* **19**:440, 1988.
423. Neckameyer WS, Quinn WG: Isolation and characterization of the gene for *Drosophila* tyrosine hydroxylase. *Neuron* **2**:1167, 1989.
424. Ichikawa S, Sasaoka T, Nagatsu T: Primary structure of mouse tyrosine hydroxylase deduced from its cDNA. *Biochem Biophys Res Commun* **176**:1610, 1991.
425. Nagatsu T, Ichinose H: Comparative studies on the structure of human tyrosine hydroxylase with those of the enzyme of various mammals. *Comp Biochem Physiol* **98**:203, 1991.
426. Brown ER, Coker GT, O'Malley KL: Organization and evolution of the rat tyrosine hydroxylase gene. *Biochemistry* **26**:5208, 1987.
427. O'Malley KL, Anhalt MJ, Martin BM, Kelsoe JR, Winfield SL, Ginns EI: Isolation and characterization of the human tyrosine hydroxylase gene: Identification of 5′ alternative splice sites responsible for multiple mRNAs. *Biochemistry* **26**:2910, 1987.
428. Kobayashi K, Kaneda N, Ichinose H, Kishi F, Nakazawa A, Kurosawa Y, Fujita K, et al: Structure of the human tyrosine hydroxylase gene: Alternative splicing from a single gene accounts for generation of four mRNA types. *J Biochem (Tokyo)* **103**:907, 1988.
429. Carrier A, Devignes MD, Renoir D, Auffray C: Chicken tyrosine hydroxylase gene: Isolation and functional characterization of the 5′ flanking region. *J Neurochem* **61**:2215, 1993.
430. Grima B, Lamouroux A, Boni C, Julien JF, Javoy-Agid F, Mallet J: A single human gene encoding multiple tyrosine hydroxylases with different predicted functional characteristics. *Nature* **326**:707, 1987.
431. Craig SP, Buckle VJ, Lamouroux A, Mallet J, Craig I: Localization of the human tyrosine hydroxylase gene to 11p15: Gene duplication and evolution of metabolic pathways. *Cytogenet Cell Genet* **42**:29, 1986.
432. Lewis DA, Melchitzky DS, Haycock JW: Four isoforms of tyrosine hydroxylase are expressed in human brain. *Neuroscience* **54**:477, 1993.
433. Le Bourdelles B, Boularand S, Boni C, Horellou P, Dumas S, Grima B, Mallet J: Analysis of the 5′ region of the human tyrosine hydroxylase gene: Combinatorial patterns of exon splicing generate multiple regulated tyrosine hydroxylase isoforms. *J Neurochem* **50**:988, 1988.
434. Sutherland C, Alterio J, Campbell DG, Le Bourdelles B, Mallet J, Haavik J, Cohen P: Phosphorylation and activation of human tyrosine hydroxylase in vitro by mitogen-activated protein (MAP) kinase and MAP-kinase-activated kinases 1 and 2. *Eur J Biochem* **217**:715, 1993.
435. Nasrin S, Ichinose H, Hidaka H, Nagatsu T: Recombinant human tyrosine hydroxylase types 1–4 show regulatory kinetic properties for the natural (6R)-tetrahydrobiopterin cofactor. *J Biochem (Tokyo)* **116**:393, 1994.
436. Alterio J, Ravassard P, Haavik J, Lecaer JP, Biguet NF, Waksman G, Mallet J: Human tyrosine hydroxylase isoforms: Inhibition by excess tetrahydropterin and unusual behavior of isoform 3 after camp-dependent protein kinase phosphorylation. *J Biol Chem* **273**:10,196, 1998.
437. Haavik J, Le Bourdelles B, Martinez A, Flatmark T, Mallet J: Recombinant human tyrosine hydroxylase isozymes: Reconstitution with iron and inhibitory effect of other metal ions. *Eur J Biochem* **199**:371, 1991.
438. Daubner SC, Fitzpatrick PF: Alleviation of catecholamine inhibition of tyrosine hydroxylase by phosphorylation at serine40, in Ayling JE, Nair MG, Baugh CM (eds): *Chemistry and Biology of Pteridines and Folates*. New York, Plenum, 1993, p 87.
439. Lazar MA, Truscott RJ, Raese JD, Barchas JD: Thermal denaturation of native striatal tyrosine hydroxylase: Increased thermolability of the phosphorylated form of the enzyme. *J Neurochem* **36**:677, 1981.
440. Thoenen H, Mueller RA, Axelrod J: Trans-synaptic induction of adrenal tyrosine hydroxylase. *J Pharmacol Exp Ther* **169**:249, 1969.
441. Lazaroff M, Patankar S, Yoon SO, Chikaraishi DM: The cyclic AMP response element directs tyrosine hydroxylase expression in catecholaminergic central and peripheral nervous system cell lines from transgenic mice. *J Biol Chem* **270**:21,579, 1995.
442. Fossom LH, Sterling CR, Tank AW: Regulation of tyrosine hydroxylase gene transcription rate and tyrosine hydroxylase mRNA stability by cyclic AMP and glucocorticoid. *Mol Pharmacol* **42**:898, 1992.
443. Tank AW, Curella P, Ham L: Induction of mRNA for tyrosine hydroxylase by cyclic AMP and glucocorticoids in a rat pheochromocytoma cell line: Evidence for the regulation of tyrosine hydroxylase synthesis by multiple mechanisms in cells exposed to elevated levels of both inducing agents. *Mol Pharmacol* **30**:497, 1986.

444. Gill M, Castle D, Hunt N, Clements A, Sham P, Murray RM: Tyrosine hydroxylase polymorphisms and bipolar affective disorder. *J Psychiatr Res* **25**:179, 1991.
445. Byerley W, Plaetke R, Hoff M, Jensen S, Holik J, Reimherr F, Mellon C, et al: Tyrosine hydroxylase gene not linked to manic-depression in seven of eight pedigrees. *Hum Hered* **42**:259, 1992.
446. Inayama Y, Yoneda H, Sakai T, Ishida T, Kobayashi S, Nonomura Y, Kono Y, et al: Lack of association between bipolar affective disorder and tyrosine hydroxylase DNA marker. *Am J Med Genet* **48**:87, 1993.
447. Korner J, Rietschel M, Hunt N, Castle D, Gill M, Nothen MM, Craddock N, et al: Association and haplotype analysis at the tyrosine hydroxylase locus in a combined German-British sample of manic depressive patients and controls. *Psychiatr Genet* **4**:167, 1994.
448. Kawada Y, Hattori M, Fukuda R, Arai H, Inoue R, Nanko S: No evidence of linkage or association between tyrosine hydroxylase gene and affective disorder. *J Affect Disord* **34**:89, 1995.
449. Oruc L, Verheyen GR, Furac I, Jakovljevic M, Ivezic S, Raeymaekers P, Van Broeckhoven C: Analysis of the tyrosine hydroxylase and dopamine D_4 receptor genes in a Croatian sample of bipolar I and unipolar patients. *Am J Med Genet* **74**:176, 1997.
450. Gasser T, Wszolek ZK, Trofatter J, Ozelius L, Uitti RJ, Lee CS, Gusella J, et al: Genetic linkage studies in autosomal dominant parkinsonism: Evaluation of seven candidate genes. *Ann Neurol* **36**:387, 1994.
451. Comings DE, Gade R, Muhleman D, Sverd J: No association of a tyrosine hydroxylase gene tetranucleotide repeat polymorphism in autism, Tourette syndrome, or ADHD. *Biol Psychiatry* **37**:484, 1995.
452. Martineau J, Herault J, Petit E, Guerin P, Hameury L, Perrot A, Mallet J, et al: Catecholaminergic metabolism and autism. *Dev Med Child Neurol* **36**:688, 1994.
453. Meloni R, Albanese V, Ravassard P, Treilhou F, Mallet J: A tetranucleotide polymorphic microsatellite, located in the first intron of the tyrosine hydroxylase gene, acts as a transcription regulatory element in vitro. *Hum Mol Genet* **7**:423, 1998.
454. Persson ML, Wasserman D, Geijer T, Jonsson EG, Terenius L: Tyrosine hydroxylase allelic distribution in suicide attempters. *Psychiatry Res* **72**:73, 1997.
455. Sander T, Harms H, Rommelspacher H, Hoeche M, Schmidt LG: Possible allelic association of a tyrosine hydroxylase polymorphism with vulnerability to alcohol-withdrawal delirium. *Psychiatr Genet* **8**:13, 1998.
456. Thibaut F, Ribeyre JM, Dourmap N, Meloni R, Laurent C, Campion D, Menard JF, et al: Association of DNA polymorphism in the first intron of the tyrosine hydroxylase gene with disturbances of the catecholaminergic system in schizophrenia. *Schizophr Res* **23**:259, 1997.
457. Wei J, Ramchand CN, Hemmings GP: Possible association of catecholamine turnover with the polymorphic $(TCAT)_n$ repeat in the first intron of the human tyrosine hydroxylase gene. *Life Sci* **61**:1341, 1997.
458. Gershon MD: The enteric nervous system. *Annu Rev Neurosci* **4**:4152, 1981.
459. Tong JH, Kaufman S: Tryptophan hydroxylase: Purification and some properties of the enzyme from rabbit hindbrain. *J Biol Chem* **250**:4152, 1975.
460. Cash CD, Vayer P, Mandel P, Maitre M: Tryptophan 5-hydroxylase: Rapid purification from whole rat brain and production of a specific antiserum. *Eur J Biochem* **149**:239, 1985.
461. Boularand S, Darmon MC, Ganem Y, Launay JM, Mallet J: Complete coding sequence of human tryptophan hydroxylase. *Nucleic Acids Res* **18**:4257, 1990.
462. Ledley FD, Hahn T, Woo SL: Selection for phenylalanine hydroxylase activity in cells transformed with recombinant retroviruses. *Somat Cell Mol Genet* **13**:145, 1987.
463. Craig SP, Boularand S, Darmon MC, Mallet J, Craig IW: Localization of human tryptophan hydroxylase (TPH) to chromosome 11p15.3-p14 by in situ hybridization. *Cytogenet Cell Genet* **56**:157, 1991.
464. Kuhn DM, Arthur RE, States JC: Phosphorylation and activation of brain tryptophan hydroxylase: Identification of serine-58 as a substrate site for protein kinase. *J Neurochem* **68**:2220, 1997.
465. Stoll J, Goldman D: Isolation and structural characterization of the murine tryptophan hydroxylase gene. *J Neurosci Res* **28**:457, 1991.
466. Nielsen DA, Goldman D, Virkkunen M, Tokola R, Rawlings R, Linnoila M: Suicidality and 5-hydroxyindoleacetic acid concentration associated with a tryptophan hydroxylase polymorphism. *Arch Gen Psychiatry* **51**:34, 1994.
467. Mann JJ, Malone KM, Nielsen DA, Goldman D, Erdos J, Gelernter J: Possible association of a polymorphism of the tryptophan hydroxylase gene with suicidal behavior in depressed patients. *Am J Psychiatry* **154**:1451, 1997.
468. Abbar M, Courtet P, Amadeo S, Caer Y, Mallet J, Baldy-Moulinier M, Castelnau D, et al: Suicidal behaviors and the tryptophan hydroxylase gene. *Arch Gen Psychiatry* **52**:846, 1995.
469. Furlong RA, Ho L, Rubinsztein JS, Walsh C, Paykel ES, Rubinsztein DC: No association of the tryptophan hydroxylase gene with bipolar affective disorder, unipolar affective disorder, or suicidal behaviour in major affective disorder. *Am J Med Genet* **81**:245, 1998.
470. Bellivier F, Leboyer M, Courtet P, Buresi C, Beaufils B, Samolyk D, Allilaire JF, et al: Association between the tryptophan hydroxylase gene and manic-depressive illness. *Arch Gen Psychiatry* **55**:33, 1998.
471. Christenson JG, Dairman W, Udenfriend S: On the identity of dopa decarboxylase and 5-hydroxytryptophan decarboxylase. *Proc Natl Acad Sci USA* **69**:343, 1972.
472. Lovenberg W, Weissbach H, Udenfriend S: Aromatic amino acid decarboxylase. *J Biol Chem* **237**:89, 1962.
473. Nagatsu T: Genes for human catecholamine-synthesizing enzymes. *Neurosci Res* **12**:315, 1991.
474. Zhu MY, Juorio AV: Aromatic L-amino acid decarboxylase: biological characterization and functional role. *Gen Pharmacol* **26**:681, 1995.
475. Sumi C, Ichinose H, Nagatsu T: Characterization of recombinant human aromatic L-amino acid decarboxylase expressed in COS cells. *J Neurochem* **55**:1075, 1990.
476. Park DH, Kim KT, Choi MU, Samanta H, Joh TH: Characterization of bovine aromatic L-amino acid decarboxylase expressed in a mouse cell line: Comparison with native enzyme. *Mol Brain Res* **16**:232, 1992.
477. O'Malley KL, Harmon S, Moffat M, Uhland-Smith A, Wong S: The human aromatic L-amino acid decarboxylase gene can be alternatively spliced to generate unique protein isoforms. *J Neurochem* **65**:2409, 1995.
478. Maras B, Dominici P, Barra D, Bossa F, Voltattorni CB: Pig kidney 3,4-dihydroxyphenylalanine (dopa) decarboxylase: Primary structure and relationships to other amino acid decarboxylases. *Eur J Biochem* **201**:385, 1991.
479. Ichinose H, Kurosawa Y, Titani K, Fujita K, Nagatsu T: Isolation and characterization of a cDNA clone encoding human aromatic L-amino acid decarboxylase. *Biochem Biophys Res Commun* **164**:1024, 1989.
480. Dominici P, Maras B, Mei G, Voltattorni B: Affinity labeling of pig kidney 3,4-dihydroxyphenylalanine (Dopa) decarboxylase with *N*-(bromoacetyl) pyridoxamine 5′-phosphate: Modification of an active-site cysteine. *Eur J Biochem* **201**:393, 1991.
481. Albert VR, Allen JM, Joh TH: A single gene codes for aromatic L-amino acid decarboxylase in both neuronal and non neuronal tissue. *J Biol Chem* **262**:9404, 1987.
482. Sumi-Ichinose C, Ichinose H, Takahashi E, Hori T, Nagatsu T: Molecular cloning of genomic DNA and chromosomal assignment of the gene for human aromatic L-amino acid decarboxylase, the enzyme for catecholamine and serotonin biosynthesis. *Biochemistry* **31**:2229, 1992.
483. Craig SP, Le Van Thai A, Weber M, Craig IW: Localisation of the gene for human aromatic L-amino acid decarboxylase (DDC) to chromosome 7p13 to p11 by in situ hybridisation. *Cytogenet Cell Genet* **61**:114, 1992.
484. Ichinose H, Sumi-Ichinose C, Ohye T, Hagino Y, Fujita K, Nagatsu T: Tissue-specific alternative splicing of the first exon generates two types of mRNAs in human aromatic L-amino acid decarboxylase. *Biochemistry* **31**:11,546, 1992.
485. Krieger M, Coge F, Gros F, Thibault J: Different mRNAs code for dopa decarboxylase in tissues of neuronal and nonneuronal origin. *Proc Natl Acad Sci USA* **89**:2161, 1991.
486. Albert VR, Lee MR, Bolden AH, Wurzburger RJ, Aguanno A: Distinct promoters direct neuronal and nonneuronal expression of rat aromatic L-amino acid decarboxylase. *Proc Natl Acad Sci USA* **89**:12,053, 1992.
487. Aguanno A, Afar R, Albert VR: Tissue-specific expression of the nonneuronal promoter of the aromatic L-amino acid decarboxylase gene is regulated by hepatocyte nuclear factor 1. *J Biol Chem* **271**:4528, 1996.
488. Le van Thai A, Coste E, Allen JM, Palmiter RD, Weber MJ: Identification of a neuron-specific promoter of human aromatic L-amino acid decarboxylase gene. *Brain Res Mol Brain Res* **17**:227, 1993.

489. Chang YT, Mues G, Hyland K: Alternative splicing in the coding region of human aromatic L-amino acid decarboxylase mRNA. *J Neurosci Lett* **202**:157, 1996.
490. Hadjiconstantinou M, Wemlinger TA, Sylvia CP, Hubble JP, Neff NH: Aromatic L-amino acid decarboxylase activity of the mouse striatum is modulated via dopamine receptors. *J Neurochem* **60**:175, 1993.
491. Zhu MY, Juorio AV, Paterson IA, Boulton AA: Regulation of striatal aromatic L-amino acid decarboxylase: Effects of blockade or activation of dopamine receptors. *Eur J Pharmacol* **238**:157, 1993.
492. Wessel T, Joh T: Parallel upregulation of catecholamine synthesizing enzymes in rat brain and adrenal gland: Effect of reserpine and correlation with immediate early gene expression. *Mol Brain Res* **15**:349, 1992.
493. Li X-M, Juorio AV, Paterson IA, Zhu M-Y: Specific irreversible monoamine oxidase B inhibitors stimulate gene expression of aromatic L-amino acid decarboxylase in PC12 cells. *J Neurochem* **59**:2324, 1992.
494. Li X-M, Juorio AV, Boulton AA: NSD-1015 alters the gene expression of aromatic L-amino acid decarboxylase in rat PC12 pheochromocytoma cells. *Neurochem Res* **18**:915, 1993.
495. Li X-M, Juorio AV, Boulton AA: Induction of aromatic L-amino acid decarboxylase mRNA by interleukin-1β and prostaglandin E_2 in PC12 cells. *Neurochem Res* **19**:591, 1994.
496. Buckland P, O'Donovan M, McGruffin P: Changes in dopa decarboxylase mRNA but not tyrosine hydroxylase mRNA levels in rat brain following antipsychotic treatment. *Psychopharmacology (Berlin)* **108**:98, 1992.
497. Wang Z, Crowe RR, Marsh JL: An SspI polymorphism for the human DOPA decarboxylase (DDC) gene on chromosome 7p. *Hum Mol Genet* **2**:2198, 1993.
498. Chang YT, Mues G, McPherson Bedell J, Marsh JL, Hyland K: Mutations in the human aromatic L-amino acid decarboxylase gene. *J Inherited Metab Dis* **21**(suppl 2):4, 1998.
499. Nagatsu T: Dopamine beta hydroxylase, in Boulton RR, Baker GB (eds): *Neuromethods I*. Clifton, NJ: Humana, 1986, p 79.
500. Kobayashi K, Kurosawa Y, Fujita K, Nagatsu T: Human dopamine beta-hydroxylase gene: Two mRNA types having different 3′-terminal regions are produced through alternative polyadenylation. *Nucleic Acids Res* **17**:1089, 1989.
501. Craig SP, Buckle VJ, Lamouroux A, Mallet J, Craig JW: Localization of the human dopamine beta hydroxylase (DBH) gene chromosome 9q34. *Cytogenet Cell Genet* **48**:50, 1988.
502. Lamouroux A, Vigny A, Faucon Biguet N, Darmon MC, Franck R, Henry JP, Mallet J: The primary structure of human dopamine-β-hydroxylase: Insights into the relationship between the soluble and the membrane-bound forms of the enzyme. *EMBO J* **6**:3931, 1987.
503. Lewis EJ, Allison S, Fader D, Claflin V, Baizer L: Bovine dopamine-β-hydroxylase cDNA: Complete coding sequence and expression in mammalian cells with vaccinia virus vector. *J Biol Chem* **265**:1021, 1990.
504. McMahon A, Geertman R, Sabban EL: Rat dopamine β-hydroxylase: Molecular cloning and characterization of the cDNA and regulation of the mRNA by reserpine. *J Neurosci Res* **25**:395, 1990.
505. McMahon A, Sabban EL: Regulation of expression of dopamine β-hydroxylase in PC12 cells by glucocorticoids and cyclic AMP analogues. *J Neurochem* **59**:2040, 1992.
506. Lamouroux A, Houhou L, Bigue NF, Serck-Hanssen G, Guibert B, Icard-Liepkalns C, Mallet J: Analysis of the human dopamine β-hydroxylase promoter: Transcriptional induction by cyclic AMP. *J Neurochem* **60**:364, 1993.
507. Hwang O, Joh TH: Effects of cAMP, glucocorticoids and calcium on dopamine β-hydroxylase gene expression in bovine chromaffin cells. *J Mol Neurosci* **4**:173, 1993.
508. Ishiguro H, Kim KT, Joh TH, Kim KS: Neuron-specific expression of the human dopamine beta-hydroxylase gene requires both the cAMP-response element and a silencer region. *J Biol Chem* **268**:17,987, 1993.
509. Kim KS, Ishiguro H, Tinti C, Wagner J, Joh TH: The cAMP-dependent protein kinase regulates transcription of the dopamine beta-hydroxylase gene. *J Neursci* **14**:7200, 1994.
510. Hwang O, Lee JD: Reduction of dopamine beta-hydroxylase gene expression by calcium in bovine chromaffin cells. *Biochem Biophys Res Commun* **211**:864, 1995.
511. Greco D, Zellmer E, Zhang Z, Lewis E: Transcription factor AP-2 regulates expression of the dopamine β-hydroxylase gene. *J Neurochem* **65**:510, 1995.
512. Hwang O, Choi HJ: Induction of gene expression of the catecholamine-synthesizing enzymes by insulin-like growth factor-I. *J Neurochem* **65**:1988, 1995.
513. Isobe K, Yukimasa N, Nakai T, Takuwa Y: Pituitary adenylate cyclase-activating polypeptide induces gene expression of the catecholamine synthesizing enzymes, tyrosine hydroxylase and dopamine β-hydroxylase, through 4′,5′-cyclic adenosine monophosphate- and protein kinase C-dependent mechanisms in cultured porcine adrenal medullary chromaffin cells. *Neuropeptides* **30**:167, 1996.
514. Kim JS, Chae HD, Joh TH, Kim KT: Stimulation of human DBH gene expression by prostaglandin E_2 in human neuroblastoma SK-N-BEC cells. *J Mol Neurosci* **9**:143, 1997.
515. Kobayashi MS, Mizuguchi T, Yamada K, Nagatsu I, Titani K, Fujita K, Hidaka H, et al: The 5′-flanking region of the human dopamine β-hydroxylase gene promotes neuron subtype-specific gene expression in the central nervous system of tansgenic mice. *Brain Res Mol Brain Res* **17**:239, 1993.
516. Hoyle GW, Mercer EH, Palmiter RD, Brinster RL: Cell-specific expression from the human dopamine β-hydroxylase promoter in transgenic mice is controlled via a combination of positive and negative regulatory elements. *J Neurosci* **14**:2455, 1994.
517. Ishiguro K, Kim KS, Joh TH: Identification of a negative regulatory element in the 5′-flanking region of the human dopamine beta-hydroxylase gene. *Brain Res Mol Brain Res* **34**:251, 1995.
518. Seo H, Yang C, Kim HS, Kim KS: Multiple protein factors interact with the *cis*-regulatory elements of the proximal promoter in a cell-specific manner and regulate transcription of the dopamine β-hydroxylase gene. *J Neurosci* **16**:4102, 1996.
519. Ichii A, Kobayashi K, Kiuchi K, Nagatsu T: Expression of two forms of human dopamine beta-hydroxylase in COS cells. *Neurosci Lett* **125**:25, 1991.
520. Cubells JF, Kobayashi K, Nagatsu T, Kidd KK, Kidd JR, Calafell F, Kranzler HR, et al: Population genetics of a functional variant of the dopamine β-hydroxylase gene (DBH). *Am J Med Genet* **74**:374, 1997.
521. Porter CJ, Nahmias J, Wolfe J, Craig IW: Dinucleotide repeat polymorphism at the human dopamine β-hydroxylase (DBH) locus. *Nucleic Acids Res* **20**:1429, 1992.
522. Wei J, Ramchand CN, Hemmings GP: Possible control of dopamine beta-hydroxylase via a codominant mechanism associated with the polymorphic $(GT)_n$ repeat at its gene locus in healthy individuals. *Hum Genet* **99**:52, 1997.
523. Wei J, Xu HM, Ramchand CN, Hemmings GP: Is the polymorphic microsatellite repeat of the dopamine β-hydroxylase gene associated with biochemical variability of the catecholamine pathway in schizophrenia? *Biol Psychiatry* **41**:762, 1997.
524. Wei J, Ramchand CN, Hemmings GP: TaqI polymorphic sites at the human dopamine β-hydroxylase gene possibly associated with biochemical alterations of the catecholamine pathway in schizophrenia. *Psychiatr Genet* **8**:19, 1998.
525. Meszaros K, Lenzinger E, Fureder T, Hornik K, Willinger U, Stompe T, Heiden AM, et al: Schizophrenia and the dopamine-β-hydroxylase gene: Results of a linkage and association study. *Psychiatr Genet* **6**:17, 1996.
526. Weyler W, Hsu YP, Breakefield XO: Biochemistry and genetics of monoamine oxidase. *Pharmacol Ther* **47**:391, 1990.
527. Chen ZY, Hotamisligil GS, Huang JK, Wen L, Ezzeddine D, Aydin-Muderrisoglu N, Powell JF, et al: Structure of the human gene for monoamine oxidase type A. *Nucleic Acids Res* **19**:4537, 1991.
528. Lan NC, Heinzman C, Gal A, Klisak I, Orth U, Lai E, Grimsby J, et al: Human monoamine oxidase A and B genes map to X_p 11.23 and are deleted in a patient with Norrie disease. *Genomics* **4**:552, 1989.
529. Levy ER, Powell JF, Buckle VJ, Hsu YP, Breakefield XO, Craig IW: Localization of human monoamine oxidase-A gene to Xp11.23-11.4 by in situ hybridization: Implications for Norrie disease. *Genomics* **5**:368, 1989.
530. Bach AW, Lan NC, Johnson DL, Abell CW, Bembeneck ME, Kwan SW, Seeburg PH, et al: cDNA cloning of human liver monoamine oxidase A and B: Molecular basis of differences in enzymatic properties. *Proc Natl Acad Sci USA* **85**:4934, 1988.
531. Kuwahara T, Takamoto S, Ito A: Primary structure of rat monoamine oxidase A deduced from cDNA and its expression in rat tissues. *Agric Biol Chem* **54**:253, 1990.
532. Ito A, Kuwahara T, Inadome S, Segara Y: Molecular cloning of a cDNA for rat liver monoamine oxidase B. *Biochem Biophys Res Commun* **157**:970, 1988.

533. Kwan SW, Bergeron JM, Abell CW: Molecular properties of monoamine oxidases A and B. *Psychopharmacology (Berlin)* **106**(suppl):S1, 1992.
534. Sablin SO, Ramsay RR: Monoamine oxidase contains a redoc-active disulfide. *J Biol Chem* **273**:14,074, 1998.
535. Gottowik J, Cesura AM, Malherbe P, Lang G, Da Prada M: Characterization of wild type and mutant forms of human monoamine oxidase A and B expressed in a mammalian cell line. *FEBS Lett* **31**:152, 1993.
536. Tsugeno Y, Ito A: A key amino acid responsible for substrate selectivity of monoamine oxidase A and B. *J Biol Chem* **272**:14,033, 1997.
537. Hsu YP, Weyler WE, Chen S, Sims KB, Rinehart WB, Utterback MC, Powell JF, et al: Structural features of human monoamine oxidase A elucidated from cDNA and peptide sequences. *J Neurochem* **51**:1321, 1988.
538. Grimsby J, Chen K, Wang LJ, Lan N, Shih JC: Human monoamine oxidase A and B genes exhibit identical exon-intron organization. *Proc Natl Acad Sci USA* **88**:3637, 1991.
539. Shih JC, Zhu QS, Grimsby J, Chen K: Identification of human monoamine oxidase (MAO) A and B gene promoters. *J Neural Transm Suppl* **41**:27, 1994.
540. Denny RM, Sharma A, Dave SK, Waguespack A: A new look at the promotor of the human monoamine oxidase A gene: Mapping transcription initiation sites and capacity to drive luciferase expression. *J Neurochem* **63**:843, 1994.
541. Zhu Q, Shih JC: An extensive repeat structure down-regulates human monoamine oxidase A promotor activity independently of an initiator-like sequence. *J Neurochem* **69**:1368, 1997.
542. Nanko S, Ueki A, Hattori M: No association between Parkinson's disease and monoamine oxidase A and B gene polymorphisms. *Neurosci Lett* **204**:125, 1996.
543. Hwang WJ, Lai ML, Tsai TT, Lai MD: Genetic polymorphism of monoamine oxidase B and susceptibility of Parkinson's disease. *Chung Hua I Hsueh Tsa Chih (Taipei)* **60**:137, 1997.
544. Costa P, Checkoway H, Levy D, Smith-Weller T, Franklin GM, Swanson PD, Costa LG: Association of a polymorphism in intron 13 of the monoamine oxidase B gene with Parkinson's disease. *Am J Med Genet* **74**:154, 1997.
545. Gade R, Muhleman D, Blake H, MacMurray J, Johnson P, Verde R, Saucier G, et al: Correlation of length of VNTR alleles at the X-linked MAOA gene and phenotypic effect in Tourette syndrome and drug abuse. *Mol Psychiatry* **3**:50, 1998.
546. Coron B, Campion D, Thibaut F, Dollfus S, Preterre P, Langlois S, Vasse T, et al: Association study between schizophrenia and monoamine oxidase A and B DNA polymorphisms. *Psychiatry Res* **62**:221, 1996.
547. Sobell JL, Lind TJ, Hebrink DD, Heston LL, Sommer SS: Screening the monoamine oxidase B gene in 100 male patients with schizophrenia: A cluster of polymorphisms in African-Americans but lack of functionally significant sequence changes. *Am J Med Genet* **74**:44, 1997.
548. Dann J, DeLisi LE, Devoto M, Laval S, Nancarrow DJ, Shields G, Smith A, et al: A linkage study of schizophrenia to markers within Xp11 near the MAOB gene. *Psychiatry Res* **70**:131, 1997.
549. Craddock N, Daniels J, Roberts E, Rees M, McGuffin P, Owen MJ: No evidence for allelic association between bipolar disorder and monoamine oxidase A gene polymorphisms. *Am J Med Genet* **60**:322, 1995.
550. Parsian A, Todd RD: Genetic association between monoamine oxidase and manic-depressive illness: Comparison of relative risk and haplotype relative risk data. *Am J Med Genet* **74**:475, 1997.
551. Hyland K: Abnormalities of biogenic amine metabolism. *J Inherited Metab Dis* **16**:676, 1993.
552. Kruesi MJP, Swedo SE, Hamburger SD, Potter WZ, Rapoport JL: Concentration gradient of monoamine metabolites in children and adolescents. *Biol Psychiatry* **24**:507, 1988.
553. Howells DW, Hyland K: Direct analysis of tetrahydrobiopterin in cerebrospinal fluid by high-performance liquid chromatography with redox electrochemistry: Prevention of autoxidation during storage and analysis. *Clin Chim Acta* **167**:23, 1987.
554. Huber C, Batchelor JR, Fuchs D, Hausen A, Lang A, Niederwieser D, Raibnegger G, et al: Immune response associated production of neopterin: Release from macrophages primarily under control of interferon gamma. *J Exp Med* **160**:310, 1984.
555. Lüdecke B, Knappskog PM, Clayton PT, Surtees RA, Clelland JD, Heales SJ, Brand MP, et al: Recessively inherited L-DOPA-responsive parkinsonism in infancy caused by point mutation (L205P) in the tyrosine hydroxylase gene. *Hum Mol Genet* **5**:1023, 1996.
556. Van den Heuvel LP, Luiten B, Smeitink JAM, Jenneke F, Van Andel DR, Steenbergen-Spanjers GCH, et al: A common point mutation in the tyrosine hydroxylase gene in autosomal recessive L-DOPA responsive dystonia (DRD) in the Dutch population. *Hum Genet* **102**:644, 1998.
557. Hoffmann GF, Surtees RAH, Wevers RA: Cerebrospinal fluid investigations for neurometabolic disorders. *Neuropediatrics* **29**:59, 1998.
558. Hyland K, Clayton P: Aromatic L-amino acid decarboxylase deficiency: Diagnostic methodology. *Clin Chem* **38**:2405, 1992.
559. Maller A, Hyland K, Milstien S, Biaggioni I, Butler IJ: Aromatic L-amino acid decarboxylase deficiency: Clinical features, diagnosis, and treatment of a second family. *J Child Neurol* **12**:349, 1997.
560. Sharpless NS, McCann DS: Dopa and 3-*O*-methyldopa in cerebrospinal fluid of parkinsonism patients during treatment with oral L-dopa. *Clin Chim Acta* **31**:155, 1971.
561. Hyland K, Surtees RAH, Rodeck C, Clayton PT: Aromatic L-amino acid decarboxylase deficiency: Clinical features, diagnosis and treatment of a new inborn error of neurotransmitter amine synthesis. *Neurology* **42**:1980, 1992.
562. Korenke CG, Christen HJ, Hyland K, Hunneman DH, Hanefeld F: Aromatic L-amino acid decarboxylase deficiency: An extrapyramidal movement disorder with oculogyric crises. *Eur J Pediatr Neurol* **1**:67, 1997.
563. Riley CM, Day RI, Greely DM, Langford WS: Central autonomic dysfunction with defective lacrimation: I. Report of five cases. *Pediatrics* **3**:468, 1949.
564. Bradbury S, Eggleston C: Postural hypotension: A report of three cases. *Am Heart J* **1**:73, 1925.
565. Shy GM, Drager G: A neurological syndrome associated with orthostatic hypotension. *Arch Neurol* **2**:511, 1960.
566. Dunnette J, Weinshilbourn RM: Inheritance of low immunoreactive human plasma dopamine hydroxylase: Radioimmunoassay studies. *J Clin Invest* **609**:1080, 1977.
567. Robertson D, Haile V, Perry SE, Robertson RM, Phillips JA, Biaggioni I: Dopamine β-hydroxylase deficiency: A genetic disorder of cardiovascular regulation. *Hypertension* **18**:1, 1991.
568. Biaggioni I, Robertson D: Endogenous restoration of noradrenaline by precursor therapy in dopamine-β-hydroxylase deficiency. *Lancet* **2**:1170, 1987.
569. Man in't Veld AJ, Boomsma F, Moleman P, Schalekamp MADH: Congenital dopamine β-hydroxylase deficiency. *Lancet* **1**:183, 1987.
570. Robertson D, Mosqueda-Garcia R, Robertson RM, Biaggioni I: Chronic hypotension: In the shadow of hypertension. *Am J Hypertens* **5**(6 pt 2):200S, 1992.
571. Robertson D, Hollister AS, Carey EL, Tung CS, Goldberg MR, Robertson RM: Increased vascular β_2-adrenoceptor responsiveness in autonomic dysfunction. *J Am Coll Cardiol* **3**:850, 1984.
572. Robertson D, Goldberg MR, Onrot J, Hollister AS, Wiley R, Thompson JG, Robertson RM: Isolated failure of autonomic noradrenergic neurotransmission: Evidence for impaired beta hydroxylation of dopamine. *N Engl J Med* **314**:1494, 1986.
573. Man in't Veld AJ, Boomsma F, Vanden Meiracker AH, Schalekamp MADH: Effect of an unnatural noradrenaline precursor on sympathetic control and orthostatic hypotension in dopamine β-hydroxylase deficiency. *Lancet* **2**:1172, 1987.
574. Johnson RH: Autonomic failure and the eyes, in Bannister R (ed): *Autonomic Failure*. Oxford: Oxford University Press, 1983, p 508.
575. Kaler SG, Holmes CS, Goldstein DS: Dopamine β-hydroxylase deficiency associated with mutations in a copper transporter gene. *Adv Pharmacol* **42**:66, 1998.
576. Brunner HG, Nelen MR, Van Zandvoort P, Abeling NGGM, Van Gennip AH, Wolters EC, Kuiper MA, et al: X-linked borderline mental retardation with prominent behavioral disturbance: Phenotype, genetic localization, and evidence for disturbed monoamine metabolism. *Am J Hum Genet* **52**:1032, 1993.
577. Abeling NGGM, Van Gennip AH, Overmars H, Van Oost B, Brunner HG: Biogenic amine metabolite patterns in the urine of monoamine oxidase A-deficient patients. *J Inherited Metab Dis* **17**:339, 1994.
578. Abeling NG, Van Gennip AH, Van Cruchten AG, Overmars H, Brunner HG: Monoamine oxidase A deficiency: Biogenic amine metabolites in random urine samples. *J Neural Transm Suppl* **52**:9, 1998.

579. Lenders JW, Eisenhofer G, Abeling NG, Berger W, Murphy DL, Kongings CH, Wagemakers LM, et al: Specific genetic deficiencies of the A and B isoenzymes of monoamine oxidase are characterized by distinct neurochemical and clinical phenotypes. *J Clin Invest* **97**:1010, 1996.
580. Vossler DG, Wyler AR, Wilkus RJ, Gardner-Walker G, Vlacek BW: Cataplexy and monoamine oxidase deficiency in Norrie disease. *Neurology* **46**:1258, 1996.
581. Grimsby J, Toth M, Chen K, Kumazawa T, Klaidman L, Adams JD, Karoum F, et al: Increased stress response and β-phenylethylamine in MAO-B-deficient mice. *Nature Genet* **17**:206, 1997.
582. Lüdecke B, Bartholomé K: Frequent sequence variant in the human tyrosine hydroxylase gene. *Hum Genet* **95**:716, 1995.
583. Ramchand CN, Clark AE, Ramchand R, Hemmings GP: Cultured human keratinocytes as a model for studying the dopamine metabolism in schizophrenia. *Med Hypotheses* **44**:53, 1995.
584. Chang YT, Mues G, Pittelkow MR, Hyland K: Cultured human keratinocytes as a peripheral source of mRNA for tyrosine hydroxylase and aromatic L-amino acid decarboxylase. *J Inherited Metab Dis* **19**:239, 1996.
585. Bräutigam C, Wavers RA, Jensen RJT, Smeitinik JAM, De Rijk-van Andel JF, Gabreels FJM, Hoffmann GF: Biochemical hallmarks of tyrosine hydroxylase deficiency. *Clin Chem* **44**:1897, 1998.
586. Zhou Q-Y, Quaife CJ, Palmiter RD: Targeted disruption of tyrosine hydroxylase gene reveals that catecholamines are essential for mouse fetal development. *Nature* **374**:640, 1995.
587. Zhou Q-Y, Palmiter RD: Dopamine-deficient mice are severely hypoactive, adipsic and aphagic. *Cell* **83**:1197, 1995.
588. Surtees R, Clayton P: Infantile parkinsonism-dystonia: Tyrosine hydroxylase deficiency. *Mov Disord* **13**:350, 1998.
589. Van Andel RFR, Wevers RA, Gabreals FJM, Smeitink JAM: Tyrosine hydroxylase deficiency: Clinical presentation, biochemistry and treatment in four Dutch cases. *Enzyme Protein* **49**:185, 1996.
590. Hyland K, Clayton PT: Aromatic amino acid decarboxylase deficiency in twins. *J Inherited Metab Dis* **13**:301, 1990.
591. Abeling NGGM, Van Gennip AH, Barth PG, Van Cruchten A, Wijburg FA: Aromatic L-amino acid decarboxylase deficiency: A new case with a mild clinical presentation and unexpected laboratory findings. *J Inherited Metab Dis* **21**:240, 1998.
592. Boomsma F, Van der Horn FAJ, Schalekamp MADH: Determination of aromatic L-amino acid decarboxylase in human plasma. *Clin Chim Acta* **159**:173, 1986.
593. Surtees R, Hyland K: 1-3,4-Dihydroxyphenylalanine (levodopa) lowers central nervous system *S*-adenosylmethionine concentrations in humans. *Neurol Neurosurg Psychiatry* **53**:569, 1990.
594. O'Connor DT, Cervenka JH, Stone RA, Levine GL, Palmer RJ, Franco-Bourland RE, Madrazo I, et al: Dopamine β-hydroxylase immunoreactivity in human cerebrospinal fluid: Properties, relationship to central noradrenergic neuronal activity and variation in Parkinson's disease and congenital dopamine β-hydroxylase deficiency. *Clin Sci* **86**:149, 1994.
595. Thomas SA, Matsumoto AM, Palmiter RD: Noradrenaline is essential for mouse fetal development. *Nature* **374**:643, 1995.
596. Mathias CJ, Bannister RB, Cortelli P, Heslop K, Polak JM, Raimbach S, Springall DR, et al: Clinical autonomic and therapeutic observations in two siblings with postural hypotension and sympathetic failure due to an inability to synthesise noradrenaline from dopamine because of a deficiency in dopamine β-hydroxylase. *Q J Med* **75**:617, 1990.
597. Biaggioni I, Goldstein DS, Atkinson T, Robertson D: Dopamine-β-hydroxylase deficiency in humans. *Neurology* **40**:370, 1990.
598. Tulen JH, Man in't Veld AJ, Mechelse K, Boomsma F: Sleep patterns in congenital dopamine β-hydroxylase deficiency. *J Neurol* **237**:98, 1990.
599. Thomas SA, Palmiter RD: Disruption of the dopamine β-hydroxylase gene in mice suggests roles for norepinephrine in motor function, learning, and memory. *Behav Neurosci* **111**:579, 1997.
600. Thomas SA, Palmiter RD: Impaired maternal behavior in mice lacking norepinephrine and epinephrine. *Cell* **91**:583, 1997.
601. Thomas SA, Palmiter RD: Thermoregulatory and metabolic phenotypes of mice lacking noradrenaline and adrenaline. *Nature* **387**:94, 1997.
602. Thomas SA, Marck BT, Palmiter RD, Matsumoto AM: Restoration of norepinephrine and reversal of phenotypes in mice lacking dopamine β-hydroxylase. *J Neurochem* **70**:2468, 1998.
603. Rea RF, Biaggioni I, Robertson RM, Haile V, Robertson D: Reflex control of sympathetic nerve activity in dopamine-beta-hydroxylase deficiency. *Hypertension* **15**:107, 1990.
604. Thompson JM, O'Callaghan CJ, Kingwell BA, Lambert GW, Jennings GL, Esler MD: Total norepinephrine spillover, muscle sympathetic nerve activity and heart-rate spectral analysis in a patient with dopamine β-hydroxylase deficiency. *J Auton Nerv Syst* **55**:198, 1995.
605. DiBona GF: Neural mechanisms in body fluid homeostasis. *Fed Proc* **45**:2871, 1986.
606. Kuchel O, Debinski W, Larochelle P: Isolated failure of autonomic noradrenergic neurotransmission. *N Engl J Med* **315**:1357, 1986.
607. Gentric A, Fouilhoux A, Caroff M, Mottier D, Jouquan J: Dopamine β-hydroxylase deficiency responsible for severe dysautonomic orthostatic hypotension in an elderly patient. *J Am Geriatr Soc* **41**:550, 1993.
608. Brunner HG, Nelen M, Breakefield XO, Ropers HH, Van Oost BA: Abnormal behaviour associated with a point mutation in the structural gene for monoamine oxidase A. *Science* **262**:578, 1993.
609. Collins FA, Murphy DL, Reiss AL, Sims KB, Lewis JG, Freund L, Karoum F, et al: Clinical, biochemical, and neuropsychiatric evaluation of a patient with contiguous gene syndrome due to a microdeletion Xp11.3 including the Norrie disease locus and monoamine oxidase (MAOA and MAOB) genes. *Am J Med Genet* **42**:127, 1992.
610. De la Chapelle A, Sankila EM, Lindlof M, Aula P, Norio R: Norrie disease caused by a gene deletion allowing carrier detection and prenatal diagnosis. *Clin Genet* **28**:317, 1985.
611. Sims KB, De la Chapelle A, Norio R, Sankila EM, Hsu YP, Rinehart WB, Corey TJ, et al: Monoamine oxidase deficiency in males with an X chromosome deletion. *Neuron* **2**:1069, 1989.
612. Chen ZY, Denney RM, Breakefield XO: Norrie disease and MAO genes: Nearest neighbors. *Hum Mol Genet* **4**:1729, 1995.
613. Cases O, Seif I, Grimsby J, Gaspar P, Chen K, Pournin S, Muller U, et al: Aggressive behavior and altered amounts of brain serotonin and norepinephrine in mice lacking MAO-A. *Science* **268**:1763, 1995.
614. Winslow JT, Miczek KA: Habituation of aggression in mice: Pharmacological evidence of catecholaminergic and serotonergic mediation. *Psychopharmacology (Berlin)* **81**:286, 1983.
615. Coccaro EF: Central serotonin and impulsive aggression. *Br J Psychiatry* **155**(suppl 8):52, 1989.
616. Troncone LRP, Tufik S: Effects of selective adrenoceptor agonists and antagonists on aggressive behavior elicited by apomorphine, DL-DOPA and fusaric acid in REM sleep deprived rats. *Physiol Behav* **50**:173, 1991.
617. Popova NK, Nikulina EM, Kulikov AV: Genetic analysis of different kinds of aggressive behavior. *Behav Genet* **23**:491, 1993.
618. Mehlman PT, Higley JD, Faucher I, Lilly AA, Taub DM, Vickers J, Suomi SJ, et al: Low CSF 5-HIAA concentrations and severe aggression and impaired impulse control in non-human primates. *Am J Psychiatry* **151**:1485, 1994.
619. Brunner HG: MAOA deficiency and abnormal behaviour: Perspectives on an association. *Ciba Found Symp* **194**:155, 1996.
620. Cohen RM, Pickar D, Garrett D, Lipper S, Gillin JC, Murphy DL: REM sleep suppression induced by selective monoamine oxidase inhibition. *Psychopharmacology (Berlin)* **78**:137, 1982.
621. Tufik S, Lindsey CJ, Carlini EA: Does REM sleep deprivation induce a supersensitivity of dopaminergic receptors in the rat brain. *Pharmacology* **16**:98, 1978.
622. Zureick JL, Meltzer HY: Platelet MAO activity in hallucinating and paranoid schizophrenia: A review and meta-analysis. *Biol Psychiatry* **24**:63, 1988.
623. Tabakoff B, Hoffman PL, Lee JM, Saito T, Willard B, De Leon-Jones F: Differences in platelet enzyme activity between alcoholics and non-alcoholics. *N Engl J Med* **318**:134, 1988.
624. Tivol EA, Shalish C, Schuback DE, Hsu YP, Breakefield XO: Mutational analysis of the human MAOA gene. *Am J Med Genet* **67**:92, 1996.
625. Cases O, Vitalis T, Seif I, De Maeyer E, Sotelo C, Gasper P: Lack of barrels in the somatosensory cortex of monoamine oxidase A-deficient mice: Role of a serotonin excess during the critical period. *Neuron* **16**:297, 1996.
626. Kim JJ, Shih JC, Chen K, Chen L, Bao S, Maren S, Anagnostaras SG, et al: Selective enhancement of emotional, but not motor, learning in monoamine oxidase A-deficient mice. *Proc Natl Acad Sci USA* **94**:5929, 1997.
627. Dhondt JL, Hayte JM, Forzy G, Delcroix M, Farriaux JP: Unconjugated pteridines in amniotic fluid during gestation. *Clin Chim Acta* **161**:269, 1986.
628. Ferre J, Naylor EW: Sepiapterin reductase in human amniotic and skin fibroblasts, chorionic villi, and various blood fractions. *Clin Chim Acta* **174**:271, 1988.

CHAPTER 79

Hypertyrosinemia

Grant A. Mitchell ▪ Markus Grompe
Marie Lambert ▪ Robert M. Tanguay

1. In humans, tyrosine is obtained from two sources, dietary intake and hydroxylation of phenylalanine. Tyrosine degradation occurs primarily in the cytoplasm of hepatocytes and is both glucogenic and ketogenic. Under most circumstances, the rate of tyrosine degradation is determined by the activity of tyrosine aminotransferase.

2. Most inborn errors of tyrosine catabolism produce hypertyrosinemia. Hypertyrosinemia is also encountered in various acquired conditions, in particular severe hepatocellular dysfunction.

3. Deficiency of cytoplasmic tyrosine aminotransferase (TAT) results in oculocutaneous tyrosinemia, characterized by palmoplantar keratosis and painful corneal erosions with photophobia (OMIM 276600). Half of reported patients have mental retardation. Ocular and cutaneous symptoms respond to dietary restriction of phenylalanine and tyrosine. Canine and mink models of TAT deficiency exist.

4. Three different conditions have been associated with dysfunction of 4-hydroxyphenylpyruvate dioxygenase (4HPPD): hereditary 4HPPD deficiency, hawkinsinuria, and transient tyrosinemia of the newborn.

5. Primary 4HPPD deficiency (OMIM 276710) has been described in at least three patients, all of whom were neurologically abnormal. The biochemical phenotype showed hypertyrosinemia and elevated urinary excretion of 4-hydroxyphenyl derivatives. A mouse model of this condition has been described.

6. Hawkinsinuria (OMIM 140350) is an autosomal dominant condition presumably caused by dysfunction of 4HPPD. It results in metabolic acidosis and failure to thrive in infancy. Hypertyrosinemia is minimal or absent. The presence in the urine of hawkinsin, an amino acid felt to be derived from an intermediate of the 4HPPD reaction, is diagnostic of this condition. Symptoms respond to dietary protein restriction and to the administration of ascorbate.

7. Transient tyrosinemia (OMIM 276500) of the newborn results from a combination of 4HPPD immaturity, elevated dietary phenylalanine and tyrosine intake, and a relative ascorbate deficiency. Improvement is spontaneous but can be accelerated by the administration of ascorbate and by dietary protein restriction. Although most children with transient neonatal tyrosinemia are asymptomatic and have normal development, some adverse effect on development cannot be eliminated.

8. A human maleylacetoacetate isomerase (MAI) cDNA has been cloned. No patients with clearly documented MAI deficiency have yet been identified.

9. Hepatorenal tyrosinemia is an autosomal recessive disease caused by deficiency of fumarylacetoacetate hydrolase (FAH) (OMIM 276700). Symptoms are highly variable and include acute liver failure, cirrhosis, hepatocellular carcinoma, renal Fanconi syndrome, glomerulosclerosis, and crises of peripheral neuropathy. Hypertyrosinemia is present in most untreated patients. The presence of elevated levels of succinylacetone in plasma or urine is diagnostic for this condition. Most patients show a partial response to dietary restriction of phenylalanine and tyrosine. Hepatic transplantation cures the liver manifestations and prevents further neurologic crises. Patients treated with NTBC, an inhibitor of 4HPPD, have not developed acute hepatic or neurologic crises, but current data do not allow conclusions on the long-term risk of hepatocellular carcinoma in NTBC-treated patients. The human *FAH* gene has been cloned and mapped to chromosome 15 q23-q25. In hepatocytes of many patients, disease-causing mutations revert to the normal sequence. Such hepatocytes form nodules with normal FAH enzyme activity. Thirty-four different *FAH* mutations have been defined. Founder mutations are known in two areas where hepatorenal tyrosinemia is frequent: The splice mutation IVS12 + 5G → A accounts for most patients in Quebec and is frequent worldwide, and W262X is common in Finland. Two murine models of FAH deficiency have been developed.

METABOLISM OF TYROSINE

General Considerations

L-Tyrosine, first purified in 1849,[1] is an aromatic amino acid of molecular weight 181.2. It is one of the least soluble amino acids (2.5 mM at 25°C in water) and forms characteristic crystals at high concentrations.[2] In this chapter, *tyrosine* refers to L-tyrosine, the only metabolically active form present in mammalian systems.

In mammals, tyrosine is derived either from hydrolysis of dietary or tissue protein or from hydroxylation of dietary or tissue phenylalanine (Fig. 79-1) and hence is considered a semiessential amino acid. Tyrosine is the starting point of synthetic pathways leading to catecholamines, thyroid hormone, and the melanin pigments. Quantitatively, however, the major fates of tyrosine are incorporation into proteins or degradation via the series of reactions shown in Fig. 79-1. The catabolic reactions are cytoplasmic and occur predominantly in hepatocytes. In the presence of excess tyrosine, physiologic degradation is controlled at the level of tyrosine aminotransferase (TAT), the first enzyme of the tyrosine catabolic pathway (see below). Tyrosine is both gluconeogenic and ketogenic. It represents one of the few sources

A list of standard abbreviations is located immediately preceding the index in each volume. Nonstandard abbreviations used in this chapter include: TAT = tyrosine aminotransferase; 4HPP = 4-hydroxyphenylpyruvic acid; SA = succinylacetone; 4HPPD = 4-hydroxyphenylpyruvic acid dioxygenase; MAA = maleylacetoacetate; MAI = maleylacetoacetate isomerase; FAH = fumarylacetoacetate hydrolase; FAA = fumarylacetoacetate; NTBC = 2-(2-nitro-4-trifluoromethylbenzoyl)-1,3-cyclohexanedione; SAA = succinylacetoacetate; ALA = delta-aminolevulinic acid.

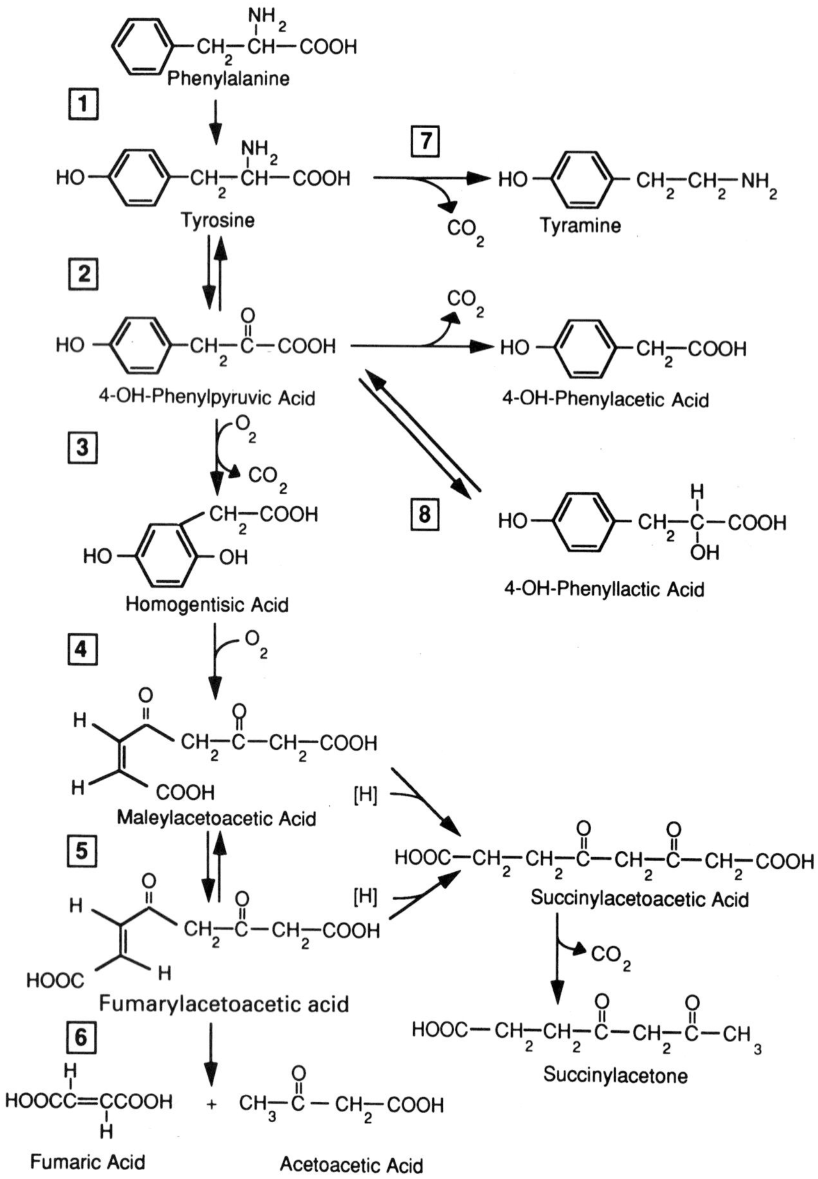

Fig. 79-1 The intermediates and enzymes of tyrosine catabolism. The numbered enzymes and their abbreviations and cofactors are (1) phenylalanine hydroxylase (tetrahydrobiopterin), (2) tyrosine aminotransferase (TAT) (pyridoxine), (3) 4-hydroxyphenylpyruvic acid dioxygenase (4HPPD) (ascorbate, oxygen), (4) homogentisic acid oxidase (iron, oxygen), (5) maleylacetoacetic acid isomerase (MAI) (glutathione), and (6) fumarylacetoacetic acid hydrolase (FAH). For reactions 7 and 8, the responsible enzymes have not been identified.

of ketone bodies independent of the 3-hydroxy-3-methylglutaryl CoA pathway (see Chap. 102).

Metabolite Levels

Typical levels of tyrosine in normal humans and mice are shown in Table 79-1. As with many amino acids, plasma tyrosine levels increase following even moderate protein ingestion,[3] decrease during sleep,[4] and are determined in part genetically.[5,6] They are not changed by moderate exercise.[3] Plasma tyrosine levels are about 10 μM lower in women than in men.[7] They are moderately decreased by pregnancy[8] and by administration of oral contraceptives.[9] A fetal-maternal gradient is present, fetal plasma tyrosine being 2.2 ± 0.5 (mean ± 1 standard deviation) times that of the mother.[2] The clearance (0.7–2.0 ml/min/1.73 m^2) and urinary concentration of tyrosine (about 2 percent of total urinary amino acids in adults) are low because of efficient tubular resorption (97–99 percent).[2]

The transamination product of tyrosine, 4-hydroxyphenylpyruvate (4HPP), is found in low concentration in plasma (< 2.8 μM)[10] and is actively cleared by the renal tubule.[10,11] Related products excreted at times of 4HPP accumulation include 4-hydroxyphenyllactate, 4-hydroxyphenylacetate, *N*-acetyltyrosine, and tyramine (see Fig. 79-1). 4-Hydroxyphenyllactate can be formed from 4HPP by lactate dehydrogenase.[12] Tyramine is formed principally by the action of gut bacteria,[13] probably with some contribution by tissue decarboxylases. Normal urinary concentrations of 4HPP, 4-hydroxyphenyllactate, and *N*-acetyltyrosine are less than 2 mmol/mol of creatinine, and of 4-hydroxyphenylacetate, 6 to 28 mmol/mol of creatinine.[14] In normal controls, succinylacetone (SA) concentrations are 0.01 to 0.14 μmol/mol of creatinine in urine and 0.005 to 0.163 μM in plasma.[15]

Enzymology

The enzymes mediating the reactions shown in Fig. 79-1 are discussed individually below. Much of this pathway was defined by the pioneering studies of W. E. Knox.[16] The genes of all the enzymes in the tyrosine catabolic pathway have been cloned. *In vitro*, the mean normal liver activity of the first enzyme discussed (TAT) is usually measured to be one-third to one-half of that of the second (4HPPD), which in turn is one-half to one-tenth that of the last enzymes of tyrosine catabolism (MAA isomerase and FAH).[17–22]

Phenylalanine Hydroxylase. Phenylalanine hydroxylase is a pteridine-dependent mixed-function oxidase located in the cytoplasm of hepatocytes. It catalyses the rate-limiting step in phenylalanine catabolism and is described in Chap. 77.

Table 79-1 Normal Levels of Tyrosine in Humans and Mice

	Age	Typical Normal Range*
Human		
Plasma (μM)	Newborn	25–103
	Child	30–90
	Adult	35–90
Cerebrospinal urine fluid (μM)	Adult	5–20
	Newborn	6–55
Urine (mmol/mol creatine)	Child	6–55
	Adult	2–23
Mouse (μM)	Adult	51±13
	Newborn	147±42

*Human values were compiled from several sources[2,7,335,336] and from values obtained locally. For individual patients, values must be compared with the normal range of the laboratory performing the analysis. Plasma tyrosine levels are from fasting individuals. For mice, values are mean ±1 standard deviation; newborn mice ($n = 4$)[240] and adult mice ($n = 14$, age $>$ 6 weeks).[242]

Tyrosine Aminotransferase

L-Tyrosine-2-oxoglutarate aminotransferase (TAT, E.C. 2.6.1.5), the first enzyme of tyrosine catabolism, has been studied extensively in rodents because of its hormone-, development-, and tissue-specific pattern of expression (reviewed in refs. 23–25) and its role as the rate-determining step of tyrosine catabolism.

The TAT gene has been characterized in humans,[26] rats,[27] and mice.[28] In humans it is located on chromosome 16q22.1-22.3,[29] spans 10.9 kb, contains 12 exons, and generates a 2.75-kb mRNA (GenBank Accession Number X55675). The predicted 454-residue peptide has a molecular weight of 50.4 kDa. TAT is a cytoplasmic dimer. It is phosphorylated, its N-terminus is acetylated, and pyridoxal-5′-phosphate is bound to Lys280.[30] Comparison with aspartate aminotransferase has identified conserved residues felt to be essential to enzyme function.[30]

TAT is a useful model for studies of hormonal regulation of gene expression. Glucocorticoids and cyclic AMP increase TAT transcription[24] by different but complementary mechanisms.[24] Under maximal induction, TAT can increase to 0.5 percent of rat hepatocyte cytoplasmic protein from a baseline level of 0.03 percent.[24] Hormone responsiveness is less well documented for human than for rodent TAT.

TAT is developmentally regulated. Although small amounts are detectable toward the end of gestation in fetal rats,[31] TAT activity increases rapidly after birth to peak at 12 hours at twice adult levels and then decreases to adult levels within 2 days.[24] In humans, TAT values are also low in the neonatal period.[32]

Since expression of TAT is strictly limited to the cytoplasm of hepatocytes,[33,34] TAT activity is a useful marker of hepatocytic differentiation. Of note, overexpression of TAT in Chinese hamster ovary cells, COS cells, and fibroblasts, using a transfected TAT cDNA with a viral promoter, produced no phenotypic effect.[35]

TAT is the rate-determining enzyme of tyrosine catabolism under most conditions.[36] Under conditions of maximal induction of TAT and tyrosine loading, 4-hydroxyphenylpyruvic acid dioxygenase (4HPPD)[36] or homogentisate oxidase[37] can become rate-limiting. Other enzymes such as aspartate aminotransferase (E.C.2.6.1.1) can transaminate tyrosine *in vitro*. Although mitochondrial aspartate aminotransferase has a high capacity for catalyzing tyrosine transamination,[33] cytoplasmic aspartate aminotransferase has little affinity for tyrosine.[33] These enzymes are felt to play a minor role in cytoplasmic tyrosine catabolism under normal conditions. The presence of marked hypertyrosinemia in untreated TAT-deficient humans and animals strongly supports this notion.

The rapid induction and short half-life (2–3 hours[24]) of TAT permit rapid fluctuations of activity in response to dietary and other stimuli. Diurnal variation of TAT is well documented in rodents. The short half-life of TAT may be due to two negatively charged PEST-like regions similar to the proline(P)-glutamate(E)-serine(S)-threonine(T) rich sequences associated with rapid degradation in other proteins.[30]

The enzymatic mechanism of tyrosine aminotransferase is felt to be similar to that of other α-aminotransferases,[23] which involves two half reactions and observes ping-pong BiBi kinetics.[38] Tyrosine and 2-oxoglutarate are the substrates for TAT *in vivo*.[23] K_m values for human TAT have been calculated[20,39]: tyrosine, 1040 μM; 2-oxoglutarate, 170 μM. The K_d value for pyridoxine-5′-pyrophosphate is 0.69 μM.[39] The TAT reaction is reversible under physiologic conditions.

4-Hydroxyphenylpyruvate Dioxygenase

4HPPD (E.C. 1.13.11.27) is an 87-kDa homodimer[40] found in the cytoplasm of hepatocytes and renal tubular cells.[41] The human 4HPPD peptide is 392 residues long.[40] 4HPPD has been purified from human,[19,42] pig,[43,44] and chicken[45] liver. Human,[46] mouse,[47] and porcine[48] cDNAs have been cloned. The enzyme is highly conserved in evolution, including in bacteria[49] and plants.[50] The human 4HPPD gene maps to chromosome 12q24-qter,[46,51] is about 21 kb in size, and contains 14 exons[52,53] (GenBank Accession Number X72389). The 5′ untranslated region contains several potential transcription factor binding elements including CRE, AP-2, and Sp1 sites. *In vitro* promoter studies revealed a possible role for cAMP in the regulation of promoter activity.[53] The C-terminus of the protein is required for enzymatic function.[54] 4HPPD is identical to the F-antigen,[48] a cytoplasmic liver protein that has been studied extensively by immunologists as a model for the induction of tolerance and autoimmunity in mice.[55,56]

The 4HPPD reaction is complex, involving the decarboxylation and oxidation of the alpha carbon of the side chain to a carboxylic acid, migration of the side chain on the benzene ring, and hydroxylation of the ring at the position from which the side chain was displaced (see Fig. 79-1). Molecular oxygen is consumed and contributes an oxygen atom to both the hydroxyl and carboxyl groups of homogentisic acid.[57] Ascorbic acid is the natural cofactor of 4HPPD, although it can be replaced *in vitro* by other reducing agents.[42] Ferrous iron is tightly bound to 4HPPD[44,58] and is catalytically important.[42] K_m values for 4HPP (40–60 μM)[34,42] and oxygen (50 μM)[42] have been calculated for the human enzyme. Substrate inhibition of 4HPPD is well documented.[59] 4HPPD is inhibited by high concentrations of the enol form of 4HPP.[60] This minor species equilibrates with the keto form of 4HPP[60] via the action of phenylpyruvate keto-enol isomerase (E.C.5.3.2.1).[16] Clues to the mechanism of 4HPPD, gleaned from studies of artificial substrates[61] and the structure of the metabolites excreted in hawkinsinuria, discussed later in this chapter, suggest that decarboxylation precedes oxidation and that an epoxide intermediate may be formed.

Homogentisic Acid Oxidase

This cytoplasmic dioxygenase (E.C.1.13.11.15) is found in liver and kidney and mediates the cleavage of the aromatic ring of homogentisic acid (see Fig. 79-1). It is described in Chap. 92. Loss of function is not associated with hypertyrosinemia.

Maleylacetoacetate Isomerase

Recently, maleylacetoacetate (MAA) isomerase was cloned as a phenylalanine inducible gene in *Aspergillus nidulans*.[62] The protein has high homology to glutathione-*S*-transferases, consistent with its requirement for reduced glutathione as a cofactor. Human and mouse cDNAs also were isolated based on nucleotide and amino acid sequence homology with *Aspergillus* sequences. The human MAA isomerase cDNA predicts a 216-residue, 24-kDa peptide (GenBank Accession Number AJ001838). Expression of the putative human maleyacetoacetate isomerase (MAI) protein in *Escherichia coli* yielded high levels of MAI activity, confirming its identity.[62]

Fumarylacetoacetate Hydrolase

Fumarylacetoacetate hydrolase (FAH) (E.C.3.7.1.2) mediates the last step of tyrosine catabolism, the hydrolytic formation of fumarate and acetoacetate. FAH is a soluble cytosolic homodimer of 46.3-kDa subunits.[63–66] It has no known cofactors. The enzyme has been purified from rat,[63,67] bovine,[68] and human liver.[65,67] Polyclonal antibodies to FAH have been used for immunodetection of the corresponding protein in human tissues and cells.[64,67,68] Human FAH has a K_m of 1.3 μM for fumarylacetoacetate[69] and is active over a wide range of pH.[69]

Enzyme assay, western blot analysis, and immunohistochemistry show that FAH is particularly abundant in liver and renal tubules but is also a housekeeping enzyme expressed in most tissues at a level approximately 2 to 5 percent of that in liver.[67,68,70] Labelle *et al.*[71] showed that anti-FAH antibodies react strongly with cerebral white matter and cultured oligodendroglia.

Following the isolation and purification of rat FAH mRNA,[72] both human[66,73] and rat[74] cDNAs were isolated and sequenced. The authenticity of the clones was confirmed by hybrid selection of mRNA,[74] *in vitro* transcription-translation,[66] and sequence homology with tryptic fragments of purified FAH.[66,73] The human cDNA has a 1257-bp open reading frame encoding 419 amino acids[66] (GenBank Accession Number M55150).

Southern blot analysis indicates that the FAH gene is present as a single copy per haploid genome in both humans[66] and rats.[74] The human FAH locus maps to 15q23-q25.[66] The human FAH gene spans 30 to 35 kb and contains 14 exons.[75] The positions of the intron-exon junctions of the human and mouse genes are identical (G Kalsey, personal communication), in contrast to earlier reports.[165]

Tyrosine Metabolism in *Aspergillus nidulans*: A Metabolic and Genetic Model for Tyrosine Catabolism

The filamentous ascomycete *A. nidulans* is an excellent model for study of the biochemistry and genetics of phenylalanine and tyrosine catabolism.[76] All six enzymes involved in phenylalanine breakdown in mammals are present in *Aspergillus.* Of note, *Aspergillus* also can metabolize phenylacetate to homogentisic acid, converging at this level with the tyrosine catabolic pathway. Two genes of tyrosine metabolism (homogentisic acid oxidase and MAI) were first cloned in *Aspergillus* by the isolation of phenylacetate-induced genes.[62,77] The human and mouse homologues were then identified by sequence homology to anonymous expressed sequence tags. The amino acid sequences are highly conserved between humans and fungus for homogentisic acid oxidase (52 percent), MAI (45 percent), and FAH (47 percent). In *Aspergillus,* these three genes are clustered within about 6 kb, and the promoters are inducible by phenylalanine and phenylacetate. Knockouts of all three genes have been generated and have distinct phenotypes. In media containing a high concentration of phenylalanine, homogentisate oxidase (HGO) knockouts grow well but accumulate red-brown pigment. MAI knockout strains grow poorly but do form small colonies, whereas FAH mutants do not grow at all. These phenotypes support the hypothesis that MAA and fumarylacetoacetate (FAA) are cytotoxic and suggest that MAA may be less toxic than FAA. The fungal mutations can be cross-complemented by expression of human genes. Thus *Aspergillus* provides a genetic system to study mutations and structure/function relationships of the enzymes of tyrosine degradation.

LABORATORY DETERMINATION OF TYROSINE AND ITS METABOLITES

Plasma tyrosine levels are usually quantitated by ion-exchange amino acid chromatography. For neonatal screening, spectrophotometric[78] or bacteriologic (Guthrie) assays can be used. 4-Hydroxyphenylpyruvate and its derivatives can be analyzed by gas chromatography–mass spectrometry.[14] The Millon test[79] was used in many early studies and can detect large amounts of tyrosine and its 4-hydroxy derivatives (i.e., tyrosyluria). The nitrosonapthol test[80] is a screening test for tyrosine, 4-hydroxyphenyllactate, and 4-hydroxyphenylacetate but not 4HPP. SA levels are often determined enzymatically[81]; a highly sensitive gas chromatography-mass spectrometry technique also has been described.[15]

DIFFERENTIAL DIAGNOSIS OF HYPERTYROSINEMIA

Several inherited and acquired conditions can cause hypertyrosinemia (Table 79-2). Most can be diagnosed by clinical history, physical examination, and readily available laboratory tests. The most common causes of fasting hypertyrosinemia are transient neonatal tyrosinemia and liver disease.

In practice, the most difficult diagnostic problem is hypertyrosinemia in the context of liver dysfunction. On the one hand, it is important that hepatorenal tyrosinemia be considered in cases of hepatic dysfunction of unknown etiology. On the other, this can lead to diagnostic problems in hepatocellular diseases with secondary hypertyrosinemia. The pattern of plasma amino acids is not particularly helpful in these patients because both tyrosine and methionine can be elevated nonspecifically in cirrhosis and in acute liver failure.[82,83]

The presence of renal tubular dysfunction in patients with hepatocellular failure is consistent with hepatorenal tyrosinemia but is also seen in other hereditary metabolic diseases such as galactosemia, hereditary fructose intolerance, and lactic acidoses, as well as glycogen storage disease type IV. Indeed, cases of galactosemia and hepatitis have been detected by neonatal tyrosine and phenylalanine screening.[84] In older children with renal Fanconi syndrome and hepatic dysfunction, Wilson disease should be considered. The presence of a family history suggestive of tyrosinemia is helpful in the diagnosis. Observation of typical neurologic crises in a patient with liver dysfunction is probably diagnostic for hepatorenal tyrosinemia. The presence of high levels of SA in blood or urine establishes the diagnosis.

A practical consideration is that plasma levels of tyrosine and of several other amino acids can be mildly elevated in nonfasting subjects. Experienced interpretation and repeated plasma amino acid chromatography should be obtained prior to initiating investigations for hypertyrosinemia, especially if the patient has none of the symptoms of the diseases described in Table 79-2. Some diseases of tyrosine catabolism and its branch pathways are not associated with hypertyrosinemia. These include albinism secondary to tyrosinase deficiency (see Chap. 221) and alkaptonuria (see Chap. 92). Hypertyrosinemia is mild or absent in hawkinsinuria.

Table 79-2 Causes of Hypertyrosinemia

1. Transient tyrosinemia of the newborn
2. Severe hepatocellular dysfunction
3. Inborn errors of tyrosine catabolism
   a. Hepatorenal tyrosinemia
   b. Oculocutaneous tyrosinemia
   c. 4HPPD deficiency
4. Other
   a. NTBC treatment
   b. Scurvy[337,338]
   c. Hyperthyroidism[338]
   d. Postprandial state

NOTE: Transient tyrosinemia of the newborn is probably still the most common cause of hypertyrosinemia, followed by hepatocellular failure and inborn errors of tyrosine catabolism. Determination of tyrosine levels is rarely of diagnostic use in the other conditions on the list. In malnutrition,[171,172] tyrosine intolerance with tyrosyluria can occur.

4-Hydroxyphenylic derivatives of tyrosine can be found in increased amounts in patients with liver disease. Urinary 4-hydroxyphenylacetic acid is frequently of gut bacterial origin and may be increased in malabsorption.[79] Patients receiving parenteral nutrition solutions containing *N*-acetyl tyrosine may excrete large amounts of this compound.[14,79]

THE BIOLOGIC EFFECTS OF HYPERTYROSINEMIA

In general, brief periods of hypertyrosinemia are well tolerated in humans and mammals. However, chronic hypertyrosinemia is associated with neurologic and developmental difficulties in numerous patients with TAT deficiency and some with 4HPPD deficiency and transient hypertyrosinemia,[85–87] although a causal link with hypertyrosinemia is not formally established. In contrast, children with hepatorenal tyrosinemia have normal intelligence, and central nervous system (CNS) signs are clinically absent. Current data do not eliminate the possibility that elevated levels of tyrosine and/or its derivatives may have noxious effects on CNS development in some patients.

In rats, massive tyrosine intake and the use of inhibitors of 4HPPD have been associated with the development of exudative keratitis and painful edema of the paws,[88,89] suggesting that the signs of oculocutaneous tyrosinemia may be directly related to increased tissue levels of tyrosine (see "Pathophysiology" under "Oculocutaneous Tyrosinemia," below). Symptoms related to branch pathways of tyrosine metabolism that lead to thyroxine, catecholamine, and melanin synthesis generally are absent in hypertyrosinemic conditions. The hepatic and renal manifestations of hepatorenal tyrosinemia are specific to that condition and not related to hypertyrosinemia.

OCULOCUTANEOUS TYROSINEMIA (TYROSINEMIA TYPE II)

Oculocutaneous tyrosinemia is caused by the autosomal recessive deficiency of TAT. It affects the skin, the ocular cornea, and the CNS. It is also known as *tyrosinemia type II, tyrosine aminotransferase deficiency, keratosis palmoplantaris with corneal dystrophy,* and *Richner-Hanhart syndrome.* It is assigned OMIM 276600.

Richner (1938)[90] and Hanhart (1947)[91] independently described this clinical syndrome and its autosomal recessive transmission. Hypertyrosinemia was associated with this presentation in 1967,[92] and in 1973, TAT deficiency was demonstrated in patients.[93] More than 50 cases have been described in patients of many different ethnic and geographic origins (e.g., Italian, German, French, Swiss, Spanish, Norwegian, American, Canadian, Australian, Arabic, Lebanese, Japanese, Turkish, and Ashkenazi Jewish[94–97]). Nearly half the reported patients are of Italian descent, and an Italian registry of the disease has been established.[98]

Pathophysiology

The current hypothesis of the corneal disease seen in tyrosinemia type II is that tyrosine crystallizes in corneal epithelial cells, disrupting their lysosomes and initiating an inflammatory response. The low solubility of tyrosine[2] may be important in this context. This aspect of oculocutaneous tyrosinemia can be reproduced in young rats fed a diet containing 10 percent tyrosine by weight.[88] In this animal model, early corneal epithelial lesions contain birefringent needle-shaped crystals thought to be tyrosine.[99] Chemotactic activity was demonstrated in supernatants of corneal organ cultures derived from tyrosine-fed rats but not in cultures from rats fed a normal diet.[100]

In contrast, neither crystal formation nor lysosomal damage has been observed on skin histology of TAT-deficient patients. It has been suggested that excessive amounts of intracellular tyrosine could enhance crosslinks between aggregated tonofilaments and modulate the number and stability of microtubules.[101] Both mechanical and regional factors also play a role in view of the confinement of the hyperkeratotic skin lesions to palms and soles and the sparing of skin grafted from other regions.[102] Strains of mink[103] and of German shepherd dogs[104] have been described in which oculocutaneous tyrosinemia and TAT deficiency are found.

Clinical Phenotype

Eye, skin, and neurologic signs are the cardinal features of the disease. The onset of ophthalmologic symptomology is usually in the first year of life but has occurred as early as the first day of life[105] and as late as 38 years of age.[97] Skin manifestations usually start after the first year but may begin by 1 month of age.[106] Either eye or skin symptoms can be the presenting complaint, and manifestations may be confined to the skin[96,107–109] or the eye.[96,110–112] The symptoms of the disease can vary among different affected family members. For instance, the brother of one symptomatic proband is totally asymptomatic at age 39 despite having persistent hypertyrosinemia.[97]

Eye signs include lacrimation, photophobia, redness, and pain, typically with exacerbations and partial remissions. On examination, there are usually central dendritic corneal erosions that stain poorly, if at all, with fluorescein. This is of clinical note because herpes simplex keratitis is an important differential diagnosis.[113] Conjunctivitis may be seen, and neovascularization may be prominent. Bacterial and viral cultures are negative. Long-term consequences include corneal opacities, decreased visual acuity, cornea plana, astigmatism, strabismus, amblyopia, and glaucoma. Rarely, nystagmus and cataracts have been reported.[110,112] Deposits in a corneal graft after lamellar keratoplasty have been reported in a patient who was not receiving dietary therapy.[114]

Skin lesions consist of painful, nonpruritic, hyperkeratotic plaques on the soles, palms, and plantar surfaces of the digits. Fingertips and the hypothenar and thenar eminences are areas of predilection. In rare cases these lesions have been preceded for years by blisters. Hyperkeratotic lesions also have been seen occasionally in other areas such as elbows, knees, and ankles.[101,109,115] Leukokeratosis of the tongue has been reported.[116] Hyperhydrosis may be associated with the hyperkeratosis.[108,115,117] Hyperpigmentation is absent. Pain may be severe enough to prevent ambulation. An intriguing observation exists of a patient who had skin from the thigh grafted onto her heel. The graft remained free of hyperkeratosis, which stopped abruptly at the graft margin.[102]

A variable degree of mental retardation occurs in less than 50 percent of patients.[94,98,118] It is not known whether cytosolic TAT deficiency can present solely as a neurologic disease.[119–121] There is no relationship between age at diagnosis and mental retardation.[120] However, it has been speculated that the degree of retardation may be related to higher values of plasma tyrosine.[98] Rarely, convulsions and microcephaly have been reported,[98] but their association with TAT deficiency is unclear. One patient had extinguished visual evoked potentials as well as developmental delay.[112] Behavioral problems also have been described.[108]

The eye, skin, and CNS are the only organs known to be affected in tyrosinemia type II. An atypical patient with cytosolic TAT deficiency and multiple congenital anomalies[92] was shown to have a small *de novo* interstitial deletion of one allele.[29] Most likely this patient had a contiguous gene syndrome.

Biochemical and Molecular Phenotypes

TAT activity is greatly reduced or absent in the supernatant of liver homogenates from the few patients in whom it has been measured. Plasma tyrosine values range from 370 to 3300 μmol/liter in untreated patients.[94,96–98,107,118] The other plasma amino acid levels are usually normal, although one untreated patient was reported to have a mildly elevated plasma phenylalanine value that returned to normal on treatment (Phe = 327 μM, Tyr = 2870 μM).[112,122] Routine renal and liver function tests are normal.

Tyrosine is the only amino acid increased in the urine of these patients. There is also an increased urinary excretion of tyrosine metabolites 4HPP, 4-hydroxyphenyllactic acid, 4-hydroxyphenylacetic acid, *N*-acetyltyrosine, and 4-tyramine. Quantitative data on urinary excretion of tyrosine metabolites are presented in previous editions.[94,95] The apparent paradox of an *increased* urinary excretion of metabolites situated downstream of the metabolic block may be explained by the ability of mitochondrial aspartate aminotransferase (E.C.2.6.1.1) to convert tyrosine to 4HPP in the presence of high circulating concentrations of tyrosine. Several tissues (e.g., liver, kidney, heart, and muscle) contain a substantial amount of aspartate aminotransferase. However, tissues other than liver and kidney lack 4HPPD activity. Presumably, significant amounts of 4HPP and its derivatives are not taken up by liver and are excreted in urine.

To date, 15 different mutations in TAT have been described. The *R57X* mutant allele, found mostly on a specific haplotype, is frequent in Italian patients.[123,124] No correlation is evident between the residual activity of the enzymes and the severity of clinical symptoms.[124]

Pathology

Light microscopy of skin biopsies may reveal hyperkeratosis, acanthosis, and parakeratosis.[94,125] Homogeneous refractile eosinophilic inclusions may be seen in the stratum corneum and upper malpighian layer.[108] These changes are not diagnostic of the disease. The following have been described on electron microscopy: lipidlike granules with 10-nm filaments and myelinlike figures intermixed with the granules,[93] keratinocytes with increased tonofibrils, and tightly packed microtubular and tonofibrillar masses.[101] Inflammatory changes are minimal.[101] Tyrosine crystals have not been seen.[101]

Conjunctival biopsy may show thickened epithelium, parakeratotic changes, and an accumulation of large inclusion bodies in the conjunctival epithelium, the fibrocytes, and the blood vessel epithelium. Subepithelial tissue may be infiltrated with plasma cells, and numerous vessels may be seen lying immediately under the epithelium. Corneal lesions may involve the epithelium, Bowman membrane, and anterior stroma. Birefringent tyrosine crystals have been seen in the corneal stroma.[126–128]

Diagnosis, Treatment, and Genetics

In a patient with a typical clinical presentation, the diagnosis is established by the finding of hypertyrosinemia. The plasma phenylalanine level is normal, and an abnormal urinary excretion of tyrosine metabolites (4HPP, 4-hydroxyphenyllactic acid, 4-hydroxyphenylacetic acid, *N*-acetyltyrosine, and 4-tyramine) is present. It is usually unnecessary to perform liver biopsy for TAT assay. Preclinical detection and treatment should be possible in areas in which neonatal screening for hypertyrosinemia is practiced.

The treatment consists of dietary restriction of tyrosine and phenylalanine to a degree sufficient to resolve eye and skin symptoms. There is no consensus as to the optimal blood level of tyrosine nor at what age the diet should be started to prevent neurologic impairment. Some authors have suggested that a blood level of tyrosine of 600 μM is a reasonable goal.[120] In order to optimize growth and meet the patient's nutritional requirements, commercial phenylalanine- and tyrosine-free supplements are used. The eye and skin lesions usually resolve after a few weeks of dietary therapy, but they recur if the diet is stopped. Oral retinoids can improve skin lesions without changing the tyrosine levels.[108,129] Tyrosine deposits in corneal grafts have been reported after lamellar keratoplasty.[114] However, such deposits after perforating keratoplasty to our knowledge have not been detected.[127] Treatment with systemic steroids should be avoided because the disease can worsen with such therapy.[127]

Although, to our knowledge, pyridoxine-responsive cases of TAT deficiency have not been described, it would be prudent to test the effect of pyridoxine administration (50–100 mg/day) early in the course of therapy.

Oculocutaneous tyrosinemia is an autosomal recessive condition. Males and females are equally affected. Consanguinity has been present in the parents of at least 20 probands.[118] The fetal effects of maternal oculocutaneous tyrosinemia are not yet well documented. Two children of an untreated mother with oculocutaneous tyrosinemia had microphthalmos and psychomotor retardation.[98] In another family, one child presented with seizures and mental retardation early in life.[130] In contrast, 15 other children of TAT-deficient mothers are doing well.[97,98,114,117,131] In view of the incidence of mental retardation in TAT-deficient patients, careful dietary control of maternal plasma tyrosine concentrations should be considered during pregnancy.[132]

DISEASES ASSOCIATED WITH ABNORMAL 4HPPD

At least three conditions are caused by dysfunction of 4HHPD. (1) Primary deficiency of 4HPPD has been documented. (2) Immaturity of 4HPPD is felt to be responsible for transient hypertyrosinemia of the newborn. (3) Hawkinsinuria is felt to arise from deficiency of an intermediate step of the 4HPPD reaction. In many cases, dysfunction of 4HPPD seems compatible with normal development, and the biochemical abnormalities respond well to therapy.

Primary Deficiency of 4HPPD (Tyrosinemia Type III)

This condition has also been called *tyrosinemia type III* and is assigned MIM 276710. Four patients have been described.[34,133–136] Three came to medical attention for neurologic problems, two for mental retardation, and one for ataxia.[133] The fourth patient was detected by neonatal screening.[135] Plasma tyrosine levels range from 355 to 640 μM, and 4HPP and 4-hyroxyphenyllactic acid are elevated in urine. Cerebrospinal fluid tyrosine concentration in one patient was 176 μM (normal, 7–41 μM). The most recently described patient[136] is a 14-year-old boy treated for 10 years with tyrosine restriction to maintain plasma tyrosine levels between 100 and 200 μM. This was associated with improvement in behavioral problems but persistent mental retardation over this period (IQ = 45 at 12 years of age), with normal results of cerebral computed tomographic scan and magnetic resonance imaging and brain stem auditory, visual, and somatosensory evoked potentials.

Hepatic histology was normal in one patient[133] and showed mild fatty degeneration in another.[134] 4HPPD activity was undetectable in the first patient.[133] Liver 4HPPD activity in the second patient was 10 percent of control values, and an increased K_m for 4-hydroxyphenylpyruvate (230 μM) was demonstrated.[34] Other enzymes of tyrosine catabolism (TAT in both patients and FAH in patient 2) were normal when measured.[34,133] In the most recent patient,[136] 4HPPD was markedly reduced in liver (0.2 nmol/min/mg of protein; normal, 10.8–18.4; $n = 3$), whereas TAT was normal and FAH activity was nearly normal (33 nmol/min/mg of protein; control range, 38.8–46.4; $n = 3$).

The relationship, if any, between 4HPPD deficiency and neurologic abnormalities remains to be established, since there is a selection bias in the way the patients were detected. The observations are worrisome, and treatment with tyrosine restriction seems indicated until further information is available. A trial of ascorbate supplementation is also reasonable.

Little can be said about the incidence of this condition because asymptomatic affected individuals may well exist. Other hypertyrosinemic patients in the literature have had metabolite profiles consistent with 4HPPD deficiency, including one[137,138] who had a tremor and moderate mental retardation and one who had mental retardation, microcephaly, and cataracts.[139] These patients were evaluated because of their neurologic findings, and hence a causal relationship between their biochemical abnormalities and neurologic symptoms cannot be proved.

Endo *et al.*[140] have described a 4HPPD-deficient mouse strain. The causal mutation is a single-base change in exon 7 that produces a stop codon and leads to skipping of exon 7 in most transcripts.[47] Murine 4HPPD deficiency is autosomal recessive and has no overt phenotypic consequences. 4HPPD activity and immunoreactive 4HPPD protein are undetectable in tissues of affected mice,[140] as is 4HPPD mRNA. The mice have hypertyrosinemia (670–1120 μM on a normal diet) and excrete massive amounts of 4-hydroxyphenylacetic, 4-hydroxyphenyllactic, and 4-hydroxyphenylpyruvic acids in comparison with congenic mice. Recently, the tyrosinemia type III mouse model has been used to demonstrate the short-term efficacy of adenoviral gene therapy.[141] Complete correction of all metabolic parameters was achieved until elimination of the adenovirally transduced cells by the immune system. Although the motor performance of 4HPPD-deficient mice is grossly normal, it will be of interest to document psychomotor development abnormalities, if any, in these mice.

Hawkinsinuria

Since the first report in 1975,[142] only five children are known to have become symptomatic with this intriguing condition, although several asymptomatic but biochemically affected family members have been described. Despite its rarity, this disease merits attention because it is treatable and because of the interesting metabolic considerations that it raises. Hawkinsinuria has been assigned OMIM 140350.

Pathophysiology. As discussed by Wilcken *et al.*,[143] the abnormal compounds produced in hawkinsinuria are felt to be derived from an intermediate of the 4HPPD reaction (Fig. 79-2). The amino acid that is diagnostic for this condition is (2-L-cystein-*S*-yl-1,4-dihydroxycyclohex-5-en-1-yl)acetic acid. Its trivial name, *hawkinsin,* is derived from the name of the family in which it was first described.[144] In isotopic loading studies in patients, hawkinsin was shown to be a metabolite of tyrosine.[145] Its structure suggests that it arises from the reaction of an epoxy intermediate with glutathione (see Fig. 79-2). The resulting depletion of glutathione could result in acceleration of glutamylcysteine synthesis and production of 5-oxoproline as in the hereditary deficiency of glutathione synthetase. 5-Oxoprolinuria has been observed in ill patients with hawkinsinuria and may explain the acidosis and hemolysis of some symptomatic infants.[143] The epoxide presumably reacts with other cell components or forms hawkinsin prior to encountering the product of the other (normal) 4HPPD allele, thus yielding a dominant phenotype. Wilcken *et al.*[143] suggested that 4-hydroxycyclohexylacetic acid, which was found in large amounts only in affected adults, may be the product of late-maturing epoxide hydrolases that may represent a detoxification mechanism in older patients. Because one normal 4HPPD allele is present in affected patients, hypertyrosinemia would be expected to be mild or absent, as is observed clinically.

The exact molecular basis of hawkinsinuria is unknown at present. It will be particularly interesting to study the effect of the mutation(s) responsible for this trait on the mechanism and subunit interactions of 4HPPD. The small number of patients with hawkinsinuria may reflect in part its benign nature under conditions of normal protein intake, which may seldom lead to medical consultation. However, the highly specific enzymatic mechanism proposed to cause hawkinsinuria would be expected to result from a limited number of mutations in 4HPPD, perhaps only one, which would be consistent with the apparent rarity of this condition.

Clinical Phenotype. The two initial patients developed metabolic acidosis and failure to thrive following weaning from breast milk.[142,143] A third was not breast fed and became symptomatic on standard formula feedings.[146] Plasma bicarbonate levels of 10 to 14 mM and blood pH values of 7.24 to 7.30 were reported. One patient[143] had a moderate hemolytic anemia. Symptoms responded to the reintroduction of breast milk or other low-protein feeds and to vitamin C supplementation. After several weeks of therapy, the diets were normalized, and the patients remained asymptomatic.[142,143] A recent abstract documents a similar patient from Germany[147] who was symptomatic until 12 months of age.

In one patient in whom microcephaly was present, "catchup" head growth was seen.[146] Several asymptomatic adults in these families had the biochemical phenotype of hawkinsinuria. All such patients for whom the information is available had been breast fed for at least 8 months, and none had suggestive symptoms in infancy.

Biochemical Phenotype. Hawkinsin is a prominent ninhydrin-positive compound that migrates in the region of phenylalanine and tyrosine on high-voltage electrophoresis of urine amino acids. On ion-exchange amino acid chromatography, hawkinsin migrates between urea and threonine.[148] Organic acid chromatography may reveal increased amounts of 4-hydroxyphenyllactic acid (e.g., 250 mmol/mol creatinine[143]) as well as 4-hydroxyphenylpyruvic

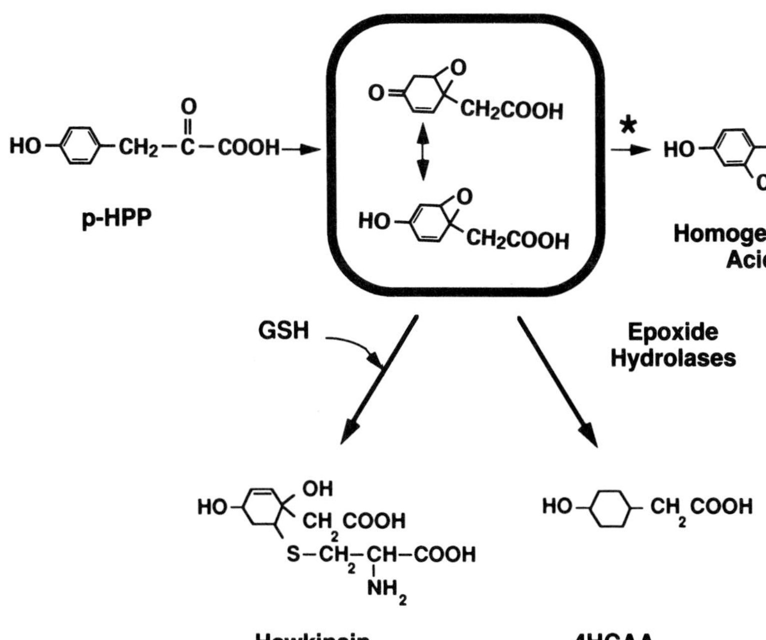

Fig. 79-2 The proposed metabolic basis of hawkinsinuria. The upper line shows the 4HPPD reaction. The epoxide compounds (enclosed within the box) are proposed to be intermediates in this reaction. In hawkinsinuria, they react either with glutathione to produce hawkinsin (*lower left*) or with epoxide hydrolases to produce 4-hydroxycyclohexylic acid (*lower right*). The defect in hawkinsinuria is hypothesized to affect the stage of the 4HPPD reaction indicated by an asterisk.

and 4-hydroxyphenylacetic acids. 5-Oxoproline (up to 20 mmol/mol creatinine[143]) may be present. 4-Hydroxycyclohexylacetic acid may be present, especially in adults. 4HPPD activity has not been reported in these patients. Hawkinsin also can be identified by iodoplatinate staining.[146] It is nitroprusside-negative. Nitroso-naphthol testing is variably positive in patients. Of note, hawkinsin has not been detected in the plasma of patients, and hypertyrosinemia (196 μM) has been reported in only one symptomatic patient.[142]

Treatment. Because the initial symptoms may be quite serious, treatment with the administration of breast milk and ascorbic acid (up to 1 g daily) should be initiated and continued for several weeks after symptoms subside, and a normal diet should be introduced progressively thereafter. Commercial infant formulas with a protein content similar to that of breast milk also may be effective in the control of symptoms.[146] Although we are not aware of manifestations in patients with hawkinsinuria after infancy, it would be prudent to follow the development of affected children and to observe them carefully for acidosis or hemolysis at times of metabolic stress.

Transient Tyrosinemia of the Newborn

Transient neonatal tyrosinemia is the most common disorder of amino acid metabolism in humans.[2] It is felt to be caused by an imbalance between the rate of tyrosine catabolism and the activity of 4HPPD, which is late to mature in the fetus and newborn. Risk factors for the development of transient tyrosinemia include prematurity, a high protein intake, and deficient vitamin C intake.[2,149] This condition, first described by Levine,[150] has been well reviewed previously.[2] Few recent studies have been reported, and its incidence may be falling because of modern neonatal feeding trends to avoid high protein intakes.

Pathophysiology. 4HPPD activity is low in the fetus and newborn of humans and other mammals,[32,41] and 4-hydroxyphenylpyruvate and its derivatives are excreted at high levels in patients with transient tyrosinemia,[2,151] consistent with a primary role for 4HPPD deficiency in transient tyrosinemia. The rapidity of the biochemical response to ascorbate supplementation suggests that 4HPPD is present but inactive within the hepatocyte. Inhibition of 4HPPD by its substrate 4HPP[59,60] may accentuate the hypertyrosinemia. Of note, tyrosine aminotransferase deficiency has been proposed as a cause of transient tyrosinemia.[32] Consistent with this, TAT is the rate-limiting step of tyrosine catabolism under normal circumstances[31,32] and shows late maturation.[32] However, the biochemical improvement of patients following administration of ascorbate, a cofactor of 4HPPD but not of tyrosine aminotransferase, suggests that most cases of transient tyrosinemia are due to immaturity of 4HPPD. Perhaps the rare variants of transient tyrosinemia that do not respond to ascorbate administration[149,152–155] are due to absence of 4HPPD protein or transient deficiency of TAT, although this is speculative.

Because of the generally benign nature of transient tyrosinemia and the localization of 4HPPD in liver and kidney only, enzymatic studies have not been performed in humans. Other primates and guinea pigs (mammals who, like humans, are unable to synthesize ascorbate) are potential models.

Transient tyrosinemia tentatively has been assigned OMIM 276500. A role for genetic factors in 4HPPD maturation is plausible but unproven. Identical twins can have discordant phenotypes.[156] Most children in studies of transient tyrosinemia received cow's milk with a protein intake of greater than 5 g/kg per day; diets providing less than 3 g/kg per day were protective.[2,156]

Diagnosis. The presence in an asymptomatic neonate of isolated hypertyrosinemia that responds to ascorbate administration or resolves spontaneously on a normal diet, together with the absence of liver, renal, or cutaneous signs, distinguishes transient tyrosinemia from other diseases discussed in this chapter.

Clinical Phenotype. Transient tyrosinemia is usually a biochemical finding in a clinically normal neonate,[157,158] although in some series hypertyrosinemia was associated with lethargy and reduced motor activity in the neonatal period.[87] Hepatorenal and cutaneous signs are absent. In one patient,[159] corneal opacities, presumably due to tyrosine crystals, were present transiently.

Some reports suggest that transient tyrosinemia may be associated with reduced intellectual prognosis in some patients.[85,86] A definitive study of this condition has not been performed. In affected individuals it is uncertain whether the developmental difficulties arose from elevated tyrosine levels or from an unknown but related neonatal phenomenon.

Biochemical Phenotype. The most specific diagnostic procedure is plasma amino acid chromatography, which reveals isolated hypertyrosinemia of a variable degree[73,157] but which may exceed 2 mM. Typically, the hypertyrosinemia peaks prior to 14 days[160,161] and resolves by 1 month. The course may be longer in premature infants, and some term neonates have prolonged hypertyrosinemia.[149,152,155] 4-Hydroxyphenyllactate is present in urine, as are 4HPP and 4-hydroxyphenylacetate. Urinary tyrosine is elevated and may form crystals. Biochemical abnormalities improve quickly following ascorbate administration. SA levels are normal in blood and urine.

Incidence. The incidence of hypertyrosinemia depends on the threshold value defined as abnormal, the age at testing, and the protein intake of the group tested. Unfortunately, detailed longitudinal studies of neonatal tyrosine levels and their relation to diet, development, and ethnicity have not been published. The following observations may provide some perspective. In the 1960s, up to 30 to 50 percent of premature newborns and 10 percent of term newborns were reported to have elevated levels of tyrosine.[2,162] Since then, newborn feeding practices have shifted from cow's milk to lower-protein formulas or breast feeding, and the mean protein intake of neonates has decreased. A reduction in the incidence of transient tyrosinemia has been reported at some centers.[163,164] In Belgium, the incidence of newborns having blood tyrosine levels above 1100 μM (20 mg/dl) at 4 to 5 days of life decreased coincident with the widespread introduction of humanized milk,[163] the percentage of neonates with birth weights under 2500 g who had hypertyrosinemia decreasing from 2.6 to 0.4 percent between 1972 and 1977. For neonates with birth weights above 2500 g, the incidence decreased from 0.7 to 0.2 percent.[163] In 1994, in Quebec, 2.4 percent of newborns had values greater than 248 μM at screening.[164] Transient tyrosinemia is particularly common in Inuits but not Native Americans of the eastern Canadian arctic and Alaska.[165] Although we have the impression that the incidence of transient tyrosinemia is falling because current feeding practices discourage high-protein intake such as cow's milk, no studies have addressed this specifically.

Treatment. Although transient neonatal tyrosinemia is probably benign in most cases, it is prudent to restrict protein intake to 2 g/kg per day and to administer ascorbic acid (50–200 mg/day orally for 1–2 weeks) to newborns identified as having transient hypertyrosinemia in order to normalize the plasma tyrosine level as quickly as possible. If the child is breast fed, we recommend continued breast feeding and administration of ascorbic acid. The serum tyrosine level begins to decrease within hours of ascorbate administration in most cases.[166] If the child has an otherwise normal examination and no family history compatible with hepatorenal tyrosinemia, he or she can be followed clinically and by a repeated tyrosine determination 2 or 3 days after the administration of ascorbic acid in order to ensure that the hypertyrosinemia is transient. In nonpremature infants or in those with any evidence of liver abnormalities, SA determination should be considered

OTHER ASPECTS OF 4HPPD METABOLISM

4HPPD inhibition by 2-(2-nitro-4-trifluoromethylbenzoyl)-1,3-cyclohexanedione (NTBC) leads to elevation in plasma tyrosine level and to urinary excretion of 4HPP and related compounds, as discussed under treatment of hepatorenal tyrosinemia.

The pioneering study of Grace Medes in 1932[167] was the first biochemical evaluation of a patient with abnormal tyrosine metabolism. The patient, a 49-year-old man of Russian Jewish descent, had myasthenia gravis but neither hepatorenal nor oculocutaneous signs and elevated urinary 4HPP excretion. Although he had no clinical evidence of oculocutaneous or hepatorenal tyrosinemia, his low excretion of urinary 4-hydroxyphenyllactate would be atypical for primary 4HPPD deficiency, as discussed in former editions of this book.[168,169] The patient remains an enigma, and his condition has been assigned a separate OMIM number (276800). For clarity and for historical reasons, we suggest reserving the term *tyrosinosis* for this entity. If another such patient is discovered, it will be of great interest to evaluate him with currently available techniques.

Hypertyrosinemia is observed in scurvy, presumably because the ascorbic acid cofactor of 4HPPD is lacking. The metabolic defect is corrected within 24 hours of ascorbate supplementation.[170] Children with marasmus may have a similar form of tyrosine intolerance.[171,172] A child with agenesis of the corpus callosum, to whom chloral hydrate was administered, transiently developed hypertyrosinemia and a pattern of urinary organic acids similar to that seen in 4HPPD deficiency.[173] However, other children receiving chloral hydrate have not shown these signs, and the same child later had a normal response to a tyrosine loading test, suggesting that this was a transient phenomenon, not necessarily related to chloral hydrate administration. The interesting family reported by Jaiswal[165] is difficult to explain in the framework of current views of tyrosinemia. The mother and all children were asymptomatic and were found fortuitously to have marked tyrosyluria. The index case had a serum tyrosine level of only 126 μM but was reported to have hepatic 4HPPD deficiency.

4HPPD is nonspecifically decreased in liver diseases, and low levels are difficult to interpret in this context. Lindblad suggested that the ratio between the activity of 4HPPD and that of other cytoplasmic hepatocyte enzymes is preserved in most causes of liver disease,[10] whereas it is selectively decreased in hepatorenal tyrosinemia. The importance of 4HPPD in hepatorenal tyrosinemia is discussed below.

MALEYLACETOACETATE ISOMERASE (MAI) DEFICIENCY

An interesting preliminary communication[174] reported a child with liver failure, renal tubular disease, and progressive psychomotor retardation detected at 9 months of age who died at the age of 1 year. The child had an elevated plasma tyrosine (680 μM) and methionine levels (1000 μM) and generalized aminoaciduria and tyrosyluria. Liver biopsy showed normal levels of 4HPPD and FAH, but liver and fibroblasts showed reduced amounts of MAI. Fibroblasts from both parents showed reduced activity of MAI. Of note, no succinylacetone was detected. This latter observation would be expected because succinylacetoacetate (SAA) is metabolized by FAH.[16] The authors named this condition *tyrosinemia type Ib*. If confirmed, this observation will be of great diagnostic and pathophysiologic interest.

However, since the cloning of the human MAA isomerase gene, several patients with a clinical phenotype similar to tyrosinemia type I but lacking SA excretion in urine (i.e., pseudotyrosinemia) have been studied by DNA sequencing of the entire gene. No mutations have been found, and thus no molecularly confirmed cases of MAI deficiency have been reported as of this writing.[175] MAI is not limited to liver and kidney.[62] Furthermore, it is plausible that other glutathione *S*-transferases may have some activity toward MAA. It is possible that the phenotype of MAI deficiency may differ from that of FAH deficiency or that there is no disease associated with deficiency.

FAH DEFICIENCY: HEPATORENAL TYROSINEMIA (TYROSINEMIA TYPE I)

Hepatorenal tyrosinemia is a clinically severe inborn error that principally affects liver, kidney, and peripheral nerve. It is also known as *FAH deficiency, tyrosinemia type I, hereditary tyrosinemia,* and *congenital tyrosinosis* and is assigned OMIM 276700. It is one of the best documented inborn errors, having been the subject of four published symposia,[176–179] with over 100 cases reports appearing in the literature (for references, see the last edition of this chapter)[165]; 123 cases have been detected by screening in the province of Quebec since 1970.[164] Van Spronsen *et al.*[180] assembled an international survey of 106 cases, and over 200 patients have been enrolled in the International NTBC trial.[164] The first report of the typical clinical and biochemical picture of hepatorenal tyrosinemia was described (as an "atypical" case) by Sakai *et al.*[181–183] in 1957. Earlier reports of probable cases exist.[184–187] Observations of porphyria-like neurologic crises[188,189] led to the discovery of increased excretion of delta-aminolevulinic acid (ALA) in patients[189–192] and to the elegant study of Lindblad *et al.*[193] in which the authors deduced the site of the deficient step in hepatorenal tyrosinemia to be FAH. This was soon confirmed enzymatically.[69,194–196]

Pathophysiology

Hepatorenal tyrosinemia is caused by a deficiency of FAH.[69,193–196] However, the mechanism by which the hepatic and renal symptoms of tyrosinemia arise is unknown. Many investigators favor the hypothesis that the final metabolites of tyrosine catabolism are toxic, possibly acting as alkylating agents and/or disrupting sulfhydryl metabolism. A body of reasoning and of circumstantial evidence is consistent with these hypotheses, which are beginning to be tested directly.

The observations include the following. Tyrosine and its early metabolites (4HPP and homogentisate; see Fig. 79-1) are present at high levels in other hereditary diseases that have no hepatic or renal symptomology and thus are unlikely to cause the hepatorenal symptoms of tyrosinemia. In contrast, the compounds immediately upstream from the FAH reaction, MAA and FAA, and their derivatives, SAA and SA, may have potent biologic activity. MAA resembles maleic acid, which can induce a renal Fanconi syndrome. Both maleylacetone and fumarylacetone can form glutathione adducts.[197] Maleic acid also can react with glutathione.[198] Free glutathione concentration was reduced to about half of normal levels when measured in one tyrosinemic liver.[17] Free sulfhydryl groups are known to be important for protection against free radicals and other toxic compounds and to be implicated in the functions of at least two enzymes known to be deficient in hepatorenal tyrosinemia, 4HPPD and methionine adenosyltransferase. When added exogenously in a mammalian cell assay, FAA, but not MAA or SA, is mutagenic, and this mutagenicity is potentiated by glutathione depletion.[199] SA can react nonenzymatically with free and protein-bound amino acids, and the majority of urinary SA in some patients may be in the form of such adducts.[200] The molecular structures of MAA and FAA predict that they may be Michael acceptors, capable of alkylating thiols, amines, and other functional groups of cellular molecules.

MAA and FAA have not been isolated as circulating or excreted metabolites. This contrasts with most inborn errors of amino acid metabolism, in which metabolites immediately preceding a metabolic block are excreted at high levels. Therefore, tyrosine metabolism may be compartmentalized, possibly within single cells, with reactive metabolites causing damage within the cell in which they were formed. If this cell-autonomous model proves correct, it will carry important implications for therapy.

4HPPD Deficiency

A secondary deficiency of hepatic 4HPPD activity (0–30 percent of normal values)[10,17,18,20,151,168,201,202] is an important factor in the biochemical phenotype of hepatorenal tyrosinemia, and 4HPPD deficiency originally was proposed as the cause of hepatorenal tyrosinemia.[18,176,201] The characteristic pattern of increased urinary organic acid excretion of 4-hydroxyphenylic acids in the absence of homogentisate can be attributed to 4HPPD deficiency. Elevation of plasma tyrosine levels in hepatorenal tyrosinemia is itself probably due to 4HPPD deficiency. FAH deficiency alone is not predicted to result in abnormal tyrosine levels (by extension from alkaptonuria, in which the metabolic block is upstream from FAH and in which normal serum tyrosine levels are found). Thus, ironically, it was the secondary inhibition of 4HPPD that directed investigators to study the tyrosine catabolic pathway in hepatorenal tyrosinemia, while diverting them for more than a decade from identifying FAH deficiency as the cause. The mechanism of 4HPPD inactivation in hepatorenal tyrosinemia is unknown, although it is tempting to speculate that sulfhydryl groups may be targets. Lindblad *et al.*[193] suggested that 4HPPD deficiency serves a protective function by reducing the production of FAA and other tyrosine metabolites downstream and found some correlation between the severity of clinical phenotype and the degree of residual hepatic 4HPPD activity. Their hypothesis is being borne out by the effectiveness of treatment with NTBC and in mice doubly mutant in both 4HPPD and FAH[203] that have no hepatic or renal symptoms.

Hypermethioninemia

A secondary deficiency of methionine adenosyltransferase (E.C.2.5.1.6) probably explains the hypermethioninemia seen in many tyrosinemic children.[21,192,204] As reviewed in the last edition of this chapter, the significance of hypermethioninemia in hepatorenal tyrosinemia, other than as a rough index of hepatic dysfunction, is uncertain. Patients with hereditary deficiency of methionine adenosyltransferase have normal development and no liver dysfunction despite circulating methionine levels in the millimolar range.[205]

The "boiled cabbage" odor observed in severe hepatorenal tyrosinemia is also found in these patients[205] and is probably due to the α-keto derivative of methionine, α-keto-δ-methiolbutyric acid.[206]

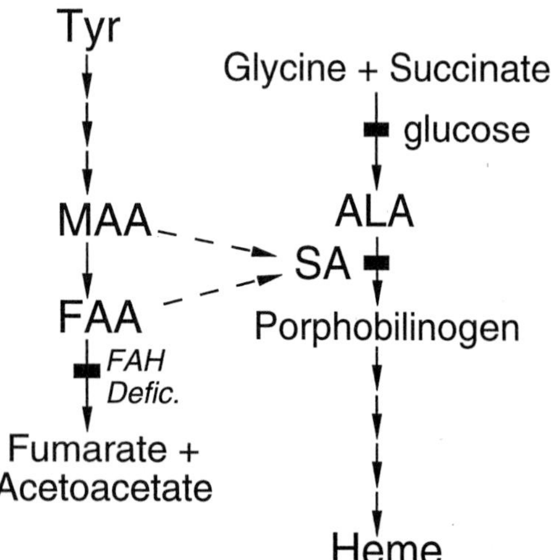

Fig. 79-3 The interrelationship between hepatorenal tyrosinemia and heme metabolism. The accumulation of succinylacetone inhibits aminolevulinic acid dehydratase, resulting in accumulation of aminolevulinic acid (ALA).

Apoptosis in Hepatocyte Death

Whatever the initial events involved in hepatocyte damage, it has been shown that apoptosis occurs in hepatocytes of FAH-deficient mice when the tyrosine catabolic pathway is activated[203] and that caspase inhibitors can markedly reduce hepatocellular damage in a mouse model of tyrosinemia[203a] and in cultured cells.[203b]

Succinylacetone

The best-established pathophysiologic mechanism in hepatorenal tyrosinemia is the role of SA in the acute episodes of porphyria-like peripheral neuropathy (Fig. 79-3). SA is the most potent known inhibitor of the porphyrin synthetic enzyme ALA dehydratase.[207] The structure of SA closely resembles that of ALA, and the K_i has been measured as 0.3 μM.[207] The inhibition is felt to be competitive[207] and does not destabilize the ALA dehydratase protein.[208] ALA dehydratase activity levels are greatly reduced in liver[208] and erythrocytes.[208] ALA is excreted at high levels in children with hepatorenal tyrosinemia.[10,64,189,191,209] ALA is neurotoxic[210–214] and is implicated in certain peripheral neuropathies such as acute intermittent porphyria, hereditary deficiency of ALA dehydratase, and lead poisoning.[215] All available clinical, biochemical, and pathologic evidence supports the notion that ALA toxicity underlies the neurologic crises of hepatorenal tyrosinemia. These crises are arguably the most severe porphyria-like condition known in humans.[215] FAH is expressed in oligodendroglia.[71] It will be interesting to examine its expression in Schwann cells as well.

SA has several other effects *in vitro* at high concentrations, including inhibition of renal tubular transport,[216–218] heme synthesis,[218,219] cell growth,[220] and noncytotoxic inhibition of immune function.[221,221a] The relationship of these effects to clinical symptoms is unknown. To some extent, SAA formation may be considered a detoxification pathway for MAA and FAA. About 8 percent of a tyrosine load administered to hepatorenal tyrosinemia patients can be recovered as SAA.[222]

Epigenic Modifiers, Revertant Nodules, and Carcinogenesis

In view of the protean manifestations of hepatorenal tyrosinemia, it will be particularly interesting to relate the clinical phenotype of the patients to the underlying FAH mutations. However, affected subjects from the same family can have different clinical presentations,[188,223–227] suggesting that factors epigenic to the FAH gene play a major role in determining the clinical phenotype.

The prediction that FAA and possibly MAA have local toxic effects within hepatocytes, including mutagenesis, is supported by the high incidence of hepatocellular carcinoma (see "Clinical Findings," below) and by the striking observation by Kvittingen of discrete liver nodules in which FAH activity is restored to normal.[228,229] The latter group subsequently showed that FAH peptide is present in such nodules and also that the sequence of one allele in cells from the nodules had mutated to the normal sequence. Presumably this is a clonal event, with revertant cells having a selective growth advantage over their neighbors, resulting in nodule formation.

This phenomenon probably explains the observation of normal FAH activity in liver biopsies of some patients discussed in the last edition of this chapter.[165] It is plausible that revertant nodules may account for some of the phenotypic differences observed among patients with the same genotype. Quantitation of the frequency of revertant nodules may provide a measure of the degree of mutagenicity of FAH deficiency within the hepatocyte. Clearly, if such a reversion could be induced in all hepatocytes, it would hold major therapeutic interest.

In the development of hepatocellular carcinoma, the relative importance of mutagenesis, apoptosis, interference with sulfhydryl metabolism, and immunosuppression[221a] remains to be determined.

Mouse Models of Hepatorenal Tyrosinemia

Two mouse models of hepatorenal tyrosinemia have been useful for the study of pathophysiology and therapeutic interventions. The first is the c^{14CoS} lethal albino mouse, one of a classic series of "lethal albino" mutants bearing large overlapping x-ray-induced deletions that include an albinism locus on chromosome 7.[230–232] Mice homozygous for the deletion die within hours of birth and display a striking hepatic phenotype. The mRNA levels of many cAMP-inducible hepatic enzymes are absent or reduced. These include TAT,[233] glucose-6-phosphatase,[230] glutamine synthetase,[230] phosphoenolpyruvate carboxykinase,[234] aldolase B, albumin, α-fetoprotein,[235,236] cyclic AMP/enhancer binding protein (C/EBP), and NADPH:meradione oxidoreductase (NIM-1). In contrast, other liver mRNAs inducible by DNA or oxidative damage are increased.[237] Histologic abnormalities are also found in both liver and kidney in these mice. Because of this down-regulation of multiple liver enzymes in the homozygous deletion, it was hypothesized that a regulatory liver gene (hepatocyte-specific developmental regulation locus = *hsdr-1*) was localized within the region.[232,236,238] In 1992, two groups reported that the mouse *Fah* gene was disrupted by the c^{14CoS} deletion, and thus FAH became a candidate for *hsdr-1*.[238,239] Subsequently, it was shown that FAH deficiency is responsible for all the major phenotypic effects of the c^{14CoS} deletion.[240,241]

The deletion in the c^{14CoS} mouse is large (4 Mb). In contrast, the second animal model was generated by a targeted gene replacement in embryonic stem cells and is mutated in exon 5 of the *Fah* gene only.[240] Both mice have a neonatal lethal phenotype. FAH-deficient mice can be rescued by administration of NTBC, a potent inhibitor of 4HPPD (see "Treatment," below).[242] NTBC abolishes the acute phenotype and permits survival with normal growth until adulthood.[242] On withdrawal of NTBC, adult mutant mice faithfully reproduce the human phenotype, including liver failure and renal tubular dysfunction. NTBC-treated mice develop hepatocellular carcinoma. In mice receiving a calculated oral dose of 4 mg/kg per day of NTBC in their drinking water, and in which phenylalanine plus tyrosine intake is restricted to the lower limit compatible with normal growth, 25 percent develop hepatocellular carcinoma between 18 and 24 months of age.[242] In contrast, Endo *et al.*[203] observed no hepatocellular carcinoma in doubly mutant mice lacking both 4HPPD and FAH. These observations have set the stage for detailed studies of pharmacologic treatment and protection of tumorigenesis in mice by use of 4HPPD inhibition.

The intense selection against FAH-deficient hepatocytes of mice has been used to advantage for gene therapy.[242a,243,243a] *In vivo* hepatic gene transfer using retroviral vectors expressing the human FAH cDNA resulted in near-complete restoration of liver function in FAH-deficient mice. Following injection into FAH-deficient mice of a first-generation adenoviral vector expressing the normal FAH gene, prolonged survival was seen in transfected cells, which formed FAH-positive nodules. However, in the neighboring nonexpressing tissue, nodules of hepatocellular carcinoma were seen frequently, supporting the notion that the hepatic disease in hepatorenal tyrosinemia is cell-autonomous.

It is important to put these results into perspective in relationship to humans. The progression of the mouse disease is much faster than that of humans, and recommended phenylalanine and tyrosine intake of mice per unit of body weight exceeds that of humans by 10- to 20-fold. Furthermore, there are important and often unknown interspecific genetic differences between humans and rodents, in the development of hepatocellular carcinoma.[243b] Even between mice and rats with hypertyrosinemia, for instance, it is notable that ocular abnormalities appear only in rats. It is necessary to employ great caution in extrapolating results from one species directly to another, particularly in a quantitative fashion. The general similarities between FAH deficiency in humans and mice, however, demonstrate that FAH-deficient mice provide an excellent model for identifying the pathophysiologic mechanisms of FAH deficiency and for initial testing of potential new therapies.

Genetics, Incidence, and Screening

Hepatorenal tyrosinemia is an autosomal recessive trait. Heterozygotes for hepatorenal tyrosinemia are asymptomatic and have normal levels of tyrosine-related metabolites. Large numbers of cases of tyrosinemia have been reported in two regions, the Saguenay-Lac St-Jean region of Quebec, Canada, and northern Europe, particularly Scandinavia and Finland. In Quebec, the increased incidence of hepatorenal tyrosinemia is based on a complex founder effect.[244–248] In a groundbreaking genealogic study, Laberge[249] traced 29 cases to a common founder couple. Subsequent studies have identified a group of possible founder couples including the one identified by Laberge,[250] suggesting that more than one couple may have introduced mutant FAH allele(s) to the region. The Saguenay-Lac St-Jean region was populated by about 5000 settlers coming largely from the nearby Charlevoix district. The Charlevoix population was itself derived from a small group of settlers near Quebec City. Furthermore, genealogic reconstructions suggest that many of them came from a few villages in northern France in the seventeenth century, and many may have been closely related to one another. Multiple social factors discouraged permanent immigration of new families to the Saguenay-Lac St-Jean region, but the large sizes of established families in the region resulted in a spectacular population growth.

In the Saguenay-Lac St-Jean region, the carrier rate for hepatorenal tyrosinemia is 1 in 20, and prior to the availability of prenatal diagnosis, 1 in 1846 live births resulted in an affected child.[245] The overall incidence of hepatorenal tyrosinemia in the province of Quebec is 1 in 16,786 live births[245,251] largely because of the high incidence in the Saguenay-Lac St-Jean region. The incidence is estimated to be 1 in 100,000 to 120,000 elsewhere in the world, including Scandinavia.[163] Lack of French-Canadian or Scandinavian ancestry does not exclude the diagnosis, since patients from a variety of ethnic backgrounds have been reported.

Screening. Neonatal screening for tyrosinemia has been underway for nearly three decades in various locations using blood samples dried on a filter paper and obtained prior to hospital discharge. Two approaches are used: screening by tyrosine levels and screening using parameters that are abnormal in hepatorenal tyrosinemia, such as methionine, succinylacetone, and ALA dehydratase levels.

Screening for hepatorenal tyrosinemia by measuring only blood tyrosine levels has the disadvantage that tyrosine levels in hepatorenal tyrosinemia overlap with those in transient tyrosinemia. In 1974, a cutoff of 414 μM (7.5 mg/dl) detected 17 of 18 patients with hepatorenal tyrosinemia, the mean age at screening was 4 days, and these levels were present in 1 percent in neonates in Quebec in the early 1970s.[78] Depending on the threshold value, unacceptable numbers of false-positive and false-negative results may be seen.[163] Repeat blood screening tests performed at 2 to 6 weeks of age in some screening programs may eliminate many false-positive results for transient tyrosinemia[163] but result in delayed treatment of newborns with hepatorenal tyrosinemia. Some patients are symptomatic by the time results become available.[180,252]

In Quebec, neonatal blood screening for tyrosinemia has been in effect since 1970 (Table 79-3). One hundred and twenty-three patients have been identified among 2,395,000 newborns. In order to reduce false-positive results, in the 1970s, only infants in whom α-fetoprotein levels also were elevated were recalled for further investigations.[253] In 1980, blood SA replaced α-fetoprotein determination on all Quebec newborns with elevated blood tyrosine levels; SA is determined using another blood spot from the original filter paper. The high specificity of SA as a marker for hepatorenal tyrosinemia permitted the use of a low threshold value for tyrosine and is felt to have permitted complete detection of

Table 79-3 Values of Tyrosine, Phenylalanine, and Succinylacetone at Screening in French-Canadian Neonates with Hepatorenal Tyrosinemia

			Level (μmol/liter)		
Date	n*	Age at Sampling (days)	Tyrosine	Phenylalanine	Succinylacetone Effect
1970–1974	18	4.2	854	227	ND†
1975–1979	29	4.1	770	206	ND
1980–1984	21	4.0	518	178	35.8
1985–1989	14	4.0	434	162	27.1
1990–1991	6	3.7	567	195	40.7
Cutoff values‡			<248	<242	Not detectable§

*Thirteen other patients identified in the 1970s are not included because of incomplete information regarding age at screening.
† ND, not done.
‡ Values above which further investigations are performed (1992).
§ Values less than 5 μM are undetectable by this technique.

SOURCE: Courtesy of André Grenier, Center hospitalier de l'Université Laval.

affected newborns for many years while eliminating false-positive results.[164]

Blood tyrosine levels at screening have continued to decline, a major factor probably being the lower average age at sampling because of early hospital discharge after birth. Because of the variable degree of biochemical abnormalities seen in hepatorenal tyrosinemia, a normal tyrosine level at the time of screening does not rule out the diagnosis in children presenting with symptoms compatible with tyrosinemia.

In 1997, the cutoff value in Quebec was lowered to 190 μM, a value exceeded by 8.3 percent of newborns. Unfortunately, 4 of 6 affected newborns, born in rapid succession that year, had values inferior to this (198, 193, 168, and 166 μM) and were missed by screening. Since April 1, 1997, tyrosine has been replaced by SA as the first-round screening test in Quebec using a modification[254] of the reported method.[81,255] Over 100,000 newborns have been tested, and 4 patients have been detected (tyrosine levels of 468, 375, 190, and 181 μM). None has been missed to our knowledge. Unlike tyrosine, the SA level is increased at birth, making SA the metabolite of choice for hepatorenal tyrosinemia screening. In Quebec, screened newborns with hepatorenal tyrosinemia begin medical treatment at an average age of 20 days.[164]

Tandem mass spectrometry screening of newborn blood spots includes methionine determination in some states. It will be of interest to test the sensitivity of this method prospectively.

Heterozygote detection is of interest in high-risk populations as well as for close relatives of affected individuals. Determination of plasma or urine metabolite profiles with or without loading with tyrosine,[256,257] 4HPP,[258] or homogentisic acid[257,259,260] is not of clinical use, although it is interesting that heterozygotes and pseudodeficient individuals often have reduced tyrosine tolerance.[257,259] Assay of FAH in leukocytes, fibroblasts, or erythrocytes is complicated by the range of activity of affected individuals and the possibility of pseudodeficiency alleles.[257,261]

Molecular testing for heterozygotes is the method of choice in populations at high risk for hepatorenal tyrosinemia type I, as in Quebec[296,297] where one or few mutations account for the majority of cases, and in families in which the mutations of the proband are known. Two approaches are possible: general population screening and so-called cascade screening (testing), i.e., successive rounds of testing of the first-degree relatives of known carriers. A detailed discussion of the ethical and public health issues surrounding molecular screening is beyond the scope of this chapter. Of note, however, is that neither approach should be initiated without proper education of the subjects undergoing testing and full consideration of the consequences in terms of genetic counseling and treatment. A pilot study of cascade screening for carriers is underway in the Saguenay-Lac St-Jean region of Quebec.

Diagnosis

Clinical. Hepatorenal tyrosinemia should be suspected in any infant or child with evidence of hepatocellular lysis, cirrhosis, or decreased hepatic synthetic function (especially perturbed coagulation studies) for which the cause is not evident. The presence of hypophosphatemic rickets and other renal tubular diseases or of typical neurologic crises[215] also suggests this diagnosis, especially if associated with abnormal hepatic function.

Metabolites. Plasma tyrosine levels are initially elevated to a variable degree in almost all symptomatic patients, although older patients with a chronic course and patients treated with low-protein diets often have normal levels of plasma tyrosine. Furthermore, hypertyrosinemia is a nonspecific finding (see Table 79-2). The same is true of plasma methionine levels, which can be markedly elevated in tyrosinemia, and of phenylalanine levels, which are often elevated at diagnosis.

The demonstration of increased amounts of SA in dried filter paper blood samples, plasma, or urine is pathognomonic for hepatorenal tyrosinemia. We have never observed a patient with hepatorenal tyrosinemia who did not have elevated levels of SA in blood and urine. However, case reports exist of patients with normal tyrosine levels and undetectable levels of SA.[262,263] We have encountered a small number of patients in whom blood SA levels are very low and in whom it is more convenient to demonstrate its presence in urine.

Enzyme Assay. In selected patients it is useful to perform FAH assays as well. FAH can be assayed in lymphocytes[34,70] and erythrocytes,[264] as well as in liver. High levels of liver FAH activity have been found in several patients, perhaps due to inadvertent sampling of revertant nodules (see above). Conversely, pseudodeficient FAH allele(s) can lead to underestimation of biologically active FAH activity,[261] being associated with no clinical symptoms and normal plasma tyrosine levels but yielding a very low activity when assayed *in vitro*. Enzyme assay results thus must be interpreted in the context of the patients' clinical and biochemical findings.

For carrier detection, enzyme assay is not recommended as a screening technique because of possible overlap with the normal range. It is being replaced by molecular testing in patients at risk for a known mutation.

Molecular. The demonstration that a patient has two mutant alleles known to cause FAH deficiency confirms the diagnosis of hepatorenal tyrosinemia.

Prenatal Diagnosis

Three methods are available for prenatal diagnosis of hepatorenal tyrosinemia: determination of SA in amniotic fluid, FAH assay, and molecular analysis in amniocytes or chorionic villi. In general, SA assay in amniotic fluid was an excellent means of prenatal diagnosis in 36 pregnancies in French-Canadians with an a priori 25 percent risk of an affected child analyzed by amniocentesis at 16 weeks' gestation.[164] In these patients, there were no false-negative results, and fetal liver FAH activity was pathologically low in all 8 patients in whom the pregnancy was terminated because of high amniotic fluid SA levels (>60 nM). We have always seen an easily identifiable separation between the ranges of normal values for amniotic fluid SA levels and those of affected pregnancies that we have followed locally (range, 250–2700 nM). In a prospective study of 10,450 pregnancies in northern Quebec for which amniocentesis was performed for other reasons, elevated SA levels were found twice (340 and 940 nM). Both pregnancies were terminated, and assay in fetal liver confirmed FAH deficiency.[165] Of note, in one affected pregnancy, amniotic fluid SA was shown to be elevated as early as 12 weeks of gestation.[265,266]

In one sample received from elsewhere, a negative result (<60 nM) was obtained on amniotic fluid, although the pregnancy later proved to be affected. Stable isotope dilution gas chromatography–mass spectrometry confirmed an amniotic succinylacetone level of 22 nM[267] (normal for this technique, 1–30 nM).[15] The patient was a genetic compound for the pathogenic E364X and IVS6 − 1g→t alleles.[267a] Although sample mixup remains a consideration in this case, it is to be expected that amniotic fluid metabolite levels may be normal in a small number of affected pregnancies given the highly variable amounts of succinylacetone excretion seen in patients with hepatorenal tyrosinemia.

It is plausible that in some cases, FAH assay in amniocytes[22,68,268] or chorionic villi[22,68,269] may detect cases that are missed by SA assay. A prospective study comparing these methods would be useful. In pregnancies at risk for which the causal mutations are known, molecular diagnosis can be performed.

CLINICAL FINDINGS

Patients with tyrosinemia traditionally were classified as either acute (i.e., "French-Canadian" type) or chronic (i.e., "Scandinavian" type). This classification can be misleading because some children with acute decompensations during the first year of life survive with a "chronic" course, and patients with the "chronic" form (defined as surviving longer than 2 years on medical treatment) remain at risk for life-threatening hepatic and neurologic crises. Clinically, we individualize the approach in each patient by assessing the aggressivity of the disease in each of the main target organs—liver, peripheral nerve, and kidney.

Statistically, the survey of van Spronsen *et al.*[180] documents that in nonscreened patients the age of onset of symptoms is an important prognostic indicator. In this series, the 1-year mortality was 60 percent for children who became symptomatic under 2 months of age, 23 percent for children presenting between 2 and 6 months of age, and 4 percent in children presenting later. In early clinical series, most patients died in infancy or early childhood, although a few survived to young adulthood. The clinical course of hepatorenal tyrosinemia possibly has been slowed by neonatal screening and early treatment and/or the shift of newborn feeding practicestoward a lower protein intake. It has been revolutionized by the advent of liver transplantation and again by the availability of NTBC.

Newborns Detected by Screening

The child is referred at about 3 weeks of age. Typically, the pregnancy and perinatal periods were normal, and the child appears healthy. Hepatomegaly of a variable degree is usually present. Blood coagulation studies are always abnormal, transaminases are usually mildly elevated (less than twice the upper limit of normal), and bilirubin level is normal. Biochemical evidence of renal tubular dysfunction may be present. Hepatic decompensation and neurologic crises may occur even in children of this age.[180,252,270] In some clinically asymptomatic patients detected by screening, we have observed biochemical findings such as markedly elevated plasma transaminases or methionine levels. Of note, 14 of 108 patients (13 percent) in the international survey became symptomatic in the first 2 weeks of life and 39 of 108 (36 percent) in the first 2 months.[180] In Quebec, the levels of tyrosine at screening in affected newborns have decreased somewhat over the past 20 years (see Table 79-3). The importance of this with respect to the clinical severity of the disease is unknown. Of 4 neonates missed by neonatal screening in 1996–1997 (see "Screening," above), 2 presented with hepatic failure at 3 and 5 months. The other 2 were detected by astute local clinicians before 2 months of age, one because of hepatomegaly and the other with hypoglycemia. These cases provide no evidence that the natural history of unscreened tyrosinemia in Quebec has changed in the last 30 years.

Hepatic Manifestations of Hepatorenal Tyrosinemia

The liver is the main organ affected in hepatorenal tyrosinemia. In the international series, 69 percent of deaths were attributable to liver failure and bleeding and 16 percent to hepatocellular carcinoma.[180] The following description is divided into three sections: acute decompensations, cirrhosis, and hepatocellular carcinoma. It should be realized, however, that all three can occur in the same patient.

A characteristic pattern of liver dysfunction is seen to some degree in all patients with hepatorenal tyrosinemia. Synthetic function is most affected. Clotting factors are often markedly reduced in comparison with other hepatic functions. Some patients with hepatorenal tyrosinemia present with bleeding but few other hepatic signs and are investigated initially for a primary hematologic problem.[165] Prothrombin and partial thromboplastin times may be extremely prolonged, even in apparently well babies detected by screening. Vitamin K supplementation does not correct these abnormalities. Serum transaminase levels are variable and may be normal or only slightly elevated, although in some crises levels of over 1000 IU/liter may be observed, indicating a more substantial degree of hepatocyte damage. Of the commonly measured hepatic function tests, serum bilirubin determination is the least sensitive indicator of dysfunction. Jaundice is rare in the early phases of hepatorenal tyrosinemia.

Acute Hepatic Crises. This is a common mode of initial clinical presentation in areas where neonatal screening is not performed. Hepatic crises may be precipitated by infections and other catabolic stresses in infants as well as in older children. The child is irritable, ill looking, and often febrile. Ascites, jaundice, and gastrointestinal bleeding are common. A "boiled cabbage" odor may be detectable.[270] Hepatomegaly of variable degree is present.

Elevations of plasma tyrosine, methionine, and often other amino acids may be observed during crises. Plasma transaminases may show acute severe increases, and hyperbilirubinemia may occur. Renal tubular dysfunction may be accentuated during this period. Although many crises resolve spontaneously, some progress to complete liver failure and hepatic encephalopathy.

Between crises, most patients have mild or moderate hepatomegaly. Some have splenomegaly. Transaminases are normal or slightly elevated, and bilirubin level is normal. α-Fetoprotein is elevated (100–400,000 ng/ml; normal, <10). Clinically, serum α-fetoprotein levels correlate roughly with the aggressivity of liver disease, as do plasma methionine levels. Hyperbilirubinemia and hyperammonemia are late signs, and their

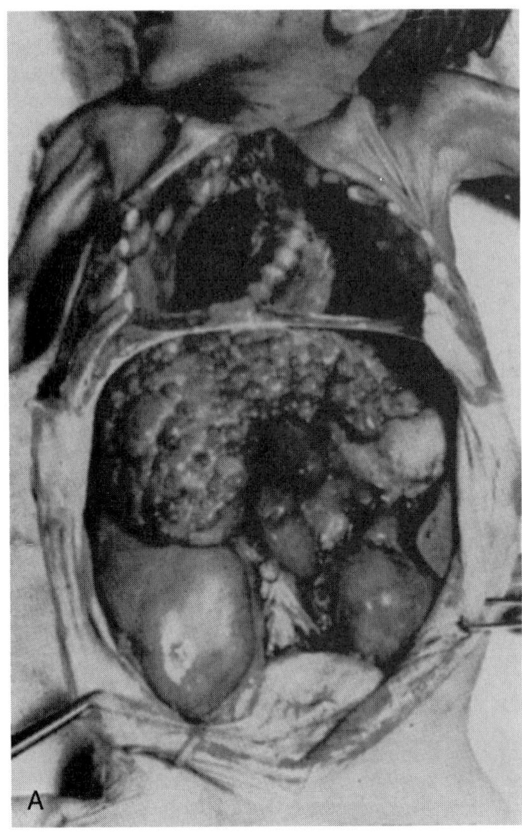

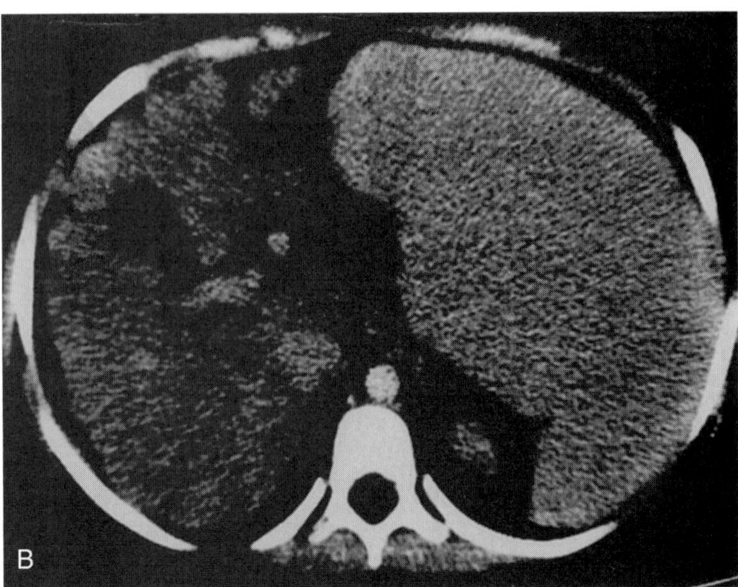

Fig. 79-4 Visceral pathology of hepatorenal tyrosinemia. *A.* Autopsy photograph showing the abdominal viscera of a child with hepatorenal tyrosinemia. Macronodular cirrhosis, splenomegaly, and nephromegaly are evident. The child also had rickets. No foci of hepatocellular carcinoma were identified. (*Reproduced with permission from Fritzell et al.*[334]) *B.* CT scan of the abdomen of a 9-year-old girl with hepatorenal tyrosinemia. Splenomegaly and extensive macronodular cirrhosis are present. At transplantation, no evidence of hepatocellular carcinoma was found.

presence increases the risk of hepatic failure and hepatic encephalopathy.

Chronic Liver Disease. Cirrhosis probably develops eventually in the natural course of all tyrosinemic patients, and the risk of hepatocellular carcinoma is extremely high. In an important early review of 42 published cases, Weinberg *et al.*[271] found that 37 percent of patients older than 2 years had liver cancer. The design and selection methods of this study suggest, however, that the incidence may have been somewhat overestimated. In the international series, the incidence was 18 percent among tyrosinemic children surviving longer than 2 years. In our experience,[165] the incidence is lower than first reported, and this may have implications when considering the urgency of liver transplantation for a child with a chronic course and no evidence of hepatic nodules on CT scan or ultrasound. In French-Canadian patients, no foci of hepatocarcinoma or dysplasia were found in resected livers in which the presence of nodules had not been detected previously by CT or ultrasound.[272,273] In 18 livers from tyrosinemic children studied histologically in the context of the Hôpital Ste-Justine liver transplantation program, 2 children (aged 44 months and 8 years) had hepatocellular carcinoma, and 1 child (aged 21 months) had dysplastic changes (3 of 18, or 17 percent).[165] Thirteen of 25 tyrosinemic children followed prior to the availability of NTBC developed no evidence of nodules on serial liver ultrasounds and CT scans.

Hepatocellular carcinoma has been reported as early as 15 months[274] in a child who presented at 5 months of age with hepatic failure and was treated subsequently with NTBC. Despite an initial 10-fold decrease of serum α-fetoprotein to 12,500 μg/liter, it rose again to 100,000 μg/liter. The child had pulmonary metastases. This is an exceptional observation. In Quebec, carcinoma has not been observed below 3 years of age. Perhaps the lower incidence of hepatocellular carcinoma in Quebec in part may reflect early screening and presymptomatic initiation of dietary therapy.

There is no noninvasive way to be sure of the nature of hepatic nodules.[275] Although the presence of hepatic nodules is worrisome, only a small minority are in fact cancerous (Fig. 79-4). Serum levels of α-fetoprotein fluctuate, particularly during liver crises, and cannot be relied on to discriminate regenerating nodules from hepatocarcinoma. For example, we observed hepatocellular carcinoma in an 8-year-old boy with an α-fetoprotein level of 87 ng/ml.[275] Nevertheless, a high degree of suspicion should be maintained when there is a significant rise of α-fetoprotein level from the usual baseline in a patient who is not recovering from a liver crisis, since this may indicate the development of a hepatocarcinoma. It has been proposed that low-attenuation nodules detected by CT scan are suggestive of hepatocarcinoma.[276] However, in our experience[275] and that of others,[276–278] neither CT, ultrasound, or angiography can reliably discriminate between all benign and malignant nodules. For CT detection, it is important to perform tomography with and without contrast enhancement, because enhancement may obscure some nodules but reveal others.[273] In our experience, the sensitivity of ultrasound is at least as high as that of CT, and no nodules have been detected by CT in patients with a normal ultrasound. However, ultrasound depends heavily on the experience of the ultrasonographer. CT scans are easier to standardize for multicenter studies. Of note, because barbiturate premedication can precipitate porphyria-like crises, we avoid its use in patients not treated with NTBC.

Neurologic Crises

The neurologic crises of hepatorenal tyrosinemia are acute episodes of peripheral neuropathy. Clinically, the crises have two phases: (1) an active period dominated by painful paresthesias, autonomic signs (e.g., hypertension, tachycardia, ileus), and sometimes progressive paralysis and (2) a period of recuperation following paralytic crises. In a series of 48 French-Canadian patients, 20 (42 percent) had crises.[215] In contrast, only 1 of 15 Norwegian patients had neurologic crises,[279] suggesting that crises are either more frequent in French-Canadians or were underreported in earlier descriptions. Much of our knowledge of the clinical aspects of neurologic crises stems from the observations of Jean Larochelle of Chicoutimi, Quebec.

Painful crises[64,188,191,192] are the most frequent neurologic variant. During the prodrome, which often occurs following a minor infection with anorexia and vomiting, the child is irritable and less active than usual. The child then develops severe pain, often in the legs. Frequently, patients adopt a position of extreme hyperextension of the trunk and neck that can be mistaken for opisthotonus[206] or meningismus. Older patients claim that this position alleviates the pain somewhat. The hypertonia also can be mistaken for tonic convulsions, but in fact, the patients are conscious. True convulsions also can be observed, often in association with severe hyponatremia.[215] It is important to note that the mental development of children with hepatorenal tyrosinemia is normal and that during crises their level of consciousness is not diminished. The excruciating pain experienced by the child, the striking postures that he or she adopts, and the frequent self-mutilation (see below) make neurologic crises very dramatic. The active phase usually lasts 1 to 7 days.

One-third of the crises were associated with weakness or paralysis.[215] In 8 of 104 crises, mechanical ventilation was necessary because of respiratory weakness, in one case for over 3 months. Electrophysiologically, there was evidence of axonal degeneration, with nerve conduction studies showing normal velocity but decreased wave amplitude and an increased threshold of stimulation progressing to absence of peripheral nerve function. Recuperation from paralytic crises is possible even after crises requiring prolonged ventilation for respiratory insufficiency. However, patients with repeated severe crises may have chronic weakness.

Other complications include laceration of the tongue and severe bruxism with avulsion of teeth. We attribute this to sensory neuropathy with oral dysesthesia. Vomiting and ileus occur frequently and can complicate nutritional management. Hypertension and sustained tachycardia are common during the early phase. Marked hyponatremia,[215] hypophosphatemia, and hypokalemia[280] can occur.

Interestingly, the neurologic crises of tyrosinemia are usually not associated with exacerbation of existing abnormalities of liver function or levels of tyrosine metabolites, except for a possible small increase in ALA.[215] Routine cerebrospinal fluid analyses are normal.[215]

Neurologic crises are a major cause of morbidity in non-NTBC-treated patients. In the international survey, 10 percent of deaths occurred during neurologic crises.[180] In 20 French-Canadian patients who experienced at least one crisis, 11 of 14 deaths occurred during crises, all associated with the complications of respiratory insufficiency.[215] All tyrosinemic children not treated by NTBC who are ill should be observed closely for signs of neurologic decompensation. In particular, respiratory insufficiency may develop rapidly, and thus children with signs suggestive of an impending neurologic crisis should be hospitalized for continuous supervision of respiratory function during the acute phase.

Renal Disease in Tyrosinemia

Some degree of renal involvement is almost always present in patients, ranging from mild tubular dysfunction to overt renal failure. Both tubular and glomerular involvement can occur.

The severity of proximal tubular dysfunction is variable and can be acutely exacerbated during periods of decompensation. In our experience and that of others,[281] long-standing tubular dysfunction may be irreversible. Hypophosphatemic rickets is the principal clinical sign of renal tubular dysfunction in hepatorenal tyrosinemia. It figured prominently in the initial clinical descriptions, and in patients with a chronic course, it may be the principal medical problem. Urinary phosphate loss is probably the main mechanism of rickets in these patients, as suggested by the frequent demonstration of hypophosphatemia and the absence of hypocalcemia or tooth-enamel hypoplasia that would suggest a vitamin D-related pathogenesis.[282] Some tyrosinemic children have renal tubular acidosis. Generalized aminoaciduria occurs more frequently than glucosuria. Evidence of proximal tubular dysfunction was present in only 7 of 25 patients evaluated at our institution. However, all patients were on a phenylalanine- and tyrosine-restricted diet when studied, which can improve renal dysfunction.

Over 80 percent of non-NTBC-treated tyrosinemic children evaluated at Ste-Justine Hospital had nephromegaly on ultrasound. Thirty-three percent had ultrasound evidence of mild to moderate nephrocalcinosis,[275] suggesting distal tubular dysfunction. Glomerular filtration rates are variable but may be decreased and should be monitored.

Other Clinical Manifestations

Although the pancreatic islet hypertrophy that frequently accompanies tyrosinemia is usually asymptomatic, several infants have had episodes of hypoglycemia. We observed a 5-month-old tyrosinemic child who did not undergo neonatal screening in whom we repeatedly documented elevated blood insulin levels in the presence of hypoglycemia. The child also had severe liver dysfunction, which may have contributed to his hypoglycemia. One tyrosinemic child had insulin-dependent diabetes mellitus, although the relationship of this condition to tyrosinemia is uncertain, and the pancreatic histology in this case was normal.[283]

Clinically significant hypertrophic cardiomyopathy has been reported in three tyrosinemic infants,[284,285] and in one it was the cause of death.[284] We have not observed this in our patients, but the physician should be alert to this possibility.

We are aware of one patient with hepatorenal tyrosinemia in whom the presence of macrosomia, hepatomegaly, and pancreatic and cardiac hypertrophy resembled the signs of maternal hyperinsulinism. In this patient and at least one other,[192] macroglossia also was present. Another patient with hepatorenal tyrosinemia had an acute episode of ataxia.[165] One patient with congenital glaucoma has been reported, and we have observed a patient with unilateral microphthalmia. It is unclear whether these latter conditions are related to tyrosinemia.

BIOCHEMICAL AND MOLECULAR PHENOTYPE

The results of routine clinical laboratory tests and tyrosine determinations and the importance of SA determination were discussed earlier. All the enzymes of tyrosine catabolism have been analyzed in patients with hepatorenal tyrosinemia. TAT activity is preserved to the same extent as unrelated hepatic enzymes[17,18,20,202,223,286]; 4HPPD activity is variably but often severely deficient (see "Pathophysiology," above); and homogentisic acid oxidase activity is normal,[17,18,286] as is MAI.[17] In liver from affected 18- to 21-week fetuses, all these enzymes were normal.[287] Enzymes unrelated to tyrosine catabolism such as aspartate aminotransferase, lactate dehydrogenase, alanine aminotransferase, glutamate dehydrogenase, and succinate dehydrogenase are reduced in proportion to the degree of hepatic involvement and have served as references by which to compare enzymes selectively diminished by tyrosinemia.[10] Catecholamine excretion is usually normal[10] and can show a normal increase in response to stress.[191]

Molecular Phenotype of Hepatorenal Tyrosinemia

There is heterogeneity among patients with hepatorenal tyrosinemia with regard to the amounts of FAH activity, immunoreactive peptide, and mRNA present in cells and tissues.[64,66–68] Four groups of patients have been defined on this basis.[290] Patients with an early onset of severe symptoms tend to have no immunologically detectable FAH peptide.[64,67,68,288] Some but not all patients with a more chronic course have immunoreactive FAH peptide.[288] Many of these findings were obtained in liver. Revertant nodules with normal FAH activity (see "Pathophysiology," above) may

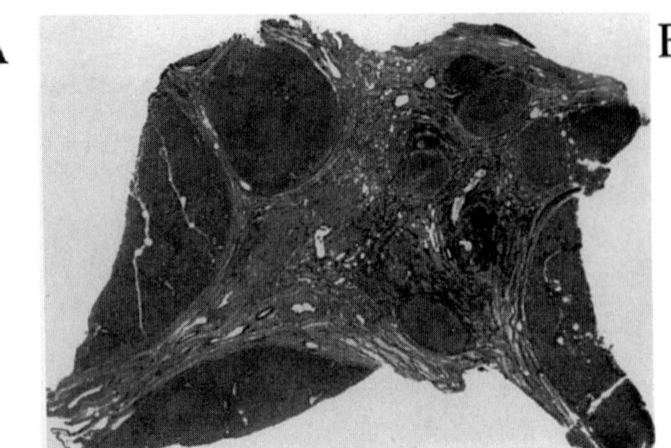

Fig. 79-5 Revertant nodules in hepatorenal tyrosinemia. Liver sample from a French-Canadian IVS12+5g→a homozygote. Masson's trichrome (*A*) and immunostaining with an antihuman FAH antibody (*B*). Several nodules express FAH (e.g., region 3). Analysis of DNA extracted from microdissected nodules confirmed the reversion of the splice mutation in one of the alleles of nodule 3 but not in regions 1 and 2, which were homozygous for the mutation. (*Reproduced from Poudrier et al.,*[303] *with permission from Academic Press.*)

provide an explanation for some mRNA-positive, CRM-positive samples, independent of the patient's germ-line genotype.

FAH Haplotypes

Haplotype analysis played a key role in demonstrating the French-Canadian founder effect,[302] as reviewed in the previous edition.[165]

Mutation Analysis in Hepatorenal Tyrosinemia

Since the first report of the missense mutation *N161* in the *FAH* mRNA, 34 *FAH* mutations have been documented in tyrosinemic patients.[289] The position of the mutations in the *FAH* gene is shown in Fig. 79-5, and some of their features are listed in Table 79-4.

There are 20 missense mutations (two of which, *Q64H* and *G337S,* alter splicing), 5 nonsense mutations, 7 mutations of splice consensus sites, 1 single-codon deletion, and 1 mutation (*N232N*) that preserves the coding sequence but affects splicing. The mutations are distributed along the length of the *FAH* gene with a slightly higher frequency in some parts of exons 8 and 13. The molecular defect causing tyrosinemia in over 50 other tyrosinemia patients remains to be uncovered.

Missense mutations in the *FAH* cDNA have been reported to influence protein instability and/or enzymatic activity; most of these mutations affect FAH amino acid residues conserved in human, rat, mouse, and *A. nidulans.*[289]

N16I was the first mutation identified as causal for the defect in FAH expression.[290] Expression of *N16I* in CV1 cells and studies of the patient's liver showed an mRNA, CRM-negative phenotype, suggesting instability of the mutated protein. This mutation has only been reported in heterozygous form in a single patient of French-Canadian origin.

The Pseudodeficiency Allele

R341W, the pseudodeficiency mutation, was found in a group of apparently healthy individuals who had very low FAH activity.[261] Normal fibroblasts of *R341W* homozygotes contain normal amounts of FAH mRNA but only small amounts of CRM.[291] Testing of this mutation by *in vitro* translation gave enzymatic activities ranging from 26 to 31 percent of normal values. The higher enzymatic activity observed in this assay as compared with that in fibroblasts (~10 percent) has been suggested to result from a greater instability of the protein *in vivo* than under the conditions of the *in vitro* test. This mutation has been reported in a British, a French, and a Pakistani family.

Splicing Mutants

Two missense mutations (*Q64H* and *G337S*) demonstrate unsuspected effects on RNA splicing. *Q64H* (192G → T) creates a donor splice site that leads to a 94-bp insertion from intron 2 immediately after the mutation, introducing premature termination codons into the FAH reading frame.[292] This is consistent with the absence of CRM in these patients.[292] *G337S* (1009G → A) is also associated with aberrant splice products in PCR-amplified *FAH* cDNA, including deletion of exon 12 or of exons 12 and 13 and a 105-bp intronic insertion leading to premature termination.[293,294] *In vitro* translation of a *G337S* construct yielded a reduced level of mutant protein and low enzymatic activities.[295] The absence of CRM in cells from patients with this mutation further suggests that the substitution may have a more severe effect *in vivo* than *in vitro*.

Population Genetics of Hepatorenal Tyrosinemia

The IVS12 + 5g → a allele accounts for over 94 percent of mutant *FAH* alleles in the Saguenay-Lac St-Jean area of Quebec[296,297] and for a substantial fraction in European patients.[298,299] Together with IVS6 − 1g → t, it accounted for 60 percent of the *FAH* alleles in 13 probands from Europe, Morocco, and Turkey.[299] The widespread distribution of the IVS12 + 5g → a and IVS6 − 1g → t alleles is suggestive of an ancient origin and warrants an initial search for these mutations in patients of unknown genotype. Both these mutations can be detected easily by simple amplification and restriction enzyme assays.[299,300] Other *FAH* mutations are prevalent in certain ethnic groups: *W262X* in Finns,[298,301] *Q64H* (192G → T) in Pakistanis,[292] and *D233V* in Turks.[292]

Genotype-Phenotype Relationships

Studies of large groups of patients[298,299] have failed to clearly associate specific genotypes with clinical severity. The clinical phenotype seems more variable in patients with splice mutations, which may reflect patient-specific variation in splicing.[295,298] Mutation reversion in the livers of patients[302,303] may contribute to phenotypic variability. To date, reversion has been documented for three mutations by sequencing of DNA from the nodule: 1009G → A, 192G → T,[229] and IVS12 + 5g → a.[228,303] Reversion also occurs for other mutations because revertant nodules have been observed in livers of patients with none of the preceding mutations.[298]

PATHOLOGY

Marked changes can occur in the viscera of patients with hepatorenal tyrosinemia (see Fig. 79-4). The liver shows a spectrum of changes. Macroscopically, it is usually enlarged and often shows severe macronodular cirrhosis (see Fig. 79-4*A*). All patients examined have had microscopic evidence of cirrhosis,[279,304] which can begin in the first weeks of life.[206]

Table 79-4 Mutations in Hepatorenal Tyrosinemia

Exon/ Intron	Mutation	Nucleotide Change	Consequence	Functional Testing: Test	mRNA	CRM	ACT	Genotype	Ethnic Origin	Note	Ref.
E1	*N16I*	47A → T	Missense	T	Normal	ND	ND	cpd	FC*		290
E2	*F62C*	185T → G	Missense	T	NT	Reduced	Reduced	hom	Japanese*		239
E2	*Q64H*	192G → T	Splice/missense	F	Splice defect	ND	NT	hom cpd	Pakistani	Reversion	292
I2	IVS2 + 1g → T	—	Splice defect	NT	—	—	—	cpd	Portuguese*		344
E5	*A134D*	401C → A	Missense	T IVT	NT —	Normal Reduced	ND ND	cpd	Norwegian Turkish		75, 340
E6	*G158D*	473G → A	Missense	NT	—	—	—	cpd	German*		344
E6	*V166G*	497T → G	Missense	NT	—	—	—	ND cpd	Unknown German Italian		298, 300, 340
E6	*R174X*	520C → T	Nonsense	NT	—	—	—	cpd?	N. Am.* (non-FC)		341
I6	IVS6 + 5g → a	—	Splice defect	NT	—	—	—	cpd	N. Am.* (non-FC)		341
I6	IVS6-1g → t	—	splice defect	L	Truncated/ complex splicing	—	—	hom cpd	Moroccan-Dutch N. Am. Europeans Turkish		298, 299, 341, 344
I6	IVS6-1g → c	—	Splice defect	NT	—	—	—	cpd?	Yogoslavian*		344
E7	*C193R*	577T → C	Missense	L	Normal	—	—	cpd	Dutch*		299
I7	IVS7-1g → a	—	Splice defect	F	ΔG	—	—	hom	Turkish*		299
E8	*G207D*	620G → A	Missense	NT	—	—	—	cpd	N. Am.*		341
E8	*N232N*	696C → T	Neutral?	L	Exon skipping	—	—	cpd	Dutch*		299
E8	*D233V*	698A → T	Missense	IVT	—	Reduced	ND	hom	Turkish		292
E8	*W234G*	700T → G	Missense	T	Normal	—	ND	cpd	American*		342
I8	IVS8-1g → c	—	Splice defect	NT	—	—	—	hom	Israeli*		344
E9	*R237X*	709C → T	Nonsense	NT	—	—	—	hom	Turkish*		299
E9	*P249T*	745C → A	Missense	NT	—	—	—	cpd	N. Am.* (non-FC)		341
E9	*P261L*	782C → T	Missense	NT	—	—	—	hom	Israeli		344

(Continued on next page)

Table 79-4 (Continued)

Exon/ Introl	Mutation	Nucleotide Change	Consequence	Functional Testing				Genotype	Ethnic Origin	Note	Ref.
				Test	mRNA	CRM	ACT				
E9	*W262X*	786G → A	Nonsense	NT IVT	— —	— Truncated protein	— ND	hom cpd	Finnish Norwegian Danish Polish	Prevalent in Finnish	292, 301, 343
E9	*Q279R*	836A → G	Missense	NT	—	—	—	cpd	German/* Irish/Polish*		Tanguay, unpublished
E10	*T294P*	880A → C	Missense	NT	—	—	—	cpd	N. Am.*		341
E12	*G337S*	1009G → A	Splice/Missense	F IVT	Aberrant splicing —	— Reduced	— Reduced	hom cpd	Northern Europe	Reversion	293–295
E12	*R341W*	1021C → T	Missense	F IVT	Normal —	Reduced Reduced	Reduced Reduced	hom cpd	British, French Pakistani	Pseudo-deficiency	291
E12	*P342L*	1025C → T	Missense	F IVT	Normal —	ND Reduced	— ND	cpd	Norwegian*		340
I12	*IVS12+5g → a*	—	Splice defect	—	Multiple splicing products	—	—	hom cpd	FC Iranian European N. Am.	Prevalent in FC Reversion	228, 293, 297, 299, 300, 303
E13	*E357X*	1069G → T	Nonsense	NT L	— ND	— —	— —	cpd	FC British Norwegian Dutch		298, 300 299
E13	*E364X*	1090G → T	Nonsense	L	ND	—	—	cpd	FC British Dutch American		298–300
E13	*DEL 366S*	1097DELCGT	Codon deletion	NT	—	—	—	cpd	Dutch, Italian		344
E13	*G369V*	1106G → T	Missense	NT	—	—	—	cpd	Morroccan		299
E13	*E381G*	1141A → G	Missense	NT	—	—	—	cpd	FC*		294
E14	*F405H*	1213TT → CA	Missense	NT	—	—	—	cpd	Portuguese*		344

NOTE: The mutations are designated using the single-letter abbreviation for amino acids, with codon 1 being the initiation methionine. The first letter corresponds to the normal residue followed by the codon number and the replacing residue. Nonsense mutations are indicated by the letter *X*. The tests for functional significance of the change are as follows: T, site-directed mutagenesis and assay by cell transfection; IVT, site-directed mutagenesis followed by *in vitro* coupled transcription translation assay; L, liver mRNA analyzed after reverse trasnscription/PCR (RT-PCR; F, fibroblast mRNA analyzed by northern blot, western blot, and enzyme activity or by RT-PCR (IVS7-lg → a). Mutations in which reversion was shown (see text) are identified.

Other Abbreviations: NT, not tested; ND, not detectable; CRM, cross-reactive material; ACT, enzyme activity; hom, homozygote; cpd genetic; compound (? indicates an unknown mutation on the second allele); FC, French Canadian. The asterisk (*) indicates that a single patient with the corresponding mutation has been reported. Reversion, revertant nodules detected in homozygotes for this mutation.

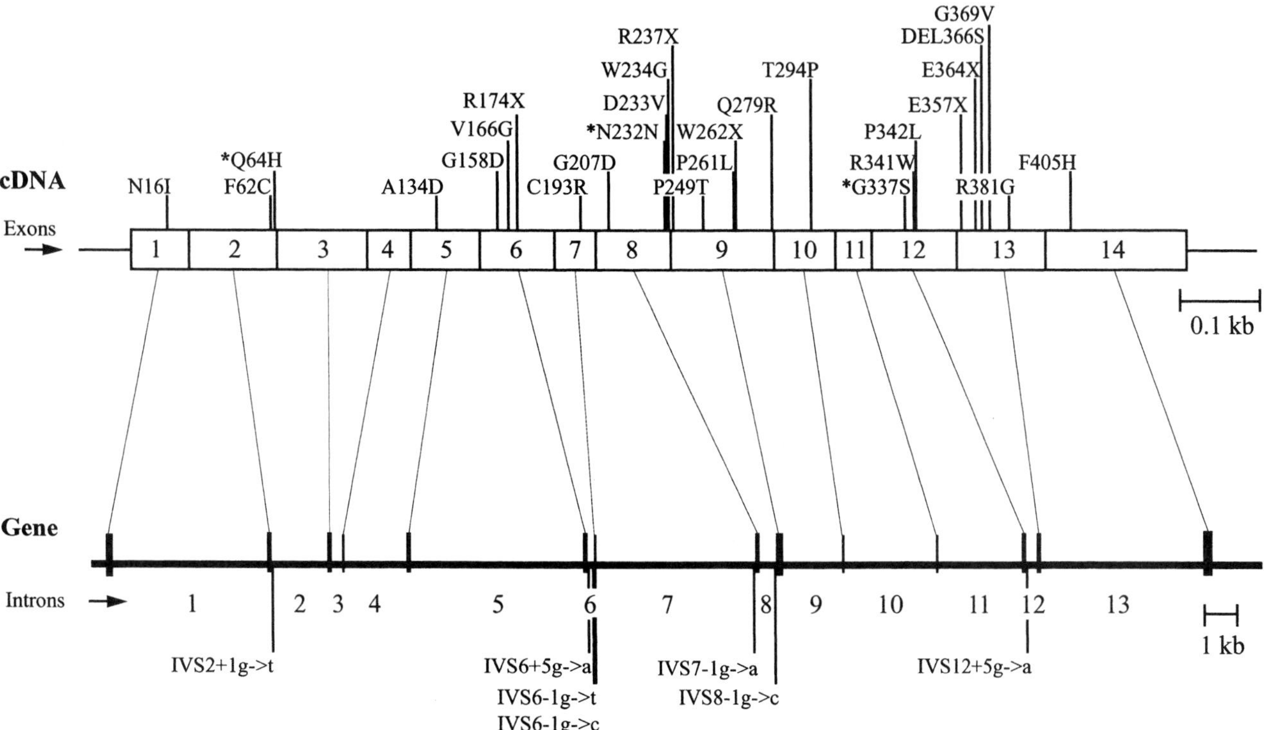

Fig. 79-6 Exon/intron structure of the human *FAH* gene and distribution of mutations. The 14 exons that are numbered in the top part of the figure. The position and name of the missense and nonsense mutations are shown. The initiation methionine codon is assigned position 1. The presence of an asterisk (*) in front of a mutation in the cDNA indicates coding sequence mutations known to alter splicing (see text). The lower portion shows the genomic organization and the positions of intronic mutations affecting splicing. The dashed lines point to the sites of the exons, which are represented by the black vertical bars.

Micronodular changes are present initially and in most patients progress to macronodular cirrhosis.[305] Patchy fat accumulation and inflammatory infiltrates can be seen.[306] In patients with a more indolent course, the liver can be completely replaced with regenerating nodules. Premalignant dysplastic changes have been reported as early as 13 months.[307] Hepatocellular carcinoma can be multifocal and may metastasize. Although biochemical changes compatible with hepatocellular dysfunction may be present prenatally,[308] no pathologic changes were observed in an affected 21-week-old fetus examined following therapeutic abortion.[304]

The kidneys are usually enlarged, up to three times their normal size (see Fig. 79-4). Microscopically, both proximal tubules and glomeruli can be altered. The tubules are swollen and show histologic and ultrastructural changes similar to those of idiopathic Fanconi syndrome.[309] Tubular dilatation and calcium deposits have been noticed as early as 3 months of age.[206] Some early reports mention glomerular abnormalities.[223,310] However, it has only recently been emphasized that glomerulosclerosis is frequent in the tyrosinemic kidney.[309,311] Although two siblings with tyrosinemia have been reported to have hyperplasia of the juxtaglomerular apparatus,[312] we have not observed this in our patients.[304] We are unaware of reports of renal neoplasms in patients with hepatorenal tyrosinemia.

Following neurologic crises, peripheral nerves show axonal degeneration with secondary demyelination,[215] indistinguishable from the changes of neuropathic porphyrias. In a French-Canadian series,[165] the histologic changes in the brain were neither constant nor specific. About one-third of these patients showed spongiosis of the white matter or of various tracts. This spongiosis was never generalized and, from one case to the other, involved different sites: optic tract, subcortical or deep cerebral or cerebellar white matter, corpus callosum, and spinal cord. In most patients, only one site was affected. Findings secondary to systemic problems are much more frequent and fall mainly into two groups: Alzheimer type II metabolic astrocytosis associated with hepatic failure and anoxic-ischemic changes. These observations are of interest in the light of recent findings of FAH expression in oligodendroglia[71] but apparently have little functional significance, since the mental development of tyrosinemic children is normal.

Other organs are affected in tyrosinemia. Pancreatic islet cell hypertrophy[206,270,306,309] occurs in many cases. One child with hepatorenal tyrosinemia died of hypertrophic cardiomyopathy,[284] and other patients with no cardiac symptoms have had similar nonspecific pathologic findings in the myocardium, including necrosis, increased numbers of mitochondria, and widening of T-tubules.[284] Bone may show the secondary changes of rickets.

MANAGEMENT

NTBC has changed the approach to management in hepatorenal tyrosinemia. Readers are referred to the preceding edition for discussion of treatment approaches prior to the discovery of NTBC.

Treatment with NTBC is effective within hours and abolishes or markedly diminishes the risk of hepatic or neurologic decompensation. Major issues now are early diagnosis, rapid availability of NTBC, the chronic effects of NTBC therapy, and the pharmacologic and economic questions common to many orphan drugs.

NTBC (2-(2-Nitro-4-Trifluoromethylbenzoyl)-1,3-Cyclohexanedione)

NTBC is a triketone compound that was developed as a herbicide. In toxicologic studies in rats, the occurrence of corneal abnormalities similar to those observed with tyrosine loading led to the search for hypertyrosinemia and subsequently to the demonstration by Sven Lindstedt and Elisabeth Holme that NTBC is a potent inhibitor of 4HPPD. In a pilot study starting in 1991 with 5 patients with hepatorenal tyrosinemia, Lindstedt and Holme observed unambiguous clinical improvement much greater than observed with any previous medical therapy.[313] NTBC was supplied by this group on an experimental basis in the context of an ongoing international study. Several abstracts and publications have described NTBC treatment.[179,314–316] A company that is seeking orphan drug status for NTBC recently has become its supplier, and the international NTBC database of Lindstedt and Holme continues to expand in collaboration with regional groups that gather and provide information.

Rationale of NTBC Therapy

NTBC inhibits 4HPPD. "Downstream" metabolites such as SA, ALA, MAA, and FAA are expected to decrease, whence the therapeutic effect. In contrast, 4HPP, 4-hydroxyphenyllactate and tyrosine are expected to increase unless the intake of dietary precursors is restricted.

Dietary Therapy

As discussed in the last edition,[165] dietary restriction of phenylalanine and tyrosine combined appears to slow the progression of hepatorenal tyrosinemia but does not eliminate acute or chronic complications, including hepatocellular carcinoma. Dietary tolerance of non-NTBC-treated patients is difficult to evaluate because no metabolites permit precise titration of intake, and the clinician must base his or her prescriptions on growth parameters and the recommended intakes for phenylalanine plus tyrosine in controls (typically overestimated to provide a margin of safety against deficiency in controls) and patients with other diseases such as oculocutaneous tyrosinemia. The secondary deficiency of 4HPPD induced by NTBC causes an increase in tyrosine levels that provides a convenient biochemical marker of dietary control.

Our current practice is to restrict phenylalanine plus tyrosine nearly completely for 24 to 48 hours following diagnosis. Initial intake in newborns is set at about 400 mg per day and then is adjusted based on serum tyrosine levels in the NTBC-treated patient. The phenylalanine plus tyrosine tolerance varies greatly among patients. Older NTBC-treated patients tolerate 15 to 70 mg/kg per day of phenylalanine plus tyrosine (median, 40; $n = 19$ patients with plasma tyrosine level <400 μM).

In the Quebec trial, we tentatively have chosen a plasma tyrosine concentration of 400 μM as a goal for treatment for the following reasons: (1) this level has not to our knowledge been associated with the development of complications in oculocutaneous tyrosinemia, (2) practically, it was approximately the level attained when pre-NTBC diets were continued in our initial patients, and (3) it has been compatible with normal growth. The level should not be considered as definitive, and further studies may reveal a more optimal target. While higher levels of plasma tyrosine may prove to be safe in some patients, the recurrent observations of mental retardation in TAT and 4HPPD deficiencies and the rare occurrence of eye complications in NTBC-treated hypertyrosinemia patients militate for continued dietary phenylalanine plus tyrosine restriction at the lowest level compatible with normal growth, at least until further data become available to address this question.

NTBC Therapy

Pharmacology. The molecular mass of NTBC is 329.2. NTBC is a reversible, tightly bound inhibitor of rat liver 4HPPD (IC_{50}, 50 nM).[317] Tyrosine hydroxylase, TAT, homogentisate oxidase, and FAH are not inhibited by NTBC at concentrations up to 100 μM.[317]

In rats, a single dose of NTBC (0.5 mg/kg; ~1.5 μmol/kg) produces marked elevations of plasma tyrosine (2500 μM) and aqueous humor (3500 μM).[89] Assay of liver 4HPPD soon after administration showed marked inhibition at all doses from 0.1 to 10 mg/kg. Corneal lesions were observed in the rats within 6 weeks following daily administration of NTBC, at a dose-dependent frequency varying from 38 to 72 percent. Following a single oral administration of either 0.3 or 30 μmol/kg of body weight of radiolabeled NTBC, the concentration of NTBC was highest in liver (2 and 49 nmol/g wet weight) and kidney (0.9 and 32 nmol/g) but was not detectable in cornea. Liver and kidney concentrations peaked at 4 to 8 hours after oral administration and declined to 4 to 20 percent of peak levels by 1 week, suggesting a long half-life. The distribution of NTBC to the CNS is not reported, although this is an important point, considering the mental retardation reported in patients with genetic 4HPPD deficiency.[136]

Experience in Humans. In humans receiving NTBC therapy for hepatorenal tyrosinemia, the current starting dose is 1.0 mg/kg per day in two divided doses. The criteria for dose adjustment are not established, but an increase in dose is indicated if SA appears in urine or other biochemical changes occur suggesting those of the pretreatment state. A technique for assay of serum NTBC levels based on 4HPPD inhibition has been developed by Lindstedt and Holme, in whose experience values greater than 50 μM have not been associated with the presence of SA in urine.[318]

Short- and Mid-Term Treatment with NTBC

The International NTBC study has more than 200 subjects including 35 from the Quebec NTBC trial. The initial results are currently being compiled. The Quebec results are also being compiled separately because of the unique characteristics of this group: Nearly all patients were detected by neonatal screening, permitting an elective start of NTBC; most are homozygous for the IVS12 + 5G → a allele; and all are closely followed in a standard fashion by a small group of physicians. In the Quebec protocol, after an initial period during which NTBC is initiated and patients are monitored in hospital, return visits are scheduled for determination of metabolites and physical examination, initially weekly but reducing to every 3 months by 6 months of treatment. Abdominal ultrasounds are performed every 6 months, and abdominal CT and isotopic glomerular filtration rate studies are done yearly. CT and ultrasound examinations are performed in the same center and scored by one person.[273] Four of 35 Quebec patients have been transplanted for preexisting liver disease after 3 to 18 months of treatment. The remaining patients have been followed for between 1 and 51 months. None has developed a neurologic or hepatic crisis after the start of therapy. In no patient have we documented a clear deterioration of the liver disease. One patient, who was transplanted for heterogeneous texture on liver ultrasound suggestive of cirrhosis, plus moderate persistent elevation of α-fetoprotein level (~70 units/liter), had a small nodule of marked hepatocellular dysplasia. Prior to transplantation, the same patient experienced the only NTBC-related complication that we have observed, the development of corneal crystals that were associated with photophobia. These resolved within 48 hours of strict limitation of phenylalanine plus tyrosine intake. In the international study, 13 patients have developed eye symptoms, including photophobia and corneal erosions.[316] There was no consistent relationship between the development of ocular symptoms and the presence of markedly high tyrosine levels.[316] In NTBC-treated patients, photophobia should lead to rapid ophthalmologic evaluation.

Long-Term Treatment with NTBC

Since it is clear that NTBC is the treatment of choice for short-term management, a number of questions have come to the fore. What is the optimal dose and the optimal metabolic parameter(s) to follow? Are there long-term side effects? To what extent does it control the development of liver cancer, cirrhosis, and kidney disease? What are the neurologic complications of treatment, if any, and how do they relate to dietary control?

Initial results of the International NTBC Trial suggest a reduction in the incidence of hepatocellular carcinoma with NTBC treatment.[316] Only detailed follow-up of a large number of patients will permit answers to these important questions, and we strongly encourage the enrollment of all new patients in the international protocol.

As mentioned earlier (see "Mouse Models of Hepatorenal Tyrosinemia," above), it is not appropriate to extrapolate the results of rodent models directly to humans. Clearly, the observation of liver cancer in FAH-deficient mice treated from birth with NTBC is strong evidence that patients must be followed carefully for the development of cancer. Further animal studies and standardized follow-up of a large number of patients are needed to resolve this important question.

Management of Acute Hepatic Decompensations

General Comments. We attempt to limit catabolism by providing sufficient energy intake with gavage supplementation or parenteral nutrition, as well as treating any intercurrent infection or complications (such as ascites and electrolyte disturbances). A reduction or cessation of phenylalanine and tyrosine intake for 24 to 48 hours is often indicated, depending on the severity of the episode. We do not stop phenylalanine and tyrosine intake completely for more than 48 hours. If the child is anorexic, continuous gavage feedings are initiated. If tolerated, oral or nasogastric feeding is preferred to intravenous administration because it permits a greater energy intake. We quickly provide intravenous alimentation, however, if the patient vomits. In all acutely ill tyrosinemic children, supplemental intravenous glucose should be administered to reduce proteolysis and to inhibit ALA deaminase. Prior to the discovery of NTBC, most acute crises resolved over the course of days to weeks, but rapid progression occurred in some. The threat of rapid deterioration is an important consideration during the initial period of NTBC treatment in patients with acute hepatic crises.

NTBC Treatment. NTBC is helpful in treatment and prevention of acute crises. Prior to beginning NTBC treatment, we rapidly obtain pretreatment blood and urine specimens plus informed consent of the parents. Marked decreases in urine SA and ALA are apparent within 24 hours of treatment.[319] This suggests that the hepatotoxic compounds specific to tyrosinemia are eliminated or greatly reduced within hours of the first dose. Our clinical impression is that the rate of clinical improvement thereafter depends on the regenerative capacity of the remaining liver tissue. Emergency liver transplantation is an option if encephalopathy develops.

Acute hepatic or neurologic complications have not been reported to occur following treatment with NTBC.

Chronic Liver Disease and Hepatocellular Carcinoma

Symptomatic therapy is of some use in coping with the problems of advanced cirrhosis, and surgery and chemotherapy are useful in palliating the complications of hepatocellular carcinoma. Liver transplantation is greatly preferred to these approaches and is best performed prior to the development of such complications. As discussed earlier (see "Chronic Liver Disease," above), it is not currently possible to reliably distinguish between malignant and benign liver nodules based on imaging or biochemical markers.

Management of Neurologic Crises

During the acute phase of a neurologic crisis, we provide analgesia for the severe pain. Narcotics are often necessary. A high level of glucose intake is also ensured because glucose inhibits the enzyme ALA synthetase reducing the production of ALA (see "Pathophysiology," above). It is necessary to provide symptomatic treatment for the hypertension, hyponatremia, hypokalemia, and hypophosphatemia that may accompany crises. Hyponatremia has been associated with convulsions in several cases. Ventilatory support and physiotherapy for muscle strengthening may be necessary during convalescence. In patients with tyrosinemia, we avoid the use of barbiturates[189] and other medications that can aggravate porphyria (see Chap. 124) prior to stabilization on NTBC.

Management of Renal Disease

Renal tubular dysfunction in tyrosinemia usually improves to some extent with dietary therapy. Rickets is the main clinical sign of tubular dysfunction in tyrosinemia. Vitamin D status should be assessed, and treatment should be individualized according to the needs of patients. The contribution of the treatment of rickets to nephrocalcinosis[320,321] is unclear, although calcification can occur in the absence of phosphate or vitamin D supplementation.[206] Some children require alkali therapy for renal tubular acidosis. No therapy has been shown to reverse the glomerular pathology of some patients. Careful evaluation of glomerular filtration rate and tubular function is necessary during assessment for hepatic transplantation.

The impact of NTBC therapy on kidney function is not clear. Established tubulopathy in older patients may be permanent. Our impression is that glomerular function does not decline during NTBC treatment, but experience is too limited to allow firm conclusions to be drawn.

Other Medical Treatments

The preceding edition reviewed the experience with *N*-acetylcysteine, aimed at increasing free glutathione levels in liver.[165] Experience to date shows no effect, but in theory, therapeutic manipulation of sulfhydryl metabolism remains an interesting option.

Organ Transplantation

Liver transplantation is felt to cure the hepatic and neurologic complications of hepatorenal tyrosinemia, and it completely changed the therapeutic approach to this disease in the last two decades. This procedure has been adapted to infants.[322–325] Children with tyrosinemia, in whom transplantation can be performed on a nonemergency basis, tend to have a good postoperative course.[180,323,326,327] It must be remembered, however, that even under optimal circumstances, liver transplantation carries a 10 to 15 percent mortality.[322] Furthermore, after transplantation, patients face a lifetime of immunosuppressive therapy with cyclosporine, the risks of which are unknown. For the stable patient, the timing of elective transplantation should be decided after weighing several factors, including the patient's current quality of life, the presence or absence of documented cirrhosis, and the local experience with pediatric hepatic transplantation. Forty-four transplanted patients were reported in the international survey,[180] and 17 have been transplanted at Ste-Justine Hospital.

We consider the presence of a hepatic nodule to be an indication for transplantation and hepatic encephalopathy as an urgent indication. As mentioned earlier, none of the radiologic characteristics of a nodule are specific enough to exclude hepatocellular carcinoma.[273] In our limited experience with children presenting with advanced liver disease, a trial of NTBC is attempted unless the child has hepatic encephalopathy. This approach usually allows transplantation to be performed on an elective basis after the patient stabilizes. Several publications document rapid improvement in the levels of tyrosine-related metabolites following hepatic transplantation.[165,325,328,329]

What is the effect of replacement of one target organ on the course of the disease in another? The question has practical importance for the treatment of hepatorenal tyrosinemia. Liver transplantation appears to cure the hepatic and neurologic complications of tyrosinemia. Its effect on renal function is less clear. Improvement in renal tubular dysfunction has been observed in some[330,331] but not all patients[281,329] following hepatic transplantation. The effect on glomerular function remains a major question. In 16 tyrosinemic patients who received hepatic transplantation in our institution, serial creatinine clearance values have been indistinguishable from those of patients transplanted for other conditions.[332] Since TAT is highly liver-specific, little tyrosine should be metabolized in the kidney following hepatic transplantation, allowing cautious optimism regarding the course of renal dysfunction in patients having had a liver transplantation. Nevertheless, SA excretion remains somewhat elevated in many transplanted patients,[328,329,333] presumably because of continuing renal production. Long-term follow-up of a number of patients will be needed before definite conclusions can be drawn, given the variable natural course of tyrosinemia and the glomerulotoxic effect of cyclosporine.

The effect of renal transplantation on hepatic function is unclear. Kvittingen *et al.*[311] reported a young adult who received a kidney transplantation without hepatic transplantation. The patient died 3 years later of complications of rejection. The patient had chronic mild cirrhosis, and no deterioration of liver function was documented after transplantation. Plasma tyrosine levels were normal. ALA excretion was not reported. Because there is no proof that renal transplantation will prevent hepatic complications such as carcinoma, we do not favor isolated renal transplantation in patients with tyrosinemia.

Combined hepatorenal transplantation should be considered in children with advanced hepatic and renal disease. To date, we have performed combined transplantation in two patients, one of whom tolerated this procedure well.[272,332] A second patient died in the immediate postoperative period of primary nonfunction of the transplanted liver. There is no evidence that combined hepatic and renal transplantation is less well tolerated than isolated transplantation of either organ,[272,332] and hepatorenal transplantation is certainly preferable immunologically to separate transplantations from unrelated donors, should renal function deteriorate following hepatic transplantation.

The question has been raised as to whether NTBC should be administered following liver transplantation to avoid the development of renal disease. We currently do not do this because (1) neither the course of renal disease following hepatic transplantation nor the effect of NTBC on renal disease are well-documented and (2) the consequences of NTBC therapy (chronic hypertyrosinemia requiring diet therapy, unknown long-term toxicity) may not be negligible. We follow renal function annually with isotopic glomerular filtration rate testing.

CONCLUSION

There has been remarkable progress over the last 4 years in the study of tyrosine metabolism and its disorders. Many questions remain, however. What are the clinical spectra of 4HPPD and MAI deficiencies? What are the neurologic consequences, if any, of chronic hypertyrosinemia? What is the molecular cause of hawkinsinuria? What is the effect of hepatic transplantation on the renal disease of hepatorenal tyrosinemia? What are the pathophysiologic mechanisms of TAT, 4HPP, and FAH deficiencies? What are the optimal dose and long-term effects of NTBC in humans with hepatorenal tyrosinemia?

ACKNOWLEDGMENTS

For discussion and sharing of results before publication, we thank F. Alvarez, J. Dubois, S. Ekberg, A. Grenier, E. Holme, J. Larochelle, and G. Sherer and our colleagues in the Quebec NTBC Study Group: J. Larochelle (Hôpital de la Sagamie, Chicoutimi), C. Scriver, E. Treacy, (Montreal Children's Hospital), D. Fenyves (CHUM, Pavillon St-Luc), F. Alvarez, L. Dallaire, J. Dubois, C. Dupuis, F. Faucher, Y. Lefevre, S. Melançon, K. Paradis, V. Phan, A. Rasquin (Hôpital Sainte-Justine), A. Grenier, R. Laframboise (CHUQ, Pavillon CHUL), K. Raymond, P. Rinaldo (Yale University School of Medicine), and E. Holme, S. Lindstedt (Sahlgren's Hospital, Gothenberg, Sweden). We thank Raffaela Ballarano for expert secretarial assistance.

REFERENCES

1. Bopp F: Einiges über albumin, caseïn und fibrin. *Ann Chem Pharm* **69**:16, 1849.
2. Scriver CR, Rosenberg LE: *Amino Acid Metabolism and Its Disorders*. Philadelphia, WB Saunders, 1973.
3. Armstrong MD, Stave U: A study of plasma free amino acid levels: I. Study of factors affecting validity of amino acid analyses. *Metab Clin Exp* **22**:549, 1973.
4. Feigin RD, Klainer AS, Beisel WR: Factors affecting circadian periodicity of blood amino acids in man. *Metab Clin Exp* **17**:764, 1968.
5. Armstrong MD, Stave U: A study of plasma free amino acid levels: IV. Characteristic individual levels of the amino acids. *Metab Clin Exp* **22**:821, 1973.
6. Armstrong MD, Stave U: A study of plasma free amino acid levels: VII. Parent-child and sibling correlations in amino acid levels. *Metab Clin Exp* **22**:1263, 1973.
7. Armstrong MD, Stave U: A study of plasma free amino acid levels: II. Normal values for children and adults. *Metab Clin Exp* **22**:561, 1973.
8. Reid DWJ, Campbell DJ, Yakymyshyn LY: Quantitative amino acids in amniotic fluid and maternal plasma in early and late pregnancy. *Am J Obstet Gynecol* **111**:251, 1971.
9. Craft IL, Peters TJ: Quantitative changes in plasma amino acids induced by oral contraceptives. *Clin Sci* **41**:301, 1971.
10. Lindblad B, Lindstedt G, Lindstedt S, Rundgren M: Metabolism of *p*-hydroxyphenylpyruvate in hereditary tyrosinaemia, in Stern J (ed): *Organic Acidurias*, Edinburgh, Churchill-Livingstone, 1972, p 63.
11. Kennaway N, Buist NRM, Fellman JH: The origin of urinary *p*-hydroxyphenylpyruvate in a patient with hepatic cytosol tyrosine aminotransferase deficiency. *Clin Chim Acta* **41**:157, 1972.
12. Woolf LI: Infants lacking *p*-hydroxyphenylpyruvate hydroxylase, in Gjessing LR (ed): *Symposium on Tyrosinosis:. In Honour of Dr Grace Medes, 2–3 June 1965*. Oslo, Norway, Scandinavian University Books, 1966, p 24.
13. Fellman JH, Roth ES, Fujita TS: Decarboxylation to tyramine is not a major route of tyrosine metabolism in mammals. *Arch Biochem Biophys* **174**:562, 1976.
14. Sweetman L: Organic acid analysis, in Hommes FA (ed): *Techniques in Diagnostic Human Biochemical Genetics: A Laboratory Manual*. New York, Wiley-Liss, 1991, p 143.
15. Jakobs C, Dorland L, Wikkerink B, Kok RM, de Jong AP, Wadman SK: Stable isotope dilution analysis of succinylacetone using electron capture negative ion mass fragmentography: An accurate approach to the pre- and neonatal diagnosis of hereditary tyrosinemia type I. *Clin Chim Acta* **171**:223, 1988.
16. Knox WE: Enzymes involved in conversion of tyrosine to acetoacetate. *Methods Enzymol* **2**:286, 1955.
17. Stoner E, Starkman H, Wellner D, Wellner VP, Sassa S, Rifkind AB, Grenier A, et al: Biochemical studies of a patient with hereditary hepatorenal tyrosinemia: Evidence of glutathione deficiency. *Pediatr Res* **18**:1332, 1984.
18. Taniguchi K, Gjessing LR: Studies on tyrosinosis: Activity of the transaminase, *para*-hydroxyphenylpyruvate oxidase, and homogentisic-acid oxidase. *Br Med J* **1**:968, 1965.
19. Lindblad B, Lindstedt G, Lindstedt S, Rundgren M: Purification and some properties of human 4-hydroxyphenylpyruvate dioxygenase, part I. *J Biol Chem* **252**:5073, 1977.
20. Whelan DT, Zannoni VG: Microassay of tyrosine-aminotransferase and *p*-hydroxyphenylpyruvic acid oxidase in mammalian liver and patients with hereditary tyrosinemia. *Biochem Med* **9**:19, 1974.
21. Berger R: Biochemical aspects of type I hereditary tyrosinemia, in Bickel H, Wachtel U (eds): *Inherited Diseases of Amino Acid Metabolism*. Stuttgart, Verlag-Thieme, 1985, p 192.
22. Kvittingen EA, Brodtkorb E: The pre- and post-natal diagnosis of tyrosinemia type I and the detection of the carrier state by assay of fumarylacetoacetase. *Scand J Clin Lab Invest Suppl* **184**:35, 1986.
23. Groenewald JV, Terblanche SE, Oelofsen W: Tyrosine aminotransferase: Characteristics and properties. *Int J Biochem* **16**:1, 1984.
24. Granner DK, Hargrove JL: Regulation of the synthesis of tyrosine aminotransferase: The relationship to mRNATAT. *Mol Cell Biochem* **53**:113, 1983.
25. Dietrich J-B: Tyrosine aminotransferase: A transaminase among others? *Cell Mol Biol* **38**:95, 1992.
26. Rettenmeier R, Natt E, Hanswalter Z, Scherer G: Isolation and characterization of the human tyrosine aminotransferase gene. *Nucl Acids Res* **18**:3853, 1990.
27. Shinomiya T, Scherer G, Schmid W, Zentgraf H, Schutz G: Isolation and characterization of the rat tyrosine aminotransferase gene. *Proc Natl Acad Sci USA* **81**:1346, 1984.
28. Müller G, Scherer G, Zentgraf H, Ruppert S, Herrmann B, Lehrach H, Schutz G: Isolation, characterization and chromosomal mapping of the mouse tyrosine aminotransferase gene. *J Mol Biol* **184**:367, 1985.
29. Natt E, Westphal EM, Toth-Fejel SE, Magenis RE, Buist NR, Rettenmeier R, Scherer G: Inherited and *de novo* deletion of the

tyrosine aminotransferase gene locus at 16q22.1q22.3 in a patient with tyrosinemia type II. *Hum Genet* **77**:352, 1987.

30. Hargrove JL, Scoble HA, Mathews WR, Baumstark BR, Biemann K: The structure of tyrosine aminotransferase: Evidence for domains involved in catalysis and enzyme turnover. *J Biol Chem* **264**:45, 1989.
31. Coufalik A, Monder C: Perinatal development of the tyrosine oxidizing system. *Biol Neonate* **34**:161, 1978.
32. Ohisalo JJ, Laskowska-Klita T, Andersson SM: Development of tyrosine aminotransferase and *p*-hydroxyphenylpyruvate dioxygenase activities in fetal and neonatal human liver. *J Clin Invest* **70**:198, 1982.
33. Hargrove JL, Mackin RB: Organ specificity of glucocorticoid-sensitive tyrosine aminotransferase isoenzymes. *J Biol Chem* **259**:386, 1984.
34. Endo F, Kitano A, Uehara I, Nagata N, Matsuda I, Shinka T, Kuhara T, et al.: Four-hydroxyphenylpyruvic acid oxidase deficiency with normal fumarylacetoacetase: A new variant form of hereditary hypertyrosinemia. *Pediatr Res* **17**:92, 1983.
35. Kohli KK, Stellwagen RH: Expression and amplification of cloned rat liver tyrosine aminotransferase in nonhepatic cells. *J Cell Physiol* **142**:194, 1990.
36. Tanaka K, Ichihara A: Control of ketogenesis from amino acids: III. In vitro and in vivo studies on ketone body formation, lipogenesis and oxidation of tyrosine by rats. *Biochim Biophys Acta* **399**:302, 1975.
37. Knox WE, Goswami MND, Lynch RD: The induction of tyrosyluria in young rats. *Ann NY Acad Sci* **111**:212, 1963.
38. Walsh C: *Enzymatic Reaction Mechanisms*. New York, WH Freeman, 1979.
39. Andersson SM, Pispa JP: Purification and properties of human liver tyrosine aminotransferase. *Clin Chim Acta* **125**:117, 1982.
40. Endo F, Awata H, Tanoue A, Ishiguro M, Eda Y, Titani K, Matsuda I: Primary structure deduced from complementary DNA sequence and expression in cultured cells of mammalian 4-hydroxyphenylpyruvic acid dioxygenase: Evidence that the enzyme is a homodimer of identical subunits homologous to rat liver-specific alloantigen F. *J Biol Chem* **267**:24235, 1992.
41. Fellman JH, Fujita TS, Roth ES: Assay, properties and tissue distribution of *p*-hydroxyphenylpyruvate hydroxylase. *Biochim Biophys Acta* **284**:90, 1972.
42. Lindstedt S, Odelhög B: 4-Hydroxyphenylpyruvate dioxygenase from human liver. *Methods Enzymol* **142**:139, 1987.
43. Buckthal DJ, Roche PA, Moorehead TJ, Forbes BJR, Hamilton GA: 4-Hydroxyphenylpyruvate dioxygenase from pig liver. *Methods Enzymol* **142**:132, 1987.
44. Roche PA, Moorehead TJ, Hamilton GA: Purification and properties of hog liver 4-hydroxyphenylpyruvate dioxygenase. *Arch Biochem Biophys* **216**:62, 1982.
45. Fellman JH: 4-Hydroxyphenylpyruvate dioxygenase from avian liver. *Methods Enzymol* **142**:148, 1987.
46. Ruetschi U, Dells'en A, Sahlin P, Stenman G, Rymo L, Lindstedt S: Human 4-hydroxyphenylpyruvate dioxygenase: Primary structure and chromosomal localization of the gene. *Eur J Biochem* **213**:1081, 1993.
47. Endo F, Awata H, Matsuda I: A nonsense mutation in the 4-hydroxyphenylpyruvic acid dioxygenase gene (*Hpd*) causes skipping of the constitutive exon and hypertyrosinemia in mouse strain III. *Genomics* **25**:164, 1995.
48. Endo F, Awata H, Tanoue A, Ishiguro M, Eda Y, Titani K, Matsuda I: Primary structure deduced from complementary DNA sequence and expression in cultured cells of mammalian 4-hydroxyphenylpyruvic acid dioxygenase. *J Biol Chem* **267**:24235, 1992.
49. Ruetschi U, Odelhog B, Lindstedt S, Barros-Soderling J, Persson B, Jornvall H: Characterization of 4-hydroxyphenylpyruvate dioxygenase: Primary structure of the Pseudomonas enzyme. *Eur J Biochem* **205**:459, 1992.
50. Norris SR, Barrette TR, DellaPenna D: Genetic dissection of carotenoid synthesis in arabidopsis defines plastoquinone as an essential component of phytoene desaturation. *Plant Cell* **7**:2139, 1995.
51. Stenman G, Roijer E, Ruetschi U, Dells'en A, Rymo L, Lindstedt S: Regional assignment of the human 4-hydroxyphenylpyruvate dioxygenase gene (*HPD*) to 12q24$\rightarrow$qter by fluorescence in situ hybridization. *Cytogenet Cell Genet* **71**:374, 1995.
52. Awata H, Endo F, Matsuda I: Structure of the human 4-hydroxyphenylpyruvic acid dioxygenase gene (*HPD*). *Genomics* **23**:534, 1994.
53. Ruetschi U, Rymo L, Lindstedt S: Human 4-hydroxyphenylpyruvate dioxygenase gene (*HPD*). *Genomics* **44**:292, 1997.
54. Lee MH, Zhang ZH, MacKinnon CH, Baldwin JE, Crouch NP: The C-terminal of rat 4-hydroxyphenylpyruvate dioxygenase is indispensable for enzyme activity. *FEBS Lett* **393**:269, 1996.
55. Oliveira DB, Nardi NB: Immune suppression genes control the anti-F antigen response in F1 hybrids and recombinant inbred sets of mice. *Immunogenetics* **26**:359, 1987.
56. Oliveira DB: F protein and immune suppression genes. *Immunol Suppl* **2**:26, 1989.
57. Lindblad B, Lindstedt G, Lindstedt S: The mechanism of enzymic formation of homogentisate from p-hydroxyphenylpyruvate. *J Am Chem Soc* **92**:7446, 1970.
58. Bradley FC, Lindstedt S, Lipscomb JD, Que L Jr, Roe AL, Rundgren M: 4-Hydroxyphenylpyruvate dioxygenase is an iron-tyrosinate protein. *J Biol Chem* **261**:11693, 1986.
59. Zannoni VG, La Du B: The tyrosine oxidation system of liver: IV. Studies on the inhibition of p-hydroxyphenylpyruvic acid oxidase by excess substrate. *J Biol Chem* **234**:2925, 1959.
60. Lindstedt S, Rundgren M: Inhibition of 4-hydroxyphenylpyruvate dioxygenase from *Pseudomonas* sp. strain P.J. 874 by the enol tautomer of the substrate. *Biochim Biophys Acta* **704**:66, 1982.
61. Pascal RA Jr, Oliver MA, Chen Y-CJ: Alternate substrates and inhibitors of bacterial 4-hydroxyphenylpyruvate dioxygenase. *Biochemistry* **24**:3158, 1985.
62. Fernandez-Canon JM, Penalva MA: Characterization of a fungal maleylacetoacetate isomerase gene and identification of its human homologue. *J Biol Chem* **273**:329, 1998.
63. Mahuran DJ, Angus RH, Braun CV, Sim SS, Schmidt DE Jr: Characterization and substrate specificity of fumarylacetoacetate fumarylhydrolase. *Biochem Cell Biol* **55**:1, 1977.
64. Tanguay RM, Laberge C, Lescault A, Valet JP, Duband JL, Quenneville Y: Molecular basis of hereditary tyrosinemia: Proof of primary defect by western blotting, in Scott W, Amhad F, Black S, Schultz J, Whelan WJ (eds): *Advances in Gene Technology: Human Genetic Disorders*. Cambridge, England, Cambridge University Press, 1984, p 250.
65. van Faassen H, van den Berg IE, Berger R: Purification of the human liver fumarylacetoacetase using immunoaffinity chromatography. *J Biochem Biophys Methods* **20**:317, 1990.
66. Phaneuf D, Labelle Y, Bérubé D, Arden K, Cavenee W, Gagné R, Tanguay RM: Cloning and expression of the cDNA encoding human fumarylacetoacetate hydrolase, the enzyme deficient in hereditary tyrosinemia: Assignment of the gene to chromosome 15. *Am J Hum Genet* **48**:525, 1991.
67. Tanguay RM, Valet JP, Lescault A, Duband JL, Laberge C, Lettre F, Plante M: Different molecular basis for fumarylacetoacetate hydrolase deficiency in the two clinical forms of hereditary tyrosinemia (type I). *Am J Hum Genet* **47**:308, 1990.
68. Berger R, van Faassen H, Taanman JW, De Vries H, Agsteribbe E: Type I tyrosinemia: Lack of immunologically detectable fumarylacetoacetase enzyme protein in tissues and cell extracts. *Pediatr Res* **22**:394, 1987.
69. Kvittingen EA, Jellum E, Stokke O: Assay of fumarylacetoacetate fumarylhydrolase in human liver-deficient activity in a case of hereditary tyrosinemia. *Clin Chim Acta* **115**:311, 1981.
70. Kvittingen EA, Halvorsen S, Jellum E: Deficient fumarylacetoacetate fumarylhydrolase activity in lymphocytes and fibroblasts from patients with hereditary tyrosinemia. *Pediatr Res* **17**:541, 1983.
71. Labelle Y, Puymirat J, Tanguay RM: Localization of cells in the rat brain expressing fumarylacetoacetate hydrolase, the deficient enzyme in hereditary tyrosinemia type 1. *Biochim Biophys Acta* **1180**:250, 1993.
72. Nicole LM, Valet JP, Laberge C, Tanguay RM: Purification of mRNA coding for the enzyme deficient in hereditary tyrosinemia, fumarylacetoacetate hydrolase. *Biochem Cell Biol* **64**:489, 1986.
73. Agsteribbe E, van Faassen H, Hartog MV, Reversma T, Taanman J-W, Pannekoek H, Evers RF, et al.: Nucleotide sequence of cDNA encoding human fumarylacetoacetase. *Nucl Acids Res* **18**:1887, 1990.
74. Labelle Y, Phaneuf D, Tanguay RM: Cloning and expression analysis of a cDNA encoding fumarylacetoacetate hydrolase: Posttranscriptional modulation in rat liver and kidney. *Gene* **104**:197, 1991.
75. Labelle Y, Phaneuf D, Leclerc B, Tanguay RM: Characterization of the human fumarylacetoacetate hydrolase gene and identification of a missense mutation abolishing enzymatic activity. *Hum Mol Genet* **2**(7):941, 1993.

76. Fernandez-Canon JM, Penalva MA: Fungal metabolic model for human type I hereditary tyrosinaemia. *Proc Natl Acad Sci USA* **92**:9132, 1995.
77. Fernandez-Canon JM, Penalva MA: Molecular characterization of a gene encoding a homogentisate dioxygenase from *Aspergillus nidulans* and identification of its human and plant homologues. *J Biol Chem* **270**:21199, 1995.
78. Grenier A, Laberge C: A modified automated fluorometric method for tyrosine determination in blood spotted on paper: A mass screening procedure for tyrosinemia. *Clin Chim Acta* **57**:71, 1974.
79. Shih VE, Mandell R, Sheinhait I: General metabolic screening tests, in Hommes FA (ed): *Techniques in Diagnostic Human Biochemical Genetics: A Laboratory Manual*. New York, Wiley-Liss, 1991, p 45.
80. Knight JA, Robertson G, Wu JT: The chemical basis and specificity of the nitrosonaphthol reaction. *Clin Chem* **29**:1969, 1983.
81. Grenier A, Lescault A: Succinylacetone, in Bergmeyer A (ed): *Methods of Enzymatic Analysis*, vol 3. Weinheim, VCH, 1985, p 73.
82. Iber FL, Rosen H, Levenson SM, Chalmers TC: The plasma amino acids in patients with liver failure. *J Lab Clin Med* **50**:417, 1957.
83. Fujinami S, Hijikata Y, Shiozaki Y, Sameshima Y: Profiles of plasma amino acids in fasted patients with various liver diseases. *Hepatogastroenterology* **37**:81, 1990.
84. David M, Michel M, Collombel C, Dutruge J, Cotte J, Jeune M: Transient hypertyrosinemia secondary to hepatic involvement: Two cases of different etiologies (galactosemia, hepatitis). *Pediatrics* **25**:459, 1970.
85. Rice DN, Houston IB, Lyon IC, Macarthur BA, Mullins PR, Veale AM, Guthrie R: Transient neonatal tyrosinaemia. *J Inherit Metab Dis* **12**:13, 1989.
86. Mamunes P, Prince PE, Thornton NH, Hunt PA, Hitchcock ES: Intellectual deficits after transient tyrosinemia in the term neonate. *Pediatrics* **57**:675, 1976.
87. Light IJ, Sutherland JM, Berry HK: Clinical significance of tyrosinemia of prematurity. *Am J Dis Child* **125**:243, 1973.
88. Martin GJ, Hueper WC: Biochemical lesions produced by diets high in tyrosine. *Arch Biochem Biophys* **1**:435, 1942.
89. Lock EA, Gaskin P, Ellis MK, McLean Provan W, Robinson M, Smith LL, Prisbylla MP, et al.: Tissue distribution of 2-(2-nitro-4-trifluoromethyl-benzoyl)cyclohexane-1,3-dione (NTBC): Effect on enzymes involved in tyrosine catabolism and relevance to ocular toxicity in the rat. *Toxicol Appl Pharmacol* **141**:439, 1996.
90. Richner H: Horhautaffektion bei Keratoma palmare et plantare heriditarium. *Klin Monatsbl Augenheilkd* **100**:580, 1938.
91. Hanhart E: Neue Sonderformen von Keratosis palmo-plantaris, u.a. eine regelmaessigdominante mit systematisieren Lipomen, ferner 2 einfach-rezessive mit Schwachsinn und z.T. mit Hornhautveraenderungen des Auges. *Dermatologica* **94**:286, 1947.
92. Campbell RA, Buist NRM, Jacinto EY, Koler RD, Hecht F, Jones RT: Supertyrosinemia (tyrosine transaminase deficiency) congenital anomalies and mental retardation. *Oral presentation, 15th* annual meeting of the Society for Pediatric Research, Los Angeles, CA, 1967.
93. Goldsmith LA, Kang E, Bienfang DC, Jimbow K, Gerald P, Baden HP: Tyrosinemia with plantar and palmar keratosis and keratitis. *J Pediatr* **83**:798, 1973.
94. Goldsmith LA: Tyrosinemia and related disorders, in Stanbury JB, Wyngaarden JB, Fredrickson DS, Goldstein JL, Brown MS (eds): *The Metabolic Basis of Inherited Disease*, 5th ed. New York, McGraw-Hill, 1983, p 287.
95. Goldsmith LA, Laberge C: Tyrosinemia and related disorders, in Scriver CR, Beaudet AL, Sly WS, Valle D (eds): *The Metabolic Basis of Inherited Disease*, 6th ed. New York, McGraw-Hill, 1989, p 547.
96. Colditz PB, Yu JS, Billson FA, Rogers M, Molloy HF, O'Halloran M, Wilcken B: Tyrosinaemia II. *Med J Aust* **141**:244, 1984.
97. Chitayat D, Balbul A, Hani V, Mamer OA, Clow C, Scriver CR: Hereditary tyrosinaemia type II in a consanguineous Ashkenazi Jewish family: Intrafamilial variation in phenotype; absence of parental phenotype effects on the fetus. *J Inherit Metab Dis* **15**:198, 1992.
98. Fois A, Borgogni P, Cioni M, Molinelli M, Frezzotti R, Bardelli AM, Lasorella G, et al.: Presentation of the data of the Italian registry for oculocutaneous tyrosinaemia. *J Inherit Metab Dis* **9**:262, 1986.
99. Gipson IK, Burns RP, Wolfe-Lande JD: Crystals in corneal epithelial lesions of tyrosine-fed rats. *Invest Ophthalmol* **14**:937, 1975.
100. Lohr KM, Hyndiuk RA, Hatchell DL, Kurth CE: Corneal organ cultures in tyrosinemia release chemotactic factors. *J Lab Clin Med* **105**:573, 1985.
101. Bohnert A, Anton-Lamprecht I: Richner-Hanhart's syndrome: Ultrastructural abnormalities of epidermal keratinization indicating a causal relationship to high intracellular tyrosine levels. *J Invest Dermatol* **79**:68, 1982.
102. Crovato F, Desirello G, Gatti R, Babbini N, Rebora A: Richner-Hanhart syndrome spares a plantar autograft. *Arch Dermatol* **121**:539, 1985.
103. Christensen K, Henriksen P, Sörensen H: New forms of hereditary tyrosinemia type II in mink: Hepatic tyrosine aminotransferase defect. *Hereditas* **104**:215, 1986.
104. Kunkle GA, Jezyk PF, West CS, Goldschmidt MH, O'Keefe C: Tyrosinemia in a dog. *J Am Anim Hosp Assoc* **20**:615, 1984.
105. Gounod N, Ogier H, Dufier J-L, Larrègue M, Saudubray J-M, De Prost Y: Tyrosinose oculo-cutanée de type II. *Ann Dermatol Venereol* **111**:697, 1984.
106. Brock DJH, Williamson DH: Purification of a diketo acid hydrolase from rat liver and its use for the enzymic determination of 3,5-dioxohexanoate (triacetate). *Biochem J* **110**:677, 1968.
107. Rehçak A, Selim MM, Yadav G: Richner-Hanhart syndrome (tyrosinaemia-II) (report of four cases without ocular involvement). *Br J Dermatol* **104**:469, 1981.
108. Fraser NG, MacDonald J, Griffiths WA, McPhie JL: Tyrosinaemia type II (Richner-Hanhart syndrome): Report of two cases treated with etretinate. *Clin Exp Dermatol* **12**:440, 1987.
109. Lestringant GG: Tyrosinemia type II with incomplete Richner-Hanhart's syndrome. *Int J Dermatol* **27**:43, 1988.
110. Gramet C, Lods F: Syndrome de Richner-Hanart sans atteinte cutanée. *Bull Soc Ophtalmol Fr* **84**:129, 1984.
111. Heidemann DG, Dunn SP, Bawle EV, Shepherd DM: Early diagnosis of tyrosinemia type II. *Am J Ophthalmol* **107**:559, 1989.
112. Roussat B, Fournier F, Beson D, Godde-Joly D: A propos de deux cas de tyrosinose de type II (syndrome de Richner-Hanhart). *Bull Soc Ophtalmol Fr* **88**:751, 1988.
113. al-Hemidan AI, al-Hazzaa SA: Richner-Hanhart syndrome (tyrosinemia type II): Case report and literature review. *Ophthalmic Genet* **16**(1):21, 1995.
114. Bardelli AM, Borgogni P, Farnetani MA, Fois A, Frezzotti R, Mattei R, Molinelli M, et al: Familial tyrosinaemia with eye and skin lesions: Presentation of two cases. *Ophthalmologica* **175**:5, 1977.
115. Goldsmith LA: Tyrosinemia II: Lessons in molecular pathophysiology. *Pediatr Dermatol* **1**:25, 1983.
116. Larregue M, De Giacomoni Ph, Bressieux J-M, Odievre M: Syndrome de Richner-Hanhart ou tyrosinose oculocutanée: A propos d'un cas. *Ann Dermatol Venereol* **106**:52, 1979.
117. Hunziker N: Richner-Hanhart syndrome and tyrosinemia type II. *Dermatologica* **160**:180, 1980.
118. Balato N, Cusano F, Lembo G, Santoianni P: Tyrosinemia type II in two cases previously reported as Richner-Hanhart syndrome. *Dermatologica* **173**:66, 1986.
119. Andersson S, Nemeth A, Ohisalo J, Strandvik B: Persistent tyrosinemia associated with low activity of tyrosine aminotransferase. *Pediatr Res* **18**:675, 1984.
120. Hervé F, Moreno JL, Ogier H, Saudubray JM, De Prost Y, Duffier JL, Charpentier C, et al: Kératite "inguérissable" et hyperkératose palmo-plantaire chronique avec hypertyrosinémie. *Arch Fr Pediatr* **43**:19, 1986.
121. deGroot GW, Dakshinamurti K, Allan L, Haworth JC: Defect in soluble tyrosine aminotransferase in skin fibroblasts of a patient with tyrosinemia. *Pediatr Res* **14**:896, 1980.
122. Lemonnier F, Charpentier C, Odievre M, Larregue M, Lemonnier A: Tyrosine aminotransferase isoenzyme deficiency. *J Pediatr* **94**:931, 1979.
123. Natt E, Kida K, Odievre M, Di Rocco M, Scherer G: Point mutations in the tyrosine aminotransferase gene in tyrosinemia type II. *Proc Natl Acad Sci USA* **89**:9297, 1992.
124. Huhn R, Stoermer H, Klingele B, Bausch E, Fois A, Farnetani M, Di-Rocco M, et al: Novel and recurrent tyrosine aminotransferase gene mutations in tyrosinemia type II. *Hum Genet* **102**:305, 1998.
125. Irons M, Levy HL: Metabolic syndromes with dermatologic manifestations. *Clin Rev Allergy* **4**:101, 1986.
126. Sammartino A, Cerbella R, Cecio A, De Crecchio G, Federico A, Fronterre A: The effect of diet on the ophthalmological, clinical and biochemical aspects of Richner-Hanhart syndrome: A morphological ultrastructural study of the cornea and the conjunctiva. *Int Ophthalmol* **10**:203, 1987.

127. Sayar RB, von Domarus D, Schäfer HJ, Beckenkamp G: Clinical picture and problems of keratoplasty in Richner-Hanhart syndrome (tyrosinemia type II). *Ophthalmologica* **197**:1, 1988.
128. Bienfang DC, Kuwabara T, Pueschel SM: The Richner-Hanhart syndrome. *Arch Ophthalmol* **94**:1133, 1976.
129. Saijo S, Kudoh K, Kuramoto Y, Horii I, Tagami H: Tyrosinemia II: Report of an incomplete case and studies on the hyperkeratotic stratum corneum. *Dermatologica* **182**:168, 1991.
130. Garibaldi LR, Durand P: Soluble tyrosine-aminotransferase (STAT) deficiency tyrosinemia: Four cases (abstract). *Pediatr Res* **14**:1428, 1980.
131. Hyanek J, Homolka J, Trnka J, Seemanova E, Cervenka J, Tresohlava Z, Kapras J, et al: Results of screening for phenylalanine and other amino acid disturbances among pregnant women. *J Inherit Metab Dis* **2**:59, 1979.
132. Francis DEM, Kirby DM, Thompson GN: Maternal tyrosinaemia II: Management and successful outcome. *Eur J Pediatr* **151**:196, 1992.
133. Giardini O, Cantani A, Kennaway NG, D'Eufemia P: Chronic tyrosinemia associated with 4-hydroxyphenylpyruvate dioxygenase deficiency with acute intermittent ataxia and without visceral and bone involvement. *Pediatr Res* **27**:25, 1983.
134. Origuchi Y, Endo F, Kitano A, Nagata N, Matsuda I: Sural nerve lesions in a case of hypertyrosinemia. *Brain Dev* **4**:463, 1982.
135. Preece MA, Rylance GW, Macdonald A, Green A, Gray RGF: A new case of tyrosinemia type III detected by neonatal screening. *J Inherit Metab Dis* **19**(suppl 1):32, 1996.
136. Cerone R, Holme E, Schiaffino MC, Caruso U, Maritano L, Romano C: Tyrosinemia type III: Diagnosis and ten-year follow-up. *Acta Paediatr* **86**(9):1013, 1997.
137. Faull KF, Gan I, Halpern B, Hammond J, Im S, Cotton RG, Danks DM, et al: Metabolic studies on two patients with nonhepatic tyrosinemia using deuterated tyrosine loads. *Pediatr Res* **11**:631, 1977.
138. Louis WJ, Pitt DD, Davies H: Biochemical studies in a patient with "tyrosinosis". *Aust NZ J Med* **4**:281, 1974.
139. Wadman SK, Sprang FJ, Maas JW, Ketting D: An exceptional case of tyrosinosis. *J Ment Defic Res* **12**:269, 1968.
140. Endo F, Katoh H, Yamamoto S, Matsuda I: A murine model for type III tyrosinemia: lack of immunologically detectable 4-hydroxyphenylpyruvic acid dioxygenase enzyme protein in a novel mouse strain with hypertyrosinemia. *Am J Hum Genet* **48**:704, 1991.
141. Kubo S, Kiwaki K, Awata H, Katoh H, Kanegae Y, Saito I, Yamamoto T, et al: In vivo correction with recombinant adenovirus of 4-hydroxyphenylpyruvic acid dioxygenase deficiencies in strain III mice. *Hum Gene Ther* **8**:65, 1997.
142. Danks DM, Tippett P, Rogers J: A new form of prolonged transient tyrosinemia presenting with severe metabolic acidosis. *Acta Paediatr Scand* **64**:209, 1975.
143. Wilcken B, Hammond JW, Howard N, Bohane T, Hocart C, Halpern B: Hawkinsinuria: A dominantly inherited defect of tyrosine metabolism with severe effects in infancy. *N Engl J Med* **305**:865, 1981.
144. Niederwieser A, Matasovic A, Tippett P, Danks DM: A new sulfur amino acid, named hawkinsin, identified in a baby with transient tyrosinemia and her mother. *Clin Chim Acta* **76**:345, 1977.
145. Niederwieser A, Wadman SK, Danks DM: Excretion of *cis*- and *trans*-4-hydroxycyclohexylacetic acid in addition to hawkinsin in a family with a postulated defect of 4-hydroxyphenylpyruvate dioxygenase. *Clin Chim Acta* **90**:195, 1978.
146. Borden M, Holm J, Leslie J, Sweetman L, Nyhan WL, Fleisher L, Nadler H, et al: Hawkinsinuria in two families. *Am J Med Genet* **44**:52, 1992.
147. Lehnert W, Stögmann W: Long-term follow-up of a new case with hawkinsinuria. Seventh International Congress of Inborn Errors of Metabolism, Vienna, 1997. Abstract.
148. Nyhan WL: Hawkinsinuria, in Nyhan WL (ed): *Abnormalities in Amino Acid Metabolism in Clinical Medicine*. Norwalk, Connecticut, Appleton-Century-Crofts, 1984, p 187.
149. Wong PWK, Lambert AM, Komrower GM: Tyrosinaemia and tyrosyluria in infancy. *Dev Med Child Neurol* **9**:551, 1967.
150. Levine SZ, Marples E, Gordon HH: A defect in the metabolism of aromatic amino acids in premature infants: The role of vitamin C. *Science* **90**:620, 1939.
151. Goodwin BL: *Tyrosine Catabolism. The Biological, Physiological, and Clinical Significance of p-Hydroxyphenylpyruvate Oxidase*. Oxford, England, Oxford University Press, 1972.
152. Bloxam HR, Day MG, Gibbs NK, Woolf II: An inborn defect in the metabolism of tyrosine in infants on a normal diet. *Biochem J* **77**:320, 1960.
153. Levy HL, Shih VE, Madigan PM, MacCready RA: Transient tyrosinemia in full-term infants. *JAMA* **209**:249, 1969.
154. Partington MW, Mathews J: The relation of plasma tyrosine level to weight gain of premature infants. *J Pediatr* **68**:749, 1966.
155. Menkes JH, Jervis GA: Developmental retardation associated with an abnormality in tyrosine metabolism. *Pediatrics* **28**:399, 1961.
156. Mathews J, Partington MW: The plasma tyrosine levels of premature babies. *Arch Dis Child* **39**:371, 1964.
157. Menkes JH, Chernick V, Ringel B: Effect of elevated blood tyrosine on subsequent intellectual development of premature infants. *J Pediatr* **69**:583, 1966.
158. Partington MW, Delahaye DJ, Masotti RE, Read JH, Roberts B: Neonatal tyrosinaemia: A follow-up study. *Arch Dis Child* **43**:195, 1968.
159. Driscoll DJ, Jabs EW, Alcorn D, Maumenee IH, Brusilow SW, Valle D: Corneal tyrosine crystals in transient neonatal tyrosinemia. *J Pediatr* **113**:91, 1988.
160. Avery ME, Clow CL, Menkes JH, Ramos A, Scriver CR, Stern L, Wasserman BP: Transient tyrosinemia of the newborn: Dietary and clinical aspects. *Pediatrics* **39**:378, 1967.
161. Partington MW: Neonatal tyrosinaemia. *Biol Neonate* **12**:316, 1968.
162. Hsia DYY, Litwack M, O'Flynn M, Jakovcic S: Serum phenylalanine and tyrosine levels in the newborn infant. *N Engl J Med* **267**:1067, 1962.
163. Halvorsen S: Screening for disorders of tyrosine metabolism, in Bickel H, Guthrie R, Hammerson G (eds): *Neonatal Screenings for Inborn Errors of Metabolism*. New York, Springer-Verlag, 1980, p 45.
164. Grenier A: Personal communication, 1998.
165. Mitchell GA, Lambert M, Tanguay RM: Hypertyrosinemia, in Scriver CR, Beaudet A, Sly W, Valle D (eds): *The Metabolic and Molecular Bases of Inherited Disease*, 7th ed. New York, McGraw-Hill, 1995, p 1077.
166. Light IJ, Berry HK, Sutherland JM: Aminoacidemia of prematurity. *Am J Dis Child* **112**:229, 1966.
167. Medes G: A new error of tyrosine metabolism: Tyrosinosis. The intermediary metabolism of tyrosine and phenylalanine. *Biochem J* **26**:917, 1932.
168. La Du B, Gjessing LR: Tyrosinosis and tyrosinemia, in Stanbury JB, Wyngaarden JB, Fredrickson DS (eds): *The Metabolic Basis of Inherited Disease*, 3d ed. New York, McGraw-Hill, 1972, p 296.
169. La Du BN, Gjessing LR: Tyrosinosis and tyrosinemia, in Stanbury JB, Wyngaarden JB, Fredrickson DS (eds): *The Metabolic Basis of Inherited Disease*, 4th ed. New York, McGraw-Hill, 1978, p 256.
170. Rogers WF, Gardner FH: Tyrosine metabolism in human scurvy. *J Lab Clin Med* **28**:1491, 1949.
171. Dhatt PS, Saini AS, Gupta I, Mehta HC, Singh H: Tyrosyluria in marasmus. *Br J Nutr* **42**:387, 1979.
172. Antener I, Verwilghen AM, Van Geert C, Mauron J: Biochemical study of malnutrition: V. Metabolism of phenylalanine and tyrosine. *Int J Vitam Nutr Res* **51**:297, 1981.
173. Watts RWE, Chalmers RA, Liberman MM, Lawson AM: Some biochemical effects of chloral hydrate in an infant with a tyrosinemia-like syndrome. *Pediatr Res* **9**:875, 1975.
174. Berger R, Michals K, Galbraeth J, Matalon R: Tyrosinemia type Ib caused by maleylacetoacetate isomerase deficiency: A new enzyme defect (abstract). *Pediatr Res* **23**:328A, 1988.
175. Fernandez-Canon JM, Grompe M: Unpublished observations, 1998.
176. *Symposium on Tyrosinosis: In Honour of Dr Grace Medes, 2–3 June 1965*. Oslo, Norway, Scandinavian University Books, 1966.
177. Symposium on tyrosinemia. *Can Med Assoc J* **97**:1051, 1967.
178. Minisymposium on tyrosinemia. *Am J Hum Genet* **47**:302, 1990.
179. SSIEM 35th Annual Symposium. *J Inherit Metab Dis* **20**(suppl 1):1, 1997.
180. van Spronsen FJ, Thomasse Y, Smit GPA, Leonard JV, Clayton PT, Fidler V, Berger R, et al: Hereditary tyrosinemia type I: A new clinical classification with difference in prognosis on dietary treatment. *Hepatology* **20**:1187, 1994.
181. Sakai K, Kitagawa T: An atypical case of tyrosinosis (1-*para*-hydroxyphenyllactic aciduria): I. Clinical and laboratory findings. *Jikei Med J* **2**:1, 1957.
182. Sakai K, Kitagawa T: An atypical case of tyrosinosis (1-*para*-hydroxyphenyllactic aciduria): II. A research on the metabolic block. *Jikei Med J* **2**:11, 1957.

183. Sakai K, Kitagawa T, Yoshioka K: An atypical case of tyrosinosis (1-*para*-hydroxyphenyllactic aciduria): III. The outcome of the patient; pathological and biochemical observations of the organ tissues. *Jikei Med J* **6**:15, 1959.
184. Van Creveld S: Levercirrhose en hydronephrose. *Maandschrift Kinder Geneesk* **3**:504, 1934.
185. Guild HG, Pierce JA, Lilienthal JL: An unfamiliar rachitic syndrome. *Am J Dis Child* **54**:1186, 1937.
186. Stowers JM, Dent CE: Studies on the mechanism of the Fanconi syndrome. *Q J Med* **16**:275, 1947.
187. Baber MD: A case of congenital cirrhosis of the liver with renal tubular defects akin to those in the Fanconi syndrome. *Arch Dis Child* **31**:335, 1956.
188. Gentz J, Lindblad B, Lindstedt S, Levy L, Shasteen W, Zetterstrom R: Dietary treatment in tyrosinemia (tyrosinosis): With a note on the possible recognition of the carrier state. *Am J Dis Child* **113**:31, 1967.
189. Kang ES, Gerald PS: Hereditary tyrosinemia and abnormal pyrrole metabolism. *J Pediatr* **77**:397, 1970.
190. Gentz J, Johansson S, Lindblad B, Lindstedt S, Zetterström R: Excretion of delta-aminolevulinic acid in hereditary tyrosinemia. *Clin Chim Acta* **23**:257, 1969.
191. Strife CF, Zuroweste EL, Emmett EA, Finelli VN, Petering HG, Berry HK: Tyrosinemia with acute intermittent porphyria: Aminolevulinic acid dehydratase deficiency related to elevated urinary aminolevulinic acid levels. *J Pediatr* **90**:400, 1977.
192. Gaull GE, Rassin DK, Solomon GE, Harris RC, Sturman JA: Biochemical observations on so-called hereditary tyrosinemia. *Pediatr Res* **4**:337, 1970.
193. Lindblad B, Lindstedt S, Steen G: On the enzymic defects in hereditary tyrosinemia. *Proc Natl Acad Sci USA* **74**:4641, 1977.
194. Fällström S-P, Lindblad B, Lindstedt S, Steen G: Hereditary tyrosinemia-fumarylacetoacetase deficiency (abstract). *Pediatr Res* **13**:78. 1979.
195. Berger R, Smit GP, Stoker-de Vries SA, Duran M, Ketting D, Wadman SK: Deficiency of fumarylacetoacetase in a patient with hereditary tyrosinemia. *Clin Chim Acta* **114**:37, 1981.
196. Gray RG, Patrick AD, Preston FE, Whitfield MF: Acute hereditary tyrosinaemia type I: Clinical, biochemical and haematological studies in twins. *J Inherit Metab Dis* **4**:37, 1981.
197. Seltzer S, Lin M: Maleylacetone cis-trans isomerase: Mechanism of the interaction of coenzyme glutathione and substrate maleylacetone in the presence and absence of enzyme. *J Am Chem Soc* **101**:3091, 1979.
198. Morgan EJ, Friedman E: Interaction of maleic acid with thiol compounds. *Biochem J* **32**:733, 1938.
199. Jorquera R, Tanguay RM: The mutagenicity of the tyrosine metabolite, fumarylacetoacetate, is enhanced by glutathione depletion. *Biochem Biophys Res Commun* **232**:42, 1997.
200. Manabe S, Sassa S, Kappas A: Hereditary tyrosinemia: Formation of succinylacetone-amino acid adducts. *J Exp Med* **162**:1060, 1985.
201. La Du BN: The enzymatic deficiency in tyrosinemia. *Am J Dis Child* **113**:54, 1967.
202. Gentz J, Heinrich J, Lindblad B, Lindstedt S, Zetterström R: Enzymatic studies in a case of hereditary tyrosinemia with hepatoma. *Acta Paediatr Scand* **58**:393, 1969.
203. Endo F, Kubo S, Awata H, Kiwaki K, Katoh H, Kanegae Y, Saito I, et al: Complete rescue of lethal albino c^{14CoS} mice by null mutation of 4-hydroxyphenylpyruvate dioxygenase and induction of apoptosis of hepatocytes in these mice by in vivo retrieval of the tyrosine catabolic pathway. *J Biol Chem* **272**(39):24426, 1997.
203a. Kubo S, Sun M, Miyahara M, Umeyama K, Urakami K-I, Yamamoto T, Jakobs C, et al: Hepatocyte injury in tyrosinemia type 1 is induced by fumarylacetoacetate and is inhibited by caspase inhibitors. *Proc Natl Acad Sci USA* **95**:9552, 1998.
203b. Jorquera R, Tanguay RM: Cyclin B-dependent kinase and caspase-1 activation precedes mitochondrial dysfunction in fumarylacetoacetate-induced apoptosis. *FASEB J* **13**: 2284, 1999.
204. Liau MC, Chang CF, Belanger L, Grenier A: Correlation of isozyme patterns of *S*-adenosylmethionine synthetase with fetal stages and pathological states of the liver. *Cancer Res* **39**:162, 1979.
205. Gahl WA, Finkelstein JD, Mullen KD, Bernardini I, Martin JJ, Backlund P, Ishak KG, et al: Hepatic methionine adenosyltransferase deficiency in a 31-year-old man. *Am J Hum Genet* **40**:39, 1987.
206. Perry TL, Hardwick DF, Dixon GH, Dolman CL, Hansen S: Hypermethioninemia: A metabolic disorder associated with cirrhosis, islet cell hyperplasia, and renal tubular degeneration. *Pediatrics* **36**:236, 1965.
207. Sassa S, Kappas A: Hereditary tyrosinemia and the heme biosynthetic pathway: Profound inhibition of delta-aminolevulinic acid dehydratase activity by succinylacetone. *J Clin Invest* **71**:625, 1983.
208. Sassa S, Fujita H, Kappas A: Succinylacetone and delta-aminolevulinic acid dehydratase in hereditary tyrosinemia: Immunochemical study of the enzyme. *Pediatrics* **86**:84, 1990.
209. Gentz J, Lindblad B, Lindstedt S, Zetterström R: Studies on the metabolism of the phenolic acids in hereditary tyrosinemia by a gas-liquid chromatographic method. *J Lab Clin Med* **74**:185, 1969.
210. Moore MR, Meredith PA: The association of delta-aminolaevulinic acid with the neurological and behavioral effects of lead exposure, in Delbert DH (ed): *Conference on Trace Substances in Environmental Health*. Columbia, University of Missouri Press, 1976, p 363.
211. Müller WE, Snyder SH: +-Aminolevulinic acid: Influences on synaptic GABA receptor binding may explain CNS symptoms of porphyria. *Ann Neurol* **2**:340, 1977.
212. Brennan MJ, Cantrill RC: Delta-aminolevulinic acid is a potent agonist for GABA autoreceptors. *Nature* **280**:514, 1979.
213. Silbergeld EK, Lamon JM: Role of altered heme synthesis in lead neurotoxicity. *Medicine* **22**:680, 1980.
214. Sima AA, Kennedy JC, Blakeslee D, Robertson DM: Experimental porphyric neuropathy: A preliminary report. *Can J Neurol Sci* **8**:105, 1981.
215. Mitchell GA, Larochelle J, Lambert M, Michaud J, Grenier A, Ogier H, Gauthier M, et al: Neurologic crises in hereditary tyrosinemia. *N Engl J Med* **322**:432, 1990.
216. Spencer PD, Medow MS, Moses LC, Roth KS: Effects of succinylacetone on the uptake of sugars and amino acids by brush border vesicles. *Kidney Int* **34**:671, 1988.
217. Roth KS, Carter BE, Moses LC, Spencer PD: On rat renal aminolevulinate transport and metabolism in experimental Fanconi syndrome. *Biochem Med Metab Biol* **44**:238, 1990.
218. Roth KS, Carter BE, Higgins ES: Succinylacetone effects on renal tubular phosphate metabolism: A model for experimental renal Fanconi syndrome. *Proc Soc Exp Biol Med* **196**:428, 1991.
219. Giger U, Meyer UA: Effect of succinylacetone on heme and cytochrome P450 synthesis in hepatocyte culture. *FEBS Lett* **153**:335, 1983.
220. Tschudy DP, Ebert PS, Hess RA, Frykholm BC, Atsmon A: Growth inhibitory activity of succinylacetone: Studies with Walker 256 carcinosarcoma, Novikoff hepatoma and L1210 leukemia. *Oncology* **40**:148, 1983.
221. Tschudy DP, Hess RA, Frykholm BC, Blaese Bethesda RM: Immunosuppressive activity of succinylacetone. *J Lab Clin Med* **99**:526, 1982.
221a. Winkelstein A, Hess RA, Leichtling KD, Jackson MO, Blaese RM, Weaver LD: Inhibition of human lymphoproliferative responses and altered lymphocyte membrane phenotype by succinylacetone. *Immunopharmacology* **24**:161, 1992.
222. Wadman SK, Duran M, Ketting D, Bruinvis L, van Sprang FJ, Berger R, Smit GP, et al: Urinary excretion of deuterated metabolites in patients with tyrosinemia type I after oral loading with deuterated L-tyrosine. *Clin Chim Acta* **130**:231, 1983.
223. Gentz J, Jagenburg R, Zetterström R: Tyrosinemia: An inborn error of tyrosine metabolism with cirrhosis of the liver and multiple renal tubular defects. *J Pediatr* **66**:670, 1965.
224. Fällström SP, Lindblad B, Steen G: On the renal tubular damage in hereditary tyrosinemia and on the formation of succinylacetoacetate and succinylacetone. *Acta Paediatr Scand* **70**:315, 1981.
225. Woolf LI: Tyrosinosis (inborn hepato-renal dysfunction). *Proc R Soc Med* **65**:814, 1965.
226. Bodegard G, Gentz J, Lindblad B, Lindstedt S, Zetterstrom R: Hereditary tyrosinemia: 3. On the differential diagnosis and the lack of effect of early dietary treatment. *Acta Paediatr Scand* **58**:37, 1969.
227. Gjessing LR, Halvorsen S: Hypermethioninaemia in acute tyrosinosis. *Lancet* **2**:1132, 1965.
228. Kvittingen EA, Rootwelt H, Brandtzaeg P, Bergan A, Berger R: Hereditary tyrosinemia type I. *J Clin Invest* **91**:1816, 1993.
229. Kvittingen EA, Rootwelt H, Berger R, Brandtzaeg P: Self-induced correction of the genetic defect in tyrosinemia type I. *J Clin Invest* **94**:1657, 1994.
230. Gluecksohn-Waelsch S: Genetic control of morphogenetic and biochemical differentiation: Lethal albino deletions in the mouse. *Cell* **16**:225, 1979.
231. Russell LB, Russell WL, Kelly EM: Analysis of the albino-locus region of the mouse: Origin and viability. *Genetics* **91**:127, 1979.

232. Niswander L, Kelsey G, Schedl A, Ruppert S, Sharan SK, Holdener KB, Rinchik EM, et al: Molecular mapping of albino deletions associated with early embryonic lethality in the mouse. *Genomics* **9**:162, 1991.
233. Schmid W, Müller G, Schütz G, Gluecksohn-Waelsch S: Deletions near the albino locus on chromosome 7 of the mouse affect the level of tyrosine aminotransferase mRNA. *Proc Natl Acad Sci USA* **82**:2866, 1985.
234. Loose DS, Shaw PA, Krauter KS, Robinson C, England S, Hanson RW, Gluecksohn-Waelsch S: Trans regulation of the phosphoenolpyruvate carboxykinase (*GTP*) gene, identified by deletions in chromosome 7 of the mouse. *Proc Natl Acad Sci USA* **83**:5184, 1986.
235. Sala-Trepat JM, Poiret M, Sellem CH, Bessada R, Erdos T, Gluecksohn-Waelsch S: A lethal deletion on mouse chromosome 7 affects regulation of liver cell-specific functions: Posttranscriptional control of serum protein and transcriptional control of aldolase B synthesis. *Proc Natl Acad Sci USA* **82**:2442, 1985.
236. Ruppert S, Boshart M, Bosch FX, Schmid W, Fournier R, Schütz G: Two genetically defined trans-acting loci coordinately regulate overlapping sets of liver-specific genes. *Cell* **61**:895, 1990.
237. Fornace AJ, Jr., Nebert DW, Hollander MC, Luethy JD, Papathanasiou M, Fargnoli J, Holbrook NJ: Mammalian genes coordinately regulated by growth arrest signals and DNA-damaging agents. *Mol Cel Biol* **9**:4196, 1989.
238. Ruppert S, Kelsey G, Schedl A, Schmid E, Thies E, Günther G: Deficiency of an enzyme of tyrosine metabolism underlies altered gene expression in newborn liver of lethal albino mice. *Genes Dev* **6**:1430, 1992.
239. Klebig ML, Russell LB, Rinchik EM: Murine fumarylacetoacetate hydrolase (*Fah*) gene is disrupted by a neonatally lethal albino deletion that defines the hepatocyte-specific developmental regulation 1 (*hsdr-1*) locus. *Proc Natl Acad Sci USA* **89**:1363, 1992.
240. Grompe M, Al-Dhalimi M, Ou CN, Burlingame T, Kennaway NG, Soriano P: Loss of fumarylacetoacetate hydrolase is responsible for the neonatal hepatic dysfunction phenotype of lethal albino mice. *Genes Dev* **7**:2298, 1993.
241. Kelsey G, Ruppert S, Beermann F, Grund C, Tanguay RM, Schütz G: Rescue of mice homozygous for lethal albino deletions: Implications for an animal model for the human liver disease tyrosinemia type I. *Genes Dev* **7**:2285, 1993.
242. Grompe M, Lindstedt S, Al-Dhalimy M, Kennaway NG, Papaconstantinou J, Torred-Ramos CA, Ou C-N, et al: Pharmacological correction of neonatal lethal hepatic dysfunction in a murine model of hereditary tyrosinaemia type I. *Nature Genet* **10**:453, 1995.
242a. Overturf M, Al-Dhalimy M, Tanguay R, Brantly M, Ou CN, Finegold, Grompe M: Hepatocytes corrected by gene therapy are selected in vivo in a murine model of hereditary tyrosinemia type I. *Nature Genet* **12**:266, 1996.
243. Overturf K, Al-Dhalimy M, Ou CN, Finegold M, Tanguay R, Lieber A, Kay M, et al: Adenovirus-mediated gene therapy in a mouse model of hereditary tyrosinemia type I. *Hum Gene Ther* **8**(5):513, 1997.
243a. Overturf K, Al-Dhalimy M, Manning K, Ou CN, Finegold M, Grompe M: Ex vivo hepatic gene therapy of a mouse model of hereditary tyrosinemia type I. *Hum Gene Ther* **9**:295, 1998.
243b. Grisham JW: Interspecies comparison of liver carcinogenesis: Implications for cancer risk assessment. *Carcinogenesis* **18**:59, 1997.
244. De Braekeleer M: Hereditary disorders in Saguenay-Lac-St-Jean (Quebec, Canada). *Hum Hered* **41**:141, 1991.
245. De Braekeleer M, Larochelle J: Genetic epidemiology of hereditary tyrosinemia in Quebec and in Saguenay-Lac-St-Jean. *Am J Hum Genet* **47**:302, 1990.
246. Gauvreau D, Bourque M: Mouvements migratoires et familles: le peuplement du Saguenay avant 1911. *Rev Histoire Am Fr* **42**:167, 1988.
247. Guillemette A, Légaré J: The influence of kinship on seventeenth-century immigration to Canada. *Continuity Change* **4**:79, 1989.
248. De Braekeleer M: Le Perche: Une province d'importance pour la population canadienne-française (abstract). *Ann ACFAS* **59**:86, 1991.
249. Laberge C: Hereditary tyrosinemia in a French Canadian isolate. *Am J Hum Genet* **21**:36, 1969.
250. Bouchard G, Laberge C, Scriver C-R: Comportements démographiques et effets fondateurs dans la population du Québec (XVIIe-XXe siècles), in *Anonymous Societe Belge de Demographie Historiens et Populations: Liber Amicorum Etienne Hélin*. Louvain-la-Neuve, Academia, 1992, p 319.
251. Bergeron P, Laberge C, Grenier A: Hereditary tyrosinemia in the province of Quebec: Prevalence at birth and geographic distribution. *Clin Genet* **5**:157, 1974.
252. Larochelle J, Mortezai A, Belanger M, Tremblay M, Claveau JC, Aubin G: Experience with 37 infants with tyrosinemia. *Can Med Assoc J* **97**:1051, 1967.
253. Grenier A, Bélanger L, Laberge C: α_1-Fetoprotein measurement in blood spotted on paper: Discriminating test for hereditary tyrosinemia in neonatal mass screening. *Clin Chem* **22**:1001, 1976.
254. Grenier A, Laberge C: Personal communication, 2000.
255. Grenier A, Laberge C: Neonatal screening for tyrosinemia type I and early sampling (abstract), in *Proceedings of the Third International Society for Neonatal Screening*. Boston, MA, Oct. 20–23, 1996.
256. Larochelle J, Privé L, Bélanger M, Bélanger L, Tremblay M, Claveau JC, Aubin G, et al: Hereditary tyrosinemia I: Clinical and biological study of 62 cases. *Pediatrics* **28**:5, 1973.
257. Kvittingen EA, Leonard JV, Pettit BR, King GS: Concentrations of succinylacetone after homogentisate and tyrosine loading in healthy individuals with low fumarylacetoacetase activity. *Clin Chim Acta* **152**:271, 1985.
258. Halvorsen S: Dietary treatment of tyrosinosis. *Am J Dis Child* **113**:38, 1967.
259. Laberge C, Lescault A, Grenier A, Morrisette J, Gagné R, Gadbois P, Halket J: Oral loading of homogentisic acid in controls and in obligate heterozygotes for hereditary tyrosinemia type I. *Am J Hum Genet* **47**:329, 1990.
260. Laberge C, Lescault A, Grenier A, Gagné R: "Effet succinylacétone" après surcharges orales d'homogentisate. *Union Med Can* **110**:621, 1981.
261. Kvittingen EA, Börresen AL, Stokke O, van der Hagen CB, Lie SO: Deficiency of fumarylacetoacetase without hereditary tyrosinemia. *Clin Genet* **27**:550, 1985.
262. Haagen AAM, Duran M: Absence of increased succinylacetone in the urine of a child with hereditary tyrosinaemia type I. *J Inherit Metab Dis* **10**(suppl 2):323, 1987.
263. Bain MD, Purkiss P, Jones M, Bingham P, Stacey TE, Chalmers RA: Dietary treatment eliminates succinylacetone from the urine of a patient with tyrosinaemia type 1. *Eur J Pediatr* **149**:637, 1990.
264. Laberge C, Grenier A, Valet JP, Morissette J: Fumarylacetoacetase measurement as a mass-screening procedure for hereditary tyrosinemia type I. *Am J Hum Genet* **47**:325, 1990.
265. Pettit BR, Kvittingen EA, Leonard JV: Early prenatal diagnosis of hereditary tyrosinaemia (letter). *Lancet* **1**:1038, 1985.
266. Jakobs C, Stellaard F, Kvittingen EA, Henderson M, Lilford R: First-trimester prenatal diagnosis of tyrosinemia type I by amniotic fluid succinylacetone determination (letter). *Prenat Diagn* **10**:133, 1990.
267. Grenier A, Cederbaum S, Laberge C, Gagné R, Jakobs C, Tanguay RM: A case of tyrosinaemia type I with normal level of succinylacetone in the amniotic fluid. *Prenat Diagn* **16**(3):239, 1996.
267a. Poudrier J, Lettre F, St-Louis M,Tanguay RM: Genotyping of a case of tyrosinemia type I with normal level of succinylacetone in amniotic fluid. *Prenat Diagn* **19**(1):61, 1999.
268. Kvittingen EA, Steinmann B, Gitzelmann R, Leonard JV, Andria G, Börresen AL, Mossman J, et al: Prenatal diagnosis of hereditary tyrosinemia by determination of fumarylacetoacetase in cultured amniotic fluid cells. *Pediatr Res* **19**:334, 1985.
269. Kvittingen EA, Guibaud PP, Divry P, Mandon G, Rolland MO, Domenichini Y, Jakobs C, et al: Prenatal diagnosis of hereditary tyrosinaemia type I by determination of fumarylacetoacetase in chorionic villus material (letter). *Eur J Pediatr* **144**:597, 1986.
270. Perry TL: Tyrosinemia associated with hypermethioninemia and islet cell hyperplasia. *Can Med Assoc J* **97**:1067, 1967.
271. Weinberg AG, Mize CE, Worthen HG: The occurrence of hepatoma in the chronic form of hereditary tyrosinemia. *J Pediatr* **88**:434, 1976.
272. Paradis K: Tyrosinemia: The Quebec experience. *Clin Invest Med* **19**(5):311, 1996.
273. Dubois J, Garel L, Patriquin H, Paradis K, Forget S, Filiatrault D, Grignon A, et al: Imaging features of type 1 hereditary tyrosinemia: A review of 30 patients. *Pediatr Radiol* **26**:845, 1996.
274. Dionisi-Vici C, Boglino C, Marcellini M, De Sio L, Inserra A, Cotugno G, Sabetta G, et al: Tyrosinemia type I with early metastatic hepatocellular carcinoma: Combined treatment with NTBC, chemotherapy and surgical mass removal (abstract). *J Inherit Metab Dis* **20**(suppl 1):3, 1997.
275. Paradis K, Weber A, Seidman EG, Larochelle J, Garel L, Lenaerts C, Roy CC: Liver transplantation for hereditary tyrosinemia: The Quebec experience. *Am J Hum Genet* **47**:338, 1990.

276. Macvicar D, Dicks-Mireaux C, Leonard JV, Wight DG: Hepatic imaging with computed tomography of chronic tyrosinaemia type 1. *Br J Radiol* **63**:605, 1990.
277. Day DL, Letourneau JG, Allan BT, Sharp HL, Ascher N, Dehner LP, Thompson WM: Hepatic regenerating nodules in hereditary tyrosinemia. *AJR* **149**:391, 1987.
278. Mieles LA, Esquivel CO, Van Thiel DH, Koneru B, Makowka L, Tzakis AG, Starzl TE: Liver transplantation for tyrosinemia: A review of 10 cases from the University of Pittsburgh. *Dig Dis Sci* **35**:153, 1990.
279. Kvittingen EA: Tyrosinaemia type I: An update. *J Inherit Metab Dis* **14**:554, 1991.
280. Bremer H, Jaenicke U, Leupold D: Urinary *p*-tyramine excretion in hypertyrosinaemia. *Clin Chim Acta* **23**:244, 1969.
281. Friedman AL, Kalayoglu M, Belzer F, Sheth K, Werlin S: Persistence of Fanconi syndrome (FS) after liver transplantation for tyrosinemia (abstract). *Pediatr Res* **23**:536A, 1988.
282. Glorieux FH: Rickets, the continuing challenge. *N Engl J Med* **325**:1875, 1991.
283. Lindberg T, Nilsson KO, Jeppsson JO: Hereditary tyrosinaemia and diabetes mellitus. *Acta Paediatr Scand* **68**:619, 1979.
284. Lindblad B, Fällström SP, Höyer S, Nordborg C, Solymar L, Velander H: Cardiomyopathy in fumarylacetoacetase deficiency (hereditary tyrosinaemia): A new feature of the disease. *J Inherit Metab Dis* **10**:319, 1987.
285. Edwards MA, Green A, Colli A, Rylance G: Tyrosinaemia type I and hypertrophic obstructive cardiomyopathy (letter). *Lancet* **1**:1437, 1987.
286. Kogut MD, Shaw KN, Donnell GN: Tyrosinosis. *Am J Dis Child* **113**:47, 1967.
287. Gagné R, Lescault A, Grenier A, Laberge C, Melançon SB, Dallaire L: Prenatal diagnosis of hereditary tyrosinaemia: Measurement of succinylacetone in amniotic fluid. *Prenat Diagn* **2**:185, 1982.
288. Kvittingen EA, Rootwelt H, van Dam T, van Faassen H, Berger R: Hereditary tyrosinemia type I: Lack of correlation between clinical findings and amount of immunoreactive fumarylacetoacetase protein. *Pediatr Res* **31**:43, 1992.
289. St-Louis M, Tanguay RM: Mutations in the fumarylacetoacetate hydrolase gene causing hereditary tyrosinemia type I: Overview. *Hum Mutat* **9**:291, 1997.
290. Phaneuf D, Lambert M, Laframboise R, Mitchell GA, Lettre F, Tanguay R: Type I hereditary tyrosinemia: Evidence for molecular heterogeneity and identification of a causal mutation in a French-Canadian patient. *J Clin Invest* **90**:1185, 1992.
291. Rootwelt H, Broodtkorb E, Kvittingen EA: Identification of a frequent pseudodeficiency mutation in the fumarylacetoacetase gene, with implications for diagnosis of tyrosinemia type I. *Am J Hum Genet* **55**:1122, 1994.
292. Rootwelt H, Berger R, Gray G, Kelly DA, Coskun T, Kvittingen EA: Novel splice, missense, and nonsense mutations in the fumarylacetoacetase gene causing tyrosinemia type 1. *Am J Hum Genet* **55**:653, 1994.
293. Rootwelt H, Kristensen T, Berger R, Hoie K, Kvittingen EA: Tyrosinemia type 1-complex splicing defects and a missense mutation in the fumarylacetoacetase gene. *Hum Genet* **94**:235, 1994.
294. St-Louis M, Poudrier J, Phaneuf D, Leclerc B, Laframboise R, Tanguay RM: Two novel mutations involved in hereditary tyrosinemia type I. *Hum Mol Genet* **4**(2):319, 1995.
295. Rootwelt H: Studies on the Molecular Genetics of Tyrosinemia Type I. Ph.D. thesis, Institute of Clinical Biochemistry, Norway, 1995.
296. Grompe M, St-Louis M, Demers SI, Al-Dhalimy M, Leclerc B, Tanguay RM: A single mutation of the fumarylacetoacetate hydrolase gene in French Canadians with hereditary tyrosinemia type I. *N Engl J Med* **331**:353, 1994.
297. Poudrier J, St-Louis M, Lettre F, Gibson K, Prévost C, Larochelle J, Tanguay RM: Frequency of the IVS12 + 5G → A splice mutation of the fumarylacetoacetate hydrolase gene in carriers of hereditary tyrosinaemia in the French-Canadian population of Saguenay-Lac-St-Jean. *Prenat Diagn* **16**:59, 1996.
298. Rootwelt H, Hoie K, Berger R, Kvittingen EA: Fumarylacetoacetate mutations in tyrosinaemia type I. *Hum Mutat* **7**:239, 1996.
299. Ploos van Amstel JK, Bergman AJ, van Beurden EA, Roijers JF, Peelen T, van den Berg IE, Poll-The BT, et al: Hereditary tyrosinemia type 1: Novel missense, nonsense and splice consensus mutations in the human fumarylacetoacetate hydrolase gene; variability of the genotype-phenotype relationship. *Hum Genet* **97**:51, 1996.
300. Grompe M, Al-Dhalimy M: Mutations of the fumarylacetoacetate hydrolase gene in four patients with tyrosinemia type I. *Hum Mutat* **2**:85, 1993.
301. St-Louis M, Leclerc B, Laine J, Salo MK, Holmberg C, Tanguay RM: Identification of a stop mutation in five Finnish patients suffering from hereditary tyrosinemia type I. *Hum Mol Genet* **3**:69, 1994.
302. Demers SI, Phaneuf D, Tanguay RM: Hereditary tyrosinemia type I: Strong association with haplotype 6 in French Canadians permits simple carrier detection and prenatal diagnosis. *Am J Hum Genet* **55**:327, 1994.
303. Poudrier J, Lettre F, Scriver CR, Larochelle J, Tanguay RM: Different clinical forms of hereditary tyrosinemia (type I) in patients with identical genotypes. *Mol Genet Metab* **64**:119, 1998.
304. Russo P: Personal communication, 1992.
305. Dehner LP, Snover DC, Sharp HL, Ascher N, Nakhleh R, Day DL: Hereditary tyrosinemia type I (chronic form): Pathologic findings in the liver. *Hum Pathol* **20**:149, 1989.
306. Prive L: Pathological findings in patients with tyrosinemia. *Can Med Assoc J* **97**:1054, 1967.
307. Manowski Z, Silver MM, Roberts EA, Superina RA, Phillips MJ: Liver cell dysplasia and early liver transplantation in hereditary tyrosinemia. *Mod Pathol* **3**:694, 1990.
308. Hostetter MK, Levy HL, Winter HS, Knight GJ, Haddow JE: Evidence for liver disease preceeding amino acid abnormalities in hereditary tyrosinemia. *N Engl J Med* **308**:1265, 1983.
309. Russo P, O'Regan S: Visceral pathology of hereditary tyrosinemia type I. *Am J Hum Genet* **47**:317, 1990.
310. Partington MW, Haust MD: A patient with tyrosinemia and hypermethioninemia. *Can Med Assoc J* **97**:1059, 1967.
311. Kvittingen EA, Talseth T, Halvorsen S, Jakobs C, Hovig T, Flatmark A: Renal failure in adult patients with hereditary tyrosinaemia type I. *J Inherit Metab Dis* **14**:53, 1991.
312. Jevtic MM, Thorp FK, Hruban Z: Hereditary tyrosinemia with hyperplasia and hypertrophy of juxta-glomerular apparatus. *Am J Clin Pathol* **61**:423, 1974.
313. Lindstedt S, Holme E, Lock EA, Hjalmarson O, Strandvik B: Treatment of hereditary tyrosinaemia type 1 by inhibition of 4-hydroxyphenylpyruvate dioxygenase. *Lancet* **340**:813, 1992.
314. Holme E, Lindstedt S: Diagnosis and management of tyrosinemia type I. *Curr Opin Pediatr* **7**:726, 1995.
315. Pronicka E, Rowinska E, Bentkowski Z, Zawadzki J, Holme E, Lindstedt S: Treatment of two children with hereditary tyrosinaemia type I and long-standing renal disease with a 4-hydroxyphenylpyruvate dioxygenase inhibitor (NTBC). *J Inherit Metab Dis* **19**(2):234, 1996.
316. Holme E, Lindstedt S: Tyrosinaemia type I and NTBC [2-(2-nitro-4-trifluoromethylbenzoyl)-1,3-cyclohexanedione]. *J Inherit Metab Dis* **21**:507, 1998.
317. Ellis MK, Whitfield AC, Gowans LA, Auton TR, McLean Provan W, Lock EA, Smith LL: Inhibition of 4-hydroxyphenylpyruvate dioxygenase by 2-(2-nitro-4-trifluoromethylbenzoyl)-cyclohexane-1,3-dione and 2-(2-chloro-4-methanesulfonylbenzoyl)-cyclohexane-1,3-dione. *Toxicol Appl Pharmacol* **133**:12, 1995.
318. Lindstedt S: Oral presentation, 35th Annual Meeting of the Society for the Study of Inborn Errors of Metabolism, Goteborg, Sweden, 1997.
319. Mitchell GA: Unpublished results, 1998.
320. Goodyer PR, Kronick JB, Jequier S, Reade TM, Scriver CR: Nephrocalcinosis and its relationship to treatment of hereditary rickets. *J Pediatr* **11**:700, 1987.
321. Verge CF, Lam A, Simpson JM, Cowell CT, Howard NJ, Silink M: Effects of therapy in X-linked hypophosphatemic rickets. *N Engl J Med* **325**:1843, 1991.
322. Whitington PF, Balistreri WF: Liver transplantation in pediatrics: Indications, contraindications, and pretransplant management. *J Pediatr* **118**:169, 1991.
323. Sokal EM, Veyckemans F, de Ville de Goyet J, Moulin D, Van Hoorebeeck N, Alberti D, Buts JP, et al: Liver transplantation in children less than 1 year of age. *J Pediatr* **117**:205, 1990.
324. Cox K, Nakazato P, Berquist W, Concepcion W, Tokunaga Y, Esquivel C: Liver transplantation in infants weighing less than 10 kilograms. *Transplant Proc* **23**:1579, 1991.
325. Flye MW, Riely CA, Hainline BE, Sassa S, Gusberg RJ, Blakemore KJ, Barwick KW, et al: The effects of early treatment of hereditary tyrosinemia type I in infancy by orthotopic liver transplantation. *Transplantation* **49**:916, 1990.

326. Starzl TE, Demetris AJ, Van Thiel D: Medical progress Liver transplantation. *N Engl J Med* **321**:1014, 1989.
327. Luks FI, St-Vil D, Hancock BJ, Laberge J-M, Bensoussan AL, Russo P, Mitchell GA, et al: Surgical and metabolic aspects of liver transplantation for tyrosinemia. *Transplantation* **56**:1376, 1993.
328. Tuchman M, Freese DK, Sharp HL, Ramnaraine ML, Ascher N, Bloomer JR: Contribution of extrahepatic tissues to biochemical abnormalities in hereditary tyrosinemia type I: Study of three patients after liver transplantation. *J Pediatr* **110**:399, 1987.
329. Tuchman M, Freese DK, Sharp HL, Whitley CB, Ramnaraine ML, Ulstrom RA, Najarian JS, et al: Persistent succinylacetone excretion after liver transplantation in a patient with hereditary tyrosinaemia type I. *J Inherit Metab Dis* **8**:21, 1985.
330. Shoemaker LR, Strife CF, Balistreri WF, Ryckman FC: Rapid improvement in the renal tubular dysfunction associated with tyrosinemia following hepatic replacement. *Pediatrics* **89**:251, 1992.
331. Flatmark A, Bergan A, Sodal G, Schrumpf E, Kvittingen EA, Jellum E, Halvorsen S: Does liver transplantation correct the metabolic defect in hereditary tyrosinemia? *Transplant Proc* **18**:67, 1986.
332. Paradis K: Personal communication, 1992.
333. Riudor E, Ribes A, Lloret J, Friden J, Holme E, Jakobs C, Martinez Ibanez V: Liver transplantation in two children with tyrosinaemia type I: Biochemical aspects. *J Inherit Metab Dis* **14**:281, 1991.
334. Fritzell S, Jagenburg OR, Schnürer L-B: Familial cirrhosis of the liver, renal, tubular defects with rickets and imparied tyrosine metabolism. *Acta Paediatr Scand* **53**:18, 1964.
335. Kamoun P, Parvy P, Rabier D: Indications et interprétation de la chromatographie des acides aminés pour le diagnostic des maladies métaboliques, in Saudubray J-M (ed): *Maladies Métaboliques*. Paris, Doin, 1992, p 1.
336. McGale EHF, Pyc IF, Stonier C: Studies of the inter-relationship between cerebrospinal fluid and plasma amino acid concentrations in normal individuals. *J Neurochem* **29**:291, 1977.
337. Rogers WF, Gardner F: Tyrosine metabolism in human scurvy. *J Clin Invest* **28**:806, 1949.
338. Rivlin RS, Melman KL, Sjoerdsma A: An oral tyrosine tolerance test in thyrotoxicosis and myxedema. *N Engl J Med* **272**:1143, 1965.
339. Awata H, Endo F, Tanoue A, Kitano A, Nakano Y, Matsuda I: Structural organization and analysis of the human fumarylacetoacetate hydrolase gene in tyrosinemia type I. *Biochim Biophys Acta* **1226**:168, 1994.
340. Rootwelt H, Chou J, Gahl WA, Berger R, Coskun T, Brodtkorb E, Kvittingen EA: Two missense mutations causing tyrosinemia type I with presence and absence of immunoreactive fumarylacetoacetase. *Hum Genet* **93**:615, 1994.
341. Timmers C, Grompe M: Six novel mutations in the fumarylacetoacetate hydrolase gene of patients with hereditary tyrosinemia type I. *Hum Mutat* **7**:367, 1996.
342. Hahn SH, Krasnewich D, Brantly M, Kvittingen EA, Gahl WA: Heterozygosity for an exon 12 splicing mutation and a W234G missense mutation in an American child with chronic tyrosinemia type I. *Hum Mutat* **6**:66, 1995.
343. St-Louis M, Poudrier J, Tanguay RM: Simple detection of a (Finnish) hereditary tyrosinemia type I mutation. *Hum Mutat* **7**:379, 1996.
344. Bergman AJIW, van den Berg IET, Brink W, Poll-The BT, Ploos van Amstel JK, Berger R: Spectrum of mutations in the fumarylacetoacetate hydrolase gene of tyrosinemia type I patients in Northern Europe and Mediterranean countries. *Hum Mutat* **12**:19, 1998.

CHAPTER 80

Disorders of Histidine Metabolism

Harvey L. Levy ▪ Robin G. Taylor ▪ Roderick R. McInnes

1. There are two known disorders of histidine metabolism: histidinemia and urocanic aciduria. Histidinemia is one of the most frequent and well known of the inborn errors of metabolism. A test for it has been included in newborn screening programs, and its incidence was about 1:12,000 in over 20 million screened infants. The frequency is particularly high in Japan (1:9600). It is an autosomal recessive trait and is due to a defect in histidase, which catalyzes the conversion of histidine to urocanic acid. This enzyme defect is most readily identified in the stratum corneum of skin. The biochemical consequences of the metabolic block include increased concentrations of histidine in blood, urine, and cerebrospinal fluid (CSF); decreased concentration of urocanic acid in blood and skin; and increased concentrations of histidine metabolites in urine. Histidinemia seems to be benign in most affected individuals, although, under certain unusual circumstances, the disorder may be harmful and produce the central nervous system disease noted in a few histidinemic patients. Dietary treatment lowers the blood histidine level but seems not to be indicated, at least for most patients, given the apparent lack of consequences of the disorder. Urocanic aciduria is an apparently autosomal recessive disorder. It is probably benign. An increased concentration of urocanic acid in urine is the only known metabolic finding.
2. The prominence of histidinemia has stimulated the study of histidase, an enzyme expressed primarily in liver and skin and regulated in a complex developmental, hormonal, and tissue-specific manner. At the molecular level, the enzyme is unusual in having a rare modified amino acid, dehydroalanine, in its active site. Full-length cDNAs of human, rat, and mouse liver histidase have been isolated. The human gene has also been cloned and characterized: It is a single-copy gene spanning approximately 25 kb and consisting of 21 exons. Several liver- and epidermis-specific transcription factor-binding sites have been identified in the 5′ flanking region. A polymorphism has been identified in exon 16. The gene has not yet been studied for mutations in histidinemic patients.
3. The deficiency of urocanic acid in histidinemia could have implications for either or both of two proposed functions of urocanic acid—as a natural sunscreen against ultraviolet (UV) light and as a mediator of ultraviolet light-induced systemic immunosuppression. As yet, there has been no evidence for impairment of either of these proposed functions in histidinemia, but further study of this question might be warranted.
4. Atypical histidinemia is a biochemically milder form of the disorder and may account for a substantial minority of persons with histidinemia. The reported individuals have been clinically normal. They have higher residual skin histidase activities and lower elevations of histidine and histidine metabolites than individuals with the classic disorder. Histidinemia may be a biochemically heterogeneous disorder, perhaps due to several allelic mutations.
5. Maternal histidinemia is probably benign. The 61 offspring from untreated pregnancies of 23 histidinemic mothers whose cases have been followed have generally been normal.
6. An animal model with the biochemical features of human histidinemia has been identified. The histidinemic mouse has a missense mutation in the coding region of the histidase structural gene that reduces the stability of the enzyme. The histidinemic mouse does not exhibit clinical abnormalities unless it is the offspring of a histidinemic mother, in which case both histidinemic (*his*/*his*) and heterozygous (*his*/+) offspring will have balance defects characterized by circling behavior and/or head tilting. This offspring effect depends on the maternal histidine level and is prevented or ameliorated if the mother is treated with a histidine-restricted diet during pregnancy. The effect is also modulated by the fetal genotype, with homozygous (*his*/*his*) fetuses more severely affected than heterozygous (*his*/+) fetuses, and by other loci, as evidenced by the decrease in the frequency of the effect in offspring when selection for high incidence of abnormalities is relaxed.
7. Histidinuria without histidinemia has been described in five children. Four were mentally retarded and two had myoclonic seizures, but an association between the histidinuria and the central nervous system manifestations has not been established. All had substantially reduced renal tubular reabsorption of histidine, with normal reabsorption of other amino acids, indicating that there is a histidine-specific transport system that is defective in this disorder. Two sibs and a third unrelated child also had evidence of an intestinal defect in histidine transport. This disorder seems to be transmitted as an autosomal recessive trait.
8. The enzyme defect in urocanic aciduria is in urocanase, which catalyzes the conversion of *trans*-urocanic acid to imidazolonepropionic acid. The defect has been proved by liver biopsy in three patients. Urocanic aciduria has been found in at least eight children. The four discovered by specific testing have been mentally retarded, but the four identified by newborn urine screening have been normal, the latter suggesting that the mental retardation may not be related to the metabolic disorder. Four of the eight children have had growth retardation. Urocanic aciduria is diagnosed on the basis of increased urocanic acid in urine with normal or only mildly increased levels of histidine and histidine metabolites.

A list of standard abbreviations is located immediately preceding the index in each volume. Additional abbreviations used in this chapter are FIGLU = formiminoglutamic acid; THF = tetrahydrofolic acid.

Interest in histidine metabolism and its disorders was sparked by the discovery of histidinemia in 1961. Ghadimi and his coworkers found increased concentrations of histidine in blood and urine from two sisters and concluded that the findings represented an inborn error of histidine metabolism.[1] One of these sisters had a speech defect, which led to the suspicion that histidinemia could cause clinical abnormalities. Subsequently, other children with histidinemia were identified when patients who had learning disabilities or other medical problems were tested. Studies of histidine metabolism in these children and in normal individuals who served as controls have elucidated the biochemical derangements in this metabolic disorder and clearly defined the normal pathways of histidine degradation in the human.

In the sixth and seventh editions of this book, this chapter included information about histidine metabolism and its disorders, notably histidinemia.[2,3] The current chapter updates that information and, in particular, describes the characteristics of the isolated cDNAs for histidase and the recently cloned human histidase gene.

METABOLISM OF HISTIDINE

Requirement for Histidine

Whether histidine is an essential amino acid for humans has been debated. Detailed information about this issue can be found in the sixth[2] and seventh[3] editions of this book. It seems clear, however, that histidine is an essential amino acid for human infants. Snyderman et al found that withdrawal of histidine from the diet of young infants resulted in a reduced rate of weight gain and a fall in nitrogen retention.[4] In addition, a rash resembling early infantile eczema developed when dietary histidine was omitted.[4–6] These workers estimated the dietary requirement of histidine for the young infant to be somewhat less than 35 mg/kg/day. The most convincing evidence that dietary histidine is required not only during infancy but also during at least early childhood comes from the results in treating histidinemia. The general experience with these patients is that the blood histidine level is lowered in direct response to the restriction of dietary histidine.[7–10]

The effect of low dietary histidine on older children and adults over long periods remains uncertain. The evidence indicates, however, that even if histidine biosynthesis occurs, it is sufficient only for basic physiological needs and is insufficient to support growth or to meet the requirements produced by physiological stress.[11,12] Thus, irrespective of biosynthesis, histidine would be an essential amino acid for the growing child and, over a period of time, for the adult.

Histidine Catabolism

In contrast to the uncertainty about endogenous histidine synthesis, the pathways of histidine utilization and catabolism in mammalian tissue are quite well understood (Fig. 80-1). The major catabolic pathway is through urocanic acid to glutamic acid, and four enzymes catalyze this sequence of reactions.

Histidase. The first reaction in this pathway is the nonoxidative deamination of L-histidine to *trans*-urocanic acid by histidase (histidine ammonia-lyase, EC 4.3.1.3). The reaction seems to involve the formation of an aminoenzyme and then release of the amino group as ammonia.[13–15] This cytosolic enzyme is expressed with high activity in the liver of all animal species and in the skin of many (but not all) mammals.[16–19] Of interest is that skin histidase is absent in amphibian, avian, and reptilian species, which suggests that its presence in mammals may have evolutionary implications.[18] Sano et al demonstrated that immunoreactive histidase is also present in renal cortex tubular epithelium, fundic mucosal glands of stomach, gastric intramuscular plexus ganglia and adrenal cortical cells.[19] This is a much broader tissue distribution than had previously been reported. Histidase is regulated in a complex developmental, hormonal, and tissue-specific manner.[18,20–23] At the molecular level, histidase has

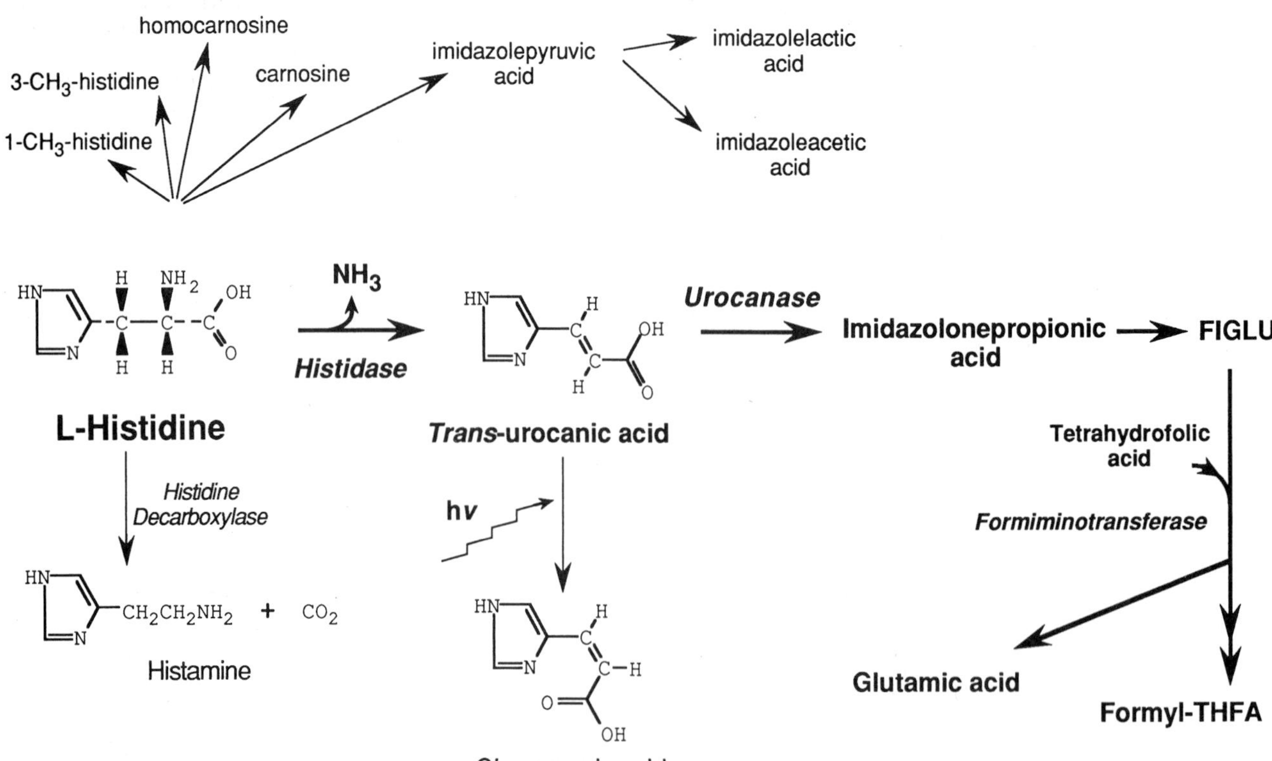

Fig. 80-1 Metabolism of L-histidine. The chemical structures of L-histidine, histamine, *trans*-urocanic acid, and *cis*-urocanic acid are shown. Enzyme names are in *italics*. The major pathway of histidine catabolism is shown in boldface type. Ultraviolet irradiation (270 to 320 nm) is indicated by hv. FIGLU, formiminoglutamic acid; THFA, tetrahydrofolic acid. (*Adapted from Taylor et al.*[32] *Used by permission.*)

proven to be unusual in having a rare modified amino acid, dehydroalanine, in its active site.[24,25] Several lines of evidence indicate that the precursor for this modified residue is serine 143 in *Pseudomonas putida* histidase and the corresponding serine 254 in rat histidase.[26–30]

Histidase has been previously reviewed by Hanson and Havir,[31] by Taylor et al,[32] and in the seventh edition of this book.[3] The K_m for L-histidine is between 0.5 and 2.0 mM at pH 8.8 to 9.2, the optimal pH for the reaction;[33–35] at physiologic pH (7.2), however, the K_m for L-histidine is greater than 2.0 mM.[35] Mammalian histidase has a molecular mass of about 200 kDa and appears to consist of three identical subunits of about 75 kDa each.[33–36] cDNAs for rat, mouse, and human liver histidase (human cDNA GenBank accession number D16626) have been isolated,[19,37–39] all of which have open reading frames of 1971 bp encoding polypeptides of 657 amino acids with predicted molecular masses of 72,165 Da, 72,212 Da, and 72,651 Da, respectively. The rat histidase cDNA detects a 2.5-kb mRNA in rat liver and skin but not in other tissues tested.[37] The human histidase gene (*HAL*) has been localized to chromosome 12q22-q24.1 by in situ hybridization.[40] The murine histidine gene (*Hal*) was localized to mouse chromosome 10C2-D1.[40] The *HAL* locus lies within a syntenic region conserved between mouse and humans, extending over the entire chromosome region 12q21-24.1 and the mouse chromosome region 10C2-D1, and containing the phenylalanine hydroxylase locus (see Chap. 77).[40]

Suchi et al cloned and characterized the human histidase gene (*HAL*). It is a single-copy gene spanning approximately 25 kb and consisting of 21 exons. Several liver- and epidermis-specific transcription factor-binding sites were identified in the 5′ flanking region, suggesting that histidase transcription may be regulated by these factors consistent with hepatic and epidermal expression. A polymorphism was identified in exon 16.[41] A tetranucleotide repeat polymorphism in intron 8 has also been described at the human histidase locus.[42]

Regulation of Histidase Expression. The developmental program of epidermal histidase differs from that of the hepatic enzyme. Histidase activity in rat epidermis peaks a few days after birth and then declines to adult levels.[43] In contrast, hepatic activity is not detectable until 4 days after birth and subsequently increases gradually until puberty. Adult females have a twofold higher level of hepatic histidase than males, owing to estrogen induction.[20–22] Other hormones, including glucocorticoids, glucagon, and triiodothyronine, also regulate hepatic histidase,[20,21,23] albeit to a lesser extent than estrogen. Dietary regulation of hepatic histidase has been demonstrated. Rats fed a high-protein diet or a histidine load show increased hepatic histidase activity.[44,45] Apart from the catabolic usefulness of increased histidase expression during periods of higher histidine intake, the significance of the other regulatory changes in histidase activity, particularly that mediated by estrogen, is unclear. However, the differences between the developmental programs of histidase in liver and epidermis could reflect differences in the metabolism of urocanic acid in these two tissues. In the liver, urocanic acid is an intermediate in the conversion of histidine to glutamic acid, whereas in the epidermis it accumulates and may be both a ultraviolet (UV) light protectant and an immunoregulator (see the sections "Urocanic Acid as a UV Protectant" and "Urocanic Acid as an Ultraviolet Light-Induced Immunoregulator").

Epidermal Histidase. A puzzling aspect of epidermal histidase expression is that histidase activity has only been reported in the stratum corneum and not in the lower layers of the skin,[46] whereas histidase immunolocalization appears to be specific to the stratum granulosum.[19] Scott's studies of histidase activity in the skin, which demonstrated 93 percent of activity in stratum corneum, took care to separate the enucleate cells of the stratum corneum from the underlying stratum granulosum.[46] Furthermore, most skin histidase assays have appeared to measure the activity only in

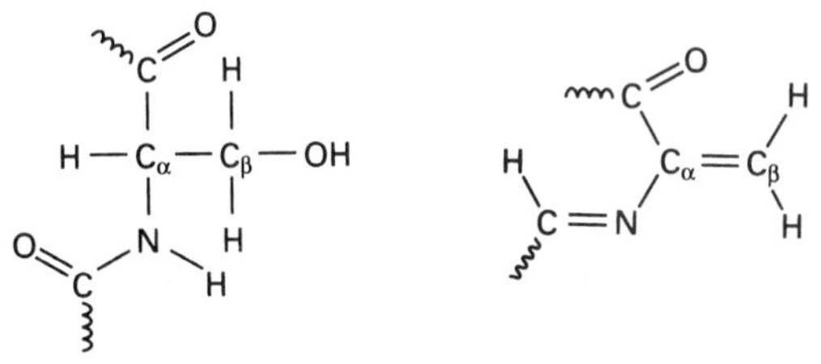

L-Serine   Dehydroalanine

Fig. 80-2 Serine, a precursor for dehydroalanine in subtilin and pyruvoyl enzymes, is shown on the left. A dehydroalanine residue containing a Schiff's base is shown on the right. The Schiff's base (C = N) is postulated to be present in histidase and phenylalanine ammonia-lyase but not in subtilin or the pyruvoyl enzymes. The α and β carbons of the amino acid residues are indicated. *Wavy lines* indicate the continuation of the polypeptide chain.

the stratum corneum.[47–49] The simplest explanation for this discrepancy is that histidase activity previously attributed to the stratum corneum is actually due to histidase in the stratum granulosum. Nevertheless, since the study that demonstrated immunoreactive histidase in stratum granulosum but not in stratum corneum did not include measurement of histidase activity in the skin,[19] there remains the possibility that histidase is present in the stratum corneum but is modified so that it is undetectable by immunochemistry while enzymatically active.

Genetic evidence (see the section "Histidase") indicates that histidase is expressed from the same gene in both skin and liver, and that the mRNA in both tissues is about 2.5 kb.[37] Thus, if there is any variation between the skin and liver enzymes, which some have reported[50,51] but which others dispute,[43] such differences may be due to alternate splicing not detectable on Northern blots.

Dehydroalanine at the Active Site. There is strong evidence for the presence of a modified amino acid, dehydroalanine (Fig. 80-2), in the active site of histidase.[52,53] The posttranslational formation of dehydroalanine is a plausible rate-limiting step in the conversion of the polypeptide to a catalytically competent form. The role of dehydroalanine in catalysis is presumed to be the activation of the amino group in histidine to form a better leaving group than $-NH_3^+$.[31] The only other enzyme known to have dehydroalanine at its active site is phenylalanine ammonia-lyase, a protein with homology to histidase[31,54–57] (see Chap. 77). In both enzymes, evidence for the presence of dehydroalanine in the active site was provided in two ways: (1) by labeling the residue with a radioactive nucleophilic reagent, resulting in inactivation of the enzyme [the products formed are consistent with the reaction of a dehydroalanine group containing a Schiff's base (see Fig. 80-2)];[24,53,56,57] and (2) by the ability of substrates and substrate analogues to prevent inactivation of histidase and phenylalanine ammonia-lyase by the nucleophilic reagents.[52,54,56]

Mechanism of Dehydroalanine Formation in Histidase. A long-standing problem in research on histidase has concerned the identity of the amino acid precursor and mechanism of formation of the dehydroalanine residue. The identity of the precursor for dehydroalanine was finally solved by Hernandez et al, who determined that the site of L-cysteine addition to dehydroalanine corresponds to serine 143 in *P. putida* histidase.[26] Previously, Klee had reported that modification of the active site dehydroalanine by L-cysteine at pH 10.5 resulted in an increase in absorbance at 340 nm.[58] After treating histidase with L-cysteine, Hernandez et al purified a tryptic peptide that absorbed at 340 nm. The peptide was further digested with V8 protease, and the 340-nm absorbing species was analyzed by tandem mass spectrometry. The fragmentation data clearly demonstrate that an excess of 141 Da is located on serine 143, indicating that it is the site of addition of L-cysteine to dehydroalanine.[26] Subsequently, serine 143 in *P. putida* histidase and the corresponding residue, serine

254 in rat histidase have been shown by in vitro mutagenesis to be essential for histidase activity.[27–30] Surprisingly, Langer et al also demonstrated that substitution of a cysteine residue for serine 143 yields fully active histidase that is indistinguishable from wild-type enzyme by any criteria assayed, including total thiol content (number of cysteines), K_m and V_{max}, and the effect of inhibitors.[29] These experiments suggest that the active site occupied by the dehydroalanine residue can be formed equally well from either serine or cysteine.

In other proteins in which dehydroalanine has been found (subtilin, thyroglobulin, and pyruvoyl enzymes such as histidine decarboxylase), the mechanism of dehydroalanine formation varies, but the process is usually self-catalyzed.[32,59–62] Expression of phenylalanine ammonia-lyase from parsley in *Escherichia coli*[63] and of rat histidase in COS-1 cells[33] and *E. coli*[19] results in the synthesis of active enzymes in cells in which neither enzyme is normally produced. These results are consistent with the generation of dehydroalanine by an autocatalytic process.

Urocanase. This cytosolic enzyme (EC 4.2.1.49) catalyzes the nonoxidative conversion of *trans*-urocanic acid to imidazolone-propionic acid by the addition of water across the double bond between the α and β carbons of urocanic acid (Fig. 80-1). Urocanase is deficient in the liver of patients with urocanic aciduria.[64,65] The bacterial enzyme is a homodimer requiring nicotinamide adenine dinucleotide (NAD).[66,67] The gene for the bacterial enzyme, cloned and sequenced in *P. putida*, has an open reading frame of 1671 nucleotides.[68] The N-terminal methionine is removed in the mature enzyme, yielding a subunit of 556 amino acids with a molecular mass of 60,771 Da. A gene that probably encodes urocanase has also been identified in the hut operon of *Bacillus subtilis* on the basis of sequence homology.[69] The mammalian enzyme does not require NAD.[70] It has been partially purified from beef liver[70] and purified from cat liver.[71] The latter enzyme, perhaps also a dimer, has an estimated molecular mass of 127,000 Da. The pH optimum for activity is 6.8 to 7.6, considerably lower than that for histidase. The K_m for urocanic acid is 1.5 μM in beef liver[70] and 7.1 μM in cat liver,[71] indicating that urocanase has a much stronger affinity for urocanic acid than does histidase for histidine. The apparent K_m of mouse and human liver urocanase for urocanic acid are 3.2 and 2.2 μM, respectively.[72] The cat liver enzyme is competitively inhibited by imidazolepropionic acid,[71] as is the bacterial enzyme.[73] Unexpectedly, glycylglycine has been found to be a highly specific inhibitor of both bacterial and bovine urocanase.[74] The mammalian enzyme has not been further characterized, nor has its gene been isolated.

Urocanase activity seems to be limited to liver. Unlike histidase, there is no detectable activity in epithelium, which explains the large amount of urocanic acid normally present in skin.[75] Nevertheless, the regulation of liver urocanase in rats has features in common with that of histidase. Urocanase activity increases with dietary protein, although not as dramatically as does histidase.[76] Thyroxine suppresses urocanase activity as it does histidase but again not to the same extent.[77] On the other hand, urocanase activity is lowered by folate deficiency in rats, whereas histidase activity is unchanged.[78] The developmental pattern of urocanase and the effect of hormones other than thyroxine on its activity have not been studied. Urocanase activity does not vary as markedly as does histidase in different strains of inbred mice.[79]

Imidazolonepropionic Acid Hydrolase. Imidazolonepropionic acid is converted to formiminoglutamic acid (FIGLU), an important intermediate that links histidine catabolism to folate metabolism (Fig. 80-1). FIGLU is a donor of formyl groups to tetrahydrofolic acid and is a marker for folic acid deficiency (see Chap. 155). The reaction involves cleavage of the imidazolone ring of imidazolonepropionate with the addition of water; it is catalyzed by imidazolonepropionate amidohydrolase (EC 3.5.2.7), an enzyme that has been identified in bacteria and mammalian liver.[80] The purified rat liver enzyme has a pH optimum 7.4 to 7.8 and a K_m of 7.0 μM for imidazolonepropionic acid.[81] The gene encoding this enzyme has not been cloned or mapped but, on the basis of sequence homology, has been putatively identified within the hut operon of *B. subtilis*.[69] The enzyme has not been studied in humans.

Formiminotransferase. This enzyme [*N*-formimino-L-glutamate: THF 5-formiminotransferase (EC 2.1.2.5)] catalyzes the formation of formiminotetrahydrofolic acid from FIGLU. Tetrahydrofolic acid is required for this reaction, and glutamic acid is liberated (Fig. 80-1). Folic acid deficiency results in a strikingly increased excretion of FIGLU in response to loading with L-histidine, presumably due to the reduction in available tetrahydrofolic acid.[82] This enzyme is described in detail in Chap. 155.

HISTIDASE DEFICIENCY (HISTIDINEMIA)

The primary disorder of histidine metabolism is histidase deficiency, more commonly known as *histidinemia*. This inborn error of metabolism blocks the conversion of histidine to urocanic acid, resulting in accumulations of histidine and histidine metabolites, as well as in a deficiency of urocanic acid (Fig. 80-1).

Enzyme Defect

In their initial report of the first two histidinemic patients, Ghadimi et al suggested that the metabolic defect was probably in an early enzymatic step in histidine metabolism, involving either histidase or urocanase.[1] Auerbach and his colleagues could not detect in urine from their patient intermediary metabolites such as urocanic acid and FIGLU, which presumably would be present and perhaps increased if the metabolic block were distal to histidase (Fig. 80-1), even after loading with histidine; in contrast, intravenous loading with urocanic acid produced large amounts of FIGLU. They concluded that the metabolic block is at the level of histidase.[83]

La Du et al verified this conclusion by identifying a deficiency of histidase activity as the enzyme defect in histidinemia. They found that skin samples (stratum corneum) from two histidinemic sibs lacked histidase activity, whereas activity was readily demonstrable in similar tissue from normal children and adults.[84] Subsequently, Auerbach et al demonstrated absence of histidase activity in liver from two other patients with histidinemia, although urocanase activity was normal or even somewhat greater than normal.[85] Accordingly, it is clear that, in histidinemia, histidase is specifically defective in two tissues that normally express this enzyme.

The defect in epidermal histidase can be readily demonstrated by a simple chromatographic analysis for urocanic acid.[86,87] Urocanic acid is normally prominent, whereas most individuals with histidinemia will have no detectable urocanic acid by this method. The absence of urocanic acid in histidinemia can also be determined by analyzing sweat.[88] With a sensitive radiochemical method,[49] however, Japanese investigators have detected measurable, albeit very low, amounts of residual skin histidase activity in most of the affected infants identified by routine newborn screening in Japan. In these studies, Matsuda et al found among 20 histidinemic children skin histidase activity of 0.48 ± 0.54 μmol/h per gram tissue compared with the normal 8.6 ± 4.3 μmol/h per gram tissue.[47] Kuroda et al found a range of 0.24 to 2.73 μmol/h per gram tissue among nine children with a normal range of 9.7 to 15.3 μmol/h per gram tissue,[89] and Ito et al found less than 0.1 to 0.2 μmol/h per gram tissue in six of seven children, compared with their relatively low control range of 1.4 to 1.5 μmol/h per gram tissue.[90] Using an equally sensitive assay, Shin et al obtained values of 1.46 ± 0.80 nmol/h per milligram protein (normal, 52.3 ± 16.5 nmol/h per milligram protein) for skin histidase activity among 24 histidinemic children from

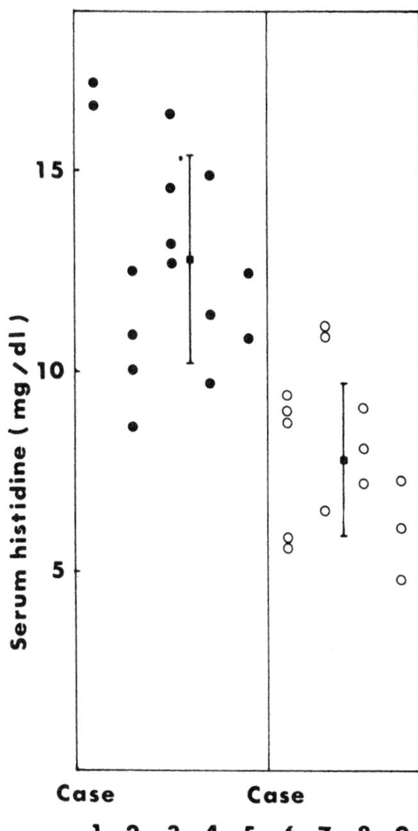

Fig. 80-3 The relationship between residual skin histidase activity and the fasting serum histidine concentration in histidinemia. *Filled circles* indicate patients with less than 10 percent (group 1) and *open circles* patients with about 20 percent (group 2) of normal skin histidase activity. *Filled squares with bars* indicate mean ± SD of the serum histidine level for each group. (*From Kuroda et al.*[89] *Used by permission.*)

Germany and Austria.[48] Thus, skin histidase activity is almost always less than 20 percent of normal in histidinemia and is usually less than 10 percent of normal. Lower skin histidase activities correlate with higher serum histidine levels (see Fig. 80-3) and lower FIGLU excretion,[47] indicating correspondence between residual skin histidase activity in vitro and histidine degradation in vivo.

Precise measurements of both skin and liver histidase activity in the same histidinemic patient have not been reported. Using a relatively insensitive assay, however, skin histidase activity and liver histidase activity was measured or estimated in 14 infants with histidinemia (R. Schön and O. Thalhammer, personal communication, 1976). Six had no detectable activity in either tissue, one had trace activity in both tissues, one had trace activity in skin but no liver activity, and six had trace activity in liver and no activity in skin.[91] These observations suggest that there is close correspondence between the skin and liver enzyme defects but that slight differences may be present in some affected individuals.

Histidinemia Without the Enzyme Defect in Skin

Four patients with persistently increased blood histidine levels and other biochemical features of histidinemia have had normal skin histidase activity and normal amounts of urocanic acid in sweat or skin.[90,92] None had liver histidase measured, so it is not known whether they have a defect in the liver enzyme without a corresponding skin enzyme defect. Three of these patients, all sibs, had unusually low elevations of histidine and a less pronounced response to histidine loading than usually observed in histidinemia.[92]

Genetics and Gene Mapping

Histidinemia is an autosomal recessive trait. The sixth edition of this book can be consulted for specific information about the genetics of this disorder.[2]

Some cases of histidinemia involving mental retardation or other abnormalities might result from a contiguous gene syndrome in which the histidase locus and genes adjacent to it are deleted. To our knowledge, there have been only three reports of cytogenetically visible deletions that include part of the region 12q22-24.1 to which the human histidase gene has been localized (see the section "Histidase").[40] One was an interstitial deletion of 12q21 to q22 in a patient with mental retardation.[93] The second was an unbalanced reciprocal translocation resulting in deletion of 12q22 to qter and duplication of 17q23 to qter in a child with severe psychomotor retardation and craniofacial malformations.[94] It is not known whether the histidase locus is deleted in either of the foregoing cases. The third patient, with a deletion of either 12q21.3-q23.2 or 12q23.2-q24.1, had short stature and developmental delay. DNA from this patient was shown by Southern blot analysis to be deleted for one copy of phenylalanine hydroxylase and insulin-like growth factor I, but not *HAL*.[95] A number of translocations of 12q have been reported but, except for the aforementioned case, all of the translocations that were unbalanced have led to duplications of 12q.[96] From the aforementioned cases, it may be concluded that large deletions of the region around the *HAL* locus have occurred, resulting in neurologic deficits, but in no case has a deletion of the *HAL* locus been demonstrated.

To determine whether contiguous gene deletions occur in patients with histidinemia, we used the human histidase cDNA to examine the histidase genes of histidinemic patients with and without mental retardation or other abnormalities (see the section "Clinical Phenotype"). Of 17 histidinemic patients, three with learning problems, we observed a partial deletion or rearrangement of the histidase gene in a patient of normal intelligence but no gross rearrangements in any other subjects (R.G. Taylor and R.R. McInnes, unpublished data). However, a larger number of patients must be examined before any conclusions can be made regarding the frequency and extent of large deletions at this locus.

Although the molecular characteristics and the precise impairment of histidase in histidinemia have not been determined, there are suggestions that at least in some patients mutations have occurred in the coding region of the histidase structural gene. Kuroda and coworkers demonstrated an altered sensitivity of skin histidase to denaturation in two patients,[97] and Shin et al found unspecified altered kinetic properties in skin histidase among the patients they studied.[48] Moreover, Suchi et al have identified heteroduplex formation in exons 7, 9, and 12 in polymerase chain reaction-amplified DNA segments from histidinemic patients. They have not yet determined whether these are histidinemia-specific mutations or nondeleterious polymorphisms.[98]

Mouse Model

A mouse model for histidase deficiency that encompasses the biochemical features of human histidinemia has been identified by Kacser and his coworkers.[99,100] Blood, urine, and tissue histidine levels are 12- to 20-fold increased, imidazole metabolites are excreted in large quantities, and histidase activity in both liver and skin is markedly reduced. Offspring from selective matings segregate as expected for an autosomal recessive trait. This mouse has no variant metabolic, metabolic, or clinical phenotype.

Histidase was compared in mutant and in normal mice.[101] Liver histidase was barely detectable in both at birth. In normal mice, liver histidase activity rose postnatally in the expected pattern of development, whereas virtually no activity appeared in the mutant mouse liver. Skin histidase activity in mutant mice was much lower at birth than in normal mice. Studies of partially purified liver histidase disclosed evidence for two components in normal liver, one with much higher activity than the other. On the basis of different patterns of heat stability and enzyme kinetics, it was concluded that the mutant mouse histidase consisted only of the very low activity component, the major component having been lost by mutation.

Taylor et al demonstrated that murine histidinemia results from a defect in the coding region of the histidase structural gene.[38] This finding followed evidence that both the murine histidase gene (*Hal*) and the murine histidinemia locus (*his*) map to the same region: mouse chromosome 10C2-D1.[40] In addition, early work had shown that affected animals have a greatly reduced abundance (less than 5 percent) of histidase protein in liver,[101] whereas the size and amount of the histidase mRNA is grossly normal.[38] To identify the molecular lesion in murine histidinemia, a full-length mouse histidase cDNA was isolated by using the rat cDNA.[37] Comparison of the mouse and rat sequences revealed 98.8 percent amino acid identity in the 657-residue open reading frame. Direct sequencing of histidase DNA amplified from histidinemic mouse mRNA by reverse transcription and the polymerase chain reaction showed a G-to-A transition at nucleotide 965 (CGA to CAA), a CpG dinucleotide on the antisense strand, resulting in the substitution of glutamine for arginine at residue 322 (R322Q). When the R322Q substitution was introduced by in vitro mutagenesis into the normal rat histidase cDNA and expressed in COS cells, the amount of histidase protein produced was 14 percent of control histidase and the enzymatic activity was 11 percent of control. These results suggest that the R322Q mutation primarily reduces the stability of the enzyme and has little effect on the specific activity.

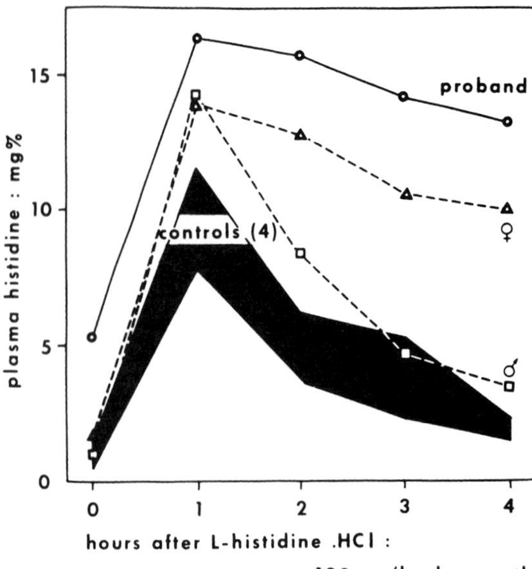

Fig. 80-5 The plasma histidine response to an L-histidine load in normal adults (*black area* of the graph), a patient with histidinemia (proband, *circles*), her mother (*triangles*), and her father (*squares*). The plasma histidine level in the patient rises much higher and remains higher up to 4 h after the load than in the controls or in either parent. The parents are intermediate between the patient and the control adults. Note that the mother has a decidedly slower clearance of histidine than the father. (*From Rosenblatt et al.*[87] *Used by permission.*)

Biochemical Features

Increased Histidine. The characteristic finding in histidinemia is a specifically increased concentration of blood histidine varying from 290 to 1420 μM (normal, 70 to 120 μM).[2,102] These are equivalent to values of 4.5 to 22.0 mg/dl (normal, 1.1 to 1.9 mg/dl). The level tends to be highest at age 1 year and slightly lower in older children and adults.[102,103] Nevertheless, the variation in the observed blood histidine concentrations among patients reflects dietary protein (histidine) intake and the degree of metabolic block much more than age. Kuroda and coworkers have shown that, in histidinemic infants and children, the serum histidine concentration rises with increasing dietary histidine (Fig. 80-4) but that, either with much dietary histidine or in the fasting state, the serum concentration is greater in those with less residual skin histidase activity (Figs. 80-3 and 80-4).[89]

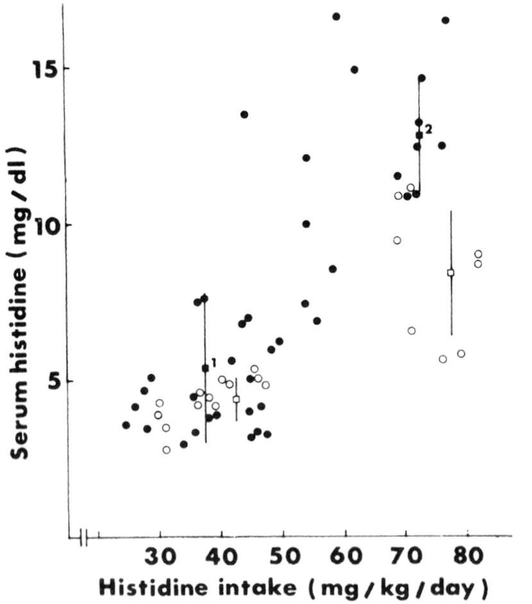

Fig. 80-4 The effect of histidine intake and the amount of residual histidase activity on serum histidine level in patients. *Filled and open circles* show values for group 1 and group 2 (see Fig. 80-3 and legend), respectively. *Filled and open squares and error bars* indicate mean and SD of serum histidine values for groups 1 and 2, respectively, at comparable diet intakes of histidine. (*From Kuroda et al.*[89] *Used by permission.*)

Oral loading with L-histidine, usually 100 mg/kg, produces a marked accentuation of the blood histidine level at 1 h with much less clearing than in normal individuals even at 4 h after the load (Fig. 80-5).

Urine histidine is markedly increased in histidinemia, reflecting overflow from the increased levels in blood. The values reported have been 2 to 6 mmol/day, representing a six- to tenfold increase over normal levels.[2] When quantified on the basis of creatinine excretion, the values have been 3 to 27 mmol/g creatinine as compared with the normal value of less than 2 mmol/g creatinine.[2,104]

Histidine is also increased in CSF. Wadman et al found a tenfold increase in CSF in one patient, with values of 142 and 129 μM compared with a normal value of 13 μM.[105] Shaw et al reported a CSF value of 48 μM in their patient, an approximately threefold elevation.[106] Notably, the CSF/plasma histidine ratio in both of these patients was normal, suggesting that the amount of histidine in brain may not be disproportionately increased in histidinemia. This finding is in contrast to disorders with severe neurologic features, such as nonketotic hyperglycinemia, in which the CSF/plasma ratio is increased because of a much greater elevation of glycine in CSF than in blood.[107] On the other hand, the CSF/plasma ratio is normal in some other neurologically important metabolic disorders, one example being phenylketonuria (PKU).[108,109]

Histidine Metabolites. The presence of histidine metabolites, particularly the products of histidine transamination (Fig. 80-1), are among the most striking biochemical findings in histidinemia. Indeed, the presence of imidazolepyruvic acid in the urine led to the discovery of histidinemia. While investigating the cause of speech delay in a 3-year-old girl, Ghadimi et al found that her urine had a positive green reaction to the addition of ferric chloride reagent, much like that in PKU. They thought she had PKU, but further study disclosed that her urine contained a large excess of histidine rather than phenylalanine.[1] Auerbach et al later identified the substance that produces the positive ferric chloride reaction in histidinemia as imidazolepyruvic acid, the immediate transamination product of histidine. They also identified other imidazole metabolites related to histidine transamination in their patient, including imidazolelactic and imidazoleacetic acids.[83]

As is true for histidine excretion, the amount of imidazole metabolites excreted is directly related to protein intake and the blood histidine concentration.[89] Imidazolepyruvic acid is not normally detectable in urine; in histidinemia, the excretion has varied from trace amounts to about 2 mmol/g creatinine.[88] Imidazolepyruvic acid is a relatively unstable compound, however, and the actual values could be higher than those recorded.[105] The quantities of other imidazole metabolites in urine from histidinemic patients, as measured by Wadman et al using column chromatography, were as follows: imidazolelactic acid, 0.4 to 5.0 mmol/g creatinine; imidazoleacetic acid, 0.1 to 2.2 mmol/g creatinine; and *N*-acetylhistidine, 0.1 to 0.6 mmol/g creatinine. The values for imidazolelactic and imidazoleacetic acids are 5- to 50-fold greater than normal, whereas those for *N*-acetylhistidine are two- to fivefold above normal.[104] In contrast to their presence in urine, these metabolites have not been detected in blood, presumably because there is little or no capacity for their renal reabsorption. Methylhistidine has also been reported to be increased in histidinemia,[110] as has carnosine[111] but not homocarnosine or anserine.

Neonates with histidinemia often lack the large quantities of histidine transamination products observed in urine from older infants and children with histidinemia.[112] Even after histidine loading, histidinemic neonates excrete much smaller quantities of imidazolepyruvic, imidazolelactic, and imidazoleacetic acids than do older children, despite excreting a comparable percentage of ingested histidine. We have explained this discrepancy on the basis of delayed postnatal maturation of histidine transaminase.[112] In some histidinemic infants, maturation of the histidine transamination system may not occur until several months of age.

A metabolite of particular interest in histidinemia is histamine, a product of histidine decarboxylation related to allergic diatheses. Imamura et al reported increased levels of histamine and its metabolites, including *N*-methylhistamine and imidazoleacetic acid conjugates, in histidinemic urine.[113] Tanabe and Sakura found that plasma histamine is also increased in histidinemia and that its level correlates positively with the plasma histidine level.[114] Thus, all of the known alternative pathways of histidine degradation (Fig. 80-1), including transamination, methylation, acetylation, and decarboxylation, seem to be activated in histidinemia. Synthesis of a histidine dipeptide, carnosine, may also be increased.[111]

Imamura et al identified *N*-ribosylhistidine in urine from normal and histidinemic children. The latter group excreted amounts seven times greater than normal. Rats fed histidine supplements increased their excretion of *N*-ribosylhistidine 30-fold.[115] Additional studies indicated that the ribosylation of histidine is mediated by a system different from imidazoleacetic acid phosphoribosyltransferase, which catalyzes the formation of ribosylimidazolylacetic acid.[116]

Decreased Urocanic Acid. Urocanic acid, the product of the histidase reaction, is normally detectable in blood but is undetectable in histidinemic patients.[117,118] The deficiency of urocanic acid is particularly striking in the skin (see the section "Enzyme Defect").

Two very different roles for epidermal urocanic acid have been proposed. One is as a natural sunscreen against UV light. The other is as a mediator of UV-induced systemic immune suppression.[119,120] Urocanic acid deficiency in histidinemia could have implications for either of these proposed functions.[32]

Urocanic Acid as an Ultraviolet Protectant. *Trans*-urocanic acid is formed from the deamination of L-histidine by histidase (Fig. 80-1) in the liver and in the epidermis.[121] In the stratum corneum, *trans*-urocanic acid ($\lambda_{max} = 275$ nm) undergoes an isomerization to *cis*-urocanic acid in UV light (Fig. 80-1),[122–125] the proportion of *cis* and *trans* isomers varying according to the UV-light exposure.[126,127]

Initial suggestions that epidermal urocanic acid may act as natural sunscreen[128,129] led to the hypothesis that the deficiency of urocanic acid in the skin renders histidinemic individuals more sensitive to sunlight and more susceptible to sunburn than others. The ability of urocanic acid to protect skin from sunburn has been demonstrated by a number of investigators,[130–134] though a recent study suggests that the protective effect of urocanic acid is very weak.[135] A study of skin erythema in two histidinemic sibs suggested increased sensitivity to UV light in one, although his affected infant brother had a normal response.[136] In a follow-up study of histidinemic adults originally identified by newborn screening, we have not found a striking increase in sensitivity to sunlight (H.L. Levy, unpublished data). Urocanic acid in the skin may also reduce photomutagenesis, since the absorption spectra of both the *cis* and *trans* isomers of urocanate overlap with the absorption spectrum of DNA.[124]

Urocanic Acid as a Ultraviolet-Induced Immunoregulator. A second role for cutaneous urocanic acid was proposed by De Fabo and Noonan, who postulated that it may act as a mediator of the systemic immunosuppression of tumor rejection observed in the week following exposure of skin to UV light.[137] Previously, two groups studying UV carcinogenesis had shown that UV irradiation is responsible not only for the formation of tumors but also for their survival.[138,139] Tumor survival was shown to be due to a UV-induced immune suppression not only at the site of UV irradiation but also systemically. Since UV light does not penetrate the epidermis,[140] the mechanism of UV-induced systemic immunosuppression is intriguing. Subsequent experiments demonstrated that T lymphocytes are involved in mediating the UV-induced immunosuppression of both tumor rejection[141–143] and delayed-type hypersensitivity to contact sensitizers.[144–152] The proposal that urocanic acid mediates UV-induced immunosuppression was based on the close fit of the absorption spectrum of urocanic acid with the observed wavelength-dependent UV immunosuppression. The initiating event of the UV-induced immunosuppression was postulated to be the UV isomerization of *trans*- to *cis*-urocanic acid.[137]

Several lines of evidence indicate that urocanic acid mediates UV-induced immunosuppression. First, UV light does not induce immunosuppression of delayed-type hypersensitivity in histidinemic mice, which have less than 10 percent of the skin urocanic acid found in wild-type (BALB/c) mice.[153] Second, Reeve et al have demonstrated that topical administration of *trans*-urocanic acid, followed by UV irradiation, results in a two- to threefold increase in the number of tumors seen in hairless mice compared with mice exposed to UV irradiation alone (the administration of *trans*-urocanic acid without UV exposure did not result in any tumor formation).[154] Third, *cis*-urocanic acid was shown to enhance tail skin graft survival in mice[155] and allogeneic heart transplants in rats.[156] In the latter experiments, permanent graft acceptance was observed in 40 percent of mice that were treated with *cis*-urocanic acid, compared with a 20 percent survival rate for rats irradiated with UV light (320 to 400 nm) and no survival for untreated rats. Fourth, suppression of delayed-type hypersensitivity by *cis*-urocanic acid has been demonstrated in a number of investigations.[149,151,157] The degree of suppression of the delayed-type hypersensitivity response depends on the doses of UV light and *cis*-urocanic acid administered,[151,152,158] and virtually complete suppression (90 to 100 percent) can be obtained.

Cellular Involvement in Immunosuppression. The mechanism of the immunosuppression mediated by *cis*-urocanic acid is uncertain. Experimental data suggest that *cis*-urocanic acid depresses the function of antigen-presenting cells of the epidermis and spleen, which in turn may have an effect on T cells.[150] This effect can be blocked in the skin by pretreatment of mice with a monoclonal antibody to *cis*-urocanic acid.[135] How *cis*-urocanic acid could produce this effect on antigen-presenting cells is unclear.

Histamine and Immunosuppression. As a first step toward understanding the molecular events involved in *cis*-urocanic acid-mediated immunosuppression, Norval et al tested the effectiveness of urocanic acid analogues in suppressing delayed-type hypersensitivity.[157] Of potential relevance to histidinemia is that histamine produces a degree of immunosuppression of delayed-type hypersensitivity equivalent to that seen with *cis*-urocanic acid. The significance of this result is uncertain, but it suggests that histamine may be able to interact with the same cellular receptors as *cis*-urocanic acid. Since histamine is known to bind to the histamine H_1 and H_2 receptors found on monocytes and some types of lymphocytes, it would be of interest to determine whether *cis*-urocanic acid is a ligand of these receptors.

Epidermal Urocanic Acid Deficiency in Histidinemia. The importance of urocanic acid in the natural environment could be studied by analyzing histidinemic individuals who have low levels of urocanic acid in the skin. As already mentioned, the decrease in epidermal urocanic acid abrogates the UV-induced immunosuppression of delayed-type hypersensitivity in histidinemic mice.[153] If, as in humans with histidinemia, these mice have increased blood histamine levels, the histamine appears to have no effect on suppression of delayed-type hypersensitivity. By analogy with histidinemic mice, therefore, histidinemic patients would be predicted to have reduced immunosuppression of delayed-type hypersensitivity and enhanced tumor rejection following UV exposure. Thus, they may be more susceptible to DNA damage after exposure to sunlight but may not be at increased risk of skin cancer because they lack *cis*-urocanic acid-mediated suppression of immune surveillance. This hypothesis could be tested by determining whether the incidence of skin cancer is significantly altered in histidinemia.

Presumably, the production of urocanic acid in the epidermis is in some way beneficial to animals. It is possible that the immunosuppression mediated by *cis*-urocanic acid is incidental to its role in protecting DNA from UV damage. On the other hand, if the immunoregulatory role of *cis*-urocanic acid is physiologically significant, then one would expect that histidinemic individuals should display the effects of low urocanic acid levels in the epidermis. Several groups have suggested that the evolutionary advantage of UV-induced immunosuppression may be to prevent autoimmune destruction of sun-damaged cells.[158,159] Consequently, a possible result of reduced epidermal urocanic acid may be a more aggressive immunologic response to UV damage of the skin. If such a response occurs, it may affect the incidence of skin disorders in histidinemic patients.

Other Biochemical Findings. These were reviewed in detail in the seventh edition of this book.[3]

Clinical Phenotype

The children identified during the first decade after the discovery of the disorder often were mentally retarded and had speech difficulties.[88] In fact, speech problems were so frequently mentioned that this was thought to be a specific clinical feature of histidinemia.[160,161] The association seemed unlikely, however, since most of those with speech impairment were mentally retarded or had low-normal intelligence.[162,163] Moreover, quite a number of individuals found to have histidinemia had normal intelligence and normal speech, suggesting that histidinemia might actually be benign and that the clinical abnormalities reported were coincidental with rather than due to the metabolic disorder.

Follow-up of children with histidinemia detected by routine neonatal urine screening in Massachusetts provided data supporting the view that histidinemia might not cause disease.[102] The 20 prospectively studied children who had been identified in this manner and their six histidinemic sibs identified by family testing, all untreated, were clinically normal. In particular, their speech was normal, and the mean IQ was essentially the same as that of their nonhistidinemic sibs (107 ± 12 versus 108 ± 11). Investigators in Los Angeles[164] and Japan[165] reached the similar conclusion that histidinemia is probably benign, also from studying histidinemic children identified by newborn screening. Specifically, the DQ/IQ scores in Japan were normal in 24 of the 25 histidinemic children.[166] Widhalm and Virmani also reported normal IQ among Austrian children with histidinemia who were identified by newborn screening, including those untreated and those treated with diet during infancy.[167] Interestingly, the 18 children who were untreated actually had a significantly higher mean IQ score at age 6 years than the 46 treated children (110 ± 18 versus 99 ± 14, $p < 0.05$). The mean blood histidine level in the newborn period before treatment and after treatment was discontinued was higher in the Austrian children who received treatment than in those who were untreated, perhaps indicating a milder form of histidinemia in those who never received treatment.[167,168] Nevertheless, given the findings from other centers (previously reviewed) and the fact that the basal blood histidine levels in the Austrian children who received treatment were not unusually high, it is doubtful that a difference in degree of histidinemia explains the higher IQ in the untreated cohort.

The results of the Japanese and Austrian studies are somewhat less clear on the question of speech difficulties in histidinemia. The Japanese investigators interpreted as reduced psycho-linguistic quotients the findings on the Illinois Test of Psycho-Linguistic Abilities in 10 histidinemia children so tested and concluded that there are difficulties in expression and auditory sequencing memory in histidinemia.[166] The absence of control subjects in this study, however, particularly because this test was applied to a Japanese-speaking population, confound interpretation of these results. The Austrian investigators reported speech disturbances in five patients.[167]

Although these studies indicate that histidinemia does not produce severe or even obvious clinical effects, the question of whether histidinemia is benign has remained. The Montreal group surveyed the published experience in histidinemic sibs identified by family screening and found, as shown in Table 80-1, that 50 percent had abnormal or impaired central nervous system development, as compared with a 13.5 percent frequency of similar impairment among the nonhistidinemic sibs.[169,170] On the other hand, a reassessment of histidinemic children identified by newborn screening in Massachusetts again indicated a normal clinical course: there were no differences from their nonhistidinemic sibs in growth and development, speech acquisition, and IQ

Table 80-1 Correlation Between Histidinemia and Central Nervous System (CNS) Phenotype in Sibs of Probands

	CNS Phenotype			
	Sibs With Histidinemia		Sibs Without Histidinemia	
Proband Phenotype	With	Without	With	Without
With CNS phenotype	11	8	5	21
Without CNS phenotype	2	5	0	11
Totals	13	13	5	32

SOURCE: From Rosenmann et al.[170] Used by permission.

Table 80-2 Psychological Assessment Scores (Mean ± SD) of Histidinemic Children and Their Age-Matched Sib Controls

WISC-R	Histidinemia ($n = 10$)	Sib Controls ($n = 10$)
Age (years)	11.2 ± 3.3	11.8 ± 3.5
Full-Scale IQ	102.8 ± 16.7	102.2 ± 13.4
Verbal IQ	98.9 ± 18.2	96.8 ± 13.4
Information	8.6 ± 2.5	8.6 ± 2.2
Vocabulary	9.7 ± 3.9	9.2 ± 3.0
Digit span	11.5 ± 3.3	9.8 ± 3.2
Arithmetic	9.7 ± 2.2	8.4 ± 1.7
Comprehension	11.7 ± 4.2	11.9 ± 3.1
Similarities	9.6 ± 4.7	9.6 ± 3.3
Performance IQ	106.2 ± 14.8	107.6 ± 12.5
Picture completion	10.2 ± 3.1	11.1 ± 1.9
Picture arrangement	10.8 ± 2.4	10.5 ± 2.9
Block design	10.7 ± 3.2	11.7 ± 3.1
Object assembly	11.1 ± 4.6	12.8 ± 3.8
Coding	10.9 ± 3.3	9.5 ± 2.6
Mazes	10.8 ± 2.4	12.6 ± 2.5

SOURCE: From Coulombe et al.[103] Used by permission.

scores (Table 80-2).[103] Since there were no biochemical differences between the histidinemic sibs in the Montreal survey and the children in the Massachusetts study, the clinical differences could not be explained on the basis of metabolic variance.[170]

In reconciling these seemingly discrepant findings, it was postulated that histidinemia is not a "disease" in humans, but that it may have a maladaptive impact on the central nervous system under certain unusual circumstances, such as perinatal hypoxia.[171] It also is possible that histidinemia, despite a consistent biochemical phenotype, may include more than one form of histidase deficiency, including a more frequent benign type and a less frequent maladaptive variant.[171] For example, the latter could be a contiguous gene-deletion syndrome (see the section "Genetics and Gene Mapping") or a locus conferring susceptibility to elevated histidine during development (see the section "Maternal Histidinemia").

Isolated neurologic and somatic abnormalities have also been reported in association with histidinemia.[2] These include cerebellar ataxia, hydrocephalus, emotional disturbances, short stature, delayed bone age, seizure disorder, recurrent infections, precocious puberty, congenital hypoplastic anemia, idiopathic thrombocytopenia purpura, and multiple congenital anomalies. Added to this list are reports of progressive myoclonus in a mentally retarded adult with histidinemia,[172] Joubert syndrome and congenital ocular fibrosis in a histidinemic infant,[173] and various abnormalities of the teeth in several affected children.[174] It is unlikely that histidinemia caused any of these findings. Tanabe and Sakura reported the frequent occurrence of atopic dermatitis among histidinemic children but also found that there was no difference in the level of histamine between patients with and without atopic dermatitis. Thus, they believe that the atopic dermatitis could not be explained by hyperhistaminemia.[114] In our follow-up of histidinemia, we have not noticed an increased frequency of allergies (H.L. Levy, unpublished data). Lucca et al reported evidence that suggested an increased frequency of heterozygosity for histidinemia in schizophrenia.[175] In a recent study, however, this group could not find a difference in frequency between those with schizophrenia and normal controls in any of the tetranucleotide repeat polymorphisms they identified in intron 8 of the histidase gene.[176]

Diagnosis

The diagnosis of histidinemia is based on finding an elevation of histidine in blood and increased excretion of histidine in the urine. The urinary metabolite imidazolepyruvic acid can usually be detected by the ferric chloride test.[88] Further information on the diagnosis of histidinemia is available in the sixth edition of this book.[2]

Treatment

Since it seems that about 99 percent of histidinemic patients do not require treatment and that only 1 percent might benefit,[171] treatment is rarely a consideration. The sixth edition of this book can be consulted for detailed information about treatment.[2] If future studies indicate that therapy should be given, this could be facilitated by enzyme replacement. Histidase has been encapsulated within cellulose-nitrate artificial cells for this purpose.[177] The encapsulation seems to protect histidase activity and to allow for substantial depletion of histidine in vitro. Studies of this system in vivo have not yet been reported.

Prevalence and Screening

Before routine newborn screening, histidinemia was considered to be a very rare inborn error. For almost a decade after its discovery, only a few cases had been identified.[88] Newborn screening dramatically altered this view by demonstrating that histidinemia is one of the most frequent of the metabolic disorders.[178] The difference can be explained by the lack of clinical abnormalities, rendering histidinemia no more frequent in populations screened for medical diagnosis than in the general population. Routine newborn screening, of course, includes many more individuals than selected populations.

Histidinemia has been most frequently identified by routine newborn screening. This screening detected affected infants on the basis of increased histidine in the newborn blood specimen[179–181] or in a newborn urine specimen.[182,183] With the exception of Quebec, where newborn urine screening continues (B. Lemieux, personal communication, 1998), histidinemia detection is no longer included in newborn screening programs.

Reported incidences of histidinemia have ranged from 1:8600 in Quebec (B. Lemieux, personal communication, 1998) to 1:90,000 in New York.[180] The composite frequency derived from these data in screening over 20 million newborns is about 1:12,000 (see Table 29-3 in the seventh edition of this book). The wide range in the reported incidence probably reflects the different sensitivities of the screening techniques more than prevalence rates. Nevertheless, the range probably also reflects ethnic differences in frequency. In Japan, until routine screening for histidinemia was discontinued in 1993, it was by far the most frequent of the inborn errors identified by neonatal screening; the incidence of 1:9600 may be compared with that of only 1:80,000 for PKU in Japan (H. Naruse, personal communication, 1998).

The original and continuing suggestion that histidinemia might produce speech difficulties has led to selective screening of children with speech disorders. This screening has failed to identify cases among 657 children in Poland[184] or among 200 children in Czechoslovakia considered to be stutterers and "clutterers."[185]

Atypical Histidinemia

There is heterogeneity in histidinemia, as there is in other inborn errors of metabolism. Anakura et al reported two sibs with histidinemia, one of whom had relatively mild biochemical abnormalities and a partial defect in skin histidase. He was clinically normal.[186] We have followed the cases of two sibs with similar findings.[102]

Studies of infants identified by newborn screening in Japan indicate that there are two groups with respect to residual skin histidase activity. One group, the larger, is characterized by activities of 0.5 μmol/h per gram tissue or less (normal 9.5 ± 4.1 μmol/h per gram tissue), and other group by activities of 1.8 to 2.7 μmol/h per gram tissue.[187] Lower fasting blood histidine levels (Fig. 80-3) and higher tolerances to dietary histidine correspond to the higher residual histidase activity in the second or atypical group.[89] Skin histidase from two sibs in the atypical group manifested heat instability; this was not present in other patients in this group or in any from the first group.[97,186] Studies in Austria of children detected by newborn screening have also indicated that there are two groups: one with blood histidine levels of 8 mg/dl or higher when on normal diets and those with lower blood histidine elevations.[167,168]

It is likely that atypical histidinemia represents a different mutant allele(s) from the one producing classic histidinemia; there may be several allelic mutations that result in histidinemia. The occurrence of both forms of histidinemia in sibships[186,187] indicates that genetic compounds of two different mutant alleles might account for some cases of atypical PKU. If so, histidinemia would be analogous to PKU and mild hyperphenylalaninemia, which may occur together in sibships as a result of different combinations of mutant alleles.[188]

MATERNAL HISTIDINEMIA

The recognition that maternal PKU causes fetal damage (see Chap.77) has led to an interest in whether other maternal inborn errors similarly affect the fetus.[189,190] Maternal histidinemia has been of particular interest, since histidinemia is one of the most frequently identified metabolic disorders.

At least 53 offspring from 21 histidinemic mothers have been reported.[165,191–196] These offspring have generally been normal and have not had the microcephaly, congenital anomalies, or mental retardation seen in offspring of women with PKU. The children in one family had lower IQ scores than their parents,[193] but we found no difference in IQ between histidinemic mothers and their children: both groups scored in the normal range (H.L. Levy, S.E. Waisbren, and D. Lobbregt, unpublished data). A follow-up study of maternal histidinemia in Massachusetts of mothers identified either by routine umbilical cord blood screening[196] or originally by routine neonatal urine screening[102] revealed no clinical abnormalities in the 21 offspring. Their mean ($\pm$ SD) IQ was 104 $\pm$ 15. Thus, no convincing evidence for an adverse fetal effect from maternal histidinemia has yet emerged.

Murine Maternal Histidinemia

Although the histidinemic mouse model does not exhibit clinical abnormalities (see the section "Mouse Model"), a balance defect characterized by circling behavior and/or head tilting is observed in offspring of histidinemic (*his*/*his*) mothers or heterozygous (*his*/+) mothers with increased plasma histidine levels induced during the second week (middle third) of pregnancy by feeding a histidine-supplemented diet.[197,198] Conversely, the offspring abnormality is prevented or substantially lessened by treating homozygous (*his*/*his*) mothers with a histidine-restricted diet and sharply reducing the plasma histidine concentration during week 2 of pregnancy. The observed behavior of the offspring is related to changes in the inner ear: abnormalities found include absence of the otoliths, enlarged or distorted cochlea, enlarged ampullae, shortened crus commune, and thin or misshapen semicircular canals.[197]

Although the offspring abnormality is clearly related to the maternal biochemical status, susceptibility to high histidine concentrations during fetal development also plays an important role. Heterozygous (*his*/+) offspring of histidinemic mothers were less severely affected than homozygous (*his*/*his*) offspring.[99] Normal (+/+) offspring produced by egg transfer into histidinemic mothers had no visible evidence of a balance defect but did show subclinical damage to the inner ear.[197] Hence, the fetal genotype at the *his* locus modulates the histidine effect. Moreover, susceptibility seems to be conferred by other loci. When selection for high incidence of these abnormalities was relaxed, the frequency of offspring with the balance defect dramatically decreased, despite no change in the maternal phenotype.[198,199]

Since susceptibility to high histidine concentrations during fetal development is an inherited trait in mice, a similar trait might be present in humans. However, this susceptibility would be observed only in the rare cases in which it is coincident with maternal histidinemia. This could explain the single report of reduced IQ in the children of one histidinemic mother,[193] whereas in other families the children have generally been normal.[196]

HISTIDINURIA

Increased urinary histidine with a normal or low blood histidine concentration has been reported in five children from four families.[200–204] Four of the children, including two sibs, were mentally retarded.[200,202,203] Since these four children were evaluated because of their clinical abnormalities, the association of histidinuria and mental retardation is likely coincidental rather than casual. Histidase activity was not determined in any of these patients. However, none excreted histidine metabolites, all had normal blood histidine levels, and the CSF histidine level was also normal in the one patient in which it was measured;[200] consequently, it is unlikely that histidase deficiency was present. The fact that three of these children had a slower response to histidine loading than did controls suggests the presence of an intestinal defect in histidine transport as well as a renal defect.[202,203] Further details on these cases are included in the sixth edition of this book[2] and elsewhere.[204]

UROCANIC ACIDURIA

Four children with urocanic acidura have been described.[64,65,205] All were mentally retarded, and the growth of at least three was retarded.[65,65]

The results of biochemical studies were consistent with a defect in urocanase (Fig. 80-1). Urocanic acid was greatly increased in urine, estimated at 10 to 50 times normal.[64,65] Histidine loading exaggerated the urocanic acid excretion and, in two patients, also led to the production of imidazolepropionic acid, a byproduct of urocanic acid.[64,205] On the other hand, metabolites such as imidazolonepropionic acid and FIGLU, which are distal to the metabolic step catalyzed by urocanase, were not present in urine after loading with histidine or urocanic acid. The presence of a urocanase deficiency in liver was proved by enzyme assay in three patients,[64,65] whereas histidase activity was normal in skin from one patient[64] and increased in liver from a second patient.[65]

It is interesting to note that all of the patients had evidence of abnormal histidine accumulation after histidine loading. In one the serum histidine response was exaggerated,[64] and in three others there was increased urinary histidine and metabolites of histidine transamination.[65,205] It is possible that these increases were the result of the huge urocanic acid elevation: although the histidase-mediated reaction is irreversible, urocanic acid is a competitive inhibitor of histidase in bacteria[206] and might similarly inhibit the mammalian enzyme in vivo. However, histidase was not inhibited in vitro in these patients.[64,65]

The mental retardation observed in the four reported cases of urocanic aciduria might not be related to the metabolic disorder. All of the patients were identified as a result of an investigation to determine the cause of their mental retardation. We identified four additional children with urocanic aciduria by routine newborn urine screening (1:250,000).[207] They have maintained normal development without dietary or other therapy. One has short stature, but several other members of her family who do not have urocanic aciduria also are short. Thus, it is likely that urocanic aciduria is benign and that the mental retardation described in reported cases is coincidental. It is also likely that urocanic aciduria is more frequent than the few identified cases would indicate. Urocanic acid is ninhydrin negative, and therefore is not identified by the usual amino acid analysis. Furthermore, urocanic acid is not soluble in ethyl acetate, the usual solvent employed in organic acid extraction of urine. Consequently, it is not identifiable by standard organic acid analysis of urine. Autosomal recessive transmission seems the most likely pattern of inheritance.

REFERENCES

1. Ghadimi H, Partington MW, Hunter A: A familial disturbance of histidine metabolism. *N Engl J Med* **265**:221, 1961.
2. Levy HL: Disorders of histidine metabolism, in Scriver CR, Beaudet AL, Sly WS, Valle D (eds): *The Metabolic Basis of Inherited Disease*, 6th ed. New York, McGraw-Hill, 1989, p 563.
3. Levy HL, Taylor RG, McInnes RR: Disorders of histidine metabolism, in Scriver CR, Beaudet AL, Sly WS, Valle D (eds): *The Metabolic and Molecular Bases of Inherited Disease*, 7th ed. New York, McGraw-Hill, 1995, p 1107.
4. Snyderman SE, Boyer A, Roitman E, Holt LE Jr, Prose PH: The histidine requirement of the infant. *Pediatrics* **31**:786, 1963.
5. Snyderman S: An eczematoid dermatitis in histidine deficiency. *J Pediatr* **66**:212, 1965.
6. Snyderman SE: The histidine requirements of infants, in Kluthe R, Katz NR (eds): *Histidine. Metabolism. Clinical Aspects. Therapeutic Use*. Stuttgart, Georg Thieme, 1978, p 2.
7. Van Sprang FJ, Wadman SK: Treatment of a patient with histidinemia. *Acta Paediatr Scand* **56**:493, 1967.
8. Corner BD, Holton JB, Norman RM, Williams PM: A case of histidinemia controlled with a low histidine diet. *Pediatrics* **41**:1074, 1968.
9. Snyderman SE, Sansaricq C, Norton PM, Manka M: The nutritional therapy of histidinemia. *J Pediatr* **95**:712, 1979.
10. Dyme IZ, Horwitz SJ, Bacchus B, Kerr DS: Histidinemia: A case with resolution of myoclonic seizures after treatment with a low-histidine diet. *Am J Dis Child* **137**:256, 1983.
11. Stifel FB, Herman RH: Is histidine an essential amino acid in man? *Am J Clin Nutr* **25**:182, 1972.
12. Albanese AA: Editorial: Histidine—Essential or not? *Nutr Rep Int* **6**:115, 1972.
13. Meister A: *Biochemistry of the Amino Acids*, 2d ed. New York, Academic, 1965.
14. Peterkofsky A: The mechanism of action of histidase: Amino-enzyme formation and partial reactions. *J Biol Chem* **237**:787, 1962.
15. Furuta T, Takahashi H, Shibasaki H, Kasuya Y: Reversible stepwise mechanism involving a carbanion intermediate in the elimination of ammonia from l-histidine catalyzed by histidine ammonia-lyase. *J Biol Chem* **267**:12,600, 1992.
16. Dhanam M, Radhakrishnan AN: Comparative studies on histidase: Distribution in tissues, properties of liver histidase and its development in rat. *Indian J Exp Biol* **14**:103, 1976.
17. Bhargava MM, Feigelson M: Studies on the mechanisms of histidase development in rat skin and liver: I. Basis for tissue specific developmental changes in catalytic activity. *Dev Biol* **48**:212, 1976.
18. Baden HP, Sviokla S, Maderson PFA: A comparative study of histidase activity in amphibian, avian, reptilian and mammalian epidermis. *Comp Biochem Physiol* **30**:889, 1969.
19. Sano H, Tada T, Moriyama A, Ogawa H, Asai K, Kawai Y, Hodgsón ME, et al: Isolation of a rat histidase cDNA sequence and expression in *Escherichia coli*: Evidence of extrahepatic/epidermal distribution. *Eur J Biochem* **250**:212, 1997.
20. Feigelson M: Multihormonal regulation of hepatic histidase during postnatal development. *Enzyme* **15**:169, 1973.
21. Lamartiniere CA, Feigelson M: Effects of estrogen, glucocorticoid, glucagon, and adenosine 3′:5′-monophosphate on catalytic activity, amount, and rate of de novo synthesis of hepatic histidase. *J Biol Chem* **252**:3234, 1977.
22. Lamartiniere CA: Neonatal estrogen treatment alters sexual differentiation of hepatic histidase. *Endocrinology* **105**:1031, 1979.
23. Armstrong EG, Feigelson M: Effects of hypophysectomy and triiodothyronine on de novo biosynthesis, catalytic activity, and estrogen induction of rat liver histidase. *J Biol Chem* **255**:7199, 1980.
24. Wickner RB: Dehydroalanine in histidine ammonia lyase. *J Biol Chem* **244**:6550, 1969.
25. Givot IL, Smith TA, Abeles RH: Studies on the mechanism of action and the structure of the electrophilic center of histidine ammonia lyase. *J Biol Chem* **244**:6341, 1969.
26. Hernandez D, Stroh JG, Phillips AT: Identification of ser^{143} as a site of modification in the active site of histidine ammonia-lyase. *Arch Biochem Biophys* **307**:126, 1993.
27. Hernandez D, Phillips AT: Ser-143 is an essential active site residue in histidine ammonia-lyase of *Pseudomonas putida*. *Biochem Biophys Res Commun* **201**:1433, 1994.
28. Langer M, Reck G, Reed J, Retey J: Identification of serine-143 as the most likely precursor of dehyroalanine in the active site of histidine ammonia-lyase: A study of the overexpressed enzyme by site-directed mutagenesis. *Biochemistry* **33**:6462, 1994.
29. Langer M, Lieber A, Retey J: Histidine ammonia-lyase mutant S143C is posttranslationally converted into fully active wild-type enzyme: Evidence for serine 143 to be the precursor of active site dehydroalanine. *Biochemistry* **33**:14,034, 1994.
30. Taylor RG, McInnes RR: Site-directed mutagenesis of conserved serines in rat histidase: Identification of serine 254 as an essential active site residue. *J Biol Chem* **269**:17,473, 1994
31. Hanson KR, Havir EA: The enzymic elimination of ammonia, in Boyer PD (ed): *The Enzymes*. New York, Academic, 1972, p 75.
32. Taylor RG, Levy HL, McInnes RR: Histidase and histidinemia: Clinical and molecular considerations. *Mol Biol Med* **8**:101, 1991.
33. Cornell NW, Villee CA: Purification and properties of rat liver histidase. *Biochim Biophys Acta* **167**:172, 1968.
34. Okamura H, Nishida T, Nakagawa H: L-Histidine ammonia-lyase in rat liver: I. Purification and general characteristics. *J Biochem* **75**:139, 1974.
35. Brand LM, Harper AE: Histidine ammonia-lyase from rat liver: Purification, properties and inhibition by substrate analogues. *Biochemistry* **15**:1814, 1976.
36. Dhanam M, Radhakrishnan AN: Purification and properties of histidine ammonia-lyase from monkey liver. *Indian J Biochem Biophys* **11**:1, 1974.
37. Taylor RG, Lambert MA, Sexsmith E, Sadler SJ, Ray PN, Mahuran DJ, McInnes RR: Cloning and expression of rat histidase: Homology to two bacterial histidases and four phenylalanine ammonia-lyases. *J Biol Chem* **265**:18,192, 1990.
38. Taylor RG, Grieco D, Clarke GA, McInnes RR, Taylor BA: Identification of the mutation in murine histidinemia (*his*) and genetic mapping of the murine histidase locus (*Hal*) on chromosome 10. *Genomics* **16**:231, 1993.
39. Suchi M, Harada N, Wada Y, Takagi Y: Molecular cloning of the cDNA encoding human histidase. *Biochim Biophys Acta* **1216**:293, 1993.
40. Taylor RG, Garcia-Heras J, Sadler SJ, Lafreniere RG, Willard HF, Ledbetter DH, McInnes RR: Localization of histidine to human chromosome region 12q22-q24.1 and mouse chromosome region 10C2-D1. *Cytogenet Cell Genet* **56**:178, 1991.
41. Suchi M, Sano H, Mizuno H, Wada Y: Molecular cloning and structural characterization of the human histidase gene (*HAL*). *Genomics* **29**:98, 1995.
42. Maffei P, Nobile M, Dibella D, Novelli E, Smeraldi E, Catalano M: Short report on DNA marker at candidate locus: Intragenic tetranucelotide repeat polymorphism at the human histidase (*HAL*) locus. *Clin Genet* **52**:194, 1997.
43. Bhargava MM, Feigelson M: Studies on the mechanisms of histidase development in rat skin and liver: II. Alterations in enzyme levels and synthetic rates during development. *Dev Biol* **48**:226, 1976.
44. Kang-Lee YAE, Harper AE: Effect of histidine intake and hepatic histidase activity on the metabolism of histidine in vivo. *J Nutr* **107**:1427, 1997.
45. Cedrangolo F, Illiano G, Servillo L, Spina AM: Histidine degradation enzymes in rat liver: Induction by high protein intake. *Mol Cell Biochem* **23**:123, 1979.
46. Scott IR: Factors controlling the expressed activity of histidine ammonia-lyase in the epidermis and the resulting accumulation of urocanic acid. *Biochem J* **194**:829, 1981.
47. Matsuda I, Matsuo K, Endo F, Uehara I, Nagata N, Jinno Y, Chikazawa S, et al: Skin histidase activity and urine formiminoglutamic acid (FIGLU) in patients with histidinemia found by screening newborn infants. *Clin Chim Acta* **119**:319, 1982.
48. Shin YS, Wegele G, Mally E, Endres W, Scheibenreiter S: A simple method for histidase assay and an alteration in the affinity of skin histidase for histidine in histidinaemia. *J Inherited Metab Dis* **6**:113, 1983.
49. Kuroda Y, Ito M, Ogawa T, Takeda E, Toshima K, Miyao M: A new sensitive method for assay of histidase in human skin and detection of heterozygotes for histidinemia. *Clin Chim Acta* **96**:139, 1979.
50. Baden HP, Gavioli L: Histidase activity in rat liver and epidermis. *J Invest Dermatol* **63**:479, 1974.
51. Allen RL, Hopewell R, Prottey C: A comparative study of hepatic and epidermal histidase in the guinea pig (*Cavia porcellus*). *Comp Biochem Physiol* **84B**:523, 1986.

52. Givot IL, Abeles RH: Mammalian histidine ammonia-lyase: In vivo inactivation and presence of an electrophilic center at the active site. *J Biol Chem* **245**:3271, 1970.
53. Consevage MW, Phillips AT: Presence and quantity of dehydroalanine in histidine ammonia-lyase from *Pseudomonas putida*. *Biochemistry* **24**:301, 1985.
54. Hanson KR, Havir EA: L-Phenylalanine ammonia-lyase: IV. Evidence that the prosthetic group contains a dehydroalanyl residue and mechanism of action. *Arch Biochem Biophys* **141**:1, 1970.
55. Emes AV, Vining LC: Partial purification and properties of L-phenylalanine ammonia-lyase from *Streptomyces verticillatus*. *Can J Biochem* **48**:613, 1970.
56. Hodgins DS: Yeast phenylalanine ammonia-lyase: Purification, properties, and the identification of catalytically essential dehydroalanine. *J Biol Chem* **246**:2977, 1971.
57. Havir EA, Hanson KR: L-Phenylalanine ammonia-lyase (maize, potato, and *Rhodotorula glutinis*): Studies of the prosthetic group with nitromethane. *Biochemistry* **14**:1620, 1975.
58. Klee CB: Stereospecific irreversible inhibition of histidine ammonia-lyase by L-cysteine. *Biochemistry* **13**:4501, 1974.
59. Recsei PA, Snell EE: Pyruvoyl enzymes. *Annu Rev Biochem* **53**:357, 1984.
60. Banerjee S, Hansen JN: Structure and expression of a gene encoding the precursor of subtilin, a small protein antibiotic. *J Biol Chem* **263**:9508, 1988.
61. Ohmiya Y, Hayashi H, Kondo T, Kondo Y: Location of dehydroalanine residues in the amino acid sequence of bovine thyroglobulin: Identification of "donor" tyrosine sites for hormonogenesis in thyroglobulin. *J Biol Chem* **265**:9066, 1990.
62. Van Poelje PD, Snell EE: Pyruvoyl-dependent enzymes. *Annu Rev Biochem* **59**:29, 1990.
63. Schulz W, Eiben H-G, Hahlbrock K: Expression in *Escherichia coli* of catalytically active phenylalanine ammonia-lyase from parsley. *FEBS Lett* **258**:335, 1989.
64. Yoshida T, Tada K, Honda Y, Arakawa T: Urocanic aciduria: A defect in the urocanase activity in the liver of a mentally retarded. *Tohoku J Exp Med* **104**:305, 1971.
65. Kalafatic Z, Lipovac, K, Jezerinac Z, Juretic D, Dumic M, Zurga B, Res L: A liver urocanase deficiency. *Metabolism* **29**:1013, 1980.
66. Egan RM, Matherly LH, Phillips AT: Mechanism of urocanase as studied by deuterium isotope effects and labeling patterns. *Biochemistry* **20**:132, 1981.
67. Matherly LH, DeBrosse CW, Phillips AT: A covalent nicotinamide adenine dinucleotide intermediate in the urocanase reaction. *Biochemistry* **21**:2789, 1982.
68. Fessenmaier M, Frank R, Retey J, Schubert C: Cloning and sequencing the urocanase gene (*hutU*) from *Pseudomonas putida*. *FEBS Lett* **286**:55, 1991.
69. Yoshida K, Sano H, Seki S, Oda M, Fujimura M, Fujita Y: Cloning and sequencing of a 2.9 kg region of the *Bacillus subtilis* genome containing the *hut* and *wapA* loci. *Microbiology* **141**:337, 1995
70. Feinberg RH, Greenberg DM: Studies on the enzymic decomposition of urocanic acid. *J Biol Chem* **234**:2670, 1959.
71. Swaine D: The effect of substrate analogues on the activity of cat liver urocanase. *Biochim Biophys Acta* **178**:609, 1969.
72. Coltorti M, Di Simone A, Budillon G: Histidine and urocanase activities of liver and plasma: Correlations between tissue enzyme levels and plasmatic increases during human and mouse viral hepatitis. *Clin Chim Acta* **13**:568, 1966.
73. Hassall H, Rabie F: The bacterial metabolism of imidazolepropionate. *Biochim Biophys Acta* **115**:521, 1966.
74. Hunter JK, Hug DH: Specific inhibition of bacterial and bovine urocanases by glycylglycine. *Peptide Res* **2**:240, 1989.
75. Zannoni VG, La Du BN: Determination of histidine α-deaminase in human stratum corneum and its absence in histidinaemia. *Biochem J* **88**:160, 1963.
76. Sahib MK, Murti CRK: Induction of histidine-degrading enzymes in protein-starved rats and regulation of histidine metabolism. *J Biol Chem* **244**:4730, 1969.
77. Neufeld E, Harell A, Chayen R: The effect of L-thyroxine on histidine metabolism. *Biochim Biophys Acta* **237**:465, 1971.
78. Baldridge RC: The metabolism of histidine: II. Effects of folic acid deficiency. *J Biol Chem* **231**:207, 1958.
79. Hanford WC, Nep RL, Arfin SM: Genetic variation in histidine ammonialyase activity in the mouse. *Biochem Biophys Res Commun* **61**:1434, 1974.
80. Rao DR, Greenberg DM: Studies on the enzymic decomposition of urocanic acid: IV. Purification and properties of 4(5)imidazolone-5(4)propionic acid hydrolase. *J Biol Chem* **236**:1758, 1961.
81. Snyder SH, Silva OL, Kies MW: The mammalian metabolism of L-histidine: IV. Purification and properties of imidazolone propionic acid hydrolase. *J Biol Chem* **236**:2996, 1961.
82. Luhby AL, Cooperman JM, Teller DN: Histidine metabolic loading test to distinguish folic acid deficiency from vit. B_{12} in megaloblastic anemias. *Proc Soc Exp Biol Med* **101**:350, 1959.
83. Auerbach VH, DiGeorge AM, Baldridge RC, Tourtellotte CD, Brigham MP: Histidinemia: A deficiency in histidase resulting in the urinary excretion of histidine and of imidazolepyruvic acid. *J Pediatr* **60**:487, 1962.
84. La Du BN, Howell RR, Jacoby GA, Seegmiller JE, Zannoni VG: The enzymatic defect in histidinemia. *Biochem Biophys Res Commun* **7**:398, 1962.
85. Auerbach VH, DiGeorge AM, Carpenter GG: Histidinemia, in Nyhan WL (ed): *Amino Acid Metabolism and Genetic Variation*. New York, McGraw-Hill, 1967, p 145.
86. Levy HL, Baden HP, Shih VE: A simple indirect method of detecting the enzyme defect in histidinemia. *J Pediatr* **75**:1056, 1969.
87. Rosenblatt D, Mohyuddin F, Scriver CR: Histidinemia discovered by urine screening after renal transplantation. *Pediatrics* **46**:47, 1970.
88. La Du BN: Histidinemia, in Stanbury JB, Wyngaarden JB, Fredrickson DS (eds): *The Metabolic Basis of Inherited Disease*, 4th ed. New York, McGraw-Hill, 1978, p 317.
89. Kuroda Y, Ogawa T, Ito M, Watanabe T, Takeda E, Toshima K, Miyao M: Relationship between skin histidase activity and blood histidine response to histidine intake in patients with histidinemia. *J Pediatr* **97**:269, 1980.
90. Ito F, Aoki K, Eto Y: Histidinemia: Biochemical parameters for diagnosis. *Am J Dis Child* **135**:227, 1981.
91. Thalhammer O: Neonatal screening for histidinemia, in Bickel H, Guthrie R, Hammersen G (eds): *Neonatal Screening for Inborn Errors of Metabolism*. Berlin, Springer-Verlag, 1980, p 59.
92. Woody NC, Snyder CH, Harris JA: Histidinemia. *Am J Dis Child* **110**:606, 1965.
93. Funderburk SJ, Sparkes RS, Klisak I, Law ML: Chromosome deletion mapping of interspersed low-copy repetitive DNA. *Am J Hum Genet* **36**:769, 1984.
94. Naccache NF, Vianna-Morgante AM, Richieri-Costa A: Brief clinical report: Duplication of distal 17q: Report of an observation. *Am J Med Genet* **17**:633, 1984.
95. Chan A, Teshima I, Polychronakos C, Holland FJ, Weksberg R: Analysis of a deletion of chromosome 12q in a patient with short stature. *Clin Invest Med* **13**:B69, 1990.
96. Ford JH, Rofe RH, Pavy RP: Translocations involving chromosome 12: I. A report of a 12,21 translocation in a woman with recurrent abortions, and a study of the breakpoints and modes of ascertainment of translocations involving chromosome 12. *Hum Genet* **58**:144, 1981.
97. Kuroda Y, Watanabe T, Ito M, Toshima K, Miyao M: Altered kinetic properties of skin histidase in two patients with histidinaemia. *J Inherited Metab Dis* **5**:73, 1982.
98. Suchi M, Harada N, Ogawa H, Kawai Y, Sano H, Mizuno H, Morishita H, et al: Molecular genetic studies on histidinemia: Isolation and expression of a full-length human histidase cDNA, characterization of the genomic structure, and mutation search among histidinemic patients, in Levy HL, Hermos RJ, Grady GF (eds.): *Proceedings: Third Meeting of the International Society for Neonatal Screening*. Boston, ISNS, 1996, p 32.
99. Kacser H, Bulfield G, Wallace ME: Histidinaemic mutant in the mouse. *Nature* **244**:77, 1973.
100. Bulfield G, Kacser H: Histidinaemia in mouse and man. *Arch Dis Child* **49**:545, 1974.
101. Wright AF, Bulfield G, Arfin SM, Kacser H: Comparison of the properties of histidine ammonia-lyase in normal and histidinemic mutant mice. *Biochem Genet* **20**:245, 1982.
102. Levy HL, Shih VE, Madigan PM: Routine newborn screening for histidinemia: Clinical and biochemical results. *N Engl J Med* **291**:1214, 1974.
103. Coulombe JT, Kammerer BL, Levy HL, Hirsch BZ, Scriver CR: Histidinaemia: Part III. Impact; a prospective study. *J Inherited Metab Dis* **6**:58, 1983.
104. Wadman SK, De Bree PK, Van der Heiden C, Van Sprang FJ: Automatic column chromatographic analysis of urinary and serum imidazoles in patients with histidinaemia and normals. *Clin Chim Acta* **31**:215, 1971.

105. Wadman SK, Van Sprang FJ, Van Stekelenburg GJ, De Bree PK: Three new cases of histidinemia: Clinical and biochemical data. *Acta Paediatr Scand* **56**:485, 1967.
106. Shaw KNF, Boder E, Gutenstein M, Jacobs EE: Histidinemia. *J Pediatr* **63**:720, 1963.
107. Levy HL, Nishimura RN, Erickson AM, Janowska SE: Hyperglycinemia: In vivo comparison of nonketotic and ketotic (propionic acidemic) forms: I. CSF glycine concentrations and blood/CSF glycine. *Pediatr Res* **6**:400, 1972.
108. Antoshechkin AG, Chentsova TV, Tatur VY, Naritsin DB, Railian GP: Content of phenylalanine, tyrosine and their metabolites in CSF in phenylketonuria. *J Inherited Metab Dis* **14**:749, 1991.
109. Snyderman SE, Sansaricq C, Norton PM, Castro JV: Plasma and cerebrospinal fluid amino acid concentrations in phenylketonuria during the newborn period. *J Pediatr* **99**:63, 1981.
110. Ghadimi H, Partington MW, Hunter A: Inborn error of histidine metabolism. *Pediatrics* **29**:714, 1962.
111. Carton D, Dhondt F, De Schrijver F, Samyn W, Kint J, Delbeke MJ, Hooft C: Histidinemia. *Helv Paediatr Acta* **25**:127, 1970.
112. Levy HL, Madigan PM, Peneva P: Evidence for delayed histidine transamination in neonates with histidinemia. *Pediatrics* **47**:128, 1971.
113. Imamura I, Watanabe T, Hase Y, Sakamoto Y, Fukuda Y, Yamamoto H, Tsuruhara T, et al: Histamine metabolism in patients with histidinemia: Determination of urinary levels of histamine, N^{t}-methylhistamine, imidazole acetic acid, and its conjugate(s). *J Biochem* **96**:1925, 1984.
114. Tanabe M, Sakura N: Hyperhistaminemia in patients with histidinemia due to increased decarboxylation of histidine. *Clin Chim Acta* **186**:11, 1989.
115. Imamura I, Watanabe T, Sakamoto Y, Wakamiya T, Shiba T, Hase Y, Tsuruhara T, et al: N^{t}-ribosylhistidine, a novel histidine derivative in urine of histidinemic patients. *J Biol Chem* **260**:10,526, 1985.
116. Imamura I, Watanabe T, Wada H: Formation of N^{t}-ribosylhistidine, a novel histidine derivative found in the urine in histidinemia, from histidine and NAD(P)+ catalyzed by an NAD(P)+ glycohydrolase system. *Biochem Biophys Res Commun* **130**:501, 1985.
117. Wilcken B, Brown DA: Histidinaemia: Evaluation of an improved method for confirmation and the implications of the diagnosis. *Aust Paediatr J* **11**:126, 1975.
118. Matsuda I, Nagata N, Endo F: Blood histidine levels during course of histidinaemia. *Lancet* **1**:162, 1982.
119. Morrison H: Photochemistry and photobiology of urocanic acid. *Photodermatology* **2**:158, 1985.
120. Norval M, Simpson TJ, Ross JA: Urocanic acid and immunosuppression. *Photochem Photobiol* **50**:267, 1989.
121. Scott IR: Factors controlling the expressed activity of histidine ammonia-lyase in the epidermis and the resulting accumulation of urocanic acid. *Biochem J* **194**:829, 1981.
122. Edlbacher S, Heitz F: Zur Kenntnis der Urocaninsaure. *Hoppe-Seylers Z Physiol Chem* **279**:63, 1943.
123. Anglin JH Jr, Bever AT, Everett MA, Lamb JH: Ultraviolet-light-induced alterations in urocanic acid in vivo. *Biochim Biophys Acta* **53**:408, 1961.
124. Morrison H, Avnir D, Bernasconi C, Fagan G: Z/E photoisomerization of urocanic acid. *Photochem Photobiol* **32**:711, 1980.
125. Morrison H, Bernasconi C, Pandey G: A wavelength effect on urocanic acid E/Z photoisomerization. *Photochem Photobiol* **40**:549, 1984.
126. Norval M. Simpson TJ, Bardshiri E, Crosby J: Quantification of urocanic acid isomers in human stratum corneum. *Photodermatology* **6**:142, 1989.
127. Pasanen P, Reunala T, Jansen CT, Rasanen L, Neuvonen K, Ayras P: Urocanic acid isomers in epidermal samples and suction blister fluid of non-irradiated and UVB-irradiated human skin. *Photodermatology* **7**:40, 1990.
128. Zenisek A, Kral JA: The occurrence of urocanic acid in human sweat. *Biochim Biophys Acta* **12**:479, 1953.
129. Zenisek A, Kral JA, Hais IM: "Sun-screening" effect of urocanic acid. *Biochim Biophys Acta* **18**:589, 1955.
130. Everett MA, Anglin JH Jr, Bever AT: Ultraviolet induced biochemical alterations in skin: I. Urocanic acid. *Arch Dermatol* **84**:717, 1961.
131. Baden HP, Pathak MA: The metabolism and function of urocanic acid in skin. *J Invest Dermatol* **48**:11, 1967.
132. Zenisek A, Hais IM, Strych A, Kral JA: Does solar irradiation affect the natural antisunburn properties of the skin? *Fr Ses Parfums* **12**:131, 1969.
133. Wadia AS, Sule SM, Mathur GP: Epidermal urocanic acid & histidase of albino guineapig following total body UV-irradiation. *Indian J Exp Biol* **13**:234, 1975.
134. Ohnishi S, Nishijima Y, Hasegawa I, Futagoishi H: Study of urocanic acid in the human skin surface (II): Geometrical isomers and sunscreen effect. *J Soc Cosmet Chem Jpn* **13**:61, 1979.
135. El-Ghorr AA, Norval M: A monoclonal antibody to *cis*-urocanic acid prevents the ultraviolet induced changes in Langerhans cells and delayed hypersensitivity responses in mice, although not preventing dendritic cell accumulation in lymph nodes draining the site of irradiation and contact hypersensitivity responses. *J Invest Dermatol* **105**:264, 1995.
136. Baden HP, Hori Y, Pathak MA, Levy HL: Epidermis in histidinemia. *Arch Dermatol* **100**:432, 1969.
137. De Fabo EC, Noonan FP: Mechanism of immune suppression by ultraviolet irradiation in vivo: I. Evidence for the existence of a unique photoreceptor in skin and its role in photoimmunology. *J Exp Med* **157**:84, 1983.
138. Fisher, MS, Kripke ML: Systemic alteration induced in mice by ultraviolet light irradiation and its relationship to ultraviolet carcinogenesis. *Proc Natl Acad Sci USA* **74**:1688, 1977.
139. Spellman CW, Daynes RA: Modification of immunological potential by ultraviolet radiation: II. Generation of suppressor cells in short-term UV-irradiated mice. *Transplantation* **24**:120, 1977.
140. Agin P, Rose AP, Lane CC, Akin FJ, Sayre RM: Changes in epidermal forward scattering absorption after UVA or UVA-UVB irradiation. *J Invest Dermatol* **76**:174, 1981.
141. Fisher MS, Kripke ML: Further studies on the tumor-specific suppressor cells induced by ultraviolet radiation. *J Immunol* **121**:1139, 1978.
142. Noonan FP, De Fabo EC, Kripke ML: Suppression of contact hypersensitivity by UV radiation and its relationship to UV-induced suppression of tumor immunity. *Photochem Photobiol* **34**:683, 1981.
143. Fisher MS, Kripke ML: Suppressor T lymphocytes control the development of primary skin cancers in ultraviolet-irradiated mice. *Science* **216**:1133, 1982.
144. Greene MI, Sy MS, Kripke ML, Benacerraf B: Impairment of antigen-presenting cell function by ultraviolet radiation. *Proc Natl Acad Sci USA* **76**:6591, 1979.
145. Noonan FP, Kripke ML, Pedersen GM, Greene MI: Suppression of contact hypersensitivity in mice by ultraviolet irradiation is associated with defective antigen presentation. *Immunology* **43**:527, 1981.
146. Howie S, Norval M, Maingay J: Exposure to low-dose ultraviolet radiation suppresses delayed-type hypersensitivity to herpes simplex virus in mice. *J Invest Dermatol* **86**:125, 1986.
147. Howie SEM, Norval M, Maingay J, Ross JA: Two phenotypically distinct T cells (Lyl+2- and Lyl-2+) are involved in ultraviolet-B light-induced suppression of the efferent DTH response to HSV-1 in vivo. *Immunology* **58**:653, 1986.
148. Howie SEM, Norval M, Maingay J: Alterations in epidermal handling of HSV-1 antigens in vitro induced by in vivo exposure to UV-B light. *Immunology* **57**:225, 1986.
149. Ross JA, Howie SEM, Norval M, Maingay J, Simpson TJ: Ultraviolet-irradiated urocanic acid suppresses delayed-type hypersensitivity to herpes simplex virus in mice. *J Invest Dermatol* **87**:630, 1986.
150. Ross JA, Howie SEM, Norval M, Maingay J: Two phenotypically distinct T cells are involved in ultraviolet-irradiated urocanic acid-induced suppression of the efferent delayed-type hypersensitivity response to herpes simplex virus, type 1 in vivo. *J Invest Dermatol* **89**:230, 1987.
151. Ross JA, Howie SEM, Norval M, Maingay J: Systemic administration of urocanic acid generates suppression of the delayed type hypersensitivity response to herpes simplex virus in a murine model of infection. *Photodermatology* **5**:9, 1988.
152. Noonan FP, De Fabo EC: Ultraviolet-B dose-response curves for local and systemic immunosuppression are identical. *Photochem Photobiol* **52**:801, 1990.
153. De Fabo EC, Noonan FP, Fisher M, Burns J, Kacser H: Further evidence that the photoreceptor mediating UV-induced systemic immune suppression is urocanic acid. *J Invest Dermatol* **80**:319, 1983.
154. Reeve VE, Greenoak GE, Canfield PJ, Boehm-Wilcox C, Gallagher CH: Topical urocanic acid enhances UV-induced tumour yield and malignancy in the hairless mouse. *Photochem Photobiol* **49**:459, 1989.
155. Gruner SV, Stoppe H, Eckert R, Sönnichsen N, Diezel W: Verlangerung der Transplantatüberlebenszeit durch eine PUVA-Behandlung des Transplantatempfangers: Bedeutung von cis-Urocäninsaure. *Dermatol Mon.schr* **176**:49, 1990.
156. Oesterwitz H, Gruner S, Diezel W, Schneider W: Inhibition of rat heart allograft rejection by a PUVA treatment of the graft recipient: Role of *cis*-urocanic acid. *Transplant Int* **3**:8, 1990.

157. Norval M, Simpson TJ, Bardshiri E, Howie SEM: Urocanic acid analogues and the suppression of the delayed type hypersensitivity response to herpes simplex virus. *Photochem Photobiol* **49**:633, 1989.
158. De Fabo EC, Noonan FP, Frederick JE: Biologically effective doses of sunlight for immune suppression at various latitudes and their relationship to changes in stratospheric ozone. *Photochem Photobiol* **52**:811, 1990.
159. Kripke ML: Photoimmunology. *Photochem Photobiol* **52**:919, 1990.
160. Witkop CJ Jr, Henry FV: Sjogren-Larsson syndrome and histidinemia: Hereditary biochemical diseases with defects of speech and oral functions. *J Speech Hear Disord* **28**:109, 1963.
161. Ghadimi H, Partington MW: Salient features of histidinemia. *Am J Dis Child* **113**:83, 1967.
162. Lott IT, Wheelden JA, Levy HL: Speech and histidinemia: Methodology and evaluation of four cases. *Dev Med Child Neurol* **12**:596, 1970.
163. Gordon N: Delayed speech and histidinaemia. *Dev Med Child Neurol* **12**:104, 1970.
164. Alfi OS, Shaw KNF, Fishler K, Wenz E: Histidinemia: Follow-up of 13 patients. *Am J Hum Genet* **30**:20A, 1978.
165. Tada K, Tateda H, Arashima S, Sakai K, Kitagawa T, Aoki K, Suwa S, et al: Intellectual development in patients with untreated histidinemia. *J Pediatr* **101**:562, 1982.
166. Ishikawa M: Developmental disorders in histidinemia: Follow-up study of language development in histidinemia. *Acta Paediatr Jpn* **29**:224, 1987.
167. Widhalm K, Virmani K: Long-term follow-up of 58 patients with histidinemia treated with a histidine-restricted diet: No effect of therapy. *Pediatrics* **94**:861, 1994.
168. Thalhammer O: Histidinemia, in Naruse H, Irie M (eds): *Neonatal Screening*. Amsterdam, Excerpta Medica, 1983, p 298.
169. Popkin JS, Scriver CR, Clow CL, Grove J: Is hereditary histidinaemia harmful? *Lancet* **1**:721, 1974.
170. Rosenmann A, Scriver CR, Clow CL, Levy HL: Histidinaemia: Part II. Impact: A retrospective study. *J Inherited Metab* Dis **6**:54, 1983.
171. Scriver CR, Levy HL: Histidinaemia: Part I. Reconciling retrospective and prospective findings. *J Inherited Metab Dis* **6**:51, 1983.
172. Duncan JS, Brown P, Marsden CD: Progressive myoclonus and histidinaemia. *Mov Disord* **6**:87, 1991.
173. Appleton RE, Chitayat D, Jan JE, Kennedy R, Hall JG: Joubert's syndrome associated with congenital ocular fibrosis and histidinemia. *Arch Neurol* **46**:579, 1989.
174. Nishino M, Arita K, Kikuchi K, Takarada T, Kinouchi A, Kamada K, Abe N, et al: Hypoplasia of tooth in children with inborn errors of metabolism. *Shoni Shikagaku Zasshi* **28**:503, 1990.
175. Lucca A, Catalano M, Valsasina R, Fara C, Smeraldi E: Biochemical investigation of histidinemia in schizophrenic patients. *Biol Psychiatry* **27**:69, 1990.
176. Nobile M, Maffei P, Nothen MM, Rietschel M, Smeraldi E, Catalano M: Association study of schizophrenia and the histidase gene. *Psychiatr Genet* **7**:107, 1997.
177. Khanna R, Chang TMS: Characterization of L-histidine ammonia-lyase immobilized by microencapsulation in artificial cells: Preparation, kinetics, stability, and in vitro depletion of histidine. *Int J Artif Organs* **13**:189, 1990.
178. Levy HL: Genetic screening. *Adv Hum Genet* **4**:1, 1973.
179. Alm J, Holmgren G, Larsson A, Schimpfessel L: Histidinaemia in Sweden: Report on a neonatal screening programme. *Clin Genet* **20**:229, 1981.
180. Amador PS, Carter TP: Historical review of newborn screening in New York state: Twenty years experience, in Carter TP, Willey AM (eds): *Genetic Disease: Screening and Management*. New York, Alan R Liss, 1986, p 343.
181. Tada K, Tateda H, Arashima S, Sakai K, Kitagawa T, Aoki K, Suwa S, et al: Follow-up study of a nation-wide neonatal metabolic screening program in Japan. *Eur J Pediatr* **142**:204, 1984.
182. Levy HL, Madigan PM, Shih VE: Massachusetts metabolic disorders screening program: I. Technics and results of urine screening. *Pediatrics* **49**:825, 1972.
183. Lemieux B, Auray-Blais C, Giguere R, Shapcott D, Scriver CR: Newborn urine screening experience with over one million infants in Quebec network of genetic medicine. *J Inherited Metab Dis* **11**:45, 1988.
184. Pieniazek D, Stecko E, Kubalska J, Krassowska A, Zychowicz K: Metabolism of histidine in children with speech abnormalities. *Acta Med Pol* **26**:27, 1985.
185. Raisova V, Hyanek J: Speech disorders associated with histidinemia and other hereditary disorders of amino acid metabolism. *Folia Phoniatr (Basel)* **38**:43, 1986.
186. Anakura M, Matsuda I, Arashima S, Fukushima N, Oka Y: Histidinemia: Classical and atypical form in siblings. *Am J Dis Child* **129**:858, 1975.
187. Kuroda Y, Watanabe T, Ito M, Takeda E, Toshima K, Miyao M: Genetic heterogeneity of histidinemia detected by screening newborn infants in Japan. *Jpn J Hum Genet* **30**:287, 1985.
188. Guldberg P, Levy HL, Koch R, Berlin CM, Francois B, Henriksen KF, Guttler F: Mutation analysis in families with discordant phenotypes of phenylalanine hydroxylase deficiency: Inheritance and expression of the hyperphenylalaninaemias. *J Inherited Metab Dis* **17**:645, 1994.
189. Levy HL: Effect of mutation on maternal-fetal metabolic homeostasis: Maternal aminoacidopathies, in Lloyd JK, Scriver CR (eds): *Genetic and Metabolic Disease in Pediatrics*. London, Butterworth, 1985, p 250.
190. Vargas JE, Levy HL: Maternal and fetal considerations in metabolic disorders. *J Jpn Soc Mass Screen* **8**(suppl 1):29, 1998.
191. Bruckman C, Berry HK, Dasenbrock RJ: Histidinemia in two successive generations. *Am J Dis Child* **119**:221, 1970.
192. Neville BGR, Harris RF, Stern DJ, Stern J: Maternal histidinaemia. *Arch Dis Child* **46**:119, 1971.
193. Lyon ICT, Gardner RJM, Veale AMO: Maternal histidinaemia. *Arch Dis Child* **49**:581, 1974.
194. Armstrong MD: Maternal histidinaemia. *Arch Dis Child* **50**:830, 1975.
195. Matsuda I, Nagata N, Endo F: A family with histidinemic parents. *J Pediatr* **103**:169, 1983.
196. Levy HL, Benjamin R: Maternal histidinemia: Study of families identified by routine cord blood screening. *Pediatr Res* **19**:250A, 1985.
197. Kacser H, Mya KM, Duncker M, Wright AF, Bulfield G, McLaren A, Lyon MF: Maternal histidine metabolism and its effect on foetal development in the mouse. *Nature* **265**:262, 1977.
198. Kacser H, Mya KM, Bulfield G: Endogenous teratogenesis in maternal histidinaemia, in Hommes FA (ed): *Models for the Study of Inborn Errors of Metabolism*. Amsterdam, Elsevier, 1979, p 43.
199. Burns JE, Kacser H: Genetic effects on susceptibility to histidine induced teratogenesis in the mouse. *Genet Res* **50**:147, 1987.
200. Kamoun PP, Parvy P, Cathelineau L, Meyer B: Renal histidinuria. *J Inherited Metab Dis* **4**:217, 1981.
201. Holmgren G, Hambraeus L, De Chateau P: Histidinemia and "normohistidinemic histidinuria": Report of three cases and the effect of different protein intakes on urinary excretions of histidine. *Acta Paediatr Scand* **63**:220, 1974.
202. Sabater J, Ferre C, Puliol M, Maya A: Histidinuria: A renal and intestinal histidine transport deficiency found in two mentally retarded children. *Clin Genet* **9**:117, 1976.
203. Nyhan WL, Hilton S: Histidinuria: Defective transport of histidine. *Am J Med Genet* **44**:558, 1992.
204. Scriver CR, Tenenhouse HS: Mendelian phenotypes as "probes" of renal transport systems for amino acids and phosphate, in Windhager E (ed): *Handbook of Physiology*. Section 8: *Renal Physiology*. New York, Oxford University Press, 1992, p 1977.
205. Van Gennip AH, Rajnherc J, De Bree PK, Wadman SK: "Urocanase deficiency" in a 7-year-old boy with psychomotor retardation, in *Soc Study IEM, Lyon, France, 6–9 September 1983*, p 119.
206. Hug DH, Roth D, Hunter J: Regulation of histidine catabolism by succinate in *Pseudomonas putida*. *J Bacteriol* **96**:396, 1968.
207. Swenson EF, Walraven C, Levy HL: A 25 year experience with newborn urine screening [abstr], in *Ninth National Neonatal Screening Symposium, April 7–11, Raleigh, NC,* 1992, p 69.

CHAPTER 81

Disorders of Proline and Hydroxyproline Metabolism

James M. Phang ▪ Chien-an A. Hu ▪ David Valle

1. **Δ^1-Pyrroline-5-carboxylate (P5C) is both the immediate precursor and the degradation product of proline and is found not only intracellularly but also circulating in plasma. P5C reductase (EC 1.5.1.2) catalyzes the conversion of P5C to proline as the committed step in biosynthesis. Proline oxidase (no EC number assigned) catalyzes the degradation of proline to P5C. Other sources of P5C are ornithine and glutamate in reactions catalyzed by ornithine-δ-aminotransferase (OAT) (EC 2.6.1.13) and P5C synthase (no EC number assigned), respectively. The P5C "outflow" is primarily to glutamate in a reaction catalyzed by P5C dehydrogenase (EC 1.5.1.12). The interconversions of P5C and proline constitute a cycle for transferring reducing-oxidizing potential between cellular organelles and between tissues.**
2. **Two inherited disorders in the degradative limb of the proline metabolic system result in hyperprolinemia. Type I hyperprolinemia (HPI) (MIM 239500) is caused by deficiency of proline oxidase, and type II hyperprolinemia (HPII) (MIM 239510) is due to a deficiency of P5C dehydrogenase; both are apparently inherited as autosomal recessive traits. Proline levels are elevated three- to fivefold in the former condition and ten- to fifteenfold in the latter. The distinguishing biochemical characteristics in HPII are high plasma P5C levels and urinary excretion of P5C.**
3. **Although the metabolic derangements in the hyperprolinemias are consistent with normal adult life, there appears to be a causal relationship between HPII and neurologic manifestations in childhood. Attempts at therapy by nutritional manipulation have been ineffective because the interconversions of the precursors makes it impossible to lower P5C or proline to any significant degree.**
4. **A newly recognized disorder apparently related to the synthetic limb of this metabolic system has been described in two sibs with mental retardation, cataracts, joint hyperlaxity, and skin hyperelasticity. The biochemical phenotype, which includes hypoprolinemia, hypocitrullinemia, hypoornithinemia, and hyperammonemia, is consistent with a deficiency of P5C synthase. No direct measurements of P5C synthase activity in tissues from these patients have been described.**
5. **4-Hydroxy-L-proline is not synthesized as the free imino acid. Rather, it is produced by hydroxylation of the third-position proline in the prevalent Gly-Pro-Pro tripeptide of the procollagen polypeptide chain. Free hydroxyproline is derived from endogenous collagen turnover and from breakdown of dietary collagen. The hydroxyproline degradation pathway resembles that of proline. Δ^1-Pyrroline-3-hydroxy-5-carboxylate, the oxidation product of hydroxyproline, is dehydrogenated to 4-erythro-hydroxy-L-glutamate. Transamination with oxaloacetate results in 4-hydroxy-2-ketoglutarate, which is then cleaved to glyoxalate and pyruvate in an aldolase reaction. The enzymes catalyzing these reactions are distinct from those for the degradation of proline, with one exception: dehydrogenation of P5C and hydroxy-P5C is catalyzed by the same enzyme, P5C dehydrogenase.**
6. **Hyperhydroxyprolinemia (MIM 237000) is an autosomal recessive trait resulting from a deficiency of hydroxyproline oxidase (no EC number assigned). This biochemical disturbance apparently has no clinical consequence. The metabolism of proline and collagen are normal.**

Because proline and hydroxyproline have only one hydrogen atom attached to the nitrogen atom inserted in a pyrrolidine ring (Fig. 81-1), they are usually referred to by the trivial name "imino acid." L-Proline is a major constituent in the extracellular pool of amino acids, rivaled in concentration only by glutamine and alanine. Hydroxy-L-proline, however, is found primarily as an oligopeptide in body fluids. The principal form of hydroxyproline in humans is 4-hydroxy-L-proline, and its major source is the degradation of dietary and endogenous collagen; 3-hydroxy-L-proline is present in much smaller amounts in body fluids, and its source is collagen found in basement membranes. In contrast to proline, free hydroxyproline is not incorporated into protein; instead, it is formed by hydroxylation of peptide-linked proline in nascent collagen polypeptide chains. Intracellular synthesis and degradation of free proline occur through metabolic pathways forming related intermediates (Fig. 81-2). Although the metabolism of free hydroxyproline occurs through analogous pathways, they are of less quantitative significance (Fig. 81-3).

Several Mendelian disorders of imino acid metabolism are known, and they have helped to elucidate the corresponding metabolic relationships in humans. The hyperprolinemias constitute two separate disorders: type I (HPI) (MIM 239500) results from deficiency of proline oxidase; type II (HPII) (MIM 239510) results from deficiency of Δ^1-pyrroline-5-carboxylate (P5C) dehydrogenase. Although these have been considered benign disorders, accumulating evidence suggests that the metabolic abnormalities, at least in HPII, cause clinical manifestations. Hyperhydroxyprolinemia (MIM 237000) is a disorder of free hydroxyproline catabolism, involving the step catalyzed by hydroxyproline oxidase. Hydroxyproline metabolism also is compromised in HPII, but only its pyrroline metabolites accumulate in this disorder. The recent identification of a new syndrome with hypoprolinemia in two sibs with presumed P5C synthase deficiency (MIM 138250) is of interest.[1,2] Additional metabolic and molecular investigation of this disorder promises to

A list of standard abbreviations is located immediately preceding the index in each volume. Additional abbreviations used in this chapter include: HPI = Type 1 hyperprolinemia; HPII = Type 2 hyperprolinemia; OAT = ornithine--aminotransferase; P5C = ^{1}-pyrroline-5-carboxylate.

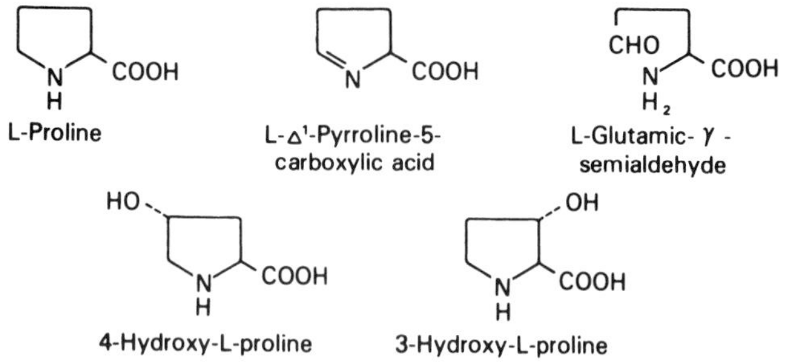

L-Proline L-Δ¹-Pyrroline-5-carboxylic acid L-Glutamic-γ-semialdehyde

4-Hydroxy-L-proline 3-Hydroxy-L-proline

Fig. 81-1 Schematic structures for proline, intermediates in the proline metabolic pathways, and the two forms of hydroxyproline found in mammalian tissues.

provide better understanding of the proline and ornithine biosynthetic pathways.

METABOLISM OF THE IMINO ACIDS

Although nonessential amino acids can be synthesized endogenously, their synthetic pathways often are not utilized to provide substrates for protein synthesis because the amino acid products are also available from dietary protein. The synthetic processes, however, may serve other metabolic functions.[3] For example, the pathways of alanine, serine, aspartate and glutamine synthesis play essential roles in fasting fuel homeostasis.[4] Proline, which can be synthesized either from glutamate or ornithine, is nonessential for full-term human infants and adults,[3,5] and conditionally indispensable for premature neonates.[6,7] As with other nonessential amino acids, the synthetic reactions and related interconversions of proline have additional metabolic functions.[8] These functions are possible, in part, because of the unique structure of proline (Fig. 81-1). Unlike other amino acids, proline has no primary amino group and is excluded from the pyridoxal-5-phosphate coenzyme-catalyzed decarboxylation and transamination reactions, which are otherwise of general importance for amino acid metabolism. Instead, proline is metabolized by reactions catalyzed by a distinctive set of enzymes with properties and regulatory mechanisms independent of those for other amino acids (Fig. 81-2).

Some of the special functions performed by proline metabolism have been elucidated in model organisms. For example, proline can serve as a defense against osmotic challenge in prokaryotes[9,10] and plants;[11,12] as a redox shuttle in insects;[13] and as a mediator of parasite-induced pathophysiology in mammalian hosts.[14] For certain cultured mammalian cells, proline appears essential for a mitogenic response.[15] Recent work with human colorectal cancer cells suggests the conversion of proline to P5C by proline oxidase may play a role in p53-induced apoptosis.[16] Although the mechanisms mediating these seemingly unrelated phenomena are not well-understood, these aspects of proline metabolism emphasize functions for this metabolic system over and above provision of proline as a substrate for protein synthesis.

In mammalian cells, one of the special functions of the proline system may include cellular regulation by redox mechanisms. Pyrroline-5-carboxylate (P5C), the intermediate common to both synthetic and degradative pathways for proline, constitutes a redox couple with proline (Fig. 81-2).[8,17] These two substances participate in a metabolic interlock linked to the NADPH/NADP$^+$ redox couple and the pentose phosphate shunt[8,18–21] (see "Metabolic Functions of the Proline Pathways" below). The interlock occurs across cellular membranes with the transfer of P5C. Similarly, when linked with the NADH/NAD$^+$ redox couple, the metabolic interlock serves as a redox shuttle. How these interlocks relate to the proline effects listed above remains unclear. Nevertheless, the enzymes of proline synthesis and degradation, and their localization and regulation, must be considered with these metabolic functions as an end-point.

Interestingly, L-proline also fulfills several of the classic criteria used to define neurotransmitters in the mammalian central nervous system including biosynthesis in synaptosomes,[22] uptake into synaptosomes by an high-affinity system,[23–25] and release after K$^+$-induced depolarization.[26] Moreover, a mammalian brain-specific proline transporter has been cloned and shown to be expressed in subpopulations of cells mediating putative glutamatergic pathways[27–29] (see "Transport of Imino Acid in Mammalian Central Nervous System" below).

Proline Synthesis

Ornithine and glutamate are the precursors of proline, with P5C or glutamic-γ-semialdehyde (the uncyclized tautomer, with which P5C is in spontaneous equilibrium) as the common intermediate.[30–35] Ornithine-δ-aminotransferase (OAT) catalyzes the conversion of ornithine to P5C, with an α-ketoacid, such as α-ketoglutarate, as the amino acceptor. OAT is localized to the mitochondrial matrix[33] and found in all tissues with the notable

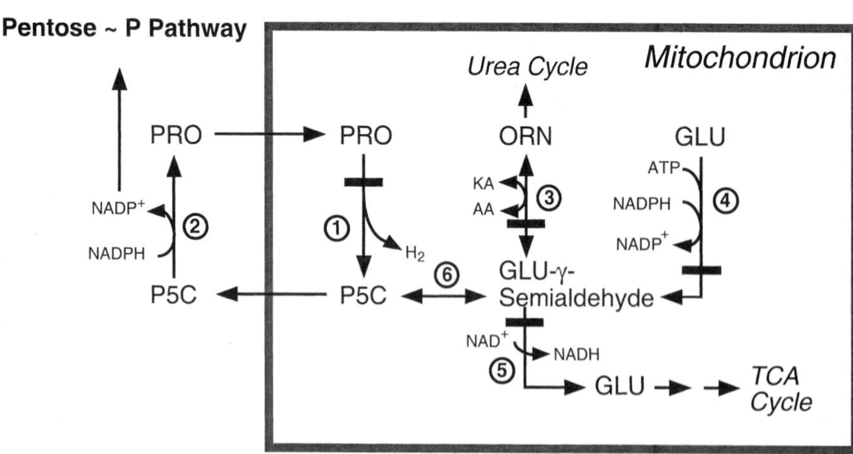

Cytosol

1. **Proline Oxidase (Type I Hyperprolinemia)**
2. **P5C Reductase**
3. **Ornithine Aminotransferase (Gyrate Atrophy)**
4. **P5C Synthase (Deficiency of P5C Synthase)**
5. **P5C Dehydrogenase (Type II Hyperprolinemia)**
6. **Non-Enzymatic**

Fig. 81-2 Composite summary of the proline metabolic pathways in mammalian tissues. The complete system is present only in certain tissues (see text). The shaded area represents mitochondria.

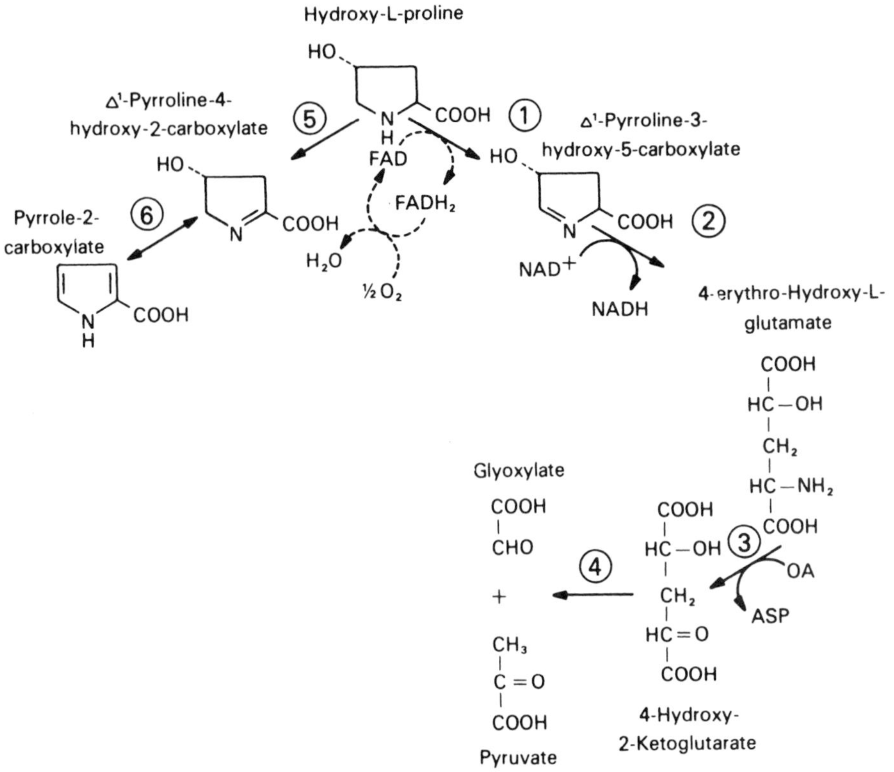

Fig. 81-3 The pathways for the degradation of 4-hydroxy-L-proline in mammalian tissues. Major pathway: Although reaction (1) is analogous to that for proline oxidation, it is catalyzed by an enzyme distinct from that for proline. Reaction (2) is catalyzed by a dehydrogenase common to the hydroxyproline and proline pathways. The enzymes are (1) hydroxy-L-proline oxidase (EC number not assigned); (2) Δ^1-pyrroline-3-hydroxy-5-carboxylate dehydrogenase (EC 1.6.1.12); (3) glutamic-oxaloacetate aminotransferase (probably EC 2.6.1.1); and (4) 4-hydroxy-2-oxoglutarate lyase (EC 4.1.3.16). Minor pathway: Reaction (5) is catalyzed by L-amino acid oxidase and reaction (6) is spontaneous. Pyrrole-2-carboxylate accumulates in the urine of patients with a defect in the major pathway at the level of the dehydrogenase (HPII).

exception of circulating erythrocytes (Table 81-1).[19,36] The biochemical and molecular features of OAT, its role in metabolism and the consequences of its deficiency, are discussed in Chap. 83.

P5C synthase, a mitochondrial inner membrane, ATP, and NADPH-dependent bifunctional enzyme, catalyzes the production of P5C from glutamate (Table 81-1). The reaction involves an initial phosphorylation of the γ-carboxyl group of glutamate catalyzed by the γ-glutamyl kinase activity of P5C synthase followed by reduction of the glutamylphosphate group to P5C catalyzed by the γ-glutamylphosphate reductase activity of P5C synthase. Interestingly, in prokaryotes and certain unicellular eukaryotes (e.g., *S. cerevisiae*) these reactions are catalyzed by two separate proteins encoded by two different genes.[37–39] In mammals, P5C synthase activity is highest in small intestinal mucosa[40–44] with measurable activity in colon, pancreas, thymus, and brain.[44]

P5C is not only a common intracellular intermediate in proline metabolism but also a constituent of human plasma. Levels fluctuate diurnally by up to tenfold, from a low of 0.2 mM in the early morning to a high of about 2.0 mM in the late evening. The peaks are associated with meals and are abolished by fasting, but the exact dietary precursor has not been established. No other amino acid shows such diurnal variations.[45]

Given that P5C is an extracellular metabolite, it is not surprising that it has a special cellular uptake mechanism. This mechanism has been shown to be a saturable, high capacity, energy-dependent system independent of sodium ion and not shared by other naturally occurring amino acids.[46] Evidence suggests that it is a group translocation mechanism linked to the oxidation of pyridine nucleotides.

P5C reductase, which catalyzes the conversion of P5C to proline with either NADH or NADPH as cofactor,[47–49] is found in

Table 81-1 Some Characteristics of Human Enzymes of Proline Metabolism

	P5C synthase	P5C reductase	OAT	Proline oxidase	P5C dehydrogenase
EC	None	EC1.5.1.2	EC2.6.1.13	None	EC1.5.1.12
Subcellular location	Mitochondrial inner membrane	Cytoplasm ? membrane assoc.	Mitochondrial matrix	Mitochondrial inner membrane	Mitochondrial matrix
Subunit size (kDa)	81	32, 35	49	63	62
Structure	Hexamer	Homopolymer	Homohexamer	Unknown	Homodimer
Cofactors	ATP, NAD(P)H	NAD(P)H	Pyridoxal phosphate	Unknown	NAD+
Activity in tissues	Small intestine mucosa, colon, pancreas, brain thymus	Ubiquitous	Ubiquitous	Liver, kidney & brain	Ubiquitous
Disease association	Hypoprolinemia	—	Gyrate atrophy	HPI	HPII
Comments	Two isoforms result from alternative splicing; short isoform inhibited by ornithine	Two isoforms encoded by separate genes	—	Inhibited by lactate	—

all tissues (Fig. 81-2; Table 81-1).[36] The enzyme has been purified from rat retina[50] and from human erythrocytes.[51] Interestingly, the turnover number of P5C reductase is several log values higher than for most "housekeeping" enzymes. Thus, despite considerable specific activity in most tissues, the abundance of enzyme protein is very low.[51] The observation that the V_{max} of P5C reductase is higher with NADH than with NADPH led originally to the conclusion that NADH is its preferred cofactor.[47,48] However, the affinity for NADPH is much higher, and the affinity for P5C also is higher in the presence of NADPH. Studies using purified reductase with differentially labeled P5C and NADPH confirmed that P5C reductase preferentially uses NADPH. In fact, differential utilization of pyridine nucleotide and regulation by oxidized $NADP^+$ suggest that the enzyme functions, in part, as a P5C-dependent NADPH dehydrogenase. The recent identification of two closely related P5C reductase genes, both encoding functional reductase enzymes, suggest that some of the kinetic differences of P5C reductase activities isolated from different tissues may reflect variable expression of the two genes in these tissues (see "Molecular Biology of Proline Metabolic Enzymes" below).[52,53] The functional linkage between the cellular entry of P5C and its reduction suggested that P5C reductase may be associated with the plasma membrane (Phang, J.M., unpublished results).

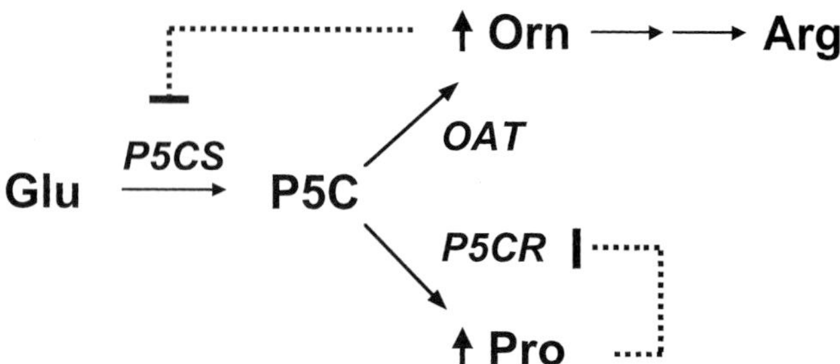

Fig. 81-4 Model for the regulation of mammalian proline and arginine biosynthesis in different tissues. The pathway for arginine biosynthesis in the small intestinal mucosa is shown above. In this tissue, the short isoform of P5C synthase predominates and is subject to feedback inhibition by ornithine. In peripheral tissues (bottom) the pathway serves to synthesize proline. In these tissues, the long isoform of P5C synthase predominates and is insensitive to ornithine. The pathway appears to be regulated by proline inhibition of P5C reductase.

Proline Degradation

The first step in proline degradation is catalyzed by proline oxidase (Fig. 81-2; Table 81-1). The enzyme is tightly bound to the mitochondrial inner membrane and is found primarily in liver, kidney, and brain. With a few exceptions, proline oxidase activity is undetectable in cultured cells.[54–57] Proline oxidase can be solubilized by treatment with detergents, but it has not been purified.[58] Functionally, electrons donated by proline enter the mitochondrial electron transport chain, probably through an intervening flavoprotein.[59]

P5C produced from proline as well as from the synthetic pathways can be degraded to glutamate by P5C dehydrogenase. This widely expressed enzyme is localized primarily to the mitochondrial matrix (Fig. 81-2; Table 81-1).[60,61] The human enzyme has been purified from liver as a "high K_m" aldehyde dehydrogenase whose preferential substrate was subsequently identified as glutamic-γ-semialdehyde; that is, P5C. Similarly, the enzyme purified from rat liver mitochondrial matrix was found to exhibit activity with other aldehydes.[62]

Metabolic Functions of the Proline Pathways

Recent advances have expanded our understanding of the regulation of this multipurpose system at a crossroads of amino acid metabolism involving interconversions of glutamate, ornithine, and proline. One important function of this system is to supply proline for protein synthesis. An increase in the activities of the enzymes of proline synthesis correlates with an increase in the demand for proline.[40] Furthermore, the flux of proline production can be directly controlled by negative feedback inhibition of P5C reductase, which catalyzes the irreversible step in proline synthesis[63] (Fig. 81-4). Additionally, proline can be utilized for hepatic gluconeogenesis and the induction of proline oxidase by glucocorticoids is consistent with this function.[58,64] A third metabolic function for proline is as a precursor for synthesis of ornithine and arginine with P5C as an intermediate (Fig. 81-2) (see "Cell-Specific Patterns of Proline and Arginine Metabolism in Small Intestine" below).

These amino acid interconversions do not, however, explain other features of proline metabolism.[59,65,66] For example, the purified P5C reductase from human erythrocytes[49] uses NADPH as the preferred cofactor. In contrast to the NADH-mediated activity, the NADPH-mediated activity is insensitive to inhibition by proline. Importantly, $NADP^+$ is a potent inhibitor of both NADH and NADPH activities.[49,51] These observations led us to propose that the regulation based on the $NADPH/NADP^+$ redox couple may be an important function of proline metabolism. Moreover, that proline and its interconversions function as a unique mechanism for redox balance and as a mediator of redox-dependent mechanisms.[8]

Unlike $NADH/NAD^+$, the $NADPH/NADP^+$ redox couple does not play a significant role in energy transfer. Its role appears to be that of a defense mechanism against deleterious redox perturbations[67] or a mediator of cellular events.[68] The latter role has received increasing attention because several transcription factors may be regulated through redox mechanism.[69,70] Because P5C reductase appears to be intimately associated with the $NADPH/NADP^+$ redox couple, we examined the effects of added P5C on metabolic pathways regulated by this redox couple. In human red cells,[19] as well as in a variety of cultured cells,[20] P5C transfers oxidizing potential across cell membranes to stimulate the flux through the oxidative arm of the pentose phosphate shunt (Fig. 81-2; see also Fig. 30-4 in the seventh edition of this work). In fact, in red cells the flux through the pentose phosphate shunt is stoichiometrically coupled to the conversion of P5C to proline.[71] By stimulating the flux through the shunt, P5C increases the production of phosphoribosyl pyrophosphate and purine nucleotides (Fig. 81-2).[35,49,71,72] In vivo studies using mouse liver also confirm that P5C stimulates phosphoribosyl pyrophosphate generation.[73,74] These studies establish that P5C, as an extracellular metabolite,[45] enters the cell through its own carrier systems[46] and transfers oxidizing potential into the cell. The effects on cellular regulation may include an interaction with growth factor postreceptor events[8,49,75] and, perhaps, with other mechanisms. A recent, interesting example of P5C as a redox mediator through the pentose phosphate shunt was demonstrated in meiotic induction in cumulus cell-enclosed mouse oocytes.[76] On the physiological level, P5C may serve as a nutritionally responsive intercellular communicator for cell regulation.

Proline and P5C may also play an important function in redox transfer between cellular compartments. Because of the cellular localization and tissue distribution of the enzymes that catalyze the interconversions of P5C and proline (i.e., proline oxidase is in the mitochondrial inner membrane, whereas P5C reductase is cytosolic), a proline-P5C cycle can be demonstrated to transfer redox potential between cellular compartments[17,76–79] and, indeed, between cells of different types (Fig. 81-2).[79] The recent observation that p53-induced apoptosis in colorectal cancer cells includes induction of proline oxidase is of special interest especially because redox mechanisms seem to be central in programmed cell death.[16] Whether proline and P5C-mediated mechanisms are directly involved in apoptosis merits additional study.

Cell-Specific Patterns of Proline and Arginine Metabolism in Small Intestine

As predicted by the early studies of Windmueller and Spaeth,[80] recent studies in pigs,[81–83] rats,[84,85] and mice[86–88] show that the epithelium of small intestine plays a crucial role in the synthesis of arginine and proline, particularly in pre- and early postnatal life[89,90] (see also Chaps. 83 and 85). Small intestine epithelial cells have the enzymatic components necessary for the *de novo* synthesis of citrulline and arginine from glutamate.[80,89,91] P5CS activity is high in small intestine mucosa[34,40,44] as is OAT, especially during the neonatal period.[88] The enzymes of the proximal urea cycle (carbamyl phosphate synthetase I [CPSI], ornithine transcarbamylase [OTC], arginine succinate synthase, and arginosuccinate lyase) are expressed in these cells and, importantly, arginase activity is low especially during the neonatal period. Thus, the epithelium of the small intestine has the enzymatic machinery to serve as an organ for citrulline and arginine synthesis. Furthermore, De Jonge et al.[85] showed that genes encoding these enzymes are highly expressed in rat small intestine during perinatal development in a spatiotemporally regulated manner. Proline also appears to be an important precursor for the intestinal synthesis of citrulline and arginine. Wu[82,83] and others[92,93] have shown relatively high activities of proline oxidase in the small intestine and enterocytes of pigs and rats.

This pathway for arginine biosynthesis is vitally important in mice. Interruption of the pathway by targeted disruption of the OAT gene is lethal in mice; affected animals are normal at birth but die between 24 and 48 h after birth despite suckling.[88] Metabolic studies in these mice show low levels of citrulline and arginine, and hyperammonemia secondary to inadequate urea cycle function. The animals can be rescued by intraperitoneal injections of arginine for the first 14 days of life. After this time growth rate slows and dietary arginine apparently is adequate for growth and metabolic homeostasis. Qualitatively similar metabolic changes have been observed in human neonates with OAT deficiency,[88] but rarely are of the extent to cause symptoms in term infants (see Chap. 83). Recent brief reports, however, suggest that in premature human infants, this pathway of arginine biosynthesis is of greater significance and that disruption (e.g., by inherited deficiency of OAT) leads to arginine deficiency and profound hyperammonemia.[94]

4-HYDROXYPROLINE METABOLISM

Biosynthesis

The principal route of 4-hydroxy-L-proline biosynthesis in mammals is the posttranslational hydroxylation of proline in nascent collagen peptides.[95] A peptidyl-proline hydroxylase catalyzes the reaction, and ferrous iron, α-ketoglutarate and O_2 are required. Collagen biosynthesis and proline hydroxylation are discussed in detail in Chap. 205. Free hydroxyproline arises exclusively from the breakdown of hydroxyproline-containing dietary or endogenous proteins and is not used in protein synthesis, as no mammalian transfer RNA for hydroxyproline has been identified.

Other than collagen, hydroxyproline is found in elastin,[96] the C1q component of complement,[97] acetylcholinesterase,[98] and several other partially characterized proteins.[99] Presumably, as in collagen, hydroxyproline in these proteins is formed posttranslationally.

Unlike 4-hydroxyproline, 3-hydroxyproline occurs at extremely low frequencies in interstitial collagen. However, in basement-membrane collagen, 3-hydroxyproline is relatively abundant (25 per 1000 residues). The ratio of 3-hydroxyproline to 4-hydroxyproline has been used to estimate the ratio of basement-membrane collagen to total collagen in tissues.[100] Formation of 3-hydroxyproline, like 4-hydroxyproline, is posttranslational and requires similar cofactors, but it is catalyzed by distinct prolyl hydroxylases.[101]

Degradation

The initial steps in the degradation of free 4-hydroxy-L-proline parallel those for proline (Fig. 81-3). Hydroxyproline is oxidized to Δ^1-pyrroline-3-hydroxy-5-carboxylate by an enzymatic mechanism similar to the one mediating proline oxidation.[99] The pyrroline product is then converted to 4-erythro-hydroxy-L-glutamate by an NAD^+-dependent dehydrogenase,[99] and hydroxyglutamate is subsequently transaminated with oxaloacetate to form 3-hydroxy-2-oxoglutarate.[102] Here the parallelism with proline ends; hydroxyoxoglutarate is cleaved to glyoxylate and pyruvate. Despite the similarities in the reactions for the degradation of the two imino acids, the analogous reactions are catalyzed by distinct enzymes, with one exception—a single enzyme catalyzes the NAD^+-dependent dehydrogenation of both P5C and pyrroline-3-hydroxy-5-carboxylate (see below).[103] Because of the low levels of 3-hydroxyproline, knowledge of its metabolism is limited, but its urinary excretion has been useful as an indication of basement-membrane turnover.[104–106]

Interaction with Proline Metabolism

That the condensation of glyoxylate and pyruvate to form 3-hydroxy-2-oxoglutarate has not been demonstrated in animals makes the *de novo* synthesis of free hydroxyproline unlikely; but the formation of hydroxyproline by reduction of the intermediate pyrroline-3-hydroxy-5-carboxylate occurs in vitro.[99] Although the existence of a common reductase for P5C and pyrroline-3-hydroxy-5-carboxylate has not been proved, it is known that each of these substances inhibits the reduction of the other to its imino acid.[99] A common enzyme catalyzing the dehydrogenation reaction for both pyrroline carboxylates has been described.[103] The affinity for P5C is higher than that for the hydroxylated analogue. The intermediates of hydroxyproline degradation could, however, affect the metabolic flux of the proline intermediates. Whether this mechanism plays a physiological role in the regulation of proline synthesis and degradation is unknown.

DISTRIBUTION OF IMINO ACIDS IN BODY FLUIDS

Free Proline

The normal values for plasma and urine proline are presented in Table 81-2. The mean plasma proline value is lower in growing children than in adults.[107] Beyond the first year of life, virtually no proline is excreted in urine.[108] Neonatal iminoglycinuria is a normal phenomenon due to immaturity of the tubular transport systems for proline reuptake (see Chap. 194). The concentration of proline in cerebrospinal fluid is low (1 to 4 μM).[108] The ratio of mean CSF/plasma proline is about 0.01. Proline is present in human amniotic fluid at an unchanging low concentration throughout pregnancy.

Free Hydroxyproline

Less than 25 percent of the hydroxyproline in plasma is in the free form; the remainder is in peptide linkage.[109,110] The

Table 81-2 Plasma Concentration of Imino Acids

State	Proline†	Hydroxyproline†
Normal*	161 (51–271)	22 (1–46)
HPI	500–2600	Normal
HPII	500–3700	Normal
Hyperhydroxyprolinemia	Normal	150–500
Lactic acidosis	300–1500	NA

†μM
*Normal values measured in children and adults after an overnight fast and expressed as mean (range). For all others, the range is provided.

age-dependent pattern of hydroxyproline excretion in urine parallels that of proline. Hydroxyproline is a negligible constituent of other body fluids.

Urinary Imino Acids in Bound Form

A large literature describes urinary excretion of peptide-bound hydroxyproline and proline.[30,111–116] The ratio of total proline to total hydroxyproline in urine ("total" meaning the sum of the free and bound fractions) rises from an average of about 1.2 in childhood to about 2.4 in adults.[112] Excretion of peptide-bound hydroxyproline increases during periods of rapid growth (infancy and adolescence), reflecting the greater rate of endogenous collagen turnover during growth.[111] Excretion of free hydroxyproline is not increased in late infancy and adolescence because renal reabsorption of imino acids is efficient after early infancy. A wide variety of proline-containing oligopeptides are found in normal urine.[112] The predominant hydroxyproline-containing peptides, prolylhydroxyproline and glycylprolylhydroxyproline, account for 60 to 75 percent of bound hydroxyproline in urine;[111] bound hydroxyproline is 96 percent of total hydroxyproline excretion after early infancy.[113]

MEMBRANE TRANSPORT OF IMINO ACIDS

Iminoglycinuria or urinary excretion of imidodipeptides is a prominent feature of the metabolic phenotype in disorders of imino acid metabolism. Interpretation of these abnormalities requires some knowledge of the renal reabsorption of these substances (see Chap. 194).

Free Imino Acids

Tissues take up L-proline and hydroxy-L-proline by stereospecific, substrate-specific, energy-coupled membrane transport systems,[117–119] which are well documented for kidney and fetal bone.[120,121] The results in kidney delineate the nature of epithelial transport of imino acids; those in fetal bone do the same for a tissue important in collagen synthesis.

In cultured cells, the uptake of proline occurs primarily through system A, which is regulated by both transinhibition and repression mechanisms as well as a variety of hormones.[117–119] Proline may be the most specific substrate for this highly regulated transport system which also transports the nonmetabolizable analogue *N*-methyl-α-aminoisobutyric acid, an imino acid.

In the kidney, proline interacts competitively with hydroxyproline and glycine on a shared carrier in the brush-border membrane of the proximal nephron,[118,119,122,123] which is responsible for uptake at concentrations in excess of 100 μM. A second system is used preferentially by imino acids at solute concentrations below 100 μM.[118,119,122,123]

In the context of human renal physiology, proline[124] and hydroxyproline[125] both have maximum rates of renal tubular absorption (T_m); T_mPro is between 180 and 300 μM/min/1.73 m^2, and T_mHypro is between 60 and 135 μM/min/1.73 m^2. The venous plasma threshold concentration at which prolinuria occurs is about 800 μM proline; for hydroxyprolinuria, it is about 400 μM hydroxyproline. The normal plasma concentration of the two imino acids is well below threshold levels; accordingly, urine is free of imino acids in healthy adults. A "combined" hyperamino-aciduria occurs when the concentration of the specific imino acid exceeds the threshold level. When either imino acid saturates the renal transport system, competition occurs for reabsorption, with displacement of the other imino acid and of glycine. The interaction of proline metabolism with apparent renal reabsorption was demonstrated in Pro/Re mice, which are deficient in proline oxidase (see "Pro/Re Mice" below). In these animals, urinary excretion of proline far exceeds the value expected from the level of proline in plasma. The explanation is that the failure to metabolize proline increases the intracellular pool of proline, which then backfluxes at the luminal membrane.[118,126,127]

Transport of Imino Acids in Mammalian Central Nervous System

L-Proline exhibits several properties similar to those of the well-characterized amino acid neurotransmitters. Circumstantial evidence, such as biosynthesis in synaptosomes,[22] uptake into synaptosomes by an high-affinity Na-dependent system,[23–25] release after K^+-induced depolarization[26] and regional distribution in brain,[24,25] implicates L-proline as a putative synaptic regulatory molecule in the plasticity of certain glutamatergic pathways. Until recently, direct evidence, supporting this role for proline such as specific high-affinity proline receptors and specific inhibitors that block proline biosynthesis, was lacking. In the last few years, however, cloning and study of a mammalian brain high-affinity L-proline transporter (PROT)[27–29,128,129] has reopened the issue of L-proline being a component in excitatory synaptic transmission. The PROT cDNA encodes a 68-kDa glycosylated protein with 12 putative transmembrane domains that exhibits 42 to 50 percent amino acid sequence identity with members of the Na- and Cl-dependent GAT1 family of plasma membrane transporters, which mediate high-affinity uptake of neurotransmitters.[119] Transient and stable expression of PROT in cultured human cells conferred Na-dependent, saturable ($K_m \approx 9.7$ μM) L-proline uptake[27,130,131] with properties corresponding to the high-affinity component of synaptosomal L-proline uptake.[24,132–134] These properties distinguish PROT from the other widely expressed Na-dependent plasma membrane carriers that transport L-proline, including the intestinal brush border "imino" carrier [135] and the system "A" and system "ASC" neutral amino acid carriers.[118,119]

Fremeau and colleagues[27,29,128] have shown that PROT mRNA is expressed by subpopulations of putative glutamatergic neurons in rat brain and the PROT transporter is localized to a subset of excitatory axon terminals forming asymmetric excitatory-type synapses.[129] These findings raise the possibility of a specialized role for PROT and its presumed natural substrate, L-proline, in the modulation of excitatory synaptic transmission in specific excitatory pathways within the central nervous system. High-affinity L-proline uptake may regulate the ability of extracellular proline to potentiate excitatory transmission at those synapses that express PROT.[136] It is also possible that, as in plants,[11,12] L-proline functions as an osmolyte, and that transport of proline by PROT is critical for osmotic homeostasis of synaptic terminals. Additionally, excitotoxic properties of proline may contribute to the possible pathophysiology of neurologic phenotypes of HPI and HPII (see below).

MOLECULAR BIOLOGY OF THE ENZYMES OF PROLINE METABOLISM

Considerable progress has been made in elucidating the molecular biology of the genes encoding the enzymes of proline metabolism since publication of the seventh edition of this book. Here, we briefly review the salient features of this work. Additional molecular details for each gene are presented in Table 81-3 and Fig. 81-5. For details regarding the molecular aspects of OAT, see Chap. 83.

P5C Synthase

Human and murine P5C synthase cDNAs were cloned by homology with the P5C synthase of the plant *Vigna aconitifolia*.[137] Mammalian P5C synthase is a bifunctional protein with an N-terminal γ-glutamyl kinase domain and a C-terminal γ-glutamyl phosphate reductase activity. In yeast, these two activities are encoded in separate genes.[138] The human cDNA can complement mutations in either of the two yeast genes, confirming the bifunctionality of the mammalian enzyme predicted by sequence similarity.[137] The full-length P5C synthase protein has 793 amino acids with an N-terminal 56- or 64-amino acid mitochondrial targeting sequence (Fig. 81-5). Consistent with the first of P5C synthase functions, the N-terminal half of the human protein has 36 percent amino acid identity with the *S. cerevisiae* γ-glutamyl

Table 81-3 Molecular Biology of Proline Metabolic Enzymes in Humans

Enzyme	GenBank accession	Map location	mRNA (kb)	ORF (bp)	Published gene structure
P5CS.long	U76542	10q24.3 to 24.6	3.6	2385	No
P5CS.short	U68758	10q24.3 to 24.6	3.6	2379	No
P5CR.1	P32322	17	1.8	957	Yes
P5CR.2	—	1	1.85	960	No
POX	U79754 AF120278.1	22q11.2	2.4	1800	No
P5CDh	U24266	1p36	3.2	1689	No

kinase and has a highly conserved 32-amino acid aspartokinase active-site motif (see Fig. 81-5). Aspartokinases catalyze phosphorylation of substrates with a carboxyl group as the nucleophilic acceptor. Interestingly, there is a cluster of 3 amino acids (-DDP-) about 50 residues N-terminal of the aspartokinase motif that are highly conserved in *Vigna* and are essential for feedback regulation of P5C synthase activity by proline.[139] Their possible function in mammalian P5C synthase remains to be determined. Finally, consistent with its function as a reductase, the C-terminal half of human P5C synthase has 48 percent amino acid identity with *S. cerevisiae* γ-glutamyl phosphate reductase and has an 11 codon NADP(H) binding-site motif.

Human P5C synthase mRNA has two splice forms: P5CS.short with an ORF of 793 codons and P5CS.long with 795 codons.[137] The two additional codons in P5CS.long result from utilization of an alternative donor splice site for an interior intron with the result that 6 bp are inserted into the mature transcript following bp +711 of P5CS.short (Fig. 81-6). This mechanism has been referred to as "exon sliding." The resulting 2-amino acid insert (-VN-) occurs immediately N-terminal to the highly conserved 32-amino acid aspartokinase active site motif in the N-terminal half of P5C synthase. The long splice form predominates in most tissues except gut, where about 90 percent of the transcripts are the short form. Expression studies in yeast and in CHO cells, which lack endogenous P5C synthase activity, show that both P5CS.short and P5CS.long confer P5C synthase activity. There is, however, a key kinetic difference between the two isoforms: the short isoform, but not the long isoform, is sensitive to noncompetitive inhibition by ornithine with a K_i under the assay conditions of $\approx$0.25 mM. This result together with the predominance of the ornithine-sensitive short isoform of P5C synthase in intestinal mucosa cells is in agreement with previous work showing that ornithine was an allosteric inhibitor of P5C synthase activity isolated from gut.[40–42]

The differences in tissue distribution and kinetic properties of the two P5C synthase isoforms provide a model to explain the physiological roles for the P5C synthase reaction in different tissues (Fig. 81-3). In gut, P5C synthase is an essential component of the pathway for arginine synthesis. Earlier we discussed the essential role of the small intestine in arginine synthesis, especially in the immediate neonatal period (see "Cell-Specific Patterns of Proline and Arginine Metabolism in Small Intestine" above). The predominance of the ornithine-sensitive short isoform of P5C synthase in this tissue provides a mechanism to regulate ornithine and arginine synthesis. In other tissues, P5C synthase is an essential component of a pathway for proline biosynthesis and redox regulation. Proline synthesis is regulated by the availability of proline from the extracellular fluid as mediated by the inhibition by proline of P5C reductase.[63] This model emphasizes the importance of P5C synthase and the intestinal mucosa in arginine synthesis. Additionally, it explains why proline synthesis apparently proceeds normally in inborn errors characterized by hyperornithinemia (gyrate atrophy and the HHH syndrome, see Chap. 83).

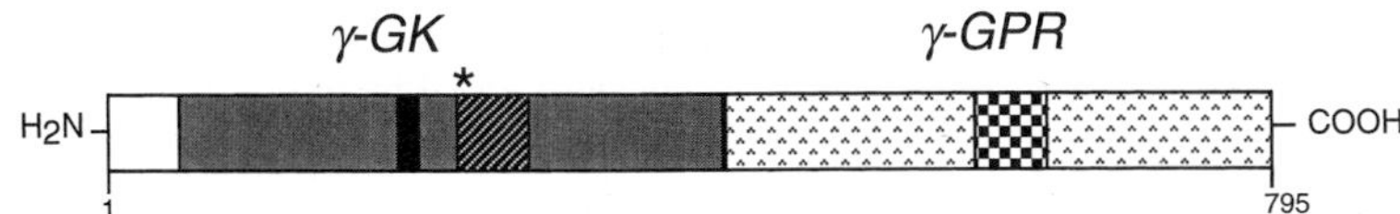

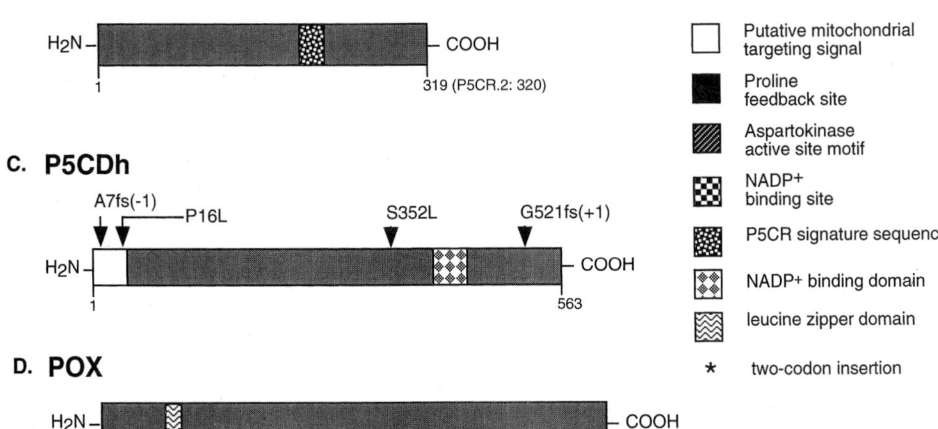

Fig. 81-5 Diagrams of the monomers of the proline metabolic enzymes showing the location of certain structural features.

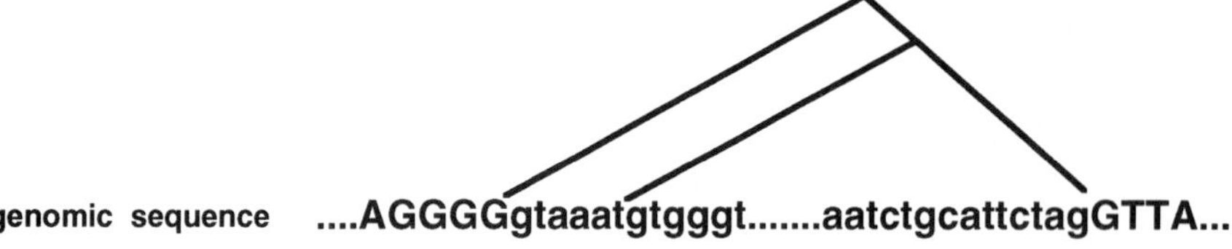
genomic sequence ....AGGGGgtaaatgtgggt.......aatctgcattctagGTTA....
+711
P5CS.short cDNA ....AGGGGGTTA....
P5CS.long cDNA ....AGGGGgtaaatGTTA....
amino acid insert V N

Fig. 81-6 Alternative use of donor splice site ("exon sliding") generates two isoforms of P5C synthase differing by a two-amino acid insert.

P5C Reductase

A human cDNA encoding P5C reductase was cloned in the pre-EST database days by complementation in a strain of *S. cerevisiae* lacking the enzyme. Dougherty and colleagues[52] utilized a human liver cDNA library cloned into a yeast expression vector.[140] Lack of P5C reductase makes the mutant yeast a proline auxotroph; transformants expressing human P5C reductase regain proline prototrophy and are able to grow on medium lacking proline. The human reductase has 32 percent amino acid identity with that of *S. cerevisiae*. Subsequently, Dougherty et al. utilized low-stringency library screening to identify a second P5C reductase cDNA also able to confer proline prototrophy to P5C reductase-deficient yeast.[53] The two genes, designated P5CR.1 and P5CR.2, respectively, map to different locations in the genome (see Table 81-3) and encode P5C reductases with 84 percent amino acid identity. Kinetic characterization of the two enzymes has not been described, but might well explain the previously observed tissue-specific differences in cofactor preference and sensitivity to feedback inhibition by proline. In this regard, the recent identification of a human leukemic lymphoblastoid line (REH cells) that expresses only P5CR.2 will be useful.[53,141] For example, Lorans and Phang[141] showed that the reductase activity in extracts of the REH cells is active with NADPH but not with NADH suggesting that the former is the cofactor for P5CR.2.

Proline Oxidase

Human and murine cDNAs encoding proline oxidase (also referred to as proline dehydrogenase) were identified by several groups on the basis of homology to *S. cerevisiae* Put1p and *Drosophila* sluggish A protein.[142–144] The 516-amino acid human protein has 51 percent and 20 percent sequence identity to the *Drosophila* and yeast orthologs, respectively.[143] Subsequent studies showed the proline oxidase structural gene is located at 22q11.2, in a region involved in the DiGeorge/CATCH 22 deletion syndromes.[143,145] This explains the observation by Jaeken of hyperprolinemia in a patient with the CATCH 22 syndrome and confirms his astute prediction that the proline oxidase gene lies within the region deleted in this contiguous gene syndrome.[146]

P5C Dehydrogenase

Human cDNAs encoding P5C dehydrogenase were cloned using peptide sequence obtained from partially purified human enzyme[147] and degenerate primer PCR.[148] The full-length human P5C dehydrogenase peptide is 563 amino acids in length and has 42 and 26 percent amino acid sequence identity with the orthologous proteins from *S. cerevisiae* and *E. coli*, respectively. Expression of the human protein rescues the growth phenotype of yeast lacking P5C dehydrogenase activity.[148] Interestingly, two human P5C dehydrogenase cDNAs were identified differing only by retention of a 1-kb intron in the 3′ untranslated sequence.[148] The longer transcript predominates in most tissues. The presence of an intron in sequence making up the 3′ untranslated sequence is unusual in mammalian transcripts occurring in less than 5 percent of reported cDNAs.[149] Whether the presence of this intron plays any role in the stability of the P5C dehydrogenase transcripts or in the consequences of P5C dehydrogenase mutations remains to be determined.

THE HYPERPROLINEMIAS

Clinical Phenotypes

There are two inherited hyperprolinemias: HPI, caused by deficiency of proline oxidase; and, HPII, caused by deficiency of P5C dehydrogenase. Information about probands in at least 14 HPI families and 8 HPII families is available.[150] In HPI, there is no categoric evidence that the inborn error is responsible for the clinical manifestations in the reported probands. However, in HPII, the study of 13 cases in 1 pedigree strongly supports a causal relationship between this metabolic disorder and neurologic manifestations (Table 81-4).

HPI. Causal relationships between proline oxidase deficiency in HPI and clinical manifestations are difficult to prove for two reasons. First, most probands with HPI were identified during the course of investigation for some clinical problem so that there is ascertainment bias. Second, and perhaps more importantly, HPI typically is a diagnosis of exclusion; that is, all cases of familial hyperprolinemia not due to a deficiency of P5C dehydrogenase (HPII) are assumed to be HPI. Unfortunately, proline oxidase activity is not expressed in normal leukocytes or cultured fibroblasts.[57] Thus, the diagnosis of HPI typically is not confirmed by direct demonstration of deficiency of proline oxidase so heterogeneity of etiology is possible, if not likely. Also, among patients who do have a primary defect at the level of proline oxidase, the amount of residual activity and its kinetic characteristics, has not been characterized.

The metabolic phenotype of HPI was discovered in a proband with Alport-like nephropathy.[151,152] There should have been no misunderstanding about the association of hyperprolinemia with the renal disease in this pedigree; the former segregated as an autosomal recessive phenotype, whereas the renal phenotype clearly segregated as an autosomal dominant trait.[151] Because individuals could have one phenotype without the other, there was no reason to presume that hyperprolinemia "caused" the nephropathy or vice versa.

Nevertheless, review of subsequent HPI cases suggests a bias associating clinical manifestations with the metabolic disorder. In 14 reported families[146,153–159] with presumed HPI, the metabolic abnormality came to attention during investigation of a clinical phenotype in the probands. The clinical features that attracted attention were not shared by all probands and included several kinds of renal disease (see, for example, the summary by Mollica and Pavone[160]), various ocular abnormalities, mental retardation, and other neurologic manifestations. One case report describes a 10-year-old boy with HPI, neurologic

Table 81-4 Personal Details and Amino Acid Profiles of Pedigree Members with Type II Hyperprolinemia

Pedigree no	Sex	Age (years)	Qualitative urinary* proline	Quantitative urinary amino acids (μM)			Serum Proline (μM)		Plasma P-5-C (μM)	Suffered from seizures	Mental handicap
				Proline	Hydroxyproline	Glycine	Fasting	Nonfasting			
Adults											
IV.17	F	31	Positive	42,100	763	19,673	1818	2047	14.75	No	No
IV.22†	M	28	Positive	29,500	518	5934	2663	2218	18.87	Grand mal	Severe
IV.42	M	36	Positive	14,211	641	3664	2257	2178	Not tested	No	No
IV.45	M	31	Positive	22,101	1145	7606	2673	2277	Not tested	Grand mal	No
IV.46	F	29	Positive	25,585	548	7050	2075	2371	22.13	Petit mal	No
IV.50	F	22	Positive	40,897	4171	20,591	2182	1951	Not tested	Grand mal	No
IV.54	F	18	Positive	25,357	1082	6119	2124	1278	29.57	Grand mal	No
Reference values				Nil	5–20	169–1298		102–336			
Children											
V.2	F	2	Positive	8718	947	3368		1193 / 1762	Not tested	No	No
V.9	F	10	Positive	6793	107	1347		2283	23.35	Grand mal	Slow
V.14	M	12	Positive	37,352	3769	15,052		1821	Not tested	Grand mal	Mild
V.16	F	10	Positive	40,215	2177	11,156		2478	Not tested	No	No
V.17	F	9	Positive	20,572	1147	7721		2210	Not tested	Grand mal	No
V.18	F	7	Positive	2102	84	1603		2713	Not tested	Grand mal	No
V.19	F	5	Positive	8279	230	3412		Not tested	Not tested	Grand mal	No
Reference values				Nil	2–22	165–1420	105–261	89–261			

*Samples of urine were random.
†Proband.
SOURCE: Flynn et al.[174] Used by permission.

manifestations, and abnormalities of central nervous system white matter.[159]

By contrast, prospective studies of HPI probands identified through newborn screening[153,155] indicate that the metabolic disorder is not necessarily associated with clinical manifestations. Contact with directors of various newborn urine screening programs (H. Levy, B. Wilcken, B. Lemieux, personal communications) corroborates this point of view. Information from "collateral" identified families[152,154,156,161–163] and from prospectively identified families[153] also shows that the metabolic disorder can be free of any associated clinical manifestations. These observations strongly suggest that HPI is a relatively benign condition in most individuals under most circumstances. Several recent observations, however, raise the possibility that proline oxidase deficiency could play a contributory rather than causative role in certain complex phenotypes. For example, Polyak et al.[16] found that proline oxidase was one of a small number of genes dramatically induced by expression of p53. This suggests that proline oxidase may play a role in certain forms of apoptosis and correspondingly, its deficiency might confer increased susceptibility for certain proliferative disorders. Additionally, the observation that the proline oxidase structural gene maps to a region of the genome (22q11.2), where several studies have localized a gene conferring increased susceptibility for schizophrenia,[164] together with the suggestion that proline may have neurotransmitter functions, suggests that proline oxidase should be considered as a candidate risk factor for schizophrenia.[142,144] Similarly, the contribution of hemizygosity for proline oxidase to the phenotypes of CATCH 22 (MIM 188400)[146] and DiGeorge/VCF syndrome (MIM 601362) phenotype deserves additional investigation.[165,166] The molecular features of the 22q11.2 region of the genome and the factors predisposing it to deletions have recently been described.[164]

HPII. In contrast to HPI, there is persuasive evidence that HPII is causally associated with neurologic manifestations. Historically, five HPII probands were identified retrospectively;[167–171] another three were discovered incidentally.[172] Asymptomatic hyperprolinemic siblings were identified in two pedigrees.[168,173] Neurologic manifestations (seizures, mental retardation) predominated in the symptomatic patients. Although the neurologic findings in these earlier studies could be due to ascertainment bias, 13 cases discovered by prospective screening of a large pedigree of Irish Travelers (nomads) identified by evaluation of a hyperprolinemic proband with seizures argue strongly for a causal relationship (Fig. 81-7).[174] The diagnosis of HPII in these individuals was based on a serum proline level greater than 1300 μM and the presence of P5C, detected as orthoaminobenzaldehyde-reactive material, in the urine in all 13 individuals (Table 81-4). Subsequent demonstration of markedly elevated plasma P5C levels and undetectable leukocyte P5C dehydrogenase activity in five of five affected members of the pedigree studied biochemically confirmed the diagnosis. Of the 13 HPII subjects in this pedigree, 9 (64 percent) had recurrent seizures; of these, 8 were grand mal and one petit mal in type. Onset of seizures was associated with febrile episodes and the seizures were severe enough to necessitate hospitalization and treatment with anticonvulsants. The incidence of seizures in unaffected members of the pedigree and in unrelated Irish Travelers was 4.2 percent, or similar to the incidence in the general population. Thus, a causal relationship between this metabolic disorder and a disposition to recurrent seizures seems highly likely. Nevertheless, even in this family, there were examples of adults with the disorder who were overtly healthy and fertile, consistent with the idea that the phenotypic consequences of HPII are highly variable.

METABOLIC AND POLYPEPTIDE PHENOTYPES OF THE HYPERPROLINEMIAS

HPI

The plasma proline concentrations in HPI are five- to tenfold increased (700 to 2400 μM) over normal (51 to 271 μM) (Table 81-2) and, on average, are lower than in HPII. Interestingly family studies show that mild hyperprolinemia (500 to 1000 μM)

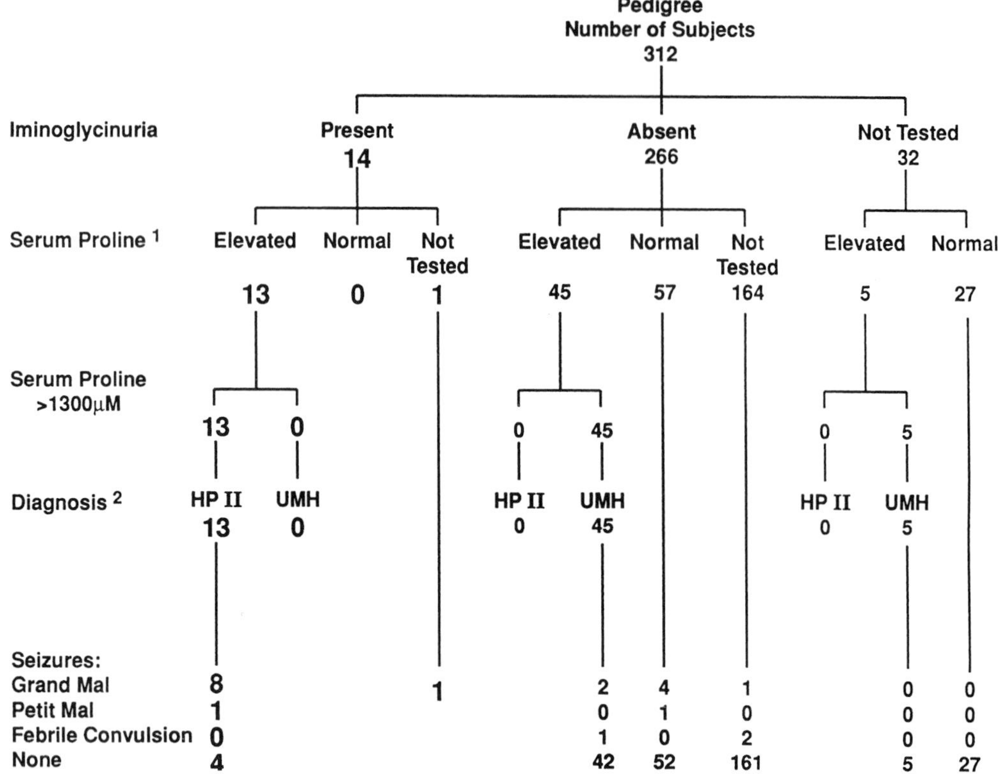

Fig. 81-7 Summary of studies of an HPII pedigree discovered in Irish Travelers. Unexplained mild hyperprolinemia (UMH) was identified, which bore no relationship to heterozygosity for HPII. (1) In this study, the normal ranges for serum proline were 102 to 336 μM for adults and 89 to 281 μM for children. (2) Thirteen individuals with serum proline levels compatible with HPII were identified. Nine of nine tested positive for orthoaminobenzaldehyde-reactive substances in the urine. Five of five tested had undetectable leukocyte P5C dehydrogenase activities and serum P5C levels, which were markedly elevated (14.8 to 29.6 μM).[174]

may be observed in HPI heterozygotes (see Fig. 81-7 in the sixth edition of this work).

Proline concentrations are also elevated in cerebrospinal fluid,[175] but the plasma:cerebrospinal fluid proline ratio is not abnormal, implying that the source of proline accumulation in cerebrospinal fluid is not the brain.[108]

Urine proline is elevated and the disorder can be detected by urine screening of newborn infants, but it must be discriminated from other inherited and physiological causes of iminoglycinuria. The mechanism of hyperprolinuria in human patients is predominately prerenal, with saturation of the reabsorption mechanism (see "Hyperaminoaciduria in the Hyperprolinemias" below).

HPI patients do not accumulate P5C in urine or plasma. This observation in the first case studied suggested that the cause of proline accumulation in HPI was either overproduction (for which there is no evidence) or decreased catabolism due to deficient proline oxidase activity. The latter was confirmed by studies of proline oxidation in the liver of the HPI proband.[175] The liver, obtained at autopsy approximately 1 h after death, was homogenized, incubated with L-proline and 4-hydroxy-L-proline and assayed for production of the corresponding pyrroline carboxylic acids as detected by the *o*-aminobenzaldehyde reaction[32,99] or with radiolabeled L-proline and DL-hydroxyproline, and assayed for the formation of labeled glutamic and γ-hydroxyglutamate. The results were compared with 23 control human liver samples obtained by biopsy or at autopsy. Conversion of proline to downstream metabolites by extracts of the liver from the HPI patient was less than 10 percent of normal. Similar studies were also performed with liver biopsy material from the father of the proband, but there was such variation in the measurement of proline oxidation in the control samples that it was not possible to document a presumed heterozygous phenotype. Oxidation of hydroxyproline was indistinguishable from normal in the proband's liver sample. This result implies that different enzymes catalyze the initial step in the oxidation of the two imino acids. Consistent with this notion, human brain has a oxidase activity for proline, but not for hydroxyproline.[175,176]

Amazingly, there are no additional published studies of proline oxidase activity in HPI. This paucity of enzyme data reflects the rarity of HPI, the lack of proline oxidase expression in accessible tissues and the benign nature of the phenotypic consequences.

HPII

In HPII homozygotes, plasma proline values almost always exceed 1500 μM (Table 81-2). Proline values in cerebrospinal fluid and urine are correspondingly greater in type II homozygotes than in type I subjects. Proline levels in HPII heterozygotes are normal.

HPII homozygotes also accumulate and excrete P5C, which can be easily identified qualitatively in urine by its reactivity with *o*-aminobenzaldehyde.[172,177–180] Quantitative determination of plasma (or serum) and urine P5C concentrations is possible by several specific assays.[181,182] The concentrations in plasma and urine of affected individuals are 10 to 40 times that of normals.[174,182] Accumulation of P5C unambiguously differentiates HPII from HPI.

HPII patients excrete a second *o*-aminobenzaldehyde-reacting substance, Δ^1-pyrroline-3-hydroxy-5-carboxylate.[172,183,184] This compound is a derivative of 4-hydroxy-L-proline. A loading test with 4-hydroxy-L-proline (100 mg/kg) markedly increases urinary Δ^1-pyrroline-3-hydroxy-5-carboxylate and is associated with attenuated clearance of hydroxyproline from plasma in HPII patients.[172,184] These results imply that P5C dehydrogenase catalyzes the second step of both the proline and hydroxyproline oxidative pathways.[103]

P5C dehydrogenase activity measured in extracts of cultured skin fibroblasts or leukocytes is severely deficient in HPII and is about half normal in obligate heterozygotes.[103,185,186] Activities of P5C reductase and OAT are normal. Catalytic activity measured in vitro with Δ^1-pyrroline-3-hydroxy-5-carboxylate as substrate is also deficient in HPII cells.[79] This result confirms that P5C dehydrogenase catalyzes the second step in the degradation of both proline and hydroxyproline. Despite this downstream defect, plasma hydroxyproline is not increased in HPII.

Molecular Aspects of the Hyperprolinemias

HPI. Although reports of cloning the human proline oxidase gene have recently appeared,[143,144] there currently are no published accounts of the mutations responsible for HPI. As described below (see "Model Organisms"), the molecular basis of the deficient proline oxidase activity in the Pro/Re mouse is a nonsense mutation[144] that truncates the reading frame, deleting the normal C-terminal 45 amino acids of murine proline oxidase (see "Model Organisms Relevant to Hyperprolinemia" below).

HPII. The P5C dehydrogenase cDNA was recently cloned and encodes a 563-amino acid monomer with an N-terminal 24-amino acid putative mitochondrial targeting sequence that is cleaved to yield a mature monomer of 539 amino acids.[148] Four HPII probands have been studied to date with identification of four mutant alleles (Fig. 81-5). Two were frameshifts: A7fs(−1), caused by deletion of a G at position +21 of the reading frame, results in premature termination 22 codons downstream in the new reading frame; G521fs(+1), caused by insertion of a T at position +1563 of the reading frame, results in termination of the new reading frame 9 codons downstream. Additionally, two missense mutations were identified: P16L, caused by a C to T transition at position +47 of the reading frame (47 C > T); and, S352L, caused by a C to T transition at position +1055 (1055 C > T). The A7fs(−1) allele, which alters the C-terminal 98 percent of the P5C dehydrogenase peptide, was assumed to be functionally significant. The remaining three alleles, G521fs(+1), P16L, and S352L, were expressed in a P5C dehydrogenase-deficient strain of yeast to determine the functional consequences of the mutations. G521fs(+1) and S35L were nonfunctional as judged by direct assay of P5C dehydrogenase activity and by lack of ability of the transformed yeast to grow on a medium with proline as the sole nitrogen source (Fig. 81-8). By these same measures, P16L was of no functional consequence and subsequent studies suggested it was a normal variant present in individuals of the same ethnicity as the proband with a frequency of about 0.01. In toto, the three functionally significant P5C dehydrogenase mutations accounted for six of the eight possible abnormal P5C dehydrogenase alleles in the four HPII probands studied. The G521fs(+1) allele was of particular interest because it is responsible for the HPII phenotype in the large Irish Traveler family that has been so informative for understanding the HPII phenotype (Fig. 81-9).

MECHANISM OF HPI AND HPII PHENOTYPES

Two observations require explanation. First, the plasma proline is higher, on average, in HPII homozygotes than in HPI homozygotes. Second, about one-third of HPI heterozygotes have hyperprolinemia, whereas HPII heterozygotes have normal plasma proline values (Table 81-2).

Quantitatively, the major metabolite that accumulates in HPII is proline, not P5C, the substrate of the deficient enzyme P5C dehydrogenase. P5C can be produced from ornithine, glutamate, and proline. The P5C pool is expanded in HPII[182] because the outflow mechanism catalyzed by P5C dehydrogenase is impaired, while synthesis is intact. Accordingly, P5C accumulates and is a substrate for P5C reductase that catalyzes conversion to proline. The total activity of P5C reductase in liver is greater than the corresponding activity of proline oxidase; moreover, the K_m values of these proline metabolic enzymes favor proline synthesis over proline degradation.[47,185] It follows that proline accumulation is greater in HPII, where P5C dehydrogenase is deficient, as compared to HPI, where the block is at the level of proline oxidase and the P5C pool is not expanded.

The finding of hyperprolinemia in HPI heterozygotes is a rare example of a metabolic phenotype occurring in the heterozygote for an autosomal recessive disorder. In this sense, HPI is a dominant trait at the metabolic level in certain families. The classic studies of Kacser and Burns offer an explanation.[187] They propose that half-normal activity (e.g., in the heterozygote) of one enzymatic component in a large metabolic network will perturb the metabolite value only minimally. On the other hand, half-normal activity of an enzyme acting alone or with only a few others results in a greater change in the concentration of the upstream metabolite. Because the defect in HPI affects the first step in proline degradation, it is essentially a one-enzyme pathway. By contrast, the defect in HPII is at the second step, downstream of a multiple branch point. It follows that half-normal activity of proline oxidase in the HPI phenotype (an assumption because no data on this point are available) could have a large effect on proline flux through its oxidative pathway, whereas the corresponding state in the HPII phenotype affects an enzyme at a different point in a network and will not significantly perturb proline homeostasis in the heterozygote.

Additionally, if future molecular and biochemical studies show that proline oxidase is a multimeric enzyme, certain mutations

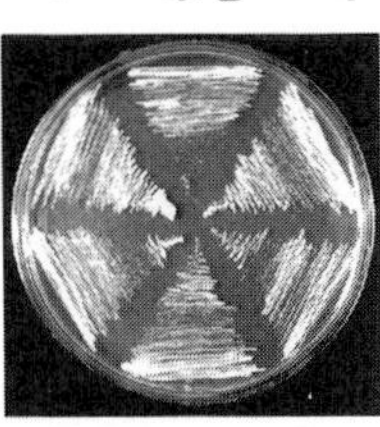

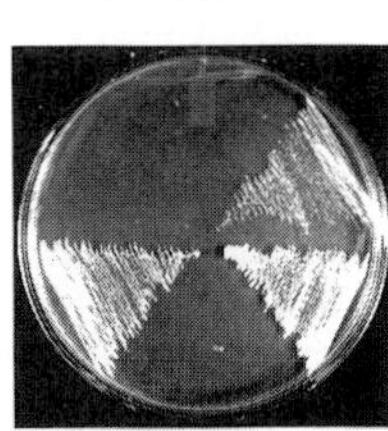

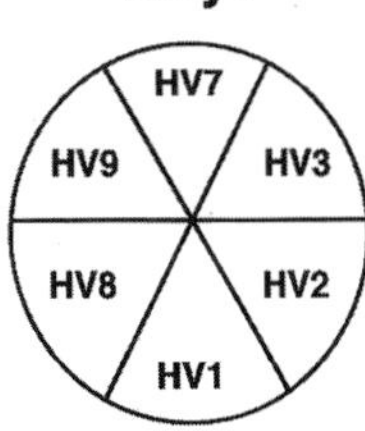

Strain	Genotype	Growth on proline	P5CDh activity* (nmol product/hr/mg protein)
MB1472	MATa *ura3-52 trp1-1 put2::TRP1*	-	0
HV1	MB1472/pSM703	-	0
HV2	MB1472/p*Sc*PUT2	++++	4.4 (4.2-4.6)
HV3	MB1472/p*Hs*P5CDhS2	+++	4.2 (4.0-4.4)
HV7	MB1472/p*Hs*P5CDh-S352L	-	0
HV8	MB1472/p*Hs*P5CDh-P16L	+++	4.3 (4.1-4.6)
HV9	MB1472/p*Hs*P5CDh-G521fs(+1)	-	0

Fig. 81-8 Expression of mutant human P5C dehydrogenase alleles in yeast. ***A***, A comparison of the growth of yeast strains expressing the indicated mutant P5C dehydrogenase alleles (HV7-9) with strains expressing vector alone (HV1), *PUT2* (HV2), the yeast ortholog of P5C dehydrogenase or wild-type human P5C dehydrogenase (HV3, pHsP5CDhS2) on medium with either ammonium sulfate or proline as sole nitrogen source. ***B***, The P5C dehydrogenase activity of extracts of these strains.

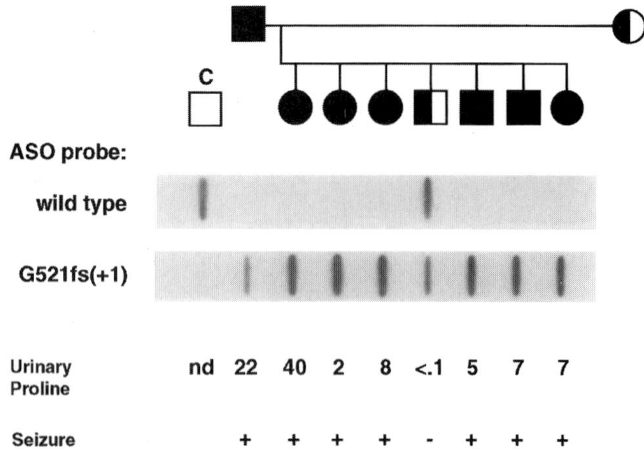

Fig. 81-9 Segregation of G521fs(+1) in a small segment of the Irish Traveler HPII pedigree by allele-specific oligonucleotide (ASO) analysis. The father and six children are all homozygous for the mutant allele; the unaffected child is heterozygous. The biochemical and clinical phenotypes are indicated below. nd = not done.

producing stable, but nonfunctional, subunits would be expected to have a dominant effect on the product of the normal allele, with the result that activity in heterozygotes would be significantly less than 50 percent. This dominant negative effect on enzyme activity would be expected to occur only for certain missense mutations, but not for mutations that result in absence of a protein product. Thus, hyperprolinemia in heterozygotes caused by this mechanism would be allele specific, occurring only in certain HPI families, and should breed true. This prediction is consistent with the observed data. The consequence of such a dominant negative effect would be more likely to be detected in plasma proline levels for the reasons proposed by Kacser and Burns (see above).[187]

Hyperaminoaciduria in the Hyperprolinemias

Whereas proline is the only amino acid with abnormal plasma concentrations in HPI and HPII, three amino acids (proline, hydroxyproline, and glycine) are increased in urine. When plasma proline exceeds 800 μM in probands, the associated "iminoglycinuria" is directly proportional to the plasma proline concentration.[124,151] This finding reflects the "combined" mechanism of hyperaminoaciduria occurring in the hyperprolinemias. Prolinuria occurs when the relevant tubular transport mechanism saturates at high substrate (proline) concentration in filtrate;[121] this saturation occurs at plasma concentrations in excess of about 800 μM. Glycine and hydroxyproline share a carrier with proline; when the latter is present at high concentration, transport of the other substrates is inhibited competitively and iminoglycinuria occurs. Hyperprolinemia was the first disorder in which the phenomenon of combined hyperaminoaciduria was recognized. The led to the identification of a renal transport system with a preference for imino acids and glycine (see Chap. 194).

Clinical Manifestations in HPII

Predictions based on the observed deficiency of P5C dehydrogenase are consistent with the metabolic phenotype of HPII patients. Plasma proline and P5C are markedly elevated and indirectly the flux of P5C through P5C reductase is apparently increased. The consequences of these metabolic abnormalities on the function of the central nervous system are uncertain, but clinical observations (see above) and the proposed role of proline as a neurotransmitter with the possibility to accentuate excitatory transmission of certain neurons (see "Transport of Imino Acid in Mammalian Central Nervous System" above) suggest they may increase the likelihood of seizures. In this context, the concentration of certain neurotransmitters in the CSF of HPII patients have been found to be elevated including γ-aminobutyric acid[188] and glutamate.[189]

In extensive studies in a single patient with HPII, abnormalities in peripheral oxygen utilization consistent with increased operation of the proline-P5C cycle were found (G.A. Fleming, A.N. Granger, J.M. Phang, unpublished observations). Bright red venous blood was noted on several occasions, and a high venous O_2 in the face of normal arterial O_2 was documented. Of more than 30 venous samples, 18 had a O_2 greater than 70 mm Hg and 8 had a O_2 of 90 mm Hg. No evidence of anatomic or functional shunting, abnormal hemoglobin, or decreased total oxygen consumption was seen. In the face of markedly decreased peripheral O_2 consumption, pyruvate:lactate ratios were normal or even increased. We interpreted these findings to signify thatincreased levels of proline and P5C facilitated the transfer of oxidizing potential to peripheral tissues in the form of P5C and of reducing potential back to the liver as proline. Thus, the redox perturbation generated by the cycle would decrease the use of O_2 for oxidizing NADH generated by glycolysis in peripheral tissues.

Differential Diagnosis of Hyperprolinemia

HPI is recognized by persistent hyperprolinemia, absence of P5C in the urine, and absence of other causes of hyperprolinemia. In particular, care should be taken to rule out lactic acidemia. Lactate inhibits proline oxidase and hyperprolinemia has been shown to be associated with lactate accumulation of multiple etiologies.[58,190] Elevated proline levels have been observed in some organic acidemias, particularly glutaric acidemia type 2.[191,192] Additionally, hyperprolinemia has been reported in the CATCH 22/ DiGeorge/Shprintzen syndromes.[146] This apparently results from hemizygosity for the proline oxidase structural gene in these syndromes, which result from variable-length deletions in the 22q11.2 region. Because the dysmorphic manifestations of these syndromes are quite variable and sometimes not detected until adulthood, a careful physical exam, as well as cytogenetic studies, including fluorescence in situ hybridization (FISH) with probes specific for the DiGeorge region, should be done before making the diagnosis of HPI. Increased urinary proline is not a sufficiently specific finding to permit the diagnosis. The associated occurrence of iminoglycinuria depends on the plasma proline value and is not an obligatory feature of the phenotype. P5C is not detected in the urine of HPI subjects.

HPII is distinguished by the coexistence of hyperprolinemia and elevated excretion of P5C in urine. The latter compound may be identified by the yellow color it produces when reacted with *o*-aminobenzaldehyde (0.5 percent, weight by volume) and trichloroacetic acid (5 percent, volume by volume) in alcohol.[32,175,193] Pyrroline-5-carboxylate can be measured in plasma by two methods:[181,182] definitive enzymatic confirmation of P5C dehydrogenase deficiency can be made on extracts from circulating leukocytes or from cultured fibroblasts.[63,185,194]

Therapy

Fortunately, because their medical consequences, as we currently understand them, appear to be modest, there is not a strong indication for treatment of the hyperprolinemias. Even in those cases of HPII in which seizures occurred during childhood, adult life appears to be symptom free.

Proline is readily synthesized from precursors. Moreover, most dietary proteins contain proline (lactalbumin is an exception).[195] Attempts at dietary therapy in probands with HPI or HPII by dietary restriction resulted in only modest control of the plasma proline value, caused no apparent harm to the subject, and made no impact on the clinical phenotype.[196–200]

In a particularly useful observation, Whelan and Connors[201] reported the outcome of two pregnancies in a woman with untreated HPI; neither child was harmed by maternal hyperprolinemia (plasma proline range 1300 to 2100 μM). Even with HPII, the Irish pedigree had four affected women who had 18 apparently normal children.[174]

MODEL ORGANISMS RELEVANT TO HYPERPROLINEMIA

Saccharomyces cerevisiae

Genes encoding all the enzymes in the proline metabolic pathway have been identified in *S. cerevisiae*, mutant strains constructed and growth phenotypes characterized.[38,39,138,202,203] Some differences from human cells are apparent. The P5C synthase activity of *S. cerevisiae* derives from two proteins, a γ-glutamyl kinase and a γ-glutamyl phosphate reductase encoded by *PRO1* and *PRO2*, respectively. Also, yeast have only a single P5C reductase gene (*PRO3*), in contrast to human cells, which have two. As in human cells, the yeast genes encoding OAT (*CARGB*), proline oxidase (*PUT1*), and P5C dehydrogenase (*PUT2*) are all single copy.

In general, yeast with mutations in the proline metabolic system have easily scorable growth phenotypes. Expression of orthologous human genes has been shown to rescue the growth phenotype of yeast deficient in OAT,[204] P5C reductase,[52] P5C dehydrogenase,[148] and P5C synthase.[137] Thus, these mutant yeast strains provide a tractable system to test the functional consequences of mutations in the corresponding human genes (Fig. 81-8).

The *Drosophila Sluggish A Mutant (slgA)*

In his pioneering studies to identify mutants of *Drosophila melanogaster* with altered behavior phenotypes,[205] Seymour Benzer and his colleagues identified a series of mutants designated "sluggish" (*slg*) because they exhibited abnormal phototaxis and movement patterns. Subsequent studies of one of these, *slgA*, showed that the responsible gene encoded proline oxidase. Homozygous *slgA* flies had free proline levels twofold over normal and proline oxidase activities of 17 $\pm$ 3 percent of control when measured at a substrate concentration of 10 mM.[206] Molecular cloning and sequencing of the *Drosophila* proline oxidase showed that it has 669 amino acids with 17 percent identity to *S. cerevisiae* and 43 percent identity to human proline oxidase.[142,143] Interestingly, behavioral studies of *slgA* mutant flies indicated that their reduced activity was caused by abnormal neural function.

The Pro/Re Mouse

A spontaneous proline oxidase-deficient mouse model, designated Pro/Re, is available for studies of the metabolic consequences of proline oxidase deficiency. Pro/Re mice were first described by Blake,[207,208] who found hyperprolinemia and hyperprolinuria associated with proline oxidase activity less than 10 percent that of control strains. Based on electrophoretic migration patterns, murine hepatic proline oxidase activity appeared to have two components, designated pro-1 and pro-2,[208] with the former deficient in the Pro/Re mice. Pro-2 may actually be hydroxyproline oxidase with some activity for proline, although this remains to be determined.[209] That proline oxidase was deficient in Pro/Re mice was defined at the molecular level when cloned cDNAs for the murine proline oxidase were identified.[142,144] A nonsense mutation (E472X; 1414 G $>$ T) truncates the C-terminal 45 amino acids of the protein. Gogos et al.[144] described a neurologic phenotype in Pro/Re mice consisting of motor retardation, learning defects, and abnormal sensorimotor gating accompanied by regional neurochemical alterations (modest but statistically significant reductions of glutamate, GABA, and aspartate) in the brain as compared to controls. The authors conclude that this neurologic phenotype results from the observed deficiency in proline oxidase.

HYPOPROLINEMIA

Nearly all recognized inborn errors of amino acid metabolism involve enzymes that function in degradative pathways (e.g., see Chap. 66). Thus, the recent report of two sibs with features suggesting deficiency of P5C synthase is of special interest.[1] These children have progressive intellectual deterioration, cataracts, joint laxity, and hyperelastic skin. Their metabolic phenotype includes subnormal plasma levels of proline (117 $\pm$ 14 μM in one and 91$\pm$ 9 μM in the other); citrulline (6 $\pm$ 1 μM in one and 6 $\pm$ 3 μM in the other, with normal being 26 $\pm$ 1 μM), and ornithine (24 $\pm$ 5 μM in one and 37 $\pm$ 4 μM in the other, with normal being 72 $\pm$ 2 μM). Additionally, they have mild fasting hyperammonemia (81 $\pm$ 9 μM in one and 79 $\pm$ 11 μM in the other, with normal being $<$50 μM). Importantly, in contrast to the normal, modest postprandial increase in plasma ammonia, in these patients, plasma ammonia fell about 15 percent after meals. This observation suggested that in the fasting state, reduced levels of urea cycle intermediates (citrulline and arginine) resulted in impaired urea cycle function. The burst of urea cycle intermediates following a meal (arginine derived from dietary protein) allowed the urea cycle to function with concomitant reduction in plasma ammonium. Preliminary analysis of the P5C synthase in these patients identified a missense mutation, L396S, that was suggested to be responsible for loss of P5C synthase function.[1] Subsequent detailed analysis, however, identified a different missense mutation (R84Q).[2] Additional study is required to clarify the etiology of this syndrome.

Although the frequency of this disorder is uncertain and likely to be rare, the metabolic abnormality in these patients could easily be overlooked. A superficial interpretation of the plasma amino acid concentrations might conclude that results were normal because of a tendency to expect abnormally *elevated* values in inborn errors of amino acid metabolism. That this disorder was recognized by Saudubray and his colleagues, reflects careful and thoughtful synthesis of subtle abnormalities of amino acid concentrations.[1] It is necessary to identify additional patients in order to determine whether all or only some of the clinical features of these two sibs are caused by the presumed deficiency of P5C synthase. Interestingly, the clinical features of these two patients fit well with those predicted by Dougherty et al. for disorders of proline biosynthesis.[52]

HYPERHYDROXYPROLINEMIA

Clinical Phenotype

Hydroxyproline is a normal constituent of plasma (normal values $<$50 μM) (Table 81-2); thus, all of humans have hydroxyprolinemia. Probands with hyperhydroxyprolinemia have plasma hydroxyproline values elevated at least five- to tenfold. At least seven probands have been reported.[210–216] The clinical phenotypes in this group are heterogenous and are likely to reflect ascertainment bias. Several reports present evidence against a causal relationship between the metabolic phenotype and clinical manifestations. Healthy hyperhydroxyprolinemic sibs have been described.[211,217] Additionally, a hyperhydroxyprolinemic girl, who was identified prospectively by routine neonatal urine screening, has been followed for more than 12 years and compared to her unaffected dizygotic twin sister without evidence of physical or cognitive deficits.[216]

Biochemical Phenotype

The concentration of 4-hydroxyproline in plasma is five- to tenfold elevated (range 140 to 500 μM) (Table 81-2). Concentrations of the other plasma amino acids are normal. The erythrocyte hydroxyproline pool is increased.[214] Hydroxyproline concentrations are not elevated in the cerebrospinal fluid.

Urinary excretion of free hydroxyproline is greatly increased (285 to 550 mg/24 h).[199,216,217] This increase is due completely to the hyperhydroxyprolinemia, because renal reabsorption of free hydroxyproline saturates normally in the hyperhydroxyprolinemia phenotype.[215] The excretion of peptide-bound hydroxyproline (about 25 to 40 mg/24 h)[175,217,218] and the profile of peptides is normal.[217] The fraction of peptide-bound hydroxyproline in relation to total hydroxyproline is diminished; this fraction is >0.95 in normal subjects and <0.15 in hyperhydroxyprolinemia probands.[175,217] If the block in free hydroxyproline oxidation is assumed to be complete, the urine data imply that about 90 percent of the hydroxyproline released during collagen turnover is degraded by the free hydroxyproline pathway in the normal state, representing a turnover of 2 g or more of collagen daily.[111]

Metabolic Studies

Loading studies with 4-hydroxy-L-proline (100 to 200 mg/kg by mouth) showed that plasma hydroxyproline increased more in subjects with hyperhydroxyprolinemia than in control subjects and remained elevated longer.[175,214,217] Up to one-half of the hydroxyproline load was excreted into urine within 24 h. Excretion of *o*-aminobenzaldehyde-reacting material (Δ^1-pyrroline-3-hydroxy-5-carboxylate is the relevant metabolite) did not increase after loading in probands; normal subjects show an increase under these conditions (see Fig. 18-8 in the sixth edition of this work).

The rise in plasma proline after a load of L-proline (100 mg/kg by mouth) is normal in hyperhydroxyprolinemia subjects.[175] Pyrrole-2-carboxylate is excreted after the ingestion of allo-hydroxy-D-proline.[175] These findings indicate that proline oxidation and D-amino acid oxidase activity (allohydroxyproline-preferring) are both normal in the hyperhydroxyprolinemia phenotype. Pyrrole-2-carboxylate is excreted in increased amounts in hyperhydroxyprolinemia.[219] This metabolite is formed from the labile intermediate Δ^1-pyrroline-4-hydroxy-2-carboxylate (see Fig. 81-3), the associated metabolic pathway perhaps disposing of any hydroxyproline accumulating in type II hyperprolinemia.[196] Metabolism of 3-hydroxyproline is not abnormal.[104]

Probable Nature of the Enzyme Defect in Hydroxyprolinemia

Direct measurements of enzymes or metabolic fluxes in vitro have not been performed in the hyperhydroxyprolinemia phenotype. The absence of Δ^1-pyrroline-3-hydroxy-5-carboxylate in urine,[175,217] and the evidence for decreased formation of this substance and other metabolites in the main degradative pathway for hydroxyproline in probands,[175,214] imply that conversion of 4-hydroxy-L-proline to Δ^1-pyrroline-3-hydroxy-5-carboxylate is impaired. Proline oxidation is normal in the hyperhydroxyprolinemia phenotype,[199] which is taken as an indication that "proline oxidase" and "hydroxyproline oxidase" are separate catalytic activities. The recent identification of two genes encoding proline oxidase and a related protein, possibly hydroxyproline oxidase, suggest that the molecular basis for deficiency of these two oxidases should soon be defined.[143,144]

Iminoaciduria in Hyperhydroxyprolinemia

Urinary excretion and endogenous renal clearance of free hydroxyproline are both increased in the hyperhydroxyprolinemia phenotype, as would be expected if the filtered load of substrate is elevated sufficiently to permit saturation of the tubular transport mechanism.[125] Renal clearance rates for proline and glycine are not elevated in probands even though hydroxyproline, proline, and glycine share a renal transport system, and even though clearance rates of hydroxyproline and glycine are likely to be raised in the hyperprolinemia phenotype (see also Chap. 194). The steady state plasma hydroxyproline concentration must exceed 400 μM for inhibition to occur;[125] plasma hydroxyproline is usually below the threshold value in the mutant phenotype.

The occurrence of hydroxyprolinuria in hydroxyproline oxidase deficiency may depend, to some extent, on impaired metabolic "runout" of hydroxyproline in renal epithelium (for a discussion of this concept, see p. 586 of the sixth edition of this work). Hydroxyproline is oxidized in the mammalian kidney,[54,99] and the free hydroxyproline content of normal mammalian kidney cortex is negligible.[124,125] A block in renal oxidation of hydroxyproline, with an increase of intracellular hydroxyproline in tubular epithelium, would inhibit net reabsorption by enhancing back-flux at the luminal membrane.

Genetics

The consanguinity of parents in some pedigrees and the appearance of the trait in both sexes and among sibs of probands indicate that hyperhydroxyprolinemia is inherited as an autosomal recessive trait.

The Heterozygous Phenotype. Parents of probands have normal plasma hydroxyproline values,[175,214,217] but clearance of hydroxyproline from plasma after a loading test is delayed in the heterozygote.[214] A heterozygous child excreted an excess of free hydroxyproline (16.5 to 18 percent of total excretion; normal, <5.2 percent.[115,217] Because hydroxyproline oxidation is physiologically attenuated in infancy[220] and this heterozygote was 2 years old, the "defect" in hydroxyproline oxidation in this subject might have been an adjunct of ontogeny and heterozygosity. Adult obligate heterozygotes have normal hydroxyproline excretion patterns.[217]

Diagnosis

Measurement of hydroxyproline in body fluids is possible with a variety of chemical and chromatographic methods (see previous editions of this text for details). The most reliable method for quantitative analysis is elution chromatography on an ion-exchange column.

The presence of hydroxyprolinuria does not in itself permit a diagnosis of hydroxyprolinemia. Hydroxyprolinuria is a normal finding for at least 3 months after birth,[108] and it is found also in hyperprolinemia and hereditary renal iminoglycinuria. Modest hyperhydroxyprolinemia (up to 100 μM) occurs as a physiological event in young infants,[220,221] and the plasma value may be even higher in infants fed formulas containing gelatin.[222] The excretion patterns of intermediates in the oxidation pathway of free hydroxyproline have not been described in immature subjects; a study of this type would identify the effect of ontogeny on hydroxyproline oxidation.

Therapy

There is no evidence that hyperhydroxyprolinemia is associated with a clinical phenotype and, therefore, there currently is no indication for therapy. Because collagen breakdown is the principal endogenous source of free hydroxyproline, it is unlikely that extracellular hydroxyproline can be lowered either by dietary limitation[175,199] or by manipulation of hydroxyproline renal excretion.[212] A diet free of hydroxyproline did not lower plasma and urine hydroxyproline values in a treated proband.[199]

ACKNOWLEDGMENTS

We thank Sandy Muscelli for assistance with the preparation of this chapter. Some of the work described in this chapter was supported by a grant from the National Eye Institute (DV; EY07814). Dr. Valle is an Investigator in the Howard Hughes Medical Institute.

REFERENCES

1. Kamoun P, Aral B, Saudubray J-M: A new inherited metabolic disease: D[1] pyrroline 5-carboxylate synthetase deficiency. *Bull Acad Natl Med* **182**:131, 1998.
2. Baumgartner MR, Hu CA, Steel JM, Kamoun P, Saudubray JM, Valle D: A mutation of Δ^1-pyrroline-5-carboxylate synthase associated with hyperammonemia, hypocitrullinemia, hypoornithinemia and hypoprolinemia. *Pediatr Res* **47**:in press, 2000.
3. Young VR, El-Khoury A: The notion of the nutritional essentiality of amino acids, revisited, with a note on the indispensable amino acid requirements in adults, in Cynober LA (ed): *Amino Acid Metabolism and Therapy in Health and Nutritional Disease*. New York, CRC Press, 1995, p 191.

4. Cahill GF Jr, Aoki TT, Smith RJ: Amino acid cycles in man. *Curr Top Cell Regul* **18**:389, 1981.
5. Hiramatsu T, Cortiella J, Marchini JS, Chapman TE, Young VR: Plasma proline and leucine kinetics: Response to 4 week with proline-free diets in young adults. *Am J Clin Nutr* **60**:207, 1994.
6. Miller RG, Keshen TH, Jahoor F, Shew SB, Jaksic T: Compartmentation of endogenously synthesized amino acids in neonates. *J Surg Res* **63**:199, 1996.
7. Miller RG, Jahoor F, Jaksic T: Decreased cysteine and proline synthesis in parenterally fed, premature infants. *J Pediatr Surg* **30**:953, 1995.
8. Phang JM: The regulatory functions of proline and pyrroline-5-carboxylic acid. *Curr Top Cell Regul* **25**:91, 1985.
9. Csonka LN: Proline over-production results in enhanced osmotolerance in Salmonella typhimurium. *Mol Gen Genet* **182**:82, 1981.
10. Brown LM, Hellebust JA: Sorbitol and proline as intracellular osmotic solutes in the green alga *Stichococcus bacillaris*. *Can J Bot* **56**:676, 1978.
11. Hu CA, Delauney AJ, Verma DPS: A bifunctional enzyme (Δ^1-pyrroline-5-carboxylate synthetase) catalyzes the first two steps in proline biosynthesis in plants. *Proc Natl Acad Sci U S A* **89**:9354, 1992.
12. KaviKishor PB, Hong Z, Miao G-H, Hu C-A, Verma DPS: Overexpression of Δ1-pyrroline-5-carboxylate synthetase increases proline production and confers osmotolerance in transgenic plants. *Plant Physiol* **108**:1387, 1995.
13. Balboni E: A proline shuttle in insect flight muscle. *Biochem Biophys Res Commun* **85**:1090, 1978.
14. Isseroff H, Sawma JT, Keino D: Fascioliasis: The role of proline in bile duct hyperplasia. *Science* **198**:1157, 1977.
15. Smith GH: Functional differentiation of virgin mouse mammary epithelium in explant culture is dependent upon extracellular proline. *J Cell Physiol* **131**:190, 1987.
16. Polyak K, Xia Y, Zweier JL, Kinzler KW, Vogelstein B: A model for p53-induced apoptosis. *Nature* **389**:300, 1997.
17. Phang JM, Yeh GC, Hagedorn CH: The intercellular proline cycle. *Life Sci* **28**:53, 1981.
18. Phang J, Downing S, Yeh G, Smith R, Williams J: Stimulation of the hexose-monophosphate pentose pathway by Δ^1-pyrroline-5-carboxylic acid in human fibroblasts. *Biochem Biophys Res Commun* **87**:363, 1979.
19. Yeh GC, Phang JM: The function of pyrroline-5-carboxylate reductase in human erythrocytes. *Biochem Biophys Res Commun* **94**:450, 1980.
20. Phang JM, Downing SJ, Yeh GC: Linkage of the HMP pathway to ATP generation by the proline cycle. *Biochem Biophys Res Comm* **93**:462, 1980.
21. Phang JM, Downing SJ, Yeh GC, Smith RJ, Williams JA, Hagedorn CH: Stimulation of the hexosemonophosphate-pentose pathway by pyrroline-5-carboxylate in cultured cells. *J Cell Physiol* **110**:255, 1982.
22. Yoneda Y, Roberts E: A new synaptosomal biosynthetic pathway of proline from ornithine and its negative feedback inhibition by proline. *Brain Res* **239**:479, 1982.
23. Hauptmann M, Wilson DF, Erecinska M: High affinity proline uptake in rat brain synaptosomes. *FEBS Lett* **161**:1983.
24. Nadler JV: Sodium-dependent proline uptake in the rat hippocampal formation: Association with ipsilateral commissural projections of CA3 pyramidal cells. *J Neurochem* **49**:1155, 1987.
25. Nadler JV, Bray SD, Evanson DA: Autoradiographic localization of proline uptake in excitatory hippocampal pathways. *Hippocampus* **2**:269, 1992.
26. Nickolson VJ: "On" and "off" responses of K^+-induced synaptosomal proline release: Involvement of the sodium pump. *J Neurochem* **38**:289, 1982.
27. Fremeau RTJ, Caron MG, Blakely RD: Molecular cloning and expression of a high affinity L-proline transporter expressed in putative glutamatergic pathways of rat brain. *Neuron* **8**:915, 1992.
28. Shafqat S, Velaz-Faircloth M, Henzi VA, Whitney KD, Yang-Feng TL, Seldin MF, Fremeau RTJ: Human brain-specific L-proline transporter: Molecular cloning, functional expression and chromosomal localization of the gene in human and mouse genomes. *Mol Pharmacol* **48**:219, 1995.
29. Velaz-Faircloth M, Guadano-Ferraz A, Henzi VA, Fremeau RT Jr: Mammalian brain-specific L-proline transporter. *J Biol Chem* **270**:15755, 1995.
30. Adams E: Metabolism of proline and of hydroxyproline. *Int Rev Connect Tissue Res* **5**:1, 1970.
31. Vogel HJ, Davis BD: Glutamic acid g-semialdehyde and Δ^1-pyrroline-5-carboxylic acid, intermediates in the biosynthesis of proline. *J Am Chem Soc* **74**:109, 1952.
32. Strecker JH: The interconversion of glutamic acid and proline 1. The formation of Δ^1-pyrroline-5-carboxylic acid from glutamic acid in *Escherichia coli*. *J Biol Chem* **225**:825, 1957.
33. Peraino C, Pitot H: Ornithine-δ-aminotransferase in the rat. I. Assay and some general properties. *Biochim Biophys Acta* **73**:222, 1963.
34. Ross G, Dunn D, Jones ME: Ornithine synthesis from glutamate in rat intestinal mucosa homogenates: Evidence for the reduction of glutamate to γ-glutamyl semialdehyde. *Biochem Biophys Res Commun* **85**:140, 1978.
35. Smith PJ, Phang JM: The importance of ornithine as a precursor for proline in mammalian cells. *J Cell Physiol* **98**:475, 1979.
36. Herzfeld A, Mezl VA, Knox WE: Enzymes metabolizing Δ^1-pyrroline-5-carboxylate in rat tissues. *Biochem J* **166**:95, 1977.
37. Deutch AH, Rushlow KE, Smith CJ: Analysis of the *Escherichia coli proBA* locus by DNA and protein sequencing. *Nucleic Acids Res* **12**:6337, 1984.
38. Li W, Brandriss MC: Proline biosynthesis in *Saccharomyces cerevisiae*: Molecular analysis of the *PRO1* gene, which encodes gamma-glutamyl kinase. *J Bacteriol* **174**:4148, 1992.
39. Pearson BM, Hernando Y, Payne J, Wolf SS, Kalogeropoulos A, Schweizer M: Sequencing of a 35.71-kb DNA segment on the right arm of yeast chromosome XV reveals regions of similarity to chromosomes I and XIII. *Yeast* **12**:1021, 1996.
40. Smith RJ, Downing SJ, Phang JM, Lodato RF, Aoki TT: Pyrroline-5-carboxylate synthase activity in mammalian cells. *Proc Natl Acad Sci U S A* **77**:5221, 1980.
41. Lodato RF, Smith RJ, Valle D, Phang JM, Aoki TT: Regulation of proline biosynthesis. The inhibition of pyrroline-5-carboxylase synthase activity by ornithine. *Metabolism* **30**:908, 1981.
42. Wakabayashi Y, Henslee JG, Jones ME: Pyrroline-5-carboxylate synthesis from glutamate by rat intestinal mucosa. *J Biol Chem* **258**:3873, 1983.
43. Wakabayashi Y, Yamada R-H, Iwashima A: Temperature- and time-dependent inactivation of pyrroline-5-carboxylate synthase: Suggestive evidence for an allosteric regulation of the enzyme. *Arch Biochem Biophys* **238**:469, 1985.
44. Wakabayashi Y, Yamada E, Hasegawa T, Yamada R: Enzymological evidence for the indispensability of small intestine in the synthesis of arginine from glutamate. I. Pyrroline-5-carboxylate synthase. *Arch Biochem Biophys* **291**:1, 1991.
45. Fleming GA, Granger A, Rogers QR, Prosser M, Ford DB, Phang JM: Fluctuations in plasma pyrroline-5-carboxylate concentrations during feeding and fasting. *J Clin Endocrinol Metab* **69**:448, 1989.
46. Mixson AJ, Phang JM: The uptake of pyrroline 5-carboxylate. Group translocation mediating the transfer of reducing-oxidizing potential. *J Biol Chem* **263**:10720, 1988.
47. Peisach J, Strecker JH: The interconversion of glutamic acid and proline. V. The reduction of Δ^1-pyrroline-5-carboxylic acid to proline. *J Biol Chem* **237**:2255, 1962.
48. Smith ME, Greenberg DM: Preparation and properties of partially purified glutamic semialdehyde reductase. *J Biol Chem* **226**:317, 1957.
49. Yeh GC, Harris SC, Phang JM: Pyrroline-5-carboxylate reductase in human erythrocytes. *J Clin Invest* **67**:1042, 1981.
50. Shiono T, Kador PF, Kinoshita JJ: Purification and characterization of rat lens pyrroline-5-carboxylate reductase. *Biochim Biophys Acta* **881**:72, 1986.
51. Merrill MJ, Yeh GC, Phang JM: Purified human erythrocyte pyrroline-5-carboxylate reductase. Preferential oxidation of NADPH. *J Biol Chem* **264**:9352, 1989.
52. Dougherty KM, Brandriss MC, Valle D: Cloning human pyrroline-5-carboxylate reductase cDNA by complementation in *Saccharomyces cerevisiae*. *J Biol Chem* **267**:871, 1992.
53. Dougherty K, Hu CA, Obie C, Valle D: Molecular cloning, characterization and functional expression of a second mammalian Δ^1-pyrroline-5-carboxylate reductase. *Am J Hum Genet* **65**:A94, 1999.
54. Taggart JV, Krakaur RG: Studies on the cyclophorase system. V. The oxidation of proline and hydroxyproline. *J Biol Chem* **177**:641, 1949.
55. Johnson AB, Strecker JH: The interconversion of glutamic acid and proline. IV. The oxidation of proline by rat liver mitochondria. *J Biol Chem* **237**:1876, 1962.
56. Kramar R, Fitscha P: Studies on the dehydrogenation of proline and hydroxyproline in animal tissue. *Enzymologia* **39**:101, 1970.
57. Downing SJ, Phang JM, Kowaloff EM, Valle D, Smith RJ: Proline oxidase in cultured mammalian cells. *J Cell Physiol* **91**:369, 1977.
58. Kowaloff EM, Phang JM, Granger AS, Downing SJ: Regulation of proline oxidase activity by lactate. *Proc Natl Acad Sci U S A* **74**:5368, 1977.

59. Meyer J: Proline transport in rat liver mitochondria. *Arch Biochem Biophys* **178**:387, 1977.
60. Small WC, Jones ME: Pyrroline 5-carboxylate dehydrogenase of the mitochondrial matrix rat liver. *J Biol Chem* **265**:18668, 1990.
61. Brunner G, Neupert W: Localization of proline oxidase and Δ^1-pyrroline-5-carboxylic acid dehydrogenase in rat liver. *FEBS Lett* **3**:283, 1969.
62. Forte-McRobbie CM, Pietruszko R: Purification and characterization of human liver "high K_m" aldehyde dehydrogenase and its identification as glutamic γ-semialdehyde dehydrogenase. *J Biol Chem* **261**:2154, 1986.
63. Valle D, Balese RM, Harris SC, Phang JM: Proline inhibition of pyrroline-5-carboxylate reductase: Alteration with lymphocyte transformation. *Nature* **253**:214, 1975.
64. Kowaloff EM, Phang JM, Granger AS, Downing SJ: Glucocorticoid induction of proline oxidase in LLC-RK1 cells. *J Cell Physiol* **97**:153, 1978.
65. Phang JM, Downing SJ, Smith RJ, Yeh GC: The inhibition of proline oxidase by long chain fatty acyl-coenzyme As. *Fed Proc* **37**:1480, 1978.
66. Kadowaki H, Patton GM, Knox WE: Proline oxidase inhibition by free fatty acids of rat pancrease. *Biochim Biophys Acta* **614**:294, 1980.
67. Kosower NS, Kosower EM: The glutathione status of cells. *Int Rev Cytol* **54**:109, 1978.
68. Eggleston LV, Krebs HA: Regulation of the pentose phosphate cycle. *Biochem J* **138**:425, 1974.
69. Abate C, Patel L, Rauscher FJ, Curran T: Redox regulation of *fos* and *jun* DNA-binding activity in vitro. *Science* **249**:1157, 1990.
70. Schreck R, Rieber P, Baeuerle PA: Reactive oxygen intermediates as apparently widely used messengers in the activation of the NF-kappa B transcription factor and HIV-1. *EMBO J* **10**:2247, 1991.
71. Yeh GC, Roth EF Jr, Phang JM, Harris SC, Nagel RL, Rinaldi A: The effect of pyrroline-5-carboxylic acid on nucleotide metabolism in erythrocytes from normal and glucose-6-phosphate dehydrogenase-deficient subjects. *J Biol Chem* **259**:5454, 1984.
72. Yeh GC, Phang JM: Pyrroline-5-carboxylate stimulates the conversion of purine antimetabolites to their nucleotide forms by a redox-dependent mechanism. *J Biol Chem* **258**:9774, 1983.
73. Boer P, Sperling O: The effect of pyrroline-5-carboxylate on R5P and PRPP generation in mouse liver in vivo. *Adv Exp Med Biol* **309**B:379, 1991.
74. Boer P, Sperling O: Stimulation of ribose-5-phosphate and 5-phosphoribosyl-1-pyrophosphate generation by pyrroline-5-carboxylate in mouse liver in vivo: Evidence for a regulatory role of ribose-5-phosphate availability in nucleotide synthesis. *Biochem Med Metab Biol* **46**:28, 1991.
75. Phang JM, Downey SJ: Synergistic stimulation of phosphoribosyl pyrophosphate by pyrroline-5-carboxylate and growth factors. *Clin Res* **33**:573A, 1985.
76. Downs SM, Humpherson PG, Leese HJ: Meiotic induction in cumulus cell-enclosed mouse oocytes: Involvement of the pentose phosphate pathway. *Biol Reprod* **58**:1084, 1998.
77. Hagedorn CH, Phang JM: Transfer of reducing equivalents into mitochondria by the interconversions of proline and Δ^1- pyrroline-5-carboxylate. *Arch Biochem Biophys* **225**:95, 1983.
78. Hagedorn CH, Phang JM: Catalytic transfer of hydride ions from NADPH to oxygen by the interconversions of proline and Δ 1-pyrroline 5-carboxylate. *Arch Biochem Biophys* **248**:166, 1986.
79. Hagedorn CH, Yeh GC, Phang JM: Transfer of Δ^1-pyrroline-5-carboxylate as oxidizing potential from hepatocytes to erythrocytes. *Biochem J* **202**:31, 1982.
80. Windmueller HG, Spaeth AE: Source and fate of circulating citrulline. *Am J Physiol* **241**:E473, 1981.
81. Wu G: An important role for pentose cycle in the synthesis of citruline and proline from glutamine in porcine enterocytes. *Arch Biochem Biophys* **336**:224, 1996.
82. Wu G, Knabe DA, Flynn NE, Yan W, Flynn SP: Arginine degradation in developing porcine enterocytes. *Am J Physiol* **34**:G913, 1996.
83. Wu G: Synthesis of citrulline and arginine from proline in enterocytes of postnatal pigs. *Am J Physiol* **272**:G1382, 1997.
84. Matsuzawa T, Kobayashi T, Tashiro K, Kasahara M: Changes in ornithine metabolic enzymes induced by dietary protein in small intestine and liver: Intestine-liver relationship in ornithine supply to liver. *J Biochem* **116**:721, 1994.
85. de Jonge WJ, Dingemanse MA, de Boer PA, Lamers WH, Moorman AF: Arginine-metabolizing enzymes in the developing rat small intestine. *Pediatr Res* **43**:442, 1998.
86. Hurwitz R, Kretchmer N: Development of arginine-synthesizing enzymes in mouse intestine. *Am J Physiol* **251**:G103, 1986.
87. Riby JE, Hurwitz RE, Kretchmer N: Development of ornithine metabolism in the mouse intestine. *Pediatr Res* **28**:261, 1990.
88. Wang T, Lawler AM, Steel G, Sipila I, Milam AH, Valle D: Mice lacking ornithine-δ-aminotransferase have paradoxical neonatal hypo-ornithinaemia and retinal degeneration. *Nat Genet* **11**:185, 1995.
89. Wu G: Intestinal mucosal amino acid catabolism. *J Nutr* **128**:1249, 1998.
90. Wu G, Morris SM: Arginine metabolism: Nitric oxide and beyond. *Biochem J* **336**:1, 1998.
91. Wakabayashi Y: The glutamate crossway, in Cynober LA (ed): *Amino Acid Metabolism and Therapy in Health and Nutritional Disease*. New York, CRC Press, 1995, p 89.
92. Murphy JM, Murch SJ, Ball RO: Proline is synthesized from glutamate during intragastric infusion but not during intravenous infusion in neonatal piglets. *J Nutr* **126**:878, 1996.
93. Samuels SE, Acton KS, Ball RO: Pyrroline-5-carboxylate reductase and proline oxidase activity in the neonatal pig. *J Nutr* **119**:1999, 1989.
94. Cleary MA, Sivakumar P, Olpin S, Wraith JE, Walter JH, Till J, Morris AA, Besley GT: Ornithine aminotransferase deficiency: Difficulties in diagnosis in the neonatal period. *J Inherit Metab Dis* **22**:69, 1999.
95. Prockop DJ: Intracellular steps in the biosynthesis of collagen, in Ramchandran GN, Reddi AH (eds): *Biochemistry of Collagen*. New York, Plenum, 1976, p 163.
96. Bentley JP, Hanson AN: The hydroxyproline of elastin. *Biochim Biophys Acta* **175**:339, 1969.
97. Porter RR, Reid KB: The biochemistry of complement. *Nature* **275**:699, 1978.
98. Anglister L, Rogozinski S, Silman I: Detection of hydroxyproline in preparations of acetylcholinesterase from the electric organ of the electric eel. *FEBS Lett* **69**:129, 1976.
99. Adams E, Goldstone A: Hydroxyproline metabolism: Enzymatic preparation and properties of Δ^1-pyrroline-3-hydroxy-5-carboxylate. *J Biol Chem* **235**:3492, 1960.
100. Man M, Adams E: Basement membrane and interstitial collagen content of whole animals and tissues. *Biochem Biophys Res Commun* **66**:9, 1975.
101. Tryggvason K, Majamaa K, Kivirikko KI: Prolyl 3-hydroxylase and 4-hydroxylase activities in certain rat and chick-embryo tissues and age-related changes in their activities in the rat. *Biochem J* **178**:127, 1979.
102. Rosso RG, Adams E: Metabolism of gamma-hydroxyglutamic acid. *J Biol Chem* **237**:3476, 1962.
103. Valle D, Goodman S, Harris S, Phang J: Genetic evidence for a common enzyme catalyzing the second step in the degradation of proline and hydroxyproline. *J Clin Invest* **64**:1365, 1979.
104. Adams E, Ramaswamy S, Lamon M: 3-Hydroxy-proline content of normal urine. *J Clin Invest* **61**:1482, 1978.
105. Bisker A, Pailler V, Randoux A, Borel JP: A new sensitive method for the quantitative evaluation of the hydroxyproline isomers. *Anal Biochem* **122**:52, 1982.
106. Chanard J, Szymanowicz A, Brunois JP, Toupance O, Melin JP, Birembaut P, Randoux A, Borel PJ: Increased renal excretion of 3-hydroxyproline in patients with active glomerular nephropathies and with polycystic renal disease. *Clin Nephrol* **17**:64, 1982.
107. Gregory DM, Sovetts D, Clow CL, Scriver CR: Plasma free amino acid values in normal children and adolescents. *Metabolism* **35**:967, 1986.
108. Scriver CR, Rosenberg LE: *Amino Acid Metabolism and Its Disorders*. Philadelphia, WB Saunders, 1973.
109. Kibrick AC, Kitagawa G, Maskaleris ML, Gaines R Jr, Milhorat AT: Hydroxyproline in human blood: Forms in which it is present. *Proc Soc Exp Biol Med* **119**:622, 1965.
110. Oye I: The amount of free hydroxyproline in human blood serum. *Scand J Clin Lab Invest* **14**:259, 1962.
111. Kivirikko KI: Urinary excretion of hydroxyproline in health and disease. *Int Rev Connect Tissue Res* **5**:93, 1970.
112. Nusgens B, Lapiere CHM: The relationship between proline and hydroxyproline urinary excretion in humans as an index of collagen metabolism. *Clin Chim Acta* **48**:203, 1973.
113. Meilman E, Urivetzky MM, Rapoprot CM: Urinary hydroxyproline peptides. *J Clin Invest* **42**:40, 1963.
114. Kivirikko KI, Laitinen O: Clinical significance of urinary hydroxyproline determinations in children. *Ann Paediatr Fenn* **11**:148, 1965.
115. Laitinen O, Nikkila EA, Kivirikko KI: Hydroxyproline in the serum and urine. Normal values and clinical significance. *Acta Med Scand* **179**:275, 1966.

116. Uitto J, Laitinen O, Lamberg BA, Kivirikko KI: Further evaluation of the significance of urinary hydroxyproline determinations in the diagnosis of thyroid disorders. *Clin Chim Acta* **22**:583, 1968.
117. Christensen HN: On the strategy of kinetic discrimination of amino acid transport systems. *J Membr Biol* **84**:97, 1985.
118. Christensen HN: Role of amino acid transport and countertransport in nutrition and metabolism. *Physiol Rev* **70**:43, 1990.
119. Palacín M, Estévez R, Zorzano A: Cystinuria calls for heteromultimeric amino acid transporters. *Curr Opin Cell Biol* **10**:455, 1998.
120. Finerman GA, Rosenberg LE: Amino acid transport in bone. Evidence for separate transport systems for neutral amino and imino acids. *J Biol Chem* **241**:1487, 1966.
121. Finerman GA, Downing S, Rosenberg LE: Amino acid transport in bone. II. Regulation of collagen synthesis by perturbation of proline transport. *Biochim Biophys Acta* **135**:1008, 1967.
122. Samarzija I, Fromter E: Electrophysiological analysis of rat renal sugar and amino acid transport. III. Neutral amino acids. *Pflugers Arch* **393**:119, 1982.
123. Foreman JW, McNamara PD, Pepe LM, Ginkinger K, Segal S: Uptake of proline by brush-border vesicles isolated from human kidney cortex. *Biochem Med* **34**:304, 1985.
124. Scriver CR, Efron ML, Schafer IA: Renal tubular transport of proline, hydroxyproline and glycine in health and in familial hyperprolinemia. *J Clin Invest* **43**:374, 1964.
125. Scriver CR, Goldman H: Renal tubular transport of proline, hydroxyproline, and glycine. II. Hydroxy-L-proline as substrate and as inhibitor in vivo. *J Clin Invest* **45**:1357, 1966.
126. Scriver CR, McInnes RR, Mohyuddin F: Role of epithelial architecture and intracellular metabolism in proline uptake and transtubular reclamation in PRO/Re mouse kidney. *Proc Natl Acad Sci U S A* **72**:1431, 1975.
127. Simell O, Scriver CR, Mohyuddin F: Structural relationships between metabolism and transport of proline in the nephron. *Pediatr Res* **10**:444, 1976.
128. Crump FT, Fremeau RT, Craig AM: Localization of the brain-specific high-affinity L-proline transporter in cultured hippocampal neurons: Molecular heterogeneity of synaptic terminals. *Mol Cell Neurosci* **13**:25, 1999.
129. Renick SE, Kleven DT, Chan J, Stenius K, Milner TA, Pickel VM, Fremeau RT Jr: The mammalian brain high-affinity L-proline transporter is enriched preferentially in synaptic vesicles in a subpopulation of excitatory nerve terminals in rat forebrain. *J Neurosci* **19**:21, 1999.
130. Fremeau RT Jr, Velaz-Faircloth M, Miller JW, Henzi VA, Cohen SM, Nadler JV, Shafqat S, Blakely RD, Domin B: A novel nonopioid action of enkephalins: Competitive inhibition of the mammalian brain high affinity L-proline transporter. *Mol Pharmacol* **49**:1033, 1996.
131. Galli A, Jayanthi LD, Ramsey IS, Miller JW, Fremeau RT Jr, DeFelice LJ: L-Proline and L-pipecolate induce enkephalin-sensitive currents in human embryonic kidney 293 cells transfected with the high-affinity mammalian brain L-proline transporter. *J Neurosci* **19**:6290, 1999.
132. Bennett JP, Logan WJ, Snyder SH: Amino acid neurotransmitter candidates: Sodium-dependent high affinity uptake by unique synaptosomal fractions. *Science* **178**:997, 1972.
133. Peterson NA, Raghupathy E: Characteristics of amino acid accumulation of synaptosomal particles isolated from rat brain. *J Neurochem* **19**:1423, 1972.
134. Balcar VJ, Johnston GAR, Stephenson AL: Transport of L-proline by rat brain slices. *Brain Res* **102**:143, 1976.
135. Stevens BR, Wright EM: Substrate specificity of the intestinal brush-border proline/sodium (IMINO) transporter. *J Membr Biol* **87**:27, 1985.
136. Cohen SM, Nadler JV: Proline-induced potentiation of glutamate transmission. *Brain Res* **761**:271, 1997.
137. Hu C-A, Lin W-W, Obie C, Valle D: Molecular enzymology of mammalian Δ^1-pyrroline-5-carboxylate synthase. *J Biol Chem* **274**:6754, 1999.
138. Brandriss MC: Proline utilization in *Saccharomyces cerevisiae*: Analysis of the cloned *PUT2* gene. *Molec Cell Biol* **3**:1846, 1983.
139. Zhang C, Lu Q, Verma DPS: Removal of feedback inhibition of Δ^1-pyrroline-5-carboxylate synthetase, a bifunctional enzyme catalyzing the first two steps of proline biosynthesis in plants. *J Biol Chem* **270**:20491, 1995.
140. Schild D, Brake AJ, Kiefer MC, Young D, Barr PJ: Cloning of three human multifunctional *de novo* purine biosynthetic genes by functional complementation of yeast mutations. *Proc Natl Acad Sci U S A* **87**:2916, 1990.
141. Lorans G, Phang JM: Proline synthesis and redox regulation: Differential functions of pyrroline-5-carboxylate reductase in human lymphoblastoid cell lines. *Biochem Biophys Res Comm* **101**:1018, 1981.
142. Lin W-W, Hu CA, Valle D: Molecular cloning of cDNAs encoding human and mouse proline oxidase, the enzyme-deficient in type I hyperprolinemia and Pro/Re mice. *Am J Hum Genet* **59**:A269, 1996.
143. Campbell HD, Webb GC, Young IG: A human homologue of the *Drosophila melanogaster sluggish-A* (proline oxidase) gene maps to 22q11.2, and is a candidate gene for type I hyperprolinaemia. *Hum Genet* **101**:69, 1997.
144. Gogos JA, Santha M, Takacs Z, Beck KD, Luine V, Lucas LR, Nadler JV, Karayiorgou M: The gene encoding proline dehydrogenase modulates sensorimotor gating in mice. *Nat Genet* **21**:434, 1999.
145. Karayiorgou M, Morris MA, Morrow B, Shprintzen RJ, Goldberg R, Borrow J, Gos A, Nestadt G, Wolyniec PS, Lasseter VK, Eisen H, Childs B, Kazazian HH, Kucherlapati R, Antonarakis SE, Pulver AE, Housman DE: Schizophrenia susceptibility associated with interstitial deletions of chromosome 22q11. *Proc Natl Acad Sci U S A* **92**:7612, 1995.
146. Jaeken J, Goemans N, Fryns JP, Farncois I, DeZegher F: Association of hyperprolinemia type I and heparin cofactor II deficiency with CATCH22 syndrome: Evidence for a contiguous gene syndrome locating the proline oxidase gene. *J Inherit Metab Dis* **19**:275, 1996.
147. Hempel J, Nicholas H, Lindahl R: Aldehyde dehydrogenases: Widespread structural and functional diversity within a shared framework. *Protein Sci* **2**:1890, 1993.
148. Hu CA, Lin W-W, Valle D: Cloning, characterization and expression of cDNAs encoding human Δ^1-pyrroline-5-carboxylate dehydrogenase. *J Biol Chem* **271**:9795, 1996.
149. Hawkins JD: A survey on intron and exon lengths. *Nucleic Acids Res* **16**:9893, 1988.
150. Phang JM, Yeh GC, Scriver CR: Disorders of proline and hydroxyproline metabolism, in Scriver CR, Beaudet AL, Sly WS, Valle D (eds): *The Metabolic and Molecular Bases of Inherited Disease*, 7th ed. New York, McGraw Hill, 1995, p 1125.
151. Scriver CR, Schafer IA, Efron ML: New renal tubular amino acid transport system and a new hereditary disorder of amino acid metabolism. *Nature* **192**:672, 1961.
152. Schafer IA, Scriver CR, Efron ML: Familial hyperprolinemia, cerebral dysfunction and renal anomalies occurring in a family with hereditary nephritis and deafness. *N Engl J Med* **267**:51, 1962.
153. Fontaine G, Farriaux JP, Dautrevaux M: Type I hyperprolinemia. Study of a familial case. *Helv Paediatr Acta* **25**:165, 1970.
154. Woody NC, Snyder CH, Harris JA: Hyperprolinemia: Clinical and biochemical family study. *Pediatrics* **44**:554, 1969.
155. Mollica F, Pavone L, Antener I: Pure familial hyperprolinemia: Isolated inborn error of amino acid metabolism without other anomalies in a Sicilian family. *Pediatrics* **48**:1971.
156. Potter JL, Waickman FJ: Hyperprolinemia. I. A study of a large family. *J Pediatr* **83**:635, 1973.
157. Fusco G, Caromagno S, Romano A, Rinaldi E, Cedrola G, Cianciaruso L, Curto A, Rosolia S, Auricchio G: Type I hyperprolinemia in a family suffering from aniridia and severe dystrophia of ocular tissues. *Opthalmologica* **173**:1, 1976.
158. Oyanagi K, Tsuchiyama A, Itakura Y, Tamura Y, Nakao T, Fujita S, Shiono H: Clinical, biochemical and enzymatic studies in type I hyperprolinemia associated with chromosomal abnormality. *Tohoku J Exp Med* **151**:465, 1987.
159. Steinlin M, Boltshauser E, Steinmann B, Wichmann W, Niemeyer G: Hyperprolinaemia type I and white matter disease: Coincidence or causal relationship? *Eur J Pediatr* **149**:40, 1989.
160. Mollica F, Pavone L: Hyperprolinaemia: A disease which does not need treatment? *Acta Paediatr* **65**:206, 1976.
161. Kopelman H, Asatoor AM, Miline MD: Hyperprolinaemia and hereditary nephritis. *Lancet* **2**:1075, 1964.
162. Perry TL, Hardwick DF, Lowry RB, Hansen S: Hyperprolinaemia in two successive generations of a North American Indian family. *Ann Hum Genet* **31**:401, 1968.
163. Hainaut H, Hariga J, Willems C, Heusden A, Chapelle P: Familial essential hyperprolinemia. *Presse Med* **79**:945, 1971.
164. Edelmann L, Pandita RK, Spiteri E, Funke B, Goldberg R, Palanisamy N, Chaganti RSK, Magenis E, Shpritzen RJ, Morrow BE: A common molecular basis for rearrangement disorders on chromosome 22q11. *Hum Mol Genet* **8**:1157, 1999.
165. Stoffel M, Karayiorgou M, Espinosa R 3rd, Beau MM: The human mitochondrial citrate transporter gene (SLC20A3) maps to chromo-

some band 22q11 within a region implicated in DiGeorge syndrome, velo-cardio-facial syndrome and schizophrenia. *Hum Genet* **98**:113, 1996.

166. Carlson C, Sirotkin H, Pandita R, Goldberg R, McKie J, Wadey R, Patanjali SR, Weissman SM, Anyane-Yeboa K, Warburton D, Scambler P, Shprintzen R, Kucherlapati R, Morrow BE: Molecular definition of 22q11 deletions in 151 velo-cardio-facial syndrome patients. *Am J Hum Genet* **61**:620, 1997.
167. Berlow S, Efron ME: A new cause of hyperprolinemia associated with the excretion of Δ^1-pyrroline-5-carboxylic acid. *Proc Soc Pediatr Res* **34**:43, 1964.
168. Simila S, Visakorpi JK: Hyperprolinemia without renal disease. *Acta Paediatr* **177**:122, 1967.
169. Emery FA, Goldie L, Stern J: Hyperprolinaemia type 2. *J Ment Defic Res* **12**:187, 1968.
170. Jeune M, Collombel C, Michel M, David M, Guibaud P, Guerrier G, Albert J: Hyperleucinisoleucinemia due to partial transamination defect associated with type 2 hyperprolinemia. Familial case of double aminoacidopathy. *Ann Pediatr* **17**:349, 1970.
171. Bellet H, Morin D, Daudet H, Dumas ML, Valette H, magnan de Bornier B, Dumas R: Type II hyperprolinaemia with renal involvement. *J Inherit Metab Dis* **14**:846, 1991.
172. Goodman SI, Mace JW, Miles BS, Teng CC, Brown SB: Defective hydroxyproline metabolism in type II hyperprolinemia. *Biochem Med* **10**:329, 1974.
173. Pavone L, Mollica F, Levy HL: Asymptomatic type II hyperprolinaemia associated with hyperglycinaemia in three sibs. *Arch Dis Child* **50**:637, 1975.
174. Flynn MP, Martin MC, Moore PT, Stafford JA, Fleming GA, Phang JM: Type II hyperprolinaemia in a pedigree of Irish Travellers (nomads). *Arch Dis Child* **64**:1699, 1989.
175. Efron ML, Bixby EM, Pryles CV: Hydroxyprolinemia. *New Engl J Med* **272**:1294, 1965.
176. Efron ML, Bixby EM, Pryles CV: Hydroxyprolinemia. II. A rare metabolic disease due to a deficiency in the enzyme "hydroxyproline oxidase." *N Engl J Med* **272**:1299, 1965.
177. Applegarth DA, Ingram P, Hingston J, Hardwick DF: Hyperprolinemia type II. *Clin Biochem* **7**:14, 1974.
178. Scriver CR, Smith RJ, Phang JM: Disorders of proline and hydroxyproline metabolism, in Stanbury JM, Wyngaarden JB, Frederickson DS (eds): *The Metabolic Basis of Inherited Disease*, 5th New York, McGraw Hill, 1983, p 360.
179. Selkoe DJ: Familial hyperprolinemia and mental retardation. A second metabolic type. *Neurology* **19**:494, 1969.
180. Simila S: Hyperprolinaemia type II. *Fla Dent J* **2**:143, 1970.
181. Mixson AJ, Granger AN, Phang JM: An assay for pyrroline-5-carboxylate based on its interaction with cysteine. *Anal Lett* **24**:625, 1991.
182. Fleming GA, Hagedorn CH, Granger AS, Phang JM: Pyrroline-5-carboxylate in human plasma. *Metabolism* **33**:739, 1984.
183. Dooley KC, Applegarth DA: Hyperprolinemia type II: Evidence of the excretion of 3-hydroxy delta 1-pyrroline 5-carboxylic acid. *Clin Biochem* **12**:62, 1979.
184. Simila S: Hydroxyproline metabolism in type II hyperprolinaemia. *Ann Clin Biochem* **16**:177, 1979.
185. Valle D, Phang JM, Goodman SI: Type II hyperprolinemia: Absent Δ^1-pyrroline-5-carboxylic acid dehydrogenase activity. *Science* **185**:1053, 1974.
186. Valle DL, Goodman SI, Applegarth DA, Shih VE, Phang JM: Type II hyperprolinemia: Δ^1-Pyrroline-5-carboxylic acid dehydrogenase deficiency in cultured skin fibroblasts and circulating lymphocytes. *J Clin Invest* **58**:598, 1976.
187. Kacser H, Burns JA: The molecular basis of dominance. *Genetics* **97**:639, 1981.
188. Felix D, Kunzle H: The role of proline in nervous transmission. In Costa E, Giacobini E, Paoletti R (eds): *Advances in Biochemical Psychopharmacology*, New York, Raven Press, 1976, p 165.
189. van Herreveld A, Fifkova E: Effects of amino acids on the isolated chicken retina and on its response to glutamate stimulation. *J Neurochem* **20**:947, 1973.
190. Marliss EB, Aoki TT, Toelos CJ, Felig P, Connon JJ, Fyner J, Huckabee WE, Cahill GF: Amino acid metabolism in lactic acidosis. *Am J Med* **52**:474, 1972.
191. Goodman SI, Reale M, Berlow S: Glutaric acidemia type II: A form with deleterious intrauterine effects. *J Pediatr* **102**:411, 1983.
192. Sweetman L, Nyhan WL, Trauner DA, Merritt A, Singh M: Glutaric aciduria type II. *J Pediatr* **96**:1020, 1980.
193. Strecker HJ: The interconversion of glutamic acid and proline. III. Δ^1-Pyrroline-5-carboxylic acid dehydrogenase. *J Biol Chem* **235**:3218, 1960.
194. Valle D, Downing SJ, Phang JM: Proline inhibition of pyrroline-5-carboxylate reductase: Differences in enzymes obtained from animal and tissue culture sources. *Biochem Biophys Res Comm* **54**:1418, 1973.
195. Blocks RJ, Bolling D: *The Amino Acid Composition of Proteins and Foods*. Springfield, IL, Charles C. Thomas, 1951.
196. Simila S: Dietary treatment in hyperprolinaemia type II. *Acta Paediatr* **63**:249, 1974.
197. Piesowicz AT: Hyperprolinaemia. *Arch Dis Child* **43**:748, 1968.
198. Harries JT, Piesowicz AT, Seakins JW, Francis DE, Wolff OH: Low proline diet in type I hyperprolinaemia. *Arch Dis Child* **46**:72, 1971.
199. Efron ML: Treatment of hydroxyprolinemia and hyperprolinemia. *Am J Dis Child* **113**:166, 1967.
200. Goyer RA, Mitchell BJ, Leonard DL: Dietary reduction of hyperprolinemia. *J Lab Clin Med* **73**:819, 1969.
201. Whelan DT, Conner WT: Maternal hyperprolinaemia. *Lancet* **2**:981, 1980.
202. Tomenchok DM, Brandriss MC: Gene-enzyme relationships in the proline biosynthetic pathway of *Saccharomyces cerevisiae*. *J Bacteriol* **169**:5364, 1987.
203. Krzywicki KA, Brandriss MC: Primary structure of the nuclear *PUT2* gene involved in the mitochondrial pathway for proline utilization in *Saccharomyces cerevisiae*. *Mol Cell Biol* **4**:2837, 1984.
204. Dougherty KM, Swanson DA, Brody LC, Valle D: Expression and processing of human ornithine-δ-aminotransferase in *Saccharomyces cerevisiae*. *Hum Mol Genet* **2**:1835, 1993.
205. Benzer S: Behavioral mutants of *Drosophila* isolated by countercurrent distribution. *Proc Natl Acad Sci U S A* **58**:1112, 1967.
206. Hayward DC, Delaney SJ, Campbell HD, Ghysen A, Benzer S, Kasparzak AB, Cotsell JN, Young IG, Gabor Miklos GL: The sluggish-A gene of *Drosophila melanogaster* is expressed in the nervous system and encodes proline oxidase, a mitochondrial enzyme involved in glutamate biosynthesis. *Proc Natl Acad Sci U S A* **90**:2979, 1993.
207. Blake RL: Hyperprolinemia and prolinuria in a new inbred strain of mice, PRO/Re. *Science* **17**:809, 1972.
208. Blake RL, Hall JG, Russell ES: Mitochondrial proline dehydrogenase deficiency in hyperprolinemic PRO/Re mice: Genetic and enzymatic analysis. *Biochem Genet* **14**:739, 1976.
209. Adams E, Frank L: Metabolism of proline and the hydroxyprolines. *Annu Rev Biochem* **49**:1005, 1980.
210. Efron ML, Bixby EM, Palattao LG, Pryles CV: Hydroxyprolinemia associated with mental deficiency. *N Engl J Med* **267**:1193, 1962.
211. Pelkonnen R, Lahdevirta J, Visakorpi JK, Kivirriko KI: Hydroxyprolinemia: A case without mental deficiency. *Scand J Clin Lab Invest* **23**:21, 1969.
212. Raine DN: Defects in renal tubular reabsorption, in Benson PF (ed): *Defects in Cellular Organelles and Membranes in Relation to Mental Retardation*. London, Churchill-Livingstone, 1971, p 43.
213. Rama Rao BS, Subhash MN, Marayanan HS: Hydroxyprolinemia: A case report. *Indian Pediatr* **11**:829, 1974.
214. Roesel RA, Blankenship PR, Lynch WR, Coryell ME, Thevaos TS, Hall WK: Hydroxyproline metabolism in two sisters with hydroxyprolinemia. *Hum Hered* **29**:364, 1979.
215. Robinson MJ, Menzies IS, Sloan I: Hydroxyprolinemia with normal development. *Arch Dis Child* **55**:484, 1980.
216. Kim SZ, Varvogli L, Waisbren SE, Levy HL: Hydroxyprolinemia: Comparison of a patient and her unaffected twin sister. *J Pediatr* **130**:437, 1997.
217. Pelkonen R, Kivirikko KI: Hydroxyprolinemia: An apparently harmless familial metabolic disorder. *N Engl J Med* **283**:451, 1970.
218. Efron ML, Bixby EM, Hockaday TDR, Smith LH Jr, Meshorer E: Hydroxyprolinemia. III. The origin of free hydroxyproline in hydroxyproinemia. Collagen turnover. Evidence for a biosynthetic pathway in man. *Biochim Biophys Acta* **165**:238, 1968.
219. Heacock AM, Adams E: Hydroxy-L-proline as a substrate for hog kidney D-amino acid oxidase. *Biochem Biophys Res Commun* **57**:279, 1974.
220. Morrow GD, Kivitikko KI, Prockop DJ: Hydroxyprolinemia and increased excretion of free hydroxyproline in early infancy. *J Clin Endocrinol Metab* **26**:1012, 1966.
221. Morrow GD, Kivirikko KI, Prockop DJ: Catabolism and excretion of free hydroxyproline in infancy. *J Clin Endocrinol Metab* **27**:1365, 1967.
222. Hyman PE, Shapiro LJ: Dietary hyperhydroxyprolinemia. *J Pediatr* **104**:595, 1984.

CHAPTER 82

Prolidase Deficiency

Peter Hechtman

1. **Prolidase deficiency (PD) (MIM 170100) is a rare, autosomal recessive, panethnic disorder associated with massive imidodipeptiduria. Undegraded dipeptides are excreted in excess of 15 mmol/day. Affected children often present with severe skin ulcers, particularly on their hands and feet. Mild to severe mental retardation occurs in approximately 75 percent of cases. Additionally, PD individuals appear to be highly susceptible to infections, some of which have been fatal. There is considerable clinical heterogeneity and at least five asymptomatic PD individuals have been identified. Three of these had severely affected sibs and two were detected in newborn screening programs.**
2. **Prolidase (imidodipeptidase, peptidase D; EC 3.4.13.9) is a ubiquitous cytosolic enzyme that catalyzes hydrolysis of dipeptides with a C-terminal proline or hydroxyproline. The enzyme is encoded by the peptidase D (*PEPD*) gene located at 19q12-q13.11. *PEPD* spans 130 kb and has 15 exons. The 2.1 to 2.2 kb mRNA is translated into a 493-amino acid protein with a predicted molecular weight of 54.3 kDa. Native prolidase is a homodimer. A second, less well-characterized enzyme able to catalyze hydrolysis of imidodipeptides is known as prolidase II. Its activity does not appear to compensate for deficiency of prolidase.**
3. **Prolidase is a metalloenzyme that is activated by Mn^{++}. The specificity and function of prolidase metal binding remains controversial. Recent reports indicate that Mn^{++} incubation affects the V_{max} but not the K_m of prolidase and that Mn^{++} also increases the thermostability of the enzyme. Some metals, such as Co^{++}, Mg^{++} and Fe^{++} stimulate enzyme activity to a lesser extent than Mn^{++}; others, such as Zn^{++}, Pb^{++}, Hg^{++} and Cd^{++}, inhibit prolidase activity.**
4. **A structural model for prolidase has been proposed based on homology modeling with crystallized *E. coli* methionine aminopeptidase. There is a "pita-bread fold" in which five amino acid residues form two metal binding sites in each subunit. This predicted stoichiometric ratio is supported by atomic absorption spectroscopy on purified, activated human prolidase. The catalytic site of prolidase is predicted to contain an arginine and an acidic amino acid.**
5. **Mutation analysis in PD individuals has identified nine *PEPD* mutations. Most are CpG mutations and only one, G448R, has been found in multiple, unrelated individuals. Expression systems for testing the functional consequences of *PEPD* mutations use COS cells or NIH3T3 cells.**
6. **Proline is a nonessential amino acid. Its biosynthesis in human tissues occurs via the action of Δ-1-pyrroline-5-carboxylic acid reductase upon glutamic semialdehyde (see Chap. 81). Both glutamic acid and arginine (via ornithine) are precursors. Studies in cultured fibroblasts have shown, however, that these sources contribute to less than 10 percent of collagen-bound proline. This suggests a role for prolidase in recycling dipeptide-bound proline back to the free amino acid pool for utilization in protein biosynthesis. Prolidase substrates can entirely satisfy the growth requirements of cultured CHO cells auxotrophic for proline.**
7. **The abundance of glycyl-L-proline (typically 15 to 35 percent of excreted dipeptide) in the urine of PD patients and the presence of hydroxyproline-containing dipeptides suggests a role for prolidase in collagen turnover. The urine of prolidase deficient patients contains high concentrations of glutamyl-L-proline and aspartyl-L-proline, dipeptides not abundant in collagen. This observation suggests that prolidase participates in the degradation of proteins other than collagen. Although prolidase is ubiquitous, both the intestine and the kidney have high prolidase activities. This suggests prolidase may be involved in the absorption of imidodipeptides. Consistent with this notion, studies in both humans and mice indicate a role for prolidase in dipeptide transport.**
8. **Laboratory diagnosis of PD is straightforward. The amino acid profile of unhydrolyzed urine samples from prolidase-deficient individuals is normal. Acid hydrolyzed specimens, however, contain massive amounts of proline, hydroxyproline, and free amino acids derived from the N-terminal position of the dipeptide. Confirmation of diagnosis by assay of prolidase activity can be performed on erythrocytes, leukocytes, or cultured fibroblasts. Small and variable activity of a second enzyme, prolidase II, may obscure the difference between markedly decreased or absent prolidase activity.**
9. **Current treatments for PD include dietary supplementation with L-proline; Mn^{++} and ascorbic acid; supplementation with essential amino acids; erythrocyte transfusions; and topical application of ointments containing L-glycine and L-proline. Despite encouraging preliminary reports, none of these therapeutic approaches has achieved consistent success.**

The investigation by Goodman et al.[1] of a patient with a "syndrome resembling lathyrism" led to the detection in urine of dipeptides, which, upon hydrolysis, yielded large amounts of proline and hydroxyproline. These peptides were subsequently shown to have the "imido" configuration (an iminoacid at the C-terminus) and to be substrates for prolidase.[2] Complete absence of this enzyme in patient's red and white blood cells was first demonstrated by Powell et al.[3]

CLINICAL PHENOTYPE

Prolidase deficiency (PD; MIM 170100) is a multisystem disorder with considerable phenotypic variability. The clinical data for this review is derived from published reports of 45 cases of PD in 31 families.[1,3–30] Because the case reports differ greatly in breadth and depth of clinical investigation, it was not possible to obtain accurate frequencies for each of the clinical features comprising

A list of standard abbreviations is located immediately preceding the index in each volume. Additional abbreviations used in this chapter include: DM = myotonic dystrophy; EGF, epidermal growth factor; OAT = ornithine--aminotransferase; pCMB = p-chloromercurobenzoate; PD = prolidase deficiency; P5C = [1] pyrroline-5-carboxylate; PDGF = platelet-derived growth factor; SLE = systemic lupus erythematosus; TGF- = transforming growth factor-beta; TNF-, tumor necrosis factor-alpha.

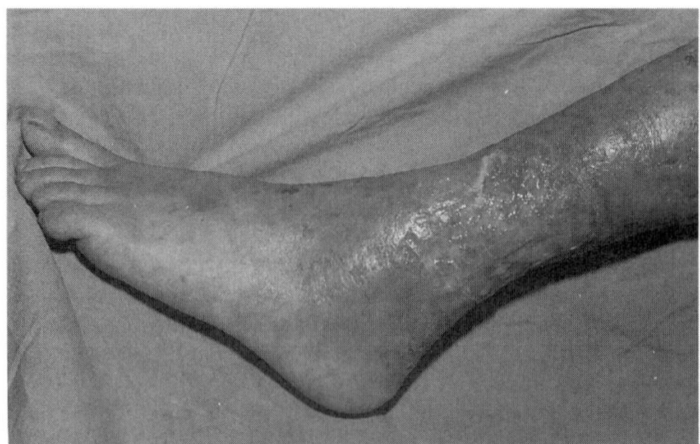

Fig. 82-1 Leg ulcers in a severely affected 12-year-old PD patient. *(Photograph courtesy of A. Klar, Dept. of Pediatrics, Bikur Cholim Hospital, Jerusalem, Israel.)*

the phenotypic spectrum. For more detailed reviews see references 8, 14, 31, and 32.

Skin and Hair

Severe, recurrent, painful skin ulcers are the hallmark of PD. Among 40 patients for whom reports are complete, 26 had active ulcers and 8 had scars due to previous ulceration or had regions of atrophic skin suggesting future ulcers. Only six reported no skin lesions. Virtually all patients with skin abnormalities were affected on the feet or lower legs. Figure 82-1 shows typical skin ulcers on the lower leg of a severely affected patient. In a few cases, ulcers also occurred on the hands and/or the gluteal area. The age of onset for skin ulcers varied between 19 months and 19 years with two-thirds of affected individuals developing lesions before puberty. In eight families with affected sib pairs or first-cousin pairs, four sib pairs experienced onset of ulcers within 3 years of each other.[11,13,19,28] There were much greater differences in age of onset in the remaining four pairs[8,9,14,22,33,34] suggesting a lack of correlation of genotype with this phenotypic feature. A variety of skin manifestations may precede the occurrence of ulcers by several years. These include scaly, erythematous, maculopapular lesions, purpura, and telangiectasias with or without photosensitivity. These lesions or rashes often have a wide distribution, whereas ulceration occurs predominantly on the feet and lower legs. Healing of ulcers may require 4 to 7 months or longer.

More than half of PD patients presenting with skin ulcers had infections of the ulcerated regions. *Pseudomonas aeruginosa* and *Staphylococcus aureus* were the most frequently reported organisms. Individual patients have been reported with skin infections by a "yeast-like fungi"[9] or by herpes.[7] Superinfections are not uncommon.[11,21,35] In several patients, appearance of ulcers was linked to trauma.[19,29,34,36] In one case, ulcers erupted at the site of skin excoriated by excessive scratching.[8]

The ulcers generally have a granular surface[8] with a necrotic base[19,28] and are encircled by thickened skin.[11] Deep ulcers over the Achilles tendon may expose and cause breakage of this tissue,[8,29] forcing the patient to use a wheelchair.[22] Amputation of severely deformed toes has been required.[37] Repeated scarring in the region of the Achilles tendon has caused contractures.[8,10,11,19,23,24]

Other areas of the body are less affected by dermatologic manifestations. In some patients, the skin of the abdomen is particularly thin, permitting visualization of the blood vessels,[11,29] and poliosis has been reported in a number of cases.[5,8,10,11,30,38]

Facies

Although many case reports refer to a "characteristic facies" there is no consensus regarding the essential features of this phenotype. For 30 families for whom such reports are available, 10 failed to mention characteristic facial features, while 8 mentioned facial dysmorphism without additional details. The 12 remaining reports[1,3,6–8,10–12,15,19,24,28] describe ocular hypertelorism (seven families), saddle nose, protruding or small lower jaw, high-arched palate, and low hair line (five families), and proptosis (two families).

Other Dysmorphic Features

Despite an emphasis on short stature in early reports, the majority of PD patients described since the mid-1980s have normal stature. Scoliosis has been reported in two patients. Five PD patients had joint laxity.

Mental Function

Some degree of mental retardation occurs in about two-thirds of PD individuals. Among the small number of patients for which psychometric measurements have been reported, the majority had mild retardation. Neither mental retardation nor its severity can be considered a fully penetrant characteristic of the genotype. In three multiplex families, sibs were discordant for mental retardation[9,28,33] and three other multiplex families contained some patients whose mental capacities were severely limited as well as others with only "borderline" impairment[11,13,16] (Mary Ampola, personal communication). A few patients, ascertained as children, showed delayed motor development or minor signs of muscular incoordination.[3,12,15,28,39]

Immune Function

The frequent occurrence of infections and splenomegaly in PD patients suggests a role for prolidase in the immune system. In addition to infections of ulcerated skin, recurrent episodes such as otitis media, sinusitis, and respiratory infections were mentioned in a majority of PD case reports. Two patients had cytomegaloviral infections. Despite the high frequency of these events, most patients had white blood cell counts within or close to normal limits. Immunoglobulin levels, however, were strikingly higher than normal in all patients for whom these values were reported.

An enlarged spleen was present in 12 patients, four of whom underwent splenectomy. Spleen size was normal in four patients and not mentioned in seven.

Shrinath et al.[26] have hypothesized that PD is a risk factor for systemic lupus erythematosus (SLE). Shared features of the two disorders include splenomegaly and skin rashes. The suggestion is intriguing because autoantibodies, which are a hallmark of SLE, can cause tissue injury by immune complex-mediated inflammatory response. Three PD patients in two families have been diagnosed with SLE.[25,40] Tests for antinuclear antibodies were positive in two additional patients,[11,23] and negative in five others.

Cause of Death

Although PD is not usually considered a fatal disorder, at least 5 of the patients in this survey died at age 50 or younger, 4 following acute respiratory infections.

Mode of Inheritance

PD is inherited as an autosomal recessive trait. Obligate heterozygotes have approximately half the normal levels of prolidase activity in erythrocytes, fibroblasts, and white cells. Males and females are affected in approximately equal numbers. Complementation analysis using fibroblasts from five PD probands indicated that a single gene is responsible for PD.[78]

LABORATORY FINDINGS

Biochemical

Occurrence of Imidodipeptiduria. PD patients have massive (10 to 30 mmol/day) imidodipeptiduria. The identification of urinary dipeptides has been performed by hydrolysis of isolated peptides with acid or prolidase followed by amino acid analysis.[1,3,5,7,9,13,20] Alternatively, the dipeptides have been identified by gas

Table 82-1 Amino Acid Analysis of 24-h Urine Samples of Two Unrelated PD Patients

	Patient 1		Patient 2	
Amino Acid	**unhydrolyzed**	**hydrolyzed**	**unhydrolyzed**	**hydrolyzed**
Proline	59*	28,800	141	30,139
Glycine	712	9,136	613	6,177
Glutamine & glutamate	418	5,400	180	4,652
Asparagine & aspartate	105	4,650	ND	5,806
Threonine	117	1,734	60	2,218
Serine	244	1,360	57	?
Isoleucine	40	1,884	0	1,711
Lysine	147	760	71	429
Valine	31	1,725	69	1,825
Leucine	?	2,694	ND	2,439
Alanine	1,189	1,156	885	1,026

*all values are μmol amino acid excreted per 24 h
ND = not detectable
? = value not considered reliable
Data from Bissonnette et al.[25] Used by permission of the *Journal of the American Academy of Dermatology.*

chromatography in combination with mass spectrometry.[7,40–42] Table 82-1 compares the identity of imidodipeptides reported by the same laboratory on two unrelated patients later shown to have different mutations (Ledoux et al., unpublished observations). Typically, glycyl-L-proline forms 15 to 35 percent of the excreted dipeptides. Little variation is seen among patients in the amount of imidodipeptide excreted (10 to 30 mmol/day) or in the relative abundance of the N-terminal amino acids (gly $>$ asx $\approx$ glx $>$ leu $>$ ile $\approx$ ala $\approx$ thr $\approx$ ser $>$ val $\approx$ phe $\approx$ tyr). Other amino acids are present in very low amounts or are undetectable. In contrast, the relative amounts of hydroxyproline-containing dipeptides appear to be quite variable with some patients having up to one-quarter of the urinary imidodipeptide as hydroxyproline compounds[3,5] and others producing very low[12,40] or completely undetectable levels of bound urine hydroxyproline.[20]

Normal individuals excrete about 30 mmol/day of nonimino acid dipeptide consisting of glutamate and glycine.[2] Freij et al.[13] reported the presence of glycyl-L-proline (24 μM) in the plasma of two related PD patients; other investigators, however, failed to detect imidodipeptides in the plasma of PD patients.

The extent of excretion of urinary dipeptides does not appear to explain the variable clinical severity of PD. In two affected sib pairs discordant for clinical severity, the clinically affected sib had imidodipeptide excretion levels only about twofold higher than the clinically unaffected sib.[9,33,43] Although this twofold difference was greater than that between pairs of PD affected sibs in which sibs had similar clinical phenotypes,[13,23,28] this variation in imidopeptide excretion is probably not biologically significant. For example, twofold differences in total dipeptide-bound proline excretion were detected in a single PD patient monitored for six consecutive days.[1]

Origins of Imidodipeptiduria. The finding of significant levels of bound hydroxyproline in the urine of the first three reported PD patients[1,3,5] together with identification of glycyl-L-proline as the most abundant urinary dipeptide suggested that PD was primarily an inborn error in collagen metabolism. Nearly all hydroxyproline is found in collagen, although small amounts of this imino acid are present in elastin and in the C1q component of complement.

Assuming that hydroxyproline is not catabolized in PD patients, Buist et al.[2] calculated a daily collagen turnover of 2.2 to 2.5 g/day based on a hydroxyproline content of 10 to 11 percent for collagen. Jackson et al.[6] challenged the assumption that hydroxyproline-containing imidodipeptides were not degraded in PD patients. He argued that the basic repeating unit of the triple helical regions of collagen contains one of the following sequences: (a) gly-pro-X; (b) gly-pro-pro; or (c) gly-X-pro. Of these three sequences, only the latter two are substrates for prolylhydroxylase, the enzyme that catalyzes the hydroxylation of the C-terminal proline. Hydroxyproline present in sequence (c) could be released from degraded protein as the N-terminal residue of an imidodipeptide and be further degraded to free hydroxyproline by a prolidase-independent mechanism. Jackson et al.[6] further proposed that the quantity of glycyl-L-proline in the urine be used as an index of collagen recycling instead of the content of peptide-bound hydroxyproline. This dipeptide sequence occurs on average 25 times in a sequence of 235 amino acids in the α_1 collagen chain. Thus, for a typical value of 7.5 mmol/day of gly-L-pro excretion the daily collagen turnover is calculated to be [7.5 mmol $\times$ (235/25) $\times$ 100 mg/mmol/ (average molecular weight for amino acids in collagen) $=$ 7.05 g/day].

Collagen is unlikely to be the exclusive source of the imidodipeptiduria in PD. Table 82-2 compares the molar percent

Table 82-2 Amino Acid Compositions of Imidodipeptides in Prolidase-Deficient Urine, Collagen, and a Protein mixture

Amino acid in dipeptide linkage	PD urine* mole %	69-Protein* mixture mole %	Dermal† collagen mole %
Aspartate + asparagine	7.4	9.3	4.8
Threonine	6.3	7.4	1.9
Serine	6.2	6.2	3.6
Glutamate + glutamine	8.5	7.0	7.2
Proline	8.1	6.4	12.0
Glycine	18.5	10.4	33.5
Alanine	5.1	8.4	10.5
Valine	6.9	4.9	2.4
Isoleucine	9.9	6.0	1.1
Leucine	9.4	6.5	2.4
Tyrosine	3.9	4.3	0.3
Phenylalanine	7.0	3.2	1.2
Lysine	0.5	5.4	3.0
Methionine	0.0	0.6	0.6
Cysteine	0.0	3.7	0.0
Histidine	1.5	4.6	0.5
Tryptophan	0.6	1.2	0.0
Arginine	0.4	3.4	4.6

*Data from Buist et al.[2]
†Data from Goodman et al.[1]

for 18 protein amino acids found in imidodipeptide linkage in the urine of a PD patient with the composition of collagen,[1] and with the composition of a mixture of 69 proteins used as an average reference standard.[2] The relative abundance of 10 of these amino acids (thr, ser, pro, ala, gly, val, ile, leu, tyr, and phe) is closer to the percent composition of the average protein mixture than to the percent composition of collagen. For four amino acids, the composition of the two protein groups is similar, and in only three cases (lys, his, and cys) is the percent composition of the urine imidodipeptide closer to the value found in collagen. It is likely, therefore, that undegraded imidodipeptides excreted into the urine of PD patients arise from collagen and other proteins.

Two studies have attempted to determine whether excreted imidodipeptides originate exclusively from either endogenous or dietary protein. Goodman et al.[1] gave a low-gelatin diet to a PD patient and found no significant change in the amount or composition of the excreted dipeptides, indicating that endogenous protein breakdown can account for all of the imidodipeptiduria. Conversely, Powell and Maniscalco[44] fed two PD patients a bolus of gelatin and found increases of 60 and 84 percent in the excretion of bound hydroxyproline indicating that dietary protein also contributes to imidodipeptiduria.

Enzyme Deficiency. Deficiency of prolidase is responsible for the clinical and biochemical phenotypes of this disorder. Enzymatic diagnoses have been variously performed on erythrocytes, leukocytes, and cultured skin fibroblasts. Discussion of the details of the enzyme assay and the properties of the enzyme are deferred to a later section.

Conversely, prolinase, which hydrolyzes dipeptides containing proline or hydroxyproline in the N-terminal position, is not deficient in PD patients. One laboratory detected a five- to eightfold elevation in plasma prolinase activity in two patients as compared to controls,[45] and a three- to fourfold elevation in fibroblast prolinase activity in three patients relative to controls.[46] The authors suggested that this rise in prolinase activity partially compensates for the prolidase deficiency by contributing proline to the intracellular pool. Others have found either no difference in erythrocytes levels of prolinase between patients and controls or a more modest elevation of prolinase activity in PD leukocytes.[3,7,9,33]

Histopathology and Electron Microscopy

Detailed ultrastructural studies of both normal and affected skin samples and underlying vasculature were performed by Pierard et al.[35] The pertinent findings included: lymphocyte infiltration around the superficial vascular plexus; inflammatory cells at the site of the ulcer; occlusion of medium sized vessels with a material whose staining properties suggested amyloid; and irregular size and orientation of collagen fibers. Based on these observations, Pierard et al. hypothesize that ulcers begin as a consequence of the degradation of the connective tissue by phagocytic neutrophils, and that the healing process is impaired by defective local circulation due to occlusion of the vasculature by amyloid deposition. However, other investigators have not consistently observed the findings on which this hypothesis is based. Arata et al.[45] also found narrowed, occluded blood vessels in affected skin, but there was no amyloid deposition and collagen fibers were of normal periodicity. Sekiya et al.,[37] examining postmortem tissue detected no morphologic abnormalities of collagen fibers and found amyloid in many organs, but not in skin, lungs, liver, and brain. Ogata et al.,[11] examining affected skin, detected irregular arrangement of collagen fibers and a "fragmented" appearance. Deposition of amyloid was confined to the capillaries. Milligan et al.[14] also noted a "shredded" appearance of collagen fibers in affected skin, and Cantatore et al.[28] detected capillary loss. A patient studied by Leoni et al.[19] had small blood vessels with thickened walls, but no occlusion, and a normal shape and distribution of collagen fibers.

The differences in collagen and vascular abnormalities found by various investigators may be ascribed to use of samples from skin regions that were in different stages of ulceration or healing. All observations, however, implicate compromised circulation in the ulceration process. The failure to detect vascular damage in biopsies of normal skin from PD patients probably means that vasculitis is not the primary cause of the dermatological manifestations.

Pasquali-Ronchetti et al.[47] performed stereological measurements on collagen and elastin fibers in unaffected skin obtained from five PD patients and age-matched controls. Their results, summarized in Table 82-3, indicate that the total amounts of collagen and elastin are not altered but for both proteins there is a greater number of smaller fibers or fiber bundles. The differences are more dramatic in the case of the elastin fibers where all patient samples showed a two- to fivefold increase in the number of fibers and a mean fiber area one-sixth to one-fourth that of the age-matched control group. Although the degree of change in bundle size and number was smaller for the collagen fibers, it is likely that these changes contribute more to the susceptibility of the skin to ulceration size because collagen is far more abundant in the

Table 82-3 Stereological Analysis on Dermal Collagen and Elastin Fibers in Prolidase-Deficient Patients and Age-Matched Controls

	Age	% Collagen ± SD	No. of fiber bundles/μ^2 10^{-2} ± SD	Bundle mean area μ^2 ± SD	% Elastin ± SD	No. of fibers/μ^2 10^{-3} ± SD	Fiber mean area μ^2 ± SD
Control							
Group A (4)	5–13	62.9 ± 2.3	2.74 ± 0.20	23.98 ± 1.51	4.02 ± 1.36	5.48 ± 0.66	7.88 ± 0.94
Group B (6)	10–19	65.8 ± 1.9	3.33 ± 0.36	22.59 ± 2.21	4.38 ± 0.65	6.39 ± 0.85	7.52 ± 0.94
Group C (4)	20–29	67.9 ± 1.9	3.13 ± 0.29	22.58 ± 1.75	4.69 ± 0.90	4.43 ± 1.19	11.41 ± 2.77
Group D (2)	30–39	60.5 ± 4.3	2.80 ± 0.35	22.37 ± 3.14	5.49 ± 0.96	5.88 ± 1.16	9.68 ± 3.67
Group E (3)	50–59	60.2 ± 5.2	3.62 ± 0.41	18.01 ± 3.43	6.70 ± 1.98	4.90 ± 0.91	13.01 ± 5.94
Patients							
1*	8	58.7 ± 2.6	4.66 ± 0.19	13.67 ± 4.68	3.28 ± 0.76	17.23 ± 4.12	1.94 ± 0.62
2	12	50.7 ± 4.4	5.87 ± 0.16	8.83 ± 2.03	2.54 ± 1.73	29.10 ± 1.94	0.86 ± 0.05
3	21	50.4 ± 0.6	5.93 ± 1.32	8.83 ± 1.78	2.50 ± 1.64	8.56 ± 0.39	2.87 ± 0.36
4	37	46.4 ± 13.1	6.66 ± 0.28	7.00 ± 2.11	3.06 ± 0.58	19.20 ± 5.74	1.80 ± 0.82
5	55	50.4 ± 1.4	3.98 ± 0.96	13.43 ± 2.42	5.46 ± 1.42	11.94 ± 2.35	4.72 ± 0.74

*Indicates asymptomatic patient.

The number of controls is shown in parentheses.

Tissue samples were all taken from femoral region.

Data adapted from Pasquali-Ronchetti et al.[47] Used by permission of *Journal of Submicroscopic Cytology and Pathology.*

dermis. These data argue strongly that PD fibroblasts produce a strikingly different type extracellular matrix than that produced by normal cells. What signals regulate this process and how these changes relate to the clinical phenotype remain to be elucidated.

BIOSYNTHESIS OF PROLINE

De Novo Biosynthesis and Salvage Pathways

Proline is a nonessential amino acid synthesized from either glutamate or arginine (via ornithine) (Fig. 82-2). Glutamate is converted to glutamic semialdehyde by the action of Δ-1-pyrroline-5-carboxylic acid synthase (P5C synthase) and ornithine is converted to the same intermediate by the action of ornithine-δ-aminotransferase (OAT). Glutamic semialdehyde is in equilibrium with its tautomer P5C, and the latter compound is converted to proline by the action of P5C reductase (see Chaps. 81 and 83).

Connective tissue cells secrete collagens in abundance. These extracellular matrix proteins contain about 25 percent imino acids. Proline produced by the *de novo* biosynthetic pathway may be insufficient for the high demand of collagen biosynthesis by these cells. Several experiments have indicated that recycling mechanisms play a major role in the reclamation of proline for synthesis of new collagen molecules. Jackson and Heininger[39] compared the decay rates of [^{3}H]-labeled proline and [$^{18}O_2$]-labeled hydroxyproline in rat skin collagen. The [^{3}H]-labeled proline is incorporated into peptide-bound proline and hydroxyproline in proportion to the content of each of these imino acids in skin collagen, whereas the [$^{18}O_2$]-label is incorporated only into hydroxyproline, which is not recyclable. The differences in decay rates of the two isotopes indicated that 50 of 54 proline residues were recycled representing an efficiency of proline conservation of 92.5 percent. Shen and Strecker[48] used tracer studies to examine the utilization of glutamate and arginine as precursors for proline in cultured human lung fibroblasts. They found that glutamate serves as a precursor for no more than 6 percent and arginine for no more than 3 percent of the imino acid residues of newly synthesized collagen. Both experiments indicate that in this cultured cell system, recycling of proline is quantitatively of much greater importance in collagen biosynthesis than is *de novo* proline synthesis.

Both prolidase and prolinase catalyze proline-releasing terminal reactions in the degradation of proteins. The ability of prolidase to perform a recycling function has been tested in cultured cell systems. Emerson and Phang[49] found that proline auxotrophic CHO cells could grow normally if supplied with imidodipeptides. Similarly, Dolenga and Hechtman[50] observed that both normal and PD cultured human skin fibroblasts had greatly reduced growth rates on proline-deficient medium. Growth rates could be restored for the normal cell lines but not for the PD cells by the addition of imidodipeptides to the medium.

PD thus represents the loss of a recycling pathway that supplies the fibroblasts with the major portion of proline used in collagen biosynthesis.

Absorption and Excretion of Proline from Protein Digestion

The movement of proline and imidodipeptides between physiological compartments can only be understood with consideration of the membrane transport of dipeptides. The observation that individuals with Hartnup disorder, an inborn error of intestinal transport of free amino acids, are asymptomatic led Tarlow et al.[51] and Asatoor and colleagues[52,53] to postulate a specialized peptide-transporting system in the intestine. Adibi et al.[54] found that 50 to 90 percent of the proline in the intestinal lumen was in peptide linkage, and Rubino et al.[55] found that when everted gut sac preparations were presented with glycyl-L-proline, they accumulated glycine in the mucosal cells more rapidly than when presented with free glycine. Ganapathy et al.[56] demonstrated the presence in intestinal and renal brush border vesicles of a saturable Na^+-independent dipeptide transport system with a K_m of about 1 mM for glycyl-L-proline. Despite extensive washing of membrane preparations, the uptake of glycyl-L-proline was strongly coupled to hydrolysis of the imide linkage and only free amino acids were detected within the vesicles. These observations strongly suggest that the bulk of amino acids are absorbed into intestinal cells in the form of dipeptides and, following intracellular peptidase catalyzed hydrolysis, are released into plasma. Nevertheless, transient accumulation of imidodipeptides in rat plasma following their presentation in the gut has been observed.[57] Peak plasma dipeptide values (0.6 mM) were reached within 10 min and were down to undetectable levels by 30 min.

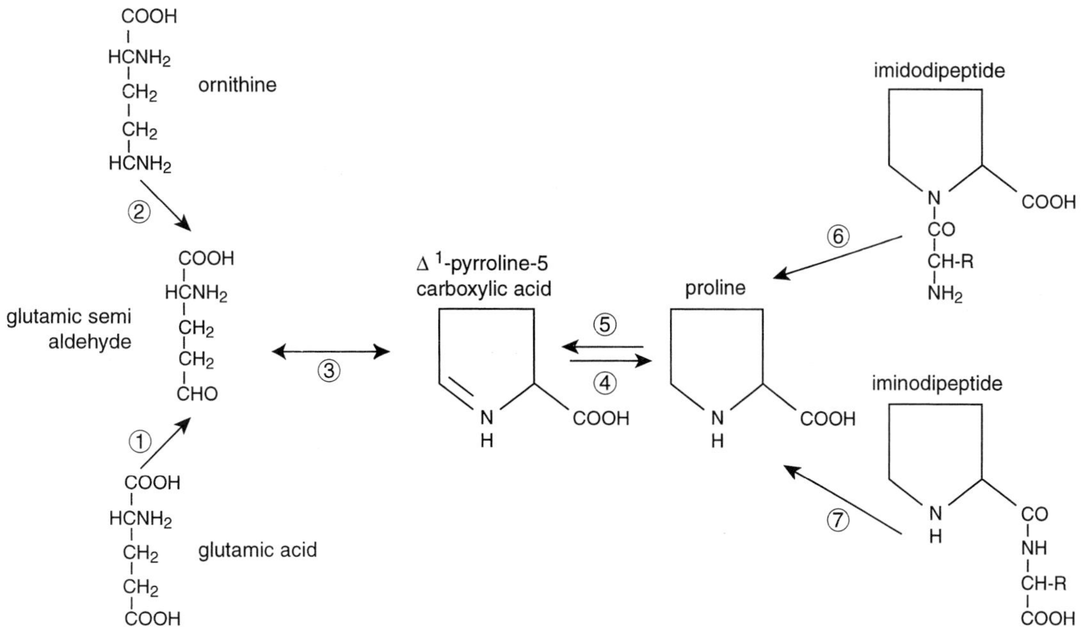

Fig. 82-2 Proline metabolic pathways. 1. P5C synthase; 2. ornithine aminotransferase; 3. spontaneous tautomerization; 4. P5C reductase; 5. proline oxidase; 6. prolidase; 7. prolinase.

The presence of a dipeptide transport system in the kidney would be difficult to reconcile with the excretion of massive amounts of imidodipeptides in PD. Such a system would be expected to reclaim filtered dipeptides returning them to the plasma either in the form of dipeptides or in the form of free amino and imino acids following prolidase-catalyzed hydrolysis in the cytoplasm of kidney cells. This problem appears to be explained by the observations of Benoit and Watten who demonstrated that even modest elevations of hydroxyproline-containing peptides in human plasma result in the predominance of imidodipeptide excretion over reabsorption in the renal tubule.[58]

Because the flux of imidodipeptide into urine is irreversible, a number of investigators have studied the interaction of peptide transport and hydrolysis in the erythrocyte. These cells can transport and hydrolyze imidodipeptides, and because they have no protein synthesis, the products of prolidase catalysis are returned to the plasma. Erythrocytes thus are able to reclaim amino and imino acids from imidodipeptides in plasma before they are lost in the urine. This rationale has lead to the use of transfusions with normal donor erythrocytes as a possible therapeutic intervention to reverse the imidodipeptiduria of PD (see "Treatment of Prolidase Deficiency" below).

King and Kuchel[58] described a saturable dipeptide transport system in erythrocytes and found that the transporter was rate-limiting for the hydrolysis of glycyl-L-proline because the V_{max} for hydrolysis of this substrate in the hemolysate was one hundred thirtyfold greater than the V_{max} for hydrolysis by intact cells. If these values pertain to cells in other organs and tissues, imidodipeptide hydrolysis at these sites will reflect the relative activity of the dipeptide transport system rather than the activity of prolidase. Additionally, these considerations indicate that the erythrocyte plays a greater role in imidodipeptide degradation than does the kidney.

Hechtman et al.[59] examined the potential role of the erythrocyte in the degradation of imidodipeptide substrates by comparing the activity of intact erythrocytes that had been "activated" by overnight incubation with Mn^{++}, to cells that had not been activated. Although they found that the rate of hydrolysis by intact cells invariably was slower than by hemolysates, their data also showed a thirtyfold increase in the V_{max} for *in situ* prolidase activity of cells in which prolidase had been activated. This result would not be predicted if dipeptide transport were the rate-limiting step in substrate hydrolysis. The activation of intact erythrocytes increased the intracellular Mn^{++} concentration from 0.014 μg/ml (a value in accord with that of Lombeck[15]) to 2.04 μg/ml.

PROPERTIES OF PROLIDASE

Discovery

An enzyme able to catalyze the hydrolysis of glycyl-L-proline was first demonstrated in extracts of intestinal mucosa by Bergmann and Fruton.[60] The first purified preparation of the enzyme was obtained from swine kidney by Davis and Smith.[61] These, and earlier investigations, established the essential catalytic features of prolidase. The unique property of prolidase is its ability to catalyze the rapid hydrolysis of a peptide bond that is a tertiary amide. Other peptidases have since been identified that hydrolyze this type of peptide bond,[62,63] but only within larger peptides or protein sequences (Fig. 82-3). Prolidase displays an absolute specificity for substrates having a free α-amino and a free α-carboxy group, and is unable to hydrolyze either substrates in which other amino acids have replaced the C-terminal imino acid or peptides that contain three or more amino acids. Prolidase has a specific requirement for Mn^{++} and is inhibited by p-chloro-mercurobenzoate (pCMB) and stimulated by glutathione. The latter observations suggested that a cysteine residue is critical for catalysis.

Enzyme Assay

Because prolidase is a relatively stable cytosolic enzyme, no special precautions are necessary in the preparation of tissue samples for enzymatic assay. Most investigators employ minor variations on the optimal conditions developed by Myara et al.[64] for assay of prolidase activity. These include a 24-h preincubation with 1 mM Mn^{++} before incubation with substrate. Preincubated samples show a 1.5- to 30-fold increase in enzymatic activity as compared to unincubated samples. The reasons for this wide variation include (a) the prolidase apo-enzyme is more labile than the holo-enzyme, thus some destruction of the former may occur during prolonged preincubations, and (b) most of the activation occurs during the first few hours of the preincubation so some activation of nonpreincubated enzyme occurs during the enzymatic reaction itself.[65] The extent of this latter effect will depend on the Mn^{++} content of the tissue used as a source of enzyme.

Prolidase assays are performed in weakly alkaline buffers (pH 7.6 to 8.0) using high (10 to 50 mM) concentrations of imidodipeptide concentrations. Following incubation at 37°, the reaction is terminated by addition of trichloroacetic acid or by heating. Released proline is quantitated using the Chinard method.[63] Alternatively, free amino acids released may be separated and quantitated using automated amino acid chromatography. An alternative method for measuring prolidase activity follows the decrease in UV absorption at 220 nm because of a decrease in the number of peptide bonds.[66] This method has the advantage of adaptation to continuous flow studies of enzymatic activity; however, it also has two disadvantages: (a) relatively pure enzyme preparations are required because large amounts of protein will increase the blank values, and (b) subsaturating amounts of substrate are required to obtain significant decreases in optical density.

The Problem of Prolidase II in Enzymatic Assays of Prolidase Activity. Prolidase II is a provisional name for a second enzyme able to catalyze the hydrolysis of imidodipeptide substrates; its activity can interfere with the estimation of prolidase activity. Except for serum which has only prolidase activity, prolidase II accounts for one-third to one-half of total prolidase activity in all tissues examined.[67] The exact contribution of prolidase II to imidodipeptide hydrolysis depends on the substrate and the tissue used as a source of enzyme. The diagnostic challenge presented by the presence of a second enzyme is to devise a means either to separate the two activities prior to enzyme assay or to utilize assay conditions that suppress prolidase II activity. Several procedures are recommended, including (a) ion exchange separation of the two enzymes;[68] (b) heating the preparation for 1 h at 48°C in the presence of Mn^{++}, which destroys most of prolidase II activity;[67] and (c) use of a substrate, glycyl-L-proline, for which prolidase II has minimal activity.[67–69] The use of serum as a source of prolidase avoids the problem, because virtually all activity in this compartment appears to derive from prolidase.[18]

Distribution of Prolidase

Hui and Lajtha undertook a systematic survey of prolidase activity in different regions of the brain and in other rat organs.[70,71] Table 82-4 shows their results. Although prolidase is a ubiquitous enzyme, the tissues with the highest specific activities are kidney and intestinal mucosa consistent with the notion that prolidase plays a transport/reclamation role in amino acid metabolism. Data from Butterworth and Priestman[67] includes other cell types, but the results from the two laboratories are difficult to compare because different substrates were employed. With this caveat, the data of Butterworth and Priestman[67] agrees with that of Hui and Lajtha[70] and indicates that pancreas, cerebral cortex, and fibroblasts are also relatively rich in prolidase. Interestingly, Hui and Lajtha[71] compared the level of prolidase activity in the rat cerebrum to the rate of protein turnover in this tissue and concluded that the enzyme was present at levels one hundred- to one thousandfold higher than is required to sustain the calculated rate of protein degradation in this organ. Regional distributions of prolidase in brain do not vary greatly and the developmental variation of activity from birth to adulthood is only about twofold.[71]

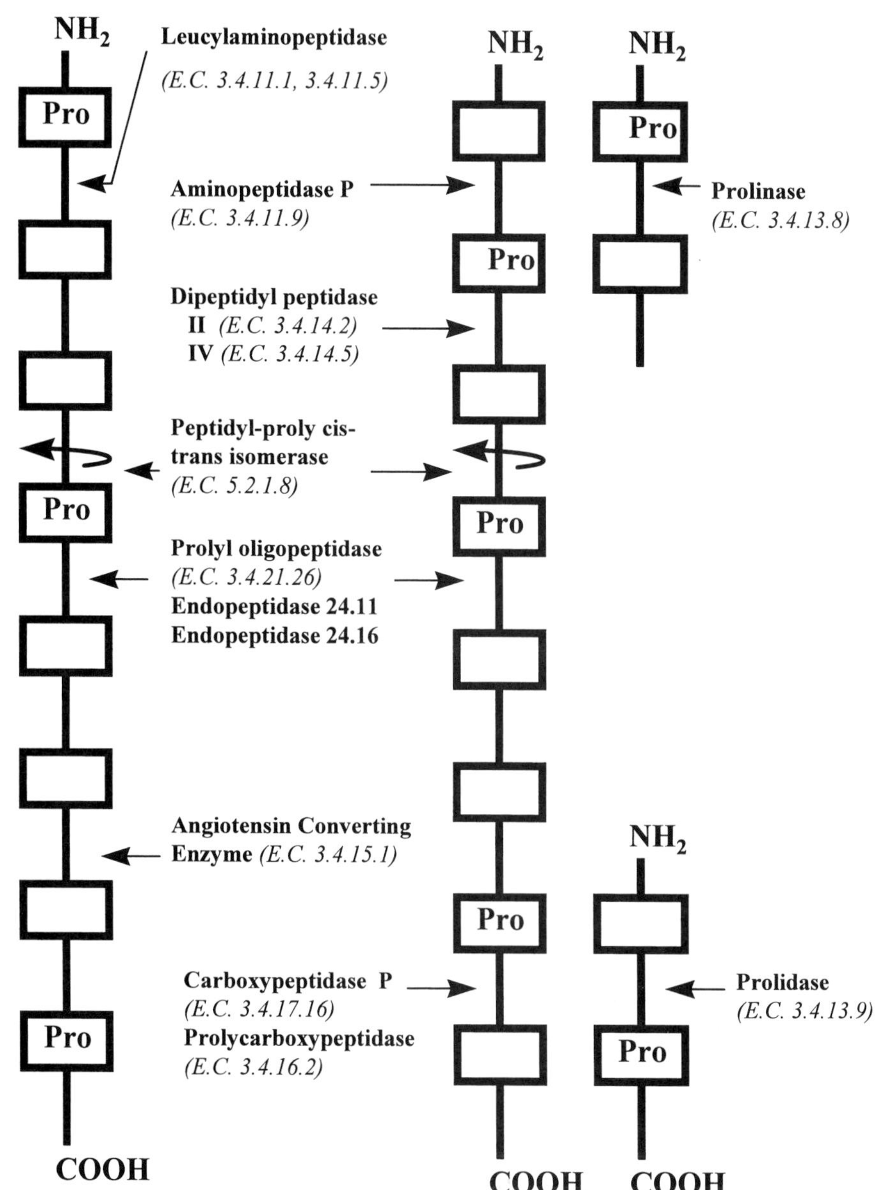

Fig. 82-3 Enzymatic hydrolysis of proline-containing peptide linkages. (*Adapted from Vanhoof et al.*[62] *Used with permission of the Federation of American Societies of Experimental Biology.*)

Enzymes with a prolidase-like function have been detected in many species of bacteria.[72,73] Of particular interest for practical reasons is the observation that a prolidase-like enzyme from *Altermonas sp.* strain JD6.5 is capable of catalyzing the hydrolysis of a group of toxic organophosphorus cholinesterase-inhibiting compounds, including pesticides and chemical nerve agents.[74]

Purification of Prolidase

Purification of prolidase from a number of mammalian and bacterial sources has been reported.[61,65,75–80] In most instances, conventional protein separation methods were used although two groups[65,77] employed pCMB-linked gels as a quasi-affinity column. Comparisons of final specific activities of different preparations are not meaningful because different assay systems were employed and some groups included a Mn^{++}-preincubation step[61,65] with the result that the final enrichment factor included both enzyme activation and enzyme purification. In general, the yield of pure enzyme is low (5 to 8 percent of starting material and 1 mg protein or less) reflecting both lability problems and the relatively low abundance of prolidase, even in tissues with the highest specific activity. These studies provided sufficient purified prolidase for characterization of catalytic properties and for the development of antisera, but not for analysis of protein structure. Recently, Carilles and Hechtman expressed human prolidase with an N-terminal hexahistidyl tag in *E. coli* and used Ni-NTA column one-step purification to achieve a homogenous preparation with a yield of 23 mg/liter of bacterial culture (unpublished).

Properties of the Purified Enzyme

Peptide hydrolysis catalyzed by porcine kidney prolidase, and probably those of other species, is specific for the *trans*-isomer of imidodipeptide substrates.[81,82] Mammalian prolidase has no activity with tripeptide substrates and has an absolute requirement for proline or hydroxyproline at the C-terminus of the peptide with a fifty- to one hundredfold preference for the former over the latter.[75,76] Substrate preference varies somewhat between species with human enzyme preparations favoring glycyl-L-proline hydrolysis over alanyl-L-proline by a factor of two- to threefold[65,76,78] and the bovine and porcine preparations favoring alanyl-L-proline.[75,77] K_ms for human prolidase substrates are in the range of 1 to 10 mM.[65,78] Mn^{++} activation may change the substrate preference.[78,79] Available data on a bacterial dipeptidase indicates some activity with nonimidodipeptide substrates and a complete absence of hydrolysis of glycyl-L-proline,[80] suggesting

Table 82-4 Distribution of Prolidase Activity in Rat Tissues

Tissues	nmol/min mg tissue	nmol/min mg protein
Kidney	31.7	161 ± 1.4
Intestinal Mucosa	21.3	139 ± 4.6
Spleen	9.94	57.4 ± 3.7
Liver	7.56	37.6 ± 1.8
Lung	4.81	36.9 ± 4.2
Heart	4.62	26.5 ± 2.0
Cervical spinal cord	2.73	29.0 ± 2.1
Sciatic Nerve	5.97	47.8 ± 1.4
Pituitary	4.15	27.0 ± 2.1
Plasma	50.8*	14.2 ± 0.8

*nmol/min/ml plasma
Data taken from Hui and Lajtha.[70] Used by permission of the *Journal of Neurochemistry*.

that this enzyme may perform very different functions than the mammalian prolidases.

For all mammalian enzyme preparations, the molecular weight of the native enzyme is 108 to 116 kDa based on Stokes radius with a subunit molecular weight of 53 to 58 kDa by SDS electrophoresis. The pI for human kidney prolidase is 4.65.[75] This value is unchanged by Mn^{++} activation (Richter and Hechtman, unpublished observations). Published amino acid compositions reveal marked differences between bovine and porcine enzymes[77] with the human enzyme having a composition closer to that of the porcine enzyme (reference 83 and Ledoux et al., unpublished observations) (Table 82-5).

Despite the requirement of prolidase for Mn^{++} ions, neither EDTA nor o-phenanthrolene inhibits activity.[77] The sulfhydryl reagent pCMB is strongly inhibitory.[61,77] Davis and Smith[61] found that Mn^{++} protected prolidase against inactivation by iodoacetamide and postulated that the Mn^{++} is bound to an –SH group. *Lactobacillus* prolidase is inhibited completely by EDTA and phenanthrolene, but only slightly by pCMB.[80]

Table 82-5 Amino Acid Composition of Prolidase from Mammalian Species (number of residues)

Amino Acid	Human†	Bovine‡	Porcine§
Lysine	32	36	37
Histidine	38	23	39
Arginine	58	35	62
Aspartic Acid*	68	93	77
Threonine	44	82	50
Serine	58	88	57
Glutamic Acid*	98	110	98
Proline	36	55	37
Glycine	82	81	103
Alanine	76	71	65
Half-cystine	26	12	39
Valine	82	62	84
Methionine	30	12	26
Isoleucine	40	43	38
Leucine	82	83	77
Tyrosine	28	48	30
Phenylalanine	44	55	45
Tryptophan	10	41	12

*Includes amide.
Data taken from.
†Endo et al.,[104]
‡Sjöström and Norén,[75] and
§Yoshimoto.[77]

Metal Activation of Prolidase and Mechanism of Catalysis

All prolidase preparations are optimally activated by Mn^{++} ions and inhibited by other ions, such as Cu^{++}, Hg^{++}, Zn^{++}, and Cd^{++}.[61,77] Variable results have been obtained with metals such as Mg^{++} and Co^{++}.[77,80,84] The role of metal ions in the catalytic reaction remains controversial. Richter et al.[65] attempted to separate the effects of Mn^{++} on enzyme activation and catalysis. They removed excess amounts of Mn^{++} following activation using dialysis or Chelex treatment. The resulting preparation was indifferent to the presence of Mn^{++} in the catalytic reaction mixture, suggesting that unbound Mn^{++} does not serve as a cosubstrate.

Human prolidase shares extensive homology with a family of peptidases. Another member of this family, *E. coli* methionine aminopeptidase, has been crystallized and a tertiary structure has been reported.[85] Homology modeling of prolidase and other related enzymes upon this three-dimensional structure reveals a common pattern within the C-terminal region of internal twofold structural symmetry referred to as the "pita-bread" fold.[86] Cobalt atoms bind to the methionine aminopeptidase structure at two sites that are defined by five amino acid residues (Fig. 82-4). The equivalent positions in prolidase are Asp 97, Asp 287, His 366, Glu 412, and Glu 452.

Mock and Liu[87] have proposed a catalytic mechanism for prolidase that requires two metal ions. One ion is postulated to chelate with both the free amino group and the carboxamide linkage, while the second ion delivers a hydroxide ion to the scissile linkage. Whatever the validity of this model may be, it takes no account of either the specificity of the metal requirement or the role of metal in producing an activated state of the enzyme.

Carilles and Hechtman (submitted) prepared homogenous human prolidase in sufficient quantity to permit analysis of its metal content by atomic absorption spectrometry and to correlate metal binding with enzymatic properties. Their findings confirmed the predictions of Bazan et al.[86] of two Mn^{++} binding sites per prolidase subunit. However, in contrast to Mock and Lui's[87] opinion that "this particular metal is not of great importance," Carilles and Hechtman found that when Zn^{++} replaced Mn^{++} catalytic activity was dramatically reduced. Activation with Mn^{++} could be performed by "nonphysiological" preincubation of purified enzyme with 1 mM divalent ion or equally *in vivo* by addition of much lower amounts of metal to the bacterial growth medium prior to harvesting of cells. Table 82-6 compares the activities of different metalloprolidases. When recombinant human prolidase was prepared after growing cells in the presence of Zn^{++} there were 4 mol of metal ion bound per subunit. The Zn^{++}-bound enzyme was thermolabile, whereas Mn-bound enzyme was thermostable. Interconversion of the Zn^{++} enzyme to the Mn^{++} enzyme was associated with little change in the K_m for imidodipeptide substrates, but with large increases in V_{max}. When expressed human prolidase was prepared from bacterial cells to which no divalent cation salts had been added, the preparation contained less than 0.1 mol of Mn^{++}/mol of prolidase subunit. A hypothetical scheme for metal activation and inhibition of prolidase is shown in Fig. 82-5.

Active Site Studies

Mock and Lui[87] proposed bidentate coordination of Mn^{++} with both amino nitrogen and carboxamide oxygen. This model is more compatible with the observation that only transisomers of imidodipeptides are hydrolyzed by prolidase than is the earlier proposal of a single site of coordination in the active site by Hui and Latha.[70] However, bidentate coordination in stereospecific fashion is equally possible with the free carboxyl group and the carboxamide oxygen. A number of compounds that lack amino groups, but which have atomic distances between the two oxygens that are identical with imidodipeptide substrates (such as

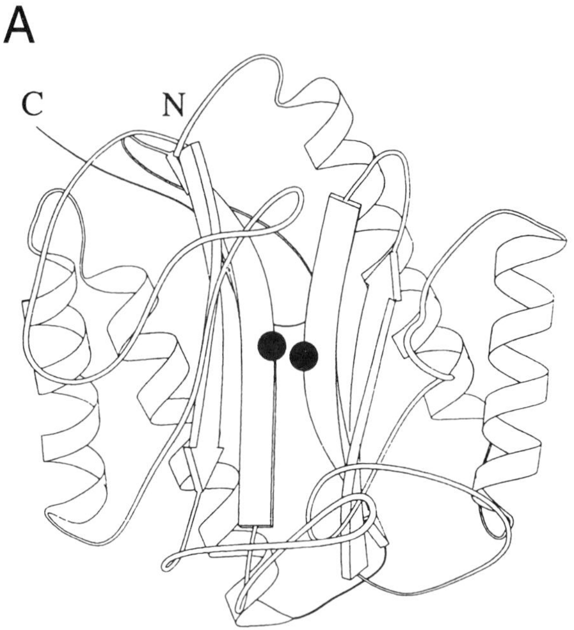

Fig. 82-4 Representations of the metal-binding region of *E. coli* aminopeptidase, an enzyme with sequence homology to human prolidase. *A,* Diagram from Bazan et al.[86] (*Used by permission of Proceedings of the National Academy of Sciences.*) *B,* Three-dimensional structure representing amino acids with contacts to metal binding sites. (*From Mock and Lui.*[87] *Used by permission of the Journal of Biological Chemistry.*)

N-benzyloxycarbonyl-L-proline), are potent competitive inhibitors of prolidase.[88] King et al.[88] also point out that bidentate coordination imposes certain size requirements on the metal atom. Thus, smaller divalent metal atoms, such as Fe^{++}, Co^{++}, Ni^{++} and Cu^{++}, are unable to accommodate bidentate coordination of substrates without significant distortion of bond angles. Figure 82-6 compares the two active site models.

Additional modeling studies on prolidase performed by Radzicka and Wolfenden[89] revealed a high binding affinity for a variety of dicarboxylic acid intermediates, a finding that is compatible with the model of Kuchel et al.[88] Although there are four atoms in imidodipeptides between the two oxygens that are hypothesized to coordinate with Mn^{++}, compounds with three atoms between the oxygens are even more potent inhibitors of prolidase than those in which the spacing between the two coordinated oxygens is identical with that of authentic prolidase substrates.

Active site amino acids have not yet been identified in prolidase. The early suggestion that a cysteine residue plays a critical role in the catalytic reaction[61] has not received much recent attention. Mock and Zhuang[90] found that the competitive inhibitor acetylproline completely or partially blocks inhibition of the enzyme by the group-specific reagents phenylglyoxal and 1-cyclohexyl-3-(2-morpholinoethyl) carbodiimide, indicating functional roles for arginine and dicarboxylic acid residues, respectively.

Table 82-6 **Metal Activation and Inhibition of Purified Human Prolidase**

Metal Ion	Single Metal Ion	Incubation with Mn^{++} and	Incubation with Zn^{++} and
	Specific Activity nmoles/min/mg		
No metal	130	19310	146
Mn^{++}	19310	—	5430
Zn^{++}	146	5430	—
Ca^{++}	1923	20171	169
Cu^{++}	87	5580	65
Co^{++}	5193	9880	239
Ni^{++}	466	10340	448
Mg^{++}	4687	18785	130

++Data from Carriles and Hechtman (submitted).

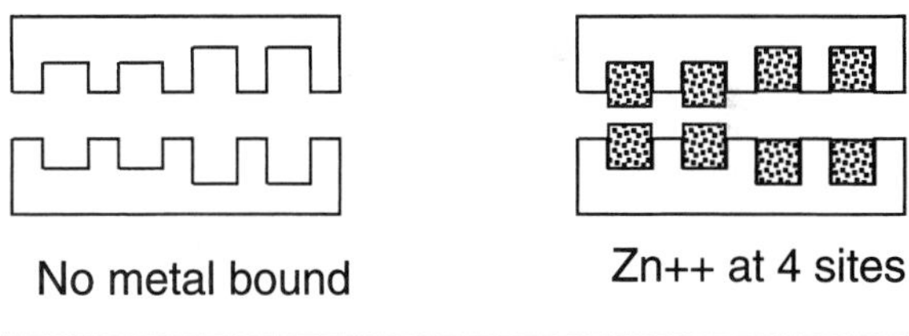

Inactive prolidase

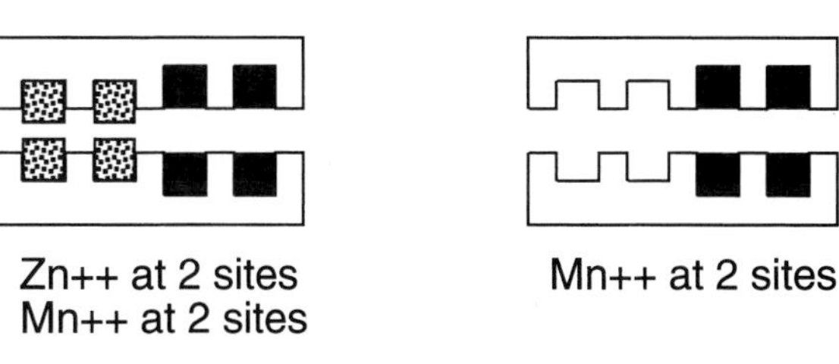

Prolidase activity half-maximal **Prolidase activity maximal**

Fig. 82-5 A hypothetical model for regulation of prolidase activity by divalent metal ions. Shallow pockets at left of subunit model represent sites at which Zn^{++} may bind and exert weak inhibition on enzyme activity. Deep pockets at right represent sites at which Mn^{++} may bind and activate the enzyme or Zn^{++} may bind and strongly inhibit catalytic activity. Data from Carriles and Hechtman (submitted).

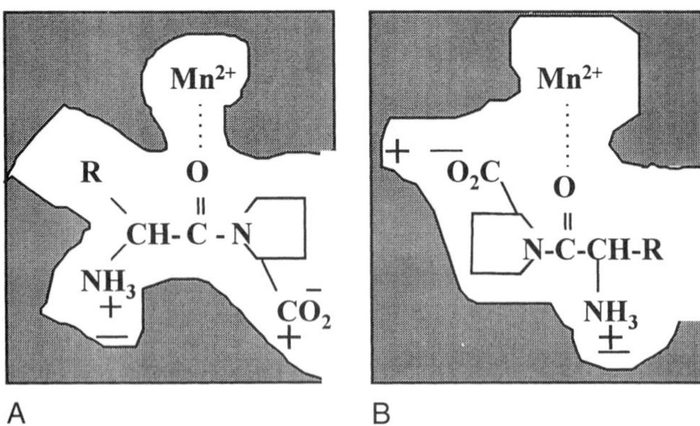

Fig. 82-6 Alternative models of the prolidase active site. *A*, Model proposed by Hui and Lajtha.[70] (Used by permission of the Journal of Neurochemistry.) B, Model proposed by King et al.[81] based on specificity of prolidase for the trans isomer of imidodipeptide substrates. (*Used by permission of the American Chemical Society.*)

Properties and Role of Prolidase II

The function of prolidase II is not yet understood. The properties of this activity have been investigated by a number of laboratories.[67–69,91,92] Prolidase II has a molecular weight of 185 kDa.[69] Most groups have found that prolidase II has a lower substrate preference for glycyl-L-proline than does prolidase, and for all substrates, prolidase II appears to have K_ms that are an order of magnitude or more higher than the corresponding values for prolidase.[69,78] The observation that an enzyme activity with properties assigned to prolidase II appears in the fibroblasts of patients who are CRM$^-$ against antihuman prolidase I antiserum indicates that prolidase II is not likely to be a posttranslational variant of prolidase.[78] Furthermore, the presence of prolidase II in cultured cells of severely affected patients[67,69,78] suggests that this enzyme does not mitigate the phenotype associated with PD.

MOLECULAR GENETICS OF THE PROLIDASE STRUCTURAL GENE *PEPD*

Mapping *PEPD*

The *PEPD* locus was mapped to chromosome 19 by McAlpine et al.,[93] an assignment that was confirmed by Brown et al.[94] A recombination study performed by O'Brien et al.[95] indicated that *PEPD* and the *DM* (myotonic dystrophy) were closely linked. Location of *DM* should, by default, also map *PEPD*. Recombination methods,[96] studies with somatic cell hybrids,[97,98] and early *in situ* hybridization studies[104] initially assigned *DM* and *PEPD* to 19p. More recent studies localized the *DM* gene to 19q13.2-13.3.[99–101] Consistent with this revision of the location of *DM*, recent studies employing somatic cell hybrids containing very small fragments of the long arm of human chromosome 19[102] and physical mapping[103] localize *PEPD* to 19q12-q13.2.

Cloning and Organization of *PEPD*

Endo and colleagues isolated prolidase cDNAs from human liver and placental cDNA libraries.[104,105] On northern blots of RNA isolated from human tissues, these cDNAs recognize a 2.1 to 2.2 kb prolidase mRNA that encodes a 493-amino acid peptide with a predicted molecular weight of 54.3 kDa. Ledoux et al.[106] cloned a human prolidase cDNA that predicted an amino acid sequence differing at seven places from that published by Endo.[104] The amino acid sequence with subsequent corrections is shown in Fig. 82-7. Although Endo et al.[104] found two potential *N*-glycosylation sites in the prolidase sequence, there is no evidence for posttranslational processing of the enzyme.[78,105] Endo et al.[107] detected the prolidase subunit immunochemically as a 56-kDa protein in extracts of liver and erythrocytes, but as a 58-kDa protein in kidney and small intestine. The explanation for this apparent size difference is unknown.

Tanoue et al.[83] showed that *PEPD* spanned more than 130 kb of genomic DNA and is comprised of 15 exons with boundaries that follow the conventional GT/AG rule (Table 82-7). There is no TATA box, but a CAAT sequence is found upstream of the transcriptional start site (−67 to −64). Seven potential binding sites for the transcription factor Sp1 (CCGCCC or GGCGGG) were identified, only four of which were upstream of the transcription start site.[105]

Identification and Expression of *PEPD* Mutations in PD Patients and Heterozygotes

The initial studies of *PEPD* mutations involved characterization of the amount of prolidase antigen and mRNA in fibroblasts from PD patients. Prolidase immunoreactive material was absent in cells from two of five patients in one study,[78] and in six of eight patients in another study.[108] There was no correlation between the amount of residual enzyme activity or the presence of prolidase immunoreactive material with the clinical severity of the disorder.

The first characterized mutation causing PD was a deletion[83] of 774 bp at the 3′ end of the gene that includes 192 bp of translated sequence encoded by exon 14.[83] This *PEPD* deletion allele produces a catalytically inactive prolidase polypeptide of 49 kDa (as compared to 54.3 kDa for wild-type prolidase). Eight other *PEPD* mutations have been identified in PD patients using RT-PCR amplification of mRNA. The mutations and their impact on the mRNA and polypeptide phenotypes are listed in Table 82-8. Two mutations (E452Δ and E452K) affect residues predicted by homology studies to be involved in the metal-binding function of prolidase.[86,106,109] A third mutation, D276N,[110] involves a residue that has been suggested to function in the catalytic process.[87] Two splice-site mutations cause deletion of exons 5 and 7 respectively from the mature mRNA.[106] The missense allele G448R appears to be the most frequent mutation and has been found in patients of Italian, Dutch, and Anglo-Saxon ancestry (Ledoux and Hechtman, unpublished observations). Five of these mutations occur at CpG dinucleotides.

Most of the mutant *PEPD* alleles listed in Table 82-8 have been expressed in BMT-10 cells,[111] NIH-3T3 cells,[110] or COS-1 cells.[112] Immunologic methods have been used to separate the mutant prolidase from the endogenous enzyme present in these cells so that the function of the mutant enzyme can be determined. For example, R184Q was associated with 7.4 percent residual activity in this system, while G278D had no enzymatic activity.[112] Interestingly, these alleles were identified in a clinically asymptomatic compound heterozygote with typical biochemical abnormalities. Similarly, E452Δ, previously shown to be associated with the lack of residual prolidase protein, was shown in these expression studies to yield a prolidase subunit that was rapidly degraded.

Identification of functionally significant *PEPD* mutations in patient samples confirmed identification of the gene responsible for PD. However, with the possible exception of the R184Q allele, which is associated with an higher residual activity than other mutations, the definition of molecular defects has not explained the clinical variability of PD. Indeed, several families have been investigated in which probands with identical genotypes have very different clinical phenotypes.

Allele Frequency and Polymorphic Variation at the *PEPD* Locus

A single study of the frequency of PD in Quebec based on systematic screening of newborn urine identified two cases for a frequency of 1 to 2 per million.[17] Interestingly, neither of these

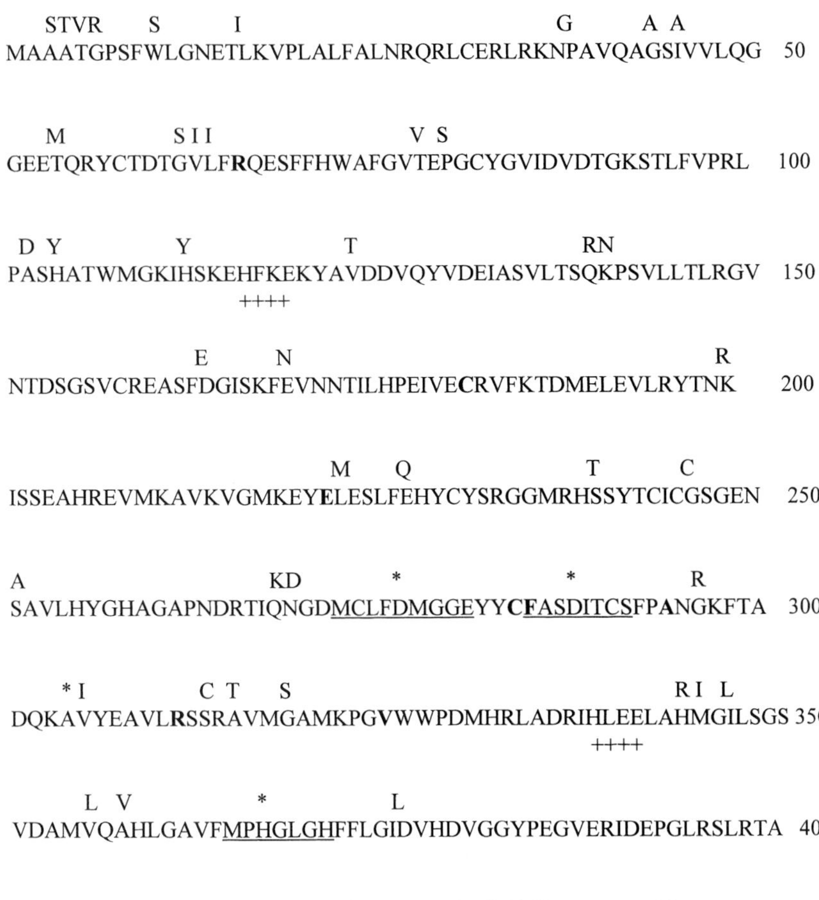

Fig. 82-7 Conceptual translation of human prolidase cDNA. Sequence data from Endo[104] and Ledoux.[109] Symbols above indicate amino acid sequence differences in mouse prolidase. Symbols indicated in bold indicate changes made in the published sequence. Underlined sequences are core β-sheet structure. Residues indicated by * are putative metal binding residues. ++++ indicates Zn^{++} binding motif.

two cases has become symptomatic in the 14 years since they were identified, suggesting that estimates based on clinical ascertainment may be low. A frequency of 1 to 2 per million predicts a few thousand cases worldwide rather than the few dozen that have actually been described. These observations suggest that PD is underdiagnosed and/or that the majority of cases are asymptomatic.

Endo and Matsuda employed a screening test for PD heterozygotes that uses dried blood samples for enzymatic analysis.[113] Testing of 1000 Japanese individuals failed to detect a single case of PD. Because the distribution of erythrocyte prolidase activity in normals is broad, this assay is not sufficiently sensitive to be used for mass heterozygote screening. For this reason, calculations of heterozygote frequency based on these results are not valid.[32,84]

Lewis and Harris reported benign electrophoretic variants of prolidase.[114] The frequencies of three genetic variants were compared in Caucasian and African-American samples[115] where it was found that both groups had a frequency for the *PEPD-1* variant >0.9 and that African-Americans had significantly higher frequencies of the minor alleles *PEPD-2* and *PEPD-3* than Caucasian populations.

High rates of sequence variation at the *PEPD* locus were detected with restriction fragment length polymorphisms. In a preliminary screen for RFLPs, Tanoue et al.[83] detected variants for the sites *Kpn*I, *Bam*HI, and *Eco*RV within the coding region of prolidase at frequencies of 0.2 to 0.3.

PATHOGENIC MECHANISMS

Is PD a Disorder of Collagen Metabolism?

Early studies of PD suggested a defect in collagen turnover.[4,6,31] Demonstration of defective collagen metabolism as a secondary consequence of PD would link two of the primary hallmarks of the disorder: excretion of large amounts of dipeptides derived from collagen and clinical/pathologic observations of connective tissue damage.

Collagen production and turnover has been measured in skin and cultured fibroblasts from PD individuals. Isemura et al.[116] examined structural features of collagen in patient dermis and found only marginal changes in the ratio of type III to type I collagen chains. They also noted some variation in the pattern of cross-linking suggested by a higher value for cross-links containing dihydroxylysinonorleucine than for age-matched controls. The single PD patient studied showed a significantly higher, although variable, level of total hydroxylysine excretion. Chamson et al.[117] and Rao et al.[118] investigated collagen production in cultured skin fibroblasts with different results. Chamson et al.[117] found significantly less collagen secreted and more collagen degraded

Table 82-7 Structure of the Human Peptidase D Gene

Exon	Size bp	Intron	Size kb	3′ exon boundary			5′ exon boundary		
1	148	1	9.5	ACC	GG			A	CCC
				thr	gly	6	6	gly	pro
2	184	2	1.6	CGC	CAG			GAG	TCC
				arg	gln	67	68	glu	ser
3	128	3	1.0	GGA	AA			G	ATC
				gly	lys	110	110	lys	ile
4	64	4	7.0	GAT	GAG			GAT	GAG
				asp	glu	131	132	ile	ala
5	48	5	4.5	ACT	TTG			CGT	GGC
				thr	leu	147	148	arg	gly
6	62	6	14.0	AGC	AA			G	TTC
				ser	lys	168	168	lys	phe
7	45	7	13.0	GAG	TG			C	CGA
				glu	cys	183	183	cys	arg
8	76	8	1.1	CGT	GAG			GTA	ATG
				arg	glu	208	209	val	met
9	47	9	>50	GAA	AG			C	CTC
				glu	ser	224	224	ser	leu
10	69	10	3.0	GGC	AG			T	GGT
				gly	ser	247	247	ser	gly
11	78	11	8.8	ATG	TG			C	CTG
				met	cys	273	273	cys	leu
12	149	12	10.5	CCA	G			GT	GAC
				pro	gly	323	323	gly	asp
13	185	13	2.7	CCA	GAG			GGC	GTG
				pro	glu	384	385	gly	val
14	192	14	1.3	GGA	GGG			GTC	CGC
				gly	gly	448	449	val	arg
15	528			AAG	TAG				
				lys	stop	493			

Adapted from Tanoue et al.[83] Used by permission of the *Journal of Biological Chemistry.*

in PD fibroblasts than did Rao et al.[118] Chamson et al.[117] also measured the size of the intracellular proline pool in relation to collagen degradation and in response to addition to the culture medium of the prolidase substrate glycyl-L-proline. They hypothesized that a decrease in the size of the proline pool is the critical regulatory signal that accelerates breakdown of collagen in cultured fibroblasts. Addition of glycyl-L-proline to control cells, surprisingly, caused a decrease in the proline pool that was associated with an increase of 2.5-fold in collagen breakdown. These conclusions should be cautiously interpreted because the bovine serum preparations used in fibroblast growth medium contain levels of prolidase activity sufficient for rapid hydrolysis of imidodipeptide[50] and because the elevation of the intracellular imidodipeptide pool predicted to occur following addition of this substrate to the medium was not documented.

In general, studies conducted with cultured skin fibroblasts are subject to the artifact of high proline and glutamate concentrations in the growth medium, which relieve cells of the need to depend on the recycling pathway. Dolenga and Hechtman[50] observed that normal human fibroblasts grew much more slowly (doubling time 80.2 ± 4.1 h) on a MEM_2-based medium (deficient in proline and glutamate) than on a MEM_1-based medium (doubling time

Table 82-8 *PEPD* Mutations Causing Prolidase Deficiency

Nucleotide change	Exon/ intron	Coding consequence	Protein phenotype	Clinical phenotype	Population	Ref
G826A	exon 12	D276N	CRM+	severe	Japanese	110
Δ774 bp	exon 14	Δ exon 14	truncated CRM	variable	Japanese	83
G1342A	exon 14	G448R	CRM+	severe	Italian, Dutch, English	106
G>A	IVS6, −2	Δ exon 7	CRM−	severe	French-Canadian	106
Δ codon 452 or 453	exon 15	E452Δ	CRM unstable	severe	Italian	106
G>C	IVS4, −1	Δ exon 5	CRM−	severe	?	106
G1354A	exon 15	E452K	CRM+	severe	Italian	109
G551A	exon 8	R184Q	CRM+	no clinical phenotype	?	112
G833A	exon 12	G278D	CRM+	?	Irish	112

55.5 ± 4.3 h) which has higher concentrations of these amino acids. Furthermore, the growth on MEM_2 could be almost doubled by supplementation of the medium with either proline or glycyl-L-proline.

The present understanding of the role of collagen turnover in the pathophysiology of PD is that an abnormality in collagen production is not the primary pathologic mechanism, but alterations in the intermediate steps of collagen turnover may occur. Significant abnormalities in the amount and type of secreted collagen or in its hydroxylation have been ruled out as secondary metabolic phenotypes in PD.

The "Toxic Substrate" Hypothesis

A role for deficiency of proline or one or more essential amino acids in the pathophysiology of PD has been difficult to establish. An alternative hypothesis is that PD results in intracellular accumulation of some imidodipeptide that interferes with critical processes necessary for normal functioning of the central nervous system, wound healing, or the mobilization of host defenses against infection. Although there is no evidence to sustain such a hypothesis, there has been no shortage of speculation on the subject.

The catalytic specificity of prolidase compared to other enzymes that cleave proline-containing linkages is shown in Fig. 82-3. Although other proteases and peptidases prefer different substrates, many of these enzymes recognize peptides with proline in the penultimate N-terminal position. These enzymes include aminopeptidase P and dipeptidyl peptidases II and IV. The role of these enzymes in the conversion of biologically inactive peptides to their active forms, or in the degradation of active peptides to inert products, is uncertain. However, there are an extraordinary number of biologically active peptides with an X-pro sequence at the N-terminus (see Table 82-9). These include peptides with immunopharmacologic, growth-enhancing vasoactive or neuroactive properties. Vanhoof et al.[62] suggested that X-pro at the N-terminus protects biologically active peptides from random degradation. Alternatively, certain propeptides may require activation by an enzyme that recognizes the X-pro N-terminal motif to achieve biologic activity. Additionally, accumulation of imidodipeptides with an X-pro N-terminus could competitively inhibit enzymes that activate or degrade bioactive peptides by a mechanism which involves recognition of the X-pro N-terminus.

Captopril (structure shown in Fig. 82-8), a structural analogue of the prolidase substrate cysteinyl-L-proline, provides a model of how such inhibition might work. Captopril is widely used for control of hypertension and congestive heart failure and was designed as a competitive inhibitor of angiotensin converting enzyme.[119,120] Ganapathy et al.[121] showed that captopril is an inhibitor of rat prolidase with a K_i in the 100 μM range, and that rats fed this drug develop imidodipeptiduria. The observation that a small number of individuals taking captopril develop adverse side effects, including cutaneous reactions such as maculopapular eruptions[122] and other lesions resembling those that occur in PD, stimulated this investigation. The explanation for this phenomenon is not known, but the experiments of Ganapathy et al.[121] point to the possibility of *in vivo* inhibition of prolidase as a potential mechanism.

N-benzyloxycarbonyl-L-proline is an analogue of prolidase substrates and a competitive inhibitor of the enzyme.[88,123] At 10 mM this compound is completely cytostatic for cultured human fibroblasts.[124]

There are few direct studies of the cellular consequences of accumulation of undegraded imidodipeptide substrates (rather than substrate analogues). PD cultured skin fibroblasts provide a potential system in which to test potential toxic properties of imidodipeptides, but must be cultured in special medium because the bovine serum typically used as a supplement contains prolidase.[50] Using a serum substitute, ITS^+ (Collaborative Research), that has undetectable prolidase activity, Dolenga and Hechman found that 5 mM glycyl-L-proline had no effect on protein synthesis or on the doubling time of cultured PD fibroblasts.[50]

Table 82-9 Partial List of Biologic Activities of Peptides Containing Proline at Position 2 or 3

Name or biologic activity	Sequence
Enhances phagocytosis by monocytes and macrophages	T-K-P-R
Prevents polymerization of fibrin and association with platelets	G-P-R-P
Drives B lymphocytes to immunoglobulin secretion	L-P-P-S-R
In vitro immunostimulating activity on macrophages and monocytes	V-E-P-I-P-Y
Immunoenhancing activity	G-P-T-G-T-G-S-K-C-P
Interleukin-1β*	A-P-V-R-S-L-N-C
Interleukin-2*	A-P-T-S-S-S-T-K
Interleukin-5*	I-P-T-E-I-P-T-S
Interleukin-6*	V-P-P-G-E-A-S-K
Interleukin-10*	S-P-G-Q-G-T-Q-S
Interleukin-13*	G-P-V-P-P-S-T-A
Granulocyte-macrophage colony-stimulating factor*	A-P-A-R-S-P-S-P
Granulocyte colony-stimulating factor*	T-P-L-G-P-A-S-S
Erythropoetin*	A-P-P-R-L-C-G-A
Insulin-like growth factor*	G-P-E-T-L-C-G-A
Tumor necrosis factor β*	L-P-G-V-L-T-P-S
Monocyte chemotactic protein I*	E-P-D-A-I-N-A-P
Granulocyte chemotactic protein II*	G-P-V-S-A-V-L-T
Growth hormone*	F-P-T-I-P-L-S-R
Prolactin*	L-P-I-C-P-G-G-A
Bradykinin	R-P-P-G-F-S-P-F-R
Substance P	R-P-K-P-Q-Q-F-F-G-L-M

*sequence of human peptide
Data taken from Vanhoof et al.[62] Used by permission of Federation of American Societies of Experimental Biology.

Prolidase and Wound Healing

The complex process of skin wound healing is becoming better understood and is the subject of several excellent reviews.[125,126] Briefly, the first stage of wound healing is the formation of a blood clot. Damaged blood vessels cause breakage of platelets that initiates the clotting cascade, which leads ultimately to thrombin-catalyzed cleavage of fibrinogen to form cross-linked fibrin fibers with embedded platelets. Factors released from disrupted platelets produce vasodilation and increased vascular permeability, and provide chemotactic signals that attract neutrophils to the site of the wound. The neutrophils dispose of contaminating bacteria and release cytokines that attract fibroblasts, keratinocytes, and macrophages. Activated macrophages engulf remaining bacteria and dying neutrophils and contribute additional cytokines including platelet-derived growth factor (PDGF), transforming growth factor-beta (TGF-β) and tumour necrosis factor-alpha (TNF-α). These cytokines are mitogenic and chemotactic for endothelial cells, and in this way promote angiogenesis. Fibroblasts migrating to the area remodel the extracellular matrix by degradation and synthesis of matrix proteins of which collagen is a principal component. Autocrine and paracrine processes regulate the balance by complex and incompletely understood processes. After laying down new extracellular matrix (ECM) fibroblasts participate in the process of wound contraction by transformation into

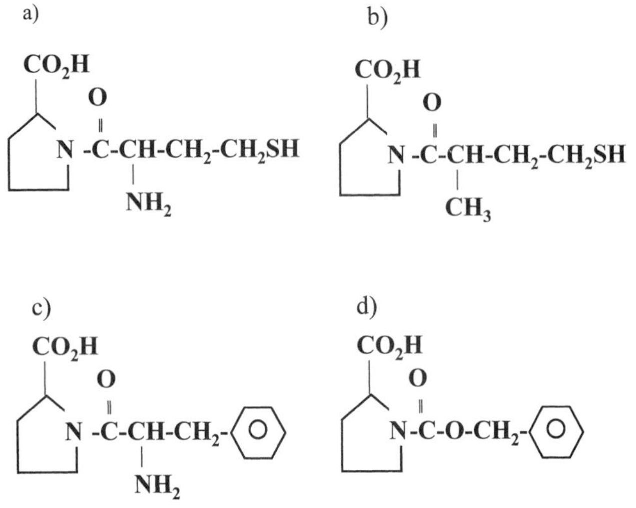

a) CO_2H O N-C-CH-CH_2-CH_2SH NH_2

b) CO_2H O N-C-CH-CH_2-CH_2SH CH_3

c) CO_2H O N-C-CH-CH_2-(O) NH_2

d) CO_2H O N-C-O-CH_2-(O)

Fig. 82-8 Structures of substrates and inhibitors of prolidase with other biologic activities. *a,* Cysteinyl-L-proline. *b,* Captopril. *c,* Phenylalanyl-L-proline. *d, N*-benzyloxy-carbonyl-L-proline (CBZ-proline).

myofibroblasts that are capable of generating contractile forces. The end-point of the healing process is reepithelialization, which involves the proliferation of keratinocytes through the fibrin clot. Key regulators of this movement appear to be members of the epidermal growth factor (EGF) family of cytokines. The migration and spread of these epithelial cells is facilitated by secretion of metalloproteases such as plasmin and collagenases that dissolve the clot material ahead of the reconstituting epidermal layer. The mechanism of scar formation (which is not a feature of wound healing in embryos) is an important and unanswered question.

Understanding the role of prolidase in the complex process of wound healing should provide insight into the pathophysiology of the skin ulcers characteristic of PD. Senboshi et al. undertook a study of the expression of prolidase mRNA in scar tissue.[127] They found that prolidase is up-regulated in hypertrophic scar tissue, and that unlike collagenase, prolidase is expressed in epidermal cells. By contrast, normal skin expressed barely detectable levels of prolidase mRNA. Prolidase is also expressed in endothelial cells of the small vessels in the region of scar tissue, an observation that the authors suggest is compatible with earlier findings by a number of investigators[11,19,35,45] showing thickening of vessel walls in PD patients. Oono and Arata[128] found that prolidase increased in skin adjacent to healing ulcers but ascribed this to fibroblast migration into the area. Using an experimental model for wound repair in with rats, Umemura et al.[129] found that at days 2 and 3 after wounding, a significant elevation of prolidase occurs.

The regulation of prolidase activity in response to the events occurring in wound healing remains a mystery. Although prolidase is a "housekeeping" enzyme, its activity in cultured fibroblasts increases over a two- to threefold range as cell density increases during the growth cycle.[130] By seeding cultured skin fibroblasts at different initial densities, Palka and Phang[131] demonstrated that cell density is not the critical variable in the up-regulation of prolidase, rather it is the interaction of ECM components with cell-surface receptors. Using an immunologic approach, they demonstrated binding of collagen to the β_1-integrin receptor effects an increase in intracellular prolidase specific activity by up to 300 percent. A possible alternative regulatory pathway is suggested by the work of Palka et al.[132] who showed that ligand binding by the mannose-6-phosphate/insulin-like growth factor II receptor enhances both chemotaxis and prolidase activity in cultured fibroblasts. In both studies, however, the extent of up-regulation of prolidase activity was modest.

The Mental Retardation Phenotype in PD

The pathophysiology of the mental retardation associated with PD is not understood. The central nervous system phenotype of certain other inborn errors of amino acid metabolism (phenylketonuria, maple syrup urine disease) may result from competitive inhibition of transport of related amino acids across the blood-brain barrier by the excessively high concentration of the offending amino acid. The consequence of this reduced uptake of certain amino acids may be impaired central nervous system protein synthesis.[133–137] While such a mechanism is unlikely in PD, it is possible that the metabolic defect also limits brain protein synthesis by reducing the availability of recycled proline to the pool of free amino acids in the brain cell. Experimental evidence supporting such a hypothesis is not available in humans; however, studies of brain protein turnover in young rats showed that the turnover of protein is 0.2 to 1.6 percent per minute.[138] The dependence of brain protein synthesis upon proline recycled from peptides has not been measured but estimation of this parameter for other amino acids has given values of 43 to 57 percent for leucine[138] and 26 percent for methionine.[139] Thus, a substantial contribution of recycling to the proline pool would certainly result in dramatic reduction of protein synthesis in PD.

Hui and Lajtha[123] has suggested an alternative model to explain the mental retardation phenomenon in PD in which the activity of neuroactive dipeptides, normally terminated by prolidase, remain undegraded. No specific neuropeptide has emerged as a candidate for the cause of mental retardation.

TREATMENT OF PROLIDASE DEFICIENCY

Amino Acid Replacement

Several therapeutic approaches for PD have been attempted, some with promising initial results but none with documented long-term improvement. The design of these strategies reflects an interpretation of the pathophysiological mechanism of PD. Some investigators, believing that the fundamental metabolic problem in PD is an insufficient supply of proline, have treated patients with oral proline supplementation either alone or in combination with other supplements. Sheffield et al.[7] used a diet supplemented with 10 g proline/day and observed elevation of plasma proline but no clinical benefit. Isemura et al.[9] found that a supplement of 4 g/day for a month had no benefit, and Ogata et al.[11] similarly found no benefit in a supplement of 6 g proline/day for a period of 6 months. Pedersen et al.[12] used a treatment regimen that included 2 g proline/day in combination with supplements of $MnCl_2$ and vitamin C. They describe improvement in IQ scores and normalization of the skin during the 9-month treatment period. A follow-up report on this same patient 13 years later indicated that long-term improvement had not occurred.[140]

Other investigators have tried an alternative dietary approach based on the hypothesis that the pathophysiology of PD involves a deficit not of proline but of the essential amino acids that form the N-terminal residues of the excreted dipeptides. Although the urinary excretion of essential amino acids in dipeptide form amounts to less than 5 percent of the recommended daily allowance for the essential amino acids, these investigators have attempted to treat patients with either intravenous or oral supplements of these nutrients. In two cases, some initial positive response was noted but it was not possible to continue the trial (V.M. der Kaloustian, personal communication) or there was no benefit (W. Rhead, personal communication).

Cofactor Supplementation

An alternative nutritional therapeutic strategy, presented by Charpentier et al.,[10,141] initially involved four components: Mn^{++}, a prolidase cofactor; ascorbate, a cofactor for the hydroxylation of proline and lysine; *N*-acetylhydroxyproline (Junetem), to replace lost hydroxyproline; and a collagenase inhibitor (Dihydan). Clinical improvement was reported with formation of scar tissue over the skin ulcers and suppression of inflammatory outbreaks.[10] The two latter components of the treatment protocol were eliminated following the observation that ascorbic acid and Mn^{++} alone reduced the imidodipeptiduria by 50 percent. The biochemical basis of this mode of therapy is uncertain. Mn^{++} is a cofactor of prolidase; however, PD erythrocytes have 2.5-fold higher level of Mn^{++} than do normal erythrocytes.[15] Measurements of Mn^{++} content have not been performed on other tissues. Nevertheless, Myara et al.[142] found that ascorbate greatly stimulated the growth of cultured PD fibroblasts. The effect of Mn on growth of deficient cells also was positive, but not as marked.

A number of other investigators have attempted to treat PD patients using variant forms of ascorbate/Mn^{++} therapy with inconsistent results. It is difficult to compare the experience of different clinical trials of this mode of therapy because each case differs with respect to the daily ascorbate load, the duration of the treatment, and the combination of ascorbate with Mn^{++} or with other therapeutic modalities. Leoni et al.[19] administered 1.18 mg/day of $MnSO_4$ and 1 g/day ascorbate for 6 months to a PD patient with no clinical improvement. Similarly, Berardesca et al.[22] and Bissonnette et al.[25] reported no improvement in patients treated with Mn^{++} and ascorbate. In contrast, two sisters with PD treated by Voigtländer et al.[23] were reported to show mild improvement with no occurrence of new ulcers. Additionally, Pedersen's patient, who was treated with oral proline plus Mn^{++} and ascorbate showed short-term improvement.[12] A patient treated by De Rijcke et al.[21] with only ascorbate (4 g/day) showed normalization of skin, but recurrence of ulcers when the treatment was discontinued at the patient's insistence. Pasolini et al.[29] reported that a patient's skin remained normal for 10 months following treatment with a combination of ascorbate, *N*-acetylhydroxyproline and diphenylhydantoin, however, there was no change in the excretion of imidodipeptides during the clinical improvement. It is difficult to draw conclusions about these widely varying outcomes of treatment with ascorbate with or without Mn^{++}. No two treatment protocols are identical and, for understandable reasons, no placebo trials were conducted. In this regard, Milligan et al.[14] remarked that a patient who was unresponsive to outpatient treatment improved considerably on hospitalization, but that ulcers returned following discharge. It is possible, therefore, that other variables, such as compliance and/or freedom of the limbs from weight bearing during the treatment course, may account for the short-term improvement. It is also possible that in some patients where the production of new skin collagen is suboptimal for nutritional reasons, stimulation of this pathway by ascorbic acid may promote healing of ulcers and formation of scar tissue.

Topical Ointments

Arata et al.[143] applied an ointment consisting of amino acid mixtures suspended in liquid paraffin kneaded into white petrolatum to the leg ulcers of a young adult with PD. After failing to achieve healing with preparations containing 1 percent, 5 percent, or 10 percent proline they reported success with a mixture containing 5 percent glycine plus 5 percent proline. Six months after treatment the treated areas of the skin remained fully epithelialized. As expected, imidodipeptiduria did not change as a result of this treatment. The authors speculate that the healing process, which is assumed to involve collagen biosynthesis, requires higher levels of these two amino acids than can easily be supplied by the circulation, and that glycine and proline, supplied in the ointment, can directly enter the pool of amino acids reserved for collagen formation.

Other investigators have had variable results using this procedure. Patients treated by Berardesca et al.[22] and Bissonnette et al.[25] did not respond to the glycine-proline ointment preparations. Jemec and Moe[140] compared treatment with the glycine-proline mixture described by Arata et al.[143] of a single ulcer on one leg with treatment of a single ulcer on the other leg with a glycine-only ointment over an 88-day course of treatment. Although the ulcer treated with the mixed ointment healed more rapidly, it was initially almost five times the area of the ulcer treated with the glycine-only ointment. Both ulcers were greatly reduced in size at the end of treatment. Following transfer to another hospital, this patient experienced a recurrence of ulcers, which were successfully treated with plasma infusions and ascorbate (G.B.E. Jemec, personal communication).

Blood Transfusion

On the rationale that normal prolidase-positive erythrocytes could reclaim proline and other peptide-bound amino acids in plasma, several investigators have attempted a treatment protocol based on transfusion of patients with normal erythrocytes; this approach has been an unequivocal failure. Lapiere,[4] Ogata et al.,[11] and Leoni et al.[19] reported no clinical improvement following transfusion. Similarly, Endo et al.[76] demonstrated that transfusion of PD patients with normal erythrocytes resulted in increasing erythrocyte prolidase levels to 35 percent of those of normal individuals but without clinical improvement or alteration of the imidodipeptiduria. Berardesca et al.[22] reported temporary improvement in ulcer healing with an intensive program involving 6 transfusions every 2 months for 1 year. The peak of prolidase activity in the patient's erythrocytes was reached 3 days after transfusion; however, imidodipeptide excretion was also maximal at this time. Eighteen months following the last transfusion, the patient's ulcers recurred.

Hechtman et al.[59] suggest that erythrocyte transfusions have failed to effect clinical and/or biochemical changes because prolidase in this cell is in an inactive or apo-enzyme form due to insufficient Mn^{++} in the erythrocyte to fully activate the enzyme. They demonstrated that erythrocyte prolidase can be activated *in vitro* by incubation with Mn^{++} salts under conditions that do not cause hemolysis but that increase the intracellular Mn^{++} concentration from 0.014 μg/ml to 2.04 μg/ml. Consequent to this change the capacity of the intact erythrocyte to hydrolyze glycyl-L-proline (V_{max}) increases from 0.36 μmol/ml RBC/h to 10 μmol/ml RBC/h. These results suggest that additional trials with Mn-loaded erythrocytes would be worthwhile provided animal studies show no detrimental effects of this approach.

REFERENCES

1. Goodman SI, Solomons CC, Muschenheim F, McIntyre CA, Miles B, O'Brien D: A syndrome resembling lathyrism associated with imidodipeptiduria. *Am J Med* **45**:152, 1968.
2. Buist NRM, Strandholm JJ, Bellinger JF, Kennaway NG: Further studies on a patient with imidodipeptiduria: A probable case of prolidase deficiency. *Metabol* **21**:1113, 1972.
3. Powell GF, Rasco MA, Maniscalo RM: A prolidase deficiency in a man with imidodipeptiduria. *Metabol* **23**:505, 1974.
4. Lapiere CM, Nusgens B: Plaies cutanèes torpides et trouble du metabolisme du collagén. *Arch Belg Dermatol Syphilig* **25**:353, 1969.
5. Powell GF, Kurosky A, Maniscalco RM: Prolidase deficiency: Report of a second case with quantitation of the excessively excreted amino acids. *J Peds* **91**:242, 1977.
6. Jackson SH, Dennis AW, Greenberg M: Imidodipeptiduria: A genetic defect in recycling collagen: A method for determining prolidase in erythrocytes. *Can Med Assoc J* **113**:759, 1975.
7. Sheffield LJ, Schlesinger P, Faull K, Halpern BJ, Schier GM, Cotton RGH, Hammond J, et al: Imidodipeptiduria, skin ulcerations and edema in a boy with prolidase deficiency. *J Pediatr* **91**:578, 1977.
8. Arata J, Umemura S, Yamamoto Y, Hagiyama M, Nohara N: Prolidase deficiency: Its dermatological manifestations and some additional biochemical studies. *Arch Dermatol* **115**:62, 1979.
9. Isemura M, Hanyu T, Gejyo F, Nakazawa R, Igarashi R, Matsuo S, Ikeda K, et al: Prolidase deficiency with imidodipeptiduria: A familial case with and without clinical symptoms. *Clin Chim Acta* **93**:401, 1979.
10. Larrègue M, Charpentier C, Laidet B, Lambert M, Bressieux J, Prigent F, Canuel C, et al: Déficit en prolidase et en manganèse A propos d'une observation: Diagnostic et traitement. *Ann Dermatol Venereol (Paris)* **109**:667, 1982.

11. Ogata A, Tanaka S, Tomoda T, Murayama E, Endo F, Kikuchi I: Autosomal recessive prolidase deficiency. *Arch Dermatol* **117**:689, 1981.
12. Pedersen PS, Christensen E, Brandt NJ: Prolidase deficiency. *Acta Paediatr Scand* **72**:785, 1983.
13. Freij BJ, Levy HL, Dudin G, Mutasim D, Deeb M, Der Kaloustian VM: Clinical and biochemical characteristics of prolidase deficiency in siblings. *Am J Med Genet* **19**:561, 1984.
14. Milligan A, Graham-Brown RAC, Burns DA, Anderson I: Prolidase deficiency: A case report and literature review. *Br J Dermatol* **12**:1405, 1989.
15. Lombeck I, Wendel U, Versieck J, van Ballenberghe L, Bremer HJ, Duran R, Wadman S: Increased manganese content and reduced arginase activity in erythrocytes of a patient with prolidase deficiency (imidodipeptiduria). *Eur J Pediatr* **14**:4571, 1986.
16. Naughten ER, Proctor SP, Levy HL, Coulombe JT, Ampola MG: Congenital expression of prolidase defect in prolidase deficiency. *Pediatr Res* **18**:259, 1984.
17. Lemieux B, Auray-Blais C, Giguere R, Shapcott D: Prolidase deficiency: Detection of cases by a newborn urinary screening programme. *J Inherit Metab Dis* **7(Suppl)**:145, 1984.
18. Ohhashi T, Ohno T, Arata J, Kodama H: Biochemical studies on prolidase in sera from control, patients with prolidase deficiency and their mother. *J Inherit Metab Dis* **11**:166, 1988.
19. Leoni A, Cetta G, Tenni R, Pasquali-Ronchetti I, Bertolini F, Guerra D, Dyne K, et al: Prolidase deficiency in two siblings with chronic leg ulcerations. *Arch Dermatol* **123**:493, 1987.
20. Wysocki SJ, Hahnel R, Mahoney T, Wilson RG, Panegyres PK: Prolidase deficiency: A patient without hydroxyproline-containing imidodipeptides in urine. *J Inherit Metab Dis* **11**:161, 1988.
21. De Rijcke S, De Maubeuge J, Laporte M, Bron D, Hariga C, Ledoux M: Déficit en prolidase: A propos d'un cas particulier. *Ann Dermatol Venereol (Paris)* **116**:309, 1989.
22. Berardesca E, Fideli D, Bellosta M, Dyne M, Zanaboni G, Cetta G: Blood transfusions in the therapy of a case of prolidase deficiency. *Br J Dermatol* **126**:193, 1992.
23. Voigtländer V, Fischer E, Larrègue M: Hereditäre Prolidasedefizienz bei zwei Schwestern mit therapieresisteneten Beingeschwüren. *Hautarzt* **39**:247, 1988.
24. Stalder JF, Myara I, Gouraud B: Cas pour diagnostic. *Ann Dermatol Venereol (Paris)* **115**:205, 1988.
25. Bissonette R, Friedmann D, Giroux J, Dolenga M, Hechtman P, Der Kaloustian VM, Dubuc R: Prolidase deficiency: A multisystemic hereditary disorder. *Am J Dermatol* **29**:818, 1993.
26. Shrinath M, Walter JH, Haeney M, Couriel JM, Lewis MA, Herrick AL: Prolidase deficiency and systemic lupus erythematosus. *Arch Dis Child* **76**:441, 1997.
27. Moulonguet I, Bamberger N, de Larrard G, Klein F, Myara I, Blanchet-Bardon C, Markuch T, et al: Ulceres de Jamb et deficit en prolidase. *Ann Dermatol Venereol (Paris)* **116**:792, 1989.
28. Cantatore FP, Papadia F, Giannico G, Simonetti S, Carrozzo M: Chronic leg ulcerations resembling vasculitis in two siblings with prolidase deficiency. *Clin Rheumatol* **12**:410, 1993.
29. Pasolini G, Pancera C, Manganoni AM, Cetta G, Zanaboni G: Ulcere agli arti inferiori da deficit di prolidasi. *Giornale Italiano Di Dermatologia E Venereologia* **123**:493, 1988.
30. Andry P, Bodmer C, Cosson C, Teillac-Hamel D, De Prost Y: Ulcères de jambes chroniques chez l'enfant avec déficit en prolidase. *Ann Dermatol Venereol (Paris)* **119**:818, 1992.
31. Der Kaloustian VM, Freij VM, Kurban AK: Prolidase deficiency: An inborn error of metabolism with major dermatological manifestations. *Dermatol* **164**:293, 1982.
32. Royce PM, Steinmann B: *Connective Tissue and Its Heritable Disorders*, ch. 18. New York, Wiley-Liss, 1993, p 533.
33. Umemura S: Studies on a patient with imidodipeptiduria. II: Lack of prolidase activity in blood cells. *Physiol Chem Phys Med* **10**:279, 1978.
34. Zanaboni G, Dyne K, Rossi A, Monafo V, Cetta G: Prolidase deficiency: Biochemical study of erythrocyte and skin fibroblast prolidase activity in Italian patients. *Haematologica* **79**:13, 1994.
35. Pierard GE, Cornil F, Lapiere CM: Pathogenesis of ulcerations in deficiency of prolidase. The role of angiopathy and of deposits of amyloid. *Am J Dermatopath* **6**:491, 1984.
36. Gray RGF, Green A, Ward AM, Anderson I, Peck DS: Biochemical and immunological studies on a family with prolidase deficiency. *J Inherit Metab Dis* **6**:143, 1983.
37. Sekiya M, Ohnishi Y, Kimura K: An autopsy case of prolidase deficiency. *Virchows Arch* **406**:125, 1985.
38. Freij BJ, Levy HL, Dudin G, Mutasim D, Deeb M, Der Kaloustian VM: Clinical and biochemical characteristics of prolidase deficiency in siblings. *Am J Med Genet* **19**:561, 1984.
39. Jackson SH, Heininger JA: Proline recycling during collagen metabolism as determined by concurrent $^{18}[O_2]$ and $^{3}[H]$ labelling. *Biochim Biophys Acta* **381**:359, 1975.
40. Johnstone RAW, Povall TJ, Baty JD, Pousset J, Charpentier C, Lemonnier A: Determination of dipeptides in urine. *Clin Chim Acta* **52**:137, 1974.
41. Kodama H, Nakamura H, Sugahara K: Liquid chromatography-mass spectrometry for the qualitative analyses of imidodipeptides in the urine of patients with prolidase deficiency. *J Chromatog* **527**:279, 1990.
42. Sugahara K, Jianying Z, Yamamoto Y, Yasuda K, Kodamoa H, Kodama H: Measurement of imidodipeptides in the serum of patients with prolidase deficiency using liquid chromatography-mass spectrometry. *Eur J Clin Chem Clin Biochem* **32**:113, 1994.
43. Kodama H, Umemura S, Shimomura S, Mizuhara S, Yamamoto Y, Arata J, Izumiya N, et al.: Studies on a patient with imidodipeptiduria. I: Identification and determination of urinary imidodipeptides. *Physiol Chem Phys Med* **8**:463, 1976.
44. Powell GF, Maniscalco RM: Bound hydroxyproline excretion following gelatin loading in prolidase deficiency. *Metabolism* **25**:503, 1976.
45. Arata J, Tada J, Yamada T, Yasutomi H, Oka E: Angiopathic pathogenesis of clinical manifestations in prolidase deficiency. *Arch Dermatol* **127**:124, 1991.
46. Miech G, Myara I, Mangeot M, Voigtlander V, Lemonnier A: Prolinase activity in prolidase-deficient fibroblasts. *J Inherit Metab Dis* **11**:266, 1988.
47. Pasquali-Ronchetti I, Quaglino D, Dyne KM, Zanaboni G, Cetta G: Ultrastructural studies on dermis from prolidase-deficient subjects. *J Submicrosc Cytol Pathol* **23**:439, 1991.
48. Shen T, Strecker HJ: Synthesis of proline and hydroxyproline in human lung fibroblasts. *Biochem J* **150**:453, 1975.
49. Emmerson KS, Phang JM: Hydrolysis of proline dipeptides completely fulfills the proline requirement in a proline-auxotrophic Chinese hamster ovary cell line. *J Nutr* **123**:909, 1993.
50. Dolenga M, Hechtman P: Prolidase deficiency in cultured human fibroblasts: Biochemical pathology and iminodipeptide-enhanced growth. *Pediatr Res* **32**:479, 1992.
51. Tarlow MJ, Seakins JW, Lloyd JK, Matthews DM, Cheng B, Thomas AJ: Intestinal absorption and biopsy transport of peptides and amino acids in Hartnup disease. *Clin Sci* **39**:18P, 1970.
52. Navab F, Asatoor AM: Studies on intestinal absorption of amino acids and a dipeptide in a case of Hartnup disease. *Gut* **113**:73, 1970.
53. Asatoor AM, Cheng B, Edwards KD, Lant AF, Matthews DM, Milne MD, Navab F, et al.: Intestinal absorption of two dipeptides in Hartnup disease. *Gut* **113**:80, 1970.
54. Adibi SA: Protein digestion in human intestine as reflected in luminal, mucosal, and plasma amino acid concentrations after meals. *J Clin Invest* **52**:1586, 1973.
55. Rubino A, Field M, Shwachman H: Intestinal transport of amino acid residues of dipeptides. I. Influx of the glycine residue of glycyl-l-proline across mucosal border. *J Biol Chem* **246**:3542, 1971.
56. Ganapathy V, Mendicino JF, Leibach FH: Transport of glycyl-proline into intestinal and renal brush border vesicles from rabbit. *J Biol Chem* **256**:118, 1981.
57. Boullin DJ, Crampton RF, Heading CE, Pelling D: Intestinal absorption of dipeptides containing glycine, phenylalanine, proline, β-alanine or histidine in the rat. *Clin Sci Mol Med* **45**:849, 1973.
58. King GF, Kuchel PW: A proton n.m.r. study of imidodipeptide transport and hydrolysis in the human erythrocyte. *Biochem J* **220**:553, 1984.
59. Hechtman P, Richter A, Corman N, Leong Y: *In situ* activation of human erythrocyte prolidase: Potential for enzyme replacement therapy in prolidase deficiency. *Pediatr Res* **24**:709, 1988.
60. Bergmann M, Fruton JS: On proteolytic enzymes. XII: Regarding the specificity of aminopeptidase and carboxypeptidase. A new type of enzyme in the intestinal tract. *J Biol Chem* **117**:189, 1937.
61. Davis NC, Smith EL: Purification and some properties of prolidase of swine kidney. *J Biol Chem* **224**:261, 1956.
62. Vanhoff G, Goossens F, De Meester I, Henriks D, Scharpé S: Proline motifs in peptides and their biological processing. *FASEB J* **9**:36, 1995.
63. Chinard FP: Photometric estimation of proline and ornithine. *J Biol Chem* **199**:91, 1952.
64. Myara I, Charpentier C, Lemonnier A: Optimal conditions for prolidase assay by proline colorimetric determination: Application to imidodipeptiduria. *Clin Chim Acta* **125**:193, 1982.

65. Richter AM, Lancaster GL, Choy FYM, Hechtman P: Purification and characterization of activated human erythrocyte prolidase. *Biochem Cell Biol* **67**:34, 1989.
66. Josefsson L, Lindberg T: Intestinal dipeptidases. I. Spectrophotometric determination of characterization of dipeptidase activity in pig intestinal mucosa. *Biochim Biophys Acta* **105**:149, 1965.
67. Butterworth J, Priestman DA: Presence in human cells and tissues of two prolidases and their alteration in prolidase deficiency. *J Inherit Metab Dis* **8**:193, 1985.
68. Myara I: Effect of long preincubation on the two forms of human erythrocyte prolidase. *Clin Chim Acta* **170**:263, 1987.
69. Ohhashi T, Ohno T, Arata J, Sugahara K, Kodama H: Characterization of prolidase I and II from erythrocytes of a control, a patient with prolidase deficiency and her mother. *Clin Chim Acta* **187**:1, 1990.
70. Hui KS, Lajtha A: Prolidase activity in brain: Comparison with other organs. *J Neurochem* **30**:321, 1978.
71. Hui KS, Lajtha A: Prolidase activity in rat brain: Developmental, regional and subcellular distribution. *Brain Res* **153**:79, 1978.
72. Yoshimoto T, Tone H, Honda T, Osatomi K, Kobayashi R, Tsuru D: Sequencing and high expression of aminopeptidase P gene from *Escherichia coli* HB101. *J Biochem* **105**:412, 1989.
73. Suga K, Kabashima T, Ito K, Tsuru D, Okamura H, Kataoka J, Yoshimoto T: Prolidase from *Xanthomonas maltophilia*: Purification and characterization of the enzyme. *Biosci Biotech Biochem* **59**:2087, 1995.
74. Cheng TC, Harvey SP, Chen GL: Cloning and expression of a gene encoding a bacterial enzyme for decontamination of organo-phosphorus nerve agents and nucleotide sequence of the enzyme. *Appl Environ Microbiol* **62**:1636, 1996.
75. Sjöström H, Norén O, Josefsson L: Purification and specificity of pig intestinal prolidase. *Biochim Biophys Acta* **327**:457, 1973.
76. Endo F, Matsuda I, Ogata F, Tanaka S: Human erythrocyte prolidase and prolidase deficiency. *Pediatr Res* **16**:227, 1982.
77. Yoshimoto T, Matsubara F, Kawano E, Tsuru D: Prolidase from bovine intestine: Purification and characterization. *J Biochem (Tokyo)* **94**:1889, 1983.
78. Boright A, Scriver CR, Lancaster GA, Choy F: Prolidase deficiency: Biochemical classification of alleles. *Am J Hum Genet* **44**:731, 1989.
79. Myara I, Cosson C, Moatti N, Lemonnier A: Human kidney prolidase-purification, preincubation properties and immunological reactivity. *Int J Biochem* **26**:207, 1994.
80. Fernandez-Espla MD, Martin-Hernandez MC, Fox PF: Purification and characterization of a prolidase from *Lactobacillus casei subsp. casei* IFPL 731. *Appl Environ Microbiol* **63**:314, 1997.
81. King GF, Middlehurst CR, Kuchel PW: Direct NMR evidence that prolidase is specific for the *trans* isomer of imidodipeptide substrates. *Biochemistry* **25**:1054, 1986.
82. Lin L, Brandts JF: Evidence suggesting that some proteolytic enzymes may cleave only the trans form of the peptide bond. *Biochemistry* **18**:43, 1979.
83. Tanoue A, Endo F, Matsuda I: Structural organization of the gene for human prolidase (peptidase D) and demonstration of a partial gene deletion in a patient with prolidase deficiency. *J Biol Chem* **265**:11306, 1990.
84. Myara I, Charpentier C, Lemonnier A: Minireview: Prolidase and prolidase deficiency. *Life Sci* **34**:1985, 1984.
85. Roderick SL, Matthews BW: Structure of the cobalt-dependent methionine aminopeptidase from *Escherichia coli*: A new type of proteolytic enzyme. *Biochemistry* **32**:3907, 1993.
86. Bazan JF, Weaver LH, Roderick SL, Huber R, Matthews BW: Sequence and structure comparison suggest that methionine aminopeptidase, prolidase, aminopeptidase P, and creatinase share a common fold. *Proc Natl Acad Sci U S A* **91**:2473, 1994.
87. Mock WL, Liu Y: Hydrolysis of picolinylprolines by prolidase: A general mechanism for the dual-metal ion-containing aminopeptidases. *J Biol Chem* **270**:18437, 1995.
88. King GF, Crossley MJ, Kuchel PW: Inhibition and active-site modelling of prolidase. *Eur J Biochem* **180**:377, 1989.
89. Radzicka A, Wolfenden R: Analogues of intermediates in the action of pig kidney prolidase. *Biochemistry* **30**:4160, 1991.
90. Mock WL, Zhuang H: Chemical modification locates guanidinyl and carboxylate groups within the active site of prolidase. *Biochem Biophys Res Commun* **180**:401, 1991.
91. Masuda S, Watanabe H, Morioka M, Fujita Y, Ageta T, Kodama H: Characteristics of partially purified prolidase and prolinase from the human prostate. *Acta Medica Okayama* **48**:173, 1994.
92. Myara I, Moatti N, Lemonnier A: Separation of two erythrocyte prolidase isoforms by fast protein liquid chromatography: Application to prolidase deficiency. *J Chromatogr A* **493**:170, 1989.
93. McAlpine PJ, Mohandas T, Roay M, Wong JL, Hamerton JL: Assignment of the peptidase D gene locus (PEPD) to chromosome 19 in man. *Cytogenet Cell Genet* **16**:204, 1976.
94. Brown S, Lalley PA, Minna JD: Assignment of the gene for peptidase S (PEPS) to chromosome 4 in man and confirmation of peptidase D (PEPD) assignment to chromosome 19. *Cytogenet Cell Genet* **22**:167, 1978.
95. O'Brien T, Ball S, Sarfarazi M, Harper PS, Robson EB: Genetic linkage between the loci for myotonic dystrophy and peptidase D. *Ann Hum Genet* **47**:117, 1983.
96. Shaw DJ, Meredith AL, Brook JD, Sarfarazi M, Harley HG, Huson SM, Bell GI, et al.: Linkage relationships of the insulin receptor gene with the complement component 3, LDL receptor, apolipoprotein C2 and myotonic dystrophy loci on chromosome 19. *Hum Genet* **74**:267, 1986.
97. Brook JD, Shaw DJ, Meredith L, Bruns GAP, Harper PS: Localisation of genetic markers on orientation of the linkage group on chromosome 19. *Hum Genet* **68**:282, 1984.
98. Lusis AJ, Heinzmann C, Sparkes RS, Scott J, Knott TJ, Geller R, Sparkes MC: Regional mapping of human chromosome 19: Organization of genes for plasma lipid transport (APOC1, -C2, and -E and LDLR) and the genes C3, PEPD, and GPI. *Proc Natl Acad Sci U S A* **83**:3929, 1986.
99. Harley HG, Walsh KV, Rundle S, Brook JD, Sarfarazi M, Kock MC, Floyd JL, et al.: Localisation of the myotonic dystrophy locus to 19q13.2-19q13.3 and its relationship to twelve polymorphic loci on 19q. *Hum Genet* **87**:73, 1991.
100. Friedrich U, Brunner H, Smeets D, Lambermon E, Ropers H: Three-point linkage analysis employing C3 and 19cen markers assigns the myotonic dystrophy gene to 19q. *Hum Genet* **75**:291, 1987.
101. Schonk D, Coerwinkel-Driessen M, van Dalen I, Oerlemans F, Smeets B, Schepens J, Hulsebos T, et al.: Definition of subchromosomal intervals around the myotonic dystrophy gene region at 19q. *Genomics* **4**:384, 1989.
102. Bachinski LL, Krahe R, White BF, Wieringa B, Shaw D, Korneluk R, Thompson LH, et al.: An informative panel of somatic cell hybrids for physical mapping on chromosome 19q. *Am J Hum Genet* **52**:375, 1993.
103. Garcia E, Elliott J, Gorvad A, Brandriff B, Gordon L, Soliman KM, Ashworth LK, et al.: A continuous high-resolution physical map spanning 17 megabases of the q12, q13.1 and q13.2 cytogenetic bands of human chromosome 19. *Genomics* **27**:52, 1995.
104. Endo F, Tanoue A, Nakai H, Hata A, Indo Y, Titani K, Matsuda I: Primary structure and gene localization of human prolidase. *J Biol Chem* **264**:4476, 1989.
105. Tanoue A, Endo F, Matsuda I: The human prolidase gene: Structure and restriction fragment length polymorphisms. *J Inherit Metab Dis* **13**:771, 1990.
106. Ledoux P, Scriver C, Hechtman P: Four novel PEPD alleles causing prolidase deficiency. *Am J Hum Genet* **54**:1014, 1994.
107. Endo F, Hata A, Indo K, Motohara K, Matsuda I: Immunochemical analysis of prolidase deficiency and molecular cloning of cDNA for prolidase of human liver. *J Inherit Metab Dis* **10**:305, 1987.
108. Endo F, Tanoue A, Kitano A, Arata J, Danks DM, Lapiere CM, Sei Y, et al.: Biochemical basis of prolidase deficiency: Polypeptide and RNA phenotypes and the relation to clinical phenotypes. *J Clin Invest* **85**:162, 1990.
109. Ledoux P: The molecular basis of prolidase deficiency. Ph D Thesis. Montreal, Quebec, Canada, McGill University, 1996, p 96.
110. Tanoue A, Endo F, Kitano A, Matsuda I: A single nucleotide change in the prolidase gene in fibroblasts from two patients with polypeptide positive prolidase deficiency. *J Clin Invest* **86**:351, 1990.
111. Tanoue A, Endo F, Akaboshi I, Oono T, Arata J, Matsuda I: Molecular defect in siblings with prolidase deficiency and absence or presence of clinical symptoms. *J Clin Invest* **87**:1171, 1991.
112. Ledoux P, Scriver CR, Hechtman P: Expression and molecular analysis of mutations in prolidase deficiency. *Am J Hum Genet* **59**:1035, 1996.
113. Endo F, Matsuda I: Screening method for prolidase deficiency. *Hum Genet* **56**:349, 1981.
114. Lewis WHP, Harris H: Human red cell peptidases. *Nature* **215**:351, 1967.
115. Fox MH, Weyer SM, Thurmon TF, Berenson GS: Genetically controlled enzymatic variation in a southern, biracial, semi-rural community: The Bogalusa Heart Study *Hum Hered* **31**:138, 1981.

116. Isemura M, Hanyu T, Ono T, Icarashi R, Sato Y, Geyjo F, Wakazawa R, et al.: Studies on prolidase deficiency with a possible defect in collagen metabolism. *Tohoku J Exp Med* **134**:21, 1981.
117. Chamson A, Voigtländer V, Myara I, Frey J: Collagen biosynthesis anomalies in prolidase deficiency: Effect of glycyl-L-proline on the degradation of newly synthesized collagen. *Clin Physiol Biochem* **7**:128, 1989.
118. Rantanen T, Palva A: Lactobacilli carry cryptic genes encoding peptidase-related proteins: Characterization of a prolidase gene (pepQ) and a related cryptic gene (orfZ) from *Lactobacillus delbrueckii subsp. Microbiology* **143**:3899, 1997.
119. Ondetti MA, Rubin B, Cushman DW: Design of specific inhibitors of angiotensin-converting enzyme: New class of orally active antihypertensive agents. *Science* **196**:441, 1977.
120. Cushman DW, Cheung HS, Sabo EF, Ondetti MA: Design of potent competitive inhibitors of angiotensin-converting enzyme. Carboxyalkanoyl and mercaptoalkanoyl amino acids. *Biochem* **16**:5484, 1977.
121. Ganapathy V, Pashley SJ, Roesel RA, Pashley DA, Leiback FH: Inhibition of rat and human prolidases by captopril. *Biochem Pharmacol* **34**:1287, 1985.
122. Vidt DG, Bravo EL, Fouad FM: Drug therapy: Captopril. *N Engl J Med* **306**:214, 1982.
123. Hui K, Lajtha A: Activation and inhibition of cerebral prolidase. *J Neurochem* **35**:489, 1980.
124. Dolenga M, Hechtman P: Cytotoxicity of carbobenzoxy-protected amino acids. *In Vitro* **28A**:300, 1992.
125. Martin P: Wound healing—Aiming for perfect skin regeneration. *Science* **276**:75, 1997.
126. Mutsaers SE, Bishop JE, McGrouther G, Laurent GJ: Mechanism of tissue repair: From wound healing to fibrosis. *Int J Biochem Cell Biol* **29**:5, 1997.
127. Senboshi Y, Oono T, Arata J: Localization of prolidase gene expression in scar tissue using *in situ* hybridization. *J Dermatol Sci* **121**:63, 1996.
128. Oono T, Arata J: Characteristics of prolidase and prolinase in prolidase-deficient patients with some preliminary studies of their role in skin. *J Dermatol* **15**:212, 1988.
129. Umemura S, Arata J, Nohara N: Prolidase activity during healing of skin burns in rats. *J Dermatol* **72**:17, 1980.
130. Myara I, Charpentier C, Gantier M, Lemonnier A: Cell density affects prolidase and prolinase activity and intracellular amino acid levels in cultured cells. *Clin Chim Acta* **150**:1, 1985.
131. Palka JA, Phang JM: Prolidase activity in fibroblasts is regulated by interaction of extracellular matrix with cell surface integrin receptors. *J Cell Biochem* **67**:166, 1997.
132. Palka JA, Karna E, Miltyk W: Fibroblast chemotaxis and prolidase activity modulation by insulin-like growth factor II and mannose-6-phosphate. *Mol Cell Biochem* **168**:177, 1997.
133. Appel SH: Inhibition of brain protein synthesis, in Lajtha A (ed): *Protein Metabolism of the Nervous System*. New York, Plenum Press, 1970, p 621.
134. Appel SH: Inhibition of brain protein synthesis: An approach to the biochemical basis of neurological dysfunction in the aminoacidurias. *Ann N Y Acad Sci* **29**:63, 1966.
135. Hughes JV, Johnson TC: Abnormal amino acid metabolism and brain protein synthesis during neural development. *Neurochem Res* **33**:81, 1978.
136. Banos G, Daniel PM, Moorhouse SR, Pratt OE: Inhibition of entry of some amino acids into the brain, with observations on mental retardation in the aminoacidurias. *Psychol Med* **4**:262, 1974.
137. Cohen SR, Lajtha A: Amino acid transport, in Lajtha A (ed): *Handbook of Neurochemistry*. New York, Plenum Press, 1972, p 543.
138. Sun Y, Deibler GE, Jehle J, Macedonia J, Dumont I, Dang T, Smith CB: Rates of local cerebral protein synthesis in the rat during normal postnatal development. *Am J Physiol* **268**:R549, 1995.
139. Grange E, Gharid A, Lepetit P, Guillaud J, Sarda N, Bobillier P: Brain protein synthesis in the conscious rat using l-[^{35}S]-methionine: Relationship of methionine-specific activity between plasma and precursor compartment and evaluation of methionine metabolic pathways. *J Neurochem* **59**:1437, 1992.
140. Jemec GBE, Moe ATT: Topical treatment of skin ulcers in prolidase deficiency. *Pediatr Dermatol* **13**:58, 1996.
141. Charpentier C, Dagbovie K, Lemonnier A, Larregue M, Johnstone RAW: Prolidase deficiency with imidodipeptiduria: Biochemical investigations and first results of attempted therapy. *J Inherit Metab Dis* **1**:77, 1981.
142. Myara I, Charpentier C, Wolfrom C, Gautier M, Lemonnier A, Larregue M, Chamson A, et al.: *In vitro* responses to ascorbate and manganese in fibroblasts from a patient with prolidase deficiency and imidodipeptiduria: Cell growth, prolidase activity and collagen metabolism. *J Inherit Metab Dis* **6**:27, 1983.
143. Arata J, Hatakenaka K, Oono T: Effect of topical application of glycine and proline on recalcitrant leg ulcers of prolidase deficiency. *Arch Dermatol* **122**:626, 1986.

CHAPTER 83

The Hyperornithinemias

David Valle ▪ Olli Simell

1. **Ornithine is a nonprotein amino acid that is the substrate or product of five enzymatic reactions and the ligand of a transmitochondrial transport protein. Two of these enzymes, ornithine-δ-aminotransferase (OAT) and ornithine decarboxylase, catalyze reactions that consume ornithine. The former catalyzes the major catabolic reaction for ornithine. The source of ornithine is arginine in dietary protein, although, under certain circumstances, *de novo* synthesis of ornithine occurs by reversal of the normal flux of the OAT reaction.**
2. **There are two distinct genetic disorders that result in hyperornithinemia: gyrate atrophy of the choroid and retina (MIM 258870) and the hyperornithinemia-hyperammonemia-homocitrullinuria (HHH) syndrome (MIM 238970).**
3. **Gyrate atrophy of the choroid and retina is a progressive chorioretinal degeneration that is inherited as an autosomal recessive trait. It is caused by a deficiency of OAT. We know of more than 150 biochemically documented cases, about one-third of which are Finnish. There is myopia, night blindness, and loss of peripheral vision starting late in the first decade, proceeding to tunnel vision and eventual blindness by the third and fourth decades. Posterior subcapsular cataracts are present in nearly all patients by the end of the second decade. The ocular fundus exhibits sharply demarcated circular areas of complete chorioretinal degeneration that start in the midperiphery and gradually extend to the posterior pole. Tubular aggregates are present in the type 2 fibers of skeletal muscle. Plasma ornithine values range from 400 to 1400 μM, and 0.5 to 10 mM of ornithine is excreted daily. Plasma glutamate, glutamine, lysine, creatine, and creatinine concentrations are modestly reduced. OAT activity in the cells and tissues of patients is from 0 to 6 percent that in control subjects, and obligate heterozygotes have intermediate values. Seven patients are known to have had *in vitro* and *in vivo* responses to pharmacologic doses of pyridoxal phosphate or pyridoxine. Additional therapeutic approaches have included an arginine-restricted diet, which in some patients has lowered plasma ornithine to normal values; administration of pharmacologic doses of L-lysine or α-aminoisobutyric acid to increase renal losses; and administration of proline or creatine. No form of therapy is unequivocally effective; however, sib pair studies with young, well-controlled patients strongly suggest that chronic reduction of plasma ornithine to values <200 μM with an arginine-restricted diet slows or stops the chorioretinal degeneration. Results in a mouse model of gyrate atrophy support this conclusion. Creatine administration has resulted in improvement of the histologic abnormalities in muscle.**
4. **Human, rat, mouse, plant, and yeast OAT cDNAs have been cloned and sequenced. The human OAT gene has been mapped to 10q26 and its structure determined. A cluster of apparently nonfunctional OAT-related sequences maps to Xp10-Xp21. In cultured fibroblasts, about 85 percent of gyrate atrophy patients express near normal amounts of normal-sized OAT mRNA, but only about 10 percent have normal amounts of normal-sized OAT protein. More than 60 mutations causing gyrate atrophy have been detected.**
5. **The HHH syndrome is an autosomal recessive inherited disorder described in more than 50 patients. The clinical symptoms are related to the hyperammonemia and resemble those of the urea cycle disorders. Visual problems or ocular fundus changes are not typical. Plasma ornithine concentrations range from 200 to 1020 μM on a self-restricted protein diet and, in general, are slightly lower than in gyrate atrophy. The pathophysiology of the disease involves diminished ornithine transport into the mitochondria with ornithine accumulation in the cytoplasm and reduced intramitochondrial ornithine causing impaired ureagenesis and orotic aciduria. OAT activity is normal. Homocitrulline is thought to originate from transcarbamylation of lysine. Its excretion is increased by lysine supplementation. The patients tolerate 1.2 to 1.5 g/kg protein daily without hyperammonemia. Ornithine or citrulline supplementation has reduced ammonia and glutamine levels in some, but not all, patients and accentuates hyperornithinemia. The long-term efficacy of this treatment is not known.**
6. **A gene (*ORNT1*), encoding a human inner mitochondrial membrane ornithine transporter, has been identified by homology with yeast and fungal mitochondrial ornithine transporters and maps to 13q14. *ORNT1* mutations have been identified in HHH patients and shown to be functionally significant.**

Ornithine is a nonprotein amino acid with an important role in the metabolism of urea, creatine, and polyamines. The pathways of ornithine metabolism are closely linked with those of proline (see Chap. 81). Together they allow the exchange of molecules between the urea (see Chap. 85) and tricarboxylic acid cycles. The major source of ornithine is arginine in dietary protein. The fates of the ornithine carbon atoms include incorporation into protein as arginine, proline, glutamate, or any of the α-ketoglutarate-derived nonessential amino acids; conversion to polyamines and γ-aminobutyric acid (GABA); and oxidation in the tricarboxylic acid cycle.

There are two inherited disorders that result in hyperorni thinemia: gyrate atrophy of the choroid and retina (MIM 258870), with symptoms limited mainly to the eye; and the hyperornithinemia-hyperammonemia-homocitrullinuria (HHH) syndrome (MIM 238970), with symptoms resulting from ammonia accumulation and protein aversion. The former condition is due to a deficiency of the mitochondrial matrix enzyme ornithine-δ-aminotransferase (OAT) (Fig. 83-1), while the basic

A list of standard abbreviations is located immediately preceding the index in each volume. Additional abbreviations used in this chapter include: 5FMOrn = 5-fluoromethylornithine; HHH = hyperornithinemia-hyperammonemia-homocitrullinuria; MCF, mitochondrial carrier family; MRS = magnetic resonance spectroscopy; NO = nitric oxide; NOS = nitric oxide synthetase; OAT = ornithine--aminotransferase; OATL = ornithine--aminotransferase-like; P5C = ^{1}-pyrroline-5-carboxylate.

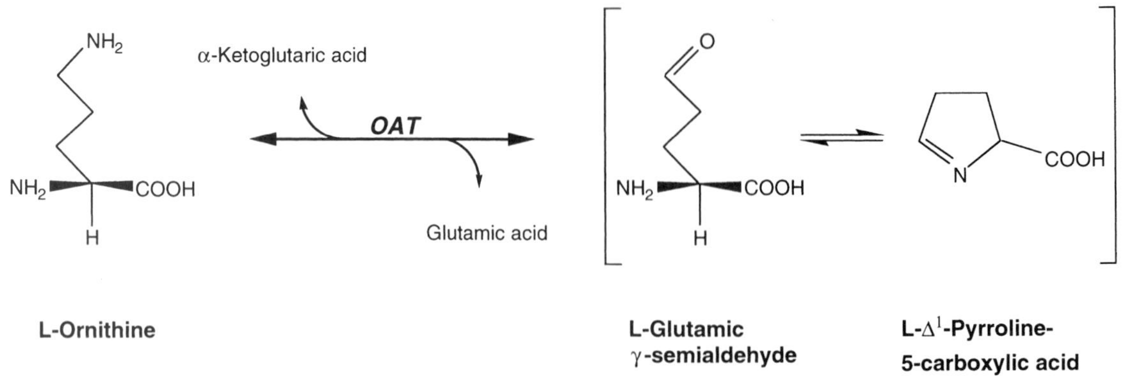

α-Ketoglutaric acid

OAT

Glutamic acid

L-Ornithine

L-Glutamic γ-semialdehyde

L-Δ^1-Pyrroline-5-carboxylic acid

Fig. 83-1 The OAT reaction. The site of the primary enzymatic defect in gyrate atrophy of the choroid and retina. L-Glutamic γ-semialdehyde and L-Δ^1 pyrroline-5-carboxylic acid are in spontaneous, nonenzymatic equilibrium.

defect in the latter is in the transporter that mediates ornithine entry into mitochondria.

ORNITHINE METABOLISM

Ornithine is a substrate or product of five enzymes and a mitochondrial transporter (Fig. 83-2). The characteristics of these proteins are listed in Table 83-1. Ornithine metabolism can be considered in four sections: the urea cycle, polyamine biosynthesis, creatine synthesis, and the OAT reaction. Depending on the physiological circumstances, the latter functions in arginine degradation, proline biosynthesis, or *de novo* ornithine synthesis.

The Urea Cycle

In most instances, ornithine serves as a catalyst in the urea cycle, providing the molecular foundation on which urea is assembled using nitrogen atoms contributed by ammonium and aspartate and a carbon atom from bicarbonate. Each molecule of ornithine converted to citrulline in the mitochondrial matrix is eventually reformed from arginine in the cytoplasm. Stoichiometric or noncatalytic utilization of ornithine in the urea cycle occurs in two special circumstances: (a) when the urea cycle is interrupted by inherited enzyme deficiencies that lead to the accumulation of citrulline, argininosuccinate, or arginine and result in the urinary loss of ornithine carbon skeletons in the form of the accumulated intermediate; and (b) when dietary arginine is less than that required for protein accretion. In the later instance, ornithine and the reactions of the urea cycle are used for arginine synthesis.

Citrulline Synthesis

Ornithine Transcarbamylase. Citrulline is formed in the mitochondrial matrix of hepatocytes and, to a much lesser extent,

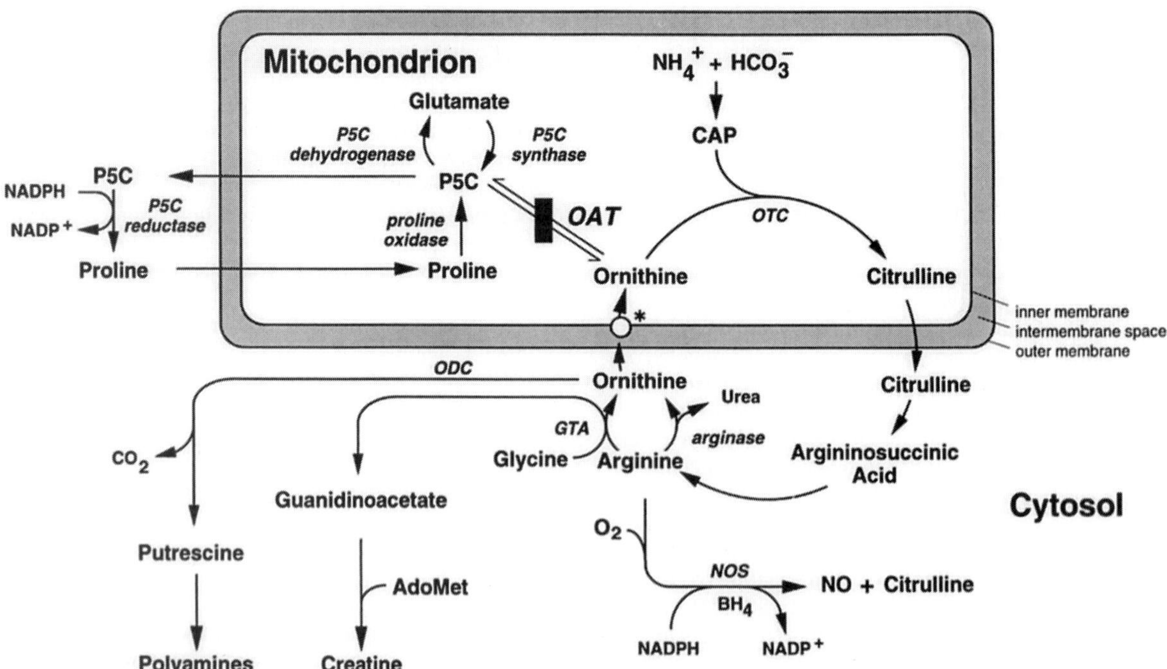

Fig. 83-2 Ornithine metabolic pathways. Not all of the enzymes shown are expressed in all cells or tissues. For example, ornithine transcarbamylase is expressed mainly in periportal hepatocytes and, to a much lesser extent, in the epithelial cells of the small intestine and renal cortex. Glycine transaminidinase is expressed mainly in kidney, pancreas, and liver (see Fig. 83-10). The black vertical rectangle signifies the site of the metabolic block in gyrate atrophy. The asterisk (*) indicates the transporter (ORNT1) that is defective in the HHH syndrome. AdoMet = S-adenosylmethionine; BH_4 = tetrahydrobiopterin; CAP = carbamyl phosphate; GTA = glycine transamidinase; NO = nitric oxide; NOS = nitric oxide synthetase; OAT = ornithine-δ-aminotransferase; ODC = ornithine decarboxylase; OTC = ornithine transcarbamylase; P5C = Δ^1 pyrroline-5-carboxylate.

Table 83-1 Enzymes of Ornithine Metabolism*

Enzyme	Subcellular Compartment	Subunit Molecular Mass, kDa	Structure	Cofactor	Kinetic Parameters	Organ or Tissue Distribution	Ref.
Ornithine aminotransferase (EC2.6.1.13)	Mitochondrial matrix	49 → 45†	Homohexamer or homotetramer	Pyridoxal phosphate	$K_{m\ orn} = 1.8$ mM $K_{m\alpha KG} = 2.7$ mM $K_{m\ PLP} = 0.7$ μM	General	147, 103, 114
Ornithine transcarbamylase (EC2.1.3.3)	Mitochondrial matrix	40 → 36†	Homotrimer	–	$K_{m\ orn} = 0.47$ mM $K_{m\ CAP} = 0.7$ mM	Primarily liver; low activity in gut	1, 8
Ornithine decarboxylase (EC4.1.1.17)	Cytoplasm	51	Monomer	Pyridoxal phosphate	$K_{m\ orn} = 0.1$ mM	General; high in rapidly dividing tissues	54, 78
Arginase (EC3.5.3.1)	Cytoplasm	30	Homotetramer	Mn^{2+}	$K_{m\ arg} = 10$ mM	Liver and erythrocytes; a second gene product expressed in kidney	40, 78
Glycine transamidinase (EC2.1.4.1)	‡	45	Homodimer	–	$K_{m\ arg} = 2.5$ mM $K_{m\ gly} = 2.5$ mM	Pancreas, kidney, liver	40, 44
Nitric oxide synthetase§ (EC1.14.23)	Membrane-bound	144	Homodimer (?)	BH_4, NADPH, FAD, FMN	$K_{m\ arg} \cong 3$ μM	Endothelial cells	27, 28

*Human sources for all. Abbreviations: αKG, α-ketoglutarate; arg, arginine; CAP, carbamyl phosphate; gly, glycine; orn, ornithine; PLP, pyridoxal phosphate; BH_4 tetrahydrobiopterin.
†Cleavage of mitochondrial signal sequence.
‡Subcellular location in human tissues not known; in rat kidney, reported to be on the cytoplasmic side of the inner mitochondrial membrane.
§The values provided are for human endothelial cell NOS; see references for data on the other two NOS isoforms.

the epithelium of the small intestine and kidney by the transfer of the carbamyl moiety of carbamyl phosphate to the δ-amino nitrogen of ornithine. The reaction is catalyzed by ornithine transcarbamylase and is markedly influenced by pH, with maximal rates between pH 8 and 9. This pH dependence suggests that zwitterionic ornithine, with an un-ionized δ-amino group (~10 percent of the total isoelectric form at physiological pH) is the actual substrate for ornithine transcarbamylase.[1,2] Although substrate specificity is high at pH 8, some homocitrulline is formed by transcarbamylation of L-lysine at pH 9.[3]

Ornithine transcarbamylase is expressed at high levels in the liver, and to a lesser extent in the epithelium of the small intestine (see Chap. 85). Like other urea cycle enzymes and OAT, ornithine transcarbamylase activity in liver is influenced by the quantity of dietary protein.[4,5] The mechanism(s) for this coordinate regulation are mainly transcriptional and appear to involve glucagon and cAMP.[6] The structure of both human and rat ornithine transcarbamylase genes and their proximal promoters has been determined.[7,8] Both genes have 10 exons. Transgenic studies indicate that sequences in 1.3 kb of the 5′ flanking region of the rat gene and in 750 bp of the 5′ flanking region of the mouse gene are sufficient to direct specific expression in liver and small intestine.[9,10] Positive effects by two transcription factors—hepatocyte nuclear factor-4 and CCAAT/enhancer binding protein—and a negative effect by another—chicken ovalbumin upstream promoter-transcription factor—are involved in achieving this pattern of expression.[11] Paradoxically, the level of expression directed by these proximal promoter sequences is higher in gut than in liver. Extensive analysis of the rat ornithine transcarbamylase promoter identified an ~110-bp enhancer element 11 kb upstream from the transcriptional start site, which modifies the activity of the proximal promoter to give higher expression in liver.[12] The enhancer contains four protein-binding sites, two for hepatocyte nuclear factor-4 and two for CCAAT/enhancer binding protein, both of which are liver-selective transcription factors.

The substrate regulation of citrulline synthesis and the ornithine transcarbamylase reaction is complex and plays an important role in the moment-to-moment synthesis of urea. Ornithine and *N*-acetylglutamate, an activator of carbamyl phosphate, are important effectors of this regulation[13–15] Ornithine acts both as a substrate for ornithine transcarbamylase and as a stimulator of carbamyl phosphate synthetase.[16–18] Within the mitochondrial matrix of hepatocytes actively synthesizing urea, ornithine concentrations are determined by ornithine entry and by the activity of ornithine transcarbamylase.[19] OAT also influences matrix ornithine concentration, but its expression is limited to a population of hepatocytes surrounding the pericentral vein of hepatic lobules that do not express ornithine transcarbamylase and are not involved in urea production.[20] Using *in vitro* studies with isolated rat liver mitochondria, Raijman and colleagues showed that ornithine exerts a regulatory effect on citrulline synthesis in the physiological range of cytoplasmic ornithine concentrations. Furthermore, their results suggested that transported ornithine is channeled directly to ornithine transcarbamylase, so that matrix ornithine concentration remains low at cytoplasmic ornithine concentrations up to 0.5 mM.[18] Similarly, carbamyl phosphate produced by matrix carbamyl phosphate synthetase is channeled to ornithine transcarbamylase.[14] Together, these observations suggest physical organization of the components of the urea cycle in the mitochondrial matrix. How this takes place is not known. Acting in concert, the regulators of citrulline synthesis provide the urea cycle with sufficient homeostatic capacity to maintain normal ammonium concentrations despite acute, large-scale changes in dietary protein intake.[21]

An X-linked deficiency of ornithine transcarbamylase has been described in humans (see Chap. 85) and in two mouse models, sparse fur (*spf*) and sparse fur-abnormal skin and hair (*spf-ash*).[22–24] In both species, affected males exhibit protein intolerance with lethargy, vomiting, hyperammonemia, coma, and orotic aciduria. Because ornithine catabolism by OAT is intact, ornithine accumulation is not a feature of ornithine transcarbamylase deficiency.

Nitric Oxide and the Nitric Oxide Synthetase Reaction. Citrulline and nitric oxide (NO) are products of a reaction catalyzed by nitric oxide synthetase (NOS) with arginine as substrate.[25–28] NO is an important messenger molecule, serving as a neurotransmitter and as a regulator of immune function and blood vessel dilation.[25–27] The affinity of NOS, a cytochrome P450 hemoprotein,[29] for arginine is much greater than that of arginase (Table 83-1). There are at least three isoforms of NOS, each encoded by different genes, one expressed constitutively in endothelial cells, one inducible in macrophages, and one expressed in discrete populations of neurons. There is some evidence for expression of NOS in photoreceptors and other retinal neurons.[30–32]

Although the NOS reaction is a quantitatively minor source of citrulline as compared to the ornithine transcarbamylase reaction, NO is a powerful regulatory molecule. How possible disturbances in its production might play a role in the pathophysiology of gyrate atrophy and urea cycle disorders remains to be determined.

Arginase. Biochemical, electrophoretic, immunologic, and genetic evidence suggests that there are at least two active arginase genes.[33–36] The cytosolic arginase of hepatic cells in ureotelic animals functions in the urea cycle and is remarkable for its activity (the highest of all the urea cycle enzymes)[37] and low substrate affinity (Table 83-1). Ornithine and lysine are weak inhibitors.[33,38] The cDNA sequence and gene structure are known.[39–41] A second form of arginase ("renal arginase"), also weakly inhibitable by ornithine, has been found in kidney, small intestine, pancreas, and mammary gland.[33,35,42,43] In most tissues, this arginase probably functions as the initial enzyme in a sequence of reactions that converts arginine to proline.[43,44]

Arginase deficiency has been described in several children with mental retardation, neuromuscular abnormalities, and hyperargininemia (see Chap. 85). Arginase activity is deficient in the erythrocytes and liver of these patients. Normal renal arginase activity was found in the kidneys of at least two of these patients[45,46] Plasma ornithine concentrations are normal or only minimally reduced, probably because renal arginase and glycine transamidinase provide alternatives for the conversion of arginine to ornithine. An interesting but so far unanswered question is whether the arginine accumulation characteristic of arginase deficiency perturbs NO production (see Fig. 83-2).[25–27]

Subcellular Compartmentation and Transport of Ornithine. Three of the urea cycle enzymes — argininosuccinate synthase, argininosuccinate lyase and arginase — are cytosolic, while two — ornithine transcarbamylase and carbamyl phosphate synthase — are in the mitochondrial matrix (Fig. 83-2). Thus, a complete turn of the urea cycle requires the transport of ornithine into and citrulline out of the mitochondria. The mitochondrial boundary is composed of inner and outer membranes with an intervening intermembrane space. The outer membrane freely admits amino acids, while the inner membrane is a true permeability barrier[47] Ornithine transport into liver mitochondria is mediated by a specific inner membrane carrier, which prefers ornithine to L-arginine or L-lysine.[48–51] There have been different views on the counterion and energy requirements for this process. Gamble and Lehninger found that mitochondria accumulated cationic L-ornithine if respiratory energy (e.g., as provided by succinate or glutamate) and a permeant proton-yielding anion (HPO_4^{2-}, H_2PO^{4-}, acetate or bicarbonate) were available.[49] Nonrespiring mitochondria were impermeable to either cationic ornithine (the prevalent form of ornithine at physiological pH) or the electroneutral analogue *N*-acetylornithine. Other studies showed that the distribution of ornithine across the mitochondrial membrane was correlated with the inner membrane pH gradient and that the intramitochondrial concentration of ornithine barely exceeded that in the medium when the catabolism of matrix ornithine by OAT was blocked by amino-oxyacetate.[48] These results suggested that cationic ornithine is transported electroneutrally in exchange for H^+, without depending on respiratory energy. Hommes and colleagues reconstituted ornithine transport into liposomes with extracts of bovine liver mitochondria and found evidence for a specific ornithine translocator, which exchanged cationic ornithine for hydrogen ions.[52]

Alternatively, McGivan proposed, on the basis of countertransport studies in intact liver mitochondria, that an ornithine/citrulline antiporter links the transmitochondrial fluxes of these urea cycle substrates.[50] More recently, Indiveri and colleagues described the purification and characterization of an ornithine/citrulline antiporter from rat liver mitochondria.[51] The purified protein had an M_r of 33.5, similar to the size of other mitochondrial metabolite transporters. In reconstituted proteoliposomes, appreciable uptake of radiolabeled ornithine from the external medium required an exchangeable *trans* substrate in the intraliposomal fluid. In proteoliposomes preloaded with a variety of possible substrates (20 mM), ornithine uptake occurred most efficiently in exchange for internal ornithine (100 percent), citrulline (82 percent), arginine (62 percent), lysine (50 percent), and γ-ornithine (32 percent). Ornithine uptake with all other *trans* substrates, including D-ornithine, was negligible (<15 percent) and the reconstituted transporter was inhibited by several sulfhydryl reagents.

Uptake of ornithine into mitochondria of nonhepatic cells may well involve different transporters. Passarella and colleagues reported evidence for an ornithine/phosphate antiporter in rat kidney mitochondria.[53] This observation is consistent with the notion that ornithine transport into mitochondria serves different purposes in different tissues; uptake into hepatic mitochondria primarily serves ureagenesis, while that into kidney and other nonhepatic mitochondria serves ornithine degradation and arginine biosynthesis.

Putrescine Biosynthesis

The physiological roles of putrescine and other polyamines are poorly understood, but, as polycations, they readily associate with nucleic acids and phospholipids. Their concentrations are tightly regulated and cellular proliferation and differentiation require polyamine biosynthesis.[54,55] Putrescine (diaminobutane) is synthesized from ornithine in an irreversible reaction catalyzed by the pyridoxal phosphate-dependent enzyme ornithine decarboxylase. Condensation of putrescine with propylamino moieties provided by decarboxy-*S*-adenosylmethionine forms the polyamines spermidine [$H_2N(CH_2)_4NH(CH_2)_3NH_2$] and spermine [$H_2N(CH_2)_3NH(CH_2)_4NH(CH_2)_3NH_2$].[54] Approximately 0.5 mM of spermidine is synthesized daily in normal adult humans.[56,57] The activities of ornithine decarboxylase and *S*-adenosylmethionine decarboxylase are thought to be the major regulatory factors in polyamine synthesis, rather than the availability of substrate,[54,55,58] although studies with 5-fluoromethylornithine (5FMOrn), an irreversible inhibitor of OAT, indicate that ornithine accumulation is associated with increased tissue levels of putrescine and urinary excretion of spermidine.[59,60] Ornithine decarboxylase activity is low in nondividing and high in rapidly proliferating cells (e.g., embryonic tissues, malignant tumors, and the stem cells of bone marrow and intestinal mucosa). A rapid and substantial ($>$ tenfold) increase in ornithine decarboxylase activity is one of the earliest events after resting cells are stimulated to proliferate and results in increased cellular levels of putrescine.[61,62] This increase in ornithine decarboxylase is due mainly to increased transcription.[62] Degradation of ornithine decarboxylase is rapid and nearly constant, with a half-life of 10 to 20 min.[54,63] A putrescine-induced 26.5-kDa protein called antizyme binds specifically to ornithine decarboxylase, stimulates an energy-dependent degradation of ornithine decarboxylase by the 26S proteasome and inhibits polyamine uptake.[54,64–66] The induction of antizyme by polyamines is independent of transcription and involves translational frameshifting (+1) producing a single, long, open reading frame from two shorter open reading frames that are 1 bp out of frame respective to each other.[64] Recent studies have identified a second antizyme (antizyme 2) that also requires translational frameshifting, inhibits polyamine uptake, and promotes ornithine decarboxylase degradation.[67,68]

A variety of specific inhibitors of ornithine decarboxylase have been used to investigate the regulation of polyamine biosynthesis, including the enzyme-activated, irreversible inhibitor DL-α-difluoromethylornithine.[69–72] This ornithine analogue does not inhibit OAT. Pharmacologic inhibition of ornithine decarboxylase results in reduced tissue polyamine levels and interferes with cell proliferation[69,73,74] and growth.[75]

Murine[76,77] and human[78] ornithine decarboxylase cDNAs have been cloned and sequenced and the organization and location of their structural genes determined.[79–81]

Putrescine is also a potential precursor of the inhibitory neurotransmitter GABA. The major source for GABA is decarboxylation of glutamic acid by glutamic acid decarboxylase.[82] However, two reaction sequences that convert putrescine to GABA have been described. One involves direct deamination by diamine oxidase (histaminase), while the other uses *N*-acetylated intermediates.[82] Thus, ornithine can serve as a precursor for GABA either by conversion to Δ^1 pyrroline-5-carboxylate (P5C) and glutamate or by decarboxylation to putrescine.[83] A significant fraction of retina GABA is derived from ornithine via putrescine in tissue,[84] and via cultured cells from embryonic chick retina.[85] By the time of hatching, however, glutamate is the major precursor of GABA.[84] In adult rat brain, ornithine may be converted to GABA in nerve terminals,[86] probably via P5C and glutamate rather than by putrescine.[83] Radioactive tracer studies with labeled ornithine and glutamate in mice suggest that the pathway for the formation of GABA from ornithine via putrescine is quantitatively minor in brain and of uncertain physiologic significance.[83] The degradation of GABA involves transamination by GABA transaminase to form succinate semialdehyde, which is further oxidized to succinate and eventually to CO_2. Thus, the conversion of putrescine to GABA provides a potential pathway for the oxidation of ornithine to CO_2 independent of OAT.

Creatine Synthesis

The first reaction in creatine synthesis, transfer of the amidino group of arginine to glycine to form guanidinoacetate and ornithine, is catalyzed by glycine transamidinase (Fig. 83-2 and Table 83-1).[87,88] Guanidinoacetate is *N*-methylated by *S*-adenosylmethionine:guanidinoacetate *N*-methyltransferase to form creatine. The transamidinase reaction is readily reversible *in vitro*, but low tissue levels of guanidinoacetate probably prevent significant reverse reaction *in vivo*.[87,89] In rats, supplementation of dietary creatine for 2 weeks reduces transamidinase activity and protein to about one-third pretreatment levels.[89,90] Immunoprecipitation of the products of *in vitro* translation reactions programmed with mRNA from these supplemented animals suggests that this decrease is due to reduced translational efficiency or reduced levels of transamidinase mRNA.[90] Ornithine is a potent competitive inhibitor of the transamidinase.[91–93]

Human and rat kidney transamidinases have been purified to homogeneity and characterized biochemically.[88,94] In humans and other mammals, both glycine transamidinase and the methyltransferase are present at high activity in renal cortex and pancreas.[87] Immunofluorescence studies in rat show prominent staining in the basilar portions of the proximal tubule cells, hepatocytes and the pancreatic islet α (glucagon-producing) cells.[95] Available data suggest that creatine is synthesized in these central organs, transported to muscle and nerve, and there phosphorylated to form creatine phosphate. The interesting possibility that other tissues, including brain, may be capable of creatine synthesis has been suggested and requires further study.[83,96,97]

Most of the total body creatine-creatine phosphate pool is located in muscle and it amounts to approximately 120 g (915 mM) in a 70-kg man. Both creatine and creatine phosphate undergo a first-order, nonenzymatic cyclization to creatinine at fractional rates of 0.011 per day and 0.026 per day, respectively.[87] Thus, in order to maintain the creatine-creatine phosphate pool, an amount of creatine equal to the amount of creatinine formed daily (approximately 2 g in an adult male) must be provided either from dietary sources or by endogenous synthesis. The relative contributions from these two sources are difficult to estimate, but studies of individuals on creatine-free diets indicate that endogenous synthesis can meet the entire requirement.[87] The relative magnitude of the synthetic pathway is indicated by the fact that creatine synthesis is quantitatively the major consumer of *S*-adenosylmethionine-donated methyl groups in the body.[57]

The OAT Pathway

OAT is a pyridoxal phosphate-requiring Ω-transaminase which catalyzes the reversible conversion of ornithine and α-ketoglutarate to P5C and glutamate (Fig. 83-1). Glutamate semialdehyde is the initial product formed by removal of the δ-amino group of ornithine; however, it cyclizes spontaneously to form P5C. Kinetic studies suggest that the cyclization is rapid and reversible.[98–100] Thus, in the subsequent discussions, we consider P5C as the reaction product, with the tacit recognition that it is in equilibrium with glutamate semialdehyde.

OAT Structure. OAT was first described in animal tissues by Quastel and Witty[101] and Meister[102] and has been purified to homogeneity from human liver,[103] rat liver,[98,104–108] and rat kidney.[109–111] The human enzyme is a homopolymer with a subunit molecular weight of 45 kDa. One molecule of cofactor pyridoxal phosphate per subunit binds to K292.[110,112,113] Although several early studies of both the human[103] and the rat[109,111] enzyme indicated that the holoenzyme was a tetramer, reinvestigation of the quaternary structure provided strong evidence that the mature enzyme is a 256-kDa homohexamer.[114] This conclusion was based on equilibrium sedimentation measurements, cross-linking experiments, and preliminary crystallographic analysis of rat liver enzyme. The native enzyme has a sedimentation coefficient ($S^\circ_{20,\omega}$) of 10 S and a frictional coefficient that is consistent with a nearly spherical structure.

Determination of the crystal structure of human OAT at a resolution of 2.5 Å confirmed these structural predictions.[115] The α_6-hexameric molecule is a trimer of three intimate dimers. Each OAT monomer contains 12 α-helices (I to XII) and 14 β-strands and can be organized into three regions: an N-terminal segment of an isolated helix and a three-stranded (A to C) antiparallel β-meander; a large central domain of eight helices and seven β-strands (a to g); and a C-terminal small domain of three helices and four β-strands (A^1 to D^1) (Fig. 83-3). The N-terminal segment is comprised of residues 38 to 79; the large domain of residues 95 to 343; and the small domain of residues 345 to 437. Loops of no standard structure connect these three regions. K292 with its covalently-linked PLP is in a loop connecting two β-strands (f and g) in the large domain.

The intimate and stable OAT dimer is held together by both hydrophobic and hydrophilic interactions that occur over approximately 5500 Å of solvent accessible surface area per monomer buried upon dimer formation. The extensive subunit contacts are between the large domains of the two monomers plus the N-terminal segment of one with the large domain of the other. These interactions are discussed extensively by Shen and colleagues.[115] The hexameric holoenzyme is formed by packing three OAT dimers in about one turn of a right-handed super helix that buries an additional 1870 $Å^2$ of subunit surface area. The structure of a second ω-aminotransferase, GABA transaminase was solved to 3.0 Å resolution by molecular replacement with the distantly related (17.4 percent amino acid identity) OAT.[116]

The Chemistry of OAT

The kinetic properties of human and rat OAT are similar, and the values for the former are provided in Table 83-1. Although this

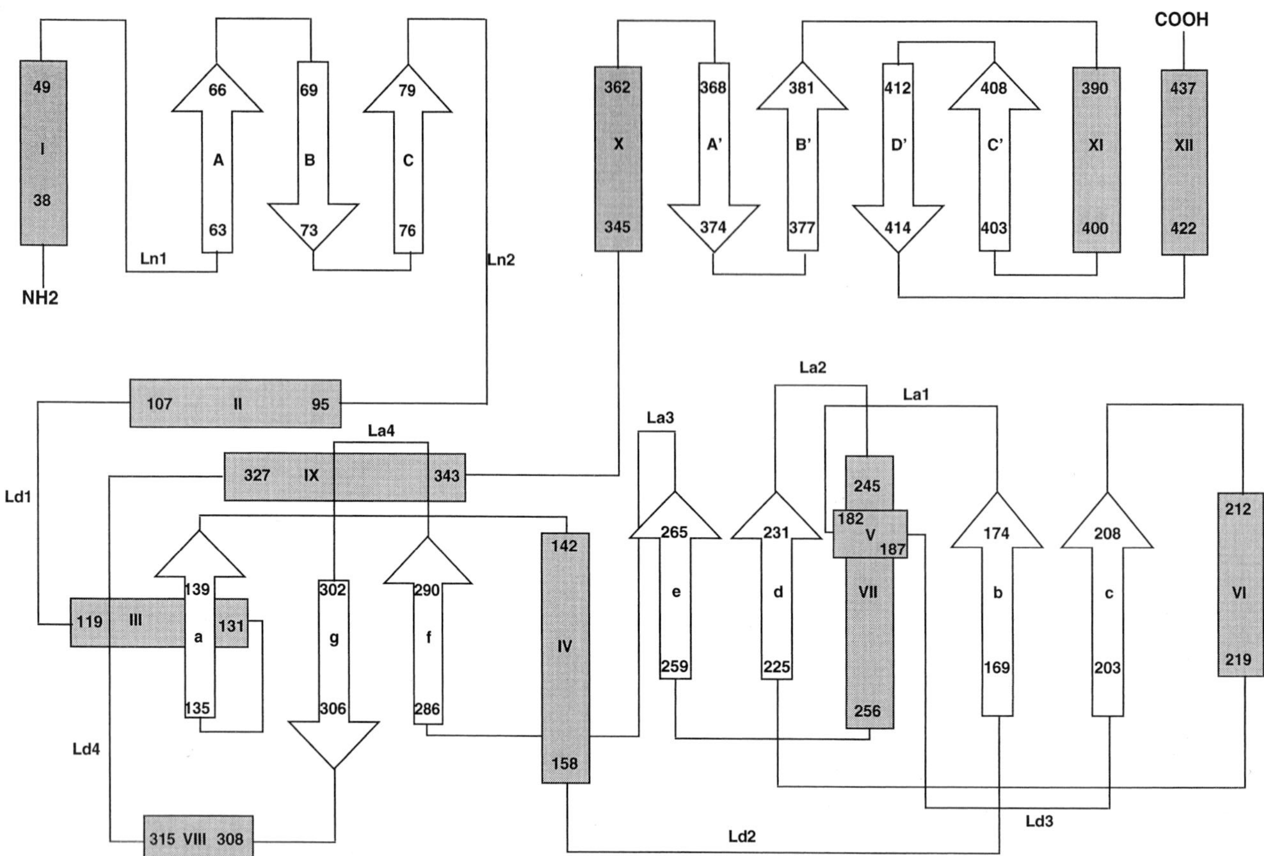

Fig. 83-3 Representation of the topography of OAT showing secondary structural elements. Only elements with more than two of the appropriate main-chain H-bonds are counted as α-helices (gray rectangles) or β-strands (arrows). The residue range of each secondary structure element is indicated. Ln1 and Ln2 = loops in the N-terminal segment; Ld1 to Ld4 = loops involved in dimer formation; La1 to La4 = loops contributing residues that line the active site.[115]

reaction is reversible,[117] the equilibrium constant favors the formation of P5C.[98] The complete reaction involves two half reactions:[112]

$$\text{Ornithine} + \text{pyridoxal} - \text{OAT} \rightarrow \text{P5C} + \text{pyridoxamine} - \text{OAT} \quad (83\text{-}1)$$

$$\text{Pyridoxamine-OAT} + \alpha\text{-ketoglutarate} \rightarrow \text{glutamate} + \text{pyridoxal-OAT} \quad (83\text{-}2)$$

The pH optimum of the overall reaction measured in the forward direction (pH 8.0 for the human enzyme) is a compromise between the more alkaline optimum of reaction (83-1) (approximately pH 9) and the more acidic optimum of reaction (83-2) (approximately pH 7). The optimum for the reverse reaction is pH 6.5.[99] The pyridoxamine enzyme is unstable and can spontaneously release its amino group, allowing the formation of P5C to exceed that of glutamate under certain conditions.[112] High concentrations of pyridoxal phosphate inhibit catalytic activity and increase the amount of bound cofactor to approximately four molecules per monomer.[112] The enzyme has high specificity for ornithine. Lysine, the one-carbon-longer homolog, has no effect on the reaction.[103] Glyoxylate and pyruvate are poor substitutes for α-ketoglutarate. High concentrations of ornithine (>25 mM) and particularly α-ketoglutarate (>3 mM) are inhibitory.[98] Other low-molecular-weight compounds that, at a concentration of 25 mM, inhibit activity of the rat enzyme by at least 40 percent in the presence of saturating ornithine concentrations include L-valine, α-ketoisovalerate, α-ketoisocaproate, GABA, and norvaline.[98,99] Additional nonspecific inhibitors include canaline, cycloserine, hydroxylamine and thiosemicarbazide.[105,118]

The search for specific inhibitors of OAT is complicated by the similarity of OAT and GABA transaminase-catalyzed reactions.[119,120] Both involve Ω-transamination of structurally related substrates. Thus, two supposedly specific, enzyme-activated, irreversible inhibitors ("suicide substrates") of GABA transaminase, 5-amino-1,3-cyclohexadienyl-carboxylic acid (gabaculine) and 4-aminohex-5-ynoic acid, also irreversibly inhibit OAT both *in vitro* and *in vivo* in mice.[121,122] The latter has been shown to bind to K292 (the pyridoxal phosphate binding residue) and to C388 of OAT.[123]

In contrast to the aforementioned compounds, 5-fluoromethylornithine (6-fluoro-2,5-diaminohexanoic acid, 5FMOrn) is a specific inhibitor of OAT.[121,124,125] 5FMOrn is an enzyme-activated irreversible inhibitor comprising a mixture of two diastereomers, each consisting of a pair of enantiomers, only one of which reacts with OAT (Fig. 83-4). With purified rat liver OAT, the K_i for 5FMOrn is 30 μM and the enzyme half-life at infinite inhibitor concentration is 4 min.[124] *In vivo* administration of 5FMOrn to mice (10 mg per kilogram body weight) resulted in ~90 percent inhibition of OAT, as compared to only 70 percent inhibition by canaline (500 mg of DL-canaline per kilogram, body weight).[124] Chronic intraperitoneal or oral administration of 5FMOrn causes an 80 to 90 percent reduction in OAT activity, ten- to twentyfold accumulation of ornithine in plasma and tissue fluid and increased synthesis of polyamines.[126,127] GABA levels are unaltered. 5FMOrn is well tolerated and has been given for as long as 53 days to mice; over this period, there was no detectable effect on the retina as measured by ophthalmoscopy, electroretinography, or histologic examination.[83,127] The accumulation of ornithine produced by 5FMOrn protects against acute intoxication with ammonium acetate[60] and against thioacetamide-induced hepatogenic encephalopathy.[128,129]

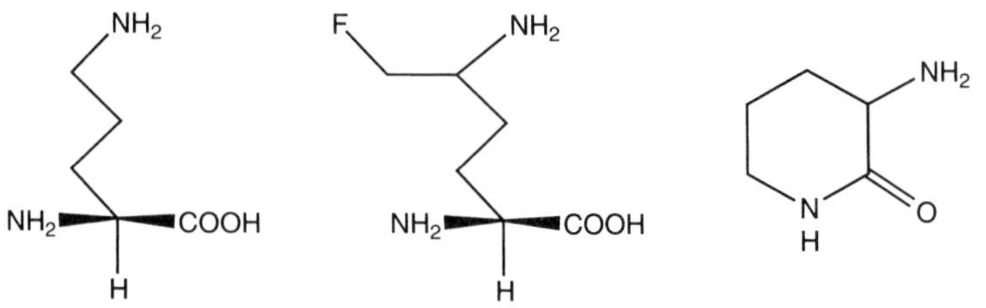

L-Ornithine 5-Fluoromethylornithine 3-Aminopiperid-2-one

Fig. 83-4 The chemical structure of L-ornithine, 5-fluoromethylornithine, an irreversible inhibitor of OAT, and 3-aminopiperid-2-one, the δ-lactam of L-ornithine found in the urine of patients with gyrate atrophy and the HHH syndrome.

OAT Assays. Three general methods of assaying OAT activity have been used.[98,130–132] One depends on the quantitative formation of a dihydroquinozolinium derivative when P5C is reacted with *o*-aminobenzaldehyde. This derivative is measured spectrophotometrically with an extinction coefficient variously reported as 2.71[98] and 2.59[100] at 441 nm. A caution in interpreting results obtained with this assay is that *o*-aminobenzaldehyde reacts with several Δ^1-pyrroline compounds, including Δ^1-pyrroline-2-carboxylate, the cyclized form of the α-keto acid of ornithine.[102,133] Thus, under certain conditions, some of the apparent product measured in this assay may not be P5C. A modification of this method using high performance liquid chromatography has increased sensitivity and specificity[134] and has been modified to measure OAT activity in peripheral lymphocytes.[135]

A second method of measuring OAT activity involves the use of radiolabeled ornithine and separation of this precursor from product P5C by ion-exchange chromatography.[130,132] This method can be adapted to either low or high substrate concentrations and has greater sensitivity and specificity than the spectrophotometric assay. The sensitivity of the assay is further enhanced by purifying commercially available, radiolabeled ornithine by ion-exchange chromatography before use. This step removes contaminants (e.g., GABA) that may be inhibitory to OAT.

A third OAT assay uses [1-^{14}C] α-ketoglutarate as the labeled substrate; glutamate decarboxylase to decarboxylate the product [1-^{14}C]glutamate; and $^{14}CO_2$ trapping to quantitate product formation.[131] This method has high sensitivity but requires dialysis of the tissue extracts before assaying to eliminate endogenous amino acids that would use α-ketoglutarate as an amino acceptor in transaminations not catalyzed by OAT.

Molecular Biology of OAT. OAT cDNAs have been isolated from libraries prepared from human liver,[136,137] human retinoblastoma (Y79) cells,[138] rat liver,[136,139,140] *Saccharomyces cerevisiae*,[141,142] and the mothbean, *Vigna aconitifolia*.[143] The human cDNA has a 1317-bp open reading frame and a 635-bp 3′ nontranslated region with a single AAUAAA poly(A) addition signal (Fig. 83-5). The lengths of the 5′ nontranslated sequence in the predominant transcripts in liver are 81 and 80 bp, depending on which transcriptional initiation site is used (see below).

The human and rat cDNAs have 84.3 percent nucleotide identity in their coding regions; both predict 439-amino-acid proteins that have 90.4 percent amino acid identity. The predicted molecular weight of the human OAT precursor is 48,534 daltons. Mueckler and Pitot noted weak homology of OAT residues 286 to 362 with the pyridoxal phosphate-binding region of aspartate aminotransferase and, on this basis, predicted that K292 is the cofactor-binding residue.[140] Subsequent direct analysis of chymotryptic and tryptic fragments of the rat enzyme by Simmaco et al.[113] and elucidation of OAT crystal structures[115] confirmed this prediction. Simmaco et al. also determined that cleavage of the mitochondrial signal peptide occurs between A25 and T26, releasing a mature OAT monomer of 414 amino acids with a molecular weight of 45,852 daltons (Fig. 83-6).

In *S. cerevisiae*[144] and certain other fungi,[145] OAT is cytoplasmic and accordingly lacks a mitochondrial signal peptide (Fig. 83-6). The 406 C-terminal residues of human OAT are 54.4

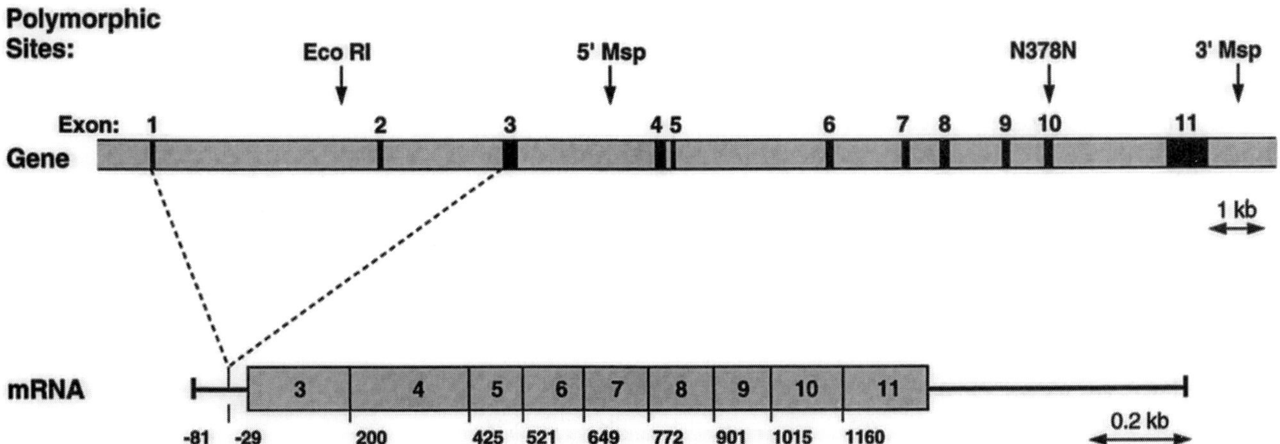

Fig. 83-5 The OAT structural gene and major mRNA transcript. The structural gene, with 11 exons, is shown above with the exons indicated as black rectangles. The positions of a polymorphic synonymous mutation, N378N, and polymorphic restriction sites are indicated above. The mRNA is below with the translated portion of the message designated by a shaded rectangle. The position of the first nucleotide in each exon, relative to the first nucleotide of the initiation codon, is indicated at the bottom. As depicted by the dashed lines, the second exon is spliced out of >98 percent of mature transcripts (see text). Note that when referring to the gene, by convention the first base in the primary transcript is +1 (see Fig. 83-7); when referring to the mRNA, the first base of the initiation methionine is +1.

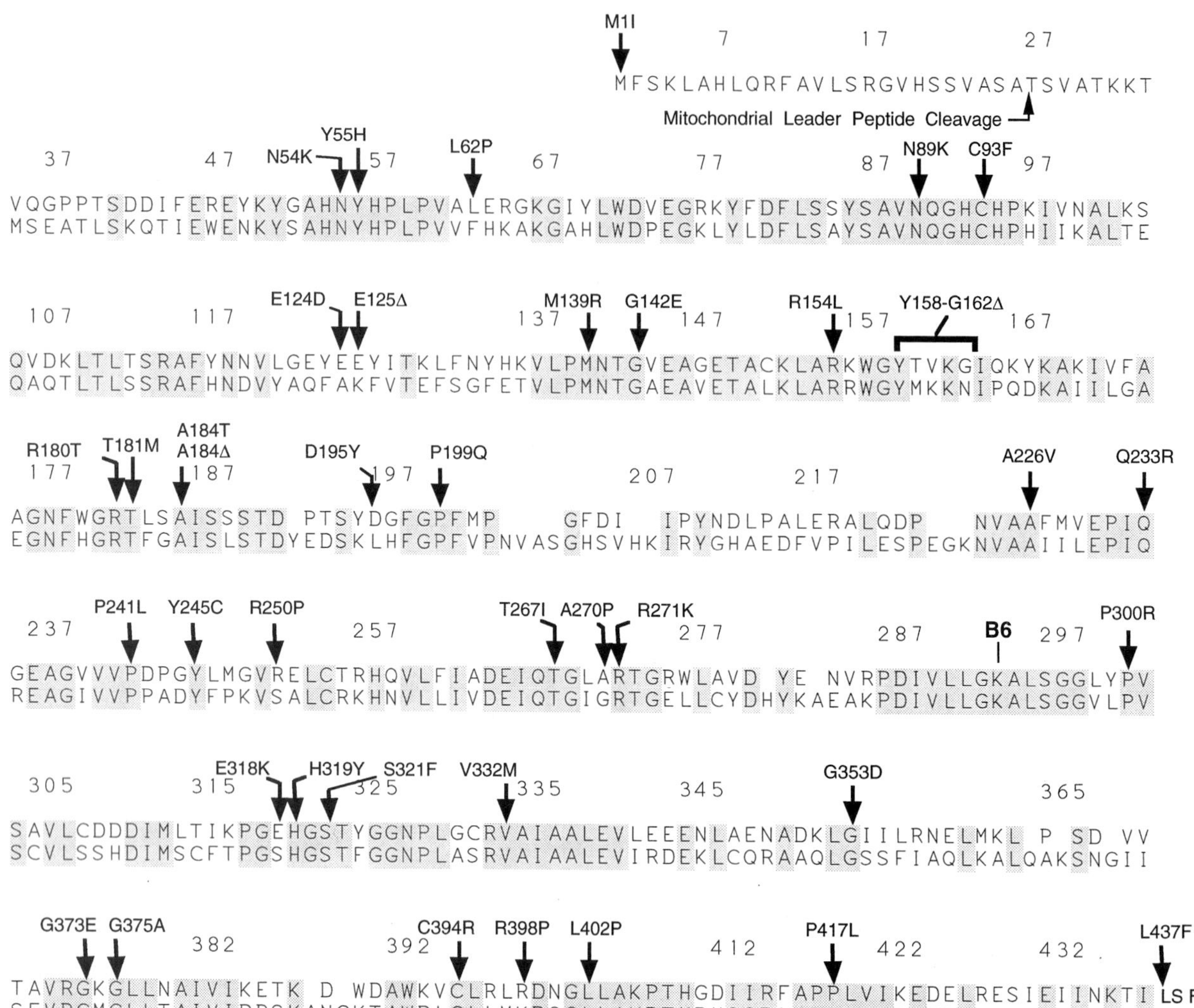

Fig. 83-6 Comparison of human and *Saccharomyces cerevisiae* OAT amino acid sequence. The 406 C-terminal residues of the human monomer (top sequence) are aligned with the yeast monomer (below). Gaps were introduced in the human sequence to maximize homology. The identities (shaded) are clustered in patches that are likely to correspond to structurally or functionally important domains of the protein. The yeast enzyme is cytoplasmic and, accordingly, has no sequence corresponding to the mitochondrial leader peptide of the human monomer. The positions of 34 missense mutations and 2 single-codon deletions (E125Δ, A184Δ) are shown by the arrows (see Table 83-5). The heavy bracket denotes a 5-codon deletion (Y158-G162Δ). B6 denotes the position of the pyridoxal phosphate-binding residue K292. Single-letter amino acid abbreviations include: A = alanine; C = cysteine; D = aspartic acid, E = glutamic acid; F = phenylalanine; G = glycine; H = histidine; I = isoleucine; K = lysine; L = leucine; M = methionine; N = asparagine; P = proline; Q = glutamine; R = arginine; S = serine; T = threonine; V = valine; W = tryptophan; Y = tyrosine.

percent identical with the *S. cerevisiae* sequence. The identities are not evenly distributed throughout the proteins but are clustered in patches of complete identity up to 13 residues in length, which presumably correspond to important structural or functional regions of the protein. The longest patch centers on the pyridoxal phosphate-binding residue, K292. Human OAT has been expressed in mutant *S. cerevisiae* lacking endogenous OAT.[146] The human enzyme is targeted to mitochondria, correctly processed, and highly active in yeast.

The human OAT structural gene has 11 exons that vary in length from 52 nucleotides (exon 1) to 793 nucleotides (exon 11) and are distributed over 21 kb of genomic DNA (Fig. 83-4).[147] Several restriction-fragment-length polymorphisms linked to the gene have been described,[147–149] and the exact positions relative to the gene structure are known for some of these sites.[147] The translational start site is in exon 3. The cofactor-binding K292 and the surrounding highly conserved 13 residues are encoded by exon 8. Primer extension studies indicate two transcriptional start sites separated by a single nucleotide and resulting in exon 1 lengths of either 52 or 51 bp.[147] Exon 2 (87 bp) is spliced out of >95 percent of the mature mRNA transcripts found in liver and was identified by homology with corresponding sequences contained in two X-linked, OAT-processed pseudogenes.[147,150] Because it is flanked by acceptable splice sites, the mechanism by which it is excluded from mature OAT mRNAs is not clear. A similar example of alternative splicing of an exon in the 5′ untranslated region with predominant expression of a transcript lacking the exon has been observed for argininosuccinate synthase.[151] Exon 2 is included in 5 to 10 percent of mature OAT mRNAs in cultured retinoblastoma cells, but these transcripts are not efficiently translated.[152–154]

The nucleotide sequence of 1.3 kb of 5′ flanking sequence of the OAT gene has been reported,[136,155] and contains elements characteristic of promoters of both housekeeping genes and genes whose expression is tissue-specific (Fig. 83-7).[155] There is a TATA box-like sequence, TTTAA, at −29 with respect to the 5′-most transcriptional initiation site and two CCAAT box-like sequences, one at −73 and a second, inverted sequence, ATTGG, at −98. The region is GC-rich (68.6 percent) with three consensus transcription factor Sp1 core sequence binding sites.[156] Other

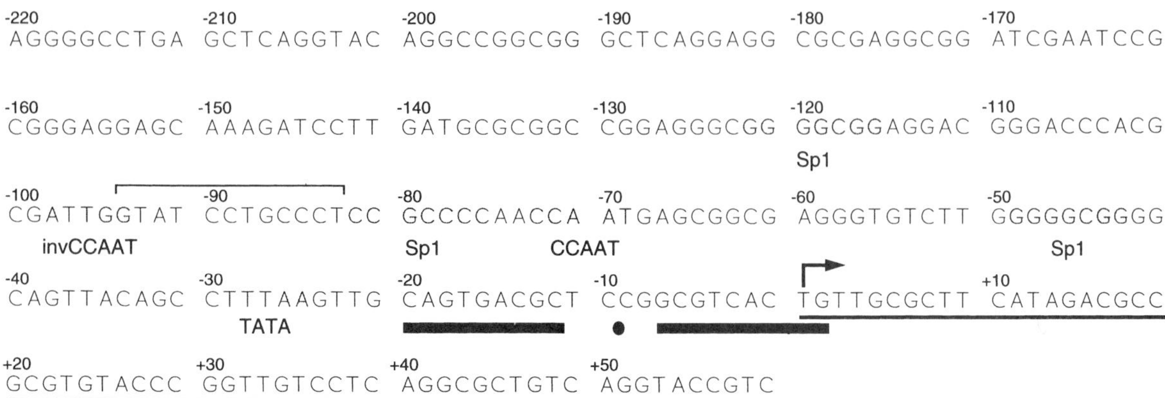

Fig. 83-7 Nucleotide sequence of exon 1 and the proximal 5′ flanking region of the human OAT gene. Exon 1, which encodes 5′ untranslated sequence, is indicated by the underline, and the most distal transcriptional start site (+1) designated by the right angle arrow. Regions of nucleotide sequence similar to known promoter elements are shaded and labeled. A 22-bp element of uncertain function with incomplete dyad symmetry at −20 is indicated by the dark underbar with the black dot denoting the center of the element. The bracket over −94 to −83 designates a sequence motif found repeatedly in the promoter of OAT and other urea cycle-related genes. invCCAAT = inverted CCAAT box.

sequences in this region of note include a region starting at −94 (5′ GTATCCTGCCCT 3′) with 10 of 12 nucleotides identical (underlined) to a consensus sequence (5′ GCANCCTGCCCT 3′) present in three urea-cycle enzymes whose 5′ regions have been characterized.[40,155] In addition, there is a 22-bp element with incomplete dyad symmetry extending from −20 to +2. Incomplete dyad symmetry is a common feature of many DNA sites that bind regulatory proteins.[157] This element also has some homology with the estrogen-responsive element of the *Xenopus vitellogenin* A2 gene.[158] Because of the close relationship of the estrogen- and glucocorticoid-responsive elements,[159] it is possible that this dyad element may play a role in either the estrogen induction of OAT in kidney or the glucocorticoid repression of glucagon-mediated OAT induction in liver (see "Regulation of OAT Activity" below).

The promoter function of the 1.3 kb of DNA flanking the 5′ end of exon 1 was examined directly using hybrid promoter/reporter gene constructs transfected into cultured liver and kidney cells.[155] Maximal expression was obtained with just 134 bp of the 5′ flanking sequence; more than 30 percent expression was obtained with constructs containing as little as 85 bp of the promoter (from −1 to −85 bp) or as much as the entire 1.3 kb. Modest (two- to fivefold) increases in expression of the −85 and −134 bp constructs were obtained by treating the cells with dibutyryl cAMP, suggesting that at least part of the information required to respond to cAMP is contained in this region of the promoter. DNase I protection experiments defined regions of protein binding in this portion of the promoter, but the responsible proteins have not been identified.

Chromosomal Localization of OAT and Related Sequences. Southern blots of human genomic DNA probed with the OAT cDNA show a complex pattern (Fig. 83-8). Several studies, including analyses of genomic DNA from rodent-human hybrid cell panels and *in situ* hybridization of human chromosome spreads, have shown that these hybridizing fragments are located in two sites: one at 10q26 that corresponds to the active structural gene, and a second at Xp11.2-p11.3 that contains multiple, apparently nonfunctional, OAT-related sequences.[147,160–163] The number of X-linked hybridizing fragments depends on the restriction enzyme but usually is two to three times the number of autosomal fragments. These OAT-related sequences are designated OATL for OAT-like. High-resolution physical mapping studies show that the X-linked OATL sequences map to two distinct intervals on Xp separated by 1 to 2 Mb: OATL1 is more telomeric (Xp11.3-p11.23); OATL2 is more centromeric (Xp11.22-Xp11.21).[163] Both OATL1 and OATL2 contain multiple copies of OAT processed pseudogenes that have undergone a variety of deletions and insertions.[150,164,165] None appears to be functional. Interestingly, the genes for several inherited retinal degenerations map near OATL1 and translocation breakpoint studies indicate that genes involved in two malignancies, synovial sarcoma and papillary renal cell carcinoma, are located in OATL1 and OATL2, respectively.[166,167] For this reason, a yeast artificial chromosome (YAC) contig has been assembled covering OATL1,[168] and YACs spanning the breakpoints for both of the malignancies have been identified.[166,167] cDNAs for several functional genes in the OATL1 contig have been isolated,[168] including one that encodes a member of the trithorax gene family.[169] Other genes in this family have been implicated in acute leukemias.[169–172] To date, however, none of the genes in the OATL1 contig has been shown to be directly involved in any of these disorders.

One additional member of the OAT gene family, a nonprocessed pseudogene designated OATL3, has been described.[162] This sequence corresponds to OAT exon 3 and its flanking intronic sequence and is localized near the functional OAT structural gene at 10q26. In this location, OATL3 could contribute to mutations of the OAT structural gene through recombination or gene conversion (see Chap. 12) but, at present, there is no evidence for such events.[162]

Tissue Distribution and Activity of OAT. OAT activity is high in adult rat kidney, liver, and small intestine.[104,173–175] The activity in neonatal small intestinal mucosa is particularly high in rat, mouse,[176,177] and pig.[178–180] The kidneys of animals exposed to estrogen (either normal females or gonadectomized males treated with estrogen) also have high activity,[173] with lower levels in pancreas, submaxillary gland, heart, brain, spleen, adrenal, lung, mammary gland, cartilage, and skeletal muscle.[42,173,175,181,182] The relative activities in several regions of the brain have been reported.[183] Similar surveys of OAT activity in various human tissues are not available.

Interestingly, the distribution of OAT activity in the liver is not uniform; in rat, mouse, and human liver, OAT is present in a thin rim of hepatocytes surrounding the central vein (Fig. 83-9).[20,184,185] Glutamine synthetase is present in the same population of hepatocytes,[186,187] while ornithine transcarbamylase and the other enzymes of the urea cycle are expressed in the periportal hepatocytes.[188–190] Thus, although OAT and ornithine transcarbamylase are coordinately and directly regulated in response to perturbations in dietary protein (see below), their positional expression in the hepatic lobule is inversely related.

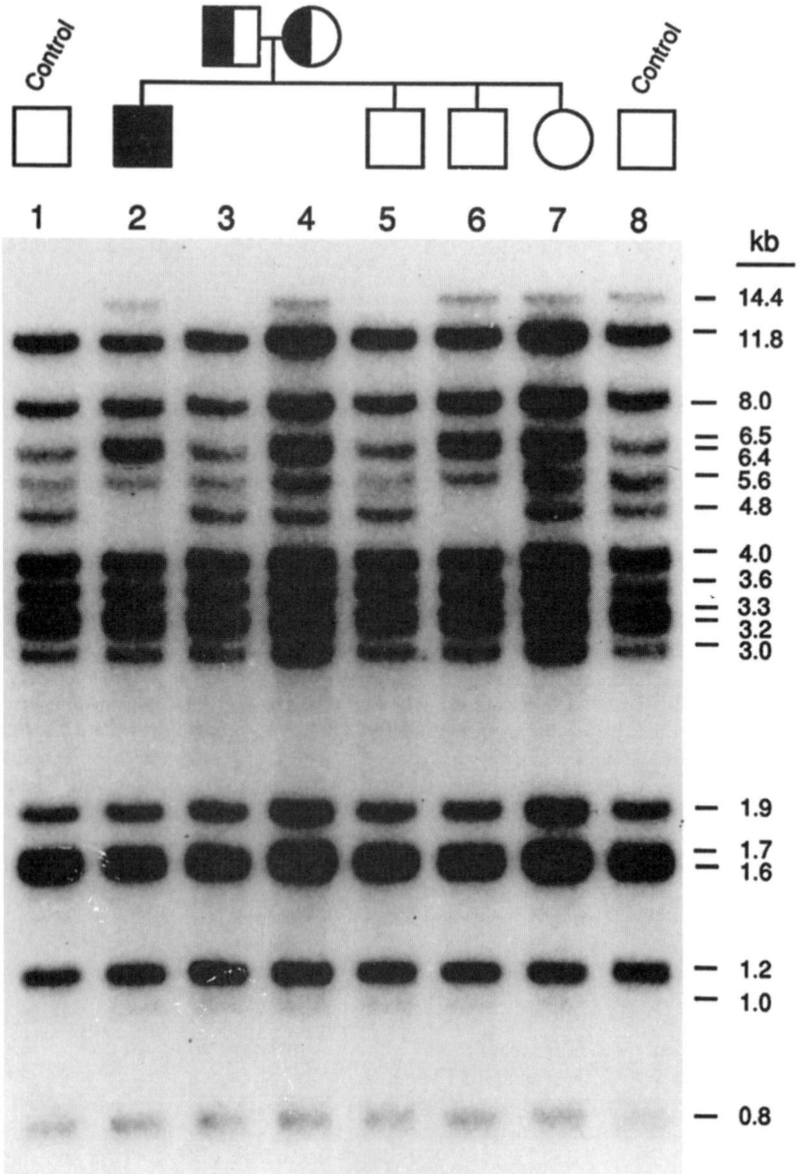

Fig. 83-8 The complicated genomic Southern blot pattern of OAT. Genomic DNA from a patient with gyrate atrophy (lane 2), his family members, and controls was digested with Pst I. The blot was hybridized to a near full-length OAT cDNA containing 15 bp of exon 1 and all of exons 3 to 11 and was washed at high stringency. The sizes of the hybridizing fragments are indicated on the right. The X-linked OAT hybridizing fragments are indicated by an asterisk following their size. These fragments are more intense in females. The remaining are from the functional OAT gene on chromosome 10. The family is segregating an X-linked, 4.8-kb/6.5-kb Pst I polymorphism which is unrelated to gyrate atrophy.

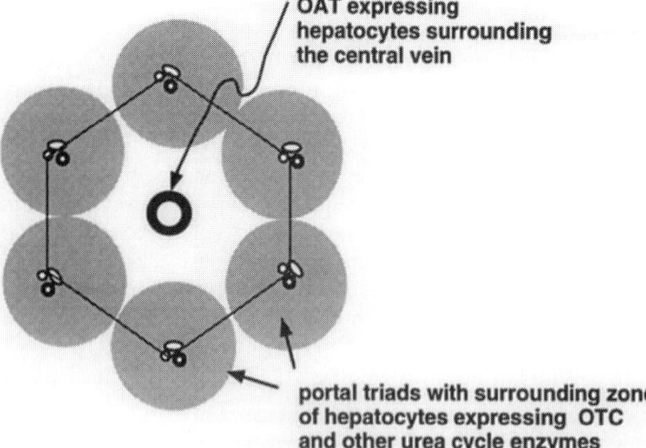

Fig. 83-9 Diagram of a hepatic lobule with a central vein surrounded by six portal triads, each containing a branch of the hepatic artery, portal vein, and bile duct. The gray-shaded zone around the triads designates the periportal hepatocytes expressing OTC and other urea-cycle enzymes. The black ring around the central vein designates the pericentral vein hepatocytes expressing OAT and glutamine synthetase.

This zonation of expression in the hepatic lobule occurs for other enzymes and is critical for establishing metabolic pathways.[188,191,192] The pattern of OAT expression in the hepatic lobule is maintained even when OAT activity is dramatically induced by increasing dietary protein.[185] Cell-cell interactions between hepatocytes and the endothelial cells of the central vein seem to play a role in establishing the high level of expression of OAT in the pericentral vein hepatocytes;[184,191–193] however, the molecular basis for this phenomenon remains to be determined. Regardless of how it is established, the pattern of OAT expression in liver has considerable effects on ornithine metabolism. In particular, OAT and ornithine transcarbamylase do not compete for ornithine in the mitochondrial matrix for the simple reason that they are expressed in different populations of hepatocytes (see "Regulation of OAT Activity" below).

OAT activity has been measured in the ocular tissues of a variety of species, including humans. Ratzlaff and Baich compared OAT activity in retinal pigment epithelium, neural retina, and liver of several vertebrates and found that in mammals and birds, the activity in pigment epithelium was 3 to 10 times higher than in neural retina or liver, while in amphibians and fish it was similar in all three tissues.[194,195] Several other studies have shown high levels of OAT activity in pigment epithelium, neural retina, ciliary body, and iris in a variety of mammals.[196–200] Immunohistochemical studies of rat ocular tissues have confirmed the presence of OAT in the epithelia of ciliary body, iris, and lens, and showed prominent immunoreactivity in pigment epithelium and Müller cells of the retina, but none in the photoreceptor cells.[201,202]

Regulation of OAT Activity. In addition to the regulation described above, OAT activity varies greatly with changes in the developmental, nutritional, and hormonal status of the organism. In rat liver and kidney, OAT activity is barely detectable prenatally or during the first two postnatal weeks, but by 30 days it has increased approximately 15-fold to adult levels.[173,203] In rat small intestine, OAT activity is 2 to 5 times higher in the first 3 weeks of life than in adult intestine or liver,[174] while, in mouse, the activity in neonatal intestine is 10 to 20 times higher than in adult liver or intestine.[176,177,204]

After the first few weeks of life, liver OAT activity in rat is markedly influenced by dietary protein, as is the case for all the enzymes directly involved in the urea cycle.[4,6,37] An increase in dietary protein from 20 to 70 percent by weight increased OAT-specific activity within 1 day, and, by 4 days, a peak activity six times higher than baseline levels was achieved. Concomitant high glucose intake prevents this induction.[108,205] Reduction of dietary protein to 5 percent causes a twofold reduction in OAT activity. Renal and small-intestinal OAT activities are not influenced by changes in dietary protein intake.[108] The increase in hepatic OAT associated with increased dietary protein may be mediated, at least in part, by glucagon, working through a cAMP-dependent mechanism. OAT activity in liver or in primary cultures of hepatocytes increases in response to glucagon[206,207] or dibutyryl cAMP.[155,208,209]

Administration of estrogen to gonadectomized rats increases renal OAT activity tenfold.[207,210–212] Thyroid hormone is necessary for, and augments, the renal estrogen response.[207] Hepatic OAT is insensitive to either estrogen or thyroid hormone. In contrast to the different responses of renal and hepatic OAT to these dietary and hormonal changes, the activity in both tissues is moderately to severely reduced in rats following subcutaneous implantation of hepatic or mammary tumors.[213]

The perturbations of OAT activity by nutritional and hormonal factors are due to quantitative changes in the amount of enzyme, which results from increased synthesis rather than decreased degradation.[117,207–209,214,215] Induction in liver results from a two- to fivefold increase in OAT mRNA and a 20-fold increase in the translational efficiency of the OAT message.[215] The induction of renal OAT by estrogen is completely accounted for by an increase in OAT mRNA.[215] The response is rapid, beginning in the first hour after estrogen administration and reaching maximal mRNA levels by 20 h.[215] Thyroid hormone also increases renal OAT mRNA levels, but more slowly.[215] Estrogen and thyroid hormone also increase OAT synthesis in retinoblastoma cells by increasing, respectively, translation and transcription.[154]

The turnover of both hepatic and renal OAT has been measured; its half-life is 0.9 to 1.9 days in liver and 4.0 days in kidney.[216,217]

Metabolic Roles of the OAT Pathway. The bridging position of the OAT reaction between the urea cycle, proline metabolism, and the tricarboxylic acid cycle results in its involvement in several different metabolic processes.[117]

Ornithine and Arginine Catabolism. The relationships that predict arginine and ornithine catabolism are shown in Fig. 83-10. In molar units, the amount of arginine catabolized to P5C (Arg_C) daily equals the amount of arginine in the diet (Arg_D) minus the sum of the arginine requirement for protein accretion (Arg_{Pro}), the ornithine requirement for polyamine synthesis (Orn_{Poly}), and the obligatory losses in urine, stool, and exfoliated skin cells of arginine (Arg_L) and ornithine (Orn_L). That is,

$$Arg_c = Arg_D - (Arg_{Pro} + Orn_{Poly} + Arg_L + Orn_L) \qquad (83\text{-}3)$$

In healthy adults who are in nitrogen balance, there is no net increase in body protein, and the amount of arginine required for protein accretion approaches zero. In contrast, both growing children and adults recovering from an episode of negative nitrogen balance will use significant arginine for Arg_{Pro}. Orn_{Poly} has not been measured directly but is estimated to be small (less than 0.5 mM/day in an adult).[56] Normally, Orn_L and Arg_L are negligible, but they become significant in patients with ornithine accumulation and overflow ornithinuria. In a healthy adult, Arg_C by way of the OAT pathway is nearly equal to Arg_D. If dietary protein equals 1.5 g protein/kg body weight/day, and if the arginine content of protein approximately equals 5 percent, then the daily OAT flux equals ~0.4 mM/kg or 28 mM in a 70-kg man.

Proline Synthesis. P5C, the immediate precursor of proline, can be synthesized either from glutamate in a reaction catalyzed by P5C synthase or from ornithine in the reaction catalyzed by OAT (Fig. 83-2). The regulation of the relative contributions of these reactions is of interest but is not well understood. Physiological concentrations of ornithine inhibit P5C synthase; thus, high ornithine concentrations should favor the OAT-mediated pathway of proline synthesis.[218] In certain cells and tissues, this pathway seems to be the preferred or only pathway of proline synthesis. For example, in hormonally stimulated rat mammary gland, arginase, OAT, and P5C reductase activities increase coordinately in response to hormonal stimulation, and arginine (via ornithine) is a major biosynthetic precursor for the proline used in milk protein synthesis.[44,181] The proline auxotrophy of Chinese hamster ovary cells is due to a deficiency of both P5C synthase and OAT.[219] Prototrophic revertants with either OAT or P5C synthase activity grow normally. Finally, the work of Ertel and Isseroff suggests that the OAT pathway is the major contributor to the tremendous proline biosynthetic capacity of the liver fluke, *Fasciola hepatica*.[220] To reiterate, in some cells and tissues the OAT-mediated pathway plays the major role in proline synthesis, although its relative contribution in most tissues that have both proline biosynthetic pathways intact and have normal substrate concentrations is still not known.

Ornithine and Arginine Synthesis. As indicated above, the flow of substrates in the OAT pathway in most tissues and physiological

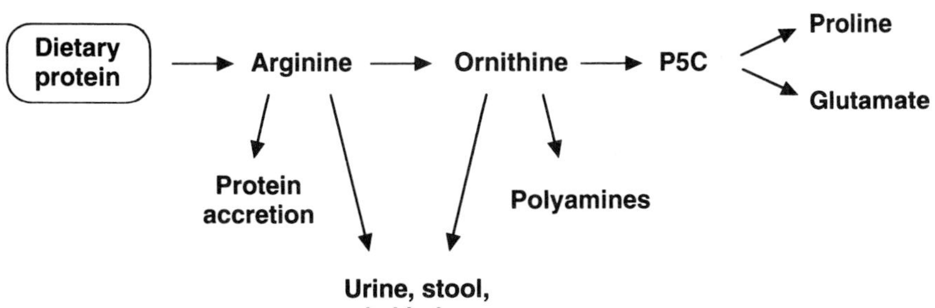

Fig. 83-10 The metabolic fates of ingested arginine.

states is toward P5C ("forward" OAT flux). The OAT reaction is reversible, however, and is an essential step in the only known pathway of *de novo* ornithine and, hence, citrulline and arginine synthesis in mammalian cells.[117,179,180] An alternative pathway of ornithine synthesis involving *N*-acetylated intermediates is present in microorganisms but has not been found in mammalian tissues.[133,221] Synthesis of ornithine from glutamate or proline has been shown to occur in mammalian tissues, particularly small intestinal mucosa,[99,102,133,222–224] and in cultured cells.[225] This *de novo* synthesis of ornithine provides a mechanism for replenishment of urea cycle intermediates and, if the urea cycle is intact, for the synthesis of arginine. Thus, when dietary arginine is insufficient to meet the requirements for protein synthesis, "reverse" OAT flux assumes major importance. This capability probably explains why arginine appears to be nonessential in full-term human infants[226] and adults[21] and why some patients with argininosuccinic acid lyase deficiency excrete more argininosuccinate than can be accounted for by arginine intake.[227,228]

The factors that favor reverse OAT flux are incompletely understood. Variation in tissue expression of ornithine-metabolizing enzymes certainly plays a role (see below), as do tissue and subcellular differences in the concentrations of the reactants.[117] Matsuzawa showed that the reverse reaction has a much lower pH optimum than the forward reaction and that it may be limited by a very low affinity for glutamate.[106] In some animals (e.g., rat, cat), arginine is essential, and failure to provide it results in growth failure, orotic aciduria, and hyperammonemia.[229,230] These animals have OAT activity, although the levels are low in cat liver and gut.[231] Thus, the presence of OAT is a necessary but not sufficient requirement for arginine synthesis.

Tissue-Specific Patterns of Ornithine Metabolism. How are the various metabolic processes described above, many of which require fluxes in opposite directions along the same pathways, choreographed? One strategy is to express the relevant enzymes in such a way that different cells or tissues contain only the components necessary for one of the metabolic pathways (Fig. 83-11). For example, only small intestine has all the enzymatic components necessary for the *de novo* synthesis of citrulline and arginine from glutamine. Expression of P5C synthetase is limited to gut; there are adequate amounts of OAT, carbamyl phosphate synthetase, *N*-acetylglutamate synthetase, and ornithine transcarbamylase; and there is virtually no arginase, so that arginine is the terminal product[117,176,178,223,232–235] Thus, an important metabolic function of small intestine is to produce arginine and its precursor citrulline. Citrulline is not taken up by hepatocytes and is converted to arginine in peripheral tissues, most notably the kidney.[236] Even in the small intestinal mucosa there are regional differences in the pattern of enzyme expression. Careful *in situ* hybridization and immunohistochemical studies in perinatal rat intestine show that there is a spatial distribution of the respective mRNAs and proteins along the villus axis. The basal enterocytes are equipped to synthesize citrulline from glutamate and proline while enterocytes in the upper half of the villus are equipped to synthesize arginine.[237]

Conversely, in the periportal hepatocytes the pattern of expression of the enzymes of ornithine metabolism is appropriate for efficient functioning of the urea cycle. All the enzymes of the urea cycle are expressed, while OAT is not expressed and so does not compete with ornithine transcarbamylase for potentially limiting amounts of ornithine in the mitochondrial matrix.[20] Arginase is present at high levels, ensuring that virtually all the arginine formed will be converted to ornithine and urea, making the pathway a true cycle.

In pericentral vein hepatocytes, OAT and glutamine synthetase are expressed without ornithine transcarbamylase or carbamyl phosphate synthetase. The affinity of glutamine synthetase for ammonium is about 10 times higher than that of carbamyl phosphate synthetase.[192] Thus, this system provides a high-affinity, low-capacity system to scavenge ammonium

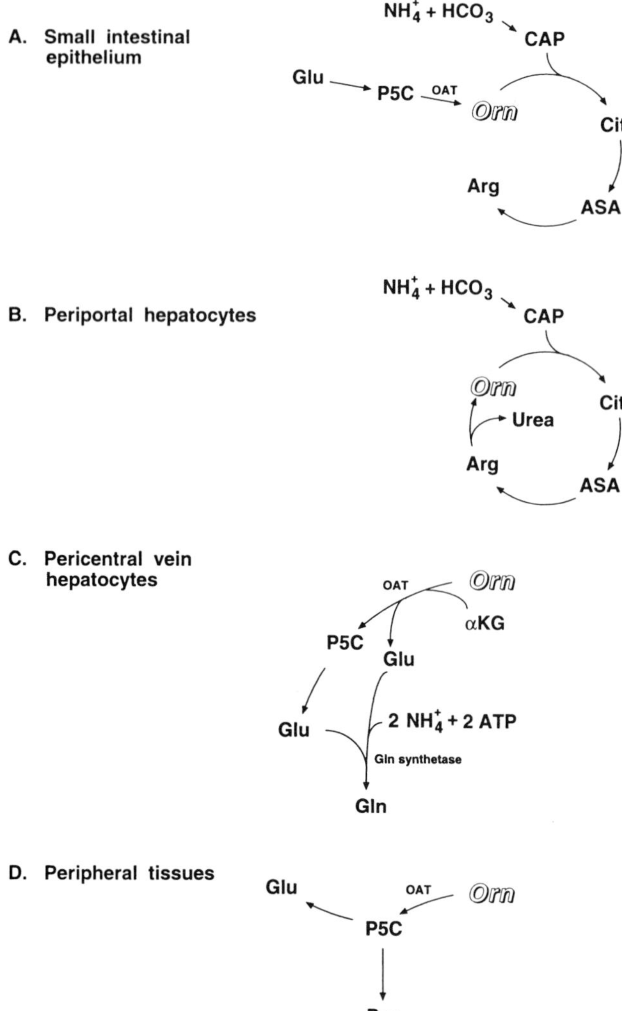

Fig. 83-11 Ornithine metabolic pathways in specified cells and tissues. The arrows indicate enzymatic reactions expressed in the indicated tissues and the usual direction of metabolic flux. The OAT and glutamine synthetase reactions are labeled for reference. (See Fig. 83-2 for names of the other enzymes.)

(Fig. 83-11). In the intact hepatic lobule, therefore, two ammonium detoxifying systems—the urea cycle and the OAT/glutamine synthetase system—are expressed sequentially along the path of blood flow: Portal blood is exposed first to hepatocytes with the high-capacity, low-affinity urea cycle and, just before efflux from the liver, to the high-affinity, low-capacity OAT/glutamine synthetase system. One salutary effect of this sequential arrangement is to maintain a low concentration of the toxic metabolite ammonium in blood leaving the liver.[20,192]

Finally, in many peripheral cells and tissues, as represented by fibroblasts, the pattern of expression of these enzymes favors the provision of amino acids for protein synthesis. Ornithine transcarbamylase, carbamyl phosphate synthetase, and arginase are not expressed; arginine is used for protein synthesis and as a precursor of NO. Expression of OAT, P5C synthase, and P5C reductase allow proline to be synthesized from either ornithine or glutamate.

DIFFERENTIAL DIAGNOSIS OF HYPERORNITHINEMIA

In normal individuals, fasting morning plasma ornithine concentrations range from 40 to 120 μM, with a mean of 60 to 80 μM. Two distinct entities are associated with significant increases in plasma ornithine concentration: gyrate atrophy of the choroid and retina, and the HHH syndrome. In patients with gyrate atrophy, visual symptoms are present by late childhood and after the first few months of life, plasma ornithine concentrations range from 400 to 1300 μM. Plasma ammonium is not elevated. In the HHH syndrome, the plasma ornithine ranges from 200 to 1100 μM and usually is lower than in gyrate atrophy. Plasma ammonium and glutamine concentrations are increased, particularly after ingestion of a protein load. Urinary excretion of ornithine and its δ-lactam (Fig. 83-4) is increased in both types of hyperornithinemia, while homocitrulline, an amino acid usually not present in urine, is found only in the HHH syndrome. Urinary excretion of orotic acid also is increased in HHH individuals.

Because only a few gyrate atrophy and HHH patients have been studied in the neonatal period, the age of onset of hyperornithinemia is not known for either. Plasma ornithine values may be normal or even subnormal in these neonates. Neonatal mice with complete deficiency of OAT caused by gene targeting (see "A Mouse Models of Gyrate Atrophy" below) have profound hypoornithinemia, hypocitrullinemia, hypoargininemia, and hyperammonemia due to the disruption of the arginine biosynthetic pathway.[177] This inability to synthesize ornithine and arginine from glutamate results from lack of "reverse" OAT function (Fig. 83-11*A*) and is fatal if the animals are not supplemented with intraperitoneal injections of arginine for the first 14 days of life. As predicted by these observations in the mouse model, one full-term infant with gyrate atrophy ingesting a mix of breast milk and standard infant formula had hypoornithinemia, hypoargininemia, and mild hyperammonemia for the first few months of life.[177] Recent preliminary reports of premature infants with gyrate atrophy with hypoornithinemia, hypoargininemia, orotic aciduria, and profound hyperammonemia indicate that neonatal metabolic phenotype similar to murine OAT deficiency occurs in low-birth-weight infants with gyrate atrophy.[238–240] Frequently these infants have been misdiagnosed as OTC deficiency or HHH syndrome. Assay of fibroblast OAT activity is indicated in infants with phenotype. Similarly, little is known about the neonatal phenotype of HHH although a few well-documented patients have had low ornithine levels in the newborn period.[241] Thus, a normal ornithine value in the neonatal period does not exclude either gyrate atrophy or the HHH syndrome.

Moderate hyperornithinemia (about three times normal) also was present in two siblings reported by Bickel et al.[242] At ages 7 and 3 years, this sister and brother had mental retardation, renal tubular dysfunction, abnormal liver function test results, and a 60 to 80 percent reduction in hepatic OAT activity, possibly because of an unexplained liver disease. At ages 15 and 9, they were severely retarded. The girl was deaf and had petit mal epilepsy. Both had normal ocular exams, normal plasma ornithine, normal liver function test results, generalized aminoaciduria, polyuria, isosthenuria, elevated serum creatinine, and hypertension. The etiology of this syndrome remains unknown.[243]

Nongenetic causes of modestly increased plasma ornithine concentrations include isoniazid therapy.[244] Spurious elevations can occur if the blood sample remains at room temperature for a prolonged period (15 min or more), owing to conversion of arginine to ornithine by erythrocyte arginase.

Most urinary amino acid screening systems yield a similar pattern of results for a group of disorders including the hyperornithinemias, cystinurias, lysinuric protein intolerance, other hyperdibasic aminoacidurias, hyperlysinemias, and, possibly, argininemia. The δ-lactam of ornithine (Fig. 83-4), which causes a faint brownish spot with ninhydrin, helps to differentiate the hyperornithinemias from other causes of dibasic aminoaciduria, although plasma amino acids have to be measured quantitatively to confirm the diagnosis.

A microfluorometric ornithine assay using two coupling enzymes (OAT and P5C reductase) has been described.[245] It can be used to measure the ornithine in a 3-mm blood-soaked filter paper and potentially is suitable for mass population screening for hyperornithinemia. Additional study of its sensitivity and reliability is necessary.

GYRATE ATROPHY OF THE CHOROID AND RETINA

Historical Note

The first description of a patient with gyrate atrophy of the choroid and retina, as defined by the characteristic appearance of the ocular fundus and a typical history of visual deterioration, was probably that of Jacobsohn in 1888.[246] His report of a case of "atypical retinitis pigmentosa" includes a striking, hand-drawn view of the fundus showing the characteristic lesions of gyrate atrophy. Cutler in 1895,[247] and Fuchs in 1896,[248] were the first ophthalmologists to recognize this condition as a distinct entity. Fuchs gave the disorder its euphonious appellation. Usher reviewed 26 cases in 1935, emphasizing the genetic aspects.[249] Several additional clinical reviews have been published.[250–254] Hyperornithinemia and ornithinuria were not recognized as the biochemical counterparts of this disorder until the report of Simell and Takki in 1973, 85 years after the initial ophthalmologic description.[255] Ironically, an earlier spark of insight into the nature of this disorder, the observation in 1960 of an abnormally large lysine-ornithine spot in the urine of a patient with gyrate atrophy, did not succeed in lighting the fires of scientific investigation.[250,251]

The Clinical Phenotype

There are about 150 biochemically confirmed cases of gyrate atrophy reported or known to us.[253–282] The major clinical problem in these patients is a slowly progressive loss of vision leading to blindness, usually by the fifth decade of life.[259,261,276–278] Myopia and decreased night vision are early symptoms, usually noted before the end of the first decade.[283] Reduced peripheral vision with constriction of the visual fields is obvious in the second decade. Virtually all patients develop posterior subcapsular cataracts late in the second decade or early in the third.[284] The combination of the cataracts and constricted visual fields may result in severe impairment during the third decade. By the fourth to fifth decades, most patients are blind. Variability in the severity of the clinical phenotype is well documented, with a few patients retaining good visual function into their sixth or seventh decade, while others experience more rapid deterioration with nearly complete loss of vision by age 20.

The changes in the ocular fundus parallel the development of the visual symptoms (Fig. 83-12). The ophthalmologic features of the childhood cases have been reviewed.[283] Younger patients often come to the attention of the ophthalmologist in late childhood, or around the time of puberty, for evaluation of myopia or decreased night vision. At this age, sharply demarcated, circular areas of chorioretinal degeneration are present in the midperiphery of the ocular fundus. There may be increased pigmentation around the margins of these lesions. When observed over time, the lesions can be seen to start as punctuate yellowish "dots" that gradually enlarge to the more typically circular areas one to two disk diameters in size.[261] In a few young patients, a diffuse depigmentation of the pigment epithelium in the mid to far periphery occurs before the development of the classic circular lesions (Fig. 83-12*A*).[283] At around the time of puberty, the retinal degeneration seems to accelerate.[261,278] The lesions enlarge, coalesce, and extend toward the posterior pole of the fundus (Fig. 83-12*B*). The margins of the lesions remain discrete and often are densely pigmented. The few choroidal vessels transversing the atrophic areas are narrowed. In some patients, additional foci of atrophy develop in the peripapillary area (Fig. 83-12*C*). By the third decade, much of the fundus is involved. Increased pigmentation is common in the macular area, while the optic disc remains pink and does not become atrophic. There are filamentous vitreous opacities. The cornea and iris are normal in appearance. In older patients, there is complete chorioretinal degeneration,

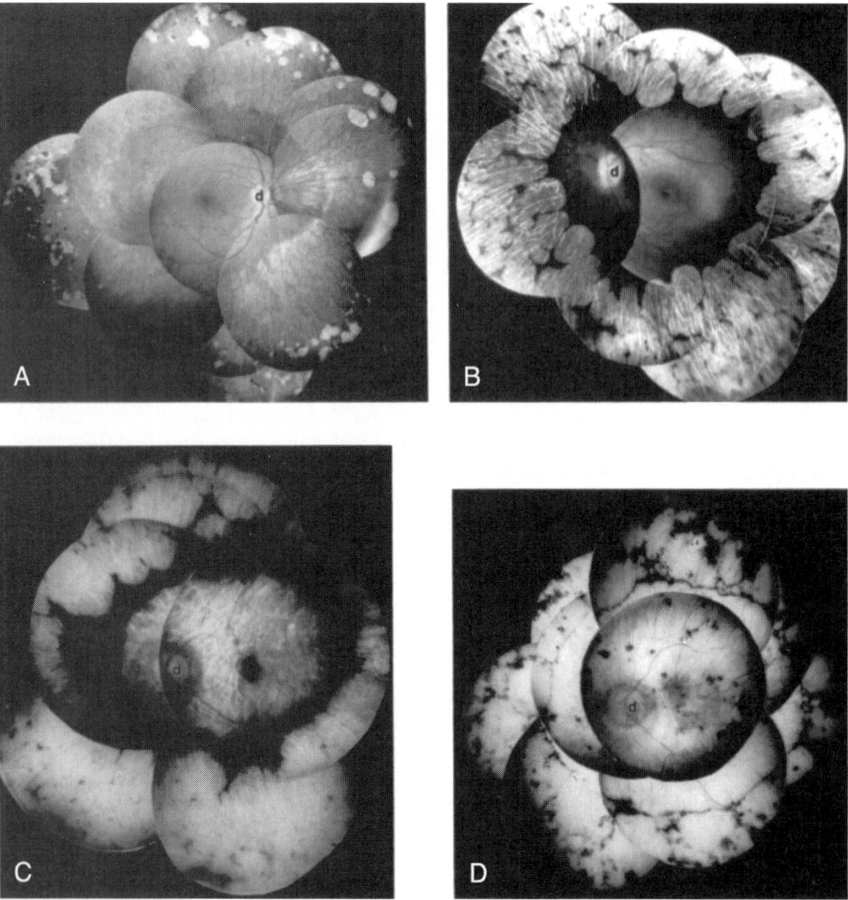

Fig. 83-12 Photographic montages of the ocular fundus of patients of various ages with gyrate atrophy. In these black-and-white photographs, the normally reddish-brown retina appears dark gray while the atrophic areas are light gray or white. The area covered by the montage, and thus the magnification of these reproductions, is different in each patient and can be judged roughly by the diameter of the optic disc. The optic disc, with its accompanying retinal vessels, is indicated in each montage with a "d." *A*, The right eye of a 6-year-old girl. There are isolated lesions in the mid- and far-periphery and circumferential diffuse thinning of the pigment in the midperiphery.[258] *B*, The left eye of a 14-year-old girl. The atrophic lesions are more prominent than in *A* and have coalesced. The posterior pole remains normal in appearance. *C*, The left eye of a 34-year-old female with much more extensive atrophy than *B*. The circumferential zone of coalesced atrophic lesions now involves most of the retina. In addition, there is a central area of atrophy surrounding the optic disc, leaving only a thin circular remnant of normal-appearing retina. *D*, The left eye of a 62-year-old male with complete chorioretinal atrophy with scattered clumps of pigment. (*All montages provided by Muriel Kaiser-Kupfer, M.D., National Eye Institute, Bethesda, MD.*)

with a few thin strands of pigmented material traversing the fundus (Fig. 83-12*D*). Early in the clinical course, the appearance of the fundus is pathognomonic for gyrate atrophy. In the final stages, the appearance is less specific and may easily be confused with the end stage of several other forms of chorioretinal degeneration, especially the X-linked disorder choroideremia (see Chap. 236).[285]

The results of the standard tests of visual function become abnormal at an irregular rate, with periods of rapid progression interspersed with periods of relatively stable function.[259,261,276–278] Visual acuity decreases gradually over several decades in some patients and abruptly over a few years in others.[278] Visual fields are progressively and concentrically reduced. Those patients with peripapillary atrophy may have ring scotoma in addition to peripheral constriction. The electroretinogram, which may be normal at a time when there are a few peripheral atrophic patches, eventually diminishes in amplitude and usually is totally extinguished well before the atrophy becomes complete.[286] Both rod and cone responses are diminished, as are the signals from the pigment epithelium.[286] The electro-oculogram, a test of rod function, is also severely diminished. Dark adaptometry is abnormal, with both an increase in the final threshold and a prolongation of the time required to reach the threshold. In some patients, fluorescein angiography has demonstrated a narrow concentric ring around the completely atrophic areas, in which an abnormally granular retinal pigment epithelium overlies a normal-appearing choroid.[252,287] This observation, plus the description of a diffuse depigmentation of the pigment epithelium in a few very young patients,[283] suggests that the initial insult in gyrate atrophy may involve the pigment epithelium.

Aside from visual impairment, patients with gyrate atrophy are for the most part asymptomatic. A few (< 10 percent) have mild proximal muscle weakness. Histologic and ultrastructural abnormalities in mitochondria and skeletal muscle fibers have been described in many patients. Mitochondria in liver and iris have shown nonspecific morphologic abnormalities, with serpiginous elongation, branching, and segmentation.[265,288] The functional significance of these abnormalities is not known. Nearly all patients studied have had histologic abnormalities of the type 2 (fast twitch) fibers in skeletal muscle (Fig. 83-13).[257,264,265,289,290] These fibers are reduced in diameter and contain accumulations of abnormally staining material demonstrable by hematoxylin-eosin, Gomori ATPase, or NADH-tetrazolium reductase techniques. The accumulations vary in size from small, subsarcolemmal deposits to large collections occupying nearly the entire cross section of the fiber. By electron microscopy, this abnormal material consists of aggregates of parallel-oriented tubules formed by one or, more typically, two concentric membranes with diameters of 50 to 70 nm for the outer and 25 nm for the inner ("tubular aggregates"; see references[291] to[293]). The type 1 fibers are normal on examination by both light and electron microscopy. They become more numerous with age in patients with gyrate atrophy, while in normal subjects the ratio remains constant with age.

Tubular aggregates are not specific for gyrate atrophy. Identical histologic abnormalities have been observed in patients with the various forms of periodic paralysis, hyperthyroidism, porphyria cutanea tarda, myasthenia gravis, myotonic dystrophy, postviral infections, and alcoholism. They have also been observed in low numbers in the muscle of apparently normal male children and adults with nonspecific muscle complaints.[291–294] Aside from patients with gyrate atrophy, they are only rarely observed in females.

In association with these histologic abnormalities, many patients with gyrate atrophy have abnormal electromyograms with short-duration, low-amplitude action potentials of the myopathic type.[289] Despite this, serum creatine phosphokinase activity and usually muscle strength are normal.[257,264,289]

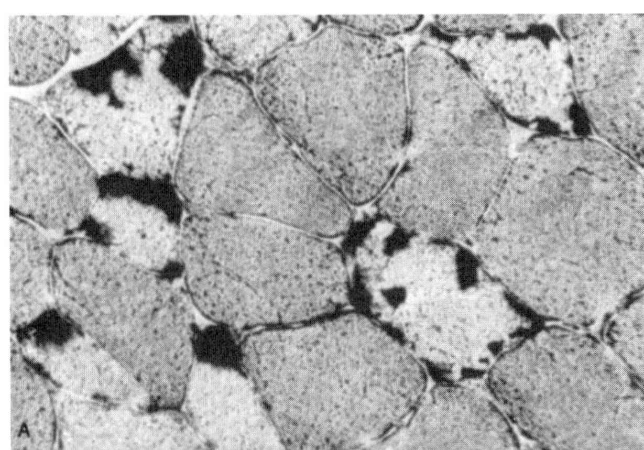

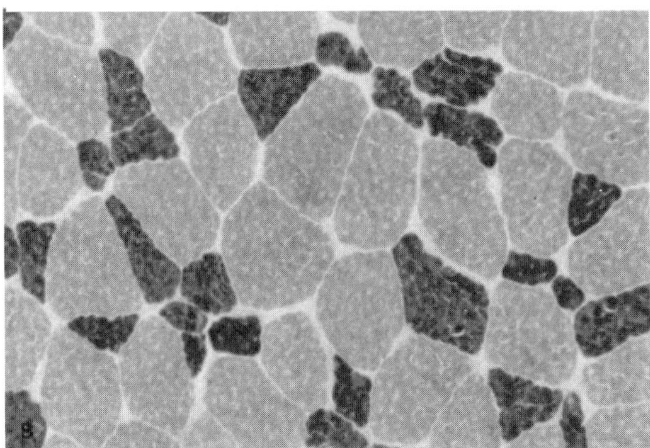

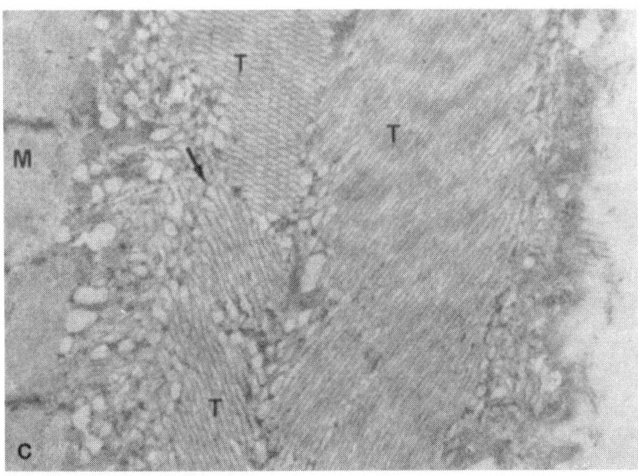

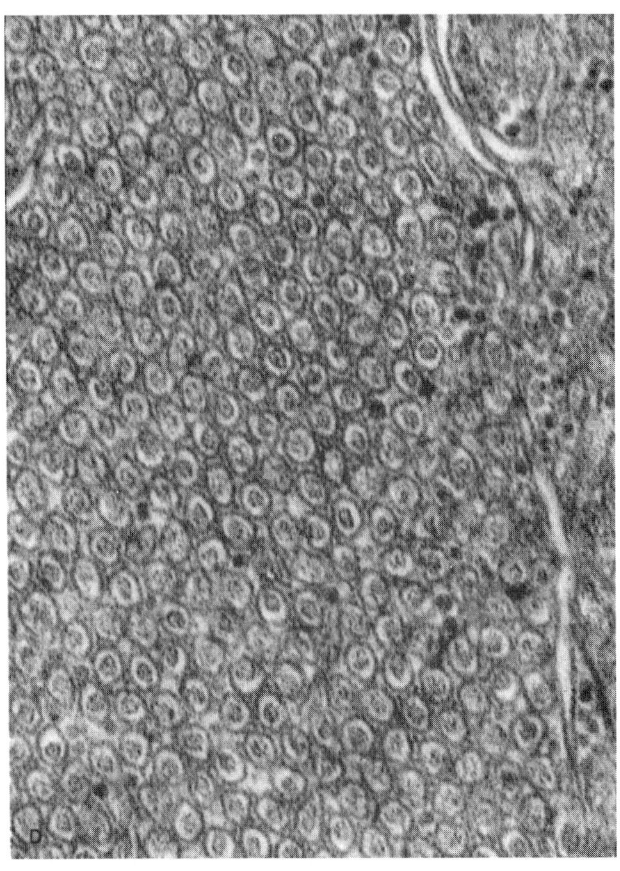

Fig. 83-13 Histologic and ultrastructural abnormalities in the skeletal muscle of gyrate atrophy patients. *A*, NADH-tetrazolium reductase stain demonstrates abnormal, irregular dark areas in the type 2 fibers which, at higher power, can be shown to be tubular aggregates. 340. *B*, ATPase stain with preincubation at pH 9.1 stains the type 2 fibers dark and demonstrates several that are atrophic with ragged borders due to lack of enzyme activity in the tubular aggregates. ×136. *C*, Ultrastructure of the tubular aggregates in the type 2 fibers showing bundles of parallel tubules (tubular aggregates). The zone between the myofibrils (M) and the regularly aligned tubules (T) consists of haphazardly oriented tubulovesicular structures. The ends of some tubules appear dilated in drumstick fashion. ×20,000. *D*, Cross-section of the tubules, most of which contain an inner tubule. ×58,000. (*From Sipila et al.,*[289] *reprinted with permission of the authors and* Neurology.)

Additional abnormalities include mild to moderate diffuse slowing on electroencephalography in one-third or less of the patients.[257,264,276] Seizures do not occur with increased frequency and most patients are of normal intelligence.[257,264] Abnormalities of scalp and body hair have been reported.[257,259,283]

Ocular Histopathology. Retinal histopathology in gyrate atrophy has been described only in one patient, a 98-year-old woman with well-documented vitamin B_6-responsive gyrate atrophy.[295] Her clinical and biochemical phenotypes were milder than those of most gyrate atrophy patients. She had useful visual acuity until the time of her death, and ophthalmoscopy showed a circular patch of relatively normal-appearing retina with a diameter of about 6 disk diameters. Her plasma ornithine was 520 μM, and she had considerable residual OAT activity in extracts of her skin fibroblasts. Histologically, there were areas of near-total atrophy of the retina with abrupt transition to areas of near-normal retina. There were some focal areas of photoreceptor atrophy with adjacent hyperplasia of the pigment epithelium. Electron microscopic examination showed some swelling of photoreceptor mitochondria. More severe mitochondrial abnormalities were present in corneal epithelium and nonpigmented ciliary epithelium. The authors concluded that these pathologic changes suggested that the primary abnormality was in the photoreceptors rather than the retinal pigment epithelium.[295]

Iridectomy samples from three gyrate atrophy patients also showed mitochondrial abnormalities in the dilator muscle and iris epithelium.[288] Ocular histopathology in a cat with gyrate atrophy

Table 83-2 Concentrations of Selected Amino Acids in Body Fluids of Patients with Gyrate Atrophy of the Choroid and Retina

	Plasma, μ*M*		Cerebrospinal Fluid, μ*M*		Aqueous Humor, μ*M*	
Amino Acid	Patients,* (*n*)	Control, † (*n*)	Patients,* (*n*)	Controls,* (*n*)	Patients,* (*n*)	Controls,* (*n*)
Ornithine	916 (51) 400–1339	75 ± 5 (22)	274 (5) 217–314	8 (5) 6–11	898 (7) 763–987	63 (4) 38–84
Lysine	84 (51) 40–160	207 ± 9 (22)	17 (5) 12–20	26 16–44 (3)	82 (7) 73–92	145 (4) 128–158
Glutamate	20 (11) 5–43	35 ± 7 (22)	–	–	–	–
Glutamine	475 (11) 322–731	669 ± 21 (22)	–	–	–	–

*Mean over range.
†Mean ± SE.

SOURCES: Data from Takki,[276] McCulloch et al..,[265] Yatziv et al,[282] Stoppoloni et al.,[275] Kennaway et al.,[290] Valle et al.,[297] Valle et al.,[298] Berson et al.[490]

showed loss of both pigment epithelium and photoreceptors to such an extent that it was not possible to determine which cell type was primarily involved.[296]

Biochemical Abnormalities

The discovery by Simell and Takki of 10-to 20-fold elevations of ornithine in plasma, cerebrospinal fluid, and aqueous humor, and of overflow ornithinuria was the first clue to the nature of the primary defect in gyrate atrophy[255,277] (Table 83-2). Modest decreases in the plasma concentrations of other amino acids, including lysine, glutamic acid, and glutamine, have been described.[254,259,265,277,282,290,297,298] Plasma lysine levels in patients eating a normal diet average about 40 percent of the normal mean and are often below normal range. Cerebrospinal fluid levels of lysine are in the low normal range.[277,297] Urinary excretion of ornithine in adult patients on a regular diet ranges from 0.5 to 10 mM/day (Table 83-3).[275,282,297,298] The excretion of arginine and lysine is also slightly increased.[275,297] An unusual compound first identified as ornithine methyl ester[290] and subsequently shown to be 3-aminopiperid-2-one, the cyclic δ-lactam of ornithine that forms spontaneously from ornithine methyl ester[272,299] (Fig. 83-4), is found in the urine of patients with gyrate atrophy and other conditions associated with hyperornithinemia. The plasma concentration of this compound is low[300] or unmeasurable,[297] suggesting that it may originate in the kidney. Small amounts of glutamylornithine also have been identified in the urine of these individuals.[301]

The plasma concentrations of creatine and its immediate precursor, guanidinoacetate are reduced in gyrate-atrophy patients.[302] Similarly, ^{31}P-magnetic resonance spectroscopy (MRS) analysis shows that phosphocreatine levels in skeletal muscle and in basal ganglia are reduced by 50 percent or more.[303,304]

The Enzyme Deficiency

The discovery of hyperornithinemia in gyrate atrophy directed attention to the enzymes of ornithine metabolism, particularly those catalyzing reactions that consume ornithine (Fig. 83-2). Deficiency of OAT has been documented in cultured skin fibroblasts,[270,279,290,305–309] in resting peripheral lymphocytes,[135] in phytohemagglutinin in stimulated lymphocytes,[308,310] in primary skeletal muscle cultures,[311] in hair roots,[312] and in liver biopsy material.[313] OAT activity measurements have been reported in fibroblasts of at least 15 gyrate atrophy patients in the literature, and in more than 50 in our own laboratory. The OAT activity in about two-thirds of the patient cell lines is undetectable (<1 percent of normal) while, in the remainder, there is residual activity up to as high as 5.7 percent of normal (Table 83-4). In our experience, the presence or absence of residual activity breeds true within a family, a result consistent with the notion that differences in residual activity reflect heterogeneity of mutant OAT alleles. Low-level OAT activity was detected in liver obtained by percutaneous biopsy from two Finnish patients.[313] The residual activity had a greatly reduced affinity for ornithine (K_m approximately 200 mM versus the normal 1.8 mM). Immunologic assays of OAT protein in fibroblasts from a number of patients provide evidence for heterogeneity, with the amount of mutant protein varying from normal to nondetectable (Fig. 83-14).[132,307,314] No evidence has been found for OAT inhibitors when gyrate atrophy and control cells or tissue extracts have been

Table 83-3 Urinary Excretion of Basic Amino Acids in Gyrate Atrophy

	Excretion, μmol/day				
	n	Ornithine	Arginine	Lysine	δ-Lactam of Ornithine
Patients*	9	3130 (490–7500)	180 (50–3800)	1300 (400–2300)	1090 (520–3100)
Controls†	14	18 ± 23	10 ± 6	155 ± 114	–

*Mean (range).
†Mean ± sd.

SOURCE: Data for patients from Valle et al.[488]; data for controls from Holmgren.[489]

Table 83-4 Ornithine-δ-Aminotransferase Activity in Cultured Skin Fibroblasts of Gyrate Atrophy Patients and Heterozygotes*

Group	n	Enzyme Activity,† nmol/(h · mg)	Percent of control
Controls	22	108.6 ± 19	100
Patients			
No activity	13	None detectable	0
Residual activity	6	1.8 (0.4–3.9)	2
Obligate heterozygotes	7	54.3 (37.8–79.4)	50

*Ornithine-δ-aminotransferase activity was assayed radioisotopically with both substrates present at 0.7 m*M* and 16 μ*M* pyriodoxal phosphate.[132] The division of patient cell lines into groups with no detectable activity and residual activity was unaffected by increasing the substrate concentrations to 15 m*M* ornithine and 2.5 m*M* α-ketoglutarate ± 0.6 m*M* pyridoxal phosphate. The ethnic origin of the patients included Finnish, English, Welsh, Scottish, Portuguese, Spanish, Japanese, and Indian.

†Expressed as mean ± SD or mean (range).

mixed.[309,310,314] Ornithine decarboxylase, the other enzyme that catalyzes an ornithine-consuming reaction, was measured and found to be normal in one patient.[310]

A few gyrate atrophy patients (< 5 percent) clearly show evidence (*in vivo* and/or *in vitro*) of partial responsiveness to pharmacologic levels of vitamin B_6. Fibroblast OAT activity in seven patients from five families increased when the concentration of pyridoxal phosphate was increased to high levels in the assay mixture.[290,308,309,315,316] At usual assay concentrations of cofactor pyridoxal phosphate (16 to 50 μM) the OAT activity in these seven cell lines ranged from undetectable to 6.5 percent of normal and increased to as much as one-third that of control subjects when the pyridoxal phosphate concentrations were between 0.6 and 4 mM. Cultured fibroblasts with appreciable OAT activity synthesize radiolabeled proline and glutamate from precursor radiolabeled ornithine (Fig. 83-2). Using this "intact cell" assay, Kennaway and her colleagues showed that OAT activity in cultured fibroblasts from her four pyridoxine-responsive patients had a higher production of proline and glutamate than did nonresponsive patients, indicating that significant residual enzyme activity was present in the pyridoxine-responsive patients.[315,317] Kinetic studies of fibroblast OAT in five pyridoxine-responsive patients showed that the K_m for pyridoxal phosphate was increased from a normal value of ~20 μM to 80 to 310 μM.[103,314,316] Six of the seven patients with an *in vitro* response had partial reductions in plasma ornithine (averaging about 50 percent) when given pharmacologic doses (500 to 1000 mg/day) of pyridoxine hydrochloride (vitamin B_6, the dietary precursor of pyridoxal phosphate).[290,308,309,316,317] Three also responded to relatively low doses (15 to 18 mg/day).[281,290,317] One patient described by Kennaway et al.[290] had an *in vitro* response without an *in vivo* response, while Valle et al.[298] described a patient with an *in vivo* response without an *in vitro* response.

OAT activity also has been assayed in cultured skin fibroblasts from at least 14 obligate heterozygotes (Table 83-4).[270,290,308,309,318] The activity ranged from 32 to 61 percent of the normal mean. A similar result was obtained in phytohemagglutinin-stimulated lymphocytes.[308,310] This approximately 50 percent reduction in activity in the cells of obligate heterozygotes provided strong genetic evidence for a primary defect in OAT as the cause of gyrate atrophy.

Molecular Defects

All defects causing gyrate atrophy appear to be in the OAT gene. All patients known to us who have typical clinical features and hyperornithinemia have had a profound deficiency of OAT activity, and complementation studies have failed to show evidence for more than one locus.[315,318,319]

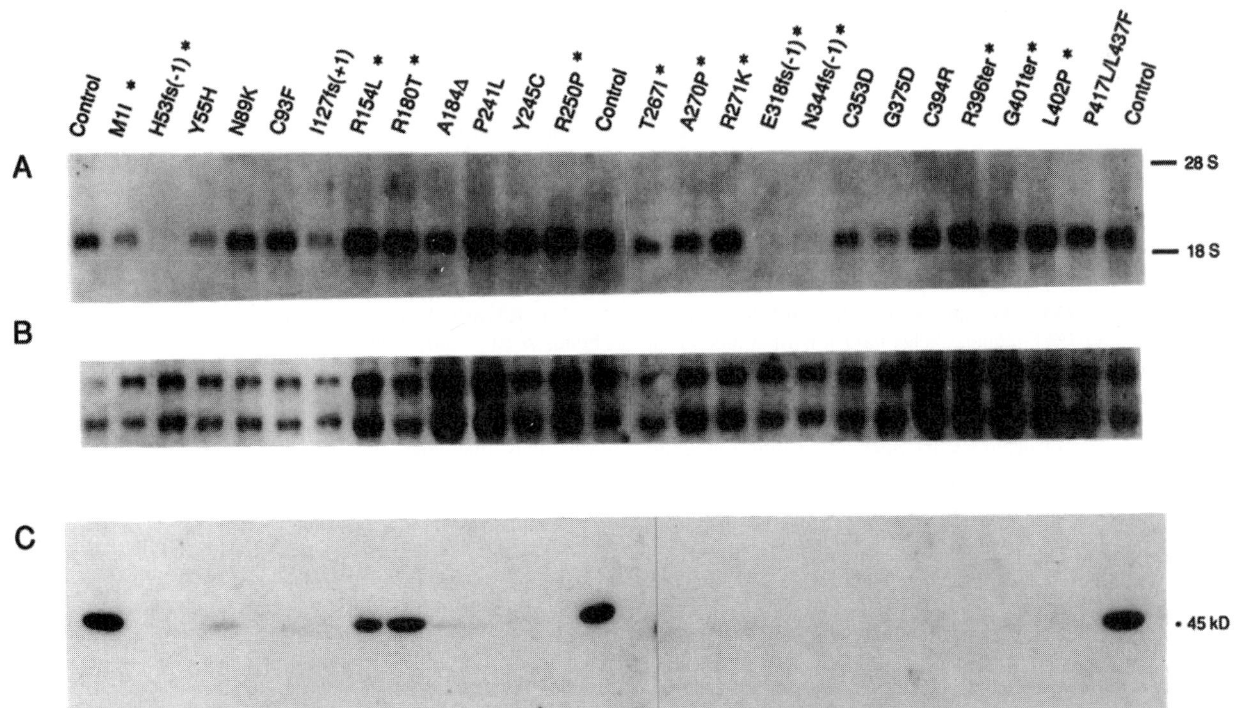

Fig. 83-14 Consequences of mutations on OAT mRNA and antigen in cultured human fibroblasts. *A*, Northern blot analysis of total cellular RNA (10 μg of RNA/lane) isolated from gyrate atrophy fibroblasts and hybridized to a human OAT cDNA probe. The positions of the 28 S and 18 S ribosomal subunits are indicated for reference. *B*, The same filter rehybridized to a mouse β-tubulin probe to control for RNA loading. *C*, Immunoblot analysis of OAT antigen in sonicates of gyrate atrophy fibroblasts (50 μg of protein/lane). (*From Brody et al.,[132] reprinted with permission of the authors and Journal of Biological Chemistry.*)

Analysis. Cloning and sequencing of human OAT cDNAs[137,138,147] and the elucidation of the gene structure[147,320] provided the necessary molecular framework for direct investigation of the mutations responsible for gyrate atrophy (Fig. 83-5). The sequence of PCR primers for each OAT exon have been published.[321] Several additional features of OAT have helped these investigations. First, OAT is expressed in cultured fibroblasts, providing an accessible and assayable source of OAT mRNA, antigen, and activity. Second, there are two excellent biologic systems for the expression of human OAT cDNAs to determine the functional consequences of any variants identified. Chinese hamster ovary cells (CHO-K1), a vigorously growing cell line, are proline auxotrophs, lacking both endogenous P5C synthase and OAT activity.[219] The molecular basis of these defects is not known, but there is no detectable OAT mRNA, antigen, or activity in these cells.[132] OAT cDNAs can be expressed in CHO-KI cells, and their protein products examined either in transient transfection assays or in stable lines selected for proline prototrophy.[322,323] An OAT-deficient strain of *S. cerevisiae* also has been described; human OAT can be expressed in these cells and the consequence of mutations on the structure and function of the protein examined.[146] Third, as mentioned above (see "Molecular Biology of OAT"), the sequence for an OAT cDNA from *S. cerevisiae* has been reported.[141] The yeast enzyme has regions of high homology with human OAT (Fig. 83-6).[147] The patches of amino acid identity in the proteins from these two distantly related organisms are likely to be important for OAT function and delineate locations where missense mutations causing gyrate atrophy can be expected to occur.[147]

OAT Alleles. Since the first report of an OAT mutation causing gyrate atrophy by Mitchell and coworkers,[324] more than 60 mutations have been reported in the OAT genes of patients with gyrate atrophy (Table 83-5). Only one is a gross change detectable by Southern blotting;[325] the remainder are subtle alterations. The subtle alterations include 36 missense mutations,[132,148,165,321,322,324,326–330] 10 nonsense mutations,[132,149,165,316,322–330] 12 microdeletions of 1 to 15 bp,[132,165,326,331,332] 1 microinsertion,[132] 2 nucleotide substitutions altering splice consensus sequences,[321,326] and 1 splice-mediated Alu insertion (G67ins, see below).[333] These mutations account for a substantial fraction of the possible OAT mutant alleles in known gyrate atrophy patients. In our own series of 92 unrelated gyrate-atrophy probands (including 31 Finn probands), 83 percent of the total possible 184 alleles and 98 percent of the 62 possible Finn alleles are accounted for by known OAT mutations.[334] Of the 57 non-Finn probands for whom we have some genotypic information, 27 (47 percent) are genetic compounds.

Consequences of OAT Mutations on OAT mRNA. At the mRNA level, most OAT mutant alleles have a normal amount of normal-sized message (Fig. 83-14). Eight alleles, however, have markedly reduced (<10 percent) levels of fibroblast OAT mRNA (Fig. 83-15).[132,329] These include three nonsense mutations and five small insertions or deletions that alter the reading frame; all are characterized by premature termination of translation in a segment of the mRNA encoded by exon 10 or by more upstream exons rather than at the normal site of translation termination in the last exon (exon 11).[132,335] In contrast, three nonsense alleles terminating translation early in exon 11 (W391ter, R396ter, and R426ter) have normal amounts of OAT mRNA. Thus, as observed with naturally occurring and induced mutations in other genes, premature termination in the terminal exon has no effect on mRNA levels, while termination in the penultimate exon or earlier is associated with markedly reduced levels of mRNA.[336–338] Studies of two of these alleles (W178ter, W275ter) have shown that this reduction in mRNA level is associated with an abnormal pattern of splicing, so that the exon containing the translation termination is spliced out of the transcript ("exon skipping") (see Chap. 12). This observation led to the hypothesis that the reading frame of maturing mRNAs somehow undergoes examination in the nucleus.[339] Splicing decisions that result in mRNAs with longer reading frames are more likely to yield transcripts that reach the cytosol.

Another OAT allele with aberrant splicing is the G67ins mutation, in which a portion of an intronic *Alu* element is spliced into the mature OAT mRNA at the site of the G67 codon. The allele was found in an Algerian patient of consanguineous origin with no detectable OAT activity and a reduced amount of a slightly larger than normal OAT mRNA.[333] The mutation is a single nucleotide substitution in an *Alu* element oriented in the direction opposite that of transcription of the OAT gene (an "antisense" *Alu*) and located in intron 3. One of several cryptic acceptor splice sites in the antisense *Alu* is activated by the mutation, with the result that 142 bp of the *Alu* sequence are inserted into the mature OAT transcript at the junction of sequence from exon 3 and 4. First recognized in OAT, splice-mediated *Alu* insertion arising from an antisense *Alu* has now been observed in more than 10 other instances (see Chap. 12).[340]

In addition to these gyrate atrophy associated mutations, a polymorphic synonymous mutation, N378N, and an intronic single nucleotide polymorphism have been described.[321,341]

Missense Mutations and OAT Structure and Function. Of the 36 OAT missense mutations, 35 occur in the portion of the human protein that has homology with *S. cerevisiae* OAT (Fig. 83-6). Of these, 27 (75 percent) alter amino acids conserved between yeast and human OAT, as compared to an overall identity of 54 percent between the two proteins. The functional significance of at least 10 of these mutations has been examined by expression of the mutant allele in CHO-K1 cells.[132,148,322,342] For the remainder, functional significance is inferred because the mutation (a) alters a conserved residue, (b) cosegregates with reduced OAT function in gyrate atrophy patients and their families, and (c) has not been detected in a large series of control subjects. Characterization of the missense mutations causing gyrate atrophy provides some insight into the structure and function of OAT. Most of these mutations ($\sim$90 percent) apparently destabilize the enzyme so that no OAT antigen is detected in immunoblots of fibroblast extracts (antigen-negative or CRM^- alleles) (Fig. 83-14).[132] Destabilizing mutations often result in the disruption of hydrophobic and electrostatic interactions in the protein core.[343] Solution of its crystal structure showed that this holds true for OAT. Shen et al. have pointed out that many of these destabilizing missense mutations occur in the domains of the OAT monomer or in the interfaces between the two monomers of the OAT dimer.[115] Most (76 percent) of these destabilizing mutations affect residues conserved between *S. cerevisiae* and human OAT (Fig. 83-6). Four of the eight missense mutations altering nonconserved residues involve proline (L62P, R250P, A270P, R398P). This imino acid forms the least-flexible peptide bond, so it is not surprising that these substitutions might be deleterious to OAT structure.[344] Most interestingly, two of the missense mutations, R180T and R154L, completely inactivate OAT function without reducing the amount of OAT antigen. Mutations that alter function without affecting stability often involve residues that participate in the active site.[343,345,346] The crystal structure of OAT shows that R180 plays a key role in substrate recognition interacting with the α-carboxylate of ornithine or the γ-carboxylate of glutamate depending on the direction of the reaction.[115] E235 and R413 are also predicted to play key roles in the active site.[115]

One OAT allele is unusual because it has two missense mutations in *cis*, P417L + L437F. To determine whether the two mutations were acting in concert or independently to inactivate OAT function, Brody et al. cloned[132] and expressed each separately: P417L is OAT antigen and activity-negative; L437F, by contrast, has no discernible effect on OAT stability or function and appears to be a neutral mutation. The P417L + L437F allele has been detected in several patients of English descent. Despite its neutrality, L437F has only been found in combination with P417L.

Table 83-5 Pathologic or Presumed Pathologic Mutations Found in the OAT Genes of GA Patients Sorted by Exon

N	Mutation	Exon	Ethnic Origin	# peds	gntyp	nt	nt change	Consequence	Fx sig	CRM	mRNA	Reference
1	M1I	3	Lebanese Maronite	3	hom	3	G>A	missense	+	0	3+	324
2	G17ter	3	Irish	1	cpd	49	G>T	nonsense	nt	0	3+	165
3	H53fs(−1)	3	Iraqi Jew	1	hom	159	deletes C	frameshift	inf	0	1+	132
4	N54K	3	English	1	?	162	C>A	missense	nt			149, 323
5	Y55H	3	Aust/ Hung/Brit	1	cpd	163	T>C	missense	nt	1+	3+	132
6	L62P	3	Nicarag	1	?	185	T>C	missense	nt			149
7	E63fs(−2)	3	English ?	1	hom	188–189	deletes AG	frameshift	inf			165
8	R64fs(−2)	3	Caucasian	1	cpd	192–3	deletes AG	frameshift	inf		5%	329
9	G67ins	3	Algerian	1	hom	200	ins 142 bp	frameshift	nt	0	1+	333
10	N89K	4	Finn	1	cpd	267	C>A	missense	nt		3+	132
11	C93F	4	Germ/It	1	cpd	278	G>T	missense	nt	0	3+	132
12	E124D	4	Italian	1	hom	372	G>T	missense	nd	?	?	165
13	E125Δ	4	Japanese	1	?	373–375	deletes GAG	deletes E 125	nt			326
14	I127fs(+1)	4	Welsh	1	cpd	380–1	ins T	frameshift	nd		?	132
15	M139R	4	Portuguese	1	?	416	T>G	missense	nt			149
16	G142E	5	Japanese	1	?	425	G>A	missense	nt			326
17	R154L	5	Eng/Germ	3	both	461	G>T	missense	+	1+	3+	132
18	Y158 -G162Δ	5	English	1	cpd	472–486	deletes 15 bp	del Y158 –G162	nt		3+	331
19	K169fs(−2)		Japanese	1	cpd	506–507	deletes 2 bp	frameshift	nt			334
20	In4acA–2G	5	English ?	2	cpd	xxx	A(−2) G	spl ste Δ	inf	0	3+	321
21	del Ex5 spl acp	5	Swedish/ Danish	1	cpd	xxx	del 9 bp	spl ste Δ; del Ex5	inf	?	?	332
22	W178ter	6	Mexican	1	hom	533	G>A	nonsense	inf	0	0	339
23	R180T	6	Finn/Amer	5	both	539	G>C	missense	+	3+	3+	333
24	T181M	6	Japanese	1	?	542	C>T	missense	nt			326
25	A184T	6	Asian Indian	1	hom	550	G>A	missense	nt			321
26	A184Δ	6	Portuguese	1	cpd	550	deletes GCT	deletes A 184	+	1+	3+	132
27	T192fs(−1)	6	Portuguese	1	hom	595–6	deletes C	frameshift	inf			334
28	D195Y	6	Japanese	1	?	583	G>T	missense	nt			326
29	P199Q	6	English	1	?	596	C>A	missense	nt			149, 327
30	Y209ter	6	Eng/Ger/Scot	1	?	627	T>A	nonsense	inf		0	329
31	del Ex6	6	English	1	cpd	int5–int6		deletes exon 6	inf		1+	325, 326
32	A226V	7	Italian	1	hom	677	C>T	missense	+		3+	324, 333
33	Q233R	7	Mexican	1	hom	698	A>G	missense	nt	0	3+	328
34	P241L	7	Germ/It	1	cpd	722	C>T	missense	nt	1+	3+	132
35	Y245C	7	English ?	1	cpd	734	A>G	missense	nt			132
36	R250P	7	French	1	?	749	G>C	missense	nt	0	?	132
37	R250 –E251Δ	7	New Zealand	1	hom	748–753	del 6 bp	2 codon deletion	nt			334
38	T267I	8	Ashk Jew; Argent	4	both	800	C>T	missense	nt	0	3+	132, 149
39	A270P	8	Portuguese	1	hom	808	G>C	missense	nt	0	3+	132
40	R271K	8	Japanese	1	hom	812	G>A	missense	+	0	3+	132
41	W275ter	8	English ?	1	cpd	840	G>A	nonsense	nt			339
42	Y299ter	8	Ital/Dutch/Irish	1	cpd	897	C>G	nonsense	inf		30%	329
43	P300R	8	Afr American	1	cpd	899	C>G	missense	nt			334
44	In8acA-2G	8	English/ German	1	?	xxx	A>G	spl ste Δ; deletes Ex9	inf			328
45	E318K	9	Eng/Scot/Irish	4	cpd	952	G>A	missense	nt	1+	2+	149, 326
46	E318fs(−1)	9	Turk (Sephardic)	1	hom	947–50	deletes G	frameshift	inf	0	1+	132
47	H319Y	9	Japanese	1	cpd	955	C>T	missense	+			330
48	S321F	9	Finn	1	cpd	962	C>T	missense	nt			334
49	V332M	9	Portuguese	1	?	994	G>A	missense	+			323
50	N334fs(−1)	10	West African	1	hom	1028–31	deletes A	frameshift	inf	0	1+	132
51	G353D	10	Spanish	3	hom	1058	G>A	missense	inf	0	3+	132
52	G373E	10	Eng/German	1	cpd	1118	G>A	missense	nt			329
53	G375A	10	Hispanic (Nicarag)	1	cpd	1124	G>C	missense	nt	0	3+	132

(Continued on next page)

Table 83-5 (Continued)

N	Mutation	Exon	Ethnic Origin	# peds	gntyp	nt	nt change	Consequence	Fx sig	CRM	mRNA	Reference
54	W391ter	11	Italian	1	hom	1171	G>A	nonsense	inf	0	2+	321
55	C394R	11	English ?	1	cpd	1180	T>C	missense	nt	0	3+	132
56	R396ter	11	East Indian	1	hom	1186	C>T	nonsense	inf	0	3+	132
57	R398ter	11	English?	1	cpd	1192	C>T	nonsense	inf		3+	316
58	R398P	11	Irish	1	cpd	1193	G>C	missense	nt	0	3+	165
59	G401ter	11	?	1	cpd	1201	G>T	nonsense	inf			132
60	L402P	11	Finn	29	both	1205	T>C	missense	+	0	3+	333
61	P417L	11	English ?	7	cpd	1250	C>T	missense	+	0	3+	132
62	R426ter	11	Japanese	1	hom	1276	C>T	nonsense	inf		90%	329
63	L437F	11	English ?	7	cpd	1311	G>T	missense	–		3+	132

Mutation nomenclature: Missense mutations are designated using the single letter abbreviations for amino acids and the codon number with codon 1 corresponding to the initiation methionine. The first letter and number indicate the normal residue and codon number with the following letter designating the replacement residue. Nonsense mutations are indicated by the suffix "ter" following the codon number. Large insertions are indicated by the suffix "ins." Small (<30 bp) insertions or deletions are indicated by "fs" (for frameshift) followed by the number of bp inserted or deleted in parentheses, e.g. E63fs(−2). The suffix "Δ" indicates deletion of a single codon, e.g. A184Δ. Splice site mutations are indicated by "In" (for intron) followed by the intron number, ac (for acceptor) or dn (for donor), the normal base, it's position relative to the splice site, and the replacement base, e.g. In4acA-2G, designates an A → G transition in the -2 position of the acceptor splice site of intron 4. Other nonstandard abbreviations: nt, not tested; 3+, normal amount; 2+, reduced; 1+, barely detectable; 0, not detectable; gntyp, genotype, nt, nucleotide; fx, functional; CRM, cross-reactive material; inf, inferred.

Thus, the two mutations are in extreme linkage disequilibrium as would be the case if they arose simultaneously in a gene conversion event but no evidence for the necessary source sequence has been reported.

Pyridoxine-Responsive Alleles. Three OAT missense mutations are of particular significance because they provide insight into the molecular basis of pyridoxine (vitamin B_6)-responsive gyrate atrophy. V332M, A226V, and E318K encode mutant enzymes with less than 2 percent of control activity when measured at standard pyridoxal phosphate concentrations (15 to 50 μM), increasing to 12 to 15 percent when the pyridoxal phosphate concentration is increased to 600 μM or more.[316,323,347] The apparent K_m of A226V OAT for pyridoxal phosphate measured at saturating concentrations of ornithine and α-ketoglutarate is 122 μM, as compared to 6 μM for wild-type enzyme.[316] Pyridoxal phosphate is covalently bound to OAT at K292.[113] Other amino acids involved in the interaction of OAT with its cofactor can be predicted from the homology of the region of OAT surrounding K292 with the corresponding region of other Ω transaminases, including ω-amino acid:pyruvate aminotransferase, a bacterial enzyme whose structure has been solved.[348–350] This comparison predicts that OAT residues E230 and D262 interact with the 3′-hydroxyl and N1 of the pyridoxal phosphate molecule, respectively (Fig. 83-16).[348] Thus, the substitution of V for A226 may in some way interfere with the interaction of E230 with the cofactor. Unfortunately, this modeling does not provide real insight on how the V332M or E318K produce a B_6-responsive OAT.

Population Distributions of Mutant OAT Alleles. Gyrate atrophy occurs throughout the world and, as discussed above, has extensive allelic heterogeneity. OAT alleles characteristic of certain ethnic groups are listed in Table 83-6. Most notably, gyrate atrophy is one of a group of genetic disorders, constituting the so-called Finnish Disease Heritage, that has higher frequencies in Finns than in other populations.[351–353] The Finnish population (4.8 million) is isolated genetically by geographic, linguistic, and cultural barriers, and is relatively homogeneous, with approximately one in five unions being consanguineous at least at the first cousin level. Despite this, even among Finns, gyrate atrophy is genetically heterogenous, with at least four mutant OAT alleles present in the population.[354] One allele, L402P, accounts for about 87 percent of the total OAT mutant genes in the Finnish population; it has only been found in Finns and is on a haplotype that is frequent in Finns.[354,355] A second allele, R180T, accounts for about 10 percent of the mutant alleles in Finns but has also been detected in American gyrate atrophy patients of non-Finnish origin. Haplotype analysis shows that this mutation has occurred at least twice, once in the ancestors of the Finn patients and once in the ancestors of the American patients.[354,355] A third allele, N89K, has been detected in one family also segregating L402P. Similarly, the fourth allele, S321F, has been detected in one family as a compound with L402P.

Pathophysiology

Biochemical Abnormalities. Deficiency of OAT explains most of the biochemical abnormalities observed in patients with gyrate atrophy. Hyperornithinemia is a direct result of the block in the OAT reaction. An adult with gyrate atrophy ingesting 1.5 g/kg/day has an arginine intake of approximately 28 mM/day. Little if any of this arginine is used for protein accretion. Arginine is converted to ornithine by arginase and, to a lesser extent, by

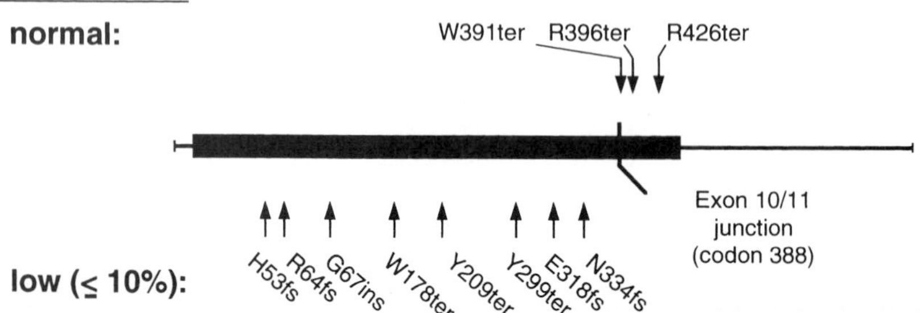

Fig. 83-15 The consequence of OAT mutations causing premature termination of translation on steady state levels of fibroblast OAT mRNA. The mature OAT transcript is shown with the thick black rectangle indicating the translated portion of the normal mRNA. (See Table 83-5 for details of the specific mutations.) All of the frame-shifting mutations terminate translation upstream (5′) of the exon 10/11 boundary.

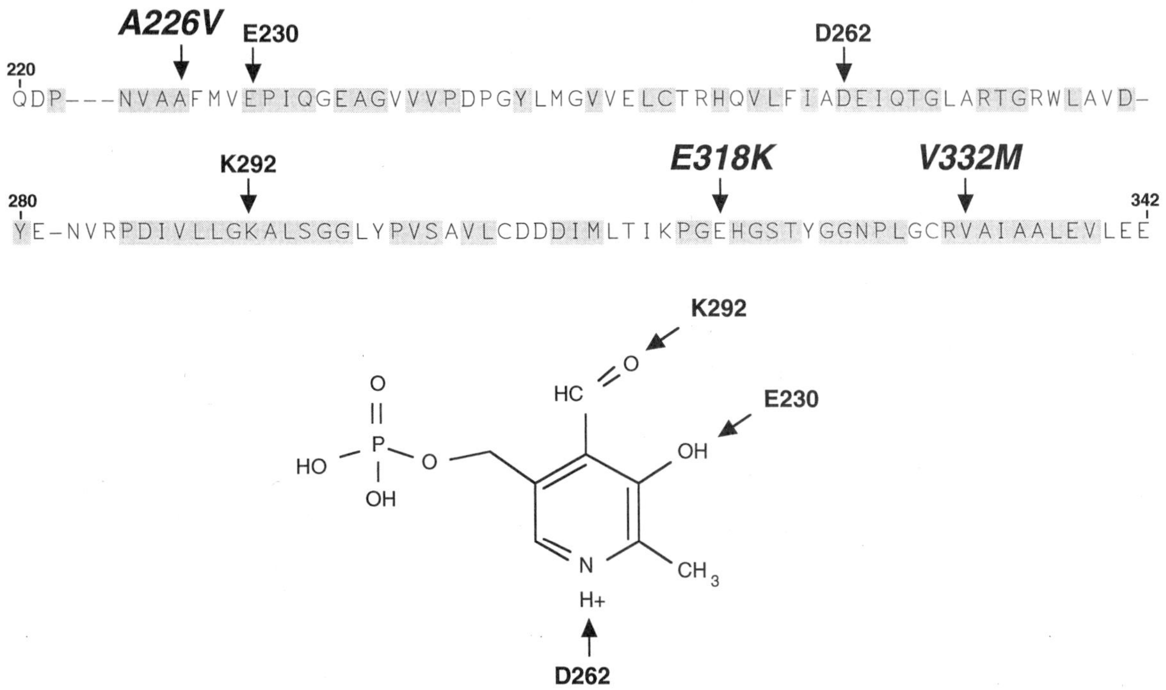

A226V E230 D262

220 QDP---NVAAFMVEPIQGEAGVVVPDPGYLMGVVELCTRHQVLFIADEIQTGLARTGRWLAVD-

K292 **E318K** **V332M**

280 YE-NVRPDIVLLGKALSGGLYPVSAVLCDDDIMLTIKPGEHGSTYGGNPLGCRVAIAALEVLEE 342

Fig. 83-16 The region of the OAT peptide around the pyridoxal phosphate binding residue, K292. The shaded residues are identical with *S. cerevisiae* OAT. In addition to K292, two residues (E230 and D262) predicted to interact noncovalently with pyridoxal phosphate based on homology of OAT to a B_6-dependent enzyme whose structure is known (ω amino acid:pyruvate transaminase) are shown. The sites of interaction of these residues with pyridoxal phosphate is indicated below. The two known pyridoxine-responsive OAT mutations (A226V, V332M) are shown in bold.

glycine transamidinase (Fig. 83-2). A fraction of the ornithine is used for the synthesis of putrescine and polyamines (an estimated 0.5 mM/day), and the remainder accumulates. Ornithine excretion increases accordingly, particularly at plasma concentrations of more than 600 μM.[298] The high renal filtered load of ornithine also results in increased renal clearances of lysine, arginine, and cystine (Table 83-3).[356]

The total urinary excretion of arginine-derived carbon skeletons (arginine, ornithine, the δ-lactam of ornithine, citrulline, and argininosuccinic acid) by patients with gyrate atrophy is much less than the estimated arginine intake (Table 83-3). Therefore, as much as 75 percent of the ingested arginine cannot be accounted for in these patients.[356] Possible explanations for this include residual OAT activity,[313] gastrointestinal losses, a greater flux to putrescine than estimated, or some unanticipated pathway for the catabolism of arginine, ornithine, or any of the urea cycle intermediates. Transamination of the α-amino group of arginine or ornithine would provide such an alternative degradation pathway, but there is no evidence that this occurs in humans.[102,357] The extent of the conversion of ornithine to putrescine by ornithine decarboxylase may have been underestimated by data from studies measuring polyamine excretion,[56,57] because putrescine may also be converted to CO_2 via GABA and succinate (Fig. 83-2). Ornithine decarboxylase is highly regulated by factors related to the growth of cells,[54] and this fact probably limits significant ornithine catabolism by this pathway. Recent studies examining the metabolic consequences of inhibition of OAT by 5MFOrn in mice do show an approximately twofold increase in tissue putrescine levels and a tenfold rise in excretion of polyamines.[60,126,127] These observations suggest that a reexamination of polyamine metabolism in gyrate atrophy is merited.

The extent of ornithine accumulation in patients with this disorder has not been determined, because the compartments in which ornithine has been measured (plasma, cerebrospinal fluid, and aqueous humor) represent only a small fraction (~10 percent) of the total body ornithine pool.[358] The major portion of the free pool of most amino acids is located in the intracellular fluid of skeletal muscle and liver. In normal humans, the intracellular ornithine concentration in muscle is five times that in plasma.[359] Lower values have been reported for rat muscle.[360,361] If the former ratio is maintained in gyrate atrophy, the total body pool of ornithine in an adult could be as high as 100 to 150 mM. A comparison of the intracellular and plasma fractions of the total body ornithine pool emphasizes the fact that a minor change in ornithine distribution can lead to a major change in plasma concentration without a change in total body ornithine. A temporary shift of ornithine from plasma to intracellular fluid may explain the transient, acute reduction of plasma ornithine in gyrate atrophy patients following a glucose load.[264,284,297]

Hyperornithinemia and intracellular ornithine accumulation also may account for some of the abnormal concentrations of other plasma metabolites. Increased renal clearance of lysine or an effect of ornithine on the catabolism or distribution of lysine are likely causes of the hypolysinemia.[297] The mechanism for the reduced levels of plasma glutamate and glutamine is not known, although it has been suggested that this effect is due to an alteration in the balance between urea precursors (glutamate, glutamine, ammonia) and urea production owing to the increased concentration of

Table 83-6 Some OAT Alleles with Ethnic Predispositions

Allele	Ethnic Group
M1I	Lebanese Maronite
R154L	English
Q233R	Hispanic
T2671	Ashkenazi Jewish
G375A	Hispanic
L402P	Finn
P417L + L437F	English

ornithine.[297] Thus, the availability of urea precursors, rather than ornithine, may limit urea production in these patients.[13]

Mechanism of the Chorioretinal Degeneration. How deficiency of OAT and subsequent ornithine accumulation leads to chorioretinal degeneration and cataract formation is not known. Any hypothesis must explain the slowly progressive nature of this disorder, the minimal involvement of other organ systems, and the apparent lack of ocular involvement in patients with the HHH syndrome. General possibilities include a toxic effect of the accumulated precursor (ornithine) or of one of its metabolites, or a deficiency of the reaction product (P5C) or one of its metabolites. The fact that OAT activity is present in retinal neurons and glia (particularly Müller cells)[201,202] and in pigment epithelium[194,196,197,199] suggests that the enzyme function may be important in these tissues but does not discriminate between these two general mechanisms.

An additional problem in understanding the mechanism of the chorioretinal degeneration is that it is not known which of the many specialized types of cells found in the retina are the first to be affected (Fig. 83-17). Attention has focused on the pigment epithelium and the photoreceptors, the two outermost cell layers of the retina (Fig. 83-17*C*).[362–366] These cells have an intimate relationship. The apices of the pigment epithelial cells interdigitate with and ensheath the outer segments of the photoreceptors, while their bases rest on Bruch's membrane, a complex structure that is composed of basement membrane components produced by both the pigment epithelium and cells in the choroid. The apical-lateral surfaces of the pigment epithelial cells are joined to one another by tight junctions, which form a zonula occludens that is the blood-retinal barrier on the outer surface of the retina.[367] The blood supply to the outermost third of the retina, including the pigment epithelium and photoreceptors, is provided by a layer of specialized, dilated capillaries, the choriocapillaris, located just beneath Bruch's membrane. Substrates such as glucose and amino acids delivered by the choriocapillaris pass through Bruch's membrane and then are transported intracellularly through the pigment epithelium to the photoreceptors. In turn, metabolites from the photoreceptors traverse the pigment epithelium, where they may undergo additional metabolism before leaving the retina. The disk-like structures in the photoreceptor outer segments are shed periodically on a circadian schedule[364] and are phagocytosed and degraded by the pigment epithelium. In addition, photoisomerized visual pigment (all-*trans*-retinol) is released from the photoreceptors, taken up by the pigment epithelium where it is either stored as retinyl esters or re-isomerized to the photosensitive form, 11-*cis*-retinaldehyde, and returned to the photoreceptors to bind with opsin to form the light-sensitive visual pigments.[365]

Because of their interdependence, damage to any of the cellular components of the retina may adversely affect others. The observations by Takki and others of areas of pigment epithelial cell damage over an intact choriocapillaris suggest that the pigment layer is the site of the initial insult in gyrate atrophy.[252,287] In support of this, Kaiser-Kupfer et al. described diffuse circumferential depigmentation of the pigment epithelium in the midperipheral and peripheral retina of young (< 10 years old) patients preceding development of the focal atrophic lesions.[283,368] Also, Kuwabara and colleagues have shown that intravitreal

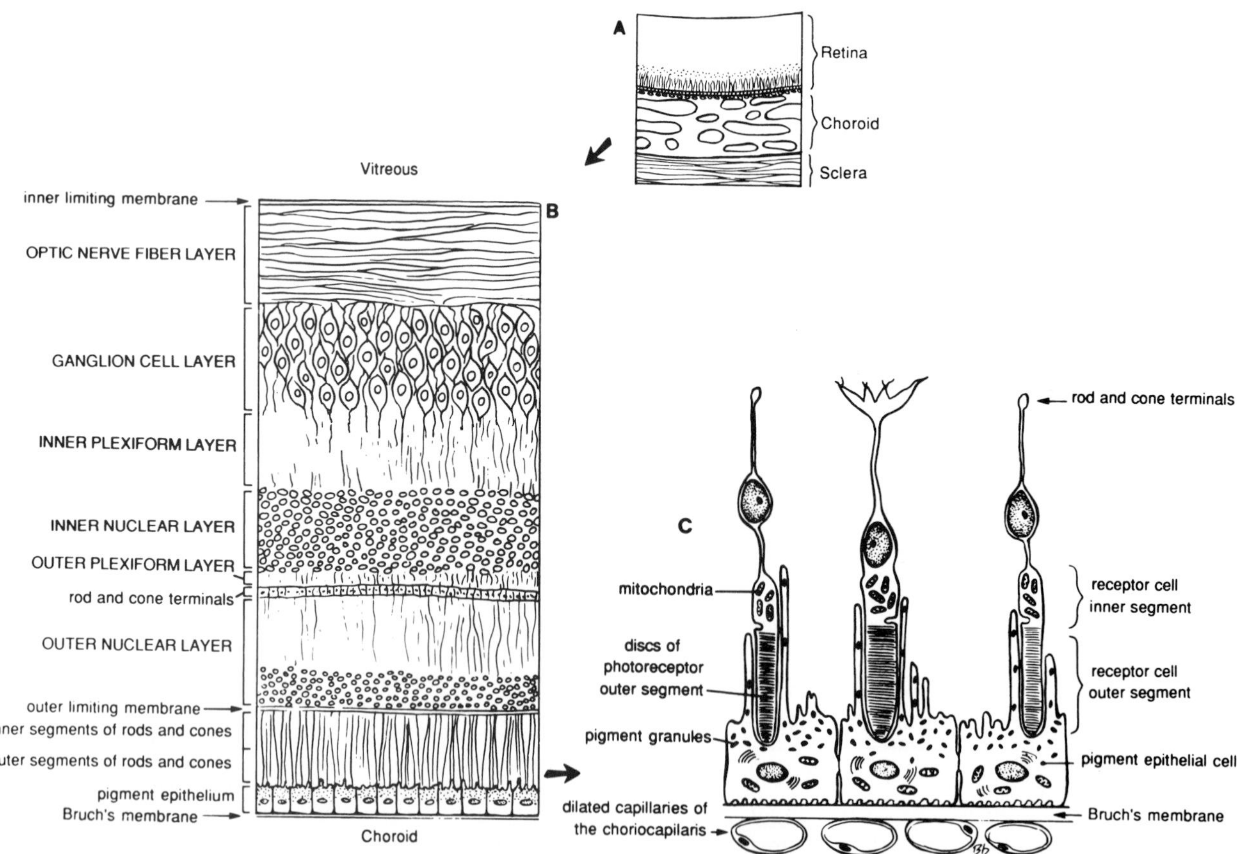

Fig. 83-17 Representation of human ocular tissues. The orientation of each diagram is the same with the inner (vitreal) surface upward and the outer (scleral) surface downward. *A*, Low-power view of a cross-section of the posterior aspect of the eye showing the relationship of the three major layers: retina, choroid, and sclera. *B*, Higher power view of the retina showing the retinal layers. *C*, Detail of the anatomic relationship of the pigment epithelium and the photoreceptor cells. Three receptor cells are shown; the one in the middle with a broad synaptic terminal is a cone. *In vivo*, each pigment epithelium cell interacts with the outer segments of many photoreceptors.[155]

injection of L-ornithine results in degeneration of the pigment epithelial cells in both rats and monkeys.[369] Finally, Ueda et al. showed that in cultured RPE cells made OAT deficient with 5-fluoromethylornithine, elevated ornithine is toxic.[370] Proline prevented the ornithine toxicity.

In support of a primary defect in the RPE, Wang et al.[371] showed that the first morphologic abnormalities in the OAT-deficient mouse are swelling and vesiculation in the RPE. Conversely, the only reported retinal histopathologic study of a patient with gyrate atrophy, a well-characterized 98-year-old woman with a relatively mild and vitamin B_6-responsive phenotype, showed areas at the margins of atrophic lesions where the pigment epithelium was hypertrophic but was preserved despite complete loss of photoreceptors, suggesting that the latter cell type is the site of initial damage (see "Ocular Histopathology" above).[295] Histopathologic studies in a cat with gyrate atrophy showed extensive involvement of the pigment epithelium, photoreceptors, neural retina, and choriocapillaris—changes so advanced that the primary site of involvement could not be determined.[296]

Two hypotheses for the pathophysiology of gyrate atrophy have been developed. Sipila and coworkers[91,289] proposed that a deficiency of creatine and creatine phosphate may account for both the histologic abnormalities in muscle and the chorioretinal degeneration. They suggest that the high ornithine concentrations inhibit glycine transamidinase, thereby reducing creatine synthesis and causing a reduction in total body creatine and creatine phosphate. Evidence supporting this hypothesis includes the well-documented sensitivity of glycine transamidinase to ornithine inhibition *in vitro*[91–93] and the observations that (a) fasting plasma guanidinoacetate, creatine, creatinine, (b) daily guanidinoacetate and creatinine excretion, and (c) the excretion of guanidinoacetate and creatine following an arginine load are all reduced in patients with gyrate atrophy as compared to normal subjects.[372,373] Additionally MRS studies show reduction by more than 50 percent of phosphocreatine levels in the skeletal muscle and basal ganglia of gyrate atrophy patients.[303,304] These observations indicate that glycine transamidinase is inhibited *in vivo* as well as *in vitro* and that there is a significant reduction of the total body creatine-creatine phosphate pool in gyrate atrophy patients. This hypothesis is consistent with the lack of ophthalmologic abnormalities in the HHH syndrome if the subcellular location of the transamidinase is within the mitochondria (Fig. 83-2).[374] The observations of histologic improvement in the muscles of gyrate atrophy patients given exogenous creatine,[375,376] of partial restoration of tissue phosphocreatine levels in a patient on an arginine-restricted diet with near normal ornithine levels,[304] and of modest improvement and/or stabilization of visual function in patients whose plasma ornithine has been reduced by means of an arginine-restricted diet[258,259,297,377,378] are in agreement with this hypothesis. Creatine excretion was low in two HHH syndrome patients on their regular diet (1.2 to 1.5 g/kg/day); however, it rose to normal levels despite pronounced hyperornithinemia, when supplements of arginine or ornithine (2 mM/kg/day) were added to the diet, suggesting that significant transamidinase activity was present.[374]

Although relatively little is known about the role of creatine and creatine phosphate in retinal function, studies in chicken retina strongly suggest that they play an important physiological function in the energy transduction of vision. Wallimann et al. found high concentrations of creatine kinase and creatine phosphate in rod and cone photoreceptor cells.[379] Two creatine kinase isoforms were identified and localized by immunofluorescence: the brain isoform was predominant and stained intensely over the inner segment of both rod and cone photoreceptors; the mitochondrial isoform was also present and was localized to the ellipsoid portion of the inner segments known to be rich in mitochondria. Creatine, creatine phosphate, and guanidinoacetate also are present in mammalian brain[87,96,380,381] but appear to cross the blood-brain barrier slowly.[382,383] Thus, local synthesis of creatine may be

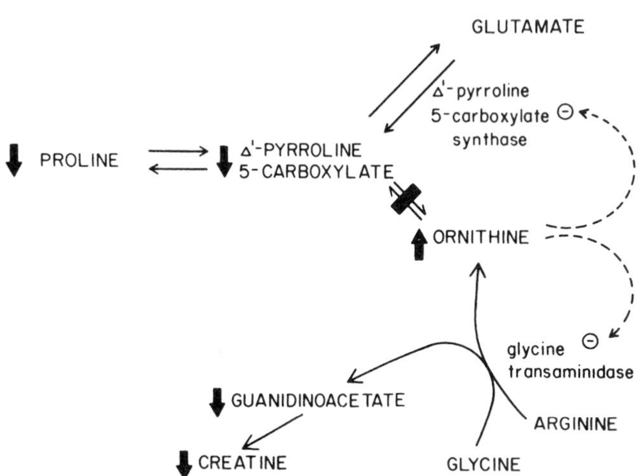

Fig. 83-18 Schematic diagram of two nonexclusive hypotheses for the pathophysiology of gyrate atrophy of the choroid and retina. In one, high ornithine concentrations inhibit glycine transamidinase, resulting in reduced synthesis of guanidinoacetate and creatine. In the other, the combination of the inherited deficiency of OAT (black rectangle) and the inhibitory effect of ornithine on Δ^1 pyrroline-5-carboxylate synthase results in decreased formation of Δ^1 pyrroline-5-carboxylate and proline.

important in brain and retina. Low glycine-transamidinase activity was found in human brain[384] but was not detected in retina.[199] Creatine phosphate also has been implicated as an important energy source for phagocytosis by peritoneal macrophages.[385] This is intriguing in view of the highly phagocytic nature of the retinal pigment epithelium, although there is no direct evidence of phagocytic abnormalities in gyrate atrophy patients. Pharmacologic agents that deplete tissues of creatine phosphate[89,382,383] and the possible reduction of creatine synthesis in other human and animal disorders[384a] provide unexploited possibilities for additional study of the role of creatine depletion in the pathophysiology of gyrate atrophy.

A second hypothesis for the pathophysiology of gyrate atrophy proposes deficient synthesis of P5C owing to the genetic deficiency of OAT and to inhibitory effects of ornithine on one isoform (the short isoform) of P5C synthase, the enzyme that catalyzes the formation of P5C from glutamate (Fig. 83-18).[386] Support for this model includes the observation that the short isoform of P5C synthase is inhibited *in vitro* by near-physiological concentrations of L-ornithine[218,386] and that ornithine in high concentrations (> 10 mM) is toxic to cells lacking OAT (gyrate atrophy fibroblasts or Chinese hamster ovary cells at concentrations tolerated by control cells).[194,387,388] This effect of ornithine is prevented by amino acids that inhibit P5C dehydrogenase, a P5C-consuming enzyme, and are partially prevented by the addition of exogenous P5C.[194,389] The hypothesis, therefore, predicts that the genetic defect in gyrate atrophy prevents the synthesis of P5C from ornithine and causes accumulation of an inhibitor (ornithine) of the alternative pathway of P5C synthesis. The reduced availability of P5C may be detrimental because of decreased proline synthesis or because it disrupts the regulatory roles that P5C and its metabolic interconversions have been shown to exert on the intracellular redox level and hexose monophosphate shunt activity.[390–394] Depending on the mechanism, cells with access to extracellular fluid proline or with the ability to synthesize P5C from proline by the proline oxidase reaction or with adequate levels of the long (ornithine-insensitive) isoform of P5C synthase are predicted to be unscathed in gyrate atrophy, thereby sparing most cells and tissues. However, retinal pigment epithelium neural retinal cells lack proline oxidase,[361] and, although the availability of proline in the extracellular fluid of retina is not known, it may be low, judging from the fact that proline crosses the blood-brain barrier poorly[395] and is virtually absent from the cerebrospinal fluid.[358] The level of expression and ratio of long to short isoform of P5C synthase in these cells remains to be determined.

Phang and his colleagues developed a sensitive, quantitative assay of P5C in biologic fluids and determined a normal human plasma value of 100 to 400 nM.[396] Pilot studies showed plasma P5C levels to be normal in gyrate atrophy patients,[397] as might be expected because the plasma compartment is exposed to tissues with proline oxidase. What is critical and as yet unknown, are the P5C and proline levels in the ocular tissues of patients with gyrate atrophy. Two additional observations support the notion of an important role for P5C in ocular metabolism: high P5C concentrations (3.3 μM or about 20 times those in plasma) were found in the aqueous humor of rabbits,[200] and P5C was shown to be a potent stimulant of lens hexose monophosphate shunt activity.[200,398]

The hypothesis involving deficient P5C synthesis would explain the lack of ocular abnormalities in the HHH syndrome based on normal P5C production from ornithine by intact OAT. The possible beneficial effects of reduced ornithine accumulation[258,259,368,377,378] would be explained as resulting from relief of the ornithine inhibition of P5C synthase. As with the first hypothesis, more information on retinal amino acid and energy metabolism in normal subjects and in patients with gyrate atrophy is required to evaluate this proposal.

Additional abnormalities of possible pathologic significance in gyrate atrophy include the modest reductions in the plasma concentrations of glutamate, glutamine, and lysine.[252,297] Of these, only lysine is reduced below the normal range. The hypolysinemia seems unlikely to be the cause of the chorioretinal degeneration because the reduced plasma levels do not indicate a true lysine deficiency[297] and because other conditions with hypolysinemia (e.g., lysinuric protein intolerance) are not associated with ocular problems.[399] However, mice receiving 5FMOrn for 3 weeks exhibited an ~50 percent reduction in brain lysine, in addition to a 22-fold increase in ornithine. This observation indicates that some effect of reduced tissue lysine cannot be dismissed and requires further study. Abnormalities of polyamines or their metabolites could also play a pathologic role in gyrate atrophy. The fragmentary available data suggest that serum spermine, spermidine, and putrescine concentrations are in the normal range in gyrate atrophy patients.[290] By contrast, animals receiving 5FMOrn exhibited modest increases in tissue putrescine levels and polyamine excretion, suggesting that further study of polyamine metabolism in gyrate atrophy also is necessary. Finally, the close chemical and metabolic relationships of ornithine with arginine, the precursor of NO, suggest that a disturbance of NO function or metabolism in the retina could result from ornithine accumulation (Fig. 83-2). In one recent study, NOS was localized to photoreceptor inner segments as well as certain amacrine cells in rabbit retina.[30] A mouse model homozygous for a knockout allele of neuronal NOS did not have morphologic alterations of the retina.[400] Despite this, investigation of NO metabolism in gyrate atrophy is warranted.

Treatment

The slow progression of the degenerative changes in gyrate atrophy and the difficulty in measuring small changes in ocular function objectively make evaluation of any therapy difficult.[269] Biochemical parameters (e.g., plasma amino acid concentrations) can be measured accurately, but until the pathophysiology is understood, there is no assurance that correcting the biochemical abnormalities in plasma will actually be beneficial. Four general approaches to the therapy of gyrate atrophy have been attempted: stimulation of residual OAT activity with pharmacologic doses of pyridoxine; correction of ornithine accumulation by reducing the intake of its precursor arginine and/or increasing renal ornithine losses; administering creatine; and administering proline.

Pyridoxine-Responsive Gyrate Atrophy. A response to pyridoxine (vitamin B_6), the precursor of the cofactor pyridoxal phosphate, should be an effective therapy regardless of the pathophysiological mechanisms, because the end result is a reduction in the accumulated precursor (ornithine) and an increased production of the reaction product (P5C). Administration of pharmacologic doses of pyridoxine hydrochloride (500 to 1000 mg/day) has been associated with a significant reduction in plasma ornithine in seven patients from six sibships.[268,269,280,281,316] The molecular basis for this phenotype has been shown for two OAT mutant alleles, V332M and A226V (see "Molecular Defects" above).[146,316,323] The actual reduction has averaged about 50 percent, although it is somewhat difficult to interpret these results because arginine intake was apparently not closely regulated during these trials. Where reported, plasma lysine returned to normal coincident with the decrease in plasma ornithine. Weleber and associates found that 15 to 20 mg/day of pyridoxine hydrochloride was just as effective as the higher dosage in some of their patients.[281] This is relevant in view of the association of peripheral neuropathy with chronic ingestion of large amounts of pyridoxine.[401,402] Fibroblast OAT activity in these patients responded *in vitro* to the addition of high concentrations of pyridoxal phosphate to the assay mixture.[290,309] In the patients followed by Weleber et al., despite initial promising results,[281] there has been mild progression of chorioretinal degeneration.[403] Similarly, two Japanese pyridoxine-responsive patients, aged 8 and 17, had some progression of their chorioretinal degeneration over 2 years while receiving 120 and 600 mg of pyridoxine, respectively.[404] Thus, the results of pyridoxine therapy in this small group of patients are disappointing. The possibility remains that at least the rate of progression has been slowed by this therapy.

Reduction of Ornithine by Nutritional Methods and/or Augmentation of Renal Losses. A second approach to the therapy of gyrate atrophy has involved correcting the ornithine accumulation by restricting dietary intake of arginine and/or by augmenting ornithine excretion. Reduction of ornithine should be beneficial if the pathophysiology of gyrate atrophy involves a direct toxic effect of ornithine or reduced synthesis of P5C, because high levels of ornithine may inhibit the alternate pathway of P5C synthesis (via P5C synthase; see "Pathophysiology" above). An arginine-restricted diet has been constructed by reducing protein intake to approximately 0.2 g/kg/day and supplying the necessary amounts of essential amino acids, calories, minerals, and vitamins.[259,269,297,298,368,378] On this regimen, plasma ornithine values have decreased two- to tenfold as ornithine is lost in the urine and consumed for polyamine synthesis. Several patients have maintained normal to near-normal ornithine values for extended periods (Fig. 83-18).[259,298] The secondary abnormalities in plasma lysine, glutamate, glutamine, and ammonia have improved coincident with the reduction in plasma ornithine. Care must be taken to avoid excessive restriction of arginine, which can lead to hypoargininemia, hypoornithinemia, and acute hyperammonemia, particularly if nitrogen intake is high.[298,378] Kaiser-Kupfer and Valle have instituted an arginine-restricted diet in more than 20 patients ranging in age from 2 to 47 years, all of whom had failed to show significant reduction in ornithine values after a 1- to 2-month trial of pharmacologic doses of pyridoxine.[258,259,377,378] A variety of problems with communication and compliance reduced the sample to 12 patients who adhered to the diet for more than 24 months. The degree of biochemical control is graded as good (plasma ornithine < 200 μM), fair (200 to 400 μM) and poor (> 400 μM). Only four patients have been consistently in the good range. Two women, both aged 34 at the time they started the diet, have had good biochemical control for more than 15 years.[405] Both had modest early improvement and subsequent stabilization in subjective and objective tests of visual function.[258,259,377] Other patients with good biochemical control have had some evidence of modest improvement or stabilization.[378] However, the disease has clearly progressed in older patients on the diet, who had control in the fair range.[259,406] Three Finnish patients, who were on the diet

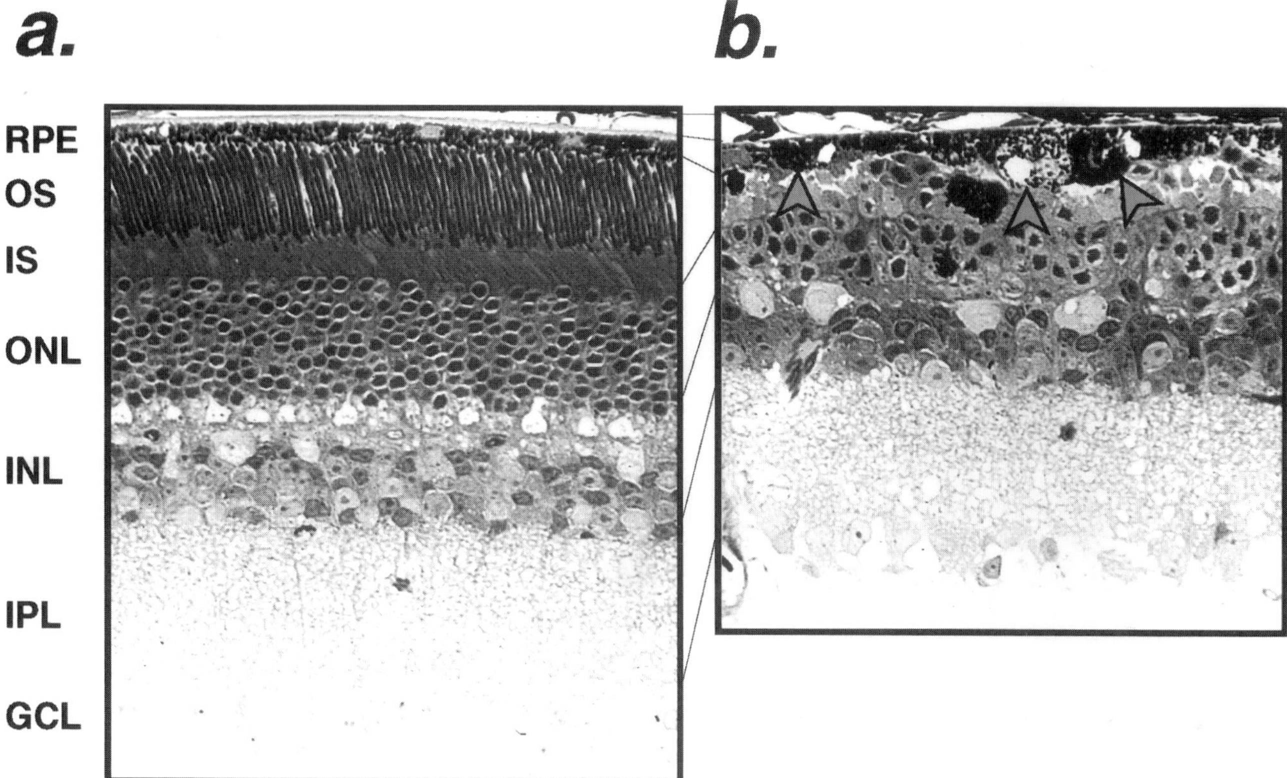

Fig. 83-19 Retinal histopathology of *Oat−/−* mice on an arginine-restricted diet (a) or a standard diet (b) at age 12 months. Note the reduced number of ONL cells and loss of IS and OS in the right panel. The arrows indicate abnormal RPE cells. GCL = ganglion cell layer; IPL = inner plexiform layer; INL = inner nuclear layer; ONL = outer nuclear layer; IS and OS = inner and outer segments, respectively, of photoreceptors.

for 3 to 5 years starting at ages 7 to 9 years, had evidence by fundus photography of enlargement of the atrophic areas, particularly in one patient.[407] The biochemical control of these patients was said to be good.

In an effort to reduce the variables that confound evaluation of this experimental treatment, Kaiser-Kupfer et al. reported 5 - to 7-year outcomes on two pairs of sibs with gyrate atrophy who were started on the diet before age 10.[368] In preliminary studies with six pairs of affected sibs, Kaiser-Kupfer et al. showed that intrafamilial phenotypic variability was less than interfamilial. This observation justified using the clinical phenotype of the older member of the sib pair at the time of diagnosis as a control for the younger, who, in each instance, was on the diet for 5 or more years by the time they reached the starting age of the older. Evaluations included psychophysical tests, electroretinography, and fundus photography. In both sib pairs, the younger had much less ocular disease than the older at the equivalent age, which has continued to the present.[408] Long-term reduction of ornithine levels with an arginine-restricted diet in the murine model of gyrate atrophy (see below) clearly prevents retinal degeneration (see Fig. 83-19).[409] These results strongly support the notion that long-term reduction of ornithine slows the progression of chorioretinal degeneration in gyrate atrophy. Furthermore, these results have implications for understanding the pathophysiological mechanism of the retinal degeneration and for the prospects for somatic gene therapy of gyrate atrophy. They suggest that it will not be necessary to express OAT in the retina to treat gyrate atrophy; rather, chronic systemic reduction of ornithine achieved by expression of OAT in any of a variety of nonocular sites should suffice.

Augmenting the renal losses of ornithine by administering compounds known to interfere with dibasic amino acid transport has been attempted alone or in combination with diet therapy. Lysine[282,297,387,410] and the nonmetabolizable amino acid α-aminoisobutyric acid[297,298] have been used for this purpose. Both have been shown to increase ornithine excretion, especially when plasma ornithine concentrations are high. As plasma ornithine concentrations decrease (particularly below 300 μM), these compounds become much less effective.[297,298] No studies of the long-term efficacy of this approach have been reported.

Creatine Administration. A third form of therapy for gyrate atrophy derives from the hypothesis that creatine deficiency plays a pathophysiological role in this disorder. Sipila and coworkers administered 1.5 g of creatine daily to seven gyrate atrophy patients for 1 year.[375] All the patients showed improvement in the histologic abnormalities in muscle; however, four patients had some progression in their ophthalmologic abnormalities documented by fundus photography. A 5-year follow-up of 13 patients treated with creatine also showed continued progress of the chorioretinal degeneration and persistent correction of the histologic abnormalities in skeletal muscle.[376] MRS spectroscopy confirms that oral creatine supplementation increases tissue levels of phosphocreatine in skeletal muscle[411] and basal ganglia.[304] These results indicate that creatine depletion does play a role in the muscle abnormalities. The progression of the ocular abnormalities despite administration of creatine suggests either that the pathophysiology of the chorioretinal degeneration has a different basis or that at the dose used an inadequate amount of creatine reached the sensitive cells in the eye.

Proline Therapy. A final experimental therapy tried for gyrate atrophy is the administration of proline, on the rationale that deficient formation of this nonessential amino acid is the major cause of the chorioretinal degeneration.[404,412] Because plasma proline concentrations are normal in gyrate atrophy, Hayasaka et al. proposed that deficient local synthesis of proline in retinal tissues is critical and cannot be compensated by normal levels of circulating proline.[404] The reasons why a local deficiency of both P5C and proline may occur in retina are discussed above under "Pathophysiology." In further support of this hypothesis, the investigators cite a patient with increased excretion of proline and the other amino acids, normal ornithine levels, and a chorioretinal degeneration resembling atypical gyrate atrophy.[404] Plasma proline was normal. How the excessive renal losses could result in chorioretinal degeneration despite normal plasma proline levels was not addressed. Chorioretinal degeneration is not a feature of iminoglycinuria (see Chap. 194). Nevertheless, these investigators treated 4 patients, aged 5 to 32, with oral proline supplements in doses ranging from 65 to 488 mg/kg/day. Plasma proline varied from unchanged to threefold increased. The youngest patient had a "minimal" increase in the atrophic area and "slight" deterioration of the electroretinogram over 5 years. An 8-year-old patient showed clear progression of the chorioretinal degeneration over 3 years, while 2 older patients, aged 23 and 32, showed no progression over 3 years. Thus, the outcome for these patients is mixed. Furthermore, because the hypothesis involving a pathologic local proline deficiency in the retina depends on a lack of entry of proline into retina from blood, it is not clear how supplemental proline can be expected to be of therapeutic benefit.

Genetics

The inheritance of gyrate atrophy is autosomal recessive. Males and females are equally affected; consanguinity is common in the reported pedigrees;[249,254,259,413] and obligate heterozygotes have partially reduced OAT activity (Table 83-4).

Gyrate atrophy is rare, with approximately 200 biochemically confirmed cases known to us. The nationality of the patients has included Finnish, Spanish, Italian, Dutch, English, Welsh, Polish, Portuguese, Japanese, Turkish, Mexican, Nicaraguan, German, Greek, and Russian.[259] One American black family with multiple affected sibs has been described briefly.[259,414] The incidence apparently is highest in Finland, with an estimated frequency of about 1 in 50,000 individuals and an estimated frequency for heterozygotes of 1 in 110 individuals. In the United States, the disorder is much rarer. A comprehensive survey of all university-affiliated ophthalmology departments in Japan yielded 15 patients.[254]

A Mouse Model of Gyrate Atrophy. Wang and colleagues produced a mouse model of gyrate atrophy by targeted disruption of the murine OAT gene.[177,371,409] The metabolic phenotype of these animals was informative and lead to better understanding of the metabolic derangements in human gyrate atrophy patients. OAT-deficient mice appear normal at birth but cease feeding, become lethargic, and die 24 to 48 h after birth. This lethal outcome was surprising in view of the apparent lack of symptoms in human neonates with gyrate atrophy. Recognizing that one of the metabolic roles of the reversible OAT reaction was to participate in the pathway for *de novo* arginine synthesis in the mucosa of the small intestine, Wang et al.[177] treated the OAT-deficient mice with L-arginine (10 mmol/kg/dose given every 12 h from birth by intraperitoneal [i.p.] injection). This treatment rescued the mice and was required only for the first 14 days of life, a time frame that correlates with the transient high expression of OAT in the intestine of normal mice. Premature discontinuation of the arginine injections invariably was followed within 24 to 48 h by the development of lethargy, onset of a high frequency tremor, and death. Administration of a single i.p. injection of arginine early in the course of this decline rescued the animals. Metabolic studies in these symptomatic animals revealed subnormal plasma ornithine, citrulline, and arginine as well as hyperammonemia and orotic aciduria. These data indicate that the net flux in the OAT reaction in the neonatal period is in the direction of ornithine synthesis rather than degradation and that the survival of the rapidly growing neonatal mouse depends on an intact OAT reaction to synthesize ornithine and arginine. This is consistent with the observations of Davis et al. who showed with metabolic balance studies that neonatal rats have an obligatory requirement for net arginine synthesis.[415] Additional information on the role of intestinal mucosal OAT in arginine biosynthesis has been reported by Matsuzawa et al.[416]

Stimulated by their observations in OAT-deficient mice, Wang et al. considered the metabolic phenotype of human neonates with gyrate atrophy.[177] Typically, gyrate atrophy patients do not come to medical attention until they develop visual symptoms in childhood, so there were no previously published data on gyrate atrophy infants. However, in a single, asymptomatic, 2-month-old human infant with gyrate atrophy ingesting breast milk supplemented with a standard infant formula, Wang et al. found hypoornithinemia, hypoargininemia, hyperglutaminemia, and mild hyperammonemia.[177] Supplementation with arginine corrected all these abnormalities and produced hyperornithinemia. These results suggest that the metabolic derangements in human infants with gyrate atrophy are qualitatively similar to those in the OAT-deficient mouse but not as severe, perhaps because of the slower growth rate of humans. The results also suggested that some gyrate atrophy patients may present with hyperammonemia and low levels of ornithine and arginine in infancy. This expectation has been confirmed. In particular, premature infants with gyrate atrophy may have profound hyperammonemia and may be misdiagnosed as OTC deficient.[238–240] At what age the direction of net flux in the OAT reaction reverses is not known, although 1- to 2-year-old gyrate atrophy patients have typical hyperornithinemia.

Post-weaning, the rescued OAT-deficient mice on a regular diet without arginine supplementation develop ornithine accumulation and lysine reduction to an extent similar to or even greater than humans with gyrate atrophy. Like humans with gyrate atrophy, these animals develop a slowly progressive retinal degeneration. At 2 months their electroretinograms are normal but by 12 months the amplitude is reduced to about 40 percent of normal. At 2 months the retinas of the OAT-deficient animals showed minimal histologic abnormalities but by 7 months the photoreceptor outer segments were shortened and markedly disorganized, particularly in the central superior and inferior retinal regions. By 10 months there was a cumulative 33 percent loss of photoreceptor cells. At the ultrastructural level, the first morphologic abnormalities were swelling of scattered RPE cells. By 7 months there was extensive degeneration of both the RPE and photoreceptors. Thus, the OAT-deficient mouse appears to be an excellent metabolic and retinal model of gyrate atrophy.[371] Future studies with these animals should be useful in understanding the retinal pathophysiology of gyrate atrophy and in developing treatments for this blinding disorder.

Subsequent studies with this model by Wang et al. showed definitively that reduction of plasma ornithine levels by restriction of dietary arginine completely prevents retinal degeneration (Fig. 83-19).[409]

HYPERORNITHINEMIA-HYPERAMMONEMIA-HOMOCITRULLINURIA (HHH) SYNDROME

In 1969, Shih and coworkers[241] described the first patient with the fascinating combination of increased plasma ornithine concentration, postprandial hyperammonemia, and homocitrullinuria. We currently know of more than 40 patients from a variety of ethnic backgrounds.[241,272,374,417–443] Autosomal recessive inheritance is suggested by the fact that several patients are from consanguineous matings and multiple cases have occurred in siblings. Increased plasma ornithine concentration differentiates the syndrome from the other urea cycle disorders, and postprandial hyperammonemia and homocitrullinuria distinguish it from gyrate atrophy.

Clinical Phenotype

The symptoms appear during the newborn period[374,417,418,424,429,441] or childhood[439] or may be delayed until late adulthood.[419,426] Pregnancy is uncomplicated, birth size normal, and the neonatal course often uneventful if the children are breast-fed. Most patients have typical histories of intermittent hyperammonemia. Many refuse to eat and have vomiting, lethargy, and even episodes of coma when fed high-protein formula or other high-protein foods. After infancy, most patients spontaneously select a low-protein diet avoiding milk and meat.

Some patients survive to adulthood relatively free of symptoms, but, usually, periods of lethargy, vomiting, ataxia, or choreoathetosis or delayed development bring the patient to medical attention during infancy or childhood. Growth is impaired, and developmental milestones are delayed. Muscle hypotonia may occur; spasticity is common later. Seizures are not uncommon; they may begin in infancy[374,419–421] and resemble infantile spasms,[241] but they often appear later.[418–421,424,433] The mental outcome has varied from low normal intelligence to severe retardation. The ocular fundi have been normal when described except in one patient, a 6-year-old French Canadian girl, who had myopia, retinal depigmentation, and chorioretinal atrophy—all changes that have been observed in gyrate atrophy.[419] The size of the liver and spleen is normal or slightly enlarged. An increased bleeding tendency was an associated feature in three patients[374,419,424] and was the leading clinical sign in one.[424]

Light microscopy of liver biopsy samples has yielded normal results, but, ultrastructurally, liver mitochondria were elongated and had bizarre shapes and a peculiar periodicity below the level of the inner limiting membrane.[419,425,444–447] The longest mitochondria contained "crystalloid" structures, probably representing elongated systems of cristae or tubules. Occasional liver samples have showed normal ultrastructure.[426] The mitochondria of cultured fibroblasts contained triangular structures resembling changes seen in the liver.[448] Loosely laminated structures resembling myelin figures have also been reported in increased numbers in the cytoplasm of the fibroblasts. Abnormal mitochondria also have been found in muscle and leukocytes.[419]

One patient, maintained on a diet of 1 g/kg/day protein restriction during her whole pregnancy, gave birth to a normal child.[419]

Biochemical Phenotype

Plasma ornithine concentrations on an unlimited diet have ranged from 200 to 1020 μM. The values overlap with those in patients with gyrate atrophy but are usually slightly lower. Restriction of protein intake diminishes hyperornithinemia, and, with extreme restrictions, the values may reach the normal range.[241,374,421] Plasma arginine is normal, lysine moderately decreased, and glutamine and alanine often increased owing to accumulation of waste nitrogen. Interestingly, protein restriction has in some instances led to a further elevation in plasma glutamine.[49,241] Fasting plasma ammonium is usually within the normal range even though the mean value is slightly higher in patients than in control subjects. Ammonia values increase after protein ingestion, and high-protein diets result in chronic hyperammonemia. Oral loading tests with 0.1 or 0.2 g of ornithine per kilogram body weight cause greater than normal increases in plasma ornithine, and the return to initial concentrations is slow. The responses of plasma citrulline and ornithine to citrulline loads, of plasma lysine to lysine loads, and of plasma and urinary homocitrulline to lysine and homocitrulline loads are indistinguishable from normal.[241,419–421,426,429,446]

Ornithinuria is highly variable (Table 83-7). Interestingly, identical plasma ornithine concentrations in patients with either the HHH syndrome or gyrate atrophy lead to higher ornithine excretions in the latter,[255,301] implying that kidney OAT has a role in ornithine reabsorption. The level of urine homocitrulline also greatly exceeds normal. Its excretion correlates weakly with lysine ingestion, and its renal tubular reabsorption is normal and is unaffected by citrulline loads.[241,418,428,446] Altogether, the regulation of homocitrulline excretion remains unclear. Urine of the patients also contains excessive amounts of the δ-lactam of ornithine, 3-amino-piperid-2-one, first believed to be ornithine methyl ester[272,418,422,446,449] and of γ-glutamylornithine, another uncommon derivative of ornithine[301] (Table 83-7). Both substances also are found in the urine of patients with gyrate atrophy. Their origin and physiological significance are unknown. Several other γ-glutamyl amino acids have been characterized in human urine.[301] Other unidentified peptides are also present in the urine of the patients with either form of hyperornithinemia, as indicated by the fact that hydrolysis of the urine significantly increases the amount of free ornithine detected (free ornithine increases from 41 to 59 percent of total ornithine in patients with the HHH syndrome, and from 76 to 83 percent in patients with gyrate atrophy).

Excretion of creatine was subnormal in two HHH syndrome patients[374] (Table 83-7). Low creatine excretion is also a feature of gyrate atrophy, supporting the hypothesis that the accumulated

Table 83-7 Urinary Excretion of Free Ornithine, Homocitrulline, Orotic Acid, 3-Amino-piperid-2-one, Polyamines, Creatine, and Creatinine by Patients with the HHH Syndrome*

	Patients			Control		
	Mean	Range	Number of Subjects	Number of Subjects	Mean	Range
Free ornithine†	656	2–8160	16	32	10	9–120
Homocitrulline	565	20–2380	21	29	20	Trace–90
Orotic acid	410	52–1520	17	21	22	< 10–130
3-Amino-piperid-1-one	294	95–459	3	6	ND‡	
γ-Glutamylornithine	34	13–67	8	8	Trace	
Polyamines, total	132**		1	1	21 ± 7††	
Creatine	16	11–21	2	1		41–104
Creatinine	113	97–130	2	1		88–132

*The data are compiled from all cases referred to in the text.[241,374,417–440] If possible, values are for samples taken while the patients were on an unlimited diet. The units are μmol/g creatinine for all except creatine and creatinine, which are in μmol per kilogram body weight per day.
†In eight patients studied for excretion of free and total hydrolyzable ornithine, free ornithine comprised 47% (41 to 59%) of total ornithine.[301]
‡ND = not detectable.
**This value is from urine collected while the patient was on an unrestricted diet.
††Mean ± SD of four controls on an unrestricted diet.

ornithine inhibits glycine transamidinase, the first enzyme in the creatine biosynthetic pathway (Fig. 83-2). Orotic acid excretion, believed to reflect carbamyl phosphate accumulation, is elevated (Table 83-7), suggesting that intramitochondrial carbamyl phosphate is underused.[374,419,420,422,427,429–433] Urinary orotate levels are often increased even though blood ammonia values are normal.[319] Urinary excretion of polyamines (total; including putrescine, cadaverine, spermidine, and spermine) was increased in the one patient studied[425,442] (Table 83-7). The excretion rates decreased markedly when the protein content of the diet was decreased, and even further when supplementary ornithine was added to the low-protein diet.

The possibility that an enzymatic deficiency causes this syndrome has been investigated, but no consistent or convincing defects have been demonstrated. The activity of carbamyl phosphate synthase is normal in the liver,[425–427,433] although an early report suggested it was moderately reduced in both liver and fibroblasts.[419] Other urea cycle enzymes measured in leukocytes and liver have been normal.[419,425–427,433] The content of *N*-acetylglutamate, an activator of carbamyl phosphate synthase, was normal in the mitochondrial pellet of liver homogenates.[427,433] The activity of OAT, the major ornithine-catabolizing enzyme, is normal in liver, fibroblasts, and other tissues of the patients.[419,421,425,427,433] Ornithine decarboxylase in cultured fibroblasts was 20 to 30 percent of the normal mean in one patient,[450] but urinary excretion of polyamines was increased in another study[425] (Table 83-6). The production of ATP by the respiring mitochondria was adequate.[427] The importance of an unknown, prominent heavy protein band in SDS-polyacrylamide gel-electrophoresis of the liver of a Japanese patient is unclear.[425]

Screening systems based on detecting an increased plasma ornithine concentration will detect patients with the HHH syndrome and those with gyrate atrophy of the choroid and retina[245] (see "Differential Diagnosis of Hyperornithinemia" above). There is, however, no practical experience of these screening methods. A potential problem is that plasma ornithine values in the HHH syndrome may be within the normal range during the newborn period, as suggested by the fact that stored blood spots from a patient with the HHH syndrome taken at 5 days and 4 weeks of age and studied several years later failed to reveal any abnormality.[241] However, hyperornithinemia, hyperammonemia, and homocitrullinuria were clearly demonstrable in another patient at the age of 19 days.[429]

Molecular Basis of the HHH Syndrome

Recent studies identified mitochondrial carrier family (MCF) proteins that transport ornithine across the inner mitochondrial membrane of *Neurospora crassa* (ARG13) and *S. cerevisiae* (ARG11).[451–453] MCF proteins are composed of approximately 300 amino acids and consist of three repeated motifs (of ~100 amino acids), each with two hydrophobic α helical segments connected by an extensive hydrophilic sequence. The topologic model of MCF proteins predicts six transmembrane segments with the N- and C-termini on one side of the membrane and the hydrophilic loops on the other.[454] They are thought to function as homodimers.[455,456] All 13 mitochondrial metabolite transporters characterized to date are MCF proteins[454,457–459] and an ornithine transporter purified from rat liver had features of an MCF protein.[51,460,461]

With this background information, Camacho et al. probed the expressed sequence-tagged (EST) database with the amino acid sequences of ARG13 and ARG11 and identified several mammalian potential orthologs. Expression of one of these (designated ORNT1) restored normal ornithine metabolism in fibroblasts from HHH patients. The human ORNT1 protein is a typical MCF protein of 301 amino acids with 95 percent identity to murine ORNT1 and 27 percent identity to ARG13 and ARG11 (Fig. 83-20). There are three repeats of approximately 100 amino acids and each repeat has 2 predicted transmembrane α-helices separated by a hydrophilic segment. Moreover, there is a typical MCF signature sequence of P-h-D/E-X-h-R/K-X-R/K-(20–30aa)-D/E-G-(4aa)-a-R/K-G (where *h* is hydrophobic and *a* is aromatic) at the C-terminus of the first transmembrane domain in each repeat.[454,462] The ORNT1 structural gene was localized to 13q14. In a survey of 11 HHH probands, these investigators identified three mutant alleles that accounted for 21 of the possible 22 mutant ORNT1 genes in this patient collection.[463] One mutant allele, F188Δ, was common in French Canadian HHH patients and was shown to encode an unstable protein with no residual function. A second mutant allele, E180K, encoded a stable protein that correctly targeted to the mitochondrion but had no residual function. The third mutant allele was a 13q14 microdeletion. These results confirmed that mutations in the ORNT1 gene are responsible for the HHH syndrome. A subsequent report by Tsujino et al. described the organization of the ORNT1 gene and identified three additional mutant alleles.[464]

Pathophysiology of the HHH Syndrome

Ammonia accumulation can be reduced or prevented *in vitro* in isolated hepatocytes and *in vivo* in animals and patients with other types of urea cycle disorders by increasing the availability of the urea cycle intermediates arginine, ornithine, or citrulline.[465–470] Accordingly, the hyperornithinemia of gyrate atrophy is associated with hypoammonemia.[297] The paradoxical combination of hyperornithinemia and hyperammonemia in the HHH syndrome has led to extensive studies on the mechanisms involved. The findings favored the original notion of Fell and coworkers that the basic defect is in the transport of ornithine across the inner mitochondrial membrane into the mitochondrial matrix.[418] This hypothesis was confirmed by the identification of ORNT1 as the gene responsible for HHH.[463] The entry of ornithine into liver mitochondria is carrier-mediated and may be dependent on respiratory energy[48–51,53,471–477] (see "Subcellular Compartmentation and Transport of Ornithine" above).

The decrease in carrier-mediated entry of ornithine into mitochondria in the HHH cells decreases citrulline synthesis and impairs ammonia detoxication. Furthermore, because OAT, the major ornithine-catabolizing enzyme, is also located in the mitochondria, diminished entry of ornithine leads to ornithine accumulation in the cytosolic and extracellular fluids. This model predicts that increasing the cytosolic ornithine might drive transmitochondrial ornithine transport and improve the patients' urea cycle function. With this rationale in mind, Fell and coworkers[418] gave their patient supplements of 6 g ornithine daily. This treatment doubled the plasma ornithine concentration and clearly reduced the plasma ammonium concentration. Other studies have supported the idea that supplementation with ornithine and arginine will reduce plasma ammonium and improve protein tolerance.[374,420,422,425,426,429,478] However, in some patients, ornithine or arginine supplementation has had little effect,[241,429] and high levels of arginine supplementation have even been deleterious.[420] In one patient, the hyperammonemia induced by alanine infusion remained unaltered even when the test was preceded by daily supplements of 6 g ornithine for 1 week and intravenous infusion of ornithine for 2 h before and during the alanine load.[429] These differences in responses to ornithine supplementation suggest that there is heterogeneity in the basic defect(s) causing this biochemical phenotype.

Several attempts have been made to directly characterize ornithine transport by the mitochondria of HHH patients. Hommes and coworkers[420,421,479] used digitonin to make the fibroblast cell membrane permeable to amino acids without damaging the mitochondria and then measured the accumulation of ornithine in the particulate fraction of such cells; this fraction is mainly composed of mitochondria. Their findings supported the view that the influx of ornithine into the mitochondria is decreased in the cells of patients with HHH syndrome. In another study of a single patient, a defect in ornithine uptake was directly demonstrated using isolated liver mitochondria.[433] Shih et al.[430] and others[422,427,429,433,446,480–483] have shown that the net capacity of

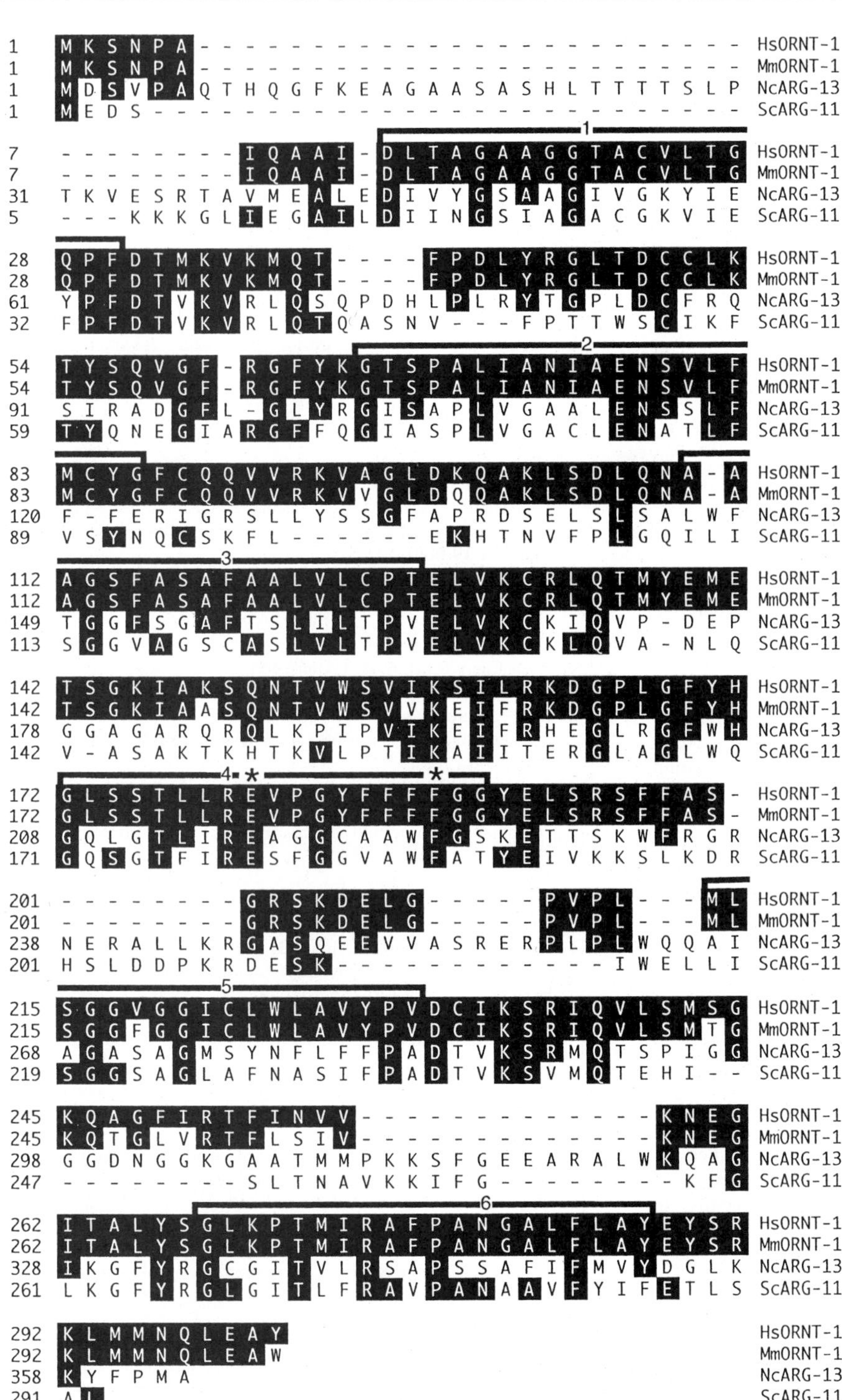

Fig. 83-20 Sequence alignment of human (Hs), mouse (Mm), *N. crassa* (Nc), and *S. cerevesiae* (Sc) MCF ornithine transporters. Amino acids identical to the human sequence are highlighted. The putative transmembrane domains are indicated by the filled lines and are numbered. Asterisks mark the sites of mutations identified in HHH patients (E180K and F188Δ).

cultured HHH fibroblasts or stimulated lymphocytes to metabolize ornithine is decreased. The cells transfer the label from 1-[^{14}C]-, 5-[^{14}C]-, or U-[^{14}C]ornithine into tissue proteins, proline, glutamate, aspartate, and CO_2 much less efficiently than do control cells, but the conversion of the labeled substrate from glutamate to proline occurs normally. In liver, citrulline synthesis by HHH syndrome mitochondria is significantly decreased.[427]

Additional indirect evidence in favor of a mitochondrial transport defect for ornithine comes from complementation assays of Shih et al.,[430,478] who have shown that heterokaryons formed from HHH syndrome and gyrate atrophy (OAT-negative) cells are able to metabolize ornithine normally. The origin of homocitrulline in these patients is uncertain. Excessive amounts of homocitrulline are also excreted by some patients with hyperlysinemia and saccharopinuria.[484–486] The hypothesis of Fell et al.[299] for the pathophysiology of this syndrome predicts that lysine uptake into mitochondria is normal and that the increased lysine:ornithine ratio in the mitochondrial matrix leads to ornithine transcarbamylase-catalyzed conversion of lysine to homocitrulline. Carter and coworkers have studied transcarbamylation of lysine more closely in digitonin-treated rat liver mitochondria.[487] Their results suggest that two separate carbamylases exist, one for ornithine and another for lysine, and that the lysine transcarbamylase is located outside the inner mitochondrial membrane. In one HHH syndrome patient, lysine supplementation was followed by a significant rise in homocitrulline excretion.[418] However, the plasma ammonium concentration increased simultaneously, suggesting that this pathway cannot be used for removal of excessive carbamyl phosphate and ammonia in these patients. In a few other patients, acute lysine loads and prolonged lysine supplementation have failed to show a clear correlation between the ingested lysine and excreted homocitrulline, leaving several questions on the metabolism of this amino acid unanswered.[422,428,446]

Treatment

Protein restriction to less than 1.2 g/kg/day prevents postprandial hyperammonemia and results in decreased concentrations of plasma ornithine. If decreased transport of ornithine into the mitochondria is the primary abnormality in this syndrome, the patients may benefit from ornithine supplementation; that is, from additional elevation of ornithine concentrations. In one patient, the addition of 6 g ornithine or 7.5 g arginine daily to the diet decreased plasma ammonium to normal or near-normal values, while fasting plasma ornithine rose to as high as 1.5 mM.[418] No immediate adverse effects of this pronounced hyperornithinemia were noted. Despite this, it would seem prudent to follow any patient with ornithine values in this range with periodic ophthalmologic examinations and electroretinograms. In a carefully conducted study by Gordon et al.,[446] an ornithine supplement given with a protein load significantly reduced hyperammonemia. Prolonged ornithine supplementation (0.5 to 1.0 mM/kg/day; i.e., 66 to 132 mg/kg/day divided into three doses) improved patients' protein tolerance and accelerated growth. Arginine and citrulline also are effective. The authors prefer citrulline which has the added benefit of consuming additional nitrogen as it is converted to arginine. Interestingly, alanine-induced hyperammonemia could not be prevented in another patient by ornithine supplement (see "Pathophysiology of the HHH Syndrome" above);[424] the minimal or even harmful effects of ornithine or arginine supplementation in some other patients[420,429] also suggest that the disease may indeed be heterogeneous. Interestingly, orotic acid excretion has been increased in several patients even when plasma ammonium levels were normal, implying that orotic aciduria is a better indicator of the impairment of ureagenesis in these patients.

Genetics

The large Canadian pedigree of Gatfield et al.,[419] with six affected subjects from both sexes, additional reports of more than one affected member in the same sibship, and the existence consanguinity in many families, strongly suggested autosomal recessive inheritance of the syndrome. This was confirmed by molecular studies of ORNT1.[463] So far, few attempts have been made to characterize the heterozygotes biochemically. In all cases studied, plasma and urine amino acid concentrations and the responses of the heterozygotes to ornithine loads were normal.[241,417,421,422]

The association of the HHH syndrome with deficiency of coagulation factors VII and X in four patients from three different ethnic backgrounds[374,419,424,443] is intriguing. Certainly, the clotting profile of all patients with this disorder should be determined.

ACKNOWLEDGMENTS

We thank Sandy Muscelli for help in the preparation of this chapter. Studies contributing to the information in this chapter were supported in part by National Eye Institute Grant EY02948 and by a grant from the Foundation Fighting Blindness. David Valle is an investigator with the Howard Hughes Medical Institute.

REFERENCES

1. Snodgrass PJ: The effects of pH on the kinetics of human liver ornithine-carbamyl phosphate transferase. *Biochemistry* **7**:3047, 1968.
2. Marshall A, Cohen PP: Ornithine transcarbamylase from *Streptococcus faecalis* and bovine liver. *J Biol Chem* **247**:1654, 1972.
3. Marshall M: Ornithine transcarbamylase from bovine liver, in Grisolia S, Baguena R, Mayor F (eds): *The Urea Cycle*. New York, Wiley, 1976, p 169.
4. Schimke RT: Adaptive characteristics of urea cycle enzymes in the rat. *J Biol Chem* **237**:459, 1962.
5. Nuzum CT, Snodgrass PJ: Urea cycle enzyme adaptation to dietary protein in primates. *Science* **172**:1042, 1971.
6. Morris SMJ, Moncman CL, Rand KD, Dizikes GJ, Cederbaum SJ, O'Brien WE: Regulation of mRNA levels for five urea cycle enzymes in rat liver by diet, cyclic AMP, and glucocorticoids. *Arch Biochem Biophys* **256**:343, 1987.
7. Hata A, Tsuzuki T, Shimada K, Takiguchi M, Mori M, Matsuda I: Isolation and characterization of the human ornithine transcarbamylase gene: Structure of the 5′-end region. *Biochem J* **100**:717, 1986.
8. Takiguchi M, Murakami T, Miura S, Mori M: Structure of the rat ornithine carbamoyltransferase gene, a large, X chromosome linked gene with an atypical promoter. *Proc Natl Acad Sci U S A* **84**:6136, 1987.
9. Murakami T, Nishiyori A, Takiguchi M, Mori M: Promoter and 11 kilobase upstream enhancer elements responsible for hepatoma cell-specific expression of the rat ornithine transcarbamylase gene. *Mol Cell Biol* **10**:1180, 1990.
10. Jones SN, Grompe M, Munir MI, Veres G, Craigen WJ, Caskey CT: Ectopic correction of ornithine transcarbamylase deficiency in sparse fur mice. *J Biol Chem* **265**:14684, 1990.
11. Kimura A, Nishiyori A, Maurakami T, Tsukamoto T, Hata S, Osumi T, Okamura R, Mori M, Takiguchi M: Chicken ovalbumin upstream promoter-transcription factor (COUP-TF) represses transcription from the promoter of the gene for ornithine transcarbamylase in a manner antagonistic to hepatocyte nuclear factor-4 (HNF-4). *J Biol Chem* **268**:11125, 1993.
12. Nishiyori A, Tashiro H, Kimura A, Akagi K, Yamamura K, Mori M, Takiguchi M: Determination of tissue specificity of the enhancer by combinatorial operation of tissue-enriched transcription factors. *J Biol Chem* **269**:1323, 1994.
13. Beliveau-Carey G, Cheung C-W, Cohen NS, Brusilow SW, Raijman L: Regulation of urea and citrulline synthesis under physiological conditions. *Biochem J* **292**:241, 1993.
14. Cohen MS, Cheung C-W, Sijuwade E, Raijman L: Kinetic properties of carbamoyl-phosphate synthase (ammonia) and ornithine carbamoyltransferase in permeabilized mitochondria. *Biochem J* **282**:173, 1992.
15. Hayase K, Yonekawa G, Yoshida A: Changes in liver concentration of *N*-acetylglutamate and ornithine are involved in regulating urea synthesis in rats treated with thyroid hormone. *J Nutr* **122**:1143, 1992.
16. Stewart PM, Walser M: Short-term regulation of ureagenesis. *J Biol Chem* **255**:5270, 1980.
17. Meijer AJ: Regulation of carbamoyl-phosphate synthase (ammonia) in liver in relation to urea cycle activity. *Biochem Sci* **4**:83, 1979.
18. Cohen MS, Cheung CW, Raijman L: Channeling of extramitochondrial ornithine to matrix ornithine transcarbamylase. *J Biol Chem* **262**:203, 1987.
19. Raijman I: Enzyme and reactant concentrations and the regulation of urea synthesis, in Grisolia S, Baguena R, Mayor F (eds): *The Urea Cycle*. New York, Wiley, 1976, p 243.
20. Kuo F, Darnell JJ: Evidence that interaction of hepatocytes with the collecting (hepatic) veins triggers position-specific transcription of the glutamine synthetase and ornithine aminotransferase genes in the mouse liver. *Mol Cell Biol* **11**:6050, 1991.
21. Carey GP, Kime Z, Rogers QR, Morris JG, Hargrove D, Buffington CA, Brusilow SW: An arginine-deficient diet in humans does not evoke hyperorotic acidemia. *J Nutr* **117**:1734, 1987.
22. De Mars R, Le Van SL, Trend BL, Russell LB: Abnormal ornithine carbamoyl transferase in mice having the sparse-fur mutation. *Proc Natl Acad Sci U S A* **73**:1693, 1976.
23. Hodges PE, Rosenberg LE: The *spf*^{ash} mouse: A missense mutation in the ornithine transcarbamylase gene also causes aberrant mRNA splicing. *Proc Natl Acad Sci U S A* **86**:4142, 1989.
24. Veres G, Gibbs R, Scherer S, Caskey C: The molecular basis of the sparse fur mouse mutation. *Science* **237**:415, 1987.
25. Lowenstein CJ, Snyder SH: Nitric oxide, a novel biologic messenger. *Cell* **70**:705, 1992.
26. Lowenstein CJ, Dinerman JL, Snyder SH: Nitric oxide: A physiologic messenger. *Ann Intern Med* **120**:227, 1994.
27. Kerwin JFJ, Heller M: The arginine-nitric oxide pathway: A target for new drugs. *Med Res Rev* **14**:23, 1994.

28. Janssens SP, Shimouchi A, Quertermous T, Bloch DB: Cloning and expression of a cDNA encoding human endothelium-derived relaxing factor/nitric oxide synthase. *J Biol Chem* **267**:14519, 1992.
29. White KA, Marletta MA: Nitric oxide synthase is a cytochrome P-450 type hemoprotein. *Biochemistry* **31**:6627, 1992.
30. Osborne NN, Barnett NL, Herrera AJ: NADPH diaphorase localization and nitric oxide synthetase activity in the retina and anterior uvea of the rabbit eye. *Brain Res* **610**:194, 1993.
31. Shiells R, Falk G: Retinal on-bipolar cells contain a nitric oxide-sensitive guanylate cyclase. *Neuro Report* **3**:845, 1992.
32. Venturini C, Knowles R, Palmer R, Moncada S: Synthesis of nitric oxide in the bovine retina. *Biochem Biophys Res Commun* **180**:920, 1991.
33. Reddi PK, Knox WE, Herzfeld A: Types of arginase in rat tissues. *Enzyme* **20**:305, 1975.
34. Soberon G, Palacios R: Arginase, in Grisolia S, Baguena R, Mayor F (eds): *The Urea Cycle*. New York, Wiley, 1976, p 221.
35. Grody WW, Dizikes GJ, Cederbaum SD: Human arginase isozymes. Isozymes. *Curr Top Biol Med Res* **13**:181, 1987.
36. Carvajai N, Cederbaum SD: Kinetics of inhibition of rat liver and kidney arginases by proline and branched chain amino acids. *Biochim Biophys Acta* **870**:181, 1986.
37. Aebi H: Coordinated changes in enzymes of the ornithine cycle and response to dietary conditions, in Grisolia S, Baguena R, Mayor E (eds): *The Urea Cycle*. New York, Wiley, 1976, p 275.
38. Bedino ST: Allosteric regulation of beef liver arginase activity by L-ornithine. *Ital J Biochem* **26**:264, 1977.
39. Haraguchi Y, Takiguchi M, Amaya Y, Kawamoto S, Matsuda I, Mori M: Molecular cloning and nucleotide sequence of cDNA for human liver arginase. *Proc Natl Acad Sci U S A* **84**:412, 1987.
40. Ohtake A, Takiguchi M, Shigeto Y, Amaya Y, Kawamoto S, Mori M: Structural organization of the gene for rat liver-type arginase. *J Biol Chem* **263**:2245, 1988.
41. Sparkes RS, Dizikes GJ, Klisak I, Grody WW, Mohandas T, Heinzmann C, Zollman S, Lusis AJ, Cederbaum SD: The gene for human liver arginase (ARG1) is assigned to chromosome band 6223. *Am J Hum Genet* **39**:186, 1987.
42. Herzfeld A, Raper SM: The heterogeneity of arginases in rat tissues. *Biochem J* **153**:469, 1976.
43. Kaysen GA, Strecker HJ: Purification and properties of arginase of rat kidney. *Biochem J* **133**:779, 1973.
44. Glass RD, Knox WE: Arginase isoenzymes of rat mammary gland, liver and other tissues. *J Biol Chem* **248**:5785, 1973.
45. Grody WW, Kern RM, Klein D, Dodson AE, Wissman PB, Barsky SH, Cederbaum SD: Arginase deficiency manifesting delayed clinical sequelae and induction of a kidney arginase isozyme. *Hum Genet* **91**:1, 1993.
46. Spector EB, Rice SCH, Cedarbaum SD: Evidence for two genes encoding human arginase. *Pediatr Res* **15**:569, 1981.
47. Klingenberg M: Metabolic transport in mitochondria. An example for intracellular membrane function. *Essays Biochem* **6**:119, 1970.
48. McGivan JD, Bradford NM, Blavis AD: Factors influencing the activity of ornithine aminotransferase in isolated rat liver mitochondria. *Biochem J* **162**:147, 1977.
49. Gamble G, Lehninger AL: Transport of ornithine and citrulline across the mitochondrial membrane. *J Biol Chem* **248**:610, 1973.
50. Bradford NM, McGivan JD: Evidence for the existence of an ornithine/citrulline antiporter in rat liver mitochondria. *FEBS Lett* **113**:294, 1980.
51. Indiveri C, Tonazzi A, Palmieri F: Identification and purification of the ornithine/citrulline carrier from rat liver mitochondria. *Eur J Biochem* **207**:449, 1992.
52. Hommes FA, Eller AG, Evans BA, Carter AL: Reconstitution of ornithine transport in liposomes with Lubrol extracts of mitochondria. *FEBS Lett* **170**:131, 1984.
53. Passarella S, Atlante A, Quagliariello E: Ornithine/phosphate antiport in rat kidney mitochondria. *Eur J Biochem* **193**:221, 1990.
54. Pegg A: Recent advances in the biochemistry of polyamines in eukaryotes. *Biochem J* **234**:249, 1986.
55. Luk GD, Casero RAJ: Polyamines in normal and cancer cells. *Adv Enzyme Regul* **26**:91, 1987.
56. Mudd SH, Poole JR: Labile methyl balances for normal humans on various dietary regimens. *Metabolism* **24**:721, 1975.
57. Mudd SH, Ebert MH, Scriver CR: Labile methyl group balances in the human. The role of sarcosine. *Metabolism* **29**:707, 1980.
58. Pegg A, Lockwood D, Williams-Ashman H: Concentrations of putrescine and polyamines and their enzymatic synthesis during androgen-induced prostatic growth. *Biochem J* **117**:17, 1970.
59. Seiler N, Grauffel C, Daune G, Gerhart F: Ornithine transaminase and ammonia toxicity. *Life Sciences* **45**:1009, 1989.
60. Seiler N, Sarhan S, Knoedgen B, Hornsperger JM, Sablone M: Enhanced endogenous ornithine concentrations protect against tonic seizures and coma in acute ammonia intoxication. *Pharmacol Toxicol* **72**:116, 1993.
61. Campbell RA, Morris DR, Bartos D, Daves GD, Bartos F: *Advances in Polyamine Research*. New York, Raven, 1978.
62. Nissley SP, Passamani J, Short P: Stimulation of DNA synthesis, cell multiplication and ornithine decarboxylase in 3T3 cells by multiplication-stimulating activity (MSA). *J Cell Physiol* **89**:393, 1976.
63. Raina A, Janne J: Physiology of the natural polyamines putrescine, spermidine and spermine. *Med Biol* **53**:121, 1975.
64. Hayashi S, Murakami Y, Matsufuji S: Ornithine decarboxylase antizyme: A novel type of regulatory protein. *TIBS* **21**:27, 1996.
65. Heller JS, Fong WE, Canellakis ES: Induction of a protein inhibitor to ornithine decarboxylase by the end products of its reaction. *Proc Natl Acad Sci U S A* **73**:1858, 1976.
66. Fong WF, Heller JS, Canellakis ES: The appearance of an ornithine decarboxylase inhibitory protein upon the addition of putrescine to cell cultures. *Biochim Biophys Acta* **428**:456, 1976.
67. Ivanov IP, Gesteland RF, Atkins JF: A second mammalian antizyme: Conservation of programmed ribosomal frameshifting. *Genomics* **52**:119, 1998.
68. Zhu C, Lang DW, Coffino P: Antizyme2 is a negative regulator of ornithine decarboxylase and polyamine transport. *J Biol Chem* **274**:26425, 1999.
69. Mamont PS, Duchesne MC, Joder-Ohlenbusch AM, Grove J: Effects of ornithine decarboxylase inhihitors on cultured cells, in Seiler N, Jung M, Koch-Weser J (eds): *Enzyme-Activated Irreversible Inhibitors*. New York, Elsevier, 1978, p 43.
70. Metcalf BW, Bey P, Danzin C, Jung MJ, Casara P, Verert PJ: Catalytic irreversible inhibition of mammalian ornithine decarboxylase (EC4 1.1 17) by substrate and product analogues. *J Am Chem Soc* **100**:2551, 1978.
71. O'Leary MH, Herreid RM: Mechanism of inactivation of ornithine decarboxylase by α-methylornithine. *Biochemistry* **17**:1010, 1978.
72. Seiler N: Polyamines. *J Chromatogr* **379**:157, 1986.
73. Fozard JR, Part ML, Prakash NJ, Grove J, Schechter PJ, Sjoerdsma A, Koch-Wester J: l-Ornithine decarboxylase: An essential role in early mammalian embryogenesis. *Science* **208**:505, 1980.
74. Porter C, Sufrin J: Interference with polyamine biosynthesis and/or function by analogs of polyamines or methionine as a potential anticancer chemotherapeutic strategy. *Anticancer Res* **6**:525, 1986.
75. Bartolome J, Huguennard J, Slotkin TA: Role of ornithine decarboxylase in cardiac growth and hypertrophy. *Science* **210**:793, 1980.
76. Kahana C, Nathans D: Isolation of cloned cDNA encoding mammalian ornithine decarboxylase. *Proc Natl Acad Sci U S A* **81**:3645, 1984.
77. Kahana C, Nathans D: Nucleotide sequence of murine ornithine decarboxylase. *Proc Natl Acad Sci U S A* **82**:1673, 1985.
78. Hickok NJ, Seppanen PJ, Gunsalus GL, Janne OA: Complete amino acid sequence of human ornithine decarboxylase deduced from complementary DNA. *DNA* **6**:179, 1987.
79. Brabant M, McConlogue L, Van Daalen Wetters T, Coffino P: Mouse ornithine decarboxylase gene: Cloning, structure and expression. *Proc Natl Acad Sci U S A* **85**:2200, 1988.
80. Katz A, Kahana C: Isolation and characterization of the mouse ornithine decarboxylase gene. *J Biol Chem* **263**:7604, 1988.
81. Moshier JA, Gilbert JD, Skunca M, Dosescu J, Almodovar KM, Luk GD: Isolation and expression of a human ornithine decarboxylate gene. *J Biol Chem* **265**:4884, 1990.
82. Baxter CF: Some recent advances in studies of GABA metabolism and compartmentation in GABA, in Roberts E, Chase T, Tower D (eds): *Nervous System Function*. New York, Raven, 1976, p 61.
83. Seiler N, Daune-Anglard G: Endogenous ornithine in search for CNS functions and therapeutic applications. *Metab Brain Dis* **8**:151, 1993.
84. DeMello FG, Bachrach U, Nirenberg M: Ornithine and glutamic acid decarboxylase activities in the developing chick retina. *J Neurochem* **27**:847, 1978.
85. DeMello MCF, Guerra-Peixe R, DeMello FC: Excitatory amino acid receptors mediate the glutamate-induced release of GABA synthesized from putrescine in cultured cells of embryonic avian retina. *Neurochem Int* **22**:249, 1993.

86. Murrin LC: Ornithine as a precursor for γ-aminobutyric acid in mammalian brain. *J Neurochem* **34**:1779, 1980.
87. Walker JB: Creatine: Biosynthesis, regulation and function. *Adv Enzymol* **50**:177, 1979.
88. Tormanen CD: Comparison of the properties of purified mitochondrial and cytosolic rat kidney transamidinase. *Int J Biochem* **22**:1243, 1990.
89. Roberts JJ, Walker JB: Higher homolog and N-ethyl analog of creatine as synthetic phosphagen precursors in brain, heart, and muscle, repressors of liver amidinotransferase and substrates for creatine catabolic enzymes. *J Biol Chem* **260**:13502, 1985.
90. McGuire DM, Gross MD, Van Pilsum JF, Towle HC: Repression of rat kidney L-arginine:glycine amidinotranferase synthesis by creatine at a pretranslational level. *J Biol Chem* **259**:12034, 1984.
91. Sipila I: Inhibition of arginine-glycine amidinotransferase by ornithine. *Biochim Biophys Acta* **613**:79, 1980.
92. Ratner S, Rochovansky O: Biosynthesis of guanidinoacetic acid. I. Purification and properties of transamidinase. *Arch Biochem Biophys* **63**:277, 1956.
93. Ratner S, Rochovansky O: Biosynthesis of guanidinoacetic acid. II. Mechanism of amidine group transfer. *Arch Biochem Biophys* **63**:296, 1956.
94. Gross MD, Eggen MA, Simon AM, Van Pilsum JF: The purification and characterization of human kidney L-arginine:glycine amidinotransferase. *Arch Biochem Biophys* **251**:747, 1986.
95. McGuire DM, Gross MD, Elde RP, Van Pilsum JF: Localization of L-arginine-glycine amidinotransferase protein in rat tissues by immunofluorescence microscopy. *J Histochem Cytochem* **34**:429, 1986.
96. DeFalco AJ, Davies RK: The synthesis of creatine by the brain of the intact rat. *J Neurochem* **7**:308, 1961.
97. Pardridge WM, Duducgian-Vartavarian L, Casanello-Ertl D, Jones MR, Kopple JD: Amino acid and creatine metabolism in adult rat skeletal muscle cells in tissue culture. *Fed Proc* **39**:1179, 1980.
98. Strecker HJ: Purification and properties of rat liver ornithine-δ-aminotransferase. *J Biol Chem* **240**:1225, 1965.
99. Matsuzawa T: Characteristics of the inhibition of ornithine-δ-aminotransferase by branched chain amino acids. *J Biochem* **75**:601, 1974.
100. Mezl VA, Knox WE: Properties and analysis of a stable derivative of pyrroline-5-carboxylase acid for use in metabolic studies. *Anal Biochem* **74**:430, 1976.
101. Quastel J, Witty R: Ornithine transaminase. *Nature* **167**:556, 1951.
102. Meister A: Enzymatic transamination reactions involving arginine and ornithine. *J Biol Chem* **206**:587, 1954.
103. Ohura T, Kominami E, Tada K, Katunuma N: Crystallization and properties of human liver ornithine aminotransferase. *J Biochem* **92**:1785, 1982.
104. Peraino C, Pitot H: Ornithine-δ-aminotransferase in the rat. I. Assay and some general properties. *Biochim Biophys Acta* **73**:222, 1963.
105. Katunuma N, Matsude Y, Tomino I: Studies on ornithine-ketoacid transaminase. I. Purification and properties. *J Biochem* **56**:499, 1964.
106. Matsuzawa T, Katsunuma T, Katunuma N: Crystallization of ornithine transaminase and its properties. *Biochem Biophys Res Commun* **32**:161, 1968.
107. Peraino C, Bunville L, Tahmaisian T: Chemical, physical and morphological properties of ornithine aminotransferase from rat liver. *J Biol Chem* **244**:2241, 1969.
108. Sanada Y, Suemori T, Katunuma N: Properties of ornithine aminotransferase from rat liver, kidney and small intestine. *Biochim Biophys Acta* **220**:42, 1970.
109. Sanada Y, Shiotani T, Okuno E, Katunuma N: Coenzyme-dependent conformational properties of rat liver ornithine aminotransferase. *Eur J Biochem* **69**:507, 1976.
110. Kalita CC, Kerman JD, Strecker HJ: Preparation and properties of ornithine-oxo-acid aminotransferase of rat kidney. *Biochim Biophys Acta* **429**:780, 1976.
111. Yip MCM, Collins RK: Purification and properties of rat kidney and liver ornithine aminotransferase. *Enzyme* **12**:187, 1971.
112. Peraino C: Functional properties of ornithine-ketoacid aminotransferase from rat liver. *Biochim Biophys Acta* **289**:117, 1972.
113. Simmaco M, John RA, Barra D, Bossa F: The primary structure of ornithine aminotransferase: Identification of active-site sequence and site of post-translational proteolysis. *FEBS Lett* **199**:39, 1986.
114. Markovic-Housley Z, Kania M, Lustig A, Vincent MG, Jansonius JN, John RA: Quaternary structure of ornithine aminotransferase in solution and preliminary crystallographic data. *Eur J Biochem* **162**:345, 1987.
115. Shen BW, Henning M, Hohenester E, Jansonius JN, Schirmer T: Crystal structure of human recombinant ornithine aminotransferase. *J Mol Biol* **277**:81, 1998.
116. Storici P, Capitani G, De Biase D, Moser M, John RA, Jansonius JN, Schirmer T: Crystal structure of GABA-aminotransferase, a target for antiepileptic drug therapy. *Biochemistry* **38**:8628, 1999.
117. Jones ME: Conversion of glutamate to ornithine and proline. Pyrroline-5-carboxylate, a possible modulator of arginine requirements. *J Nutr* **115**:509, 1985.
118. Kito K, Sanada Y, Katunuma N: Mode of inhibition of ornithine aminotransferase by L-canaline. *J Biochem* **83**:201, 1978.
119. Jung MJ, Seiler N: Enzyme activated irreversible inhibitors of L-ornithine:2-oxoacid aminotransferase. *J Biol Chem* **253**:7431, 1978.
120. John RA, Jones ED, Fowler LJ: Enzyme-induced inactivation of transaminases by acetylenic and vinyl analogues of 4-aminobutyrate. *Biochem J* **177**:721, 1979.
121. Daune G, Seiler N: Interrelationships between ornithine, glutamate and GABA. II. Consequences of inhibition of GABA-T and ornithine aminotransferase in brain. *Neurochem Res* **13**:69, 1988.
122. Alonso E, Rubio V: Participation of ornithine aminotransferase in the synthesis and catabolism of ornithine in mice. *Biochem J* **259**:131, 1989.
123. DeBiase D, Simmaco M, Barra D, Bossa F, Hewlins M, John RA: Mechanism of inactivation and identification of sites of modification of ornithine aminotransferase by 4-aminohex-5-ynoate. *Biochem* **30**:2239, 1991.
124. Bolkenius FN, Knodgen B, Seiler N: DL-Canaline and 5-fluoromethylornithine. *Biochem J* **268**:409, 1990.
125. Seiler N, Grauffel C, Daune G, Gerhart F: Ornithine aminotransferase activity, liver ornithine concentration and acute ammonia intoxication. *Life Sci* **45**:1009, 1989.
126. Seiler N, Daune G, Bolkenius FN, Knodgen B: Ornithine aminotransferase activity. Tissue ornithine concentrations and polyamine metabolism. *Int J Biochem* **21**:425, 1989.
127. Daune-Anglard G, Bonaventure N, Seiler N: Some biochemical and pathophysiological aspects of long-term elevation of brain ornithine concentrations. *Pharmacol Toxicol* **73**:29, 1993.
128. Seiler N, Sarhan S, Knodgen B: Inhibition of ornithine aminotransferase by 5-fluoromethylornithine: Protection against acute thioacetamide intoxication by elevated tissue ornithine levels. *Pharmacol Toxicol* **70**:373, 1992.
129. Sarhan S, Knodggen B, Grauffel C, Seiler N: Effects of inhibition of ornithine aminotransferase on thioacetamide-induced hepatogenic encephalopathy. *Neurochem Res* **18**:539, 1993.
130. Phang J, Downing S, Valle D: A radioisotopic assay for ornithine-δ-aminotransferase. *Anal Biochem* **55**:272, 1973.
131. Wong PTH, McGeer ER, McGeer PL: A sensitive radiometric assay for ornithine aminotransferase. Regional and subcellular distributions in rat brain. *J Neurochem* **36**:501, 1981.
132. Brody LC, Mitchell GA, Obie C, Michaud J, Steel G, Fontaine G, Robert M-F, Kaiser-Kupfer MI, Valle D: Ornithine-δ-aminotransferase mutations causing gyrate atrophy: Allelic heterogeneity and functional consequences. *J Biol Chem* **267**:3302, 1992.
133. Adams E, Frank L: Metabolism of proline and the hydroxyprolines. *Annu Rev Biochem* **49**:1005, 1980.
134. O'Donnell JJ, Sandman RP, Martin SR: Assay of ornithine aminotransferase by high-performance liquid chromatography. *Anal Biochem* **90**:41, 1978.
135. Heinänen K, Näntö-Salonen K, Leino L, Pulkki K, Heinonen O, Valle D, Simell O: Gyrate atrophy of the choroid and retina: Lymphocyte ornithine-δ-aminotransferase activity in different mutations and carriers. *Pediatr Res* **44**:381, 1998.
136. Mitchell GA, Valle D, Willard H, Steel G, Suchanek M, Brody L: Human ornithine-δ-aminotransferase (OAT): Cross-hybridizing fragments mapped to chromosome 10 and Xpll.1-21.1. *Am J Hum Genet* **39**:163A, 1986.
137. Ramesh V, Shaffer MM, Allaire JM, Shih VE, Gusella JF: Investigation of gyrate atrophy using a cDNA clone for human ornithine aminotransferase. *DNA* **5**:493, 1986.
138. Inana G, Totsuks S, Redmond M, Dougherty T, Nagle J, Shiono R, Ohura T, Kominami E, Katunuma N: Molecular cloning of human aminotransferase mRNA. *Proc Natl Acad Sci U S A* **83**:1203, 1986.
139. Himeno M, Mueckler MM, Gonzales FJ, Pitot HC: Cloning of DNA complementary to ornithine aminotransferase mRNA. *J Biol Chem* **257**:4669, 1982.

140. Mueckler MM, Pitot HC: Sequence of the precursor to rat ornithine aminotransferase deduced from a cDNA clone. *J Biol Chem* **260**:12993, 1985.

141. Degols G: Functional analysis of the regulatory region adjacent to the carg B gene of *Saccharomyces cerevisiae*: Nucleotide sequence, gene fusion experiments and *cis*-dominant regulatory mutation analysis. *Eur J Biochem* **169**:193, 1987.

142. Degols G, Jauniaus JC, Wiami JM: Molecular characterization of transposable-element associated mutations that lead to constitutive L-ornithine aminotransferase expression in *Saccharomyces cerevisiae*. *Eur J Biochem* **165**:289, 1987.

143. Delauney AJ, Hu C-A, Kavi Kishor PB, Verma DP: Cloning of ornithine-δ-aminotransferase cDNA from *Vigna aconitifolia* by *trans*-complementation in *Escherichia coli* and regulation of proline biosynthesis. *J Biol Chem* **268**:18673, 1993.

144. Jauniaus JC, Urrestarazu LA, Wiame JM: Arginine metabolism in *Saccharomyces cerevisiae*: Subcellular localization of the enzymes. *J Bacteriol* **133**:1096, 1978.

145. Davis RH, Weiss RL: Novel mechanisms controlling arginine metabolism in Neurospora. *Trends Biochem Sci* **13**:101, 1988.

146. Dougherty KM, Swanson DA, Brody LC, Valle D: Expression and processing of human ornithine-δ-aminotransferase in *Saccharomyces cerevisiae*. *Hum Mol Genet* **2**:1835, 1993.

147. Mitchell GA, Looney JE, Brody LC, Steel G, Suchanek M, Engelhardt JF, Willard HF, Valle D: Human ornithine-δ–aminotransferase: cDNA cloning and analysis of the structural gene. *J Biol Chem* **263**:14288, 1988.

148. Ramesh V, Benoit L, Crawford P, Harvey P, Shows T, Shih V, Gusella J: The ornithine aminotransferase (OAT) locus: Analysis of RFLPs in gyrate atrophy. *Am J Hum Genet* **42**:365, 1988.

149. Ramesh V, Gusella J, Shih V: Molecular pathology of gyrate atrophy of the choroid and retina due to ornithine aminotransferase deficiency. *Mol Biol Med* **8**:81, 1991.

150. Looney J, Mitchell G, Brody L, Suchanek M, Steel G, Willard H, Valle D: Ornithine aminotransferase (OAT) hybridizing regions on the X chromosome: Integration of at least one processed gene on X and subsequent genomic duplication has generated multiple OAT-hybridizing fragments. *Am J Hum Genet* **41**:A226, 1987.

151. Freytag SO, Beaudet AL, Bock HGO, O'Brien WE: Molecular splicing of the human argininosuccinate synthetase gene. Occurrence of alternative mRNA splicing. *Mol Cell Biol* **4**:1978, 1984.

152. Fagan RJ, Sheffield WP, Rozen R: Regulation of ornithine aminotransferase in retinoblastomas. *J Biol Chem* **264**:20513, 1989.

153. Fagan RJ, Lazaris-Karatzas A, Sonenberg N, Rozen R: Translational control of ornithine aminotransferase. *J Biol Chem* **266**:16518, 1991.

154. Fagan RJ, Rozen R: Translational control of ornithine-δ–aminotransferase (OAT) by estrogen. *Mol Cell Endocrin* **90**:171, 1993.

155. Engelhardt JF, Steel G, Valle D: Transcriptional analysis of the human ornithine aminotransferase promoter. *J Biol Chem* **266**:752, 1991.

156. Kadonaga JT, Jones KA, Tijian R: Promoter-specific activation of RNA polymerase H transcription by Spl. *Trends Biochem Sci* **11**:10, 1986.

157. Pabo CO, Sauer RT: Protein-DNA recognition. *Annu Rev Biochem* **53**:293, 1984.

158. Klein-Hitpass L, Schorpp M, Wagner U, Ryffel GU: An estrogen-responsive element derived from the 5′ flanking region of the *Xenopus vitellogenin* A2 gene functions in transfected human cells. *Cell* **46**:1053, 1986.

159. Klock G, Strahle U, Schutz G: Oestrogen and glucocorticoid responsive elements are closely related but distinct. *Nature* **329**:734, 1987.

160. Ramesh V, Eddy R, Bruns G, Shih V, Shows T, Gusella J: Localization of the ornithine aminotransferase gene and related sequences on two human chromosomes. *Hum Genet* **76**:121, 1987.

161. Barrett DJ, Bateman JB, Sparkes RS, Mohandas T, Klisak I, Inana G: Chromosomal localization of human ornithine aminotransferase gene sequences to 10q26 and Xpll.2. *Invest Ophthalmol Vis Sci* **28**:1037, 1987.

162. Geraghty MT, Kearns WG, Pearson PL, Valle D: Isolation and characterization of an ornithine aminotransferase-related sequence (OATL3) mapping to 10q26. *Genomics* **17**:510, 1993.

163. Lafreniere R, Geraghty M, Valle D, Shows T, Willard H: Ornithine aminotransferase-related sequences map to two nonadjacent intervals on the human X chromosome short arm. *Genomics* **10**:276, 1991.

164. Mitchell GA, Valle D, Suchanek M, Steel G, Brody L, Looney J, Willard H: Ornithine aminotransferase (OAT): Evidence for a dispersed gene family with member(s) localized to Xpll.l-Xp21.1. *Pediatr Res* **21**:292A, 1987.

165. Geraghty MT, Brody LC, Mitchell GA, Valle D: Unpublished observations.

166. Suijkerbuijk RF, Meloni AM, Sinke RJ, deLeeuw B, Wilbrink M, Janssen HAP, Geraghty MT, Monaco AP, Sandberg AA, Geurts Van Kessel A: Identification of a yeast artificial chromosome that spans the human papillary renal cell carcinoma-associated t(X;1) breakpoint in Xp11.2. *Cancer Genet Cytogenet* **7**:164, 1993.

167. deLeeuw B, Suijkerbuijk RF, Balesmans M, Sinke RJ, de Jong B, Molenaar WM, Meloni AM, Sandberg AA, Geraghty MT, Hofker M, Ropers HH, Geurts Van Kessel A: Sublocalization of the synovial sarcoma-associated t(X;18) chromosomal breakpoint in Xp11.2 using cosmid cloning and fluorescence *in situ* hybridization. *Oncogene* **8**:1457, 1993.

168. Geraghty MT, Brody LC, Martin LS, Marble M, Kearns W, Pearson P, Monaco AP, Lehrach H, Valle D: The isolation of cDNAs from OATL1 at Xp11.2 using a 480 kb YAC. *Genomics* **16**:440, 1993.

169. Mazo AM, Huang DH, Mozer BA, Dawid IB: The trithorax gene, a *trans*-acting regulator of the bithorax complex in *Drosophila*, encodes a protein with zinc-binding domains. *Proc Natl Acad Sci U S A* **87**:2112, 1990.

170. Parry P, Djabali M, Bower M, Khristich J, Waterman M, Gibbons B, Young B, Evans G: Structure and expression of the human trithorax-like gene 1 involved in acute leukemias. *Proc Natl Acad Sci U S A* **90**:4738, 1993.

171. Ford AM, Ridge SA, Cabrera ME, Mahmoud H, Steel CM, Chan LC, Greaves M: *In utero* rearrangements in the trithorax-related oncogene in infant leukemias. *Nature* **363**:358, 1993.

172. Nakamura T, Alder H, Gu Y, Prasad R, Canaani O, Kamada N, Gale RP, Lange B, Crist WM, Nowell PC, Croce CM, Canaani E: Genes on chromosomes 4, 9 and 19 involved in 11q23 abnormalities in acute leukemia share sequence homology and/or common motifs. *Proc Natl Acad Sci U S A* **90**:4631, 1993.

173. Herzfeld A, Knox WE: The properties, developmental formation and estrogen induction of ornithine aminotransferase in rat tissues. *J Biol Chem* **243**:3227, 1968.

174. Herzfeld A, Raper S: Enzymes of ornithine metabolism in adult and developing rat intestine. *Biochim Biophys Acta* **428**:600, 1976.

175. Herzfeld A, Raper S: Amino acid metabolizing enzymes in rat submaxillary gland, normal or neoplastic, and in pancreas. *Enzyme* **21**:471, 1976.

176. Riby JE, Hurwitz RE, Kretchmer N: Development of ornithine metabolism in the mouse intestine. *Pediatr Res* **28**:261, 1990.

177. Wang T, Lawler AM, Steel G, Sipila I, Milam AH, Valle D: Mice lacking ornithine-δ–aminotransferase have paradoxical neonatal hypoornithinaemia and retinal degeneration. *Nat Genet* **11**:185, 1995.

178. Wu G, Knabe DA, Flynn NE: Synthesis of citrulline from glutamine in pig enterocytes. *Biochem J* **299**:115, 1994.

179. Wu G, Morris SM: Arginine metabolism: Nitric oxide and beyond. *Biochem J* **336**:1, 1998.

180. Wu G, Knabe DA, Flynn NE, Yan W, Flynn SP: Arginine degradation in developing porcine enterocytes. *Am J Physiol* **34**:G913, 1996.

181. Mezl VA, Knox WE: Metabolism of arginine in lactating rat mammary gland. *Biochem J* **166**:105, 1977.

182. Smith RJ, Phang JM: Proline metabolism in cartilage: The importance of proline biosynthesis. *Metabolism* **27**:685, 1978.

183. Matsuzawa T, Obara Y: Amino acid synthesis from ornithine: Enzymes and quantitative comparison in brain slices and detached retinas from rats and chicks. *Brain Res* **413**:314, 1987.

184. Kuo F, Hwu W, Valle D, Darnell JJ: Colocalization in pericentral hepatocytes in adult mice and similarity in developmental expression pattern of ornithine aminotransferase and glutamine synthetase mRNA. *Proc Natl Acad Sci U S A* **88**:9468, 1991.

185. Hwu W, Valle D: Unpublished results.

186. Kuo C, Darnell JJ: Mouse glutamine synthetase is encoded by a single gene that can be expressed in a localized fashion. *J Mol Biol* **208**:45, 1989.

187. Fahrner J, Labruyere WT, Gaunitz C, Moorman AFM, Gebhardt R, Lamers WH: Identification and functional characterization of regulatory elements of the glutamine synthetase gene from rat liver. *FEBS Lett* **213**:1067, 1993.

188. Jungermann K, Katz N: Functional specialization of different hepatocyte populations. *Ann Rev Physiol* **69**:708, 1989.

189. Meijer AJ, Lamers WH, Chamuleau RAFM: Nitrogen metabolism and ornithine cycle function. *Physiol Rev* **70**:701, 1990.

190. Moorman AM, De Boer PAJ, Das AT, Labruyere WT, Charles R, Lamers WH: Expression patterns of mRNAs for ammonia-metabolizing enzymes in the developing rat: The ontogenesis of hepatocyte heterogeneity. *Biochem J* **22**:457, 1990.
191. Gebhardt R: Metabolic zonation of the liver: Regulation and implications for liver function. *Pharmac Ther* **53**:275, 1992.
192. Haussinger D, Lamers WH, Moorman AFM: Hepatocyte heterogeneity in the metabolism of amino acids and ammonia. *Enzyme* **46**:72, 1992.
193. Gebhardt R: Comments: Cell-cell interactions: Clues to hepatocyte heterogeneity and beyond? *Hepatology* **16**:843, 1992.
194. Baich A: Effect of methionine on the accumulation of ornithine by Chinese hamster cells in culture. *Biochim Biophys Acta* **756**:238, 1983.
195. Ratzlaff K, Batch A: Comparison of ornithine activities in the pigment epithelium and retina of vertebrates. *Comp Biochem Physiol* **88B**:35, 1987.
196. Hayakasa S, Shiono T, Takaku Y, Mizuno K: Ornithine ketoacid aminotransferase in the bovine eye. *Invest Ophthalmol* **19**:1457, 1980.
197. Hayasaka S, Matsuzawa T, Shiono T, Mizuno K, Ishiguro I: Enzymes metabolizing ornithine-proline pathway in the bovine eye. *Exp Eye Res* **34**:635, 1982.
198. Valle D, Kaiser-Kupfer M: Gyrate atrophy of the choroid and retina, in Daenti D (ed): *Clinical, Structural, and Biochemical Advances in Hereditary Eye Disorders*. New York, Alan R. Liss, 1982, p 123.
199. Rao GN, Cotler E: Ornithine delta-aminotransferase activity in retina and other tissues. *Neurochem Res* **9**:555, 1984.
200. Fleming GA, Steel G, Valle D, Granger A, Phang JM: The aqueous humor of rabbit contains high concentrations of pyrroline-5-carboxylase. *Metabolism* **35**:933, 1986.
201. Kasahara M, Matsuzawa T, Kokubo M, Gushiken Y, Tashiro K, Koide T, Watanabe H, Katanuma N: Immunohistochemical localization of ornithine aminotransferase in normal rat tissues by Fab-′ horseradish peroxidase conjugates. *J Histochem Cytochem* **34**:1385, 1986.
202. Takahashi O, Ishiguro S-I, Mito T, Hayasaka S, Shiono T, Mizuno K, Ohura T, Tada K: Immunocytochemical localization of ornithine aminotransferase in rat ocular tissues. *Invest Ophthalmol Vis Sci* **28**:1617, 1987.
203. Raiha N, Kekomaki M: Studies on the development of ornithine-ketoacid aminotransferase activity in rat liver. *Biochem J* **108**:521, 1968.
204. Wang T, Steel G, Valle D: Unpublished results.
205. Peraino C, Pitot H: Studies on the induction and repression of enzymes in rat liver. *J Biol Chem* **239**:4308, 1964.
206. Lyons RT, Pitot HC: The regulation of ornithine aminotransferase synthesis by glucagon in the rat. *Arch Biochem Biophys* **174**:262, 1976.
207. Lyons RT, Pitot HC: Hormonal regulation of ornithine aminotransferase biosynthesis in rat liver and kidney. *Arch Biochem Biophys* **180**:472, 1977.
208. Merrill MJ, Pitot HC: Regulation of ornithine aminotransferase by cyclic AMP and glucose in primary cultures of adult rat hepatocytes. *Arch Biochem Biophys* **237**:373, 1985.
209. Merrill MJ, Mueckler MM, Pitot HC: Levels of ornithine aminotransferase messenger RNA under conditions of cyclic AMP induction in cultured hepatocytes. *J Biol Chem* **260**:11248, 1985.
210. Ikeda M, Okada M: Effect of pyridoxine deficiency on ornithine aminotransferase in rat kidney and liver. *J Nutr Sci Vitaminol* **31**:553, 1985.
211. Ikeda M, Okada M: Regulation of ornithine aminotransferase in rat kidney by estradiol and pyridoxine. *J Nutr Sci Vitaminol* **32**:23, 1986.
212. Wu C: Estrogen induction of ornithine aminotransferase in rat kidney slices. *Biochem Biophys Res Commun* **82**:782, 1978.
213. Matthaei KI, Williams JF: Ornithine aminotransferase turnover in host tissues of tumor-bearing rats. *J Natl Cancer Inst* **79**:805, 1987.
214. Mueckler MM, Moran S, Pitot HC: Transcriptional control of ornithine aminotransferase synthesis in rat kidney by estrogen and thyroid hormone. *J Biol Chem* **259**:2302, 1984.
215. Mueckler MM, Merrill MJ, Pitot HC: Translational and pretranslational control of ornithine aminotransferase synthesis in rat liver. *J Biol Chem* **258**:6109, 1983.
216. Ip MM, Chee PY, Swick RW: Turnover of hepatic mitochondrial ornithine aminotransferase and cytochrome oxidase using ^{14}C-carbonate as tracer. *Biochim Biophys Acta* **354**:29, 1974.
217. Augustine SL, Swick RW: Turnover of total proteins and ornithine aminotransferase during liver regeneration in rats. *Am J Physiol* **238**:46, 1980.
218. Lodato RF, Smith RJ, Valle D, Phang JM, Aoki TT: Regulation of proline biosynthesis. The inhibition of pyrroline-5-carboxylase synthase activity by ornithine. *Metabolism* **30**:908, 1981.
219. Valle D, Downing S, Harris S, Phang J: Proline biosynthesis: Multiple defects in Chinese hamster ovary cells. *Biochem Biophys Res Commun* **53**:1130, 1973.
220. Ertel J, Isseroff H: Proline in fascioliasis. I. Comparative activities of ornithine-δ-aminotransferase and proline oxidase in Fasciola and in mammalian livers. *J Parasitol* **60**:574, 1974.
221. Smith AD, Benziman M, Strecker HJ: The formation of ornithine from proline in animal tissues. *Biochem J* **104**:557, 1967.
222. Ross G, Dunn D, Jones ME: Ornithine synthesis from glutamate in rat intestinal mucosa homogenates: Evidence for the reduction of glutamate to ?gamma;-glutamyl semialdehyde. *Biochem Biophys Res Commun* **85**:140, 1978.
223. Windmueller HG, Spaeth AE: Intestinal metabolism of glutamine and glutamate from the lumen as compared to glutamine from blood. *Arch Biochem Biophys* **171**:662, 1975.
224. Fuller MF, Reeds PJ: Nitrogen cycling in the gut. *Annu Rev Nutr* **18**:385, 1998.
225. Valle D, Phang JM, Downing SJ: Unpublished observations.
226. Snyderman SE, Boyer A, Holt LE: The arginine requirement of the infant. *Am J Dis Child* **97**:78, 1959.
227. Moser HW, Efron ML, Brown H, Diamond R, Neuman CG: Argininosuccinic aciduria. Report of two new cases and demonstration of intermittent elevation of blood ammonia. *Am J Med* **42**:9, 1967.
228. Brusilow S, Batshaw M: Personal communication.
229. Morris JG, Rogers QR: Ammonia intoxication in the near-adult cat as a result of a dietary deficiency of arginine. *Science* **199**:431, 1978.
230. Morris JG, Rogers QR: Arginine: An essential amino acid for the cat. *J Nutr* **108**:1944, 1978.
231. Stewart PM, Walser M, Batshaw M, Valle D: Effects of arginine-free meals on ureagenesis in cats. *Am J Physiol* **241**:310, 1981.
232. Wakabayashi Y, Henslee JG, Jones ME: Pyrroline-5-carboxylate synthesis from glutamate by rat intestinal mucosa. *J Biol Chem* **258**:3873, 1983.
233. Wakabayashi Y, Yamada E, Hasegawa T, Yamada R: Enzymological evidence for the indispensability of small intestine in the synthesis of arginine from glutamate. I. Pyrroline-5-carboxylate synthase. *Arch Biochem Biophys* **291**:1, 1991.
234. Yamada E, Wakabayashi Y: Development of pyrroline-5-carboxylate synthase and *N*-acetylglutamate synthase and their changes in lactation and aging. *Arch Biochem Biophys* **291**:15, 1991.
235. Cynober L: Can arginine and ornithine support gut functions? *Gut* **35**:S42, 1994.
236. Featherston WR, Rogers QR, Freedland RA: Relative importance of kidney and liver in synthesis of arginine by the rat. *Am J Physiol* **224**:127, 1973.
237. De Jonge WJ, Dingemanse MA, de Boer PA, Lamers WH, Moorman AF: Arginine-metabolizing enzymes in the developing rat small intestine. *Pediatr Res* **43**:442, 1998.
238. Cleary MA, Sivakumar P, Olpin S, Wraith JE, Walter JH, Till J, Morris AA, Besley GT: Ornithine aminotransferase deficiency: Difficulties in diagnosis in the neonatal period. *J Inherit Metab Dis* **22**:69, 1999.
239. Dorland L, Mandel R, Hemmes AM, Duran M, de Vries WB, Brink W, Roeleveld ABC, de Koning TJ, Shih VE, Berger R, Poll-The BT: A patient diagnosed as HHH without HH. *J Inherit Metab Dis* **22**:7, 1999.
240. Webster M, Allen J, Rawlinson D, Brown A, Olpin S, Leonard JV: Ornithine aminotransferase deficiency presenting with hyperammonaemia in a premature newborn. *J Inherit Metab Dis* **22**:80, 1999.
241. Shih V, Efron ML, Moser HW: Hyperornithinemia, hyperammonemia, and homocitrullinuria. A new disorder of amino acid metabolism associated with myoclonic seizures and mental retardation. *Am J Dis Child* **117**:83, 1969.
242. Bickel H, Feist D, Muller H, Quadbeck G: Ornithinamie, eine weiter aminosaurenstoif-Wechselsturung mit hirnschadigung. *Dtsch Med Wochenschr* **47**:2247, 1968.
243. Grubner R: Personal communications.
244. Perry T, Hansen S: Biochemical effects in man and rat of three drugs which can increase brain GABA content. *J Neurochem* **30**:679, 1978.
245. Fujimura Y, Matsuzawa T, Kawamura M, Tada K, Mizuno K: Mass screening of urea cycle diseases. A new mass screening method of hyperornithinemia by using two coupling enzymes. *Tohoku J Exp Med* **141**:257, 1983.

246. Jacobsohn E: Ein fall von Retinitis pigmentosa atypica. *Klin Monatsbl Augenheilkd* **26**:202, 1888.
247. Cutler CW: Drei ungewohnliche Falle von Retinochorioideal degeneration. *Arch Augenheilkd* **30**:117, 1895.
248. Fuchs E: Ueher zwei der retinitis pigmentosa verwandte Krankheiten (retinitis punctata albescens und atrophia gyrata chorioideae et retinae). *Arch Augenheilkd* **32**:111, 1896.
249. Usher CH: The Bowman Lecture—On a few hereditary eye affections. *Trans Ophthalmol Soc UK* **55**:164, 1935.
250. Kurstjens J: Choroideremia and gyrate atrophy of the choroid and retina. Brief historical review. *Doc Ophthalmol* **19**:1, 1965.
251. Francois J: Heredity of the choroidal dystrophies. *Adv Ophthalmol* **35**:1, 1978.
252. Takki K: Gyrate atrophy of the choroid and retina associated with hyperornithinemia. *Thesis*. University of Helsinki, 1975.
253. Kaiser-Kupfer MI, Valle D, Bron AJ: Clinical and biochemical heterogeneity in gyrate atrophy. *Am J Ophthalmol* **89**:219, 1980.
254. Hayasaka S, Shiono T, Mizuno K, Sasayama C, Akiya S, Tanaka Y, Hayakawa M, Miyake Y, Ohba N: Gyrate atrophy of the choroid and retina: I5 Japanese patients. *Br J Ophthalmol* **70**:612, 1986.
255. Simell O, Takki K: Raised plasma ornithine and gyrate atrophy of the choroid and retina. *Lancet* **1**:1031, 1973.
256. Kaiser-Kupfer MI, Valle D, Del Valle LA: A specific enzyme defect in gyrate atrophy. *Am J Ophthalmol* **85**:200, 1978.
257. Kaiser-Kupfer MI, Kuwabara T, Askansas V, Brody L, Takki K, Dvoretzky I, Engel WK: Systemic manifestations of gyrate atrophy of the choroid and retina. *Ophthalmology* **88**:302, 1981.
258. Kaiser-Kupfer MI, De Monasterio F, Valle D, Walser M, Brusilow SW: Visual results of a long-term trial of a low-arginine diet in gyrate atrophy of the choroid and retina. *Ophthalmology* **88**:307, 1981.
259. Kaiser-Kupfer MI, Valle D: Clinical, biochemical and therapeutic aspects of gyrate atrophy, in Osbourne N, Chader J (eds): *Progress in Retinal Research*. Oxford, Pergamon, 1986, p 179.
260. Hodes DT, Mushin AS, Laurance BM, Oberholzer VG, Briddon A: Hyperornithinemia with gyrate atrophy of the choroid and retina in two siblings. *J Royal Soc Med* **73**:588, 1980.
261. Francois J: Gyrate atrophy of the choroid and retina. *Ophthalmologica (Basel)* **178**:311, 1979.
262. Jaeger W, Kettler JV, Lutz P, Hilsdorf C: Differential diagnosis of gyrate atrophy of the choroid and retina (gyrate atrophy of the choroid and retina with and without hyperornithinemia). *Metab Pediatr Ophthalmol* **3**:189, 1979.
263. Iannetti F: Hyperornithinemia in the gyrate atrophy of the retina and choroid. *Ann Ottal Clin Ocul* **12**:555, 1976.
264. McCulloch C, Marliss EB: Gyrate atrophy of the choroid and retina with hyperornithinemia. *Am J Ophthalmol* **80**:1047, 1975.
265. McCulloch JC, Arshinoff SA, Marliss EB, Parker JA: Hyperornithinemia and gyrate atrophy of the choroid and retina. *Ophthalmology* **85**:918, 1978.
266. Akiya S, Ohsava M, Ogata T: Gyrate atrophy of the choroid and retina. Long-term observation of two brothers of gyrate atrophy of the choroid and retina with hyperornithinaemia. *Acta Soc Ophthalmol Jpn* **81**:310, 1978.
267. Bakker HD, Abeling NGGM, Van Schooneveld MJ, Wanders RJA, Van Gennip AH: A far advanced case of gyrate atrophy in a 12 year old girl. *J Inherit Metab Dis* **14**:379, 1991.
268. Berson EL, Schmidt SY, Shih VE: Ocular and biochemical abnormalities in gyrate atrophy of the choroid and retina. *Ophthalmology* **85**:1018, 1978.
269. Berson EL, Shih VE, Sullivan PL: Ocular findings in patients with gyrate atrophy on pyridoxine and low-protein, low-arginine diets. *Ophthalmology* **88**:311, 1981.
270. O'Donnell JJ, Sandman RP, Martin SR: Gyrate atrophy of the retina: Inborn error of L-ornithine:2-oxoacid aminotransiferase. *Science* **200**:200, 1978.
271. Douglas EP: Hyperprolinaemia and gyrate atrophy of the choroid and retina in members of the same family. *Br J Ophthalmol* **69**:588, 1985.
272. Oberholzer VG, Briddon A: 3-Amino-2-piperidone in the urine of patients with hyperornithinemia. *Clin Chim Acta* **87**:411, 1978.
273. Rinaldi E, Stoppoloni GP, Savastano S, Russo S, Cotticelli L: Gyrate atrophy of choroid associated with hyperornithaenemia: Report of the first case in Italy. *J Pediatr Ophthalmol Strabismus* **16**:133, 1979.
274. Steel D, Wood CM, Richardson J, McCarthy J: Anterior subcapsular plaque cataract in hyperornithinaemia gyrate atrophy—A case report. *Br J Ophthalmol* **76**:762, 1992.
275. Stoppoloni G, Prisco F, Santinelli R, Tolone C: Hyperornithinemia and gyrate atrophy of choroid and retina. *Helv Paediatr Acta* **33**:429, 1978.
276. Takki K: Gyrate atrophy of the choroid and retina associated with hyperornithinemia. *Br J Ophthalmol* **58**:3, 1974.
277. Takki K, Simell O: Gyrate atrophy of the choroid and retina with hyperornithinemia. *Birth Defects* **12**:373, 1976.
278. Takki K, Milton RC: The natural history of gyrate atrophy of the choroid and retina. *Ophthalmology* **88**:292, 1981.
279. Trijbels JMF, Sengers RCA, Bakkeren JAJM, DeKort AFM, Dutman AF: L-Ornithine-ketoacid-transferase deficiency in cultured fibroblasts of a patient with hyperornithinemia and gyrate atrophy of the choroid and retina. *Clin Chim Acta* **79**:371, 1977.
280. Weleber RG, Kennaway NG, Buist NR: Vitamin B6 in management of gyrate atrophy of choroid and retina. *Lancet* **2**:1213, 1978.
281. Weleber RG, Kennaway NG: Clinical trial of vitamin B6 for gyrate atrophy of the choroid and retina. *Ophthalmology* **88**:316, 1981.
282. Yatziv S, Statter M, Merin S: Metabolic studies in two families with hyperornithinemia and gyrate atrophy of choroid and retina. *J Lab Clin Med* **93**:749, 1979.
283. Kaiser-Kupfer MI, Ludwig IH, DeMonasterio FM, Valle D, Krieger I: Gyrate atrophy of the choroid and retina. Early findings. *Ophthalmology* **92**:394, 1985.
284. Kaiser-Kupfer MI, Kuwabara T, Uga S, Takki K, Valle D: Cataracts in gyrate atrophy: Clinical and morphologic studies. *Invest Ophthalmol Vis Sci* **24**:432, 1983.
285. Krill AE: Clinical characteristics, in Krill A (ed): *Krill's Hereditary Retinal and Choroidal Diseases*. New York, Harper & Row, 1977, p 1012.
286. Raitta C, Carlson S, Vannas-Sulonen K: Gyrate atrophy of the choroid and retina: ERG of the neural retina and the pigment epithelium. *Br J Ophthalmol* **74**:363, 1990.
287. Vannas Sulonen K: Progression of gyrate atrophy of the choroid and retina: A long-term follow-up by fluorescein angiography. *Acta Ophthalmol* **65**:101, 1987.
288. Vannas Sulonen K, Vannas A, O'Donnell JJ, Sipila I, Wood I: Pathology of iridectomy specimens in gyrate atrophy of the retina and choroid. *Acta Ophthalmol* **61**:9, 1983.
289. Sipila I, Simell O, Rapola J, Sainio K, Tuuteri L: Gyrate atrophy of the choroid and retina with hyperornithinemia: Tubular aggregates and type 2 fiber atrophy in muscle. *Neurology* **29**:996, 1979.
290. Kennaway NG, Weleber RG, Buist NRM: Gyrate atrophy of the choroid and retina with hyperornithinemia. Biochemical and histologic studies and response to vitamin B6. *Am J Hum Genet* **32**:529, 1980.
291. Engel WK, Bishop DW, Cunningham GG: Tubular aggregates in type II muscle fibers: Ultrastructural and histochemical correlation. *J Ultrastruct Res* **31**:507, 1970.
292. Niakan E, Harati Y, Danon MJ: Tubular aggregates: Their association with myalgia. *J Neurol Neurosurg Psychiatry* **48**:882, 1985.
293. Maron BJ, Ferrans VJ: Aggregates of tubules in human cardiac muscle cells. *J Mal Cell Cardiol* **6**:249, 1974.
294. Rosenberg NL, Neville IH, Ringel SP: Tubular aggregates: their association with neuromuscular diseases, including the syndrome of myalgias/cramps. *Arch Neurol* **42**:973, 1985.
295. Wilson DJ, Weleber RG, Green WR: Ocular clinicopathologic study of gyrate atrophy. *Am J Ophthalmol* **111**:24, 1991.
296. Valle D, Boison A, Jezyk J, Aguirre G: Gyrate atrophy of the choroid and retina in a cat. *Invest Ophthalmol Vis Sci* **20**:251, 1981.
297. Valle D, Walser M, Brusilow S, Kaiser-Kupfer M: Gyrate atrophy of the choroid and retina: Amino acid metabolism and correction of hyperornithinemia with an arginine deficient diet. *J Clin Invest* **65**:371, 1980.
298. Valle D, Walser M, Brusilow S, Kaiser-Kupfer M, Takki KB: Gyrate atrophy of the choroid and retina. Biochemical considerations and experience with an arginine-restricted diet. *Ophthalmology* **88**:325, 1981.
299. Fell V, Pollitt RJ: 3-Aminopiperid-2-one, an unusual metabolite in the urine of a patient with hyperammonaemia, hyperornithinaemia and homocitrullinuria. *Clin Chim Acta* **87**:405, 1978.
300. Oberholzer VG: Personal communication.
301. Roesel RA, Coryell ME, Blankenship PR, Hommes FA: γ-Glutamylornithine excretion in patients with hyperornithinemia. *Clin Chim Acta* **140**:133, 1984.
302. Sipilä I, Valle D: Low guanidinoacetic acid and creatine concentrations in gyrate atrophy of the choroid and retina (GA), in DeDeyn PP, Marcscau N, Stalon V, Qureshi LA (eds): *Guanidino Compounds in Biology and Medicine*. London, John Libbey, 1992, p 379.

303. Heinänen K, Näntö-Salonen K, Komu M, Erkintalo M, Heinonen O, Pulkki K, Valtonen M, Kikoskelainen E, Alanen A, Simell O: Muscle creatine phosphate in gyrate atrophy of the choroid and retina with hyperornithinemia (GA): Clues to pathogenesis. *Eur J Clin Invest* **29**:426, 1999.
304. Näntö-Salonen K, Komu M, Lundbom N, Heinänen K, Alanen A, Sipilä I, Simell O: Reduced brain creatine in gyrate atrophy of the choroid and retina with hyperornithinemia. *Neurology* **53**:303, 1999.
305. Kennaway NG, Weleber RG, Buist NRM: Gyrate atrophy of the choroid and retina: Deficient activity of ornithine-ketoacid aminotransferase in cultured skin fibroblasts. *N Engl J Med* **297**:1180, 1977.
306. O'Donnell JJ, Sandman RP, Martin SR: Deficient L-ornithine:2-oxoacid aminotransferase activity in cultured fibroblasts from a patient with gyrate atrophy of the retina. *Biochem Biophys Res Commun* **79**:3696, 1977.
307. Ohura T, Kominami E, Tada K, Katunuma N: Gyrate atrophy of the choroid and retina: Decreased ornithine aminotransferase concentration in cultured skin fibroblasts from patients. *Clin Chim Acta* **136**:29, 1984.
308. Hayasaka S, Saito T, Nakajima H, Takaku Y, Shiono T, Mizuno K, Ohmura K, Tada K: Gyrate atrophy with hyperornithinaemia: Different types of responsiveness to vitamin B6. *Br J Ophthalmol* **65**:478, 1981.
309. Shih VE, Berson EL, Mandell R, Schmidt SY: Ornithine ketoacid transaminase deficiency in gyrate atrophy of the choroid and retina. *Am J Hum Genet* **30**:174, 1978.
310. Valle D, Kaiser-Kupfer M, Del Valle L: Gyrate atrophy of the choroid and retina: Deficiency of ornithine aminotransferase in transformed lymphocytes. *Proc Natl Acad Sci U S A* **74**:5159, 1977.
311. Askansas V, Valle D, Kaiser-Kupfer MI, Takki K, Engel WK, Blumenkopf B: Cultured muscle fibers of gyrate atrophy patients. Tubules, ornithine toxicity and L-ornithine-2-oxoacid aminotransferase deficiency. *Neurology* **30**:368, 1980.
312. Jansses AJM, Plakke T, Trijbels FJM, Sengers RCA, Monnens LAH: l-Ornithine ketoacid-transaminase assay in hair roots of homozygotes and heterozygotes for gyrate atrophy. *Clin Chim Acta* **3**:213, 1981.
313. Sipila I, O'Donnell JJ, Simell O: Gyrate atrophy of the choroid and retina with hyperornithinemia: Characterization of mutant liver-L-ornithine:2-oxoacid aminotransferase kinetics. *J Clin Invest* **67**:1805, 1981.
314. Kennaway NG, Stankova L, Wertz MK, Weleber RG: Gyrate atrophy of the choroid and retina (GA). Characterization of heterogeneity and mechanism of response to vitamin B6. *Am J Hum Genet* **41**:A9, 1987.
315. Wirtz MK, Kennaway NG, Weleber RG: Heterogeneity and complementation analysis of fibroblasts from vitamin B6 responsive and non-responsive patients with gyrate atrophy of the choroid and retina. *J Inherit Metab Dis* **8**:71, 1985.
316. Michaud J, Mitchell GA, Thompson GN, Brody LC, Steel G, Fontaine G, Schappert K, Keith CG, Valle D: Pyridoxine-responsive gyrate atrophy of the choroid and retina: Clinical and biochemical correlates of the mutation A226V. *Am J Hum Genet* **56**:616, 1995.
317. Weleber RG, Wirtz MK, Kennaway NG: Gyrate atrophy of the choroid and retina: Clinical and biochemical heterogeneity and response to vitamin B6. *Birth Defects* **18**:219, 1982.
318. Valle D, Boison A, Kaiser-Kupfer M: Complementation analysis of gyrate atrophy of the choroid and retina. *Pediatr Res* **13**:427, 1979.
319. Shih VE, Mandell R, Jacoby LB, Berson EL: Genetic-complementation analysis in fibroblasts from gyrate atrophy and the syndrome of hyperornithinemia, hyperammonemia and homocitrullinuria. *Pediatr Res* **15**:569, 1981.
320. Zintz C, Inana G: Analysis of the human ornithine aminotransferase gene family. *Exp Eye Res* **50**:759, 1990.
321. Michaud J, Brody LC, Steel G, Fontaine G, Martin LS, Valle D, Mitchell GA: Strand-separating conformational polymorphism (SSCP) analysis: Efficacy of detection of point mutations in the human ornithine-δ-aminotransferase gene. *Genomics* **13**:389, 1992.
322. Mitchell GA, Brody LC, Sipila I, Looney JE, Wong C, Engelhardt JF, Patel AS, Steel G, Obie C, Kaiser-Kupfer MI, Valle D: At least two mutant alleles of ornithine-δ-aminotransferase cause gyrate atrophy of the choroid and retina in Finns. *Proc Natl Acad Sci U S A* **86**:197, 1989.
323. Ramesh V, McClatchey A, Ramesh N, Benoit L, Berson E, Shih V, Gusella J: Molecular basis of ornithine aminotransferase deficiency in B6-responsive and nonresponsive forms of gyrate atrophy. *Proc Natl Acad Sci U S A* **85**:3777, 1988.
324. Mitchell GM, Brody LC, Looney J, Steel G, Suchanek M, Dowling C, Der Kaloustian V, Kaiser-Kupfer MI, Valle D: An initiator codon mutation in ornithine-δ-aminotransferase causing gyrate atrophy. *J Clin Invest* **81**:630, 1988.
325. Akaki Y, Hotta Y, Mashima Y, Murakimi A, Kennaway NG, Weleber RG, Inana G: A deletion in the ornithine aminotransferase gene in gyrate atrophy. *J Biol Chem* **267**:12950, 1992.
326. Mashima Y, Weleber RG, Kennaway NG, Shiono T, Inana G: Detection of point mutations in the ornithine aminotransferase gene in gyrate atrophy using PCR, denaturing gradient gel electrophoresis and direct sequencing. *Am J Hum Genet* **50**:A197, 1991.
327. Kaufman DL, Ramesh V, McClatchey AI, Menkes JH, Tobin AJ: Detection of point mutations associated with genetic diseases by an exon scanning technique. *Genomics* **8**:656, 1990.
328. Park JK, Herron BJ, O'Donnell JJ, Shih VE, Ramesh V: Three novel mutations of the ornithine aminotransferase (OAT) gene in gyrate atrophy. *Genomics* **14**:553, 1992.
329. Mashima Y, Murakami A, Weleber RG, Kennaway NG, Clarke L, Shiono T, Inana G: Nonsense-codon mutations of the ornithine aminotransferase gene with decreased levels of mutant mRNA in gyrate atrophy. *Am J Hum Genet* **51**:81, 1992.
330. Shiono T, Hotta Y, Inana G, Chambers C, Inouye L, Filpula D, Pulford S: Molecular genetics of gyrate atrophy: point mutation affecting processing of the ornithine aminotransferase precursor, in Yoshida T, Wilson J (eds): *Molecular Approaches to the Study and Treatment of Human Diseases*. New York, Elsevier, 1992, p 57.
331. Park JK, O'Donnell JJ, Shih VE, Gusella JF, Ramesh V: A 15-bp deletion in exon 5 of the ornithine aminotransferase (OAT) locus associated with gyrate atrophy. *Hum Mut* **1**:293, 1992.
332. McClatchey AI, Kaufman DL, Berson EL, Tobin AJ, Shih VE, Gusella JF, Ramesh V: Splicing defect at the ornithine aminotransferase (OAT) locus in gyrate atrophy. *Am J Hum Genet* **47**:790, 1990.
333. Mitchell GA, Labuda D, Fontaine G, Saudubray J-M, Bonnefont J-P, Lyonnet S, Brody L, Steel G, Obie C, Valle D: Splice-mediated insertion of an Alu sequence inactivates ornithine-δ-aminotransferase: A new role for Alu in human mutation. *Proc Natl Acad Sci U S A* **88**:815, 1991.
334. Valle D, Mitchell GA: Unpublished observations.
335. Mashima Y, Weleber RG, Kennaway NG, Inana G: A single base change at a splice acceptor site in the ornithine aminotransferase gene causes abnormal RNA splicing in gyrate atrophy. *Hum Genet* **90**:305, 1992.
336. Belgrader P, Cheng J, Maquat LE: Evidence to implicate translation by ribosomes in the mechanism by which nonsense codons reduce the nuclear level of human triosephosphate isomerase mRNA. *Proc Natl Acad Sci U S A* **90**:482, 1993.
337. Bach G, Moskowitz SM, Tieu PT, Matynia A, Neufeld EF: Molecular analysis of Hurler syndrome in Druze and Muslim Arab patients in Israel: Multiple allelic mutations of the *IDUA* gene in a small geographic area. *Am J Hum Genet* **53**:330, 1993.
338. Carothers AM, Urlaub G, Grunberger D, Chasin LA: Splicing mutants and their second site suppressors at the dihydrofolate reductase locus in Chinese hamster ovary cells. *Mol Cell Biol* **13**:5085, 1993.
339. Dietz HC, Valle D, Francomano CA, Rendzior RJ, Pyeritz RE, Cutting GR: The skipping of constitutive exons *in vivo* induced by nonsense mutations. *Science* **259**:680, 1993.
340. Makalowski A, Mitchell G, Labuda D: Alu sequences in the coding regions of mRNA: A source of protein variability. *Trends Genet* **10**:188, 1994.
341. Martin LS, Mitchell GA, Brody LC, Valle D: A polymorphic synyomous mutation in human ornithine-δ-aminotransferase. *Nucleic Acids Res* **19**:1962, 1991.
342. Hotta Y, Inana G: Gene transfer and expression of human ornithine aminotransferase. *Invest Ophthalmol Vis Sci* **30**:1024, 1989.
343. Pakula AA, Sauer RT: Genetic analysis of protein stability and function. *Annu Rev Genet* **23**:289, 1989.
344. Schulz GE, Schirmer: *Principles of Protein Structure*. New York, Springer-Verlag, 1978.
345. Bowie JU, Reidhaar-Olson JF, Lim WA, Sauer RT: Deciphering the message in protein sequences: Tolerance to amino acid substitutions. *Science* **247**:1306, 1990.
346. Knowles JR: Tinkering with enzymes: What are we learning? *Science* **236**:1252, 1987.
347. Mashima Y, Weleber RG, Kennaway NG, Inana G: Genotype-phenotype correlation of a pyridoxine-responsive form of gyrate atrophy. *Ophthal Genet* **20**:219, 1999.

348. Yonaha K, Nishie M, Aibara S: The primary structure of ω-amino acid: Pyruvate aminotransferase. *J Biol Chem* **267**:12506, 1992.
349. Watanabe N, Sakabe K, Sakabe N, Higashi T, Sasaki K, Aibara S, Morita Y, Yonaha K, Toyama S, Fukutani H: Crystal structure analysis of ω-amino acid: Pyruvate aminotransferase with a newly developed Weissenberg camera and an imaging plate using synchrotron radiation. *J Biochem* **105**:1, 1989.
350. Watanabe N, Yonaha K, Sakabe K, Sakabe N, Aibara S, Morita Y: Crystal structure of ω-amino acid: Pyruvate aminotransferase, in Fukui T, Kagamiyama H, Soda K, Wada H (eds): *Enzymes Dependent on Pyridoxal Phosphate and Other Carbonyl Compounds as Cofactors*. Osaka, Japan, Pergamon Press, 1990. p 121.
351. Nevanlinna HR: Rare hereditary diseases and markers in Finland: An introduction, in Eriksson A, Forsius H, Nevanlinna H, Workman P, Norio R (eds): *Population Structure and Genetic Disorders*. London, Academic Press, 1980, p 569.
352. de la Chapelle A: Disease gene mapping in isolated human populations: The examples of Finland. *J Med Genet* **30**:857, 1993.
353. Peltonen L, Jalanko A, Varilo T: Molecular genetics of the Finnish disease heritage. *Hum Mol Genet* **8**:1913, 1999.
354. Sipila I, Valle D, Mitchell G, Brody L: Hyperornitinemia ja pyororappeuma (gyrata-atrofia) eli HOGA-tauti. Suomalalsesta taudista ornitliniaminotransferaasin geenidefektlin. *Duodecim* **110**:681, 1994.
355. Valle D, Mitchell GA, Sipila I, Simell O: Unpublished results.
356. Inana G, Hotta Y, Inouye L, Zintz C, Shiono T: Single point mutation and amino acid change in ornithine aminotransferase from a gyrate atrophy patient. *Invest Ophthalmol Vis Sci* **29**:14, 1988.
357. Stetten MR: Mechanism of the conversion of ornithine into proline and glutamic acid *in vivo*. *J Biol Chem* **189**:499, 1951.
358. Scriver CR, Rosenberg LE: *Amino Acid Metabolism and Its Disorders*, Philadelphia, WB Saunders, 1973.
359. Bergstrom J, Furst P, Noree LO, Vinnars E: Intracellular free amino acid concentration in human muscle tissue. *J Appl Physiol* **36**:693, 1974.
360. Gopalakrishna R, Nagarajan B: A modified method for estimation of ornithine in biological samples. *Anal Biochem* **101**:472, 1980.
361. Matsuzawa T, Ishiguro I: Hyperornithinemia with gyrate atrophy and enzymes involved in ornithine metabolism of the eye. *Biochem Int* **1**:179, 1980.
362. Cohen AI: The retina and optic nerve, in Moses R (ed): *Adler's Physiology of the Eye*. St Louis, CW Mosby, 1975, p 367.
363. Zinn KM, Marmor MF: *The Retinal Pigment Epithelium*. Cambridge, MA, Harvard University Press, 1979.
364. Besharse JC: Photosensitive membrane turnover: Differentiated membrane domains and cell-cell interaction, in Adler R, Farber D (eds): *The Retina: A Model for Cell Biology Studies*. New York, Academic Press, 1986, p 297.
365. Clark VM: The cell biology of the retinal pigment epithelium, in Adler R, Farber D (eds): *The Retina: A Model for Cell Biology Studies*. New York, Academic Press, 1986, p 129.
366. Dowling JM: *The Retina: An Approachable Part of the Brain*. Cambridge, MA, Harvard University Press, 1987.
367. Rodieck RW: *The Vertebrate Retina*. San Francisco: WH Freeman, 1973.
368. Kaiser-Kupfer MI, Caruso RC, Valle D: Gyrate atrophy of the choroid and retina: Chronic reduction of ornithine slows retinal degeneration. *Arch Ophthalmol* **109**:1539, 1991.
369. Kuwabara T, Ishikawa Y, Kaiser-Kupfer M: Experimental model of gyrate atrophy in animals. *Ophthalmology* **88**:331, 1981.
370. Ueda M, Masu Y, Ando A, Maeda H, Del Monte MA, Uyama M, Ito S: Prevention of ornithine cytotoxicity by proline in human retinal pigment epithelial cells. *Invest Ophthalmol Vis Sci* **39**:820, 1998.
371. Wang T, Milam AH, Steel G, Valle D: A mouse model of gyrate atrophy of the choroid and retina: Early retinal pigment epithelium damage and progressive retinal degeneration. *J Clin Invest* **97**:2753, 1996.
372. Sipila I, Simell O, Arjomaa P: Gyrate atrophy of the choroid and retina with hyperornithinemia. Deficient formation of guanidinoacetic acid from arginine. *J Clin Invest* **66**:684, 1980.
373. Sipila I, Valle D, Brusilow SW, Kaiser-Kupfer MI: Defective creatine metabolism in gyrate atrophy of the choroid and retina. *Pediatr Res* **17**:226A, 1984.
374. Dionisi Vici C, Bachmann C, Gambarara M, Colombo JP, Sabetta G: Hyperornithinemia-hyperammonemia-homocitrullinuria syndrome: Low creatine excretion and effect of citrulline, arginine, or ornithine supplement. *Pediatr Res* **22**:364, 1987.
375. Sipila I, Rapola J, Simell O, Vannas A: Supplementary creatine as a treatment for gyrate atrophy of the choroid and retina. *N Engl J Med* **304**:867, 1981.
376. Vannas Sulonen K, Sipila J, Vannas A, Simell O, Rapola J: Gyrate atrophy of the choroid and retina. A five-year follow-up of creatine supplementation. *Ophthalmology* **92**:1719, 1985.
377. Kaiser-Kupfer MI, De Monasterio FM, Valle D, Walser M, Brusilow S: Gyrate atrophy of the choroid and retina: Improved visual function following reduction of plasma ornithine by diet. *Science* **210**:1128, 1980.
378. McInnes RR, Arshinoff SA, Bell L, Marliss EB, McCulloch JC: Hyperornithinaemia and gyrate atrophy of the retina. Improvement of vision during treatment with a low-arginine diet. *Lancet* **1**:513, 1981.
379. Walliman T, Wegmann G, Moser H, Huber R, Eppenberger HM: High content of creatine kinase in chicken retina: Compartmentalized localization of creatine kinase isoenzymes in photoreceptor cells. *Proc Natl Acad Sci U S A* **83**:3816, 1986.
380. Matsumoto M, Kobayashi K, Mori A: Distribution of guanidino compounds in bovine brain. *J Neurochem* **32**:645, 1979.
381. Mori A, Katayama Y, Higashidate S, Kimura S: Fluorometrical analysis of guanidino compounds in mouse brain. *J Neurochem* **32**:643, 1979.
382. Woznicki DT, Walker JB: Formation of a supplemental long time-constant reservoir of high energy phosphate by brain *in vivo* and *in vitro* and its reversible depletion by potassium depolarization. *J Neurochem* **33**:75, 1979.
383. Woznicki DT, Walker JB: Utilization of cyclocreatine phosphate and analogue of creatine phosphate by mouse brain during ischemia and its sparing action on brain energy reserves. *J Neurochem* **34**:1247, 1980.
384. Methfessel J: Zur organ-und subzellularverteilung der transamidinase bei mensch und ratte. *Acta Biol Med Ger* **35**:309, 1976.
384a. Harvey JC: Reduced renal arginine-glycine transamidinase activity in myotonic goats and in patients with myotonic muscular dystrophy. *Johns Hopkins Med J* **125**:270, 1969.
385. Loike JD, Kozler VF, Silverstein SC: Increased ATP and creatine phosphate turnover in phagocytosing mouse peritoneal macrophages. *J Biol Chem* **254**:9558, 1979.
386. Hu C-A, Lin W-W, Obie C, Valle D: Molecular enzymology of mammalian Δ^1-pyrroline-5-carboxylate synthase. *J Biol Chem* **274**:6754, 1999.
387. Valle D, Boison A, Kaiser-Kupfer M: Increased sensitivity of gyrate atrophy fibroblasts to ornithine toxicity. *Pediatr Res* **13**:426, 1979.
388. Valle D, Askanas V, Kaiser-Kupfer M, Takki K, Engel K: Increased sensitivity of gyrate atrophy fibroblasts and cultured muscle cells to ornithine toxicity. *Pediatr Res* **14**:1980.
389. Valle D, Boison AP, Phang JM, Smith RJ, Kaiser-Kupfer MI: Unpublished observations.
390. Hagedorn CH, Phang JM: Transfer of reducing equivalents into mitochondria by the interconversions of proline and $\Delta^?$? pyrroline-5-carboxylate. *Arch Biochem Biophys* **225**:95, 1983.
391. Hagedorn CH, Phang JM: Catalytic transfer of hydride ions from NADPH to oxygen by the interconversions of proline and delta L-pyrroline 5-carboxylate. *Arch Biochem Biophys* **248**:166, 1986.
392. Phang J, Downing S, Yeh G, Smith R, Williams J: Stimulation of the hexose-monophosphate pentose pathway by $\Delta^\bullet$-pyrroline-5-carboxylic acid in human fibroblasts. *Biochem Biophys Res Commun* **87**:363, 1979.
393. Yeh GC, Harris SC, Phang JM: Pyrroline-5-carboxylate reductase in human erythrocytes. *J Clin Invest* **67**:1042, 1981.
394. Yeh GC, Phang JM: Pyrroline-5-carboxylate stimulates the conversion of purine antimetabolites to their nucleotide forms by a redox-dependent mechanism. *J Biol Chem* **258**:9774, 1983.
395. Oldendorf WH: Brain uptake of radiolabeled amino acids, amines and hexoses after arterial injection. *Am J Physiol* **221**:1629, 1971.
396. Fleming GA, Hagedorn CH, Granger AS, Phang JM: Pyrroline-5-carboxylate in human plasma. *Metabolism* **33**:739, 1984.
397. Fleming GA, Phang JM, Valle D: Unpublished observations.
398. Shiono T, Kador PF, Kinoshita JH: Stimulation of the hexose monophosphate pathway by pyrroline-5-carboxylate reductase in the lens. *Exp Eye Res* **41**:767, 1985.
399. Rajantie J, Simell O, Perheentupa J: Lysinuric protein intolerance. Basolateral transport defect in renal tubuli. *J Clin Invest* **67**:1078, 1981.
400. Huang PL, Dawson TM, Bredt DS, Snyder SH, Fishman C: Targeted disruption of the neuronal nitric oxide synthase gene. *Cell* **75**:1273, 1993.

401. Schaumburg H, Kaplan J, Windebank A, Vick N, Rasmus S, Pleasure D, Brown MJ: Sensory neuropathy from pyridoxine abuse. A new mega vitamin syndrome. *N Engl J Med* **309**:445, 1983.
402. Dalton K, Dalton MJ: Characteristics of pyridoxine overdose neuropathy syndrome. *Acta Neurol Scand* **76**:8, 1987.
403. Weleber R: Personal communications. 1988.
404. Hayasaka S, Saito T, Nakajima H, Takahashi O, Mizuno K, Tada K: Clinical trials of vitamin B6 and proline supplementation for gyrate atrophy of the choroid and retina. *Br J Ophthalmol* **69**:283, 1985.
405. Valle D, Simell O: The hyperornithinemias, in Scriver CR, Beaudet AL, Sly WS, Valle D (eds): *The Metabolic and Molecular Bases of Inherited Disease*. New York, McGraw Hill, 1995, p 1147.
406. Berson EL, Hanson AH, Rosner B, Shih VE: A two-year trial of low protein, low-arginine diets or vitamin B6 for patients with gyrate atrophy. *Birth Defects* **18**:209, 1982.
407. Vannas Sulonen K, Simell O, Sipila I: Gyrate atrophy of the choroid and retina. The ocular disease progresses in juvenile patients despite normal or near normal plasma ornithine concentration. *Ophthalmology* **94**:1428, 1987.
408. Kaiser-Kupfer MI, Valle D: Unpublished observations.
409. Wang T, Steel G, Milam AH, Valle D: Correction of ornithine accumulation prevents retinal degeneration in a mouse model of gyrate atrophy of the choroid and retina. *Proc Natl Acad Sci U S A* **97**:1224, 2000.
410. Giordano D, DeSanto NG, Pluvio M, Santinelli R, Stoppoloni G: Lysine in treatment of hyperornithinemia. *Nephron* **22**:97, 1978.
411. Heinänen K, Näntö-Salonen K, Komu M, Erkintalo M, Alanen A, Heinonen OJ, Pulkki K, Nikoskelainen E, Sipilä I, Simell O: Creatine corrects muscle ^{31}P spectrum in gyrate atrophy with hyperornithinaemia. *Eur J Clin Invest* **29**:1060, 1999.
412. Saito T, Hayasaka S, Yabata K, Omura K, Mizuno K, Tada K: Atypical gyrate atrophy of the choroid and retina and iminoglycinuria. *Tohoku J Exp Med* **135**:331, 1981.
413. Takki K, Simell O: Genetic aspects in gyrate atrophy of the choroid and retina with hyperornithinemia. *Br J Ophthalmol* **58**:907, 1974.
414. Pai GS, VanRens GH, Mayfield RK, Chambers JK, Genco PV, Valle D: Lipoatrophic diabetes and gyrate atrophy of the retina and choroid in a black sibship. *Am J Hum Genet* **40**:A14, 1987.
415. Davis TA, Fiorotto ML, Reeds PJ: Amino acid composition of body and milk proteins change during the suckling period in rats. *J Nutr* **123**:947, 1993.
416. Matsuzawa T, Kobayashi T, Tashiro K, Kasahara M: Changes in ornithine metabolic enzymes induced by dietary protein in small intestine and liver: Intestine-liver relationship in ornithine supply to liver. *J Biochem* **116**:721, 1994.
417. Wright T, Pollitt R: Psychomotor retardation, epileptic and stuporous attacks, irritability and ataxia associated with ammonia intoxication, high blood ornithine levels and increased homocitrulline in the urine. *Proc R Soc Med* **66**:221, 1973.
418. Fell V, Pollitt RJ, Sampson GA, Wright T: Ornithinemia, hyperammonemia, and homocitrullinuria. A disease associated with mental retardation and possibly caused by defective mitochondrial transport. *Am J Dis Child* **127**:752, 1974.
419. Gatfield PD, Taller E, Wolfe DM, Haust DM: Hyperornithinemia, hyperammonemia, and homocitrullinuria associated with decreased carbamyl phosphate synthetase I activity. *Pediatr Res* **9**:488, 1975.
420. Hommes FA, Roesel RA, Metoki K, Hartlage PL, Dyken PR: Studies on a case of HHH-syndrome (Hyperammonemia, hyperornithinemia, homocitrullinuria). *Neuropediatrics* **17**:48, 1986.
421. Hommes FA, Ho CK, Roesel RA, Coryell ME: Decreased transport of ornithine across the inner mitochondrial membrane as a cause of hyperornithinaemia. *J Inherit Metab Dis* **5**:41, 1982.
422. Rodes M, Ribes A, Pineda M, Alvarez L, Fabregas I, Fernandes Alvarez E, Coude FX, Grimber G: A new family affected by the syndrome of hyperornithinaemia, hyperammonaemia and homocitrullinuria. *J Inherit Metab Dis* **10**:73, 1987.
423. Rennert OM, Garnica AD, Chan WY: Hyperornithinemia and hyperammonemia. A rare disorder of ammonia metabolism, in Preisign R, Bircher J, Baumgartner G (eds): *The Liver: Quantitative Aspects of Structure and Function*. Aulendorf, Editio Cantor, 1976, p 298.
424. Simell O, Mackenzie S, Clow CL, Scriver CR: Ornithine loading did not prevent induced hyperammonemia in a patient with HHH syndrome. *Pediatr Res* **19**:1283, 1985.
425. Shimizu H, Eto Y, Maekawa K, Sasaki H, Tanaka T, Suzuki T: Biochemical and morphological studies in hyperornithinemia associated with hyperammonemia and homocitrullinuria. *Jikeikai Med J* **34**:227, 1987.
426. Oyanagi K, Tsuchiyama A, Itakura Y, Sogawa H, Wagatsuma K, Nakao T: The mechanism of hyperammonaemia and hyperornithinaemia in the syndrome of hyperornithinaemia, hyperammonaemia with homocitrullinuria. *J Inherit Metab Dis* **6**:133, 1983.
427. Inoue I, Koura M, Saheki T, Kayanuma K, Uono M, Nakajima M, Takeshita K, Koike R, Yuasa T, Miyatake T, Sakoda K: Abnormality of citrulline synthesis in liver mitochondria from patients with hyperornithinaemia, hyperammonaemia and homocitrullinuria. *J Inherit Metab Dis* **10**:277, 1987.
428. Gjessing LR, Lunde HA, Undrum T, Broch H, Alme A, Lie SO: A new patient with hyperornithinaemia, hyperammonaemia and homocitrullinuria treated early with low-protein diet. *J Inherit Metab Dis* **9**:186, 1986.
429. Ogier H, Poll-The BT, Rabier D, Bonte JB, Charpentier C, Shih VE, Saudubray JM: Neonatal onset form of HHH syndrome: Three years clinical course and therapeutic attempts. Personal communication, 1988.
430. Shih VE, Mandell R, Herzfeld A: Defective ornithine metabolism in cultured skin fibroblasts from patients with the syndrome of hyperornithinemia, hyperammonemia and homocitrullinuria. *Clin Chim Acta* **118**:149, 1982.
431. Zamboni G, Marradi P, Praderio R, Dall'Agnola A: Hyperornithinemia with hyperammonemia and homocitrullinuria in two brothers. *Acta Med Auxol* **14**:121, 1982.
432. Kirsch SE, McInnes RR: Control of hyperammonemia in the 3H syndrome by ornithine administration. *Pediatr Res* **20**:267, 1986.
433. Koike R, Fujimori K, Yuasa T, Miyatake T, Inoue I, Saheki T: Hyperornithinemia, hyperammonemia, and homocitrullinuria. Case report and biochemical study. *Neurology* **37**:1813, 1987.
434. Koike R, Fujimori K, Yuasa T, Miyatake T: Hyperornithinemia, hyperammonemia and homocitrullinuria syndrome in a family. *Rinsho Shinkeigaku* **27**:465, 1987.
435. Endo T, Saito A, Sakamoto S, Yachi A: A case with hyperornithinemia, hyperammonemia, and homocitrullinuria. *Jpn J Med* **21**:253, 1982.
436. Haass C, Pedicino R, Sabetta G, Panero A, Colarizzi P: Hyperornithinemia, hyperammonemia and homocitrullinuria (HHH syndrome) with neonatal onset and favourable evolution. *Ital J Pediatr* **12**:143, 1986.
437. Halvorsen S: Personal communication, 1988.
438. Otten A, Buerger U, Bachmann C, Hillig U, Wolf H: Late diagnosis of and therapeutical approach to the HHH syndrome. *Abstracts of the Third International Symposium on Inborn Error of Metabolism in Humans*, Munich, 1984.
439. Lemay J, Lambert M, Mitchell G, Vanasse M, Valle D, Arbour J, Dube J, Flessas J, Laberge M, Lafleur L, Orquin J, Qureshi I, Dery R: HHH syndrome: Neurologic, ophthalmologic and psychological evaluation of six patients. *J Pediatr* **121**:725, 1992.
440. Sabetta G, Lombardi M, Castro M, Scapaticci A, Giampaolo R, D'Ippoliti M, Lucidi V: Iperammoniemia, iperornitinemia, omocitruilinuria: Descrizione di un caso. *Agg Pediatr* **31**:479, 1980.
441. Shih VE, La Framboise R, Mandell R, Pichette J: Neonatal form of the hyperornithinaemia, hyperammonaemia and homocitrullinuria (HHH) syndrome and prenatal diagnosis. *Prenat Diagn* **12**:717, 1992.
442. Shimizu H, Maekawa K, Eto Y: Abnormal urinary excretion of polyamines in HHH syndrome. *Brain Dev* **12**:533, 1990.
443. Smith L, Lambert MA, Brochu P, Jasmin G, Qureshi IA, Seidman EG: Hyperornithinemia, hyperammonemia, homocitrullinuria (HHH) syndrome: Presentation as acute liver disease with coagulopathy. *J Pediatr Gastroent Nutr* **15**:431, 1992.
444. Haust DM, Gordon BA: Letter to the editor: Ultrastructural changes in the mitochondria in disorders of ornithine metabolism. *Pediatr Res* **14**:1411, 1980.
445. Haust DM, Gatfield PD, Gordon BA: Ultrastructure of hepatic mitochondria in a child with hyperornithinemia, hyperammonemia, and homocitrullinuria. *Hum Pathol* **12**:212, 1981.
446. Gordon BA, Gatfield DP, Haust DM: The hyperornithinemia, hyperammonemia, homocitrullinuria syndrome: An ornithine transport defect remediable with ornithine supplements. *Clin Invest Med* **10**:329, 1987.
447. Winters MS, Perez-Atayade AR, Levy ML, Shih VE: Unique hepatic ultrastructural changes in a patient with hyperornithinemia, hyperammonemia and homocitrullinuria. *Pediatr Res* **14**:583, 1980.

448. Metoki K, Hommes FA, Dyken P, Kelloes C, Trefz J: Ultra-structural changes in fibroblast mitochondria of a patient with HHH-syndrome. *J Inherit Metab Dis* **7**:147, 1984.
449. Gordon BA, Gatfield PD, Taller E: Ornithine methyl ester. An unusual metabolite encountered in the urine of patients with a urea cycle disorder characterized by hyperammonemia, hyperornithinemia, and homocitrullinuria. *Clin Biochem* **10**:78, 1977.
450. Shih VE, Mandell R: Metabolic defect in hyperornithinemia. *Lancet* **2**:1522, 1974.
451. Liu Q, Dunlap JC: Isolation and analysis of the *arg-113* gene of *Neurospora crassa*. *Genetics* **143**:1163, 1996.
452. Crabeel M, Soetens O, De Rijcke M, Pratiwi R, Pankiewicz R: The *ARG11* gene of *Saccharomyces cerevisiae* encodes a mitochondrial integral membrane protein required for arginine biosynthesis. *J Biol Chem* **271**:25011, 1996.
453. Palmieri L, De Marco V, Iacobazzi V, Palmieri F, Runswick MJ, Walker JE: Identification of the yeast ARG-11 gene as a mitochondrial ornithine carrier involved in arginine biosynthesis. *FEBS Lett* **410**:447, 1997.
454. Palmieri F: Mitochondrial carrier protein. *FEBS Lett* **346**:48, 1994.
455. Krämer R: Structural and functional aspects of the phosphate carrier from mitochondria. *Kidney Int* **49**:947, 1996.
456. Schroers A, Burkovski A, Wohlrab H, Krämer R: The phosphate carrier from yeast mitochondria. *J Biol Chem* **273**:14269, 1998.
457. Palmieri F, Indiveri C, Bisaccia F, Iacobazzi V: Mitochondrial metabolite carrier proteins: Purification, reconstitution and transport studies. *Methods Enzymol* **260**:349, 1995.
458. Mouali̇j B, Duyckaerts C, Lamotte-Brasseur J, Sluse FE: Phylogenetic classification of the mitochondrial carrier family of *Saccharomyces cerevisiae*. *Yeast* **13**:573, 1997.
459. Nelson DR, Felix CM, Swanson JM: Highly conserved charge-pair networks in the mitochondrial carrier family. *J Mol Biol* **277**:285, 1998.
460. Indiveri C, Palmieri L, Palmieri F: Kinetic characterization of the reconstituted ornithine carrier from rat liver mitochondria. *Biochim Biophys Acta* **1188**:293, 1994.
461. Indiveri C, Tonazzi A, Stipani I, Palmieri F: The purified and reconstituted ornithine/citrulline carrier from rat liver mitochondria: Electrical nature and coupling of the exchange reaction with H^+ translocation. *Biochem J* **327**:349, 1997.
462. Kuan J, Saier MHJ: The mitochondrial carrier family of transport proteins: Structural, functional and evolutionary relationships. *Crit Rev Biochem Mol Biol* **28**:209, 1993.
463. Camacho JA, Obie C, Biery B, Goodman BK, Hu C-A, Almashanu S, Steel G, Caey R, Lombard M, Mitchell GA, Valle D: Hyperornithinemia-hyperammonemia-homocitrullinuria (HHH) syndrome is caused by mutations in a gene encoding a mitochondrial ornithine transporter. *Nature Genet* **22**:151, 1999.
464. Tsujino S, Kanazawa N, Ohashi T, Eto Y, Saito T, Kira J; Yamada T: Three novel mutations (G27E, insAAC, R179X) in the ORNT1 gene of Japanese patients with HHH syndrome. *Ann Neurol* **200**:625, 2000.
465. Briggs S, Freedland RA: Effect of ornithine and lactate on urea synthesis in isolated hepatocytes. *Biochem J* **160**:205, 1976.
466. Brusilow SW, Batshaw MM: Arginine therapy of argininosuccinase deficiency. *Lancet* **1**:124, 1979.
467. Greenstein JP, Winitz M, Gullino P, Birnbaum SM, Otey MC: Studies on the metabolism of amino acids and related compounds *in vivo*. III. Prevention of ammonia toxicity by arginine and related compounds. *Arch Biochem Biophys* **64**:342, 1956.
468. Nathans D, Fahey JL, Ship AG: Sites of origin and removal of blood ammonia formed during glycine infusion: Effect of L-arginine. *J Lab Clin Med* **51**:124, 1958.
469. Rajantie J, Simell O, Rapola J, Perheentupa J: Lysinuric protein intolerance: A two-year trial of dietary supplementation therapy with citrulline and lysine. *J Pediatr* **97**:927, 1980.
470. Simell O, Perheentupa J, Rapola J, Visakorpi JK, Eskelin LE: Lysinuric protein intolerance. *Am J Med* **59**:229, 1975.
471. Aronson DL, Diwan JJ: Uptake of ornithine by rat liver mitochondria. *Biochemistry* **20**:7064, 1981.
472. Bryla J, Harris EJ: Accumulation of ornithine and citrulline in rat liver mitochondria in relation to citrulline formation. *FEBS Lett* **72**:331, 1976.
473. Hommes F, Kitchings L, Eller AG: The uptake of ornithine and lysine by rat liver mitochondria. *Biochem Med* **30**:313, 1983.
474. Metoki K, Hommes FA: A possible rate limiting factor in urea synthesis by isolated hepatocytes. The transport of ornithine into hepatocytes and mitochondria. *Int J Biochem* **16**:1155, 1984.
475. Metoki K, Hommes FA: The uptake of ornithine and lysine by isolated hepatocytes and fibroblasts. *Int J Biochem* **16**:833, 1984.
476. Raijman L: Citrulline synthesis in rat tissues and liver content of carbamoyl phosphate and ornithine. *Biochem J* **138**:225, 1974.
477. Shih VE: Regulation of ornithine metabolism. *Enzyme* **26**:254, 1981.
478. Shih VE, Mandell R: Defective ornithine metabolism in the syndrome of hyperornithinaemia, hyperammonaemia and homocitrullinuria. *J Inherit Metab Dis* **4**:95, 1981.
479. Metoki K, Hommes FA: The pH of mitochondria of fibroblasts from a hyperornithinaemia, hyperammonaemia, homocitrullinuria syndrome patient. *J Inherit Metab Dis* **7**:9, 1984.
480. Oyanagi K, Aoyama T, Tsuchiyama A, Nakao T, Uetsuji N, Wagatsuma K, Tsugawa S: A new type of hyperlysinaemia due to a transport defect of lysine into mitochondria. *J Inherit Metab Dis* **9**:313, 1986.
481. Gray RGF, Hill SE, Pollitt RJ: Reduced ornithine catabolism in cultured fibroblasts and phytohaemagglutinin-stimulated lymphocytes from a patient with hyperornithinaemia, hyperammonaemia and homocitrullinuria. *Clin Chim Acta* **118**:141, 1982.
482. Gray RGF, Hill SE, Pollitt RJ: Studies on the pathway from ornithine to proline in cultured skin fibroblasts with reference to the defect in hyperornithinaemia with hyperammonaemia and homocitrullinuria. *J Inher Metab Dis* **6**:143, 1983.
483. Botschner J, Smith DW, Simell O, Scriver CR: Comparison of ornithine metabolism in hyperornithinaemia-hyperammonaemia-homocitrullinuria syndrome, lysinuric protein intolerance and gyrate atrophy fibroblasts. *J Inher Metab Dis* **12**:33, 1989.
484. Carson NA, Scally BG, Neill DW, Carre IJ: Saccharopinuria: A new inborn error of lysine metabolism. *Nature* **218**:679, 1968.
485. Simell O, Visakorpi JK, Donner M: Saccharopinuria. *Arch Dis Child* **47**:52, 1972.
486. Simell O, Sipila I, Rajantie J: Hyperlysinemia with hyperammonemia and homocitrullinuria. *Pediatr Res* **14**:174, 1980.
487. Carter AL, Eller AG, Rufo S, Metoki K, Hommes FA: Further evidence for a separate enzymic entity for the synthesis of homocitrulline, distinct from the regular ornithine transcarbamylase. *Enzyme* **32**:26, 1984.
488. Valle D, Walser M, Brusilow SW, Kaiser-Kupfer MI: Unpublished observations.
489. Holmgren G: Effect of low, normal and high dietary protein intake on urinary amino acid excretion and plasma aminogram I children. *Nutr Metab* **16**:223, 1974.
490. Berson EL, Schmidt SY, Rabin AR: Plasma amino acids in hereditary retina disease: Ornithine, lysine and taurine. *Br J Ophthalmol* **60**:142, 1976.

CHAPTER 84

Guanidinoacetate Methyltransferase Deficiency

Kurt von Figura ■ Folker Hanefeld
Dirk Isbrandt ■ Sylvia Stöckler-Ipsiroglu

1. Guanidinoacetate methyltransferase (GAMT)-deficiency (MIM 601240) is a disease of creatine biosynthesis. Creatine is synthesized in a two-step mechanism from glycine, arginine, and methionine. In the first reaction, guanidinoacetate and ornithine are formed by arginine: glycine aminidinotransferase. In the second reaction, catalyzed by GAMT, S-adenosylmethionine donates the methyl group for formation of creatine from guanidinoacetate.

2. GAMT-deficiency manifests during the first months of life as developmental delay or arrest. Neurologic symptoms are heterogeneous, including muscular hypotonia and weakness, poor head control, involuntary extrapyramidal movements, epilepsy, and, in older patients, autistic behavior. Abnormal signals in the globus pallidus, as observed on MRI scans, may provide an important clue for diagnosis.

3. Diagnosis of the disease is based on the demonstration of excessive amounts of guanidinoacetate in body fluids, the deficiency of creatine/phosphocreatine in brain, and the absence of GAMT activity in fibroblasts, lymphocytes, or amniotic fluid cells.

4. GAMT deficiency is an autosomal recessive disorder. Two GAMT deficiency alleles have been characterized, which account for four of the six alleles in the three patients analyzed so far. The two alleles give rise to transcripts that encode truncated or elongated, presumably nonfunctional polypeptides.

5. The bulk of creatine is synthesized in liver, pancreas, and kidney; released into the blood; and taken up by cells via creatine transporters. In tissues with highly fluctuating demand for energy, such as muscle and brain, the creatine/phosphocreatine system serves as a temporal and spatial energy buffering system. Some of the abnormalities observed in GAMT deficiency can be explained by the deficiency of high-energy phosphate in such cells, while others appear to be related to the accumulation of guanidinoacetate.

6. Oral supplementation of creatine in GAMT deficiency patients partially restores the creatine/phosphocreatine in brain and has beneficial effects on the clinical manifestations. The elevation of guanidinoacetate in plasma is largely refractory to oral supplementation of creatine, which may explain the persistence of some of the clinical symptoms.

HISTORY

As early as 1928, Hunter[1] wrote in his monograph on creatine and creatinine, "creatine, in fact, is probably not a waste product but an essential tissue constituent with a special function." The chemical was first described and named "creatine" by Chevreul[2] in 1835 and von Liebig[3] in 1847, and its biosynthesis and metabolism were clarified over a period of more than 100 years.[4] Around 1930 it became apparent that oral supplementation increases the creatine/phosphocreatine pool in animals and humans,[1,5] and phosphocreatine, which diminishes during electrical stimulation of muscle,[6] was recognized as a key intermediate of skeletal muscle metabolism.[7]

Although there are ample biochemical publications on the role of creatine in energy metabolism of different tissues and the creatine transport systems, little attention was paid to these topics in clinical medicine. The concentration of the end-product, creatinine, in plasma and its excretion in urine has been used as an indicator of kidney function: High concentrations of creatinine in plasma indicate impairment, while low levels are considered to reflect normal renal function. The significance of low creatine and creatinine concentrations as disease markers became obvious with the discovery of the first inherited metabolic defect of creatine synthesis, reported by Stöckler et al. in 1994.[8]

The index patient with GAMT deficiency[8] (MIM 601240) was born after an uneventful pregnancy at 41 weeks of gestation (birth weight 3405 g, length 51 cm). The neonatal period and early development were normal. At 4–6 months, dystonic postures beginning in his left arm were noticed; he lost the ability to turn from the prone to the supine position and was unable to crawl or sit at the age of 11 months. His head control was poor, and he had roving eye movements with a tonic squint. Although there was no severe muscular weakness, he was hypotonic. All tendon reflexes were present, and the plantar reflexes were flexor.

Over the next months, global developmental delay became more evident, with an abnormal dyskinetic movement pattern, failing head control, and irregular eye movements. Seizure-like head drops were observed in the prone position. The electroencephalogram showed a peculiar pattern of intermittent runs of high-voltage slow activity (1.5–3 s) intermingled with few spikes. The biochemical investigations done at different stages of the child's development revealed hyperammonemia, orotic aciduria, and hyperornithinemia. Urinary excretion of dicarboxylic acids, 3-methylglutaronic acid, and methylmalonic acid were elevated.

These laboratory abnormalities led to a number of diagnostic considerations and specialized investigations on fibroblasts and muscle tissue. All proved inconclusive. One constant finding, however, the very low creatinine concentrations in plasma (0.08–0.1 mg/dl) and in urine, escaped attention. In retrospect it became clear that the hyperornithinemia was an artifact due to improper sample handling and the apparent increased excretion of dicarboxylic acids was due to normalization of the absolute amounts with an abnormally low creatinine value. The latter seemed almost too banal to be considered seriously as the clue to the underlying biochemical defect. Head ultrasound and computerized tomography were normal at the age of 6 months. MRI of the brain, first performed at age 12 months demonstrated a high level of signal in globus pallidus bilaterally, proving morphologic alteration of a structure known to be of particular vulnerability and explaining many of the clinical symptoms. At this time

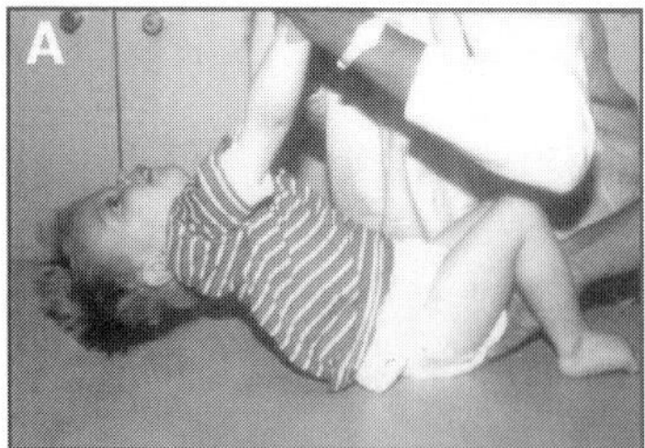

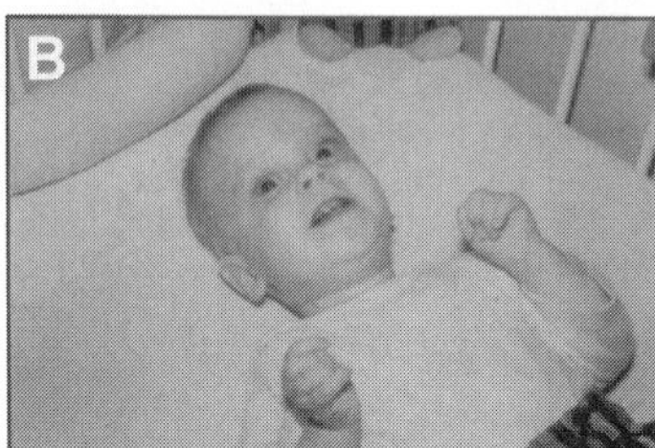

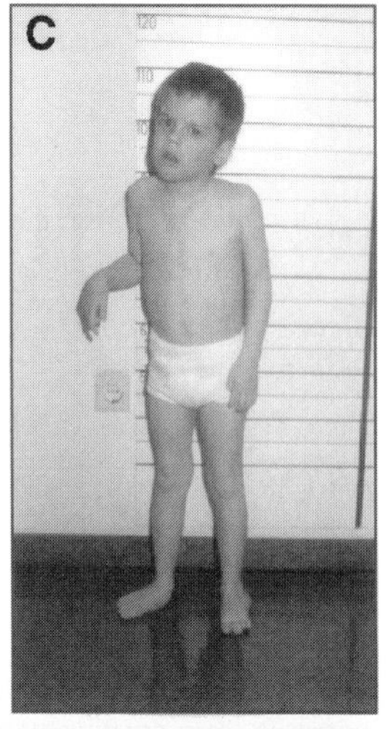

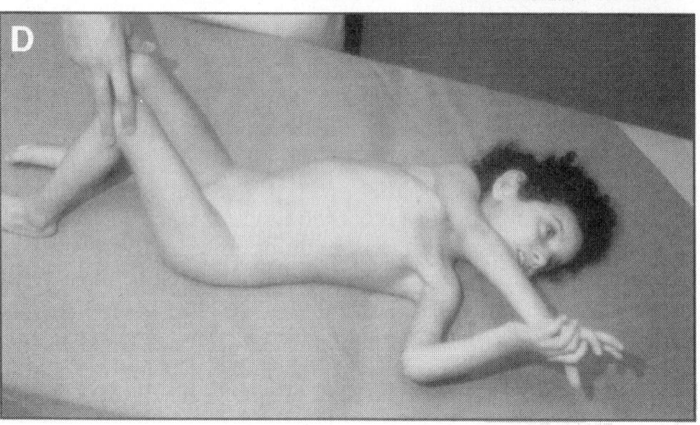

Fig. 84-1 Two patients with GAMT deficiency. (A–C) The index patient. Oral supplementation with creatine was started at the age of 23 months. (A) Severe muscular hypotonia and weakness at 9 months. (B) Dystonia at 22 months. (C) Considerable improvement of motor abilities after treatment with creatine at $5\frac{1}{2}$ years. (D) The second patient with GAMT deficiency at the age of 4 years. (*Courtesy of Prof. Rating, Heidelberg.*)

MR-spectroscopy (MRS) of the brain showed a spectrum lacking a creatine signal and having an elevated guanidinoacetate peak. Such a spectrum had never been seen or described in the literature. The combination of high guanidinoacetate with deficient creatine suggested a block in creatine synthesis at the level of the transformation of guanidinoacetate to creatine. Further evidence for this hypothesis was obtained by feeding the child with arginine, a precursor of guanidinoacetate, which resulted in an increase of guanidinoacetate as measured by MRS without restoring the missing creatine signal. Oral supplementation with creatine monohydrate resulted in appearance of a creatine signal and a decrease in guanidinoacetate. The patient's condition improved with respect to muscle tone, dyskinetic movements, and mental and motor development. Within 6 months of institution of oral creatine supplementation, the patient was able to sit unsupported. The electroencephalogram normalized, and the globus pallidus showed a normal signal on MRI. Since the age of 5 years he has been able to walk without ataxia or dyskinetic movements. His muscle tonus is still low, and at the age of 6 years he still does not speak. Despite the marked progress in motor development, he shows some autistic features, with self-injurious behavior (Fig. 84-1, A–C).

Subsequent studies confirmed the postulated lack of GAMT activity in liver and identified the molecular defect.[9]

CLINICAL MANIFESTATIONS

Since this first observation, three more patients with creatine deficiency have been discovered using MRS.[10–12] Their clinical findings are summarized in Table 84-1 and Fig. 84-1. From these observations, the clinical phenotype of GAMT appears to be a progressive encephalopathy with onset during the first months of life, characterized by muscular hypotonia, dyskinetic movements, and dysphagia. Intially delayed, development may arrest and even regress in some patients. Loss of active speech was also observed in all patients. Autistic, self-injurious behavior is present in almost all. Peripheral nerves, vision, and hearing are not affected. The tendon reflexes are normal. Dysmorphic features or organomegaly are absent. Liver, kidney, and cardiac function are normal. The hematopoetic system is not affected, and parameters of somatic growth, including head circumference, are within the normal range.

LABORATORY FINDINGS

Although clinical manifestations of GAMT deficiency may be very heterogeneous, some specific pathologic laboratory parameters were observed in all known patients (Table 84-2). Creatinine excretion in 24-h urine (9–12 μmol/kg/d) and concentrations in plasma (3.3–7.0 μmol/L) and cerebrospinal fluid (<1.0 μmol/L) were clearly below the lower normal limits (71–177 μmol/kg/d, 18–25 μmol/L, and 29–40.5 μmol/L, respectively). Creatinine concentrations in random urine samples (1060–2060 μmol/L) were in the low normal range (1800–4400 μmol/L). Consequently, the excretion of all metabolites whose concentrations are

Table 84-1 Clinical Manifestations of GAMT Deficiency

Parameter	Patient			
	1	2	3	4
Sex/origin	male/German	female/Kurdish	male/Welsh	male/Dutch
Age at onset	4 months	6 months	6 weeks	?
Age at diagnosis	22 months	3 years, 8 months	5 years	3 years
Developmental arrest	+	+	+	+
Hypotonia	+	+	+	?
Dyskinesia	+	+	–	–
Reflexes	normal	normal	normal	?
Seizures	?	+	+	–
Mental retardation	mild	severe	severe	severe
Autism/self-injurious behavior	+	–	+	+
Active speech	none	none	none	none
Reference	8	10	11	12

Table 84-2 Laboratory Findings in GAMT Deficiency

Parameter	Effect
Creatinine/creatine (plasma, urine, CSF)	decreased
Guanidinoacetate (plasma, urine, CSF)	elevated
Electroencephalography	abnormal
Nerve conductance velocity	normal
Brainstem auditory evoked potentials	normal
Visual evoked potential	normal
Magnetic resonance imaging (globus pallidus)	abnormal
Magnetic resonance spectroscopy	
creatine/phosphocreatine	absent
guanidinoacetate	elevated

routinely normalized to that of creatinine appeared to be elevated. Urinary creatine concentrations were also low.[8,13]

The most prominent and consistent abnormality was the elevation of guanidinoacetate in urine (2224–3987 μmol/L, normal 63–429 μmol/L), plasma (12.9–20.7 μmol/L, normal 0.83 ± 0.31 μmol/L) and especially in cerebrospinal fluid (10.6–12.7 μmol/L, normal 0.055 ± 0.032 μmol/L).[13] Mild hyperammonemia and hyperuricemia were detected in some of the patients. Normal values were obtained for all other routine laboratory parameters, among them blood cell count, serum electrolytes, glucose, urea, liver aminotransferases, creatine kinase, lactate dehydrogenase, and blood coagulation tests. Despite the initial report of modest hyperornithinemia and hypoargininemia, the levels of these and all other amino acids in plasma and urine are normal. In the cerebrospinal fluid, intermittently elevated lactate concentrations were detected in one patient, probably because of high seizure activity. When examined by echocardiography, cardiac function was normal. Histologic examination of liver specimens from two patients yielded a normal cytoarchitecture but fat droplets and signs of mild steatosis. Muscle histology in a third patient was completely normal.

The electroencephalogram was abnormal in all patients, showing some symmetric intermediate slow activity intermingled with spikes (Fig. 84-2). Neurophysiologic examination of auditory and visual evoked potentials revealed no abnormalities.

Cranial MRI in three patients demonstrated abnormal signal intensities in the globus pallidus (Fig. 84-3), a structure affected in several metabolic disorders.[14] *In vivo* MRS demonstrated the complete absence of creatine and phosphocreatine and the accumulation of guanidinoacetate in the brain of all patients with GAMT deficiency (Fig. 84-4).

CREATINE METABOLISM AND FUNCTION

Phosphocreatine and its immediate precursor, creatine, are degraded nonenzymatically to creatinine. The fractional rates for these reactions are 2.6 and 1.1 percent/day for phosphocreatine and creatine, respectively. Creatinine is excreted in the urine. A normal adult excretes 1.5 to 2 g creatinine daily, which is generated from a pool of 120 g phosphocreatine and creatine.[4] Phosphocreatine and creatine lost due to formation of creatinine must be replenished from dietary sources and *de novo* synthesis. On average, about half of the creatine is replaced by endogenous synthesis. It should be noted that vegetarian diets are poor in creatine, because plants, together with microorganisms and most invertebrates, do not contain creatine. The biosynthesis of creatine in mammals comprises the two steps shown in Fig. 84-5.[15]

Arginine:glycine amidinotransferase (AT, EC 2.1.4.1) catalyzes the first of the two reactions, the transfer of the amidino group from arginine to glycine, to form guanidinoacetate, the precursor of creatine, and ornithine. This reaction is thought to be the rate-limiting step of creatine biosynthesis.[16] In humans, the highest activity levels of AT are found in pancreas,[17,18] kidney,[19–2021] and liver.[22] AT is also detectable in heart, lung, spleen, muscle, brain, testis, and thymus; in rat, collective AT activity in these organs may approach the activity in pancreas and kidney.[23] In kidney, AT is localized in the intermembrane space of mitochondria.[24] AT was isolated from the cytosol, but it is likely that this reflects release from mitochondria during the isolation procedure.[25] The localization of AT in the mitochondrial intermembrane space separates this reaction from the other major arginine-consuming reactions, including cleavage by arginase to urea and ornithine, conversion by NO synthase into citrulline and NO, and transfer to arginyl-tRNA, which all occur in the cytosol. Human AT is synthesized as a precursor of 423 amino acids. The N-terminal 37 residues are cleaved after transport to the mitochondrial intermembrane space, yielding a mature protein of

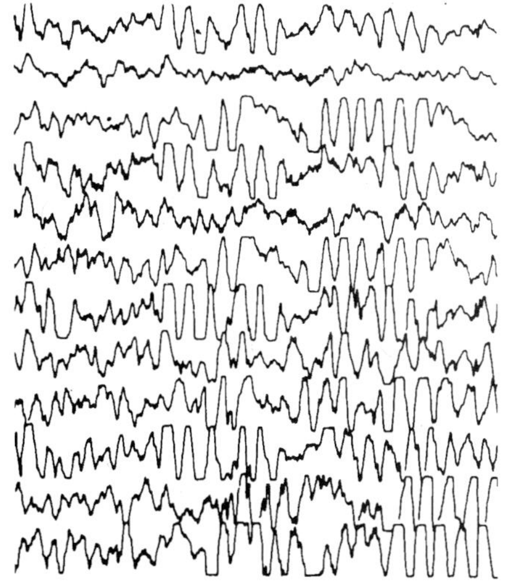

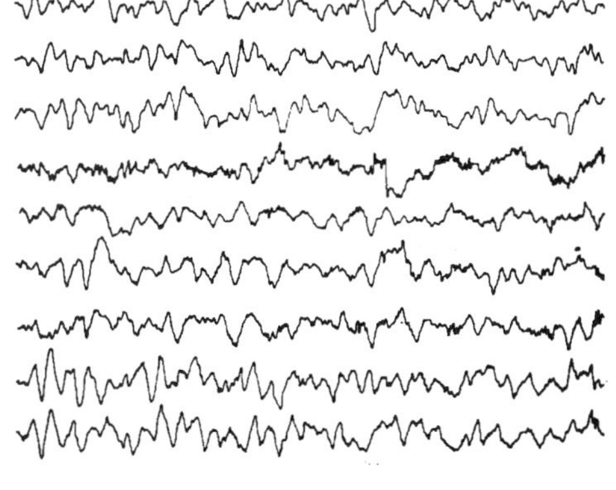

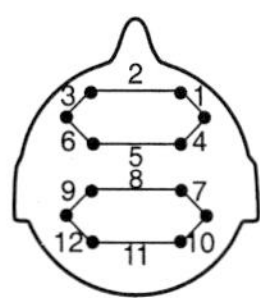

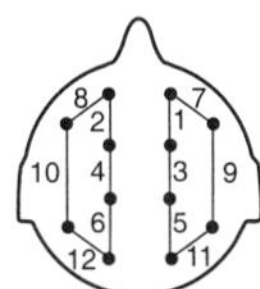

Fig. 84-2 Electroencephalography of the index patient. (Left) At the age of 22 months, prior to treatment. (Right) At the age of 25 months, after 2 months of oral supplementation with creatine.

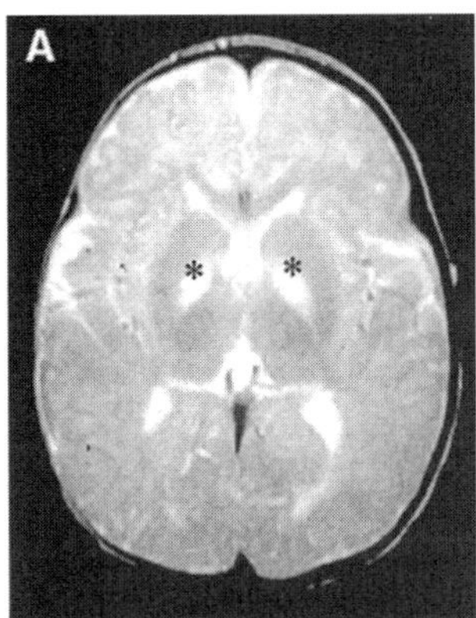

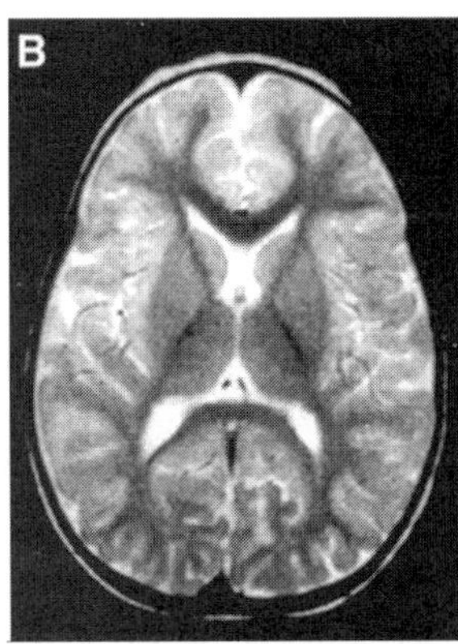

Fig. 84-3 Magnetic resonance imaging of the index patient. (A) At the age of 12 months there is bilateral abnormal signal hyperintensity in the globus pallidus before treatment (asterisks). (B) At the age of 35 months, after 12 months of supplementation with oral creatine, there is complete normalization. (Axial T_2-weighted magnetic resonance imaging scans, TR = 3500 msec, TE = 20 msec).

386 residues. A second form of AT has been reported, which carries five additional residues at its N-terminus. Both forms are likely to be encoded by a single gene[26] localized to chromosome 15q15.3.[27] AT exists as a dimer. The crystal structure of AT has shown that the active site, with a catalytic triad Cys-His-Asp, is accessible through a narrow channel. The catalytic mechanism consists of two half-reactions. In the first the amidino group is transferred from arginine onto the sulfur of the active-site cysteine residue. The resulting ornithine has to diffuse out of the active-site channel before glycine can enter. In the second half-reaction, the amidino group is transferred onto the glycine.[28]

AT is the key enzyme for regulation of creatine biosynthesis. Expression of AT is repressed by creatine[25,29] and induced by thyroxine and growth hormone.[30] Furthermore, AT is inhibited by ornithine, one of its reaction products.[31]

S-adenosyl-L-methionine:guanidinoacetate N-methyltransferase (guanidinoacetate methyltransferase [GAMT, EC 2.1.1.2]) catalyzes the second step of creatine biosynthesis. GAMT is expressed ubiquitously,[20,32] with activity highest in liver[20,33] and pancreas[17] and lower in kidney.[20,21] Other cell types, including neuronal, ovary, Sertoli, and epididymal epithelial cells contain appreciable amounts of GAMT.[32,34] GAMT is a cytosolic protein and has been purified to homogeneity from various nonhuman sources.[35,36]

The cDNA for human GAMT predicts a protein of 236 amino acids[37] with more than 80 percent homology to GAMT in rat[38] and mouse.[39] The human GAMT gene is localized on chromosome 19p13.3,[39,40] spans about 5 kb, and comprises six exons. The mouse and rat GAMT genes have a similar organization.[39,41]

GAMT binds S-adenosylmethionine and guanidinoacetate with apparent K_m values in the range of 1.2–6.7 μM and 31–98 μM,[32,36,38] respectively. Chemical modification and site-directed mutagenesis have identified several residues critical for catalytic activity. Glycine 67 and 69 and aspartate 134 are critical for binding of S-adenosylmethionine, and tyrosine 136 stabilizes this binding.[41–43] Integrity of cysteine 15 is crucial for the activity of GAMT and may be involved in the binding of guanidinoacetate.[45,46] Mechanistically, GAMT obeys an ordered BiBi mechanism in which S-adenosylmethionine binds first and guanidinoacetate second.[44]

The major sites of creatine biosynthesis in humans are liver, pancreas, and kidney. Dietary experiments in humans suggest that the availability of arginine and glycine limits the biosynthesis of guanidinoacetate.[47] In agreement with the rate-limiting role of the AT reaction, feeding of guanidinoacetate increases the synthesis of creatine.[48,49] In humans, the biosynthesis of creatine accounts for about 70 percent or more of the total utilization of methionine through S-adenosylmethionine.[50]

If *de novo* synthesis of creatine isinadequate because of low AT activity, cells expressing GAMT can synthesize creatine from guanidinoacetate obtained from the extracellular fluid. Guanidinoacetate occurs in the plasma at concentrations in the micromolar range. A significant fraction may derive from kidney, where the activity of GAMT relative to that of AT is lower than in liver and pancreas. The reported mean values for guanidinoacetate in plasma or serum vary between 0.8 and 5.0 μMol/l.[13,51–53] Guanidinoacetate can be internalized against a concentration gradient. The concentration of guanidinoacetate in cells is not

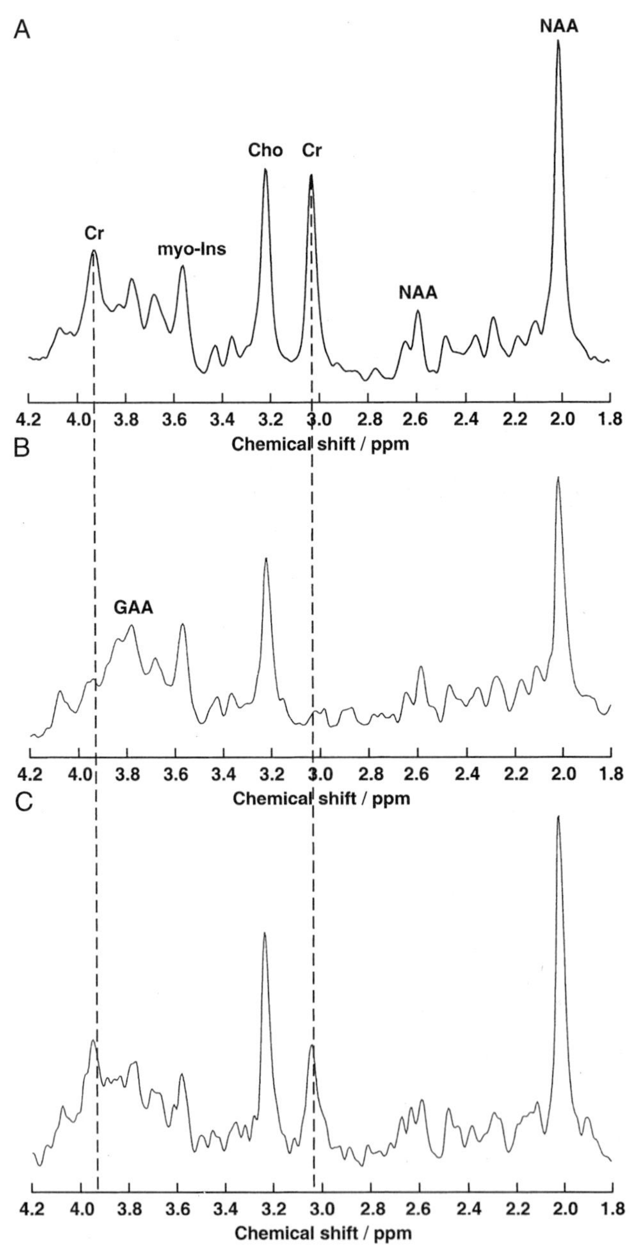

Fig. 84-4 Proton magnetic resonance spectroscopy of white matter. (A) Controls (averaged from 20 healthy 2- to 5-year-old children). (B) The index patient at 22 months. (C) The index patient at 41 months, after 18 months of oral substitution with creatine. (STEAM, TR/TE/TM = 6000/20/30 msec, 64 accumulations.) Cho = choline; Cr = creatine; GAA = guanidinoacetate; myo-Ins = myo-inositol; NAA = N-acetylaspartate.

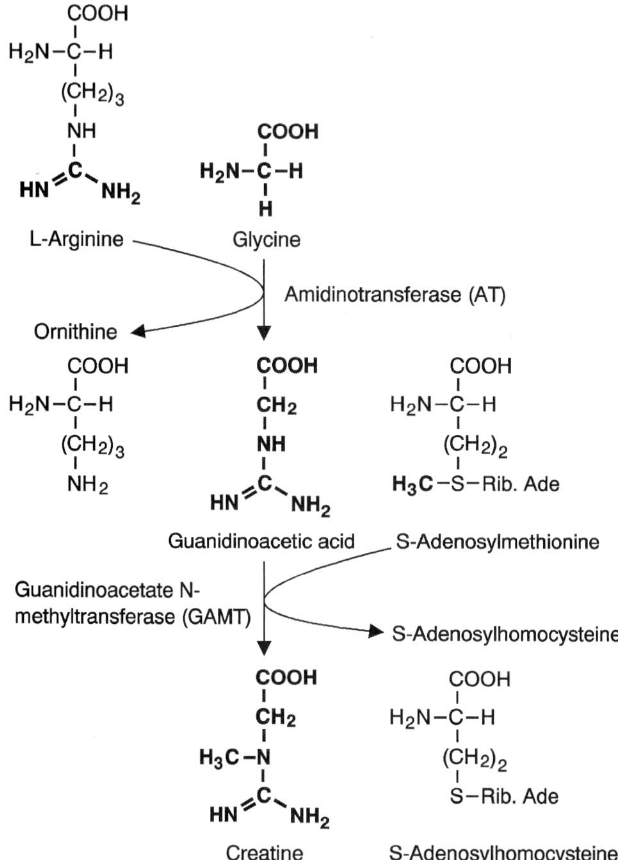

Fig. 84-5 Pathway of creatine synthesis. Building blocks of creatine are indicated by bold letters.

known. In cultured fibroblasts and neuroblastoma cells, synthesis of creatine from extracellularly derived guanidinoacetate can maintain the intracellular pool of creatine and phosphocreatine.[32] The traditional view is that the site of biosynthesis of creatine and the site of its use are separated. Synthesis takes place mainly in liver and pancreas, while the highest accumulations are in tissues with a high energy demand, such as skeletal muscle and brain. It should be noted, however, that the substantial degrees of activity of AT outside of liver, pancreas, and kidney; the availability of guanidinoacetate in the extracellular fluid; and the appreciable activity levels of GAMT in skeletal muscle and neuronal cells could allow substantial amounts of creatine to be synthesized locally.[32] Inhibition of creatine uptake reduces the creatine/phosphocreatine pool in brain only to half of normal values, indicating that brain depends only partially on creatine from outside sources.[54]

Tissues that synthesize creatine in significant amounts, such as liver and pancreas, do not contain high levels of creatine kinase, and vice versa. The separation of sites of creatine synthesis from sites of use as phosphocreatine requires development of mechanisms for efflux of creatine from organs in which it is synthesized and its uptake in organs where it is utilized.

Little is known about the efflux of creatine. Creatine is efficiently retained in muscle[55–58] and is lost only after conversion of creatinine.[55] Creatine efflux from erythrocytes occurs through a non-protein-dependent, nonactive process.[59] Fibroblasts and neuroblastoma cells retain most of the creatine synthesized from [^{14}C]guanidinoacetate, while hepatoma cells release more than 95 percent of the creatine they synthesize.[32] This suggests carrier-mediated egress of creatine from some cells, such as hepatocytes.

The concentration of creatine in human plasma is 10–100 μM.[3,60–62] Creatine uptake has been studied in a variety of tissues and shown to be specific, saturable, Na^+- and energy-dependent, and concentrative.[59,61–66] Two molecules of Na^+ are transported for every creatine molecule; values K_m for creatine and Na^+ are 15–50 μM and 55 mM, respectively. At creatine concentrations far above physiological levels, additional transport mechanisms contribute to uptake of creatine.[67] Uptake of creatine by the Na^+-dependent transporter is competitively inhibited by β-guanidinopropionate with a K_i of about 20 μM and abolished if Na^+ is replaced by Li^+. The gene for the human creatine transporter has been mapped to chromosome Xq28[68] and a second gene for a testis-specific isoform to chromosome 16p11.2.[69] The cDNA for the human creatine transporter predicts a polypeptide of 635 amino acids with 12 putative transmembrane proteins[70] and over 95 percent homology to the corresponding transporters in rabbit[71,72] and rat.[73,74] The creatine transporter belongs to a family of Na^+-driven transporters for GABA, dopamine, serotonin, glycine, proline, catecholamine, and taurine.[71] Expression of the creatine transporter is high in skeletal and cardiac muscle and kidney; moderate in brain, placenta, and lung; and below the limit of detection in liver and pancreas.[70,72] Multiple isoforms of the creatine transporter have been isolated that may originate from alternative splicing.[75]

The expression of the creatine transporter is regulated by creatine. Physiological creatine concentrations reduce expression by about half from that present in the absence of creatine. Creatine appears to induce the synthesis of a repressor of the creatine transporter gene.[65] Contrary to early reports, thyroxine increases creatine uptake by muscle.[76–79]

Conversion of creatine to phosphocreatine consumes ATP and provides a reservoir for high-energy phosphate. The reverse reaction maintains ATP at sites of ATP consumption. This reversible interconversion of creatine and creatine phosphate is catalyzed by creatine kinases (EC 2.7.3.2). The five known creatine kinase isoenzymes are expressed in a tissue-specific manner and have different intracellular locations. The cytosolic isoenzymes exist as homo- or heterodimers of M (muscle) and/or B (brain) subunits. The MM isoenzyme is found predominantly in skeletal and cardiac muscle. The BB isoenzyme is highest in brain and is also present in smooth muscle cells, renal epithelium, intestine and uterus, spermatozoa, and the photoreceptor cells of the retina. During embryonic development, the BB isoenzyme is also the predominant creatine kinase in skeletal and cardiac muscle.[80–82] The heterodimeric MB isoenzyme is mainly found in adult heart.[83] Additionally, there are two mitochondrial isoenzymes in the mitochondrial intermembrane space in the form of either dimers or octamers. They are concentrated at sites where the inner and outer membrane are in close apposition.[80] The sarcomeric mitochondrial isoenzyme is expressed in skeletal muscle together with the cytosolic MM isoenzyme, while in other cells the ubiquitous mitochondrial isoenzyme is expressed together with the cytosolic B subunit. In cardiac muscle, all five isoenzymes are found and the ratio between them is developmentally regulated.[84] The cell type specificity of the expression is exemplified by the Purkinje cells, which in several species share the creatine kinase isoenzyme pattern with skeletal muscle rather than with other brain cells.[85,86]

The creatine kinases catalyze a near-equilibrium reaction, with the majority of creatine (>70 percent) being phosphorylated.[87,88] In tissues like skeletal muscle, the level of phosphocreatine can reach 30 mM and more and exceed that of adenine nucleotides by one order of magnitude. In other tissues, such as brain, smooth muscle, and kidney, phosphocreatine is in the range of 1–10 mM. This correlates with lower activity of creatine kinase, which in smooth muscle and in brain is about a thirtieth of that in skeletal muscle and a sixth of that in cardiac muscle.[84]

In cells with a rapidly changing demand for energy and high levels of phosphocreatine, such as fast-twitch muscle, the phosphocreatine/creatine kinase system functions as an energy buffering system. Phosphocreatine serves as a local fuel for rapid rephosphorylation of ADP, thereby sustaining a rather constant level of ATP at the expense of phosphocreatine. It has been calculated that a decrease of ATP by 30 μM is accompanied by an increase of creatine by 4 mM.[89] This function of the creatine/phosphocreatine system has also been referred to as a *temporal energy buffer.*

Another still debated but probably universal function of the creatine/phosphocreatine system is that of a shuttle for high-energy phosphate, also referred to as a *spatial energy buffer.* This function can also be fulfilled with more moderate phosphocreatine levels, as occur in cardiac and smooth muscle and in nonmuscle tissues. The shuttle hypothesis[90–92] takes into account the dual localization of creatine kinase isoenzymes in the cytosol and at the outer surface of the inner mitochondrial membrane. The essential feature of this concept is that phosphocreatine and creatine rather than ATP and ADP shuttle between the sites of ATP consumption and ATP formation. The equilibrium constants of the mitochondrial isoenzyme favor the formation of phosphocreatine, those of the cytosolic isoenzymes the consumption of phosphocreatine. The cytosolic isoenzymes are in a close spatial and functional relationship with the ATPases associated with the myofibrils, the sarcoplasmic reticulum, and the plasma membrane, as well as with glycolytic enzyme complexes,[93] while the mitochondrial isoenzymes are in close proximity to the ATP/ADP translocase of the inner mitochondrial membranes and are associated with porins of the outer mitochondrial membrane.[80] Local regeneration of ATP at the site of ATP consumption has several advantages. It minimizes changes of the ATP/ADP ratio, which controls the activity of many key enzymes of metabolism; it avoids the need to transport ADP, most of which is bound to cytosolic proteins and not free to diffuse, to mitochondria; and it minimizes pH changes associated with changes of the ATP/ADP ratio. The role of creatine as an acceptor of high-energy phosphate at the outer surface of the inner mitochondrial membrane also implies a key function for creatine as a regulator of respiration. In muscle, ATP is regenerated at the expense of phosphocreatine in the initial burst of energy consumption during contraction, and re-formation of phosphocreatine at the expense of ATP is inhibited. This regulation is mediated by an AMP-activated protein kinase. The lowering of the phosphocreatine/creatine ratio following the initial burst of energy demand activates the kinase, which in turn inactivates MM creatine kinase by phosphorylation. This prevents ATP consumption for regeneration of phosphocreatine while ATP is still being utilized for contraction. At the same time, the protein kinase activates ATP production from fatty acid oxidation.[94]

New insights concerning the function of the different creatine kinase isoenzymes came from the analysis of mice lacking one or two of the isoenzymes due to targeted gene disruption. Mice with a deficiency of cytosolic MM creatine kinase have normal levels of phosphocreatine and ATP in skeletal muscle under resting conditions. They generate normal absolute muscle tension but lack burst activity.

The high-energy phosphate exchange between phosphocreatine and ATP is reduced by a factor of at least 20, in spite of a normal decrease of phosphocreatine during muscle exercise.[95] Facilitation of adenine nucleotide transport between mitochondrial and cytosolic ATPases and an increase in cytosolic ATP production are believed to contribute to compensation for the loss of MM-creatine kinase.[96,97] Furthermore, expression of BB-creatine kinase in muscle can functionally replace that of the MM isoenzyme.[98] Null alleles for the gene encoding the cytosolic B creatine kinase isoenzyme were not transmitted from chimeric mice to their offspring.[99] Mice deficient in the ubiquitous or the sarcomeric mitochondrial creatine kinase are viable and fertile and exhibit no overt abnormality in the phenotype.[100,101] In mice with a combined deficiency of the cytosolic creatine kinase and the sarcomeric mitochondrial creatine kinase, the phosphocreatine in muscle can no longer serve to regenerate ATP, even under the most strenuous conditions, such as complete anoxia. The tetanic force output and the release of Ca^{2+}, as well as sequestration, are significantly impaired in these animals. Contrary to expectation, the phosphocreatine level was almost normal. A series of compensatory mechanisms, including adenylate kinase mediating ATP ↔ ADP exchange, relocation of mitochondria and changes of glycolysis may contribute to the remarkable preservation of basal functions in skeletal muscle deficient in cytosolic and mitochondrial creatine kinase.[102,103]

ENZYME DEFECT

The low levels of creatine/phosphocreatine, the accumulation of guanidinoacetate in brain, and the corresponding changes in the body fluids in the index case were suggestive of a block of creatine biosynthesis at the level of GAMT. Determination of GAMT activity in a cytosolic extract of liver revealed a profound deficiency of GAMT in two patients,[9] with residual activity of 4 percent in the index patient[8] and <2 percent in a second patient.[10] The presence of an inhibitor causing the deficiency of GAMT activity was excluded.

MOLECULAR DEFECT

Two GAMT-deficiency alleles have been characterized so far. One has a single base substitution at nt 327 (327G>A), and the other has a 13-bp insertion following nt 309 (309ins13). The index patient was a compound heterozygote for these two alleles; a second was homozygous for the 327G>A allele,[9] and a third patient was heterozygous for the 327G>A allele, with his second allele yet to be identified.[104]

Transcripts of the two alleles were detectable in liver, leukocytes, and fibroblasts. Each of these two mutant GAMT alleles gives rise to two transcripts. G327 occupies the position −1 of the 5′ splice site of intron 2. A G in this position is critical for the stability of the base pairing with U1snRNA and is a frequent location of mutations of 5′ splice sites.[105,106] Consequently, the 327G>A substitution leads to skipping of exon 2 or to the use of a cryptic 5′ splice site within intron 2. Both processed transcripts contain premature translation termination codons that result in synthesis of nonfunctional, truncated polypeptides.

The 13-bp insertion in the 309ins13 allele is a direct repeat, which suggests that it may have arisen from slipped mispairing during DNA replication. In addition to the transcript with the 13-nt insertion, a second transcript resulting from the use of the cryptic 5′ splice site in intron 2 is produced from this mutant allele. The former encodes a truncated nonfunctional polypeptide lacking critical residues located in the C-terminal half of GAMT; the latter encodes a polypeptide that may retain some catalytic activity. The frameshift introduced by the 13-nt insertion is corrected by a 44-nt insertion introduced by utilization of the downstream cryptic 5′ splice site. This results in a mutant GAMT polypeptide in which residues 105–110 are replaced by a novel sequence of 24 residues.[9] It remains to be determined if the low GAMT activity in the liver of the index patient, who has one 309ins13 allele, is due to residual activity of the GAMT polypeptide with this 24-residue insert.

INHERITANCE AND INCIDENCE

GAMT deficiency is inherited as an autosomal recessive trait. The four known cases of GAMT deficiency occurred in families of German, Kurdish, Welsh, and Dutch origin.[8–12] The parents of the Kurdish patient are first cousins. As might be expected from consanguinity of the parents, the patient was homozygous for the 327G>A allele. The same allele was also found in the two other compound heterozygous patients, one of whom also had the 309ins13 allele.[9]

The first clinical description of GAMT deficiency dates back to 1994. In this initial report, the diagnostic hallmarks of the disease and the beneficial effect of oral creatine substitution were described.[8] In spite of wide attention to this report, only three further patients with GAMT deficiency have been diagnosed as of May 1998.[10,11,104] The small number of patients identified in the past 6 years argues for a low incidence of GAMT deficiency. However, the diagnosis may be overlooked in a substantial fraction of patients because of the nonspecificity and variability of the clinical symptoms (muscular hypotonia and involuntary extrapyramidal movements in the index patient,[8] intractable epilepsy in two other patients,[11] and severe autism in a fourth patient[12]) and the lack of a specific screening method. Greater physician attention to low plasma creatinine values may increase the number of recognized cases.

PATHOPHYSIOLOGY

The immediate metabolic consequences predicted from a deficiency of GAMT are accumulation of guanidinoacetate and a decrease in creatine. If the latter cannot be compensated for by dietary creatine, either because intake is inadequate or because circulating creatine is not efficiently delivered to the appropriate cells, phosphocreatine levels will fall. A decrease of the creatine/phosphocreatine pool will reduce the formation and urinary excretion of creatinine.

Since creatine regulates its own synthesis by repressing AT, the activity of the latter increases. De-repression of AT increases formation of guanidinoacetate and the formation of ornithine. The accumulation of guanidinoacetate may also lead to formation of unusual guanidino compounds, which may be toxic to certain cells. The blockage of the GAMT-catalyzed reaction also increases the availability of S-adenosylmethionine, since this reaction normally consumes about 70 percent of this metabolite.

Most of these expected metabolic changes have been observed in the patients with GAMT deficiency. There is a reduction of creatine/phosphocreatine in brain and body fluids and an increase of guanidinoacetate and ornithine in body fluids. Oral supplementation with creatine partially corrected the deficiency of phosphocreatine in brain and normalized urinary creatinine and plasma ornithine levels. The levels of guanidinoacetate in plasma remained high, suggesting that the expected repression of AT by the increased creatine levels was not sufficient to lower the formation of guanidinoacetate to an extent that would decrease its accumulation. The normalization of the plasma ornithine concentration indicates, however, that oral supplementation of creatine does reduce the metabolic flux through the AT-catalyzed reaction.

The improvement of clinical and biochemical parameters by creatine supplementation helps to correlate some of the clinical symptoms of GAMT deficiency with the underlying metabolic derangements. The muscular weakness prominent in GAMT deficiency is improved considerably by oral supplementation with creatine.[8,10,11] It is therefore likely that this clinical feature results from deficiency of creatine/phosphocreatine. The effect of oral creatine supplementation on the level of phosphocreatine in skeletal muscle and on muscular performance is well established.[107–110] It should be noted, however, that creatine/phosphocreatine levels in muscle have not yet been studied in GAMT-deficient patients. Thus, it remains to be determined to what extent the hypotonia is due to alterations in muscle or to alterations in the central nervous system.

In two of the four patients with GAMT deficiency, extrapy ramidal symptoms manifesting as dyskinetic-dystonic involuntary movements were a key feature. While in one case the extrapyramidal symptoms responded well to oral supplementation with creatine,[8] this was less evident in another case.[10] The less favorable response in the latter patient has tentatively been ascribed to this patient's older age when creatine supplementation was initiated and to a more profound deficiency of GAMT. This therapeutic result supports the hypothesis that deficiency of phosphocreatine is a major factor in development of the extrapyramidal symptoms.

The importance of the creatine/phosphocreatine system as a source for high-energy phosphate in brain is suggested by several observations. The concentration of phosphocreatine in brain is 4–6 mM, or about 2–3 times higher than that of ATP.[111] The phosphocreatine/ATP ratio and the activity of creatine kinase show developmental changes and regional differences, with higher creatine kinase activities and phosphocreatine/ATP levels in white than in gray matter.[112,113] Recent determinations of the creatine kinase–catalyzed flux with localized ^{31}P-NMR saturation transfer measurements confirmed a higher flux in the white than in the gray matter.[114] These differences are also observed at the cellular level. Astroglial cells are the only type of brain cell known to synthesize creatine from glycine, arginine, and methionine.[115] A fraction of the guanidinoacetate synthesized by astrocytes is released and may be utilized by other brain cells for synthesis of creatine. The activity of creatine kinase in glial cells is higher than that in neuronal cells,[116,117] and their phosphocreatine/ATP ratio is three times higher than that in neurons.[118] Additionally, creatine uptake by astroglial cells is much higher than uptake by neuronal cells.[66] Compared to activity in astroglia and neurons, the activity of cytosolic creatine kinase is highest in oligodendrocytes, where it is related to myelinogenesis.[119] The rapid decrease in phosphocreatine caused by hypoxia,[120–123] seizures,[124] and pharmacologic stimulation of ion channels,[125] while ATP remains rather constant, supports the role of phosphocreatine in regenerating ATP in brain.[126,127] In addition, phosphocreatine may have also a more direct function, as indicated by its ATP-independent stimulation of L-glutamate uptake by synaptic vesicles.[128,129]

All four GAMT-deficient patients had pathologic electroencephalograms, and three had abnormal MRI signal intensities in the globus pallidus. Epileptic seizures were prominent in two.[10,11] It is tempting to relate these alterations to the accumulation of guanidinoacetate, a compound with known neurotoxicity and convulsive activity.[130–133] The epilepsy was refractory to oral supplementation of creatine in one patient,[10] while in the other two patients the pathologic electroencephalograms[8] and the seizures[11] responded to creatine supplementation and the changes in the globus pallidus disappeared. In the two patients in whom the guanidinoacetate levels in plasma and urine were monitored during oral supplementation with creatine, they remained high.[10,13] Because the electroencephalograms improved almost to normal in one of these patients but continued to show abnormal hypersynchronous activity in the other, it is likely that guanidinoacetate is only one of several factors contributing to the development of abnormal electrical activity and seizures.

Finally, in all GAMT-deficient patients, clinical manifestations were absent at birth and developed only after the first month and sometimes significantly later (Table 84-1). This may reflect the fetus' receiving supplementation with creatine across the placenta. In rat, creatine is transported across the placenta by an active process.[134] The asymptomatic interval may correspond to the period that can be covered by the creatine/phosphocreatine pool of the neonate. The creatine content of breast milk is 40–275 μmol/L[135] and therefore supplies less than 5 mg/kg/day of creatine. The beneficial effect of oral supplementation in patients with Becker type muscular dystrophy persists for up to six weeks after withdrawal,[136] suggesting that over this time frame the endogenous creatine/phosphocreatine pool, which decreases by 2 percent daily due to formation of creatinine, becomes depleted below a critical threshold.

DIAGNOSIS

The clinical phenotype of GAMT deficiency, as assembled from the first four patients, is quite variable. It may be represented as a progressive encephalopathy with onset during the first months of life and including muscular hypotonia and/or weakness, dyskinetic movements, swallowing difficulties, seizures, and autistic behavior (Table 84-1).

Table 84-3 GAMT Activity in Cultured Cells

Proband	EBV-transformed lymphoblasts	Fibroblasts
	(nmol/mg×h)*	
Patient 1[8]	<0.1	<0.1
3[11]	<0.1	nd
4[12]	nd	<0.1
Heterozygote of (brother pt. 1)	0.23	nd
Controls	0.61–0.84 (m=8)	0.38–0.56 (m=7)

*The values for the controls give the range; nd = not determined. (*Adapted from Jeas et al.*[145])

Abnormal MRI signals in the basal ganglia, particularly in the globus pallidus, seem to be characteristic, although these are observed in many metabolic diseases. The electroencephalogram may show hypersynchronous activity with intermittent multifocal-spike slow waves, whereas investigation of evoked responses and nerve conduction velocity are normal.

Creatinine levels in plasma at or below the lower normal limit and low excretion of creatinine in 24 h urine permit an easy screening method that usually only requires the critical review of already obtained laboratory results. The concentrations of creatinine and other guanidino compounds are best measured in plasma and CSF. The determination of creatinine in collected urine should be preferred to random urine samples, since very concentrated urine, such as that obtained in the first voided morning sample, may have concentrations of creatinine at the lower normal limit. In routine metabolic screening, the excretion of metabolites is often normalized to creatinine. This will result in artifically elevated values in GAMT deficiency, which may mislead the investigator.

The detection of elevated guanidinoacetate levels in random urine samples is specific for GAMT deficiency[13] and is a result of the characteristic enormous accumulation of guanidinoacetate in body fluids. A variety of methods for the determination of guanidino compounds in CSF, plasma, and urine have been developed, including chromatographic,[20,53,137–139] colorimetric,[140–142] and *in vitro* [^{1}H] MRS[143] techniques. Presently, *in vivo* [^{1}H] MRS is the most sensitive and noninvasive method for the detection of creatine deficiency and guanidinoacetate accumulation in the brain and should be applied whenever available.[144] The method of choice for the diagnosis of GAMT deficiency, however, is the determination of guanidinoacetate in urine,[138,139] for its convenience, sensitivity, and specificity.

The clinical diagnosis of GAMT deficiency should be confirmed by determination of GAMT activity. Absence of GAMT activity was first demonstrated in liver biopsy samples, in which the highest GAMT activity is normally observed.[123] GAMT activity can also be reliably measured in fibroblasts and EBV-transformed lymphoblasts (Table 84-3). The GAMT activity in cultured amniotic cells is in the range of that in EBV-transformed lymphoblasts, suggesting that prenatal diagnosis is feasible.[145]

Identification of the molecular defect completes the diagnostic evaluation.

TREATMENT

Symptoms of creatine deficiency develop only after a normal neonatal period, when creatine pools are being progressively depleted. Consequently, it is essential to identify patients with GAMT deficiency as early as possible in order to initiate creatine therapy before irreversible damage occurs.

Systemic creatine deficiency can be treated successfully by oral supplementation with creatine monohydrate, which is well absorbed and replenishes body creatine pools. In three patients with GAMT deficiency creatine doses ranging from 350 mg to 2 g/kg/day were used. At high doses, crystals of creatine in urine were noted.[146] No serious side effects have been observed to date. In athletes, healthy volunteers, and patients with muscle disorders receiving up to 20 g creatine per day, a slight increase in body weight was noticed.[108,136,147–151] Doses higher than 10 g/day may be useless, since the bulk of the administered creatine is excreted in the urine.[136]

The concentration of creatinine in plasma and the amount of daily creatinine excretion in urine serve as markers for successful creatine replacement. Both, however, mainly reflect normalization of muscle creatine pools. The restoration of the creatine pool and the decline of guanidinoacetate in the brain are best monitored by [^{1}H]- or [^{31}P]-MR spectroscopy.

Determination of creatine concentrations in plasma and urine is not suitable for monitoring therapy, because it reflects only intestinal absorption. Although guanidinoacetate concentration in the brain, as measured with [^{1}H]-MR spectroscopy, declined during therapy, its concentration in plasma and urine remained nearly unchanged.[10,11,152] Therefore, the determination of guanidinoacetate concentration is also not useful for follow-up control.

MRS studies can show the course of correction of abnormal signal intensities during therapy. The electroencephalogram gives some additional information about seizure activity but does not play an important role in monitoring treatment.

Three previously reported patients have benefited from creatine supplementation to different degrees; none has returned to a normal developmental level (Table 84-4 and Fig. 84-1). This may be explained by the delay in institution of creatine supplementation.

In the index patient, muscle tone improved with treatment; the extrapyramidal symptoms, swallowing problems, and postprandial vomiting disappeared. Seizurelike drop attacks of the head were no longer observed, and after some time, the patient was able to use his hands normally. He learned to sit and crawl, and since the age of 5 years he has been able to walk freely, without ataxia or dyskinetic movements. Despite this remarkable progress in motor development, no active speech has developed, and he continues to show some autistic features and self-injurious behavior. Repeated examination revealed normalization of initially pathologic MRI and MRS findings (Figs. 84-3, 84-4). The electroencephalogram normalized during treatment and no longer shows any seizure activity (Fig. 84-2). Creatine supplementation replenished the total creatine/phosphocreatine body pool to control levels, as indicated by the normal urinary excretion of creatinine (Fig. 84-6). The plasma concentration and urinary excretion of guanidinoacetate have remained high, reflecting the deficiency of GAMT (Fig. 84-6). The guanidinoacetate signal in brain disappeared, while the

Table 84-4 Response to Oral Supplementation of Creatine

Parameter	Effect		
	Patient 1[8]	Patient 2[10]	Patient 3[11]
Hypotonia	improved	(unchanged)	improved
Dyskinesia	disappeared	slightly decreased	(not present)
Seizures	controlled	resistant	controlled
MRI	normalized	(unchanged)	normalized
Developmental progress	accelerated	accelerated	accelerated
Mental retardation	mild	severe	severe
Active speech	no	no	no

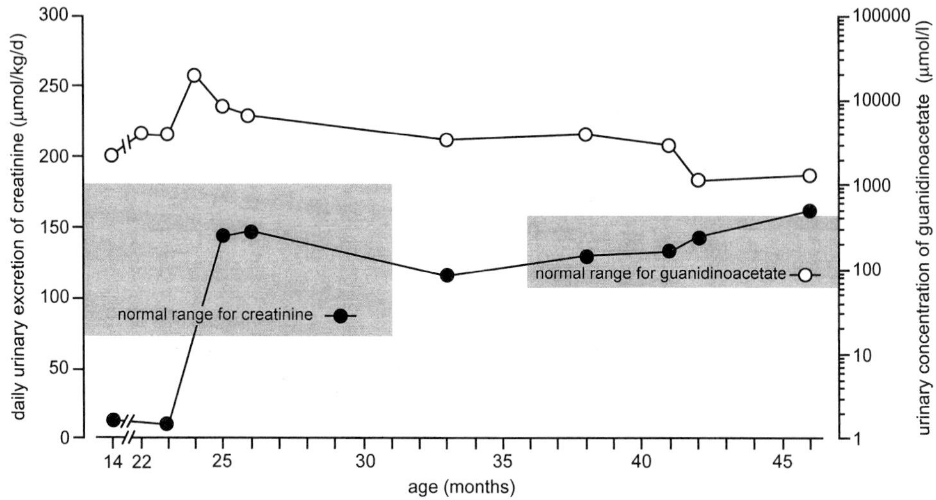

Fig. 84-6 Daily excretion of creatinine (filled circles) and concentration of guanidinoacetate (open circles) in the urine of the index patient. Oral supplementation with creatine was started at the age of 23 months. The mean values ± SD for controls are indicated by the shaded area.

creatine/phosphocreatine concentration in gray (Fig. 84-7) and white matter reached no more than two-thirds of control values. The inability to fully correct the creatine/phosphocreatine deficit in brain may reflect compromised creatine uptake into the CNS. Guanidinoacetate, which remained high in the patient's plasma, may competitively inhibit uptake of creatine. In muscle, however, guanidinoacetate inhibits uptake of creatine, with a K_i of 3 mM,[153] a concentration more than a hundred fold higher than that observed in the patients. Furthermore, it should be noted that the loading of the brain pool is a protracted process, in the case of the index patient requiring creatine supplementation for more than a year.

Creatine supplementation in the patient of Welsh origin resulted in an acceleration of developmental progress, in cessation of the epileptic seizures, and in normalization of the globus pallidus, as well as in considerable improvement of his behavior.[11] The patient of Kurdish origin was almost refractory to therapy and did not show a change in the frequency of epileptic seizures.[10]

Owing to the short time that has elapsed since GAMT deficiency was discovered and to the variability of the patients' symptoms, the long-term prognosis of the disease and the long-term effects of creatine therapy remain to be determined.

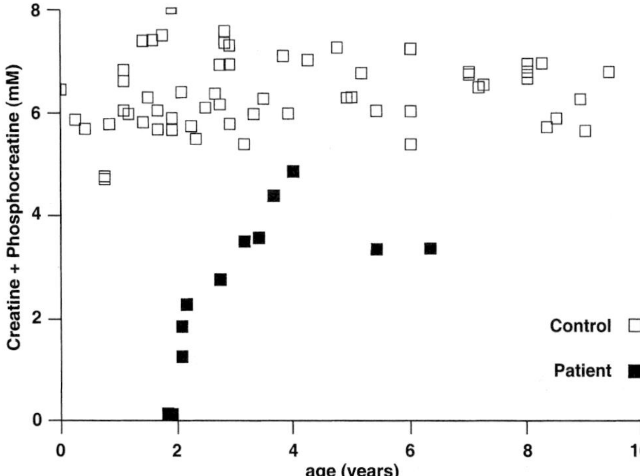

Fig. 84-7 Creatine/phosphocreatine in gray matter of healthy controls (open squares) and of the index patient (filled squares) as determined by MRS. Oral supplementation with creatine was started at the age of 23 months.

ADDENDUM

Since submission of this chapter in August 1998 four new patients have been diagnosed, three of which are reported in ref. [154] and [155]. Patient 4 in Table 84-1 and Table 84-3 is patient 1 in ref.[155]

REFERENCES

1. Hunter A: Creatine and creatinine. London, Lougmans Greene and Co, 1928.
2. Chevreul 1832 cited in Rose WC: The metabolism of creatine and creatinine. *Annu Rev Biochem* 187, 1933.
3. Von Liebig J: Über die Bestandteile der Flüssigkeiten des Fleisches. *Ann Chem Pharm* **52**:257, 1847.
4. Walker JB: Creatine: Biosynthesis, regulation and function. *Adv Enzymol* **50**:177, 1979.
5. Rose WC: The metabolism of creatine and creatinine. *Annu Rev Biochem* 187, 1933.
6. Fiske CH, Subbarow Y: Phosphocreatine. *J Biol Chem* **81**:629, 1929.
7. Lundsgaard E: Weitere Untersuchungen über Muskelkontraktionen ohne Milchsäurebildung. *Biochem Z* **227**:51, 1930.
8. Stöckler S, Holzbach U, Hanefeld F, Marquardt I, Helms G, Requart M, Hänicke W, Frahm J: Creatine deficiency in the brain: A new, treatable inborn error of metabolism. *Pediatr Res* **36**:409, 1994.
9. Stöckler S, Isbrandt D, Hanefeld F, Schmidt B, von Figura K: Guanidinoacetate methyltransferase deficiency: The first inborn error of creatine metabolism in man. *Am J Hum Genet* **58**:914, 1996.
10. Schulze A, Hess T, Wevers R, Mayatepek E, Bachert P, Marescau B, Knopp MV: Creatine deficiency syndrome caused by guanidinoacetate methyltransferase deficiency: Diagnostic tools for a new inborn error of metabolism. *J Pediatr* **131**:626, 1997.
11. Ganesan V, Johnson A, Connelly A, Eckhardt S, Surtees RA: Guanidinoacetate methyltransferase deficiency: New clinical features. *Pediatr Neurol* **17**:155, 1997.
12. Van der Knaap M, Jacobs C, personal communication.
13. Stöckler S, Marescau B, De Deyne PP, Trijbels JMF, Hanefeld F: Guanidino compounds in guanidinoacetate methyltransferase deficiency, a new inborn error of creatine synthesis. *Metabolism* **46**:1189, 1997.
14. Barkovich AJ: Pediatric neuroimaging 2d ed. New York, Raven, 1996.
15. Borsook H, Dubnoff JW: The formation of glycamine in animal tissues. *J Biol Chem* **138**:389, 1941.
16. Carison M, van Pilsum JF: S-Adenosylmethionine:guanidinoacetate N-methyltransferase activities in livers from rats with hormonal deficiencies or excesses. *Proc Soc Exp Biol Med* **143**:1256, 1973.
17. Walker JB, Walker MS: Formation of creatine from guanidinoacetate in pancreas. *Proc Soc Exp Biol Med* **101**:807, 1959.
18. Walker JB: Role of pancreas in biosynthesis of creatine. *Proc Soc Exp Biol Med* **98**:7, 1958.
19. Sorenson RL, Stout LE, Brelje TC, van Pilsum JF, McGuire DM: Evidence for the role of pancreatic acinar cells in the production of ornithine and guanidinoacetic acid by L-arginine:glycine amidinotransferase. *Pancreas* **10**:389, 1995.

20. Van Pilsum JF, Stephens GC, Taylor D: Distribution of creatine, guanidinoacetate and the enzymes for their biosynthesis in the animal kingdom. *Biochem J* **126**:325, 1972.
21. Koszalka TR: Extrahepatic creatine synthesis in the rat. *Arch Biochem Biophys* **122**:400, 1967.
22. Walker JB: Formaminidine group transfer in extracts of human pancreas, liver and kidney. *Biochim Biophys Acta* **73**:241, 1963.
23. Van Pilsum JF, Olsen B, Taylor D, Rozycki T, Pierce JC: Transamidinase activities, *in vitro*, of tissues from various mammals and from rats fed protein-free, creatine supplemented and normal diets. *Arch Biochem Biophys* **100**:520, 1963.
24. Magri E, Balboni G, Grazi E: On the biosynthesis of creatine. Intramitochondrial localization of transamidinase from rat kidney. *FEBS Lett* **55**:91, 1975.
25. Mc Guire DM, Gross MD, Van Pilsum JF, Towle HC: Repression of rat kidney L-arginine:glycine amidinotransferase synthesis by creatine at a pretranslational level. *J Biol Chem* **259**:12034, 1984.
26. Humm A, Fritsche E, Mann K, Gönl U, Huber R: Recombinant expression and isolation of human L-arginine:glycine amidinotransferase and identification of its active site cysteine residue. *Biochem J* **322**:771, 1997.
27. Fougerousse F, Bronx O, Richard I, Allamand V, deSouza AP, Boürg N, Breuguier L, Devand C, Pastürand P, Roüdaüt C: Mapping of a chromosome 15 region involved in limb girdle muscular dystrophy. *Hum Mol Genet* **3**:285, 1994.
28. Humm A, Fritsche E, Steinbacher S, Huber R: Crystal structure and mechanism of human L-arginine:glycine amidinotransferase: A mitochondrial enzyme involved in creatine biosynthesis. *EMBO J* **16**:3373, 1997.
29. Guthmiller P, Van Pilsum JF, Boen JR, McGuire DM: Cloning and sequencing of rat kidney L-arginine:glycine amidinotransferase. *J Biol Chem* **269**:17556, 1994.
30. McGuire DM, Tormanen CD, Segal IS, Van Pilsum JF: The effect of growth hormone and thyroxine on the amount of L-arginine:glycine amidinotransferase in kidneys of hypophysectomized rat. *J Biol Chem* **255**:1152, 1980.
31. Sipilä I, Simell O, Arjoma P: Gyrate atrophy of the choroid and retina with hyperornithinemia. *J Clin Invest* **6**:684, 1980.
32. Daly MM: Guanidinoacetate methyltransferase activity in tissues and cultured cells. *Arch Biochem Biophys* **238**:576, 1985.
33. Cantoni GL, Vignos PJ Jr: Enzymatic mechanism of creatine biosynthesis. *J Biol Chem* **209**:647, 1954.
34. Lee H, Ogawa H, Fujikoka M, Gerton GL: Guanidinoacetate methyltransferase in the mouse: Extensive expression in Sertoli cells of the testis and in microvilli of caput epididymis. *Biol Reprod* **50**:152, 1994.
35. Im YS, Chiang K, Cantoni GL: Guanidinoacetate methyltransferase: Purification and molecular properties. *J Biol Chem* **254**:11047, 1979.
36. Ogawa H, Ishiguro Y, Fujioka M: Guanidinoacetate methyltransferase from rat liver: Purification, properties and evidence for the involvement of sulfhydryl groups of activity. *Arch Biochem Biophys* **226**:265, 1983.
37. Isbrandt D, von Figura K: Cloning and sequence analysis of human guanidinoacetate N-methyltransferase cDNA. *Biochim Biophys Acta* **1264**:265, 1995.
38. Ogawa H, Date T, Gomi T, Konishi K, Pitot HC, Cantoni GL, Fujioka M: Molecular cloning, sequence analysis and expression in *Escherichia coli* of the cDNA for guanidinoacetate methyltransferase from rat liver. *Proc Natl Acad Sci USA* **85**:694, 1988.
39. Jenne DE, Olsen AS, Zimmer M: The human guanidinoacetate methyltransferase (GAMT) gene maps to a syntenic region on 19p 13.3 homologous to band C of mouse chromosome 10, but GAMT is not mutated in jittery mice. *Biochem Biophys Res Commun* **238**:723, 1997.
40. Chae YJ, Chung CE, Kim BJ, Lee MK, Lee H: The gene encoding guanidinoacetate methyltransferase (GAMT) maps to human chromosome 19 at band p13.3 and to mouse chromosome 10. *Genomics* **49**:162, 1998.
41. Ogawa H, Fujioka M: Nucleotide sequence of the rat guanidinoacetate methyltransferase gene. *Nucleic Acids Res* **16**:8715, 1988.
42. Hamahata A, Takata Y, Gomi T, Fujikoka: Probing the S-adenosylmethionine-binding site of rat guanidinoacetate methyltransferase. *Biochem J* **317**:141, 1996.
43. Takata Y, Fujioka M: Identification of a tyrosine residue in rat guanidinoacetate methyltransferase that is photolabeled with S-adenosylmethionine. *Biochemistry* **31**:4369, 1992.
44. Takata Y, Konishi K, Gomi T, Fujioka M: Rat guanidinoacetate methyltransferase. Effect of site-directed alteration of an aspartic acid residue that is conserved across most mammalian L-adenosylmethionine-dependent methyltransferases. *J Biol Chem* **269**:5537, 1994.
45. Fujioka M, Konishi K, Takata Y: Recombinant rat liver guanidinoacetate methyltransferase: Reactivity and function of sulfhydryl groups. *Biochemistry* **27**:7658, 1988.
46. Konishi K, Fujioka M: Reversible inactivation of recombinant rat liver guanidinoacetate methyltransferase by glutathione disulfide. *Arch Biochem Biophys* **289**:90, 1991.
47. Borsook H, Dubnoff JW, Lilly JC, Marriott W: The formation of glycamine in man and its urinary excretion. *J Biol Chem* **138**:405, 1941.
48. Stetten D Jr, Grail GF: Effect of dietary choline, ethanolamine, serine, cysteine, homocysteine, and guanidoacetic acid on the liver lipids of rats. *J Biol Chem* **144**:175, 1942.
49. Walker JB, Wang SH: Tissue repressor concentration and target enzyme level. *Biochim Biophys Acta* **81**:435, 1964.
50. Mudd SH, Poole JR: Labile methyl balances for normal humans on various dietary regimens. *Metabolism* **24**:721, 1975.
51. De Deyn P, Marescau B, Lornoy W, Becaus I, Lowenthal A: Guanidino compounds in uraemic dialysed patients. *Clin Chim Acta* **157**:143, 1986.
52. Marescau B, De Deyn PP, Holvoet J, Nagels G, Saxena V, Mahler L: Guanidino compounds in serum and urine of cirrhotic patients. *Metabolism* **44**:584, 1995.
53. Yasuda M, Sugahara K, Zhang J, Ageta T, Nakayama K, Shuin T, Kodama H: Simultaneous determination of creatinine, creatine and guanidinoacetate acid in human serum and urine using liquid chromatography-atmospheric pressure chemical ionization mass spectrometry. *Analyt Biochem* **253**:231, 1997.
54. Holtzman D, McFarland E, Moerland T, Koutcher J, Kushmerick M, Neuringer L: Brain creatine phosphate and creatine kinase in mice fed an analogue of creatine. *Brain Res* **438**:68, 1989.
55. Bloch K, Schoenheimer R, Rittenberg D: Rate of formation and disappearance of body creatine in normal animals. *J Biol Chem* **138**:155, 1941.
56. Otten JV, Fitch CD, Wheatley JB, Fischer VW: Thyrotoxic myopathy in mice: Accentuation by creatine transport inhibitor. *Metabolism* **35**:481, 1986.
57. Meyer RA: Linear dependence of muscle phosphocreatine kinetics on total creatine content. *Am J Physiol* **257** (*Cell Physiol* 26):C1149, 1989.
58. Fitch CD, Sinton DW: A study of creatine metabolism in diseases causing muscle wasting. *J Clin Invest* **43**:444, 1964.
59. Ku CP, Passow H: Creatine and creatinine transport in old and young human red blood cells. *Biochim Biophys Acta* **600**:212, 1980.
60. Marescau B, De Deyn P, Wiechert P, van Gorp L, Lowenthal A: Comparative study of guanidino compounds in serum and brain of mouse, rat, rabbit and man. *J Neurochem* **46**:717, 1986.
61. Loike JD, Somes M, Silverstein SC: Creatine uptake, metabolism and efflux in human monocytes and macrophages. *Am J Physiol* **251**:C128, 1986.
62. Bennett SE, Bevington A, Walls J: Active accumulation of creatine by cultured rat myoblasts. *Biochem Soc Trans* **19**:172S, 1991.
63. Clark JF, Odoom J, Tracey I, Dunn J, Boehm EA, Paternostro G, Radda GK: Experimental observations of creatine phosphate and creatine metabolism, in Conway MA, Clark JF (eds.) *Creatine and Creatine Phosphate*. San Diego and New York, New York, Academic, 1996, p 33.
64. Fitch CD, Shields RP, Payne WF, Dacus JF: Creatine metabolism in skeletal muscle. III. Specificity of the creatine entry process. *J Biol Chem* **243**:2024, 1968.
65. Loike JD, Zalutsky DL, Kaback E, Miranda AF, Silverstein SC: Extracellular creatine regulates creatine transport in rat and human muscle cells. *Proc Natl Acad Sci USA* **85**:807, 1988.
66. Möller A, Hamprecht B: Creatine transport in cultured cells of rat and mouse brain. *J Neurochem* **52**:544, 1989.
67. Daly MM, Seifter S: Uptake of creatine by cultured cells. *Arch Biochem Biophys* **203**:317, 1980.
68. Gregor P, Nash SR, Caron MG, Seldin MF, Warren ST: Assignment of the creatine transporter gene (SLC6A8) to human chromosome Xq28 telomeric to G6PD. *Genomics* **25**:332, 1995.
69. Iyer GS, Krahe R, Goodwin LA, Doggett NA, Siciliano MJ, Funanage VL, Proujansky R: Identification of a testis-expressed creatine transporter gene at 16p11.2 and confirmation of the linked locus to Xa28. *Genomics* **34**:143, 1996.
70. Sora I, Richman J, Santoro G, Wei G, Wang Y, Vanderah T, Horvath R, Nguyen M, Waite S, Roeske WR, Yamamüra HI: The cloning and expression of a human creatine transporter. *Biochem Biophys Res Commun* **204**:419, 1994.

71. Guimbal C, Kilimann MW: A Na(+)-dependent creatine transporter in rabbit brain, muscle, heart, and kidney. cDNA cloning and functional expression. *J Biol Chem* **268**:8418, 1993.
72. Nash SR, Giros B, Kingsmore SF, Rochelle JM, Suter ST, Gregor P, Seldin MF, Caron MG: Cloning, pharmacological characterization, and genomic localization of the human creatine transporter. *Receptors Channels* **2**:165, 1994.
73. Schloss P, Mayser W, Betz H: The putative rat choline transporter CHOT1 transports creatine and is highly expressed in neural and muscle-rich tissues. *Biochem Biophys Res Commun* **198**:637, 1994.
74. Saltarelli MD, Bauman AL, Moore KR, Bradley CC, Blakely RD: Expression of the rat brain creatine transport *in situ* and in transfected HeLa cells. *Dev Neurosci* **18**:524, 1996.
75. Barnwell LE, Chandhuri G, Townsel JG: Cloning and sequencing of a cDNA encoding a novel member of the human brain GABA/noradrenaline neurotransmitter transporter family. *Gene* **159**:287, 1995.
76. Seppet EK, Adoyaan AJ, Kallikorm AP, Chernousova GB, Lyulina NV, Sharov VG, Severin VV, Popovich MI, Saks VA: Hormone regulation of cardiac energy metabolism. Creatine transport across cell membranes of euthyroid and hyperthyroid rat heart. *Biochem Med* **34**:267, 1985.
77. Odoom JE, Kemp GK, Radda GK: Control of intracellular creatine concentration in a mouse myoblast cell line. *Biochem Soc Trans* **21**:441S, 1993.
78. Dinking JS, Coker R, Fitch CD: Creatine metabolism in hyperthyroidism. *Proc Soc Exp Biol Med* **100**:118, 1959.
79. Fitch CD, Coker R, Dinning JS: Metabolism of creatine-1-C14 by vitamin E-deficient and hyperthyroid rats. *Am J Physiol* **198**:1232, 1960.
80. Wallimann T, Wyss M, Brdiczak D, Nicolay K, Eppenberger HM: Intracellular compartmentalization, structure and function of creatine kinase isoenzymes in tissues with high and fluctuating energy demands: The phosphocreatine circuit for cellular energy homeostasis. *Biochem J* **281**:21, 1992.
81. Friedman DL, Perryman MB: Compartmentalization of multiple forms of creatine kinase in the distal nephron of the rat kidney. *J Biol Chem* **266**:22404, 1991.
82. Ishida Y, Riesinger T, Wallimann T, Paul RJ: Compartmentation of ATP synthesis and utilization in smooth muscle: Roles of aerobic glycolysis and creatine kinase. *Mol Cell Biochem* **133/134**:39, 1994.
83. Perriard JC, Perriard ER, Eppenberger HM: Detection and relative quantitation of RNA for creatine kinase isoenzymes in RNA from myogenic cell cultures and embryonic chicken tissues. *J Biol Chem* **253**:6529, 1989.
84. Clark JF, Field M, Ventura-Clapier R: An introduction to the cellular creatine kinase system in contractile tissue, in Conway MA, Clark JF (eds.) *Creatine and Creatine Phosphate*. New York, Academic, 1996, p 51.
85. Hemmer W, Wallimann T: Functional aspects of creatine kinase in brain. *Dev Neurosci* **15**:249, 1993.
86. Kaldis P, Hemmer W, Zanolla E, Holtzmann D, Wallimann T: "Hot spots" of creatine kinase localization in brain: Cerebellum, hippocampus and choroid plexus. *Dev Neurosci* **18**:542, 1996.
87. Beis I, Newsholme EA: The contents of adenine nucleotides, phosphagens and some glycolytic intermediates in resting muscles from vertebrates and invertebrates. *Biochem J* **152**:23, 1975.
88. Shoubridge EA, Radda GK: A ^{31}P-nuclear magnetic resonance study of skeletal muscle metabolism in rats depleted of creatine with the analogue β-guanidino proprionic acid. *Biochim Biophys Acta* **805**:79, 1984.
89. Brdiczka D: Function of the outer mitochondrial compartment in the regulation of energy metabolism. *Biochim Biophys Acta* **1187**:264, 1994.
90. Jacobus WE, Lehninger AL: Creatine kinase of rat heart mitochondria: Coupling of creatine phosphorylation to electron transport. *J Biol Chem* **248**:4803, 1973.
91. Bessmann SP, Geiger PJ: Transport of energy in muscle: The phosphoryl-creatine shuttle. *Science* **211**:448, 1981.
92. Bessmann SP, Carpenter CL: The creatine-creatine phosphate energy shuttle. *Annu Rev Biochem* **54**:831, 1985.
93. Sharov VG, Saks VA, Smirnov VN, Chazov El: An electron microscopic histochemical investigation of the localization of creatine phosphokinase in heart cells. *Biochim Biophys Acta* **468**:495, 1977.
94. Ponticos M, Lu QL, Morgan JE, Hardie DG, Partridge TA, Carling D: Dual regulation of the AMP-activated protein kinase provides a novel mechanism for the control of creatine kinase in skeletal muscle. *EMBO J* **17**:1688, 1998.
95. van Deursen J, Heerschap A, Oerlemans F, Ruitenbeek W, Jap P, ter Laak H, Wieringa B: Skeletal muscle of mice deficient in muscle creatine kinase lack burst activity. *Cell* **74**:621, 1993.
96. Ventura-Clapier R, Kuznetsov AV, d'Albis A, van Deursen J, Wieringa B, Veksler VI: Muscle creatine kinase-deficient mice. I. Alterations in myofibrillar function. *J Biol Chem* **270**:19914, 1995.
97. Veksler VI, Kuznetsov AV, Anflous K, Mateo P, van Deursen J, Wieringa B, Ventura-Clapier R: Muscle creatine kinase-deficient mice. II. Cardiac and skeletal muscle exhibit tissue-specific adaptation of the mitochondrial function. *J Biol Chem* **270**:19921, 1995.
98. Roman BB, Wieringa B, Koretsky AP: Functional equivalence of creatine kinase isoforms in mouse skeletal muscle. *J Biol Chem* **272**:17790, 1997.
99. van Deursen J, Wieringa B: Approaching the multifaceted nature of energy metabolism: Inactivation of the cytosolic creatine kinases via homologous recombination in mouse embryonic stem cells. *Mol Cell Biochem* **133/134**:263, 1994.
100. Steeghs K, Oerlemans F, Wieringa B: Mice deficient in ubiquitous mitochondrial creatine kinase are viable and fertile. *Biochim Biophys Acta* **1230**:130, 1995.
101. Steeghs K, Heerschap A, de Haan A, Ruitenbeek W, Oeriemans F, van Deursen J, Perryman B, Pette D, Brückwilder M, Koüdijs J, Jap P, Wieringa B: Use of gene targeting of compromising energy homeostasis in neuromuscular tissues: The role for sarcomeric mitochondrial creatine kinase. *J Neurosci Method* **71**:29, 1997.
102. Steeghs K, Benders A, Oerlemans F, de Haan A, Heerschap A, Ruitenbeek W, Jost C, van Deürsen J, Perryman B, Pette D, Brückwilder M, Koüdijs J, Jap P, Veerkawp J, Wieringa B: Altered Ca^{2+} responses in muscles with combined mitochondrial and cytosolic creatine kinase deficiencies. *Cell* **89**:93, 1997.
103. Watchko JF, Daood MJ, Sieck GC, LaBella JJ, Ameredes BT, Koretsky AP, Wieringa B: Combined myofibrillar and mitochondrial creatine kinase deficiency impairs mouse diaphragm isotonic to function. *J Appl Physiol* **82**:1416, 1997.
104. Isbrand D, personal communication.
105. Zhuang Y, Weiner AM: A compensatory base change in U1snRNA suppresses a 5′ splice site mutation. *Cell* **46**:827, 1986.
106. Weber S, Aebi M: *In vitro* splicing of mRNA precursors: 5′ cleavage site can be predicted from the interaction between the 5′ splice region and the 5′ terminus of U1snRNA. *Nucleic Acids Res* **16**:471, 1988.
107. Harris RC, Söderlund K, Hultman E: Elevation of creatine in resting and exercised muscles of normal subjects by creatine supplementation. *Clin Sci* **83**:367, 1992.
108. Hultman E, Söderlund K, Timmons JA, Cederblad G, Greenhaff PL: Muscle creatine loading in man. *Am J Appl Physiology* **81**:232, 1996.
109. Greenhaff PL, Casey A, Short AH, Harris R, Söderlund K, Hultman E: Influence of oral creatine supplementation on muscle torque during repeated bouts of maximal voluntary exercise in man. *Clin Sci* **84**:565, 1993.
110. Earnest CP, Snell PG, Rodriguez R, Almada AL: The effect of creatine monohydrate ingestion on anaerobic power indices, muscular strength and body composition. *Acta Physiol Scand* **153**:207, 1995.
111. Erecinska M, Silver IA: ATP and brain function. *J Cerebr Blood Flow Metabol* **9**:2, 1989.
112. Kato K, Suzuki F, Shimizu A, Shinohara H, Semba R: Highly sensitive immunoassay for rat brain-type creatine kinase: Determination in isolated Purkinje cells. *J Neurochem* **46**:1783, 1986.
113. Tsuji MK, Mulkern RV, Cook CU, Meyers RL, Holtzman D: Relative phosphocreatine and nucleotide triphosphate concentrations in cerebral gray and white matter measured *in vivo* by ^{31}P nuclear magnetic resonance. *Brain Res* **707**:146, 1996.
114. Holtzman D, Mulkern R, Tsuji M, Cook C, Meyers R: Phosphocreatine and creatine kinase systems in gray and white matter of the developing piglet brain. *Dev Neurosci* **18**:535, 1996.
115. Dringen R, Verleysdonk S, Hamprecht B, Willker W, Leibfritz D, Brand A: Metabolism of glycine in primary astroglial cells: Synthesis of creatine, serine and glutathione. *J Neurochem* **70**:836, 1998.
116. Wilson CD, Shen W, Molloy GR: Expression of the brain creatine kinase gene is low in neuroblastoma cell lines. *Dev Neurosci* **19**:375, 1997.
117. Molloy GR, Wilson CD, Benfield PA, deVellis J, Kuma S: Rat brain creatine kinase messenger RNA levels are high in primary cultures of brain astrocytes and oligodendrocytes and low in neurons. *J Neurochem* **59**:1925, 1992.
118. Brand A, Richter-Landsberg C, Leibfritz D: Multinuclear NMR studies on the energy metabolism of glial and neuronal cells. *Dev Neurosci* **15**:289, 1993.

119. Manos P, Bryan GK: Cellular and subcellular compartmentation of creatine kinase in brain. *Dev Neurosci* **15**:271, 1993.
120. La Manna JC, Haxhiu MA, Kutina-Nelson KL, Pundik S, Erokwu B, Yeh ER, Lust WD, Cherniack NS: Decreased energy metabolism in brain stem during central respiratory depression in response to hypoxia. *J Appl Physiol* **81**:1772, 1996.
121. Espanol MT, Litt L, Chang LH, James TL, Weinstein PR, Chan PH: Adult rat brain-slice preparation for nuclear magnetic resonance spectroscopy studies of hypoxia. *Anesthesiology* **84**:201, 1996.
122. Cohen Y, Chang LH, Litt L, Kim F, Severinghaus JW, Weinstein PR, Davis RL, Germano I, James TL: Stability of brain intracellular lactate and ^{31}P-metabolite levels at reduced intracellular pH during prolonged hypercapnia in rats. *J Cereb Blood Flow Metab* **10**:277, 1990.
123. Pettigrew LC, Grotta JC, Rhoades HM, Reid C, McCandless DW: Regional depletion of adenosine triphosphate, phosphocreatine, and glucose in ischemic hippocampus. *Metab Brain Dis* **3**:185, 1988.
124. Ingvar M, Soderfeldt B, Folbergrova J, Kalimo H, Olsson Y, Siesjo BK: Metabolic, circulatory, and structural alterations in the rat brain induced by sustained pentylenetetrazole seizures. *Epilepsia* **25**:191, 1984.
125. Jacquin T, Gillet B, Fortin G, Pasquier C, Beloeil JC, Champagnat J: Metabolic action of N-methyl-D-aspartate in newborn rat brain *ex vivo*: ^{31}P magnetic resonance spectroscopy. *Brain Res* **497**:296, 1989.
126. Prichard JW, Alger JR, Behar KL, Petroff OAC, Shulman RG: Cerebral metabolic studies *in vivo* by ^{31}P NMR. *Proc Natl Acad Sci USA* **80**:2746, 1983.
127. Petroff OAC, Prichard JW, Behar KL, Alger JR, Shulman RG: *In vivo* phosphorus nuclear magnetic resonance spectroscopy in status epilepticus. *Ann Neurol* **16**:168, 1984.
128. Xu CJ, Klunk WE, Kanfer JN, Xiong Q, Miller G, Pettegrew JW: Phosphocreatine-dependent glutamate uptake by synaptic vesicles. A comparison with ATP-dependent glutamate uptake. *J Biol Chem* **271**:13435, 1996.
129. Xu CJ, Kanfer JN, Klunk WE, Xiong Q, McClure RJ, Pettegrew JW: Effect of phosphomonoesters, phosphodiesters, and phosphocreatine on glutamate uptake by synaptic vesicles. *Mol Chem Neuropathol* **32**:89, 1997.
130. Hirayasu Y, Morimoto K, Otsuki S: Increase of methylguanidine and guanidinoacetic acid in the brain of amygdala-kindled rats. *Epilepsia* **32**:761, 1991.
131. Shimizu Y, Morimoto K, Kuroda S, Mori A: Sustained increase of methylguanidine in rats after amygdala or hippocampal kindling. *Epilepsy Res* **21**:11, 1995.
132. Shiraga H, Watanabe Y, Mori A: Guanidino compound levels in the serum of healthy adults and epileptic patients. *Epilepsy Res* **8**:142, 1991.
133. Mori A, Kolmo M, Masumizu T, Noda Y, Packer L: Guanidino compounds generate reactive oxygen species. *Biochem Mol Biol Int* **40**:135, 1996.
134. Davis BM, Miller RK, Breut RL, Koszalka TR: Materno-fetal transport of creatine in the rat. *Biol Neonate* **33**:43, 1978.
135. Hülsmann J, Manz F, Wember T, Schöch G: Die Zufuhr von Kreatin und Kreatinin mit Frauenmilch und Säuglingsmilchpraeparation. *Klin Pädiatr* **199**:292, 1987.
136. Hanefeld F, unpublished.
137. Huang SM, Huang YC: Chromatography and electrophoresis of creatinine and other guanidino compounds. *J Chromatogr* **429**:235, 1988.
138. Marescau B, Deshmukh DR, Kockx M, Possemiers I, Qureshi IA, Wiechert P, De Deyn PP: Guanidino compounds in serum, urine, liver, kidney, and brain of man and some ureotelic animals. *Metabolism* **41**:526, 1992.
139. Hunneman DH, Hanefeld F: GC-MS determination of guanidinoacetate in urine and plasma. *J Inherit Metab Dis* **20**:450, 1997.
140. Schulze A, Mayatepek E, Rating D, Bremer HJ: Sakaguchi reaction: A useful method for screening guanidinoacetate-methyltransferase deficiency. *J Inherit Metab Dis* **19**:706, 1996.
141. Shirokane Y, Utsushikawa M, Nakajima M: A new enzymic determination of guanidinoacetic acid in urine. *Clin-Chem* **33**:394, 1987.
142. Shirokane Y, Nakajima M, Mizusawa K: A new enzymatic assay of urinary guanidinoacetic acid. *Clin Chim Acta* **202**:227, 1991.
143. Wevers RA, Engelke U, Wendel U, de Jong JG, Gabreëls FJ, Heerschap A: Standardized method for high-resolution 1H-NMR of cerebrospinal fluid. *Clin Chem* **41**:744, 1995.
144. Frahm J, Hanefeld F: Localized proton magnetic resonance spectroscopy of brain disorders in childhood, in Bachelard H (ed) *Advances in Neurochemistry*. Vol 8. New York, Plenum, 1997 p 329.
145. Jeas J, Mühl A, Stöckler-Jpsiroglu S: Guanidinoacetate methyltransferase (GAHT) deficiency: non-invasive enzymatic diagnosis of newly recognized inborn error of metabolism. *Clin Chim Acta* **290**:179, 2000.
146. Rating P, personal communication.
147. Andrews R, Greenhaff P, Curtis S, Perry A, Cowley AJ: The effect of dietary creatine supplementation on skeletal muscle metabolism in congestive heart failure. *Eur Heart J* **19**:617, 1998.
148. Clark JF: Creatine: A review of its nutritional applications in sport. *Nutrition* **14**:322, 1998.
149. Mujika I, Padilla S: Creatine supplementation as an ergogenic acid for sports performance in highly trained athletes. A critical review. *Int J Sports Med* **18**:491, 1997.
150. Tarnopolsky MA, Roy BD, MacDonald JR: A randomized, controlled trial of creatine monohydrate in patients with mitochondrial cytopathies. *Muscle Nerve* **20**:1502, 1997.
151. Maughan RJ: Creatine supplementation and exercise performance. *Int J Sport Nutr* **5**:94, 1995.
152. Stöckler S, Hanefeld F, Frahm J: Creatine replacement therapy in guanidinoacetate methyltransferase deficiency, a novel inborn error of metabolism. *Lancet* **348**:789, 1996.
153. Fitch CD, Shields RP, Payne WF, Dacus JM: Creatine metabolism in skeletal muscle. III. Specificity of the creatine entry process. *J Biol Chem* **243**:2024, 1968.
154. Bianchi MC, Tosetti M, Fornai F, Alessandri MG, Cipriani P, de Vito G, Canapicchi R: Reversible brain creatine deficiency in two sisters with normal blood creatine level. *Ann Neurol* **47**:511, 2000.
155. van der Knaap MS, Verhoeven NM, Maaswinkel-Mooij P, Pouwels PJW, Onkenhot W, Peeters EA, Stöckler-Ipsiroglu S, Jakobs C: Mental retardation and behavioral problems as presenting signs of a creatine synthesis defect. *Ann Neurol* **47**:540, 2000.

CHAPTER 85

Urea Cycle Enzymes

Saul W. Brusilow ▪ Arthur L. Horwich

1. **The urea cycle, which consists of a series of five biochemical reactions, has two roles. In order to prevent the accumulation of toxic nitrogenous compounds, the urea cycle incorporates nitrogen not used for net biosynthetic purposes into urea, which serves as the waste nitrogen product in mammals. The urea cycle also contains several of the biochemical reactions required for the *de novo* synthesis of arginine.**
2. **Urea cycle disorders are characterized by the triad of hyperammonemia, encephalopathy, and respiratory alkalosis (the earliest objective evidence of encephalopathy). Five well-documented diseases (each with considerable genetic and phenotypic variability) have been described, each representing a defect in the biosynthesis of one of the normally expressed enzymes of the urea cycle. Four of these five diseases—deficiencies of carbamyl phosphate synthetase (CPS) (OMIM 237300), ornithine transcarbamylase (OTC) (OMIM 311250), argininosuccinic acid synthetase (AS) (OMIM 215700), and argininosuccinate lyase (AL) (OMIM 207900)—are characterized by signs and symptoms induced by the accumulation of precursors of urea, principally ammonium and glutamine. The most dramatic clinical presentation of these four diseases occurs in full-term infants with no obstetric risk factors who appear normal for 24 to 48 hours and then exhibit progressive lethargy, hypothermia, and apnea all related to very high plasma ammonium levels.**
3. **Milder forms of these diseases occur; they may present with signs of encephalopathy at any age from infancy to adulthood. The most common of these late-onset diseases occurs in female carriers of a mutation at the OTC locus of one of their X chromosomes. The late-onset cases present with respiratory alkalosis and episodic mental status changes progressing, if not emergently treated, to cerebral edema, brainstem compression, and death. The acute encephalopathy is characterized by brain edema and swollen astrocytes, the cause of which is attributed to intraglial accumulation of glutamine resulting in osmotic shifts of water into the cell. Axons, dendrites, synapses, and oligodendroglia are normal. A fifth disease, arginase deficiency (OMIM 107830), is characterized by a clinical picture consisting of progressive spastic quadriplegia and mental retardation; symptomatic hyperammonemia, which can be life-threatening, occurs neither as severely or as commonly as in the other four diseases. Apart from OTC deficiency, which is inherited as an X-linked disorder, the other four diseases are inherited as autosomal-recessive traits. Carrier status of OTC mutations in women is determined by pedigree analysis and molecular methods. For fetuses at risk, antenatal diagnosis is available by a number of methods, particular to each disease, including enzyme analysis of fibroblasts cultured from aminocytes, as well as molecular (DNA) methods.**
4. **Molecular genetic analysis of the urea cycle enzymes has addressed their structure and expression and has permitted DNA-based diagnosis of deficiency, in many cases by direct analysis of mutations. Using the cloned complementary DNA as probes, expression in liver of RNA for all the enzymes has been observed to be increased severalfold by starvation. RNA coding for the 160-kDa subunit of the CPS I homodimer is detected almost exclusively in the liver and translates a precursor protein representing the product of fusion of two ancestral prokaryotic subunits, joined with an N-terminal mitochondrial targeting sequence. Few mutations have been identified in this large coding sequence in affected pedigrees so far, but a restriction fragment-length polymorphism (RFLP) in the human CPS locus is useful in prenatal diagnosis of deficiency. OTC is also expressed principally in the liver, and its subunit is also translated as a precursor, comprising an N-terminal mitochondrial targeting sequence that functions via an α-helical structure and net positive charge, joined with a mature portion that resembles prokaryotic transcarbamylases. Mitochondrial import requires the action of a variety of components in the cytosol to maintain an import-competent conformation, in the outer mitochondrial membrane for recognition of the precursor, in both outer and inner membrane for protein translocation, and in the matrix for proteolytic processing and folding to the active conformation. Gene deletions have been observed in approximately 15 percent of affected males. More than 100 different single base substitutions have been identified, producing amino acid substitution in many cases, involving either of the two domains of the OTC subunit. In other cases, splicing is affected, either destabilizing the messenger RNA (mRNA) or frameshifting the subunit. Prenatal diagnosis can be offered to most women who are established as heterozygous carriers by pedigree analysis, allopurinol testing, or DNA analysis, using direct DNA analysis of fetal DNA where the mutation is known, or using RFLPs. Recombinant OTC retroviruses have transduced cultured hepatocytes of mice with inherited OTC deficiency, and recombinant OTC adenoviruses have been injected into newborn mutant animals with evidence of rescue of deficiency. These gene transfer experiments aim toward achieving stable long-term OTC expression. Argininosuccinate synthetase (AS) is programmed from a single locus, but a large number of homologous processed**

A list of standard abbreviations is located immediately preceding the index in each volume. Nonstandard abbreviations used in this chapter include: AL = argininosuccinate lyase; AS = argininosuccinic acid synthetase; Can^r = canavanine resistant; CAT = chloramphenicol acyltransferase; CP = carbamyl phosphate; CPS = carbamyl phosphate synthetase 1; HHH = hyperammonemia, hyperornithinemia, homocitrullinuria syndrome; LPI = lysinuric protein intolerance syndrome; LTR = long terminal repeat; MIP = mitochondrial intermediate processing peptidase; MPP = matrix processing peptidase; NAG = *N*-acetylglutamate; OTC = ornithine transcarbamylase; PBF = presequence binding factor.

pseudogenes are localized throughout the genome. Expression of AS mRNA has been studied in cultured cells, where the level of mRNA is greatly increased in response to canavanine treatment and repressed by the presence of arginine. The AS coding sequence has been successfully transferred into both cultured cells and mouse bone marrow cells as an approach to AS deficiency of supplying enzyme activity outside the liver. Analysis of AS mutations reveals considerable heterogeneity in the position of mutation, with most composed of codon substitutions that produce unstable protein products. Where direct mutation analysis is not possible, a number of polymorphisms at the AS locus enable linkage study of affected pedigrees. Human AL is similar to avian δ-crystallins, in which a virtually identical protein is apparently used as a structural component. Analysis of AL mutants also reveals considerable heterogeneity. Arginase in human liver and red cells is a cytosolic enzyme distinct from a second mitochondrial-localized enzyme. Deficient patients have shown heterogeneity in the site of mutation. Two RFLPs at the locus have been identified.

5. **Treatment requires restriction of dietary protein intake and activation of other pathways of waste nitrogen synthesis and excretion. For patients deficient in CPS, OTC, and AS, treatment with sodium phenylbutyrate activates the synthesis of phenylacetylglutamine, which has a dual effect. By providing a new vehicle for waste nitrogen excretion, which suppresses residual urea synthesis in the late-onset group, a reserve urea synthetic capacity is generated that may support nitrogen homeostasis when required. In patients deficient in AS and argininosuccinase, supplementation of the diet with arginine promotes the synthesis of citrulline in the former and argininosuccinate in the latter, both of which serve as waste nitrogen products.**

   Outcome of treatment of neonatal-onset disease has been disappointing. Even those neonates treated prospectively prior to the onset of hyperammonemia are at high risk for neurologic deficits. Parents should be realistically counseled as to the likely outcome if the infant is rescued. Treatment of late-onset disease appears to preserve the neurologic status found at the start of therapy.

The urea cycle serves two purposes: (1) it contains, in part, the biochemical reactions required for the *de novo* biosynthesis and degradation of arginine, and (2) it incorporates nitrogen atoms not retained for net biosynthetic purposes into urea, which serves as a waste nitrogen product. Campbell's review[1] of the comparative biochemistry of nitrogen metabolism describes other waste nitrogen products (ammonium and purines) found in other animals.

It also has been proposed[2] that the urea cycle plays an important role in the disposal of bicarbonate and hence on pH homeostasis. A number of arguments against this view have been offered.[3] Perhaps the strongest case against this function of the urea cycle can be found in patients with complete, or nearly so, defects in one of the enzymes of the urea cycle; apart from respiratory alkalosis related to the stimulatory effect of ammonium on respiration, these patients have little evidence of a disorder of pH homeostasis. For example, 28 ornithine transcarbamylase (OTC)-deficient neonates who presented with hyperammonemia had a respiratory alkalosis as manifested by the following blood gases: pH 7.5; pCO_2, 24 torr; HCO_3, 19.3 mM.[4] As shown in Fig. 85-1, a respiratory alkalosis develops very early in the course of untreated hyperammonemia in an OTC-deficient neonate. Furthermore, a decrease in ureagenesis caused by partial hepatectomy did not influence acid–base balance.[5] These data suggest that hepatic urea synthesis plays little or no role in maintaining acid–base balance, as has been proposed.[6]

A defect in the ureagenic pathway has two consequences: arginine becomes an essential amino acid[7] (except in arginase deficiency, where the enzyme defect results in a failure of degradation of arginine) and nitrogen atoms accumulate in a variety of molecules, the pattern of which varies according to the specific enzymatic defect, although plasma levels of ammonium and glutamine are increased in all urea cycle disorders not under metabolic control.

WASTE NITROGEN DISPOSAL

The biochemical pathway of urea synthesis is described in Fig. 85-2 and in Table 85-1. Waste nitrogen disposal is far more complex, requiring interorgan, intrahepatic, and cellular compartmentation relationships in the conversion to urea of nitrogen not used for net biosynthetic purposes. Although it has been known for decades that ammonium and aspartate are the sources of nitrogen for ureagenesis, the pathways from amino acid nitrogen to ammonium and aspartate have been less clear.

Intrahepatic Sources of Nitrogen for Ureagenesis

It was proposed on theoretical grounds[15] that intramitochondrial ammonium for the carbamyl phosphate synthetase (CPS) reaction was derived from the oxidative deamination of glutamate by glutamate dehydrogenase (Fig. 85-3). Although this interpretation is commonly accepted, attempts to verify this hypothesis in respiring mitochondria have repeatedly shown that the vast portion of glutamate is not deaminated but rather transaminated,[16,17] suggesting that glutamate may not be the principal precursor for citrulline biosynthesis. The virtual absence of experimental evidence supporting the hypothesis that oxidative deamination of glutamate via glutamate dehydrogenase is a source of ammonium for the biosynthesis of citrulline and urea has led some researchers to conclude that, "studies of glutamate dehydrogenase in liver have failed to yield any clear consensus of the role of this enzyme"[18] or "it is still not possible to define the role of this enzyme in animal tissues."[19] Krebs also has reviewed this subject.[20]

Jungermann[21] reviewed the role of metabolic zonation in the liver as it pertains to nitrogen homeostasis. It is proposed that periportal hepatocytes predominantly contain enzymes that catalyze transamination reactions and ureagenesis, whereas perivenous hepatocytes predominantly contain enzymes that catalyze the amidation or deamination of glutamate to glutamine or ammonium and ketoglutarate, respectively.

Cooper et al.[22] suggested that no more than 20 percent (and possible much less) of the α-amino moiety of liver glutamate is deaminated *in vivo*, but rather it is predominantly transaminated to aspartate and incorporated into urea. These studies were done in a series of three experiments in which each of ^{13}N-labeled glutamate, alanine, and glutamine (amide) was injected into the portal vein, after which the liver was freeze-clamped at intervals of 5 to 60 s and the distribution of the label described. Aspartate and urea were promptly labeled after ^{13}N-alanine and ^{13}N-glutamate were injected but not after ^{13}N-glutamine (amide). Ammonium and citrulline were not labeled, suggesting that little glutamate was deaminated. The absence of incorporation of glutamine nitrogen into the urea cycle in these *in vivo* experiments does not support the glutamine channeling hypothesis of Meijer.[23] The rapidity of nitrogen exchange among the linked transaminases in these and other studies[22] was striking—within 10 s of the injection of the labeled amino acids or ammonium. In previous studies[24] these investigators showed that intraportal vein injection of ^{13}N-ammonium resulted in labeling of citrulline.

From these studies it may be concluded that although glutamate may be deaminated, it may not be a major source of ammonium for the CPS reaction. As described below, extrahepatic glutamine metabolism provides the single most important source of ammonium for the CPS reaction. However, within the liver there are a number of other amino acids that are deaminated and

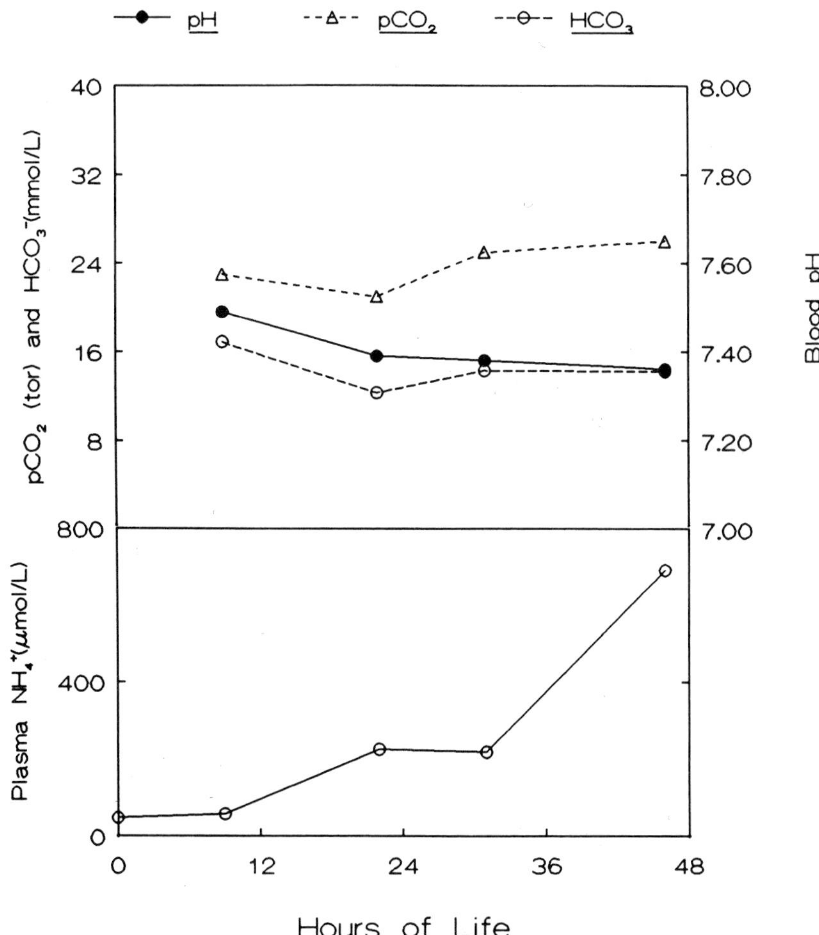

Fig. 85-1 Course of blood pH, PCO_2, plasma bicarbonate, and ammonium concentration of untreated OTC-deficient neonate. Early onset and persistence of hyperventilation and respiratory alkalosis are apparent.

may provide ammonium for ureagenesis (e.g., histidine, tryptophan, threonine, and lysine).

Extrahepatic Sources of Nitrogen for Ureagenesis

Intestine. In a series of studies of the metabolism of the perfused rat intestine, Windmueller and Spaeth[25,26] showed not only that glutamine carbon atoms were an important respiratory fuel but also that glutamine nitrogen was converted to the urea precursors ammonium, citrulline, and alanine, all of which were released into the portal circulation (Fig. 85-3). Whereas alanine and ammonium are taken up by the liver, citrulline apparently is not but rather is transported to the kidney, where it is converted to arginine.[27]

Kidney. Rat kidney uptake of citrulline is approximately equivalent to its rate of intestinal release.[27,28] This observation is compatible with the report that anephric animals incorporate little citrulline into liver.[29] In confirmation of the absence of a large role of the liver in citrulline metabolism are the findings in patients with urea cycle disorders who have undergone orthotopic liver transplantation; plasma citrulline levels are undetectable or nearly so, similar to the pretransplant values.[30,31]

That the kidney may be an extrahepatic source of ammonium is suggested by the observation that the ammonium concentration of the renal vein exceeds that of the renal artery; a consequence of renal glutaminase activity. Thus, the kidney may supply ammonium directly for the CPS reaction and, as described above, generate another waste nitrogen atom by catalyzing the synthesis of arginine from citrulline and aspartate via renal argininosuccinic acid synthetase (AS).

Muscle. Because glutamine is constantly being extracted from the circulation by the intestine, a potent source of glutamine must be found elsewhere. The most likely source of glutamine is muscle; several studies have shown a net release of glutamine from muscle *in vivo*[32,33] and *in vitro*.[34] The biosynthetic pathway for muscle glutamine synthesis is not entirely clear, although glutamine synthetase does play a role.[32] The source of ammonium for amidation is also unclear; purine nucleotide deamination is a possibility.[35,36] Alanine production by muscle, via transamination of pyruvate, represents another important nitrogen precursor for ureagenesis.

Figure 85-3 presents an integrated view of the interorgan relationships required for synthesis of urea. Muscle appears to be the starting point of waste nitrogen disposal via transamination of amino acid nitrogen to alanine and glutamate and thence amidation of glutamate to produce glutamine.

THE BIOCHEMISTRY OF THE UREA CYCLE

The enzymes, substrates, and cofactors required for ureagenesis are described in Fig. 85-2 and Tables 85-1 and 85-2. CPS, a mitochondrial matrix enzyme, catalyzes the biosynthesis of carbamyl phosphate (CP) from ammonium and bicarbonate; *N*-acetylglutamate [NAG; synthesized from glutamate and acetyl coenzyme A (CoA)] is an allosteric cofactor for this enzyme and may be an important regulator of ureagenesis. OTC, also a mitochondrial matrix enzyme, catalyzes the biosynthesis of citrulline from ornithine and CP (see Chapter 83 for a discussion of the mitochondrial import of ornithine). Citrulline is exported to

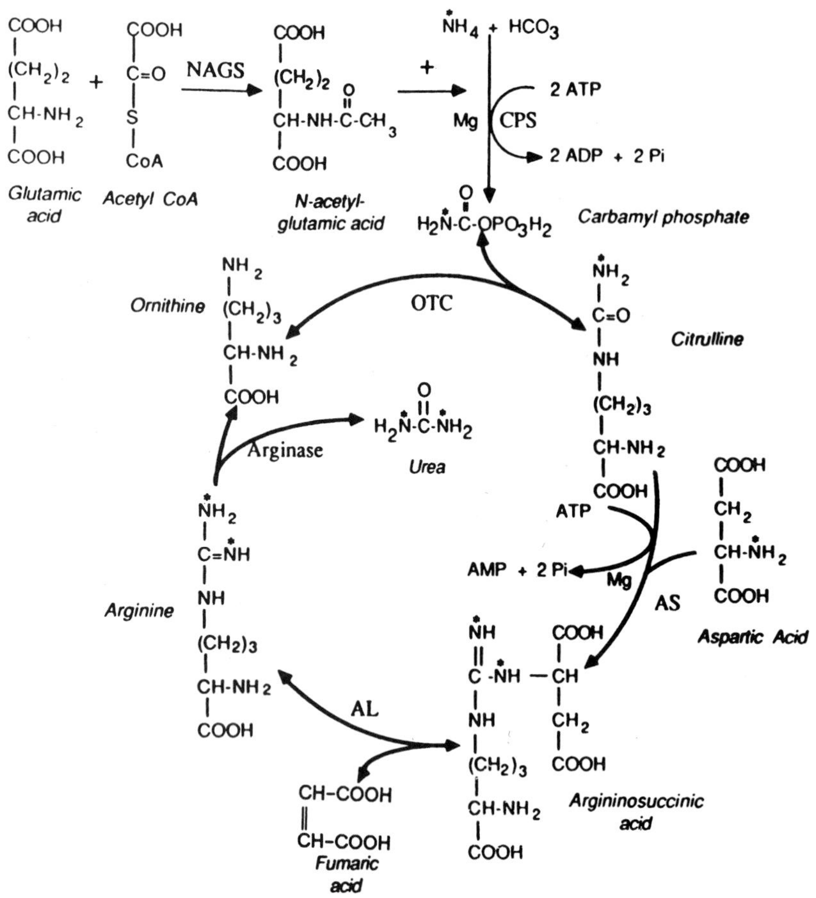

Fig. 85-2 Substrates, products, and cofactors required for ureagenesis. The asterisks denote waste nitrogen atoms. AS = argininosuccinic acid synthetase; AL = argininosuccinase; CPS = carbamyl phosphate synthetase; NAGS = *N*-acetylglutamate synthetase; OTC = ornithine transcarbamylase.

Table 85-1 The Enzymes of the Urea Cycle*

Enzyme	Compartment	Activity	M_r	pH opt	K_m, mM	Equilibrium Constant	Tissue Distribution
N-acetyl glutamate synthetase, EC 2.3.11	Mitochondrial matrix	0.30–1.49	200,000	8.5	Glu, 3.0 Ac CoA 0.7 Arg, 0.01	Irreversible	Liver, intestine, kidney (trace), spleen
Carbamyl phosphate Synthetase EC 6.3.4.16	Mitochondrial matrix	279†	310,000 dimer	6.8–7.6	NH_4, 0.8 HCO_3, 6.7 Mg ATP, 1.1 NAG, 0.1	Irreversible	Liver, intestine, kidney (trace)
Ornithine transcarbamylase, EC 2.1.3.3	Mitochondrial matrix	6600	108,000 trimer	7.7	CP, 0.16 Orn, 0.40	$\frac{(\text{Cit})(\text{p})}{(\text{Orn})(\text{CP})} = 10^5$	Liver, intestine, kidney (trace)
Argininosuccinic acid synthetase, EC 6.3.4.5	Cytosol	90	185,000 tetramer	8.7	Asp, .03 Cit, .03	$\frac{(\text{ASA})(\text{AMP})(\text{Mg PP})(2\text{H})}{(\text{Cit})(\text{Asp})(\text{Mg ATP})} = 0.89^{\ddagger}$	Liver, kidney, fibroblasts, brain (trace)
Argininosuccinase, EC4.3.2.1	Cytosol	220	173,200 tetramer	7.5	Asp, 0.017 Cit, 0.016 ATP, 0.041	$\frac{(\text{Arg})(\text{fumarate})}{(\text{ASA})} = 11.4 \times 10^{-3}$	Liver, kidney, brain, fibroblasts
Arginase, EC 3.5.3.1	Cytosol	86,600	107,000 tetramer	9.5	Arg, 10.5	Irreversible	Liver, erythrocytes, kidney, lens, brain (trace)

*Enzyme activity is expressed as micromoles per hour per gram wet weight. Apart from the equilibrium constants, the values described are those of human liver.

†The monomers may have substantial catalytic activity.[11]

‡AT pH = 7.0.

SOURCE: Table assembled from Ratner,[4] Snodgrass,[9] Meijer and Hensgens,[10] Jackson, et al.,[11] Beaudet et al.,[12] Lusty,[13] and Bachman et al.[14]

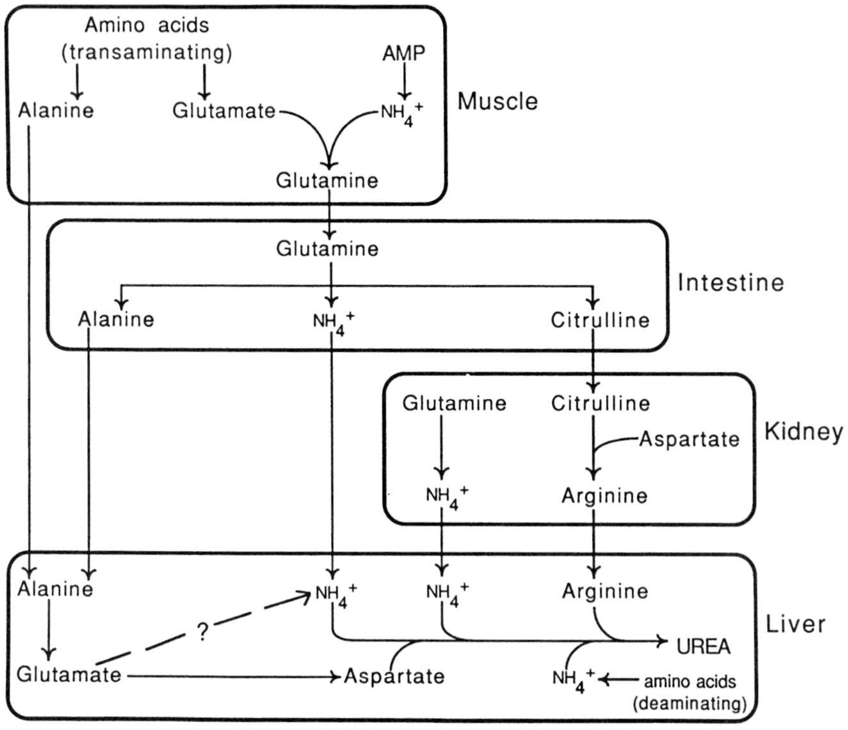

Fig. 85-3 Pathways of waste nitrogen synthesis from amino acids. Muscle, by virtue of its production of alanine and glutamine, is the major source of nitrogen destined for incorporation into urea. The role of the intestines, kidney, and liver are outlined as described in the text.

the cytosol, where it condenses with aspartate via AS to form argininosuccinate, which is cleaved to arginine and fumarate by argininosuccinase. Arginine is subsequently hydrolyzed by arginase to urea and ornithine, the latter again to be transcarbamylated to citrulline.

Studies of urea cycle enzyme activities in the human fetus reveal activity by 10 to 13 weeks of gestation; at approximately 20 weeks of gestation, enzyme activity is similar to that found at birth, which may be 50 to 90 percent of adult values.[37,38]

Although the mutant enzymes are mainly characterized by a reduction of their activity under all conditions, a number of other biochemical characteristics have been reported, principally for OTC. K_m mutants for both substrates have been found, as well as sensitivity to other factors, pH, temperature, and substrates.[39–46]

Also relevant to inborn errors of ureagenesis is the understanding that the α and the ω nitrogen atoms of ornithine do not normally serve as waste nitrogen products. Only ammonium nitrogen and aspartate nitrogen (Fig. 85-2) (derived from the free amino acid pool) constitute waste nitrogen atoms, which are incorporated into urea, argininosuccinate, and arginine.

Regulation of Ureagenesis

In humans the synthesis of urea is a function of nitrogen intake. On high nitrogen intakes (100 g protein), urinary urea nitrogen accounts for over 80 percent of dietary nitrogen, whereas on low nitrogen intakes (42 g protein), urinary urea nitrogen accounts for 46 percent of dietary nitrogen. The physiologic, biochemical, and molecular mechanisms accounting for this regulation are incompletely understood.[47]

Table 85-2 Concentration of Urea Cycle Intermediates in Rat Liver

	μmol per g wet weight
Carbamyl phosphate	0.001
Ornithine	0.2–0.6
Citrulline	0.03–0.1
Aspartate	0.3–3.5
Argininosuccinate	0.034
Arginine	0.02–0.1

SOURCE: Data taken from Meijer and Hensgens,[10] except for carbamyl phosphate, which was taken from Cooper et al.[24]

Although it has been demonstrated in rats[48] and primates[49] that there is a coordinated increase in all hepatic urea cycle enzyme activities when dietary nitrogen is increased, the regulatory factors accounting for these specfic events are complex. The quality of dietary nitrogen and energy intake may play a role,[50] perhaps by affecting transcriptional factors.[51,52] Hormonal factors also play a role.[47,52,54] Much attention has been focused on the role of small molecular weight substrates (ammonia, pH, and amino acids, especially arginine, ornithine, and glutamine). NAG, the product of glutamate and acetyl CoA via NAG synthetase, an intramitochondrial matrix enzyme (Fig. 85-2), is known to be an arginine-sensitive allosteric activator of CPS.[9,55–58]

MOLECULAR ANALYSIS OF UREA CYCLE ENZYMES*

Carbamyl Phosphate Synthetase

Molecular analysis of mammalian CPS I has enabled prediction of the structure of this large hepatic mitochondrial enzyme and revealed it to be the product of fusion of two ancestral functional domains that sequentially catalyze glutamine amide transfer and synthesis of CP. The contemporary mammalian enzyme functions

*GenBank Accession number:

CPS1: Human cDNA NM_001875

OTC: Human cDNAs K02100, D00230
Human exons D00221, D00229
Mouse cDNA, includes Spf/ash M17030

AS: Human cDNA NM_000050
Human exons L00079, L00084
Human exons AH002610

AL: Human cDNAs NH_000048, M57638

Arginase 1: Human cDNA NM_000045
Human exons X12662, X12669

Arginase 2: Human cDNAs NM_001172, U82256, D86724, U75667

as a dimer of 160-kDa subunits. In liver this protein constitutes as much as 15 to 30 percent of mitochondrial protein and 4 percent of total cell protein. This is a feature of stability of the enzyme, rather than a high rate of synthesis; the messenger RNA (mRNA) is of moderately low abundance. However, because the mRNA encoding the subunit is necessarily large, enrichment for it was accomplished in a straightforward manner using sucrose gradient fractionation of polyA$^+$ mRNA from rat liver.[59] A complementary DNA (cDNA) clone synthesized from the enriched mRNA was identified by hybrid-selected translation, and this clone was in turn used to identify additional rat and human cDNA clones. Northern analysis using these cDNAs identifies a 5-kb mRNA in liver. Developmental analysis of CPS mRNA in rat liver revealed its first appearance late in gestation at day 17, an increase to 30 to 40 percent of adult levels over the following 3 to 4 days, then a decline at the time of birth followed by a slow increase over a 3-week period to adult levels.

Treatment of rats with dibutyryl cyclic adenosine monophosphate (cAMP) or dexamethasone led to a twofold increase of CPS RNA in liver, and starvation for 5 days led to a 37-fold increase in RNA.[60] When levels of CPS RNA were examined in rat hepatoma cells, the line 5123D was found to contain levels twofold higher than in normal adult liver, whereas the line 3924A was devoid of CPS RNA.[61]

Sequence analysis of the cloned rat CPS cDNA indicates that the corresponding mRNA contains a 5′-untranslated sequence of 139 bases, an open reading frame of 4500 nucleotides, and a 3′-untranslated sequence of 905 nucleotides, followed by a polyA tract.[62] The rat cDNA was used as a hybridization probe to isolate human cDNA clones that exhibited similar-sized untranslated regions and encoded a subunit precursor with 94 percent identity to the rat subunit.[63] The coding sequences for the CPS I subunit precursors encode at the N-terminus 38 residues that comprise a cleavable leader peptide that directs the precursor to mitochondria. When this coding domain and 55 codons from the mature portion of the rat cDNA were joined with the distal two thirds of the coding sequence for the mature subunit of OTC, the *in vitro*–synthesized hybrid protein was directed to isolated mitochondria[64] (see later section on Mitochondrial Import). Like other mitochondrial signal peptides analyzed to date, the CPS leader is highly basic in overall amino acid composition, containing four arginine residues, four lysine residues, and a single aspartate residue.

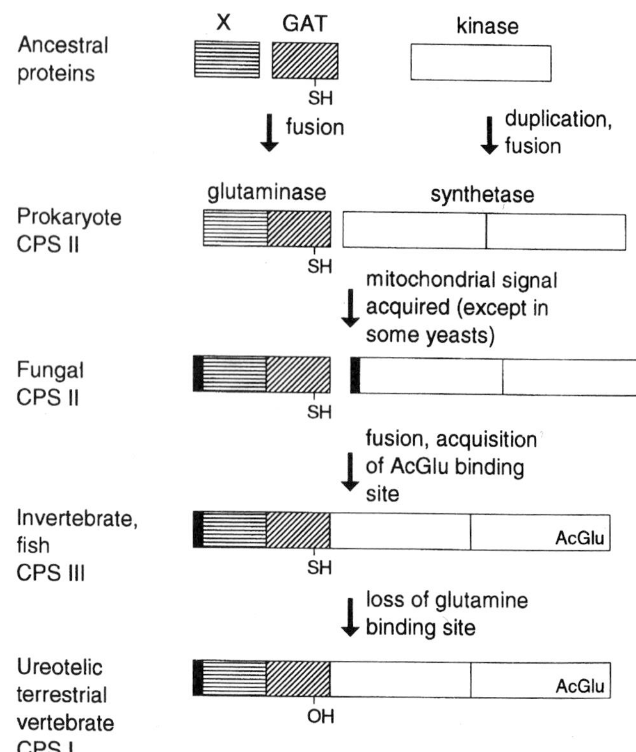

Fig. 85-4 Evolution of CPS enzymes. Steps are shown of gene duplication (open bar), fusion, signal attachment (black bar), loss of active site sulfhydryls (SH), and acquisition of *N*-acetylglutamate allosteric activation sites (AcGlu) that have produced the various modern-day enzymes. Note that, consistent with the immediate relationship of types III and I CPS enzymes (lower two bars), the intron–exon organization of CPS III from the pufferfish (fugu) and from rat CPS I have been found to be identical.[68] Notably, however, the fugu gene spans only 21 kb, whereas the rat spans 88 kb. (*Reprinted with permission from Hong J, Salo WL, Lusty CJ, Anderson PM: Carbamyl phosphate synthetase III, an evolutionary intermediate in the transition between glutamine-dependent and ammonia-dependent carbamyl phosphate synthetases.* J Mol Biol *243:131, 1994.*)

Mature Subunit: An Evolutionary Fusion. The mature portion of the rat CPS I precursor is strikingly homologous along its length to the CPS enzyme from *Escherichia coli* and yeast (both termed type II), with 42 percent and 45 percent identity at the amino acid level, respectively,[65,66] and to the enzyme from shark liver (type III), with 72 percent identity.[67] The type II enzymes are composed of two different subunits encoded by separate genes (Fig. 85-4). The small subunit catalyzes transfer of the amide nitrogen from glutamine, as ammonia, to a catalytic center for CP synthesis located on the large subunit (see Fig. 85-5 for partial reactions). The large subunit is composed of two homologous halves, the apparent product of an ancient gene duplication.[69] By itself, this subunit can catalyze synthesis of CP from ammonia, bicarbonate, and adenosine triphosphate (ATP).[65] The shark and mammalian enzymes (types III and I, respectively) represent a precise gene fusion of the glutamine amide transfer domain corresponding to the small subunit, at the N-terminus, with the synthetase domain, corresponding to the large subunit, at the C-terminus.[62,66] Whereas the shark enzyme, like the bacterial and fungal, employs the amide of glutamine as a nitrogen donor, the mammalian type I enzyme uses ammonium. Accordingly, whereas the glutamine hydrolytic site in *E. coli*, yeast, and shark contains a reactive cysteine residue,[67,70] in the mammalian enzyme, which fails to catalyze glutamine hydrolysis, the cysteine is absent. Although the hydrolytic site is lost, two ATP-binding sites present in the CPS catalytic centers of type II and III enzymes are retained in the mammalian enzyme and are highly conserved in sequence. Mutation of one of these, involving the substitution E841K, abolished synthesis of CP.[71] Bicarbonate-dependent ATP hydrolysis was stimulated, whereas synthesis of ATP from adenosine diphosphate (ADP) and CP was suppressed (Figs. 85-4 and 85-5). E841 was thus suggested to be essential to phosphorylation of carbamate. The effect on HCO_3^--dependent ATPase activity suggested interaction between the two catalytic ATP sites, coupling formation of enzyme-bound carbamate with its phosphorylation.[71] The catalytic ATP sites were tentatively localized in the rat liver enzyme using the ATP analogue 5′-fluoro-sulfonylbenzoyladenosine.[72] Two sites were located, one in each of the duplicated synthetase domains, and were differentially affected by the allosteric activator NAG. Likewise, an ultraviolet photoaffinity labeling study by the same group using ^{32}P-ATP labeled the two synthetase domains[73] (see also Guy and Evans[74] for a study of the homologous synthetase subdomains of CPS II, which, remarkably, confer CPS activity when joined individually with the amide transfer domain, but they form noncovalent dimers).

Carbamyl phosphate synthetase enzymes are subject to allosteric regulation. In the case of the *E. coli* enzyme, the regulators are uridine monophosphate (UMP), inosine monophosphate (IMP), and cytidine monophosphate (CMP), and competition for these regulators was examined using a fluorescent analogue.[75] Photoaffinity labeling with ^{14}C UMP identified a specific lysine.[76] The mammalian mitochondrial enzyme, as well as the type III fish enzyme, is activated by NAG. A photoaffinity compound, *N*-chloroacetyl L-[^{14}C]glutamate, could be bound to

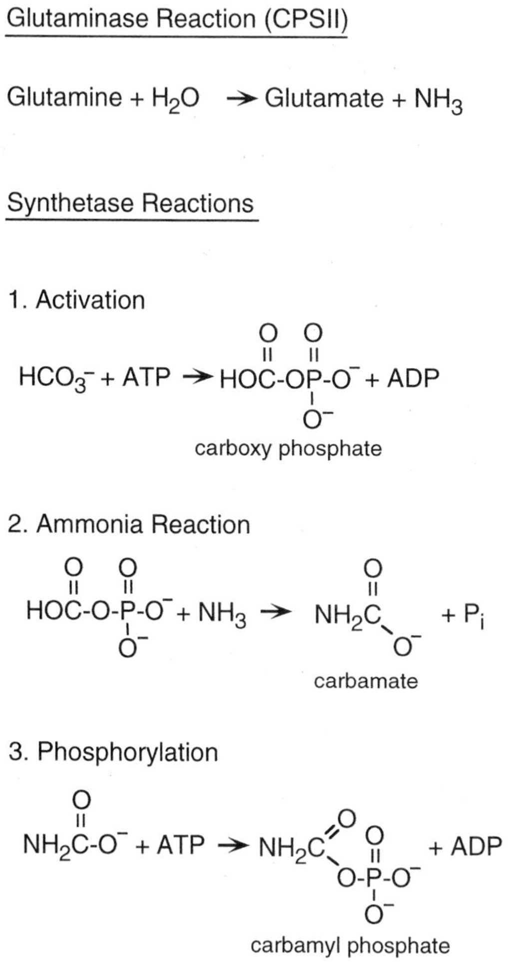

Glutaminase Reaction (CPSII)

$$\text{Glutamine} + H_2O \rightarrow \text{Glutamate} + NH_3$$

Synthetase Reactions

1. Activation

$$HCO_3^- + ATP \rightarrow HOC(=O)\text{-}O\text{-}P(=O)(O^-)\text{-}O^- + ADP$$

carboxy phosphate

2. Ammonia Reaction

$$HOC(=O)\text{-}O\text{-}P(=O)(O^-)\text{-}O^- + NH_3 \rightarrow NH_2C(=O)O^- + P_i$$

carbamate

3. Phosphorylation

$$NH_2C(=O)\text{-}O^- + ATP \rightarrow NH_2C(=O)\text{-}O\text{-}P(=O)(O^-)\text{-}O^- + ADP$$

carbamyl phosphate

Fig. 85-5 Partial reactions of carbamyl phosphate synthetase enzymes. In the first reaction, performed by the amide transfer domain (see Fig. 85-4, glutaminase), glutamine is hydrolyzed to produce ammonia, which is then transferred to the other domain, the CPS catalytic center, for the third reaction (ammonia reaction). Note that the first reaction is mediated by CPS II and III enzymes, whereas CPS I uses ammonium as a donor and does not perform glutamine hydrolysis (although, nevertheless, CPS I has preserved its amide transfer domain). In the second reaction (activation), performed by the catalytic domain, bicarbonate is activated by ATP to form carboxy phosphate, a transient intermediate, which in turn reacts with ammonia in the third (ammonia) reaction to form carbamate, which in the fourth reaction (phosphorylation) is phosphorylated to produce carbamyl phosphate. Two ATPs are consumed: one in activation and one in phosphorylation of carbamate. (*Adapted with permission from Guy HI, Evans DR: Function of the major synthetase subdomains of carbamyl-phosphate synthetase.* J Biol Chem *271:13762, 1996.*)

the mammalian mitochondrial enzyme and was competed by NAG. The site of binding could be localized after irradiation, using limited proteolysis, to the C-terminal 20 kDa.[77] This argues that the NAG binding site is not evolved from the N-terminally situated glutamine substrate binding site (corresponding to the small subunit in *E. coli*) (however, see McCudden and Powers-Lee,[78] who observed carbodiimide-activated ^{14}C-NAG to identify multiple sites including two in the N-terminus and two near the ATP sites). Structural requirements on the part of NAG for binding have been examined,[77,79] and, in general, analogues binding with high affinity acted as activators.

Structure of *E.coli* CPS A major recent advance in mechanistic understanding of CPS comes from the determination of the crystal structure of the E.coli enzyme at 2.1 Å resolution by Holden, Rayment, and their colleagues.[600] This reveals an α/β heterodimer

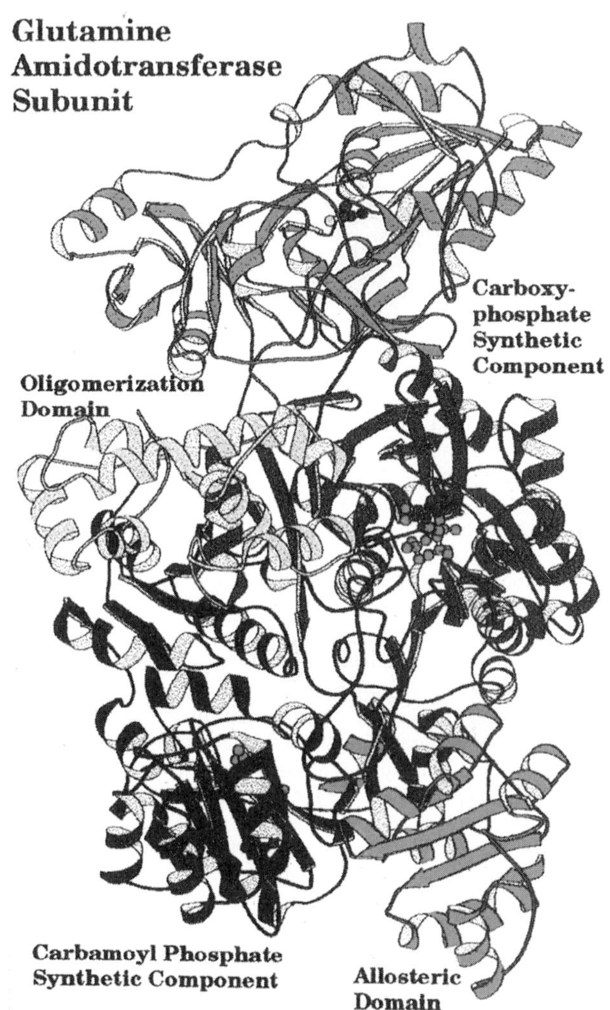

Fig. 85-5a Ribbon model of *E.coli* carbamyl phosphate synthetase α/β heterodimer, showing the small amidotransferase subunit (top) and the larger synthetase subunit composed of four individual domains (below). A molecular tunnel of ~100 Å is projected to run from the small subunit active site into the carboxy phosphate active site and then into the carbamyl phosphate synthetic site (see text for discussion). The active site cysteine in the small subunit and ADP molecules in the two synthetic domains in the large subunit are shown in ball and stick representation. (*With permission.*)

with an amidotransferase subunit of 42 kDa and a larger synthetase subunit of 118 kDa, itself divided into four domains (Fig. 85-5a). In the small subunit, a catalytic triad composed of a cysteine,[269] a glutamate, and a histidine mediates the hydrolysis of glutamine to produce an NH_3 molecule. This product appears to transfer through a tunnel identified between the small subunit active site and the carboxy phosphate synthetic site in the large subunit. This latter site in the crystal structure contains resolvable ADP and P_i; presumably the terminal phosphate marks the site of the formation of carboxy phosphate. This site, able to stabilize carboxy phosphate, may also function as the site for the reaction with ammonia, forming carbamate. The carbamate product must then in turn transfer through a second limb of the identifiable tunnel ($>$ 100 Å in net length) to reach the carbamyl phosphate synthetic site. While these two phosphorylation sites, one producing carboxy phosphate and the other producing carbamyl phosphate, lie in subdomains with shared primary structure and essentially the same structural fold (with the subdomains related to each other by a local two-fold symmetry axis), the subdomains differ at the active sites. For example, the terminal phosphate is not visible in the carbamyl phosphate synthetic site. The positions of critical metals in these active sites also differ. Two additional domains also comprise the large subunit, an oligomerization domain, enabling conversion of the $\alpha\beta$ heterodimer to $(\alpha\beta)_4$ tetramers, and the allosteric domain, binding IMP via a Rossmann fold or ornithine via a different site, but also contributing to oligomerization.

Transcriptional Regulation. The human CPS I gene has been localized to chromosome 2q35 by fluorescence *in situ* hybridization.[80,81] Initial analysis of the 5′ flanking portion of the gene indicated a TATA sequence at −30 bases.[82,83] A flanking promoter region between −34 and −150 has been observed to contain four functional segments: an element rich in GAG (−34 to −68), composed of a direct repeat of the sequence GAGGAGGGG; and three adjoining elements (−79 to −150), termed I, II, and III.[84] In transient transfections of H4IIEC3 rat hepatoma cells, the GAG element was found to be sufficient to activate the otherwise inactive TATA element, producing an activity similar to that of the entire −157 segment. Analyses of sites I to III in isolation indicated sites I and III in the absence of II to have a suppressive effect on GAG activation, whereas site II had an antisuppressive action. In gel shift assays, GAG-containing oligonucleotide formed a complex that migrated differently from those formed using sites I, II, or III oligonucleotides; moreover GAG oligonucleotide did not compete with sites I, II, or III, whereas any of the latter competed with each other. In a further study by the same group the 5′ flanking region up to −13.4 kb was analyzed and found to confer cell type–specific activation when joined with the GAG element, producing activation of an attached reporter in the hepatoma cell line but not in fibroblast or neural-derived cell lines.[85] The responsible region was defined as lying between −10.8 and −9.4 kb, and could be directly joined to the GAG element to produce full activation; it was observed to provide orientation-independent enhancement.

Ornithine Transcarbamylase.

Molecular genetic analysis of human OTC has involved characterization of a large X chromosome–localized gene that encodes a subunit precursor that is posttranslationally imported by mitochondria. The gene is expressed specifically in liver and gut, and, like the other urea cycle genes, is subject to heterogeneous mutation. In the liver, the OTC mRNA comprises approximately 0.05 to 0.1 percent of polyA^+ mRNA, and cloning of this moderate abundance mRNA was facilitated by the preparation of immunoaffinity-enriched OTC mRNA from rat liver.[86] This enabled preparation of rat OTC cDNA clones[87] and, in turn, the isolation, by homology, of cDNA clones encoding the human OTC precursor.[88] Subsequent analysis of genomic clones, identified using cloned cDNA, indicated that the human OTC gene spans a region of greater than 85 kb and contains 10 exons.[89] Using somatic cell hybrids and *in situ* hybridization, the gene was localized to band p2.1 of the X chromosome,[90] approximately 12 cM proximal to the Duchenne's muscular dystrophy locus. Genes affected in chronic granulomatous disease, Norrie's disease, retinitis pigmentosa, glycerol kinase deficiency, and adrenal hypoplasia all lie nearby, and occasional chromosomal deletions can involve both OTC and some or all of these neighboring loci, leading to clinical presentation of both OTC deficiency and the other disorders. The OTC gene is subject to X-chromosome inactivation in females, elegantly demonstrated by the presence of patches of activity observed on *in situ* enzyme assay in the liver of a female heterozygous for OTC deficiency.[91] A more recent study, using anti-OTC antibody staining of sparse-fur Ash OTC mutant heterozygous mice, observed extreme variegation of mosaic patches, potentially reflecting complex patterns of cellular migration following random X-inactivation of a few primordial liver cells.[92] Interestingly, X-inactivation at the OTC locus has been shown, in the case of OTC in mice, to reverse with advancing age.[93]

Transcriptional Regulation. The cloned rat cDNA has been used to measure levels of OTC mRNA during development by dot-blot analysis. RNA was first detected on day 14 of rat development at a level of 40 percent of adult levels and increased to a peak at day 20, decreased at the time of birth, then increased to adult levels during the second week after birth.[94] When adult rats were starved for 5 days, the level of RNA increased sixfold. No change in RNA levels was observed following treatment with dibutyryl cAMP or dexamethasone.

The 5′ regions of mammalian OTC genes have been studied.[95–97] The human and mouse sequences extending from the translational start codon to a position 500 bases upstream are 80 percent identical, and homology of approximately 40 percent extends further upstream through an additional 150 bases. In the case of the mouse gene, several transcriptional start sites have been identified, using procedures of S1 nuclease mapping and primer extension analysis, with a major initiation site identified 136 bases upstream from the translational initiation codon. At a position 25 bases further upstream, a sequence TAACAA is found, and at a position 153 bases upstream, the sequence ATAAATA was identified. Whether these TATA-like sequences function as transcriptional regulatory elements remains to be determined. A multiplicity of transcriptional start sites has been observed for the human OTC message using the two procedures of S1 nuclease mapping and primer extension, with the most common sites at positions 95, 120, 150, 161, and 166 bases upstream from the translational start codon. Thus, transcription of the human OTC gene appears to initiate not at a particular site but within a region of about 70 bases.

In functional analyses, when an 800-bp segment of the 5′ flanking region of mouse OTC was joined with the chloramphenicol acetyltransferase (CAT) gene and introduced into the human hepatoma line HepG2, which expresses OTC enzyme activity at a very low level, CAT activity was readily detected, whereas none was observed when the promoterless plasmid pSV0CAT was transferred or when the same construct placing the 5′ flanking region in the reverse orientation was transferred.[96] Similar observations detecting expression in HepG2 cells but not Chinese hamster ovary cells were made with 1.3 kb of 5′ rat OTC sequence.[97] Evidence for an upstream enhancer was obtained in transient expression assays with 11 kb of 5′ flank.[97] At the position 11 kb upstream, a 230-base enhancer segment was delimited, containing four protected areas seen by footprint analysis. Requirement in the intact animal for such an extensive flanking sequence or for intron sequences was suggested by failure to observe expression of human OTC minigenes carrying as much as 6 kb of 5′ flank joined with cDNA in transgenic mice. Stringent tissue-specific regulation of OTC is supported by the observations that few hepatomas express the gene, that primary cultures of hepatocytes generally lose OTC activity within 24 h, and that although hepatoma cells expressing other liver-specific genes could be selected in culture, OTC expression could only be obtained by fusion with hepatocytes.[98] It thus appears that both the promoter region and upstream enhancer are liver specific. Involvement of the liver-specific factor HNF-4, a member of the steroid receptor superfamily, was suggested by DNA binding studies and cotransfection analyses in HepG2 cells, recognizing two sites in the promoter and two in the enhancer.[99] The stimulatory action at these sites was opposed by the related, ubiquitously expressed factor COUP-TF.

Coding Sequences. The messenger RNAs encoded by human,[88] rat,[100] and mouse OTC[101,102] genes are approximately 1600 nucleotides in length, including approximately 150 bases of 5′-untranslated sequence, 1062 bases of sequence encoding the subunit precursor, and, as defined for rat OTC, 360 bases of 3′-untranslated sequence. The coding portion of the OTC subunit precursor includes a leader portion containing 32 codons and a mature portion composed of 322 codons. The latter region is much more highly conserved, with 93 percent homology between rats and humans, whereas the former exhibits only 72 percent homology between these two species, indicating perhaps less evolutionary constraint on it, permitting divergence.[100] Interestingly, the first exon of both human and mouse OTC genes contains the first 26 codons of the leader portion,[95,96] which, as detailed below, provides sufficient information to direct mitochondrial localization of the OTC precursor. Thus, this exon conceivably could have arisen independently in evolution to direct mitochondrial localization.

Mitochondrial Import. OTC has been used as a model for elucidating how cytosolically synthesized precursor proteins are imported into mitochondria. Like other precursors, it is translated in the cytosol and imported into the mitochondria posttranslationally.[103] Import involves a series of molecular interactions:

1. Chaperone interactions in the cytosol that maintain a "loose" protein conformation necessary for translocation through the mitochondrial membranes
2. Specific recognition of an N-terminal "leader peptide" in the precursor by a receptor complex in the mitochondrial outer membrane
3. Translocation in an extended protein conformation through translocation complexes in the outer and inner mitochondrial membranes
4. Proteolytic processing of the leader, mediated, in the case of OTC, in two sequential steps by two peptidases in the matrix space
5. Folding to native form mediated by the Hsp60 chaperonin complex and a cooperating Hsp10 component

These steps are described below and in Fig. 85-6.

Cytosolic Factors. During and after translation, the OTC precursor is stabilized in non-native form in the cytosol by several cytosolic components that maintain the precursor in an import-competent "loose" conformation.[104] This includes a member of the cytosolic Hsp70 family[105] and a member of the family of the cooperating component, dnaJ.[106,107] A requirement for cytosolic ATP[108–110] reflects at least in part the requirement by Hsp70 for ATP in order to release bound polypeptides and recycle, following hydrolysis, to a state with high affinity for non-native polypeptide. In particular, with *in vitro* import studies, translating precursor OTC (pOTC) in reticulocyte lysate and importing the newly made protein into isolated rat liver mitochondria, Terada and coworkers[111] observed that if pOTC was translated in a lysate from which hsp70 had been depleted (by antibody capture), import was blocked and could not be restored by readdition of the chaperone once synthesis was completed. In similar depletion experiments with the mammalian cytosolic DnaJ homologues Hdj1 and Hdj2, the Hdj2 was found to also be required during pOTC synthesis for enabling import competence of the precursor, and Hdj2 is presumed to be the cooperating partner of HsP70 in facilitating import-competent conformation[112] (see Bukau and Horwich[113] for a review of cooperation between Hsp70 and DnaJ components).

A factor was isolated from reticulocyte lysate that could bind the precursor of but not the mature form of OTC.[114] The so-called presequence binding factor (PBF) was required for import of OTC precursor from reticulocyte lysate into isolated mitochondria: import was blocked when lysate was depleted of PBF by treatment with pOTC-sepharose, and restored by readdition of the purified factor. In the depleted lysate, pOTC was found as a monomer, whereas in the presence of PBF, pOTC was found in a 7-9S complex. Although import of aspartate transaminase (AST) and malate dehydrogenase from reticulocyte lysate also appeared to require PBF, the rat 3-oxoacyl CoA thiolase did not. Additional biochemical and genetic studies should indicate whether PBF, acting in cooperation with cytosolic Hsp70 in maintenance of import-competent conformation, is essential for protein import.

A second cytosolic component also has been identified, called mitochondrial import stimulation factor (MSF), which is a heterodimer of 30- and 32-kDa subunits as purified from rat liver cytosol via affinity capture by a presequence-containing protein that recognizes mitochondrial presequences and maintains import-competent conformation of precursor proteins in an ATP-dependent manner.[115] Concerning its action on conformation, purified MSF was shown to be able to mediate ATP-dependent disaggregation of 40S complexes of preadrenodoxin that are import incompetent, enabling import. Associated with this, the preadrenodoxin converted from a trypsin-resistant to -sensitive conformation. So far, no homologue of this component has been found in yeast or *Neurospora*, so a formal genetic test of its action remains to be carried out.

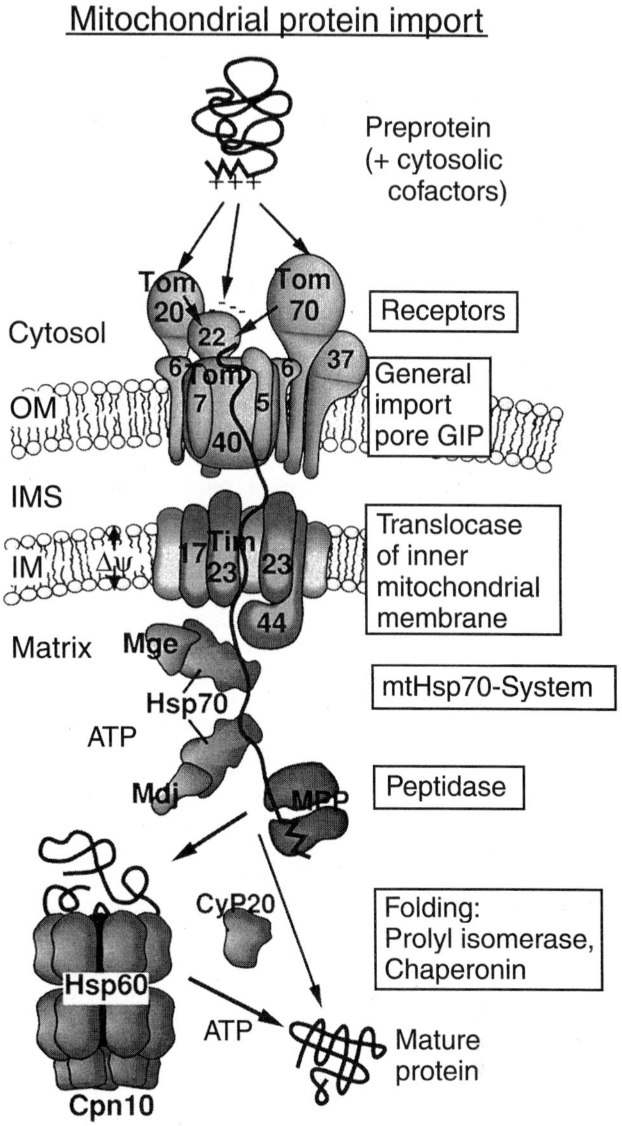

Fig.85-6 Protein import into mitochondria. Pathway of import of a mitochondrial precursor protein (top, with its N-terminal targeting peptide designated by positive charges), involving recognition by outer membrane receptor complex (Tom20, 70, 22; negatively charged surfaces), translocation through the outer membrane (Tom40, 5, 6, 7), recognition by Tim23 in the inner membrane and translocation through the inner membrane complex (Tim17, 23), assisted by Hsp70 and Tim44, processing of the signal peptide by MPP, and ATP-dependent folding assisted by Hsp70, Mdj, and Hsp60/Cpn10. $\Delta\psi$ designates the electrochemical gradient across the inner mitochondrial membrane, necessary for translocation of the N-terminal signal peptide across the membrane.

Recognition and Translocation of pOTC by Mitochondria Requires an N-terminal Signal Peptide. Most mitochondrial proteins destined for the matrix, inner membrane, or intermembrane space are translated with N-terminal cleavable peptides, typically composed of 20 to 60 amino acids, rich in basic and hydroxylated residues while devoid of acidic residues. The OTC leader peptide, for example, is 32 residues in size and contains four arginine residues and no acidic ones. It was shown to contain all the information to direct mitochondrial localization: when joined with either of two proteins normally localized in the cytosol, the fusion protein was directed into mitochondria.[116,117] Features within the leader peptide responsible for both mitochondrial localization and proteolytic processing were identified by testing the behavior of mutant OTC precursors both in intact cells and following incubation with isolated rat liver mitochondria. The mid-portion of the human OTC leader peptide from residues 8 to 22 was found to be both necessary and sufficient to direct mitochondrial localization of the precursor.[118] Basic residues, comprising four arginines identically positioned in the human, rat, and mouse OTC leader peptides, play a critical functional role; neutral substitution strongly reduces the extent of import. Arg 23, positioned in the mid-portion, is important to import and essential for proteolytic processing.[119] Based on effects of various substitutions at this position, the residue appears to participate in a functional secondary structure, probably an α helix.[118] The presence of such a structure is supported by studies with synthetic peptides; a peptide containing residues 1 to 27 was shown to exhibit α-helical structural properties in circular dichroism (CD) analysis, particularly in the presence of cardiolipin, an anionic phospholipid unique to mitochondrial membranes. The peptide competed for uptake of both OTC precursor and two other matrix-targeted precursors by isolated mitochondria. In contrast, a peptide containing residues 16 to 27 failed to block uptake.[120] Concerning the arrangement of positively charged side chains on an α-helical secondary structure, when putative α-helical domains of the OTC leader or other leader peptides are plotted in helical wheel projections, the positive charges generally locate to one side of the helix while the opposite side remains uncharged.[121,122] This so-called amphiphilic character appears to be critical to interaction of the signal peptide with the recognition and translocation components. Mutational analysis indicates that loss of positive charge or insertion of negative charge impairs import; additionally, alterations disrupting the putative α-helix character have a similar effect.[118,123,124] Net positive charge also could be necessary for an electrostatic interaction between the leader peptide and the electrochemical gradient across the mitochondrial inner membrane, which is relatively charge negative inside; this could result in "electrophoresis" of the signal domain across the membranes.[121,122] It might be predicted that natural mutation affecting the leader peptide of OTC could produce failure of the precursor to enter mitochondria, and because the precursor form of OTC is both biologically inactive and subject to rapid proteolytic turnover in the cytosol, this would lead to the clinical features of OTC deficiency. Such a mutation potentially producing such a defect, R26Q, has been reported[125] in a pedigree with several males affected with neonatal symptomatology, but the level of hepatic OTC RNA encoding this mutant subunit was found to be virtually nondetectable, indicating that this mutation likely destabilizes RNA and affects the position 26 codon; thus, the primary defect in this mutant appears to lie at the level of transcription as opposed to posttranslational events.

Receptor and Translocation Complexes. Identification of receptor and translocation complexes has employed biochemical, immunologic, and genetic tools and has been performed in baker's yeast and *Neurospora crassa*.[126–128] Given the highly evolutionarily conserved nature of those components of the import apparatus identified to date,[129,130] the studies in these systems almost certainly reveal the workings of the mammalian equivalents. To summarize the course of import (Fig. 85-6), precursor proteins are first recognized at the mitochondrial surface by an outer membrane receptor complex, most likely via electrostatic interaction between the signal peptide and clusters of negative charges in the receptor components. The signal peptide and precursor are then translocated, with the signal peptide leading the way via further electrostatic interactions with negative charges, down a chain of subsequently interacting components.[131–133] First there is transfer from the outer membrane receptor complex to the physically associated outer membrane insertion–translocation complex. Subsequently, the translocated precursor transfers to an inner membrane translocation complex. This complex makes direct physical contact with the outer membrane translocation complex at so-called contact sites between the mitochondrial outer and inner membranes. Formation of such sites of contact between the outer and inner membrane translocation machineries seems to be directed by the presence of the translocating precursor because coimmunoprecipitation of the machineries did not occur in the absence of the precursor.[30] Translocation through both membranes at the same time, occurring as a concerted event, is thus probably the normal mode of import, although this does not appear to be absolutely required.[135]After engaging the inner membrane complex, in cooperation with the electrochemical potential gradient across the inner membrane (negative at the inside aspect), the signal peptide traverses the inner membrane. At the matrix aspect of the inner membrane, chaperone components recognize the entering chain and promote the later, ATP-dependent stages of translocation into the matrix compartment. Proteins targeted to the inner membrane are in some cases transported to the matrix, then reexported, but, alternatively, and perhaps in general, are directed partway to the matrix by a signal peptide, then halt further transfer through the action of a transmembrane segment, and exit the import apparatus to reside in the inner membrane. In some cases the "stopped" protein, with most of its mass residing in the intermembrane space, is cleaved by an intermembrane space protease and comes to reside in the intermembrane space. In contrast with the cleavable precursors, the large family of inner membrane carrier proteins lack N-terminal signal peptides but follow the same pathway through the outer membrane apparatus to the inner membrane where a separate but structurally related inner membrane translocation complex recognizes and inserts the carrier proteins into the inner membrane.[136–138]

Concerning the outer membrane receptor and translocation system, coimmunoprecipitation and cross-linking studies have identified eight proteins of 70, 40, 37, 22, 20, 8, 7, and 5 kDa, termed Tom (translocator of the outer membrane) components[126–130] (Fig. 85-6). The Tom20–Tom22 complex functions as a heterodimeric import receptor with a preference for presequence-containing precursor proteins[139] that would include pOTC. Indeed import of pOTC into rat liver mitochondria was blocked by antibodies against the mammalian Tom20 or by incubation with an excess of the cytosolic domain of Tom20.[140] The Tom70–Tom37 complex functions as a receptor system with a preference for proteins with internal targeting information, like the abundant inner membrane ATP–ADP carrier protein.[126–128] Additional experiments suggest that the Tom70–Tom37 complex also might have preference for precursors that require cytosolic ATP (and presumably chaperone action) for delivery to the organelles; for example, in a "mixed species" experiment, precursors interacting with mammalian MSF prefer Tom70–Tom37 for entering isolated yeast mitochondria.[141]One member each of the two receptor complexes, Tom20 and Tom70, respectively, is anchored to the outer membrane via a hydrophobic N-terminal anchor sequence, while the remaining portion is exposed to the cytosol.[142,143] These two components and the respective complexes are linked to each other, however, via 35-residue tetratricopeptide repeats in their cytosolic portions.[144] Concerning the Tom20–Tom22 complex, both members display a cluster of negative charges in their cytosolically exposed domains that can directly interact with positively charged presequences of precursor proteins. Tom22, however, appears to be the central clearinghouse component for both receptor systems, because it is essential in yeast, whereas the other three receptor components are not.[131,145–148] In functional terms, proteins bound initially to Tom70–Tom37 have been observed to transfer to the

Tom22–Tom20 receptor before translocating through the outer membrane. Mutational alteration of the tetratricopeptide repeat in Tom20 blocked such transfer, indicating a requirement for physical association.[144] In turn, proteins transferred to or initially bound at Tom22–Tom20 are relayed via their positive presequences through the essential Tom20 component to a small component, Tom5, a 50-amino acid protein, that is negatively charged at its N-terminus and anchored in the outer membrane via its C-terminus.[132] Tom5 appears to lie at the gateway of, or is a part of, the general insertion pore (GIP), because it is stably associated with the central component of GIP, Tom40. Thus, there appears to be a binding relay mechanism at the outer membrane, at its outer *cis* face, that feeds the precursor protein into the GIP site (composed of Tom40, Tom6, and Tom7) for translocation through the outer membrane. Additional acidic binding sites reside at the inside, *trans*, aspect of the outer membrane. For example, the C-terminus of Tom22, which protrudes into the intermembrane space, is negatively charged, and deletion of this region reduced translocation by three- to eightfold.[149] Likewise, the outer aspect of the inner membrane machinery component, Tim23, has exposed acidic domains. Thus, acidic sites in the import pathway that bind the positively charged signal peptide, could drive protein transport, an acidic chain mechanism.[132,133] The directionality of such transfer could be dictated by progressively increasing avidity, as reflected in studies of binding and transfer of precursor proteins between the cytosolic domain of Tom20, the intermembrane space domain of Tom22, and that of Tim23 carried out *in vitro*.[150]

The intact TOM complex has recently been isolated by digitonin-solubilization of *Neurospora* outer mitochondrial membranes and affinity capture through a 6 His-tagged Tom22.[151] It fractionates as a 600-kDa complex that contains multiple copies of the pore protein Tom40, and by electron microscopy appears as a 140 Å diameter complex with two or three electron-dense "holes" approximately 20 Å in diameter. When inserted into lipid bilayers, the TOM complex produces cation-selective conductance (in three increments of 0.3 nanoSiemens, suggesting open, half-opened, and closed states). The TOM complex inserted into proteoliposomes reconstituted their ability to incorporate outer membrane proteins, but the liposomes also could translocate an N-terminal presequence peptide. The isolation of the TOM complex in a functional state should now enable detailed structural and functional analysis.

The inner membrane translocation (TIM) complex also has been identified and characterized by genetic, coimmunoprecipitation, and cross-linking studies, and is composed of at least five proteins of 23, 17, 33, 14, and 44 kDa, termed Tim components (Fig. 85-6).[152–159] Tim17 and Tim23 share homologous C-terminal hydrophobic regions that span the inner membrane three to four times; in addition, Tim23 exposes a negatively charged N-terminal region of 100 amino acids to the intermembrane space, which participates in the acidic chain that can recognize presequences. Interspersed with the negative charges in the distal half of this region is a heptad repeat motif (leucine zipper) that enables coiled-coil dimerization of Tim23.[160] Such dimerization was shown to be dependent on the presence of the electrochemical potential gradient across the inner membrane, and dissociation of the dimer was triggered by binding of a presequence to the acidic cluster and maintained during passage of the translocating protein. Thus, the N-terminus of Tim23 serves as a voltage-sensing gate to the inner membrane channel. Both Tim17 and Tim23 can be cross-linked to a translocating precursor at a point where the presequence has not fully traversed the inner membrane.[158] The two channel proteins were isolatable as a high-molecular-weight complex with two additional proteins, Tim33 and Tim14, also stably associated, and with a third protein, Tim44, loosely associated.[159] Tim44, like Tim17 and Tim23, proves to be an essential component, but it is a hydrophilic protein with no membrane-spanning segments, which localizes at the matrix aspect of the TIM complex through specific association with it.

The TIM complex plays an active role in the early step of inner membrane translocation, during which the presequence engages the complex, at the Tim23 gate as described. The electrochemical potential gradient is required both for this initial interaction with the TIM complex and for passage of the presequence across the inner membrane, possibly through an electrophoretic action.[161] After presequence passage, a passive role is played by the TIM complex: antibodies to Tim23 or Tim17, which could block the early steps, had no effect at this point.[159] Similarly, the electrochemical potential gradient is not required for completion of translocation.[161] Rather, at this stage, matrix-localized Hsp70, in some cases in cooperation with Tim44, acts to energetically drive the protein across the inner membrane.[162,163] This chaperone-dependent step, like others directed by Hsp70, is ATP dependent, such that with depletion of matrix ATP, precursor proteins cannot complete translocation across the inner membrane; moreover, under such conditions, in the absence of tight binding by the TIM channel itself, the precursor can slide back out of the channel and is no longer coprecipitable with the complex.[159] In the presence of ATP, however, a precursor engaged in the translocation machinery (experimentally trapped there by virtue of a tightly folded domain in its mature portion) can be cross-linked to Tim17, Tim23, Tim44, and Hsp70, as well as with Tom40, reflecting its extension through both outer and inner membrane machineries.

The mechanism of mitochondrial Hsp70-directed translocation into the matrix has been a subject of considerable study. The role in translocation was originally recognized by study of yeast mutants affecting this component, where deficiency led to impairment of import, with precursors remaining uncleaved and at positions spanning the mitochondrial membranes.[164,165] Several studies indicated direct physical interaction between the matrix-localized Hsp70 and the newly entering polypeptide chains.[165,166] Hsp70 proteins generally have been shown to interact with polypeptide chains occupying extended conformations, binding to short hydrophobic stretches.[167,168] Here, the translocating chain apparently occupies such a conformation, with approximately 50 residues sufficient to span across the outer and inner membrane translocation machineries between cytosol and matrix space.[169] Relative to the action of Hsp70 inside the matrix, binding to the entering chain, a Brownian ratchet type of translocation mechanism was proposed, with Hsp70 inside providing a directional forward matrix-directed movement to a chain that is otherwise diffusing randomly backward or forward.[170] A force-generating aspect of Hsp70 in generating such forward movement, and particularly in directing unfolding of structured portions of the chain remaining in the cytosol, was emphasized by a motor model.[171] Recent studies suggest that Hsp70 can interact with either Tim44 at the matrix aspect of the TIM complex, or directly with the Tim23–Tim17 channel, to bind translocating chains as they emerge at the matrix aspect of the inner membrane. The ATP-dependent interaction of Hsp70 and Tim44 appears to be necessary, and motorlike in their role, for import of precursors with tightly folded mature domains, facilitating their unfolding and passage.[164] In this action, Hsp70 can bind to a Tim44 molecule bearing a segment of translocating polypeptide.[162] Transfer to Hsp70 then occurs, and either concerted or subsequent nucleotide-driven dissociation of Hsp70 from Tim44 advances the chain into the matrix. Tim44 can then bind or cooperate with Hsp70 to bind a more C-terminal segment of chain, with cycles of such interaction producing progressive forward movement into the matrix. The action of Hsp70 in this context serves also to favor unfolding and translocation of domains of the precursor protein residing in the cytosol.[172]

Proteolytic Maturation. Following translocation into the matrix, precursor proteins are proteolytically processed to mature size and folded and assembled into active forms. For matrix-localized proteins, proteolytic removal of the leader domain in the matrix space may be needed to render membrane translocation nonreversible, but it also may be required for folding and assembly of newly imported subunits. That is, many precursor proteins cannot assume native form until their presequences are removed. Many precursor proteins are processed in a single step, using the soluble matrix-processing protease (MPP), composed of two structurally related subunits of approximately 50 kDa, α and β [formerly known as MPP and processing enhancing protein (PEP)].[173–175] Other precursors, including pOTC, require two processing steps, the first by MPP, leaving an intermediate form with a characteristic N-terminal octapeptide, followed by a second, mediated by a distinct so-called intermediate peptidase. In the case of MPP, as isolated from mammalian and yeast mitochondria, the α and β subunits are associated,[176,177] but in *N. crassa* the two subunits are not stably associated even though they are both required.[174,178] Nevertheless, α and β subunits of the rat enzyme are readily exchangeable.[179] The sequences of α and β subunits were originally identified in yeast and *Neurospora*,[180–182] but subsequently they were also determined from mammalian sources.[183,184] Both α and β subunit genes are essential in yeast, indicating that mitochondrial protein import, an essential function, is critically dependent on this processing step. α and β subunits themselves are translated as larger precursors with N-terminal targeting peptides. The newly made protease components thus appear to be proteolytically matured by preexisting components, reflecting that mitochondria cannot be formed *de novo* but are begotten from preexisting organelles.[205] Cleavage mediated by the MPP processing enzyme is divalent metal dependent. Concerning the site recognized, the substrate precursor proteins are often cleaved by the protease after the residue following an arginine.[185,186] Additionally, residues C-terminal to the processing site are important, with a preference noted by several workers for an aromatic residue at the P_1' position.[174,187] Concerning the nature of the specific roles of the α and β subunits, α has been shown to cross-link preferentially to a precursor,[188] suggesting a role in recognition, whereas β contains an HXXEH metal-binding motif identified by mutational analysis to be essential for proteolytic activity, indicating a role in catalysis.[179]

The first structural insights into the action of MPP has come from the crystal structure of the bovine cytochrome bc_1 complex,[189] which includes at its matrix aspect the components known as Core I and Core II, which are homologous to β and α subunits of MPP, respectively, as well as the 78-residue presequence peptide of the Rieske Fe/S protein, which after its proteolytic cleavage from the mature portion of the Fe/S protein (which localizes in the intermembrane space), remains a part of the bc_1 complex, known as subunit 9, and remains sandwiched between Core I and Core II, as if to record that it was the Core I–Core II heterodimer unit that was responsible for the proteolytic processing event. It seems likely that this is the case, although purified bc_1 complex does not exhibit MPP activity. Consistent with the earlier cross-linking data suggesting a role for α subunit in precursor recognition, subunit 9 turns out to be most closely associated with Core II, with a C-terminal two-stranded β sheet in subunit 9 forming an extension of a β sheet in Core II. The nature of the catalytic action remains unclear, however, because the putative HXXEH sites of Core I and Core II, neither precisely conserved and neither occupied with metal, both lie distant from the C-terminus of subunit 9. On the other hand, the N-terminus of the Fe/S mature protein lies near the putative site in Core I. Thus, it seems possible that after putative cleavage by Core I, there is a conformational rearrangement that displaces the subunit 9 cleavage product.

In the case of OTC, malate dehydrogenase, and several other proteins entering the matrix, an additional step of proteolytic processing is performed subsequent to the MPP step, mediated by a second so-called mitochondrial intermediate processing peptidase (MIP).[190] For these precursors, the first event of processing leaves an N-terminal octapeptide that usually contains a hydrophobic residue at position 1 and a serine or threonine residue at position 4.[186] Specificity of MIP as an octapeptidase was supported by the observation that a synthetic octapeptide could inhibit processing activity *in vitro* of MIP but not MPP.[191] The octapeptide may serve the purpose of acting as a spacer in proteins whose mature N-terminus needs to occupy a conformation that would not be compatible with MPP recognition or cleavage while present in a precursor form.[192] The octapeptidase enzyme was first purified from rat liver and identified as a single 75-kDa polypeptide that could cleave intermediate forms of OTC or MDH to mature size *in vitro* in a reaction dependent on divalent cations. Sequence analysis of cDNA encoding rat MIP and expression *in vitro* revealed it to contain an N-terminal cleavable presequence. Homology to several additional peptidases was noted, centering around the metal binding motif HEXXH.[193] A more extended motif has subsequently been identified, $FHEXGHXXHX_{12}GX_5DXXEXPSX_3EX$, present in a collective of bacterial peptidases.[194] A yeast homologue of the rat enzyme was subsequently identified by hybridization, which when disrupted led to failure to grow on nonfermentable carbon sources, associated with defects of complexes III and IV and failure of both cytochrome oxidase subunit IV and the iron sulfur protein to be converted from intermediate form to mature form.[195] Further study revealed effects on maturation of a number of additional imported components, including a component of the ribosome (protein S28), the EF-Tu homologue, and a single-stranded binding protein (RIM1), involved in DNA replication. Concerning this last defect, in addition to the respiratory defects in the setting of MIP deficiency, a loss of mitochondrial DNA was also observed.[196]

Chaperonin-Mediated Protein Folding. Imported subunits of OTC require folding and assembly in the matrix space to produce the active homotrimer because, like other mitochondrial precursor proteins, the enzyme subunits enter the organelles in extended conformations. This process had been thought to occur spontaneously until a mutant of yeast was discovered[197] in which expressed human OTC subunits were imported and processed to mature size but failed to produce enzyme activity. The subunits failed to bind to a substrate affinity column containing the analogue δ-*N*-phosphonoacetyl-L-ornithine, further indicating that the active trimer had not been formed. Additional study showed that the OTC subunits were present in insoluble aggregates. Similar effects were observed on endogenous imported yeast mitochondrial matrix proteins, including the α subunit of the F_1 ATPase,[197] and the subunits of ketoglutarate dehydrogenase and lipoamide dehydrogenase.[198] Biogenesis of the conservatively sorted Rieske iron–sulfur protein that is first imported to the matrix space and then reexported across the inner membrane was also affected. This monomeric protein, which usually undergoes two steps of matrix processing during biogenesis, was found in a once-cleaved intermediate form in the matrix space.[197] This suggested an involvement in this yeast mutant of polypeptide chain folding as distinct from a role in assembly of subunits into oligomeric proteins.

The component affected in the yeast mutant proved to be an abundant matrix protein called heat-shock protein 60 (Hsp60), comprising approximately 1 percent of mitochondrial protein.[197] This component was originally identified in the mitochondria of *Tetrahymena thermophila* as a protein that was induced approximately twofold in response to heat treatment.[199] Hsp60 is a homooligomeric tetradecamer—in the electron microscope it appeared as two stacked rings each containing seven identical radially arranged subunits.[200] The complexes appeared in side views as cylinders that are about the size of ribosomes, approximately 145 Å in height and 135 Å in diameter, with central cavities within the rings measuring approximately 45 Å in diameter. The function of Hsp60 proved to be essential at all temperatures; yeast deleted of the Hsp60 gene was not viable at any temperature.[197,201] The involvement of Hsp60 function in protein folding was further demonstrated using the small monomeric enzyme dihydrofolate reductase (DHFR).[202] When imported into mitochondria in the absence of ATP, via an attached presequence domain, DHFR became stably associated with Hsp60 complex. The bound protein could be shown to occupy a non-native conformation by both its sensitivity to protease and its recognition by an antiserum that reacts specifically with non-native forms of DHFR. When ATP was added to the mitochondrial mixture, the DHFR was released from Hsp60 and exhibited native-like protease resistance, indicating that ATP was required for steps of folding or release from the complex.

Hsp60 function has been shown to be required for the folding or assembly of a substantial number of mitochondrial proteins reaching the matrix space. In addition to those mentioned, a recent survey by two-dimensional gel analysis and mass spectrometric identification of imported precursors that become insoluble in mif4 mitochondria adds substantially to the list.[203] The study also identifies other proteins that are not significantly affected by deficiency of Hsp60 and that apparently do not require chaperonin action to reach native form, at least in the isolated organelles used in the study. Interestingly, among those proteins that are affected is the imported subunit of Hsp60 itself, in agreement with an early study showing that cells conditionally defective for Hsp60 function could import and proteolytically process wild-type Hsp60 subunits induced at restrictive temperature, but could not fold and assemble them to produce new Hsp60 complex.[204] Thus, in the same way that mitochondria were unable to be formed *de novo*[205] but rather are derived from preexistent organelles, this folding machine inside of them also cannot be formed *de novo* but is dependent on preexisting complex for its own biogenesis. Thus, the machine cannot self-assemble.

Further studies of the mechanism of Hsp60 action have been facilitated by the presence in the bacterial cytoplasm of a homologous component, the GroEL protein. Also an essential gene,[206] in this case as much as fivefold induced by heat shock,[207] *groE* was originally identified as the operon affected in mutant *E. coli* that could grow instead of lysing following infection with bacteriophage λ.[208,209] In particular, aggregated abnormal-looking phage head structures were observed in these strains. More recently, temperature-sensitive lethal mutations affecting *groEL* have been produced that affect not only λ phage biogenesis but also folding of newly translated monomeric and oligomeric cytoplasmic proteins.[210] Also, coprecipitation studies with anti-GroEL antibodies suggest that 10 to 15 percent of newly translated bacterial protein becomes associated with GroEL.[211] The *groE* operon encodes not only GroEL, which is 60 percent identical to Hsp60 in amino acid sequence[201] and also found as a tetradecameric double-ring structure,[212] but also the GroES protein, a single seven-member dome-shaped ring 80 Å in diameter and 30 Å in height, composed of identical 10-kDa subunits.[213,214] *In vitro* experiments with the two components purified from overproducing *E. coli* have reconstituted folding of a number of proteins,[215–218] including mammalian OTC,[219] after dilution from denaturant. The process involves binding of non-native polypeptide, with a stoichiometry of one polypeptide per GroEL complex, followed by folding, mediated by ATP and GroES. Binding involves capture of a non-native conformation, typically in a collapsed, globular state, in the central cavity of a GroEL ring.[220–222] Recent crystallographic and functional studies of GroEL indicate that such recognition is mediated by hydrophobic interactions between the apical (end portion) surface of the central cavity (Fig. 85-7) and exposed hydrophobic surface of the non-native protein substrate.[223–227] The hydrophobic surface exposed in the non-native state of a protein becomes buried to the interior in the native state and thus is no longer recognizable, explaining the selective binding by GroEL of non-native states. Such binding of non-native forms is likely to be multivalent, with the non-native protein contacted by a number of the seven surrounding apical hydrophobic binding sites. This effectively prevents access of hydrophobic surfaces in the non-native substrate with those of another non-native protein, thus preventing multimolecular aggregation, generally an irreversible event.[228] Binding may in some cases be associated with partial unfolding, rescuing a protein out of a kinetically trapped state.[229] Alternatively, and more likely in most cases, GroEL may have higher affinity for somewhat less-folded conformations, and binding thus serves to shift an equilibrium between various non-native forms toward a more unfolded state[230] (for a review of binding and effects on conformation, see Fenton and Horwich[222]).

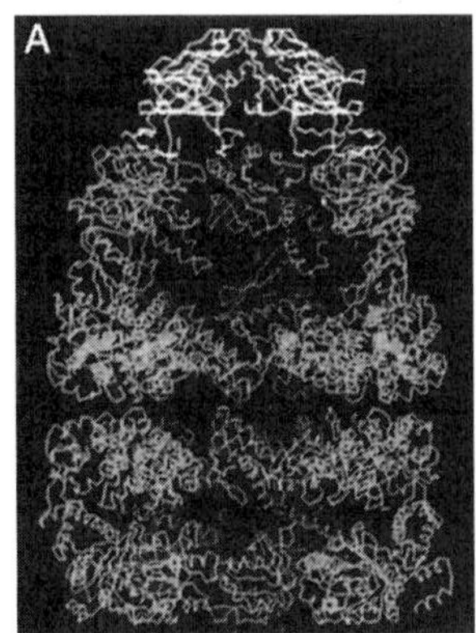

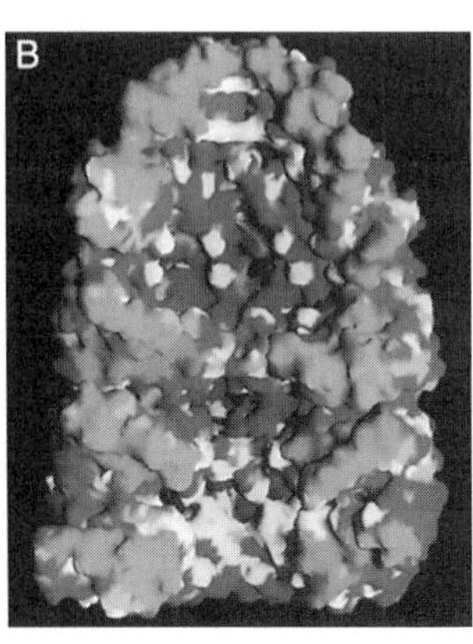

Fig. 85-7 Architecture of the bacterial chaperonin/cochaperonin, GroEL/GroES, closely homologous to mitochondrial Hsp60/Hsp10, in a folding-active conformation. A cutaway ribbon diagram is shown in A. GroES is shown in white and GroEL in gray. Note the elongation of the GroES-bound *cis* GroEL ring, in which polypeptide folding takes place, reflecting rigid body movements of the GroEL apical peptide-binding domains (upward and clockwise; compare with apical domains of the unbound ring; see Fig. 85-8). This movement produces a change in character of the central cavity, shown in B, wherein hydrophobic residues (shown in white), initially used to capture a non-native polypeptide in an open ring, are replaced by hydrophilic ones (dark gray). This is associated with eviction of polypeptide into the encapsulated cavity and with favoring burial of hydrophobic surfaces in the folding substrate protein and exposure of its hydrophilic surfaces, favoring production of the native state. (*Reprinted with permission from Xu Z, Horwich AL, Sigler PB: The crystal structure of the asymmetric* GroEL–GroES–ADP$_7$ *chaperonin complex.* Nature *388:741, 1997.*)

Following polypeptide binding, the presence of ATP and GroES produces the native state. The nature of this reaction has become more clear with the results of structural and functional studies summarized below. But it must first be pointed out that chaperonins do not appear to perform true chemical catalysis of folding because the rates of folding *in vitro* in the presence of GroEL–GroES or Hsp60–Hsp10 do not appear significantly different from those in their absence. In some cases, the rate of folding is slower. In structural terms, the steric information governing polypeptide folding resides in the primary structure of a polypeptide, as recognized by Anfinsen and co-workers. Molecular chaperones in general do not appear to provide such information, but, rather, provide kinetic assistance to the folding process, which under physiologic conditions (e.g., temperature of 37°C) is prone to missteps off the pathway. Such kinetic assistance is essential in the cell. In the absence of such assistance, as in the genetic mutants mentioned above, many proteins fail to reach the native state.

The nature of the folding reaction mediated by GroEL–GroES became more clear with the identification of the folding-active state as a *cis* ternary complex, in which polypeptide is sequestered in the central cavity of a GroEL ring underneath bound GroES (Fig. 85-7).[231–233] This folding-active state is formed when ATP and GroES become bound to the same GroEL ring containing bound polypeptide. ATP binds cooperatively to the equatorial domains of the seven subunits of the ring[222,234,235] and initiates allosteric en bloc movement of its apical domains (transmitted through the hinge-like intermediate domains) (Fig. 85-8),[236] presumably enabling GroES to bind to the apical domains. Association of GroES effectively stabilizes the apical domains seven-valently in a fully open and twisted topology (Figs. 85-7 and 85-8) and closes off the central cavity, sequestering polypeptide in the cavity.[231,236–238] A crystallographic study of a GroEL–GroES–ADP$_7$ complex[238] has revealed at 3-Å resolution the large

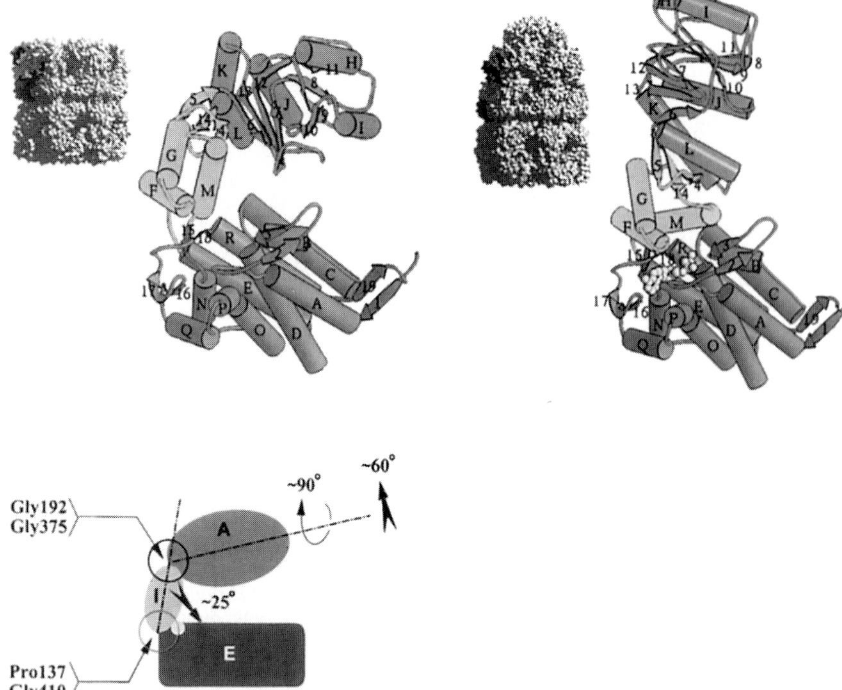

Fig. 85-8 Rigid body movements of GroEL subunits in the ring bound by nucleotide and cochaperonin. The GroEL subunit of an unliganded complex (left) and from the *cis* ring of an asymmetric GroEL–GroES complex (right) is shown, in each case next to a space-filling model of the respective assembly, in which the indicated subunit is in black. The rigid body movements of the unliganded subunit that occur upon GroES binding are shown schematically below. In the top panels, helices are indicated by lettering. Bottom panel: A = apical domain; I = intermediate domain; E = equatorial domain. (*Reprinted with permission from Xu Z, Horwich AL, Sigler PB: The crystal structure of the asymmetric* GroEL–GroES–ADP$_7$ *chaperonin complex.* Nature *388:741, 1997.*)

en bloc conformational changes of the apical domains associated with GroES binding, involving 60-Å elevation of the hydrophobic binding surface and 90-Å clockwise rotation, removing the binding surface from facing the central cavity. At this point the surface makes hydrophobic contact, in part with a mobile loop segment extending from each contacting GroES subunit (particularly, through an IVL apolar region), while the remaining portion forms a new interface with the apical domain of the neighboring subunit. The net effect of this dramatic apical movement is that polypeptide is driven off of the hydrophobic binding surface into the central channel, which ultimately has "new" walls with a hydrophilic character. Such a switch in the character of the cavity walls to hydrophilic favors burial of hydrophobic surfaces of the substrate protein and exposure of its hydrophilic surface, overall promoting formation of the native state. Thus, the GroEL machine functions most essentially in assisting polypeptide folding by alternately switching its cavity surface from a hydrophobic state to a hydrophilic character.

The role of nucleotide is to direct the GroEL–GroES machine through the respective polypeptide-accepting and folding-active conformational states. This reaction cycle is diagrammed in Fig. 85-9. Briefly:

1. Polypeptide is accepted into the open (*trans*) ring of an asymmetric GroEL–GroES complex (see third panel of Fig. 85-9, bottom ring), which is the species predominantly populated under physiologic conditions.[239,240] Notably, adenine nucleotide is required for GroES binding, with ATP the favored nucleotide[213,241]; ATP binds and hydrolyzes cooperatively within a ring (e.g., top ring in first two panels of Fig. 85-9) but anticooperatively with respect to the opposite ring.[234,235,242] However, once ATP turns over within the seven subunits of a *cis* ring, seven ATPs (as well as polypeptide) can enter the opposite unoccupied ring (third panel Fig. 85-9), triggering an allosteric change that evicts ADP, GroES, and polypeptide ligands from the *cis* ring (third and fourth panels, Fig. 85-9).[243,244] The presence of non-native polypeptide, which can bind to the *trans* ring in addition to ATP (third panel), has been observed to further accelerate the discharge of the *cis*-bound ligands (Rye HS et al., unpublished observation).
2. GroES binds to the ATP-polypeptide–bound *trans* ring, ordering the formation of a new folding-active *cis* complex (first and fourth panels of Fig. 85-9) (Rye HS et al., unpublished observation).
3. Folding proceeds in the *cis* ternary GroEL–GroES–ATP complex for approximately 15 s (23°C), after which ATP hydrolyzes in the *cis* ring (first panel, Fig. 85-9). This weakens the highly energetic *cis* ATP complex (resistant to dissociation even by 0.4 M guanidine HCl), priming the *cis* complex for dissociation driven by ATP binding to the opposite ring.[244] Significantly, the *cis* ATP hydrolysis event is the slow step in the reaction cycle. Thus, the folding-active state is both the most stable and longest lived state in the reaction.
4. ATP hydrolysis in the *cis* ring not only weakens the *cis* complex, priming it for dissociation, but gates entry of ATP and polypeptide into what was the unoccupied (*trans*) ring, commencing formation of a new folding-active *cis* complex. The machine thus alternates its folding-active state back and forth between rings, efficiently expending seven ATPs for each folding-active cycle. That is, one round of ATP is used simultaneously to discharge the previous folding-active complex and establish a new one.
5. In any given folding-active cycle (half-life 15 s at 23°C), by the time the *cis* complex is dissociated and polypeptide is evicted from the central cavity, a substrate protein may have reached the native state or a state "committed" to reaching native form, that is, a state that is no longer recognizable by GroEL and that proceeds to native form in the bulk solution (fourth panel of Fig. 85-9). Alternatively, it may have failed to reach native form or a committed state and leaves the cavity in a non-native state that can be rebound by another molecule of GroEL.[243,245–249] (In some cases, non-native protein may rebind to the same GroEL molecule, because it may be the most physically proximal). Rebound molecules may occupy the same conformation originally bound, indicating that each round of interaction with GroEL is likely to be an all-or-none trial at reaching the native state.[245] Multiple such trials are apparently required for many polypeptides before all of the species reach native form. For example, in a given folding cycle, less than 5 percent of molecules of rhodanese or malate dehydrogenase

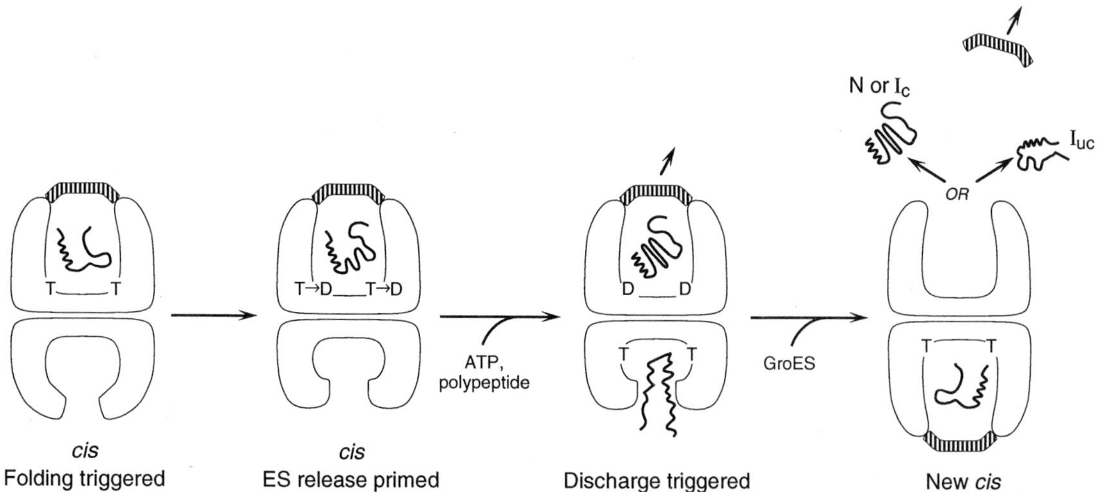

Fig. 85-9 GroEL–GroES reaction cycle. Rings alternate in formation of folding-active *cis* complexes. Folding is triggered upon ATP/GroES binding to the same (*cis*) ring as polypeptide, releasing it into the GroES-encapsulated, enlarged, and now hydrophilic cavity. This very stable complex is the longest-lived state of the system in the presence of non-native protein, and it is weakened by hydrolysis in the *cis* ring, priming it for dissociation. ATP hydrolysis in the *cis* ring allows for entry of ATP and non-native polypeptide into the *trans* ring, producing rapid *cis* complex dissociation. Subsequent binding of GroES to the *trans* ring produces a new *cis* complex. Thus GroEL rings alternate back and forth as folding-active, expending only one round of ATP per folding cycle, with ATP employed simultaneously to produce a new *cis* complex while dissociating the previous one.

reach the native state.[232,245,249] Thus GroEL can expend several hundred ATP molecules to enable folding of such proteins. This, however, represents only a fraction of the cost of translating these chains. Instead of rebinding to GroEL, released non-native forms can be bound by another chaperone (e.g., the Hsp70 class of chaperone[250]) or can be recognized and cleaved by a protease, the latter of which would be necessary for removal of proteins that are irreversibly damaged.[251] Such a process of kinetic partitioning is likely to be operative in the cell, with the fate of any given non-native protein determined by the relative affinities for it of the various chaperones and proteases and by their concentrations.

The expectation from studies of GroE-mediated folding was that a GroES-like Hsp10 component would be present in the mitochondrial matrix, and indeed such a component has been uncovered in both mammalian[252,253] and yeast mitochondria.[254,255] In the mammalian studies, a component capable of associating with GroEL and promoting release of ribulose bisphosphate carboxylase (Rubisco) was isolated from bovine liver[252]; in another study, a heat-inducible 10-kDa component was observed in mitochondria of a hepatoma cell line, and proved on primary structural analysis to be approximately 30 percent identical to GroES.[253] Using the purified component and Hsp60, Hartman et al.[253] reconstituted ATP-mediated folding of OTC diluted from guanidine. Correspondingly, in yeast, the homologous Hsp10 has been shown to be an essential component[254,255] that assists Hsp60 in mediating folding, as observed in intact organelles of such imported endogenous proteins as the α subunit of the matrix-processing peptidase and the Rieske iron-sulfur protein, as well as in heterologously imported mammalian OTC. A more recent two-dimensional gel/mass spectrometry survey of imported proteins insoluble in Hsp10 temperature-sensitive yeast mitochondria included many of the same substrates as identified for Hsp60, including Hsp60 subunits themselves. Concerning mammalian Hsp60, it has been of interest that the mammalian version, in contrast with chaperonins from other sources, is isolated from tissue or cultured cells, or from expressing bacteria, as a single ring.[256] Although it has seemed possible that folding-active *cis* complexes can be produced and discharged in the absence of association of a second ring,[257] such behavior, based on substantially lower affinity of Hsp10 for Hsp60 once *cis* hydrolysis produces an ADP-bound ring (vs. higher affinity of ADP-bound GroES for GroEL), would differ substantially from that of all of the other chaperonins examined to date. Indeed, upon exposure of the mammalian Hsp60 assembly to ATP, EM studies reveal it to form double-ring structures efficiently, suggesting that association of the second ring may in fact occur during the cycle of this chaperonin as well, required here also for communication of allosteric signals discharging the folding-active ring.

Ornithine Transcarbamylase Mature Enzyme. From the cloned cDNA, the sequence of the mature portion of the OTC subunit was predicted. This revealed two motifs highly conserved with prokaryotic transcarbamylases: an N-terminal one including residues 53 to 62, potentially involved with binding of the substrate CP, and a second, C-terminal one including residues 268 to 273, potentially involved with binding ornithine.[87] Support for these assignments came initially from structural similarity to the other trimeric transcarbamylase from *E. coli*, aspartate transcarbamylase (ATC), whose three-dimensional structure has been extensively examined crystallographically, and from a domain-swapping experiment in which the N-terminal homologous domains of both ATC and OTC, comprising so-called polar domains, and shown to be involved with the shared action of CP binding, were swapped and the OTC–ATC fusion was observed to rescue a pyrimidine auxotrophic strain deleted of ATCase coding sequences for growth in the absence of pyrimidine.[258]

More recently, crystal structures of *E. coli* and human OTC enzymes have been solved,[259–261] yielding information about both catalysis and effects of human mutations. The *E. coli* enzyme has been studied both in an unliganded state and liganded with the transition state analogue δ-N-phosphonoacetyl-L-ornithine (PALO), whereas the human enzyme has been studied in the liganded state, at 1.8-Å resolution (Fig. 85-10). The structures of the *E. coli* and human enzymes are nearly isomorphous except for an additional loop in the bacterial subunit (in the ornithine-binding domain, believed to prevent the bacterial subunit from binding to the ATCase regulatory subunit) and an extension of 10 amino acids in the human enzyme not present in the bacterial protein, which might have a role in interaction with the mitochondrial inner membrane.[261] The OTC subunit exhibits an α/β fold, with the human subunit composed of 14 α helices and 9 β strands, folded into two domains, an N-terminal polar domain (aa 33–168 and

A

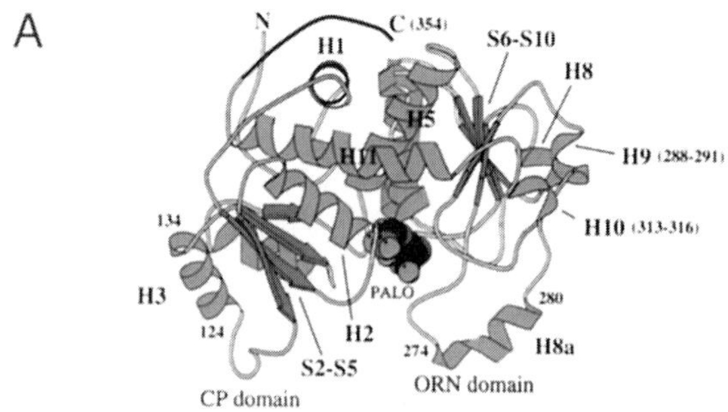

B

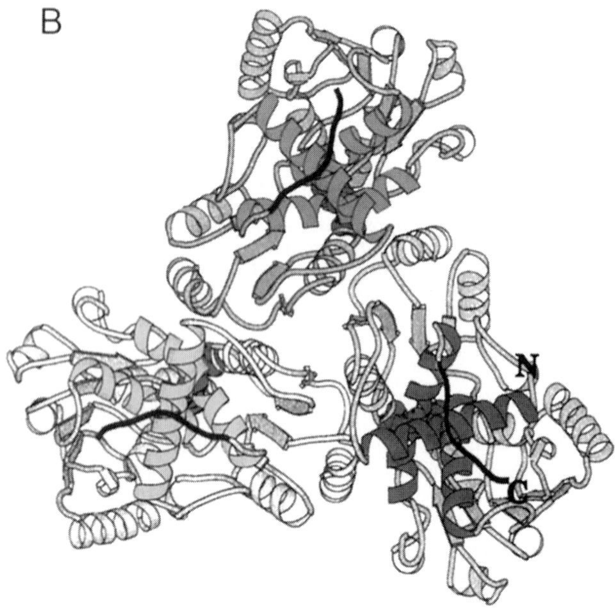

Fig. 85-10 Architecture of the human OTC enzyme in the 1.85 Å crystal structure. A: OTC subunit, showing polar CP binding domain and equatorial ornithine binding domain. PALO substrate is shown at the interface between the two domains. The domain can be oriented with respect to the intact trimer shown in B by comparing the position of the C-terminal segment, shown in black. H = helical domains; S = β-strands. (*Reprinted with permission from Shi D, Morizono H, Ha Y, Aoyagi M, Tuchman M, Allewell NM: 1.85 X resolution crystal structure of human ornithine transcarbamoylase complexes with N-phosphoacetyl-L-ornithine: Catalytic mechanism and correlation with inherited deficiency.* J Biol Chem *273:34247, 1998.*)

345–354), predominantly α helical, but including a four-stranded β sheet that binds CP, and a C-terminal equatorial domain, containing a central five-stranded β sheet flanked by α helices, that binds ornithine (aa 183–322) (Fig. 85-10A). The two domains are connected through two long crossed α helices, H5 and H11. The homotrimer of these subunits forms a "cup" approximately 50 Å deep and 90 Å across whose deepest, central point lies on a threefold symmetry axis (Fig. 85-10B, looking at the bottom of the cup). The walls of the cup are composed of the polar domains at the bottom and equatorial domains higher up. The major contacts between subunits are formed between the polar domains, residues 89 to 94 in one subunit, contacting residues 110 to 122 from a neighbor—a salt bridge between R94 and E122 is highly conserved. In the PALO-bound structures, three molecules of the PALO transition state analogue are resolved, one in each of the three active sites of the homotrimer. Each active site is composed mostly of residues from the individual monomer, but there is cooperation from the neighboring subunit, showing that monomers of OTC are enzymatically inactive. Concerning substrate contacts (Fig. 85-11), the contacts with PALO indeed are formed with the highly conserved residues predicted earlier to be involved: the absolutely-conserved STRT (aa 90–93) segment forms stabilizing contacts with the negatively charged phosphate oxygens, both through side chains of S90 and R92 and main chain NH contacts of T91 and R92. Contacts are also formed between side chains of H117 and R141 and phosphate oxygen. The latter residue is absolutely conserved, and it also contacts the carbonyl oxygen of PALO as do the side chains of absolutely conserved H168 and R330. In the equatorial domain, contacts with ornithine are similarly formed with absolutely conserved residues: N199, D263, and S267, as well as a main chain contact with M268 (see Fig. 85-15). A catalytic mechanism has been proposed (Fig. 85-12)[261] in which the thiolate anion of absolutely conserved C303 (favored by close proximity of the side chain of D263) accepts a proton from the δ-amino group of ornithine, enabling nucleophilic attack by the δ nitrogen on the carbonyl carbon of CP. This forms a tetrahedral intermediate in which the δ nitrogen is again positively charged, whereas the carbonyl oxygen of CP is negatively charged. Breakdown of the intermediate to form citrulline and inorganic phosphate is associated with departure of the δ-nitrogen proton, either ligating to the leaving phosphate or to nearby His.[174] Associated with ligand binding and catalysis are domain movements appreciated from comparison of unliganded and liganded structures of the *E. coli* enzyme:[259,260] the two domains move toward each other in the liganded state to enclose the PALO ligand, with the major movement involving a loop in the equatorial domain containing aa 232 to 256 (*E. coli* numbering), which swings toward the CP binding domain. The ornithine binding domain also rotates approximately 9 Å relative to the CP binding domain.

The effects of natural human mutation on the OTC enzyme should now be possible to resolve, with the availability of a high-resolution structure. Caution must be taken, however, insofar as many of the single-residue substitution mutants may fail to reach a native fold, preventing extrapolation to the native, assembled, structure. Expression studies will be necessary to distinguish those subunits that can be properly folded and assembled from those that are misfolded and that ultimately either aggregate or are proteolytically turned over (in the cytosol or inside mitochondria). Such studies might best be carried out in *E. coli* expressing mature mutant human OTC subunits, as has been accomplished already for several mutants by Tuchman and colleagues.[308] Indeed there is considerable homology of the folding machinery and reducing environment of the bacterial cytoplasm to the mitochondrial matrix, and expression of OTC mature subunits at high levels is not difficult to achieve. Thus, this affords straightforward initial conclusions about mutant subunits. Alternatively, expression of mutant precursor in COS cells can be informative[301] and particularly useful where an issue is raised about RNA processing/stability, translation, precursor stability, or mitochondrial import. However, COS cell expression probably will not be of much use in an attempt to characterize a folded/assembled mutant homotrimer because levels of expression will be insufficient to garner sufficient material to conduct kinetic studies *in vitro*. To date, only a few human OTC substitution mutants have been analyzed using this method. In their early COS cell studies of the R141Q mutant, it turned out that Nussbaum and co-workers examined a catalytically crucial residue. We know now that this is an absolutely conserved active site residue, which forms contacts with both phosphate and carbonyl oxygens of PALO in the crystal structure (see Fig. 85-14). Presumably the glutamine mutation can form a homotrimer that has no significant affinity for the substrate CP. The data of Lee and Nussbaum are consistent with this possibility, because upon expression of the mutant in COS cells, they found that protein was made that had a specific activity of less than 1 percent wild-type.[262] Of course, expression in the bacterial system would now allow purification and direct kinetic characterization. Such studies by Tuchman and co-workers, using expression in *E. coli*, recently examined the R277W and R277Q mutants,[308] which clinically exhibit late onset and have recurred in a number of pedigrees. Mutation at this strongly conserved

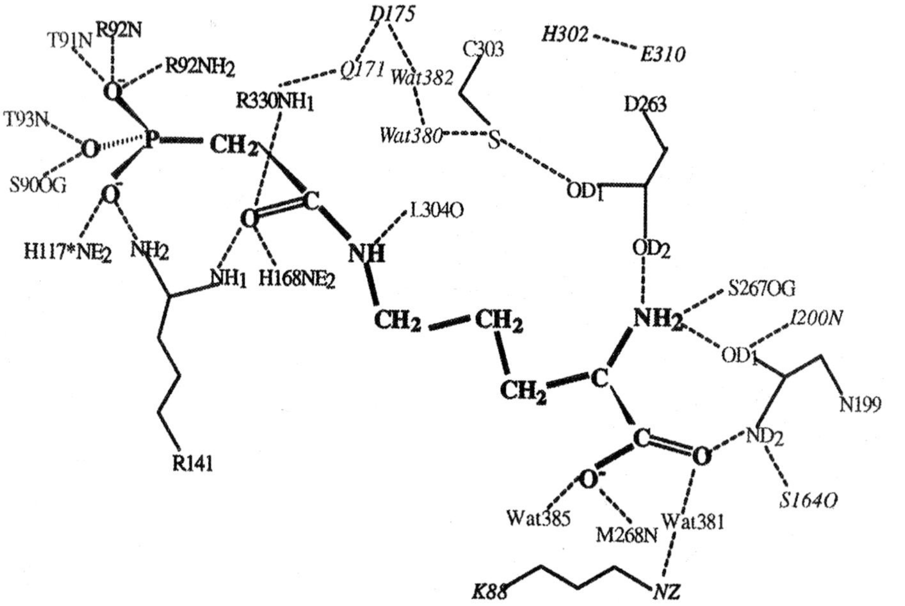

Fig. 85-11 Interaction of the bisubstrate analogue, PALO, with active site of OTC subunit in crystal structure of complex with human OTC. PALO is shown in bold. H117 derives from an adjacent subunit, designated by asterisk. (*Reprinted with permission from Shi D, Morizono H, Ha Y, Aoyagi M, Tuchman M, Allewell NM: 1.85 X resolution crystal structure of human ornithine transcarbamoylase complexes with N-phosphoacetyl-L-ornithine: Catalytic mechanism and correlation with inherited deficiency.* J Biol Chem *273:34247, 1998.*)

residue, which lies in the loop region of the equatorial domain that moves in association with substrate binding, was indeed found to produce a large decrease in affinity of the purified mutant homotrimers for ornithine.

Transfer of Cloned OTC Sequences into Cultured Cells and Animals

DNA-Mediated Transfer. The OTC precursor has been expressed in a variety of settings. Overexpression in *E. coli* produced a substrate used in a variety of *in vitro* import experiments employing isolated mitochondria. Expression in mammalian cells resulted in import into mitochondria and processing and folding/assembly to produce the mature active enzyme, indicating that the steps of import and biogenesis are ubiquitously present, even though the enzyme subunit is normally transcribed in liver and gut. In mammalian cells, the level of expression of transfected SV40-driven human OTC cDNA was approximately 1 percent of the activity in normal liver, but coamplification of the transfected segment with a DHFR segment resulted in an approximately hundredfold increase of both copy number and activity, the latter reaching the level of normal liver.[263] When human OTC cDNA was programmed from a galactose (GAL) 1 operon promoter in yeast, this also resulted in targeting of precursor to mitochondria, and biogenesis of the enzyme recapitulated the steps observed in mammalian cells, indicating the conserved nature of protein import into mitochondria and serving as the basis of a genetic screen that enabled isolation of components involved with protein import.[264]

In addition to cell transfer, germline transfer experiments have been conducted in mice. Both heterologous promoter segments and an OTC promoter have been used. In one study, SV40 promoter and splice and polyA signals were joined with rat cDNA and the fragment injected into fertilized eggs of spf^{ash} (sparse fur/abnormal skin and hair) homozygous females that had been mated with C57BL males.[265] A normal-appearing male was detected in one litter and found to have normal levels of urinary orotic acid. This animal sired additional correct-appearing males, whose levels of hepatic OTC activity proved to be near normal. Low levels of activity also were observed in spleen and lung.

In an additional study, correction of OTC deficiency of the sparse fur strain was accomplished by introduction into the germline of a segment containing 750 bp of 5′ flanking sequence from the mouse OTC gene, the human OTC cDNA, and an SV40 splice signal. Two lines of mice with multicopy head-to-tail transgenes exhibited expression of RNA and enzymatic activity confined to the small intestine, but this enabled clinical correction with elimination of orotic aciduria and normal fur.[266] Likewise, in another study transferring 1.3 kb of 5′ flanking sequence from the rat OTC gene adjoined with rat OTC cDNA into spf^{ash} mice, only a doubling of liver activity was observed, but intestinal activity was increased sixfold.[267] This pattern of expression was associated with normal hair growth and normal orotic acid excretion. The results of the foregoing transgenic studies suggest that so far we do not have a clear understanding of the sequences necessary for normal expression of OTC in both liver and gut.

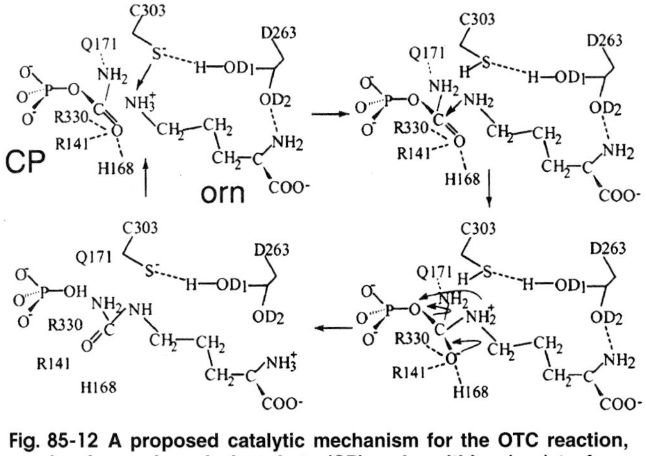

Fig. 85-12 A proposed catalytic mechanism for the OTC reaction, condensing carbamyl phosphate (CP) and ornithine (orn) to form citrulline. (*Reprinted with permission from Shi D, Morizono H, Ha Y, Aoyagi M, Tuchman M, Allewell NM: 1.85 resolution crystal structure of human ornithine transcarbamoylase complexes with N-phosphoacetyl-L-ornithine: Catalytic mechanism and correlation with inherited deficiency.* J Biol Chem *273:34247, 1998.*)

Virally Mediated Transfer. Expressible OTC cDNA also has been transferred by viral transduction with a view to possible somatic gene therapy. Two viral vector systems have been used, retroviruses and adenoviruses, the latter of which have received much more intense study over the past few years. A focus of attention on adenoviruses is at least in part due to lack of requirement of adenovirus transduction for a mitotically active tissue target, as compared with such a requirement by retroviruses. An OTC retrovirus experiment should be mentioned, however, in which a simple long terminal repeat (LTR)-OTC-LTR virus was prepared from a previously designed viral genome called δ-N2.[268] Recombinant ecotropic virus at a titer greater than 10^6/mL was used to infect primary cultures of hepatocytes prepared by collagenase perfusion from *spf* or *spf*^{ash} livers. Efficient infection could be achieved, with at least 30 to 40 percent of cells in the target population harboring a proviral genome. RNA expression of the introduced human sequence reached levels similar to that of human liver. Enzyme activity, however, was only slightly increased over that of the mutant background and reached a level 2 weeks after infection no greater than 3 percent of wild type. The nature of the possible block at the level of translation is unknown. Clearly, this problem would need resolution before any protocols of transplanting infected cells could be usefully pursued. Such protocols have to date involved transfer of cells corrected by infection in culture into the portal vein for targeting into the hepatic parenchyma. For example, a sufficient number of low density lipoprotein (LDL) receptor–deficient hepatocytes was infected with LDL receptor virus and reintroduced into the liver of a Watanabe rabbit deficient in the receptor to enable at least transient lowering of serum cholesterol.[269]

The feasibility of adenovirus as an agent of delivering expressible OTC cDNA directly into an animal was demonstrated as early as 1990. Stratford-Perricaudet et al. produced a recombinant adenovirus bearing rat OTC cDNA joined with the adenovirus major late promoter.[270] The recombinant virus was shown to produce the expected adenovirus–OTC chimeric RNA and OTC enzymatic activity both in the virus producer cell line and after infection of HeLa cells. The level of activity corresponded to that observed following transfection of HeLa cells with SV40-driven human OTC cDNA, approximately 1 percent of normal hepatic activity. Remarkably, however, intravenous injection of virus into newborn *spf*^{ash} mice (produced by mating homozygous affected females with affected males) resulted in production in 4 of 14 animals of near-normal levels of OTC activity measured at 1 or 2 months. Where such activity was observed, animals exhibited evidence of clinical correction, with normal-appearing fur. Whether the enzyme produced is derived entirely from the adenovirus promoter remains unproven, but adenovirus–OTC transcripts could be detected by PCR amplification of cDNA prepared from the livers of two animals 15 months after injection. Both animals exhibited reduction of orotic aciduria as compared with uninjected controls, and one animal exhibited hepatic OTC activity at a level 50 percent of normal. A subsequent study infected 6- to 10-week-old *spf*/y or *spf*^{ash} mice by intravenous injection with E1-deleted viruses bearing a segment joining the CMV promoter with mouse OTC cDNA.[271] Here, with E1 deletion alone, there was initial augmentation of hepatic OTC activity and correction of orotic aciduria, but these effects were lost after 28 days. In contrast, when an E2a temperature-sensitive lesion was introduced in addition to E1 deletion, substantial activity was still present at 28 days, and orotic aciduria remained corrected until approximately 6 weeks postinjection. Associated with this increased period of expression, there was a reduction in hepatic inflammation as compared with that incurred by the virus bearing only E1 deletion. It was presumed that residual expressed viral protein induces both humoral and cellular immune responses that are associated with both inflammation and extinction of expression.

Short-term expression and correction of orotic aciduria, as well as occurrence of normal hair growth, were reported in another study, where a recombinant E1 deletion–E3 mutant adenovirus with a hybrid SV40-HIV LTR (R-U5) promoter was injected into the liver of newborn *spf*^{ash} mice.[272] It was suggested that such virus treatment might be used clinically in the setting of acute decompensation. In this context, in a further study, the E1-deleted E2a-CMV-OTC adenovirus conferred a degree of protection of *spf*/y mice against behavioral and biochemical abnormalities following NH_4Cl challenge, when supplied intravenously 1 to 14 days prior to the challenge.[273] It would seem, however, that if 24 h is required for acquisition of effect of injected virus, other therapies would need to be instituted during this time in an acute clinical situation. Since this is often a critical period, requiring lowering of plasma ammonia within hours to subvert CNS toxicity, the utility of supplying recombinant adenovirus in the setting of acute decompensation seems uncertain.

In another study aiming toward longer-term therapy, Kiwaki et al.[274] injected 8-week-old *spf*^{ash} mice intravenously with an E1,E3-deleted adenovirus bearing human OTC cDNA adjoined to a hybrid promoter composed of β-actin promoter–CMV–IE enhancer. This promoter functioned more strongly in cells and animals than the SV40-HIV LTR promoter. In the short term, animals exhibited substantial levels of hepatic OTC activity associated with correction of orotic aciduria. But as in the other studies, extinction of expression occurred, here observed at approximately 2 months, associated with development of neutralizing antibody against virus. Further injection did not produce resurrection of activity. In retrospect, the success of the initial Stratford-Perricaudet study was potentially a function of targeting 1-day-old animals, which may exhibit tolerance to injected virus. More generally, it has been realized that the major barrier to clinical utilization of OTC adenoviruses for long-term correction is immune reaction against expressed viral components, involving both humoral immunity and cytotoxic T cells. An approach to overcoming this involves the use of recombinant adenoviruses devoid of all viral coding sequences.[275–279] Impressively, a single intravenous injection of such a virus bearing the human α_1-antitrypsin gene into 6- to 10-week-old mice resulted in stable hepatic expression and normal liver architecture over 10 months at the time of the report.[280]

In summary, with a new generation of recombinant adenoviruses, devoid of viral coding sequences, it may be possible to accomplish long-term transduction of sequences programmed for expression. In the case of OTC, it is not yet clear which arrangement of promoter, cDNA, or genomic sequences will allow such expression. Beyond this, issues of safety still must be addressed. It will be crucial to develop a means to generate recombinant virus stocks that are devoid of any helper that could recombine with the therapeutic genome to produce a replication-competent virus. It will also be desirable to develop a means of delivery that will be specific to hepatic tissue, avoiding, for example, the problem of germline infection. Whether intrahepatic injection, as above, will be required, as opposed to simple IV injection, seems unresolved at present.

Several additional aspects of therapy with OTC adenoviruses have been considered. In one study, infecting primary cultures of hepatocytes from affected patients, interference with production of activity was reported between endogenous mutant subunits and input wild-type subunits, occurring potentially at the level of assembly of mixed trimers.[272] Thus, consideration of the particular OTC-deficient allele involved may dictate the level of expression ultimately needed for correction. The issue of germline infection by injected adenovirus also has been addressed, in a primate study, where baboons were injected intravenously in the hepatic artery or its branches followed by inspection of tissues for viral DNA as measured by PCR.[281] Higher doses but not lower doses of an E1-E4–deleted vector led to gonadal infection.

OTC Deficiency. The isolation of cloned human OTC sequences enabled DNA-based diagnosis of OTC deficiency using nonhepatic cells, including amniocytes and fibroblasts, which do not express the enzyme. Similarly, DNA-based diagnosis has enabled identification of asymptomatic female carriers in affected pedigrees. In particular, PCR analysis of the 10 exons of the gene has allowed direct identification in both affected probands and asymptomatic carrier females, enabling straightforward pedigree analysis. Where mutation cannot be identified in the setting of enzyme deficiency, for example, due to unidentifiable intron mutation or promoter mutations, biochemical studies, particularly allopurinol testing of suspected female heterozygotes, can be conducted. In these cases, biochemical information can then be coupled with RFLP testing for informative DNA analysis.

Strategies of Molecular Analysis of Pedigrees. The considerable heterogeneity of mutation at the OTC locus is one component addressed in the molecular analysis of OTC pedigrees. Recent tabulation of the mutations occurring at this locus[328] indicates that large deletions of one exon or more account for approximately 7 percent of patients, small deletions or insertions account for 9 percent of patients, and all of the remaining patients harbor single base substitutions, approximately 15 percent of which involve splicing. A few base changes are recurrent, and turn out to affect CpG dinucleotide "hot spots." Direct identification of mutation in probands has been addressed by PCR amplification of the 10 OTC exons, including intron–exon boundaries, from genomic DNA, followed by either chemical cleavage or single-strand conformational polymorphism to localize a mutation, ultimately followed by direct DNA sequencing, to identify the abnormality.[282,292] Where a deleterious mutation can be unambiguously distinguished from a polymorphism — for example, by its recurrence among the 100 or more mutations now known (Table 85-3; see also a locus-specific mutation database as http://www.peds.umn.edn/otc/),[293–329] by its causing premature translational termination or frameshift, or by drastic substitution of a conserved residue — this allows molecular analysis of individuals at risk. In some cases, such a distinction may not be straightforward, requiring expression studies in either *E. coli*[308] or COS cells,[262] in which a mutant cDNA can be shown to be defective in producing OTC enzyme activity. A substantial percentage of OTC mutations may be directly identified by the foregoing strategies, but occasionally these approaches fail to identify lesions in promoter or intron regions. Thus, even with direct mutation identification, biochemical testing and RFLP analysis remain available as evaluation modes for pedigrees where mutations cannot be identified but where hepatic enzymatic deficiency has been demonstrated.

Origin of Mutation. The ability to identify specific mutations in probands and their relatives has allowed an assessment of where new mutations arise. Tuchman and colleagues noted that only 2 of 28 male probands had sporadic mutations (i.e., approximately 95 percent inherited mutation from their mother), whereas 12 of 15 female probands were sporadic mutations; that is, approximately 80 percent represented new mutations.[330] Thus, the ratio of occurrence of new mutation in sperm is estimated to be 50 times the rate of occurrence in egg. This suggests a 9 out of 10 chance that the mother of an affected male is a carrier versus a 2 out of 10 chance for the mother of an affected female. More recently, however, it was found that 33 percent of mothers of singleton males do not carry the mutation found in their affected son,[476] suggesting that new mutations may occur in the egg more frequently than supposed.

The occurrence of somatic and gonadal mosaicism can have obvious importance both in interpreting phenotype and estimating risks. In the percentage of cases where the mother of a proband is identified as not carrying the mutant allele of the proband, one must nonetheless consider the possibility of gonadal mosaicism. Such an occurrence has been observed, with multiple affected males of a somatically normal female.[476a] In the setting of only one case, it is difficult to provide accurate risk assessment, but a figure of 1 percent or less might seem appropriate for female gonadal mosaicism in the setting of an affected male, lack of mutation in maternal somatic tissue, and maternal biochemical normality. This is probably an overestimate, particularly in the face of the low mutation rate in egg. Indeed, gonadal mosaicism might be more favored in males, with multiple affected daughters. Such a pedigree has been reported in which three daughters were severely affected with OTC deficiency (due to the mutation L148F), but instead of observing the mother to be mosaic, the

Table 85-3 Human OTC Mutations

Mutations	Pres.	Ref.
M1V ex1	F	319
R23X ex1 TaqI	N	334
R26Q ex	N	282
IVS1 + 1G > T	F	324
IVS1 + 3G > A	L	297
IVS1 + 4 RsaI	N	302
IVS1 + 5G > A	N	324
Q32Xex2	F	319
G39C ex2	N	321
R40H ex2	L	295, 301, 308, 314
R40C ex2	L	309
L43F ex2	F	319
T44I ex2	L	317
L45P ex2	N	282
L45V ex2	F	328
K46R ex2 polymorphism		282
N47ins G, fs, term	N	320
N47I ex2	N	324
G50X ex2MspI	F	283
G50R ex2 MspI	L	324
Y55D ex2	L	312
M56T ex2	L	324
S60L ex2	F	322
L63P	F	319
63fster	N	321
IVS2 + 1-4ag-aa > acc	N	292
IVS2 + 1 g > a	E	318
G79E ex3	N	292
delL81 ex3	F	322
G83R ex3 DdeI	N	324
E87K ex3MseI	L	283
K88N ex3	L	284
S90Rex3	F	328
R92X ex3 TaqI	N	334
R92Q ex3 TaqI	N	334
T93A ex3	L	311
R94T ex3	L	292
IVS3 + 1GA	N	297
IVS3 + 1-5gtaagdel	F	324
G100D ex4	F	319
L101F ex4 polymorphism		311
A102E EspI	N	322
L111P ex4 polymorphism		334
H117L ex4	L	293
H117R ex4	L	327
120fster ex4	N	321
E5-8delsomatic mosiac	L	335
T125M ex4	N	298
D126G ex4	N	194
R129H + splerr = spfash	F,L	295, 329
R129L + splerr	L	322
IVS4-2 ag-tg acc spl err	N	285
132ins Tfs,term ex5	N	293
135delG,fs,term	N	292
H136R	L	310, 316
L139S ex5	F	329
R141X ex5TaqI	N	286
R141Q ex5TaqI	N	305, 317, 335
R141P ex5TaqI	F	324
L144X ex5	F	311
L148F ex5	L	307
E154X ex	N	282
I159T ex5	F	297
N161S ex5	F	322
G162R ex	N	283

(Continued on next page)

Table 85-3 (Continued)

Mutations	Pres.	Ref.
S164X ex5	N	326
Y167X ex	N	297, 320
H168Q ex5 FokI	L	324
I172M ex	N	294
A174P ex	F	282
D175V ex5	F	324
Y176C ex5	L	299
delT178&L79	N	320
T178M	N	309
Q180H ex5	L,N	320, 322
IVS5 + 1G > C	E	318
IVS5 + 2T > C	N	325
E181G ex6	N	328
H182L ex6	N	293
Y183C ex6	N	287
Y183D	FN	319
G188R	N	298
S192R ex6	N	288
W193X ex6	N	320
G195R ex6	F	295
D196V ex6	N	288
D196Y ex6	N	328
G197E ex6	F	328
del199/200TA,fs	N	295
L201P ex6	N	320
H202Y ex6	L	324
S203C ex6	F,N	293
M206R ex6	N	329
S207R ex6	N	320
A208T CfoI	L	295, 306, 324
A209V ex6	F	297
M213K	F	319
H214Y ex6	N	317
215ins T, fs, term	N	293
Q216E ex6	N	282
P220A ex6	L	299
K221 AAG > AAA	L	318
IVS6 + 1G > T	E	318
IVS6insgtt > gtta	F	311
IVS6gt > gc	F	324
delex7-9som.mosaic	L	336
delex 7,8	N	333
222delGfs,term	F	324
P225L ex7MspI	N	289
P225R ex7	N	313
P225T ex7	L	295
239GAG > GAAsplerr	F	324
IVS7gt-gc,ex7del	N	285
IVS7gta-gtg,ex7del	N	285
IVS7del	N	321
T242I ex8 Kpn	L	324
L244Q ex8	N	321
del244-247fs ex8	F	321
T247K ex8	N	311
H255P ex8	N	328
D263N ex8	F	324
D263G ex8	F	328
T264A ex8	L	288
T264I ex8	L	320
S267R ex8	L	320
M268T ex8 NlaIII	L	288
G269E ex8	N	296
Q270R ex8 pmorphism		292
delE272/273	L	300
R277W ex8	L	288, 290, 308, 309, 315
R277Q ex8NlaIV	L	295, 308

Table 85-3 (Continued)

Mutations	Pres.	Ref.
IVS8G > T	N	318
IVS8GT > AT MboII	N	Tuchman unpublished observations
delex9	N	333
294δT, fs, term CfoI	N	287
297delTG	F	303
H302L ex9	F	298
H302Y orn bind.	N	299
H302Q	L	324
C303R ex9	N	321
C303Y ex9	F	324
L304F ex9	L	290
delE309	L	295
E310X ex9MboII	N	287
R320L ex9TaqI	N	334
R320X ex9	N	317
R330G ex9	F	324
W332X ex9	N	294
IVS9 + 1G > T	N	324
A336S ex1	L	Tuchman, unpublished observations
V337L ex1	L	323
V339L ex1	N	324
S340P ex1	F	319
T343K ex10	F	299
Y345D ex10	F	292
Y345C ex10	N	328
Q348X ex10	F	319
F354C ex10 FsiI	L	324

Human OTC mutations are listed along with the time of presentation (Pres.) and reference (Ref.) for the case studies. The exon affected (ex.) or intron involved (IVS) is indicated. Where followed by numbers, this indicates the nucleotides in an intron that are affected by mutation. Where a restriction enzyme is diagnostic of the mutation, it is indicated. The time of presentation is designated: N, neonatal; L, late-onset; E, early-onset (first few months of life); F, affected female.

father was found to carry the mutation in his lymphocytes and sperm.[307] Whereas usually patients are mosaic in either the germline or in somatic tissue, in this case, evidently there was mosaicism in both lineages, arguing for very early postzygotic occurrence of the mutation.

Deletion Defects. In general, the larger defects exhibit neonatal disease in affected males. Rozen and colleagues conducted initial Southern blot analyses of genomic DNA from affected males and identified gene deletion in four cases of approximately 50 examined.[331,332] Three of these deletions involved only a portion of the OTC gene, whereas a fourth involved complete deletion of the gene but not of two anonymous flanking X-chromosomal loci, L128 and 754. Of the four deletions, two were shown to be inherited from a heterozygous female, whereas one had arisen *de novo*. Additional deletions were reported in 3 of 13 male probands examined.[333] One was deleted of the entire gene, a second was missing exons 7 and 8, and a third had deletion of exon 9. An additional study observed three gene deletions from a series of 18 patients.[334] Somatic mosaicism for intragenic OTC deletion also has been recognized in two cases, both presenting with late-onset symptoms of OTC deficiency. In one case, deletion involved exons 5 to 8, and in a second case, exons 7 to 9 were deleted.[335,336] Larger cytogenetically detectable deletions also have been observed. A kindred has been described with an interstitial deletion in the Xp21 region with OTC deficiency, glycerol kinase deficiency, and congenital adrenal hypoplasia.[337] An interstitial deletion of Xp21 in a mildly retarded woman who had a history of dietary protein intolerance and urinary orotic acid elevation with dietary protein challenge also has been described.[338] A number of more recently reported small deletions, affecting a single exon or involving one or two residues, are indicated in Table 85-3. Some of these may be compatible with residual enzyme activity; for example, deletions of either E272+E273 or of Q309 were compatible with a late presentation.[295,300] Finally, deletion can affect the interpretation of RFLP analyses at the OTC locus: what may appear as null RFLP alleles that raise a question about maternity or paternity in fact prove to be deletions that remove the marker entirely.[339]

Mouse Mutants. A strain of mouse OTC mutant (*spf*^{ash}) exhibits abnormal RNA processing. Affected males exhibit a level of mRNA, immunoreactive protein, and enzymatic activity approximately 10 percent of normal, and the enzyme itself exhibits normal kinetic parameters.[340–342] G $\rightarrow$ A transition was found in the last nucleotide of exon 4, leading both to a reduced level of normal-sized mRNA due to reduced splicing at the donor site and to the presence of an elongated mRNA that used a cryptic donor site 48 bases downstream in the intron.[343] These alterations are reflected at the protein level in production of two OTC proteins that target to mitochondria: one a protein from the correctly spliced mRNA, bearing the substitution R129H, that appears at 10 percent of normal levels and exhibits a normal specific activity, and a second protein elongated by 16 amino acids, produced from the misspliced RNA, that fails to be assembled into an active trimeric enzyme. The exact mutation of *spf*^{ash} has been reported in a female heterozygote[295] and subsequently in two Spanish families.[329] In the latter report an affected male had 1.3 percent residual activity but was developing normally. A second mouse OTC mutant strain (*spf*) bears the substitution H85N and exhibits somewhat greater than normal amounts of a normal-sized enzyme with decreased specific activity.[344]

Argininosuccinic Acid Synthetase

Molecular studies of human AS have revealed striking dispersion of AS pseudogenes, interesting regulation of transcription, and heterogeneity of mutation. The original isolation of AS cDNA clones was facilitated by the availability of a human cultured cell line, which when grown in medium containing the arginine analogue canavanine produced high levels of AS mRNA.[345] cDNA clones derived from this RNA subsequently were used to isolate and characterize AS genomic sequences and to perform the initial molecular analyses of mutations causing AS deficiency.

The active AS gene localizes to chromosome 9q34[235] near ABO and *abl* and is 63 kb in size, with 16 exons. It encodes a major mRNA of approximately 1600 bases[346,347] and a minor species of 2700 bases that transcribes beyond the polyA site of the major RNA. Both RNAs contain an open reading frame of 1236 bases encoding a subunit of the homotetrameric enzyme of approximately 46,400 daltons.[348] The 5′-untranslated sequence of the AS message comprises 102 bases, and at a position 27 bases upstream from the translational start codon there are three in-frame tandem arginine codons. These were originally postulated to influence the half-life of the AS message, possibly by interacting with arginyl transfer RNA. This hypothetical interaction could explain arginine-mediated repression of AS expression, but subsequent studies demonstrated that this repression also occurs in minigenes that lack these sequences.[349] Levels of AS mRNA in adult rat liver increase 24-fold following starvation for 5 days, and they increase 5-fold in response to treatment with either dibutyryl cAMP or dexamethasone.[60,350]

Transcriptional Regulation. The 5′ flanking region of the AS gene has been analyzed and found to contain several putative regulatory sequences.[346,351,352] In addition to a TATAA sequence at position −30, there are three GGCGGGG heptanucleotides similar to the consensus SP1 binding sequence, at positions −116 to −110 and −97 to −91 on the noncoding strand and −71 to −77 on the coding strand. These sequences could be shown to bind purified SP1 *in vitro*.[353] Deletion of sequences to the 5′-most heptanucleotide had no effect on expression of AS from a minigene plasmid construction introduced into RPMI 2650 cells. However, partial deletion of the heptanucleotide reduced expression 12-fold, and complete deletion reduced expression 50-fold. Targeted mutations at the individual heptanucleotide sites that should abolish SP1 binding led in each case to reduction of transcription and collectively to greater-than-additive effects, suggesting synergistic action of the SP1 sites in transcriptional activation.[353] At positions −137 to −129 there is the sequence TGTGAACGC, which resembles an element found in the promoter regions of yeast genes that are derepressed during general amino acid starvation. Deletion of this region from a minigene construct produced a loss of arginine regulation. Further upstream, at −470, is an octameric sequence, AGAAGTGA, which is also found in the 5′ flanking region of the genes encoding factor VIII and albumin.

These various upstream sequences may contribute to the observed pattern of AS expression. The GC-rich elements, usually found in housekeeping genes, appear to play a role in the low-level expression of AS observed in nonhepatic tissues. The TATAA sequence and octameric element are features of genes expressed in a tissue-specific manner, and these may contribute to the approximately 100-fold higher level of expression of AS observed in the liver as compared with other tissues. Tissue-specific extinguisher (TSE), a factor responsible for liver-specific expression of AS as well as several other genes, has been identified by somatic cell hybrid studies examining extinction of AS expression on fusion of hepatoma cells with fibroblasts.[354] The TSE factor was first mapped to a several megabase segment of chromosome 17 and then TSE1 cDNA was isolated, in one case by subtractive hybridization[355] and in another by candidate transfection.[356] The cDNA was identified as encoding the regulatory subunit, RIα, of cAMP-dependent protein kinase. RIα levels correlated with extinguisher activity in various hybrid lines, with hepatic cells expressing at least 50-fold less than other tissue types. This finding implies that AS is positively regulated through the PKA–CREB pathway and that a target CRE element must be present. Of course, this draws attention to the nature of hepatic regulation of RIα itself.

Within the AS gene, the first two exons encode a 5′-untranslated sequence, and the translational initiation codon is situated in exon 3. Alternative splicing of these exons occurs in transcripts from human and baboon cells. In human cells, exons 1 and 3 are joined, deleting the second exon from most of the AS mRNA. In contrast, the second exon is retained in most of the AS mRNA found in baboon[346] and in mouse cells.[357]

Pseudogenes. In addition to the transcriptionally active AS locus, a remarkable number of pseudogenes with homology to cloned human AS cDNA has been detected, mapping to 14 different loci,[358–360] including two loci on chromosome 9 at positions distant from the active gene, two loci on the X chromosome, and one locus on the Y chromosome. Genomic DNA clones of these pseudogenes have been analyzed; all are approximately 2 kb in size and are devoid of introns.[361] Three pseudogenes analyzed in detail have been discovered to contain small insertions or deletions, and multiple termination codons were found in all three reading frames. Two of the three had adenine-rich regions at the 3′-terminus and were flanked by nearly perfect direct repeats. These features are typical of processed pseudogenes, which probably arise from reverse transcription of a messenger RNA followed by integration of the copied sequences into genomic DNA. It has been proposed that the multiplicity of the dispersed processed AS sequences could have arisen in part from the replication of an intermediate molecule prior to integration.[361]

Canavanine Resistance — Transcription Regulation of transcription of the AS gene has been examined in cultured human lymphoblastoid cell lines (RPMI 2650). Consistent with previous observations concerning arginine-mediated repression of AS enzyme activity, when wild-type RPMI 2650 cells were grown in the presence of citrulline instead of arginine, a sevenfold increase of AS mRNA was observed. In variants of either the RPMI 2650 cells[362] or of cultured human lymphoid lines[363] selected for resistance to the arginine analogue canavanine (Can^r cells) both AS mRNA and AS enzyme were present at a level nearly 200-fold greater than wild-type cells grown in arginine. This level of expression corresponds to that observed in normal liver. The basis of canavanine resistance remains unresolved. Resistance clearly correlates with an increased level of both the AS mRNA and enzyme, and these features, once selected for, are apparently stable, being maintained in the absence of the analogue. At the DNA level, neither alteration in AS gene copy number, as would occur with gene amplification, nor rearrangement of the active gene, has been observed.[345]

The mechanism governing the increased RNA level could be *trans*-acting, suggested by S1 analysis of RNA from Can^r human lymphoblasts isolated from an individual heterozygous for a mutation in the AS gene. Increased levels of both the normal and mutant transcript were observed.[364] The apparent *trans* effect appears to be positively acting, as suggested by a cell fusion experiment in which RPMI 2650 cells were fused with Can^r cells. The level of AS message in the hybrids was equal to that of the Can^r parent. Thus, the increased level of mature AS mRNA could result from increased gene transcription, increased stability of nuclear RNA, or altered nuclear RNA processing. Concerning the last possibility, it seemed conceivable that alternate RNA processing could increase the percentage of AS mRNA containing exon 2 sequences and that this species might be more stable than mRNA lacking this exon; however, examination of Can^r cells revealed predominant elevation in the level of mRNA lacking exon 2 sequences.[346] One study suggested that it is increased AS transcription that occurs in Can^r cells. When nuclear runoff transcription was measured in isolated nuclei, the rate of transcription was at least 100 times greater in Can^r cells than in RPMI 2650 parental cells.[365] Yet attempts to define *cis*-acting sequences responsible for canavanine resistance using gene transfer into RPMI 2650 cells, seeking to isolate Can^r derivatives, have been unsuccessful.[349,363,365] Furthermore, when minigene constructs joining the AS 5′ flanking region with a CAT reporter sequence were transferred into both parental cells and Can^r cells, the level of CAT activity detected in the two cell types was similar. The analyzed constructs included as much as 3 kb of 5′ flanking sequence and the first four exons of the gene. Finally, more recently, a further study comparing run-on transcription between isolated nuclei from RPMI 2650 and Can^{r}1 cells found no difference in transcription initiation or elongation.[366] Instead, a posttranscriptional mechanism was suggested by observation that the stability of the nuclear AS transcripts was drastically reduced in the RPMI 2650 cells but not the Can^{r}1 cells. That is, in a 45-min reaction, virtually no AS RNA was detectable in the RPMI 2650 nuclei, whereas a high level was detected in the Can^{r}1 nuclei. A *trans*-acting mechanism was proposed to be involved. Consistent with this, both AS alleles were found to be involved in the transcriptional overexpression observed in Can^{r}1 cells. Also, when cells were treated with cycloheximide, production of AS nuclear RNA was inhibited.

Although transfected minigenes failed to express CAT at higher levels in Can^r cells, repression of CAT activity by addition of arginine to the growth medium (as compared with citrulline) was observed.[349,363] This effect could be observed when a minigene construct was used that contained as little as 150 bp of AS 5′ flanking sequence. Interestingly, the same pattern of repression of AS in the presence of amino acid is observed for leucine.[365] More generally, AS may be but one enzyme regulated in the same fashion as the general amino acid control system of *Saccharomyces cerevisiae*.[367] Although metabolite regulation of AS has been suggested to be a regulatory effect distinct from canavanine resistance, it is of note that neither the level of steady-state AS mRNA nor the level of run-on transcript is subject to such regulation in Can^r cells (as distinct from the results with transfected CAT minigenes). Correspondingly, levels of enzyme activity were not affected.[365] Absence of metabolite regulation of AS in Can^r cells is consistent with an alteration of AS sequences or chromatin structure leading to constitutive high levels of AS expression. In sum, the nature of activation of AS in Can^r cells remains an unresolved and fascinating issue.

Gene Transfer. Expression of transferred AS sequences has been accomplished in a variety of studies. In one type of study in cell culture, Chinese hamster cell lines — which lack AS enzymatic activity and are unable to grow in medium substituting citrulline for arginine — have been used as the recipient. When metaphase chromosomes derived from a lymphoid line that overproduces AS were transferred into AS-deficient Chinese hamster cells, stable transformants were isolated that could grow in citrulline-containing medium.[368] In most cases these transformants expressed human AS, although several transformants apparently activated expression of the hamster enzyme. In a second type of transfer experiment, genomic DNA derived from Can^r human cells was used for calcium phosphate–mediated transfection of the Chinese hamster line.[369] Transformants were isolated that could grow in citrulline-containing medium. Blot analyses with cloned human AS sequences as a probe confirmed transfer of approximately 80 kb of hybridizable sequence and identified in five of six cases a normal human AS mRNA transcript corresponding in size to the larger of the two human AS mRNAs. In the sixth case, a transcript corresponding in size to the larger AS mRNA of rodent cells was detected, presumed to be the product of activation of the hamster AS gene.

Gene transfer also has been performed using recombinant retroviruses containing the cloned human AS cDNA sequence.[370,371] Such virus-mediated transfer of AS could have potential utility for correcting deficiency of enzyme activity in citrullinemia. Introduction of a functional cDNA into either hepatic or nonhepatic cell types might exert a therapeutic effect. In the case of nonhepatic cells, because the substrate citrulline can cross plasma membranes, it is conceivable that its entry into extrahepatic cells containing transferred AS could result in its efficient metabolism. Product argininosuccinate could be further metabolized in these same cells, or because this intermediate also can cross membranes, it could be subsequently metabolized in the liver.

In the retrovirus studies, initial experiments used recombinant ecotropic viruses carrying AS cDNA sequences to infect XC cell lines devoid of AS activity, permitting selection for transduction of AS by ability of transformants to grow in citrulline-containing (arginine-free) medium. Blot analysis of the transformants revealed the presence of the recombinant proviral genome. This genome also contained the bacterial *Neo* gene, which encodes neomycin phosphotransferase, an enzyme that confers resistance to the neomycin analogue G418. Assay of AS activity in the virus transformants revealed a level approximately 10 percent that of normal human liver. In addition to programming expression of AS using ecotropic viruses, an amphotrophic retrovirus with a simplified structure, placing the AS cDNA between two LTRs, has been used to infect both XC cells and immortalized human citrullinemic fibroblasts.[372] AS activity was readily detected in these cells by means of incorporation of added ^{14}C citrulline into total cell protein.

Long-term expression of AS has been observed in mice after bone marrow transplantation with retrovirus-transduced marrow cells.[371] The marrow cells were cocultivated with lethally irradiated producer cells, then isolated on Percoll gradients and injected into lethally irradiated recipients. When amphotropic virus was used, increased AS activity could be detected in peripheral blood for periods of 4 to 6 weeks but then declined. By contrast, when ecotropic virus was used, a stable increase was observed for the lifetime of the animals. The level of activity in blood could be correlated with the percentage of granulocyte–macrophage spleen colonies that contained the recombinant AS segment.

More recently, a mouse model for citrullinemia has been produced, carrying a homologous recombination-generated disruption of the AS gene, that offers an excellent target for testing gene transfer strategies.[373] These animals develop hyperammonemia (2680 ± 970 μM by 16 h) and die within 24 h of birth. Plasma citrulline was elevated 64-fold over normal; aspartic acid was elevated 30-fold; and arginine was 42 percent of normal. These features closely resemble those of severely affected humans, validating this as an animal model.

AS Deficiency

With cloned AS sequences, it has been possible to conduct molecular analyses of citrullinemia patients. Blot analysis of genomic DNA has been made difficult by the profusion of pseudogenes, but cloned intron probes have been of help. Gross deletions were not observed in Southern blot analysis of genomic DNA derived from 11 cell lines.[374] In early studies, three polymorphisms were detected in the AS locus, with the enzymes *Hind* III, *Sph* I, and *Pst* I,[375] and a highly polymorphic microsatellite variable number of tandem repeats (VNTR) [GT repeat; nine alleles, polymorphic information content (PIC) = 0.79] was also found.[376]

Analysis of patients with classical citrullinemia at the RNA and genomic levels reveals two common mutations in Japanese patients, accounting for approximately 70 percent of alleles in Japan, but no such homogeneity in American patients.[361] The collective of mutations identified to date in both populations is presented in Fig. 85-13. The two common Japanese lesions involve an A → G base change at the −2 position in intron 6, affecting the splice acceptor site and leading to deletion of exon 7, accounting for approximately 50 percent of Japanese alleles,[378,380] and the substitution R304W, accounting for another approximately 20 percent of Japanese alleles.[377–379] Expression of the latter substituted protein in *E. coli* yielded an enzyme with specific activity approximately 1 percent of normal, and a K_m for the substrate citrulline increased by four orders of magnitude.[379] The considerable number of additional alleles identified, coming from various genetic compounds of Japanese or American origin, have been analyzed initially at the RNA level by RT-PCR sequence analysis, but in many cases, particularly where splicing is affected, by exon amplification and sequencing.[377] Diagnosis using various primer pairs and restriction digestion is indicated in Fig. 85-13, and reference to study of the particular alleles is as designated.

Although citrullinemia patients producing protein with abnormal kinetics have been designated type I and those with little or no protein have been designated type III,[374] in Japan a third class of patients with adult-onset hepatic AS enzyme deficiency with normal AS mRNA[383] and a reduced amount of AS protein with normal kinetic properties, has been reported, termed type II. This defect appears to lie outside of the AS locus because, even in consanguineous families, no homozygosity of markers was consistently observed at this locus in affected patients.[384] An mRNA differential display comparing hepatic mRNA of type II with normal mRNA showed a strong increase of mRNA for pancreatic secretory trypsin inhibitor, an acute phase protein that is primarily expressed in pancreas but also in liver and ectopically in various tumors.[385] The relationship of this increase to the deficiency of AS protein is unclear, but the induction of the trypsin inhibitor as detected in serum may be useful as a diagnostic marker.

Deficiency of AS also has been reported in a strain of dairy cattle in Australia, with AS mRNA at levels less than 5 percent of

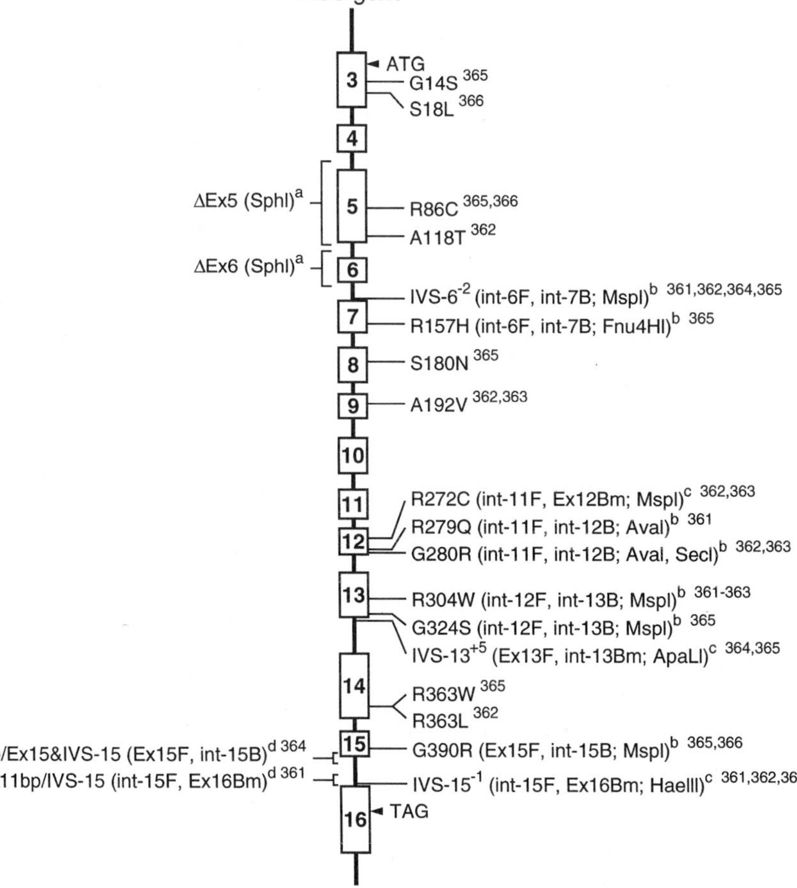

Fig. 85-13 Mutations in the argininosuccinate synthetase gene and their DNA diagnoses. Those detected by RFLP analysis are designated with a superscript "a"; those detected by PCR and restriction digestion by "b"; by modified PCR and restriction digestion by "c"; by PCR and size of product by "d." Exons are numbered in the boxes. Primers and restriction enzymes are shown in parentheses. References to the mutation study follow. (*Reprinted with permission from Kakinoki H, Kobayashi K, Terazono H, Nagata Y, Saheki T: Mutations and DNA diagnoses of classical citrullinemia. Hum Mutat 9:250, 1997.*)

normal. Both amplified cDNA and genomic sequences reveal a nonsense mutation changing Arg 86 to a stop codon.[386]

Argininosuccinate Lyase

Molecular study of argininosuccinate lyase has revealed a structural as well as a catalytic function to this protein in some species and, like the other enzymes of the urea cycle, substantial heterogeneity in human mutation. cDNA clones encoding both human[387] and rat[388] AL were originally isolated using antibody screening of λgt11 libraries followed by confirmation of identity using hybridization-selected mRNA translation. The human cDNA contains an open reading frame encoding a subunit of the homotetrameric enzyme of 463 amino acids, predicting a size of approximately 52 kDa. The predicted subunit has the same number of residues as the previously analyzed yeast enzyme and shares 56 percent of its amino acids with that enzyme. Complementation studies as well as more recent crystallographic analyses indicate that there are four active sites present in each homotetramer, with the active site in each "corner" of the homotetramer contributed to by three of the subunits.

Relationship to Crystallins. Remarkably, human AL has approximately 60 percent homology with a protein found in abundance in the lenses of birds and reptiles — crystallin.[389] In ducks, there are two closely related crystallins, apparently the product of gene duplication, and both are highly similar to AL of humans. Surprisingly, when duck lenses were assayed for AL activity, an enormous amount was detected.[390,391] This observation was consistent with a dual role of AS as both a catalyst and a structural component. Apparently the thermodynamic stability and ability of the enzyme to accumulate to high intracellular concentration without precipitation, allowing transparency, made AL as well as several other enzymes attractive for utilization as a major protein of the lens (see Simpson et al.[392] concerning supramolecular packing of δ-crystallin). Remarkably, the high level of AL enzyme activity is tolerated by lens metabolism, perhaps as a feature of compartmentalization or regulation within the lens cells.[393]

Although dual function is observed for δ-crystallins of duck, following gene duplication there has been some divergence of the two δ-crystallins. Only one of the gene products, δD2, has retained enzymatic activity.[394] By contrast, δD1-crystallin appears to have evolved as a structural component, because it lacks AL activity. The structural basis for the lack of activity of δD1 has been suggested from crystallographic studies comparing a δD2-crystallin from duck with enzymatically inactive turkey δD1-crystallin: the N-terminal tail and a loop at aa 76–91 (in domain 1) differ significantly between the two structures, and this may produce failure of δD1 to bind substrate, as was observed for an H91N δD2 mutant.[395] This evolution of the δD1 subunit, remaining assembly competent but unable to recognize substrate, would account for the observation that activity of δD1/2 heterotetramers naturally formed in the duck lens and experimentally separated by isoelectric focusing is directly proportional to the number of δD2 polypeptides in any given heterotetramer.[396] An even further evolutionary divergence from an AL active form has occurred in chickens, in which δD1-crystallin is the major species found in the lens and lacks AL activity, whereas δD2-crystallin is only a minor species (1 percent of δD1) in the lens and confers only a low level of AL activity.[397] However, high expression of AL activity in avian lens seems likely to have been present before the duplication event, because a lens-specific enhancer has been identified in the same intron (intron 3) of both chicken genes.[398]

The common evolutionary path of the mammalian and avian AL gene is supported by the observation that the genomic organization of the chicken genes with respect to exon–intron boundaries is identical to that of the rat AL gene.[399] Although δD-crystallins are present in most avian species, they are apparently not required for a functional lens — the chimney swift lacks them entirely.[400] Conversely, it should be noted that birds lack a urea cycle; however, they require a functional AL gene product in order to carry out arginine biosynthesis.

Transcriptional Expression. The mRNA species observed in Northern analysis of rat liver mRNA using the human cDNA as probe was approximately 2 kb in size. A somewhat larger 5′-untranslated sequence was detected in a brain cDNA bearing the same coding sequence.[401] Rat AL mRNA increased 12-fold following starvation for 5 days and 2-fold following treatment with dibutyryl cAMP but did not change following dexamethasone treatment.[60] In isolated late fetal hepatocytes, dexamethasone increased AL mRNA levels whereas insulin prevented the effect. Administration of cortisol to fetuses *in utero* was without effect, but insulin depletion increased AL mRNA levels.[402] Levels of AL mRNA also have been measured in rat hepatoma lines and are variable, but correlated with amounts of enzyme activity.[403] Southern analysis of somatic cell hybrids confirmed the previous localization of the human AL gene to chromosome 7, although the 5′ portion of the human cDNA hybridized with sequences on chromosome 22.[404] Whether this latter genomic sequence represents a truncated pseudogene is unknown.

AL Deficiency

McInnes and co-workers have conducted complementation studies of AL deficiency using fibroblast lines derived from patients. Lines from 28 patients were fused in pairwise combinations and AL activity examined in the heterokaryons.[405] All the mutants mapped to a single major complementation group, but extensive interallelic complementation was observed, separating the mutants into 12 subgroups. This suggested the presence of at least 12 allelic mutations and indicated extensive genetic heterogeneity at the AL locus, like the other urea cycle loci examined. The cell lines were further examined at the protein level by blot analysis of extracts. The quantity of immunoreactive protein did not correlate with the amount of residual enzyme activity, consistent with the presence of at least one class of mutant with catalytically inactive protein. In some of the lines, immunoreactivity was detected in smaller molecular size species, suggesting degradation of unstable translation product.

The conclusions drawn from complementation and immunoblot studies were supported by PCR amplification, cloning, and sequence analysis of RNA from the AL-deficient fibroblasts.[406] Six different mutations were observed in four independent lines in an initial study: three were missense mutations (R111W, Q286R, and R193Q), one was a nonsense mutation (Q454X), and two were exon deletions. Additional site-directed changes were tested in yeast cells devoid of endogenous AL activity. A further consanguineous mutant was found to exhibit an R95C substitution.[407] When this cDNA was expressed in COS cells, normal levels of RNA were observed, but only a small amount of AL protein was detected, associated with less than 1 percent normal activity.

Subsequently, mutational analysis has focused on cell strains that either frequently complemented others or that complemented with a high degree of restoration of activity.[408] Q286R was found in the former category, whereas D87G produced the latter action. When these mutations were introduced into AL cDNA and expressed in COS cells alone, less than 0.01 percent and 4.5 percent specific activity was detected, respectively, but when introduced together, on separate encoding plasmids, a specific activity of approximately 30 percent of wild type was recovered. The basis to this intragenic complementation has been determined from crystallographic studies of δ-crystallin and AL, respectively.[409,410] It was known from the primary structures of δ-crystallin, AL, and other tetramers catalyzing a reaction homologous to that of AL (e.g., fumarase, aspartase, adenylosuccinase) that there are three highly conserved regions (12, 12, and 18 residues in size) that are intolerant of mutation and believed to be involved in catalysis. In the crystal structures of δ-crystallin (2.5 Å) and AL (4 Å), these regions indeed contribute to four sites,

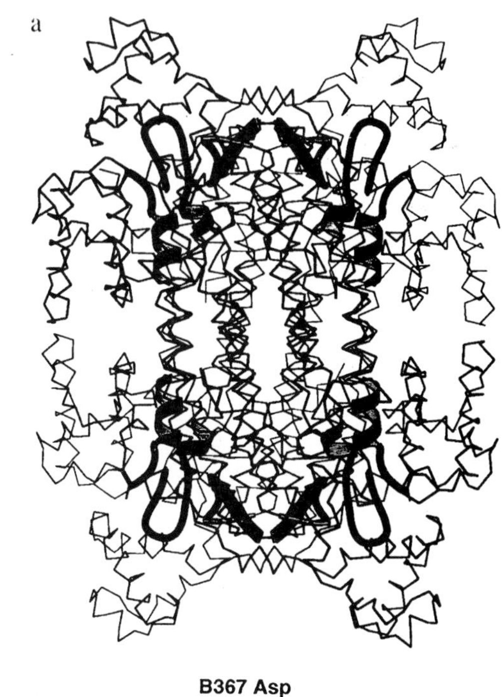

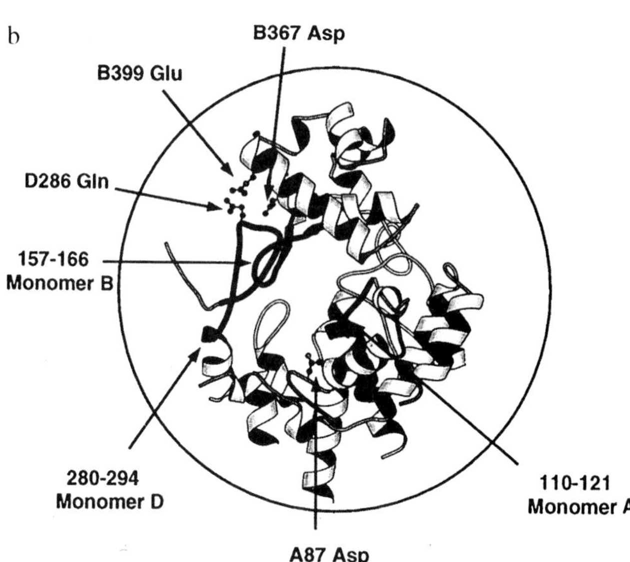

Fig. 85-14 Structural features of human argininosuccinate lyase, determined from the 4 Å crystal structure. A: General architecture illustrated in ribbons trace, showing the pair of dimers, with black regions indicating conserved residues. B: An active site region (of four per tetramer), contributed by residues from three adjacent monomers. See text and Turner et al.[410] for discussion of potential catalytic mechanism. (*Reprinted with permission from Turner MA, Simpson A, McInnes RR, Howell PL: Human argininosuccinate lyase: A structural basis for intragenic complementation. Proc Natl Acad Sci U S A 94:9063, 1997.*)

one in each of the "corners" of the tetramer (Fig. 85-14). Each site is composed of the three highly conserved regions, one region deriving from each of three separate subunits. Supporting the notion that this is the active site, cocrystals of fumarase complexed with inhibitors reveal the inhibitors in these sites.[411] The catalytic mechanism of AL has been speculated in relation to its active site[410]; a sequence of proton abstraction with production of a carbanion intermediate, followed by proton addition, is probable. A histidine (160, in conserved region 2) has been proposed to mediate proton abstraction; a lysine (287, in conserved region 3) has been proposed as potentially stabilizing the carbanion.[410] The identity of the proton donor is unclear. Nevertheless, with this information, taking intragenic complementation into consideration, the nature of complementation by the 87 and 286 mutations is suggested to arise not from the coadjustment of two nonfunctional regions in the same active site, but rather to arise from the production of active sites that have neither mutant 87 nor 286 regions contributing to them (Fig. 85-15).[410] In particular, in a 1:3 homotetramer there will be one active site, whereas in two of the three potential arrangements of 2:2 tetramers there will be two active sites. The overall expected activity of this collective of tetramers would be approximately 25 percent, approximating the 30 percent observed in the COS cell reconstruction experiment.[412] Although this model thus seems likely to explain intragenic complementation, the other model, invoking activity from a doubly mutant active site, does not seem entirely excluded. Kinetic data, showing that the affinities for substrates and inhibitors of the 87/287 mutant reconstruction is unchanged from wild type, would provide strong additional support for the model that it is nonmutant active sites that are restoring activity.

Arginase

The terminal enzyme of the urea cycle is a homotrimeric enzyme that hydrolyzes arginine to produce urea plus ornithine. It exhibits tissue-specific expression in liver and erythrocytes and exhibits the same large degree of heterogeneity of human mutation. cDNA clones encoding rat liver arginase have been synthesized from mRNA enriched for the arginase species by polysome immunopurification.[414] These were in turn used to isolate human liver arginase cDNA clones.[415] cDNA clones have been verified as encoding arginase by hybrid-selected translation, directing synthesis of the 35-kDa enzyme subunit. This subunit expressed from cloned cDNA in *E. coli* was further characterized and exhibited chemical, immunologic, and catalytic properties identical to those of arginase from human erythrocytes.[416] Thus, the hepatic and red cell versions of the enzyme appear identical. These enzymes were found as trimers. The structure of the rat liver enzyme has recently been determined crystallographically at 2.1 Å resolution, revealing the homotrimer of three 35-kDa monomers, with each subunit containing an active site.[417]

When the cloned rat cDNA was used to probe hepatic polyA+ RNA, a species of approximately 1700 bases was identified. Because 1000 bases is sufficient to encode the 35-kDa enzyme subunit, the mRNA is predicted to contain approximately 700 bases of untranslated sequence. When mRNA from tissues other than liver and red cells was examined, negligible amounts of mRNA were detected. In particular, in human embryonic kidney cells, which contain high levels of mitochondrial arginase activity, no hybridization was observed, consistent with the idea that hepatic cytosolic arginase and renal mitochondrial arginase are encoded by two separate genes with substantially different structures.[419] In support of this idea, isozyme studies indicated that in patients deficient in the hepatic red cell enzyme activity (termed AI), activity of the kidney enzyme (AII) was elevated fourfold.[420] Subsequently, cDNAs encoding the AII enzyme have been isolated from *Xenopus laevis*, HepG2 cells, and human kidney, encoding a 38-kDa protein homologous along its length to the AI enzyme except for the addition of a 32-residue mitochondrial targeting peptide at its N-terminus.[421–423] In the mature portion of the protein, the active site histidine and aspartate residues of the AII enzyme are absolutely conserved with AI, indicating that the catalytic mechanism of this enzyme is the same. Because the AII enzyme from human kidney is 58 percent identical to type I human enzyme and 71 percent identical to the *Xenopus* enzyme, it was suggested that arginase gene duplication occurred before the divergence of mammals and amphibians.[421,423] mRNA for the AII enzyme was detected ubiquitously in human and mouse tissues. The functional role of AII is unclear, but a role in downregulating nitric oxide synthesis by removal of arginine substrate by AII was supported by Gotoh et al.,[422] who observed that LPS induction of a macrophage-like cell line caused simultaneous induction of iNOS and AII. A potential role of AII in glutamate and proline synthesis, by hydrolyzing arginine to

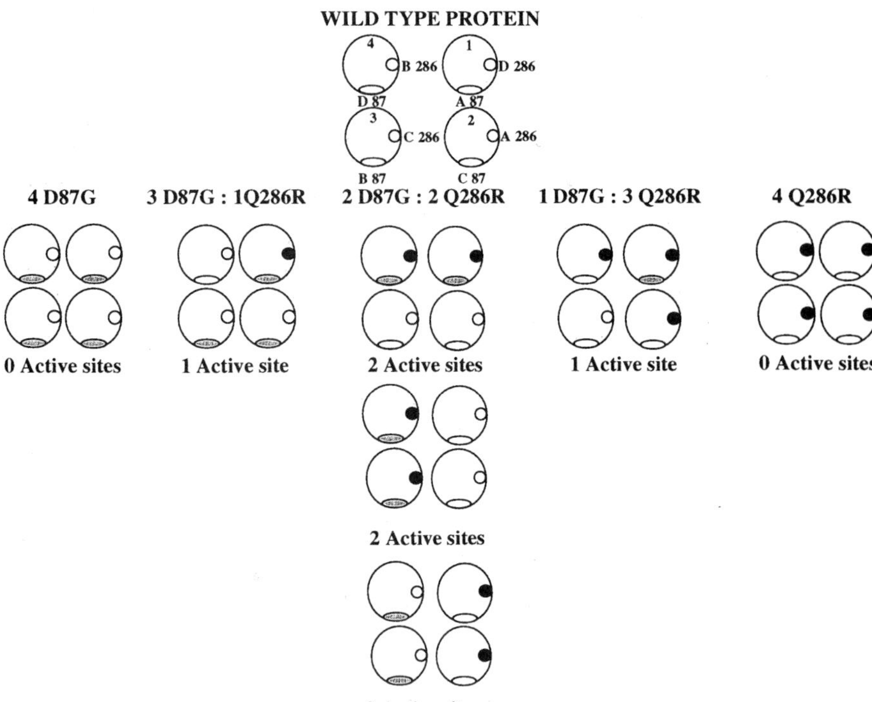

Fig. 85-15 Intragenic complementation: possible combinations of active sites of D87G:Q286R producing intragenic complementation of the AL tetramer. Each circle represents an active site and the circle within represents D87 status, whereas the oval within represents Q286 status, with open indicating wild type and black or shaded indicating mutant. There are four monomers, designated A through D. For 2 × 87:2 × 286, there are three ways to combine the monomers that will give rise to either two or zero native active sites; for 3:1 and 1:3, the monomer bearing the mutation also must be considered, giving rise to different possible solutions. Thus, overall, the combinations have a degeneracy of 1:4:6:4:1. (*Reprinted with permission from Turner MA, Simpson A, McInnes RR, Howell PL: Human argininosuccinate lyase: A structural basis for intragenic complementation. Proc Natl Acad Sci U S A 94:9063, 1997.*)

ornithine (followed by ornithine aminotransferase-mediated conversion to P5C) also has been suggested, in relation to varying levels of different isoforms of the AII enzyme, correlating with different collagen syntheses in developing tadpoles.[421]

The level of hepatic (type I) arginase mRNA in adult rats increased 24-fold following 5 days of starvation; 7-fold following treatment with dibutyryl cAMP; and 2-fold following dexamethasone treatment.[60] When mRNA from H4 hepatoma cells was examined, as predicted from the presence of hepatic arginase enzyme activity in this cell line, a substantial level of arginase mRNA was detected. Hydrocortisone treatment of these cells increased the level of detectable enzyme activity; correspondingly, the level of hybridizable mRNA was increased. Southern blot analysis of rat and mouse genomic DNA conducted with the rat liver cDNA probe revealed a simple pattern suggesting the presence of a single gene whose size is not greater than 15 kb. When the human cDNA clone was used to probe human genomic DNA, a hybridization pattern suggesting a single gene was observed. Using somatic cell hybrids, this locus was mapped to band q23 of chromosome 6.[424] Human genomic sequences were isolated and analyzed, revealing a gene 11.5 kb in size containing eight exons.[425] Twenty-eight bases upstream from the hepatic cap site, a TATA-like sequence was identified. A site resembling those binding CTF–NF1 was identified at −72. Glucocorticoid response elements, cAMP response elements, and enhancer core sequences were also observed. A DNase I–protected area was observed and contained these binding sites; also, several hypersensitive sites were observed in hepatic nuclear extracts. *In vitro* transcription using hepatic nuclear extracts revealed accurate transcriptional initiation and was more efficient than with brain extracts.[425] Deletion analysis showed that the DNase I–protected areas at −90 to −51 exerted positive regulation. Factors bound to these sites were shown to be CTF–NF1 and C-EBP, respectively, by oligonucleotide competition analysis. In a further study, the factors binding to two footprinted regions, designated A at −90 and B at −55, were assessed using cotransfection of plasmids encoding various factors with one joining the arginase promoter, −299 to +37, to CAT.[426] Both the C-EBPs (α, β, or γ) and the albumin D-element binding protein (also a B-zip protein) stimulated transcription, with C-EBPβ the strongest stimulator. Recombinant C-EBPβ protein bound to both area A and area B in gel shift assays, although the latter was speculated to be primarily responsible for C-EBP–mediated activation. By contrast, the promoter was inhibited by HNF-4, found to be mediated through site B.

A glucocorticoid-responsive element was identified by transient transfection of hepatoma cells, localizing to a 233 base segment positioned 11 kb downstream from the transcription start, spanning the junction of intron 7 and exon 8.[427] A number of protein binding sites were identified in this region, two of which appear to be recognized by C-EBP family members. This element could confer glucocorticoid responsiveness when adjoined with a herpes simplex virus thymidine kinase promoter in rat hepatoma H4IIE cells.[428] As might be predicted, footprinting of the two C-EBP regions changed upon steroid treatment, and supershift assays showed that C-EBPβ is one of the components bound. Induction of arginase mRNA by glucocorticoid is delayed in its response; this appears to be at least in part the result of initial induction of C-EBPβ mRNA and protein followed by binding to the 233 base element.

Structure of Hepatic Arginase, and Proposed Mechanism of Its Action, Involving a Manganese Binuclear Cluster in the Active Site. Our understanding of the mechanism of arginase-mediated arginine hydrolysis, particularly the mechanism of a binuclear metal cluster in catalysis, has been advanced considerably by the determination of the crystal structure of the rat liver enzyme at 2.1 Å by the Christianson group.[417] A Mn^{2+}-Mn^{2+} cluster was found in each subunit at the bottom of an active site cleft that is 15 Å deep (Fig. 85-16). A water molecule was found to bridge between the two metal ions (Figs. 85-17 and 85-18). The observed spin coupling previously observed between the two Mn^{2+} metals[429,430] was accountable by three types of ligand interactions, a bidentate one with Asp 124 (Fig. 85-17), a monodentate with Asp 232 (with Oδ1 coordinated *anti* and *syn* with metals A and B, respectively), and the solvent molecule. Further inspection of the active site cleft[417] suggested that Glu 277 could form a salt link with the guanidinium group of arginine, positioning the electrophilic guanidinium carbon directly over the solvent molecule, which is likely to be the nucleophile (as hydroxide) in the reaction (Fig. 85-18). A tetrahedral intermediate is thus formed that collapses upon proton transfer to the ε-amino group of ornithine.

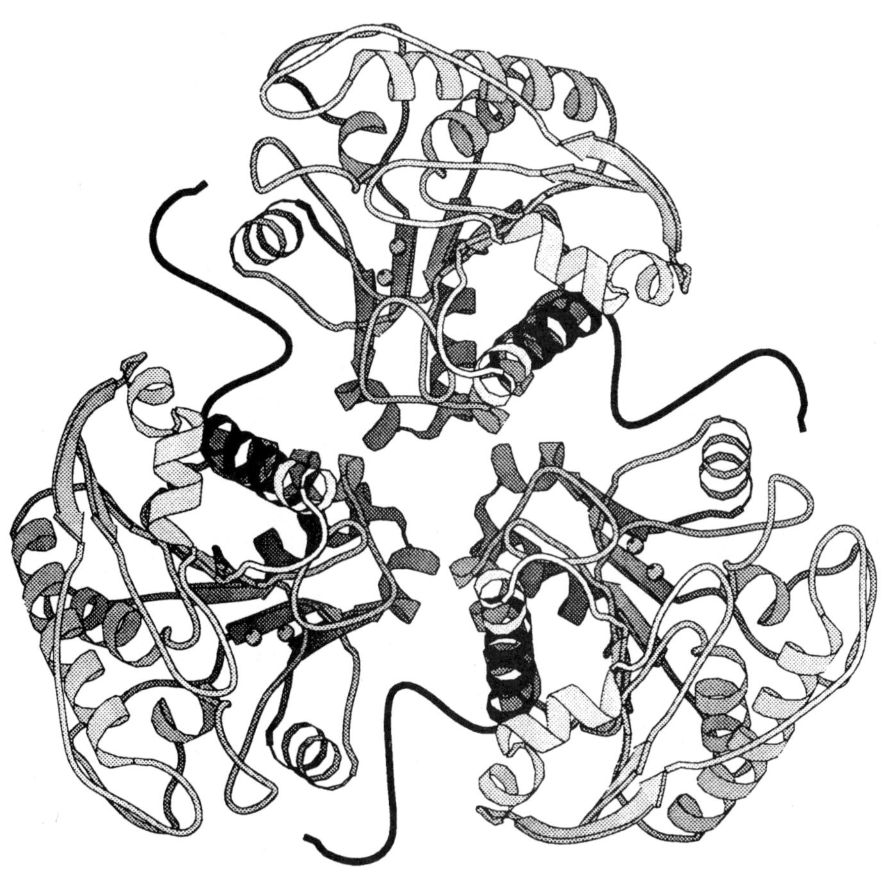

Fig. 85-16 Ribbon diagram of the human arginase homotrimer. The Mn^{2+}-Mn^{2+} cluster in the active site of each monomer is shown as a pair of spheres. The C-terminus of each monomer forms an S shaped oligomerization motif. (*Repinted with permission from Kanyo ZF, Scolnick LR, Ash DE, Christianson DW: Structure of a unique binuclear manganese cluster in arginase. Nature 383:554, 1996.*)

This step of transfer is likely to be mediated by Asp 128. Subsequently, the nearby side chain of His 141 may shuttle a further proton from the solvent onto the ε-amino group of ornithine. Finally, urea dissociates and another water molecule enters the active site to be ionized by the metal cluster.

In addition to spin-labeling studies, support for this mechanism is provided by mutational studies. For example, Cavalli et al.[431] changed each of the three highly conserved histidines in the active site (H101, H126, and H141) to asparagine (Figs. 85-17 and 85-18). They also measured activity in the presence or absence of chelator and examined the effect of diethyl pyrocarbonate (DEP), known to inactivate the enzyme by modifying a single histidine side chain. Replacement of H101N and H126N had only modest effects on activity, but chelator abolished activity of these enzymes, supporting the notion that these His residues are normally ligands to the binuclear center (and that asparagine serves as a weaker ligand) and that both metals are essential for activity. By contrast, activity of the H141N substitution was more substantially reduced (in the presence of metal), although not completely (to 10 percent of wild type). This substitution, however, was unaffected by addition of chelator. Nevertheless, the 141 substitution was resistant to DEP inactivation, whereas substitution at the other two sites left the enzyme sensitive to DEP. These results are consistent with a role of His 141 in facilitating the reaction, but it is not essential—a proton can apparently be directly extracted from solvent onto ornithine. In a further structural and functional analysis of both wild-type and H101N enzymes, Scolnick et al.[432] observed that removal of $Mn^{2+}{}_{A}$, either by extensive dialysis/chelator treatment of the wild-type enzyme or by substitution of the 101 side chain ligand, compromised both catalysis and thermostability. Crystallographic analyses directly confirmed reduced occupancy of site A metal under these conditions.

Arginase Deficiency

The majority of identified arginase-deficient pedigrees have been screened at the molecular level.[433] Only 2 of 15 affected patients had detectable arginase protein in Western blot analysis of red cell

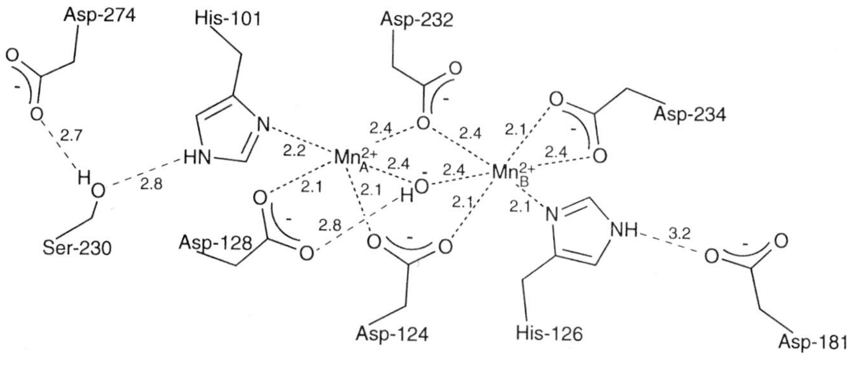

Fig. 85-17 View of the Mn^{2+}-Mn^{2+} binuclear cluster. Hydrogen bonds are indicated by dashed lines. (*Reprinted with permission from Ash DE, Scolnick LR, Kanyo ZF, Vockley JG, Cederbaum SD, Christianson DW: Molecular basis of hyperargininemia: Structure–function consequences of mutations in human liver arginase.* Mol Genet Metab *64:243, 1998.*)

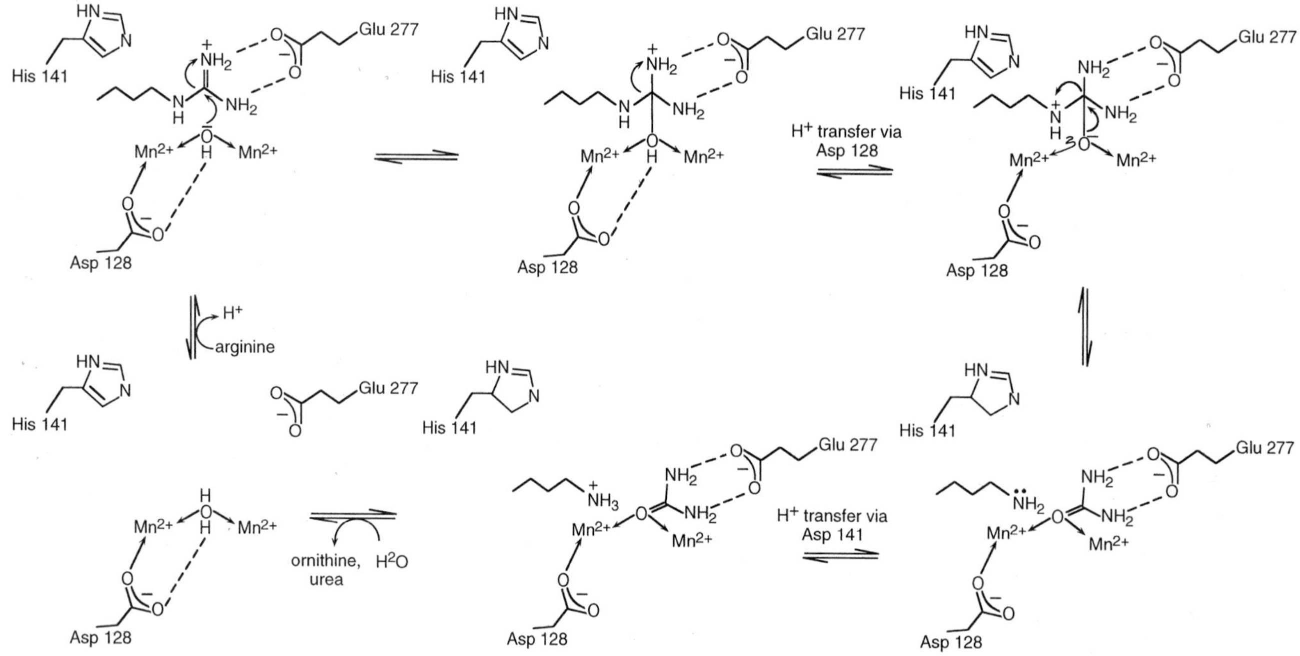

Fig. 85-18 **Proposed mechanism of arginase-catalyzed hydrolysis of arginine by metal-activated solvent. α-amino group and α-carboxylate of the arginine substrate are not shown. (*Reprinted with permission from Kanyo ZF, Scolnick LR, Ash DE, Christianson DW: Structure of a unique binuclear manganese cluster in arginase.* Nature *383:554, 1996.*)**

extracts. At the DNA level, Southern analysis did not identify gross gene deletion in any of these patients. However, a *Taq* I cleavage site was missing in three patients. In two of these, the alteration was identified by PCR amplification of genomic sequences and sequence determination. One patient was homozygous for R291X, and another was heterozygous for T290S. In a second study,[434] cloned genomic sequences from the offspring of a nonconsanguineous mating revealed a compound comprising an allele with a 4-base deletion in exon 3 leading to frameshift at residue 87 and termination 45 residues beyond, and an allele with a 1-base deletion in exon 2 producing a frameshift at residue 26 and termination 5 residues beyond. In further studies of Japanese patients by this group,[435] the mutations W122X, G235R, and L282FS were detected; these products were inactive when expressed in *E. coli*. Even more significantly, they were not detectable in erythrocytes from the patients, most likely reflecting instability. An additional study observed substitutions D128G and H141L,[436] the latter affecting the residue indicated to facilitate proton abstraction at the catalytic site. In a further patient study, I11T, with 10 percent residual activity, and G138V changes were observed, but splice mutants also were detected at the donor site of intron 1 and acceptor site of intron 4.[437] It thus appears that human arginase deficiency, like the other urea cycle defects, is produced by a variety of mutational alterations.

DNA diagnosis thus will rely for the most part on exon amplification and sequencing to directly identify the alleles involved. However, also of potential use are a *Pvu* II RFLP within the arginase locus that has been reported,[413] as well as a dinucleotide repeat polymorphism, with heterozygosity of 47 percent and a PIC of 0.43.[438]

INBORN ERRORS OF UREA SYNTHESIS

Epidemiology

Until relatively recently, urea cycle disorders were thought mainly to be rare diseases of the newborn infant and therefore to be of principal interest to neonatologists. However, the experience at this center over the past 20 years suggests that urea cycle disorders occur at later ages and are more common than previously thought. Table 85-4 describes the distribution of 545 cases referred to The Johns Hopkins Hospital; OTC deficiency constitutes 61 percent of the cases, arginase less than 1 percent and the remainder almost evenly divided at 10 to 13 percent of the cases. An estimate of the absolute incidence of each of these diseases may be calculated by combining these data with argininosuccinase deficiency screening performed at 4 weeks of age,[439] which showed an incidence of 1 per 70,000 live births. These calculations (oversimplified as they may be) revealed that incidence of urea cycle disorders is 1 per 8000 and that OTC deficiency had an incidence of 1 per 14,000 (Table 85-5). These data are similar to those of many commonly recognized diseases; for example, childhood leukemia has an incidence of 1 per 25,000,[440] end-stage renal disease has an incidence of 1 per 100,000.[441]

The distribution of cases of OTC deficiency is shown in Table 85-6. There were 50 percent more late-onset cases than neonatal cases; late-onset cases in males represented 33 percent of these and 20 percent of all late-onset cases.

The clinical presentation of patients with CPS, OTC, AS, and AL deficiencies is virtually identical, but with great variability within and among these diseases. The clinical manifestations may appear in the neonatal period and be fatal, or they may appear any

Table 85-4 Distribution of Urea Cycle Cases Referred to the Johns Hopkins Hospital from 1974 to 1994

Enzyme Deficiency	Number of Cases Referred
Carbamyl phosphate synthetase	69
Ornithine transcarbamylase	334
Argininosuccinic acid synthetase	74
Argininosuccinase	57
Arginase	11
Total	545

Reprinted from Brusilow S, Maestri NE: Urea cycle disorders: diagnosis, pathophysiology, therapy, in Barness LA, DeVivo DC, Kaback MM, Morrow G, Oski FA, Rudolph AM (eds): *Advances in Pediatrics.* Chicago, Mosby, 1996 v 43, p 127; with permission.

Table 85-5 Estimation of the Incidence of Each Urea Cycle Disorder Based on Its Incidence Relative to Argininosuccinase Deficiency

Enzyme Deficiency	Incidence
Carbamyl phosphate synthetase	1 per 62,000
Ornithine transcarbamylase	1 per 14,000
Argininosuccinate synthetase	1 per 57,000
Argininosuccinase	1 per 70,000
Arginase	1 per 363,000
All urea cycle disorders	1 per 8200

Reprinted from Brusilow S, Maestri NE: Urea cycle disorders: diagnosis, pathophysiology, therapy, in Barness LA, DeVivo DC, Kaback MM, Morrow G, Oski FA, Rudolph AM (eds): *Advances in Pediatrics.* Chicago, Mosby, 1996 v 43, p 127; with permission.

time thereafter with varying degrees of severity. The similarity of clinical presentation is related to hyperammonemia, which is common to all these diseases. Their variability is presumably a function of the different mutations (and hence enzyme activity) responsible for them. The variability in severity also may be related to other genomic factors as well as the metabolic consequences of the various enzyme deficiencies; for example, AL deficiency of a degree similar to OTC deficiency may not be as severe a disease because newly synthesized argininosuccinate may serve as a waste nitrogen product. An exception to this general rule exists in the female who carries an OTC mutant allele on one X chromosome; variability in expression in such females is related also to the proportion of hepatocytes in which the normal (or mutant) allele is on the active X chromosome. The other diseases—CPS, AS, and AL deficiencies—are inherited as autosomal-recessive characteristics. These diseases can be distinguished from one another only by appropriate laboratory studies, although a pedigree with evidence of X-linked transmission will suggest a diagnosis of OTC deficiency. AL deficiency has two distinguishing features: severe hepatomegaly in the early-onset form and a hair abnormality (trichorexis nodosa) in the late-onset form. Similar hair abnormalities also have been described in AS deficiency.

Because of the dramatic clinical presentation of these diseases in the neonatal period and the long-term consequences of neonatal hyperammonemia, it is convenient to divide CPS, OTC, AS, and AL deficiencies into two clinical groups: one group presenting in the neonatal period and a second group presenting any time thereafter. It should be recognized, however, that this is an arbitrary division of a continuous spectrum imposed by different mutations and other genomic factors.

Table 85-6 Distribution of Cases of Ornithine Transcarbamylase Deficiency

Distribution	Number of Cases
Neonatal onset	134
Late onset	200
Males	
< 18 yr	61
> 18 yr	5
Females	
< 18 yr	102
> 18 yr	21
Unknown age	11
Total cases	334

Reprinted from Brusilow S, Maestri NE: Urea cycle disorders: diagnosis, pathophysiology, therapy, in Barness LA, DeVivo DC, Kaback MM, Morrow G, Oski FA, Rudolph AM (eds): *Advances in Pediatrics.* Chicago, Mosby, 1996 v 43, p 127; with permission.

The Neonatal-Onset Group

The clinical course of the neonatal group of these diseases is monotonous in its regularity. The infant, almost always the product of a full-term normal pregnancy with no prenatal or perinatal risk factors and normal labor and delivery, appears to be normal for at least 24 h. Sometime between 24 and 72 h (occasionally several days later) the infant becomes lethargic and requires stimulation for feeding. Within hours, additional signs and symptoms may develop, including vomiting, increasing lethargy, and hypothermia. Notwithstanding the rarity of sepsis in the clinical setting of a full-term infant with no apparent risk factors, a misdiagnosis of sepsis is made half the time.[4,442]

The initial laboratory finding of a respiratory alkalosis (the earliest objective indication of encephalopathy and a constant finding in neonatal hyperammonemia prior to the onset of hemodynamic problems) is often unrecognized. Other routine laboratory data are uninformative except for the serum urea nitrogen, which may be as low as 1 mg/dl. Without intervention, the encephalopathy progresses, requiring mechanical ventilation. A diagnosis of intracranial hemorrhage is often considered if a bulging fontanel and increasing head size are noted; however, a CT scan of the head will reveal cerebral edema. If the plasma ammonium level is not measured, the infant's death will be ascribed to sepsis, intracranial hemorrhage, or some other disease commonly associated with prematurity, even though the patient is a full-term infant. Regrettably, the family history is often neglected. A history of consanguinity, neonatal sib deaths, or neonatal male deaths on pedigree analysis is frequently omitted only to be discovered after a diagnosis is made.

The finding of an increased plasma ammonium level will direct diagnostic efforts toward an inborn error of metabolism. The differential diagnosis of hyperammonemia in a neonate is limited to urea cycle enzyme deficiencies, an increasing number of organic acidemias, transient hyperammonemia of the newborn (a poorly understood disease characterized by symptomatic pulmonary disease within the first 24 h of life and severe hyperammonemia[442,443]), and herpes simplex.[444,445] Figure 85-19 demonstrates that by combining the clinical characteristics with plasma amino acid values and urinary orotate excretion, transient hyperammonemia of the newborn, the organic acidemias (as a group) and the individual urea cycle enzyme defects can be distinguished from one another.

Diagnosis

Plasma amino acid analysis measured by automated quantitative column chromatography provides sufficient information to make a confident diagnosis of a deficiency of AS or AL.[446] The former is characterized by plasma citrulline levels (normal levels, 10–20 μM) between 1000 and 5000 μM, and the latter is characterized by the presence of high concentrations of argininosuccinate and its anhydrides, neither of which is normally found in plasma. (An important technical point should be noted in analyzing amino acid chromatograms in infants in hyperammonemic encephalopathy. Unless the retention time of argininosuccinate is known, it may not be recognized because it may cochromatograph with normally occurring amino acids.) Plasma citrulline levels are moderately increased in argininosuccinase deficiency (100–300 μM).

Because citrulline is a product of CPS and OTC, it is undetectable or nearly so in plasma after 24 h of life in hyperammonemic neonates suffering a deficiency in one of those enzymes. CPS and OTC can usually be distinguished by the level of urinary orotate; high levels occur in OTC deficiency as a consequence of diversion of accumulated mitochondrial CP to the cytosolic pyrimidine synthetic pathway. Other pyrimidines, including uracil, uridine, and pseudouridine, have been found in the urine of patients with OTC deficiency.[447,448]

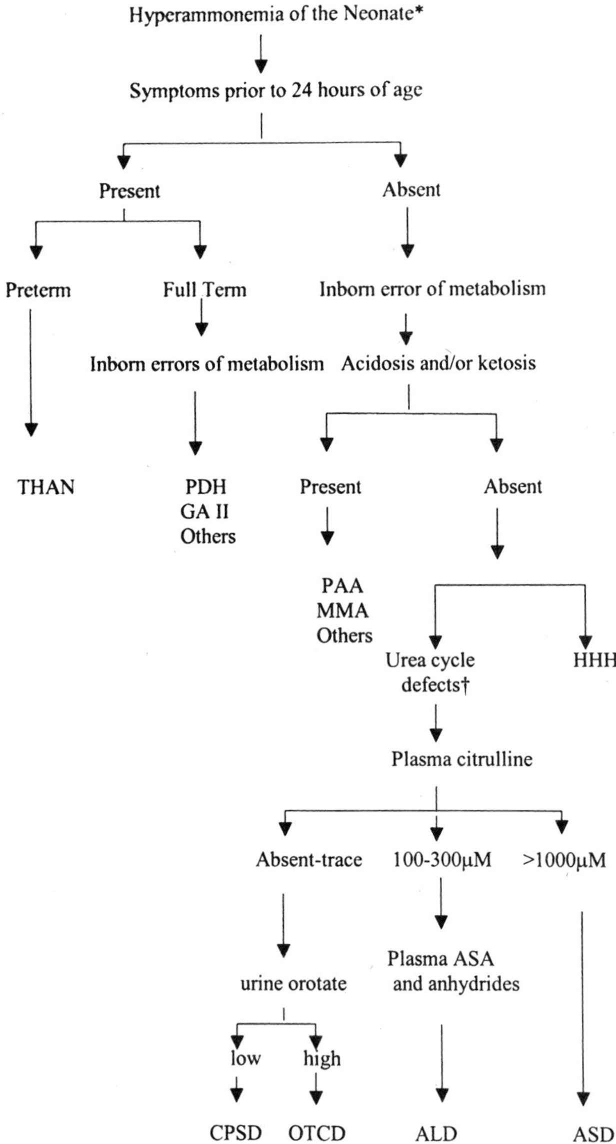

Fig. 85-19 Diagnostic flow chart for neonatal hyperammonemia. Symptomatic hyperammonemia prior to 24 hours of age occurs in two groups: transient hyperammonemia of the newborn (THAN) and those inborn errors in which the pathophysiology may reside in product deficiency. A second group includes those inborn errors of metabolism (urea cycle disorders among them) in which symptoms develops after 24 hours of age, usually following hospital discharge.[4] In this group the pathophysiology is presumably a consequence of the accumulation of a toxic product. *Neonatal herpes simplex may present with severe hyperammonemia[444,445], †a respiratory alkalosis regularly occurs early in the course in urea cycle disorders.[4] Abbreviations: HHH, hyperornithinemia, hyperammonemia, homocitrullinemia syndrome (see Chap. 83); PDH, pyruvate dehydrogenase deficiency; GA II glutaric acidemia type II; PAA, propionic acidemia: MMA, methylmalonic acidemia.

Other abnormalities plasma amino acid levels in include increased plasma glutamine and alanine levels and decreased levels of ornithine and arginine. It may be useful in some cases of OTC deficiency to further establish the diagnosis by detecting the mutation at the OTC locus.

The diagnosis of CPS deficiency is initially made by exclusion; however, because such a diagnosis implies a lifetime commitment to an artificial diet and burdensome medication, it may be appropriate to measure CPS activity in liver obtained by percutaneous biopsy. No complications have been encountered with needle biopsy of liver in these infants after metabolic control is established.

An attempt to make a diagnosis of symptomatic urea cycle defects by discontinuing therapy or protein loading is strongly discouraged; the risks of hyperammonemic encephalopathy outweigh those of liver biopsy. Measurement of CPS and OTC activity on intestinal samples obtained by biopsy may be useful, although experience is limited.[449–451]

Although patients with propionic and methylmalonic acidemia have clinical presentations similar to those with urea cycle defects, there are usually three features that distinguish them: acidosis with ketosis rather than a respiratory alkalosis, high plasma glycine levels, and abnormal urinary metabolites that can be detected by gas chromatography/mass spectroscopy (GC/MS).

There are an increasing number of inborn errors that are associated with severe hyperammonemia (e.g., medium-chain acyl CoA dehydrogenase deficiency, 3-hydroxy,3-methylglutaryl CoA lyase deficiency, pyruvate carboxylase deficiency, glutaric acidemia II, lysinuric protein intolerance). Careful clinical assessment accompanied by appropriate laboratory studies (including plasma lactate and pyruvate as well as analysis of urine by GC/MS) should provide a diagnosis.

NAG Synthetase Deficiency

There are a number of reports[13,452–457] that attempt to describe the phenotype of NAG synthetase deficiency (OMIM 237310). These reports do not provide a clear description of the clinical or biochemical phenotype. The reported major characteristics include severe hyperammonemia, mild hyperammonemia associated with paradoxically deep encephalopathy, recurrent diarrhea and acidosis, movement disorder, hypoglycemia, hyperornithemia, and unexpectedly normal plasma arginine and citrulline levels as well as normal liver NAG content. Diagnosis has relied on assay of liver enzyme activity.[456]

That NAG synthetase deficiency is rarely seen in North America is suggested by our findings that during the diagnosis of 31 patients who presented with the phenotype of CPS and (presumably) NAG synthetase deficiency (e.g., hyperammonemia, acitrullinemia/hypocitrullinemia, and absent orotic aciduria), all 31 had low to undetectable levels of hepatic CPS activity.

The Late-Onset Group

Among the four diseases CPS, OTC, AS, and AL deficiencies, there are few phenotypic differences apart from the hair abnormality in AL deficiency and perhaps AS deficiency as well (hepatomegaly does not appear to be as constant a finding in late-onset AL deficiency as in the neonatal form) and rarely orotic acid crystalluria in OTC deficiency.[458] The variability in age of onset, severity, and degree of residual enzyme activity is similar among the four enzyme deficiencies; there are cases that present from the first year of life to adulthood.[458–466] Figure 85-20 shows an unusual late-onset OTC pedigree in which males appear to have their first episode in the first to fourth decade of life.[464–466] Male-to-female transmission is another unusual characteristic of this pedigree.

The large number of girls in the late-onset group is a consequence of symptomatic OTC deficiency in females, in whom the mutant allele is expressed on the active X chromosome in a preponderance of hepatocytes. The variability of phenotypic expression in females is quite wide.[467–469]

In infants these episodes may be associated with weaning from breast milk or changing from low-protein milk formula to cow's milk; in older children and adults the symptoms may be related to high-protein meals. In all patients, infection may precipitate symptoms, although not infrequently an episode may occur with no obvious cause. The milder episodes will often abate with cessation of protein intake or intravenous infusion of glucose. Many of these patients select a low-protein diet.

It should be emphasized that patients with urea cycle disorders, in whom hyperammonemia develops, rarely present abruptly with

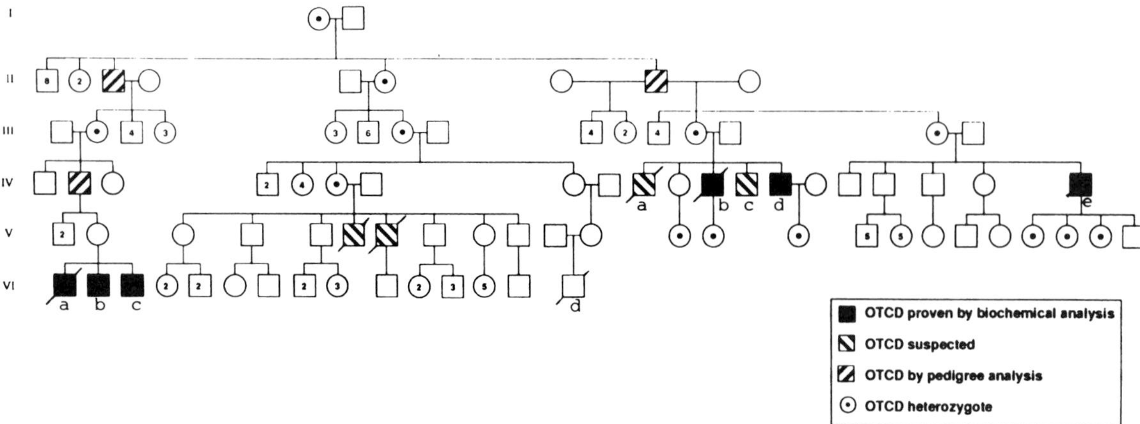

Fig. 85-20 Unusual late-onset OTC deficiency pedigree demonstrating male-to-female transmission.[466] Patient VI-a had multiple episodes of hyperammonemia starting at 9 years of age; his hepatic OTC activity was 7 percent of normal. He died in hyperammonemic coma at 19 years of age. Patients VI-b and VI-c have had episodes of hyperammonemia (starting in childhood) associated with orotic aciduria. Patient VI-d died from liver failure at 9 months of age; he had normal hepatic OTC activity. Patient V-a had a positive allopurinol test result. Patient IV-a died of "encephalitis." Patient IV-b died during his first episode of hyperammonemic coma at 44 years of age. Patient IV-c is mentally retarded. Patient IV-d had an episode of hyperammonemic encephalopathy diagnosed as Reye's syndrome at 30 years of age.[464] Patient IV-e had multiple episodes of hyperammonemia and had hepatic OTC activity that was 26 percent of normal.[313] Both patients IV-d and IV-e had positive allopurinol test results. There is no known consanguinity, nor are the female spouses in the pedigree related.

such neurologic manifestations as apnea, seizures, or loss of consciousness, unless they had sustained brain damage during previous episodes of hyperammonemia. Rather, as described below, hyperammonemia results in the appearance over several days of symptoms and signs attributed to the cerebral cortex, only after which may be followed by seizures or other sudden neurologic manifestations. Whether the reports[470,471] describing sudden strokes in a girl with OTC deficiency are relevant to OTC deficiency and second case in a girl with CPS deficiency are specific to urea cycle disorders or have some other explanation is unclear.

The major symptoms of these episodes of hyperammonemia include vomiting, an abnormal mental status as manifested by lethargy, progressive somnolence, irritability, agitation, combativeness, disorientation, ataxia, and amblyopia. Seizures, delayed physical growth, and developmental delay are common, although there are reports of normal development.[461] Apart from hyperammonemia, routine laboratory studies often reveal a respiratory alkalosis, an early sign of encephalopathy. Diagnostic delay and error are common; the median delay of diagnosis was 16 months. Symptoms have been attributed to colic, gastroenteritis, cyclical vomiting, hyperactivity, encephalitis, Reye's syndrome, epilepsy, anicteric hepatitis, drug toxicity, glioma, and child abuse.[467]

Diagnosis of Late-Onset Urea Cycle Disorders

For patients presenting with hyperammonemia encephalopathy who do not have severe liver disease or malignancy[472,473] the diagnostic possibilities include CPS, OTC, AS, and AL deficiencies; the hyperammonemia, hyperornithinemia, and homocitrullinemia (HHH) syndrome; lysinuric protein intolerance (LPI); a large number of inherited organic acidemias; Reye's syndrome; and ammoniagenesis in an infected distended bladder or ureter.[474] A syndrome that almost completely mimics late-onset OTC deficiency occurs in rare cases of hepatocellular carcinoma.[475] Such patients (two additional patients have been identified here) present with hyperammonemic encephalopathy, orotic aciduria, hyperglutaminemia, and no evidence of liver failure. Unless a hepatocellular carcinoma is detected, this syndrome cannot be distinguished from OTC deficiency.

Plasma amino acid analyses will be diagnostic for AS deficiency (citrulline levels of over 1500 μM), AL deficiency (high concentrations of argininosuccinate and its anhydrides and citrulline levels of 100 to 300 μM), and the HHH syndrome (high concentrations of ornithine and homocitrulline). The organic acidemias will be suggested by the presence, early in the course, of a metabolic acidosis in contrast to the respiratory alkalosis associated with the hyperammonemia in urea cycle disorders. Analysis of urine by GC/MS will usually result in a specific diagnosis of an organic acidemia.

Late-onset CPS deficiency and OTC deficiency cannot be distinguished from each other by amino acid analysis, but the latter is characterized by large increases in urinary orotate, a measurement that is particularly important during hyperammonemic episodes. Pedigree analysis may be helpful. If CPS deficiency is suggested by exclusion, it is recommended that it be confirmed by CPS assay on liver obtained by biopsy because of the therapeutic implications of making this diagnosis. If, as often is the case, orotic acid has not been measured, mutational analysis may be helpful in distinguishing OTC from CPS deficiency. The allopurinol test[476] also may be useful if mutational analysis is unsuccessful. Measurement of hepatic CPS and OTC activity, if properly done, should be definitive for the CPS deficiency, but may be ambiguous for OTC deficiency in women, because the liver is a mosaic of hepatocytes. It has been demonstrated in fatal cases of late-onset OTC deficiency in females that there may be great variability in OTC activity in liver biopsy samples taken from the same liver.[477] For example, 10 samples with a mean weight of 16.8 mg obtained from the liver of a woman with OTC deficiency who died during an episode of hyperammonemic encephalopathy had a range of OTC activity of 3.1 to 16.1 percent of normal values (mean ± SD, 10.2 ± 5 percent). Similarly, in a girl with OTC deficiency who died, the range of 10 measurements of OTC activity (mean sample size of 12.7 mg) was 4.8 to 27.0 percent of normals (mean ± SD, 12.7 ± 8 percent). It has been reported[478] (and we have made a similar observation) that *in vivo* OTC activity may be normal in symptomatic females. These data suggest that detection of very low levels (if properly done) may be helpful in the diagnostic process, but higher levels may be difficult to interpret. Detection of mutations at the OTC locus may be the diagnostic procedure of choice.

Reye's syndrome, which now is rare, may be distinguished by the absence of orotate aciduria and the presence of high liver transaminase levels as well as increased plasma lysine levels.[479]

Table 85-7 Plasma Amino Acid and Ammonia Levels in Carrier Women as Compared with Control Women

	Carriers (n = 75) Mean (SD)	Noncarriers (n = 95) Mean (SD)	IP Mean (SD)
Glutamine	702 (167)	558 (84.4)	<0.001
Citrulline	22.5 (11.6)	31.2 (12.8)	<0.001
Arginine	62.4 (20.3)	85.5 (23.1)	<0.001
Alanine	439 (128)	334 (84.4)	<0.001
Ammonia	27.6 (3.76)	25.5 (2.46)	0.001

All values are μM.

LPI is characterized by increased urinary excretion, principally of lysine, but also of ornithine and arginine.

The Phenotype of Asymptomatic Carriers

An epidemiologic study[476] compared 74 asymptomatic carriers of OTC deficiency with 96 related noncarrier female relative and found similar educational characteristics, anthropometric measurements, medical and pregnancy histories and no evidence of an increased incidence of migraine headaches.

The study confirmed the previously suggested[469,480] plasma amino acid and ammonia differences between the two groups as shown in Table 85-7; carriers had significantly higher glutamine, ammonia, and alanine values and lower citrulline and arginine values. Carriers also differed from the control group in other aspects of nitrogen metabolism; as compared with noncarriers, they excreted less urea (4.88 g vs. 6.05 g/day, $p = 0.006$), and less total urinary nitrogen (6.04 vs. 7.29 g/day, $p = 0.007$). These nitrogen balance data provide quatititative support for the clinical observation that many carriers are protein avoiders.

Some unknown small number of carriers are at risk for symptomatic hyperammonemia in the postpartum period.[480] Four to eight days following a normal pregnancy and perinatal period, a typical hyperammonemic encephalopathy episode develops that, if not treated, results in severe cerebral edema, brain stem compression, and death.

In all 10 such cases referred to this laboratory, the fetus was not an OTC-deficient male. Based on an early report[480] that included five such cases (an additional five such cases are now known), it was proposed that postpartum hyperammonemia in carriers was a consequence of the departure of the urea synthetic capacity provided *in utero* by the fetus and the failure of the woman's partially OTC-deficient liver to compensate for the metabolic stress accompanying the puerperium.

A simplified allopurinol test was developed to establish OTC carrier status in women at risk for being a carrier[476] in the event that molecular techniques are unsuccessful. The sensitivity and specificity were 0.927 and 1.0, respectively, when 24-h orotidine excretion was measured.

Hyperammonemic Encephalopathy: A Disorder of Astrocyte Organic Osmolyte Homeostasis

Hyperammonemia. Unlike patients with decompensated liver disease in which ammonium is only one of several putative toxins,[481] ammonium appears to be the only cause of the acute encephalopathy seen in urea cycle defects (apart from arginase deficiency). Therefore, hyperammonemic encephalopathy as a pathophysiologic entity may be different from hepatic encephalopathy; only the former will be discussed here.

Voorhies et al.[482] have produced a very instructive clinical model of hyperammonemic encephalopathy during a 24-h period in awake primates. All the clinical signs and symptoms found in hyperammonemic patients were reproduced in those experiments. Plasma levels of ammonia were varied over a fivefold range, during which the animals had the progressive behavioral, physiologic, biochemical, electroencephalographic, and neuropathologic changes found in hyperammonemic patients.

At low levels of hyperammonemia the animals exhibited decreased spontaneous activity, disinterest in surroundings, lethargy, and vomiting. These symptoms were associated with slight increases in intracranial pressure and evidence of hyperventilation and a respiratory alkalosis. As the plasma ammonium level increased, all these signs and symptoms worsened: somnolence progressing to seizures, absence of corneal reflexes, apnea, and progressive increase in intracranial pressure. Electroencephalographic changes included slow-wave appearance correlating with the clinical and biochemical status. Several animals with high ammonium levels exhibited burst suppression and long periods of isoelectricity.

Gross neuropathologic changes included brain swelling, flattening of cortical gyri, and herniation of cerebellar tonsils. Light and electron microscopy revealed astrocyte swelling with pleomorphic mitochondria. Of particular importance was the absence of pathologic changes in neurons, axons, dendrites, oligodendroglia, and synapses.

It is apparent from this study and from clinical observations that brain swelling often leading to increased intracranial pressure is a primary physiologic response to hyperammonemia and that neurologic symptoms occur in the absence of neuronal pathology. It may be inferred from these data that the brain swelling is a consequence of swelling of the astrocyte, the only brain cell found to be affected. Because of the intimate relationship of the astrocyte processes with cerebral capillaries and venules, it is not surprising to learn that alterations of cerebral blood flow are commonly found in experimental hyperammonemia.[483–485]

Glutamine: An Astrocyte Organic Osmolyte. It has become increasingly evident that cell volume (glial cells among them) is, to a large degree, determined by intracellular organic osmolyte metabolism.[485a,485b,485c] Because astrocytes are rich in glutamine synthetase, it has been suggested[472,486,487] that the cerebral edema associated with hyperammonemia is a consequence of the osmotic effects of an increased glutamine content of the astrocyte leading to astrocyte swelling. If this were true, then the many other theories accounting for hyperammonemic encephalopathy[481,488,489] could be explained as phenomena secondary to gross alterations of astrocyte size and function and their effects on the functions of adjacent structures (blood vessels, neurons, axons, dendrites, ependyma, and synapses) and could be responsible for the many metabolic and neurochemical abnormalities associated with hyperammonemia.

In the first of a series of experiments done to support the hypothesis, Takahashi et al.[490] demonstrated that the cerebral edema associated with hyperammonemia can be prevented by preventing glutamine accumulation in the brain, suggesting that hyperammonemia is necessary but not sufficient to produce cerebral edema. Table 85-8 summarizes their results; it shows that *in vivo*, the increase in brain water and decrease in brain specific gravity produced by hyperammonemia can be prevented by inhibiting glutamine synthetase activity, thereby preventing glutamine accumulation.

It was later demonstrated that not only can brain glutamine accumulation and the resulting cerebral edema in hyperammonemic states be prevented by methionine sulfoximine (MSO), but the astrocyte swelling associated with hyperammmonemia is also prevented by MSO.[491] Astrocytes in culture behave similarly[492]; swelling in hyperammonemic media is prevented by MSO. It has been shown that hyperammonemia-induced astrocyte swelling may be ameliorated by downregulation of intracellular organic regulatory osmolytes, notably myoinositol.[493]

These data support the hypothesis that ammonia-induced astrocyte glutamine accumulation creates an osmotic gradient that causes a shift of water into the astrocyte, resulting in cerebral edema and increased intracranial pressure, the typical clinical findings in hyperammonemic urea cycle enzyme-deficient patients.

Table 85-8 Plasma Ammonium Levels and Cortical Tissue Water and Biochemical Measurements in Four Groups of Rats*

	Control (Group I)	Control + MSO (Group II)	Ammonium Infusion (Group III)	Ammonium Infusion + MSO (Group IV)
Plasma NH_4 (μM)	29 ± 3	87 ± 7†	601 ± 38†	908 ± 196†
Glutamine synthetase activity, units	38.8 ± 0.8	14.2 ± 0.6†	39.0 ± 0.3	14.1 ± 0.2†‡
Cortical glutamine mmol/kg wet wt	5.6 ± 0.4	1.8 ± 0.4†	18.8 ± 0.4†	2.6 ± 0.4†‡
Cortical specific gravity	1.0452 ± 0.0003	1.0462 ± 0.0003	1.0424 ± 0.003†	1.0446 ± 0.0003‡
Fractional water content of cortex	0.783 ± 0.003	0.782 ± 0.004	0.804 ± 0.003	0.784 ± 0.005‡

Values are means ± SE.
*Control, control plus methionine sulfoximine (MSO) a glutamin synthetase inhibitor, ammonium infused rats and ammonium infused plus MSO treated rats. These studies demonstrate that inhibition of brain glutamin accumulation prevents cerebral edema in hyperammonemic rats.
†0.01 from control group I.
‡ < 0.01 between group III (non-MSO) and group IV (MSO).

However, it appears that cerebral edema may not be the only deleterious effect of glutamine accumulation. Figure 85-21 shows that hyperammonemia causes extracellular potassium concentration to increase; but that increase is attenuated[494] when glutamine synthetase in inhibited.

Pial arteriolar responsiveness to hypocapnia is impaired during hyperammonemia, but this impairment is prevented by glutamine synthetase inhibition.[495] Because pial arterioles are not surrounded by astrocyte end feet, these studies suggest that glutamine or astrocyte dyfunction in some way plays a role in vascular reactivity during hyperammonemia.

Although neurotransmitter dyshomeostasis is clearly responsible for the clinical manifestations of hyperammonemic encephalopathy, there is evidence to suggest that brain neurotransmitter accumulation may be a secondary effect of the consequences of astrocyte glutamine accumulation. For example, the neutral amino acid precursors of serotonin that accumulate in the brains of hyperammonemic animals are prevented by MSO.[496] That neurochemicals by themselves are not responsible for cerebral edema may be adduced by the absence of any neurochemical experimental model that mimics the signs, symptoms, and neuropathology found in hyperammonemic humans or animals. Glutamatergic neurotransmiters do not appear to affect astrocytes, but rather, their pathologic affect appears to be confined to neurons.[497] This theory does not, of course, exclude the fact, as previously noted, that neurotransmitters are the final common pathway accounting for the symptomatology and that therapy directed at the neurochemical abnormality may be beneficial in treating symptoms.

Figure 85-22 describes a pathway that would account for the pathophysiology of hyperammonemic encephalopathy. It suggests that hyperammmonia results in astrocyte glutamine accumulation and astrocyte swelling as well as astrocyte dyfunction.

Glutamine also has been implicated as a factor in hyperammonemic encephalopathy in patients. It has been demonstrated that plasma glutamine levels increase prior to hyperammonemia[498] and that there is a strong correlation between plasma glutamine and ammonium levels (Figs. 85-23 and 85-24).[499] Interpretation of plasma glutamine levels in treated patients must take into account the diurnal variations associated with treatment (Fig. 85-25). The importance of glutamine is supported by the strong relationship between hyperammonemia, neurologic dysfunction, and cerebrospinal glutamine concentration observed in hepatic encephalopathy.[500] During hyperammonemic encephalopathy, cerebrospinal glutamine concentrations in patients with OTC deficiency[501] and AS deficiency[502] are extraordinarily high—6300 and 8660 μM, respectively (normal, 614 ± 241 μM). Further support for this

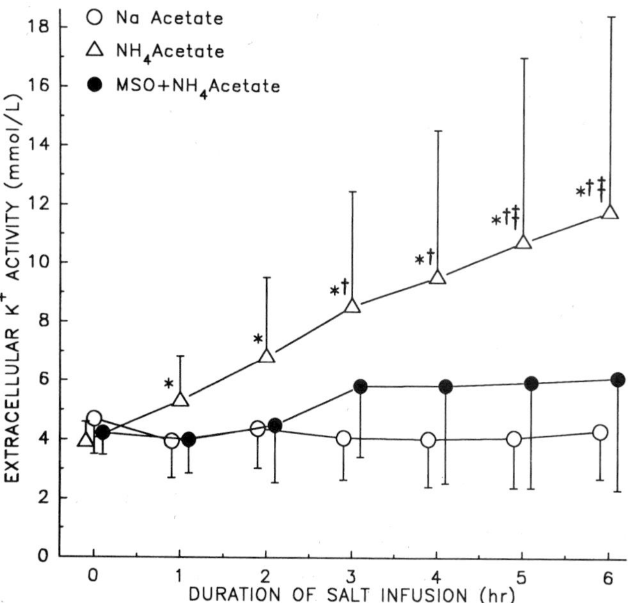

Fig. 85-21 Cortical extracellular K^+ activity (±SD) in groups of rats during intravenous infusion of sodium acetate (n = 8), ammonium acetate (n = 9), and ammonium acetate after MSO pretreatment (n = 8). *p = 0.05 baseline value within group; †p = 0.05 from sodium acetate group at that time; ‡p>0.05 from MSO + ammonium acetate group at that time. (*Reprinted with permission from Sugimoto H, Koehler RC, Wilson DA, Brusilow SW, Traystman RJ: Methionine sulfoximine, a glutamine synthetase inhibitor, attenuates increased extracellular potassium activity during acute hyperammonemia.* J Cereb Blood Flow Metab *17:44, 1997.*)

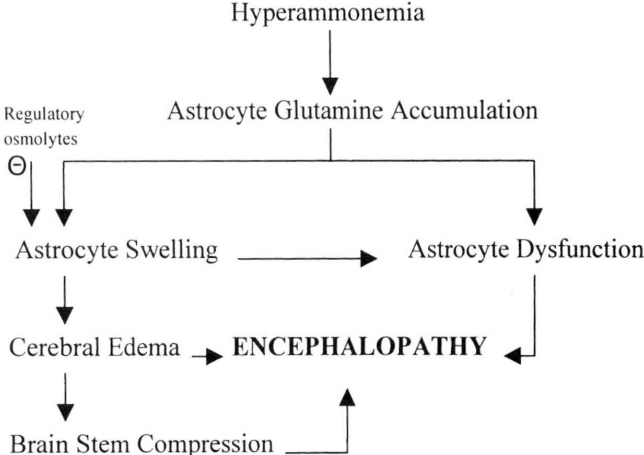

Fig. 85-22 Diagrammatic representation of the pathophysiology responsible for hyperammonemic encephalopathy. The primary event is activation by ammonia of glutamine synthetase within the astrocyte, leading to the accumulation of glutamine within the astrocyte. This has a dual effect: (1) glutamine serves as an intracellular osmolyte, causing entry of water and astrocyte swelling and cerebral edema, and (2) the swollen astrocyte or the high glutamine concentration causes astrocyte dysfunction.

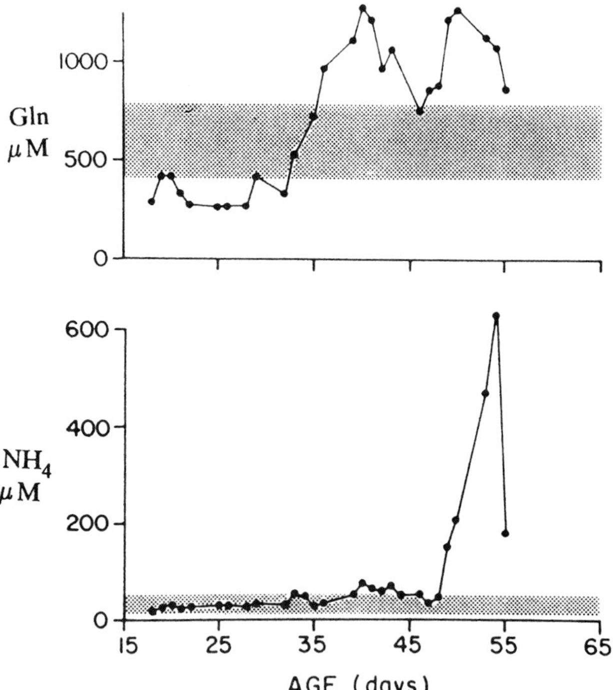

Fig. 85-23 Plasma glutamine and ammonium levels in an infant male with OTC deficiency demonstrating the accumulation of glutamine prior to the onset of severe hyperammonemia. (*Reprinted ith permission from Batshaw ML, Walser M, Brusilow SW: Plasma α-ketoglutarate in urea cycle enzymopathies and its role as a harbinger of hyperammonemic coma.* Pediatr Res *14:1316, 1980.*)

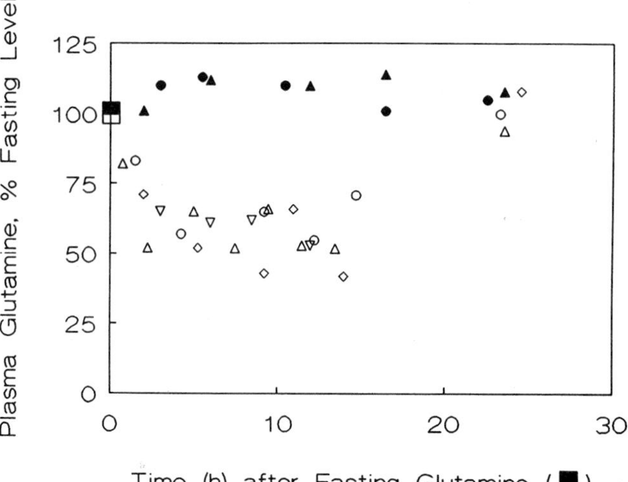

Fig. 85-25 The effect of drug therapy (open symbols) compared with no drug therapy (closed symbols) on the 24-h course of plasma glutamine levels in patients with urea cycle disorders. Fasting levels (μM) for untreated patients were ● = 1030, ▲ = 1110 and for treated patients were △ = 670, ▽ = 1260, □ = 1210, and ○ = 1300. (*Modified with permission from Brusilow SW: Phenylacetylglutamine may replace urea as a vehicle for waste nitrogen excretion.* Pediatr Res *29:147, 1991.*)

theory was obtained in patients with OTC deficiency whose hyperammonemic encephalopathy was shown to be related to brain glutamine accumulation as measured by magnetic resonance spectroscopy.[503] Were it generally available, magnetic resonance spectroscopy would be a desirable noninvasive clinical method to evaluate the degree of brain glutamine accumulation and thereby judge the degree of metabolic control.[503,504]

It has been well documented that ammonium is rapidly incorporated into brain glutamine and that the astrocyte is the site of this incorporation.[505,506] The observation that hyperammonemia activates the synthesis and accumulation of astrocyte glutamine via glutamine synthetase, an ATP-dependent reaction, casts doubt on the ATP depletion theory of hyperammonemic encephalopathy.

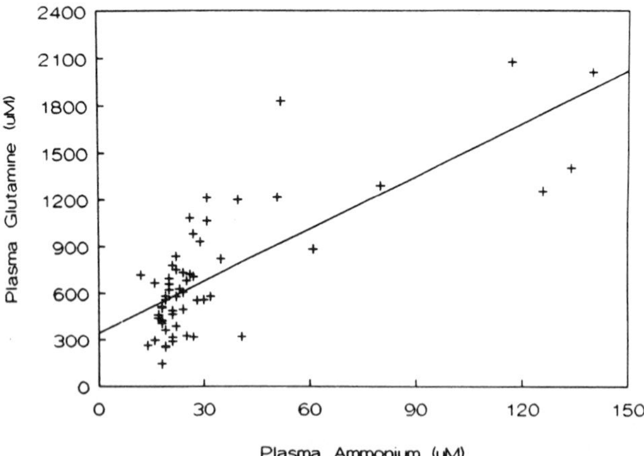

Fig. 85-24 Relationship between plasma glutamine and ammonium concentrations. For all values, the Pearson correlation coefficient between glutamine and ammonia is 0.77 ($p < 0.001$). For plasma ammonium values less than 30 μM, $p = 0.436$; $p < 0.0001$.

Arginine Requirement

The essentiality of dietary arginine for patients with the neonatal form of hyperammonemia was demonstrated,[7] where it was found that removal of arginine from the diet of affected patients (CPS, OTC, AS, or AL deficiencies) promptly resulted in nitrogen accumulation as ammonium or glutamine or both, and orotic aciduria in OTC deficiency and AL deficiency. Citrulline but not ornithine could substitute for arginine.

Except for patients with urea cycle defects (apart from arginase deficiency), arginine is a nonessential amino acid in humans, unlike other animals (carnivores and rodents) who, when challenged with an arginine-free diet have one or more of the following: hyperammonemia, orotic aciduria, or reduced growth rate.[507–509] Infants grow normally on arginine-free diets,[510,511] and adults maintain nitrogen balance[512] and do not have hyperammonemia or orotic aciduria.[513] This difference in arginine metabolism between humans and lower species has important consequences in relating data obtained in lower species to humans.

Substrate Accumulation

Because patients with AS deficiency have plasma concentrations of citrulline as high as 5000 μM (normal limits, 15 to 30 μM), citrulline itself is a candidate neurotoxin. A similar argument has been made for argininosuccinate and its anhydrides in patients with AL deficiency. Evaluation of the potential toxicity of these two compounds has been difficult because of the confounding effect of persistent low-grade hyperammonemia and repeated episodes of hyperammonemic encephalopathy. The use of benzoate, phenylacetate, phenylbutyrate, and arginine in AS deficiency and arginine in AL deficiency has permitted the long-term developmental evaluation with the complications of hyperammonemia minimized.

In the case of AS deficiency, a number of patients in whom hyperammonemia has been prevented show no deterioration of development while maintaining very high concentrations of citrulline in plasma. That argininosuccinate is not toxic may be concluded from the long-term follow-up of 12 patients with treated late-onset AL deficiency; there was no deterioration of intellectual function despite high plasma levels of argininosuccinate and its anhydrides.[514]

The role of arginine accumulation in arginase deficiency is discussed separately under the section on Arginase Deficiency.

Pathology of Urea Cycle Defects

The Brain. Analysis of the morbid anatomy of the brain of patients with urea cycle defects is hampered not only by genetic and clinical heterogeneity within each of these diseases but also by artifacts induced by variable agonal periods. Interpretation of the relative effect of acute and chronic metabolic alterations also is difficult, particularly when superimposed on children of varying ages and varying nutritional states. Furthermore, the pathologic features of the brain in urea cycle defects are described in scattered reports of varying thoroughness.[515–528]

By and large it appears that there are few differences in the neuropathology of deficiencies of CPS, OTC, AS, and AL when onset, severity, and age of death are considered. Acute hyperammonemia of the newborn resulting in death in the first week of life is associated with brain swelling and Alzheimer type II astrocytes in the cortex and brain stem with few other changes. Occasionally, neuronal abnormalities are seen; more rarely, cystic necrosis may be noted at the junction of the cortical white and gray matter. However, neuronal changes in this group of patients are either absent or mild. CT scanning of the brain is useful in describing the extent of brain destruction.[529,530]

The Liver. There are varying degrees of portal fibrosis in AL deficiency survivors and girls with OTC deficiency.[531,532]Although a single case of severe liver fibrosis in AL deficiency has been reported,[533] a review of liver biopsy specimens in five cases revealed considerable variability, with very mild portal fibrosis being the most common finding.[532] One child with AL deficiency, who was rescued from neonatal hyperammonemic encephalopathy, had normal liver architecture after 8 years of treatment.

Electron microscopic examination of liver occasionally reveals abnormalities such as pleomorphic mitochondria with swollen cristae and dense matrixes as well as pathologic changes in the endoplasmic reticulum.[534,535] It appears that these ultrastructural changes in CPS, OTC, and AL deficiencies may not be found unless hyperammonemia is present, except perhaps in AL deficiency, in which these abnormalities were noted while the patient was under good metabolic control. Similar electron microscopic findings have been described in mice in whom hyperammonemia was induced by urease injection.[535] Liver function, particularly synthetic function, is normal, although increased transaminase levels are not uncommon during but not limited to episodes of hyperammonemia.

Measurement of Plasma Ammonium Levels

Interpretation of plasma ammonium measurements is hampered by the absence of peer-reviewed comparative studies of the accuracy and reproducibility of any of the various methods in use, particularly as applied to the intensive care environment.

TREATMENT OF UREA CYCLE DEFECTS

The goal of therapy of urea cycle defects is to provide a diet sufficient in protein, arginine, and energy to promote growth and development while preventing the metabolic perturbations associated with those diseases—hyperammonemia and hyperglutaminemia. Thus, successful therapy can be judged by anthropometric and nutritional assessment and maintenance of normal plasma ammonium and glutamine levels. Measurement of plasma glutamine level may be the best single guide to effective therapy because it appears to be a harbinger of hyperammonemia (Figs. 85-19 and 85-20)[498,499] and may reflect the fundamental pathophysiology of hyperammonemic encephalopathy.

It appears that glutamine represents a storage form of nitrogen that can offer substantial short-term "buffering" of ammonium. Maintenance of plasma glutamine levels at normal or near-normal levels, if possible, is an important goal of therapy.

There are three components of nitrogen metabolism to consider in designing therapy: nitrogen intake, nitrogen retention in protein (which will vary with growth rate), and nitrogen excretion. Early recommendations for therapy included the manipulation of dietary nitrogen to reduce the requirement for waste nitrogen synthesis via the urea cycle. This was attempted by providing low-protein diets, essential amino acid diets,[536] or a combination of essential amino acids and several of their nitrogen-free analogues.[537] These approaches failed for patients with the severe enzyme deficiencies.

The explanation for the failure of dietary therapy probably resides in the mechanism for maintenance of nitrogen balance and nitrogen retention.[538,539] When nitrogen intake falls below a threshold level, the positive balance between protein degradation (which normally is approximately 6.6 g/kg/day in infants) and protein synthesis (which normally is approximately 7.0 g/kg/day) will become negative; protein degradation will exceed protein synthesis, and growth failure will ensue. Because the amount of nitrogen intake required for growth exceeds nitrogen retention, there must be a mechanism to excrete the nitrogen not retained. To the extent that there is residual ureagenic capacity, there will be a residual degree of dietary nitrogen tolerance. In the absence or near absence of residual ureagenesis, some other pathway of waste nitrogen excretion will be necessary to prevent nitrogen accumulation.

It should be noted that during the first months of life, dietary nitrogen tolerance in patients with defective ureagenesis will be substantially greater than in later years because the requirement for urea synthesis in the rapidly growing infant is only 19 percent of nitrogen intake as compared with over 80 percent in children and adults.[540]

Treatment of Argininosuccinase Deficiency

Because argininosuccinic acid contains the same two nitrogen atoms destined for urea synthesis, and because its renal clearance is the same as the glomerular filtration rate, it was proposed[541,542] that argininosuccinate might serve as a waste nitrogen product in patients with argininosuccinase deficiency (Fig. 85-26 and Table 85-9). To promote argininosuccinate biosynthesis in these patients, it is necessary to provide large amounts of exogenous arginine because the major pathway for arginine biosynthesis is impaired via argininosuccinase. Secondly, although ornithine may be synthesized *de novo* via ornithine aminotransferase, the equilibrium of this reaction greatly favors ornithine degradation; although adequate to supply the daily arginine requirement, it appears that the reverse reaction cannot supply sufficient ornithine to permit adequate argininosuccinic acid synthesis for maintaining nitrogen homeostasis.

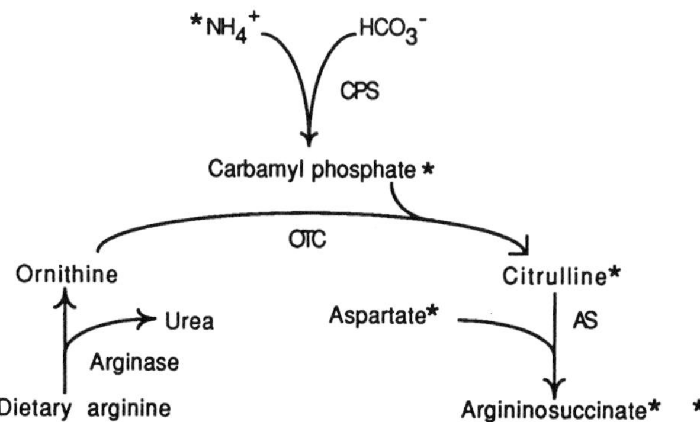

Fig. 85-26 Pathway of waste nitrogen synthesis in patients with ALD when treated as described in Table 85-9. Supplementary dietary arginine supports the continued synthesis of argininosuccinate and hence its excretion as a waste nitrogen product. Asterisks denote the number of waste nitrogen atoms contained in various substrates and products.

The estimated arginine dose in these patients is approximately 3 mmol/kg/day (Table 85-9). If, after hydrolysis to ornithine, stoichiometric amounts of argininosuccinic acid were synthesized from this arginine intake, 112 mg/kg of waste nitrogen would be available for excretion, equivalent to the nitrogen content found in 0.7 g/kg/day of dietary protein. With this new pathway of waste nitrogen synthesis, patients with argininosuccinase deficiency can tolerate between 1.25 and 1.75 g of dietary protein/kg/day, the larger and smaller amount recommended for infants and older children, respectively.

When the partition of urinary nitrogen was measured in two AL-deficient patients[540] treated as described above, 40 and 42 percent of urinary nitrogen was derived from argininosuccinate. In these calculations it is assumed that only two of four argininosuccinate nitrogen atoms were waste nitrogen, the remaining two having been derived from the arginine supplement. For the same reason, urea nitrogen (all, or nearly all, of which is derived from hydrolysis of dietary arginine) is excluded from calculation of urinary waste nitrogen.

Neither high-dose arginine therapy nor the resulting high plasma levels of argininosuccinate and its anhydrides appear to be harmful; a long-term follow-up of 12 patients with AL deficiency who were so treated showed no deterioration in intellectual or psychomotor function.[514] It also has been observed that the hair abnormality is corrected by arginine therapy.[543] On a theoretical basis, phenylbutyrate therapy should be helpful in the treatment of AL deficiency, much as it is in deficiencies of CPS, OTC, and AS.

Citrate has been recommended for treatment of AL deficiency[544] based on the assumption that there is a significant and not easily replaceable loss of tricarboxylic acid cycle substrate via oxaloacetate. This argument ignores the capacity of the anaplerotic pathway for oxaloacetate biosynthesis via pyruvate carboxylase; this pathway is 10-fold greater than the potential loss of oxaloacetate incorportated into argininosuccinate.[540] Episodes of hyperammonemia are uncommon in AL deficiency; they promptly resolve when treated with intravenous arginine, as described below (Table 85-9).

Treatment of CPS and OTC Deficiency

Unlike the treatment of AS deficiency or AL deficiency, in which nitrogen-rich intermediates can be exploited as waste nitrogen products, therapy for CPS deficiency and OTC deficiencies must rely on activation of latent biochemical pathways whose products can serve as substitutes for urea (Table 85-9). That such potentially useful pathways exist was shown long ago,[545,546] when the administration of benzoate or phenylacetic acid resulted in decreased urea nitrogen excretion, the decrease accounted for by the respective appearance of hippurate nitrogen, and phenylacetylglutamine nitrogen in the urine. It was first shown in 1980 that these pathways may be useful in patients with defective ureagenesis.[547]

Figure 85-27 shows the pathways whereby nitrogen can be diverted from urea synthesis to amino acid acylation and acetylation products after administration of benzoate or phenylbutyrate, respectively. Benzoate and phenylacetate* (the β oxidation product of phenylbutyrate) are esterified to their CoA esters via medium-chain fatty acyl CoA ligase. A glycine-specific enzyme, benzoyl CoA:glycine acyltransferase (EC 2.3.1.13) catalyzes the formation of the peptide bond required for hippurate biosynthesis. Another enzyme, specific for glutamine, phenylacetyl CoA:glutamine acetyltransferase (EC 2.3.1.68) catalyzes the formation of the peptide bond required for phenyacetylglutamine biosynthesis. These enzymes are located in the mitochondrial matrix of liver and kidney.[548–550] The enzyme activity in the kidney appears to be greater than that in the liver, suggesting that when corrected for weight both organs have approximately equal conjugating ability.

Virtually all mammals, including primates, convert benzoate to hippurate. However, there is considerable species specificity in the

*Oral phenylacetate is not an acceptable medical product because of its repugnant odor.

Table 85-9 Recommended Management of Patients with Neonatal Onset Urea Cycle Disorders*

Carbamyl Phosphate Synthetase or Ornithine Transcarbamylase Deficiency

Diet	g/kg/d	or	$g/m^2/d$
Essential amino acids†	0.7*		
Protein	0.7*		

(Patients with late onset disease including females heterozygous for OTCD initially receive a diet containing the age determined minimal daily natural protein requirement which may be increased as tolerated. Essential amino acids are rarely necessary.) Caloric supplementation with protein free diet powder

Medication		
Sodium phenylbutyrate‡	0.45–0.60	9.9–13.0
Citrulline§	0.17	3.8

Argininosuccinic Acid Synthetase Deficiency

Diet	
Protein	1.25–2.00

Caloric supplementation with Mead Johnson protein-free diet powder (4.9 calorie/g)

Medication		
Sodium phenylbutyrate‡	0.45–0.60	9.9–13.0
Arginine (free base)	0.40–0.70	8.8–15.4

Argininosuccinase Deficiency

Diet	
Protein	1.25–2.00

Caloric supplementation with Mead Johnson protein free diet powder (4.9 calorie/g)

Medication		
Arginine (free base)	0.40–0.7	8.8–15.4

*The goal of therapy is to promote growth and development. To achieve this end, fasting plasma levels of ammonium, branched chain amino acids, arginine, and serum plasma protein should be maintained within normal limits and plasma glutamine at levels less than 1000 μM if possible. Interpretation of the plasma glutamine in patients being treated with drugs requires awareness that during a 24-h period, plasma glutamine levels dramatically decrease during the day only to increase after an overnight fast (Fig. 85-25). The dose of 0.7 g each of essential amino acids and protein represents an average intake for the average patient with neonatal-onset CPS deficiency or OTC deficiency. The degree to which nitrogen intake is partitioned into natural protein and essential amino acids is a function of age, residual enzyme activity, and dose of sodium phenylbutyrate. It has become apparent that infants with neonatally expressed disorders may tolerate as much as 2 g/kg/d of natural protein in the first few months of life (plasma ammonium and amino acid levels should decrease as the infant's growth rate decreases and therefore require reduction of nitrogen intake). After 6 months of age, the final nitrogen intake for these neonatally expressed disorders is derived from 0.7 g/kg of natural protein and 0.7 g/kg of essential amino acids as noted in the table. Some patients may require a lower intake of essential amino acids and protein.

†Mixtures containing 80% essential amino acids are available commercially.

‡The precise dose of sodium phenylbutyrate will depend on clinical circumstances. The highest dose is recommended for all patients, although the lower dose may suffice for patients with significant residual enzyme activity. Because phenylbutyrate on a molar basis is twice as effective as benzoate, the use of oral benzoate is no longer included in this FDA-approved protocol.

In some patients with the late-onset form of CPS and OTC deficiency, arginine (free base) may be substituted for citrulline (whose cost is three to four times that of arginine).

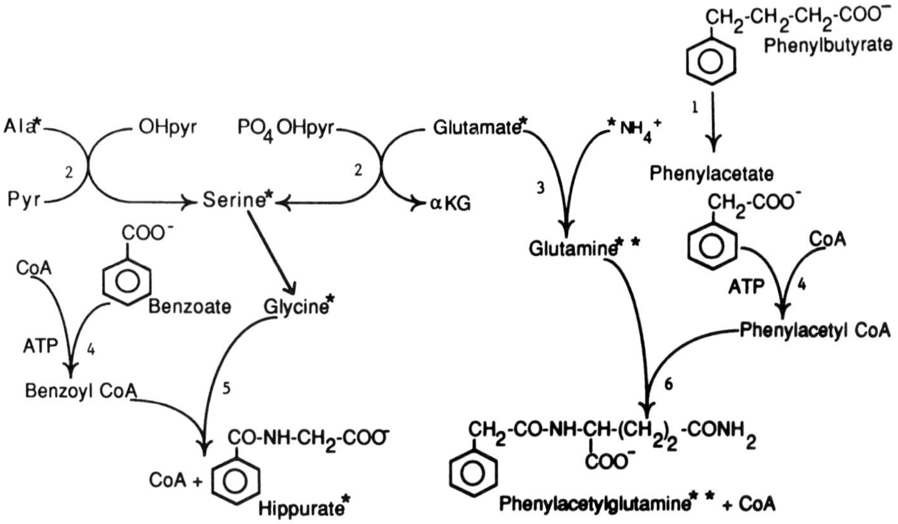

Fig. 85-27 Pathways of waste nitrogen synthesis in patients with CPS, OTC, and AS deficiencies. Asterisks denote nitrogen atoms destined for waste nitrogen excretion in hippurate and phenylacetylglutamine. The enzymatic reactions are numbered: 1 = β-oxidation; 2 = transamination; 3 = glutamine synthetase; 4 = medium-chain fatty acyl CoA ligase; 5 = benzoyl CoA:glycine acyltransferase; 6 = phenylacetyl CoA:glutamine acetyl-transferase; α-KG = α-ketoglutarate; Ala = alanine; OH pyr = hydroxypyruvate; PO_4OH = pyrophosphohydroxypyruvate; Pyr = pyruvate.

metabolism of phenylacetate.[551] Humans and Old World monkeys synthesize the glutamine conjugate but not the glycine conjugate. Only baboons and chimpanzees are similar to humans in that they conjugate virtually all administered phenylacetate with glutamine.

As glycine is incorporated into hippurate, it is resynthesized from serine, which in turn is the product of two transamination reactions with alanine or glutamate as the nitrogen donor. As glutamine is incorporated into phenylacetylglutamine it is resynthesized via amidation of glutamate by ammonia via glutamine synthetase. The net result of benzoate and phenylacetate administration is a flux of nitrogen from the usual urea precursors—ammonium, alanine, and glutamate—to glycine or glutamine, after which they are respectively conjugated to yield hippurate and phenylacetylglutamine. Presumably the ammonium that ordinarily serves as a substrate for ureagenesis in the mitochondria matrix of the hepatocyte is diverted to glutamate synthesis via glutamate dehydrogenase and then to glutamine via glutamine synthetase.

Quantitative Aspects of Waste Nitrogen Synthesis as Hippurate or Phenylacetylglutamine

Children or adults receiving a low but adequate protein intake excrete 40 to 45 percent of their dietary nitrogen as urea nitrogen.[540] Thus, a child receiving 1.25 g/kg/day of protein has the obligatory requirement to synthesize 93 mg/kg/day of waste nitrogen as urea. This requirement can be met by patients with the neonatal form of CPS deficiency and OTC deficiency if they receive 600 mg/kg/day of sodium phenylbutyrate (the prodrug for phenylacetate), which if completely conjugated with glutamine will lead to the excretion of 90 mg/kg/day of phenylacetylglutamine nitrogen.

These theoretical considerations were confirmed in an 8-year-old boy with the neonatal form of CPS deficiency.[552] Benzoate has been abandoned in the long-term treatment of these diseases because its conjugation product, hippurate, contains only one nitrogen atom. Furthermore, it has been suggested that as much as 23 percent of benzoate given to humans may be converted to its glucuronide[553] and thus may serve no useful purpose for these diseases. Phenylacetate also has been abandoned because of its unacceptable sensory characteristics. Table 85-9 describes current drug and nutritional therapy of urea cycle disorders. Figure 85-28, shows the intraday pharmacokinetics of phenylbutyrate.

Dietary Aspects of Treatment of the Neonatal Form of CP and OTC Deficiencies

Notwithstanding the establishment of new pathways of waste nitrogen synthesis and excretion, some manipulation of dietary nitrogen intake is necessary to reduce the requirement for waste nitrogen synthesis for patients with the neonatal forms of CPS and OTC deficiencies. The current recommended dietary protocol

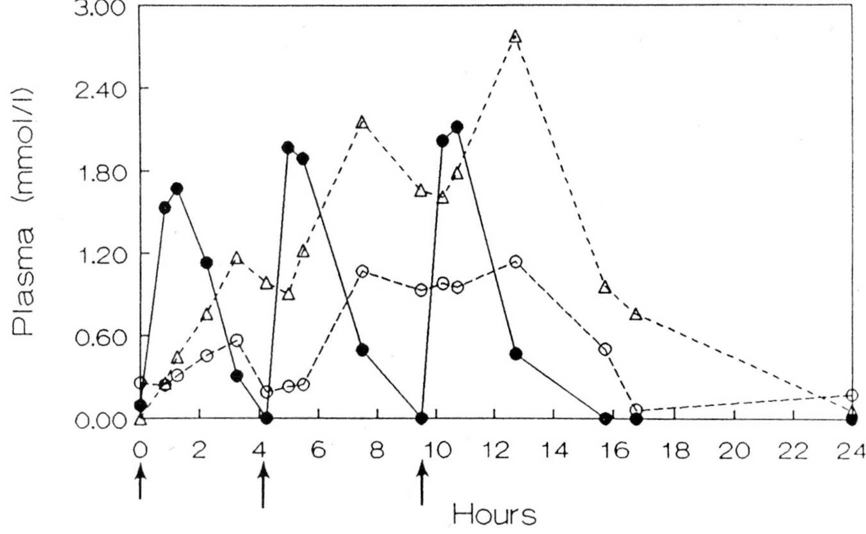

Fig. 85-28 Precursor–product relationships during the oral administration of 625 mg/kg/day of sodium phenylbutyrate in three divided doses (arrows) to a 4-year-old girl with CPS deficiency. ● = phenylbutyrate; Δ = phenylacetate; ○ = phenylacetylglutamine.

includes 0.7 g/kg/day of food protein and 0.7 g/kg/day of an essential amino acid mixture, although in the first 6 months of life the infant may tolerate a natural protein intake of up to 1.75 g/kg/day. The essential amino acids offer two advantages. They ensure a high-quality nitrogen intake, and they only contain 11 to 12 percent nitrogen as compared with whole protein, of which 16 percent is nitrogen. The diet is supplemented with citrulline, which serves as a source of arginine but contributes one less nitrogen atom to the free amino pool than does arginine. However, for patients with late-onset disease, arginine is an acceptable substitute for citrulline because of the increased nitrogen tolerance of these patients. As growth rate slows and protein accretion declines, the nitrogen tolerance of patients with CPS and OTC deficiencies may decrease. It may then be advisable to modify the quantity of dietary protein nitrogen intake to the minimum levels compatible with growth. Table 85-9 summarizes currently recommended therapy.

Treatment of AS Deficiency (Neonatal Form)

The therapy of AS deficiency exploits citrulline as a waste nitrogen product by a mechanism similar to that used in AL deficiency. The diet is supplemented with arginine to stimulate citrulline synthesis and excretion. As a waste nitrogen product, citrulline has two disadvantages as compared with argininosuccinate: it has only one waste nitrogen atom (derived from CP), and its renal clearance at high plasma citrulline levels is 20 percent of the glomerular filtration rate. However, it appears that when phenylbutyrate is added to supplementary dietary arginine, sufficient waste nitrogen capacity is achieved to permit a natural diet with protein intake limited to 1.75 g/kg/day. Figure 85-28 describes the pathways of waste nitrogen synthesis and excretion in AS deficiency and Table 85-5 summarizes therapy.

Liver Transplantation

Although allogeneic orthotopic liver transplantation has been performed in patients with inborn errors of metabolism,[554–556] the indications for transplantation in such patients have been the consequences of global liver failure. However, the use of liver transplantation as a form of enzyme replacement is an option for patients with the neonatal form of CPS deficiency and OTC deficiency.[557–559] Because survival of such patients who survive the neonatal period and are treated medically is approximately 90 percent at 1 year of age,[4] liver transplantation may justifiably be delayed until then.

Rescue from Neonatal Hyperammonemic Encephalopathy

Before attempting the rescue and treatment of a neonate with severe neonatal hyperammonemic encephalopathy, parents should be thoroughly counseled about the severe medical burden imposed by these diseases and disappointing survival and neurodevelopmental outcome.[4,530] This center has found it useful to suggest that parents discuss these options with others who have dealt with this problem.

Should neonatal rescue be attempted, hemodialysis is the most effective method of lowering the plasma ammonia level; it results in a reduction of plasma ammonium levels within a matter of hours,[560–562] as compared with peritoneal dialysis or arteriovenous hemofiltration,[563] which may require 24 h to have an effect.[564–567] The clearance of ammonium and amino acids by conventional hemodialysis is not only more timely but also is approximately 10 times greater than by peritoneal dialysis or arteriovenous hemofiltration.[563] Other less effective hemodialytic techniques should be avoided. Because exchange transfusion is useful in removing toxins principally confined to the vascular space, it has no role in the removal of ammonium and amino acid accumulation, which are distributed through total body water. It is likely that dialytic procedures exert their principal effect by promptly removing the major nitrogen accumulation product glutamine.[567] Stoichiometric considerations and experience suggest that benzoate and phenylacetate by themselves will not be effective in controlling the accumulated nitrogen in severe neonatal hyperammonemia. It may be useful, however, to supply arginine in the doses described in Tables 85-9 and 85-10. Prompt and repeated hemodialysis appears to be the most effective method of rapidly reducing the plasma ammonium level seen in severely encephalopathic neonates. As plasma ammonium approaches levels three to four times the upper limits of normal, treatment with intravenous benzoate and phenylacetate followed by oral sodium phenylbutyrate is recommended. However, intravenous arginine should be included in the daily fluid requirement of patients with CPS, OTC, and AS deficiencies, the last requiring high doses (Table 85-10).

Treatment of Late-Onset Urea Cycle Defects (Including Females with Symptomatic OTC Deficiency)

It appears that many patients with late-onset urea cycle disorders who have had documented evidence of one or more episodes of hyperammonemic encephalopathy suffer some degree of brain damage or death.[468,568,569]

Thus, the goals of treatment of patients with late-onset disease are similar to those described earlier for the more severe form of the disease: normal growth; maintenance of normal plasma levels of ammonium, glutamine, and arginine in OTC-deficient heterozygotes; and the absence of orotic aciduria.

Although in mild cases it may be possible to maintain metabolic control using dietary means alone, the use of phenylbutyrate confers special advantages to these patients, all of whom have residual ureagenic activity. Treatment of patients with late-onset disease with the protocol described in Table 85-9 has a dual effect. Not only does the administration of phenylbutyrate provide an additional pathway for waste nitrogen excretion, it suppresses residual endogenous urea synthesis, which then is available as a reserve waste nitrogen pathway in the event it is needed.[570] For example, Fig. 85-29 shows the effect of phenylbutyrate on net urea nitrogen synthesis before and after an increase in dietary protein. It is apparent that urea nitrogen synthesis, which is suppressed by phenylbutyrate activation of phenylacetylglutamine nitrogen synthesis, becomes available when additional waste nitrogen synthesis is required to maintain nitrogen homeostasis.

Intercurrent Hyperammonemia

Despite attempts to maintain adequate nutrition with diet and arginine or citrulline supplements and high-dose phenylbutyrate therapy, patients with urea cycle disorders are at constant risk for life-threatening or brain-damaging intercurrent hyperammonemia. The early signs and symptoms of hyperammonemia — irritability, lethargy, vomiting, behavioral changes, and a respiratory alkalosis — are indications for monitoring plasma ammonium and glutamine levels. We suggest that for symptomatic patients who have plasma ammonium levels three times the upper limit of normal, the protocol described in Table 85-10 should be started.[571] The best time to abort a potentially serious episode of hyperammonemia is at the earliest stages; once cerebral edema has occurred, with or without increased intracranial pressure, management becomes increasingly difficult especially if hemodynamic problems ensue. We regard increasing hyperammonemia in this setting as a medical emergency equivalent to hemodynamic instability secondary to blood and fluid loss.

Full clinical recovery from hyperammonemic encephalopathy may be prompt but also take up to a week — the duration a function of the depth and duration of encephalopathy. Not an uncommon complication of encephalopathy and cerebral edema, cortical blindness was first reported in an adult man with OTC deficiency.[572] Fortunately, it appears to be transitory, although two patients have suffered permanent loss of visual activity. During the recovery phase of hyperammonemic encephalopathy, cortical blindness may be detected by optokinetic tests or mirror following.

Table 85-10 Protocols for Management of Intercurrent Hyperammonemia in Patients with Urea Cycle Disorders

Early Diagnosis and Therapy

This is the most important aspect of intercurrent by hyperammonemia. Delays are disastrous. A plasma ammonium level should be done as an emergency procedure on any child with these diseases who exhibits lethargy or vomiting of any degree. Parents should be taught that such symptoms are emergencies demanding immediate medical attention.

If the ammonium level approaches three times the upper limits of normal, the ammonium level should be repeated and venous plasma obtained for electrolytes, pH, P_{CO_2} and quantitative amino acids. Without waiting for the repeat ammonium value, the appropriate regimen described in Table 85-1 should be followed as an emergency procedure. Repeat priming doses are not recommended. These intravenous drugs are extremely toxic when given in greater than recommended doses.

The drugs may cause one or two vomiting episodes , usually toward the end of the 90 minute treatment period. *Recent preliminary experience with Zofran (ondansetron HCl, Glaxo), a serotonin 5-HT$_3$ receptor blocking agent, suggests that the nausea and vomiting may be preventable. The dose of Zofran is 0.15 mg/kg given intravenously during the first 15 min of the priming infusion. By using Zofran it has been possible to include enteral calories during the primary infusion.*

Respiratory alkalosis may occur or be exacerbated during therapy with these drugs.

All dietary or intravenous nitrogen intake should be discontinued. Because reduction of body protein breakdown is desirable, a high parenteral caloric intake should be provided from 10% to 15% glucose and Intralipid; for infants the goal should be 80–100 cal/kg/d and proportionately less for older children. If the patient can tolerate enteral feedings, he should be given a formula consisting of 14 g of Mead Johnson Product 80056 in 100 mL of water, which supplies 20 cal/ounce.

The hemodialysis team should be alerted. To avoid delays in establishing emergency vascular access, it may be most efficient to rely upon your cardiologists or intensivists to place the lines.

Plasma levels of ammonium, electrolytes, pH and P_{CO_2} should be measured shortly after completion of the priming infusion and every 8 h thereafter until plasma ammonium levels are normal or near normal.

If intracranial pressure is elevated, conventional osmotherapy with mannitol should begin. Corticosteroids may be contraindicated because they induce negative nitrogen balance. Hyperventilation also may be inadvisable because in the hyperammonemic state the decrease in cerebral blood flow associated with hypocapnia is abolished and in some regions of the brain there is a paradoxical increase in blood flow.[484,484a]

When the ammonium level is stable at normal or near normal levels, oral medication may be gradually added as the intravenous medication is reduced. Two or three days are usually required to restore the patient to his or her previous entered nutritional and oral medications.

Carbamyl Phosphate Synthetase or Ornithine Transcarbamylase Deficiency

Priming infusion: to be given over 90 min in 25–35 mL per kg of 10% glucose or for older patients 400–600 mL per m^2 of 10% glucose. Zofran, a potent antiemetic, may be given intravenously (O.15 mg/kg) during the first 15 min of the priming infusion. *All orders for these drugs should be independently reviewed; there have been several cases of overdose because of improperly written orders or erroneous calculations.*[571c]

	g/kg per dose	or	g/m^2 per dose
Sodium benzoate*	0.250		5.5
Sodium phenylacetate*	0.250		5.5
10% Arginine HCl†	0.210 (2 mL/kg)		4.0

Sustaining infusion: drugs to be diluted in 25–35 mL per kg of 10% glucose or 400–600 mL per m^2 of 10% glucose and this volume to be infused over 24 h. The drugs are given in addition to daily maintenance fluid requirements.

	g/kg per day	or	g/m^2 per day
Sodium benzoate*	0.250		5.5
Sodium phenylacetate*	0.250		5.5
10% Arginine HCl†	0.210 (2 mL/kg)		4.0

Hemodialysis should be started as an emergency procedure if the plasma ammonium level does not significantly decrease within 8 h. Repeat priming doses are not recommended. If hemodialysis is necessary it should be done with the largest catheters consistent with the patient's size (ammonium clearance is approximately equal to blood flow). Because both peritoneal dialysis and continuous arteriovenous hemofilteration produce ammonium clearances 10% that of hemodialysis, hemodialysis is the treatment of choice.

Argininosuccinic Acid Synthetase Deficiency

Priming infusion: to be given over 90 min in 25–35 mL per kg of 10% glucose or for older patients 400–600 mL per m^2 of 10% glucose. Zofran, a potent antiemetic, may be given intravenously (0.15 mg/kg) during the first 15 min of the priming infusion. *All orders for these drugs should be independently reviewed; there have been several cases of overdose because of improperly written orders or erroneous calculations.*[571a]

	g/kg per dose	or	g/m^2 per dose
Sodium benzoate*	0.250		5.5
Sodium phenylacetate*	0.250		5.5
10% Arginine HCl†	0.660 (6 mL/kg)		12.0

Sustaining infusion: drugs to be diluted in 25–35 mL per kg of 10% glucose or 400–600 mL per m^2 of 10% glucose and this volume infused over 24 h. The drugs are given in addition to daily maintenance fluid requirements.

	g/kg/day	or	g/m^2 per day
Sodium benzoate*	0.250		5.5
Sodium phenylacetate*	0.250		5.5
10% Arginine HCl†	0.660 (6 mL/kg)		12.0

Hemodialysis should be started as an emergency procedure if the plasma ammonium level does not significantly decrease within 8 h. Repeat priming doses are not recommended. If hemodialysis is necessary it should be done with the largest catheters consistent with the patient's size (ammonium clearances are approximately equal to blood flow). Because both peritoneal dialysis and continuous arteriovenous hemofilteration produce ammonium clearances 10% that of hemodialysis, hemodialysis is the treatment of choice.

Argininosuccinase Deficiency

Priming infusion: to be given over 90 minutes in 25–35 mL per kg of 10% glucose or 400–600 mL per m^2 of 10% glucose.

	g/kg/dose	or	g/m^2/dose
10% Arginine HCl†	0.660 (6 mL/kg)		12.0

(Continued on next page)

Table 85-10 Protocols for Management of Intercurrent Hyperammonemia in Patients with Urea Cycle Disorders (Continued)

Sustaining infusion: drugs to be diluted in 25–35 mL per kg of 10% glucose or 400–600 mL per m^2 of 10% glucose and this volume infused over 24 h. Arginine is given in addition to daily maintenance fluid requirements.

	g/kg/dose	or	g/m²/dose
10% Arginine HCl†	0.660 (6 mL/kg)		12.0

Hemodialysis should be started as an emergency procedure if the plasma ammonium level does not significantly decrease within 8 h. Repeat priming doses are not recommended. If hemodialysis is necessary it should be done with the largest catheters consistent with the patient's size (ammonium clearance is approximately equal to blood flow). Because both peritoneal dialysis and continuous arteriovenous hemofilteration produce ammonium clearances 10% that of hemodialysis, hemodialysis is the treatment of choice.

*One gram of sodium benzoate contains 160 mg of sodium. One gram of sodium phenylacetate contains 147 mg of sodium. Because urine potassium loss is enhanced by the excretion of the nonreabsorbable anions (hippurate and phenylacetylglutamine), the plasma potassium levels should be monitored and treated with necessary.

†Because a hyperchloremic acidosis may ensure after high-dose arginine HCl, plasma levels of chloride and bicarbonate should be monitored and appropriate amounts of bicarbonate be administered.

NOTE: 10% Arginine HCl is available as a sterile, pyrogen free solution from Kabivitrun, Clayton, North Carolina.

The mechanism of cortical blindness following hyperammonemia is unclear, but we hypothesize that the cerebral edema associated with hyperammonemia may compress the posterior cerebral arteries against the tentorial rim and thereby impair, to varying degrees, circulation to the visual cortex. Lyle[573] has described reversible cortical visual impairment caused by such a mechanism.

Prevention of Neonatal Hyperammonemia in Infants at Risk

For neonates in whom an antenatal diagnosis of a urea cycle was made or who are at risk because of a previously affected sib, a diagnostic and therapeutic protocol has been developed that is effective in establishing an early diagnosis and preventing symptomatic neonatal hyperammonemia.[574] The protocol relies on the prevention of hyperammonemia and the differential diagnostic value of the plasma citrulline or argininosuccinate level at 60 h of age. The therapeutic protocol begins within hours of birth and is similar to that described in Table 85-8 with a modification that excludes dietary protein for the first 24 h. Although the outcome of these infants is much better than of those treated after hyperammonemic encephalopathy has ensued, the results are disappointing in that most such patients have some development impairment; only a few demonstrate anticipated normal developmental status. This outcome of prospective therapy coupled with the immense burden of caring for such children suggest that realistic counseling should be offered to parents contemplating such a program.

Outcome of Therapy

Neonatal Onset. For those infants rescued from severe neonatal hyperammonemia, the neurodevelopmental outlook is disappointing[530]; virtually all patients suffer severe brain damage. A later study of neonatal-onset AS deficiency,[575] treated as described earlier, revealed that 11 of 15 patients were classified as severely to profoundly developmentally delayed; the remaining 4 patients had IQ measurements in the borderline to mildly developmentally delayed categories. A small study of prospective therapy[443] of neonates at risk revealed a better outcome, but neurologic abnormalities were common.

Of 72 OTC-deficient neonates for whom the age of death was known, 32 died during the neonatal period despite rescue attempts. Of the 40 survivors, the median survival was 3.83 years; the oldest survivor was 16 years (Fig. 85-30). Survival of neonatal-onset AS deficiency was much better; the cumulative survival rate at 5 and 10 years of age was 87.5 and 72 percent, respectively.

Physicians should be aware of these outcomes in reproductive counseling or discussions about attempts to rescue a severely hyperammonemic neonate.

Late Onset. A study of 32 girls with OTC deficiency[576] treated as described earlier was much more encouraging; while on treatment with phenylbutyrate they had fewer hyperammonemic episodes and were at reduced risk for further cognitive decline.

Antenatal Diagnosis

All five inborn errors of ureagenesis can be diagnosed antenatally. The techniques for doing so vary widely and include measurement of an abnormal metabolite in amniotic fluid, analysis of DNA from chorionic villus or amniocytes, and enzyme or *in utero* liver biopsy samples.

For fetuses at risk for CPS deficiency and when DNA is available from an affected member of the family, RFLP analysis may be the simplest method of establishing a diagnosis. There are four intragenic polymorphisms and four useful flanking markers. Mutational analysis of the large coding sequence is also available.

For fetuses at risk for OTC deficiency, the diagnostic procedure of choice is targeted sequencing (when the mutation has previously been identified) or sequencing all exons at the OTC locus. RFLP analysis is also highly sensitive if a mutation can be linked to an informative polymorphism.

The role of prenatal diagnosis and pregnancy termination of female fetuses at risk is controversial because it requires an estimate of the likelihood of the fetus to become symptomatic.

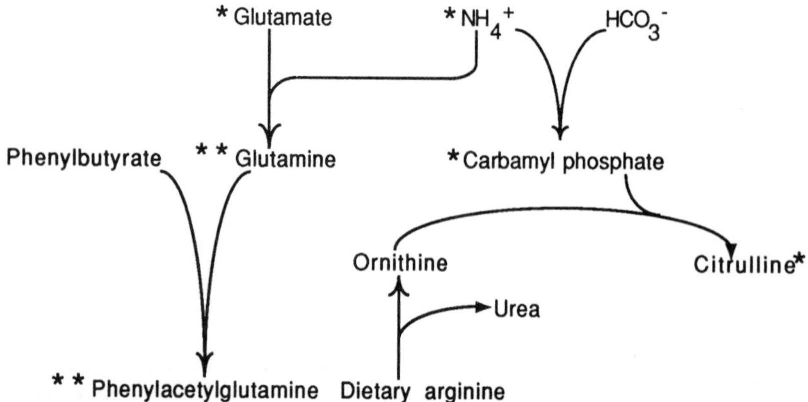

Fig. 85-29 The pathways of waste nitrogen synthesis in patients with AS deficiency when treated as described in Table 32-5[JCJ61]. Supplementary dietary arginine supports the continued synthesis of citrulline and hence its excretion as a waste nitrogen product. Phenylbutyrate functions as described in Fig. 85-10. The asterisks denote nitrogen atoms destined for waste nitrogen excretion in citrulline and phenylacetylglutamine.

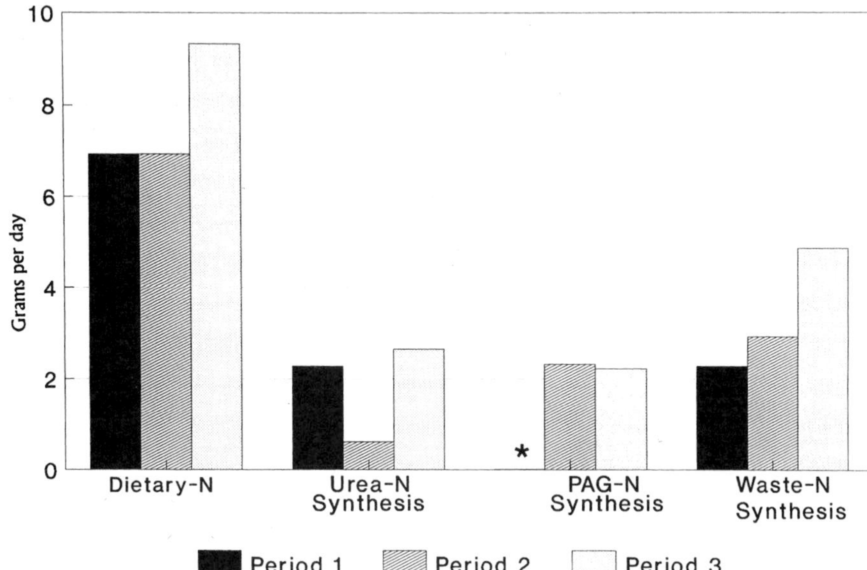

Fig. 85-30 The effect of phenylbutyrate therapy on nitrogen homeostasis: dietary nitrogen, net urea nitorgen synthesis, and phenylacetylglutamine (PAG) nitrogen synthesis in an adult patient with OTC deficiency. Period 1 (3 days), low-protein diet only; period 2 (3 days), same as period 1 with 45 g of sodium phenylbutyrate added (16.5 g/day); period 3 (3 days), same as period 2 with 45 g dietary protein added (15 g/day). The experiment demonstrates that treatment with phenylbutyrate suppresses urea nitrogen synthesis, which is increased when nitrogen intake is increased. It also shows that PAG nitrogen synthesis is equal to the patient's urea nitrogen synthesis when untreated during period 1. Waste nitrogen synthesis is the sum of urea nitrogen and PAG nitrogen synthesis. The asterisk denotes a control value of PAG nitrogen synthesis of 0.023 g/3 days (0.007 g/day).

Estimating the risk of a female fetus being symptomatic may be done by analogy to the biochemical findings of late-onset males. Fifteen late-onset males had hepatic OTC activities of 4.3 percent of normal with a large standard deviation of 4.9 percent.[466] In females this would suggest that the likelihood of such a skewed distribution of hepatocytes containing the active mutant allele would occur with a probability of 0.05 to 0.10, assuming that inactivation of each X chromosome was random. Thus a female carrier fetus might have a 5–10% risk of being symptomatic.

As discussed in the section of this chapter devoted to molecular aspects of AS, mutational analysis is available, but curiously, there are no citations describing its use for prenatal diagnosis. Classical biochemical techniques[11] relying on the incorporation of ^{14}C citrulline into amniocyte-derived fibroblast protein appear to be the most commonly used prenatal test for AS deficiency.

There are two reliable biochemical techniques available for antenatal diagnosis of AL deficiency: measurement of enzyme activity in cultured amniocytes[577] and measurement of argininosuccinic acid levels in amniotic fluid.[577,578] Molecular approaches are also available for identifying an AL-deficient fetus (see section on AL Mutations).

For fetuses at risk for arginase deficiency, measurement of fetal erythrocyte arginase activity appears to be the most satisfactory technique notwithstanding the availability of a few intragenic markers.

Heterozygote Identification in OTC-Deficient Pedigrees

Pedigree Analysis. A woman can be identified as an obligate heterozygote if she has had one or more children with OTC deficiency or if there is another case of OTC deficiency elsewhere in the pedigree. Although it is highly likely that a woman is a heterozygote if she has had two affected children, gonadal mosaicism cannot be completely excluded as an explanation for transmission of a mutant gene.

The most direct test for ascertaining carrier is by mutation analysis, the sensitivity for which may be as high as 90 percent (see earlier section on OTC Deficiency). The allopurinol test[476] may be helpful in conjunction with RFLP analysis if mutational analysis is unsuccessful.

The protein tolerance test[579–582] has been abandoned because the high-protein meal is often repugnant to many carriers, and it carries the risk of hyperammonemia. The alanine tolerance test also has been abandoned because of its low specificity[583,584] and the risk of hyperammonemia.

ARGINASE DEFICIENCY

Clinical Manifestations

The clinical manifestations of arginase deficiency (OMIM 107830) are strikingly different from those of CPS, OTC, AS, and ALD deficiencies.[585–587] The major symptoms of arginase deficiency, all of which are progressive, include spastic tetraplegia with the lower limbs affected much more severely than the upper limbs, seizures, psychomotor retardation, hyperactivity, growth failure, and, in one reported case, athetosis. Symptomatic hyperammonemia progressing to encephalopathy may occur, but plasma ammonium levels are three to four times normal values, with levels rarely as high as six times normal.

Although there is phenotypic variability, with some cases presumably asymptomatic at 4 years of age, close inspection of reported cases suggests that clinical manifestations occur early in the first year of life; they include irritability, unconsolable crying, anorexia, vomiting, and delayed developmental milestones. One report[588] described a proband with less than 2 percent hepatic arginase activity but with a plasma arginine level of 170 μM—far below other reported cases. The infant was extremely protein intolerant and died at 49 days of age.

Laboratory Abnormalities

The most prominent laboratory findings include mild hyperammonemia, hyperargininemia as high as 1500 μM, hyperaminoaciduria (arginine, lysine, cystine, ornithine), and orotic aciduria. Plasma glutamine levels may be increased. The increased concentration of many amino acids in cerebrospinal fluid is striking. The very high arginine concentration is understandable; however, no hypothesis readily serves to explain the high cerebrospinal fluid concentrations of ornithine, aspartate, threonine, glycine, and methionine. As has been noted,[586] no pattern characteristic of shared transport systems in brain is apparent.

In addition to orotic aciduria noted above, other pyrimidines are excreted in the urine in greater amounts than normal (i.e., uracil and uridine).[589] The mechanism of pyrimidinuria is unclear. It has been suggested that intramitochondrial ornithine deficiency may be a consequence of the reduced hydrolysis of arginine. As a

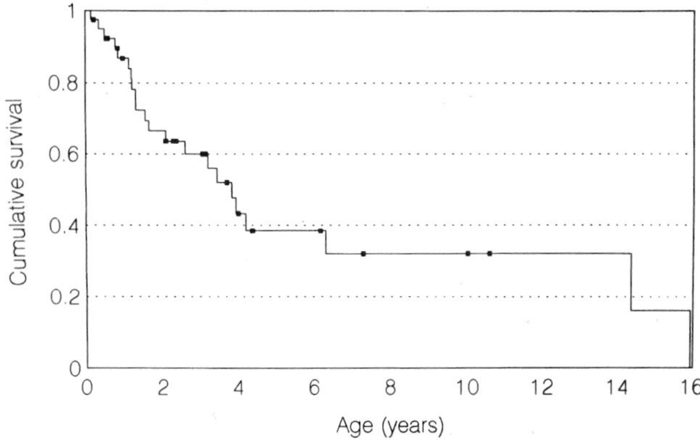

Fig. 85-31 Long-term survival of 40 infants who survived their neonatal hyperammonemic episode. Each small square represents length of time surviving patients were monitored (time until they were censored). Patients were censored at their age of orthotopic liver transplantation, when they were lost to follow-up, or when this study ended.

result, the flux through the OTC reaction may be limited by the relative unavailability of ornithine. The biochemical consequences would then be similar to that found in OTC deficiency: accumulation and diffusion of intramitochondrial CP into the cytosol and stimulation of pyrimidine biosynthesis. Curiously, ornithine administration has no effect on orotic aciduria in arginase deficiency.[590] Another explanation for mitochondrial CP overproduction and hence pyrimidine overproduction assumes that high intramitochondrial arginine levels inappropriately activate NAG synthetase, thereby overstimulating CPS activity.[591] There is little direct evidence to support either of these explanations.

Although large amounts of monosubstituted guanidino compounds are found in the urine of arginase-deficient patients,[592–594] most of these are not a result of amidino group donation by arginine, but rather are derivatives of arginine itself: keto-guanidinovaleric acid (the keto analogue of arginine), N-acetylarginine, and argininic acid. Of the urinary monosubstituted guanidino groups that are a result of amidino group donation by arginine, guanidinoacetic acid (the normal reaction product of arginine and glycine via glycine transamidinase) is excreted in the largest amount, followed by guanidinobutyric acid.

Pathophysiology and Treatment

The pathophysiology is in some way related to the known laboratory abnormalities described above: episodic mild hyperammonemia, hyperargininemia, and perhaps high plasma and tissue levels of monosubstituted guanidino compounds. Impaired neurotransmitter metabolism has been described in arginase deficiency.[595] That arginine is the substrate for nitric oxide synthetase raises the question whether overproduction of nitric oxide may play a role in the pathophysiology.[596] Regardless of which one or combination of these factors is culpable, it appears that the restriction of dietary protein and thereby dietary nitrogen may be beneficial. Reduced nitrogen intake will inevitably lead to reduced flux through the attenuated urea cycle and hence reduce arginine biosynthesis. Artificial diets devoid of arginine have been used in an attempt to reduce plasma arginine levels.[590,597,598] These studies are flawed in that nitrogen intake was not constant during the arginine-replete and arginine-deficient study periods. In one of these studies,[597] biochemical improvement was noted when 0.9 g/kg/day of an essential amino acid arginine-free diet was compared to a diet containing 0.9 g/kg/day of protein without recognizing that the essential amino acid mixtures used contained 11 percent nitrogen, whereas natural protein contains 16 percent nitrogen. A similar flaw is noted in a study in which the nitrogen-free analogues of several essential amino acids supplemented an essential amino acid arginine-free diet.[590] In formulating dietary treatment of arginase deficiency, it is important to remember that virtually all dietary nitrogen is available for *de novo* synthesis of arginine. This amount is considerably greater than the small amount of arginine residues in dietary protein.

Only preliminary data are available to support the use of benzoate and phenylacetate in arginase deficiency. On theoretical grounds, any diversion of nitrogen from ureagenesis (and hence argininogenesis) should lower plasma arginine levels as well as improve waste nitrogen synthetic capacity. Sodium benzoate at a dose of 375 mg/kg/day led to a reduction of plasma arginine level from 500 to 300 μM in a patient on a very low protein diet (0.5 g/kg/day).[599] The substitution of high-dose phenylbutyrate for benzoate should have the salutary effect of diverting twice as much nitrogen from argininogenesis, thereby both permitting a more adequate diet and maintaining a more normal plasma arginine level.

REFERENCES

1. Campbell JW: *Comparative Biochemistry of Nitrogen Metabolism*. London, Academic, 1970.
2. Bean ES, Atkinson DE: Regulation of the rate of urea synthesis in liver by extracellular pH. *J Biol Chem* **259**:1552, 1984.
3. Walser M: Roles of urea production, ammonium excretion, and amino acid oxidation in acid-base balance. *Am J Physiol* **250**:F181, 1986.
4. Maestri NE, Clissold DB, Brusilow S: Neonatal onset ornithine transcarbamylase deficiency: A retrospective analysis. *J Pediatr* **134**:268, 1999.
5. Almdal T, Vilstrup H, Bjerrum K, Kristenson LO: Decrease in ureagenesis by partial hepatectomy does not influence acid-base balance. *Am J Physiol* **254**:F696, 1989.
6. Haussinger D: Liver regulation of acid-base balance. *Miner Electrolyte Metabolism* **23**:249, 1997.
7. Brusilow SW: Arginine, an indispensable amino acid for patients with inborn errors of urea synthesis. *J Clin Invest* **74**:2144, 1984.
8. Ratner S: Enzymes of arginine and urea synthesis, in Meister A (ed): *Advances in Enzymology*. Vol. 39. New York, John Wiley, 1973, p 1.
9. Snodgrass PJ: Biochemical aspects of urea cycle disorders. *Pediatrics* **68**:273, 1981.
10. Meijer AJ, Hensgens HESJ: Ureogenesis, in Sies H (ed): *Metabolic Compartmentation*. London, Academic, 1982, p 259.
11. Jackson MJ, Beaudet AL, O'Brien WE: Mammalian urea cycle enzymes. *Annu Rev Genet* **20**:431, 1986.
12. Beaudet AL, O'Brien WE, Bock HGO, Freytag SO, Su TS: The human argininosuccinate synthetase locus and citrullinemia, in Harris H, Hirschhorn K (eds): *Advances in Human Genetics*. New York, Plenum, 1986, p 161.
13. Lusty CJ: Catalytically active monomer and dimer forms of rat liver carbamoyl-phosphate synthetase. *Biochemistry* **20**:3665, 1981.
14. Bachmann C, Krahenbuhl S, Colombo JP, Schubiger G, Jaggi KH, Tonz O: *N*-Acetylglutamate synthetase deficiency: A disorder of ammonia detoxication. *New Engl J Med* **304**:543, 1981.
15. Braunstein AE: Les voies principales de l'assimilation et dissimilation de l'azote chez les animaux. *Adv Enzymol* **19**:335, 1957.
16. De Hann EJ, Tager JM, Slater EC: Factors affecting the pathway of glutamate oxidation in rat-liver mitochondria. *Biochim Biophys Acta* **131**:1, 1967.
17. Charles R, Tager JM, Slater ED: Citrulline synthesis in rat-liver mitochondria. *Biochim Biophys Acta* **131**:29, 1967.
18. Frieden C: The regulation of glutamate dehydrogenase, in Grisolia S, Baguena R, Mayor F (eds): *The Urea Cycle*. New York, John Wiley, 1976, p 59.
19. McCarthy AD, Tipton KF: Glutamate dehydrogenase, in Hertz L, Kvamme E, McGeer E, Schousbee A (eds): *Glutamate and GABA in the Central Nervous System*. New York, Alan R. Liss, 1983, p 19.
20. Krebs HA, Hems R, Lund P, Halliday D, Read WWC: Sources of ammonia for mammalian urea synthesis. *Biochem J* **176**:733, 1978.
21. Jungermann K: Functional heterogeneity of periportal and perivenous hepatocytes. *Enzyme* **35**:161, 1986.
22. Cooper JL, Nieves E, De Ricco SF, Gebhard AS: Short term metabolic fate of (^{13}N) ammonia, L-(^{13}N) alanine, L-(^{13}N) glutamate, and L-(amide ^{13}N) glutamine in normal rat liver *in vivo*. *J Hepatol* **4**(suppl):12, 1987.
23. Meijer AJ: Channeling of ammonia from glutaminase to carbamoyl-phosphate synthetase in liver mitochondria. *FEBS Lett* **3040**:249, 1985.

24. Cooper JL, Nieves E, Coleman AE, Filc-De Recco S, Gelbard AS: Short-term fate of [^{13}N] ammonia in rat liver *in vivo*. *J Biol Chem* **262**:1073, 1987.
25. Windmueller HG: Glutamine utilization by the small intestine, in Meister A (ed): *Advances in Enzymology*. New York, John Wiley, 1982, p 201.
26. Windmueller HG, Spaeth AE: Respiratory fuels and nitrogen metabolism *in vivo* in small intestine of fed rats. *J Biol Chem* **255**:107, 1980.
27. Featherston WE, Rogers QR, Freeland RA: Relative importance of kidney and liver in synthesis of arginine by the rat. *Am J Physiol* **224**:127, 1973.
28. Dhanakoti SN, Brosman JT, Hertzberg GR, Brosman ME: Renal arginine synthesis: Studies *in vitro* and *in vivo*. *Am J Physiol* **259**:E437, 1990.
29. Windmueller HG, Spaeth AE: Source and fate of circulating citrulline. *Am J Physiol* **241**:E473, 1981.
30. Tuchman M: Persistent acitrullinemia after liver transplantation for carbamoylphosphate synthetase deficiency. *New Engl J Med* **320**:1498, 1989.
31. Rabier D, Narcy C, Parvy JB, Saudubray JM, Kamoun P: Arginine remains an essential amino acid after liver transplantation in urea cycle enzyme deficiencies. *J Inherit Metab Dis* **14**:277, 1991.
32. Marliss EB, Aoki TT, Pozefsky T, Most AS, Cahill GF Jr: Muscle and splanchnic glutamine and glutamate metabolism in postabsorptive and starved man. *J Clin Invest* **50**:814, 1971.
33. Ruderman NB, Berger M: The formation of glutamine and alanine in skeletal muscle. *J Biol Chem* **249**:5500, 1974.
34. Garber AJ, Karl IE, Kipnis DM: Alanine and glutamine release from skeletal muscle. *J Biol Chem* **251**:826, 1976.
35. Lowenstein JM: Ammonia production in muscle and other tissues: The purine nucleotide cycle. *Physiol Rev* **52**:382, 1972.
36. Brady TG, O'Donovan CI: A study of the tissue distribution of adenosine deaminase in six mammal species. *Comp Biochem Physiol* **14**:101, 1965.
37. Raiha NCR, Suihkonen J: Development of urea-synthesizing enzymes in human liver. *Acta Paediatr Scand* 57:121, 1968.
38. Baig MMA, Swamy HM, Hassan SI, Zaman TU, Ayesha Q, Devi BG: Studies on urea cycle enzyme levels in the human fetal liver at different gestational ages. *Pediatr Res* **31**:143, 1992.
39. Tedesco TA, Mellman WJ: Argininosuccinate synthetase activity and citrulline metabolism in cells cultured from a citrullinemic subject. *Proc Natl Acad Sci U S A* **57**:829, 1967.
40. Matsuda I, Arashima S, Nambu H, Takekoshi Y, Anakura M: Hyperammonemia due to a mutant enzyme of ornithine transcarbamylase. *Pediatrics* **48**:595, 1971.
41. Saudubray JM, Cathelineau L, Laugier JM, Charpentier C, Lejune JA, Mozziconacci P: Hereditary ornithine transcarbamylase deficiency. *Acta Paediatr Scand* **64**:464, 1975.
42. Heiden CVD, Desplanque J, Bakker HD: Some kinetic properties of liver ornithine carbamoyl transferase (OTC) in a patient with OTC deficiency. *Clin Chim Acta* **80**:519, 1977.
43. Qureshi IA, Letarte J, Ouellet R: Study of enzyme defect in a case of ornithine transcarbamylase deficiency. *Diabetes Metab* **4**:239, 1978.
44. Briand P, Francois B, Rabier D, Cathelineau L: Ornithine transcarbamylase deficiencies in human males; kinetic and immunochemical classification. *Biochim Biophys Acta* **704**:10, 1982.
45. Francois B, Brian P, Cathelineau L: Immunochemical assay in 16 boys with ornithine transcarbamylase deficiency. *Adv Exp Med Biol* **153**:53, 1982.
46. Matsuda I, Nagata N, Ohyanagi K, Tsuchiyama A, Yamamoto H, Hase Y, Kodama H, Kai Y: Biochemical heterogeneity of ornithine carbamoyl transferase (OTC) in patients with OTC deficiency. *Jpn J Hum Genet* **29**:327, 1984.
47. Morris SM. Regulation of enxymes of urea and arginine synthesis. *Annu Rev Nutr* **12**:81, 1992.
48. Schimke RT: Adaptive characteristics of the urea cycle enzymes in the rat. *J Biol Chem* **237**:459, 1962.
49. Nuzum CT, Snodgrass PJ: Urea cycle enzyme adaptation to dietary protein in primates. *Science* **172**:1042, 1972.
50. Das TK, Waterlow JC: The rate of adaptation of urea cycle enzymes, aminotransferases and glutamic dehydrogenase to changes in dietary protein intake. *Br J Nutr* **32**:353, 1974.
51. Marten NW, Sladek FM, Straus DS: Effect of dietary protein restriction on liver transcription factors. *Biochem J* **317**:361, 1996.
52. Tillman JB, Dhahbi JM, Mote PL, Walford RL, Spindler SR: Dietary calorie restriction in mice induces carbamyl phosphate synthetase I gene transcription tissue specifically. *J Biol Chem* **271**:3500, 1996.
53. Cohen PP: Regulation of the ornithine-urea cycle enzymes, in Waterlow JC, Stephen JML (eds): *Nitrogen Metabolism in Man*. London, Applied Science, 1981, p 215.
54. Grofte T, Wolthers T, Jensen SA, Moller N, Jorgensen JO, Tygstrup N, Orskov H, Vilstrup H: Effects of growth hormone and insulin-like growth factor-1 singly and in combination on *in vivo* capacity of urea synthesis, gene expression of urea cycle enzymes, and organ nitrogen contents in rats *Hepatology* **25**:964, 1997
55. Cohen NS, Cheung CW, Raijman L: Channeling of extramitochondrial ornithine to matrix ornithine transcarbamylase. *J Biol Chem* **262**:203, 1987.
56. Cheung CW, Cohen NS, Raijman L: Channeling of urea cycle intermediates *in situ* in permeabilized hepatocytes. *J Biol Chem* **264**:4038, 1989.
57. Walser M: Urea cycle disorders and other hyperammonemia syndromes, in Stanbury JB, Wyngaarden JB, Fredrickson DS, Goldstein JL, Brown MS (eds): *The Metabolic Basis of Inherited Disease*, 5th ed. New York, McGraw-Hill, 1983, p 402.
58. Meijer AJ: Regulation of carbamoylphosphate synthetase (ammonia) in liver in relation to urea cycle activity, in Ochs RS, Hanson RW, Hall Z (eds): *Metabolic Regulation*. New York, Elsevier, 1985, p 171.
59. Adcock MW, O'Brien WE: Molecular cloning of cDNA for rat and human carbamyl phosphate synthetase I. *J Biol Chem* **259**:13471, 1984.
60. Morris SM, Moncman CL, Rand KD, Dizikes GJ, Cederbaum SD, O'Brien WE: Regulation of in mRNA levels for five urea cycle enzymes in rat liver by diet, cyclic AMP and glucocorticoids. *Arch Biochem Biophys* **256**:343, 1987.
61. Ryall J, Rachubinski RA, Nguyen M, Rozen R, Broglie KE, Shore GC: Regulation and expression of carbamyl phosphate synthetase I mRNA in developing rat liver and Morris hepatoma 5123D. *J Biol Chem* **259**:9172, 1984.
62. Nyunoya H, Broglie KE, Widgren EE, Lusty CJ: Characterization and derivation of the gene coding for mitochondrial carbamyl phosphate synthetase I of rat. *J Biol Chem* **260**:9346, 1985.
63. Haraguchi Y, Uchino T, Takiguchi M, Endo R, Mori M, Matsuda I: Cloning and sequence of a cDNA encoding human carbamyl phosphate synthetase I: Molecular analysis of hyperammonemia. *Gene* **107**:335, 1991.
64. Nyunoya H, Argan C, Lusty CJ, Shore GC: Import and processing of hybrid proteins by mammalian mitochondria *in vitro*. *J Biol Chem* **261**:800, 1986.
65. Rubino SD, Nyunoya H, Lusty CJ: *In vivo* synthesis of carbamyl phosphate from NH_3 by the large subunit of *Escherichia coli* carbamyl phosphate synthetase. *J Biol Chem* **262**:4382, 1987.
66. Nyunoya H, Broglie KE, Lusty CJ: The gene coding for carbamoyl-phosphate synthetase I was formed by fusion of an ancestral glutaminase gene and a synthetase gene. *Proc Natl Acad Sci U S A* **82**:2244, 1985.
67. Hong J, Salo WL, Lusty CJ, Anderson PM: Carbamyl phosphate synthetase III, an evolutionary intermediate in the transition between glutamine-dependent and ammonia-dependent carbamyl phosphate synthetases. *J Mol Biol* **243**:131, 1994.
68. Schofield JP, Elgar G, Greystrong J, Lye G, Deadman R, Micklem G, King A, Brenner S, Vaudin M: Regions of human chromosome 2 (2q32-q35) and mouse chromosome 1 show synteny with the pufferfish genome (*Fugu rubripes*). *Genomics* **45**:158, 1997.
69. Lawson FS, Charlebois RL, Dillon JA: Phylogenetic analysis of carbmoylphosphate synthetase genes: Complex evolutionary history includes an internal duplication within a gene which can root the tree of life. *Mol Biol Evol* **13**:970, 1996.
70. Rubino SD, Nyunoya H, Lusty CJ: Catalytic domains of carbamyl phosphate synthetase. Glutamine-hydrolyzing site of *Escherichia coli* carbamyl phosphate synthetase. *J Biol Chem* **261**:111320, 1986.
71. Guillou F, Liao M, Garcia-Espana A, Lusty CJ: Mutational analysis of carbamyl phosphate synthetase. Substitution of Glu841 leads to loss of functional coupling between the two catalytic domains of the synthetase subunit. *Biochemistry* **31**:1656, 1992.
72. Potter MD, Powers-Lee SG: Location of the ATP gamma-phosphate-binding sites on rat liver carbamoyl-phosphate synthetase I. Studies with the ATP analog 5′-p-fluorosulfonylbenzoyladenosine. *J Biol Chem* **267**:2023, 1992.

73. Potter MD, Powers-Lee SG: Direct photoaffinity labeling of rat liver carbamoyl phosphate synthetase I with ATP. *Arch Biochem Biophys* **306**:377, 1993.
74. Guy HI, Evans DR: Function of the major synthetase subdomains of carbamyl-phosphate synthetase. *J Biol Chem* **271**:13762, 1996.
75. Kasprzak AA, Villafranca JJ: Interactive binding between the substrate and allosteric sites of carbamoyl-phosphate synthetase. *Biochemistry* **27**:8050, 1988.
76. Cervera J, Bendala E, Britton HG, Nassif BJ, Lusty CJ, Rubio V: Photoaffinity laveling with UMP of lysine 992 of carbamyl phosphate synthetase from *Escherichia coli* allows identification of the binding site for the pyrimidine inhibitor. *Biochemistry* **35**:7247, 1996.
77. Rodriguez-Aparicio LB, Guadalajara AM, Rubio V: Physical location of the site for *N*-acetyl-L-glutamate, the allosteric activator of carbamoyl phosphate synthetase, in the 20-kilodalton COOH-terminal domain. *Biochemistry* **28**:3070, 1989.
78. McCudden CR, Powers-Lee SG: Required allosteric effector site for *N*-acetylglutamate on carbamoyl-phosphate synthetase I. *J Biol Chem* **271**:18285, 1996.
79. Britton HG, Garcia-Espana A, Goya P, Rozas I, Rubio V: A structure–reactivity study of the binding of acetylglutamate to carbamoyl phosphate synthetase I. *Eur J Biochem* **188**:47, 1990.
80. Hoshide R, Soejima H, Ohta T, Niikawa N, Haraguchi Y, Matsuura T, Endo F, Matsuda I: Assignment of the human carbamyl phosphate synthetase I gene (*CPSI*) to 2q35 by fluorescence *in situ* hybridization. *Genomics* **28**:124, 1995.
81. Summar ML, Dasouki MJ, Schofield PJ, Krishnamani MR, Vnencak-Jones C, Tuchman M, Mao J, Phillips JA 3rd: Physical and linkage mapping of human carbamyl phosphate synthetase I (CPSI) and reassignment from 2p to 2q35. *Cytogenet Cell Genet* **71**:266, 1995.
82. Howell BW, Lagacé M, Shore GC: Activity of the carbamyl phosphate synthetase I promoter in liver nuclear extracts is dependent on a *cis*-acting C/EBP recognition element. *Mol Cell Biol* **9**:2928, 1989.
83. Lagacé M, Goping IS, Mueller CR, Lazzaro M, Shore GC: The carbamyl phosphate synthetase promoter contains multiple binding sites for C/EBP-related proteins. *Gene* **118**:231, 1992.
84. Goping IS, Shore GC: Interactions between repressor and anti-repressor elements in the carbamyl phosphate synthetase I promoter. *J Biol Chem* **269**:3891, 1994.
85. Goping IS, Lamontagne S, Shore GC, Nguyen M: A gene-type-specific enhancer regulates the carbamylphosphate synthetase I promoter by cooperating with the proximal GAG activating element. *Nucleic Acids Res* **23**:1717, 1995.
86. Kraus JP, Rosenberg LE: Purification of low-abundance messenger RNAs from rat liver by polysome immunoabsorption. *Proc Natl Acad Sci U S A* **79**:4051, 1982.
87. Horwich AL, Kraus JP, Williams K, Kalousek F, Konigsberg W, Rosenberg LE: Molecular cloning of the cDNA coding for rat ornithine transcarbamylase. *Proc Natl Acad Sci U S A* **80**:4258, 1983.
88. Horwich AL, Fenton WA, Williams KR, Kalousek F, Kraus JP, Doolittle RF, Konigsberg W, Rosenberg LE: Structure and expression of a complementary DNA for the nuclear coded precursor of human mitochondrial ornithine transcarbamylase. *Science* **224**:1068, 1984.
89. Hata A, Tsuzuki T, Shimada K, Takiguchi M, Mori M, Matsuda I: Isolation and characterization of the human ornithine transcarbamylase gene: Structure of the 5′ end region. *J Biochem* **100**:717, 1986.
90. Lindgren V, De Martinville B, Horwich AL, Rosenberg LE, Francke U: Human ornithine transcarbamylase locus mapped to band Xp21.1, near the Duchenne muscular dystrophy locus. *Science* **226**:698, 1984.
91. Ricciuti FC, Gelehrter TD, Rosenberg LE: X-chromosome inactivation in human liver: Confirmation of X-linkage of ornithine transcarbamylase. *Am J Hum Genet* **28**:32, 1976.
92. Mrozek JD, Holzknecht RA, Butkowski RJ, Mauer SM, Tuchman M: X-chromosome inactivation in the liver of female heterozygous OTC-deficient *sparse-fur^{ash}* mice. *Biochem Med Metab Biol* **45**:333, 1991.
93. Holliday R: X chromosome reactivation and aging. *Nature* **37**:311, 1989.
94. McIntyre P, Graf L, Mercer JFB, Wake SA, Hudson P, Hoogenraad N: The primary structure of the imported mitochondrial protein, ornithine transcarbamylase from rat liver: mRNA levels during ontogeny. *DNA* **4**:147, 1985.
95. Hata A, Tsuzuki T, Shimada K, Takiguchi M, Mori M, Matsuda I: Isolation and characterization of the human ornithine transcarbamylase gene: Structure of the 5′ end region. *J Biochem* **100**:717, 1986.
96. Veres G, Craigen WJ, Caskey CT: The 5′flanking region of the ornithine transcarbamylase gene contains DNA sequences regulating tissue-specific expression. *J Biol Chem* **261**:7588, 1986.
97. Murakami T, Nishiyori A, Takiguchi M, Mori M: Promoter and 11-kilobase upstream enhancer elements responsible for hepatoma cell-specific expression of the rat ornithine transcarbamylase gene. *Mol Cell Biol* **10**:11180, 1990.
98. Farmer AA, Gross SJ: BWTG3 hepatoma cells can acquire phenylalanine hydroxylase, cystathionine synthetase and *CPS-1* without genetic manipulation, but activation of the silent *OTC* gene requires cell fusion with hepatocytes. *J Cell Sci* **98**(part 4):533, 1991.
99. Kimura A, Nishiyori A, Murakami T, Tsukamoto T, Hata S, Osumi T, Okamura R, Mori M, Takiguchi M: Chicken ovalbumin upstream promoter-transcription factor (COUP-TF) represses transcription from the promoter of the gene for ornithine transcarbamylase in a manner antagonistic to hepatocyte nuclear factor-f (HNF-4). *J Biol Chem* **268**:11125, 1993.
100. Kraus JP, Hodges PE, Williamson CL, Horwich AL, Kalousek F, Williams KR, Rosenberg LE: A cDNA clone for the precursor of rat mitochondrial ornithine transcarbamylase: Comparison of rat and human leader sequences and conservation of catalytic sites. *Nucleic Acids Res* **13**:943, 1985.
101. Hodges PE, Rosenberg LE: The spfash mouse: A missense mutation in the ornithine transcarbamylase gene also causes aberrant mRNA splicing. *Proc Natl Acad Sci U S A* **86**:4142, 1984.
102. Veres G, Gibbs RA, Scherer SE, Caskey CT: The molecular basis of the sparse fur mouse mutation. *Science* **237**:415, 1987.
103. Conboy JG, Rosenberg LE: Posttranslational uptake and processing of in vitro synthesized ornithine transcarbamoylase precursor by isolated rat liver mitochondria. *Proc Natl Acad Sci U S A* **78**:3073, 1981.
104. Murakami K, Amaya Y, Takiguchi M, Ebina Y, Mori M: Reconstitution of mitochondrial protein transport with purified ornithine carbamoyltransferase precursor expressed in *Escherichia coli. J Biol Chem* **263**:18437, 1988.
105. Deshaies RJ, Koch BD, Werner-Washburne M, Craig EA, Schekman R: A subfamily of stress proteins facilitates translocation of secretory and mitochondrial precursor polypeptides. *Nature* **332**:800, 1988.
106. Murakami H, Pain D, Blobel G: 70-kD heat shock–related protein is one of at least two distinct cytosolic factors that stimulate protein import into mitochondria. *J Cell Biol* **263**:18437, 1988.
107. Sheffield WP, Shore GC, Randall SK: Mitochondrial precursor protein. Effects of 70-kilodalton heat shock protein on polypeptide folding, aggregation, and import competence. *J Biol Chem* **265**:11069, 1990.
108. Pfanner N, Tropschug M, Neupert W: Mitochondrial protein import: Nucleoside triphosphates are involved in conferring import-competence to precursors. *Cell* **49**:815, 1987.
109. Chen WJ, Douglas MG: Phosphodiester bond cleavage outside mitochondria is required for the completion of protein import into the mitochondrial matrix. *Cell* **49**:651, 1987.
110. Eilers M, Oppliger W, Schatz G: Both ATP and an energized inner membrane are required to import a purified precursor protein into mitochondria. *EMBO J* **6**:1073, 1987.
111. Terada K, Ohtsuka K, Imamoto N, Yoneda Y, Mori M: Role of heat shock cognate 70 protein in import or ornithine transcarbamylase precusor into mammalian mitochondria. *Mol Cell Biol* **15**:3708, 1995.
112. Terada K, Kanazawa M, Bukau B, Mori M: The human DnaJ homogue dj2 facilitates mitochondrial protein import and luciferase refolding. *J Cell Biol* **139**:1089, 1997.
113. Bukau B, Horwich AL: The Hsp70 and Hsp60 chaperone machines. *Cell* **92**:351, 1998.
114. Murakami K, Tanase S, Morino Y, Mori M: Presequence binding factor-dependent and independent import of proteins into mitochondria. *J Biol Chem* **267**:13119, 1992.
115. Hachiya N, Alam R, Sakasegawa Y, Sakaguchi M, Mihara K, Omura T: A mitochondrial import factor purified from rat liver cytosol is an ATP-dependent conformational modulator for precursor proteins. *EMBO J* **12**:1579, 1993.
116. Horwich AL, Kalousek F, Hellman I, Rosenberg LE: A leader peptide is sufficient to direct mitochondrial import of a chimeric protein. *EMBO J* **4**:1129, 1985.
117. Nyunoya H, Argan C, Lusty CJ, Shore GC: Import and processing of hybrid proteins by mammalian mitochondria *in vitro. J Biol Chem* **268**:800, 1986.
118. Horwich AL, Kalousek F, Fenton WA, Pollack RA, Rosenberg LE: The ornithine transcarbamylase leader peptide directs mitochondria:

Definition of critical regions and residues in the leader peptide. *Cell* **44**:451, 1986.

119. Isaya G, Fenton WA, Hendrick JP, Furtak K, Kalousek F, Rosenberg LE: Mitochondrial import and processing of mutant human ornithine transcarbamylase precursors in cultured cells. *Mol Cell Biol* **8**:5150, 1988.
120. Gillespie LL, Argan C, Taneja AT, Hodges RS, Freeman KB, Shore GC: A synthetic signal peptide blocks import of precursor proteins destined for the mitochondrial inner membrane or matrix. *J Biol Chem* **260**:16045, 1985.
121. Horwich AL, Kalousek F, Fenton WA, Furtak K, Pollock RA, Rosenberg LE: The ornithine transcarbamylase leader peptide directs mitochondrial import through both its midportion structure and net positive charge. *J Cell Biol* **105**:669, 1987.
122. Von Heijne G: Mitochondrial targeting sequences may form amphiphilic helices. *EMBO J* **5**:1335, 1986.
123. Bedwell DM, Strobel SA, Yun K, Jongweard GD, Emr SD: Sequence and structural requirements of a mitochondrial protein import signal defined by saturation cassette mutagenesis. *Mol Cell Biol* **9**:1014, 1989.
124. Lemire BD, Fankhauser C, Baker A, Schatz G: The mitochondrial targeting function of randomly generated peptide sequences correlate with predicted helical amphiphilicity. *J Biol Chem* **264**:20206, 1989.
125. Grompe M, Muzny DM, Caskey CT: Scanning detection of mutations in human ornithine transcarbamylase by chemical mismatch cleavage. *Proc Natl Acad Sci U S A* **86**:5888, 1989.
126. Pfanner N, Meijer M: The Tom and Tim machine. *Curr Biol* **7**:100, 1997.
127. Haucke V, Schatz G: Import of proteins into mitochondria and chloroplasts. *TICB* **7**:103, 1997.
128. Neupert W: Protein import into mitochondria and chlorplasts. *Ann Rev Biochem* **66**:863, 1997.
129. Goping IS, Millar DG, Shore GC: Identification of the human mitochondrial protein import receptor, huMas20p. Complementation of Δmas20 in yeast. *FEBS Lett* **373**:45, 1995.
130. Wada J, Kanwar YS: Characterization of mammalian translocase of inner mitochondrial membrane (Tim44) isolated from diabetic newborn mouse kidney. *Proc Natl Acad Sci U S A* **95**:144, 1998.
131. Keibler M, Keil P, Schneider H, van der Klei IJ, Pfanner N, Neupert W: The mitochondrial receptor complex: A central role of MOM22 in mediating preprotein transfer from receptors to the general insertion pore. *Cell* **74**:483, 1993.
132. Dietmeier K, Honlinger A, Bomer U, Dekker PJT, Eckerskorn C, Lottspeich F, Kubrich M, Pfanner N: Tom5 functionally links mitochondrial preprotein receptors to the general import pore. *Nature* **388**:195, 1997.
133. Schatz G: Just follow the acid chain. *Nature* **388**:121, 1997.
134. Horst M, Hilfilker-Rothenfluh S, Oppliger W, Schatz G: Dynamic interaction of the protein translocation systems in the inner and outer membranes of yeast mitochondria. *EMBO J* **14**:2293, 1995.
135. Segui-Real B, Kispal G, Lill R, Neupert W: A dynamic model of the mitochondrial protein import machinery. *Cell* **68**:999, 1992.
136. Sirrenberg C, Bauer MR, Guiard B, Neupert W, Brunner M: Import of carrier proteins into the mitochondrial inner membrane mediated by Tim22. *Nature* **384**:582, 1996.
137. Koehler CM, Jarosch E, Tokatlidis K, Schmid K, Schweyen RJ, Schatz G: Import of mitochondrial carriers mediated by essential proteins of the intermembrane space. *Science* **279**:369, 1998.
138. Sirrenberg C, Endres M, Folsch H, Stuart RA, Neupert W, Brunner M: Carrier protein import mitochondria mediated by the intermembrane proteins Tim10/Mrs11 and Tim12/Mrs5. *Nature* **391**:912, 1998.
139. Mayer A, Nargang FE, Neupert W, Lill R: MOM22 is a receptor for mitochondrial targeting sequences and cooperates with MOM19. *EMBO J* **14**:4202, 1995.
140. Terada K, Kanazawa M, Yano M, Hanson B, Hoogenraad N, Mori M: Participation of the import receptor Tom20 in protein import into mammalian mitochondria: analyses *in vitro* and in cultured cells. *FEBS Lett* **403**:309, 1997.
141. Hachiya N, Mihara K, Suda K, Horst M, Schatz G, Lithgow T: Reconstitution of the initial steps of mitochondrial protein import. *Nature* **376**:705, 1995.
142. Schneider H, Sollner T, Dietmeier K, Eckerskorn C, Lottspeich F, Trulzsch B, Neupert W, Pfanner N: Targeting of the master receptor MOM19 to mitochondria. *Science* **254**:1659, 1991.
143. Hase T, Riezman H, suda K, Schatz G: Import of proteins into mitochondria: Nucleotide sequence of the gene for a 70 kg protein of the yeast mitochondrial outer membrane. *EMBO J* **2**:2169, 1983.
144. Haucke V, Horst M, Schatz G, Lithgow T: The Mas20p and Mas70p subunits of the protein import receptor of yeast mitochondria interact via the tetratricopeptide repeat motif in Mas20p: evidence for a single hetero-oligomeric receptor. *EMBO J* **15**:1231, 1996.
145. Ramage L, Junne T, Hahne K, Lithgow T, Schatz G: Functional cooperation of mitochondrial protein import receptors in yeast. *EMBO J* **12**:4115, 1993.
146. Lithgow T, Junne T, Suda K, Gratzer S, Schatz G: The mitochondrial outer membrane protein Mas22p is essential for protein import and viability of yeast. *Proc Natl Acad Sci U S A* **91**:11973, 1994.
147. Gratzer S, Lithgow T, Bauer RE, Lamping E, Paltauf F, Kohlwein SD, Haucke V, Junne T, Schatz G, Horst M: Mas37p, a novel receptor subunit for protein import into mitochondria. *J Cell Biol* **129**:25, 1995.
148. Honlinger A, Kibrich M, Moczko M, Gartner F, Mallet L, Bussereau F, Eckerskorn C, Lottspeich F, Dietmeier K, Jacquet M, Pfanner N: The mitochondrial receptor complex: Mom22 is essential for cell viability and directly interacts with preproteins. *Mol Cell Biol* **15**:3382, 1995.
149. Bolliger L, Junne T, Schatz G, Lithgow T: Acidic receptor domains on both sides of the outer membrane mediate translocation of precursor proteins into yeast mitochondria. *EMBO J* **14**:6318, 1995.
150. Komiya T, Rospert S, Koehler C, Looser R, Schatz G, Mihara K: Interaction of mitochondrial targeting signals with acidic receptor domains along the protein import pathway: evidence for the "acid chain" hypothesis. *EMBO J* **17**:3886, 1998.
151. Kunkele K-P, Heins S, Dembowski M, Nargang FE, Benz R, Thieffry M, Walz J, Lill R, Nussberger S, Neupert W: The preprotein translocation channel of the outer membrane of mitochondria. *Cell* **93**:1009, 1998.
152. Maarse AC, Bloom J, Grivell LA, Meijer M: *MPII*, an essential gene encoding a mitochondrial membrane protein, is probably involved in protein transport into yeast mitochondria. *EMBO J* **11**:3619, 1992.
153. Scherer PE, Manning-Kreig U, Jeno P, Schatz G, Horst M: Identification of a 45-K Da protein at the protein import site of the yeast mitochondrial inner membrane. *Proc Natl Acad Sci U S A* **89**:11920, 1992.
154. Dekker PJT, Keil P, Rassow J, Maarse AC, Pfanner N, Meijer M: Identification of MIM23, a putative component of the protein import machinery of the mitochondrial inner membrane. *FEBS Lett* **33**:66, 1993.
155. Blom J, Kubrich M, Rassow J, Voos W, Dekker PJT, Maarse AC, Meijer M, Pfanner N: The essential yeast protein MIM44 (encoded by MPII) involved in an early step of preprotein translocation across the mitochondrial inner membrane. *Mol Cell Biol* **13**:7364, 1993.
156. Emtage JLT, Jensen RE: MAS6 encodes an essential inner membrane component of the yeast mitochondrial protein import pathway. *J Cell Biol* **122**:1003, 1993.
157. Ryan KR, Menold MM, Garrett S, Jensen RE: SMSI, a high-copy suppressor of the yeast mass mutant, encodes an essential inner membrane protein required for mitochondrial protein import. *Mol Biol Cell* **5**:529, 1994.
158. Kubrich M, Keil P, Rassow J, Dekker PJT, Blom J, Meijer M, Pfanner N: The polytopic mitochondrial inner membrane proteins MIM17 and MIM23 operate at the same preprotein import site. *FEBS Lett* **349**:222, 1994.
159. Berthold J, Bauer MF, Schneider HC, Klaus C, Dietmeier K, Neupert W, Brunner M: The MIM complex mediates preprotein translocation across the mitochondrial inner membrane and couples it on the mt-Hsp 70/ATP driving system. *Cell* **81**:1085, 1995.
160. Bauer MR, Sirrenberg C, Neupert W, Brunner M: Role of Tim23 as voltage sensor and presequence receptor in protein import into mitochondria. *Cell* **87**:33, 1996.
161. Schleyer M, Neupert W: Transport of proteins into mitochondria: Translocational intermediates spanning contact sites between outer and inner membranes. *Cell* **43**:339, 1985.
162. Schneider HC, Bertold J, Bauer MF, Dietmeier K, Guiard B, Brunner M, Neupert W: Mitochondrial Hsp70/MIM44 complex facilitates protein import. *Nature* **371**:768, 1994.
163. Bomer U, Maarse AC, Martin F, Geissler A, Merline A, Schonfisch B, Meijer M, Pfanner N, Rassow J: Separation of structural and dynamic functions of the mitochondrial translocase: Tim44 is crucial for the inner membrane import sites in translocation of tightly folded

domains, but not of loosely folded preproteins. *EMBO J* **17**:4226, 1998.
164. Craig EA, Kramer J, Shilling J, Werner-Washburne M, Holmes S, Kosic-Smithers J, Nicolet CM: SSCI, an essential member of the yeast hsp70 multigene family encodes a mitochondrial protein. *Mol Cell Biol* **9**:3000, 1989.
165. Kang PJ, Ostermann J, Shilling J, Neupert W, Craig EA, Pfanner N: Requirement for hsp70 in the mitochondrial matrix for translocation and folding of precursor proteins. *Nature* **348**:137, 1990.
166. Scherer PE, Krieg UC, Hwang ST, Vestweber D, Schatz G: A precusor protein partly translocated into yeast mictochondria is bound to a 70 kd mitochondrial stress protein. *EMBO J* **9**:4315, 1990.
167. Flynn GC, Pohl J, Flocco MT, Rothman JE: Peptide-binding specificity of the molecular chaperone BiP. *Nature* **353**:726, 1991.
168. Rudiger S, Germeroth L, Schneider-Mergener J, Bukau B: Substrate specificity of the DnaK chaperone determined by screening cellulose-bound peptide libraries. *EMBO J* **16**:1501, 1997.
169. Rassow J, Hartl FU, Guiard B, Pfanner N, Neupert W: Polypeptides traverse the mitochondrial envelope in an extended state. *FEBS Lett* **275**:190, 1990.
170. Neupert W, Hartl FU, Craig EA, Pfanner N: How do polypeptides cross the mitochondrial membranes? *Cell* **63**:447, 1990.
171. Glick BS: Can Hsp70 proteins act as force-generating motors? *Cell* **80**:11, 1995.
172. Matouschek A, Azem A, Ratliff K, Glick BS, Schmid K, Schatz G: Active unfolding of precursor proteins during mitochondrial protein import. *EMBO J* **16**:6727, 1997.
173. Geli V: Functional reconstitution in *Escherichia coli* of the yeast mitochondrial matrix peptidase from its two inactive subunits. *Proc Natl Acad Sci U S A* 90:6247, 1993.
174. Arretz M, Schneider H, Guiard B, Brunner M, Neupert W: Characterization of the mitochondrial processing peptidase of *Neurospora crassa*. *J Biol Chem* **269**:4959, 1994.
175. Saavedra-Alanis VM, Rysavy P, Rosenberg LE, Kalousek F: Rat liver mitochondrial processing peptidase. *J Biol Chem* **269**:9284, 1994.
176. Ou WJ, Ito A, Okazaki H, Omura T: Purification and characterization of a processing protease from rat liver mitochondria. *EMBO J* **8**:2605, 1989.
177. Yang M, Jensen RE, Yaffe MP, Oppliger W, Schatz G: Import of proteins into yeast mitochondria: The purified matrix processing protease contains two subunits which are encoded by the nuclear *MAS1* and *MAS2* genes. *EMBO J* **7**:3857, 1989.
178. Hawlitschek G, Schneider H, Schmidt B, Tropschug M, Hartl FU, Neupert W: Mitochondrial protein import: identification of processing peptidase and of PEP, a processing enhancing protein. *Cell* **53**:795, 1988.
179. Kitada S, Shimokata K, Niidome T, Ogishima T, Ito A: A putative metal-binding site in the β subunit of rat mitochondrial processing peptidase is essential for its catalytic activity. *J Biochem* **117**:1148, 1995.
180. Pollock RA, Hartl FU, Cheng MY, Ostermann J, Horwich A, Neupert W: The processing peptidase of yeast mitochondria: The two co-operating components MPP and PEP are structurally related. *EMBO J* **7**:3493, 1988.
181. Jensen RE, Yaffe MP: Import of proteins into yeast mitochondria: The nuclear *MAS2* gene encodes a component of the processing protease that is homologous to the *MAS1*-encoded subunit. *EMBO J* **7**:3863, 1988.
182. Schneider H, Arretz M, Wachter E, Neupert W: Matrix processing peptidase of mitochondria. *J Biol Chem* **265**:9881, 1990.
183. Kleiber J, Kalousek F, Swaroop M, Rosenberg LE: The general mitochondrial matrix processing protease from rat liver: Structural characterization of the catalytic subunit. *Proc Natl Acad Sci U S A* **87**:7987, 1990.
184. Paces V, Rosenberg LE, Fenton WA, Kalousek F: The β subunit of the mitochondrial processing peptidase from rat liver: Cloning and sequencing of a cDNA and comparison with a proposed family of metallopeptidases. *Proc Natl Acad Sci U S A* **90**:5355, 1993.
185. Von Heijne G, Steppuhn J, Herrmann RG: Domain structure of mitochondrial and chloroplast targeting peptides. *Eur J Biochem* **180**:535, 1989.
186. Hendrick JP, Hodges PE, Rosenberg LE: Survey of amino-terminal proteolytic cleavage sites in mitochondrial precursor proteins: Leader peptides cleaved by two matrix proteases share a three-amino acid motif. *Proc Natl Acad Sci U S A* **86**:4056, 1989.
187. Ogishima T, Niidome T, Shimokata K, Kitada S, Ito A: Analysis of elements in the substrate required for processing by mitochondrial processing peptidase. *J Biol Chem* **270**:30322, 1995.
188. Yang M, Geli V, Oppliger W, Suda K, James P, Schatz G: The MAS-encoded processing protease of yeast mitochondria. *J Biol Chem* **266**:6416, 1991.
189. Iwata S, Lee JW, Okada K, Lee JK, Iwata M, Rasmussen B, Link TA, Ramaswamy S, Jap B: Complete structure of the 11-subunit bovine mitochondrial cytochrome bc_1 complex. *Science* **281**:64, 1998.
190. Kalousek F, Hendrick JP, Rosenberg LE: Two mitochondrial matrix proteases act sequentially in the processing of mammalian matrix enzymes. *Proc Natl Acad Sci U S A* **85**:7536, 1988.
191. Isaya G, Kalousek F, Rosenberg LE: Amino terminal octapeptides function as recognition signals for the mitochondrial intermediate peptidase. *J Biol Chem* **267**:7904, 1992.
192. Isaya G, Kalousek F, Fenton WA, Rosenberg LE: Cleavage of precursors by the mitochondrial processing peptidase requires a compatible mature protein or an intermediate octapeptide. *J Cell Biol* **113**:65, 1991.
193. Isaya G, Kalousek F, Rosenberg LE: Sequence analysis of rat mitochondrial intermediate peptidase: Similarity to zinc metallopeptidases and to a putative yeast homologue. *Proc Natl Acad Sci U S A* **89**:8317, 1992.
194. Isaya G, Sakati WR, Rollins RA, Shen GP, Hanson LC, Ullrich RC, Novotny CP: Mammalian mitochondrial intermediate peptidase: structure/function analysis of a new homologue from *Schizophyllum commune* and relationship to thimet oligopeptidase. *Genomics* **28**:450, 1995.
195. Isaya G, Miklos D, Rollins RA: *MIP1*, a new yeast gene homologous to the rat mitochondrial intermediate peptidase gene, is required for oxidative metabolism in *Saccharomyces cerevisiae*. *Mol Cell Biol* **14**:5603, 1994.
196. Branda SS, Isaya G: Prediction and identification of new natural substrates of the yeast mitochondrial intermediate peptidase. *J Biol Chem* **270**:27366, 1995.
197. Cheng MY, Hartl FU, Martin J, Pollock RA, Kalousek F, Neupert W, Hallberg EM, Hallberg RL, Horwich AL: Mitochondrial heat-shock protein hsp 60 is essential for assembly of proteins imported into yeast mitochondria. *Nature* **337**:620, 1989.
198. Glick BS, Brandt A, Cunningham K, Muller S, Hallberg RL, Schatz G: Cytochromes cl and b2 are sorted to intermembrane space of yeast mitochondria by a stop transfer mechanism. *Cell* **69**:809, 1992.
199. McMullen TW, Hallberg RL: A normal mitochondrial protein is selectively synthesized and accumulated during heat shock in *Tetrahymena thermophila*. *Mol Cell Biol* **7**:4414, 1987.
200. McMullen TW, Hallberg RL: A highly evolutionary conserved mitochondrial protein is structurally related to the protein encoded by the *Escherichia coli groEL* gene. *Mol Cell Biol* **8**:371, 1988.
201. Reading DS, Hallberg RL, Myers AM: Characterization of the yeast *HSP60* gene coding for a mitochondrial assembly factor. *Nature* **337**:655, 1989.
202. Ostermann J, Horwich AL, Neupert W, Hartl FU: Protein folding in mitochondria requires complex formation with hsp60 and ATP hydrolysis. *Nature* **341**:125, 1989.
203. Dubaquie Y, Looser R, Funfschilling U, Jeno P, Rospert S: Identification of *in vivo* substrates of the yeast mitochondrial chaperonins reveals overlapping but non-identical requirement for hsp60 and hsp10. *EMBO J* **17**:5868, 1998.
204. Cheng MY, Hartl FU, Horwich AL: The mitochondrial chaperonin hsp60 is required for its own assembly. *Nature* **348**:455, 1990.
205. Luck DJL: Formation of mitochondria in *Neurospora crassa*. *J Cell Biol* **24**:461, 1965.
206. Fayet O, Ziegelhoffer T, Georgopoulos C: The groEs and groEL heat shock gene products of *Escherichia coli* are essential for bacterial growth at all temperatures. *J Bacteriol* **171**:1379, 1989.
207. Neidhardt FC, Van Bogelen RA, Vaughn VA: The genetics and regulation of heat-shock proteins. *Ann Rev Genet* **18**:295, 1984.
208. Georgopoulos CP, Hendrix RW, Casjens SR, Kaiser AD: Host participation in bacteriophage lambda head assembly. *J Mol Biol* **76**:45, 1973.
209. Sternberg N: Properties of a mutant of *Escherichia coli* defective in bacteriophage λ head formation (groE). *J Mol Biol* **76**:45, 1973.
210. Horwich AL, Low KE, Fenton WA, Hirschfield IN, Furtak K: Folding in vivo of bacterial cytoplasmic proteins: Role of *GroEL*. *Cell* **74**:909, 1993.

211. Ewalt KL, Hendrick JP, Houry WA, Hartl FU: *In vivo* observation of polypeptide flux through the bacterial chaperonin system. *Cell* **90**:491, 1997.
212. Hendrix RW: Purification and properties of groE, a host protein involved in bacteriophage assembly. *J Mol Biol* **129**:375, 1979.
213. Chandresekhar GN, Tilly K, Wollford C, Hendrix R, Georgopoulos C: Purification and properties of the groES morphogenetic protein of *Escherichia coli*. *J Biol Chem* **261**:12414, 1986.
214. Hunt FJ, Weaver AJ, Landry SJ, Gierasch L, Deisenhofer J: The crystal structure of the *GroES* co-chaperonin at 2.8 X resolution. *Nature* **379**:37, 1996.
215. Goloubinoff P, Christeller JT, Gatenby AA, Lorimer GH: Reconstitution of active dimeric ribulose bisphosphate carboxylase from an unfolded state depends on two chaperonin proteins and Mg-ATP. *Nature* **342**:884, 1989.
216. Martin J, Langer T, Boteva R, Chramel A, Horwich AL, Hartl FU: Chaperonin-mediated protein folding at the surface of groEL through a "molten-globule" like intermediate. *Nature* **352**:36, 1991.
217. Buchner J, Schmidt M, Fuchs M, Jaenicke R, Rudoph R, Schmid FX, Kiefhaber T: *GroE* facilitates refolding of citrate synthase by suppressing aggregation. *Biochemistry* **30**:1586, 1991.
218. Badcoe IG, Smith CJ, Wood S, halsall DJ, Holbrook JJ, Lund P, Clarke AR: Binding of a chaperonin to the folding intermediates of lactate dehydrogenase. *Biochemistry* **30**:9195, 1991.
219. Zheng X, Rosenberg LE, Kalousek F, Fenton WA: GroEL, GroES, and ATP-dependent folding and spontaneous assembly of ornithine transcarbamylase. *J Biol Chem* **268**:7489, 1993.
220. Langer T, Pfeifer G, Martin J, Baumeister W, Hartl FU: Chaperonin-mediated protein folding: groES binds to one end of the groEL cylinder which accommodates the protein substrate within its central cavity. *EMBO J* **11**:4757, 1992.
221. Braig K, Hainfeld J, Wall J, Furuya F, Simon M, Horwich AL: Polypeptide bound to the chaperonin groEL binds within its central cavity. *Proc Natl Acad Sci U S A* **90**:3978, 1993.
222. Fenton WA, Horwich AL: GroEL-mediated protein folding. *Protein Sci* **6**:743, 1997.
223. Braig K, Otwinowski Z, Hedge R, Boisvert DC, Joachimiak A, Horwich AL, Sigler PB: The crystal structure of the bacterial chaperonin *GroEL* at 2.8 X. *Nature* **371**:578, 1994.
224. Fenton WA, Kashi Y, Furtak K, Horwich AL: Residues in chaperonin *GroEL* required for polypeptide binding and release. *Nature* **371**:614, 1994.
225. Itzhaki LS, Otzen DE, Fersht AR: Nature and consequences *GroEL*–protein interactions. *Biochemistry* **34**:14581, 1995.
226. Lin Z, Schwarz FP, Eisenstein E: The hydrophobic nature of *GroEL*-substrate binding. *J Biol Chem* **270**:1011, 1995.
227. Buckle AM, Zahn R, Fersht AR: A structural model for *GroEL*-polypeptide recognition. *Proc Natl Acad Sci U S A* **94**:3571, 1997.
228. Ranson NA, Dunster NJ, Burston SG, Clarke AR: Chaperonins can catalyze the reversal of early aggregation steps when a protein misfolds. *J Mol Biol* **250**:581, 1995.
229. Zahn R, Perrett S, Stenberg G, Fersht AR: Catalysis of amide proton exhange by the molecular chaperones *GroEL* and *SecB*. *Science* **271**:642, 1996.
230. Walter S, Lorimer GH, Schmid FX: A thermodynamic coupling mechanism for *GroEL*-mediated unfolding. *Proc Natl Acad Sci U S A* **93**:9425, 1996.
231. Weissman JS, Hohl CM, Kovalenko O, Kashi Y, Chen S, Braig K, Saibil HR, Fenton WA, Horwich AL: Mechanisms of *GroEL* action: productive release of polypeptide from a sequestered position under *GroES*. *Cell* **83**:577, 1995.
232. Mayhew M, da Silva ACR, Martin J, Erdjument-Bromage H, Tempst P, Hartl FU: Protein folding in the central cavity of the *GroEL-GroES* chaperonin complex. *Nature* **379**:420, 1996.
233. Weissman JS, Rye HS, Fenton WA, Beechem JM, Horwich AL: Characterization of the active intermediate of a GroEL-GroES–mediated protein folding reaction. *Cell* **84**:481, 1996.
234. Gray TE, Fersht AR: Cooperativity in ATP hydrolysis by *GroEL* is increased by *GroES*. *FEBS Lett* **292**:254, 1991.
235. Bochkareva ES, Lissin NM, Flynn GC, Rothman JE, Girshovich AS: Positive cooperativity in the functioning of molecular chaperone *GroEL*. *J Biol Chem* **267**:254, 1991.
236. Roseman AM, Chen S, White H, Braig K, Saibil HR: The chaperonin ATPase cycle: mechanism of allosteric switching and movements of substrate-binding domains in *GroEL*. *Cell* **87**:241, 1996.
237. Chen S, Roseman AM, Hunter AS, Wood SP, Burston SG, Ranson NA, Clarke AR, Saibil HR: Location of a folding protein and shape changes in *GroEL–GroES* complexes imaged by cryo-electron microscopy. *Nature* **371**:261, 1994.
238. Xu Z, Horwich AL, Sigler PB: The crystal structure of the asymmetric *GroEL–GroES–ADP*$_7$ chaperonin complex. *Nature* **388**:741, 1997.
239. Burston SG, Ranson NA, Clarke AR: The origins and consequences of asymmetry in the chaperonin reaction cycle. *J Mol Biol* **249**:138, 1995.
240. Hayer-Hartl M, Martin J, Hartl F-U: Asymmetrical interaction of *GroEL* and *GroES* in the ATPase cycle of assisted protein folding. *Science* **269**:836, 1995.
241. Jackson GS, Staniforth RA, Halsall DJ, Atkinson T, Holbrook JJ, Clarke AR, Burston SG: Binding and hydrolysis of nucleotides in the chaperonin catalytic cycle: Implications for the mechanism of assisted protein folding. *Biochemistry* **32**:2554, 1993.
242. Yifrach O, Horovitz AL: Nested cooperativity in the ATPase activity of the oligomeric chaperonin *GroEL*. *Biochemistry* **34**:5303, 1995.
243. Todd MJ, Viitanen PV, Lorimer GH: Dynamics of the chaperonin ATPase cycle: Implications for facilitated protein folding. *Science* **265**:659, 1994.
244. Rye HS, Burston SG, Fenton WA, Beechem JM, Xu Z, Sigler PB, Horwich AL: Distinct actions of *cis* and *trans* ATP within the double ring of the chaperonin *GroEL*. *Nature* **388**:792, 1997.
245. Weissman JS, Kashi Y, Fenton WA, Horwich AL: GroEL-mediated protein folding proceeds by multiple rounds of binding and release of nonnative forms. *Cell* 78:693, 1994.
246. Taguchi H, Yoshida M: Chaperonin releases the substrate protein in a form with tendency to aggregate and ability to rebind to chaperonin. *FEBS Lett* **359**:195, 1995.
247. Smith KE, Fisher MT: Interactions between the *GroE* chaperonins and rhodanese. Multiple intermediates and release and rebinding. *J Biol Chem* **270**:21517, 1995.
248. Burston SG, Weissman JS, Farr GW, Fenton WA, Horwich AL: Release of both native and non-native proteins from a *cis*-only *GroEL* ternary complex. *Nature* **383**:96, 1996.
249. Ranson NA, Burston SG, Clarke AR: Binding, encapsulation and ejection: Substrate dynamics during a chaperonin-assisted folding reaction. *J Mol Biol* **266**:656, 1997.
250. Buchberger A, Schroder H, Hesterkamp T, Schonfeld HJ, Bukau B: Substrate shuttling between the DnaK and *GroEL* systems indicates a chaperone network promoting protein folding. *J Mol Biol* **261**:328, 1996.
251. Kandror O, Busconi L, Sherman M, Goldberg AL: Rapid degradation of an abnormal protein in *Escherichia coli* involves the chaperones *GroEL* and *GroES*. *J Biol Chem* **269**:23575, 1994.
252. Lubben TH, Gatenby AA, Donaldson GK, Lorimer GH, Viitanen PV: Identification of a *groEs*-like chaperonin in mitochondria that facilitates protein folding. *Proc Natl Acad Sci U S A* **87**:7683, 1990.
253. Hartman DJ, Hoogenraad NJ, Condron R, Hoj PB: Identification of a mammalian 10-kDa heat shock protein, a mitochondrial chaperonin 10 homologue essential for assisted folding of trimeric ornithine transcarbamyoylase *in vitro*. *Proc Natl Acad Sci U S A* **89**:3394, 1992.
254. Rospert S, Glick BS, Jeno P, Schatz G, Todd MJ, Lorimer GH, Viitanen PV: Identification and functional analysis of chaperonin 10, the *GroES* homolog from yeast mitochondria. *Proc Natl Acad Sci U S A* **90**:10967, 1993.
255. Hohfeld J, Hartl FU: Role of the chaperonin cofactor Hsp10 in protein folding and sorting in yeast mitochondria. *J Cell Biol* **126**:305, 1994.
256. Viitanen PV, Lorimer GH, Seetheram R, Gupta RS, Oppenheim J, Thomas JO, Cowan NJ: Mammalian mitochondrial chaperonin 60 functions as a single toroidal ring. *J Biol Chem* **267**:695, 1992.
257. Nielsen KL, Cowan NJ: A single ring is sufficient for productive chaperonin-mediated folding *in vivo*. *Mol Cell* **2**:93, 1998.
258. Houghton JE, O'Donovan GA, Wild JR: Reconstruction of an enzyme by domain substitution effectively switches substrate specificity. *Nature* **338**:172, 1989.
259. Jin L, Seaton BA, Head JF: Crystal structure at 2.8 X resolution of anabolic ornithine transcarbamylase from *Escherichia coli*. *Nature Struct Biol* **4**:622, 1997.
260. Ha Y, McCann MT, Tu[illegible]hman M, Allewell NM: Substrate-induced conformational change [illegible] a trimeric ornithine transcarbamylase. *Proc Natl Acad Sci U S A* [illegible]9550, 1997.
261. Shi D, Morizono H, Ha Y, Aoyagi M, Tuchman M, Allewell NM: 1.85 X resolution crystal structure of human ornithine transcarbamoylase complexes with *N*-phosphoacetyl-L-ornithine: Catalytic mechanism

and correlation with inherited deficiency. *J Biol Chem* **273**:34247, 1998.

262. Lee J, Nussbaum RL: An arginine to glutamine mutation in residue 109 of human ornithine transcarbamylase completely abolishes enzyme activity in Cos cells. *J Clin Invest* **84**:1762, 1989.
263. Horwich AL, Fenton WA, Figaira FA, Fox JE, Kolansky D, Mellman IS, Rosenberg LE: Expression of amplified DNA sequences for ornithine transcarbamylase in HeLa cells: Arginine residues may be required for mitochondrial import of enzyme precursor. *J Cell Biol* **10**:1515, 1985.
264. Cheng MY, Pollock RA, Hendrick JP, Horwich AL: The cytoplasmically-synthesized subunit precursor of human mitochondrial ornithine transcarbamylase can be imported and prroteolytically processed to an enzymatically active form by mitochondria of *S. cerevisiae*. *Proc Natl Acad Sci U S A* **84**:4063, 1987.
265. Cavard C, Grimber G, Dubois N, Chasse JF, Bennoun M, Minet-Thuriaux M, Kamoun P, Briand P: Correction of mouse ornithine transcarbamylase deficiency by gene transfer into the germ line. *Nucleic Acid Res* **16**:2099, 1988.
266. Jones SN, Grompe M, Munir MI, Veres G, Craigen WJ, Caskey CT: Ectopic correction of ornithine transcarbamylase deficiency in sparse fur mice. *J Biol Chem* **265**:14684, 1990.
267. Shimada T, Noda T, Tashiro M, Murakami T, Takiguchi M, Mori M, Yamamura K, Saheki T: Correction of ornithine transcarbamylase (OTC) deficiency in spf-ash mice by introduction of rat *OTC* gene. *FEBS Lett* **279**:198, 1991.
268. Grompe M, Jones SN, Loul-segal, Caskey CT: Retroviral mediated gene transfer of human ornithine transcarbamylase into primary hepatocytes of spf and spf-ash mice. *Hum Gene Ther* **3**:35, 1992.
269. Wilson JM, Chowdhury NR, Grossman M, Wajsman R, Epstein A, Mulligan JC, Chowdhury JR: Temporary amelioration of hyperlipidemia in low density lipoprotein receptor-deficient rabbits transplanted with genetically modified hepatocytes. *Proc Natl Acad Sci U S A* **87**:8437, 1990.
270. Stratford-Perricaudet LD, Levrero M, Chasse JF, Perricaudet M, Briand P: Evaluation of the transfer and expression in mice of an enzyme-encoding gene using a human adenovirus vector. *Hum Gene Ther* **1**:241, 1990.
271. Ye X, Robinson MB, Batshaw ML, Furth EE, Smith I, Wilson JM: Prolonged metabolic correction in adult ornithine transcarbamylase-deficient mice with adenoviral vectors. *J Biol Chem* **271**:3639, 1996.
272. Morsy MA, Zhao JZ, Ngo TT, Warman AW, O'Brien WE, Gaham FL, Caskey CT: Patient selection may affect gene therapy success. *J Clin Invest* **97**:826, 1996.
273. Ye X, Robinson MB, Pabin C, Quinn T, Jawad A, Wilson J, Batshaw ML: Adenovirus-mediated *in vitro* gene transfer rapidly protects ornithine transcarbamylase-deficient mice from an ammonium challenge. *Pediatr Res* **41**:527, 1997.
274. Kiwaki K, Kanegae Y, Saito I, Komaki S, Nakamura K, Miyazaki JI, Endo F, Matsuda I: Correction of ornithine transcarbamylase deficiency in adult spf^{ash} mice and in OTC-deficient human hepatocytes with recombinant adenoviruses bearing the CAG promoter. *Hum Gene Ther* **7**:821, 1996.
275. Kochanek S, et al: A new adenoviral vector: Replacement of all viral coding sequences with 28 kb of DNA independently expressing both full-length dystrophin and β-galactosidase. *Proc Natl Acad Sci U S A* **93**:5731, 1996.
276. Fisher KJ, Choi H, Burda J, Chen SJ, Wilson JM: Recombinant adenovirus deleted of all viral genes for gene therapy of cystic fibrosis. *Virology* **217**:11, 1996.
277. Parks RJ, Chen L, Anton M, Sankar U, Rudnicki MA, Graham FL: A helper-dependent adenovirus vector system: Removal of helper virus by Cre-mediated excision of the viral packaging signal. *Proc Natl Acad Sci U S A* **93**:13565, 1996.
278. Chen HH, Mack LM, Kelly R, Ontell M, Kochanek S, Clemens PR: Persistence in muscle of an adenoviral vector that lacks all viral genes. *Proc Natl Acad Sci U S A* **94**:1645, 1997.
279. Hardy S, Kitamura M, Harris-Stansil T, Dai Y, Phipps ML: Construction of adenovirus vectors through Cre-lox recombination. *J Virol* **71**:1842, 1997.
280. Schiedner G, Morral N, Parks RJ, Wu Y, Koopmans SC, Langston C, Graham FL, Beaudet AL, Kochanek S: Genomic DNA transfer with a high-capacity adenovirus vector results in improved *in vivo* gene expression and decreased toxicity. *Nat Genet* **18**:180, 1998.
281. Raper SE, Haskal ZJ, Ye X, Pugh C, Furth EE, Gao GP, Wilson JM: Selective gene transfer into the liver of non-human primates with El-deleted, E2A-defective, or E1–E4 deleted recombinant adenoviruses. *Hum Gene Ther* **9**:671, 1998.
282. Grompe M, Muzny DM, Caskey CT: Scanning detection of mutations in human ornithine transcarbamylase by chemical mismatch cleavage. *Proc Natl Acad Sci USA* **86**:5888, 1989.
283. Feldmann D, Rozet JM, Pelet A, Hentzen D, Briand P, Hubert P, Largilliere C, Rabier D, Farriaux JP, Munnich A: Site-specific screening for point mutations in ornithine transcarbamylase deficiency. *J Med Genet* **29**:471, 1992.
284. Tuchman M: Mutations and polymorphisms in the human ornithine transcarbamylase gene. *Hum Mutat* **2**:174, 1993.
285. Carstens RP, Fenton WA, Rosenberg LE: Identification of RNA splicing errors resulting in human ornithine transcarbamylase deficiency. *Am J Hum Genet* **48**:1105, 1991.
286. Hata A, Setoyama C, Shimada K, Takeda E, Kuroda Y, Akaboshi I, Matsuda I: Ornithine transcarbamylase deficiency resulting from a C-to-T substitution in exon 5 of the onrithine transcarbamylase gene. *Am J Hum Genet* **45**:123, 1989.
287. Reish O, Plante RJ, Tuchman M: Three new mutations in the ornithine transcarbamylase gene associated with acute neonatal hyperammonemia. *Biochem Med Metab Biol* **50**:169, 1993.
288. Matsuura T, Hoshide R, Setoyama C, Shimada K, Hase Y, Yanagawa T, Kajita M, Matsuda I: Four novel gene mutations in five Japanese male patients with neonatal or late onset OTC deficiency: application of PCR-single-strand conformation polymorphisms for all exons and adjacent introns. *Hum Genet* **92**:49, 1993.
289. Hentzen D, Pelet A, Feldman D, Rabier D, Berthelot J, Munnich A: Fatal hyperammonemia resulting from a C to T mutation at a *Msp*I site of the ornithine transcarbamylase gene. *Hum Gene* **88**:153, 1991.
290. Finkelstein JE, Francomano CA, Brusilow SW, Traystman MD: Use of denaturing gradient gel electophoresis for detection of mutation and prospective diagnosis in late onset ornithine transcarbamylase deficiency. *Genomics* **7**:167, 1990.
291. Tsai MY, Holzknecht RA, Tuchman M: Single-strand conformational polymorphism and direct sequencing applied to carrier testing in families with ornithine transcarbamylase deficiency. *Hum Genet* **91**:321, 1993.
292. Tuchman M, Holzknecht RA, Gueron AB, Berry SA, Tsai MY: Six new mutations in the ornithine transcarbamylase gene detected by single-strand conformation polymorphism. *Pediatr Res* **32**:600, 1992.
293. Tuchman M, Plante RJ, Giguere Y, Lemieux B: The ornithine transcarbamylase gene: New "private" mutations in four patients and study of a polymorphism. *Hum Mutat* **3**:318, 1994.
294. Matsuura T, Hoshide R, Kiwaki K, Komaki S, Koike E, Endo F, Oyanagi K, Suzuki Y, Kato I, Ishikawa K, Yoda H, Kamitani S, Sakaki Y, Matsuda I: Four newly identified ornithine transcarbamylase (OTC) mutations (D126G, R129H,I172M, and W332X) in Japanese male patients with early-onset OTC deficiency. *Hum Mutat* **3**:402, 1994.
295. Tuchman M, Plante RJ, McCann MT, Qureshi AA: Seven new mutations in the human ornithine transcarbamylase gene. *Hum Mutat* **4**:57, 1994.
296. Zimmer KP, Matsuura T, Colombo JP, Koch HG, Ullrich K, Deufel T, Harms E, Matsuda I: A novel point mutation at codon 269 of the ornithine transcarbamylase (OTC) gene causing neonatal onset of OTC deficiency. *J Inherit Metab Dis* **18**:356, 1995.
297. Garcia-Perez MA, Paz Briones PS, Garcia-Munnoz MJ, Rubio V: A splicing mutation, a nonsense mutation (Y167X) and two missense mutations (I159T and A209V) in Spanish patients with ornithine trascarbamylase deficiency. *Hum Genet* **96**:549, 1995.
298. Gilbert-Dussardier B, Segues B, Rozet JM, Rabier D, Calvas P, deLumley L, Bonnefond JP, Munnich A: Partial duplication (dup TCAC178) and novel point mutations (T125M, G188R, A209V, and H302L) of the ornithine transcarbamylase gene in congenital hyperammonemia. *Hum Mutat* **8**:74, 1996.
299. Leibundgut EO, Wermuth B, Colombo JP, Liechti-Gallati S: Ornithine transcarbamylase deficiency: Characterization of gene mutations and polymorphisms. *Hum Mutat* **8**:333, 1996.
300. Segues B, Veber PS, Rabier D, Calvas P, Saudubray JM, Gilbert-Dussardier B, Bonnefont JP, Munnich A: A 3-base pair in-frame deletion in exon 8 (delGlu272/273) of the ornithine transcarbamylase gene in late-onset hyperammonemic coma. *Hum Mutat* **8**:373, 1996.
301. Matsuda I, Matsuura T, Nishiyori A, Komaki S, Hoshide R, Matsumoto T, Funakoshi M, Kiwaki K, Endo F, Hata A, Shimadzu M, Yoshino M: Phenotypic variability in male patients carrying the mutant ornithine transcarbamylase (OTC) allele, Arg40His, ranging

from a child with an unfavourable prognosis to an asymptomatic older adult. *J Med Genet* **33**:645, 1996.
302. Hoshide R, Matsuura T, Sagara Y, Kobo T, Shimadzu M, Endo F, Matsuda I: Prenatal monitoring in a family at high risk for ornithine transcarbamylase (OTC) deficiency: a new mutation of an A-to-C transversion in position +4 or intron 1 of the *OTC* gene that is likely to abolish enzyme activity. *Am J Med Genet* **64**:459, 1996.
303. Schimanski U, Krieger D, Horn M, Stremmel W, Wermuth B, Theilmann L: A novel two-nucleotide deletion in the ornithine transcarbamylase gene causing fatal hyperammonemia in early pregnancy. *Hepatology* **24**:1413, 1996.
304. van Diggelen OP, Zzaremba J, He W, Keulemans JL, Boer AM, Reuser AJ, Ausems MG, Smeitink JA, Kowalczyk J, Pronicka E, Rokicki D, Tarnowska-Dziduszko E, Kneppers AL, Bakker E: Asymptomatic and late-onset ornithine transcarbamylase (OTC) deficiency in males of a five-generation family, caused by an A208T mutation. *Clin Genet* **50**:310, 1996.
305. Ahrens MJ, Berry SA, Whitley CB, Markowitz DJ, Plante RJ, Tuchman M: Clinical and biochemical heterogeneity in females of a large pedigree with ornithine transcarbamylse deficiency due to the R141Q mutation. *Am J Med Genet* **66**:311, 1996.
306. Ausems MG, Bakker E, Berger R, Duran M, van Diggelen OP, Keulemans JL, de Valk HW, Kneppers AL, Dorland L, Eskes PF, Beemer FA, Poll-The BT, Smeitink JA: Asymptomatic and late-onset ornithine transcarbamylase deficiency caused by a A208T mutation: Clinical, biochemical and DNA analyses in a four-generation family. *Am J Med Genet* **68**:236, 1997.
307. Komaki S, Matsuura T, Oyanagi K, Hoshide R, Kiwaki K, Endo F, Shimadzu M, Matsuda I: Familial lethal inheritance of a mutated paternal gene in females causing X-linked ornithine transcarbamylase (OTC) deficiency. *Am J Med Genet* **68**:177, 1997.
308. Morizono H, Listrom CD, Rajagopal BS, Aoyagi M, McCann MT, Allewell NM, Tuchman M: "Late onset" of ornithine transcarbamylase deficiency: Function of three purified recombinant mutant enzymes. *Hum Mol Genet* **6**:963, 1997.
309. Leibundgut EO, Liechti-Gallati S, Colombo JP, Wermuth B: Ornithine transcarbamylase deficiency: New sites with increased probability of mutation. *Hum Genet* **95**:191, 1995.
310. Vella S, Steiner F, Schlumbom V, Zurbrugg R, Wiesmann UN, Schaffner T, Wermuth B: Mutation of ornithine transcarbamylase (H136R) in a girl with severe intermittent orotic aciduria but normal enzyme activity. *J Inherit Metab Dis* **20**:517, 1997.
311. Tuchman M, Plante RJ: Mutations and polymorphisms in the human ornithine transcarbamylase gene:mutation update addendum. *Hum Mutat* **5**:293, 1995.
312. Nishiyori A, Yoshino M, Tananari Y, Matsuura T, Hoshide R, Mastuda I, Mori M, Kato H: Y55D mutation in ornithine transcarbamylase associated with late-onset hyperammonemia in a male. *Hum Mutat* **8**(suppl 1):131, 1998.
313. Garcia-Perez MA, Climent C, Briones P, Vilaseca MA, Rodes M, Rubio V: Missense mutation in codon 225 of ornithine transcarbamylase (OTC) result in decreased amounts of OTC protein: a hypothesis on the molecular mechanism of OTC deficiency. *J Inherit Metab Dis* **20**:769, 1997.
314. Nishiyori A, Yoshino M, Kato H, Matsuura T, Hoshide R, Matsuda I, Kuno T, Miyazaki S, Hirose S, Kuromaru R, Mori M: The R40H mutation in a late onset type of human ornithine transcarbamylase deficiency in male patients. *Hum Genet* **99**:171, 1997.
315. Morizono H, Tuchman M, Rajagopal BS, McCann MT, Listrom CD, Yuan X, Venugopal D, Barany G, Allewell NM: Expression, purification and kinetic characterization of wild-type human ornithine transcarbamylase and a recurrent mutant that produces "late-onset" hyperammonemia. *Biochem J* **322**:625, 1997.
316. Vells S, Steiner F, Schlumbom V, Zurbrugg R, Wiesmann UN, Schaffner T, Wermuth B: Mutation of ornithine transcarbamylase (H136R) in a girl with severe intermittent orotic aciduria but normal enzyme activity. *J Inherit Metab Dis* **20**:517, 1997.
317. Yoo HW, Kim GH, Lee DH: Identification of new mutations in the ornithine transcarbamylase (*OTC*) gene in Korean families. *J Inherit Metab Dis* **19**:31, 1996.
318. Oppliger Leibundgut E, Wermuth B, Colombo JP, Liechti-Gallati S: Identification of four novel splice site mutations in the ornithine transcarbamylse gene. *Hum Genet* **97**:209, 1996.
319. Oppliger Leibundgut E, Liechti-Gallati S, Colombo JP, Wermuth B: Ornithine transcarbamylase deficiency: Ten new mutations and high proportion of *de novo* mutations in heterozygous females. *Hum Mutat* **9**:409, 1997.
320. Shimadzu M, Matsumoto H, Matsuura T, Kobayashi K, Komaki S, Kiwaki K, Hoshide R, Endo F, Saheki T, Matsuda I: Ten novel mutations of the ornithine transcarbamylase (*OTC*) gene in OTC deficiency. *Hum Mutat* **8**(suppl 1):5, 1998.
321. Calvas P, Segues B, Rozet JM, Rabier D, Bonnefond JP, Munnich A: Novel intragenic deletions and point mutations of the ornithine transcarbamylase gene in cogenital hyperammonemia. *Hum Mutat* **8**(suppl 1):81, 1998.
322. Tuchman M, Morizono H, Reish O, Yuan X, Allewell NM: The molecular basis of ornithine transcarbamylase deficiency: modelling of the human enzyme and the effects of mutations. *J Med Genet* **32**:680, 1995.
323. Matsuda I, Tanase S: The ornithine transcarbamylase (*OTC*) gene: Mutations in 50 Japanese families with OTC deficiency. *Am J Med Genet* **71**:378, 1997.
324. Tuchman M, Morizono H, Rajagopal BS, Plante RJ, Allewell NM: Identification of "private" mutations in patients with ornithine transcarbamylase deficiency. *J Inherit Metab Dis* **20**:525, 1997.
325. Matsuura T, hoshide R, Komaki S, Kiwaki K, Endo F, Nakamura S, Jitosho T, Matsuda I: Identification of two new aberrant splicings in the ornithine carbamoyltransferase (*OTC*) gene in patients with OTC deficiency. *J Inherit Metab Dis* **18**:273, 1995.
326. Hoshide R, Matsuura T, Komaki S, Koike E, Ueno I, Matsuda I: Specificity of PCR-SSCP for detection of the mutant ornithine transcarbamylase (*OTC*) gene in patients with OTC deficiency. *J Inherit Metab Dis* **16**:857, 1993.
327. Satoh Y, Sannomiya Y, Ohtake A, Takayanagi M, Niimi H: Molecular characterization of four different mutant alleles of *OTC* gene in four unrelated patients with ornithine transcarbamylase deficiency. *J Jpn Pediatr Soc* **96**:1855, 1992.
328. Tuchman M, Morizono H, Rajagopal BS, Plante RJ, Allewell NM: The biochemical and molecular spectrum of ornithine transcarbamylase deficiency. *J Inherit Metab Dis* **21**(suppl):40, 1998.
329. Garcia-Perez MA, Sanjurjo P, Rubio V: Demonstration of the spf-ash mutation in Spanish patients with ornithine transcarbamylase deficiency of moderate severity. *Hum Genet* **95**:183, 1995.
330. Tuchman M, Matsuda I, Munnich A, Malcolm S, Strautnieks S, Briede T: Proportions of spontaneous mutations in males and females with ornithine transcarbamylase deficiency. *Am J Med Genet* **55**:67, 1995.
331. Rozen R, Fox J, Fenton WA, Horwich AL, Rosenberg LE: Gene deletion and restriction fragment length polymorphism at the human ornithine transcarbamylase locus. *Nature* **313**:815, 1985.
332. Rozen R, Fox JE, Hack AM, Fenton WA, Horwich AL, Rosenberg LE: DNA analysis for ornithine transcarbamylase deficiency. *J Inherit Metab Dis* **9**:49, 1986.
333. Suess PJ, Tsai MY, Hozknecht RA, Horowitz M, Tuchman M: Screening for gene deletions and known mutations in 13 patients with ornithine transcarbamylase deficiency. *Biochem Med Metab Biol* **47**:250, 1992.
334. Grompe M, Caskey CT, Fenwick RG: Improved molecular diagnostics for ornithine transcarbamylase deficiency. *Am J Hum Genet* **48**:212, 1991.
335. Maddalena A, Sosnoski DM, Berry GT, Nussbaum RL: Mosaicism for an intragenic deletion in a boy with mild ornithine transcarbamylase deficiency. *New Engl J Med* **319**:999, 1988.
336. Legius E, Baten E, Stul M, Marynen P, Cassiman JJ: Sporadic late onset ornithine transcarbamylase deficiency in a boy with somatic mosaicism for an intragenic deletion. *Clin Genet* **38**:155, 1990.
337. Old JM, Purvis-Smith S, Wilcken S, Fearson P, Williamson R, Briand PL, Howard NJ, Hammond J, Cathelineau L, Davies KE: Prenatal exclusion of ornithine transcarbamylase deficiency by direct gene analysis. *Lancet* **1**:73, 1984.
338. Francke U: Random X inactivation resulting in mosaic nullisomy of region Xp21.3 associated with heterozygosity for ornithine transcarbamylase deficiency and for chronic granulomatous disease. *Cytogenet Cell Genet* **38**:298, 1984.
339. Segues B, Rozet MJ, Gilbert B, Saugier-Veber P, Rabier D, Saudubray JM, Carre M, Rouleau FP, Menget A, Bonardi JM: Apparent segregation of null alleles ascribed to deletions of the ornithine transcarbamylase gene in congenital hyperammonemia. *Prenat Diagn* **15**:757, 1995.
340. De Mars R, Le Van SL, Trend BL, Russell LB: Abnormal ornithine carbamoyltransferase in mice having the sparse-fur mutation. *Proc Natl Acad Sci U S A* **73**:1693, 1976.
341. Briand P, Miura S, Mori M, Cathelineau L, Kamoun P, Tatibana M: Cell-free synthesis and transport of precursors of mutant ornithine

carbamoyltransferases into mitochondria. *Biochim Biophys Acta* **760**:389, 1983.
342. Rosenberg LE, Kalousek F, Orsulak MD: Biogenesis of ornithine transcarbamylase in spfash mutant mice: Two cytoplasmic precursors, one mitochondrial enzyme. *Science* **222**:426, 1983.
343. Hodges PE, Rosenberg LE: The spfash mouse: A missense mutation in the ornithine transcarbamylase gene also causes aberrant mRNA splicing. *Proc Natl Acad Sci U S A* **86**:4142, 1984.
344. Veres G, Gibbs RA, Scherer SE, Caskey CT: The molecular basis of the sparse fur mouse mutation. *Science* **237**:415, 1987.
345. Su TS, Bock HGO, O'Brien WE, Beaudet AL: Cloning of cDNA for argininosuccinate synthetase mRNA and study of enzyme over production in a human cell line. *J Biol Chem* **256**:11826, 1981.
346. Freytag SO, Beaudet AL, Bock HGO, O'Brien WE: Molecular structure of the human argininosuccinate synthetase gene: Occurrence of alternative mRNA splicing. *Mol Cell Biol* **4**:1978, 1984.
347. Su TS, Lin LH: Analysis of a splice acceptor site mutation which produces multiple splicing abnormalities in the human argininosuccinate synthetase locus. *J Biol Chem* **265**:19716, 1990.
348. Bock HGO, Su TS, O'Brien WE, Beaudet AL: Sequences for human argininosuccinate synthetase cDNA. *Nucleic Acids Res* **11**:6505, 1983.
349. Boyce FM, Anderson MG, Rusk CD, Freytag SO: Human argininosuccinate synthetase minigenes are subject to arginine-mediated repression but not to *trans* induction. *Mol Cell Biol* **6**:1244, 1986.
350. Morris SM, Kepka DM, Sweeney WE, Avner ED: Abundance of mRNAs encoding urea cycle enzymes in fetal and neonatal mouse liver. *Arch Biochem Biophys* **269**:175, 1990.
351. Jinno Y, Nomiyama H, Matuo S, Shimada K, Matsuda I: Structure of the 5′ end region of the human argininosuccinate synthetase gene. *J Inherit Dis* **8**:157, 1985.
352. Jinno Y, Matuo S, Nomiyama H, Shimada K, Matsuda I: Novel structure of the 5′ end region of the human argininosuccinate synthetase gene. *J Biochem* **98**:1395, 1985.
353. Anderson GM, Freytag SO: Synergistic activation of a human promoter *in vivo* by transcription factor Sp1. *Mol Cell Biol* **11**:1935, 1991.
354. Thayer MJ, Fournier RE: Hormonal regulation of TSE1-repressed genes: Evidence for multiple genetic controls in extinction. *Mol Cell Biol* **9**:2837, 1989.
355. Jones KW, Shapero MH, Chevrette M, Fournier REK: Subtractive hybridization cloning of a tissue-specific extinguisher: TSE1 encodes a regulatory subunit of protein kinase A. *Cell* **66**:849, 1991.
356. Boshart M, Weih F, Nichols M, Schutz G: The tissue-specific extinguisher locus TSE1 encodes a regulatory subunit of cAMP-dependent protein kinase. *Cell* **66**:849, 1991.
357. Surh LC, Beaudet AL, O'Brien WE: Molecular characterization of the murine argininosuccinate synthetase locus. *Gene* **99**:181, 1991.
358. Su TS, Nussbaum RL, Airpart S, Ledbetter DH, Mohandas T, O'Brien WE, Beaudet AL: Human chromosomal assignments for 14 argininosuccinate synthetase pseudogenes: Cloned DNAs as reagents for cytogenetic analysis. *Am J Hum Genet* **36**:954, 1984.
359. Beaudet A, Su TS, O'Brien WE: Dispersion of argininosuccinate synthetase-like human genes to multiple autosomes and the X chromosome. *Cell* **30**:287, 1982.
360. Daiger SP, Wildin RS, Su TS: Sequences on the human Y chromosome homologous to the autosomal gene for argininosuccinate synthetase. *Nature* **298**:682, 1983.
361. Freytag SO, Bock HGO, Beaudet AL, O'Brien WE: Molecular structures of human argininosuccinate synthetase pseudogenes. Evolutionary and mechanistic implications. *J Biol Chem* **259**:3160, 1984.
362. Su TS, Beaudet AL, O'Brien WE: Increased translatable messenger ribonucleic acid for argininosuccinate synthetase in canavanine-resistant human cells. *Biochemistry* **20**:2956, 1981.
363. Amos JA, Fleming BC, Gusella JF, Jacoby LB: Relative argininosuccinate synthetase mRNA levels and gene copy number in canavanine-resistant lymphoblasts. *Biochem Biophys Acta* **782**:247, 1984.
364. Jackson MJ, O'Brien WE, Beaudet AL: Arginine-mediated regulation of an argininosuccinate synthetase minigene in normal and canavanine-resistant human cells. *Mol Cell Biol* **6**:2257, 1986.
365. Jackson MJ, Allen SJ, Beaudet AL, O'Brien WE: Metabolite regulation of argininosuccinate synthetase in cultured human cells. *J Biol Chem* **263**:16388, 1988.
366. Tsai TF, Su TS: A nuclear post-transcriptional event responsible for overproduction of argininosuccinate synthetase in a canavanine-resistant variant of a human epithelial cell line. *Eur J Biochem* **229**:233, 1995.
367. Hinnebusch AG: Mechanism of gene regulation in the general control of amino acid biosynthesis in *S. cerevisiae*. *Microbiol Rev* **52**:248, 1988.
368. Hudson LD, Erbe RW, Jacoby LB: Expression of human argininosuccinate synthetase gene in hamster transferents. *Proc Natl Acad Sci U S A* **77**:4234, 1980.
369. Su TS, O'Brien WE, Beaudet AL: Genomic DNA-mediated gene transfer for argininosuccinate synthetase. *Somat Cell Mol Genet* **10**:601, 1984.
370. Wood PA, Partridge CA, O'Brien WE, Beaudet AL: Expression of human argininosuccinate synthetase after retroviral-mediated gene transfer. *Somat Cell Mol Genet* **12**:493, 1986.
371. Demarquoy J, Herman GE, Lorenzo I, Trentin J, Beaudet AL, O'Brien WE: Long-term expression of human argininosuccinate synthetase in mice following bone marrow transplantation with retrovirus-transduced hematopoietic stem cells. *Hum Gene Ther* **3**:3, 1992.
372. Wood PA, Herman GE, Chao CYJ, O'Brien WE, Beaudet AL: Retrovirus mediated gene transfer of argininosuccinate synthetase into cultured rodent cells and human citrullinemic fibroblasts. *Cold Spring Harb Symp Quant Biol* **51**(part II):1027, 1986.
373. Patejunas G, Bradley A, Beaudet AL, O'Brien WE: Generation of a mouse model for citrullinemia by targeted disruption of the argininosuccinate synthetase gene. *Somat Cell Mol Genet* **20**:55, 1994.
374. Su TS, Bock HO, Beaudet AL, O'Brien WE: Molecular analysis of argininosuccinate synthetase deficiency in human fibroblasts. *J Clin Invest* **70**:1334, 1982.
375. Northrup H, Lathrop M, Lu SY, Daiger SP, Beaudet AL, O'Brien WE: Multilocus linkage analysis with the human argininosuccinate synthetase gene. *Genomics* **5**:442, 1989.
376. Kwiatkowski DJ, Nygaard TG, Schuback DE, Perman S, Trugman JM, Bressman SB, Burke RE, Brin MF, Ozelius L, Breakefield XO, Fahn S, Kramer PL: Identification of a highly polymorphic microsatellite VNTR within the argininosuccinate synthetase locus: Exclusion of the dystonia gene on 9q32-34 as the cause of dopa-responsive dystonia in a large kindred. *Am J Hum Genet* **48**:121, 1991.
377. Kakinoki H, Kobayashi K, Terazono H, Nagata Y, Saheki T: Mutations and DNA diagnoses of classical citrullinemia. *Hum Mutat* **9**:250, 1997.
378. Kobayashi K, Shaheen N, Terazono H, Saheki T: Mutations in argininosuccinate synthetase mRJNA of Japanese patients, causing classical citrullinemia. *Am J Hum Genet* **55**:1103, 1994.
379. Shaheen N, Kobayashi K, Terazono H, Fukushige T, Horiuchi M, Saheki T: Characterization of human wild-type and mutant argininosuccinate synthetase proteins expressed in bacterial cells. *Enzyme Protein* **48**:251, 1994.
380. Kobayashi K, Kakinoki H, Fukushige T, Shaheen N, Terzono H, Saheki T: Nature and frequency of mutations in the argininosuccinate synthetase gene that cause classical citrullinemia. *Hum Genet* **96**:454, 1995.
381. Kobayashi K, Jackson MJ, Tick DB, O'Brien WE, Beaudet AL: Heterogeneity of mutations in argininosuccinate synthetase causing human citrullinemia. *J Biol Chem* **265**:11361, 1990.
382. Kobayashi K, Rosenbloom C, Beaudet AL, O'Brien WE: Additional mutations in argininosuccinate synthetase causing citrullinemia. *Mol Biol Med* **8**:95, 1991.
383. Saheki T, Kobayashi K, Ichiki H, Matuo S, Tatsuno M, Imamura Y, Inoue I, Noda T, Hagihara S: Molecular basis of enzyme abnormalities in urea cycle disorders. Recent advances in inborn errors of metabolism. Proceedings of the 4th International Congress. *Enzyme* **38**:227, 1987.
384. Kobayashi K, Shaheen N, Kumashiro R, Tanikawa K, O'Brien WE, Beaudet AL, Saheki T: A search for the primary abnormality in adult-onset type II citrullinemia. *Am J Hum Genet* **53**:1024, 1993.
385. Kobayashi K, Nakata M, Terazono H, Shinsato T, Saheki T: Pancreatic secretory trypsin inhibitor gene is highly expressed in the liver of adult-onset type II citrullinemia. *FEBS Lett* **372**:69, 1995.
386. Dennis JA, Healy PJ, Beaudet AL, O'Brien WE: Molecular definition of bovine argininosuccinate synthetase deficiency. *Proc Natl Acad Sci U S A* **86**:7947, 1989.

387. O'Brien WE, McInnes R, Kalumcuk K, Adcock M: Cloning and sequence analysis of cDNA for human argininosuccinate lyase. *Proc Natl Acad Sci U S A* **83**:7211, 1986.
388. Lambert MA, Simard LR, Ray PN, McInnes RR: Molecular cloning of cDNA for rat argininosuccinate lyase and its expression in rat hepatoma cell lines. *Mol Cell Biol* **6**:1722, 1986.
389. Wistow G, Piatigorsky J: Recruitment of enzymes as lens structural proteins. *Science* **236**:154, 1987.
390. Piatigorsky J, O'Brien WE, Norman BL, Kalumuck K, Wistow GJ, Borras T, Nickerson JM, Wawrousek EF: Gene sharing by δ-crystallin and argininosuccinate lyase. *Proc Natl Acad Sci U S A* **85**:3479, 1988.
391. Lee HJ, Chiou SH, Chang GG: Biochemical characterization and kinetic analysis of duck delta-crystallin with endogenous argininosuccinate lyase activity. *Biochem J* 283:597, 1992.
392. Simpson A, Moss D, Slingsby C: The avian eye lens protein delta-crystallin shows a novel packing arrangement of tetramers in a supramolecular helix. *Structure* **3**:403, 1995.
393. Piatigorsky J, Wistow GJ: Enzyme/crystallins: Gene sharing as an evolutionary strategy. *Cell* **57**:197, 1989.
394. Barbosa P, Wistow GJ, Cialkowski M, Piatigorsky J, O'Brien WE: Expression of duck lens delta-crystallin cDNAs in yeast and bacterial hosts. Delta 2-crystallin is an active argininosuccinate lyase. *J Biol Chem* **266**:22319, 1991.
395. Abu-Abed M, Turner MA, Vallee F, Simpson A, Slingsby C, Howell PL: Structural comparison of the enzymatically active and inactive forms of δ-crystallin and the role of histidine 91. *Biochemistry* **36**:14012,
396. Piatigorsky J, Horwitz J: Characterization and enzyme activity of argininosuccinate lyase/delta-crystallin of the embryonic duck lens. *Biochim Biophys Acta* **1295**:158, 1996.
397. Kondoh H, Araki I, Yasuda K, Matsubasa T, Mori M: Expression of the chicken "delta 2-crystallin" gene in mouse cells: Evidence for encoding of argininosuccinate lyase. *Gene* **99**:267, 1991.
398. Hayashi S, Goto K, Okada TS, Kondoh H: Lens-specific enhancer in the third intron regulates expression of the chicken δD-1-crystallin gene. *Genes Dev* **1**:818, 1987.
399. Matsubasa T, Takiguchi M, Amaya Y, Matsuda I, Mori M: Structure of the rat argininosuccinate lyase gene: Close similarity to chicken delta-crystallin genes. *Proc Natl Acad Sci U S A* **86**:592, 1989.
400. Wistow G, Anderson A, Piatigorsky J: Evidence for neutral and selective processes in the recruitment of enzyme-crystallins in avian lenses. *Proc Natl Acad Sci U S A* **87**:6277, 1990.
401. Kawamoto S, Kaneko T, Mizuki N, Ohsuga A, Fukushima J, Amaya Y, Mori M, Iluda K: Molecular cloning and nucleotide sequence of rat brain argininosuccinate lyase cDNA with an extremely long 5′-untranslated sequence: Evidence for the identity of the brain and liver enzymes. *Brain Res Mol Brain Res* **5**:235, 1989.
402. Husson A, Renouf S, Fairand A, Buquet C, Benamar M, Vaillant R: Expression of argininosuccinate lyase mRNA in foetal hepatocytes. Regulation by glucocorticoids and insulin. *Eur J Biochem* **192**:677, 190.
403. Lambert MA, Simard LR, Ray PN, McInnes RR: Molecular cloning of cDNA for rat argininosuccinate lyase and its expression in rat hepatoma cell lines. *Mol Cell Biol* **6**:1722, 1986.
404. O'Brien WE, McInnes R, Kalumuck K, Adcock M: Cloning and sequence analysis of cDNA for argininosuccinate lyase. *Proc Natl Acad Sci U S A* **83**:7211, 1986.
405. McInnes RR, Shih V, Chilton S: Interallelic complementation in an inborn error of metabolism: Genetic heterogeneity in argininosuccinate lyase deficiency. *Proc Natl Acad Sci U S A* **81**:4480, 1984.
406. Barbosa P, Cialkowski M, O'Brien WE: Analysis of naturally occurring and site-directed mutations in the argininosuccinate lyase gene. *J Biol Chem* **266**:5286, 1991.
407. Walker DC, McCloskey DA, Simard LR, McInnes RR: Molecular analysis of human argininosuccinate lyase: Mutant characterization and alternative splicing of the coding region. *Proc Natl Acad Sci U S A* **87**:9625, 1990.
408. Walker DC, Christodoulou J, Craig HJ, Simard LR, Ploder L, Howell PL, McInnes RR: Intragenic complementation at the human argininosuccinate lyase locus. *J Biol Chem* **272**:6777, 1997.
409. Simpson A, Bateman O, Driessen H, Lindley P, Moss D, Mylvaganam S, Narebor E, Slingsby C: The structure of avian eye lens δ-crystallin reveals a new fold for a superfamily of oligomeric enzymes. *Nature Struct Biol* **1**:724, 1994.
410. Turner MA, Simpson A, McInnes RR, Howell PL: Human argininosuccinate lyase: A structural basis for intragenic complementation. *Proc Natl Acad Sci U S A* **94**:9063, 1997.
411. Weaver TM, Levitt DG, Donnelly MI, Wilkens Stevens PP, Banaszak LJ: The multisubunit active site of fumarase C from *Escherichi coli*. *Nature Struct Biol* **2**:654, 1995.
412. Walker DC, Christodoulou J, Craig HJ, Simard LR, Ploder L, Howell PL, McInnes RR: Intragenic complementation at the human argininosuccinate lyase locus. *J Biol Chem* **272**:6777, 1997.
413. Kidd JR, Dizikes GJ, Grody WW, Cederbaum SD, Kidd KK: A *Pvu*11 RFLP for the human liver arginase (*ARG1*) gene. *Nucleic Acids Res* **14**:9544, 1986.
414. Dizikes GJ, Spector EB, Cederbaum SD: Cloning of rat liver arginase cDNA and the elucidation of the regulation of arginase gene expression in H4 rat hepatoma cells. *Somat Cell Mol Genet* **12**:375, 1986.
415. Dizikes GJ, Grody WW, Kern RM, Cederbaum SD: Isolation of human arginase cDNA and absence of homology between the two arginase genes. *Biochem Biophys Res Commun* **141**:53, 1986.
416. Ikemoto M, Tabata M, Miyake T, Kono T, Mori M, Totani M, Murachi T: Expression of human liver arginase in *Escherichia coli*. Purification and properties of the product. *Biochem J* **270**:697, 1990.
417. Kanyo ZF, Scolnick LR, Ash DE, Christianson DW: Structure of a unique binuclear manganese cluster in arginase. *Nature* **383**:554, 1996.
418. Ash DE, Scolnick LR, Kanyo ZF, Vockley JG, Cederbaum SD, Christianson DW: Molecular basis of hyperargininemia: Structure–function consequences of mutations in human liver arginase. *Mol Genet Metab* **64**:243, 1998.
419. Grody WW, Dizikes GJ, Cederbaum SD: Human arginase isozymes, in *Isozymes: Current Topics in Biological and Medical Research*. New York, Alan R. Liss, 1993.
420. Grody WW, Argyle C, Kern RM, Dizikes GJ, Spector EB, Strickland AD, Klein D, Cederbaum SD: Differential expression of the two human arginase genes in hyperargininemia. Enzymatic, pathologic, and molecular analysis. *J Clin Invest* **83**:602, 1989.
421. Paterton D, Shi YB: Thyroid hormone-dependent differential regulation of multiple arginase genes during amphibian metamorphosis. *J Biol Chem* **269**:25328, 1994.
422. Gotoh T, Sonoki T, Nagasaki A, Terada K, Takiguchi M, Mori M: Molecular cloning of cDNA for nonhepatic mitochondrial arginase (arginase II) and comparison of its induction with nitric oxide synthase in amurine macrophage-like line. *FEBS Lett* **395**:119, 1996.
423. Morris SM, Bhamidipati D, Kepaka-Lenhart D: Human type II arginase: Sequence analysis and tissue-specific expression. *Gene* **193**:157, 1997.
424. Sparkes RS, Dizikes GJ, Klisak I, Grody WW, Mohandas T, Heinzmann C, Sollman S, Lusis AJ, Cederbaum SD: The gene for human liver arginase (ARG1) is assigned to chromosome band 6q23. *Am J Hum Genet* **39**:186, 1986.
425. Takiguchi M, Mori M: *In vitro* analysis of the rat liver-type arginase promoter. *J Biol Chem* **266**:9186, 1991.
426. Chowdhury S, Gotoh T, Mori M, Takiguchi M: *In vitro* analysis of the rat liver type arginase promoter. *J Biol Chem* **266**:9186, 1991.
427. Gotoh T, Haraguchi Y, Takiguchi M, Mori M: The delayed glucocorticoid-responsive and hepatoma cell-selective enhancer of the rat arginase gene is located around intron 7. *Biochemistry* **115**:778, 1994.
428. Gotoh T, Chowdhury S, Takiguchi M, Mori M: The glucocorticoid-responsive gene cascade. Activation of the rat arginase gene through induction of C/EBPbeta. *J Biol Chem* **272**:3694, 1997.
429. Reczkowdki RS, Ash DE: EPR evidence for binnclear Mn (II) centers in rat liver arginase. *J Am Chem Soc* **114**:10992, 1992.
430. Khangulov SV, Pessiki PJ, Barynin VV, Ash DE, Dismukes GC: Determination of the metal ion separation and energies of the three lowest electronic states of dimanganese (II,II) complezes and enzymes: Catalase and liver arginase. *Biochemistry* **34**:2015, 1995.
431. Cavalli RC, Burke CJ, Kawamoto S, Soprano DR, Ash DE: Mutagenesis of rat liver arginase expressed in *Escherichia coli*: Role of conserved histidines. *Biochemistry* **33**:10652, 1994.
432. Scolnick LR, Kanyo ZF, Cavalli RC, Ash DE, Christianson DW: Altering the binuclear manganese cluster of arginase diminishes thermostability and catalytic function. *Biochemistry* **36**:10558, 1997.
433. Grody WW, Klein D, Dodson AE, Kern RM, Wissman PB, Goodman BK, Bassand P, Marescau B, Kang SS, Leonard JV, Cederbaum SD: Molecular genetic study of human arginase deficiency. *Am J Hum Genet* **50**:1281, 1992.
434. Haraguchi Y, Aparicio JM, Takiguchi M, Akaboshi I, Yoshino M, Mori M, Matsuda I: Molecular basis of argininemia. Identification of

two discrete frame-shift deletions in the liver-type arginase gene. *J Clin Invest* **86**:347, 1990.

435. Uchino T, Haraguchi Y, Aparicio JM, Mizutani N, Higashikawa M, Naitoh H, Mori M, Matsuda I: Three novel mutations in the liver-type arginase gene in three unrelated Japanese patients with argininemia. *Am J Hum Genet* **51**:1406, 1992.
436. Vockley JG, Tabor DE, Kern RM, Goodman BK, Wissmann PB, Kang DS, Grody WW, Cederbaum SD: Identification of mutations (D128G, H141L) in the liver arginase gene of patients with hyperargininemia. *Hum Mutat* **4**:150, 1994.
437. Uchino T, Snyderman SE, Lambert M, Qureshi IA, Shapira SK, Sansaricq C, Smit LM, Jakobs C, Matsuda I: Molecular basis of phenotypic variation in patients with argininemia. *Hum Genet* **96**:255, 1995.
438. Meloni R, Fougerousse F, Roudaut C, Beckmann JS: Dinucleotide repeat polymorphism at the human liver arginase gene (*ARG1*). *Nucleic Acids Res* **20**:1166, 1992.
439. Levy HL, Coulombe JT, Shih VE: Newborn urine screening, in Bickel H, Gunthrie R, Hammersen G (eds): *Neonatal Screening for Inborn Errors of Metabolism*. Berlin, Springer-Verlag, 1980, p 89.
440. Young JL, Miller RW: Incidence of malignant tumors in U.S. children. *J Pediatr* **86**:254, 1975.
441. Pediatric end stage renal disease. *Am J Kidney Dis* **16**(suppl 2):65, 1990.
442. Hudak ML, Jones MD, Brusilow SW: Differentiation of transient hyperammonemia of the newborn and urea cycle enzyme defects by clinical presentation. *J Pediatr* **107**:712, 1985.
443. Ballard RA, Vinocur B, Reynolds JW, Wennberg RP, Merritt A, Sweetman L, Nyhan WL: Transient hyperammonemia of the preterm infant. *New Engl J Med* **29**:920, 1978.
444. Barnes PM, Wheldon DB, Eggerding C, Marshall WC, Leonard JV: Hyperammonaemia and disseminated herpes simplex infection in the neonatal period. *Lancet* **2**:1362, 1982.
445. Schutze GE, Edwards MS, Adham BI, Belmont JW: Hyperammonemia and neonatal herpes simplex pneumonitis. *Pediatr Infect Dis J* **9**:749, 1990.
446. Batshaw ML, Thomas GH, Brusilow SW: New approaches to the diagnosis and treatment of inborn errors of urea synthesis. *Pediatrics* **68**:290, 1981.
447. Webster DR, Simmons HA, Barry DMJ, Becroft DMO: Pyrimidine and purine metabolites in ornithine carbamoyl transferase deficiency. *J Inherit Metab Dis* **4**:27, 1981.
448. Van Gennip AH, Van Bree-Blom EJ, Grift J, De Bree PK, Wadman SK: Urinary purines and pyrimidines in patients with hyperammonemia of various organs. *Clin Chim Acta* **104**:227, 1980.
449. Hoogenraad NJ, Mitchell JD, Don NA, Sutherland TM, McCleary AD: Detection of carbamyl phosphate synthetase 1 deficiency using duodenal biopsy samples. *Arch Dis Child* **55**:292, 1980.
450. Matsushima A, Orit T: The activity of carbamoyl-phosphate synthetase I and ornithine transcarbamylase (OTC) in the intestine and screening for OTC deficiency in the rectal mucosa. *J Inherit Metab Dis* **4**:83, 1978.
451. Nagata N, Endo F, Matsuda I: Ornithine carbamoyltransferase (OTC) in jejunal mucosa, as a reference of the liver OTC. *Clin Chim Acta* **134**:155, 1983.
452. Bachmann C, Brandis M, Weissenbarth-Reidel E, Burghard R, Colombo JP: *N*-acetylglutamate synthetase deficiency, a second patient. *J Inherit Metab Dis* **11**:191, 1991.
453. Elpeleg ON, Colombo JP, Amir N, Bachmann C, Hurvitz H: Late-onset form of partial *N*-acetylglutamate synthetase deficiency. *Eur J Pediatr* **149**:634, 1990.
454. Pandya AL, Koch R, Hommes FA, Williams JC: *N*-acetylglutamate synthetase deficiency: Clinical and laboratory observations. *J Inherit Metab Dis* **14**:685, 1991.
455. Vockley J, Vockley CMW, Lei SP, Tuchman M, Wu TC, Lin CY, Seashore M: Normal *N*-acetylglutamate concentration measured in liver from a new patient with *N*-acetylglutamate synthetase deficiency: Physiologic and biochemical implications. *Biochem Med Metab Biol* **47**:38, 1992.
456. Tuchman M, Holzknecht RA: Human hepatic *N*-acetylglutamate content and *N*-acetylglutamate synthase activity. *Biochem J* **271**:325, 1990.
457. Burlina AB, Bachmann C, Wermuth B, Bordugo A, Ferrari V, Columbo JP, Zacchelo F: Partial *N*-acetylglutamate synthetase deficiency: A new case with uncontrollable movement disorders. *J Inherit Metab Dis* **15**:395, 1992.
458. Macleod P, Mackenzie S, Schriver CR: Partial ornithine carbamyl transferase deficiency: An inborn error of the urea cycle presenting as orotic aciduria in a male infant. *Can Med Assoc J* **107**:405, 1972.
459. Call G, Seay AR, Sherry R, Qureshi IA: Clinical features of carbamyl phosphate synthetase-I deficiency in an adult. *Ann Neurol* **16**:92, 1984.
460. Granot E, Lotan C, Lijovetzky G, Matoth I, Shvil Y, Yatziv S: Partial carbamyl phosphate synthetase deficiency, simulating Reye's syndrome, in a 9-year-old-girl. *Isr J Med Sci* **22**:463, 1986.
461. Yudkoff M, Yang W, Snodgrass PJ, Segal S: Ornithine transcarbamylase deficiency in a boy with normal development. *J Pediatr* **96**:441, 1980.
462. Oizumi J, Ng WG, Koch R, Shaw KNF, Sweetman L, Velazquez A, Donnell GN: Partial ornithine transcarbamylase deficiency associated with recurrent hyperammonemia, lethargy and depressed sensorium. *Clin Genet* **25**:538, 1984.
463. Tallan HH, Shaffner F, Taffet SL, Schneidman K, Gaull GE: Ornithine carbamoyltransferase deficiency in an adult male: Significance of hepatic ultrastructure in clinical diagnosis. *Pediatrics* **71**:224, 1983.
464. Dimagno EP, Lowe JE, Snodgrass PJ, Jones JD: Ornithine transcarbamylase deficiency—a cause of bizarre behavior in a man. *New Engl J Med* **315**:744, 1986.
465. McMurray WC, Rathbun JC, Mohyuddin F, Koegler SJ: Citrullinuria. *Pediatrics* **32**:347, 1963.
466. Finkelstein JE, Hauser ER, Leonard CO, Brusilow SW: Late onset transcarbamylase deficiency in male patients. *J Pediatr* **117**:897, 1990.
467. Rowe PC, Valle D, Brusilow SW: Inborn errors of metabolism in children referred with Reye's syndrome. *JAMA* **260**:3167, 1988.
468. Arn PH, Hauser ER, Thomas GH, Herman G, Hess D, Brusilow SW: Hyperammonemia in women with a mutation at the ornithine carbamoyltransferase locus: A cause of postpartum coma. *New Engl J Med* **322**:1652, 1990.
469. Brusilow SW: Inborn errors of urea synthesis, in Lloyd JK, Scriver CR (eds): *Genetic and Metabolic Disease in Pediatrics*. London, Butterworths, 1985, p 140.
470. Christadolu J, Qureshi IA, McInnes RR, Clarke JTR: Ornithine transcarbamylase deficiency presenting with stroke-like episodes. *J Pediatr* **122**:423, 1993.
471. Sperl W, Felber S, Skladal D, Wermuth B: Metabolic stroke in carbamyl phosphate synthetase deficiency. *Neuropediatrics* **28**:229, 1997.
472. Watson AJ, Karp JE, Walker WG, Chambers T, Risch VR, Brusilow SW: Transient idiopathic hyperammonemia in adults. *Lancet* **2**:1271, 1985.
473. Mitchell RB, Wagner JE, Karp JE, Watson JA, Brusilow SW, Przepeorka D, Storb R, Santos GW, Burke PJ, Saral R: Syndrome of idiopathic hyperammonemia after high-dose chemotherapy: Review of nine cases. *Am J Med* **85**:662, 1988.
474. Samtoy B, DeBeukelaer MM: Ammonia encephalopathy secondary to urinary tract infection with *Protein mirabilis*. *Pediatrics* **65**:294, 1980.
475. Jeffers LJ, Dubow RA, Zieve L, Reddy R, Livingstone AS, Neimark S, Viamonte M, Schiff ER: Hepatic encephalopathy and orotic aciduria associated with hepatocellular carcinoma in a noncirrhotic liver. *Hepatology* **8**:78, 1988.
476. Maestri NE, Lord CR, Glynn M, Bale A, Brusilow SW: The phenotype of ostensibly healthy women who are carriers for ornithine transcarbamylase deficiency. *Medicine* **77**:389–397, 1998.

476a. Bowling F, McGown I, Mcgill S, Cowley D, Tuchman M: Maternal gonadal mosaicism causing ornithine transcarbamylase deficiency. *Am J Med Genet* **85**:452, 1999.

477. Brusilow SW, Maestri NE: The phenotype of women who have a mutation at the ornithine transcarbamylase locus. In, Effects of Genetic Disorders on Pregnancy Outcome, Platt L, Koch R, DeLa Cruz F, eds. Parthenon Publishing Group, New York, NY, pp 979–995, 1996.
478. Stuadt M, Wermuth B, Freisinger P, Hassler A, Pontz BF: Symptomatic ornithine transcarbamylase deficiency (point mutation H202P) with normal in vitro activity. *J Inherit Metab Dis* **21**:71, 1998.
479. Hilty MD, Romshe CA, Delamater PV: Reye's syndrome and hyperaminoaciduria. *J Pediatr* **84**:362, 1974.
480. Arn PH, Hauser ER, Thomas GH, Herman G, Hess D, Brusilow SW: Hyperammonemia in women with a mutation at the ornithine transcarbamylase locus. *New Engl Med* **322**:1652, 1990.

481. Fraser CL, Arieff A: Hepatic encephalopathy. *New Engl J Med* **313**:865, 1985.
482. Voorhies TM, Ehrlich ME, Duffy TE, Petito CK, Plum F: Acute hyperammonemia in the young primate: Physiologic and neuropathologic correlates. *Pediatr Res* **17**:971, 1983.
483. Gjedde A, Lockwood AH, Duffy TE, Plum F: Cerebral blood flow and metabolism in chronically hyperammonemic rats: Effect of an acute ammonia challenge. *Ann Neurol* **3**:325, 1978.
484. Barzilay Z, Britten AG, Koehler RC, Dean MJ, Traystman R: Interaction of CO_2 and ammonia on cerebral blood flow and O_2 consumption in dogs. *Am J Physiol* **248**:H507, 1985.
484a. Takahashi H, Koehler RC, Hirata T, Brusilow SW, Traytsman RJ: Restoration of cerebrovascular CO_2 responsitivity by glutamine synthesis inhibition in hyperammonemic rats. *Circ Res* **71**:1220, 1992.
485. Chodobski A, Szmydynger-Chodobska J, Urbanska A, Szczepanska-Sadowska E: Intracranial pressure, cerebral blood flow and cerebrospinal fluid formation during hyperammonemia in cat. *J Neurosurg* **65**:86, 1986.
485a. Strange K: Maintenance of cell volume in health and disease. *Pediatr Nephrol* **7**:689, 1993.
485b. McManus ML, Churchwell KB, Strange K: Regulation of cell volume in health and disease. *N Engl J Med* **333**:1260, 1995.
485c. Kirk K, Strange K: Functional properties and physiological role of organic solute channels. *Annu Rev Physiol* **60**:719, 1998.
486. Brusilow SW: Inborn errors of urea synthesis, in Lloyd JK, Scriver CR (eds): *Genetic and Metabolic Disease in Pediatrics*. London, Butterworths, 1985, p 140.
487. Brusilow SW, Traystman R: Hepatic encephalopathy. *New Engl J Med* **314**:768, 1986.
488. Hindfelt B: Ammonia intoxication and brain energy metabolism, in Kleinberger G, Deutsch G (eds): *New Aspects of Clinical Nutrition*. Basel, Karger, 1983, p 474.
489. Felyso V. Grau E, Minana M, Grisolia S: Hyperammonemia decreases protein-kinase-C–dependent phosphorylation of microtubule-associated protein 2 and increases its binding to tubulin. *Eur J Biochem* **214**:243, 1993.
490. Takahashi H, Koehler RC, Brusilow SW, Traystman RJ: Inhibition of brain glutamine accumulation prevents cerebral edema in hyperammonemic rats. *Am J Physiol* **26**:H825, 1991.
491. Willard-Mack CL, Koehler RC, Hirata T, Cork LC, Takahashi H, Traystman RJ, Brusilow SW: Inhibition of glutamine synthetase reduces ammonia-induced astrocyte swelling in rat. *Neuroscience* **71**:598, 1996.
492. Norenberg MD, Isaacks RE, Dombro RS, Bender AS: Prevention of ammonia-induced toxicity in astrocytes by L-methionine-DL-sulfoximine, In Capocaccia L, Merle M, Riggio O (eds): *Advances in Encephalopathy and Metabolic Nitrogen Exchange*. Boca Raton, FL, CRC Press, 1995, p 176.
493. Zwingmann C, Brand A, Richter-Landsberg C, Leibfritz D: Multinuclear NMR spectroscopy studies on NH_4Cl-induced metabolic alterations and detoxification processes in primary astrocytes and glioma cells. *Dev Neurosci* **20**:417, 1998.
494. Sugimoto H, Koehler RC, Wilson DA, Brusilow SW, Traystman RJ: Methionine sulfoximine, a glutamine synthetase inhibitor, attenuates increased extracellular potassium activity during acute hyperammonemia. *J Cereb Blood Flow Metab* **17**:44, 1997.
495. Hirata T, Kawaguchi T, Brusilow SW, Traystman RJ, Koehler RC: Preserved hypocapnic pial arteriolar constriction during hyperammonemia by glutamine synthetase inhibition. *Am J Physiol* **276**:H1, 1999.
496. Jonung T, Rigotti P, Jeppsson B, James JH, Peters JC, Fischer JE: Methionine sulfoximine prevents the accumulation of large neutral amino acids in brain of hyperammonemic rats. *J Surg Res* **36**:349, 1984.
497. Choi DW: Glutamate neurotoxicity and diseases of the nervous system. *Neuron* **1**:623, 1988.
498. Batshaw ML, Walser M, Brusilow SW: Plasma α-ketoglutarate in urea cycle enzymopathies and its role as a harbinger of hyperammonemic coma. *Pediatr Res* **14**:1316, 1980.
499. Maestri NE, McGowan KD, Brusilow SW: Plasma glutamine concentration: A guide in the management of urea cycle disorders. *J Pediatr* **121**:259, 1992.
500. Ansley JD, Isaacs JW, Reekers LF, Kutner MH, Nordlinger BM, Rudman D: Quantitative tests of nitrogen metabolism in cirrhosis: Relation to other manifestations of liver disease. *Gastroenterology* **75**:572, 1978.
501. Levin B, Abraham VG, Oberholzer VG, Burgens EA: Hyperammonemia: A deficiency of liver ornithine transcarbamylase, occurrence in mother and child. *Arch Dis Child* **44**:152, 1969.
502. Van Der Zee SPM, Trijbels JMF, Monnens LAH, Hommes FA, Schretlen EDAM: Citrullinaemia with rapidly fatal neonatal course. *Arch Dis Child* **46**:874, 1971.
503. Connelly A, Cross JH, Gadian DG, Hunter JV, Kirkham RJ, Leonard JV: Magnetic resonance spectroscopy shows increased brain glutamine in ornithine carbamoyl transferase deficiency. *Pediatr Res* **33**:77, 1993.
504. Ross BD, Danielsen ER, Bluml S. Proton magnetic resonance spectroscopy: The new gold standard for diagnosis of clinical and subclinical hepatic encephalopathy. *Dig Dis* **14**:30, 1996.
505. Cooper AJL, Vergara F, Duffy TE: Cerebral glutamine synthetase, in Hertz E, Krammer E, McGeer EG, Schousbee A (eds): *Glutamine, Glutamate, and GABA in the Central Nervous System*. New York, Alan R. Liss. 1983, p 77.
506. Duffy TE, Plum F, Cooper AJL: Cerebral ammonia metabolism in vivo, in Hertz E, Krammer E, McGeer EG, Schousbee A (eds): *Glutamine, Glutamate, and GABA in the Central Nervous System*. New York, Alan R. Liss. 1983, p 3717.
507. Visek WJ: Arginine needs, physiological state and usual diets. A reevaluation. *J Nutr* **116**:36, 1986.
508. Morris JG: Nutritional and metabolic responses to arginine deficiency in carnivores. *J Nutr* **115**:524, 1985.
509. Visek WJ: Arginine and disease states. *J Nutr* **115**:532, 1985.
510. Snyderman SE, Boyer A, Holt EL: The arginine requirement of the infant. *Am J Dis Child* **97**:192, 1959.
511. Nakagawa I, Takahashi T, Suzuki T, Kobayashi K: Amino acid requirements of children: Minimal needs of tryptophan arginine and histidine based on nitrogen balance methods. *J Nutr* **80**:305, 1963.
512. Rose WC, Haines WJ, Warner DT: The amino acid requirements of man. V. The role of lysine, arginine and tryptophan. *J Biol Chem* **206**:421, 1954.
513. Carey GP, Kime Z, Rogers QR, Morris JG, Hargrove D, Buffington CA, Brusilow SW: An arginine-deficient diet in humans does not evoke hyperammonemia or orotic aciduria. *J Nutr* **117**:1734, 1987.
514. Widhalm K, Koch S, Scheibenreiter S, Knoll E, Colombo JP, Bachmann C, Thalhammer O: Long-term follow-up of 12 patients with late-onset variant of argininosuccinic acid lyase deficiency: No impairment of intellectual and psychomotor development during therapy. *Pediatrics* **89**:1182, 1992.
515. Krauer-Mayer B, Keller M, Hottinger A: Ober den frauenmilchinduzierten icterus prolongatus des neugeborenen. *Helv Paediatr Acta* **23**:68, 1968.
516. Hopkins IJ, Connely JF, Dawson AG, Hird FJR, Madison TG: Hyperammonemia due to ornithine transcarbamylase deficiency. *Arch Dis Child* **44**:143, 1969.
517. Levin B, Abraham JM, Oberholzer VG, Burgess EA: Hyperammonemia: A deficiency of liver ornithine transcarbamylase. *Arch Dis Child* **33**:152, 1969.
518. Bruton CJ, Corsellis JAN, Russell A: Hereditary hyperammonemia. *Brain* **93**:423, 1970.
519. Vidailhet Levin B, Dautrevaux M, Paysant P, Gelot S, Badonnel LY, Pierson M, Neimann N: Citrullinemie. *Arch Fr Pediatr* **28**:521, 1971.
520. Martin JJ, Schlote W: Central nervous system lesions in disorders of amino-acid metabolism. *J Neurol Sci* **15**:49, 1972.
521. Ebels EJ: Neuropathological observations in a patient with carbamylphosphate synthetase deficiency and in two sibs. *Arch Dis Child* **47**:47, 1972.
522. Wick H, Bachmann C, Baumgartner R, Brechbuhler T, Colombo JP, Wiesmann U, Mihatsch MJ, Ohnacker H: Variants of citrullinaemia. *Arch Dis Child* **48**:636, 1973.
523. Leibowitz J, Thoene J, Spector E, Nyhan W: Citrullinemia. *Arch Pathol Anat Histol* **377**:249, 1978.
524. Martin JJ, Fariaux JP, De Jonghe P: Neuropathology of citrullinaemia. *Arch Neuropathol (Berl)* **56**:303, 1982.
525. Kornfeld M, Woodfin BM, Papile L, Davis LE, Bernard LR: Neuropathology of ornithine carbamyl transferase deficiency. *Acta Neuropathol (Berl)* **65**:261, 1985.
526. Lewis PD, Miller AL: Argininosuccinic aciduria. *Brain* **93**:413, 1970.
527. Solitare GB, Shih VE, Nelligan DJ, Dolan TF Jr: Argininosuccinic aciduria: Clinical, biochemical, anatomical and neuropathological observations. *J Ment Defic Res* **13**:153, 1969.
528. Harding BN, Leonard JV, Eerdohazi M: Ornithine carbamoyl transferase deficiency: A neuropathological study. *Eur J Pediatr* **141**:215, 1984.

529. Kendall BE, Kingsley DPE, Leonard JV, Lingham S, Oberholzer VG: Neurological features and computed tomography of the brain in children with ornithine carbamoyl transferase deficiency. *J Neurol Neurosurg Psychiatry* **46**:28, 1983.
530. Msall M, Batshaw ML, Suss R, Brusilow SW, Mellits ED: Neurologic outcome in children with inborn errors of urea synthesis. *New Engl J Med* **310**:1500, 1984.
531. Labrecque DR, Latham PS, Riely CA, Hsia YE, Klatskin G: Heritable urea cycle enzyme deficiency-liver disease in 16 patients. *J Pediatr* **94**:580, 1979.
532. Flick JA, Latham PS, Perman J, Brusilow SW: Hepatic involvement in argininosuccinase deficiency. *Pediatr Res* **20**:239A, 1986.
533. Zimmerman A, Bachmann C, Baumgartner R: Severe liver fibrosis in argininosuccinic aciduria. *Arch Pathol Lab Med* **110**:136, 1986.
534. Capistrano-Estrada S, Marsden DL, Nyhan WL, Newbury RO, Krous HF, Tuchman M: Histopathological findings in a male with late-onset ornithine transcarbamylase deficiency. *Pediatr Pathol* **14**:235, 1994.
535. O'Conner JE, Renau-Piqueras J, Gisolia S: Effects of urease-induced hyperammonemia in mouse liver. *Virchows Arch [B]* **46**:187, 1984.
536. Snyderman SE, Samsaricq C, Phansalklar SV, Schacht RG, Norton PM: The therapy of hyperammonemia due to ornithine transcarbamylase deficiency in a male neonate. *Pediatrics* **56**:65, 1975.
537. Brusilow S, Batshaw M, Walser M: Use of keto acids in inborn errors of urea synthesis, in Winick M (ed): *Nutritional Management of Genetic Disorders*. New York, John Wiley, 1979, p 65.
538. Young VR, Steffee WP, Pencharz PB, Winterer JC, Scrimshaw NS: Total human body protein synthesis in relation to protein requirements at various ages. *Nature* **253**:192, 1975.
539. Bier DM, Young VR: Assessment of whole-body protein-nitrogen kinetics in the human infant, in Foman SJ, Heird WC (eds): *Energy and Protein Needs During Infancy*. New York, Academic, 1986, p 107.
540. Brusilow SW: Treatment of urea cycle disorders, in Desnick RJ (ed): *Treatment of Genetic Disease*. New York, Churchill Livingstone, 1991, pp 79.
541. Brusilow SW, Batshaw ML: Arginine therapy of argininosuccinase deficiency. *Lancet* 1:124, 1979.
542. Brusilow SW, Valle DL, Batshaw ML: New pathways of nitrogen excretion in inborn errors of urea synthesis. *Lancet* **2**:452, 1979.
543. Kvedar JC, Baden HP, Baden LA, Shih VE, Kolodny EH: Dietary management reverses grooving and abnormal polarization of hair shafts in argininosuccinase deficiency. *Am J Med Genet* **40**:211, 1991.
544. Iafolla AK, Gale DS, Roe CR: Citrate therapy in argininosuccinate lyase deficiency. *J Pediatr* **117**:102, 1990.
545. Lewis HB: Studies in the synthesis of hippuric acid after benzoate ingestion in man. *J Biol Chem* **18**:225, 1914.
546. Shiple GJ, Sherwin CP: Synthesis of glycocoll and glutamine in the human organisms. I. Synthesis of glycocoll and glutamine in the human organism. *J Am Chem Soc* **44**:618, 1922.
547. Brusilow W, Tinker J, Batshaw ML: Amino acid acylation: A mechanism of nitrogen excretion in inborn errors of urea synthesis. *Science* **207**:659, 1980.
548. Webster LT, Siddiqui UA, Lucas SV, Strong JM, Mieyal JJ: Identification of separate Acyl-CoA:glycine and Acyl-CoA:L-glutamine *N*-acyltransferase activities in mitochondrial fractions from liver of rhesus monkey and man. *J Biol Chem* **251**:3352, 1976.
549. Killenberg PG, Webster LT: Conjugation by peptide bond formation, in Jakoby WB (ed): *Enzymatic Basis of Detoxication*. Vol. 2. New York, Academic, 1980, p 141.
550. Moldave K, Meister A: Synthesis of phenylacetylglutamine by human tissue. *J Biol Chem* **229**:463, 1957.
551. James OM, Smith RL, Williams RT, Reidenberg M: The conjugation of phenylacetic acid in man, sub-human primates and some non-primate species. *Proc R Soc Lond [Biol]* **182**:25, 1972.
552. Brusilow SW: Phenylacetylglutamine may replace urea as a vehicle for waste nitrogen excretion. *Pediatr Res* **29**:147, 1991.
553. Snapper I, Saltzman A: Quantitative aspects of benzoylglucaronate formation in normal individuals and in patients with liver disorders. *Am J Med* **2**:327, 1947.
554. Malatack JJ, Iwatsuki S, Gartner JC, Roe T, Finegold DN, Shaw BW, Zitelli BJ, Starzl TE: Liver transplantation for type I glycogen storage disease. *Lancet* **1**:1073, 1983.
555. Lewis HJ, Bontempo FA, Spero JA, Ragni MV, Starzl TE: Liver transplantation in a hemophiliac. *New Engl J Med* **312**:1189, 1985.
556. Tuchman M, Freese DK, Sharp HL, Rammaraine M, Ascher N, Bloomer JR: Contribution of extrahepatic tissues to biochemical abnormalities in hereditary tyrosinemia type I: Study of three patients after liver transplantation. *J Pediatr* **110**:401, 1987.
557. Todo S, Starzl TE, Tzakis A, Benkov KJ, Kalousek F, Saheki T, Tanikawa K, Fenton WA: Orthotopic liver transplantation for urea cycle enzyme deficiency. *Hepatology* **15**:419, 1992.
558. Goss JA, Seu P, Dulkanchainun TS, Yanni GS, McDiarmid SV, Busuttil RW: The role of orthotopic liver transplantation in the treatment of ornithine transcarbamylase deficiency. *Liver Transplant Surg* **4**:350, 1998.
559. Whitington PF, Alonso EM, Boyle JT, Molleston JP, Rosenthal P, Edmund, JC, Millis JM: Liver transplantation for the treatment of urea cycle disorders. *J Inherit Metab Dis* **21**:112, 1998.
560. Wiegand C, Thompson T, Bock GH, Mathis RK, Kjellstrand CM, Mauer SM: The management of life-threatening hyperammonemia: A comparison of several therapeutic modalities. *J Pediatr* **96**:142, 1980.
561. Donn SM, Swartz RD, Thoene JG: Comparison of exchange transfusion, peritoneal dialysis and hemodialysis for the treatment of hyperammonemia in an anuric newborn infant. *J Pediatr* **95**:67, 1979.
562. Kiley JE, Pender JC, Welch HF, Welch CS: Ammonia intoxication treated by hemodialysis. *New Engl J Med* **259**:1156, 1958.
563. Neu AM, Christenson MJ, Brusilow SW: Hemodialysis for inborn errors of metabolism, in Nissenson AR, Fine AR (eds): *Dialysis Therapy*, 2nd ed. Philadelphia, Hanley & Belfus, 1992, p 371.
564. Herrin JT, McCredie DA: Peritoneal dialysis in the reduction of blood ammonia levels in a case of hyperammonemia. *Arch Dis Child* **44**:149, 1969.
565. Batshaw ML, Brusilow SW: Treatment of hyperammonemic coma caused by inborn errors of urea synthesis. *J Pediatr* **97**:893, 1980.
566. Siegel NJ, Brown RS: Peritoneal clearance of ammonia and creatinine in a neonate. *J Pediatr* **82**:1044, 1973.
567. Rutledge SL, Havens PL, Haymond MW, McClean RH, Kan JS, Brusilow SW: Neonatal hemodialysis: Effective therapy for the encephalopathy of inborn errors of metabolism. *J Pediatr* **116**:125, 1990.
568. Rowe PC, Newman SL, Brusilow SW: Natural history of symptomatic partial ornithine transcarbamylase deficiency. *New Engl J Med* **314**:541, 1986.
569. Batshaw ML, Msall M, Beaudet AL, Trojak J: Risk of serious illness in heterozygotes for ornithine transcarbamylase deficiency. *J Pediatr* **108**:236, 1986.
570. Brusilow SW, Finkelstein JE: Restoration of nitrogen homeostasis in a man with partial ornithine transcarbamylase deficiency. *Metabolism* **42**:1336, 1993.
571. Brusilow SW, Danney M, Waber L, Batshaw M, Burton B, Levitsky L, Roth K, McKeethren C, Ward J: Treatment of episodic hyperammonemia in children with inborn errors of urea synthesis. *New Engl J Med* **310**:1630, 1984.
571a. Praphanphoj V, Boyadjiev SA, Waber LJ, Brusilow SW, Geraghty MT: Three cases of intravenous sodium benzoate and sodium phenylacetate toxicity occurring in the treatment of acute hyperammonemia. *J Inherited Metab Dis* **23**:129, 2000.
572. Snebold NG, Ruzzo JF III, Lessell S, Pruett RC: Transient visual loss in ornithine transcarbamylase deficiency. *Am J Ophthalmol* **104**:407, 1987.
573. Lyle DJ: Eye symptoms produced by tentorial herniation from increased intracranial pressure. *XVII Concilium Ophthalmologicum* **3**:845, 1954.
574. Maestri NE, Hauser ER, Bartholomew D, Brusilow SW: Prospective treatment of urea cycle disorders. *J Pediatr* **119**:923, 1992.
575. Maestri NE, Clissold DB, Brusilow SW: Long-term survival of patients with argininosuccinate synthetase deficiency. *J Pediatr* **127**:929, 1995.
576. Maestri NE, Brusilow SW, Clissold DB, Bassett S: Long-term treatment of girls with ornithine transcarbamylase deficiency. *New Engl J Med* **335**:855, 1996.
577. Fleisher LD, Rassen DK, Desnick RJ, Salwen HR, Rogers P, Bean M, Guall GE: Argininosuccinic aciduria: Prenatal studies in a family at risk. *Am J Hum Genet* **31**:349, 1979.
578. Goodman SI, Mace JW, Turner B, Garrett WJ: Antenatal diagnosis of argininosuccinic aciduria. *Clin Genet* **4**:236, 1973.
579. Hokanson JR, O'Brien WE, Idemoto J, Schafer IA: Carrier detection in ornithine transcarbamylase deficiency. *J Pediatr* **93**:75, 1978.
580. Ng WG, Oizumi J, Koch R, Shaw KNF, McLaren J, Donnel GN, Carter M: Carrier detection of urea cycle disorders. *Pediatrics* **68**:448, 1981.

581. Hann EA, Danks DM, Grimes A: Carrier detection in ornithine transcarbamylase deficiency. *J Inherit Metab Dis* **5**:37, 1982.
582. Becroft DMO, Barry DMJ, Webster DR, Simmons HA: Failure of protein loading tests to identify heterozygosity for ornithine carbamoyltransferase deficiency. *J Inherit Metab Dis* **7**:157, 1984.
583. Batshaw ML, Naylor EW, Thomas GH: False positive alanine tolerance test results in heterozygote detection of urea cycle disorders. *J Pediatr* **115**:595, 1989.
584. MacKenzie AE, MacLeod HL, Hans M, Heick C, Korneluk RG: False positive results from the alanine loading test for ornithine carbamoyltransferase deficiency heterozygosity. *J Pediatr* **115**:605, 1989.
585. Terheggen HG, Schwenk A, Lowenthal A, Van Sandh M, Colombo JP: Argininaemia with arginase deficiency. *Lancet* **2**:748, 1969.
586. Cederbaum SD, Shaw KNF, Spector EB, Verity MA, Snodgrass PJ, Sugarman GI: Hyperargininemia with arginase deficiency. *Pediatr Res* **13**:827, 1979.
587. Iyer R, Jenkinson CP, Vockley JC, Kern RM, Grody WW, Cederbaum S: The human arginases and arginase deficiency. *J Inherit Metab Dis* **21**:86, 1998.
588. Jorda A, Rubio V, Portoles M, Vilas J, Garcia-Pino J: A new case of arginase deficiency in a Spanish male. *J Inherit Metab Dis* **9**:393, 1986.
589. Naylor EW, Cederbaum SD: Urinary pyrimidine excretion in arginase deficiency. *J Inherit Dis* **4**:207, 1981.
590. Cederbaum SD, Moedjono SJ, Shaw KNF, Carter M, Naylor E, Walzer M: Treatment of hyperargininaemia due to arginase deficiency with a chemically defined diet. *J Inherit Dis* **5**:95, 1982.
591. Bachmann C, Colombo JP: Diagnostic value of orotic acid excretion in heritable disorders of the urea cycle and in hyperammonemia due to organic acidurias. *Eur J Pediatr* **134**:109, 1980.
592. Wiechert P, Mortelmans J, Lavinha F, Clara R, Terheggen HG, Lowenthal A: Excretion of guanidino-derivatives in urine of hyperargininemic patients. *J Hum Genet* **24**:61, 1976.
593. Marescau B, Pintens J, Lowenthal A, Terheggen HG: Excretion of keto-δ-guanidinovaleric acid and its cyclic form in patients with hyperargininemia. *Clin Chim Acta* **98**:35, 1979.
594. Marescau B, Lowenthal A: Isolation and identification of some guanidino compounds in the urine of patients with hyperargininaemia by liquid chromatography, thin-layer chromatography and gas chromatography mass spectrometry. *J Chromatogr* **224**:185, 1981.
595. Hyland K, Smith I, Clayton PT, Leonard JV: Impaired neurotransmitter amine metabolic deficiency. *J Neurol Neurosurg Psychiatry* **48**:1189, 1985.
596. Mori M, Gotoh T, Nagasaki A, Takiguchi M, Sonoki T: Regulation of the urea cycle enzyme genes in nitric oxide synthesis. *J Inherit Metab Dis* **21**:59, 1998.
597. Snyderman SE, Sansaricq C, Chen WJ, Norton P, Phansalkar SV: Argininemia. *J Pediatr* **90**:563, 1977.
598. Snyderman SE, Sansaricq C, Norton PM, Goldstein F: Brief clinical and laboratory observations. *J Pediatr* **95**:61, 1979.
599. Qureshi IA, Letarte J, Ouellet R, Batshaw ML, Brusilow SW: Treatment of hyperargininemia with sodium benzoate and arginine restricted diet. *J Pediatr* **104**:473, 1984.
600. Thoden JB, Raushel FM, Benning MM, Rayment I, Holden HM: The structure of carbamoyl phosphate synthetase determined to 2.1 Å resolution. *Acta Crystallogr D Biol Crystallogr* **55**:8, 1999.

CHAPTER 86

Errors of Lysine Metabolism

Rody P. Cox

1. **Familial hyperlysinemia is an autosomal recessive disease caused by a defect in the bifunctional protein α-aminoadipic semialdehyde synthase. The two associated enzyme activities, lysine-ketoglutarate reductase and saccharopine dehydrogenase, normally initiate the degradation of lysine by removal of the ε amino group. In familial hyperlysinemia, both activities are reduced to 10 percent of normal or less, causing hyperlysinemia and lysinuria, frequently accompanied by a relatively mild saccharopinuria. The condition appears to be benign. A variant, saccharopinuria, has been described in which 30 percent of lysine-ketoglutarate activity was retained and the saccharopine dehydrogenase activity was undetectable. Saccharopinuria was prominent, exceeding the associated lysinuria. Experience with the variant is too limited to know if this metabolic abnormality causes disease.**
2. **Removal of the α amino group of lysine constitutes a minor pathway for lysine degradation in most tissues, with pipecolic acid as a product. Hyperpipecolatemia is regularly observed in familial hyperlysinemia as an overflow phenomenon. It is also a common concomitant of Zellweger syndrome, as the result of a defect in peroxisome formation and the consequent deficiency of L-pipecolic acid oxidase activity. A convincing example of a patient with hyperpipecolatemia as a primary defect has not been reported. The hyperpipecolatemia in Zellweger syndrome becomes manifest after the major symptoms are already evident, suggesting that it is not a significant contributing factor.**

This chapter is devoted to inherited metabolic diseases of the first enzymatic steps in lysine degradation. Familial hyperlysinemia and saccharopinuria are the most prominent and most clearly elucidated abnormalities. Hyperpipecolatemia has received considerable attention and also will be discussed briefly. Sporadic reports of hyperlysinemia of uncertain etiology and lysinuria in the absence of hyperlysinemia will not be considered. The latter generally results from transport defects, often as part of a dibasic amino acid transport defect, and is discussed in Chap. 193.

METABOLISM OF LYSINE

Lysine is an essential six-carbon dibasic amino acid.[1] L-Lysine uptake into cells is generally efficient. Saturable and unsaturable transport systems have been described, as well as a sodium-independent carrier of the $y+$ type that is specific for L-lysine.[2,3] In common with other amino acids, an excess of lysine beyond that needed for protein synthesis is degraded through the Krebs cycle after removal of amino groups, yielding energy. Early workers in intermediary metabolism noted that the keto acid of lysine could not replace the amino acid in the diet and correctly concluded that lysine did not participate in classic transamination. The initial steps in the degradation of lysine remained uncertain, however, until relatively recently.

A list of standard abbreviations is located immediately preceding the index in each volume.

Saccharopine Pathway

It is now recognized that the major pathway for the degradation of lysine involves transfer of the ε amino group to α-ketoglutarate through the stable intermediate saccharopine.[4–6] The end result of transamination is thereby achieved, although by a different mechanism. Two enzymatic steps are involved, which are carried out by a bifunctional enzyme, aminoadipic semialdehyde synthase[7] (Fig. 86-1). The two activities contained in the synthase are lysine-ketoglutarate reductase and saccharopine dehydrogenase. In the first step, saccharopine is formed as a ligand between lysine and α-ketoglutarate. In the second step, saccharopine is cleaved to α-aminoadipic acid semialdehyde and glutamic acid, completing the transfer of the ε amino group. The aldehyde is oxidized to α-aminoadipic acid. Subsequent steps in this degradative pathway involve transamination of the α amino group to form α-ketoadipic acid and successive decarboxylations to form first glutaryl coenzyme A (CoA) and then crotonyl CoA, which, in turn, is oxidized to acetyl CoA. The metabolism distal to α-aminoadipic acid and genetic defects thereof (α-ketoadipic acidemia and glutaric acidemia type I) are discussed in Chap. 95.

Pipecolic Acid Pathway

The pipecolic acid pathway was long believed to be the major degradative pathway for lysine[8,9] (see Fig. 86-1). It is now recognized that its capacity is inadequate for the large amounts of L-lysine that must be degraded with normal dietary intake. It functions as an overflow pathway for L-lysine and as the major pathway for D-lysine. L-Lysine metabolism by the pipecolic acid pathway appears to be prominent in the brain.[10–12] The saccharopine pathway is active in fetal rat brain but gradually diminishes and is negligible in the adult. In rat liver, the saccharopine pathway gradually increases during development and is the major pathway for lysine degradation in liver.[12] Pipecolic acid binds to the γ-aminobutyric acid (GABA) receptor as an agonist and modulates the function of that neurotransmitter.[12,13] The initial step in the pipecolic acid pathway is removal of the α amino group of lysine by oxidative deamination. The keto acid undergoes a condensation to form a piperideine compound and is reduced to pipecolic acid. L-Pipecolic acid is the product of both L- and D-lysine. Pipecolic acid is oxidized to α-aminoadipic semialdehyde, joining the saccharopine pathway.

Bifunctional α-Aminoadipic Semialdehyde Synthase

Investigation of patients with familial hyperlysinemia revealed that the two sequential degradative activities, lysine-ketoglutarate reductase and saccharopine dehydrogenase, were consistently defective.[6,15] It was postulated that both enzyme activities might reside in one protein. This hypothesis was challenged by the report that two separate enzymes had been isolated from rat liver.[16] Studies of bovine and baboon liver, however, have provided convincing evidence of a single bifunctional protein.[7] The relative activities of lysine-ketoglutarate reductase and saccharopine dehydrogenase remained constant throughout extensive purification to apparent homogeneity. Activity staining of a native gel demonstrated that both activities (reductase and dehydrogenase) migrate the same distance toward the anode, providing further

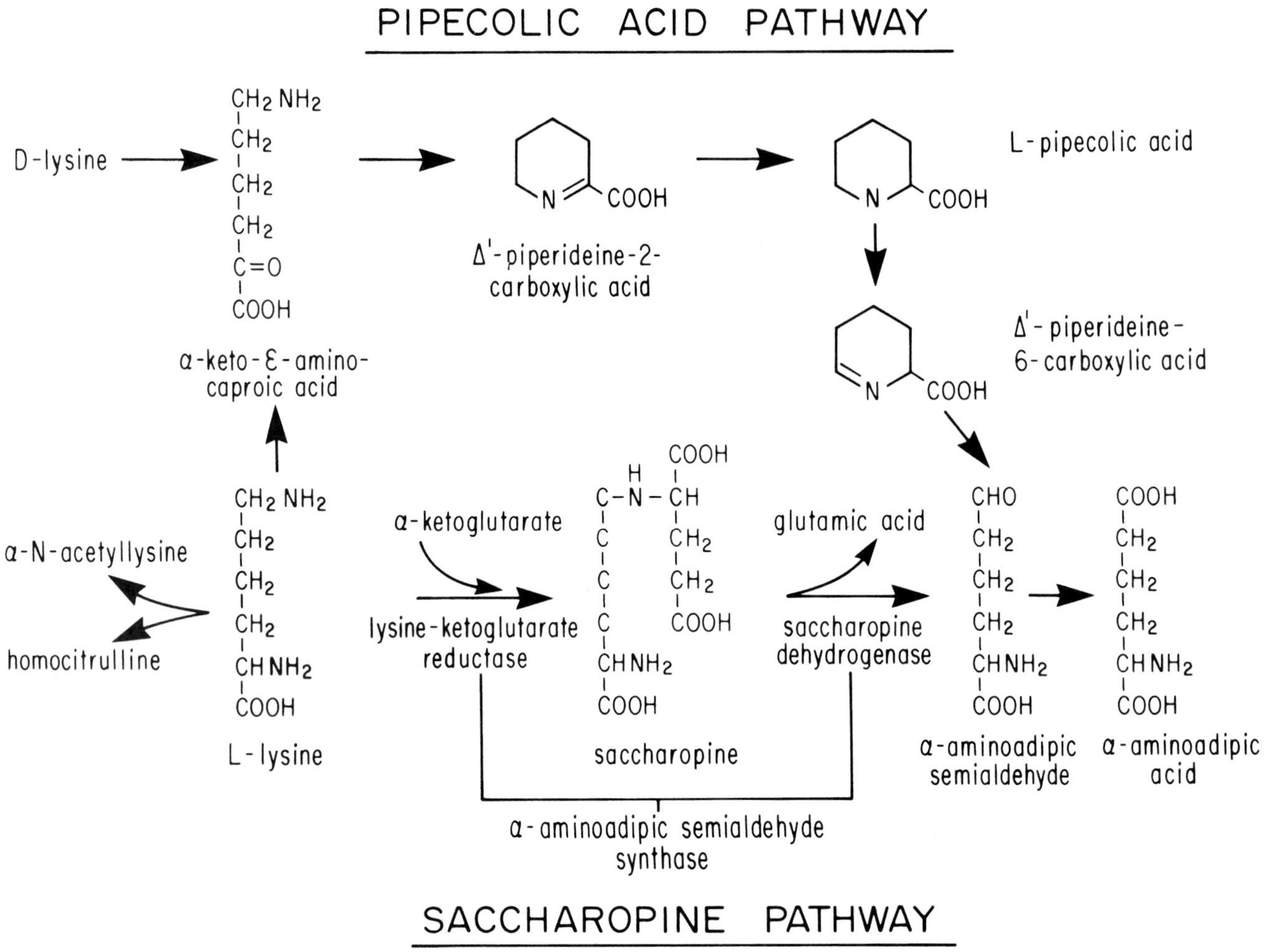

PIPECOLIC ACID PATHWAY

D-lysine

α-keto-ε-amino-caproic acid

Δ'-piperideine-2-carboxylic acid

L-pipecolic acid

Δ'-piperideine-6-carboxylic acid

α-N-acetyllysine

homocitrulline

L-lysine

α-ketoglutarate

lysine-ketoglutarate reductase

saccharopine

glutamic acid

saccharopine dehydrogenase

α-aminoadipic semialdehyde

α-aminoadipic acid

α-aminoadipic semialdehyde synthase

SACCHAROPINE PATHWAY

Fig. 86-1 Metabolism of lysine.

evidence that the purified synthase is a single protein. Electrophoresis on sodium dodecyl sulfate (SDS)-polyacrylamide gel yielded a single protein band with a molecular weight of 115,000. The synthase has a molecular weight of 468,000 and appears to exist as a tetramer of a 115-kDa polypeptide. The domains for lysine ketoglutarate reductase and saccharopine dehydrogenase can be separated by diethylaminoethyl (DEAE)-Biogel column chromatography following limited digestion with elastase without loss of activity.[17] The isolated reductase and dehydrogenase domains appear to exist in multiple aggregates consisting of peptide fragments of 62,700 and 49,200 Da, respectively. The results indicate that the reductase and dehydrogenase domains of the aminoadipic semialdehyde synthase are separately folded and functionally independent.

Covalent linkage of functionally related enzymes is not uncommon in eukaryotic organisms, presumably providing an evolutionary advantage. In bacteria and fungi, lysine-ketoglutarate reductase and saccharopine dehydrogenase are represented by two separate proteins with molecular weights of 49,000 and 73,000 Da, respectively.[18,19] However, in *Caenorhabditis elegans*, the two enzyme activities are covalently linked, indicating an early evolutionary fusion of the genes (Stephen Gould, personal communication, Johns Hopkins University, 1998). One possible advantage of linkage of enzymes is the more efficient use of substrate as a result of "channeling." Bound intermediates are subjected to sequential enzymatic reactions while being protected from dilution and competing reactions. The kinetic advantages of substrate channeling were elegantly demonstrated for indole conversion to tryptophan by tryptophan synthase.[20] Covalent linkage also maintains the component enzymes in equimolar amounts, adding to the efficiency of the system.

There may be similarities between hereditary orotic aciduria (see Chap. 113) and familial hyperlysinemia. Orotic aciduria type I exhibits a combined deficiency of orotate phosphoribosyl transferase and orotidine-5′-phosphate decarboxylase, the last two sequential steps in the *de novo* synthesis of uridine. In orotic aciduria type II, the second activity, the decarboxylase, is deficient, whereas the transferase activity is nearly normal.[21] A bifunctional enzyme, uridine monophosphate (UMP) synthase ($M_r = 51{,}500$), has both activities.[22,23] The efficiency of channeling of orotidine-5′-monophosphate, the product of the first enzyme and the substrate of the second, was tenfold greater with the bifunctional protein than when the two enzyme activities were separated.[24]

Multifunctional proteins also have been described for fatty acid synthetase[25,26] and the carbamyl phosphate synthetase–aspartate carbamyltransferase–dehydrogenase (CAD) complex.[27]

Recently, a full-length human gene encoding the bifunctional α-aminoadipic semialdehyde synthase has been cloned.[27a] The genomic structure consists of 24 exons scattered over 68 kb and maps to chromosome 7q31-32. The cDNA has an open reading frame of 2781 bp that is predicted to encode a protein with 927 amino acids. The 5′ end of the cDNA is homologous to the yeast saccharopine dehydrogenase, and the 3′ end of the cDNA is similar to the yeast lysine-ketoglutarate reductase. The cDNA on northern blot analysis cross-hybridizes to transcripts that are highly expressed in liver and to a lesser extent in most other tissues. The genomic DNA from a hyperlysinemic patient (JJa), who is the progeny of a consanguineous mating, had a homozygous out-of-frame 9-bp deletion in exon 15 that resulted in a premature stop codon at position 534 of the protein.[27a]

FAMILIAL HYPERLYSINEMIA

Biochemical Defect

Lysine-ketoglutarate reductase and saccharopine dehydrogenase activities are distributed widely in human tissues.[28,29] The skin fibroblast grown in tissue culture proved a convenient approach to study of the biochemical defect. Both enzyme activities were grossly deficient in patients with familial hyperlysinemia.[6,15] Retrograde splitting of saccharopine to yield lysine also was greatly reduced. It is uncertain whether this reaction is catalyzed by a distinct enzyme, saccharopine oxidoreductase, or reflects the reversibility of lysine-ketoglutarate reductase activity. Liver obtained at autopsy from a hyperlysinemic patient had the same enzyme deficiencies.[6]

The magnitude of the defect in lysine metabolism was estimated in two subjects by administering [^{14}C]lysine and collecting exhaled $^{14}CO_2$.[30] Under conditions of normal dietary intake, the amount of labeled carbon dioxide collected from two hyperlysinemic patients was about 10 percent of that in two control subjects (Fig. 86-2). Furthermore, the controls had a reserve capacity to handle excesses of lysine. Following administration of an acute load of lysine, the amount of lysine degraded to CO_2 increased twofold without increasing the fraction excreted into the urine.

An unusual patient with familial hyperlysinemia, presenting with "cystinuria," was detected by careful examination of urine.[31] Cystine overlies saccharopine in the usual chromatographic systems. By oxidizing cystine to cysteic acid, it was revealed that the patient had saccharopinuria rather than cystinuria. Excesses of saccharopine were unexpected because saccharopine is distal to the defect in lysine-ketoglutarate activity. To confirm this observation, the tentatively identified saccharopine was isolated from the urine and heated to 110°C for 5 hours. A new compound appeared with the chromatographic characteristics of pyrosaccharopine. Of an additional six subjects with the double enzymatic activity defect characteristic of familial hyperlysinemia, four had a detectable saccharopinuria. A reasonable explanation of this unexpected finding is that residual lysine-ketoglutarate reductase activity permits the synthesis of small amounts of saccharopine, and a more complete defect in saccharopine dehydrogenase activity prevents its metabolic disposal.

Clinical Presentation

The initial observation is generally an impressive lysinuria detected during biochemical studies of a patient with presumed metabolic disease, often with neurologic symptoms. Measurement of plasma amino acid levels shows the lysine to be considerably elevated, regularly exceeding 680 mM in classic cases and often reaching twice that concentration. Screening of other family members may reveal asymptomatic individuals with the same biochemical findings. Both sexes are affected, and consanguinity of parents has been reported, indicating autosomal recessive inheritance. Confirmation of the diagnosis is by enzymatic studies on the skin fibroblast.

Diagnosis

Normal skin fibroblasts effectively degrade lysine to carbon dioxide. It was therefore possible to reproduce the studies originally performed *in vivo* by incubating skin fibroblasts with [^{14}C]lysine.[15] In skin fibroblasts from seven subjects with enzymatically confirmed diagnoses of familial hyperlysinemia, 5 to 10 percent of the normal amount of radioactive CO_2 was liberated (Table 86-1). In the presence of significant hyperlysinemia in the patient, a reduction in the degradation of lysine to CO_2 can be assumed to involve a defect in either or both of the first two enzymatic steps in the saccharopine pathway. Hyperlysinemia has not been reported in defects below α-aminoadipic acid or as the result of defects in the pipecolic acid pathway.

Specific diagnoses require assays for lysine-ketoglutarate reductase and saccharopine dehydrogenase activities. These tests are not available in most laboratories, and the latter requires a substrate that is not commercially available. Fortunately, there should be few instances in which these specific assays are clinically necessary.

Evolution of $^{14}CO_2$. Skin fibroblasts are grown to confluence. Cells from about 38 cm^2 of growing surface are transferred to a flat-bottomed vial, the medium removed following centrifuging, and replaced with 0.225 ml of Krebs-Ringer phosphate buffer. To this is added 0.025 ml of DL-[^{14}C]lysine labeled in the 2 position, 20 mCi/ml in 0.08 M NaCl. The cells are incubated for 4 hours at 35°C under oxygen with gentle agitation. CO_2 is collected in a center well containing 0.1 ml 1 N NaOH. The well contents are transferred to a scintillant to determine radioactivity.[15] Prior to incubation, the radioactive substrate is freed of volatile impurities by bubbling with N_2 at pH 3.

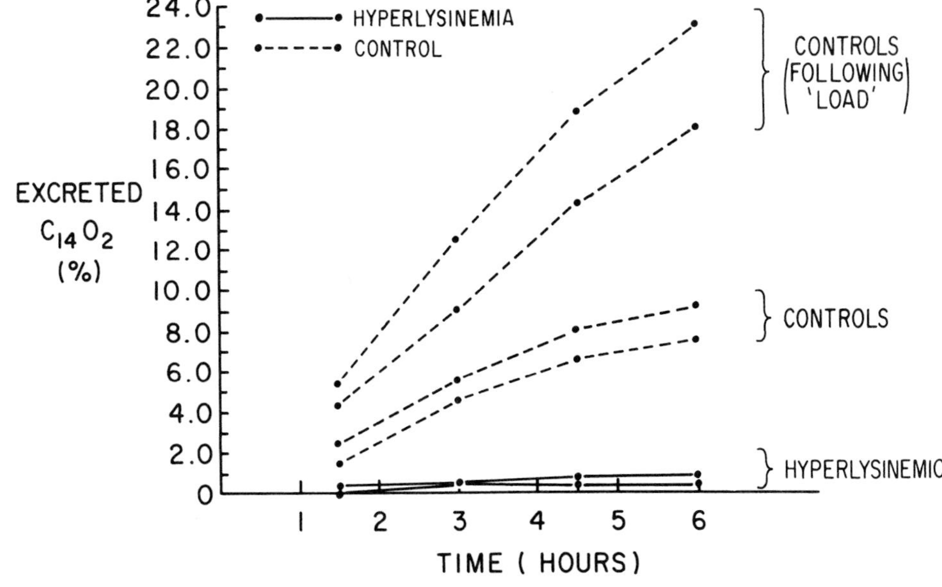

Fig. 86-2 Cumulative excretion of $^{14}CO_2$ following administration of [U-^{14}C]lysine. [^{14}C]Lysine was injected into two control and two hyperlysinemic subjects, and the $^{14}CO_2$ expired was measured. The control subjects also were loaded with 150 mg/kg of the lysine base prior to injection of [^{14}C]lysine and the measurements repeated. The cumulative excretion of radioactive CO_2 is presented as a percentage of administered radioactivity. (*From Woody et al.,[30] by permission of American Journal of Diseases of Children.*)

Table 86-1 Metabolism of Skin Fibroblasts*

Hyperlysinemia Patients	Lysine-Ketoglutarate Reductase†	Saccharopine Dehydrogenase‡	CO_2 Evolution§ (Lysine-2-^{14}C)
1	0	0	—
2	0	0	0.08
3	27	0	0.17
4	0	0	0.03
5	4	0	0.27
6	26	9	0.12
7	35	5	0.06
Mean	13	2	0.12
Range	0–35	0–9	0.03–0.27
Controls			
Number	8	6	12
Mean	357	95.3	2.75
Range	240–402	63–164	0.92–6.0

* Lysine-ketoglutarate reductase and saccharopine dehydrogenase activities were assayed in homogenates and mitochondrial preparations, respectively, as described in the text. The formation of CO_2 was measured following the incubation of intact fibroblasts with [2,^{14}C]lysine.
† Activity, pmol/min per milligram cell protein.
‡ Activity, pmol/min per milligram mitochondrial protein.
§ $^{14}CO_2$ evolved/min per milligram protein.
SOURCE: Adapted from Dancis *et al.*[15] by permission of The University of Chicago Press.

Lysine-Ketoglutarate Reductase. Fibroblasts are disrupted by repetitive freeze-thawing. Approximately 4 million cells are incubated with L-[U-^{14}C]lysine (0.5 M, 1.0 mmol), $MgCl_2$ (0.05 mmol), potassium α-ketoglutarate (2 mmol), potassium phosphate, pH 7.1 (10 mmol), NADPH (1.5 mmol), and water to a final volume of 1 ml.[5,6] Incubation is for 60 minutes, with shaking, at 30°C under a stream of N_2. Incubation is terminated by adding 5 mmol saccharopine in 0.05 ml of water and placing the tubes in boiling water for 5 minutes. The reaction mixture is centrifuged and the supernatant subjected to high-voltage electrophoresis. The saccharopine area is eluted, and saccharopine is isolated by ion-exchange chromatography. Radioactivity is measured, and the synthesis of saccharopine is calculated.

Saccharopine Dehydrogenase. The reaction mixture contains 0.1 ml sonicated mitochondria from skin fibroblasts, 0.5 mmol NAD^+ in 0.02 ml Tricine-NaOH buffer, pH 8.9, saccharopine [U-^{14}C]glutaryl, 0.1 mCi, 0.1 mmol in water to 0.25 ml.[5,6] Incubation is with agitation for 60 minutes at 25°C. The reaction is stopped by adding 0.1 ml of 10 mM glutamate solution and 0.05 ml of 1 N HCl. Radioactive glutamic acid is measured by reacting with glutamic decarboxylase. The substrate, radioactive saccharopine, is synthesized as described previously.

Prognosis

Several of the patients with familial hyperlysinemia were detected as a result of diagnostic studies for neurologic damage and mental retardation. The relation of the metabolic defect to the clinical manifestations was therefore uncertain. To avoid this bias, a study was conducted of patients identified during routine newborn screening or because of family surveys of affected individuals.[32] Ten subjects were located who met these criteria and in whom the diagnosis of familial hyperlysinemia had been confirmed by enzymatic assays of skin fibroblasts. In none was any damage observed that was attributable to the hyperlysinemia.

One patient was particularly impressive in confirming the absence of toxicity of extremely high concentrations of lysine. A normal infant was born to a woman with familial hyperlysinemia. Lysine is rapidly transferred across the placenta, establishing levels in fetal blood that are slightly higher than in the mother. It can be safely assumed, therefore, that the fetus was exposed to severe hyperlysinemia during the susceptible periods of development without ill effect. Periodically, there are reports of familial hyperlysinemia associated with neurologic deficits[34] or other disorders; however, these associations appear to be fortuitous.

Similar information is not available for the variant, saccharopinuria.

Treatment

The preceding observations make it clear that hyperlysinemia of considerable magnitude can be tolerated without ill effect. They do not establish that hyperlysinemia is always benign. The question of dietary control therefore must be addressed.

Lysine is present in high concentration in most natural foods. A simple low-lysine diet cannot be devised. By reducing protein intake from the high levels that are customary in American diets, it is possible to lower the plasma lysine concentration from approximately 1400 mM to about 680 to 800 mM. Further reductions toward normal can be accomplished only by substituting a mixture of purified amino acids restricted in lysine for dietary protein.

The weight of the evidence at present is against subjecting the family to the financial and psychological burdens of strict dietary control. Some parents and physicians have chosen to limit protein intake; most have avoided any restrictions.

Saccharopinuria

In 1968, a retarded 22-year-old woman was reported with saccharopinuria and a less severe lysinemia.[33] It appeared reasonable at that time to attribute the metabolic defect to the second step in lysine degradation, saccharopine dehydrogenase, with familial hyperlysinemia resulting from a deficiency in the first step, lysine-ketoglutarate reductase. The subsequent recognition that both enzyme activities were defective in familial hyperlysinemia and that saccharopinuria also was observed made the distinction between the two entities less certain. It should be emphasized, however, that the magnitude of the saccharopinuria is considerably less in familial hyperlysinemia and that it is overshadowed by the lysinuria, whereas the reverse was true in the patient with saccharopinuria. The lysine/saccharopine ratios in urine have ranged from 56 to 185 in familial hyperlysinemia,[31] whereas it was 0.33 in the reported case of saccharopinuria. Enzyme studies done on the patient's fibroblasts at a later date revealed that the lysine-ketoglutarate reductase activity was reduced to one-third the normal level, and no saccharopine dehydrogenase activity was

Table 86-2 Pipecolatemia in Zellweger Syndrome*

Patient	Age	Plasma Pipecolic Acid, μM
B. Su	4 days	7.8
M. Ja	10 days	7.7
B. Fl	2 mos	17.0
	4 mos	60.0
S. Ha	2 mos	24.0
	4 mos	245.0
A. Cu	$3\frac{1}{2}$ wks	15.0
	$4\frac{1}{2}$ wks	19.0
	$5\frac{1}{2}$ wks	36.0
	$6\frac{1}{2}$ wks	50.0
	2 mos	38.0
	$2\frac{1}{2}$ mos	51.0

*The plasma pipecolic acid concentration in the normal newborn infant is 12 ± 5.6 μM and 2.1 ± 1.6 μM in children and adults. The normal range has not been defined for the first months of life. In Zellweger syndrome, pipecolic acid concentrations increase to abnormal levels after birth.

SOURCE: From Lam *et al.*[41] by permission of The University of Chicago Press.

detected.[35] Given the many significant similarities between familial hyperlysinemia and saccharopinuria, it would appear more useful to consider the latter a variant rather than a discrete entity. A second case of saccharopinuria has been reported in which the enzymatic defects have not been as clearly defined.[36] Recently, a third patient with prominent saccharopinuria as a variant form of familial hyperlysinemia was described in Japan.[36a]

The diagnosis of saccharopinuria was made in each instance in the course of investigations of neurologic deficits. The relation of the metabolic anomaly to the symptoms is therefore uncertain.

At the molecular level, the relation between familial hyperlysinemia and saccharopinuria may be explained on the basis of polarity mutations of a bifunctional enzyme. Defects near the origin of the protein are likely to affect both enzyme activities, whereas those nearer the termination may preferentially affect saccharopine dehydrogenase. Whether a similar mechanism applies to orotic aciduria types I and II is not known. Transferase and decarboxylase activities of the bifunctional UMP synthase are differentially affected by conformational changes in the protein (see Chap. 113).

HYPERPIPECOLATEMIA

Pipecolic acid is not detected in normal plasma with routine ion-exchange chromatography. By modifying the ninhydrin reaction to intensify the color and making additional relatively minor alterations in technique, circulating pipecolic acid can be consistently detected in normal subjects.[37] The plasma concentration is 12 ± 5.6 mM at birth. It decreases during the first few months to 2.1 ± 1.6 mM and is maintained at that level into adulthood. The consistency with which pipecolic acid is formed in the absence of lysine excesses and the preservation of the pathway in a variety of animal species[38] suggest that it may have a physiologic function.

In familial hyperlysinemia, the plasma pipecolic acid concentration is elevated many times. In seven patients, the mean concentration was 31.9 ± 10.7 mM, as compared with normal of 2.1 mM. In the same patients, the lysine concentration was 1009 ± 240 mM. It is evident that the capacity to synthesize pipecolic acid is very limited and that degradation is even more limited. It is also clear that concentrations of this magnitude are tolerated without ill effect.[32]

Interest in hyperpipecolatemia has revived recently because of Zellweger syndrome (see Chap. 129). Increased plasma concentrations of pipecolic acid are regularly found in the absence of hyperlysinemia, excluding "overflow" as the mechanism and suggesting a defect in degradation.[39,40] Excesses of L-pipecolic acid appear in the urine consistent with an interruption in the normal catabolic pathway.[41] The association of hyperpipecolatemia and absence of peroxisomes in Zellweger syndrome[42] led to the presumption that the enzyme responsible for pipecolic acid oxidation resides in the peroxisome. Confirmation has come from purification and characterization of peroxisomal L-pipecolic acid oxidase from monkey liver.[43] Peroxisomal L-pipecolic acid oxidation is deficient in liver from Zellweger syndrome patients.[44] In rabbits and rodents, L-pipecolic acid oxidation activity is associated with mitochondria, whereas in monkeys and humans, the activity is associated with peroxisomes.[45,46]

A limited number of observations suggest that the plasma concentration of pipecolic acid is within normal limits at birth in Zellweger syndrome and increases with age to distinctly abnormal concentrations, as has been observed in other aminoacidopathies (Table 86-2). The full spectrum of the major manifestations of Zellweger syndrome was observed before pathologic concentrations were reached, making it questionable that the hyperpipecolatemia contributes significantly to the disease.[47]

Recognition of a patient with a specific defect in pipecolic acid metabolism would clarify the issue. Previously reported patients with hyperpipecolatemia with associated neuropathy and hepatomegaly probably were unrecognized examples of Zellweger syndrome.

REFERENCES

1. Montgomery R, Conway TW, Spector AA: *Biochemistry: A Case-Oriented Approach*, 5th ed. St. Louis, Mosby, 1990, p 354.
2. Bowring MA, Foreman JW, Lee J, Segal S: Characteristics of lysine transport by isolated rat renal cortical tubule fragments. *Biochim Biophys Acta* **901**:23, 1987.
3. Kudo Y, Boyd CA: Characterization of amino acid transport system in human placental basal membrane vesicles. *Biochim Biophys Acta* **1021**:169, 1990.
4. Higashino K, Fujiaka M, Takakazu A, Yamamura Y: Metabolism of lysine in rat liver. *Biochem Biophys Res Commun* **29**:95, 1967.
5. Dancis J, Hutzler J, Cox RP, Woody NC: Familial hyperlysinemia with lysine-ketoglutarate reductase insufficiency. *J Clin Invest* **48**:1447, 1969.
6. Dancis J, Hutzler J, Woody NC, Cox RP: Multiple enzyme defects in familial hyperlysinemia. *Pediatr Res* **10**:686, 1976.
7. Markovitz PJ, Chuang DT, Cox RP: Familial hyperlysinemias: Purification and characterization of the bifunctional aminoadipic semialdehyde synthase with lysine-ketoglutarate reductase and saccharopine dehydrogenase activities. *J Biol Chem* **259**:11643, 1984.
8. Rothstein M, Miller LL: The conversion of lysine to pipecolic acid in the rat. *J Biol Chem* **211**:851, 1954.
9. Kim S, Benoiton L, Paik WJ: ε-Alkyl-lysinase: Purification and properties of the enzyme. *J Biol Chem* **239**:3790, 1964.
10. Chang YF:Lysine metabolism in rat brain: The pipecolic acid-forming pathway. *J Neurochem* **30**:347, 1978.
11. Giacobini E, Nomura Y, Schmidt-Glenewinkel T: Pipecolic acid: Origin, biosynthesis and metabolism in brain. *Cell Mol Biol* **26**:135, 1980.
12. Rao VV, Pan X, Chang YF: Developmental changes of L-lysine-ketoglutarate reductase in rat brain and liver. *Comp Biochem Physiol* **103B**:221, 1992.
13. Charles AK: Pipecolic acid receptors in rat cerebral cortex. *Neurochem Res* **11**:521, 1986.
14. Gutilerrez MC, Delgado-Coello BA: Influence of pipecolic acid on the release and uptake of [^{3}H]GABA from brain slices of mouse cerebral cortex. *Neurochem Res* **14**:405, 1989.
15. Dancis J, Hutzler J, Cox RP: Familial hyperlysinemia: Enzyme studies, diagnostic methods, comments on terminology. *Am J Hum Genet* **31**:290, 1979.
16. Noda C, Ichihara A: Purification and properties of L-lysine-α-ketoglutarate reductase from rat liver mitochondria. *Biochim Biophys Acta* **525**:307, 1978.
17. Markovitz PJ, Chuang DT: The bifunctional bovine amino-adipic semialdehyde synthase in lysine degradation: Separation of reductase

and dehydrogenase domain by limited proteolysis. *J Biol Chem* **262**:9353, 1987.
18. Saunders PP, Broquist HP: Saccharopine, an intermediate of the aminoadipic acid pathway of lysine biosynthesis. *J Biol Chem* **241**:3435, 1966.
19. Jones EE, Broquist HP: Saccharopine, an intermediate of the aminoadipic acid pathway of lysine biosynthesis: III Aminoadipic semialdehyde-glutamate reductase. *J Biol Chem* **241**:3430, 1966.
20. Anderson KS, Miles EW, Johnson KA: Serine modulates substrate channeling in tryptophan synthase: A novel intersubunit triggering mechanism. *J Biol Chem* **266**:8020, 1991.
21. Fox RM, O'Sullivan WJ, Firkin BG: Orotic aciduria: Differing enzyme patterns. *Am J Med* **47**:332, 1969.
22. Brown GK, O'Sullivan WJ: Subunit structure of the orotate phosphoribosyltransferase-orotidylate decarboxylase complex from human erythrocytes. *Biochemistry* **16**:3235, 1977.
23. McClard RW, Black MJ, Livingstone LR, Jones ME: Isolation and initial characterization of the single polypeptide that synthesizes uridine 5′-monophosphate from orotate in Ehrlich ascites carcinoma: Purification by tandem affinity chromatography of uridine 5′-monophosphate synthase. *Biochemistry* **19**:4699, 1980.
24. Pragobpol S, Gero AM, Lee CS, O'Sullivan WJ: Orotate phosphoribosyltransferase and orotidylate decarboxylase from *Crithidia luciliae:* Subcellular location of the enzymes and a study of substrate channeling. *Arch Biochem Biophys* **230**:285, 1984.
25. Wakil SJ, Stoops JK, Joshi VC: Fatty acid synthesis and its regulation. *Annu Rev Biochem* **52**:537, 1983.
26. Schweizer E, Kniep B, Castorp H, Holzner U: Pantethine-free mutants of the yeast fatty-acid synthase complex. *Eur J Biochem* **39**:353, 1973.
27. Coleman PF, Suttle DP, Stark GR: Purification from hamster cells of the multifunctional protein that initiates *de novo* synthesis of pyrimidine nucleotides. *J Biol Chem* **252**:6379, 1977.
27a. Sackstedar KA, Biery BJ, Morrell JC, Geisbrecht BV, Cox RP, Gersghty MT: Characterization of the gene encoding α-aminoadipic semialdehyde synthase. *Am J Hum Genet* **65**(Suppl):429, 1999.
28. Hutzler J, Dancis J: Lysine-ketoglutarate reductase in human tissues. *Biochim Biophys Acta* **377**:42, 1975.
29. Hutzler J, Dancis J: Conversion of lysine to saccharopine by human tissues. *Biochim Biophys Acta* **158**:62, 1968.
30. Woody NC, Hutzler J, Dancis J: Further studies of hyperlysinemia. *Am J Dis Child* **112**:577, 1966.
31. Cederbaum SD, Shaw KNF, Dancis J, Hutzler J, Blaskovics JC: Hyperlysinemia with saccharopinuria due to combined lysine-ketoglutarate reductase and saccharopine dehydrogenase deficiencies presenting as cystinuria. *J Pediatr* **95**:234, 1979.
32. Dancis J, Hutzler J, Ampola JG, Shih VE, Van Gelderen HH, Kirby LT, Woody NC: The prognosis of hyperlysinemia: An interim report. *Am J Hum Genet* **35**:438, 1983.
33. Carson NAJ, Scally BG, Nell DW, Carre IJ: Saccharopinuria: A new inborn error of lysine metabolism. *Nature* **218**:679, 1968.
34. Yiannikas C, Cordato D: Familial hyperlysinemia in a patient presenting with progressive spastic paraparesis. *Neurology* **47**:846, 1996.
35. Fellows FCI, Carson NAJ: Enzyme studies in a patient with saccharopinuria: A defect of lysine metabolism. *Pediatr Res* **8**:42, 1974.
36. Simell O, Johansson T, Aula P: Enzyme defect in saccharopinuria. *J Pediatr* **82**:54, 1973.
36a. Higashino K: Saccharopinuria, a variant form of familial hyperlysinemia. *Ryoikibetsu Shokogun Shirizu* **18**:191, 1998.
37. Hutzler J, Dancis J: The determination of pipecolic acid: Method and results of hospital survey. *Clin Chim Acta* **128**:75, 1983.
38. Dancis J, Hutzler J: Comparative rates of metabolism of pipecolic acid metabolism in several animal species. *Comp Biochem Physiol [B]* **73**:1011, 1982.
39. Danks DM, Tippet P, Adams C, Campbell P: Cerebro-hepato-renal syndrome of Zellweger. *J Pediatr* **86**:382, 1975.
40. Trijbels JMF, Monnens LAH, Bakkeren JAJM, Van Raay-Selton AHJ, Corstiaensen JMB: Biochemical studies in the cerebro-hepato-renal syndrome of Zellweger: A disturbance in the metabolism of pipecolic acid. *J Inherit Metab Dis* **2**:39, 1979.
41. Lam S, Hutzler J, Dancis J: L-Pipecolaturia in Zellweger syndrome. *Biochim Biophys Acta* **882**:254, 1986.
42. Goldfischer S, Moore CL, Johnston AB, Spiro AJ, Valsamis MP, Wismewski HK, Ritch RH, et al: Peroxisomal and mitochondrial defects in the cerebro-hepato-renal syndrome. *Science* **182**:62, 1983.
43. Mihalik SJ, McGuinness M, Watkins PA: Purification and characterization of peroxisomal L-pipecolic acid oxidase from monkey liver. *J Biol Chem* **266**:32768, 1991.
44. Mihalik SJ, Moser HW, Watkins PA, Danks DM, Poulos A, Rhead WJ: Peroxisomal L-pipecolic acid oxidation is deficient in liver from Zellweger syndrome patients. *Pediatr Res* **25**:548, 1989.
45. Mihalik SJ, Rhead WJ: L-Pipecolic acid oxidation in the rabbit and cynomolus monkey: Evidence for differing organellar locations and cofactor requirements in each species. *J Biol Chem* **264**:2509, 1989.
46. Dancis J, Hutzler J: Unpublished observations, 1991.
47. Dancis J, Hutzler J: The significance of hyperpipecolatemia in Zellweger syndrome. *Am J Hum Genet* **38**:707, 1986.

CHAPTER 87

Maple Syrup Urine Disease (Branched-Chain Ketoaciduria)

David T. Chuang ▪ Vivian E. Shih

1. Maple syrup urine disease (MSUD) or branched-chain ketoaciduria is caused by a deficiency in activity of the branched-chain α-keto acid dehydrogenase (BCKD) complex. This metabolic block results in the accumulation of the branched-chain amino acids (BCAAs) leucine, isoleucine, and valine, and the corresponding branched-chain α-keto acids (BCKAs). Based on the clinical presentation and biochemical responses to thiamine administration, MSUD patients can be divided into five phenotypes: classic, intermediate, intermittent, thiamine-responsive, and dihydrolipoyl dehydrogenase (E3)-deficient. Classic MSUD has a neonatal onset of encephalopathy and is the most severe and most common form. Variant forms of MSUD generally have the initial symptoms by 2 years of age. The levels of the BCAAs, particularly leucine, are greatly increased in plasma and urine. The presence of alloisoleucine is diagnostic of MSUD. Activity of the BCKD complex in skin fibroblasts or lymphoblast cultures is reduced, and ranges from less than 2 percent of normal in the classic form to 30 percent of normal in the variant forms. The E3-deficient MSUD presents a combined deficiency of BCKD, pyruvate dehydrogenase, and α-ketoglutarate dehydrogenase complexes. This is the result of E3 being a common component of the three mitochondrial multienzymes. An animal model in Polled Hereford calves has been described.
2. MSUD is an autosomal recessive metabolic disorder of panethnic distribution. The worldwide frequency based on routine screening data from 26.8 million newborns is approximately 1 in 185,000. In the inbred Old Order Mennonite population of Lancaster and Lebanon Counties, Pennsylvania, MSUD occurs in approximately 1 in 176 newborns.
3. The BCAAs comprise about 35 percent of the indispensable amino acids in muscle, and 40 percent of the performed amino acids required by mammals. The catabolic pathways for BCAAs begin with the transport of these amino acids into cells by the system L transporter located in the cytosolic membrane. Inside the cell, BCAAs undergo reversible transamination by the cytosolic or mitochondrial isoforms of the branched-chain amino acid aminotransferase (BCAT) in the respective compartment to produce the BCKAs α-ketoisocaproate (KIC) from leucine, α-keto-β-methylvalerate (KMV) from isoleucine, and α-ketoisovalerate (KIV) from valine. BCKAs synthesized in the cytosol are translocated by the specific BCKA transporter into mitochondria, where oxidative decarboxylation of the three BCKAs is catalyzed by the single BCKD multienzyme complex. These reactions generate the respective branched-chain acyl-CoAs that are further metabolized via separate pathways. The end products of leucine catabolism are acetyl-CoA and acetoacetate. BCAAs, as a group, are both ketogenic and glucogenic. They are the precursor for fatty acids and cholesterol synthesis through acetyl-CoA. These amino acids are also substrates for energy production via succinyl-CoA and acetoacetate.
4. The oxidation of BCAAs occurs primarily in liver, kidney muscle, heart, brain, and adipose tissue. There is evidence that transamination is rate limiting in the catabolism of BCAAs in rat liver, where BCAT activity is low. Based on the rat model, a significant proportion of BCKAs appears to originate from skeletal muscle, and circulates to the liver where it is oxidized. However, recent studies confirm that the BCKD complex activity in human liver is markedly lower than that in rat liver. The results support the view that skeletal muscle is the major site for both BCAA transamination and oxidation in humans.
5. The human BCKD complex is loosely associated with the inner membrane of the mitochondria. This multienzyme complex is a macromolecule (molecular mass 4×10^6 daltons) comprising three catalytic components: a thiamine pyrophosphate (TPP)-dependent decarboxylase, or E1, with an $\alpha_2\beta_2$ structure; a transacylase, or E2, that contains 24 lipoate-bearing polypeptides; and a dehydrogenase, or E3, that is flavoprotein of homodimeric structure. In addition, the BCKD complex contains two regulatory enzymes, a kinase and a phosphatase, that control activity of the complex through a reversible phosphorylation (inactive)/dephosphorylation (active) mechanism. The BCKD complex is organized around the E2 cubic core, to which E1, E3, the specific kinase, and the specific phosphatase are attached through ionic interactions. The crystal structure of human E1 has recently been determined at 2.7 Å resolution.
6. Full-length cDNAs encoding E1α, E1β, E2, E3, and the specific kinase of mammalian BCKD complex have been cloned. Using these probes, the human BCKD genes were assigned to different chromosomes: E1α (gene symbol *BCKDHA*) to chromosome 19q13.1-q13.2; E1β (gene symbol *BCKDHB*) to 6p21-p22; E2 (gene symbol *DBT*) to 1p31; and E3 (gene symbol *DLD*) to 7q31-q32. The genomic structure including the regulatory-promoter regions of E1α, E1β, E2, E3, and the kinase genes of the mammalian BCKD complex have been characterized. The human E1α gene (>55 kb) consists of 9 exons. The human E1β (>100 kb) and E2 (68 kb) genes and the rat kinase (6 kb) gene each contains

A list of standard abbreviations is located immediately preceding the index in each volume. Additional abbreviations used in this chapter include: BCAAs = branched-chain amino acids; BCAT = branched-chain amino acid aminotransferase; BCKAs = branched-chain -keto acids; BCKD = branched-chain -keto acid dehydrogenase; DPNH = 2,4-dinitrophenylhydrazine; E1 = branched-chain -keto acid decarboxylase; E2 = dihydrolipoyl transacylase; E3 = dihydrolipoyl dehydrogenase; KIV = -ketoisovalerate; KIC = -ketoisocaproate; KMV = -keto--methylvalerate; MSUD = maple syrup urine disease; TPP = thiamine pyrophosphate.

11 exons. The human E3 gene (approximately 20 kb) comprises 14 exons.

7. **The genetic heterogeneity in MSUD demonstrated previously by complementation studies can now be explained by the six loci that contribute to the human BCKD complex. Four molecular phenotypes based on the affected locus of the BCKD complex are classified. Type IA (MIM 248600) refers to mutations in E1α gene; type IB (MIM 248611) refers to mutations in E1β gene; type II (MIM 248610) refers to mutations in E2 gene; and type III (MIM 246900) refers to mutations in E3 gene. Sixty-three mutations in all four phenotypes have been identified, and some have been characterized. The type IA defect in Mennonite MSUD patients is a homozygous Tyr-393 to Asn substitution in the E1α subunit that impairs the assembly with E1β. The adverse effects of type IA and type IB MSUD mutations on the catalysis and assembly of the human $\alpha_2\beta_2$ heterotetramer can now be explained at the three-dimensional structure level. A strong correlation between type II mutations and the thiamine-responsive clinical phenotype has been demonstrated.**
8. **The majority of untreated classic patients die within the early months of life from recurrent metabolic crisis and neurologic deterioration. Treatment involves both long-term dietary management and aggressive intervention during acute metabolic decompensation. Advances in both aspects of treatment have considerably reduced the morbidity, mortality, and length of initial hospitalization for patients. The age of diagnosis and the subsequent metabolic control are the most important determinants of long-term outcome. Patients in whom treatment is initiated after 14 days of age rarely achieve normal intellect.**
9. **There have been five successful pregnancies in two intermediate MSUD patients. The major concerns are the stress of pregnancy on metabolic homeostasis and the rapidly changing nutritional requirements during the course of pregnancy and after delivery. These parameters require careful monitoring.**

CATABOLISM OF BCAAs AND BCKAs

Overview

The three essential amino acids (leucine, isoleucine, and valine) are classified as branched-chain amino acids (BCAAs). They are neutral aliphatic amino acids, each with a branched methyl group in the side chain. BCAAs constitute about 35 percent of the essential amino acids in muscle, and 40 percent of the preformed amino acids required by mammals.[1] The fates of the carbon skeletons of BCAAs include incorporation into proteins and oxidative degradation in mitochondria. The catabolism of BCAAs has been a subject of intense interest because of their nutritional, biochemical, and clinical significance. It was observed that after ingestion of protein, the BCAAs contribute to more than 60 percent of the increase in amino acid concentration in human blood.[2] BCAAs are metabolized by skeletal muscle as an alternative energy source,[3,4] and are also actively oxidized in kidney,[5] heart,[6,7] adipose tissue,[8] and brain.[9] In liver or hepatocytes, the branched-chain α-keto acids (BCKAs) derived from BCAAs are rapidly catabolized to yield ketone bodies and succinyl-CoA.[10–12] Adipose tissue and muscle utilize acetyl-CoA produced from leucine for the synthesis of long-chain fatty acids and cholesterol.[13] Leucine appears to also have an important role in promoting protein synthesis,[14,15] inhibiting its degradation,[16] and stimulating insulin secretion.[17–20] Clinically, BCAA infusions counteract the catabolic state observed in sepsis[21] and severe trauma.[22] In patients with liver cirrhosis,[23] hepatic encephalopathy,[24] and chronic renal failure,[25] plasma BCAAs levels are decreased. Dietary supplements with BCAAs or BCKAs restore nitrogen balance and ameliorate the pathophysiological disturbances.[23–25] The area of therapeutic applications of BCAAs and BCKAs is reviewed elsewhere.[26–28]

Degradative Pathways

The oxidation of BCAAs begins with the transport of these amino acids into cells through the Na^+-independent system L transporter in the plasma membrane.[29–31] In the cell, the BCAAs undergo three initial common steps: transamination, oxidative decarboxylation, and dehydrogenation (Fig. 87-1).[32] The first transamination step is catalyzed by BCAA aminotransferases (BCATs), which are either cytosolic or mitochondrial,[33] to produce BCKAs. The BCKAs comprise α-ketoisocaproate (KIC), α-keto-β-methylvalerate (KMV), and α-ketoisovalerate (KIV) that are derived from leucine, isoleucine, and valine, respectively. The cytosolic BCKAs are transported across the mitochondrial membrane by the BCKA transporter.[34] The latter is distinct from the pyruvate transporter, and is regulated by external and matrix pH.[34,35] The three BCKAs compete for uptake by the reconstituted BCKAs transporter.[36] There is evidence to suggest that the transporter is the mitochondrial isoform of BCAT.[37] The second step, oxidative decarboxylation of BCKAs, is catalyzed by the single mitochondrial BCKD complex.[38,39] The reaction products of KIC, KMV, and KIV are isovaleryl-CoA, α-methylbutyryl-CoA and isobutyryl-CoA, respectively. These branched-chain acyl-CoAs then undergo a third common step: dehydrogenation by specific acyl-CoA dehydrogenases. The dehydrogenation of isovaleryl-CoA is catalyzed by isovaleryl-CoA dehydrogenase,[40] and α-methylbutyryl-CoA and isobutyryl-CoA by α-methyl branched-chain acyl-CoA dehydrogenase.[41] After these steps, the degradative pathway for each BCKA diverge (see Chap. 93). Leucine yields acetyl-CoA and acetoacetate as end products, and is, therefore, a ketogenic amino acid (Fig. 87-1). Valine produces succinyl-CoA and is, accordingly, glucogenic. Succinyl-CoA enters the Krebs cycle, and is eventually converted to glucose by gluconeogenesis.[42] Isoleucine is both lipogenic and glucogenic because it is metabolized to acetyl-CoA and succinyl-CoA.

Interorgan Relationships

Oxidation of BCAAs involves extensive interplay of metabolites between muscle and liver in the rat. This is due to the nonuniform distribution of BCATs and the BCKD complex among organs and tissues.[43] In rat skeletal muscle, BCAT activity is high,[43,44] but the BCKD complex activity is low.[43–45] A reverse situation exists in rat liver with respect to levels of the two enzyme activities.[43] Both rat liver[10–12,46,47] and heart[6,47] degrade BCKAs at high rates, and in hepatectomized rats leucine oxidation is decreased.[48] This led to the prevailing view, based on the rat model, that the primary role of muscle is transamination of BCAAs, which provides the major source of circulating BCKAs.[4,49,50] BCKAs are transported to liver, kidney, and heart, where they are oxidized.[10,43,49] However, the interorgan shuttling of BCAA metabolites may not occur in humans. A recent study showed that actual BCKD complex activity in human liver is similar to that in skeletal muscle (Table 87-1).[51] The results confirm an earlier observation that BCKD-complex activity in human liver and kidney is markedly lower than in the rat counterparts, but activity in skeletal muscle is similar between the two species.[52] It is noteworthy that the human liver exhibits twice as high BCAT activity as human skeletal muscle, as also shown in Table 87-1. This finding suggests that human liver is capable of oxidizing BCAAs in situ and does not depend on BCAT activity in skeletal muscle for the conversion of BCAAs to BCKAs. Because skeletal muscle comprises 40 percent of body mass, this tissue is likely the major site for BCAA oxidation in humans.

Moreover, in skeletal muscle, anaerobic glycolysis and respiration are active. This results in the production of pyruvate and α-ketoglutarate. These substrates are converted to alanine and glutamic acid by transamination of the amino groups from

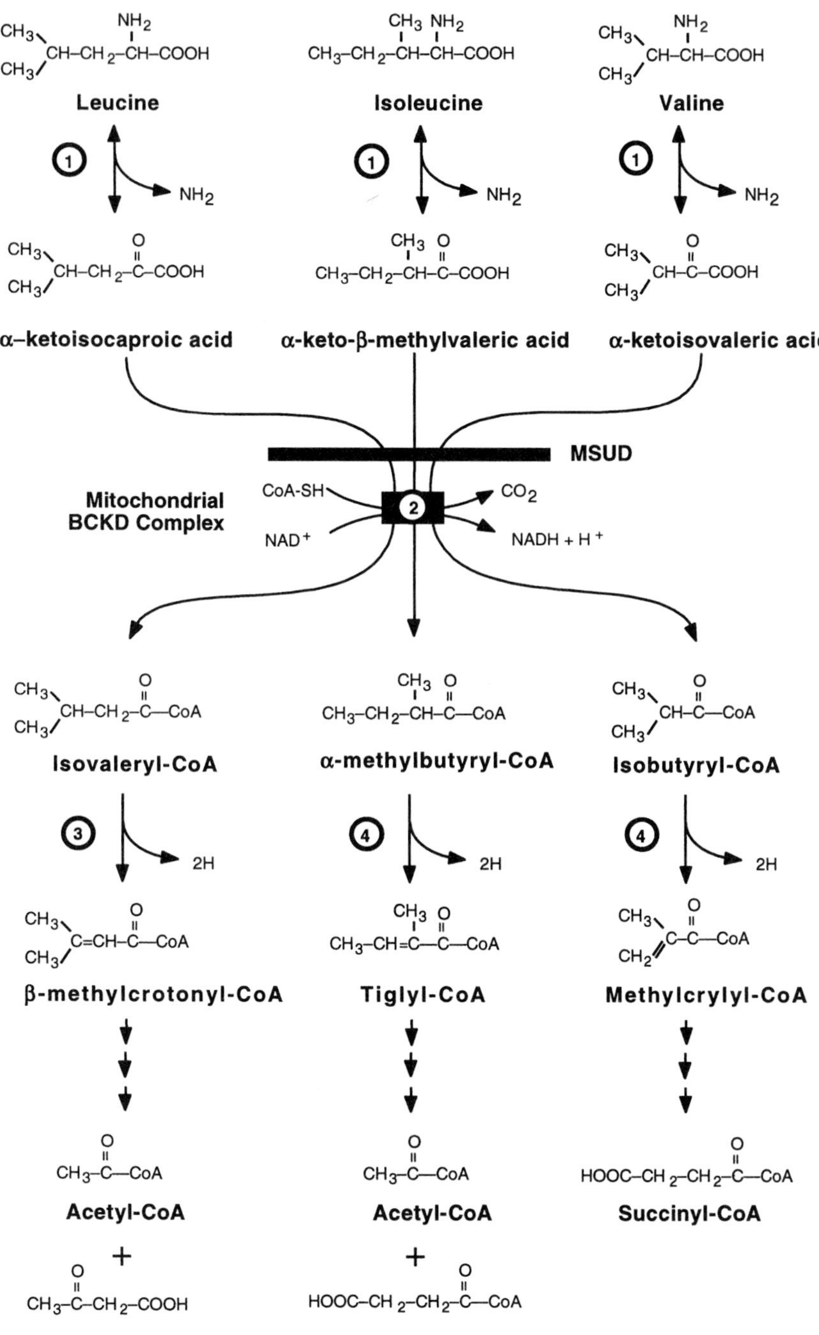

Fig. 87-1 **Catabolic pathways for the branched-chain amino acids (BCAAs) leucine, isoleucine, and valine. The first three common reactions are catalyzed by the following enzymes: reversible transamination by BCAA aminotransferases (1), oxidative decarboxylation of BCKAs and esterification of CoASH by the single mitochondrial branched-chain α-keto acid dehydrogenase (BCKD) complex (2), and dehydrogenation by isovaleryl-CoA dehydrogenase (3) or α-methyl branched-chain acyl-CoA dehydrogenase (4). After these steps, the degradation pathway for each amino acid diverges (see Chap. 93). As end products, leucine yields acetyl-CoA and acetoacetic acid, isoleucine produces acetyl-CoA and succinyl-CoA, and valine is converted exclusively to succinyl-CoA. The solid horizontal bar (center) depicts the metabolic block imposed by MSUD mutations in the BCKD complex.**

BCAAs.[10,43,49,53–55] Alanine circulates to the liver, where it is converted to pyruvate by the alanine aminotransferase. The amino group from alanine is converted to urea by the hepatic urea cycle. Pyruvate is a substrate for gluconeogenesis,[42] and glucose formed is returned to muscle. This completes the so-called glucose-alanine cycle,[56–58] which exemplifies interactions between muscle, blood, and liver. This cycle appears to play an important role in maintaining blood glucose homeostasis by production of alanine from BCAAs. A similar mechanism exists in adipose tissue, where glutamine, as well as alanine and glutamate, are produced from leucine.[59] This was proposed to be the route in this tissue for the disposal of amino groups from BCAAs through transamination.[59]

Regulation

The oxidation of BCAAs and BCKAs is tightly regulated (for review see Harper et al.[1]) The plasma concentrations of BCAAs and BCKAs are elevated in starvation[50,60,61] and in clinical conditions such as diabetes mellitus,[62–64] obesity,[60,65] and MSUD.[50] Epinephrine (10^{-5} M to 10^{-6} M) and glucagon (2×10^{-8} M to 5×10^{-9} M) were shown to stimulate BCAA oxidation in the heart and hemidiaphragms of rats.[66] Oxidation of BCAAs is accelerated in muscles from fasted and diabetic rats.[66–69] Insulin decreases the oxidation of BCKAs in striated muscle of fed rats, whereas in starvation the hormone increases oxidative decarboxylation of the keto acids.[5,61,67,69,70] In humans, insulin produces a decrease in plasma BCKAs and BCAAs,[71] with clinical implications. Clofibrate administration was reported to augment BCAA oxidation in muscle,[72] but inhibit their degradation in liver.[73] Carnitine,[74–76] ketone bodies,[66] hexanoate, and octanoate[6,77] increase the oxidation of leucine by skeletal muscle, whereas pyruvate[6] and decanoate[77] exert inhibitory effects. The regulation of BCKA oxidation was shown to be at the BCKD

Table 87-1 Distribution of Branched-chain Aminotransferase (BCAT) and Branched-Chain α-Ketoacid Dehydrogenase (BCKD) Complex Activities in Human Tissues

Tissue	BCAT	BCKD Complex Actual†	BCKD Complex Total‡	%Active§
	mU/g wet wt			
Heart	387 ± 23 (14)*	3.3 ± 0.5 (6)	8.2 ± 0.8 (6)	40
Skeletal muscle	124 ± 14 (10)	1.3 ± 0.3 (11)	4.9 ± 0.9 (6)	26
Brain	510 ± 49 (5)	6.4 ± 0.7 (5)	10.9 ± 0.8 (5)	59
Liver	248 ± 32 (9)	4.2 ± 0.41 (7)	14.8 ± 1.3 (7)	28
Kidney	880 ± 48 (5)	15.9 ± 2.6 (5)	110.9 ± 8.6 (5)	14
Stomach	447 (1)	1.8 (1)	4.8 (1)	38
Small intestine	241 ± 11 (3)	0.7 ± 0.1 (3)	1.6 ± 0.2 (3)	44
Colon	253 ± 23 (4)	2.3 ± 0.2 (4)	5.7 ± 0.3 (4)	40
Adipose	84 (2)	1.1 (2)	2.7 (2)	41

The data are expressed as mean ± SEM with n = number of determinations.
†Actual activity refers to BCKD activity without dephosprhorylation by broad-specificity phosphatase.
‡Total activity denotes activity of fully dephosphorylated (activated) BCKD complex measured after incubation of the tissue extract with broad-specificity phosphatase.
§% activity BCKD represents the ratio of actual activity to total activity × 100.
SOURCE: Suryawan.[51] Used by permission.

complex step by using the inhibitors oleate and palmitoyl carnitine.[78] The metabolism of KIC in isolated rat hepatocytes is inhibited by fatty acids, KIV, KMV, and pyruvate.[46] The mechanism of regulation for BCAA and BCKA oxidation was not fully elucidated in these earlier studies. However, it is now clear that these controls are exerted by alteration in activity state or degree of phosphorylation of the BCKD complex (see "Regulation of the Mammalian BCKD Complex" below).[79]

Transamination of BCAAs: The Aminotransferases

BCAT catalyzes the reversible transamination of BCAAs leucine, isoleucine, and valine to produce the corresponding BCKAs (Fig. 87-1). BCAT activity is widely distributed in different human organs and tissues (Table 87-1). Mammalian BCAT exists in two isoforms — mitochondrial and cytosolic.[44,80] The mitochondrial isoform of BCAT is widely distributed in rat[81] and human[51] tissues, whereas the cytosolic isoform is predominantly expressed in the brain.[51,81]

The rat heart mitochondrial BCAT has been purified more than 1300-fold in Hutson's laboratory to apparent homogeneity.[82] The ratio of enzyme activity with the three BCAAs remained constant throughout the purification procedure. The purified enzyme appears to be a monomer of 43 kDa. Antiserum prepared against the rat heart BCAT did not recognize any protein in the rat brain cytosol.[82] The results indicate that rat brain and heart BCATs are immunologically distinct. Further studies suggest that the rat heart BCAT is a bifunctional protein catalyzing both BCAA transamination and BCKA transport.[37] The physiological implications for the role of the mitochondrial BCAT in BCKA transport are presently not clear. It may facilitate efflux and the concomitant reamination of unoxidized BCKAs in mitochondria. The cytosolic BCAT of rat brain has also been purified.[83] The cytosolic enzyme is homodimer with a monomer molecular mass of 47 kDa. Comparison of tryptic peptide maps of the cytosolic and mitochondrial BCATs from rat brain and heart, respectively, confirmed that they are different gene products.[83] cDNAs for both mitochondrial and cytosolic isoforms of rat and human BCAT have been cloned;[84,85] the human mitochondrial BCAT was assigned to chromosome 19 and the human cytosolic BCAT to chromosome 12. Recently, human mitochondrial and cytosolic BCATs have been expressed in *E. coli*.[86] Both isoforms of BCAT require reducing equivalent for maximal activity. Titration of –SH groups show that the no disulfide bonds are present in mitochondrial BCAT while at least two disulfide bonds are present in the cytosolic isoform.

THE BRANCHED-CHAIN α-KETOACID DEHYDROGENASE COMPLEX

The BCAA can be transaminated in the cytosol by the cytosolic BCAT, and the resulting BCKAs (KIC, KMV, and KIV) are transported across the inner mitochondrial membrane on a specific keto acid transporter[34,36] into the matrix space. Alternatively, the BCAAs can enter the mitochondria presumably by neutral amino acid carrier,[87] and are then converted into BCKAs by the mitochondrial BCAT.[88–90] The oxidative decarboxylation of the BCKAs in mitochondria is catalyzed by the BCKD complex, which is associated with the inner membrane of this organelle.[91,92] The reaction is irreversible and constitutes the first committed step in the oxidation of the BCAAs.

Purification of the BCKD Complex

The concomitant elevation of the three BCKAs in the urine of MSUD patients prompted the early speculation that a single enzyme catalyzed the decarboxylation of the three BCKAs.[93] This hypothesis was supported by nutritional studies of Wohlhueter and Harper in 1970,[94] which showed the enzyme activities in rat liver for the decarboxylation of the three BCKAs were coinduced by feeding the animal with casein. In contrast, Connelly et al. isolated from bovine liver an enzyme preparation that was capable of catalyzing the oxidation of KIC and KMV, but not KIV.[95,96] The physiological significance of this enzyme was questioned, because the K_m values (3.5 mM for KIC and 2.5 mM for KMV) were much higher than the normal concentrations of BCKAs in plasma, which are in the <0.1 mM range.[49,50] Differential decarboxylation with each of the three keto acids was observed in mitochondria from livers of hypophysectomized rats,[97,98] and in enriched leukocyte and cattle liver homogenates.[99] These findings and those of Connelly et al.[95,96] prompted controversies as to whether there was more than one enzyme catalyzing the decarboxylation of the three BCKAs.

The subsequent purification of the mammalian mitochondrial BCKD complex with high specific activity was largely unsuccessful. Parker and Randle[100,101] and Danner et al.[39,102] were able to purify the BCKD complex from rat and bovine liver mitochondria with an approximately twenty-fivefold increase in specific activity. Kinetic parameters and the copurification of enzyme activity with each of the three BCKAs strongly suggested the presence of a single BCKD complex. The product stoichiometry for the oxidative decarboxylation of the three BCKAs was CO_2 : acyl-CoA : NADH = 1 : 1 : 1.[39] In 1978, the BCKD complex was

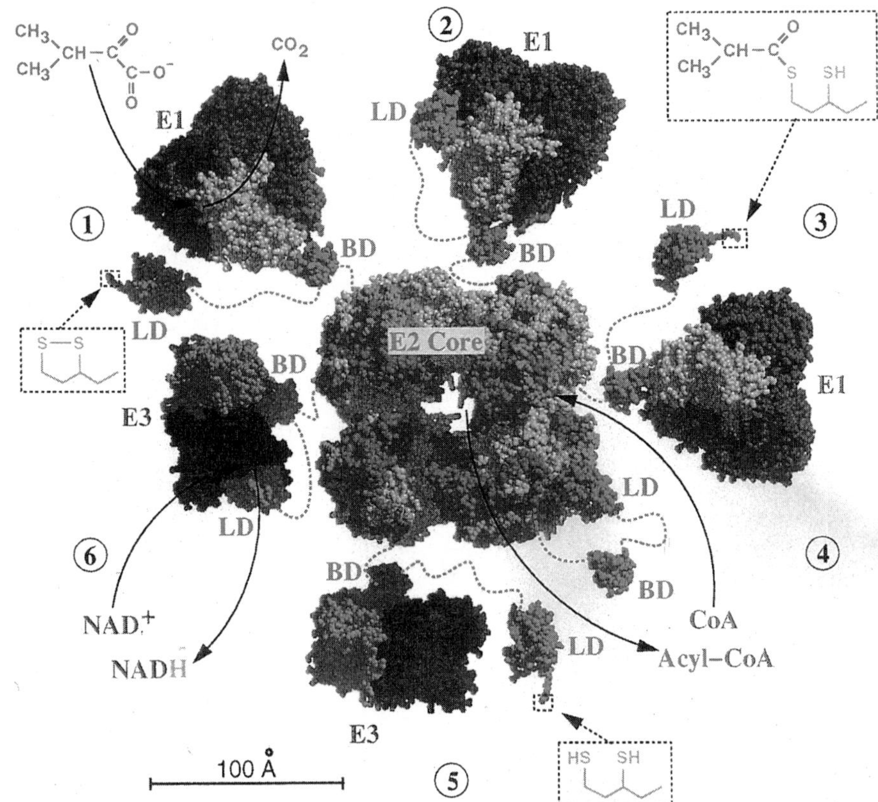

Fig. 87-2 Structural organization and individual component reactions of the human BCKD complex. The macromolecular structure (4 × 10^6 daltons in size) is organized around a cubic transacylase (E2) core (based on the structure of *Azotobacter* pyruvate dehydrogenase E2),[152] to which a decarboxylase (E1) (based upon *Pseudomonas* BCKD E1 structure)[124] and a dehydrogenase (E3) (according to the structure of *Azotobacter* pyruvate dehydrogenase E3)[165] are attached through ionic interactions. E2 of the BCKD complex contains 24 identical subunits with each polypeptide made up of three folded domains: lipoyl (LD), E1/E3-binding (BD), and the E2 core domains that are linked by flexible regions. E1$\alpha_2\beta_2$ heterotetramers or E3 homodimers are attached to BD. The BCKD kinase and BCKD phosphatase (not shown) presumably bind to LD. E1 catalyzes the TPP-mediated oxidative decarboxylation of BCKAs. The TPP-hydroxyacyl moiety is transferred to a reduced lipoyl prosthetic group (in the box) on LD. The flexible LD carries S-acyl dihydrolipoamide to the active site in the E2 core to generate acyl-CoA. The reduced lipoyl moiety on LD is oxidized by E3 on BD with concomitant reduction of NAD^+. *(From Aevarsson et al.*[124] *Reproduced by permission.)*

purified to apparent homogeneity, for the first time, by Reed and associates from mitochondria of bovine kidney.[38] High specific activity (12 units/mg protein with KIV) of the enzyme complex was achieved by the addition of exogenous dihydrolipoyl dehydrogenase (E3) in the assay mixture. The BCKD complex was shown to oxidize the three BCKAs (KIV, KIC, and KMV) as well as α-ketobutyrate and pyruvate. The K_m values were 40, 50, 37, 56, and 1,000 μM, respectively.[38] The ratio of specific activity for the three BCKAs (KIV : KIC : KMV = 2.0 : 1.5 : 1.0) remained constant for each step of the purification. The result established unequivocally that a single mitochondrial multienzyme complex catalyzes the oxidative decarboxylation of the three α-keto acids derived from leucine, isoleucine, and valine. The purified bovine BCKD complex was later shown to also catalyze the oxidative decarboxylation of D-methytlthio-α-ketobutyrate, a transamination product of methionine[103] with a K_m value of 67 μM.

The mammalian BCKD complex was later purified from rabbit liver,[104] beef liver,[105,106] rat kidney,[107–109] human liver,[110] and *Pseudomonas aeruginosa*[111] to apparent homogeneity. In most of these purification procedures, Triton X-100 (1 to 5 percent, v/v) was used to efficiently extract the BCKD complex from mitochondria. These enzyme preparations were similar in component composition and the size of subunits. Antibodies prepared against the bovine E1 and E2 components inhibit the overall reaction, and cross-react with the corresponding human, murine, ovine, and avian subunits.[112–116]

Macromolecular Organization and Component Reactions

The mammalian BCKD complex is a member of the highly conserved α-keto acid dehydrogenase complexes comprising pyruvate dehydrogenase complex (PDC), α-ketoglutarate dehydrogenase complex (α-KGDC), and the BCKD complex with similar structure and function.[117,118] The mammalian BCKD complex consists of three catalytic components: a heterotetrameric ($\alpha_2\beta_2$) branched-chain α-keto acid decarboxylase, or E1, a homo-24 meric dihydrolipoyl transacylase, or E2, and a homodimeric dihydrolipoamide dehydrogenase, or E3. E1 and E2 components are specific for the BCKD complex, whereas the E3 component is common among the three α-keto acid dehydrogenase complexes (Fig. 87-2). In addition, the mammalian BCKD complex contains two regulatory enzymes: the specific kinase and the specific phosphatase that regulate activity of the BCKD complex through phosphorylation (inactivation)/dephosphorylation (activation) cycles (Fig. 87-2).[117,119] The six subunits that make up the mammalian BCKD complex are shown in Table 87-2. The BCKD complex is organized around the cubic E2 core, to which 12 copies of E1, 6 copies of E3, the kinase and the phosphatase are attached

Table 87-2 Component Enzymes and Subunit Composition of the Mammalian Branched-Chain α-Ketoacid Dehydrogenase (BCKD) Complex

Component	Molecular mass (daltons)	Prosthetic group (P) and cofactor (C)
BCKA decarboxylase (E1)	1.7 × 10^5 (α_2 β_2)	TPP (C)
αSubunit	46,500	Mg^{2+} (C)
β Subunit	37,200	
Dihydrolipoyl transacylase (E2)	1.1 × 10^6 (α_{24})	Lipoic acid (P)
Subunit	46,518*	
Dihydrolipoyl dehydrogenase (E3)	1.1 × 10^5	FAD (C)
Submit	55,000	
BCKD kinase	43,000	Mg^{2+} (C)
Subunit	43,000	
BCKD phosphatase	4.6 × 10^5	None
Subunit	33,000	

*Calculated from the amino acid composition deduced from a bovine E2 cDNA. The E2 subunit migrates anomalously as a 52-kDa species in SDS-PAGE. TPP = thiamine pyrophosphate.

through ionic interactions (Fig. 87-2).[117] The molecular mass of the BCKD multienzyme complex is estimated to be 4×10^6 daltons. The purified bovine E1-E2 subcomplex has a sedimentation coefficient ($S_{20,w}$) of 40 *S*.[38] The E3 component has low affinity for the E2 core, and is usually lost during purification.[38,110,112] The E1-E2 subcomplex purified from bovine liver[120] and kidney[38,121] and from rat liver[108] was dissociated into individual E1 and E2 components in the presence of 1 M NaCl. High specific activity of E1 and E2 was maintained when these components are separated at neutral pH by gel filtration.[121] Separated E1 and E2 components can be assayed independently using component enzyme assays.[120,122] Self-assembly of E1 and E2 was readily achieved by mixing these components in vitro.[121] In the study by Ono et al.,[108] the entire BCKD complex was reconstituted by incubating E1, E2, and E3 in vitro.

The reaction steps catalyzed by the three enzyme components are also shown in Fig. 87-2. The E1 component catalyzes a thiamine pyrophosphate (TPP)-mediated decarboxylation of the α-keto acids and the subsequent reduction of the lipoyl moiety, which is covalently bound to E2. The reduced lipoyl moiety plus the lipoyl domain serves as a "swinging arm" to transfer the acyl group from E1 to CoA, giving rise to acyl-CoA. Finally, the E3 component with a tightly bound flavin adenine dinucleotide (FAD) reoxidizes the dihydrolipoyl residue of E2 with NAD^+ as the ultimate electron acceptor.[123] The net or overall reaction is the production of branched-chain acyl-CoA, CO_2, and NADH from BCKAs (Reaction 1).

$$\mathrm{RCO\text{-}COOH + CoA\text{-}SH + NAD^+} \\ \rightarrow \mathrm{RCO\text{-}S\text{-}CoA + CO_2 \uparrow + NADH + H^+} \quad \text{(Reaction 1)}$$

The E1 Component. The mammalian E1 component contains two α and two β subunits with $M_r = 45{,}500$ and 37,800, respectively, as deduced from amino acid composition (Table 87-2). The E1 component has an apparent $M_r = 166{,}600$ and requires potassium ions, $MgCl_2$, and TPP for activity.[122] The crystal structures of *Pseudomonas putida*[124] and human[125] E1 components were recently determined. The overall $\alpha_2\beta_2$ heterotetrameric structure of human E1 is shown in Fig. 87-3. The tetrahedral arrangement dictates that each subunit is in contact with other three subunits. Subunits α, α′, β, and β′ are designated such that the α subunit and the β subunit when combined correspond to one polypeptide of the related dimeric yeast transketolase[126] and are equivalent to the αβ heterodimeric assembly intermediate of human E1.[127] The prominent features in the structure are the crossover of the N-terminal tails of the α-subunit and the C-terminal extensions of the same subunit that provide interactions with the β subunits. The small C-terminal extension of the α subunit is critical for the $\alpha_2\beta_2$ assembly of human E1 and is the site of the prevalent Mennonite mutation (Y393N-α) (see "Type IA MSUD Mutations" below).

The binding pocket for cofactor TPP is located at the interface between α and β′ or α′ and β subunits (Fig. 87-3, upper panel). The TPP-binding motif, Gly-Asp-Gly(X)$_{28-30}$N[126] in the α subunit forms an integral part of the cofactor binding fold. Residues Glu76-β′ and Ser162-α are bound to N1′ and the C4′ amino group of the aminopyridine ring, respectively. These two active-site residues directly participate in the TPP-mediated decarboxylation reaction. The coordination of the Mg^{2+} ion and the interactions of TPP with amino acid residues from the α and the β subunits that are conserved in the TPP-binding superfamily[128,129] and are present in the human E1 component. K^+-ion-binding sites are found in both the α and the β subunits. These novel K^+ ion coordinations play important roles in stabilizing the TPP-binding fold as well as in maintaining the integrity of the E1 heterotetramer. The results explain the requirement of the K^+ or Rb^+ ion, but not Na^+, for preserving E1 activity in heat activation[130] or during purification.[131,132] The phosphorylation sites Ser292-α and Ser302-α[133,134] are located close to the active site. The conserved His291 binds to a phosphate group in cofactor TPP, and may have a direct role in catalysis, as suggested by the *Pseudomonas* E1 structure[124] and an earlier study.[135] The C-terminal end of the β subunit binds to the E2 component, confirming the topology previously deduced from sedimentation studies[136] and dark-field electron microscopy.[137] The human E1 structure has provided explanations for most, if not all, of MSUD missense mutations identified to date that affect the α and the β subunits, as described in a later section.

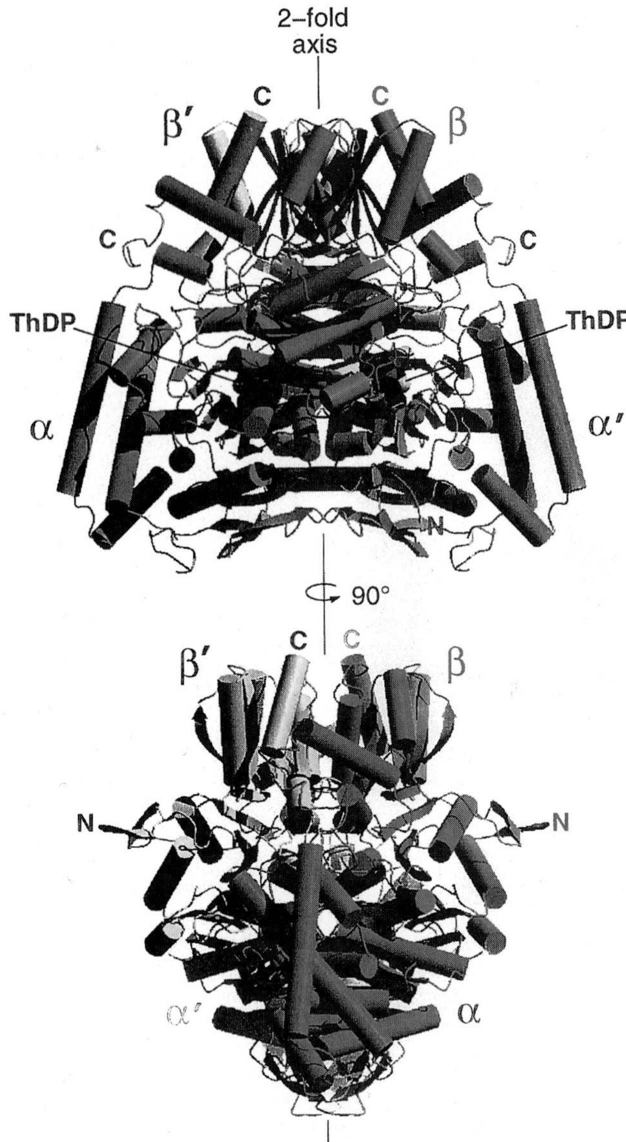

Fig. 87-3 Crystal structure of the E1 heterotetramer of human BCKD. The upper and lower panels depict two structures with orientations rotated 90° relative to each other along the vertical axis. The secondary structural elements are represented by cylinders (helices) and arrows (β strands). The designation of α, α′, β, and β′ subunits is such that α | β and α′ | β′ form an individual heterodimeric intermediate during $\alpha_2\beta_2$ assembly and each corresponds to a subunit in the yeast transketolase homodimer. N- and C-termini of each subunit are indicated. ThDP depicts the two moles of cofactor thiamine diphosphate bound to an E1 heterotetramer. (*From Aevarsson et al.*[125] *Reproduced by permission.*)

The E2 Component. The E2 subunits carry covalently linked lipoic acid at Lys-44 that facilitates the acyl transfer reaction[105,106,138,139] and participates in active site coupling.[140,141] The results of limited proteolysis show that the E2 chain contains a compact inner core that confers a highly assembled 24-mer structure and the active site.[120] The deduced primary structures indicate that the mature mammalian E2 subunit consists of three folded domains (5′ to 3′)-lipoyl-bearing, E1/E3 binding, and inner-core domains.[142–145] These folded domains are linked together by flexible hinge regions that are rich in proline residues or that are negatively charged amino acids. The flexible linkers between domains allow the lipoyl-bearing domain to sequentially visit the E1, E2, and E3 active sites (Fig. 87-2). Site-directed mutagenesis of His-391 residue in the inner-core domain of the bovine BCKD-E2 to an Asn or Gln residue results in complete loss of the transacylase activity of E2.[146] The results support Guest's thesis that His-391 acts as a general base in the acyl transfer reaction.[147] A later study shows that Ser-338 is hydrogen-bonded to the negatively charged tetrahedral transition state, and that Ala-348 plays a key role in acyl-CoA specificity.[148] The E2 domain structure is conserved in all E2 proteins of α-keto acid dehydrogenase complexes from bacteria, yeast, and mammals. The only variation is in the number of lipoate-bearing domains, ranging from one to three.[149] In the mammalian BCKD complex, a single lipoyl-bearing domain is present to carry one lipoic acid moiety.[138,139] The E2 subunit migrates as a 52-kDa species in SDS gels,[36] whereas the molecular mass based on the deduced amino acid composition is 46,158 daltons for the mature bovine E2 subunit.[142] The higher apparent molecular mass for E2 as determined by SDS-PAGE is presumably due to an anomalous migration caused by the acidic lipoyl-bearing domain.[150,151] The molecular mass of the bovine E2 24-mer is 1.1×10^6 daltons, as measured by sedimentation equilibrium analysis.[118,142] None of the three-dimensional structures of the E2 domains from the BCKD complex have been determined as yet. However, the crystal structure of the assembled inner core of E2p in the related pyruvate dehydrogenase complex from *Azotobacter vinelandii* has been solved at 2.6 Å resolution.[152] The 24 identical subunits are assembled into 8 trimers, each occupying one corner of a hollow cube. The active site resides on the interface formed by two neighboring subunits in a trimer. CoA must enter the 29 Å-long active-site channel from the inside of the cube, and lipoamide enters from the outside. This active-site structure is conserved in the 60-meric E2p inner-core of pyruvate dehydrogenase complex from *Bacillus stearothermophilus* and *Enterococcus faecalis*.[153] The structure of the lipoyl-bearing domain of the *Bacillus* pyruvate dehydrogenase complex, as determined by NMR spectroscopy, comprises two four-stranded β-sheets, which form a flat β-barrel around a well-defined hydrophobic core.[154] The lipoylated lysine residue is prominently situated on a tight turn at the corner of one of the β-sheets for interactions with E1. The structure of the inner lipoyl-bearing domain of human pyruvate dehydrogenase complex was recently determined.[155] The chain fold of the E1/E3-binding domain of the *E. coli* α-ketoglutarate dehydrogenase complex was also determined by NMR spectroscopy.[156] The remarkably small domain of 35 amino acids is made up of two parallel helices—a five-residue helix-like turn and an irregular loop. The structures of E2 domains of the related pyruvate and α-ketoglutarate dehydrogenase complexes serve as a basis for modeling of their counterparts in the human BCKD complex.

E2 components of the human BCKD and pyruvate dehydrogenase complex are major M2 autoantigens in primary biliary cirrhosis.[157] High titers against epitopes of the lipoyl-bearing domains of the three mitochondrial α-ketoacid dehydrogenase complexes are present in plasma of these patients.[155,158] Interestingly, sera from patients with idiopathic dilated cardiomyopathy also react with the E2 component of the BCKD complex.[159] The mechanism for these autoimmune responses to these proteins is currently unknown.

The E3 Component. The native pig heart E3 is a homodimer with a molecular weight of 110 kDa (Table 87-2);[160] it has high affinity for FAD. The amino acid sequences of human[161,162] and porcine[161] E3 subunits deduced from cDNAs show extensive homologies with human erythrocyte glutathione reductase and mercuric reductase.[161] Mature and precursor forms of human E3 have been expressed in *E. coli*.[163] Site-directed mutagenesis indicates that His-452 and Glu-557 are important for the binding dihydrolipoamide, by analogy with the crystal structure of human glutathione reductase.[164] The first E3 crystal structure described is that of *Azotobacter vinelandii* E3.[165] Each of the two identical subunits consists of four domains: FAD-binding, NAD-binding, the central domain, and the interface domain. The active site is located in the interface between the two subunits. The flavin ring of FAD bound to each subunit combines with an adjacent disulfide bridge to form a redox center, which transfers electrons from dihydrolipoamide to NAD^+. Recently, the crystal structure of eukaryotic E3 from yeast was determined.[166] The active site consists of FAD, Cys-44, and Cys-49 from one subunit and His-457 from the other subunit. The overall structure is similar to those of the prokaryotic enzymes.

Regulatory Enzymes: Kinase and Phosphatase

The early study by Reed and associates[38] reported that the activity of the bovine BCKD complex was not regulated by a reversible phosphorylation-dephosphorylation mechanism. In contrast, studies by Parker and Randle[167,168] and by Odessey[169] showed that the BCKD complex from mitochondria of rat heart and skeletal muscle, respectively, can be inactivated by ATP. This prompted a series of investigations in the early 1980s[104,170–174] that led to the conclusion that the mammalian BCKD complex is modulated by posttranslational phosphorylation-dephosphorylation, similar to the mammalian pyruvate dehydrogenase complex[117,175,176] (Fig. 87-4). Ser-292 (site 1) and Ser-302 (site 2) of the E1α subunit can be phosphorylated with a concomitant inactivation of the BCKD complex.[177–180] The phosphorylation of site 1 alone is sufficient to completely inhibit the overall reaction.[178,179]

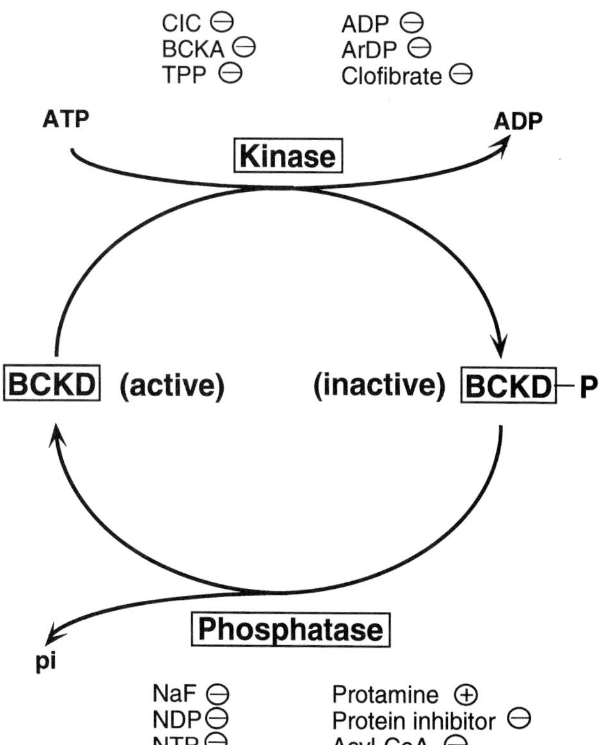

Fig. 87-4 Regulation of the BCKD complex by the phosphorylation-dephosphorylation cycle. Phosphorylation of the E1α subunit at Ser292 by BCKD kinase in the presence of ATP results in the inactivation of the BCKD complex. Removal of the phosphate group on E1 reverts the BCKD complex to the active form. Inhibitors (−) and activators (+) for each enzyme are shown. CIC = α-chloroisocaproate; ArDP = arylidenepyruvate; NDP = nucleoside diphosphate; NTP = nucleoside triphosphate.

Site-directed mutagenesis studies showed that a negative charge at site 1 alone is responsible for kinase-mediated inactivation of E1 and that site 2 is not involved in regulation by phosphorylation.[181] The sequences flanking the two phosphorylated serine residues on E1α[133,180] are highly conserved between rats,[134] cows,[182] and humans.[116,183] The BCKD kinase was purified to apparent homogeneity from rat liver and heart,[184] and from bovine kidney.[185] The subunit of the purified enzyme has a molecular mass of 43 to 44 kDa. The isolated kinase was inhibited by α-chloroisocaproate and dichloroacetate, with 50 percent inhibition at 14 μM and 1.8 mM, respectively,[185] confirming earlier studies with these compounds.[186,187] In addition, partially purified kinase preparations is inhibited by the three BCKAs, TPP, ADP,[188] octanoate, branched chain acyl-CoAs,[189] and arylidenepyruvates.[190] The BCKD kinase is associated with the E2 core[121] and probably binds to the lipoyl-bearing domain by analogy with pyruvate dehydrogenase kinases.[191]

The amino acid sequence deduced from a cDNA for the rat BCKD-kinase aligned with a high degree of similarity with subdomains of prokaryotic histidine protein kinases, but not eukaryotic serine/threonine protein kinases.[192] The recombinant BCKD-kinase is capable of autophosphorylation at a serine residue, but cannot transfer the resultant seryl phosphate group to E1.[193] Therefore, despite the sequence similarity to prokaryotic histidine protein kinases, the mitochondrial rat BCKD-kinase does not phosphorylate E1 via a histidine residue-mediated phosphotransfer reaction.

Dephosphorylation of the phosphorylated E1 by a specific phosphatase restores the activity of the BCKD complex.[175,194] The BCKD phosphatase was partially purified from bovine kidney, and shown to be different from the pyruvate dehydrogenase phosphatase.[195] A broad-specificity cytosolic phosphatase can dephosphorylate and reactivate the phosphorylated BCKD complex.[196] This mechanism, however, is not physiologically relevant because the BCKD complex is located in mitochondria. The catalytic component of the BCKD phosphatase has been highly purified from bovine kidney mitochondria.[197] It consists of a single polypeptide chain with an apparent M_r of 33,000 as estimated by SDS gel electrophoresis. The BCKD phosphatase has an apparent M_r of 460,000, and is dissociated into its catalytic subunits, by treatment with 6 M urea, with no apparent change in activity. A heat- and acid-stable protein inhibitor of the BCKD phosphatase was purified from bovine kidney mitochondria.[198,199] The highly purified inhibitor protein has an apparent molecular mass of 36 kDa. It is a noncompetitive inhibitor of the BCKD phosphatase with an inhibitor constant (K_i) of 0.13 nM.[199] The inhibition can be partially reversed by Mg^{2+} and spermine. This inhibitor protein is different from the cytosolic protein phosphatase inhibitors 1 and 2.[198] The BCKD phosphatase is inhibited by nucleoside triphosphates and diphosphates, but not by nucleoside monophosphates.[195] The enzyme is also inhibited by 50 mM fluoride,[194] but unlike the pyruvate dehydrogenase complex phosphatase, it is active in the absence of divalent ions such as Ca^{2+}, Mn^{2+}, or Mg^{2+}.[118,195] A loose attachment of the BCKD phosphatase to the E2 core has been speculated, similar to the pyruvate dehydrogenase complex phosphatase,[118] but this has not been established.

Import and Assembly of BCKD Complex

Mitochondrial proteins are encoded by nuclear genes, synthesized in the cytosol and imported into mitochondria, where folding and assembly occurs.[200] Earlier in vitro translation studies confirmed that larger precursor polypeptides of mammalian mitochondrial α-keto acid dehydrogenase complexes are imported into mitochondria and processed into smaller mature forms.[201] Amino acid sequences deduced from cDNA show that mammalian E1α, E1β, E2, and E3 precursor polypeptides contain relatively long mitochondrial targeting presequences of 45, 50, 61, and 35 residues, respectively.[142,161,182,202] The significance of these long presequences remains to be elucidated. Import rate measurements show that the relative rates for BCKD subunits to enter mitochondria are E1α > E2 > E1β.[203] The results suggest that the import of the E1β subunit is rate limiting in biogenesis of the BCKD complex. In transfection studies, plasmids carrying cDNA for E1α and E2 have been introduced into MSUD cells deficient in the corresponding subunits.[204–206] The processed mature E1α and E2 subunits are capable of assembly with the other normal endogenous subunits inside mitochondria to restore BCKD complex activity. Using the similar transfection approach, a later study suggests that the amount of E1β subunit is limiting in the assembly of the BCKD complex.[207]

Mature E2 subunits were expressed in *E. coli* and shown to assemble into a cubic 24-mer.[208] The recombinant E2 possessed transacylase activity when assayed in the presence of exogenous hydrolipoamide and isovaleryl-CoA. However, the recombinant 24-mer is essentially devoid of bound lipoic acid. Mitochondrial extract prepared from beef liver catalyzes the incorporation of DL-[2-^{3}H]lipoic acid into recombinant apo E2. The lipoyltransferase for the related H protein of glycine decarboxylase complex has been purified from bovine liver mitochondria.[209] The partially purified enzyme utilizes lipoyl AMP, but not lipoic acid and ATP, for the lipoylation of the apo H protein. The mammalian lipoylation system consists of two components: a lipoate-activating enzyme that catalyzes the formation of lipoate AMP from lipoic acid and ATP and a lipoyltransferase. Interestingly, bovine lipoate-activating enzyme and lipoyltransferase together lipoylate lipoyl-bearing domains of E2p and E2k of mammalian pyruvate and α-ketoglutarate dehydrogenase complexes, respectively, as efficiently as H protein, but the lipoylation rate of E2 of the BCKD complex is extremely slow.[210] The bacterial lipoylation enzyme, LplA from *E. coli* has also been cloned and expressed[211] with full activity.[212]

Chaperone-Mediated Folding of E1 and E2 Components

An active recombinant E1 component of the mammalian BCKD complex was expressed in *E. coli*.[131] This was achieved by coexpression of mature E1α and E1β subunits on the same plasmid, which was transformed into a bacterial cell. In vitro incubation of individually expressed recombinant E1α and E1β subunits did not result in assembly of a functional E1. In a later study, cotransformation of a second plasmid overexpressing bacterial chaperonins GroEL and GroES resulted in an increase of 500 times in the specific activity of E1[132] compared to the single transformant of E1 subunits. The results strongly suggest bacterial chaperonins promote folding and assembly of heterotetramers ($\alpha_2\beta_2$) of mammalian E1 in *E. coli*. Chaperonins GroEL and GroES are homologues of mitochondrial heat-shock proteins Hsp60 and Hsp10.[213] Assembly intermediate also requires GroEL/GroES and Mg-ATP for dimerization to form the active $\alpha_2\beta_2$ heterotetramer of E1. The obligatory interaction of the heterodimeric intermediate with GroEL/GroES appears to be the rate-limiting step in E1 assembly. Evidence suggests that the chaperonins promote dissociation/reassociation cycles of the heterodimeric intermediate. This iterative annealing step is essential for priming the assembly intermediate for subsequent $\alpha_2\beta_2$ assembly of E1.[214]

Regulation of the Mammalian BCKD Complex

There are currently three levels of mechanisms known to regulate the activity of the mammalian BCKD complex: inhibition by products and substrate analogues, reversible phosphorylation-dephosphorylation, and regulation of gene expression. These are discussed individually.

Inhibition by Products and Substrate Analogues. The BCKD complexes purified from bovine kidney,[38] bovine liver,[102] and rat liver[100] are subject to feedback inhibition by branched-chain acyl CoA and NADH. In isolated rat liver hepatocytes, elevation of the mitochondrial NADH : NAD^+ ratio by addition of oleate suppresses the oxidative decarboxylation of KIC.[12] Decarboxylation of KIC in perfused rat liver is inhibited by pyruvate through an increase of the mitochondrial NADH : NAD^+ efflux through the BCKD complex.[78] Carnitine stimulates the oxidation of BCKA[74–76] by increasing the formation of branched-chain acyl carnitine.[215] It was proposed that depletion of branched-chain acyl CoA removes product inhibition of the BCKD complex, thereby increasing the BCKA flux through this step. This mechanism is supported by studies with the perfused rat liver, which showed that the rate of [1-^{14}C]KIV decarboxylation is enhanced by coinfusion of L(−)carnitine, although [1-^{14}C]KIC decarboxylation is unaffected.[46] The purified bovine BCKD complex is inhibited by clofibrate, phenylpyruvate,[216] and the arylidenepyruvates.[188] These compounds appear to be substrate analogues because of their structural resemblance to BCKAs.

Phosphorylation-Dephosphorylation. It is firmly established that the activity of the BCKD complex is predominantly regulated by this covalent modification.[80,118,175,176] The activity state of the complex in different tissues is determined by the ratio of the phosphorylated form (inactive) to the fully dephosphorylated (maximally active) form.[79] By using a broad-specificity phosphatase to dephosphorylate the BCKD complex, Harris and associates showed that virtually all of the rat liver enzyme is in the active (dephosphorylated) form.[196] The same study showed that the enzyme was 10 to 20 percent active in the heart, and 70 to 80 percent active in the kidney under various nutritional states and in diabetes. Wagenmakers et al.,[70] by preincubating mitochondria with kinase or phosphatase inhibitors, later found that the enzyme complex was 6 percent active in skeletal muscle of fed rats, 7 percent in heart, 20 percent in diaphragm, 40 percent in kidney, 60 percent in brain, and 98 percent in liver. Results similar to the latter study were obtained by Patston and associates in tissues of fed normal rats.[217] However, recent measurements using the broad-specificity phosphatase show that percent active BCKD in human tissues is significantly different from that in the rat, with 40 percent in heart, 26 percent in skeletal muscle, and only 28 percent in liver of humans (Table 87-1).[51] The human kidney has the lowest percent active BCKD at 14 percent, but highest total BCKD activity per gram wet weight among the tissues studied. In rat adipose tissue, leucine activates the BCKD complex, presumably by inhibiting the kinase through KIC.[218] Dietary clofibrate at low concentrations increases activity state of the liver BCKD complex of rats fed a protein-deficient diet by inhibiting the kinase, but causes no induction of BCKD subunit content and mRNAs.[219] A later study shows that clofibrate reduces mRNA and protein level of the BCKD kinase in rat liver, but is without effect in skeletal muscle.[220] Octanoate increases the oxidation of leucine in skeletal muscle by increasing the activity state (percent dephosphorylated form) of the BCKD complex.[221] This study also shows that perfusion of rat hind limb with glucose, leucine, and octanoate results in a 150-fold increase in the activity of the muscle BCKD complex. Fluoride, a known inhibitor of the BCKD phosphatase,[194] largely abolishes the increase in enzyme activity in isolated hepatocytes with kinase inhibitors, presumably by preventing dephosphorylation of the enzyme complex.[222] Diet and hormones also play an important role in modulating the activity of the BCKD complex through phosphorylation-dephosphorylation. Rats fed low-protein diets show low hepatic BCKD complex activity.[119,217,223,224] The decrease in hepatic enzyme activity is accompanied by a reduction in the activity state of the enzyme complex compared to fed rats.[119,224] The decrease in activity state was later shown to result from an increase in the amounts of the BCKD kinase protein and mRNA in rat liver.[225] Feeding rats with a high-protein diet increases the BCKD complex activity fourfold postprandially in skeletal muscle.[226] Immunochemical studies demonstrate convincingly that liver and muscle mitochondria from rats fed with a high-protein diet contain mostly, if not all, the dephosphorylated form of the E1α subunit of the BCKD complex.[227] In contrast, mitochondria from rats fed with a low-protein diet contain predominantly a phosphorylated form of the enzyme complex. Starvation and diabetes stimulate the activity of the BCKD complex in skeletal muscle[228,229] by increasing the proportion of active or dephosphorylated enzyme. Starvation also caused mild progressive increases in plasma BCAA, which may inhibit the specific kinase, and account for activation of the enzyme complex.[229] The increase in BCKD activity in mitochondria of diabetic rats cannot be reversed by ATP, suggesting that mechanisms other than phosphorylation-dephosphorylation may be involved.[228] Administration of glucagon or adrenaline (200 μg/100 g body weight) resulted in a fourfold increase in the percent active BCKD complex in the liver of rats fed low-protein diets.[230] Similar effects on the activity state occurs with insulin and cAMP, but to a lesser extent.[230] In contrast, infusion of glucagon (0.35 μM) and adrenaline (0.5 μM) results in transient decreases in the amount of active BCKD complex in hearts from rats fed *ad libitum*.[231] Cortisone treatment for 2 to 5 days of fed rats causes the doubling of the percent active enzyme complex in skeletal muscle.[226] The increase in BCKD complex activity correlated with a rise in the concentration of leucine in plasma and muscle, which may account for, in part, the inhibition of the specific kinase.[226] A recent study shows that glucocorticoids cause a marked reduction in the BCKD mRNA level in rat hepatoma cells and rat liver with a concomitant increase in the activity state of the BCKD complex in hepatoma cells.[232] Glucocorticoids and/or acidification significantly increase the activity state of the BCKD complex in pig kidney cells expressing the hormone receptor.[233] The activity state of the BCKD complex in rat muscle is also elevated in acute uremia[234] and by physical training.[235]

Regulation of BCKD Gene Expression. The activity of the enzyme complex is increased ten- to twentyfold during differentiation of Swiss mouse 3T3-L1 preadipocytes into adipocytes.[236,237] The increase in total activity during differentiation is accompanied by concomitant increases in component (E1, E2, and E3) activities[236] and subunit mRNA and protein content.[182] Glucose is implicated to regulate the E1α mRNA level in pancreatic islets and rat insulinoma cells.[238] These studies suggest the control of the BCKD complex activity by modulating the expression of BCKD subunit genes. In this context, dexamethasone and a cAMP analog 8-(4-chlorophenythio) adenosine 3′,5′-monophosphate, increase the relative abundance of E1α (3.2-fold), E1β (2.9-fold), and E2 (1.6-fold) subunits of the rat BCKD complex, without significant effects on the activity state of the enzyme complex.[239] By comparison, the induction of subunit mRNAs is less stoichiometric at 7.4-, 21.7-, and 4.8-fold for E1α, E1β, and E2 mRNAs, respectively. Noncoordinate regulation of BCKD subunit mRNAs also occurs in rats fed with different percent protein diets.[240,241] In contrast, coordinate changes among BCKD subunits were observed in developing murine tissues and during 3T3-L1 adipocyte differentiation. Insulin reduces the E1α mRNA and protein levels in H4IIEC3 cells, but has no apparent effects on the abundance of E1β and E2 mRNA.[242] Half-lives of E1α and E2 mRNAs are not altered by insulin. The accumulative evidence to date supports the thesis that the actual regulation of BCKD subunit gene expression is at translational and posttranslational steps.[239] The latter step is complex as it involves possible coordination of BCKD subunit folding and assembly by mitochondrial chaperonins Hsp60 and Hsp10, as suggested by in vivo[132] and in vitro reconstitution studies with the E1 heterotetramer.[243,214]

Molecular Genetics of the Mammalian BCKD Complex

The powerful approach of molecular biology has provided an impetus for understanding structure, function, and molecular genetics of the BCKD complex.[228,242,244,245] Except for the specific phosphatase all the subunits have been cloned. At the time of this writing, the protein database (NBCI Blast Search) contains 7 E1α, 6 E1β, 7 E2, 65 E3, and 3 kinase cDNA sequences of the BCKD complex. The amino acid sequences deduced from these cDNAs have facilitated the analysis of the domain structures and functions of the subunits comprising this multienzyme complex. Highly specific cDNA probes allowed chromosome localization of the human genes encoding specific subunits of the BCKD complex. Moreover, the genes encoding the unique human BCKD subunits E1α, E1β, and E2, including the promoter region, have been isolated and characterized. The genes for the human E3 and the rat BCKD kinase have also been cloned and their promoter regions investigated. The following sections provide an account of the advances in the molecular genetics of the mammalian BCKD complex.

Chromosomal Localization of BCKD Genes. The human E1α gene (*BCKDHA*) was initially localized to chromosome 19[246] and later regionally mapped to 19q13.1-q13.2 by *in situ* hybridization.[247] The human E1β gene (*BCKDHB*) was localized to human chromosome 6[248,249] and regionally assigned to chromosome 6p21-p22 also by *in situ* hybridization.[248] The human E2 gene (*DBT*) was localized to chromosome 1.[250,251] The gene was regionally assigned to chromosome 1p31 by *in situ* hybridization[248] and to 1p22 to centromere by PCR amplification.[252] The human E3 gene *(DLD)* was regionally assigned to 7q31-q32.[253]

Isolation and Characterization of Human BCKD Genes. The human E1α gene (GenBank L08634) contains 9 exons and spans at least 55 kb. The size of intron 1 is uncertain, but it is larger than 20 kb.[254,255] Exon 1 contains multiple transcription-initiation sites at bases +1, +18, and +22. Sequencing of the 5′-flanking region disclosed the absence of a canonical TATA box. Several sets of "CAAT"-box-like sequences and Spl binding sites are present. The luciferase reporter assay with deletion constructs in HepG2 cells indicates that the region for high-level transcription is located between bases −320 and −115. Extension of the 5′-end of the insert to beyond base −320 markedly reduces promoter activity, suggesting the presence of inhibitory elements in the region upstream of base −320. Assays in CHO cells show that the region of high-level transcription lies between bases −909 and −115. The variation in the region for high-level transcription in HepG2 and CHO cells may represent cell-type specific differences in the E1α gene promoter function.

The human E1β gene (GenBank D90382 to D90391) spans over 100 kb with the sizes of introns 3 and 6 not determined and was originally reported to contain 10 exons.[249] However, a later study determined that the human E1β gene actually comprises 11 exons.[256] The previously undescribed exon 11 codes for a 3′-untranslated region, and is absent in one of the isolated human E1β cDNAs due to alternate splicing. A single transcription initiation site is located 47 nucleotides upstream of the initiation Met codon. Two "CAAT"-box-like sequences are present at bases −39 and −75, but there was also no "TATA"-box-like sequence. There are three sets of sequences homologous to the transcription factor Sp1-binding sites and two sets of sequences resembling the enhancer core sequence.

The structural organization of the human E2 gene (GenBank X15069, X68104) has also been determined by characterization of overlapping genomic clones.[257] The single-copy human E2 gene spans approximately 68 kb and comprises 11 exons. Exon 11 is 2239 bp in length and encodes the entire 3′-untranslated region of 2074 bp in the human E2 mRNA. Sequencing of the region flanking exon 8 reveals the presence of a cryptic 3′-acceptor splice site located 370 bases upstream of exon 8, which results in alternate splicing of intron 7.[258] In addition, two polyadenylation signals are present in the intronic sequence downstream of exon 8, which promotes truncation by RNA processing. Sequence analysis of the promoter regulatory region showed the presence of a "CAAT"-box-like sequence at base −537; the "TATA"-box-like sequence, however, is again absent. Promoter assays using human hepatoma cells (HepG2) and mouse preadipocytes (3T3-L1) showed that a 4.1-kb *Pst*I fragment upstream of the transcription start site confers high expression of the luciferase reporter gene. An intronless E2 pseudogene was also isolated.[257] It corresponds to the complete mitochondrial presequence and the lipoyl-bearing domain that are encoded by exons I through IV of the functional E2 gene. The E2 pseudogene contains multiple base changes, deletions, and insertions, and is flanked by short direct repeats. The data indicate that the E2 pseudogene is a retroposon, and may represent an ancestral gene for the lipoyl-bearing domain.

The promoter regulatory region of the human E3 gene (GenBank L13761) has been cloned and partially characterized.[259] The gene comprises 14 exons and is approximately 20 kb in length.[260] A "CAAT"-box-like sequence is present at −39 bp in the TATA-less human E3 promoter.[260] Deletion of a promoter element between −769 and −1223 bp resulted in a threefold increase in chloramphenicol acetyltransferase reporter activity. These results suggest that a negative regulatory element is present between bases −769 and −1223 of the human E3 promoter.[259]

The above studies describe genomic structures for the four catalytic subunits of the BCKD complex. This information has facilitated mutational analysis of MSUD patients, including mutations in exonic and intronic sequences, as well as the promoter regulatory region. It is noteworthy that the human E1α, E1β, E2, and E3 gene promoters invariantly lack canonical TATA boxes. Multiple copies of CAAT boxes and Sp1-binding sequences are present in these genes (E1α, E1β, and E2) of the human BCKD complex. These features are common to the promoters of housekeeping genes.[261] The isolation of the promoter regulatory regions of the genes encoding subunits of the human BCKD complex also offers the opportunity to investigate the control of expression of these genes.

Isolation and Characterization of Rodent BCKD-Kinase Genes. The gene for the rat BCKD-kinase (GenBank U36774) isolated from a P1 genomic library contains 11 exons and spans 6 kb, with the region encoding 5′-untranslated region interrupted by intron 1.[262] The region between bases −58 and +21 is indispensable for basal activity of the TATA-less rat kinase promoter.[263] Moreover, binding of Sp1 or Sp1-like proteins to a nonconsensus Sp1 sequence (ACAACTCCCA) plays a major role in transactivating basal expression of the rat BCKD-kinase gene. Down-regulation of the rat kinase gene has been demonstrated in rat hepatoma H4IIE cells in the rat liver.[232] The glucocorticoid-responsive elements are not located in the −6.5 kb promoter region examined. It is proposed that glucocorticoids and nutritional stimuli regulate the rat BCKD-kinase gene in the liver by a repression/derepression cycle.[232] A TATA-less murine E2 gene promoter has also been isolated, and initial characterization shows that promoter region between bases −65 and −40 is important for regulating E2 gene expression.[264]

MAPLE SYRUP URINE DISEASE (BRANCHED CHAIN KETOACIDURIA)

Historical Perspective

In 1954, Menkes, Hurst, and Craig reported four cases of familial cerebral degenerative disease with the onset in the first week of life and death occurring within 3 months.[265] The urine of these sibs had an odor resembling maple syrup. Westall et al. subsequently studied another patient and found that the levels of BCAAs leucine, isoleucine, and valine were greatly elevated.[266] The new syndrome was called maple syrup urine disease (MSUD).[266] The BCKAs (KIC, KIV, and KMV) derived from the three BCAAs were isolated from the urine of MSUD patients and identified as 2,4-dinitrophenylhydrazones.[267] The results suggested that catabolic pathways of the BCAAs were blocked at the decarboxylation of the respective α-keto acids. Therefore, the disease was alternately called 'branched-chain ketoaciduria'[268] or branched-chain ketonuria.[269] In 1960, Dancis et al. demonstrated that the decarboxylation of [1-^{14}C] BCKAs is deficient in white blood cells from MSUD patients.[270] The transamination of BCAA appeared to

Table 87-3 Clinical and Biochemical Phenotypes in MSUD

Clinical phenotype	Prominent clinical features	Biochemical features	Decarboxylation activity,* % of normal
Classic	Neonatal onset, poor feeding, lethargy, increased/decreased tone, ketoacidosis, and seizures	Markedly increased alloisoleucine, BCAA, and BCKAS	0–2
Intermediate	Failure to thrive, often no ketoacidosis, devlopmental delay	Persistently increased alloisoleucine, BCAA,and BCKA	3–30
Intermittent	Normal early devlopement, episodic ataxia/ketoacidosis precipitated by infection or stress; episodes can be fatal, usually normal intellect	Normal BCAA when asymptomatic	5–20
Thiamine-responsive	Similar to intermediate MSUD	Decreased BCKA and/or BCAA with thiamine therapy	2–40
Lipoamide dehydrogenase (E3) deficiency	Usually no neonatal symptoms, failure to thrive, hypotonia, lactic acidosis, developmental delay, movement disorder, progressive deterioration	Moderative increased BCAA, BCKA; elevated α-ketoglutarate and pyruvate	0–25

*Most commnly measured in intact peripheral blood leukocytes or cultured fibroblasts or lymphoblasts with [1-^{14}C]-labeled BCAA or BCKA as substrate.

be unaffected in these cells. Variant forms of MSUD were later described that were milder in their clinical manifestations and had episodic symptoms related to infection, increased dietary protein, and stress.[269,271–274] Attempts at dietary therapy were initiated but were largely unsuccessful.[275] In 1964, Snyderman and associates described a more rigorous and successful dietary approach for the treatment of MSUD by restricting dietary BCAAs.[276] In 1971, Scriver and associates reported a new thiamine-responsive form of MSUD in which the hyperaminoacidemia was completely corrected by thiamine in pharmacologic dosage without recourse to dietary restrictions.[277] This completed the initial phase of the history of MSUD in which the phenotypes were defined, the metabolic block was identified, and dietary treatment was devised. The recognition of this disorder focused attention on the importance of BCAA metabolism, and provided the basis for extensive investigation in the 1970s into the metabolic defect of this disease at the cell-culture level.

It is remarkable that Menkes, in as early as 1959, recognized the complexity of the enzyme system involved in MSUD.[277] He postulated that a single multienzyme system is responsible for the decarboxylation of the three BCKAs, based on the concomitant accumulation of these α-keto acids in the urine of MSUD patients. Complementation studies in heterokaryons derived by fusing fibroblasts from unrelated MSUD patients indicated that multiple gene products were involved.[278–280] A breakthrough in the enzymology of MSUD occurred in 1978, when the branched chain α-keto acid dehydrogenase (BCKD) complex was purified to homogeneity from bovine kidney mitochondria by Reed and associates.[38] The specific kinase[184] and phosphatase[197] for the BCKD complex were later purified to homogeneity. These results indicate that six genetic loci contribute to the synthesis and assembly of the complex, and explain the genetic heterogeneity defined by earlier complementation studies.

The molecular genetics of MSUD dawned in the late 1980s with cloning of cDNA for the catalytic subunits (E1α, E1β, and E2) of the mammalian BCKD complex. The availability of the cDNA permitted chromosomal localization of the gene for the three unique subunits of the complex[247–249,251] and the elucidation of genomic structure of the three specific human BCKD genes.[249,255,257] The cDNA sequence and results of limited proteolysis defined the domain structure of the E2 subunit. To date, 63 MSUD mutations in E1α, E1β, E2, and E3 loci have been identified and some characterized, including the prevalent Y393N-α mutation in the Mennonite kindred.[281,282] An animal model for MSUD in Polled Hereford calves was described[283,284] and its mutation identified.[285] The information provided by MSUD mutations has allowed prenatal and carrier detection at the gene level. As more MSUD mutations are identified, their origin and population distributions can be addressed. Stable correction of the BCKD complex deficiency in MSUD cells has been demonstrated by retroviral-mediated gene transfer.[286,287] These studies provide a basis for the development of gene therapy for MSUD. Very recently, the crystal structure of the human E1 heterotetramer was determined.[118] Most, if not all, of MSUD mutations in E1 subunits can now be explained from the structure/function perspective of this enzyme component. It is anticipated that the progress made in understanding the molecular and biochemical basis of MSUD will ultimately lead to the development of effective gene and drug therapeutics for this important metabolic disorder.

Clinical Phenotypes

Based on the mode of clinical presentation and biochemical responses to thiamine administration, MSUD patients can be divided into five clinical and biochemical phenotypes—classic, intermediate, intermittent, thiamine-responsive, and dihydrolipoyl dehydrogenase (E3)-deficient MSUD (Table 87-3). Their phenotypes are described in the following subsection. Categorization of the variant cases reported in the literature is sometimes difficult because of a lack of uniform criteria. The clinical phenotype of the animal model is also described.

Classic MSUD. In the original family with MSUD reported by Menkes,[265] four sibs died in the newborn period. MSUD with a neonatal onset of encephalopathy is now considered the classic form, and represents the most severe and most common form of this disease. The levels of the BCAA, particularly leucine, are greatly increased in the blood, cerebrospinal fluid, and urine, and the presence of alloisoleucine is diagnostic of MSUD (see "Screening and Diagnosis" below). In classic MSUD, 50 percent or more of the BCKAs are derived from leucine. The activity of the BCKD complex in skin fibroblasts or lymphoblast cultures is usually less than 2 percent of normal. Affected newborns appear normal at birth, and symptoms usually develop between 4 and 7 days of age. Breast-feeding may delay onset to the second week of life. Lethargy and poor sucking with little interest in feeding are usually the first signs. This is followed by weight loss and progressive neurologic signs of alternating hypertonia and hypotonia with dystonic extension of the arms resembling decerebrate posturing. Ketosis and the maple syrup or burnt sugar odor becomes obvious at this time. Hypoglycemia is reported, but it is not a prominent feature.[288,289] Seizures and coma ensue, leading to death if untreated. Bulging fontanel and pseudotumor cerebri are occasionally observed.[290–292]

The prognosis is poor in the untreated patient. The majority of patients die within the early months of life from recurrent metabolic crisis and neurologic deterioration, often precipitated by infection or other stresses, such as vaccination or surgery. Sudden death has occurred in two infants with MSUD. One died at 6 days of age before the results of newborn screening became available (RJ Evans, personal communication, March 26, 1992). One 7-day-old infant had a sudden cardiopulmonary arrest and the diagnosis of MSUD was made by the characteristic amino acid pattern in postmortem tissue.[293] Surviving patients suffer from severe neurologic damage, including mental retardation, spasticity, and, occasionally, cortical blindness. One exceptional patient survived until 13 years of age.[294] Although early treatment has greatly improved the outlook for these infants, there can be complications. Sudden onset of transient ataxia lasting 30 min to 1 h occurred in patients who apparently had good metabolic control.[289] During ketonemia, patients have experienced visual hallucinations. Even with treatment some patients have died of uncontrollable brain edema.[288,289,295] Pancreatitis has been reported in patients with several organic acidemias, including MSUD.[296,297] One patient suffered from transient retinopathy associated with pancreatitis.[298]

Intermediate MSUD. Patients with the intermediate form of MSUD have persistent elevations of BCAA and neurologic impairment, but do not have catastrophic illness in the neonatal period. Many do not have episodes of acute metabolic decompensation. The residual enzyme activity in intermediate MSUD is generally greater than in the classic form, and ranges from 3 to 30 percent of normal. Three patients have been reported with immeasurable or markedly reduced activity of the BCKD complex.[299–301] The first intermediate patient, a 19-month-old female, was described by Schulman et al. in 1970.[302] This patient was noted to have an odor resembling maple syrup in her urine during evaluation for mental retardation. She consumed a normal diet and had normal physical growth, but her developmental milestones were substantially delayed. She also had mild hypertelorism, iron-deficiency anemia, hyperuricemia, and mild systemic acidosis. Markedly increased levels of BCAAs and BCKAs in serum and urine were consistently present. Protein restriction reduced serum BCAAs and urate concentrations. Significant acidosis did not occur with BCAA loading. Thiamine at 100 mg/day for 1 week had no effect on the BCAA levels. The patient had 15 to 25 percent residual BCKD complex activities in both leukocytes and cultured fibroblasts.

There are now approximately 20 reported patients in the intermediate category. Most were diagnosed between age 5 months and 7 years during evaluation for developmental delay and/or seizures;[300,303–307] several had episodes of ketoacidosis;[300,301,308–310] but acute encephalopathy was rare.[299,301] Three patients first presented with ophthalmoplegia during the neonatal period.[311–314] One patient with borderline low intelligence as the only clinical finding was diagnosed at 19 years of age.[300] She excreted only one-third the amount of ketoacids excreted by Schulman's patient. The excretion pattern of BCKAs in this patient and in one other patient[309] was different from that seen in classic MSUD in that 75 to 80 percent of the BCKAs were derivatives of isoleucine.

Intermittent MSUD. Patients with the intermittent form of MSUD show normal early development, with normal growth and intelligence. However, they are at risk for acute metabolic decompensation during stressful situations. While asymptomatic, their laboratory data, including plasma BCAA levels, are normal. Activity of BCKD complex in these patients ranges from 5 to 20 percent of normal. In two cases, the activity was reduced to the levels seen in classic MSUD.[273,315] In 1961, Morris et al. described the first patient (a 24-month-old female) with the intermittent MSUD variant phenotype.[271] Recurrent episodic ataxia, lethargy, and semicoma developed in this previously asymptomatic female following otitis media at age 16 months. Maple syrup odor was noted during one of these episodes, and increased urine BCAA and BCKA confirmed the diagnosis. A younger male sib had no aberrant clinical or laboratory abnormality until his first acute episode at 10.5 months of age. Both patients benefited from dietary protein restriction. The older child was normal in growth and development at 9 years,[269] but her younger brother died from postoperative bleeding and metabolic decompensation after tonsillectomy at 4.5 years of age.[316]

There are many reported patients with intermittent MSUD.[269,272,273,289,315–328] The initial symptoms generally appear between 5 months and 2 years of age in association with otitis media or other infection, but may appear as late as the fifth decade of life.[324] Episodes of acute behavioral change and unsteady gait may progress to seizures and stupor or coma. The amino acid and organic acid profiles at these times are characteristic of MSUD. Patients have died during these episodes.[269,271,273,315,316,329] In one family, one patient was diagnosed at 2 years of age with recurrent ketoacidosis, and her younger sib had lethargy and opisthotonos during the neonatal period.[319] There is one unusual case of valine-toxic intermittent MSUD.[329] Correct diagnosis is important for appropriate treatment and for preventing recurrent attacks.

Thiamine-Responsive MSUD. A number of putative thiamine-responsive patients have been reported. The lack of uniform criteria in therapeutic trials makes it difficult to assess the degree of thiamine dependency and to compare different patients. In general, these patients did not have acute neonatal illness, and their early clinical course was similar to that of intermediate MSUD. The first patient (WG-34) described by Scriver et al.[330] was studied for developmental delay at the age of 11 months. Her plasma BCAA concentrations were five times greater than normal, and alloisoleucine was detected. These levels fell abruptly to normal with thiamine 10 mg/day for 4 days while on a constant protein diet. There was a rebound of the BCAA levels during one of the two trials of thiamine withdrawal.[330,331] A combined treatment of long-term thiamine administration and a protein-restricted diet was continued, and her BCAA levels were maintained near normal over the years. The patient had five episodes of metabolic decompensation in the first decade, one of which required peritoneal dialysis.[331] She had an IQ of 85, graduated from high school, and is now married.[288] Measurements with skin fibroblasts showed 30 to 40 percent of residual BCKD complex activity.[332] An additional eight patients[333–339] have been reported. Duran et al.[333] administered thiamine to a 7-year-old patient on a low-protein diet. They found that 1000 mg/day reduced BCKA excretion, but this high dose of thiamine had little effect on the plasma BCAA levels. The patient had no further episodes of metabolic decompensation. He had apparently normal mental and physical development at age 18.[340] Fernhoff[336] and Elsas[337,338] and their colleagues have described five patients whose clinical course is consistent with the intermediate variant and whose BCKD complex activity is in the range of 2.7 to 9.4 percent of normal. The plasma BCAA and BCKA concentrations in these patients showed a significant decrease after thiamine at 100 to 150 mg/day. However, achieving the full effect required approximately 3 weeks. The patient described by Pueschel et al.[341] was treated with a low-protein diet and thiamine until 6 years of age. He remained in good health on a normal diet, with only occasional mildly elevated BCAAs. His IQ was 108 at age 16.[289] This patient's newborn blood specimen, obtained on the third day of life, was normal (HL Levy, personal communication). Thiamine-responsive patients are heterogeneous, and a wide range of dosage between 10 to 1000 mg a day has been administered with limited success. None have been treated with thiamine alone; all patients have been treated with combined therapy of dietary BCAA restriction and thiamine for metabolic control.

Dihydrolipoyl Dehydrogenase (E3)-Deficient MSUD. E3 deficiency is a rare disorder; less than 20 patients have been described.[342–348,374] The clinical phenotype is similar to intermediate MSUD, but is accompanied by severe lactic acidosis. The urine organic acid profile exhibits abnormalities of both lactic acidosis and MSUD. Lactate, pyruvate, α-ketoglutarate, α-hydroxyisovalerate, and α-hydroxyglutarate are all increased. Hyperalaninemia secondary to pyruvate accumulation is often present. BCAAs are mildly to moderately increased in the plasma as compared with classic MSUD patients, and alloisoleucine was observed in one patient with E3 deficiency.[344] These patients have a combined deficiency of the BCKD, pyruvate, and α-ketoglutarate dehydrogenase complexes.

E3-deficient patients have a relatively uneventful first few months of life; however, a brief neonatal mild metabolic acidosis has been observed in two patients. After the development of persistent lactic acidosis between age 8 weeks and 6 months, the course was marked by progressive neurologic deterioration, including hypotonia, developmental delay, and movement disorder. The neuropathology showed myelin loss and cavitation in discrete areas of the basal ganglia, thalami, and brain stem, resembling Leigh encephalopathy.[343,345] The results of several treatments that included pharmacologic doses of thiamine, biotin, and lipoic acid, and dietary restriction of fat and BCAA have generally been disappointing.[342,345a,345]

Unclassified MSUD. There are at least four unusual families in which both a parent and child are affected.[273,317,321,324,349] In some families, there is more than one clinical phenotype present.[317,321,349,350] It appears that there are at least two different mutant alleles segregating in each family and that the variant patients are compound heterozygotes.

Animal Model. A severe encephalopathy has been described in association with abnormal BCAA metabolism in Polled Hereford inbred calves in Australia[283,351] and in horned Hereford calves in Canada.[284] This bovine metabolic disorder has many similarities to human MSUD, and it may serve as an animal model. The majority of affected calves are dull at birth; some develop sluggishness, intermittent opisthotonos, and disorganized limb paddling within 2 to 3 days. Death usually occurs within 5 days of life. The urine has a "bitter sweet odor of burnt sugar" and a positive 2,4-dinitrophenylhydrazine (DPNH) test.

The major neuropathologic finding is extensive status spongiosus throughout the white matter.[283,284,352] Electron microscopy shows myelin edema with splitting of the myelin sheath at the intraperiod line.[353] Neurotransmitter studies showed reduced concentrations of the transmitter amino acids glutamate, aspartate, and GABA, as well as a 50 percent loss in number of postsynaptic GABA receptors as assessed from [^{3}H] diazepam binding.[354] Markedly increased BCAAs have been found in serum, cerebrospinal fluid, and brain tissue. A severe deficiency of the BCKD activity has been confirmed in an affected calf by measurement of $^{14}CO_2$ from [1-^{14}C] leucine with intact fibroblasts and from α-[1-^{14}C] KIC with disrupted fibroblasts.[351]

An autosomal recessive inheritance is suggested by breeding experiments. Comparison of this animal model with human MSUD shows that there are some differences. Affected calves have been stillborn or born with neurologic symptoms suggesting prenatal metabolic defects. In contrast, patients with MSUD appear normal at birth by both clinical and laboratory examination; symptoms develop toward the end of the first week of life.

Molecular Phenotypes: The Affected Loci

As described above, the human BCKD complex consists of three catalytic components and two regulatory enzymes that are encoded by six genetic loci (Table 87-2). Mutations in any one of these loci could theoretically produce the MSUD phenotype. Enzyme assays for each component (E1, E2, or E3) were developed using model reactions or by enzyme reconstitution.[121,122,355–357] This enabled the detection of deficiencies in E1[355,358] or E3.[345] The component assays on purified E1 and E2 components are reliable, but are difficult with cell-culture homogenates because of low sensitivity.[357] Assays of E3 are sensitive for both purified enzyme[160] and cell-culture material.[345,356]

The availability of specific antibodies and cDNA probes has allowed the use of more direct molecular approaches to identify the mutant locus in MSUD. A deficiency in the E2 subunit was first determined in a classic MSUD patient by western blotting.[114] Deficiencies in other catalytic subunits (E1α, E1β, and E3) were later detected by western and/or northern blot analysis.[115,116,319,359,360] The advantage of these two methods is that they can detect the reduction or absence of mRNA and/or protein for a specific subunit as compared with normal. A limitation is the inability to detect point mutations and small deletions or insertions, which do not grossly affect abundance and size of the mutant polypeptide. In this situation, a vector carrying a normal cDNA for each of the four catalytic subunits can be transfected into MSUD cells, preferably into cultured lymphoblasts because they proliferate rapidly. Transfected cells are selected for antibiotic resistance. The restoration of decarboxylation of [1-^{14}C] KIV in transfected MSUD cells by one of the vectors identifies the mutant locus.[204,206,361] The cDNA-mediated complementation, albeit laborious, may be required if northern and western blot analysis and component assays are uninformative.[116] One can screen for known mutations in MSUD cells using allele-specific oligonucleotide (ASO) probes.[281,282,285,359] If the patient is a heterozygote for a known mutation, it is highly probable that the second mutation involves the same locus.

Based on the subunits of the human BCKD complex that are shown to be affected, MSUD can be classified into four molecular phenotypes. These consist of types IA, IB, II, and III, referring to deficiencies in E1α, E1β, E2, and E3 subunits, respectively. The numbering system of these four types corresponds to that of the affected catalytic subunit. Although not yet described, type IV and type V are reserved for lesions in the BCKD kinase and BCKD phosphatase, respectively. The classification of molecular phenotypes shows the genetic heterogeneity of MSUD and provides a convenient way to indicate the subunit and the corresponding locus responsible for the disorder. The molecular phenotype is distinct from the genotype, which describes the combinations of mutant alleles that exhibit Mendelian inheritance. After the affected locus is identified by the methods described above, one can focus on the analysis of mutations in the implicated gene. The relationship between the molecular and clinical phenotypes cannot be fully assessed until more patients are studied. Nonetheless, more than one clinical phenotype was observed within each affected locus (Table 87-4). This is expected because different mutations in the same subunit may exert dissimilar effects on the stability and function of the polypeptide, leading to varying degrees of clinical manifestations.

Molecular Genetic Basis of MSUD

The molecular cloning of cDNA and genes for the subunits of the BCKD complex has facilitated the identification of mutations in MSUD. The advent of PCR[362] further accelerated the detection of mutations at the DNA level. Molecular defects in E1α, E1β, E2, and E3 genes of MSUD patients have been described, and the functional significance of these mutations, in some cases, have been studied. Few MSUD mutations are reported, as compared with some other single-gene disorders such as phenylketonuria (see Chap. 77). Table 87-4 summarizes the 63 mutations that have been described to date in the BCKD complex genes of MSUD patients, under the classification of the molecular phenotype. The majority of the mutations reported affect the E1 α (type IA) or E2 (type II) locus. The associated clinical phenotype is that described for homozygous or compound-heterozygous patients. With respect to compound heterozygotes, the clinical type may vary, depending on the interaction between the two mutant alleles.

Table 87-4 Mutations in the BCKD Genes of MSUD Patients

Molecular phenotype	Affected locus	MSUD allele[†]	Gene/protein alteration	Clinical phenotype[‡]	Ethnic origin	Reference
IA	E1α	144insC	Frame shift after Pro-(−7)	C, I	French Canadian, Caucasian	371
IA	E1α	M64T	ATG → ACG	I	Caucasian	371
IA	E1α	R114W	CGG → TGG	C	Japanese	365
IA	E1α	538delC	Frame shift after Pro-125	C	Thai	371
IA	E1α	Q145K	CAG → AAG	C	Japanese	365
IA	E1α	T166M	ACG → ATG	C	Thai	371
IA	E1α	IVS5-1g → c	Exon 6 deletion	C	Middle Eastern	416
IA	E1α	G204S	GGC → AGC	I/M	French Canadian	364
IA	E1α	A208T	GCT → ACT	C	Japanese	365
IA	E1α	R220W	CGG → TGG	C	African American	364
IA	E1α	N222S	AAT → AGT	C	Caucasian	364
IA	E1α	A240P	GCA → CCA	C	Caucasian	364
IA	E1α	R242X	CGA → TGA	C	Israeli	512
IA	E1α	G245R*	GGG → AGG	I	Hispanic-Mexican	364
IA	E1α	887del8	Frameshift After Ala-241	C	Caucasian	513
IA	E1α	R252H	CGC → CAC	I	Caucasian	371
IA	E1α	T265R	ACA → AGA	C	French Canadian	364
IA	E1α	I281T	ATC → ACC	C	Japanese	365
IA	E1α	F364C	TTC → TGC	I	Hispanic-Mexican	364
IA	E1α	Y368C	TAT → TGT	I	Caucasian	371, 513
IA	E1α	Y393N*	TAC → AAC	C	Mennonite, Caucasian, Italian	204, 281, 282, 381
IA	E1α	Q(−6)X	CAG → TAG	C	Polled Hereford calves	285
IB	E1β	52insG	Frameshift after Gly-(−33)	C	Japanese	365
IB	E1β	92del11*	Frameshift after Gly-(−21)	C	Japanese,Italian	365, 367, 381
IB	E1β	N126Y	AAC → TAC	C	Unknown	369
IB	E1β	H156R	CAT → CGT	C	Japanese	365
IB	E1β	IVS5 + 1G → T	Skipping of exons 5 and 6	C	Japanese	366
IB	E1β	954delT	Frameshift after Ser-268	C	Japanese	365
IB	E1β	R274X	CGA → TGA	C	Unknown	369
II	E2	I37M	ATC → ATG	I/M	Japanese	514
II	E2	90delAT*	Frameshift after Asn-(−38) in presequence	C, T,I/M	Caucasian	205
II	E2	354del7	Frame shift after Ser-51	I	Puerto Rican	371
II	E2	E27del	3-bp in frame deletion	C	Mexican-American	244
II	E2	P73L	CCA → CTA	C	Greek	371
II	E2	P73R	GGT → CGT	Unknown	Unknown	371
II	E2	D76Y	GAC → TAC	C	African-American	371
II	E2	I77T	CAT → TAT	C	Mexican-American	244
II	E2	IVS4del[−3.2 kb : −14]*	17-bp insertion at base 450 (Frameshift after Lys-83)	T, I,C	Caucasian, French Canadian	370, 372
II	E2	IVS4del[−15 : −4]	10-bp insertion at base 450 (Frameshift after Lys-83)	I	Caucasian	372
II	E2	501delAC	Frameshift after His-100)	I	Caucasian	371
II	E2	IVS5del[−1 : +1]	ATgt → A–T (Skipping of exon 5)	T	Caucasian	372
II	E2	E163X*	GAA → TAA	C,	African-American, Caucasian	205
II	E2	15–20 kb Alu deletion	Coding stops after Lys-196	C, T	Unknown	252
II	E2	F215C*	TTT → TGT	T,I,I/M	Caucasian, French Canadian, Mennonite	370,372
II	E2	R230G	CGA → GGA	T	Caucasian	371
II	E2	R240C*	CGT → TGT	T, I/M	Caucasian	371,372
II	E2	K252N	AAG → AAC	I/M	Caucasian, Middle Eastern	372
II	E2	K278K*	AAGgt → AAAgt (Skipping of exon 8)	I/M, T	Caucasian	251,371
II	E2	IVS8-700a → G	126-bp insertion at base 1033 (Frameshift after Lys-278)	I/M	Japanese	514
II	E2	IVS8del+1g	Skipping of exon 8	T	Japanese	368
II	E2	H281T	CAT → TAT	T	Caucasian	371
II	E2	G292R	GGT → CGT	T	Netherlands	371

Table 87-4 (Continued)

Molecular phenotype	Affected locus	MSUD allele†	Gene/protein alteration	Clinical phenotype‡	Ethnic origin	Reference
II	E2	G323S	GGT → AGT	I/M	Indian, Japanese	371,514
II	E2	IVS9-7a → g	6-bp insertion at base 1225 (Ser-342 stop)	C	Moroccan	372
II	E2	IVS10del[−9:+1]	21-bp deletion at base 1297 (Ala-367 → Asn-373) deletion	C	American Indian, Spanish	372
II	E2	X422L	TGA → TTA (7 extra amino acids at C-term)	M	Japanese	514
III	E3	Y35X*	TAC → TAAC	E3-deficient	Ashkenazi Jews	374
III	E3	K37E	AAA → GAA	E3-deficient	Japanese	373
III	E3	G229C*		E3-deficient	Ashkenazi Jews	374
III	E3	P453L	CCG → CTG	E3-deficient	Japanese	373
III	E3	R460G	AGA → GGA	E3-deficient	NA	515

*Frequent alleles that are present in three or more unrelated MSUD subjects.
†Terminology for MSUD alleles is based on recommendations by the Ad Hoc Committee on Mutation Nomenclature.[516]
C = Classic; I = Intermediate; I/M = Intermittent; T = Thiamine-responsive

Type IA MSUD Mutations. To date there have been 22 reported type IA mutations affecting the E1α subunit that occur in MSUD patients worldwide. A prominent feature associated with type IA mutations is that 90 percent of them (18 of 22) are missense mutations. Moreover, with a few exceptions, type IA mutations cause the severe classic form of MSUD. The most prevalent type IA mutation is the Y393N that was originally detected in a heterozygous Italian classic MSUD patient.[359] This first described MSUD allele was later shown to be present in homozygous Mennonite MSUD patients.[281,282] The identification of this mutation in Mennonites is significant, because the incidence of MSUD in this community is 1:176 live births.[363] The unusually high frequency of this allele in the homozygous state[363] in the Mennonite population suggests a founder effect. A second type IA mutation of ethnic significance is the G245R. This allele is segregated in the homozygous state in three of four unrelated Hispanic-Mexican patients with intermediate MSUD.[364] It should be noted that four of the type IA mutations (R114W, Q145K, A208T, I281T) are relatively frequent alleles that occur in the Japanese population.[365] Other type IA alleles are distributed among French Canadian, Hispanic-Mexican, Thai, Middle Eastern, African-American, and Caucasian populations. The Q(−6)X allele is present in homozygous Polled Hereford calves.[285]

Type IB Mutations. There are currently 7 known type IB mutations altering the E1β subunit. The majority of type IB mutations are present in Japanese classic MSUD patients as described by Matsuda's group.[365,366] The 92del11 allele is relatively frequent as it is present in several Japanese and Italian classic patients.[365,367,368] It is of interest that a G to T base change in the intron 5 splice junction causes skipping of exons 5 and 6.[366] Two new mutations (N126Y and R274X) are recently reported, but their ethnic origins are unknown.[369]

Type II Mutations. Presently, there are 28 type II MSUD mutations that impair the E2 core of the BCKD complex. A distinct characteristic of type II MSUD is related to its milder clinical phenotype than the phenotypes of type IA or type IB. The majority of type II patients manifest intermediate or intermittent MSUD phenotype, and several of these patients have been reported to respond to thiamine treatments. Unlike type IA mutations, only 43 percent of type II belong to the missense category. The F215C mutation[370] occurs in one allele of the original thiamine-responsive patient described by Scriver and associates.[330] This allele is one of the two prevalent type II missense alleles, and segregates among French Canadians and other ethnic groups.[371] The second frequent missense type II allele is E163X, which is present in African-Americans and Caucasians.[205] There are four type II missense alleles (P73L, P73R, D76Y, and I77T) in the lipoic acid-bearing domain. Interestingly, these mutations affect stability of the E2 subunit but are without effect on lipoic acid incorporation.[371] The 90delAT mutation is present in a compound heterozygous state in several MSUD patients. Skipping of exon 8 caused by a primary base alteration at the splice junction in a type II MSUD allele was described in a Japanese patient.[368] It is of interest that a silent AAG to AAA codon alteration at the 3′ end of exon 8 also results in the skipping of this exon.[252]

A prominent and novel feature of type II MSUD mutations involves deletions of internal intronic segments that lead to secondary insertions/deletions through utilization of new or cryptic splice sites.[372] These secondary mutations were initially detected by RT-PCR and direct sequencing of the mutant E2 transcript. One of these type II alleles is the IVS4del[−3.2kb:−14], which carries a 3.2-kb deletion in intron 4, resulting in 17-bp intronic insertion in the E2 mRNA. The 17-bp insertion was originally detected in a mutant E2 cDNA from Scriver's thiamine-responsive patient.[370] However, the postulated large intronic deletion was not confirmed until genomic DNA from a homozygous French Canadian patient was available. This allowed detection of the 3.2-kb deletion in intron 4 by long PCR and nucleotide sequencing. The IVS4del[−15:−4] mutation results in a 10-bp insertion of intronic sequences at exon 5. The consequence of IVS5del[−1:+1] mutation is the expected deletion of entire exon 5 in the E2 transcript. The A to G transition in the IVS9-7A to G allele creates a new 3′ splice site in intron 9, resulting in a 6-bp insertion harboring a stop codon in exon 10 of a homozygous patient. Another example of intronic deletion is the loss of 10 bp 5′ to exon 11 which results in the removal of the 3′-ag splice site and the first 5′ base of exon 11. As a consequence, a cryptic 3′ splice site located in exon 11 is used, causing the deletion of 21 bp in the mutant E2 mRNA. This allele, designated as IVS10del[−9:+1], occurs in a homozygous type II MSUD patient. The accumulated data indicate that the E2 locus of the human BCKD complex is prone to splicing errors, caused either by primary exonic mutations or large internal intronic alterations.

Type III Mutations. There are 5 known type III mutations that affect the common E3 subunit of α-ketoacid dehydrogenase complexes; all of them are missense mutations. The K37E and the P453L alleles are detected in a compound heterozygous Japanese patients.[373] The recently described G229C mutation is a predominant allele in Ashkenazi Jews in that 12 of the 14 mutant E3 alleles carry this mutation.[374]

Biochemical Mechanisms for MSUD. As described above, the human BCKD complex is a multiprotein component enzyme complex. Intricate protein-to-protein interactions are required for the catalytic function of the BCKD complex.[92,117,118] Considerable genetic heterogeneity in MSUD has been demonstrated (see "Molecular Phenotypes: The Affected Loci," above), and mutations in different subunits are known (see Table 87-4). However, the progress in understanding the biochemical consequences of MSUD mutations has been slow, due to the complexity and low abundance of the enzyme complex in tissues. In earlier studies, kinetic analysis of the mutant enzyme complex and each component was carried out.[114,319,355,356] Results from these early investigations showed that the mutant BCKD complex had reduced affinity for BCKAs.[114,340,355] This provided a basis to explain the accumulation of BCAAs and BCKAs in plasma and urine.[58,266,267] Recent determination of the x-ray crystal structure of the human E1 component has provided a basis for understanding the effects of MSUD mutations on the structure/function and assembly of the BCKD complex. The following subsection describes our current understanding of the biochemical mechanisms underlying MSUD.

Structural Perspectives of Type IA and Type IB Mutations. There are 19 known missense mutations that cause amino acid substitution in the E1α and E1β subunits of the human E1 heterotetramer (Table 87-4). Based on the human E1 structure, these mutations can be classified into three subgroups. Group 1 contains mutations affecting cofactor TPP-binding. As described above, the TPP-binding pocket in human E1 is formed by $\alpha \mid \beta'$ and $\alpha' \mid \beta$ subunit interactions (Fig. 87-3). The most notable mutation in this group, N222S-α, is involved in coordinating to the Mg^{2+} ion (Fig. 87-5). Asn-222 provides a ligand to the metal ion through the side-chain carbonyl group, which cannot be replaced by the hydroxyl group of the Ser side chain. R114W-α and R220W-α are two similar mutations in that each wild-type residue binds to a phosphate groups of TPP through ionic interactions. Replacement of either residue with an aromatic Trp residue disrupts the charge interaction required for tight TPP binding. An intriguing mutation is the T166M-α, which is involved in the ligation to K^+ in one of the novel metal ion-binding sites. Because K^+ binding stabilizes the TPP-binding pocket, a disruption of the metal ion coordination by T166M-α interferes with cofactor binding.

Group 2 encompasses mutations that impair subunit interactions. The most notable mutations in this group are the Y393N-α, F364C-α and Y368C-α mutations. These wild-type aromatic residues are located in the so-called Mennonite region, or C-terminal portion of the E1α subunit. It was previously shown that the Y393N-α mutation in homozygous Mennonite MSUD patients interferes with $\alpha_2\beta_2$ E1 assembly, resulting in preferential degradation of the E1β subunit.[21] The human E1 structure discloses that Tyr-393 and Phe-364 in the α subunit are hydrogen-bonded to residues in the β' subunit (Fig. 87-6). Mutations in these aromatic residues abolish the $\alpha \mid \beta'$ or $\alpha' \mid \beta$ interactions that are necessary for dimerization of the $\alpha\beta$ heterodimeric intermediates. This results in permanently locked inactive heterodimers as shown in an earlier study.[127] The Y368C-α mutation is related to the interaction between $\alpha \mid \beta$ and $\alpha' \mid \beta'$ subunit interactions. The substitution with a Cys residue is likely to impede the formation of the heterodimeric intermediate during E1 assembly. Other mutations in the E1α subunit that belong to this group are A209D-α, A240P-α, G245R-α, and R252H-α. The two known type IB missense mutations, H156R-β and N126Y-β, also alter E1 subunit interactions. His156-β is critical for homologous $\beta \mid \beta'$ interactions. The side chain of His156-β in one β subunit is, like a knob, embedded in a pocket formed by residues in the other β subunit. Substitution of His-156 with an

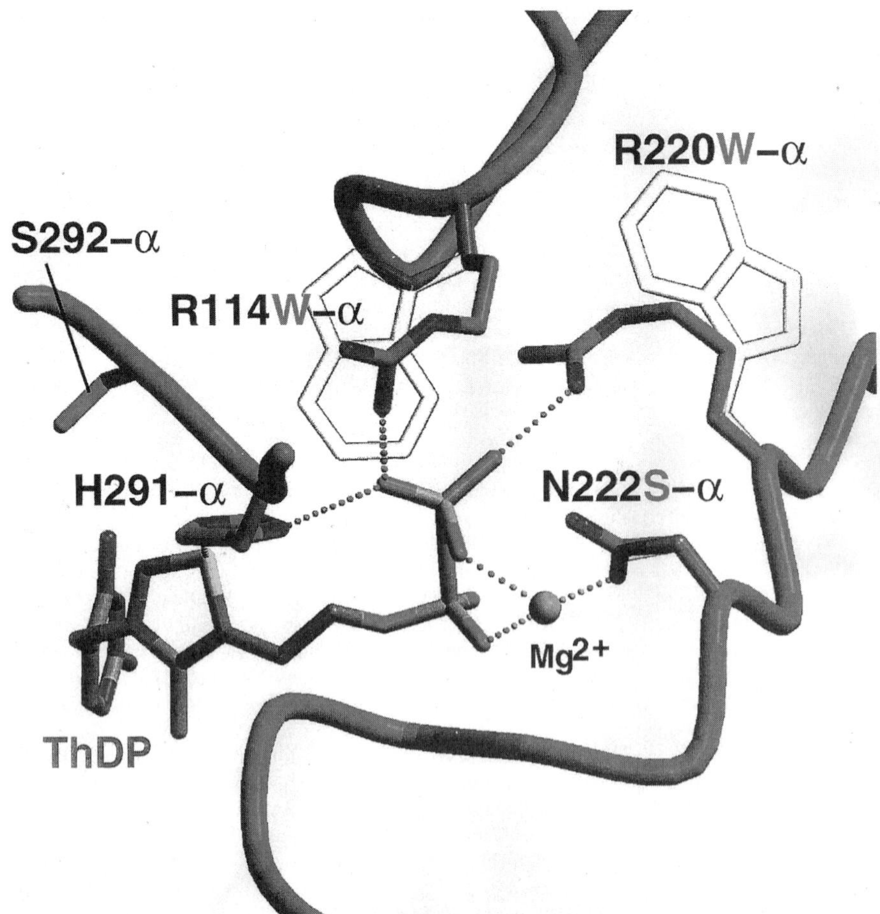

Fig. 87-5 Type IA (E1α) missense mutations affecting cofactor binding. N222S-α is involved in coordination with the Mg^{2+} ion. Asn222-α is the last residue in the thiamine diphosphate (ThDP)-binding motif Gly-Asp-Gly$(X)_{22-30}$NN. Substitution with a Ser residue in the N222S-α mutation abolishes a ligand provided by the carbonyl group of the wild-type residue. R114W-α and R220W-α are similar in that each wild-type residue interacts with an oxygen atom in the terminal phosphate group in ThDP. Replacement in each case with an aromatic Trp residue disrupts the interaction, resulting in the inability of human E1 to bind the cofactor. Ser292-α is site 1 for phosphorylation by the BCKD kinase. His291-α may be involved in catalysis,[124] in addition to coordinating with the cofactor terminal phosphate group. (*From Aevarsson et al.*[125] *Reproduced by permission.*)

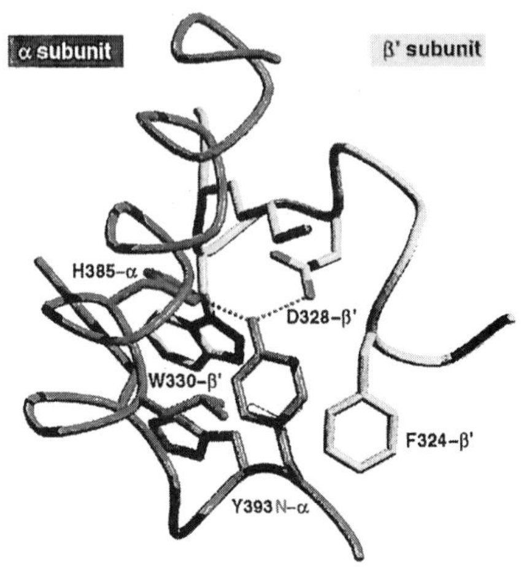

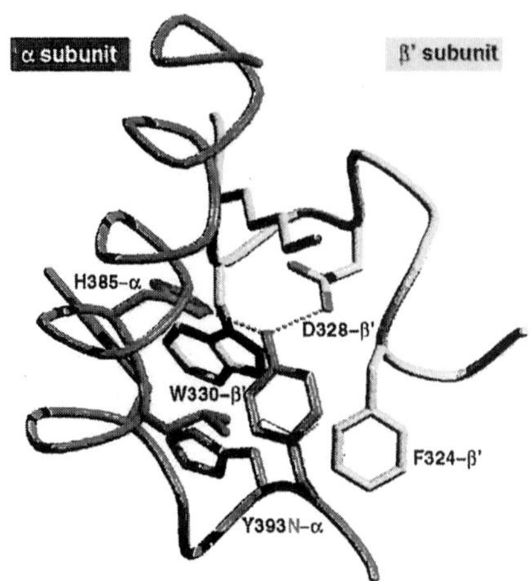

Fig. 87-6 Stereo view of the Y393N-α mutation affecting subunit interactions. This type IA MSUD mutation prevalent in the Mennonite population is located at the interface between the small C-terminal domain of the α subunit and the β' subunit. Tyr393-α is packed in between the side chains of Phe324-β and Trp330-β'. The hydroxyl group of Tyr393-α makes hydrogen bond with side chains of His385-α and Asp328-β'. The Y393N-α mutation disrupts $\alpha | \beta'$ and $\alpha' | \beta$ subunit interfaces, resulting in inability of $\alpha\beta'$ and $\alpha'\beta$ heterodimers to assemble into a functional $\alpha_2\beta_2$ heterotetramer of E1. See Fig. 87-3 for the designation of E1 subunits. *(From Aevarsson et al.*[125] *Reproduced by permission.)*

Arg residue disrupts the normal hydrogen bonding between H156-β and residues on the β' subunit. These adverse effects prevent association between the two β subunits during the $\alpha_2\beta_2$ assembly of human E1.

Group 3 comprises mutations affecting the hydrophobic core of E1. The T265R-α and I281T-α mutations in the E1α subunit are adjacent to each other and are in the hydrophobic core of the human E1. Introduction of a large and charged Arg side chain in T265R-α, or of a polar Thr side chain in I281T-α, disrupts the packing of the hydrophobic core, resulting in a dysfunctional E1. Other mutations in this group are G204S-α, A208T-α, and M64T-α. The identification of missense mutations affecting the hydrophobic core of the E1α subunits raises the possibility for development of chemical therapeutics. Small molecules, such as osmolytic electrolytes (e.g., trimethylamine N-oxide), have been used to correct the temperature-sensitive folding defects of Δ508 mutation in CFTR in cell culture.[375] These compounds exert their beneficial effects by increasing hydrophobic packing on tight binding to the protein. It remains to be seen whether this approach will ameliorate the MSUD phenotype due to mutations in the hydrophobic core.

Strong Correlation Between Thiamine-Responsive MSUD and Type II (E2) Mutations. Since the first description of a thiamine-responsive MSUD patient (WG-34) by Scriver and associates,[330] the biochemical mechanism for this clinical phenotype has been a subject of intense interest.[331] It was speculated that the E1 component was defective as it uses TPP, a derivative of thiamine for decarboxylation of BCKAs. There are conflicting reports, however, as to whether the BCKD complex from WG-34 has a reduced affinity or elevated K_m for the cofactor TPP.[332,376] A kinetic study proposes that the reduced affinity for the cofactor of the mutant BCKD complex accounts for beneficial effects of thiamine supplements in the patient's diet.[332] Other studies suggest that saturating TPP concentrations are capable of stabilizing the BCKD complex by attenuating the turnover of the enzyme complex.[333,377–379] However, a very recent report shows that excess dietary thiamine does not induce greater amounts of the BCKD complex in rat liver, nor do the resultant elevations in mitochondrial TPP levels affect the stability of the BCKD complex or the activity of its kinase.[377]

On the other hand, the discovery that the E2 component is deficient in Scriver's thiamine-responsive patient (WG-34) was unexpected.[370] This finding was later confirmed by nucleotide sequencing, which showed that the sequences of both the E1α and E1β subunits in WG-34 are normal.[378] As described above, the WG-34 thiamine-responsive patient was shown to carry F215C and IVSdel[−3.2 kb : −14] type II MSUD mutations in the E2 subunit.[372] Another thiamine-responsive patient was later studied by whole-body [1-^{13}C]-leucine oxidation while on a BCAA-restricted diet; thiamine supplements at 200 mg/day increased her rate of $^{13}CO_2$ release from undetectable to 14.2 percent of normal levels.[379] This patient is compound-heterozygous for the K278K and the 15- to 20-kb deletion alleles.[251] Two additional documented thiamine-responsive patients have also been studied.[333,341] Both patients were found to carry type II mutations; one is compound-heterozygous for the P73R and G292R substitutions and the other carries a R223G substitution and the IVSdel[−3.2kb : −14] deletion.[371] A survey of the known MSUD mutations in Table 87-4 shows that 10 of the 27 type II alleles, including the aforementioned, are associated with the thiamine-responsive phenotype. These data establish a good correlation between the thiamine-responsive phenotype and the type II MSUD mutations. Equally important, thus far none of the type IA (E1α-deficient) MSUD patients exhibit a thiamine-responsive phenotype. It should also be noted that 10 other type II mutations in Table 87-4 are related to the milder intermediate or intermittent phenotype. These patients are not reported to be thiamine-responsive. Nevertheless, the recommendation is that these type II MSUD patients should receive thiamine supplements in their diets, which on a long-term basis may prove beneficial.

The biochemical mechanism for thiamine response in type II MSUD patients remains unknown. Because a normal E1 component is present in these patients, TPP may exert its residual effects by augmenting residual E1 activity. The requirement for high doses of thiamine may be explained by a reduced affinity of E1 for TPP in the absence of a normal E2 component. Additional biochemical studies are needed to substantiate or differentiate these possibilities.

Genetics

MSUD is an autosomal recessive metabolic disorder of panethnic distribution. The worldwide frequency based on routine screening data from 26.8 million newborns is approximately 1 in 185,000[380] (EW Naylor, personal communication, February 11, 1993). This frequency includes both the classic and certain variant forms of MSUD. Apparently, a number of patients with the intermediate phenotype have been missed because the infant is on a low-protein diet.[381] The frequency in a Georgia population appears to be significantly higher at 1 in 84,000. This value is based on virtually 100 percent compliance with routine screening of 756,163 newborns over an 8-year period.[382] In countries where consanguineous marriage is common (Saudi Arabia, Turkey, Spain, and India), the frequency is also higher. MSUD is highly prevalent in the inbred Mennonite population of Lancaster and Lebanon counties, Pennsylvania, occurring in approximately 1 in 176 newborns.[363] A large Mennonite kindred has been reported from Pennsylvania.[383] Eight families were studied with 70 members and 12 classic MSUD patients. Transmission is clearly autosomal recessive. All the Mennonite patients studied so far have had the classic

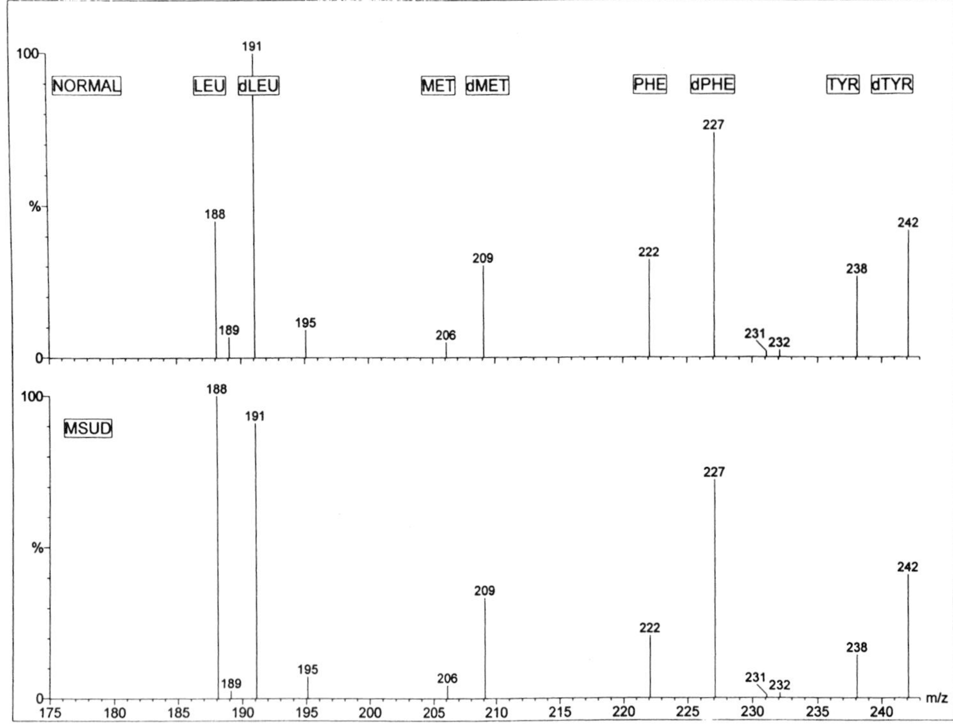

Fig. 87-7 MS-MS amino acid profile of blood on filter paper from two newborns, showing a normal pattern (top) and a maple syrup urine disease pattern (bottom). Leu = ion signal m/z 188, including leucine, isoleucine, and allo-isoleucine; dLeu = internal standard [$^2H_3$] Leucine. A deuterated internal standard is included for each amino acid (dMet, dPhe, dTyr). ***(Courtesy of Thomas Zytkovicz, New England Newborn Screening Program.)***

phenotype due to a single gene mutation in the E1α subunit.[204,281,282,383] In a study of 20 patients, Marshall and DiGeorge[363] were able to trace the lineage of all of them to one ancestral couple who emigrated from Europe early in the eighteenth century.

Screening and Diagnosis

Routine Newborn Screening. Newborn screening for MSUD has traditionally been performed by Guthrie bacterial inhibition assay. However, in the past few years, with advances in technology, automated tandem mass spectrometry has become the state-of-the-art technique for newborn screening. For the diagnosis of MSUD, the blood filter paper specimens are subjected to a solvent extraction and a butyl ester derivatization procedure. The fragmentation pattern of the protonated molecular ions of leucine and its isomers are similar and the signal at m/z 188 measures the sum of these isomers (Fig. 87-7). Because the three isomers—leucine, isoleucine, and alloisoleucine—are all elevated in this disorder, a high concentration of the total ions, and a high ratio in reference to phenylalanine, is diagnostic of MSUD in newborns.

A blood leucine level greater than 4 mg/dl, or a level of 3 to 4 mg/dl (305 mM) in the first 24 h of life, requires immediate notification of the infant's physician. Patients with classic MSUD, the intermediate form, and E3 deficiency[384] can usually be detected by screening in the newborn period. It is unlikely that patients with the intermittent form can be detected, as their blood BCAA levels are normal when asymptomatic. Thiamine-responsive MSUD cases have been missed by newborn screening.[380]

Amino Acid and Organic Acid Analysis. When the patient presents with clinical symptoms, the diagnosis can be made easily by amino acid analysis or organic acid profiling. The BCAAs are greatly increased in the blood, cerebrospinal fluid, and urine, and the presence of alloisoleucine is pathognomonic for MSUD. The elevated "methionine" peak initially identified in the urine of MSUD patients[385] was later shown to be L-alloisoleucine.[276,386] The formation of L-alloisoleucine occurs through racemization of L-isoleucine and a keto-enol tautomerization and transamination of KMV by the BCAA aminotransferase.[276,387–390] This metabolite has a delayed clearance, and high levels persist in the plasma for several days following an episode of decompensation. It is detectable in classic MSUD patients at all times. A low plasma alanine is consistently found during metabolic decompensation and is secondary to the consumption of alanine for reamination of the increased BCKAs and for gluconeogenesis. In encephalopathic patients, the blood: cerebrospinal fluid ratios of BCAAs and of BCKAs, as well as the concentrations of alanine, glutamine, and lysine, are reduced.[275,391,392] The urine 2,4-dinitrophenylhydrazine (DNPH) test is a simple test for α-keto acids and is useful for preliminary screening.[393] It is usually positive when the plasma leucine is approximately 700 mM or higher. The urine is mixed with an equal amount of the reagent (0.1 percent DNPH in 2 N HC1), and a yellow precipitate within 10 min is a positive reaction. Acidification of the urine also intensifies the maple syrup odor.

Gas chromatographic-mass spectroscopy (GC-MS) analysis of urine and plasma organic acids as their oxime-trimethylsilyl (TMS)[394] or quinoxalinol derivatives gives characteristic profiles.[395,396] The hydroxy analogue of the valine keto acid, α-hydroxyisovalerate is the major hydroxylated metabolite in urine and is diagnostic of MSUD, whereas most of the KIC and KMV are excreted as the keto acids with only small amounts of the α-hydroxy analogues. The major keto acid accumulated in blood is KIC due to low renal clearance and inefficient hydroxylation.[391,397–399] During the acute phase, large increases of ketones are found in both the blood and the urine. In patients with the intermittent form of MSUD, the metabolic profile is normal during remission, and the diagnosis can be made only when the patient is symptomatic. A twofold increase of the BCAAs in response to fasting for 3 to 4 days is known to occur in normal individual,[382] and in ketotic hypoglycemia.[365] Such transient elevations of BCAAs without the appearance of alloisoleucine should not be mistaken for MSUD. Mild-to-moderate elevation of the BCAA in association with increases of lactate, pyruvate, α-ketoglutarate, and the BCKAs and their hydroxy derivatives is diagnostic of E3 deficiency.[400,401]

A close linear relationship between elevated BCAA and BCKA level in plasma has been observed in plasma from MSUD patients, and adequate monitoring of therapy can be accomplished by the determination of plasma BCAAs.[394,398] Early detection is possible in infants at high risk for MSUD, such as sibs of known patients, using quantitative amino acid analysis of a few drops of blood collected in a capillary tube or on filter paper. Five of seven infants with the classic form who were studied had clearly elevated BCAAs and detectable alloisoleucine within 24 h of life, irrespective of type of feeding.[289,402,403] However, alloisoleucine, the marker for MSUD, may not appear until as long as the sixth day of life despite elevated leucine level.[404,405] A trace amount of alloisoleucine was detected in the cord plasma of one newborn whose MSUD was diagnosed prenatally (U Caruso and R Cerone, personal communication, February 1, 1993). Urine metabolic screening is less sensitive than plasma amino acid analysis for the early diagnosis of MSUD. Changes in urine amino acids may be minimal even when the plasma BCAAs are already two to four times above normal. A distinctive odor of maple syrup or burnt sugar is easily detected on a wet diaper, or in earwax (H Morton, unpublished observation), but the odor is less obvious in urine from older patients. The chemical responsible for the odor, a mystery for many years, has recently been identified as sotolone (4,5-dimethyl-3-hydroxy-2[5H]-furanone) and is probably derived from isoleucine or alloisoleucine.[406] In breast-fed newborns, a sweet urine odor from spices or curry in the maternal diet may be confused with maple syrup.[407] Cleaning the umbilical cord with Betadine also may leave an odor that resembles maple syrup.

Cell-Culture and Whole-Body Studies. The direct determination of MSUD requires enzymatic studies of cells or cell cultures from patients. Postmortem material was largely unsatisfactory because of the instability of the BCKD complex.[268,408] Leukocytes from MSUD subjects were previously used to demonstrate deficiency in decarboxylation of [1-^{14}C]-labeled leucine, isoleucine, and valine.[93,270] The leukocyte population, however, consists of several cell types that contribute to variability of the decarboxylation rate. Moreover, fresh preparations must be assayed. Cultured skin fibroblasts[357,409] and lymphoblasts[280,410] are suitable for diagnostic studies, as they are relatively homogeneous cell populations. Decarboxylation of [1-^{14}C]-labeled BCAAs was conveniently used as substrate for assays of cultured fibroblasts due to their stability and low background activity. Micromethods using as few as 5000 to 50,000 cultured fibroblasts or 200 ml of blood have been described.[411,412]

BCKAs, on the other hand, are more direct substrates than BCAAs for measuring BCKD complex activity.[356,413] They do not require aminotransferase reaction in the cell. The disadvantage of using BCKAs is their instability and high background $^{14}CO_2$ release. [1-^{14}C]-labeled BCKA can be readily prepared from [1-^{14}C]-labeled BCAA, as described by Rudiger et al.,[414] using L-amino acid oxidase. Activity of the BCKD complex can be measured either by intact[332,357,415,416] or disrupted cell assay.[332,357,359,367,413,416] The former is carried out by incubating harvested cells in isotonic saline buffer with 1 mM [1-^{14}C]-labeled BCKAs.[313,340] Decarboxylation of [1-^{14}C]-labeled pyruvate or α-ketoglutarate can be used as a control. The disrupted cell assay allows measurement of the BCKD complex activity in vitro. The enzymatic assay is carried out in the presence of cofactors NAD^+, CoA, TPP, and $MgCl_2$.[332] The cells are disrupted by freezing and thawing, and the inclusion of 1 to 2 percent fetal-calf serum in the assay mixture is important for inhibiting proteolysis of the enzyme complex. Alternatively, mitochondrial inner membranes, where the BCKD complex resides, were prepared from cultured fibroblasts for enzymatic assay.[413] The measurement of BCKD activity using disrupted cells or inner membrane preparations is difficult, and not recommended for routine diagnosis. Nonetheless, the enzymatic assay is needed to establish the deficiency of the BCKD complex in MSUD cells. For diagnostic purposes, the enzymatic assay should be carried out at low BCKA concentrations (<1 mM). The mutant BCKD complex from MSUD cells exhibits significant residual activity at high α-keto acid concentrations.[356,417,418] The total activity of the BCKD complex in cultured fibroblasts can be measured by incubating cells with the kinase inhibitor α-chloroisocaproate prior to the disrupted cell assay.[358,419] The preincubation results in dephosphorylation of the enzyme complex by the intrinsic phosphatase, while the kinase reaction is blocked.

Heterozygote detection by assaying both intact leukocytes and cultured skin fibroblasts for leucine or BCKA decarboxylation has largely been unsatisfactory because of the overlap in the rate of $^{14}CO_2$ production from obligate heterozygotes and controls.[411] Assay of the individual components of the BCKD complex, using a disrupted cell suspension, may allow better discrimination between heterozygotes and normals.[358] In families in which the mutations are known, and for inbred populations such as the Mennonites, allele-specific oligonucleotide (ASO) probing using DNA prepared from blood or cultured cells can detect carriers.[205,281,282,359]

Elsas et al.[420] assessed whole-body leucine oxidation by a noninvasive breath test. They quantified $^{13}CO_2$ in expired air after an oral dose of a stable isotope labeled L-[1-^{13}C]-leucine. The cumulative oxidation of oral leucine at 60 and 90 min in six adult obligate heterozygotes was significantly different from controls. Schadewaldt et al.[421] reexamined this experimental approach and observed considerable interindividual and intraindividual variability. They concluded that the noninvasive breath test yielded only limited information on whole body leucine oxidation.

Prenatal Diagnosis. Direct analysis of tissue from CVS and cells cultured from CVS or amniotic fluid can be used reliably for prenatal diagnosis,[422] but the use of uncultured amniotic fluid cells is not reliable.[423] The BCKD complex activity in cultured amniocytes and chorionic villus is in the same range as in cultured skin fibroblasts.[358,411] Prenatal diagnosis of MSUD has been achieved using intact amniocytes cultured from midtrimester (week 14 to 18 of gestation) amniotic fluid by measurement of decarboxylation of [1-^{14}C]-labeled BCKA,[411,424,425] or BCAA,[423,426–428] in cell suspensions, or in monolayers on microtiter plates. In two cases in which the amniocyte culture was epithelioid and slow growing, the diagnosis was uncertain. At birth, one infant was affected[403] and another was unaffected (VE Shih, unpublished observation). First-trimester diagnosis of MSUD using direct CVS has been accomplished in two fetuses by incubation of tissue with [1-^{14}C] leucine as substrate.[422] A DNA-based prenatal diagnosis for MSUD with a CVS at risk for a known mutation has been reported.[416] Although there is clearly an advantage to early prenatal diagnosis, the safety of CVS is an issue,[429] and early transabdominal amniocentesis at approximately 11 weeks may be an alternative.[429] Molecular diagnosis by detection of known mutations in fetuses at risk should be possible by ASO probing of amplified DNA prepared directly from amniocytes, and a primer-specified restriction analysis has been described for the common mutation among Mennonite MSUD patients[383] (see Table 87-4). Attempts to achieve prenatal diagnosis of MSUD by determining the concentrations of BCAAs and the α-keto acids and their corresponding α-hydroxyacids in amniotic fluid were uniformly unsuccessful.[423,430–432] Prenatal diagnosis for the purpose of starting treatment may not be necessary, as the diagnosis of MSUD can be achieved by plasma amino acid analysis in the first day or two of life.

Neuroradiologic Findings

Neuroradiologic studies in untreated patients often reveal abnormalities that correspond well to the underlying neuropathology of this disease. In a series of 10 infants with the classic form and 2 with variant forms of MSUD studied by Brismar et al.,[433] 26 CT scans and 13 MRI studies were performed. Both untreated and treated patients between ages 3 days and 27 months were studied. Their findings are representative of the early encephalopathic changes, which have also been observed by other investigators (Fig. 87-8). The CT scans were within normal limits in two 3-day-old asymptomatic patients, who were identified because of older

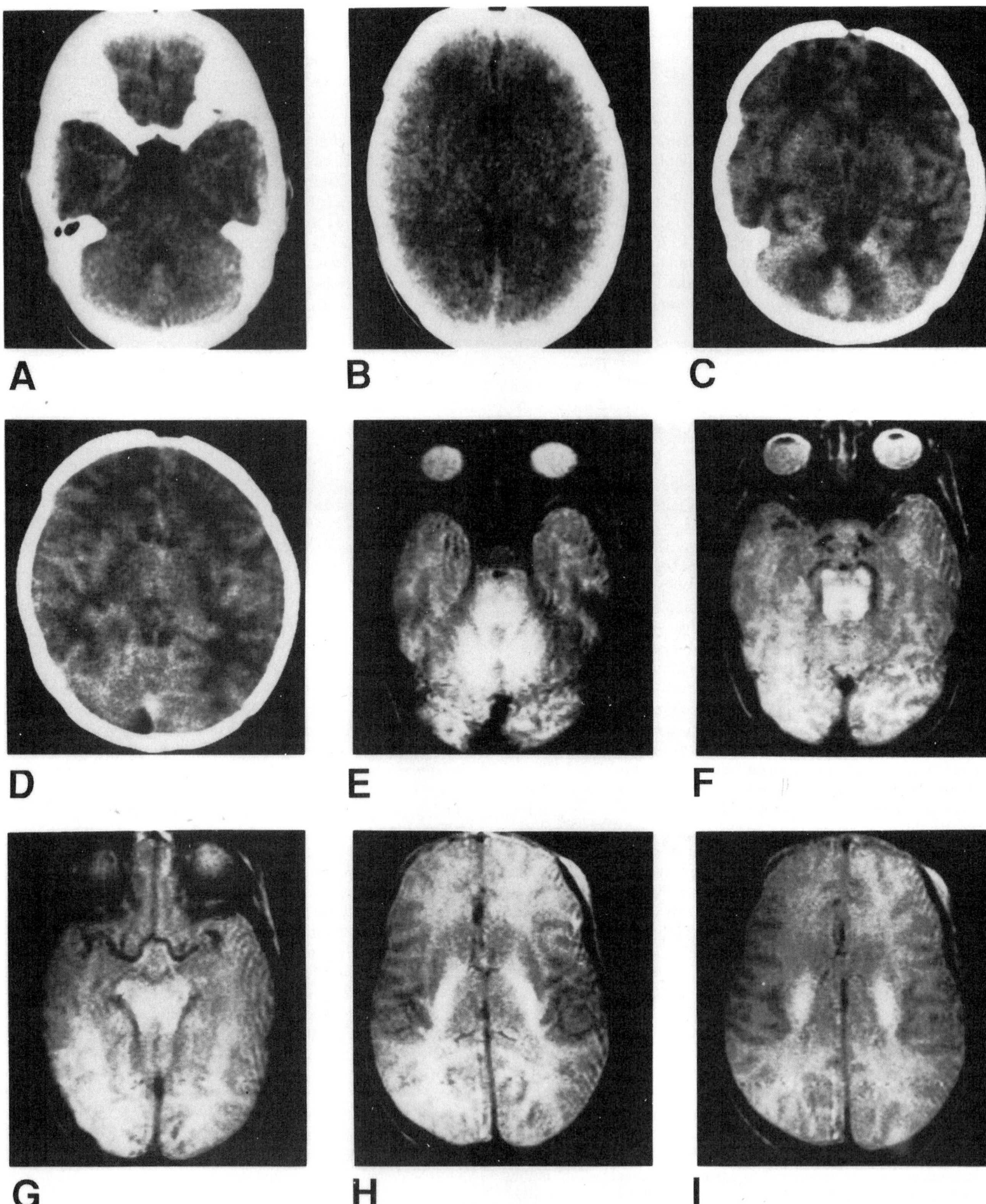

Fig. 87-8 Serial imaging studies of the brain from an infant male with classic MSUD. *A* and *B*, CT scan at age 3 days, before any symptoms had developed; findings are normal for age. *C* and *D*, Repeat CT scans 6 days later when the infant exhibited severe convulsions and myoclonus; findings are a severe generalized edema. *E* through *I*, T2-weighted axial MRI (2000/90) at age 22 days, which clear shows the distribution of severe intense localized edema. (*From Brismar et al.*[433] *Used with permission.*)

affected sibs (Figs. 87-8A and 87-8B). Neurologic symptoms developed in one of these infants after treatment with a restricted diet for 2 days. A second CT scan performed at 9 days of age showed severe diffuse generalized edema (Figs. 87-8C and 87-8D). Similar radiologic findings were observed in four untreated patients examined between 2 and 6 weeks of age. In addition to the generalized edema, a unique localized intense edema involving the cerebellar deep white matter, the dorsal brain stem, the cerebral peduncles, the posterior limb of the internal capsule, and the posterior aspect of the centrum semiovale was found in 9 of the 10 patients studied (Figs. 87-8E through I). This pattern of edema was considered characteristic of MSUD by Brismar and colleagues[433] and was most prominent in the third week. The intense edema diminished after the third month to two small low-density (or high-T2-intensity on MRI) lesions dorsally in the brain stem. The generalized edema also disappeared, and low-attenuation changes were limited to periventricular white matter. Hypodensity was also observed in globus pallidus and thalamus, affecting the white matter tracts in these regions. These changes are indicators of hypomyelination. The acute phase was followed by widening of the sulci over the frontal lobes and of the interhemispheric and Sylvian fissures indicating cerebral atrophy.[415] In untreated variant patients, the imaging findings are similar to those in classic patients.[288,303,304,434,435] Findings suggestive of acute brain edema usually improve or resolve following short-term treatment.[436,437] Imaging studies of classic MSUD patients following long-term treatment (>10 years) may show changes suggestive of dysmyelination[288,436] depending on the degree of metabolic control over the years, however, some treated patients have had normal neuroradiologic examinations.[288,289,436]

Magnetic Resonance Spectroscopy

Localized proton magnetic resonance spectroscopy (1H-MRS) of the brain is a noninvasive method for studying the metabolic changes in disorders such as MSUD. Three patients (ages 9 years, 3.5 years, and newborn), all in acute metabolic decompensation, had a small inverted signal at a chemical shift of 0.9 to 1.0 ppm, which corresponds to the methyl residue of the BCAA and BCKA.[437–439] Follow-up studies in two patients showed that the disappearance of the resonance corresponded with clinical improvement.[437,439]

Neuropathology

Morphologic Changes. MSUD is a white-matter disease, and histopathologic studies confirm the abnormalities detected by imaging studies. The spongy changes in white matter and delayed myelination are not specific to MSUD, as they have also been observed in other metabolic disorders.[440,441] Severe brain edema is usually seen in MSUD patients who died during acute metabolic crisis.[288,295,440,442] In untreated cases, myelin deficiency and striking spongy degeneration of the white matter are prominent findings. A delay in myelination involves mainly the tracts normally myelinated after birth. The pyramidal tracts of the spinal cord, the myelin around the dentate nuclei, the corpus callosum, and the cerebral hemispheres are most affected. The reduction of oligodendrocytes parallels the extent of myelin deficiency. A moderate degree of astrocytic hypertrophy in the white matter was observed in all untreated as well as in some treated patients. Impressive alterations are also present in the cerebellum, where extensive necrosis of the granular-cell layer with preservation of the molecular and Purkinje cell layers was present. Considerable nerve-cell loss was present in the pontine nuclei and substantia nigra.[272] There is no evidence of myelin degradation, although dysmyelination has been reported.[288,443] The neurons and axons are usually well preserved. Golgi studies of the brain from a 6-year-old patient who died of cerebral edema showed aberrant orientation of neurons together with abnormalities of dendrites and dendritic spines.[442] Evidence suggestive of minor disturbance of neuronal migration also has been reported in three other patients.[440,444,445] In treated patients, the neuropathologic changes may be similar but of a lesser degree or the examination may be normal[288,440,446] (VE Shih, unpublished data).

Neurochemical Changes. The most prominent change in untreated subjects is the reduction of myelin lipids (cerebrosides, proteolipids, and sulfatides).[447,448] This finding corroborates the morbid anatomy of delayed myelination. These chemical changes are quite variable, but are less striking in very young patients. Normal values of brain lipids were reported in a 12-day-old patient.[447] Significant reduction of white matter lipids, particularly cerebrosides and proteolipids, were found in three other untreated patients who died at age 17 days,[449] 25 days,[448] and 20 months.[448] In contrast, the concentrations of these lipids were within normal ranges in most treated patients.[443,448,450,451] In one treated subject, abnormal protein and lipid composition of the cerebral myelin was described.[443] Free amino acids in the brain from a 25-day-old infant with untreated MSUD showed marked elevation of BCAAs and significant reduction of glutamate, glutamine, and GABA.[448,452]

EEG Findings. An unusual comb-like rhythm of 5 to 9 Hz spindle-like sharp waves over the central regions has been found in newborns with classic MSUD between the ages of 2 and 3 weeks, and is believed to be characteristic of MSUD.[288,453–456] Other major abnormalities include multiple shifting spikes and sharp waves with suppression bursts, and excessive delta activity is usually found when the infants are encephalopathic. These changes improve once the plasma BCAA levels are normalized. Leucine loading has provoked EEG abnormalities in an asymptomatic adult MSUD patient.[457]

Neuropathophysiology. The BCAAs, in particular leucine, are rapidly transported into the brain and actively metabolized. Yudkoff[458] proposed a leucine-glutamate cycle that plays an important role in maintaining a steady supply of glutamate, a major excitatory neurotransmitter for interneuronal communication. The BCAAs are nitrogen donors for glutamate synthesis in astrocytes, a major site of BCAA transamination. The amino group is transferred to α-ketoglutarate to yield glutamate. This amino acid is in turn converted to glutamine. By ^{15}N-labeled BCAA studies, at least one-third of the amino groups of brain glutamate are derived from BCAAs. The BCKAs may be released from astrocytes to the extracellular fluid and taken up by neurons. Although neurons can oxidize KIC, it is preferentially reaminated to leucine. The flux of the reverse transamination in rat cortical synaptosomes is several times greater than the rate of nitrogen transfer from leucine to glutamate. This is in contrast to the flux in astrocytes, which is mainly for glutamate synthesis. In the leucine oxidative pathway, acetoacetyl-CoA is generated for ketone synthesis or for cleavage to acetyl-CoA to enter the tricarboxylic acid cycle.

In MSUD, the excess BCAAs and their ketoacids interfere with the neuronal and astrocytic metabolism. By using a microdialysis technique, Parini et al. and Fukutomi et al.[459,460] showed that by perfusion with leucine and KIV, they created a microenvironment similar to that found in MSUD. The infusion of leucine resulted in an increase of large neutral amino acids in the extracellular space, thereby a decreased concentration in neurons. The infusion of KIC caused an elevenfold increase of leucine and two- to threefold increase of the other large neutral amino acids in the extracellular space. This pattern is consistent with active transamination of KIC to leucine. These changes could affect biosynthesis of serotonin and catecholamines, and alter the homeostasis of the leucine/glutamate cycle and the glutamate/glutamine cycle in brain.

Treatment

The management of hereditary deficiencies in the degradative pathway for essential amino acids requires limited intake of the specific amino acid(s) to that required for growth and development. This minimizes the accumulation of intermediates that damage organs, particularly the nervous system. Administration of individual BCAAs to patients with MSUD revealed that increased leucine was associated with the appearance of neurologic symptoms, whereas increased isoleucine led to an intensifying of the distinct maple syrup odor.[276] Valine loading does not have any clinical effects, except in one unusual patient with intermittent MSUD[329] who developed irritability, lethargy, acidosis, and hypoglycemia. Based on these observations, leucine and/or its ketoacid are considered the neurotoxic metabolites in MSUD, and the plasma leucine concentration is an important criterion for monitoring treatment.

There are two aspects to the treatment: long-term management and therapy during acute metabolic decompensation. Results of long-term management have shown that there is a positive correlation between good metabolic control and intellectual achievement. Life-long dietary treatment is necessary as potentially fatal episodes of decompensation may occur during periods of dietary indiscretion or stress, such as infection, fever, or other intercurrent illness at any age. Prompt therapy to reduce plasma levels of the toxic metabolites may require peritoneal dialysis or hemodialysis. Future developments, including liver transplantation and somatic gene therapy, may correct the underlying metabolic defect.

Long-Term Dietary Management. The principles of dietary management are to normalize the concentrations of blood BCAAs by limiting the intake of these three essential amino acids, while providing nutrition adequate to maintain growth and development in young patients. A trial of thiamine therapy, 50 to 300 mg/day for at least 3 weeks,[337] is advisable in every newly diagnosed patient to determine thiamine-responsiveness. Dietary treatment should continue throughout the patient's life.[457] Dietary therapy was first used in England. Gelatin was chosen as a source of BCAAs because of its relatively low BCAA content (leucine, 3.6 percent; isoleucine, 1.6 percent; valine, 2.8 percent) and was given with a supplement of modified casein hydrolysate from which most of the BCAAs had been removed by a cation exchange column.[275,461] In the United States, Snyderman et al. developed a synthetic formula in which the protein requirement was supplied in the form of a mixture of individual amino acids based on the amino acid composition of breast milk minus the BCAAs.[276] Carbohydrate, fat, and a mixture of minerals and vitamins were used to provide the remaining nutrients. This diet made it possible to adjust the intake of each of the BCAAs, guided by the patient's plasma levels.

Commercial medical diets have since been developed for MSUD, based on Snyderman's synthetic formula.[276] The prescribed diet for MSUD infants consists of a BCAA-free formula, prepared at 20 to 24 kcal/oz with an intake of 2 to 3 g amino acids/kg/day. The requirement for leucine is satisfied by a calculated amount of standard formula for infants and of natural foods in older patients. The isoleucine and valine content in natural food, especially cow's milk, is often low relative to leucine, and supplementation of these as free amino acids is often necessary to maintain normal plasma levels. Plasma BCAA levels should be kept as close to the normal range as possible, avoiding the situation of a high leucine level with low isoleucine and valine. A relaxed treatment protocol may not be adequate to prevent brain damage.[288] It is advisable to monitor the plasma BCAA levels weekly in the first 6 to 12 months of life. Later, the interval between testing can be gradually extended. Home monitoring of urine BCKAs by DNPH test is a useful adjunct in older patients.[462]

Patients with intermediate MSUD should be treated in a similar manner to those with the classic form. In some patients with high residual enzyme activity, protein restriction without supplements of the synthetic formula may be adequate. Because the BCAA levels are not elevated in patients with the intermittent form of MSUD, except during acute episodes, these patients can generally be treated with a reduction of protein intake during periods of stress. The daily BCAA requirement varies considerably with age, growth rate, and the severity of the enzyme defect. It is highest in the first 6 months of life. The leucine requirement in patients with classic MSUD stabilizes at approximately 2 to 3 years of life, and remains fairly constant during the first decade. The daily leucine requirement is in the range of 300 to 600 mg. The optimal intake of BCAA for MSUD patients should be individualized and is often only two-thirds to one-half of the recommended requirements for normal children.[457,463–469] A system similar to that used for dietary control of diabetic patients uses leucine equivalents and exchange lists.[470,471] When a patient is on a semisynthetic diet, there is a risk of nutritional imbalance and every effort should be make to include adequate amounts of vitamins, minerals, and trace elements. Insufficient intake of isoleucine or leucine resulting in an altered ratio of plasma leucine to isoleucine is associated with dermatologic complications. Papillary eruptions around the mouth have been described with an apparently mild deficiency of isoleucine.[472] Severe deficiency is associated with a generalized rash resembling acrodermatitis enteropathica[473] or with extensive dermatitis in the perineal region. Deficiency of valine or leucine is also manifested as a papillary and macular rash over the trunk or in some cases in the diaper area. It is indistinguishable in appearance from common "heat rash" or "allergic rash." The dermatitis typically disappears within 24 to 48 h after increase in the intake of these amino acids.

It is well known that infection often precipitates acute decompensation with complications. Animal studies have shown that amino acid imbalance, especially excessive leucine, and malnutrition have immunosuppressive effects.[474] During infection, and occasionally during the incubation period, tolerance to food protein is lower.[475] Behavioral changes and loss of appetite are often the first signs of metabolic perturbation. Immediate reduction of dietary protein and substitution of BCAA-free synthetic formulas and protein-free foods are instituted to ensure adequate caloric intake. Such nutritional changes can prevent the rise of plasma BCAAs and BCKAs to toxic levels. Prompt treatment of bacterial infection also prevents further deterioration. Oral bicarbonate administration in the form of citric acid-sodium citrate may be used at home as symptomatic relief. Measles and smallpox vaccinations have precipitated acute ketoacidosis 8 to 10 days after inoculation in two patients with undiagnosed and untreated MSUD.[310,328] On the other hand, routine childhood immunizations have been administered without complications to infants under good metabolic control.[289,461] Pharmacologic doses of thiamine, 10 to 1000 mg/day, in conjunction with moderate restriction of protein intake, may be effective in preventing episodes of ketoacidosis in thiamine-responsive patients.[340]

Acute-Phase Management. Marked accumulation of the BCAAs and their ketoacids leads to acute deterioration of cerebral functions. This is a life-threatening situation, and aggressive treatment is imperative. Clinical improvement is not possible until tissue catabolism is reversed. There are two aspects to management of this metabolic crisis: rapid removal of the putative toxic metabolites and minimizing the catabolic state and/or promoting anabolism. Experience suggests that promoting anabolism may be the one most important factor in acute-phase management. The best results have been achieved by a regimen that combines all or most of these measures.

For metabolite removal, peritoneal dialysis was first used in 1969 with significant improvement in the neurologic status within hours.[446,476,477] The advantage of peritoneal dialysis is that it is relatively simple to implement, however, other studies have suggested that continuous venovenous hemofiltration may be more effective in BCAA/BCKA clearance.[478,479] These invasive procedures are very effective in reducing the BCAAs and their keto acids from very high levels (3 to 5 mM) to approximately 1 mM, but are minimally effective below that level.[457,464,479,480] The choice of procedure depends on the availability and expertise at each locale. They are useful for the initial treatment of severe metabolic decompensation to rapidly dispose of toxic metabolites. For high-risk infants whose diagnosis is made in the first 3 days of life before severe metabolic crisis develops, aggressive nutritional therapy may eliminate the need for invasive procedures.

There are several approaches to treatment of the catabolic state in MSUD and promoting anabolism. Parenteral nutrition therapy[481–483] can be used alone in anorexic patients in mild metabolic decompensation, or in combination with other therapy in severe metabolic decompensation. The preparation consists of a BCAA-free L-amino acid mixture in combination with glucose, lipid, electrolytes, and vitamins to provide balanced nutrition. The composition of the amino acid mixture is modeled after that of the MSUD formula or that of standard total parenteral nutrition but with the omission of the BCAAs. The plasma concentrations of isoleucine and valine will drop faster than leucine during treatment. Thus, it is necessary to replace these two amino acids after 1 or 2 days of treatment. When the ratio of plasma leucine to isoleucine is high, the response to treatment is poor. Raising the isoleucine and valine levels facilitates the normalization of plasma leucine level.[484] One MSUD patient with the rare complication of chronic pancreatitis and a pancreaticopleural fistula, was successfully treated with MSUD-modified total parenteral nutrition for 45 days, until resolution of his fistula.[296]

Insulin and other treatments have been used in MSUD to stimulate anabolism. A large glucose infusion combined with subcutaneous regular insulin can result in a rapid decline of blood leucine.[464,481,485] A fall in plasma amino acids has been observed following the administration of human growth hormone.[486] Morton studied a teenaged patient who developed a hypercatabolic state following brain surgery that was unresponsive to insulin infusion and MSUD hyperalimentation, even with a high caloric intake of 180 kcal/kg/day.[487] He hypothesized that the abnormal hypermetabolic state was most likely related to catecholamine release secondary to the surgery on the brain stem. Within 24 h after the addition of IV propranolol (a catecholamine antagonist), the blood leucine level declined from 2135 to 915 mM and to nearly normal (229 mM) in the next 24-h period. Another patient in metabolic decompensation was treated similarly and also responded favorably.

Nyhan et al.[488] developed enteral (nasogastric) amino acid mixtures devoid of BCAAs but rich in alanine for patients in metabolic crisis. The composition was modified daily to include sufficient isoleucine and valine to maintain a normal plasma level. The preparations were used in combination with intravenous glucose and electrolytes during three acute episodes in two patients, a 2-year-old boy and a 9-year-old boy, and both responded well. Parini et al.[489] used continuous nasogastric feeding of a normal to high caloric BCAA-free diet to treat four neonates with decompensation. The initial blood leucine levels of 3.0 to 3.3 mM were reduced to <0.5 mM in 7 to 12 days. The long-term consequences of this slow response in the newborn period are still unknown. On the other hand, nasogastric feeding of BCAA-free formula to anorexic patients during subsequent episodes has effectively corrected metabolic ketoacidosis in a few days.

Management of Surgery. Surgery is a stressful situation that can precipitate a metabolic crisis in patients with MSUD.[316] There are three case reports describing such occurrences after major surgery and all patients recovered with proper management. One 2-year-old patient with MSUD deteriorated neurologically after open-heart surgery for the repair of tetralogy of Fallot. She was successfully treated with peritoneal dialysis and parenteral nutrition.[490] Another 17-year-old woman with classic MSUD underwent spondylodesis in two stages for progressive scoliosis. Insulin was necessary to stabilize the plasma leucine level after the first surgery.[491] An 8-year-old patient with the intermediate form of MSUD recovered from surgery for hip dislocation complicated by moderate increase of plasma leucine.[492] A 1-year-old and a 5-year-old patient had smooth recoveries from minor surgery.[493]

Liver Transplantation and Organ Donation. Two patients with classic MSUD, treated by diet therapy from the first week of life with normal development received orthotopic liver transplant because of liver failure caused by fulminant hepatitis A virus infection in one patient[478] and vitamin A intoxication in the other.[494] These patients have remained metabolically and neurologically stable on an unrestricted diet for more than 2 years. Alloisoleucine was still detectable in plasma at a low level in the first patient, but was not detectable in the other patient, except with catabolic stress. It appears that the KMV remaining in muscle exceeds the capacity of the muscle residual BCKD complex activity and is converted to alloisoleucine.[387] This finding supports the experimental data that although most of the keto acids are exported to the liver, there is normally a significant amount of BCAA decarboxylation occurring in the skeletal muscle.[80] This study adds MSUD to the list of inborn errors of metabolism that have been corrected by liver transplantation, and such therapy might be considered for severe cases of the classic form.

Information regarding the suitability of organ donation by patients with inborn errors of metabolism is limited. A recent experience of successful transplantation of kidney, pancreas, cornea, and long bones from a 22-year-old patient, who was well treated for his MSUD and in good health before the terminal episode of encephalopathy, highlights the potential for organ donation from patients with this and other inborn errors of metabolism.[495]

Somatic Gene Therapy. MSUD appears to be a suitable disease for attempting somatic gene therapy because increasing enzyme activity by a few percent can alter the phenotype from classic to intermittent.[274] Moreover, as described above, the BCKAs from skeletal muscle circulate in plasma.[10,49,50] These keto acids may be degraded by genetically reconstituted endothelial cells or hepatocytes with significant BCKD complex activity. Studies on the transfer of normal E1α[204] and E2[205,206] cDNA into MSUD cells have restored near-normal BCKD complex activity to cells deficient in these subunits. These experiments used a plasmid for transient expression to correct the MSUD phenotype. The results show that the recombinant normal subunit is imported into mitochondria, where the mature peptide is capable of assembling with other endogenous normal subunits to form a functional BCKD complex. A stable gene transfer into MSUD cells has been reported.[286] In this preliminary study, a normal E1α cDNA was inserted into a modified Maloney murine leukemia retroviral vector, and the packaged recombinant virus was used to transduce cultured E1α-deficient lymphoblasts from a Mennonite MSUD patient. Stable chromosomal integration and persistent restoration of the BCKD complex activity were achieved. A later study shows that type II MSUD with a deficient E2 subunit can also be stably corrected by retroviral-mediated transfer of a normal E2 cDNA into cultured fibroblasts derived from the patient.[287] Decarboxylation of [1-^{14}C] leucine in transduced MSUD cells was restored to 93 percent of the normal level. Stable expression and correct targeting of the recombinant normal E2 protein to mitochondria were demonstrated. These studies may represent the first step for developing somatic gene therapy in animal models,[283,284] and subsequently in MSUD patients.

Pregnancy in MSUD

There are only a few reports of successful pregnancies in women with organic acidemias.[496,497] MSUD women who were treated early have only recently reached reproductive age. A major concern for MSUD women is the stress of pregnancy on metabolic homeostasis in conjunction with rapidly changing nutritional requirements during the course of the pregnancy. These parameters require careful monitoring. Van Calcar et al.[497] recently described a successful pregnancy in a 25-year-old woman with classic MSUD who was treated from the age of 11 days. In the first 6 years of life, she required 11 hospitalizations for metabolic decompensation.[470] Despite these complications, her IQ was greater than 100 but her visual motor skills were below average. When evaluated at 11 weeks of gestation, her blood BCAA levels were normal. In the first trimester, her diet consisted of 1.2 g/kg/day total protein, 0.6 g of food protein, and 0.6 g protein equivalents from BCAA-free formula. This diet was similar to her usual diet except that the protein equivalents from the BCAA-free formula were increased from 0.4 to 0.6 g/kg/day. In the second trimester, an increased food protein intake of 0.8 g/kg/day was necessary to maintain low-normal blood BCAA levels. Carnitine supplementation was required at 50 mg/kg/day to maintain normal blood levels. In the thirty-seventh week of gestation, she was hospitalized for dietary adjustment because of slow fetal growth and low plasma-free carnitine. Her daily food protein intake was increased to 1.5 g/kg and carnitine to 150 mg/kg. The patient gave birth to a 2.6-kg girl following an uneventful labor and delivery, and the infant has no detectable congenital anomalies. The infant was developmentally normal at 2 years of age and growing at the fifth percentile (SC Van Calcar, personal communication, December 10, 1992). After delivery, the mother's daily total protein intake was reduced to 1 g/kg food protein and 0.6 g/kg BCAA-free formula. The postpartum course was complicated by the development of dizziness and lethargy 9 days after delivery. These symptoms were associated with a plasma leucine level above 1 mM. It appears that the combination of a higher-than-usual protein intake after delivery and the involutional changes of the uterus generate extra nitrogenous products. The BCAAs exceeded the patient's limited capacity for their disposal. Similar postpartum metabolic decompensation has been observed in patients with urea cycle disorders.[498] Thus, the postpartum period is a critical time, and additional protein restriction may be advisable. Five successful pregnancies have also been reported in two patients with intermittent MSUD.[317,324] At the time of their pregnancies these women were undiagnosed, and they received no dietary treatment for their MSUD. There were no acute or postpartum complications.

Outcome

Dietary therapy for MSUD was initiated in 1959.[275,276,499] Advances during the past 10 years, in both long-term nutritional therapy and acute-phase management, have considerably reduced the morbidity, mortality, and length of initial hospitalization. The team approach to management and parental understanding and cooperation are essential for successful metabolic control. One of the earliest successfully treated patients with classic MSUD was diagnosed shortly after birth because of an affected older sib.[461,500–502] Her plasma BCAAs and urine BCKAs rose markedly on the fourth day of life. The elevated BCAAs and BCKAs preceded her clinical symptoms of poor feeding and sluggish Moro reflex. Dietary therapy was begun on the sixth day and carefully monitored. Despite a number of episodes of metabolic relapse in the first decade, the patient continued to have normal growth and development. At the last follow-up she was well at age 27 years, employed full-time, and led an apparently normal life (DP Brenton, personal communication, August 1988).

The outcome following treatment in over 150 patients with classic MSUD and over 25 patients with the variant forms of MSUD has now been reported[288,289,457,463,503–509] (K Aoki, personal communication, 1992). Most patients were detected by routine newborn screening or were diagnosed by laboratory testing based on clinical suspicion. A small number of patients were prospectively treated because of previously affected sibs. In terms of intelligence, approximately one-third of the classic MSUD patients had IQ scores greater than 90 and one-third had IQ scores between 70 and 90. In most studies, only the full-scale IQ score is reported. When both performance and verbal scores are available, the verbal scores have been consistently higher than the performance scores.[289,506,510] The discrepancy between the two scores is not surprising because cerebellar dysfunction is often an early sign of acute metabolic decompensation. Short attention span and minor learning disabilities — for example, difficulty with visual-motor integrative abilities — were observed even in patients with normal intellect who were treated soon after birth.[289,496,506] Poor intellectual outcome is often associated with neurologic sequelae such as spasticity and quadriplegia.[457,503] Approximately one-fifth of the classic MSUD patients died, the majority during acute complications precipitated by infection. Cerebral edema has occurred in patients in acute metabolic crisis, as well as during the recovery phase, and can be fatal. This complication is often the cause of death in preschool-aged patients.[288,289,295,442,511] Acute metabolic encephalopathy is less likely to occur after the first 5 or 6 years of life. Older patients tolerate stress much better, particularly if effective biochemical control is maintained.

Several Factors Affect the Long-Term Outlook for MSUD Patients. The age at diagnosis and the subsequent course are the most important determinants. Treatment initiated before 10 days of age gives the best results, and only a few patients treated after 14 days of age achieved normal intellect (Fig. 87-9).[289,457,506,507,509] Diagnosis at a younger age is usually also associated with a milder neonatal course. The impact of the degree of severity of the acute neonatal and subsequent metabolic complications is unfortunately difficult to quantitate. Chronic mild to moderate elevations of the

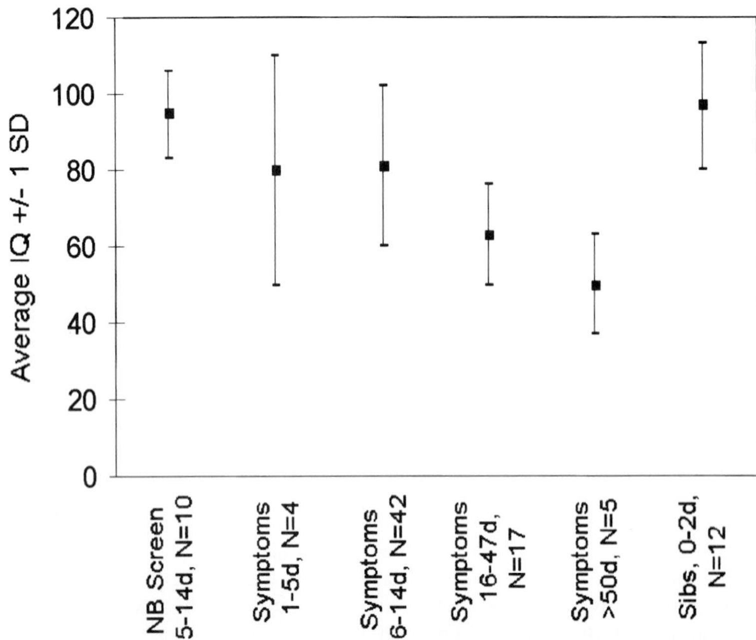

Fig. 87-9 Long-term intellectual outcome in MSUD patients. IQ vs. age at which treatment was initiated.

BCAAs/BCKAs have been associated with dysmyelinating changes in brain by imaging studies,[288] thus demonstrating the importance of good metabolic control.

ACKNOWLEDGMENTS

This work was supported, in part, by Grants DK-26758 and NS-05096 from the National Institutes of Health, Grant I-1286 from the Robert A. Welch Foundation, and the Scott C. Foster Endowed Fund for Genetic Research on MSUD at the Massachusetts General Hospital.

REFERENCES

1. Harper AE, Miller RH, Block KP: Branched-chain amino acid metabolism. *Annu Rev Nutr* **4**:409, 1984.
2. Wahren J, Felig P, Hagenfeldt L: Effect of protein ingestion on splanchnic and leg metabolism in normal man and in patients with diabetes mellitus. *J Clin Invest* **57**:987, 1976.
3. Odessey R, Goldberg AL: Oxidation of leucine by rat skeletal muscle. *Am J Physiol* **223**:1376, 1972.
4. Hutson SM, Cree TC, Harper AE: Regulation of leucine and α-ketoisocaproate metabolism in skeletal muscle. *J Biol Chem* **253**:8126, 1978.
5. Goldberg AL, Odessey R: Oxidation of amino acids by diaphragms from fed and fasted rats. *Am J Physiol* **223**:1384, 1972.
6. Buse MG, Biggers JF, Friderici KH, Buse JF: Oxidation of branched chain amino acids by isolated hearts and diaphragms of the rat. The effect of fatty acids, glucose, and pyruvate respiration. *J Biol Chem* **247**:8085, 1972.
7. Sans RM, Jolly WW, Harris RA: Studies on the regulation of leucine catabolism. III. Effects of dichloroacetate and 2-chloropropionate on leucine oxidation by the heart. *J Mol Cell Cardiol* **12**:1, 1980.
8. Goodman HM: Site of action of insulin in promoting leucine utilization in adipose tissue. *Am J Physiol* **233**:E97, 1977.
9. Chaplin ER, Goldberg AL, Diamond I: Leucine oxidation in brain slices and nerve endings. *J Neurochem* **26**:701, 1976.
10. Krebs HA, Lund P: Aspects of the regulation of the metabolism of branched-chain amino acids. *Adv Enzyme Regul* **15**:375, 1977.
11. Crabb DW, Harris RA: Studies on the regulation of leucine catabolism in the liver. Stimulation by pyruvate and dichloroacetate. *J Biol Chem* **253**:1481, 1978.
12. Williamson JR, Walajtys-Rode E, Coll KE: Effects of branched chain α-ketoacids on the metabolism of isolated rat liver cells. I. Regulation of branched chain α-ketoacid metabolism. *J Biol Chem* **254**:11511, 1979.
13. Rosenthal J, Angel A, Farkas J: Metabolic fate of leucine: A significant sterol precursor in adipose tissue and muscle. *Am J Physiol* **226**:411, 1974.
14. Odessey R, Khairallah EA, Goldberg AL: Origin and possible significance of alanine production by skeletal muscle. *J Biol Chem* **249**:7623, 1974.
15. Chua B, Siehl DL, Morgan HE: Effect of leucine and metabolites of branched chain amino acids on protein turnover in heart. *J Biol Chem* **254**:8385, 1979.
16. Buse MG, Reid SS: Leucine. A possible regulator of protein turnover in muscle. *J Clin Invest* **56**:1250, 1975.
17. Yalow RS, Berson SA: Immunoassay of endogenous plasma insulin in man. *J Clin Invest* **39**:1157, 1960.
18. Panten U, Kriegstein EV, Poser W, Schonborn J, Hasselblatt A: Effects of l-leucine and α-ketoisocaproic acid upon insulin secretion and metabolism of isolated pancreatic islets. *FEBS Lett* **20**:225, 1972.
19. Lenzen S: Effects of α-ketocarboxylic acids and 4-pentenoic acid on insulin secretion from the perfused rat pancreas. *Biochemical Pharmacology* **27**:1321, 1978.
20. Hutton JC, Sener A, Herchuelz A, Atwater I, Kawazu S, Boschero AC, Somers G, Devis G, Malaisse WJ: Similarities in the stimulus-secretion coupling mechanisms of glucose- and 2-keto acid-induced insulin release. *Endocrinology* **106**:203, 1980.
21. Mizock BA: Branched-chain amino acids in sepsis and hepatic failure. *Arch Intern Med* **145**:1284, 1985.
22. Freund HR, Lapidot A, Fischer JE: The use of branched-chain amino acids in the injured-septic patient, in Walser M, Williamson J (eds): *Metabolism and Clinical Implications of Branched Chain Amino and Ketoacids*. New York, Elsevier/North-Holland, 1981, p 527.
23. Rosen HM, Yoshimura N, Hodgman JM, Fischer JE: Plasma amino acid patterns in hepatic encephalopathy of differing etiology. *Gastroenterology* **72**:483, 1977.
24. Fischer JE, Rosen HM, Ebeid AM, James JH, Keane JM, Soeters PB: The effect of normalization of plasma amino acids on hepatic encephalopathy in man. *Surgery* **80**:77, 1976.
25. Mitch WE, Collier VU, Walser M: Treatment of chronic renal failure with branched-chain ketoacids plus the other essential amino acids or their nitrogen-free analogues, in Walser M, Williamson J (eds): *Metabolism and Clinical Implications of Branched Chain Amino and Ketoacids*. New York, Elsevier/North Holland, 1981, p 587.
26. Walser M: Therapeutic aspects of branched-chain amino and keto acids. *Clin Sci* **66**:1, 1984.
27. Sax HC, Talamini MA, Fischer JE: Clinical use of branched-chain amino acids in liver disease, sepsis, trauma, and burns. *Arch Surg* **121**:358, 1986.
28. Morgan MY: Branched chain amino acids in the management of chronic liver disease. Facts and fantasies. *J Hepatol* **11**:133, 1990.
29. Oxender DL, Christensen HN: Distinct mediating systems for the transport of neutral amino acids by the Ehrlich cell. *J Biol Chem* **238**:3686, 1963.
30. LeCam A, Freychet P: Neutral amino acid transport. Characterization of the A and the L systems in isolating rat hepatocytes. *J Biol Chem* **252**:148, 1977.
31. Prentki M, Renold AE: Neutral amino acid transport in isolated rat pancreatic islets. *J Biol Chem* **258**:14239, 1983.
32. Meister A: *Biochemistry of the Amino Acids*, 2d ed. New York, Academic Press, 1965, p 729.
33. Desantiago S, Torres N, Suryawan A, Tovar AR, Hutson SM: Regulation of branched-chain amino acid metabolism in the lactating rat. *J Nutr* **128**:1165, 1998.
34. Hutson SM, Rannels SL: Characterization of a mitochondrial transport system for branched chain α-keto acids. *J Biol Chem* **260**:14189, 1985.
35. Hutson SM: pH regulation of mitochondrial branched chain α-keto acid transport and oxidation in rat heart mitochondria. *J Biol Chem* **262**:9629, 1987.
36. Hutson SM, Roten S, Kaplan RS: Solubilization and functional reconstitution of the branched-chain α-keto acid transporter from rat heart mitochondria. *Proc Natl Acad Sci U S A* **87**:1028, 1990.
37. Hutson SM, Hall TR: Identification of the mitochondrial branched chain aminotransferase as a branched chain α-keto acid transport protein. *J Biol Chem* **268**:3084, 1993.
38. Pettit FH, Yeaman SJ, Reed LJ: Purification and characterization of branched chain α-keto acid dehydrogenase complex of bovine kidney. *Proc Natl Acad Sci U S A* **75**:4881, 1978.
39. Danner DJ, Lemmon SK, Besharse JC, Elsas LJ: Purification and characterization of branched chain α-ketoacid dehydrogenase from bovine liver mitochondria. *J Biol Chem* **254**:5522, 1979.
40. Ikeda Y, Tanaka K: Isovaleryl-CoA dehydrogenase from rat liver. *Methods Enzymol* **166**:374, 1988.
41. Ikeda Y, Tanaka K: 2-Methyl branched-chain acyl-CoA dehydrogenase from rat liver. *Methods Enzymol* **166**:360, 1988.
42. Hers HG, Hue L: Gluconeogenesis and related aspects of glycolysis. *Annu Rev Biochem* **52**:617, 1983.
43. Shinnick FL, Harper AE: Branched-chain amino acid oxidation by isolated rat tissue preparations. *Biochim Biophys Acta* **437**:477, 1976.
44. Ichihara A, Koyama E: Transaminase of branched-chain amino acids. I. Branched-chain amino acids α-ketoglutarate transaminase. *J Biochem (Tokyo)* **59**:160, 1966.
45. Dancis J, Hutzler J, Levitz M: Tissue distribution of branched chain keto acid decarboxylase. *Biochim Biophys Acta* **52**:60, 1961.
46. Patel TB, DeBuysere MS, Barron LL, Olson MS: Studies on the regulation of the branched-chain α-keto acid dehydrogenase in the perfused rat liver. *J Biol Chem* **256**:9009, 1981.
47. Buffington CK, DeBuysere MS, Olson MS: Studies on the regulation of the branched chain α-keto acid dehydrogenase in the perfused rat heart. *J Biol Chem* **254**:10453, 1979.
48. Noda C, Ichihara A: Control of ketogenesis from amino acids. IV. Tissue specificity in oxidation of leucine, tyrosine, and lysine. *J Biochem (Tokyo)* **80**:1159, 1976.
49. Livesey G, Lund P: Enzymic determination of branched-chain amino acids and 2-oxoacids in rat tissues. Transfer of 2-oxoacids from skeletal muscle to liver in vivo. *Biochem J* **188**:705, 1980.
50. Hutson SM, Harper AE: Blood and tissue branched-chain amino acids and α-keto acid concentrations: Effect of diet, starvation, and disease. *Am J Clin Nutr* **34**:173, 1981.

51. Suryawan A, Hawes JW, Harris RA, Shimomura Y, Jenkins AE, Hutson SM: A molecular model of human branched-chain amino acid metabolism. *Am J Clin Nutr* **68**:72, 1998.
52. Khatra BS, Chawla RK, Sewell CW, Rudman D: Distribution of branched chain α-keto acid dehydrogenases in primate tissues. *J Clin Invest* **59**:558, 1977.
53. Chang TW, Goldberg AL: The origin of alanine produced in skeletal muscle. *J Biol Chem* **253**:3677, 1978.
54. Adibi SA: Roles of branched chain amino acids in metabolic regulation. *J Lab Clin Med* **95**:475, 1980.
55. Goldberg AL, Chang TW: Regulation and significance of amino acid metabolism in skeletal muscle. *Fed Proc* **37**:2301, 1978.
56. Harris RA, Crabb DW, San RM: Studies on the regulation of leucine metabolism. II. Mechanism responsible for dichloroacetate stimulation of leucine oxidation by the liver. *Arch Biochem Biophys* **190**:8, 1978.
57. Felig P: Amino acid metabolism in man. *Annu Rev Biochem* **44**:933, 1975.
58. Snell K, Duff DA: Branched-chain amino acid metabolism and alanine formation in rat muscles in vitro. Mitochondrial-cytosolic interrelationships. *Biochem J* **225**:737, 1985.
59. Tischler ME, Goldberg AL: Leucine degradation and release of glutamine and alanine by adipose tissue. *J Biol Chem* **255**:8074, 1980.
60. Adibi SA: Influence of dietary deprivations on plasma concentration of free amino acids of man. *J Appl Physiol* **25**:52, 1968.
61. Hutson SM, Zapalowski C, Cree TC, Harper AE: Regulation of leucine and α-ketoisocaproic acid metabolism in skeletal muscle. Effects of starvation and insulin. *J Biol Chem* **255**:2418, 1980.
62. Felig P, Marliss E, Ohman JL, Cahill GF Jr: Plasma amino acid levels in diabetic ketoacidosis. *Diabetes* **19**:727, 1970.
63. Aoki TT, Assal J-P, Manzano FM, Kozak GP, Cahill GF: Plasma and cerebrospinal fluid amino acid levels in diabetic ketoacidosis before and after corrective therapy. *Diabetes* **24**:463, 1975.
64. Carlsten A, Hallgren B, Jagenburg R, Svanborg A, Werko L: Amino acids and free fatty acids in plasma in diabetes. I. The effect of insulin on the arterial levels. *Acta Med Scand* **179**:361, 1966.
65. Felig P, Marliss E, Cahill GF Jr: Plasma amino acid levels and insulin secretion in obesity. *N Engl J Med* **281**:811, 1969.
66. Buse MG, Biggers JF, Drier C, Buse JF: The effect of epinephrine, glucagon, and the nutritional state on the oxidation of branched chain amino acids and pyruvate by isolated hearts and diaphragms of the rat. *J Biol Chem* **248**:697, 1973.
67. Paul HS, Adibi SA: Leucine oxidation in diabetes and starvation: Effects of ketone bodies on branched-chain amino acid oxidation in vitro. *Metabolism* **27**:185, 1978.
68. Buse MG, Herlong HF, Wiegand DA: The effect of diabetes, insulin, and the redox potential on leucine metabolism by isolated rat hemidiaphragm. *Endocrinology* **98**:1166, 1976.
69. Aftring RP, Manos PN, Buse MG: Catabolism of branched-chain amino acids by diaphragm muscles of fasted and diabetic rats. *Metabolism* **34**:702, 1985.
70. Wagenmakers AJM, Schepens JTG, Veldhuizen JAM, Veerkamp JH: The activity state of the branched-chain 2-oxo acid dehydrogenase complex in rat tissues. *Biochem J* **220**:273, 1984.
71. Schauder P, Schroder K, Matthaei D, Henning HV, Langenbeck U: Influence of insulin on blood levels of branched chain keto and amino acids in man. *Metabolism* **32**:323, 1983.
72. Paul HS, Adibi SA: Leucine oxidation and protein turnover in clofibrate-induced muscle protein degradation in rats. *J Clin Invest* **65**:1285, 1980.
73. Wagenmakers AJM, Veerkamp JH, Schepens JTG, Van Moerkerk HTB: Effect of clofibrate on branched-chain amino acid metabolism. *Biochem Pharmacol* **34**:2169, 1985.
74. Bieber LL, Choi YR: Isolation and identification of aliphatic short-chain acylcarnitines from beef heart. Possible role for carnitine in branched-chain amino acid metabolism. *Proc Natl Acad Sci U S A* **74**:2795, 1977.
75. Paul HS, Adibi SA: Effect of carnitine on branched-chain amino acid oxidation by liver and skeletal muscle. *Am J Physiol* **234**:E494, 1978.
76. Van Hinsbergh VW, Veerkamp JH, Engelen PJM, Ghijsen WJ: Effect of L-carnitine on the oxidation of leucine and valine by rat skeletal muscle. *Biochem Med* **20**:115, 1978.
77. Paul HS, Adibi SA: Assessment of effect of starvation, glucose, fatty acids and hormones on α-decarboxylation of leucine in skeletal muscle of rat. *J Nutr* **106**:1079, 1976.
78. Corkey BE, Martin-Requero A, Walajtys-Rode E, Williams RJ, Williamson JR: Regulation of the branched chain α-ketoacid pathway in liver. *J Biol Chem* **257**:9668, 1982.
79. Harris RA, Paxton R, Powell SM, Goodwin GW, Kuntz MJ, Han AC: Regulation of branched-chain α-ketoacid dehydrogenase complex by covalent modification. *Adv Enzyme Regul* **25**:219, 1986.
80. Kadowaki H, Knox WE: Cytosolic and mitochondrial isozymes of branched-chain amino acid aminotransferase during development of the rat. *Biochem J* **202**:777, 1982.
81. Hutson SM: Subcellular distribution of branched-chain aminotransferase activity in rat tissues. *J Nutr* **118**:1475, 1988.
82. Wallin R, Hall TR, Hutson SM: Purification of branched chain aminotransferase from rat heart mitochondria. *J Biol Chem* **265**:6019, 1990.
83. Hall TR, Wallin R, Reinhart GD, Hutson SM: Branched chain aminotransferase isoenzymes. Purification and characterization of the rat brain isoenzyme. *J Biol Chem* **268**:3092, 1993.
84. Hutson SM, Bledsoe RK, Hall TR, Dawson PA: Cloning and expression of the mammalian cytosolic branched chain aminotransferase isoenzyme. *J Biol Chem* **270**:30344, 1995.
85. Bledsoe RK, Dawson PA, Hutson SM: Cloning of the rat and human mitochondrial branched chain aminotransferases (BVATm). *Biochim Biophys Acta* **1339**:9, 1997.
86. Davoodi J, Drown PM, Bledsoe RK, Wallin R, Reinhart GD, Hutson SM: Overexpression and characterization of the human mitochondrial and cytosolic branched-chain aminotransferases. *J Biol Chem* **273**:4982, 1998.
87. LaNoue KF, Schoolwerth AC: Metabolite transport in mitochondria. *Annu Rev Biochem* **48**:871, 1979.
88. Ogawa K, Yokojima A, Ichihara A: Transaminase of branched chain amino acids. VII. Comparative studies on isozymes of ascites hepatoma and various normal tissues of rat. *J Biochem (Tokyo)* **68**:901, 1970.
89. Aki K, Ogawa K, Ichihara A: Transaminases of branched chain amino acids. IV. Purification and properties of two enzymes from rat liver. *Biochim Biophys Acta* **159**:276, 1968.
90. Aki K, Yokojima A, Ichihara A: Transaminase of branched chain amino acids. VI. Purification and properties of the hog brain enzyme. *J Biochem (Tokyo)* **65**:539, 1969.
91. Danner DJ, Elsas LJII: Subcellular distribution and cofactor function of human branched chain α-ketoacid dehydrogenase in normal and mutant cultured skin fibroblasts. *Biochem Med* **13**:7, 1975.
92. Yeaman SJ: The mammalian 2-oxoacid dehydrogenase: A complex family. *Trends Biochem Sci* **11**:293, 1986.
93. Dancis J, Hutzler J, Levitz M: The diagnosis of maple syrup urine disease (branched-chain ketoaciduria) by the in vitro study of the peripheral leukocyte. *Pediatrics* **32**:234, 1963.
94. Wohlhueter RM, Harper AE: Coinduction of rat liver branched chain α-keto acid dehydrogenase activities. *J Biol Chem* **245**:2391, 1970.
95. Connelly JL, Danner DJ, Bowden JA: Branched chain α-keto acid metabolism. I. Isolation, purification, and partial characterization of bovine liver α-ketoisocaproic: α-keto- β-methylvaleric acid dehydrogenase. *J Biol Chem* **243**:1198, 1968.
96. Bowden JA, Connelly JL: Branched chain α-keto acid metabolism. II. Evidence for the common identity of α-ketoisocaproic acid and α-keto-β-methyl-valeric acid dehydrogenases. *J Biol Chem* **243**:3526, 1968.
97. Sullivan SG, Dancis J, Cox RP: Modulation of branched-chain α-keto acid decarboxylase activity in rat liver mitochondria by hypophysectomy. *Arch Biochem Biophys* **176**:225, 1976.
98. Sullivan SG, Dancis J, Cox RP: Transient and long-term differential modulations of branched-chain α-keto acid decarboxylase activity in hypophysectomized rats. *Biochim Biophys Acta* **539**:135, 1978.
99. Goedde HW, Hufner M, Mohlenbeck F, Blume KG: Biochemical studies on branched-chain oxoacid oxidases. *Biochim Biophys Acta* **132**:524, 1967.
100. Parker PJ, Randle PJ: Branched chain 2-oxo-acid dehydrogenase complex of rat liver. *FEBS Lett* **90**:183, 1978.
101. Parker PJ, Randle PJ: Partial purification and properties of branched-chain 2-oxo acid dehydrogenase of ox liver. *Biochem J* **171**:751, 1978.
102. Danner DJ, Lemmon SK, Elsas LII: Substrate specificity and stabilization by thiamine pyrophosphate of rat liver branched chain α-keto acid dehydrogenase. *Biochem Med* **19**:27, 1978.
103. Jones SMA, Yeaman SJ: Oxidative decarboxylation of 4-methylthio-2-oxobutyrate by branched-chain 2-oxo acid dehydrogenase complex. *Biochem J* **237**:621, 1986.
104. Paxton R, Harris RA: Isolation of rabbit liver branched chain α-ketoacid dehydrogenase and regulation by phosphorylation. *J Biol Chem* **257**:14433, 1982.

105. Heffelfinger SC, Sewell ET, Danner DJ: Identification of specific subunits of highly purified bovine liver branched-chain ketoacid dehydrogenase. *Biochemistry* **22**:5519, 1983.
106. Chuang DT, Hu C-WC, Ku LS, Niu WL, Myers DE, Cox RP: Catalytic and structural properties of the dihydrolipoyl transacylase component of bovine branched-chain α-keto acid dehydrogenase. *J Biol Chem* **259**:9277, 1984.
107. Odessey R: Purification of rat kidney branched-chain oxo acid dehydrogenase complex with endogenous kinase activity. *Biochem J* **204**:353, 1982.
108. Ono K, Hakozaki M, Kimura A, Kochi H: Purification, resolution, and reconstruction of rat liver branched-chain α-keto acid dehydrogenase complex. *J Biochem (Tokyo)* **101**:19, 1987.
109. Shimomura Y, Paxton R, Ozawa T, Harris RA: Purification of branched chain α-ketoacid dehydrogenase complex from rat liver. *Anal Biochem* **163**:74, 1987.
110. Ono K, Hakozaki M, Nishimaki H, Kochi H: Purification and characterization of human liver branched-chain α-keto acid dehydrogenase complex. *Biochem Med Metab Biol* **37**:133, 1987.
111. McCully V, Burns G, Sokatch JR: Resolution of branched-chain oxo acid dehydrogenase complex of *Pseudomonas aeruginosa* PAO. *Biochem J* **233**:737, 1986.
112. Heffelfinger SC, Sewell ET, Danner DJ: Antibodies to bovine liver branched-chain 2-oxo acid dehydrogenase cross-react with this enzyme complex from other tissues and species. *Biochem J* **213**:339, 1983.
113. Danner DJ, Armstrong N, Heffelfinger SC, Sewell ET, Priest JH, Elsas LJ: Absence of branched chain acyl-transferase as a cause of maple syrup urine disease. *J Clin Invest* **75**:858, 1985.
114. Indo Y, Kitano A, Endo F, Akaboshi I, Matsuda I: Altered kinetic properties of branched-chain α-keto acid dehydrogenase complex due to mutation of the β-subunit of the branched chain α-keto acid decarboxylase (E1) component in lymphoblastoid cells derived from patients with maple syrup urine disease. *J Clin Invest* **80**:63, 1987.
115. Fisher CW, Chuang JL, Griffin TA, Lau KS, Cox RP, Chuang DT: Molecular phenotypes in cultured maple syrup urine disease cells. Complete E1α cDNA sequence and mRNA and subunit contents of the human branched chain α-keto acid dehydrogenase complex. *J Biol Chem* **264**:3448, 1989.
116. Eisenstein RS, Miller RH, Hoganson G, Harper AE: Phylogenetic comparisons of the branched-chain α-ketoacid dehydrogenase complex. *Comp Biochem Physiol B Biochem Mol Biol* **97**:719, 1990.
117. Reed LJ, Damuni Z, Merryfield ML: Regulation of mammalian pyruvate and branched-chain α-keto acid dehydrogenase complexes by phosphorylation-dephosphorylation. *Curr Top Cell Regul* **27**:41, 1985.
118. Yeaman SJ: The 2-oxo acid dehydrogenase complexes: Recent advances. *Biochem J* **257**:625, 1989.
119. Harris RA, Paxton R, Goodwin GW, Powell SM: Regulation of the branched-chain 2-oxo acid dehydrogenase complex in hepatocytes isolated from rats fed on a low-protein diet. *Biochem J* **234**:285, 1986.
120. Chuang DT, Hu C-WC, Ku LS, Markovitz PJ, Cox RP: Subunit structure of the dihydrolipoyl transacylase component of branched-chain α-keto acid dehydrogenase complex from bovine liver. Characterization of the inner transacylase core. *J Biol Chem* **260**:13779, 1985.
121. Cook KG, Bradford AP, Yeaman SJ: Resolution and reconstitution of bovine kidney branched-chain 2-oxo acid dehydrogenase complex. *Biochem J* **225**:731, 1985.
122. Chuang DT: Assays for E1 and E2 components of the branched-chain keto acid dehydrogenase complex. *Methods Enzymol* **166**:146, 1988.
123. Oliver RM, Reed LJ: Multienzyme complexes, in Harris J (ed): *Electron Microscopy of Proteins*, vol 2. London, Academic Press, 1982, p 1.
124. Aevarsson A, Seger K, Turley S, Sokatch JR, Hol WGJ: First picture of all the major components of 2-oxo acid dehydrogenase multienzyme complexes obtained by the crystal structure of 2-oxoisovalerate dehydrogenase. *Nature Str Biol* **6**:902, 1999.
125. Aevarsson A, Chuang J, Wynn M, Truley S, Chuang D, Hol WGJ: Crystal structure of human branched-chain α-ketoacid dehydrogenase and the molecular basis of multienzyme complex deficiency in maple syrup urine disease. *Structure* **8**:277, 2000.
126. Hawkins CF, Borges A, Perham RN: A common structural motif in thiamin pyrophosphate-binding enzymes. *FEBS Lett* **255**:77, 1989.
127. Wynn RM, Davie JR, Chuang JL, Cote CD, Chuang DT: Impaired assembly of E1 decarboxylase of the branched-chain α-ketoacid dehydrogenase complex in type IA maple syrup urine disease. *J Biol Chem* **273**:13110, 1998.
128. Lindqvist Y, Schneider C, Ermler U, Sundstrom M: Three-dimensional structure of transketolase, a thiamine diphosphate-dependent enzyme, at 2.5 Å resolution. *EMBO J* **11**:2373, 1992.
129. Schneider G, Lindquist Y: Crystallography and mutagenesis of transketolase: Mechanistic implications for enzyme thiamin catalysis. *Biochim Biophys Acta* **1385**:3807, 1998.
130. Shimomura Y, Kuntz MJ, Suzuki M, Ozawa T, Harris RA: Monovalent cations and inorganic phosphate alter branched-chain α-ketoacid dehydrogenase-kinase activity and inhibitor sensitivity. *Arch Biochem Biophys* **266**:210, 1988.
131. Davie JR, Wynn RM, Cox RP, Chuang DT: Expression and assembly of a functional E1 component (α2β2) of mammalian branched-chain α-ketoacid dehydrogenase complex in *Escherichia coli*. *J Biol Chem* **267**:16601, 1992.
132. Wynn RM, Davie JR, Cox RP, Chuang DT: Chaperonins groEL and gro ES promote assembly of heterotetramers (α_2 β_2) of mammalian mitochondrial branched-chain α-keto acid decarboxylase in Escherichia coli. *J Biol Chem* **267**:12400, 1992.
133. Cook KG, Bradford AP, Yeaman SJ, Aitken A, Fearnley IM, Walker JE: Regulation of bovine kidney branched-chain 2-oxoacid dehydrogenase complex by reversible phosphorylation. *Eur J Biochem* **145**:587, 1984.
134. Zhang B, Kuntz MJ, Goodwin GW, Harris RA, Crabb DW: Molecular cloning of a cDNA for the E1 subunit of rat liver branched chain α-ketoacid dehydrogenase. *J Biol Chem* **262**:15220, 1987.
135. Hawes JW, Schnepf RJ, Jenkins AE, Shimomura Y, Popov KM, Harris RA: Roles of amino acid residues surrounding phosphorylation site 1 of branched-chain α-ketoacid dehydrogenase (BCKDH) in catalysis and phosphorylation site recognition by BCKDH kinase. *J Biol Chem* **270**:31071, 1995.
136. Wynn RM, Chuang JL, Davie JR, Fisher CW, Hale MA, Cox RP, Chuang DT: Cloning and expression in *Escherichia coli* of mature E1β subunit of bovine mitochondrial branched-chain α-keto acid dehydrogenase complex. Mapping of the E1β-binding region on E2. *J Biol Chem* **267**:1881, 1992.
137. Hackert ML, Xu W-X, Oliver RM, Wall JS, Hainfeld JF, Mullinax TR, Reed LJ: Branched-chain α-keto acid dehydrogenase complex from bovine kidney: Radial distribution of mass determined from dark-field electron micrographs. *Biochemistry* **28**:6816, 1989.
138. Hu C-WC, Griffin TA, Lau KS, Cox RP, Chuang DT: Subunit structure of the dihydrolipoyl transacylase component of branched-chain α-keto acid dehydrogenase complex from bovine liver. Mapping of the lipoyl-bearing domain by limited proteolysis. *J Biol Chem* **261**:343, 1986.
139. Hummel KB, Litwer S, Bradford AP, Aitken A, Danner DJ, Yeaman SJ: Nucleotide sequence of a cDNA for branched chain acyltransferase with analysis of the deduced protein structure. *J Biol Chem* **263**:6165, 1988.
140. Collins JH, Reed LJ: Acyl group and electron pair relay system: A network of interacting lipoyl moieties in the pyruvate and α-ketoglutarate dehydrogenase complexes from *Escherichia coli*. *Proc Natl Acad Sci U S A* **74**:4223, 1977.
141. Danson MJ, Fersht AR, Perham RN: Rapid intramolecular coupling of active sites in the pyruvate dehydrogenase complex of *Escherichia coli*: Mechanism for rate enhancement in a multimeric structure. *Proc Natl Acad Sci U S A* **75**:5386, 1978.
142. Griffin TA, Lau KS, Chuang DT: Characterization and conservation of the inner E2 core domain structure of branched-chain α-keto acid dehydrogenase complex from bovine liver. Construction of a cDNA encoding the entire transacylase (E2b) precursor. *J Biol Chem* **263**:14008, 1988.
143. Lau KS, Griffin TA, Hu C-WC, Chuang DT: Conservation of primary structure in the lipoyl-bearing and dihydrolipoyl dehydrogenase binding domains of mammalian branched-chain α-keto acid dehydrogenase complex: Molecular cloning of human and bovine transacylase (E2) cDNAs. *Biochemistry* **27**:1972, 1988.
144. Danner DJ, Litwer S, Herring WJ, Pruckler J: Construction and nucleotide sequence of a cDNA encoding the full-length preprotein for human branched chain acyltransferase. *J Biol Chem* **264**:7742, 1989.
145. Nobukuni Y, Mitsubuchi H, Endo F, Matsuda I: Complete primary structure of the transacylase (E2b) subunit of the human branched chain α-keto acid dehydrogenase complex. *Biochem Biophys Res Commun* **161**:1035, 1989.

146. Griffin TA, Chuang DT: Genetic reconstruction and characterization of the recombinant transacylase (E2b) component of bovine branched-chain α-keto acid dehydrogenase complex. Implication of histidine 391 as an active site residue. *J Biol Chem* **265**:13174, 1990.
147. Guest JR: Functional implications of structural homologies between chloramphenicol acetyltransferase and dihydrolipoamide acetyltransferase. *FEMS Microbiol Lett* **44**:417, 1987.
148. Meng M, Chuang DT: Site-directed mutagenesis and functional analysis of the active-site residues of the E2 component of bovine branched-chain α-keto acid dehydrogenase complex. *Biochemistry* **33**:12879, 1994.
149. Russell GC, Guest JR: Sequence similarities within the family of dihydrolipoamide acyltransferases and discovery of a previously unidentified fungal enzyme. *Biochim Biophys Acta* **1076**:225, 1991.
150. Bleile DM, Hackert ML, Pettit FH, Reed LJ: Subunit structure of dihydrolipoyl transacetylase component of pyruvate dehydrogenase complex from bovine heart. *J Biol Chem* **256**:514, 1981.
151. Guest JR, Lewis HM, Graham LD, Packman LC, Perham RN: Genetic reconstruction and functional analysis of the repeating lipoyl domains in the pyruvate dehydrogenase multienzyme complex of *Escherichia coli*. *J Mol Biol* **185**:743, 1985.
152. Mattevi A, Obmolova G, Schulze E, Kalk KH, Westphal AH, de Kok A, Hol WGJ: Atomic structure of the cubic core of the pyruvate dehydrogenase multienzyme complex. *Science* **255**:1544, 1992.
153. Izard T, Aevarsson A, Allen MD, Westphal AH, Perham RN, De Kok A, Hol WGJ: Principles of quasi-equivalence and euclidean geometry govern the assembly of cubic and dodecahedral cores of pyruvate dehydrogenase complexes. *Proc Natl Acad Sci U S A* **96**:1240, 1999.
154. Dardel F, Davis AL, Laue ED, Perham RN: The three-dimensional structure of the lipoyl domain from Bacillus stearothermophilus pyruvate dehydrogenase multienzyme complex. *J Mol Biol* **229**:1037, 1993.
155. Bassendine MF, Jones DEJ, Yeaman SJ: Biochemistry and autoimmune response to the 2-oxoacid dehydrogenase complexes in primary biliary cirrhosis. *Semin Liver Dis* **17**:49, 1997.
156. Robien MA, Clore GM, Omichinski JG, Perham RN, Appella E, Sakaguchi K, Gronenborn A: Three-dimensional solution structure of the E3-binding domain of the dihydrolipoamide succinyltransferase core from the 2-oxoglutarate dehydrogenase multienzyme complex of Escherichia coli. *Biochemistry* **31**:3463, 1992.
157. Gershwin ME, Mackay IR: Primary biliary cirrhosis: Paradigm or paradox for autoimmunity. *Gastroenterology* **100**:822, 1991.
158. Van de Water J, Cooper A, Surh CD, Coppel R, Danner D, Ansari A, Dickson R, Gershwin ME: Detection of autoantibodies to recombinant mitochondrial proteins in patients with primary biliary cirrhosis. *N Engl J Med* **320**:1377, 1989.
159. Ansari AA, Neckelmann N, Villinger F, Leung P, Danner DJ, Brar SS, Zhao S, Gravanis MB, Mayne A, Gershwin ME, Herskowitz A: Epitope mapping of the branched chain alpha-ketoacid dehydrogenase dihydrolipoyl transacylase (BCKD-E2) protein that reacts with sera from patients with idiopathic dilated cardiomyopathy. *J Immunol* **153**:4754, 1994.
160. Sakurai Y, Fekuyoshi Y, Hamada M, Hayakawa T, Koike M: Mammalian α-keto acid dehydrogenase complexes. VI. Nature of the multiple forms of pig heart lipoamide dehydrogenase. *J Biol Chem* **245**:4453, 1970.
161. Otulakowski G, Robinson BH: Isolation and sequence determination of cDNA clones for porcine and human lipoamide dehydrogenase: Homology to other disulfide oxidoreductases. *J Biol Chem* **262**:17313, 1987.
162. Pons G, Raefsky-Estrin C, Carothers DJ, Pepin RA, Javed AA, Jesse BW, Ganapathi MK, Samols D, Patel MS: Cloning and cDNA sequence of the dihydrolipoamide dehydrogenase component of human α-ketoacid dehydrogenase complexes. *Proc Natl Acad Sci U S A* **85**:1422, 1988.
163. Kim H, Liu T-C, Patel MS: Expression of cDNA sequences encoding mature and precursor forms of human dihydrolipoamide dehydrogenase in *Escherichia coli*. Differences in kinetic mechanisms. *J Biol Chem* **266**:9367, 1991.
164. Kim H, Patel MS: Characterization of two site-specifically mutated human dihydrolipoamide dehydrogenases (His-452 → Gln and Glu-457 → Gln). *J Biol Chem* **267**:5128, 1992.
165. Mattevi A, Schierbeek AJ, Hol WGJ: The refined crystal structure of lipoamide dehydrogenase from *Azotobacter vinelandii* at 2.2 Å resolution. *J Mol Biol* **220**:975, 1991.
166. Toyoda T, Suzuki K, Sekiguchi T, Reed LJ, Takenaka A: Crystal structure of eucaryotic E3, lipoamide dehydrogenase from yeast. *J Biochem (Tokyo)* **123**:668, 1998.
167. Parker PJ, Randle PJ: Inactivation of rat heart branched-chain 2-oxoacid dehydrogenase complex by adenosine triphosphate. *FEBS Lett* **95**:153, 1978.
168. Parker PJ, Randle PJ: Active and inactive forms of branched-chain 2-oxoacid dehydrogenase complex in rat heart and skeletal muscle. *FEBS Lett* **112**:186, 1980.
169. Odessey R: Reversible ATP-induced inactivation of branched-chain 2-oxo acid dehydrogenase. *Biochem J* **192**:155, 1980.
170. Odessey R: Direct evidence for the inactivation of branched-chain oxo-acid dehydrogenase by enzyme phosphorylation. *FEBS Lett* **121**:306, 1980.
171. Lau KS, Fatania HR, Randle PJ: Inactivation of rat liver and kidney branched chain 2-oxoacid dehydrogenase complex by adenosine triphosphate. *FEBS Lett* **126**:66, 1981.
172. Hughes WA, Halestrap AP: The regulation of branched-chain 2-oxo acid dehydrogenase of liver, kidney and heart by phosphorylation. *Biochem J* **196**:459, 1981.
173. Fatania HR, Lau KS, Randle PJ: Inactivation of purified ox kidney branched chain 2-oxoacid dehydrogenase complex by phosphorylation. *FEBS Lett* **132**:285, 1981.
174. Patel TB, Olson MS: Evidence for the regulation of the branched chain α-keto acid dehydrogenase multienzyme complex by a phosphorylation/dephosphorylation mechanism. *Biochemistry* **21**:4259, 1982.
175. Randle PJ, Fatania HR, Lau KS: Regulation of the mitochondrial branched-chain 2-oxoacid dehydrogenase complex of animal tissues by reversible phosphorylation, in Cohen P (ed): *Enzyme Regulation by Reversible Phosphorylation—Further Advances*. Amsterdam, Elsevier, 1984, p 1.
176. Harris RA, Paxton R: Regulation of branched chain α-ketoacid dehydrogenase complex by phosphorylation-dephosphorylation. *Fed Proc* **44**:305, 1985.
177. Lau KS, Phillips CE, Randle PJ: Multi-site phosphorylation in ox-kidney branched-chain 2-oxoacid dehydrogenase complex. *FEBS Lett* **160**:149, 1983.
178. Cook KG, Lawson R, Yeaman SJ: Multi-site phosphorylation of bovine kidney branched-chain 2-oxoacid dehydrogenase complex. *FEBS Lett* **157**:59, 1983.
179. Paxton R, Kuntz M, Harris RA: Phosphorylation sites and inactivation of branched-chain α-ketoacid dehydrogenase isolated from rat heart, bovine kidney, and rabbit liver, kidney, heart, brain and skeletal muscle. *Arch Biochem Biophys* **244**:187, 1986.
180. Cook KG, Lawson R, Yeaman SJ, Aitken A: Amino acid sequence at the major phosphorylation site on bovine kidney branched-chain 2-oxoacid dehydrogenase complex. *FEBS Lett* **164**:47, 1983.
181. Zhao Y, Hawes J, Popov KM, Jaskiewicz J, Shimomura Y, Crabb DW, Harris RA: Site-directed mutagenesis of phosphorylation sites of the branched chain α-ketoacid dehydrogenase complex. *J Biol Chem* **269**:18583, 1994.
182. Hu C-WC, Lau KS, Griffin TA, Chuang JL, Fisher CW, Cox RP, Chuang DT: Isolation and sequencing of a cDNA encoding the decarboxylase (E1) precursor of bovine branched-chain α-keto acid dehydrogenase complex. Expression of E1α mRNA and subunit in maple syrup urine disease and 3T3-L1 cells. *J Biol Chem* **263**:9007, 1988.
183. Zhang B, Crabb DW, Harris RA: Nucleotide and deduced amino acid sequence of the E1α subunit of human liver branched-chain α-ketoacid dehydrogenase. *Gene* **69**:159, 1988.
184. Shimomura Y, Nanaumi N, Suzuki M, Popov KM, Harris RA: Purification and partial characterization of branched-chain α-ketoacid dehydrogenase kinase from rat liver and rat heart. *Arch Biochem Biophys* **283**:293, 1990.
185. Lee HY, Hall TB, Kee SM, Tung HY, Reed LJ: Purification and properties of branched-chain α-keto acid dehydrogenase kinase from bovine kidney. *Biofactors* **3**:109, 1991.
186. Harris RA, Paxton R, DePaoli-Roach AA: Inhibition of branched chain α-ketoacid dehydrogenase kinase activity by α-chloroisocaproate. *J Biol Chem* **257**:13915, 1982.
187. Paxton R, Harris RA: Clofibric acid, phenylpyruvate, and dichloroacetate inhibition of branched-chain α-ketoacid dehydrogenase kinase in vitro and in perfused rat heart. *Arch Biochem Biophys* **231**:58, 1984.
188. Lau KS, Fatania HR, Randle PJ: Regulation of the branched chain 2-oxoacid dehydrogenase kinase reaction. *FEBS Lett* **144**:57, 1982.

189. Paxton R, Harris RA: Regulation of branched-chain α-ketoacid dehydrogenase kinase. *Arch Biochem Biophys* **231**:48, 1984.
190. Lau KS, Cooper AJL, Chuang DT: Inhibition of the bovine 2-oxo acid dehydrogenase complex and its kinase by arylidenepyruvates. *Biochim Biophys Acta* **1038**:360, 1990.
191. Radke GA, Ono K, Ravindran S, Roche TE: Critical role of a lipoyl cofactor of the dihydrolipoyl acetyltransferase in the binding and enhanced function of the pyruvate dehydrogenase kinase. *Biochem Biophys Res Commun* **190**:982, 1993.
192. Popov KM, Zhao Y, Shimomura Y, Kuntz MJ, Harris RA: Branched-chain α-ketoacid dehydrogenase kinase. Molecular cloning, expression, and sequence similarity with histidine protein kinases. *J Biol Chem* **267**:13127, 1992.
193. Davie JR, Wynn RM, Meng M, Huang Y, Aalund G, Chuang DT, Lau KS: Expression and characterization of branched-chain α-ketoacid dehydrogenase kinase from the rat. *J Biol Chem* **270**:19861, 1995.
194. Fatania HR, Patston PA, Randle PJ: Dephosphorylation and reactivation of phosphorylated purified ox-kidney branched-chain dehydrogenase complex by co-purified phosphatase. *FEBS Lett* **158**:234, 1983.
195. Damuni Z, Merryfield ML, Humphreys JS, Reed LJ: Purification and properties of branched-chain α-keto acid dehydrogenase phosphatase from bovine kidney. *Proc Natl Acad Sci U S A* **81**:4335, 1984.
196. Harris RA, Paxton R, Parker RA: Activation of the branched-chain α-ketoacid dehydrogenase complex by a broad specificity protein phosphatase. *Biochem Biophys Res Commun* **107**:1497, 1982.
197. Damuni Z, Reed LJ: Purification and properties of the catalytic subunit of the branched-chain α-keto acid dehydrogenase phosphatase from bovine kidney mitochondria. *J Biol Chem* **262**:5129, 1987.
198. Damuni Z, Lim Tung HY, Reed LJ: Specificity of the heat-stable protein inhibitor of the branched-chain α-keto acid dehydrogenase phosphatase. *Biochem Biophys Res Commun* **133**:878, 1985.
199. Damuni Z, Humphreys JS, Reed LJ: A potent, heat-stable protein inhibitor of [branched-chain α-keto acid dehydrogenase]-phosphatase from bovine kidney mitochondria. *Proc Natl Acad Sci U S A* **83**:285, 1986.
200. Hartl FU, Pfanner N, Nicholson DW, Neupert W: Mitochondrial protein import. *Biochim Biophys Acta* **988**:1, 1989.
201. Lindsay JG: Targeting of 2-oxo dehydrogenase complexes to the mitochondrion. *Ann N Y Acad Sci* **573**:254, 1989.
202. Nobukuni Y, H M, Endo F, Asaka J, Oyama R, Titani K, Matsuda I: Isolation and characterization of a complementary DNA clone coding for the E1β subunit of the bovine branched-chain α-ketoacid dehydrogenase complex: Complete amino acid sequence of the precursor protein and its proteolytic processing. *Biochemistry* **29**:1154, 1990.
203. Sitler TL, McKean MC, Peinemann F, Jackson E, Danner DJ: Import rate of the E1β subunit of human branched chain α-ketoacid dehydrogenase is a limiting factor in the amount of complex formed in the mitochondria. *Biochim Biophys Acta* **1404**:385, 1998.
204. Fisher CR, Chuang JL, Cox RP, Fisher CW, Star RA, Chuang DT: Maple syrup urine disease in Mennonites. Evidence that the Y393N mutation in E1α impedes assembly of the E1 component of branched-chain α-keto acid dehydrogenase complex. *J Clin Invest* **88**:1034, 1991.
205. Fisher CW, Fisher CR, Chuang JL, Lau KS, Chuang DT, Cox RP: Occurrence of a 2-bp (AT) deletion allele and a nonsense (G-to-T) mutant allele at the E2 (DBT) locus of six patients with maple syrup urine disease: Multiple-exon skipping as a secondary effect of the mutations. *Am J Hum Genet* **52**:414, 1993.
206. Litwer S, Herring WJ, Danner DJ: Reversion of the maple syrup urine disease phenotype of impaired branched chain α-ketoacid dehydrogenase complex activity in fibroblasts from an affected child. *J Biol Chem* **264**:14597, 1989.
207. McConnell BB, McKean MC, Danner DJ: Influence of subunit transcript and protein levels on formation of a mitochondrial multienzyme complex. *J Cellular Biochem* **61**:118, 1996.
208. Griffin TA, Wynn RM, Chuang DT: Expression and assembly of mature apotransacylase (E2b) of bovine branched-chain α-keto acid dehydrogenase complex in Escherichia coli. Demonstration of transacylase activity and modification by lipoylation. *J Biol Chem* **265**:12104, 1990.
209. Fujiwara K, Okamura-Ikeda K, Motokawa Y: Expression of mature bovine H-protein of the glycine cleavage system in *Escherichia coli* and in vitro lipoylation of the apo form. *J Biol Chem* **267**:20011, 1992.
210. Fujiwara K, Okamura-Ikeda K, Motokawa Y: Lipoylation of acyltransferase components of α-ketoacid dehydrogenase complexes. *J Biol Chem* **271**:12932, 1996.
211. Morris TW, Reed KE, Cronan JE Jr: Identification of the gene encoding lipoate-protein ligase A of *Escherichia coli*. *J Biol Chem* **269**:16091, 1994.
212. Chuang JL, Davie JR, Wynn RM, Chuang DT: Production of recombinant mammalian Holo-E2 and E3 and reconstitution of functional BCKD complex with recombinant E1. *Methods Enzymol* **324**:192, 2000.
213. Hartl FU, Martin J, Neupert W: Protein folding in the cell: The role of molecular chaperones Hsp70 and Hsp60. *Annu Rev Biophys Biomol Struct* **21**:293, 1992.
214. Wynn RM, Song J, Chuang DT: GroEL/GroES promote dissociation/reassociation cycles of a heterodimeric intermediate during $\alpha_2\ \beta_2$ protein assembly. *J Biol Chem* **275**:2786, 2000.
215. May ME, Aftring RP, Buse MG: Mechanism of the stimulation of branched chain oxoacid oxidation in liver by carnitine. *J Biol Chem* **255**:8394, 1980.
216. Danner DJ, Sewell ET, Elsas LJ: Clofibric acid and phenylpyruvic acid as biochemical probes for studying soluble bovine liver branched-chain ketoacid dehydrogenase. *J Biol Chem* **257**:659, 1982.
217. Patston PA, Espinal J, Randle PJ: Effects of diet and alloxan-diabetes on the activity of branched-chain 2-oxo acid dehydrogenase complex and of activator protein in rat tissues. *Biochem J* **222**:711, 1984.
218. Frick GP, Tai L-R, Blinder L, Goodman HM: l-Leucine activates branched chain α-keto acid dehydrogenase in rat adipose tissue. *J Biol Chem* **256**:2618, 1981.
219. Zhao Y, Jaskiewicz J, Harris RA: Effects of clofibric acid on the activity and activity state of the hepatic branched-chain 2-oxo acid dehydrogenase complex. *Biochem J* **285**:167, 1992.
220. Paul HS, Liu W, Adibi SA: Alteration in gene expression of branched-chain keto acid dehydrogenase kinase but not in gene expression of its substrate in the liver of clofibrate-treated rats. *Biochem J* **317**:411, 1996.
221. Paul HS, Adibi SA: Mechanism of increased conversion of branched chain keto acid dehydrogenase from inactive to active form by a medium chain fatty acid (octanoate) in skeletal muscle. *J Biol Chem* **267**:11208, 1992.
222. Han AC, Goodwin GW, Paxton R, Harris RA: Activation of branched-chain α-ketoacid dehydrogenase in isolated hepatocytes by branched-chain α-ketoacids. *Arch Biochem Biophys* **258**:85, 1987.
223. Dixon JL, Harper AE: Effects on plasma amino acid concentrations and hepatic branched-chain α-keto acid dehydrogenase activity of feeding rats diets containing 9 or 50% casein. *J Nutr* **114**:1025, 1984.
224. Harris RA, Powell SM, Paxton R, Gillim SE, Nagae H: Physiological covalent regulation of rat liver branched-chain α-ketoacid dehydrogenase. *Arch Biochem Biophys* **243**:542, 1985.
225. Popov KM, Zhao Y, Shimomura Y, Jaskiewicz J, Kedishvili NY, Irwin J, Goodwin GW, Harris RA: Dietary control and tissue specific expression of branched-chain α-ketoacid dehydrogenase kinase. *Arch Biochem Biophys* **316**:148, 1995.
226. Block KP, Richmond WB, Mehard WB, Buse MG: Glucocorticoid-mediated activation of muscle branched-chain α-keto acid dehydrogenase in vivo. *Am J Physiol* **252**:E396, 1987.
227. Miller RH, Eisenstein RS, Harper AE: Effects of dietary protein intake on branched-chain keto acid dehydrogenase activity of the rat. Immunochemical analysis of the enzyme complex. *J Biol Chem* **263**:3454, 1988.
228. Paul HS, Adibi SA: Role of ATP in the regulation of branched-chain α-keto acid dehydrogenase activity in liver and muscle mitochondria of fed, fasted, and diabetic rats. *J Biol Chem* **257**:4875, 1982.
229. Aftring RP, Miller WJ, Buse MG: Effects of diabetes and starvation on skeletal muscle branched-chain α-keto acid dehydrogenase activity. *Am J Physiol* **254**:E292, 1988.
230. Block KP, Heywood BW, Buse MG, Harper AE: Activation of rat liver branched-chain 2-oxo acid dehydrogenase in vivo by glucagon and adrenaline. *Biochem J* **232**:593, 1985.
231. Hildebrandt EF, Buxton DB, Olson MS: Acute regulation of the branched-chain 2-oxo acid dehydrogenase complex by adrenaline and glucagon in the perfused rat heart. *Biochem J* **250**:835, 1988.
232. Huang Y, Chuang DT: Down-regulation of rat mitochondrial branched-chain 2-oxoacid dehydrogenase kinase gene expression by glucocorticoids. *Biochem J* **339**:503, 1999.
233. Wang X, Jurkovitz C, Price SR: Regulation of branched-chain ketoacid dehydrogenase flux by extracellular pH and glucocorticoids. *Am J Physiol* **272**:C2031, 1997.

234. Price SR, Reaich D, Marinovic AC, England BK, Bailey JL, Caban R, Mitch WE, Maroni BJ: Mechanisms contributing to muscle wasting in acute uremia: Activation of amino acid catabolism. *J Am Soc Nephrol* **9**:439, 1998.
235. Fujii H, Tokuyama K, Suzuki M, Popov KM, Zhao Y, Harris RA, Nakai N, Murakami T, Shimomura Y: Regulation by physical training of enzyme activity and gene expression of Branched-chain 2-oxo acid dehydrogenase complex in rat skeletal muscle. *Biochim Biophys Acta* **1243**:277, 1995.
236. Chuang DT, Hu C-WC, Patel MS: Induction of the branched-chain 2-oxo acid dehydrogenase complex in 3T3-L1 adipocytes during differentiation. *Biochem J* **214**:177, 1983.
237. Frerman FE, Sabran JL, Taylor JL, Grossberg SE: Leucine catabolism during the differentiation of 3T3-L1 cells. Expression of a mitochondrial enzyme system. *J Biol Chem* **258**:7087, 1983.
238. MacDonald MJ, McKenzie DI, Kaysen JH, Walker TM, Moran SM, Fahien LA, Towle HC: Glucose regulates leucine-induced insulin release and the expression of the branched chain ketoacid dehydrogenase E1α subunit gene in pancreatic islets. *J Biol Chem* **266**:1335, 1991.
239. Chicco AG, Adibi SA, Liu W, Morris SM Jr, Paul HS: Regulation of gene expression of branched-chain keto acid dehydrogenase complex in primary cultured hepatocytes by dexamethasone and a cAMP analog. *J Biol Chem* **269**:19427, 1994.
240. Chinsky JM, Bohlen LM, Costeas PA: Noncoordinated responses of branched-chain alpha-ketoacid dehydrogenase subunit genes to dietary protein. *Faseb J* **8**:114, 1994.
241. Zhao Y, Popov KM, Shimomura Y, Kedishvili NY, Jaskiewicz J, Kuntz MJ, Kain J, Zhang B, Harris RA: Effect of dietary protein on the liver content and subunit composition of the branched-chain alpha-ketoacid dehydrogenase complex. *Arch Biochem Biophys* **308**:446, 1994.
242. Zhang B, Zhao Y, Harris RA, Crabb DW: Molecular defects in the E1α subunit of the branched-chain α-ketoacid dehydrogenase complex that cause maple syrup urine disease. *Mol Biol Med* **8**:39, 1991.
243. Chuang JL, Wynn RM, Song J, Chuang DT: GroEL/GroES-dependent reconstitution of α_2 β_2 tetramers of human mitochondrial branched chain α-ketoacid decarboxylase. *J Biol Chem* **274**:10395, 1999.
244. Chuang DT, Fisher CW, Lau KS, A GT, Wynn RM, Cox RP: Maple syrup urine disease: Domain structure, mutations and exon skipping in the dihydrolipoyl transacylase (E2) component of the branched-chain α-keto acid dehydrogenase complex. *Mol Biol Med* **8**:49, 1991.
245. Cox RP, Chuang DT: Maple syrup urine disease. Clinical and molecular genetic considerations, in Rosenberg R, Prusiner S, DiMauro S, Barchi R (eds): *The Molecular and Genetic Basis of Neurological Disease*. London, Butterworths, 1992, p 189.
246. Crabb DW, Deaven LL, Luedemann M, Zhang B, Harris RA: Assignment of the gene for the E1α subunit of branched chain α-ketoacid dehydrogenase to chromosome 19. *Cytogenet Cell Genet* **50**:40, 1989.
247. Fekete G, Plattner R, Crabb D, Zhang B, Harris RA, Heerema N, Palmer CG: Localization of the human gene for the E1α subunit of branched chain keto acid dehydrogenase (BCKDHA) to chromosome 19q13.1 $\rightarrow$ q13.2. *Cytogenet Cell Genet* **50**:236, 1989.
248. Zneimer SM, Lau KS, Eddy RL, Shows TB, Chuang JL, Chuang DT, Cox RP: Regional assignment of two genes of the human branched-chain α-keto acid dehydrogenase complex: The E1β gene (BCKDHB) to chromosome 6p21-22 and the E2 gene (DBT) to chromosome 1p31. *Genomics* **10**:740, 1991.
249. Mitsubuchi H, Nobukuni Y, Endo F, Matsuda I: Structural organization and chromosomal localization of the gene for the E1β subunit of human branched chain α-keto acid dehydrogenase. *J Biol Chem* **266**:14686, 1991.
250. Lau KS, Eddy RL, Shows TB, Fisher CW, Chuang DT, Cox RP: Localization of the dihydrolipoamide branched-chain transacylase gene (DBT) of the human branched-chain keto acid dehydrogenase complex to chromosome 1. *Cytogenet Cell Genet* **56**:33, 1991.
251. Herring WJ, Litwer S, Weber JL, Danner DJ: Molecular genetic basis of maple syrup urine disease in a family with two defective alleles for branched chain acyltransferase and localization of the gene to human chromosome 1. *Am J Hum Genet* **48**:342, 1991.
252. Herring WJ, McKean M, Dracopoli N, Danner DJ: Branched chain acyltransferase absence due to an Alu-based genomic deletion allele and an exon-skipping allele in a compound heterozygote proband expressing maple syrup urine disease. *Biochim Biophys Acta* **1138**:236, 1992.
253. Scherer SW, Otulakowski G, Robinson BH, Tsui LC: Localization of the human dihydrolipoamide dehydrogenase (DLD) to 7q31-q32. *Cytogenet Cell Genet* **56**:176, 1991.
254. Dariush N, Fisher CW, Cox RP, Chuang DT: Structure of the gene encoding the entire mature E1α subunit of human branched-chain α-keto acid dehydrogenase complex. *FEBS Lett* **284**:34, 1991.
255. Chuang JL, Cox RP, Chuang DT: Characterization of the promoter-regulatory region and structural organization of E1α gene (BCKDHA) of human branched-chain α-keto acid dehydrogenase complex. *J Biol Chem* **268**:8309, 1993.
256. Chuang JL, Cox RP, Chuang DT: Maple syrup urine disease: The E1β gene of human branched-chain α-ketoacid dehydrogenase complex has 11 rather than 10 exons, and the 3′ UTR in one of the two E1β mRNAs arises from intronic sequences. *Am J Hum Genet* **58**:1373, 1996.
257. Lau KS, Herring WJ, Chuang JL, McKean M, Danner DJ, Cox RP, Chuang DT: Structure of the gene encoding dihydrolipoyl transacylase (E2) component of human branched chain α-keto acid dehydrogenase complex and characterization of an E2 pseudogene. *J Biol Chem* **267**:24090, 1992.
258. Lau KS, Lee J, Fisher CW, Cox RP, Chuang DT: Premature termination of transcription and alternative splicing in the human transacylase (E2) gene of the branched-chain α-ketoacid dehydrogenase complex. *FEBS Lett* **279**:229, 1991.
259. Johanning GL, Morris JI, Madhusudhan KT, Samols D, Patel MS: Characterization of the transcriptional regulatory region of the human dihydrolipoamide dehydrogenase gene. *Proc Natl Acad Sci U S A* **89**:10964, 1992.
260. Feigenbaum AS, Robinson BH: The structure of the human dihydrolipoamide dehydrogenase gene (DLD) and its upstream elements. *Genomics* **17**:376, 1993.
261. Martini G, Toniolo D, Vulliamy T, Luzzatto L, Dono R, Viglietto G, Paonessa G, D'Urso M, Persico MG: Structural analysis of the X-linked gene encoding human glucose 6-phosphate dehydrogenase. *EMBO J* **5**:1849, 1986.
262. Huang Y, Chuang DT: Structural organization of the rat branched-chain 2-oxo acid dehydrogenase kinase gene and partial characterization of the promoter-regulatory region. *Biochem J* **313**:603, 1996.
263. Huang Y, Chuang DT: Mechanism for basal expression of rat mitochondrial branched-chain-2-oxo-acid dehydrogenase. *Biochem J* **334**:713, 1998.
264. Costeas PA, Chinsky JM: Isolaiton of the murine branched-chain α-ketoacid dehydrogenase E2 subunit promoter region. *Biochim Biophys Acta* **1399**:111, 1998.
265. Menkes JH, Hurst PL, Craig JM: A new syndrome: Progressive familial infantile cerebral dysfunction associated with an unusual urinary substance. *Pediatrics* **14**:462, 1954.
266. Westall RG, Dancis J, Miller S: Maple syrup urine disease. *Am J Dis Child* **94**:571, 1957.
267. Menkes JH: Maple syrup disease. Isolation and identification of organic acids in the urine. *Pediatrics* **23**:348, 1959.
268. Dancis J, Levitz M, Westall RG: Maple syrup urine disease: Branched-chain keto-aciduria. *Pediatrics* **25**:72, 1960.
269. Dancis J, Hutzler J, Rokkones T: Intermittent branched-chain ketonuria. Variant of maple-syrup-urine disease. *N Engl J Med* **276**:84, 1967.
270. Dancis J, Hutzler J, Levitz M: Metabolism of the white blood cells in maple-syrup-urine disease. *Biochim Biophys Acta* **43**:342, 1960.
271. Morris MD, Lewis BD, Doolan PD, Harper HA: Clinical and biochemical observations on an apparent non-fatal variant of branched-chain ketoaciduria (maple syrup urine disease). *Pediatrics* **28**:918, 1961.
272. Kiil R, Rokkones T: Late manifesting variant of branched-chain ketoaciduria (maple syrup urine disease). *Acta Paediatr* **53**:356, 1964.
273. Goedde HW, Langenbeck U, Brackertz D, Keller W, Rokkones T, Halvorsen S, Kiil R, Merton B: Clinical and biochemical-genetic aspects of intermittent branched-chain ketoaciduria. Report of two Scandinavian families. *Acta Paediatr Scand* **59**:83, 1970.
274. Dancis J, Hutzler J, Snyderman SE, Cox RP: Enzyme activity in classical and variant forms of maple syrup urine disease. *J Paediatr* **81**:312, 1972.
275. Dent CE, Westall RG: Studies in maple syrup urine disease. *Arch Dis Child* **36**:259, 1961.
276. Snyderman SE, Norton PM, Roitman E, Holt LE Jr: Maple syrup urine disease, with particular reference to dietotherapy. *Pediatrics* **34**:454, 1964.

277. Menkes JH: Maple syrup disease. Investigations into the metabolic defect. *Neurology* **9**:826, 1959.
278. Lyons LB, Cox RP, Dancis J: Complementation analysis of maple syrup urine disease in heterokaryons derived from cultured human fibroblasts. *Nature* **243**:533, 1973.
279. Singh S, Willers I, Goedde HW: Heterogeneity in maple syrup urine disease: Aspects of cofactor requirement and complementation in cultured fibroblasts. *Clin Genet* **11**:277, 1977.
280. Jinno Y, Akaboshi I, Matsuda I: Complementation analysis in lymphoid cells from five patients with different forms of maple syrup urine disease. *Hum Genet* **68**:54, 1984.
281. Matsuda I, Nobukuni Y, Mitsubuchi H, Indo Y, Endo F, Asaka J, Harada A: A T-to-A substitution in the E1α subunit gene of the branched-chain α-ketoacid dehydrogenase complex in two cell lines derived from Mennonite maple syrup urine disease patients. *Biochem Biophys Res Commun* **172**:646, 1990.
282. Fisher CR, Fisher CW, Chuang DT, Cox RP: Occurrence of a Tyr393 $\rightarrow$ Asn (Y393N) mutation in the E1α gene of the branched-chain α-keto acid dehydrogenase complex in maple syrup urine disease patients from a Mennonite population. *Am J Hum Genet* **49**:429, 1991.
283. Harper PA, Healy PJ, Dennis JA: Maple syrup urine disease as a cause of spongiform encephalopathy in calves. *Vet Rec* **119**:62, 1986.
284. Baird JD, Wojcinski ZW, Wise AP, Godkin MA: Maple syrup urine disease in five Hereford calves in Ontario. *Can Vet J* **28**:505, 1987.
285. Zhang B, Healy PJ, Zhao Y, Crabb DW, Harris RA: Premature translation termination of the pre-E1α subunit of the branched chain α-ketoacid dehydrogenase as a cause of maple syrup urine disease in Polled Hereford calves. *J Biol Chem* **265**:2425, 1990.
286. Koyata H, Cox RP, Chuang DT: Stable correction of maple syrup urine disease in cells from a Mennonite patient by retroviral-mediated gene transfer. *Biochem J* **295**:635, 1993.
287. Mueller GM, McKenzie LR, Homanics GE, Watkins SC, Robbins PD, Paul HS: Complementation of defective leucine decarboxylation in fibroblasts from a maple syrup urine disease patient by retrovirus-mediated gene transfer. *Gene Ther* **2**:461, 1995.
288. Treacy E, Clow CL, Reade TR, Chitayat D, Mamer OA, Scriver CR: Maple syrup urine disease: Interrelations between branched-chain amino-, oxo- and hydroxyacids; implications for treatment; associations with CNS dysmyelination. *J Inherit Metab Dis* **15**:121, 1992.
289. Shih VE, Levy HL, Herrin JT, McGrail K, Pueschel S, Ampola M: Outcome of MSUD patients detected by newborn screening following long-term treatment. (Unpublished.)
290. Mikati MA, Dudin GE, Der Kaloustian VM, Benson PF, Fensom AH: Maple syrup urine disease with increased intracranial pressure. *Am J Dis Child* **136**:642, 1982.
291. Mantovani JF, Naidich TP, Prensky AL, Dodson SE, Williams JC: MSUD: Presentation with pseudotumor cerebri and CT abnormalities. *J Pediatr* **96**:279, 1980.
292. Lungarotti MS, Calabro A, Signorini E, Garibaldi LR: Cerebral edema in maple syrup urine disease. *Am J Dis Child* **136**:648, 1982.
293. Hallock J, Morrow GD, Karp LA, Barness LA: Postmortem diagnosis of metabolic disorders. The finding of maple syrup urine disease in a case of sudden and unexpected death in infancy. *Am J Dis Child* **118**:649, 1969.
294. Donnell GN, Lieberman E, Shaw KNF, Koch R: Hypoglycemia in maple syrup urine disease. *Am J Dis Child* **113**:60, 1967.
295. Riviello JJ Jr, Rezvani I, Digeorge AM, Foley CM: Cerebral edema causing death in children with maple syrup urine disease. *J Pediatr* **119**:42, 1991.
296. Friedrich CA, Marble M, Maher J, Valle D: Successful control of branched-chain amino acids (BCAA) in maple syrup urine disease using elemental amino acids in total parenteral nutrition during acute pancreatitis. *Am J Hum Genet* **51**:A350, 1992.
297. Kahler SG, Woolf DA, Leonard JV, Zaritsky A, Lawless ST, Sherwood WG: Pancreatitis and organic acidurias — An under-recognized association [Abstract]? *Fifth International Congress Inborn Errors of Metabolism*, Pacific Grove, CA, June 1-5 1990, W5.4.
298. Danias J, Raab EL, Friedman AH: Retinopathy associated with pancreatitis in a child with maple syrup urine disease. *Br J Ophthalmol* **82**:841, 1998.
299. Muller H, Bickel H, Feist D, Lutz P: Maple syrup urine disease with an intermittent relatively benign course. *Verlauf Dtsch Med Wochenschr* **96**:1552, 1971.
300. Fischer MH, Gerritsen T: Biochemical studies on a variant of branched chain ketoaciduria in a 19-year-old female. *Pediatrics* **48**:795, 1971.
301. Gonzalez-Rios MDC, Chuang DT, Cox RP, Schmidt K, Knopf K, Packman S: A distinct variant of intermediate maple syrup urine disease. *Clin Genet* **27**:153, 1985.
302. Schulman JD, Lustberg TJ, Kennedy JL, Museles M, Seegmiller JE: A new variant of maple syrup urine disease (branched chain ketoaciduria). Clinical and biochemical evaluation. *Am J Med* **49**:118, 1970.
303. Verdu A, Lopez-Herce J, Pascual-Castroviejo I, Martinez-Bermejo A, Ugarte M, Garcia MJ: Maple syrup urine disease variant form: Presentation with psychomotor retardation and CT scan abnormalities. *Acta Paediatr Scand* **74**:815, 1985.
304. Rittinger O, Bachmann C, Irnberger T, Pilz P, Walter GF, Wendel U, Plochl E: The intermediate form of maple syrup disease. *Klin Padiatr* **198**:37, 1986.
305. Kalyanaraman K, Chamukuttan S, Arjundas G, Gajanan N, Ramamurthi B: Maple syrup urine disease (branched-chain ketoaciduria) variant type manifesting as hyperkinetic behaviour and mental retardation. Report of two cases. *J Neurol Sci* **15**:209, 1972.
306. Weiss L, Noonan SN, Hyde T: An unusual variant of maple syrup urine disease. *Am J Hum Genet* **27**:93A, 1975.
307. Stoppoloni G, Santinelli R, Tolone C, Prisco F: Dietary treatment in a case of maple syrup urine disease, mild variant. *Ital J Pediatr* **2**:395, 1976.
308. Velazquez A, Montiel F, Shaw KN, Carnevale A, Del Castillo V: Maple syrup urine disease. Genetic heterogeneity, heterozygote diagnosis and new therapeutic approach. *Rev Invest Clin* **33**:273, 1981.
309. Duran M, Tielens AG, Wadman SK, Stigter JC, Kleijer WJ: Effects of thiamine in a patient with a variant form of branched-chain ketoaciduria. *Acta Paediatr Scand* **67**:367, 1978.
310. Van Der Horst JL, Wadman SK: A variant form of branched-chain keto aciduria. *Acta Paediatr Scand* **60**:594, 1971.
311. Chhabria S, Tomasi LG, Wong PW: Ophthalmoplegia and bulbar palsy in variant form of maple syrup urine disease. *Ann Neurol* **6**:71, 1979.
312. MacDonald JT, Sher PK: Ophthalmoplegia as a sign of metabolic disease in the newborn. *Neurology* **27**:971, 1977.
313. Hurwitz LJ, Carson NA, Allen IV, Chopra JS: Congenital ophthalmoplegia, floppy baby syndrome, myopathy, and aminoaciduria. Report of a family. *J Neurol Neurosurg Psychiatry* **32**:495, 1969.
314. Zee DS, Freeman JM, Holtzman NA: Ophthalmoplegia in maple syrup urine disease. *J Pediatr* **84**:113, 1974.
315. Valman HB, Patrick AD, Seakins JW, Platt JW, Gompertz D: Family with intermittent maple syrup urine disease. *Arch Dis Child* **48**:225, 1973.
316. Morris MD, Fisher DA, Fiser R: Late-onset branched-chain ketoaciduria (maple syrup urine disease). *Lancet* **86**:149, 1966.
317. Zaleski LA, Dancis J, Cox RP, Hutzler J, Zaleski WA, Hill A: Variant maple syrup urine disease in mother and daughter. *Can Med Assoc J* **109**:299, 1973.
318. Gretter TE, Lonsdale D, Mercer RD, Robinson C, Shamberger RJ: Maple syrup urine disease variant. Report of a case. *Cleve Clin Q* **39**:129, 1972.
319. Indo Y, Akaboshi I, Nobukuni Y, Endo F, Matsuda I: Maple syrup urine disease: A possible biochemical basis for the clinical heterogeneity. *Hum Genet* **80**:6, 1988.
320. Holmgren G, Brundin A, Gustavson KH, Sjogren S, Kleijer WJ, Niermeijer MF: Intermittent neurological symptoms in a girl with a maple syrup urine disease (MSUD) variant. *Neuropediatrics* **11**:377, 1980.
321. Saudubray JM, Amedee-Manesme O, Munnich A, Ogier H, Depondt E, Charpentier C, Coude FX, Rey F, Frezal J: Heterogeneity of leucinosis. Correlations between clinical manifestations, protein tolerance and enzyme deficiency. *Arch Fr Pediatr* **39**:735, 1982.
322. Boisse J, Saudubray JM, Pham HT, Charpentier C, Castets M, Lemonnier A, Jerome H, Mozziconacci P: The intermittent variant of leucinosis (study of a new case). *Arch Fr Pediatr* **28**:161, 1971.
323. Irwin WC, Martel SB, Goluboff N: Intermittent branched chain ketonuria (variant of maple syrup urine disease). *Clin Biochem* **4**:52, 1971.
324. Ellingsen LIEI, Haugstad S, Holm H: Tailoring of the diet for the individual in maple syrup urine disease: Long-term home dietary treatment of an adult patient with MSUD by monitoring of daily intake with a personal computer. A case report. *Hum Nutr Appl Nutr* **39**:130, 1985.
325. Pueschel SM: Thiamine non-responsive intermittent branched-chain ketoaciduria in a Laotian child. *J Inherit Metab Dis* **9**:72, 1986.

326. Fritsch G, Langenbeck U, Wendel U, Lehnert W, Plam W, Steger W: [Intermittent maple syrup urine disease in a 12-year-old boy: Clinical aspects, diagnosis and treatment.] Knaben: Klinik, Diagnostik und Therapie. *Klin Padiatr* **195**:351, 1983.
327. Stastna M, Wendel S, Verner P, Zemen J, Kozich V, Hyanek J, Rytir Z, Nemcova DV: Intermittent form of MSUD in brother and sister. Paper presented at the Society for the Study of Inborn Errors of Metabolism Annual Symposium 1992.
328. Steen-Johnsen J, Vellan EJ, Gjessing LR: Maple syrup urine disease variant — Amino acid pattern and problems of treatment during acute attacks. *Acta Paediatr Scand Suppl* **206**:71, 1970.
329. Zipf WB, Hieber VC, Allen RJ: Valine-toxic intermittent maple syrup urine disease: A previously unrecognized variant. *Pediatrics* **63**:286, 1979.
330. Scriver CR, Mackenzie S, Clow CL, Delvin E: Thiamine-responsive maple-syrup-urine disease. *Lancet* **1**:310, 1971.
331. Scriver CR, Clow CL, George H: So-called thiamin-responsive maple syrup urine disease: 15-year follow-up of the original patient. *J Pediatr* **107**:763, 1985.
332. Chuang DT, Ku LS, Cox RP: Thiamin-responsive maple syrup urine disease: Decreased affinity of the mutant branched-chain α-ketoacid dehydrogenase for α-ketoisovalerate and thiamin pyrophosphate. *Proc Natl Acad Sci U S A* **79**:3300, 1982.
333. Duran M, Tielens AGM, Wadman SK, Stigter JCM, Kleijer WJ: Effects of thiamine in a patient with a variant form of branched-chain ketoaciduria. *Acta Paediatr Scand* **67**:367, 1978.
334. Elsas L, Blocker T, Wheeler F, Pask B, Perl D, Trusler S: Variant "classical" maple syrup urine disease: Co-factor response. *Clin Res* **20**:43, 1972.
335. Pueschel SM, Bresnan MJ, Shih VE, Levy HL: Thiamine-responsive intermittent branched-chain ketoaciduria. *J Pediatr* **94**:628, 1979.
336. Fernhoff PM, Lubitz D, Danner DJ, Dembure PP, Schwartz HP, Hillman R, Bier DM, Elsas LJ: Thiamine response in maple syrup urine disease. *Pediatr Res* **19**:1011, 1985.
337. Elsas L, Danner D, Lubitz D, Fernhoff P, Dembure P: Metabolic consequences of inherited defects in branched chain alpha-ketoacid dehydrogenase: Mechanism of thiamine action, in M W, Williamson J (eds): *Metabolism and Clinical Implications of Branched Chain Amino and Ketoacids*. New York, Elsevier/North Holland, 1981, p 369.
338. Elsas LJII, Danner DJ: The role of thiamin in maple syrup urine disease. *Ann N Y Acad Sci* **378**:404, 1982.
339. Kodama S, Seki A, Hanabusa M, Morisita Y, Sakurai T: Mild variant of maple syrup urine disease. *Eur J Pediatr* **124**:31, 1976.
340. Duran M, Wadman SK: Thiamine-responsive inborn errors of metabolism. *J Inherit Metab Dis* **8(Suppl 1)**:70, 1985.
341. Pueschel SM, Bresnan MJ, Shih VE, Levy HL: Thiamine-responsive intermittent branched-chain ketoaciduria. *J Pediatr* **94**:628, 1979.
342. Matalon R, Stumpf DA, Michals K, Hart RD, Parks JK, Goodman SI: Lipoamide dehydrogenase deficiency with primary lactic acidosis: Favorable response to treatment with oral lipoic acid. *J Pediatr* **104**:65, 1984.
343. Robinson BH, Taylor J, Kahler SG, Kirkman HN: Lactic acidemia, neurologic deterioration and carbohydrate dependence in a girl with dihydrolipoyl dehydrogenase deficiency. *Eur J Pediatr* **136**:35, 1981.
344. Taylor J, Robinson BH, Sherwood WG: A defect in branched-chain amino acid metabolism in a patient with congenital lactic acidosis due to dihydrolipoyl dehydrogenase deficiency. *Pediatr Res* **12**:60, 1978.
345. Robinson BH, Taylor J, Sherwood WG: Deficiency of dihydrolipoyl dehydrogenase (a component of the pyruvate and α-ketoglutarate dehydrogenase complex): A cause of congenital chronic lactic acidosis in infancy. *Pediatr Res* **11**:1198, 1977.
345a. Sakaguchi Y, Yoshino M, Aramaki S, Yoshida I, Yamashita F, Kuhara T, Matsumoto I, Hayashi T: Dihydrolipoyl dehydrogenase deficiency: A therapeutic trial with branched-chain amino acid restriction. *Eur J Pediatr* **145**:271, 1986.
346. Matuda S, Kitano A, Sakaguchi Y, Yoshino M, Saheki T: Pyruvate dehydrogenase subcomplex with lipoamide dehydrogenase deficiency in a patient with lactic acidosis and branched chain ketoaciduria. *Clin Chim Acta* **140**:59, 1984.
347. Haworth JC, Perry TL, Blass JP, Hansen S, Urquhart N: Lactic acidosis in three sibs due to defects in both pyruvate dehydrogenase and alpha-ketoglutarate dehydrogenase complexes. *Pediatrics* **58**:564, 1976.
348. Munnich A, Saudubray JM, Taylor J, Charpentier C, Marsac C, Rocchiccioli F, Amedee-Manesme O, Coude FX, Frezal J, Robinson BH: Congenital lactic acidosis, α-ketoglutaric aciduria and variant form of maple syrup urine disease due to a single enzyme defect: Dihydrolipoyl dehydrogenase deficiency. *Acta Paediatr Scand* **71**:167, 1982.
349. Frezal J, Amedee-Manesme O, Mitchell G, Heuertz S, Rey F, Rey J, Saudubray JM: Maple syrup urine disease: Two different forms within a single family. *Hum Genet* **71**:89, 1985.
350. Langenbeck U: Two different forms of maple syrup urine disease in a single family. *Hum Genet* **72**:279, 1986.
351. Harper PA, Dennis JA, Healy PJ, Brown GK: Maple syrup urine disease in calves: A clinical, pathological and biochemical study. *Aust Vet J* **66**:46, 1989.
352. Harper PA, Healy PJ, Dennis JA: Maple syrup urine disease (branched chain ketoaciduria). *Am J Pathol* **136**:1445, 1990.
353. Harper PA, Healy PJ, Dennis JA: Ultrastructural findings in maple syrup urine disease in Poll Hereford calves. *Acta Neuropathol (Berl)* **71**:316, 1986.
354. Dodd PR, Williams SH, Gundlach AL, Harper PA, Healy PJ, Dennis JA, Johnston GA: Glutamate and gamma-aminobutyric acid neurotransmitter systems in the acute phase of maple syrup urine disease and citrullinemia encephalopathies in newborn calves. *J Neurochem* **59**:582, 1992.
355. Rudiger HW, Langenbeck U, Schulze-Schencking M, Goedde HW, Schuchmann L: Defective decarboxylase in branched chain ketoacid oxidase multienzyme complex in classic type of maple syrup urine disease. *Humangenetik* **14**:257, 1972.
356. Chuang DT, Niu W-L, Cox RP: Activities of branched-chain 2-oxo acid dehydrogenase and its components in skin fibroblasts from normal and classical-maple-syrup-urine-disease subjects. *Biochem J* **200**:59, 1981.
357. Chuang DT, Cox RP: Enzyme assays with mutant cell lines of maple syrup urine disease. *Methods Enzymol* **166**:135, 1988.
358. Chuang DT, Ku LS, Kerr DS, Cox RP: Detection of heterozygotes in maple-syrup-urine disease: Measurements of branched-chain α-ketoacid dehydrogenase and its components in cell cultures. *Am J Hum Genet* **34**:416, 1982.
359. Zhang B, Edenberg HJ, Crabb DW, Harris RA: Evidence for both a regulatory mutation and a structural mutation in a family with maple syrup urine disease. *J Clin Invest* **83**:1425, 1989.
360. Eisenstein RS, Hoganson G, Miller RH, Harper AE: Altered phosphorylation state of branched-chain 2-oxo acid dehydrogenase in a branched-chain acyltransferase deficient human fibroblast cell line. *J Inherit Metab Dis* **14**:37, 1991.
361. Nobukuni Y, Mitsubuchi H, Ohta K, Akaboshi I, Indo Y, Endo F, Matsuda I: Molecular diagnosis of maple syrup urine disease: Screening and identification of gene mutations in the branched-chain α-ketoacid dehydrogenase multienzyme complex. *J Inherit Metab Dis* **15**:827, 1992.
362. Saiki RK, Gelfand DH, Stoffel S, Scharf SJ, Higuchi R, Horn GT, Mullis KB, Erlich HA: Primer-directed enzymatic amplifications of DNA with a thermostable DNA polymerase. *Science* **239**:487, 1988.
363. Marshall L, DiGeorge A: Maple syrup urine disease in the old order Mennonites. *Am J Hum Genet* **33**:139A, 1981.
364. Chuang JL, Davie JR, Chinsky JM, Wynn RM, Cox RP, Chuang DT: Molecular and biochemical basis of intermediate maple syrup urine disease. Occurrence of homozygous G245R and F364C mutations at the E1α locus of Hispanic-Mexican patients. *J Clin Inves* **95**:954, 1995.
365. Nobukuni Y, Mitsubuchi H, Hayashida Y, Ohta K, Indo Y, Ichiba Y, Endo F, Matsuda I: Heterogeneity of mutations in maple syrup urine disease (MSUD): screening and identification of affection E1α and E1β subunits of the branched-chain α-keto-acid dehydrogenase multienzyme complex. *Biochim Biophys Acta* **1225**:64, 1993.
366. Hayshida Y, Mitsubuchi H, Indo Y, Ohta K, Endo F, Wada Y, Matsuda I: Deficiency of the E1β subunit in the branched-chain α-keto acid dehydrogenase complex due to a single base substitution of the intron 5, resulting in two alternatively spliced mRNAs in a patient with maple syrup urine disease. *Biochim Biophys Acta* **1225**:317, 1994.
367. Nobukuni Y, Mitsubuchi H, Akaboshi I, Indo Y, Endo F, Yoshioka A, Matsuda I: Maple syrup urine disease. Complete defect of the E1β subunit of the branched chain α-ketoacid dehydrogenase complex due to a deletion of an 11-bp repeat sequence which encodes a mitochondrial targeting leader peptide in a family with the disease. *J Clin Invest* **87**:1862, 1991.
368. Mitsubuchi H, Nobukuni Y, Akaboshi I, Indo Y, Endo F, Matsuda I: Maple syrup urine disease caused by a partial deletion in the inner E2 core domain of the branched chain α-keto acid dehydrogenase complex due to aberrant splicing. A single base deletion at a 5′-splice

donor site of an intron of the E2 gene disrupts the consensus sequence in this region. *J Clin Invest* **87**:1207, 1991.

369. McConnell BB, Burkholder B, Danner DJ: Two new mutations in the human E1β subunit of branched chain α-ketoacid dehydrogenase associated with maple syrup urine disease. *Biochim Biophys Acta* **1361**:263, 1997.
370. Fisher CW, Lau KS, Fisher CR, Wynn RM, Cox RP, Chuang DT: A 17-bp insertion and a Phe215 $\rightarrow$ Cys missense mutation in the dihydrolipoyl transacylase (E2) mRNA from a thiamine-responsive maple syrup urine disease patient WG-34. *Biochem Biophys Res Commun* **174**:804, 1991.
371. Chuang JL, Cox RP, Chuang DT: Manuscript in preparation. 2000.
372. Chuang JL, Cox RP, Chuang DT: E2 transacylase-deficient (Type II) maple syrup urine disease, aberrant splicing of E2 mRNA caused by internal intronic deletions and association with thiamine-responsive phenotype. *J Clin Invest* **100**:736, 1997.
373. Liu T-C, Kim H, Arizmendi C, Kitano A, Patel MS: Identification of two missense mutations in a dihydrolipoamide dehydrogenase-deficient patient. *Proc Natl Acad Sci U S A* **90**:5186, 1993.
374. Shaag A, Saada A, Berger I, Mandel H, Joseph A, Feigenbaum A, Elpeleg ON: Molecular basis of lipoamide dehydrogenase deficiency in Ashkenazi Jews. *Am J Med Genet* **82**:177, 1999.
375. Brown CR, Hong-Brown LQ, Welch WJ: Correcting temperature-sensitive protein folding defects. *J Clin Invest* **99**:1432, 1997.
376. Danner DJ, Wheeler FB, Lemmon SK, Elsas LJII: In vivo and in vitro response of human branched chain α-ketoacid dehydrogenase to thiamine and thiamine pyrophosphate. *Pediatr Res* **12**:235, 1978.
377. Blair PV, Kobayashi RK, Edwards HMIII, Shay NF, Baker DH, Harris RA: Dietary thiamin level influences levels of its diphosphate form and thiamin-dependent enzymic activities of rat liver. *J Nutr* **129**:641, 1999.
378. Zhang B, Wapner RS, Brandt IK, Harris RA, Crabb DW: Sequence of the E1α subunit of branched chain α-ketoacid dehydrogenase in two patients with thiamine-responsive maple syrup urine disease. *Am J Human Genet* **46**:843, 1990.
379. Ellerine NP, Herring WJ, Elsas IILJ, McKean MC, Klein PD, Danner DJ: Thiamin-responsive maple syrup urine disease in a patient antigenically missing dihydrolipoamide acyltransferase. *Biochem Med Metabol Biol* **49**:363, 1993.
380. Naylor EW: Newborn screening for maple syrup urine disease (branched-chain ketoaciduria), in Bickel H, Guthrie R, Hammersen G (eds): *Neonatal Screening for Inborn Errors of Metabolism*. Berlin, Springer-Verlag, 1980, p 19.
381. Parrella T, Iolascon SS, Sartore M, Heidenreich R, Diamond G, Ponzone A: Maple syrup urine disease (MSUD): Screening for known mutations in Italian patients. *J Inherit Metab Dis* **17**:652, 1994.
382. Danner DJ, Elsas LJII: Disorders of branched chain amino acid and keto acid metabolism, in Scriver C, Beaudet A, Sly W, Valle D (eds): *The Metabolic Basis of Inherited Disease*, 6th ed. New York, McGraw-Hill, 1989, p 671.
383. Mitsubuchi H, Matsuda I, Nobukuni Y, Heidenreich R, Indo Y, Endo F, Mallee J, Segal S: Gene analysis of Mennonite maple syrup urine disease kindred using primer-specified restriction map modification. *J Inherit Metab Dis* **15**:181, 1992.
384. Yoshino M, Koga Y, Yamashita F: A decrease in glycine cleavage activity in the liver of a patient with dihydrolipoyl dehydrogenase deficiency. *J Inherit Metab Dis* **9**:399, 1986.
385. Dancis J, Levitz M, Miller S, Westall RG: Maple syrup urine disease. *Br Med J* **1**:91, 1959.
386. Norton PM, Roitman E, Snyderman SE, Holt LE Jr: A new finding in maple-syrup-urine disease. *Lancet* **1**:26, 1962.
387. Matthews DE, Ben-Galim E, Haymond MW, Bier DM: Alloisoleucine formation in maple syrup urine disease: Isotopic evidence for the mechanism. *Pediatr Res* **14**:854, 1980.
388. Mamer OA, Reimer MLJ: On the mechanisms of the formation of L-alloisoleucine and the 2-hydroxy-3-methylvaleric acid stereoisomers from l-isoleucine in maple syrup urine disease patients and in normal humans. *J Biol Chem* **267**:22141, 1992.
389. Schadewaldt P, Hammen HW, Dalle-Feste C, Wendel U: On the mechanism of L-alloisoleucine formation: Studies on a healthy subject and in fibroblasts from normals and patients with maple syrup urine disease. *J Inherit Metab Dis* **13**:137, 1990.
390. Wendel U, Langenbeck U, Seakins JW: Interrelation between the metabolism of L-isoleucine and L-allo-isoleucine in patients with maple syrup urine disease. *Pediatr Res* **25**:11, 1989.
391. Shigematsu Y, Kikuchi K, Momoi T, Sudo M, Kikawa Y, Nosaka K, Kuriyama M, Haruki S, Sanada K, Hamano N: Organic acids and branched-chain amino acids in body fluids before and after multiple exchange transfusions in maple syrup urine disease. *J Inherit Metab Dis* **6**:183, 1983.
392. Sansaricq C, Smith L, Faruki M: Cerebrospinal fluid in maple syrup urine disease (MSUD). *Pediatr Res* **25**:202A, 1989.
393. Thomas GH, Howell RR: *Selected Screening Tests for Genetic Metabolic Diseases*. Chicago, Year Book, 1973, p 9.
394. Lancaster G, Mamer OA, Scriver CR: Branched-chain alpha-keto acids isolated as oxime derivatives: Relationship to the corresponding hydroxy acids and amino acids in maple syrup urine disease. *Metabolism* **23**:257, 1974.
395. Tanaka K, West-Dull A, Hine DG, Lynn TB, Lowe T: Gas-chromatographic method of analysis for urinary organic acids. II. Description of the procedure, and its application to diagnosis of patients with organic acidurias. *Clin Chem* **26**:1847, 1980.
396. Langenbeck U, Hoinowski A, Mantel K, Mohring H-U: Quantitative gas chromatography and single-ion detection of aliphatic α-keto acids from urine as their *O*-trimethylsilylquinoxalinol derivatives. *J Chromatogr* **143**:39, 1977.
397. Langenbeck U, Wendel U, Mench-Hoinowski A, Kuschel D, Becker K, Przyrembel H, Bremer H: Correlations between branched-chain amino acids and branched-chain alpha-keto acids in blood in maple syrup urine disease. *Clin Chim Acta* **88**:283, 1978.
398. Snyderman SE, Goldstein F, Sansaricq C, Norton PM: The relationship between the branched chain amino acids and their alpha-ketoacids in maple syrup urine disease. *Pediatr Res* **18**:851, 1984.
399. Langenbeck U: Pathobiochemical and pathophysiologic analysis of the MSUD phenotype, in Adibi S, Fekl W, Langenbeck U, Schauder P (eds): *Branched Chain Amino and Keto Acids in Health and Disease*. Basel, Karger, 1984, p 315.
400. Yoshida I, Sweetman L, Nyhan WL: Metabolism of branched-chain amino acids in fibroblasts from patients with maple syrup urine disease and other abnormalities of branched-chain ketoacid dehydrogenase activity. *Pediatr Res* **20**:169, 1986.
401. Kuhara T, Shinka T, Inoue Y, Matsumoto M, Yoshino M, Sakaguchi Y, Matsumoto I: Studies of urinary organic acid profiles of a patient with dihydrolipoyl dehydrogenase deficiency. *Clin Chim Acta* **133**:133, 1983.
402. Wendel U, Lombeck I, Bremer HJ: Maple-syrup-urine disease. *N Engl J Med* **308**:1100, 1983.
403. Romano C, Cerone U, Caruso A, Gandolfo M, Cotellessa G: Maple syrup urine disease (MSUD): Prenatal diagnosis vs branched-chain amino acid levels during the first two days of life. *Perspect Inherit Metab Dis* **6**:121, 1986.
404. Digeorge AM, Rezvani I, Garibaldi LR, Schwartz M: Prospective study of maple-syrup-urine disease for the first four days of life. *N Engl J Med* **307**:1492, 1982.
405. Shih VE: Maple-syrup-urine disease. *N Engl J Med* **310**:596, 1984.
406. Podebrad F, Heil M, Reichert S: 4,5-Dimethyl-3-hydroxy-2[5H]-furanone (sotolone)—The odour of maple syrup urine disease. *J Inherit Metab Dis* **22**:107, 1999.
407. Hauser GJ, Chitayat D, Berns L, Braver D, Muhlbauer B: Peculiar odours in newborns and maternal prenatal ingestion of spicy food. *Eur J Pediatr* **144**:403, 1985.
408. Patrick AD: Maple syrup urine disease. *Arch Dis Child* **36**:269, 1961.
409. Dancis J, Jansen V, Hutzler J, Levitz M: The metabolism of leucine in tissue culture of skin fibroblasts of maple-syrup-urine disease. *Biochim Biophys Acta* **77**:523, 1963.
410. Skaper SD, Molden DP, Seegmiller JE: Maple syrup urine disease: Branched-chain amino acid concentrations and metabolism in cultured human lymphoblasts. *Biochem Genet* **14**:527, 1976.
411. Wendel U, Wohler W, Goedde HW, Langenbeck U, Passarge E, Rudiger HW: Rapid diagnosis of maple syrup urine disease (branched chain ketoaciduria) by micro-enzyme assay in leukocytes and fibroblasts. *Clin Chim Acta* **45**:433, 1973.
412. Fensom AH, Benson PF, Baker JE: A rapid method for assay of branched-chain keto acid decarboxylation in cultured cells and its application to prenatal diagnosis of maple syrup urine disease. *Clin Chim Acta* **87**:169, 1978.
413. Elsas LJ, Priest JH, Wheeler FB, Danner DJ, Pask BA: Maple syrup urine disease: Coenzyme function and prenatal monitoring. *Metabolism* **23**:569, 1974.
414. Rudiger HW, Langenbeck U, Goedde HW: A simplified method for the preparation of 14C-labelled branched-chain α-oxo acids. *Biochem J* **126**:445, 1972.
415. Schadewaldt P, Beck K, Wendel U: Analysis of maple syrup urine disease in cell culture: Use of substrates. *Clin Chim Acta* **184**:47, 1989.

416. Chuang J, Chuang D: Diagnosis and Mutational Analysis of Maple Syrup Urine Disease Using Cell Cultures. *Methods Enzymol* **324**:413, 2000.
417. Wendel U, Wentrup H, Rudiger HW: Maple syrup urine disease: Analysis of branched chain ketoacid decarboxylation in cultured fibroblasts. *Pediatr Res* **9**:709, 1975.
418. Dancis J, Hutzler J, Cox RP: Maple syrup urine disease: Branched-chain keto acid decarboxylation in fibroblasts as measured with amino acids and keto acids. *Am J Hum Genet* **29**:272, 1977.
419. Toshima K, Kuroda Y, Yokota I, Naito E, Ito M, Watanabe T, Takeda E, Miyao M: Activation of branched-chain α-ketoacid dehydrogenase complex by α-chloroisocaproate in normal and enzyme-deficient fibroblasts. *Clin Chim Acta* **147**:103, 1985.
420. Elsas LJ, Ellerine NP, Klein PD: Practical methods to assess whole body leucine oxidation in maple syrup urine disease. *Pediatr Res* **33**:445, 1993.
421. Schadewaldt P, Wendel U: Metabolism of branched-chain amino acids in maple syrup urine disease. *Eur J Pediatr* **156(Suppl 1)**:S62, 1997.
422. Kleijer WJ, Horsman D, Mancini GM, Fois A, Boue J: First-trimester diagnosis of maple syrup urine disease on intact chorionic villi. *N Engl J Med* **313**:1608, 1985.
423. Dancis J: Maple syrup urine disease and congenital hyperuricemia, in Dorfman A (ed): *Antenatal Diagnosis*, Chicago, University of Chicago Press, 1972, p 123.
424. Wendel U, Rudiger HW, Passarge E, Mikkelsen M: Maple syrup urine disease: Rapid prenatal diagnosis by enzyme assay. *Humangenetik* **19**:127, 1973.
425. Wendel U, Gamm G, Claussen U: Maple syrup urine disease: Alpha-ketoisocaproate decarboxylation activity in different types of cultured amniotic fluid cells. *Prenat Diagn* **1**:235, 1981.
426. Potashnik R, Carmi R, Sofer S, Bashan N, Abeliovich D: Maple syrup urine disease in a Bedouin tribe: Pre- and postnatal diagnosis. *Isr J Med Sci* **23**:886, 1987.
427. Wendel U, Claussen U: Antenatal diagnosis of maple-syrup-urine disease. *Lancet* **1**:161, 1979.
428. Cox RP, Hutzler J, Dancis J: Antenatal diagnosis of maple-syrup-urine disease. *Lancet* **2**:212, 1978.
429. Jorgensen FS, Bang J, Lind AM, Christensen B, Lundsteen C, Philip J: Genetic amniocentesis at 7–14 weeks of gestation. *Prenat Diagn* **12**:277, 1992.
430. Wendel U, Claussen U, Langenbeck U: Pattern of branched-chained alpha-keto acids in amniotic fluid. *Clin Chim Acta* **102**:267, 1980.
431. O'Neill RT, Morrow GD, Hammel D, Auerbach VH, Barness LA: Diagnostic significance of amniotic fluid amino acids. *Obstet Gynecol* **37**:550, 1971.
432. Sweetman L: Prenatal diagnosis of the organic acidurias. *J Inherit Metab Dis* **7(Suppl 1)**:18, 1984.
433. Brismar J, Aqeel A, Brismar G, Coates R, Gascon G, Ozand P: Maple syrup urine disease: Findings on CT and MR scans of the brain in 10 infants. *AJNR Am J Neuroradiol* **11**:1219, 1990.
434. Suzuki S, Naito H, Abe T, Niehei K: Cranial computed tomography in a patient with a variant form of maple syrup urine disease. *Neuropediatrics* **14**:102, 1983.
435. Uziel G, Savoiardo M, Nardocci N: CT and MRI in maple syrup urine disease. *Neurology* **38**:486, 1988.
436. Taccone A, Schiaffino MC, Cerone R, Fondelli MP, Romano C: Computed tomography in maple syrup urine disease. *Eur J Radiol* **14**:207, 1992.
437. Sperl W, Felber S, Widschwendter M, Zaknun J, Wendel U: 1H NMR imaging and spectroscopy during metabolic decompensation in maple syrup urine disease. Society for the Study of Inborn Errors of Metabolism Annual Symposium, 1991.
438. Heindel W, Kugel H, Wendel U, Roth B: Magnetic resonance spectroscopy reflects maple syrup urine disease [Abstract]. *29th Society for the Study of Inborn Errors of Metabolism Annual Symposium*, London, 1991.
439. Wang Z, Bogdan AR, Detre JA, Gusnard DA, Zimmerman RA: In vivo 1H MRS studies of pediatric metabolic diseases [Abstract]. *Proceedings of the 10th Society of Magnetic Resonance in Medicine Meeting*, 1991.
440. Diezel PB, Martin K: Die Ahornsirupkrankheit mit familiaren Befall. *Virchows Arch [A]* **337**:425, 1964.
441. Feigin I, Budzilovich G, Pena C: The infantile spongy degeneration. *J Neuropathol Exp Neurol* **27**:158, 1968.
442. Kamei A, Takashima S, Chan F, Becker LE: Abnormal dendritic development in maple syrup urine disease. *Pediatr Neurol* **8**:145, 1992.
443. Taketomi T, Kunishita T, Hara A, Mizushima S: Abnormal protein and lipid compositions of the cerebral myelin of a patient with maple syrup urine disease. *Jpn J Exp Med* **53**:109, 1983.
444. Silberman J, Dancis J, Feigin I: Neuropathological observations in maple syrup urine disease. *Arch Neuro* **l5**:351, 1961.
445. Linneweh F, Solcher H: On the effect of dietetic prophylaxis on the myelogenesis of leucinosis (maple syrup urine disease). *Klin Wochenschr* **43**:926, 1965.
446. Gaull GE: Pathogenesis of maple syrup urine disease: Observation during dietary management and treatment of coma by peritoneal dialysis. *Biochem Med* **3**:130, 1969.
447. Menkes JH, Philippart M, Fiol RE: Cerebral lipids in maple syrup disease. *J Pediatr* **66**:584, 1965.
448. Prensky AL, Moser HW: Brain lipids, proteolipids, and free amino acids in maple syrup urine disease. *J Neurochem* **13**:863, 1966.
449. Woolf L: Recent work on phenylketonuria and maple syrup disease. *Proc R Soc Med* **55**:824, 1962.
450. Menkes JH, Solcher H: Maple syrup disease. Effects of dietary therapy on cerebral lipids. *Arch Neurol* **16**:486, 1967.
451. Voyce MA, Montgomery JN, Crome L, Bowman J, Ireland JT: Maple syrup urine disease. *J Ment Defic Res* **11**:231, 1967.
452. Prensky AL, Moser HW: Changes in the amino acid composition of proteolipids of white matter during maturation of the human nervous system. *J Neurochem* **14**:117, 1967.
453. Estivill E, Sanmarti FX, Vidal R, Alvira R, Liarraga I, Linares J: Comb-like rhythm: An EEG pattern peculiar to leucinosis. *Ann Esp Pediatr* **22**:123, 1985.
454. Iinuma K, Saito T, Wada Y, Onuma A, Takamatsu N: Electro-encephalograms in a case of maple syrup urine disease: Their relation to serum levels of branched-chain amino acids. *Tohoku J Exp Med* **120**:191, 1976.
455. Trottier A, Metrakos K, Geoffroy G, Andermann F: A characteristic EEG finding in newborns with maple syrup urine disease (branched-chain keto aciduria). *Electroencephalogr Clin Neurophysiol* **38**:108, 1975.
456. Tharp BR: Unique EEG pattern (comb-like rhythm) in neonatal maple syrup urine disease. *Pediatr Neurol* **8**:65, 1992.
457. Snyderman SE: Treatment outcome of maple syrup urine disease. *Acta Paediatr Jpn* **30**:417, 1988.
458. Yudkoff M: Brain metabolism of branched-chain amino acids. *Glia* **21**:92, 1997.
459. Huang Y, Zielke RH, Tildon JT: Elevation of amino acids in the interstitial space of the rat brain following infusion of large neutral amino and keto acids by microdialysis: Leucine infusion. *Dev Neurosci* **18**:415, 1996.
460. Zielke HR, Huang Y, Tildon JT: Elevation of amino acids in the interstitial space of the rat brain following infusion of large neutral amino and keto acids by microdialysis: alpha-Ketoisocaproate infusion. *Dev Neurosci* **18**:420, 1996.
461. Westall RG: Dietary treatment of a child with maple syrup urine disease (branched-chain ketoaciduria). *Arch Dis Child* **38**:485, 1963.
462. Lundquist TG, Morton DH: Use of a branched-chain ketoacid precipitation test to monitor maple syrup urine disease. *Unpublished*, 1993.
463. Clow CL, Reade TM, Scriver CR: Outcome of early and long-term management of classical maple syrup urine disease. *Pediatrics* **68**:856, 1981.
464. Wendel U: Acute and long-term treatment of children with maple syrup urine disease, in Adibi S, Fekl W, Langenbeck U, Schauder P (eds): *Branched Chain Amino and Keto Acids in Health and Disease*. Basel, Karger, 1984, p 335.
465. Elsas LJII, Acosta PB: Nutrition support of inherited metabolic diseases, in Shils M, Young V (eds): *Modern Nutrition in Health and Disease*. Philadelphia, Lea & Febiger, 1988, p 1337.
466. Kindt E, Halvorsen S: The need of essential amino acids in children. An evaluation based on the intake of phenylalanine, tyrosine, leucine, isoleucine, and valine in children with phenylketonuria, tyrosine amino transferase defect, and maple syrup urine disease. *Am J Clin Nutr* **33**:279, 1980.
467. Ruch T, Kerr D: Decreased essential amino acid requirements without catabolism in phenylketonuria and maple syrup urine disease. *Am J Clin Nutr* **35**:217, 1982.
468. Parsons HG, Carter RJ, Unrath M, Snyder FF: Evaluation of branched-chain amino acid intake in children with maple syrup urine disease and methylmalonic aciduria. *J Inherit Metab Dis* **13**:125, 1990.

469. Goodman SI, Pollak S, Miles B, O'Brien D: The treatment of maple syrup urine disease. *J Pediatr* **75**:485, 1969.
470. Smith BA, Waisman HA: Leucine equivalency system in managing branched chain ketoaciduria. *J Am Diet Assoc* **59**:342, 1971.
471. Bell L, Chao E, Milne J: Dietary management of maple syrup urine disease: Extension of equivalency systems. *J Am Diet Assoc* **74**:357, 1979.
472. Diliberti JH, Digeorge AM, Auerbach VH: Abnormal leucine/isoleucine ratio and the etiology of acrodermatitis enteropathica-like rash in maple syrup urine disease (MSUD). *Pediatr Res* **7**:154, 1973.
473. Marshall JR, Gracy RW, Kester MV: Maple syrup urine disease: Response to dietary modifications. *J Am Osteopath Assoc* **79**:98, 1979.
474. Chevalier P, Aschkenasy A: Hematological and immunological effects of excess dietary leucine in the young rat. *Am J Clin Nutr* **30**:1645, 1977.
475. Thompson GN, Francis DE, Halliday D: Acute illness in maple syrup urine disease: Dynamics of protein metabolism and implications for management. *J Pediatr* **119**:35, 1991.
476. Sallan SE, Cottom D: Peritoneal dialysis in maple syrup urine disease. *Lancet* **2**:1423, 1969.
477. Rey F, Rey J, Cloup M, Feron JF, Dore F, Labrune B, Frezal J: Traitement d'urgence d'une form algue de leucinose par dialyse peritoneale. *Arch Fr Pediatr* **26**:133, 1969.
478. Rutledge SL, Havens PL, Haymond MW, McLean RH, Kan JS, Brusilow SW: Neonatal hemodialysis: Effective therapy for the encephalopathy of inborn errors of metabolism. *J Pediatr* **116**:125, 1990.
479. Jouvet P, Poggi F, Rabier D: Continuous venovenous haemodiafiltraion in the acute phase of neonatal maple syrup urine disease. *J Inherit Metab Dis* **20**:463, 1997.
480. Wendel U, Becker K, Przyrembel H, Bulla M, Manegold C, Mench-Hoinowski A, Langenbeck U: Peritoneal dialysis in maple-syrup-urine disease: Studies on branched-chain amino and keto acids. *Eur J Pediatr* **134**:57, 1980.
481. Berry GT, Heidenreich R, Kaplan P, Levine F, Mazur A, Palmieri MJ, Yudkoff M, Segal S: Branched-chain amino acid-free parenteral nutrition in the treatment of acute metabolic decompensation in patients with maple syrup urine disease. *N Engl J Med* **324**:175, 1991.
482. Townsend I, Kerr DS: Total parenteral nutrition therapy of toxic maple syrup urine disease. *Am J Clin Nutr* **36**:359, 1982.
483. Shih VE, Herrin JT, Erickson AM: Hyperalimentation and peritoneal dialysis during acute metabolic decompensation in maple syrup urine disease. *Pediatr Res* **9**:355, 1975.
484. Rogers QR, Spolter PD, Harper AE: Effect of leucine-isoleucine antagonism on plasma amino acid pattern of rats. *Arch Biochem Biophys* **97**:497, 1962.
485. Wendel U, Langenbeck U, Lombeck I, Bremer HJ: Maple syrup urine disease—Therapeutic use of insulin in catabolic states. *Eur J Pediatr* **139**:172, 1982.
486. Hatcher GW: Maple syrup urine disease. *Proc R Soc Med* **61**:287, 1968.
487. Morton H: MSUD news from the Clinic for Special Children. *Maple Syrup Urine Disease* **10**:9, 1992.
488. Nyhan WL, Rice-Kelts M, Klein J: Treatment of the acute crisis in Maple syrup urine disease. *Arch Pediatr Adolesc Med* **152**:593, 1998.
489. Parini R, Sereni LP, Bagozzi DC: Continuous feeding as the only treatment in neonatal maple syrup urine disease. *Society for the Study of Inborn Errors of Metabolism Annual Symposium*, 1991.
490. Fukutomi M, Kitamura S, Kawachi K: Successful repair and postoperative management of tetralogy of Fallot in a patient with maple syrup urine disease. *Heart Vessels* **8**:48, 1993.
491. Biggemann B, Zass R, Wendel U: Postoperative metabolic decompensation in maple syrup urine disease is completely prevented by insulin. *J Inherit Metab Dis* **16**:912, 1993.
492. Koga Y, Iwanaga T, Yoshida I: Maple syrup urine disease: Nutritional management by intravenous hyperalimentation and uneventful course after surgical repair of dislocation of the hip. *J Inherit Metab Dis* **21**:177, 1998.
493. Kahraman S, Ercan M, Akkus O: Anaesthetic management in maple syrup urine disease. *Anaesthesia* **51**:575, 1996.
494. Kaplan P, Mazur AM, Smith R: Transplantation for maple syrup urine disease (MSUD) and methylmalonic acidopathy (MMA). *J Inherit Metab Dis* **20**:37, 1997.
495. Shih VE, Stewart B: Organ donation by a maple syrup urine disease patient. *J Inherit Metab Dis* **18**:367, 1995.
496. Shih VE, Aubry RH, Degrande G, Bursky SF, Tanaka K: Maternal isovaleric acidemia. *J Pediatr* **105**:77, 1984.
497. Van Calcar SC, Harding CO, Davidson SR, Barness LA, Wolff JA: Case reports of successful pregnancy in women with maple syrup urine disease and propionic acidemia. *Am J Med Genet* **44**:641, 1992.
498. Arn PH, Hauser ER, Thomas GH, Herman G, Hess D, Brusilow SW: Hyperammonemia in women with a mutation at the ornithine carbamoyltransferase locus: A cause of postpartum coma. *N Engl J Med* **322**:1652, 1990.
499. Snyderman SE: Medical and nutritional aspects of maple syrup urine disease, in Koch R, Shaw K, Durkin F (eds): *Maple Syrup Urine Disease Issues and Perspectives*. San Diego, Department of Health, Education, and Welfare, 1977, p 18.
500. Westall RG: Dietary treatment of maple syrup urine disease. *Am J Dis Child* **113**:58, 1967.
501. Brenton DP, Creed HM, Cummings J, Cusworth DC: Synthetic diets in human disease. *Nutrition (Lond)* **27**:184, 1973.
502. Moser HW: Maple syrup urine disease, in Klawans HL (ed): *Metabolic and Deficiency Diseases of the Nervous System*. Amsterdam, North-Holland, 1977, p 53.
503. Naughten ER, Jenkins J, Francis DE, Leonard JV: Outcome of maple syrup urine disease. *Arch Dis Child* **57**:918, 1982.
504. Committee for improvement of Hereditary Disease Management: Management of maple syrup urine disease in Canada. *Can Med Assoc J* **115**:1005, 1976.
505. Rousson R, Guibaud P: Long-term outcome of organic acidurias: Survey of 105 French cases (1967-1983). *J Inherit Metab Dis* **7**:10, 1984.
506. Nord A, Van Doorninck WJ, Greene C: Developmental profile of patients with maple syrup urine disease. *J Inherit Metab Dis* **14**:881, 1991.
507. Kaplan P, Mazur A, Field M, Berlin JA, Berry GT, Heidenreich R, Yudkoff M, Segal S: Intellectual outcome in children with maple syrup urine disease. *J Pediatr* **119**:46, 1991.
508. Aoki K, Wada Y: Outcome of the patients detected by newborn screening in Japan. *Acta Paediatr Jpn* **30**:429, 1988.
509. Hilliges C, Awiszus D, Wendel U: The intellectual performance of patients with maple syrup urine disease (MSUD). *SSIEM Twenty-Eighth Annual Symposium*, 1990.
510. Nyhan WL, Wulfeck BB, Tallal P, Marsden DL: *Metabolic Correlates of Learning Disability*. La Jolla, CA, University of California-San Diego, 1989, p 1.
511. Levin ML, Scheimann A, Lewis RA, Beaudet AL: Cerebral edema in maple syrup urine disease. *J Pediatr* **122**:167, 1993.
512. Chinsky J, Appel M, Almashanu S, Costeas P, Ambulos N Jr, Carmi R: A nonsense mutation (R242X) in the branched-chain α-keto acid dehydrogenase E1α subunit gene (BCKDHA) as a cause of maple syrup urine disease. *Hum Mutat* **12**:136, 1998.
513. Chuang JL, fisher CR, Cox RP, Chuang DT: Molecular basis of maple syrup urine disease: Novel mutations at the E1α locus that impair E1 ($\alpha_2\beta_2$) assembly or decrease steady-state E1α mRNAlevels of branched-chain α-ketoacid dehydrogenase complex. *Am J Hum Genet* **55**:297, 1994.
514. Tsuruta M, Mitsubuchi H, Mardy S, Miura Y, Hayashida Y, Kinugasa A, Ishitsu T, Matsuda I, Indo Y: Molecular basis of intermittent maple syrup urine disease: Novel mutations in the E2 gene of the branched-chain α-keto acid dehydrogenase comlex. *J Hum Genet* **43**:91, 1998.
515. Hong YS, Kerr DS, Craigen WJ, Tan J, Pan Y, Lusk M, Patel MS: Identification of two mutations in a compound heterozygous child with dihydrolipoamide dehydrogenase deficiency. *Hum Mol Genet* **5**:1925, 1996.
516. Ad Hoc Committee on Mutation Nomenclature: Update on nomenclature for human gene mutations. *Hum Mutat* **8**:197, 1996.

CHAPTER 

Disorders of Transsulfuration

S. Harvey Mudd ▪ Harvey L. Levy ▪ Jan P. Kraus

1. **The complete transcription unit of *MAT1A*, the gene encoding the catalytic subunit of the two isozymes of methionine adenosyltransferase (MAT I and MAT III) expressed solely in nonfetal mammalian liver, has recently been characterized. It spans approximately 20 kbp and contains nine exons. Forty-eight patients with isolated hypermethioninemia have been shown to have deficiencies of the combined activity of these isozymes (MAT I/III deficiency). Most were ascertained during routine screening of newborns for hypermethioninemia or family screening. Seventeen mutations in *MAT1A* have been identified in these patients. Most patients have some residual activity of MAT I/III and are clinically well, but a few with complete MAT I/III deficiency have developed demyelination of the brain. MAT activities in tissues other than liver are normal, consistent with the functioning of the MAT isozyme(s) encoded by the separate gene, *MAT2A*. The residual activity of MAT in liver, the normal activities in nonhepatic tissues, and the high tissue concentrations of methionine together provide for synthesis by these individuals of virtually normal amounts of *S*-adenosylmethionine (AdoMet).**
2. **Cystathionine β-synthase (CBS) deficiency is the most frequently encountered cause of homocystinuria. In addition to Hcy, methionine and a variety of other metabolites of homocysteine accumulate in the body or are excreted in the urine of such patients. More than 600 cases of proven or presumptive CBS deficiency have been studied. Dislocation of the optic lens, osteoporosis, thinning and lengthening of the long bones, mental retardation, and thromboembolism affecting large and small arteries and veins are the most common clinical features. Affected patients vary widely in the extent to which they manifest these abnormalities or the rate at which they become apparent.**
3. **CBS deficiency is inherited as an autosomal recessive trait, but available evidence suggests considerable genetic heterogeneity. Some patients have small residual activities of CBS, whereas others have no such activities detected by even the most sensitive methods. Pyridoxine-responsive individuals generally have milder, or more slowly developing, manifestations than do those not responsive to pyridoxine.**
4. **A full-length CBS cDNA has been cloned. It is over 2500 bp long and encodes a polypeptide of 551 amino acids. Using this cDNA, 92 mutations in the CBS gene have been demonstrated in more than 300 alleles from individuals with CBS deficiency. Recently, the entire human CBS gene has been cloned and sequenced. It spans approximately 28 kbp, including 5 kbp of 5′-flanking sequence, and contains 23 exons. The CBS polypeptide is encoded by exons 1 to 16. Two alternatively used promoters have been identified approximately 5 kbp upstream from the initiator codon.**
5. **Routine screening of newborns for hypermethioninemia has been used to identify individuals with CBS deficiency. Striking regional differences in the rates of detection are present. The CBS deficiency of most detected individuals has been unresponsive to pyridoxine treatment, and it is virtually certain that a significant portion of CBS-deficient individuals, especially those responsive to pyridoxine, are being missed by current screening programs.**
6. **Management of CBS-deficient patients emphasizes amelioration of the characteristic biochemical abnormalities. Most patients detected during early infancy have been treated with low-methionine, cystine-supplemented diets. Excellent, statistically validated, beneficial effects have been demonstrated for such regimens in preventing mental retardation and dislocation of optic lenses. Less definitive data suggest there may also be a reduction in the occurrence of initial thromboembolic events and in the incidence of seizures. Methionine-restricted diets are usually less acceptable to patients detected after infancy. Pyridoxine is used for those responsive to this vitamin, perhaps accompanied by less stringent methionine dietary restriction. Betaine is useful for vitamin B_6-nonresponsive patients in whom dietary management is unsatisfactory. The latter regimens have been statistically proven to markedly reduce the frequencies of initial vascular events.**
7. **γ-Cystathionase deficiency leads to persistent excretion of large amounts of cystathionine in the urine, as well as to accumulation of cystathionine in body tissues and fluids. *N*-Acetylcystathionine and a variety of additional cystathionine metabolites are also excreted. The clinical status of proven or presumptive γ-cystathionase-deficient patients suggests that no clinical abnormalities are characteristically associated with this disorder. The deficiency is inherited as an autosomal recessive trait. Considerable genetic heterogeneity is likely to exist among known patients, one manifestation of which is responsiveness to pyridoxine of the cystathioninuria associated with γ-cystathionase deficiency.**

The transsulfuration pathway converts the sulfur atom of methionine into the sulfur atom of cysteine. This pathway is the chief route of disposal of methionine and explains why cysteine is not an essential amino acid in normal human adults. Intimately

A list of standard abbreviations is located immediately preceding the index in each volume. Additional abbreviations used in this chapter include: AdoHcy = *S*-adenosylhomocysteine; AdoMet = *S*-adenosyl-L-methionine; vitamin B_6 = pyridoxine; CBS = cystathionine β-synthase; MAT = methionine adenosyltransferase; MTHFR = methylenetetrahydrofolate reductase; PLP = pyridoxal 5′-phosphate. For homocysteine and related compounds, the term homocysteine designates only the sulfhydryl amino acid, HS-R, where R = $-CH_2CH_2CH(NH_2)COOH$; homocystine designates only the disulfide RS-SR; and homocysteine-cysteine mixed disulfide is RS-SCys, where Cys = $-CH_2CH(NH_2)COOH$. Hcy is used in circumstances where several homocysteine-related compounds may contribute to the total under discussion. tHcy designates the total amount of homocysteine that would be formed after treatment of such a mixture with a reducing reagent that cleaves all disulfide bonds. In plasma, tHcy consists of homocysteine moieties bound to protein cysteines by disulfide linkages (RS-SPr, where Pr = protein), homocystine, homocysteine-cysteine mixed disulfide, homocysteine, and small amounts of other disulfides, such as homocysteine-cysteinylglycine disulfide. Plasma free Hcy designates non-protein-bound forms and is commonly taken to be the quantity (2 × homocystine plus homocysteine-cysteine disulfide). tCys is used to designate the totality of cysteine formed upon treatment with a disulfide-reducing agent.

CH_3-S-$CH_2CH_2CH(NH_2)COOH$

Methionine

$HOOCCH(NH_2)CH_2$-S-$CH_2CH_2CH(NH_2)COOH$

Cystathionine

H-S-$CH_2CH_2CH(NH_2)COOH$

Homocysteine

$HOOCCH(NH_2)CH_2CH_2$-S-S-$CH_2CH_2CH(NH_2)COOH$

Homocystine

H-S-$CH_2CH(NH_2)COOH$

Cysteine

$HOOCCH(NH_2)CH_2$-S-S-$CH_2CH(NH_2)COOH$

Cystine

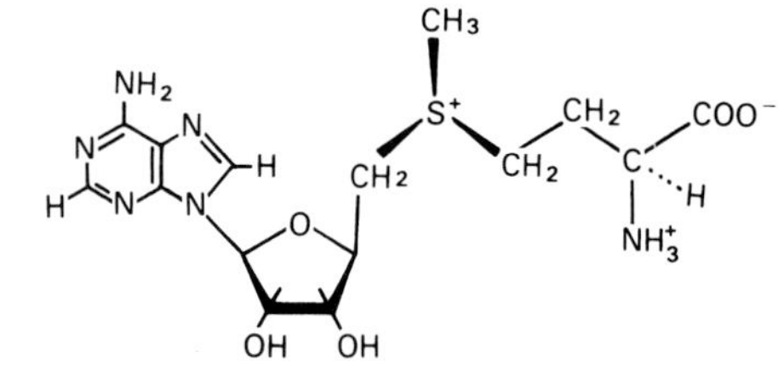

S-Adenosylmethionine

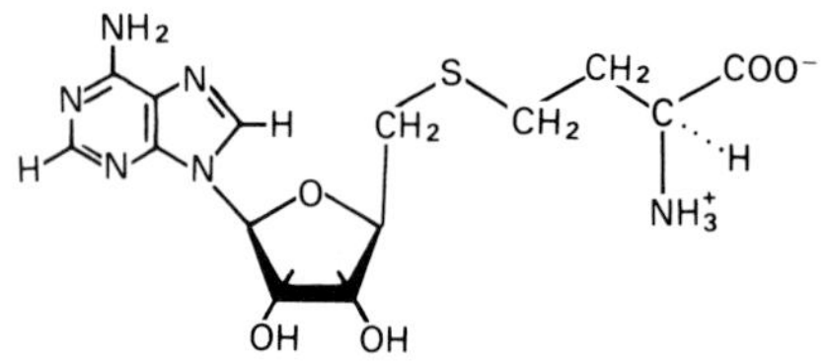

S-Adenosylhomocysteine

$(CH_3)_3N^+CH_2CH_2OH$

Choline

$(CH_3)_3N^+CH_2COOH$

Betaine

Fig. 88-1 Structural formulas of compounds of interest. The naturally occurring amino acids illustrated each have the absolute L configuration at the α-carbon atom. In naturally occurring AdoMet, the dominant absolute configuration at the asymmetric sulfonium pole is S, i.e., viewed from where the sulfur atom obscures the lone electron pair the adenosyl, the 3-amoni-3-carboxypropyl, and the methyl groups are arranged in counterclockwise order.[1] AdoMet and AdoHcy are shown in the favored *anti* conformation at the N(9)–C(1′) bond, i.e., with the ribose pointed away from, rather than toward, the purine ring.[2–4]

related are two additional metabolic sequences: the transmethylation reactions, whereby the methyl group of methionine is ultimately transferred to form any of a host of methylated compounds, and the reformation of methionine by methylation of homocysteine. Structural formulas of the relevant compounds are shown in Fig. 88-1.

METABOLISM OF METHIONINE, HOMOCYSTEINE, AND CYSTATHIONINE

The pertinent reactions of the transsulfuration pathway and related areas of metabolism are summarized in Fig. 88-2. At least nine specific genetic disorders have been recognized that affect one of the reactions shown. In this chapter, primary coverage is given to three disorders that involve reactions (1), (4), and (5). Limitations of space and in the number of references have necessitated emphasis on recent developments and citations. Citations to many of the original contributions in areas that have not changed greatly since the last version of this chapter[6] can be found there, in earlier versions,[7–9] or in the reviews cited in this chapter.

AdoMet Formation

The gateway to the transsulfuration pathway is the formation of AdoMet, reaction (1), catalyzed by MAT (ATP–L-methionine *S*-adenosyltransferase; EC 2.5.1.6). In this unusual reaction, the adenosyl moiety of ATP is transferred to methionine, forming a sulfonium bond between the 5′-carbon atom of the ribose and the sulfur atom of the amino acid. The tripolyphosphate that results from transfer of the adenosyl portion of ATP remains bound to the enzyme that, by virtue of a second catalytic activity, cleaves the tripolyphosphate to inorganic phosphate and pyrophosphate. With certain forms of MAT, this tripolyphosphatase activity is specifically and markedly stimulated by AdoMet. Removal of tripolyphosphate assists in making the synthesis of AdoMet essentially irreversible under physiological conditions.[10] MAT activity requires both divalent and monovalent cations. The animal enzyme has a rather strict substrate specificity for ATP and a somewhat broader specificity for methionine.[9]

Mammals possess at least two different structural genes for MAT, termed in a recent consensus nomenclature *MAT1A* and *MAT2A*[11] and located in humans on chromosomes 10q22[12] and 2p11.2,[13] respectively. The complete transcription units of *MAT1A* from mouse[14] and humans[15] have recently been characterized. Each spans approximately 20 kbp and contains nine exons. *MAT1A* and *MAT2A* encode catalytic subunits, α1 and α2, that, in humans, are 84 percent identical in their amino acid sequences[16] and, in rats, 85 percent identical.[17] The sequences of the human and rat α1-subunits are 95 percent identical,[18] and the α2 -subunits

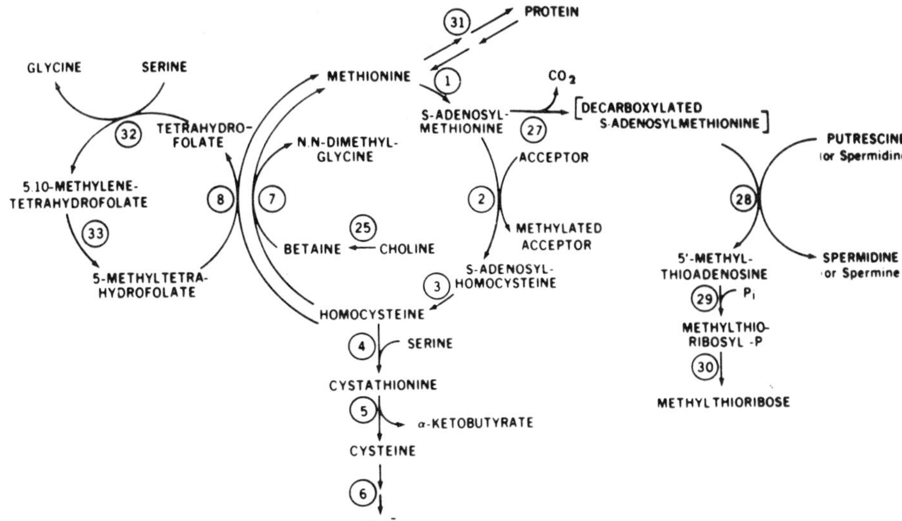

Fig. 88-2 The metabolism of methionine, homocysteine, and cystathionine. ***(From Poole.[5] Used by permission.)***

are 99 percent identical.[16] *MAT1A* is expressed solely in nonfetal liver to form two native holoenzymes: a tetramer, MAT I $(\alpha 1)_4$; and a dimer, MAT III $(\alpha 1)_2$. *MAT2A* is expressed in many tissues, including fetal liver and, to a small extent, nonfetal liver. The resulting holoenzymes, termed generally MAT II, are composed of $\alpha 2$-subunits, or modified such subunits, $\alpha 2'$, together with another subunit, β, encoded by a different gene and presumed to be regulatory.[11,19]

MAT I and MAT III differ markedly in their kinetic properties: for example, MAT III has a relatively high K_m for methionine, a high V_{max}, and at low methionine concentration its activity is stimulated manyfold by dimethylsulfoxide. MAT I has a lower K_m for methionine and is little affected by dimethylsulfoxide.[9,20–23] MAT III is activated by AdoMet, whereas MAT I is inhibited.[19] The tripolyphosphatase activity of both isozymes, however, is markedly stimulated by AdoMet.[24] Forms of MAT II have low K_ms for methionine, are not stimulated by dimethylsulfoxide,[9] and are inhibited by AdoMet at concentrations that might occur physiologically.[25–27] Further details about these enzymes and their regulation can be found in previous versions of this chapter[6–9] and in recent papers and reviews.[28–31]

Individuals with inactivating mutations in *MAT1A* that lead to deficiencies in the combined activity of MAT I and MAT III (termed *MAT I/III activity* when the specific contributions of MAT I and MAT III have not been clarified) are discussed in the section "MAT I/III Deficiency."

Methyl Transfer Reactions

Because of its sulfonium bonds, AdoMet may be regarded as a *high energy* compound. Many methyl transfers originate from AdoMet. In addition, this compound, after decarboxylation, is the source of the 3-carbon moieties of the polyamines, spermidine, and spermine.[32] Liver cytosol and mitochondria may contain kinetically distinguishable pools of AdoMet.[33] Details of the biochemical mechanisms involved in methyl group transfer have been reviewed.[34] An assessment has been made of the relative quantitative demands made by each of the transmethylation reactions likely to occur in normal humans on the available supply of AdoMet.[5,35] All of these reactions produce a common sulfur-containing product, *S*-adenosylhomocysteine (AdoHcy). Many AdoMet-dependent methyltransferases are strongly inhibited by AdoHcy, and it has been calculated that when the ratio of AdoMet to AdoHcy is 4:1 a variety of methyltransferases will be inhibited by 10 to 60 percent.[36] Because the tissue concentrations of AdoHcy rise markedly within seconds following death, and the AdoMet concentration may change also,[37,38] to obtain valid measurements of these metabolites in tissues such samples must be processed or frozen extremely rapidly.[39] Representative values for adult rat liver from studies in which such precautions were specified to have been taken were AdoMet, 60 to 85 nmol/g,[37] 84 ± 11 nmol/g,[39] or 64 ± 10 nmol/g (SE);[38] and, AdoHcy, 10 to 15 nmol/g,[37] 13 ± 7 nmol/g, or 13 ± 5 (SE).[38] The corresponding AdoMet/AdoHcy ratios were 6:1, 6.5:1, and 4.9:1,[37–39] making it unlikely that severe inhibition of most transmethylation reactions is occurring at these physiological concentrations.

AdoHcy Hydrolysis

AdoHcy is further metabolized by a hydrolase (EC 3.3.1.1) that cleaves the thioether to homocysteine and adenosine. The mammalian enzyme is a tetramer, composed of four subunits, each weighing 47 kDa.[40–42] The human gene is on chromosome 20.[43] Several pseudogenes have been identified.[44] In mice, a lethal mutation includes a deletion of the gene encoding AdoHcy hydrolase.[45] The amino acid sequences of this enzyme from rat[46] and human[47,48] livers are 97 percent identical.[48] The crystal structure of the human placental enzyme has been reported[49] and a molecular model of the active site proposed.[50] Each subunit of the enzyme contains 1 equivalent of tightly bound NAD^+. During the catalytic cycle, the NAD^+ is reduced to NADH, with concomitant oxidation of the 3′-hydroxyl of AdoHcy to a keto group. After homocysteine is eliminated, the enzyme-bound NADH reduces the keto group back to a hydroxyl before release of adenosine. AdoHcy hydrolase activity is widely distributed in mammalian tissues. Although the equilibrium of the reaction favors AdoHcy accumulation, in vivo both its products—homocysteine and adenosine—are normally rapidly removed, so that the hydrolase functions overall in the cleavage direction.[9] Three sibs with hypermethioninemia and markedly decreased activities of hepatic activity of AdoHcy hydrolase have been described, but the fact that AdoHcy hydrolase activity was normal in cultured fibroblasts[51] indicates they did not have primary inactivating mutation(s) in this enzyme, nor have other humans been described with AdoHcy hydrolase mutations. The biologic effects of inhibitors of this activity have been reviewed extensively.[52]

Homocysteine Methylation

Homocysteine lies at an important metabolic branch point. It may be either converted to cystathionine through the transsulfuration pathway [Fig. 88-2, reaction (4)] or methylated to form methionine [reactions (7) and (8)], thus completing the sulfur conservation cycle. Homocysteine is methylated in mammals by use of either betaine or 5-methyltetrahydrofolic acid as methyl donor.

Betaine-dependent methylation of homocysteine is catalyzed by two enzymes: betaine-homocysteine methyltransferase (EC 2.1.1.5) and dimethylthetin-homocysteine methyltransferase (EC 2.1.1.3) (so called because it catalyzes at a higher rate with the nonphysiological substrate, dimethylacetothetin, than with betaine). The relative contributions of these two enzymes to overall betaine-dependent homocysteine methylation is unclear.[53] Betaine-homocysteine methyltransferase of human liver has been purified to apparent homogeneity.[54,55] It is a hexamer[56] of subunits containing 406 amino acid residues with M_r 44,969,[57] encoded by a gene on chromosome 5q13.1–q15[58] and expressed only in liver and kidney.[59] The organization of the human gene has been characterized.[59a] The amino acid sequence of the subunit shows six regions of homology with a B_{12}-dependent *Escherichia coli* enzyme that catalyzes the transfer of a methyl group from N^5-methyltetrahydrofolate to homocysteine.[57] Both of these enzymes contain zinc essential for enzymatic activity.[56,56a,60] Rat liver betaine-homocysteine methyltransferase activity is increased both by diets containing excessive methionine and by those devoid of methionine.[61] The highest levels of expression are attained with methionine restriction accompanied by the presence of a methyl donor (choline, betaine, dimethylacetothetin, or dimethylpropiothetin) in the diet.[56,59a] In pig liver or kidney, however, only minimal activity changes occur under similar dietary regimens.[62] Rat liver activity is inactivated by AdoMet or AdoHcy.[63] The K_ms of the human enzyme, expressed in *E. coli*, were 2200 μM for betaine and 4 μM for homocysteine,[56] in contrast to the corresponding values of 23 and 32 μM for the purified porcine liver enzyme.[57] The ability of the human enzyme to compete for homocysteine may then be markedly affected by the availability of betaine.

No mammalian mutants defective in betaine-dependent methylation of homocysteine have yet been described. Recently, Lundberg et al reported proton nuclear magnetic resonance (NMR) measurements of urinary betaine and *N,N*-dimethylglycine, a product of the transfer of a methyl group from betaine to homocysteine, in 17 normal controls and 13 patients with premature vascular disease and abnormal postmethionine-load elevations of plasma free Hcy. None of the patients had high urinary betaine and low *N,N*-dimethylglycine as might have been expected had they had impaired betaine-homocysteine methyltransferase.[64]

The alternative methyl donor for homocysteine methylation is 5-methyltetrahydrofolic acid. Several groups of patients with genetic defects ultimately affecting this reaction are now recognized. N^5-Methyltetrahydrofolate-dependent methylation of homocysteine is catalyzed by a cobalamin (B_{12})-containing enzyme, N^5-methyltetrahydrofolate-homocysteine methyltransferase (methionine synthase: EC 2.1.1.13).[65] The gene for human methionine synthase is on chromosome 1q43 and encodes an enzyme 1265 amino acids long.[66] The reaction involves the intermediate formation of an enzyme-bound methylcobalamin.[65] Patients with mutations in this gene comprise the *cblG* complementation group. The phenotype includes megaloblastic anemia, elevation of plasma tHcy (totality of the homocysteinyl moieties), homocystinuria, and hypomethioninemia.[66,67] Other patients with similar phenotypes fall into the *cblE* complementation group and have functional deficiencies of methionine synthase due to limitation in the ability to maintain the cobalamin associated with this enzyme in a proper state of reduction.[68] A cDNA for methionine synthase reductase, a flavoprotein defective in *cblE* patients, has recently been cloned and characterized.[69] Additional patients with elevated plasma tHcy and homocystinuria are unable to carry out the N^5-methyltetrahydrofolate-dependent methylation of homocysteine because of either defective release of cobalamin from lysosomes (*cblF*),[70–72] a primary inability to form methylcobalamin and adenosylcobalamin (*cblC* and *cblD* groups),[73,74] or inability to form the cosubstrate, N^5-methyltetrahydrofolate, because of lack of activity of 5,10-methylenetetrahydrofolate reductase (MTHFR) [EC 1.1.99.15; reaction (33), Fig. 88-2].[75] These patients are discussed in Chap. 155 dealing with disorders of folic acid and B_{12} metabolism.

Cystathionine Synthesis

In the metabolism of homocysteine, the major alternative to methylation is condensation with serine to form the thioether cystathionine. The reaction is catalyzed by cystathionine β-synthase [CBS; L-serine hydrolyase (adding homocysteine); EC 4.2.1.22]. The locus for human CBS was mapped to chromosome 21 by study of Chinese hamster-human cell hybrids,[76] an assignment corroborated by in situ hybridization studies using a cDNA probe for CBS.[77] The gene has subsequently been localized more precisely to the subtelomeric region of band 21q22.3 of chromosome 21,[78] where the gene for α-A-crystallin, a major structural protein of the ocular lens, is also found. Synteny of these two loci is conserved in mice on chromosome 17,[79] in rats on chromosome 20,[87] and in cows in syntenic group U10.[80]

To clone the cDNA for CBS, a plasmid library was prepared using rat liver CBS mRNA purified to homogeneity by immunopurification.[77] A partial CBS cDNA clone was isolated and used, in turn, to isolate full-length cDNA clones.[80,81] Each was shown by sequencing to relate to peptides found in purified CBS. Among the resulting cDNA inserts, four different types, I through IV, were found. Catalytic activity was observed for types I and III expressed in Chinese hamster ovary (CHO) cells and in *E. coli.* Rat type-I and III isoforms differ by the alternative usage of exon 16 (present in the former, but absent in the latter) that encodes an additional 14 amino acids. The presence of exon 16 leads to a threefold reduction in the half-life of the type-I enzyme, without altering its kinetic and catalytic properties.[82] The cDNA with the longest continuous reading frame, type I, was used as a probe to screen a rat genomic library, and genomic inserts were identified that together enabled reconstruction of the organization of the entire rat CBS gene. It is approximately 25 kbp long, with the coding sequence broken into 18 exons.[81,83] Using the rat CBS cDNA as a probe, several human CBS cDNAs were isolated from liver and skin fibroblast libraries.[84] The full-length human cDNA is 2554 nucleotides long and encodes a polypeptide of 551 amino acids.† Recently, additional human CBS cDNAs were isolated encoding the most upstream portions of the 5′-UTR. The 5′-UTR of human CBS mRNA is formed by one of five alternatively used exons, designated −1a to −1e, and one invariably present, exon 0, whereas the 3′-UTR is encoded by exons 16 and 17.[85] Interestingly, intron 16 appears to be retained in the 3′-UTR of most of the fibroblast and liver mRNA of every individual.[84]

A preliminary description of the exon-intron organization of the human CBS gene has been reported.[86] Very recently, the entire human CBS gene was cloned and sequenced.[88] A total of 28,046 nucleotides were reported that in addition to the CBS gene contain approximately 5 kbp of 5′-flanking sequence. The human CBS gene contains 23 exons, and the CBS polypeptide is encoded in exons 1 to 16. Exon 15, the human homologue of rat exon 16, is alternatively spliced and appears to be incorporated in relatively few mature human CBS mRNA molecules. The organization of the human CBS gene and its restriction map is illustrated in Fig. 88-3. While the exon-intron organization of the human CBS gene in the protein-coding region is perfectly conserved with the rat and mouse CBS genes, this is not the case for the genomic organization of the untranslated regions.[81,83,85,88]

At least two alternatively used promoters in the human gene are upstream of exons −1a and −1b. They are GC rich (some 80 percent) and contain numerous putative binding sites for Sp1, Ap1, Ap2 and c-myb, but lack the classical TATA box. To evaluate the relative levels of the −1a and −1b promoter activities, reporter constructs were generated by cloning the promoter regions of approximately 400 bp into a luciferase reporter vector. Following

†The human CBS cDNA sequence was deposited under the GenBank accession number L19501. Subsequently, other CBS cDNA sequences were deposited with the following numbers: L14577, X82166, and L00972.

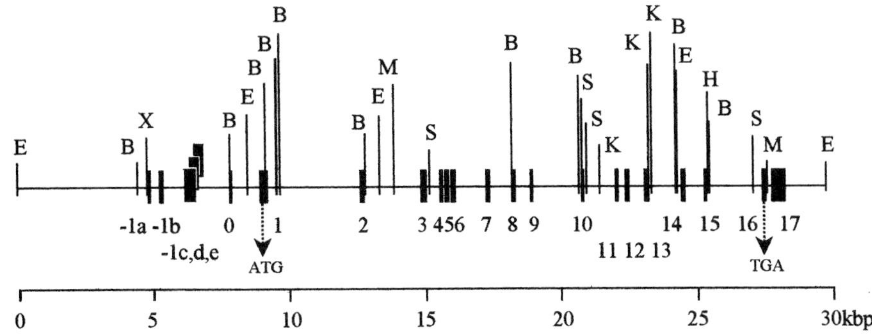

Fig. 88-3 Genomic organization of the human cystathionine β-synthase (CBS) gene. All exons, including the alternatively used exons-1a, b, c, d, e and 15 are represented by *solid boxes*. The beginning and the end of the coding region are indicated by the codons ATG and TGA, respectively. The restriction sites are B, BamH I; E, EcoR I; H, Hind III; K, Kpn I; M, Mlu I; S, Sfi I; and X, Xba I.

transfection of the reporter constructs into COS 7 and HepG cells, analysis of luciferase activity in these cells indicated that both of these regions contain all of the sequences essential for promoter activity, with the −1b promoter activity being approximately 7- to 10-fold stronger than that of −1a.[88]

The CBS locus contains an unusually high number of *Alu* repeats that may predispose this gene to deleterious rearrangements. Additionally, a number of DNA sequence repeats and single-base variations that are polymorphic in North American and European Caucasians have been reported.[84,88] Sebastio et al[89] described an insertion of 68 bp in exon 8 (844ins68) in an allele from a CBS-deficient patient that also contained the frequent I278T mutation. Subsequently, the 844ins68 was shown[90–92a] to be a polymorphism occurring in up to 13.5 percent of Caucasian alleles and to be prevalent among the Brazilian and African blacks studied (mutant heterozygotes, 37.7 percent; and homozygotes, 4 percent), but to be absent, or virtually absent, in Asians and Amerinds.[92a] In all carriers, the 844ins68 mutation cosegregated in *cis* with the 833T → C mutation leading to I278T.[92a] The insertion duplicates the intron-7 acceptor splice site and may lead to two alternatively spliced transcripts. If the upstream splice site is used, the resulting mRNA will contain the I278T mutation and a stop codon. If, on the other hand, the downstream site is used, the I278T mutation and part of the insertion are spliced out, leaving a completely normal CBS transcript. Further experiments showed that only the normal CBS mRNA is detectable in the cytoplasm, whereas both forms are present in a nuclear RNA fraction, suggesting the abnormal transcript is degraded before it leaves the nucleus.[90] A recent study[93,93a] found a prevalence of 16.8 percent of 844ins68 heterozygotes among patients with peripheral arterial occlusive disease, compared with 11.0 percent in controls ($P < 0.07$), but no elevation of tHcy due to such heterozygosity. This possible association merits further investigation.

The primary translational product of both the human and the rat CBS gene is a polypeptide with molecular weight of 63 kDa.[94] In fresh liver extracts, the enzyme is found predominantly as a tetramer of this subunit, whereas after a procedure in which the enzyme is first "aged" at 4° for 7 days and then purified, CBS is isolated as a dimer of a 48-kDa subunit.[94,95] The reduction in size, caused by limited proteolysis, is accompanied by a significant increase in catalytic activity at physiologic concentrations of homocysteine.

CBS has been purified from several vertebrate livers[95] (for other references, see Kraus et al[96]). The human CBS cDNA was used in various expression vectors to express the human enzyme in *E. coli*,[97] in yeast,[98] and in CHO cells.[84] Recently, large amounts of the recombinant human CBS were purified from *E. coli* and characterized.[97,99] Each subunit of CBS binds, in addition to the two substrates, three additional ligands: pyridoxal 5′-phosphate (PLP), AdoMet (an allosteric activator), and, surprisingly, heme, the function of which in the enzyme is unknown.[99] It has recently been suggested (see ref 228) that the heme may have a catalytic role in activating homocysteine similar to the action of zinc in the enzymes involved in the remethylation of homocysteine.[56,56a,60] The activity of the enzyme correlates with its heme saturation. The presence of heme is required for PLP binding, and the amount of PLP bound is limited by the heme content.[99] CBS depends fully on the presence of PLP for activity.[96,100,101] Recently, it was unequivocally demonstrated that the residue in CBS forming a Schiff base with PLP is Lys 119.[102]

The active core of the enzyme was generated by limited digestion with trypsin from the full-length CBS or, alternatively, by expression of a truncated CBS cDNA in *E. coli*. This active core, extending from Glu 37 to Arg 413, forms a dimer of 45-kDa subunits. The dimer is about twice as active as the tetramer. It binds both PLP and heme cofactors, but is no longer activated by AdoMet.[103] This 45-kDa active core is the portion of CBS most homologous with the evolutionarily related enzymes isolated from plants, yeast, and bacteria (see below). Similar results were observed when human CBS cDNA containing a premature stop codon in position 409 was expressed in a CBS-deficient yeast. The enzyme lacking the carboxy-terminal 143 amino acids was twice as active as the wild-type enzyme. Surprisingly, when any one of several human inactivating pathogenic mutations were expressed in yeast in *cis* with this truncation, CBS activity was restored sufficiently to permit growth of the yeast on medium lacking cysteine. For some mutations, activities expressed in vitro were near wild-type levels.[104]

The displacement of the OH group of serine by homocysteine proceeds with retention of configuration.[105] CBS can catalyze alternative β-replacement reactions in which sulfide is a substrate or a product[106] according to the general scheme:

$$XCH_2CH(NH_2)COOH + YH \rightarrow XH + YCH_2CH(NH_2)COOH$$

where X = OH or SH and Y = SH or S-alkyl

The active core of human CBS shares a high degree of structural similarity (52 percent if conservative replacements are counted) with the related *O*-acetylserine sulfhydrases (cysteine synthases) from plants and bacteria.[81,107] These enzymes catalyze the synthesis of cysteine from sulfide and acetylserine. It was suggested that during evolution the capacity to synthesize cystathionine was acquired by broadening the substrate specificity of such enzymes to include homocysteine as well as inorganic sulfide.[81]

Deficiency of CBS activity is the most frequently encountered genetic disorder of transsulfuration and is described in a subsequent section ("CBS Deficiency").

Cystathionine Cleavage

The transsulfuration sequence is completed by cleavage of cystathionine to cysteine and α-ketobutyrate [reaction (5)], catalyzed by γ-cystathionase [L-cystathionine cysteine-lyase (deaminating]; EC 4.4.1.1). The gene for human γ-cystathionase has been provisionally mapped to chromosome 16.[108] Studies of cDNA derived from human liver mRNA have shown two clones coding for hepatic γ-cystathionase. One encodes a catalytic subunit with a 44 amino acid deletion compared with the corresponding sequence from rat liver,[108a] whereas the other encodes an undeleted sequence with 82 percent amino acid identity to the rat liver enzyme.[109] The native enzyme is a tetramer[106,110] containing four molecules of PLP bound at two types of sites that differ in their affinities for coenzyme and their reactivities with substrates and inhibitors.[106,110] In the liver of B_6-deficient rats, the proportion of γ-cystathionase present as apoenzyme increases dramatically, but the total holoenzyme activity is unchanged, because under these conditions there is an increase in the concentration of the mRNA encoding this enzyme and an increase in its rate of synthesis, balanced by an increased rate of its lysosomal degradation.[111]

Mammalian γ-cystathionase has several catalytic activities in addition to cystathionine cleavage, including the ability to catalyze cysteine desulfhydration:[112]

$$\text{cysteine} + H_2O \rightarrow \text{pyruvate} + NH_3 + H_2S$$

However, the recombinant human enzyme has recently been shown to have relatively little activity toward either cysteine or cystine.[112a] Other activities are summarized elsewhere.[7] Individuals with genetically determined defects of γ-cystathionase activity are discussed in the section "γ-Cystathionase Deficiency."

Quantitative Relationships Among Transmethylation, Transsulfuration, and Homocysteine Methylation

Some information about the quantitative relationships among methyl transfer reactions, transsulfuration, and homocysteine methylation has been provided by studies of normal young adults maintained in metabolic steady states on varying defined intakes of methionine and choline. These studies showed that utilization of methyl groups is normally accounted for chiefly by creatine-creatinine formation. This reaction consumes more AdoMet than all other transmethylations together. Male subjects utilize more methyl groups for methyl transfer reactions than they consume in a normal diet in the form of methionine. The difference in methyls is made up from two sources: (1) Conversion to betaine of choline moieties ingested in the diet. Total choline intake in an adult probably is equivalent to 5.0 to 8.3 mmol/day, but only a portion will be bioavailable.[113] Thus, dietary intake of choline may limit the amount of betaine-dependent homocysteine methylation occurring under normal conditions. (2) De novo formation of methyl groups through the tetrahydrofolate-dependent pathway. The latter methyls are also used to methylate homocysteine. To the extent that homocysteine is methylated, the portion of this compound diverted at any given moment to cystathionine is decreased. In male subjects on normal diets, at least 47 percent of the available homocysteine is methylated. Nevertheless, in the steady-state metabolic condition, the intake of methionine sulfur is balanced by metabolism of an equivalent amount of homocysteine sulfur through the transsulfuration pathway. These observations indicate that during its passage through the body the average homocysteinyl moiety cycles more than once between methionine and homocysteine. For males on normal diets, the calculated mean of such cycles is at least 1.9, whereas, for females, it is at least 1.5.[5] Extension of such studies to a subject unable to remove sarcosine metabolically because of a genetic defect in her sarcosine-oxidizing system permitted a slight upward revision, to 2.0, of the minimal estimate for the number of times the average homocysteinyl moiety cycles in the human female. The results suggest also that, when the dietary intake of labile methyl moieties exceeds the amount required for creatine formation and for other ongoing methyl transfer reactions, the excess is disposed of by methylation of glycine, forming sarcosine, which, in normal humans, is then converted to a 1-carbon fragment at the formaldehyde oxidation level, with regeneration of the glycine.[35] Many of these conclusions have been quantitatively confirmed and extended by means of stable-isotope-tracer studies.[114–116]

Tissue- and Age-Dependent Variations in Enzyme Patterns

The patterns just described apply only to the total body metabolism of young adults. The distributions and the specific activities of the pertinent enzymes are such that the bulk of this metabolism must occur in the liver. It is likely that gross departures from the specified patterns occur locally in other tissues. The relevant evidence has been reviewed in detail elsewhere.[8,117] In brief, available results suggest that almost all human tissues have some capacity to convert methionine to homocysteine, but that the apportionment of homocysteine to the transsulfuration or remethylation pathways may vary markedly from tissue to tissue.[118] The fetus probably directs a relatively larger proportion of available homocysteine through the N^5-methyltetrahydrofolate-dependent methylation pathway than in the direction of cystathionine synthesis, with concomitant increases in methylneogenesis and conservation of the homocysteine moiety. Measurements of betaine have shown that this compound is present in the urine 1 day after birth, and that excretion reaches a maximum of nearly 1.5 mol/mol creatinine at 2 to 3 months of age and then declines to less than 0.2 mol/mol creatinine after 1 year. During part, if not most, of the neonatal period, betaine excretion may exceed the choline intake, providing further evidence of the importance of folate-dependent homocysteine methylation at this stage.[119]

Because fetal tissues and placenta lack γ-cystathionase activity, it has been suggested that cyst(e)ine may be an essential amino acid at this stage of life.[120,121]

Methionine Transamination

An alternative for methionine degradation other than by transsulfuration is the transamination pathway.[122–126] Methionine and 4-methylthio-2-oxobutyrate are interconverted by transamination. Glutamine transaminase may play a major role in catalyzing this reaction,[127,128] but other transaminases may participate also.[129–131] 4-Methylthio-2-oxobutyrate arises also as a product of the metabolism of 5′-methylthioadenosine, formed, in turn, as a result of polyamine synthesis. It has been proposed that in the cytoplasm under normal physiological conditions the function of the transamination reaction in question is to convert the keto acid to methionine.[131] Alternatively, 4-methylthio-2-oxobutyrate may be oxidatively decarboxylated to CO_2 and 3-methylthiopropionate,[124] a reaction catalyzed by branched-chain keto acid dehydrogenase,[128,132] but not by pyruvate or α-ketoglutarate dehydrogenases.[132] Disposal of excess methionine by these steps may occur chiefly in mitochondria.[131] 3-Methylthiopropionate may be further degraded to CO_2, sulfate, methanethiol, and H_2S.[125]

Normal human subjects excrete a daily mean of approximately 55 μmol of 4-methylthio-2-oxobutyrate, accompanied by 10 μmol of 4-methylthio-2-hydroxybutyrate.[133] Following ingestion of 7 to 20 mmol of D-, but not L-methionine, increased amounts of 4-methylthio-2-oxobutyrate[134] and 3-methylthiopropionate[135] are excreted in the urine, and dimethylsulfide becomes elevated in the breath.[136] Increased amounts of methionine transamination products are present in plasma and urine of patients with severe hypermethioninemia due to either MAT I/III deficiency[137] or CBS deficiency.[138] However, when the transsulfuration pathway is blocked, the transamination pathway does not catabolize methionine at a rate sufficient to prevent biochemical abnormalities, as shown by the facts that MAT I/III-deficient patients accumulate greatly elevated concentrations of methionine (see the section "MAT I/III Deficiency," below), and that CBS-deficient patients can convert methionine sulfur to sulfate at rates only far below the normal maximum capacity.[138]

Additional Pathways Involving Homocysteinyl-tRNA

Jakubowski and his colleagues have presented convincing evidence that homocysteine may be activated by the mammalian protein synthetic apparatus to form homocysteinyl-tRNA. Such "mis-activated" homocysteine is efficiently edited so that it does not enter proteins but rather is converted to homocysteine thiolactone.[139,140] It has been suggested that homocysteinylation of cellular proteins (particularly at lysine residues) by homocysteine thiolactone may play a role in the pathophysiology of conditions in which excess homocysteine accumulation accelerates the rate of such mis-activation."[140]

Another pathway also involves activation of homocysteine to form homocysteinyl-tRNA, in this instance with the initiator tRNA that functions to place methionine in the N-terminal position of proteins undergoing synthesis. Such activated homocysteine is then methylated, the resultant methionine moiety becomes N-terminal and is then released after chain initiation, thereby contributing to the cellular methionine pool.[141]

MAT I/III DEFICIENCY

Causes of Hypermethioninemia

Aside from protein synthesis, the major pathway for methionine metabolism is initiated by conversion of methionine to AdoMet (Fig. 88-2). Impairment of this conversion leads to abnormal methionine accumulation and hypermethioninemia, as borne out by studies of patients with MAT I/III deficiency (discussed below). Hypermethioninemia may occur also in generalized liver disease, tyrosinemia I, cystathionine β-synthase deficiency, or in infants fed diets either rich in protein or supplemented with DL-methionine. For further discussion of the latter situations, see a previous version of this chapter.[6]

Recent results have made it apparent that the most common genetic cause of persistent isolated hypermethioninemia (i.e., abnormal elevation of plasma methionine in the absence of tyrosinemia I, CBS deficiency, or liver disease) is deficiency of MAT I/III activity.

Ascertainment

Isolated hypermethioninemia has been described, to date, in at least 61 individuals,[12,15,137,142–162] most of whom have been discovered as a result of the screening of newborn children for abnormal elevations of plasma methionine to identify individuals with homocystinuria due to deficient CBS activity.

Diagnosis of MAT I/III Deficiency

Studies of MAT Activity in Liver. Assay of hepatic MAT activity has been reported for a total of 15 individuals with isolated hypermethioninemia. For eight patients, such studies produced convincing evidence of deficient activity of MAT in liver.[142,143,146,150,152] In each case, there was some detectable MAT activity in liver. Although the liver extracts were not chromatographed to separate the three isozyme forms of MAT (I, II, and III) present in nonfetal liver, the residual activities were lower relative to control values when assayed at high methionine concentrations. For example, MAT activities in liver extracts from two patients were 39 percent of the mean control value when assayed at 6 μM methionine, 26 to 28 percent when assayed at 100 μM methionine, and only 7 to 8 percent when assayed at 1000 μM methionine.[143,152] Activity of patients was not stimulated by dimethylsulfoxide.[152] These results suggested that the predominant loss of activity was of MAT III, the isozyme with the highest K_m for methionine and the form that is greatly stimulated by dimethylsulfoxide.[163,164] Furthermore, MAT activities in fibroblasts, red blood cells, or lymphoid cells of these patients were normal when tested,[146,153,165] indicating that MAT II, encoded by the separate gene, *MAT2A*, was not affected. These results left unclear whether the small activities found in the livers of these patients were due solely to MAT II, or whether there were also some residual MAT I/III activities.

For certain cases, assay of MAT activity in liver produced results that, at first, were confusing with respect to the etiology of the isolated hypermethioninemia of the patients in question. Thus, in two Japanese pedigrees, the affected members had MAT activities in liver extracts within, or even slightly above, the reference range when assayed at the intermediate concentration of 131 μM methionine.[149,151] Initially, these results were interpreted as demonstrating normal MAT activity in liver.[151] However, for the single members of each pedigree tested, the K_ms for methionine were found to be 111 and 174 μM (reference K_m, 714 to 800 μM), and the V_{max}s were 3.44 and 10.4 nmol/mg protein/h (reference V_{max}, 7.7 to 9.1 nmol/mg protein/h).[151] It was subsequently pointed out that, at least for the first family, these data were consistent with a partial deficiency of the MAT isozymes in liver with the highest K_ms and V_{max}s (i.e., MAT I and III), as had been found in the aforementioned patients.[137] Indeed, Nagao and Oyanagi have now found that in both these pedigrees the isolated hypermethioninemia is attributable to the R264H mutation in *MAT1A*[157,159] that is now known to cause partial loss of MAT I/III activity and mild hypermethioninemia inherited as a Mendelian dominant trait[158] (see below).‡

A $7\frac{1}{2}$-year-old Serbo-Croatian girl with mental deficiency and myopathy represents an example of isolated hypermethioninemia that may not be due to MAT I/III deficiency, despite plasma methionine concentrations of 69 to 700 μM, the latter value being higher than has been observed in any individual proven to be heterozygous for the R264H mutation and within the range of hypermethioninemia noted in patients with proven more severe sorts of MAT I/III deficiency (see below). MAT activity in liver of this girl was found to be 274 nmol/mg protein/h (reference range, 130 ± 68)[147] when assayed under conditions that appear to have included a methionine concentration of at least 10 mM,[165] conditions used to demonstrate MAT deficiency in livers of four other patients studied in the same laboratory.[146] Whereas these findings suggest that deficient activity of MAT in her liver did not cause the isolated hypermethioninemia of this girl, more stringent testing of this conclusion by molecular genetic study of her *MAT1A* gene has not been performed.

When early experience with hypermethioninemic patients gave rise to the impression that they were not severely affected clinically, liver biopsy for diagnostic purposes came often to be considered not to be justified, and such studies have not been performed on most of these patients ascertained recently.

Hepatic activities of AdoHcy hydrolase, γ-cystathionase, betaine-homocysteine methyltransferase, and N^5-methyltetrahydrofolate-homocysteine methyltransferase have been normal in patients with deficient MAT activity in liver. Hepatic CBS was moderately low in two, and questionably low in another, of the four patients in whom this enzyme was assayed.[6]

Inactivating Mutations in *MAT1A*. Identification of mutations in *MAT1A* has contributed greatly to clarification of the most frequent etiology of isolated hypermethioninemia.[12,15,157–160,166] Genomic DNA from individuals with isolated hypermethioninemia has been examined by polymerase chain reaction amplification of each of the nine *MAT1A* exons and the corresponding exon-intron junctions, followed by SSCP analysis or complete sequencing of the resulting material. By these means, *MAT1A* mutations have been identified in five individuals[12,15,160] in whom deficient MAT activity in liver had been demonstrated by enzyme assay.[146,152] Further study of individuals with isolated hypermethioninemia for whom the diagnosis had not been established by assay of MAT in liver have defined *MAT1A* mutations in 38 additional persons[12,157–159,161] to bring the total of individuals with known *MAT1A* mutations to 43. To date, 17 mutations have been identified in 58 alleles from 18 pedigrees (Table 88-1). Most of these mutations have been expressed and shown to decrease MAT activity severely in mammalian and/or bacterial systems.

‡ Some of the aforementioned patients have been reported upon more than once. For details on the sequence of reports and on the results of the assays of MAT activity in liver discussed in this paragraph, see the report by Mudd et al.[162]

Table 88-1 Published Mutations in *MAT1A*

Mutation*	Exon	Activity (%)†	Refs.
Point mutations			
113G > A(S38N)	II	0	166
164C > A(A55D)	II	6	15
595C > T(R199C)	VI	11	12
791C > T(R264C)	VII	0	166
792G > A(R264H)	VII	1	157–159
914T > C(L305P)	VII	16	15
966T > G(I322M)	VIII	11	15
1006G > A(G336R)	VIII	23	166
1031A > C(E344A)	VIII	12	166
1068G > A(R356Q)	VIII	53	12
1070C > T(P357L)	VIII	22	15
1132G > A(G378S)	IX	0.2	12
Insertions			
539ins TG(185X)	V	ND‡	12,160
827insG(351X)	VII	0	12
Deletions			
255delCA (92X)	III	0	166
1043delTG(350X)	VIII	0	12
Possible splicing disruption			
292G↓gt > A↓gt	III	ND	166

*The nomenclature system recommended for human gene mutations by Antonarakis et al[167] has been used, listing both the nucleotide change and the amino acid change. X, site of newly generated stop codon.

†Activity when expressed, percent of wild type.

‡Not determined.

The point mutations generally have had some residual activity, whereas those truncating mutations tested have had virtually none.[12,15,158] Both patients homozygous for a given mutation and those who are compound heterozygotes have been identified. To date, studies have not been carried out to determine the effect of particular *MAT1A* mutations on the kinetic properties, the tripolyphosphatase activity, or the ability to be stimulated by dimethylsulfoxide of the mutant enzymes, nor to assess possible effects of many of these mutations on the distribution of mutant MAT α1 -subunits between the dimeric and the tetrameric (and perhaps other) forms.

Assay of Plasma AdoMet. Loehrer et al showed that after administration of an oral dose of L-methionine (0.1 g/kg body weight) to control human subjects the concentration of AdoMet in their plasma rose within hours to as high as almost ninefold the preload concentration. These authors suggested that this increase "probably reflects liver metabolism of methionine."[168] In the latter organ the AdoMet concentration increased to 442 percent of the control value 30 min after administration of 0.1 g/kg L-methionine intraperitoneally to experimental rats, whereas in adrenal, heart, spleen, kidney, lung, and brain the mean increase was to only 159 percent (range, 127 to 221 percent).[169]

Gaull et al found that the concentration of AdoMet in the liver of an MAT I/III-deficient patient was not elevated.[146] In a similar patient, Gahl et al found a liver concentration of AdoMet of 18 μmol/kg wet weight (below the reference range) in spite of a plasma methionine concentration of 716 μM and a liver concentration of this amino acid of 4.8 nmol/mg protein (control value, 1.6 nmol/mg protein).[152] Together, these results indicated it might be possible to provide evidence of a deficient ability to form AdoMet in liver of patients with MAT I/III deficiency by assay of plasma AdoMet. A recently published method[170] has been used to measure the plasma AdoMet concentrations in 12 patients with isolated hypermethioninemia. In these patients, with concurrent plasma methionine concentrations ranging from 1510 down to 52 μM, plasma AdoMet concentrations ranged from 48.2 to 89.2 nM, in no instance rising above the reference ranges of 89.2 ± 5.9 nM for children and 93.6 ± 9.0 nM for adults.[171]

The hypermethioninemic patients in whom plasma AdoMet has been assayed include nine in whom MAT I/III deficiency has been proven by identification of inactivating mutations in *MAT1A*[12,15,160,166] and three for whom neither assay of MAT activity in liver nor identification of inactivating mutations in *MAT1A* have been reported. For the latter three, the failure of plasma AdoMet to rise above normal even in the face of elevations of plasma methionine supports a diagnosis of MAT I/III deficiency.[162]

Categorization of Patients with Isolated Hypermethioninemia with Respect to MAT I/III Deficiency

From the results just described, among 61 patients with isolated hypermethioninemia,[162] strong evidence for MAT I/III deficiency has been presented for eight by assay of MAT activity in liver, 43 by identification of mutations in *MAT1A*, and 12 by assay of plasma AdoMet. Because some patients have been studied by more than one of these means, there is overlap, and the total number with strong supportive evidence comes to 48. For 12, none of the aforementioned studies have been carried out and, for one, liver assay suggests a diagnosis other than MAT I/III deficiency.

Patterns of Inheritance

Most of the mutations described in Table 88-1 for which evidence is available are inherited as Mendelian recessives, with heterozygotes having little or no abnormal elevation of plasma methionine. For example, among ten individuals proven to be heterozygous for either R199C, I322M, or 539insTG (185X), the mean plasma methionine concentration was 32 μM, with a range (19 to 57 μM) that included at most very mild elevations above the reference range (upper end, 35 to 45 μM in most laboratories).[162] A striking exception is the R264H mutation. Among 28 heterozygotes for this mutation the mean plasma, methionine was 188 μM, with a range from 45 to 400 μM, so that virtually all these individuals had at least mild hypermethioninemia.[162] In three large pedigrees, heterozygosity for this mutation has been shown to track with mild hypermethioninemia for as many as four generations.[158,159] As is true of virtually all the point mutations identified to date, the amino acid altered by the R264H mutation is highly conserved during evolution, from bacteria through higher plants and mammals. Crystallographic studies have shown that the homologous residue in *E. coli* MAT is involved in a salt bridge that through polar interactions forms a spherical tight dimer. These dimers associate to a peanut-shaped tetrameric enzyme.[172,173] A strong positive charge at human position 264 is needed for dimerization.[158] That negative subunit interaction may be responsible for the dominance of the R264H mutation has been demonstrated by Chamberlin et al, who showed that R264H *MAT1A* cDNA was virtually inactive when transfected into COS-1 cells. When wild-type (R264) and mutant (R264H) *MAT1A* cDNAs were cotransfected, MAT activity was only about half that which would have been contributed by the amount of wild-type cDNA used for transfection, suggesting that the R264H mutant subunit can dimerize with the R264 wild-type *MAT1A* subunit, but the resultant heterodimer retains little enzymatic activity.[158]

Of the 43 persons with isolated hypermethioninemia for whom mutations in *MAT1A* have been identified (Table 88-1), 15 are homozygotes or compound heterozygotes for point or truncating mutations, whereas 28 are heterozygotes for R264H. The predominance of the latter mutation among detected hypermethioninemic individuals presumably reflects, not a markedly greater allele frequency of the R264H mutation, but rather the enhanced detectability of the heterozygous state. Indeed, there seems to be a reasonable possibility that, with the cutoff concentrations used for identification of hypermethioninemia in current screening programs of newborns, many individuals heterozygous for R264H may be being missed.

Metabolic Aspects

Plasma Methionine. Plasma methionine concentrations vary widely among affected individuals, but have ranged from a low of near 50 μM to as high as 2500 μM. Elevations of methionine have tended to be higher in those with truncating lesions, but there has not been a very strong correlation between the rises of plasma methionine and the decreases in expressed MAT activity, perhaps because elevations of plasma methionine are markedly affected by the dietary intake of methionine.[137] As already detailed, individuals heterozygous for the R264H mutation in *MAT1A* have MAT activities in their livers that usually fall within the reference range when assayed at low methionine concentration. These persons clearly have only relatively mild hypermethioninemia.

In addition to abnormal elevations of methionine, the plasma and urine of these patients contain high concentrations of methionine sulfoxide[146] (demonstrated in one case to be solely the L-methionine-*d* -sulfoxide enantiomer[153]).

Capacity to Synthesize AdoMet. As already mentioned, patients with inactivating mutations of *MAT1A* have normal activities of MAT II. That such activity may contribute a very significant ability to synthesize AdoMet is suggested by a balance study carried out by Gahl et al[153] on an individual now proven to be homozygous for a 539insTG mutation in *MAT1A*.[160] The encoded protein is truncated at residue 185 (of the 395 residues in the wild-type subunit) and is thus likely to have very little, if any, MAT activity. Nevertheless, this patient was demonstrated to be forming at least 14.9 mmol/day of AdoMet, an amount normal for men on normal diets. Indeed, the abnormal elevation of methionine could be regarded as being due not so much to an abnormally low flux into AdoMet, but rather to a continuation of the conversion of homocysteine back to methionine that would normally be down-regulated when AdoMet raises.

Methionine Transamination as a Spillover Pathway. Intermediates of the methionine transamination pathway rise above normal in plasma and urine of individuals with isolated hypermethioninemia, but only when the plasma methionine is 300 to 350 μM, or higher.[137] Thus, methionine transamination appears to become important as a spillover only when plasma methionine is almost 10-fold elevated. Further, there appeared to be an age-dependent utilization of this pathway, so that elevation of transamination metabolites occurred only minimally prior to about 0.9 years of age.[137] Dimethylsulfide is volatile, and a portion of this compound formed appears in respiratory air, accounting for the malodorous breath of some hypermethioninemic persons.[137,153]

Hypermethioninemia and Elevated Serum Folate. The concentrations of serum folate were markedly increased in the three patients studied by Uetsuji and colleagues, as much as 30-fold above the upper limit of normal.[149,151] Evidence suggests that these patients were heterozygous for the R264H dominant mutation in *MAT1A*,[157] but whether the abnormality of serum folate is related to the abnormality in MAT I/III has not been clarified.[157] Persistent abnormal elevation of serum folate has not been observed in affected members of three additional pedigrees carrying the R264H *MAT1A* mutation.[137,156,158,159]

Clinical Aspects

It is a reasonable expectation that the type and severity of any clinical consequences among individuals with evidence of MAT I/III deficiency might be a function of the extent of the underlying enzyme loss. Certainly for individuals heterozygous for R264H, it is clear that no apparently associated clinical manifestations have been described, even among those who are elderly.[137,156–159]

For homozygotes or compound heterozygotes for more severe MAT I/III deficiency, the picture is less clear. To date, most of these individuals have been clinically well, but only 20 are known and many are still young. Thus, 12 were below age 8 years at last follow-up. Of these, a boy ascertained by newborn screening [patient 7 (Mudd et al[137])], in spite of being normal neurologically at age 4.2 years, was found upon magnetic resonance imaging (MRI) to have brain demyelination.[174] Evidence has been reported that this child is homozygous for a mutation in *MAT1A* that may disrupt the normal splicing of the pre-mRNA and yield a truncated, inactive protein.[166] In agreement with the possibility he has a severe deficit in MAT I/III activity, he persistently has extremely high plasma methionine concentrations, yet with a concurrent plasma methionine of 1510 μM, his plasma AdoMet concentration was only 51.5 nM. Five of the 20 patients were between 8 and 20 years of age. Two have developed brain demyelination: (1) A girl [patient C (Surtees et al[155])] ascertained by newborn screening had neurologic abnormalities and MRI evidence of brain demyelination at age 11 years.[155] She is homozygous for 827insG in *MAT1A* and so produces a protein truncated at residue 351 and devoid of activity upon expression.[12] Her cerebrospinal fluid (CSF) contained an elevated concentration of methionine, but AdoMet was abnormally low. During treatment with oral AdoMet, the CSF AdoMet rose, and the neurologic signs and the MRI-visualized demyelination both improved.[155] (2) A girl ascertained because of dystonia was found by MRI at age 11 to have "myelination arrest" [patient 8 (Mudd et al[137])]. This girl has another truncating lesion, 1043delTG (350X), that again encodes a protein devoid of activity when expressed.[12] The remaining three patients are ages 24, 24, and 43 years [patients 1 and 2 (Mudd et al[137]) and Mr C (Gahl et al[152,160])] and are clinically free of manifestations that can be attributed to MAT I/III deficiency.

Is There a Cause-and-Effect Relationship Between Severe Deficiency of MAT I/III and Brain Demyelination? That three individuals with complete, or at least likely to be very severe, deficiencies of MAT I/III have developed brain demyelination strongly suggests there may be a cause-and-effect relationship. This possibility is supported both by the beneficial effect of AdoMet for the hypermethioninemic patient of Surtees et al[155] and by the fact that patients with other metabolic abnormalities that lead to subnormal AdoMet in the brain are prone to demyelination.[155,175] However, demyelination has not been a constant feature in subjects homozygous for truncating *MAT1A* mutations. Two individuals homozygous for 539insTG (185X) are clinically well and had normal brain MRIs at ages of 43 years[160] and 6.3 years [patient 3 (Mudd et al[137,176])]. It appears that a presumptive virtually complete lack of MAT I/III activity may be compatible with clinical well-being at least to age 43 years. MAT II activity may be sustaining.

Results obtained with experimental animals suggest connection between deficient MAT activity and myelin abnormalities. Administration of cycloleucine (1-aminocyclopentane carboxylic acid), an inhibitor of MAT, causes abnormalities of myelin in the brains of mice[177,178] or rats[179] against which AdoMet protects.[179] However, it is not clear that these effects can be attributed solely to inhibition of MAT I/III activity. The concentrations of cycloleucine required for 50 percent inhibition of MATs I, II, and III of rat liver are, respectively, 0.29, 0.18, and 2.50 mM.[180]

Is There a Liver-Brain Connection? In either bovine[181] or rat brain,[17] MAT II is the isozyme expressed. The K_m for methionine of MAT in extracts from human parietal cortex was reported to be 11.4 μM,[182] and, in those from human caudate nucleus, 7.5 μM.[183] Both values are low enough to indicate the isozyme in question is MAT II. If humans, like the animals studied, express MAT I/III solely in nonfetal liver and only MAT II in brain, how might a MAT I/III deficiency in liver lead to brain demyelination? One possibility is that there is normally a quantitatively important transport of AdoMet from liver to brain. This would be the most simple explanation of the low CSF AdoMet observed in the patient of Surtees et al who developed demyelination[155] and would be compatible with the evidence that liver may export AdoMet into the plasma[168] and with the recent finding that AdoMet has an affinity for the nucleoside-carrier system of rat brain endothelial cells in the range of the K_m values for thymidine and other substrates.[184] If a deficiency in the export of AdoMet from liver to plasma is the cause of the demyelination, then patients with demyelination might be expected to have lower plasma AdoMet concentrations than those without demyelination. However, the plasma AdoMet concentrations of the two patients with brain demyelination tested [patient C (Surtees et al[155]) and patient 7 (Mudd et al[137])] have now been found to be 70.9 and 51.5 nM, respectively. Although these are each somewhat below the reference range, lower values have been observed in other patients who have not developed demyelination.[171] These observations provide no firm indication that deficient export of AdoMet from liver is the sole cause of brain demyelination in MAT I/III-deficient patients.

Another possibility is that some methylated compound synthesized in liver in an AdoMet-dependent reaction is normally furnished by liver to brain. One compound that fits these criteria is choline, normally chiefly synthesized in liver as phosphatidylcholine and present in very large quantities in brain both as phosphatidylcholine and sphingomyelin (discussed more fully by Chamberlin et al[12]). Assays of both free and phospholipid-bound choline[185,186] have now been carried in plasmas from 12 MAT I/III-deficient patients.[187] Most values for free choline were below 11.4 μM, the mean of the reference range, but within 1 standard error (±3.7 μM) of this mean.[188] The value for patient C of Surtees et al[155] was only 6.8 μM, but two other patients without demyelination had similarly low values. Thus, the available results appear not to support deficient plasma choline as a sole cause of the demyelination. Dietary intake of choline and/or choline derivatives, accompanied by synthesis of AdoMet generated by MAT II, appears to be sufficient to maintain plasma choline and phosphatidylcholine at least at marginal levels in these patients.

Maternal MAT I/III Deficiency. One pregnancy has been followed in a woman with proven MAT I/III deficiency, an apparent homozygote for the I322M point mutation [patient 2 (Mudd et al[137])]. The woman, age 23 years at the time of pregnancy, is clinically well (present age, 24 years). No problems occurred during pregnancy. Plasma methionine concentrations, measured at 6- to 10-week intervals, ranged from 318 to 354 μM ($n = 6$), close to the last prepregnancy value of 336 μM. A normal boy was delivered without difficulty and has developed normally to at least age 1 year.[189]

CYSTATHIONINE β-SYNTHASE DEFICIENCY

Patients with greatly elevated concentrations of homocystine in their urine were first reported in 1962.[190,191] Within 2 to 3 years, further cases had been discovered, the chief clinical manifestations had been outlined,[9] and the enzyme defect had been shown to be deficient activity of CBS.[192]

Homocysteine and Its Derivatives in Normal Plasma

In normal human plasma, some 20 to 30 percent of the total homocysteinyl moieties occur in non-protein-bound forms,[193–195] with perhaps one-tenth this amount as the reduced sulfhydryl, homocysteine,[194,196,197] and nine-tenths as disulfides presumably formed by chemical oxidation occurring in vivo in the plasma itself. Because in normal plasma cysteine is the predominant sulfhydryl,[196] after oxidation most non-protein-bound plasma homocysteinyl moieties end as the mixed disulfide, homocysteine-cysteine.[198,199] The remaining 70 to 80 percent of the total homocysteinyl moieties of normal human plasma are bound to protein as mixed disulfides with protein cysteines.[200] Two sorts of artifacts may obscure the original distribution of homocysteinyl moieties in plasma. First, in deproteinized samples processed in the usual manner, the -SH form oxidizes almost entirely to -S-S-forms.[201] Second, when plasma is stored without prior deproteinization, homocysteinyl moieties originally not bound to protein become so bound.[193,200,202] A number of methods have now been described that circumvent these artifacts, enabling measurement of the tHcy present in a plasma sample.[6,203,204] The normal range for plasma tHcy in adults is 5 to 15 μM, with a mean near 10 μM. Women have lower concentrations than men, and tHcy increases with age and especially after menopause.[205] Children have slightly lower values than adults.[206,207]

In plasma, tHcy may be considered to be in a steady state so that import is balanced by export. Proliferating cells export more Hcy than do stationary cells, but the major portion of the approximately 1.2 millimoles exported daily from cells to plasma seems to originate chiefly in hepatocytes. This is only 5 to 10 percent of the homocysteine normally produced each day[208] (see the section "Quantitative Relationships Among Transmethylation, Transsulfuration, and Homocysteine," above). This input of Hcy is balanced by renal excretion only to the extent of about 6 μmol/day—i.e., only about 0.5 percent of the input. The remainder appears to be cleared by the tissues.[208] Measurements of arteriovenous differences across the kidneys of rats[209] and dogs[210] have shown that these organs remove considerable amounts of Hcy from the plasma, far more than is accounted for by urinary excretion, indicating that renal metabolism is occurring[209–212] (chiefly by the transsulfuration rather than the remethylation pathway[212,212a]). Humans with chronic renal failure have abnormal elevations of plasma tHcy[213,214] and clear tHcy from the plasma abnormally slowly, suggesting that renal metabolism of Hcy is important in humans, as well.[208,215] The latter conclusion, however, may not apply as strongly to fasting humans with normal plasma concentrations of tHcy. In a recent study, Van Guldener and colleagues measured plasma tHcy and free Hcy in renal arterial and venous blood in 20 subjects with normal renal function. No significant differences were observed. An arteriovenous difference of 0.43 μM for plasma tHcy could be excluded with 95 percent confidence.[216] For a maximal normal renal plasma flow of approximately 600 ml/min,[217] such a difference would correspond to only 0.37 millimoles/day.

Causes of Elevated Plasma Hcy and/or Homocystinuria

A great many advances have now made it clear that not only deficient activity of CBS, but also genetic defects that impair the N^5-methyltetrahydrofolate-dependent conversion of homocysteine to methionine, may lead to abnormal accumulation of Hcy in the plasma (elevated plasma tHcy) and, perhaps, to the appearance of excessive homocystine in the urine. Among these are mutations that severely inactivate the activity of MTHFR, and the cblC, cblD, cblE, cblF, and cblG mutations that impact more or less directly on the activity of N^5-methyltetrahydrofolate-homocysteine methyltransferase (methionine synthase) (detailed briefly above in the section "Homocysteine Methylation" and covered in Chap. 155). In contrast to most cases of CBS deficiency, hypermethioninemia is absent in the latter conditions.

The technology for measurement of homocysteine and its derivatives in the plasma has been developed, so that the quantity determined by most modern methods is plasma tHcy, the sum of all homocysteine moieties arising after treatment of a sample with a reagent that cleaves disulfide bonds and so liberates homocysteine from not only the free disulfides, homocystine and homocysteine-cysteine mixed disulfide, but also the major portion of homocysteine that normally exists bound as a mixed disulfide to protein cysteines. Extensive utilization of such methodology (see, for example, Refsum et al[205]) has revealed that many additional conditions may lead to (usually less severe) elevations of plasma tHcy. Such conditions have been reviewed extensively (see, for example, Refsum et al,[205] Van den Berg and Boers,[218] Bakker and Brandjes,[219] and Pietrzik and Brönstrup[220]) and include homozygosity for the 677C→T mutation leading to thermolability of MTHFR (Chap. 155), Immerslund syndrome, transcobalamin II abnormalities,[6] renal disease,[221] deficiencies of folate or B_{12},[205] and treatment with a variety of drugs including folate antagonists, nitrous oxide,[205] drugs that may interfere with B_6 function,[6] and others.[6,205] Standardized loading with methionine may elicit abnormal elevations of plasma tHcy in subjects without fasting elevations[205,218] and, of relevance to CBS deficiency, may be particularly useful in suggesting heterozygosity for this deficiency.[205,218]

The Genetic Defect and Genetic Heterogeneity

Numerous homocystinuric patients have now been found to have deficient activity of CBS in extracts of liver and/or extracts of fibroblasts cultured from skin. CBS activity was found also to be abnormally low in brain, in phytohemagglutinin-stimulated lymphocytes, and in long-term cultures of lymphocytes from such patients, as well as in cultured amniotic fluid cells and chorionic villi.[9]

Residual CBS in patients with a deficiency of this enzyme has been found to differ both from normal CBS and between different affected individuals in numerous ways:[9] (1) The amounts of residual CBS activity in cultured fibroblasts have ranged from none detected up to 10 percent of mean control activity. (2) The stimulation of CBS activities in crude fibroblast extracts by addition of PLP in vitro has varied and has not always correlated with the in vivo response of the patient to B_6. (3) Affinities of residual CBS activity for PLP have usually been lower than that of control and have differed markedly among affected patients.[222] (4) Immunologically cross-reacting material may or may not be detectable in fibroblasts cultured from deficient individuals, without correlation between the amount of cross-reacting antigen and clinical course of the disease.[223,224] (5) The CBS subunit was indistinguishable in size from that of control in 15 of 17 cell lines from affected individuals, but two mutant lines had no detectable cross-reacting material. For one of these lines, derived from a mildly affected patient (no. 366; see below), CBS subunits were detected upon in vitro translation of mRNA prepared from his fibroblasts. The subunit encoded on the maternal allele was of normal size (63 kDa), while the paternal allele produced a smaller polypeptide with an apparent molecular weight of 56 kDa.[223] This patient was also the first one whose mutations were subsequently determined at the DNA level (see below).

Nature of the Cystathionine β-Synthase Mutations

Cloning of human CBS cDNA[84] has permitted a detailed definition of the mutations in individual patients. In an initial study, a mutation-screening system based on expression of hybrid CBS cDNAs in an *E. coli*-expression system was devised.[224,225] These hybrid cDNAs consist of different segments of patient cDNA in the context of an otherwise normal CBS cDNA sequence. Pathogenic mutation(s) in the test segment extinguishes CBS activity in the transformed *E. coli* host. Reverse transcription of fibroblast mRNA from patient 366 into cDNA, and the utilization of the *E. coli*-screening system, enabled the demonstration in the maternal allele of a T-to-C transition at bp 833 that led to a change of ile 278 to thr, and, in the paternal allele, of an in-frame deletion of exon 12 (46 amino acids).[225] The finding of the deletion[225] appropriately explained the presence of the abnormal polypeptide detected 8 years earlier.[223] Following this study, a large number of mutations in the CBS gene have been identified both at the cDNA level and the genomic DNA level.[226,] (see also ref 613) Figure 88-4 shows the location of the known CBS mutations (as of March 1999) along the CBS gene.

More than 300 individual homocystinuric alleles have been studied, and 92 mutations were detected. (see ref 613) Table 88-2 lists the mutations by type: missense, nonsense, deletions, insertions, and splicing and linked mutations (see also refs 227–257). The nucleotide changes at the cDNA level are indicated, together with effects on the coding region. Whenever known, the ethnic origins of the patients are shown, as are the relevant citations. Clearly, the majority of the mutations are private missense mutations. The mutations I278T and G307S, on the other hand, represent more than half the affected alleles. The I278T mutation is a panethnic mutation detected in the majority of European populations. In some countries (e.g., the Netherlands), it accounts for nearly half the affected alleles. Screening of 500 consecutive Danish newborns revealed that this mutation (not linked to the aforementioned 844ins68 polymorphism[92a]) occurred with a surprisingly high prevalence of 1.4 percent of heterozygotes.[257a] The G307S mutation is undoubtedly the leading cause of homocystinuria in Ireland (71 percent of affected alleles).[258] It has also been detected frequently in U.S. and Australian patients of "Celtic" origin, including families with Irish, Scottish, English, French, and Portuguese roots. A finding of this mutation in Norway[245] may, however, indicate that this allele originated there and spread elsewhere. The G307S mutation has not been detected in Italy, the Netherlands, Germany, or the Czech Republic. The third most frequent alteration is a splice mutation in intron 11, IVS 11-2 A>C, that results in skipping of the entire exon 12. Surprisingly, although it was found in Germany in about 20 percent of affected chromosomes of German and Turkish origin,[256] it was never detected in Italy and the Netherlands in nearly 70 alleles studied. The remaining cases originate from Central and Eastern Europe. In addition, several splicing mutations as well as insertions and deletions have been found. To date, mutations linked to another mutation on the same allele have been found in nine isolated cases. Most of these mutations have been reproduced separately by in vitro mutagenesis, and each was found to be deleterious to CBS activity

Most Mutations Are Found in the Conserved Active Core of Cystathionine β-Synthase. Figure 88-5 compares the human CBS amino acid sequence to the rat enzyme and to the sequences of *O*-acetylserine lyase (cysteine synthase) from bacteria and plants. Exons 2 to 7 are the most highly conserved. Exon 3 contains lysine 119, which was recently shown to be the PLP-binding residue.[102] About a quarter of the missense mutations identified so far are located in exon 3. In most cases, the human mutation changes an amino acid conserved between the human and rat CBS and, in many cases, a residue shared between all the enzymes has been altered. For example, the frequently seen I278T and G307S mutations change absolutely conserved isoleucine and glycine residues, respectively.

Genotype and Vitamin-(AU36)B_6 Responsiveness

The majority of homocystinuric patients are compound heterozygotes, with the exception of I278T/I278T and G307S/G307S homozygotes. The I278T mutation usually confers B_6 responsiveness, whether in homozygotes or compound heterozygotes (Table 88-3). The clinical phenotype in many of these patients appears to be mild[248] with the exception of a group of Dutch patients reported by Kluijtmans et al.[233] In addition to the I278T mutation, the A114V, R266K, R336H, K384E, and L539S mutations also appear to correlate with pyridoxine responsiveness in vivo. On the other hand, the R121L, R125Q, C165Y, E176K, T191M, T257M, and T262M mutations, and the frequent G307S mutation, in one or two copies, appear to be incompatible with pyridoxine responsiveness. Accordingly, patients carrying the G307S mutation seem to have moderate to severe phenotypes, except for those who have been treated since birth.[258] Recently, a first patient was identified who is a compound heterozygote for the I278T and G307S mutations. This patient is B_6 nonresponsive.[453]

Lack of Correlation Between In Vitro and In Vivo Observations. A number of CBS-deficient patients have no measurable

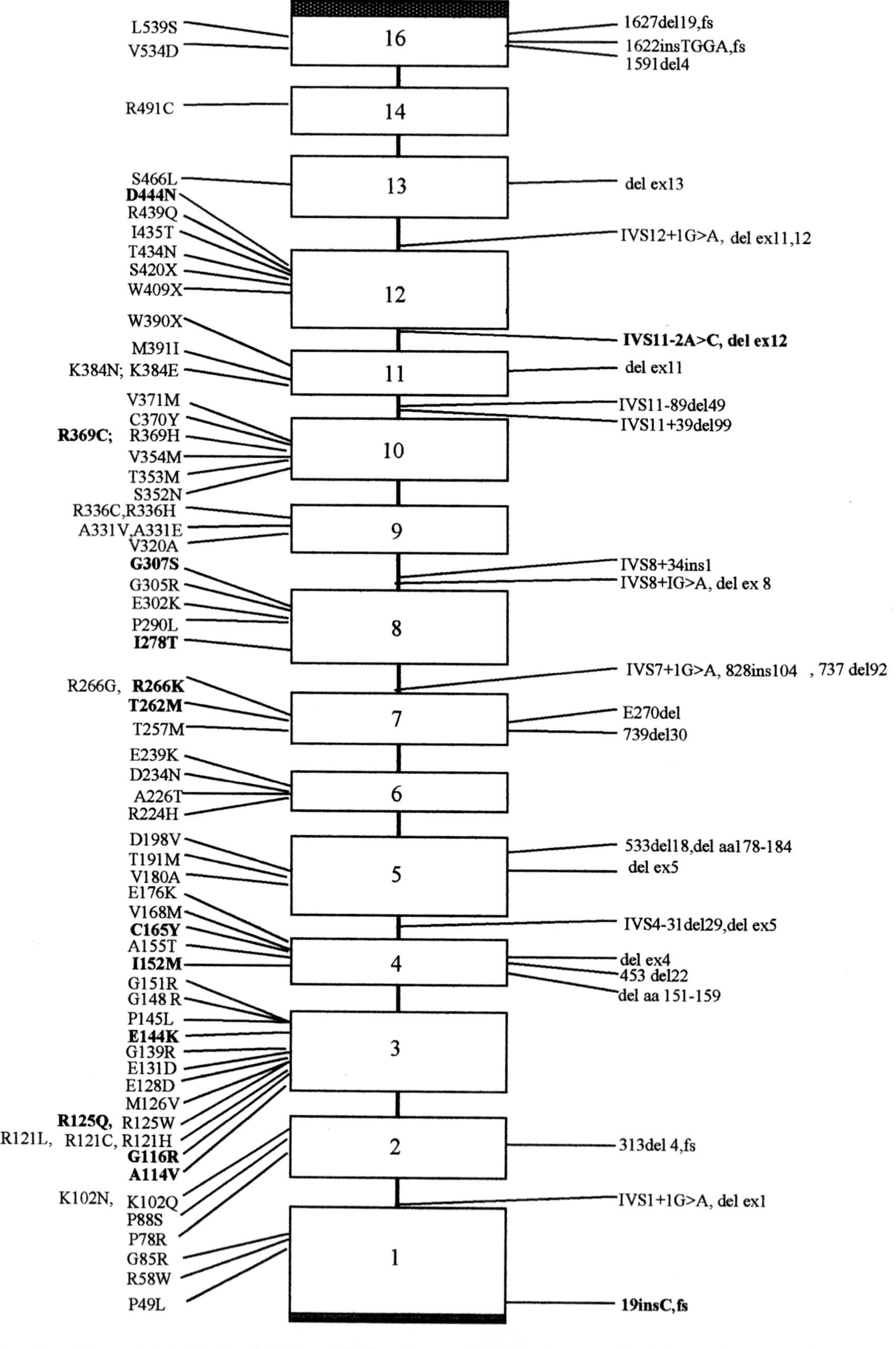

Fig. 88-4 Location of human cystathionine β-synthase (CBS) mutations. The exons in the coding region are drawn to scale, but the introns are not. The *shaded areas* are parts of 5′- and 3′-untranslated regions of CBS mRNA found in exon 1 and exon 16, respectively. The mutations shown on the *left* are missense and nonsense, and the mutations on the *right* are deletions, insertions, and splicing aberrations. The mutations shown in **bold** were detected in three or more alleles.

Table 88-2 List of Cystathionine β-Synthase (CBS) Mutations*

Nucleotide Change†	Effect on Coding Region‡	No. of Alleles	Ancestry§	Refs.
Missense Mutations				
146 C > T	P49L	1	Italian	227
172 C > T	R58W	1	Italian	249
233 C > G	P78R	1	Irish	224
253 G > A	G85R	1	Danish	614
262 C > T	P88S	1	Italian	89
304 A > C	K102Q	2	Arabian	229
306 G > C	K102N	1	Irish	224
341 C > T	A114V	6	Italian, Irish/German	230, 249
346 G > A	G116R	3	Italian	231
361 C > T	R121C	2	Norwegian/Irish/German	232
362 G > A	R121H	1	African American	232
362 G > T	R121L	2	Chinese	232
373 C > T	R125W	1	Dutch	233
374 G > A	R125Q	5	Italian, Portugese, Irish	89, 234, 235
376 A > G	M126V	1	Italian	249
384 G > C	E128D	1	French	236
393 G > C	E131D	1	Irish	234
415 G > A	G139R	1	Italian/Irish	237
430 G > A	E144K	3	*Australian*, English	237–239
434 C > T	P145L	1	Irish/German	230
442 G > A	G148R	1	Japanese	615
451 G > A	G151R	2	African American	232
456 C > G	I152M	3	Dutch	233
463 G > A	A155T	2	Czech	240
494 G > A	C165Y	5	Dutch, *South African*	239, 241
502 G > A	V168M	1	ND	242
526 G > A	E176K	2	Slovak	243
539 T > C	V180A	1	Dutch	233
572 C > T	T191M	2	Spanish	244
593 A > T	D198V	1	Irish/Italian, *Scandinavian*	232
671 G > A	R224H	1	ND	242
676 G > A	A226T	1	African American	104
700 G > A	D234N	1	*Puerto Rican*	232
715 G > A	E239K	1	Irish	224
770 C > T	T257M	2	Italian	89
785 C > T	T262M	6	Norwegian, Irish/French/English, Italian	232
796 A > G	R266G	1	Japanese	615
797 G > A	R266K	7	Norwegian	245
833 T > C	I278T	66	Panethnic	225
869 C > T	P290L	1	Spanish	246
904 G > A	E302K	1	Italian	249
913 G > A	G305R	1	Italian	90, 247
919 G > A	G307S	73	Irish, French/Scottish, English, Portuguese, Norwegian, African American	248
959 T > C	V320A	2	Norwegian	245
992 C > A	A331E	1	*Australian*	238
992 C > T	A331V	1	ND	242
1006 C > T	R336C	1	English	249
1007 G > A	R336H	2	*North African*	250
1055 G > A	S352N	1	*Haitian*	232
1058 C > T	T353M	2	*Australian*, African American	238
1060 G > A	V354M	1	Portuguese	250
1105 C > T	R369C	3	Norwegian, Dutch	233, 245
1106 G > A	R369H	2	Irish	251
1109 G > A	C370Y	1	Italian/Polish	252
1111 G > A	V371M	2	Dutch	241
1150 A > G	K384E	2	French	253
1152 G > C	K384N	2	Lebanese	254
1173 G > T	M391I	1	German	254
1301 C > A	T434N	1	Dutch	233
1304 T > C	I435T	1	Danish	614
1316 G > A	R439Q	2	English/German, *Australian*	238, 252

(Continued on next page)

Table 88-2 (Continued)

Nucleotide Change†	Effect on Coding Region‡	No. of Alleles	Ancestry§	Refs.
1330 G > A	D444N	5	Dutch, *Venezuelan*, German, Danish	255
1397 C > T	S466L	1	Danish	614
1471 C > T	R491C	2	Dutch	233
1601 T > A	V534D	1	French	250
1616 T > C	L539S	2	French	253
Nonsense mutations				
1170 G > A	W390X	1	French Canadian/English	232
1226 G > A	W409X	1	Slovak	243
1259 C > G	S420X	1	*North African*	250
Deletions, insertions, and splicing mutations¶				
19insC	fs, stop at aa36	3	Czech, Slovak	229
IVS1 + 1G > A	Idel209(del ex 1) or 153del57	1	French/Scottish, English/Welsh	232, 239, 254
313del4	313del 4,fs	1	French Canadian/English	232
452del 27;	del aa 151–159	1	Italian	227
452del 80	del ex 4	1	*Haitian*	232
532del 135	del ex 5	1	ND	254
453del22	fs, del aa 165–172	1	Danish	616
IVS4-31 del 29	del ex 5	2	Arabian	229
533 del 18	del aa 178–184	1	German/Polish/French	232
739del 30	del aa 247–256	1	German	256
808del3	del E270	1	German	256
IVS7 + 1 G > A	828ins 104, 737del92	1	Czech	240
IVS8 + 1 G > A	829 del 126(del ex 8)	1	Danish	614
IVS8 + 34ins1	L539S	1	ND	232
IVS11 + 39del99	?	1	Czech	243
IVS11-89del49	?	1	Italian	246
1146 del 78	del ex 11	1	ND	242
IVS11-2 A > C	1224del 135 (del ex 12)	13	Jewish, German, Slovak, Czech, *Austrian*, Turkish	225, 243, 256
IVS 12 + 1 G > A	wt;del ex 12; del ex 11, 12	1	ND	257
1359del 109	del ex 13	2	Turkish	254
1591del4	1591del TTCG, fs	1	Japanese	615
1622ins4	1622ins TGGA, fs	1	*South African*	239
1627del 19	fs, stop at aa 568	2	Arabian	229
Linked mutations				
[146 C > T; IVS11-89del49]	[P49L;?]	1	Italian	227, 246
[172C > T, 341 C > T]	[R58W, A114V]	1	Italian	249
[233 C > G, 306 G > C]	[P78R, K102N]	1	Irish	224
[304 A > C; IVS4-31del29]	[K102Q;del ex5]	2	Arabian	229
[374 G > A; 393 G > C]	[R125Q;E131D]	1	Irish	234
[430 G > A; 1316 G > A]	[E144K;R439Q]	1	*Australian*	238
[919 G > A; 1601 T > A]	[G307S;V534D]	1	French	250
[1105 C > T;1471 C > T]	[R369C;R491C]	2	Dutch	233
[IVS7 + 1G > A;IVS11 + 39del99]	[828ins 104, fs;?]	1	Czech	243

*Additional information can be found at http://www.uchsc.edu/sm/cbs.

†The A in the initiator codon for Met was designated as number 1 in the CBS cDNA sequence; the CBS cDNA sequence is accessible under GenBank L19501.

‡Predicted amino acid changes or observed alternatively spliced mRNA isoforms are given.

§The ethnicity of the patient is shown if known. In some cases, *italics* is used to indicate the country of patient's origin. *Slashes* indicate ethnic origin of patient's parents, commas indicate separate alleles.

¶In some cases the causative mutation at the genomic level was not determined. Some of the splicing mutations lead to multiple mRNA isoforms.

NOTE: For splicing mutations for which the primary defect in genomic DNA has been determined, the locations of causative mutations are shown within the adjacent introns (IVS).

ABBREVIATIONS: ND, not determined; fs = Frameshift.

activity in their fibroblasts, and the CBS subunits themselves are undetectable in fibroblast extracts of some of these individuals. Many of these patients, however, are B_6 responsive. Aforementioned patient 366 had no detectable fibroblast CBS protein, but clinically had a very mild B_6-responsive homocystinuria. Furthermore, although pyridoxine responsiveness is absolutely constant within sibships, the clinical phenotype is often not. For example, three siblings have been described[224] who have an identical genotype, with E239K on the maternal allele and two mutations, P78R and K102N, on the paternal allele. The brother has normal intelligence and has had a single episode of venous thrombosis of the calf at the age of 34 years. In contrast, his sisters are mentally retarded and have suffered from skeletal abnormalities and other clinical complications from early ages. Their asymptomatic mother also lacks detectable CBS subunits in her fibroblasts. She is, however, a heterozygote and has one normal allele and one carrying the E239K mutation.[224] Other examples of significant differences in the clinical phenotype within sibships are the pairs ArD and AnD, N4a and N4b, LM and AM, JC and MC, and N6a and N6b (see http://www.uchsc.edu/sm/cbs). Taken together,

```
              →1                              Q →2
              ▼       R      R  S             PN ▼        V R
CBS   HS 68 TAPAKSPKILPDILKKIGDTPMVRINKIGKKFGLKCELLAKCEFFNAGGS  117
CBS   RN 65 TVPTKSPKILPDILRKIGNTPMVRINRISKNAGLKCELLAKCEFFNAGGS  114
CYSK  EC  1 ---SKIFED-NSLT--IGHTPLVRLNRIGNG---R--ILAKVESRNPSFS   39
CYSK  ST  1 ---SKIYED-NSLT--IGHTPLVRLNRIGNG---R--ILAKVESRNPSFS   39
CSYN  SO  1 MVEEKAFIA-KDVTELIGKTPLVYLNTVADGCVAR--VAAKLEGMEPCSS   47
               .*       ..  **.**.* .* ...    .  . ** *  ..  *
               L
               H   W                          →3
               C   QV D  D       R     KL  R  RM             Y
CBS   HS    VKDRISLRMIEDAERDGTLKPGDT-IIEPTSGNTGIGLA-LAAAVRGYRCI  166
CBS   RN    VKDRISLRMIEDAERAGTLKPGDT-IIEPTSGNTGIGLA-LAAAVKGYRCI  163
CYSK  EC    VKCRIGANMIWDAEKRGVLKPGVE-LVEPTSGNTGIALAYVAAA-RGYKLT   88
CYSK  ST    VKCRIGANMIWDAEKRGVLKPGVE-LVEPTNGNTGIALAYVAAA-RGYKLT   88
CSYN  SO    VKDRIGFSMITDAEKSGLITPGESVLIEPTSGNTGIGLAFIAAA-KGYKLI   97
            ** **. .** ***. * ..** .  .***.*****.**  *** .**. .
                     →4
             M       K▼  A          M      V
CBS   HS    IVMPEKMSSEKVDVLRALGAEIVRTPTNARFDSPESHVGVAWRLKNEIPN  216
CBS   RN    IVMPEKMSMEKVDVLRALGAEIVRTPTNARFDSPESHVGVAWRLKNEIPN  213
CYSK  EC    LTMPETMSIERRKLLKALGANLVLTEGAKGMKGA-IQKAEE-IVASNPEK  136
CYSK  ST    LTMPETMSIERRKLLKALGANLVLTEGAKGMKGA-IQKAEE-IVASDPQK  136
CSYN  SO    ITMPASMSLERRTILRAFGAELILTDPAKGMKGA-VQKAEE-IRDKTPNS  145
            ..**..** *. ..*.*.**... *  .  ....  . . .    ..  .
                →5                     →6                    G
                 ▼ H T       N    K     ▼           M    M   K
CBS   HS    SHILDQYRNASNPLAHYDTTADEILQQCDGKLDMLVASVGTGGTITGIAR  266
CBS   RN    SHILDQYRNASNPLAHYDDTAEEILQQCDGKVDMLVASAGTGGTITGIAR  263
CYSK  EC    YLLLQQFSNPANPEIHEKTTGPEIWEDTDGQVDVFIAGVGTGGTLTGVSR  186
CYSK  ST    YLLLQQFSNPANPEIHEKTTGPEIWEDTDGQVDVFISGVGTGGTLTGVTR  186
CSYN  SO    YIL-QQFENPANPKVHYETTGPEIWKGTGGKIDIFVSGIGTGGTITGAGR  194
              . .*. *..**  * ..*. ** .  .*..*..... *****.** .*
                     →7
               ΔQ    ▼ T              L           K  R S
CBS   HS    KLKEKCPGCRIIGV--DP-EGSILAEPEELNQTEQTTYEVEGIGYDFIPT  313
CBS   RN    KLKEKCPGCKIIGV--DP-EGSILAEPEELNQTEQTAYEVEGIGYDFIPT  310
CYSK  EC    YIKGTKGKTDLISVAVEPTDSPVIAQALAGEEIKPGPHKIQGIGAGFIPA  236
CYSK  ST    YIKGTKGKTDLITVAVEPTDSPVIAQALAGEEIKPGPHKIQGIGAGFIPG  236
CSYN  SO    YLKEQNPDVKLIGL--EPVESAV----LSGG--KPGPHKIQGLGAGFIPG  236
             .*.      .*.. .*  ....     . .  ........*.* .***.
               →8            E    H         →9
                ▼ A          V    C          ▼    NMM
CBS   HS    VLDRTVVDKWFKSNDEEAFTFARMLIAQEGLLCGGSAGSTVAVAVKAAQE  363
CBS   RN    VLDRAVVDRWFKSNDDDSFAFARMLISQEGLLCGGSSGSAMAVAVKAAQE  360
CYSK  EC    NLDLKLVDKVIGITNEEAISTARRLMEEEGILAGISSGAAVAAALKLQED  286
CYSK  ST    NLDLKLIDKVVGITNEEAISTARRLMEEEVFLAGISSGAAVAAALKLQED  286
CSYN  SO    VLDVNIIDEVVQISSEESIEMAKLLALKEGLLVGISSGAAAAAAIKVAKR  286
             **  ..*     ....... *.  * .* .* * *.*.. *.*.*  ..
                 C              →10N                      →11
                 HY   M          ▼ E     XI                ▼X
CBS   HS    LQEGQRC---VVILPDSVRNYMTKFLSDRWMLQKGFLKEEDLTEKKPWWW  410
CBS   RN    LKEGQRC---VVILPDSVRNYMSKFLSDKWMLQKGFMKEE-LSVKRPWWW  406
CYSK  EC    --ESFTNKNIVVILPSSGE-------------------------------  303
CYSK  ST    --ESFTNKNIVVILPSSGE-------------------------------  303
CSYN  SO    -PE-NAGKLIVAVFPSFGE-------------------------------  303
              *       *...*
```

Fig. 88-5 Evolutionary conservation of the active core of cystathionine β-synthase (CBS) and mutations. CBS HS, human CBS; CBS RN, rat CBS; CYSK EC, *Escherichia coli O*-acetylserine lyase; CYSK ST, *Salmonella typhimurium O*-acetylserine lyase; CYSN SO, spinach cysteine synthase. *Asterisks* signify absolute conservation of amino acid residues, and *dots* show conservative replacements. Approximate positions of introns are indicated by *solid, numbered triangles*. The human CBS mutations are noted above the sequences by *bold letters*.

these observations indicate that the absence of detected CBS protein in fibroblasts does not preclude an in vivo response to pyridoxine, and that an identical CBS genotype does not always result in the same phenotype, even within a family.

Mode of Inheritance

CBS deficiency is inherited as an autosomal recessive trait, as shown both by pedigree studies and by studies of enzymes in parents of affected children. Obligate heterozygous individuals have had 22 to 47 percent of mean control CBS activity in extracts of liver and 0 to 45 percent in extracts of cultured fibroblasts.[9] Thus, in each tissue, obligate heterozygotes have had less than 50 percent of the mean control specific activity of the affected enzyme. This decrease below 50 percent activity may be due to negative interaction between mutant and normal subunits combined in "hybrid" enzyme molecules.[7]

Metabolic Sequelae

The primary metabolic consequence of a deficient activity of CBS is a tendency for homocysteine to accumulate intracellularly. Under such conditions, mammalian cells export homocysteine[263] and, in the plasma, the tendency to intracellular accumulation is reflected by abnormal concentrations of a variety of homocysteine derivatives. Untreated CBS-deficient patients have been found to have fasting plasma concentrations of free homocystine up to 200 μM. Cysteine-homocysteine mixed disulfide is also present. Another mixed disulfide occurring abnormally is homocysteine-cysteinylglycine. This replaces the normally occurring cystinylglycine, presumably as a result of oxidation of a mixture originally containing homocysteine and cysteinylglycine. CBS-deficient patients have an increase in protein-bound homocysteine as well as plasma free Hcy, and, indeed, protein-bound homocysteine may be the more sensitive indicator of an elevation of plasma tHcy.[9] Homocysteine appears to compete very favorably with cysteine for protein-binding sites.[264–266] As plasma tHcy increases, the contribution of plasma free Hcy rises disproportionately,[266–268] so that Hcy becomes by far the most abundant sulfhydryl species in plasma, exceeding cysteine and cysteinylglycine.[268] The relationship between free homocystine and tHcy in plasma is triphasic: (1) when tHcy was less than 60 μM, an increase in free homocystine was minimal; (2) as tHcy ranged from 60 to 150 μM, free homocystine rose between less than 1 and 20 μM, indicating

Table 88-3 Genotype and Vitamin-B_6 Responsiveness in Cystathionine β-Synthase (CBS) Deficiency

Cell Line	Genotype		B_6†	Refs.
419	19insC(fs, K36X)	19insC(fs, K36X)	−	229
LT	A114V	A114V	+	89
R600	R121L	R121L	−	232
SGo	R125Q	R125Q	−	235
AP	C165Y	C165Y	−	233
428	E176K	E176K	−	243
S	T191M	T191M	−	244
NO	T257M	T257M	−	89
N2	T262M	T262M	−	245
N1,N4a*, N4b, N9	R266K	R266K	+	245
RB, C110, MP, 426, PA, CG, M	I278T	I278T	+	237, 260
AB, B-H, H.B/G, JU, GE, W.S/J	I278T	I278T	+	233
L209, L188	I278T	I278T	+	248
NM, MW	I278T	I278T	+	254
NM	I278T	I278T	+	89
426	I278T	I278T	+	240
RS*, SS	I278T	P88S	+	89
LM*, AM	I278T	G116R	+	259
L264	I278T	G139R	+	237
L265	I278T	E144K	+	237
JC*, MC	I278T	I152M	+	233
403	I278T	A155T	+	240
HvE(RD55)	I278T	C165Y	+	241
GC	I278T	G305R	+	90, 247
IWa	I278T	T353M	−	238
N6a*, N6b	I278T	R369C	+	245
AC	I278T	C370Y	+	252
JM, JR	I278T	V371M	+	233
DS	I278T	R439Q	+	252
366	I278T	IVS11-2A > C, del ex12	+	225
427	I278T	IVS11-2A > C, del ex12	±	240
TD	I278T	IVS11-2A > C, del ex12	+	261
ST, FH	G307S	G307S	−	262
N10	G307S	G307S	−	245
MGL 166, MGL246	G307S	G307S	−	232
AP, DA	G307S	G307S	−	260
7215	R336H	R336H	+	236
P465	K384E	K384E	+	253
P325	L539S	L539S	+	253

*Sibling pairs.
†A ± indicates some response to pyridoxine treatment with Hcy concentrations remaining above 50 μM.
NOTE: Additional information can be found at http://www.uchsc.edu/sm/cbs.

that only a portion of the total continued to bind to protein; and (3) as tHcy rose from 150 to 250 μM, there was an equal increase in free homocystine above 20 μM, indicating that the binding capacity for Hcy had been exceeded.[268a]

A second characteristic feature of CBS deficiency is the presence of abnormal concentrations of methionine in plasma. Normally, fasting human plasma contains less than 35 μM methionine. Untreated CBS-deficient patients have been reported with fasting plasma concentrations of methionine up to 2000 μM.[9] Such elevations are presumably due to enhanced rates of homocysteine methylation brought about by increased concentrations of the latter. This effect has been directly demonstrated in a study of a CBS-deficient patient by using stable isotope and continuous-infusion methodology. The control ratio of the rate of homocysteine remethylation relative to the rate of transsulfuration was 0.96, whereas in the patient the ratio was 2.25 at a time when his plasma tHcy was elevated to 92 μM.[269] Factors affecting the rate of homocysteine methylation affect the balance between the accumulation of methionine and Hcy. For example, there is evidence suggesting that some CBS-deficient patients in the newborn period may accumulate relatively more methionine and less homocystine than do most adult patients.[270] Perhaps such observations will be explained by a carryover of the relatively high activities of N^5-methyltetrahydrofolate-homocysteine methyltransferase found in the fetus into the first weeks or months of extrauterine life.[271] Conversely, some untreated older CBS-deficient patients (as many as 6 percent[272]) even in the presence of elevated Hcy in plasma and urine did not have plasma methionine concentrations above normal.[9] Enhanced methionine/homocystine ratios may be brought about in some patients by administration of betaine or its metabolic precursor choline,[6] thus providing more substrate for betaine-homocysteine methyltransferase. Treatment with folic acid leads to similar shifts in the methionine-Hcy balance, probably by increasing the rate of N^5-methyltetrahydrofolate-dependent homocysteine methylation.[9]

Abnormal accumulations of methionine and Hcy occur not only in plasma, but also in other body fluids, such as CSF[273–275] and aqueous humor.[276]

Renal tubular reabsorption of methionine is very efficient and, even at moderate elevations of plasma methionine, the urinary excretion of this amino acid may be within normal limits. Homocystine is reabsorbed less well, and, in patients with severe untreated CBS deficiency, more than 1 mmol of this disulfide may be excreted each day.[9]

The metabolically active form of homocystine is the sulfhydryl homocysteine. The presence in tissues of relatively large concentrations of reduced glutathione,[277] as well as an enzyme that catalyzes a disulfide interchange between glutathione and homocysteine,[278] ensures that intracellularly homocysteine will predominate over homocystine. Few analyses of tissue amino acids have been reported for CBS-deficient patients.[8] In general, methionine concentrations were reported to be abnormally elevated in liver, brain, and erythrocytes, but not in cultured skin fibroblasts.[9] Homocystine was usually not detected. In rat tissues in vivo, almost half the total homocysteinyl moieties are bound to protein by disulfide bonds.[279] After death of the animal, or removal of tissue, free homocysteinyl moieties quickly become protein bound.[280] Postmortem rises occur rapidly in AdoHcy concentrations.[37–39] In view of these artifactual changes, the earlier studies of tissue amino acids in CBS-deficient patients should probably be regarded as nondefinitive.

A number of derivatives of homocysteine and methionine are also present in abnormally elevated amounts in plasma or urine of CBS-deficient patients. These compounds have been described in detail elsewhere.[7] A recent addition to this list is homocysteine thiolactone, formed following the "mis-activation" of homocysteine to homocysteinyl-tRNA, a reaction that occurs more rapidly in CBS-deficient cells than in control cells.[140] The thiolactone is hydrolyzed rapidly, but evidence has been reported that it is also incorporated into proteins by acylation of side-chain amino groups of lysine residues. Such protein acylation has been suggested as a possible contributor to the pathologic consequences of homocysteine accumulation.[140]

Compounds metabolically distal to the block at CBS would be expected to form at abnormally slow rates in patients with deficiency of this enzyme. Evidence compatible with this expectation has emerged from studies of cystathionine, cyst(e)ine, and sulfate. Again, these studies have been summarized in detail elsewhere.[8] Most noteworthy in relation to possible harmful effects is the tendency for plasma tCys to be decreased in CBS-deficient patients.[266,268]

Finally, several additional metabolic sequelae of CBS deficiency have been reported: Plasma ornithine concentrations are elevated two- to threefold above normal, without accompanying overflow ornithinuria.[281] Plasma copper is increased about 1.4-fold, with corresponding increases in ceruloplasmin concentrations.[282] Neither of these effects is understood mechanistically. While on folate therapy, CBS-deficient patients have slightly lower-than-normal plasma serine concentrations. It was proposed that under these conditions folate-dependent methylation of homocysteine is proceeding faster than normal, leading to depletion of serine, the ultimate source of the 1-carbon unit required for this reaction.[283]

The Pyridoxine Effect and Its Mechanism

In 1967, Barber and Spaeth reported that three CBS-deficient patients responded to very high doses of pyridoxine (250 to 500 mg daily), with decreases of plasma methionine levels to normal and virtual elimination of homocystine from plasma and urine.[284] This observation has since been extended to many additional patients by many authors. During the response to B_6, there are decreases in a number of additional compounds formed proximal to the metabolic block at CBS and increases in compounds distal to the block.[7] Some CBS-deficient patients are not responsive to pyridoxine. In a large international survey, virtually equal proportions of patients were judged to be responsive and nonresponsive.[272] There is ample evidence that the pyridoxine-induced response is not due to correction of a preexisting vitamin-B_6 deficiency or to alleviation of a defect in vitamin-B_6 metabolism that might limit the ability of responsive patients to form PLP, the form of vitamin B_6 active as a cofactor for CBS.[7] The biochemical response to B_6 may not be manifest in folate-depleted patients until after folate replenishment,[285,286] presumably thereby enabling optimal functioning of N^5-methyltetrahydrofolate-dependent homocysteine remethylation. Such depletion may explain the apparent failure of some potentially responsive patients to respond to B_6 treatment. Therefore, to be most readily interpretable, the effect of B_6 must be studied in the presence of adequate folate.

B_6-responsive patients are not uniform. Some patients in response continue to have slight elevations of homocystine in plasma or urine, whereas others do not.[9] Brenton and Cusworth defined three classes of pyridoxine responsiveness, including a group intermediate between those who display little or no response and those with very clear responses.[287] Approximately 13 percent of patients may show such intermediate responses.[272] Even those patients who respond most favorably are clearly not restored to biochemical normality, continuing to have abnormal rises of plasma and urinary homocystine after methionine loads, delayed restoration of plasma methionine to basal concentrations, and maximal capacities for transsulfuration far below normal.[9]

Pyridoxine responsiveness is constant within sibships,[272] indicating not only that the capacity to respond to B_6 is genetically determined, but also that the genetic determinant governing responsiveness is closely linked with, or identical to, that determining CBS deficiency itself. The simplest interpretation is that the same mutation that makes an individual CBS deficient determines also whether he or she will be B_6 responsive. A single alteration of apoenzyme structure might well determine both properties.

Studies of CBS activities support the hypothesis that responsiveness or nonresponsiveness may be determined by the specific properties of the mutant enzyme molecule. There is a strong correlation between the presence of detected residual activity of CBS in liver extracts and clinical responsiveness to B_6 and between absence of any detected residual hepatic activity and nonresponsiveness.[6] As already mentioned, exceptions to this generalization have been found, particularly when considering CBS activity in cultured fibroblasts.

Quantitatively, the residual activities of CBS in extracts of fibroblasts cultured from B_6-responsive patients have varied from about 0.1 to 10 percent of mean control values.[9] When potentially B_6-responsive patients were receiving normal dietary intakes of B_6, their liver extracts, assayed in the presence of ample PLP, have usually had residual activities ranging from 1 to 9 percent of mean control values (in one case, 31 percent). When the same patients were receiving large dietary intakes of B_6, the CBS-specific activities in their liver extracts were enhanced 1.3- to 4.5-fold.[9]

Taken together, these results suggest that, in most patients, B_6 responsiveness is based on the presence of at least a small residual activity of mutant CBS, the steady-state amount of which is enhanced somewhat when a patient is taking large doses of B_6. CBS-deficient patients are unable to convert methionine sulfur to sulfate at a maximal rate even close to normal.[138] However, because there is normally a large excess of this capacity over the usual dietary intake of methionine of 8 to 12 mmol/day,[138] even a markedly diminished capacity may be very important in providing an ability to metabolize almost all the methionine in a normal diet by conversion ultimately to sulfate. Compounds metabolically proximal to the block at CBS account for only a minor portion of excretory sulfur. Thus, for untreated CBS-deficient patients on relatively normal diets, homocystine, homocysteine-cysteine mixed disulfide, AdoHcy, 5-amino-4-imidazole carboxamide-5′-*S*-homocysteinylribonucleoside, methionine, methionine sulfoxide, homolanthionine, and other minor abnormal compounds together may account (very approximately) for 2 to 3 mg-atom of daily urinary sulfur.[7] In patients with small, but detectable, residual activities of CBS, at least 2.5 to 4.0 mmol of methionine sulfur is converted to cysteine daily,[288] and this pathway would explain formation of an almost equivalent amount of sulfate. B_6-responsive CBS-deficient patients increase their maximal capacities to convert methionine sulfur to sulfate when given therapeutic doses of B_6.[289] These quantitative considerations are thus fully compatible with the suggestion that a modest increase in the residual CBS activity of a deficient patient might provide the increased capacity to metabolize methionine that drastically diminishes the accumulation of homocysteine and related metabolites and might thus account for the favorable metabolic response to vitamin treatment.[7,290,291] This formulation leaves unexplained the mechanism of response in those responsive patients for whom CBS activity has not been detected in cultured fibroblasts. Either these negative findings for fibroblasts do not accurately reflect the situation in the livers of such patients, or some mutant forms of the enzyme are extremely unstable in crude extracts.

The molecular properties of mutant CBSs crucial in conferring B_6 responsiveness remain obscure. Because heme incorporation into CBS may be a prerequisite for PLP binding, and the amount of PLP bound to the enzyme is limited by its heme saturation,[99] certain CBS mutations might interfere with binding of heme and thus indirectly affect the interaction of the enzyme with PLP. The mere presence of some residual CBS activity is not sufficient, as proven by the finding of clinically nonresponsive patients with readily detected residual activities. With enzymes from responsive patients, restoration of near-normal activity by high concentrations of PLP in vitro, such as would take place if the mutations affected only the K_m for this cofactor, has never occurred. Some of the largest observed enhancements of activity by addition of PLP in vitro have occurred with enzymes from clinically nonresponsive patients.[9] Lipson and coworkers[222] suggested that those patients whose cells contain a mutant synthase with a moderately reduced affinity for PLP (two- to fivefold) are able to increase cellular PLP content sufficiently after B_6 supplementation so that CBS activity rises above that critical value needed to prevent accumulation of homocysteine. B_6 nonresponsiveness, on the other hand, may be observed for one of two general reasons: either because the cell contains no residual CBS activity or because the cell contains a mutant CBS whose affinity for PLP is so reduced (20- to 70-fold) that, despite any feasible B_6 supplementation, the cell is unable to increase PLP content enough to stimulate appreciable formation of synthase holoenzyme. When cell extracts are prepared and these cellular barriers are obviated, much higher concentrations of PLP can be added, thereby creating the possibility that cells from a patient who does not respond in vivo may contain residual CBS activity markedly stimulated by addition of PLP.

Clinical and Pathologic Manifestations

Homocystinuria due to CBS deficiency is accompanied by an abundance and variety of clinical and pathologic abnormalities. Four organ systems show major involvement: the eye, and the skeletal, vascular, and central nervous systems. Other organs, including the liver, hair, and skin, may also be involved (Table 88-4). Data from an international survey of the natural history of CBS deficiency in more than 600 affected individuals indicated that the risk of developing a manifestation of the disease increases with age and that B_6-responsive patients usually are more mildly affected than B_6-nonresponsive patients. It should be noted that our present picture of the clinical features may be influenced by ascertainment bias, a possibility that has been discussed in detail elsewhere.[272] The following sections summarize the abnormalities in the major organ systems involved. For more details as to the clinical phenotypes and the pathologic findings, see the previous version of this chapter.[6]

Table 88-4 Clinical Abnormalities in Cystathionine β-Synthase (CBS) Deficiency

- I. Eye
  - A. Frequent
    1. Ectopia lentis
    2. Myopia
  - B. Less frequent
    1. Glaucoma
    2. Optic atrophy
    3. Retinal degeneration
    4. Retinal detachment
    5. Cataracts
    6. Corneal abnormalities
- II. Skeletal system
  - A. Frequent
    1. Osteoporosis
    2. Biconcave ("codfish") vertebrae
    3. Scoliosis
    4. Increased length of long bones
    5. Irregular, widened metaphyses
    6. Metaphyseal spicules
    7. Abnormal size and shape of epiphyses
    8. Growth arrest lines
    9. Pes cavus
    10. High-arched palate
  - B. Less frequent
    1. Arachnodactyly
    2. Enlarged carpal bones
    3. Abnormal bone age
    4. Pectus carinatum or excavatum
    5. Genu valgum
    6. Kyphosis
    7. Short fourth metacarpal
- III. Central nervous system
  - A. Frequent
    1. Mental retardation
    2. Psychiatric disturbances
  - B. Less frequent
    1. Seizures
    2. Abnormal EEG
    3. Extrapyramidal signs
- IV. Vascular system
  - A. Frequent
    1. Vascular occlusions
    2. Malar flush
    3. Livedo reticularis
- V. Other involvement
  - A. Fair, brittle skin
  - B. Thin skin
  - C. Fatty changes in liver
  - D. Inguinal hernia
  - E. Myopathy
  - F. Endocrine abnormalities
  - G. Reduced clotting factors

SOURCE: For citations to the original literature, see Mudd et al.[9]

Eye: Ectopia Lentis. Probably the most consistent finding in CBS deficiency is ectopia lentis (dislocation of the ocular lens). Fraying and disruption of the zonular fibers leads to loosening of the lens and, eventually, to dislocation. Iridodonesis (quivering of the iris) is a frequent sign that the lens has dislocated. Myopia appears as the lens loosens, allowing for passive spherical deformation (spherophakia). The myopia becomes marked when lenticular subluxation occurs.[292] Ectopia lentis has been noted as early as age 4 weeks in one patient.[9] However, time-to-event graphs for untreated patients showed a lag of approximately 2 years after birth before an appreciable frequency of dislocation was noted (Fig. 88-6). After this age, B_6-nonresponsive patients had a higher rate of dislocation than did B_6-responsive patients. Although the great majority of untreated patients eventually develop dislocated lenses, normal results on ophthalmologic

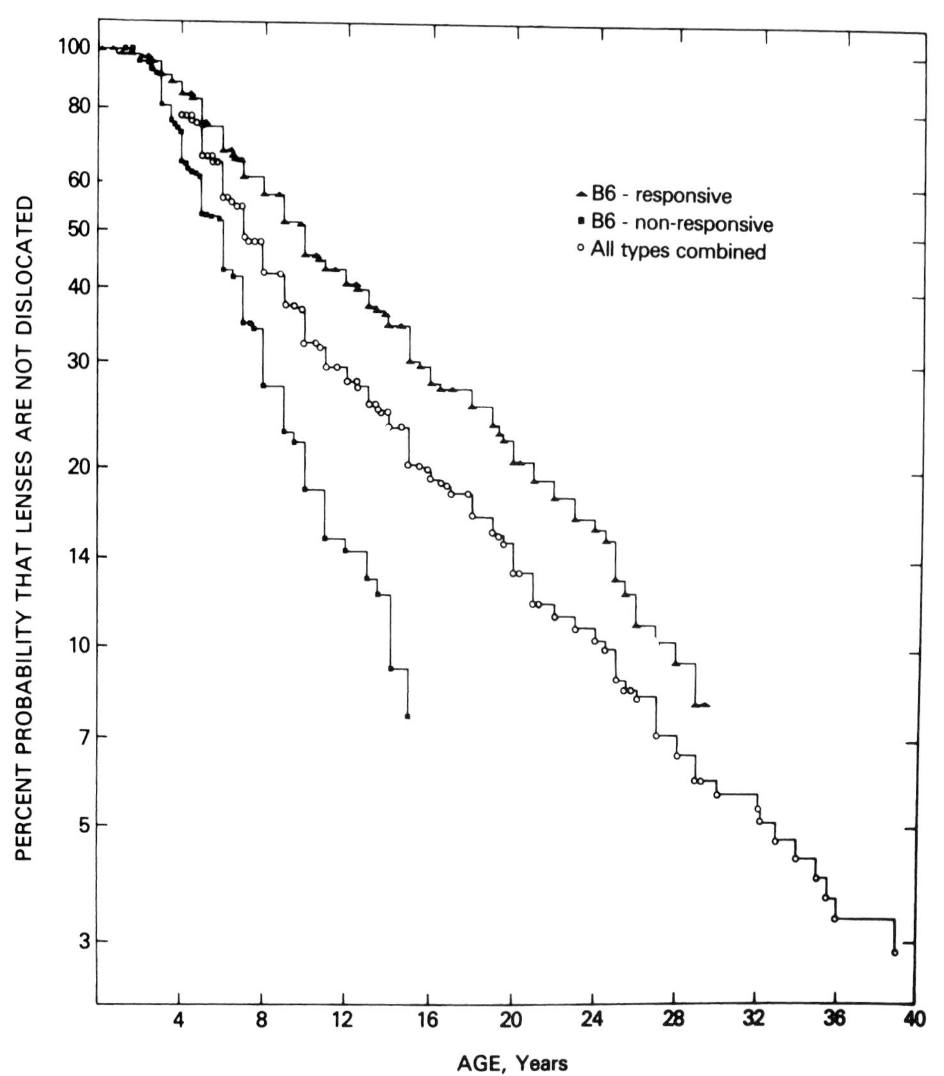

Fig. 88-6 Time-to-event graphs for lens dislocation in untreated patients. Patients were removed from the at-risk groups upon commencement of any therapy. (*From Mudd et al.*[272] *Used by permission.*)

examination at any age should not be a reason to reject the diagnosis of this disease.

A frequent complication of ectopia lentis is acute pupillary block glaucoma due to anterior dislocation of the lens. Other complications are listed in Table 88-4.

Skeletal System: Osteoporosis. This is the most consistent skeletal change. Osteoporosis is most common in the spine, followed by the long bones. A lateral radiograph of the lumbar spine may be the most efficient indicator of osteoporosis in CBS deficiency. Time-to-event graphs for radiologic evidence of spinal osteoporosis in untreated patients indicate that osteoporosis had been detected in at least 50 percent of patients by the end of the second decade of life, appearing earlier in B_6-nonresponsive patients than in patients responsive to B_6 (Fig. 88-7). Scoliosis is also frequent, perhaps as a consequence of spinal osteoporosis.

There are a large number of other skeletal abnormalities (Table 88-4). Notable among these is dolichostenomelia (thinning and lengthening of the long bones), which produces tall and thin individuals who are often considered to have a *marfanoid* appearance. Pectus carinatum, pes cavus, and genu valgum are also frequent.

Vascular System: Thromboembolism. A major cause of morbidity, and the most frequent cause of death, in CBS deficiency is thromboembolism. Vascular occlusion can occur in any vessel, including the portal vein,[293] and at any age, including infancy.[294] In an international survey,[272] 158 (of a total of 629) patients were reported to have had a total of 253 thromboembolic events. Among these events, 51 percent involved peripheral veins (of which about a quarter resulted in pulmonary embolism), 32 percent were cerebrovascular accidents, 11 percent affected peripheral arteries, 4 percent produced myocardial infarctions, and 2 percent fell into none of these categories. The occurrence of clinically apparent thromboembolism depends on age and pyridoxine responsiveness (Fig. 88-8). Untreated B_6-responsive patients seemed to be at little risk until the age of 12 years, with increasing risk thereafter, so that by age 20 years the cumulative risk for a thromboembolic event was about 25 percent. Untreated B_6-nonresponsive patients had a cumulative risk of 25 percent by age 15 years. Ultrasonographic detection has shown that many patients have signs of early vascular disease even in the absence of symptoms of ischemia.[295] Pregnancy and the postpartum state seem to increase the risk of thromboembolism (see the section "Maternal Cystathionine β-Synthase Deficiency," below). The postoperative state may also increase the risk of thromboembolism, although an international survey disclosed only 14 postoperative thromboembolic events among 241 major surgical procedures,[272] far fewer than earlier anecdotal reports had suggested.[9] These data indicate that, given proper attention,[296] the great majority of operations in patients with CBS deficiency may be conducted without vascular complications.

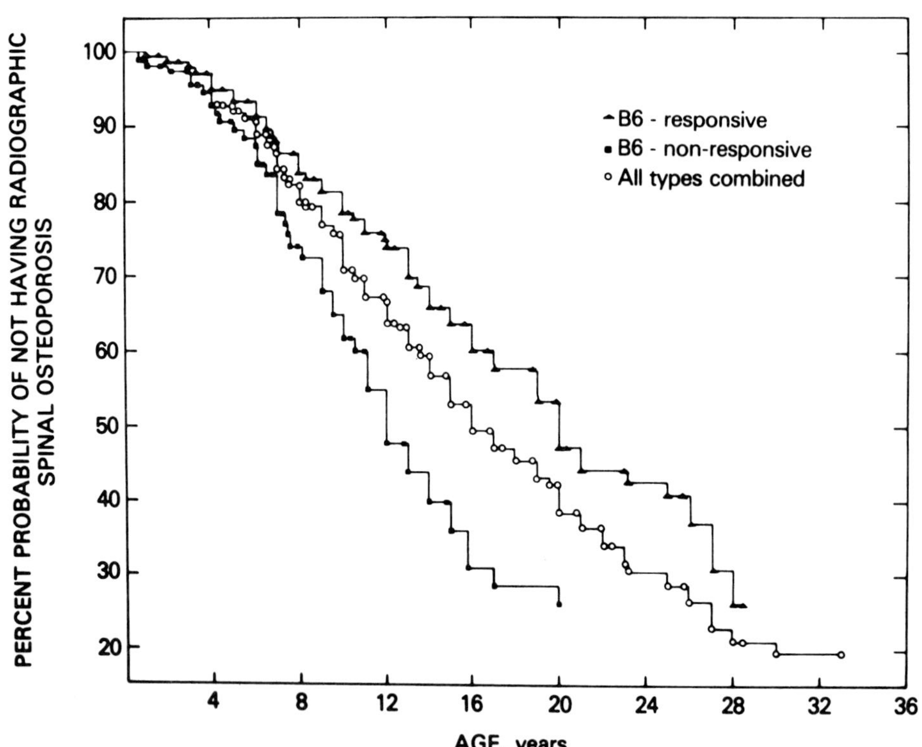

Fig. 88-7 Time-to-event graphs for radiologic spinal osteoporosis in untreated patients. (*From Mudd et al.*[272] *Used by permission.*)

Central Nervous System

Mental Retardation. The most frequent abnormality of the central nervous system is mental retardation, which is often the first recognized sign of CBS deficiency, presenting as developmental delay during the first or second year of life. Nevertheless, the cognitive capability of patients not treated from the newborn period varies widely. In an international survey, IQ scores ranged from 10 to 138 (Fig. 88-9), with the median of the cumulative frequency curves at approximately 64.[272] The distribution for B-responsive patients was shifted toward higher IQs (median, 78) than was found in B_6-nonresponsive patients (median, 56). The Italian Collaborative Study Group on Homocystinuria has also reported a significantly higher frequency of mental retardation among those nonresponsive to B_6.[227]

Neurologic Abnormalities. About 21 percent of patients with CBS deficiency not treated from early infancy have had seizures, most often grand mal type.[272] Other neurologic features have

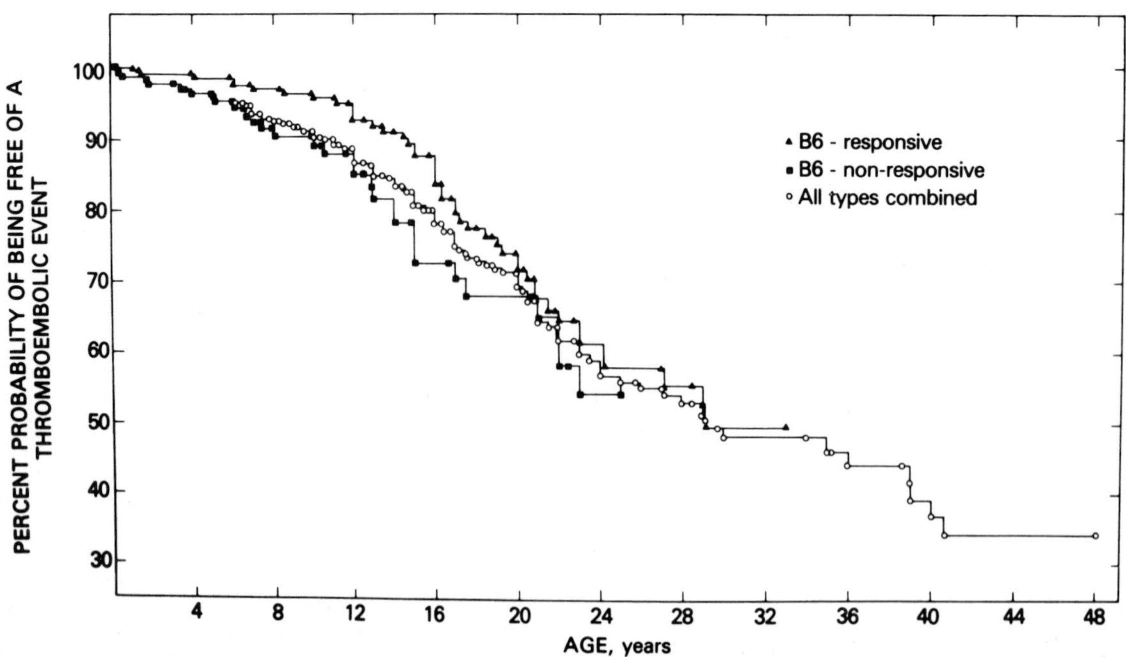

Fig. 88-8 Time-to-event graphs for initial clinically detected thromboembolic event in untreated patients. (*From Mudd et al.*[272] *Used by permission.*)

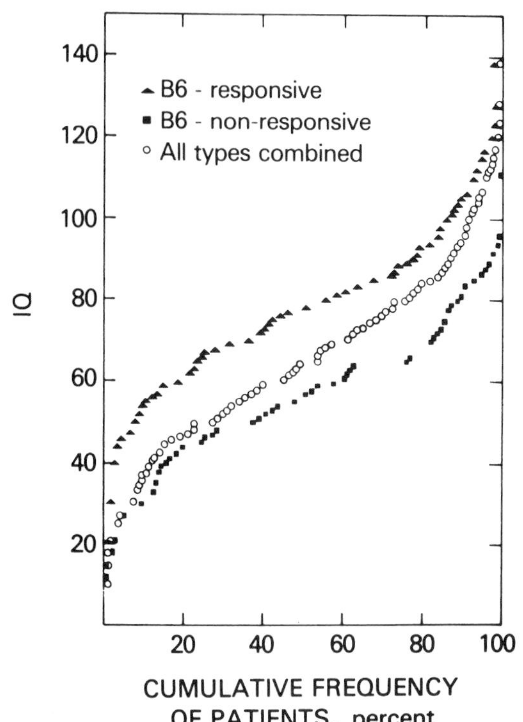

Fig. 88-9 Distribution of IQs among patients not detected by newborn screening (*From Mudd et al.*[272] *Used by permission.*)

included abnormal electroencephalograms and extrapyramidal disturbances (Table 88-4). Focal neurologic signs suggest the presence of a cerebrovascular occlusion.

Psychiatric Abnormalities. Mental illness has been reported frequently among individuals with CBS deficiency. In an investigation of 63 such patients, clinically significant psychiatric disorders were present in 51 percent.[297] Four diagnostic categories predominated: personality disorders (19 percent), disorders of behavior (17 percent), episodic depression (10 percent), and obsessive-compulsive disorder (5 percent). Although anecdotal reports have suggested that schizophrenia might be common among CBS-deficient patients, it may, in fact, be uncommon. Psychiatric problems may be more frequent among B_6-nonresponsive patients.[227]

Other Involvement. Abnormalities in other systems have been reported (Table 88-4). The Minnesota group called attention to, and examined the origin of, the hypopigmentation in CBS deficiency.[298] They studied two patients who had blond hair, unlike the darker hair of unaffected family members. Both patients were B_6 responsive and, when their plasma tHcy and free Hcy levels decreased with treatment, their hair darkened; the hair of one patient who discontinued treatment reverted again to blond.[299] The investigators found that tyrosinase activity in melanoma cells was decreased when the cells were grown in the presence of homocysteine, but that this effect could be reversed by the addition of copper to the growth media. They concluded that the hypopigmentation in CBS deficiency is due to reduced melanin production caused by the inhibition of tyrosinase when homocysteine chelates copper from this copper-containing enzyme.[298]

Spontaneous pneumothorax has also been described as a complication of CBS deficiency.[300]

Maternal Cystathionine *β*-Synthase Deficiency. Unlike maternal hyperphenylalaninemia where there is risk only to the fetus (teratogenicity) (see Chap. 77), pregnancy in CBS deficiency may well confer increased risk for maternal thromboembolism, especially post partum, but seems to have only very limited teratogenic potential.

Thromboembolic events have been reported previously in four pregnancies, all occurring post partum. These include multiple arterial occlusions,[301] ileofemoral thrombophlebitis,[302] extensive thromboses of the superior sagittal sinus and cortical veins resulting in death,[303] and a cavernous sinus thrombosis.[304] Two of the women were B_6 responsive,[301,304] one was B_6 nonresponsive,[302] and in one the response to pyridoxine was unknown.[303] We have encountered thrombophlebitis during the third trimester in a B_6-responsive woman who was untreated during her pregnancy.[305] Most pregnancies of women with CBS deficiency, however, have apparently proceeded without mishap. The 11 pregnancies known to Wildig et al[306] and Walter[307] were without vascular complications, and six of the seven pregnancies that we followed were also without such complications.[305] Maternal CBS deficiency might predispose pregnant women to preeclampsia, since plasma tHcy has been reported to be significantly increased in nulliparas with preeclampsia compared to nulliparas without preeclampsia (although not higher than the plasma tHcy concentrations in nonpregnant women).[308] Preeclampsia complicated one reported B_6-responsive maternal CBS-deficient pregnancy;[304] two of the pregnancies in our series, one in a B_6-nonresponsive woman and the other in a B_6-responsive woman;[305] and one of the nine pregnancies followed by Wildig et al[306] and Walter.[307] Again, however, most pregnancies in CBS deficiency have progressed without obstetric complications.

The available data on outcome of pregnancies in women with CBS deficiency are summarized in Table 88-5. For other citations to original literature, see Mudd et al.[9] Not included in this table are pregnancies ended by elective abortion.[272,304] Most of the conceptions have occurred in B_6-responsive women, and very few of the living offspring have had abnormalities recognized at birth or during infancy. The relatively few children from these pregnancies whose cases have been followed into childhood have also seemed to do well, with normal growth and development in most instances.[305,306] Among the 11 pregnancies in B_6-nonresponsive women known to us, eight have resulted in liveborn offspring. Six of these offspring, including one born prematurely, are normal, although only one was beyond early infancy when last reported.[306] Two, however, have had abnormalities: in one, now age 12 years, colobomas of the irides and choroid, intellectual delay, spina bifida and tethered spinal cord with fatty filum, and undescended testes that required surgical correction;[305,309] and, in the other, congenital heart disease due to transposition of the great vessels.[307] Thus, caution in predicting normal outcomes for pregnancies in B_6-nonresponsive women may be in order.

The data of Table 88-5 indicate that among B_6-responsive women the incidence of fetal loss (ectopic pregnancies, spontaneous abortions, and stillbirths combined) was 25 (44 percent) of 57 when the patient was untreated, and 9 (19 percent) of 48 when the patient was given B_6, suggesting this treatment may exert a beneficial effect on excessive fetal loss. That these results may not be representative of the expectations for most patients, however, is shown by the fact that the above data are strongly influenced by outcomes from three women who between them had 22 stillbirths or spontaneous abortions, and only two normal births.[272] Removal of the data for these apparently exceptional individuals would leave the great majority of B_6-responsive patients for whom the incidence of fetal loss was 5 (14 percent) of 37 in the absence of B_6 treatment and 7 (16 percent) of 44 during such therapy. These frequencies of fetal loss are within the range expected in the general population.[315] For most B_6-responsive patients, therefore, it seems there might not be increased fetal loss, even when untreated. This question, however, is as yet unsettled. Ectopic pregnancies and spontaneous abortions have also occurred in B_6-nonresponsive women (Table 88-5).

Table 88-5 Outcomes of Pregnancies in Cystathionine β-Synthase (CBS)-Deficient Women

	Therapy During Pregnancy				
	Pyridoxine-Responsive		Pyridoxine-Nonresponsive	Intermediate Response	Response Unknown
	None	Vitamin B_6	Folate	None	None
Full-term, normal child	28	37[a]	5[b]	5	11[c]
Child with abnormality	4[d]	1[e]	2[f]	—	—
Premature birth	—	1[g]	1[h]	1[i]	2[j]
Stillborn	5	2	—	—	2[k]
Spontaneous abortion	19	6	1[l]	3	1
Ectopic pregnancy	1	1	2[l]	—	—
Totals	57	48	11	9	16

[a]Includes one patient treated also with betaine.
[b]Includes one patient also treated with aspirin until one week before delivery and dipyridamole until 2 weeks before delivery; one patient who was poorly compliant on a methionine-restricted diet and also received aspirin from 18 weeks of gestation until delivery, but did not receive folate; and a third patient who did not receive therapy during any of three pregnancies (she was diagnosed following these pregnancies).
[c]Includes one patient who was not specified as either treated or not treated.
[d]One offspring with coloboma of iris but otherwise normal at age 4; one offspring with fused sagittal suture and mental retardation; one offspring with birth microcephaly; and one offspring with Beckwith-Wiedmann syndrome.
[e]One child with trisomy 21.
[f]Includes one patient treated also with betaine until 13 weeks of gestation and aspirin from 20 weeks of gestation. The offspring had congenital heart disease due to transposition of the great vessels. The offspring of the other pregnancy in question had colobomas of irides and choroid, undescended testes, psychomotor delay, seizures, and neural tube defect.
[g]Normal offspring delivered at 33 weeks.
[h]Patient treated also with betaine and vitamin B_6 from 12 weeks of gestation to delivery. A normal infant was born prematurely at 36 weeks of gestation.
[i]Died of hyaline membrane disease.
[j]Intrauterine growth retardation prompted cesarean sections at 31 weeks of gestation (the baby survived) and at 29 weeks (the baby died at 1 week of necrotizing enterocolitis secondary to umbilical artery thrombosis presumably initiated by an umbilical artery catheter).
[k]One offspring stillborn at 28 weeks and one hydrocephalic offspring, stillborn as a result of a decompression procedure done to enable delivery.
[l]Patients did not receive folate or any other therapy during any of these pregnancies.
SOURCES: References 298,299,304–307, and 309–314. For other citations to original literature, see Mudd et al.[9]

Paternal Cystathionine β-Synthase Deficiency. All but one of the 38 recognized conceptions involving CBS-deficient men resulted in apparently normal offspring.[9]

Pathophysiology

Perhaps no aspect of CBS deficiency has remained so obscure as the intermediate steps by which the enzyme deficiency leads to the specific clinical manifestations associated with it. As early as 4 years after the discovery of this disease, McKusick included it among the "heritable disorders of connective tissue."[316] This classification has been continued ever since, up through a recent international nosology in which homocystinuria was listed among the "heritable disorders of connective tissue secondary to metabolic defects."[317] The many recent advances in knowledge of the structure and biosynthesis of the components of connective tissue, and clinical and genetic aspects of their primary diseases, now make possible a reanalysis of CBS deficiency in the light of these advances. In the following sections, we discuss the pathophysiology of the four major clinical manifestations of CBS deficiency: dislocation of the optic lenses, osteoporosis and other abnormalities of bone, the thromboembolic diathesis, and mental retardation.

Dislocation of the Optic Lenses. Pathologic studies show that degenerative changes in the zonular fibers that hold the optic lens in place suspended from the ciliary body are the immediate cause of the ectopia lentis that is such a characteristic manifestation of CBS deficiency.[318] Studies in several laboratories revealed some time ago that these fibers are devoid of hydroxylysine and hydroxyproline and are resistant to collagenase. Thus, collagen is not one of their important components.[9] As shown initially by Raviola, and elaborated by Streeten and her colleagues, and others, zonular fibers are ultrastructurally similar to the elastin-associated microfibrils of widespread tissue distribution. Immunologic studies support the same conclusion. Biochemically, the total protein of zonular fibers is characterized by an exceptionally high content of half-cystine residues, from 38 to 83 per 1000 amino acid residues. Elastin itself is absent (for details on the foregoing, see citations in Mudd et al[6]). In 1986, Sakai and coworkers described a 350-kDa glycoprotein that they called *fibrillin*, and that they showed by immunologic studies is localized to ocular zonule and to elastin-associated and other non-elastin-associated microfibrils.[319] Both chemical and sequence analyses show that fibrillin is rich in cyst(e)ine residues (see Chap. 207). Disulfide bonds are important in maintaining the structural integrity of fibrillin multimers in tissue.[320] A variety of evidence now indicates that genetic defects in the fibrillin gene on chromosome 15[321] account for most cases of Marfan syndrome (see Chap. 207). Together, these findings suggest that a possible explanation for dislocation of the optic lenses in CBS deficiency is disruption or abnormality of fibrillin structure, as is likewise the cause of the frequent occurrence of lens dislocation in Marfan syndrome.

A mechanism for such disruption was suggested by Irreverre et al as long ago as 1967.[322] These workers found dislocated optic lenses in the first patient identified with sulfite oxidase deficiency, and this has turned out to be a frequent complication when the activity of this enzyme is deficient (see Chap. 128). They pointed out that, in both CBS- and sulfite oxidase-deficient patients, protein disulfide bridges may be broken, in the first instance by homocysteine-dependent disulfide exchange

$$\text{HSHcy} + \text{PrCyS-SCyPr} \rightarrow \text{PrCyS-SHcy} + \text{HSCyPr}$$

and, in the second instance, by the closely analogous reaction of sulfite-dependent sulfitolysis

$$H_2SO_3 + \text{PrCyS-SCyPr} \rightarrow \text{PrCyS-}SO_3H + \text{HSCyPr}$$

Fibrillin, being rich in disulfide bonds, is a reasonable participant in such reactions and is known to be solubilized by sulfhydryl reagents.[320] Chemical analyses of zonular material from CBS-deficient patients have not been reported, so direct evidence bearing upon this hypothesis is lacking. The hypothesis has the advantage that it accounts on a unified basis, namely, defects of fibrillin, for the lens dislocation in three genetic diseases in which this feature is common.

With respect to the lens, CBS deficiency differs from Marfan syndrome in several respects. In CBS deficiency, dislocation occurs relatively late (Fig. 88-6), is progressive, occurs in an inferior or inferonasal direction, and many or most zonular fibers ultimately break completely. In Marfan syndrome, dislocation occurs relatively early (in 62 children studied prospectively, the mean age of dislocation was 2.7 years, with a range of 2 months to 6 years), progresses slowly, if at all, occurs in a superotemporal direction, and, as a rule, the zonular fibers are stretched rather than broken.[6] These differences suggest that in Marfan syndrome the extent of the abnormality of fibrillin may be largely fixed at the time of initial formation of the fibrils, whereas in CBS deficiency fibrillin is normal at the time of formation, but, as time passes in the presence of an ongoing chemical insult it slowly weakens and ultimately ruptures, with the lens dislocating downward due to gravity.

Zonular fibers contain proteins other than fibrillin. Thus, hypotheses alternative to the one just presented are possible, involving either disruption of disulfide bridges if such bonds play an important role in the structure of these proteins or in their assembly into microfibrils; or inhibition of lysyl oxidase (see the section "Osteoporosis and Other Abnormalities of Bone," below) if covalent *crosslinking* dependent on the action of this enzyme is important in microfibrillar structure.[6]

Osteoporosis and Other Abnormalities of Bone. Osteoporosis, kyphoscoliosis, pigeon breast, genu valgum, and excessively long extremities with a decreased upper segment/lower segment ratio were among the bony abnormalities that led McKusick to classify CBS deficiency as a disease of connective tissue.[323] Scoliosis, anterior chest deformities, and disproportionately long legs are features of Marfan syndrome,[324] and perhaps these abnormalities may result from damage to fibrillin in both Marfan syndrome and CBS deficiency.

An alternative possibility for CBS deficiency, namely, defective crosslinking of collagen, was first suggested by Harris and Sjoerdsma,[325] and has attracted a great deal of experimental attention. Many collagen molecules are composed of three polypeptide chains bound together by intermolecular crosslinks (see Chap. 206). An essential step in crosslinking is the lysyl oxidase-catalyzed formation of aldehydic groups by oxidation of terminal amino groups of lysyl or hydroxylysyl residues in collagen monomers. These aldehydes form crosslinks both by Schiff-base formation with amino groups of lysine or hydroxylysine on other chains and by aldol condensation between two aldehydes. These crosslinks undergo further *maturation* reactions, producing crosslinks embodied within the primary structure of collagen fibrils. Prominent among these crosslinks are two forms of 3-hydroxypyridinium derivatives: hydroxylysylpyridinoline, incorporating three residues of hydroxylysine; and lysylpyridinoline, incorporating two residues of hydroxylysine and one of lysine (see the review by Eyre et al[326]). Increased solubility of dermal collagen, suggestive of poor crosslinking, occurred in patients[327] and in experimental rats[328] treated with penicillamine, a compound that, like homocysteine, has neighboring free sulfhydryl and amino groups. The mechanism was thought to be the formation of a thiazolidine-type complex between aldehydic groups and penicillamine, with consequent interference with crosslinking.[329] Similar complexing occurs between aldehydic groups and homocysteine, in that case forming a thiazine ring.[330] Increased solubility of dermal collagen was demonstrated in four of six CBS-deficient patients investigated,[325,331] and decreased amounts of the aldehyde, ε-hydroxynorleucine, and aldehyde-derived crosslink compounds in each of the three studied.[331] In vitro, homocysteine was shown to interfere with the formation of collagen crosslinks, prevent insolubilization of fibrils, inhibit lysyl oxidase, and, perhaps, to delay the synthesis of more complex collagen mature crosslinks.[6] In view of the recent evidence that excess formation of homocysteine thiolactone may occur in CBS deficiency,[139,140] of special interest is the finding that this thiolactone irreversibly inhibits lysyl oxidase by derivatizing and reducing the active-site carbonyl cofactor of this enzyme.[331a] Direct evidence bearing on the McKusick hypothesis of deficient collagen crosslinking in patients with CBS deficiency has been reported by Lubec and coworkers.[332] In ten patients with elevated tHcy (nine with CBS deficiency and one with the thermolabile form of methylenetetrahydrofolate reductase), measurements were made of plasma levels of carboxy-terminal propeptide of type-I procollagen, *N*-terminal propeptide of procollagen type III, and serum carboxy-terminal telopeptide of collagen type I. The first two are indicators of the rate of synthesis of collagen types I and III, respectively, and were normal in the patients. The third is an indicator of collagen type-I crosslinkage, and was significantly decreased in the patients: patient mean, 1.14 μg/liter (SD 0.24); control mean, 3.29 μg/liter (SD 0.32). These results were interpreted as indicating that the bone manifestations of homocystinuria are not due to a deficit in collagen synthesis, but rather perhaps suggest a reduction in collagen crosslinking.[332]

Alternative hypotheses of possible disruption of disulfide crosslinking of collagens that might help explain the kyphoscoliosis and deformities of the sternum and long bones seen in patients with CBS deficiency have been discussed elsewhere.[6] Because collagen type I does not contain significant cysteine residues required for disulfide crosslinking, such hypotheses would appear not to apply to collagen type I.[332] A second candidate may be collagen type VI, a compound that is a constituent of bone, albeit a quantitatively minor one, at present of uncertain function.[333] Structurally, collagen type VI is a nonfibrillar heterotrimer assembled in tetramers that in turn form linear aggregates described as beaded filaments. These complex assemblies are stabilized by disulfide bonds, not by lysine-derived crosslinks like most other collagens (see Chap. 206).

Thrombosis and Atherosclerosis. Thromboembolism is a major feature of CBS deficiency (see the section "Clinical and Pathologic Manifestations," above). This complication is related to changes in vascular walls[6] and, very likely, to a clotting diathesis.[334,335] Thromboembolism is not a prominent manifestation in Marfan syndrome[324] (see also Chap. 207), osteogenesis imperfecta, or other primary disorders of collagen biosynthesis and structure (see also Chaps. 134 and 206). Apparently, events of this kind are chiefly attributable to abnormalities of neither fibrillin nor collagen. As initially observed by McCully[336,337] and subsequently confirmed by others,[338,339] children dying of defects in homocysteine methylation that produce elevations of plasma Hcy, but not hypermethioninemia, have often had vascular pathology similar in many important respects to the abnormalities of arteries and perivascular connective tissue found in patients with CBS deficiency. Cardiovascular lesions resembling those seen in atherosclerosis were found in sheep following a 34-week period of induced cobalt-vitamin-B_{12} deficiency.[340] These findings suggest that Hcy, or its derivatives other than methionine, may be the principal contributor(s) to the vascular damage of CBS deficiency.[9]

Many investigations have been conducted to define the cause(s) of the abnormal clotting and atherosclerotic tendencies of CBS-deficient patients, but no coherent, generally accepted view has emerged. Presently, evidence exists suggesting that effects on platelets, endothelium, nonendothelial vascular cells, coagulation disorders, or possibly even damage to lipoprotein(a) or other lipoproteins may contribute. These lines of evidence are reviewed in turn below.

Platelets. In early studies, McDonald et al reported increased adhesiveness of the platelets from a majority of hyperhomocystinemic patients.[340a] However, these results were not reproduced when other methods of measuring adhesiveness were used,[6] and, more recently Stamler et al reported data demonstrating that homocysteine does not cause platelet aggregation directly. These authors concluded that their data "provide no evidence that the thrombotic tendencies associated with elevated plasma tHcy derive from a direct effect of homocysteine or its oxidized derivatives on platelets.[341] Likewise, Ammar et al found no evidence that homocysteine stimulated platelet activation as measured by expression of a specific marker for such activation: P-selectin.[342]

In 1982, Graeber and coworkers showed that homocystine (1 mM) or DL-homocysteine (1 mM), added in vitro, altered arachidonic acid metabolism of normal platelets so that two cyclogenase products — 12-hydroxy-5,8,10-heptadecatrienoic acid and the proaggregatory thromboxane A_2 (measured as its stable end product, thromboxane B_2) — increased significantly from control levels. Methionine, cysteine, or cystine did not have similar effects. These workers suggested that changes in arachidonic acid metabolism might contribute to the thrombotic diathesis of patients with CBS deficiency.[343] Both Strisciuglio et al[343a] and Coppola et al[344] observed abnormally high urinary excretion of thromboxane in CBS-deficient patients, but the latter authors suggested the abnormality was due to something other than high biosynthesis by the platelets.

Other abnormalities of platelets, such as those affecting their interactions with ADP, or ADP-induced aggregation, have been found in occasional patients but have been absent in larger numbers of additional patients.[9] Reported morphologic abnormalities detected by electron microscopy of platelets from CBS-deficient patients[345,346] were not confirmed.[347]

Endothelial Cellular Effects. Studies of both intact organisms (human patients and various animals) and of in vitro endothelial cellular preparations have suggested effects of homocysteine on endothelium. Possible desquamation of endothelial cells in CBS-deficient patients and in experimental animals following intravenous injections of homocystine, chronic infusion of DL-homocysteine, or homocysteine thiolactone, and the appearance of occasional microscopic foci of intimal degeneration and mural thickening in renal arterioles of two pigs maintained on B_6-deficient diets that produced severe elevations of tHcy have been discussed previously.[6] Evidence has been presented that endothelial cellular damage may result from exposure to homocysteine,[348] especially in the presence of copper,[349] and that this damage may be mediated by production of hydrogen peroxide.[6] Thrombomodulin and von Willebrand factor, markers of endothelial damage, were reported to be elevated in two sibs with CBS deficiency but to normalize with treatment.[350] Dudman et al incubated human arterial endothelial cells for 24 h in medium containing 16% fetal calf serum[351] and various concentrations of homocysteine. At 3.8 ± 1.7 mM homocysteine, 50 percent cellular detachment was observed. Since homocysteine was more effective than equimolar cysteine, but was autoxidized substantially more slowly than cysteine, it was concluded that the rate-limiting step in induction of cellular detachment in this medium was not hydrogen peroxide production. These authors advanced several reasons to question the endothelial cell detachment model as a valid explanation of the early atherosclerosis in patients with homocystinuria, among them the facts that homocysteine at concentrations found in the plasma of homocystinuric patients did not cause discernible endothelial desquamation, that evidence of endothelial desquamation has been absent from reports of postmortem pathology in homocystinuric patients, and that the rate of desquamation observed in vitro was less than the proportion of endothelial cells turned over daily in some regions of normal rat aorta.[352]

In recent reviews Lentz[353,354] mentions a variety of effects of homocysteine on cultured endothelial cells in vitro. All required relatively high concentrations of homocysteine, ranging from 50 to 5000 μM. Among these effects, the following showed some specificity for homocysteine and were not produced to the same extent by cysteine or (where tested) by homocystine or methionine: (1) activation of coagulation factor V,[355] (2) impaired activation of protein C,[356–358] (3) induction of tissue factor activity,[359] (4) impaired binding of tissue plasminogen activator,[360,361,361a] (5) decreased activity of glutathione peroxidase,[362] and (6) inhibition of growth and p21^{ras} methylation.[363] (7) Additional, similarly specific effects reported by Upchurch et al include the stimulation of endothelial nitric oxide production by homocysteine in the presence of bradykinin[364] and induction of a family of acute translational response genes through a protein synthesis-dependent transcriptional mechanism. The latter was said to occur at a homocysteine concentration as low as 5 μM.[364a] For the other effects listed, no such specificity for homocysteine was demonstrated: (8) altered secretion of von Willebrand factor,[365] (9) impaired synthesis of heparin sulfate,[366] (10) decreased availability of nitric oxide,[341,362] (11) decreased production of prostacyclin[367] (see also citations in Mudd et al[6] regarding prostacyclin production), and (12) induction of stress-response genes.[368]

Difficulties pertain to these in vitro studies of homocysteine-dependent effects on endothelial cells for two major reasons: First, because plasma tCys normally exceeds plasma tHcy by more than 20-fold,[196] it is especially important to demonstrate specificity for homocysteine and its derivatives over cysteine and its derivatives. Further, Strydom has advanced mechanistic reasons why formation of a disulfide bond with homocysteine may be more disruptive than formation of a similar bond with cysteine.[369] For these reasons, the relevance of the studies in which no specificity for homocysteine as compared to cysteine has been demonstrated may be especially questioned. Second, significant changes have usually been observed following treatment for relatively short periods with concentrations of homocysteine far higher than occur in CBS-deficient patients. At present, it is not possible to predict from such studies the effects of exposures to lower concentrations maintained for much longer periods.

The evidence implicating increased activation of factor V and impaired activation of protein C merits special interest because factor V in its activated form, Va, interacts with factor Xa to accelerate conversion of prothrombin to thrombin and thus promote coagulation.[370,371] Moreover, factor Va is inactivated by activated protein C, itself formed from protein C on the surface of endothelial cells by the action of thrombin, the conformation of which has been modified through combination with calcium and the endothelial surface glycoprotein, thrombomodulin. This protein C-dependent regulation is thought to play an important role in normal anticoagulation.[372] A mutation in factor V, factor V Leiden, replaces glutamine with arginine at position 506, a site of proteolytic cleavage normally attacked by activated protein C, thus rendering activated factor V Leiden resistant to activated protein C. This mutation attains carrier rates as high as 15 percent among some European populations[373] and is a major risk factor for venous thrombosis.[374] Mandel et al studied several patients with severe elevations of plasma tHcy due to CBS deficiency or other genetic conditions who, in addition, were homozygous or heterozygous for factor V Leiden. These patients were shown to be at greatly increased risk for early thrombotic disease.[375] Ridker et al, in a study of venous thromboembolism not related to surgery, trauma, or cancer, found the relative risk associated with mild elevation of plasma tHcy (above 17.25 μM) to be 2.43, that associated with heterozygosity for factor V Leiden to be 2.87, and that associated with both together to be 21.8 ($P = 0.0004$).[376] Cattaneo et al found that, among 77 patients with deep-vein thrombosis, there was overrepresentation of coexisting factor V Leiden mutations and homozygosity for the 677C → T mutation in methylenetetrahydrofolate reductase that leads to thermolability and mild elevations of plasma tHcy. They concluded that homozygosity for the 677C → T increases the risk associated with factor V Leiden.[377] Although heterozygosity for factor V Leiden is clearly not a prerequisite for the occurrence of thromboembolism in either CBS deficiency[378,379,] (see also ref 468a) or in the presence of milder elevations of plasma tHcy,[378] and even though an interaction between factor V Leiden and elevated plasma tHcy in causing venous thrombosis has not been found in some studies,[380,381] a deleterious interaction might be envisioned if indeed homocysteine accelerates activation of factor V and retards activation of protein C. Protein C antigen was moderately low in plasma of two of three CBS-deficient patients,[382] but activated protein C was not low in patients with mild elevations of plasma tHcy and at least one episode of deep-vein thrombosis.[383] Lentz et al observed that monkeys with plasma tHcy raised from a mean normal of 4.0 ± 0.2 μM to 10.6 ± 2.6 after being fed a diet enriched in methionine, depleted in folate, and free of choline had impaired endothelium-dependent activation of protein C.[384]

Attempts have been made to assess endothelial dysfunction as assessed by impaired endothelium-dependent vasodilatation in intact humans with either severe[385] or mild elevations of plasma tHcy of either natural occurrence[386–388] or following acute[388,389–391] or chronic methionine loading.[391] Such dysfunction was detected in most of the studies,[385–390] but not in one.[391] Similar dysfunction was observed by Lentz et al in their studies of monkeys on the modified diets described in the preceding paragraph.[384]

An early study by De Groot et al[392] raised the question of whether endothelial cells from persons with CBS deficiency are abnormally susceptible to Hcy-induced injury. These workers found that, when endothelial cells from an obligate heterozygote for CBS deficiency were cultured in the presence of 10 mM homocystine, the viability and function of these cells were affected more markedly than were those of cells from a normal subject. However, subsequent studies have shown that endothelial cells from a homozygous CBS-deficient patient were normal with regard to homocysteine export and endothelial function as measured by a number of markers.[393] Indeed, there is controversy as to whether normal human endothelial cells have CBS activity.[394–396] If not, there is no obvious reason why CBS deficiency should affect the sensitivity of endothelial cells to Hcy damage.

Effects on Nonendothelial Vascular Cells. Homocysteine has been found to promote DNA synthesis in,[397] and growth of,[398,399] vascular smooth muscle cells. Induction of cyclin A gene expression, increased cyclin A protein[400] and increased cyclin-dependent kinase,[400,401,401a] and enhancement of the mitogenic response to platelet-derived growth factor, presumably by disturbing the activity of antioxidant enzymes,[399] have been mentioned as possible mediators of this effect. Additional effects of homocysteine on arterial smooth muscle cells include stimulation of collagen synthesis,[402] induction of the synthesis of a serine elastase that breaks down elastin,[403] production of phospholipids, activation of protein kinase C, induction of c-fos and c-myb,[404] and increased nitric oxide production by NF-*kB*-dependent transcriptional activation of *Nos2*, the inducible form of nitric oxide synthase.[405] Higher concentrations of homocysteine were used in most of these studies than are likely to occur even in patients with severe elevations of tHcy, and, with the exception of the effect on cyclin-dependent kinase,[401] specificity for homocysteine over cysteine was not demonstrated. Brown and coworkers[405a] postulated that some of the aforementioned sequence of signal transduction effects could be downstream of a receptor activated by homocysteine and found that, indeed, homocysteine activated a kinase for mitogen-activated protein (MAP-kinase), a point of convergence for proliferative signaling. An exceptionally low concentration of 0.5 μM brought about 50 percent of the maximal effect. Homoserine was almost as potent as homocysteine, suggesting an -SH group is not needed for this effect, and the effect was blocked by MP-801, an NMDA (*N*-methyl-D-aspartate) receptor blocker. Especially intriguing is a recent study by Tyagi[405b] that demonstrated that homocystine (half-maximal effect at 5 μM), but not homocysteine or cysteine at comparable or higher concentrations, stimulated proliferation and collagen synthesis of cultured human vascular smooth muscle cells. At least some of these effects on vascular smooth muscle cells appear to provide plausible means by which homocysteine and/or homocystine might promote atherosclerotic and other vascular wall changes.

Hosoki et al showed that hydrogen sulfide is produced in ileum, portal vein, and thoracic aorta, in part by the action of CBS upon cysteine. Hydrogen sulfide caused relaxation of smooth muscle in these areas and, in lower concentrations, strongly enhanced the relaxing effect of nitric oxide on thoracic aorta. Cysteine or glutathione had neither of these relaxing effects.[406] These findings raise the possibility that diminished ability to form hydrogen sulfide might contribute to functional vascular abnormalities in CBS deficiency.

Coagulation Disorders. Low antithrombin activity (51 to 74 percent of mean control) has been reported in some, but not all, homocystinuric patients.[6] Decreased antithrombin activity has not been clearly associated with elevated plasma tHcy, since antithrombin activity has both remained low in the face of a dietary-induced decrease in plasma and urine homocystine, and returned to normal during pyridoxine administration, which did not decrease homocystinemia.[9] In patients treated with methotrexate, there was no decrease in plasma antithrombin III in those who developed the most markedly elevated plasma tHcy.[407] Since studies of many families with inherited deficiencies of antithrombin III have shown that decreases in this factor to 40 to 50 percent of normal are associated with severe tendencies to thrombosis,[9] the moderate decreases reported in at least some CBS-deficient patients could be clinically significant.

A single early report described a clotting abnormality due to activation of the Hageman factor (factor XII) by homocystine.[408] This finding has not been reported in other patients.[8] Homocystine-related decreases in proconvertin (factor VII) to 20 to 45 percent of normal have been reported in several CBS-deficient patients.[9,382] Activation of factor VII by tissue thromboplastin is thought to initiate the extrinsic coagulation pathway.[409] Although deficiency of this factor is not contradictory to the occurrence of thromboembolism,[409,410] no mechanism has been suggested whereby such a deficiency might contribute in a positive way to a clotting diathesis.

Lipoprotein(a). Lipoprotein(a) refers to a family of plasma lipoprotein particles, elevated concentrations of which are correlated with an increased risk of cardiovascular disease. Their structure includes a disulfide bridge between apolipoprotein(a) [apo(a)] and apo B-100, as well as 14 to 38 kringles (triple-looped, disulfide crosslinked domains), the number of the latter being determined by a series of allelic structural genes for apo(a).[411] Harpel and coworkers found that lipoprotein(a) binds to immobilized fibrin and fibrinogen, that the affinity of this binding is enhanced 3.7-fold by plasmin treatment of the fibrinogen,[412] and that addition of 2 mM homocysteine results in a further threefold increase.[413] It was suggested this binding may potentiate incorporation of lipoprotein(a) into the vessel wall, thereby providing a mechanism to explain the association between thrombosis, coronary atherosclerosis, and increased blood concentrations of lipoprotein(a) and, further, that homocysteine may play a role in this process. Because of its high content of structurally important disulfide bonds, lipoprotein(a) may well be sensitive to disruption by sulfhydryl compounds. Glutathione could replace homocysteine in bringing about the effect in question. Cysteine was not tried.[413] Thus, at present, there is no evidence of specificity for homocysteine in this sequence.

Other Lipoproteins. Another possible role for sulfur-containing amino acids in atherogenesis was suggested by Heinecke et al,[414] who found that cultured monkey arterial smooth muscle cells bring about a cystine-dependent modification of low-density lipoprotein (LDL) such that the modified material was taken up and degraded less well by cells utilizing the receptor for native LDL, but better by cells utilizing the scavenger receptor. Modification of LDL so that it is better taken up by macrophages via the scavenger pathway may well enhance the atherogenicity of this substance.[6] However, cystine was much more effective than homocystine in causing production of the superoxide thought to mediate the modification of LDL in question.[415] Furthermore, any proposal that lipid uptake into vessel walls plays an important role in the atherosclerotic abnormalities associated with CBS deficiency must contend with the observation by McCully that there is a lack of lipid in these lesions that "indicates a dissociation of intimal injury and abnormal connective tissue synthesis from filtration and binding of lipids in these rapidly progressive examples of arteriosclerosis."[416]

Vascular Changes Seen in Experimental Animals on High-Methionine Diets. Minipigs with elevated tHcy due to being fed a high-methionine diet manifested hypertension and extended reactive hyperemia with arteries that had expanded volumetric compliance, curtailed stiffness, and prevalence of the viscous wall component. In vessel walls, there was splitting and fragmentation of elastic lamina and smooth muscle hypertrophy, hyperplasia, and migration, with insignificant lipid deposition within the lesions. These changes mimic those observed in patients with severe elevations of plasma tHcy.[417] Rats on high-methionine diets developed thickening of the intima and media of the aorta due to smooth muscle cell hypertrophy,[418] considerable loss of aortic endothelium and degeneration, with dissolution of cells of the media,[419] potentiated platelet aggregation in response to ADP, and thrombin-induced thromboxane synthesis.[420]

Possible Mechanisms of Damage due to Homocystinuria. Among the mechanisms whereby homocysteine might bring about its thromboembolic-promoting effects, two are receiving increasing experimental attention:[354]

1. *Oxidant stress.* Under certain conditions, oxidation of homocysteine may generate reactive species of oxygen, for example, superoxide anion, hydrogen peroxide, or hydroxyl radical,[415,421,422] and it has repeatedly been suggested that these species may lead to endothelial cellular damage, lipid peroxidation, inhibition of nitric oxide-related cerebrovascular responses[423] and perhaps other harmful effects.[6,415,422,424,425] Pigs with elevated plasma tHcy due to intermittent exposure to nitrous oxide had increased malondialdehyde, a major secondary product of oxidation of polyunsaturated fatty acids, as well as decreased linoleic and linolenic acids.[426] Similarly, rabbits fed methionine-enriched diets had elevations of thiobarbituric acid-reactive substances (TBARS), a less specific indicator of malondialdehyde.[427] However, studies of patients with CBS deficiency with severely elevated plasma tHcy[428,429] or plasma free Hcy[430] have found no evidence of elevations in high-density lipoprotein (HDL) cholesteryl ester hydroperoxides (the major form of plasma lipid peroxides),[430] of the extent of oxidation of LDL (as measured by total diene production),[428] of TBARS,[428,429] or of the extent of oxidation of either LDL or HDL.[429] In one study, however, increased plasma TBARS were detected in human volunteers after methionine loads.[431] The total concentration of tHcy plus tCys in the CBS-deficient patients studied by Córdoba-Porras et al[429] was slightly lower than in controls due to the decrease in tCys. These authors suggested that this lowering may contribute to the normal findings in CBS-deficient patients with regard to lipid peroxidation.[429]

2. *Inhibition of transmethylation reactions.* Whenever intracellular homocysteine is abnormally elevated, elevation of AdoHcy may be expected to occur because the equilibrium of AdoHcy hydrolase favors formation of the latter thioether. This rise in AdoHcy will tend to inhibit a variety of methyltransferases. As mentioned earlier, when the ratio of AdoMet to AdoHcy falls from the normal value of 4.9 to 6.5:1 to 4:1, a variety of methyltransferases will likely be inhibited by 10 to 60 percent.[36,52] A direct demonstration of such inhibition was reported by Wang et al,[363] who found that incubation of endothelial cells with 10 to 50 μM homocysteine (but not cysteine) inhibited DNA synthesis and caused growth arrest in the G_1 phase. Decreased carboxyl methylation was observed of $p21^{ras}$, a G_1 regulator, the activity of which is regulated in part by methylation. The extent to which other methyltransferases are inhibited when homocysteine accumulates remains, in most instances, to be defined.

Summary. Despite many studies, no single mechanism has been definitively shown to lead to the atherosclerotic/thrombotic diathesis present in the several diseases that are associated with elevated plasma tHcy. At present, various lines of evidence suggest effects on platelets, endothelial cells, nonendothelial vascular cells, soluble factors, and possibly even lipoprotein(a) or other lipoproteins. None of these abnormalities can be regarded as unequivocally established, nor are they mutually exclusive. More than one may certainly make some contribution.

Excellent long-term outcomes are now being reported for treated CBS-deficient patients (see the section "Management and Outcomes," below). Nevertheless, these patients continue to have elevations of plasma tHcy far greater than the increase of, for example, 5 μM above the normal mean near 10 μM estimated in a recent meta-analysis to increase the odds ratio for arteriosclerotic vascular disease by 1.6-fold. Such an increase in risk is about the same as that conferred by an increase of 0.5 mM of total cholesterol.[432] The excellent outcomes in CBS-deficient patients still carrying more severe elevations of plasma tHcy indicate that these elevations may be withstood for considerable periods without thromboembolic events necessarily occurring. One may speculate that perhaps confounding variables protect such patients.[433] For example, one might consider the possibilities that methionine, a structural analogue, may compete with homocysteine at the site(s) at which the latter causes damage,[433] that the elevation of methionine in the presence of intact MAT I/III activity will lead to elevated AdoMet and thus to restoration of the AdoMet/AdoHcy ratio to less inhibitory levels, and/or, as already mentioned, that the decrease in tCys that accompanies CBS deficiency is protective by mitigating the rise in total intracellular and/or plasma sulfhydryl concentrations that would otherwise occur. In remethylation defects, on the other hand, methionine tends to be low, or low normal, and neither cystathionine nor cysteine and its derivatives are low, so that any postulated protection by high methionine, elevated AdoMet, and/or low tCys would not be expected.

Neurologic Abnormalities and Mental Retardation. The absence of mental retardation, convulsions, or other consistent neurologic difficulties in patients with Marfan syndrome[324] (see Chap. 207), or primary disorders of collagen biosynthesis and structure (Chap. 206) suggest that the central nervous system abnormalities of patients with CBS deficiency are not attributable to defects of either fibrillin or collagen. An alternative possibility—that a chemical abnormality of the central nervous system might contribute to the neurologic difficulties and mental retardation of such individuals — has been raised with respect to several compounds, as discussed next.

Cystathionine. This thioether acid is present in higher concentrations in normal human brain (possibly in neurons) than in either brains of other species or other human tissues. Investigations of a possible neurotransmitter role for cystathionine have been inconclusive. The three autopsy brain specimens examined from CBS-deficient patients were grossly deficient in cystathionine, although the possibility remains that CBS-deficient patients with some residual activity of this enzyme may accumulate significant amounts of cystathionine in brain. A reasonably convincing indication that cystathionine is not needed for physiological brain function would be provided by identification of individuals lacking any residual CBS activity, yet of normal intelligence. Several well-documented descriptions of B_6-nonresponsive patients with normal IQ values are strong evidence in this regard.[9]

Hcy and Methionine. Very high intraperitoneal doses of DL-homocysteine induce tonic-clonic grand mal seizures. Homocysteine thiolactone, applied locally, produced excitation of neurons and, injected intraperitoneally, induced generalized convulsive status epilepticus in rats with motor cortex cobalt lesions. Methionine enhances the homocysteine-induced seizures. Vitamin B_6 also enhances homocysteine-induced convulsions, and some evidence has been reported in support of the possibility that a synergistic effect of PLP and homocysteine in blocking the postsynaptic γ-aminobutyric acid receptor might explain the seizure activity.[9] Homocysteine administered to rodent neocortical tissues trapped adenosine as AdoHcy. Since "adenosine is predominantly depressant in cerebral actions," possibly "the convulsive conditions and mental changes associated with administered homocysteine and with homocystinuria are due to cerebral adenosine concentrations being diminished."[434]

AdoHcy and AdoMet. As just explained, an untreated CBS-deficient patient with hypermethioninemia and elevated plasma tHcy may be expected to have increases in tissue concentrations of both AdoMet and AdoHcy, and the ratio of AdoMet to AdoHcy may affect the rate of a variety of transmethylation reactions. AdoMet, applied iontophoretically to rat sensorimotor cortex, increased the rate of spontaneous firing of neurons. Increases in brain AdoHcy of mice have been shown to decrease the rates of methylation of proteins and phosphatidylethanolamine derivatives and the activities of catechol *O*-methyltransferase and histamine *N*-methyltransferase in undialyzed tissue extracts. The functional results of any such effects that may occur in patients with elevated plasma tHcy remain unknown.[9]

Homocysteic and Homocysteine Sulfinic Acids. It is now generally accepted that glutamate, aspartate and other *excitatory amino acids* may produce several important effects in the mammalian central nervous system by acting as agonists for certain neuronal receptors. Excessive activation of such receptors can produce neuronal injury and death. A subtype of these, termed *NMDA receptors* because of the agonist action of *N*-methyl-D-aspartic acid, is abundant and well characterized. L-Homocysteic acid and L-homocysteine sulfinic acid each are potent agonists acting at the glutamate-binding site of NMDA receptors and exert cytotoxic effects on neurons in tissue preparations or in culture. The pattern of such toxicity, as well as its blockade by NMDA receptor antagonists, strongly suggests the neuronal damage in question is due to excessive stimulation of NMDA receptors.[6,435] Bouvier et al calculated that homocysteate and homocysteine sulfinate are both far more potent neuronal excitotoxins than is, for example, glutamate itself.[436] Homocysteate and homocysteine sulfinate were both identified by Ohmori et al in urine from homocystinuric patients but not in urine from normal subjects.[437] McCully reported that significant amounts of radioactive homocysteine sulfinate and homocysteate were formed during incubation of extracts of normal guinea pig liver with radioactive homocysteine thiolactone, but that extracts from scorbutic animals formed virtually no homocysteate. It was proposed that homocysteate was formed by an ascorbate-dependent chemical oxidation.[438] Considerations similar to those just outlined led Schwarz and Zhou to suggest that "the central nervous system symptoms of patients with homocystinuria can be explained by NMDA receptor overstimulation by L-homocysteic acid."[439] A wider role for homocysteate as a normal endogenous NMDA agonist has been suggested by Do and colleagues [439a], who reported in a series of papers that small quantities of homocysteate, identified chromatographically, were released from rat brain slices during K^+-dependent depolarization. Kilpatrick and Mozley reported also the extraction and chromatographic determination of homocysteate from normal rat brain.[440] However, these results, and the others mentioned earlier, appear to be subject to criticism because of the possibility that oxidation of homocysteine occurred during sample preparation and/or storage.[6,441] More recently, improved methodology has enabled the demonstration of homocysteate and/or homocysteine sulfinate in the plasma of rats chronically fed homocysteine thiolactone sufficient to double the control concentration of tHcy in plasma,[442] in the CSF of children treated with methotrexate when tHcy in that fluid rose above 0.355 μM,[443] and even in normal human serum (means of 677 nM for homocysteine sulfinate and 34 nM for homocysteate).[444] The availability of such methodology may facilitate evaluation of the suggested role for neuroexcitatory homocysteine derivatives, or even of homocysteine itself,[445] in such phenomena as the neuronal damage of homocystinuria,[445] homocysteine-induced convulsions in experimental animals,[446,447] and the neuropsychiatric manifestations associated with folate, cobalamin, and B_6 deficiencies.[448] Alleviation by baclofen of polymyoclonus and ataxia in a CBS-deficient patient was postulated perhaps to have taken place through suppression of the excitotoxic action of homocysteic acid.[449] That the relationship between plasma tHcy and plasma homocysteic acid is not a simple one, however, is indicated by a recent report[401a] that, although plasma homocysteic acid in a group of ten patients with homocystinuria (mean plasma tHcy, approx. 130 μM) was slightly elevated above control levels to, perhaps, 10 μM (both numerical values read only approximately from Fig. 1 in reference 401a), there was no significant correlation between the concentrations of these compounds.

Hydrogen Sulfide. Recent evidence indicates that H_2S is produced in rat brain largely by the activity of CBS, acting as a cysteine desulfhydrase (see the equation in the section "Cystathionine Synthesis"), and that physiological concentrations of H_2S selectively enhance NMDA receptor-mediated responses and facilitate the induction of hippocampal long-term potentiation.[450] The consequences of CBS deficiency for this role of H_2S remain to be defined.

Alternative Possibility. An alternative to the chemical causation of the central nervous system dysfunction in CBS deficiency is that repeated cerebral vascular thromboses produce many infarctions of the brain, too small individually to come to clinical attention but together sufficient to produce the abnormalities in question.[451] If this hypothesis were true, an increased frequency of focal neurologic signs would be expected among patients with mental retardation. Cerebrovascular occlusions in infancy and early childhood do result in mental retardation,[452] but most patients with mental retardation have no focal neurologic signs.

Possible Experimental Animal Models

A difficulty that has stood in the way of elucidation of the pathophysiology of CBS deficiency is the lack of available experimental animal models for this enzyme defect. Several recent developments suggest this situation may change in the near future: Kraus has produced transgenic mice with the human CBS gene "to see if pathological and biochemical correlations between the phenotype of these mice and their level of expression of CBS" can be found.[80,453] In addition, Watanabe et al produced a CBS knockout mouse in which exons 3 and 4 were excised from the mouse CBS gene by homologous recombination.[454] Surprisingly, total CBS deficiency in mice is highly deleterious, with more than 80 percent of the animals dying at a postnatal age of 8 weeks. Although the levels of tHcy measured in these mice are comparable to those of human patients, the mice die of liver disease. Heterozygotes had liver CBS activity equal to 42 percent of that in wild type, and plasma tHcy increased twofold above normal to about 14 μM, but clinically these heterozygotes did not manifest thrombi or other major abnormalities. However, preliminary results have shown that in response to methacholine the mesenteric microvessels of both the heterozygotes and homozygotes display a paradoxical vasoconstriction, in contrast to the dilatation shown by wild-type mice.[455] Further experiments will show the extent to which this animal model will elucidate the pathophysiology of human CBS deficiency.

Diagnosis

The presence of one or more of the typical clinical signs may lead to a suspicion of CBS deficiency. Cruysberg et al have emphasized the frequency of delayed diagnosis of CBS deficiency.[292] In their series of 34 patients who came to diagnosis at a mean age of 24 years, there was a mean delay of 11 years between the first major sign of the disease and a definitive diagnosis of CBS deficiency. They pointed out that myopia in excess of 5 diopters is extremely rare in children less than 5 years of age and uncommon even in adults. Thus, this finding, by itself, should raise the suspicion of ectopia lentis, perhaps due to CBS deficiency, and lead to appropriate laboratory tests. Moreover, they suggested that in addition to ectopia lentis, *myopia plus* or myopia of 1 diopter or more associated with signs of systemic disease such as vascular events, skeletal abnormalities, or central nervous system involvement should especially alert examiners to the possibility of CBS deficiency. However, definitive diagnosis is based on the presence of certain characteristic biochemical abnormalities.

The most consistent biochemical finding is homocystinuria.[456] No patient in the untreated state and beyond the period of early infancy has yet been described who did not have this abnormality. The presence of homocystine is most easily suspected when the urinary cyanide-nitroprusside reaction is positive.[9] Since this test detects most disulfides, it may be positive in other disulfidurias (e.g., cystinuria and β-mercaptolactate-cysteinuria). Consequently, homocystine must be specifically identified. In CBS-deficient individuals, quantitative amino acid analysis may reveal the presence of abnormal amounts of other sulfur-containing compounds, including homocysteine-cysteine mixed disulfide, homolanthionine, AdoHcy, and 5-amino-4-imidazole-carboxyamide-5′-*S*-homocysteinylribonucleoside.[8]

False negative results can be encountered in testing for homocystinuria. Some individuals with the B_6-responsive form of CBS deficiency may show marked response to relatively low intakes of B_6, even as little as 2 mg pyridoxine daily.[457] Thus, an affected individual with this type of responsiveness who ingests as little as one vitamin tablet daily might have negative reactions to screening tests for homocystinuria. (Most general vitamin preparations contain 2 to 5 mg pyridoxine hydrochloride in each tablet or capsule.) In view of the possibility of false negative screening results, all individuals with a clinical problem that strongly suggests the diagnosis of CBS deficiency, but whose results on screening for homocystinuria are negative, should be questioned about dietary intake with particular attention to supplemental vitamin ingestion. Any supplemental B_6 should be discontinued and the patient retested in 2 to 4 weeks by assay of plasma tHcy (or homocystine in the urine by column chromatography so that the presence of a small amount of excretory homocystine will not be overlooked).

The presence of homocystinuria is not sufficient to establish the diagnosis of CBS deficiency. Not only is homocystinuria noted in other disorders, but it may also be seen as an artifact of bacterial contamination of urine in cystathioninuria.[458,459] Consequently, amino acids in the plasma or serum should be measured in all suspected individuals. In CBS deficiency, this measurement should reveal elevated plasma tHcy, usually accompanied by a markedly reduced concentration of cystine. Furthermore, an increased concentration of methionine is found in most patients. Hypermethioninemia is an important finding since, in the metabolic defects in homocysteine methylation that are alternative causes of homocystinuria, the blood methionine concentration is low or normal (see Chap. 155).

A word of caution is in order with regard to homocystine in the analysis of plasma or serum amino acids. Homocystine readily undergoes disulfide exchange with sulfhydryl-containing compounds, including protein cysteine, forming disulfides with these thiols and gradually disappearing as a free amino acid. This disappearance may take place even in frozen specimens. Thus, delay in deproteinizing plasma or serum in preparation for quantitative amino acid analysis can result in the binding of most or all of the Hcy to protein and its not being detected in this analysis. We are aware of delay in the diagnosis of CBS deficiency in at least three patients as a result of this phenomenon.[460] Moreover, Applegarth et al have pointed out that plasma tHcy must reach a level of at least 50 μM, or about four times above the upper limit of normal, before any free homocystine is detectable in plasma even with immediate deproteinization[461] (see also Bonham et al[268a]). Consequently, the preferred procedure to identify increased Hcy in blood is to measure plasma tHcy.[460–463]

Direct enzyme assay confirms the diagnosis of CBS deficiency. This activity can be assayed in liver biopsy specimens,[464] cultured skin fibroblasts,[465] phytohemagglutinin-stimulated lymphocytes,[466] or long-term established lines of such cells.[467] CBS activities in extracts of cultured fibroblasts below the ranges for control subjects and heterozygotes have, with rare exceptions, been correlated with other indications of CBS deficiency.[9]

Once the diagnosis of CBS deficiency is established biochemically, it is important to determine whether the patient is responsive or nonresponsive to B_6. Those responsive to B_6 may be metabolically controlled with B_6 only, or with B_6 and moderately reduced intake of methionine, a great advantage since this avoids the difficulty of imposing a diet severely restricted in methionine (see the section "Management and Outcomes," below). To investigate responsiveness of CBS-deficient patients, Kluijtmans et al[233] gave B_6 for 6 weeks in doses of 750 mg/day to adults and 200 to 500 mg/day to children. Those in whom plasma free Hcy decreased to below 20 μM, or plasma tHcy decreased to below 50 μM, were classified as B_6 responsive. Wilcken and Wilcken[311] also ascertained B_6 responsiveness on the basis of a plasma free Hcy level consistently below 20 μM, but while the patients were receiving B_6 in a dose of only 100 to 200 mg/day. Yap and Naughten[468] determined B_6 responsiveness in infants on the basis of "a rapidly falling methionine level and clearing of free homocystine from the plasma" while the patient received 150 mg B_6/day for 3 days.

Management and Outcomes

Medical management of CBS deficiency has two major aims: (1) control or elimination of biochemical abnormalities with the goal of preventing clinical disease, halting the progression of existing clinical defects, or ameliorating clinical manifestations that may be reversible; and (2) supportive treatment of complications.

From experience with other metabolic diseases, as well as from present understanding of the pathophysiology of CBS deficiency, it is reasonable to assume that one or more of the biochemical abnormalities characteristic of this disease is responsible for its clinical complications and that optimal treatment should aim to minimize these biochemical abnormalities. Whenever possible, therapy to achieve biochemical control should begin before clinical complications occur, since many of these complications are irreversible. Even before clinical effects are recognizable, tissue damage may have occurred. Thus, maximal benefit from therapy may be possible only when the disorder is detected in the newborn period, either as a result of known disease in the family or through routine neonatal screening. Since management will usually differ according to the type of patient, it may be helpful to consider separately the management of patients in three categories: (1) pyridoxine-responsive individuals detected after the newborn period, (2) patients diagnosed as newborns, and (3) patients not responsive to pyridoxine and detected after the newborn period.

Pyridoxine-Responsive Patients Detected After the Newborn Period. The administration of relatively large amounts of pyridoxine, usually orally in the form of pyridoxine hydrochloride, has been effective in reducing, but usually not completely normalizing, the biochemical abnormalities in many patients with CBS deficiency.[233,284,311,313] Wilcken and Wilcken reported plasma free Hcy levels consistently below 20 μM in 17 B_6-responsive patients (pretreatment levels not provided);[311] and Kluijtmans et al observed reductions in the mean plasma free Hcy level from 116 to 160 μM at diagnosis to 13 to 23 μM on B_6 therapy.[233] Although the latter values are still elevated, they represent reductions of 67 to 90 percent.[233] The majority of these patients also maintained plasma tHcy below 50 μM (reference range, approx. 5 to 15 μM) and reductions of 33 to 56 percent in plasma methionine. Such responses probably depend on residual CBS activity (see the section "The Pyridoxine Effect and Its Mechanism," above). The doses of B_6 administered have varied considerably. Barber and Spaeth used doses of 250 to 500 mg/day,[284] Gaull et al used 800 to 1200 mg/day,[469] and Kluijtmans et al used 750 mg/day in adults and at least 200 mg/day in children.[233] An occasional patient has responded to doses as low as 25 mg/day[470] or even lower. According to Perry, a patient should not be considered unresponsive until a dose of 500 to 1000 mg/day has been given for several weeks.[451] However, Wilcken and Wilcken have used no more than 200 mg/day and concluded that maximal response is probably reached at 100 mg/day given in two divided doses.[311]

The effectiveness of pyridoxine in preventing initial clinically detected thromboembolic events has been validated statistically in several studies.[233,272,311] Only four such events occurred among 135 B_6-responsive patients treated with B_6, whereas the time-to-event curve for untreated patients (Fig. 88-8) indicated that, were such treatment without effect, 20 thromboembolic events would have been expected, a statistically significant decrease ($P < 0.001$).[272] Wilcken and Wilcken encountered only two vascular events during 281 patient-years of treatment in 17 B_6-responsive patients, in contrast to the 11 such events expected in the absence of treatment[311] (calculated on the basis of the previously published time-to-event curves[272]). Kluijtmans et al[233] also encountered only two vascular events during 378 patient-years of treatment. For prevention of thromboembolism alone, therefore, B_6 treatment is strongly indicated for B_6-responsive patients diagnosed at any age. A similar analysis suggested that pyridoxine treatment may reduce the frequency of lens dislocation.[272] Finally, improvement in behavior and in IQ has been reported in several late-treated B_6-responsive patients.[471]

Whether pyridoxine therapy alone can be considered adequate treatment for patients who are B_6 responsive, or should be combined with a methionine-restricted diet, cystine supplementation, or other measures, is not settled by existing data. *A priori* considerations support methionine restriction for patients incompletely responsive to pyridoxine, since this may further correct the biochemical abnormalities. Even patients with maximum B_6 responsiveness have reduced tolerance to methionine as measured by methionine loading tests.[287,289,474] Such patients may in theory experience abnormal episodic increases in methionine or Hcy concentrations following protein ingestion. Some methionine restriction or the use of small, frequent feedings might be prudent.[289] Wilcken et al demonstrated that betaine treatment will blunt the plasma Hcy response to methionine loading in B_6-responsive patients and suggested that betaine should be added to the treatment regimen of pyridoxine and folic acid in B_6-responsive patients so that Hcy accumulation will be normal throughout the day during normal dietary intake[475] (see also the section "Patients Not Responsive to Pyridoxine and Detected after the Newborn Period," below).

Safety of Pyridoxine. Safety issues arising from the use of pyridoxine have been reviewed.[476] Sensory neuropathy with ataxia has been reported in otherwise normal adults ingesting large amounts of pyridoxine. The reviewers concluded that doses up to 500 mg/day for up to 2 years appear to be safe, but that daily doses exceeding 1000 mg/day, or total doses of 1000 g or more, are *high-risk regimens* for development of neurologic changes. Such abnormalities improved dramatically following withdrawal of pyridoxine, but in some instances minor changes persisted. Ludolph et al found among eight late-treated homocystinuric patients a frequency and extent of extrapyramidal dysfunction "greater than expected,"[477] slight impairment of propioception in five, paresthesias of the feet in two, and abnormal sural nerve conduction in four of the five clinically affected patients. Seven of these patients had received doses of 900 to 1200 mg/day pyridoxine for periods of 4 to 22 years,[478] but there was no clear correlation of neurologic abnormalities with dose. Sensory neuropathy induced by high-level pyridoxine consumption was included among the possible reasons for the observed deficits. Mpofu et al, however, found no signs or symptoms suggestive of neuropathy by neurologic examination and electrophysiological studies of 17 patients with homocystinuria treated with 200 to 500 mg/day pyridoxine for 7 to 24 years, so that total doses received were 511 to 3833 g [mean, 2085 ± 1035 (SD)].[479] Twelve of the compliant patients had received totals exceeding 1000 g (1533 to 3833 g). Wilcken and Wilcken have not encountered B_6-related complications with doses up to 200 mg/day during 281 patient-years.[311]

We have knowledge of two infants who, 1 to 2 weeks after commencement of a daily dose of 500 mg pyridoxine hydrochloride at age 2 to 3 weeks, became apneic and unresponsive and required respiratory support.[480,481] Each had been identified because of hypermethioninemia discovered during routine newborn screening and started on pyridoxine pending definitive diagnosis. One is now known to be CBS deficient, whereas the other has MAT I/III deficiency. Computed axial tomography and MRI ruled out focal neurologic lesions in both. After discontinuation of the pyridoxine, both improved dramatically within days and recovered completely within weeks. Although concurrent enteroviral infection is a possible explanation of the neurologic abnormalities in one of these infants, the similarity of their cases suggests they may have been suffering from acute toxicity associated with pyridoxine administration. Four infants with pyridoxine-responsive neonatal seizures have been observed to become unresponsive and apneic shortly after receiving 5 to 50 mg pyridoxine intramuscularly[482–484] or 50 mg orally.[485] Although it is uncertain whether the mechanism is the same in each of these cases, prudence suggests limiting the oral dose of pyridoxine for young infants to considerably less than 500 mg daily. In agreement, recently a report appeared of a 1-month-old Japanese girl with CBS deficiency who, 8 days after being placed on a daily dose of 500 mg pyridoxine hydrochloride, developed acute respiratory failure requiring immediate respiratory ventilation, with myoglobinuria and an extremely high value of creatine phosphokinase, attributed possibly to rhabdomyolysis. Vitamin B_6 was discontinued the same day, and the patient's clinical status and laboratory abnormalities indicative of rhabdomyolysis normalized within a few weeks.[485a]

Administration of 500 mg/kg pyridoxine to male rats daily for 6 weeks was accompanied by decreases in absolute and relative weights of testis, epididymis, prostate gland, and seminal vesicle and decreased sperm counts.[486] To our knowledge, no report has been published about infertility following megadoses of pyridoxine to people.

Treatment with the pyridoxine derivative, PLP, was associated with the appearance of liver dysfunction in a child with pyridoxine-nonresponsive CBS deficiency. The dose had been started 2 months earlier at 500 mg/day and increased gradually. Signs and symptoms of hepatotoxicity appeared 4 days after increase of the PLP to 1000 mg/day, disappeared upon its withdrawal, and did not recur during therapy with pyridoxine hydrochloride, even at doses up to 1800 mg/day.[487]

Patients Detected as Newborns. The great majority of patients detected by newborn screening have been B_6 nonresponsive (see the section "Prevalence and Screening," below). Consequently, with few exceptions, these patients have been treated by methionine-restricted diets (see below). However, dietary treatment is difficult and a major event in the life of the infant and his or her family, and it is thus important to determine that an infant is not B_6 responsive before beginning dietary therapy and to do so while avoiding, on the one hand, risk of brain damage due to continuation of abnormally high metabolite levels and, on the other, the chance of causing B_6 toxicity. Thus, following confirmation of CBS deficiency, while continuing a normal diet the infant should be given vitamin B_6 in a dose of 250 mg/day for 4 to 6 days with daily assays of plasma methionine, homocystine, and/or tHcy. The child should be carefully monitored clinically with particular attention to respiratory status and responsiveness (see foregoing section on vitamin-B_6 toxicity). Published evidence suggests that most fully B_6-responsive patients will show at least a partial biochemical response within such a period,[284,284a,286,287,289] although attainment of the full potential response may require a longer time.[286] Should substantial reductions in methionine, homocystine, and tHcy be observed, the dose of B_6 should promptly be reduced in decrements of 50 mg/day to determine the lowest dose that produces the maximal biochemical response. The infant may then be treated with that amount. However, monitoring of plasma levels should continue at least weekly to determine whether the infant is fully responsive to B6 or requires either a lower protein intake or a methionine-restricted diet.

Should amino acid analyses not be available on a daily basis, an alternative would be to conduct the B_6 challenge with daily collection of plasma specimens, each prepared with immediate separation of red cells (and rapid deproteinization if free homocystine is to be determined[460]) and delivered to an outside laboratory as soon as possible. Pending receipt of the results, the infant could begin the methionine-restricted diet with adjustment accordingly when the challenge results become known.

The methionine-restricted diets are designed to reduce the accumulation of methionine, Hcy, and their metabolites, and, through supplementation with L-cystine to increase cysteine. Cysteine is an essential amino acid for some, but not all, patients with CBS deficiency.[288] The different types of methionine-restricted diets that have been used were mentioned in a previous edition of this text.[8] Currently, proprietary medical products based on a methionine-free synthetic mixture supplemented with cystine are in virtually exclusive use.[488] At least four such products are available.[9] The methionine requirement is met during infancy by adding small amounts of breast milk[468] or standard proprietary formula[489] and, later, by adding low-protein foods in carefully controlled quantities.[313,489] The desired amount of dietary methionine is judged by maintenance of blood methionine levels within or near the normal range (20 to 40 μM) and by the absence, or near absence, of homocystine in blood.[489] Yap and Naughten reported median plasma homocystine levels of 4 to 11 μM in children treated with diets and 5.5 to 18 μM in adolescents and young adults. One exception was an adult with a median plasma homocystine of 48 μM.[468] Walter et al recommend a plasma free Hcy concentration below 10 μM for good control.[313]

Methionine restriction, started in early infancy, has been effective in preventing or delaying a number of serious problems. Among 16 B_6-nonresponsive children ascertained by newborn screening and treated with diet from early ages who were reported in an international survey, the mean IQ was 94 ± 4, approximately 35 points above the mean IQ of B_6-nonresponsive patients who were untreated or late treated.[272] Among an additional 23 early-treated B_6-nonresponsive children for whom only qualitative estimates of mental capabilities were available, 19 (82 percent) were estimated to have average or above-average intelligence, and only four (17 percent) were retarded. Early dietary treatment seemed also to delay or prevent dislocation of the lens in some patients.[272] Dietary therapy may also prevent seizures.[272] In this study, early-treated patients were still too young as a group for evaluation of the effects of diet on thromboembolism or osteoporosis.[272]

These previous data[272] have been confirmed and extended by recent reports of long-term follow-up of patients identified in the newborn period by routine or at-risk screening. Eleven such B_6-nonresponsive patients in Manchester, England, treated with diet from the newborn period, attained a median IQ of 100 (range, 84 to 117), significantly better than the median of 58 (range, 20 to 86) among B_6 nonresponders diagnosed after infancy.[313] A twelfth patient was developmentally normal at age 4 years.[307] None of these 12 patients have eye or skeletal abnormalities.[307] In Ireland, 18 of 21 B_6-nonresponsive patients have had no complications, including absence of ectopia lentis (although three have developed increasing myopia), no radiologic evidence of osteoporosis, and no mental handicap with age-appropriate education standards. Thromboembolic events have not occurred.[468] Among the Irish study group, had the patients not been treated, at least 16 thromboembolic events would have been expected during the 403.9 patient years of treatment.[468a] Of the three patients who have been noncompliant to the diet, one developed osteoporosis and reduced IQ, another developed ectopia lentis and reduced IQ, and the third developed iridodonesis.[468] The value of early detection and treatment is further supported by a recent report in which a detailed comparison of the ophthalmic abnormalities observed in a group of early-detected and treated patients (Irish and British; B_6 responsive and B_6 nonresponsive) with those in a group of late-detected patients showed that the former group had far fewer and less severe problems.[468b]

Most of the relatively few B_6-responsive individuals detected by newborn screening have been treated by methionine restriction, in some instances accompanied by B_6. A few have been treated solely with B_6. The limited data available indicate that most such patients treated in these ways will attain normal, or near normal, intelligence.[272]

As discussed in the next section, the methyl donor, betaine, is frequently used to lower Hcy levels in older children and adults with CBS deficiency in whom dietary therapy is unacceptable. Whether betaine should also be considered as additional treatment for diet-treated infants not in metabolic control, perhaps because of poor compliance with the diet, is an issue. Because brain lacks betaine-homocysteine methyltransferase activity,[489a] a concern in the use of betaine has been that it might not lower brain Hcy, perhaps an especially important consideration for the developing infantile brain. However, Surtees et al[496] have shown that betaine therapy alone results in substantial lowering of CSF tHcy concomitant with reduction in plasma tHcy (see the details in next section), suggesting that much of the central nervous system Hcy may be derived from blood. If so, betaine could have a role in the treatment of infants with CBS deficiency. Nevertheless, it may be prudent to exhaust efforts toward dietary compliance and metabolic control before considering addition of betaine. Should betaine be added, the recommended dose is 200 to 250 mg/kg/day. It is available as an approved drug on prescription.[§]

§Cystadane (betaine anhydrous powder) from Chronimed Pharmacy, Minnetonka, Minnesota (telephone 1-800-900-4267).

Patients Not Responsive to Vitamin B_6 and Detected After the Newborn Period. This category of patients offers the most difficult therapeutic challenge. Methionine restriction through dietary control has often been attempted, but acceptance of the restrictive and unpalatable diet by older children or adults is difficult to achieve.[6,313] When accepted, methionine restriction in older patients has often ameliorated biochemical abnormalities.[9] When such patients have been very strictly managed, the results, although not published in detail, appear promising in terms of prevention of thromboembolic events.[490] Anecdotal evidence suggestive of developmental improvement or improvement in school performance has been reported.[471] However, perhaps because of difficulties in compliance, no statistically significant evidence of the effectiveness of methionine restriction in prevention of initial thromboembolic events was forthcoming in an international survey.[272]

There has been a relatively recent upsurge of interest in the use of the methyl donor, betaine, as a treatment especially promising in late-detected B_6-nonresponsive patients.[9] This compound,[491] or its metabolic precursor, choline,[492] was early shown to lower Hcy, with concomitant rise in methionine concentrations, in patients with CBS deficiency. The mechanism of this effect is presumed to be an increase in the rate of homocysteine methylation through betaine-homocysteine methyltransferase by making available more of the methyl donor for this reaction (Fig. 88-2). This redistribution of metabolites may be desirable on the assumption that methionine and its derivatives make lesser contributions to the pathophysiology of CBS deficiency than do homocysteine and its metabolites, an assumption that appears reasonable in light of available knowledge. It has been suggested, also, that such redistribution might enhance methionine degradation through the transamination pathway (in which the defective step at CBS is bypassed).[493]

All reported B_6-nonresponsive patients have shown a reduction in plasma Hcy, and most have shown a rise in methionine in response to betaine treatment.[313,491–494] CSF tHcy, which was substantially increased before betaine treatment, significantly decreased during such treatment (mean values, 1.18 μM vs 0.32 μM; reference value, ± 0.10 μM).[496] Plasma cystine also rises,[491,494] usually in parallel with the reduction in Hcy.[267]

The most notable clinical response to betaine has been the absence of vascular events in treated patients. Wilcken and Wilcken reported that, during 258 patient-years of treatment in 15 B_6-nonresponsive patients, no vascular event occurred.[311] In the absence of treatment, at least ten such events would have been expected.[272] Improved behavior and reduction in mood disturbance have also been reported in some,[493–495,497] but not all,[497] patients in response to betaine therapy. In one study, vertebral body bone density was unchanged in five B_6-nonresponsive patients over a 2-year period of alternate on/off betaine treatment.[498]

The dose of betaine used has been 6 to 9 g/day in two divided doses for adults[311] or 200 to 250 mg/kg/day in two or three divided doses for children.[313,496] No adverse effects of betaine given in the recommended dose of 6 to 9 g/day[311] have been noted, with the occasional exception of a detectable body odor.[495] There have been no changes in liver, renal, or hematopoietic function.[495] Betaine has also been given during two pregnancies without evidence of teratogenic effect. However, a third pregnancy in which betaine treatment was continued to 13 gestational weeks resulted in an offspring with congenital heart disease due to transposition of the great vessels (Table 88-5).

Finally, it is noted that some physicians are now routinely giving pyridoxine even to apparently "nonresponsive" patients.[311,475]

Additional Measures. Folate depletion has been noted in a number of CBS-deficient patients.[285,472] In two of these depleted patients, therapy with folate alone reduced the excretion of homocystine and increased the excretion of methionine.[472] In other patients, therapy with folate in combination with vitamin B_{12} and pyridoxine resulted in a lower concentration of homocystine, with little or no increase in the methionine concentration.[285,311] Folate repletion may be necessary to permit a pyridoxine response. Conversely, CBS deficiency may exacerbate folate deficiency from other causes, for example, nutritional deprivation.[473] Clinicians treating CBS-deficient patients currently appear to be following a variety of practices with respect to folate and B_{12} supplementation. Yap and Naughten, dealing with relatively young Irish patients, almost all of whom are B_6 nonresponsive, gave folate or B_{12} only if the patient was found to be deficient in these factors.[468] At Boston Children's Hospital, CBS-deficient children after 2 years of age are given folate (1 mg/day) with supplemental B_{12} as indicated by monitoring of serum B_{12}. Wilcken and Wilcken gave all patients, B_6 responsive or not, folic acid (5 mg/day) and B_6 (100 to 200 mg/day), and gave most patients intermittent hydroxocobalamin twice yearly.[311] If folate is given in relatively large doses, it may be advisable to monitor the B_{12} status, or to give a B_{12} supplement, especially with older patients, to avoid the possibilities of masking the megaloblastic anemia and/or accelerating the neurologic abnormalities associated with B_{12} deficiency.[498a,498b]

Several additional approaches to possible melioration of some of the biochemical abnormalities in CBS deficiency have been considered but not attempted in patients.[8] These include replenishment of cystathionine by direct administration, promotion of the synthesis of this compound through administration of homoserine together with cysteine, and enhancement of the excretion of homocystine by administration of arginine, α-aminobutyric acid, or dibasic amino acids.[9]

Medical therapies directed toward reducing or eliminating the thrombotic tendency, but that do not affect the basic biochemical abnormalities, have also been reviewed.[8,9] Dipyridamole, an inhibitor of platelet function, either alone or in combination with aspirin, corrected the decreased platelet survival times reported in some patients.[499] Attempts by such means to prevent further thrombotic episodes in patients who had experienced thromboembolism have met with mixed results, one group reporting success,[499] another lack of success.[302,500] Data from an international survey were insufficient to enable evaluation of the long-term benefits of dipyridamole, aspirin, or both in preventing thrombotic complications.[272] Sulfinpyrazone, also an inhibitor of platelet function, reduced arterial damage and normalized platelet survival in baboons given homocystine,[499] but use of this compound has not been reported in patients with CBS deficiency. Finally, some authors have suggested that patients avoid activities associated with an increased risk of thromboembolism, for example, use of oral contraceptives, perhaps even pregnancy.[9] A small, but statistically significant rise in fasting plasma tHcy has been demonstrated during the low-hormonal phase of the treatment cycle in normal women taking a monophasic sub-50 oral contraceptive,[501] but data are lacking as to the effect of contraceptives on Hcy concentrations in CBS-deficient patients themselves.

Complications. The supportive treatment of clinical complications in CBS-deficient patients is essentially the same as the treatment of these complications when due to other causes.[9] An exception is the avoidance of surgery whenever possible. The danger of thromboembolism has been said to be increased postoperatively in CBS deficiency,[502] although the data from an international survey,[272] reviewed in the section on "Clinical and Pathologic Manifestations," did not provide strong support for this conclusion. A few patients have died of thromboembolism following ocular surgery. Ocular complications of surgery, including marked and prolonged vitreous hemorrhage, vitreous loss, and retinal detachment, have been reported.[9] Gerding has described a novel surgical procedure that might reduce the possibility of these complications by allowing for minimal invasive removal of the lens, preservation of the anterior vitreous cortex, and implantation of an artificial intraocular lens.[503] There has been a report of an acute schizophrenic episode experienced by a CBS-deficient girl following eye surgery and lasting 6 days.[504]

Should surgery be necessary, the risk of thromboembolism may be lessened by increasing hydration with intravenous fluids preoperatively and postoperatively.[505,506] Intravenous pyridoxine has been given during surgery in at least two cases without untoward effects.[507] The data from an international survey[272] showed that, when suitable precautions (such as those mentioned previously) are taken, the great majority of surgical procedures performed on CBS-deficient patients do not lead to thromboembolic complications.

Acute glaucoma due to pupillary block by the dislocated lens can usually be treated medically.[508,509] Initially, the pupil should be fully dilated with any suitable mydriatic and the lens repositioned from the anterior chamber by pressure on the cornea. Should this fail, a peripheral iridectomy may be performed. Following any of these procedures, miosis should be maintained constantly so as to prevent the lens from again dislocating anteriorly.[508]

Prevalence and Screening

To date, most screening of newborns for CBS deficiency has relied on the detection of hypermethioninemia. In previous compilations of data for such screening, CBS deficiency had been detected with a frequency of between 1:200,000 and 1:335,000.[8,9] This chapter in the previous edition included a table (Table 35-4) that provided screening data from several countries throughout the world.[6] Several lines of evidence indicate these frequencies are very likely an underestimate of the true rate of occurrence of CBS deficiency. First, hypermethioninemia may not be present during the first few days of life when the blood specimen is customarily collected for screening.[8,473,510,511] This possibility has been enhanced because current practices of infant feeding have led progressively to lower protein intake,[512] and because the newborn blood specimen is now often collected earlier in the neonatal period than was formerly the case.[513] Second, there are differences among programs in the extent of hypermethioninemia required to trigger further testing.[514] This may lead to missed cases and account for some of the apparent differences in reported rates of detection. Third, not all cases of CBS deficiency identified in newborn-screening programs have been reported in a manner that would have led to their inclusion in screening data for CBS deficiency.[515] Fourth, screening of newborns for hypermethioninemia has only recently begun in at least one area—New South Wales, Australia—in which the relatively high frequency of 1:60,000 for CBS deficiency has been estimated.[516] Fifth, and perhaps most important, relatively few B_6-responsive patients have been identified by newborn screening. Among those detected by newborn screening in Manchester, England, all 12 infants,[313] in Ireland all 21 infants,[468] and in the United States the 17 patients on whom data were available[517] have been B_6 nonresponsive. The sole B_6-responsive infant to have come to attention in New England through routine screening had a normal blood methionine concentration in the specimen obtained at 4 days of age but an increased concentration in a second specimen obtained at 4 weeks of age. At that time, collection of the latter specimen was a routine procedure in the screening program.[270] In an international survey,[272] of the 55 patients who had been both discovered by screening of newborns and classified with respect to pyridoxine responsiveness, only 13 percent were B_6 responsive, whereas 78 percent were nonresponsive and 9 percent were intermediate in response. These frequencies were quite different from those for the patients in the total survey population. Among the 529 classified as to pyridoxine response, 43.7 percent were judged to be responsive, 43.7 percent nonresponsive, and 12.7 percent intermediate in response. Thus, the evidence strongly suggests that the B_6-responsive form of CBS deficiency, the most readily treatable form, is being preferentially missed by newborn screening as currently carried out. In agreement, a DNA-based screening of newborns in Denmark showed 1.4 percent of them to be heterozygous for the I278T mutation.[257a] This value corresponds to a homozygote frequency of approximately 1:20,000, a significantly higher incidence than the aforementioned figure of detection frequency of 1:200,000 to 1:335,000.

An alternative to screening newborns for hypermethioninemia to identify CBS deficiency would be to detect elevated Hcy in blood or urine. No such method for newborn screening is available. Even if available, neonates may not accumulate Hcy sufficiently increased above normal to be identifiable on that basis.[518] Screening urine of neonates for homocystine has been even less reliable than screening blood for hypermethioninemia as a means of identifying CBS deficiency. In Australia, only one case was discovered among 700,000 infants tested by the screening of urine; one case is known to have been missed.[519] No cases were discovered by this means in Massachusetts.[520] Homocystine may be absent from the urine of neonates with CBS deficiency[521] or present in such low concentrations as to go undetected by the usual screening methods.[270,518] However, an assay that uses a fluorescent thiol reagent, dansylaminophenylmercuric acetate, to form a fluorescent derivative of homocysteine after reduction of urinary homocystine with metabisulfite might be sufficiently sensitive and specific to be effective for urine screening of newborns.[522] The method was reported to be "about a thousand times more sensitive than the modified cyanide-nitroprusside test"[523] and, in a preliminary study, was used successfully to "easily detect" homocystine in urine samples from each of four children with homocystinuria. There were no false positives among 98 samples from normal subjects and patients with various other disorders.

Discouragement over the low rate of detection and the need for a separate assay to screen for the disorder has led to the discontinuation of screening for CBS deficiency in many newborn-screening programs.[514] This is unfortunate, since newborn detection and early treatment is clearly beneficial (see the section "Management and Outcomes," above). The need for a separate screening assay is no longer an adequate objection to screening for this disorder. The technology of tandem mass spectrometry adapted for newborn screening enables screening for multiple metabolites, including methionine, by a single test.[524] Thus, screening for CBS deficiency can now be combined with newborn screening for PKU, maple syrup urine disease, and many organic acid and fatty-acid oxidation disorders in a single procedure.[525] It is likely that within the next few years this will be the predominant technique used in newborn screening for inborn errors of metabolism.

Heterozygotes

Identification. Methods aimed at identifying heterozygotes have used three approaches: enzyme assays, metabolite measurements, a combination of both, or genotyping methodology:

Enzyme Assays

1. *Liver.* Of the eight obligate heterozygotes for whom specific activities of hepatic CBS have been determined, seven had values below the control range, whereas one barely overlapped the low end of the control range.[6]
2. *Phytohemagglutinin-stimulated lymphocytes.* CBS activities in extracts of phytohemagglutinin-stimulated lymphocytes grown from 17 obligate heterozygotes were below the control range for 14, whereas three overlapped this range.[6]
3. *Long-term cultured lymphocytes.* CBS activity in extracts from long-term cultured lymphocytes from three obligate heterozygotes did not overlap with normal activities.[6]
4. *Cultured fibroblasts.* Results of assays of CBS activities in extracts of fibroblasts cultured from obligate heterozygotes have been published for more than 70 individuals. As was the case for the other tissues, the mean specific activity of CBS for obligate heterozygotes was less than 50 percent of the mean control specific activity. Cumulatively, values for close to half

of the obligate heterozygotes overlapped the control range.[6] Thus, enzyme assays may provide tentative identification of some, but not all, heterozygotes. Both false negative and false positive results (see below) may be obtained.[6]

Metabolite Concentrations. Early studies of methionine and/or homocystine in urine or plasma, and of urinary sulfate excretion after oral L-methionine loads failed to develop criteria that could conclusively and reliably distinguish obligate heterozygotes from control subjects.[6] More recently, measurements in a number of laboratories of either protein-bound homocysteine or of tHcy in plasma have consistently encountered overlap between obligate heterozygotes and normals.[6,259]

Boddie and colleagues presented evidence that determination of the ratio of tHcy to tCys may be a better discriminant,[526] but further experience with this approach has not yet been forthcoming.

Measurements of postmethionine-load plasma free Hcy or tHcy have been quite successful, especially if account is taken of menopausal status and the results are combined with measurements of CBS activity in cultured fibroblasts.[6,527,528] However, difficulties remain in the interpretation of the results of each of these measurements.[6] Differing mutations within the CBS gene may affect the results of each of these measurements differently.[259,528]

Genotyping. Genotyping may be a useful adjunct for the identification of heterozygotes for CBS deficiency. At the moment, such methodology is most useful for the detection of the two most prevalent CBS mutations, I278T and G307S,[528] but methodology is now under development that may enable practical extension of this approach to a number of additional CBS mutations.

Mild Elevations of Plasma tHcy and Possible Risks for Heterozygotes. In 1976, Wilcken and Wilcken[529] investigated methionine tolerance in male subjects under age 50 years who had angiographic evidence of ischemic heart disease but were free of known risk factors for such disease. Seven of 25 patients, but only one of 22 control subjects, had peak postmethionine plasma concentrations of homocysteine-cysteine mixed disulfide that were elevated to the same extent as had been reported at that time for obligate heterozygotes for CBS deficiency.[530] Since that pioneering study, a great number of studies have explored possible relationships between mild elevation of plasma tHcy (with or without methionine loading) and coronary artery, cerebrovascular, or peripheral vascular disease, as well as venous thrombosis. A complete review of these studies is beyond the scope of this chapter, but see, for example, references 205, 432, and 531–536. Together, these studies have led to wide acceptance of the conclusion that relatively mild elevation of plasma tHcy is an independent risk factor for early vascular disease. However, it may be noted that recently accumulated evidence indicates that, although homozygosity for the C677T mutation in the methylenetetrahydrofolate reductase gene that confers thermolability to this enzyme is a common cause of mildly elevated plasma tHcy, such homozygosity does not increase cardiovascular risk.[536a,536b] It was suggested that the mild elevations of tHcy frequently found in vascular disease patients are not causally related to the pathogenesis of the vascular disease but rather may be an epiphenomenon resulting from well-established risk factors such as male sex, age, smoking, blood pressure, elevated cholesterol, and lack of exercise.[536a]

Because the elevations of Hcy in many of the aforementioned studies were of similar magnitude to those observed in obligate heterozygotes for CBS deficiency after methionine loading, the possibilities arose that such heterozygosity might (1) enhance the risk of early vascular disease and (2) account for a significant proportion of early vascular disease in some populations. Subsequent observations have produced evidence that both these possibilities are unlikely:

1. With respect to the risk for obligate heterozygotes, a questionnaire study of parents and grandparents in 203 families with CBS-deficient children revealed no statistically significant increases in the incidence of heart attacks or strokes in these relatives compared with the incidences in similar relatives of children with either impaired phenylalanine tolerance or new-mutation achondroplastic dwarfism. The data were sufficiently sensitive to virtually exclude an increase in the cardiovascular risk for heterozygotes for CBS deficiency of as much as fivefold and to make improbable a relative risk of as much as threefold. Fewer than 5 percent of such heterozygotes were likely to have a thromboembolic episode by age 50.[537] Clarke studied 25 parents of CBS-deficient patients by noninvasive ultrasound assessment of the extracranial neck arteries. Both male parents and age-matched male controls had only minor endothelial plaques in 58 percent of the cases. There was a slight excess prevalence (38 percent compared to 28 percent) of plaques in female parents compared to age-matched controls, but this was not statistically significant, and it was concluded that there was no excess vascular disease in the obligate heterozygotes.[538] Rubba et al used ultrasound to study 12 parents of CBS-deficient patients and one sister in whom enzyme determination "indicated a low CBS activity." Their mean age was 46 years. Overt clinical atherosclerotic disease among these subjects was not mentioned, save for one who had signs of previous deep-venous thrombosis. Seven of the 13 heterozygotes had evidence of wall abnormalities or partial stenoses in their iliac arteries, compared to 2 of 47 age-matched controls ($P < 0.01$); 6 of 13 had non-flow-reducing carotid lesions compared to 3 of 47 among controls ($P < 0.05$).[295] In more recent noninvasive studies, however, no abnormalities were found in the brachial arteries of 14 obligate heterozygous adults.[385] Moreover, 23 heterozygotes 18 to 50 years of age had no clinical evidence of disease in coronary, peripheral, and cerebral arteries, and the distribution of intima-media thickness was similar to that found in 12 control subjects.[539] Similarly, a later study of carotid artery intima-media thickness found values among 15 obligate heterozygotes to be similar to those of control subjects, whereas homozygosity was associated with carotid wall hypertrophy.[539a] Most recently, it was reported that, among 36 parents of Irish CBS-deficient patients with an age range of 34 to 74 years (median, 51.5 years), all had been free of thromboembolic events save for one man with pulmonary embolism subsequently diagnosed and treated for connective tissue disease.[468a] Taken together, these studies suggest that most obligate heterozygotes for CBS deficiency will not have overt clinical atherosclerotic disease by middle age.

2. There is strong evidence that heterozygotes for CBS deficiency do not account for a significant proportion of patients with early vascular disease, even those who have accompanying mildly abnormal postmethionine-load elevations of plasma tHcy. In two early studies of patients with premature vascular disease and abnormal elevations of Hcy after methionine loading, assays of CBS activities in cultured fibroblasts appeared to indicate that many were heterozygotes for CBS deficiency.[540,541] However, the enzyme assay results in question were found not to be reproducible when repeated on a number of subjects from these two studies.[542–544] Nordström and Kjellström studied CBS activity in cultured fibroblasts as a function of the age of the donor at the time of cell donation. In control subjects, there was a tendency for activity to decrease with donor age (statistically significantly in the first study,[544a] but not significantly in the second[544b]). In comparisons of fibroblasts from older subjects, no significant decrease in CBS activities between controls and patients with atherosclerotic disease, or those who had suffered a deep-vein thrombosis, were observed, although a nonstatistically significant tendency in this direction was found in fibroblasts from the younger age groups.[544a,544b] These results suggest that in any future studies of CBS activity in patients with thromboembolic disease it will be imperative to control for the age of the cell donors.

Several studies have used molecular genetic methods to seek more directly for CBS mutations in patients with thromboembolic disease: Kozich et al were unable to find any inactivating mutations in the coding regions of four subjects with elevations of postmethionine-load plasma tHcy, peripheral arterial occlusive disease, and low CBS activities in cultured fibroblasts. Their results implied that the low CBS activities resulted from altered enzyme expression rather than mutations in coding regions.[545] Among 111 Irish subjects with premature vascular disease, no heterozygotes for the G307S mutation were found,[546] although this mutation accounts for 71 percent of the CBS mutations in that population.[258] The I278T mutation that predominates among the Dutch was not found in 60 such patients with cardiovascular disease.[543] Similarly, a search by Evers et al for the G307S mutation, the IVS11-2 A > C mutation, or mutations at Lys 119 (the PLP binding site) failed to show abnormalities among 27 subjects selected for such studies because of elevated plasma tHcy (tHcy > 15.6 μM) from a group of 125 patients with recent ischemic stroke.[546a] Finally, it has been pointed out by Daly et al that the known proportion of heterozygotes in studied populations is too low to account for the number of observed patients with premature vascular disease and mild elevations of plasma tHcy.[547] An exception to these generally negative results is a report by Dudman et al that the mean CBS activity of fibroblasts cultured from 15 patients with premature vascular disease and impaired homocysteine metabolism detected by methionine loading was 3.68 ± 2.52 nmol/h/mg protein, whereas the mean for fibroblasts from 31 healthy adults was 7.61 ± 4.49 nmol/h/mg protein. However, the scatter of normal values was such that it was not possible to identify individuals heterozygous for CBS deficiency,[548] and later sequencing of CBS cDNA from four of these patients showed that only one was heterozygous for a CBS missense mutation. It was suggested that down-regulation of CBS might explain the depressed CBS activities.[549]

Recently, two studies have been performed that had the potential to reveal mutations of the CBS gene, including those located in noncoding DNA sequences, that affect CBS expression, and the possible association of such mutations with elevation of plasma tHcy and/or increased risk for cardiovascular disease. Kluijtmans and coworkers studied two synonymous polymorphisms, 699C > T and 1080T > C,[84] in the CBS gene in 184 patients with arterial occlusive disease and 87 controls to evaluate the possibility that these were in linkage disequilibrium with functional mutations.[550] Postmethionine-load plasma tHcy concentrations were significantly elevated in individuals with the 699TT genotype as compared to those with 699CC ($P = 0.02$). A similar, but statistically marginally significant, difference was observed between those with the 1080CC and 1080TT genotypes ($P = 0.08$). The authors suggested there may be one or more molecular defects in the CBS gene predisposing individuals to elevated plasma tHcy after methionine loading, but the molecular basis of this association remained to be elucidated. However, no differences were observed between cases and controls for either polymorphism in genotype and haplotype distribution, nor in allele frequencies. De Stefano et al found only slight, statistically insignificant differences in the fasting plasma tHcy values of 785 healthy young European males between those with the differing alleles of the aforementioned polymorphisms or an additional polymorphism, 1985C > T.[550a]

For the moment, the observations from the Kluitjmans study[550] may be similar to those for heterozygotes for inactivating mutations in the coding regions of CBS: both situations lead to mild elevations of plasma tHcy, most marked after methionine loading, but the available evidence suggests that neither are strong risk factors for early vascular disease. Furthermore, there are similarities also to the situation for treated CBS-deficient patients who continue to have (somewhat more marked) elevations of plasma tHcy but to date have been surprisingly free of thromboembolic events. If protective factors (such as those already discussed in the summary portion of the section "Thrombosis and Atherosclerosis," above) are at work in such treated patients, perhaps they may also be present in the heterozygotes and in the individuals with elevated plasma tHcy studied by Kluijtmans et al.[550]

Mild elevation of plasma tHcy has recently been implicated in neural tube defects.[551] However, as is the case for premature vascular disease, the mutant CBS G307S allele was not found at increased frequency among individuals with neural tube defects, nor mothers of such individuals. The same was true of the 68-bp insertion/I278T allele.[552] However, when this insertion coexists with the C677T mutation that leads to thermolability of methylenetetrahydrofolate reductase, there may be some increased risk of spina bifida.[553]

Reproductive Fitness. The obstetrical history of eight women obligate heterozygotes revealed that they had had 34 pregnancies, 4 (12 percent) of which ended in spontaneous abortion. Mean birth weight for the remaining 30 babies was not significantly different from that for the general population. Among the 30 infants, there were three perinatal deaths,[554] a finding of uncertain significance.

Prenatal Diagnosis

Prenatal diagnosis of CBS deficiency is feasible in both the first and the second trimesters of pregnancy. Extracts of cells cultured from amniotic fluid contain readily detectable activity of CBS,[465,555,556] and several pregnancies at risk have been investigated with this method.[8] Fowler and colleagues reported the first diagnosis of an affected fetus[557] and have subsequently identified a second case.[463] In another pregnancy in which the activity of CBS in cultured amniotic cells was lower than could confidently be attributed to a heterozygous fetus, assay of phytohemagglutinin-stimulated fetal lymphocytes obtained in gestational week 23 enabled the exclusion of CBS deficiency.[558] The catalytic activity of CBS in chorionic villi is insufficient for direct assay of the enzyme.[559] Using extracts of cells grown in tissue culture from chorionic villi, however, one CBS-deficient fetus and two unaffected fetuses have been identified before gestational week 12.[560] Options for prenatal diagnosis of CBS deficiency and remethylation defects that lead to homocystinuria have recently been reviewed.[463]

γ-CYSTATHIONASE DEFICIENCY

In 1959, Harris and his colleagues described a 64-year-old, mentally retarded woman who excreted more than 2 mmol of cystathionine daily in her urine.[561] Their studies of this patient, her relatives, and other patients with severe mental retardation led these workers to postulate that the patient had a genetically determined deficiency of γ-cystathionase activity, but that the metabolic disorder might have been only fortuitously associated with mental retardation.

Cystathioninuria

Cystathioninuria or hypercystathioninemia may be due to either underutilization or overproduction of cystathionine. Genetically determined impairment of γ-cystathionase activity often leads to massive cystathioninuria, as discussed below. A much more modest extent of cystathioninuria is often observed in premature infants and others with low birth weights who are fed protein- or methionine-enriched diets.[9] Transient cystathioninuria was detected in 123 of 35,809 apparently normal infants screened at age 6 weeks in Australia.[562] These findings may be explained by the observations that γ-cystathionase is absent in fetal liver tissue but appears in the liver of newborns.[120]

Nongenetic causes of impaired cystathionine utilization include vitamin B_6 deficiency, thyrotoxicosis, and generalized liver disease.[6,9] Both CBS and γ-cystathionase activities are PLP dependent,, but in vitamin B_6-deficient rats the γ-cystathionase holoenzyme contents of the tissues are much more decreased than are the CBS holoenzyme contents.[6] In vitamin B_6-deficient humans, cystathionine synthesis may continue at a rate such that homocystine may be absent from the urine or present only in trace amounts, whereas cystathionine excretion may become quite marked.[563] Vitamin B_6-deficient rats and pigs do have marked rises of plasma Hcy.[9]

Cystathionine is overproduced when a normal amount of CBS is provided with an abnormally elevated concentration of its substrate, homocysteine, as occurs when N^5-methyltetrahydrofolate-homocysteine methyltransferase is unable to function normally. Thus, cystathioninuria/hypercystathioninemia has been noted in patients with genetically determined deficiency of methylenetetrahydrofolate reductase,[564] with cblC mutations,[565] and with dietary deficiencies of vitamin B_{12}[566,567] or folate.[567] The accompanying homocystinuria/elevated plasma tHcy of such patients, and usually the relative mildness of their elevations of cystathionine, provide means of distinguishing them from those with γ-cystathionase deficiency. Moreover, the presence of cystathioninuria distinguishes them from patients with CBS deficiency.

Many functional neural tumors contain relatively high concentrations of cystathionine, and patients with these tumors are cystathioninuric. Since nervous tissue contains relatively more CBS than γ-cystathionase activity, this form of cystathioninuria may represent a local imbalance between production and utilization. Similar imbalances could account for the cystathioninuria reported in some cases of hepatoblastoma.[9]

An unusual type of moderate familial cystathioninuria was suggested by Frimpter and colleagues to be due to a renal defect affecting the transport of this amino acid.[568,569]

The Genetic Defect and Genetic Heterogeneity

Deficient activity of γ-cystathionase in liver and/or in long-term lymphoid cell lines has now been demonstrated in at least ten cystathioninuric individuals. The deficiency was most marked when cell extracts were assayed without added PLP.[6,9] Assays of γ-cystathionase activity in cultured skin fibroblasts is of questionable use because the activity in question has been detected only inconstantly in control cell lines,[6] although the presence of some γ-cystathionase activity is suggested by the report that control fibroblast cultures did form small amounts of ^{35}S-cysteine (detected as ^{35}S-cysteic acid) from ^{35}S-homocysteine.[570]

Homoserine dehydratase activities in the livers of γ-cystathionase-deficient patients are also very low.[571,572] This finding indicates that human γ-cystathionase possesses also homoserine dehydratase activity, as is true of the analogous enzyme from rat liver,[573,574] and that the genetic mutation, or mutations, in the patients studied had affected both activities. No reports have appeared of measurements in γ-cystathionase-deficient patients of the further alternative reactions catalyzed by this enzyme, including cysteine desulfhydrase,[112] homocysteine desulfhydrase,[575] and L-diaminopropionate ammonia lyase.[576]

Several additional enzyme activities involved in sulfur amino acid metabolism have been studied in tissues of cystathioninuric individuals. MAT and CBS activities were normal in extracts of a single γ-cystathionase-deficient liver.[571] Activities of AdoMet decarboxylase and of N^5-methyltetrahydrofolate-homocysteine methyltransferase were within the control ranges in extracts of four lines of γ-cystathionase-deficient, long-term lymphoid cells.[577]

Although enzyme studies have been carried out in relatively few γ-cystathionase-deficient subjects, the data available indicate differences in the properties of the residual activities of γ-cystathionase (when present) and those of normal γ-cystathionase, and between the residual γ-cystathionase activities of different affected individuals: (1) Residual γ-cystathionase activities have in some cases been stimulated more by the addition of PLP to the assay reaction mixture than was control γ-cystathionase activity;[577–579] in other cases, such high stimulation did not occur.[571,580,581] (2) Residual γ-cystathionase activities from two deficient individuals were reported to be sensitized to heat inactivation by PLP, whereas normal γ-cystathionase was stabilized.[582] (3) Immunologic studies of long-term lymphoid lines have shown the absence in one line of γ-cystathionase-deficient cells of material that cross-reacted with rabbit antibody to control human hepatic γ-cystathionase, whereas three such lines did have cross-reacting material. These cross-reacting materials had weak γ-cystathionase activities in the presence of PLP. More detailed immunologic studies suggested there might be differences between the cross-reacting materials of these three lines.[577,579] As with CBS deficiency, these results strongly suggest genetic heterogeneity among the lesions that produce γ-cystathionase deficiency and that most mutations causing deficient activity of γ-cystathionase lie in the structural gene for this enzyme.

Additional Patients Without Enzyme Data

As just discussed, γ-cystathionase deficiency has been clearly demonstrated in at least ten cystathioninuric patients. Without pyridoxine treatment, and on unrestricted diets, these patients excreted from 1000 to 5800 μmol cystathionine daily in their urine. A search of published and unpublished records[8] revealed at least 37 additional patients with cystathionine excretions comparable to the excretions of those proven to be γ-cystathionase deficient.[9] As discussed previously in more detail,[6] in what follows the patients with proven γ-cystathionase deficiency as well as the 37 additional patients with presumptive deficiency are referred to as the γ-cystathionase-deficient group.

Mode of Inheritance

Although no quantitative assays of γ-cystathionase activity in livers of obligate heterozygotes have been published, studies of long-term cultured lymphoid lines do suggest an autosomal recessive mode of inheritance.[577] The γ-cystathionase-specific activities in extracts of such cells cultured from five parents of γ-cystathionase-deficient children ranged from 11.2 to 18.9 nmol/mg protein per hour (assayed in the presence of 0.25 mM PLP), with a mean of 15.8 ± 1.5 (SE). A total of 21 control lymphocyte lines had a mean specific activity of 25.8 ± 1.7, with a range from 12.5 to 47.5; three cystathioninuric patients, offspring of the parents in question, had specific activities ranging from 3.6 to 7.3. Thus, the parents had intermediate values, but there was extensive overlap with the lower end of the control range.

Cystathionine excretions, measured in a number of parents of γ-cystathionase-deficient subjects under various experimental conditions, are not inconsistent with autosomal recessive inheritance.[7] In general, such parents on normal diets have had at most very moderate elevations of cystathionine compared to those of normal adults,[6,583] whereas those receiving oral methionine loads have tended to have more abnormal postload increases in cystathionine excretion.

Metabolic Sequelae

γ-Cystathionase-deficient patients not only excrete abnormal amounts of cystathionine in their urine but accumulate elevated concentrations of this amino acid in their body fluids and tissues. Plasma cystathionine concentrations have been presented for 17 pyridoxine-responsive patients. In 16, the concentrations were definitely elevated, ranging from 10 to 60 μM,[9] whereas none was detected in one patient.[584] Two B_6-nonresponsive patients had plasma cystathionine concentrations of 6 to 80 μM.[585,586] Although cystathionine has not been detected in normal human serum or plasma by most conventional methods, recent application of gas chromatographic/mass spectrometric methodology detected a mean concentration of cystathionine in normal human serum of 140 nM, with a range of 65 to 301 nM.[567]

Cystathionine concentrations in CSF have been 10, 1, and 0.5 μM, and "not detected."[9] Control values were not listed, but only traces (i.e., <1 μM) of cystathionine are present in normal CSF.[587]

Tissues from one patient, obtained post mortem, were examined for cystathionine. The concentrations were: liver, 1.3

to 2.0 μmol/g (control range, 0.05 to 0.9); kidney, 0.56 to 0.82 μmol/g (none detected in control kidney); and frontal lobe of brain, 2.6 to 3.0 μmol/g (control range, 0.22 to 0.35).[561,588] A liver biopsy specimen from a patient not responsive to B_6 contained 9.6 μmol/g.[589]

In addition to cystathionine, most γ-cystathionase-deficient patients excrete substantial amounts of *N*-acetylcystathionine.[9] Published values range from 134 to 474 μmol/day.

A number of additional sulfur-containing compounds have been identified in urine from two cystathioninuric sisters studied intensively by Kodama and associates.[590] These compounds fall into three groups:

1. *Cystathionine sulfoxide*. Small amounts of this oxidation product of cystathionine were isolated from a large pooled urine sample. It is not certain whether the sulfoxide was formed in vivo or during the isolation procedure.[590]

2. *Compounds formed from either cystathionine or* N-*acetylcystathionine by transamination, followed by either reduction, decarboxylation, or cyclization*. The structure of these compounds and the pathways proposed for their formation have been detailed previously.[7] More recently, *N*-acetyl-*S*-(3-oxo-3-carboxy-*n*-propyl)cysteine, *S*-(3-oxo-3-carboxy-*n*-propyl)cysteine, *S*-(2-oxo-2-carboxyethyl)homocysteine, cyclic cystathionine sulfoxide, and cyclic *N*-acetylcystathionine have been added to this list.[591–593] The sulfoxides in question may arise by oxidation of the corresponding cystathionine derivatives.[593] Two enzymic reactions of the proposed pathways have been studied in vitro: A bovine kidney transaminase acting upon cystathionine to form *S*-(2-oxo-2-carboxyethyl)-homocysteine was highly purified and its properties studied.[594] The keto compound may be reduced to the corresponding hydroxy analogue by lactate dehydrogenase, or it may undergo cyclization to a cystathionine ketimine.[595] The latter compound has been detected as a normal metabolite in human brain.[596]

3. *Very minor amounts of* S-*(3-hydroxy-3-carboxy-*n-*propylthio)-homocysteine and* S*(β-carboxyethylthio)-homocysteine*.[597] These compounds are present in homocystinuric urine and are thought to derive from Hcy.[8] Their presence in cystathioninuric urine is unexplained.

Little evidence has emerged to suggest that γ-cystathionase-deficient patients have functional lacks of sulfur-containing metabolites formed distal to the metabolic block. In contrast to the decreased plasma cystine concentrations often found in CBS-deficient patients, plasma cystine concentrations have been reported as normal in γ-cystathionase-deficient subjects.[9] Possible explanations for this difference have been discussed,[7] but there are ample reasons to believe that at least those γ-cystathionase-deficient individuals with detected residual activities of this enzyme retain the capacity to form substantial amounts of cysteine,[7] although the metabolic pathway by which this occurs has not been clarified.

A convenient experimental animal model in which to study the metabolic sequelae of decreased γ-cystathionase activity is provided by the use of propargylglycine, an irreversible inhibitor of γ-cystathionase.[598] Following injection of this substance into mice[598] or rats,[599] hepatic γ-cystathionase activity decreased rapidly,[598,599] whereas CBS activity was unaffected in either liver[599] or brain.[600,601] The treated rats accumulated cystathionine in both cytosol and mitochondria of liver[602] and in brain,[600,601] and excreted large amounts of cystathionine, *N*-acetylcystathionine, and secondary products formed by the aforementioned pathways: *S*-(carboxymethyl)homocysteine, *S*-(2-hydroxy-2-carboxyethyl)-homocysteine, *S*-(3-hydroxy-3-carboxy-*n*-propyl)cysteine, and *S*-(β-carboxyethyl)cysteine.[599,603] The same compounds, as well as the *N*-acetyl derivatives of the latter two, accumulated in liver, kidney, and serum.[599,604] Other compounds more recently identified in urine include perhydro-1,4-thiazepine-3,5-dicarboxylic acid, cystathionine mono-oxo acids, cystathionine ketimines, cystathionine sulfoxide, and *N*-acetylcystathionine sulfoxide.[605] The pattern of appearance of these metabolites suggests that the major pathway in propargylglycine-treated rats is monodeamination of cystathionine with subsequent formation of cystathionine ketimines and perhydro-1,4-thiazepine-3,5-dicarboxylic acid.[605a]

The Pyridoxine Effect and Its Mechanism

γ-Cystathionase deficiency provided the first instance in which, in a human, the major biochemical abnormality due to a defined enzyme defect was clearly shown to be alleviated by administration of large doses of pyridoxine.[606] The majority of γ-cystathionase-deficient patients encountered (33 of the 37 classified in this respect) respond to high intakes of vitamin B_6 with major decreases in urinary cystathionine excretion. Four patients have shown little or no response. The decrease in urinary cystathionine excretion may be accompanied by an increase in urinary sulfate[606] or by an increase in the ratio of urinary sulfate to total urinary sulfur,[607] although the increment in sulfate is small compared with the basal rate of sulfate excretion and has not been detected in all studies.[608]

Although cystathioninuria is a prominent manifestation of vitamin-B_6 deficiency,[563,609] the response in γ-cystathionase-deficient patients is not attributable to correction of a preexisting deficiency of this vitamin.[7] The factors affecting pyridoxine responsiveness or nonresponsiveness in γ-cystathionase-deficient patients are strongly reminiscent of the analogous situation in CBS-deficient patients. Thus, (1) responsiveness or nonresponsiveness in γ-cystathionase deficiency has so far been constant within sibships,[8] and (2) there is a correlation between the presence of detected residual activity of γ-cystathionase and clinical responsiveness to B_6 and between the absence of detected residual activity and nonresponsiveness. Adequately sensitive assays have demonstrated low residual activities of γ-cystathionase in liver extracts of three of three B_6-responsive subjects studied (although no activities were detected in a separate family of three γ-cystathionase-deficient B_6-responsive sibs when assays were performed that required at least 6 percent of control activity for detection). With cultured cells, activities were detected in one fibroblast line and three long-term lymphoid lines from four B_6-responsive individuals but not in the single lymphoid line studied from a B_6-nonresponsive subject. Residual γ-cystathionase activities in tissue extracts from B_6-responsive subjects have shown variable enhancements upon addition of PLP to enzyme assay mixtures, ranging from 1.3-fold to as much as 50-fold. In no instance has γ-cystathionase activity been restored to normal by even the highest concentration of PLP.[9]

A considerable body of evidence suggests that normal humans have a large reserve capacity of γ-cystathionase in comparison to the amount of cystathionine metabolized during intake of a normal diet.[7] As already discussed, pyridoxine responsiveness in γ-cystathionase deficiency probably depends on the presence of at least a small residual activity of the deficient enzyme. The steady-state activity of this enzyme is presumably enhanced somewhat when a patient is taking large doses of B_6 and becomes sufficient to metabolize the cystathionine arising from a normal methionine intake without accumulation severe enough to produce cystathioninuria. The molecular mechanism (or mechanisms) of the enhancement requires further clarification.

Clinical Manifestations

Following the discovery of γ-cystathionase deficiency in a mentally retarded individual,[561] the search for cystathioninuric patients was initially concentrated on the mentally retarded. The resulting ascertainment bias may have fostered the early impression that γ-cystathionase deficiency is a cause of mental abnormalities. In addition to mental retardation, a wide assortment of other clinical aberrations has been found occasionally in individuals with presumptive γ-cystathionase deficiency. Among these are convulsions, hypoplastic genitalia, acromegaly, thrombocytopenia, urinary calculi, nephrogenic diabetes insipidus, and insulin-dependent diabetes mellitus.[8] It is doubtful, however, that any clinical abnormalities result specifically from γ-cystathionase deficiency. Among the 26 known γ-cystathionase-deficient patients for whom ascertainment bias may be expected to be minimal, only five have clinical aberrations that could be related to the metabolic disorder, and for four of these either additional cystathioninuric sibs are normal, or sibs without severe γ-cystathionase deficiency are equally affected clinically.[8] Even among the four known individuals with B_6-nonresponsive cystathioninuria, in whom the biochemical defect may be more complete than in those with B_6-responsive cystathioninuria, only one is mentally retarded, and he was ascertained by screening conducted because of mental retardation. No clinical information has been published about one, and the remaining two were normal at last follow-up at ages 1[610] or 25 years.[507]

Maternal γ-Cystathionase Deficiency. We are aware of two pregnancies in a woman with B_6-nonresponsive γ-cystathionase deficiency followed by us since infancy.[458,507] The first pregnancy was uncomplicated. Plasma and urinary cystathionine levels were 14 μM and 1706 μmol/g creatinine, respectively, during the pregnancy. The baby girl was normal at birth and has continued to grow and develop normally with a mental development index of 112 at age 1 year and a normal score on the Vineland Adaptive Behavior Scales at age 2 years. This woman has now had a second pregnancy, also uncomplicated, during which her plasma and urinary cystathionine levels were 9 μM and 1647 μmol/g creatinine, respectively.

Diagnosis

The characteristic finding in γ-cystathionase deficiency is a specific cystathioninuria readily demonstrable by amino acid analysis. In γ-cystathionase deficiency, metabolites of cystathionine may be present, most notably *N*-acetylcystathionine (see the section "Metabolic Sequelae," above), but homocystine will be absent. Should the latter be present also, the presence of a homocysteine methylation defect should be considered rather than γ-cystathionase deficiency.

It is important that the urine examined for cystathioninuria be clean and contain preservative (such as thymol or toluene) that inhibits bacterial growth. Microorganisms contain β-cystathionase, an enzyme that cleaves cystathionine to homocysteine and pyruvate. Thus, in a contaminated urine sample, cystathionine may be converted to Hcy, and confusion may result.[458]

Cystathioninuria per se does not establish the diagnosis of inherited γ-cystathionase deficiency. Whenever cystathioninuria is discovered, the alternative causes of this abnormality mentioned and detailed previously[6] should be ruled out. When cystathioninuria has been established as persistent and of an apparently primary nature, a trial of supplemental pyridoxine may be given to establish whether the disorder is vitamin B_6-responsive. Initially, oral pyridoxine hydrochloride in amounts of 100 mg/day should be administered. If there is no decrease in urinary cystathionine after 2 weeks, the dose of pyridoxine hydrochloride may be increased by 100 mg and the urine examined for cystathionine at the end of another 2 weeks.

Although the diagnosis can be confirmed by measurement of γ-cystathionase activity in liver obtained by biopsy, even the small risk entailed in a liver biopsy militates against such confirmation of this probably benign disorder. Enzymatic analysis of a cultured lymphoid cell line is an alternative means of diagnosis.[9]

Management

Since γ-cystathionase deficiency is probably a benign disorder, no specific management is indicated. For individuals responsive to pyridoxine, oral pyridoxine hydrochloride can be given in daily doses of 100 mg, or somewhat more, without known risk.[611] The amount necessary can best be judged by titration aimed at elimination or substantial reduction of the cystathioninemia/uria. Possibly a low-methionine diet would also reduce the accumulation of cystathionine. Such a diet might be considered for B_6-nonresponsive patients if further experience indicates they are at risk for specific clinical complications.

Prevalence and Screening

In Australia, screening of 1,000,000 infants disclosed three subjects with persistent cystathioninuria severe enough to lead to a presumptive diagnosis of γ-cystathionase deficiency, a prevalence of 1:333,000.[612] In Quebec, screening of more than one million newborns by thin-layer chromatography of urine collected between 14 and 21 days of age ascertained eight with cystathioninuria, an incidence of 1:124,000.[612a] In Massachusetts, among 1,028,581 newborns screened by paper chromatography of urine, 14 children with persistent severe cystathioninuria were discovered, a prevalence of 1:73,000.[520]

REFERENCES

1. Cornforth JW, Reichard SA, Talalay P, Carrell HL, Glusker JP: Determination of the absolute configuration at the sulfonium center of *S*-adenosylmethionine: Correlation with the absolute configuration of the diasteromeric *S*-carboxymethyl-(*S*)-methionine salts. *J Am Chem Soc* **99**:7292, 1977.
2. Klee WA, Mudd SH: The conformation of ribonucleosides in solution: The effect of structure on the orientation of the base. *Biochemistry* **6**:988, 1967.
3. Follmann H, Gremels G: Adenine nucleosides in solution: Stabilization of the *anti*-conformation by C-5′ substituents. *Eur J Biochem* **47**:187, 1974.
4. Ishida T, Morimoto H, Inoue M, Fujiwara T, Tomita KI: Three-dimensional x-ray crystal structure of *S*-adenosyl-L-homocysteine, a potent inhibitor of *S*-adenosylmethionine-dependent methyltransferases. *J C S Chem Comm* **1**:671, 1981.
5. Mudd SH, Poole JR: Labile methyl balances for normal humans on various dietary regimens. *Metabolism* **24**:721, 1975.
6. Mudd SH, Levy HL, Skovby F: Disorders of transsulfuration, in Scriver CR, Beaudet AL, Sly WS, et al (eds): *The Metabolic and Molecular Bases of Inherited Disease*, 7th ed. New York, McGraw-Hill, 1995, p 1279.
7. Mudd SH, Levy HL: Disorders of transsulfuration, in Stanbury JB, Wyngaarden JB, Frederickson DS (eds): *The Metabolic Basis of Inherited Disease*, 4th ed. New York, McGraw-Hill, 1978, p 458.
8. Mudd SH, Levy HL: Disorders of transsulfuration, in Stanbury JB, Wyngaarden JB, Frederickson DS, et al (eds): *The Metabolic Basis of Inherited Disease*, 5th ed. New York, McGraw-Hill, 1983, p 522.
9. Mudd SH, Levy HL, Skovby F: Disorders of transsulfuration, in Scriver CR, Beaudet AL, Sly WS, et al (eds): *The Metabolic Basis of Inherited Disease*, 6th ed. New York, McGraw-Hill, 1989, p 693.
10. Mudd SH: The adenosyltransferases, in Boyer PD (ed): *The Enzymes*: Part A, vol 8, 3d ed. New York, Academic, 1973, p 121.
11. Kotb M, Mudd SH, Mato JM, Geller AM, Kredich NM, Chou JY, Cantoni GL: Consensus nomenclature for the mammalian methionine adenosyltransferase genes and gene products. *Trends Genet* **13**:51, 1996.
12. Chamberlin ME, Ubagai T, Mudd SH, Wilson WG, Leonard JV, Chou JY: Demyelination of the brain is associated with methionine adenosyltransferase I/III deficiency. *J Clin Invest* **98**:1021, 1996.
13. De la Rosa J, Ostrowski J, Hryniewicz MM, Kredich NM, Kotb M, LeGros HL Jr, Valentine M, et al: Chromosomal localization and catalytic properties of the recombinant α subunit of human lymphocyte methionine adenosyltransferase. *J Biol Chem* **270**:21,860, 1995.
14. Sakata SF, Shelly LL, Ruppert S, Schutz G, Chou JY: Cloning and expression of murine *S*-adenosylmethionine synthetase. *J Biol Chem* **268**:13,978, 1993.
15. Ubagai T, Lei K-J, Huang S, Mudd SH, Levy HL, Chou JY: Molecular mechanisms of an inborn error of methionine pathway: Methionine adenosyltransferase deficiency. *J Clin Invest* **96**:1943, 1995.
16. Horikawa S, Tsukada K: Molecular cloning and developmental expression of a human kidney *S*-adenosylmethionine synthetase. *FEBS Lett* **312**:37, 1992.
17. Horikawa S, Sasuga J, Shimizu K, Ozasa H, Tsukada K: Molecular cloning and nucleotide sequence of cDNA encoding the rat kidney *S*-adenosylmethionine synthetase. *J Biol Chem* **265**:13,683, 1990.

18. Horikawa S, Tsukada K: Molecular cloning and nucleotide sequence of cDNA encoding the human liver *S*-adenosylmethionine synthetase. *Biochem Int* **25**:81, 1991.
19. Kotb M, Geller AM: Methionine adenosyltransferase: Structure and function. *Pharmacol Ther* **59**:125, 1993.
20. Liau MC, Chang CF, Belanger L, Grenier A: Correlation of isozyme patterns of *S*-adenosylmethionine synthetase with fetal stages and pathological states of the liver. *Cancer Res* **39**:162, 1979.
21. Kunz GL, Hoffman JL, Chia C-S, Stremel B: Separation of rat liver methionine adenosyltransferase isozymes by hydrophobic chromatography. *Arch Biochem Biophys* **202**:565, 1980.
22. Suma Y, Shimizu K, Tsukada K: Isozymes of *S*-adenosylmethionine synthetase from rat liver: Isolation and characterization. *J Biochem (Tokyo)* **100**:67, 1986.
23. Cabrero C, Puerta J, Alemany S: Purification and comparison of two forms of *S*-adenosyl-L-methionine synthetase from rat liver. *Eur J Biochem* **170**:299, 1987.
24. Shimizu K, Maruyama I, Iijima S, Tsukada K: Tripolyphosphatase associated with *S*-adenosylmethionine synthetase isozymes from rat liver. *Biochim Biophys Acta* **883**:293, 1986.
25. Sullivan DM, Hoffman JL: Fractionation and kinetic properties of rat liver and kidney methionine adenosyltransferase isozymes. *Biochemistry* **22**:1636, 1983.
26. Geller AM, Kotb MYS, Jernigan HM Jr, Kredich NM: Purification and properties of rat lens methionine adenosyltransferase. *Exp Eye Res* **43**:997, 1986.
27. Kotb M, Kredich NM: Regulation of human lymphocyte *S*-adenosylmethionine synthetase by product inhibition. *Biochim Biophys Acta* **1039**:253, 1990.
28. Mato JM, Alvarez L, Ortiz P, Pajares MA: *S*-Adenosylmethionine synthesis: Molecular mechanisms and clinical implications. *Pharmacol Ther* **73**:265, 1997.
29. Hiroki T, Horikawa S, Tsukada K: Structure of the rat methionine adenosyltransferase 2A gene and its promoter. *Eur J Biochem* **250**:653, 1997.
30. Mingorance J, Alvarez L, Pajares MA, Mato JM: Recombinant rat liver *S*-adenosyl-L-methionine synthetase tetramers and dimers are in equilibrium. *Int J Biochem Cell Biol* **29**:485, 1997.
31. Shimizu-Saito K, Horikawa S, Kojima N, Shiga J, Senoo H, Tsukada K: Differential expression of *S*-adenosylmethionine synthetase isozymes in different cell types of rat liver. *Hepatology* **26**:424, 1997.
32. Tabor H, Rosenthal SM, Tabor CW: The biosynthesis of spermidine and spermine from putrescine and methionine. *J Biol Chem* **233**:907, 1958.
33. Farooqui JZ, Lee HW, Kim S, Paik WK: Studies on compartmentation of *S*-adenosyl-L-methionine in *Saccharomyces cerevisiae* and isolated rat hepatocytes. *Biochim Biophys Acta* **757**:342, 1983.
34. Mudd SH: Biochemical mechanisms in methyl group transfer, in Fishman WH (ed): *Metabolic Conjugation and Metabolic Hydrolysis*, vol 3. New York, Academic, 1973, p 297.
35. Mudd SH, Ebert MH, Scriver CR: Labile methyl group balances in the human: The role of sarcosine. *Metabolism* **29**:707, 1980.
36. Cantoni GL, Richards HH, Chiang PK: Inhibitors of *S*-adenosylhomocysteine hydrolase and their role in the regulation of biological methylation, in Usdin E, Borchardt RT, Creveling CR (eds): *Transmethylation*. New York, Elsevier/North-Holland, 1979, p 155.
37. Hoffman DR, Cornatzer WE, Duerre JA: Relationship between tissue levels of *S*-adenosylmethionine, *S*-adenosylhomocysteine, and transmethylation reactions. *Can J Biochem* **57**:56, 1979.
38. Helland S, Ueland PM: Effect of 2′-deoxycoformycin infusion on *S*-adenosylhomocysteine hydrolase and the amount of *S*-adenosylhomocysteine and related compounds in tissues of mice. *Cancer Res* **43**:4142, 1983.
39. Finkelstein JD, Kyle WE, Harris BJ, Martin JJ: Methionine metabolism in mammals: Concentration of metabolites in rat tissues. *J Nutr* **112**:1011, 1982.
40. Richards HH, Chiang PK, Cantoni GL: Adenosylhomocysteine hydrolase: Crystallization of the purified enzyme and its properties. *J Biol Chem* **253**:4476, 1978.
41. Doskeland SO, Ueland PM: Comparison of some physicochemical and kinetic properties of *S*-adenosylhomocysteine hydrolase from bovine liver, bovine adrenal cortex and mouse liver. *Biochim Biophys Acta* **708**:185, 1982.
42. Fujioka M, Takata Y: *S*-Adenosylhomocysteine hydrolase from rat liver: Purification and some properties. *J Biol Chem* **256**:1631, 1981.
43. Hershfield MS, Francke U: The human genes for *S*-adenosylhomocysteine hydrolase and adenosine deaminase are syntenic on chromosome 20. *Science* **216**:739, 1982.
44. Merta A, Aksamit RR, Kasir J, Cantoni GL: The gene and pseudogenes of rat *S*-adenosyl-L-homocysteine hydrolase. *Eur J Biochem* **229**:575, 1995.
45. Miller MW, Duhl DMJ, Winkes BM, Arredondo-Vega F, Saxon PJ, Wolff GL, Epstein CJ, et al: The mouse *lethal nonagouti* (a^x) mutation deletes the *S-adenosylhomocysteine hydrolase* (*Ahcy*) gene. *EMBO J* **13**:1806, 1994.
46. Ogawa H, Gomi T, Mueckler MM, Fujioka M, Backlund PS, Aksamit RR, Unson CG, et al: Amino acid sequence of *S*-adenosyl-L-homocysteine hydrolase from rat liver as derived from the cDNA sequence. *Proc Natl Acad Sci USA* **84**:719, 1987.
47. Arredonondo-Vega FX, Charlton JA, Edwards YH, Hopkinson DA, Whitehouse DB: Isozyme and DNA analysis of human *S*-adenosyl-L-homocysteine hydrolase (AHCY). *Ann Hum Genet* **53**:157, 1989.
48. Coulter-Karis DE, Hershfield MS: Sequence of full length cDNA for human *S*-adenosylhomocysteine hydrolase. *Ann Hum Genet* **53**:169, 1989.
49. Turner MA, Dole K, Yuan C-S, Hershfield MS, Borchardt RT, Howell PL: Crystallization and preliminary X-ray analysis of human placental *S*-adenosylhomocysteine hydrolase. *Acta Crystallogr* **D53**:339, 1997.
50. Yeh JC, Borchardt RT, Vedani A: A molecular model for the active site of *S*-adenosyl-L-homocysteine hydrolase. *J Comput Aided Mol Des* **5**:213, 1991.
51. Labrune P, Perignon JL, Rault M, Brunet C, Lutun H, Charpentier C, Saudubray JM, et al: Familial hypermethioninemia partially responsive to dietary restriction. *J Pediatr* **117**:220, 1990.
52. Chiang PK: Biological effects of inhibitors of *S*-adenosylhomocysteine hydrolase. *Pharmacol Ther* **77**:115, 1998.
53. Klee WA, Richards HH, Cantoni GL: The synthesis of methionine by enzymic transmethylation: VII. Existence of two separate homocysteine methylpherases in mammalian liver. *Biochim Biophys Acta* **54**:157, 1961.
54. Skiba WE, Taylor MP, Wells MS, Mangum JH, Awad WM Jr: Human hepatic methionine biosynthesis: Purification and characterization of betaine-homocysteine *S*-methyltransferase. *J Biol Chem* **257**:14,944, 1982.
55. Shi X, Millian N, Garrow T: Purification of human recombinant betaine-homocysteine methyltransferase (BHMT) expressed in *Escherichia coli* (*E. coli*) [abstr]. *FASEB J* **11**:A609, 1997.
56. Garrow TA, Millian NS, Park EI, et al: The influence of nutrition on rat betaine-homocysteine methyltransferase expression and preliminary characterization of recombinant human BHMT as a zinc metalloenzyme, in Mato JM, Caballero A (eds): *Methionine Metabolism: Molecular Mechanisms and Clinical Implications*. Madrid, CSIC, 1998, p 63.
56a. Millian NS, Garrow TA: Human betaine-homocysteine methyltransferase is a zinc metalloenzyme. *Arch Biochem Biophys* **356**:93, 1998.
57. Garrow TA: Purification, kinetic properties, and cDNA cloning of mammalian betaine-homocysteine methyltransferase. *J Biol Chem* **271**:22,831, 1996.
58. Sunden SLF, Renduchintala MS, Park EI, Miklasz SD, Garrow TA: Betaine-homocysteine methyltransferase expression in porcine and human tissues and chromosomal localization of the human gene. *Arch Biochem Biophys* **345**:171, 1997.
59. Park EI, Renduchintala MS, Garrow TA: Diet-induced changes in hepatic betaine-homocysteine methyltransferase activity are mediated by changes in the steady-state level of its mRNA. *Nutr Biochem* **8**:541, 1997.
59a. Park EI, Garrow TA: Interaction between dietary methionine and methyl donor intake on rat liver betaine-homocysteine methyltransferase gene expression and organization of the human gene. *J Biol Chem* **274**:7816, 1999.
60. Goulding CW, Matthews RG: Cobalamin-dependent methionine synthase from *Escherichia coli*: Involvement of zinc in homocysteine activation. *Biochemistry* **36**:15,749, 1997.
61. Finkelstein JD, Harris BJ, Martin JJ, Kyle WE: Regulation of hepatic betaine-homocysteine methyltransferase by dietary methionine. *Biochem Biophys Res Commun* **108**:344, 1982.
62. Emmert JL, Webel DM, Biehl RR, Griffiths MA, Garrow LS, Garrow TA, Baker DH: Hepatic and renal betaine-homocysteine methyltransferase activity in pigs as affected by dietary intakes of sulfur amino acids, choline, and betaine. *J Anim Sci* **76**:606, 1998.

63. Finkelstein JD, Martin JJ: Inactivation of betaine-homocysteine methyltransferase by adenosylmethionine and adenosylethionine. *Biochem Biophys Res Commun* **118**:14, 1984.
64. Lundberg P, Dudman NPB, Kuchel PW, Wilcken DEL: ^{1}H NMR determination of urinary betaine in patients with premature vascular disease and mild homocysteinemia. *Clin Chem* **41**:275, 1995.
65. Taylor RT, Weissbach H: N^5-Methyltetrahydrofolate-homocysteine methyltransferases, in Boyer PD (ed): *The Enzymes: Part B*, vol 9, 3d ed. New York, Academic, 1973, p 121.
66. Leclerc D, Campeau E, Goyette P, Adjalla CE, Christensen B, Ross M, Eydoux P, et al: Human methionine synthase: cDNA cloning and identification of mutations in patients of the *cblG* complementation group of folate/cobalamin disorders. *Hum Mol Genet* **5**:1867, 1996.
67. Gulati S, Baker P, Li YN, Fowler B, Kruger W, Brody LC, Banerjee R: Defects in human methionine synthase in cblG patients. *Hum Mol Genet* **5**:1859, 1996.
68. Fowler B, Schutgens RBH, Rosenblatt DS, Smit GPA, Lindemans J: Folate-responsive homocystinuria and megaloblastic anemia in a female patient with functional methionine synthase deficiency (cblE disease). *J Inherited Metab Dis* **20**:731, 1997.
69. Leclerc D, Wilson A, Dumas R, Gafuik C, Song D, Watkins D, Heng HHQ, et al: Cloning and mapping of a cDNA for methionine synthase reductase, a flavoprotein defective in patients with homocystinuria. *Proc Natl Acad Sci USA* **95**:3059, 1998.
70. Rosenblatt DS, Cooper BA, Pottier A, Lue-Shing H, Matiaszuk N, Grauer K: Altered vitamin B_{12} metabolism in fibroblasts from a patient with megaloblastic anemia and homocystinuria due to a new defect in methionine biosynthesis. *J Clin Invest* **74**:2149, 1984.
71. Shih VE, Axel SM, Tewksbury JC, Watkins D, Cooper BA, Rosenblatt DS: Defective lysosomal release of vitamin B_{12} (cblF): A hereditary cobalamin metabolic disorder associated with sudden death. *Am J Med Genet* **33**:555, 1989.
72. Vassiliadis A, Rosenblatt DS, Cooper BA, Bergeron JJM: Lysosomal cobalamin accumulation in fibroblasts from a patient with an inborn error of cobalamin metabolism (cblF complementation group): Visualization by electron microscope radiography. *Exp Cell Res* **195**:295, 1991.
73. Cooper BA, Rosenblatt DS: Inherited defects of vitamin B_{12} metabolism. *Annu Rev Nutr* **7**:291, 1987.
74. Fenton WA, Rosenberg LE: Inherited disorders of cobalamin transport and metabolism, in Scriver CR, Beaudet AL, Sly WS, et al (eds): *The Metabolic Basis of Inherited Disease*, 6th ed. New York, McGraw-Hill, 1989, p 2065.
75. Rosenblatt DS: Inherited disorders of folate transport and metabolism, in Scriver CR, Beaudet AL, Sly WS, et al (eds): *The Metabolic Basis of Inherited Disease*, 6th ed. New York, McGraw-Hill, 1989, p 2049.
76. Skovby F, Krassikoff N, Francke U: Assignment of the gene for cystathionine β-synthase to human chromosome 21 in somatic cell hybrids. *Hum Genet* **65**:291, 1984.
77. Kraus JP, Williamson CL, Firgaira FA, Yang-Feng TL, Münke M, Francke U, Rosenberg LE: Cloning and screening with nanogram amounts of immunopurified mRNAs: cDNA cloning and chromosomal mapping of cystathionine β-synthase and the β subunit of propionyl-CoA carboxylase. *Proc Natl Acad Sci USA* **83**:2047, 1986.
78. Münke M, Kraus JP, Ohura T, Francke U: The gene for cystathionine β-synthase (CBS) maps to the subtelomeric region on human chromosome 21q and to proximal mouse chromosome 17. *Am J Hum Genet* **42**:550, 1988.
79. Stubbs L, Kraus J, Lehrach H: The α-A-crystallin and cystathionine β-synthase genes are physically very closely linked in proximal mouse chromosome 17. *Genomics* **7**:284, 1990.
80. Kraus JP: Molecular analysis of cystathionine β-synthase: A gene on chromosome 21. *Prog Clin Biol Res* **360**:201, 1990.
81. Swaroop M, Bradley K, Ohura T, Tahara T, Roper MD, Rosenberg LE, Kraus JP: Rat cystathionine β-synthase: Gene organization and alternative splicing. *J Biol Chem* **267**:11,455, 1992.
82. Roper MD, Kraus JP: Rat cystathionine β-synthase: Expression of four alternatively spliced isoforms in transfected cultured cells. *Arch Biochem Biophys* **298**:514, 1992.
83. Roper MD, Straubhaar JR, Kraus E, Sokolová J, Hrebicek M, Kraus JP: Comparison of the 5′ end of the rat and mouse cystathionine β-synthase genes. *Mamm Genome* **7**:754, 1996.
84. Kraus JP, Le K, Swaroop M, Ohura T, Tahara T, Rosenberg LE, Roper MD, et al: Human cystathionine β-synthase cDNA: Sequence, alternative splicing and expression in cultured cells. *Hum Mol Genet* **2**:1633, 1993.
85. Bao L, Vlcek C, Paces V, Kraus JP: Identification and tissue distribution of human cystathionine beta-synthase messenger-RNA isoforms. *Arch Biochem Biophys* **350**:95, 1998.
86. Chassé JF, Paul V, Escañez R, Kamoun P, London J: Human cystathionine β-synthase: Gene organization and expression of different 5′ alternative splicing. *Mamm Genome* **8**:917, 1997.
87. Locker JGT, Gill TJ III, Kraus JP, Ohura T, Swaroop M, Riviere M, Islam MQ, et al: The rat MHC and cystathionine β-synthase are syntenic on chromosome 20. *Immunogenetics* **31**:271, 1990.
88. Kraus JP, Oliveriusova J, Sokolova J, Kraus E, Vlcek C, de Franchis R, Maclean KN, et al: The human cystathionine β-synthase (CBS) gene: Complete sequence, alternative splicing and polymorphisms. *Genomics* **52**:312, 1998.
89. Sebastio G, Sperandeo MP, Panico M, de Franchis R, Kraus J, Andria G: The molecular basis of homocystinuria due to cystathionine β-synthase deficiency in Italian families, and report of four novel mutations. *Am J Hum Genet* **56**:1324, 1995.
90. Sperandeo MP, de Franchis R, Andria G, Sebastio G: A 68-bp insertion found in a homocystinuric patient is a common variant and is skipped by alternative splicing of the cystathionine β-synthase mRNA. *Am J Hum Genet* **59**:1391, 1996.
91. Tsai MY, Bignell M, Schwichtenberg K, Hanson NQ: High prevalence of a mutation in the cystathionine β-synthase gene. *Am J Hum Genet* **59**:1262, 1996.
92. Kluijtmans LAJ, Boers GHJ, Trijbels FJM, Van Lith-Zanders HMA, Van den Heuvel LPWJ, Blom HJ: A common 844INS68 insertion variant in the cystathionine β-synthase gene. *Biochem Mol Med* **62**:23, 1997.
92a. Franco RF, Elion J, Lavinha J, Krishnamoorthy R, Tavella MH, Zago MA: Heterogeneous ethnic distribution of the 844ins68 in the cystathionine β-synthase gene. *Hum Hered* **48**:338, 1998.
93. Orendac M, Muskova B, Richterova F, Zvarova J, Stefek M, Zaykova E, Stribrny J, et al: Mutation C677T in the MTHFR gene and polymorphism 844ins68bp in the CBS gene: Risk factors for peripheral arterial occlusive disease. *Neth J Med* **52**(suppl):S47, 1998.
93a. Orendac M, Muskova B, Richterova F, Zvarova J, Stefek M, Zaykova E, Kraus JP, et al: Is the common 844ins68 polymorphism in the cystathionine β-synthase gene associated with atherosclerosis? *J Inherited Metab Dis* **22**:674, 1999.
94. Skovby F, Kraus JP, Rosenberg LE: Biosynthesis of human cystathionine β-synthase in cultured fibroblasts. *J Biol Chem* **259**:583, 1984.
95. Kraus JP, Rosenberg LE: Cystathionine β-synthase from human liver: Improved purification scheme and additional characterization of the enzyme in crude and pure form. *Arch Biochem Biophys* **222**:44, 1983.
96. Kraus JP, Packman S, Fowler B, Rosenberg LE: Purification and properties of cystathionine β-synthase from human liver. *J Biol Chem* **253**:6523, 1978.
97. Bukovska G, Kery V, Kraus JP: Expression of human cystathionine β-synthase in *Escherichia coli*: Purification and characterization. *Protein Exp Purif* **5**:442, 1994.
98. Kruger WD, Cox DR: A yeast system for expression of human cystathionine β-synthase: Structural and functional conservation of the human and yeast genes. *Proc Natl Acad Sci USA* **91**:6614, 1994.
99. Kery V, Bukovska G, Kraus JP: Transsulfuration depends on heme in addition to pyridoxal 5′-phosphate: Cystathionine β-synthase is a heme protein. *J Biol Chem* **269**:25283, 1994.
100. Kimura H, Nakagawa H: Studies on cystathionine synthetase: Characteristics of purified rat liver enzyme. *J Biochem (Tokyo)* **69**:711, 1971.
101. Brown FC, Gordon PH: Cystathionine synthase from rat liver: Partial purification and properties. *Can J Biochem* **49**:484, 1971.
102. Kery V, Poneleit L, Meyer J, Manning M, Kraus JP: Binding of pyridoxal 5′-phosphate to the heme protein human cystathionine β-synthase. *Biochemistry* **38**:2716, 1999.
103. Kery V, Poneleit L, Kraus JP: Trypsin cleavage of human cystathionine β-synthase into an evolutionary conserved active core: Structural and functional consequences. *Arch Biochem Biophys* **355**:222, 1998.
104. Shan X, Kruger WD: Correction of disease-causing *CBS* mutations in yeast. *Nat Genet* **19**:91, 1998.
105. Borcsok E, Abeles RH: Mechanism of action of cystathionine synthase. *Arch Biochem Biophys* **213**:695, 1982.
106. Braunstein AE, Goryachenkova EV: The β-replacement-specific pyridoxal-*P*-dependent lyases. *Adv Enzymol* **56**:1, 1984.

107. Kraus JP: Molecular basis of phenotype expression in homocystinuria. *J Inherited Metab Dis* **17**:383, 1994.
108. Donald LJ, Wang HS, Hamerton JL: Assignment of the gene for cystathionase (CTH) to human chromosome 16. *Cytogenet Cell Genet* **32**:268, 1982.
108a. Erickson PF, Maxwell IH, Su L-J, Baumann M, Glode LM: Sequence of cDNA for rat liver cystathionine γ-lyase and comparison of deduced amino acid sequence with related *Escherichia coli* enzymes. *Biochem J* **269**:335, 1990.
109. Lu Y, O'Dowd BF, Orrego H, Israel Y: Cloning and nucleotide sequence of human liver cDNA encoding for cystathionine γ-lyase. *Biochem Biophys Res Commun* **189**:749, 1992.
110. Churchich JE: Pyridoxal phosphate enzymes catalyzing γ elimination or replacement, in Dolphin D, Poulson R, Avramovic O (eds): *Vitamin B_6: Pyridoxal Phosphate—Chemical, Biochemical, and Medical Aspects (Part B)*. New York, John Wiley and Sons, 1986, p 311.
111. Sato A, Nishioka M, Awata S, Nakayama K, Okada M, Horiuchi S, Okabe N, et al: Vitamin B_6 deficiency accelerates turnover of cystathionase in rat liver. *Arch Biochem Biophys* **330**:409, 1996.
112. Loiselet J, Chatagner F: Purification et étude de quelques propriétés de la cystéine désulfurase "soluble" (cystathionase) du foie de rat. *Bull Soc Chim Biol* **47**:33, 1965.
112a. Steeghorn C, Clausen T, Sondermann P, Jacob U, Worbs M, Marinkovic S, Huber R, et al: Kinetics and inhibition of recombinant human cystathionine γ-lyase: Toward the rational control of transsulfuration. *J Biol Chem* **274**:12,675, 1999.
113. Zeisel SH: Choline deficiency. *J Nutr Biochem* **1**:332, 1990.
114. Storch KJ, Wagner DA, Burke JF, Young VR: Quantitative study in vivo of methionine cycle in humans using [methyl-$^2H_3$]- and [1-^{13}C]methionine [abstr]. *Am J Physiol* **255**:E322, 1988.
115. Storch KJ, Wagner DA, Young VR: Methionine kinetics in adult men: Effects of dietary betaine on L-[$^2H_3$-methyl-1-^{13}C]methionine. *Am J Clin Nutr* **54**:386, 1991.
116. Young VR, Yu Y-M, Fukagawa NK, Raguso CA: Methionine kinetics and balance, in Graham I, Refsum H, Rosenberg IH, et al (eds): *Homocysteine Metabolism: From Basic Science to Clinical Medicine*. Boston, Kluwer Academic, 1997, p 11.
117. Finkelstein JD: The metabolism of homocysteine: pathways and regulation. *Eur J Pediatr* **157**(suppl 2):S40, 1998.
118. Mudd SH: Homocystinuria and homocysteine metabolism: Selected aspects, in Nyhan WL (ed): *Heritable Disorders of Amino Acid Metabolism*. New York, John Wiley and Sons, 1974, p 429.
119. Davies SEC, Woolf DA, Chalmers RA, Rafter JEM, Iles RA: Proton NMR studies of betaine excretion in the human neonate: Consequences for choline and methyl group supply. *J Nutr Biochem* **3**:523, 1992.
120. Sturman JA, Gaull GE, Räihä NCR: Absence of cystathionase in human fetal liver: Is cystine essential? *Science* **169**:74, 1970.
121. Viña J, Vento M, García-Sala F, Puertes IR, Gascó E, Sastre J, Asensi M, et al: l-Cysteine and glutathione metabolism are impaired in premature infants due to cystathionase deficiency. *Am J Clin Nutr* **61**:1067, 1995.
122. Case GL, Benevenga NJ: Evidence for *S*-adenosylmethionine independent catabolism of methionine in the rat. *J Nutr* **106**:1721, 1976.
123. Mitchell AD, Benevenga NJ: The role of transamination in methionine oxidation in the rat. *J Nutr* **108**:67, 1978.
124. Steele RD, Benevenga NJ: Identification of 3-methylthiopropionic acid as an intermediate in mammalian methionine metabolism in vitro. *J Biol Chem* **253**:7844, 1978.
125. Steele RD, Benevenga NJ: The metabolism of 3-methylthiopropionate in rat liver homogenates. *J Biol Chem* **254**:8885, 1979.
126. Asche GL, Benevenga NJ, Haas LG: Metabolism of L-methionine (MET) and 3-methylthiopropionate (MTP) by the pig. *FASEB J* **2**:A1765, 1988.
127. Livesey G, Lund P: Methionine metabolism via the transamination pathway in rat liver. *Biochem Soc Trans* **8**:540, 1980.
128. Livesey G: Metabolism of "essential" 2-oxo acids by liver and a role for branched-chain oxo acid dehydrogenase in the catabolism of methionine, in Walser M, Williamson JR (eds): *Metabolism and Clinical Implications of Branched Chain Amino and Ketoacids*. New York, Elsevier, 1980, p 143.
129. Cooper AJL: Biochemistry of sulfur-containing amino acids. *Annu Rev Biochem* **52**:187, 1983.
130. Livesey G: Methionine degradation: "Anabolic and catabolic." *Trends Biochem Sci* **9**:27, 1984.
131. Scislowski PWD, Pickard K: Methionine transamination: Metabolic function and subcellular compartmentation. *Mol Cell Biochem* **129**:39, 1993.
132. Jones SMA, Yeaman SJ: Oxidative decarboxylation of 4-methylthio-2-oxobutyrate by branched-chain 2-oxo acid dehydrogenase complex. *Biochem J* **237**:621, 1986.
133. Mårtensson J: The occurrence of 4-methylthio-2-hydroxybutyrate in human urine. *Anal Biochem* **154**:43, 1986.
134. Kaji H, Saito N, Murao M, Ishimoto M, Kondo H, Gasa S, Saito K: Gas chromatographic and gas chromatographic-mass spectrometric studies on α-keto-γ-methyl-thiobutyric acid in urine following ingestion of optical isomers of methionine. *J Chromatogr* **221**:145, 1980.
135. Kaji H, Saito K, Saito N, Hisamura M, Ishimoto M, Kondo H: Simple gas chromatographic analysis of 3-methylthiopropionate in human urine. *J Chromatogr* **272**:166, 1983.
136. Kaji H, Hisamura M, Saito N, Murao M: Biochemical aspect of dimethyl sulfide breath test in the studies on methionine metabolism. *Res Commun Chem Pathol Pharmacol* **32**:515, 1981.
137. Mudd SH, Levy HL, Tangerman A, Boujet C, Buist N, Davidson-Mundt A, Hudgins L, et al: Isolated persistent hypermethioninemia. *Am J Hum Genet* **57**:882, 1995.
138. Laster L, Mudd SH, Finkelstein JD, Irreverre F: Homocystinuria due to cystathionine synthase deficiency: The metabolism of L-methionine. *J Clin Invest* **44**:1708, 1965.
139. Jakubowski H, Goldman E: Synthesis of homocysteine thiolactone by methionyl-tRNA synthetase in cultured mammalian cells. *FEBS Lett* **317**:237, 1993.
140. Jakubowski H: Metabolism of homocysteine thiolactone in human cell cultures: Possible mechanism for pathological consequences of elevated homocysteine levels. *J Biol Chem* **272**:1935, 1997.
141. Antonio CM, Nunes MC, Refsum H, Abraham AK: A novel pathway for the conversion of homocysteine to methionine in eukaryotes. *Biochem J* **328**:165, 1997.
142. Gaull GE, Tallan HH: Methionine adenosyltransferase deficiency: New enzymatic defect associated with hypermethioninemia. *Science* **186**:59, 1974.
143. Finkelstein JD, Kyle WE, Martin JJ: Abnormal methionine adenosyltransferase in hypermethioninemia. *Biochem Biophys Res Commun* **66**:1491, 1975.
144. Gout J-P, Serre J-C, Dieterlen M, Antener I, Frappat P, Bost M, Beaudoing A: Une nouvelle cause d'hypermethioninemie de l'enfant: Le deficit en *S*-adenosyl-methionine-synthetase. *Arch Fr Pediatr* **34**:416, 1977.
145. Guizar-Vazquez J, Sanchez-Aguilar G, Velazquez A, Fragoso R, Rostenberg I, Alejandre I: Hipermetioninemia: A propósito de un caso en un matrimonio consanguíneo. *Bol Med Hosp Infant Mex* **37**:1237, 1980.
146. Gaull GE, Tallan HH, Lonsdale D, Przyrembel H, Schaffner F, Von Bassewitz DB: Hypermethioninemia associated with methionine adenosyltransferase deficiency: Clinical, morphological and biochemical observations on four patients. *J Pediatr* **98**:734, 1981.
147. Gaull GE, Bender AN, Vulovic D, Tallan HH, Schaffner F: Methioninemia and myopathy: A new disorder. *Ann Neurol* **9**:423, 1981.
148. Congdon PJ, Haigh D, Smith R, Green A, Pollitt RJ: Hypermethioninaemia and 3-hydroxyisobutyric aciduria in an apparently healthy baby. *J Inherited Metab Dis* **4**:79, 1981.
149. Tsuchiyama A, Oyanagi K, Nakata F, Uetsuji N, Tsugawa S, Nakao T, Mori M: A new type of hypermethioninemia in neonates. *Tohoku J Exp Med* **138**:281, 1982.
150. Hase Y, Sawada Y, Tsuruhara T, Kobayashi Y, Ohtake H, Miyagi T, Oura T, et al: Hypermethioninemia associated with hepatic methionine adenosyltransferase deficiency: Report of two cases. *Acta Paediatr Jpn* **26**:565, 1984.
151. Uetsuji N: Genetical and biochemical studies in patients with congenital hypermethioninemia. *J Clin Pediatr (Sapporo)* **34**:167, 1986.
152. Gahl WA, Finkelstein JD, Mullen KD, Bernardini I, Martin JJ, Backlund P, Ishak KG, et al: Hepatic methionine adenosyltransferase deficiency in a 31-year-old man. *Am J Hum Genet* **40**:39, 1987.
153. Gahl WA, Bernardini I, Finkelstein JD, Tangerman A, Martin JJ, Blom HK, Mullen KD, et al: Transsulfuration in an adult with hepatic methionine adenosyltransferase deficiency. *J Clin Invest* **81**:390, 1988.
154. Boujet C, Joannard A, Favier A: Urinary metabolic profiles in a case of methionine adenosyl transferase deficiency, in *Symposium, Society*

for the Study of Inborn Errors of Metabolism, UK, Birmingham, 1990.
155. Surtees R, Leonard J, Austin S: Association of demyelination with deficiency of cerebrospinal-fluid *S*-adenosylmethionine in inborn errors of methyl-transfer pathway. *Lancet* **338**:1550, 1991.
156. Blom HJ, Davidson AJ, Finkelstein JD, Luder AS, Bernardini I, Martin JJ, Tangerman A, et al: Persistent hypermethioninaemia with dominant inheritance. *J Inherited Metab Dis* **15**:188, 1992.
157. Nagao M, Oyanagi K: Molecular characterization of persistent hypermethioninemia with dominant inheritance [abstr 61], in *39th Meeting of the Japanese Society of Inherited Metabolic Disease, Nov 14–16, 1996*, Tokyo, Japan 40, 1996.
158. Chamberlin ME, Ubagai T, Mudd SH, Levy HL, Chou JY: Dominant inheritance of isolated hypermethioninemia is associated with a mutation in the human methionine adenosyltransferase 1A gene. *Am J Hum Genet* **60**:540, 1997.
159. Nagao M, Oyanagi K: Genetic analysis of isolated persistent hypermethioninemia with dominant inheritance. *Acta Paediatr Jpn* **39**:601, 1997.
160. Hazelwood S, Bernardini I, Tangerman A, Guo J, Shotelersuk V, Mudd SH, Gahl WA: Lack of brain demyelination in a patient homozygous for a mutation encoding a severely truncated methionine adenosyltransferase I/III. *Am J Med Genet* **75**:395, 1998.
161. Nagao M: Personal communication, 1997.
162. Mudd SH, Chamberlin ME, Chou JY: Isolated persistent hypermethioninemia: Genetic, metabolic, and clinical aspects, in Mato JM (ed): *Methionine Metabolism: Molecular Mechanisms and Clinical Implications*. Madrid, CSIC, 1998, p1.
163. Hoffman JL, Kunz GL: Differential activation of rat liver methionine adenosyltransferase isozymes by dimethylsulfoxide. *Biochem Biophys Res Commun* **77**:1231, 1977.
164. Okada G, Teraoka H, Tsukada K: Multiple species of mammalian *S*-adenosylmethionine synthetase: Partial purification and characterization. *Biochemistry* **20**:934, 1981.
165. Tallan HH, Cohen PA: Methionine adenosyltransferase: Kinetic properties of human and rat liver enzymes. *Biochem Med* **16**:234, 1976.
166. Chamberlin ME, Ubagai T, Mudd SH, Thomas J, Pao VY, Nguyen TK, Greene CL, Thomas JA, et al: Methionine adenosyltransferase I/III deficiency: Novel mutations and clinical variations. *Am J Hum Genet* **66**:347, 2000.
167. Antonarakis SE, and the Nomenclature Working Group: Recommendations for a nomenclature system for human gene mutations. *Hum Mutat* **11**:1, 1998.
168. Loehrer FMT, Haefeli WE, Angst CP, Browne G, Frick G, Fowler B: Effect of methionine loading on 5-methyltetrahydrofolate, *S*-adenosylmethionine and *S*-adenosylhomocysteine in plasma of healthy humans. *Clin Sci* **91**:79, 1996.
169. Baldessarini RJ: Alterations in tissue levels of *S*-adenosylmethionine. *Biochem Pharmacol* **15**:741, 1966.
170. Wagner C, Capdevila A: Measurement of plasma *S*-adenosylmethionine and *S*-adenosylhomocysteine as their fluorescent isoindoles *Anal Biochem* **265**:180, 1998.
171. Wagner C, Capdevila A, Mudd SH: Unpublished observations, 1998.
172. Takusagawa F, Kamitori S, Misaki S, Markham GD: Crystal structure of *S*-adenosylmethionine synthetase. *J Biol Chem* **271**:136, 1996.
173. Takusagawa F, Kamitori S, Markham GD: Structure and function of *S*-adenosylmethionine synthetase: Crystal structures of *S*-adenosylmethionine synthetase with ADP, BrADP, and PP_i at 2.8 Å resolution. *Biochemistry* **35**:2586, 1996.
174. Thomas JA, Freehauf C, Greene CL: Personal communication, 1997.
175. Surtees R: Demyelination and inborn errors of the single carbon transfer pathway. *Eur J Pediatr* **157**(suppl 2):S118, 1998.
176. Wilson WG: Personal communication, 1998.
177. Gandy G, Jacobson W, Sidman R: Inhibition of a transmethylation reaction in the central nervous system: An experimental model for subacute combined degeneration of the cord. *J Physiol (Lond)* **233**:1P, 1973.
178. Lee C-C, Surtees R, Duchen LW: Distal motor axonopathy and central nervous system myelin vacuolation caused by cycloleucine, an inhibitor of methionine adenosyltransferase. *Brain* **115**:935, 1992.
179. Bianchi R, Calzi F, Bellasio R, Savaresi S, Galbete JL, Tsankova V, Tacconi MT: Role of methyl groups in myelination [abstr]. *J Periph Nerv Syst* **2**:84, 1997.
180. Lombardini JB, Sufrin JR: Chemotherapeutic potential of methionine analogue inhibitors of tumor-derived methionine adenosyltransferases. *Biochem Pharmacol* **32**:489, 1983.
181. Mitsui K, Teraoka H, Tsukada K: Complete purification and immunochemical analysis of *S*-adenosylmethionine synthetase from bovine brain. *J Biol Chem* **263**:11,211, 1988.
182. Gomes-Trolin C, Löfberg C, Trolin G, Oreland L: Brain ATP:L-methionine *S*-adenosyltransferase (MAT), *S*-adenosylmethionine (SAM) and *S*-adenosylhomocysteine (SAH): Regional distribution and age-related changes. *Eur Neuropsychopharmacol* **4**:469, 1994.
183. Gomes-Trolin C, Gottfries CG, Regland B, Oreland L: Influence of vitamin B_{12} on brain methionine adenosyltransferase activity in senile dementia of the Alzheimer's type. *J Neural Transm* **103**:861, 1996.
184. Reichel A, Chishty M, Begley DJ, Nunn P, Abbott NJ: Carrier-mediated transport of *S*-adenosylmethionine across the blood-brain barrier in vitro. *J Physiol (Lond)* **505P**:48P, 1997.
185. Jenden DJ, Roch M, Booth RA: Simultaneous measurement of endogenous and deuterium-labeled tracer variants of choline and acetylcholine in subpicomole quantities by gas chromatography/mass spectrometry. *Anal Biochem* **55**:438, 1973.
186. Freeman JJ, Choi RL, Jenden DJ: Plasma choline, its turnover and exchange with brain choline. *J Neurochem* **24**:729, 1975.
187. Jenden DJ, Mudd SH: Unpublished observations, 1998.
188. Buchman AL, Dubin M, Jenden D, Moukarzel A, Roch MH, Rice K, Gornbein J, et al: Lecithin increases plasma free choline and decreases hepatic steatosis in long-term total parenteral nutrition patients. *Gastroenterology* **102**:1363, 1992.
189. Mudd SH, Tangerman A, Levy HL, Jenden DJ, Wagner C, Capdevila A, Kotb M: Unpublished observations, 1998.
190. Field CMB, Carson NAJ, Cusworth DC, Dent CE, Neill DW: Homocystinuria: A new disorder of metabolism [abstr], in *Abstracts of the Tenth International Congress of Pediatrics (Lisbon) 274*, 1962.
191. Carson NAJ, Neill DW: Metabolic abnormalities detected in a survey of mentally backward individuals in Northern Ireland. *Arch Dis Child* **37**:505, 1962.
192. Mudd SH, Finkelstein JD, Irreverre F, Laster L: Homocystinuria: An enzymatic defect. *Science* **143**:1443, 1964.
193. Refsum H, Helland S, Ueland PM: Radioenzymic determination of homocysteine in plasma and urine. *Clin Chem* **31**:624, 1985.
194. Araki A, Sako Y: Determination of free and total homocysteine in human plasma by high-performance liquid chromatography with fluorescence detection. *J Chromatogr* **422**:43, 1987.
195. Andersson A, Brattström L, Israelsson B, Isaksson A, Hamfelt A, Hultberg B: Plasma homocysteine before and after methionine loading with regard to age, gender, and menopausal status. *Eur J Clin Invest* **22**:79, 1991.
196. Mansoor MA, Svardal AM, Ueland PM: Determination of the in vivo redox status of cysteine, cysteinylglycine, homocysteine, and glutathione in human plasma. *Anal Biochem* **200**:218, 1992.
197. Mansoor MA, Svardal AM, Schneede J, Ueland PM: Dynamic relation between reduced, oxidized and protein-bound homocysteine and other thiol components in plasma during methionine loading in healthy men. *Clin Chem* **38**:1316, 1992.
198. Gupta VJ, Wilcken DEL: The detection of cysteine-homocysteine mixed disulphide in plasma of normal fasting man. *Eur J Clin Invest* **8**:205, 1978.
199. Wilcken DEL, Gupta VJ: Cysteine-homocysteine mixed disulphide: Differing plasma concentrations in normal men and women. *Clin Sci* **57**:211, 1979.
200. Kang S-S, Wong PWK, Becker N: Protein-bound homocyst(e)ine in normal subjects and in patients with homocystinuria. *Pediatr Res* **13**:1141, 1979.
201. Perry TL, Hansen S, MacDougall L, Warrington PD: Sulfur-containing amino acids in the plasma and urine of homocystinurics. *Clin Chim Acta* **15**:409, 1967.
202. Perry TL, Hansen S: Technical pitfalls leading to errors in the quantitation of plasma amino acids. *Clin Chim Acta* **25**:53, 1969.
203. Ueland PM, Refsum H, Stabler SP, Malinow MR, Andersson A, Allen RH: Total homocysteine in plasma or serum: Methods and clinical applications. *Clin Chem* **39**:1764, 1993.
204. Refsum H, Fiskerstrand T, Guttormsen AB, Ueland PM: Assessment of homocysteine status. *J Inherited Metab Dis* **20**:286, 1997.
205. Refsum H, Ueland PM, Nygård O, Vollset SE: Homocysteine and cardiovascular disease. *Annu Rev Med* **49**:31, 1998.
206. Reddy MN: Reference ranges for total homocysteine in children [abstr]. *Clin Chim Acta* **262**:153, 1997.
207. Vilaseca MA, Moyano D, Ferrer I, Artuch R: Total homocysteine in pediatric patients. *Clin Chem* **43**:690, 1997.

208. Refsum H, Guttormsen AB, Fiskerstrand T, Ueland PM: Hyperhomocysteinemia in terms of steady-state kinetics. *Eur J Pediatr* **157**(suppl 2):S45, 1998.
209. Bostom A, Brosnan JT, Hall B, Nadeau MR, Selhub J: Net uptake of plasma homocysteine by the rat kidney in vivo. *Atherosclerosis* **116**:59, 1995.
210. Brosnan JT, Hall B, Selhub J, Nadeau MR, Bostom AG: Renal metabolism of homocysteine in vivo [abstr]. *Biochem Soc Trans* **23**:470S, 1995.
211. House JD, Brosnan ME, Brosnan JT: Renal homocysteine metabolism. *Contrib Nephrol* **121**:79, 1997.
212. House JD, Brosnan ME, Brosnan JT: Characterization of homocysteine metabolism in the rat kidney. *Biochem J* **328**:287, 1997.
212a. House JD, Brosnan ME, Brosnan JT: Renal uptake and excretion of homocysteine in rats with acute hyperhomocysteinemia. *Kidney Int* **54**:1601, 1998.
213. Bostom AG, Shemin D, Lapane KL, Miller JW, Sutherland P, Nadeau M, Seyoum E, et al: Hyperhomocysteinemia and traditional cardiovascular disease risk factors in end-stage renal disease patients on dialysis: A case-control study. *Atherosclerosis* **114**:93, 1995.
214. Bostom AG, Shemin D, Verhoef P, Nadeau MR, Jaques PF, Selhub J, Dworkin L, et al: Elevated fasting total plasma homocysteine levels and cardiovascular disease outcomes in maintenance dialysis patients. *Arterioscler Thromb Vasc Biol* **17**:2554, 1997.
215. Guttormsen AB, Ueland PM, Svarstad E, Refsum H: Kinetic basis of hyperhomocysteinemia in patients with chronic renal failure. *Kidney Int* **52**:495, 1997.
216. Van Guldener C, Donker AJM, Jakobs C, Teerlink T, de Meer K, Stehouwer CDA: No net renal extraction of homocysteine in fasting humans. *Kidney Int* **54**:166, 1998.
217. Arendshorst WJ, Navar LG: Renal circulation and glomerular hemodynamics, in Schrier RW, Gottschalk CW (eds): *Diseases of the Kidney*, vol 1, 5th ed. Boston, Little, Brown, 1993, p 65.
218. Van den Berg M, Boers GHJ: Homocystinuria: What about mild hyperhomocysteinaemia? *Postgrad Med J* **72**:513, 1996.
219. Bakker RC, Brandjes DPM: Hyperhomocysteinemia and associated disease. *Pharm World Sci* **19**:126, 1997.
220. Pietrzik K, Brönstrup A: Causes and consequences of hyperhomocysteinemia. *Int J Vitam Nutr Res* **67**:389, 1997.
221. Bostom AG, Lathrop L: Hyperhomocysteinemia in end-stage renal disease: Prevalence, etiology, and potential relationship to arteriosclerotic outcomes. *Kidney Int* **52**:10, 1997.
222. Lipson MH, Kraus J, Rosenberg LE: Affinity of cystathionine β-synthase for pyridoxal 5′-phosphate in cultured cells: A mechanism for pyridoxine-responsive homocystinuria. *J Clin Invest* **66**:188, 1980.
223. Skovby F, Kraus JP, Rosenberg LE: Homocystinuria: Biogenesis of cystathionine β-synthase subunits in cultured fibroblasts and in an in vitro translation system programmed with fibroblast messenger RNA. *Am J Hum Genet* **36**:452, 1984.
224. De Franchis R, Kozich V, McInnes RR, Kraus JP: Identical genotypes in siblings with different homocystinuric phenotypes: Identification of three mutations in cystathionine β-synthase using an improved bacterial expression system. *Hum Mol Genet* **3**:1103, 1994.
225. Kozich V, Kraus JP: Screening for mutations by expressing patient cDNA segments in *E. coli*: Homocystinuria due to cystathionine β-synthase deficiency. *Hum Mutation* **1**:113, 1992.
226. Kraus JP: Biochemistry and molecular genetics of cystathionine β-synthase deficiency. *Eur J Pediatr* **157**(suppl 2):S50, 1998.
227. De Franchis R, Sperandeo MP, Sebastio G, Andria G, and the Italian Collaborative Study Group on Homocystinuria: Clinical aspects of cystathionine β-synthase deficiency: How wide is the spectrum? *Eur J Pediatr* **157**(suppl 2):S67, 1998.
228. Taoka S, Ohja S, Shan X, Kruger WD, Banerjee R: Evidence for heme-mediated redox regulation of human cystathionine β-synthase. *J Biol Chem* **273**:25,179, 1998.
229. Kozich V, Janosik M, Sokolova J, Mandel H, Kraus JP: Different molecular consequences of intronic and exonic deletions in the CBS gene [abstr]. *J Inherited Metab Dis* **20**(suppl 1):P2.10, 1997.
230. Kozich V, de Franchis R, Kraus JP: Molecular defect in a patient with pyridoxine-responsive homocystinuria. *Hum Mol Genet* **2**:815, 1993.
231. Sperandeo MP, de Franchis R, Amato M, Lucariello S, Candito M, Gatti R, Andria G, et al: Heterogeneity of cystathionine β-synthase gene mutations in Italy [abstr]. *J Inherited Metab Dis* **19**(suppl 1):39, 1996.
232. Shih VE: Unpublished observations, 1998.
233. Kluijtmans LAJ, Boers GHJ, Kraus JP, Van den Heuvel LPWJ, Cruysberg JRM, Trijbels FJM, Blom HJ: The molecular basis of cystathionine β-synthase deficiency in Dutch patients with homocystinuria: Effect of CBS genotype on biochemical and clinical phenotype, and on response to treatment. *Am J Hum Genet* **65**:59, 1999.
234. Marble M, Geraghty MT, de Franchis R, Kraus JP, Valle D: Characterization of a cystathionine β-synthase allele with three mutations *in cis* in a patient with B_6 nonresponsive homocystinuria. *Hum Mol Genet* **3**:1883, 1994.
235. Gordon R: Unpublished observations, 1998.
236. Coudé M, Aupetit J, Zabot MT, Kamoun P, Chadefaux-Vekemans B: Four novel mutations at the cystathionine β-synthase locus causing homocystinuria. *J Inherited Metab Dis* **21**:823, 1998.
237. Shih VE, Fringer JM, Mandell R, Kraus JP, Berry GT, Heidenreich RA, Korson MS, et al: A missense mutation (I278T) in the cystathionine β-synthase gene prevalent in pyridoxine-responsive homocystinuria and associated with mild clinical phenotype. *Am J Hum Genet* **57**:34, 1995.
238. Dawson PA, Cox AJ, Emmerson BT, Dudman NPB, Kraus JP, Gordon RB: Characterisation of five missense mutations in the cystathionine beta-synthase gene from three patients with B_6-nonresponsive homocystinuria. *Eur J Hum Genet* **5**:15, 1997.
239. Gordon RG, Cox AJ, Dawson PA, Emmerson BT, Kraus JP, Dudman NPB: Mutational analysis of the cystathionine β-synthase gene: A splicing mutation, two missense mutations and an insertion in patients with homocystinuria [abstr]. *Hum Mutat* **11**:332, 1998.
240. Kozich V: Unpublished observations, 1998.
241. Kluijtmans LAJ, Blom HJ, Boers GHJ, Van Oost BA, Trijbels FJM, Van den Heuvel LPWJ: Two novel missense mutations in the cystathionine β-synthase gene in homocystinuric patients. *Hum Genet* **96**:249, 1995.
242. Kruger WD, Cox DR: A yeast assay for functional detection of mutations in the human cystathionine β-synthase gene. *Hum Mol Genet* **4**:1155, 1995.
243. Kozich V, Janosik M, Sokolova J, Oliveriusova J, Orendac M, Kraus JP, Elleder D: Analysis of CBS alleles in Czech and Slovak patients with homocystinuria: Report on three novel mutations E176K, W409X and 1223 + 37 del99. *J Inherited Metab Dis* **20**:363, 1997.
244. Kluijtmans LAJ: Unpublished observations, 1998.
245. Kim CE, Gallagher PM, Guttormsen AB, Refsum H, Ueland PM, Ose L, Folling I, et al: Functional modeling of vitamin responsiveness in yeast: A common pyridoxine-responsive cystathionine β-synthase mutation in homocystinuria. *Hum Mol Genet* **6**:2213, 1997.
246. Sperandeo MP, Panico M, Pepe A, Candito M, de Franchis R, Kraus JP, Andria G, et al: Molecular analysis of patients affected by homocystinuria due to cystathionine β-synthase deficiency: Report of a new mutation in exon 8 and a deletion in intron 11. *J Inherited Metab Dis* **18**:211, 1995.
247. Sperandeo MP, de Franchis R, Pepe A, Mandato C, Amato M, Andria G, Sebastio G: A 68 bp insertion in the coding region of the cystathionine beta-synthase gene is polymorphic in the general population and is skipped by an alternative splicing of the mRNA [abstr]. *Am J Hum Genet* **59**:A1654, 1996.
248. Hu FL, Gu Z, Kozich V, Kraus JP, Ramesh V, Shih VE: Molecular basis of cystathionine β-synthase deficiency in pyridoxine responsive and nonresponsive homocystinuria. *Hum Mol Genet* **2**:1857, 1993.
249. De Franchis R, Kraus E, Kozich V, Sebastion G, Kraus JP: Four novel mutations in the cystathionine β-synthase gene: The effect of a second linked mutation on the severity of the homocystinuric phenotype. *Hum Mutation* **13**:453, 1999.
250. Coudé M, Aral B, Zabot MT, Aupetit J, Kamoun P, Chadefaux-Verkemans B: Four mutations at the cystathionine β-synthase locus causing homocystinuria [abstr]. *Ir J Med Sci* **16**(suppl 15):4, 1995.
251. Valle DL: Unpublished observations, 1998.
252. Tsai MY, Wong PWK, Garg U, Hanson NQ, Schwichtenberg K: Two novel mutations in the cystathionine β-synthase gene of homocystinuric patients. *Mol Diagn* **2**:129, 1997.
253. Aral B, Coudé M, London J, Aupetit J, Chassé J-F, Zabot M-T, Chadefaux-Vekemans B, et al: Two novel mutations (K384E and L539S) in the C-terminal moiety of the cystathionine β-synthase protein in two French pyridoxine-responsive homocystinuria patients. *Hum Mutat* **9**:81, 1997.
254. Koch HG: Unpublished observations, 1998.
255. Kluijtmans LAJ, Boers GHJ, Stevens EMB, Renier WO, Kraus JP, Trijbels JMF, Van den Heuvel LPWJ, et al: Defective cystathionine

β-synthase regulation by S-adenosylmethionine in a partially pyridoxine responsive homocystinuria patient. *J Clin Invest* **98**:285, 1996.

256. Koch HG, Ullrich K, Deufel T, Harms E: High prevalence of a splice site mutation in the cystathionine β-synthase gene causing pyridoxine nonresponsive homocystinuria [abstr], in *Sixth International Congress, Inborn Errors of Metabolism, Milan, May 27–31*, Milan, Italy, 1994.
257. Tsai MY, Wong PWK, Garg U, Hanson NQ, Schwichtenberg K: Identification of a splice site mutation in the cystathionine β-synthase gene resulting in variable and novel splicing defects of pre-mRNA. *Biochem Mol Med* **61**:9, 1997.
257a. Gaustadnes M, Ingerslev J, Rütiger N: Prevalence of congenital homocystinuria in Denmark. *N Engl J Med* **340**:1513, 1999.
258. Gallagher PM, Ward P, Tan S, Naughten E, Kraus JP, Sellar GC, McConnell DJ, et al: High frequency (71%) of cystathionine β-synthase mutation G307S in Irish homocystinuria patients. *Hum Mutat* **6**:177, 1995.
259. Sperandeo MP, Candito M, Sebastio G, Rolland MO, Turc-Carel C, Giudicelli H, Dellamonica P, et al: Homocysteine response to methionine challenge in four obligate heterozygotes for homocystinuria and relationship with cystathionine β-synthase mutations. *J Inherited Metab Dis* **19**:351, 1996.
260. Tsai MY, Hanson NQ, Bignell MK, Schwichtenberg KA: Simultaneous detection and screening of $T_{833}C$ and $G_{919}A$ mutations of the cystathionine β-synthase gene by single-strand conformational polymorphism. *Clin Biochem* **29**:473, 1996.
261. Tsai MY: Unpublished observations, 1998.
262. Dawson PA, Cochran DAE, Emmerson BT, Kraus JP, Dudman NPB, Gordon RB: Variable hyperhomocysteinaemia phenotype in heterozygotes for the Gly307Ser mutation in cystathionine β-synthase. *Aust NZ J Med* **26**:180, 1996.
263. Christensen B, Refsum H, Vintermyr O, Ueland PM: Homocysteine export from cells cultured in the presence of physiological or superfluous levels of methionine: Methionine loading of non-transformed, transformed, proliferating, and quiescent cells in culture. *J Cell Physiol* **146**:52, 1991.
264. Malloy MH, Rassin DK, Gaull GE: Plasma cyst(e)ine in homocyst(e)inemia. *Am J Clin Nutr* **34**:2619, 1981.
265. Smolin LA, Benevenga NJ: The use of cyst(e)ine in the removal of protein-bound homocysteine. *Am J Clin Nutr* **39**:730, 1984.
266. Wiley VC, Dudman NPB, Wilcken DEL: Interrelations between plasma free and protein-bound homocysteine and cysteine in homocystinuria. *Metabolism* **37**:191, 1988.
267. Wiley VC, Dudman NPB, Wilcken DEL: Free and protein-bound homocysteine and cysteine in cystathionine β-synthase deficiency: Interrelations during short- and long-term changes in plasma concentrations. *Metabolism* **38**:734, 1989.
268. Mansoor MA, Ueland PM, Aarsland A, Svardal A: Redox status and protein binding of plasma homocysteine and other aminothiols in patients with homocystinuria. *Metabolism* **42**:1481, 1993.
268a. Bonham JR, Moat SJ, Allen JC, Powers HJ, Tanner MS, McDowell I, Bellamy MF: Free homocystine may be a poor measure of control in homocystinuria. *J Inherited Metab Dis* **20**(suppl 1):20, 1997.
269. Barshop BA, Steiner RD: Stable isotope studies of methionine metabolism in homocystinuria [abstr]. *J Invest Med* **46**:130A, 1998.
270. Levy HL, Shih VE, MacCready RA: Screening for homocystinuria in the newborn and mentally retarded population, in Carson NAJ, Raine DN (eds): *Inherited Disorders of Sulphur Metabolism*. London, Churchill Livingstone, 1971, p 235.
271. Mudd SH, Levy HL, Morrow G III: Deranged B_{12} metabolism: Effects on sulfur amino acid metabolism. *Biochem Med* **4**:193, 1970.
272. Mudd SH, Skovby F, Levy HL, Pettigrew KD, Wilcken B, Pyeritz RE, Andria G, et al: The natural history of homocystinuria due to cystathionine β-synthase deficiency. *Am J Hum Genet* **37**:1, 1985.
273. Carson NAJ, Dent CE, Field CMB, Gaull GE: Homocystinuria: Clinical and pathological review of ten cases. *J Pediatr* **66**:565, 1965.
274. Kennedy C, Shih VE, Rowland LP: Homocystinuria: A report in two siblings. *Pediatrics* **36**:736, 1965.
275. Tada K, Yoshida T, Hirono H, Arakawa T: Homocystinuria: Amino acid pattern of the liver. *Tohoku J Exp Med* **92**:325, 1967.
276. Curtius H-CH, Martenet AC, Anders PW: Bestimmung von freien Aminosauren im Augenkammerwasser des Menschen bei Homocystinurie-patienten und Kontrollfallen. *Clin Chim Acta* **19**:469, 1968.
277. Jocelyn PC: Glutathione metabolism in animals, in Crook EM (ed): *Glutathione*. Cambridge, Cambridge University Press, 1959, p 43.
278. Racker E: Glutathione-homocystine transhydrogenase. *J Biol Chem* **217**:867, 1955.
279. Svardal A, Refsum H, Ueland PM: Determination of in vivo protein binding of homocysteine and its relation to free homocysteine in the liver and other tissues of the rat. *J Biol Chem* **261**:3156, 1986.
280. Ueland PM, Helland S, Broch OJ, Schanche JS: Homocysteine in tissues of the mouse and rat. *J Biol Chem* **259**:2360, 1984.
281. Perry TL: Mild elevations of plasma ornithine in homocystinuria. *Clin Chim Acta* **117**:97, 1981.
282. Dudman NPB, Wilcken DEL: Increased plasma copper in patients with homocystinuria due to cystathionine β-synthase deficiency. *Clin Chim Acta* **127**:105, 1983.
283. Dudman NPB, Tyrrell PA, Wilcken DEL: Homocysteinaemia: Depressed plasma serine levels. *Metabolism* **36**:198, 1987.
284. Barber GW, Spaeth GL: Pyridoxine therapy in homocystinuria. *Lancet* **1**:337, 1967.
284a. Carson NAJ, Carré IJ: Treatment of homocystinuria with pyridoxine: A preliminary study. *Arch Dis Child* **44**:387, 1969
285. Morrow G III, Barness LA: Combined vitamin responsiveness in homocystinuria. *J Pediatr* **81**:946, 1972.
286. Wilcken B, Turner B: Homocystinuria: Reduced folate levels during pyridoxine treatment. *Arch Dis Child* **48**:58, 1973.
287. Brenton DP, Cusworth DC: The response of patients with cystathionine synthase deficiency to pyridoxine, in Carson NAJ, Raine DN (eds): *Inherited Disorders of Sulphur Metabolism*. London, Churchill Livingstone, 1971, p 264.
288. Poole JR, Mudd SH, Conerly EB, Edwards WA: Homocystinuria due to cystathionine synthase deficiency: Studies of nitrogen balance and sulfur excretion. *J Clin Invest* **55**:1033, 1975.
289. Mudd SH, Edwards WA, Loeb PM, Brown MS, Laster L: Homocystinuria due to cystathionine synthase deficiency: The effect of pyridoxine. *J Clin Invest* **49**:1762, 1970.
290. Mudd SH: Diseases of sulphur metabolism: Implications for the methionine-homocysteine cycle, and vitamin responsiveness. *Ciba Found Symp* **72**:239, 1980.
291. Mudd SH: Vitamin-responsive genetic abnormalities. *Adv Nutr Res* **4**:1, 1982.
292. Cruysberg JRM, Boers GHJ, Trijbels JMF, Deutman AF: Delay in diagnosis of homocystinuria: Retrospective study of consecutive patients. *BMJ* **313**:1037, 1996.
293. Hong HS, Lee HK, Kwon KH: Homocystinuria presenting with portal vein thrombosis and pancreatic pseudocyst: A case report. *Pediatr Radiol* **27**:802, 1997.
294. Kerrin D, Eaton DM, Livingston J, Henderson M, Smith M: Homocystinuria presenting with sagittal sinus thrombosis in infancy. *J Child Neurol* **11**:70, 1996.
295. Rubba P, Faccenda F, Pauciullo P, Carbone L, Mancini M, Strisciuglio P, Carrozzo R, et al: Early signs of vascular disease in homocystinuria: A noninvasive study by ultrasound methods in eight families with cystathionine-β-synthase deficiency. *Metabolism* **39**:1191, 1990.
296. Parris WCV, Quimby CW: Anesthetic considerations for the patient with homocystinuria. *Anesth Analg* **61**:708, 1982.
297. Abbott MH, Folstein SE, Abbey H, Pyeritz RE: Psychiatric manifestations of homocystinuria due to cystathionine β-synthase deficiency. *Am J Med Genet* **26**:959, 1987.
298. Reish O, Townsend D, Berry SA, Tsai MY, King RA: Tyrosinase inhibition due to interaction of homocyst(e)ine with copper: The mechanism for reversible hypopigmentation in homocystinuria due to cystathionine β-synthase deficiency. *Am J Hum Genet* **57**:127, 1995.
299. Reish O, Berry SA, King RA: Spontaneous hair hyperpigmentation in response to vitamin intake in pregnancy: A clue for homocystinuria. *Am J Obstet Gynecol* **173**:1640, 1995.
300. Bass HN, LaGrave D, Mardach R, Cederbaum SD, Fuster CD, Cherry M: Spontaneous pneumothorax in association with pyridoxine-responsive homocystinuria. *J Inherited Metab Dis* **20**:831, 1997.
301. Newman G, Mitchell JRA: Homocystinuria presenting as multiple arterial occlusions. *Q J Med* **210**:251, 1984.
302. Schulman JD, Mudd SH, Shulman NR, Landvater L: Pregnancy and thrombophlebitis in homocystinuria. *Blood* **56**:326, 1980.
303. Constantine G, Green A: Untreated homocystinuria: A maternal death in a woman with four pregnancies—Case report. *Br J Obstet Gynaecol* **94**:803, 1987.
304. Calvert SM, Rand RJ: A successful pregnancy in a patient with homocystinuria and a previous near-fatal postpartum cavernous sinus thrombosis. *Br J Obstet Gynaecol* **102**:751, 1995.
305. Vargas JE, Rodriquez-Anza S, Shih VE, Waisbren SE, Kurczynski T, Roeder E, Rosengren S, et al: Unpublished observations, 1998.

306. Wildig K, Walter JH, Wraith EW: Outcome in maternal homocystinuria [abstr], in *67th Annual Meeting of the British Paediatric Assocociation*, 1995.
307. Walter JH: Personal communication, 1998.
308. Rajkovic A, Catalano PM, Malinow MR: Elevated homocyst(e)ine levels with preeclampsia. *Obstet Gynecol* **90**:168, 1997.
309. Rodriquez-Anza S, Levy HL: Unpublished observations, 1992.
310. Kurczynski TW, Zacher R: Personal communication, 1992.
311. Wilcken DEL, Wilcken B: The natural history of vascular disease in homocystinuria and the effects of treatment. *J Inherited Metab Dis* **20**:295, 1997.
312. Rand RJ, Parker D: Puerperal cavernous sinus thrombosis: A complication of homocystinuria. *Hosp Update* **16**:167, 1990.
313. Walter JH, Wraith JE, White FJ, Bridge C, Till J: Strategies for the treatment of cystathionine β-synthase deficiency: The experience of the Willink Biochemical Genetics Unit over the past 30 years. *Eur J Pediatr* **157**(suppl 2):S71, 1998.
314. Wilcken B: Personal communication, 1994.
315. Shapiro S, Jones EW, Densen PM: A life table of pregnancy terminations and correlates of fetal loss. *Milbank Mem Fund Q* **70**:7, 1962.
316. McKusick VA: *Heritable Disorders of Connective Tissue*, 3d ed. St Louis, CV Mosby, 1966, p 150.
317. Beighton P, de Paepe A, Hall JG, Hollister DW, Pope FM, Pyeritz RE, Steinmann B, et al: Molecular nosology of heritable disorders of connective tissue. *Am J Med Genet* **42**:431, 1992.
318. Streeten BW: Pathology of the lens, in Albert D, Jakobiec F (eds): *Principles and Practice of Ophthalmology: Clinical Practice*, vol 4. Philadelphia, WB Saunders, 1994, p 2180.
319. Sakai LY, Keene DR, Engvall E: Fibrillin, a new 350-kD glycoprotein, is a component of extracellular microfibrils. *J Cell Biol* **103**:2499, 1986.
320. Sakai LY: Disulfide bonds crosslink molecules of fibrillin in the connective tissue space, in Tamburro A, Davidson J (eds): *Elastin: Chemical and Biological Aspects*. Galatina, Italy, Congedo, 1990, p 213.
321. Magenis RE, Maslen CL, Smith L, Allen L, Sakai LY: Localization of the fibrillin (FBN) gene to chromosome 15, band q21.1. *Genomics* **11**:346, 1991.
322. Irreverre F, Mudd SH, Heizer WD, Laster L: Sulfite oxidase deficiency: Studies of a patient with mental retardation, dislocated ocular lenses, and abnormal urinary excretion of *S*-sulfo-l-cysteine, sulfite, and thiosulfate. *Biochem Med* **1**:187, 1967.
323. McKusick VA: *Heritable Disorders of Connective Tissue*, 4th ed. St Louis, CV Mosby, 1972, p 224.
324. Pyeritz RE: The Marfan syndrome, in Royce PM, Steinmann B (eds): *Connective Tissue and Its Heritable Disorders: Molecular, Genetic, and Medical Aspects*. New York, Wiley-Liss, 1993, p 437.
325. Harris ED Jr, Sjoerdsma A: Collagen profile in various clinical conditions. *Lancet* **2**:707, 1966.
326. Eyre DR, Paz MA, Gallop PM: Cross-linking in collagen and elastin. *Annu Rev Biochem* **53**:717, 1984.
327. Harris ED Jr, Sjoerdsma A: Effect of penicillamine on human collagen and its possible application to treatment of scleroderma. *Lancet* **2**:996, 1966.
328. Nimni ME: A defect in the intramolecular and intermolecular cross-linking of collagen caused by penicillamine: I. Metabolic and functional abnormalities in soft tissues. *J Biol Chem* **243**:1457, 1968.
329. Deshmukh K, Nimni ME: A defect in the intramolecular and intermolecular cross-linking of collagen caused by penicillamine: II. Functional groups involved in the interaction process. *J Biol Chem* **244**:1787, 1969.
330. Jackson SH: The reaction of homocysteine with aldehyde: An explanation of the collagen defects in homocystinuria. *Clin Chim Acta* **45**:215, 1973.
331. Kang AH, Trelstad RL: A collagen defect in homocystinuria. *J Clin Invest* **52**:2571, 1973.
331a. Liu G, Nellaiappan K, Kagan HM: Irreversible inhibition of lysyl oxidase by homocysteine thiolactone and its selenium and oxygen analogues: Implications for homocystinuria. *J Biol Chem* **272**:32,370, 1997.
332. Lubec B, Fang-Kircher S, Lubec T, Blom HJ, Boers GHJ: Evidence for McKusick's hypothesis of deficient collagen cross-linking in patients with homocystinuria. *Biochim Biophys Acta* **1315**:159, 1996.
333. Keene DR, Sakai LY, Burgeson RE: Human bone contains type III collagen, type VI collagen, and fibrillin: Type III collagen is present on specific fibers that may mediate attachment of tendons, ligaments, and periosteum to calcified bone cortex. *J Histochem Cytochem* **39**:59, 1991.
334. D'Angelo A, Selhub J: Homocysteine and thrombotic disease. *Blood* **90**:1, 1997.
335. Rosendaal FR: Risk factors for venous thrombosis: Prevalence, risk and interaction. *Semin Hematol* **34**:171, 1997.
336. McCully KS: Vascular pathology of homocysteinemia: Implications for the pathogenesis of arteriosclerosis. *Am J Pathol* **56**:111, 1969.
337. McCully KS: Homocystinuria, arteriosclerosis, methylmalonic aciduria, and methyltransferase deficiency: A key case revisited. *Nutr Rev* **50**:7, 1992.
338. Kanwar YS, Manaligod JR, Wong PWK: Morphologic studies in a patient with homocystinuria due to 5,10-methylenetetrahydrofolate reductase deficiency. *Pediatr Res* **10**:598, 1976.
339. Baumgartner R, Wick H, Ohnacker H, Probst A, Maurer R: Vascular lesions in two patients with congenital homocystinuria due to different defects of remethylation. *J Inherited Metab Dis* 3:101, 1980.
340. Mohammed R, Lamand M: Cardiovascular lesions in cobalt-vitamin B12 deficient sheep. *Ann Rech Vet* **17**:447, 1986.
340a. McDonald L, Bray C, Field C, Love F, Davies B: Homocystinuria, thrombosis, and the blood-platelets. *Lancet* **1**:745, 1964.
341. Stamler JS, Osborne JA, Jaraki O, Rabbani LE, Mullins M, Singel D, Loscalzo J: Adverse vascular effects of homocysteine are modulated by endothelium-derived relaxing factor and related oxides of nitrogen. *J Clin Invest* **91**:308, 1993.
342. Ammar T, Tabakin B, Bronheim D: Effect of homocysteine on platelet function using flow cytometry [abstr]. *Anesth Analg* **82**:SCA101, 1996.
343. Graeber JE, Slott JH, Ulane RE, Schulman JD, Stuart MJ: Effect of homocysteine and homocystine on platelet and vascular arachidonic acid metabolism. *Pediatr Res* **16**:490, 1982.
343a. Strisciuglio P, Di Minno G, Margaglione M, Cirillo F, Davi G, Cerbone AM, Grandone E, et al: Monocyte superoxide anion generation and in vivo activation of platelets in homocystinuria.. *Am J Hum Genet* **49**(Suppl):166, 1991. (Abstract)
344. Coppola A, Albisinni R, Madonna P, Pagano A, Cerbone AM, Di Minno G: Platelet and monocyte variables in homocystinuria due to cystathionine-β-synthase deficiency. *Haematologica (Pavia)* **82**:189, 1997.
345. Gröbe H, Von Bassewitz DB: Thromboembolische Komplikationen und Thrombocytenanomalien bei Homocystinurie. *Z Kinderheilkd* **112**:309, 1972.
346. Gröbe H, Balleisen L, Stahl K: Platelet function and morphology in homocystinuria. *Pediatr Res* **13**:72, 1979.
347. Uhlemann ER, Tenpas JH, Lucky AW, Schulman JD, Mudd SH, Shulman NR: Platelet survival and morphology in homocystinuria due to cystathionine synthase deficiency. *N Engl J Med* **295**:1283, 1976.
348. Wall RT, Harlan JM, Harker LA, Striker GE: Homocysteine induced endothelial cell injury in vitro: A model for the study of vascular injury. *Thromb Res* **18**:113, 1980.
349. Starkebaum G, Harlan JM: Endothelial cell injury due to copper-catalyzed hydrogen peroxide generation from homocysteine. *J Clin Invest* **1370**, 1986.
350. Schienle HW, Seitz R, Nawroth P, Rohner I, Lerch L, Krumpholz B, Krauss G, et al: Thrombomodulin and ristocetincofactor in homocystinuria: A study of two siblings. *Thromb Res* **77**:79, 1995.
351. Dudman NPB, Hicks C, Lynch JF, Wilcken DEL, Wang J: Homocysteine thiolactone disposal by human arterial endothelial cells and serum in vitro. *Arterioscler Thromb* **11**:663, 1991.
352. Dudman NPB, Hicks C, Wang J, Wilcken DEL: Human arterial endothelial cell detachment in vitro: Its promotion by homocysteine and cysteine. *Arteriosclerosis* **91**:77, 1991.
353. Lentz SR: Minireview: Homocysteine and vascular dysfunction. *Life Sci* **61**:1205, 1997.
354. Lentz SR: Mechanisms of thrombosis in hyperhomocysteinemia. *Curr Opin Hematol* **5**:343, 1998.
355. Rodgers GM, Kane WH: Activation of endogenous factor V by a homocysteine-induced vascular endothelial cell activator. *J Clin Invest* **77**:1909, 1986.
356. Rodgers GM, Conn MT: Homocysteine, an atherogenic stimulus, reduces protein C activation by arterial and venous endothelial cells. *Blood* **75**:895, 1990.

357. Lentz SR, Sadler JE: Inhibition of thrombomodulin surface expression and protein C activation by the thrombogenic agent homocysteine. *J Clin Invest* **88**:1906, 1991.
358. Hayashi T, Honda G, Suzuki K: An atherogenic stimulus homocysteine inhibits cofactor activity of thrombomodulin and enhances thrombomodulin expression in human umbilical vein endothelial cells. *Blood* **79**:2930, 1992.
359. Fryer RH, Wilson BD, Gubler DB, Fitzgerald LA, Rodgers GM: Homocysteine, a risk factor for premature vascular disease and thrombosis, induces tissue factor activity in endothelial cells. *Arterioscler Thromb* **13**:1327, 1993.
360. Hajjar KA: Homocysteine-induced modulation of tissue plasminogen activator binding to its endothelial cell membrane receptor. *J Clin Invest* **91**:2873, 1993.
361. Hajjar KA, Mauri L, Jacovina AT, Zhong F, Mirza UO, Padovan JC, Chait BT: Tissue plasminogen activator binding to the annexin II tail domain: Direct modulation by homocysteine. *J Biol Chem* **273**:9987, 1998.
361a. Hajjar KA, Jacovina AT: Modulation of annexin II by homocysteine: Implications for atherothrombosis. *J Invest Med* **46**:364, 1998.
362. Upchurch GR Jr, Welch GN, Fabian AJ, Freedman JE, Johnson JL, Keaney JF Jr, Loscalzo J: Homocyst(e)ine decreases bioavailable nitric oxide by a mechanism involving glutathione peroxidase. *J Biol Chem* **272**:17,012, 1997.
363. Wang H, Yoshizumi M, Lai K, Tsai J-C, Perrella MA, Haber E, Lee M-E: Inhibition of growth and p21^{ras} methylation in vascular endothelial cells by homocysteine but not cysteine. *J Biol Chem* **272**:25,380, 1997.
364. Upchurch GR Jr, Welch GN, Fabian AJ, Pigazzi A, Keaney JF Jr, Loscalzo J: Stimulation of endothelial nitric oxide production by homocyst(e)ine. *Atherosclerosis* **132**:177, 1997.
364a. Chacko G, Ling Q, Hajjar KA: Induction of acute translational response genes by homocysteine: Elongation factors-122α, -β, and γ. *J Biol Chem* **273**:19,840, 1998.
365. Lentz SR, Sadler JE: Homocysteine inhibits von Willebrand factor processing and secretion by preventing transport from the endoplasmic reticulum. *Blood* **81**:683, 1993.
366. Nishinaga M, Ozawa T, Shimada K: Homocysteine, a thrombogenic agent, suppresses anticoagulant heparan sulfate expression in cultured porcine aortic endothelial cells. *J Clin Invest* **92**:1381, 1993.
367. Wang J, Dudman NPB, Wilcken DEL: Effects of homocysteine and related compounds on prostacyclin production by cultured human vascular endothelial cells. *Thromb Haemost* **70**:1047, 1993.
368. Kokame K, Kato H, Miyata T: Homocysteine-respondent genes in vascular endothelial cells identified by differential display analysis: GRP78/BiP and novel genes. *J Biol Chem* **271**:29,659, 1996.
369. Strydom AJC: The amino acid homocysteine as a atherogenic risk factor: A mechanistical proposition [abstr]. *Ir J Med Sci* **164**(suppl15):19, 1995.
370. Jackson CM: Biochemistry of prothrombin activation, in Bloom AL, Thomas DP (eds): *Haemostasis and Thrombosis*. London, Churchill Livingstone, 1981, p 140.
371. Jackson CM: Mechanisms of prothrombin activation, in Colman RW, Hirsh J, Marder VJ, et al (eds): *Hemostasis and Thrombosis: Basic Principles and Clinical Practice*. Philadelphia, JB Lippincott, 1982, p 100.
372. Esmon CT: The regulation of natural anticoagulant pathways. *Science* **235**:1348, 1987.
373. Rees DC, Cox M, Clegg JB: World distribution of factor V Leiden. *Lancet* **346**:1133, 1995.
374. Zöller B, Hillarp A, Berntorp E, Dahlbäck B: Activated protein C resistance due to a common factor V gene mutation is a major risk factor for venous thrombosis. *Annu Rev Med* **48**:45, 1997.
375. Mandel H, Brenner B, Berant M, Rosenberg N, Lanir N, Jakobs C, Fowler B, et al: Coexistence of hereditary homocystinuria and factor V Leiden: Effect on thrombosis. *N Engl J Med* **334**:763, 1996.
376. Ridker PM, Hennekens CH, Selhub J, Miletich JP, Malinow MR, Stampfer MJ: Interrelation of hyperhomocyst(e)inemia, factor V Leiden, and risk of future venous thromboembolism. *Circulation* **95**:1777, 1997.
377. Cattaneo M, Tsai MY, Bucciarelli P, Taioli E, Zighetti ML, Bignell M, Mannucci PM: A common mutation in the methylenetetrahydrofolate reductase gene (C677T) increases the risk for deep-vein thrombosis in patients with mutant factor V (factor V:Q^{506}) [abstr]. *Blood* **88**(suppl 1):285a, 1996.
378. Kluijtmans LAJ, Boers GHJ, Verbruggen B, Trijbels FJM, Nováková IRO, Blom HJ: Homozygous cystathionine β-synthase deficiency, combined with factor V Leiden or thermolabile methylenetetrahydrofolate reductase in the risk of venous thrombosis. *Blood* **91**:2015, 1998.
379. Quéré I, Lamarti H, Chadefaux-Vekemans B: Thrombophilia, homocystinuria, and mutation of the factor V gene. *N Engl J Med* **335**:289, 1996.
380. Kluijtmans LAJ, den Heijer M, Reitsma PH, Heil SG, Blom HJ, Rosendaal FR: Thermolabile methylenetetrahydrofolate reductase and factor V Leiden in the risk of deep-vein thrombosis. *Thromb Haemost* **79**:254, 1998.
381. D'Angelo A, Fermo I, D'Angelo SV: Thrombophilia, homocystinuria, and mutation of the factor V gene. *N Engl J Med* **335**:289, 1996.
382. Brattström L, Israelsson B, Tengborn L, Hultberg B: Homocysteine, factor VII and antithrombin III in subjects with different gene dosage for cystathionine β-synthase. *J Inherited Metab Dis* **12**:475, 1989.
383. Cattaneo M, Martinelli I, Faioni E, Franchi F, Zighetti ML, Mannucci PM, Bianchi A: High plasma concentrations of activated protein C in patients with deep vein thrombosis and hyperhomocysteinemia [abstr]. *Br J Haematol* **93**(suppl 2):8, 1996.
384. Lentz SR, Sobey CG, Piegors DJ, Bhopatkar MY, Faraci FM, Malinow MR: Vascular dysfunction in monkeys with diet-induced hyperhomocyst(e)inemia. *J Clin Invest* **98**:24, 1996.
385. Celermajer DS, Sorensen K, Ryalls M, Robinson J, Thomas O, Leonard JV, Deanfield JE: Impaired endothelial function occurs in the systemic arteries of children with homozygous homocystinuria but not in their heterozygous parents. *J Am Coll Cardiol* **22**:854, 1993.
386. Tawakol A, Omland T, Gerhard M, Wu JT, Creager MA: Hyperhomocyst(e)inemia is associated with impaired endothelium-dependent vasodilation in humans. *Circulation* **95**:1119, 1997.
387. Woo KS, Chook P, Lolin YI, Cheung ASP, Chan LT, Sun YY, Sanderson JE, et al: Hyperhomocyst(e)inemia is a risk factor for arterial endothelial dysfunction in humans. *Circulation* **96**:2542, 1997.
388. Bellamy MF, McDowell IFW: Putative mechanisms for vascular damage by homocysteine. *J Inherited Metab Dis* **20**:307, 1997.
388a. Bellamy MF, McDowell IFW, Ramsey MW, Brownlee M, Bones C, Newcombe RG, Lewis MJ: Hyperhomocysteinemia after an oral methionine load acutely impairs endothelial function in healthy adults. *Circulation* **98**:1948, 1998.
389. Kanani PM, Sinkey CA, Knapp H, Haynes WG: Acute induction of moderate hyperhomocyst(e)inemia produces endothelial dysfunction in healthy humans [abstr]. *Circulation* **96**(suppl 1):I-418, 1997.
390. Chambers JC, McGregor A, Jean-Marie J, Kooner JS: Acute hyperhomocysteinaemia and endothelial dysfunction. *Lancet* **351**:36, 1998.
391. Hanratty CG, McAuley DF, McGurk C, Young IS, Johnston GD: Homocysteine and endothelial vascular function. *Lancet* **351**:1288, 1998.
392. De Groot PG, Willems C, Boers GHJ, Gonsalves MD, Van Aken WG, Van Mourik JA: Endothelial cell dysfunction in homocystinuria. *Eur J Clin Invest* **13**:405, 1983.
393. Van der Molen EF, Hiipakka MJ, Van Lith-Zanders H, Boers GHJ, Van den Heuvel LPWJ, Monnens LAH, Blom HJ: Homocysteine metabolism in endothelial cells of a patient homozygous for cystathionine β-synthase (CS) deficiency. *Thromb Haemost* **78**:827, 1997.
394. Wang J, Dudman NPB, Wilcken DEL, Lynch JF: Homocysteine catabolism: Levels of three enzymes in cultured human vascular endothelium and their relevance to vascular disease. *Atherosclerosis* **97**:97, 1992.
395. Jacobsen DW, Savon SR, DiCorleto PE: Metabolism of homocysteine by vascular cells and tissues: Is the transsulfuration pathway active? [abstr]. *Ir J Med Sci* **164**(suppl 15):10, 1995.
396. Jacobsen DW, Savon SR, Stewart RW, Robinson K, Green R, Kottke-Mamhant K, DiCorleto PE: Limited capacity for homocysteine catabolism in vascular cells and tissues: A pathophysiologic mechanism for arterial damage in hyperhomocyst(e)inemia [abstr]. *Circulation* **92**(suppl):I-228, 1995.
397. Tang L, Mamotte CDS, Van Bockxmeer FM, Taylor RR: The effect of homocysteine on DNA synthesis in cultured human vascular smooth muscle. *Atherosclerosis* **136**:169, 1998.
398. Tsai J-C, Perrella MA, Yoshizumi M, Hsieh C-M, Haber E, Schlegel R, Lee M-E: Promotion of vascular smooth muscle cell growth by homocysteine: A link to atherosclerosis. *Proc Natl Acad Sci USA* **91**:6369, 1994.

399. Nishio E, Watanabe Y: Homocysteine as a modulator of platelet-derived growth factor action in vascular smooth muscle cells: A possible role for hydrogen peroxide. *Br J Pharmacol* **122**:269, 1997.
400. Tsai J-C, Wang H, Perrella MA, Yoshizumi M, Sibinga NES, Tan LC, Haber E, et al: Induction of cyclin A gene expression by homocysteine in vascular smooth muscle cells. *J Clin Invest* **97**:146, 1996.
401. Lubec B, Labudova O, Hoeger H, Muehl A, Fang-Kircher S, Marx M, Mosgoeller W, et al: Homocysteine increases cyclin-dependent kinase in aortic rat tissue [abstr]. *Circulation* **94**:2620, 1996.
401a. Fritzer-Szekeres M, Blom H, Boers GHJ, Szekeres T, Lubec B: Growth promotion by homocysteine but not by homocysteic acid: A role for excessive growth in homocystinuria or proliferation in hyperhomocysteinemia. *Biochim Biophys Acta* **1407**:1, 1998.
402. Majors A, Ehrhart LA, Pezacka EH: Homocysteine as a risk factor for vascular disease: Enhanced collagen production and accumulation by smooth muscle cells. *Arterioscler Thromb Vasc Biol* **17**:2074, 1997.
403. Jourdheuil-Rahmani D, Rolland PH, Rosset E, Branchereau A, Garçon D: Homocysteine induces synthesis of a serine elastase in arterial smooth muscle cells from multi-organ donors. *Cardiovasc Res* **34**:597, 1997.
404. Dalton ML, Gadson PF Jr, Wrenn RW, Rosenquist TH: Homocysteine signal cascade: Production of phospholipids, activation of protein kinase C, and the induction of c-fos and c-myb in smooth muscle cells. *FASEB J* **11**:703, 1997.
405. Welch GN, Upchurch GR Jr, Farivar RS, Pigazzi A, Vu K, Brecher P, Keaney JF Jr, et al: Homocysteine-induced nitric oxide production in vascular smooth-muscle cells by NF-*k*B-dependent transcriptional activation of *Nos2*. *Proc Assoc Am Physicians* **110**:22, 1998.
405a. Brown JC III, Rosenquist TH, Monaghan DT: ERK2 activation by homocysteine in vascular smooth muscle cells. *Biochem Biophys Res Commun* **251**:669, 1998.
405b. Tyagi SC: Homocystine redox receptor and regulation of extracellular matrix components in vascular cells. *Am J Physiol* **43**:C396, 1998.
406. Hosoki R, Matsuki N, Kimura H: The possible role of hydrogen sulfide as an endogenous smooth muscle relaxant in synergy with nitric oxide. *Biochem Biophys Res Commun* **237**:527, 1997.
407. Bienvenu T, Chadefaux B, Ankri A, Leblond V, Coude M, Salehian B, Binet JL, et al: Antithrombin III activity is not related to plasma homocysteine concentrations. *Haemostasis* **21**:65, 1991.
408. Ratnoff OD: Activation of Hageman factor by L-homocystine. *Science* **162**:1007, 1968.
409. Munnich A, Saudubray JM, Dautzenberg MD, Parvy P, Ogier H, Girot R, Manigne P, et al: Diet-responsive proconvertin (factor VII) deficiency in homocystinuria. *J Pediatr* **102**:730, 1983.
410. Palareti G, Salardi S, Piazzi S, Legnani C, Poggi M, Grauso F, Caniato A, et al: Blood coagulation changes in homocystinuria: Effects of pyridoxine and other specific therapy. *J Pediatr* **109**:1001, 1986.
411. Scanu AM: Lipoprotein(a): A genetic risk factor for premature coronary heart disease. *JAMA* **267**:3326, 1992.
412. Harpel PC, Gordon BR, Parker TS: Plasmin catalyzes binding of lipoprotein (a) to immobilized fibrinogen and fibrin. *Proc Natl Acad Sci USA* **86**:3847, 1989.
413. Harpel PC, Chang VT, Borth W: Homocysteine and other sulfhydryl compounds enhance the binding of lipoprotein(a) to fibrin: A potential biochemical link between thrombosis, atherogenesis, and sulfhydryl compound metabolism. *Proc Natl Acad Sci USA* **89**:10,193, 1992.
414. Heinecke JW, Kawamura M, Suzuki L, Chait A: Oxidation of low density lipoprotein by thiols: Superoxide-dependent and -independent mechanisms. *J Lipid Res* **34**:2051, 1993.
415. Heinecke JW, Rosen H, Suzuki LA, Chait A: The role of sulfur-containing amino acids in superoxide production and modification of low density lipoprotein by arterial smooth muscle cells. *J Biol Chem* **262**:10,098, 1987.
416. McCully KS: Homocysteine theory of arteriosclerosis: Development and current status. *Arterioscler Rev* **11**:157, 1983.
417. Rolland PH, Friggi A, Barlatier A, Piquet P, Latrille V, Faye MM, Guillou J, et al: Hyperhomocysteinemia-induced vascular damage in the minipig: Captopril-hydrochlorothiazide combination prevents elastic alterations. *Circulation* **91**:1161, 1995.
418. Fau D, Peret J, Hadjiisky P: Effects of ingestion of high protein or excess methionine diets by rats for two years. *J Nutr* **118**:128, 1988.
419. Matthias D, Becker C-H, Riezler R, Kindling PH: Homocysteine induced arteriosclerosis-like alterations of the aorta in normotensive and hypertensive rats following application of high doses of methionine. *Atherosclerosis* **122**:201, 1996.
420. Durand P, Lussier-Cacan S, Blache D: Acute methionine load-induced hyperhomocysteinemia enhances platelet aggregation, thromboxane biosynthesis, and macrophage-derived tissue factor activity in rats. *FASEB J* **11**:1157, 1997.
421. Loscalzo J: The oxidant stress of hyperhomocyst(e)inemia. *J Clin Invest* **98**:5, 1996.
422. Stamler JS, Slivka A: Biological chemistry of thiols in the vasculature and in vascular-related disease. *Nutr Rev* **54**:1, 1996.
423. Zhang F, Slungaard A, Vercellotti GM, Iadecola C: Superoxide-dependent cerebrovascular effects of homocysteine. *Am J Physiol* **274**:R1704, 1998.
424. Blundell G, Jones BG, Rose FA, Tudball N: Homocysteine mediated endothelial cell toxicity and its amelioration. *Atherosclerosis* **122**:163, 1996.
425. Welch GN, Loscalzo J: Homocysteine and atherothrombosis. *N Engl J Med* **338**:1042, 1998.
426. Young PB, Kennedy S, Molloy AM, Scott JM, Weir DG, Kennedy DG: Lipid peroxidation induced by hyperhomocysteinaemia in pigs. *Atherosclerosis* **129**:67, 1997.
427. Toborek M, Kopieczna-Grzebieniak E, Drózdz M, Wieczorek M: Increased lipid peroxidation as a mechanism of methionine-induced atherosclerosis in rabbits. *Atherosclerosis* **115**:217, 1996.
428. Blom HJ, Kleinveld HA, Boers GHJ, Demacker PNM, Hak-Lemmers HLM, te Poele-Pothoff MTWB, Trijbels JMF: Lipid peroxidation and susceptibility of low-density lipoprotein to in vitro oxidation in hyperhomocysteinaemia. *Eur J Clin Invest* **25**:149, 1995.
429. Córdoba-Porras A, Sánchez-Quesada JL, González-Sastre F, Ordóñez-Llanos J, Blanco-Vaca F: Susceptibility of plasma low- and high-density lipoproteins to oxidation in patients with severe hyperhomocysteinemia. *J Mol Med* **74**:771, 1996.
430. Dudman NPB, Wilcken DEL, Stocker R: Circulating lipid hydroperoxide levels in human hyperhomocysteinemia: Relevance to development of arteriosclerosis. *Arterioscler Thromb* **13**:512, 1993.
431. Domagala TB, Libura M, Szczeklik A: Hyperhomocysteinemia following oral methionine load is associated with increased lipid peroxidation. *Thromb Res* **87**:411, 1997.
432. Boushey CJ, Beresford SAA, Omenn GS, Motulsky AG: A quantitative assessment of plasma homocysteine as a risk factor for vascular disease: Probable benefits of increasing folic acid intakes. *JAMA* **274**:1049, 1995.
433. Mudd SH: Cystathionine β-synthase deficiency: Metabolic aspects, in Rosenberg IH, Graham I, Ueland P, et al (eds): *International Conference on Homocysteine Metabolism: From Basic Science to Clinical Medicine*. Norwell, MA, Kluwer Academic, 1995, p 77.
434. McIlwain H, Poll JD: Interaction between adenosine generated endogenously in neocortical tissues, and homocysteine and its thiolactone. *Neurochem Int* **7**:103, 1985.
435. Flott-Rahmel B, Schürmann M, Schluff P, Fingerhut R, Musshoff U, Fowler B, Ullrich K: Homocysteic and homocysteine sulphinic acid exhibit excitotoxicity in organotypic cultures from rat brain. *Eur J Pediatr* **157**(suppl 2):S112, 1998.
436. Bouvier M, Miller BA, Szatkowski M, Attwell D: Electrogenic uptake of sulphur-containing analogues of glutamate and aspartate by Müller cells from the salamander retina. *J Physiol (Lond)* **444**:441, 1991.
437. Ohmori S, Kodama H, Ikegami T, Mizuhara S, Oura T, Isshiki G, Uemura I: Unusual sulfur-containing amino acids in the urine of homocystinuric patients: III. Homocysteic acid, homocysteine sulfinic acid, *S*-(carboxymethylthio)homocysteine, and *S*-(3-hydroxy-3-carboxy-*n*-propyl)homocysteine. *Physiol Chem Phys* **4**:286, 1972.
438. McCully KS: Homocysteine metabolism in scurvy, growth and arteriosclerosis. *Nature* **231**:391, 1971.
439. Schwarz S, Zhou G-Z: *N*-Methyl-d-aspartate receptors and CNS symptoms of homocystinuria. *Lancet* **337**:1226, 1991.
439a. Do KQ, Grandes P, Hansel C, Jiang ZP, Klancnik J, Streit P, Tschopp P, et al: Sulphur containing excitatory amino acids: Release, activity and localization. *Mol Neuropharmacol* **2**:39, 1992.
440. Kilpatrick IC, Mozley LS: An initial analysis of the regional distribution of excitatory sulphur-containing amino acids in the rat brain. *Neurosci Lett* **72**:189, 1986.
441. Waller SJ, Kilpatrick IC, Chan MWJ, Evans RH: The influence of assay conditions on measurement of excitatory dibasic sulphinic and sulphonic alpha-amino acids in nervous tissue. *J Neurosci Methods* **36**:167, 1991.

442. Frauscher G, Karnaukhova E, Muehl A, Hoeger H, Lubec B: Oral administration of homocysteine leads to increased plasma triglycerides and homocysteic acid: Additional mechanisms in homocysteine induced endothelial damage? *Life Sci* **57**:813, 1995.

443. Quinn CT, Greiner JC, Bottiglieri T, Hyland K, Farrow A, Kamen BA: Elevation of homocysteine and excitatory amino acid neurotransmitters in the CSF of children who receive methotrexate for the treatment of cancer. *J Clin Oncol* **15**:2800, 1997.

444. Santhosh-Kumar CR, Deutsch JC, Kolhouse JC, Hassell KL, Kolhouse JF: Measurement of excitatory sulfur amino acids, cysteine sulfinic acid, cysteic acid, homocysteine sulfinic acid, and homocysteic acid in serum by stable isotope dilution gas chromatography-mass spectroscopy and selected ion monitoring. *Anal Biochem* **220**:249, 1994.

445. Lipton SA, Kim W-K, Choi Y-B, Kumar S, D'Emilia DM, Rayudu PV, Arnelle DR, et al: Neurotoxicity associated with dual actions of homocysteine at the *N*-methyl-D-aspartate receptor. *Proc Natl Acad Sci USA* **94**:5923, 1997.

446. Folbergrova J: NMDA and not non-NMDA receptor antagonists are protective against seizures induced by homocysteine in neonatal rats. *Exp Neurol* **130**:344, 1994.

447. Folbergrova J: Anticonvulsant action of both NMDA and non-NMDA receptor antagonists against seizures induced by homocysteine in immature rats. *Exp Neurol* **145**:442, 1997.

448. Santhosh-Kumar CR, Hassell KL, Deutsch JC, Kolhouse JF: Are neuropsychiatric manifestations of folate, cobalamin and pyridoxine deficiency mediated through imbalances in excitatory sulfur amino acids? *Med Hypotheses* **43**:239, 1994.

449. Awaad Y, Sansaricq C, Moroney J, Fish I, Kyriakakos A, Snyderman SE: Baclofen in the treatment of polymyoclonus and ataxia in a patient with homocystinuria. *J Child Neurol* **10**:294, 1995.

450. Abe K, Kimura H: The possible role of hydrogen sulfide as an endogenous neuromodulator. *J Neurosci* **16**:1066, 1996.

451. Perry TL: Homocystinuria, in Nyhan WL (ed): *Heritable Disorders of Amino Acid Metabolism*. New York, John Wiley and Sons, 1974, p 395.

452. Dunn HG, Perry TL, Dolman CL: Homocystinuria. *Neurology* **16**:407, 1966.

453. Kraus JP: Unpublished observations, 1998.

454. Watanabe M, Osada J, Aratani Y, Kluckman K, Reddick R, Malinow MR, Maeda N: Mice deficient in cystathionine β-synthase: Animal models for mild and severe homocyst(e)inemia [abstr]. *Proc Natl Acad Sci USA* **92**:1585, 1995.

455. Loscalzo J: Personal communication, 1998.

456. Isherwood DM: Homocystinuria: Early diagnosis and intervention reduces risk of visual impairment and thromboembolism. *BMJ* **313**:1996.

457. Mudd SH, Poole JR, Siggers DC: Unpublished observations, 1981.

458. Levy HL, Mudd SH, Uhlendorf BW, Madigan PM: Cystathioninuria and homocystinuria. *Clin Chim Acta* **58**:51, 1975.

459. Levy HL, Mudd SH: Homocystinuria due to bacterial contamination in pyridoxine-unresponsive cystathioninemia [abstr]. *Pediatr Res* **7**:162, 1973.

460. Smith KL, Bradley L, Levy HL, Korson MS: Inadequate laboratory technique for amino acids analysis resulting in missed diagnoses of homocystinuria. *Clin Chem* **44**:897, 1998.

461. Applegarth DA, Vallance HD, Seccombe D: Are patients with homocystinuria being missed? *Eur J Pediatr* **154**:589, 1995.

462. McDowell I, Bradley D: Delay in diagnosis of homocystinuria: Total rather than free homocysteine is better for screening. *BMJ* **314**:370, 1997.

463. Fowler B, Jakobs C: Post- and prenatal diagnostic methods for the homocystinurias. *Eur J Pediatr* **157**(suppl 2):S88, 1998.

464. Finkelstein JD, Mudd SH, Irreverre F, Laster L: Homocystinuria due to cystathionine synthetase deficiency: The mode of inheritance. *Science* **146**:785, 1964.

465. Uhlendorf BW, Mudd SH: Cystathionine synthase in tissue culture derived from human skin: Enzyme defect in homocystinuria. *Science* **160**:1007, 1968.

466. Goldstein JL, Campbell BK, Gartler SM: Cystathionine synthase activity in human lymphocytes: Induction by phytohemagglutinin. *J Clin Invest* **51**:1034, 1972.

467. Fleisher LD, Beratis NG, Tallan HH, Hirschhorn K, Gaull GE: Homocystinuria due to cystathionine synthase (CS) deficiency: Investigations in cultured long-term lymphocytes, fetal skin fibroblasts and amniotic fluid cells [abstr]. *Pediatr Res* **8**:388, 1974.

468. Yap S, Naughten E: Homocystinuria due to cystathionine beta-synthase deficiency in Ireland: 25 years experience of a newborn screened and treated population with reference to clinical outcome and biochemical control. *J Inherited Metab Dis* **21**:738, 1998.

468a. Yap S, O'Donnell KA, O'Neill C, Mayne PD, Thornton P, Naughten E: Factor V Leiden (arg506gln), a confounding genetic risk factor but not mandatory for the occurrence of venous thromboembolism in homozygotes and obligate heterozygotes for cystathionine β-synthase deficiency *Thromb Haemost* **81**, 502, 1999.

468b. Taylor RH, Burke J, O'Keefe M, Beighi B, Naughten E: Ophthalmic abnormalities in homocystinuria: The value of screening. *Eye* **12**:427, 1998.

469. Gaull GE, Rassin DK, Sturman JA: Pyridoxine-dependency in homocystinuria. *Lancet* **2**:1302, 1968.

470. Hollowell JG Jr, Coryell ME, Hall WK, Findley JK, Thevaos TG: Homocystinuria as affected by pyridoxine, folic acid, and vitamin B_{12}. *Proc Soc Exp Biol Med* **129**:327, 1968.

471. Gröbe H: Homocystinuria (cystathionine synthase deficiency): Results of treatment in late-diagnosed patients. *Eur J Pediatr* **135**:199, 1980.

472. Carey MC, Fennelly JJ, Fitzgerald O: Homocystinuria: II. Subnormal serum folate levels, increased folate clearance and effects of folic acid therapy. *Am J Med* **45**:26, 1968.

473. Wagstaff J, Korson M, Kraus JP, Levy HL: Severe folate deficiency and pancytopenia in a nutritionally deprived infant with homocystinuria caused by cystathionine beta-synthase deficiency. *J Pediatr* **118**:569, 1991.

474. Gaull GE, Rassin DK, Sturman JA: Enzymatic and metabolic studies of homocystinuria: Effects of pyridoxine. *Neuropaediatrie* **1**:199, 1969.

475. Wilcken DEL, Dudman NPB, Tyrrell PA: Homocystinuria due to cystathionine β-synthase deficiency: The effects of betaine treatment in pyridoxine-responsive patients. *Metabolism* **34**:1115, 1985.

476. Bendich A, Cohen M: Vitamin B_6 safety issues. *Ann NY Acad Sci* **585**:321, 1990.

477. Ludolph AC, Ullrich K, Bick U, Fahrendorf G, Przyrembel H: Functional and morphological deficits in late-treated patients with homocystinuria: A clinical, electrophysiologic and MRI study. *Acta Neurol Scand* **83**:161, 1991.

478. Ludolph AC, Masur H, Oberwittler C, Koch HG, Ullrich K: Sensory neuropathy and vitamin B6 treatment in homocystinuria. *Eur J Pediatr* **152**:271, 1993.

479. Mpofu C, Alani SM, Whitehouse C, Fowler B, Wraith JE: No sensory neuropathy during pyridoxine treatment in homocystinuria. *Arch Dis Child* **66**:1081, 1991.

480. Korson MS, Asamoah A, Levy HL: Unpublished observations, 1992.

481. Greene CL, Abenur JE, Davidson-Mundt A: Personal communication, 1992.

482. Garty R, Yonis Z, Braham J, Steinitz K: Pyridoxine-dependent convulsions in an infant. *Arch Dis Child* **37**:21, 1962.

483. Heeley A, Pugh RJP, Clayton BE, Shepherd J, Wilson J: Pyridoxol metabolism in vitamin B6-responsive convulsions of early infancy. *Arch Dis Child* **53**:794, 1978.

484. Bankier A, Turner M, Hopkins IJ: Pyridoxine dependent seizures: A wider clinical spectrum. *Arch Dis Child* **58**:415, 1983.

485. Kroll JS: Pyridoxine for neonatal seizures: An unexpected danger. *Dev Med Child Neurol* **27**:377, 1985.

485a. Shoji Y, Takahashi T, Sato W, Shoji Ya, Takada G: Acute life-threatening event with rhabdomyolysis after starting on high-dose pyridoxine therapy in an infant with homocystinuria. *J Inherited Metab Dis* **21**:439, 1998.

486. Mori K, Kaido M, Fujishiro K, Inoue N, Koide O: Effects of megadoses of pyridoxine on spermatogenesis and male reproductive-organs in rats. *Arch Toxicol* **66**:198, 1992.

487. Yoshida I, Sakaguchi Y, Nakano M, Yamashita F, Hitoshi T: Pyridoxal phosphate-induced liver injury in a patient with homocystinuria. *J Inherited Metab Dis* **8**:91, 1985.

488. Task Force on Dietary Management of Metabolic Disorders: Report to FDA, Contract 22372-2304 Committee on Nutrition, American Academy of Pediatrics, 1985.

489. Acosta PB, Elsas LJ II: Nutrition support of vitamin B6-responsive homocystinuria. *Metab Currents* **15**:13, 1992.

489a. McKeever MP, Weir DG, Molloy A, Scott JM: Betaine-homocysteine methyltransferase: Organ distribution in man, pig and rat and subcellular distribution. *Clin Sci* **81**:551, 1991.

490. Carson NAJ: Homocystinuria: Clinical and biochemical heterogeneity, in Cockburn F, Gitzelmann R (eds): *Inborn Errors of Metabolism in Humans*. London, England, MTP, 1982, p 53.
491. Komrower GM, Sardharwalla IB: The dietary treatment of homocystinuria, in Carson NAJ, Raine DN (eds): *Inherited Disorders of Sulphur Metabolism*. London, Churchill Livingstone, 1971, p 254.
492. Perry TL, Hansen S, Love DL, Crawford LE, Tischler B: Treatment of homocystinuria with a low-methionine diet, supplemental cystine, and a methyl donor. *Lancet* **2**:474, 1968.
493. Smolin LA, Benevenga NJ, Berlow S: The use of betaine for the treatment of homocystinuria. *J Pediatr* **99**:467, 1981.
494. Wilcken DEL, Wilcken B, Dudman NPB, Tyrrell PA: Homocystinuria: The effects of betaine in the treatment of patients not responsive to pyridoxine. *N Engl J Med* **309**:448, 1983.
495. Wilcken DEL, Wilcken B: The long term outcome in homocystinuria, in Rosenberg IH, Graham I, Ueland P, et al (eds): *International Conference on Homocysteine Metabolism: From Basic Science to Clinical Medicine*. Norwell, MA, Kluwer Academic, 1997, p 51.
496. Surtees R, Bowron A, Leonard J: Cerebrospinal fluid and plasma total homocysteine and related metabolites in children with cystathionine β-synthase deficiency: The effect of treatment. *Pediatr Res* **42**:577, 1997.
497. Berlow S, Bachman RP, Berry GT, Donnell GN, Grix A, Levitsky LL, Hoganson G, et al: Betaine therapy in homocystinemia. *Brain Dysfunction* **2**:10, 1989.
498. Gahl WA, Bernardini I, Chen S, Kurtz D, Horvath K: The effect of oral betaine on vertebral body bone density in pyridoxine-nonresponsive homocystinuria. *J Inherited Metab Dis* **11**:291, 1988.
498a. Johnston RB Jr: Folic acid: New dimensions of an old friendship. *Adv Pediatr* **44**:231, 1997.
498b. Rothenberg SP: Increasing the dietary intake of folate: Pros and cons. *Semin Hematol* **36**:65, 1999.
499. Harker LA, Slichter SJ, Scott CR, Ross R: Homocystinemia: Vascular injury and arterial thrombosis. *N Engl J Med* **291**:537, 1974.
500. Schulman JD, Agarwal B, Mudd SH, Shulman NR: Pulmonary embolism in a homocystinuric patient during treatment with dipyridamole and acetylsalicylic acid. *N Engl J Med* **299**:661, 1978.
501. Steegers-Theunissen RPM, Boers GHJ, Steegers EAP, Trijbels FJM, Thomas CMG, Eskes TKAB: Effects of sub-50 oral contraceptives on homocysteine metabolism: A preliminary study. *Contraception* **45**:129, 1992.
502. Francois J: Homocystinuria, in Winkelman JE, Crone RA. (eds): *Perspectives in Ophthalmology*, vol 2. Amsterdam, Excerpta Medica, 1970, p 81.
503. Gerding H: Ocular complications and a new surgical approach to lens dislocation in homocystinuria due to cystathionine-β-synthetase deficiency. *Eur J Pediatr* **157**(suppl 2):S94, 1998.
504. Eschweiler GW, Rosin R, Thier P, Giedke H: Postoperative psychosis in homocystinuria. *Eur Psychiatry* **12**:98, 1997.
505. Frost PM: Anaesthesia and homocystinuria. *Anaesthesia* **35**:918, 1980.
506. Fuks AB, Kaufman E, Galili D, Garfunkel A: Comprehensive dental treatment under general anesthesia for patients with homocystinuria. *J Dent Child* **47**:340, 1980.
507. Levy HL: Unpublished observations, 1998.
508. Elkington AR, Freedman SS, Jay B, Wright P: Anterior dislocation of the lens in homocystinuria. *Br J Ophthalmol* **57**:325, 1973.
509. Lieberman TW, Podos SM, Hartstein J: Acute glaucoma, ectopia lentis and homocystinuria. *Am J Ophthalmol* **61**:252, 1966.
510. Tada K, Tateda H, Arashima S, Sakai K, Kitagawa T, Aoki K, Suwa S, et al: Follow-up study of a nation-wide neonatal metabolic screening program in Japan. *Eur J Pediatr* **142**:204, 1984.
511. Sardharwalla IB: Personal communication, 1992.
512. Whiteman PD, Clayton BE, Ersser RS, Lilly P, Seakins JWT: Changing incidence of neonatal hypermethioninaemia: Implications for the detection of homocystinuria. *Arch Dis Child* **54**:593, 1979.
513. Doherty LB, Rohr FJ, Levy HL: Detection of phenylketonuria in the very early newborn blood specimen. *Pediatrics* **87**:240, 1991.
514. Naughten ER, Yap S, Mayne PD: Newborn screening for homocystinuria: Irish and world experience. *Eur J Pediatr* **157**(suppl 2):S84, 1998.
515. Naruse H: Personal communication, 1992.
516. Wilcken B, Hammond J: Homozygous cystathionine β-synthase deficiency (CSD) and homocysteine remethylating disorders: Relative incidence in New South Wales [abstr]. *Ir J Med Sci* **164**(suppl 15):23, 1995.
517. Berry HK: Newborn screening for homocystinuria [abstr]. *Am J Hum Genet* **57**:A321, 1995.
518. Snyderman SE, Sansaricq C: Newborn screening for homocystinuria. *Early Hum Dev* **48**:203, 1997.
519. Wilcken B, Turner G: Homocystinuria in New South Wales. *Arch Dis Child* **53**:242, 1978.
520. Swenson EF, Walraven C, Levy HL: A 25 year experience with newborn urine screening [abstr], in *9th National Neonatal Screening Symposium, April 7–11, Raleigh, North Carolina*, 69, 1992.
521. Watanabe T, Kuroda Y, Naito E, Ito M, Takeda E, Toshima K, Miyao M, et al: Urinary homocystine levels in a newborn infant with cystathionine synthase deficiency. *Eur J Pediatr* **146**:436, 1987.
522. Maddocks JL, MacLachlan J: Application of new fluorescent thiol reagent to diagnosis of homocystinuria. *Lancet* **2**:1043, 1991.
523. Spaeth GL, Barber GW: Prevalence of homocystinuria among the mentally retarded: Evaluation of a specific screening test. *Pediatrics* **40**:586, 1967.
524. Chace DH, Hillman SL, Millington DS, Kahler SG, Adam BW, Levy HL: Rapid diagnosis of homocystinuria and other hypermethioninemias from newborns' blood spots by tandem mass spectrometry. *Clin Chem* **42**:349, 1996.
525. Champion MP, Turner C, Bird S, Dalton RN: Delay in diagnosis of homocystinuria: Neonatal screening avoids complications of delayed treatment. *BMJ* **314**:369, 1997.
526. Boddie AM, Steen MT, Sullivan KM, Pasquali M, Dembure PP, Coates RJ, Elsas LJ II: Cystathionine-β-synthase deficiency: Detection of heterozygotes by ratios of homocysteine to cysteine and folate. *Metabolism* **47**:207, 1997.
527. Boers GHJ, Fowler B, Smals AGH, Trijbels FJM, Leermakers AI, Kleijer WJ, Kloppenborg PWC: Improved identification of heterozygotes for homocystinuria due to cystathionine synthase deficiency by the combination of methionine loading and enzyme determination in cultured fibroblasts. *Hum Genet* **69**:164, 1985.
528. Tsai MY, Garg U, Key NS, Hanson NQ, Suh A, Schwichtenberg K: Molecular and biochemical approaches in the identification of heterozygotes for homocystinuria. *Atherosclerosis* **122**:69, 1996.
529. Wilcken DEL, Wilcken B: The pathogenesis of coronary artery disease: A possible role for methionine metabolism. *J Clin Invest* **57**:1079, 1976.
530. Sardharwalla IB, Fowler B, Robins AJ, Komrower GM: Detection of heterozygotes for homocystinuria: Study of sulphur-containing amino acids in plasma and urine after L-methionine loading. *Arch Dis Child* **49**:553, 1974.
531. Malinow MR: Plasma homocyst(e)ine: A risk factor for arterial occlusive diseases. *J Nutr* **126**:1238S, 1996.
532. Graham IM, Daly LE, Refsum HM, Robinson K, Brattström LE, Ueland PM, Palma-Reis RJ, et al: Plasma homocysteine as a risk factor for vascular disease: The European Concerted Action Project. *JAMA* **277**:1775, 1997.
533. Boers GHJ: Hyperhomocysteinemia as a risk factor for arterial and venous disease: A review of evidence and relevance. *Thromb Haemost* **78**:520, 1997.
534. Fermo I, Vigano'D'Angelo S, Paroni R, Mazzola G, Calori G, D'Angelo A: Prevalence of moderate hyperhomocysteinemia in patients with early-onset venous and arterial occlusive disease. *Ann Intern Med* **123**:747, 1995.
535. Den Heijer M, Koster T, Blom HJ, Bos GMJ, Briët E, Reitsma PH, Vandenbroucke JP, et al: Hyperhomocysteinemia as a risk factor for deep-vein thrombosis. *N Engl J Med* **334**:759, 1996.
536. Nygård O, Nordrehaug JE, Refsum H, Ueland PM, Farstad M, Vollset SE: Plasma homocysteine levels and mortality in patients with coronary artery disease. *N Engl J Med* **337**:230, 1997.
536a. Brattström L, Wilcken DEL, Öhrvik J, Brudin L: Common methylenetetrahydrofolate reductase gene mutation leads to hyperhomocysteinemia but not to vascular disease: The result of a meta-analysis. *Circulation* **98**:2520, 1998.
536b. Verhoeff BJ, Trip MD, Prins MH, Kastelein JJP, Reitsma PH: The effect of a common methylenetetrahydrofolate reductase mutation on levels of homocysteine, folate, vitamin B12 and on the risk of premature atherosclerosis. *Atherosclerosis* **141**:161, 1998.
537. Mudd SH, Havlik R, Levy HL, McKusick VA, Feinleib M: A study of cardiovascular risk in heterozygotes for homocystinuria. *Am J Hum Genet* **33**:883, 1981.
538. Clarke R: The Irish experience, in Robinson K (ed): *Homocysteinaemia and Vascular Disease: Proceedings on an EC Comac Epidemiology Expert Group Workshop, 1989*. Luxembourg, Commission of the European Communities, CD-NA-12834-EN-C, 1990, p 41.

539. De Valk HW, Van Eeden MKG, Banga JD, Van der Griend R, De Groot E, Haas FJLM, Meuwissen OJAT, et al: Evaluation of the presence of premature atherosclerosis in adults with heterozygosity for cystathionine-β-synthase. *Stroke* **27**:1134, 1996.
539a. Megnien J-L, Gariepy J, Saudubray J-M, Nuoffer J-M, Denarie N, Levenson J, Simon A: Evidence of carotid artery wall hypertrophy in homozygous homocystinuria. *Circulation* **98**:2276, 1998.
540. Boers GHJ, Smals AGH, Trijbels FJM, Fowler B, Bakkeren JAJM, Schoonderwaldt HC, Kleijer WJ, et al: Heterozygosity for homocystinuria in premature peripheral and cerebral occlusive arterial disease. *N Engl J Med* **313**:709, 1985.
541. Clarke R, Daly L, Robinson K, Naughten E, Cahalane S, Fowler B, Graham I: Hyperhomocysteinemia: An independent risk factor for vascular disease. *N Engl J Med* **324**:1149, 1991.
542. Engbersen AMT, Franken DG, Boers GHJ, Stevens EMB, Trijbels FJM, Blom HJ: Thermolabile 5,10-methylenetetrahydrofolate reductase as a cause of mild hyperhomocysteinemia. *Am J Hum Genet* **56**:142, 1995.
543. Kluijtmans LAJ, Van den Heuvel LPWJ, Boers GHJ, Frosst P, Stevens EMB, Van Oost BA, Den Heijer M, et al: Molecular genetic analysis in mild hyperhomocysteinemia: A common mutation in the methylenetetrahydrofolate reductase gene is a genetic risk factor for cardiovascular disease. *Am J Hum Genet* **58**:35, 1996.
544. Fowler B: Disorders of homocysteine metabolism. *J Inherited Metab Dis* **20**:270, 1997.
544a. Nordström M, Kjellström T: Age dependency of cystathionine beta-synthase activity in human fibroblasts in homocyst(e)inemia and atherosclerotic disease. *Atherosclerosis* **94**:213, 1992.
544b. Nordström M, Kjellström T: Age and cystathionine β-synthase activity in cultured fibroblasts from patients with arterial and venous vascular disease. *Atherosclerosis* **139**:231, 1998.
545. Kozich V, Kraus E, de Franchis R, Fowler B, Boers GHJ, Graham I, Kraus JP: Hyperhomocysteinemia in premature arterial disease: Examination of cystathionine β-synthase alleles at the molecular level. *Hum Mol Genet* **4**:623, 1995.
546. Gallagher PM, Meleady R, Shields DC, Tan KS, McMaster D, Rozen R, Evans A, et al: Homocysteine and risk of premature coronary heart disease: Evidence for a common gene mutation. *Circulation* **94**:2154, 1996.
546a. Evers S, Koch HG, Grotemeyer KH, Ullrich K, Deufel T, Harms E: Hyperhomocysteinemia in ischemic stroke is not due to mutations of the cystathionine-beta-synthase gene [abstr]. *Cerebrovasc Dis* **6**(suppl 2):19, 1996.
547. Daly L, Robinson K, Tan KS, Graham IM: Hyperhomocysteinaemia: A metabolic risk factor for coronary heart disease determined by both genetic and environmental influences? *Q J Med* **86**:685, 1993.
548. Dudman NPB, Wilcken DEL, Wang J, Lynch JF, Macey D, Lundberg P: Disordered methionine/homocysteine metabolism in premature vascular disease. *Arterioscler Thromb* **13**:1253, 1993.
549. Dudman NPB, Guo X-W, Gordon RB, Dawson PA, Wilcken DEL: Human homocysteine catabolism: Three major pathways and their relevance to development of arterial occlusive disease. *J Nutr* **126**:1295S, 1996.
550. Kluijtmans LAJ, Verhoef P, Boers GHJ, Den Heijer M, Van den Heuvel LPWJ, Trijbels FJM, Blom HJ: Cystathionine β-synthase and mild hyperhomocysteinemia: An association study. PhD thesis, University of Nijmegen, Nijmegen, The Netherlands, 1998.
550a. De Stefano V, Dekou V, Nicaud V, Chasse JF, London J, Stansbie D, Humphries SE, et al: Linkage disequilibrium at the cystathionine β synthase (CBS) locus and the association between genetic variation at the CBS locus and plasma levels of homocysteine. *Ann Hum Genet* **62**:481, 1998.
551. Eskes TKAB: Neural tube defects, vitamins and homocysteine. *Eur J Pediatr* **157**(suppl 2):S139, 1998.
552. Ramsbottom D, Scott JM, Molloy A, Weir DG, Kirke PN, Mills JL, Gallagher PM, et al: Are common mutations of cystathionine β-synthase involved in the aetiology of neural tube defects? *Clin Genet* **51**:39, 1997.
553. De Franchis R, Mandato C, Buoninconti A, Sperandeo MP, Capra V, De Marco P, Ricci R, et al: Risk factors for neural tube defects: Analysis of common genetic variants of methylenetetrahydrofolate reductase and cystathionine β-synthase [abstr]. *Am J Hum Genet* **61**(suppl):861, 1997.
554. Burke G, Robinson K, Refsum H, Stuart B, Drumm J, Graham I: Intrauterine growth retardation, perinatal death, and maternal homocysteine levels. *N Engl J Med* **326**:69, 1992.
555. Mudd SH: Discussion, in Carson NAJ, Raine DN (eds): *Inherited Disorders of Sulphur Metabolism*. London, Churchill Livingstone, 1971, p 311.
556. Fleisher LD, Longhi RC, Tallan HH, Beratis NG, Hirschhorn K, Gaull GE: Homocystinuria: Investigations of cystathionine synthase in cultured fetal cells and the prenatal determination of genetic status. *J Pediatr* **85**:677, 1974.
557. Fowler B, Borresen AL, Boman N: Prenatal diagnosis of homocystinuria. *Lancet* **2**:875, 1982.
558. Fensom AH, Benson PF, Crees MJ, Ellis M, Rodeck CH, Vaughan RW: Prenatal exclusion of homocystinuria (cystathionine β-synthase deficiency) by assay of phytohaemagglutinin-stimulated fetal lymphocytes. *Prenatal Diagn* **3**:127, 1983.
559. Fowler B, Giles L, Cooper A, Sardharwalla IB: Chorionic villus sampling: Diagnostic uses and limitations of enzyme assays. *J Inherited Metab Dis* **12**(suppl 1):105, 1989.
560. Kraus JP: Unpublished observations, 1986.
561. Harris H, Penrose LS, Thomas DHH: Cystathioninuria. *Ann Hum Genet* **23**:442, 1959.
562. Lyon ICT, Procopis PG, Turner B: Cystathioninuria in a well baby population. *Acta Paediatr Scand* **60**:324, 1971.
563. Park YK, Linkswiler H: Effect of vitamin B_6 depletion in adult man on the excretion of cystathionine and other methionine metabolites. *J Nutr* **100**:110, 1970.
564. Shih VE, Salam MZ, Mudd SH, Uhlendorf BW, Adams RD: A new form of homocystinuria due to $N^{5,10}$-methylene tetrahydrofolate reductase deficiency [abstr]. *Pediatr Res* **6**:135, 1972.
565. Levy HL, Mudd SH, Schulman JD, Dreyfus PM, Abeles RH: A derangement in B_{12} metabolism associated with homocysteinemia, cystathioninemia, hypomethioninemia, and methylmalonic aciduria. *Am J Med* **48**:390, 1970.
566. Higginbottom MC, Sweetman L, Nyhan WL: A syndrome of methylmalonic aciduria, homocystinuria, megaloblastic anemia and neurologic abnormalities in a vitamin B_{12}-deficient breast-fed infant of a strict vegetarian. *N Engl J Med* **299**:317, 1978.
567. Allen RH, Stabler SP, Savage DG, Lindenbaum J: Metabolic abnormalities in cobalamin (vitamin B_{12}) and folate deficiency. *FASEB J* **7**:1344, 1993.
568. Frimpter GW: Cystathioninuria in a patient with cystinuria. *Am J Med* **46**:832, 1969.
569. Frimpter GW, Greenberg AJ: Renal clearance of cystathionine in homozygous and heterozygous cystathioninuria, cystinuria, and the normal state. *J Clin Invest* **46**:975, 1967.
570. Fowler B: Transsulphuration and methylation of homocysteine in control and mutant human fibroblasts. *Biochim Biophys Acta* **721**:201, 1982.
571. Finkelstein JD, Mudd SH, Irreverre F, Laster L: Deficiencies of cystathionase and homoserine dehydratase activities in cystathioninuria. *Proc Natl Acad Sci USA* **55**:865, 1966.
572. Kint JA, Carton D: New evidence for the identity of homoserine deaminase and cystathionase in human liver. *Arch Int Physiol Biochim* **79**:202, 1971.
573. Matsuo Y, Greenberg DM: A crystalline enzyme that cleaves homoserine and cystathionine: IV. Mechanism of action, reversibility, and substrate specificity. *J Biol Chem* **234**:516, 1959.
574. Pascal TA, Tallan HH, Gillam BM: Hepatic cystathionase: Immunochemical and electrophoretic studies of the human and rat forms. *Biochim Biophys Acta* **285**:48, 1972.
575. Roisin M-P, Chatagner F: Purification et étude de quelques propriétés de l'homocystéine désulfhydrase du foie de rat: Identification à la cystathionase. *Bull Soc Chim Biol* **51**:481, 1969.
576. Mushahwar IK, Koeppe RE: Rat liver L-diaminopropionate ammonia lyase: Identification as cystathionase. *J Biol Chem* **248**:7407, 1973.
577. Pascal TA, Gaull GE, Beratis NG, Gillam BM, Tallan HH: Cystathionase deficiency: Evidence for genetic heterogeneity in primary cystathioninuria. *Pediatr Res* **12**:125, 1978.
578. Frimpter GW: Cystathioninuria: Nature of the defect. *Science* **149**:1095, 1965.
579. Pascal TA, Gaull GE, Beratis NG, Gillam BM, Tallan HH, Hirschhorn K: Vitamin B_6-responsive and -unresponsive cystathioninuria: Two variant molecular forms. *Science* **190**:1209, 1975.
580. Hooft C, Carton D, De Schryver F: Cystathioninemia in three siblings, in Allan JD, Holt KS, Ireland JT, et al (eds): *Enzymopenic Anaemias, Lysosomes and Other Papers*. London, Churchill Livingstone, 1969, p 200.
581. Hooft C: Personal communication, 1975.

582. Pascal TA, Beratis NG, Tallan HH, Gaull GE: Cystathionase deficiency: The effect of cofactor on the stability of normal and abnormal enzyme from lymphoid cell lines. *Enzyme* **24**:265, 1979.
583. Endres W, Seibold H: Renal excretion of cystathionine and creatinine in humans at different ages. *Clin Chim Acta* **87**:425, 1978.
584. Shaw KNF, Lieberman E, Koch R, Donnell GN: Cystathioninuria. *Am J Dis Child* **113**:119, 1967.
585. Tada K, Yoshida T, Yokoyama Y, Sato T, Nakagawa H, Arakawa T: Cystathioninuria not associated with vitamin B_6 dependency: A probably new type of cystathioninuria. *Tohoku J Exp Med* **95**:235, 1968.
586. Levy HL, Mudd SH, Madigan PM: Pyridoxine-unresponsive cystathioninemia [abstr]. *Pediatr Res* **7**:162, 1973.
587. Perry TL, Jones RT: The amino acid content of human cerebrospinal fluid in normal individuals and in mental defectives. *J Clin Invest* **40**:1363, 1961.
588. Brenton DP, Cusworth DC, Gaull GE: Homocystinuria: Biochemical studies of tissues including a comparison with cystathioninuria. *Pediatrics* **35**:50, 1965.
589. Tada K, Yosdhida T, Arakawa T: Free amino acid pattern in the liver from the patients with amino acid disorders: Postmortem diagnosis of inborn errors of amino acid metabolism. *Tohoku J Exp Med* **101**:223, 1970.
590. Kodama H, Ishimoto Y, Shimomura M, Hirota T, Ohmori S: Isolation of two new sulfur-containing amino acids from the urine of a cystathioninuric patient. *Physiol Chem Phys* **7**:147, 1975.
591. Okada T, Takechi T, Wakiguchi H, Kurashige T, Sugahara K, Kodama H: Identification of new cystathionine mono-oxo acids, *S*-(3-oxo-3-carboxy-*n*-propyl)cysteine and *S*-(2-oxo-2-carboxyethyl)homocysteine in the urine of a patient with cystathioninuria. *Arch Biochem Biophys* **305**:385, 1993.
592. Zhang J, Masuoka N, Ubaka T, Sugahara K, Kodama H: Identification of *N*-acetyl-*S*-(3-oxo-3-carboxy-*n*-propyl)cysteine in the urine of a patient with cystathioninuria using LC/APCI-MS. *J Inherited Metab Dis* **18**:675, 1995.
593. Zhang J, Sugahara K, Sagara Y, Hashimoto K, Masuoka N, Kodama H: Identification of cyclic cystathionine sulfoxide and *N*-acetylcyclic cystathionine in the urine of a patient with cystathioninuria using liquid chromatography-mass spectrometry with an atmospheric pressure chemical ionization interface system. *Metabolism* **45**:1312, 1996.
594. Ricci G, Nardini M, Federici G, Cavallini D: The transamination of L-cystathionine, L-cystine and related compounds by a bovine kidney transaminase. *Eur J Biochem* **157**:57, 1986.
595. Cavallini D, Ricci G, Duprè S, Pecci L, Costa M, Matarese RM, Pensa B, et al: Sulfur-containing cyclic ketimines and imino acids. *Eur J Biochem* **202**:217, 1991.
596. Fontana M, Brunori A, Costa M, Antonucci A: Detection of cystathionine ketimine and lanthionine ketimine in human brain. *Neurochem Res* **22**:821, 1997.
597. Kodama H, Ikegama T, Hirayama K, Mizuhara S: Effect of pyridoxine treatment of a cystathioninuric patient on the urinary excretion of some unusual sulfur-containing amino acids. *Clin Chim Acta* **51**:29, 1974.
598. Abeles RH, Walsh CT: Acetylenic enzyme inactivators: Inactivation of γ-cystathionase, in vitro and in vivo, by propargylglycine. *J Am Chem Soc* **95**:6124, 1973.
599. Kodama H, Mikasa H, Sasaki K, Awata S, Nakayama K: Unusual metabolism of sulfur-containing amino acids in rats treated with DL-propargylglycine. *Arch Biochem Biophys* **225**:25, 1983.
600. Kodama H, Ikeda H, Awata S, Nakayama K: Cystathionine accumulation in various regions of brain of dl-propargylglycine-treated rats. *J Neurochem* **44**:1207, 1985.
601. Kodama H, Sasaki K, Mizobuchi N, Kikuchi R: Contents of cystathionine and taurine in various cerebellar regions of dl-propargylglycine-treated rats. *J Neurochem* **51**:1046, 1988.
602. Ohta J, Ubuka T, Kodama H, Sugahara K, Yao K, Masuoka N, Kinuta M: Increase in cystathionine content in rat liver mitochondria after DL-propargylglycine administration. *Amino Acids* **9**:111, 1995.
603. Kodama H, Sasaki K, Ageta T: Effect of propargylglycine on cystathionine metabolism in rats. *Biochem Int* **4**:195, 1982.
604. Mizobuchi N, Ageta T, Kodama H: Quantification of DL-propargylglycine and identification of cystathionine metabolites in various tissues of DL-propargylglycine-treated rats. *J Clin Biochem Nutr* **8**:121, 1990.
605. Machida Y, Zhang J, Hashimoto K, Wakiguchi H, Kurashige T, Masuoka N, Ubuka T, et al: Identification of perhydro-1,4-thiazepine-3,5-dicarboxylic acid, cysthathionine mono-oxo acids, cystathionine ketimines, cystathionine sulfoxide and *N*-acetylcystathionine sulfoxide in the urine sample of D,L-propargylglycine treated rats. *Physiol Chem Phys Med NMR* **27**:203, 1996.
605a. Zhang J, Zhang M, Ma D, Sugahara K, Kodama H: Metabolism of cystathionine, *N*-acetylcystathionine, perhydro-1,4-thiazepine-3,5-dicarboxylic acid, and cystathionine ketimine in the liver and kidney of D,L-propargylglycine-treated rats.
606. Frimpter GW, Haymovitz A, Horwith M: Cystathioninuria. *N Engl J Med* **268**:333, 1963.
607. Frimpter GW, Kozlowski KK, Horwith M: Distribution of sulfur in urine of patients with cystathioninuria before and during administration of pyridoxine. *Metabolism* **25**:355, 1976.
608. Scott CR, Dassell SE, Clark SH, Chang-Teng C, Swedberg KR: Cystathioninemia: A benign genetic condition. *J Pediatr* **76**:571, 1970.
609. Scriver CR, Hutchinson JH: The vitamin B_6 deficiency syndrome in human infancy: Biochemical and clinical observations. *Pediatrics* **31**:240, 1963.
610. Levy HL, Shih VE: Unpublished observations, 1987.
611. Berlow S: Studies in cystathioninemia. *Am J Dis Child* **112**:135, 1966.
612. Wilcken B, Smith A, Brown DA: Urine screening for aminoacidopathies: Is it beneficial? *J Pediatr* **97**:492, 1980.
612a. Lemieux B, Auray-Blais C, Giguère R, Shapcott D, Scriver CR: Newborn urine screening experience with over one million infants in the Quebec Network of Genetic Medicine. *J Inherited Metab Dis* **11**:45, 1988.
613. Kraus JP, Janosik M, Kozich V, Mandell R, Shih V, Sperandeo MP, Sebastio G, et al: Cystathionine β-synthase mutations in homocystinuria. *Hum Mutat* **13**:362, 1999.
614. Gaustadnes M: Unpublished observations, 1998.
615. Ohura T: Unpublished observations, 1998.
616. Gaustadnes M, Kluijtmans LAJ, Jensen OK, Rasmussen K, Heil SG, Kraus JP, Blom HJ, et al: Detection of a novel deletion in the cystathionine β-synthase (CBS) gene using an improved genomic DNA based method. *FEBS Lett* **431**:175, 1998.

CHAPTER 89

Sarcosinemia

C. Ronald Scott

1. **Sarcosinemia is a phenotype characterized by increased concentration of sarcosine (N-methylglycine) in plasma and increased excretion of sarcosine in urine. Sarcosinemia occurs because of a defect in the conversion of sarcosine to glycine that is catalyzed by sarcosine dehydrogenase. A deficiency of sarcosine dehydrogenase can occur because of a genetic alteration in the apoenzyme, a dysfunction of a necessary electron transfer flavoprotein, or a severe deficiency of folic acid.**
2. **The formation and degradation of sarcosine occur in liver and kidney tissue. Sarcosine is formed enzymatically from dimethylglycine by dimethylglycine dehydrogenase (EC 1.5.99.2) and converted to glycine by sarcosine dehydrogenase (EC 1.5.99.1). A small fraction of sarcosine may be generated from glycine by the enzyme glycine methyltransferase (EC 2.1.1.20)**
3. **It was originally reported that sarcosinemia was causally related to mental retardation or neurologic problems. It is most probable that sarcosinemia is a "benign" condition that is unrelated to neurologic symptoms or significant clinical problems.**
4. **Sarcosinemia that occurs from a genetic deficiency of sarcosine dehydrogenase activity is inherited as an autosomal recessive condition. The incidence of sarcosinemia found in newborn screening programs that evaluate urine specimens has varied from 1/350,000 (New England) to 1/28,000 (Quebec). Detection of heterozygotes by sarcosine loading studies is unreliable. The gene for human sarcosine dehydrogenase has been cloned and is located on chromosome 9q34.**
5. **A mouse with the phenotype of sarcosinemia and sarcosinuria has been identified. In the mouse, sarcosinemia has occurred from a deficiency of sarcosine dehydrogenase activity in liver mitochondria. The phenotype is genetically transmitted as an autosomal recessive trait, and the gene has been mapped to chromosome 2 within 15 to 18 cM of the centromere.**

INTRODUCTION

Sarcosinemia (MIM 268900) is a rare and controversial disorder. Originally described in 1966 in a child with mental retardation, it was assumed that sarcosinemia, in a manner similar to that seen in phenylketonuria, was responsible for the child's neurologic symptoms.[1] In the following years, additional persons were identified with sarcosinemia; some had symptoms of mental disorder, others had congenital defects, and still others were clinically normal. It was subsequently proposed that the finding of sarcosinemia in individuals with neurologic symptoms most likely occurred because of ascertainment bias, i.e., only persons with clinical problems routinely underwent evaluation for alterations in plasma or urine amino acid concentrations. This concept of sarcosinemia being a benign condition is currently the most prevalent belief, but some doubt remains, based on family data and the fact that more than a single biochemical mechanism may account for elevated concentrations of sarcosine in biologic fluid.

The enzymatic error in the most common phenotype of sarcosinemia is in the activity of sarcosine dehydrogenase. Precise and convincing enzymatic data are lacking in these patients because of the rarity of the clinical condition and the ethical limitations imposed in obtaining liver or kidney tissue for biochemical evaluation. Genetic data are consistent with an autosomal recessive mode of inheritance. The gene for sarcosine dehydrogenase has been localized to 9q34.

Sarcosinemia is similar to hyperphenylalaninemia or homocystinuria in that more than a single enzyme alteration may exist for the biochemical phenotype. Sarcosinemia may be caused by one of four possible mechanisms: defects involving 1) the sarcosine dehydrogenase apoenzyme, 2) an electron transfer flavoprotein (ETF), 3) a peroxisomal oxidase, 4) a severe folate deficiency. A mouse model of sarcosinemia due to a deficiency of sarcosine dehydrogenase has been identified.

BIOCHEMISTRY OF SARCOSINE

Sarcosine is a unique amino acid whose role in intermediary metabolism is primarily as a single step in "one-carbon" metabolism. Structurally, sarcosine (N-methylglycine) is a glycine molecule that is modified by the addition of a methyl group attached to its nitrogen atom. The compound is normally undetectable in biologic fluids and is not a component of mammalian protein. Sarcosine is formed from the oxidative demethylation of N,N-dimethylglycine. The methyl group is removed at the oxidative level of "active" formaldehyde. In the identical manner in which it is formed from N,N-dimethylglycine, sarcosine is oxidized by the removal of the methyl group to form glycine and an active one-carbon fragment (Fig. 89-1). These two sequential steps are believed to be carried out by two separate enzymatic proteins, dimethylglycine dehydrogenase and sarcosine dehydrogenase.[2,3] The two consecutive oxidative demethylation steps that produce the active one-carbon fragments account for the majority of one-carbon groups available for the formation of an active one-carbon fragment.[4] These one-carbon groups react with tetrahydrofolate to form the intermediate N^5,N^{10}-methylenetetrahydrofolate. This activated intermediate of folic acid is available for formation of the 3-carbon of serine by condensation with glycine and for other intermediary processes.

BIOCHEMISTRY OF DIMETHYLGLYCINE DEHYDROGENASE AND SARCOSINE DEHYDROGENASE

The reactions that form sarcosine and subsequently oxidize it to glycine occur within the mitochondria.[3,5] The formation of sarcosine is catalyzed by dimethyglycine dehydrogenase (EC 1.5.99.2) and requires folate as a cofactor.[5] The oxidation of sarcosine is performed by sarcosine dehydrogenase (EC 1.5.99.1) and also requires a folate derivative as a cofactor. Both enzymes

A list of standard abbreviations is located immediately preceding the index in each volume. Additional abbreviations used in this chapter include: ETF = electron transfer flavoprotein; PMS = phenozinemethosulfate; Tm = tubular maximum; ENU = ethylnitrosourea.

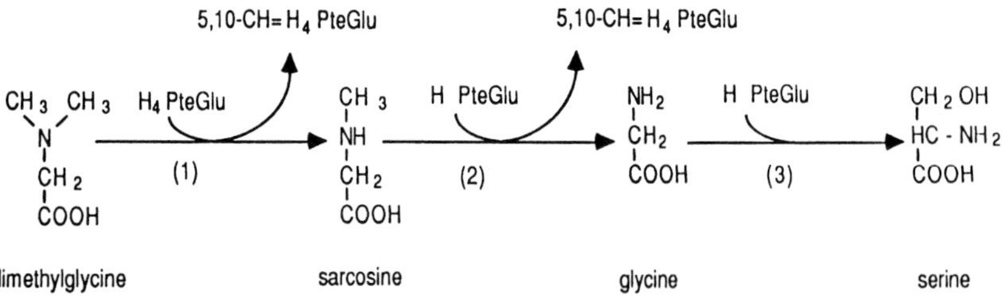

Fig. 89-1 The formation and degradation of sarcosine. 1) Dimethylglycine dehydrogenase. 2) Sarcosine dehydrogenase. 3) Serine hydroxymethylase.

are flavoproteins with molecular weights of 90,000 for dimethylglycine dehydrogenase and 105,000 for sarcosine dehydrogenase.[6] In isolated rat liver, these proteins and glycine-N-methyltransferase are the major folate-binding proteins.[7–9] The primary folate bound to the enzymes is tetrahydropteroylpentaglutamate.[6,9] Their affinity for this compound is $K_d = 0.2$ μM, followed by less strong binding by tetrahydrofolate and its 5-formyl and 5-methyl derivatives. The reduced folates bind a hundredfold tighter than folate or methyltrexate. Kinetic properties indicate that 1 mole of folate is bound per mole of protein.[10] Similarly, electrophoretic studies show that 1 mole of flavin is bound covalently to 1 mole of protein. Dimethylglycine dehydrogenase demonstrates substrate binding and activity for both dimethylglycine and sarcosine. The activity with sarcosine, however, is only 25 percent of that with dimethylglycine. The K_m for dimethylglycine is 0.05 m*M*.[10] Other compounds (N-methylalanine and ξ-N-methylglycine) are significantly poorer substrates. Substrate specificities are assayed with an artificial electron acceptor, phenozinemethosulfate (PMS), in the presence of a dye reduction system (2,6-dichloroindophenol).

It has been demonstrated that dimethylglycine dehydrogenase from rat liver is uniquely found in the mitochondrial fraction and that the FAD cofactor is covalently bound at the riboflavin 8α position to Nπ of histidine.[11] A cDNA clone from rat hepatocytes has been isolated that has an open reading frame for a polypeptide of 96,059 Da with an apparent 43-amino-acid-leader peptide.[12]

Sarcosine dehydrogenase and dimethylglycine dehydrogenase have similar binding properties for folates, although the specific properties of the latter enzyme with various folates have not been reported. Sarcosine dehydrogenase does bind sarcosine specifically and does not oxidize other N-methyl amino acids. The K_m for sarcosine is 0.5 m*M*.[10]

A second system for sarcosine oxidation may exist in the peroxisome. In bacteria, sarcosine oxidase exists as a monomeric protein, and a similar enzyme has been identified in rabbit liver and in mouse liver and kidney.[13,14] In the rabbit and the mouse, this enzyme is a monomer of approximately 40,000 Da and contains a peroxisomal targeting sequence. In addition to using sarcosine as a substrate, it also degrades L-pipecolic acid and L-proline. A similar enzyme in humans has not been identified.

FORMATION OF "ACTIVE" FORMALDEHYDE

"Active" formaldehyde is formed in the reactions of dimethyl or sarcosine dehydrogenase. The methyl group released by these reactions is used preferentially for incorporation into the three-carbon of serine.[4] This particular carbon atom participates preferentially in linked enzymatic reactions and is called an *active* formaldehyde. Blakely[15] demonstrated that the cosubstrate required by serine hydroxymethyltransferase in the conversion of serine from glycine required 5,10-methylene tetrahydrofolate, which is converted from the released methyl group in a separate enzymatic step. The addition of dimethylglycine to its dehydrogenase, prepared with bound [^{3}H]tetrahydrofolate, results in the formation of 5,10-methylene tetrahydrofolate directly. Thus, this compound is formed directly on the protein, without undergoing a separate enzymatic reaction. It was postulated that serine hydroxymethylase may be located close to the aforementioned enzymes on the mitochondrial membrane and have a selective advantage in gaining access to the 5,10-methylene tetrahydrofolate that is formed by the enzymatic action of dimethylglycine and sarcosine dehydrogenase (Fig. 89-2).

SARCOSINE FORMATION FROM GLYCINE

An alternative mechanism for the formation of sarcosine has been proposed.[16] Measurement of the incorporation of the methyl carbon of methionine into sarcosine and serine indicates that 5 to 14 percent of the 1-methyl-[^{14}C]methionine in the diet of humans is converted to sarcosine. In this reaction, methionine is metabolized to S-adenosylmethionine, and this compound reacts with glycine to form sarcosine and S-adenosylhomocysteine. The enzyme for this reaction is S-adenosylmethionine:glycine methyltransferase (EC 2.1.1.20). It is present in liver, kidney, and pancreas of the adult rabbit and rat.[17,18] It is postulated that glycine methyltransferase functions to remove a physiological excess of methyl groups (from S-adenosylmethionine) by forming sarcosine, which in turn is recycled back to glycine.[17] Glycine methyltransferase is a major folate-binding protein in rat liver, whose rate of activity is increased by phosphorylation by a protein kinase and inhibited when it is coupled with its natural folate

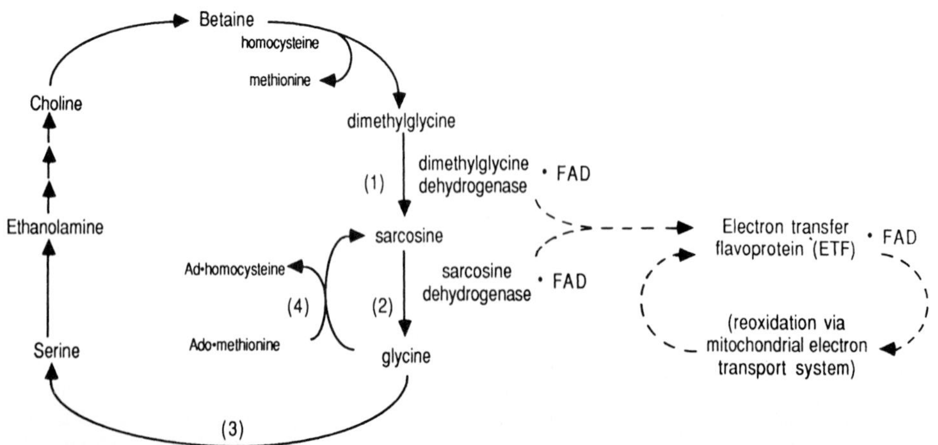

Fig. 89-2 Pathway of the "one-carbon cycle" with sarcosine as an intermediate. Sarcosine may also be formed from glycine (reaction 4). The electron transfer flavoprotein (ETF) accepts electrons from dimethylglycine dehydrogenase and sarcosine dehydrogenase and in turn is reoxidized by the mitochondrial electron transport system. 1) Dimethylglycine dehydrogenase. 2) Sarcosine dehydrogenase. 3) Serine hydroxymethylase. 4) S-Adenosylmethionine:glycine methyltransferase. (*Modified from Mudd et al.,*[19] *with permission.*)

ligand, 5-methyltetrahydropteroylpentaglutamate.[8] This regulatory step in sarcosine formation is important in regulating the ratio of S-adenosylmethionine to S-adenosylhomocysteine. The existence of this pathway in humans has not been confirmed.

PHYSIOLOGICAL FLUX OF GLYCINE

In a careful clinical study, Mudd and co-workers[19] have measured the rate at which the methyl moiety of methionine is oxidized through the sarcosine pathway. They evaluated two patients with sarcosinemia and sarcosinuria and measured the contribution of methionine, choline, and glycine to the excretion of sarcosine. They concluded that at a basal metabolic rate, approximately 2 mmol/24 h of sarcosine is formed from choline and excreted in the urine. An increased contribution to sarcosine formation through the one-carbon cycle did not occur until the total labile methyl intake approached or exceeded 13 mmol/24 h. The incremental increase in sarcosine synthesis above the basal rate was most likely due to glycine methylation as a mechanism for removing "excess" labile methyl groups, a process that is shared by both glycine methyltransferase and the sarcosine oxidizing system.

In measuring the flux of the methyl group from methionine, it was estimated that 10.2 mmol/24 h was used for creatine, 1.4 mmol/24h for transmethylation reactions, 0.5 mmol/24 h for polyamine synthesis, and 2.0 mmol/24 h for sarcosine formation. The total estimated use of labile methyl groups comes to 14.1 mol/24 h. When the labile methyl intake from dietary sources exceeds this total, the excess is largely used for the formation of sarcosine. The latter response most likely takes place from the methylation of glycine.

RENAL TRANSPORT OF SARCOSINE

Under normal physiological conditions, the existence of sarcosine outside of the liver parenchyma must be quite transitory. An independent renal transport mechanism for sarcosine has not been identified. Glorieux and colleagues[20] have studied the renal tubular reabsorption of sarcosine in rat kidney, in normal humans, and in persons with sarcosinemia. There are several renal transport systems for related amino acids in humans.[21,22] The measurement of sarcosine uptake in rat kidney slices *in vitro*[20] showed that it is partitioned between low-K_m and high-K_m systems (Fig. 89-3) and competes with proline and glycine for uptake. These events occur in the slice predominantly at the basolateral membrane.

Similar studies of sarcosine transport have not been performed with human kidney. Renal tubular reabsorption of sarcosine *in vivo* has been measured in normal persons and in two patients with sarcosinemia.[20] In the latter, there was clear evidence that the majority of the filtered sarcosine is reabsorbed in a high-capacity system that is shared by glycine, proline, and hydroxyproline. The estimate for the tubular maximum (Tm) for filtered sarcosine was 160 µmol/min/1.73 m^2.[20]

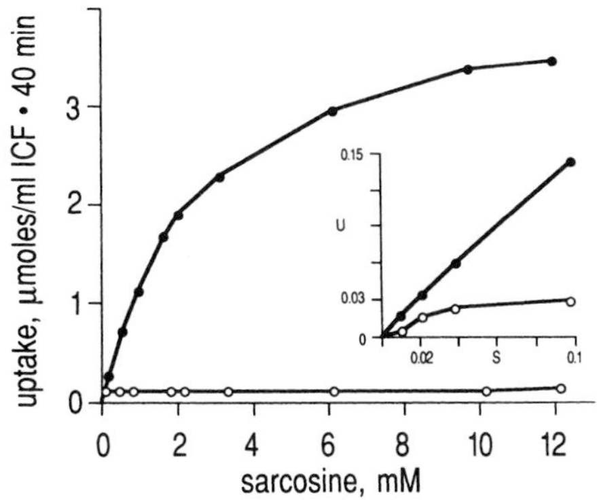

Fig. 89-3 Michaelis plot of sarcosine uptake by rat kidney assigned to low-K_m (○) and high-K_m (•) systems. The major fraction of sarcosine uptake is achieved by the high-K_m system. The K_m values are 0.1 millimolars and 3.0 millimolars for the low- and high-K_m systems, respectively. *(From Glorieux et al.,[20] with permission.)*

TRANSMEMBRANE TRANSPORT OF SARCOSINE

The mechanism by which sarcosine is transported across cellular membranes is becoming clearer. A human glycine transporter system, GlyT-1, has been cloned and sequenced.[23] It is located on chromosome 1p31.3 and has an open reading frame of 1914 nucleotides. The expressed protein possesses 12 putative transmembrane domains, contains 638 amino acids, and is a Na^+/Cl^--dependent transporter. It has several isoforms derived from alternative splicing, each isoform being expressed differently in various tissues. The glycine uptake on this system has a K_m of 80 to 90 µM and is competitively inhibited by sarcosine with a similar potency ($K_i = 80$ to 90 µM). Thus, it is likely that sarcosine and glycine share this same system for transport.

GlyT-1 is strongly expressed in human brain and kidney; GlyT-1c, an isoform of GlyT-1, is expressed only in brain, while GlyT-1a is apparently the only subtype expressed in peripheral tissue. A similar glycine transporter (GlyT-2) has also been cloned, sequenced, and expressed. GlyT-2 is specifically localized to spinal cord, brain stem, and cerebellum but, unlike GlyT-1, shows no inhibition by sarcosine.[24] There is no evidence that this system is involved in sarcosine transport. Thus, it is plausible that some patients with high levels of sarcosine in brain or CSF may have inhibition of the GlyT-1 system that regulates the rapid flux of glycine concentrations involved in neurotransmission.

AN ANIMAL MODEL FOR SARCOSINEMIA

A mouse (*sar*) has been identified that has a deficiency of sarcosine dehydrogenase in liver and has the phenotype of sarcosinemia and sarcosinuria.[25] The mouse was identified within a program using ethylnitrosourea (ENU) by intraperitoneal injection to induce random mutations in male BTBR mice. Urine from the generational progeny of these mutagenized mice was screened for amino acids, and increased excretion of sarcosine was identified in two male siblings. Subsequent breeding allowed selection of a small colony of mice with sarcosinemia (*sar/sar*). The same laboratory subsequently localized the gene for sarcosine dehydrogenase in the mouse to chromosome 2, approximately 15 to 18 cM from the centromere,[26] a region homologous to the region 9q33-q34 of the human genome. The gene localization was performed by the use of polymorphic markers in intersubspecific crosses between females of an inbred strain of mice (*sar/sar*) and a male of an inbred strain (MAI/Pas,2). The pattern of inheritance was autosomal recessive.

The mean sarcosine concentration in the plasma of *sar/sar* mice was 785 ± 153 µM, and that in urine was 102 ± 58 µmol/g creatinine. Sarcosine is normally undetectable in the blood or urine of mice. Sarcosine dehydrogenase activity in mitochondria prepared from liver tissue was 0.54 ± 0.61 µmol 10^{-6}/min per mg protein as compared to 3.14 ± 1.20 µmol 10^{-6} /min per mg protein in preparations from unaffected mice.

No behavioral symptoms or pathology have been observed in the sarcosinemic mice. This particular animal model may have value for the study of one-carbon metabolism in mammals and as a model system for hepatic cell or gene transplantation.

METABOLIC DEFECTS CAUSING SARCOSINEMIA

In humans, the finding of increased sarcosine in blood or urine is a rare event. The phenotype of sarcosinemia or sarcosinuria can occur on the basis of at least three recognized mechanisms: 1) an apparent defect in the holoenzyme of sarcosine dehydrogenase, 2) a mutation in the electron transfer flavoprotein that is shared by sarcosine dehydrogenase, dimethylglycine dehydrogenase, and other acyl dehydrogenases, and 3) severe folate deficiency. If a sarcosine oxidase exists in human peroxisomes, a deficiency of this enzyme may also contribute to the phenotype of sarcosinemia and sarcosinuria.

CLINICAL PHENOTYPE

The original report of sarcosinemia described an infant with mental retardation, hypertonia, and tremors, having an excess of sarcosine in the urine and elevated levels of sarcosine (15 to 31 mM) in plasma.[1] Because the child had mental retardation, it was proposed that the abnormality in sarcosine metabolism was responsible for the mental retardation and perhaps contributed to his other neurologic problems. This concept was reinforced by the finding within the family of an older sibling with similar plasma values of sarcosine and an estimated IQ of 81. Another older sibling existed, without sarcosinemia, who appeared physically and neurologically normal with an IQ of 101. The oldest boy in this family, however, was physically normal and unaffected with sarcosinemia; his IQ was 81.

In the 5 years following the original description of sarcosinemia, there were five additional reports of sarcosinemic children with clinical problems. Hagge and coworkers[27] reported a child born to Indonesian parents who were first cousins. This child had hepatomegaly but no signs of mental or neurologic abnormalities. Scott and coauthors[28] evaluated a child with mental retardation and growth failure; Willems and associates[29] describe two siblings with an unspecified form of dwarfism, and Glorieux and colleagues[20] reported their evaluations of a child with short stature with normal intelligence. Because of the variation in clinical phenotype and lack of consistent association between sarcosinemia and mental retardation, Scott and co-workers originally proposed that sarcosinemia was a benign condition that had erroneously been implicated as the cause of clinical abnormalities because of ascertainment bias.[28] Another report tends to confirm the concept that sarcosinemia is a benign condition unrelated to neurologic alterations. Levy *et al.*[30] identified three patients through the newborn screening program in Massachusetts. Clinical and intellectual evaluations between the ages of 3.8 years and 15 years showed they had full-scale IQ scores between 89 and 111 and were free of neurologic problems.

The literature documents a total of 21 patients with sarcosinemia and sarcosinuria associated with putative deficiency of sarcosine dehydrogenase activity. Fifteen were detected because of clinical symptoms; three were identified by screening of urine amino acids in newborns; and three were siblings of original probands. Over 30 patients with confirmed sarcosinemia have now been identified in the Quebec urine screening program.[31] Some of these patients have now been followed for almost 20 years. There are no manifestations of disease in this cohort of patients. However, since the disorder clusters in this population and probably reflects the effect of founder effect and genetic drift, it may not be representative of all patients with sarcosinemia. There is no indication that the cause of sarcosinemia in these patients is anything other than sarcosine dehydrogenase deficiency (Laframboise R and Scriver CR, personal communication, 1992).

There is, however, some lingering doubt that sarcosinemia is completely benign. This is based on four bits of evidence: 1) The mean IQ of siblings of affected individuals who were detected because of neurologic symptoms is only 74 (Group II, Table 89-1). This may have occurred because of low parental IQ or because sarcosine does have some influence on intellectual development. 2) Blom and Fernandes[32] have proposed that some patients may have symptoms of chronic vomiting and poor weight gain as a consequence of their sarcosinemia. Vomiting and poor weight gain have been seen in several of the patients detected with sarcosinemia. Blom and Fernandes report a lessening of clinical symptoms with long-term folic acid therapy. 3) More than a single enzymatic defect may be responsible for sarcosinemia. If such a defect should also include dimethylglycine dehydrogenase, then elevations of both dimethylglycine and sarcosine could occur and theoretically give rise to a different clinical phenotype than the one observed from sarcosine dehydrogenase deficiency. 4) In rabbit and mouse liver, sarcosine has been shown to be oxidized by a peroxisomal enzyme. This enzyme contains a covalently bound

Table 89-1 Summary of Laboratory and Clinical Data of Patients Reported with Sarcosinemia Attributable to a Defect in Sarcosine Dehydrogenase*

	Number of Patients	Concentration of Sarcosine in Plasma *μ mol/L*	Urinary Excretion of Sarcosine *μ mol/24 h*	Urinary Excretion of Sarcosine *μ mol/mmol*† Creatinine	IQ	Clinical Problems	References
Group 1– Patients ascertained because of neurologic symptoms	9	157–540	1150–5570	170–5080	20–100 (x̄ = 55)	Mental retardation, growth delay, vomiting, hypertension, hypoactivity, cranial synostosis, syndactyly, blindness, Usher syndrome, cardiomyopathy	1, 28, 38, 42, 44, 45, 46
Group 2– Sibs of patients in Group 1	3	53–326	5320–7891	723	x̄ = 74) (est)	Mild mental retardation	1, 29, 42
Group 3– Patients ascertained without neurologic symptoms or from newborn screening program	9	80–760	864–6740	237–1062	89–116 (x̄ = 103)	None, or vomiting, dyslexia, small size, enlarged liver	20, 27, 29, 30, 32

*When the patients are separated by means of ascertainment, it suggests that the sarcosinemia phenotype is probably independent of mental retardation.
†An estimate of 24-h excretion of sarcosine can be approximated by assuming 1 g creatinine is excreted in 24 h by adults. Sarcosine (μmol/mmol creatinine) may be multiplied by 8.85 to estimate μmol/g creatinine.

flavin and is capable of metabolizing L-pipecolic acid, L-proline, and sarcosine.[13,14] It is not yet confirmed that a similar enzyme exists in humans.

PHENOTYPIC COMPARISON TO DIMETHYLGLYCINURIA

Moolenaar and colleagues[32a] reported a 3-year-old male with a lifelong complaint of having a "fish odor." He was otherwise in good health. By the use of NMR spectroscopy and GC/MS, they documented a 100-fold elevation of dimethylglycine in serum (221 μM) and a 20-fold elevation in urine (449 mmol/mol creatinine). There was no apparent elevation of sarcosine in blood and urine, nor abnormalities in folate values. They cloned the cDNA for human dimethylglycine dehydrogenase and compared the sequence to that obtained from their proband. The affected male had a His → Arg alteration occurring near the putative flavin binding site.

The preliminary clinical data for dimethylglycine dehydrogenase deficiency suggests that except for the "fish odor," similar to trimethylaminuria, it has a benign clinical phenotype with no apparent neurologic component.

LABORATORY DATA

Sarcosine is not normally detectable in plasma or in urine. In patients with sarcosinemia, the concentration in blood ranged from 53 μM to 760 μM and urinary excretion from 864 μmol/24 h to 7900 μmol/24 h. The actual quantity of sarcosine excreted in a 24-h period appears to be related to the person's age, body mass, and dietary intake of methyl groups.

Two reports document the concentration of sarcosine in CSF of affected patients: 5 μM in a 2-year-old male[28] and 17 μM in a 5.8-year-old male.[30] Sarcosine is not normally detectable in spinal fluid.

Reports of hematologic and biochemical assays in patients with sarcosinemia are scant. It is assumed that such parameters have been measured but are not abnormal.

SARCOSINE LOADING STUDIES

Six patients were studied in oral sarcosine loading studies.[1,20,27,28,29,33] If the conversion of sarcosine to glycine is impaired, the rise in plasma sarcosine should be greater than normal and the rise in plasma glycine less. Loading studies in all patients produced this response. Sarcosine concentration peaked at 1 to $1\frac{1}{2}$ h and remained elevated for 5 to 8 h after ingestion. In a 3-month-old infant evaluated by Willems,[29] plasma values did not reach their maximum until 3 h after administration. This slow rise may have been related to a slower rate of intestinal absorption of sarcosine in young infants, since a control child of 3 months, unaffected with sarcosinemia, also had a delay in the rise of her serum sarcosine until 3 h after administration.

Glorieux and coworkers calculated the half-life of plasma sarcosine in an affected individual to be over 6 h.[20] In four normal persons, it was about $1\frac{1}{2}$ h. The patient with sarcosinemia showed no rise in plasma glycine following sarcosine administration. Patients reported by Scott *et al.*[28] and by Kang *et al.*[33] showed a modest rise in plasma glycine following sarcosine administration (Fig. 89-4).

THE ENZYMATIC ERROR

Quantitative data on enzyme activity from patients with sarcosinemia are scarce. The conversion from sarcosine to glycine requires sarcosine dehydrogenase apoenzyme and the ability to transfer the generated electron to an electron transfer flavoprotein (ETF). Many steps in this reaction could theoretically be defective. The apoenzyme itself could be affected, or the ability to transfer the electron to its flavoprotein could be impaired. The flavoprotein

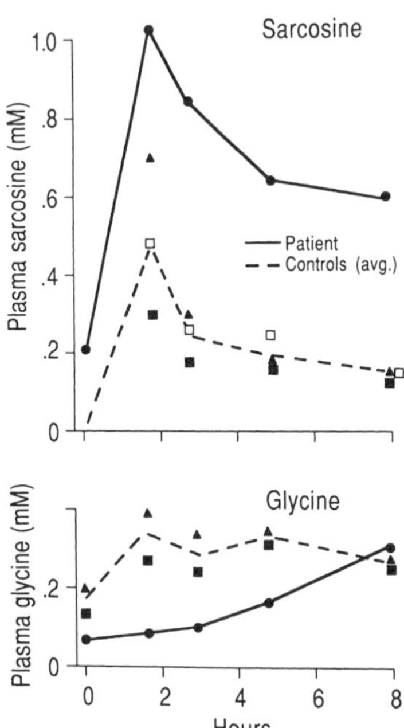

Fig. 89-4 Typical response of plasma sarcosine and glycine concentrations to oral ingestion of 100 mg/kg of sarcosine in a child with sarcosinemia. (*From Scott et al.,*[28] *with permission.*)

could be altered in its abundance, stability, configuration, or unique ability to bind or accept electrons from sarcosine dehydrogenase. Because of the rarity of the disorder, it is likely that no single mutation is shared by the majority of the patients affected with sarcosinemia. Defects of electron transport, however, should affect both sarcosine and dimethylglycine dehydrogenases.

Gerritsen measured the activity of sarcosine dehydrogenase in a liver biopsy.[34] He found deficient sarcosine dehydrogenase activity. The assay was performed in a manner that did not clarify whether the lesion was in the apoenzyme for sarcosine dehydrogenase or in the ETF.*

Subsequently, a second child affected with sarcosinemia had a liver biopsy to measure sarcosine dehydrogenase activity.[35] This assay utilized a mitochondrial-enriched preparation that included PMS as an electron acceptor. The specific activity of sarcosine dehydrogenase in this patient was normal. It was concluded that the defect in this particular patient must exist "in or distal to the flavoprotein that acts as the natural electron acceptor." No specific data on fatty acid metabolism were given for this patient, an important point in view of subsequent findings that the ETF serving sarcosine dehydrogenase and dimethylglycine dehydrogenase also functions as the electron acceptor for fatty acyl-CoA dehydrogenase. Patients with severe deficiencies of this ETF have glutaric aciduria and may excrete sarcosine in their urine.[36] Attempts to measure the enzymatic activity of sarcosine dehydrogenase in tissues other than liver have not been successful. Sarcosine oxidation occurs only in liver and kidney; no enzyme activity was detected in skin fibroblasts or peripheral leukocytes.[20,28,37]

GENETICS

The precise chromosomal locus of human sarcosine dehydrogenase (SARDH) was delineated by Eschenbrenner and Jorns.[37a] The gene is located on chromosome 9q34 and is at least 75.3 kb long.

*In a previous review article, it was indicated that the *in vitro* assay system used by Gerritsen included PMS as an electron acceptor in the assay.[34] In a personal communiction to H. Mudd,[19] Gerritsen clarified this point, indicating that PMS was not utilized in the assay mixture. Thus, the defect could have involved either the apoenzyme or the ETF.

The protein has a predicted mass of 99 505 Da (including covalently bound FAD) and exhibits 89% homology to rat liver sarcosine dehydrogenase and 35% homology to rat liver dimethylglycine dehydrogenase. The authors identified cDNAs that correspond to alternately sliced and polyadenylated transcripts. The adult human liver clone corresponds to the full-length cDNA and is assembled from 21 exons. Exon 2 contains the first in-frame methionine codon, the ADP-binding motif and the presumed flavin attachment site. The first 22 residues in the deduced amino acid sequence exhibit features expected for a mitochondrial targeting sequence. The putative human SARDH is highly expressed in adult and fetal liver, with lower expression in adult pancreas and kidney and in fetal kidney. Pedigree studies indicate an autosomal recessive pattern of inheritance. Males and females are affected, and siblings of probands are sometimes affected; at least three of 12 siblings had sarcosinuria and sarcosinemia. Kang *et al.*[33] proposed their patient was the offspring of a homozygous (father) × heterozygous (mother) mating. The parents of the individual reported by Hagge *et al.*[27] were first cousins, and the parents of the case reported by Christensen *et al.*[38] were an uncle and niece.

INCIDENCE OF SARCOSINEMIA

The incidence of sarcosinemia has been estimated by Levy *et al.*[30] as one in 350,000 live births, ascertained by amino acid screening of urine from newborns (source population: approximately 1×10^6 newborns). The incidence is 1 in 28,000 newborns in Quebec (same method of ascertainment and similar sample size),[31] the latter incidence is explained by founder effect and genetic drift in a portion of the Quebec population (Laframboise R, Scriver CR, personal communication, 1992).

HETEROZYGOTE DETECTION

Heterozygote detection has been attempted by means of sarcosine loading. The assumption is that persons heterozygous for a deficiency of sarcosine dehydrogenase activity may have limited capacity to clear sarcosine from their plasma and that there may be an increased excretion of sarcosine in the urine. Ten obligate heterozygotes have been studied in this manner. Four of eight obligate heterozygotes showed an elevation in the concentration of sarcosine in their plasma following sarcosine ingestion that was considered above the normal range. Glorieux and associates[20] also measured the rate of sarcosine disappearance from the plasma, two obligate heterozygotes showed a slightly prolonged half life (mean value 2.2 h, compared to 1.6 h in controls). These data suggest that the measurement of serum sarcosine concentration following the oral ingestion of sarcosine is not a reliable indicator of the heterozygous state, since only 60 percent of obligate heterozygotes could be detected by this technique.

Quantitation of sarcosine in the urine following sarcosine ingestion has been reported in the parents of five patients. Six of eight heterozygotes showed increased excretion of urinary sarcosine compared to control values established for each study. Two of the heterozygotes showed such increased excretion even though their plasma values remained within the control range. Two of the individuals with normal urinary excretion and normal plasma sarcosine concentrations following sarcosine loading studies were fathers of patients. In each case the possibility of nonpaternity was not excluded.[1,29]

Glorieux and coworkers[20] have reported urinary excretion of sarcosine in terms of renal clearance values for the parents of an affected child. Their renal clearance rates were 9.4 and 9.7 μmol/min per 1.73 m^2, which compared favorably with values of 3.6 to 50.6 μmol/min per 1.73 m^2 for normal adults. There was no obvious alteration in the tubular reabsorptive function of sarcosine in these parents.

It is not unexpected that the measurement of sarcosine in the blood or urine may not be a reliable indicator of heterozygosity for sarcosinemia. This is a common problem in using biochemical or physiological measurements in attempting to ascertain genotype. Because of genetic heterogeneity for recessive disorders and variations in biochemical fluxes that exist between individuals, it is unlikely that clear boundaries can be drawn between "normal" persons and "heterozygotes" for a specific trait. For an excellent review see McGill *et al.*[39]

SARCOSINEMIA FROM GLUTARIC ACIDEMIA TYPE II

Sarcosinemia and sarcosinuria occur in patients with deficiency of either the ETF or ETF:ubiquinone oxidoreductase (ETF:QO). Young children with genetic defects of the ETF are classified as having glutaric acidemia type II (see Chap. 103). They have recurrent hypoglycemia, metabolic acidosis without ketosis, and significant excretion of specific organic acids in the urine.[40,41] The urinary organic acid profile reveals lactic, glutaric, 2-hydroxyglutaric, and dicarboxylic acids.[36,40,41] The presence of 2-hydroxyisovaleric acid may give rise to an odor of "sweaty feet." If the deficiency of the ETF is incomplete and allows partial activity of dimethylglycine dehydrogenase and sarcosine dehydrogenase, small quantities of sarcosine may be formed and detectable in serum and urine.[30,40,41] Such quantities are usually on the order of less than 20 μM in plasma and less than 300 μM in urine. The majority of patients with glutaric acidemia type II have not been noted to have detectable sarcosinemia or sarcosinuria.

Glutaric acidemia type II is inherited as an autosomal recessive condition and has been detected prenatally by analysis of organic acids in amniotic fluid and by biochemical evaluation of cultured cells from amniotic fluid.[41]

SARCOSINEMIA ASSOCIATED WITH FOLATE DEFICIENCY

A deficiency of folic acid is associated with sarcosinemia and sarcosinuria. Tippett and Danks[42] reported a child of 11 months who became folate deficient on a diet of goat's milk alone. Her urine sarcosine concentration was reported as 145 and 368 μmol/mmol creatinine. The sarcosinuria disappeared upon correction of her folate deficiency. Sarcosinemia and sarcosinuria have also been observed in an infant with severe folate deficiency secondary to congenital folate malabsorption. This male infant had sarcosine values of 14 μM in plasma and 185 μM in urine. His sarcosinemia became undetectable after correction of his folate deficiency (Scott CR, unpublished observation).

The actual spectrum of sarcosine concentrations in patients with various reasons for having folate deficiency has been difficult to quantify because of the insensitivity of the amino acid analyzer for quantifying low levels of sarcosine. A report[43] describing the development of a GC/MS method for sarcosine and N,N-dimethylglycine detection has improved the sensitivity of quantitation of these compounds and found them statistically elevated in folate deficiency. In 28 patients with various causes of inadequate folate levels, the mean value of sarcosine was 5.6 ± 1.0 μM, compared to 1.4 ± 0.6 μM in 60 normal persons ($P < 0.001$). N,N-dimethyl glycine concentrations were even higher, at 55.5 μM (normal = 3.6 ± 1.4 μM; $P < 0.001$).

The authors postulate that the increased levels of plasma sarcosine in folate deficiency occur through accelerated synthesis of sarcosine by glycine N-methyltransferase and simultaneous slowing of its conversion to glycine by sarcosine dehydrogenase. Folate deficiency would lead to low levels of 5-CH_3-tetrahydrofolate, resulting in decreased binding to glycine-N-methyltransferase and an inappropriate increase in its activity. Low levels of 5-CH_3-tetrahydrofolate would decrease the activity of sarcosine dehydrogenase by limiting its availability as a cofactor.

Further evidence of the effect of serum folate concentrations on the conversion of sarcosine to glycine is implied in a case report by Blom and Fernandes.[32] The conversion of sarcosine to glycine improved after prolonged folate therapy, with a lowering of the concentration of sarcosinemia in serum.

ACKNOWLEDGMENT

We thank MS Jorns (ref. 37a) for advance notice of the cloned human gene.

REFERENCES

1. Gerritsen T, Waisman HA: Hypersarcosinemia: An inborn error of metabolism. *N Engl J Med* **275**:66, 1966.
2. Hoskins DD, MacKenzie CG: Solubilization and electron transfer flavoprotein requirement of mitochondrial sarcosine dehydrogenase and dimethylglycine dehydrogenase. *J Biol Chem* **236**:177, 1961.
3. Frisell WR, MacKenzie CG: Separation and purification of sarcosine dehydrogenase and dimethylglycine dehydrogenase. *J Biol Chem* **237**:94, 1962.
4. MacKenzie CG, Abeles RH: Production of active formaldehyde in the mitochondrial oxidation of sarcosine. *J Biol Chem* **222**:145, 1956.
5. Frisell WR, Cronin JR, MacKenzie CG: Coupled flavoenzymes in mitochondrial oxidation of N-methyl groups. *J Biol Chem* **237**:2975, 1962.
6. Wittwer AJ, Wagner C: Identification of the folate binding proteins of rat liver mitochondria as dimethylglycine dehydrogenase and sarcosine dehydrogenase: Purification and folate-binding characteristics. *J Biol Chem* **256**:4102, 1981.
7. Wittwer AJ, Wagner C: Identification of folate binding protein of mitochondria as dimethylglycine dehydrogenase. *Proc Natl Acad Sci USA* **77**:4484, 1980.
8. Wagner C, Decha-Umphai W, Corbin J: Phosphorylation modulates the activity of glycine N-methyltransferase, a folate binding protein. *J Biol Chem* **264**:9638,1989.
9. Wittwer AJ, Wagner C: Identification of the folate-binding proteins of rat liver mitochondria as dimethylglycine dehydrogenase and sarcosine dehydrogenase: Flavoprotein, nature and enzymatic properties of the purified proteins. *J Biol Chem* **256**:4109, 1981.
10. Porter DH, Cook RJ, Wagner C: Enzymatic properties of dimethylglycine dehydrogenase and sarcosine dehydrogenase from rat liver. *Arch Biochem Biophys* **243**:396, 1985.
11. Cook RJ, Misono KS, Wagner C: The amino acid sequence of the flavin-peptides of dimethylglycine dehydrogenase and sarcosine dehydrogenase from rat liver mitochondria. *J Biol Chem* **260**:12998, 1985.
12. Lang H, Polster M, Brandsch R: Rat liver dimethylglycine dehydrogenase: Flavinylation of the enzyme in hepatocytes in primary culture and characterization of a cDNA clone. *Eur J Biochem* **198**:793, 1991.
13. Reuber BE, Karl C, Reimann SA, Mihalik SJ, Dodi G: Cloning and functional expression of a mammalian gene for a peroxisomal sarcosine oxidase. *J Biol Chem* **272**:6766, 1997.
14. Herbst R, Barton JL, Nicklin MJ: A mammalian homolog of the bacterial monomeric sarcosine oxidases maps to mouse chromosome 11, close to Cryba1. *Genomics* **46**:480, 1997.
15. Blakley RL: A spectrophotometric study of the reaction catalysed by serine transhydroxymethylase. *Biochem J* **77**:459, 1960.
16. Mitchell AD, Benevenga NJ: The role of transamination in methionine oxidation in the rat. *J Nutr* **108**:67, 1978.
17. Kerr SJ: Competing methyltransferase systems. *J Biol Chem* **247**:4248, 1972.
18. Heady JE, Kerr SJ: Purification and characterization of glycine N-methyltransferase. *J Biol Chem* **248**:69, 1973.
19. Mudd SH, Ebert MH, Scriver CR: Labile methyl group balances in the human: The role of sarcosine. *Metabolism* **29**:707, 1980.
20. Glorieux FH, Scriver CR, Delvin E, Mohyuddin F: Transport and metabolism of sarcosine in hypersarcosinemic and normal phenotypes. *J Clin Invest* **50**:2313, 1971.
21. Scriver CR, Efron ML, Schafer IA: Renal tubular transport of proline, hydroxyproline and glycine in health and in familial hyperprolinemia. *J Clin Invest* **43**:374, 1964.
22. Scriver CR: Renal tubular transport of proline, hydroxyproline and glycine: III. Genetic basis for more than one mode of transport in human kidney. *J Clin Invest* **47**:823, 1968.
23. Kim K-M, Kingsmore SF, Han H, Yang-Feng TL, Godinot N, Seldin MF, Caron MG, Giros B: Cloning of the human glycine transporter type 1: Molecular and pharmacological characterization of novel isoform variants and chromosomal localization of the gene in the human and mouse genomes. *Mol Pharmacol* **45**:608, 1994.
24. Liu Q-R, López-Corcuera B, Mandiyan S, Nelson H, Nelson N: Cloning and expression of a spinal cord- and brain-specific glycine transporter with novel structural features. *J Biol Chem* **268**:22802, 1993.
25. Harding CO, Williams P, Pflanzer DM, Colwell RE: Sar: A genetic mouse model for human sarcosinemia generated by ethylnitrosourea mutagenesis. *Proc Natl Acad Sci USA* **89**:2644, 1992.
26. Brunialti AL, Harding CO, Wolff JA, Guénet JL: The mouse mutation sarcosinemia (sar) maps to chromosome 2 in a region homologous to human 9q33-q34. *Genomics* **36**:182, 1996.
27. Hagge W, Brodehl J, Gellissen K: Hypersarcosinemia. *Pediat Res* **1**:409, 1967.
28. Scott CR, Clark SH, Teng CC, Swedberg KR: Clinical and cellular studies of sarcosinemia. *J Pediatr* **77**:805, 1970.
29. Willems C, Heusden A, Hainaut A: Hypersarcosinémie avec sarcosinurie: Etude d'une nouvelle famille. *J Genet Hum* **19**:101, 1971.
30. Levy HL, Coulombe JT, Benjamin R: Massachusetts Metabolic Disorders Screening Program: III. Sarcosinemia. *Pediatrics* **74**:509, 1984.
31. Lemieux B, Auray-Blais C, Giguère R, Shapcott D, Scriver CR: Newborn urine screening experience with over one million infants in the Quebec Network of Genetic medicine. *J Inher Metab Dis* **11**:45, 1988.
32. Blom W, Fernandes J: Folic acid dependent hypersarcosinemia. *Clin Chim Acta* **91**:117, 1979.

32a. Moolenaar SH, Poogi-Bach J, Engelke UFH, Corstiaensen JMB, Heerschap A, De Jong JGN, Binzak BA, Vockley J, Wevers RA: Defect in dimethylglycine dehydrogenase, a new inborn error of metabolism: NMR spectroscopy study. *Clin Chem* **45**(4):459, 1999.

33. Kang ES, Seyer J, Todd TA, Herrera C: Variability in the phenotypic expression of abnormal sarcosine metabolism in a family. *Hum Genet* **64**:80, 1983
34. Gerritsen T: Sarcosine dehydrogenase deficiency, the enzyme defect in hypersarcosinemia. *Helv Paediatr Acta* **27**:33, 1972.
35. Scott CR. Sarcosinemia, in Nyhan WL (ed): *Heritable Disorders of Amino Acid Metabolism*. New York, Wiley, 1974, p 324.
36. Goodman SI, McCabe ERB, Fennessey PV, Mace JW: Multiple acyl-CoA dehydrogenase deficiency (glutaric aciduria type II) with transient hypersarcosinemia and sarcosinuria: Possible inherited deficiency of an electron transfer flavoprotein. *Pediatr Res* **14**:12, 1980.
37. Rehberg ML, Gerritsen T: Sarcosine metabolism in the rat. *Arch Biochem Biophys* **127**:661, 1968.

37a. Eschenbrenner M, Jorns MS: Cloning and mapping of the cDNA for human sarcosine dehydrogenasè, a flavoenzyme defective in patients with sarcosinemia. *Genomics* **59**:300, 1999.

38. Christensen E, Brandt NJ, Rosenberg T: Sarcosinaemia in a patient with Usher syndrome. *J Inher Metab Dis* **12**:487,1989.
39. McGill JJ, Mettler G, Rosenblatt DS, Scriver CR: Detection of heterozygotes for recessive alleles: Homocyst(e)inemia: Paradigm of pitfalls in phenotypes. *Am J Med Genet* **36**:45, 1990.
40. Sweetman L, Nyhan WL, Trauner DA, Merritt TA, Singh M: Glutaric aciduria type II. *J Pediatr* **96**:1020, 1980.
41. Bennett MJ, Curnock DA, Engel PC, Shaw L, Gray RGF, Hull D, Patrick AD, Pollitt RJ: Glutaric aciduria (type II): Biochemical investigation and treatment of a child diagnosed prenatally. *J Inher Metab Dis* **7**:57, 1984.
42. Tippett P, Danks DM: The clinical and biochemical findings in three cases of hypersarcosinemia and one case of transient hypersarcosinuria associated with folic acid deficiency. *Helv Paediatr Acta* **29**:261, 1974.
43. Allen RH, Stabler SP, Lindenbaum J: Serum betaine, *N,N*-dimethylglycine and *N*-methylglycine levels in patients with cobalamin and folate deficiency and related inborn errors of metabolism. *Metabolism* **42**:1448, 1993.
44. Minami R, Olek K, Wardenbach P: Hypersarcosinemia with craniostenosis-syndactylism syndrome. *Hum Genet* **28**:167, 1975.
45. Sewell AC, Krille M, Wilhelm I: Sarcosinaemia in a retarded, amaurotic child. *Eur J Pediatr* **144**:508, 1986.
46. Meissner T, Mayatepek E: Sarcosinemia in a patient with severe progressive neurological damage and hypertrophic cardiomyopathy. *J Inher Metab Dis* **20**:717, 1997.

CHAPTER 90

Nonketotic Hyperglycinemia

Ada Hamosh ▪ Michael V. Johnston

1. **Nonketotic hyperglycinemia (NKH) is an inborn error of glycine degradation in which large quantities of glycine accumulate in all body tissues, including the central nervous system. The diagnosis is established by calculating the cerebrospinal fluid/plasma glycine concentration ratio. A value of greater than 0.08 is diagnostic. Confirmation of the diagnosis requires measurement of the activity of the glycine cleavage system in liver tissue.**
2. **Most patients have the neonatal phenotype, presenting in the first few days of life with lethargy, hypotonia, and myoclonic jerks, and progressing to apnea, and often to death. Those who regain spontaneous respiration develop intractable seizures and profound mental retardation.**
3. **A minority of NKH patients develop symptoms somewhat later in life. In the infantile form, patients present with seizures and have various degrees of mental retardation after a symptom-free interval and seemingly normal development for up to 6 months. In the mild-episodic form, patients present in childhood with mild mental retardation and episodes of delirium, chorea, and vertical gaze palsy during febrile illness. In the late onset form, patients present in childhood with progressive spastic diplegia and optic atrophy, but intellectual function is preserved and seizures have not been reported.**
4. **Transient NKH has been described in six newborns with symptoms indistinguishable from those of the neonatal phenotype. Plasma and CSF glycine concentrations initially are identical to those seen in neonatal NKH, but return to normal by 8 weeks of age. Five of the six infants had no neurologic sequelae after 6 months to 13 years of followup. One had severe developmental delay at age 9 months.**
5. **Glycine is a neurotransmitter. It is inhibitory in the spinal cord and brain stem, which effect is probably responsible for the apnea and hiccuping seen early in the disease course. Glycine is excitatory in the cortex at the *N*-methyl-D-aspartate receptor channel complex. Excessive stimulation at this site probably explains the intractable seizures and brain damage seen in this disorder.**
6. **The primary biochemical defect in NKH is in the glycine cleavage system, an intramitochondrial enzyme complex with four components: the P protein (a pyridoxal phosphate-dependent glycine decarboxylase); the H protein (a lipoic acid containing hydrogen-carrier protein); the T protein (a tetrahydrofolate-dependent protein), and the L protein (lipoamide dehydrogenase). Defects in the P, H, and T proteins have been identified in NKH. Over 80 percent of patients with the neonatal phenotype have a defect in the P protein. Later onset cases are more likely to have defects in the H or T proteins.**
7. **The gene for the human P protein, GLDC (MIM 238300), maps to chromosome 9p13 or 9p23–24 and consists of 25 exons spanning over 135 kb. It encodes an mRNA of 3783 nt and a protein of 1020 amino acids. The human H protein gene, GCSH (MIM 238330), encodes a mRNA of 1192 nt and a precursor protein of 173 amino acids, which is cleaved to mature protein of 125 amino acids. Three pseudogenes for H protein are known, but none are mapped. The human T protein gene, AMT (MIM 238310), maps to chromosome 3q21.1–21.2 and consists of 9 exons spanning 6 kb. It encodes a mRNA of 1209 nt and a precursor protein of 403 amino acids, which is cleaved to a mature protein of 376 amino acids.**
8. **NKH is inherited as an autosomal recessive trait. Its incidence is unknown except in Finland, where a founder effect has resulted in an incidence of 1 in 12,000 live births in one county. Prenatal diagnosis is possible by measuring glycine cleavage activity using chorionic villus samples. The enzyme is not expressed in amniocytes. DNA diagnosis is feasible in families where the specific mutation(s) is known.**
9. **No effective treatment exists, but several experimental therapies directed at decreasing the glycine concentration and blocking its effect at the *N*-methyl-D-aspartate receptor are under investigation.**

The study of patients with nonketotic hyperglycinemia (NKH) has led to the elucidation of the glycine cleavage system, which catalyzes the major reaction of glycine degradation.[1] This complex involves the products of at least four genes; to date, defects in three have been described in patients with the various NKH phenotypes.[2–4]

Although glycine plays many roles in intermediary metabolism, the symptoms of NKH seem to relate to glycine's function as a neurotransmitter. In the brain stem and spinal cord, glycine is an inhibitory neurotransmitter.[5] In contrast, in the cortex, it is an excitatory agonist of the *N*-methyl-D-aspartate (NMDA)-type glutamate receptor-channel complex.[6] Thus, NKH can be regarded as a member of the growing class of inborn errors of neurotransmission.

The first patient, a $5\frac{1}{2}$-year-old with intractable seizures and severe developmental delay, was described in 1965 by Gerritsen and colleagues.[7] Since then, over 150 patients have been reported. Most present in the first few days of life with severe neurologic abnormalities, including lethargy, hypotonia, myoclonic jerks, and apnea progressing to coma and death, or profound mental retardation and intractable seizures.[8] A few milder cases have been described.[9–16] The phenotype is consistent with perturbation of both the inhibitory and the stimulatory roles of glycine in the central nervous system.

GLYCINE METABOLISM

Glycine is structurally the simplest of amino acids. In addition to an amino group and a carboxyl group, the alpha carbon has two symmetric hydrogens.[17] Therefore, there are no D- and L-stereoisomers. An average adult American diet contains 3 to 5 g of glycine per day.[17] In addition, glycine is easily synthesized from serine. Glycine can be converted to glucose via pyruvate and is therefore glycogenic. The glycine pool is approximately 80 mg/kg body weight.[8] The rate of glycine turnover is about 1 g/kg per day.[17] Normal glycine concentrations in various body fluids are shown in Table 90-1.

Glycine is an important constituent of proteins, providing more than a fourth of the amino acid residues of abundant structural proteins such as collagen, elastin, and gelatin, where its small size

Table 90-1 Glycine Concentrations (μM) in Plasma and Corebrospinal Fluid

	Normal Newborn (n)	Neonatal NKH (n)	Atypical NKH (n)
Plasma	56 – 308 (20)*	920 – 1827 (7)*	447,793 (2)*
	204 ± 83 (10)†	780 ± 276 (5)†	
CSF	2.9 – 10.4 (20)*	83 – 280 (7)*	42,72 (2)*
	4.0 ± 2.1 (10)†	88 ± 41 (5)†	
CSF/Plasma	0.024; 0.012 – 0.040 (20)‡	0.136; 0.09 – 0.25 (7)‡	0.094 – 0.097 (2)*

*Range or individual values; data from Hayasaka *et al.*[142]
†Values as mean ± 1 SD; data from von Wendt *et al.*[143]
‡Values as mean followed by range; data from Tada and Hayasaka.[101]

is useful for minimizing steric interference and thus allowing the alpha-helical structure essential to these proteins. Glycine also plays an important synthetic role in metabolism (Fig. 90-1). Its carbon skeleton is incorporated into purines, glutathione, creatine, and δ-aminolevulinate, the precursor of porphyrin and heme.[8]

Approximately 1 g of glycine is used daily in various conjugation reactions, which play a role in detoxification.[17] Glycine is conjugated with benzoic acid to form hippurate, and with salicylates to form salicyluric acid, both of which are excreted in the urine.[17] Choline is conjugated with glycine to form the bile acid, glycocholate, which is excreted into the intestine.[17] In certain inborn errors, glycine conjugation is prominent. For example, patients with isovaleric acidemia excrete large quantities of isovalerylglycine,[18] while those with medium chain acyl CoA dehydrogenase deficiency excrete phenylpropionyl glycine.[19]

Minor pathways in degradation of glycine include oxidation to glyoxylate by glycine oxidase, and condensation with acetyl-CoA to form aminoacetone.[8]

Ingested labeled glycine is rapidly converted into labeled serine by serine hydroxymethylase, a ubiquitous cytoplasmic enzyme.[8] This reaction is reversible, and, under normal physiological conditions, the net flow is from serine to glycine[8] as shown in the following reaction:

$$\mathrm{HOCH_2CHNH_2COOH + CO_2 + NH_3}$$
$$\mathrm{\rightarrow 2\ NH_2CH_2COOH + H_2O}$$

The glycine-serine interconversion was initially thought to be the main pathway of glycine catabolism, but studies of NKH patients have shown otherwise.[1] Nevertheless, in the fasting state, the glycine-serine interconversion is an important source of serine and pyruvate.

The Glycine Cleavage System

The major pathway for the catabolism of both glycine and serine is the glycine cleavage system (GCS) (Fig. 90-2). The GCS is a four-peptide complex located in the inner mitochondrial membrane of the liver, kidney, brain, and placenta.[1] The enzyme complex is similar to the pyruvate dehydrogenase and α-ketoglutarate dehydrogenase complexes (Chap. 100). The overall reaction catalyzed by the GCS complex (where THF is tetrahydrofolate) is:

$$\mathrm{HOOCCH_2NH_3 + THF + NAD+ \leftrightarrow N5, N10}$$
$$\mathrm{= CH_2 - THF + NH_3 + CO_2 + NADH}$$

The individual steps of this reaction are shown in Fig. 90-2. The first is catalyzed by P protein, a pyridoxal phosphate-dependent 120-kDa glycine decarboxylase, and by H protein, a lipoic-acid containing hydrogen carrier protein. H protein is small (15 kDa), acidic, and heat-stable. The action of P and H proteins liberates the carboxyl group of glycine as CO_2. The next step is catalyzed by T protein, a tetrahydrofolate-dependent 34-kDa protein, which liberates the amino group of glycine as NH3 and transfers the alpha carbon of glycine to THF, forming 5,10-methylene THF. Finally, the L protein, a lipoamide dehydrogenase of 110 kDa, and NAD+ reoxidize the dithiol form of H protein to the disulfide form. The proteins of the complex are easily dissociated, except the P and L proteins, which are tightly bound.[1] The stoichiometry of the complex is not known.

Regulating GCS Activity

The activity of hepatic GCS is regulated by a variety of hormones. Most importantly, liver GCS activity increases in response to glucagon.[20] A high-protein diet results in high levels of glucagon and increased glucagon/insulin ratio, which result in increased GCS flux.[20] Postprandial secretion of glucagon increases the levels of intracytosolic cAMP and free calcium, which in turn increase GCS flux.[20] Other hormones that are α-agonists, such as norepinephrine, epinephrine, phenylephrine, and vasopressin,

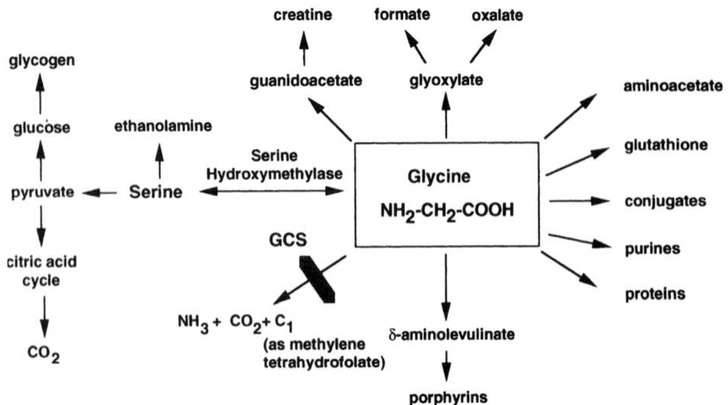

Fig. 90-1 Metabolic pathways of glycine.

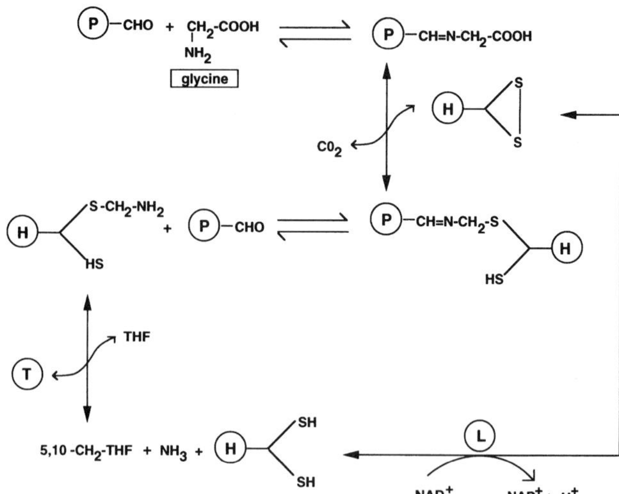

Fig. 90-2 The glycine cleavage system. Circles designate proteins with the active group shown. THF is tetrahydrofolate. In the presence of P and H proteins, glycine is decarboxylated and the remaining aminoethyl group binds to the reduced lipoic acid on the H protein. T protein is required to release ammonia and transfer the α carbon of glycine to THF, forming 5,10-CH2-THF. L protein is necessary to regenerate the correct form of the H protein.

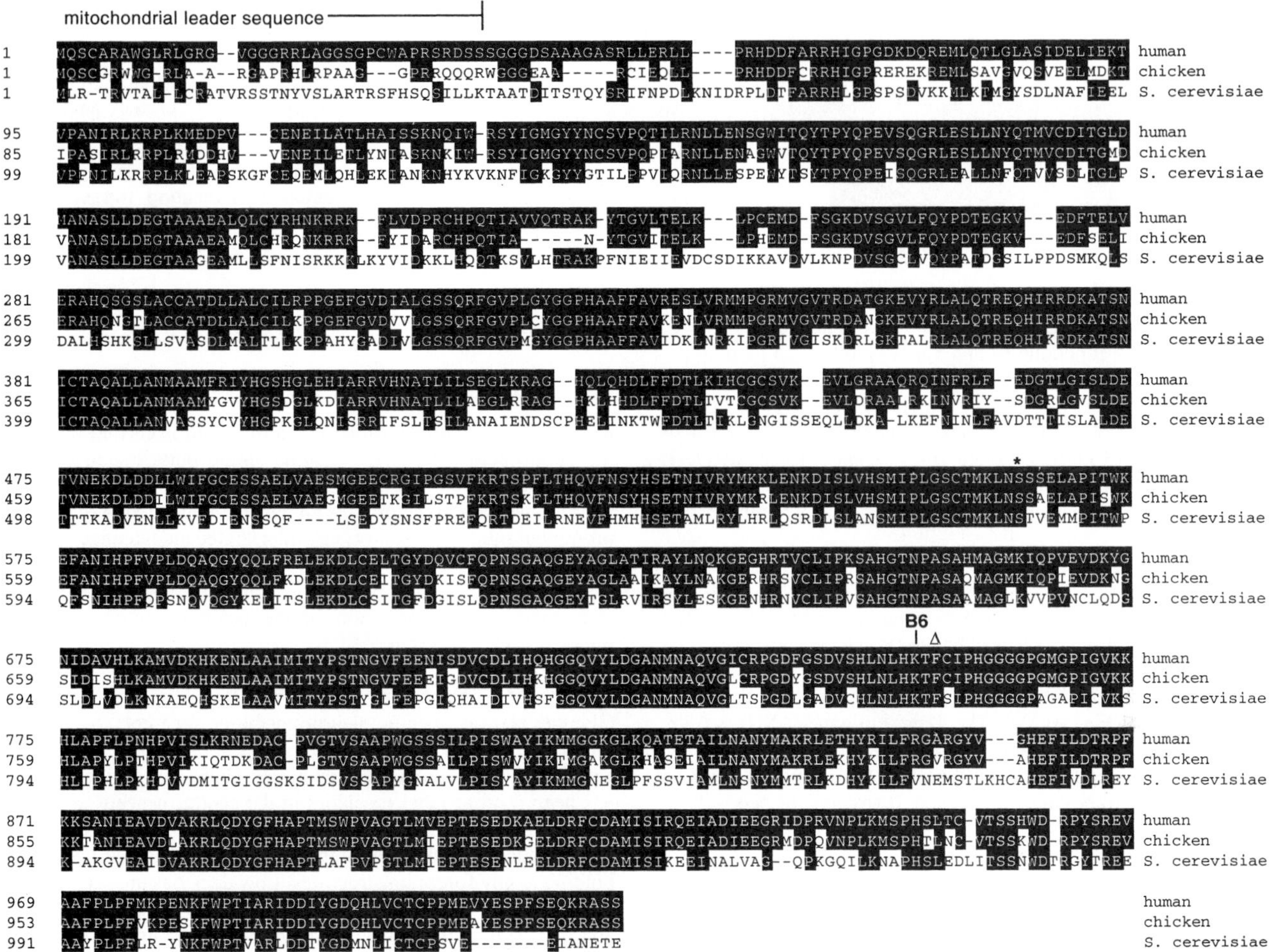

Fig. 90-3 Alignment of human, bovine, and *S. cerevisiae*[3] P protein (or glycine decarboxylase) amino acid sequence. Identical residues are indicated in black. B6 above the line indicates the pyridoxal phosphate-binding site at lysine 754. The asterisk denotes the common Finnish mutation, S564I. The triangle indicates the phenylalanine at residue 756.

also result in elevated cytosolic calcium and increased GCS flux.[21] Studies of isolated mitochondria have confirmed that the activation is modulated through calcium.[22] Calcium's effect depends on the presence of inorganic phosphorous, which is needed not merely as a permeant anion nor in relation to its use in oxidative phosphorylation. Replacement of phosphorous with acetate or thiocyanate does not restore the calcium effect and rotenone, which inhibits mitochondrial respiration, does not affect the increased GCS flux in the presence of calcium and phosphorous.[22]

In contrast to serine hydroxymethylase, which is active at high levels from birth, the GCS is not fully active in the newborn rat.[23] In 2-day-old rat pups, the GCS activity was only 29 percent of the adult activity, and increased steadily with age. Rat pup plasma glycine levels were highest at 2 days and fell by half at 14 days. Serine levels were constant. A similar developmental profile of the GCS could account for transient NKH (see below), but human studies have not been performed.

THE MOLECULAR BIOLOGY OF THE GLYCINE CLEAVAGE SYSTEM

The P Protein

A human P protein cDNA was simultaneously isolated by Kure *et al.* from a human placenta γgt 11 library using an antibody against the rat P protein and by Kume *et al.* from human liver cDNA library using an antibody against the chicken P protein.[24,25] The 3.8-kb mRNA has a 3060 nt open reading frame preceded by 150 nt 5′-untranslated sequence and followed by 532 nt 3′-untranslated sequence ending in a poly-A tail. The 1020 amino acid protein has a predicted molecular mass of 112 kDa (Fig. 90-3). There is a 40-amino acid N-terminal mitochondrial target sequence that is cleaved on entry into the mitochondria leaving a 980-amino acid mature protein. The chicken cDNA has also been cloned and predicts a mature protein with 84 percent amino acid identity with the human protein. The human P protein gene, GLDC, is a single-copy gene that maps to chromosome 9p13[26] or 9p23−3427. This localization was originally suggested by identification of a patient with 9p − syndrome and NKH.[28] Its genomic structure has been analyzed.[29] It spans more than 135 kb and is composed of 25 exons.[29] A second gene with homology to glycine decarboxylase, which is a processed pseudogene, maps to chromosome 3q12.[27]

The H Protein

Koyata and Hiraga first isolated the human H protein cDNA from a human liver cDNA library.[30,31] The 1.2-kb cDNA has a 519-bp open reading frame, which is preceded by a 93-bp 5′-untranslated sequence and followed by either a 17-bp or a 522-bp 3′-untranslated sequence ending in a poly-A tail. Northern analysis performed with labeled H protein cDNA against liver total RNA revealed two transcripts: a 1.4-kb mRNA that used the downstream poly(A) site and, 50 times less abundant, an 0.9-kb mRNA that used the upstream poly(A) site.[30] The 173-amino acid protein has a predicted molecular mass of 19 kDa (Fig. 90-4). There is a 48-amino acid N-terminal mitochondrial target sequence, which is cleaved on entry into the mitochondria, leaving a 125-amino acid (14-kDa) mature protein. The human and chicken H proteins are

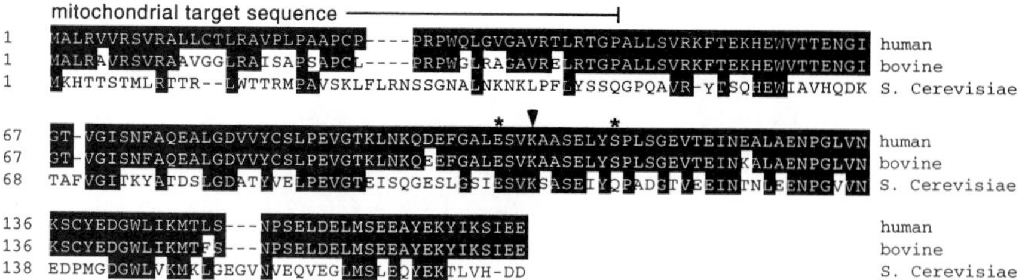

Fig. 90-4 Alignment of human, bovine, and *S. cerevisiae* H protein amino acid sequence.[4] Identical residues are indicated in black. The triangle denotes lysine 107, the lipoamide-binding site, flanked by two asterisks indicating the conserved surrounding region.

highly homologous, with 86 percent amino acid identity; 11 of the 18- amino acid substitutions are conservative. There are conserved cysteine residues at codons 85 and 138, one of which participates in intermolecular disulfide bond formation. The lipoic acid binding site is at lysine 107. The complete genomic organization of the human H protein gene, GCSH, has not been elucidated, but it is known to span 13 kb of genomic DNA.[30] There is one active H protein gene. Three related sequences, which are apparently processed pseudogenes, have been identified by Southern blot analysis.

The T Protein

The human T protein cDNA and its gene have been cloned. The cDNA has a 1209-bp open reading frame which encodes a 403-amino acid precursor protein, which is ultimately processed to a 376-amino acid mature protein after cleavage of the mitochondrial target sequence (Fig. 90-5).[32] The T protein gene, AMT, is 6 kb, consists of 9 exons, and maps to chromosome 3q21.1–21.2.[33] The amino acid sequence of human T protein has 90 percent and 68 percent identity to bovine and chicken T proteins, respectively.[32]

Expression

Molecular studies of the tissue-specific expression of the various components of the GCS have been performed in the chicken.[34] Glycine decarboxylase (P protein) gene expression is exclusively tissue-specific, occurring only in the brain, kidney, and liver. The relative levels of glycine decarboxylase mRNA are liver 1.0, kidney 0.23, and brain 0.03. The H protein gene is expressed in a coordinated fashion with the P protein; that is, there is a linear relationship between H protein and P protein in the tissues where P protein is expressed, but H protein transcription is always present at a basal level. The mechanism of this coupled expression is unknown. The H and T proteins are also expressed at a basal level in many other tissues, such as heart, spleen, and skeletal muscle, where glycine decarboxylase mRNA is undetectable.[34] The purpose of this low-level transcription in other tissues is unknown.

GLYCINE AS A NEUROTRANSMITTER

Most synaptic neurotransmission in the brain is carried out using the amino acids glutamate, gamma amino butyric acid (GABA) and glycine as neurotransmitters.[35] The most prominent excitatory neurotransmitter in the brain is glutamate, while GABA is the most prominent inhibitory neurotransmitter.[36] Recent evidence suggests that glycine plays an important role in neurotransmission, being predominantly inhibitory in the spinal cord and mediating excitatory neurotransmission in the cerebral cortex and other regions of the forebrain.[5,6,37]

Inhibitory Actions of Glycine

Glycine acts at specific neurotransmitter receptors to play an inhibitory role in the brain stem and spinal cord.[38] The drug strychnine, a specific antagonist at the inhibitory glycine receptor, has been used to label receptors in the central nervous system of animals and humans.[6] Autoradiographic studies of specific [^{3}H]strychnine binding to inhibitory receptors showed no specific binding to any forebrain structures. Low densities are seen in most of the mid-brain, with higher amounts in the periaqueductal gray and the oculomotor nuclei. Relatively high binding is present in the pons, medulla, and upper cervical spinal cord, especially in specific nuclei such as those of the trigeminal and hypoglossal nerves. In human brain, some of the highest densities are in the substantia gelatinosa of the trigeminal nucleus in the medulla oblongata. High levels of binding also are seen in the substantia gelatinosa and ventral horns of the spinal cord. In the spinal cord, intrinsic glycinergic neurons are thought to play an important role in maintaining normal muscle tone. In experimental models, these glycine-containing interneurons are especially vulnerable to hypoxic injury.[39] This lesion is associated with spasticity or

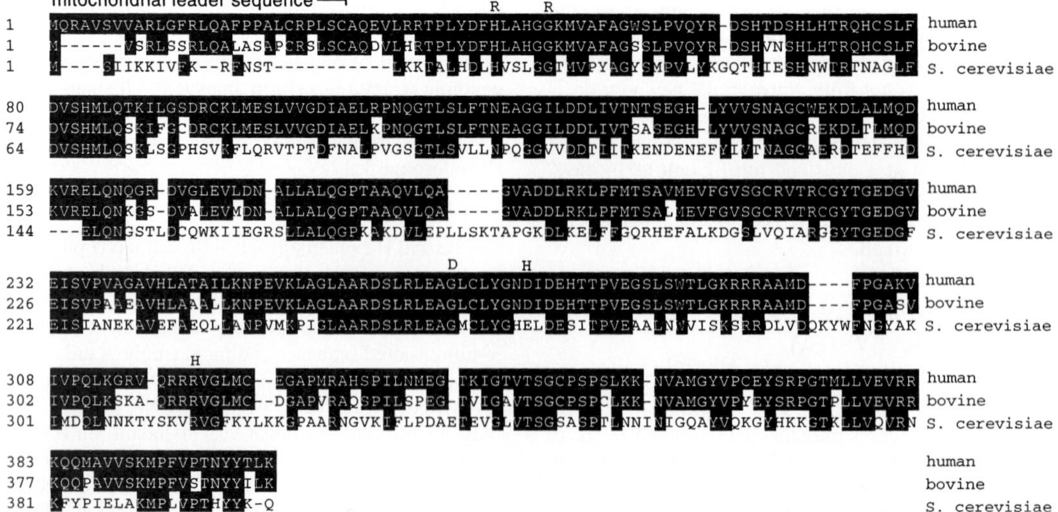

Fig. 90-5 Alignment of human, bovine, and *S. cerevisiae*[5] T protein (or aminomethyl transferase) amino acid sequence. Identical residues are indicated in black. Missense mutations H42R, G47R, G269D, D276H, and R320H are indicated above the line.

increased muscle tone. The strychnine-sensitive inhibitory glycine receptor has been purified from several mammalian species, and subunits have been cloned.[40] In polled Hereford calves with an autosomal recessive deficiency of inhibitory glycine receptors, skeletal muscle myoclonic jerks occur both spontaneously and in response to sensory stimuli.[41] The function of glycine as a major inhibitory transmitter in the spinal cord and brain stem may be enhanced in NKH, producing hypertonia, suppression of respiration, intermittent ophthalmoplegia, and abnormal reflex activity, such as hiccuping.

Electrophysiologically, glycine's inhibitory effects are due to enhanced chloride permeability in postsynaptic neurons, a mechanism similar to the one observed for GABA.[42] Strychnine poisons the nervous system and produces myoclonic jerks both spontaneously and in response to stimuli.[43] A role of glycine in the spinal cord and brain stem is also suggested by the stimulation of dorsal roots, which causes release of glycine in perfused spinal cord.[38] Less is known about the high affinity uptake system for glycine in the synaptosome, but it may be similar to the high affinity uptake for other amino acid neurotransmitters.[44]

Excitatory Neurotransmission

Until recently, it was thought that glycine's primary action on the central nervous system was through the inhibitory receptor. However, exploration of the function of the more numerous excitatory glutamate receptors demonstrated that glycine serves as a co-agonist for the *N*-methyl-D-aspartate (NMDA) type glutamate receptor and is capable of modulating its activity (Fig. 90-6).[6,45,46]

Three major types of neurotransmitter receptors mediate the excitatory actions of glutamate.[47,48] The receptors are defined according to the ability of well-characterized rigid analogues to activate them. These three major types are the NMDA type glutamate receptor, the α-amino-3-hydroxy-5-methyl-4-isoxazole propionic acid (AMPA) receptor, and the so-called metabotropic glutamate receptor that stimulates formation of second messengers. The AMPA receptor mediates most of the fast excitatory neuronal activity, while the NMDA type glutamate receptor activates prolonged electrical depolarizations. In addition, the NMDA receptor is distinct in being blocked at negative membrane potentials by magnesium.[49] A reduction in membrane potential toward a more positive potential produced by membrane stimulation with AMPA receptors makes it easier for the NMDA receptor channel to open and pass calcium. These features of the receptor-channel complex make it suitable for several special activities. For example, the NMDA receptor-channel complex appears to participate in a form of simple learning whereby synaptic depolarization is facilitated by a previous increase in excitatory activity.[50] Through this process, previous neuronal input may facilitate or strengthen neurotransmission through the NMDA receptor-channel complex. The NMDA receptor-channel complex is thought to play an important role in a number of developmental processes, including the shaping of ocular dominance columns by ocular experience, control of neuronal migration, and pruning of redundant synapses in the postnatal period.[51] However, overstimulation of the NMDA receptor-channel complex can be quite stressful for neurons and, in some cases, excessive calcium conduction mediated by these channels can lead to so-called excitotoxic neuronal death.[52] Antagonists of the NMDA receptor-channel complex have been shown to prevent excitotoxic injury.

An excitatory glycine site, called the glycine B receptor, is an important component of the NMDA receptor channel complex.[53–56] A strychnine-insensitive high affinity glycine-binding site with K_d in the range of 100 to 200 nM is found throughout the central nervous system with a distribution that matches the distribution of NMDA receptors.[57] The site is blocked by kynurenic acid, an endogenous metabolite of tryptophan, as well as by other antagonists, including HA966 (a GABA analogue) and CNQX (6-cyano-7-nitroquinoxaline-2,3-dione). The glycine site is an allosteric binding site on the NMDA receptor-channel complex. Glycine binding enhances binding of glutamate to the NMDA binding site.[58] The converse is also true; glycine binding is enhanced by NMDA and depressed by competitive antagonists of glutamate at the NMDA site. Glycine also increases the association rate constant of antagonists, such as MK-801, within the NMDA receptor-channel complex. In addition, there may be an absolute requirement for glycine in order for glutamate to activate the NMDA receptor channel. The glycine modulatory site is an intrinsic part of the cloned NMDA receptor-channel complex.[59] Electrophysiologic evaluation of glycine's action using whole-cell and patch-clamp studies revealed an estimated K_d of 80 nM—significantly lower than the value of 150 nM estimated in the presence of NMDA. The glycine modulatory site follows a developmental curve similar to that followed by the NMDA channel site.[51] It is noteworthy that the concentrations of glycine needed for binding to the excitatory receptor reach saturation at much lower levels (100 to 300 nM) than those required for binding to the inhibitory glycine site which has an EC_{50} of 90 to 100 μM.

The main effect of the binding of glycine to its receptor on the NMDA receptor-channel complex is to increase the frequency of channel openings once glutamate (or NMDA) is bound to the receptor.[56–58] Several studies suggest that glycine modulates NMDA neurotransmission and high levels of glycine may enhance excitotoxic events. Glycine has been shown to potentiate NMDA responses in rat hippocampal neurons and in neurocortical slices.[60,61] In tissue culture, addition of 100 to 3000 μM of glycine potentiated neuronal loss in a concentration dependent manner.[62] In organotypic slice cultures of hippocampus from neonatal rats, addition of a high concentration (10 mM) of glycine for 30 min caused marked hyperexcitability and neurotoxicity. Lower concentrations (4 mM) for 24 h also caused neuronal damage.[63] The NMDA antagonists MK-801 (10 μM) and APV (D-2-amino-5-phosphonopentanoic acid, 100 μM) inhibited neuronal damage, but antagonists of the AMPA receptor did not. In animal models, intraventricularly administered glycine potentiated seizures in animals treated with strychnine to block inhibitory glycine receptors.[64] In addition, in animals pretreated with subconvulsive doses of strychnine, glycine-enhanced NMDA mediated convulsions. These results suggest that glycine accumulation might have two important effects on the NMDA receptor-channel complex. At moderately elevated levels, the amino acid may disrupt normal impulse traffic through the NMDA receptor-channel complex

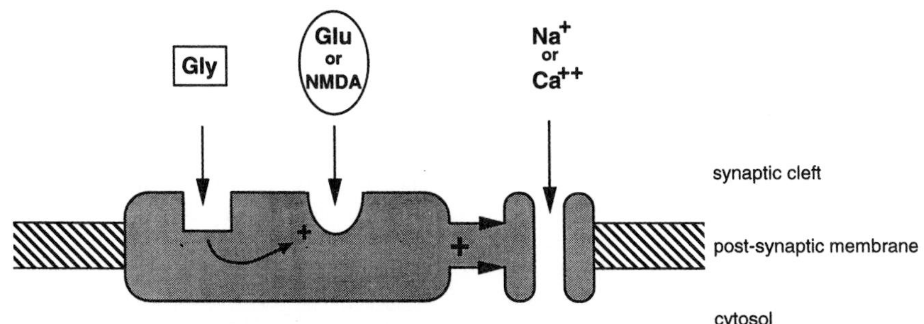

Fig. 90-6 The *N*-methyl-D-aspartate type glutamate receptor channel. This type of glutamate receptor is defined by the ability of the rigid analogue *N*-methyl-D-aspartate (NMDA) to activate it.

and thereby disrupt important developmental events. At high levels, glycine may produce overactivation of the NMDA receptor-channel complex, resulting in seizures and brain injury.

In the immature brain, the NMDA receptor-channel complex is especially active.[51] Injection of NMDA into the immature brain produces more injury and seizures than in the adult brain. These events appear to be activated to serve important developmental roles in the developing brain. Therefore, an increase in glycine may be especially apt to disrupt development in the perinatal brain. Information about the excitatory role of glycine leads to a better understanding of the common occurrence of seizures in clinical NKH.

NONKETOTIC HYPERGLYCINEMIA

As with other inborn errors, NKH has a broad spectrum of clinical phenotypes. Five different phenotypes have been described: neonatal, infantile, mild-episodic, late onset, and transient. The available family data indicate that these phenotypes breed true in families.

Neonatal NKH

The vast majority of cases of NKH fall into this category, and patients with this phenotype have a remarkably stereotyped presentation. Over 150 cases have been reported in the literature.[65–82] Most patients were products of uncomplicated, full-term pregnancies. No external congenital malformations have been recorded, and the infants were average for gestational age in all growth parameters. In a review of 53 NKH patients, the symptom-free interval ranged from 6 h to 8 days, with 66 percent of patients symptomatic by 48 h.[66] Patients develop lethargy and profound hypotonia, and refuse to feed. Wandering eye movements and intermittent ophthalmoplegia are frequent.[47] Most patients have normal to increased deep-tendon reflexes. As the encephalopathy progresses to coma, the infants develop frequent segmental myoclonic jerks, apneic episodes, and hiccups. Most infants require assisted ventilation in the first weeks of life.

Routine laboratory studies of children with NKH are remarkably normal, given the severe neurologic abnormalities. Hematologic parameters are normal, with no anemia, leukopenia, neutropenia, or thrombocytopenia. The electrolyte levels are normal, without evidence of metabolic acidosis. The anion gap is normal, and there is no ketosis. There may be respiratory acidosis secondary to inadequate respiratory effort. Urine organic acids are normal. The only consistent abnormality is elevation of glycine concentrations in urine, plasma, and cerebrospinal fluid (CSF).

There is a single case report of neutropenia with NKH.[78] Two cases of NKH have been reported in which the patients had significant metabolic acidosis, similar to that seen in methylmalonic acidemia or propionic acidemia, but normal urine organic acids.[83] It is essential to analyze urine organic acids when considering the diagnosis of NKH to differentiate it from other causes of hyperglycinemia (see "Differential Diagnosis of NKH" below).

Because an assay of the GCS is not routinely available, and because the enzyme is not expressed in readily accessible cells or tissues, the diagnosis is established at the substrate level by simultaneously determining CSF and plasma glycine concentrations, and by calculating the CSF/plasma glycine ratio.[84,85] Although plasma and urine glycine concentrations are usually elevated, this is not always the case. Plasma glycine concentrations in NKH range from high normal to values eight times the normal mean and four times the upper limit of normal. Urine glycine concentrations are usually elevated, but interpretation is difficult because of the physiologic hyperglycinuria that is characteristic of the newborn infant. For this reason, urinary glycine determinations are not useful in the diagnosis of NKH. CSF glycine concentration is elevated (15 to 30 times normal) to a much greater extent than plasma glycine concentration; hence, the abnormally high value for the CSF/plasma ratio. A CSF/plasma glycine ratio of > 0.08 is considered diagnostic of NKH. Definitive diagnosis can be established by determining the hepatic glycine cleavage system activity, but this procedure requires a liver biopsy and usually is not feasible in a critically ill neonate.

Even with respiratory support, approximately 30 percent of patients die in the neonatal period.[65,86] Those who survive usually regain spontaneous respiration by 3 weeks of age, and have been reported to live for several months to 22 years. The transient nature of the respiratory failure is in keeping with the observations of De Groot and colleagues who showed that when exposed to elevated central nervous system glycine concentrations, animals experienced less toxicity after the first week of life.[87]

Most patients regain the suck reflex, but many must be gavage fed. Untreated patients develop refractory seizures by age 12 months but rarely before age 3 months. The seizure pattern evolves, beginning as myoclonic jerks and progressing to infantile spasms, partial motor seizures, and/or tonic extension. Severe psychomotor retardation with little adaptive or social behavior is the uniform outcome. Spastic quadriplegia often replaces the initial hypotonia.

The electroencephalogram has been described and reviewed by Markand and colleagues in 46 patients with NKH.[65,66,70,73,75,76,79] In the first 2 weeks of life, the electroencephalogram is characterized by a burst-suppression pattern (Fig. 90-7). A burst-suppression pattern on electroencephalogram of a neonate is not diagnostic of NKH but is highly suggestive, because its most common cause is NKH. Severe metabolic encephalopathy can give rise to burst-suppression pattern and has been reported in neonatal adrenoleukodystrophy, N^5N^{10}-methylenetetrahydrofolate reductase deficiency, citrullinemia, molybdenum cofactor deficiency, and Ohtahara syndrome (early infantile epileptic encephalopathy). A burst-suppression pattern has also been reported in brain dysplasias such as dentato-olivary dysplasia, Aicardi syndrome, and hemimeganencephaly.

As the NKH infant ages, the background activity changes to high-voltage slow waves. By 3 months, the EEG is consistent with typical or atypical hypsarrhythmia. The EEG usually does not correlate with the patient's clinical activity; that is, an infantile spasm may not be reflected in a simultaneous EEG abnormality. After 1 year of age, the sleeping and awake EEGs differ: hypsarrhythmia is routine in sleep, but the awake tracing reveals a slow background with lack of normal wake and sleep components and frequent independent multifocal spike discharges.

All patients (aged 2 weeks to 4 years) studied with brain stem auditory evoked response (BAER) had prolonged latencies, which suggests slowed conduction along the brain stem auditory pathway.[70] Visual evoked responses were abnormal in three of five patients studied.[70]

Patients with neonatal NKH may experience *in utero* brain damage.[68,71,74] Of 16 NKH patients whose brains were examined either at autopsy or by computed tomography, 6 had dysgenesis of the corpus callosum, ranging from excessive thinness (1 to 2 mm, rather than the usual 5 to 8 mm) to complete agenesis.[71] Because the corpus callosum develops between the eleventh and twentieth weeks of gestation, this finding implies significant ongoing *in utero* insults and emphasizes the difficulty in treating this disorder.

Agenesis of the corpus callosum is not specific for NKH and has been described in several other inborn errors of metabolism, including pyruvate dehydrogenase deficiency, pyruvate carboxylase deficiency, Zellweger syndrome, neonatal adrenoleukodystrophy, Menkes syndrome, and glutaric aciduria type II.[71] The outcome for infants with each of these disorders is poor.

Consistent with the idea that glycine toxicity has a prenatal onset is the observation that mothers of infants with NKH frequently report abnormal fetal movements, which are interpreted as persistent *in utero* "hiccups." Von Wendt and colleagues studied two unrelated newborns with a positive family history of NKH prior to the onset of symptoms.[74] At birth, both had normal

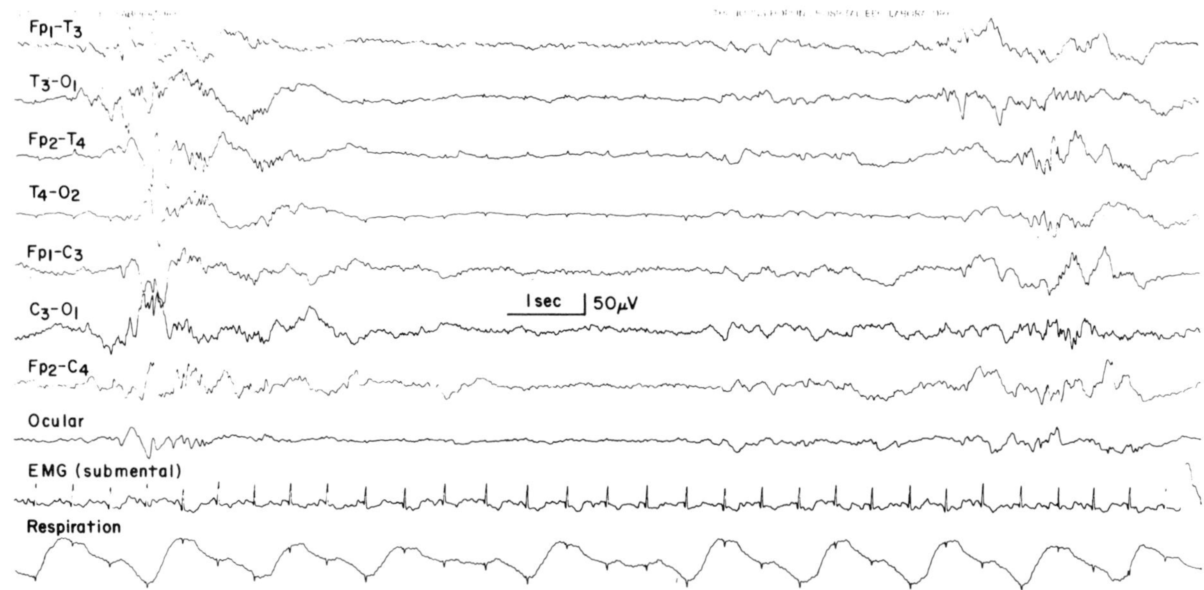

Fig. 90-7 Electroencephalogram of an untreated 4-day-old male with NKH.

plasma glycine levels but markedly elevated CSF glycine levels, which worsened over the first 24 h. Both also had abnormal EEGs before the onset of symptoms. One had a partial burst-suppression pattern at 30 min of age, and the other had the classic burst-suppression pattern at 2 h of age.

Proton MR spectroscopy was used to evaluate two patients with neonatal NKH.[88] Neither had delayed myelination or hypoplasia of the corpus callosum by routine MRI. The proton spectrum indicated a large glycine signal at 3.55 ppm. The signal was of similar intensity in the parieto-occipital white matter and the basal ganglia. The calculated concentration of brain glycine was 4.0 to 4.8 mM for the first patient and gradually declined from 7.4 to 2.3 mM for the second patient after institution of benzoate therapy at 150 to 300 mg/kg per day. This decline in brain glycine content was associated with improved clinical status, but not with changes in CSF or plasma glycine concentration. Heindel and colleagues suggest that proton MR spectroscopy can be used to follow brain glycine content nonivasively.[88]

At autopsy, infants with NKH have spongiform degeneration of the white matter, which is normally well myelinated at birth.[69,73,81] There is diffuse vacuolation of the myelin. If they die much after the neonatal period, the white matter areas that normally myelinate after birth have thin myelin. Electron microscopy of areas of spongy myelinopathy reveals that the vacuoles are formed by splitting of the myelin lamellae.[73] Spongy leukodystrophy is seen in other metabolic disorders, particularly aminoacidopathies such as phenylketonuria and propionic acidemia. Although the idea has not been proved, it is thought that an imbalance of brain amino acid components interferes with proper myelin synthesis.

Atypical NKH

There are several reports of patients who have the diagnostic criterion for NKH of an elevated CSF/plasma glycine ratio but who did not present with disease in the neonatal period. Infantile NKH has been described in several children who had normal growth and development until at least 6 months of age.[13,14] Other than the delay in onset of disease, these patients are very similar to those with neonatal NKH, except that they present with seizures and tend to survive, being spared the profound apnea and hypotonia that is typical of neonatal NKH. One 39-year-old man was recently described.[144] Mental retardation in infantile NKH is not as profound as in the neonatal variety. One patient was described with a neurodegenerative course following 6 months of normal growth and development.[89]

Mild-episodic NKH was described in four children with mild mental retardation and episodes of agitated delirium, chorea, and vertical gaze palsy precipitated by febrile illness.[9,15,16] In one patient, the CSF/plasma glycine ratio was 0.06 and liver GCS activity was 0.4 nM/mg protein per hour (control 2.1 to 4.6 nM/mg protein per hour), suggesting residual activity, given that all cases of neonatal NKH had undetectable GCS activity.[16]

Late onset NKH has been described in seven patients in four sibships.[10–12] Three brothers and one unrelated individual of Lebanese origin developed progressive spastic paraparesis and optic atrophy with onset between 2 and 33 years.[10,90] These patients are intellectually intact and have not developed seizures. Two sibs of unspecified ethnic origin were described with mild mental retardation and choreoathetosis.[14] A 24-year-old African-American male with severe developmental delay and rare seizures also has been described.[12] Biochemically, the CSF glycine in these late onset cases has ranged from 21 to 101 μM, with CSF/plasma glycine ratios that are above normal, but in some cases, below the level seen in neonatal NKH. The hepatic glycine cleavage activity has not been described in these patients, except in one case, in which the P protein activity was only 3.5 percent of normal, which is similar to that found in neonatal NKH cases.[12]

Transient NKH

Six patients have been described with the fascinating phenotype of transient NKH.[72,91–93] At presentation, these patients were clinically indistinguishable from patients with neonatal NKH, with elevated CSF/plasma glycine ratios diagnostic of NKH and a burst-suppression pattern on the electroencephalogram. By 2 to 8 weeks of age, their plasma and CSF glycine levels had returned to normal. Five of these patients had no apparent neurologic sequelae at ages 6 months to 13 years,[72,91,93] but one had "bilateral subcortical atrophy with deficient myelination of the inner white matter" detected by magnetic resonance imaging[92] at 3 months and by 9 months of age was severely retarded. The etiology of transient NKH is presumably related to immaturity of the glycine cleavage system in both the liver and the brain. Recurrence of transient NKH in a family has not been reported; thus, evidence for a genetic etiology is lacking.

Biochemical Features

Patients with NKH may have urinary and plasma glycine levels 2 to 8 times normal (see Table 90-1). CSF glycine concentration is 15 to 30 times normal (see Table 90-1). Glycine metabolism in the

Table 90-2 The Differential Diagnosis of Hyperglycinemia and Hyperglycinuria

Hyperglycinemia
Nonketotic
nonketotic hyperglycinemia
valproate therapy
D-glyceric acidemia
Ketotic
methylmalonic acidemia
propionic acidemia
isovaleric acidemia
β-ketothiolase deficiency
Hyperglycinuria
Benign (transient immaturity of renal glycine reabsorption)
Familial iminoglycinuria
Type I hyperprolinemia (iminoglycinuria)
Type II hyperprolinemia (iminoglycinuria)
Nonketotic hyperglycinemia

central nervous system depends on GCS activity. There appears to be some correlation between CSF glycine concentration and clinical phenotype—the higher the CSF glycine concentration, the more severe the disease. The strongest correlation, however, is with the CSF/plasma glycine ratio. The normal ratio consistently is less than 0.02; patients with atypical NKH have ratios around 0.09, whereas neonatal patients have ratios ranging from 0.2 to 0.3 (see Table 90-1).

The high CSF glycine concentration reflects brain glycine content, which is markedly elevated in this disorder.[85] In four NKH patients, brain glycine content was 2 to 4 times normal (normal is 2.0 to 2.2 μM/g wet weight).[84,85,94] Brain glycine content was not elevated in patients with other forms of hyperglycinemia. This suggests that GCS flux is normally significant in the central nervous system.

Differential Diagnosis of NKH

Several disorders are associated with hyperglycinemia and/or hyperglycinuria (see Table 90-2). It is critical to establish the correct diagnosis, as therapy and prognosis are dramatically different. In 1961, Childs and colleagues described the first patient with "ketotic hyperglycinemia" who subsequently was found to have propionic acidemia.[90] The child had severe metabolic acidosis, ketosis, intermittent neutropenia, and thrombocytopenia, and mental retardation, which is now known to be the usual course for untreated patients with propionic acidemia (see Chap. 94). Methylmalonic acidemia (Chap. 94), isovaleric acidemia (Chap. 93), and *β*-ketothiolase deficiency (Chap. 93) can have similar presentations. Patients with organic acidemias due to defects in the branched chain amino acid catabolic pathways develop hyperglycinemia as a secondary process (Chap. 93). The organic acids that accumulate interfere with the hepatic glycine cleavage system.[95] CSF and brain glycine content are normal in these disorders, which distinguishes them from NKH.[85]

The rare disorder D-glyceric acidemia also is associated with nonketotic hyperglycinemia.[96] The first reported case was in a 2-year-old boy who had severe hypotonia from birth and developed seizures and choreoathetotic movements in addition to severe mental retardation. Glycine concentrations were elevated in the urine, plasma and CSF. Urinary excretion of D-glyceric acid ranged between 1.5 and 2.5 g per day, allowing diagnosis by analysis of urine organic acids.

The most common cause of hyperglycinemia is administration of the anticonvulsant valproate (sodium dipropylacetate, Depakene).[97] In 13 children receiving valproate therapy, mean plasma glycine was 427 μM, compared to 237 μM in control subjects. CSF glycine concentration was normal in two patients receiving valproate. Valproate reduces the quantity of the rat hepatic GCS, presumably by interfering with enzyme synthesis.[98] The diagnosis of NKH cannot be established in the presence of valproate therapy.

Urinary glycine excretion is increased in newborns and particularly in premature infants because of the immaturity of the renal glycine transport system.[99] Urine glycine is also markedly elevated in patients with familial iminoglycinuria (Chap. 194) and types I and II hyperprolinemia (Chap. 81), along with urine proline and hydroxyproline. The imino acids and glycine share a common renal carrier. Patients with types I and II hyperprolinemia have an elevated plasma proline concentration. Excessive excretion of proline leads to saturation of the renal carrier and overflow iminoglycinuria. Familial iminoglycinuria and type I hyperprolinemia are asymptomatic; type II hyperprolinemia may be asymptomatic or may be associated with seizures and mental retardation.

To establish the diagnosis of NKH, it is essential to determine the plasma and CSF amino acids, to calculate the CSF/plasma glycine ratio, and to analyze urine organic acids by gas chromatography/mass spectroscopy to rule out hyperglycinemia secondary to organic acidemias.

The Biochemical Defect in NKH

Ando and colleagues performed the first *in vivo* studies of glycine metabolism.[18] Patients and control subjects were given intravenous injection of ^{14}C-labeled glycine, labeled at either the 1 carbon or 2 carbon. Depending on which of these substrates was used, either expired air was collected and $^{14}CO_2$ measured, or serine was isolated from plasma and degraded, and the ^{14}C at the 3 carbon was measured. Virtually no $^{14}CO_2$ was formed in patients given [1-^{14}C] glycine, and no specific activity was found at the 3 carbon of serine. These results indicated a defect in the conversion of the 1 carbon of glycine to CO_2 and of the 2 carbon of glycine to the 3 carbon of serine, suggesting a block in the GCS.

Similar observations were made in liver homogenates and in brain sections from patients with NKH.[4,100,101] The specific diagnosis of NKH can be made by measuring glycine cleavage activity by the decarboxylation assay from [1-^{14}C] glycine in liver biopsy samples. In the neonatal form of NKH, overall GCS activity is usually very low or undetectable ($\leq$7 percent of normal), while in the atypical forms, some residual activity is present. In two patients with atypical disease, hepatic GCS activity was 25 percent of the control level.[3] Kure and colleagues reported that the GCS is activated in lymphocytes transformed with Epstein-Barr virus.[102] In control-transformed lymphocytes, the overall GCS activity (0.93 + 0.27 nM [^{14}C]CO_2 formed/mg protein per hour) is approximately 20 percent of the level in control liver specimens (3.9 to 5.2 nM [^{14}C]CO_2 formed/mg protein per hour). The overall GCS activity and specific P protein activity was undetectable in the transformed lymphocytes of six patients with NKH.[102] Transformed lymphocytes were also used to diagnose atypical NKH with residual GCS activity due to partial T-protein function.[103] Others were unable to confirm the diagnosis in 6 of 23 NKH patients by measuring GCS activity in lymphoblasts (4 of the 6 patients had undetectable GCS activity in liver biopsy specimens); 2 of 15 control lymphoblast samples were below the range of the other control samples (Derek Applegarth, personal communication).

Patients with NKH have been found to have defects in the activity of specific components of the GCS by assays of the glycine-[$^{14}CO_2$] exchange reaction in the presence of excessive amounts of the other components.[2,3,101] Of a series of 30 patients with neonatal NKH, 26 had specific defects in the P protein, and the remainder had defects in the T protein, all with undetectable activity.[94,101] Of three atypical patients, two had defects in the T protein and one had a defect in the H protein.[3,101]

In several patients with neonatal NKH and agenesis of the corpus callosum, P protein activity was undetectable and no P protein was found by immunoprecipitation.[65,94] While this is a potentially interesting association, it is important to note that not all patients with agenesis of the corpus callosum have been studied for specific defects and that there are patients with undetectable P protein activity who do not have agenesis of the corpus callosum.

Only one patient with deficient H protein activity has been identified.[3] The patient had atypical NKH and features of progressive degeneration of the central nervous system. In this patient, the H protein was missing the lipoic acid moiety that is usually covalently bound to it. Defects in L protein (lipoamide dehydrogenase) activity have not been reported in patients with NKH. This may be because L protein is also the E3 moiety of the pyruvate dehydrogenase, α-ketoglutarate dehydrogenase, and branched-chain α-ketoacid dehydrogenase complexes so that affected patients would have symptoms and biochemical abnormalities of all four disorders.[104] This hypothesis is supported by studies in mice; heterozygous disruption of murine dihydrolipoamide dehydrogenase resulted in a 50 percent reduction of all four enzyme complexes.[105] Homozygous disruption caused perigastrulation lethality.[105]

Molecular Defects

Seventy percent of the NKH genes of Finnish origin have a particular missense mutation in the P protein—S564I—which is caused by a G-to-T substitution at nucleotide 1691[106] (see Fig. 90-3). Expression studies of the P protein S564I allele in COS 7 cells showed that it encodes a functionally inactive protein.[106] The Ser564 is the amino terminal residue of the decapeptide between Ser564 and Trp573, which is imperfectly repeated between Ser807 and Trp815.[26] These two decapeptide repeats flank the pyridoxal phosphate-binding site at Lys754. A Japanese patient with neonatal NKH was found to have an in-frame 3 bp deletion (TCT), which results in deletion of the Phe756 (F756Δ).[24] No P protein activity was detected when the F756Δ allele was expressed in COS 7 cells.[24] Because of the proximity of Phe756 to Lys754, the mutation was thought to prevent binding of pyridoxal phosphate.

Mutations in the T-protein gene have been identified in both typical and atypical NKH patients[107–109] (see Fig. 90-5). One patient with neonatal NKH was homozygous for a G → A transition, leading to a Gly-to-Asp substitution at residue 269 (G269D).[107] Another mutation, an A → G transition, leading to a His-to-Arg substitution at residue 42 (H42R), is responsible for neonatal NKH in homozygosity in a large, inbred, Israeli-Arab kindred.[109] Three children affected with neonatal NKH were compound heterozygous for a frameshift mutation in exon 1, 183delC, and a G → C transversion at position 955, leading to an Asp-to-His substitution at residue 276 (D276H). The aspartic acid residue at 276 is invariant in human, bovine, chicken, and peas, and is replaced by glutamic acid in *Escherichia coli*, suggesting that an acidic amino acid may be required at this site.[108] The Gly at position 269 and the His at position 42 are invariant in human, bovine, chicken, and *E. coli* T-protein.[107,109] The atypical patient had mild developmental delay but was treated with strychnine and benzoate. She is a compound heterozygote for two G → A transitions, one leading to a Gly-to-Arg substitution at codon 47 (G47R), and the other leading to an Arg-to-His substitution at codon 320 (R320H). Ala and Leu replace the Gly at position 47 and the Arg at position 320, respectively, in *E. coli,* which suggests that these amino acids may be less essential to T-protein function.

No specific molecular defects in H protein have been described. There is evidence for a rearranged H protein gene in one patient with NKH, but the multiple pseudogenes have interfered with exact description of the rearrangement.[31]

Genetics

NKH is an autosomal recessive condition of unknown frequency. It has been reported to be very rare,[8] but the speed and severity of symptoms suggests that the reported frequency may be spuriously low owing to underdiagnosis of infants with neonatal NKH.

A founder effect has resulted in a very high frequency of NKH in northern Finland, where the incidence is 1 in 12,000 live births.[86] The incidence in all of Finland is 1 in 55,000.

Accurate assessment of the carrier state is still not available except by liver biopsy. It was thought that quantitation of $^{14}CO_2$ after intravenous administration of [1-^{14}C] glycine revealed abnormal kinetics in obligate heterozygotes. However, extensive studies of this technique revealed significant overlap with the normal range, precluding use of this technique. If GCS activity is reliably expressed in transformed lymphocytes, analysis of these cells should allow accurate determination of the carrier state, which will greatly facilitate genetic counseling in areas of high incidence.[110]

Prenatal Diagnosis

Accurate prenatal diagnosis has been available for NKH since 1990.[111] The GCS is active in the placenta, so chorionic villus biopsy specimens collected and immediately frozen at −80°C can be used to assay GCS activity. Tada and colleagues have performed prenatal diagnosis on 31 at-risk pregnancies.[26] In 23 cases, GCS activity was normal and an unaffected infant was born. In eight cases, GCS activity was undetectable in chorionic villus samples. In these cases, termination of pregnancy was elected and absent GCS activity was confirmed in liver and brain of each aborted fetus. Toone and colleagues report similar results in 47 cases.[112,113] Less than 10 percent of fetuses may have residual enzyme activity making accurate prenatal diagnosis impossible (Derek Applegarth, personal communication). DNA diagnosis can be used in cases where the mutation is known.

Measurement of glycine/serine ratios in the amniotic fluid was once suggested to be diagnostic.[114] However, the range of values included in the affected group of fetuses was found to overlap the range in the control group.[115] This method should not be used.

THERAPY

Many therapeutic strategies have been tried in an effort to ameliorate the intractable seizures and relentless brain damage characteristic of this disorder, but none of these approaches has been consistently effective.

Problems relating to judging the efficacy of any therapy for NKH include the considerable phenotypic variation of the disease, which is not understood at the molecular level, and the lack of any clinical scoring methods for these patients. We do not understand which, or if, patients suffer such severe prenatal damage that any postpartum treatment is unlikely to be effective. We cannot distinguish which of the patients who present with the classical neonatal phenotype have not suffered prenatal damage and might respond well to stringent efforts to reduce glycine levels and antagonize overstimulation of the NMDA receptor-channel complex, either directly at the glycine site or at the channel pore itself.

Glycine Reduction

Reduction of tissue glycine levels by administration of glycine-free or glycine-serine-free diets resulted in reduced plasma and urine glycine concentrations but had no effect on seizure frequency or developmental progress.[65,76,77] Benzoate, which conjugates with glycine to form hippurate, which is excreted in the urine, has been used extensively. While several studies using benzoate at doses ranging from 150 to 750 mg/kg per day achieved both a reduction in plasma glycine to normal and a partial reduction of CSF glycine concentrations, as well as somewhat improved arousal and decreased seizure frequency, none has achieved improvement in developmental progress.[8,65,84,87,116] The only exception to this was an unusual patient with classical symptoms of NKH and initial CSF and plasma glycine of 124 and 1200 μM, respectively, at 3 days, but of 13 and 1400 μM, respectively at 7 days.[117] She was started on benzoate (250 mg/kg per day) and improved dramatically. At 2 years, 3 months, she was developmentally normal, despite CSF and plasma glycines of 74 and 585 μM, respectively.

Single Carbon Donors

Several investigators have used various single carbon donors in an attempt to correct the presumed deficiency of single carbon units in this disease.[65,82,118] Some used methionine in conjunction with dietary restriction of glycine and serine; no clinical effect was seen.[65] Others used leucovorin, folate, and/or choline with or without dietary or pharmacologic (benzoate or salicylate) measures to reduce glycine levels; again, there was no change in seizure frequency or developmental progress.[82,118]

Receptor Blockade

A better understanding of the role of glycine as both an excitatory and an inhibitory neurotransmitter has led to new therapeutic strategies for treating infants with NKH. The high levels of glycine probably produce seizures through an NMDA-mediated excitotoxic mechanism.[64] Conventional anticonvulsant agents (phenytoin and phenobarbital), which act by enhancing inhibition, are not effective in NKH. Valproate may be specifically contraindicated in NKH because it can cause hyperglycinemia in patients without NKH by interfering with GCS activity in the liver.[97,98] Some workers have reported an increased seizure frequency in NKH patients on valproate therapy, while others have reported no change in glycine concentration and improved seizure control.[119,120]

Knowledge of glycine's role as an inhibitory neurotransmitter in the brain stem and spinal cord led to bold attempts to block this receptor with its antagonist strychnine.[121–126] While some studies reported improved respiratory effort and arousal,[121,125,126] others saw no clinical response.[122–124] Long-term use of strychnine may actually have deleterious effects because it allows the extra glycine to activate the NMDA receptor-channel complex, potentially resulting in worsened seizures and brain damage. Diazepam used in conjunction with benzoate and folic acid reportedly controlled intractable seizures in two female infants with NKH.[127] Whether this effect was due to the diazepam, owing to its ability to enhance GABAergic inhibition, or to benzoate, is unclear because both agents were used simultaneously.

Several recent studies have employed antagonists of the NMDA receptor-channel complex, either in isolation or coupled with benzoate to reduce tissue glycine concentrations. The use of ketamine, an anesthetic NMDA channel blocker, in a 9-month-old infant with intractable seizures and no interactive skills resulted in decreased irritability, and improved voluntary movements and electroencephalogram.[110] Ketamine (5 mg/kg per day orally) and benzoate (250 mg/kg per day orally) were used in two newborns with neonatal NKH.[117] Each had a normal EEG at 2 months and no seizures, but IQ was approximately 50 at 14 and 10 months of age, respectively.

The antitussive, dextromethorphan, and its major metabolite, dextrorphan, are moderately potent antagonists of the NMDA channel. [^{3}H]Dextrorphan binds to a site within the channel of the NMDA receptor,[64] and dextromethorphan inhibits NMDA induced convulsion in an animal model.[128] Dextromethorphan was used alone at very high doses (35 mg/kg per day; normal antitussive dose is 3 mg/kg per day) in a 9-week-old infant.[129] The patient's seizures (myoclonic jerks and flexor spasms) stopped and the electroencephalogram normalized. At 6 months, the dextromethorphan was stopped for 24 h; the patient developed somnolence, hypotonia, and myoclonic jerks progressing to flexor spasms. The electroencephalogram showed multifocal spikes superimposed over extremely slow background activity. Reintroduction of dextromethorphan at 35 mg/kg per day resulted in recovery over 24 h.

We have treated four patients with a combination of benzoate at doses of 500 to 750 mg/kg per day and dextromethorphan at doses of 5 to 22 mg/kg per day with follow-up of 3 months to 8 years.[130,131] One patient was diagnosed at 4 days and has been treated with benzoate at 750 mg/kg per day and dextromethorphan at 5 mg/kg per day for 3.5 years.[131] He is seizure free; his EEG was normal after starting therapy until 18 months of age, since then diffuse slowing and unusually high voltage has been observed. Magnetic resonance imaging has shown delayed but steadily progressing myelination. Developmentally, he is delayed but only in the moderate range except for a severe expressive language delay. At 8 years, he runs, follows two-step commands, and can sign several words. A second patient with neonatal NKH was not diagnosed until 7 months of age. At that time, she was in status epilepticus with an electroencephalogram consistent with hypsarrhythmia and was severely hypotonic. Benzoate and dextromethorphan at similar doses resulted in cessation of seizure activity and improvement of the electroencephalogram to diffuse slowing without focal discharges. At 3 years, seizures resumed. They were initially responsive to felbamate, which was subsequently discontinued because of potential toxic side effects. Carbamazepine was modestly helpful; lamotrigine was somewhat more effective. Topiramate has been successful in completely eliminating seizures at 6 years. Her magnetic resonance imaging shows only mildly delayed myelination. Developmentally, she functions at the 8-month level. A third patient developed seizures at 3 months with spike and sharp waves on EEG. MRI was normal. CSF and plasma glycine were diagnostic. Treatment with benzoate (500 mg/kg per day) and dextromethorphan (7.5 mg/kg per day) eliminated seizures within 2 weeks. At 6 years, he is hyperactive, runs, but has no language. A fourth patient was diagnosed at 5 days of age with myoclonic jerks and typical burst-suppression pattern on electroencephalogram and elevated CSF and plasma glycine levels. Benzoate at 500 mg/kg per day resulted in arousal and suck reflex with normalization of the EEG and plasma glycine concentrations. Dextromethorphan was started at 5 mg/kg per day. He did well until 6 weeks of age, when increased irritability and poor feeding were noted. Shortly thereafter seizures occurred despite normal plasma glycine concentrations and a CSF glycine concentration of only 20 μM. Elevation of the dextromethorphan dose up to 22 mg/kg per day and the addition of phenytoin resolved the seizures briefly. The EEG had deteriorated to hypsarrhythmia. The patient continued to have breakthrough seizures, including one that lead to prolonged apnea, which resulted in brain death and the patient expiring at 12 weeks of age. Thus, our results with combined benzoate and dextromethorphan therapy are inconsistent.

Zammarchi and colleagues reported treatment starting at 65 hours of age with 500 mg/kg per day of benzoate and 7.5 to 40 mg/kg per day of dextromethorphan, although initially of significant clinical benefit, but was ultimately unable to prevent intractable seizures, severe neurologic abnormalities, and death at 5 months of age in an infant with neonatal NKH, delayed myelination, and severe hypoplasia of the corpus callosum.[132] They postulated that prenatal brain damage, or differences in the pharmacokinetics of dextromethorphan metabolism, may be responsible for the lack of response in their patient. Alternatively, Tada and Kure reported improvement in two patients using dextromethorphan alone.[29] Alemzadeh and Matteson report an infant with NKH, myoclonic seizures, hypsarrhythmia, and nystagmus in whom 0.25 mg/kg per day of dextromethorphan caused resolution of nystagmus and improvement of the EEG.[133] Their patient was already being treated with protein restriction (1.5 g/kg per day), benzoate (400 mg/kg per day), arginine (400 mg/kg per day), benzodiazepam (0.4 mg/kg per day), folic acid (1 mg per day), carnitine (25 mg/kg per day), and phenobarbital (5 mg/kg per day), which had improved tone and resolved clinical seizures, although the EEG remained markedly abnormal. The addition of 1 mg/kg per day of dextromethorphan led to anorexia, but a dose of 0.25 mg/kg per day resolved the nystagmus and improved the EEG. Whether this child was exquisitely sensitive to dextromethorphan, or whether the dextromethorphan had synergistic effects with the many other pharmacologic interventions in this patient, remains to be studied.

There are extreme variations in dextromethorphan metabolism. Plasma dextromethorphan clearance is influenced by the cytochrome P450 isoform, debrisoquine hydroxylase (CYP2D6).[134] The poor metabolizer phenotype is inherited as an autosomal recessive trait and has a prevalence of 7 to 8 percent in mixed-race North Americans.[135] Arnold and colleagues reported two patients, one an extensive metabolizer, the other a poor metabolizer of dextromethorphan.[136] In both cases, plasma dextromethorphan levels of 50 to 100 ng/ml were temporally associated with anticonvulsant efficacy. Arnold observed that cimetidine, an inhibitor of hepatic P450 activity, increased plasma dextromethorphan levels by 1.9-fold in the extensive metabolizer.[136] Plasma and CSF concentrations of both dextromethorphan and its metabolite, dextrorphan, should be measured to ensure that a measurable but nontoxic level is achieved.

Some patients on high-dose benzoate treatment develop carnitine deficiency. Van Hove and colleagues observed this in three of four patients[137] and Arnold in one of two patients;[136] we have not observed carnitine deficiency in four patients. Plasma carnitine levels should be monitored in NKH patients receiving benzoate.

Matsuo and colleagues reported a 10-point increase in IQ following use of 150 mg/kg per day of tryptophan in a 4.5-year-old girl with neonatal onset of atypical NKH.[138] Except for transient anorexia, no side effects were seen. The proposed mechanism is that high doses of tryptophan lead to increased levels of kynurenic acid, which is an endogenous antagonist of the NMDA receptor. Higher CSF levels of kynurenic acid and 5-HIAA were observed after initiation of treatment.

Several new anticonvulsants, which act at the NMDA receptor, may be useful in the future. For example, felbamate acts to block the NMDA-activated cation channel, and possibly also blocks the glycine receptor.[139,140] Felbamate also potentiates GABA-mediated inhibitory responses.[140] Unfortunately, use of this drug is limited by a high incidence of bone marrow and liver complications. Topiramate, a drug that preferentially blocks AMPA receptors, may be useful in some patients with persistent seizures.[141] It will be important to study the effect of these agents in NKH patients to determine whether agents that are more potent blockers of NMDA receptors than dextromethorphan can give a better outcome.

To date, the different therapeutic trials have involved one or a few patients. We must first develop a better understanding of the phenotypic variability of this disease and develop stringent methodsfor studying various therapeutic interventions on sufficient numbers of patients to allow accurate assessment of clinical effect.

The long-term outcome of patients with severe neonatal NKH remains poor: at least moderate mental retardation, and often seizures, are the norm despite treatment with any or all of the drugs listed above. Apnea, which is such a prominent feature in the early neonatal period, usually resolves by 3 weeks of age, so there is a limited opportunity for withdrawal of support, should that be the parents' wishes. Alternatively, patients surviving the neonatal period, while at risk of death from sudden onset of intractable seizures, are not certain of it. It is essential that patients receive appropriate medical care, including nutritional support, anticonvulsant therapy, and developmental interventions, such as occupational, physical, and speech therapies.

REFERENCES

1. Kikuchi G: The glycine cleavage system: Composition, reaction mechanism, and physiological significance. *Mol Cell Biochem* **1**:169, 1973.
2. Hayasaka K, Tada K, Kikuchi G, Winter S, Nyhan WL: Nonketotic hyperglycinemia: Two patients with primary defects of P-protein and T-protein, respectively, in the glycine cleavage system. *Pediatr Res* **17**:967, 1983.
3. Sinclair DA, Hong SP, Dawes IW: Specific induction by glycine of the gene for the P-subunit of glycine decarboxylase from *Saccharomyces cerevisiae*. *Mol Microbiol* **19**:611, 1996.
4. Nagarajan L, Storms RK: Molecular characterization of GCV3, the *Saccharomyces cerevisiae* gene coding for the glycine cleavage system hydrogen carrier protein. *J Biol Chem* **272**:4444, 1997.
5. Mc Neil JB, Zhang F-R, Taylor BV, Sinclair DA, Pearlman RE, Bognar AL: Cloning and molecular characterization of the GCV1 gene encoding the glycine cleavage T-protein from *Saccharomyces cerevisiae*. *Gene* **186**:13, 1997.
6. Ascher P, Johnson JW: The NMDA receptor, its channel and its modulation by glycine, in Watkins JC, Collinridge GL (ed): *The NMDA Receptor*. Oxford, UK, Oxford University Press, 1989, p 109.
7. Gerritsen T, Kaveggia E, Waisman HA: A new type of idiopathic hyperglycinemia with hypo-oxaluria. *Pediatrics* **36**:882, 1965.
8. Nyhan WL: Nonketotic hyperglycinemia, in Scriver CR, Beaudet al, Sly WS, Valle D (eds): *The Metabolic Basis of Inherited Disease*. New York, McGraw-Hill, 1989, p 743.
9. Frazier DM, Summer GK, Chamberlin HR: Hyperglycinuria and hyperglycinemia in two siblings with mild developmental delay. *Am J Dis Child* **132**:777, 1978.
10. Steinman GS, Yudkoff M, Berman PH, Blazer-Yost B, Segal S: Late-onset nonketotic hyperglycinemia and spinocerebellar degeneration. *J Pediatr* **94**:907, 1979.
11. Bank WJ, Morrow G: A familial spinal cord disorder with hyperglycinemia. *Arch Neurol* **27**:136, 1972.
12. Singer HS, Valle D, Hayasaka K, Tada K: Nonketotic hyperglycinemia: Studies in an atypical variant. *Neurology* **39**:286, 1989.
13. Holmgren G, Blomquist HK: Non-ketotic hyperglycinemia in two sibs with mild psycho-neurological symptoms. *Neuropediatrics* **8**:67, 1977.
14. Flannery DB, Pellock J, Bousounis D, Hunt P, Nance C, Wolf B: Nonketotic hyperglycinemia in two retarded adults: A mild form on infantile nonketotic hyperglycinemia. *Neurology* **33**:1064, 1983.
15. Nightingale S, Barton ME: Intermittent vertical supranuclear ophthalmoplegia and ataxia. *Mov Disord* **6**:76, 1991.
16. Steiner RD, Sweetser DA, Rohrbaugh JR, Dowton B, Toone JR, Applegarth DA: Nonketotic hyperglycinemia: Atypical clinical and biochemical manifestations. *J Pediatr* **128**:243, 1996.
17. Scriver CR, Rosenberg LE: Glycine, in Scriver CR (ed): *Amino Acid Metabolism and Its Disorders*. Philadelphia, WB Saunders, 1973, p 400.
18. Ando T, Klingberg WG, Ward AN, Rasmussen K, Nyhan WL: Isovaleric acidemia presenting with altered metabolism of glycine. *Pediatr Res* **5**:478, 1971.
19. Rinaldo P, O'shea JJ, Coates PM, Hale DE, Stanley CA, Tanaka K: Medium-chain acyl-CoA dehydrogenase deficiency: Diagnosis by stable isotope dilution analysis of urinary *n*-hexanoyl glycine and 3-phenylpropionyl glycine. *N Engl J Med* **319**:1308, 1988.
20. Jois M, Hall B, Fewer K, Brosnan JT: Regulation of hepatic glycine catabolism by glucagon. *J Biol Chem* **264**:3347, 1989.
21. Jois M, Hall B, Brosnan JT: Stimulation of glycine catabolism in isolated perfused rat liver by calcium mobilizing hormones and in isolated rat liver mitochondria by submicromolar concentrations of calcium. *J Biol Chem* **265**:1246, 1990.
22. Jois M, Ewart S, Brosnan JT: Regulation of glycine metabolism in rat liver mitochondria. *Biochem J* **283**:435, 1992.
23. Kalbag SS, Palekar AG: Postnatal development of the glycine cleavage system in rat liver. *Biochem Med Metab Biol* **43**:128, 1990.
24. Kure S, Narisawa K, Tada K: Structural and expression analyses of normal and mutant mRNA encoding glycine decarboxylase: Three-base deletion in mRNA causes nonketotic hyperglycinemia. *Biochem Biophys Res Commun* **174**:1176, 1991.
25. Kume a, Koyata H, Sakakibara T, Ishiguro Y, Kure S, Hiraga K: The glycine cleavage system: Molecular cloning of the chicken and human glycine decarboxylase cDNAs and some characteristics involved in the deduced protein structures. *J Biol Chem* **266**:3323, 1991.
26. Tada K, Kure S: Nonketotic hyperglycinemia: molecular lesion and pathophysiology. *Int Pediatr* **8**:52, 1993.
27. Isobe M, Koyata H, Sakakibara T, Momoi-Isobe K, Hiraga K: Assignment of the true and processed gene for human glycine decarboxylase to 9p23–24 and 4q12. *Biochem Biophys Res Commun* **203**:1483, 1994.
28. Burton BK, Pettenati MJ, Block SM, Bensen J, Roach ES: Nonketotic hyperglycinemia in a patient with the 9p- syndrome. *Am J Med Genet* **32**:504, 1989.
29. Tada K, Kure S: Nonketotic hyperglycinemia: molecular lesion, diagnosis, and pathophysiology. *J Inherit Metab Dis* **16**:691, 1993.
30. Koyata H, Hiraga K: The glycine cleavage system: Structure of a cDNA encoding human H-protein, and partial characterization of its

gene in patients with hyperglycinemias. *Am J Hum Genet* **48**:351, 1991.

31. Koyata H, Hiraga K: Partial structure of the human H-protein gene. *Biochem Biophys Res Commun* **178**:1072, 1991.
32. Hayasaka K, Nanao K, Takada F, Okamura-Ikeda K, Motokawa Y: Isolation and sequence determination of cDNA encoding human T-protein of the glycine cleavage system. *Biochem Biophys Res Commun* **192**:766, 1993.
33. Nanao K, Takada G, Takahashi E, Seki N, Komatsu Y, Okamua-Ikeda K, Motokawa Y, Hayasaka K: Structure and chromosomal localization of the gene encoding human T-protein of the glycine cleavage system. *Genomics* **19**:27, 1994.
34. Kure S, Koyata H, Kume a, Ishiguro Y, Hiraga K: The glycine cleavage system. The coupled expression of the glycine decarboxylase gene and the H-protein gene in the chicken. *J Biol Chem* **266**:3330, 1991.
35. Greenamyre JT: The role of glutamate in neurotransmission and in neurologic disease. *Arch Neurol* **43**:1058, 1986.
36. Probst A, Cortes R, Palacios JM: The distribution of glycine receptors in the human brain. A light microscopic autoradiographic study. *Neuroscience* **17**:11, 1986.
37. Krnjevic K: Chemical nature of synaptic neurotransmission in vertebrates. *Physiol Rev* **54**:418, 1974.
38. Zorbin MA, Wamsley JK, Kiehor MJ: Glycine receptor: light microscopic localization with ^{3}H-strychnine. *J Neurosci* **1**:532, 1981.
39. Davidoff RA, Graham LT, Shank RP, Werman R, Aprison MH: Changes in amino acid concentrations associated with loss of spinal interneurons. *J Neurochem* **14**:1025, 1967.
40. Grenningloh G, Rienitz a, Schmitt B, Methfessel C, Zensen M, Beyreuther K, Gundelfinger ED, Betz H: The strychnine-binding subunit of the glycine receptor shows homology with nicotinic acetylcholine receptors. *Nature* **328**:215, 1987.
41. Gundlach AL, Dodd PR, Grabara CSG, Watson WEJ, Johnston GAR, Harper PAW, Dennis JA, Healy PJ: Deficit of spinal cord glycine/strychnine receptors in inherited myoclonus of Poll Hereford calves. *Science* **241**:1807, 1988.
42. Alger BE: GABA and glycine: Post-synaptic actions, in Rogawski MA, Barker JL (ed): *Neurotransmitter Actions in the Vertebrate Nervous System*. New York, Plenum, 1985, p 33.
43. Bradley K, Easton EM, Eccles JC: An investigation of primary or direct inhibition. *J Physiol* **122**:474, 1953.
44. Curtis DR, Duggan AW, Johnston GAR: The specificity of strychnine as a glycine antagonist in the mammalian spinal cord. *Exp Brain Res* **12**:547, 1971.
45. Johnson JW, Ascher P: Equilibrium and kinetic study of glycine action on the NMDA receptor in cultured mouse brain neurons. *J Physiol* **455**:339, 1992.
46. Thomson AM: Glycine modulation of the NMDA receptor channel complex. *Trends Neurosci* **12**:349, 1989.
47. Macdonald JT, Sher PK: Ophthalmoplegia as a sign of metabolic disease in the newborn. *Neurolology* **27**:971, 1977.
48. Young AB, Fagg GE: Excitatory amino acid receptors in the brain: Membrane binding and receptor autoradiographic approaches. *Trends Pharm Sci* **11**:126, 1990.
49. Mayer ML, Westbrook GL: The physiology of excitatory amino acids in the vertebrate central nervous system. *Prog Neurobiol* **28**:197, 1987.
50. Collingridge GL, Bliss TV: NMDA receptors—their role in long-term potentiation. *Trends Neurosci* **10**:288, 1987.
51. McDonald JW, Johnston MV: Physiological and pathophysiological roles of excitatory amino acids during central nervous system development. *Brain Res Rev* **15**:41, 1990.
52. Choi DW: Glutamate neurotoxicity and diseases of the nervous systems. *Neuron* **1**:623, 1988.
53. Jansen KLR, Dragunow M, Faull LM: ^{3}H-glycine binding sites, NMDA and PCP receptors have similar distribution in the human hippocampus: An autoradiographic study. *Brain Res* **482**:174, 1989.
54. Ransom RW, Stec NL: Cooperative modulation of ^{3}H-MK-801 binding to the NMDA receptor-ion channel complex by l-glutamate, glycine, and polyamines. *J Neurochem* **51**:830, 1988.
55. Kessler M, Terramani T, Lynch G, Baudry M: A glycine site with NMDA receptors: Characterization and identification of a new class of antagonists. *J Neurochem* **52**:1319, 1989.
56. Thiels E, Weisz DJ, Berger TW: In vivo modulation of NMDA receptor-dependent long-term potentiation by the glycine modulatory site. *Neuroscience* **46**:501, 1992.
57. Huetner JE: Competitive antagonism of glycine at the NMDA receptor. *Biochem Pharm* **41**:9, 1991.
58. Kemp JA, Leeson PD: The glycine site of the NMDA receptor—Five years on. *Trends Pharm Sci* **14**:20, 1993.
59. Mariyoshi K, Masu M, Ishii T, Shigemoto R, Mizuno N, Makanishi S: Molecular cloning and characterization of the rat NMDA receptor. *Nature* **354**:31, 1991.
60. Thomson AM, Walker VE, Flynn DM: Glycine enhancer NMDA-receptor mediated synaptic potentials in neocortical slices. *Nature* **338**:422, 1989.
61. Johnson JW, Ascher P: Glycine potentiates the NMDA response in cultured mouse brain neurons. *Nature* **325**:529, 1987.
62. Sklow B, Goldberg MP, Choi DW: High concentration of glycine potentiate cortical neuronal injury produced by combined oxygen-glucose deprivation in vivo. *Neurology* **41**(Suppl):227, 1991.
63. Newell DW, Barth a, Ricciardi TN, Malouf AT: Glycine causes increased excitability and neurotoxicity by activation of NMDA receptors in the hippocampus. *Exp Neurol* **145**:235, 1997.
64. Larson AA, Beitz AJ: Glycine potentiates strychnine-induced convulsions: Role of NMDA receptors. *J Neurosci* **8**:3822, 1988.
65. Langan T, Pueschel SM: Nonketotic hyperglycinemia: clinical, biochemical, and therapeutic considerations. *Curr Prob Pediatr* **13**:5, 1983.
66. Dalla Bernardina B, Aicardi J, Goutieres F, Plouin P: Glycine encephalopathy. *Neuropaediatrics* **10**:209, 1979.
67. Von Wendt L, Simila S, Hirvasniemi a, Suvanto E: Nonketotic hyperglycinemia: A clinical analysis of 19 Finnish patients. *Monogr Hum Genet* **9**:58, 1978.
68. Rogers T, Al-Rayess M, O'Shea P, Ambler MW: Dysplasia of the corpus callosum in identical twins with nonketotic hyperglycinemia. *Pediatr Pathol* **11**:897, 1991.
69. Schuman RM, Leech RW, Scott R: The neuropathology of the nonketotic and ketotic hyperglycinemias: Three cases. *Neurology* **28**:139, 1978.
70. Markand ON, Garg BP, Brandt IK: Nonketotic hyperglycinemia: Electroencephalographic and evoked potential abnormalities. *Neurology* **32**:151, 1982.
71. Dobyns WB: Agenesis of the corpus callosum and gyral malformations are frequent manifestations of nonketotic hyperglycinemia. *Neurology* **39**:817, 1989.
72. Schiffmann R, Boneh a, Ergaz Z, Glick B: Nonketotic hyperglycinemia presenting with pinpoint pupils and hyperammonemia. *Isr J Med Sci* **28**:91, 1992.
73. Scher MS, Bergman I, Ahdab-Barmada M, Fria T: Neurophysiological and anatomical correlations in neonatal nonketotic hyperglycinemia. *Neuropediatrics* **17**:137, 1986.
74. Von Wendt L, Simila S, Saukkonen A-L, Koivisto M, Kouvalainen K: Prenatal brain damage in nonketotic hyperglycinemia. *Am J Dis Child* **135**:1072, 1981.
75. Seppalainen AM, Simila S: Electroencephalographic findings in three patients with nonketotic hyperglycinemia. *Epilepsia* **12**:101, 1971.
76. Reploh H, Grobe H, Dickmann L, Palm D, Bassewitz DBV, Jennett W: The clinical findings in a patient with nonketotic hyperglycinemia. *Z Kinderheilk* **114**:191, 1973.
77. Ziter FA, Bray PF, Madsen JA, Nyhan WL: The clinical findings in a patient with nonketotic hyperglycinemia. *Pediatr Res* **2**:250, 1968.
78. Baumgartner R, Ando T, Nyhan WL: Nonketotic hyperglycinemia. *J Pediatr* **75**:1022, 1969.
79. Plochl E, Rittinger O, Doringer E, Laubichler W: Neonatale form einer nicht-ketotischen hyperglycinamie bei blutsverwandten eltern. *Klin Padiatr* **203**:455, 1991.
80. Kolvraa S, Brandt NJ, Christensen E: Nonketotic hyperglycinemia: Clinical, biochemical and therapeutic aspects. *Acta Paediatr Scand* **68**:629, 1979.
81. Slager UT, Berggren RL, Marubayashi S: Nonketotic hyperglycinemia: Report of a case and review of the clinical, chemical, and pathological changes. *Ann Neurol* **1**:399, 1977.
82. Trijbels JMF, Monnens LAH, Van Der Zee SPM, Vrenken JAT, Sengers RCA, Schretlen EDAM: A patient with nonketotic hyperglycinemia: Biochemical findings and therapeutic approaches. *Pediatr Res* **8**:598, 1974.
83. Okken A, De Groot CJ, Hommes FA: Nonketotic hyperglycinemia. *J Pediatr* **77**:164, 1970.
84. Scriver CR, White A, Sprague W, Horwood SP: Plasma-CSF glycine ratios in normal and nonketotic hyperglycinemia subjects. *N Engl J Med* **293**:778, 1975.
85. Perry TL, Urquhart N, Maclean J, Evans ME, Hansen S, Davidson AGF, Applegarth DA, MacLeod PJ, Lock JE: Nonketotic hyperglycinemia. *N Engl J Med* **292**:1269, 1975.

86. Von Wendt L, Hirvasniemi A, Simila S: Nonketotic hyperglycinemia: A genetic study of 13 Finnish families. *Clin Genet* **15**:411, 1979.
87. De Groot CJ, Hommes FA, Touwen BCL: The altered toxicity of glycine in nonketotic hyperglycinemia. *Hum Hered* **27**:178, 1977.
88. Heindel W, Kugel H, Roth B: Noninvasive detection of increased glycine content by proton MR spectroscopy in the brains of two infants with nonketotic hyperglycinemia. *Am J Neuroradiol* **14**:629, 1993.
89. Trauner DA, Page T, Greco C, Sweetman L, Kulovich S, Nyhan WL: Progressive neurodegenerative disorder in a patient with nonketotic hyperglycinemia. *J Pediatr* **98**:272, 1981.
90. Childs B, Nyhan WL, Borden M, Bard L, Cooke RE: Idiopathic hyperglycinemia and hyperglycinuria, a new disorder of amino acid metabolism. *Pediatrics* **27**:522, 1961.
91. Luder AS, Davidson A, Goodman SI, Greene CL: Transient nonketotic hyperglycinemia in neonates. *J Pediatr* **114**:1013, 1989.
92. Eyskens FJM, Van Doorn JWD, Marlen P: Neurologic sequelae in transient nonketotic hyperglycinemia of the neonate. *J Pediatr* **121**:620, 1992.
93. Zammarchi E, Donati MA, Ciani F: Transient neonatal nonketotic hyperglycinemia: A 13-year follow-up. *Neuropediatrics* **26**:328, 1995.
94. Tada K: Nonketotic hyperglycinemia: Clinical and metabolic aspects. *Enzyme* **38**:27, 1987.
95. Hayasaka K, Tada K: Effects of the metabolites of the branched-chain amino acids and cysteamine on the glycine cleavage system. *Biochem* **6**:225, 1983.
96. Brandt NJ, Rasmussen K, Brandt S, Kolvraa S, Schonheyder F: d-Glyceric acidaemia, and nonketotic hyperglycinaemia. *Acta Paediatr Scand* **65**:17, 1976.
97. Belkinsopp WK, DuPont PA: Dipropylacetate (valproate) and glycine metabolism. *Lancet* **2**:617, 1977.
98. Kochi H, Hawasaka K, Hiraga K, Kikuchi G: Reduction of the level of glycine cleavage system in the rat liver resulting from administration of dipropylacetic acid: An experimental approach to hyperglycinemia. *Arch Biochem Biophys* **198**:589, 1979.
99. Brodehl J, Gellissen K: Endogenous renal transport of free amino acids in infancy and childhood. *Pediatrics* **42**:395, 1968.
100. De Groot CJ, Troelstra JA, Hommes FA: Nonketotic hyperglycinemia: An in vitro study of the glycine-serine conversion in liver of three patients and the effect of dietary methionine. *Pediatr Res* **4**:238, 1970.
101. Tada K, Hayasaka K: Non-ketotic hyperglycinaemia: Clinical and biochemical aspects. *Eur J Pediatr* **146**:221, 1987.
102. Kure S, Narisawa K, Tada K: Enzymatic diagnosis of nonketotic hyperglycinemia with lymphoblasts. *J Pediatr* **120**:95, 1992.
103. Christodoulu J, Kure S, Hayasaka K, Clarke JTR: Atypical nonketotic hyperglycinemia confirmed by assay of the glycine cleavage system in lymphoblasts. *J Pediatr* **123**:100, 1993.
104. Yoshino M, Koga Y, Yamashita F: A decrease in glycine cleavage activity in the liver of a patient with dihydrolipoyl dehydrogenase deficiency. *J Inherit Metab Dis* **9**:399, 1986.
105. Johnson MT, Yang H-S, Magnuson T, Patel MS: Targeted disruption of the murine dihydrolipoamide dehydrogenase gene (Dld) results in perigastrulation lethality. *Proc Natl Acad Sci U S A* **94**:14512, 1997.
106. Kure S, Takayanagi M, Narisawa K, Tada K, Leisti J: Identification of a common mutation in Finnish patients with nonketotic hyperglycinemia. *J Clin Invest* **90**:160, 1992.
107. Nanao K, Okamura-Ikeda K, Motokawa Y, Danks DM, Baumgartner ER, Takada G, Hayasaka K: Identification of the mutations in the T-protein gene causing typical and atypical nonketotic hyperglycinemia. *Hum Genet* **93**:655, 1994.
108. Kure S, Shinka T, Sakata Y, Osamu N, Takayanagi M, Tada K, Matsubara Y, Narisawa K: A one base deletion (183delC) and a missense mutation (D276H) in the T protein gene from a Japanese family with nonketotic hyperglycinemia. *J Hum Genet* **43**:135, 1998.
109. Kure S, Mandel H, Rolland MO, Sakata Y, Shinka T, Drugan A, Boneh A, Tada K, Matsubara Y, Narisawa K: A missense mutation (His42Arg) in the T-protein gene from a large Israeli-Arab kindred with nonketotic hyperglycinemia. *Hum Genet* **102**:430, 1998.
110. Ohya Y, Ochi N, Mizutani N, Hayakawa C, Watanabe K: Nonketotic hyperglycinemia: Treatment with NMDA antagonist and consideration of neuropathogenesis. *Pediatr Neurol* **7**:65, 1991.
111. Hayasaka K, Fueki N, Aikawa J: Prenatal diagnosis of non-ketotic hyperglycinemia: Enzymatic analysis of the glycine cleavage system in chorionic villi. *J Pediatr* **116**:444, 1990.
112. Toone JR, Applegarth DA, Levy HL: Prenatal diagnosis of non-ketotic hyperglycinemia. *J Inherit Metab Dis* **15**:713, 1992.
113. Toone JR, Applegarth DA, Levy HL: Prenatal diagnosis of NKH: Experience in 50 at-risk pregnancies. *J Inherit Metab Dis* **17**:342, 1994.
114. Garcia-Castro JM, Isales-Forsythe BS, Levy HL, Shih VE, Lao-Velez CR, Gonzalez-Rios MDC, Reyes de Torres LC: Prenatal diagnosis of nonketotic hyperglycinemia. *N Engl J Med* **306**:79, 1982.
115. Mesavage C, Nance CS, Flannery DB, Weiner DL, Suchy SF, Wolf B: Glycine/serine ratios in amniotic fluid: An unreliable indicator for the prenatal diagnosis of nonketotic hyperglycinemia. *Clin Genet* **23**:354, 1983.
116. Wolff JA, Kulovich S, Qiao C-N, Nyhan WL: The effectiveness of benzoate in the management of seizures in nonketotic hyperglycinemia. *Am J Dis Child* **140**:596, 1986.
117. Boneh a, Degani Y, Harari M: Prognostic clues and outcome of early treatment of nonketotic hyperglycinemia. *Pediatr Neurol* **15**:137, 1996.
118. Spielberg SP, Lucky AW, Schulman JD, Kramer LI, Hefter L, Goodman SI: Failure of leucovorin therapy in nonketotic hyperglycinemia. *J Pediatr* **89**:681, 1976.
119. MacDermot K, Nelson W, Weinberg JA, Schulman JD: Valproate in nonketotic hyperglycinemia. *Pediatrics* **65**:624, 1980.
120. Simila S, Von Wendt L, Linna S-L, Saukkonen A-L, Huhtaniemi I: Dipropylacetate and hyperglycinemia. *Neuropediatrics* **10**:158, 1979.
121. Arneson D, Ch'ien LT, Chance P, Wilroy RS: Strychnine therapy in nonketotic hyperglycinemia. *Pediatrics* **63**:369, 1979.
122. Gitzelmann R, Steinmann B, Cuenod M: Strychnine for the treatment of nonketotic hyperglycinemia. *N Engl J Med* **298**:1424, 1978.
123. MacDermot KD, Nelson W, Reichert CM, Schulman JD: Attempts at use of strychnine sulfate in the treatment of nonketotic hyperglycinemia. *Pediatrics* **65**:61, 1980.
124. Von Wendt L, Simila S, Saukkonen A-L, Koivisto M: Failure of strychnine treatment during the neonatal period in three Finnish children with nonketotic hyperglycinemia. *Pediatrics* **65**:1166, 1980.
125. Warburton D, Boyle RJ, Keats JP, Vohr B, Peuschel S, Oh W: Nonketotic hyperglycinemia: Effects of therapy with strychnine. *Am J Dis Child* **134**:273, 1980.
126. Gitzelmann R, Steinmann B, Otten a, Dumermuth G, Herdan M, Reubi JC, Cuenod M: Nonketotic hyperglycinemia treated with strychnine, a glycine receptor antagonist. *Helv Paediat Acta* **32**:517, 1977.
127. Matalon R, Naidu S, Hughes JR, Michals K: Nonketotic hyperglycinemia: Treatment with diazepam — a competitor for glycine receptors. *Pediatrics* **71**:581, 1983.
128. Ferkany JW, Borosky DB, Pontecorro MJ: Dextromethorphan inhibits NMDA-induced convulsions 2. *Eur J Pharm* **151**:151, 1988.
129. Schmitt B, Steinmann B, Gitzelmann R, Thun-Hohenstein L, Mascher H, Dumermuth G: Nonketotic hyperglycinemia: Clinical and electrophysiologic effects of dextromethorphan, an antagonist of the NMDA receptor. *Neurology* **43**:421, 1993.
130. Hamosh A, Maher JF, Bellus GA, Rasmussen SA, Johnston MV: Long-term use of high-dose benzoate and dextromethorphan for the treatment of nonketotic hyperglycinemia. *J Pediatr* **132**:709, 1998.
131. Hamosh A, McDonald JW, Valle D, Francomano CA, Niedermeyer E, Johnston MV: Dextromethorphan and high-dose benzoate therapy for nonketotic hyperglycinemia in an infant. *J Pediatr* **121**:131, 1992.
132. Zammarchi E, Kure S, Hayasaka K, Clarke JTR: Failure of early dextromethorphan and sodium benzoate therapy in an infant with nonketotic hyperglycinemia. *Neuropediatrics* **25**:274, 1994.
133. Alemzadeh RMK: Efficacy of low-dose dextromethorphan in the treatment of nonketotic hyperglycinemia. *Pediatrics* **97**:924, 1996.
134. Jacqz-Aigrain E, Funck-Brentano C, Cresteil T: CYP2D6- and CYP31-dependent metabolism of dextromethorphan in humans. *Pharmacogenetics* **3**:197, 1993.
135. Woodworth JR, Dennis SRK, Moore L, Rotenberg KS: The polymorphic metabolism of dextromethorphan. *J Clin Pharmacol* **27**:139, 1987.
136. Arnold GL, Griebel ML, Valentine JL, Koroma DM, Kearns GL: Dextromethorphan in nonketotic hyperglycinemia: Metabolic variation confounds the dose-response relationship. *J Inherit Metab Dis* **20**:28, 1997.
137. Van Hove JL, Kishnani P, Muenzer J, Wenstrup RJ, Summar ML, Brummond MR, Lachiewicz AM, Millington DS, Kahler SG:

Benzoate therapy and carnitine deficiency in non-ketotic hyperglycinemia. *Am J Med Genet* **59**:444, 1995.

138. Matsuo S, Inoue F, Takeuchi Y, Yoshioka H, Kinugasa a, Sawada T: Efficacy of tryptophan for the treatment of nonketotic hyperglycinemia: a new therapeutic approach for modulating the *N*-methyl-D-aspartate receptor. *Pediatrics* **95**:142, 1995.

139. McCabe RT, Wasterlain CG, Kucharczyk N: Evidence for anticonvulsant and neuroprotectan action of felbamate mediated by strychnine-insensitive glycine receptors. *J Pharmacol Exp Ther* **264**:1248, 1993.

140. Rho J, Donevan SD, Rogawski MA: Mechanism of action of the anticonvulsant felbamate: opposing effects on NMDA and GABA receptors. *Ann Neurol* **35**:229, 1994.

141. Marson AG, Kadir ZA, Hutton JA, Chadwick DW: The new antiepileptic drugs: A systematic review of the efficacy and tolerability. *Epilepsia* **38**:859, 1997.

142. Hayasaka K, Tada K, Fueki N, Nakamura Y, Nyhan Wl, Schmidt K, Packman S, Seashore MR, Haan E, Danks DM, Schutgens RBH: Nonketotic hyperglycinemia: Analyses of glycine cleavage system in typical and atypical cases. *J Pediatr* **110**:873, 1987.

143. von Wendt L, Similä S, Hirvasniemi A, Suvanto E: Altered levels of various amino acids in blood plasma and cerebrospinal fluid of patients with nonketotic hyperglycinemia. *Neuropädiatrie* **9**:360, 1978.

144. Wraith JE: Non-kinetic hyperglycinaemia: Prolonged survival in a patient with a mild variant. *J Inherit Metab Dis* **19**:695, 1996.

CHAPTER 91

Disorders of β- and γ-Amino Acids in Free and Peptide-Linked Forms*

K. Michael Gibson ▪ Cornelis Jakobs

1. **Five β- or γ-amino acids occur in free forms in mammalian (including human) tissues and body fluids: β-alanine and R-β-AiB are pyrimidine catabolites of uracil and thymine, respectively; S-β-AiB is a catabolite of L-valine; β-leucine is a precursor of α-leucine; and γ-aminobutyric acid (GABA) is a derivative of L-glutamate and, to a minor extent, of L-ornithine via putrescine.**
2. **β-alanine and GABA also occur as imidazole dipeptides that are products of carnosine synthetase activity. The major dipeptides are carnosine (β-alanyl-L-histidine), anserine (β-alanyl-1-methyl-L-histidine, not itself a constituent of human tissues), and homocarnosine (β-aminobutyryl-L-histidine, present only in the brain in humans).**
3. **GABA is a major inhibitory neurotransmitter; β-alanine and carnosine may also have neurotransmitter functions. Carnosine (and anserine) may act as an intracellular buffer and antioxidant in skeletal muscle during anaerobic glycolysis.**
4. **Several disorders of β-alanine metabolism are known, notably:**
   - **4.1 Dihydropyrimidine dehydrogenase (EC 1.3.1.2) deficiency (autosomal recessive) is a disorder of uracil and thymine catabolism (affecting endogenous synthesis of β-alanine and R-β-AiB). One form is an *inborn error of metabolism* with onset early in life and featuring one or more of the following symptoms: convulsions, psychomotor retardation, hypertonicity, microcephaly, autism, and growth retardation. The *pharmacogenetic* form presents following exposure to the anticancer agent 5-fluorouracil. Clinical manifestations include myelosuppression, gastrointestinal and cutaneous findings, and neurologic toxicity, occasionally with fatal outcome. Enzyme activity is negligible in the inborn error of *metabolism* and up to half normal in the pharmacogenetic form. Circadian fluctuation in enzyme activity may significantly influence enzyme activity determination.**
   - **4.2 Dihydropyrimidinuria (dihydropyrimidinase [EC 3.5.2.2] deficiency) is recognized by urinary excretion of excessive dihydrouracil and dihydrothymine. The clinical course is characterized by neurologic abnormalities, although two asymptomatic patients with dihydropyrimidinuria have been identified. Inheritance is likely autosomal recessive, and liver biopsy is necessary for enzymatic confirmation of the defect. Probands would be expected to manifest toxicity to 5-fluorouracil.**
   - **4.3 NMR spectroscopy revealed the presence of ureidopropionate (N-carbamyl-β-alanine) and ureidobutyrate (N-carbamyl-β-amino isobutyric acid) in urine of an 11-month-old girl who presented with developmental delay, dystonia, scoliosis, and microcephaly. A novel enzyme assay using [^{14}C]-N-carbamyl-β-alanine in homogenate of biopsied liver derived from the patient confirmed β-alanine synthase deficiency. Two frameshift alleles were detected in the relevant gene using genomic DNA derived from the patient.**
   - **4.4 Hyper-β-alaninemia (two cases) is associated with impaired neurologic development. Elevated levels of β-alanine and GABA may occur in urine, plasma, and/or CSF. Complex hyperaminoaciduria (β-alanine, GABA, β-AiB, and taurine) in the index case was explained by combined saturation and inhibition of a β-amino acid-preferring transport system in the nephron. The enzyme defect (β-alanyl-α-ketoglutarate transaminase, EC 2.6.1.19 or 2.6.1.22; tentatively identified in the second proband) would be expected to have an effect on GABA metabolism secondarily. Pharmacologic doses of pyridoxine (precursor of the transaminase cofactor) ameliorated the metabolic phenotype in the index proband and the clinical phenotype in the second.**
   - **4.5 Another disorder with impaired β-alanine catabolism has a characteristic urine metabolite pattern consistent with combined malonic/methylmalonic semialdehyde dehydrogenase deficiency. Impaired oxidation of β-alanine has been demonstrated in skin fibroblasts derived from two of four patients. A single (putative) pathologic allele has been identified in one patient.**
5. **Hyper-β-AiBuria is a benign "metabolic polymorphism" present in human populations (5 to 10 percent in Caucasians, 40 to 95 percent in Asian populations). R-β-AiB is the form excreted. The enzyme deficiency is hepatic R-β-AiB-pyruvate transaminase (EC 2.6.1.40), inherited as an (incompletely) autosomal recessive trait; heterozygotes can have modestly elevated β-AiB excretion, with their enzyme activity intermediate between that of low**

*The authors have drawn substantively from the earlier version of this chapter (MMBID 7th Edition, Vol 1, Chapter 38, pp. 1349–1368) and gratefully acknowledge the significant contribution of the preceding primary author, Dr. Charles R. Scriver.

A list of standard abbreviations is located immediately preceding the index in each volume. Nonstandard abbreviations used in this chapter include: AiB = aminoisobutyric acid; GAD = glutamic acid decarboxylase; 4-HBA = 4-hydroxybutyric acid; PLP = pyridoxal 5′-phosphate; PET = positron emission tomography; SSADH = succinic semialdehyde dehydrogenase.

excretors (homozygous normal) and high excretors (homozygous mutant).

6. **There are three disorders of GABA metabolism (putative and proven):**
   6.1 **The diagnosis of pyridoxine (vitamin B_6) dependency with seizures is dependent upon a seizure disorder, refractive to all conventional anticonvulsants, that responds to pharmacologic doses of pyridoxine. Inheritance is autosomal recessive, and there are neonatal and delayed-onset forms. Pathogenesis is believed to be related to altered central nervous system glutamate/GABA ratios, perhaps the result of defective association of pyridoxal 5′-phosphate with glutamic acid decarboxylase (GAD). Molecular characterization of the different mammalian forms of GAD (so-called GAD_{65} and GAD_{67}) failed to identify a disease-linked mutation in a cohort of patients. Mice lacking both forms of GAD (GAD_{67}-/- and GAD_{65}-/-) manifest significantly decreased GAD activities and central nervous system GABA content, and increased seizure activity with decreased PLP-inducible apo-GAD reservoirs.**

   6.2 **GABA transaminase deficiency, a rare disorder, is associated with seizures and profound psychomotor retardation. Distinctive clinical and metabolic phenotypes seem to differentiate the disorder from hyper-β-alaninemia despite the fact that both conditions appear to have impaired GABA and β-alanine homeostasis. Deficiency of the GABA-α-ketoglutarate transaminase (EC 2.6.1.19) has thus far been documented in white cells derived from two patients, with autosomal recessive inheritance. The human cDNA is available, and a single disease-associated allele has been identified in one patient.**

   6.3 **Deficiency of succinic semialdehyde dehydrogenase (EC 1.2.1.24), also called 4-hydroxybutyric aciduria, is associated with retardation in mental, motor, and language development and with muscular hypotonia (>150 cases known). Early development may be normal or delayed. The principal metabolic derivative (4-hydroxybutyrate) of the deficient enzyme's natural substrate accumulates in patient physiological fluids. Deficient dehydrogenase activity is readily demonstrated in white cells using fluorometric assays. The relevant human gene maps to chromosome 6p22, and inheritance is autosomal recessive.**

7. **Two disorders of dipeptide catabolism, serum carnosinase (EC 3.4.13.3) deficiency and "homocarnosinosis," are apparently one disorder. Although neurologic signs occur in some patients, the majority are healthy. The association of clinical disease with the metabolic disorder is either coincidental or a consequence of unidentified variables in environment and/or genotype. Both disorders involve deficient serum carnosinase activity, more extreme in homocarnosinosis. Serum and cytosolic carnosinases are different enzymes; tissue carnosinase activity is normal in probands. Homocarnosine accumulation in CSF is explained by deficiency of serum carnosinase activity. The phenotype (serum carnosinase deficiency; "homocarnosinosis") is autosomal recessive. Heterozygotes have partial enzyme deficiency but no metabolic abnormalities. Serum carnosinase activity is normally low in infancy, which may lead to an erroneous diagnosis of hereditary serum carnosinase deficiency.**

This chapter describes three areas of human metabolism. They involve: (1) the oxidation of β-alanine, β-aminoisobutyric acid (β-AiB), and their associated pyrimidines; (2) the principal metabolic pathway of γ-aminobutyric acid (GABA), but not the interactions at the associated synaptic GABA receptors (see Chap. 90); and (3) metabolism of the corresponding β-alanine and GABA-containing dipeptides carnosine, anserine, and homocarnosine.

Interindividual (genetic) variation affects disposal of each metabolite described here (Table 91-1). Some phenotypes reflect ontogeny as well as mutation (e.g., carnosinemia); others reflect genetic polymorphism at the population level (e.g., hyper-β-AiBuria; "electromorph" GABA transaminase variation). The remainder are the result of rare alleles. Four of the diseases affect β-alanine metabolism, three affect GABA oxidation, and two are probably a single disorder affecting the metabolism of carnosine and homocarnosine.

In only five of these disorders, dihydropyrimidine dehydrogenase deficiency, dihydropyrimidinase deficiency, pyridoxine dependency with seizures (presumed to result from deficiency of one ([or more?]) isoforms of glutamic acid decarboxylase in brain), GABA-transaminase deficiency, and succinic semialdehyde dehydrogenase deficiency (SSADH), have the relevant genes been cloned. This chapter, like its predecessor (Chap. 90),[1] describes "inborn errors of metabolism" awaiting more information about the molecular biology and genetics of the corresponding phenotypes. The detailed biochemical background is available in the primary literature.[2–4]

β- AND γ-AMINO METABOLITES

Five β- or γ-aminomonocarboxylic acids occur in free or peptide-linked forms in mammals (Fig. 91-1). β-Alanine and R-β-AiB are derivatives of the pyrimidines uracil and thymine, respectively.[2] S-β-AiB is the transamination product of S-methylmalonic acid semialdehyde, a metabolite of L-valine.[2]

GABA is the decarboxylation product of l-glutamic acid.[3] It has a neurotransmitter function in central nervous system, and a metabolic role both in brain and in some extraneural tissues, notably pancreas and kidney.

Mammalian tissues contain the dipeptides carnosine (β-alanyl-L-histidine) and anserine (β-alanyl-1-methyl-L-histidine)[2]; human tissues contain carnosine only. GABA occurs to a minor extent in peptide linkage as homocarnosine (β-aminobutyryl-L-histidine). β- and γ-amino acids do not appear in proteins. GABA (and perhaps β-alanine and carnosine) functions as a neurotransmitter.

β-Leucine, a precursor of α-L-leucine,[4] has no inherited disorder of its own metabolism in humans, and its plasma level is not increased in a major Mendelian disorder of leucine metabolism, maple syrup urine disease (see Chap. 87). However, plasma β-leucine is modestly elevated in pernicious anemia (24.7±12.4 μM; normal value 4.8±3.1 μM), because leucine 2,3-aminomutase, which converts β-leucine to α-leucine, requires adenosylcobalamin as a coenzyme.[4]

β-ALANINE

Neurotransmitter Role and Normal Metabolism

While it is widely accepted that GABA, glutamate, and glycine function as neurotransmitters in the mammalian central nervous system, the role of β-alanine as a neurotransmitter remains somewhat controversial. Historically, three criteria are applicable in identifying brain neurotransmitters, namely presynaptic localization, Ca^{2+}-dependent release or release on stimulation of specific neuronal pathways, and identification of postsynaptic receptors.[5] β-alanine fulfills these criteria, although it is present in low concentrations in brain. Kinetic data suggest that GABA, β-alanine, and glycine are taken up by the same family of vesicular transporters and that all three inhibit each other competitively.[5–8] In studies of the glycine receptor in chick sympathetic neurons, however, β-alanine was only half as effective as glycine in triggering inward currents in voltage-clamped cells.[9] Thus,

Table 91-1 Mendelian Phenotypes Affecting β- and γ-Amino Acid Metabolism

Disorder	MIM	Locus	Enzyme	EC*
Dihydropyrimidine dehydrogenase deficiency	274270	1p22–q21	Dihydrouracil dehydrogenase ($NADP^+$)	1.3.1.2
Dihydropyrimidinase deficiency (dihydropyrimidinuria)	222748	8q22	Dihydropyrimidinase	3.5.2.2
β-Alanine synthase deficiency	–	?	β-Alanine synthase (β-ureido propionase)	3.5.1.6
Hyper-β-alaninemia	237400	?	β-alanine, α-ketoglutarate aminotransferase	2.6.1.22§ or 2.6.1.19§
Methylmalonate semialdehyde dehydrogenase deficiency	236795	14q24.3	Methylmalonic acid semialdehyde dehydrogenase (acylating)	1.2.1.27, 1.2.1.18‡
Hyper-β-aminoisobutyric aciduria	210100	?	D-(*R*)-3-Aminoisobutyrate, pyruvate aminotransferase	2.6.1.40
Pyridoxine dependency with seizures	266100	10p11.23 or 2q31 (?)	Glutamic acid decarboxylase (GAD_{65}/GAD_{67}?)†	4.1.1.15
GABA-transaminase deficiency	137150	?	4-Aminobutyrate, α-ketoglutarate aminotransferase	2.6.1.19§
4-Hydroxybutyric aciduria (SSADH deficiency)	271980	6p22	Succinic semialdehyde dehydrogenase (SSADH)	1.2.1.24
Homocarnosinosis and/or carnosinemia	236130 212200	18q†	Serum carnosinase	3.4.13.3¶

* Enzyme classification number from International Union of Biochemists (1984).
† The variant phenotype and disease locus are provisional.
‡ Studies in cultured fibroblasts indicate a combined semialdehyde dehydrogenase deficiency also affecting malonic semialdehydes in addition to methylmalonic acid semialdehyde.
§ Mendelian phenotypes imply that MIM 237400 and MIM 137150 involve different aminotransferases (see Table 91-2).
¶ Separate EC numbers have not been assigned to serum and tissue carnosinases.

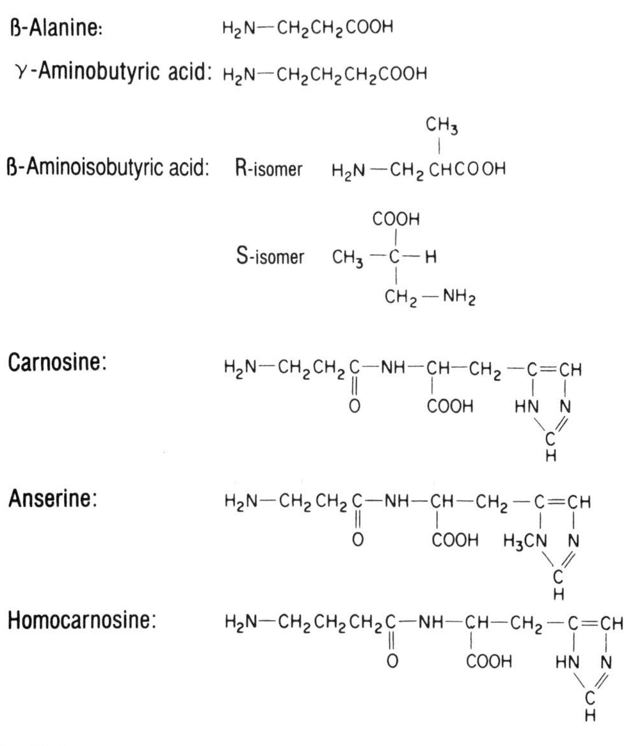

ß-Alanine: $H_2N{-}CH_2CH_2COOH$

γ-Aminobutyric acid: $H_2N{-}CH_2CH_2CH_2COOH$

ß-Aminoisobutyric acid: R-isomer $H_2N{-}CH_2CH(CH_3)COOH$

S-isomer $CH_3{-}C(COOH)(H){-}CH_2{-}NH_2$

Carnosine: $H_2N{-}CH_2CH_2C(=O){-}NH{-}CH(COOH){-}CH_2{-}C{=}CH$ (imidazole ring: HN, N, C–H)

Anserine: $H_2N{-}CH_2CH_2C(=O){-}NH{-}CH(COOH){-}CH_2{-}C{=}CH$ (imidazole ring: H_3CN, N, C–H)

Homocarnosine: $H_2N{-}CH_2CH_2CH_2C(=O){-}NH{-}CH(COOH){-}CH_2{-}C{=}CH$ (imidazole ring: HN, N, C–H)

Fig. 91-1 Molecular structures of compounds (and related substances) involved in the disorders discussed in the text of this chapter.

although the preponderance of the data suggests a role for β-alanine as a neurotransmitter in mammalian brain, the current evidence is not completely convincing.

β-Alanine is an endogenous derivative of uracil and a precursor of the oxidative substrate acetyl-coenzyme A (acetyl-CoA) (Fig. 91-2). R-β-AiB, the metabolic analogue of β-alanine, is derived from thymine. Enzymes controlling pyrimidine catabolism are active toward the metabolites of both pathways. β-Ureidopropionase, new name β-alanine synthase [reaction (4), Fig. 91-2], is located predominantly in liver, where it catalyzes production of both β-alanine and R-β-AiB from their pyrimidine precursors. The moment-to-moment size of the free β-amino acid pool reflects the balance among pyrimidine salvage in dividing cells, catabolism in quiescent cells, dietary intake of pyrimidines, and delivery of precursors to liver.[2]

Aspartate decarboxylation and hydrolysis of carnosine and anserine are minor sources of free β-alanine [reactions (24) and (25) in Fig. 91-2]. Since bacteria are the principal sites of the former reaction, microbial metabolism in large intestine could be an extraneous source of β-alanine in humans. Mammals also form small amounts of β-alanine through the action of cysteine sulfinate decarboxylase and glutamate decarboxylase on the relevant precursors.[2]

Disposal of β-alanine is achieved by two routes. The first involves incorporation of the free amino acid into carnosine or anserine [reaction (26), Fig. 91-2]. The other involves transamination to yield malonic acid semialdehyde [reactions (5) and (6)]. Further metabolism is complex: formation of malonyl-CoA is not important in humans; decarboxylation of the semialdehyde [reactions (7) and (8)] generates acetyl products. Several aminotransferases are involved in the metabolism of β-alanine,

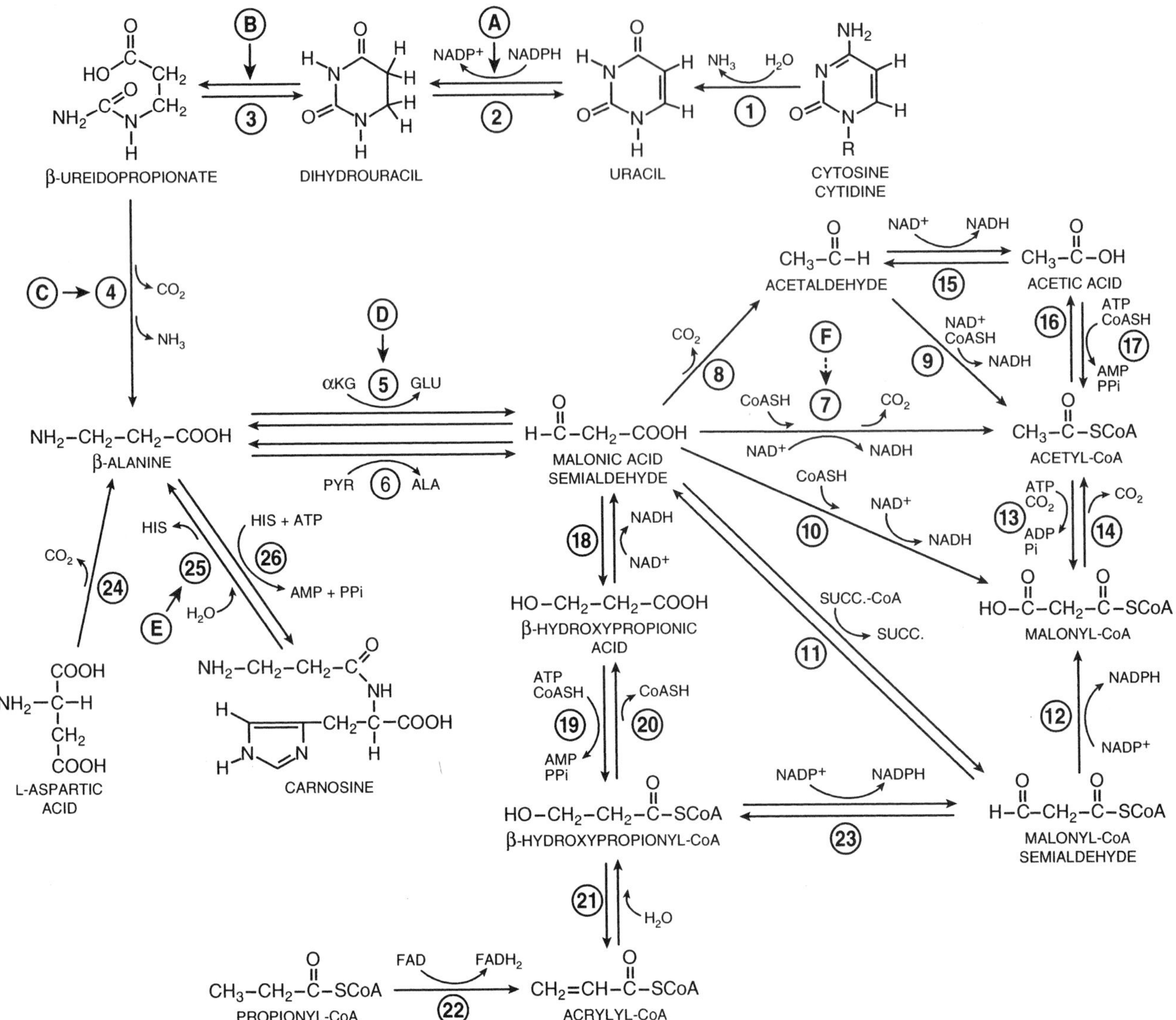

Fig. 91-2 Formation and metabolism of β-alanine. The circled numbers indicate enzymes or metabolic processes: 1 = cytosine ring deamination; 2 = dihydropyrimidine dehydrogenase; 3 = dihydropyrimidinase; 4 = β-alanine synthase; 5 = β-alanine-α-ketoglutarate transaminase; 6 = β-alanine-pyruvate transaminase; 7 = malonate semialdehyde dehydrogenase (acetylating); 8 = nonenzymatic or (?) malonate semialdehyde decarboxylase; 9 = acetaldehyde dehydrogenase; 10 = as 9 (?); 11 = succinylacetoacetyl-CoA transferase; 12 = malonate semialdehyde dehydrogenase; 13 = acetyl-CoA carboxylase; 14 = malonyl-CoA decarboxylase; 15 = aldehyde dehydrogenase; 16 = acetyl-CoA hydrolase; 17 = acetyl-CoA synthetase; 18 = 3-hydroxypropionate dehydrogenase; 19 = acyl-CoA synthetase (?); 20 = 3-hydroxypropionate dehydrogenase; 21 = enoyl-CoA hydratase (crotonase); 22 = butyryl-CoA dehydrogenase; 23 = 3-hydroxypropionyl-CoA dehydrogenase (?); 24 = aspartate decarboxylase (in bacteria) or a minor activity of mammalian cysteine sulfinate decarboxylase and glutamate decarboxylase; 25 = carnosinase; 26 = carnosine synthetase. The circled letters indicate confirmed (solid arrows) or putative (interrupted arrow) enzyme deficiencies: A = dihydropyrimidine dehydrogenase deficiency (hyperuracil-, thyminuria); B = dihydropyrimidinase deficiency; C = β-alanine synthase deficiency; D = hyper-β-alaninemia E = serum carnosinase deficiency (carnosinemia); F = shared disorders of β-alanine and β-AiB catabolism.[101,102] *(Pathway diagram reproduced from Griffith,[2] with permission.)*

β-AiB, and GABA (Table 91-2), a fact to be taken into consideration when trying to identify the enzyme deficiency in the associated disorders.

Disorders of β-Alanine Metabolism

Dihydropyrimidine Dehydrogenase Deficiency. Albeit a disorder of pyrimidine catabolism [MIM (McKusick) 274270], known also as combined uraciluria-thyminuria, it is also one of β-amino acid metabolism, in that formation of β-alanine and R-β-AiB from pyrimidine precursors is potentially impaired. The extent of the contribution of impaired β-amino acid production to the associated clinical phenotype is unknown.

Dihydropyrimidine dehydrogenase deficiency has two clinical forms. One form is an inborn error of metabolism with onset early in life. At least 33 patients have been reported,[10] with considerable phenotypic heterogeneity. Neurologic manifestations appear prominent, including convulsions and mental retardation.[11] Associated findings include growth retardation, dysmorphia, microcephaly, motor retardation, hypertonia, autistic features, and hyperreflexia.[10,12–26] A family history of epileptic disease may be present. Bilateral hydroceles, hypohydrotic ectodermal dysplasia, and hepatosplenomegaly were observed in two cases.[21,27] In one patient, ocular findings included bilateral microphthalmia, iris and choroid colobomas, and nystagmus.[24,28] Asymptomatic family members of affected probands have been identified as having enzyme deficiency, suggesting that it may be prudent to screen family members of affected probands.[21,26,29–31]

In the pharmacogenetic form, onset of symptomatology follows exposure to 5-fluorouracil, a widely used chemotherapeutic agent. The therapeutic target of 5-fluorouracil is thymidylate kinase.[32]

Table 91-2 Aminotransferases Relevant to β- and γ-Amino Acid Metabolism

EC Number	Primary Substrate	Other Substrates	Keto Acid Acceptor
2.6.1.18	β-Alanine	—	Pyruvate
2.6.1.19	GABA	β-Alanine RS-β-AiB	α-Ketoglutarate
2.6.1.22	S-β-AiB	β-Alanine GABA	α-Ketoglutarate
2.6.1.40	R-β-AiB	—	Pyruvate
2.6.1.61	R-β-AiB	—	α-Ketoglutarate

The clinical efficacy of 5-fluorouracil is decreased by substantial (>90 percent) metabolism through dihydropyrimidine dehydrogenase and concomitant short plasma half-life (~10 min).[33,34] Inhibitors of dihydropyrimidine dehydrogenase (5-benzyloxybenzyluracil, 5-ethynyluracil) have been coadministered to enhance 5-fluorouracil efficacy.[33] The activity of xenobiotic metabolizing enzymes, such as dihydropyrimidine dehydrogenase, is genetically influenced such that a fixed percentage of the population exhibits reduced enzyme activity.[35] In the pharmacogenetic form, clinical manifestations for 17 reported patients include myelosuppression, gastrointestinal effects, and cutaneous and, infrequently, neurologic toxicity.[36–39] At least five patients have died from treatment-related toxicity.[34,39,40] In two instances, 5-fluorouracil toxicity was associated with osteogenesis imperfecta.[37,38] In cancer patients, the differential diagnosis of dihydropyrimidine dehydrogenase deficiency should be entertained in any patient experiencing unexplained severe diarrhea, mucositis, and myelosuppression following the first doses of 5-fluorouracil.[39,41] Clinical manifestations reflect impaired disposal of 5-fluorouracil.[42–46]

Metabolic Phenotype. The pyrimidine catabolic pathway is the only route for production of β-alanine in mammals.[47] In both forms of the disorder, excess uracil, thymine, and 5-hydroxymethyluracil (a metabolite of thymine) accumulate in urine, the preferred biologic fluid for screening. Dihydropyrimidines do not accumulate in either form. In both forms of the disease, pyrimidine metabolites are also elevated in plasma and cerebrospinal fluid.[27,39,40] Gas chromatographic-mass spectrometric analysis may be employed to detect up to 300-fold elevated pyrimidine metabolites in urine.[10,48] Variable extraction efficiencies and smaller accumulation of pyrimidine analogues indicate that HPLC methodology is the method of choice for quantitation in plasma and cerebrospinal fluid.[49,50]

Plasma half-lives of 5-fluorouracil are increased in patients manifesting toxicity in the pharmacogenetic form (120–5430 min; control <20 min).[33,35,39] Davies and coworkers[51] reported the utility of determining urinary uracil levels to screen for dihydropyrimidine dehydrogenase deficiency as well as hemizygotes/heterozygotes for ornithine carbamoyl transferase deficiency. The pyrimidine and urea cycle synthetic routes share a common intermediate, carbamoyl phosphate (for additional details, see Chapter 85). Consistent elevations in urinary uracil (in comparison to urinary pseudouridine) were identified in "asymptomatic" carriers and hemizygotes with ornithine carbamoyl transferase deficiency, even when urinary orotic acid was undetectable. Pseudouridine, a component of tRNA, does not share the N-glycosidic linkage typical of nucleosides but rather employs a carbon-5 base linkage to the C-1 of the ribose sugar (i.e., 5-(1′-ribosyl)-uracil). Uracil concentrations show considerable age-dependent variation, as does pseudouridine, which is unrelated to pyrimidine metabolism and employed as an endogenous internal marker.[51] The ratio of uracil to pseudouridine corrects for age-dependent variation in excretion. In the differential diagnosis of dihydropyrimidine dehydrogenase deficiency (and dihydropyrimidinuria, see Dihydropyrimidinuria below), thymine excretion is also elevated in dihydropyrimidinuria.

Enzyme Phenotype. Dihydropyrimidine dehydrogenase catalyzes the first, and rate-limiting, step in pyrimidine catabolism.[52] Enzyme activity can be determined in blood cells (monocytes, lymphocytes, platelets, and granulocytes), skin fibroblasts, and liver.[53,54] For population analysis, long-term storage of polymorphonuclear cells appears feasible.[55] Decreased amounts of dihydropyrimidine dehydrogenase cross-reactive material (CRM) were identified in skin fibroblasts from a proband using a polyclonal antibody directed against the purified human protein.[54] The activity of NADPH- and NADH-linked dihydropyrimidine dehydrogenase was equally decreased in fibroblasts derived from a proband with combined uraciluria-thyminuria,[56] suggesting clinical heterogeneity might be associated with differential expression of the two enzymes.

In the inborn error of metabolism form, residual dihydropyrimidine dehydrogenase is uniformly absent (<5 percent of control levels).[11,24,32,45,54,56] Equally low or much higher residual enzyme activities are detected in the pharmacogenetic form.[45] In a study of 185 patients with head and neck cancer, Etienne and coworkers[57] defined dihydropyrimidine dehydrogenase deficiency in the pharmacogenetic form as enzyme activity <0.1 nmol/min-mg protein. This "threshold" of activity has gained general acceptance.[27,38–40] Two patients with severe 5-fluorouracil toxicity manifested 24–57 percent of control dihydropyrimidine dehydrogenase activity.[37] Parents of patients with the inborn error of metabolism form have intermediate enzyme activities, although values in some are considerably less than half normal, perhaps compatible with a dominant negative phenotype effect.[14,16,42] Although demonstration of heterozygosity by enzyme assay is influenced by circadian rhythm, intermediate values of dihydropyrimidine dehydrogenase activity appear sufficient to induce 5-fluorouracil toxicity in the pharmacogenetic form of the disease.[29,58] A child with medulloblastoma had fluctuating uraciluria-thyminuria and partial enzyme activity in leukocytes, suggesting heterozygosity.[59] The metabolic profile appeared during chemotherapy; no exposure to 5-fluorouracil was mentioned. This case suggests that a heterozygote might express the metabolic phenotype under "load" conditions unrelated to 5-fluorouracil.

Dihydropyrimidine dehydrogenase manifests a circadian rhythm (and interindividual variability), with peak at 1 AM and trough at 1 PM., on average, and enzyme activity levels varying up to sixfold.[27,32,33] Circadian variability of plasma 5-fluorouracil correlates with circadian fluctuations of enzyme activity in lymphocytes.[35] Population studies of dihydropyrimidine dehydrogenase activity suggest an estimate of heterozygosity approximating 3 percent.[57] Application of Hardy-Weinberg equilibrium to this heterozygote frequency suggests 1 in 1000 births may be homozygous for mutant dihydropyrimidine dehydrogenase alleles.[47] The fact that each individual exhibits a unique profile of circadian rhythm for dihydropyrimidine dehydrogenase activity limits the significance of enzyme determination for prediction of 5-fluorouracil pharmacokinetics.[46] On the other hand, enzyme estimates permit identification of a low proportion (up to 3 percent, all heterozygotes) of patients at risk of developing 5-fluorouracil-related toxicity, and perhaps alteration of the choice of chemotherapeutic intervention.[44,57,60]

Recent results suggest that it may be prudent to screen patients with tumors for activity of dihydropyrimidine dehydrogenase deficiency prior to institution of 5-fluorouracil therapy. Lu *et al.*[60a] found that 21 of 360 patients with breast cancer were dihydropyrimidine dehydrogenase deficient by assay of peripheral blood mononuclear cells, arguing in favor of individualization of 5-fluorouracil dose. Similarly, 19 of 53 patients undergoing chemotherapy in different French institutions manifested significant dihydropyrimidine dehydrogenase deficiency.[60b] As expected, toxicity (mainly neurotoxicity) of 5-fluorouracil directly correlated with residual dihydropyrimidine dehydrogenase activity. Partial dihydropyrimidine dehydrogenase deficiency can also lead to severe 5-fluorouracil toxicity in patients with cancer.[60c] The development of new fluoropyrimidine drugs to inhibit dihydropyrimidine dehydrogenase may overcome some of the difficulties associated with dihydropyrimidine dehydrogenase variation (both diurnal and hereditary).[60d] Katonia and coworkers have recommended determination of dihydropyrimidine dihydrogenase activity in patients, prior to implementation of 5-fluorouracil-based chemotherapy, based on their studies in patients with colorectal cancer.[60e,60f]

Genetics. Both forms of dihydropyrimidine dehydrogenase deficiency are compatible with autosomal recessive inheritance. Consanguinity is prevalent among affected families,[14,17,21,42] implying either locus heterogeneity, rarity of mutant alleles, or both. The cDNA encoding human dihydropyrimidine dehydrogenase was recently cloned.[52] The mature protein is a dimer of weight-identical subunits with M_r = 111 kDa, encoding 1025 amino acids.[31] The human protein is encoded by a single gene mapped to chromosome 1 (1p22-q21), spanning 950 kb and consisting of 23 exons (Genbank accession number U09178).[61,62] All intron-exon boundaries conform to the canonical GT-AG rule.[62] Description of the physical map has facilitated mutation screening of affected probands.

At least eleven disease-associated alleles have thus far been identified in dihydropyrimidine dehydrogenase deficiency in addition to several polymorphisms.[62a–62d]. An RNA-splicing abnormality (GT → AT substitution at a consensus 5′-splicing site) results in deletion of a 165-bp exon from the mature cDNA and a loss of amino acids 581–635 from the primary amino acid sequence. This mutation has been characterized extensively, with high prevalence in patients of Northern European descent.[10,11,26,28,29,47,58,58a–58d] Other defects include a 4-bp deletion (del TCAT, nucleotides 295–298), a single base pair deletion at position 1897 ((Δc 1897); a T → C substitution at bp 85, resulting in substitution of arginine for cysteine at amino acid 29 of the polypeptide sequence; and a T → C substitution at bp 703, resulting in substitution of tryptophan for arginine at position 235 of the amino acid sequence.[10,31] The latter two missense mutations, and others, result in a recombinant dihydropyrimidine dehydrogenase enzyme without measurable enzyme activity.[63,63b] Expression of R886H, R235W, V995F, V335L, and E386X mutations in *Escherichia coli* results in significantly decreased dihydropyrimidine dehydrogenase activities.[63b,63c] A point mutation at codon 974 (aspartic acid to valine) was detected in a patient who experienced severe 5-fluorouracil toxicity.[64] Attempts thus far to correlate genotype with phenotype have been unrewarding.[63]

Limited population screening by ethnic group for the exon-skipping mutation was of interest.[58] This allele was present in the Finnish (2.2 percent of 90 alleles analyzed) and Taiwanese (2.7 percent of 72 alleles) subjects. No mutant alleles were detected in British (60 alleles), Japanese (10 alleles), or African-American (40 alleles) subjects. Identification of 4–5 percent of Finnish and Taiwanese individuals as carriers of the splicing mutation is consistent with previous estimates of 3 percent heterozygosity in the general population. No mutations in codon 974 were detected in 303 individuals (606 alleles) represented by 29 Scottish blood donors with low dihydropyrimidine dehydrogenase activity or in 274 control American donors.[64]

Diagnosis. Defects of pyrimidine metabolism, including dihydropyrimidine dehydrogenase deficiency, dihydropyrimidinase (EC 3.5.2.2.), β-alanine synthase, β-aminoisobutyric aciduria, and hyper-β-alaninuria, can be identified by amino acid determination.[48,65–67] The method involves isolation of pyrimidine metabolites, their conversion to the corresponding amino acids by acid hydrolysis, and determination of amino acid content in the sample at each stage of the method. GC/MS analysis of urinary trimethylsilylated organic acid extracts is also valuable,[10] although HPLC techniques remain the method of choice for accurate quantification.

Duran and coworkers[49] and Simmonds and colleagues[68] summarized clinical findings in which screening for purine and pyrimidine disorders appeared warranted. Renal stones of unknown origin, gouty arthritis, mental retardation with neurologic deficits (autism, cerebral palsy, deafness), immune deficiency of unknown origin, unexplained hemolytic anemia, failure to thrive, susceptibility to recurrent infection, self-mutilation, muscle weakness, hyper- or hypotonicity, microcephaly, dysmorphia, and an inability to walk or talk were all identified as clinical findings suggestive of abnormal purine/pyrimidine metabolism.

Prenatal diagnosis was positive[69] in a fetus in a documented sibship;[19] amniotic fluid at 16 weeks contained excesses of thymine and uracil, and diagnosis was confirmed by enzyme assay.[69]

Animal Model. Certain inbred strains of mice express variants of pyrimidine metabolism; one has rapid degradation, the other slow degradation of uracil.[70] A single pair of alleles (gene symbol Pd for pyrimidine degrading), designated Pda (slow rate) and Pdb (fast rate), was postulated to control together the first three steps of uracil catabolism [reactions (2), (3), and (4) in Fig. 91-2].

β-Alanine Synthase (β-ureidopropionase[E.C. 3.5.1.6]) Deficiency. A single female patient has been described.[70a,70b] Clinical findings included severe developmental delay, dystonic movements, scoliosis, and microcephaly at 11 months of age.

Metabolic Phenotype. Apparently, small increases in dihydrothymine/dihydrouracil were found in urine of the patient; normal activities of dihydropyrimidine dehydrogenase and dihydropyrimidinase suggested a defect in β-alanine synthase [reaction (4), Fig. 91-2; reaction (3), Fig. 91-4], which catalyzes formation of β-alanine and β-aminoisobutyric acid. NMR spectroscopy of the patient's urine revealed increased ureidopropionic and ureidoisobutyric acids.[70c] Following hydrolysis, GC/MS analysis confirmed the presence of both species. Quantitative values were not available.

Enzyme Phenotype. Van Gennip and coworkers developed a novel radiometric assay for β-alanine synthase (BAS) in liver homogenate,[70b] since this enzyme does not appear to be present in peripheral cells. BAS activity was determined following conversion of [^{14}C]-N-carbamyl-β-alanine to $^{14}CO_2$, which was quantified by liquid scintillation spectrophotometry. BAS activity in control liver homogenates (n = 10) was 35–165 nmol/h/mg protein and undetectable in homogenate of liver derived from the patient. Further verification was obtained by monitoring flux of [4-^{14}C]-thymine to dehydrothymine, N-carbamyl-β-aminoisobutyric acid and β-aminoisobutyric acid (Fig. 91-4) employing HPLC with on-line detection of radioactivity. In control liver homogenates, all products were observed; conversely, liver homogenate from the patient accumulated dihydrothymine and N-carbamyl-β-aminoisobutyric, whereas β-aminoisobutyric acid was completely absent.

Genetics. Molecular genetic analysis of the BAS gene revealed two different splice-site mutations in the patient's genomic DNA. Analysis of cDNA revealed 170 and 172 bp deletions, resulting in frameshifts. Compound heterozygosity (parental analyses were not reported) suggests autosomal-recessive inheritance.

Dihydropyrimidinuria (Dihydropyrimidinase [EC 3.5.2.2] Deficiency). Dihydropyrimidinuria is rare, thus far reported in only seven patients.[71–78,78a.] Dihydropyrimidinase (EC 3.5.2.2.) deficiency was documented in three (see below). The index case presented with seizures and subsequent normal development.[71–73] Henderson and coworkers[79] reported a male patient in whom seizures, microcephaly, global developmental delay, and spastic quadriplegia were associated with choreiform movements of the upper limbs and inability to sit unaided. Asymptomatic dihydropyrimidinuria was reported in an 11-month-old female, a 37-year-old male, and an adult Japanese female.[74,75,76b] At 18 months, the female remained asymptomatic.[80] These patients were identified by mass screening (urine from 2237 infants and 1132 adults, all healthy at sampling) for pyrimidine disorders in Japan; incidence of dihydropyrimidinuria in Japan is estimated at 1/10,000[76b].

Dihydropyrimidinuria and liver dihydropyrimidinase deficiency were identified in a Turkish boy who also had congenital microvillus atrophy (McKusick 251850).[76] Intractable diarrhea was accompanied by electrolyte imbalance and disturbed renal tubular function. Cholestasis was noted at 2 weeks of age and rapidly led to liver cirrhosis; septicemia was the cause of death at 7 months.

Two patients of different nationalities manifested a comparable clinical course,[77,78] characterized by a severe neurodegenerative process. These patients showed dysmorphia, intractable seizures with severe developmental delay, increasing microcephaly, and pyramidal/choreic signs. Imaging studies indicated neuronal atrophy, delayed myelination, and cerebral cortical atrophy.

Although few patients with dihydropyrimidinuria have been reported, heterogeneity appears substantial. Neurologic findings are unlikely to be directly related to concentration of dihydropyrimidines in physiological fluids, because asymptomatic cases had concentrations comparable to those of patients with severe neurologic symptomatology. On the other hand, quantitation of pyrimidine metabolites has not been performed routinely in CSF; increased central nervous system metabolite levels could be closely linked to neurologic sequelae. Other factors may be involved in phenotype development, such as environmental influences, modifier genes, or additional gene loci. Conversely, the genotype in Japanese patients may yield a dihydropyrimidinase protein with substantial residual enzyme activity.

Metabolic Phenotype. Urine concentrations of dihydropyrimidine analogues (dihydrouracil and dihydrothymine) were elevated up to 65-fold in both symptomatic and asymptomatic patients; combined uracil/thymine excretion was elevated up to 25-fold.[74,76,78,80] Dihydropyrimidines were up to 50-fold increased in plasma and CSF, with much smaller accumulations of uracil and thymine.[74,76,78] These findings are consistent with a defect at the of dihydropyrimidinase (step 3 in Fig. 91-2 and step 2 in Fig. 91-4).

Loading tests in the index patients indicated a block in uracil and thymine catabolic pathways at the level of dihydropyrimidinase.[72,73] In an asymptomatic adult male, uracil loading (10 mg/kg) resulted in a peak blood dihydrouracil of 192 μmol/liter (control < 25) with a significantly prolonged transit time.[75] Eight hours postload, blood uracil was still elevated 17-fold in comparison to control levels. There were no reported adverse reactions to the load.

Enzyme Phenotype. Enzyme diagnosis requires liver biopsy, because cultured skin fibroblasts and blood leukocytes do not express dihydropyrimidinase activity.[72] Quantitation of enzyme activity is achieved in homogenates by monitoring release of $^{14}CO_2$ from [2-^{14}C] dihydrouracil with concomitant HPLC analysis of pyrimidine intermediates.[77] For two patients, activity was undetectable, while in a third case residual activity approximated 5 percent of control values.[76,78]

Genetics. Inheritance is likely autosomal recessive, based upon three observations: 1) sex distribution between patients (4 male : 3 female); 2) occurrence of the disease in families with clinically unaffected offspring; and 3) the fact that consanguineous matings resulted in the birth of all five symptomatic patients.[78] The last implies locus heterogeneity, rarity of mutant alleles, or both. The relevant human gene has been cloned (rat gene sequence, Genbank accession number D63704).[81] The occurrence of dihydropyrimidinase deficiency and congenital microvillus atrophy in the same patient may represent a contiguous gene syndrome that could assist in chromosomal localization, which has recently been localized to 8q22.[76,76a] Human dihydropyrimidinase spans >80 kb contained in 10 exons.[76] Mutation screening in one symptomatic/five asymptomatic patients with dihydropyrimidinuria revealed one frameshift and five missense mutations. Two related Japanese adults were homozygous for a Q334R substitution; a Caucasian patient presenting with epilepsy, dysmorphic features, and severe developmental delay was homozygous for a W360R substitution. Expression analysis verified that all alleles reduced dihydropyrimidinase activity significantly.[76]

Diagnosis. Gas chromatography-mass spectrometry should identify increased quantities of the relevant dihydropyrimidines,[79] although HPLC methodology is preferable for accurate quantification. [76] ^{1}H-nuclear magnetic resonance has shown great utility in detection of pyrimidine and dihydropyrimidine metabolites in urine and CSF from two patients.[76,78] Two patients with confirmed microvillus atrophy had normal urine concentrations of pyrimidines.[76] Patients with dihydropyrimidinase deficiency would be expected to be at increased risk for adverse response to 5-fluorouracil therapy, as would patients with dihydropyrimidine dehydrogenase deficiency. To assess 5-fluorouracil toxicity, a uracil loading test was performed on parents of two adult Japanese probands.[76b] Urine dihydrouracil in parents were several times higher than the same values in control after loading, indicating heterozygosity in the parents and suggesting that homozygotes might be at risk for 5-fluorouracil toxicity.[76b]

Pathogenesis. The patient described by Putman and colleagues[78] manifested a clinical course consistent with a progressive neurodegenerative disease. Evoked potentials suggested delayed central conduction and maturation, while imaging results were consistent with neuronal degeneration. Because catabolism of uracil is the only known pathway for generation of β-alanine in mammals, it could be argued that decreased production of the inhibitory neurotransmitter in dihydropyrimidinase-deficient patients plays a role in disease pathogenesis.[78] The role of increased dihydropyrimidine levels in the central nervous system in relation to pathogenesis remains unclear. Cerebrospinal fluid concentrations of dihydrouracil and dihydrothymine were highly elevated in two patients. Dihydropyrimidine levels were not evaluated in the CSF from asymptomatic patients, although urine and blood levels were elevated.

Hyper-β-Alaninemia. This disorder is very rare, with only two reported cases.[82,83] It has provided useful insight on renal handling of β-amino acids, and there is doubt it is different from the disorder known as GABA transaminase deficiency (see below).

The original proband,[82] born to nonconsanguineous parents, was diagnosed at 2 months of age; he died in his 5th month with an uncontrolled seizure disorder punctuated by extreme somnolence. Linear growth was normal. There was persistent lethargy from birth. The Moro and sucking reflexes were impaired, and the infant was continuously somnolent and hypotonic between seizures, which appeared at the 7th week of life. All anticonvulsant therapy attempted was ineffective. At autopsy, the brain was edematous, small for age (470 g; normal, 620 (±71 g), the cerebral ventricles were enlarged, and demarcation of white matter was blurred. Beading of myelin sheaths was the only significant abnormality observed by microscopy.

Pyridoxine-responsive hyper-β-alaninemia was reported in a patient presenting with intermittent seizures, lethargy, and Cohen syndrome (MIM 216550). The last is characterized by hypotonia; hyporeflexia; mid-childhood obesity; mental deficit; and facial, oral, ocular, and limb anomalies. In the proband, intermittent episodes of weakness and lethargy occurred at least monthly, frequently associated with changes in diet or physical activity. She had two generalized tonic-clonic seizures during acute illness, with interictal EEG demonstrating slow background and

Table 91-3 Concentrations of β-Alanine, Carnosine, and GABA in Postmortem Tissues of a Patient with Hyper-β-Alaninemia[82]

Tissue	Source*	Wet Weight, μmol/g		
		β-Alanine	Carnosine	GABA
Brain	Patient	0.20	0.39	3.83†
	Control	0	0.2	0.82
Muscle‡	Patient	0.07–0.11	36–45	0.02
	Control	0.01	6.6–6.8	0
Liver	Patient	0.36	0	0.02
	Control	0.16	0	0
Kidney	Patient	1.12	0	0.24
	Control	—	—	0.03–0.45§

* Postmortem control is an age-matched, male patient with Werdnig-Hoffman disease. Tissues from patient and control were obtained 2 and 3 h, respectively, after death.
† Values indicate total (bound and free) GABA in occipital cortex, deproteinized with picric acid. The patient's value is high for his age compared with control and published data on infants and children.[308] The wide range of published control values[308–310] reflects techniques of tissue preparation and an age effect, since GABA content of human brain increases during infancy.[308]
‡ Deltoid and rectus abdominis.
§ Values obtained from Whelan et al.[311] and Zachmann et al.[312]

paroxysmal activity in the frontoparietal areas. During a 2-year period of clinical observation, there were no further episodes of seizures or somnolence while she received oral pyridoxine (100 mg/d). No toxic or side effects of pyroxidine were reported.

Metabolic Phenotype. β-alanine levels in the index patient[82] were 20 to 51 μM in plasma, 45 μM in CSF, and up to 100 times normal in urine. The normal concentrations of β-alanine are < 14 μM in plasma, < 0.06 μM in CSF, and < 10 μmol/g of total nitrogen in urine.[84,85] In the patient with Cohen syndrome, plasma β-alanine reached a maximum of 51 μM during a 12-h fast, with elevated urine β-alanine of 28 μmol/24 hours. Fifteen hours after fasting, urine β-alanine rose to 44 mmol/mol creatinine (normal < 1). Under nonprovocative conditions, β-alanine was not detected in CSF or plasma.[83]

Free GABA was also elevated in the index patient's plasma (1 to 7 μM; normal, < 0.5 (μM), urine (25 to 400 (mol/g total nitrogen; normal, 0), and CSF (1 to 2 μM; normal, < 0.12 (μM). Tissues examined 2 h after death had increased levels of β-alanine, GABA, and carnosine (Table 91-3). During life, the urine contained greatly elevated amounts of taurine, β-AiB (isomer not identified), and GABA; carnosine levels in plasma, urine, and CSF were not known to be elevated in life. In the patient with Cohen syndrome, GABA was increased in urine after fasting (8 mmol/mol creatinine; normal, undetected); trace amounts of GABA were detected in CSF under baseline conditions. No mention was made of taurine, β-AiB, or carnosine levels in physiological fluids of the second proband. Free and total plasma L-carnitine were low in this patient.[83] Experimental hyper-β-alaninuria was induced in rats by injection with 2-aminooxyacetic acid, a potent transminase inhibitor.[83a] The data suggested involvement of β-alanine aminotransferase in hyper-β-alaninemia (Table 91-2).

Mechanism of Hyperaminoaciduria in Hyper-β-Alaninemia. Urine and plasma concentrations of β-alanine were directly proportional in the index proband (Fig. 91-3A). Urine β-AiB and plasma β-alanine were also directly proportional (Fig. 91-3B), without a corresponding increase in plasma β-AiB. Urine taurine was influenced by its own plasma concentration but was also directly proportional to the filtered load of β-alanine (Fig. 91-3C). The findings imply combined prerenal and renal mechanisms for the selective hyperaminoaciduria:[86] overflow for the β-alanine component and competition among shared substrates on a β-amino-acid-preferring renal transport system.[87–89] Various studies since have identified a renal membrane carrier with preference for β-amino acids (including taurine) located in the renal brush-border membrane of the proximal tubule.[90–92]

The cause of excessive GABA excretion in urine is of special interest in these patients. GABA reabsorption in the proximal nephron is accommodated by a low-capacity, GABA-preferring carrier in the brush-border membrane that tolerates inhibition by β-alanine.[92,93] Reabsorption of filtered GABA on this carrier could have been inhibited by β-alanine in these patients; the same carrier also would have undergone some saturation at the elevated filtered load of GABA. However, GABA excretion in the probands was not proportional to β-alanine excretion,[82,83] implying that the source of urinary GABA was not in filtrate alone. Backflux from an expanded pool in epithelial cells might have been an additional source, since it is now known that GABA is synthesized in kidney (see below). The anomaly of GABA excretion in these patients may be consistent with the (putative) variant enzyme phenotype.

Enzyme Phenotype. Impaired transamination of β-alanine is a reasonable explanation for the associated metabolic phenotype. In

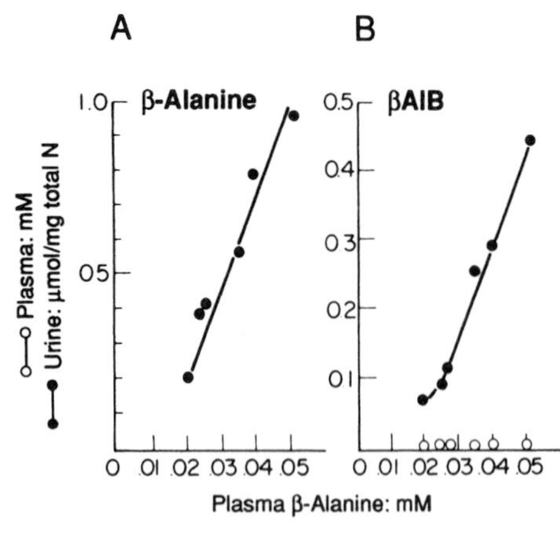

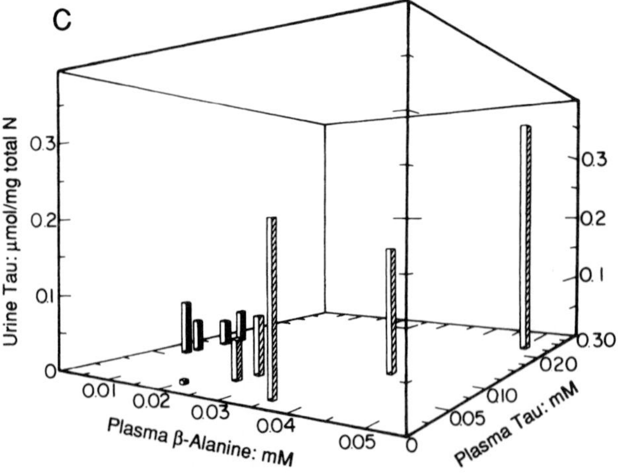

Fig. 91-3 Excretion of β-amino compounds (A, β-alanine; B, β-aminoisobutyric acid [β-AiB]; C, taurine) in relation to plasma concentration of β-alanine in the index patient with hyper-β-alaninemia. The direct relationship indicates that hyper-β-aminoaciduria reflects interaction at a tubular transport site selective for these compounds. This specific aminoaciduria is of the "combined" type, representing overflow (β-alanine) and renal (β-AiB and taurine) mechanisms, the latter by virtue of competitive inhibition by β-alanine. (*Reproduced from Scriver et al.,*[82] *with permission.*)

the absence of excess malonic semialdehyde in urine,[82] the block would be expected at the transamination step [reactions (5) and (6) in Fig. 91-2]. Two features fit this hypothesis: 1) pyridoxine treatment apparently improved the chemical phenotype *in vivo* in the index proband[82] and ameliorated the clinical phenotype in the patient with Cohen syndrome,[83] and pyridoxal-5-phosphate is the coenzyme for aminotransferases; and 2) β-alanine, GABA, and S-β-AiB all transaminate with α-ketoglutarate on particular transaminases (see Table 91-2) present in liver and brain.[94–97]

The particular transaminase involved (EC 2.6.1.18, 2.6.1.19, or 2.6.1.22) could perhaps be identified indirectly by identifying the predominant β-AiB isomer excreted in the index proband with hyper-β-alaninemia. Because GABA accumulation was a feature in both probands, it is unlikely that the specific β-alanine pyruvate aminotransferase (EC 2.6.1.18) is deficient. Moreover, β-alanine may inhibit the GABA α-ketoglutarate transaminase (EC 2.6.1.19) secondarily.

Consistent with the above observations, fibroblasts from the proband with Cohen syndrome demonstrated β-alanyl-α-ketoglutarate transaminase (AKT; EC 2.6.1.19 or 2.6.1.22) activity that was decreased to 70 percent of control values for assays supplemented with 0.02 mM pyridoxine.[83] This activity increased more than twofold when assays were supplemented with 0.1 mM pyridoxine. In addition, the cytotoxic effect of β-alanine on the growth characteristics of cultured fibroblasts was assessed. For patient cells, 25–50 mM β-alanine yielded a 50-percent reduction in cell survival; comparable reduction in cell survival for control cells was achieved at >100 mM β-alanine. β-Alanine toxicity was abolished when skin fibroblasts from the patient were supplemented with 0.1 mM pyridoxine.

There remain the problems of distinguishing between GABA transaminase deficiency (MIM 137150) and hyper-β-alaninemia (MIM 237400) and determining whether they involve different enzymes or the same affected enzyme with different disease phenotypes. This index proband with hyper-β-alaninemia had impaired somatic growth from birth; GABA-transaminase-deficient patients had accelerated growth. Paradoxically, all of these patients had a seizure disorder.

Pathogenesis. In the index patient, complex hyperaminoaciduria was explained by renal overflow and reabsorption mechanisms; neurologic findings were explained by the agonist effect of β-alanine on GABA receptors. The characteristics of hypotonia, hyporeflexia, somnolence, and lethargy in the probands were associated with elevated levels of known (or probable) inhibitory neurotransmitters (β-alanine, GABA, and carnosine) in body fluids and tissues. An additional explanation for seizures and encephalopathy in hyper-β-alaninemia may reside in the agonist effect of β-alanine on the glycine and N-methyl-D-aspartate receptors.[82,83]

The metabolic profile of the two probands was clearly different, perhaps suggesting different primary lesions or variant phenotypes of the same abnormality. A concern in the patient with Cohen syndrome was the absence of metabolites without provocative fasting, perhaps suggesting mobilization and breakdown of endogenous carnosine. Moreover, the reduction in AKT activity in fibroblasts was only partial, perhaps the result of other transaminases' consuming assay substrates. On the other hand, the patient's clinical response to pyridoxine administration, and that of her fibroblasts *in vitro*, argued in favor of an alteration in one or more transaminase activities acting on β-alanine. The benign clinical course in the second proband may have been a function of her low metabolite excretion, high residual enzyme activity, and favorable response to pyridoxine.

Diagnosis and Treatment. The combination of hyper-β-alaninemia with related hyperaminoaciduria (β-AiB, taurine, carnosine, and/or GABA) is suggestive but not diagnostic of the disorder. Plasma levels of β-alanine and GABA are similar in hyper-β-alaninemia and GABA-transaminase deficiency, but β-alanine levels in CSF were a hundredfold higher in the index proband with hyper-β-alaninemia than in the patient with GABA-transaminase deficiency (Table 91-4).

Table 91-4 Metabolite Concentrations (μM) in Disorders of β-Alanine and GABA Metabolism

	Hyper-β-alaninemia (Index Proband)	GABA Transaminase Deficiency	Controls
β-Alanine			
Plasma	20–51	23	<14
CSF	45	0.48	<0.06
GABA			
Plasma	1–7	2.9	<0.50
CSF	1–2	4.8	<0.12

SOURCE: Data taken from Scriver et al.[82] (for hyper-β-alaninemia) and Gibson et al.,[129] Jaeken et al.,[130] and Jaeken[184] (for GABA transaminase deficiency).

Hyper-β-alaninemia with hyper-β-aminoaciduria occurs in the presence of certain drugs that inhibit the relevant transaminase (e.g., isoniazid, aminooxyacetic acid, and (γ-vinyl GABA).[98–100] The associated metabolic abnormality resembles that of the congenital disorder. The acquired finding supports the hypothesis that transaminase activity can be deficient in the congenital condition.

Conventional quantitative amino acid analysis will identify hyper-β-alaninuria.[82] Amino acid screening methods should recognize the urine phenotype if it is expressed in the early newborn period. No newborn urine screening program has yet reported a case of hyper-β-alaninuria. Pharmacologic doses of pyridoxine improved the metabolic phenotype in the index proband and ameliorated the clinical phenotype in the second patient.

Malonate/Methylmalonate Semialdehyde Dehydrogenase Deficiency (Putative). Deficient activities of malonate and methylmalonate semialdehyde dehydrogenases [see reaction (7) in Fig. 91-2, reaction (5) in Fig. 91-4, and reaction (8), Fig. 91-5] were implicated in an otherwise healthy male who had excessive urinary excretion of β-alanine, 3-hydroxypropionate, *RS*-β-AiB, 3-hydroxyisobutyrate, and *S*-2-(hydroxymethyl) butyrate.[101,102] *S*-2-(hydroxymethyl) butyrate and 3-hydroxypropionate putatively derive from ethylmalonate and malonate semialdehydes, respectively. In three additional patients, phenotypic heterogeneity ranged from an uneventful clinical course to congenital malformations associated with failure to thrive, hypotonia, and infantile spasms.[103–106] All patients manifested increased urinary excretion of 3-hydroxyisobutyric acid, which is believed to arise from enzymatic reduction of accumulated methylmalonate semialdehyde.[106a]

Enzyme Phenotype. In one patient, β-alanine and β-aminoisobutyric acid were persistently elevated in urine and plasma.[104] The putative defect resides in the catabolic pathway of β-alanine, β-AiB, and L-valine (and perhaps β-alloisoleucine, which eventually produces ethylmalonate semialdehyde).[105] Direct enzymatic verification of the enzyme defect is hampered by the extreme instability of the relevant semialdehyde substrates. The defect has been inferred from substantially reduced intact cell oxidation of β-alanine and L-valine.[102,105] The differences in metabolite patterns and clinical course distinguish "putative" combined semialdehyde dehydrogenase deficiency from hyper-β-alaninemia.

Genetics. There has been confusion based on metabolic phenotypes and their correlation with (putative) methylmalonate semialdehyde dehydrogenase (MMSDH) deficiency. The proband of Pollitt and coworkers[102,104] had a complex metabolite profile described above, the proband described by Gibson *et al.*[105] manifested 3-hydroxyisobutyric and lactic acidurias, and a

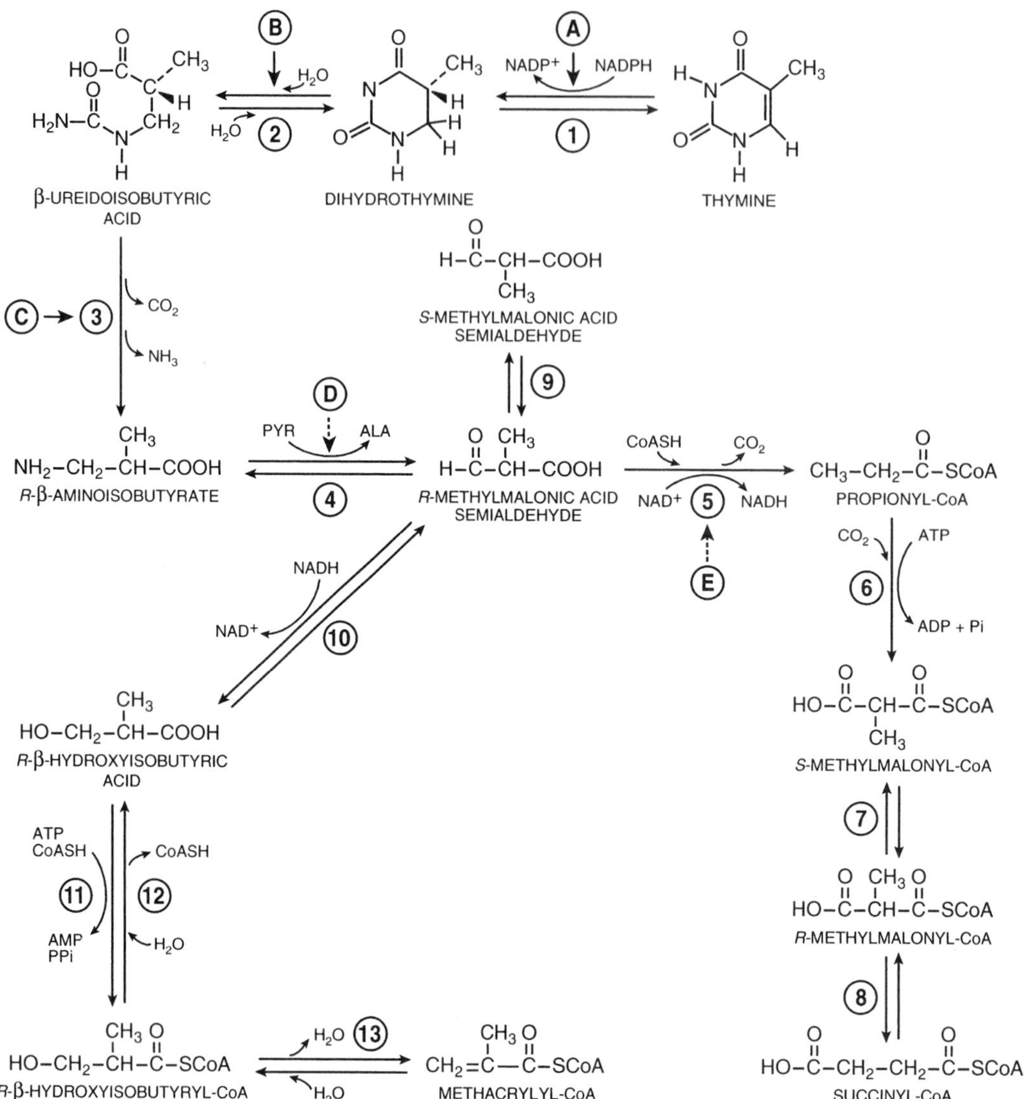

Fig. 91-4 Formation and metabolism of R-β-aminoisobutyrate (R-β-AiB). The circled numbers indicate enzymes or metabolic processes: 1 = dihydropyrimidine dehydrogenase; 2 = dihydropyrimidinase; 3 = β-alanine synthase; 4 = β-aminoisobutyrate-pyruvate transaminase; 5 = methylmalonate semialdehyde dehydrogenase (acetylating) (?); 6 = propionyl-CoA carboxylase; 7 = methylmalonyl-CoA racemase; 8 = methylmalonyl-CoA mutase; 9 = nonenzymatic; 10 = 3-hydroxyisobutyrate dehydrogenase; 11 = an acyl-CoA synthetase (?); 12 = 3-hydroxyisobutyryl-CoA hydrolase; 13 = nonenzymatic for R-isomers (?). The circled letters indicate confirmed (solid arrow) and putative (interrupted arrows) enzyme deficiencies: A = dihydropyrimidine dehydrogenase deficiency; B = dihydropyrimidinase deficiency; C = β-alanine synthase deficiency; D = hyper-β-AiBuria; E = a shared disorder of β-alanine and β-AiB catabolism.[101,102] *(Pathway diagram reproduced from Griffith,[2] with permission.)*

proband described by Roe *et al.*[105a]manifested mild methylmalonic aciduria and developmental delay. Based on significantly decreased oxidation of radiolabeled L-valine and β-alanine, MMSDH deficiency was suggested in two of three probands.[101,102,105] Similar oxidation studies were normal in fibroblasts derived from the proband described by Roe and coworkers,[105a] for whom the diagnosis of MMSDH deficiency was based on *in vivo* oxidation of [$^2H_8$]-valine and [$^2H_4$]-thymine.

To clarify these conflicting reports, Chambliss and coworkers[105b,105c] completed cDNA and genomic cloning of human MMSDH and undertook mutation analysis in peripheral cells obtained from the above probands. Human MSSDH is divided into 12 exons spanning at least 23 kb, and maps to chromosome 14q24.3. Genomic and cDNA PCR analysis revealed that the patient described earlier by Pollitt and coworkers[101,102] was homozygous for a single nucleotide change, G1336A leading to a G446R substitution. This glycine is absolutely conserved from human to bacteria; the patient's mother was heterozygous for this substitution (no specimens could be obtained from the patient's father). Ding *et al.*[105d] reported a complex insertion/deletion mutation in the MSSDH gene derived from fibroblasts of the proband reported earlier by Roe and coworkers.[105a] These analyses were not confirmed by work by Chambliss *et al.*,[105b,105c] in which no abnormality of the MSSDH-coding region was detected in fibroblasts derived from this patient[105a,105d] nor in the patient described earlier by Gibson *et al.*[105] These results suggest that the complex metabolite profile detected in the proband of Pollitt and coworkers,[101,102] and later identified in another patient,[103] reflects MMSDH deficiency.

β-AMINOISOBUTYRIC ACID (β-AIB)

Normal Metabolism

The classic discussion by Sutton[107] and a general review[2] cover relevant source literature. β-AiB, a nonprotein amino acid, has a

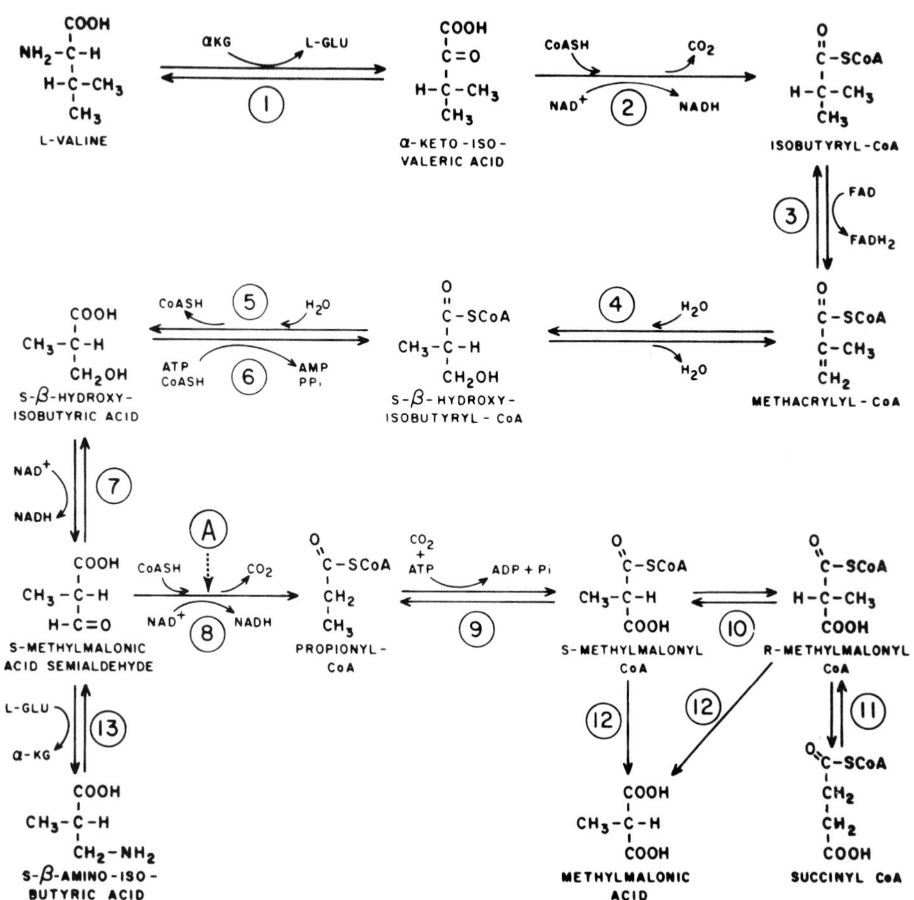

Fig. 91-5 Relationship between L-valine catabolism and S-β-amino-isobutyrate (S-β-AiB) metabolism. The circled numbers indicate the following enzymes: 1 = branched-chain amino acid transaminase(s); 2 = branched-chain α-keto acid dehydrogenase; 3 = isobutyryl-CoA dehydrogenase; 4 = enoyl-CoA hydratase; 5 = 3-hydroxyisobutyryl-CoA hydrolase; 6 = an acyl-CoA synthetase (?); 7 = 3-hydroxyisobutyrate dehydrogenase; 8 = methylmalonate semialdehyde dehydrogenase (acylating); 9 = propionyl-CoA carboxylase; 10 = methylmalonyl-CoA racemase; 11 = methylmalonyl-CoA mutase; 12 = thioester hydrolase (?); 13 = S-β-aminoisobutyrate-α-ketoglutarate transaminase. Disorders of valine oxidation (A)[101,102,104,105] *may affect reaction 13. step. (Pathway diagram reproduced from Griffith,[2] with permission.)*

stable chiral structure at the α-carbon. The *R*-isomer [old name, D-(−)-β-AiB] derives from thymine (Fig. 91-4); the *S*-isomer [L-(+)-β-AiB] from L-valine (Fig. 91-5). Early clinical studies[107] placed little emphasis on the chiral form; chromatographic resolution of enantiomers shows that human urine contains *R*-β-AiB almost exclusively, whereas the plasma isomer is mostly *S*-β-AiB.[108]

The first, second, and third steps of thymine catabolism leading to *R*-β-AiB formation (Fig. 91-4) correspond to the second, third, and fourth steps of cytosine/uracil catabolism yielding β-alanine (Fig. 91-2). Accordingly, the balance between salvage and catabolism of pyrimidines will influence *R*-β-AiB pool size. β-Ureidoisobutyric acid and its precursors must be transported to the liver to form R-β-AiB because β-ureidopropionase is active only in the liver. Catabolism of R-β-AiB is glycogenic [reactions (4) to (8), Fig. 91-4]. The relevant transamination reaction (step 4) has pyruvate as acceptor (EC 2.6.1.40). Methylmalonate semialdehyde dehydrogenase (step 5) may act only on the *S*-isomer. Racemization of the *R* to the *S* form of the substrate can occur either by a nonenzymatic reaction [reaction (9), Fig. 91-4] or by a reversible pathway and through the nonchiral intermediate methacrylyl-CoA.

L-Valine is a distant precursor of *S*-β-AiB (see Fig. 91-5). A transamination reaction which uses α-ketoglutarate as acceptor (step 13) is involved in the formation of the β-AiB isomer; the transaminase (EC 2.6.1.22) accepts GABA and β-alanine.

Disorders of β-Aminoisobutyric Acid Metabolism

Dihydropyrimidine Dehydrogenase, Dihydropyrimidinase, and β-Alanine Synthase Deficiencies. Endogenous synthesis of *R*-β-AiB is supposedly impaired in the face of dihydropyrimidine dehydrogenase and dihydropyrimidinase, and β-alanine synthase deficiencies.[13,15,36,67,70a,70b,71,72] What bearing any abnormality of β-AiB synthesis might have on pathogenesis of the associated clinical phenotype is unknown.

Hyper-β-AiBuria. Crumpler et al.[109] identified elevated urine β-AiB in about 1 in 20 healthy Caucasians, and by family studies Harris showed the trait was recessive.[110] *R*-β-AiB is the isomer excreted in excess,[111] and the associated impairment of β-AiB catabolism affects only *R*-β-AiB.112 A particular pyruvate-requiring transaminase (see Table 91-2) (EC 2.6.1.40) is affected.[113–115] Genetic high excretors have less than 10 percent of normal transaminase activity.[115] The enzyme data, obtained from liver samples at autopsy, are compatible with studies *in vivo*.[116,117] High excretors have impaired ability to degrade exogenous loads of R-β-AiB or thymine;[116] loading with *R*-β-AiB increases its excretion in both high excretors[116] and low excretors;[117] loading with L-valine does not increase β-AiB excretion in the high-excretor phenotype.[116] The responses to loads of thymine and *R*-β-AiB imply that the transamination step is rate-limiting in both normal subjects and genetic high excretors; in the low-excretor phenotypes, urinary β-AiB is related inversely to enzyme activity.[115] High β-AiB excretors have normal β-alanine and GABA homeostasis.

Plasma β-AiB is slightly elevated in the high-excretor phenotype.[118] The renal tubule handles the two isomers of β-AiB by different mechanisms.[112] *S*-β-AiB is filtered at the normal low plasma load (< 3 μM)[118] and then absorbed, albeit inefficiently. *R*-β-AiB is both filtered by the glomerulus and "secreted" by tubule cells.[112] Accordingly, renal clearance of β-AiB can exceed the glomerular filtration rate in high excretors. Assuming the transaminase for the *R*-isomer is present in tubule cells, there would be a contiguous cellular source for urinary *R*-β-AiB, in addition to the augmented filtered load, in the hyperexcreting individual.

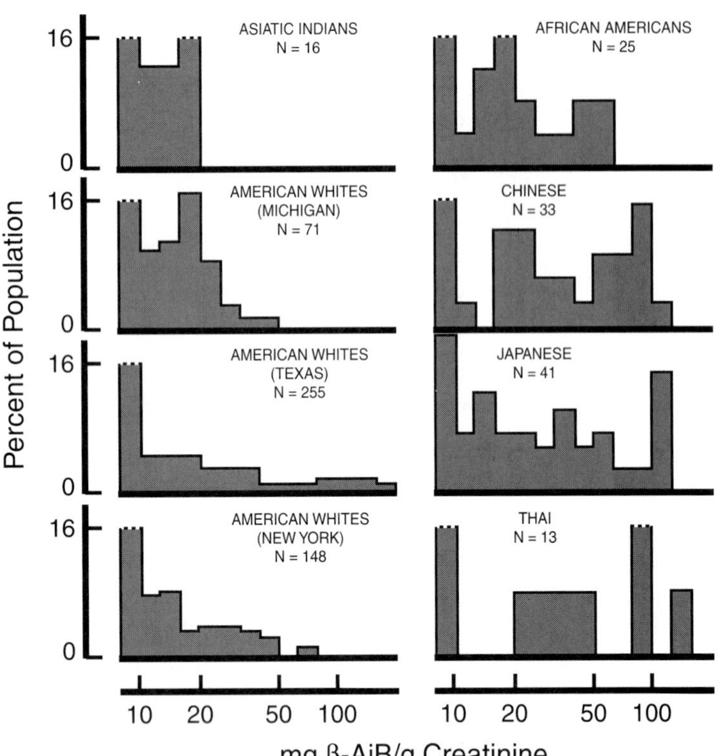

Fig. 91-6 Frequency distributions of urine β-AiB excretion in human populations. Phenotype values in "nonexcretors" are below 20 mg/g creatinine. (*Reproduced, slightly modified, from Sutton,[107] with permission.*)

Genetics of Hyper-β-AiBuria. A clear definition of the hyperexcretor phenotype is elusive, yet classification of the phenotype and interpretation of its inheritance depends on finding a hyperexcretor. An early definition for the high-excretor trait stated that the β-AiB spot should have greater intensity than the β-alanine spot on a two-dimensional paper chromatogram of urine amino acids;[110] this amount is equivalent to >70 mg/g creatinine. Column chromatography discriminates normal excretors from hyperexcretors at 20 to 50 mg/g creatinine; 20 mg/g creatinine is widely used now as the threshold value.

Both Mendelian and acquired factors influence β-AiB excretion, among them age (higher excretion in children) and gender (higher in females).[108,119] Nongenetic factors that increase catabolism may explain why putative heterozygotes could have an "incompletely" recessive phenotype.[115,119,120] Whether allelic heterogeneity (none as yet identified) along with polygenic and multifactorial components explains the interindividual variance in this quantitative trait is not yet known.

The metabolic trait has been treated as a genetic polymorphism[96,120–122] at a single locus with nonrandom distribution in human populations[93,122] (Fig. 91-6); the highest frequencies of the trait are found in Micronesians, the lowest in Caucasians. Simpson and Norton[121] used the "admirably detailed data on excretion" of β-AiB for complex segregation analysis. Their intention was to isolate the codominant, single-locus, polymorphic system from other factors contributing to the quantitative trait. They concluded that the high-excretor phenotype, when segregating in families in a high-excretor population (Japanese), was determined by an incompletely recessive gene plus other familial factors with the following parameters: gene frequency, 0.6; dominance, 0.2; polygenic heritability, 0.1. Events that contribute to the quantitative trait, such as catabolism, confound attempts to compare individuals, to do linkage studies, and to identify disease associations.[121]

Diagnosis. Urine of high excretors contains the *R*-isomer of β-AiB predominantly. However, not every high excretor has the genetic form.[107] β-AiB excretion is increased by catabolism, in neoplastic states,[123] in Down syndrome, and when somatic growth increases the turnover of pyrimidines. In these circumstances, the *R*-isomer is excreted primarily.[109] β-AiB excretion can be used to monitor clinical progress and response to treatment of certain neoplasms.[2]

Elevated β-AiB excretion has been detected in Asian and Amerindian populations,[124] in selected populations deriving from the town of Asbest, Russia,[125] in certain Lithuanian children suffering CMV infection and atherosclerosis,[126] in an adult Japanese male with megaloblastic anemia,[127] and in certain Japanese workers experiencing long-term exposure to heavy metals in the workplace.[128] Whether these cases represent genetic forms or sporadic instances of secondary β-AiB elevation remains to be determined.

β-AiB excretion is also increased in disorders of L-valine catabolism with differing clinical phenotypes. In one the clinical course is mild[101–103]; the other manifests as brain dysgenesis.[104] In both, there is an apparent deficiency of methylmalonate semialdehyde dehydrogenase (step 8, Fig. 91-5). Although it has not been ascertained as such, *S*-β-AiB should be the isomer excreted in this disorder.

γ-AMINOBUTYRIC ACID (GABA)

GABA functions both as a metabolic intermediate in neural and extraneural tissues[3] and as a neurotransmitter in neural tissue. Discussion here is limited to the metabolic pathway (Fig. 91-7). Its role as neurotransmitter is discussed in Chap. 90. There are four inborn errors of GABA-related metabolism[129,130]—three confirmed and one putative (pyridoxine dependency with seizures). Hyper-β-alaninemia constitutes a fifth disorder, either primary or secondary. The conditions discussed in this section are pyridoxine dependency with seizures (MIM 266100), GABA transaminase deficiency (MIM 137150), and succinic semialdehyde dehydrogenase deficiency or 4-hydroxybutyric aciduria (MIM 271980). Homocarnosinosis (MIM 236130) also impairs the metabolism of GABA, but in its dipeptide form (homocarnosine); it is described later.

The traits affecting metabolism of free GABA are each associated with cerebral dysfunction. GABA concentrations in

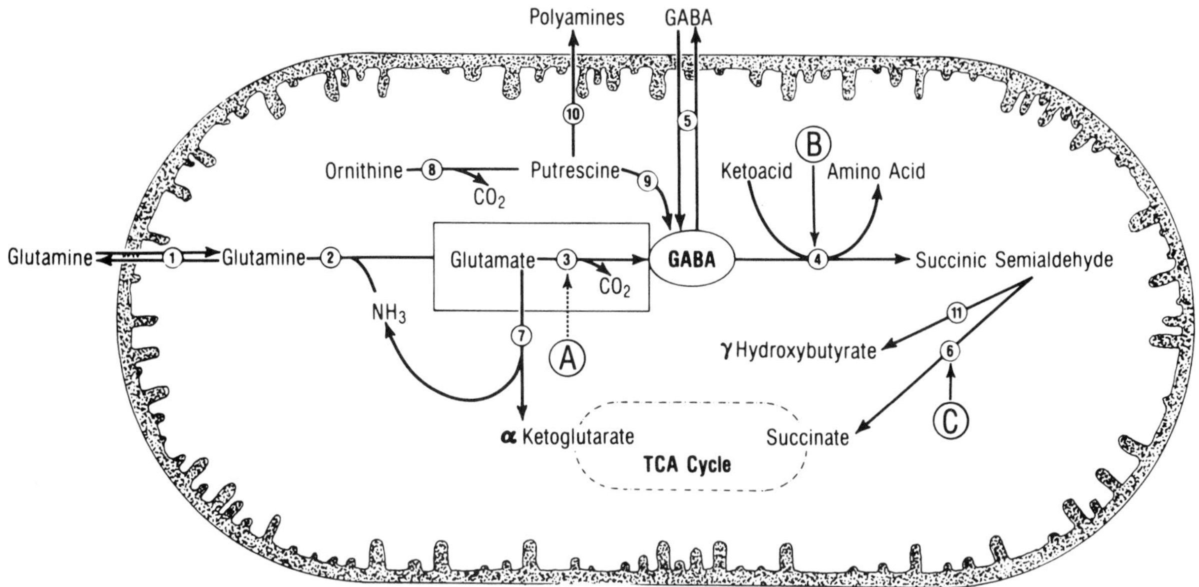

Fig. 91-7 Metabolism of γ-aminobutyric acid (GABA). Circled numbers indicate enzymes or metabolic processes: 1 = glutamine transport across the inner mitochondrial membrane; 2 = phosphate-dependent glutaminase and ammonia formation; 3 = glutamate decarboxylase and GABA formation (this step is intramitochondrial in kidney and extramitochondrial in brain); 4 = GABA transaminase regenerates glutamate in brain by utilizing α-ketoglutarate as cosubstrate (in kidney, pyruvate may be utilized as well, with net disposal of glutamate by the GABA pathway); 5 = GABA transport (incompletely characterized); 6 = succinic semialdehyde dehydrogenase and succinate formation (commits the carbon chain to oxidative metabolism via the tricarboxylic acid cycle); 7 = glutamate dehydrogenase (major pathway of glutamate disposal during renal ammoniagenesis); 8 = ornithine decarboxylase and putrescine formation; 9 = GABA formation from putrescine (details of the pathway are not fully studied); 10 = polyamine formation from putrescine; 11 = γ-hydroxybutyrate formation (biochemical details and metabolic role not fully studied). Circled letters indicate confirmed (solid arrows) or putative (interrupted arrow) deficiency of enzyme activity: A = putative pyridoxine dependency with seizures; B = GABA-transaminase (α-ketoglutarate-requiring) deficiency; C = succinic semialdehyde dehydrogenase deficiency (4-hydroxybutyric aciduria). (*Reproduced from Rozen et al.,[3] by permission.*)

brain are partially reflected in CSF.[130] GABA concentrations in normal CSF (Table 91-5) serve as a reference point here. Levels are low in pyridoxine dependency (putative glutamic acid decarboxylase deficiency), elevated in GABA transaminase deficiency, and perhaps raised in succinic semialdehyde dehydrogenase deficiency.[130] Significant differences between neural and nonneural tissues in the initial step of the GABA pathway, involving its synthesis by glutamic acid decarboxylase, are relevant for the understanding of pyridoxine dependency.

Normal Metabolism. GABA is found predominantly in brain (Table 91-6), where up to one third of synapses probably employ it as an inhibitory neurotransmitter. GABA is found also in extraneural tissues, notably kidney and pancreas islet β-cells (see Tables 91-6 and 91-7). Extraneural GABA is dependent on synthesis in situ, not on interorgan transport.

GABA is made from ornithine, putrescine (derived from spermine and spermidine), and L-glutamate in mammalian tissues (see Fig. 91-7). The latter is the more important source, and the pathway is initiated by glutamate decarboxylation. Native human brain glutamic acid decarboxylase (GAD, EC 4.1.1.15), requires pyridoxal-5-phosphate as coenzyme; the apoenzyme has multiple molecular forms in brain.[131] Distributions of GAD and GABA are similar in brain, and they are found in gray matter predominantly. The presence and characteristics of GAD have been investigated in numerous nonneural tissues, including liver, kidney, pancreas, testis, ova, adrenal, sympathetic ganglia, gastrointestinal tract, and circulating erythrocytes.[132] In some tissues, one form of GAD predominates. GABA-transaminase, the first of two GABA catabolic enzymes, has been localized in most of the same tissues via histochemical and/or immunochemical methods. Identification of these enzymes argues in favor of a metabolic role for GABA in these nonneural tissues.

GABA acts on neurons by modifying the transmembrane potential difference. It binds to two classes of synaptic receptors. The $GABA_A$ receptor, the more important species, is blocked by

Table 91-5 GABA Concentration in Human Cerebrospinal Fluid

Form of GABA	Mean	Range, μM (n = 20)
Total	9.2	5.3–10.1
Free	0.07*	0.04–0.14 (10th–90th centile)
Homocarnosine	7.6	4.0–8.7
Unidentified	0.5	0–2

*Mean values for free GABA rise about fourfold, to levels shown, in the first year of life. Age-related frequency distribution data are available (see Carchon HA et al., *Clin Chim Acta* 201:83–88, 1991).

SOURCE: Adapted from Jaeken.[184]

Table 91-6 Distribution of GABA in Mammalian Tissues

	GABA (nmol/g Wet Weight)		
	Human	Rat	Mouse
Brain	1850–5690	1900	2610
Ovary	—	590	—
Pancreas	562	41	4
Kidney	440	180	33
Liver	—	30	15
Heart	—	20	—
Testes	—	0	—
Plasma	0.9	0.8	0.5
Thyroid	—	0	—
Muscle	—	0	—

Table 91-7 Localization of GABA and GABA Metabolic Enzymes in Mammalian Nonneural Tissues

		GAD			
Tissue	GABA	GAD_{65}	GAD_{67}	GABA-T	SSADH
Liver	+	(+)	(+)	+	+
Kidney	+	(+)	(+)	+	+
Heart	+	(+)	(+)	+	+
Spleen	+	(+)	(+)	(?)	+
Ovary	+	(+)	(+)	+	(?)
Oviduct	+	+	+	+	(?)
Uterus	+	(+)	(+)	+	(?)
Testes	+	–	+	+	(?)
Pancreas	+	+	+	+	(?)
Sympathetic ganglia	+	(+)	(+)	+	(?)
Adrenal gland	+	(+)	(+)	+	+
Gastrointestinal tract	+	(+)	(+)	+	+
Blood vessels	+	(+)	(+)	+	(?)
Erythrocytes	(?)	(+)	(+)	(?)	(?)
Platelets	(?)	(+)	(+)	+	+
Lymphocytes	(?)	(?)	(?)	+	+
Fibroblasts	(?)	(?)	(?)	(?)	+
Amniocytes	(?)	(?)	(?)	+	+
Chorion tissue	(?)	(?)	(?)	+	+

+, present; (+), present, but predominant molecular form, if any, not determined; –, not present; (?), not determined.

SOURCE: Tillakaratne et al.[132]

the antagonist bicuculline and possesses high-affinity, sodium-independent binding of GABA; the receptor modulates chloride ion permeability in synaptic membranes.[133] The $GABA_B$ receptor species is less abundant, is bicuculline-insensitive, and appears to regulate potassium channel activity.[134]

GABA disposal is a postsynaptic event in brain. Catabolism is initiated after removal of GABA from the synaptic cleft by uptake on a high-affinity system. A transport system with lower affinity has also been identified in glial cells. GABA also supports oxidative metabolism by its conversion to succinate in brain and extraneural tissues (see Fig. 91-7). Two mitochondrial matrix enzymes are required: an α-ketoglutarate-requiring GABA-transaminase (EC 2.6.1.19) and succinic semialdehyde dehydrogenase (EC 1.2.1.24).

Extraneural Metabolism of GABA

GABA metabolism in extraneural tissues is relevant to the interpretation of pyridoxine dependency and hyper-β-alaninemia. For example, GABA synthesis in human kidney is about 30 percent as active by tissue weight as it is in brain. The properties of renal GAD and GABA transaminase differ from those of the corresponding brain enzymes.[3] Accordingly, it is likely that different genes control GABA metabolism in brain and in kidney.

A GAD gene was mapped to human chromosome 2q and mouse chromosome 2; this gene is presumed to be GAD1,[135] the putative "neurotransmitter" species of decarboxylase. Expressed nucleotide sequences for human brain and pancreatic GAD are significantly different.[136] Rat brain is a source of two polypeptides with glutamic acid decarboxylase activity (GAD_{65}, GAD_{67}), two mRNAs, and two cDNAs.[136] Two cDNAs were also obtained from human brain;[137] rat and human cDNAs are very similar (91 percent) in their coding regions.[137] The human GAD_{65} (Genbank accession number M81882) encodes a polypeptide of 585 amino acids (M_r = 65,000); the GAD_{67} (Genbank accession number M81883) cDNA encodes 594 residues (M_r = 67,000). The source of the molecular heterogeneity lies in two different nuclear genes.[137,138] In bacterial expression systems the two genes have GAD activities.[136,137] The smaller GAD_{65} enzyme is undersaturated with coenzyme in the native state and is located in the synaptosome; the larger native GAD_{67} enzyme is saturated with coenzyme and is located in the cell body.[138] GAD_{65} and GAD_{67} are found also in pancreas, for example.[138] The corresponding human genes for GAD_{65} and GAD_{67} have been assigned to chromosomes 10p11.23 and 2q31, respectively.[137]

Renal GABA synthesis is initiated by an enzyme with properties that differ significantly from those of the corresponding enzyme in brain.[3,139] Renal GAD activity and GABA concentration are high in deep cortex and outer medulla (rat kidney); GAD is enriched in isolated rat proximal tubules relative to whole cortex and glomeruli.[139] Accordingly, the renal tubule is equipped with mechanisms to provide cellular GABA independent of the inefficient but specific transport systems for GABA in kidney.[93]

The renal GABA pathway permits net disposal of glutamate because renal GABA transaminase uses pyruvate[140] (might it be the β-alanine-pyruvate transaminase? see Table 91-2), whereas the brain GABA transaminase uses α-ketoglutarate specifically.[3] The renal GABA transaminase is apparently confined to proximal tubule cells of outer medulla.[134] The renal GABA pathway in rat accounts for about one quarter of glutamate disposal,[141] acting as a passive arbiter of this process during ammoniagenesis.[140] Renal GABA content and GAD activity increase in parallel during ontogeny.[142] Together these findings indicate that GAD properties in brain and kidney are probably quite different and that GABA plays different roles in the two tissues. Accordingly, it could be unwise to measure renal GAD activity as a surrogate for brain GAD. Moreover, autoimmune diseases have been tentatively identified that involve GAD of pancreas (insulin-dependent diabetes mellitus) and GAD of brain (stiff-man syndrome), a finding that can be taken as further evidence for the existence of tissue-specific isomeric forms of GAD.[136,137]

Disorders of γ-Aminobutyric Acid Metabolism

Pyridoxine Dependency with Seizures. This autosomal recessive disease (MIM 266100) may be a disorder of GABA synthesis,[143] but the evidence that brain GAD activity is deficient in affected patients remains controversial.

The diagnosis of pyridoxine dependency with seizures is dependent upon the presence of a seizure disorder, refractive to all conventional anticonvulsants, that responds to pharmacologic doses of pyridoxine.[144–146,146a,146b] Less than 100 probands have been reported. Additional clinical features in nine cases included high-pitched shrill cry, jitteriness, nonparalytic squint, hypothermia, abnormal tone, hepatomegaly, abdominal distension, macrocephaly, cortical visual agnosia, limb hypertonia, and neonatal dystonia.[144,147,148] Later in life, some developed delayed speech and severe articulatory dyspraxia. Although one patient had severe global delay, pyridoxine dependency with seizures appeared associated with specific rather than global learning difficulties, especially expressive language.[144] Additional features that may assist in the differential diagnosis include abnormal intrauterine movement, hypotonia, resistance to other anticonvulsants, lethargy (+/− apnea), and a positive family history.[143,144]

Poor developmental progress despite early therapeutic intervention may correlate with persistent EEG abnormalities, the latter possibly related to increased levels of the excitatory neurotransmitter glutamate.[144,148,149] Baumeister and coworkers[149] suggested that the dose of pyridoxine administered be sufficient to: 1) resolve seizures and 2) lower CSF glutamate below a threshold neurotoxic level of 100 μM. These authors postulated that accumulated glutamate hyperexcites the N-methyl-D-aspartate receptor, leading to cell death and ultimately developmental delays.

Continued description of probands reveals additional clinical features of the disorder. A variant late-onset form of the disease exists, with seizures beginning as late as 2 years of age.[144,150–153] The majority of cases, however, are of the early onset form. Intervention with pharmacologic doses of pyridoxine (10–1000 mg/d) ameliorates seizures, and therapy may be lifelong.[144] Hecht[155a] reported serial MRI scans in two patients that revealed progressive dilation of the ventricular system, atrophy of the cortex and subcortical white matter, and an increase in ventricle-to-brain ratio (VBR). These authors suggested that these abnormalities were related to chronic excitotoxicity due to GABA/glutamate cerebral imbalances.

Some patients with seizures resistant to conventional anticonvulsants, who also have low levels of GABA in CSF, are not responsive to pyridoxine.[130] In addition, these patients manifest elevated N-acetyl aspartate levels in CSF and respond to clonazepam (Canavan disease?), which may be confused with the metabolic phenotype of "classical" pyridoxine dependency with seizures.

Imaging Abnormalities. Recent findings suggest pyridoxine dependency with seizures are associated with altered neurologic status. Baxter and coworkers[144] reported on a cohort of six patients. Cerebellar findings included dysplasia and hypoplasia of the right hemisphere in two patients, generalized atrophy of cerebral gray and white matter in three, gliosis in three, intracerebral hemorrhage in three, and neuronal dysplasia in two. Individual patient findings included periventricular hyperintensity with cortical atrophy and nonspecific neuronal degeneration. CT studies in one case revealed hypodensity of the white matter in the frontal/occipital lobes, suggesting myelination abnormalities.[154] Shih and coworkers[155] reported an elegant and thorough analysis of a patient using EEG, evoked potentials, MRI, and positron emission tomography (PET) analysis. In this patient, MRI revealed diffuse atrophy, with probable cortical and axonal dysfunction; evoked potentials indicated bilaterally absent cortical potentials with altered myelin or axonal formation; and PET suggested global cortical hypometabolism with a prominence of bilateral subcortical structures.

There are reports of pyridoxine toxicity, however, in adults and during use in pregnancy.[144a,144b]Shih and coworkers[155] suggested that pyridoxine dependency with seizures was associated with diffuse structure/function abnormalities characterizing a generalized disease process. Pyridoxine therapy in one case resulted in a sensory neuropathy, characterized by absent sensory action potentials in median and ulnar nerves. These findings were consistent with earlier work in animals, in which pyridoxine application resulted in a distal neuropathy.[156]

Metabolic Phenotype. Although pyridoxine metabolism appears normal, the majority of data in patients (and animals) suggests an alteration in glutamate and GABA levels associated with pyridoxine-dependent seizures.[143,157] Brain glutamate content was raised and GABA content decreased in an affected proband.[158] CSF glutamate level was elevated 200-fold in another proband, decreasing to normal only with pyridoxine administration in excess of that required to control seizures.[149] The thalamic glutamate:GABA ratio was increased in pyridoxine-starved rats in comparison to control animals, with a corresponding reduction of seizure threshold in response to picrotoxin or pentylenetetrazole application.[159] Altered glutamate:GABA ratios in various brain regions were similarly increased in epilepsy-prone BALB/c mice.[160] Inclusion of pyridoxine in the diet abolished enhanced sensitivity to chemical convulsants and normalized amino acid ratios in the majority of brain regions. Although these observations in animals are consistent with findings in human probands, suggesting an abnormality in a pyridoxine-dependent enzyme system, they can be considered only suggestive, since the animals required application of a convulsive stimulus for the induction of seizures (in the presence or absence of pyridoxine), whereas probands with pyridoxine dependency and seizures manifest spontaneous convulsive activity.[160]

Enzyme and Molecular Phenotype. The concept that pyridoxine dependency with seizures is the result of altered cofactor binding to GAD apoenzyme remains controversial.[142,143,161] The original study by Yoshida and colleagues[161] investigated GAD activity in kidney homogenate derived from a proband. Because renal and brain GAD enzymes are not identical, the relevance of these findings is in question. Gospe and coworkers[162] evaluated GABA synthesis in fibroblasts from a patient with pyridoxine dependency and seizures. Pyridoxal 5′-phosphate (PLP)-independent GAD activity was similar in control and patient fibroblasts; the patient's PLP-dependent GAD activity was reduced in comparison to that of controls. No further confirmatory enzyme studies have been reported.

Bu and colleagues[163] sequenced all 16 exons encoding GAD_{65} and GAD_{67} in a cohort of 22 patients with classic (seven patients) or atypical (15 patients) forms of pyridoxine-dependent seizures. No defects were identified in coding regions, leading these investigators to conclude that most patients with pyridoxine dependency and seizures do not have mutations in either form of GAD. Conversely, noncoding (regulatory?) regions may carry mutations that were not characterized in this study. Kure *et al.*[163a] studied two families with pyridoxine-dependent seizures using transcribed GAD mRNA ectopically transcribed in immortalized cultured lymphoblasts. All alterations in GAD_{65} and GAD_{67} were found to be common polymorphisms, which suggested an etiologic mechanism other than a K_M mutant for GAD as the cause of pyridoxine-dependent seizures in their patients.

The advent of transgenic murine models has provided new approaches to the study of pyridoxine dependency with seizures. Mice lacking GAD_{67} (so-called GAD_{67}-/- mice) died from cleft palate in the newborn period.[164] GAD activities and GABA contents were reduced to 20 and 7 percent of control values, respectively, in cerebral cortex, without structural defects. Heterozygote mice had intermediate GAD and GABA levels in comparison to control and affected mice. Conversely, GAD_{65}-deficient mice (so-called GAD_{65}-/- mice) had normal brain GABA content with lowered threshold-to-seizure induction by chemical agents (picrotoxin, pentylenetetrazol) and no upregulation of GAD_{67}.[165] These observations provide evidence for an integral role for GAD_{67} in the control of brain GABA content. In an unrelated study, GAD_{65}-/- mice had PLP-inducible apo-GAD reservoirs that were significantly decreased and developed spontaneous seizures resulting in increased mortality.[166,166a–166d] Continued analyses in these murine transgenic models may provide important insight into human pyridoxine dependency with seizures.

Pathogenesis. Data from human and animal studies suggest an alteration in PLP binding to GAD as the underlying metabolic lesion in pyridoxine dependency with seizures, yet confirmatory enzyme studies of GAD activity in probands have not been reported.

Clues to pathogenesis may be gleaned from other "model" systems. For example, seizures induced by theophylline and isoniazid overdose, in addition to magnesium-dependent audiogenic seizures in the mouse, are responsive to pharmacologic doses of pyridoxine.[167–174] Pathogenesis in all of these instances may relate to depressed GABA levels, presumably corrected through interconversion of apo-GAD to holo-GAD via PLP binding. Isoniazid (a compound structurally similar to pyridoxine) overdose leads to formation of isoniazid-pyridoxal hydrazones, resulting in lowered GABA levels through increased production of apo-GAD.[171] In addition to GABA, pyridoxine is involved in metabolism of numerous amine synaptic transmitters, including noradrenaline, adrenaline, tyramine, dopamine, and serotonin.[168] Intracellular transport of PLP is mediated through conversion of PLP to pyridoxal by pyridoxal kinase.[167] Formation of pyridoxal adducts, altered metabolism of other synaptic transmitters, and intracellular transport of PLP may all play a role in the pathogenesis of pyridoxine dependency with seizures.

Variant γ-Aminobutyric Acid Transaminase Phenotypes

γ-Aminobutyric acid, α-ketoglutarate aminotransferase (EC 2.6.1.19) is a dimeric homopolymer[175] for which pyridoxal phosphate is the coenzyme. Specific activity in human tissues is highest in liver; intermediate in brain, kidney, and pancreas; and least in other tissues (heart, testis, spinal cord, intestine). The enzyme transaminates GABA and β-alanine equally well.[175] Several cDNAs have been cloned from mammalian species, although a chromosome assignment in humans has not been reported.[15,176–179] These cDNAs (Genbank accession numbers: rat enzyme U29701, human enzyme U80226) encode signal peptides of 27–28 amino acids, consistent with mitochondrial localization for the mature protein.[178,180] Pyridoxal-5′ phosphate binds to lysine residue 330.[180,181]

GABA transaminase is polymorphic (three alleles), expressed as electromorphic variation without loss of activity;[122,175,182] allele 1 (slow band) is the most prevalent (frequency >0.5) in European and Asian populations.

γ-Aminobutyric Acid Transaminase Deficiency. Deficiency of GABA transaminase is rare. It has been reported[183] in two Flemish sibs (female and male) and an unrelated Hispanic male (WL Nyhan, personal communication). The two siblings presented with accelerated linear growth (99th centile since birth), severe psychomotor retardation, a seizure disorder, hypotonia, and hyperreflexia. Treatment with pyridoxine or picrotoxin had no beneficial effect. Both sibs died, the brother at 1 year of age and the sister at $2\frac{1}{2}$ years.[129] Leukodystrophy was found in the brains at autopsy. The third patient presented with seizures from birth, severe hypotonia, brainstem dysfunction, and a burst-suppression EEG pattern. MRI revealed cerebellar hypoplasia and agenesis of the corpus callosum. Deep tendon reflexes were pathologically brisk with clonus. Growth parameters were normal.

In the siblings, levels of GABA and β-alanine were elevated in CSF and plasma[183] (see Table 91-4). Homocarnosine was increased fourfold in CSF;[129] unidentified GABA conjugates were present also. Urine metabolites,[130,184] notably GABA, β-alanine, and β-AiB, did not resemble the pattern in hyper-β-alaninemia. Elevated fasting plasma growth hormone (8–38 ng/ml; normal, <5 ng/ml) was attributed to the growth hormone-releasing effect of GABA[185] and probably explained the excessive rate of growth in the patients. In the third patient, quantitative metabolite data were lacking, although GABA concentrations in urine, plasma, and CSF were said to be elevated (WL Nyhan, personal communication).

Activity of GABA transaminase in a liver biopsy sample from one affected sib was about 15 percent of normal relative to that in 10 controls;[183] activity in lymphocytes and transformed lymphocytes was about 2 percent of normal.[186] In the third patient, activity in transformed lymphocytes approximated 25 percent of control values (KM Gibson, LK Medina-Kauwe, and WL Nyhan, unpublished results).

Kinetic parameters of GABA transaminase are similar in lymphocytes, platelets, and brain, but the specific activity is much higher in brain.[129] On this basis, it was assumed that brain GABA transaminase activity is deficient in the affected patients. A diagnosis of GABA transaminase deficiency cannot be accomplished in cultured skin fibroblasts, because these cells do not express the enzyme.[187] GABA transaminase is present in chorionic villus tissue.[188] Immunoblot analysis of GABA transaminase protein from tissues or peripheral cells of affected patients has not been reported. These studies may require the use of antibodies raised against only the human protein, as there is evidence indicating that GABA-T in human brain is immunologically distinct from that in other mammalian brains.[189]

The parents of the affected sibs had GABA transaminase levels only 15 percent and 37 percent of normal in their lymphocytes. Whereas these data imply the phenotype is autosomal recessive, the skewed gene dose effect in the heterozygote is compatible with a dominant negative effect on the homodimeric enzyme.[190]

A single causative mutation has been identified in one of two Flemish siblings, a G→A transition at nucleotide 754 of the coding region. This missense mutation results in conversion of arginine to lysine at amino acid 220.[179] The father of the patient carried this allele, while the mother did not, indicating that the patient was a compound heterozygote. Bacterial expression of the mutant cDNA produced an intact recombinant GABA transaminase protein with a 75 percent reduction of enzymatic activity in comparison to control.

Two Different Transaminase-Deficient Phenotypes?

The clinical and metabolic phenotypes of GABA transaminase deficiency and hyper-β-alaninemia β-alanine α-ketoglutarate transaminase) are different. Linear growth is normal or increased in GABA transaminase deficiency and decreased in hyper-β-alaninemia. β-Alanine levels in CSF are a hundredfold higher in hyper-β-alaninemia than in GABA-transaminase deficiency (see Table 91-4). The existence of two diseases implies that the transaminases for GABA and β-alanine are different enzymes, each sharing the alternative substrate and each encoded by a different gene.

Succinic Semialdehyde Dehydrogenase Deficiency (4-Hydroxybutyric Aciduria). Jakobs and coworkers described the index case of γ-hydroxybutyric aciduria in 1981.[191] Since then, more than 150 cases have been identified and more than 60 of them reported.[192–207] Succinic semialdehyde dehydrogenase (SSADH, EC 1.2.1.24) activity is deficient (see Fig. 91-7), impairing the predominant oxidative conversion of succinic semialdehyde (SSA) to succinic acid, in response to which SSA is reduced to 4-hydroxybutyric acid (4-HBA, Fig. 91-7) in a reaction catalyzed by 4-hydroxybutyrate dehydrogenase (EC 1.1.1.61). All patients manifest mild to severe retardation of intellectual, motor, speech, and language development.[194,198,208] Many present with hypotonia and some with nonprogressive truncal and appendicular ataxia.[194] Ataxia, when present, appears to resolve with age.[208] For some patients, associated manifestations include oculomotor apraxia, microcephaly or macrocephaly, hyporeflexia or hyperreflexia, hyperkinesis, somnolence, seizures, and autistic features.[193,194,209–211] Three related patients (including an adult) displayed aggressive behavior.[194] Male and female sibs (who presented with generalized seizures, slowing on the electroencephalogram, and elevated creatine kinase activity) manifested nonspecific myopathy and ragged-red fibers in biopsied muscle.[209,212] Choreoathetosis developed in two unrelated patients in the first year; magnetic resonance imaging in both showed bilateral globus pallidus abnormalities, which resolved in one and progressed in the other.[196–197] Basal ganglia abnormalities were detected in two siblings with undetectable SSADH activity.[213]

In a recent survey of 23 patients, seizures and ataxia were not prominent features, being reported in less than 50 percent of patients. Moreover, the data implied the existence of subcategories of SSADH deficiency, differentiated by the course of early development. Rahbeeni and coworkers described six patients (three families) in Saudi Arabia.[200,201] Severe global delay, hypotonia, and seizures were present in all; three patients had choreoathetosis, two each manifested optical atrophy and myoclonus, and one displayed severe dystonia. In comparison to the cases of the other patients, the clinical course appeared both more severe and more progressive. Phenotypic heterogeneity is substantial, even within sibships.[202,202a]

Metabolic Phenotype. The biochemical hallmark of SSADH deficiency is the accumulation of 4-HBA in physiological fluids without an accompanying metabolic acidosis.[214] Concentrations of 4-HBA are determined by combined GC/MS and, more accurately, by using a stable-isotope dilution assay employing D_6-4-HBA as internal standard.[215] Concentrations of 4-HBA in patients range from twofold to 800-fold normal in urine, fourfold to 200-fold in plasma, and a 100-fold to 1200-fold in CSF in comparison with control ranges.[194,215] Urinary 4-HBA excretion appears to decrease with age in patients but is still elevated relative to that in controls.[194,208,215] This finding was especially evident in an adult patient whose urinary excretion was only twice the upper limit of the control range,[194] reflecting perhaps the changing ratio of brain size to body weight. A similar age-dependent decrease in levels of an accumulated metabolite has been observed in hawkinsinuria,[216] in which disease symptoms occur only in infancy (when metabolite levels are high) and disappear by adulthood.

In addition to 4-HBA, other compounds are detected at elevated levels in affected patients. Urinary metabolites indicative of β-oxidation of excess 4-HBA include 3,4-dihydroxybutyric, 3-oxo-4-hydroxybutyric, and glycolic acids.[191,195,197,198,210,211,217] Increased urinary 2,4-dihydroxybutyric (and its lactone) and 3-hydroxypropionic acid levels indicate metabolism of 4-HBA by α-oxidation.[217] Threo- and erythro-4,5-dihydroxyhexanoic acids (and the corresponding lactones) have been identified in the urine of some patients.[198,217] Brown and coworkers propose that these compounds are condensation products of SSA with a two-carbon intermediate in pyruvate metabolism. Dicarboxylic aciduria in 4-HBA may indicate a secondary inhibition of mitochondrial fatty acid β-oxidation by SSA or its derivatives.[193,217]

Whereas dicarboxylic aciduria and 3-hydroxypropionic aciduria may reflect disorders of fatty acyl-CoA or propionyl-CoA metabolism, the presence of increased 4-HBA assists in the differential diagnosis of SSADH deficiency.

Patients may have excess glycine in urine, plasma, and CSF.[193,196,197,209,211] Although glycolic acid may be metabolized to glycine, a significant increase in the glycine pool arising from the glycolic acid produced by β-oxidation of 4-HBA seems unlikely.[193] The cause of the glycine abnormality in SSADH-deficient patients remains unclear.

Two unrelated patients manifested increased concentrations of homovanillic acid in CSF, suggesting increased dopamine turnover in the nigrostriatal system.[196] The widening scope of metabolic aberrations suggests that SSADH deficiency has deleterious effects on intermediary metabolism of peripheral tissues as well as on the central nervous system.

Recent studies have verified the difficulty of accurately quantifying 4-HBA in urine from affected patients and the variable excretion pattern of the compound.[218–220] In the urine of an affected newborn, the level of 4-HBA was only twice the upper limit of levels in controls.[218] In a sampling for quality assessment of screening laboratories, fully 50 percent of responding laboratories failed to identify 4-HBA in the urine of an affected patient.[219] More recently, our laboratory has investigated five patients in whom the metabolite profile in urine suggested SSADH deficiency associated with only slight (or no) increase in 4-HBA excretion.[220] In two of five patients, SSADH activity was decreased in comparison to that in controls; it was normal in the remaining three. These results indicate that urinary 4-HBA may not be completely pathognomonic for SSADH deficiency and may be only marginally increased in some patients.

Enzyme Phenotype. SSADH activity in peripheral lymphocytes or cultured lymphoblasts, measured by radiometric or spectrofluorometric assay,[192,221] is 10 percent of normal in probands; there is a tendency for intact cells to have higher levels of activity than cell extracts.[192,194,221] SSADH activity is intermediate between patient and control values in extracts of lymphocytes and lymphoblasts from parents of probands, indicating autosomal recessive inheritance.[192,198,221] Parental consanguinity in several families supports this mode of inheritance.[192,194,211] SSADH activity is low, but measurable, in cultured skin fibroblasts and can be measured in cultured amniocytes and biopsied chorionic villus tissue.[188,215,220] Prenatal diagnosis has been accurately performed using a combination of isotope-dilution MS to assess quantities of 4-HBA in amniotic fluid with determination of SSADH activity in amniocytes or biopsied chorionic villus.[207]

Therapeutic Intervention. In SSADH deficiency, therapeutic intervention with the antiepileptic vigabatrin (γ-vinyl GABA; Sabril), an irreversible GABA-transaminase inhibitor, remains the sole treatment modality, but long-term clinical efficacy is questionable.[195,222,223] Several patients have developed seizures, at which time the dosage was decreased or alternative experimental therapie applied.[204–206,224] In those patients for whom therapy was clinically useful, there were variable improvements in manageability, consciousness, attention span, and ataxia. In other patients, vigabatrin has not provided any improvement in clinical outlook.[225] Other drugs, such as the 4-HBA receptor antagonist NCS-382 or the $GABA_B$ receptor antagonist, may be more relevant, but clinical trial data on the use of these agents are lacking.[224] Methylphenidate, administered to a patient to offset daytime somnolence, improved alertness and central auditory processing.[226] This drug was ineffective in another patient with hyperkinesis controlled only by thioridazine.[210]

Expressed Genotype. SSADH was purified to apparent homogeneity from rat and human brain.[227] Immunologic and electrophoretic characterization of purified human SSADH indicates a homotetrameric protein with subunit M_r of 58. Prenatal diagnosis of SSADH deficiency was undertaken in the family of a proband from Turkey.[228] Elevated 4-HBA was detected in amniotic fluid, and deficient SSADH activity was demonstrated in cultured amniocytes. SSADH activity was undetectable in homogenates of brain, liver, and kidney derived from the affected fetus but ranged from 0.2 to 1.4 nmol/min/mg protein in control fetal tissue homogenates.[229] SSADH CRM was not detected in homogenates of affected fetal tissues by Western immunoblot using polyclonal antibodies raised against purified rat brain SSADH. Conversely, homogenates of control fetal liver and kidney displayed an immunoreactive band at M_r 58 kDa; SSADH CRM was not detected in homogenates of control fetal brain but was detected in homogenates of control adult brain. These data verify SSADH deficiency in affected organ tissues. Moreover, SSADH in liver and kidney appears to share immunologic identity with the enzyme in brain. SSADH deficiency in liver and kidney may be responsible for some of the abnormal metabolite findings in patients and indicates that the disease is systemic.[132,230]

Availability of purified mammalian SSADH protein has permitted cloning of the relevant cDNAs encoding rat and human SSADH (Genbank accession number Y11192).[231,232] The human gene maps to chromosome 6p22.[232,233] Mutation analysis has thus far identified two exon-skipping mutations at consensus splice sites in four patients from two families.[233] Heterozygosity in family members for these splicing errors providing further evidence for autosomal recessive transmission has recently been identified.[233a] Thus far, there is no clear phenotype/genotype correlation, because most mutations are private within the families studied.

Pathogenesis. The pharmacology of 4-HBA has been reviewed.[224,234] Developed as an anesthetic by the pharmaceutical industry in the 1960s, 4-HBA proved to have adverse effects that precluded its clinical use. 4-HBA, a normal brain metabolite, is found in substantial quantities in peripheral organs of animals, but its role there is unclear.[234,235] 4-HBA is being used now in the treatment of narcolepsy[236] and alcohol-withdrawal syndrome.[237] Illicit use allegedly produces a "high," and there are reports of toxicity.[238] Pharmacologic doses of 4-HBA induce drowsiness, hypotonia, and seizurelike activity similar to symptoms observed for SSADH-deficient patients.[208] The age-related decrease of 4-HBA excretion in SSADH deficiency[194] may coincide with variation in clinical status. Younger patients manifest somnolence and have high 4-HBA concentrations in physiological fluids; older patients have lower 4-HBA concentrations, with a tendency toward hyperactivity or aggressive behavior or both.[194] 4-HBA may act on excitatory receptors at low concentrations and on inhibitory receptors at high concentrations.

Comparison of clinical and biochemical findings in patients with existing neuropharmacologic data in animals and humans indicates that 4-HBA contributes to the pathogenesis of SSADH deficiency.[224] Whether these effects are mediated by 4-HBA, by GABA following metabolic interconversion, or synergistically by both compounds remains to be determined.

CARNOSINE AND OTHER IMIDAZOLE DIPEPTIDES

β-Alanyl-Dipeptide Synthesis

The majority of β-alanine in the human body occurs as the dipeptide carnosine.[2,239] Skeletal muscle, but not cardiac muscle, contains carnosine,[240,241] and it is present in brain, particularly in the primary olfactory pathways; its concentration there is maintained by intact pathways for synthesis and hydrolysis of the dipeptide. It may play a role in brain as a neurotransmitter.[242,243]

Carnosine is synthesized by carnosine synthetase, an enzyme that requires ATP during the formation of an intermediate enzyme: β-alanyl-adenylate complex. L-Histidine is then united with β-alanine, and the dipeptide (β-alanyl-L-histidine) is released from the enzyme.[244–248]

Skeletal muscle of birds and certain species of mammals, notably the rabbit, rat, and whale, contains anserine (β-alanyl-1-methyl-L-histidine) (see Fig. 91-1). This dipeptide is normally absent from human tissues and body fluids, and its appearance there is an artifact of diet[249] and serum carnosinase deficiency. The methyl group of anserine is added to carnosine by the enzyme *S*-adenosylmethionine:carnosine *N*-methyltransferase.[250]

The physiological functions of β-alanyl-imidazole dipeptides are not completely understood.[251] They may serve as buffers to stabilize the pH of muscle contracting anaerobically[235,248] and as antioxidants.[251–253] Carnosine and anserine are potent in vitro activators of myosin ATPase in concentrations comparable to those found in skeletal muscle.[254] The dipeptides also chelate copper.[253,255]

Coenzyme A. β-Alanine is a constituent of coenzyme A in its pantothenate moiety (see Fig. 91-1). Since incorporation into pantothenic acid does not occur in mammalian tissues, pantothenate is an essential human nutrient.

β-Alanyl-Dipeptide Catabolism. Carnosine is hydrolyzed by two isozymes in humans: tissue (cytosolic) carnosinase and serum carnosinase; they have the same EC number (3.4.13.3). Tissue carnosinases of human and nonhuman tissues differ in their respective properties.[256–258] The tissue enzyme is a metalloprotein, and although it is activated in vitro by both manganese and zinc, the native enzyme uses zinc.[257]

Cytosolic carnosinase activity is present in most human tissues[259,260] at high levels in kidney, liver, spleen, and brain and low levels in skeletal muscle and heart. Human cytosolic carnosinase ($M_r \approx 90{,}000$) has an in vitro pH optimum of 9.5 and a K_m value of 10 mM for carnosine. This carnosinase does not hydrolyze anserine or homocarnosine[260] (Table 91-8). Prolinase (see Chap. 90) and cytosolic carnosinase are the same enzyme;[261] it has broad specificity as a dipeptidase, and the name "human cytosolic nonspecific dipeptidase" has been proposed for it.

Serum and cytosolic carnosinases are indeed different enzymes[258] (see Table 91-8). The former has a higher molecular weight, a lower pH optimum *in vitro* and a different K_m value for carnosine. Human serum carnosinase hydrolyzes anserine and carnosine equally well; it hydrolyzes homocarnosine very poorly.[258] Under ideal assay conditions,[258] the normal adult

Table 91-8 Properties of Human Carnosinases (EC 3.4.13.3)

Property	Cytosolic Carnosinase	Serum Carnosinase
Relative dipeptide-hydrolyzing activity (%)	Carnosine, 100 Anserine, 0 Homocarnosine, 0	Carnosine, 100 Anserine, 100 Homocarnosine, 4
Relative molecular weight (M_r)	90,000	160,000
Cysteine-containing enzyme	Yes	No
pH optimum, *in vitro*	9.5	8.5
Isoelectric point	5.6	4.7
K_m (*mM*)		
Carnosine	10 mM	4.0 mM
Homocarnosine	—	0.4 mM
Activated by	Mn^{2+}, dithiothreitol	Cd^{2+}, citrate
Inhibited by	EDTA, p-Hydroxymercuribenzoate	EDTA, dithiothreitol

SOURCE: Adapted from data by Lenney et al.[258–260]

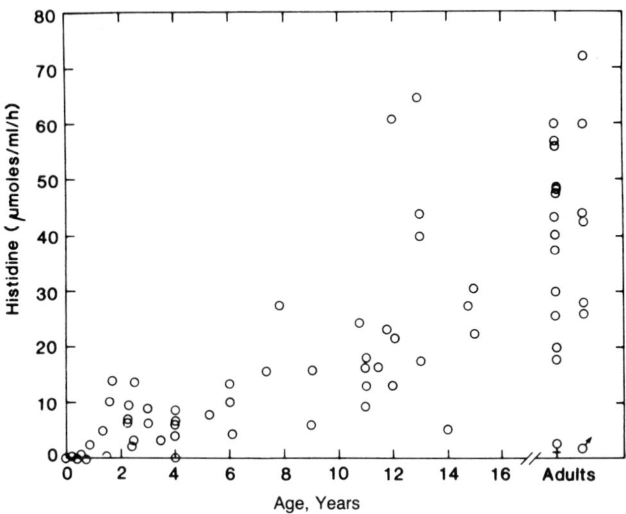

Fig. 91-8 Relationship between serum carnosinase activity (measured by histidine release from carnosine) and age in human controls. (*Reproduced from Lenney et al.,*[258] *with permission.*)

human serum enzyme hydrolyzes carnosine (42 μmol/ml serum per hour) about seventeenfold faster than reported for other assays. Serum carnosinase activity is low in infancy (Fig. 91-8) and increases gradually to reach adult values by adolescence.[258,262,263] CSF contains some carnosinase activity of the serum type.[260]

Related Imidazole Dipeptides. Homocarnosine (γ-aminobutyryl-L-histidine, Fig. 91-1), was isolated first from bovine brain[264] and later from brain of other mammalian species, including humans.[265] It is a brain-specific dipeptide. Homocarnosine and carnosine in brain are both synthesized by carnosine synthetase in glial cells.[266,267] Homocarnosine is hydrolyzed by serum carnosinase but not by the cytosolic enzyme.[260]

Human brain contains 100 times more homocarnosine than carnosine.[243,268] Homocarnosine concentrations are highest in the dentate and inferior olivary nuclei (> 1 mM), intermediate in the substantia nigra and globus pallidus, and lowest in the frontal cortex, caudate nucleus, and nucleus accumbens[268,269]; concentrations are higher in adults than in infants.[269] The physiological role of brain homocarnosine is unknown, although there is evidence that specific neuronal tracts of the human central nervous system may produce GABA from homocarnosine via hydrolysis by serum carnosinase.[270]

Homoanserine (γ-aminobutyryl-L-methylhistidine) occurs in bovine brain,[271] α-β-alanyl)-lysine in rabbit muscle,[272] and α-γ-aminobutyryl)-lysine[273] and γ-aminobutyryl-cystathionine[274] in brain of several mammalian species. Their roles are unknown. Dipeptides containing GABA, other than homocarnosine, occur in human brain and CSF at low concentrations,[130] notably, γ-aminobutyryl-lysine, γ-aminobutyryl-cystathionine, *N*-carboxyethyl-GABA, and 2-pyrrolidinone. Hydrolysis of these peptides during analysis of CSF and brain yields spurious free GABA values.[130]

Imidazole Dipeptides in Physiological Fluids: Relation to Diet

Carnosine, anserine, and homocarnosine are not detectable in normal fasting plasma, nor are they found in significant amounts in normal urine of adults. Urine contains many unidentified ninhydrin-reacting compounds, some of which are β-alanine and imidazoles in peptide linkage.[275] Normal persons who consume large amounts of carnosine or anserine — when they eat fowl or rabbit, for example[249,276–279] — excrete these dipeptides intact in the urine, presumably because they escape complete hydrolysis and are cleared rapidly by kidney; they also excrete free β-alanine[249] and 1-methylhistidine.[249,277,278] Renal clearance of 1-methylhistidine is normally high,[280,281] and large amounts of urinary 1-methylhistidine can provoke a green ferric chloride reaction.[249] Diet-induced carnosinuria occurs more rapidly in infants than in adults as a consequence of the low serum carnosinase activity in infants[258,262,263,282–284] (see Fig. 91-8).

Homocarnosine is present in CSF of normal subjects; concentrations are higher in infants[285] than in adults.[286] The mean concentration of homocarnosine is on the order of 1 μM in adults and 8 μM in normal infants and young children. Homocarnosine values and serum carnosinase activity are age-related and inversely related to each other.

Disorders of Dipeptide Metabolism

Serum Carnosinase Deficiency. Numerous patients[263,282,287–296] have been reported with persistent carnosinuria and serum carnosinase deficiency (MIM 274270). The disorder is autosomal recessive.

Neurologic signs were reported in about half the cases. Since clinical manifestations are not uniformly associated with the biochemical phenotype,[263,295] the former may reflect an ascertainment bias. Asymptomatic family members with serum carnosinase deficiency have been ascertained through symptomatic probands,[263,290,295] and a proband with serum carnosinase deficiency and normal development was identified during newborn urine screening.[292] Whether the infantile cases with neurologic disease[282,287,289,292,294,295] had hereditary serum carnosinase deficiency is unclear, because enzyme activity is normally low in the human infant (see Fig. 91-8).

Metabolite Patterns. Carnosine excretion by children and adults eating normal diets is negligible (< 20 nmoles/g creatinine);[297] excretion increases following meals rich in imidazole dipeptides (see above). Persistent dipeptiduria during a meat-free diet is a significant finding compatible with serum carnosinase deficiency. The principal source of urinary carnosine in such a person will be turnover of endogenous dipeptide pools; excretion rates are 0.5 to 1 mmoles/g creatinine.[263,287,289]

Anserine appears in the urine of persons with serum carnosinase deficiency only after eating foods containing the dipeptide. Normal persons excrete L-methylhistidine after ingesting anserine;[249] persons with serum carnosinase deficiency excrete little or no L-methylhistidine.[263,287,289]

Normal subjects have no carnosine in fasting serum;[287] persons with serum carnosinase deficiency have measurable amounts.[263,287,293]

Persons with serum carnosinase deficiency can have normal amounts of homocarnosine in CSF.[281,287,295]

An adolescent proband with hereditary serum carnosinase deficiency had elevated tissue levels of carnosine.[282,287]

Serum Carnosinase Activity. Several methods have been devised to assay serum carnosinase activity. The preferred method[258] was used to obtain the normal values depicted in Fig. 91-8. Age-related controls must be used to interpret serum carnosinase activity in putative cases. Several subjects[282,287,289,292,294,295] classified originally as having hereditary serum carnosinase deficiency probably had the normal age-related "deficiency" of serum carnosinase. Serum activity may be low in other diseases, for example, in urea cycle disorders,[283] the muscular dystrophies,[284] and hepatic cirrhosis or hepatoma.[298]

Parents of probands with "hereditary" serum carnosinase deficiency have partial deficiency of enzyme activity,[263,289,291] hence the assumption that the phenotype is autosomal recessive.

Homocarnosinosis (Putative Severe Serum Carnosinase Deficiency)

Homocarnosinosis has been the subject of several reports;[296,299–301] there is only one known affected family. A

Norwegian woman, healthy at age 72, and three of her four children had elevated homocarnosine levels in CSF; the three children with the metabolic finding had progressive spastic paraplegia (onset between 6 and 29 years of age), progressive mental deterioration, and retinal pigmentation.

Metabolic Phenotype. Homocarnosine values in CSF were much elevated (50 to 75 μM; normal value for age, 1.3 ± 1.5 μM), but carnosine levels were not increased — a puzzling observation. The affected subjects also excreted substantial amounts of carnosine on a meat-free diet and of anserine after eating meat.[296,302] At autopsy, the brain of one affected offspring had elevation of homocarnosine levels to four times normal.[301]

Serum Carnosinase Deficiency and Homocarnosinosis: One Disorder?

Serum carnosinase deficiency and "homocarnosinosis" are now treated as one disorder. Homocarnosine pools in CSF and brain are presumably in equilibrium with each other. Impaired hydrolysis of homocarnosine (by serum carnosinase) should cause the dipeptide to rise in both compartments. But why are carnosine levels not also increased? The neurologic abnormalities in "homocarnosinosis" are thought not to be related to the metabolic disorder. Serum from patients with homocarnosinosis does, however, contain an immunoreactive protein indistinguishable from the carnosinase band seen in normal serum, suggesting the production of an inactive form of carnosinase in these patients.[303]

Diagnosis of Serum Carnosinase Deficiency.

Dipeptiduria can be detected by partition or column chromatography (see Scriver and Gibson[1] for details). Subjects should receive a meat- and fowl-free diet for several days before their urine is collected. If dipeptiduria persists on a meat-free diet, and if dietary loading with anserine does not produce L-methylhistidinuria (the normal response), serum carnosinase activity should be measured by the preferred method.[258] The effect of age must be considered to interpret the result (see Fig. 91-8).

Treatment. If serum carnosinase deficiency is not causally related to neurologic disease,[296] treatment is not indicated. Normal donor plasma, infused into a subject with serum carnosinase deficiency over a 45-h period, induced a prompt increase of serum carnosinase activity and a fall in urine carnosine.[289] The effect of the infusion was brief. The observation has metabolic but no clinical interest.

Lunde et al.[304] treated two "homocarnosinosis" patients with a diet very low in histidine for 2.5 years. Histidine values in body fluids fell, and homocarnosine values in CSF were 91 percent of pretreatment values after 6 months. There was no associated clinical improvement.

Genetics of Serum Carnosinase Deficiency. Parental consanguinity in some families,[287–289] the occurrence of multiple affected sibs in others,[263,295] and partial enzyme deficiency in parents of probands[263,289,291] are all compatible with autosomal recessive inheritance. A recent report identified serum carnosinase deficiency in a 2-year-old girl with 18q− syndrome, suggesting that the gene for serum carnosinase resides in this portion of the genome.[305]

Neurologic disease, sometimes associated with serum carnosinase deficiency, may have an independent cause or may have a multifactorial origin in affected probands. Accordingly, Wassif and colleagues investigated serum carnosinase activity in five groups of patients with neurologic disease. This activity was not reduced in patients with idiopathic epilepsy or motor neuron disease but was significantly reduced in patients with Parkinson disease or multiple sclerosis and following a cerebrovascular accident, including acute stroke.[306,307] This reduction may result from anoxic damage to carnosine-producing cells or disruption of the blood-brain barrier. At present, the neurologic prognosis for a prospectively identified patient with serum carnosine deficiency is unclear.

REFERENCES

1. Scriver CR, Gibson KM: Disorders of β- and γ-amino acids in free and peptide-linked forms, in Scriver CR, Beaudet AL, Sly WS, Valle D (eds): *The Metabolic Basis of Inherited Disease* 7th ed. New York, McGraw-Hill, 1995, p 1349.
2. Griffith OW: β-amino acids: Mammalian metabolism and utility as amino-acid analogues. *Annu Rev Biochem* **55**:855, 1986.
3. Rozen R, Goodyer PR, Scriver CR: GABA and taurine: What are metabolites like this doing in places like that? in Freinkel N (ed.): *Contemporary Metabolism* vol 2. New York, Plenum, 1982, p 189.
4. Poston JM: β-leucine and the β-keto pathway of leucine metabolism. *Adv Enzymol* **58**:173, 1986.
5. Fyske EM, Fonnum F: Amino acid neurotransmission: Dynamics of vesicular uptake. *Neurochem Res* **21**:1053, 1996.
6. Strange PG: The structure and mechanism of neurotransmitter receptors: Implications for the structure and function of the central nervous system. *Biochem J* **249**:309, 1988.
7. Jursky F, Tamura S, Tamura A, Mandiyan S, Nelson H, Nelson N: Structure, function and brain localization of neurotransmitter transporters. *J Exper Biol* **196**:283, 1994.
8. Peterson WM, Miller SS: Identification and functional characterization of a dual GABA/taurine transporter in bullfrog retinal pigment epithelium. *J Gen Physiol* **106**:1089, 1995.
9. Boehm S, Harvey RJ, Vonholst A, Rohrer H, Betz H: Glycine receptors in cultured chick sympathetic neurons are excitatory and trigger neurotransmitter release. *J Physiol (Lond)* **504**:683, 1997.
10. Van Gennip AH, Abeling NG, Vreken P, van Kuilenburg AB: Inborn errors of pyrimidine degradation: Clinical, biochemical and molecular aspects. *J Inherit Metab Dis* **20**:203, 1997.
11. Holopainen I, Pulkki K, Heinonen OJ, Näntö-Salonen K, Haataja L, Greter J, Holme E, et al: Partial epilepsy in a girl with a symptom-free sister: First two Finnish patients with dihydropyrimidine dehydrogenase deficiency. *J Inherit Metab Dis* **20**:719, 1997.
12. Van Gennip AH, Kamerling JP, De Bree PK, Wadman SK: Linear relationship between *R* and *S* enantiomorphs of β-amino-isobutyric acid in human urine. *Clin Chim Acta* **116**:261, 1981.
13. Bakkeren JAJM, De Abreu RA, Sengers RCA, Gabreels FJM, Maas JM, Renier WO: Elevated urine, blood and cerebrospinal fluid levels of uracil and thymine in a child with dihydrothymine dehydrogenase deficiency. *Clin Chim Acta* **140**:247, 1984.
14. Berger R, Stoker-De Vries SA, Wadman SK, Duran M, Beemer FA, Debree PK, Van Der Woude JK: Dihydropyrimidine dehydrogenase deficiency leading to thymine-uraciluria: An inborn error of pyrimidine metabolism. *Clin Chim Acta* **141**:227, 1984.
15. Wadman SK, Beemer FA, Debree PK, Duran M, van Gennip AH, Ketting D, van Sprang FJ: New defects of pyrimidine metabolism. *Adv Exp Med Biol* **165**:109, 1984.
16. Wadman SK, Berger R, Duran M, De Bree PK, Stoker-De Vries SA, Beemer FA, et al: Dihydropyrimidine dehydrogenase deficiency leading to thymine-uraciluria: An inborn error of pyrimidine metabolism. *J Inherit Metab Dis* **2**:113, 1985.
17. Wilcken B, Hammond J, Berger R, Wise G, James C: Dihydropyrimidine dehydrogenase deficiency — a further case. *J Inherit Metab Dis* **2**:115, 1985.
18. Van Gennip AH, Bakker HD, Zoetekomer A, Abeling NGGM: A new case of thymine-uraciluria. *Klin Wochenschr* **65**(Suppl):14, 1987.
19. Brockstedt M, Jakobs C, Smit L, van Gennip AH: A new case of dihydropyrimidine dehydrogenase deficiency. *J Inherit Metab Dis* **13**:121, 1991.
20. Adolph KJ, Fung E, McLeod DR, Morgan K, Snyder FF: Dihydropyrimidine dehydrogenase deficiency in a Hutterite newborn. *Adv Exp Med Biol* **309B**:311, 1991.
21. Henderson MJ, Jones S, Walker P, Duley J, Simmonds HA: Heterogeneity of symptomatology in two male siblings with thymine uraciluria. *J Inherit Metab Dis* **18**:85, 1995.
22. Fernandez-Salguero P, Gonzalez FJ, Etienne MC, Milano G, Kimura S: Correlation between catalytic activity and protein content for the polymorphically expressed dihydropyrimidine dehydrogenase in human lymphocytes. *Biochem Pharmacol* **50**:1015, 1995.
23. Van Gennip AH, Abeling NG, Stroomer AEM, van Lenthe H, Bakker HD: Clinical and biochemical findings in six patients with pyrimidine degradation defects. *J Inherit Metab Dis* **17**:130, 1994.

24. Bakker HD, Rubio Gozalbo ME, van Gennip AH: Dihydropyrimidine dehydrogenase deficiency presenting with psychomotor retardation and ocular abnormalities. *J Inherit Metab Dis* **17**:640, 1994.
25. Van Gennip AH, Abeling NGGM, Vreken P, van Kuilenburg ABP: Genetic metabolic disease of pyrimidine metabolism: Implications for diagnosis and treatment. *Int Pediatr* **12**:28, 1997.
26. Vreken P, Van Kuilenburg ABP, Meinsma R, Smit GPA, Bakker HD, De Abreu RA, van Gennip AH: A point mutation in an invariant splice donor site leads to exon skipping in two unrelated Dutch patients with dihydropyrimidine dehydrogenase deficiency. *J Inherit Metab Dis* **19**:645, 1996.
27. Milano G, Etienne MC: Individualizing therapy with 5-fluorouracil related to dihydropyrimidine dehydrogenase: Theory and limits. *Ther Drug Monit* **18**:335, 1996.
28. Meinsma R, Fernandez-Salguero P, van Kuilenburg ABP, van Gennip AH, Gonzalez FJ: Human polymorphism in drug metabolism: Mutation in the dihydropyrimidine dehydrogenase gene results in exon skipping and thymine uracilurea. *DNA Cell Biol* **14**:1, 1995.
29. Fernandez-Salguero PM, Sapone A, Wei X, Holt JR, Jones S, Idle JR, Gonzalez FJ: Lack of correlation between phenotype and genotype for the polymorphically expressed dihydropyrimidine dehydrogenase in a family of Pakistani origin. *Pharmacogenetics* **7**:162, 1997.
30. Vreken P, van Kuilenburg AB, Meinsma R, van Gennip AH: Identification of novel point mutations in the dihydropyrimidine dehydrogenase gene. *J Inherit Metab Dis* **20**:335, 1997.
31. Vreken P, van Kuilenburg AB, Meinsma R, De Abreu RA, Van Gennip AH: Identification of a four-base deletion (delTCAT296–299) in the dihydropyrimidine dehydrogenase gene with variable clinical expression. *Hum Genet* **100**:263, 1997.
32. Lu Z, Zhang R, Diasio RB: Population characteristics of hepatic dihydropyrimidine dehydrogenase activity, a key metabolic enzyme in 5-fluorouracil chemotherapy. *Clin Pharmacol Ther* **58**:512, 1995.
33. Khor SP, Amyx H, Davis ST, Nelson D, Baccanari DP, Spector T: Dihydropyrimidine dehydrogenase inactivation and 5-fluorouracil pharmacokinetics: Allometric scaling of animal data, pharmacokinetics and toxicodynamics of 5-fluorouracil in humans. *Cancer Chemother Pharmacol* **39**:233, 1997.
34. Milano G, Etienne MC: Potential importance of dihydropyrimidine dehydrogenase (DPD) in cancer chemotherapy. *Pharmacogenetics* **4**:301, 1994.
35. Fleming RA, Milano GA, Gaspard MH, Bargnoux PJ, Thyss A, Plagne R, Renée N, et al: Dihydropyrimidine dehydrogenase activity in cancer patients. *Eur J Cancer* **29A**:740, 1993.
36. Tuckman M, Stoeckeler JS, Kiang DT, O'Dea RF, Ramaraine ML, Mirkin BL: Familial pyrimidinemia and pyrimidinuria associated with severe fluorouracil toxicity. *N Engl J Med* **313**:245, 1985.
37. Lyss AP, Lilenbaum RC, Harris BE, Diasio RB. Severe 5-fluorouracil toxicity in a patient with decreased dihydropyrimidine dehydrogenase activity. *Cancer Investigation* **11**:239, 1993.
38. Beuzeboc P, Pierga JY, Stoppa-Lyonnet D, Etienne MC, Milano G, Pouillart P: Severe 5-fluorouracil toxicity possibly secondary to dihydropyrimidine dehydrogenase deficiency in a breast cancer patient with osteogenesis imperfecta. *Eur J Cancer* **32A**:369, 1996.
39. Morrison GB, Bastian A, De la Rosa T, Diasio RB, Takimoto CH: Dihydropyrimidine dehydrogenase deficiency: A pharmacogenetic defect causing severe adverse reactions to 5-fluorouracil-based chemotherapy. *Oncol Nurs Forum* **24**:83, 1997.
40. Houyau P, Gay C, Chatelut E, Canal P, Roche H, Milano G: Severe fluorouracil toxicity in a patient with dihydropyrimidine dehydrogenase deficiency. *J Natl Cancer Inst* **85**:1602, 1993.
41. Risso ME, Hasson NK, Lum BL: Dihydropyrimidine dehydrogenase deficiency: A potential etiology for 5-fluorouracil-induced neurotoxicity. *Pharmacotherapy* **17**:847, 1997.
42. Diasio RB, Beavers TL, Carpenter J: Familial deficiency of dihydropyrimidine dehydrogenase. *J Clin Invest* **81**:47, 1988.
43. Vesell ES: Genetic host factors: Determinants of drug response. *N Engl J Med* **313**:261, 1985.
44. Lu Z, Zhang R, Diasio RB: Dihydropyrimidine dehydrogenase activity in human peripheral blood mononuclear cells and liver: Population characteristics, newly identified deficient patients, and clinical implication in 5-fluorouracil chemotherapy. *Cancer Res* **53**:5433, 1993.
45. Harris BE, Carpenter JT, Diasio RB: Severe 5-fluorouracil toxicity secondary to dihydropyrimidine dehydrogenase deficiency: A potentially more common pharmacogenetic syndrome. *Cancer* **68**:499, 1991.
46. Milano G, Etienne MC: Dihydropyrimidine dehydrogenase (DPD) and clinical pharmacology of 5-fluorouracil [Review]. *Anticancer Res* **14**:2295, 1994.
47. Gonzalez FJ, Fernandez-Salguero P: Diagnostic analysis, clinical importance and molecular basis of dihydropyrimidine dehydrogenase deficiency. *Trends Pharmacol Sci* **16**:325, 1995.
48. Van Gennip AH, Busch S, Elzinga L, Stroomer AEM, van Cruchten A, Scholten EG, Abeling NGGM: Application of simple chromatographic methods for the diagnosis of defects in pyrimidine degradation. *Clin Chem* **39**:380, 1993.
49. Duran M, Dorland L, Meuleman EE, Allers P, Berger R: Inherited defects of purine and pyrimidine metabolism: Laboratory methods for diagnosis. *J Inherit Metab Dis* **20**:227, 1997.
50. Gamelin E, Boisdroncelle M. Larra F, Robert J: A simple chromatographic method for the analysis of pyrimidines and their dihydrogenated metabolites. *Journal of Liquid Chromatography and Related Technologies* **20**:3155, 1997.
51. Davies PM, Fairbanks LD, Duley JA, Simmonds HA: Urinary uracil concentrations are a useful guide to genetic disorders associated with neurological deficits and abnormal pyrimidine metabolism. *J Inherit Metab Dis* **20**:328, 1997.
52. Yokota H, Fernandez-Salguero P, Furuya H, Lin K, McBride OW, Podschun B, Schnackerz KD, et al: cDNA cloning and chromosome mapping of human dihydropyrimidine dehydrogenase, an enzyme associated with 5-fluorouracil toxicity and congenital thymine uraciluria. *J Biol Chem* **269**:23192, 1994.
53. Van Kuilenburg AB, Blom MJ, Van Lenthe H, Mul E, van Gennip AH: The activity of dihydropyrimidine dehydrogenase in human blood cells. *J Inherit Metab Dis* **20**:331, 1997.
54. Diasio RB, van Kuilenburg ABP, Lu Z, Zhang R, van Lenthe H, Bakker HD, van Gennip AH: Determination of dihydropyrimidine dehydrogenase (DPD) in fibroblasts of a DPD deficient pediatric patient and family members using a polyclonal antibody to human DPD. *Adv Exp Med Biol* **370**:7, 1994.
54a. Van Kuilenburg AB, van Lenthe H, Blom MJ, Mul EP, van Gennip AH: Profound variation in dihydropyrimidine dehydrogenase activity in human blood cells: major implications for the detection of partly deficient patients. *Br J Cancer* **79**:620, 1999.
55. McMurrough J, McLeod HL: Analysis of the dihydropyrimidine dehydrogenase polymorphism in a British population. *Br J Clin Pharmacol* **41**:425, 1996.
56. Van Gennip AH, van Lenthe H, Abeling NGGM, Bakker HD, van Kuilenburg AB: Combined deficiencies of NADPH- and NADH-dependent dihydropyrimidine dehydrogenases, a new finding in a family with thymine-uraciluria. *J Inherit Metab Dis* **18**:185, 1995.
57. Etienne MC, Lagrange JL, Dassonville O, Fleming R, Thyss A, Renée N, Schneider M, et al: Population study of dihydropyrimidine dehydrogenase in cancer patients. *J Clin Oncol* **12**:2248, 1994.
58. Wei X, McLeod HL, McMurrough J, Gonzalez FJ, Fernandez-Salguero P: Molecular basis of the human dihydropyrimidine dehydrogenase deficiency and 5-fluorouracil toxicity. *J Clin Invest* **98**:610, 1996.
58a. Van Kuilenburg ABP, Vreken P, Beex LVAM, De Abreu RA, van Gennip AH: Severe 5-fluorouracil toxicity caused by reduced dihydropyrimidine dehydrogenase activity due to heterozygosity for a G → A point mutation. *J Inherit Metab Dis* **21**:280, 1998.
58b. Christensen E, Cezanne I, Kjærgaard S, Hørlyk H, Faurholt Pedersen V, Vreken P, van Kuilenburg ABP, van Gennip AH: Clinical variability in three Danish patients with dihydropyrimidine dehydrogenase deficiency all homozygous for the same mutation. *J Inherit Metab Dis* **21**:272, 1998.
58c. Van Kuilenburg AB, Vreken P, Beex LV, Meinsma R, van Lenthe H, De Abreu RA, van Gennip AH: Heterozygosity for a point mutation in an invariant splice donor site of dihydroyprimidine dehydrogenase and severe 5-fluorouracil related toxicity. *Eur J Cancer* **33**:2258, 1997.
58d. Van Kuilenburg AB, Vreken P, Abeling NG, Bakker HD, Meinsma R, van Lenthe H, De Abreau RA, Smeitink JA, Kayserili H, Apak MY, Christensen E, Holopainen I, Pulkki K, Riva D, Botteon G, Holme E, Tulinius M, Kleijer WJ, Beemer FA, Duran M, Niezen-Koning KE, Smit GP, Jakobs C, Smit LM, van Gennip AH, et al: Genotype and phenotype in patients with dihydropyrimidine dehydrogenase deficiency. *Hum Genet* **104**:1, 1999.
59. Berglund G, Greter J, Lindstedt S, Steen G, Waldenstrom J, Wass U: Urinary excretion of thymine and uracil in a two-year-old child with a malignant tumor of the brain. *Clin Chem* **25**:1325, 1979.

60. Tateishi T, Nakura H, Watanabe M, Tanaka M, Kumai T, Kobayashi S: Preliminary examination of the influence of incubation time or cytosolic protein concentration on dihydropyrimidine dehydrogenase activity. *Clin Chim Acta* **252**:1, 1996.

60a. Lu Z, Zhang R, Carpenter JT, Diasio RB: Decreased dihydropyrimidine dehydrogenase activity in a population of patients with breast cancer: implication for 5-fluorouracil-based chemotherapy. *Clin Cancer Res* **4**:325, 1998.

60b. Milano G, Etienne MC, Pierrefite V, Barberi-Heyob M, Deporte-Fety R, Renee N: Dihydropyrimidine dehydrogenase deficiency and fluorouracil-related toxicity. *Br J Cancer* **79**:627, 1999.

60c. Van Gennip AH, Vreken P, van Lenthe H, Haasjes J, van Kuilenburg ABP: Partial dihydropyrimidine dehydrogenase deficiency: An example of an important pharmacogenetic syndrome [abstract P114]. *J Inherit Metab Dis* **22**(Suppl):118, 1999.

60d. Diasio RB: The role of dihydropyrimidine dehydrogenase (DPD) modulation in 5-FU pharmacology. *Oncology* **12**(10 Suppl 7):23, 1998.

60e. Katona C, Kralovanszky J, Rosta A, Pandi E, Fonyad G, Toth K, Jeney A: Putative role of dihydropyrimidine dehydrogenase in the toxic side effect of 5-fluorouracil in colorectal cancer patients. *Oncology* **55**:468, 1998.

60f. Shehata N, Pater A, Tang SC: Prolonged severe 5-fluorouracil-associated neurotoxicity in a patient with dihydropyrimidine dehydrogenase deficiency. *Cancer Invest* **17**:201, 1999.

61. Takai S, Fernandez-Salguero P, Kimura S, Gonzalez FJ, Yamada K: Assignment of the human dihydropyrimidine dehydrogenase gene (DPYD) to chromosome region 1p22 by fluorescence in situ hybridization. *Genomics* **24**:613, 1994.

62. Johnson MR, Wang K, Tillmanns S, Albin N, Diasio RB: Structural organization of the human dihydropyrimidine dehydrogenase gene. *Cancer Res* **57**:1660, 1997.

62a. Wei X, Elizondo G, Sapone A, McLeod HL, Raunio H, Fernandez-Salguero P, Gonzalez FJ: Characterization of the human dihydropyrimidine dehydrogenase gene. *Genomics* **51**:391, 1998.

62b. Ridge SA, Sludden J, Brown O, Robertson L, Wei X, Sapone A, Fernandez-Salguero PM, Gonzalez FJ, Vreken P, van Kuilenburg AB, van Gennip AH, McLeod HL: Dihydropyrimidine dehydrogenase pharmacogenetics in Caucasian subjects. *Br J Clin Pharmacol* **46**:151, 1998.

62c. Ridge SA, Sludden J, Wei X, Sapone A, Brown O, Hardy S, Canney P, Fernandez-Salguero P, Gonzalez FJ, Cassidy J, McLeod HL: Dihydropyrimidine dehydrogenase pharmacogenetics in patients with colorectal cancer. *Br J Cancer* **77**:497, 1998.

62d. Vreken P, van Kuilenburg AB, Meinsma R, van Gennip AH: Dihydropyrimidine dehydrogenase deficiency. Identification of two novel mutations and expression of missense mutations in *E. Coli*. *Adv Exp Med Biol* **431**:341, 1998.

63. Vreken P, van Kuilenburg AB, Meinsma R, van Gennip AH: Dihydropyrimidine dehydrogenase (DPD) deficiency: Identification and expression of missense mutations C29R, R886H and R235W. *Hum Genet* **101**:333, 1997.

63a. Van Kuilenburg ABP, Vreken P, Riva D, Botteon G, Abeling NGGM, Bakker HD, van Gennip AH: Clinical and biochemical abnormalities in a patient with dihydropyrimidine dehydrogenase deficiency due to homozygosity for the C29R mutation. *J Inherit Metab* **22**:191, 1999.

63b. Vreken P, van Kuilenburg ABP, Miensma R, Beemer FA, Duran M, van Gennip AH: Dihydropyrimidine dehydrogenase deficiency: A novel mutation and expression of missense mutations in *E. coli*. *J Inherit Metab Dis* **21**:276, 1998.

63c. Kouwaki M, Hamajima N, Sumi S, Nonaka M, Sasaki M, Dobashi K, Kidouchi K, Togari H, Wada Y: Identification of novel mutations in the dihydropyrimidine dehydrogenase gene in a Japanese patient with 5-fluorouracil toxicity. *Clin Cancer Res* **4**:2999, 1998.

64. Ridge SA, Brown O, McMurrough J, Fernandez-Salguero P, Evans WE, Gonzales FJ, McLeod HL: Mutations at codon 974 of the DPYD gene are a rare event. *Br J Cancer* **75**:178, 1997.

65. Van Gennip AH, Driedijk PC, Elzinga A, Abeling NGGM: Screening for defects of dihydropyrimidine degradation by analysis of amino acids in urine before and after acid hydrolysis. *J Inherit Metab Dis* **15**:413, 1992.

66. Jaeken J: Cerebrospinal fluid as a tool in the diagnosis of neurometabolic diseases: Amino acid analysis before and after acid hydrolysis. *Eur J Pediatr* **153**:S86, 1994.

67. Van Gennip AH, Busch S, Schotten EG, Abeling NGGM: Simple method for the quantitative analysis of dihydropyrimidines and N-carbamyl-β-amino acids in urine. *Proc Soc Study Inborn Errors Metab* **29**:P40, 1991.

68. Simmonds HA, Duley JA, Fairbanks LD, McBride MB: When to investigate for purine and pyrimidine disorders: Introduction and review of clinical and laboratory indications. *J Inherit Metab Dis* **20**:214, 1997.

69. Jakobs C, Stellaard F, Smit LME, van Vugt JMG, Duran M, Berger R, Rovers P: The first prenatal diagnosis of dihydropyrimidine dehydrogenase deficiency. *Eur J Pediatr* **150**:291, 1991.

70. Dagg CP, Coleman DL, Fraser GM: A gene affecting the rate of pyrimidine degradation in mice. *Genetics* **49**:979, 1964.

70a. Moolenaar SH, Göhlich-Ratmann G, Assmann B, Engelke U, Bräutigam C, van Gennip AH, de Jong JGN, Voit T, Hoffmann GF, Vreken P, Wevers RA: Ureidopropionase deficiency: a novel inborn error of metabolism discovered with NMR spectoscopy [abs. O10]. *J Inherit Metab Dis* **22**(Suppl 1):5, 1999.

70b. Van Gennip AH, Van Lenthe H, Assmann B, Gehlich-Ratmann G, Hoffmann GF, Brõutigam C, Vreken P, Wevers RA, van Kuilenburg ABP: Confirmation of the enzyme defect in the first case of β-alanine synthase deficiency [abs. P143]. *J Inherit Metab Dis* **22**(Suppl 1):117, 1999.

70c. Wevers RA, Engelke U, Rotteveel JJ, Heerschap A, De Jong JG, Abeling NG, van Gennip AH, De Abreu RA: 1H NMR spectroscopy of body fluids in patients with inborn errors of purine and pyrimidine metabolism. *J Inherit Metab Dis* **20**:345, 1997.

71. Wadman SK, Duran M, Dorland L: Biochemical diagnosis of inherited metabolic diseases, in Kotyk A (ed): *Highlights of Modern Biochemistry* vol 2. VSP Zeist, 1989, p 1379.

72. Duran M, Rovers P, De Bree PK, Schreuder CH, Beukenhorst H, Dorland L, Berger R: Dihydropyrimidinuria: A new inborn error of pyrimidine metabolism. *J Inherit Metab Dis* **14**:367, 1991.

73. Duran M, Rovers P, de Bree PK, Schreuder CH, Beukenhorst H, Dorland L, Berger R: Dihydropyrimidinuria. *Lancet* **336**:817, 1990.

74. Ohba S, Kidouchi K, Sumi S, Imaeda M, Takeda N, Yoshizumi H, Tatematsu A, et al: Dihydropyrimidinuria: The first case in Japan. *Adv Exp Med Biol* **370**:383, 1994.

75. Hayashi K, Kidouchi K, Sumi S, Mizokami M, Orito E, Kumada K, Ueda R, et al: Possible prediction of adverse reactions to pyrimidine chemotherapy from urinary pyrimidine levels and a case of asymptomatic adult dihydropyrimidinuria. *Clin Cancer Res* **2**:1937, 1996.

76. Assmann B, Hoffmann GF, Wagner L, Bräutigam C, Seyberth HW, Duran M, Van Kuilenburg ABP, et al: Dihydropyrimidinase deficiency and congenital microvillus atrophy: Coincidence or genetic relation? *J Inherit Metab Dis* **20**:681, 1997.

76b. Hamajima N, Kouwaki M, Vreken P, Matsuda K, Sumi S, Imaeda M, Ohba S, Kidouchi K, Nonaka M, Tamaki N, Endo Y, De Abrou R, Rotteveel J, van Kuilenburg A, van Gennip A, Togari H, Wada Y: Dihydropyrimidinase deficiency structural organization chromosomal localization, and mutation analysis of the human dihydropyrimidinase gene. *Am J Hum Genet* **63**:717, 1998.

76b. Sumi S, Imaeda M, Kidouchi K, Ohba S, Hamajima N, Kodama K, Togari H, Wada Y: Population and family studies of dihydropyrimidinuria; prevalence, inheritance mode, and risk of fluorouracil toxicity. *Am J Med Genet* **78**:336, 1998.

77. van Gennip AH, de Abreu RA, van Lenthe H, Bakkeren J, Rotteveel J, Vreken P, van Kuilenburg ABP: Dihydropyrimidinase deficiency: Confirmation of the enzyme defect in dihydropyrimidinuria. *J Inherit Metab Dis* **20**:339, 1997.

78. Putman MM, Rotteveel JJ, Wevers RA, van Gennip AH, Bakkeren JA, De Abreu RA: Dihydropyrimidinase deficiency, a progressive neurological disorder? *Neuropediatrics* **28**:106, 1997.

78a. Van Gennip AH, De Abreu RA, Vreken P, Van Kuilenburg AB: Clinical and biochemical aspects of dihydropyrimidinase deficiency. *Adv Exp Med Biol* **431**:125, 1998.

79. Henderson MJ, Ward K, Simmonds HA, Duley JA, Davies PM: Dihydropyrimidinase deficiency presenting in infancy with severe developmental delay. *J Inher Metab Dis* **16**:574, 1993.

80. Sumi S, Kidouchi K, Hayashi K, Ohba S, Wada Y: Dihydropyrimidinuria without clinical symptoms. *J Inherit Metab Dis* **19**:701, 1996.

81. Hamajima N, Matsuda K, Sakata S, Tamaki N, Sasaki M, Nonaka M: A novel gene family defined by human dihydropyrimidinase and three related proteins with differential tissue distribution. *Gene* **180**:157, 1996.

82. Scriver CR, Pueschel S, Davies E: Hyper-β-alaninemia associated with β-aminoaciduria and γ-aminobutyricaciduria, somnolence and seizures. *N Engl J Med* **274**:636, 1966.

83. Higgins JJ, Kaneski CR, Bernardini I, Brady RO, Barton NW: Pyridoxine-responsive hyper-β-alaninemia associated with Cohen's syndrome. *Neurology* **44**:1728, 1994.
83a. Kurozumi Y, Abe T, Yao WB, Ubuka T: Experimental beta-alaninuria induced by (aminooxy) acetate. *Acta Med Okayama* **53**:13, 1999.
84. Dickinson JC, Rosenblum H, Hamilton PB: Ion exchange chromatography of the free amino acids in the plasma of the newborn infant. *Pediatrics* **36**:2, 1965.
85. Scriver CR, Rosenberg LE: *Amino Acid Metabolism and Its Disorders* Philadelphia, Saunders, 1973.
86. Scriver CR: The use of human genetic variation to study membrane transport of amino acids in kidney. *Am J Dis Child* **117**:4, 1969.
87. Gilbert JB, Lorene YK, Rogers L, Williams RJ: The increase in urinary taurine after intraperitoneal administration of amino acids in the mouse. *J Biol Chem* **235**:1055, 1960.
88. Wilson OH, Scriver CR: Specificity of transport of neutral and basic amino acids in rat kidney. *Am J Physiol* **213**:185, 1967.
89. Goldman H, Scriver CR: A transport system in mammalian kidney with preference for β-amino compounds. *Pediatr Res* **1**:212A, 1967.
90. Hammerman M, Sacktor B: Transport of β-alanine in renal brush-border membrane vesicles. *Biochim Biophys Acta* **509**:338, 1978.
91. Rozen R, Tenenhouse HS, Scriver CR: Taurine transport in renal brush-border membrane vesicles. *Biochem J* **180**:245, 1979.
92. Dantzler WH, Silbernagl S: Renal tubular reabsorption of taurine γ-aminobutyric acid (GABA) and β-alanine studied by continuous microperfusion. *Pflugers Arch* **367**:123, 1976.
93. Goodyer PR, Rozen R, Scriver CR: A γ-aminobutyric acid-specific transport mechanism in mammalian kidney. *Biochim Biophys Acta* **818**:45, 1985.
94. Tamaki N, Aoyama H, Kubo K, Ikeda T, Hama T: Purification and properties of β-alanine aminotransferase from rabbit liver. *J Biochem* **92**:1009, 1982.
95. Buzenet AM, Fages C, Bloch-Tardy M, Gonnard P: Purification and properties of 4-aminobutyrate 2-ketoglutarate aminotransferase from pig liver. *Biochim Biophys Acta* **522**:400, 1978.
96. Maitre M, Ciesielski L, Cash C, Mandel P: Purification and studies on some properties of the 4-aminobutyrate-2-ketoglutarate transaminase from rat brain. *Eur J Biochem* **52**:157, 1975.
97. Schousboe A, Wu J-Y, Roberts E: Purification and characterization of the 4-aminobutyrate-2-ketoglutarate transaminase from mouse brain. *Biochemistry* **12**:2868, 1973.
98. Perry TL, Hansen S: Biochemical effects in man and rat of three drugs which can increase brain GABA content. *J Neurochem* **30**:679, 1978.
99. Brandt NJ, Christensen E: β-Aminoaciduria induced by γ-vinyl GABA. *Lancet* **1**:450, 1984.
100. Schechter PJ, Lewis PJ, Newberne JW: γ-Vinyl GABA, GABA and β-alanine transamination. *Lancet* **B**:737, 1984.
101. Pollitt RJ, Green A, Smith R: Excessive excretion of β-alanine and of 3-hydroxypropionic, R- and S-3-aminoisobutyric, R- and S-3-hydroxyisobutyric and S-2-(hydroxymethyl) butyric acids probably due to a defect in the metabolism of the corresponding malonic semialdehydes. *J Inherit Metab Dis* **8**:75, 1985.
102. Gray RG, Pollitt RJ, Webley J: Methylmalonic semialdehyde dehydrogenase deficiency: Demonstration of defective valine and β-alanine metabolism and reduced malonic semialdehyde dehydrogenase activity in cultured fibroblasts. *Biochem Med Metab Biol* **38**:121, 1987.
103. Boulat O, Benador N, Girardin E, Bachmann C: 3-Hydroxyisobutyric aciduria with a mild clinical course. *J Inherit Metab Dis* **18**:204, 1995.
104. Ko FJ, Nyhan WL, Wolff J, Barshop B, Sweetman L: 3-Hydroxyisobutyric aciduria: An inborn error of valine metabolism. *Pediatr Res* **30**:322, 1991.
105. Gibson KM, Lee CF, Bennett MJ, Holmes B, Nyhan WL: Combined malonic, methylmalonic and ethylmalonic acid semialdehyde dehydrogenase deficiencies: An inborn error of β-alanine, L-valine and L-alloisoleucine metabolism? *J Inherit Metab Dis* **16**:563, 1993.
105a. Roe CR, Struys E, Kok RM, Roe DS, Harris RA, Jakobs C: Methylmalonic semialdehyde dehydrogenase deficiency: psychomotor delay and methylmalonic aciduria without metabolic decompensation. *Mol Genet Metab* **65**:35, 1998.
105b. Chambliss KL, Gray RGF, Rylance G, Pollitt RJ, Gibson KM: Molecular characterization of methylmalonate semialdehyde dehydrogenase deficiency. *J Inherit Metab Dis*. **23**:497, 2000.
105c. Chambliss KL, Gray RGF, Rylance G, Pollitt RJ, Gibson KM: Molecular characterization of methylmalonate semialdehyde dehydrogenase (MMSDH) deficiency [Abstract P97]. *J Inherit Metab Dis* **22**(Suppl 1):85, 1999.
105d. Ding J-H, Yang B-Z, Wilkinson JK, Chambliss KL, Roe CR: Molecular basis of methylmalonic semialdehyde dehydrogenase (MMSDH) deficiency. [Abstract P112]. *J Inherit Metab Dis* **22**(Suppl 1):93, 1999.
106. Chitayat D, Meagher-Villemure K, Mamer OA, O'Gorman A, Hoar DI, Silver K, Scriver CR: Brain dysgenesis and congenital intracerebral calcification associated with 3-hydroxyisobutyric aciduria. *J Pediatr* **121**:86, 1992.
106a. Sasaki M, Kimura M, Sugai K, Hoshimoto T, Yamaguchi S: 3-Hydroxyisobutyric aciduria in two brothers. *Pediatr Neurol* **18**:253, 1998.
107. Sutton HE: β-Aminoisobutyric aciduria, in Stanbury JB, Wyngaarden B, Fredrickson DS (eds): *The Metabolic Basis of Inherited Disease*. New York, McGraw-Hill, 1st ed, 1960, p 729.
108. Solem E, Jellum E, Eldjarn L: The absolute configuration of β-aminoisobutyric acid in human serum and urine. *Clin Chim Acta* **50**:393, 1974.
109. Crumpler HR, Dent CE, Harris H, Westall RG: β-Aminoisobutyric acid (α-methyl-β-alanine): A new amino acid, obtained from human urine. *Nature* **617**:307, 1951.
110. Harris H: Family studies on the urinary excretion of β-aminoisobutyric acid. *Ann Eugenics* **18**:43, 1953.
111. Kakimoto Y, Armstrong MD: The preparation and isolation of D-(−)-β-aminoisobutyric acid. *J Biol Chem* **236**:3283, 1961.
112. Armstrong MD, Yates K, Kakimoto Y, Taniguchi K, Kappe T: Excretion of β-aminoisobutyric acid by man. *J Biol Chem* **238**:1447, 1963.
113. Kakimoto Y, Kanazawa A, Taniguchi K, Sano I: β-aminoisobutyrate-α-ketoglutarate transaminase in relation to β-aminoisobutyric aciduria. *Biochim Biophys Acta* **156**:374, 1968.
114. Kakimoto Y, Taniguchi K, Sano I: D-β-Aminoisobutyrate: Pyruvate aminotransferase in mammalian liver and excretion of β-aminoisobutyrate by man. *J Biol Chem* **244**:335, 1969.
115. Taniguchi K, Takehiko T, Kakimoto Y: Deficiency of β-aminoisobutyrate: Pyruvate aminotransferase in the liver of genetic high excretors of D-β-aminoisobutyrate. *Biochim Biophys Acta* **279**:475, 1972.
116. Gartler SM: A metabolic investigation of urinary β-aminoisobutyric acid excretion in man. *Arch Biochem* **80**:400, 1959.
117. Solem E: The absolute configuration of β-aminoisobutyric acid formed by degradation of thymine in man. *Clin Chim Acta* **53**:183, 1974.
118. Solem E, Agarwal DP, Goedde HW: The determination of β-aminoisobutyric acid in human serum by ion-exchange chromatography. *Clin Chim Acta* **59**:203, 1975.
119. Yanai J, Kakimoto Y, Tsujio T, Sano I: Genetic study of β-aminoisobutyric acid excretion by Japanese. *Am J Hum Genet* **21**:115, 1969.
120. Scriver CR, Rosenberg LE: *Amino Acid Metabolism and Its Disorders*. Philadelphia, Saunders, 1973.
121. Simpson SP, Norton NE: Complex segregation analysis of the locus from β-aminoisobutyric acid excretion (BAIB). *Hum Genet* **59**:64, 1981.
122. Roychoudhury AK, Nei M: *Human Polymorphic Genes: World Distribution* New York, Oxford University Press, 1988, p 260.
123. Kvist E, Sjolin K-E, Iversen J, Nyholm K: Urinary excretion patterns of pseudouridine and β-aminoisobutyric acid in patients with tumours of the urinary bladder. *Scand J Urol Nephrol* **27**:45, 1993.
124. Richard JJ, Ruedas E, Nirde P: Probable genetic independence of four hereditary characteristics peculiar to Mongoloid populations [French]. *Rom J Morphol Embryol* **42**:3, 1996.
125. Spistyn VA, Afanas'eva IS, Alekseeva NV: Ecogenetic aspects of the study of phenotypes and levels in β-aminoisobutyric acid excretion [Russian]. *Genetika* **29**:1871, 1993.
126. Spistyn VA, Stakishaitis DV, Preiksha RA: Genetic dimorphism in β-aminoisobutyric acid excretion in patients with atherosclerosis of the coronary artery and in groups at risk for atherosclerosis in the Lithuanian population. *Genetika* **29**:1861, 1993.
127. Konjiki O, Yoneda Y, Sato Y, Oosawa Y, Imamura Y, Takasaki M: A case of megaloblastic anemia with abnormally high urine level of β-aminoisobutyric acid. *Nippon Ronen Igakkai Zasshi* **30**:65, 1993.
128. Tomokuni K, Ichiba M, Hirai Y: Urinary N-acetyl-β-d-glucosaminidase and β-aminoisobutyric acid in workers occupationally exposed to metals such as chromium, nickel, and iron. *Int Arch Occup Environ Health* **65**:19, 1993.

129. Gibson KM, Nyhan WL, Jaeken J: Inborn errors of GABA metabolism. *Bioessays* **4**:24, 1986.
130. Jaeken J, Casaer P, Haegele KD, Schechter PJ: Review: Normal and abnormal central nervous system GABA metabolism in childhood. *J Inherit Metab Dis* **13**:793, 1990.
131. Martin DL: Regulatory properties of brain glutamate decarboxylase. *Cell Mol Neurobiol* **7**:237, 1987.
132. Tillakaratne NJK, Medina-Kauwe L, Gibson KM. Gamma-aminobutyric acid (GABA) metabolism in mammalian neural and nonneural tissues. *Comp Biochem Physiol* **112A**:247, 1995.
133. Schofield PR, Darlison MG, Fujita N, Burt DR, Stephenson FA, Rodriguez H, Rhee LM, et al: Sequence and functional expression of the GABA receptor shows a ligand-gated receptor super-family. *Nature* **328**:221, 1988.
134. Van Gelder NM: A possible enzyme barrier for γ-aminobutyric acid in the central nervous system. *Prog Brain Res* **29**:259, 1967.
135. Brilliant MH, Szaba G, Katarova Z, Kozak CA, Glazer TM, Greenspan RJ, Hausmans DE: Sequences homologous to glutamic acid decarboxylase cDNA are present on mouse chromosomes 2 and 10. *Genomics* **6**:115, 1990.
136. Cram DS, Barnett LD, Joseph JL, Harrison LC: Cloning and partial nucleotide sequence of human glutamic acid decarboxylase cDNA from brain and pancreatic islets. *Biochem Biophys Res Commun* **176**:1239, 1991.
137. Bu D-F, Erlander MG, Hitz BC, Tillakaratne JK, Kaufman DL, Wagner-McPherson CB, Evans GA, et al: Two human glutamate decarboxylases, 65-kDa GAD and 67-kDa GAD, are each encoded by a single gene. *Proc Natl Acad Sci USA* **89**:2115, 1992.
138. Erlander MG, Tillakaratne NJK, Feldblum S, Patel N, Tobin AJ: Two genes encode distinct glutamate decarboxylases. *Neuron* **7**:91, 1991.
139. Goodyer PR, Mills M, Scriver CR: Properties of γ-aminobutyric acid synthesis by rat renal cortex. *Biochim Biophys Acta* **716**:348, 1982.
140. Goodyer PR, Lancaster G, Villeneuve M, Scriver CR: The relationship of γ-aminobutyric acid metabolism to ammoniagenesis in renal cortex. *Biochim Biophys Acta* **633**:191, 1980.
141. Lancaster GA, Mohyuddin F, Scriver CR, Whelan DT: A γ-aminobutyrate pathway in mammalian kidney cortex. *Biochim Biophys Acta* **297**:229, 1973.
142. Lancaster GA, Mohyuddin F, Scriver CR: Ontogeny of L-glutamic acid decarboxylase and γ-aminobutyric acid concentration in human kidney. *Pediatr Res* **9**:484, 1975.
143. Scriver CR, Whelan DT: Glutamic acid decarboxylase (GAD) in mammalian tissue outside the central nervous system, and its possible relevance to hereditary vitamin B_6 dependency with seizures. *Ann NY Acad Sci* **166**:83, 1969.
144. Baxter P, Griffiths P, Kelly T, Gardner-Medwin D: Pyridoxine-dependent seizures: Demographic, clinical, MRI and psychometric features, and the effect of dose on intelligence quotient. *Dev Med Child Neurol* **38**:998, 1996.
144a. Veresova S, Kabova R, Velisek L: Proconvulsant effects induced by pyridoxine in young rats. *Epilepsy Res* **29**:259, 1998.
144b. South M: Neonatal seizures after use of pyridoxine in pregnancy [research letter] *Lancet* **353**:1940, 1999.
145. Haenggeli CA, Girardin E, Paunier L: Pyridoxine-dependent seizures, clinical and therapeutic aspects. *Eur J Pediatr* **150**:452, 1991.
146. Mikati MA, Trevathan E, Krishnomoorthy KS, Lombroso CT: Pyridoxine-dependent epilepsy: EEG investigations and long-term follow-up. *Electroencephalogr Clin Neurophysiol* **78**:215, 1991.
146a. Gospe SM Jr: Current perspectives on pyridoxine-dependent seizures. *J Pediatr* **132**:919, 1998.
146b. Ebinger M, Schultze C, König S: Demographics and diagnosis of pyridoxine-dependent seizures [letter]. *J Pediatr* **134**:795, 1999.
147. Tanak R, Okumara M, Arima J, Yamakura S, Momoi T: Pyridoxine-dependent seizures: A report of a case with atypical clinical features and abnormal MRI scans. *J Child Neurol* **7**:24, 1992.
148. Singh UK, Sinha RK: Pyridoxine-dependent seizures. *Indian Pediatr* **33**:121, 1996.
149. Baumeister FAM, Gesel W, Shin YS, Egger J: Glutamate in pyridoxine-dependent epilepsy: Neurotoxic glutamate concentration in the cerebrospinal fluid and its normalization by pyridoxine. *Pediatrics* **94**:318, 1994.
150. Bankier A, Turner M, Hopkins IJ: Pyridoxine-dependent seizures — a wider clinical spectrum. *Arch Dis Child* **58**:415, 1983.
151. Goutieres F, Aicardi J: Atypical presentations of pyridoxine-dependent seizures: A treatable cause of intractable epilepsy in infants. *Ann Neurol* **17**:117, 1985.
152. Chou M-L, Wang H-S, Hung P-C, Sun P-C, Huang S-C: Late-onset pyridoxine-dependent seizures: Report of two cases. *Acta Paed Sin* **36**:434, 1995.
153. Salih MAM, Kabiraj M, Gascon GG, Jarallah ASA, Al-Zamil FA: Typical and atypical presentations of pyridoxine-dependent seizures. *Saudi Medical Journal* **16**:347, 1995.
154. Jardin LB, Pires RF, Martins CES, Vargas CR, Vizioli J, Kliemann FAD, Giugliani R: Pyridoxine-dependent seizures associated with white matter abnormalities. *Neuropediatrics* **25**:259, 1994.
155. Shih JJ, Kornblum H, Shewmon DA: Global brain dysfunction in an infant with pyridoxine dependency: Evaluation with EEG, evoked potentials, MRI, and PET. *Neurology* **47**:824, 1996.
155a. Gospe SM Jr, Hecht ST: Longitudinal MRI findings in pyridoxine-dependent seizures. *Neurology* **51**:74, 1998.
156. McLachlan RS, Brown WF: Pyridoxine dependent epilepsy with iatrogenic sensory neuronopathy. *Can J Neurol Sci* **22**:50, 1995.
157. Kurleman G, Loscher W, Dominick HC, Palm GD: Disappearance of neonatal seizures and low CSF GABA levels after treatment with vitamin B_6. *Epilepsy Res* **1**:152, 1987.
158. Lott IT, Coulombe T, Di Paolo RV, Richardson EP, Levy HL: Vitamin B_6-dependent seizures: Pathology and chemical findings in brain. *Neurology* **28**:47, 1978.
159. Sharma SK, Bolster B, Dakshinamurti K: Picrotoxin and pentylene tetrazole induced seizure activity in pyridoxine-deficient rats. *J Neurol Sci* **121**:1, 1994.
160. Dolina S, Peeling J, Sutherland G, Pillay N, Greenberg A: Effect of sustained pyridoxine treatment of seizure susceptibility and regional brain amino acid levels in genetically epilepsy-prone BALB/c mice. *Epilepsia* **34**:33, 1993.
161. Yoshida T, Tada K, Arakawa T: Vitamin B_6-dependency of glutamic acid decarboxylase in the kidney from a patient with vitamin B_6-dependent convulsions. *Tohoku J Exp Med* **104**:195, 1971.
162. Gospe SM Jr, Olin KL, Keen CL: Reduced GABA synthesis in pyridoxine-dependent seizures. *Lancet* **343**:1133, 1994.
163. Bu D-F, Christodoulou J, Murrell MJ, Ploder L, Gibson W, Tobin AJ, McInnes RR: Pyridoxine-responsive epilepsy appears not to be caused by mutations in the GAD1 and GAD2 genes. *Am J Hum Genet* 57(Suppl):A177, 1995.
163a. Kure S, Sakata Y, Miyabayashi S, Takahashi K, Shinka T, Matsubara Y, Hoshino H, Narisawa K: Mutation and polymorphic market analysis of 65 K- and 67 K-glutamate decarboxylase genes in two families with pyridoxine-dependent epilepsy. *J Hum Genet* **43**:128, 1998.
164. Asad H, Kawamura Y, Maruyama K, Kume H, Ding R-G, Kanbara N, Kuzume H, et al: Cleft palate and decreased brain γ-aminobutyric acid in mice lacking the 67-kDa isoform of glutamic acid decarboxylase. *Proc Natl Acad Sci USA* **94**:6496, 1997.
165. Asad H, Kawamura Y, Maruyama K, Kume H, Ding R-G, Ju FY, Kanbara N, et al: Mice lacking 65 kDa isoform of glutamic acid decarboxylase (GAD65) maintain normal levels of GAD67 and GABA in their brains but are susceptible to seizures. *Biochem Biophys Res Commun* **229**:891, 1996.
166. Kash SF, Johnson RS, Tecott LH, Noebels JL, Mayfield RD, Hanahan D, Baekkeskov S: Epilepsy in mice deficient in the 65-kDa isoform of glutamic acid decarboxylase. *Proc Natl Acad Sci USA* **94**: 14060, 1997.
166a. Kash SF, Condie BG, Baekkeskov S: Glutamate decarboxylase and GABA in pancreatic islets: Lessons from knock-out mice. *Horm Metab Res* **31**:340, 1999.
166b. Kash SF, Tecott LH, Hodge C, baekkeskov S: Increased anxiety and altered responses to anxiolytics in mice deficient in the 65-kDa isoform of glutamic acid decarboxylase. *Proc. Natl Acad Sci U S A* **96**:1698, 1999.
166c. Ji F, Kanbara N, Obata K: GABA and histogenesis in fetal and neonatal mouse brain lacking both the isoforms of glutamic acid decarboxylase. *Neurosci Res* **33**:187, 1999.
166d. Ji F, Obata K: Development of the GABA system in organotypic culture of hippocampal and cerebellar splices from a 67-kDa isoform of glutamic acid decarboxylase (GAD_{67})-deficient mice. *Neurosci Res* **33**:233, 1999.
167. Glenn GM, Krober MS, Kepy P, McCarty J, Weir M: Pyridoxine as therapy in theophylline-induced seizures. *Vet Human Toxicol* **37**:342, 1995.
168. Asnis DS, Bhat JG, Melchert AF: Reversible seizures and mental status changes in a dialysis patient on isoniazid preventative therapy. *Ann Pharmacother* **27**:444, 1993.
169. Alvarez FG, Guntupalli KK: Isoniazid overdose: Four case reports and review of the literature. *Intensive Care Med* **21**:641, 1995.

170. Blowey DL, Johnson D, Verjee Z: Isoniazid-associated rhabdomyolysis. *Am J Emerg Med* **13**:543, 1995.
171. Shah BR, Santucci K, Sinert R, Steiner P: Acute isoniazid neurotoxicity in an urban hospital. *Pediatrics* **95**:700, 1995.
172. Aggarwal P: INH-induced neurotoxicity [Letter]. *J Assoc Physicians India* **42**:429, 1994.
173. Villar D, Knight MK, Holding J, Barret GH, Buck WB: Treatment of acute isoniazid overdose in dogs. *Vet Human Toxicol* **37**:473, 1995.
174. Bac P, Herrenknecht C, Binet P, Durlach J: Audiogenic seizures in magnesium-deficient mice: Effects of magnesium pyrrolidone-2-carboxylate, magnesium acetyltaurinate, magnesium chloride and vitamin B-6. *Magnes Res* **6**:11, 1993.
175. Jeremiah S, Povey S: The biochemical genetics of human γ-aminobutyric acid transaminase. *Ann Hum Genet* **45**:231, 1981.
176. Park J, Osei YD, Churchich JE: Isolation and characterization of recombinant mitochondrial 4-aminobutyric aminotransferase. *J Biol Chem* **268**:7636, 1993.
177. Osei YD, Churchich JE: Screening and sequence determination of a cDNA encoding the human brain 4-aminobutyrate aminotransferase. *Gene* **155**:185, 1995.
178. Medina-Kauwe LK, Tillakaratne NJK, Wu J-Y, Tobin AJ: A rat brain cDNA encodes enzymatically active GABA transaminase and provides a molecular probe for GABA-catabolizing cells. *J Neurochem* **62**:1267, 1994.
179. Medina-Kauwe LK, Nyhan WL, Gibson KM, Tobin AJ: Identification of a familial mutation associated with GABA transaminase deficiency disease. *Neurobiology of Disease* **5**:89, 1998.
180. Kwon OS, Park JH, Churchich JE: Brain 4-aminobutyrate aminotransferase: Isolation and sequence of a cDNA encoding the enzyme. *J Biol Chem* **267**:7215, 1992.
181. Kim YT, Song YH, Churchich JE: Recombinant brain 4-aminobutyrate aminotransferase: Overexpression, purification, and identification of Lys-330 at the active site. *Biochim Biophys Acta* **1337**:248, 1997.
182. Bhattacharya SP, Saha N, Wee KP: γ-Aminobutyric acid transaminase (GABAT) polymorphism among ethnic groups in Singapore — with report of a new allele. *Am J Hum Genet* **37**:358, 1985.
183. Jaeken J, Casaer P, Decock P, Corbeel L, Eeckels R, Eggermont E, Schecter PJ, et al: Gamma-aminobutyric acid-transaminase deficiency: A newly recognized inborn error of neurotransmitter metabolism. *Neuropediatrics* **15**:165, 1984.
184. Jaeken J: Disorders of neurotransmitters, in Fernandes J, Saudubray J-M, Tada K (eds): *Inborn Metabolic Diseases: Diagnosis and Treatment*. Berlin, Springer-Verlag, 1990, p 637.
185. Racagni G, Apud JA, Cocchi D, Locatelli V, Muller EE: Mini-review: GABAergic control of anterior pituitary hormone secretion. *Life Sci* **31**:823, 1992.
186. Gibson KM, Sweetman L, Nyhan WL, Jansen I, Jaeken J: Demonstration of 4-aminobutyric acid aminotransferase deficiency in lymphocytes and lymphoblasts. *J Inherit Metab Dis* **8**:204, 1985.
187. Gibson KM, Sweetman L, Nyhan WL, Jakobs C, Rating D, Siemes H, Hanefeld F: Succinic semialdehyde dehydrogenase deficiency: An inborn error of γ-aminobutyric acid metabolism. *Clin Chim Acta* **133**:33, 1983.
188. Sweetman FR, Gibson KM, Sweetman L, Nyhan WL, Chin H, Swartz W, Jones OW: Activity of biotin-dependent and GABA metabolizing enzymes in chorionic villus samples: Potential for 1st trimester prenatal diagnosis. *Prenat Diagn* **6**:187, 1986.
189. Choi EY, Jang SH, Choi SY: Human brain GABA transaminase is immunologically distinct from those of other mammalian brains. *Neurochem Int* **28**:597, 1996.
190. Scriver CR: The salience of Garrod's "molecular groupings" and "inborn factors in disease." *J Inherit Metab Dis* **12**:9, 1989.
191. Jakobs C, Bojasch M, Moench E, Rating D, Siemes H, Hanefeld F: Urinary excretion of γ-hydroxybutyric acid in a patient with neurological abnormalities. *Clin Chim Acta* **111**:169, 1981.
192. Pattarelli PP, Nyhan WL, Gibson KM: Oxidation of [U-^{14}C]succinic semialdehyde in cultured human lymphoblasts: Measurement of residual succinic semialdehyde dehydrogenase activity in 11 patients with 4-hydroxybutyric aciduria. *Pediatr Res* **24**:455, 1988.
193. Gibson KM, Goodman SI, Frerman FE, Glasgow AM: Succinic semialdehyde dehydrogenase deficiency associated with combined 4-hydroxybutyric and dicarboxylic acidurias: Potential for clinical misdiagnosis based on urinary organic acid profiling. *J Pediatr* **114**:607, 1989.
194. Jakobs C, Smit LME, Kneer J, Michael T, Gibson KM: The first adult case with 4-hydroxybutyric aciduria. *J Inherit Metab Dis* **13**:341, 1990.
195. Jaeken J, Casaer P, De Cock P, Francois B: Vigabatrin in GABA metabolism disorders. *Lancet* **1**:1074, 1989.
196. De Vivo DC, Gibson KM, Resor LD, Steinschneider M, Aramaki S, Cote L: 4-Hydroxybutyric acidemia: Clinical features, pathogenetic mechanisms, and treatment strategies. *Ann Neurol* **24**:304, 1988.
197. Shih VE, Younes MC, Gotoff JM, Dooling EC, Gibson K: Transient increase in CSF glycine in a patient with succinic semialdehyde dehydrogenase (SSADH) deficiency [Abstract]. *Am J Hum Genet* **47**:A166, 1990.
198. Onkenhout W, Maaswinkel-Mooij PD, Poorthuis BJHM: 4-Hydroxybutyric aciduria: Further clinical heterogeneity in a new case. *Eur J Pediatr* **149**:194, 1989.
199. Jakobs C, Jaeken J, Gibson KM: Inherited disorders of GABA metabolism. *J Inherit Metab Dis* **16**:704, 1993.
200. Rahbeeni Z, Ozand PT, Rashed M, Gascon GG, Nasser MA, Odaib AA, Subramanayam SB, et al: 4-Hydroxybutyric aciduria. *Brain Dev* **16**(Suppl):64, 1994.
201. Worthen HG, Ashwal AA, Ozand PT, Garawi S, Rahbeeni Z, Odaib AA, Subramanayam SB, et al: Comparative frequency and severity of hypoglycemia in selected organic acidemias, branched chain amino acidemia, and disorders of fructose metabolism. *Brain Dev* **16**(Suppl):81, 1994.
202. Gibson KM, Doskey AE, Rabier D, Jakobs C, Morlat C: Differing clinical presentations of succinic semialdehyde dehydrogenase deficiency in adolescent siblings from Lifu Island, New Caledonia. *J Inherit Metab Dis* **20**:370, 1997.
202a. Peters H, Cleary M, Boneh A: Succinic semialdehyde dehydrogenase deficiency in siblings: Clinical heterogeneity and response to early treatment. *J Inherit Metab Dis* **22**:198, 1999.
203. Gibson KM, Christensen E, Jakobs C, Fowler B, Clarke MA, Hammersen G, Raab K, et al: The clinical phenotype of succinic semialdehyde dehydrogenase deficiency (4-hydroxybutyric aciduria): Case reports of 23 new patients. *Pediatrics* **99**:567, 1997.
204. Matern D, Lehnert W, Gibson KM, Korinthenberg R: Seizures in a boy with succinic semialdehyde dehydrogenase deficiency treated with vigabatrin γ-vinyl-GABA). *J Inherit Metab Dis* **19**:313, 1996.
205. Uziel G, Bardelli P, Pantaleoni C, Rimoldi M, Savoiardo M: 4-Hydroxybutyric aciduria: Clinical findings and vigabatrin therapy. *J Inherit Metab Dis* **16**:520, 1993.
206. Gibson KM, Jakobs C, Ogier H, Hagenfeldt L, Eeg-Olofsson KE, Eeg-Olofsson O, Aksu F, et al: Vigabatrin therapy in six patients with succinic semialdehyde dehydrogenase deficiency. *J Inherit Metab Dis* **18**:143, 1995.
207. Gibson KM, Baumann C, Ogier H, Rossier E, Vollmer B, Jakobs C: Pre- and postnatal diagnosis of succinic semialdehyde dehydrogenase deficiency using enzyme and metabolite assays. *J Inherit Metab Dis* **17**:732, 1994.
208. Hodson AK, Gibson KM, Jakobs C: Developmental resolution of ataxia in succinic semialdehyde dehydrogenase deficiency. *Ann Neurol* **28**:438, 1990.
209. Roesel RA, Hartlage PL, Carroll JE, Hommes FA, Blankenship PR, Gibson KM: 4-Hydroxybutyric aciduria and glycinuria in two siblings [Abstract]. *Am J Hum Genet* **41**:A16, 1987.
210. Gibson KM, Hoffmann G, Nyhan WL, Aramaki S, Thompson JA: 4-Hydroxybutyric aciduria in a patient without ataxia or convulsions. *Eur J Pediatr* **147**:529, 1988.
211. Haan EA, Brown GK, Mitchell D, Danks DM: Succinic semialdehyde dehydrogenase deficiency — a further case. *J Inherit Metab Dis* **8**:99, 1985.
212. Hodson AK, Hartlage P, Roesel A, Gibson M: Succinic semialdehyde dehydrogenase deficiency: seizures and ragged-red fibers. *Cleveland Clin J Med* **56**(Suppl, Part 2):278, 1989.
213. Fletcher JM, Keenan RJ, Harrison JR, Johnson DW, Thomas DG: Basal ganglia abnormalities in sibs with succinic semialdehyde dehydrogenase deficiency [Abstract]. *J Inherit Metab Dis* **19** (Suppl):49, 1996.
214. Gibson KM, Jansen IV, Sweetman L, Nyhan WL, Johnson DA, Thompson JA, Goodman SI: Heterogeneity of clinical manifestations in 4-hydroxybutyric aciduria. *Ann Neurol* **20**:141, 1986.
215. Gibson KM, Aramaki S, Sweetman L, Nyhan WL, De Vivo DC, Hodson AK, Jakobs C: Stable isotope dilution analysis of 4-hydroxybutyric acid: An accurate method for quantification in physiological fluids and the prenatal diagnosis of 4-hydroxybutyric aciduria. *Biomed Environ Mass Spectrom* **19**:89, 1990.

216. Nyhan WL: *Abnormalities in Amino Acid Metabolism in Clinical Medicine.* Norwalk, CT, Appleton-Century-Crofts, 1984, p 187.
217. Brown GK, Cromby CH, Manning NJ, Pollitt RJ: Urinary organic acids in succinic semialdehyde dehydrogenase deficiency: Evidence of α-oxidation of 4-hydroxybutyric acid, interaction of succinic semialdehyde with pyruvate dehydrogenase and possible secondary inhibition of mitochondrial β-oxidation. *J Inherit Metab Dis* **10**:367, 1987.
218. Pitt JJ, Hawkins R, Cleary M, Eggington M, Thorburn DR, Warwick L: Succinic semialdehyde dehydrogenase deficiency: Low excretion of metabolites in a neonate. *J Inherit Metab Dis* **20**:39, 1997.
219. Bonham JR, Downing M, Pollitt RJ, Manning NJ, Carpenter KH, Olpin SE, Allen JC, et al: Quality assessment of urinary organic acid analysis. *Ann Clin Biochem* **31**:129, 1994.
220. Gibson KM, Sweetman L, Kozich V, Pijackova A, Tscharre A, Cortez A, Eyskens G, et al: Unusual enzyme findings in five patients with metabolic profiles suggestive of succinic semialdehyde dehydrogenase deficiency (4-hydroxybutyric aciduria). *J Inherit Metab Dis* 1998, In press.
221. Gibson KM, Lee CF, Chambliss KL, Kamali V, Francois B, Jaeken J, Jakobs C: 4-Hydroxybutyric aciduria: Application of a fluorometric assay to the determination of succinic semialdehyde dehydrogenase activity in extracts of cultured human lymphoblasts. *Clin Chim Acta* **196**:219, 1991.
222. Jakobs C, Michael T, Jaeger E, Jaeken J, Gibson KM: Further evaluation of vigabatrin therapy in 4-hydroxybutyric aciduria. *Eur J Pediatr* **265**:447, 1991.
223. Gibson KM, De Vivo DC, Jakobs C: Vigabatrin therapy in patient with succinic semialdehyde dehydrogenase deficiency. *Lancet* **2**:1105, 1989.
224. Gibson KM, Hoffmann GF, Hodson AK, Bottiglieri T, Jakobs C: 4-Hydroxybutyric acid and the clinical phenotype of succinic semialdehyde dehydrogenase deficiency, an inborn error of GABA metabolism. *Neuropediatrics* **29**:14, 1998.
225. Dietz B, Aksu F, Agiugah G, Witting W, Aygen S, Lehnert W, Jakobs C: Vigabatrin therapy in a 7-year-old boy with succinic semialdehyde dehydrogenase deficiency. *Monatsschrift Kinderheilkunde* **144**:797, 1996.
226. Daly DM, Hodson A, Gibson KM: Central auditory processing in a patient with SSADH deficiency. *Soc Neurosci Absts* **17**(Part I):892, 1991.
227. Chambliss KL, Gibson KM: Succinic semialdehyde from mammalian brain: Subunit analysis using polyclonal antiserum. *Int J Biochem* **24**:1493, 1992.
228. Jakobs C, Ogier H, Rabier D, Gibson KM: Prenatal detection of succinic semialdehyde dehydrogenase deficiency (4-hydroxybutyric aciduria). *Prenat Diagn* **13**:150, 1993.
229. Chambliss KL, Lee CF, Ogier H, Rabier D, Jakobs C, Gibson KM: Enzymatic and immunological demonstration of normal and defective succinic semialdehyde dehydrogenase activity in fetal brain, liver and kidney. *J Inherit Metab Dis* **16**:523, 1993.
230. Chambliss KL, Zhang Y-A, Rossier E, Vollmer B, Gibson KM: Enzymatic and immunologic identification of succinic semialdehyde dehydrogenase in rat and human neural and nonneural tissues. *J Neurochem* **65**:851, 1995.
231. Chambliss KL, Caudle DL, Hinson DD, Moomaw CR, Slaughter CA, Jakobs C, Gibson KM: Molecular cloning of the mature NAD(+)-dependent succinic semialdehyde dehydrogenase from rat and human: cDNA isolation, evolutionary homology, and tissue expression. *J Biol Chem* **270**:461, 1995.
232. Trettel F, Malaspina P, Jodice C, Novelletto A, Slaughter CA, Caudle DL, Hinson DD, et al: Human succinic semialdehyde dehydrogenase: Molecular cloning and chromosomal localization. *Adv Exp Med Biol* **414**:253, 1997.
233. Chambliss KL, Hinson DD, Trettel F, Malaspina P, Novelletto A, Jakobs C, Gibson KM: Two exon skipping mutations as the molecular basis of succinic semialdehyde dehydrogenase deficiency (4-hydroxybutyric aciduria). *Am J Hum Genet* **63**:399, 1998.
233a. Hogema BM, Jakobs C, Oudejans CBM, Schutgens RB, Grompe M, Gibson KM. Mutation analysis in succinic semialdehyde dehydrogenase (SSADH) deficiency (4-hydroxybutyric aciduria). *Amer J Hum Genet* **65**:A238, 1999.
234. Mamelak M: γ-Hydroxybutyrate: An endogenous regulator of energy metabolism. *Neurosci Biobehav Rev* **13**:187, 1989.
235. Hochachka PW, Mommsen TP: Protons and anaerobiosis. *Science* **219**:1393, 1983.
236. Mamelak M, Scharf M, Woods M: Treatment of narcolepsy with γ-hydroxybutyrate: A review of the clinical and sleep laboratory findings. *Sleep* **9**:285, 1986.
237. Gallimberti L, Gentile N, Cibin M, Fadda F, Canton G, Ferri M, Ferrara SD, et al: Gamma-hydroxybutyric acid for treatment of alcohol withdrawal syndrome. *Lancet* **2**:787, 1989.
238. Centers for Disease Control: Multistate outbreak of poisonings associated with illicit use of hydroxybutyrate [Editorial]. *JAMA* **265**:447, 1991.
239. Crush KC: Carnosine and related substances in animal studies. *Comp Biochem Physiol* **34**:3, 1970.
240. Schmidt G, Cubiles R: Comparative studies on occurrence of carnosine-anserine fraction in skeletal muscle and heart. *Arch Biochem Biophys* **58**:227, 1955.
241. Reddy WJ, Hegsted DM: Measurement and distribution of carnosine in rat. *J Biol Chem* **237**:705, 1962.
242. Margolis FL: Carnosine in the primary olfactory pathway. *Science* **184**:909, 1974.
243. Sakai M, Ashihara M, Nishimura T, Nagatsu I: Carnosine-like immunoreactivity in human olfactory mucosa. *Acta Otolaryngol* **109**:450, 1990.
244. Kalyankar GD, Meister A: Enzymatic synthesis of carnosine and related β-alanyl and γ-aminobutyryl peptides. *J Biol Chem* **234**:3210, 1959.
245. Stenesh JJ, Winnick T: Carnosine-anserine synthetase of muscle: Partial purification of the enzyme and further studies of β-alanyl peptide synthesis. *Biochem J* **77**:575, 1960.
246. McManus JR, Benson MS: Studies on the formation of carnosine and anserine in pectoral muscle of the developing chick. *Arch Biochem Biophys* **119**:444, 1967.
247. Duvigneaud V, Behrens O: Carnosine and anserine. *Ergeb Physiol* **41**:917, 1939.
248. Davey CL: Significance of carnosine and anserine in striated skeletal muscle. *Arch Biochem Biophys* **89**:303, 1960.
249. Davies E, Scriver CR: 1-Methylhistidinuria in man: A festive index [Abstract]. *Proc Soc Pediatr Res* 134, 1967.
250. McManus IR: Enzymatic synthesis of anserine in skeletal muscle by N-methylation of carnosine. *J Biol Chem* **237**:1207, 1962.
251. Boldyrev AA, Severin SE: The histidine containing dipeptides, carnosine and anserine: Distribution properties and biological significance. *Adv Enzyme Regul* **30**:175, 1990.
252. Araoma OI, Laughton MJ, Halliwell B: Carnosine, homocarnosine and anserine: Could they act as antioxidants in vivo? *Biochem J* **264**:863, 1989.
253. Kohen R, Misgav R, Ginsburg I: The SOD-like activity of copper:carnosine, copper:anserine and copper:homocarnosine complexes. *Free Radic Res Commun* **12-13**(Part I):179, 1991.
254. Avena RM, Bowen WJ: Effects of carnosine and anserine on muscle adenosine triphosphatases. *J Biol Chem* **244**:1600, 1969.
255. Brown CE, Antholine WE: Evidence that carnosine and anserine may participate in Wilson's disease. *Biochem Biophys Res Comm* **92**:470, 1980.
256. Hanson HT, Smith EL: Carnosinase: An enzyme of swine kidney. *J Biol Chem* **179**:789, 1949.
257. Rosenberg A: Purification and some properties of carnosinase of swine kidney. *Arch Biochem Biophys* **88**:83, 1960.
258. Lenney JF, George RP, Weiss AM, Kucera CM, Chan PWH, Rinzler GS: Human serum carnosinase: Characterization, distinction from cellular carnosinase, and activation by cadmium. *Clin Chim Acta* **123**:221, 1982.
259. Lenney JF, Peppers SC, Kucera-Orallo M, George RP: Characterization of human tissue carnosinase. *J Biochem* **228**:653, 1985.
260. Lenney JF: Carnosinase and homocarnosinosis. *J Oslo City Hosp* **35**:27, 1985.
261. Lenney JF: Human cytosolic carnosinase: Evidence of identity with prolinase and non-specific dipeptidase. *Biol Chem Hoppe Seyler* **371**:167, 1990.
262. Van Munster PJJ, Trijbels JMF, Van Heeswijk PJ, Schut-Jansen B, Moerkerk C: A new sensitive method for the determination of serum carnosinase activity using L-carnosine-(1-^{14}C) β-alanyl as substrate. *Clin Chim Acta* **29**:243, 1970.
263. Murphy WH, Lindmark DG, Patchen LI, Housler ME, Harrod EK, Mosovich L: Serum carnosinase deficiency concomitant with mental retardation. *Pediatr Res* **7**:601, 1973.
264. Pisano JJ, Wilson JD, Cohen L, Abraham D, Udenfriend S: Isolation of γ-aminobutyrylhistidine (homocarnosine) from brain. *J Biol Chem* **236**:499, 1961.

265. Abraham D, Pisano JJ, Udenfriend S: The distribution of homocarnosine in mammals. *Arch Biochem Biophys* **99**:210, 1962.
266. Skaper SD, Das S, Marshall FD: Some properties of a homocarnosine-carnosine synthetase isolated from rat brain. *J Neurochem* **21**:1429, 1973.
267. Bauer K, Hallermayer K, Salnikow J, Kleinkauf H, Hamprecht B: Biosynthesis of carnosine and related peptides by glial cells in primary culture. *J Biol Chem* **257**:3593, 1982.
268. Kish SJ, Perry TL, Hansen S: Regional distribution of homocarnosine, homocarnosine-carnosine synthetase and homocarnosinase in human brain. *J Neurochem* **32**:1629, 1979.
269. Perry TL: Cerebral amino acid pools, in Lajtha A (ed): *Handbook of Neurochemistry* 2d ed, vol 1. New York, Plenum, 1982, p 151.
270. Jackson MC, Scollard DM, Mack RJ, Lenney JF: Localization of novel pathway for the liberation of GABA in the human CNS. *Brain Res Bull* **33**:379, 1994.
271. Nakajima T, Wolfgram F, Clark WG: The isolation of homoanserine from bovine brain. *J Neurochem* **14**:1107, 1967.
272. Matsuoka M, Nakajima T, Sano I: Identification of α-(β-alanyl)-lysine in rabbit muscle. *Biochim Biophys Acta* **177**:169, 1969.
273. Nakajima T, Kakimoto Y, Kumon A, Matsuoka M, Sano I: α-γ-Aminobutyryl-lysine in mammalian brain: Its identification and distribution. *J Neurochem* **16**:417, 1969.
274. Perry TL, Hansen S, Schier GM, Halpern B: Isolation and identification of γ-aminobutyryl-cystathionine from human brain and CSF. *J Neurochem* **29**:791, 1977.
275. Westall RG: The amino acids and other ampholytes of urine: Unidentified substances expected in normal human urine. *Biochem J* **60**:247, 1955.
276. Block WD, Hubbard RW, Steele BF: Excretion of histidine and histidine derivatives by human subjects ingesting protein from different sources. *J Nutr* **85**:419, 1965.
277. Hubbard RW, Block WD: Urinary excretion of 1-methylhistidine and histidine in human subjects on low and high protein intake. *Fed Proc* **22**:320, 1963.
278. Butts JH, Fleshler B: Anserine, a source of 1-methylhistidine in urine of man. *Proc Soc Exp Biol Med* **118**:722, 1965.
279. Gardner ML, Illingworth KM, Kelleher J, Wood D: Intestinal absorption of the intact dipeptide carnosine in man, and comparison with intestinal permeability to lactulose. *J Physiol* **439**:411, 1991.
280. Cusworth DC, Dent CE: Renal clearances of amino acids in normal adults and in patients with aminoaciduria. *Biochem J* **74**:550, 1960.
281. Scriver CR, Davies E: Endogenous renal clearance rates of free amino acids in pre-pubertal children. *Pediatrics* **32**:592, 1965.
282. Perry TL, Hansen S, Love DL: Serum-carnosinase deficiency in carnosinemia. *Lancet* **1**:1229, 1968.
283. Burgess EA, Oberholzer VG, Palmer T, Levin B: Plasma carnosinase deficiency in patients with urea cycle defects. *Clin Chim Acta* **61**:215, 1975.
284. Bando K, Shimotsuji T, Toyoshima H, Hayashi C, Miyai K: Fluorometric assay of human serum carnosinase activity in normal children, adults and patients with myopathy. *Ann Clin Biochem* **21**:510, 1984.
285. Perry TL, Hansen S, Stedman D, Love D: Homocarnosine in human cerebrospinal fluid: An age-dependent phenomenon. *J Neurochem* **15**:1203, 1968.
286. Perry TL, Hansen S, Kennedy J: CSF amino acids and plasma-CSF amino acid ratios in adults. *J Neurochem* **24**:587, 1975.
287. Perry TL, Hansen S, Tischler B, Bunting R, Berry K: Carnosinemia: A new metabolic disorder associated with neurologic disease and mental defect. *N Engl J Med* **277**:1219, 1967.
288. Perry TL: Carnosinemia, in Nyhan WL (ed): *Heritable Disorders of Amino Acid Metabolism*. New York, Wiley, 1974, p 293.
289. Van Heeswijk PJ, Trijbels JMF, Schretlen E, Van Munster PJJ, Monnens LAH: A patient with a deficiency of serum-carnosinase activity. *Acta Paediatr Scand* **58**:584, 1969.
290. Terplan KL, Cares HL: Histopathology of the nervous system in carnosinase enzyme deficiency with mental retardation. *Neurology* **22**:644, 1972.
291. Fleischer LD, Rassin DK, Wisniewski K, Salwen HR: Carnosinase deficiency: A new variant with high residual activity. *Pediatr Res* **14**:269, 1980.
292. Gordon EDJR, Coulombe JT, Sepe SJ, Levy HL: A variant of carnosinemia with normal serum carnosinase activity in an infant. *Pediatr Res* **11**:456, 1977.
293. Leininger ML, Chapoy P, Charvet J, Vovan L, Louchet E: La carnosinémie: prémiére observation française. *Pédiatrie* **35**:341, 1980.
294. Hartlage PL, Roesel RA, Eller G, Hommes FA: Serum carnosinase deficiency: Decreased affinity of the enzyme for the substrate. *J Inherit Metab Dis* **5**:13, 1982.
295. Cohen M, Hartlage PL, Krawiecki N, Roesel RA, Carter AL, Hommes FA: Serum carnosinase deficiency: A non-disabling phenotype? *J Ment Defic Res* **29**:383, 1985.
296. Gjessing LR, Lunde HA, Morkrid L, Lenney JF, Sjasstad O: Inborn errors of carnosine and homocarnosine metabolism. *J Neural Transm* **29**(Suppl):91, 1990.
297. Tocci PM, Bessman SP: Histidine peptiduria, in Nyhan WL (ed): *Amino Acid Metabolism and Genetic Variation*. New York, McGraw-Hill, 1967, p 161.
298. Bando K, Ichihara K, Toyoshima H, Shimotuji T, Koda K, Hayashi C, Miyai K: Decreased activity of carnosinase in serum of patients with chronic liver disorders. *Clin Chem* **32**:1563, 1986.
299. Gjessing LR, Sjaastad O: Homocarnosinosis: A new metabolic disorder associated with spasticity and mental retardation. *Lancet* **2**:1028, 1974.
300. Sjaastad O, Berstad J, Gjesdahl P, Gjessing L: Homocarnosinosis: A familial disorder associated with spastic paraplegia, progressive mental deficiency, and retinal pigmentation. *Acta Neurol Scand* **53**:275, 1976.
301. Perry TL, Kish SJ, Sjaastad O, Gjessing LR, Nesbakken R, Schrader H, Loken AC: Homocarnosinosis: Increased content of homocarnosine and deficiency of homocarnosinase in brain. *J Neurochem* **32**:1637, 1979.
302. Lunde H, Sjaastad O, Gjessing L: Homocarnosinosis: Hypercarnosinuria. *J Neurochem* **38**:242, 1982.
303. Jackson MC, Lenney JF: Homocarnosinosis patients and great apes have a serum protein that cross-reacts with human serum carnosinase. *Clin Chim Acta* **205**:109, 1992.
304. Lunde HA, Gjessing LR, Sjaastad O: Homocarnosinosis: Influence of dietary restriction of histidine. *Neurochem Res* **11**:825, 1986.
305. Willi SM, Zhang Y, Hill JB, Phelan MC, Michaelis RC, Holden KR: A deletion in the long arm of chromosome 18 in a child with serum carnosinase deficiency. *Pediatr Res* **41**:210, 1997.
306. Wassif WS, Sherwood RA, Amir A, Idowu B, Summers B, Leigh N, Peters TJ: Serum carnosinase activities in central nervous system disorders. *Clin Chim Acta* **225**:57, 1994.
307. Butterworth RJ, Wassif WS, Sherwood RA, Gerges A, Poyser KH, Garthwaite J, Peters TJ, et al: Serum neuron-specific enolase, carnosinase, and their ratio in acute stroke: An enzyme test for predicting outcome? *Stroke* **27**:2064, 1996.
308. Okamura N, Otsuku S, Kameyama A: Studies on free amino acids in human brain. *J Biochem* **47**:315, 1960.
309. Tallan HH: A survey of the amino acids and related compounds in nervous tissue, in Holden JT (ed): *Amino Acid Pools: Distribution, Formation, and Function of Free Amino Acids*. New York, Elsevier, 1962, p 471.
310. Palo J, Saifer A, Mazelis F: Free amino acids in Tay-Sachs and normal human gray matter. *Clin Chim Acta* **22**:327, 1968.
311. Whelan DT, Scriver CR, Mohyuddin F: Glutamic acid decarboxylase and γ-aminobutyric acid in mammalian kidney. *Nature* **224**:916, 1969.
312. Zachmann M, Tocci P, Nyhan WL: The occurrence of γ-aminobutyric acid in human tissues other than brain. *J Biol Chem* **241**:1355, 1966.

PART 9

ORGANIC ACIDS

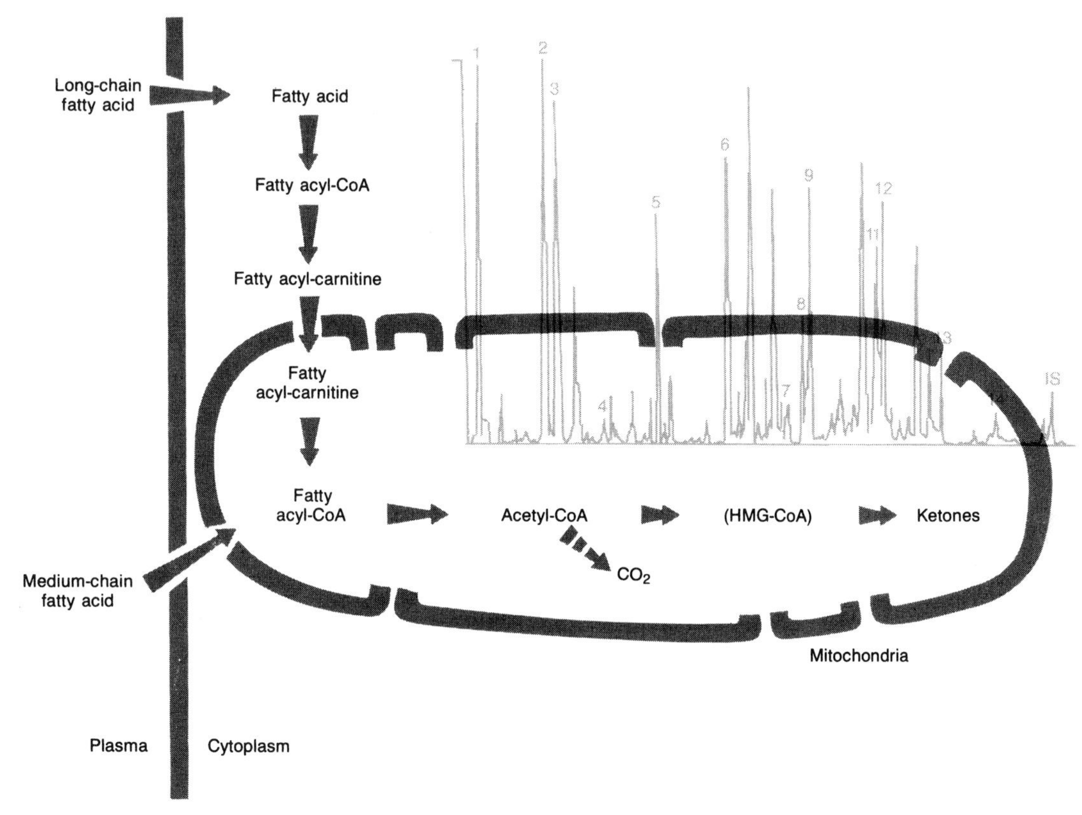

CHAPTER 92

Alkaptonuria

Bert N. La Du

1. **Alkaptonuria (MIM 203500; gene symbol *AKU*) is a rare, hereditary, metabolic disease in which homogentisic acid, an intermediary product in the metabolism of phenylalanine and tyrosine, cannot be further metabolized. The metabolic defect causes a characteristic triad of homogentisic aciduria, ochronosis, and arthritis.**
2. **The cause of the disease is a constitutional lack of the enzyme homogentisic acid oxidase. This enzyme normally exists primarily in the liver and kidney. It requires oxygen, ferrous iron, and sulfhydryl groups to open the ring of homogentisic acid.**
3. **The condition is inherited as an autosomal recessive disease. No metabolic method for the detection of heterozygotes has been devised; mutation analysis for this purpose is feasible. The molecular basis of alkaptonuria has been demonstrated to be defects in the gene coding for homogentisic acid oxidase (symbol *HGO*). The *AKU* and *HGO* genes are the same and map to human chromosome 3q21-q23; the nucleotide sequence (GenBank U63008) is divided into 14 exons over 60 kb of genomic DNA.**
4. **The relationships between the metabolic defect and the complications ochronosis and arthritis remain a challenging research problem of the future. Even though the lack of homogentisic acid oxidase is the ultimate cause of these complications, the mechanisms that bring them about are unknown.**

Alkaptonuria is a rare, hereditary, metabolic disease in which the enzyme homogentisic acid oxidase is missing. Because of this defect, homogentisic acid produced during the metabolism of phenylalanine and tyrosine cannot be further metabolized; instead, it accumulates and is excreted in the urine.

If urine containing homogentisic acid is allowed to stand for some time, it gradually turns dark as the acid is oxidized to a melaninlike product (Fig. 92-1). The polymerization is speeded by alkali, which explains why washing diapers of alkaptonuric infants with soap tends to make the stains more intense instead of removing them.

It is not surprising that such an obvious sign as dark urine led to the early recognition of this disease. Several persons reported in the medical literature of the sixteenth and seventeenth centuries who continually passed dark urine are presumed to have had alkaptonuria.[1] It is of interest that an Egyptian mummy dated approximately 1500 BC showed the characteristic x-ray changes of alkaptonuria—that is, extensive intervertebral disk calcification and narrowing of the hip and knee joints. Spectral analysis of pigment obtained from the hip region of the mummy resembled closely the reference pigment obtained by oxidation of homogentisic acid.[2] Although it was not possible to identify homogentisic acid in the tissues, this may well be the earliest case of alkaptonuria.

Boedeker described the first patient in whom the diagnosis was made with certainty in 1859.[3] He recognized that the reducing properties of his patient's urine were different from those of urine containing glucose (e.g., it did not reduce bismuth hydroxide), and he observed the darkening of the urine when alkali was added. He used the property of avid oxygen uptake in alkaline solution to give the substance the name "alcapton."[3] Two years later,[4] Boedeker spelled it "Alkapton," and since then, this condition has been known as *Alkaptonurie* in the German literature and as *alcaptonurie* in the French literature.

Boedeker precipitated homogentisic acid from alkaptonuric urine as the lead salt,[3,4] but was unable to determine its exact chemical structure. He did note the similarity of its behavior in alkali with that of known hydroxyphenols. Wolkow and Baumann[6] identified the substance as 2,5-dihydroxyphenylacetic acid and named it "homogentisic acid" because of its close structural similarity to gentisic acid (2,5-dihydroxybenzoic acid).

Once the aromatic structure of homogentisic acid was known suggestions were made about possible sources of this unusual urinary product. Tyrosine and phenylalanine, as aromatic components of the dietary proteins were, of course, the primary suspects (Fig. 92-2). In 1891, Wolkow and Baumann[6] demonstrated that feeding extra tyrosine, or a diet high in protein, greatly increased the amount of homogentisic acid excreted by an alkaptonuric patient. This initiated a series of clinical investigations by several groups to determine the pathway by which phenylalanine and tyrosine were metabolized to homogentisic acid. Numerous chemicals suspected of being intermediary compounds in this metabolic pathway were fed to alkaptonuric subjects. The expectation was that only compounds in the metabolic sequence would increase the excretion of homogentisic acid, but those not intermediate would fail to do so. Based on such studies, Neubauer suggested a scheme of tyrosine metabolism in 1909,[7] the first such scheme for any amino acid. He revised it slightly in 1928 to incorporate some additional data[8] (Fig. 92-3). Except for a few minor modifications, his basic scheme has remained unchanged for the past 70 years.

Studies on alkaptonuria have been of great importance in the development of ideas about diseases of metabolism. As a result of his studies on alkaptonuria, Sir Archibald Garrod developed his concept of inheritable metabolic diseases. In 1908, he discussed alkaptonuria in one of the Croonian Lectures,[1] and in the following year he expanded his ideas more completely in his classic book *Inborn Errors of Metabolism*.[9] He thought of alkaptonuria as a metabolic "freak" or "sport," comparable to a structural abnormality, rather than as a disease in the usual sense. He felt that patterns of metabolism varied in each individual according to the hereditary background and that alkaptonuria and the other inborn errors of metabolism represented extreme examples of such variant possibilities.[10] He suspected that these variations ultimately might depend on differences in the activity of specific enzymes, anticipating by many years the conclusion of Beadle and Tatum[11] that a single defective gene is correlated with a metabolic block in one enzymatic reaction.

In 1909, Garrod[9] wrote of the probable defect in alkaptonuria:

> **We may further conceive that the splitting of the benzene ring in normal metabolism is the work of a special enzyme, that in congenital alcaptonuria this enzyme is wanting, whilst in disease its working may be partially or even completely inhibited. The experiments of G. Embden and others upon perfusion of the liver suggest that organ as the most probable seat of the change.**

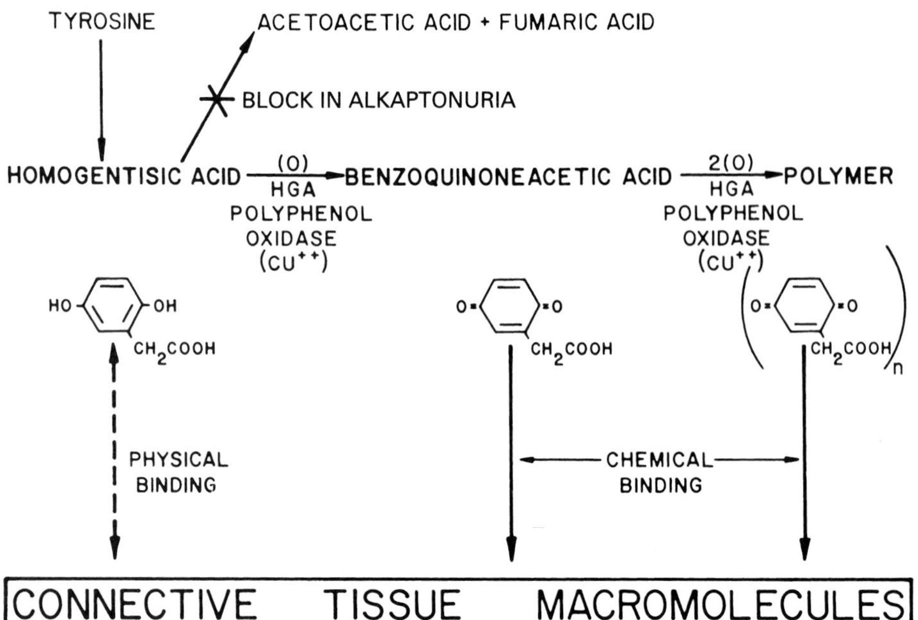

Fig. 92-1 Postulated scheme for the formation of ochronotic pigment in alkaptonuria. (*From Zannoni et al.*[5] *Used by permission.*)

Garrod's supposition that a specific enzyme is missing in alkaptonuria was supported through the years by many types of circumstantial evidence and was confirmed in 1958 by direct biochemical assay of alkaptonuric liver preparations.[12]

CLINICAL FEATURES

The cardinal features of alkaptonuria are signs due to the presence of homogentisic acid in the urine, pigmentation of cartilage and other connective tissues, and nearly always, in later years, arthritis.[13] The metabolic disorder does not appear to reduce the normal life span of affected subjects.[14]

Urinary Changes

According to the usual textbook description, people with alkaptonuria give a history of dark urine or urine which turns dark on standing. It should be emphasized that in a large number of alkaptonuric patients this finding is not observed. Many patients have never noted any abnormality in the color of their urine during childhood,[15–17] and diagnosis has been made only after they sought treatment for arthritis during their later years.[16–21] In some earlier cases, diagnosis followed a false positive test for diabetes[16,20] or the finding of the unusual and distinctive x-ray changes in the spine.[22] In others, the disease was not suspected until a surgical procedure revealed marked pigmentation of the cartilage.[23]

Alkaptonuric individuals on a normal diet void urine that at first is not an abnormal color and that may not darken for many hours if it remains at an acid pH. This is true even for patients with extensive ochronosis. It appears, therefore, that in instances in which freshly voided urine turns dark quickly, additional factors must be involved. Two factors that favor rapid darkening are the

CH_2CHNH_2COOH Phenylalanine — OH, CH_2CHNH_2COOH Tyrosine — OH, CH_2COOH, OH Homogentisic acid

Fig. 92-2 Formulas of phenylalanine, tyrosine, and homogentisic acid.

excretion of alkaline urine and a lower concentration than normal of vitamin C and possibly other reducing agents that are usually present in urine. It is well-known that vitamin C protects homogentisic acid against oxidation, and in the past, vitamin C was suggested as a therapeutic agent because of this property.[24]

The unusual findings in alkaptonuric urine can all be attributed to one abnormal constituent: homogentisic acid. No abnormal amino acid pattern[25] or other tyrosine metabolic products are found.[26] It has been reported that an alkaptonuric patient excreting about 7 g of homogentisic acid also excreted about 0.5 mg of gentisic acid per day.[27] The conversion of small amounts of homogentisic acid to gentisic acid has been demonstrated in homogenates of rabbit liver.[28,29]

Most of the diagnostic tests for alkaptonuria by urinalysis are based on the detection of homogentisic acid through its unusual chemical properties. Its ease of oxidation results in a gradual darkening of the urine downward from the surface until the entire sample is dark brown; this darkening is greatly accelerated by alkali. Further evidence of its ease of oxidation is the behavior of alkaptonuric urine in its reaction with Benedict's sugar reagent. Homogentisic acid not only reduces the copper reagent to yield a yellow-orange precipitate, but it also undergoes darkening because of the alkalinity of the reagent. The net effect is an orange precipitate in a muddy brown solution. The reduction of molybdate is the basis of the Briggs test, commonly used to follow the urinary excretion of homogentisic acid.[30] Reduction of silver in photographic paper emulsion has been used as a qualitative test[31] and as the basis of a quantitative method to measure this acid.[32] Homogentisic acid is not fermented by yeast, and it does not fluoresce under ultraviolet light.

A presumptive diagnosis of alkaptonuria can be made based on these nonspecific tests, but a more specific means for its identification is desirable. In many cases, homogentisic acid has been isolated from the urine after precipitation as the lead salt,[26,33] and the product shown to have the correct chemical composition and melting point. Paper chromatography of the urine directly, or of the product obtained by extracting acidified urine with ether, furnishes a simple technique to identify homogentisic acid.[34] A specific enzymatic method has been developed[35] that permits the quantitative analysis of homogentisic acid in urine, blood, and other tissues.[35,36] Rapid analysis of homogentisic acid in urine and plasma is also now possible using an HPLC method.[37] A stable isotope dilution gas chromatography-mass spectroscopic method permits the measurement of homogentisic acid in normal human

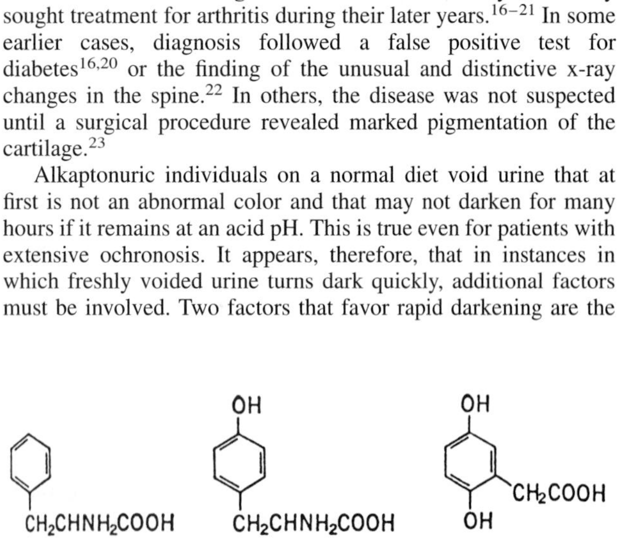

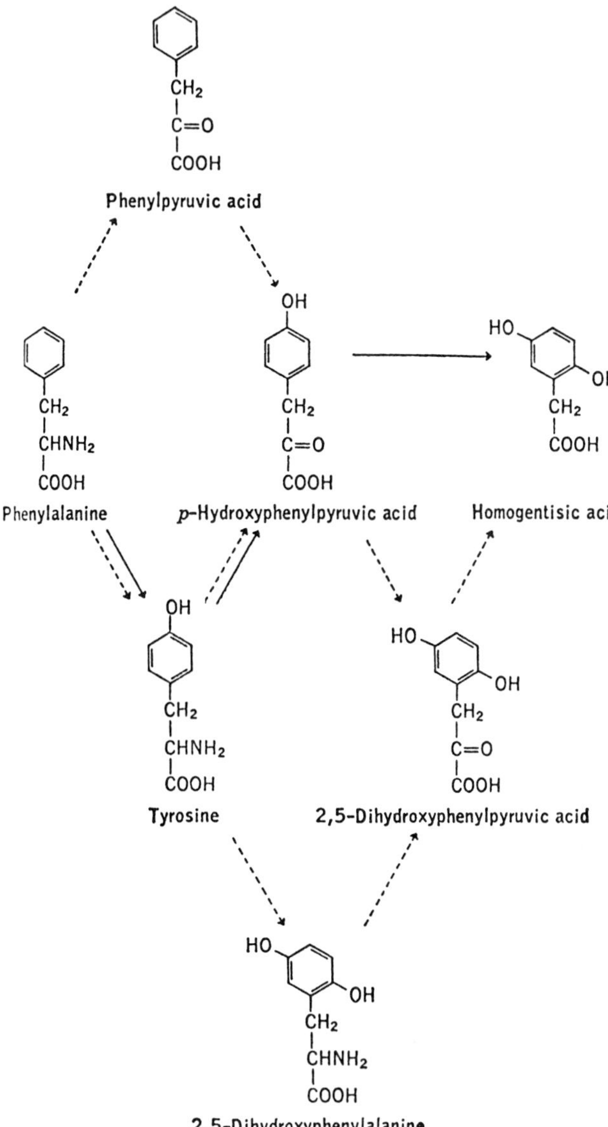

Fig. 92-3 Scheme of phenylalanine and tyrosine metabolism to homogentisic acid based on feeding experiments with alkaptonuric patients. The dotted arrows show various pathways considered possible by Neubauer;[8] the solid arrows indicate the pathway as it is viewed today. (*From Neubauer et al.[8] Used by permission.*)

plasma; the levels are reported to be 2.4 to 12 ng/ml, or about 1/1000th of those found in alkaptonuric plasma.[38]

Ochronosis

In 1866 Virchow described a peculiar type of generalized pigmentation in the connective tissues of a 67-year-old man.[39] The pigment was gray to bluish black grossly, but ochre microscopically, and for this reason, he named the condition "ochronosis." Although the patient's clinical history was not known, it is very likely that Virchow described for the first time the generalized pigmentation that gradually develops in alkaptonuric individuals. Actually, it was not until nearly 40 years later that Albrecht, in 1902,[40] clearly demonstrated the connection between ochronosis and alkaptonuria. Not long thereafter, Osler diagnosed ochronosis clinically for the first time in two alkaptonuric brothers.[41] He recognized that the pigmentation of the scleras and ears were signs of the same metabolic abnormality that had previously been detected only by changes in the urine.

Perhaps it is not unexpected that such a delay occurred in the clinical recognition of ochronotic pigmentation as a feature of alkaptonuria. Generally, the earliest change that can be detected externally is a slight pigmentation of the scleras or the ears, but these changes are rarely noticeable before the alkaptonuric patient is 20 to 30 years old. Pigmentation of the eye is found about midway between the cornea and outer and inner canthi, at the site of the insertions of the rectus muscles (Fig. 92-4). In addition, a more diffuse pigmentation may involve the conjunctiva and cornea.[42] The typical pigmentary changes in the ear cartilages similarly occur only after longstanding alkaptonuria. The cartilage is slate blue or gray, and feels irregular and thickened. It is first seen in the concha and the antihelix, and later in the tragus.

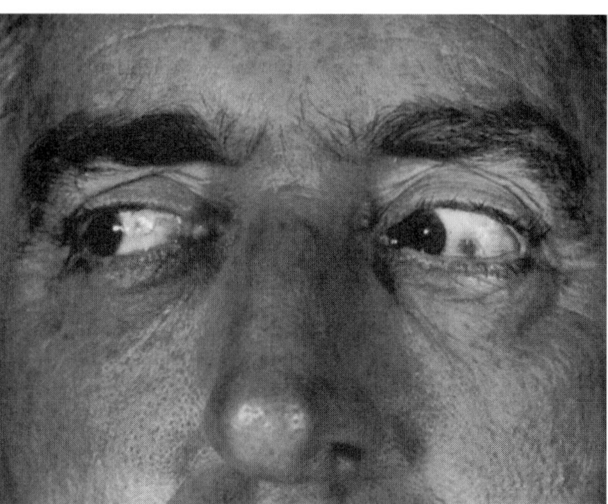

Fig. 92-4 The bilateral deposition of ochronotic pigment in the scleras, best seen in the left eye. (*From Bunim et al.[43] Used by permission.*)

It is sometimes reported that a dusky discoloration, corresponding to the underlying tendons, can be seen through the skin over the hands. The prominence of this pigmentation is variable, and in many instances, it is scarcely evident at all. The pigment appears in perspiration; clothing near the axillary regions may be stained, and the skin may have a brownish discoloration in the axillary and genital regions.[22]

In contrast to these rather minimal findings, the pigmentation observed in the tissues of an elderly alkaptonuric patient at operation or at postmortem is indeed striking.[39,44–47] Cartilage in many areas, particularly the costal, laryngeal, and tracheal cartilage, is densely pigmented and is described as being coal black in some areas. Pigmentation is also present throughout the body in fibrous tissues, fibrocartilage, tendons, and ligaments (Fig. 92-5). To a lesser degree, it is also found in the endocardium, the intima of the larger vessels, in various organs, such as kidney and lung, and in the epidermis. Microscopic examination shows the pigment to be deposited both intercellularly and intracellularly, and it may be either granular or homogeneous.[48] Electron microscopy of alkaptonuric synovial membranes,[49] hip joint tissue,[50] and articular cartilage[51] shows in greater detail the fragments of cartilage stained with pigment derived from homogentisic acid. Like melanin, the ochronotic pigment is bleached when treated for 24 h with hydrogen peroxide, and it is soluble in alkali, but only slightly soluble in hydrochloric acid. Thus, in many of its chemical characteristics the ochronotic pigment resembles melanin arising from 3,4-dihydroxyphenylalanine (dopa). Unfortunately, there is no specific stain to distinguish the ochronotic pigment of alkaptonuria from melanin derived from other sources. Although Fitzpatrick and Lerner[52] state that Becker's silver stain for melanin is not darkened by ochronotic pigment and that the latter is stained intensely black with polychrome methylene blue, Cooper and Moran[46] compared the staining properties of ochronotic pigment and melanin, employing a number of special stains. They concluded that no

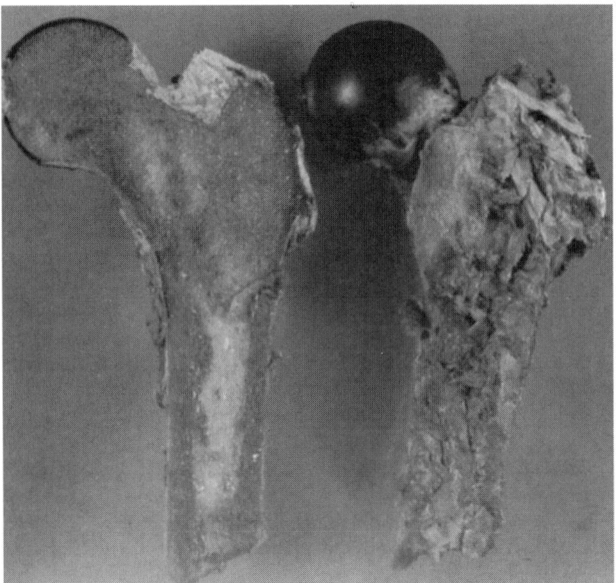

Fig. 92-5 Ochronotic pigmentation of the femur of a 56-year-old alkaptonuric patient. (*Courtesy of Dr. H. W. Edmonds of the Washington Hospital Center, Washington, DC.*)

specific differentiation could be made with any of the stains used. The Nile blue stains of Lillie best detected both pigments.[53]

The pigment deposited in ochronosis is presumably a polymer derived from homogentisic acid, but its exact chemical structure has not yet been determined. It is possible that some other constituents, in addition to homogentisic acid, are included in the product, just as melanin obviously contains more than a polymerized dopa unit—that is, a considerable quantity of sulfur.[54]

The formation of the pigment in the tissues may be entirely nonenzymatic, like the darkening of alkaptonuric urine. Solutions of pure homogentisic acid, made alkaline and aerated with air or oxygen, form a dark-brown product that has an ultraviolet absorption peak at 250 μm.[55] Unfortunately, the pigment deposited in the tissues of an alkaptonuric patient with ochronosis has not been analyzed in the same way, and so the relevance of the model polymerization to the *in vivo* process has not been established. Milch and Titus[56] suggested that because polymerization of pure homogentisic acid solutions does not proceed at neutral pH and low partial pressure of oxygen (as occurs in cartilage), it is likely that if molecular oxygen is involved in vivo, it involves the participation of an enzyme system present locally. This conclusion assumes not only that the composition steps of formation of the ochronotic pigment would be the same in vivo as in solutions of pure homogentisic acid, but that the pigment is both formed and deposited within the cartilage. It is not possible today to say to what degree enzymes play a role in the synthesis of the ochronotic pigmentation in alkaptonuria, although on the basis of their specificity, it seems reasonable to exclude the enzymes involved in the synthesis of melanin by way of dopa.

Mammalian (human, rabbit, and guinea pig) skin and cartilage contain an enzyme called "homogentisic acid polyphenol oxidase," which catalyzes the oxidation of homogentisic acid to an ochronotic-like pigment.[5] Benzoquinoneacetic acid has been identified as an intermediary metabolite in the oxidation. The enzyme is a copper protein, but it is clearly distinguished from tyrosinase by the finding that tyrosine, dopa, and other catechols are not substrates for this polyphenol oxidase. Earlier studies by La Du and Zannoni[57] demonstrated that p-quinones, such as benzoquinoneacetic acid, could form 1,4 addition products with sulfhydryl groups, and Stoner and Blivaiss[58] observed similar derivatives with the amino groups of glycine. Binding and chemical reactions of benzoquinone (or polymers derived from the acid) with the connective tissues may produce important chemical changes that alter tissue constituents and lead to ochronosis and ochronotic arthritis.[25] A possible scheme for the enzymatic oxidation of homogentisic acid and the formation of ochronotic pigment in the connective tissues of alkaptonuric patients is given in Fig. 92-1.

When Ochronosis is Not Due to Homogentisic Acid

Clinically, ochronosis due to alkaptonuria might be confused with the pigmentation of the skin, nail beds, conjunctivas, and cartilage seen in persons who have taken Atabrine for many months.[59,60] Of course, the history and the failure to find homogentisic acid in the urine should establish the diagnosis.

Another type of acquired ochronosis is that secondary to the prolonged use of carbolic acid dressings for chronic cutaneous ulcers.[61–66] This pigmentation is reversible and recedes after medication is discontinued, but carbolic acid dressings are rarely used today. A related chemical, hydroquinone, is the active ingredient in a number of skin-lightening creams and lotions. Long-term use of these preparations leads to a chemically induced ochronosis.[67–69] Associated inflammatory changes in the treated skin produce papular lesions that persist, although the hyperpigmentation gradually fades after hydroquinone treatment is discontinued.

It is possible that melanotic tumors might cause a generalized ochronosis also, but it is unlikely that a patient with such a condition would survive long enough for this complication to become evident.[68] In one case of alkaptonuria, the ochronotic pigment in the eye was misdiagnosed as a melanosarcoma, and the eye was removed.[70]

On the other hand, instances in which alkaptonuria, unaccompanied by ochronosis, have been diagnosed with certainty are extremely rare. From the nature and completeness of the metabolic defect, one expects that ochronosis would develop to some degree in all alkaptonuric patients if they live to middle age. A less than complete block in the pathway, due to a variant form of the condition, might also cause homogentisic aciduria without much tissue pigmentation. The two patients with alkaptonuria, who did not have ochronosis at autopsy,[71,72] had extensive tuberculosis. No mention was made of ochronotic changes in their connective tissues, but it is unlikely that they would have gone unnoticed if they were present to the degree found in most alkaptonuric patients.

Arthritis

"Ochronotic arthritis" is a regular manifestation of longstanding alkaptonuria. From the case reports in the literature, it appears that alkaptonuric arthritis occurs at an earlier age and is more severe in males than in females,[73] even though the sex incidence of alkaptonuria is roughly equal. This sex difference in ochronotic arthritis is reminiscent of the similar preponderance of gouty arthritis in males. Hench[74] has stated that ochronotic arthritis resembles rheumatoid arthritis clinically, but is like osteoarthritis roentgenographically. The earliest symptom observed is usually some degree of limitation of motion of the hip, knee joints, or, occasionally, the shoulders. There are nearly always periods of acute inflammation that may resemble rheumatoid arthritis, and later there is usually rather marked limitation of motion and ankylosis in the lumbosacral region.

X-rays may reveal changes considered almost pathognomonic of alkaptonuria.[22] The vertebral bodies of the lumbar spine show degeneration of the intervertebral disks with a narrowing of the space and dense calcification of the remaining disk material (Fig. 92-6). This is accompanied to a variable degree by fusion of the vertebral bodies. From the x-ray changes in the lumbar spine alone, it is often possible to be reasonably certain of the diagnosis of alkaptonuria. In contrast to rheumatoid spondylitis, little osteophyte formation and minimal calcification of the intervertebral ligaments are present. The large peripheral joints involved also differ from osteoarthritis in that the degenerative

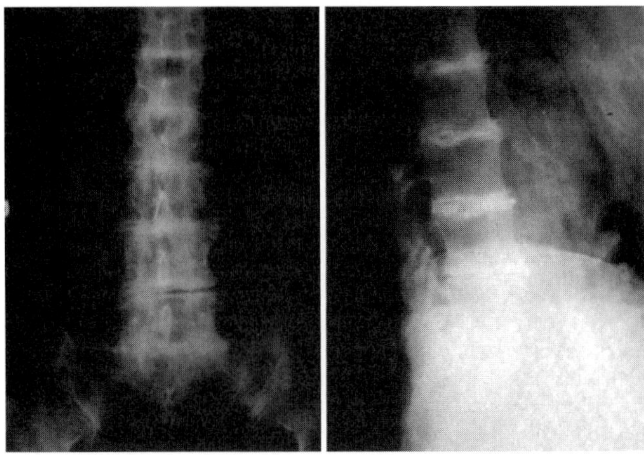

Fig. 92-6 Roentgenograms of the spine showing the typical narrowing and calcification of the intervertebral disks. (*From Bunim et al.*[43] *Used by permission.*)

joint changes in ochronotic arthritis are most commonly in the shoulder and hip, whereas such joints as the sacroiliac may be completely spared.

Calcification of the ear cartilage is another sign of the disease that may be observed on x-ray films. The large joints affected generally show degenerative osteoarthritic changes with calcified deposits most commonly in the muscle tendons around the large joints. Occasionally, free intra-articular bodies are found.[75] In contrast, the smaller joints usually show little or no abnormality.

The common occurrence of arthritis in the general population and the long period before its onset in patients with alkaptonuria no doubt account for the failure of the earlier investigators to appreciate the regular association of arthritis with alkaptonuria. The first case described by Boedeker was reported to have neuralgia of the lower lumbar spine. The early investigators considered alkaptonuria a completely benign disease without symptoms and of clinical importance only in that it might be misdiagnosed as diabetes. A review of the earlier case reports shows that in most instances osteoarthritis was mentioned, and, indeed, arthritis develops in nearly all alkaptonuric patients during their later years. The arthritic complications are often severe and painful and may lead to a completely bedridden existence in later life.

The relationship between the deposition of pigment in the connective tissue and the degenerative changes that occur in some areas of the connective tissues, particularly the cartilage and the intervertebral disks, remains unknown. It has been proposed that the pigment acts as a chemical irritant to accelerate a degenerative process in the cartilage, leading to changes similar to those in osteoarthritis.[19,75] The intra-articular injection of homogentisic acid into the knee joints of rabbits produced local lesions in cartilage and the soft tissues resembling those seen in alkaptonuria.[76] It is also possible that either the ochronotic pigment or homogentisic acid itself inhibits some of the enzyme systems involved in cartilage metabolism. Greiling[77] has shown that low concentrations of the pigment prepared by treating homogentisic acid with alkali inhibit the action of hyaluronidase on chondroitin sulfuric acid and on hyaluronic acid, but homogentisic acid does not act as an inhibitor at the same concentrations. Dihlmann et al.[78] extended these studies to show the inhibition of several additional enzymes, particularly glutamic dehydrogenase, hexokinase, and malate dehydrogenase by the oxidized, polymerized product of homogentisic acid.

Inhibition of lysyl hydroxylase[79] may be particularly important, because it would reduce the amount of hydroxylysine and the number of cross-linkage bonds, which are essential for the tensile strength of collagen fibers. Reducing agents, such as ascorbic acid and 1,4-dithiothreitol, competitively protect against inhibition of lysyl hydroxylase in the chick embryo, so the actual inhibitory agent may be an oxidation product of homogentisic acid, such as benzoquinoneacetic acid.

In recent years, it has been possible, using the techniques of molecular biology, to discover a number of molecular mutations that affect the structure of collagen,[80] some of which are responsible for hereditary forms of arthritis.[81] Whether homogentisic acid or its metabolites are responsible for inducing a similar type of change to reduce the cross-linkage in collagen structure and reduce its resistance to shearing stress in alkaptonuric subjects remains to be established. If the arthritic complications could be prevented or greatly reduced, the major clinical detriment of this disorder would be eliminated.

Other workers have evaluated the effects of homogentisic acid on articular chondrocytes.[82] Cytotoxic effects were noted with rabbit adult articular chondrocytes at homogentisic acid concentrations of 5 μg/ml or above; effects were seen with fetal articular chondrocytes at concentrations of 1 μg/ml. Another laboratory[83] has shown that hyaline cartilage incubated with the polymerized products of homogentisic acid oxidation develops an increased hardness and decreased elasticity. It is suggested that these changes, along with mechanical stress to the large joints, lead to cartilage destruction.[84]

Other Findings in Alkaptonuria

In addition to the features mentioned above, other complications seem to occur in alkaptonuric patients with a greater frequency than might be anticipated in the general population. The relationship between ochronosis and cardiovascular disease is not clearly established, but a review of the case histories of alkaptonuric patients indicates that there is a high incidence of heart disease.[20] In 1910, Beddard[64] tabulated the autopsy findings in 11 patients with ochronosis (none due to treatment with phenol) and found that 8 had chronic mitral and aortic valvulitis, 1 had an aortic aneurysm, and 1 had an aneurysm of the left ventricle. Other investigators[44,85] have noted generalized arteriosclerosis and calcification in the heart valves and of the annulus of the aortic and mitral valves.[45,86] Myocardial infarction was a common cause of death in this group.

Other complications regularly found in alkaptonuric patients are ruptured intervertebral disks,[87] prostatitis,[15,20,88,89] and renal stones.[89] Clinical case reports on new cases of alkaptonuria should be encouraged so that additional phenomena related to this metabolic disease are revealed. One patient with alkaptonuria with polycythemia,[90] one with nephrocalcinosis,[91] and one with severe renal disease called "ochronotic nephrosis,"[46] remain isolated examples, presumably because of chance association with other diseases. Remember that conditions that favor the expression of alkaptonuria, such as consanguineous marriages, would also favor the manifestation of other recessive but unrelated traits.

SYNTHESIS AND DEGRADATION OF HOMOGENTISIC ACID

Biosynthesis

In mammals most of the dietary phenylalanine and tyrosine is oxidized to acetoacetic acid by enzyme systems localized primarily in the liver and kidney. The scheme of this metabolic pathway is shown in Fig. 92-7. Reviews of phenylalanine and tyrosine metabolism[92–94] (see also Chaps. 77 and 79) may be consulted for the detailed experimental evidence supporting each of the steps in this scheme. As mentioned above, the scheme is based on the earlier studies with alkaptonuric patients and many animal experiments in vivo. It has been revised and extended particularly during the past 45 years by a large number of experiments on tyrosine metabolism in vitro. These include studies with isotopically labeled phenylalanine and tyrosine to determine the fate of each of the carbon atoms in the aromatic ring and the side chain[95–99] and the distribution of the isotope in the

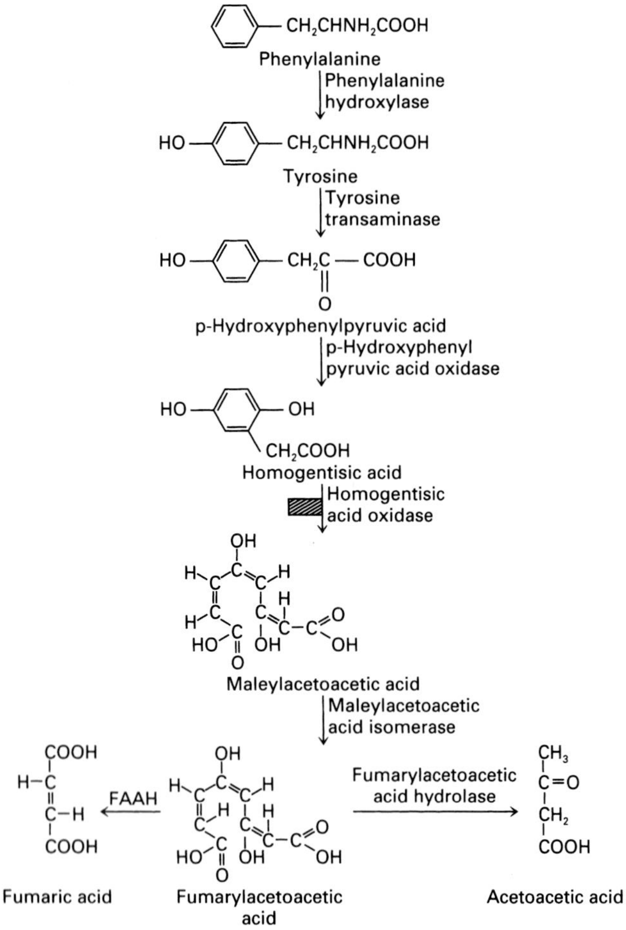

Fig. 92-7 Enzymatic steps in the oxidation of phenylalanine and tyrosine to acetoacetic acid. → = block in alkaptonuria.

products—CO_2, acetoacetic acid, and fumaric acid. These experiments showed that two of the four carbon atoms of acetoacetic acid were derived from carbon atoms 2 and 3 of the side chain, and that the other two came from the ring. Furthermore, the position of the isotope from the ring carbon atoms indicated that the side chain must have migrated during the oxidation (Fig. 92-8), in agreement with the scheme postulated earlier by Neubauer[8] (see Fig. 92-3), to account for the 2,5-dihydroxyphenyl

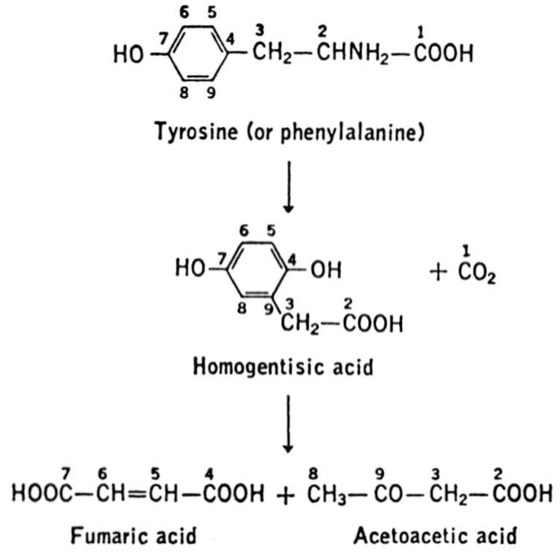

Fig. 92-8 Fate of each of the carbon atoms of phenylalanine or tyrosine based on experiments with the amino acids labeled with isotopic carbon.

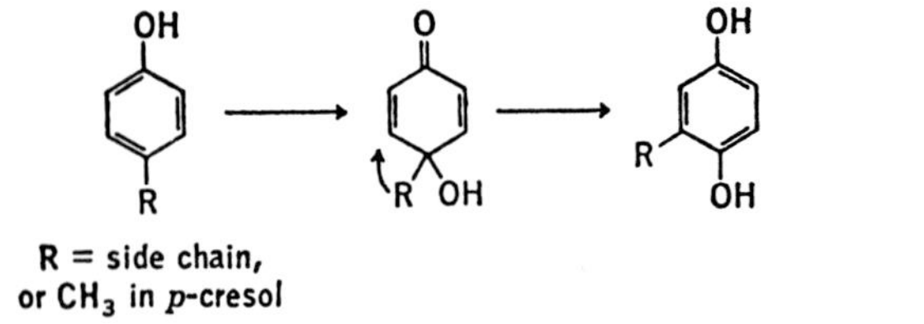

Fig. 92-9 Formation of quinol intermediate and migration of the substituent (CH_3 in *p*-cresol or side chain) in *p*-hydroxyphenylpyruvic acid oxidation.

intermediary product, homogentisic acid, from the 4-hydroxyphenyl substrates. This rearrangement was believed to involve a quinol intermediate with a migration of the side chain (Fig. 92-9), so that the hydroxylation of the ring, migration, and the oxidative decarboxylation of the side chain all take place as a complex, single step.[101–103] Although there was once some debate about homogentisic acid being a normal intermediary compound in this scheme,[104–106] this is no longer questioned.

The present scheme of tyrosine oxidation is therefore very much like Neubauer's scheme (see Fig. 92-3) in the steps leading to the formation of homogentisic acid, with the notable exception that neither 2,5-dihydroxyphenylalanine nor 2,5-dihydroxyphenylpyruvic acid is considered an intermediate. Both compounds produced extra homogentisic acid when fed to alkaptonuric patients,[7,32] but they were found to be inactive as substrates when tested with mammalian liver preparations, which oxidize tyrosine or *p*-hydroxyphenylpyruvic acid to homogentisic acid.[34,107–109] These results also exclude the alternative pathway suggested by Neuberger in 1947, in which tyrosine would be oxidized first to 2,5-dihydroxyphenylalanine and then either through 2,5-dihydroxyphenylpyruvic acid or 2,5-dihydroxyphenylethylamine to homogentisic acid.[110]

Metabolic Defect in Alkaptonuria

Even though Garrod suggested in 1909[9] that the metabolic defect in alkaptonuria was the absence of the liver enzyme catalyzing the oxidation of homogentisic acid, other possible explanations were suggested from time to time by other investigators. However, the direct analysis of the enzymes involved in tyrosine metabolism in biopsied normal and alkaptonuric liver showed that only homogentisic acid oxidase was missing in alkaptonuric liver, and that all the other enzymes involved in tyrosine metabolism to acetoacetic acid were present with about the same activity as in normal liver[12,43] (Table 92-1). Evidence was also obtained that the lack of activity was not due to the presence of inhibitor or to the lack of any known cofactor.[12] It is now reasonable to define the defect in alkaptonuria as the failure to synthesize active homogentisic acid

Table 92-1 Activity of Tyrosine Oxidation Enzymes in Alkaptonuric and Nonalkaptonuric Human Liver Homogenate

	Enzyme Activity μM Substrate Oxidized (h·g) Liver	
Enzymes	Nonalkaptonuric	Alkaptonuric
Tyrosine transaminase	36	32
p-Hydroxyphenylpyruvic acid oxidase	67	46
Homogentisic acid oxidase	268	< 0.048
Maleylacetoacetic acid isomerase*	960	780
Fumarylacetoacetic acid hydrolase	288	222

*Units calculated as Δ log density (h·0.1 g) wet weight liver.[111]

SOURCE: From La Du et al.[12]

oxidase and to attribute all the findings in alkaptonuria to this specific enzymatic defect. Whether these individuals form a catalytically inactive protein, differing perhaps only slightly in structure from active homogentisic acid oxidase, or whether they produce no protein at all resembling the enzyme, is still unknown, but molecular biology techniques are beginning to answer such questions.

Later, the opportunity to obtain autopsy samples of kidney tissue from two alkaptonuric patients made it possible to show that homogentisic acid oxidase is also absent in alkaptonuric kidney, but that the other enzymes involved in the oxidation of tyrosine to acetoacetic acid can easily be detected.[112] Homogentisic acid oxidase could be demonstrated in nonalkaptonuric human kidney autopsy samples. Thus, the genetic defect in alkaptonuria is not limited to the synthesis of homogentisic acid oxidase in liver; it appears to affect the synthesis of the enzyme wherever it is normally present. This is of theoretical interest from the viewpoint of the genetic control and tissue specificity of enzymes, and it may be of some practical value in the detection of the carrier trait in relatives of alkaptonuric patients. It might be possible to show a decreased amount of enzyme in carriers of the trait by a direct assay of the enzymes in a tissue more accessible than liver or kidney, rather than to determine it indirectly by the reduced rate of metabolism of homogentisic acid in an oral tolerance test.

[^{14}C]Carboxyl-labeled homogentisic acid injected intravenously in two alkaptonuric patients was over 90 percent excreted in the urine without change. In contrast, only 3.2 percent was excreted by a control patient, and over 95 percent was oxidized to $^{14}CO_2$ within 12 h.[113] The results support the conclusions from earlier enzymatic studies in vitro and metabolic balance studies in vivo that the enzymatic block is essentially complete in alkaptonuria.

The metabolic abnormality in alkaptonuria is present essentially from birth. Garrod noted, in 1901,[114] that staining of the diapers was scarcely evident 38 h after birth, although after 52 h they were deeply stained and continued to be thereafter. The reason for the delay in the excretion of homogentisic acid in newborn alkaptonuric patients is probably that the enzyme systems involved in tyrosine oxidation are not completely developed at birth, but increase in activity during the first few days after birth.[115] Once established, the defect continues relentlessly throughout life. No therapeutic agent has been found that substantially alters the degree of the defect. The amount of homogentisic acid excreted per day is usually from 4 to 8 g; changing the content of phenylalanine and tyrosine in the diet can alter it. In starvation there is a marked decrease in homogentisic acid excretion,[116] as would be expected, although Mittleback[117] showed that on a diet very low in protein, the alkaptonuric patient continued to excrete some homogentisic acid, presumably from the breakdown of tissue proteins.

Homogentisic Acid Oxidase

The enzymatic step that is missing in alkaptonuria is the further metabolism of homogentisic acid by an oxidative cleavage of the ring to yield maleylacetoacetic acid,[118] which, in turn, is isomerized enzymatically to fumarylacetoacetic acid[111,119,120] (see Fig. 92-7). The next step is hydrolysis to fumaric and acetoacetic acids by an enzyme that appears to be the same as that shown to hydrolyze a number of α-γ-diketo acids by Meister and Greenstein[121] and to hydrolyze triacetic acid.[122,123]

In 1950, Suda and Takeda[124] solubilized an enzyme from a strain of *Pseudomonas* adapted to tyrosine, which catalyzed the oxidation of homogentisic acid; they named it "homogentisicase." They also studied the properties of a similar enzyme from rabbit liver.[125] Homogentisicase, or, as it more generally called, "homogentisic acid oxidase," has been purified to some degree in several laboratories, and many of its properties have been described.[118,126–128] It belongs to the class of oxygenases. In the cleavage of the benzene ring, both oxygen atoms come from atmospheric oxygen, as indicated in experiments with ^{18}O.[129] The enzyme contains essential sulfhydryl groups and requires ferrous iron,[125,130] as do several of the other oxygenases involved in ring cleavage reactions, such as pyrocatechase,[131,132] hydroxyanthranilate oxidase,[133] and protocatechuic acid oxidase[134,135] (see Mason,[136] p. 126). No other cofactors are clearly implicated in this reaction. Although Suda and Takeda[125] presented evidence that one did exist in 1950, it now appears that a protective effect of glutathione may account for the earlier results.[137] There is also general agreement that the previously suggested requirement for ascorbic acid in this enzyme system[138] is an indirect one due to the requirement for ferrous iron. The only function that has been demonstrated for ascorbic acid in this reaction is to maintain iron in the reduced form.[125,139] Homogentisic acid oxidase activity in isolated rat hepatocytes depends on the oxygen tension.[140] The enzyme is inhibited by various quinones,[127] by sulfhydryl-binding agents,[130] and by metal-chelating agents such as α,α'-dipyridyl and o-phenoanthroline,[141] which reacts with ferrous iron.

Homogentisic acid oxidase activity can be measured manometrically, because the oxidation requires the uptake of two atoms of oxygen,[142,143] or spectrophotometrically,[142] by following the absorption of the product maleylacetoacetic acid at 330 nm, provided that product is stable and not further metabolized under the assay conditions. The enzyme is found in the soluble fraction of liver and kidney,[144] as are all the mammalian enzymes involved in the conversion of tyrosine to acetoacetic acid.[145] Homogentisic acid oxidase activity is highest in liver; there is less activity in kidney; and no significant activity has been found in any of the other tissues so far examined,[128,146] such as blood, salivary glands, germinal α epithelium, and muscle. This general distribution pattern has been found in rats, rabbits, guinea pigs, and pigeons.[128] In humans, too, it is highest in liver,[12] with appreciable activity also present in kidney.[112] The liver of the toad *Buffo marinus* has homogentisic acid oxidase activity as high as that found in mammalian liver.[147] The presence of the enzyme in some microorganisms adapted to tyrosine was mentioned above.[124,148]

The optimal pH for this enzyme is about 7,[125,126] and it is specific for homogentisic acid. Closely related compounds, such as o-hydroxyphenylacetic acid, *p*-hydroxyphenylacetic acid, and gentisic acid, are not oxidized,[126] nor are homogentisic acid ethyl ester and homogentisic acid lactone. The quinone formed by oxidizing homogentisic acid[149] does not appear to be an intermediate in the oxidation;[126] in fact, this quinone is an inhibitor of the enzyme.[7,126,150] The requirement for ferrous iron is apparently specific because other bivalent metals, such as Co^{++}, Zn^{++}, Mg^{++}, and Mn^{++}, cannot replace it.[125,150]

A report in the German literature[151] that gentisic acid was less well metabolized in an alkaptonuric patient than in a normal person led Garrod to conclude that the enzyme system defective in alkaptonuria must also catalyze the oxidation of some other 2,5-dihydroxyphenyl compounds.[1] The specificity of the enzyme rules out this possibility, and the reason for the results in the original study is not known. Perhaps more gentisic acid is excreted as the free acid, and less is conjugated in the alkaptonuric patient because of some inhibitory effect of homogentisic acid on gentisate conjugation. However, in one attempt to confirm this finding, the excretion of free gentisic acid was found to be about the same in an alkaptonuric patient as in nonalkaptonuric persons.[142]

Low concentrations of homogentisic acid have been identified in the urine and serum of nonalkaptonuric subjects by gas chromatography-mass spectrometry[152] following the administration of high doses of salicylates. Of course, gentisic acid is a normal minor metabolite of salicylate, but the presence of homogentisic acid is unexpected. The authors suggest that gentisic acid, or one of the other salicylate metabolites, inhibits homogentisic acid oxidase sufficiently to account for this finding.

Intermittent Alkaptonuria

There are a few reports in the literature of intermittent alkaptonuria, or instances in which it is reported that alkaptonuria has spontaneously disappeared.[44] In view of the finding that alkaptonuria is associated with the lack of a specific enzyme, it is difficult to imagine how this hereditary condition would undergo intermittent exacerbations and remissions or a spontaneous cure. Perhaps some of these cases of "alkaptonuria" were misdiagnosed and have some other reducing substances present in the urine. Other cases may be examples in which some agent, such as those described below (which can induce experimental alkaptonuria) in animals, has altered the activity of the enzymatic pathway, with resultant homogentisic acid excretion. Any further cases of alkaptonuria of this type should be carefully investigated with the specific methods now available to establish beyond reasonable doubt that homogentisic acid is the reducing substance excreted in the urine. In 1948, Fishberg reported[107] that a patient with autotoxic enterogenous cyanosis excreted up to 0.5 g of benzoquinoneacetic acid per day, the quinone corresponding to homogentisic acid. The amount excreted varied in inverse ratio to the ascorbic acid excretion. She also found, based on nonspecific tests, that patients with both rheumatic fever and scurvy excrete a similar quinone capable of producing methemoglobinemia. These results have been questioned by Consden et al.,[153] who found no benzoquinoneacetic acid excreted in scorbutic guinea pigs or in patients with rheumatic fever. They suggest that bacterial activity in the urine leading to nitrite formation may have been responsible for the results of the qualitative tests employed by Fishberg. The excretion of benzoquinoneacetic acid in the case of enterogenous cyanosis cannot be dismissed so easily. They suggest that the primary metabolite might have been homogentisic acid that was oxidized to the quinone by nitrite arising from bacterial activity. Others have found nitrite in the urine and blood of patients with enterogenous cyanosis.[154]

Metabolism of Homogentisic Acid

Under normal conditions no significant amounts of homogentisic acid are present in the urine, and, until recently,[38] none could be detected in normal plasma.[38] Leaf and Neuberger[155] found that feeding as much as 5 g homogentisic acid to normal adults produced no homogentisic aciduria. However, they found a transitory alkaptonuria following the intravenous injection of either 0.3 g or 1.0 g homogentisic acid. In these experiments, the plasma concentration never rose above 15 mg/100 ml plasma, and it returned to normal values within 30 min.

One might expect to find elevated plasma levels of homogentisic acid in alkaptonuric patients in view of the large quantity of this acid excreted per day. Neuberger et al.[26] found, however, that in a 7-year-old alkaptonuric girl, the fasting plasma level was not more than about 3 mg/100 ml plasma, and that this level did not increase significantly following the oral administration of 3 g L-phenylalanine. Nevertheless, within 6 h approximately 85 percent of the given amino acid could be accounted for as extra homogentisic acid in the urine. Neuberger et al. made a very significant observation regarding the excretion of homogentisic acid during this investigation. The plasma clearance data indicated that unless a large fraction of the urinary homogentisic acid was both synthesized and excreted within the kidney, glomerular filtration alone could not begin to account for the rapid rate of homogentisic acid excretion. In fact, its clearance approached 400 to 500 ml/min, about equal to the renal blood flow. Even though it is unusual for a normally occurring intermediate to be actively secreted by the kidney, it is not unusual for homogentisic acid. This conclusion is in agreement with the earlier observation of Katsch and Metz[156] that intravenous homogentisic acid given to an alkaptonuric subject did not increase the plasma concentration significantly.

Experiments using an enzymatic assay to estimate plasma homogentisic acid have confirmed these conclusions.[35] Alkaptonuric and nonalkaptonuric individuals were found to excrete homogentisic acid rapidly after oral administration, and the renal clearance data indicated active secretion by the kidney. The possibility[26] that there might be an important difference in the renal handling of homogentisic acid between normal individuals and alkaptonuric patients can be dismissed.

It appears that two factors serve to keep the plasma, and presumably the tissue, concentrations of homogentisic acid at a low level: the great capacity to metabolize this acid in the liver and kidney and the rapid renal tubular secretion of homogentisic acid. Even in the alkaptonuric patient, the renal mechanism is capable of effectively lowering the plasma level when extra homogentisic acid is given. This defense mechanism may be highly significant in view of the many years required for ochronosis to appear. It is quite possible that in the alkaptonuric person the tissues are only occasionally flooded with homogentisic acid and that this event has to be repeated many times over a period of years before tissue pigmentation occurs to a significant extent. Benzoquinoneacetic acid may be an intermediate in this process.

Experimental Alkaptonuria and Ochronosis

Spontaneous alkaptonuria has very rarely been reported in species other than human beings. A recent study describes a wild-caught Cynomolgus male monkey with this condition. The urine contained appreciable amounts of homogentisic acid, which was identified by gas chromatography-mass spectrometric analysis.[157] Another recent report mentions the finding of a mutant mouse with undetectable liver homogentisic acid oxidase and with homogentisic aciduria but no pigment deposits in the tissues. The authors suggest that the lack of ochronosis in the tissues might be explained by the presence of relatively high concentrations of endogenously produced ascorbic acid.[158] In contrast, there is an earlier paper by Lewis[159] describing a rabbit with urine that darkened on exposure to air and showed some other qualitative tests for homogentisic acid. The latter compound was never isolated or positively identified, and the rabbit died without offspring. There are also a few reports of generalized ochronosis in bones and connective tissues of cattle, dogs, and horses in which the tissues are described as being as black as coal; but, again, homogentisic acid was not identified in the urine of these animals with certainty.[18,160,161] Experimental alkaptonuria has been produced in rats and mice by feeding large quantities of phenylalanine or tyrosine (Table 92-2). It is also reported that vitamin C-deficient guinea pigs fed extra phenylalanine[139,162] or tyrosine[139] excreted homogentisic acid, as well as *p*-hydroxyphenylpyruvic acid and *p*-hydroxyphenyllactic acid. Other workers, however, have found only the latter two compounds and no homogentisic acid in similar experiments with vitamin C-deficient guinea pigs.[163] It should be noted that in some experiments of this type the claim has been made that homogentisic acid was excreted, even though the analytic methods employed would not distinguish between *p*-hydroxyphenylpyruvic acid and homogentisic acid.[164]

Experimental alkaptonuria has been produced in rats and mice by feeding large quantities of phenylalanine and tyrosine (see Table 92-2). There is also a report of transitory homogentisic acid excretion after feeding a human volunteer large amounts of L-tyrosine.[165]

Another type of experimental alkaptonuria has been induced in rats by a diet deficient in the sulfur-containing amino acids.[166] This was not corrected by giving ascorbic acid but was reversed by giving cysteine.[167] In this type of experimental alkaptonuria, proportionately less *p*-hydroxyphenylpyruvic acid is excreted than in the type that responds to ascorbic acid.

In addition to the above methods, the finding that homogentisic acid oxidase requires ferrous iron and can be inhibited by α,α'-dipyridyl was used by Suda and Takeda[125] to induce experimental alkaptonuria in guinea pigs. They injected α,α'-dipyridyl and fed extra tyrosine. The excretion of homogentisic acid in these animals was not corrected by administration of vitamin C.

In another investigation, it was found that human volunteers on a vitamin C-deficient diet for several months with frank scorbutic symptoms did not excrete increased amounts of urinary phenols when given 20 g tyrosine orally.[177] This is further evidence that there is no direct requirement for ascorbic acid in homogentisic

Table 92-2 Methods of Producing Experimental Alkaptonuria

Agent	Species	Comment	Reference
Feeding L-phenylalanine	Rats		168–170
	Mice		171
	Guinea pig	Excreted HGA and PHPP on vitamin C-deficient diet; defect corrected by vitamin C	139, 162
Feeding L-tyrosine	Rats	Believed by authors to be due to adaptive increase in tyrosine transaminase activity, but decrease in homogentisic acid oxidase activity also found	172
	Guinea pigs	On vitamin C-deficient diet; other workers find only PHPP or PHPL, but no HGA	138, 173, 163
		Defect corrected by ascorbic acid or folic acid	139, 173, 174
	Human beings	Large doses over 1 day; 50 g; 150 g; little or no HGA excreted	165
Diet deficient in sulfur amino acids	Rats	Effects reversed by cysteine, not by ascorbic acid	166, 167
	Rats	Effects reversed by tryptophan	175
Diet deficient in α, α′-Dipyridyl	Guinea pigs	Defect not altered by ascorbic acid	125, 176

HGA = homogentisic acid; PHPP = *p*-hydroxyphenylpyruvic acid; PHPL = *p*-hydroxyphenyllactic acid.

acid oxidation. It can be concluded that the majority of instances of experimental alkaptonuria are either the result of direct inhibition of homogentisic acid oxidase or are due to an imbalance in the various enzyme reactions sufficient to cause an accumulation of homogentisic acid and its urinary excretion.

Lin and Knox[172] reported that in experimental alkaptonuria in rats induced by a diet supplemented with extra tyrosine, no homogentisic acid was excreted for the first 3 or 4 days. Following this initial lag period, the degree of homogentisic acid excretion increased during the next several weeks. They attribute the gradual increase in intensity of the alkaptonuria to an adaptive increase in tyrosine transaminase activity. They believe that this type of alkaptonuria occurs because the relative rate of homogentisic acid formation overbalances the rate of homogentisic acid degradation. Their data also show a significant decrease in liver homogentisic acid oxidase in the experimental group, and this may contribute to the resulting alkaptonuria.

It is of interest to recall that the activity of the enzymes in the pathway following homogentisic acid oxidase was approximately normal in alkaptonuric liver (see Table 92-1). Because the only known endogenous source of maleylacetoacetic acid is the oxidation of homogentisic acid, it appears that normal levels of the isomerase are maintained in the absence of any substrate, and it is a constitutive rather than an adaptive enzyme.

Attempts to produce experimental alkaptonuria and ochronosis in animals by feeding special diets have met with very limited success. In most instances, the inhibition of homogentisic acid oxidase has been inadequate, and only a small fraction of the normal activity is sufficient to prevent the accumulation of the acid and deposition of ochronotic pigment. Prolonged feeding of L-tyrosine has produced some degree of ochronotic pigmentation of the connective tissues in animals. Bondurant and Henry[178] maintained rats on a diet supplemented with 12 percent tyrosine for 40 days. Gross examination of the dissected knee and hip joints revealed no structural abnormalities, but these tissues showed the deposition of pigment in the articular cartilage of the head of the femur and in opposing tibial and patellar surfaces of the knee joint. Microscopic examination showed focal accumulations of dark-brown pigment in the cytoplasm of chondrocytes in the epiphyseal cartilage in some animals.

Blivaiss et al.[179] induced experimental ochronosis in 4-week-old rats by supplementing their diet with 8 percent tyrosine for as long as 28 months. After this time, there were ochronotic-like pigment deposits in cartilage, such as the joint capsules, condyles, sternum, and trachea. Pathologic changes were found in the articular cartilage, which included abnormal alignment of chondrocytes with pigment inclusion, fibrillation, and fragmentation, as well as bone denudation. By histochemical techniques, they found an increase in nonsulfated acid mucopolysaccharides in the connective tissues. The histochemical changes were similar to those observed in the patella of a patient with alkaptonuria.

HEREDITARY ASPECTS

The first paper describing the inheritance of alkaptonuria was that of Garrod in 1902,[10] in which he presented evidence that this condition is congenital and familial, and that it occurs more often in families in which there are consanguineous marriages. He suggested that alkaptonuria might be transmitted as a single, recessive, Mendelian trait. He believed that homogentisic acid arose in the normal course of tyrosine metabolism and that consanguineous marriages brought to light a recessive defect in this metabolic process. In 1902, Bateson and Saunders[180] also suggested that the inheritance of a rare recessive factor might explain the incidence of alkaptonuria. These studies on the mode of transmission of alkaptonuria were among the first on hereditary metabolic diseases.

During the subsequent years, several examples were recorded in which direct transmission (i.e., parent and offspring affected) of alkaptonuria occurred, but Garrod believed these to be examples of a heterozygous individual mating with a homozygous alkaptonuric, not a dominant form of the disorder. As more family histories were described, the general conclusion about the recessive nature of the disease remained unchallenged.

In 1932, Hogben et al.[181] carefully summarized all the known cases of alkaptonuria reported to that time. Again, the recessive character of the disease was confirmed in nearly all the families, and it was observed that at least half of the affected individuals were offspring of consanguineous matings. Although there was an unequal sex distribution in their cases — 100 males and 46 females — the authors did not consider this to be an indication that the condition was semilethal in females. They noted that males were more often the probands in affected families and suggested that the higher incidence in males might be explained by the more frequent medical examination of males. They also noted that among infants there were slightly more females than males, in agreement with this explanation. Nevertheless, it is frequently stated in medical texts that the incidence of alkaptonuria is twice as high in males as in females. The paper by Hogben et al.[181] is obviously the source of this information.

Among the families reviewed by Hogben et al.[181] there were a few in which a dominant form of alkaptonuria had to be considered. In a family studied by Pieter,[182] the author felt compelled to conclude that a dominant type of alkaptonuria existed. In the end, such a conclusion depends on the predicted opportunity for marriage between homozygous and heterozygous individuals, and the frequency of the heterozygote in the general population, or, perhaps more exactly, the incidence of the

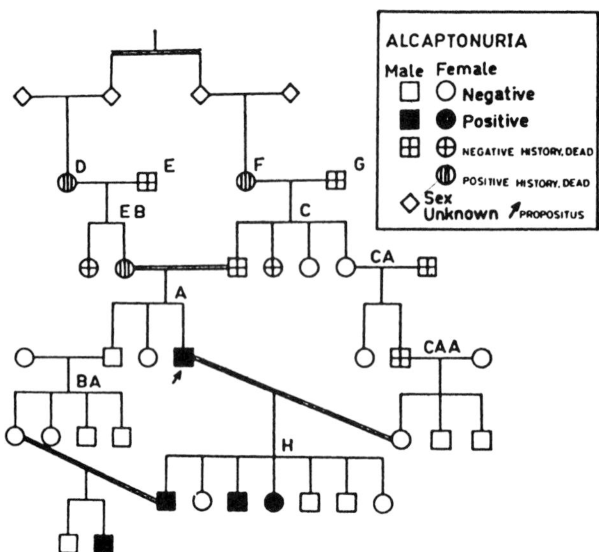

Fig. 92-10 Alkaptonuria in a Lebanese family. (*From Khachadurian and Abu Feisal.*[184] *Used by permission.*)

heterozygote within a selected population. The incidence of alkaptonuria in the general population can be only roughly estimated. At least 1000 cases have been described, but this is a conservative number, because new cases are generally not reported unless there are some other special features present. It is reasonable to assume, however, that alkaptonuria is less rare than was believed 50 years ago. It has been reported[183] that in a study in Northern Ireland by A. C. Stephenson, the incidence of alkaptonuria was from 3 to 5 per million individuals. This would give a considerably higher incidence of heterozygous individuals in the general population than assumed by Hogben et al.[181]

Remember that in the families in which direct transmission of alkaptonuria has been found the number of consanguineous marriages was very high. An excellent example of this is the kindred described by Khachadurian and Abu Feisal.[184] In this Lebanese family, there were eight alkaptonuric patients in five successive generations (Fig. 92-10). Careful investigations, however, showed that the grandmothers of the propositus were first cousins and that at least three consanguineous marriages existed in this family. This pedigree is particularly instructive because it illustrates how a recessive trait can appear to be dominant unless the entire family pedigree is known.

At present most, if not all, cases appear to represent the inheritance of a single autosomal recessive gene. This is supported by the biochemical finding that a single enzyme system is inactive in this condition and that only one clinical form of alkaptonuria is known. The few cases in which it has been considered as possibly a dominant form have not shown any clinical differences from the majority of cases.

An unusually high incidence of alkaptonuria has been observed in the Trencin District of Czechoslovakia, near the Slovakian-Bohemian border.[185] Nearly 200 alkaptonuric individuals have been identified among the 16,000 inhabitants.[186,187] Genetic analysis of the affected families shows a concentration of alkaptonuric patients within specific localities, and the authors propose that the most reasonable explanation is a founder effect, with genetic drift and inbreeding in the specific isolated hamlets of that region.[188]

The suggestion by Milch[189,190] that alkaptonuria is inherited as a dominant trait with incomplete penetrance seems unnecessarily complicated to explain the data at hand.[183] In fact, although the possibility of a dominant type of alkaptonuria cannot be excluded, no convincing evidence for it has yet been presented.

That a rare disease with recessive inheritance may be encountered more frequently in selected inbred populations complicates the estimation of the incidence of heterozygotes in the general population. It would be most helpful if a diagnostic test were available to detect the carrier state. In view of the nature of the enzymatic defect in alkaptonuric individuals, one might hope to find approximately half the normal amount of enzyme in the tissues of heterozygous individuals, as is apparently the situation in phenylketonuria and galactosemia. However, heterozygous carriers of alkaptonuria do not excrete homogentisic acid after an oral loading dose of L-tyrosine,[191] and measurements of the ability to metabolize homogentisic acid by an oral homogentisic acid tolerance test have so far shown no difference between relatives of alkaptonuric patients and normal controls.[192] These results may be due to the tremendous capacity of the liver (see Table 92-1) to metabolize this acid. Perhaps even when this reserve has been reduced to half, it may still not be exceeded by an oral tolerance test. In fact, assuming a liver weight of 1500 g, and assuming that the liver homogentisic acid oxidase is as efficient in vivo as under assay conditions in vitro, it can be calculated that the normal adult liver can metabolize over 1600 g of homogentisic acid per day.

In studies related to hereditary tyrosinemia, Laberge et al.[193] gave 25 to 100 mg/kg of homogentisic acid to four adult control subjects and two who were obligatory carriers of tyrosinemia as an oral tolerance test. The doses of homogentisic acid were rapidly cleared from the plasma, and excreted as free homogentisic acid and as a thioether conjugate, primarily of glutathione. The latter pathway is still another alternative system for removal of homogentisic acid, even if the level of homogentisic acid oxidase were reduced to half in heterozygous carriers of alkaptonuria.

MOLECULAR BIOLOGY OF THE GENETIC DEFECT

In the last few years, considerable progress has been made in our understanding of the genetic defect in alkaptonuria at a molecular level (see commentary by Scriver).[194] There was evidence from the coinheritance of alkaptonuria and other Mendelian diseases in some families, which indicated that chromosome 3 was the probable location of the gene causing alkaptonuria. Homozygosity mapping with polymorphic markers in two consanguineous families indicated the most likely region to be 3q2 (combined lod score = 4.3).[195] Another group also assigned the alkaptonuria gene (symbol, *AKU*) to human chromosome 3q.[196] Further supporting evidence came from another source,[197] which recently mapped the murine alkaptonuria gene (symbol, aku) to mouse chromosome 16 in a region of synteny between human chromosome 3 and that mouse chromosome.

The structural gene for human homogentisic acid oxidase (*HGO*) was finally cloned in 1996 by a research group in Madrid.[198] The nucleotide sequence (cDNA) is listed under these accession numbers at GenBank: U63008 and AF000573 (*HGO*) and AF045167 (*AKU*). These investigators also demonstrated that mutations of the *HGO* gene were associated with the alkaptonuria phenotype, and followed the expected segregation within the alkaptonuric family members. The same Spanish laboratory also showed that the *HGO* gene mapped to human chromosome 3q21-q23, the location of the *AKU* locus.[198] Their unusual approach to cloning the human *HGO* gene began by first cloning the homologous *HGO* gene in *Aspergillus nidulans* after induction by growing the mold on phenylalanine.[199] As described in fascinating detail by Scazzocchio,[200] the success of the Spanish group with the *Aspergillus* genetic analysis led to similar success cloning the human *HGO* gene using probes derived from the mold HGO and a spectrophotometric method to measure homogentisic acid by its absorption after conversion to maleylacetoacetic acid.[201]

The human *HGO* gene contains 14 exons extending over nearly 60 kb of DNA. There seems to be only one copy of the gene.[198] Two pedigrees were analyzed for mutations that might be expected to result in the loss of catalytic function. One mutation, P230S, was present in both parents of family M and in one parent of

A

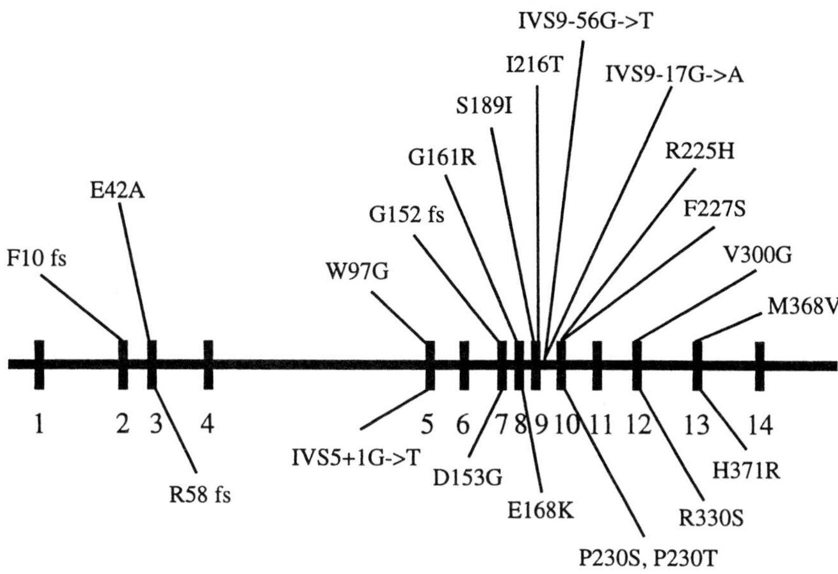

B

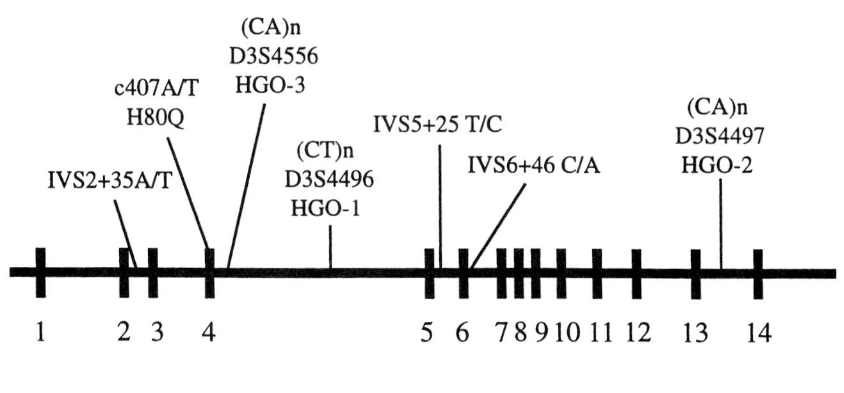

Fig. 92-11 Location of sites of mutations causing alkaptonuria (A) and polymorphisms (B) in the human homogentisic acid oxidase (HGO) gene. Twelve mutations and the polymorphic sites were reported by Beltran-Valero de Bernabe et al.,[205] two by Gerhig Schmidt et al.,[204] one by Higashino et al.,[206] and three by Peterson et al.[207] The 14 exons of the HGO gene are located roughly to scale on the diagrams. Modified from Figure 1 of Beltran-Valero de Bernabe et al.[205] with permission and valuable assistance from Dr. S. Rodriguez de Cordoba.

family S. Another mutation, V300G, was present in the other parent of family S. The affected children all had either a double dose of P230S, or were compound heterozygotes with both of these mutations. Expression experiments in *E. coli* of the wild type and P230S mutant forms of human *HGO* showed that this single amino acid change in the protein structure resulted in a complete loss of enzymatic activity.[198]

A more complete description of the human *HGO* gene has been published from the same Spanish laboratory[202] with further details about the regulatory regions' intronic and exonic characteristics. Several simple sequence repeats (SSR) in the introns were polymorphic in their Spanish population sample, and these markers will be very useful in tracing particular *HGO* mutations in different ethnic groups and geographic areas in the future.

Researchers at the University of Würtzberg have reported the cloning of the mouse *HGO* gene.[203] In collaboration with Slovak investigators at the Komensky University, they used the high degree of homology (93 percent) between human and mouse *HGO* to independently clone the human *HGO* gene.[204] They found the same 14 introns and coding sequence published by the Spanish group.[198] In four alkaptonuric patients of the Slovakian region, they found two novel mutations: G481A, in exon 8, and a single base insertion in exon 7 (454-457insG), which leads to a stop codon 21 codons downstream.[204] The elevated prevalence of alkaptonuria in Slovakia (up to 1 in 19,000) will be explored with these new molecular probes to determine founder effects and the distribution of *HGO* mutations in this selected population.

The Spanish laboratory has reported on the *HGO* mutations in 14 representative alkaptonuric subjects from 6 European countries, Algeria, and Turkey. Point mutations believed to produce nonfunctional enzymes were identified in 11 of the 14 exons, and several intronic defects were believed to be responsible for this metabolic disorder.[205]

Analyses of structural mutations associated with alkaptonuria in Japanese[206] and Finnish[207] subjects were recently reported. These mutations, and those found in the Slovak alkaptonuric individuals, are illustrated in Fig. 92-11.

The associated polymorphisms and repetitive sequences found to be associated with the *HGO* gene and its mutations permit the designation of several distinct haplotypes; five of the most representative have been characterized so far. These haplotypes will be very useful in exploring the long history and migration of alkaptonuria mutation carriers in different populations throughout the world.

TREATMENT

Attempts to treat alkaptonuria have been directed either toward correcting the underlying metabolic defect or preventing or reversing the pigmentation and arthritis changes. Galdston et al.[44] administered several vitamins, brewers' yeast, tyrosinase, insulin, and adrenocortical extract without altering the amount of homogentisic acid excreted by an alkaptonuric patient. Several groups have studied the effectiveness of vitamin C.[27,44,208,209] Although it corrects the alkaptonuria induced in guinea pigs by feeding large amounts of tyrosine,[138] it does not change the defect in the hereditary type of alkaptonuria.

Other agents, such as vitamin B_{12},[210] cortisone,[3,211,212] and phenylbutazone,[213] are without influence on the metabolic defect. Cope and Kassander's[214] report that cortisone corrected the metabolic error is difficult to interpret, because the authors claim this was a case of ochronosis without homogentisic acid in the urine.

In the past, it has been suggested that dietary phenylalanine and tyrosine be reduced to decrease the output of homogentisic acid. A severe restriction of the intake of these amino acids is not practical except for brief periods and might be dangerous to the patient if continued very long, but treatment with NTBC, the inhibitor of *p*HPPA oxidase (see Chapter 79), is an alternative, in principle.

Because from a practical standpoint the important consequence of the metabolic defect is that it leads to arthritic changes and pigmentation, effective therapeutic measures could be aimed at preventing or correcting these complications. It is possible, as Sealock et al. have pointed out, that increased tissue concentrations of ascorbic acid might prevent the deposition of ochronotic pigment, even though this treatment does not alter the basic metabolic defect.[24]

Murray et al.'s[79] observation that ascorbic acid protects lysyl hydroxylase from inhibition (via benzoquinoneacetic acid?) leads to the obvious suggestion that prolonged maintenance of relatively high tissue concentrations of ascorbic acid might delay, and possibly reduce, the degree of pathologic changes in the connective tissues. At least, extended clinical experience giving 1 g or so of ascorbic acid per day in divided doses is worth investigating.[215] It has been claimed that an alkaptonuric patient with arthritis had symptomatic improvement after taking 2 g of ascorbic acid per day.[216] Megadoses of ascorbic acid, however, should probably be avoided and could be counterproductive; at very high levels, ascorbic acid may compete with, and compromise the active secretion of homogentisic acid in the kidney.

The recent advances in our understanding of the molecular defect in alkaptonuria will no doubt encourage the application of genetic engineering to replace the missing enzyme by recombinant techniques. While it may be possible to achieve such a result at some time in the future, it is important now to be aware of the potential toxicity of some of the intermediary compounds that occur later in the tyrosine metabolism pathway—maleylacetoacetic acid and fumarylacetoacetic acid (see Fig. 92-7 and Chap. 79). Extensive conversion of homogentisic acid to these other metabolites in inappropriate environments, where these compounds may not be easily further metabolized, might lead to a greater toxicity for the patient than that experienced from homogentisic acid.[217]

REFERENCES

1. Garrod AE: The Croonian lecturers on inborn errors of metabolism. Lecture II. Alkaptonuria. *Lancet* **2**:73, 1908.
2. Stenn FF, Milgram JW, Lee SL, Weigand RJ, Veis A: Biochemical identification of homogentisic acid pigment in an ochronotic Egyptian mummy. *Science* **197**:566, 1977.
3. Boedeker C: Über das Alcapton; ein neuer Beitrag zur Frage: Welche Stoffe des Harns können Kupfer-reduction bewirken? *Rat Med* **7**:130, 1859.
4. Boedeker C: Das Alkapton; ein Beitrag zur Frage: Welche Stoffe des Harns können aus einer alkalischen Kupferoxydlösung Kupferoxydul reduciren? *Ann Chem Pharmacol* **117**:98, 1861.
5. Zannoni VG, Lomtevas N, Goldfinger S: Oxidation of homogentisic acid to ochronotic pigment in connective tissue. *Biochim Biophys Acta* **177**:94, 1969.
6. Wolkow M, Baumann E: Über das Wesen der Alkaptonurie. *Z Physiol Chem* **15**:228, 1891.
7. Neubauer O: Über den Abbau der Aminosaüren in gesunden und kranken Organismus. *Dtsch Arch Klin Med* **95**:211, 1909.
8. Neubauer O: Intermediärer Eiweisstoffwechsel. *Handb Norm Pathol Physiol* **5**:671, 1928.
9. Garrod AE: *Inborn Errors of Metabolism*. London, Frowde, Hodder & Stoughton, 1909.
10. Garrod AE: The incidence of alkaptonuria: A study in chemical individuality. *Lancet* **2**:1616, 1902.
11. Beadle GW, Tatum EL: Genetic control of biochemical reactions in neurospora. *Proc Natl Acad Sci U S A* **27**:499, 1941.
12. La Du BN, Zannoni VG, Laster L, Seegmiller JE: The nature of the defect in tyrosine metabolism in alcaptonuria. *J Biol Chem* **230**:251, 1958.
13. O'Brien WM, La Du BN, Bunim JJ: Biochemical, pathological and clinical aspects of alcaptonuria, ochronosis and ochronotic arthropathy. *Am J Med* **34**:813, 1963.
14. Srsen S, Vondräcek J, Srsnova K, Sväc J: Analyza dlzky zivota alkaptonurickych pacientov. [Analysis of the life span of alcaptonuric patients.] *Cas Lek Cesk* **124**:1288, 1985.
15. Cooper PA: Alkaptonuria with ochronosis. *Proc R Soc Med* **44**:917, 1951.
16. Minno AM, Rogers JA: Ochronosis: Report of a case. *Ann Intern Med* **46**:179, 1957.
17. Yules JH: Ochronotic arthritis: Report of a case. *Bull N Engl Med Center* **16**:168, 1954.
18. Martin WJ, Underdahl LO, Mathieson DR: Alkaptonuria: Report of 3 cases. *Proc Staff Meet Mayo Clin* **27**:193, 1952.
19. Crissey RE, Day AJ: Ochronosis: A case report. *J Bone Joint Surg [Am]* **32**:688, 1950.
20. Smith HP, Smith HP Jr: Ochronosis: Report of two cases. *Ann Intern Med* **42**:171, 1955.
21. Hammond G, Powers HW: Alkaptonuric arthritis: Report of a case. *Lahey Clin Bull* **11**:18, 1958.
22. Pomeranz MM, Friedman LJ, Tunick IS: Roentgen findings in alcaptonuric ochronosis. *Radiology* **37**:295, 1941.
23. Rose GK: Ochronosis. *Br J Surg* **44**:481, 1957.
24. Sealock RR, Gladston M, Steele JM: Administration of ascorbic acid to an alkaptonuric patient. *Proc Soc Exp Biol Med* **44**:580, 1940.
25. La Du BN, Zannoni VG: Ochronosis, in Wolman M (ed): *Pigments in Pathology*. New York, Academic, 1969, p 465.
26. Neuberger A, Rimington C, Wilson JMG: Studies on alcaptonuria II. Investigations on a case of human alcaptonuria. *Biochem J* **41**:438, 1947.
27. Sakamoto Y, Nakamura K, Inamori I, Ikeda S, Ichihara K: On the formation of gentisic acid. II. *J Biochem (Tokyo)* **44**:849, 1957.
28. Ichihara K, Ikeda S, Sakamoto Y: On the formation of gentisic acid from homogentisic acid by the liver extract. *J Biochem (Tokyo)* **43**:129, 1956.
29. Kanda M, Watanabe H, Nakata Y, Higashi T, Sakamoto Y: The formation of gentisic acid from homogentisic acid. IV. *J Biochem (Tokyo)* **55**:65, 1964.
30. Briggs AP: A colorimetric method for the determination of homogentisic acid in urine. *J Biol Chem* **51**:453, 1922.
31. Fishberg EH: The instantaneous diagnosis of alkaptonuria on a single drop of urine. *JAMA* **119**:882, 1942.
32. Neuberger A: Studies on alcaptonuria. I. The estimation of homogentisic acid. *Biochem J* **41**:431, 1947.
33. Medes G: Modification of Garrod's method for preparation of homogentisic acid from urine. *Proc Soc Exp Biol Med* **30**:751, 1933.
34. Knox WE, Lemay-Knox M: The oxidation in liver of L-tyrosine to acetoacetate through *p*-hydroxyphenylpyruvate and homogentisic acid. *Biochem J* **49**:686, 1951.
35. Seegmiller JE, Zannoni VG, Laster L, La Du BN: An enzymatic spectrophotometric method for the determination of homogentisic acid in plasma and urine. *J Biol Chem* **236**:774, 1961.
36. La Du BN, O'Brien WM, Zannoni VG: Studies on ochronosis. I. The distribution of homogentisic acid in guinea pigs. *Arthritis Rheum* **5**:81, 1962.
37. Bory C, Boulieu R, Chantin C, Mathieu M: Diagnosis of alcaptonuria: Rapid analysis of homogentisic acid by HPLC. *Clin Chim Acta* **189**:7, 1990.

38. Deutsch JC, Santhosh-Kumar CR: Quantitation of homogentisic acid in normal human plasma. *J Chromatogr B Biomed Sci Appl* **677**:147, 1996.
39. Virchow R: Ein Fall von allgemeiner Ochronose der Knorpel und knorpelähnlichen Theile. *Arch Pathol Anat* **37**:212, 1866.
40. Albrecht H: Ueber Ochronose. *Heilkd* **23**:366, 1902.
41. Osler W: Ochronosis: The pigmentation of cartilages, sclerotics, and skin in alkaptonuria. *Lancet* **1**:10, 1904.
42. Smith JW: Ochronosis of the sclera and cornea complicating alkaptonuria: Review of the literature and report of four cases. *JAMA* **120**:1282, 1942.
43. Bunim JJ, McGuire JS Jr, Hilbish TF, Laster L, La Du BN Jr, Seegmiller JE: Alcaptonuria: Clinical staff conference at the National Institutes of Health. *Ann Intern Med* **47**:1210, 1957.
44. Galdston M, Steele JM, Dobriner K: Alcaptonuria and ochronosis with a report of three patients and metabolic studies in two. *Am Med* **13**:432, 1952.
45. Lichtenstein L, Kaplan L: Hereditary ochronosis: Pathological changes observed in two necropsied cases. *Am J Pathol* **30**:99, 1954.
46. Cooper JA, Moran TJ: Studies on ochronosis. *AMA Arch Pathol* **64**:46, 1957.
47. O'Brien WM, Banfield WG, Sokoloff L: Studies on the pathogenesis of ochronotic arthropathy. *Arthritis Rheum* **4**:137, 1961.
48. Gaines JJ Jr: The pathology of alkaptonuric ochronosis. *Hum Pathol* **20**:40, 1989.
49. Kutty MK, Iqbal QM, Teh EC: Ochronotic arthropathy: An electron microscopical study with a view on pathogenesis. *Arch Pathol* **98**:55, 1974.
50. Gaucher A, Faure G, Netter P, Floquet J, Duheille J: Synovial membrane from ochronotic arthropathy of the hip joint. *Z Rheumatol* **39**:231, 1980.
51. Mohr W, Wessinghage D, Lenschow E: Die Ultrastruktur von hyalinen Knorpel und Gelenkkapselgewebe bei der alkaptonischen Ochronose. *Z Rheumatol* **39**:55, 1980.
52. Fitzpatrick TB, Lerner AB: Biochemical basis of human melanin pigmentation. *AMA Arch Dermatol* **69**:133, 1954.
53. Lillie RD: A Nile blue staining technic for the differentiation of melanin and lipofuscins. *Stain Technol* **31**:151, 1956.
54. Morner KAH: Zur Kenntnis von den Farbostoffen der melanotischen Geschwulste. *Z Physiol Chem* **11**:66, 1887.
55. Milch RA, Titus ED, Loo TL: Atmospheric oxidation of homogentisic acid: Spectrophotometric studies. *Science* **126**:209, 1957.
56. Milch RA, Titus ED: Studies of alcaptonuria: Absorption spectra of homogentisic acid-chondroitin sulfate solutions. *Arthritis Rheum* **1**:566, 1958.
57. La Du BN, Zannoni VG: Oxidation of homogentisic acid catalyzed by horseradish peroxidase. *Biochim Biophys Acta* **67**:281, 1963.
58. Stoner R, Blivaiss BB: Homogentisic acid metabolism: A 1,4-addition reaction of benzoquinone-2-acetic acid with amino acids and other biological amines. *Fed Proc* **24**:656, 1965.
59. Sugar HS, Waddell WW: Ochronosis-like pigmentation associated with the use of atabrine. *Ill Med J* **89**:234, 1946.
60. Ludwig GD, Toole JF, Wood JC: Ochronosis from quinacrine (atabrine). *Ann Intern Med* **59**:378, 1963.
61. Pick L: Ueber die Ochronose. *Berl Klin Wochenschr* **43**:591, 1906.
62. Reid E, Osler W, Garrod AE: On ochronosis. *Q J Med* **1**:199, 1908.
63. Pope FM: A case of ochronosis: With a note on the relationship of alkaptonuria to ochronosis by A.E. Garrod. *Lancet* **1**:24, 1906.
64. Beddard AP: Ochronosis associated with carboluria. *Q J Med* **3**:329, 1910.
65. Beddard AP, Pulmtre CM: A further note on ochronosis associated with carboluria. *Q J Med* **5**:505, 1912.
66. Brogren N: Case of exogenetic ochronosis from carbolic acid compresses. *Acta Derm Venereol (Stockh)* **32**:258, 1952.
67. Findlay GH, De Beer HA: Chronic hydroquinone poisoning of the skin from skin-lightening cosmetics. *S Afr Med J* **57**:187, 1980.
68. Tidman MJ, Horton JJ, MacDonald DM: Hydroquinone-induced ochronosis-light and electron microscopic features. *Clin Exp Dermatol* **11**:224, 1986.
69. Phillips JI, Isaacson C, Carman H: Ochronosis in black South Africans who used skin lighteners. *Am J Dermatopathol* **8**:14, 1986.
70. Skinsnes OK: Generalized ochronosis: Report of an instance in which it was misdiagnosed as melanosarcoma, with resultant enucleation of an eye. *Arch Pathol* **45**:552, 1948.
71. Fürbringer P: Beobachtungen über einen Fall von Alkaptonurie. *Berl Klin Wochenschr* **12**:330, 1875.
72. Von Moraczewski W: Ein Fall von Alkaptonurie. *Centr Inn Med* **17**:177, 1896.
73. Harrold AJ: Alkaptonuric arthritis. *J Bone Joint Surg Br* **38**:532, 1956.
74. Hench PS: Rheumatism and arthritis: Review of American and English literature of recent years. 9th Rheumatism review. *Ann Intern Med* **28**:310, 1948.
75. Sutro CJ, Anderson ME: Alkaptonuric arthritis: Cause for free intra-articular bodies. *Surgery* **22**:120, 1947.
76. Moran TJ, Yunis EJ: Studies on ochronosis. 2. Effects of injection of homogentisic acid and ochronotic pigment in experimental animals. *Am J Pathol* **40**:359, 1962.
77. Greiling H: Beitrag zur Entstehung der Ochronose bei Alkaptonurie. *Klin Wochenschr* **35**:889, 1957.
78. Dihlmann W, Greiling H, Kisters R, Stuhlsatz IW: Biochemische und radiologische Untersuchungen zur Pathogense der Alkaptonurie. *Dtsch Med Wochenschr* **95**:839, 1970.
79. Murray JC, Lindberg KA, Pinnell SE: In vitro inhibition of chick embryo lysyl hydroxylase by homogentisic acid. *J Clin Invest* **59**:1071, 1977.
80. Prockop DJ: Mutations that alter the structure of type I collagen. *J Biol Chem* **265**:15349, 1990.
81. Knowlton RG, Katzenstein PL, Moskowitz RW, Weaver EJ, Malemud CJ, Pathria MN, Jimenez SA, Prockop DJ: Genetic linkage of a polymorphism in the type II procollagen gene (COL2A1) to primary osteoarthritis associated with mild chondrodysplasia. *N Engl J Med* **322**:526, 1990.
82. Kirkpatrick CJ, Mohr W, Mutschler W: Experimental studies on the pathogenesis of ochronotic arthropathy. *Virchows Arch* **47**:347, 1984.
83. Eberle P, Mohr W, Claes L: Biomechanische Untersuchungen zur Pathogenese der ochronotischen Arthropathie. *Z Rheumatol* **43**:249, 1984.
84. La Du BN: Alcaptonuria and ochronotic arthritis. *Mol Biol Med* **8**:31, 1991.
85. Coodley EL, Greco AJ: Clinical aspects of ochronosis, with report of a case. *Am J Med* **8**:816, 1950.
86. Vlay SC, Hartman AR, Culliford AT: Alkaptonuria and aortic stenosis. *Ann Intern Med* **104**:446, 1986.
87. Eisenberg H: Alkaptonuria, ochronosis, arthritis, and ruptured intervertebral disk. *AMA Arch Intern Med* **86**:79, 1950.
88. Oppenheimer BS, Kline BS: Ochronosis, with a study of an additional case. *Arch Intern Med* **29**:732, 1922.
89. Young HH: Calculi of the prostate associated with ochronosis and alkaptonuria. *J Urol* **51**:48, 1944.
90. Rosenbaum H, Reveno WS: Polycythemia and alkaptonuria. *Harper Hosp Bull* **10**:36, 1952.
91. Goldberg BH, Penso JS, Stern LM, Bergstein JM: Alcaptonuria and nephrocalcinosis. *J Pediatr* **88**:518, 1976.
92. Lerner AB: Metabolism of phenylalanine and tyrosine. *Adv Enzymol* **14**:73, 1953.
93. Meister A: *Biochemistry of the Amino Acids*, 2nd ed. New York, Academic, 1965.
94. Zannoni VG, Malawista SE, La Du BN: Studies on ochronosis. II. Studies on benzoquinoneacetic acid, a probable intermediate in the connective tissue pigmentation of alcaptonuria. *Arthritis Rheum* **5**:547, 1962.
95. Schepartz B, Gurin S: The intermediary metabolism of phenylalanine labeled with radioactive carbon. *J Biol Chem* **180**:663, 1949.
96. Weinhouse S, Millington RH: Ketone body formation from tyrosine. *J Biol Chem* **175**:995, 1948.
97. Weinhouse S, Millington RH: Ketone body formation from tyrosine. *J Biol Chem* **181**:645, 1949.
98. Dische R, Rittenberg D: The metabolism of phenylalanine-4-C14. *J Biol Chem* **211**:199, 1954.
99. Lerner AB: On the metabolism of phenylalanine and tyrosine. *J Biol Chem* **181**:281, 1949.
100. Bamberger E: Über das Verhalten paraalkylierter Phenole gegen das Carosches Reagens. *Berl Dtsch Chem Ges* **36**:2028, 1903.
101. Schweizer J, Lattrell R, Heckler E: Conversion of *p*-hydroxyphenylpyruvic acid into homogentisic acid: Possible participation of *p*-quinol intermediates. *Experientia* **31**:1267, 1975.
102. Saito I, Chujo Y, Shimazu H, Yamane M, Matsuura T, Cahnmann HJ: Nonenzymatic oxidation of *p*-hydroxyphenylpyruvic acid with singlet oxygen to homogentisic acid. A model for the action of *p*-hydroxyphenylpyruvate hydroxylase. *J Am Chem Soc* **97**:5272, 1975.
103. Leinberger R, Hull WE, Simon H, Retey J: Steric course of the NIH shift in the enzymic formation of homogentisic acid. *Eur J Biochem* **117**:311, 1981.

104. Dakin HD: The chemical nature of alkaptonuria. *J Biol Chem* **9**:151, 1911.
105. Dakin HD: Experiments relating to the mode of decomposition of tyrosine and of related substances in the animal body. *J Biol Chem* **8**:11, 1910.
106. Wakeman AJ, Dakin ID: The catabolism of phenylalanine, tyrosine, and of their derivatives. *J Biol Chem* **9**:139, 1911.
107. Fishberg EH: Excretion of benzoquinoneacetic acid in hypovitaminosis C. *J Biol Chem* **172**:155, 1948.
108. La Du BN, Zannoni VG: The tyrosine oxidation system of liver. II. Oxidation of *p*-hydroxyphenylpyruvic acid to homogentisic acid. *J Biol Chem* **217**:777, 1955.
109. Edwards SW, Hsia DYY, Knox WE: The first oxidative enzyme of tyrosine metabolism, *p*-hydroxyphenylpyruvate oxidase. *Fed Proc* **14**:206, 1955.
110. Neuberger A: Synthesis and resolution of 2:5-dihydroxyphenylalanine. *Biochemistry* **43**:599, 1948.
111. Knox SWE, Edwards SW: The properties of maleylacetoacetate, the initial product of homogentisate oxidation in liver. *J Biol Chem* **216**:489, 1955.
112. Zannoni VG, Seegmiller JE, La Du BN: Nature of the defect in alcaptonuria. *Nature* **193**:952, 1962.
113. Lustberg TJ, Schulman JD, Seegmiller JE: Metabolic fate of homogentisic acid-1-14C (HGA) in alcaptonuria and effectiveness of ascorbic acid in preventing experimental ochronosis. *Arthritis Rheum* **12**:678, 1969.
114. Garrod AD: About alkaptonuria. *Lancet* **2**:1484, 1901.
115. Kretchmer O, Levine SZ, McNamara H, Barnett HL: Certain aspects of tyrosine metabolism in the young. I. The development of the tyrosine oxidizing system in human liver. *J Clin Invest* **32**:236, 1956.
116. Braid F, Hickmans EM: Metabolic study of an alkaptonuric infant. *Arch Dis Child* **4**:389, 1929.
117. Mittelbach F: Ein Beitrag zur Kenntnis der Alkaptonurie. *Dtsch Arch Klin Med* **71**:50, 1901.
118. Knox WE, Edwards SW: Homogentisate oxidase of liver. *J Biol Chem* **216**:479, 1955.
119. Edwards SW, Knox WE: Homogentisate metabolism: The isomerization of maleylacetoacetate by an enzyme which requires glutathione. *J Biol Chem* **220**:79, 1956.
120. Ravdin RG, Crandall DI: The enzymatic conversion of homogentisic acid to 4-fumarylacetoacetic acid. *J Biol Chem* **189**:137, 1951.
121. Meister A, Greenstein JP: Enzymatic hydrolysis of 2,4-diketo acids. *J Biol Chem* **175**:573, 1948.
122. Witter RF, Stotz E: The metabolism in vitro of triacetic acid and related diketones. *J Biol Chem* **176**:501, 1948.
123. Connors WM, Stotz E: The purification and properties of a triacetic acid-hydrolyzing enzyme. *J Biol Chem* **178**:881, 1949.
124. Suda M, Takeda Y: Metabolism of tyrosine. I. Application of successive adaptation of bacteria for the analysis of the enzymatic breakdown of tyrosine. *J Biochem (Tokyo)* **37**:375, 1950.
125. Suda M, Takeda Y: Metabolism of tyrosine. II. Homogentisicase. *J Biochem (Tokyo)* **37**:381, 1950.
126. Crandall DI: Homogentisic acid oxidase. II. Properties of the crude enzyme in rat liver. *J Biol Chem* **212**:565, 1955.
127. Schepartz B: Inhibition and activation of the oxidation of homogentisic acid. *J Biol Chem* **205**:185, 1953.
128. Crandall DI, Halikis DN: Homogentisic acid oxidase. I. Distribution in animal tissues and relation to tyrosine metabolism in rat kidney. *J Biol Chem* **208**:629, 1954.
129. Crandall DI, Yasunobu K, Krueger RC, Mason HS: Oxygen transfer by homogentisate oxidase. *Fed Proc* **17**:207, 1958.
130. Crandall DI: The ferrous ion activation of homogentisic acid oxidase and other aromatic ring-splitting oxidases, in McElroy WD, Glass HB (eds): *Symposium on Amino Acid Metabolism.* Baltimore, MD, Johns Hopkins University Press, 1955, p 867.
131. Suda M, Hashimoto K, Matsuoka H, Kamahora T: Further studies on pyrocatecase. *J Biochem (Tokyo)* **38**:289, 1951.
132. Stanier RY, Ingraham JL: Protocatechuic acid oxidase. *J Biol Chem* **210**:799, 1954.
133. Long CL, Hill HN, Weinstock IM, Henderson LM: Studies of the enzymatic transformation of 3-hydroxyanthranilate to quinolinate. *J Biol Chem* **211**:405, 1954.
134. MacDonald DL, Stanier RY, Ingraham JL: The enzymatic formation of *β*-carboxymuconic acid. *J Biol Chem* **210**:809, 1954.
135. J Dagley S, Patel MD: Microbial oxidation of p-cresol and protocatechuic acid. *Biochem J* **60**:35, 1955.
136. Mason HS: Mechanisms of oxygen metabolism. *Adv Enzymol* **19**:79, 1957.
137. Suda M: Homogentisic acid oxidizing enzyme. *Med J Osaka Univ (Suppl)* **8**:57, 1958.
138. Sealock RR, Silberstein HE: The control of experimental alcaptonuria by means of vitamin C. *Science* **90**:571, 1939.
139. Sealock RR, Silberstein HE: The excretion of homogentisic acid and other tyrosine metabolites by the vitamin C-deficient guinea pig. *J Biol Chem* **135**:251, 1940.
140. Jones DP, Mason HS: Metabolic hypoxia: Accumulation of tyrosine metabolites in hepatocytes at low pO_2. *Biochem Biophys Res Commun* **80**:477, 1978.
141. Schepartz B: Intermediate steps in tyrosine metabolism. *Fed Proc* **12**:265, 1953.
142. La Du B: Unpublished observations, 1998.
143. Edwards SW, Knox WE: Homogentisate oxidase from rat liver, in Colowick SP, Kaplan NO (eds): *Methods in Enzymology.* New York, Academic, 1955, vol 2, p 292.
144. Crandall DL: L-Tyrosine oxidation in rat kidney. *Fed Proc* **13**:195, 1954.
145. Knox WE: *p*-Hydroxyphenylpyruvate enol-keto tautomerase, in Colowick SP, Kaplan NO (eds): *Methods in Enzymology.* New York, Academic, 1955, vol 2, p 287.
146. Lin ECC, Knox WE: Specificity of the adaptive response of tyroxine-*α*-ketoglutarate transaminase in the rat. *J Biol Chem* **233**:1186, 1958.
147. La Du BN, Zannoni VG: Unpublished observations, 1998.
148. Jones JD, Smith BS, Evans WC: Homogentisic acid, an intermediate in the metabolism of tyrosine by the aromatic ring-splitting microorganisms. *Biochem J* **51**:11, 1952.
149. Mörner CT: Weitere Beitrage Beiträge zur Chemie der Homogentisinsäure. *Z Physiol Chem* **78**:306, 1912.
150. Crandall DI: Properties and distribution of homogentisic acid oxidase. *Fed Proc* **12**:192, 1953.
151. Neubauer O, Falta W: Über das Schicksal einiger aromatischer Säuren bei der Alkaptonurie. *Z Physiol Chem* **42**:81, 1904.
152. Montgomery JA, Mamer OA: Profiles in altered metabolism. II: Accumulation of homogentisic acid in serum and urine following acetylsalicylic acid ingestion. *Biomed Mass Spectrom* **5**:331, 1978.
153. Consden R, Forbes HAW, Glynn LE, Stanier WM: Observations on the oxidation of homogentisic acid in urine. *Biochem J* **50**:274, 1951.
154. Evans AS, Enzer N, Eder HA, Finch CA: Hemolytic anemia with paroxysmal methemoglobinemia and sulfhemoglobinemia. *AMA Arch Intern Med* **86**:22, 1950.
155. Leaf G, Neuberger A: The preparation of homogentisic acid and of 2:5-dihydroxyphenylethylamine. *Biochem J* **43**:606, 1948.
156. Katsch G, Metz E: Der Nachweis der Homogentisinsäure in Serum des Alkaptonurikers. *Dtsch Arch Klin Med* **157**:143, 1927.
157. Johnson EH, Miller RL: Alcaptonuria in a Cynomolgus monkey *(Macaca fascicularis)*. *J Med Primatol* **22**:428, 1993.
158. Kamoun P, Coude M, Forest M, Montagutelli X, Guenet JL: Ascorbic acid and alcaptonuria. *Eur J Pediatr* **151**:149, 1992.
159. Lewis JH: Alcaptonuria in a rabbit. *J Biol Chem* **70**:659, 1926.
160. Poulsen V: Über Ochronose bei Menschen und Tieren. *Beitr Pathol Anat* **48**:346, 1910.
161. Nilsson N-G, Grabell I: A case of bovine ochronosis. *Acta Vet Scand* **18**:426, 1978.
162. Papageorge E, Lewis HB: Experimental alcaptonuria in the white rat. *J Biol Chem* **123**:211, 1938.
163. Painter HA, Zilva SS: The influence of L-ascorbic acid on the disappearance of the phenolic group of L-tyrosine in the presence of guinea pig liver suspension. *Biochem J* **46**:542, 1950.
164. Malakar MC, Banerjee SN: Effect of glycine or choline chloride on the excretion of homogentisic acid by the tyrosine-fed and scorbutic guinea pigs. *Ann Biochem Exp Med* **15**:69, 1955.
165. Abderhalden E: Bildung von Homogentisinsäure nach Aufnahme grosser Mengen von L-Tyrosin per os. *Z Physiol Chem* **77**:454, 1912.
166. Glynn LE, Himsworth HP, Neuberger A: Pathological states due to deficiency of the sulfur-containing amino acids. *Br J Exp Pathol* **26**:326, 1945.
167. Neuberger A, Webster TA: Studies on alcaptonuria. 3. Experimental alcaptonuria in rats. *Biochem J* **41**:449, 1947.
168. Butts J, Dunn MS, Hallman LF: Studies in amino acid metabolism. IV. Metabolism of DL-phenylalanine and DL-tyrosine in the normal rat. *J Biol Chem* **123**:711, 1938.
169. Lanyar F: Über experimentelle Alkaptonurie bei der weissen Maus. *Z Physiol Chem* **275**:225, 1942.

170. Lanyar F: Über experimentelle Alkaptonurie bei der weissen Ratte. *Z Physiol Chem* **278**:155, 1943.
171. Sealock RR, Perkinson JD Jr, Basinski DH: Further analysis of the role of ascorbic acid in phenylalanine and tyrosine metabolism. *J Biol Chem* **140**:153, 1941.
172. Lin ECC, Knox WE: Role of enzymatic adaptation in production of experimental alkaptonuria. *Proc Soc Exp Biol Med* **96**:501, 1957.
173. Woodruff CW, Cherrington ME, Stockell AK, Darby WJ: The effect of pteroylglutamic acid and related compounds upon tyrosine metabolism in the scorbutic guinea pig. *J Biol Chem* **178**:861, 1949.
174. Woodruff CW, Darby WJ: An in vivo effect of pteroylglutamic acid upon tyrosine metabolism in the scorbutic guinea pig. *J Biol Chem* **172**:851, 1948.
175. Woodford VR, Quan L, Cutts F: Experimental alkaptonuria in the rat induced by tryptophan deficiency. *J Biol Chem* **45**:791, 1967.
176. Suda M, Takeda Y, Sujishi K, Tanaka T: Metabolism of tyrosine. III. Relation between homogentisicase, ferrous ion, and L-ascorbic acid in experimental alcaptonuria of guinea pig. *J Biochem (Tokyo)* **38**:297, 1951.
177. Bartley W, Krebs HA, O'Brien JRP: *Vitamin C Requirement of Human Adults*. Medical Research Council, Special Report Series. London, HM Stationery Office, 1953, vol 280, p 27.
178. Bondurant RE, Henry JB: Pathogenesis of ochronosis in experimental alkaptonuria of the white rat. *Lab Invest* **14**:62, 1965.
179. Blivaiss BB, Rosenberg EF, Kutuzov H, Stoner R: Experimental ochronosis: Induction in rats by long-term feeding with L-tyrosine. *AMA Arch Pathol* **82**:45, 1966.
180. Bateson W, Saunders ER: *Report of the Evolution Committee of the Royal Society (London)*. **1**:133, 1902.
181. Hogben L, Worrall RL, Zieve I: The genetic basis of alkaptonuria. *Proc R Soc Edinb [Biol]* **52**:264, 1932.
182. Pieter H: Une famille d'alcaptonuriques. *Presse Med* **33**:1310, 1925.
183. Knox WE: Sir Archibald Garrod's "Inborn errors of metabolism." II. Alkaptonuria. *Am J Hum Genet* **10**:95, 1958.
184. Khachadurian A, Abu Feisal K: Alkaptonuria: Report of a family with seven cases appearing in four successive generations with metabolic studies in one patient. *J Chron Dis* **7**:455, 1958.
185. Cervenansky J, Sitaj S, Urbanek T: Alkaptonuria and ochronosis. *J Bone Joint Surg Am* **41**:1169, 1959.
186. Srsen S, Cisarik F, Pasztor L, Harmecko L: Alkaptonuria in the Trečin District of Czechoslovakia. *Am J Med Genet* **2**:159, 1978.
187. Srsen S: *Alkaptonuria*. Czechoslovakia, Osveta, 1984.
188. Srsen S: Analysis of the causes of the relatively frequent incidence of alkaptonuria in Slovakia. *Cas Lek Ces* **122**:1585, 1983.
189. Milch RA: Direct inheritance of alcaptonuria. *Metabolism* **4**:513, 1955.
190. Milch RA: Inheritance of alcaptonuria. *Bull Hosp J Dis* **18**:103, 1957.
191. Roth M, Felgenhauer WR: Recherche de l'excretion d'acide homogentisique urinaire chez des heterozygotes pour l'alcaptonurie. *Enzymol Biol Clin* **9**:53, 1968.
192. La Du B: Unpublished observations, 1998.
193. Laberge CA, Lescault A, Grenier A, Gagne R: Ëffet succinylacetonë après surcharges orales d'homogentisate. *Union Med Can* **110**:621, 1981.
194. Scriver CR: Alkaptonuria: such a long journey. *Nat Genet* **14**:5, 1996.
195. Pollak MR, Chou Y-HW, Cerda, JJ, Steinmann B, La Du BN, Seidmann JG, Seidman CE: Homozygosity mapping of the gene for alkaptonuria to chromosome 3q2. *Nat Genet* **5**:201, 1993.
196. Jonocha S, Wolz W, Srsen S, Srsnova K, Montagutelli X, Guenet JL, Grimm T, Kress W, Muller CR: The human gene for alkaptonuria (AKU) maps to chromosome 3q. *Genomics* **19**:5, 1994.
197. Montagutelli X, Lalouette A, Coude M, Kamoun P, Forest M, Guenet J-L: aku, a mutation of the mouse homologous to human alkaptonuria, maps to chromosome 16. *Genomics* **19**:9, 1994.
198. Fernandez-Canon JM, Granadino B, Beltran-Valero de Bernabe D, Renedo M, Fernandez-Ruiz E, Penalva MA, Rodriguez de Cordoba S: The molecular basis of alkaptonuria. *Nat Genet* **14**:19, 1996.
199. Fernandez-Canon JM, Penalva MA: Molecular characterization of a gene encoding a homogentisate dioxygenase from *Aspergillus nidulans* and identification of its human and plant homologues. *J Biol Chem* **270**:21199, 1995.
200. Scazzochio C: Alkaptonuria: from humans to moulds and back. *Trend Genet* **13**:125,1997.
201. Fernandez-Canon JM, Penalva MA: Spectrophotometric determination of homogentisate using *Aspergillus nidulans* homogentisate dioxygenase. *Anal Biochem* **245**:218, 1997.
202. Granadino B, Beltran-Valero de Bernabe D, Fernandez-Canon JM, Penalva MA, Rodriquez de Cordoba S: The human homogentisate 1,2-dioxygenase (HGO) gene. *Genomics* **43**:115,1997.
203. Schmidt SR, Gehrig A, Koehler MR, Schmid M, Muller CR, Kress W: Cloning of the homogentisate 1,2-dioxygenase gene, the key enzyme of alkaptonuria in mouse. *Mamm Genone* **8**:168,1997.
204. Gehrig Schmidt SR, Muller CR, Srsen S, Srsnova K, Kress W: Molecular defects in alkaptonuria. *Cytogenet Cell Genet* **76**:14, 1997.
205. Beltran-Valero de Bernabe D, Granadino B, Chiarelli I, Porfirio B, Mayatepek E, Aquaron R, Moore MM, et al.: Mutation and polymorphism analysis of the human homogentisate 1,2-dioxygenase gene in alkaptonuria patients. *Am J Hum Genet* **62**:776, 1998.
206. Higashino K, Liu W, Ohkawa T, Yumamoto T, Fukui K, Olmo M, Imanishi H, Iwasaki A, Amuro Y, Hada T: A novel point mutation associated with alkaptonuria. *Clin Genet* **53**:228, 1998.
207. Peterson P, Beltran-Valero de Bernabe D, Krohn K, Ranki A, Rodriguez de Cordoba S: HGO mutations in Finnish alkaptonuria patients. *Am J Hum Genet* **63**:A272, 1998.
208. Mosonyi L: A propos del'alcaptonurie et de son traitement. *Presse Med* **47**:708, 1939.
209. Diaz CJ, Mendoza HC, Rodriguez JS: Alkapton, Aceton und Kohlehydratmangel. *Klin Wochenschr* **18**:965, 1939.
210. Flaschentrager B, Halawani A, Nabeh I: Alkaptonurie und Vitamin B12. *Klin Wochenschr* **32**:131, 1954.
211. Black RL: Use of cortisone in alkaptonuria. *JAMA* **155**:968, 1954.
212. Suzman MM: The clinical application of corticotropin and cortisone therapy: A report of 247 cases. *S Afr Med J* **27**:195, 1953.
213. Biggs TG Jr, Cannon E Jr: Ochronosis: Report of a case. *J La State Med Soc* **105**:395, 1953.
214. Cope CB, Kassander P: Cortisone in ochronotic arthritis. *JAMA* **150**:997, 1952.
215. Woff JA, Barshop B, Nyhan WL, Leslie J, Seegmiller JE, Gruber H, Garst M, Winter S, Michals K, Matalon R: Effects of ascorbic acid in alkaptonuria: Alterations in benzoquinone acetic acid and an ontogenic effect in infancy. *Pediatr Res* **26**:140, 1989.
216. Pradeep JK, Kehinde EO, Daar AS: Symptomatic response to ascorbic acid. *Br J Urol* **77**:319, 1996.
217. La Du BN: Are we ready to cure alkaptonuria? *Am J Hum Genet* **62**:765, 1998.

CHAPTER 93

Branched Chain Organic Acidurias

Lawrence Sweetman ▪ Julian C. Williams

1. *Metabolism of the Branched Chain Organic Acids.* The essential branched chain amino acids, leucine, isoleucine, and valine, are transaminated to the 2-oxo branched chain organic acids and oxidatively decarboxylated to form branched chain acyl coenzyme A (CoA) products. The branched chain amino acid and organic acid disorder maple syrup urine disease, caused by a deficiency of branched chain α-ketoacid dehydrogenase, is described in Chap. 87. Isovaleryl-CoA, derived from leucine; 2-methylbutyryl-CoA, derived from isoleucine; and isobutyryl-CoA, derived from valine, are metabolized by separate pathways to intermediates, which enter the general metabolism. Defects in these pathways cause 10 known metabolic disorders, called branched chain organic acidurias (see Table 93-1).
   Propionic acidemia and methylmalonic acidemia are disorders of propionic acid degradation derived in part from the catabolism of isoleucine and valine, but they are described separately in Chap. 94. Inherited deficiencies of all four enzymes of the catabolism of isovaleryl-CoA derived from leucine are known: isovaleric acidemia (isovaleryl-CoA dehydrogenase deficiency), isolated biotin-unresponsive 3-methylcrotonyl-CoA carboxylase deficiency, 3-methylglutaconic aciduria (3-methylglutaconyl-CoA hydratase deficiency), and 3-hydroxy-3-methylglutaryl-CoA lyase deficiency. Mevalonic aciduria, due to a defect in the biosynthesis of cholesterol and isoprenoids from 3-hydroxy-3-methylglutaryl-CoA, is also considered a branched chain organic aciduria in this chapter. One inherited disorder of the catabolism of 2-methylbutyryl-CoA derived from isoleucine is known: mitochondrial acetoacetyl-CoA thiolase deficiency. Five disorders of the catabolism of isobutyryl-CoA derived from valine are known: isobutyryl-CoA dehydrogenase deficiency; 3-hydroxyisobutyryl-CoA deacylase deficiency; 3-hydroxyisobutyric aciduria; methylmalonic semialdehyde dehydrogenase deficiency with combined 3-hydroxyisobutyric, 3-aminoisobutyric, 3-hydroxypropionic, β-alanine, and 2-ethyl-3-hydroxybutyric aciduria; and a new form of mild methylmalonic aciduria related to methylmalonic semialdehyde metabolism. A new disorder, ethylmalonic encephalopathy, with increased excretion of ethylmalonic acid, isobutyrylglycine, and 2-methylbutyrylglycine, may be due to a deficiency or inhibition of short-branched chain acyl-CoA dehydrogenase affecting the catabolism of both valine and isoleucine. Although not a branched chain organic aciduria, malonic aciduria due to malonyl-CoA decarboxylase deficiency is described in this chapter.
2. *Isovaleric Acidemia (Isovaleryl-CoA Dehydrogenase Deficiency, MIM 243500).* Isovaleryl-CoA dehydrogenase deficiency may present either in the neonatal period as an acute episode of severe metabolic acidosis and moderate ketosis with vomiting, which may lead to coma and death, or as a chronic intermittent form with episodes of metabolic acidosis. Infants who survive an acute neonatal episode go on to exhibit the chronic form. Neutropenia, thrombocytopenia, or, rarely, pancytopenia often occurs with acidotic episodes. The "odor of sweaty feet" due to isovaleric acid is usually present during acute episodes. The major abnormal metabolite findings are large elevations of isovalerylglycine in urine and of isovalerylcarnitine in plasma. Treatment with leucine restriction and carnitine and/or glycine generally results in normal development if no permanent neurologic damage has occurred during the initial presentation.
3. *Isolated 3-Methylcrotonyl-CoA Carboxylase Deficiency (MIM 210200).* The isolated deficiency of 3-methylcrotonyl-CoA carboxylase is not responsive to biotin and is distinct from the biotin-responsive multiple carboxylase deficiencies that are due to a deficiency of biotinidase or holocarboxylase synthetase described in Chap. 156. Patients typically present with acute metabolic acidosis, hypoglycemia, and carnitine deficiency. The major abnormal metabolites are 3-hydroxyisovaleric acid in urine and 3-hydroxyisovalerylcarnitine in plasma. Treatment with carnitine and restriction of leucine usually results in normal development.
4. *3-Methylglutaconic Aciduria.* At least four types of this disorder are known. Type I (MIM 250950), with a deficiency of 3-methylglutaconyl-CoA hydratase, has diverse and nonspecific clinical symptoms. The major urinary metabolites are 3-methylglutaconic and 3-hydroxyisovaleric acids. Dietary treatment has not proven to be of definite benefit, but carnitine supplementation and modest leucine restriction may be mildly beneficial.
   Type II (Barth syndrome, MIM 302060), or X-linked, 3-methylglutaconic aciduria is associated with dilated cardiomyopathy, neutropenia, and growth retardation, with normal activity of 3-methylglutaconyl-CoA hydratase. Excretion rates of 3-methylglutaconic acid and 3-methylglutaric acid are only moderately increased, and that of 3-hydroxyisovaleric acid is normal. The basic biochemical abnormality is unknown, and the clinical outcome is variable. Specific dietary restriction has not been effective.
   Type III (Costeff optic atrophy syndrome, MIM 258501) includes optic atrophy, choreoathetosis, spastic

A list of standard abbreviations is located immediately preceding the index in each volume. Nonstandard abbreviations used in this chapter include: ETF = electron transfer flavoprotein.

paraparesis, cerebellar ataxia, and nystagmus, with mild 3-methylglutaconic aciduria (normal 3-hydroxyisovaleric acid) and normal activity of 3-methylglutaconyl-CoA hydratase.

Type IV (MIM 250951), or the "unclassified" form, with mild 3-methylglutaconic aciduria and normal activity of 3-methylglutaconyl-CoA hydratase, is a clinically heterogeneous group of disorders with variable psychomotor retardation, hypertonicity, hypotonia, optic atrophy, dysmorphic features, seizures, cardiomyopathy, and hepatic dysfunction. Some patients have elevated lactic or citric acid cycle intermediates, and some have abnormalities of the mitochondrial electron transport chain. The basic biochemical defect(s) is unknown, and no effective treatment has been found.

5. *3-Hydroxy-3-methylglutaryl-CoA Lyase Deficiency (MIM 246450).* One-third of patients present in the neonatal period, and two-thirds present between 3 and 11 months of age with severe hypoglycemia and metabolic acidosis (but with little or no ketosis), hyperammonemia, vomiting, and hypotonia, which may progress to coma and death. The symptoms resemble those of Reye syndrome. Treatment by restriction of leucine and fat, avoidance of fasting, and carnitine supplementation generally leads to normal development. 3-Hydroxy-3-methylglutaryl-CoA lyase deficiency is a disorder of branched chain amino acid (leucine) metabolism; its diagnosis from the major abnormal metabolites in urine, 3-hydroxy-3-methylglutaric, 3-methylglutaconic, and 3-hydroxyisovaleric acids, is described in this chapter. But this disorder is also one of ketone body metabolism, and therefore its clinical, biochemical, and molecular aspects are described in detail in Chap. 102.
6. *Mevalonic Aciduria (Mevalonate Kinase Deficiency, MIM 251170).* Patients with the severe form of mevalonic aciduria present in the neonatal period with dysmorphic features, anemia, hepatosplenomegaly, gastroenteropathy, failure to thrive, and severe developmental delay. Patients with a milder form show poor muscle development, hypotonia, ataxia, and elevated creatine kinase. There is no metabolic acidosis, and although the defect is in cholesterol biosynthesis, blood cholesterol may be normal. The only abnormal metabolite finding is an extremely elevated amount of mevalonic acid in urine and plasma. No effective therapy is yet available.
7. *Mitochondrial Acetoacetyl-CoA Thiolase Deficiency (MIM 203750).* In patients with mitochondrial acetoacetyl-CoA thiolase deficiency, intermittent episodes of severe metabolic acidosis and ketosis begin during the first 2 years of life. These are accompanied by vomiting (often with hematemesis), diarrhea, and coma, which may progress to death. Deficiency of this thiolase is a disorder of branched chain amino acid (isoleucine) metabolism, and diagnosis from detection in urine of the major abnormal metabolites, 2-methyl-3-hydroxybutyric acid, 2-methylacetoacetic acid, and tiglylglycine, is described in this chapter. But this disorder is also one of ketone body metabolism, and therefore clinical, biochemical, and molecular aspects are described in detail in Chap. 102.
8. *Isobutyryl-CoA Dehydrogenase Deficiency?* A patient presenting with anemia and dilated cardiomyopathy at 11 months of age had low carnitine levels and an elevation of a four-carbon (butyryl/isobutyryl)acylcarnitine. When fibroblasts were incubated with [^{13}C]valine, [^{13}C]isobutyrylcarnitine accumulated, suggesting an isolated deficiency of isobutyryl-CoA dehydrogenase. Treatment with carnitine reversed the cardiomyopathy.
9. *3-Hydroxyisobutyryl-CoA Deacylase Deficiency (MIM 250620).* In a single patient with a deficiency of 3-hydroxyisobutyryl-CoA deacylase, there were congenital malformations and a lack of neurologic development without acidosis. The major abnormal urinary metabolites are not organic acids but the amino acids *S*-(2-carboxypropyl)-cysteine and *S*-(2-carboxypropyl)-cysteamine, which are formed by addition of cysteine to methacrylyl-CoA, the precursor of 3-hydroxyisobutyryl-CoA. No treatment is known.
10. *3-Hydroxyisobutyric Aciduria (MIM 236795).* A number of patients have presented with 3-hydroxyisobutyric aciduria, which may be due to a deficiency of 3-hydroxyisobutyrate dehydrogenase or to a secondary inhibition of this enzyme. Symptoms can include repeated episodes of ketoacidosis and lactic acidemia, failure to thrive, dysmorphic features, brain dysgenesis, malformations, and hypotonia. There is a high rate of excretion of 3-hydroxyisobutyric acid. Treatment with carnitine and valine restriction may be beneficial.
11. *Methylmalonic Semialdehyde Dehydrogenase Deficiency with Combined 3-Hydroxypropionic, β-Alanine, 3-Hydroxyisobutyric, and 3-Aminoisobutyric Aciduria.* In one individual with no clinical symptoms and another with mild symptoms, a deficiency of an uncharacterized semialdehyde dehydrogenase acting on both methylmalonic semialdehyde and malonic semialdehyde led to elevated excretion levels of 3-hydroxyisobutyric, 3-aminoisobutyric, 2-ethyl-3-hydroxybutyric, and 3-hydroxypropionic acids, together with β-alanine.
12. *Methylmalonic Aciduria Related to Methylmalonic Semialdehyde Dehydrogenase Deficiency.* A patient with developmental delay and no episodes of metabolic acidosis excreted moderate amounts of methylmalonic acid. Methylmalonyl-CoA mutase was normal, and there was no indication of a cobalamin disorder. Patients with deficient activity of methylmalonyl-CoA metabolism have elevated propionylcarnitine levels, which this patient did not, suggesting that the elevated methylmalonic acid levels were derived not from methylmalonyl-CoA but rather from methylmalonic semialdehyde. In vivo studies of the metabolism of labeled valine and thymine to isomers of 3-hydroxyisobutyric acid and 3-aminoisobutyric acid suggest a defect in methylmalonic semialdehyde dehydrogenase.
13. *Ethylmalonic Aciduria Encephalopathy (MIM 602473).* This disorder may be due to a deficiency or a secondary inhibition of a short-branched chain acyl-CoA dehydrogenase affecting both valine and isoleucine catabolism. Patients present with neonatal hypotonia, severe progressive pyramidal dysfunction and spastic diplegia, orthostatic acrocyanosis with distal swelling, chronic diarrhea, and diffuse petechiae. The outcome has been severe mental retardation or death. Biochemical abnormalities include lactic acidemia and increased excretion of ethylmalonic acid, 2-methylbutyrylglycine, and isobutyrylglycine. Therapeutic intervention has been unsuccessful.
14. *Malonic Aciduria (Malonyl-CoA Decarboxylase Deficiency, MIM 248360).* Fifteen patients have been reported with malonic aciduria, generally accompanied by lesser excretions of methylmalonic acid. Most have had developmental delay, many are hypotonic, and some have had hypoglycemia, metabolic acidosis, cardiomyopathy, or gastrointestinal distress. Eight of the patients have been documented to have a deficiency of malonyl-CoA decarboxylase, two had normal activity, and in the others, enzyme activity was not determined. Treatment with

carnitine and a high-carbohydrate diet low in long chain fatty acids with medium chain triglyceride supplementation has had some success.

CATABOLISM OF THE BRANCHED CHAIN AMINO ACIDS AS BRANCHED CHAIN ORGANIC ACIDS

Transamination and Oxidative Decarboxylation

The initial step in the catabolism of the three branched chain amino acids, leucine, valine, and isoleucine (and also alloisoleucine derived from isoleucine), is reversible transamination to the branched chain 2-oxo acids, as described in Chap. 87. A deficiency of a transaminase would cause elevation of the amino acid with no elevation of the corresponding 2-oxo acid or other organic acid metabolites. The second step in the catabolism of the branched chain amino acids is irreversible oxidative decarboxylation of the 2-oxo acids by branched chain 2-oxo acid dehydrogenase, with formation of branched chain acyl-CoA thioesters with one less carbon than the parent amino and 2-oxo acids, as described in Chap. 87. A deficiency of branched chain 2-oxo acid dehydrogenase causes maple syrup urine disease, with elevation of all of the branched chain amino acids and branched chain 2-oxo acids, because the transamination is reversible. Branched chain 2-hydroxy acids may be elevated due to reduction of the elevated branched chain 2-oxo acids, but no other organic acid metabolites of the branched chain 2-oxo acids are elevated.

General Aspects of Branched Chain Acyl-CoA Metabolism

The branched chain acyl-CoA thioesters derived from the three branched chain amino acids are metabolized in a series of steps to simple organic acid intermediates that enter the general metabolism. A distinguishing feature of deficiencies of any of these enzymes is that only branched chain organic acid metabolites are elevated, without elevation of the branched chain amino acids or branched chain 2-oxo acids, because the reaction of branched chain 2-oxo acid dehydrogenase is not reversible. In contrast, many of the catabolic reactions of the branched chain acyl-CoA thioesters after the initial acyl-CoA dehydrogenase reactions are reversible, and as a general consequence, deficiency of an enzyme can cause elevation of metabolites of many of the intermediates proximal to the deficiency. The elevated acyl-CoA thioesters can also be metabolized by multiple secondary pathways to produce a variety of additional metabolites.

Diagnosis of Branched Chain Organic Acidurias by Analysis of Urinary Organic Acids and Acylcarnitines in Plasma or Dried Blood Spots

The rapid differential diagnosis of these disorders is best accomplished by determination of an abnormal pattern of urinary organic acids determined by GC/MS.[1–3] Quantitative analysis is of value because the patterns include elevation of normal urinary constituents as well as the presence of metabolites not usually detected in normal individuals.[3] Although the metabolites are often extremely elevated in acute episodes, at other times the elevation may be very modest and need to be distinguished from normal levels. A diagnosis rarely depends on the level of a single compound but rather on a pattern of elevation of a group of organic acids. Defects in sequential enzymes in the catabolic pathways of the branched chain amino acids often have overlapping patterns of metabolite elevation because of reversibility of the steps above the enzymatic deficiencies.

Some of the organic acidurias may present clinically as features resembling Reye syndrome, and analysis of urinary organic acids is helpful in the differential diagnosis. The organic acids in urine of patients with Reye syndrome are generally normal, but there may be either a) nonspecific elevation of 3-hydroxybutyric and acetoacetic acids with secondary elevation of dicarboxylic acids or b) elevation of lactic and pyruvic acids with normal tricarboxylic acid cycle intermediates.[1]

Another very useful diagnostic technique that is complementary to urinary organic acid analysis is identification of elevated acylcarnitines by tandem MS.[4,5] Many of the intermediates in the catabolism of branched chain amino acids are CoA esters, and most of these are in equilibrium with the corresponding acylcarnitines. An enzymatic block often results in elevation of acylcarnitines in blood and plasma. Urinary acylcarnitine profiles obtained by tandem MS are more complex and less diagnostic than plasma or blood profiles. Although tandem MS does not distinguish between isomers such as isovalerylcarnitine and 2-methylbutyrylcarnitine or isobutyrylcarnitine and butyrylcarnitine, it is a useful screening technique in combination with GC/MS of urinary organic acids. It has the added advantage that it can be performed on dried blood spots obtained for routine neonatal screening, leading to very early diagnosis of many of the branched chain organic acidurias.[5]

Metabolic Effects of Enzyme Deficiency and Implications for Therapy

Diagnostic evaluation of a patient with a potential inborn error of intermediary metabolism centers on the detection of abnormal levels of a physiological compound(s) or, more rarely, on the identification of an abnormal metabolite(s). Accumulation of such compounds prior to the block in an enzymatic pathway suggests the specific enzymatic deficiency and is usually presumed to be the cause of the primary pathologic effects, that is, toxicity of the accumulated substrate. In addition to direct toxicity, much of the physiological abnormality may result from endogenous compensatory mechanisms, such as increased fatty acid oxidation and ketogenesis to provide fuel replacement for a blocked gluconeogenic pathway. Failure of a substrate to proceed normally along a pathway may also result in an alteration in the availability of reducing equivalents or of an intermediate necessary for synthetic or regulatory functions. In the organic acidemias, accumulation of acyl-CoAs inhibits function of the urea cycle, resulting in hyperammonemia, and alters the availability of free CoA, thus affecting the CoA-carnitine exchange mechanism across the mitochondrial membrane and catabolism of other acyl moieties from fatty acid and amino acid oxidation. The primary paradigm of therapeutic intervention in both the acute and the chronic state is to lower the levels of the accumulated metabolite. Secondary therapeutic methods focus on correcting the physiological effects of the metabolite's elevation; this should never become the sole or primary goal of intervention.

As the branched chain amino acids cannot be synthesized in humans, increased flux through a catabolic pathway can result only via exogenous protein intake or endogenous degradation of protein. Thus, the goal of minimizing flux through the affected pathway is achieved by regulating intake of the offending essential amino acid(s) to the minimum necessary for new protein synthesis (i.e., obligatory maintenance protein turnover and in infants that necessary for growth) and by minimizing catabolic breakdown (i.e., gluconeogenesis induced by fasting, infection, or iatrogenic amino acid deficiency). In our experience it is the latter mechanism of endogenous catabolism that is the major culprit not only in acute crises but also in chronic failure to thrive and its concomitant increased frequency of recurrent crises. Although selective amino acid restriction is important in the management of many of these disorders, in the past it could be achieved only by restriction of total protein intake, resulting in a chronic borderline catabolic state. Currently, the advent of specialized foods selectively deficient in a given amino acid(s) permits limitation of the offending agent to that necessary for anabolic functions while not limiting other amino acids. Specific data on dietary protocols and age-related requirements for each amino acid have been published.[6] This results in improved growth and fewer and less severe episodes of catabolic decompensation associated with fasting or infection. The importance of providing adequate amino acid intake is also seen in the acute crises in which protein intake is totally eliminated and energy is provided solely by intravenous glucose. Although this is very effective in limiting endogenous catabolism via an increased insulin:glucagon ratio, invariably within 3 to 5 days protein breakdown escapes this restraint and the patient deteriorates or the previous improvement is arrested. Provision of exogenous amino acids in judicious amounts at this time results in further improvement. The limited availability of intravenous amino acid solutions selectively deficient in a specific amino acid(s) is unfortunate, as supplementation in the acutely ill child at the onset of catabolic crises may be of great benefit.

In addition to decreasing the levels of accumulated metabolites via regulation of substrate flux through the affected pathway, removal of these metabolites by dialysis in the acute stage has long been a mainstay of treatment. Long-term removal of metabolites by means of selective agents may also have an important role. As in the choice of peritoneal dialysis versus hemodialysis, controlled blind trials have not been performed, but accrued clinical experience suggests that in some disorders provision of specific compounds, such as benzoate for the urea cycle defects, glycine in isovaleric acidemia, and carnitine in organic acidemias with elevated acylcarnitine levels, may be of benefit. The evidence for the first two is convincing, and that for the latter is accumulating. Organic acidemias frequently result in increased levels of acyl-CoA derivatives and acylcarnitines. This results in decreased availability of free CoA and carnitine. Acylcarnitine derivatives are not reabsorbed in the renal tubule. This leads to a further decrease in carnitine, which may impair substrate transport across the mitochondrial membrane and subsequent energy generation. Provision of exogenous carnitine corrects this deficiency and may also shift the acyl-CoA:CoA ratio to free up CoA. It is our impression that given otherwise identical clinical management, exogenous carnitine decreases the frequency and severity of crises in patients with organic acidemia who have low free carnitine levels in plasma and ongoing urinary losses of acylcarnitine.

In summary, acute management of crises in the organic acidemias requires: (1) elimination of intake of the offending amino acid(s) in the short term; (2) provision of adequate caloric intake, usually with glucose, which also serves to suppress endogenous protein degradation and ketogenesis; (3) dialysis as needed; (4) correction of fluid and electrolyte abnormalities; (5) maintenance of cerebral function with adequate perfusion, oxygenation, and glucose; (6) avoidance of cerebral edema; (7) provision of vitamin cofactors as indicated; and (8) use of selective chemical detoxicants, such as glycine and carnitine. It should be pointed out that failure to adhere to the above goals as the primary therapy results in the endogenous generation of far more acid equivalents than can be corrected by the use of sodium bicarbonate. As in the current recommendations for the use of sodium bicarbonate in cardiac arrest, the primary focus is on correcting the underlying problem and not on treating a laboratory value. Sodium bicarbonate is indicated only at arterial pH values that impair cardiac function and is used sparingly in conjunction with the above guidelines. Long-term therapy focuses on provision of the minimum amount of the restricted amino acid(s) necessary for growth and of a surfeit of the other amino acids and calories by means of a combination of natural protein and specialized formulas. Long-term use of carnitine and/or glycine is of benefit in some disorders. Avoidance of a chronic catabolic state and quick intervention during acute catabolic crises is essential.

DISORDERS OF LEUCINE CATABOLISM

Catabolism of Leucine

The normal pathway for the catabolism of leucine to the common metabolic intermediates acetoacetic acid and acetyl-CoA is shown in Fig. 93-1. Inherited deficiencies of each of the six enzymes in the pathway are known. The four disorders of leucine catabolism considered to be branched chain organic acidurias in this chapter are isovaleric acidemia, isolated 3-methylcrotonyl-CoA carboxylase deficiency, 3-methylglutaconyl-CoA hydratase deficiency, and 3-hydroxy-3-methylglutaryl-CoA lyase deficiency (Table 93-1). The enzymes of the catabolic pathway for leucine are located in the mitochondria, and their relevant properties are summarized below.

Isovaleryl-CoA Dehydrogenase. The first step of branched chain organic acid metabolism of leucine is the irreversible dehydrogenation of isovaleryl-CoA to 3-methylcrotonyl-CoA, catalyzed by isovaleryl-CoA dehydrogenase (see Fig. 93-1). The identification of a dehydrogenase specific for isovaleryl-CoA is an example of how the discovery of an inherited disorder and its detailed characterization can elucidate normal metabolic pathways. It had been thought that a single acyl-CoA dehydrogenase, "butyryl-CoA or green acyl-CoA dehydrogenase," was responsible for the dehydrogenation of short-chain acyl-CoAs in fatty acid oxidation and that of isovaleryl-CoA in leucine catabolism.[7] The identification of the inherited disorder isovaleric acidemia without elevation of other short-chain acids led Tanaka and colleagues to propose the existence of a dehydrogenase specific for isovaleryl-CoA.[8] Rhead and Tanaka confirmed this by demonstrating a deficiency of isovaleryl-CoA dehydrogenase with normal activity of butyryl-CoA dehydrogenase in mitochondria from fibroblasts of patients with isovaleric acidemia.[9] Further confirmation came from separation of isovaleryl-CoA dehydrogenase and butyryl-CoA dehydrogenase in pig liver[10] and from isolation from rat liver mitochondria and characterization of isovaleryl-CoA dehydrogenase[11] and four other acyl-CoA dehydrogenases that are immunologically distinct.[12] Human isovaleryl-CoA dehydrogenase has also been purified from liver and characterized.[13]

Isovaleryl-CoA dehydrogenase is synthesized on cytosolic free polysomes as a subunit precursor of 45 kDa.[14] It is processed to a 43-kDa subunit during importation into the mitochondria, where four identical subunits form a tetrameric enzyme of 172 kDa located in the matrix or on the inner face of the mitochondrial membrane.[11,15] It is a flavin enzyme with approximately one mole of FAD per subunit. Electrons from the FAD are accepted by ETF[16] and transmitted to coenzyme Q in the mitochondrial electron transport chain by ETF dehydrogenase, an iron-sulfur flavoprotein,[17] as described in Chap. 103. In rat tissues, isovaleryl-CoA dehydrogenase is most active in heart, with lesser amounts of activity in liver, kidney, and skeletal muscle in decreasing order.[18] The activity is also present in normal human fibroblasts in culture.[9]

Isovaleryl-CoA dehydrogenase purified from human liver has a K_m for isovaleryl-CoA of 14 μM.[13] With substrates at 100 μM, the activity, as compared with 100 percent for isovaleryl-CoA, is 37 percent for valeryl-CoA, 22 percent for hexanoyl-CoA, 18 percent for butyryl-CoA, and 6 percent for 2-methylbutyryl-CoA. The product with isovaleryl-CoA as substrate, 3-methylcrotonyl-CoA, is a competitive inhibitor with a K_i of 100 μM for the rat enzyme.[11] The stereochemistry of the dehydrogenation reaction has been shown with isotopically labeled compounds to involve removal of the 2-pro-R hydrogen of isovaleryl-CoA[19] with anti-elimination of hydrogens from C-2 and C-3.[20]

The cDNA for isovaleryl-CoA dehydrogenase from the rat has been cloned and sequenced (GenBank M34192).[21] The cDNA of 2.104 kb includes a 30-amino-acid leader peptide and a 394-amino-acid mature peptide.[22] There is considerable sequence homology to the fatty acid acyl-CoA dehydrogenases. Clones of cDNA for rat isovaleryl-CoA dehydrogenase were used in human-rodent somatic hybrids to assign the gene to human chromosome 15q14-q15.[21] The cDNA for human isovaleryl-CoA dehydrogenase has been cloned and shown to have amino acid residues 89.6 percent identical with those of the rat enzyme.[23] Northern-blot analysis of human liver and fibroblast mRNA for isovaleryl-CoA dehydrogenase gave three different sizes: 4.6, 3.8, and 2.1 kb. A high level of expression in *Escherichia coli* of the cDNA for human isovaleryl-CoA dehydrogenase was obtained by modifying

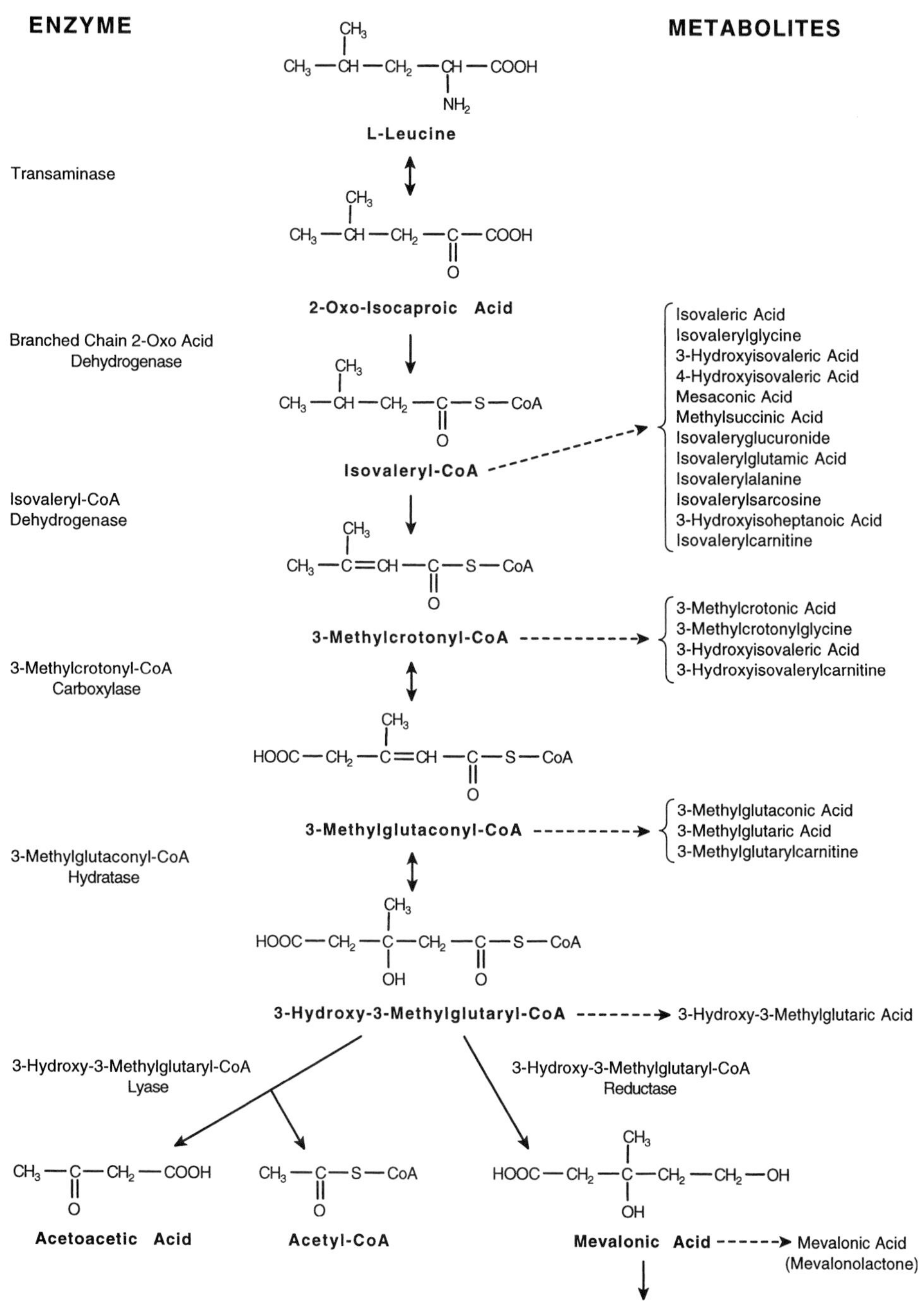

Fig. 93-1 Catabolism of leucine. The structures and names of the intermediates in the pathway for catabolism of leucine are shown in the center with solid arrows indicating enzymatic reactions. The names of the enzymes are on the left, and the metabolites that may be elevated due to a deficiency of these enzymes is shown by dashed arrows to the right.

the nucleotide sequence at the 5′-end for *E. coli* codon usage without changing the amino acid sequence.[24] The substrate specificity of this expressed enzyme is similar to that of the enzyme purified from human liver. With substrates at 50 μM, the activity, as compared with 100 percent for isovaleryl-CoA, is 46 percent for valeryl-CoA, 21 percent for butyryl-CoA, 15 percent for hexanoyl-CoA, and 0 for isobutyryl-CoA.[25] Using this high-level expression and specific mutations, glutamate at position 254 was identified as the active site catalytic base responsible for abstracting the C-2 proton from the isovaleryl-CoA substrate.[25]

The structure of the purified expressed human isovaleryl-CoA dehydrogenase was determined by x-ray diffraction at 2.6 Å resolution and the glutamate at 254 confirmed to be the catalytic base.[26] G374 and A375 in the substrate binding pocket are important for the branched chain specificity of the enzyme. Tyrosine rather than glycine is present at this position in all other acyl-CoA dehydrogenases.

3-Methylcrotonyl-CoA Carboxylase. The product of isovaleryl-CoA dehydrogenase, 3-methylcrotonyl-CoA, is carboxylated at the four-carbon by 3-methylcrotonyl-CoA carboxylase to form 3-methylglutaconyl-CoA (see Fig. 93-1). The reaction, extensively studied for the bacterial enzyme, utilizes ATP and bicarbonate, and the product is (E)-3-methylglutaconyl-CoA (i.e., a trans double bond).[27] The reaction is reversible. Highly purified 3-methylcrotonyl-CoA carboxylase from bovine kidney mitochondria[28,29] has an approximate size of 835 kDa and may be composed of six protomers. There are two nonidentical subunits, the A-subunit of 61 kDa and the B-subunit of 73.5 kDa, which contains covalently bound biotin;[28,29] it is likely that the protomer is AB. As in all carboxylases, biotin is attached by an amide bond with an epsilon amino group of lysine, as described in Chap. 156. The enzyme is associated with the inner membrane of the mitochondria.[30] Normal human fibroblasts and lymphocytes express 3-methylcrotonyl-CoA carboxylase activity (Chap. 156).

Table 93-1 Features of Branched Chain Organic Acidurias

Disorder	Occurrence*	Clinical Presentation	Prominent Metabolites	Comments
Isovaleric acidemia, isovaleryl-CoA dehydrogenase deficiency	> 70 cases	Half with acute neonatal, half with infantile chronic intermittent presentation: vomiting, acidosis, ketosis, mild hyperammonemia, hypocalcemia, transient bone marrow suppression, lethargy, and coma	Urine: Isovalerylglycine, during episodes 3-hydroxyisovalerate, isovalerylglucuronide, 4-hydroxyisovalerate. Plasma, blood: Isovaleric acid, isovalerylcarnitine	"Sweaty feet odor" during episodes. Usually normal development with leucine restriction and treatment with carnitine and/or glycine.
3-Methylcrotonyl-CoA carboxylase deficiency	> 25 cases	May include episodes of vomiting, acidosis, hypoglycemia, hypotonia, and coma; some patients have no clinical symptoms	Urine: 3-Hydroxyisovalerate, 3-methylcrotonylglycine, 3-hydroxyisovalerylcarnitine Plasma, blood: 3-Hydroxyisovaleryl-carnitine but very low free carnitine	Distinct from multiple carboxylase deficiency; does not respond to biotin. Normal development with protein restriction and carnitine.
3-Methylglutaconic aciduria type I: 3-Methylglutaconyl-CoA hydratase deficiency	8 cases	Speech retardation, acidosis with intercurrent infection, hypotonia, and hepatomegaly	Urine: 3-Methylglutaconate, 3-hydroxyisovalerate	Diagnosis requires assay of hydratase.
3-Methylglutaconic aciduria type II: Barth syndrome	> 30 cases	X-linked dilated cardiomyopathy, skeletal myopathy, neutropenia, and growth retardation	Urine: 3-Methylglutaconate, 3-methylglutarate; 3-Hydroxyisovalerate not elevated	Normal hydratase. Abnormal G4.5 protein, function unknown.
3-Methylglutaconic aciduria type III: Costeff optic atrophy syndrome	> 39 cases	Infantile bilateral optic atrophy, choreiform movements, cerebellar ataxia, and mild spasticity	Urine: 3-Methylglutaconate, 3-methylglutarate. 3-Hydroxyisovalerate not elevated	Normal hydratase. Found in Iraqi Jewish patients
3-Methylglutaconic aciduria type IV: "unclassified"	> 20 cases	Variable; psychomotor retardation, neurodegeneration with hypotonia, seizures, optic atrophy, deafness, hepatic dysfunction, cardiomyopathy, and failure to thrive, usually without acidosis	Urine: 3-Methylglutaconate, 3-methylglutarate; 3-Hydroxyisovalerate not elevated	Normal hydratase. Some have abnormal mitochondrial electron transport chain, Pearson syndrome.
3-Hydroxy-3-methylglutaryl-CoA lyase deficiency	> 40 cases	Neonatal, infantile, or childhood presentation; vomiting, hypotonia, lethargy, coma, acidosis, and hyperammonemia, hypoglycemia without ketosis	Urine: 3-Hydroxy-3-methylglutarate; 3-methylglutaconate, 3-hydroxyisovalerate. Plasma, blood: 3-Methylglutarylcarnitine	Often presents like Reye syndrome. Deficient ketogenesis. Covered in detail in Chap. 102.
Mevalonic aciduria, mevalonate kinase deficiency	19 cases	Variable; may include dysmorphic features, failure to thrive, gastroenteropathy, hepatosplenomegaly, anemia, and death	Urine: Mevalonate Plasma: Mevalonate	Low or normal blood cholesterol. No acidosis.
Mitochondrial acetoacetyl-CoA thiolase deficiency	> 20 cases	Infantile presentation; intermittent acidosis, ketosis, vomiting, diarrhea, and coma	Urine: 2-Methyl-3-hydroxybutyrate, 2-methylacetoacetate, sometimes tiglylglycine Plasma, blood: tiglylcarnitine	Normal development with protein restriction. Defect of ketone body metabolism. Covered in detail in Chap. 102.
Isobutyryl-CoA dehydrogenase deficiency?	1 case	Anemia, dilated cardiomyopathy	Plasma, blood: 4-Carbon acylcarnitine, low free carnitine	Cardiomyopathy reversed by carnitine.
3-Hydroxyisobutyryl-CoA deacylase deficiency	1 case	Malformations, failure to thrive, delayed neurologic development, and death	*S*-(2-carboxypropyl)-cysteine, *S*-(2-carboxypropyl)-cysteamine	No abnormal organic acids.

Table 93-1 (Continued)

Disorder	Occurrence*	Clinical Presentation	Prominent Metabolites	Comments
3-Hydroxyisobutyric aciduria	10 cases	Infantile presentation; acidosis, ketosis, lactic acidemia, failure to thrive, dysmorphic features, brain dysgenesis, malformations, and hypotonia	Urine: 3-Hydroxyisobutyrate, half with lactate	
Methylmalonic semialdehyde dehydrogenase deficiency with 3-amino and 3-hydroxy aciduria	2 cases	No or mild clinical symptoms	3-Hydroxyisobutyrate, 3-aminoisobutyrate, 3-hydroxypropionate, β-alanine, 2-ethyl-3-hydroxypropionate	No acidosis; coincident hypermethioninemia in one case.
Methylmalonic semialdehyde dehydrogenase deficiency with mild methylmalonic aciduria	1 case	Developmental delay, seizures	Urine: Moderate methylmalonate, no other acids Plasma, blood: No elevation of propionylcarnitine	No metabolic decompensation.
Ethylmalonic aciduria encephalopathy	19 cases	Neonatal hypotonia, severe progressive pyramidal dysfunction, spastic diplegia, orthostatic acrocyanosis, petechiae, diarrhea	Urine: Ethylmalonate, methylsuccinate, isobutyrylglycine, 2-methylbutyrylglycine. Plasma: Lactate, isobutyrylcarnitine, isovalerylcarnitine, 2-methylbutyrylcarnitine	Metabolite profile can be similar to that of multiple acyl-CoA dehydrogenase deficiency, but without glutarate.
Malonic aciduria, malonyl-CoA decarboxylase deficiency	16 cases	Developmental delay, hypotonia, variable hypoglycemia, acidosis, lactic acidemia, cardiomyopathy	Urine: Malonate, lesser elevation of methylmalonate Plasma, blood: Malonylcarnitine	Two cases, normal enzyme activity, one with methylmalonate > malonate.

* Incidences are uncertain because of the lack of general population screening and reporting of new cases.

3-Methylcrotonyl-CoA carboxylase requires Mg^{2+} and is activated fourfold to fivefold over baseline levels by K^+ and NH_4^+.[29] The K_m values of bovine kidney 3-methylcrotonyl-CoA carboxylase are 82 μM for ATP, 1.8 μM for bicarbonate, and 75 μM for 3-methylcrotonyl-CoA. As compared with 3-methylcrotonyl-CoA, with a relative velocity of 100 percent, other CoA esters that are substrates are: (2Z)-3-ethylcrotonyl-CoA, with a K_m of 22 μM and a relative velocity of 44 percent; trans-crotonyl-CoA, with a K_m of 225 μM and a relative velocity of 27 percent; and acetoacetyl-CoA, with a K_m of about 17 μM and a relative velocity of 12 percent.[29] Tiglyl-CoA, which is 2-methylcrotonyl-CoA, is also believed to be a substrate for 3-methylcrotonyl-CoA carboxylase, because most patients with disorders of isoleucine catabolism in whom tiglyl-CoA accumulates also excrete (E)-2-methylglutaconic acid.[31] Butyryl-CoA and propionyl-CoA are not substrates but are weak competitive inhibitors, with K_i values of 1.6 mM and 1.78 mM, respectively.[29]

3-Methylglutaconyl-CoA Hydratase. The product of 3-methylcrotonyl-CoA carboxylase, 3-methylglutaconyl-CoA, is hydrated by a specific enzyme, 3-methylglutaconyl-CoA hydratase, to 3-hydroxy-3-methylglutaryl-CoA (see Fig. 93-1). Purified crotonase that hydrates crotonyl-CoA and other 2,3-unsaturated monocarboxylic acid CoA esters has been reported to hydrate 3-methylglutaconyl-CoA,[32] but this activity was removed by repeated recrystallization of crotonase.[33] The specific 3-methylglutaconyl-CoA hydratase has been purified fiftyfold from sheep liver[33] and one hundredfold from beef liver.[34] The enzyme is presumably localized in the mitochondria, as are the other enzymes of leucine catabolism. Its activity is expressed in normal human fibroblasts and lymphocytes.[35]

3-Methylglutaconyl-CoA hydratase is highly specific for its unsaturated dicarboxylic acid substrate and does not hydrate the related monocarboxylic acid compounds crotonyl-CoA and 3-methylcrotonyl-CoA.[33]

Human fibroblast 3-methylglutaconyl-CoA hydratase has a K_m for (E)-3-methylglutaconyl-CoA of 6.9 μM, while the lymphocyte K_m is 9.4 μM.[35] The reaction is reversible, with a K_m for dehydration of 3-hydroxy-3-methylglutaryl-CoA of 100 μM for the sheep liver enzyme.[33] At equilibrium, the ratio of the hydrated product, 3-hydroxy-3-methylglutaryl-CoA, to the substrate, 3-methylglutaconyl-CoA, is 5.5.[33] The stereochemistry of the dehydration of 3-hydroxy-3-methylglutaryl-CoA by 3-methylglutaconyl-CoA hydratase has been determined.[36] The product is (E)-3-methylglutaconyl-CoA, which would therefore also be the substrate isomer for hydration. The addition and elimination of water are syn, in contrast to most enzymatic dehydrations, which are anti.[36] The stereoisomeric product of 3-methylglutaconyl-CoA hydratase is (3S)-3-hydroxy-3-methylglutaryl-CoA.

3-Hydroxy-3-Methylglutaryl-CoA Lyase. The product of 3-methylglutaconyl-CoA hydratase, 3-hydroxy-3-methylglutaryl-CoA, is cleaved by 3-hydroxy-3-methylglutaryl-CoA lyase to acetoacetic acid and acetyl-CoA (see Fig. 93-1). In addition to a role in the catabolic pathway for leucine, the lyase has an important role in ketone body synthesis; the enzymatic and molecular aspects of the lyase are covered in detail in Chap. 102.

Isovaleric Acidemia: Isovaleryl-CoA Dehydrogenase Deficiency

Since the first reports of isovaleric acidemia by Tanaka and colleagues in 1966[8] and 1967,[37] more than 70 cases have been reported. Because new cases of organic acidemias are not routinely reported once a "threshold level" is reached, the incidence is difficult to estimate in the absence of newborn screening data or population studies for carrier frequency utilizing molecular techniques. Isovaleric acidemia has been identified in various ethnic and racial groups. The literature on the earlier cases has been thoroughly reviewed,[38,39] and here reference will be made primarily to cases reported since 1980. Isovaleric acidemia was the first inherited organic acid disorder to be diagnosed by GC/MS of metabolites, which has become the major technique for identification and diagnosis of new as well as recognized disorders.[1–3] Tandem MS has also become useful for diagnosis of isovaleric acidemia by detecting elevated C-5 acylcarnitine (isovalerylcarnitine).[4]

Clinical Aspects. Two clinically different presentations of isovaleric acidemia have been reported, with about half the patients presenting with an acute severe neonatal illness and about half with a chronic intermittent form. The biochemical defect, a deficiency of isovaleryl-CoA dehydrogenase activity, is the same in both forms as, determined by in vitro enzyme assay. As in the other organic acidemias, the difference in clinical presentation may be not a consequence of differing severity of the causative mutation but a result of the timing of application of catabolic stress or other factors.

With the acute form, the infants are well at birth, but within a few days (usually 3 to 6, but it may be as early as the first day of life or as late as 14 days of age) begin to refuse feeding and to vomit, becoming dehydrated, listless, and lethargic. They are often hypothermic and may have tremors or twitching and convulsions.[40] A foul "odor of sweaty feet" due to elevated isovaleric acid is commonly noticed. Metabolic acidosis with mild to moderate ketonuria and lactic acidemia is typical, and more recently reported patients have been noted to have significant hyperammonemia of 200 to 1200 μM.[41–44] Thrombocytopenia and neutropenia[41,44–46] and pancytopenia[44,47] are common, as is hypocalcemia.[41,45] The typical progression is that patients become cyanotic and lapse into a coma followed by death. The cause of death may be severe metabolic acidosis, cerebral edema, hemorrhage,[41,42,48] or infection. More than half the patients initially reported with the acute form did not survive, but with rapid diagnosis and recent improvements in therapy, such as administration of glycine[40,43,46,47] and carnitine (see Treatment below), outcomes have been much more favorable. If the patient survives the acute neonatal episode, the subsequent course is that of the chronic intermittent form, and further development may be normal.[40,43,46,47]

Magnetic resonance spectroscopy for cerebral ^{31}P and ^{1}H was performed at 108 h of age in an infant with acute metabolic encephalopathy due to isovaleric acidemia.[49] It showed elevated levels of glutamate+glutamine, an increased ratio of lactate to N-acetylaspartate, and a severely reduced ratio of phosphocreatine to inorganic phosphate, indicating a major impairment of oxidative phosphorylation. On treatment, the neurologic abnormalities normalized, and magnetic resonance spectroscopy was normal at 18 days of age. At 1 year of age, neurologic assessment was normal.

Clinical features of the chronic intermittent form of isovaleric acidemia are well illustrated by the first two patients reported,[37,50] as well as by more recent cases.[51] The first episode of illness usually occurs during the first year of life. Episodes often follow upper respiratory infections or increased intake of protein-rich foods. The recurrent episodes typically involve vomiting, lethargy progressing to coma, acidosis with ketonuria, and the characteristic "odor of sweaty feet" due to elevated isovaleric acid levels. The episodes resolve with protein restriction and infusion of glucose. Additional symptoms that may occur with episodes include diarrhea, thrombocytopenia, neutropenia, pancytopenia,[52] and in some cases alopecia[52–54] and hyperglycemia; the last may be erroneously thought to be diabetic ketoacidosis [55,56] Hyperglycemia can occur in many organic acidemias, and sometimes the same patient has it one time and not another. It probably is due not to the disease but to stress-induced hormonal effects. As in most of the organic acidemias, the frequency of catabolic episodes is highest during infancy and subsequently decreases because of fewer infections and decreased protein intake, which naturally occur with normal growth. Most patients with chronic intermittent isovaleric acidemia have normal psychomotor development, but some have developmental delay and mild[37,50] or even severe[57] mental retardation. Many patients develop a natural aversion to protein-rich foods.[54] Currently, biochemical diagnostic services are more generally available, so that a diagnosis of isovaleric acidemia often is made with the first episode. Combining early diagnosis with protein restriction and administration of glycine and carnitine has improved the chances of normal development considerably. The oldest patient, now more than 30 years old,[37,50] although mildly retarded, had only two mild episodes of dizziness, blurred vision, and unsteady gait as a teenager. She tolerated a pregnancy with little difficulty, and there were no adverse effects on the offspring.[50]

Abnormal Metabolites. Isovaleric acidemia derives its name from the elevated concentrations of isovaleric acid found in the blood of patients.[8] The normal concentrations of isovaleric acid in plasma are less than 10 μM. During remission patients may have concentrations of isovaleric acid from normal to 10 times normal (10 to 50 μM), but during severe episodes the levels rise as high as 100 to 500 times normal (600 to 5000 μM). Isovaleric acid has the "odor of sweaty feet." This odor is generally not noticeable during remission but can be quite pronounced during catabolic episodes. The amount of isovaleric acid in the urine of patients is much less than that in plasma, with excretion rates ranging from 8 to 300 μmol/day (normal less than 2 μmol/day).

The major metabolite of isovaleryl-CoA that accumulates because of the deficiency of isovaleryl-CoA dehydrogenase is not the deacylation (hydrolysis) product isovaleric acid but rather an amide product produced by conjugation with the amino group of glycine — isovalerylglycine.[58] This reaction is catalyzed by the mitochondrial enzyme glycine N-acylase, which also forms benzoylglycine (hippuric acid) from benzoyl-CoA.[59,60] A variety of acyl-CoAs are substrates for the bovine liver enzyme, which has a K_m for isovaleryl-CoA of 180 μM, about 20 times that for benzoyl-CoA but with comparable maximum velocities for these two substrates.[59] Human liver glycine N-acylase has a K_m for isovaleryl-CoA of 672 μM.[60] The excretion of isovalerylglycine by patients with isovaleric acidemia ranges from 2000 to 15,000 μmol/day, compared with normal excretions of less than 15 μmol/day. Excretion is highest during acute episodes but is still very high during remission. Isovalerylglycine appears to be a nontoxic, readily excreted conjugate. The capacity of the glycine N-acylase appears to be adequate to remove the amount of isovaleryl-CoA usually produced by the patients, so little is deacylated to isovaleric acid. However, during acute episodes, when the amount of isovaleryl-CoA is greatly increased by catabolic crisis, the capacity of glycine N-acylase is exceeded, and free isovaleric acid becomes elevated. A second metabolite of isovaleric acid that was identified early is 3-hydroxyisovaleric acid.[61] This is excreted in abnormal amounts only during acute episodes, when it can be as high as 3000 μmol/day, or about 40 percent as much as isovalerylglycine. It is thought to arise from ω-1 oxidation of elevated free isovaleric acid.

As shown in Fig. 93-1, a large number of additional metabolites of isovaleryl-CoA have now been identified in the urine of patients with isovaleric acidemia. 4-Hydroxyisovaleric acid is believed to be formed by ω-oxidation of free isovaleric acid[48,62,63] and can be further oxidized to methylsuccinic acid and then dehydrogenated to mesaconic acid (methylfumaric acid). These oxidation products are elevated only during acute episodes. Isovaleryl-CoA can also form a number of different conjugation products, including isovalerylglucuronide,[64,65] isovalerylglutamic acid,[66] isovalerylalanine,[67] isovalerylsarcosine,[67] and isovalerylcarnitine.[52] Isovaleryl-CoA can also be condensed with acetyl-CoA by 3-oxothiolase to form 3-hydroxyisoheptanoic acid.[68] Of these metabolites, which are significantly elevated in the urine of patients with isovaleric acidemia only during acute episodes, only isovalerylglucuronide and isovalerylcarnitine are of importance, and their excretion levels are usually a small fraction of that of isovalerylglycine. However, in plasma or dried blood spots, elevated isovalerylcarnitine (C5 acylcarnitine) is of considerable diagnostic importance.

Although presence of the amino acid alloisoleucine in plasma or urine is generally considered diagnostic for maple syrup urine disease, slight elevations (2 to 10 μM) in plasma of three patients with isovaleric acidemia have been reported.[69] Alloisoleucine may be formed from 2-oxo-3-methylvaleric acid when elevated levels are caused by inhibition of branched chain 2-oxoacid dehydrogenase by isovaleryl-CoA.[70]

Enzyme Deficiency. The oxidation of [1-^{14}C]isovaleric acid to $^{14}CO_2$ in leukocytes[8] and the oxidation of [2-^{14}C]leucine to $^{14}CO_2$ in fibroblasts[71,72] is markedly deficient in patients with isovaleric acidemia. A sensitive assay for isovaleryl-CoA dehydrogenase was developed based on the release of tritium from [2,3-^{3}H]isovaleryl-CoA, with equilibration of the label into water.[10] The activity in mitochondria isolated from fibroblasts of patients with isovaleric acidemia was shown to be about 13 percent of normal.[9] With an improved tritium release assay, the residual activity in nine patients ranged from 0 to 3.5 percent of normal, and the amount of residual activity did not correlate with the degree of clinical severity.[73] The K_m for isovaleryl-CoA from normal fibroblasts was 22 μM. A deficiency of isovaleryl-CoA dehydrogenase in the fibroblasts of a patient with isovaleric acidemia has also been demonstrated by a fluorescent ETF-linked assay.[74]

Genetics. Isovaleric acidemia shows autosomal recessive inheritance. The gene for isovaleryl-CoA dehydrogenase has been assigned to human chromosome 15q14-q15 by Southern-blot analysis of DNA from human-rodent somatic-cell hybrids and by in situ hybridization.[21] Both the acute neonatal presentation and the chronic intermittent form can occur in the same family, suggesting that the clinical heterogeneity is caused in part by nongenetic factors. Genetic complementation studies of fibroblasts showed no complementation among 12 patients with isovaleric acidemia, half of whom had the severe form and half of whom had the mild intermittent form, indicating involvement of a single locus.[75] This is consistent with the fact that the enzyme is a homopolymer of four identical subunits.[11]

Molecular heterogeneity of isovaleryl-CoA dehydrogenase in fibroblasts from 15 patients with isovaleric acidemia was shown by labeling of the proteins with [^{35}S]methionine, precipitation of the enzyme with antirat isovaleryl-CoA dehydrogenase antiserum, and sodium dodecyl sulfate-polyacrylamide gel electrophoresis (SDS-PAGE).[76] The labeling was done both in the presence of rhodamine 6G to prevent processing into mitochondria, in order to determine the size of the newly synthesized precursor enzyme, and without rhodamine 6G to determine the size of the mature processed enzyme in the mitochondria. Five classes of variant enzymes were found, about half being class I with normal 45-kDa precursor and 43-kDa mature sizes, suggesting that they have point mutations and are processed normally. Class II had a smaller (42-kDa) precursor, and very little was processed into a smaller (40-kDa) mature form. Class III was synthesized as a 43-kDa precursor and processed to a 41-kDa mature form. Class IV was synthesized as a 42-kDa precursor and processed to a 40-kDa mature form. No immunoprecipitable protein was detected with class V mutants. Two cell lines were found to be compound heterozygotes for classes I and II. In Northern blots, the three normal sizes of isovaleryl-CoA dehydrogenase mRNA, 4.6, 3.8, and 2.1 kb, were found in fibroblasts of class I, II, III, and IV mutants, suggesting that these mutants are due to point mutations or small deletions.[23] To further characterize the mutations, the isovaleryl-CoA dehydrogenase coding region from mutant fibroblast cDNA was amplified by PCR and sequenced.[77] Two class I mutants contained different missense mutations. One showed a single mutant allele in cDNA, with a T-to-C substitution at position 125 leading to a leucine to proline change at position 13 of the mature enzyme. In contrast to the case in cDNA, two different alleles were found in genomic DNA. This new class VI mutant is not expressed at the mRNA level and may be transcriptionally defective or result in an unstable mRNA. A class III mutant had a single base deletion at position 1179, leading to a frameshift resulting in incorporation of eight abnormal amino acids followed by a premature termination codon. No abnormalities were found in the cDNA sequence of a class V mutant, which may be due to a deficiency in translation of the mRNA.

One class II mutant has been characterized in detail by PCR and sequencing.[78] The cDNA had a 90-bp deletion caused by an error in RNA splicing, resulting in an in-frame deletion of 30 amino acids beginning with leucine 20 of the mature isovaleryl-CoA dehydrogenase. This explains the smaller size of the precursor and mature forms of this mutant enzyme. Although the mutant precursor protein was cleaved by purified mitochondrial leader peptidases at a normal rate, binding to the surface of mitochondria and import into mitochondria was 30 percent of normal.[78]

Eight mutations in seven patients with isovaleric acidemia have been found to cause abnormal processing of the RNA for isovaleryl-CoA dehydrogenase.[79] Three of the point mutations result in abnormal splicing of the RNA and deletion of exon 2 in the cDNA.

Diagnosis. The diagnosis of isovaleric acidemia requires the analysis of organic acids, because the clinical features are common to a number of the organic acidurias. An "odor of sweaty feet" during acute episodes may be suggestive of isovaleric acidemia but must be distinguished from the similar odor that can occur in glutaric aciduria type II due to the accumulation of butyric, isobutyric, 2-methylbutyric, and isovaleric acids. The odor is generally not present during remission and is not always noticeable during episodes. The possibility of isovaleric acidemia should be considered in neonates or older infants with any combination of refusal to feed, vomiting, lethargy, coma, metabolic acidosis, ketosis, hyperammonemia, hypocalcemia, neutropenia, thrombocytopenia, and pancytopenia. Analysis of volatile short-chain acids in plasma demonstrating elevation of isovaleric acid without elevation of other short-chain acids suggests a diagnosis of isovaleric acidemia. 3-Methylbutyrolactone derived from elevated 4-hydroxyisovaleric acid found in acutely ill patients with isovaleric acidemia may also be detected by analysis of volatile short-chain acids.[63] However, accurate analysis of the plasma short-chain acids is difficult, often not readily available, and possibly unable to provide a diagnosis of other organic acidurias if the patient does not have isovaleric acidemia. Therefore, it is preferable to analyze the urine for nonvolatile organic acids, because isovalerylglycine, but not isovaleric acid, is always highly elevated in urine of patients with isovaleric acidemia, and most other organic acidemias can be distinguished by their characteristic urinary nonvolatile organic acid profiles.[1–3,80] The urinary acid profile diagnostic of isovaleric acidemia during an acute episode shows a very large elevation of isovalerylglycine (2000 to 9000 mmol/mol of creatinine) together with lesser elevations of 3-hydroxyisovaleric acid (1000 to 2000 mmol/mol of creatinine). Significant but much smaller amounts (20 to 300 mmol/mol of creatinine) of the minor metabolites, 4-hydroxyisovaleric acid, mesaconic acid, methylsuccinic acid, 3-hydroxyisoheptanoic acid, isovalerylglutamic acids, isovalerylglucuronide, isovalerylalanine, and isovalerylsarcosine, may be seen. In addition, nonspecific large elevations of lactic, 3-hydroxybutyric, and acetoacetic acids are often seen. During remission, the only diagnostic organic acid commonly seen is a large amount of isovalerylglycine (1000 to 3000 mmol/mol of creatinine).

High-field proton NMR is a promising technique for the rapid diagnosis of organic acidurias by direct analysis of a small aliquot of urine; it can readily detect isovalerylglycine.[81–83] Isovaleric acidemia may be especially amenable to diagnosis by NMR because it is the only disorder in which isovalerylglycine is very highly elevated in urine whether the patient is acutely ill or in remission.

The analysis of carnitine esters in blood and urine is a complementary approach to the analysis of organic acids for the diagnosis of isovaleric acidemia. The acyl-CoAs are in equilibrium with their acylcarnitines, and these are present in plasma and readily excreted in the urine. Isovalerylcarnitine in small amounts (10 to 20 mmol/mol of creatinine) has been identified by tandem MS in the urine of a patient with isovaleric acidemia during remission.[52] On oral administration of 100 mg/kg of L-carnitine, the excretion of isovalerylcarnitine rose to 3200 mmol/mol of creatinine, suggesting that administration of carnitine would increase the reliability of the diagnosis of isovaleric acidemia by assay of acylcarnitines in urine. Electrospray tandem MS of plasma or dried blood spots for elevated C5 acylcarnitine (isovalerylcarnitine) is a useful diagnostic test for isovaleric acidemia that can also be used for newborn screening. Although tandem MS does not distinguish isomers of C5 acylcarnitines, elevation of only C5 is most likely due to isovalerylcarnitine. Another C5 acylcarnitine, 2-methylbutyrylcarnitine, may be elevated together with isovalerylcarnitine in multiple acyl-CoA dehydrogenase deficiency, but this is usually accompanied by elevated C4 acylcarnitine in this disorder.

Diagnosis of isovaleric acidemia from assay of the metabolites can be confirmed by assay of fibroblasts for a deficiency of isovaleryl-CoA dehydrogenase by either the tritium release[73] or the fluorometric[74] assay. Unfortunately, the enzyme assay is not readily available.

Prenatal diagnosis of isovaleric acidemia can be accomplished by assay of isovaleryl-CoA dehydrogenase activity by fluorometric assay, by macromolecular labeling from [1-^{14}C]isovaleric acid in cultured amniocytes, or by stable isotope dilution analysis of elevated isovalerylglycine in amniotic fluid following amniocentesis.[84] Isovalerylglycine was undetectable in 10 normal amniotic fluids and measured only 0.04 μM in one other normal fluid. It was highly elevated at 3.50 and 6.02 μM in the amniotic fluids from two pregnancies with fetuses affected with isovaleric acidemia. It was also slightly elevated at 0.11 μM in amniotic fluids from three pregnancies at risk for isovaleric acidemia but with unaffected fetuses. In 18 pregnancies at risk for isovaleric acidemia, two were found to have highly elevated isovalerylglycine by stable isotope dilution GC/MS of amniotic fluid at 14–17 weeks.[85] The results of affected fetuses were confirmed by incorporation of labeled isovaleric acid into macromolecules. Thus, the precise quantification of isovalerylglycine in amniotic fluid by stable isotope dilution analysis provides rapid and accurate prenatal diagnosis of isovaleric acidemia. Analysis of isovalerylglycine in maternal urine is not suitable for prenatal diagnosis. The finding of isovalerylglycine in human amniotic fluid with an affected fetus at 12 weeks[85] suggests that glycine N-acylase is active early in human fetal development, in contrast to the rabbit and rat, in which the activity appears perinatally.[86] First-trimester prenatal diagnosis of isovaleric acidemia has also been accomplished by incorporation of labeled isovaleric acid in both fresh chorionic villi (CV) and cultured CV cells.[85]

A new method for prenatal diagnosis of isovaleric acidemia is electrospray ionization tandem MS analysis of acylcarnitines in amniotic fluid. Five unaffected at-risk pregnancies had isovalerylcarnitine levels of 0.59–0.99 μM, similar to levels in 24 controls (0.13–0.71 μM), while five affected pregnancies had highly elevated levels of isovalerylcarnitine (3.12–12.0 μM).[87] The ratio of C5-acylcarnitine to C3-acylcarnitine shows an even larger difference between affected and unaffected pregnancies.

Treatment. Patients with isovaleric acidemia have been treated during acute episodes with nonspecific procedures appropriate for a number of organic acidurias: glucose infusion to provide calories and reduce endogenous protein catabolism and, perhaps unnecessarily, bicarbonate infusion to control the acidosis.[38,39] Treatment during recovery and remission generally consists of restriction of natural dietary protein to age-adjusted leucine requirements and supplementation with a leucine-free medical food as a source of other amino acids. This has been effective in decreasing the frequency of episodes, although the wide variation in frequency of episodes among untreated patients and the decreasing frequency with age make it difficult to evaluate accurately the true effectiveness of this versus newer modes of therapy. The two newer approaches to treatment, administration of glycine and carnitine, were designed to enhance the removal of isovaleryl-CoA as nontoxic, readily excreted products, isovalerylglycine and isovalerylcarnitine.

Glycine is required for the synthesis of isovalerylglycine by glycine N-acylase, and its concentration may be rate limiting, especially when isovaleryl-CoA is highly elevated during an acute episode. The concentration of glycine in the plasma of patients with isovaleric acidemia tends to decrease during acute episodes, suggesting that insufficient amounts of glycine are available for isovalerylglycine synthesis.[88] Normal tissue levels of glycine are far below the reported K_m for glycine of the enzyme: 3 mM for the beef liver enzyme[59] and 500 mM for the human liver enzyme.[60] Increasing the concentration of glycine would be expected to increase the rate at which isovaleryl-CoA is conjugated with glycine to isovalerylglycine. When 250 mg/kg of body weight of glycine was given orally with a leucine challenge to a patient with isovaleric acidemia, the usual rise in plasma isovaleric acid was prevented and the excretion of isovalerylglycine doubled.[88] Long-term therapy with 250 mg/kg per day of glycine (divided into three doses) and a protein intake of 1.5 g/kg per day led to improved weight gain but did not prevent two acute episodes, although their duration was greatly shortened with rectal administration of 200 mg/kg of glycine every 6 h.[88] Two infants were treated with 250 mg/kg of glycine by nasogastric tube, with rapid decreases in metabolite levels but much slower clinical response.[40] Continued oral treatment with 800 mg per day of glycine and 1.5 g/kg of protein resulted in normal development without additional episodes. Similar experiences have been reported.[89,90] It has been suggested that the optimal amount of glycine is 150 mg/kg per day when patients are stable on a leucine-restricted diet but that this can be increased to 600 mg/kg per day when isovaleric acid is elevated.[91] A detailed quantitative description of the effects of glycine on the metabolites of isovaleric acid during an acute episode has been reported.[53] Benzoic acid, which as its CoA metabolite competes with isovaleryl-CoA for glycine N-acylase, prevents the beneficial effect of glycine.[53] Salicylic acid derived from aspirin is also a substrate for glycine N-acylase and could also interfere with the synthesis of isovalerylglycine. Therefore, the administration of aspirin would appear to be contraindicated in isovaleric acidemia.

Many patients with isovaleric acidemia were found to have a deficiency of total carnitine and a high percentage of esterified carnitine in plasma and in urine.[51,52,92,93] Some patients have increased urinary excretion of total carnitine with an abnormally high percentage of esterified carnitine.[51,94] These facts can be accounted for by the equilibrium between isovaleryl-CoA and isovalerylcarnitine catalyzed by carnitine acetyltransferase and continued loss of isovalerylcarnitine into urine at a rate greater than can be compensated for by carnitine synthesis. In a patient who had been treated with oral L-carnitine, changing to intravenous L-carnitine or acetyl-L-carnitine at increasing doses (up to 60 mg/kg per day carnitine or 76 mg/kg per day acetylcarnitine in four divided doses) did not increase the excretion of isovalerylcarnitine but did decrease the excretion of isovalerylglycine by as much as 50 percent.[95] It was suggested that this may have been due to decreased protein degradation, a major source of leucine for catabolism. In a single patient not routinely treated with carnitine, treatment for 4 weeks with 100 mg/kg per day of L-carnitine in two divided doses resulted in improvement of exercise tolerance, with increased oxygen uptake at the anaerobic threshold.[96] It was not determined whether exercise tolerance was normal before treatment with carnitine.

The relative effectiveness of carnitine and glycine in treatment of isovaleric acidemia has been compared.[52,92,97,98] Prior to treatment with carnitine, a patient excreted an amount of isovalerylcarnitine only 0.4 percent that of isovalerylglycine. Treatment orally with 100 mg/kg of carnitine resulted in a 10-percent decrease in isovalerylglycine excretion and a rise in isovalerylcarnitine to 50 percent of that of isovalerylglycine.[52] When given with a leucine challenge, equal doses (2 mmol/kg) of glycine or carnitine were similarly effective, as judged by the total excretion of isovalerylglycine and isovalerylcarnitine. Continued treatment was with 25 mg/kg per 6 h of L-carnitine without glycine, with satisfactory results. Another patient has been treated with moderate restriction of protein to 2 g/kg per day and administration of L-carnitine 40 mg/kg per day in three divided doses.[92] Isovalerylglycine excretion remained much higher than that of acylcarnitines, but the patient has grown normally and tolerated an intercurrent illness without ketoacidosis. Administration of carnitine while this patient was receiving glycine resulted not only in an increase in isovalerylcarnitine excretion but also in a doubling of the excretion of isovalerylglycine.[92] Detailed analyses of carnitine and esterified carnitine in the plasma and urine of a patient treated with various amounts of carnitine have been reported.[51] Two patients receiving 40–50 mg/kg per day of oral glycine were treated with doses of oral L-carnitine ranging from 25 to 100 mg/kg per day.[97] The excretion of isovalerylcarnitine was a small fraction of that of isovalerylglycine, but the excretion of isovalerylglycine increased with the dose of carnitine. The metabolite excretion of a patient receiving carnitine alone, glycine alone, or glycine plus carnitine and after a load of leucine on each of the treatments was evaluated.[98] Isovalerylglycine was the dominant metabolite with all three treatments. A load of leucine did not increase isovalerylglycine excretion during glycine treatment but did increase it markedly during treatment with carnitine or carnitine plus glycine. All of the above studies suffer from lack of a common protocol, varying doses and diets, small patient number and different patient ages, i.e., different metabolic and growth rates. Thus, it is difficult to determine whether glycine or carnitine is more effective for the long-term management of isovaleric acidemia, but the removal of isovaleric acid as isovalerylglycine with endogenously produced glycine is clearly of primary importance. Restricting the amount of isovaleric acid that must be disposed of by moderate restriction of dietary leucine is also valuable. Treatment with L-carnitine seems appropriate to prevent carnitine deficiency from developing and to provide a second route of isovaleric acid disposal, independent of glycine. During an acute episode, additional treatment with glycine to maximize removal as both isovalerylglycine and isovalerylcarnitine would appear to be the most effective therapeutic modality.

One study of the catabolism of L-($^2H_3$-methyl)-leucine to isovalerylglycine, isovalerylcarnitine, and 3-hydroxyisovaleric acid in a patient with isovaleric acidemia questioned the value of restriction of dietary protein in this disorder.[99] In this study, the amount of labeled leucine given was equivalent to the amount of leucine in a low-protein diet of 0.75 g/kg per day. For each of the three urinary metabolites, less than 10 percent was labeled, indicating that more than 90 percent of the labeled leucine was incorporated into protein. The continued excretion of labeled metabolites after the labeled leucine was stopped reflected turnover of proteins into which the labeled leucine had been incorporated. Thus, at this low, and probably inadequate, level of protein intake, the major source of isovaleric acid is the turnover of protein, and the value of protein restriction was questioned. Many patients with isovaleric acidemia have been restricted to 1.5 to 2.0 g/kg per day of protein, and further studies are needed to determine the fraction of leucine directly metabolized to isovaleric acid metabolites as a function of protein intake. Restriction of total protein makes little sense in light of the availability of low-leucine medical foods. Rather, a low-leucine diet with at least a normal total protein and caloric intake is more logical and in our experience has resulted in lower morbidity.

Other Aspects. The mechanism of the toxicity of isovaleric acid is not established, but it is an inhibitor of succinate:CoA ligase in the tricarboxylic acid cycle and inhibits liver but not muscle mitochondrial oxygen consumption with glutamic, 2-oxoglutaric, and succinic acids.[100] Isovaleric acid is an inhibitor of granulopoietic progenitor cell proliferation in bone marrow cultures with half-maximal inhibition at 1.6 mM, and this may account for the neutropenia frequently seen in isovaleric acidemia.[101]

Isolated Deficiency of 3-Methylcrotonyl-CoA Carboxylase Distinction from Multiple Carboxylase Deficiency

The isolated deficiency of 3-methylcrotonyl-CoA carboxylase, which is not responsive to treatment with biotin, must be distinguished from the biotin-responsive multiple-carboxylase deficiencies, which are due to disorders of biotin metabolism (biotinidase deficiency and holocarboxylase synthetase deficiency) and affect all four of the biotin-dependent carboxylases, as discussed in Chap. 156. In all these disorders, the major abnormal urinary metabolites are 3-hydroxyisovaleric acid and 3-methylcrotonylglycine, due to a deficiency of 3-methylcrotonyl-CoA carboxylase. In the multiple-carboxylase deficiencies, these are accompanied by small elevations of methylcitric and 3-hydroxypropionic acids — metabolites characteristic of propionyl-CoA carboxylase deficiency. Therefore, the differential diagnosis of isolated 3-methylcrotonyl-CoA carboxylase deficiency depends on careful quantitative analysis of urinary organic acid profiles, on assay of fibroblasts or leukocytes for a deficiency of this enzyme with normal activities of the other carboxylases, or on assay of biotinidase in plasma. It is difficult to determine whether some of the earlier-described patients had an isolated deficiency of 3-methylcrotonyl-CoA carboxylase, because the possibility of multiple carboxylase deficiency was not always ruled out.

More than 25 patients with clear indications of isolated 3-methylcrotonyl-CoA carboxylase deficiency have been reported.

Clinical Aspects. Patients with an isolated deficiency of 3-methylcrotonyl-CoA carboxylase usually have normal growth and development until they present with an acute episode between 6 months and 3 years of age, although presentation has been as early as the neonatal period[102–104] and as late as 5 years of age.[105] A number of siblings of affected patients have been clinically normal, suggesting that the degree of catabolic stress is an important factor.[106,107] The presentation is often similar to that of Reye syndrome or 3-hydroxy-3-methylglutaryl-CoA lyase deficiency. The episodes frequently follow minor infections and involve feeding difficulty, vomiting, lethargy, apnea, muscle hypotonia, or hyperreflexia. Infantile spasms or seizures may occur.[102,104,108,109] Several patients have had neutrophilia, although this may have been due to infection or a nonspecific consequence of stress-related epinephrine release.[110,111] One older patient had loss of scalp hair.[105] Two patients showed fatty changes in the liver resembling those of Reye syndrome.[112–114] One patient died from cardiac arrest,[108] one from cerebral edema,[112] and one from cardiocirculatory crisis.[102]

As GC/MS analysis of urinary organic acids became more widely used to investigate possible metabolic disorders, patients with a wider range of clinical symptoms were found to have 3-methylcrotonyl-CoA carboxylase deficiency. Some had failure to thrive in the neonatal period[103,115] or presented with developmental delay,[116] familial hypotonia,[107] or even hypertonia.[115] One patient was diagnosed because of studies for lethargy following a minor head trauma.[117] An asymptomatic newborn was diagnosed with 3-methylcrotonyl-CoA carboxylase deficiency during investigation for maple syrup urine disease because of an elevated leucine on neonatal screening.[118] Four adult women with no or few clinical symptoms were found to have 3-methylcrotonyl-CoA carboxylase deficiency during follow-up of elevated 3-hydroxyisovalerylcarnitine levels found on neonatal screening of their babies by tandem MS.[119] Three patients had clinically asymptomatic sibs who were also found to have 3-methylcrotonyl-CoA carboxylase deficiency by analysis of urinary organic acids. Thus, the clinical course of this disorder ranges from severe to apparently clinically benign. The lack of symptoms should not lull the clinician into a false sense of security, as in other organic acidemias acute decompensation and death have occurred with the first severe catabolic episode in the second decade of life.

Typical laboratory findings during an acute episode are severe hypoglycemia (blood glucose <1 mM), hyperammonemia, elevated hepatic transaminases, mild metabolic acidosis, and moderate ketonuria.[109-114] The levels of free carnitine in plasma are extremely low, from 0.7 to 5 μM (normal, >20 μM), and the ratio of carnitine esters to free carnitine is elevated.[107,109,111,114]

Abnormal Metabolites. The characteristic abnormal urinary metabolites seen in deficiency of 3-methylcrotonyl-CoA carboxylase are 3-hydroxyisovaleric acid and 3-methylcrotonylglycine.[105,111] Excretion can be extremely elevated, from 460 to 59,000 mmol/mol of creatinine for 3-hydroxyisovaleric acid[110,114] and from 70 to 3700 mmol/mol of creatinine for 3-methylcrotonylglycine.[109,111] 3-Methylcrotonylglutamic acid was detected in the urine of one patient.[114]

The major fate of 3-methylcrotonyl-CoA that accumulates in this disorder is not deacylation to 3-methylcrotonic acid but appears to be hydration to 3-hydroxyisovaleryl-CoA catalyzed by crotonase (enoyl-CoA hydratase)[32,120,121] and then deacylation to 3-hydroxyisovaleric acid. The K_m of ox liver crotonase for crotonyl-CoA is 20 μM, and at equilibrium the level of the hydrated product is 3.5 times that of the unsaturated substrate. 3-Methylcrotonyl-CoA is a substrate, and although it is hydrated at 14 percent of the rate of crotonyl-CoA, the equilibrium would favor 3-hydroxyisovaleryl-CoA. An alternative fate is conjugation with glycine catalyzed by glycine N-acylase.[59] The K_m for 3-methylcrotonyl-CoA is 14 μM for the bovine liver enzyme, which is comparable to the K_m for benzoyl-CoA and 10 times lower than the K_m for isovaleryl-CoA.[59] The maximum velocities are comparable for the three substrates. Excretion of more 3-hydroxyisovaleric acid than 3-methylcrotonylglycine by these patients may reflect higher activity of crotonase than of glycine N-acylase rather than substrate affinities of the two enzymes. 3-Hydroxyisovaleric acid has been shown to be highly elevated at 166 μM in the plasma (normal <2 μM) and 285 μM in the CSF (normal <2 μM) of a patient with 3-methylcrotonyl-CoA carboxylase who had severe neurologic abnormalities.[122] Another patient with only mild developmental delay had 3-hydroxyisovaleric acid levels of 600 μM in plasma and 540 μM in CSF.[106]

The severe secondary deficiency of free carnitine in plasma and the elevated ratio of esterified carnitine to free carnitine suggested that an abnormal carnitine ester is excreted by patients with a deficiency of 3-methylcrotonyl-CoA carboxylase. This would be expected to be 3-methylcrotonylcarnitine, but this accounted for only 2% of the total urinary acylcarnitine as determined by HPLC in the urine of six patients.[123] Instead, the major acylcarnitine in plasma, urine and cultured fibroblasts was identified as 3-hydroxyisovaleryl-carnitine by tandem MS[124] and in urine by tandem MS and GC/MS.[123] This is unusual, since hydroxyacyl carnitines are not generally elevated in other organic acid disorders. Carnitine acetyltransferase does not convert 3-hydroxyisovaleryl-CoA to a carnitine ester, suggesting that 3-methylcrotonyl-CoA forms 3-methylcrotonylcarnitine, which is then hydrated to 3-hydroxyisovalerylcarnitine.[123]

Enzyme Deficiency. Fibroblasts from two sibs had only 2 percent of normal incorporation of [1-^{14}C]isovaleric acid into macromolecules in cultured fibroblasts.[125] Patients have a severe deficiency of 3-methylcrotonyl-CoA carboxylase both in leukocytes, whether the patients were treated with biotin or not, and in fibroblasts cultured with different concentrations of biotin, while the activity levels of the other carboxylases were normal.[102,104,105,110] This confirms the lack of response to biotin, consistent with a genetic defect in apo-3-methylcrotonyl-CoA carboxylase. The activities of 3-methylcrotonyl-CoA carboxylase in cultured fibroblasts of patients are generally 0 to 2 percent of normal.[106,109,111,113,118] A patient with only moderately elevated excretion of 3-hydroxyisovaleric acid and 3-methylcrotonylglycine had a partial deficiency of 3-methylcrotonyl-CoA carboxylase.[115]

Genetics. This disorder is inherited as an autosomal recessive trait.

Diagnosis. The possibility of a deficiency of 3-methylcrotonyl-CoA carboxylase should be considered in patients with the typical signs of an organic aciduria and especially those with hypoglycemia or symptoms of Reye syndrome. It should also be considered in patients with hypotonia, seizures, or developmental delay. A very low plasma free carnitine may also suggest this disorder. The diagnosis can be made by finding a high excretion (500 to 7000 mmol/mol of creatinine) of 3-hydroxyisovaleric acid and 50 to 4000 mmol/mol of creatinine of 3-methylcrotonylglycine.[105,107,109-111,113,114] These elevations occur without elevation of isovalerylglycine or of the distal metabolites of leucine, 3-methylglutaconic acid, or 3-hydroxy-3-methylglutaric acid and without the modest elevation of 3-hydroxypropionic, methylcitric, and lactic acids seen in multiple carboxylase deficiency. Ketotic patients excrete moderately elevated amounts of 3-hydroxybutyric and acetoacetic acids and may have secondary elevation of dicarboxylic acids.[109,110] It should be noted that the modest elevations of 3-hydroxyisovaleric acid ranging from 50 to 200 mmol/mol of creatinine (normal: 1 to 20 mmol/mol of creatinine) that are seen in patients with severe ketosis of any cause[126] are generally lower than the excretion levels in patients with 3-methylcrotonyl-CoA carboxylase deficiency. Also, 3-methylcrotonylglycine is not elevated secondary to ketosis.

3-Methylcrotonyl-CoA carboxylase deficiency can also be diagnosed by analysis of plasma or dried blood spots for acylcarnitines by tandem MS, which shows a large elevation of 3-hydroxyisovalerylcarnitine.[124] 3-Methylcrotonylcarnitine may or may not be present. Patients with 3-hydroxy-3-methylglutaryl-CoA lyase deficiency also may have elevated 3-hydroxyisovalerylcarnitine, but this is accompanied by 3-methyl glutarylcarnitine.[127] Patients with multiple carboxylase deficiency may also have elevated 3-hydroxyisovalerylcarnitine, but this would usually be accompanied by elevated propionylcarnitine. Neonatal screening by tandem MS analysis of dried blood spots can readily detect elevated 3-hydroxyisovalerylcarnitine and suggest 3-methylcrotonyl-CoA carboxylase deficiency. An unexpected finding of this neonatal screening was the identification of four Amish/Mennonite babies with elevated 3-hydroxyisovalerylcarnitine who had normal activity of 3-methylcrotonyl-CoA carboxylase, but whose mothers were found to have a deficiency of this enzyme.[119] The transfer of 3-hydroxyisovalerylcarnitine from the mothers to the babies was not through breast milk (where this metabolite is not detected), since some of the babies were fed formula. Presumably it was transferred through the placenta.

For definitive diagnosis of isolated 3-methylcrotonyl-CoA carboxylase deficiency and exclusion of multiple carboxylase deficiency, a deficit of the former with normal activity of at least one other carboxylase should be shown in leukocytes, regardless of treatment with biotin, or in fibroblasts, regardless of the concentration of biotin in the culture medium.[105,110,111]

Heterozygotes for isolated 3-methylcrotonyl-CoA carboxylase deficiency cannot be reliably diagnosed by assay of the enzyme in leukocytes or cultured fibroblasts because its activity is usually within the normal range.[105,111,114]

Prenatal diagnosis of this disorder should be possible by stable isotope dilution analysis for elevated 3-hydroxyisovaleric acid in amniotic fluid, as has been shown for multiple carboxylase deficiency due to an abnormal holocarboxylase synthetase.[128] Prenatal diagnosis by assay for a deficiency of 3-methylcrotonyl-CoA carboxylase in CV samples or cultured amniocytes should also be possible.[129]

Treatment. Treatment of acute episodes with glucose and correction of acidosis and long-term treatment with restriction of dietary leucine have been effective, resulting in normal development. Biotin at 10 to 20 mg per day was without clinical effect and did not alter excretion of 3-hydroxyisovaleric acid and 3-methylcrotonylglycine,[105,109] as would be expected for a defect in the 3-methylcrotonyl-CoA carboxylase apoprotein, unlike the response in multiple carboxylase deficiency, in which the defect is in biotin metabolism.

Because patients with 3-methylcrotonyl-CoA carboxylase deficiency have a severe secondary deficiency of free carnitine in plasma, treatment with 75 to 100 mg/kg per day of oral L-carnitine is important to correct this deficiency, although it has little effect on urinary organic acid excretion levels.[109,111,114,123,130] Before treatment with carnitine, 3-hydroxyisovalerylcarnitine accounts for 2 percent of the total excretion of 3-hydroxyisovaleric acid, 3-methylcrotonylglycine, and 3-hydroxyisovalerylcarnitine and after treatment it accounts for 11 percent of the total.[123]

To increase detoxification of 3-methylcrotonyl-CoA, patients have been treated with glycine to increase excretion of 3-methylcrotonylglycine. One patient treated with 500 mg of glycine twice daily in addition to biotin and carnitine has remained clinically well.[114] Carnitine and glycine treatments were compared in a patient whose major metabolite was 3-methylcrotonylglycine.[130] Carnitine increased 3-hydroxyisovalerylcarnitine excretion, but it remained less than 20 percent of 3-methylcrotonylglycine excretion. Treatment with glycine increased 3-methylcrotonylglycine excretion more than twofold, with the maximum effect at 175 mg glycine/kg per day. Glycine also increased the levels of free and total carnitine in plasma in a dose-related manner. The excretion of 3-hydroxyisovaleric acid was not affected by either carnitine or glycine. Although combined therapy with glycine and carnitine was not tried, it may be the most effective treatment during metabolic crisis, but whether the combined therapy is best for chronic therapy is unknown. Long-term treatment with modest leucine restriction and oral L-carnitine generally appears to be sufficient for normal growth and development, assuming no catastrophic episodes occur with infection.

3-Methylglutaconic Aciduria

This is a clinically heterogeneous group of disorders with one feature in common: increased excretion of 3-methylglutaconic acid, which is associated with neurologic or cardiac abnormalities in some of the forms.[131,132] Patients with 3-methylglutaconic aciduria have been classified into the following four types, which will be discussed separately in the following sections:[133]

Type I: 3-Methylglutaconyl-CoA hydratase deficiency: a primary enzyme deficiency

Type II: Barth syndrome: X-linked cardiomyopathy, neutropenia, and growth retardation

Type III: Costeff optic atrophy syndrome: optic atrophy, choreoathetosis, spastic paresis, cerebellar ataxia, nystagmus, autosomal recessive inheritance

Type IV: Unclassified, variable clinical features including neurologic and cardiac abnormalities

The elevated excretion of 3-methylglutaconic acid in Type I clearly results from a block in the catabolic pathway for leucine. In the other three types, the source of 3-methylglutaconic acid is unknown; it does not appear to come from leucine and is presumably a secondary phenomenon due to a number of different primary metabolic defects.

3-Methylglutaconic aciduria has also been reported during pregnancy. Two women with toxemia of pregnancy excreted moderately elevated amounts of 3-methylglutaconic acid, which had no effect on the infants, who were normal at birth and had normal development.[134] In a study of 25 pregnancies of mothers who had had previous children with microcephaly and severe psychomotor retardation, in six pregnancies there was moderate elevation of 3-methylglutaconic acid (19–40 mmol/mol creatinine, normal 0–5) and 3-methylglutaric acid (2–15 mmol/mol creatinine, normal 0–2).[135] However, modest elevation of these organic acids may be normal during pregnancy, since 13 of 18 normal pregnant women had elevations of 3-methylglutaconic acid compared to nonpregnant women in another study.[136] On the hypothesis that increased excretion of 3-methylglutaconic acid in pregnancy might be due to increased steroid synthesis, 3-methylglutaconic acid levels were determined in patients with congenital adrenal hyperplasia who had increased steroid synthesis.[137] No increase in 3-methylglutaconic or 3-methylglutaric acid was seen.

3-Methylglutaconic Aciduria Type I: 3-Methylglutaconyl-CoA Hydratase Deficiency

Eight patients in seven families have been shown to have 3-methylglutaconic aciduria with a deficiency of 3-methylglutaconyl-CoA hydratase. The clinical symptoms range from minimal to severe. All the patients excrete large amounts of 3-methylglutaconic acid and in addition have high excretion rates of 3-hydroxyisovaleric acid, which is not seen in the other types of 3-methylglutaconic aciduria.

Clinical Aspects. In the first family, two brothers were diagnosed at ages 5 and 7 with speech retardation as the only clinical symptom.[138] One had a 1-day episode of coma at age 1 year and had mild psychomotor retardation at 2 years. On fasting for 18 hours, hypoglycemia and compensated metabolic acidosis occurred in one sib but not the other. A male patient in the second family was diagnosed at 4 months of age when he presented with bronchiolitis, mild hyperchloremic acidosis, and gastroesophageal reflux.[139] The fourth patient was a Chinese boy with normal growth, mild microcephaly, and speech retardation who presented with vomiting, seizures, and coma during an adenovirus respiratory infection.[140] He had acidosis, low blood glucose, and hyperammonemia and was initially thought to have Reye syndrome. Another patient had psychomotor retardation, failure to thrive, spastic quadraplegia, dystonia, and atrophy of the basal ganglia.[141] A female patient presented with vomiting, insomnia, and irritability after birth but developed normally until 1 year of age, when crying fits, self-mutilation, poor feeding, and hepatomegaly were noted.[142] Clinical symptoms resolved upon treatment with L-carnitine. Another patient required cardiopulmonary resuscitation at birth and at six months had severe acidosis, developmental delay, and dystonic cerebral dystonia.[143] A premature male had delayed psychomotor development and frequent respiratory infections in infancy, severe hypotonia at one year of age, and by two years of age, lumbar scoliosis and seizures.[143]

Abnormal Metabolites. The major abnormal metabolite excreted is 3-methylglutaconic acid, at levels ranging between 250 and 1150 mmol/mol of creatinine (normal, <6 mmol/mol of creatinine).[138,143] Two isomers are found in urine, corresponding to the E (trans) and Z (cis) isomers. 3-Hydroxyisovaleric acid, also elevated at 50 to 400 mmol/mol of creatinine (normal, 0 to 16 mmol/mol of creatinine), is derived from reversibility of the pathway to 3-methylcrotonyl-CoA and hydration. Very small amounts of 3-methylglutaric acid (5 to 20 mmol/mol of creatinine, normally undetectable) derived from hydrogenation of 3-methylglutaconyl-CoA were excreted. The product of 3-methylglutaconyl-CoA hydratase, 3-hydroxy-3-methylglutaric acid, was excreted in normal amounts (5 to 15 mmol/mol of creatinine). The levels of the three abnormal metabolites changed in parallel, increasing twofold with a high-protein diet (4 g/kg per day) or fasting, decreasing to half with a low-protein diet (1.5 g/kg per day), and increasing threefold with a challenge of 100 mg/kg of leucine.[138] One patient had elevated 3-methylglutaric only when ill with an intercurrent viral infection.[139] Tandem MS showed the presence of 3-methylglutaconylcarnitine and 3-methylglutarylcarnitine in the urine of one patient.[142]

Enzyme Deficiency. The incorporation of [1-^{14}C]isovaleric acid into macromolecules in intact fibroblasts of the two affected sibs was only moderately decreased, to 55 to 65 percent of normal,[125] and the oxidation of [U-^{14}C]leucine to $^{14}CO_2$ in lymphoblasts of the third patient was 39 percent of that in normal lymphoblasts.[139] The activity of 3-methylglutaconyl-CoA hydratase in fibroblasts from the first two sibs was markedly deficient, at only 3 percent of normal.[35] The enzyme activity in lymphoblasts of the third patient was 17 percent of normal.[139] Activity of the hydratase in fibroblasts of the fourth patient was 25 percent of normal.[140] Deficient activity of 3-methylglutaconyl-CoA hydratase in fibroblasts, measured by the incorporation of labeled sodium bicarbonate into 3-hydroxybutyryl-CoA, has been summarized for all patients.[143]

Genetics. Most but not all patients with a deficiency of 3-methylglutaconyl-CoA hydratase are male, consistent with autosomal recessive inheritance.

Diagnosis. The presenting clinical symptoms are diverse and rather nonspecific, as described above. Diagnosis of 3-methylglutaconic aciduria can be made by quantitative analysis of urinary organic acids finding a large elevation of 3-methylglutaconic acid (500 to 1000 mmol/mol of creatinine). It should be noted that with the use of trimethylsilyl derivatives, in addition to the two peaks for the E and Z isomers of the di-trimethylsilyl derivatives, smaller peaks of tris-trimethylsilyl are formed by the addition of trimethylsilyl and oxytrimethylsilyl across the double bond.[3] In addition to the highly elevated 3-methylglutaconic acid levels, in 3-methylglutaconic aciduria Type I there is high elevation of 3-hydroxyisovaleric acid (100 to 250 mmol/mol of creatinine), only slight elevation of 3-methylglutaric acid, and normal excretion of 3-hydroxy-3-methylglutaric acid. A different pattern of metabolite excretion is seen in patients with 3-methylglutaconic aciduria without a deficiency of 3-methylglutaconyl-CoA hydratase: elevated excretion of 3-methylglutaconic acid and 3-methylglutaric acid, but no elevation of 3-hydroxyisovaleric acid excretion. To distinguish these patients more accurately, it is necessary to assay the activity of 3-methylglutaconyl-CoA hydratase in leukocytes or cultured fibroblasts.[35,139,143,144] It is not known whether heterozygotes can be diagnosed by finding intermediate activities of 3-methylglutaconyl-CoA hydratase in leukocytes or cultured fibroblasts.

Prenatal diagnosis should be possible by GC/MS analysis of elevated 3-hydroxyisovaleric acid[128,145] and 3-methylglutaconic acid[145,146] in amniotic fluid. 3-Methylglutaconyl-CoA hydratase is likely to be expressed in cultured normal amniocytes, and assay for a deficiency of this enzyme should be suitable for prenatal diagnosis.

Treatment. It is not known whether leucine restriction is of clinical benefit in this disorder, but since excretion of the metabolites varies in proportion to protein intake, it might be worthwhile to evaluate modest restriction of leucine. Some patients have low carnitine levels in plasma and have responded well to carnitine supplementation.[143] Treatment with L-carnitine normalized the feeding difficulties, insomnia, and hepatomegaly of one patient.[142]

3-Methylglutaconic Aciduria Type II: Barth Syndrome with Normal 3-Methylglutaconyl-CoA Hydratase

More than 30 male patients with Barth syndrome have been reported, with mild elevations of 3-methylglutaconic acid but with normal 3-methylglutaconyl-CoA hydratase activity.[132,147]

Clinical Aspects. Barth syndrome[148] is characterized by dilated cardiomyopathy, skeletal myopathy, growth failure, and moderate to severe neutropenia.[147] Cardiac dysfunction is attributable to biventricular dilatation and hypertrophy with a decreased left ventricular shortening fraction. Lipid deposition exists in cardiac and skeletal muscle, along with variably low plasma and muscle carnitine levels. Ketone and dicarboxylic acid production on fasting are normal. Mildly decreased cholesterol levels are common, and some patients demonstrate mild lactic acidosis and/or hypoglycemia. Abnormal mitochondrial ultrastructure has been reported in some patients, but it is not universal and the changes are nonspecific. Frequent bacterial infections occur in some patients. Although motor function is severely impaired, cognitive development is usually normal. In a study of six patients in four families, it was noted that the cardiomyopathy and frequency and severity of bacterial infections decreased with age and that the older patients had similar facial appearances, due to a facial myopathy.[149]

Abnormal Metabolites. Most but not all patients showed small but significantly increased excretion of 3-methylglutaconic and 3-methylglutaric acids, with the sum of these two being 29 to 93 mmol/mol of creatinine, compared with normal excretion of less than 16 mmol/mol of creatinine.[147,149] Most patients also had modest elevations of 2-ethyl-3-hydroxypropionic acid (2-ethylhydracrylic acid) of 2 to 33 mmol/mol of creatinine, compared with normal excretion (less than 3 mmol/mol of creatinine). They did not have increased excretion of 3-hydroxyisovaleric acid.

Enzyme Deficiency. The basic enzyme defect is unknown. The activity of 3-methylglutaconyl-CoA hydratase is not deficient in these patients.[132] The excretion of 3-methylglutaconic acid and 3-methylglutaric acid is not affected by varying protein in the diet or by a leucine challenge.[147] This suggests that the source of these acids is not leucine. It had been hypothesized that the source of 3-methylglutaconic acid in patients now classified as having X-linked cardiomyopathy or "unspecified" 3-methylglutaconic aciduria might be the recycling of intermediates of the cholesterol biosynthetic pathway secondary to a block in this pathway.[131] This "mevalonic acid shunt" involves conversion of dimethylallyl pyrophosphate to 3-methylcrotonic acid and thence to 3-methylglutaconic acid.[150,151] However, the activity of the first four enzymes of the cholesterol biosynthetic pathway and the synthesis of cholesterol from acetate have been shown to be normal in fibroblasts of these patients.[132] Thus, the elevation of 3-methylglutaconic acid appears to be secondary to some other, as yet undetermined defect.

There is evidence of partial deficiencies of complexes I and IV in the mitochondrial electron transport chain in muscle[148,149] or fibroblasts[152] of some patients. A deficiency of three respiratory chain enzymes was found in muscle of a child with Barth syndrome who did not survive.[153]

Genetics. This is an X-linked recessive disorder. The gene was assigned by linkage analysis to distal Xq28, linked to the DXS52 marker.[152,154] A novel gene in this region, G4.5 (GenBank X92762), is expressed at high levels in cardiac and skeletal muscle, and mutations have been identified in this gene in four families with Barth syndrome.[155] The four unique mutations were identified in both affected males and carrier mothers. Each introduces a stop codon in the open reading frame. The gene has a complex pattern of expression, with different RNAs depending on splicing. Two forms differing in the region encoded by exons 5, 6, and 7 or by the 5′-end were more abundant. The gene has no similarities to other known genes, and the functions of the proteins it encodes are unknown. Further characterization of the G4.5 gene in 14 Barth syndrome pedigrees showed that each had a unique mutation and that nine of the mutations would be expected to disrupt the protein products.[156] The importance of exon 8 is suggested by the finding of four missense mutations in this exon. No correlation was found between the location or type of mutation and the clinical and biochemical phenotype. The mutation 985C > T in the G4.5 gene, which was present in one of the above pedigrees, has been found in another pedigree.[153]

Female carriers of Barth syndrome are healthy, which could be due to selection against cells with the mutant allele on the active X chromosome. Analysis of obligate heterozygotes showed a markedly skewed pattern of X inactivation in 11 of 16 carriers.[157] In seven cases studied, the parental origin of the inactive X chromosome was maternal.

Diagnosis. This disorder may be suspected in patients with dilated cardiomyopathy, neutropenia, and growth retardation;[147] with dilated cardiomyopathy, skeletal myopathy, neutropenia, and abnormal mitochondrial structure;[148] or with a similar cardiomyopathy with endocardial fibroelastosis.[158] Careful quantitative analysis of urinary organic acids by GC/MS is needed to determine accurately the very small elevation levels of 3-methylglutaconic and 3-methylglutaric acids. The total of these is 29 to 93 mmol/mol of creatinine, which is only two to six times the upper normal limit of 16 mmol/mol of creatinine.[147] Some patients do not have elevation of 3-methylglutaconic acid.[149] 2-Ethyl-3-hydroxypropionic acid levels may range from normal to 10 times the normal excretion of 3 mmol/mol of creatinine. 3-Hydroxyisovaleric acid and 3-hydroxy-3-methylglutaric acid are not elevated in these patients.

In a pregnancy in which three maternal uncles were retrospectively diagnosed with Barth syndrome, a fetal echocardiogram showed cardiac abnormalities in the male fetus, possibly suggesting Barth syndrome, which were confirmed after birth.[159] Urinary organic acids showed elevated 3-methylglutaconic and 3-methylglutaric, which together with the growth delay and dilated cardiomyopathy confirmed the diagnosis of Barth syndrome.

Now that the gene G4.5 has been identified as causing Barth syndrome, analysis of mutations in this gene may be a definitive method of diagnosis that should also be useful in carrier detection and prenatal diagnosis.

Treatment. Although one patient had a low plasma total carnitine level and episodic hypoglycemia that responded to carnitine supplementation, there was no effect on cardiac function, muscle weakness, or neutropenia.[147] Similarly, the dilated cardiomyopathy typical of this disorder has not been carnitine-responsive in other patients. In one patient, treatment with carnitine was associated with rapid cardiac deterioration, which reversed with large doses of intravenous pantothenic acid.[160] Changing to treatment with an oral vitamin preparation containing large amounts of racemic pantothenol resulted in gross heart failure, which was reversed by intravenous pantothenic acid; cardiac function continued to improve with 50 mg of pantothenate three times a day. Pantothenic acid is the precursor of coenzyme A, and treatment with large amounts of pantothenate may increase coenzyme A levels and affect 3-methylglutaconyl-CoA metabolism.

3-Methylglutaconic Aciduria Type III: Costeff Optic Atrophy Syndrome and Normal 3-Methylglutaconyl-CoA Hydratase

A new variant of 3-methylglutaconic aciduria has been identified in Iraqi-Jewish patients with a syndrome of infantile bilateral optic atrophy, choreoathetosis, spastic paraparesis, and cerebellar ataxia.[161,162]

Clinical Aspects. This syndrome is characterized by infantile bilateral optic atrophy, nystagmus, and an early-onset choreiform movement disorder with later development of mild spasticity in half of the patients and mild mental retardation in some.[161,162] The course of the disease is nonprogressive beyond childhood.

Abnormal Metabolites. 3-Methylglutaconic acid is moderately elevated in urine at 10 to 200 mmol/mol creatinine, together with lesser elevation of 3-methylglutaric acid and no elevation of 3-hydroxyisovaleric or 2-ethyl-3-hydroxypropionic acid.[162,163]

Enzyme Studies. The activity of 3-methylglutaconyl-CoA hydratase is normal.[163] The basic enzyme defect is not known.

Genetics. The inheritance is autosomal recessive, based on the ratio of 23 female to 16 male patients.[133] The syndrome has been linked to chromosome 19q13.2-13.3 by a shared segment analysis.[164] Although the gene for muscle type creatine kinase maps within this region, no mutations were found in this gene.

Diagnosis. This syndrome appears to be found only in Iraqi-Jews; the clinical diagnosis by optic atrophy and chorea is confirmed by finding elevated 3-methylglutaconic acid in the urine of these patients.

Treatment. No effective treatment has been found.

3-Methylglutaconic Aciduria Type IV: "Unclassified" with Normal 3-Methylglutaconyl-CoA Hydratase Levels

This is a clinically very heterogeneous group, with many patients described, whose symptoms can include psychomotor retardation, spasticity, hypertonicity, hypotonicity, failure to thrive, seizures, optic atrophy, deafness, cardiomyopathy, and hepatic dysfunction.[131–133] The elevation of 3-methylglutaconic acid may be secondary to a variety of primary causes, some of which seem to be in energy metabolism.

Clinical Aspects. Clearly this is a nonspecific group of patients whose only common feature is the increased excretion of 3-methylglutaconic acid and normal 3-methylglutaconyl-CoA hydratase. Both males and females are affected. Clinical manifestations include: (1) neonatal hyperammonemia; (2) severe psychomotor retardation, microcephaly, hypotonia, and/or spasticity; (3) cardiomyopathy with respiratory chain abnormalities,[165–167] and (4) no clinical abnormality in two adult women.[134,146] Aplastic anemia and dysmorphic features with congenital heart disease have occurred in isolated cases.[132,146] Ten cases with diverse clinical symptoms were reported in Saudi Arabia.[168] Hepatic dysfunction may occur.[169] Patients may have Pearson syndrome with hematologic disorders, lactic acidemia, and abnormalities of the electron transport chain with mitochondrial DNA deletions.[170] All of these symptoms are seen in patients with various types of mitochondrial dysfunction, and in our experience, increased excretion of 3-methylglutaconic acid is usually present in patients with proven mitochondrial defects. Until the heterogeneity can be resolved by delineation of the basic biochemical defect, further clinical classification appears to be fruitless.

Abnormal Metabolites. All patients were noted to have elevated excretion of 3-methylglutaconic acid and 3-methylglutaric acid without elevated excretion of 3-hydroxyisovaleric acid and 3-hydroxy-3-methylglutaric acid.[131] The excretion rates of 3-methylglutaconic acid ranged widely: 25 to 65 mmol/mol of creatinine in two sibs[171] and two adults,[134] 70 to 600 in most other cases,[172–174] and as high as 1600 in a single case.[131] These rates are generally lower than those of patients with a deficiency of 3-methylglutaconyl-CoA hydratase. The excretion of 3-methylglutaric acid is usually 20 to 50 percent of that of 3-methylglutaconic acid.[131] In some patients, the two elevated urinary metabolites increased with a leucine challenge[171,175,176] and decreased in parallel when protein intake was reduced or stopped.[173] However, in others a high-protein diet or a leucine challenge failed to increase the excretion of the metabolites.[173,174,177] With fasting there was a normal ketogenic response,[172,178] and with an acidotic episode, ketosis also occurred.[174] The parents of patients did not show any elevation of the metabolites.[171,172] Some patients also had high excretion of 2-oxoglutaric acid[131,173,174,178] or elevated blood lactic acid.[174,175,176,178]

Analysis of urinary acylcarnitines by tandem MS showed elevated 3-methylglutarylcarnitine in two patients with 3-methylglutaconic aciduria and the presence of 3-methylglutaconylcarnitine, which increased following treatment with carnitine in one.[142]

Enzyme Studies. The oxidation of [2-^{14}C]leucine[172,174] or [1-^{14}C]isovaleric acid[172] was normal in cultured fibroblasts. Extensive fibroblast metabolism and enzyme studies in one case showed that there were no abnormalities in fatty acid or pyruvate oxidation or in many tricarboxylic acid cycle and mitochondrial enzymes.[174] The activity of 3-methylglutaconyl-CoA hydratase was normal in the cultured fibroblasts of all patients studied[131,132] and was also normal in liver and kidney tissues in one patient.[132] The basic enzyme defect is currently unknown.

An earlier hypothesis was that the increased 3-methylglutaconic acid might come from the "mevalonic acid shunt,"[150,151] secondary to a block in cholesterol biosynthesis.[131] This appears to be ruled out by the normal activity of the first four enzymes of the cholesterol biosynthetic pathway and the normal synthesis of cholesterol from acetate in fibroblasts.[132]

The lactic acidemia or elevated 2-oxoglutarate and tricarboxylic acid cycle intermediates in some patients suggest that the elevation of 3-methylglutaconic acid and 3-methylglutaric acid may be secondary to disturbances of mitochondrial energy metabolism. One patient with severe neurologic symptoms and lactic acidemia was found to be deficient in pyruvate and malate oxidation in muscle and had low activities of succinate: cytochrome c oxidoreductase and reduced NADH:O_2 oxidoreductase.[175] Another patient with lactic acidemia and increased tricarboxylic acid cycle intermediates in urine had elevated body temperature following mild physical activity as in Luft disease, which may suggest uncoupled mitochondria.[178] The activities of a number of mitochondrial enzymes were normal in fibroblasts. 3-Methylglutaconic aciduria occurs with deficiencies of respiratory chain complexes I, III, IV, and V in muscle;[167] partial deficiency of complexes II and III in fibroblasts;[165] deficiency of complexes I and IV in muscle;[166] and deficiency of mitochondrial ATP-synthase.[179] 3-Methylglutaconic aciduria and elevated tricarboxylic acid cycle intermediates can occur in Pearson syndrome with mitochondrial DNA deletions.[170]

Thus, 3-methylglutaconic aciduria may be a general secondary effect of energy metabolism.

Genetics. Since male and female sibs have been affected, this group of disorders is likely to involve nuclear DNA as well as mitochondrial DNA in its inheritance, as is the case for disorders of mitochondrial function.

Diagnosis. The clinical features of patients with "unspecified" 3-methylglutaconic aciduria are diverse, and the elevated urinary metabolites are generally found during analysis of organic acids as part of a general metabolic evaluation. Patients have an elevation of 3-methylglutaconic acid of 25 to 1600 mmol/mol of creatinine, with about 20 to 50 percent as much 3-methylglutaric acid and normal excretion of 3-hydroxyisovaleric acid and 3-hydroxy-3-methylglutaric acid. Some patients also have high excretion of 2-oxoglutaric acid, lactic acid, or tricarboxylic acid cycle intermediates. Assay of 3-methylglutaconyl-CoA hydratase in fibroblasts is not necessary to distinguish patients with a deficiency of this enzyme (type I) from those with type IV "unclassified" 3-methylglutaconic aciduria. Patients with normal excretion of 3-hydroxyisovaleric acid have normal activity of the hydratase, unlike those with a deficiency of the hydratase, who excrete elevated amounts of 3-hydroxyisovaleric acid.[131]

Diagnosis of heterozygotes is not possible because metabolite excretions are normal and the affected enzyme is unknown.

Prenatal diagnosis may be possible by analysis of the levels of 3-methylglutaconic acid and 3-methylglutaric acid in amniotic fluid. In one pregnancy at risk for 3-methylglutaconic aciduria, the metabolite levels were normal and the infant was not affected.[146] It is not known whether the levels will be significantly elevated in amniotic fluid with an affected fetus. A concern about attempting prenatal diagnosis by measurement of 3-methylglutaconic acid in amniotic fluid is the unknown effect of maternal 3-methylglutaconic aciduria that appears to be associated with pregnancy.[136]

Treatment. No effective treatment has been found. Since the elevation of 3-methylglutaconic and 3-methylglutaric acids appears to be secondary to undetermined primary defects, perhaps in energy metabolism, it is difficult to suggest logical approaches to treatment. Restriction of leucine does not appear to be of benefit.

3-Hydroxy-3-Methylglutaric Aciduria: 3-Hydroxy-3-Methylglutaryl-CoA Lyase Deficiency

This disorder not only is a defect in the catabolism of leucine but also has an important role in ketone body metabolism; therefore, the clinical, enzymologic, and molecular aspects are described in detail in Chap. 102. However, the diagnosis is usually made from the characteristic abnormal organic aciduria involving leucine metabolites, which is described here.

Diagnosis. The possibility of 3-hydroxy-3-methylglutaryl-CoA lyase deficiency should be considered in neonates and infants presenting with symptoms resembling Reye syndrome, neurologic dysfunction (such as obtundation, combativeness, and/or posturing), tachypnea, vomiting, hypoglycemia, hyperammonemia, hepatomegaly, and elevated transaminases in blood but without ketosis. Nonketotic hypoglycemia or hypoketotic hypoglycemia should be an immediate clinical indication to consider this disorder. A number of other organic acidurias can also present as symptoms similar to those of Reye syndrome, and it is important to analyze the urinary organic acids in all patients with these symptoms. Patients with Reye syndrome do not have the elevations in the urinary organic acids that are found in 3-hydroxy-3-methylglutaric aciduria.

Abnormal Metabolites. The characteristic abnormal metabolites in urine include 3-hydroxy-3-methylglutaric acid, derived from hydrolysis of the 3-hydroxy-3-methylglutaryl-CoA that accumulates due to deficiency of the lyase. This metabolite is derived both from the catabolism of leucine and from the ketone body synthetic pathway from fatty acid oxidation (Fig. 93-1). The average concentration of 3-hydroxy-3-methylglutaric acid in urine is about 1300 mmol/mol of creatinine (range, 200 to 4000) when the patients are well and rises to 11,000 mmol/mol of creatinine (range, 1500 to 19,000) during metabolic crises. This is very high compared to the normal excretion of 3-hydroxy-3-methylglutaric acid, 50 to 90 mmol/mol of creatinine in the first months of life, which decreases to less than 20 mmol/mol of creatinine by age 3 years.[180] It should be noted that with the use of trimethylsilyl derivatives, not all of the 3-hydroxy-3-methylglutaric acid is converted to the tris-trimethylsilyl derivative, and significant amounts may be present as the di-trimethylsilyl derivative.[181]

Because of the reversibility of 3-methylglutaconyl-CoA hydratase, the excretion of 3-methylglutaconic acid can be comparable to that of 3-hydroxy-3-methylglutaric acid in affected patients. About 10 percent of the 3-methylglutaconyl-CoA is hydrogenated to 3-methylglutaric acid. Because of the reversibility of 3-methylcrotonyl-CoA carboxylase reaction or inhibition by high concentrations of its product 3-methylglutaconyl-CoA, accumulated 3-methylcrotonyl-CoA is hydrated, leading to a high elevation of 3-hydroxyisovaleric acid, to about 30 to 100 percent of the 3-hydroxy-3-methylglutaric acid levels. When patients are severely ill, the 3-hydroxyisovaleric acid level tends to increase dramatically and 3-methylcrotonylglycine may also be elevated.[182–184] Two-dimensional NMR can detect 3-hydroxyisovaleric, 3-methylglutaconic, and 3-hydroxy-3-methylglutaric acids in urine and may be useful for rapid diagnosis.[185] The diagnosis of 3-hydroxy-3-methylglutaryl-CoA lyase deficiency cannot be made with certainty from the elevations of urinary metabolites alone but must be demonstrated by direct assay of the enzyme in leukocytes or fibroblasts.

Elevation of 3-methylcrotonic acid in urine has been reported,[186] but the presence of both this compound (also called 3-methyl-2-butenoic acid) and an isomer, 3-methyl-3-butenoic acid, have been shown to be artifacts resulting from decarboxylation of 3-methylglutaconic acid in the GC analysis of 3-methylcrotonic acid.[187,188] It has also been suggested that 3-methylcrotonic acid levels can rise as an artifact of dehydration of 3-hydroxyisovaleric acid in the GC analysis. There is often secondary elevation of glutaric (up to 3000 mmol/mol of creatinine) and adipic (up to 1100 mmol/mol of creatinine) acids when the patients are acutely ill.[182,187,189–191] The glutaric acid elevation may arise from inhibition of glutaryl-CoA dehydrogenase by 3-methylglutaryl-CoA or 3-methylglutaconyl-CoA. Some patients have had high elevation of lactic acid during severe episodes,[191] as is common in any of the organic acidemias during crises with cardiovascular dysfunction. It should be noted that these patients have a greatly diminished capacity to synthesize ketone bodies and consequently have inappropriately low levels of acetoacetic acid and 3-hydroxybutyric acid even when fasting or acutely ill.

In common with many other organic acidurias, 3-hydroxy-3-methylglutaric aciduria has been found to cause elevated ratios of acylcarnitine to free carnitine in urine.[192] 3-Methylglutarylcarnitine has been identified by tandem MS in urine.[193] No carnitine derivatives of 3-hydroxy-3-methylglutaric or 3-methylglutaconic acids were detected, even though these acids are more highly elevated in urine than 3-methylglutaric acid. Tandem MS also shows elevation of 3-methylglutarylcarnitine, and in addition, 3-hydroxyisovalerylcarnitine, in plasma.[124] This suggests that lyase deficiency should be detectable by tandem MS newborn screening of dried blood spots.

Mevalonic Aciduria: Mevalonate Kinase Deficiency (See Addendum)

Nineteen patients with mevalonic aciduria are known. Although this disorder is the first recognized defect in the biosynthesis of cholesterol and isoprenoids, it is considered a branched chain organic aciduria because the initial substrate for this pathway is 3-hydroxy-3-methylglutaryl-CoA, which is an intermediate in the mitochondrial pathway for leucine catabolism.

Pathway for Mevalonate and Cholesterol Biosynthesis. The relevant portions of the pathway for the biosynthesis of cholesterol are shown in Fig. 93-2, and the regulatory aspects are discussed more fully in Chap. 120. Although this pathway was previously thought to be localized in the cytoplasm, over the last 8 years most of the pathway has been shown to be present in peroxisomes. A cytoplasmic acetoacetyl-CoA thiolase (not shown in Fig. 93-2) interconverts acetyl-CoA and acetoacetyl-CoA, which are then condensed by a cytoplasmic 3-hydroxy-3-methylglutaryl-CoA synthase to form 3-hydroxy-3-methylglutaryl-CoA.[194] As described in Chap. 102, these cytosolic enzymes responsible for the synthesis of 3-hydroxy-3-methylglutaryl-CoA for cholesterol biosynthesis are distinct from the mitochondrial enzymes that are involved in ketone body synthesis.

The first step of isoprenoid biosynthesis involves peroxisomal 3-hydroxy-3-methylglutaryl-CoA reductase, which reductively decarboxylates the CoA thioester group of the substrate with NADP to release carbon dioxide, CoA, and 3-R-mevalonic acid.[195] This enzyme is highly regulated in its activity by phosphorylation and dephosphorylation. Its rate of degradation may be affected by oxygenated sterols.[195] Its synthesis is controlled at the transcriptional level by end products of isoprenoid biosynthesis and in particular by sterols.[195–197] The reductase reaction is not reversible.

The second step is phosphorylation of the 5-hydroxy group of mevalonic acid with ATP by mevalonate kinase to form 3-R-mevalonic acid-5-phosphate.[198–200] The porcine liver enzyme is a homodimer of 98 kDa[199] or 104 kDa[200] with a subunit 52 kDa.[200] The rat liver enzyme is a homodimer of 86 kDa with a subunit of 39.9 kDa.[201] The porcine liver enzyme has a K_m for (RS)-mevalonic acid of 19 μM,[199] as compared with 271 μM for the rat enzyme.[201] It is inhibited by geranyl pyrophosphate and farnesyl pyrophosphate.[202] Rat liver mevalonate kinase is now known to be predominantly localized in the peroxisomes, although it is easily solubilized during cell fractionation.[203] The activity is decreased in fibroblasts from patients with a deficiency of peroxisomes.

A 1.7-kb rat liver cDNA for mevalonate kinase has been cloned and sequenced.[204] It codes for a protein of 395 amino acids and 41.99 kDa and an mRNA of 2 kb. The levels of mRNA and enzyme activity in rat liver are increased by inhibitors of 3-hydroxy-3-methylglutaryl-CoA reductase and decreased by a diet with 5 percent cholesterol. The human cDNA for mevalonate kinase has been cloned, coding for a 396-amino-acid protein of 42.45 kDa (GenBank M88468).[205] The gene has been localized to human chromosome 12.[205]

The next reaction is phosphorylation of mevalonic acid-5-phosphate with ATP by mevalonic acid-5-phosphate kinase to form mevalonic acid-5-pyrophosphate.[198] The human cDNA for phosphomevalonate kinase has been cloned and shown to have a peroxisomal targeting sequence.[206] Mevalonic acid-5-pyrophosphate is decarboxylated and dehydrated in an ATP-requiring irreversible reaction by mevalonic acid pyrophosphate decarboxylase to form isopentenyl pyrophosphate. This is in equilibrium with dimethylallyl pyrophosphate, which has the branched five-carbon isoprene structure. Isopentenyl pyrophosphate and dimethylallyl pyrophosphate are condensed to form the 10-carbon isoprenoid farnesyl pyrophosphate. At this point there are branch points to the other isoprenoid end products, dolichol, ubiquinone, heme A, and, via geranyl pyrophosphate and squalene, cholesterol. These end products serve a variety of functions in human metabolism. Cholesterol is an important component of plasma membranes and is a precursor of steroid hormones and bile acids. Dolichol is involved in the synthesis of glycoproteins. Ubiquinone is a component of the electron transport chain in mitochondria.

A mevalonic acid shunt (see Fig. 93-2) can recycle mevalonic acid produced from cytosolic 3-hydroxy-3-methylglutaryl-CoA to 3-hydroxy-3-methylglutaryl-CoA in the mitochondria, where it can be cleaved to acetoacetate and acetyl-CoA for ketone body synthesis. Alternatively, these molecules can be transferred to the cytosol for fatty acid synthesis, and ultimately a portion can be oxidized to carbon dioxide.[150,151] This pathway involves the hydrolysis of dimethylallyl pyrophosphate by phosphatases to form dimethylallyl alcohol (3-methylcrotonaldehyde), which is oxidized sequentially by alcohol and aldehyde dehydrogenases to 3-methylcrotonic acid.[207] After formation of the CoA derivative in the mitochondria, 3-methylcrotonyl-CoA is carboxylated to 3-methylglutaconyl-CoA, hydrated to 3-hydroxy-3-methylglutaryl-CoA, and cleaved to acetoacetic acid and acetyl-CoA by the enzymes of the leucine catabolic pathway. The kidneys account for about half the shunting of mevalonic acid to pathways not leading to isoprenoid synthesis in the rat.[208] In humans, the excretion rate of endogenously produced *R*-mevalonic acid is 1.7 μmol per day, or 29 percent of the glomerular filtration rate,[209] and in perfused rat kidneys, the excretion rate is 40 to 50 percent of the glomerular

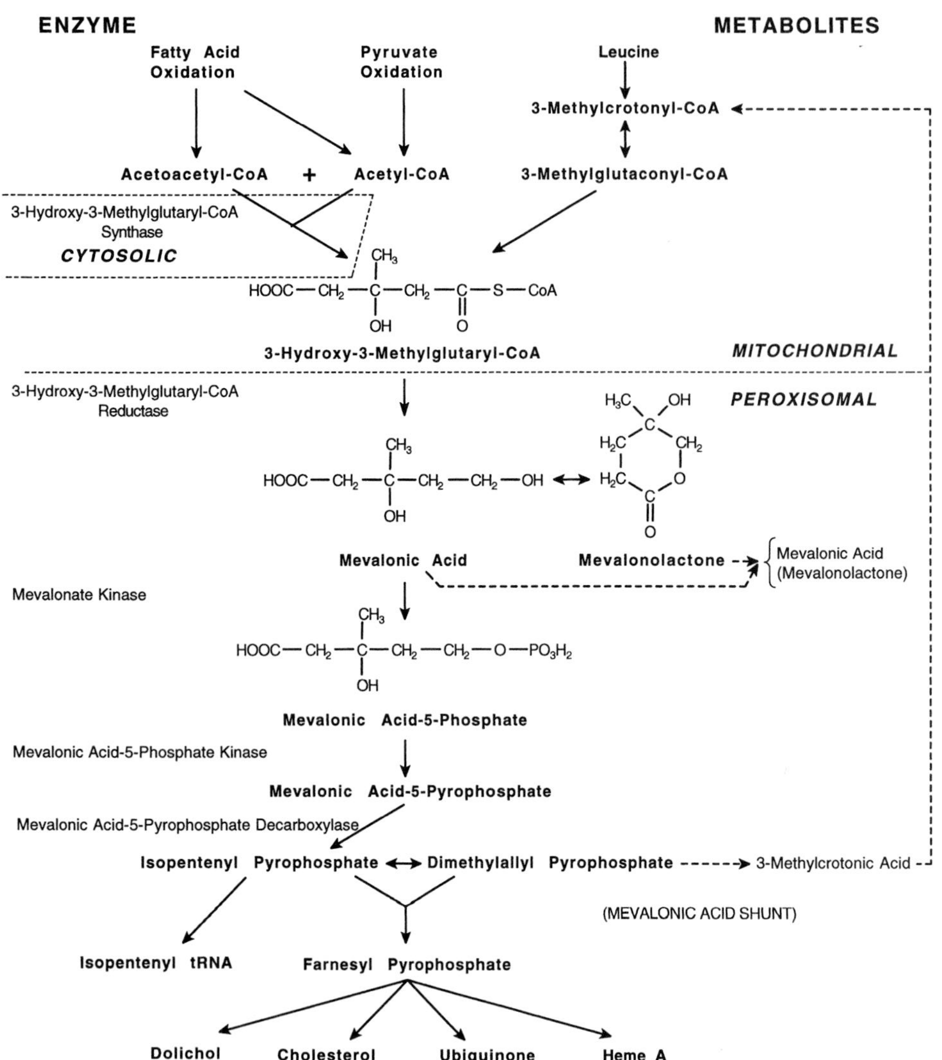

Fig. 93-2 Metabolism of mevalonic acid and early steps in the biosynthesis of cholesterol. The structures and names of the intermediates in the synthetic pathway for mevalonic acid and cholesterol and other isoprenoids are shown in the center, with the names of the enzymes on the left and the metabolites that may be elevated due to a deficiency of mevalonate kinase shown on the right. 3-Hydroxy-3-methylglutaryl-CoA is derived from fatty acid oxidation, pyruvate oxidation, and leucine catabolism in the mitochondria and also synthesized in the cytosol, although its conversion to isoprenoids and sterols takes place in the peroxisomes. Arrows indicate enzymes and metabolites as in Fig. 93-1.

filtration rate.[210] Both mevalonic acid and mevalonolactone are readily taken up by cells, but the circulating form in plasma is the salt of mevalonic acid, because there is a serum enzyme that catalyzes hydrolysis of the lactone.[211] In humans the concentrations of mevalonic acid in plasma are about 50 to 100 nanomolars and show a circadian rhythm.[212] It has been suggested that the intracellular concentration of mevalonic acid is proportional to its rate of synthesis by the highly regulated 3-hydroxy-3-methylglutaryl-CoA reductase and hence is proportional to the rate of cholesterol biosynthesis. The assumption that a constant small fraction of this intracellular mevalonic acid diffuses into the plasma would explain the excellent linear correlation between plasma mevalonic acid concentrations and cholesterol biosynthetic rates.[212]

Clinical Aspects. Of the 19 known patients with mevalonic aciduria, 11 have had the clinical and biochemical features of their disease summarized.[213] There is considerable clinical heterogeneity among patients with mevalonic aciduria, ranging from severe, fatal disease to milder symptoms. Most patients show severe failure to thrive, psychomotor retardation, hypotonia, and recurrent crises of high fever with rash, vomiting, or diarrhea.[214–218] About half the patients have had ataxia, cerebellar atrophy, splenomegaly, and dysmorphic features.[216,217,219–221] Anemia and hepatosplenomegaly with cholestatic liver disease were seen in two patients.[218] Dysmorphic features include dolichocephaly, a triangular face, down-slanted eyes, and large, posteriorly rotated, low-set ears.[214]

Six patients had cataracts.[214,217,221] Mevalonic acid has been shown to cause cataracts in young rat lenses in culture, apparently via an increase in the permeability of cell membranes.[222]

Mevalonic aciduria has been fatal in 4 of 11 of the cases.[213] Patients have died at ages ranging from 6 months[215] and 21 months[214] to 4 years.[216]

One patient had considerably milder symptoms, with hypotonia, cerebellar ataxia, poor muscle development, and elevated creatine kinase levels in blood.[219,220] A recent patient had minimal clinical symptoms.[223] He was well until 21 days of age, when he developed fever, diarrhea, and emesis requiring hospitalization for a month with persistent diarrhea and acidosis. At 9 months he had a skin rash, and development was normal at 11 months. His excretion of mevalonic acid was much less than that of other patients, and there was considerable residual activity of mevalonate kinase. The clinical severity tends to correlate with the degree of elevation of mevalonic acid in urine.

Systemic metabolic acidosis is not a usual feature of mevalonic aciduria despite the very high production of mevalonic acid, due to the high renal clearance of mevalonic acid. Although the basic defect is in isoprenoid and cholesterol biosynthesis, in general the levels of cholesterol are normal or only slightly low in serum, and steroid profiles are normal.

Abnormal Metabolites. The striking biochemical abnormality in this disorder is the extremely high elevation of mevalonic acid in urine. Normal excretion in children is less than 0.3 mmol/mol of creatinine.[214] Patients with the severe phenotype excreted 3000 to

56,000 mmol/mol of creatinine,[214,215,221] or 10,000 to 200,000 times the normal excretion. The patient with a milder phenotype excreted 900 to 1700 mmol/mol of creatinine,[219] but this is still 3000 to 6000 times normal. The patient with the mildest phenotype excreted only 50 to 70 mmol/mol of creatinine.[223] Unlike the other branched chain organic acidurias due to defects in catabolic pathways, in which metabolite excretion shows large increases with acidotic episodes, mevalonic aciduria is due to a defect in an anabolic pathway, and each patient showed fairly constant excretion of mevalonic acid. The very high production of mevalonic acid in these patients is due to a lack of feedback inhibition and repression of 3-hydroxy-3-methylglutaryl-CoA reductase caused by decreased synthesis of end products. This results in overproduction of mevalonic acid, which is readily cleared by the kidneys.

In the severely affected patients, the plasma levels of mevalonic acid were highly elevated, at 440 μM,[214] 70 to 542 μM,[215] and 38 μM[216] as compared with normal levels of less than 0.04 μM.[224] Although these levels are 1000 to 13,000 times normal, the absolute levels of mevalonic acid are not high enough to cause metabolic acidosis. In the very mildly affected patient, mevalonic acid was only 1.3 μM in plasma, but this is still 30 times normal.[223]

No abnormal metabolites other than mevalonic acid have been detected in the urine of these patients, suggesting that it is rapidly cleared by the kidneys and is not metabolized.

Enzyme Deficiency. The high excretion of mevalonic acid in the urine of the patients suggested three possible enzymes that may be deficient: mevalonate kinase, mevalonic acid-5-phosphate kinase, and mevalonic acid-5-pyrophosphate decarboxylase (see Fig. 93-2). An assay for mevalonate kinase with [5-^{3}H]mevalonolactone and ATP and separation of the phosphorylated products can provide information about all these enzyme activities.[225] Lysates of fibroblasts, lymphocytes, or lymphoblasts from all patients were found to be markedly deficient in the synthesis of both mevalonic acid-5-phosphate and mevalonic acid-5-pyrophosphate, showing that mevalonate kinase was deficient.[214–216,219–221] The residual activity of mevalonate kinase ranged from 1 to 15 percent of normal, and the amount did not correlate with the clinical severity, although the patient with very mild symptoms did have the highest residual activity at 15%.[223] The cells of patients were able to metabolize *R*-[2-^{14}C]mevalonic-acid-phosphate and *R*-[2-^{14}C]mevalonic-acid-5-pyrophosphate normally, indicating that the second kinase and the decarboxylase were normal.[214]

Heterozygotes have intermediate levels of mevalonate kinase activity in fibroblasts or lymphoblasts.[214,216,220,226,227]

Cell Metabolism Studies. Although the severe deficiency of mevalonate kinase in cells of the patients would be expected to interfere with cholesterol synthesis, the normal levels of cholesterol in blood of the patients suggested that cholesterol synthesis is not significantly impaired. The incorporation of [5-^{3}H]mevalonolactone into cholesterol in intact fibroblasts was studied with cells grown with fetal-calf serum (cholesterol and LDL present) and with delipidated serum (LDL and cholesterol removed).[214] In the delipidated medium, in which cholesterol synthesis should be maximal, patients' fibroblasts synthesized about 33 percent as much cholesterol as normal. In the medium with serum, in which cholesterol synthesis is depressed by half in normal cells, the patients' fibroblasts synthesized cholesterol at 45 percent of the normal rate. Similarly, incorporation of [2-^{14}C]acetate into cholesterol by the patients' fibroblasts was 89 percent of normal with delipidated serum and 41 percent of normal with normal serum.[228] Thus, the cells are able to synthesize considerable amounts of cholesterol, but in the absence of exogenous cholesterol, the cells cannot increase synthesis to the same extent as normal cells. The fibroblasts of the patients up-regulate 3-hydroxy-3-methylglutaryl-CoA reductase to compensate for the deficiency of mevalonate kinase. The activity is about six times normal in the patients' cells cultured with fetal-calf serum,[229] which apparently raises the concentration of mevalonic acid sufficiently to compensate in large part for the low activity of mevalonate kinase, thereby yielding almost normal rates of cholesterol synthesis.

Although the synthesis and levels of cholesterol may be normal in the patients, it is possible that there are deficiencies of other products of the pathway, such as dolichol or ubiquinone. The levels of cholesterol and dolichol phosphate were somewhat low at 60 percent of normal in the liver of an abortus with mevalonic aciduria.[230]

Five patients with mevalonate kinase deficiency were found to have increased excretion of leukotriene E_4.[231] The excellent linear correlation between levels of mevalonic acid and leukotriene suggested that increased cysteinyl leukotriene levels may be involved in the pathophysiology of this disorder. It has since been demonstrated that the peroxisomal degradation of cysteinyl leukotrienes was not impaired in mevalonic aciduria.[232]

Genetics. Mevalonic aciduria is an autosomal recessive disorder.[226] The human cDNA for mevalonate kinase has been cloned and sequenced and the gene localized to human chromosome 12.[205] A single base substitution (A > C) at nucleotide 902 resulting in a change of asparagine to threonine at residue 301 (N301T) was detected in one patient with mevalonic aciduria.[205] This patient[214] is a compound heterozygote for this mutation, which was found in the father and a sibling but not the mother. Identification of carriers of this mutation was extended to a larger number of members of the pedigree.[233] This mutation has not been found in other patients with mevalonic aciduria. A mutation in mevalonate kinase, a G > A transversion at nucleotide 1000 of the coding region of the cDNA, results in the substitution of threonine for alanine at position 334.[234] Two patients in one family were homozygous for this mutation, and a patient in another family was heterozygous for it. Kinetic analysis of the expressed mutant cDNA mevalonate kinase showed that it had a normal K_m for ATP, a thirtyfold elevation in the K_m for mevalonic acid, and a V_{max} only 1.4% of normal. Another mutation has been identified in a patient who is homozygous for a missense mutation causing the amino acid change I268T.[235]

Diagnosis. Clinical features suggesting the possibility of mevalonic aciduria include failure to thrive, anemia, gastroenteropathy, hepatosplenomegaly, psychomotor retardation, hypotonia, ataxia, cataracts, and dysmorphic features. The patients generally do not have acidosis or low serum cholesterol. The diagnosis can be easily made by analysis of the urinary organic acids in which mevalonic acid shows an overwhelmingly large peak. With most acidic extraction procedures, mevalonolactone is formed, and with trimethylsilylation, a monotrimethylsilyl derivative of mevalonolactone is the major derivative, although some tris-trimethylsilyl of mevalonic acid may be seen. In addition, a variety of other minor derivatives may be formed.[236] If the derivatization is with methylation, mevalonolactone does not form a methyl ester and may be missed unless a polar GC column is used that will show mevalonolactone and its dehydration product. Accurate quantification of mevalonic acid is difficult due to the interconversion of the acid and the lactone and is best accomplished by stable isotope dilution GC/MS.[224,236] Excretion levels of mevalonic acid have ranged from 900 to 56,000 mmol/mol of creatinine in affected patients (except for the mildest case, with 50 to 70 mmol/mol creatinine) as compared with normal excretions of less than 0.3 mmol/mol creatinine. The diagnosis should be confirmed by assay of mevalonate kinase in fibroblasts or lymphocytes, since there is the possibility that some patients with mevalonic aciduria may have a defect in either of the two subsequent enzymes in the metabolic pathway, phosphomevalonate kinase and mevalonate diphosphate decarboxylase.

Heterozygotes can be diagnosed by assay of mevalonate kinase in fibroblasts or lymphocytes, where the activity is less than 80 percent of normal and often less than 50 percent of normal.[214–216,223,226]

Mevalonic aciduria can be diagnosed prenatally by stable isotope dilution analysis of mevalonic acid in amniotic fluid.[224,236] Mevalonic acid was elevated three-thousandfold in the amniotic fluid with an affected fetus at 16 weeks of gestation, with a concentration of 272 μM as compared with normal concentrations of less than 0.08 μM.[236] Prenatal diagnosis can also be accomplished by demonstrating a deficiency of mevalonate kinase in cultured amniocytes.[214]

Treatment. A suitable treatment has not been developed. On the hypothesis that the elevated mevalonic acid levels might be toxic, a trial of low doses of a 3-hydroxy-3-methylglutaryl-CoA reductase inhibitor to lower mevalonic acid levels was done with two patients.[213] The trials were discontinued because both patients developed severe clinical crises with myopathic changes, elevated CPK levels, worsened ataxia, diarrhea, and vomiting. The levels of mevalonic acid in plasma and urine decreased, as did the blood cholesterol. Therefore, it appears that the clinical symptoms are related to a deficiency of sterol and isoprenoid products rather than to the elevation of mevalonic acid itself. If the failure to thrive is exacerbated by poor intestinal absorption of nutrients, parenteral nutrition may be of benefit. A high-cholesterol diet might compensate for decreased capacity to synthesize cholesterol. Treatment with ubiquinone might be considered, since its synthesis may be impaired, as suggested by low levels of ubiquinone-10 in four of six patients studied.[213] However, there was no lactic acidemia or abnormality of muscle mitochondria in the patients, as might be expected if the mitochondrial electron transport chain were compromised. Treatment of two patients in clinical crisis with corticosteroids yielded a dramatic response.

DISORDERS OF ISOLEUCINE CATABOLISM

Catabolism of Isoleucine: The *S*-Pathway

The normal pathway for the catabolism of isoleucine is in the mitochondria via intermediates with the *S*-stereochemical configuration to the common metabolic intermediates acetyl-CoA and succinyl-CoA, as shown in Fig. 93-3. Inherited deficiencies of five of the eight enzymes in the pathway are known. Mitochondrial acetoacetyl-CoA thiolase deficiency is a branched chain organic acid disorder involving the catabolism of isoleucine via the *S*-pathway. The diagnosis is generally made from the abnormal pattern of elevations of urinary organic acids and is described in this chapter. Thiolase deficiency is also a disorder of ketone body metabolism and is described in detail in Chap. 102. Two other disorders of the terminal steps of isoleucine catabolism, propionic acidemia and methylmalonic acidemia, are described in Chap. 94. Ethylmalonic encephalopathy may be due to a defect in 2-methylbranched chain acyl-CoA dehydrogenase in the *S*-pathway of isoleucine catabolism and formation of ethylmalonic acid via the *R*-pathway for isoleucine catabolism; it is described in this chapter. No patients have been identified with an inherited deficiency of either of two of the enzymes of isoleucine catabolism, tiglyl-CoA hydratase and 2-methyl-3-hydroxybutyryl-CoA dehydrogenase, which would be expected to lead to branched chain organic acidurias.

Isoleucine has two asymmetric carbons and can be converted to a slight extent to a diastereoisomer (via the 2-oxo acid intermediate), alloisoleucine. The catabolism of alloisoleucine proceeds via a minor pathway, the *R*-pathway, which results in different end products than does the major *S*-pathway for isoleucine. The *R*-pathway will be described later.

2-Methylbranched Chain Acyl-CoA Dehydrogenase. The first step of branched chain organic acid metabolism of isoleucine is the irreversible dehydrogenation of 2-methylbutyryl-CoA to tiglyl-CoA (which could also be called 2-methylcrotonyl-CoA), catalyzed by 2-methylbranched chain acyl-CoA dehydrogenase (see Fig. 93-3). This enzyme is distinct from the dehydrogenases acting on the straight-chain acyl-CoA dehydrogenases of fatty acid β-oxidation and also from isovaleryl-CoA dehydrogenase in the leucine catabolic pathway.[12] 2-Methylbranched chain acyl-CoA dehydrogenase has been purified from rat liver mitochondria.[237] It is composed of four identical subunits of 41.5 kDa, each containing one FAD, to form an approximately 170-kDa enzyme. Electrons from the FAD are transferred to ETF and then to the electron transport chain by ETF dehydrogenase in the same manner as for isovaleryl-CoA dehydrogenase.

The enzyme catalyzes the dehydrogenation of the ethyl group of *S*-2-methylbutyryl-CoA derived from isoleucine to tiglyl-CoA in the major *S*-pathway. It catalyzes equally well the dehydrogenation of isobutyryl-CoA (which is 2-methylpropionyl-CoA) derived from valine to form methacrylyl-CoA, hence its name.[237] The dehydrogenation of butyryl-CoA is 5 percent of that for *S*-2-methylbutyryl-CoA. The maximum rate of dehydrogenation of the methyl group of *R*-2-methylbutyryl-CoA derived from alloisoleucine to 2-ethylacrylyl-CoA is only 22 percent of that with the *S*-isomer. This reaction leads to the minor *R*-catabolic pathway, as described later. Other acyl-CoAs are not substrates. The K_m values for the substrates are 20 μM for *S*-2-methylbutyryl-CoA and 89 μM for isobutyryl-CoA. At equilibrium, the ratio of product to substrate is 4 with *S*-2-methylbutyryl-CoA as substrate and 1 with isobutyryl-CoA as substrate. Tiglyl-CoA, the product of the enzyme with *S*-2-methylbutyryl-CoA as substrate, is a potent competitive inhibitor of the enzyme, with a K_i of 7 μM with *S*-2-methylbutyryl-CoA as substrate and 3 μM with isobutyryl-CoA as substrate. Moderate inhibition is also found with butyryl-CoA, valeryl-CoA, and crotonyl-CoA, but not with propionyl-CoA, isovaleryl-CoA, or 3-methylcrotonyl-CoA.

The cDNA for the rat precursor short-branched chain acyl-CoA dehydrogenase has been cloned[238] It is 84 percent identical (93 percent similar) to the human cloned enzyme. The rat cDNA for the mature subunit was expressed in *E. coli* and its substrate specificity determined; it is somewhat different from that of the enzyme purified from rat liver mitochondria. The activities as percentages of that with *S*-2-methylbutyryl-CoA are *R*-2-methylbutyryl-CoA, 61 percent; isobutyryl-CoA, 37 percent; butyryl-CoA, 25 percent; 2-ethylhexanoyl-CoA, 8.6 percent; hexanoyl-CoA, 8.4 percent; and valproyl-CoA, 37 percent. Thus, the expressed cloned rat enzyme has less activity with isobutyryl-CoA and more with butyryl-CoA than the purified rat liver enzyme.

The cDNA for the human precursor short-branched chain acyl-CoA dehydrogenase has been cloned.[239] The 1.3-kb cDNA (GenBank U12778) encodes a precursor protein of 431 amino acids, which can be processed in vitro to a mature protein of 399 amino acids with a molecular weight of 43.7. It has homology with other acyl-CoA dehydrogenases, with the highest homology being 38 percent to short-chain acyl-CoA dehydrogenase. When the mature cDNA is expressed in *E. coli*, activity levels relative to *S*-2-methylbutyryl-CoA are butyryl-CoA, 55 percent; hexanoyl-CoA, 66 percent; octanoyl-CoA, 9 percent; isobutyryl-CoA, 27 percent; isovaleryl-CoA, 10 percent; and 2-methylhexanoyl-CoA, 50 percent.[239] Thus, the human enzyme has considerably more activity with the short straight chain substrates, butyryl-CoA and hexanoyl-CoA, than the rat enzyme. The relatively low activity with isobutyryl-CoA (in the valine pathway) raises the possibility that there may be another enzyme acting on this substrate. The human enzyme has very little activity with valproyl-CoA, unlike the rat enzyme.[238] Human short-branched chain acyl-CoA dehydrogenase RNA was present in all human tissues tested, with the highest activity in liver and kidney.[238] Interestingly, two transcripts of poly(A) RNA of 2.7 and 6.5 kb were found in the human but not the rat, making this enzyme unlike all other acyl-CoA dehydrogenases, in which a single transcript is seen in both species.

Tiglyl-CoA Hydration. Although the possibility of a hydratase specific for tiglyl-CoA has not been excluded, it is believed that

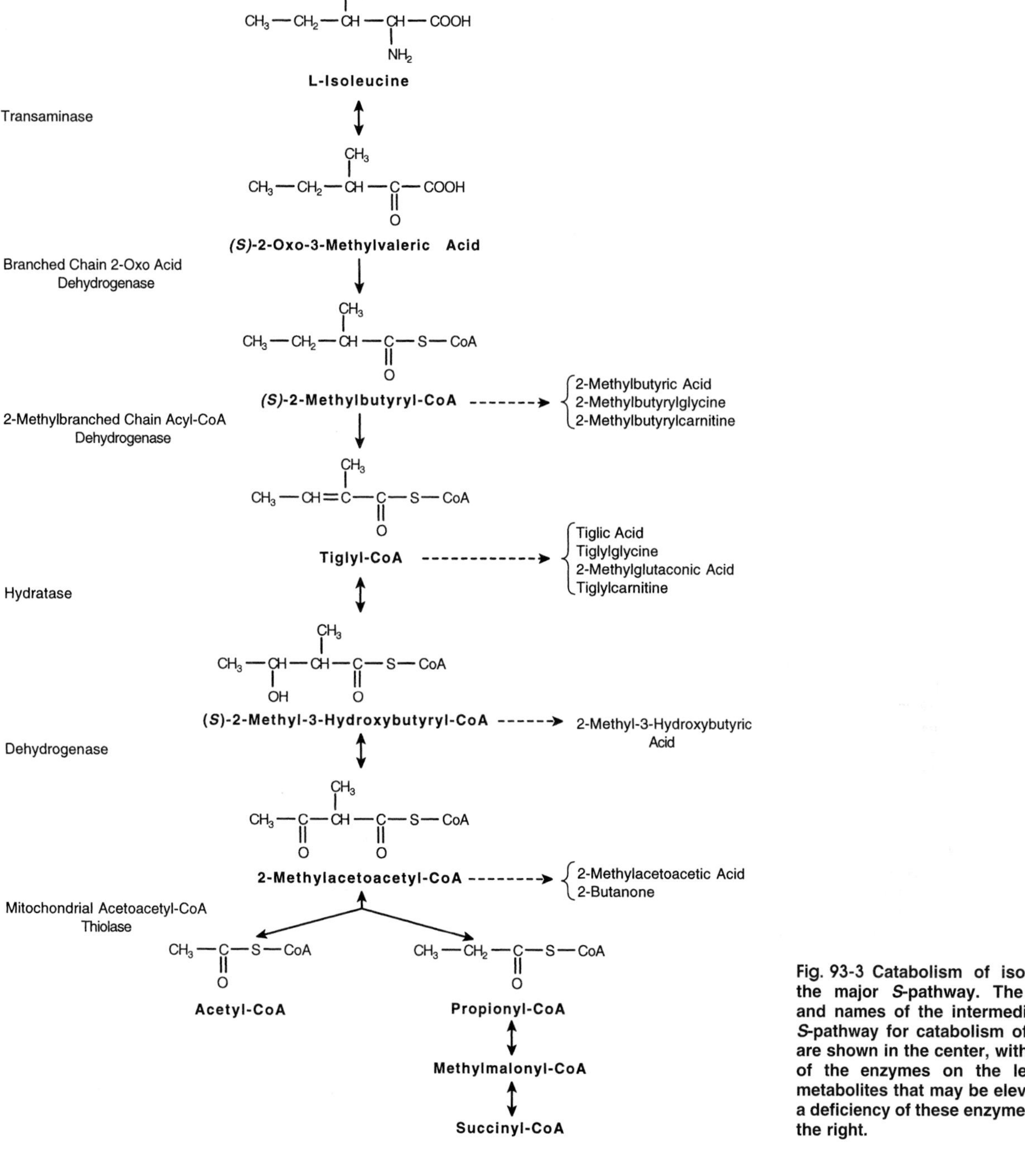

Fig. 93-3 Catabolism of isoleucine via the major *S*-pathway. The structures and names of the intermediates in the *S*-pathway for catabolism of isoleucine are shown in the center, with the names of the enzymes on the left and the metabolites that may be elevated due to a deficiency of these enzymes shown on the right.

tiglyl-CoA is hydrated to 2-methyl-3-hydroxy-butyryl-CoA by crotonase.[32] The crystallized enzyme purified from bovine liver is a 164-kDa hexamer of identical subunits[240] that hydrates tiglyl-CoA much more slowly than crotonyl-CoA, but the kinetic constants have not been reported. Sonicated human liver hydrates tiglyl-CoA at 11 percent of the rate of hydration of crotonyl-CoA.[241]

2-Methyl-3-Hydroxybutyryl-CoA Dehydrogenase. The oxidation of 2-methyl-3-hydroxybutyryl-CoA to 2-methylacetoacetyl-CoA is catalyzed by a hydroxyacyl-CoA dehydrogenase (see Fig. 93-3). This may be the dehydrogenase that acts on short or medium straight chain 3-hydroxyacyl-CoA substrates in fatty acid β-oxidation, but the possibility of a specific dehydrogenase for this 2-methylbranched substrate has not been excluded.

Mitochondrial Acetoacetyl-CoA Thiolase. 3-Oxothiolases catalyze the reversible thiolytic cleavage of a 3-oxoacyl-CoA with a CoA to form an acyl-CoA with two fewer carbons and acetyl-CoA.[242] Thus, mitochondrial acetoacetyl-CoA thiolase interconverts 2-methylacetoacetyl-CoA to propionyl-CoA plus acetyl-CoA (see Fig. 93-3 in isoleucine catabolism and acetoacetyl-CoA to two acetyl-CoAs in fatty acid oxidation. The acetyl-CoA produced by 2-methylacetoacetyl-CoA thiolase enters the general tricarboxylic acid cycle metabolism of the mitochondria. The other product, propionyl-CoA, is first carboxylated to methylmalonyl-CoA, racemized, then isomerized to succinyl-CoA before entering the tricarboxylic acid cycle. These reactions and the disorders propionic acidemia and methylmalonic acidemia, resulting from deficiencies of the enzymes, are described in Chap. 94.

Mitochondrial acetoacetyl-CoA thiolase has a major role in ketone body metabolism, and therefore its enzymatic properties and molecular aspects are described in detail in Chap. 102.

Deficiency of Mitochondrial Acetoacetyl-CoA Thiolase

This deficiency is a disorder in the catabolism of isoleucine, and the diagnosis is usually made from the characteristic abnormal organic aciduria involving isoleucine metabolites. Deficiency of this thiolase also has an important effect on ketone body metabolism, and therefore its clinical, enzymologic, and molecular aspects are described in detail in Chap. 102.

Diagnosis and Abnormal Metabolites. The diagnosis of mitochondrial acetoacetyl-CoA thiolase deficiency should be considered in children presenting with recurrent episodes of severe ketosis and acidosis but without chronic ketosis.

There are considerable variations in the patterns and amounts of abnormal organic acids excreted by patients with a deficiency of mitochondrial acetoacetyl-CoA thiolase. In addition, several of the metabolites (2-methylacetoacetic acid, 2-butanone, and tiglylglycine) can be difficult to analyze quantitatively by the routine methods for urinary organic acids, requiring use of special analytical techniques. Thus, the information on excretion of these metabolites is fragmentary, and it is difficult to specify a typical quantitative profile. The elevated urinary metabolite most characteristic of a deficiency of mitochondrial acetoacetyl-CoA thiolase is 2-methyl-3-hydroxybutyric acid.[243–247] This is often accompanied by elevation of 2-methylacetoacetic acid and its decarboxylation product 2-butanone. 2-Methylacetoacetic acid is generally not the most elevated metabolite, although it is the substrate for the defective enzyme and might be expected to be most elevated. Rather, due to the reversible reaction of 3-hydroxyacyl-CoA dehydrogenase and the normally high ratio of NADH to NAD, the reduced compound 2-methyl-3-hydroxybutyric acid is more elevated. Most patients also excrete elevated amounts of tiglylglycine, but some patients do not.[243,244,246] This compound can be elevated due to the accumulation of 2-methyl-3-hydroxybutyryl-CoA, which is in equilibrium with its dehydrated form, tiglyl-CoA. Tigly-CoA is a substrate for glycine N-acylase, which forms tiglylglycine.[59] The excretion of these metabolites of isoleucine increases during episodes and is accompanied by high elevation of acetoacetic acid and 3-hydroxybutyric acid. During ketotic episodes, there is also secondary elevation of dicarboxylic acids such as adipic acid, which occurs in any ketotic subject.

The normal excretion of 2-methyl-3-hydroxybutyric acid is 1 to 9 mmol/mol of creatinine, which can increase to as high as 200 mmol/mol of creatinine during ketosis of any cause.[126] When well, patients with 2-methylacetoacetyl-CoA thiolase deficiency often have excretion rates of 2-methyl-3-hydroxybutyric acid of 200 to 1000 mmol/mol of creatinine, which increase to 1000 to 14,400 mmol/mol of creatinine during acute catabolism, with high protein intake, or with a challenge of isoleucine.[243–247] However, more mildly affected patients can have excretion rates in the normal range or up to 70 mmol/mol of creatinine when well and show increases that are still within the normal range or up to 300 mmol/mol of creatinine when ill or when challenged with isoleucine.[246,248,249] There are very few reports of the quantities of 2-methylacetoacetic acid excreted, but these are often about one-tenth to one-fourth of those of 2-methyl-3-hydroxybutyric acid,[243,250] although there may be more 2-methylacetoacetic acid during a challenge with isoleucine.[244] 2-Methylacetoacetic acid may not be detectable by routine organic acid analysis in mildly affected patients, even with an isoleucine challenge.[246,248,249] Tiglylglycine levels as high as 7000 mmol/mol of creatine have been reported,[244,246,247] but some patients do not excrete tiglylglycine[243,246] except following a load of isoleucine.[246] 2-Butanone has not been quantified in the urine of patients and was not detectable in some.[244] Small amounts of 2,3-dimethyl-3-hydroxyglutaric acid (3 to 8 mmol/mol of creatinine) have been detected.[245,251] This presumably arises from condensation of elevated 2-methylacetoacetyl-CoA with acetyl-CoA catalyzed by mitochondrial 3-hydroxy-3-methylglutaryl-CoA synthase to form 2,3-dimethyl-3-hydroxyglutaryl-CoA.

The diagnosis of most severely affected patients can be done easily by analysis of urinary organic acids finding highly elevated excretion of 2-methyl-3-hydroxybutyric acid (100 to 14,000 mmol/mol of creatinine), 2-methylacetoacetic acid (25 to 250 mmol/mol of creatinine), and tiglylglycine (70 to 7,000 mmol/mol of creatinine). However, some patients do not have more than trace amounts of 2-methylacetoacetic acid, and others do not excrete tiglylglycine. Elevation of only 2-methyl-3-hydroxybutyric acid during a ketotic episode is not diagnostic, because of the secondary elevation of this acid to levels as high as 200 mmol/mol of creatinine in patients with ketosis for any reason.[126] 2-Methylacetoacetic acid can also be elevated secondary to ketosis of any cause. The continued elevation of 2-methyl-3-hydroxybutyric acid or 2-methylacetoacetic acid between ketotic episodes is strongly suggestive of a deficiency of mitochondrial acetoacetyl-CoA thiolase. There are mildly affected patients who do not have clearly diagnostic elevation of any of the metabolites on routine urinary organic acid analysis during or between episodes.[246,249] These patients can be diagnosed by an oral challenge with 100 mg/kg of isoleucine. Earlier we had suggested on the basis of routine analysis of organic acids that elevation of tiglylglycine even without elevation of 2-methylacetoacetic acid after the challenge was indicative of a deficiency of mitochondrial acetoacetyl-CoA thiolase.[246] More sensitive and accurate methods for the specific quantification of the metabolites showed that elevation of tiglylglycine after an isoleucine challenge is not unique to those with mitochondrial acetoacetyl-CoA thiolase deficiency but also occurs in other subjects with ill-defined metabolic problems.[252] Similarly, 2-methyl-3-hydroxybutyric acid also increases in control subjects after an isoleucine challenge, although not as much as in the patients. An elevation of the sum of 2-methylacetoacetic acid and 2-butanone, its decarboxylation product, following a challenge with isoleucine appears to be a specific diagnostic response to an isoleucine challenge in patients with mitochondrial acetoacetyl-CoA thiolase deficiency.[252]

Catabolism of Isoleucine: The *R*-Pathway

Some of the enzymes of the *S*-pathway of isoleucine catabolism can act on the *R*-isomers, giving rise to different end products for the two isomers (Fig. 93-4). Isoleucine is transaminated to *S*-2-oxo-3-methylvaleric acid. Until the 1990s this was believed to undergo a slow interconversion to *R*-2-oxo-3-methylvaleric acid via a keto-enol tautomerization.[253] This was thought to occur only to a slight extent with the usual rapid flux through the oxo acid dehydrogenase to *S*-2-methylbutyryl-CoA, and hence the *R*-pathway was expected to be very minor in normal subjects. Significant amounts of the *R*-isomer of 2-oxo-3-methylvaleric acid do form in patients with maple syrup urine disease, in which the catabolism of the oxo acid is deficient, and this is transaminated to alloisoleucine.[254] However, these patients cannot oxidize the *R*-2-oxo-3-methylvaleric acid to *R*-2-methylbutyric acid, so that the *R*-pathway does not function even though the precursor is elevated.

When normal subjects are loaded with L-isoleucine, alloisoleucine does increase moderately in plasma.[255] Mamer [256] pointed out that keto-enol tautomerism of 2-oxo-3-methylvaleric acid to interconvert the *R* and *S* forms occurs only at a high pH and does not occur at physiological pH. He proposed that in the action of transaminase on isoleucine, the intermediate *S*-ketimine can form the *R*-ketimine via tautomerism of an intermediate enamine. The *R*-ketimine could revert to alloisoleucine or form *R*-2-oxo-3-methylvaleric acid. Recent studies with L-[^{13}C]-isoleucine in vivo in normal subjects showed that the kinetics of formation of labeled *S*- and *R*-2-oxo-3-methylvaleric acid were the same, suggesting that formation of the *R*-oxo acid is an inevitable byproduct of the

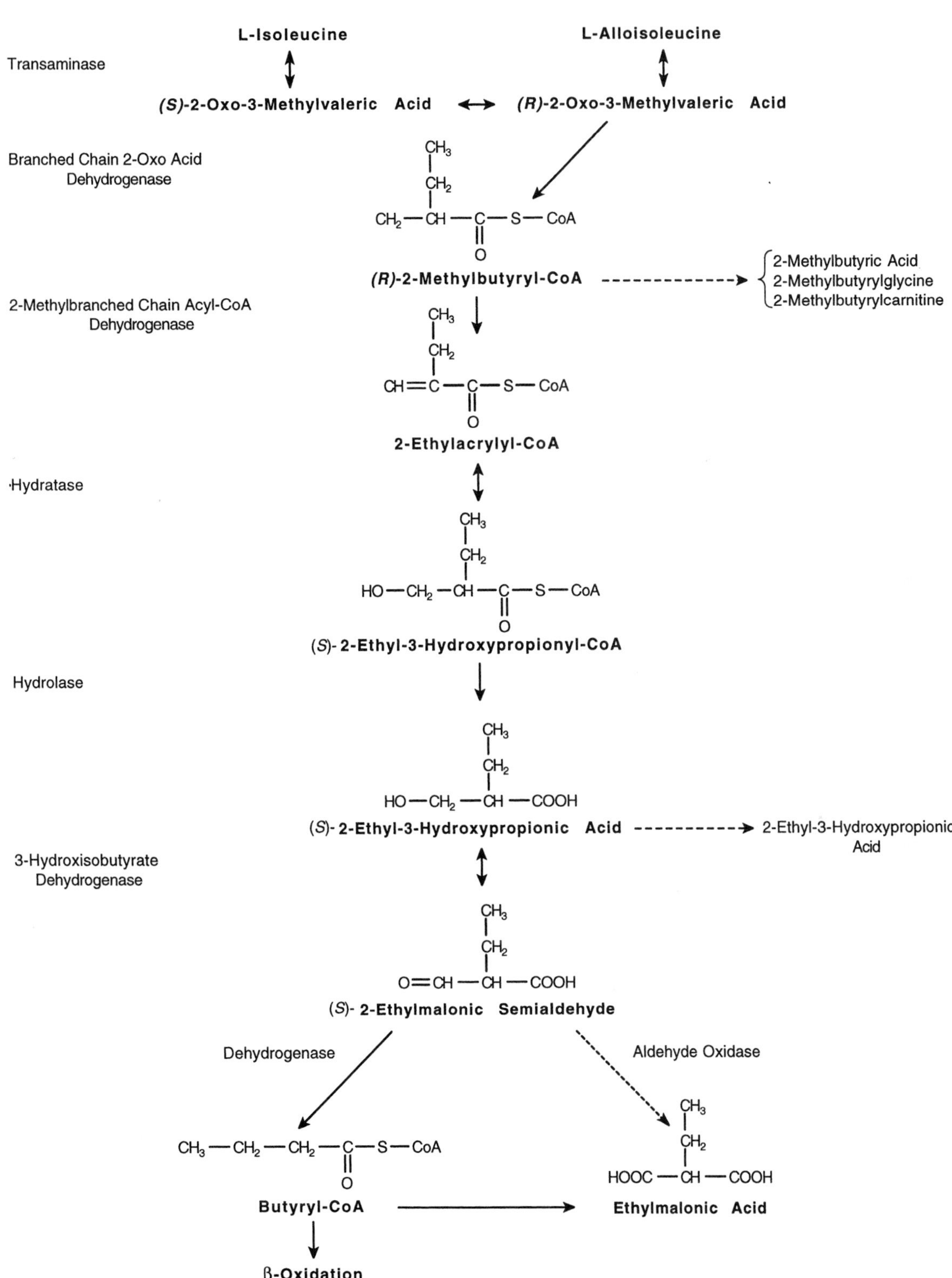

Fig. 93-4 Catabolism of isoleucine via the minor *R*-pathway. The structures and names of the intermediates in the *R*-pathway for catabolism of isoleucine are shown in the center, with the names of the enzymes on the left and the metabolites that may be elevated due to a deficiency of these enzymes shown on the right.

transamination of isoleucine.[257] This is consistent with Mamer's hypothesis that the *R*-oxo acid is formed by the transaminase. Thus, the production of the *R*-isomer is likely to be much greater than the previously proposed slow keto-enol tautomerism of the *S*-isomer, and therefore, the *R* pathway for isoleucine metabolism may be more important than previously thought.

R-2-oxo-3-methylvaleric acid is oxidatively decarboxylated by branched chain 2-oxoacid dehydrogenase to *R*-2-methylbutyryl-CoA. This is a substrate for 2-methylbranched chain acyl-CoA dehydrogenase, producing 2-ethylacrylyl-CoA as the product (Fig. 93-4). The activity of the purified rat dehydrogenase for the *R*-isomer is about 20 percent of the rate for the *S*-isomer in the

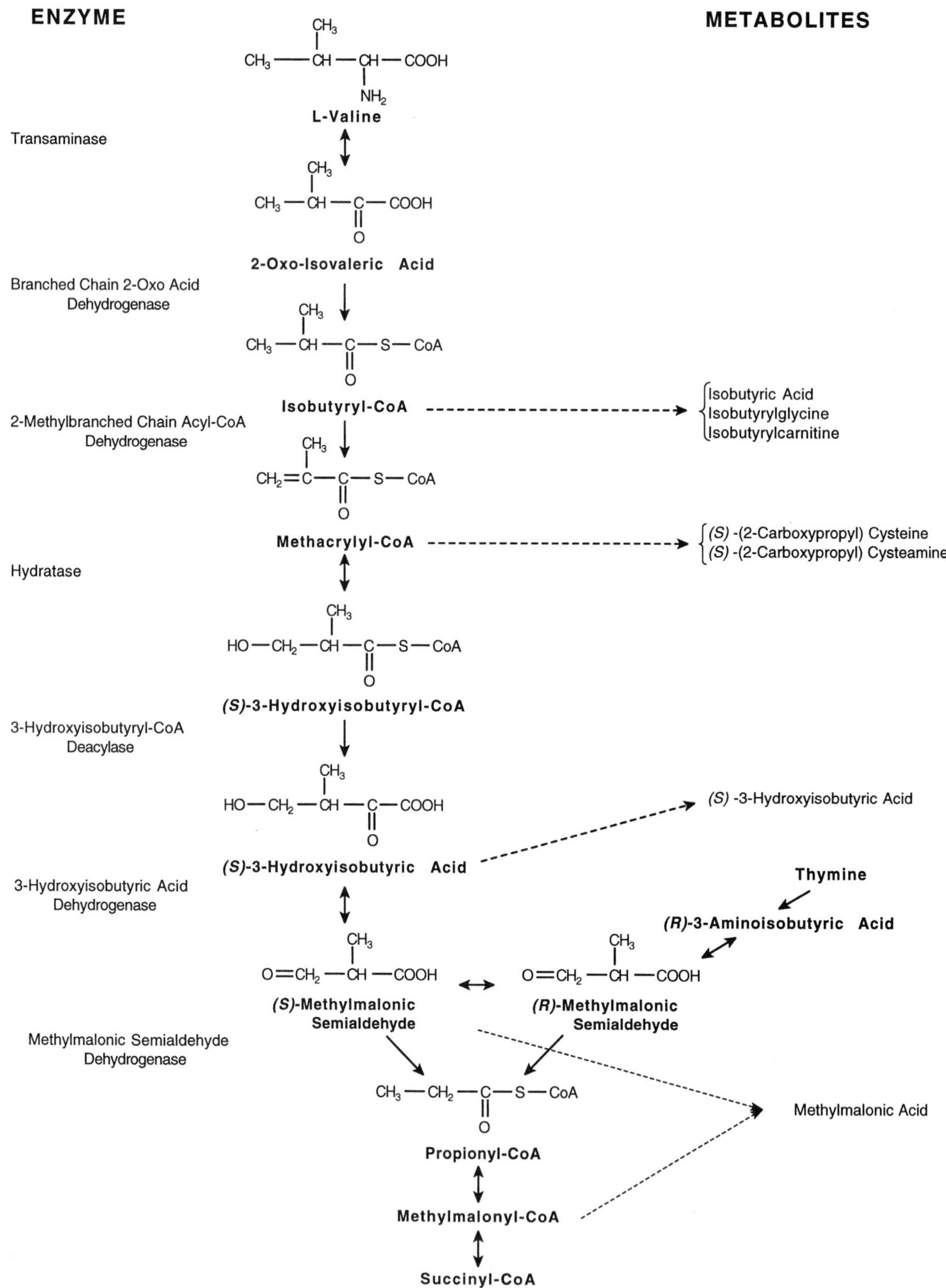

Fig. 93-5 Catabolism of valine and its convergence with catabolism of thymine. The structures and names of the intermediates in the pathway for catabolism of valine are shown in the center, with the names of the enzymes on the left and the metabolites that may be elevated due to a deficiency of these enzymes shown on the right.

main *S*-pathway for isoleucine catabolism.[237] The rat short-branched chain acyl-CoA dehydrogenase expressed from the cloned cDNA shows higher activity with the *R*-2-methylbutyryl-CoA, 60 percent of that of the *S*-isomer.[238] The relative activity of the human expressed cDNA for *R*-2-methylbutyryl-CoA has not been reported.[238,239]

The product of the dehydrogenation of *R*-2-methylbutyryl-CoA is 2-ethylacrylyl-CoA, which is a homologue of methacrylyl-CoA in the valine pathway and is metabolized similarly (Fig. 93-4 and Fig. 93-5). 2-Ethylacrylyl-CoA is hydrated to *S*-2-ethyl-3-hydroxypropionyl-CoA, presumably by crotonase. The CoA ester is deacylated to *S*-2-ethyl-3-hydroxypropionic acid, perhaps by

3-hydroxyisobutyryl-CoA deacylase, which acts on the homologous substrates, 3-hydroxyisobutyryl-CoA in the valine catabolic pathway and 3-hydroxypropionyl-CoA.[258]

3-Hydroxyisobutyrate dehydrogenase, which forms methylmalonic semialdehyde in the valine pathway, oxidizes *S*-2-ethyl-3-hydroxypropionic acid to ethylmalonic semialdehyde (Fig. 93-4).[259] In the valine pathway, methylmalonate semialdehyde dehydrogenase decarboxylates methylmalonic semialdehyde and esterifies the semialdehyde to form propionyl-CoA (Fig. 93-5).[259] This enzyme purified from rat liver also metabolizes malonic semialdehyde to acetyl-CoA but does not oxidize ethylmalonic semialdehyde to butyryl-CoA.[259] Ethylmalonic acid is a product of the metabolism of *R*-2-methylbutyric acid and may be formed by direct oxidation of ethylmalonic semialdehyde to ethylmalonic acid. It may also be oxidatively decarboxylated to form butyryl-CoA by some enzyme other than methylmalonic semialdehyde dehydrogenase. Although butyryl-CoA is normally metabolized by short chain acyl-CoA dehydrogenase to acetyl-CoA, when elevated it can be carboxylated by propionyl-CoA carboxylase to ethylmalonyl-CoA, which may be hydrolyzed to ethylmalonic acid. Ethylmalonyl-CoA can also be isomerized to form methylsuccinyl-CoA, which may be hydrolyzed to methylsuccinic acid.

The *R*-pathway was proposed based on the different excretion levels of the intermediate 2-ethyl-3-hydroxypropionic acid (ethylhydracrylic acid) by patients with various defects in isoleucine catabolism.[260] When an isoleucine load is given to a normal subject, ethylmalonic acid excretion is increased.[260] The pathway was demonstrated by administering deuterium-labeled *R*-2-methylbutyric acid to animals and identifying deuterium-labeled 2-ethyl-3-hydroxypropionic acid as the major labeled urinary metabolite and also deuterium-labeled ethylmalonic acid.[261,262] The pathway was shown to proceed primarily from 2-ethyl-3-hydroxypropionic acid through butyryl-CoA to ethylmalonic acid by administration of stable isotopically labeled *RS*-2-methylbutyric acid to hypoglycin-treated rats and analyzing the isotopic composition of labeled urinary ethylmalonic acid.[263] Thus, the direct oxidation of ethylmalonic semialdehyde to ethylmalonic acid is minor compared to the pathway through butyryl-CoA. The enzyme that forms butyryl-CoA from ethylmalonic semialdehyde has not been identified.

DISORDERS OF VALINE CATABOLISM

Catabolism of Valine

The normal pathway for the catabolism of valine is shown in Fig. 93-5. Inherited deficiencies of six of the enzymes are known. Of the five known disorders of valine metabolism considered to be branched chain organic acidurias, only four, isobutyryl-CoA dehydrogenase deficiency, 3-hydroxyisobutyryl-CoA deacylase deficiency, 3-hydroxyisobutyric aciduria (possibly due to a deficiency of 3-hydroxyisobutyrate dehydrogenase), and methylmalonic semialdehyde dehydrogenase deficiency, will be described in this chapter (see Table 93-1). Two others, propionic acidemia and methylmalonic acidemia, are described in Chap. 94. There have been no patients described with an inherited deficiency of one of the enzymes, methacrylyl-CoA hydratase. The enzymes of the valine catabolic pathway and their relevant properties are described below.

2-Methylbranched Chain Acyl-CoA Dehydrogenase. This enzyme has been described under 2-methylbranched chain acyl-CoA dehydrogenase in "Disorders of Isoleucine Catabolism," because it has the same function in the catabolism of both 2-methylbutyryl-CoA from isoleucine and isobutyryl-CoA (2-methylpropionyl-CoA) from valine.[237] The product of the dehydrogenation of isobutyryl-CoA is methacrylyl-CoA (see Fig. 93-5). The relative activity of the purified rat liver mitochondrial 2-methylbranched chain acyl-CoA dehydrogenase for isobutyryl-CoA is 92 percent of that for *S*-2-methylbutyryl-CoA at high concentrations of substrate, but the K_m for isobutyryl-CoA is 4.5 times higher than that for *S*-2-methylbutyryl-CoA, and at equilibrium, the ratio of product to substrate is 1 with isobutyryl-CoA compared with 4 for *S*-2-methylbutyryl-CoA.[237] This suggests that the activity of this enzyme at physiological concentrations of the substrates may be less for isobutyryl-CoA than it is for *S*-2-methylbutyryl-CoA.

The rat cDNA for this enzyme, described as short-branched chain acyl-CoA dehydrogenase, was cloned and the cDNA for the mature subunit expressed in *E. coli*.[238] The relative activity of this expressed enzyme for isobutyryl-CoA was 37 percent of that for *S*-2-methylbutyryl-CoA, in contrast to the relative activity of 92 percent for the enzyme purified from rat liver mitochondria. In addition, the expressed cDNA enzyme had 25 percent activity with butyryl-CoA compared with *S*-2-methylbutyryl-CoA, whereas the purified mitochondrial enzyme had only 5 percent activity with butyryl-CoA.

The cloned human cDNA for the mature subunit of short-branched chain acyl-CoA dehydrogenase was expressed in *E. coli* and had relative activities of 27 percent for isobutyryl-CoA, 55 percent for butyryl-CoA, and 100 percent for *S*-2-methylbutyryl-CoA.[239] The relatively low activity for isobutyryl-CoA and the higher activity for butyryl-CoA raise the possibility that there may be another dehydrogenase acting on isobutyryl-CoA.

Methacrylyl-CoA Hydratase. Purified bovine liver crotonase can hydrate methacrylyl-CoA to 3-hydroxyisobutyryl-CoA.[32,120,121] Human liver sonicates hydrate methacrylyl-CoA at 6 percent of the rate of hydration of crotonyl-CoA, and human fibroblast sonicates can hydrate methacrylyl-CoA.[241] In addition, in aqueous solution there is reversible nonenzymatic hydration of methacrylyl-CoA to 3-hydroxyisobutyryl-CoA so that these compounds are in equilibrium.[264,265]

3-Hydroxyisobutyryl-CoA Deacylase (Hydrolase). Unlike the pathway for catabolism of leucine and the *S*-pathway for catabolism of isoleucine, in which all of the intermediates are CoA esters, in the catabolism of valine, the portion of the pathway between 3-hydroxyisobutyryl-CoA and propionyl-CoA involves the free acids rather than CoA esters (Fig. 93-5).[264] Thus, a specific deacylase is required to hydrolyze 3-hydroxyisobutyryl-CoA to 3-hydroxyisobutyric acid.[265] The enzyme has been partially purified from pig heart and shows a high substrate specificity for 3-hydroxyisobutyryl-CoA and 3-hydroxypropionyl-CoA.[265] The reaction is irreversible. Highly purified rat liver 3-hydroxyisobutyryl-CoA hydrolase has a molecular weight of 36,000 and is a monomer.[258] It has a very narrow substrate specificity, acting on 3-hydroxypropionyl-CoA at 57 percent of the rate for S-3-hydroxyisobutyryl-CoA and at less than 1 percent for a large number of other acyl-CoA compounds.[258] The K_m for *S*-3-hydroxyisobutyryl-CoA was 6 μM, and the turnover number of 266 is higher than that of other enzymes in the valine pathway. The stereoisomer of 3-hydroxyisobutyric acid produced from isobutyric acid in rats has been shown to be the *S*(+)-isomer.[266]

The deacylase is present in human liver and cultured fibroblasts.[241] The human 3-hydroxyisobutyryl-CoA hydrolase has been cloned and sequenced.[267] It has 1146 bp coding a protein of 352 amino acids, a molecular weight of 39,398, and a 28-amino-acid mitochondrial leader sequence. The purified recombinant human mature enzyme expressed in *E. coli* had the highest activity with *S*-3-hydroxyisobutyryl-CoA, 54 percent as much activity with 3-hydroxypropionyl-CoA, and less than 1 percent with other tested acyl-CoA compounds. Western blotting showed the human tissue distribution to be liver $=$ kidney $>$ heart $\gg$ muscle $=$ brain. Interestingly, the human amino acid sequence has no similarity to sequences of other thioester hydrolases but rather has homology to the enoyl-CoA hydratase/isomerase superfamily of enzymes.[267]

3-Hydroxyisobutyric Acid Dehydrogenase. The *S*-3-hydroxyisobutyric acid produced by the deacylation of *S*-3-hydroxyisobutyryl-CoA is oxidized with NAD as substrate to form methylmalonic semialdehyde (see Fig. 93-5).[268,269] The enzyme has been purified two hundredfold from pig kidney[268] and eighteen hundredfold from rabbit liver.[269] The latter is 74-kDa and is a homodimer of 34-kDa subunits. The rabbit liver enzyme is highly specific for *S*-3-hydroxyisobutyric acid, with a K_m of 61 μM, and for NAD, with a K_m of 23 μM.[269] *R*-3-hydroxyisobutyric acid is a poor substrate, with a K_m of 1440 μM. The enzyme is very sensitive to inhibition by NADH, with a K_i of 5.7 μM. The enzyme also acts on *S*-2-ethyl-3-hydroxypropionic acid (in the *R*-pathway for isoleucine catabolism) to form ethylmalonic semialdehyde.[269] The reaction is reversible, and the equilibrium constant of 0.036 favors reduction of methylmalonic semialdehyde to 3-hydroxyisobutyric acid.[269] Hexadeuterated isobutyric acid administered to humans leads to the expected excretion of *S*-3-hydroxyisobutyric acid labeled with five deuterium atoms.[270] However, it also leads to considerable excretion of *S*-3-hydroxyisobutyric acid labeled with four deuterium atoms and about 20 percent as much *R*-3-hydroxyisobutyric acid labeled with four deuterium atoms.[270] The former can be accounted for by oxidation to *S*-methylmalonic semialdehyde with loss of a deuterium atom and reduction back to *S*-3-hydroxyisobutyric acid with four deuterium atoms catalyzed reversibly by 3-hydroxyisobutyric acid dehydrogenase. *S*-Methylmalonic semialdehyde can undergo spontaneous keto-enol tautomerism, causing racemization to a mixture of *S*- and *R*-methylmalonic semialdehyde and reduction of the latter to form *R*-3-hydroxyisobutyric acid.

The cDNA for rat liver 3-hydroxyisobutyrate dehydrogenase has been cloned (GenBank J04628) and sequenced.[271] It has 1038 bp, coding for a 300-amino-acid mature protein of 31.6 kDa. On Northern blots, a 2-kb mRNA was found at high levels in rat kidney, moderate levels in heart and liver, and low levels in skeletal muscle.

Methylmalonic Semialdehyde Dehydrogenase. The carboxyl group of *S*-methylmalonic semialdehyde is decarboxylated to carbon dioxide, and the aldehyde group is oxidized with NAD to a carboxylic acid group that forms a thioester with CoA to produce propionyl-CoA in a complex reaction catalyzed by methylmalonic semialdehyde dehydrogenase. The enzyme has been purified from bacteria[272] and also purified six hundredfold from rat liver.[259] The enzyme from the latter is about 250 kDa, suggesting a tetramer of 58-kDa subunits. The enzyme has a K_m of 5.3 μM for methylmalonic semialdehyde, 150 μM for NAD, and 30 μM for CoA and is inhibited by NADH, with a K_i of 3.1 μM. It also acts on malonic semialdehyde (derived from the catabolism of uracil), with a K_m of 4.5 μM, to form acetyl-CoA with a maximum velocity about fourfold higher than that for methylmalonic semialdehyde. The enzyme has a small amount of activity with succinic semialdehyde but very little activity with ethylmalonic semialdehyde derived from the *R*-pathway of isoleucine catabolism. Both *S*-methylmalonic semialdehyde and *R*-methylmalonic semialdehyde in a racemic mixture are metabolized by purified methylmalonic semialdehyde dehydrogenase.[259] At one time the catabolic pathway of valine was thought to involve direct oxidation of methylmalonic semialdehyde to methylmalonic acid. Studies of the in vivo metabolism of [2-^{13}C]valine and [2,3-^{13}C]valine to methylmalonic acid in a patient with methylmalonic acidemia, using NMR analysis of urinary methylmalonic acid, clearly demonstrated that the carboxyl group of methylmalonic semialdehyde was lost, as expected, from metabolism by methylmalonic semialdehyde dehydrogenase to propionyl-CoA with subsequent carboxylation to methylmalonic acid.[273] More-extensive studies in rats with stable isotopically labeled isobutyric acid also demonstrated the same pathway.[274] Studies of the metabolism of deuterium-labeled *S*(+)-3-hydroxyisobutyric acid and [^{13}C]bicarbonate with rat liver mitochondria also demonstrated decarboxylation of the carboxyl group of methylmalonic semialdehyde.[275] Analysis of the products of purified rat liver methylmalonic semialdehyde dehydrogenase confirmed that the product with methylmalonic semialdehyde was propionyl-CoA and the product with malonic semialdehyde was acetyl-CoA.[259]

The rat liver cDNA for methylmalonic semialdehyde dehydrogenase has been cloned and sequenced.[276] It codes for a 32-amino-acid-leader peptide and a mature 55.33-kDa enzyme of 503 amino acids. An mRNA of 3.8 kb was found in rat tissues, with progressively decreasing amounts in kidney, liver, heart, and brain. The human liver cDNA has also been cloned (GenBank M93405) and shows 97.7 percent homology with the rat cDNA.[276]

Convergence at Methylmalonic Semialdehyde of the Valine and Thymine Pathways. As described immediately above, the catabolism of valine produces *S*-methylmalonic semialdehyde. Also shown in Fig. 93-5 are the terminal steps of degradation of thymine, a pyrimidine. The *R*-3-aminoisobutyric acid derived from oxidation and cleavage of thymine is transaminated to *R*-methylmalonic semialdehyde. Racemic *S*- and *R*-methylmalonic semialdehyde are metabolized to propionyl-CoA by the same enzyme, methylmalonic semialdehyde dehydrogenase. Either both the *S* and *R* isomers are substrates, or they are spontaneously interconverted at a physiological pH due to the acidic nature of the chiral hydrogen alpha to two oxo groups. It is also possible that there is an enzyme in vivo that catalyzes the racemization of the *S*- and *R*- isomers of methylmalonic semialdehyde. Like thymine, uracil is degraded to a 3-amino acid, *β*-alanine, which is transaminated to malonic semialdehyde, which is oxidized to acetyl-CoA by the same methylmalonic semialdehyde dehydrogenase. Thus, a deficiency of this enzyme would be expected to cause the accumulation of malonic semialdehyde and both *S*- and *R*-methylmalonic semialdehyde. Because of the reversible reactions of the transaminases and 3-hydroxyisobutyric acid dehydrogenase, one might expect accumulation of *β*-alanine and 3-hydroxypropionic acid from malonic semialdehyde and *S*- and *R*-3-aminoisobutyric acid and *S*- and *R*-3-hydroxyisobutyric acid from methylmalonic semialdehyde.

Propionyl-CoA and Methylmalonyl-CoA Metabolism. The further metabolism of propionyl-CoA derived from valine (and thymine) is by carboxylation to methylmalonyl-CoA and isomerization to succinyl-CoA, as described in Chap. 94. Because the formation of propionyl-CoA from methylmalonic acid semialdehyde is irreversible, none of the intermediates of the valine catabolic pathway prior to propionyl-CoA accumulate in patients with propionic acidemia or methylmalonic acidemia.

Isolated Isobutyryl-CoA Dehydrogenase Deficiency?

One patient was recently described who may have an isolated deficiency of a specific isobutyryl-CoA dehydrogenase in the valine pathway but normal activity of short-branched chain acyl-CoA dehydrogenase for 2-methylbutyryl-CoA in the isoleucine pathway.[277]

Clinical Aspects and Abnormal Metabolites. The female infant presented at 11 months with anemia and dilated cardiomyopathy. Plasma carnitine levels were very low: 5 μM free carnitine and 6 μM total carnitine. After treatment with L-carnitine (200 mg/kg per day), analysis of plasma acylcarnitines showed a markedly elevated 4-carbon acylcarnitine (butyryl- and/or isobutyryl-carnitine) level. Urinary organic acids did not show elevation of butyrylglycine or isobutyrylglycine.

Enzyme Deficiency. To determine which four-carbon acylcarnitine was elevated and to attempt to identify the site of an enzyme deficiency, cultured skin fibroblasts were studied for the metabolism of labeled palmitic acid and labeled branched chain amino acids to labeled acylcarnitines by tandem MS. Incubation of intact fibroblasts from the patient with labeled palmitic acid did not cause elevation of labeled butyrylcarnitine as is seen in short chain acyl-CoA dehydrogenase (SCAD) deficiency, excluding this possibility. Incubation with labeled valine caused high elevation of labeled isobutyrylcarnitine, suggesting a deficiency of isobutyryl-CoA dehydrogenase, while incubation with labeled isoleucine did not cause elevation of labeled 2-methylbutyrylcarnitine. These results suggest a deficiency of a dehydrogenase specific for isobutyryl-CoA and not a deficiency of short-branched chain acyl-CoA dehydrogenase, which acts on butyryl-CoA, isobutyryl-CoA, and 2-methylbutyryl-CoA. Confirmation will depend upon isolation and characterization of a specific isobutyryl-CoA dehydrogenase from human tissues.

Genetics. The mode of inheritance is unknown.

Diagnosis. Analysis of acylcarnitines in plasma or dried blood spots showing elevation of a four-carbon acylcarnitine with normal urine organic acids may suggest this disorder.

Treatment. Continued treatment of the patient with carnitine reversed the cardiomyopathy, and growth and development were normal at 27 months of age.

3-Hydroxyisobutyryl-CoA Deacylase Deficiency

Only one patient has been identified with this disorder.[241,278]

Clinical Aspects. The male infant had dysmorphic features at birth, poor feeding, failure to thrive, lack of development of motor skills, hypotonia, and absence of neurologic development.[241] The infant died at 3 months of age, and other findings included vertebral abnormalities, tetralogy of Fallot, and agenesis of the cingulate gyrus and corpus callosum. It is unknown whether the congenital malformations are a result of the biochemical defect in methacrylyl-CoA metabolism, but methacrylate esters are teratogenic in rats.[279]

Abnormal Metabolites. Although this is considered to be a disorder of branched chain organic acid metabolism of valine, no abnormal organic acids are excreted, because the accumulated intermediates react with cysteine derivatives to yield unusual sulfur amino acids. High-voltage electrophoresis of urine showed two unusual amino acids on staining with ninhydrin, and both were positive for sulfur by the iodoplatinate reagent. These were identified as *S*-(2-carboxypropyl)-cysteine and *S*-(2-carboxypropyl)-cysteamine.[278] The former has been identified as a trace component in urine of normal children.[280] Both compounds were detected in tissues from the patient at levels of 1 to 10 nmol/g of tissue.[241] The cysteine adduct is presumably derived from the addition of cysteine across the double bond of methacrylyl-CoA, an intermediate in the catabolism of valine, and the cysteamine adduct could be formed by the decarboxylation of the cysteine adduct. The addition of cysteine and cysteamine to methacrylyl-CoA occurs spontaneously in neutral aqueous solutions.[241] Methacrylyl-CoA would accumulate in tissues of the patient due to the equilibrium between 3-hydroxyisobutyryl-CoA and methacrylyl-CoA catalyzed by crotonase as a result of the demonstrated deficiency of 3-hydroxyisobutyryl-CoA deacylase.

Enzyme Deficiency. Fibroblasts of the patient, but not of normal controls, produced both labeled *S*-(2-carboxypropyl)-cysteine and *S*-(2-carboxypropyl)-cysteamine from either [^{35}S]cysteine or [^{14}C]valine, and the oxidation of [2-^{14}C]valine to $^{14}CO_2$ was markedly deficient in fibroblasts of the patient, indicating a defect in valine catabolism.[241] A deficiency of crotonase could lead to an accumulation of methacrylyl-CoA and the abnormal sulfur amino acids, but crotonase was normal in the liver and fibroblasts of the patient. 3-Hydroxyisobutyryl-CoA deacylase was shown to be severely deficient in the patient, with 4 percent of normal activity in liver and 20 percent of normal activity in fibroblasts.[241] Fibroblasts of the parents had 40 to 55 percent of normal activity.

Genetics. This is presumably an autosomal recessive disorder, because both parents had activities of 3-hydroxyisobutyryl-CoA deacylase of about 50 percent of normal, as would be expected for heterozygotes.[241]

Diagnosis. The diagnosis should be considered in infants with dysmorphic features and skeletal and cardiac malformations, but it is not known whether these will be consistent features of the disorder. There is no acidosis or abnormalities of organic acids in this disorder, but two unusual amino acids can be detected by high-voltage electrophoresis or thin-layer chromatography of urinary amino acids, with abnormal spots detected by ninhydrin, confirmed as containing sulfur by reaction with iodoplatinate.[278] It may be possible to detect these amino acids with an amino acid analyzer, but retention data have not been reported. Trace amounts of *S*-(2-carboxypropyl)-cysteine are detected in the urine of children, but high elevation of this and *S*-(2-carboxypropyl)-cysteamine is unique to the deficiency of 3-hydroxyisobutyryl-CoA deacylase.[278] The identity of these compounds can be confirmed by MS.[278] The diagnosis can be confirmed by assay for a deficiency of 3-hydroxyisobutyryl-CoA deacylase in cultured fibroblasts.[241] Heterozygotes can be diagnosed by intermediate levels of activity of the enzyme in fibroblasts. Prenatal diagnosis should be possible, because the enzyme activity is expressed in normal cultured amniocytes and amniocytes from a fetus at risk for this disorder had heterozygous levels of enzyme activity.[241]

Treatment. Treatment has not been attempted and would likely be ineffective if damage occurs in utero, as suggested by the congenital malformations.

3-Hydroxyisobutyric Aciduria: Deficient Activity of 3-Hydroxyisobutyrate Dehydrogenase?

Twelve patients have been reported with increased excretion of 3-hydroxyisobutyric acid, suggesting deficient activity of 3-hydroxyisobutyric acid dehydrogenase or methylmalonic semialdehyde dehydrogenase in the valine pathway. Elevated methylmalonic semialdehyde due to a deficiency of the semialdehyde dehydrogenase would be expected to cause an elevation of 3-hydroxyisobutyric acid because of the reversible nature of 3-hydroxyisobutyrate dehydrogenase reactions but would also be expected to cause elevated 3-aminoisobutyric acid levels due to the reversibility of the transaminase reaction (see Fig. 93-5). Moreover, a deficiency of methylmalonic semialdehyde dehydrogenase would also be expected to cause the accumulation of malonic semialdehyde as well as methylmalonic semialdehyde,[259] which would cause elevated 3-hydroxypropionic acid and 3-aminopropionic acid levels.

Two of the 12 patients with increased excretion of 3-hydroxyisobutyric acid had elevated 3-aminoisobutyric acid, 3-hydroxypropionic acid, and 3-aminopropionic acid levels, consistent with the abnormal metabolite pattern expected for methylmalonic semialdehyde dehydrogenase deficiency, and discussed later under that heading. The eight other patients with elevated 3-hydroxyisobutyric acid but without the elevation of the two 3-amino acids that is most consistent with deficient activity of 3-hydroxyisobutyrate dehydrogenase will be discussed here.

Clinical Aspects. One patient presented with malformations, massive acidosis, and hypotonia.[281] Another patient had dysmorphic features, with a small triangular face, long philtrum, and small, low ears.[282] There were bilateral simian creases, clinodactyly of the fifth fingers, and mild bilateral syndactyly of the second and third toes. The patient had failure to thrive, with recurrent episodes of vomiting, lactic acidosis, ketoacidosis, and dehydration.[282] At 10 years of age his intelligence was normal. Twins presented at 5 months with infantile spasms.[283] One died at 4 years of age following influenza, seizures, fever, and disseminated intravascular coagulopathy. The other twin had static encephalopathy, microcephaly, and infrequent seizures. Another set of twins (males) had congenital brain dysgenesis and intracerebral calcification.[284] Dysmorphic features included triangular face, short sloped forehead, long philtrum, hypoplastic molar areas, and micrognathia. There were bilateral Sidney lines, cortical thumbs, and bilateral clinodactyly of the fourth and fifth toes. The twins were hypotonic, with poor limb movements and absent suck reflex; they died of respiratory failure at 4 and 18 days. Two male siblings with repeated episodes of vomiting and ketoacidosis had motor delay and mild hypotonia with normal mental development and no dysmorphic features.[285] One sib died at 4 years of age with severe ketoacidosis. The other showed focal white matter abnormalities in the MRI. A patient with poor weight gain, microcephaly, and bilateral cataracts had a sibling with similar but milder symptoms with the same 3-hydroxyisobutyric aciduria.[286] The clinical features of these two patients from a consanguineous marriage may not be related to 3-hydroxybutyric aciduria, because four cousins from a consanguineous marriage had clinical features without 3-hydroxybutyric aciduria.

Abnormal Metabolites. All patients excreted increased amounts of 3-hydroxyisobutyric acid, typically ranging from 60 to 390 mmol/mol of creatinine but reaching as high as 10,000 mmol/mol of creatinine during acute episodes. One patient also excreted lesser but still abnormal amounts of 3-hydroxypropionic, 2-ethyl-3-hydroxypropionic (ethylhydracrylic), and 3-hydroxyisovaleric acids.[281] Another patient consistently excreted 2-ethyl-3-hydroxypropionic acid.[287] Lactic acid was highly elevated in the urine of five of the patients. Two patients had elevated urinary 3-hydroxybutyric, 3-hydroxypropionic, and 2-ethyl-3-hydroxypropionic acids and elevated *β*-alanine but not 3-aminoisobutyric in plasma. 3-Aminopropionic *β*-alanine) and 3-aminoisobutyric acids were not elevated in the plasma or urine of any of the other patients. *S*-(2-carboxypropyl)-cysteine was detected in the urine of only one patient.[281] Free carnitine was low in plasma, and the ratio of esterified to free carnitine was high in one patient.[282]

In three patients given a valine load, 3-hydroxyisobutyric acid increased to 1100 to 2800 mmol/mol of creatinine.[281–283] Methylmalonic semialdehyde was not detected. One patient became lethargic, vomited with a challenge of valine, and had very high excretion of 3-hydroxybutyric and lactic acids.[282]

Enzyme Deficiency. The basic enzyme deficiency has not yet been determined for these patients with 3-hydroxyisobutyric aciduria. A prime candidate is 3-hydroxyisobutyric acid dehydrogenase, although a deficiency of methylmalonic semialdehyde dehydrogenase might be possible, because 3-hydroxyisobutyric acid levels in urine would be expected to be higher than those of methylmalonic semialdehyde due to the reversibility of 3-hydroxyisobutyrate dehydrogenase reactions and the normal redox state. The lack of elevation of 3-aminopropionic and 3-aminoisobutyric acids, which would be expected to be formed by transamination of the corresponding semialdehydes, makes a deficiency of methylmalonic semialdehyde very unlikely. Fibroblasts from one set of twins had normal activity levels for the valine pathway enzymes: methacrylyl-CoA hydratase, 3-hydroxyisobutyryl-CoA deacylase, 3-hydroxyisobutyrate dehydrogenase, and methylmalonic semialdehyde dehydrogenase.[283] Oxidation of [2-^{14}C]-valine was normal in fibroblasts from one and 42 percent of normal in the other twin. These results suggest that the defect in valine metabolism may not be expressed in fibroblasts. In fibroblasts from another patient, activity of 3-hydroxyisobutyrate dehydrogenase was normal, but oxidation of [U-^{14}C]-valine was low at 8 percent of the control mean and oxidation of *β*-[1-^{14}C]-alanine was 26 percent of the control mean, although the oxidations overlapped the control range.[287] The authors suggested that these results could indicate a deficiency of methylmalonic semialdehyde dehydrogenase, but this is difficult to reconcile with the lack of elevation of 3-aminoisobutyric and 3-aminopropionic acids and the consistent elevation of 3-hydroxypropionic acid in this patient.[282]

The inability to demonstrate a deficiency in cultured fibroblasts of 3-hydroxyisobutyrate dehydrogenase, the most likely enzyme deficiency to explain the organic aciduria, raises the interesting possibility that 3-hydroxyisobutyric aciduria may be due to a secondary deficiency rather than a primary deficiency of 3-hydroxyisobutyrate dehydrogenase. This enzyme is highly sensitive to inhibition by NADH,[269] and an abnormally reduced state of the redox potential could manifest itself primarily as an inhibition of this enzyme, causing 3-hydroxyisobutyric to be elevated. Inhibition of this enzyme would also account for the elevation of 2-ethyl-3-hydroxypropionic acid seen in some patients, since this metabolite in the *R*-pathway for isoleucine is also a substrate for 3-hydroxyisobutyrate dehydrogenase. Most of the patients had elevated lactic acid, which would be consistent with an increase in NADH. There are many causes of an abnormally elevated NADH/NAD ratio, and it would be interesting to explore this in patients with 3-hydroxyisobutyric aciduria. The high elevation of 3-hydroxyisobutyric acid seen during normal ketosis may also be due to inhibition of 3-hydroxyisobutyrate dehydrogenase by NADH.[269]

Genetics. The mode of inheritance has not been determined. Five of the patients were male, but the sex of the other three was not reported.

Diagnosis. The possibility of 3-hydroxyisobutyric aciduria should be considered in infants with dysmorphic features, brain dysgenesis, malformations, hypotonia, failure to thrive, lactic acidemia, or episodes of acidosis, ketosis, and vomiting. Elevations as high as 2500 mmol 3-hydroxyisobutyric acid/mol of creatinine can occur nonspecifically in ketosis of any cause.[126] Therefore, the diagnosis of 3-hydroxyisobutyric aciduria cannot be made during a ketotic episode. In addition, the trimethylsilyl derivatives of 3-hydroxybutyric acid and 3-hydroxyisobutyric acid coelute in many GC/MS analyses of urinary organic acids, making quantitation of 3-hydroxyisobutyric acid difficult unless the unique fragment at an m/z (mass/charge ratio) of 177 is used for quantitation. Elevated excretion of 3-hydroxyisobutyric acid of 60 to 600 mmol/mol of creatinine when the patient is not ketotic suggests this disorder. Patients with 3-hydroxyisobutyric aciduria may also have elevated lactic acid or increased excretion of other 3-hydroxy acids but no increased excretion of 3-aminopropionic and 3-aminoisobutyric acids. The excretion of 3-hydroxyisobutyric acid increases with a valine load,[281–283] but this can cause a severe clinical response and is not recommended.[282]

Prenatal diagnosis may be possible, because 3-hydroxyisobutyric acid was elevated at 7 μM (normal, 0.9 to 2.4 μM) in amniotic fluid of affected twins.[284]

Treatment. Two patients were treated with a low-protein diet (0.75 and 2.0 g/kg per day) and carnitine (100 mg/kg), which resulted in a marked reduction in the frequency and severity of acidotic episodes.[282,285]

Methylmalonic Semialdehyde Dehydrogenase Deficiency: Mild or Benign Clinical Features with Combined 3-Hydroxypropionic, 3-Aminopropionic (*β*-Alanine), 3-Hydroxyisobutyric, 3-Aminoisobutyric (*β*-Aminoisobutyric), and 2-Ethyl-3-Hydroxypropionic Aciduria. A child has been reported with a pattern of metabolites explained by a deficiency of methylmalonic semialdehyde dehydrogenase.[288,289] Another patient, recently described as having 3-hydroxyisobutyric aciduria, had a similar pattern of elevated 3-hydroxy and 3-amino acids.[290] Both patients had minor clinical abnormalities.

Clinical Aspects. The first male infant had episodes of diarrhea and vomiting at 3 weeks and again at 9 months of age.[288] A low-methionine diet was given starting at 3 weeks of age and was discontinued at 3 years of age. Loading studies with methionine had no clinical effect. At 4 years of age, on a regular diet, he was clinically well and development was normal. The second male presented at 2 years of age with vomiting, lethargy, and an episode of tonic-clonic movements. Other than a previous febrile convulsion, he has been clinically well.[290]

Abnormal Metabolites. The first infant was found to have hypermethioninemia by newborn screening.[289] He had persistent hypermethioninemia higher than 1000 μM and elevated excretion of hydroxy and amino acids as described below, but the methionine elevation is probably not related to these, because a cousin has hypermethioninemia without elevation of the other metabolites. The hypermethioninemia in these children may be due to a deficiency of methionine adenosyltransferase deficiency, which is generally clinically benign.

The first child had high excretion levels of the three-carbon compounds 3-aminopropionic acid, also known as *β*-alanine (100 to 400 mmol/mol of creatinine) and 3-hydroxypropionic acid (500 to 1000 mmol/mol of creatinine), the four-carbon compounds 3-aminoisobutyric acid also known as *β*-aminoisobutyric acid (1000 to 3000 mmol/mol of creatinine), and 3-hydroxybutyric acid (3000 to 4000 mmol/mol of creatinine), and the five-carbon compound 2-ethyl-3-hydroxypropionic acid also known as ethylhydracrylic acid or 2-hydroxymethylbutyric acid (3000 mmol/mol of creatinine), but no detectable 2-ethyl-3-aminopropionic acid.[288,289] 3-Aminoisobutyric acid was greatly elevated in plasma, at 30 μM as compared to normal levels of 1.8 to 4.5 μM, and the plasma 3-aminopropionic acid level was 6 μM. The second child had somewhat lower excretion rates of the same 3-hydroxy and 3-amino acids, which were considerably higher during the initial ketotic episodes.[290] The 3-amino acids were also elevated in plasma, as were 3-hydroxypropionic and 3-hydroxyisobutyric acids when he was ketotic.

The metabolites of the first child were further characterized as to their chiral configuration. The 3-aminoisobutyric acid was about equally composed of the *S*- and *R*-isomers, while normally the *R*/*S* ratio is about 95.[291] 3-Hydroxyisobutyric acid was about 75 percent *S*- and 25 percent *R*-isomer, and all of the 2-ethyl-3-hydroxypropionic acid was the *S*-isomer.[289] These metabolite elevations are consistent with a deficiency of a dehydrogenase acting on malonic semialdehyde, methylmalonic semialdehyde, and ethylmalonic semialdehyde.[289]

The precursors of the urinary metabolites were identified by loading studies with valine, which is normally metabolized to *S*-3-hydroxyisobutyric acid,[270] and thymine, which is normally metabolized to *R*-3-aminoisobutyric acid,[292,293] together with about 5 percent as much *S*-3-aminoisobutyric acid.[291] Loading studies in the patient had no effect on the excretion of 3-hydroxypropionic acid, which is a minor metabolite of propionic acid, or on the excretion of 3-aminopropionic acid, which comes from degradation of uracil and the peptides carnosine and anserine. Loading with valine caused a large increase in excretion of *S*-3-hydroxyisobutyric acid and had little effect on the excretion of 3-aminoisobutyric acid and no effect on the ratio of *R*:*S*-3-aminoisobutyric acid. The plasma 3-aminoisobutyric acid (largely the *S*-isomer) doubled with the load of valine. This suggests that a small proportion of *S*-methylmalonic semialdehyde derived from valine was transaminated to *S*-3-aminoisobutyric acid and retained in plasma because of efficient renal reabsorption of this isomer.[292,293] Loading with thymine did not increase the level of plasma 3-aminoisobutyric acid, which is efficiently excreted, and caused a large increase in the amount of *R*-3-aminoisobutyric acid but not of 3-hydroxyisobutyric acid in urine. The presence of *R*-3-hydroxybutyric acid in the urine is probably due to some transamination of *R*-3-aminoisobutyric acid to R-methylmalonic semialdehyde and reduction. The excreted *S*-2-ethyl-3-hydroxypropionic acid presumably arises from a block at ethylmalonic semialdehyde in the minor *R*-pathway of isoleucine metabolism.

Enzyme Studies. From the metabolite elevations, it is likely that there is a deficiency of a dehydrogenase acting on malonic semialdehyde, methylmalonic semialdehyde, and ethylmalonic semialdehyde to form acetyl-CoA, propionyl-CoA, and butyryl-CoA, respectively. Malonic semialdehyde and methylmalonic semialdehyde are excellent substrates for methylmalonic semialdehyde dehydrogenase purified from rat liver.[259] Thus, a deficiency of this enzyme would account for the elevation of all of the metabolites (see Fig. 93-5) except 2-ethyl-3-hydroxypropionic acid (see Fig. 93-4). Ethylmalonic semialdehyde is not a substrate for the rat enzyme, so a deficiency of this enzyme would not be expected to cause elevated 2-ethyl-3-hydroxypropionic acid levels. However, it appears that human methylmalonic semialdehyde dehydrogenase has a substrate specificity different from that of the rat enzyme and can utilize ethylmalonic semialdehyde as a substrate, so that a deficiency causes increased 2-ethyl-3-hydroxypropionic acid excretion.

The metabolism of valine and *β*-alanine have been studied in intact fibroblasts from the first patient.[294] The oxidation of [1-^{14}C]valine to $^{14}CO_2$ was normal, but the oxidation of [2-^{14}C]valine to $^{14}CO_2$ was undetectable, indicating a severe block in valine metabolism below the level of isobutyryl-CoA. The oxidation of *β*-[1-^{14}C]alanine was only 7 percent of normal. The label in the 2-position of valine would be metabolized to the 1-position of methylmalonic semialdehyde, the label in the 1-position of *β*-alanine would be metabolized to the 1-position of malonic semialdehyde, and both would yield labeled carbon dioxide if methylmalonic semialdehyde dehydrogenase were active. Thus, the lack of production of labeled carbon dioxide from these two substrates strongly indicates a deficiency of methylmalonic semialdehyde dehydrogenase in this patient. However, assay of malonic semialdehyde dehydrogenase in lysed fibroblasts by decarboxylation of labeled malonic semialdehyde derived from *β*-alanine did not show as severe a deficiency (about 50 to 60 percent of control levels), although much of this activity could be spontaneous decarboxylation of the unstable malonic semialdehyde.

Genetics. The mode of inheritance is unknown. Both patients were male.

Diagnosis. There are no clinical symptoms clearly associated with this biochemical disorder, and it may be benign. The diagnosis may be made by the detection of the elevated urinary amino acids *β*-alanine and 3-aminoisobutyric acid and the elevated urinary organic acids 3-hydroxypropionic acid, 3-hydroxyisobutyric acid, and 2-ethyl-3-hydroxypropionic acid. Elevation of 3-hydroxyisobutyric acid without elevation of the two 3-amino acids suggests 3-hydroxybutyric aciduria rather than methylmalonic semialdehyde dehydrogenase deficiency.

Treatment. No treatment is indicated at this time, as the two affected subjects are well and developing normally.

Methylmalonic Semialdehyde Dehydrogenase Deficiency: More Severe Clinical Presentation and a Different Biochemical Phenotype of Only Mildly Elevated Methylmalonic Acid

One patient with atypical mild methylmalonic acidemia has a clinical and biochemical phenotype very different from that of the patients in the preceding section, although studies suggest an abnormality of methylmalonic semialdehyde dehydrogenase.

Clinical Aspects and Abnormal Metabolites. The male infant had recurrent emesis at 18 months of age due to malrotation of the gut, which was corrected surgically at 22 months of age along with removal of a Meckel's diverticulum.[295] He was developmentally delayed at 20 months of age. His clinical course has been characterized by seizures and developmental delay without metabolic decompensation.

Organic acid analysis of urine showed a moderate methylmalonic aciduria of 20 to 55 (μmol/kg per day, compared with the average of 1157 (μmol/kg per day for a patient with methylmalonyl-CoA mutase deficiency. Plasma methylmalonic acid averaged 8.5 μM, compared with 400 μM in a patient with mutase deficiency. There was no elevation of malonic, ethylmalonic, 3-hydroxypropionic, 3-aminopropionic, or 3-aminoisobutyric acids in urine.

Propionylcarnitine was not elevated in plasma or urine, unlike the case in patients with methylmalonyl-CoA mutase deficiency. The activity of methylmalonyl-CoA mutase was normal, as was incorporation of labeled propionate in cultured fibroblasts. He had normal transcobalamin II and serum vitamin B_{12} binding capacity, and treatment with cyanocobalamin and hydroxocobalamin did not affect plasma or urine methylmalonic acid levels. Treatment with carnitine did not change plasma or urine methylmalonic acid concentrations Treatment with carnitine also did not increase plasma levels of propionylcarnitine nor urine excretion of propionylcarnitine, in contrast to its effect in patients with methylmalonyl-CoA mutase deficiency or cobalamin defects, who have large increases of propionylcarnitine levels upon treatment with carnitine. Thus, there was no evidence for a defect in propionic acid metabolism, methylmalonyl-CoA mutase, or cobalamin metabolism to account for the elevated methylmalonic acid levels.

Metabolism Studies. The lack of elevation of propionylcarnitine and the moderate methylmalonic acidemia suggested that the methylmalonic acid was not derived from propionyl-CoA via methylmalonyl-CoA but may have come from oxidation of methylmalonic semialdehyde. However, a deficiency of methylmalonic semialdehyde dehydrogenase that could elevate methylmalonic semialdehyde for oxidation to methylmalonic acid would also be expected to cause increased excretion of 3-hydroxyisobutyric, 3-hydroxypropionic, 3-aminopropionic, and 3-aminoisobutyric acids, which was not observed in this patient. Normally the ratio of *R*-3-aminoisobutyric acid (derived from thymine) to *S*-3-aminoisobutyric acid (derived from valine) is about 95.[291] Due to a relative increase in *S*-3-aminoisobutyric acid, the patient had an *R*/*S* ratio of 0.7.

The patient was infused with deuterium-labeled valine and deuterium-labeled thymine, and his excretion levels of labeled products compared to those of a methylmalonyl-CoA mutase-deficient patient. The atypical methylmalonic acidemia patient showed much greater excretion of labeled *S*- and *R*-3-hydroxyisobutyric acid and labeled *S*-3-aminoisobutyric acid after labeled valine than did the mutase patient. This suggests a block in the area of methylmalonic semialdehyde dehydrogenase with interconversion of the accumulated *S*-methylmalonic semialdehyde to *S*- and *R*-3-hydroxyisobutyric and *S*- and *R*-3-aminoisobutyric acids.

It is difficult to understand why this patient normally excretes only moderate amounts of methylmalonic acid and not of the 3-hydroxy and 3-amino acids excreted in large amounts by the patients described above for the mild/benign form of this disorder, when both types of patients are believed to have a deficiency of methylmalonic semialdehyde dehydrogenase. One possibility is that his abnormal methylmalonic semialdehyde dehydrogenase has a normal affinity for methylmalonic semialdehyde and can catalyze a partial reaction that oxidizes methylmalonic semialdehyde to methylmalonic acid but has a lower rate of decarboxylation to form a propionic acid intermediate or decreased ability to transfer this intermediate to CoA to form propionyl-CoA. If the majority of the methylmalonic semialdehyde and all of the malonic semialdehyde were metabolized to propionyl-CoA and acetyl-CoA, respectively, this could account for the lack of elevation of 3-hydroxy and 3-amino acids derived from the semialdehydes and the modest elevation of methylmalonic acid without elevation of malonic acid. Further studies of the mechanism of the complex reaction catalyzed by methylmalonic semialdehyde and the substrate specificity of the human enzyme should help provide answers to these questions.

Genetics. The mode of inheritance is unknown.

Diagnosis. This atypical methylmalonic acidemia may be suggested by developmental delay and seizures with moderate elevation of methylmalonic acid and no elevation of propionylcarnitine or of 3-hydroxyisobutyric, 3-hydroxypropionic, 2-ethyl-3-hydroxypropionic, 3-aminopropionic, and 3-aminoisobutyric acids.

Treatment. A treatment has not been developed.

Ethylmalonic Aciduria Encephalopathy: Possible Secondary Deficiency of Short-Branched Chain Acyl-CoA Dehydrogenase?

Four unrelated Italian patients were identified with encephalopathy and a pattern of metabolite excretions including ethylmalonic acid and branched chain acylglycines and acylcarnitines suggestive of a deficiency of short-methylbranched chain acyl-CoA dehydrogenase in the catabolic pathways of both valine and isoleucine.[296–298] Subsequently a total of 19 patients from Italy, Spain, Saudi Arabia, Canada, and the United States have been reported.

Clinical Aspects. The Italian patients presented with neonatal hypotonia followed by severe progressive pyramidal dysfunction, mental retardation, orthostatic acrocyanosis with distal swelling, chronic diarrhea, recurrent petechiae, and abnormal brain MRI.[296–298] Two patients died suddenly at age 2 years, and the others have severe mental retardation. MRI showed areas of hyperintensity in the cerebellar white matter and the caudate and lenticular nuclei. The patients had chronic lactic acidemia and repeated metabolic decompensation with metabolic acidosis but not ketosis and normal blood glucose and ammonia levels.[298–300] In a patient from Spain with similar clinical features, there were a large number of bilateral lesions in many areas of the brain on MRI.[299] Five patients from Saudi Arabia had similar clinical features but did not have chronic diarrhea.[300] In addition, all of these patients had retinal lesions. Three of them died following the sudden appearance of severe lesions in the basal ganglia, putamen, and caudate. Of three sibs in an American Hispanic family with similar clinical features, a girl had dysmorphic features, hepatomegaly, and gross hematuria and died at 15 months of age.[301] Two Canadian sibs with clinical features similar to those of the Italian patients had structural abnormalities on MRI of the brain and spine, tethered cord in one and cerebellar ectopia in the other.[302] These symptoms are similar to those seen in mitochondrial disorders, and in our experience elevated ethylmalonic acid is common in proven mitochondrial defects. Thus, this "disease" is similar to 3-methylglutaconic aciduria type IV.

Abnormal Metabolites. Ethylmalonic acid was the most elevated urinary metabolite, at 60 to 930 mmol/mol of creatinine (normal < 17 mmol/mol of creatinine).[298] This was accompanied by smaller elevations of its metabolite, methylsuccinic acid, at 2 to 200 mmol/mol creatinine (normal < 12 mmol/mol of creatinine). Ethylmalonic acid may be derived from carboxylation of elevated butyryl-CoA by propionyl-CoA carboxylase or from the *R*-pathway of isoleucine catabolism. The excretion of lactic acid was consistently elevated, and the 2-ethyl-3-hydroxypropionic acid level was elevated during acute episodes. There were no elevations of glutaric or other dicarboxylic acids of 6 to 10 carbons.[298] However, some of the Saudi Arabian patients had elevated glutaric and adipic acids and thus a pattern of excretion resembling that in multiple acyl-CoA dehydrogenase deficiency.[300] Lactic and pyruvic acids were consistently elevated in blood, and the ratio of lactic to pyruvic acid was elevated.[298,299,303]

Acylglycines derived from butyryl-CoA and from the acyl-CoA compounds in the catabolism of leucine, isoleucine, and valine were also generally excreted in increased amounts: isobutyrylglycine, 0 to 160 mmol/mol of creatinine (normal, < 8 mmol/mol of creatinine); isovalerylglycine, 0 to 90 mmol/mol of creatinine (normal, < 10 mmol/mol of creatinine); n-butyrylglycine, 2 to 170 mmol/mol of creatinine (normal, < 2 mmol/mol of creatinine); and 2-methylbutyrylglycine, 0 to 18 mmol/mol of creatinine (normal, < 5 mmol/mol of creatinine).[298] There was no elevation of hexanoylglycine, phenylpropionylglycine, or suberylglycine.

Isobutyrylcarnitine was the major increased acylcarnitine in urine, and 2-methylbutyrylcarnitine and isovalerylcarnitine were also generally elevated. Excretion increased upon treatment with carnitine. Isobutyryl-, isovaleryl-, and 2-methylbutyryl-carnitine were found in plasma of three patients and butyryl- and hexanoyl-carnitine in two.[298]

The pattern of urinary metabolite elevations in ethylmalonic aciduria encephalopathy has considerable similarity to that of multiple acyl-CoA dehydrogenase deficiency (MADD) due to ETF or ETF dehydrogenase deficiency; these include elevation of ethylmalonic acid and of acylglycines and acylcarnitines derived from the branched chain amino acids. However, glutaric, 2-hydroxyglutaric, and other dicarboxylic acids that are prominent in the latter are not elevated in ethylmalonic aciduria encephalopathy.

Loading studies with isoleucine have been performed to elucidate the origins of ethylmalonic acid and other possible metabolites of isoleucine. Oral loading with 100 mg isoleucine/kg body weight in two patients increased the excretion of ethylmalonic acid, although the increase was not significant,[298] and a load of 150 mg/kg in another patient also increased ethylmalonic acid excretion.[303] This suggests that the metabolism of isoleucine through the *R*-pathway is not the major source of ethylmalonic acid, leaving butyryl-CoA as a possible source. However, methylsuccinic acid excretion was moderately increased after the isoleucine challenges. 2-Methylbutyrylglycine was increased above normal after the challenges with isoleucine[298,303] and the increase in tiglylglycine was minimal and less than normal in one patient,[303] suggesting decreased activity of short-methylbranched acyl-CoA dehydrogenase. 2-Ethyl-3-hydroxypropionic acid (the precursor of ethylmalonic acid in the *R*-pathway for isoleucine catabolism) levels were increased in all three patients after the isoleucine load.

Enzyme Deficiency. The basic enzyme defect is still not known. Studies in cultured fibroblasts have shown normal oxidation of myristic, palmitic, octanoic, and butyric acids and of isoleucine, leucine, and valine.[298–300,303,304] The activity levels of short-, medium-, long-, and 2-methylbranched chain acyl-CoA dehydrogenases were normal in fibroblasts.[298,299] These results rule out a deficiency of ETF or ETF dehydrogenase.

Studies of the possible causes of the lactic acidemia showed normal electron chain transport activities in cultured fibroblasts and normal or slightly reduced cytochrome c oxidase.[298–300,303] Muscle biopsies have shown normal activity levels of the respiratory chain complexes except for cytochrome c oxidase, which is partially deficient in some but not all patients studied.[298,299,303,304] A deficiency of muscle cytochrome c oxidase has also been found in patients with abnormal excretion of ethylmalonic acid and branched chain acylglycines, with or without increased glutaric acid excretion and clinical phenotypes different from that of ethylmalonic aciduria encephalopathy.[305,306]

Genetics. Both males and females are affected, but the mode of inheritance has not been determined.

Diagnosis. The possibility of this disorder involving both valine and isoleucine catabolism should be considered in patients with lactic acidemia, hypotonia, spastic diplegia, orthostatic acrocyanosis with distal swelling, and diarrhea.[296] The pattern of organic acid metabolites in urine with highly elevated ethylmalonic acid and isobutyrylglycine, together with elevation of methylsuccinic acid, butyrylglycine, isovalerylglycine, and 2-methylbutyrylglycine and elevated C4 and C5 acylcarnitines in plasma and urine but without elevation of glutaric or 2-hydroxyglutaric acid appears to be diagnostic. Multiple acyl-CoA dehydrogenase deficiency should be ruled out by fatty acid oxidation studies or assay for ETF and ETF dehydrogenase.

Treatment. An effective treatment is not known. Riboflavin and carnitine have been without benefit. A diet low in branched chain amino acids would theoretically be appropriate.

Malonic Aciduria: Malonyl-CoA Decarboxylase Deficiency

Fifteen patients with malonic aciduria (and usually a lesser elevation of urine methylmalonic acid) have been reported. Eight patients have been shown to have a deficiency of malonyl-CoA decarboxylase in mitochondria, two were shown to have normal activity of this enzyme, and activity in the rest has not yet been determined. Although this is not a disorder of branched chain amino acid metabolism, it is included here because the organic aciduria includes methylmalonic acid derived from the catabolism of isoleucine and valine in addition to the malonic aciduria. The source of mitochondrial malonyl-CoA is believed to be acetyl-CoA, which is carboxylated to malonyl-CoA by propionyl-CoA carboxylase, which is not completely specific for propionyl-CoA.

Clinical Aspects. The clinical features are variable, but most patients have had developmental delay in early childhood. Other clinical symptoms, variably present in 20 to 40 percent of the cases, include seizures, hypotonia, diarrhea, vomiting, metabolic acidosis, hypoglycemia, ketosis and lactic acidemia, and hypertrophic cardiomyopathy.[307–317]

MRI of the brain has been abnormal in some cases, with enlarged ventricles[313] or frontotemporal atrophy and hypodense areas,[311] but normal in others.[316]

One patient died in the neonatal period,[315] and two infants died.[311,317]

Abnormal Metabolites. The major abnormality in the urinary organic acids is highly elevated malonic acid levels, together with moderately elevated methylmalonic acid. Patients with a deficiency of malonyl-CoA decarboxylase commonly have malonic acid excretion levels of 200 to 300 mmol/mol creatinine (normal < 8 mmol/mol creatinine), but excretions can range from 20 to 2000 mmol/mol creatinine depending on the diet and metabolic status.[307–309,311–313,315] A carbohydrate load increased malonic acid excretion compared with a protein load.[307] In another patient, lower excretion levels of malonic acid were found with a high-carbohydrate diet than with a high-fat diet.[308] Treatment of another patient with carnitine and a high-carbohydrate, low-fat diet had no consistent effect on malonic acid excretion.[312] In addition to the malonic aciduria, excretion of methylmalonic acid is usually elevated, ranging from 30 to 300 mmol/mol creatinine (normal < 12 mmol/mol creatinine),[307–309,311,313,315] but can be normal.[312] The increased methylmalonic acid excretion is believed to be due to inhibition of methylmalonyl-CoA mutase by elevated malonyl-CoA.

One patient with normal activity of malonyl-CoA decarboxylase had elevation of urinary malonic and methylmalonic acids similar to that in patients lacking this enzyme activity but also had high excretion levels of 3-hydroxy-3-methylglutaric and succinic acids.[311] Another patient with normal activity of malonyl-CoA decarboxylase excreted much more methylmalonic acid than malonic acid.[314] The excretion of both malonic and methylmalonic acids increased with a high-protein diet.

Plasma total carnitine and acylcarnitine were low in one patient.[313] Elevated malonylcarnitine has been found in plasma, dried blood spots, and urine.[310,312,316]

Enzyme Deficiency. A deficiency of malonyl-CoA decarboxylase has been shown in fibroblasts or lymphocytes of eight patients with malonic aciduria.[307–310,312,313,317] The activity was normal in a patient who had elevated 3-hydroxy-3-methylglutaric and succinic acids[311] and in a patient who excreted much more methylmalonic acid than malonic acid.[314]

Genetics. Both males and females are affected, and the relatively common consanguinity found in families with malonic aciduria is consistent with autosomal recessive inheritance.

The human gene for malonyl-CoA decarboxylase has been cloned for comparison with the gene for this enzyme in the goose, which shows 77 percent homology with the human.[318] The gene has a peroxisomal targeting sequence, and subcellular localization indicates the enzyme is present in both mitochondria and peroxisomes. Two different homozygous mutations resulting in premature stop codons have been identified.

Diagnosis. The possibility of malonic aciduria may be considered in patients with the relatively nonspecific features of developmental delay, hypotonia, or cardiomyopathy. Analysis of urinary organic acids shows elevated malonic acid, typically 220 to 300 mmol/mol creatinine (range 20 to 2000 mmol/mol creatinine), and lesser elevations of methylmalonic acid, typically 30 to 300 mmol/mol creatinine. Malonic aciduria does not have other abnormally elevated organic acids that are seen in methylmalonic aciduria due to mutase deficiency or cobalamin defects. Diagnosis of malonic aciduria can also be made by tandem MS to detect acylcarnitines in plasma or urine showing elevated C3-dicarboxylic acylcarnitine (malonylcarnitine) without elevation of propionylcarnitine. Malonylcarnitine is elevated in dried blood spots of affected patients, suggesting the possibility of detection of malonic aciduria in newborn screening by tandem MS.[316]

Treatment. A clearly effective treatment has not been developed. In one study, a high-carbohydrate, low-fat diet decreased the excretion of malonic and methylmalonic acids.[308] In another patient, treatment with carnitine and a high-carbohydrate, low-fat diet had no effect on malonic acid excretion.[312] A high-carbohydrate, low-fat diet together with carnitine supplementation in one patient did result in normalization of acidosis and liver size and cessation of vomiting, although hypotonia and developmental delay remained.[313]

Malonyl-CoA has an important regulatory role in fatty acid metabolism, and many of the patients with proven malonyl-CoA decarboxylase deficiency have abnormal brain myelination, mental retardation, microcephaly, and low cholesterol levels. We have hypothesized that a normal total fat intake may be important for normal brain development but that long chain fatty acids may play a role in the development of cardiomyopathy in this disorder. A male sibling of a reported patient[312] was born with severe cardiomyopathy, low cholesterol levels, and elevated malonic and methylmalonic acids in urine. The patient was placed on carnitine supplementation and a diet with low long chain fatty acid but normal total fat intake via medium chain triglycerides. On this regimen, malonic acid excretion increased from 316 to 1457 mmol/mol creatinine, serum cholesterol increased from 98 to 136 mmol/mol creatinine, and left ventricular function became normal. At 21 months he has a normal head circumference, normal cognitive and motor development, and a normal physical exam without any neurologic abnormalities. Unlike his retarded sibling, his brain MRI shows normal myelination.

ADDENDUM

Mevalonic Aciduria

A syndrome of hyperimmunoglobulinema D and periodic fever was initially identified in a group of Dutch patients.[319] The clinical features of 50 patients with this syndrome have been summarized.[320] Most were from Europe (56% from the Netherlands), and the existence of multiple affected family members suggested that the condition is inherited. The onset of episodic fevers usually begins in infancy with episodes lasting several days occurring at one to two month intervals throughout life. During episodes of fever, most patients have abdominal pain, diarrhea, and skin lesions, and many have vomiting and headaches. Most patients also have lymphadenopathy, polyarthralgia, and arthritis.

Patients with this syndrome of hyperimmunoglobulinemia D and periodic fever were recently found to have elevations of mevalonic acid in urine during the episodes of fever but not between episodes.[321] The elevations of mevalonic acid were far less than the continuously high elevations previously seen in patients with mevalonic aciduria due to a deficiency of mevalonate kinase. However, molecular analysis for mutations in the mevalonate kinase gene identified a number of mutations in patients with hyperimmunoglobulinemia D and episodic fever, with diminished activity of mevalonate kinase and decreased mevalonate kinase protein in fibroblasts.[321,322] Clinical symptoms that are common to both patients with the syndrome of elevated IgD with episodic fever and the previously described patients with mevalonate kinase deficiency include recurrent crises with fever, lymphadenopathy, arthralgia, and a skin rash.[213] Patients with these symptoms should be examined for possible deficiency of mevalonate kinase activity or mutations in the mevalonate kinase gene. They may also be diagnosed by finding elevated mevalonic acid in urine during episodes of fever, but with the intermittent nature of mevalonate excretion, enzymatic or molecular diagnosis is likely to be more reliable.

ACKNOWLEDGMENT

Special thanks to Veronica Tran for assistance with the references.

REFERENCES

1. Chalmers RA, Lawson AM: *Organic Acids in Man: The Analytical Chemistry, Biochemistry, and Diagnosis of the Organic Acidurias.* London, Chapman & Hall, 1982.
2. Goodman SI, Markey SP: *Diagnosis of Organic Acidemias by Gas Chromatography-Mass Spectrometry.* New York, Liss, 1981.
3. Sweetman L: Organic acid analysis, in Hommes FA (ed): *Techniques in Diagnostic Human Biochemical Genetics: A Laboratory Manual.* New York, Wiley-Liss, 1991, p 143.
4. Millington DS, Kodo N, Norwood DL, Roe CR: Tandem mass spectrometry: A new method for acylcarnitine profiling with potential for neonatal screening for inborn errors of metabolism. *J Inherit Metab Dis* **13**:321, 1990.
5. Rashed MS, Bucknall MP, Little D, Awad A, Jacob M, Alamoudi M, Alwattar M, et al.: Screening blood spots for inborn errors of metabolism by electrospray tandem mass spectrometry with a microplate batch process and a computer algorithm for automated flagging of abnormal profiles. *Clin Chem* **43**:1129, 1997.
6. Acosta PB: *Nutrition Support Protocols.*Columbus, OH, Ross Laboratories, 1989.
7. Beinert H: Acyl dehydrogenases from pig and beef liver and beef heart, in Colowick SP, Kaplan NO (eds): *Methods in Enzymology vol V.* New York, Academic Press, 1962 p 546.
8. Tanaka K, Budd MA, Efron ML, Isselbacher KJ: Isovaleric acidemia: A new genetic defect of leucine metabolism. *Proc Natl Acad Sci USA* **56**:236, 1966.
9. Rhead WJ, Tanaka K: Demonstration of a specific mitochondrial isovaleryl-CoA dehydrogenase deficiency in fibroblasts from patients with isovaleric acidemia. *Proc Natl Acad Sci USA* **77**:580, 1980.
10. Rhead WJ, Hall CL, Tanaka K: Novel tritium release assays for isovaleryl-CoA and butyryl-CoA dehydrogenases. *J Biol Chem* **256**:1616, 1981.
11. Ikeda Y, Tanaka K: Purification and characterization of isovaleryl coenzyme A dehydrogenase from rat liver mitochondria. *J Biol Chem* **258**:1077, 1983.
12. Ikeda Y, Dabrowski C, Tanaka K: Separation and properties of five distinct acyl-CoA dehydrogenases from rat liver mitochondria. *J Biol Chem* **258**:1066, 1983.

13. Finocchiaro G, Ito M, Tanaka K: Purification and properties of short chain acyl-CoA, medium chain acyl-CoA, and isovaleryl-CoA dehydrogenases from human liver. *J Biol Chem* **262**:7982, 1987.
14. Ikeda Y, Fenton WA, Tanaka K: In vitro translation and post-translational processing of four mitochondrial acyl-CoA dehydrogenases. *Fed Proc* **43**:2024, 1984.
15. Ikeda Y, Keese SM, Fenton WA, Tanaka K: Biosynthesis of four rat liver mitochondrial acyl-CoA dehydrogenases: in vitro synthesis, import into mitochondria, and processing of their precursors in a cell-free system and in cultured cells. *Arch Biochem Biophys* **252**:662, 1987.
16. Mckean MC, Beckmann JD, Frerman FE: Subunit structure of electron transfer flavoprotein. *J Biol Chem* **258**:1866, 1983.
17. Ruzicka FJ, Beinert H: A new iron-sulfur flavoprotein of the respiratory chain. *J Biol Chem* **252**:8440, 1977.
18. Rhead WJ, Dubiel B, Tanaka K: The tissue distribution of isovaleryl CoA dehydrogenase in the rat, in Walser M, Williamson JR (eds): *Metabolism and Clinical Implications of Branched Chain Amino and Ketoacids*. New York, Elsevier/North Holland, 1981, p 47.
19. Aberhart DJ, Tann CH: Substrate stereochemistry of isovaleryl-CoA dehydrogenase: elimination of the 2-pro-R hydrogen in biotin-deficient rats. *Bioorg Chem* **10**:200, 1981.
20. Aberhart DJ, Finocchiaro G, Ikeda Y, Tanaka K: Substrate stereochemistry of isovaleryl-CoA dehydrogenase. II. Steric course of C-3 hydrogen elimination. *Bioorg Chem* **14**:170, 1986.
21. Kraus JP, Matsubara Y, Barton D, Yang-Feng TL, Glassberg R, Ito M, Ikeda Y, et al.: Isolation of cDNA clones coding for rat isovaleryl-CoA dehydrogenase and assignment of the gene to human chromosome 15. *Genomics* **1**:264, 1987.
22. Matsubara Y, Indo Y, Naito E, Ozasa H, Glassberg R, Vockley J, Ikeda Y, et al.: Molecular cloning and nucleotide sequence of cDNAs encoding the precursors of rat long chain acyl-coenzyme A, short chain acyl coenzyme A, and isovaleryl-coenzyme A dehydrogenases: Sequence homology of four enzymes of the acyl-CoA dehydrogenase family. *J Biol Chem* **264**:16321, 1989.
23. Matsubara Y, Ito M, Glassberg R, Satyabhama S, Ikeda Y, Tanaka K: Nucleotide sequence of messenger RNA encoding human isovaleryl coenzyme A dehydrogenase and its expression in isovaleric acidemia fibroblasts. *J Clin Invest* **85**:1058, 1990.
24. Mohsen A-WA, Vockley J: High-level expression of an altered cDNA encoding human isovaleryl-CoA dehydrogenase in *Escherichia coli*. *Gene* **160**:263, 1995.
25. Mohsen A-WA, Vockley J: Identification of the active site catalytic residue in human isovaleryl-CoA dehydrogenase. *Biochemistry* **34**:10146, 1995.
26. Tiffany KA, Roberts DL, Wang M, Paschke R, Mohsen A-WA, Vockley J, Kim J-JP: Structure of human isovaleryl-CoA dehydrogenase at 2.6 Å resolution: Structural basis for substrate specificity. *Biochem* **36**:8455, 1997.
27. Lynen F, Knappe J, Lorch E, Jutting G, Ringelmann E, Lachance JP: Zur biochemischen Funktion des Biotins. II. Reinigung und Wirkungsweise der beta-Methyl-crotonyl-Carboxylase. *Biochem Z* **335**:123, 1961.
28. Lau EP, Cochran BC, Munson L, Fall RR: Bovine kidney 3-methylcrotonyl-CoA carboxylase and propionyl-CoA carboxylases: Each enzyme contains nonidentical subunits. *Proc Natl Acad Sci USA* **76**:214, 1979.
29. Lau EP, Cochran BC, Fall RR: Isolation of 3-methylcrotonyl-coenzyme A carboxylase from bovine kidney. *Arch Biochem Biophys* **205**:352, 1980.
30. Hector ML, Cochran BC, Logue EA, Fall RR: Subcellular localization of 3-methylcrotonyl-coenzyme A carboxylase in bovine kidney. *Arch Biochem Biophys* **199**:28, 1980.
31. Duran M, Bruinvis L, Ketting D, Kamerling JP, Wadman SK, Schutgens RBH: The identification of (E)-2-methylglutaconic acid, a new isoleucine metabolite, in the urine of patients with beta-ketothiolase deficiency, propionic acidaemia and methylmalonic acidaemia. *Biomed Mass Spectrom* **9**:1, 1982.
32. Stern JR, Del Camplillo A: Enzymes of fatty acid metabolism: II. Properties of crystalline crotonase. *J Biol Chem* **218**:985, 1956.
33. Hilz H, Knappe J, Ringelmann E, Lynen F: Methylglutaconase, eine neue Hydratase, die am Stoffwechsel verzweigter Carbonsauren beteiligt ist. *Biochem Z* **329**:476, 1958.
34. Villanueva VR, Lynen F: Une nouvelle méthode de préparation de la méthylglutaconase à partir du foie de boeuf. *C R Acad Sci Paris* **270**:3318, 1970.
35. Narisawa K, Gibson KM, Sweetman L, Nyhan WL, Duran M, Wadman SK: Deficiency of 3-methylglutaconyl-coenzyme A hydratase in two siblings with 3-methylglutaconic aciduria. *J Clin Invest* **77**:1148, 1986.
36. Messner B, Eggerer H, Cornforth JW, Mallaby R: Substrate stereochemistry of the hydroxymethylglutaryl-CoA lyase and 3-methylglutaconyl-CoA hydratase reactions. *Eur J Biochem* **53**:255, 1975.
37. Budd MA, Tanaka K, Holmes LB, Efron ML, Crawford JD, Isselbacher KJ: Isovaleric acidemia—clinical features of a new genetic defect of leucine metabolism. *N Engl J Med* **277**:321, 1967.
38. Tanaka K, Rosenberg LE: Disorders of branched chain amino acid and organic acid metabolism, in Stanbury JB, Wyngaarden JB, Fredrickson DS, Goldstein JL, Brown MS (eds): *The Metabolic Basis of Inherited Disease 5th ed*. New York, McGraw-Hill, 1983, p 440.
39. Tanaka K: Inborn errors of branched-chain amino acid metabolism, in Odessy R (ed): *Problems and Potential of Branched-Chain Amino Acids in Physiology and Medicine*. New York, Elsevier, 1986, p 201.
40. Cohn RM, Yudkoff M, Rothman R, Segal S: Isovaleric acidemia: Use of glycine therapy in neonates. *N Engl J Med* **299**:996, 1978.
41. Fischer AQ, Challa VR, Burton BK, McLean WT: Cerebellar hemorrhage complicating isovaleric acidemia: A case report. *Neurology* **31**:746, 1981.
42. Mendiola J, Robotham JL, Liehr JG, Williams JC: Neonatal lethargy due to isovaleric acidemia and hyperammonemia. *Texas Med* **80**:52, 1984.
43. Wilson WG, Audenaert SM, Squillaro EJ: Hyperammonaemia in a preterm infant with isovaleric acidemia. *J Inherit Metab Dis* **7**:71, 1984.
44. Hou JW, Wang TR: Isovaleric acidemia: Report of one case. *Acta Paed Sin* **31**:262, 1990.
45. Newman CGH, Wilson BDR, Callaghan P, Young L: Neonatal death associated with isovaleric acidemia. *Lancet* **2**:439, 1967.
46. Beauvais P, Peter MO, Barbier B: Forme néo-natale de l'acidémie isovalérique. *Arch Fr Pediatr* **42**:531, 1985.
47. Kelleher JF, Yudkoff M, Hutchison R, August CS, Cohn RM: The pancytopenia of isovaleric acidemia. *Pediatrics* **65**:1023, 1980.
48. Truscott RJW, Malegan D, McCairns E, Burke D, Hick L, Sims P, Halpern B, et al.: New metabolites in isovaleric acidemia. *Clin Chim Acta* **110**:187, 1981.
49. Lorek AK, Penrice JM, Cady EB, Leonard JV, Wyatt JS, Iles RA, Burns SP, et al.: Cerebral energy metabolism in isovaleric acidaemia. *Arch Dis Child* **74**:F211, 1996.
50. Shih VE, Aubry RH, DeGrande G, Gursky SF, Tanaka K: Maternal isovaleric acidemia. *J Pediatr* **105**:77, 1984.
51. Mayatepek E, Kurczynski TW, Hoppel CL: Long-term L-carnitine treatment in isovaleric acidemia. *Pediatr Neurol* **7**:137, 1991.
52. Roe CR, Millington DS, Maltby DA, Kahler SG, Bohan TP: L-Carnitine therapy in isovaleric acidemia. *J Clin Invest* **74**:2290, 1984.
53. Shigematsu Y, Sudo M, Momoi T, Inoue Y, Suzuki Y, Kameyama J: Changing plasma and urinary organic acid levels in a patient with isovaleric acidemia during an attack. *Pediatr Res* **16**:771, 1982.
54. Gerdes AM, Gregersen N, Ludvigsson P, Guttler F: A Scandinavian case of isovaleric acidemia. *J Inherit Metab Dis* **11**:218, 1988.
55. Williams KM, Peden VH, Hillman RE: Isovaleric acidemia appearing as diabetic ketoacidosis. *Am J Dis Child* **135**:1068, 1981.
56. Attia N, Sakati N, Al Ashwal A, Al Saif R, Rashed M, Ozand PT: Isovaleric acidemia appearing as diabetic ketoacidosis. *J Inherit Metab Dis* **19**:85, 1996.
57. Duran M, Bruinvis L, Ketting D, Wadman SK, Van Pelt BC, Batenburg-Plenter AM: Isovaleric acidemia presenting with dwarfism, cataract and congenital abnormalities. *J Inherit Metab Dis* **5**:125, 1982.
58. Tanaka K, Isselbacher KJ: The isolation and identification of N-isovalerylglycine from urine of patients with isovaleric acidemia. *J Biol Chem* **242**:2966, 1967.
59. Bartlett K, Gompertz D: The specificity of glycine-N-acylase and acylglycine excretion in the organic acidaemias. *Biochem Med* **10**:15, 1974.
60. Gregersen N, Kolvraa S, Mortensen PB: Acyl-CoA:glycine N-acyltransferase: In vitro studies on the glycine conjugation of straight- and branched-chained acyl-CoA esters in human liver. *Biochem Med Metab Biol* **35**:210, 1986.
61. Tanaka K, Orr JC, Isselbacher KJ: Identification of beta-hydroxyisovaleric acid in the urine of a patient with isovaleric acidemia. *Biochim Biophys Acta* **152**:638, 1968.
62. Lehnert W, Niederhoff H: 4-Hydroxyisovaleric acid: A new metabolite in isovaleric acidemia. *Eur J Pediatr* **136**:281, 1981.

63. Shigematsu Y, Kikawa Y, Sudo M, Kikuchi K, Ohta S, Okamata M: A simple method of determining 4-hydroxyisovaleric acid and its level in a patient with isovaleric acidemia. *Clin Chim Acta* **138**:333, 1984.
64. Dorland L, Duran M, Wadman SK, Niederwieser A, Bruinvis L, Ketting D: Isovalerylglucuronide, a new urinary metabolite in isovaleric acidemia: Identification problems due to rearrangement reactions. *Clin Chim Acta* **134**:77, 1983.
65. Hine DG, Tanaka K: The identification and the excretion pattern of isovaleryl glucuronide in the urine of patients with isovaleric acidemia. *Pediatr Res* **18**:508, 1984.
66. Lehnert W: Excretion of N-isovalerylglutamic acid in isovaleric acidemia. *Clin Chim Acta* **116**:249, 1981.
67. Lehnert W: N-isovalerylalanine and N-isovalerylsarcosine: Two new minor metabolites in isovaleric acidemia. *Clin Chim Acta* **134**:207, 1983.
68. Lehnert W: 3-Hydroxyisoheptanoic acid: A new metabolite in isovaleric acidemia. *Clin Chim Acta* **113**:101, 1981.
69. Rabier D, Parvy P, Bardet J, Saudubray JM, Kamoun P: Alloisoleucine in isovaleric acidemia. *J Inherit Metab Dis* **15**:154, 1992.
70. Petit FH, Yeaman SJ, Reed LJ: Purification and characterization of branched chain alpha-keto acid dehydrogenase complex of bovine kidney. *Proc Natl Acad Sci USA* **75**:4881, 1978.
71. Shih VE, Mandell R, Tanaka K: Diagnosis of isovaleric acidemia in cultured fibroblasts. *Clin Chim Acta* **48**:437, 1973.
72. Tanaka K, Mandell R, Shih VE: Metabolism of [1-^{14}C] and [2-^{14}C]leucine in cultured skin fibroblasts from patients with isovaleric acidemia. *J Clin Invest* **58**:164, 1976.
73. Hyman DB, Tanaka K: Isovaleryl-CoA dehydrogenase activity in isovaleric acidemia fibroblasts using an improved tritium release assay. *Pediatr Res* **20**:59, 1986.
74. Frerman FE, Goodman SI: Fluorometric assay of acyl-CoA dehydrogenases in normal and mutant human fibroblasts. *Biochem Med* **33**:38, 1985.
75. Dubiel B, Dabrowski C, Wetts R, Tanaka K: Complementation studies of isovaleric acidemia and glutaric aciduria type II using cultured skin fibroblasts. *J Clin Invest* **72**:1543, 1983.
76. Ikeda Y, Keese SM, Tanaka K: Molecular heterogeneity of variant isovaleryl-CoA dehydrogenase from cultured isovaleric acidemia fibroblasts. *Proc Natl Acad Sci USA* **82**:7081, 1985.
77. Vockley J, Parimoo B, Tanaka K: Molecular characterization of four different classes of mutations in the isovaleryl-CoA dehydrogenase gene responsible for isovaleric acidemia. *Am J Hum Genet* **49**:147, 1991.
78. Vockley J, Nagao M, Parimoo B, Tanaka K: The variant human isovaleryl-CoA dehydrogenase gene responsible for type II isovaleric acidemia determines an RNA splicing error, leading to the deletion of the entire second coding exon and the production of a truncated precursor protein that interacts poorly with mitochondrial import receptors. *J Biol Chem* **267**:2494, 1992.
79. Vockley J, Andersn BD, Willard JM, Seelan RS, Smith DI, Liu W: Abnormal splicing of IVD RNA in isovaleric acidemia caused by amino acid altering point mutations in the IVD gene: A novel molecular mechanism for disease. *Am J Hum Genet* **63**:A14, 1998.
80. Tanaka K, West-Dull A, Hine DG, Lynn TB, Lowe T: Gas-chromatographic method of analysis for urinary organic acids. II. Description of the procedure, and its application to diagnosis of patients with organic acidurias. *Clin Chem* **26**:1847, 1980.
81. Yamaguchi S, Koda N, Eto Y, Aoki K: Quick screening and diagnosis of organic acidemia by NMR urinalysis. *J Pediatr* **106**:620, 1985.
82. Iles RA, Hind AJ, Chalmers RA: Use of proton nuclear magnetic resonance spectroscopy in detection and study of organic acidurias. *Clin Chem* **31**:1795, 1985.
83. Lehnert W, Hunkler D: Possibilities of selective screening for inborn errors of metabolism using high-resolution 1H-FT-NMR spectrometry. *Eur J Pediatr* **145**:260, 1986.
84. Hine DG, Hack AM, Goodman SI, Tanaka K: Stable isotope dilution analysis of isovalerylglycine in amniotic fluid and urine and its application for the prenatal diagnosis of isovaleric acidemia. *Pediatr Res* **20**:222, 1986.
85. Kleijer WJ, Van Der Kraan M, Huijmans JGM, Van Der Heuvel CMM, Jakobs C: Prenatal diagnosis of isovaleric acidaemia by enzyme and metabolite assay in the first and second trimesters. *Prenat Diagn* **15**:527, 1995.
86. James MO, Bend JR: Perinatal development of, and effect of chemical pretreatment on, glycine N-acyltransferase activities in liver and kidney of rabbit and rat. *Biochem J* **172**:293, 1978.
87. Shigematsu Y, Hata I, Nakai A, Kikawa Y, Sudo M, Tanaka Y, Yamaguchi S, et al.: Prenatal diagnosis of organic acidemias based on amniotic fluid levels of acylcarnitines. *Pediatr Res* **39**:680, 1996.
88. Krieger I, Tanaka K: Therapeutic effects of glycine in isovaleric acidemia. *Pediatr Res* **10**:25, 1976.
89. Velazquez A, Prieto EC: Glycine in acute management of isovaleric acidemia. *Lancet* **1**:313, 1980.
90. Yudkoff M, Cohn RM, Pushak R, Rothman R, Segal S: Glycine therapy in isovaleric acidemia. *J Pediatr* **92**:813, 1978.
91. Naglak M, Salvo R, Madsen K, Dembure P, Elsas L: The treatment of isovaleric acidemia with glycine supplement. *Pediatr Res* **24**:9, 1988.
92. De Sousa C, Chalmers RA, Stacey TE, Tracey BM, Weaver CM, Bradley D: The response to L-carnitine and glycine therapy in isovaleric acidaemia. *Eur J Pediatr* **144**:451, 1986.
93. Stanley CA, Hale DE, Whiteman DEH, Coates PM, Yudkoff M, Berry GT, Segal S: Systemic carnitine (carn) deficiency in isovaleric acidemia (IVA). *Pediatr Res* **17**:296A, 1983.
94. Chalmers RA, Roe CR, Stacey TE, Hoppel CL: Urinary excretion of L-carnitine and acylcarnitines by patients with disorders of organic acid metabolism: Evidence for secondary insufficiency of L-carnitine. *Pediatr Res* **18**:1325, 1984.
95. van Hove JLK, Kahler SG, Millington DS, Roe DS, Chace DH, Heales SJ, Roe CR: Intravenous L-carnitine and acetyl-L-carnitine in medium chain acyl CoA dehydrogenase deficiency and isovaleric acidemia. *Pediatr Res* **35**:96, 1994.
96. Lee PJ, Harrison EL, Jones MG, Chalmers RA, Leonard JV, Whipp BJ: Improvement in exercise tolerance in isovaleric acidaemia with L-carnitine therapy. *J Inherit Metab Dis* **21**:136, 1998.
97. Itoh T, Ito T, Ohba S, Sugiyama N, Mizuguchi K, Yamaguchi S, Kidouchi K: Effect of carnitine administration on glycine metabolism in patients with isovaleric acidemia: Significance of acetylcarnitine determination to estimate the proper carnitine dose. *Tohoku J Exp Med* **179**:101, 1996.
98. Fries MH, Rinaldo P, Schmidt-Sommerfeld E, Jurecki E, Packman S: Isovaleric acidemia: Response to a leucine load after three weeks of supplementation with glycine, L-carnitine, and combined glycine-carnitine therapy. *J Pediatr* **129**:449, 1998.
99. Millington DS, Roe CR, Maltby DA, Inoue F: Endogenous catabolism is the major source of toxic metabolites in isovaleric acidemia. *J Pediatr* **110**:56, 1987.
100. Bergen BJ, Stumpf DA, Haas R, Parks JK, Eguren LA: A mechanism of toxicity of isovaleric acid in rat liver mitochondria. *Biochem Med* **27**:154, 1982.
101. Hutchison RJ, Bunnell K, Thoene JG: Suppression of granulopoietic progenitor cell proliferation by metabolites of the branched-chain amino acids. *J Pediatr* **106**:62, 1985.
102. Bannwart C, Wermuth B, Baumgartner R, Suormala T, Wiesmann UN: Isolated biotin-resistant deficiency of 3-methylcrotonyl-CoA carboxylase presenting as a clinically severe form in a newborn with fatal outcome. *J Inherit Metab Dis* **15**:863, 1992.
103. Murayama K, Kimura M, Yamaguchi S, Shinka T, Kodama K: Isolated 3-methylcrotonyl-CoA carboxylase deficiency in a 15-year-old girl. *Brain Dev* **19**:303, 1997.
104. Lehnert W, Niederhoff H, Suormala T, Baumgartner R: Isolated biotin-resistant 3-methylcrotonyl-CoA carboxylase deficiency: Long-term outcome in a case with neonatal onset. *Eur J Biochem* **155**:568, 1996.
105. Beemer FA, Bartlett K, Duran M, Ghneim HK, Wadman SK, Bruinvis L, Ketting D: Isolated biotin-resistant 3-methylcrotonyl-CoA carboxylase deficiency in two sibs. *Eur J Pediatr* **138**:351, 1982.
106. Mourmans J, Bakkeren J, de Jong J, Wevers R, van Diggelen OP, Suormala T, Baumgartner R, et al.: Isolated (biotin-resistant) 3-methylcrotonyl-CoA carboxylase deficiency: Four sibs devoid of pathology. *J Inherit Metab Dis* **18**:643, 1995.
107. Elpeleg ON, Havkin S, Barash V, Jakobs C, Glick B, Shaley RS: Familial hypotonia of childhood caused by isolated 3-methylcrotonyl-coenyzme A carboxylase deficency. *J Pediatr* **121**:407, 1992.
108. Finnie MDA, Cottrall K, Seakins JWT, Snedden W: Massive excretion of 2-oxoglutaric acid and 3-hydroxyisovaleric acid in a patient with a deficiency of 3-methylcrotonyl-CoA carboxylase. *Clin Chim Acta* **73**:513, 1976.
109. Tsai MY, Johnson DD, Sweetman L, Berry SA: Two siblings with biotin-resistant 3-methylcrotonyl-coenzyme A carboxylase deficiency. *J Pediatr* **115**:110, 1989.
110. Bartlett K, Bennett MJ, Hill RP, Lashford LS, Pollit RJ, Worth HGJ: Isolated biotin-resistant 3-methylcrotonyl-CoA carboxylase deficiency presenting with life-threatening hypoglycemia. *J Inherit Metab Dis* **7**:182, 1984.

111. Gitzelmann R, Steinmann B, Niederwieser A, Fanconi S, Suormala T, Baumgartner R: Isolated (biotin-resistant) 3-methylcrotonyl-CoA carboxylase deficiency presenting at age 20 months with sopor, hypoglycemia and ketoacidosis. *J Inherit Metab Dis* **10**(suppl 2):290, 1987.
112. Kobori JA, Johnston K, Sweetman L: Isolated 3-methylcrotonyl CoA carboxylase deficiency presenting as a Reyes-like syndrome. *Pediatr Res* **25**:142A, 1989.
113. Layward EM, Tanner MS, Pollit RJ, Bartlett K: Isolated biotin-resistant 3-methylcrotonyl-CoA carboxylase deficiency presenting as a Reye syndrome-like illness. *J Inherit Metab Dis* **12**:339, 1989.
114. Rolland MO, Divry P, Zabot MT, Guibaud P, Gomez S, Lachaux A, Loras I: Isolated 3-methylcrotonyl-CoA carboxylase deficiency in a 16-month-old child. *J Inherit Metab Dis* **14**:838, 1991.
115. Tuchman M, Berry SA, Thuy LP, Nyhan WL: Partial methylcrotonyl-coenzyme A carboxylase deficiency in an infant with failure to thrive, gastrointestinal dysfunction, and hypertonia. *Pediatrics* **91**:664, 1993.
116. Yap S, Monavari AA, Thorton P, Naughten E: Late-infantile 3-methylcrotonyl-CoA carboxylase deficiency presenting as global developmental delay. *J Inherit Metab Dis* **21**:175, 1998.
117. Pearson MA, Aleck KA, Heidenreich RA: Benign clinical presentation of 3-methylcrotonylglycinuria. *J Inherit Metab Dis* **18**:640, 1995.
118. Ihara K, Kuromaru R, Inoue Y, Kuhara T, Matsumoto I, Yoshino M, Fukushige J: An asymptomatic infant with isolated 3-methylcrotonyl-coenzyme A carboxylase deficiency detected by newborn screening for maple syrup urine disease. *Eur J Pediatr* **156**:713, 1997.
119. Gibson KM, Bennett MJ, Naylor EW, Morton DH: 3-Methylcrotonyl-coenzyme A carboxylase deficiency in Amish/Mennonite adults identified by detection of increased acylcarnitines in blood spots of their children. *J Pediatr* **132**:519, 1998.
120. Steinman HM, Hill RL: Bovine liver crotonase (enoyl coenzyme A hydratase). *Methods Enzymol* **35**:136, 1975.
121. Stern JR: Crotonase, in Boyer PD, Lardy H, Myrback K (eds): *The Enzymes vol 5, 2d ed.* New York, Academic Press, 1961, p 511.
122. Duran M, Baumgartner ER, Suormala TM, Bruinvis L, Dorland L, Smeitink JAM, Poll-The BT: Cerebrospinal fluid organic acids in biotinidase deficiency. *J Inherit Metab Dis* **16**:513, 1993.
123. Röschinger W, Millington DS, Gage DA, Huang Z-H, Iwamoto T, Yano S, Packman S, et al.: 3-Hydroxyisovalerylcarnitine in patients with deficiency of 3-methylcrotonyl CoA carboxylase. *Clin Chim Acta* **240**:35, 1995.
124. van Hove JLK, Rutledge SL, Nada MA, Kahler SG, Millington DS: 3-Hydroxyisovalerylcarnitine in 3-methylcrotonyl-CoA carboxylase deficiency. *J Inherit Metab Dis* **18**:592, 1995.
125. Sovik O, Sweetman L, Gibson KM, Nyhan WL: Genetic complementation analysis of 3-hydroxy-3-methylglutaryl-coenzyme A lyase deficiency in cultured fibroblasts. *Am J Hum Genet* **36**:791, 1984.
126. Landaas S: Accumulation of 3-hydroxyisobutyric acid, 2-methyl-3-hydroxybutyric acid and 3-hydroxyisovaleric acid in ketoacidosis. *Clin Chim Acta* **64**:143, 1975.
127. Millington DS, Norwood DL, Kodo N, Roe CR, Inoue F: Application of fast atom bombardment with tandem mass spectrometry and liquid chromatography/mass spectrometry to the analysis of acylcarnitines in human urine, blood, and tissue. *Anal Biochem* **180**:331, 1989.
128. Jakobs C, Sweetman L, Nyhan WL, Packman S: Stable isotope dilution analysis of 3-hydroxyisovaleric acid in amniotic fluid: Contribution to the prenatal diagnosis of inherited disorders of leucine catabolism. *J Inherit Metab Dis* **7**:15, 1984.
129. Sweetman FR, Gibson MK, Sweetman L, Nyhan WL: Activity of biotin-dependent and GABA metabolizing enzymes in chorionic villus samples: Potential for 1st trimester prenatal diagnosis. *Prenat Diagn* **6**:187, 1986.
130. Rutledge SL, Berry GT, Stanley CA, van Hove JLK, Millington DS: Glycine and L-carnitine therapy in 3-methylcrotonyl-CoA carboxylase deficiency. *J Inherit Metab Dis* **18**:299, 1995.
131. Gibson KM, Nyhan WL, Sweetman L, Narisawa K, Lehnert W, Divry P, Robinson BH, et al.: 3-Methylglutaconic aciduria: A phenotype in which activity of 3-methylglutaconyl-coenzyme A hydratase is normal. *Eur J Pediatr* **148**:76, 1988.
132. Gibson KM, Sherwood WG, Hoffmann GF, Stumpf DA, Dianzani I, Schutgens RBH, Barth PG, et al.: Phenotypic heterogeneity in the syndromes of 3-methylglutaconic aciduria. *J Pediatr* **118**:885, 1991.
133. Gibson KM, Elpeleg ON, Jakobs C, Costeff H, Kelley RI: Multiple syndromes of 3-methylglutaconic aciduria. *Pediatr Neurol* **9**:120, 1993.
134. Kuhara T, Matsumoto I, Saiki K, Takabayashi H, Kuwabara S: 3-Methylglutaconic aciduria in two adults. *Clin Chim Acta* **207**:151, 1992.
135. de Koning TJ, Duran M, Dorland L, Berger R, Poll-The BT: Maternal 3-methylglutaconic aciduria associated with abnormalities in offspring. *Lancet* **348**:887, 1996.
136. Walsh R, Conway H, Roche G, Naughten E, Mayne PD: 3-Methylglutaconic aciduria in pregnancy. *Lancet* **349**:776, 1997.
137. Walsh R, Conway H, Roche G, Costigan C, Mayne PD: What is the origin of 3-methylglutaconic acid? *J Inherit Metab Dis* **21**:51, 1998.
138. Duran M, Beemer FA, Tibosch AS, Bruinvis L, Ketting D, Wadmans SK: Inherited 3-methylglutaconic aciduria in two brothers—another defect of leucine metabolism. *J Pediatr* **101**:551, 1982.
139. Gibson KM, Lee CF, Wappner RS: 3-Methylglutaconyl-coenzyme-A hydratase deficiency: A new case. *J Inherit Metab Dis* **15**:363, 1992.
140. Hou JW, Wang TR: 3-Methylglutaconic aciduria presenting as Reye syndrome in a Chinese boy. *J Inherit Metab Dis* **18**:645, 1995.
141. Shoji Y, Takahashi T, Sawaish Y, et al. A severe form of 3-methylglutaconic aciduria type I. *Proc 39th Meeting Jap Inherit Metab Dis* **48**, 1996.
142. Jooste S, Erasmus E, Mienie LJ, de Wet WJ, Gibson KM: The detection of 3-methylglutarylcarnitine and a new dicarboxylic conjugate, 3-methylglutaconylcarnitine, in 3-methylglutaconic aciduria. *Clin Chim Acta* **230**:1, 1994.
143. Gibson KM, Wappner RS, Jooste S, Erasmus E, Mienie LJ, Gerlo E, Desprechins B, et al.: Variable clinical presentation in three patients with 3-methylglutaconyl-coenzyme A hydratase deficiency. *J Inherit Metab Dis* **21**:631, 1998.
144. Narisawa K, Gibson KM, Sweetman L, Nyhan WL: 3-Methylglutaconyl-CoA hydratase, 3-methylcrotonyl-CoA carboxylase and 3-hydroxy-3-methylglutaryl-CoA lyase deficiencies: A coupled enzyme assay useful for their detection. *Clin Chim Acta* **184**:57, 1989.
145. Chalmers RA, Mistry J, Penketh R, McFadyen IR: First trimester prenatal diagnosis of 3-hydroxy-3-methylglutaric aciduria. *J Inherit Metab Dis* **12**(suppl 2):283, 1989.
146. Chitayat D, Chemke J, Gibson KM, Mamer OA, Kronick JB, McGill JJ, Rosenblatt B, et al.: 3-Methylglutaconic aciduria: A marker for as yet unspecified disorders and the relevance of prenatal diagnosis in a "new" type ("type 4"). *J Inherite Metab Dis* **15**:204, 1992.
147. Kelley RI, Cheatham JP, Clark BJ, Nigro MA, Powell BR, Sherwood GW, Sladky JT, et al.: X-linked dilated cardiomyopathy with neutropenia, growth retardation, and 3-methylglutaconic aciduria. *J Pediatr* **119**:738, 1991.
148. Barth PG, Scholte HR, Berden JA: An X-linked mitochondrial disease affecting cardiac muscle, skeletal muscle and neutrophil leukocytes. *J Neurol Sci* **62**:327, 1983.
149. Christodoulou J, McInnes RR, Jay V, Wilson G, Becker LE, Lehotay DC, Platt B-A, et al.: Barth synrome: Clinical observations and genetic linkage studies. *Am J Med Genet* **50**:255, 1994.
150. Edmond J, Popjak G: Transfer of carbon atoms from mevalonate to n-fatty acids. *J Biol Chem* **249**:66, 1974.
151. Brady PS, Scofield RF, Schumann WC, Ohgaku S, Kumaran K, Margolis M, Landau BR: The tracing of the pathway of mevalonate's metabolism to other than sterols. *J Biol Chem* **257**:10742, 1982.
152. Barth PG, Van Den Bogert C, Bolhuis PA, Scholte HR, van Gennip AH, Schutgens RBH, Ketel AG: X-linked cardioskeletal myopathy and neutropenia (Barth syndrome): Respiratory-chain abnormalities in cultured fibroblasts. *J Inherit Metab Dis* **19**:157, 1996.
153. Carragher F, Kirk J, FitzPatrick D, Heales S, Land J, Tonolio D: 3-Methylglutaconic aciduria and reduced activity of mitochondrial respiratory chain enzymes in a patient with Barth syndrome. *J Inherit Metab Dis* **21**:78, 1998.
154. Ades LC, Gedeon AK, Wilson MJ, Latham M, Partington MW, Mulley JC, Nelson J, et al.: Barth syndrome: Clinical features and confirmation of gene localization to distal Xq28. *Am J Med Genet* **45**:327, 1993.
155. Bione S, Adamo P, Maestrini E, Gedeon AK, Bolhuis PA, Toniolo D: A novel X-linked gene, G4.5, is responsible for Barth syndrome. *Nat Genet* **12**:385, 1996.
156. Johnston J, Kelley RI, Feigenbaum A, Cox GF, Iyer GS, Funanage VL, Proujansky R: Mutation characterization and genotype-phenotype correlation in Barth syndrome. *Am J Hum Genet* **61**:1053, 1997.
157. Orstavik KH, Orstavik RE, Naumova AK, D'Adamo P, Gedeon A, Bolhuis PA, Barth PG, et al.: X chromosome inactivation in cariers of Barth syndrome. *Am J Hum Genet* **63**:1457, 1998.
158. Neustein HB, Lurie PR, Dahms B, Takahashi M: An X-linked cardiomyopathy with abnormal mitochondria. *Pediatrics* **64**:24, 1979.

159. Cardonick EH, Kuhlman K, Ganz E, Pagatto LT: Prenatal clinical expression of 3-methylglutaconic aciduria: Barth syndrome. *Prenat Diagn* **17**:983, 1997.
160. Östman-Smith I, Brown G, Johnson A, Land JM: Dilated cardiomyopathy due to type II X-linked 3-methylglutaconic aciduria: Successful treatment with pantothenic acid. *Br Heart J* **72**:349, 1994.
161. Costeff H, Gadoth N, Apter N, Prialnic M, Savir H: A familial syndrome of infantile optic atrophy, movement disorder, and spastic paraplegia. *Neurology* **39**:595, 1989.
162. Zeharia A, Elpeleg ON, Mukamel M, Weitz R, Ariel R, Mimouni M: 3-Methylglutaconic aciduria—A new variant. *Pediatrics* **89**:1080, 1992.
163. Elpeleg ON, Costeff H, Joseph A, Shental Y, Weitz R, Gibson KM: 3-Methylglutaconic aciduria in the Iraqi-Jewish "optic atrophy plus" (Costeff) syndrome. *Dev Med Child Neurol* **36**:167, 1994.
164. Nystuen A, Costeff H, Elpeleg ON, Apter N, Bonné-Tamir B, Mohrenweiser H, Haider N, et al.: Iraqi-Jewish kindreds with optic atrophy plus (3-methylglutaconic aciduria type 3) demonstrate linkage disequilibrium with the CTG repeat in the 3′ untranslated region of the myotonic dystrophy protein kinase gene. *Hum Mol Genet* **6**:563, 1997.
165. Ruesch S, Krühenbühl S, Kleinle S, Liechti-Gallati S, Schaffner T, Wermuth B, Weber J, et al.: Combined 3-methylglutaconic and 3-hydroxy-3-methylglutaric aciduria with endocardial fibroelastosis and dilatative cardiomyopathy in male and female siblings with partial deficiency of complex II/III in fibroblasts. *Enzyme Protein* **49**:321, 1996.
166. Ibel H, Endres W, Hadorn H-B, Deufel T, Paetzke I, Duran M, Kennaway NG, et al.: Multiple respiratory chain abnormalities associated with hypertrophic cardiomyopathy and 3-methylglutaconic aciduria. *Eur J Pediatr* **152**:665, 1993.
167. Besley GTN, Lendon M, Broadhead DM, Till J, Heptinstall LE, Phillips B: Mitochondrial complex deficiencies in a male with cardiomyopathy and 3-methylglutaconic aciduria. *J Inherit Metab Dis* **18**:221, 1995.
168. Al Aqeel A, Rashed M, Ozand PT, Brismar J, Gascon GG, Al-Odaib A, Dabbagh O: 3-Methylglutaconic aciduria: Ten new cases with a possible new phenotype. *Brain Dev* **16**:23, 1994.
169. Broide E, Elpeleg ON, Lama R: Type IV 3-methylglutaconic (3-MGC) aciduria: A new case presenting with hepatic dysfunction. *Pediatr Neurol* **17**:353, 1997.
170. Gibson KM, Bennett MJ, Mize CE, Jakobs C, Rotig A, Munnich A, Lichter-Konecki U, et al.: 3-Methylglutaconic aciduria associated with Pearson syndrome and respiratory chain defects. *J Pediatr* **121**:940, 1992.
171. Greter J, Hagberg B, Steen G, Soderhjelm U: 3-Methylglutaconic aciduria: Report on a sibship with infantile progressive encephalopathy. *Eur J Pediatr* **129**:231, 1978.
172. Hagberg B, Hjalmarson O, Lindstedt S, Ransnäs L, Steen G: 3-Methylglutaconic aciduria in two infants. *Clin Chim Acta* **134**:59, 1983.
173. Lehnert W, Scharf J, Wendel U: 3-Methylglutaconic and 3-methylglutaric aciduria in a patient with suspected 3-methylglutaconyl-CoA hydratase deficiency. *Eur J Pediatr* **143**:301, 1985.
174. Haan EA, Scholem RD, Pitt JJ, Wraith JE, Brown GK: Episodes of severe metabolic acidosis in a patient with 3-methylglutaconic aciduria. *Eur J Pediatr* **146**:484, 1987.
175. Bakkeren JAJM, Sengers RCA, Ruitenbeek W, Trijbels JMF: 3-Methylglutaconic aciduria in a patient with a disturbed mitochondrial energy metabolism. *Eur J Pediatr* **151**:313, 1992.
176. Largilliere C, Vallee L, Cartigny B, Dubos JP, Gibson KM, Nuyts JP, Farriaux JP: 3-Methylglutaconic aciduria: Neonatal onset with lactic acidosis. *J Inherit Metab Dis* **12**:333, 1989.
177. Divry P, Vianey-Liaud C, Mory O, Ravussin JJ: 3-Methylglutaconic aciduria: Familial neonatal form with fatal onset. *J Inherit Metab Dis* **10**(suppl 2):286, 1987.
178. Elpeleg ON, Meiron D, Barash V, Hurwitz Y, Tal I, Amir N: 3-Methylglutaconic aciduria with persistent metabolic acidosis and "uncoupling episodes." *J Inherit Metab Dis* **13**:235, 1990.
179. Holme E, Greter J, Jacobson C-E, Lindstedt S, Nilsson KO, Oldfors A, Tulinius M: Mitochondrial ATP-synthase deficiency in a child with 3-methylglutaconic aciduria. *Pediatr Res* **32**:731, 1992.
180. Lippe G, Galsigna L, Rancesconi M, Zorzi C, Deana R: Age-dependent excretion of 3-hydroxy-3-methylglutaric acid (HMG) and ketone bodies in the urine of full-term and pre-term newborns. *Clin Chim Acta* **126**:291, 1982.
181. Mills GA, Hill MAW, Buchanan R, Corina DL, Walker V: 3-Hydroxy-3-methylglutaric aciduria: A possible pitfall in diagnosis. *Clin Chim Acta* **204**:131, 1991.
182. Wilson WG, Cass MB, Sovik O, Gibson MK, Sweetman L: A child with acute pancreatitis and recurrent hypoglycemia due to 3-hydroxy-3-methylglutaryl-CoA lyase deficiency. *Eur J Pediatr* **142**:289, 1984.
183. Faull KF, Bolton PD, Halpern B, Hammond J, Danks DM: The urinary organic acid profile associated with 3-hydroxy-3-methylglutaric aciduria. *Clin Chim Acta* **73**:553, 1976.
184. Wysocki SJ, Hahnel R: 3-Methylcrotonylglycine excretion in 3-hydroxy-3-methylglutaric aciduria. *Clin Chim Acta* **86**:101, 1978.
185. Iles RA, Jago JR, Williams SR, Chalmers RA: 3-Hydroxy-3-methylglutaryl-CoA lyase deficiency studied using 2-dimensional proton nuclear magnetic resonance spectroscopy. *FEBS Lett* **203**:49, 1986.
186. Wysocki SJ, Wilkinson SP, Hahnel R, Wong CYB, Panegyres PK: 3-Hydroxy-3-methylglutaric aciduria, combined with 3-methylglutaconic aciduria. *Clin Chim Acta* **70**:399, 1976.
187. Duran M, Ketting D, Wadman SK, Jakobs C, Schutgens RBH, Veder HA: Organic acid excretion in a patient with 3-hydroxy-3-methylglutaryl-CoA lyase deficiency: facts and artefacts. *Clin Chim Acta* **90**:187, 1978.
188. Jakobs C, Bojasch M, Duran M, Ketting D, Wadman SK, Leupold D: 3-Methyl-3-butenoic acid: An artefact in the urinary metabolic pattern of patients with 3-hydroxy-3-methylglutaryl-CoA lyase deficiency. *Clin Chim Acta* **106**:85, 1980.
189. Divry P, Rolland MO, Teyssier J, Cotte J, Formosinho Fernandes MC, Tavares De Almeida I, Da Silveira C: 3-Hydroxy-3-methylglutaric aciduria combined with 3-methylglutaconic aciduria: A new case. *J Inherit Metab Dis* **4**:173, 1981.
190. Zoghbi HY, Spence JE, Beaudet AL, O'Brien WE, Goodman CJ, Gibson KM: Atypical presentation and neuropathological studies in 3-hydroxy-3-methylglutaryl-CoA lyase deficiency. *Ann Neurol* **20**:367, 1986.
191. Green CL, Cann HM, Robinson BH, Gibson KM, Sweetman L, Holm J, Nyhan WL: 3-Hydroxy-3-methylglutaric aciduria. *J Neurogenet* **1**:165, 1984.
192. Chalmers RA, Roe CR, Tracey BM, Stacey TE, Hoppel L, Millington DS: Secondary carnitine insufficiency in disorders of organic acid metabolism: Modulation of acyl-CoA/CoA ratios by L-carnitine in vivo. *Biochem Soc Trans* **11**:724, 1983.
193. Roe CR, Millington DS, Maltby DA: Identification of 3-methylglutarylcarnitine: A new diagnostic metabolite of 3-hydroxy-3-methylglutaryl-coenzyme A lyase deficiency. *J Clin Invest* **77**:1391, 1986.
194. Clinkenbeard KD, Reed WD, Mooney RA, Lane MD: Intracellular localization of the 3-hydroxy-3-methylglutaryl coenzyme A cycle enzymes in liver. *J Biol Chem* **250**:3108, 1975.
195. Schroepfer GJ, Jr.: Sterol biosynthesis. *Ann Rev Biochem* **50**:585, 1981.
196. Goldstein JL, Brown MS: Progress in understanding the LDL receptor and HMG-CoA reductase, two membrane proteins that regulate the plasma cholesterol. *J Lipid Res* **25**:1450, 1984.
197. Brown MS, Goldstein JL: Multivalent feedback regulation of HMG CoA reductase, a control mechanism coordinating isoprenoid synthesis and cell growth. *J Lipid Res* **21**:505, 1980.
198. Levy HR, Popjak G: Studies on the biosynthesis of cholesterol. X. Mevalonic kinase and phosphomevalonic kinase from liver. *Biochem J* **75**:417, 1960.
199. Beytia E, Dorsey JK, Marr J, Cleland WW, Porter JW: Purification and mechanism of action of hog liver mevalonic kinase. *J Biol Chem* **245**:5450, 1970.
200. Lee CS, O'Sullivan WJ: An improved purification procedure, an alternative assay and activation of mevalonate kinase by ATP. *Biochim Biophys Acta* **747**:215, 1983.
201. Tanaka RD, Schafer BL, Lee LY, Freudenberger JS, Mosley ST: Purification and regulation of mevalonate kinase from rat liver. *J Biol Chem* **265**:2391, 1990.
202. Dorsey JK, Porter JW: The inhibition of mevalonic kinase by geranyl and farnesyl pyrophosphates. *J Biol Chem* **243**:4667, 1968.
203. Biardi L, Sreedhar A, Zokaei A, Vartak NB, Bozeat RL, Shackelford JE, Keller G-A, et al.: Mevalonate kinase is predominantly localized in peroxisomes and is defective in patients with peroxisome deficiency disorders. *J Biol Chem* **269**:1197, 1994.
204. Tanaka RD, Lee LY, Schafer BL, Kratunis VJ, Mohler WA, Robinson GW, Mosley ST: Molecular cloning of mevalonate kinase and regulation of its mRNA levels in rat liver. *Proc Natl Acad Sci USA* **87**:2872, 1990.
205. Schafer BL, Bishop RW, Kratunis VJ, Kalinowski SS, Mosley ST, Gibson KM, Tanaka RD: Molecular cloning of human mevalonate

kinase and identification of a missense mutation in the genetic disease mevalonic aciduria. *J Biol Chem* **267**:13229, 1992.
206. Chambliss KL, Slaughter CA, Schreiner R, Hoffmann GF, Gibson KM: Molecular cloning of human phosphomevalonate kinase and identification of a consensus peroxisomal targeting sequence. *J Biol Chem* **271**:17330, 1996.
207. Cristophe J, Popjak G: Studies on the biosynthesis of cholesterol: XIV. The origin of prenoic acids from allyl pyrophosphates in liver enzyme systems. *J Lipid Res* **2**:244, 1961.
208. Edmond J, Fogelman AM, Popjak G: Mevalonate metabolism: Role of the kidneys. *Science* **193**:154, 1976.
209. Kopito RR, Brunengraber H: (R)-Mevalonate excretion in human and rat urines. *Proc Natl Acad Sci USA* **77**:5738, 1980.
210. Brunengraber H, Weinstock SB, Story DL, Kopito RR: Urinary clearance and metabolism of mevalonate by the isolated perfused rat kidney. *J Lipid Res* **22**:916, 1981.
211. Wiley MH, Huling S, Siperstein MD: Conversion of mevalonolactone to its open-chain salt by a serum enzyme. *Biochem Biophys Res Commun* **88**:605, 1979.
212. Parker TS, Mcnamara DJ, Brown CD, Kolb R, Ahrens EH, Jr., Alberts AW, Tobert J, et al.: Plasma mevalonate as a measure of cholesterol synthesis in man. *J Clin Invest* **74**:795, 1984.
213. Hoffmann GF, Charpentier C, Mayatepek E, Mancini J, Leichsenring M, Gibson KM, Divry P, et al.: Clinical and biochemical phenotype in 11 patients with mevalonic aciduria. *Pediatrics* **91**:915, 1993.
214. Hoffmann G, Gibson KM, Brandt IK, Bader PI, Wappner RS, Sweetman L: Mevalonic aciduria—An inborn error of cholesterol and nonsterol isoprene biosynthesis. *N Engl J Med* **314**:1610, 1986.
215. de Klerk JBC, Duran M, Dorland L, Brouwers HAA, Bruinvis L, Ketting D: A patient with mevalonic aciduria presenting with hepatosplenomegaly, congenital anaemia, thrombocytopenia and leukocytosis. *J Inherit Metab Dis* **11(Suppl 2)**:233, 1988.
216. Kozich V, Gibson KM, Zeman J, Nemecek J, Hoffmann GF, Pehal F, Hyanek J, et al.: Mevalonic aciduria. *J Inherit Metab Dis* **14**:265, 1991.
217. Mancini J, Philip N, Chabrol B, Divry P, Rolland MO, Pinsard N: Mevalonic aciduria in 3 siblings: A new recognizable metabolic encephalopathy. *Pediatr Neurol* **9**:243, 1993.
218. Hinson DD, Rogers ZR, Hoffmann GF, Schachtele M, Aberhart DJ, Fingerhut R, Kohlschutter A, et al.: Hematological abnormalities and cholestatic liver disease in two patients with mevalonate kinase deficiency. *Am J Med Genet* **78**:408, 1998.
219. Berger R, Smit GPA, Schierbeek H, Bijsterveld K, Le Coultre R: Mevalonic aciduria: An inborn error of cholesterol biosynthesis? *Clin Chim Acta* **152**:219, 1985.
220. Gibson KM, Hoffmann G, Nyhan WL, Sweetman L, Berger R, Le Coultre R, Smit GPA: Mevalonate kinase deficiency in a child with cerebellar ataxia, hypotonia and mevalonic aciduria. *Eur J Pediatr* **148**:250, 1988.
221. Divry P, Rolland MO, Zabot MT, Mancini J, Philip N, Pinsard N: Mevalonate kinase deficiency in 2 siblings. *SSIEM, Proceedings 29th Ann Symp,* London P146, 1991.
222. Cenedella RJ, Sexton PS: Probing cataractogenesis associated with mevalonic aciduria. *Curr Eye Res* **17**:153, 1998.
223. Gibson KM, Hoffmann GF, Sweetman L, Buckingham B: Mevalonate kinase deficiency in a dizygotic twin with mild mevalonic aciduria. *J Inherit Metab Dis* **20**:391, 1997.
224. Hoffmann GF, Sweetman L: An improved chemical ionization assay for mevalonic acid. *Biomed Environ Mass Spectrom* **19**:517, 1990.
225. Harwood HJ, Jr., Rodwell VW: HMG-CoA reductase kinase: Measurement of activity by methods that preclude interference by inhibitors of HMG-CoA reductase activity or by mevalonate kinase. *J Lipid Res* **23**:754, 1982.
226. Gibson KM, Hoffmann G, Nyhan WL, Sweetman L, Brandt IK, Wappner RS, Bader PI: Mevalonic aciduria: Family studies in mevalonate kinase deficiency, an inborn error of cholesterol biosynthesis. *J Inherit Metab Dis* **10(Suppl 2)**:282, 1987.
227. Gibson KM, Lohr JL, Broock RL, Hoffmann G, Nyhan WL, Sweetman L, Brandt IK, et al.: Mevalonate kinase in lysates of cultured human fibroblasts and lymphoblasts: Kinetic properties, assay conditions, carrier detection and measurement of residual activity in a patient with mevalonic aciduria. *Enzyme* **41**:47, 1989.
228. Hoffmann G, Gibson KM, Nyhan WL, Sweetman L: Mevalonic aciduria: Pathobiochemical effects of mevalonate kinase deficiency on cholesterol metabolism in intact fibroblasts. *J Inherit Metab Dis* **11(Suppl 2)**:229, 1988.
229. Gibson KM, Hoffmann G, Schwall A, Broock RL, Aramaki S, Sweetman L, Nyhan WL, et al.: 3-Hydroxy-3-methylglutaryl coenzyme A reductase activity in cultured fibroblasts from patients with mevalonate kinase deficiency: Differential response to lipid supplied by fetal bovine serum in tissue culture medium. *J Lipid Res* **31**:515, 1990.
230. Keller RK, Simonet WS: Near normal levels of isoprenoid lipids in severe mevalonic aciduria. *Biochem Biophys Res Commun* **152**:857, 1988.
231. Mayatepek E, Hoffmann GF, Bremer HJ: Enhanced urinary excretion of leukotriene E_4 in patients with mevalonate kinase deficiency. *J Pediatr* **123**:96, 1993.
232. Mayatepek E, Tiepelmann B, Hoffmann G: Enhanced excretion of urinary leukotriene E_4 in mevalonic aciduria is not caused by an impaired peroxisomal degradation of cysteinyl leukotrienes. *J Inherit Metab Dis* **20**:721, 1997.
233. Goebel-Schreiner B, Schreiner R, Hoffmann GF, Gibson KM: Segregation of the N301T mutation in the family of the index patient with mevalonate kinase deficiency. *J Inherit Metab Dis* **18**:197, 1995.
234. Hinson DD, Chambliss KL, Hoffmann GF, Krisans S, Keller RK, Gibson KM: Identification of an active site alanine in mevalonate kinase through characterization of a novel mutation in mevalonate kinase deficiency. *J Biol Chem* **272**:26756, 1997.
235. Houten SM, Waterham HR, Romeeijn GJ, Gibson KM, Poll-The BT, Duran M, de Klerk JBC, et al.: Mevalonate kinase deficiency: Enzymatic and molecular basis in two patients with classical mevalonic aciduria. *J Inherit Metab Dis* **21**:51, 1998.
236. Hoffmann GF, Sweetman L, Bremer HJ, Hunneman DH, Hyanek J, Kozich V, Lehnert W, et al.: Facts and artefacts in mevalonic aciduria: Development of a stable isotope dilution GCMS assay for mevalonic acid and its application to physiological fluids, tissue samples, prenatal diagnosis and carrier detection. *Clin Chim Acta* **198**:209, 1991.
237. Ikeda Y, Tanaka K: Purification and characterization of 2-methyl-branched chain acyl-coenzyme A dehydrogenase, an enzyme involved in the isoleucine and valine metabolism, from rat liver mitochondria. *J Biol Chem* **258**:9477, 1983.
238. Willard J, Vicanek C, Battaile KP, Van Veldhoven PP, Fauq AH, Rozen R, Vockley J: Cloning of a cDNA for short/branched chain acyl-coenzyme A dehydrogenase from rat and characterization of its tissue expression and substrate specificity. *Arch Biochem Biophys* **331**:127, 1996.
239. Rozen R, Vockley J, Zhou L, Milos R, Willard J, Fu K, Vicanek C, et al.: Isolation and expression of a cDNA encoding the precursor for a novel member (ACADSB) of the acyl-CoA dehydrogenase gene family. *Genomics* **24**:280, 1994.
240. Hass GM, Hill RL: The subunit structure of crotonase. *J Biol Chem* **244**:6080, 1969.
241. Brown GK, Hunt SM, Scholem R, Fowler K, Grimes A, Mercer JFB, Truscott RM, et al.: Beta-hydroxyisobutyryl coenzyme A deacylase deficiency: A defect in valine metabolism associated with physical malformations. *Pediatrics* **70**:532, 1982.
242. Middleton B: The existence of ketoacyl-CoA thiolases of differing properties and intracellular location in ox liver. *Biochem Biophys Res Commun* **46**:508, 1972.
243. Daum RS, Scriver CR, Mamer OA, Delvin E, Lamm P, Goldman H: An inherited disorder of isoleucine catabolism causing accumulation of alpha-methylacetoacetate and alpha-methyl-beta-hydroxybutyrate, and intermittent metabolic acidosis. *Pediatr Res* **7**:149, 1973.
244. Schutgens RBH, Middleton B, v.d. Blij JF, Oorthuys JWE, Veder HA, Vulsma T, Tegelaers WHH: Beta-ketothiolase deficiency in a family confirmed by in vitro enzymatic assays in fibroblasts. *Eur J Pediatr* **139**:39, 1982.
245. Bennett MJ, Littlewood JM, Macdonald A, Pollitt RJ, Thompson J: A case of beta-ketothiolase deficiency. *J Inherit Metab Dis* **6**:157, 1983.
246. Middleton B, Bartlett K, Romanos A, Gomez Vasquez J, Conde C, Cannon RA, Lipson M, et al.: 3-Ketothiolase deficiency. *Eur J Pediatr* **144**:586, 1986.
247. Merinero B, Pérez-Cerda C, García MJ, Carrasco S, Lama R, Ugarte M, Middleton B: Beta-ketothiolase deficiency: Two siblings with different clinical conditions. *J Inherit Metab Dis* **10(Suppl 2)**:276, 1987.
248. Halvorsen S, Stokke O, Jellum E: A variant form of 2-methyl-3-hydroxybutyric and 2-methylacetoacetic aciduria. *Acta Paediatr Scand* **68**:123, 1979.
249. Leonard JV, Middleton B, Seakins JWT: Acetoacetyl CoA thiolase deficiency presenting as ketotic hypoglycemia. *Pediatr Res* **21**:211, 1987.
250. Hillman RE, Keating JP: Beta-ketothiolase deficiency as a cause of the "ketotic hyperglycinemia syndrome." *Pediatrics* **53**:221, 1974.

251. Pollitt RJ: The occurrence of substituted 3-methyl-3-hydroxyglutaric acids in urine in propionic acidaemia and in beta-ketothiolase deficiency. *Biomed Mass Spectrom* **10**:253, 1983.
252. Aramaki S, Lehotay D, Sweetman L, Nyhan WL, Winter SC, Middleton B: Urinary excretion of 2-methylacetoacetate, 2-methyl-3-hydroxybutyrate and tiglylglycine after isoleucine loading in the diagnosis of 2-methylacetoacetyl-CoA thiolase deficiency. *J Inherit Metab Dis* **14**:63, 1991.
253. Weinberg RB, Walser M: Racemization and amination of the keto-analog of isoleucine in the intact dog. *Biochem Med* **17**:164, 1977.
254. Mathews DE, Ben-Galim E, Haymond MW, Bier DM: Alloisoleucine formation in maple syrup urine disease: Isotopic evidence for the mechanism. *Pediatr Res* **14**:854, 1980.
255. Schadewaldt P, Hammen HW, Dalle-Feste C, Wendel U: On the mechanism of L-alloisoleucine formation: Studies on a healthy subject and in fibroblasts from normals and patients with maple syrup urine disease. *J Inherit Metab Dis* **13**:137, 1990.
256. Mamer OA: The earliest steps in L-isoleucine catabolism: Rediscovering the wheel. *Proc Jap Soc Biomed Mass Spectrom* **9**:15, 1992.
257. Schadewaldt P, Hammen HW, Bodner A, Wendel U: On the mechanism of L-alloisoleucine formation in vivo: ^{13}C-Transfer into isoleucine metabolites after oral application of L-[^{13}C]isoleucine. *J Inherit Metab Dis* **20(Suppl 1)**:19, 1997.
258. Shimomura Y, Murakami T, Fujitsuka N, Nakai N, Sato Y, Sugiyama S, Shimomura N, et al.: Purification and partial characterization of 3-hydroxyisobutyryl-coenzyme A hydrolase in rat liver. *J Biol Chem* **269**:14248, 1994.
259. Goodwin GW, Rougraff PM, Davis EJ, Harris RA: Purification and characterization of methylmalonate-semialdehyde dehydrogenase from rat liver: Identity to malonate dehydrogenase. *J Biol Chem* **264**:14965, 1989.
260. Mamer OA, Tjoa SS: 2-Ethylhydracrylic acid: A newly described urinary organic acid. *Clin Chim Acta* **55**:199, 1974.
261. Mamer OA, Tjoa SS: 2-Ethyl-3-deuterohydracrylic acid, the major urinary metabolite of 2-trideuteromethylbutyric acid by a new metabolic pathway. *Biomed Mass Spectrom* **2**:133, 1975.
262. Mamer OA, Tjoa SS, Scriver CR, Klassen GA: Demonstration of a new mammalian isoleucine catabolic pathway yielding an R series of metabolites. *Biochem J* **160**:417, 1976.
263. Baretz BH, Lollo CP, Tanaka K: Metabolism in rats in vivo of RS-2-methylbutyrate and n-butyrate labeled with stable isotopes at various positions. *J Biol Chem* **254**:3468, 1979.
264. Robinson WG, Nagle R, Bachhawat BK, Kupiecki FP, Coon MJ: Coenzyme A thiol esters of isobutyric, methacrylic, and beta-hydroxyisobutyric acids as intermediates in the enzymatic degradation of valine. *J Biol Chem* **224**:1, 1957.
265. Rendina G, Coon MJ: Enzymatic hydrolysis of the coenzyme A thiol esters of beta-hydroxypropionic and beta-hydroxyisobutyric acids. *J Biol Chem* **225**:523, 1957.
266. Amster J, Tanaka K: Isolation and identification of S(+)-3-hydroxyisobutyric acid in the urine of rats loaded with isobutyric acid. *Biochem Biophys Acta* **585**:643, 1979.
267. Hawes JW, Jaskiewicz J, Shimomura Y, Huang B, Bunting J, Harper ET, Harris RA: Primary structure and tissue-specific expression of human β-hydroxyisobutyryl-coenzyme A hydrolase. *J Biol Chem* **271**:26430, 1996.
268. Robinson WG, Coon MJ: The purification and properties of beta-hydroxyisobutyric dehydrogenase. *J Biol Chem* **225**:511, 1957.
269. Rougraff PM, Paxton R, Kuntz MJ, Crabb DW, Harris RA: Purification and characterization of 3-hydroxyisobutyrate dehydrogenase from rabbit liver. *J Biol Chem* **263**:327, 1988.
270. Manning NJ, Pollitt RJ: Tracer studies of the interconversion of R- and S-methylmalonic semialdehydes in man. *Biochem J* **231**:481, 1985.
271. Rougraff PM, Zhang B, Kuntz MJ, Harris RA, Crabb DW: Cloning and sequence analysis of a cDNA for 3-hydroxyisobutyrate dehydrogenase: Evidence for its evolutionary relationship to other pyridine nucleotide-dependent dehydrogenases. *J Biol Chem* **264** :5899, 1989.
272. Bannerjee D, Sanders LE, Sokatch JR: Properties of purified methylmalonate semialdehyde dehydrogenase of *Pseudomonas aeruginosa*. *J Biol Chem* **245**:1828, 1970.
273. Tanaka K, Armitage IA, Ramsdell HS, Hsia YE, Lipsky SR, Rosenberg LE: [^{13}C]Valine metabolism in methylmalonic acidemia using nuclear magnetic resonance: Propionate as an obligate intermediate. *Proc Natl Acad Sci USA* **72**:3692, 1975.
274. Baretz BH, Tanaka K: Metabolism in rats in vivo of isobutyrates labeled with stable isotopes at various positions: Identification of propionate as an obligate intermediate. *J Biol Chem* **253**:4203, 1978.
275. Yoshino M, Sweetman L, Nyhan WL, Craig JC, Gruenke L: Metabolism of deuterated 3-hydroxyisobutyrate in rat liver. *Proc Jap Soc Biomed Mass Spectrom* **5**:97, 1981.
276. Kedishvili NY, Popov KM, Rougraff PM, Zhao Y, Crabb DW, Harris RA: CoA-dependent methylmalonate semialdehyde dehydrogenase, a unique member of the aldehyde dehydrogenase superfamily: cDNA cloning, evolutionary relationships, and tissue distribution. *J Biol Chem* **267**:19724, 1992.
277. Roe CR, Cederbaum SD, Roe DS, Mardach R, Galindo A, Sweetman L: Isolated isobutyryl-CoA dehydrogenase deficiency: An unrecognized defect in human valine metabolism. *Mol Genet Metab* **65**:264, 1998.
278. Truscott RJW, Malegan D, McCairns E, Halpern B, Hammond J, Cotton RGH, Mercer JFB, et al.: Two new sulphur-containing amino acids in man. *Biomed Mass Spectrom* **8**:99, 1981.
279. Singh RR, Lawrence WH, Autian J: Embryonic-fetal toxicity and teratogenic effects of a group of methacrylate esters in rats. *J Dent Res* **51**:1632, 1972.
280. Ohmori S, Shimomura T, Azumi T, Mizuhara S: S-(β-carboxy-n-propyl)-L-cysteine and S-(β-carboxyethyl)L-cysteine in urine. *Biochem Z* **343**:9, 1965.
281. Mienie LJ, Erasmus E: Biochemical studies on a patient with a possible 3-hydroxyisobutyrate dehydrogenase deficiency. *Fifth Int Cong Inborn Errors of Metabolism* OC2.7, 1990.
282. Ko FJ, Nyhan WL, Wolff J, Barshop B, Sweetman L: 3-Hydroxyisobutyric aciduria: An inborn error of valine metabolism. *Pediatr Res* **30**:322, 1991.
283. Brewster M, Goodman S, Rhead W, Brown G, Collie W, Bornhofen J: Valine-related 3-hydroxyisobutyric aciduria in twins. *Soc Inherit Metab Dis* P8, 1991.
284. Chitayat D, Meagher-Villemure M, Mamer OA, O'Gorman A, Hoar DI, Silver K, Scriver CR: Brain dysgenesis and congenital intracerebral calcification associated with 3-hydroxyisobutyric aciduria. *J Pediatr* **121**:86, 1992.
285. Sasaki M, Kimura M, Sugai K, Hashimoto T, Yamaguchi S: 3-Hydroxyisobutyric aciduria in two brothers. *Pediatr Neurol* **18**:253, 1998.
286. Allen JT, Brown AY, Hamilton-Shields J, Pennock CA, Ewart-Clarke DL: Two cases of 3-hydroxyisobutyric aciduria with multiple clinical abnormalities. *J Inherit Metab Dis* **21**:53, 1998.
287. Gibson KM, Lee CF, Bennett MJ, Holmes B, Nyhan WL: Combined malonic, methylmalonic, and ethylmalonic acid semialdehyde dehydrogenase deficiencies: An inborn error of β-alanine, L-valine, and L-alloisoleucine metabolism? *J Inherit Metab Dis* **16**:563, 1993.
288. Congdon PJ, Haigh D, Smith R, Green A, Pollitt RJ: Hypermethioninaemia and 3-hydroxyisobutyric aciduria in an apparently healthy baby. *J Inherit Metab Dis* **4**:79, 1981.
289. Pollitt RJ, Green A, Smith R: Excessive excretion of beta-alanine and of 3-hydroxypropionic, R- and S-3-aminobutyric, R- and S-3-hydroxyisobutyric and S-2-(hydroxymethyl)butyric acids probably due to a defect in the metabolism of the corresponding malonic semialdehydes. *J Inherit Metab Dis* **8**:75, 1985.
290. Boulat O, Benador N, Girardin E, Bachmann C: 3-Hydroxyisobutyric aciduria with a mild clinical course. *J Inherit Metab Dis* **18**:204, 1995.
291. van Gennip AH, Kamerling JP, de Bree PK, Wadman SK: Linear relationship between the R- and the S-enantiomers of beta-aminoisobutyric acid in human urine. *Clin Chim Acta* **116**:261, 1981.
292. Solem E, Jellum E, Eldjarn L: The absolute configuration of beta-aminoisobutyric acid in human serum and urine. *Clin Chim Acta* **50**:393, 1974.
293. Solem E: The absolute configuration of beta-aminoisobutyric acid formed by degradation of thymine in man. *Clin Chim Acta* **53**:183, 1974.
294. Gray RGF, Pollitt RJ, Webley J: Methylmalonic semialdehyde dehydrogenase deficiency: Demonstration of defective valine and beta-alanine metabolism and reduced malonic semialdehyde dehydrogenase activity in cultured fibroblasts. *Biochem Med Metab Biol* **38**:121, 1987.
295. Roe CR, Struys E, Kok RM, Roe DS, Harris RA, Jakobs C: Methylmalonic semialdehyde dehydrogenase deficiency: Psychomotor delay and methylmalonic aciduria without metabolic decompensation. *Mol Genet Metab* **65**:35, 1998.

296. Burlina AB, Zacchello F, Dionisi-Vici C, Bertini E, Sabetta G, Bennett MJ, Hale DE, et al.: New clinical phenotype of branched-chain acyl-CoA oxidation defect. *Lancet* **338**:1522, 1991.
297. Burlina AB, Bennett MJ, Dionisi-Vici C, Gabrielli O, Rinaldo P, Schmidt-Sommerfeld E, Hale DE, et al.: Studies on four patients with evidence for a new defect in branched-chain amino acid metabolism. *Pediatr Res* **31**:131A, 1992.
298. Burlina AB, Dionisi-Vici C, Bennett MJ, Gibson KM, Servidei S, Bertini E, Hale DE, et al.: A new syndrome with ethylmalonic aciduria and normal fatty acid oxidation in fibroblasts. *J Pediatr* **124**:79, 1994.
299. García-Silva MT, Ribes A, Campos Y, Garavaglia B, Arenas J: Syndrome of encephalopathy, petechiae, and ethylmalonic aciduria. *Pediatr Neurol* **17**:165, 1997.
300. Ozand PT, Rashed M, Millington DS, Sakati N, Hazza S, Rahbeeni Z, Al-Odaib A, et al.: Ethylmalonic aciduria: An organic acidemia with CNS involvement and vasculopathy. *Brain Dev* **16(Suppl)**:12, 1994.
301. Chen E, Jurecki ER, Rinaldo P, Keilman C, Packman S, Johnston K: Nephrotic syndrome and dysmorphic facial features in a new family of three affected siblings with ethylmalonic encephalopathy. *Am J Hum Genet* **55**:A2000, 1994.
302. Nowaczyk MJM, Blasser SI, Clarke JTR: Central nervous system malformations in ethylmalonic encephalopathy. *Am J Med Genet* **75**:292, 1998.
303. Nowaczyk MJM, Lehotay DC, Platt B-A, Fisher L, Tan R, Phillips H, Clarke JTR: Ethylmalonic and methylsuccinic aciduria in ethylmalonic encephalopathy arise from abnormal isoleucine metabolism. *Metabolism* **47**:836, 1998.
304. Garavaglia B, Colamaria V, Carrara F, Tonin P, Rimoldi M, Uziel G: Muscle cytochrome c oxidase deficiency in two Italian patients with ethylmalonic aciduria and peculiar clinical phenotype. *J Inherit Metab Dis* **17**:301, 1994.
305. Christensen E, Brandt NJ, Schmalbruch H, Kamieniecke Z, Herz B, Ruitenbeek W: Muscle cytochrome c oxidase deficiency accompanied by a urinary organic acid pattern mimicking multiple acyl-CoA dehydrogenase deficiency. *J Inherit Metab Dis* **16**:553, 1993.
306. Lehnert W, Ruitenbeek W: Ethylmalonic aciduria associated with progressive neurologic disease and cytochrome c oxidase deficiency. *J Inherit Metab Dis* **16**:557, 1993.
307. Brown G, Scholem RD, Bankier A, Danks DM: Malonyl CoA decarboxylase deficiency. *J Inherit Metab Dis* **7**:21, 1984.
308. Haan EA, Scholem RD, Croll HB, Brown GK: Malonyl coenzyme A decarboxylase deficiency. *Eur J Pediatr* **144**:567, 1986.
309. MacPhee GB, Logan RW, Mitchell JS, Howells DW, Tsotis E, Thorburn DR: Malonyl coenzyme A decarboxylase defiency. *Arch Dis Child* **69**:433, 1993.
310. Matalon R, Michaels K, Kaul R, Whitman V, Rodriguez-Novo J, Goodman S, Thorburn DR: Malonic aciduria and cardiomyopathy. *J Inherit Metab Dis* **16**:571, 1993.
311. Ozand PT, Nyhan WL, Al Aqeel A, Christodoulou J: Malonic aciduria. *Brain Dev* **16(Suppl)**:7, 1994.
312. Yano S, Sweetman L, Thorburn DR, Mofidi S, Williams JC: A new case of malonyl coenzyme A decarboxylase deficiency presenting with cardiomyopathy. *Eur J Pediatr* **156**:382, 1997.
313. Krawinkel MB, Oldigs HD, Santer R, Lehnert W, Wendel U, Schaub J: Association of malonyl-CoA decarboxylase deficiency and heterozygote state for haemoglobin C disease. *J Inherit Metab Dis* **17**:636, 1994.
314. Gregg AR, Warman AW, Thorburn DR, O'Brien WE: Combined malonic and methylmalonic aciduria with normal malonyl-coenzyme A decarboxylase activity: A case supporting multiple aetiologies. *J Inherit Metab Dis* **21**:382, 1998.
315. Buyukgebiz B, Jakobs C, Scholte HR, Huijmans JGM, Kleijer WJ: Fatal neonatal malonic aciduria. *J Inherit Metab Dis* **21**:76, 1998.
316. Henderson MJ, Evans CE, Kumar V, Pourfarzam M: Malonic aciduria presenting with developmental delay, malonylcarnitine increased in blood spots. *J Inherit Metab Dis* **21(Suppl 2)**:53, 1998.
317. Gibson KM, Cohen J, Waber L, Bennett MJ: Fatal infantile malonyl-CoA decarboxylase (MACAD) deficiency in a patient with malonic aciduria and hypertrophic cardiomyopathy. *Am J Hum Genet* **63**:A267, 1998.
318. Fitzpatrick DR, Thorburn DR, Tolmie J, Hill A, Christodoulou J: The molecular basis of malonyl-CoA decarboxylase deficiency. *J Inherit Metab Dis* **21**:52, 1998.
319. van der Meer JW, Vossen JM, Radl J, van Nieuwkoop JA, Meyer CJ, Lobatto S, van Furth R: Hyperimmunoglobulinaemia D and periodic fever: a new syndrome. *Lancet* 1087, 1984.
320. Drenth JP, Haagsma CJ, van der Meer JW: Hyperimmunoglobulinemia D and periodic fever syndrome. The clinical spectrum in a series of 50 patients. International Hyper-IgD Study Group. *Medicine* (Baltimore) **73**:133, 1994.
321. Houten SM, Kuis W, Duran M, de Koning TJ, van Royen-Kerkhof A, Romeijn GJ, Frenkel J, et al.: Mutations in MVK, encoding mevalonate kinase, cause hyperimmunoglobulinaemia D and periodic fever syndrome. *Nat Genet* **22**:175, 1999.
322. Drenth JP, Cuisset L, Grateau G, Vasseur C, van de Velde-Visser SD, de Jong JG, Beckmann JS et al.: Mutations in the gene encoding mevalonate kinase cause hyper-IgD and periodic fever syndrome. International hyper-IgD study group. *Nat Genet* **22**:178, 1999.

CHAPTER 94

Disorders of Propionate and Methylmalonate Metabolism

Wayne A. Fenton ▪ Roy A. Gravel ▪ David S. Rosenblatt

1. Propionyl coenzyme A (CoA)—formed in the catabolism of several essential amino acids (isoleucine, valine, methionine, threonine), odd-chain fatty acids, and cholesterol—is metabolized primarily by enzymatic conversion to methylmalonyl CoA, which is subsequently isomerized to succinyl CoA. This sequence depends on the activity of several enzymes (see Fig. 94-2): propionyl CoA carboxylase, methylmalonyl CoA racemase, and methylmalonyl CoA mutase. Propionyl CoA carboxylase requires biotin as a cofactor, whereas methylmalonyl CoA mutase requires adenosylcobalamin (AdoCbl), a cobalamin (Cbl; vitamin B_{12}) coenzyme.
2. Propionyl CoA carboxylase and methylmalonyl CoA mutase are oligomeric enzymes. Propionyl CoA carboxylase is composed of nonidentical subunits (α and β); biotin binds to the α subunit. The holocarboxylase contains six α and six β subunits ($\alpha_6\beta_6$). The α subunit is encoded by a gene on chromosome 13 (NM_000282) in humans, the β subunit by a gene on chromosome 3 (NM_000532). Methylmalonyl CoA mutase is a dimer of identical subunits (α_2), encoded by a gene on chromosome 6 (NM_000255).
3. Inherited deficiency of propionyl CoA carboxylase activity in humans results from genetically distinct defects at four loci. Isolated deficiency is caused by mutations at the α and β loci coding for the carboxylase subunits. Deficiency of multiple biotin-dependent carboxylases occurs in two forms: one resulting from deficiency of holocarboxylase synthase (the enzyme that attaches biotin to apocarboxylase subunits), the other from deficiency of biotinidase (the enzyme that cleaves biotin from the lysine residue in the carboxylase to which the biotin is attached). Multiple carboxylase deficiency is discussed in detail in Chapter 156.
4. Isolated deficiency of propionyl CoA carboxylase, a major cause of the ketotic hyperglycinemia syndrome, results in the accumulation of propionate in blood and of 3-hydroxypropionate, methylcitrate, tiglylglycine, and unusual ketone bodies in urine. Two complementation groups, *pccA* (OMIM 232000) and *pccBC* (OMIM 232050) have been defined among propionyl CoA carboxylase–deficient patients. These groups correspond to mutations affecting genes coding for the α subunit and the β subunit, respectively, of the carboxylase apoprotein. Clinically, the disorder is characterized by severe metabolic ketoacidosis, which often appears in the neonatal period and requires vigorous alkali therapy and protein restriction. Oral antibiotic therapy to reduce gut propionate production also may prove useful.
5. Multiple carboxylase deficiency (OMIM 253270) leads to impaired activity of four biotin-dependent enzymes: acetyl CoA carboxylase, propionyl CoA carboxylase, 3-methylcrotonyl CoA carboxylase, and pyruvate carboxylase. The clinical hallmarks of this disorder include ketoacidosis, a diffuse erythematous rash, alopecia, seizures, hypotonia, and developmental retardation (see Chapter 156).
6. Inherited deficiency of methylmalonyl CoA mutase activity in humans is caused by mutations at many different loci. Isolated deficiency results from mutations at the apomutase locus (OMIM 251000) and at two loci coding for gene products required, specifically for the biosynthesis of AdoCbl. Combined deficiency of mutase and of the other major Cbl-dependent enzyme in mammalian cells, methionine synthase (formally, N^5-methyltetrahydrofolate:homocysteine methyltransferase), results from inherited defects in Cbl transport and from three distinct defects in the intracellular pathway of Cbl coenzyme synthesis affecting the synthesis of both AdoCbl and methylcobalamin (MeCbl), the coenzyme required by methionine synthase. These several defects in intracellular Cbl metabolism are discussed in detail in Chapter 155.
7. Neonatal or infantile metabolic ketoacidosis is the clinical hallmark of isolated methylmalonyl CoA mutase deficiency. Cells from some apomutase-deficient children have no functional mutase (designated mut^0); cells from others contain a structurally altered mutase with reduced affinity for AdoCbl and with reduced stability (mut^-). Such children exhibit methylmalonic acidemia and methylmalonic aciduria that do not respond to Cbl supplementation but can sometimes be treated with dietary protein restriction. Carnitine, as well as oral antibiotic therapy to reduce gut flora, may be effective as well.
8. Two abnormalities in AdoCbl synthesis only, designated *cblA* (OMIM 251100) and *cblB* (OMIM 251110), lead to impaired methylmalonyl CoA mutase activity and are characterized by a clinical and chemical picture virtually identical to that seen in apomutase-deficient children. In most *cblA* patients and some *cblB* patients, pharmacologic supplements of CN-Cbl or hydroxocobalamin (OH-Cbl) produce distinct reductions in methylmalonate accumulation and offer a valuable therapeutic adjunct to dietary protein limitation.

A list of standard abbreviations is located immediately preceding the index in each volume. Nonstandard abbreviations used in this chapter include: AdoCbl = adenosylcobalamin; *cbl* = cobalamin metabolism locus (*cblA*, *cblB*, etc.); Cbl = cobalamin; CN-Cbl = cyanocobalamin; CoA = coenzyme A; CPS I = carbamylphosphate synthetase I; DMB = dimethyl benzimidazoyl; H_4folate = tetrahydrofolate; IF = intrinsic factor; MeCbl = methylcobalamin; Me-H_4folate = N^5-methyltetrahydrofolate; *mut* = methylmalonyl CoA mutase locus; OH-Cbl = hydroxocobalamin; OLCFA = odd-numbered long-chain fatty acids; *pcc* = propionyl CoA carboxylase locus; TC (I, II, or III) = transcobalamin (I, II, or III).

9. **Three other distinct defects—*cblC* (OMIM 277400), *cblD* (OMIM 277410), and *cblF* (OMIM 277380)—lead to impaired synthesis of both AdoCbl and MeCbl and, accordingly, to deficient activity of both methylmalonyl CoA mutase and methionine synthase. Such children have methylmalonic aciduria and homocystinuria. Most children with a *cblC* mutation appear to be more severely affected clinically than the two known sibs in the *cblD* group, although a number of *cblC* patients have had an onset of disease in adult life. Major clinical problems in *cblC* patients include failure to thrive, developmental retardation, and such hematologic abnormalities as megaloblastic anemia and macrocytosis. The precise defect in the *cblC* and *cblD* patients is not yet known, but it involves an early step in the intracellular metabolism of cobalamins. The defect in *cblF* cells involves impaired efflux of free Cbl from lysosomes. Therapy includes protein restriction, pharmacologic doses of OH-Cbl, and betaine supplementation.**
10. **The discriminating biochemical features of the known forms of inherited methylmalonic acidemia are shown in Table 94-4.**
11. **All of the disorders of propionate and methylmalonate metabolism for which there are adequate data are inherited as autosomal-recessive traits. Heterozygotes for the following defects can be detected biochemically: *pccA*, *mut⁰*, *mut⁻*, and *cblB*. Genetic complementation analyses with somatic cell heterokaryons have been particularly useful in demonstrating genetic heterogeneity and in confirming the existence of autosomal-recessive inheritance among the propionic acidemias and the methylmalonic acidemias. Precise molecular defects have been described for *pccA*, *pccBC*, *mut⁰*, and *mut⁻* patients.**
12. **Prenatal detection of fetuses with propionyl CoA carboxylase deficiency, methylmalonyl CoA apomutase deficiency, and defective synthesis of AdoCbl or of both coenzymes is best done using assays in cultured amniotic cells and gas chromatographic/mass spectroscopic determinations on amniotic fluid or maternal urine.**

Methylmalonic acid and its immediate precursor, propionic acid, are detectable in only trace amounts in normal human blood, urine, and cerebrospinal fluid. The minuscule quantities of these compounds in extracellular fluids have obscured the key role that these acids play in human metabolism. Biochemists investigating animal nutrition have been interested in propionate metabolism for many years because ruminants derive most of their energy requirements from the oxidation of propionate and acetate produced by bacterial fermentation in their rumens.[1] Although propionate and methylmalonate are of little quantitative importance in humans as direct sources of energy, these acids, found intracellularly largely as their coenzyme A (CoA) esters, are vital intermediates in the catabolism of fat and protein.

Several independent, and seemingly unrelated, lines of evidence drew the attention of the physician and the clinical investigator to the study of propionate and methylmalonate metabolism. In 1959 and 1960, several groups reported that adenosylcobalamin (AdoCbl), one of the coenzyme forms of cobalamin (Cbl) (vitamin B_{12}), is an essential cofactor in the enzymatic conversion of L-methylmalonyl CoA to succinyl CoA.[2–4] Shortly thereafter, patients with acquired Cbl deficiency were shown to excrete large amounts of methylmalonic acid in their urine.[5,6] The methylmalonic aciduria was rapidly reversed by administration of physiologic doses of Cbl and was attributed to an acquired block in methylmalonate catabolism caused by inadequate amounts of the needed Cbl coenzyme.

In 1961, Childs and associates[7] described a young boy with recurrent attacks of severe ketoacidosis who had elevated concentrations of glycine and several other amino acids in his blood and urine. A series of detailed metabolic studies demonstrated that the attacks were precipitated by protein feeding and more specifically by ingestion of the branched chain amino acids, methionine and threonine. Because elevation in plasma glycine level was the most striking biochemical abnormality, the disorder was called ketotic hyperglycinemia. Later evidence has established that this disorder is caused by an inherited defect in the catabolism of propionate, not by a primary abnormality in glycine utilization or biosynthesis.[8,9]

Since 1967, a number of critically ill children have been described who draw these seemingly disparate observations together and focus attention on the enzymes and coenzymes that participate in the pathway responsible for the formation of propionate and its conversion to succinate. Oberholzer,[10] Stokke,[11] and their colleagues described infants with profound metabolic acidosis and hyperglycinemia (or hyperglycinuria) who excreted huge amounts of methylmalonic acid in their urine, but who were not Cbl deficient. Subsequently, Rosenberg and his colleagues[8] reported that urine from the index patient with ketotic hyperglycinemia and from his affected sister contained no methylmalonic acid. This observation indicated that primary methylmalonic acidemia and ketotic hyperglycinemia were different disorders with identical clinical manifestations.[3]

The latter group and Lindblad et al.[12,13] also described children with ketoacidosis and methylmalonic acidemia who were not Cbl deficient, but who responded to administration of pharmacologic doses of cyanocobalamin (CN-Cbl) or its coenzyme with a marked decrease in concentration of urinary methylmalonic acid. The index patient[8] was subsequently shown to suffer from a primary defect in AdoCbl synthesis,[14,15] not from a defect of the apoenzyme that catalyzes the conversion of methylmalonyl CoA to succinyl CoA.

These observations and others, which will be discussed in detail subsequently, emphasize that numerous inherited abnormalities in the metabolic pathway for propionate and methylmalonate occur and that these defects lead to profound illness and, in many cases, death due to a disturbed acid-base balance or developmental failure. The study of these disorders has led to important insights in our understanding of the role of this pathway in humans and has illustrated, once again, that a group of clinically identical disorders can be produced by several different mutations affecting the synthesis of related apoenzymes and coenzymes. Several reviews of this subject matter have been published.[16–21]

BIOCHEMICAL PATHWAYS

Propionate Metabolism

Formation of Propionate and Methylmalonate. Most of the propionic acid used by ruminant animals is formed by bacterial fermentation in the rumen.[1] By contrast, nonruminant mammals derive most of their propionate from the catabolism of lipid and protein. As noted in Fig. 94-1, catabolism of the branched chain amino acid isoleucine leads to the formation of propionyl CoA, as does the degradation of methionine and threonine.[22] Studies with [^{13}C]valine in a patient with methylmalonic acidemia[23] and with the valine catabolite [^{13}C]isobutyrate in rats[24] indicate that valine is also a propionate precursor and is not catabolized directly to methylmalonyl CoA, as had been suggested. Catabolism of these amino acids accounts for much of the propionate formed in humans; data presented by Thompson et al.[25] indicate that their contribution is on the order of 50 percent in patients with inborn errors of propionate or methylmalonate metabolism. Other sources of propionate include β-oxidation of fatty acids with an odd number of carbon atoms, which ultimately leads to the formation of 1 mole of propionyl CoA per mole of fatty acid.[25–27] Degradation of the side chain of cholesterol also leads to the synthesis of propionyl CoA, but this pathway appears to be of little quantitative significance.[28] Finally, there have been suggestions

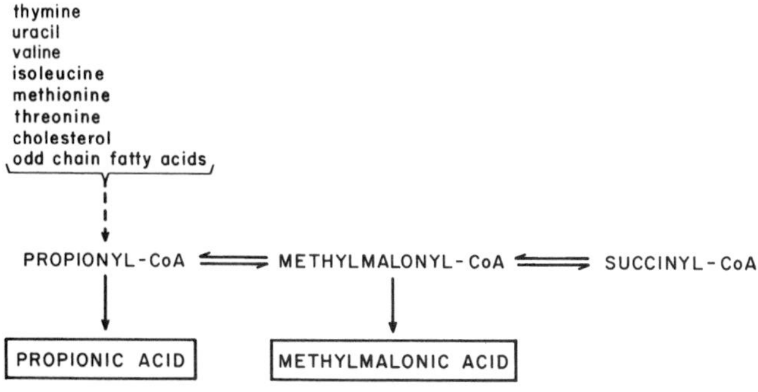

Fig. 94-1 Precursors of and the major catabolic pathway for propionate and methylmalonate. The free acids are derived from their CoA esters by hydrolysis. A number of clinical disorders arise from errors at various steps in these pathways. Broken arrows indicate the presence of several reactions.

that gut bacteria may contribute a substantial amount of propionate, at least under some circumstances. These findings are based on the ability of oral antibiotics to decrease urine[29] and plasma[25] propionate concentrations in some propionic and methylmalonic acidemia patients. From stable isotope studies in patients with methylmalonic aciduria and propionic aciduria, Leonard estimated that about 50 percent of propionate production is due to amino acid catabolism, 25 percent is due to the odd chain fatty acid catabolism, and 25 percent is due to bacterial activity in the gut.[30]

Methylmalonyl CoA is synthesized essentially only from propionyl CoA (Fig. 94-1). Propionate has long been known to be glycogenic in animals,[31] but the pathway by which propionate is converted to carbohydrate became clear only when Lardy and Adler demonstrated that liver mitochondria contain enzymes that synthesize succinate from propionate.[31] The discovery in 1955 that methylmalonate is an intermediate in the formation of succinate from propionate (Fig. 94-1) provided an important further step in the characterization of this pathway.[32,33]

Kaziro and Ochoa first defined the individual steps of propionate catabolism in animal tissues and characterized the enzymes involved.[26] Propionyl CoA, formed either by the degradative reactions discussed above or by the enzymatic esterification of propionate itself,[34] may be considered the precursor of this reaction sequence (Fig. 94-2). Three enzymatic reactions are responsible for the conversion of propionyl CoA to succinyl CoA. The first involves the carboxylation of propionyl CoA to methylmalonyl CoA,[34,35] a reaction catalyzed by propionyl CoA carboxylase (EC 6.4.1.3). Although two stereoisomers of methylmalonyl CoA exist, only the D form is produced in the carboxylation reaction.[36,37] This isomer is not a substrate for the subsequent mutase reaction and must be racemized to the L configuration by another enzyme, methylmalonyl CoA racemase (EC 5.1.99.1).[38] The third reaction, catalyzed by methylmalonyl CoA mutase (EC 5.4.99.2), isomerizes L-methylmalonyl CoA to succinyl CoA.[39] The latter compound enters the tricarboxylic acid cycle and is ultimately glycogenic because of its conversion to pyruvate by way of oxaloacetate. The sum of these reactions may be written as follows:

$$\text{Propionate} + \text{ATP} \rightarrow \text{pyruvate} + 4\text{H}^+ + \text{ADP} + \text{P}_i$$

In bacteria, propionate is formed from pyruvate by reversal of the reaction sequence just described,[26] but in mammalian systems the equilibrium of the system is far in the direction of propionate catabolism, rather than biosynthesis.

Apoenzymes

Propionyl CoA Carboxylase. This enzyme, first crystallized from pig heart,[40] has been purified to homogeneity from bovine kidney[41] and human liver.[42,43] The enzyme is composed of nonidentical subunits (α and β): the required cofactor, biotin, is bound exclusively to the larger (α) subunit. The molecular masses of the human enzyme are 750 to 800 kDa for the native form, 72 kDa for the α subunit, and 56 kDa for the β subunit. In the enzyme from *Mycobacterium smegmatis*, each mole contains 6 moles of biotin.[44] This suggests that the native enzyme is a hexamer of protomers, each protomer containing a single α and a single β subunit. The size of the human enzyme implies a similar structure, namely an $(\alpha\beta)_6$ quaternary structure.

The carboxylation of propionyl CoA occurs in a two-step reaction.[26] In the first step, which requires adenosine triphosphate (ATP) and Mg^{2+} and is stimulated by K^+, bicarbonate is attached to the ureido (N^1) nitrogen of biotin in the apoenzyme–biotin complex (Fig. 94-3), forming a carboxybiotin–apoenzyme intermediate. This complex, in turn, reacts with propionyl CoA to transfer the carboxyl group from biotin to the second carbon of propionyl CoA, forming D-methylmalonyl CoA. As with other biotin-catalyzed carbon dioxide fixation reactions, the biotin molecule is directly responsible for the transfer of the carboxyl group.[45]

The complementary DNAs (cDNAs) for the α and β subunits have been cloned from human[46–48] and rat liver[49–51] libraries. A 2.9-kb messenger RNA (mRNA) codes for the α chain and a major 2.0-kb mRNA codes for the β chain.[46,50] Based on the sequence of the full-length cDNAs, the human α chain contains 703 amino acids[52] and the β chain 539 amino acids.[53,54] As is the case for most nuclear-encoded mitochondrial proteins, the α and β subunits are synthesized on free cytoplasmic polyribosomes as larger precursors, bearing cleavable N-terminal leader peptides.[55] The N-terminus of the mature human α subunit has been determined and implicates a leader peptide of 26 amino acids.[48] In studies on the rat enzyme, the positively charged leader peptides of both subunits were shown to direct mitochondrial uptake and processing *in vitro*.[51,56] Assembly of the mature α and β subunits into the oligomeric holoenzyme is expected to occur after mitochondrial import and removal of the leader peptides have occurred.

The polypeptide sequences of the α and β subunits have revealed a number of highly conserved regions by comparison with related enzymes from bacteria to mammals. Most striking is the near universal tetrapeptide, Ala-Met-Lys-Met, that defines the biotin-binding site (Lys residue) of the α subunit.[47,51] In addition, the α subunit contains a recognizable biotin carboxylase domain

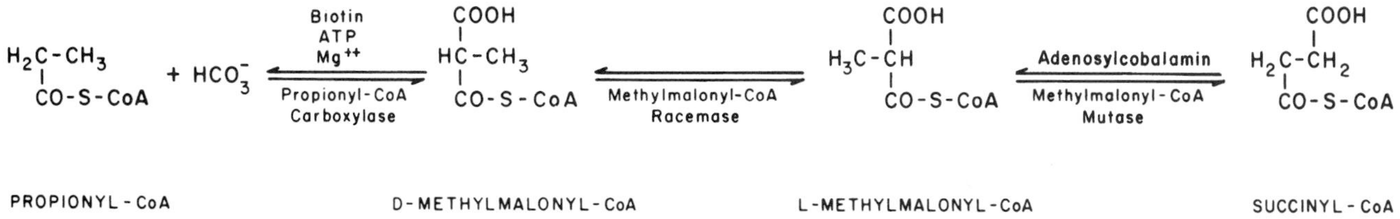

$H_2C{-}CH_3$ / $CO{-}S{-}CoA$ + HCO_3^- ⇌ (Biotin, ATP, Mg^{++}; Propionyl-CoA Carboxylase) COOH / $HC{-}CH_3$ / $CO{-}S{-}CoA$ ⇌ (Methylmalonyl-CoA Racemase) COOH / $H_3C{-}CH$ / $CO{-}S{-}CoA$ ⇌ (Adenosylcobalamin; Methylmalonyl-CoA Mutase) COOH / $H_2C{-}CH_2$ / $CO{-}S{-}CoA$

PROPIONYL-CoA — D-METHYLMALONYL-CoA — L-METHYLMALONYL-CoA — SUCCINYL-CoA

Fig. 94-2 Enzymatic details of the major catabolic pathway for propionyl CoA and methylmalonyl CoA. Succinyl CoA has several metabolic fates, including oxidation through the tricarboxylic acid cycle and condensation with glycine to form δ-aminolevulinic acid. Two coenzymes act in the reaction sequence: biotin, in the carboxylation of propionyl CoA, and adenosylcobalamin (AdoCbl), in the isomerization of methylmalonyl CoA to succinyl CoA.

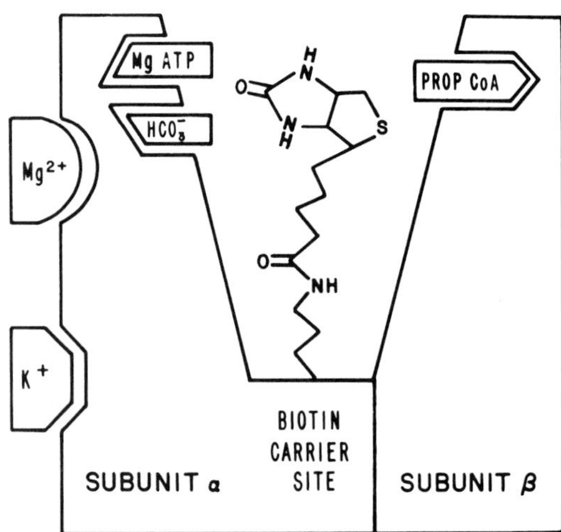

Fig. 94-3 A model for the mammalian propionyl CoA carboxylase protomer containing two nonidentical subunits (α and β), a biotin carrier site on the α subunit, and multiple substrate and effector sites.

and, within it, an ATP binding site[57]; the β subunit contains sequences related to carboxybiotin and propionyl CoA binding domains (Fig. 94-3) . Expression of the C-terminal 67 amino acids of the human α subunit in *Escherichia coli* results in its biotinylation by the bacterial biotin ligase, BirA, or by coexpressed human holocarboxylase synthase.[58]

The human *PCCA* gene, encoding the α subunit, has been mapped to chromosome 13q32.[46,59] The *PCCA* gene is at least 100 kbp long, but its intron–exon organization remains to be elucidated. The *PCCB* gene, encoding the β subunit, is on chromosome 3q13.3-q22[46,49] and has been positioned within a YAC contig containing the blepharophimosis-ptosis-epicanthus inversus syndrome locus.[60] The *PCCB* gene contains 15 exons, ranging in size from 57 to 183 bp.[61]

Methylmalonyl CoA Racemase. This enzyme owes its discovery to the observation that methylmalonyl CoA synthesized chemically is a substrate for the mutase reaction (Fig. 94-2), whereas methylmalonyl CoA formed enzymatically from the carboxylation of propionyl CoA will not react with the mutase unless it is first heated. Ultimately, the demonstration that heating converts D-methylmalonyl CoA to DL-methylmalonyl CoA led to the conclusion that only the L form of the ester will react with the mutase enzyme. This interpretation was confirmed by separating mutase activity from racemase activity using Sephadex chromatography.[26,38,62] The racemase has been purified extensively from sheep liver.[38] It has no known cofactor requirements and catalyzes the conversion of D- to L-methylmalonyl CoA by inducing a shift in the α-hydrogen atom.[38,62]

Methylmalonyl CoA Mutase. In 1955, Flavin et al.[32] and Katz and Chaikoff[33] observed independently that the isomerization of methylmalonyl CoA to succinyl CoA was catalyzed by an enzyme found in sheep kidney and rat liver. The chemical analogy between this isomerization reaction and the isomerization of glutamate to β-methylaspartate in bacteria,[63] along with the demonstration by Barker and his colleagues[64,65] that a coenzyme form of Cbl was needed for the latter reaction, led to the finding in several laboratories that a Cbl coenzyme is also required for the isomerization of methylmalonyl CoA.[2–4] The enzyme, originally called *methylmalonyl CoA isomerase* but now designated *methylmalonyl CoA mutase*, was first crystallized from sheep kidney and bacteria. More recently, it has been purified to homogeneity from human placenta[66] and human liver.[67] From both human sources, the enzyme appears to be a dimer (145 to 150 kDa) of identical subunits (72 to 77 kDa). The holoenzyme contains 1 mole AdoCbl per mole of subunit,[67] the Cbl cofactor being very tightly bound to the apoenzyme (K_m of the purified, expressed human enzyme for AdoCbl is 5×10^{-8} M).[68] Under certain conditions, the human enzyme displays complex kinetics with regard to the binding of methylmalonyl CoA and AdoCbl, leading to the thesis that the active sites of the dimeric enzyme are not equivalent.[69] In this regard, it is significant that hydroxocobalamin (OH-Cbl) appears to act as both a competitive and an irreversible inhibitor of human mutase.[69]

As indicated in Figure 94-2, the isomerization reaction could occur by exchange of a hydrogen for either the free carboxyl group or the CoA-carboxyl moiety of methylmalonyl CoA. Studies using isotopically labeled substrate demonstrated convincingly that it is the CoA-carboxyl group that is transferred[70] through an intramolecular isomerization.[71,72] The role of the Cbl coenzyme in this reaction has been established by electron paramagnetic resonance and ultraviolet (UV)-visible spectroscopy. As suggested by Halpern,[73] AdoCbl serves as the source of a pair of free radicals, generated initially by homolysis of the cobalt–carbon bond. Although no evidence for such radicals has been obtained with holoenzyme alone, in the presence of substrate, a tightly exchange-coupled free radical pair can be observed.[74,75] One electron is clearly on cob(II)alamin, as further identified by its UV-visible spectrum.[76] The nature of the other radical species is less clear, but isotope effect data suggest that it is substrate derived, rather than a radical form of the 5′-deoxyadenosyl group.[76] For mutase from *Propionibacterium shermanii*, about 20 to 25 percent of the cofactor is present in a radical form under steady-state conditions, and stopped-flow kinetic observations suggest that homolysis is much faster than the overall reaction.[76] This implies that a later, slow step (such as product release) must be rate controlling, a conclusion supported by tritium isotope effect studies[77] and rationalized by structural investigations of the enzyme.

The mutase subunit is synthesized as a larger cytoplasmic precursor, bearing a 3- to 4-kDa cleavable leader peptide.[78] In a cell-free system, the precursor is imported by mitochondria via an energy-dependent mechanism and cleaved to its mature form by a divalent cation-dependent protease (the mitochondrial processing peptidase). In intact cells, the precursor is rapidly (half-life = 6–9 min) converted to its mature form.[78]

Both cDNA and genomic DNA encoding human mutase have been cloned, as have the corresponding murine sequences.[79–82] The cDNA sequence predicts a leader peptide 32 amino acids long that is strongly positively charged (4 Arg, 2 Lys, 1 Glu).[80,82] Analysis of Southern blots of DNA from human/hamster somatic cell hybrids and *in situ* hybridization, using the mutase cDNAs as probes, mapped the human gene for mutase and the MUT locus to region 6p12-p21.2[83] and uncovered one highly informative restriction fragment length polymorphism.[79]

Mutase from *P. shermanii* has been purified, cloned, and overexpressed in *E. coli*. It is an αβ heterodimer with a single active subunit (α) that binds one molecule of AdoCbl.[84,85] The α subunit is about 60 percent identical (75 percent similar) to the human enzyme, with many of the nonconservative substitutions occurring in the N-terminal region.[86] Several forms of *P. shermanii* mutase have been crystallized and their radiographic structures solved (PDB codes 1REQ–5REQ).[87–89] Based on these, mutase consists of two major domains, with an N-terminal region involved in subunit–subunit interaction and an interdomain linker (see Fig. 94-10). The first domain is a $(\beta\alpha)_8$ TIM barrel, with the substrate binding site threaded through its center. The second domain is the so-called Cbl-binding domain, by virtue of its close sequence and structural homology with the Cbl-binding domain of methionine synthase.[90] It is a $(\beta\alpha)_5$ barrel that has a groove for binding the 5,6-dimethylbenzimidazolyl (DMB) side chain of Cbl, the stabilized histidine side chain that displaces the DMB from the lower axial position of the Cbl, and interaction sites for the lower face of the corrin ring. The interface between these domains

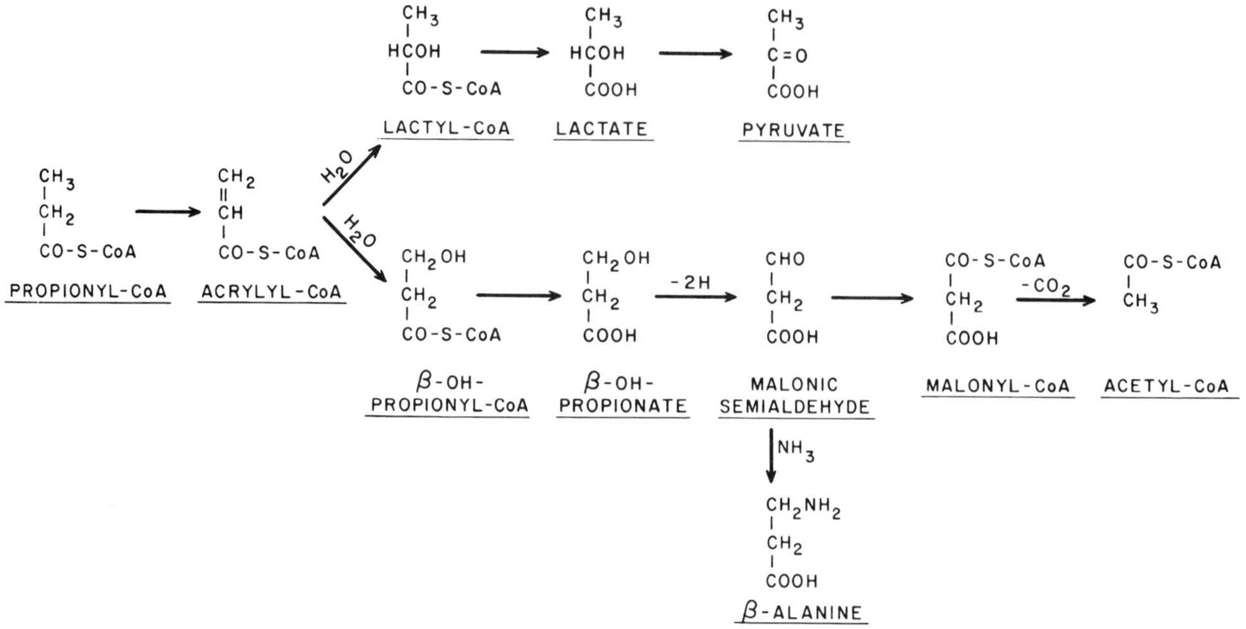

Fig. 94-4 Minor pathways of propionate catabolism. Note that both pathways can ultimately generate acetyl CoA. The significance of these minor pathways is discussed in the text.

accommodates the upper face of the corrin and the 5′-deoxyadenosyl group.

Comparison of substrate-free and substrate-bound structures indicates both how substrate and product come and go from the active site and how the enzyme protects the radicals at its active site.[88] In the substrate-free (open) conformation, four of the $\beta\alpha$ pairs in the first domain have moved as a rigid body, relative to the other four and the second domain, to split open the TIM barrel and provide access to the active site and the binding sites for the pantotheine chain of the substrate. In the bound (closed) configuration, however, the domain has come back together to close the active site around the methylmalonyl group, the rest of the substrate blocks access through the middle of the barrel, the active site cavity is reduced in volume, and the binding site for the 5′-deoxyadenosyl group is destroyed. Thus, the substrate-triggered conformational change appears to simultaneously drive homolysis of the cobalt–carbon bond while sequestering the radicals formed at the active site, permitting a free-radical rearrangement protected from the surrounding aqueous environment. Because a corresponding opening of the TIM barrel must occur before product can be released, it has been suggested that this is likely the slow step in the overall forward reaction.[88]

Alternative Pathways of Propionate Metabolism

Although the catabolism of propionate to succinate through methylmalonate is the major pathway for propionate utilization in mammalian systems, alternative pathways exist. Propionyl CoA can replace acetyl CoA as a "primer" for long-chain fatty acid synthesis[91] and lead to the formation of odd-chain fatty acids, notably heptanoate, nonanoate, and undecanoate. There are also alternative catabolic mechanisms, one of which is described in Fig. 94-4.[26] The first step in this sequence involves the formation of an α,β-unsaturated fatty acid, acrylyl CoA, which is subsequently hydrated, leading to the formation of either lactyl CoA or β-OH-propionyl CoA. The former compound is hydrolyzed to lactate, thus providing a second means by which propionate may be converted to pyruvate. Catabolism of β-OH-propionyl CoA leads ultimately to the synthesis of acetyl CoA or β-alanine, compounds discussed in Chapter 91. In addition, propionyl CoA may condense with oxaloacetate to form methylcitrate in a reaction analogous to the biosynthesis of citric acid from acetyl CoA and oxaloacetate.[92] These alternative pathways are of little quantitative importance in normal subjects but become much more prominent in patients with blocks in the major pathway of propionate metabolism.[93–95]

Coenzymes

Biotin. Biotin is widely distributed in plants and animal tissues and is readily synthesized by a variety of microorganisms. It was first isolated from egg yolk in 1936 by the Dutch biochemist Kogl,[96] and its structure was defined soon thereafter by du Vigneaud and colleagues.[97] Our understanding of this water-soluble cofactor is inextricably linked with the evolution of our knowledge concerning avidin, an egg white protein that binds biotin very tightly. Comprehensive reviews on biotin[98,99] and on biotin-dependent enzymes[100,101] exist. The reader is referred to Chapter 156 for further discussion of biotin.

Structure and Function. Biotin is the essential cofactor of the four bicarbonate-utilizing carboxylases in mammals. Structurally, it is composed of fused imidazole and thiophene rings to which is attached an *n*-valeric acid side chain; it has a molecular mass of 244 daltons. It is covalently attached to carboxylases through a linkage between the carboxyl group and the ε-amino group of a lysine residue in a well-defined biotin-binding domain, which is highly conserved among carboxylases from bacteria to mammals (Fig. 94-3).[102] Its role is to act as the carboxyl carrier in the carboxylation of substrate molecules (Fig. 94-5).

The four biotin-dependent carboxylases are enzymes of intermediary metabolism.[103] One of these, acetyl CoA carboxylase, occurs in two forms[104,105] and is a cytosolic enzyme. It catalyzes the key step in long-chain fatty acid biosynthesis, the formation of malonyl CoA from acetyl CoA. The three other biotin-dependent carboxylases are found in the mitochondrial matrix, where they catalyze critical steps in amino acid and organic acid metabolism. Pyruvate carboxylase is a key enzyme of gluconeogenesis; β-methylcrotonyl CoA carboxylase and propionyl CoA carboxylase are involved in the catabolism of amino acids, and the latter also performs the final step in the oxidation of fatty acids of odd-numbered chain lengths and cholesterol.

All four carboxylases are biotinylated by the same enzymatic reaction (reviewed in Chapter 156). This is confirmed genetically by the inherited metabolic disorder biotin-responsive multiple carboxylase deficiency, in which the activity of all four biotin-dependent carboxylases is impaired.[106] The responsible enzyme,

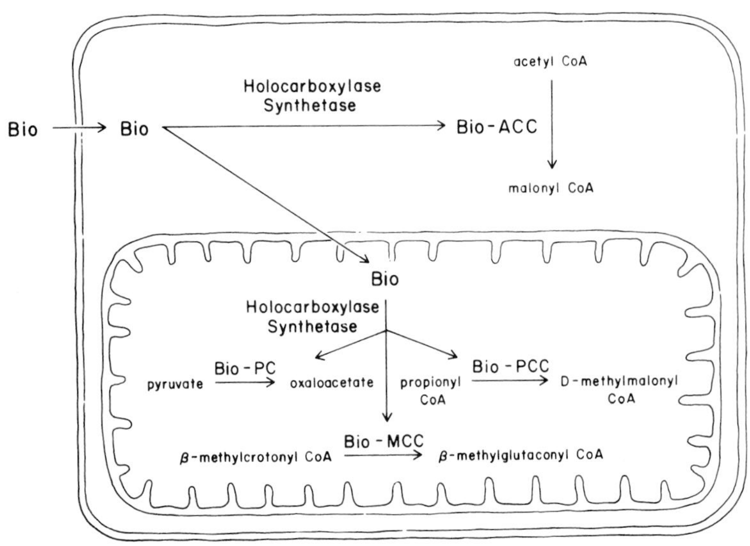

Fig. 94-5 Schematic representation of biotin uptake and metabolism by tissue cells. Neither the mechanism by which biotin is transported across the plasma membrane nor that by which it enters the mitochondrion is well understood. Abbreviations: bio = biotin; ACC = acetyl CoA carboxylase; PC = pyruvate carboxylase; MCC = β-methylcrotonyl CoA carboxylase; PCC = propionyl CoA carboxylase.

holocarboxylase synthase, has been purified from bovine liver and is found in both the mitochondria and cytosol.[107,108] Although mitochondrial apocarboxylases are expected to be biotinylated subsequent to their import, it has been shown experimentally that biotinylation of the α subunit of propionyl CoA carboxylase can be accomplished in either compartment.[109] Holocarboxylase synthase shows a striking ability to cross species barriers and is fully interchangeable with the orthologous *E. coli* biotin ligase BirA, with which it shares sequence similarity across its biotin binding region.[110,111] Either enzyme will biotinylate the *E. coli* biotin carboxyl carrier protein, a component of the bacterial acetyl CoA carboxylase, or the 67–amino acid, biotin-carrier component of the human propionyl CoA carboxylase α subunit.[58,111,112]

Biotin remains bound to the carboxylases until they are degraded. On proteolysis of the enzymes, biotin is released from small biotinylated peptides or from biocytin (biotinyl lysine) by the enzyme biotinidase. The latter enzyme, widely distributed in tissues and most abundant in serum, has been purified to homogeneity.[113,114] In addition to its biocytin hydrolase activity, the enzyme has been shown to have a biotinyl-transferase activity in which biotin is transferred from biocytin to lysine-containing acceptors, including poly-lysine and histones, the latter suggesting a novel physiologic role for biotin.[115,116] (discussed in detail in Chapter 156).

Absorption and Distribution. It seems likely that free biotin is formed in the intestinal lumen, either by enzymatic hydrolysis of ingested, protein-bound biotin or by release from intestinal microorganisms. Biotinidase may play a role in releasing biotin from foods.[117] Saturable, carrier-mediated, sodium-dependent systems for biotin transport and absorption have been demonstrated in human[118] and rat[119] intestine and in human intestinal brush-border membranes.[120] In addition, a second, sodium-independent system has been described in basolateral membrane vesicles from human intestine,[121] thus accounting for both intestinal absorption and release into the portal circulation. Although nonmediated transport can occur, particularly at low pH, it seems likely that the mediated system predominates at physiologic biotin concentrations and pH. Biotin in blood appears to be largely free.[122] Although experiments in cultured cell systems have been rather uninformative concerning the mechanism of cellular transport, basolateral membrane vesicles prepared from rat[123] or human[124] liver show a sodium-dependent, carrier-mediated transport, as do brush-border membrane vesicles from human placenta,[125] suggesting that biotin transport is generally a mediated process.

Biotin Deficiency. Spontaneous biotin deficiency has almost never been reported in humans, probably because the daily requirement is very small (estimated at ~120 mg/day) and because intestinal microorganisms synthesize sufficient amounts of the cofactor even in the absence of nutritional sources. Biotin deficiency has been reported, however, in patients with the short bowel syndrome being fed exclusively by parenteral alimentation.[126] Experimental biotin deficiency has been produced in animals and humans by ingestion of large amounts of egg white, which contains the potent biotin binder avidin.[127] Under these conditions, cutaneous pallor, dermatitis, depression, lassitude, muscle pains, hyperesthesia, and finally anemia and electrocardiographic changes developed in four experimental human subjects. All these symptoms and signs were reversed rapidly by administration of 150 to 300 mg biotin daily for several days. In animals, experimental biotin deficiency has been shown to produce decreased activity of biotin-dependent carboxylases in tissues.[98–100]

Cobalamin (Vitamin B_{12}). The structure and function of this compound have intrigued students of human biology since 1926, when Minot and Murphy demonstrated that oral administration of crude liver extract was effective in the treatment of pernicious anemia.[128] In 1948, this anti-pernicious anemia factor was isolated from liver and kidney[129,130] and was named vitamin B_{12}. Administration of as little as 1 μg of the vitamin daily was shown to prevent relapse of pernicious anemia. Although the vitamin is widely distributed in animal tissues, there is strong evidence that it is synthesized only in microorganisms found in soil, water, or the rumen and intestine of animals. For further information on Cbl, the reader is referred to Chapter 155. For comprehensive reviews of Cbl chemistry and metabolism, the reader is referred elsewhere.[131]

Structural Features. The isolation of vitamin B_{12} culminated in the elucidation of its three-dimensional structure by Hodgkin and co-workers using x-ray crystallographic techniques.[132] Vitamin B_{12}, or, as it is now officially designated, cobalamin, is composed of a central cobalt atom (Co) surrounded by a planar corrin ring and a complex side chain extending down from the corrin plane consisting of a 5,6-dimethylbenzimidazolyl phosphoribosyl moiety (Fig. 94-6). The benzimidazole is linked to the Co atom through one of its nitrogens, whereas the phosphate is bonded to the D ring of the corrin. The molecule is completed by coordinate linkage of one of several different radicals to the Co nucleus from above the corrin plane. Thus, CN-Cbl or, more strictly, α-(5,6-dimethylbenzimidazolyl)-cobamide cyanide, is formed by the

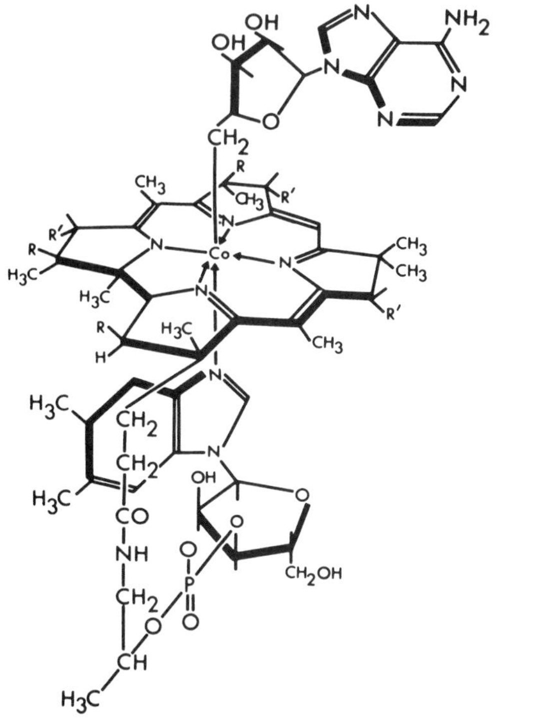

Fig. 94-6 **Structure of adenosylcobalamin (AdoCbl). R = CH_2CONH_2; R′ = $CH_2CH_2CONH_2$. Other radicals that may be coordinately linked to the cobalt atom include CH_3 (methylcobalamin), OH^- (hydroxocobalamin), and CN^- (cyanocobalamin). (Reprinted with permission from Babior BM: Cobamides as cofactors: Adenosylcobamide dependent reactions, in: *Cobalamin Biochemistry and Pathophysiology*. New York, Wiley, 1975, p 141.)**

attachment of a cyanide radical to the Co atom. Although this compound is the most common commercial form of the vitamin, it is an artifact of isolation and does not occur naturally in microorganisms, plants, or animal tissues. Many other cobalamins can be formed by replacement of the cyanide radical, but only four have been isolated from mammalian tissue: OH-Cbl, glutathionylcobalamin (GSCbl), methylcobalamin (MeCbl), and AdoCbl. The latter two compounds are unique for two reasons: They are the only two compounds in nature known to have a direct carbon–cobalt bond, and they are the only two forms of Cbl known to act as specific coenzymes in mammalian systems.

The structure and nomenclature of the cobalamins are further complicated by oxidation and reduction of the Co atom. In OH-Cbl, the Co atom is trivalent [cob(III)alamin], and this compound has been called vitamin B_{12a}. When the Co is reduced to a divalent state [cob(II)alamin], the molecule is called vitamin B_{12r} and, in the monovalent state [cob(I)alamin], it is called vitamin B_{12s}. These oxidation-reduction states are important because there appear to be specific reductase enzymes that sequentially convert cob(III)alamin to cob(I)alamin, with cob(II)alamin acting as an intermediate.[133] The Co atom must be reduced to its monovalent state prior to formation of MeCbl or AdoCbl.

Cobalamin Coenzymes. In 1958, Barker and his colleagues demonstrated that the glutamate mutase reaction in *Clostridium tetanomorphum* required vitamin B_{12}[63] and, more specifically, that the active coenzyme form of the vitamin was AdoCbl.[64,65] One year later, Smith and Monty reported that the analogous isomerization of methylmalonyl CoA to succinyl CoA was defective in the liver of Cbl-deficient rats.[2] They suggested that Cbl is a cofactor for the latter isomerization system, a thesis borne out by Gurnani et al.[3] and Stern and Friedmann,[4] who showed *in vitro* that the activity of methylmalonyl CoA mutase in liver from Cbl-deficient animals could be restored to normal by the addition of AdoCbl, but

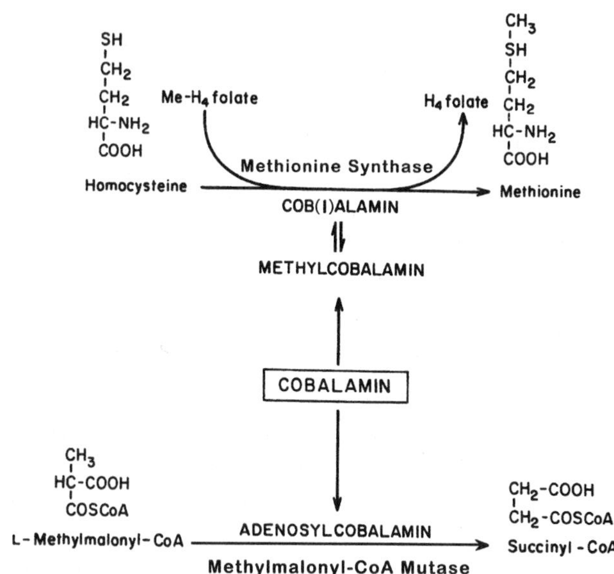

Fig. 94-7 Reactions catalyzed by cobalamin coenzymes in mammalian tissues. Note the specificity of adenosylcobalamin for the isomerization of methylmalonyl CoA and of methylcobalamin for the methylation of homocysteine. Me-H_4folate = N^5-methyltetrahydrofolate; H_4folate = tetrahydrofolate.

not by CN-Cbl or other vitamin B_{12} analogues (Fig. 94-7). For several years, because AdoCbl was the only known coenzyme form of vitamin B_{12}, it was designated *coenzyme* B_{12}.

In 1966, Weissbach and his colleagues[134] demonstrated that MeCbl is a cofactor in the complex reaction by which homocysteine is methylated to methionine (Fig. 94-7). This reaction requires *S*-adenosylmethionine and N^5-methyltetrahydrofolate (Me-H_4folate), as well as the methionine synthase apoenzyme and MeCbl. The mechanism of homocysteine methylation probably involves the following sequence: Me-H_4folate is converted to tetrahydrofolate (H_4 folate) by transferring its methyl group to a reduced Cbl prosthetic group on the methionine synthase holoenzyme; in turn, the methyl group is transferred from MeCbl to homocysteine, leading to the formation of methionine[135,136] (see Chapter 155).

The conversion of methylmalonyl CoA to succinyl CoA and the methylation of homocysteine to methionine are the only Cbl-dependent reactions that have been demonstrated conclusively in mammalian systems. Poston reported that AdoCbl acts as a cofactor in the enzymatic reaction by which α-leucine is isomerized to β-leucine,[137] but this has not been confirmed in other laboratories. In microorganisms, several other enzymes require AdoCbl[138,139]: glutamate mutase, diol dehydrase, glycerol dehydrase, ethanolamine ammonia-lyase, and ribonucleotide reductase. In addition, MeCbl is involved in the formation of methane and acetic acid and the fermentation of lysine in bacteria.

Cbl Absorption and Distribution. The Cbl vitamins have a unique and highly specialized mechanism of intestinal absorption that has been reviewed in detail.[140–142] The ability to transport physiologic quantities of the vitamin depends on the combined action of gastric, ileal, and pancreatic components. The gastric substance, called intrinsic factor (IF) by Castle,[138] who first demonstrated its existence, is a glycoprotein, synthesized by gastric parietal cells, that binds cobalamins in the intestinal lumen after they have been released from dietary protein by acid and peptic hydrolysis. Subsequently, the IF–Cbl complex interacts through its protein moiety with a specific ileal receptor protein, called cubilin.[143] The vitamin is transcytosed across the ileal epithelial cells and appears in the portal blood bound to transcobalamin II (TC II), the transport protein for newly absorbed vitamin.[140,144,145] When labeled Cbl is administered intravenously or orally, most of it is immediately bound to TC II and disappears from the plasma in a few hours.[146,147] Two other Cbl-binding proteins, transcobalamin I (TC I) and transcobalamin III (TC III), are also found in serum. TC I and TC III are glycoproteins of the R-binder, or haptocorrin, family, which carry the majority of Cbl found in plasma, but their physiologic role is unclear. For example, only a small fraction of newly absorbed Cbl binds to TC I, and this component turns over very slowly. MeCbl is the major circulating Cbl species, accounting for 60 to 80 percent of total plasma Cbl; OH-Cbl and AdoCbl make up the remainder.[148] Because over 90 percent of total plasma Cbl is bound to TC I, it is clear that most of the circulating MeCbl travels with this R-binder. This Cbl distribution pattern is puzzling, particularly in the face of evidence indicating that AdoCbl accounts for approximately 70 percent of total hepatic Cbl, whereas MeCbl constitutes a mere 1 to 3 percent.[148] A preponderance of AdoCbl is also present in such other tissues as erythrocytes, kidney, and brain. The physiologic significance of these widely different fractional amounts of Cbl compounds in extracellular and intracellular compartments remains obscure.

Transcobalamin II facilitates Cbl uptake by mammalian tissues. Finkler and Hall[149] showed that CN-Cbl bound to TC II was accumulated by HeLa cells much more rapidly than free CN-Cbl or CN-Cbl bound to TC I, IF, or other binding proteins. Such TC II–mediated uptake has been subsequently confirmed in a variety of cell types, both *in vivo* and in culture.[141] These findings, coupled with the observations *in vivo* that TC II disappeared from plasma as TC II–Cbl was absorbed[150] and appeared in lysosomal fractions of hepatic[151] and kidney[152] cells, led to the proposal that the circulating TC II–Cbl complex is recognized by a specific, widely distributed plasma membrane receptor, a hypothesis supported by considerable experimental evidence. Youngdahl-Turner and associates[153] showed that the complex binds to a specific, high-affinity ($K_a \sim 10^{-10}$ M) cell surface receptor on cultured skin fibroblasts, that the TC II–Cbl complex is internalized intact via adsorptive endocytosis,[154] and that the degradation of TC II and release of Cbl from the complex occur as a result of lysosomal protease activity.[153,154] Cbl then exits from the lysosome and is either converted to MeCbl and bound to the methionine synthase in the cytosol or enters the mitochondrion, where, after reduction and adenosylation, it is bound to methylmalonyl CoA mutase (Fig. 94-8).[155,156]

The intricate process just described is surely the most widely distributed physiologic means by which mammalian cells obtain Cbl, but it is not the only one. Hepatocytes, for instance, contain a surface receptor for asialoglycoproteins, and this receptor interacts with TC I–Cbl (and perhaps TC III–Cbl) complexes, thereby providing a second potential means by which this particular tissue obtains Cbl.[157] There is also evidence that at least some tissues are capable of taking up free (unbound) Cbl if the concentration of unbound vitamin is increased to sufficiently high concentrations. In cultured fibroblasts, this uptake process for free Cbl is saturable, Ca^2 independent, and sensitive to inhibitors of protein synthesis and sulfhydryl reagents.[158] Its functional role under most circumstances is probably negligible, however.

Coenzyme Biosynthesis and Compartmentation. Because methylmalonyl CoA mutase, the mammalian enzyme dependent on AdoCbl, is a mitochondrial protein,[159] whereas the MeCbl-dependent methionine synthase is cytoplasmic,[160] it becomes important to relate the cellular biology of the vitamin to its cellular and molecular chemistry. The chemical pathway of AdoCbl synthesis was defined initially in bacteria.[133,161] Three enzymes are required for coenzyme synthesis: two reductases and an adenosyltransferase. The reductases are flavoproteins that require NAD as a cofactor. The first (EC 1.6.99.8) is responsible for converting cob(III)alamin (i.e., OH-Cbl) to cob(II)alamin, and the second (EC 1.6.99.9) for catalyzing the further reduction to cob(I)alamin. The latter compound and ATP are substrates for an adenosyltransferase (EC 2.5.1.17), which completes the synthesis of AdoCbl. Neither of the reductases has been purified extensively, but the adenosyltransferase has. It has an optimal pH of 8, requires Mn^{2+}, and has a K_m of 1×10^{-5} M for cob(I)alamin and 1.6×10^{-5} M for ATP.[161] The biosynthetic steps leading to MeCbl formation are somewhat analogous, likely involving reduction followed by methylation directly by the methionine synthase apoenzyme.[162,163]

Evidence has accumulated that indicates that mammalian cell metabolism of Cbl may proceed by a very similar set of reactions (Fig. 94-8). In 1964, Pawalkiewicz et al.[164] showed that human liver and kidney homogenates could convert CN-Cbl to AdoCbl. Several years later, AdoCbl synthesis from OH-Cbl was observed in HeLa cell extracts incubated with ATP and a reducing system that presumably bypassed the enzymatic reduction of OH-Cbl [cob(III)alamin] to cob(I)alamin.[165] Subsequently, Mahoney and Rosenberg[166] demonstrated the synthesis of both AdoCbl and MeCbl by intact human fibroblasts growing in a tissue culture medium containing OH-[^{57}Co]Cbl. This system was subsequently characterized in cell extracts.[167,168] As with the HeLa cell system, chemical reductants were employed to bypass both Cbl

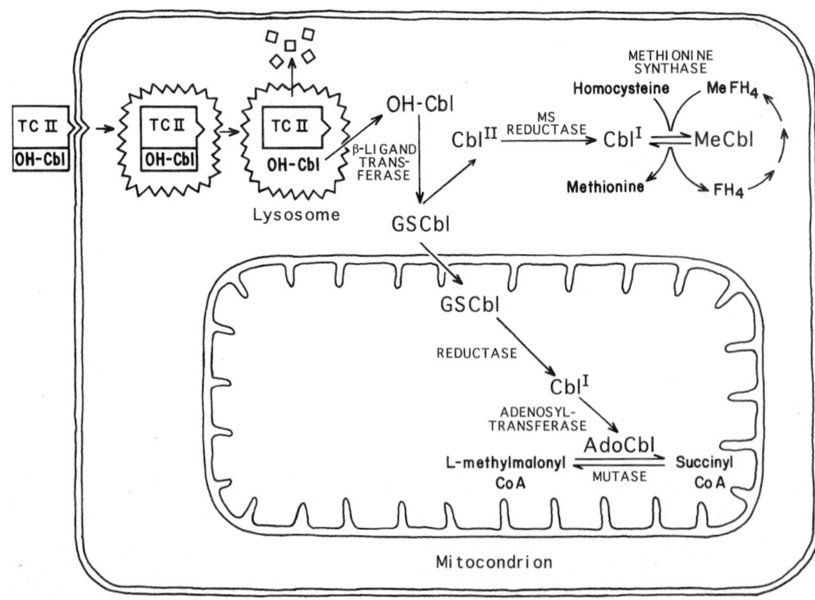

Fig. 94-8 General pathway of the cellular uptake and subcellular compartmentation of Cbl, and of the intracellular distribution and enzymatic synthesis of Cbl coenzymes. TC II = transcobalamin II; OH-Cbl = hydroxocobalamin; GSCbl = glutathionylcobalamin; MeCbl = methylcobalamin; MeFH$_4$ = methyltetrahydrofolate; FH$_4$ = tetrahydrofolate; AdoCbl = adenosylcobalamin; Cbl^{III}, Cbl^{II}, Cbl^{I} = cobalamins with cobalt valence of 3$^+$, 2$^+$, and 1$^+$, respectively.

reductases.[168] Such extracts synthesized AdoCbl, thereby demonstrating that the adenosyltransferase found in bacteria also exists in normal human cells. These experiments also revealed that the adenosyltransferase was mitochondrial in location, implying that both the synthesis and cofactor activity of AdoCbl take place in this organelle. In contrast, MeCbl synthesis takes place in the cytosol in conjunction with the methionine synthase reaction (Fig. 94-8).

Metabolic Abnormalities in Cbl Deficiency. The biochemical abnormalities in plasma and urine of patients with Cbl deficiency reflect the dysfunction of the enzymes dependent on Cbl coenzymes. The first relevant observation in this context was the demonstration by Cox and White[5] and by Barness and his colleagues[6] that methylmalonic acid excretion in the urine was distinctly increased in Cbl-deficient patients with classic pernicious anemia. The methylmalonic aciduria in these patients was reversed rapidly by administration of physiologic doses of Cbl, indicating that repletion of Cbl restored the methylmalonyl CoA mutase reaction to normal. Later, Cox et al. reported that patients with Cbl deficiency also have distinctly increased amounts of propionic acid in the urine, this abnormality again being reversed by treatment.[169] Interestingly, they also found excessive amounts of acetic acid in the urine of Cbl-deficient subjects. The mechanism of this abnormality is not clear, because acetate does not participate in the major pathway of propionate catabolism. The finding could reflect increased utilization of the alternative pathways of propionate metabolism in the face of a block in the major pathway, because each of the alternative routes leads eventually to the formation of acetyl CoA (Fig. 94-4). Excessive excretion of homocystine also has been documented in Cbl-deficient patients,[170,171] as has combined methylmalonic aciduria and homocystinuria.[172] The latter report is particularly interesting because it documents congenital but not hereditary Cbl deficiency, in this instance due to acquired Cbl deficiency in the offspring of a strictly vegetarian mother who also was deficient in the vitamin. A number of such cases have now been reported.[21]

DISEASE STATES

The Propionic Acidemias

In 1961, Childs et al.[7] described a male infant with episodic metabolic ketoacidosis, protein intolerance, and remarkably elevated plasma glycine concentration. Several hundred children with similar clinical and biochemical findings have since been described. Many of these children were subsequently found to have methylmalonic acidemia[173]; a few had β-ketothiolase deficiency (see Chapter 93). However, the patient described by Childs et al., and many reported subsequently, had propionic acidemia due to a primary and specific deficiency of propionyl CoA carboxylase activity (Fig. 94-2). This conclusion was derived independently from the description of a patient with massive propionate accumulation in blood,[174] from another with impaired propionate oxidation in leukocytes[9] and defective carboxylase activity in fibroblast extracts,[175] and from a third with both propionic acidemia and defective carboxylase activity.[176] We now recognize that propionyl CoA carboxylase deficiency also occurs in children with inherited abnormalities in biotin metabolism, leading to the deficiency of multiple biotin-dependent carboxylases (see Chapter 156). Hence, we must now use the term *propionic acidemias* to refer to this heterogeneous group of related inborn errors. As will be discussed subsequently, a similar heterogeneity exists among the methylmalonic acidemias.

Propionyl CoA Carboxylase Deficiency. ***Clinical Manifestations.*** As mentioned above, this disorder was originally referred to as ketotic hyperglycinemia. E.G., the patient described by Childs and Nyhan and their colleagues,[7,177,178] presented with dehydration, lethargy, and coma on the first day of life. He was found to be severely ketoacidotic and responded slowly to massive alkali replacement. The clinical course was characterized by recurrent attacks of ketoacidosis, precipitated by infections or protein ingestion, and by developmental retardation, electroencephalographic (EEG) abnormalities, and osteoporosis. The patient had episodic neutropenia and thrombocytopenia prior to death at age 7. A sister (A.G.) also became ketotic and acidotic during the first 4 days of life, but the course of her condition has been modified dramatically because of the extensive experience gained in studying her brother. Although she has had mild attacks of ketoacidosis during intercurrent infections, maintenance on a low-protein diet has resulted in little need for hospital care and normal somatic and mental development up to 15 years of age.[179]

In 1968, Hommes and his colleagues[174] described a male infant with hyperventilation, areflexia, and grunting at 60 h of age. There was a profound metabolic acidosis (arterial pH 6.98), and despite administration of massive amounts of sodium bicarbonate and *tris*(hydroxymethyl)-aminomethane, the infant died on the fifth day of life. Leukocytes and platelets were normal. Postmortem examination showed only a fatty liver and degeneration of Purkinje cells and the granular layer of the cerebellum.

Subsequent descriptions of patients with propionic acidemia have confirmed that most patients present in the newborn period with severe metabolic acidosis manifested by refusal to feed, vomiting, lethargy, and hypotonia; dehydration, seizures, and hepatomegaly occur less often.[180,181] Other patients have presented later, either with acute encephalopathy or episodic ketoacidosis or with developmental retardation apparently uncomplicated by attacks of ketosis or acidosis.[182,183] A 5-year-old boy presented with a fatal necrosis of the basal ganglia without either metabolic acidosis or hyperammonemia.[184] Propionic acidemia has been identified in a 29-year-old man who presented initially with adult-onset chorea and dementia.[185] Still other children, with almost complete deficiency of propionyl CoA carboxylase activity as measured in extracts of cultured fibroblasts, have had no clinical abnormalities whatever and have been identified only during family studies.[186,187] No satisfactory explanation for this striking lack of clinical enzymatic correlation exists at present.

Based on a survey of 65 patients with propionic acidemia, Wolf et al.[181] reported that the clinical course of symptomatic patients is characterized by repeated relapses, usually precipitated by excessive protein intake, constipation, or intercurrent infection. Treatment of these children has been quite difficult, and neurologic sequelae have been common. Among the neurologic complications often observed, developmental delay, focal and general seizures, cerebral atrophy, and EEG abnormalities have been the most prominent. Surtees et al.[183] also have reported a high prevalence of neurologic sequelae, including dystonia, severe chorea, and pyramidal signs, particularly in patients who survive longer. The cranial computer tomographic and magnetic resonance imaging findings in propionic acidemia were reviewed by Bergman et al., who showed spectroscopic abnormalities, specifically an increase in glutamine/glutamate, even when the patients appeared to be stable.[188] Walter et al. described 11 newborn patients with elevated blood ammonia levels and neurologic symptoms; only 4 had clinically important acidosis.[189] Leukopenia and thrombocytopenia, perhaps due to marrow suppression by one or more of the toxic metabolites produced, is also not uncommon. Parathyroid hormone resistance and B-cell lymphopenia was described in a 7-week-old patient.[190]

Biochemical Abnormalities. Childs and Nyhan[7,177,178,191] studied their index patient extensively. Because of the hyperglycinemia, they focused their attention on the pathways of glycine formation and utilization but found no consistent abnormalities. Normal hemoglobin concentration in the peripheral blood indicated that the pathway from glycine to δ-aminolevulinic acid was not blocked. Slices of the patient's liver incorporated [^{14}C]glycine into protein and carbon dioxide as well as slices of rat liver did. Salicylate and benzoate were normally conjugated with glycine, and the glutathione concentration of whole blood was normal. Although the rate of conversion of tritiated glycine to serine *in vivo* was slower than in controls, this difference may have reflected the enlarged glycine pool rather than a specific block in the conversion of glycine to serine.[191]

Moreover, several observations suggested an abnormality in the catabolism of the branched chain amino acids, methionine, and threonine. Plasma concentrations of valine, isoleucine, and leucine were elevated intermittently; administration of leucine, valine, isoleucine, threonine, and methionine each precipitated attacks of ketoacidosis, but no other amino acids were toxic. Menkes[192] reported that the urine contained large amounts of butanone (a four-carbon ketone that is a by-product of isoleucine catabolism) and the longer chain ketones, pentanone and hexanone. These long-chain ketones were not detected in the urine of patients with ketosis due to diabetes, starvation, or ketogenic diets. Because isoleucine, valine, threonine, and methionine are all precursors of propionate, a defect in propionate metabolism seemed likely, but patient E.G. died before any other studies of propionate catabolism could be performed. Subsequently, Hsia et al.[9] demonstrated a striking defect in propionate catabolism in A.G., the affected sister of E.G. When leukocytes isolated from her peripheral blood were incubated with [3-^{14}C]propionate, negligible quantities of $^{14}CO_2$ were evolved as compared with values in controls, but her cells oxidized methylmalonate and succinate normally. Identical findings were obtained using fibroblasts grown in tissue culture. These data showed that the primary metabolic defect in E.G. and A.G. was in the conversion of propionyl CoA to D-methylmalonyl CoA, a reaction catalyzed by propionyl CoA carboxylase. This conclusion was confirmed subsequently by direct assay of carboxylase activity in fibroblast extracts.[175]

In their child with lethal neonatal acidosis, Hommes et al.[174] found that the serum propionic acid concentration was 400 mg/dl (5.4 mM), a value more than 100 times that reported in normal infants. The liver contained fatty acids with 15 and 17 carbon atoms in addition to the even-chain fatty acids found in control livers. From these data, Hommes et al. also postulated a defect in propionyl CoA carboxylation in their patient.

Subsequent investigations have confirmed and extended these early findings. Analysis of body fluids in several additional patients[92–94,176] showed that propionate accumulation in blood and urine occurs regularly, its magnitude being related to the severity of the clinical course and the time at which sampling is performed. Ando and colleagues[92] have stressed that other propionate derivatives also accumulate in urine. These include methylcitrate, which is probably formed from the intramitochondrial condensation of propionyl CoA with oxaloacetate[92]; propionylglycine, which results from the conjugation of propionate with glycine[93]; β-hydroxypropionate, an intermediate in one of the alternative pathways of propionate catabolism[94] (Fig. 94-4); and tiglic acid,[193] an isoleucine catabolite several steps proximal to the block. Although the exact amounts of these compounds in urine have not always been determined, they appear to account for a small fraction of the propionate pool that accumulates *in vivo* in this disease. Their presence may be important in mitigating the toxic effects of propionate excess. Wendel et al. showed elevated levels of odd-numbered fatty acids (OLCFA) in the erythrocyte lipids of five patients with propionic acidemia and suggested that OLCFA levels reflect the continuous burden of propionyl CoA toxicity within cells and could serve as a means of evaluating the quality of long-term metabolic control.[194]

Other compounds, not directly concerned with the propionate pathway, also have been found in significantly increased amounts. In addition to hyperglycinemia and hyperglycinuria, which were discussed earlier, marked hyperammonemia has been documented in several patients,[181,195] and a distinct correlation between plasma propionate and blood ammonia has been noted in two patients.[196]

The Enzymatic Defect. The molecular pathology of propionic acidemia is both complex and interesting. Cell extracts from a number of affected patients share a common finding, namely, reduction in propionyl CoA carboxylase activity to 1 to 5 percent of that in controls.[197–199] Because the enzyme is composed of two independently encoded enzyme subunits, the causative mutations will necessarily occur in one of two genes. This was first illustrated in complementation experiments in which fibroblast heterokaryons formed between pairs of affected cell lines were assayed for recovery of functional propionyl CoA carboxylase by fixation of ^{14}C-propionate.[200–202] Two major complementation groups, *pccA* and *pccBC*, were identified, the latter group showing intragroup complementation (subgroups *pccB* and *pccC*) compatible with the occurrence of interallelic complementation (see Fig. 94-11). It was shown subsequently that patients in the *pccA* group have a primary defect in the *PCCA* gene encoding the α subunit of propionyl CoA carboxylase, whereas patients in the *pccBC* group and subgroups have defects of the *PCCB* gene encoding the β subunit.[203,204]

There are several unusual features of mutant fibroblast lines from patients belonging to the different complementation groups. First, many individuals in the *pccA* group lack detectable α subunit protein; when this is the case, they invariably lack detectable β subunits as well.[203,205] This has been explained by the inherent instability and consequent degradation of the β subunit in the absence of α subunit with which to assemble to form the native enzyme. Among α-minus/β-minus cell lines, some lack α subunit mRNA but contain β subunit mRNA, confirming the assignment of the *pccA* complementation group to mutations of the *PCCA* gene.[204] Second, a number of *pccBC* or subgroup fibroblasts lack β subunits but have α subunits. These have unstable β subunit protein due to mutation, although β subunit protein is present in at least some cases.[205,206] Importantly, the small amount of residual propionyl CoA carboxylase activity observed in extracts of most mutant fibroblasts appears to be present even in those with absent α or β subunits. This suggests that the "background" activity is due to the minimal activity of other carboxylases acting on propionyl CoA as substrate, not to propionyl CoA carboxylase itself.[207] A third unusual feature of propionic acidemia is that many heterozygotes of the *pccBC* group or subgroups have propionyl CoA carboxylase activity indistinguishable from that in controls, whereas obligate heterozygotes of the *pccA* group have the expected 50 percent of control activity.[199] This has proved to be due to relative differences in the synthesis of the enzyme subunits. It has been shown that β subunits are synthesized in four- to fivefold excess over α subunits, so that heterozygotes for null-type β subunit mutations still have more than enough wild-type β subunits to interact with the limiting amount of α subunits to form normal amounts of carboxylase enzyme.[205] Conversely, any reduction in the amount of α subunit, as in *pccA* heterozygotes, is directly reflected in a proportionate reduction in carboxylase activity.[199] All three of these features of mutant cell lines can be used diagnostically to identify the affected gene, but caution is warranted because patients with point mutations in either gene may have both subunits present, despite having a defective holoenzyme.

Pathologic Physiology. A defect in the carboxylation of propionate provides a satisfactory explanation for many of the findings reported in this disorder. This defect would be expected to lead to an elevated concentration of propionate in the blood and an inability of leukocytes to catabolize propionate to carbon dioxide. Because isoleucine, valine, threonine, and methionine are precursors of propionate, such a block also should lead to the observed protein and specific amino acid intolerance. The appearance of long, odd-chain fatty acids in the liver suggests that when propionyl CoA carboxylation is blocked, odd-chain fatty acid biosynthesis may be augmented because propionyl CoA is the "primer" for such compounds. Finally, the presence of such compounds as butanone, methylcitrate, β-hydroxypropionate, propionylglycine, and tiglic acid very likely results from reversal of reactions proximal to the primary carboxylase block or from increased utilization of alternative pathways.

It is not at all clear from the foregoing, however, why some patients have a severe and often life-threatening course, and others are only mildly affected clinically. Major differences in dietary protein uptake and quality, in the contributions of gut bacteria to total propionate load, or in the activity of alternative mechanisms for propionate disposal are possible explanations for the wide clinical spectrum, but the prominent intrafamilial differences in severity are not easily explained this way.[186] Furthermore, several other features of the disease are not adequately explained by the block in propionate catabolism. The ketosis produced in E.G. by leucine is not understood, because this amino acid is not catabolized to propionate. However, it is ketogenic in normal subjects, suggesting that its effect in E.G. was nonspecific. The cause for the hyperglycinemia seen in many, but not all, of these patients also has not been adequately defined. Because the infant described by Hommes et al.[174] with massive propionic acidemia never demonstrated signs of hyperglycinemia, the latter cannot be ascribed simply to the acidosis or ketosis. Numerous theses have been put forth in explanation. For example, one or more products of isoleucine catabolism may interfere with glycine cleavage or glycine–serine interconversion.[191,208,209] Ando et al.[92] speculated that methylcitrate cleavage in the cytosol may yield propionate and glyoxylate, the latter being used as a substrate for glycine overproduction. Impaired glycine conjugation systems have been suggested, but no data in support of this notion have been forthcoming. Because plasma glycine concentration may increase in sick children with negative nitrogen balance of many causes,[210] the hyperglycinemia may be nonspecific. The hyperammonemia often observed in this disorder has been the subject of considerable investigation. It appears likely that this secondary but clinically important finding results from inhibition of the first enzyme of the urea cycle, mitochondrial carbamyl phosphate synthetase (CPS I), by the organic acids and CoA esters that accumulate intramitochondrially behind the block in propionyl CoA carboxylation. This conclusion rests on data from studies with experimental animals and animal tissues. For example, propionate inhibits ureagenesis in rat liver slices when ammonia, but not citrulline or aspartate, is the nitrogen-donating substrate.[211] Administration to rats of sufficiently large amounts of propionate or methylmalonate to produce hyperammonemia is associated with a marked decrease in hepatic concentration of *N*-acetyl glutamate,[212] the required allosteric effector of CPS I, probably by competitively inhibiting *N*-acetyl glutamate synthetase.[213] That such CPS I inhibition occurs *in vivo* as well as *in vitro* is supported by case reports that describe selective impairment of CPS I activity in the livers of patients with propionic acidemia[214] or methylmalonic acidemia.[215]

Genetics. As a prelude to mutation identification in propionic acidemia, it is first necessary to identify the affected gene. This is most readily done by conducting complementation tests and determining whether the affected patient belongs in the *pccA* or *pccBC* group or a subgroup. Determination of the subgroup (e.g., *pccB* or *pccC* vs. *pccBC*) is not specifically required, but does provide insight into the functional impact of mutations affecting the β subunit (see Fig. 94-11). Alternatively, as described above, demonstration of some of the peculiarities of propionyl CoA carboxylase activity or of mRNA or enzyme subunit expression can also reveal the affected gene. Thus, the demonstration of normal enzyme activity in parents of an affected child would be compatible with mutations in the *PCCB* gene, although obtaining the converse, 50 percent activity, does not necessarily implicate the *PCCA* gene. Absence of both α and β subunits by Western blotting does identify the *PCCA* gene as responsible for the disease. Other more straightforward findings, such as absence or abnormality of one of the two mRNA species or polypeptide, also will identify the affected gene. Performing the required experiments is worthwhile because there is a great diversity of mutations in the *PCCA* gene, and although the *PCCB* gene shows bias toward a small number of mutations that account for about 30 to 60 percent of alleles in different populations, there remains a large diversity of mutations that account for the rest.

Mutations in the* PCCA *Gene. Nineteen disease-causing mutations have been identified in the *PCCA* gene, eight of which fail to produce a complete α subunit. There are four splicing mutations, two nonsense mutations and two small deletions causing frameshifts. All four splicing mutations cause exon skipping. Three of them—1771IVS-2del9, 1824IVS+3del4, and 1824IVS+3insCT—affect the same exon.[216] The nonsense mutations, R288X and S537X, and the small deletions, 700del5 and 1115del4, are expected to produce truncated proteins. However, fibroblasts from a patient homozygous for 1115del4 failed to show mRNA by Northern blot, although it could be detected by reverse transcriptase polymerase chain reaction (RT-PCR). A similar finding was made for a patient heteroallelic for R288X and 700del5, indicating that both mutant mRNA species are unstable.[217] These results suggest a propensity for mutations disrupting normal mRNA translation to produce mRNA-minus outcomes, as has been noted for other genes.

An unusual finding in patient cells with mRNA destabilizing mutations at both alleles is the detection of an RT-PCR product showing an 84 bp insertion at nucleotide 1209, containing two in-frame stop codons.[217] The insertion is an anomalous exon derived by aberrant splicing within the adjacent intron. The cryptic transcript is part of the background "noise" of abnormal mRNAs occurring at very low level in normal cells. Cell lines in which the 84 bp insertion is detected as a predominant (but low-level) species share at both alleles severely deleterious mutations, which are consistent with rendering the normally structured mRNA species unstable and rapidly degraded. In a study of 12 mutant cell lines, 4 showed the characteristic transcript. The mutations included a splicing mutation (1671IVS + 5G$\rightarrow$C), a nonsense mutation (R288X, three occurrences), and two small deletions (700del5, 1115del4) causing frameshifts.[217] Screening for the 84 bp insertion by RT-PCR may provide a diagnostic benefit, given the high proportion of such cell lines.

The remaining mutations cause amino acid substitutions, which are expected to produce inactive or unstable α subunits, although most have yet to be evaluated in expression experiments. Two subunits with point mutations, G643R and Cdel687, have been expressed in *E. coli* and shown to abolish biotin binding.[57] Another mutation, M348K, has been shown to reduce the intramitochondrial stability of the mutant α chain without appreciably affecting its import.[218] This α chain failed to be biotinylated, as also was found for two other nearby mutations, D343G and G354V, and one near the N-terminus, A50P,[57] indicating that all four mutations likely result in unstable α chains *in vivo*, accounting for the lack of biotinylation, because the biotin binding domain is far removed toward the C-terminus of the protein.

Mutations in the* PCCB *Gene. Twenty-eight disease-causing mutations have been identified in the *PCCB* gene. There are 16 missense mutations, three nonsense, three insertions, and one complex insertion/deletion (ins/del). Five other mutations cause disease through disruption of normal splicing. The most frequent mutation in white individuals is ins/del,[219–221] present in 32 percent of alleles of mixed white heritage. A similar value also was obtained in a study involving 29 patients of Spanish or Latin American heritage.[61] Two other mutations have been found in significant frequency in the same populations. These are 1170insT and E168K, with combined frequencies of 14 percent and 17 percent, respectively, in Spanish and Latin American patients.[61,222] The remaining mutations occur singly or have been found in only two or three patients among whites.

Six mutation have been identified among Japanese patients. Two of them, R410W and T428I, appear to be prevalent, occurring in 25 and 31 percent of alleles, respectively.[221,223] There are also two splicing mutations (IVS4+3del4 and IVS12+3del8), both of which result in exon skipping; one nonsense mutation (R499X), and one other point mutation (R165W).[54,223,224] Of these, R410W and R165W also have been found in whites.[61,225]

The ins/del mutation is a complex mutation resulting from a deletion of 14 nucleotides and their replacement by 12 nucleotides unrelated to those that were lost. The outcome is the loss of an *Msp* I site, which has been used diagnostically, and generation of a frameshift that results in the production of an unstable, truncated protein.[220] The origin of the ins/del is not obvious, but it is attractive to speculate that it is derived from duplication of nine nucleotides just upstream of the site, with random filling of three more nucleotides.[219] The R410W mutation occurs in the same location and also results in loss of the *Msp* I site. This leaves ambiguous the results of diagnosis by *Msp* I digestion of PCR products. Dot blotting can be used to distinguish these possibilities,[219] or PCR products that show at least one allele not cleaved by *Msp* I can be sequenced.

Two amino acid substitutions, L519P and R512C, are unusual in that they are associated with apparently absolute deficiency of β subunits.[61] Both are present in patients with null-type second alleles (1170insT and ins/del, respectively) and both patients' cells are negative for the β subunit by Western blot. Other point mutations, including R44P, G131R, R165W, E168K, R410W, and A497V are associated with unstable β subunits, which appear reduced in quantity and may show smaller-sized fragments by Western blot.[61,223] The abundance of β subunit mutations that are CRM negative (in the presence of detectable α subunit) highlights the affected gene (*PCCB*) and focuses the analysis for mutations.

The identification of mutations in the *PCCB* gene has made it possible to assess the basis of interallelic complemention that defines the *pccB* and *pccC* subgroups. Each complementing cell line would have one, if homozygous, or two candidate mutations that could be responsible for the interallelic complementation observed between mutant subgroups. The identity of the complementing allele in several cell lines was determined by microinjecting β subunit cDNA plasmids containing the candidate mutations into fibroblasts of each subgroup and assaying for recovery of ^{14}C-propionate metabolism by autoradiography.[225,226] The results paralleled the original complementation results, and the distribution of complementing alleles shows a pattern suggestive of functional domains within the β subunit. For example, two mutations from the *pccB* subgroup in the N-terminal half of the protein, dupKICK140 and P228L, are both complementing alleles. These mutations reside in the putative carboxybiotin binding domain by homology with related sequences in the 12S subunit of *P. shermanii* transcarboxylase. Similarly, two complementing alleles from the *pccC* subgroup, Idel408 and R410W, are close together in the C-terminal half of the protein. They are located in a region of high homology with the propionyl CoA binding site of the *P. shermanii* 12S subunit. These findings suggest the importance of β–β interactions in the enzyme and indicate the benefit of determining subgroup complementation within the *PCCB* gene as a way of assessing functional characteristics of the enzyme.

A particular difficulty for investigating the impact of mutations is the requirement for a two-subunit expression system and successful biotinylation to obtain functional propionyl CoA carboxylase. So far, this has been achieved in only one instance. Kelson et al.[227] coexpressed cDNAs encoding the α and β subunits in *E. coli*, along with the chaperonin proteins GroES and GroEL to facilitate folding and assembly, and obtained fully assembled, biotinylated propionyl CoA carboxylase. Using this system, they evaluated the Japanese T428I mutation in the β subunit and showed that it resulted in complete obliteration of enzyme activity.

Diagnosis and Mutation Analysis. A defect in propionate carboxylation must be considered in any child in whom ketosis or acidosis develops in the neonatal period. Other inborn errors of metabolism must be ruled out, as must the more common causes of acidosis in the newborn period. Determinations of propionic acid and its metabolites in blood or urine and studies of propionyl CoA carboxylase activity in leukocyte or fibroblast extracts are required for definitive diagnosis. The enzymatic test is, in fact, the only absolutely specific one, because propionate accumulation can occur in patients with defects of methylmalonate metabolism as well as in those with propionyl CoA carboxylase deficiency. Such assays on cord blood leukocytes should allow immediate diagnosis in a high-risk newborn. Prenatal diagnosis has been accomplished reliably by measuring carboxylase activity in cultured amniotic fluid cells[228] or chorionic villous biopsies,[229] by measuring [^{14}C]propionate fixation in amniotic fluid cells,[230] or by measuring methylcitrate in amniotic fluid.[231]

The identification of the specific gene defect, in *PCCA* or *PCCB*, responsible for the enzyme deficiency is important for monitoring future pregnancies and to contribute to genotype–phenotype correlations. The gene assignment can be achieved most unequivocally through complementation analysis. However, this is an esoteric procedure that is not readily available in most laboratories.[200–202] Other methods can be used that take advantage of some of the peculiarities of each complementation group, although the techniques do not apply universally. For example, estimation of PCC activity in parents' fibroblasts will indicate *PCCB* gene mutations if the activity is within the normal range, although this does not apply in all cases of β subunit defects.[199] Western blot, or ^{3}H-biotin labeling in the case of the α subunit, will indicate defects of the *PCCA* gene, if both the α and β subunits are absent, or implicate the *PCCB* gene if only the β subunit is absent, reduced in quantity, or partially degraded.[205] Finally, Northern blot or semiquantitative RT-PCR will identify the defective gene if the level or mobility of one or the other mRNA species is adversely affected.[204]

After identification of the defective gene, cell lines can be analyzed for mutation by conventional techniques. In the *PCCB* gene, it is worthwhile to first screen for common mutations. These include ins/del, which appears widespread, and 1170insT and E168K, which are frequent in Spanish and Latin American populations.[61,219–221] In Japanese patients, the common mutations include R410W and T428I.[221,223] When screening for the ins/del by loss of the *Msp* I site, it should be recalled that R410W is also associated with loss of the same site. Although ins/del has not been observed in Japanese patients, R410W and R165W do occur in both Japanese and white individuals. It would be important to confirm the mutation by sequencing if it is identified through loss of the *Msp* I site. The *PCCA* gene does not have predominant mutations. Because a number of patients have had null mutations on both alleles, however, it is worthwhile to test for the characteristic 84-bp insertion detectable by RT-PCR in patients with absent or unstable mRNA.[217]

For determining the identity of unknown mutations, genomic DNA can be analyzed in the case of the *PCCB* gene. With the structure of the *PCCB* gene completed, it is possible to amplify each of the 15 exons and flanking intronic sequences for analysis of PCR products.[61] Alternatively, RT-PCR and sequencing have been used to identify mutations at the mRNA level[222,223] and to examine the effect of splicing mutations.[54,224] In the case of the *PCCA* gene, where complete genomic structure is still lacking, analysis of overlapping cDNA segments generated by RT-PCR has been the method of choice.[57,217,218]

Treatment. A low-protein diet (0.5–1.5 g/kg per day) or one selectively reduced in the content of propionate precursors appears to be the best treatment for the disorder at this time. Such diets will minimize the number of attacks of ketoacidosis but will not necessarily prevent them or allow normal development in all patients. Because fasting has been shown to increase the excretion of propionate metabolites in patients, frequent feeding has been recommended.[27] Attacks of ketoacidosis should be treated vigorously by withdrawing all dietary protein and administering sodium bicarbonate parenterally; glucose is also required to avoid catabolism. Acute attacks, particularly those accompanied by hyperammonemia, have been treated with peritoneal dialysis.[232] Total parenteral nutrition also has been used to treat critically ill patients.[233] Because propionyl CoA carboxylase requires biotin as a coenzyme and because some patients' cells show a biotin-dependent increase in enzyme activity,[234] it is possible that certain patients could improve when given supplementary biotin, but no clear example of a biotin-responsive patient with isolated propionyl CoA carboxylase deficiency has yet been documented. On the other hand, dramatic biotin responsiveness has been described in several children in whom propionyl CoA carboxylase deficiency is part of the constellation now called multiple carboxylase deficiency (see Chapter 156).

Two additional therapeutic adjuncts deserve mention. Roe and Bohan reported marked, transient clinical improvement in a child with propionic acidemia given a single oral dose (100 mg/kg) of L-carnitine.[173] Because this child's urinary hippurate concentration increased markedly after carnitine, because free plasma carnitine was reduced in three other patients with propionic acidemia,[235] and because urinary propionylcarnitine was present in large amounts in such patients,[235] these workers proposed that patients with propionic acidemia have a relative carnitine deficiency. Subsequently, Wolff et al.[236] observed that L-carnitine supplements significantly reduced the ketogenic response to fasting in patients with propionic acidemia. Thus, it appears that long-term L-carnitine supplementation in these patients warrants serious consideration. To date, no results of long-term treatment with carnitine have been published.

The recognition that gut bacteria may contribute significantly to propionate production in at least some individuals[25] has led to the suggestion that specific antimicrobial therapy may be of clinical benefit to some children with propionic acidemia by reducing the total amount of propionate in their serum and tissues.[237] Metronidazole (10 mg/kg) has been reported to reduce fecal propionate substantially, concomitant with a reduction in the anaerobic bacterial count.[237] Plasma propionate also decreased by 50 to 60 percent in two patients, whereas urinary excretion of propionate metabolites was reduced by an average of 34 percent in four.[237] No comment was made on the effect of this treatment on the clinical status of these patients. Others have reported using a similar treatment, but also without any firm evidence of clinical efficacy[183] (see the later subsection on Diagnosis and Treatment under the section on The Methylmalonic Acidemias). Further study is clearly required to establish whether such therapy improves the management of acute episodes of metabolic decompensation or provides any long-term benefit with respect to growth, mental development, or neurologic outcome for this condition.

In a retrospective study of 17 patients (12 early-onset, 5 late-onset) from a single hospital over 20 years, 7 patients died (5 early-onset, 2 late-onset).[238] The neurologic outcome of the surviving patients was felt to be satisfactory, and was even better for early-onset patients. The investigators felt that other treatments such as liver transplantation or somatic gene therapy could improve the quality of life of propionic acidemia patients in the future.

Not unexpectedly, successful application of therapy, particularly in mildly affected patients, is leading to the survival of women with propionic acidemia into their child-bearing years. One report documents a relatively uneventful pregnancy and delivery in a woman mildly affected with propionic acidemia treated with protein restriction and carnitine supplementation.[239] Other such pregnancies are likely to occur; each will need to be handled individually according to the mother's specific clinical and biochemical status.

Multiple Carboxylase Deficiency. In 1971, Gompertz et al.[240] reported a male infant (J.R.) thought to have specific deficiency of the mitochondrial, biotin-dependent enzyme, β-methylcrotonyl CoA carboxylase (Fig. 94-5). This infant developed a diffuse, erythematous skin rash at 5 weeks of age and was admitted to the hospital at 5 months of age because of a worsening rash, recurrent vomiting, irritability, and a mild metabolic acidosis. His urine, which smelled like "tomcats' urine," was analyzed for organic acids and was found to contain large excesses of β-methylcrotonylglycine, tiglylglycine, and β-hydroxyisovaleric acid. When he was given 10 mg biotin (about 100 times the estimated human requirement) by mouth daily for several days, the rash, vomiting, irritability, and abnormal urine metabolites all disappeared dramatically. Several years later, it became clear that J.R. had multiple — not specific — carboxylase deficiency. His reanalyzed urine contained metabolites characteristic of propionyl CoA carboxylase deficiency, as well as β-methylcrotonyl CoA carboxylase deficiency[241]; his cultured fibroblast extracts were deficient in pyruvate carboxylase,[202] as well as in propionyl CoA and β-methylcrotonyl CoA carboxylase[242,243]; and supplementation of the fibroblast growth medium with biotin led to complete correction of the deficiency of all three biotin-dependent enzymes.[202,242,243] Subsequently, more than 50 children with multiple carboxylase deficiency have been described.[106] These children are now known to suffer from defects in one of two steps in biotin metabolism: the transfer of biotin to apocarboxylases, catalyzed by holocarboxylase synthase[244–247]; or the hydrolysis of biocytin, the biotin-containing product of degraded holocarboxylases, to release biotin, catalyzed by biotinidase.[248–250]

As a group, children with holocarboxylase synthase deficiency tend to present in the first days or weeks of life with feeding difficulties, hypotonia, lethargy, and seizures; some have a diffuse skin rash or alopecia.[106] The first described patient with multiple carboxylase deficiency, J.R., proved to have a defect in holocarboxylase synthase. Early studies showed that his enzyme had a reduced affinity for biotin when assayed *in vitro*.[251,252] This was confirmed by the identification of a point mutation in the biotin-binding region of the enzyme and the production of a biotin-responsive mutant enzyme when it was expressed in *E. coli*.[253,254] Several additional mutations have been identified in patients, many of them clustering within the biotin-binding region of the enzyme.[253–257]

A second, larger group of children is deficient in biotinidase activity.[248–250] These children usually present later in life (mean age of onset 3 months) with a variety of neurologic problems (seizures, hypotonia, developmental delay, hearing loss, optic atrophy). Although a large number of mutations have been identified in the biotinidase gene, several are highly prevalent and account for the majority of alleles in patients.[258–260]

Both groups respond dramatically to biotin supplements (10 mg daily) with prompt and sustained clinical improvement. Thus, multiple carboxylase deficiency differs markedly from isolated propionyl CoA carboxylase deficiency in response to biotin and, hence, in long-term prognosis. It should be emphasized, however, that the clinical presentations may be very similar. For this reason, urinary metabolite identification is of important therapeutic significance.

For more information on multiple carboxylase deficiency, the reader is referred to Chapter 156.

The Methylmalonic Acidemias

In 1967, Oberholzer,[10] Stokke,[11] and their colleagues described critically ill infants with profound metabolic ketoacidosis and developmental retardation who accumulated huge amounts of methylmalonate in their blood and urine. These children had none of the hematologic or neurologic stigmata of Cbl deficiency, failed to respond to Cbl supplements, and excreted much larger amounts of methylmalonate than those observed in patients with pernicious anemia.[6,7] They were presumed to have a congenital defect of methylmalonyl CoA racemase or of the methylmalonyl CoA mutase apoenzyme (Fig. 94-2). Shortly thereafter, Rosenberg,[261] Lindblad,[12,13] and their co-workers reported children with similar clinical presentations whose methylmalonic aciduria responded dramatically to pharmacologic but not physiologic amounts of CN-Cbl or AdoCbl. Such children were found subsequently to have a primary defect of AdoCbl synthesis that resulted in impaired mutase activity.[14,15] The array of different biochemical and clinical disturbances of methylmalonate metabolism was broadened still further in 1969 and 1970, when Mudd,[262] Goodman,[263] and their associates described children with methylmalonic aciduria whose clinical and chemical findings differed from those described above. Ketoacidosis was not present, and the increased methylmalonate excretion was accompanied by homocystinuria, cystathioninuria, and hypomethioninemia. This biochemical constellation was interpreted as evidence for defective synthesis of both Cbl coenzymes, with secondary impairment of AdoCbl-dependent methylmalonyl CoA mutase and MeCbl-dependent methionine synthase (Fig. 94-7). These early descriptions, coupled with a body of data to be discussed below, have demonstrated that there are many different biochemical bases for inherited forms of methylmalonic acidemia: two distinct defects of the mutase apoenzyme, one producing complete mutase deficiency (*mut*^{0}), the other partial deficiency (*mut*$^-$); two distinct defects of AdoCbl synthesis, one probably due to deficiency of a mitochondrial Cbl reductase (*cblA*), the other to deficiency of mitochondrial cob(I)alamin adenosyltransferase (*cblB*); and three distinct defects of both AdoCbl and MeCbl synthesis due to abnormal cytosolic or lysosomal metabolism of cobalamins (*cblC*, *cblD*, and *cblF*). Patients with lesions producing methylmalonic acidemia only (*mut*^{0}, *mut*$^-$, *cblA*, *cblB*) share many clinical features and will be discussed as a group; discussion of the other group of patients whose lesions produce methylmalonic acidemia and homocystinuria (*cblC*, *cblD*, and *cblF*) will follow.

Methylmalonyl CoA Mutase Deficiency. ***Clinical and Laboratory Presentation.*** More than 100 children with isolated mutase deficiency have been documented. Although, as mentioned above, there are four known etiologies for such deficiency, the clinical findings in affected patients from the four groups are remarkable more for their similarities than for their differences. Matsui et al. surveyed[264] the natural history in 45 such patients: 15 were *mut*^{0}; 5 were *mut*$^-$, 14 were *cblA*, and 11 were *cblB*. There were approximately equal numbers of males and females in each group. Information was obtained from questionnaires completed by the patients' physicians, published reports, unpublished communications, and personal experience. The most common signs and symptoms at the onset of clinical difficulty were lethargy, failure to thrive, recurrent vomiting, dehydration, respiratory distress, and muscular hypotonia (Table 94-1). Little interclass difference was observed for these major clinical manifestations or for such less common ones as developmental retardation, hepatomegaly, or coma. Patients in the *mut*^{0} class, however, presented earlier than those in the other groups (Fig. 94-9). Whereas 80 percent of children in the *mut*^{0} class became ill during the first week of life, less than half the children in the three other groups presented during this interval. Furthermore, clinical onset occurred in 90 percent of *mut*^{0} patients before the end of the first month, whereas onset beyond the first month was observed in an appreciable fraction of patients in each of the other groups. A survey of 20 *mut* patients has reached similar conclusions.[265]

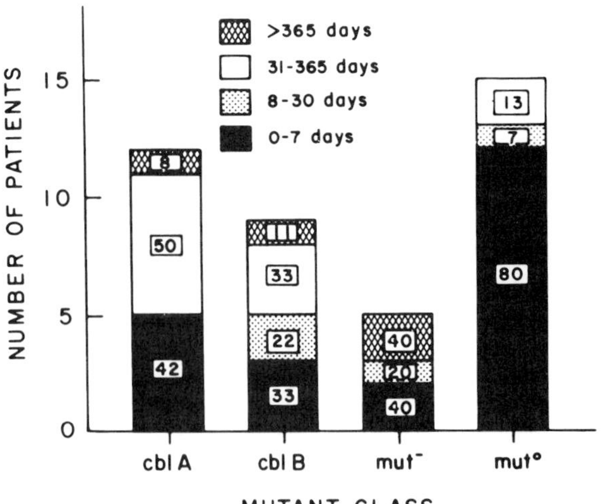

Fig. 94-9 Age at clinical onset in 45 patients with methylmalonic acidemia. Inset numbers denote percentages of patients in each group. (*Reprinted with permission from Matsui SM, Mahoney MJ, Rosenberg LE: The natural history of the inherited methylmalonic acidemias. New Engl J Med 308:857, 1983.*)

The laboratory findings in affected patients at the time that methylmalonic acidemia (with or without aciduria) was first documented are shown in Table 94-2. As expected, serum Cbl concentrations were routinely normal. Metabolic acidosis, with blood pH values as low as 6.9 and serum bicarbonate concentrations as low as 5 mEq/L, was observed in the majority of patients in all four groups. Ketonemia or ketonuria was found in 80 percent of patients, with hyperammonemia being only slightly less common, occurring in 70 percent of affected patients. Leukopenia, thrombocytopenia, and anemia were the only other manifestations that were noted in 50 percent or more of this group of patients. Earlier case reports[266] reported that hypoglycemia occurs in about 40 percent of affected patients. Inadvertently, this parameter was not assessed in this survey.

It should be mentioned that mutase deficiency is not always associated with serious clinical consequences. Ledley et al.[267] reported eight children, between the ages of 18 months and 13 years, who had methylmalonate accumulation in blood and urine,

Table 94-1 Clinical Presentation in 45 Patients wth Methylmalonic Acidemia

Signs and Symptoms at Onset	Mutant Class				
	cblA	*cblB*	*mut*$^-$	*mut*^{0}	Total
Lethargy	78	83	100	85	84
Failure to thrive	75	86	40	77	73
Recurrent vomiting	58	86	80	77	73
Dehydration	64	86	100	62	71
Respiratory distress	89	67	50	55	67
Muscular hypotonia	44	57	33	91	63
Developmental retardation	36	33	25	65	47
Hepatomegaly	11	67	0	57	41
Coma	50	29	40	38	40

Numerical values represent percentages of patients in each group. Reprinted with permission from reference 264.

Table 94-2 Laboratory Findings in 45 Patients with Methylmalonic Acidemia

Findings at Clinical Onset	Mutant Class				
	cblA	*cblB*	*mut*$^-$	*mut*^{0}	Total
Normal serum cobalamin	100	100	100	100	100
Metabolic acidosis	100	88	100	85	92
Ketonemia/ketonuria	78	67	100	85	81
Hyperammonemia	50	83	80	75	71
Hyperglycinemia/glycinuria	70	83	40	70	68
Leukopenia	70	45	60	62	60
Anemia	10	45	0	58	55
Thrombocytopenia	75	45	40	40	50

Numerical values represent percentages of patients in each group. Reprinted with permission from reference 264.

but had no symptoms. Presumably, these apomutase-deficient patients have an enzyme defect so "leaky" that homeostasis is not compromised. At least some of these individuals continued to be symptom free 7 years after the initial report.[268]

Another report determined that patients, initially ascertained by a newborn screening program with methylmalonic aciduria urine levels of less than 1400 mmoles/mmole creatinine, had normal somatic and cognitive outcomes.[269]

Conversely, another group of patients appear to have methylmalonic acidemia without a demonstrable defect in mutase activity, at least as measured in cultured cells. Although the elevations of methylmalonate are relatively mild as compared with mutase-deficient patients, they are chronic and usually are discovered on laboratory workup for failure to thrive or developmental retardation.[270] Because Cbl metabolism also appears to be normal in this group, the cause of the disease remains an enigma. Roe et al. have described a patient with psychomotor delay, methylmalonic aciduria without episodes of metabolic acidosis, and methylmalonic semialdehyde dehydrogenase deficiency.[271] It is possible that others in this group have the same defect.

***Chemical Abnormalities* In Vivo.** Large amounts of methylmalonic acid have been found in the urine or blood of all reported patients. Whereas normal children and adults excrete less than 0.04 mmole (5 mg) methylmalonate daily, children with isolated methylmalonic acidemia have excreted from 2.1 to 49 mmoles (240 to 5700 mg) in a 24-h period. Their plasma concentrations of methylmalonate, almost undetectable in normal subjects, have ranged from 0.22 to 2.9 mM (2.6–34 mg/dl). In the few patients in whom it was measured, the cerebrospinal fluid concentration of methylmalonate equaled that of plasma (for references to early case reports, the reader is referred elsewhere[266]). It is important to note that patients with mild, late-onset, or "benign"[267] disease may have much lower levels, particularly when clinically asymptomatic.[267,268] No relationship between the quantities of methylmalonate accumulated in body fluids and the etiology of mutase deficiency (i.e., apoenzyme vs. coenzyme deficiency) has been reported. Methylmalonate is surely the major, but not the only, abnormal metabolite found in body fluids of these patients. Because propionyl CoA carboxylation is reversible, propionate and some of its precursors (butanone) or metabolites (β-hydroxypropionate and methylcitrate) also accumulate in blood and urine,[8,92,93,272,273] although their amounts are small compared with that of methylmalonate.

Several groups have studied the relationship between protein or amino acid loading and methylmalonate accumulation in these patients. Without exception, administration of protein or amino acids known to be precursors of propionate and methylmalonate, such as methionine, threonine, valine, or isoleucine, has resulted in augmented methylmalonate accumulation and, in some instances, ketosis or acidosis.[8,10–12] When Cbl-responsive patients are given supplements of this vitamin, such augmentation by methylmalonate precursors is lessened considerably.[274] All these findings suggest that patients with discrete defects at the mutase step have a major block in the utilization of methylmalonyl CoA that is expressed as methylmalonate accumulation.

Localization of Enzymatic Defects. Because the conversion of propionate to succinate is blocked in each of the methylmalonic acidemias, an early screening test for these disorders measured the ability of intact peripheral blood leukocytes or cultured fibroblasts to oxidize [^{14}C]propionate to $^{14}CO_2$ and compared this with the oxidation of [^{14}C]succinate to $^{14}CO_2$.[261] By including estimation of [^{14}C]methylmalonate oxidation as well, this test can distinguish between deficiency of propionyl CoA carboxylase and of methylmalonyl CoA mutase. Incorporation of [^{14}C]propionate into trichloroacetic acid–precipitable material by intact cultured cells has replaced the more cumbersome $^{14}CO_2$ evolution technique.[230,275] Further discrimination among the methylmalonic acidemias has depended on studies of Cbl uptake and AdoCbl formation by intact cultured fibroblasts, on assays of mutase activity in cell extracts, and on genetic complementation studies with cultured cell heterokaryons.

Table 94-3 Methylmalonyl CoA Mutase Activity in Liver Homogenates from Patients with Methylmalonic Acidemia

Subjects	Enzymatic Activity* Without Added AdoCbl	With Added AdoCbl (4×10^{-5} M)
Controls (3)	535–866	799–1058
Patients		
1	1	3
2	8	33
3	3	7
4	80	1368

*Assayed by measuring conversion of DL-[^{3}H]methylmalonyl CoA to [^{3}H]succinyl CoA. Values expressed as picomoles of succinate formed per milligram protein per 30 min.

Reprinted with permission from reference 276.

Mutase Apoenzyme Deficiency. Morrow and colleagues[276] provided the first evidence *in vitro* for apoenzyme abnormalities and for biochemical heterogeneity among the methylmalonic acidemias. In four patients who had died, they studied mutase activity in liver homogenates by measuring the conversion of DL-[^{3}H]methylmalonyl CoA to [^{3}H]succinyl CoA (Table 94-3). Activity was barely detectable in three and showed no response when AdoCbl was added at concentrations sufficient to saturate the normal enzyme. In the fourth, mutase activity was restored to control values by AdoCbl. These findings were interpreted as evidence for a mutase apoenzyme defect in the first three patients and for defective AdoCbl synthesis in the fourth. These findings were confirmed subsequently in studies with cultured fibroblasts.[277] Cells from the first three patients synthesized AdoCbl normally but had much reduced mutase activity in extracts regardless of the amount of AdoCbl added; cells from the fourth had a distinct defect in AdoCbl synthesis.

Subsequently, it has become clear that two general types of apomutase defects exist. In one type, designated mut^0 and constituting about two thirds of the *mut* complementation group, mutase activity in extracts of cultured fibroblasts is undetectable (<0.1 percent of control), even when assayed in the presence of AdoCbl concentrations greatly in excess of that normally required to saturate the enzyme.[277–279] When CRM was sought by radioimmunoassay under steady-state conditions in cell lines from 21 such patients, 12 had no immunologically identifiable mutase protein (CRM$^-$), whereas 9 had reduced amounts of CRM ranging from 1 to 40 percent of that found in control extracts.[280] In a follow-up study,[281] cells from this group of patients were pulse labeled to determine how amounts of newly synthesized mutase protein, detected by specific immunoprecipitation, compared with the CRM values obtained under steady-state conditions. As expected, all CRM$^+$ mutants had easily detectable newly synthesized mutase. Of 11 CRM$^-$ lines, however, 5 had amounts of newly synthesized mutase ranging from barely detectable to nearly half that seen in controls. Thus, some apomutase mutations lead to the synthesis of unstable mutase proteins, which are rapidly degraded intracellularly. One other result of this study bears mention. Using a pulse-chase experimental protocol, mitochondrial import and cleavage of the apomutase precursor were studied in control lines and in 38 lines from *mut* mutants that synthesized mutase protein. In one of the 38 mutant lines, an N-terminal deletion resulted in failure of the mutant mutase to be taken up by mitochondria.[281,282] All the others underwent normal mitochondrial uptake and processing.

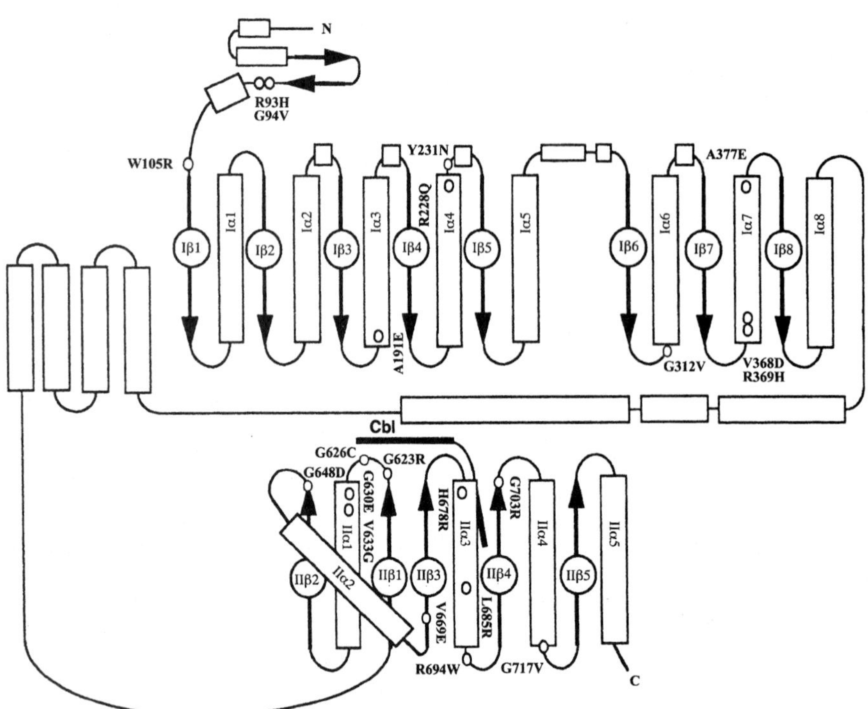

Fig. 94-10 Schematic representation of the secondary structure of human methylmalonyl CoA mutase, predicted by homology modeling based on the radiographic structure of the *P. shermanii* mutase α subunit. Helices are denoted by rectangles, β strands by bold arrows, and coils or turns by a thin line. For each of the two main domains, the βα pairs are labeled. The AdoCbl is represented by the horizontal thick line labeled Cbl (the position of the corrin ring) attached to an almost vertical thick line indicating the DMB side chain as it extends into the Cbl-binding domain. The approximate positions of a number of characterized missense mutations determined in *mut* patients are indicated on the structure by small ellipses. Although many mutations affecting AdoCbl binding are located in the Cbl-binding domain, several, including R93H, Y231N, and R369H, are in the N-terminal $(\beta\alpha)_8$ barrel domain. (Redrawn with permission from Thoma NH, Leadley PF: Homology modelling of human methylmalonyl-CoA mutase: A structural basis for point mutations causing methylmalonic aciduria. *Protein Sci* 5:1922, 1996.)

The second type, designated *mut*⁻, involves a structurally abnormal mutase apoenzyme. The mutant apoenzymes in extracts of these cells retain maximally 2 to 75 percent of control activity, have a K_m for AdoCbl approximately 200 to 5000 times normal, show a normal K_m for methylmalonyl CoA, and exhibit increased thermolability relative to control enzyme.[278,279,283] By radioimmunoassay, the amount of immunologically reactive mutase protein in these extracts ranges from 20 to 100 percent of control.[280] Because pairwise crosses between mut^0 and mut^- generally yield noncomplementing heterokaryons and because there are affected individuals who appear to be mut^0/mut^- compound heterozygotes, both mutant types reflect abnormalities of the locus coding for the apomutase structural gene.[278,279] The identification of nonsense and missense mutations within the mutase gene that lead to absent enzyme or abnormal enzyme kinetics have firmly established this conclusion.

Ledley and his colleagues first described the molecular changes in *mut* patients. They surveyed a number of patient fibroblasts and found no evidence for gross rearrangements at the genomic level, but reductions in mRNA in some lines.[284] A number of point mutations were described, including nonsense changes that lead to a mut^0 phenotype,[282] missense mutations that also generate a mut^0 phenotype,[285,286] and a missense mutation that generates a mut^- phenotype.[287] Each of these changes was confirmed as a mutation causing deficiency of mutase activity by expressing the variant protein, either in a mut^0 fibroblast line[285,286] or in *Saccharomyces cerevisiae* cells.[287] Interestingly, one of the mut^0 lines was able to complement a number of the other mut^0 and mut^- lines, although not all,[286] an example of interallelic complementation. To date, 28 mutations and 2 benign sequence changes have been identified, some of which have been characterized by expression in cultured cells or in *E. coli*.[68,288,289] A common mutation (G717V) was found in five black patients of African and African-American ancestry,[290,291] and in a series of patients from Japan, six patients carried the same mutation (E117X).[292]

Figure 94-10 is a linear representation of the structure of human mutase,[86] based on the crystal structure of the *P. shermanii* homologue.[87] On it are indicated the locations of a number of the missense mutations in mutase identified so far. The effects of some of these on mutase activity have been rationalized in terms of the predicted three-dimensional structure of the human enzyme.[68,86,289,293] The easiest to explain are the mut^0 mutations G630E and G703R, affecting residues that line the binding pocket for the DMB side-chain of AdoCbl. Although both change flexible glycine residues to charged ones, the main effect is to introduce bulky side chains into the narrow binding pocket, effectively blocking access to it and preventing AdoCbl binding.[293] Some changes in the Cbl-binding domain (G623R, G626C) appear to affect the positioning of His627, whose side-chain provides the essential bottom ligand to the bound AdoCbl,[86,293] whereas others likely affect the position or interaction of the βα strands that form the Cbl-binding domain. One of these, G717V, results in a highly unstable protein, in addition to modifying AdoCbl binding.[68] Mutations in the N-terminal TIM barrel, particularly those producing a mut^- phenotype, are less easily explained. W105R appears to affect the substrate channel in the TIM barrel, whereas A377E, V368D, and R369H are in the likely dimer interface. The interaction between dimerization or dimer stability and AdoCbl binding, revealed by the mut^- phenotype of R369H,[68] remains unexplained.

Even less apparent is an explanation of the interallelic complementation supported by two mutations in the N-terminus of mutase, R93H and G94V. R93H was identified in homozygous form in a cell line that showed interallelic complementation with a

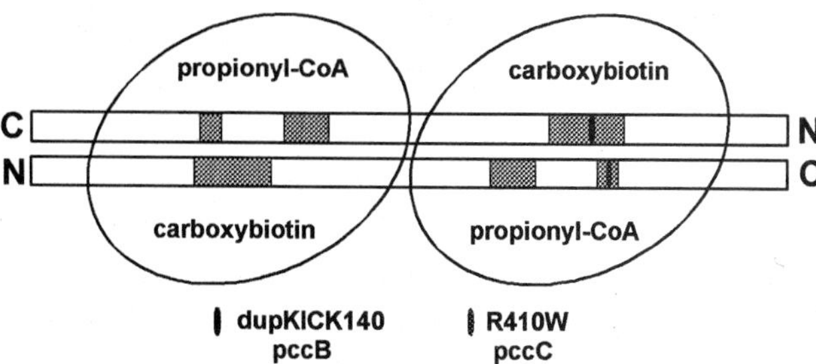

Fig. 94-11 Model for interallelic complementation between *pccB* and *pccC* mutations causing propionic acidemia. The schematic shows a pair of β subunits aligned head to toe so that two functional domains are produced, with the carboxybiotin site coming from one subunit and the propionyl CoA binding site coming from the other. In the case in which each β subunit contains complementing mutations—near the N-terminus of one subunit for dupKICK140 and near the C-terminus of the other subunit for R410W—the outcome is that only one of the two functional sites is inactivated. The second functional site retains activity despite the presence of a mutation on each subunit.

number of other *mut* lines,[286] and G94V was found in heterozygous form in a cell line that appeared to show interallelic complementation with the G717V mutation *in vivo*.[68] Subsequent *in vitro* experiments with mutant proteins expressed in *E. coli* have confirmed its ability to complement a range of other *mut* cell lines (J. Janata and W. Fenton, unpublished observations). This region of mutase is the least homologous between the human and *P. shermanii* enzymes. In the bacterial enzyme, this region forms a long element that wraps around the TIM domain of the other subunit, and thus appears to be involved with subunit–subunit interactions. How this relates to AdoCbl binding (G94V is mut^-)[68] and how these mutations modify the effects of mutations in the distant Cbl-binding domain to produce interallelic complementation are questions that may only be answered by crystal structures of the human enzyme and these mutant versions.

It seems clear from the available structures, however, that complementation is not simply a matter of bringing together unaffected regions from each subunit of a mutase dimer to form one "normal" active site,[293] as may be the case for the β subunits of PCC (Fig. 94-11). The active site of mutase is clearly contained in a single subunit, with no possibility for sharing elements of it between subunits.[87] Moreover, the combined active site model predicts that the kinetic parameters of the restored site should be the same as wild type. This is not what is observed *in vivo* for the complementing G94V/G717V pair, where the "complemented," presumably heterodimeric, enzyme has a K_m at least 10-fold lower than either of its homodimeric parents, but 100-fold higher than wild type.[68] Similar results have been obtained *in vitro* by combining the individually expressed mutant enzymes (J. Janata and W. Fenton, unpublished observations), suggesting a more complex mechanism for restoration of activity upon interallelic complementation between mutase mutants.

Finally, it should be mentioned that the only patient thus far reported to have methylmalonyl CoA racemase deficiency[294] has been restudied and shown conclusively to be a mut^- mutant biochemically and genetically.[17]

Defective Synthesis of AdoCbl. A series of observations by Rosenberg,[14] Mahoney,[15] and their colleagues on the fibroblasts of the index patient with Cbl-responsive methylmalonic acidemia led to the demonstration of a primary defect in AdoCbl synthesis in intact cells, resulting in a deficiency of mutase activity. Although intact cells were unable to convert OH-[^{57}Co]Cbl to Ado[^{57}Co]Cbl, cell-free extracts from this line synthesized AdoCbl normally when incubated with OH-[^{57}Co]Cbl, ATP, and a reducing system designed to bypass the Cbl reductases (Fig. 94-8). Subsequent biochemical[167] and genetic complementation[295–297] studies have differentiated two mutant classes among patients defective in AdoCbl synthesis. One class, which contains the index Cbl-responsive patient, is designated *cblA*, and may be due to a deficiency of one of the mitochondrial Cbl reductases, perhaps an NADPH-linked aquacobalamin reductase.[298] Complementation has been demonstrated between several *cblA* lines, raising the possibility of interallelic complementation in this disorder as well.[299] The second, designated *cblB*, has been shown to result from a specific deficiency of cob(I)alamin adenosyltransferase.[168]

Pathophysiology. All studies *in vivo* and *in vitro* in patients with methylmalonic acidemia due to specific methylmalonyl CoA mutase deficiency indicate that the primary block in the conversion of methylmalonyl CoA to succinyl CoA explains the accumulation of methylmalonate in blood and urine; the augmentation of methylmalonate excretion and the precipitation of ketosis by protein, amino acids, or propionate; and the excretion of long-chain ketones formed in the catabolism of branched chain amino acids. However, the primary block does not explain several important physiologic disturbances: the acidosis, hypoglycemia, hyperglycinemia, and hyperammonemia. Oberholzer et al.[10] pointed out that the concentration of methylmalonate in the blood (no more than 3 mM) could not alone explain the acidosis and suggested other possibilities. They proposed that an accumulation of CoA, "trapped" intracellularly as methylmalonyl CoA, could lead to an insufficiency of this widely utilized coenzyme and, secondarily, to impaired carbohydrate metabolism and subsequent acidosis. Alternatively, they suggested that an excess of methylmalonyl CoA, a known inhibitor of pyruvate carboxylase,[300] could interfere with gluconeogenesis and lead directly to hypoglycemia and indirectly to excessive catabolism of lipid, with ketosis and acidosis. Halperin et al.[301] showed that methylmalonate inhibited the transmitochondrial shuttle of malate and argued that impairment of this key step in gluconeogenesis could lead to hypoglycemia. As discussed earlier for deficiencies of β-ketothiolase and propionyl CoA carboxylase, the mechanism of the hyperglycinemia and hyperammonemia so often observed in children with any one of these disorders probably reflects inhibition of the intramitochondrial glycine cleavage enzyme and of CPS I, respectively, by the accumulated organic acids or their CoA esters.[208,209,211–215] Thus, as shown in Fig. 94-12, each of the major secondary biochemical abnormalities in the propionic and methylmalonic acidemias can be explained satisfactorily by inhibition of specific intramitochondrial processes by the accumulated organic acids and esters.

As a further consideration, about half the reported patients with isolated methylmalonic acidemia also show pancytopenia.[264] One report suggests that methylmalonate inhibits growth of marrow stem cells in a concentration-dependent fashion.[302]

By comparing and contrasting the findings in patients with isolated mutase deficiency with those in patients with Cbl deficiency (as in classic pernicious anemia), it has been possible to shed some light on the mechanism responsible for the hematologic and neurologic abnormalities in the latter disorder. Thus, the absence of megaloblastic anemia in any patient with isolated mutase deficiency militates against any involvement of this enzyme in the typical megaloblastosis seen in Cbl deficiency. Similarly, the cerebellar and posterior column abnormalities so often encountered in Cbl-deficient patients have never been observed in patients with methylmalonic acidemia due to specific mutase dysfunction. Therefore, the notion that neurologic dysfunction in pernicious anemia reflects aberrant incorporation of odd-chain or branched-chain fatty acids into myelin because of a block in the propionate pathway has little to recommend it. It appears likely, then, that abnormalities in the Cbl-dependent methionine synthase account for the hematologic and neurologic

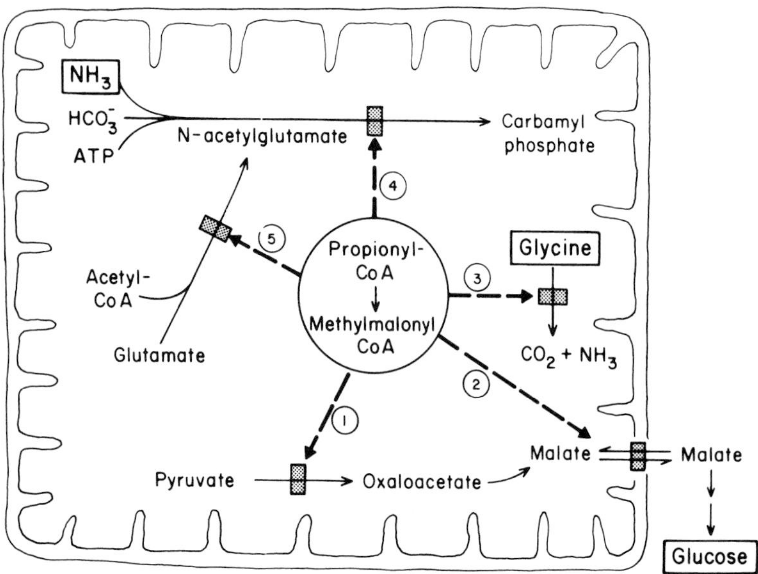

Fig. 94-12 Proposed mechanisms of hypoglycemia, hyperglycinemia, and hyperammonemia in patients with inherited deficiencies of β-ketothiolase (see Chapter 93), propionyl CoA carboxylase, or methylmalonyl CoA mutase. Inhibitory effects of the enlarged intramitochondrial pools of acyl CoA esters (such as propionyl CoA) or their respective free acids on selected mitochondrial functions are shown by the numbered dashed lines corresponding to the following enzymatic or shuttle-mediated reactions: (1) pyruvate carboxylase; (2) the transmitochondrial malate shuttle; (3) the glycine cleavage enzyme; (4) carbamyl phosphate synthetase I; and (5) *N*-acetylglutamate synthetase.

abnormalities in Cbl-deficient patients. This matter will be discussed further when we consider that group of patients with methylmalonic acidemia and homocystinuria.

Genetic Considerations. Each of the four etiologic bases for specific methylmalonyl CoA mutase deficiency (mut^0, mut^-, *cblA*, and *cblB*) is almost certainly inherited as an autosomal-recessive trait. This conclusion is based on the following findings. First, approximately equal numbers of affected males and females are encountered in each group.[264] Second, no instance of vertical transmission from affected parent to affected child has been reported. Third, interclass heterokaryons formed between cell lines from different etiologic groups (i.e., $mut^0 \times cblA$) complement each other, whereas intraclass heterokaryons (i.e., $mut^0 \times mut^0$) generally do not (with the exception of interallelic complementation); thus, each mutant class behaves as a recessive in culture.[295–297] Fourth, cell lines from heterozygotes for the mut^0, mut^-, and *cblB* mutations show partial mutase apoenzyme deficiency[279] and partial adenosyltransferase deficiency,[168] respectively. And fifth, among a large group of *mut* mutants studied, some have inherited a genetically different mutant allele from each parent, thereby being compound heterozygotes rather than true homozygotes.[279,284,285]

It is not possible to define with any precision the prevalence of these disorders in the general population. A survey of newborns in Massachusetts has suggested that methylmalonic acidemia may occur in 1:48,000 infants.[303] A similar survey in Quebec yielded 1:61,000 infants.[304] Because this study screened urines from infants 3 to 4 weeks of age and because it is known that many children with methylmalonic acidemia die in the first week of life from ketoacidosis or hyperammonemia or both, the true prevalence must be greater.

Diagnosis, Treatment, and Prognosis. Because simple colorimetric assays for urinary methylmalonate and more complex gas chromatography–mass spectrometry assays for serum and urinary methylmalonate are now available, it should no longer be difficult to make a diagnosis of methylmalonic acidemia once this condition is considered. Other sources of neonatal or infantile ketoacidosis must be ruled out. If excessive amounts of methylmalonate are found in the urine, Cbl deficiency can be excluded by direct measurement of serum Cbl concentration. Confirmation and etiologic designation (i.e., *mut* or *cbl*) depend on studies with cultured cells and extracts therefrom.[17,305] Prenatal detection of methylmalonic acidemia has been accomplished in two ways: by measurement of methylmalonate in amniotic fluid and maternal urine at mid-trimester[306,307] and by studies of mutase activity and Cbl metabolism in cultured amniotic fluid cells.[295,307,308] Assays of [^{14}C]propionate utilization[230] in uncultured chorionic villous biopsy specimens have proven unsatisfactory, however.[309] Mutase apoenzyme[307,308] and AdoCbl synthesis[230,306] deficiencies have been identified prenatally.

Two treatment regimens for children with methylmalonic acidemia exist and should be used in tandem. A diet restricted in protein (or a special formula restricted in amino acid precursors of methylmalonate) should be instituted as soon as life-threatening problems such as ketoacidosis, hypoglycemia, or hyperammonemia have been addressed; and supplementary Cbl (1–2 mg CN-Cbl or, preferably, OH-Cbl intramuscularly daily for several days) should be given as soon as the diagnosis of methylmalonic acidemia is made (or even seriously considered). Such measures should decrease the circulating concentrations of methylmalonate and propionate. Even Cbl-unresponsive children with delayed development have been shown to improve markedly when treated with careful dietary protein restriction.[310,311] As discussed above for patients with propionyl CoA carboxylase deficiency, Roe and associates[235,312,313] have pointed out that L-carnitine supplements may be a useful therapeutic adjunct in patients with methylmalonic acidemia, presumably by repleting intracellular and extracellular stores of free carnitine that are depleted in affected patients because of exchange with excess methylmalonyl CoA and propionyl CoA. Likewise, oral antibiotic therapy may prove useful here as well. Thompson and his colleagues report that three patients showed subjective improvement in alertness and appetite following brief metronidazole therapy[237]; longer treatment periods have resulted in significant improvements in other patients, including decreased number and severity of acidotic episodes, increased appetite, decreased vomiting, growth acceleration, and improved behavior.[29,314] Total parenteral nutrition also has been used in at least one reported case.[233]

The previously mentioned survey[264] suggests that both the response to Cbl supplements and the long-term outcome in affected patients depend considerably on the nature of the biochemical lesion causing the methylmalonic acidemia. As shown in Figure 94-13, essentially none of the children designated mut^0 or mut^- responded to Cbl supplements with a distinct decrease in blood or urinary methylmalonate, whereas over 90 percent of the *cblA* and about 40 percent of the *cblB* patients showed such a response. Given the complete absence of mutase activity in cells from the mut^0 group, it is not surprising that they

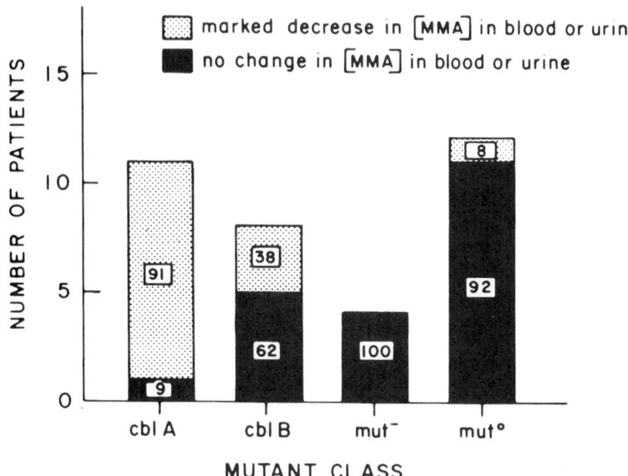

Fig. 94-13 Biochemical response to cobalamin supplementation in 45 patients with methylmalonic acidemia. *MMA* refers to the concentration of methylmalonate. The supplementation protocol generally used 1 mg CN-Cbl parenterally daily for 7 to 14 days. Inset numbers denote the percentage of patients in each group. (*Reprinted from Matsui SM, Mahoney MJ, Rosenberg LE: The natural history of the inherited methylmalonic acidemias. New Engl J Med 308:857, 1983.*)

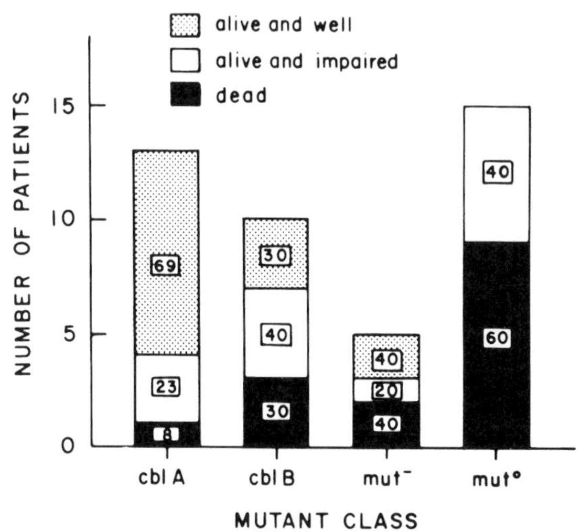

Fig. 94-14 Long-term outcome in 45 patients with methylmalonic acidemia. The ages of the patients surveyed ranged from a few weeks to 14 years. (*Reprinted with permission from Matsui SM, Mahoney MJ, Rosenberg LE: The natural history of the inherited methylmalonic acidemias. New Engl J Med 308:857, 1983.*)

were regularly Cbl-unresponsive *in vivo*. The disappointing absence of response in four *mut*$^-$ patients presumably means that even parenteral Cbl supplements could not drive tissue concentrations of AdoCbl sufficiently high to increase significantly their mutase holoenzyme activity. The fraction (60 percent) of *cblB* patients unresponsive to Cbl supplements presumably has such complete adenosyltransferase deficiency that AdoCbl synthesis cannot be augmented by Cbl supplements, as it apparently can in the *cblB* patients with leaky mutations that permit responsiveness *in vivo*. Patients in the *cblA* group were uniformly responsive, suggesting either that the responsible mutations are generally leaky, thereby allowing mass action to result in more AdoCbl synthesis, or that alternative pathways of Cbl reduction that require high substrate concentrations exist in cells. It should be emphasized that clinical responsiveness *in vivo* does not mean complete correction of mutase deficiency. Even in a patient whose clinical improvement is dramatic, Cbl administration only reduces, rather than eliminates, methylmalonate excretion. Studies with cultured cells from a variety of patients with methylmalonic acidemia[17,297] suggest that raising holomutase activity to only 10 percent of normal values by supplementing the growth medium with OH-Cbl results in distinct augmentation of propionate pathway activity (or, conversely, in a distinct decrease in the magnitude of the metabolic block). Some patients in the *cblB* group, unresponsive to CN-Cbl or OH-Cbl *in vivo*, might be expected to respond to AdoCbl itself, but published reports on two patients suggest that this logical alternative is ineffective.[315,316]

The long-term outlook for affected patients is revealing. As noted in Fig. 94-14, the *mut*^{0} group has the poorest prognosis, with 60 percent deceased and 40 percent distinctly impaired developmentally at the time of the survey. Shevell et al. reported similar findings.[265] In sharp contrast, the *cblA* patients (i.e., the group biochemically most responsive to Cbl supplements) had the best outcome: 70 percent were alive and well at ages up to 14 years. The *cblB* and *mut*$^-$ groups were intermediate, with about equal fractions in each group being found in the alive and well, the alive and impaired, or the deceased category.

It is interesting, albeit anecdotal, that the index patient in the *cblA* group (now over 30 years old) discontinued Cbl supplements at age 9 years despite advice to the contrary. In the ensuing years, his development and general health have remained excellent despite the high concentration of methylmalonate in his blood and his continued excretion of very large amounts of methylmalonate.

Perhaps, as in some other inherited metabolic disorders, treatment of methylmalonic acidemia is most critical during the early years of life, making expert clinical management in the early weeks or months of life most important. There have been several reports of "metabolic stroke" in patients following episodes of metabolic decompensation.[317–319] Three of the patients[317,318] belonged to the Cbl-responsive *cblA* group, but were not being treated at the time. Extrapyramidal signs, particularly dystonia, were accompanied by bilateral lucencies of the globus pallidus and persisted after the acute crisis had passed. In one case, the dystonia has been gradually progressive over a period of 7 years without visible progression of the neurologic lesions.[319]

Another complication of long-term survival of some methylmalonic acidemia patients is chronic renal failure.[320] One report has indicated that 8 of 12 non–Cbl-responsive patients (1–9 years of age) had a reduced glomerular filtration rate, with five severely affected.[321] In one of these, "greatly improved metabolic control" over a period of 18 months led to increased, but still impaired, renal function.[321] Significantly, the index *cblA* patient referred to above returned for treatment of moderate renal dysfunction due to biopsy-proven interstitial nephritis. We do not yet know what impact better metabolic control and Cbl supplementation may have in this and similar cases.

A 7-year-old boy with *mut*$^-$ methylmalonic aciduria developed persistent lactic acidosis and multiorgan failure. He was shown to have glutathionine deficiency and responded to treatment with high-dose ascorbate.[322]

The feasibility of prenatal therapy with Cbl supplements also has been demonstrated. Ampola et al.[307] showed that administration of Cbl supplements to a woman carrying a Cbl-responsive, affected fetus resulted in significant reduction in maternal excretion of methylmalonate. Other cases also have been reported.[323,324] However, the value of this regimen over one in which therapy is instituted immediately postnatally remains to be established.

Because of the poor prognosis of early-onset severe methylmalonic aciduria, liver transplantation has been attempted in a limited number of patients.[325–328] Although liver transplantation appears to protect against acute metabolic decompensation, biochemical correction is incomplete and it is not certain that there will be complete protection against the renal and neurologic complications. Finally, it must be noted that preliminary steps have been taken toward somatic gene therapy for mutase deficiency.[329,330] Besides all the usual questions of safety and long-term stability of response that surround somatic gene therapy, two important issues remain unanswered for mutase: How much activity must be restored *in vivo* to normalize the biochemical hallmarks of the disease? And, does correction of the defect in the liver, for example, lead to reversal or amelioration of the pathologic changes in other organ systems, such as the kidneys, and overall clinical improvement? Much work remains to be done before we can address these problems.

Combined Deficiency of Methylmalonyl CoA Mutase and Methionine Synthase. ***Clinical and Laboratory Presentations.*** Many patients with inherited combined methylmalonic acidemia and homocystinuria have been the subject of individual case reports.[263,331–347] Cells from these children comprise three biochemically and genetically distinct complementation groups, designated *cblC*, *cblD*, and *cblF*.[167,295,296,348]

Clinical findings have varied widely among the more than 100 known patients in the *cblC* group, including some who have been diagnosed only in adult life. In a review of 50 patients, 44 had onset in the first year of life and 6 had onset after 6 years of age.[349] The median age of onset was 1 month, and the range was from birth to 14 years. Thirteen of the early-onset patients died, with a mean age of death at 9.6 months and a range of 1 to 47 months. The early-onset patients had feeding difficulties, hypotonia, failure to thrive, seizures, microcephaly, developmental delay, cortical atrophy, hydrocephalus, nystagmus, pigmentary retinopathy, and decreased visual acuity. Blood findings included megaloblastic anemia, thrombocytopenia, leukopenia, and neutropenenia. In some patients there was renal failure, sometimes with a hemolytic-uremic syndrome. The later-onset patients presented in childhood or adolescence with acute neurologic findings, which included decreased cognitive performance, confusion, dementia, delirium, myelopathy, and tremor. Only one late-onset patient in this series had pigmentary retinopathy. Hematologic abnormalities were seen in half the late-onset patients. Significantly, serum Cbl and folate concentrations are generally normal in *cblC* patients.

Neither of the two brothers in the *cblD* group[263] had any clinically significant problems until later in life. The older brother came to medical attention because of severe behavioral pathology and moderate mental retardation at 14 years of age. He also had a poorly defined neuromuscular problem involving his lower extremities. His then 2-year-old brother was asymptomatic, although biochemically affected. No hematologic abnormalities were noted in either sib.

Five patients have been reported in the *cblF* group. The first two (both female) were small for gestational age and had methylmalonic aciduria, poor feeding, growth retardation, and persistent stomatitis.[344,345] One had minor facial anomalies, dextrocardia, and abnormal Cbl absorption from the gut. The other had a persistent rash, macrocytosis, and elevated homocysteine and died suddenly despite a good biochemical response to Cbl treatment. A male *cblF* patient had recurrent stomatitis in infancy, arthritis at age 4, and confusion, disorientation, and a pigmentary dermatitis at age 10.[347] Another boy had aspiration pneumonia at birth, hypotonia, lethargy, hypoglycemia, thrombocytopenia, and neutropenia. A native Canadian girl was diagnosed at 6 months of age because of anemia, failure to thrive, developmental delay, recurrent infections, low serum Cbl, and Cbl malabsorption.[346] As a group, the *cblF* patients have responded well to treatment with Cbl.

***Chemical Abnormalities* In Vivo.** In addition to the methylmalonic aciduria and homocystinuria that characterize the *cblC*, *cblD*, and *cblF* groups of patients, some have shown hypomethioninemia and cystathioninuria. This constellation of chemical abnormalities, plus the normal serum Cbl values, led to the proposal[262,331] that these children suffered from a defect in cellular metabolism of Cbl such that both Cbl-dependent enzyme activities (mutase and methionine synthase; see Fig. 94-7) were deficient. The methylmalonic aciduria in these children is distinctly less severe than that encountered in children with isolated mutase deficiency. It is important to note that elevations of homocystine may be unremarkable in some *cblC* patients, even when acutely ill. One of the *cblF* patients had no detectable homocystinuria despite a cellular deficit in methionine synthase activity,[344] although all the others have shown homocystinuria.[345–347] Moreover, neither hyperglycinemia nor hyperammonemia has been reported in any of the *cblC*, *cblD*, or *cblF* patients.

Localization of Defective Cellular Metabolism of Cbl. It has long been clear that patients in the *cblC* and *cblD* groups have a defect in cellular metabolism of Cbl. This conclusion is based on the following data: total Cbl content of liver, kidney, and cultured fibroblasts is markedly reduced[262,332,350,351]; the ability of cultured cells to retain ^{57}Co-labeled CN-Cbl[352] or to convert ^{57}Co-labeled CN-Cbl or OH-Cbl to AdoCbl and MeCbl is markedly impaired[15,296]; activity of methylmalonyl CoA mutase and methionine synthase in cultured cells is deficient, such deficiency being improved by supplementation of the growth medium with OH-Cbl[296,297,353]; and the mutase and methionine synthase apoenzymes in cells from affected patients appear to be normal.[262,263,296,297,354] The precise nature of the metabolic defect in the *cblC* and *cblD* classes remains elusive, but some progress has been made. Because these mutant cells demonstrate normal receptor-mediated adsorptive endocytosis of the TC II–Cbl complex and normal intralysosomal hydrolysis of TC II,[17,153,154,296] perusal of Fig. 94-8 makes it clear that the defects in the *cblC* and *cblD* cells affect some step or steps subsequent to cellular uptake, common to the synthesis of both coenzymes, and prior to the binding of the Cbl coenzymes to their respective apoproteins. Significantly, *cblC* (and, to a lesser extent, *cblD*) cells use CN-Cbl less well than OH-Cbl[353,355] and are unable to convert CN-Cbl to OH-Cbl, a step shown in normal cells to be a metabolic prerequisite for the synthesis of both AdoCbl and MeCbl.[355] The latter results have been interpreted as evidence for a defect in a cytosolic cob(III)alamin reductase, which is required for reducing the trivalent cobalt of Cbl prior to alkylation.[355] In both *cblC* and *cblD* fibroblast extracts, partial deficiencies of CN-Cbl β-ligand transferase and microsomal cob(III)alamin reductase have been described by Pezacka.[356,357] Watanabe and colleagues have described a partial deficiency of a mitochondrial NADH-linked aquacobalamin reductase in *cblC* fibroblast extracts.[298] The suggestion that glutathionyl Cbl may be an intermediate in the reductive pathway[358] provides another potential site for the mutation in one of these groups. Finally, it should be pointed out that the distinction between the *cblC* and *cblD* classes is based first and foremost on complementation studies that define the two classes as unique,[296] although essentially only one example of *cblD* exists. The biochemical differences between them appear to be quantitative rather than qualitative, with the *cblC* group having more severe metabolic derangements (and, at the same time, more severe clinical involvement) than the sibs designated *cblD*. Thus, the possibility must be considered that *cblD* is an allele of *cblC* that shows interallelic complementation.

Studies using cultured fibroblasts from two patients in the *cblF* group are of particular interest. As with cells from *cblC* and *cblD* patients, both mutase and methionine synthase activities were impaired, and AdoCbl and MeCbl contents were reduced. In contrast to the *cblC* and *cblD* mutants, however, the *cblF* cells accumulated unmetabolized, non–protein-bound CN-Cbl in lysosomes.[359] These findings indicate that *cblF* cells are deficient in the mediated process by which Cbl vitamers exit from lysosomes after being taken up by receptor-mediated endocytosis.

The biochemical features of patient fibroblasts that distinguish the various methylmalonic acidemias are summarized in Table 94-4.

Table 94-4 Salient Biochemial Features of Cultured Fibroblasts from Patients with the Various Methylmalonic Acidemias

	Mutant Class						
Biochemical Parameter	*mut*⁰	*mut*⁻	*cblA*	*cblB*	*cblC*	*cblD*	*cblF*
Studies with intact cells							
[^{14}C]propionate oxidation	−	−	−	−	−	−	−
[^{14}C]MeH_4F fixation	+	+	+	+	−	−	−
MeCbl synthesis	+	+	+	+	−	−	−
AdoCbl synthesis	+	+	−	−	−	−	−
Conversion of CN-Cbl to OH-Cbl	+	+	+	+	−	±	−
Lysosomal efflux of free Cbl	+	+	+	+	+	+	−
Enzyme activities in cell extracts*							
Mutase holoenzyme	−	−	−	−	−	−	nt
Mutase total enzyme	−	±	+	+	+	+	nt
Met synthase holoenzyme	+	+	+	+	−	−	−
Met synthase total enzyme	+	+	+	+	±	±	±
Cob(I)alamin adenosyltransferase	+	+	+	−	+	+	+

**Holoenzyme* is defined as that enzyme activity measured in the absence of added cofactor; *total enzyme* is that activity measured in the presence of saturating concentrations of cofactor. Abbreviations: + = normal; − = markedly deficient or undetectable; ± = partially deficient; nt = not tested; MeH_4F = N^5-methyltetrahydrofolate; MeCbl = methylcobalamin; AdoCbl = adenosylcobalamin; CN-Cbl = cyanocobalamin; OH-Cbl = hydroxocobalamin.

Pathophysiology. The megaloblastic anemia so commonly observed in the *cblC* patients almost surely reflects the enzymatic disturbance of methionine synthase. This can be stated with some assurance because patients with isolated methylmalonyl CoA mutase deficiency (*mut*^{0}, *mut*$^-$, *cblA*, *cblB*) more severe than that encountered in the *cblC* patients exhibit no such hematologic dysfunction. The early and severe central nervous system abnormalities encountered in the *cblC* group probably reflect the methionine synthase abnormality as well, in that such patients do not have the severe metabolic ketoacidosis that probably accounts for the neurologic problems in patients with mutase deficiency only. Thus, patients with severe, inherited dysfunction in the

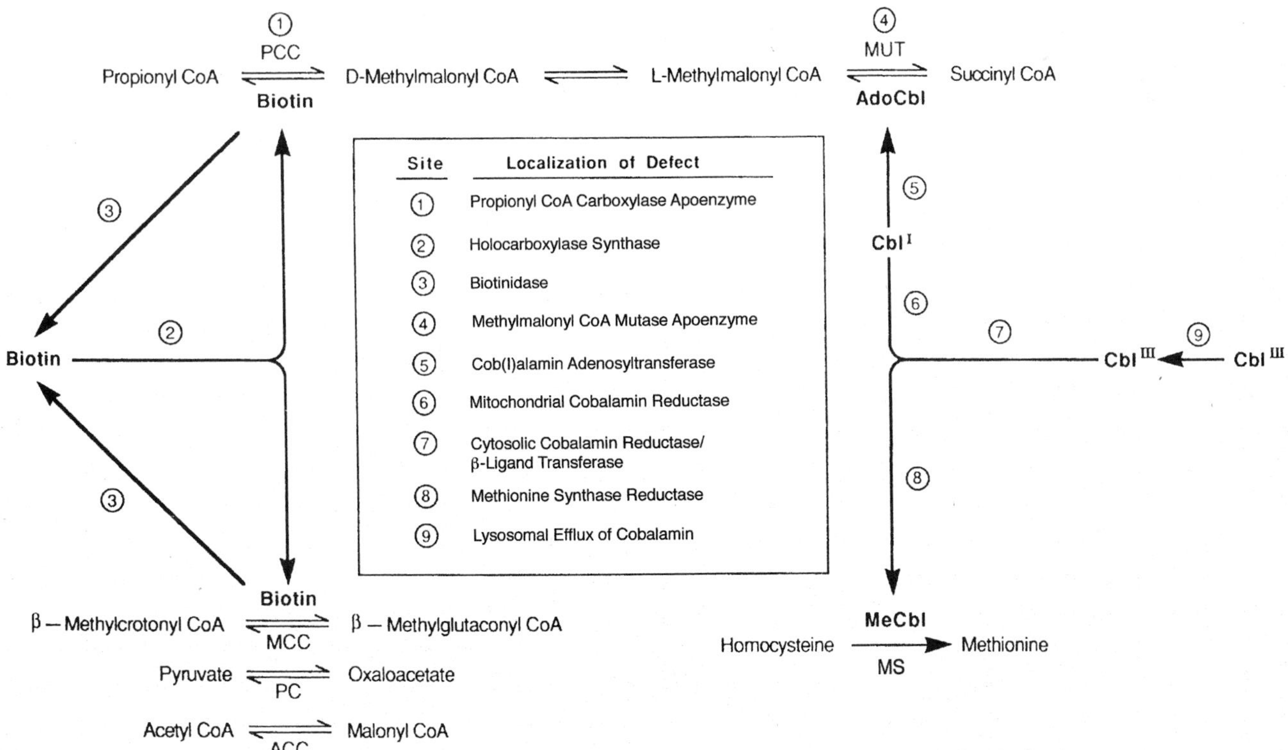

Fig. 94-15 Summary scheme of inherited defects of propionate and methylmalonate metabolism. The circled numbers and their key signify the nine general sites at which abnormalities have been identified. Abbreviations: PCC = propionyl CoA carboxylase; MCC = β-methylcrotonyl CoA carboxylase; PC = pyruvate carboxylase; ACC = acetyl CoA carboxylase; MUT = methylmalonyl CoA mutase; Cbl^{III} = cob(III)alamin (e.g., OH-Cbl); Cbl^{I} = cob(I)alamin; AdoCbl = adenosylcobalamin; MeCbl = methylcobalamin; MS = methionine synthase.

synthesis of both Cbl coenzymes resemble closely patients with exogenous Cbl deficiency, both groups having prominent hematologic and neurologic manifestations resulting from the blocked methionine synthase system.

Genetic Considerations. Because equal numbers of affected males and affected females exist in the *cblC* group, because females have been as seriously affected as males, and because cells from affected patients behave as recessives in complementation studies,[295] it seems safe to predict that this disorder is inherited as an autosomal-recessive trait. The mode of inheritance of the *cblD* and the *cblF* mutations cannot yet be defined with certainty, because of the paucity of known patients. Identification of heterozygotes for *cblC*, *cblD*, or *cblF* has not yet been accomplished. One additional contribution of the somatic cell genetic studies used to characterize these disorders deserves mention. The locus coding for the human methionine synthase structural gene was originally mapped to chromosome 1 using human–hamster hybrids.[354] This assignment has been confirmed with the cloning of the gene.[360–363]

Diagnosis, Treatment, and Prognosis. The combination of methylmalonic aciduria, homocystinuria, and normal serum Cbl concentrations is the triad needed to distinguish patients in the *cblC*, *cblD*, or *cblF* groups from those with isolated mutase deficiency, with other causes of homocystinuria such as cystathionine synthase deficiency or $N^{5,10}$-methylenetetrahydrofolate reductase deficiency, with Cbl deficiency, or with the *cblE* and *cblG* mutations affecting only methionine synthase (see Chapters 88 and 155). Such distinctions, easily confirmed by cell studies, are critical because appropriate therapy depends on them. Whereas exogenous Cbl deficiency will respond dramatically to physiologic amounts of Cbl and certain forms of homocystinuria will respond to supplements of pyridoxine or folate, successful treatment of *cblC*, *cblD*, or *cblF* patients may demand administration of very large amounts (up to 1 mg daily) of OH-Cbl.[263,333,335–337,344] Such treatment has resulted in dramatic decreases in urinary methylmalonate (and less dramatic decreases in urinary homocystine) in patients who have received it.[364] Supplementation with betaine can reduce homocysteine levels and restore methionine, although the clinical effects of this treatment are unclear.[365] Early diagnosis and prompt institution of therapy with Cbl supplements (and betaine) may be the only way to change the outcome of these patients, which, at least in the case of the *cblC* group, has been dismal thus far.[366] Documentation of experience with such treatments will be particularly important in assessing the clinician's ability to modify the natural history of these disorders.

OVERVIEW

The panorama of variants leading to methylmalonic aciduria is shown in Fig. 94-15, juxtaposed to those seen in inherited forms of propionic acidemia.

REFERENCES

1. Marston HR, Allen SH, Smith RM: Primary metabolic defect supervening on vitamin B_{12} deficiency in the sheep. *Nature* **190**:1085, 1961.
2. Smith RM, Monty KJ: Vitamin B_{12} and propionate metabolism. *Biochem Biophys Res Commun* **1**:105, 1959.
3. Gurnani S, Mistry SP, Johnson BC: Function of vitamin B_{12} in methylmalonate metabolism. 1. Effect of a cofactor form of B_{12} on the activity of methylmalonyl-CoA isomerase. *Biochim Biophys Acta* **38**:187, 1960.
4. Stern JR, Friedmann DC: Vitamin B_{12} and methylmalonyl-CoA isomerase. I. Vitamin B_{12} and propionate metabolism. *Biochem Biophys Res Commun* **2**:82, 1960.
5. Cox EV, White AM: Methylmalonic acid excretion: Index of vitamin-B_{12} deficiency. *Lancet* **2**:853, 1962.
6. Barness LA, Young D, Mellman WJ, Kahn SB, Williams WJ: Methylmalonate excretion in patients with pernicious anemia. *New Engl J Med* **268**:144, 1963.
7. Childs B, Nyhan WL, Borden M, Bard L, Cooke RE: Idiopathic hyperglycinemia and hyperglycinuria: New disorder of amino acid metabolism I. *Pediatrics* **27**:522, 1961.
8. Rosenberg LE, Lilljeqvist A-C, Hsia YE: Methylmalonic aciduria: An inborn error leading to metabolic acidosis, long-chain ketonuria and intermittent hyperglycinemia. *New Engl J Med* **278**:1319, 1968.
9. Hsia YE, Scully KJ, Rosenberg LE: Defective propionate carboxylation in ketotic hyperglycinaemia. *Lancet* **1**:757, 1969.
10. Oberholzer VC, Levin B, Burgess EA, Young WF: Methylmalonic aciduria: An inborn error of metabolism leading to chronic metabolic acidosis. *Arch Dis Child* **42**:492, 1967.
11. Stokke O, Eldjarn L, Norum KR, Steen-Johnsen J, Halvorsen S: Methylmalonic aciduria: A new inborn error of metabolism which may cause fatal acidosis in the neonatal period. *Scand J Clin Lab Invest* **20**:313, 1967.
12. Lindblad B, Olin P, Svanberg B, Zetterstrom R: Methylmalonic acidemia. *Acta Paediatr Scand* **57**:417, 1968.
13. Lindblad B, Lindstrand K, Svanberg B, Zetterstrom R: The effect of cobamide coenzyme in methylmalonic acidemia. *Acta Paediatr Scand* **58**:178, 1969.
14. Rosenberg LE, Lilljeqvist AC, Hsia YE, Rosenbloom FM: Vitamin B_{12} dependent methylmalonicaciduria: defective B_{12} metabolism in cultured fibroblasts. *Biochem Biophys Res Commun* **37**:607, 1969.
15. Mahoney MJ, Rosenberg LE, Mudd SH, Uhlendorf BW: Defective metabolism of vitamin B_{12} in fibroblasts from children with methylmalonicaciduria. *Biochem Biophys Res Commun* **44**:375, 1971.
16. Fenton WA, Rosenberg LE: Disorders of propionate and methylmalonate metabolism, in Scriver CR, Beaudet AL, Sly WS, Valle D (eds): *The Metabolic and Molecular Bases of Inherited Disease*. New York, McGraw-Hill, 1995, p 1423.
17. Willard HF, Rosenberg LE: Inherited deficiencies of human methylmalonyl CoA mutase: Biochemical and genetic studies in cultured skin fibroblasts, in Hommes FA (ed): *Models for the Study of Inborn Errors of Metabolism*. Amsterdam, Elsevier North-Holland, 1979, p 297.
18. Rosenberg LE: The inherited methylmalonic acidemias: A model system for the study of vitamin metabolism and apoenzyme-coenzyme interactions (Milner Lecture), in Belton NR, Toothill C (eds): *Transport and Inherited Disease*. Lancaster, England, MTP, 1981, p 3.
19. Wolf B, Feldman GL: The biotin dependent carboxylase deficiencies. *Am J Hum Genet* **34**:699, 1982.
20. Rosenblatt DS, Fenton WA: Inborn errors of cobalamin metabolism, in Banerjee R (eds): *Chemistry and Biology of B_{12}*. New York, Wiley, 1999, p 367.
21. Rosenblatt DS, Whitehead VM: Cobalamin and folate deficiency: Acquired and hereditary disorders in children. *Semin Hematol* **36**:1, 1999.
22. Meister A: *Biochemistry of the Amino Acids*. New York, Academic, 1965.
23. Tanaka K, Armitage IM, Ramsdell HS, Hsia YE, Lipsky SR, Rosenberg LE: [^{13}C]Valine metabolism in methylmalonicacidemia using nuclear magnetic resonance: Propionate as an obligate intermediate. *Proc Natl Acad Sci U S A* **72**:3692, 1975.
24. Baretz BH, Tanaka K: Metabolism in rats *in vivo* of isobutyrates labelled with stable isotopes at various positions: Identification of propionate as an obligate Intermediate. *J Biol Chem* **253**:4203, 1978.
25. Thompson GN, Walter JH, Bresson J-L, Ford GC, Lyonnet SL, Chalmers RA, Saudubray J-M, Leonard JV, Halliday D: Sources of propionate in inborn errors of propionate metabolism. *Metabolism* 39:1133, 1990.
26. Kaziro Y, Ochoa S: The metabolism of propionic acid. *Adv Enzymol* **26**:283, 1964.
27. Thompson GN, Chalmers RA: Increased urinary metabolite excretion during fasting in disorders of propionate metabolism. *Pediatr Res* **27**:413, 1990.
28. Danielsson H: Present status of research on catabolism and excretion of cholesterol. *Adv Lipid Res* **1**:335, 1963.
29. Bain MD, Jones M, Borriello SP, Reed PJ, Tracey BM, Chalmers RA, Stacey TE: Contribution of gut bacterial metabolism to human metabolic disease. *Lancet* **1**:1078, 1988.
30. Leonard JV: Stable isotope studies in propionic and methylmalonic acidaemia. *Eur J Pediatr* **156**(suppl):67, 1997.
31. Lardy HA, Adler J: Synthesis of succinate from propionate and bicarbonate by soluble enzymes from liver mitochondria. *J Biol Chem* **219**:935, 1956.

32. Flavin M, Ortiz PJ, Ochoa S: Metabolism of propionic acid in animal tissues. *Nature* **176**:823, 1955.
33. Katz J, Chaikoff IL: The metabolism of propionate by rat liver slices and the formation of isosuccinic acid. *J Am Chem Soc* **77**:2659, 1955.
34. Flavin M, Ochoa S: Metabolism of propionic acid in animal tissues. I. Enzymatic conversion of propionate to succinate. *J Biol Chem* **229**:965, 1957.
35. Tietz A, Ochoa S: Metabolism of propionic acid in animal tissues. V. Purification and properties of propionyl Carboxylase. *J Biol Chem* **234**:1394, 1959.
36. Sprecher M, Clark MJ, Sprinson DB: The absolute configuration of methylmalonyl-CoA and stereochemistry of the methylmalonyl-CoA mutase reaction. *Biochem Biophys Res Commun* **15**:581, 1964.
37. Retey J, Lynen F: The absolute configuration of methylmalonyl-CoA. *Biochem Biophys Res Commun* **16**:358, 1964.
38. Mazumder R, Sasakawa T, Kaziro Y, Ochoa S: Metabolism of propionic acid in animal tissues. IX. Methylmalonyl coenzyme A racemase. *J Biol Chem* **237**:3065, 1962.
39. Beck WS, Flavin M, Ochoa S: Metabolism of propionic acid in animal tissues. III. Formation of Succinate. *J Biol Chem* **229**:997, 1957.
40. Kaziro Y, Ochoa S, Warner RC, Chen J: Metabolism of propionic acid in animal tissues. VIII. Crystalline propionyl carboxylase. *J Biol Chem* **236**:1917, 1961.
41. Lau EP, Cochran BC, Munson L, Fall RR: Bovine kidney 3-methylcrotonyl-CoA and propionyl-CoA carboxylases: Each enzyme contains nonidentical subunits. *Proc Natl Acad Sci U S A* **76**:214, 1979.
42. Kalousek F, Darigo MD, Rosenberg LE: Isolation and characterization of propionyl-CoA carboxylase from normal human liver: Evidence for a protomeric tetramer of nonidentical subunits. *J Biol Chem* **255**:60, 1980.
43. Gravel RA, Lam KF, Mahuran D, Kronis A: Purification of human liver propionyl-CoA carboxylase by carbon tetrachloride extraction and monomeric avidin affinity chromatography. *Arch Biochem Biophys* **201**:669, 1980.
44. Haase FC, Beegen H, Allen SHK: Propionyl-coenzyme A carboxylase of *Mycobacterium smegmatis*: An electron microscopic study. *Eur J Biochem* **140**:147, 1984.
45. Mistry SP, Dakshinamurti K: Biochemistry of biotin. *Vitam Horm* **22**:1, 1964.
46. Lamhonwah AM, Barankiewics TJ, Willard HF, Mahuran DJ, Quan F, Gravel RA: Isolation of cDNA clones coding for the α and β chains of human propionyl-CoA carboxylase: Chromosomal assignments and DNA polymorphisms associated with PCCA and PCCB genes. *Proc Natl Acad Sci U S A* **83**:4864, 1986.
47. Lamhonwah AM, Quan F, Gravel RA: Sequence homology around the biotin-binding site of human propionyl-CoA carboxylase and pyruvate carboxylase. *Arch Biochem Biophys* **254**:631, 1987.
48. Lamhonwah AM, Mahuran D, Gravel RA: Human mitochondrial propionyl-CoA carboxylase: Localization of the N-terminus of the pro- and mature alpha chains in the deduced primary sequence of a full-length cDNA. *Nucleic Acids Res* **17**:4396, 1989.
49. Kraus JP, Williamson CL, Firgaira FA, Yang-Feng TL, Munke M, Francke U, Rosenberg LE: Cloning and screening with nanogram amounts of immunopurified messenger RNAs: cDNA cloning and chromosomal mapping of cystathionine β-synthase and the β-subunit of propionyl CoA carboxylase. *Proc Natl Acad Sci U S A* **83**:2047, 1986.
50. Kraus JP, Firgaira F, Novotny J, Kalousek F, Williams KR, Williamson C, Ohura T, et al.: Coding sequence of the precursor of the β subunit of rat propionyl-CoA carboxylase. *Proc Natl Acad Sci U S A* **83**:8049, 1986.
51. Browner MF, Taroni F, Sztul E, Rosenberg LE: Sequence analysis, biogenesis, and mitochondrial import of the α-subunit of rat liver propionyl-CoA carboxylase. *J Biol Chem* **264**:12680, 1989.
52. Stankovics J, Ledley FD: Cloning of functional alpha propionyl CoA carboxylase and correction of enzyme deficiency in pccA fibroblasts. *Am J Hum Genet* **52**:144, 1993.
53. Lamhonwah AM, Leclerc D, Loyer M, Clarizio R, Gravel RA: Correction of the metabolic defect in propionic acidemia fibroblasts by microinjection of a full-length cDNA or RNA transcript encoding the propionyl-CoA carboxylase beta subunit. *Genomics* **19**:500, 1994.
54. Ohura T, Ogasawara M, Ikeda H, Narisawa K, Tada K: The molecular defect in propionic acidemia: Exon skipping caused by an 8-bp deletion from an intron in the PCCB allele. *Hum Genet* **92**:397, 1993.
55. Rosenberg LE, Fenton WA, Horwich AL, Kalousek F, Kraus JP: Targeting of nuclear-encoded proteins to the mitochondrial matrix: Implications for human genetic defects. *Ann N Y Acad Sci* **488**:99, 1986.
56. Kraus JP, Kalousek F, Rosenberg LE: Biosynthesis and mitochondrial processing of the β subunit of propionyl CoA carboxylase from rat liver. *J Biol Chem* **258**:7245, 1983.
57. Campeau E, Dupuis L, Leon-del-Rio A, Gravel R: Coding sequence mutations in the alpha subunit of propionyl-CoA carboxylase in patients with propionic acidemia. *Mol Genet Metab* **67**:1, 1999.
58. Leon-del-Rio A, Gravel RA: Sequence requirements for the biotinylation of carboxyl-terminal fragments of human propionyl-CoA carboxylase alpha subunit expressed in *Escherichia coli*. *J Biol Chem* **269**:22964, 1994.
59. Kennerknecht I, Suormala T, Barbi G, Baumgartner ER: The gene coding for the alpha-chain of human propionyl-CoA carboxylase maps to chromosome band 13q32. *Hum Genet* **86**:238, 1990.
60. Piemontese MR, Memeo E, Carella M, Amati P, Chomel JC, Bonneau D, Cao A, et al.: A YAC contig spanning the blepharophimosis-ptosis-epicanthus inversus syndrome and propionic acidemia loci. *Eur J Hum Genet* 5:171, 1997.
61. Rodriguez-Pombo P, Hoenicka J, Muro S, Perez B, Perezcerda C, Richard E, Desviat LR, et al.: Human propionyl-CoA carboxylase beta subunit gene—Exon-intron definition and mutation spectrum in Spanish and Latin American propionic acidemia. *Am J Hum Genet* **63**:360, 1998.
62. Overath P, Kellerman GM, Lynen F, Fritz HP, Keller HJ: Zum Mechanismus der Umlagerung von Methylmalonyl-CoA in Succinyl-CoA. II. Verusche zur Wirkungweise von Methylmalonyl-CoA-Isomerase und Methylmalonyl-CoA-Racemase. *Biochem Z* **335**:500, 1962.
63. Barker HA, Smyth RD, Wawszkiewicz EJ, Lee MN, Wilson RM: Enzymatic preparation and characterization of an a-L-b-methylaspartic acid. *Arch Biochem Biophys* **78**:468, 1958.
64. Barker HA, Weissbach H, Smyth RD, Toohey J: A coenzyme containing pseudovitamin B_{12} Isolation and properties of B_{12} coenzymes containing benzimidazole or dimethylbenzimidazole. *Proc Natl Acad Sci U S A* **45**:521, 1959.
65. Weissbach H, Toohey J, Barker HA: Isolation and properties of B_{12} coenzymes containing benzimidazole or dimethylbenzimidazole. *Proc Natl Acad Sci U S A* **45**:521, 1959.
66. Kolhouse JF, Utley C, Allen RH: Isolation and characterization of methylmalonyl-CoA mutase from human placenta. *J Biol Chem* **255**:2708, 1980.
67. Fenton WA, Hack AM, Willard HF, Gertler A, Rosenberg LE: Purification and properties of methylmalonyl CoA mutase from human liver. *Arch Biochem Biophys* **214**:815, 1982.
68. Janata J, Kogekar N, Fenton WA: Expression and kinetic characterization of methylmalonyl-CoA mutase from patients with the *mut*$^-$ phenotype: Evidence for naturally occurring interallelic complementation. *Hum Mol Genet* **6**:1457, 1997.
69. Willard HF, Rosenberg LE: Interactions of methylmalonyl CoA mutase from normal human fibroblasts with adenosylcobalamin and methylmalonyl CoA: Evidence for nonequivalent active sites. *Arch Biochem Biophys* **200**:130, 1980.
70. Eggerer H, Stadtman ER, Overath P, Lynen F: Zum Mechanismus der durch Cobalamin-Coenzyme katalysierten Umlagerung von Methylmalonyl-CoA in Succinyl-CoA. *Biochem Z* **333**:1, 1960.
71. Kellermeyer RW, Wood HG: Methylmalonyl isomerase: A study of the mechanism of isomerization. *Biochemistry* **1**:1124, 1962.
72. Phares EF, Long MV, Carson SF: An intramolecular rearrangement in the methylmalonyl isomerase reaction as demonstrated by positive and negative mass analysis of succinic acid. *Biochem Biophys Res Commun* **8**:142, 1962.
73. Halpern J: Mechanisms of coenzyme B_{12}-dependent rearrangements. *Science* **227**:869, 1985.
74. Zhao Y, Abend A, Kunz M, Such P, Retey J: Electron paramagnetic resonance studies of the methylmalonyl-CoA mutase reaction. *Eur J Biochem* **225**:891, 1994.
75. Padmakumar R, Banerjee R: Evidence from electron paramagnetic resonance spectroscopy of the participation of radical intermediates in the reaction catalyzed by methylmalonyl-coenzyme A mutase. *J Biol Chem* **270**:9295, 1995.
76. Padmakumar R, Banerjee R: Evidence that cobalt–carbon bond homolysis is coupled to hydrogen atom abstration from substrate in methylmalonyl-CoA mutase. *Biochemistry* **36**:3713, 1997.
77. Meier TW, Thoma NH, Leadlay PF: Tritium isotope effects in adenosylcobalamin-dependent methylmalonyl-CoA mutase. *Biochemistry* **35**:11791, 1996.

78. Fenton WA, Hack AM, Helfgott D, Rosenberg LE: Biogenesis of the mitochondrial enzyme methylmalonyl-CoA mutase: Synthesis and processing of a precursor in a cell-free system and in cultured cells. *J Biol Chem* **259**:6616, 1984.
79. Ledley FD, Lumetta M, Nguyen PN, Kolhouse JF, Allen RH: Molecular cloning of L-methylmalonyl-CoA mutase: Gene transfer and analysis of *mut* cell lines. *Proc Natl Acad Sci U S A* **85**:3518, 1988.
80. Jansen R, Kalousek F, Fenton WA, Rosenberg LE, Ledley FD: Cloning of full-length methylmalonyl-CoA mutase from a cDNA library using the polymerase chain reaction. *Genomics* **4**:198, 1989.
81. Nham S-U, Wilkemeyer MF, Ledley FD: Structure of the human methylmalonyl-CoA mutase (*MUT*) locus. *Genomics* **8**:710, 1990.
82. Wilkemeyer MF, Crane AM, Ledley FD: Primary structure and activity of mouse methylmalonyl-CoA mutase. *Biochem J* **271**:449, 1990.
83. Ledley FD, Lumetta MR, Zoghli HY, Van Tuinen P, Ledbetter SA, Ledbetter DH: Mapping of human methylmalonyl CoA mutase (MUT) locus on chromosome 6. *Am J Hum Genet* **42**:839, 1988.
84. Francalanci F, Davis NK, Fuller JQ, Murfitt D, Leadlay PF: The subunit structure of methylmalonyl-CoA mutase from *Propionibacterium shermanii. Biochem J* **236**:489, 1986.
85. Marsh EN, McKie N, Davis NK, Leadlay PF: Cloning and structural characterization of the genes coding for adenosylcobalamin-dependent methylmalonyl-CoA mutase from *Propionibacterium shermanii. Biochem J* **260**:345, 1989.
86. Thoma NH, Leadley PF: Homology modelling of human methylmalonyl-CoA mutase: A structural basis for point mutations causing methylmalonic aciduria. *Protein Sci* **5**:1922, 1996.
87. Mancia F, Keep NH, Nakagawa A, Leadley PF, McSweeney S, Rasmussen B, Bosecke P, Diat O, Evans PR: How coenzyme B_{12} radicals are generated: The crystal structure of methylmalonyl-coenzyme A mutase at 2 A resolution. *Structure* **4**:339, 1996.
88. Mancia F, Evans PR: Conformational changes on substrate binding to methylmalonyl CoA mutase and new insights into the free radical mechanism. *Structure* **6**:711, 1998.
89. Thoma NH, Meier TW, Evans PR, Leadlay PF: Stabilization of radical intermediates by an active-site tyrosine residue in methylmalonyl-CoA mutase. *Biochemistry* **37**:14386, 1998.
90. Drennan CL, Huang S, Drummond JT, Matthews RG, Ludwig ML: How a protein binds B_{12}: A 3.0 A X-ray structure of B_{12}-binding domains of methionine synthase. *Science* **266**:1669, 1994.
91. Lynen F: Biosynthesis of saturated fatty acids. *Fed Proc* **20**:941, 1961.
92. Ando T, Rasmussen K, Wright JM, Nyhan WL: Isolation and identification of methylcitrate, a major metabolic product of propionate in patients with propionic acidemia. *J Biol Chem* **247**:2200, 1972.
93. Rasmussen K, Ando T, Nyhan WL, Hull D, Cotton D, Wadlington W, Kilroy AW: Excretion of propionylglycine in propionic acidemia. *Clin Sci* 42:665, 1972.
94. Ando T, Rasmussen K, Nyhan WL, Hull D: 3-Hydroxypropionate: Significance of β-oxidation of propionate in patients with propionic acidemia and methylmalonic acidemia. *Proc Natl Acad Sci U S A* **69**:2807, 1972.
95. Thompson GN, Walter JH, Bresson JL, Ford GC, Bonnefont JP, Chalmers RA, Saudubray JM et al.: Substrate disposal in metabolic disease: A comparison between rates of *in vivo* propionate oxidation and urinary metabolite excretion in children with methylmalonic acidemia. *J Pediatr* **115**:735, 1989.
96. Kogl F, Tonis, B: Uber das Bios-Problem. Darstellung und Krystallisiertem biotin aus Eigelb. *Z Physiol Chem* **242**:43, 1936.
97. du Vigneaud V, Hoffmann K, Melville DB: On the structure of biotin. *J Am Chem Soc* **64**:188, 1942.
98. Sebrell WH, Harris RS: Biotin, in *The Vitamins: Chemistry, Physiology, Pathology Methods*. New York, Academic, 1978, p 261.
99. Murthy PNA, Mistry SP: Biotin. *Prog Food Nutr Sci* **2**:405, 1977.
100. Moss J, Lane MD: The biotin-dependent enzymes. *Adv Enzymol* **35**:321,1971.
101. Wood HG, Barden RE: Biotin enzymes. *Annu Rev Biochem* **46**:385, 1978.
102. Chapman-Smith A, Cronan JE: Molecular biology of biotin attachment to proteins. *J Nutr* **129**(suppl):477, 1999.
103. Samols D, Thornton CG, Murtif VL, Kumar GK, Haase FC, Wood HG: Evolutionary conservation among biotin enzymes. *J Biol Chem* **263**:6461, 1988.
104. Ha J, Daniel S, Kong IS, Park CK, Tae HJ, Kim KH: Cloning of human acetyl-CoA carboxylase cDNA. *Eur J Biochem* **219**:297, 1994.
105. Ha J, Lee JK, Kim KS, Witters LA, Kim KH: Cloning of human acetyl-CoA carboxylase-beta and its unique features. *Proc Natl Acad Sci U S A* **93**:11466, 1996.
106. Baumgartner ER, Suormala T: Multiple carboxylase deficiency: Inherited and acquired disorders of biotin metabolism. *Int J Vitam Nutr Res* **67**:377, 1997.
107. Chiba Y, Suzuki Y, Aoki Y, Ishida Y, Narisawa K: Purification and properties of bovine liver holocarboxylase synthetase. *Arch Biochem Biophys* **313**:8, 1994.
108. Hiratsuka M, Sakamoto O, Li X, Suzuki Y, Aoki Y, Narisawa K: Identification of holocarboxylase synthetase (HCS) proteins in human placenta. *Biochim Biophys Acta* **1385**:165, 1998.
109. Ohta T, Iwata T, Kayukawa Y, Okada T: Daily activity and persistent sleep-wake schedule disorders. *Prog Neur Psychopharm Biol Psychiatr* **16**:529, 1992.
110. Suzuki Y, Aoki Y, Ishida Y, Chiba Y, Iwamatsu A, Kishino T, Niikawa N, et al.: Isolation and characterization of mutations in the human holocarboxylase synthetase cDNA. *Nat Genet* **8**:122, 1994.
111. Leon-del-Rio A, Leclerc D, Akerman B, Wakamatsu N, Gravel RA: Isolation of a cDNA encoding human holocarboxylase synthetase by functional complementation of a biotin auxotroph of *Escherichia coli. Proc Natl Acad Sci U S A* **92**:4626, 1995.
112. Suzuki Y, Aoki Y, Sakamoto O, Li X, Miyabayashi S, Kazuta Y, Kondo H, et al.: Enzymatic diagnosis of holocarboxylase synthetase deficiency using apo-carboxyl carrier protein as a substrate. *Clin Chim Acta* **251**:41, 1996.
113. Craft DV, Goss NH, Chandramouli N, Wood HG: Purification of biotinidase from human plasma and its activity on biotinyl peptides. *Biochemistry* **24**:2471, 1985.
114. Chauhan J, Dakshinamurti K: Purification and characterization of human serum biotinidase. *J Biol Chem* **261**:4268, 1986.
115. Hymes J, Fleischhauer K, Wolf B: Biotinylation of histones by human serum biotinidase: Assessment of biotinyl-transferase activity in sera from normal individuals and children with biotinidase deficiency. *Biochem Molec Med* **56**:76, 1995.
116. Hymes J, Wolf B: Human biotinidase isn't just for recycling biotin. *J Nutr* **129**(suppl):485, 1999.
117. Wolf B, Heard GS, McVoy JS, Raetz HM: Biotinidase deficiency: The possible role of biotinidase in the processing of dietary protein-bound biotin. *J Inherit Metab Dis* **7**:121, 1984.
118. Said HM, Redha R, Nylander W: Biotin transport in the human intestine: Site of maximum transport and effect of pH. *Gastroenterology* **95**:1312, 1988.
119. Bowman BB, Selhub J, Rosenberg IH: Intestinal absorption of biotin in the rat. *J Nutr* **116**:1266, 1986.
120. Said HM, Redha R, Nylander W: A carrier-mediated, Na^+ gradient-dependent transport for biotin in human intestinal brush-border membrane vesicles. *Am J Physiol* **253**:G631, 1987.
121. Said HM, Redha R, Nylander W: Biotin transport in basolateral membrane vesicles of human intestine. *Gastroenterology* **94**:1157, 1988.
122. Mock DM, Malik ML: Distribution of biotin in human plasma: Most of the biotin is not bound to protein. *Am J Clin Nutr* **56**:427, 1992.
123. Said HM, Korchid S, Horne DW, Howard M: Transport of biotin in basolateral membrane vesicles of rat liver. *Am J Physiol* **259**:G865, 1990.
124. Said HM, Hoefs J, Mohammadkhani R, Horne DW: Biotin transport in human liver basolateral membrane vesicles: A carrier-mediated, Na^+ gradient-dependent process. *Gastroenterology* **102**:2120, 1992.
125. Grassl SM: Human placental brush-border membrane Na^+-biotin cotransport. *J Biol Chem* **267**:17760, 1992.
126. Mock DM, Delorimer AA, Liebman WM, Sweetman L, Baker H: Biotin deficiency: An unusual complication of parenteral alimentation. *New Engl J Med* **304**:820, 1981.
127. Sydenstricker VP, Singal SA, Briggs AP, DeVaughn NM: Preliminary observations on "egg white injury" in man and its cure with a biotin concentrate. *Science* **95**:1976, 1942.
128. Minot GR, Murphy LP: Treatment of pernicious anemia by a special diet. *JAMA* **87**:470, 1926.
129. Smith EL: Purification of anti-pernicious anemia factors from liver. *Nature* **161**:638, 1948.
130. Rickes EL, Brink NG, Koniuszy FR, Wood TR, Folkers K: Crystalline vitamin B_{12}. *Science* **107**:396, 1948.
131. Banerjee R (ed): *Chemistry and Biochemistry of B_{12}*. New York, Wiley, 1999.
132. Hodgkin DC, Kamper J, Mackay M, Pickworth J, Trueblood KN, White JG: Structure of vitamin B_{12}. *Nature* **178**:64, 1956.
133. Walker GA, Murphy S, Heunnekens F: Enzymatic conversion of vitamin B_{12} to adenosyl-B_{12}: Evidence for the existence of two separate reducing systems. *Arch Biochem Biophys* **134**:95, 1969.

134. Weissbach H, Taylor R: Role of vitamin B_{12} in methionine biosynthesis. *Fed Proc* **25**:1649, 1966.
135. Taylor RT, Weissbach H: Enzymatic synthesis of methionine: Formation of a radioactive cobamide enzyme with N^5methyl-^{14}C-tetrahydrofolate. *Arch Biochem Biophys* **119**:572, 1967.
136. Taylor RT, Weissbach H: *Escherichia coli* B N^5-methyltetrahydrofolate-homocysteine vitamin-B_{12} transmethylase: Formation and photolability of a methylcobalamin enzyme. *Arch Biochem Biophys* **123**:109, 1968.
137. Poston JM: Leucine 2,3-aminomutase, an enzyme of leucine catabolism. *J Biol Chem* **251**:1859, 1976.
138. Castle WB, Townsend WC, Heath CW: Observations on the etiologic relationship of achylia gastrica to pernicious anemia. III. The nature of the reaction between normal human gastric juice and beef muscle leading to clinical improvement and increased blood formation similar to the effect liver feeding. *Am J Med Sci* **180**:305, 1930.
139. Babior BM: Cobamides as cofactors: Adenosylcobamide dependent reactions, in: *Cobalamin Biochemistry and Pathophysiology*. New York, Wiley, 1975, p 141.
140. Donaldson RM Jr: Intrinsic factor and the transport of cobalamin, in Johnson LR (ed): *Physiology of the Gastrointestinal Tract*. New York, Raven, 1981.
141. Sennett C, Rosenberg LE, Mellman IS: Transmembrane transport of cobalamin in prokaryotic and eukaryotic cells. *Annu Rev Biochem* **50**:1053, 1981.
142. Seetharam B: Gastrointestinal absorption and transport of cobalamin (vitamin B_{12}), in Johnson LR (ed): *Physiology of the Gastrointestinal Tract*. New York, Raven, 1994, p 1997.
143. Moestrup SK, Kozyraki R, Kristiansen M, Kaysen JH, Rasmussen HH, Brault D, Pontillon F, et al.: The intrinsic factor-vitamin B_{12} receptor and target of teratogenic antibodies is a megalin-binding peripheral membrane protein with homology to developmental proteins. *J Biol Chem* **273**:5235, 1998.
144. Allen RH: Human vitamin B_{12}-transport proteins. *Prog Hematol* **9**:57, 1975.
145. Ellenbogen LE: Uptake and transport of cobalamins. *Int Rev Biochem* **27**:45, 1979.
146. Hall CA, Finkler AE: The dynamics of transcobalamin. II. A vitamin B_{12} binding substance in plasma. *J Lab Clin Med* **65**:459, 1965.
147. Hom BL: Plasma turnover of ^{57}cobalt-vitamin B12 bound to transcobalamin I and II. *Scand J Haematol* **4**:321, 1967.
148. Linnell JC: The fate of cobalamins in vivo, in Babior BM (ed): *Cobalamin: Biochemistry and Pathophysiology*. New York, Wiley, 1975, p 287.
149. Finkler AE, Hall CA: Nature of the relationship between vitamin B_{12} binding and cell uptake. *Arch Biochem Biophys* **120**:79, 1967.
150. Tan CH, Hansen HJ: Studies on the site of synthesis of transcobalamin II. *Proc Soc Exp Biol Med* **127**:740, 1968.
151. Pletsch QA, Coffey JW: Properties of the proteins that bind vitamin B_{12} in subcellular fractions of rat liver. *Arch Biochem Biophys* **151**:157, 1972.
152. Newmark P, Newman GE, O'Brien JRP: Vitamin B_{12} in the rat kidney: Evidence of an association with lysosomes. *Arch Biochem Biophys* **141**:121, 1970.
153. Youngdahl-Turner P, Rosenberg LE, Allen RH: Binding and uptake of transcobalamin II by human fibroblasts. *J Clin Invest* **61**:133, 1978.
154. Youngdahl-Turner P, Mellman IS, Allen RH, Rosenberg LE: Protein mediated vitamin uptake: Adsorptive endocytosis of the transcobalamin II-cobalamin complex by cultured human fibroblasts. *Exp Cell Res* **118**:127, 1979.
155. Mellman IS, Youngdahl-Turner P, Willard HF, Rosenberg LE: Intracellular binding of radioactive hydroxocobalamin to cobalamin-dependent apoenzymes in rat liver. *Proc Natl Acad Sci U S A* **74**:916, 1977.
156. Kolhouse JF, Allen RH: Recognition of two intracellular cobalamin binding proteins and their identification as methylmalonyl-CoA mutase and methionine synthase. *Proc Natl Acad Sci U S A* **74**:921, 1977.
157. Burger RL, Schneider RJ, Mehlman CS, Allen RH: Human plasma R-type vitamin B_{12} binding protein. II. The role of transcobalamin I, transcobalamin III and the normal granulocyte vitamin B_{12}-binding protein in the plasma transport of vitamin B_{12}. *J Biol Chem* **250**:7707, 1975.
158. Berliner N, Rosenberg LE: Uptake and metabolism of free CN-Cbl by cultured human fibroblasts from controls and a patient with transcobalamin II deficiency. *Metabolism* **30**:230, 1981.
159. Frenkel EP, Kitchens RL: Intracellular localization of hepatic propionyl-CoA carboxylase and methylmalonyl-CoA mutase in humans and normal and vitamin B_{12} deficient rats. *Br J Haematol* **31**:501, 1975.
160. Wang FK, Koch J, Stokstad EL: Folate coenzyme pattern, folate linked enzymes and methionine biosynthesis in rat liver mitochondria. *Biochem Z* **246**:458, 1967.
161. Vitols E, Walker GA, Huennekens FM: Enzymatic conversion of vitamin B_{12} to a cobamide coenzyme, a (5,6-dimethylbenzimidazolyl) deoxyadenosylcobamide (adenosyl-B_{12}). *J Biol Chem* **241**:1455, 1966.
162. Ertel R, Brot N, Taylor R, Weissbach H: Studies on the nature of the bound cobamide in *E. coli* N^5-methyltetrahydrofolate-homocysteine transmethylase. *Arch Biochem Biophys* **126**:353, 1968.
163. Taylor RT, Weissbach H: *E. coli* B N^5-methyltetrahydrofolate-homocysteine methyltransferase: Sequential formation of bound methylcobalamin with S-adenosyl-L-methionine and N^5-methyltetrahydrofolate. *Arch Biochem Biophys* **129**:728, 1969.
164. Pawalkiewicz J, Gorna M, Fenrych W, Magas S: Conversion of cyanocobalamin *in vivo* and *in vitro* into its coenzyme form in humans and animals. *Ann N Y Acad Sci* **112**:641, 1964.
165. Kerwar SS, Spears C, McAuslan B, Weissbach H: Studies on vitamin B_{12} metabolism in HeLa cells. *Arch Biochem Biophys* **142**:231, 1971.
166. Mahoney MJ, Rosenberg LE: Synthesis of cobalamin coenzymes by human cells in tissue culture. *J Lab Clin Med* **78**:302, 1971.
167. Mahoney MJ, Hart AC, Steen VD, Rosenberg LE: Methylmalonicacidemia: Biochemical heterogeneity in defects of 5′-deoxyadenosylcobalamin synthesis. *Proc Natl Acad Sci U S A* **72**:2799, 1975.
168. Fenton WA, Rosenberg LE: The defect in the cbl B class of human methylmalonic acidemia: Deficiency of cob(I)alamin adenosyltransferase activity in extracts of cultured fibroblasts. *Biochem Biophys Res Commun* **98**:283, 1981.
169. Cox EV, Robertson-Smith D, Small M, White AM: The excretion of propionate and acetate in vitamin B_{12} deficiency. *Clin Sci* **35**:123, 1968.
170. Shipman RT, Townley RRW, Danks DM: Homocystinuria, addisonian pernicious anaemia, and partial deletion of a G chromosome. *Lancet* **2**:693, 1969.
171. Hollowell JG Jr, Hall WK, Coryell ME, McPherson JJ, Hahn DA: Homocystinuria and organic aciduria in a patient with vitamin-B_{12} deficiency. *Lancet* **2**:1428, 1969.
172. Higginbottom MC, Sweetman L, Nyhan WL: A syndrome of methylmalonic aciduria, homocystinuria, megaloblastic anemia and neurologic abnormalities in a vitamin B_{12}-deficient breast-fed infant of a strict vegetarian. *New Engl J Med* **299**:317, 1978.
173. Morrow G, Barness LA, Auerbach VH, Di George AM, Ando T, Nyhan WL: Observations on the coexistence of methylmalonic acidemia and glycinemia. *J Pediatr* **74**:680, 1969.
174. Hommes FA, Kuipers JRG, Elema JD, Janse JF, Jonxis JJP: Propionicacidemia, a new inborn error of metabolism. *Pediatr Res* **2**:519, 1968.
175. Hsia YE, Scully KJ, Rosenberg LE: Inherited propionyl-CoA carboxylase deficiency in "ketotic hyperglycinemia." *J Clin Invest* **50**:127, 1971.
176. Gompertz D, Storrs CN, Bau DCK, Peters TJ, Hughes EA: Localization of enzyme defect in propionicacidemia. *Lancet* **1**:1140, 1970.
177. Nyhan WL, Borden M, Childs B: Idiopathic hyperglycinemia: A new disorder of amino acid metabolism. II. The concentrations of other amino acids in the plasma and their modification by the administration of leucine. *Pediatrics* **27**:539, 1961.
178. Childs B, Nyhan WL, Brandt IK, Hsia YE, Clement DH, Provence SA: Further observations of a patient with hyperglycinemia Propionicacidemia (ketotic hyperglycinemia): Dietary treatment results in normal growth and development. *Pediatrics* **53**:391, 1974.
179. Brandt IK, Hsia YE, Clement DH, Provence SA: Propionic acidemia (ketotic hyperglycinemia): Dietary treatment results in normal growth and development. *Pediatrics* **53**:391, 1974.
180. Nyhan WL, Ando T, Rasmussen K: Ketotic hyperglycinemia in Stern J, in Toothill C (eds): *Organic Acidurias*. London, Churchill Livingstone, 1972, p 1.
181. Wolf B, Hsia YE, Sweetman L, Gravel R, Harris DJ, Nyhan WL: Propionic acidemia: A clinical update. *J Pediatr* **99**:835, 1981.
182. Mahoney MJ, Hsia YE, Rosenberg LE: Propionyl-CoA carboxylase deficiency (propionicacidemia): A cause of non-ketotic hyperglycinemia. *Pediatr Res* **5**:395, 1971.
183. Surtees RAH, Matthews EE, Leonard JV: Neurologic outcome of propionic acidemia. *Pediatr Neurol* **8**:333, 1992.
184. Perez-Cerda C, Merinero B, Marti M, Cabrera JC, Pena L, Garcia MJ, Gangoiti J, et al.: An unusual late-onset case of propionic acidaemia:

Biochemical investigations, neuroradiological findings and mutation analysis. *Eur J Pediatr* **157**:50, 1998.
185. Sethi KD, Ray R, Roesel RA, Carter AL, Gallagher BB, Loring DW, Hommes FA: Adult-onset chorea and dementia with propionic acidemia. *Neurology* **39**:1343, 1989.
186. Wolf B, Paulsen EP, Hsia YE: Asymptomatic propionyl CoA carboxylase deficiency in a 13-year-old girl. *J Pediatr* **95**:563, 1979.
187. Inoue Y, Matsumoto I: Urinary acid profiles of asymptomatic propionyl CoA carboxylase deficiency. *J Pediatr* **113**:787, 1988.
188. Bergman AJIW, Van Der Knaap MS, Smeitink JAM, Duran M, Dorland L, Valk J, Poll-The BT: Magnetic resonance imaging and spectroscopy of the brain in propionic acidemia: Clinical and biochemical considerations. *Pediatr Res* **40**:404, 1996.
189. Walter JH, Wraith JE, Cleary MA: Absence of acidosis in the initial presentation of propionic acidaemia. *Arch Dis Child (Fetal and Neonatal Edition)* **72**:F197, 1995.
190. Griffin TA, Hostoffer RW, Tserng KY, Lebovitz DJ, Hoppel CL, Mosser JL, Kaplan D, et al.: Parathyroid hormone resistance and B cell lymphopenia in propionic acidemia. *Acta Paediatr* **85**:875, 1996.
191. Nyhan WL, Childs B: Hyperglycinemia. V. The miscible pool and turnover rate of glycine and the formation of serine. *J Clin Invest* **43**:2404, 1964.
192. Menkes JH, Idiopathic hyperglycinemia: Isolation and identification of three previously undescribed urinary ketones: *J Pediatr* **69**:413, 1966.
193. Nyhan WL, Ando T, Rasmussen K, Wadlington W, Kilroy AW, Cottom D, Hull D: Tiglic aciduria in propionic-acidemia. *Biochem J* **126**:1035, 1972.
194. Wendel U, Eissler A, Sperl W, Schadewaldt P: On the differences between urinary metabolite excretion and odd-numbered fatty acid production in propionic and methylmalonic acidaemias. *J Inher Metab Dis* **18**:584, 1995.
195. Hsia YE: Inherited hyperammonemic syndromes. *Gastroenterology* **67**:347, 1974.
196. Wolf B, Hsia YE, Tanaka K, Rosenberg LE: Correlation between serum propionate and blood ammonia concentrations in propionic acidemia. *J Pediatr* **93**:471, 1978.
197. Hsia YE, Scully KJ, Rosenberg LE: Human propionyl CoA carboxylase: Some properties of the partially purified enzyme in fibroblasts from controls and patients with propionic acidemia. *Pediatr Res* **13**:746, 1979.
198. Wolf B, Hsia YE, Rosenberg LE: Biochemical differences between mutant propionyl-CoA carboxylases from two complementation groups. *Am J Hum Genet* **30**:455, 1978.
199. Wolf B, Rosenberg LE: Heterozygote expression in propionyl coenzyme A carboxylase deficiency: Differences between major complementation groups. *Clin Invest* **62**:931, 1978.
200. Gravel RA, Lam K-F, Scully KJ, Hsia YE: Genetic complementation of propionyl-CoA carboxylase deficiency in cultured human fibroblasts. *Am J Hum Genet* **29**:378, 1977.
201. Wolf B, Willard HF, Rosenberg LE: Kinetic analysis of genetic complementation in heterokaryons of propionyl CoA carboxylase-deficient human fibroblasts. *Am J Hum Genet* **32**:16, 1980.
202. Saunders M, Sweetman L, Robinson B, Roth K, Cohn R, Gravel RA: Biotin-response organicaciduria: Multiple carboxylase defects and complementation studies with propionicacidemia in cultured fibroblasts. *J Clin Invest* **64**:1695, 1979.
203. Lamhonwah AM, Lam KF, Tsui F, Robinson B, Saunders ME, Gravel RA: Assignment of the α and β chains of human propionyl-CoA carboxylase to genetic complementation groups. *Am J Hum Genet* **35**:889, 1983.
204. Lamhonwah AM, Gravel RA: Propionic-acidemia: Absence of alpha chain mRNA in fibroblasts from patients of the pccA complementation group. *Am J Hum Genet* **41**:1124, 1987.
205. Ohura T, Kraus JP, Rosenberg LE: Unequal synthesis and differential degradation of propionyl CoA carboxylase subunits in cells from normal and propionic acidemia patients. *Am J Hum Genet* **45**:33, 1989.
206. Ohura T, Miyabayashi S, Narisawa K, Tada K: Genetic heterogeneity of propionic acidemia: Analysis of 15 Japanese patients. *Hum Genet* **87**:41, 1991.
207. Kalousek F, Orsulak MD, Rosenberg LE: Absence of cross-reacting material in isolated propionyl CoA carboxylase deficiency: Nature of residual carboxylating activity. *Am J Hum Genet* **35**:409, 1983.
208. Hillman RE, Sowers LH, Cohen JL: Inhibition of glycine oxidation in cultured fibroblasts by isoleucine. *Pediatr Res* **7**:945, 1973.
209. Hillman RE, Otto EF: Inhibition of glycine-serine interconversion in cultured human fibroblasts by products of isoleucine catabolism. *Pediatr Res* **8**:941, 1974.
210. Snyderman SE, Holt CE, Norton PM, Roitman E, Phansalkar SV: The plasma aminogram. I. Influence of the level of protein intake and a comparison of whole protein and amino acid diets. *Pediatr Res* **2**:131, 1968.
211. Glasgow AM, Chase HP: Effect of propionic acid on fatty acid oxidation and ureagenesis. *Pediatr Res* **10**:683, 1976.
212. Stewart PM, Walser M: Failure of the normal ureagenic response to amino acids in organic acid loaded rats: A proposed mechanism for the hyperammonemia of propionic and methylmalonic acidemia. *J Clin Invest* **66**:484, 1980.
213. Coude FX, Sweetman L, Nyhan WL: Inhibition by propionyl CoA of *N*-acetylglutamate synthetase in rat liver mitochondria. *J Clin Invest* **64**:1544, 1979.
214. Kirkman HN, Kiesel JL: Congenital hyperammonemia. *Pediatr Res* **3**:358, 1969.
215. Harris DJ, Yang BJ-Y, Snodgrass PJ: Carbamyl phosphate synthetase deficiency: A possible transient phenocopy of dysautonomia [Abstract]. *Am J Hum Genet* **29**:52, 1977.
216. Richard E, Desviat LR, Perez-Cerda C, Ugarte M: Three novel splice mutations in the PCCA gene causing identical exon skipping in propionic acidemia patients. *Hum Genet* **101**:93, 1997.
217. Campeau E, Dupuis L, Leclere D, Gravel RA: Detection of a normally rare transcript in propionic acidemia patients with mRNA destabilizing mutations in the PCCA gene. *Hum Mol Genet* **8**:107, 1999.
218. Richard E, Desviat LR, Perez B, Perez-Cerda C, Ugarte M: Genetic heterogeneity in propionic acidemia patients with alpha-subunit defects. Identification of five novel mutations, one of them causing instability of the protein. *Biochim Biophys Acta* **1453**:351, 1999.
219. Lamhonwah AM, Troxel CE, Schuster S, Gravel RA: Two distinct mutations at the same site in the PCCB gene in propionic acidemia. *Genomics* **8**:249, 1990.
220. Tahara T, Kraus JP, Rosenberg LE: An unusual insertion/deletion in the gene encoding the β-subunit of propionyl-CoA carboxylase is a frequent mutation in caucasian propionic acidemia. *Proc Natl Acad Sci U S A* **87**:1372, 1990.
221. Tahara T, Kraus JP, Ohura T, Rosenberg LE, Fenton WA: Three independent mutations in the same exon of the PCCB gene: Differences between caucasian and Japanese propionic acidaemia. *J Inherit Metab Dis* **16**:353, 1993.
222. Hoenicka J, Rodriguez-Pombo P, Perez-Cerda C, Muro S, Richard E, Ugarte M: New frequent mutation in the PCCB gene in Spanish propionic acidemia patients. *Hum Mutat* **12**:1, 1999.
223. Ohura T, Narisawa K, Tada K: Propionic acidaemia: Sequence analysis of mutant mRNAs from Japanese beta subunit-deficient patients. *J Inherit Metab Dis* **16**:863, 1993.
224. Ohura T, Narisawa K, Tada K, Iinuma K: A novel splicing mutation in propionic acidemia associated with a tetranucleotide direct repeat in the PCCB gene. *Hum Genet* **95**:707, 1995.
225. Gravel RA, Akerman BR, Lamhonwah A-M, Loyer M, Leon-del-Rio A, Italiano I: Mutations participating in interallelic complementation in propionic acidemia. *Am J Hum Genet* **55**:51, 1994.
226. Loyer M, Leclerc D, Gravel RA: Interallelic complementation of beta-subunit defects in fibroblasts of patients with propionyl-CoA carboxylase deficiency microinjected with mutant cDNA constructs. *Hum Mol Genet* **4**:1035, 1995.
227. Kelson TL, Ohura T, Kraus JP: Chaperonin-mediated assembly of wild-type and mutant subunits of human propionyl-CoA carboxylase expressed in *Escherichia coli*. *Hum Mol Genet* **5**:331, 1996.
228. Gompertz D, Goodey PA, Thom H, Russell G, Johnston AW, Mellor DH, MacLean MW, et al.: Prenatal diagnosis and family studies in case of propionicacidemia. *Clin Genet* **8**:244, 1975.
229. Chadefaux B, Augereau C, Rabier D, Rocchiccioli F, Boué J, Oury JF, Kamoun P: Prenatal diagnosis of propionic acidaemia in chorionic villi by direct assay of propionyl-CoA carboxylase. *Prenat Diagn* **8**:161, 1988.
230. Willard HF, Ambani LM, Hart AC, Mahoney MJ, Rosenberg LE: Rapid prenatal and postnatal detection of inborn errors of propionate, methylmalonate, and cobalamin metabolism: A sensitive assay using cultured cells. *Hum Genet* **34**:277, 1976.
231. Sweetman L, Weyler W, Shafai T, Young PE, Nyhan WL: Prenatal diagnosis of propionic acidemia. *JAMA* **242**:1048, 1979.
232. Gortner L, Leupold D, Pohlandt F, Bartmann P: Peritoneal dialysis in the treatment of metabolic crises caused by inherited disorders of organic and amino acid metabolism. *Acta Paediatr Scand* **78**:706, 1989.
233. Kahler SG, Millington DS, Cederbaum SD, Vargas J, Bond LD, Maltby DA, Gale DS, Roe CR: Parenteral nutrition in propionic and methylmalonic acidemia. *J Pediatr* **15**:235, 1989.

234. Wolf B: Reassessment of biotin-responsiveness in "unresponsive" propionyl CoA carboxylase deficiency. *J Pediatr* **97**:964, 1980.
235. Roe CR, Millington DS, Maltby DA, Bohan TP: L-carnitine enhances excretion of propionyl coenzyme A as propionylcarnitine in propionic acidemia. *J Clin Invest* **73**:1785, 1984.
236. Wolff JA, Carroll JE, Thuy LP, Prodanos C, Haas R, Nyhan WL: Carnitine reduces fasting ketogenesis in patients with disorders of propionate metabolism. *Lancet* **1**:289, 1986.
237. Thompson GN, Chalmers RA, Walter JH, Bresson JL, Lyonnet SL, Reed PJ, Saudubray JM, et al.: The use of metronidazole in management of methylmalonic and propionic acidaemias. *Eur J Pediatr* **149**:792, 1990.
238. Van der Meer SB, Poggi F, Spada M, Bonnefont JP, Ogier H, Hubert P, Depondt E, et al.: Clinical outcome and long-term management of 17 patients with propionic acidaemia. *Eur J Pediatr* **155**:205, 1996.
239. Van Calcar SC, Harding CO, Davidson SR, Barness LA, Wolff JA: Case reports of successful pregnancy in women with maple syrup urine disease and propionic acidemia. *Am J Med Genet* **44**:641, 1992.
240. Gompertz D, Draffan GH, Watts JL, Hull D: Biotin-responsive methylcrotonyl-glycinuria. *Lancet* **2**:22, 1971.
241. Sweetman L, Bates SP, Hull D, Nyhan WL, Saunders M, Robinson B, Roth K, et al.: Propionyl-CoA carboxylase deficiency in a patient with biotin-responsive 3-methylcrotonyl-glycinuria biotin-response organicaciduria: Multiple carboxylase defects and complementation studies with propionicacidemia in cultured fibroblasts. *Pediatr Res* **64**:1695, 1979.
242. Bartlett K, Gompertz D: Combined carboxylase defect: Biotin-responsiveness in cultured fibroblasts. *Lancet* **2**:804, 1976.
243. Weyler W, Sweetman L, Maggie DC, Nyhan WL: Deficiency of propionyl-CoA carboxylase and methylcrotonyl-CoA carboxylase in a patient with methylcrotonylglycinuria. *Clin Chim Acta* **76**:321, 1977.
244. Buri BJ, Sweetman L, Nyhan WL: Mutant holocarboxylase synthetase: Evidence for the enzyme defect in early infantile biotin-responsive multiple carboxylase deficiency. *J Clin Invest* **68**:1491, 1981.
245. Ghneim HK, Bartlett K: Mechanism of biotin-responsive combined carboxylase deficiency. *Lancet* **1**:1187, 1982.
246. Saunders ME, Sherwood WG, Duthie M, Surh L, Gravel RA: Evidence for a defect of holocarboxylase synthetase activity in cultured lymphoblasts from a patient with biotin-responsive multiple carboxylase deficiency. *Am J Hum Genet* **34**:590 1982.
247. Burri BJ, Sweetman L, Nyhan WL: Heterogeneity of holocarboxylase synthetase in patients with biotin-responsive multiple carboxylase deficiency. *Am J Hum Genet* **37**:426, 1985.
248. Wolf B, Brier RE, Allen RJ, Goodman SI, Kien CL: Biotinidase deficiency: The enzymatic defect in late-onset multiple carboxylase deficiency. *Clin Chim Acta* **131**:272, 1983.
249. Gaudry M, Munnich A, Agoier H, Marsac C, Marquet A, Saudubray JM, Mitchell G, et al.: Deficient liver biotinidase activity in multiple carboxylase deficiency. *Lancet* **2**:397, 1983.
250. Wolf B, Heard GS, Secor Mcvoy JR, Grier RE: Biotinidase deficiency. *Ann N Y Acad Sci* **447**:529, 1985.
251. Burri BJ, Sweetman L, Nyhan WL: Mutant holocarboxylase synthetase: Evidence for the enzyme defect in early infantile biotin-responsive multiple carboxylase deficiency. *J Clin Invest* **68**:1491, 1981.
252. Burri BJ, Sweetman L, Nyhan WL: Heterogeneity of holocarboxylase synthetase in patients with biotin-responsive multiple carboxylase deficiency. *Am J Hum Genet* **37**:426, 1985.
253. Dupuis L, Leon-del-Rio A, Leclerc D, Campeau E, Sweetman L, Saudubray JM, Herman G, et al.: Clustering of mutations in the biotin-binding region of holocarboxylase synthetase in biotin-responsive multiple carboxylase deficiency. *Hum Mol Genet* **5**:1011, 1996.
254. Dupuis L, Campeau E, Leclerc D, Gravel RA: Mechanism of biotin responsiveness in biotin-responsive multiple carboxylase deficiency. *Mol Genet Metab* **66**:80, 1999.
255. Aoki Y, Suzuki Y, Sakamoto O, Li X, Takahashi K, Ohtake A, Sakuta R, et al.: Molecular analysis of holocarboxylase synthetase deficiency: A missense mutation and a single base deletion are predominant in Japanese patients. *Biochim Biophys Acta* **1272**:168, 1995.
256. Sakamoto O, Suzuki Y, Aoki Y, Li X, Hiratsuka M, Yanagihara K, Inui K, et al.: Molecular analysis of new Japanese patients with holocarboxylase synthetase deficiency. *J Inherit Metab Dis* **21**:873, 1998.
257. Aoki Y, Suzuki Y, Li X, Sakamoto O, Chikaoka H, Takita S, Narisawa K: Characterization of mutant holocarboxylase synthetase (HCS): A K_m for biotin was not elevated in a patient with HCS deficiency. *Pediatr Res* **42**:849, 1997.
258. Pomponio RJ, Hymes J, Reynolds TR, Meyers GA, Fleischhauer K, Buck GA, Wolf B: Mutations in the human biotinidase gene that cause profound biotinidase deficiency in symptomatic children — molecular, biochemical, and clinical analysis. *Pediatr Res* **42**:840, 1997.
259. Norrgard KJ, Pomponio RJ, Swango KL, Hymes J, Reynolds TR, Buck GA, Wolf B: Mutation (Q456H) is the most common cause of profound biotinidase deficiency in children ascertained by newborn screening in the United States. *Biochem Mol Med* **61**:22, 1997.
260. Pomponio RJ, Reynolds TR, Cole H, Buck GA, Wolf B: Mutational hotspot in the human biotinidase gene causes profound biotinidase deficiency. *Nat Genet* **11**:96, 1995.
261. Rosenberg LE, Lilljeqvist A, Hsia YE: Methylmalonic aciduria: Metabolic block localization and vitamin B_{12} dependency. *Science* **162**:805, 1968.
262. Mudd SH, Levy HL, Abeles RH: A derangement in B_{12} metabolism leading to homocystinemia, cystathioninemia and methylmalonicaciduria. *Biochem Biophys Res Commun* **35**:121, 1969.
263. Goodman SI, Moe PG, Hammond KB, Mudd SH, Uhlendorff BW: Homocystinuria with methylmalonic aciduria: Two cases in a sibship. *Biochem Med* **4**:500, 1970.
264. Matsui SM, Mahoney MJ, Rosenberg LE: The natural history of the inherited methylmalonic acidemias. *New Engl J Med* **308**:857, 1983.
265. Shevell MI, Matiaszuk N, Ledley FD, Rosenblatt DS: Varying neurological phenotypes among *mut*^{0} and *mut*$^-$ patients with methylmalonylCoA mutase deficiency. *Am J Med Genet* **45**:619, 1993.
266. Rosenberg LE: Disorders of propionate, methylmalonate and cobalamin metabolism, in Stanbury JB, Wyngaarden JB, Fredrickson DS (eds): *The Metabolic Basis of Inherited Disease*, 4th ed. New York, McGraw-Hill, 1978, p 411.
267. Ledley FD, Levy HL, Shih VE, Benjamin R, Mahoney MJ: Benign methylmalonic aciduria. *New Engl J Med* **311**:1015, 1984.
268. Shapira SK, Ledley FD, Rosenblatt DS, Levy HL: Ketoacidotic crisis as a presentation of benign methylmalonic aciduria. *J Pediatr* **119**:80, 1991.
269. Sniderman LC, Lambert M, Giguere R, Auray-Blais C, Lemieux B, Laframboise R, Rosenblatt DS, et al.: Outcome of individuals with low-moderate methylmalonic aciduria detected through a neonatal screening program. *J Pediatr* **134**:680, 1999.
270. Mayatepek E, Hoffmann GF, Baumgartner R, Schulze A, Jacobs C, Trefz FK, Bremer HJ: Atypical vitamin B_{12}-unresponsive methylmalonic aciduria in a sibship with severe progressive encephalopathy: a new genetic disease? *Eur J Pediatr* **155**:398, 1996.
271. Roe CR, Struys E, Kok RM, Roe DS, Jakobs C: Methylmalonic semialdehyde dehydrogenase deficiency: Psychomotor delay and methylmalonic aciduria without metabolic decomposition. *J Inher Metab Dis* **21**:54, 1998.
272. Ando T, Rasmussen K, Nyhan WL, Donnell GN, Barnes ND: Propionicacidemia in patients with ketotic hyperglycinemia. *J Pediatr* **78**:827, 1971.
273. Stokke O, Jellum E, Eldjarn L, Schnitler R: The occurrence of hydroxy-*n*-valeric acid in a patient with propionic and methylmalonic acidemia. *Clin Chim Acta* **45**:391, 1973.
274. Hsia YE, Scully K, Lilljeqvist A-CH, Rosenberg LE: Vitamin B_{12} dependent methylmalonicaciduria. *Pediatrics* **46**:497, 1970.
275. Morrow G, Revsin B, Mathews C, Giles H: A simple rapid method for prenatal detection of defects in propionate metabolism. *Clin Genet* **10**:218, 1976.
276. Morrow G 3rd, Barness LA, Cardinale GJ, Abeles RH, Flaks JG: Congenital methylmalonic acidemia: Enzymatic evidence for two forms of the disease. *Proc Natl Acad Sci U S A* **63**:191, 1969.
277. Morrow G, 3rd, Mahoney MJ, Mathews C, Lebowitz J: Studies of methylmalonyl coenzyme A carbonylmutase activity in methylmalonic acidemia. I. Correlation of clinical, hepatic, and fibroblast data. *Pediatr Res* **9**:641, 1975.
278. Willard HF, Rosenberg LE: Inherited deficiencies of human methylmalonyl CoA mutase activity: Reduced affinity of mutant apoenzyme for adenosylcobalamin. *Biochem Biophys Res Commun* **78**:927, 1977.
279. Willard HF, Rosenberg LE: Inherited methylmalonyl CoA mutase apoenzyme deficiency in human fibroblasts: Evidence for allelic heterogeneity, genetic compounds, and codominant expression. *J Clin Invest* **65**:690, 1980.
280. Kolhouse JF, Utley C, Fenton WA, Rosenberg LE: Immunochemical studies on cultured fibroblasts from patients with inherited methylmalonic acidemia. *Proc Natl Acad Sci U S A* **78**:7737, 1981.
281. Fenton WA, Hack AM, Kraus JP, Rosenberg LE: Immunochemical studies of fibroblasts from patients with methylmalonyl-CoA mutase

apoenzyme deficiency: Detection of a mutation interfering with mitochondrial import. *Proc Natl Acad Sci U S A* **84**:1421, 1987.
282. Ledley FD, Jansen R, Nham SU, Fenton WA, Rosenberg LE: Mutation eliminating mitochondrial leader sequence of methylmalonyl-CoA mutase causes *mut*^{0} methylmalonic aciduria. *Proc Natl Acad Sci U S A* **87**:3147, 1990.
283. Morrow G III, Revsin B, Clark R, Lebowitz J, Whelen DT: A new variant of methylamlonic acidemia: Defective coenzyme-apoenzyme binding in cultured fibroblasts. *Clin Chem Acta* **85**:67, 1978.
284. Ledley FD, Crane AM, Lumetta M: Heterogeneous alleles and expression of methylmalonyl CoA mutase in *mut* methylmalonic acidemia. *Am J Hum Genet* **6**:539, 1990.
285. Jansen R, Ledley FD: Heterozygous mutations at the MUT locus in fibroblasts with methylmalonic acidemia identified by Polymerase Chain Reaction and cDNA cloning. *Am J Hum Genet* **47**:808, 1990.
286. Raff ML, Crane AM, Jansen R, Ledley FD, Rosenblatt DS: Genetic characterization of a MUT locus mutatation discriminating heterogeneity in *mut*^{o} and *mut*$^-$ methymalonic aciduria by interallelic complementation. *J Clin Invest* **87**:203, 1991.
287. Crane AM, Jansen R, Andrews ER, Ledley FD: Cloning and expression of a mutant methylmalonyl coenzyme A mutase with altered cobalamin affinity that causes *mut*$^-$ methylmalonic aciduria. *J Clin Invest* **89**:385, 1992.
288. Ledley FD, Rosenblatt DS: Mutations in mut methylmalonic acidemia: Clinical and enzymatic correlations. *Hum Mut* **9**:1, 1997.
289. Adjalla CE, Hosack AR, Gilfix BM, Sun S, Chan A, Evans S, Matiaszuk NV, et al.: Seven novel mutations in mut methylmalonic aciduria. *Hum Mut* **11**:270, 1998.
290. Adjalla CE, Hosack AR, Matiaszuk NV, Rosenblatt DS: A common mutation among blacks with mut$^-$ methylmalonic aciduria. *Hum Mut Suppl* **1**:248, 1998.
291. Crane A, Martin LS, Valle D, Ledley FD: Phenotype of disease in three patients with identical mutations in methylmalonyl CoA mutase. *Hum Genet* **89**:259, 1992.
292. Ogasawara M, Matsubara Y, Mikami H, Narisawa KK: Identification of two novel mutations in the methylmalonyl-CoA mutase gene with decreased levels of mutant mRNA in methylmalonic acidemia. *Hum Mol Genet* **3**:867, 1994.
293. Drennan CL, Matthews RG, Rosenblatt DS, Ledley FD, Fenton WA, Ludwig ML: Molecular basis for dysfunction of some mutant forms of methylmalonyl-CoA mutase: Deductions from the structure of methionine synthase. *Proc Natl Acad Sci U S A* **93**:5550, 1996.
294. Kang ES, Snodgrass PJ, Gerald PS: Methylmalonyl coenzyme A racemase defect: Another cause of methylmalonic aciduria. *Pediatr Res* **6**:875, 1972.
295. Gravel RA, Mahoney MJ, Ruddle FH, Rosenberg LE: Genetic complementation in heterokaryons of human fibroblasts defective in cobalamin metabolism. *Proc Natl Acad Sci U S A* **72**:3181, 1975.
296. Willard HF, Mellman IS, Rosenberg LE: Genetic complementation among inherited deficiencies of methylmalonyl-CoA mutase activity: Evidence for a new class of human cobalamin mutant. *Am J Hum Genet* **30**:1, 1978.
297. Willard HF, Rosenberg LE: Inborn errors of cobalamin metabolism: Effect of cobalamin supplementation in culture on methylmalonyl CoA mutase activity in normal and mutant human fibroblasts. *Biochem Genet* **17**:57, 1979.
298. Watanabe F, Saido H, Yamaji R, Miyatake K, Isegawa Y, Ito A, Yubisui T, et al.: Mitochondrial NADH- or NADP-linked aquacobalamin reductase activity is low in human skin fibroblasts with defects in synthesis of cobalamin coenzymes. *J Nutr* **126**:2947, 1996.
299. Cooper BA, Rosenblatt DS, Watkins D: Methylmalonic aciduria due to a new defect in adenosylcobalamin accumulation by cells. *Am J Hematol* **34**:115, 1990.
300. Utter MF, Keech DB, Scrutten ML: A possible role for acetyl-CoA in the control of gluconeogenesis, in Webber G (ed): *Advances in Enzyme Regulation*. Vol. 2. New York, Pergamon, 1964, p 49.
301. Halperin ML, Schiller CM, Fritz IB: The inhibition by methylmalonic acid of malate transport by the dicarboxylate carrier in rat liver mitochondria: A possible explanation for hypoglycemia in methylmalonic aciduria. *J Clin Invest* **50**:2276, 1971.
302. Inoue S, Krieger I, Sarnaik A, Ravindranath Y, Fracassa M, Ottenbreit MJ: Inhibition of bone marrow stem cell growth *in vitro* by methylmalonic acid: A mechanism for pancytopenia in a patient with methylmalonic acidemia. *Pediatr Res* **15**:95, 1981.
303. Coulombe JT, Shih VE, Levy HL: Massachusetts Metabolic Disorders Screening Program. II. Methylmalonic aciduria. *Pediatrics* **67**:26, 1981.
304. MacMahon M: Requesting vitamin B_{12} and folate assays. *Lancet* **346**:973, 1995.
305. Rosenblatt DS, Cooper BA: Inherited disorders of vitamin B_{12} metabolism. *Blood Rev* **1**:177, 1987.
306. Morrow G, Schwartz RH, Hallock JA, Barness LA: Prenatal detection of methylmalonic acidemia. *J Pediatr* **77**:120, 1970.
307. Ampola MG, Mahoney MJ, Nakamura E, Tanaka K: Prenatal therapy of a patient with vitamin B_{12} responsive methylmalonic acidemia. *New Engl J Med* **293**:313, 1975.
308. Mahoney MJ, Rosenberg LE, Linblad B, Waldenstrom J, Zetterstrom R: Prenatal diagnosis of methylmalonic aciduria. *Acta Paediatr Scand* **64**:44, 1975.
309. Hack AM, Fenton WA: Unpublished results.
310. Nyhan WL, Fawcett N, Ando T, Rennert OM, Julius RL: Response to dietary therapy in B_{12} unresponsive methylmalonic acidemia. *Pediatrics* **51**:539, 1973.
311. Satoh T, Narisawa K, Igarashi Y, Saitoh T, Hayasaka K, Ichinohazama Y, Onodera H, Tada K, Oohara K: Dietary therapy in two patients with vitamin B_{12}-unresponsive methylmalonic acidemia. *Eur J Pediatr* **135**:305, 1981.
312. Roe CR, Bohan TP: L-carnitine therapy in propionic acidemia. *Lancet* **1**:1411, 1982.
313. Roe CR, Hoppel CL, Stacey TE, Chalmers RA, Tracey BM, Millington DS: Metabolic response to carnitine in methylmalonic aciduria. *Arch Dis Child* **58**:916, 1983.
314. Koletzko B, Bachmann C, Wendel U: Antibiotic therapy for improvement of metabolic control in methylmalonic aciduria. *J Pediatr* **117**:99, 1990.
315. Batshaw ML, Thomas GH, Cohen SR, Matalon R, Mahoney MJ: Treatment of the cbl B form of methylmalonic acidaemia with adenosylcobalamin. *J Inherit Metab Dis* **7**:65, 1984.
316. Chalmers RA, Bain MD, Mistry J, Tracey BM, Weaver C: Enzymologic studies on patients with methylmalonic aciduria: Basis for a clinical trial of deoxyadenosylcobalamin in a hydroxocobalamin-unresponsive patient. *Pediatr Res* **30**:560, 1991.
317. Korf B, Wallman JK, Levy HL: Bilateral lucency of the globus pallidus complicating methylmalonic acidemia. *Ann Neurol* **20**:364, 1986.
318. Morrow G III, Burkel GM: Long-term management of a patient with vitamin B_{12}-responsive methylmalonic acidemia. *J Pediatr* **96**:425, 1980.
319. Thompson GN, Christodoulou J, Danks DM: Metabolic stroke in methylmalonic acidemia. *J Pediatr* **115**:499, 1989.
320. Rutledge SL, Geraghty M, Mroczek E, Rosenblatt D, Kohout E: Tubulointerstitial nephritis in methylmalonic aciduria. *Pediatr Nephrol* **7**(1):81, 1993.
321. Walter JH, Michalski A, Wilson WM, Leonard JV, Barratt TM, Dillon MJ: Chronic renal failure in methylmalonic acidaemia. *Eur J Pediatr* **148**:344, 1989.
322. Treacy E, Arbour L, Chessex P, Graham G, Kasprzak L, Casey K, Bell L, et al.: Glutathione deficiency as a complication of methylmalonic acidemia, response to high ascorbate. *J Pediatr* **129**:445, 1996.
323. Van der Meer SB, Spaapen LJM, Fowler B, Jakobs C, Kleijer WJ, Wendel U: Prenatal treatment of a patient with vitamin B_{12}-responsive methylmalonic acidemia. *J Pediatr* **117**:923, 1990.
324. Evans MI, Duquette DA, Rinaldo P, Bawle E, Rosenblatt DS, Whitty J, Quintera RA, Johnson MP: Modulation of B_{12} dosage and response in fetal treatment of methylmalonic aciduria (MMA): Titration of treatment dose to serum and urine MMA. *Fetal Diagn Ther* **12**:21, 1997.
325. Leonard JV: The management and outcome of propionic and methylmalonic acidaemia. *J Inherit Metab Dis* **18**:430, 1995.
326. Nicolaides P, Leonard J, Surtees R: Neurological outcome of methylmalonic acidaemia. *Arch Dis Child* **78**:508, 1998.
327. Wilcken B, Carpenter K, Dorney S, Shun A: Liver transplantation in methylmalonic aciduria. *J Inherit Metab Dis* **21**:42, 1998.
328. McKiernan PJ, Preece MA, Leonard JV, Mayer AD, Buckels JAC: Liver transplantation in infancy for severe methylmalonic acidaemia. *J Inherit Metab Dis* **21**:42, 1998.
329. Adams RM, Soriano HE, Wang M, Darlington G, Steffen D, Ledley FD: Transduction of primary human hepatocytes with amphotropic and xenotropic retroviral vectors. *Proc Natl Acad Sci U S A* **89**:8981, 1992.
330. Stankovics J, Andrews E, Wu G, Ledley FD: Overexpression of human methylmalonyl CoA mutase (MCM) in mouse liver after *in vivo* gene delivery using asialoglycoprotein complexes [Abstract]. *Am J Hum Genet* **51**:177, 1992.
331. Levy HL, Mudd SH, Schulman JD, Dreyfus PM, Abeles RH: A derangement in B_{12} metabolism associated with homocystinemia,

cystathioninemia, hypomethioninemia and methylmalonic aciduria. *Am J Med* **48**:390, 1970.

332. Dillon MJ, England JM, Gompertz D, Goodey PA, Grant DB, Hussein HA, Linnell JC, et al. Mental retardation, megaloblastic anemia, methylmalonic aciduria and abnormal homocysteine metabolism due to an error in vitamin B_{12} metabolism. *Clin Sci Mol Med* **47**:43, 1974.
333. Anthony M, McLeay AC: A unique case of derangement of vitamin B_{12} metabolism. *Proc Aust Assoc Neurol* **13**:61, 1976.
334. Baumgartner ER, Wick H, Maurer R, Egli N, Steinmann B: Congenital defect in intracellular cobalamin metabolism resulting in homocystinuria and methylmalonic aciduria. I. Case report and histopathology. *Helv Paediatr Acta* **34**:465, 1979.
335. Carmel R, Bedros AA, Mace JW, Goodman SI: Congenital methylmalonic aciduria-homocystinuria with megaloblastic anemia: Observations on response to hydroxocobalamin and on the effect of homocysteine and methionine on the deoxyuridine suppression test. *Blood* **55**:570, 1980.
336. Shinnar S, Singer HS: Cobalamin C mutation (methylmalonic aciduria and homocystinuria) in adolescence: A treatable cause of dementia and myelopathy. *New Engl J Med* **311**:451, 1984.
337. Mitchell GA, Watkins D, Melancon SB, Rosenblatt DS, Geoffroy G, Orquin J, Homsy MB, et al.: Clinical heterogeneity in cobalamin C variant of combined homocystinuria and methylmalonic aciduria. *J Pediatr* **108**:410, 1986.
338. Cogan DG, Schulman J, Porter RJ, Mudd SH: Epileptiform ocular movements with methylmalonic aciduria and homocystinuria. *Am J Ophthalmol* **90**:251, 1980.
339. Linnell JC, Miranda B, Bhatt HR, Dowton SB, Levy HL: Abnormal cobalamin metabolism in a megaloblastic child with homocystinuria, cystathioninuria and methylmalonic aciduria. *J Inherit Metab Dis* **6**(Suppl 2):137, 1983.
340. Mamlock RJ, Isenberg JN, Rassin DN: A cobalamin metabolic defect with homocystinuria, methylmalonic aciduria and macrocytic anemia. *Neuropediatrics* **17**:94, 1986.
341. Ravindranath Y, Krieger I: Vitamin B_{12} (Cbl) and folate interrelationship in a case of homocystinuria-methylmalonic (HC-MMA)-uria due to genetic deficiency. *Pediatr Res* **18**:247a, 1984.
342. Ribes A, Vilaseca A, Briones P, Maya A, Sabater J, Pascual P, Alvarez L, Ros J, Gonzalez Pascual E. Methylmalonic aciduria with homocystinuria. *J Inherit Metab Dis* **7**:129, 1984.
343. Robb RM, Dowton SB, Fulton AB, Levy HL: Retinal degeneration in vitamin B_{12} disorder associated with methylmalonic aciduria and sulfur amino acid abnormalities. *Am J Ophthalmol* **97**:691, 1984.
344. Rosenblatt DS, Laframboise R, Pichette J, Langevin P, Cooper BA, Costa T: New disorder of vitamin B_{12} metabolism (cobalamin F) presenting as methylmalonic aciduria. *Pediatrics* **78**:51, 1986.
345. Shih VE, Axel SM, Tewksbury JC, Watkins D, Cooper BA, Rosenblatt DS: Defective lysosomal release of vitamin B_{12} (cblF): A hereditary metabolic disorder associated with sudden death. *Am J Med Genet* **33**:555, 1989.
346. Wong LTK, Rosenblatt DS, Applegarth DA, Davidson AGF: Diagnosis and treatment of a child with cblF disease [Abstract]. *Clin Invest Med* **15**(suppl):111, 1992.
347. MacDonald MR, Wiltse HE, Bever JL, Rosenblatt DS: Clinical heterogeneity in two patients with cblF disease [Abstract]. *Am J Hum Genet* **51**:353, 1992.
348. Watkins D, Rosenblatt DS: Failure of lysosomal release of vitamin B_{12}: A new complementation group causing methylmalonic aciduria (cblF). *Am J Hum Genet* **39**:404, 1986.
349. Rosenblatt DS, Aspler AL, Shevell MI, Pletcher BA, Fenton WA, Seashore MR: Clinical heterogeneity and prognosis in combined methylmalonic aciduria and homocytinuria (cblC). *J Inherit Met Dis* **20**:528, 1997.
350. Linnell JC, Matthews DM, Mudd SH, Uhlendorf BW, Wise IJ: Cobalamins in fibroblasts cultured from normal control subjects and patients with methylmalonic aciduria. *Pediatr Res* **10**:179, 1976.
351. Baumgartner ER, Wick H, Linnell JC, Gaull GE, Bachmann C, Steinmann B: Congenital defect in intracellular cobalamin metabolism resulting in homocystinuria and methylmalonic aciduria. II. Biochemical investigations. *Helv Paediatr Acta* **34**:483, 1979.
352. Rosenberg LE, Patel L, Lilljeqvist A: Absence of an intracellular cobalamin binding protein in cultured fibroblasts from patients with defective synthesis of 5′-deoxyadenosylcobalamin and methylcobalamin. *Proc Natl Acad Sci U S A* **72**:4617, 1975.
353. Mudd SH, Uhlendorf BW, Hinds KR, Levy HL: Deranged B_{12} metabolism: Studies of fibroblasts grown in tissue culture. *Biochem Med* **4**:215, 1970.
354. Mellman IS, Lin P-F, Ruddle FH, Rosenberg LE: Genetic control of cobalamin binding in normal and mutant cells: Assignment of the gene for 5-methyltetrahydrofolate: L-homocysteine S-methyltransferase to human chromosome 1. *Proc Natl Acad Sci U S A* **76**:405, 1979.
355. Mellman IH, Willard HF, Youngdahl-Turner P, Rosenberg LE: Cobalamin coenzyme synthesis in normal and mutant human fibroblasts: Evidence for a processing enzyme activity deficient in cblC cells. *J Biol Chem* **254**:11847, 1979.
356. Pezacka EH: Identification and characterization of two enzymes involved in the intracellular metabolism of cobalamin: Cyanocobalamin beta-ligand transferase and microsomal cob(III)alamin reductase. *Biochim Biophys Acta* **1157**:167, 1993.
357. Pezacka EH, Rosenblatt DS: Intracellular metabolism of cobalamin. Altered activities of β-axial-ligand transferase and microsomal cob(III)alamin reductase in cblC and cblD fibroblasts, in Bhatt HR, James VHT, Besser GM, Bottazzo GF, Keen H (eds): *Advances in Thomas Addison's Diseases*. London, Bristol, Journal of Endocrinology, 1994, p 315.
358. Pezacka E, Green R, Jacobsen DW: Glutathionylcobalamin as an intermediate in the formation of cobalamin coenzymes. *Biochem Biophys Res Commun* **169**:443, 1990.
359. Vassiliadis A, Rosenblatt DS, Cooper BA, Bergeron JJ: Lysosomal cobalamin accumulation in fibroblasts from a patient with an inborn error of cobalamin metabolism (cblF complementation group): Visualization by electron microscope radioautography. *Exp Cell Res* **195**:295, 1991.
360. Leclerc D, Campeau E, Goyette P, Adjalla CE, Christensen B, Ross M, Eydoux P, et al.: Human methionine synthase: cDNA cloning and identification of mutations in patients of the cblG complementation group of folate/cobalamin disorders. *Hum Mol Genet* **5**:1867, 1996.
361. Li YN, Gulati S, Baker PJ, Brody LC, Banerjee R, Kruger WD: Cloning, mapping and RNA analysis of the human methionine synthase gene. *Hum Mol Genet* **5**:1851, 1996.
362. Gulati S, Baker P, Li YN, Fowler B, Kruger WD, Brody LC, Banerjee R: Defects in human methionine synthase in cblG patients. *Hum Mol Genet* **5**:1859, 1996.
363. Chen LH, Liu M, Hwang H, Chen L, Korenberg J, Shane B: Human methionine synthase: cDNA cloning, gene localization and expression. *J Biol Chem* **272**:3628, 1997.
364. Bellini C, Cerone R, Bonacci W, Caruso C, Magliano CP, Serra G, Fowler B, et al.: Biochemical diagnosis and outcome of 2 years treatment in a patient with combined methylmalonic aciduria and homocystinuria. *Eur J Pediatr* **151**:818, 1992.
365. Bartholomew DW, Batshaw ML, Allen RH, Roe CR, Rosenblatt D, Valle DL, Francomano CA: Therapeutic approaches to cobalamin-C methylmalonic acidemia and homocystinuria. *J Pediatr* **112**:32, 1988.
366. Kashani SA, Cooper BA: Endogenous folate of normal fibroblasts using high-performance liquid chromatography and modified extraction procedure. *Anal Biochem* **146**:40, 1985.

CHAPTER 95

Organic Acidemias Due to Defects in Lysine Oxidation: 2-Ketoadipic Acidemia and Glutaric Acidemia

Stephen I. Goodman ▪ Frank E. Frerman

1. **2-Ketoadipic acid, an intermediate in the metabolism of L-lysine, hydroxy-L-lysine, and L-tryptophan, undergoes successive oxidative decarboxylations by 2-ketoadipic dehydrogenase and glutaryl-CoA dehydrogenase to form glutaryl-CoA and crotonyl-CoA, respectively.**
2. **Deficiency of 2-ketoadipic dehydrogenase causes 2-ketoadipic acidemia (OMIM 245130), a condition characterized by accumulation and excretion of 2-ketoadipic, 2-aminoadipic, and 2-hydroxyadipic acids, probably without adverse phenotypic effects.**
3. **Deficiency of glutaryl-CoA dehydrogenase causes glutaric acidemia type I (OMIM 231670), a disorder characterized clinically by dystonia and dyskinesia appearing during the first years of life, chemically by excretion of glutaric and 3-hydroxyglutaric acids in urine, and pathologically by neuronal degeneration of the caudate and putamen. CT and MRI scans often show frontotemporal atrophy and/or arachnoid cysts before the onset of symptoms.**
4. **Glutaryl-CoA dehydrogenase deficiency is inherited as an autosomal recessive trait. More than 60 pathogenic mutations have been identified in the GCD gene (19p13.2), and because no one mutation is prominent outside of inbred groups, most GA1 patients are heterozygous for two different mutant alleles. Identification of heterozygous carriers, while possible by demonstration of activity of intermediate enzymes in cultured fibroblasts and peripheral leukocytes, is most accurately done by mutation analysis.**
5. **Striatal damage and neurologic phenotype do not develop in all patients, and there is evidence that early supplementation with L-carnitine, vigorous treatment of intercurrent infections with fluids, glucose and insulin, and (perhaps) dietary restriction of lysine and tryptophan can prevent their development in most instances.**
6. **Prenatal diagnosis is possible and is based on demonstrating increased concentrations of glutaric acid in amniotic fluid, deficiency of glutaryl-CoA dehydrogenase in cultured amniocytes or (probably) material obtained by CVS, or, in appropriate families, by mutation analysis.**

BIOCHEMISTRY

Steps in the conversion of L-lysine to 2-ketoadipic acid and defects in this pathway have been discussed in Chap. 86. 2-Ketoadipic acid, which is also an intermediate in the oxidation of hydroxy-L-lysine and L-tryptophan, is converted to crotonyl-CoA, an intermediate in fatty acid oxidation, by the sequential action of two enzymes, 2-ketoadipic dehydrogenase and glutaryl-CoA dehydrogenase (Fig. 95-1) Inherited defects in these proteins cause 2-ketoadipic acidemia and glutaric acidemia, respectively.

2-Ketoadipic dehydrogenase is a mitochondrial enzyme and has not been separated from 2-ketoglutaric acid dehydrogenase (EC 1.2.4.1), the citric acid cycle enzyme that forms succinyl-CoA.[1] The enzyme has at least three subunits analogous to those of pyruvate dehydrogenase (see Chap. 100): a thiamine-containing E-1 subunit that decarboxylates 2-ketoadipic acid to active glutaraldehyde (and possibly also 2-ketoglutaric acid to active succinaldehyde), an E-2 transacetylase, and an E-3 lipoamide dehydrogenase. It is likely that the E-3 subunit is the same protein as the E-3 subunits of pyruvate dehydrogenase and of branched-chain ketoacid dehydrogenase, and it may also form part of the glycine cleavage enzyme. Electrons from 2-ketoadipic dehydrogenase are transferred into the respiratory chain via NADH:ubiquinone oxidoreductase (Complex I).

Glutaryl CoA dehydrogenase (EC 1.3.99.7) is one of nine primary flavoprotein dehydrogenases of the mitochondrial matrix whose electrons are transferred to ubiquinone in the respiratory chain via ETF and ETF:ubiquinone oxidoreductase. Disorders of these enzymes, and the enzymes themselves, are discussed in Chaps. 89, 93, 101.

All preparations of glutaryl-CoA dehydrogenase (GCD), whether from *Pseudomonas fluorescens*,[2] *Paracoccus denitrificans*,[3,4] or mammalian mitochondria,[5,6] catalyze the oxidative decarboxylation of glutaryl-CoA to crotonyl-CoA. The paracoccal and mammalian enzymes are homotetramers, with each subunit containing one equivalent of noncovalently bound FAD.[3,6] Human GCD cDNA (GenBank accession number U69141) has been cloned and overexpressed in *Escherichia coli*. The mature subunit has a molecular weight of approximately 43.5 and is targeted to the mitochondrial matrix by a typical N-terminal leader sequence.[7]

A list of standard abbreviations is located immediately preceding the index in each volume. Nonstandard abbreviations used in this chapter include: ETF = electron transfer flavoprotein; GAD = glutamic acid decarboxylase; GCD = glutaryl-CoA dehydrogenase; MCAD = medium-chain acyl-CoA dehydrogenase; MCPA-CoA = methylene(cyclopropyl)acetyl-CoA; QA = quinolinic acid; SCAD = short-chain acyl-CoA dehydrogenase.

L-TRYPTOPHAN
L-LYSINE
HYDROXY-L-LYSINE
α-AMINOADIPIC ACID ① α-KETOADIPIC ACID ② GLUTARYL-CoA ③ CROTONYL-CoA → → 2 ACETYL-CoA
CoA, CO_2, NAD, NADH+H⁺, CO_2, FAD, FAD·2H

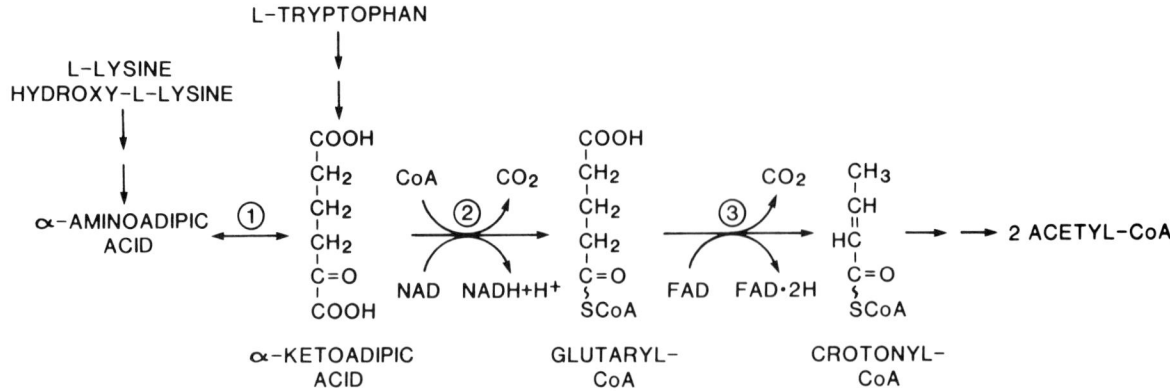

Fig. 95-1 Synthesis and oxidation of 2-ketoadipic acid in mammals. (1) Transaminase, (2) 2-ketoadipic dehydrogenase, (3) glutaryl-CoA dehydrogenase.

The three-dimensional structure of expressed human GCD has been resolved to 2.6 Å by x-ray crystallography,[8] and the GCD subunit has the same domain structure as other acyl-CoA dehydrogenases.[9] There is also appreciable sequence homology between the amino acid sequences of GCD and medium-chain acyl-CoA dehydrogenase (MCAD), particularly in areas defined by crystal structure to be important in substrate and FAD binding.[7] Glu376 in MCAD, the catalytic base that removes an α-proton to initiate catalysis, is conserved in GCD as Glu370. The position of this residue relative to substrate is the same as in MCAD and is not in the orientation found in isovaleryl-CoA and long-chain acyl-CoA dehydrogenases.[10,11] The structural similarities of GCD and MCAD also make it likely that GCD binds to ETF through salt bridges and hydrogen bonds to amino acid side chains in the C-terminal domain of the α-ETF subunit and to a few side chains in the β-subunit.[12]

The redox behavior of GCD differs somewhat from that of medium- and short-chain acyl-CoA dehydrogenases. Like MCAD and short-chain acyl-CoA dehydrogenase (SCAD), paracoccal and human GCD stabilize an anionic semiquinone of FAD in the presence of bound product (crotonyl-CoA); free MCAD and SCAD, however, stabilize a neutral semiquinone, but free GCD does not stabilize appreciable amounts of either an anionic or a neutral semiquinone. Also unlike MCAD and SCAD, human and bacterial GCD do not show appreciable long-wavelength absorbance when reduced with substrate under anaerobic conditions.[4,13]

Expressed human GCD has K_ms values of 4.2 μM and 1.1 μM for glutaryl-CoA and ETF, respectively, and a turnover number of 14.3/sec when assayed fluorometrically at 25°C.[7] The stoichiometry of the reaction is one glutaryl-CoA molecule oxidized per two equivalents of ETF semiquinone formed (Fig. 95-2). At 37°C, assayed with methylene blue as the electron acceptor and measurement of $^{14}CO_2$ release, the turnover number is 14/sec.[6] At high concentrations, hexanoyl-, octanoyl-, butyryl-, and isovaleryl-CoA, alternative substrates for oxidation, competitively inhibit decarboxylation of glutaryl-CoA.[6]

Glutaconyl-CoA may be a transient enzyme-bound intermediate in the reaction, as some data suggest that it can be decarboxylated by a partially purified preparation of glutaryl-CoA dehydrogenase from *Pseudomonas fluorescens*.[14] However, when radiolabeled glutaryl-CoA is oxidized by the mammalian enzyme, the only radiolabeled reaction products are crotonyl-CoA and carbon dioxide; glutaconyl-CoA (and 3-hydroxyglutaryl-CoA) is not detected.[5,6]

Investigation of the chemical mechanism of glutaryl-CoA dehydrogenase[2] suggests initial formation of an α-carbanion as the result of proton abstraction by a base catalyst on the enzyme, followed by transfer of the β-hydrogen as a hydride ion to FAD, yielding a glutaconyl-CoA intermediate (Fig. 95-3). An initial proton abstraction of this type is apparently common in the mechanisms of acyl-CoA dehydrogenases.[9] Carbon dioxide is not released from the intermediate in the absence of an electron acceptor for the reduced flavin.[2] The proton of the ω-methyl group of the crotonyl-CoA product is apparently derived from the α-proton, since solvent protons are not incorporated into this position, while the β-proton of the substrate exchanges with solvent via the flavin.[2] A similar proton shift occurs when MCAD catalyzes the conversion of 3,4-pentadienoyl-CoA to 2,4-pentadienoyl-CoA without net oxidation, probably by forming an N5 covalent adduct of the flavin.[15]

GCD is inhibited by methylene(cyclopropyl)acetyl-CoA (MCPA-CoA),[16] the hypoglycin A metabolite responsible for Jamaican vomiting sickness. The transient α-carbanion created by oxidation of MCPA-CoA leads to opening of the cyclopropyl ring, forming a compound that reacts covalently and irreversibly with the enzyme-bound flavin. MCPA-CoA thus acts as an active site directed inhibitor.[17]

GCD activity can be measured in several ways. The simplest and most sensitive assay uses (1,5-^{14}C)glutaryl-CoA as substrate (Fig. 95-4) and measures release of $^{14}CO_2$.[5] Another radioassay measures the release of tritium from carbon-3 of [2,3,4-^{3}H] glutaryl-CoA as it equilibrates with solvent water.[16] In both assays artificial electron acceptors are used to regenerate the oxidized dehydrogenase. GCD activity can also be assayed by following the disappearance of ETF flavin fluorescence as it becomes reduced to the semiquinone.[6] This assay, though far less sensitive, is potentially sensitive to alterations of the GCD domain that interacts with ETF.

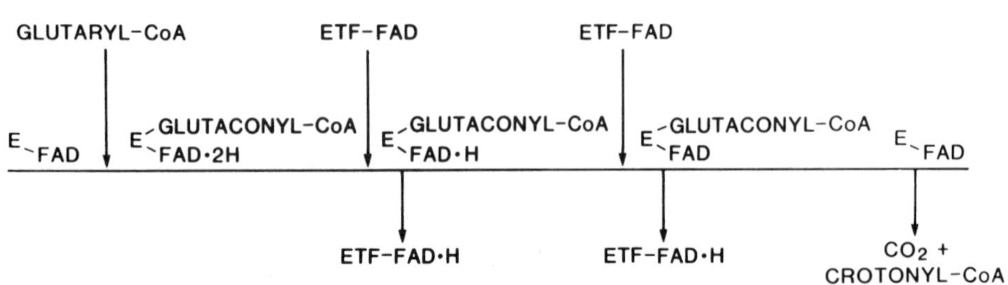

Fig. 95-2 Catalytic mechanism of glutaryl-CoA dehydrogenase. The sequence in which carbon dioxide and crotonyl-CoA leave the protein is not known.

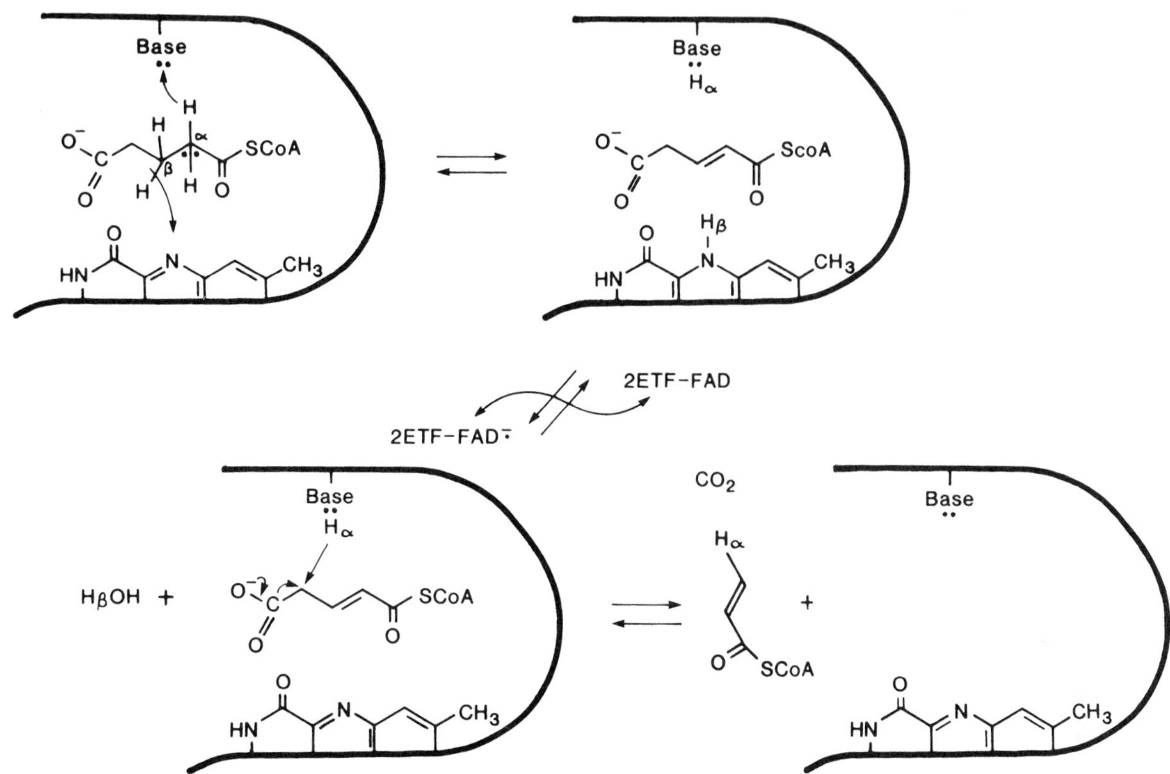

Fig. 95-3 Proton transfers during catalysis by glutaryl-CoA dehydrogenase, showing exchange of β-proton with solvent and transfer of α-proton to ω-carbon of crotonyl-CoA.

Glutaryl-CoA can be oxidized to glutaconyl-CoA in peroxisomes.[18] The enzyme responsible for the reaction, glutaryl-CoA oxidase, has an apparent K_m about fiftyfold higher and a V_{max} about fivefold lower than those of glutaryl-CoA dehydrogenase but is otherwise not well characterized. Shuttling of glutaryl-CoA between the mitochondrion and peroxisome has not been demonstrated in the normal state, and peroxisomal oxidation probably does not contribute actively to normal oxidation of lysine and tryptophan.[19] The question of whether shuttling might occur when the intracellular glutaryl-CoA concentration is elevated, as it is in GCD deficiency, has not been resolved.

2-KETOADIPIC ACIDEMIA

2-Ketoadipic acidemia (OMIM 245130) is an inborn error of lysine, tryptophan, and hydroxylysine metabolism that may have no clinical significance. It is probably due to deficiency of the E-1 or E-2 component of 2-ketoadipic acid dehydrogenase and is manifested by the accumulation and excretion of 2-aminoadipic, 2-ketoadipic, and 2-hydroxyadipic acids. Inheritance is probably autosomal recessive.

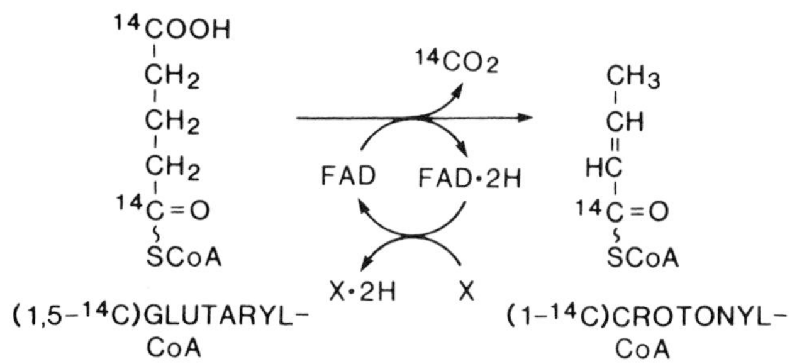

^{14}COOH – CH$_2$ – CH$_2$ – CH$_2$ – ^{14}C=O – SCoA
(1,5-^{14}C)GLUTARYL-CoA
$^{14}CO_2$
FAD FAD·2H
X·2H X
CH$_3$ – CH = HC – ^{14}C=O – SCoA
(1-^{14}C)CROTONYL-CoA

Fig. 95-4 Assay of glutaryl-CoA dehydrogenase by $^{14}CO_2$ release from [15-^{14}C]glutaryl-CoA. In most assays X = methylene blue or phenazine methosulfate.

Several affected individuals have been described. These include a 14-month-old girl with hypotonia, intermittent metabolic acidosis, and motor and developmental delay;[20] a 14-year-old retarded boy and his normal sister;[21] a 9-year-old boy with a mild learning disability and his normal brother;[22,23] a 10-year-old retarded girl;[24] a 9-year-old male with psychomotor retardation and a history of seizures;[25] and a 7-year-old girl with developmental delay and cerebellar ataxia.[26] Three additional siblings, initially detected by a newborn screening program,[27] were apparently normal at 12, 17, and 19 years of age.[28] These observations suggest that the condition is not deleterious and that the large number of individuals with developmental delay and other neurologic symptoms are accounted for by sampling bias.

Almost all probands were identified when prominent spots of 2-aminoadipic acid were noted on amino acid chromatography of urine, with subsequent investigations demonstrating 2-aminoadipic acidemia and increased urine concentrations of 2-ketoadipic and 2-hydroxyadipic acids. 2-Hydroxyglutaric acid is observed in urine in some patients, possibly because 2-ketoglutaric dehydrogenase and 2-ketoadipic dehydrogenase are the same enzyme. Small amounts of glutaric acid are also detected in the urine, almost certainly because of spontaneous decarboxylation of 2-ketoadipic acid.[25]

The accumulated metabolites suggest a block in 2-ketoadipic dehydrogenase, and intact mutant fibroblasts are almost totally unable to oxidize 2-amino[l-^{14}C]adipic and 2-keto[l-^{14}C]adipic acid to $^{14}CO_2$,[25,29] but a defect in 2-ketoadipic dehydrogenase has not been demonstrated directly. If 2-ketoadipic dehydrogenase and 2-ketoglutaric dehydrogenase are indeed the same, it is not clear how so central a defect can produce so mild a phenotype. This may indicate that the two enzymes are different.

Because the condition may have no clinical consequences, treatment and antenatal diagnosis may be of little import, although protein restriction to 1.5 g/kg per day is reported to have produced some clinical improvement in one patient, perhaps leading to improved interaction between the child and his parents.

Inheritance as an autosomal recessive trait is inferred from the pedigrees, and there is no evidence that heterozygous carriers can be distinguished from control subjects. The incidence is not known.

GLUTARIC ACIDEMIA TYPE I

Glutaric acidemia type I (GA1, OMIM 231670) is characterized clinically by dystonia and dyskinesia in childhood; pathologically by striatal degeneration, in particular of the caudate and putamen; and biochemically by tissue deficiency of glutaryl-CoA dehydrogenase. Large amounts of glutaric and 3-hydroxyglutaric acids are usually present in urine. The disorder is transmitted as an autosomal recessive trait. Treatment with L-carnitine and prompt treatment of catabolic events with intravenous fluids, glucose, and insulin may prevent neurologic symptoms in patients without striatal damage at diagnosis, but the effect of treatment with riboflavin and dietary restriction of glutarigenic amino acids (lysine and tryptophan) in such patients is much less clear.

Clinical Phenotype[30–48]

Macrocephaly at or appearing shortly after birth is common. A period of apparently normal development averaging 1 year is typical; although soft neurologic signs such as irritability and jitteriness are often present, symptoms rarely if ever have their onset after 5 years of age. The disease usually presents as an acute encephalopathic episode during a respiratory or gastrointestinal illness, with the sudden onset of hypotonia, loss of head control, and seizures, followed by opisthotonus, grimacing, fisting, tongue thrusting, rigidity, and dystonia (Fig. 95-5); recovery is slow and incomplete. Neurologic symptoms may then remain static, in which case the condition resembles extrapyramidal cerebral palsy, or may progress slowly, punctuated by episodes of ketosis, vomiting, hepatomegaly, and encephalopathy (coma and convulsions) associated with infection. In some patients motor delay, hypotonia, dystonia, and dyskinesia develop gradually during the first few years of life. Whatever the type of onset, there is relative preservation of intellect. Episodes of high fever in patients with severe dystonia may be due to constant and unabated activity of large skeletal muscles. Patients with severe neurologic impairment may survive well into adult life or may succumb during the first decade with intercurrent illnesses or Reye syndrome-like episodes; the latter become less frequent with age. Some enzyme-deficient individuals, including the occasional sibling of a severely affected child, do not develop neurologic manifestations.[40,42]

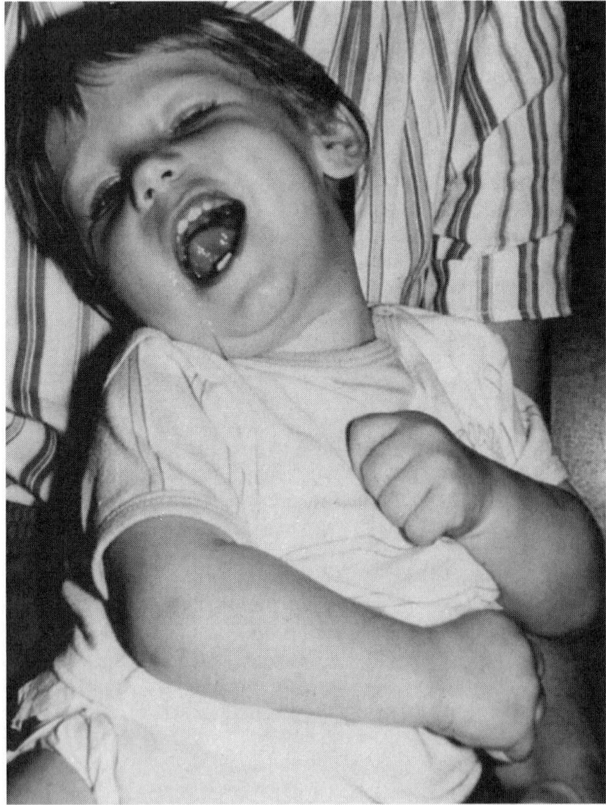

Fig. 95-5 A 13-month-old boy with glutaric acidemia, showing dystonia of face, tongue, neck, back, arms, and hands. This child did not have abnormal urine organic acids (*Courtesy of Dr. I. Bergman.*)

Most routine laboratory studies, including serum electrolytes and pH, are normal except during acute episodes, when acidosis, hypoglycemia, ketonemia and ketonuria, hyperammonemia, and mild parenchymal liver disease may appear.[34,49,50] Routine studies on CSF may show slightly increased protein or may be normal. Amino acids in blood and urine are usually normal, but during acute episodes serum 2-aminoadipic acid may be greatly elevated and the urine may show generalized aminoaciduria, with special prominence of glutamine, glutamic acid, 2-aminoadipic acid, and saccharopine.[34,49] Similar changes have been described in patients with typical Reye syndrome and are not diagnostic. Serum L-carnitine is almost always very low at diagnosis, with an increased esterified fraction, and increased glutarylcarnitine can be demonstrated in plasma and urine.[38,39,41,42,45]

Urine organic acids are usually abnormal (Fig. 95-6), showing large quantities of glutaric acid (up to 22 mg/mg creatinine; normal less than 15 μg/mg creatinine) and lesser amounts of 3-hydroxyglutaric acid (up to 0.7 mg/mg creatinine) and (occasionally) glutaconic acid.[51] Excretion of glutaconic acid may become prominent, exceeding that of 3-hydroxyglutaric acid, during episodes of ketosis.[34,49,50]

Glutaric acid concentrations are also increased in blood and CSF[30,31] but may be demonstrable only by stable isotope dilution GC/MS. Glutaric acid in urine, blood, and CSF is elevated in some patients only when they are acutely ill[39,41,43,44] but is normal in other patients even during catabolic episodes. A few patients are known in whom glutaric acid was elevated only in CSF at diagnosis.[48,52]

Neuroradiologic Phenotype (Fig. 95-7)

The neuroradiologic findings in GA1 have been reviewed by Brismar and Ozand.[53] CT and MRI scans often show collections of fluid over the frontal lobes and at the base of the brain, with atrophy of the frontal and temporal lobes and failure of the temporal lobes to cover the insular region. In some instances the extracerebral fluid collections in the Sylvian region are in arachnoid (or subdural) cysts.[54,55] These changes may be present at birth and have been observed in otherwise clinically normal infants in whom the diagnosis was made during evaluation for macrocephaly.[46,56,57] White matter changes may be observed in association with these abnormalities. Subdural hematomas have been noted in several patients,[58–61] possibly because the fluid collections between the brain and cranium stretch the bridging vessels, making them more vulnerable to minor trauma. Changes in the basal ganglia, in particular atrophy of the caudate and putamen, are rarely present at birth but can develop within a few days or weeks of an encephalopathic episode.[62] The globus pallidus and the thalamus are usually spared.

Anatomic Pathology

The striatum bears the brunt of neurotoxicity in GA1. Moderate fatty changes in neurons in the caudate and increased numbers of astrocytes in the putamen were observed in two severely affected patients who died at about 1 year of age.[37,39] Changes in the basal ganglia were much more marked in older patients,[49,63–65] all of whom showed severe neuronal loss and extensive fibrous gliosis in the caudate and putamen (Fig. 95-8). Some also showed degeneration of the globus pallidus and spongy degeneration of cortical white matter; in one case this was due to splitting of myelin sheaths.[65]

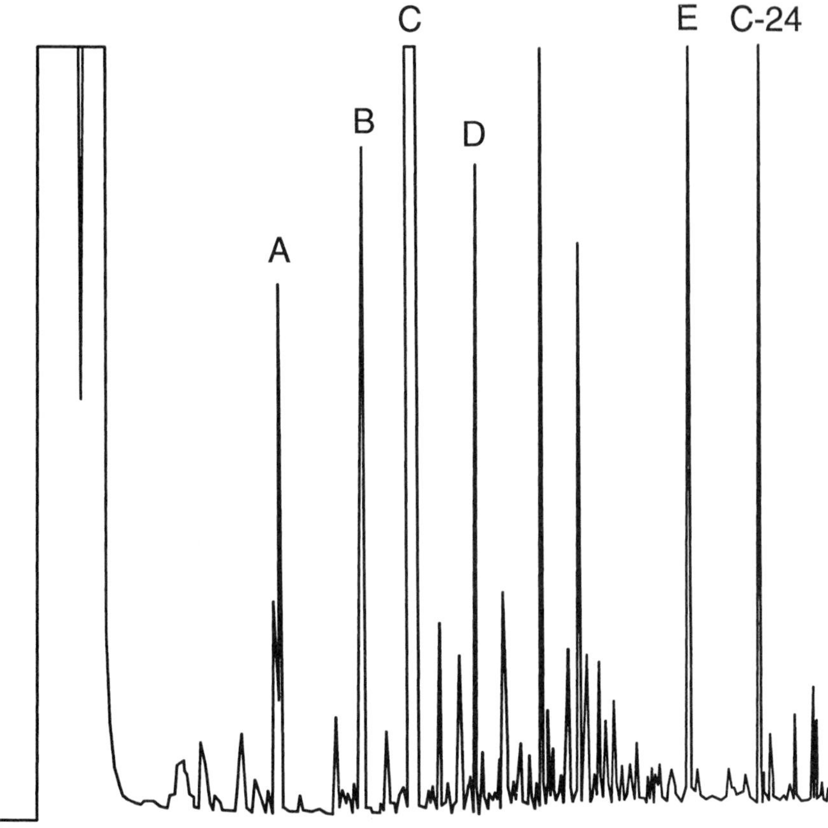

Fig. 95-6 Urine organic acids in glutaric acidemia. A = dimethylmalonic acid (internal standard), B = succinic acid, C = glutaric acid, D = 3-hydroxyglutaric acid, and E = hippuric acid. (*Goodman, unpublished.*)

Most autopsied patients have also shown microvesicular fatty infiltration of liver parenchymal cells, cells of the proximal renal tubule, and myocardial cells.[37,39,49] These changes are not pathognomonic and are seen in several other disorders, including Reye syndrome, other organic acidemias, and disorders of the urea cycle.

Molecular Basis of Disease

GCD cDNA from pig, human, and mouse has been cloned and characterized, as have the human (GenBank accession number U69141) and murine (GenBank accession number U18992) GCD genes.[7,66,67] The human gene has been mapped to chromosome 19p13.2,[68] is about 7 kb long, and contains 11 exons.[69] More than 60 pathogenic GCD mutations have been found in GA1 patients (Fig. 95-9),[70] but there is no single common mutation except in inbred populations like Island Lake Indians in Canada (IVS1+5G > T)[71] and the Old Order Amish in Lancaster County in Pennsylvania (A421V).[69] The most common mutation outside of these populations is R402W,[69] which accounts for fewer than 20 percent of mutant alleles; most patients are compound heterozygotes for mutations found in comparatively few individuals.

There is no apparent correlation between genotype and clinical severity. Patients in populations in which single mutations

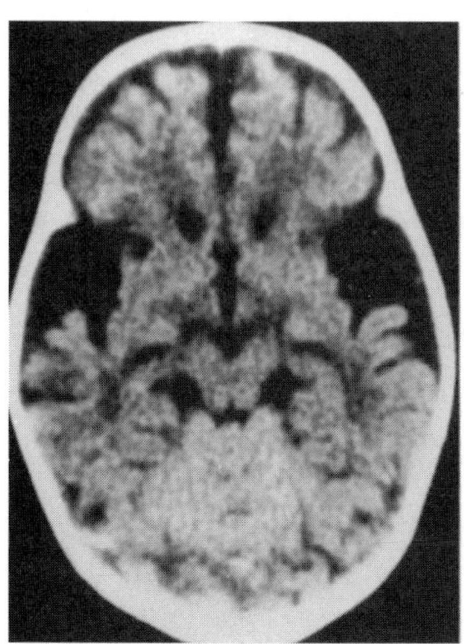

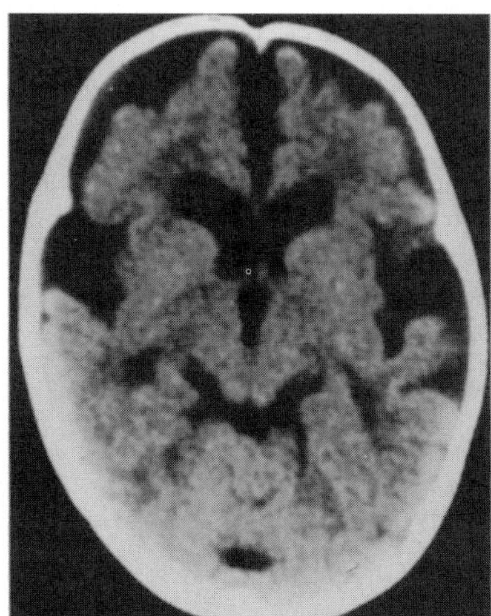

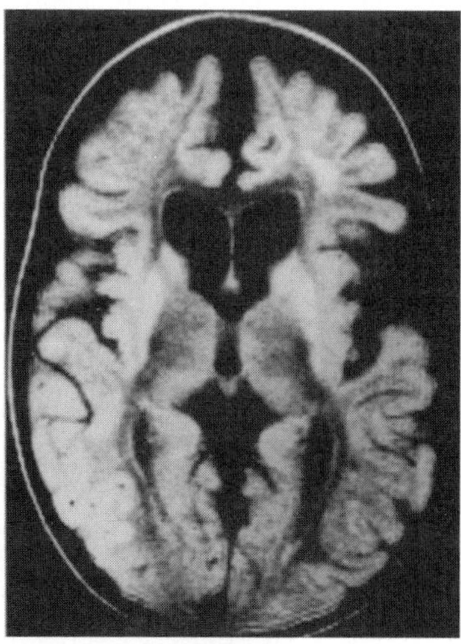

Fig. 95-7 CT and MRI scans of brain in glutaric acidemia. Left: CT scan of 10-month-old boy, 3 months after the onset of movement disorder, showing loss of cerebral volume, most notable in the temporal lobes, and widening of Sylvian fissures. (*Courtesy of Dr. I. Bergman.*) Middle: CT scan of a 5-month-old boy without movement disorder but with abnormal urine organic acids and glutaryl-CoA dehydrogenase deficiency, showing the same changes. (*Courtesy of Dr. S. Seshia.*) Right: MRI scan of a 3-year-old girl showing cortical atrophy, dilated lateral ventricles, and shrinkage and increased intensity of the caudate and putamen, suggesting fibrosis.

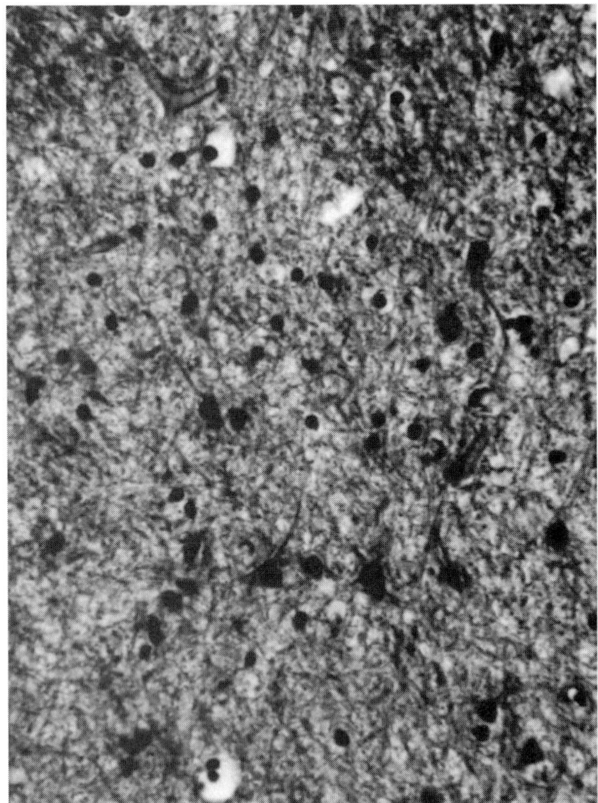

Fig. 95-8 Histologic section of the caudate nucleus from a 10-year-old boy with glutaric acidemia, showing almost total neuronal loss and replacement by gliotic tissue. H & E; original magnification × 300. (*Courtesy of Dr. M. D. Norenberg.*)

predominate show a variety of clinical phenotypes,[43,44] and in other populations sibships contain GCD-deficient individuals who are clinically unaffected.[40,42] This is true even when unaffected and affected sibs are homozygous for a mutation that terminates translation upstream of the substrate binding site.[72] It appears that, whatever the responsible mutation(s), GCD deficiency confers a high but not absolute risk for developing striatal damage in infancy or childhood.

Specific mutations do, however, correlate with the presence and/or severity of organic aciduria. The R227P allele has been associated with little or no excretion of glutaric acid,[73] even in heterozygous patients, and there may be a similar association with A293T, G178R, and R88C.[70] The reason for this is not clear, as GCD containing any of these substitutions produces stable subunits with very low specific activity when expressed in *E. coli*. The possibility that intragenic complementation may occur between particular mutations has not been examined.

Pathogenesis

The excretion of glutaric acid is probably due to accumulation of glutaryl-CoA behind deficient glutaryl-CoA dehydrogenase, whose activity varies from 0 to 10 percent of normal in most GA1 patient tissues, and subsequent hydrolysis to the free acid by intracellular thioesterases. Glutaconyl-CoA, the presumed source of 3-hydroxyglutaric acid, is not produced by mutant GCD[16,49] but may be formed from accumulated glutaryl-CoA by MCAD in mitochondria or by glutaryl-CoA oxidase in peroxisomes.[18] Because 3-hydroxyglutaric acid is not excreted in glutaric acidemia type II, in which MCAD and other mitochondrial dehydrogenases are deficient and in which peroxisomal glutaryl-CoA oxidase is presumably normal, its origin in GA1 is more likely to be MCAD or a related mitochondrial enzyme.

Glutaric acid concentrations have been increased in all tissues that have been examined at death, including brain. The concentration of glutaric acid in brain may be different in different areas; in one patient it was 0.67 μmol/g wet weight in frontal

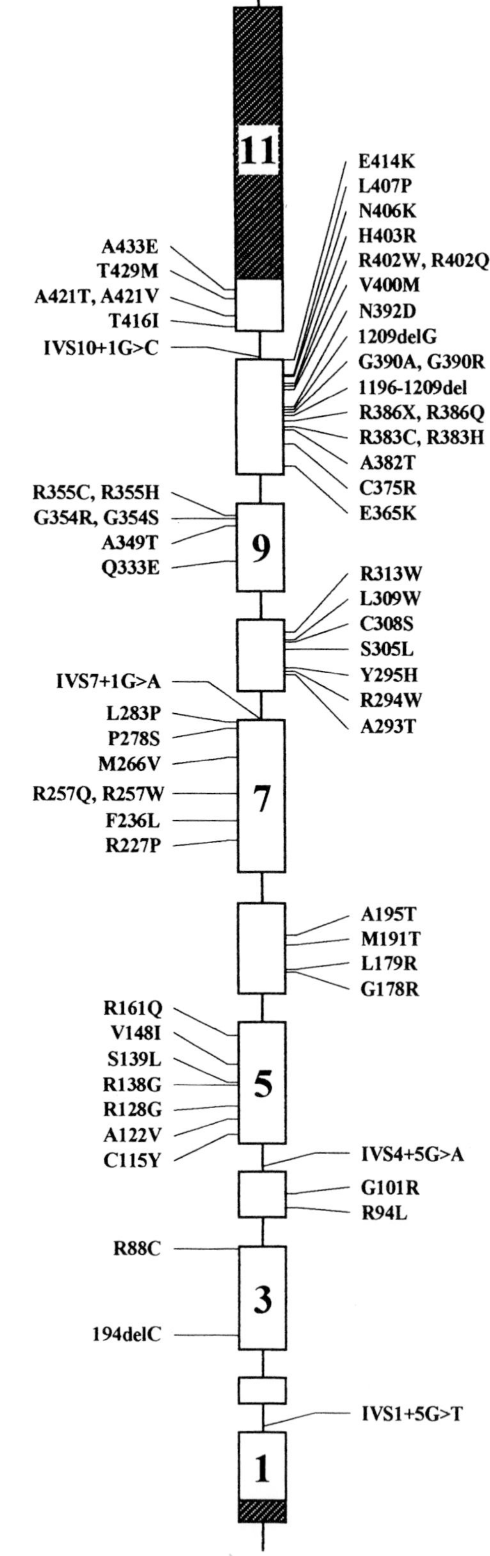

Fig. 95-9 Pathogenic mutations in glutaryl-CoA dehydrogenase. (*Reprinted by permission of John Wiley & Sons, Inc. from Goodman SI, Stein DE, Schlesinger S, Christensen E, Schwartz M, Greenberg CR, Elpeleg O: Glutaryl-CoA dehydrogenase mutations in glutaric acidemia (type 1): Review and report of thirty novel mutations. (Hum Mutat* 12: 141, 1998.))

cortex and 1.25 μmol/g wet weight in basal ganglia.[63] In another patient, the glutaric acid concentration in frontal cortex was 0.83 μmol/g wet weight (normal = undetected).[49] Glutaconic acid has not been detected in brain, even when large amounts of the compound were being excreted in urine just before death.[49]

The concentrations of γ-aminobutyric acid (GABA) were extremely low in the caudate (0.60 μmol/g wet weight; normal = 3.03 ± 0.83) and putamen (0.87 μmol/g wet weight; normal = 5.69 ± 0.75) of one patient and correlated with severe deficiency of neuronal glutamate decarboxylase in these areas. Enzyme activities, and the concentrations of GABA, were much nearer to the normal range in frontal, occipital, and cerebellar cortex.[63]

Any theory to explain the pathogenesis of GA1 must explain the particular vulnerability of the striatum, and in particular the caudate and putamen, to neuronal degeneration; why striatal damage rarely if ever occurs after 5 years of age; and why it occurs in patients with only minimal elevations of abnormal metabolites in blood and CSF. No theory has been put forth that addresses all these points adequately. Nonetheless, several studies have examined the possibility that striatal degeneration in some way relates to accumulation of glutaric acid or one of its derivatives.

Different effects of accumulated metabolites on striatal cultures have been noted. One study showed that glutaric acid caused neurodegenerative changes in cortical-striatal cultures and that, unlike kainic acid and quinolinic acid, glutaric acid toxicity did not require prior synapse formation but occurred even before synapses were well established.[74,75] Another study on the effects of glutaric, 3-hydroxyglutaric, and glutaconic acids on cultures from rat hippocampus, cortex, and striatum showed only a reversible cytotoxic effect from 5 mM glutaric and glutaconic but also showed that 3-hydroxyglutaric acid produced concentration-dependent toxicity starting at 1.5 mM.[76] This effect could be reduced by glutamate receptor antagonists, suggesting that an excitotoxic mechanism is involved.

Glutaric, glutaconic, and 3-hydroxyglutaric acids competitively inhibit neuronal glutamic acid decarboxylase (GAD), the enzyme responsible for GABA biosynthesis, and the K_i of glutarate (1.3×10^{-3} molar)[77] approximates the concentration in which it is found in brain in glutaric acidemia. The low concentrations of GABA found in the caudate and putamen in one patient[63] are consistent with such an effect, but it is not known if inhibition of GAD alone could produce neuronal damage and loss. Further, decreased GAD activity and GABA concentration in the striatum may be secondary to cell death from some other cause, as it is in Huntington chorea.[78]

Evidence is accumulating that excitotoxicity plays a major role in the pathogenesis of disorders such as Huntington disease, and glutaric and/or 3-hydroxyglutaric acid might cause cell death in the striatum if it excited excessively one or all classes of glutamate receptors. High affinity uptake of glutamic acid by rat synaptosomes is inhibited 80 percent by 10 mM glutaric acid[79] but not at all by 0.1 mM,[80] but it is not known if the 1.0 to 1.5 mM concentrations found in brain in glutaric acidemia can inhibit glutamate uptake and thus cause high and possibly stimulatory concentrations of the neurotransmitter to be retained in the synaptic cleft. The effects of 3-hydroxyglutaric and glutaconic acid have not been studied.

Another possible pathogenetic mechanism involves quinolinic acid (QA), an intermediate in tryptophan metabolism in brain (Fig. 95-10). QA is a potent neurotoxin when injected into the CNS of experimental animals,[81] and neurones are so sensitive to its effects that even endogenous concentrations may be toxic.[82] A block in glutaryl-CoA dehydrogenase could shunt tryptophan down the kynurenine pathway, particularly when viral infections provoke the production of the α- and γ-interferons that induce indolamine-2,3-dioxygenase.[83]

Whatever the toxic compound(s), the limited time during which the striatum can apparently be damaged suggests particular vulnerability of a receptor that is spatially and temporally regulated, i.e., that is present in the striatum only for a limited time during development. Glutamate receptors that fit this model have been described in the rat.[84]

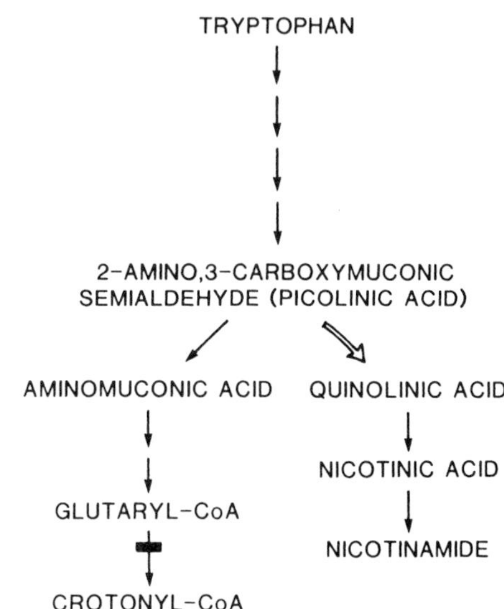

Fig. 95-10 The two pathways of tryptophan metabolism in brain, one through glutaryl-CoA and one through quinolinic acid.

The cause of the fatty changes seen at autopsy in the liver, kidneys, and heart is also unknown, but they may merely be due to nonspecific mitochondrial toxicity. The observation of severe ketosis during Reye syndrome-like episodes in this condition suggests that carnitine deficiency, if present, does not seriously limit the capacity of the liver to oxidize long-chain fatty acids. It is also possible that glutaconic acid, which is excreted in large amounts during ketotic episodes, is a mitochondrial toxin; excretion may rise during ketotic episodes because the enoyl-CoA intermediates of fatty acid oxidation competitively inhibit hydration of glutaconyl-CoA to 3-hydroxyglutaryl-CoA. Whatever its cause, the accumulation of 2-aminoadipic acid and saccharopine observed during acute episodes appears to relate more to general mitochondrial dysfunction than to back-up of metabolites proximal to glutaryl-CoA, because the same abnormalities have been described in Reye syndrome.[85,86]

Genetics

Pedigree analysis, which shows that males and females are affected with approximately equal frequency, and enzyme analysis, showing partial GCD deficiency in cells from obligate heterozygotes, establish inheritance of GA1 as an autosomal recessive trait.[87,88] Heterozygous carriers are clinically normal, and two carriers did not excrete detectable glutaric acid even after oral loads of L-lysine.[30] There has not been enough experience with carrier detection based on GCD activity in leukocytes or fibroblasts to be certain about its reliability in carrier detection, but the elucidation of pathogenic mutations in the GCD gene and the development of rapid and accurate methods for mutation screening, e.g., allele specific hybridization, now permit carriers to be identified with certainty in families and populations in which disease-causing mutations are known.

Incidence

Well over 200 patients have been detected since GA1 was first described in 1975, and the condition is certainly one of the more common organic acidemias. There are no accurate figures about incidence, however, because the disorder is very often misdiagnosed as "dystonic cerebral palsy" and because it is not usually screened for in newborns. Screening for glutarylcarnitine in dried blood spots from newborns by tandem MS has detected nine confirmed patients in about 450,000 livebirths,[89] but most of them were from the Old Order Amish community in Lancaster County, a population in which the condition is especially frequent.[44] The incidence of disease in the Island Lake Indians in Canada is on the order of 1:225 livebirths,[71] and the incidence in Sweden may be about the same as that of phenylketonuria there, i.e., about 1 in 30,000 livebirths.[90]

Diagnosis and Screening

In most cases the diagnosis is made on the basis of increased glutaric and 3-hydroxyglutaric acids in urine and confirmed by finding deficiency of glutaryl-CoA dehydrogenase in cultured fibroblasts. The diagnosis is almost certain if 3-hydroxyglutaric acid is identified, as it has not been found in any other condition. Increased urine glutaric acid may also be found in the setting of glutaric acidemia type II (Chap. 103), glutaryl-CoA oxidase deficiency,[91] α-aminoadipic acidemia,[25] short-gut syndrome,[92] unusual intestinal flora,[93] and use of infant formulas that contain medium-chain triglycerides. Because glutaric acid concentrations in urine, blood, and cerebrospinal fluid may be normal, GCD assay and/or mutation analysis should be carried out whenever the condition is strongly suspected on clinical or neuroradiologic grounds.

GCD activity in fibroblasts (or leukocytes) is usually less than 5 to 10 percent of normal in affected patients, whether measured by decarboxylation of [1,5-^{14}C]glutaryl-CoA[30] or by tritium release from [2,3,4-^{3}H]glutaryl-CoA,[16] but can be as high as 30 percent of normal in patients with the R227P/V400M genotype.[73,94] This amount of enzyme activity is not unusual in heterozygous carriers, and positive diagnosis of such patients may be possible only by mutation analysis.

A rationale for newborn screening comes from the observation that treatment can prevent development of striatal damage if begun before the onset of symptoms[61] (see below). Other than in populations with one prevalent mutation, in which screening for GA1 might be done by mutation analysis, the only test available that appears to have the required sensitivity and specificity is to measure glutarylcarnitine in dried blood spots from newborns by tandem MS. A program based on this methodology has been initiated in a US population comprised in part of the Old Order Amish, in whom the disease's incidence is particularly high. While false positive results with this technique are expected to be rare, and have not been detected, there are still too little data available to know the incidence of the disease in the population at large and the frequency of false negative results. It is, however, expected that GA1 will increasingly be the focus of newborn screening programs.

Prenatal Diagnosis

Prenatal diagnosis of an affected fetus has been achieved on several occasions, in some cases by demonstrating increased glutaric acid levels in amniotic fluid and in others by showing enzyme deficiency in cultured cells or directly in chorionic villus samples. One affected fetus showed increased glutaric acid in amniotic fluid (4.35 to 13.3 μg/ml; normal < 0.39) and decreased GCD activity in cultured amniotic cells; the diagnosis was confirmed by the presence of large amounts of glutaric acid in fetal liver (17 μg/g wet weight), brain (112 μg/g wet weight), and kidney (70.2 μg/g wet weight) and by decreased GCD activity in liver and kidney. Minimal and possibly insignificant changes were observed in the striatum.[95] Four other affected fetuses have been detected by assaying GCD activity in chorionic villus samples directly and/or in cultured chorionic cells.[96] Prenatal diagnosis by mutation analysis, while possible, has not yet been reported.

It may be that measuring glutaric acid in amniotic fluid is predictive only when the proband in the family consistently excretes large amounts of glutaric acid and that enzyme assay and/or mutation analysis is necessary in other instances.

Treatment

There is increasing evidence that striatal degeneration can be prevented in many patients by treatment with L-carnitine (100 mg/kg per day) and by prompt and vigorous treatment of intercurrent illnesses with fluids, insulin, and glucose.[61,97] Without treatment, almost all patients with GA1 develop an incapacitating dystonic-dyskinetic disorder, but more than 80 percent of patients treated in this way have developed normally.[61,97] The role of protein, or lysine and tryptophan, restriction in treatment is not clear, but few patients have been helped by diet alone. Results of treatment when striatal damage is present at the time of diagnosis are less favorable, although it is possible that further damage is prevented.[61]

Observations that glutaric, glutaconic, and 3-hydroxyglutaric acid inhibit neuronal GAD[77] and that GAD activity and GABA concentrations are low in the basal ganglia of glutaric acidemia patients[63] have prompted treatment with pharmacologic agents that increase GABA concentrations in brain. Those that have been tried are baclofen, valproic acid, and vigabatrin.

It was originally thought that baclofen, i.e., β-(4-chlorophenyl)GABA, activated GABA receptors, but it has since been learned that it activates neurons that are normally inhibited by this neurotransmitter.[98,99] Whatever effect it has in this disorder may thus not relate to a GABA-like function. Baclofen therapy has been tried in several patients, with variable effect. In some patients there has been no effect whatever,[37] but Brandt *et al.* have reported significant improvement in two of three Danish patients given 2 mg/kg per day, even when administration was controlled in a double blind fashion.[100] Effects varying from none to questionable have been observed in several additional patients, but we know of no other case in which the effects were as dramatic as those noted in the Danish patients.

Valproic acid therapy has also been tried in several patients, with the rationale that the drug causes selective increase of GABA in synaptic areas by inhibiting GABA transaminase or succinic semialdehyde dehydrogenase or by inhibiting GABA uptake by glial cells and nerve endings. Some improvement on valproic acid has been noted in one patient in the literature,[36] but many researchers feel that, because it competes with glutaryl-CoA for esterification with carnitine, valproic acid should be avoided whenever possible.[45]

There is one brief report of significant clinical improvement, and increased concentrations of GABA and glutaric acid in CSF, following the use of vigabatrin (γ-vinyl-GABA) at an oral dose of 35 to 50 mg/kg per day.[101]

GLUTARYL-COENZYME A OXIDASE DEFICIENCY

Glutaryl-CoA oxidase deficiency has been described once, in an 11-month-old girl with β-thalassemia and mild glutaric aciduria.[91] Glutaric acid was the sole abnormal metabolite in urine and was raised only slightly by oral lysine loading. The enzyme deficiency in this patient was not thought to have had adverse consequences.

REFERENCES

1. Hirashima M, Hayakawa T, Koike M: Mammalian α-keto acid dehydrogenase complexes. II. An improved procedure for the preparation of 2-oxoglutarate dehydrogenase complex from pig heart muscle. *J Biol Chem* **242**:902, 1976.
2. Gomes B, Fendrich G, Abeles RH: Mechanism of action of glutaryl-CoA and butyryl-CoA dehydrogenases: Purification of glutaryl-CoA dehydrogenase. *Biochemistry* **20**:1481, 1981.
3. Husain M, Steenkamp DJ: Partial purification and chracterization of glutaryl-coenzyme A dehydrogenase, electron transfer flavoprotein, and electron transfer flavoprotein-Q oxidoreductase from *Paracoccus denitrificans*. *J Bacteriol* **163**:709, 1985.
4. Byron CM, Stankovich MT, Husain M: Spectral and electrochemical properties of glutaryl-CoA dehydrogenase from *Paracoccus denitrificans*. *Biochemistry* **29**:3691, 1990.
5. Besrat A, Polan CE, Henderson LM: Mammalian metabolism of glutaric acid. *J Biol Chem* **244**:1461, 1969.
6. Lenich AC, Goodman SI: The purification and characterization of glutaryl-coenzyme A dehydrogenase from porcine and human liver. *J Biol Chem* **261**:4090, 1986.

7. Goodman SI, Kratz LE, DiGiulio KA, Biery BJ, Goodman KE, Isaya G, Frerman FE: Cloning of glutaryl-CoA dehydrogenase cDNA, and expression of wild-type and mutant enzymes in *Escherichia coli*. *Hum Mol Genet* **4**:1493, 1995.
8. Kim J-JP, Wang M, Paschke R, Goodman SI, Biery BJ, Frerman FE: The crystal structure of human glutaryl-CoA dehydrogenase, in Ghisla S, Kroneck P, Macheroux P, Sund H (eds): *Flavins and Flavoproteins*. Berlin, Rudolph Weber, in press.
9. Thorpe C, Kim J-JP: Structure and mechanism of action of the acyl-CoA dehydrogenases. *FASEB J* **9**:718, 1995.
10. Tiffany KA, Roberts DL, Wang M, Paschke R, Mohsen AW, Vockley J, Kim JJ: Structure of human isovaleryl-CoA dehydrogenase at 2.6 Å resolution: Structural basis for substrate specificity. *Biochemistry* **36**:8455, 1997.
11. Djordjevic S, Dong Y, Paschke R, Frerman FE, Strauss AW, Kim JJ: Identification of the catalytic base in long chain acyl-CoA dehydrogenase. *Biochemistry* **33**:4258, 1994.
12. Roberts DL, Frerman FE, Kim JJ: Three-dimensional structure of human electron transfer flavoprotein to 2.1-Å resolution. *Proc Natl Acad Sci USA* **93**:14355, 1996.
13. Goodman SI, Frerman FE: Unpublished observations.
14. Numa S, Ishimura Y, Nakazawa T, Okazaki T, Hayaishi O: Enzymic studies on the metabolism of glutarate in *Pseudomonas*. *J Biol Chem* **239**:3915, 1964.
15. Wenz A, Ghisla S, Thorpe C: Reaction of general acyl-CoA dehydrogenase with 3,4-pentadienoyl-CoA in flavins and flavoproteins, in Massey V, Williams CH (eds): *Developments in Biochemistry vol 21*. New York, Elsevier/North-Holland, 1982, p 605.
16. Hyman DB, Tanaka K: Specific glutaryl-CoA dehydrogenating activity is deficient in cultured fibroblasts from glutaric aciduria patients. *J Clin Invest* **73**:778, 1984.
17. Wenz A, Thorpe C, Ghisla S: Inactivation of general acyl-CoA dehydrogenase from pig kidney by a metabolite of hypoglycin A. *J Biol Chem* **256**:9809, 1981.
18. Vamecq J, van Hoof F: Implications of a peroxisomal enzyme in the catabolism of glutaryl-CoA. *Biochem J* **221**:203, 1984.
19. Vamecq J, Libert R, van Hoof F, de Hoffmann E, Vallée L, Cartigny B, Nuyts JP, et al: Peroxisomes and glutaric aciduria type I. *Arch Int Physiol Biochim* **94**:B49, 1986.
20. Przyrembel H, Bachmann D, Lombeck I, Becker K, Wendel U, Wadman SK, Bremer HJ: Alpha-ketoadipic aciduria, a new inborn error of lysine metabolism: Biochemical studies. *Clin Chim Acta* **58**:257, 1975.
21. Wilson RW, Wilson CM, Gates SC, Higgins JV: α-Ketoadipic aciduria: A description of a new metabolic error in lysine-tryptophan degradation. *Pediat Res* **9**:522, 1975.
22. Fischer MH, Gerritsen T, Opitz JM: α-Aminoadipic aciduria, a non-deleterious inborn metabolic defect. *Humangenetik* **24**:265, 1974.
23. Fischer MH, Brown RR: Tryptophan and lysine metabolism in alpha-aminoadipic aciduria. *Am J Med Genet* **5**:35, 1980.
24. Casey RE, Zaleski WA, Philp M, Mendelson IS, MacKenzie SL: Biochemical and clinical studies of a new case of α-aminoadipic aciduria. *J Inher Metab Dis* **1**:129, 1978.
25. Duran M, Beemer FA, Wadman SK, Wendel U, Janssen B: A patient with α-ketoadipic and α-aminoadipic aciduria. *J Inher Metab Dis* **7**:61, 1984.
26. Vianey-Liaud C, Divry P, Cotte J, Teyssier G: α-Aminoadipic and α-ketoadipic aciduria: Detection of a new case by a screening program using two dimensional thin layer chromatography of amino acids. *J Inher Metab Dis* **8** suppl 2:133, 1985.
27. Wilcke B, Smith A, Brown DA: Urine screening for aminoacidopathies: Is it beneficial? *J Pediatr* **97**:492, 1980.
28. Wilcken B: Personal communication.
29. Wendel U, Rüdiger HW, Przyrembel H, Bremer HJ: Alpha-aminoadipic aciduria: Degradation studies with fibroblasts. *Clin Chim Acta* **58**:271, 1975.
30. Goodman SI, Markey SP, Moe PG, Miles BS, Teng CC: Glutaric aciduria; A "new" disorder of amino acid metabolism. *Biochem Med* **12**:12, 1975.
31. Gregersen N, Brandt NJ, Christensen E, Gron I, Rasmussen K, Brandt S: Glutaric aciduria: Clinical and laboratory findings in two brothers. *J Pediatr* **90**:740, 1977.
32. Kyllerman M, Steen G: Intermittently progressive dyskinetic syndrome in glutaric aciduria. *Neuropädiatrie* **8**:397, 1977.
33. Brandt NJ, Brandt S, Christensen E, Gregersen N, Rasmussen K: Glutaric aciduria in progressive choreo-athetosis. *Clin Genet* **13**:77, 1978.
34. Floret D, Divry P, Dingeon N, Monnet P: Acidurie glutarique: Une nouvelle observation. *Arch Fr Pediatr* **36**:462, 1979.
35. Dunger DB, Snodgrass GJAI: Glutaric aciduria type I presenting with hypoglycaemia. *J Inher Metab Dis* **7**:122, 1984.
36. Stutchfield P, Edwards MA, Gray RGF, Crawley P, Green A: Glutaric aciduria type I misdiagnosed as Leigh's encephalopathy and cerebral palsy. *Devel Med Child Neurol* **27**:514, 1985.
37. Bennett MJ, Marlow N, Pollitt RJ, Wales JKH: Glutaric aciduria type I: Biochemical investigations and postmortem findings. *Eur J Pediatr* **145**:403, 1986.
38. Seccombe DW, James L, Booth F: L-Carnitine treatment in glutaric aciduria type I. *Neurology* **36**:264, 1986.
39. Bergman I, Finegold D, Gartner JC, Zitelli BJ, Claassen D, Scarano J, Roe CR, et al.: Acute profound dystonia in infants with glutaric acidemia. *Pediatrics* **83**:228, 1989.
40. Amir N, Elpeleg O, Shalev RS, Christensen E: Glutaric aciduria type I: Clinical heterogeneity and neuroradiologic features. *Neurology* **37**:1654, 1987.
41. Lipkin PH, Roe CR, Goodman SI, Batshaw ML: A case of glutaric acidemia type I: Effect of riboflavin and carnitine. *J Pediatr* **112**:62, 1988.
42. Amir N, Elpeleg ON, Shalev RS, Christensen E: Glutaric aciduria type I: Enzymatic and neuroradiologic investigations of two kindreds. *J Pediatr* **114**:983, 1989.
43. Haworth JC, Booth FA, Chudley AE, deGroot GW, Dilling LA, Goodman SI, Greenberg CR, et al.: Phenotypic variability in glutaric aciduria type I: Report of fourteen cases in five Canadian Indian kindreds. *J Pediatr* **118**:52, 1991.
44. Morton DH, Bennett MJ, Seargeant LE, Nichter CA, Kelley RI: Glutaric aciduria type I: A common cause of episodic encephalopathy and spastic paralysis in the Amish of Lancaster County, Pennsylvania. *Am J Med Genet* **41**:89, 1991.
45. Hoffmann GF, Trefz FK, Barth PG, Bohles H-J, Biggemann B, Bremer HJ, Christensen E, et al.: Glutaryl-CoA dehydrogenase deficiency: A distinct encephalopathy. *Pediatrics* **88**:1194, 1991.
46. Hoffmann GF, Trefz FK, Barth PG, Bohles H-J, Lehnert W, Christensen E, Valk J, et al.: Macrocephaly: An important indication for organic acid analysis. *J Inher Metab Dis* **14**:329, 1991.
47. Kyllerman M, Skjeldal OH, Lundberg M, Holme I, Jellum E, von Dobeln U, Fossen A, et al.: Dystonia and dyskinesia in glutaric aciduria type I: Clinical heterogeneity and therapeutic considerations. *Mov Disord* **9**:22, 1994.
48. Merinero B, Pérez-Cerdá C, Font LM, García MJ, Aparicio M, Lorenzo G, Martínez Pardo M, Garzo C, Martinez-Bermejo A, Pascual Castroviejo I, Christensen E, Ugarte M: Variable clinical and biochemical presentation of seven Spanish cases with glutaryl-CoA-dehydrogenase deficiency. *Neuropediatrics* **26**:238, 1995.
49. Goodman SI, Norenberg MD, Shikes RH, Breslich DJ, Moe PG: Glutaric aciduria: Biochemical and morphologic considerations. *J Pediatr* **90**:746, 1977.
50. Gregersen N, Brandt NJ: Ketotic episodes in glutaryl-CoA dehydrogenase deficiency (glutaric aciduria). *Pediatr Res* **13**:977, 1979.
51. Stokk O, Goodman SI, Thompson JA, Miles BS: Glutaric aciduria: Presence of glutaconic and β-hydroxyglutaric acids in urine. *Biochem Med* **12**:386, 1975.
52. Campistol J, Ribes A, Alvarez L, Christensen E, Millington DS: Glutaric aciduria type I: Unusual biochemical presentation. *J Pediatr* **121**:83, 1992.
53. Brismar J, Ozand PT: CT and MR of the brain in glutaric acidemia type I: A review of 59 published cases and a report of 5 new patients. *Am J Neuroradiol* **16**:675, 1995.
54. Hald JK, Nakstad PH, Skjeldal OH, Stromme P: Bilateral arachnoid cysts of the temporal fossa in four children with glutaric aciduria type 1. *Am J Neuroradiol* **12**:407, 1991.
55. Jamjoom ZAB, Okamoto E, Jamjoom A-HB, Al-Hajery O, Abu-Melha A: Bilateral arachnoid cysts of the sylvian region in female siblings with glutaric aciduria type I. *J Neurosurg* **82**:1078, 1995.
56. Yager JY, McClarty BM, Seshia SS: CT-scan findings in an infant with glutaric aciduria type I. *Develop Med Child Neurol* **30**:808, 1988.
57. Iafolla AK, Kahler SG: Megalencephaly in the neonatal period as the initial manifestation of glutaric aciduria type I. *J Pediatr* **114**:1004, 1989.
58. Osaka H, Kimura S, Nezu A, Yamazaki S, Saitoh K, Yamaguchi S: Chronic subdural hematoma, as an initial manifestation of glutaric aciduria type-1. *Brain Dev* **15**:125, 1993.
59. Drigo P, Burlina AB, Battistella PA: Subdural hematoma and glutaric aciduria type 1. *Brain Dev* **15**:460, 1993.

60. Woefle J, Kreft B, Emons D, Haverkamp F: Subdural hemorrhage as an initial sign of glutaric aciduria type 1: A diagnostic pitfall. *Pediatr Radiol* **26**:779, 1996.
61. Hoffmann GF, Athanassopoulos S, Burlina AB, Duran M, de Klerk JBC, Lehnert W, Leonard JV, et al.: Clinical course, early diagnosis, treatment, and prevention of disease in glutaryl-CoA dehydrogenase deficiency. *Neuropediatrics* **27**:115, 1996.
62. Superti-Furga A, Hoffmann GF: Glutaric aciduria type 1 (glutaryl-CoA-dehydrogenase deficiency): Advances and unanswered questions. *Eur J Pediatr* **156**:821, 1997.
63. Leibel RL, Shih VE, Goodman SI, Bauman ML, McCabe ERB, Zwerdling RG, Bergman I, et al.: Glutaric acidemia: A metabolic disorder causing progressive choreoathetosis. *Neurology* **30**:1163, 1980.
64. Chow CW, Haan EA, Goodman SI, Anderson RM, Evans WA, Kleinschmidt-DeMasters BK, Wise G, et al.: Neuropathology in glutaric acidaemia type I. *Acta Neuropathol* **76**:590, 1988.
65. Soffer D, Amir N, Elpeleg ON, Gomori JM, Shalev RS, Gottschalk-Sabag S: Striatal degeneration and spongy myelinopathy in glutaric acidemia. *J Neurol Sci* **107**:199, 1992.
66. Goodman SI, Kratz LE, Frerman FE: Pork and human cDNAs encoding glutaryl-CoA dehydrogenase, in Coates PM, Tanaka K (eds): *New Developments in Fatty Acid Oxidation*. New York, Wiley-Liss, 1992, p 169.
67. Koeller DM, DiGiulio KA, Angeloni SV, Dowler LL, Frerman FE, White RA, Goodman SI: Cloning, structure, and chromosome localization of the mouse glutaryl-CoA dehydrogenase gene. *Genomics* **8**:508, 1995.
68. Greenberg CR, Duncan AMV, Gregory CA, Singal R, Goodman SI: Assignment of human glutaryl-CoA dehydrogenase (GCDH) to the short arm of chromosome 19 (19p13.2) by in situ hybridization and somatic cell hybrid analysis. *Genomics* **21**:289, 1994.
69. Biery BJ, Stein DE, Morton DH, Goodman SI: Gene structure and mutations of glutaryl-coenzyme A dehydrogenase: Impaired association of enzyme subunits due to an A421V substitution causes glutaric acidemia (type I) in the Amish. *Am J Human Genet* **59**:1006, 1996.
70. Goodman SI, Stein DE, Schlesinger S, Christensen E, Schwartz M, Greenberg CR, Elpeleg O: Glutaryl-CoA dehydrogenase mutations in glutaric acidemia (type 1): Review and report of thirty novel mutations. *Hum Mutat* **12**:141, 1998.
71. Greenberg CR, Reimer D, Singal R, Triggs-Raine B, Chudley AE, Dilling LA, Philipps S, et al.: A G-to-T transversion at the +5 position of intron 1 in the glutaryl-CoA dehydrogenase gene is associated with the Island Lake variant of glutaric acidemia type 1. *Hum Mol Genet* **4**:493, 1995.
72. Anikster Y, Shaag A, Joseph A, Mandel H, Ben-Zeev B, Christensen E, Elpeleg ON: Glutaric aciduria type I in the Arab and Jewish communities in Israel. *Am J Hum Genet* **59**:1012, 1996.
73. Christensen E, Ribes A, Busquets C, Pineda M, Duran M, Poll-The BT, Greenberg CR, et al.: Compound heterozygosity in the glutaryl-CoA dehydrogenase gene with R227P in one allele is associated with no or very low free glutarate excretion. *J Inher Metab Dis* **20**:383, 1997.
74. Whetsell WO, Schwarcz R: The organotypic tissue culture model of corticostriatal system used for examining amino acid neurotoxicity and its antagonism: Studies on kainic acid, quinolinic acid and (−)2-amino-7-phosphonoheptanoic acid. *J Neural Transm* **Suppl 19**:53, 1983.
75. Whetsell WO: The use of organotypic tissue culture for study of amino acid neurotoxicity and its antagonism in mammalian CNS. *Clin Neuropharm* **7**(suppl 1):452, 1984.
76. Flott-Rahmel B, Falter C, Schluff P, Fingerhut R, Christensen E, Jakobs C, Musshoff U, et al.: *J Inher Metab Dis* **20**:387, 1997.
77. Stokke O, Goodman SI, Moe PG: Inhibition of brain glutamate decarboxylase by glutarate, glutaconate, and β-hydroxyglutarate: Explanation of the symptoms in glutaric aciduria? *Clin Chim Acta* **66**:411, 1976.
78. Appel SH: Membrane defects in Huntington's disease, in Chase TN, Wexler NS, Barbeau A (eds): *Huntington's Disease, Advances in Neurology, Vol 23.* New York, Raven, 1979, p 387.
79. Bennett JP, Logan WJ, Snyder SH: Amino acids as central nervous transmitters: The influence of ions, amino acid analogues, and ontogeny on transport systems for L-glutamic and L-aspartic acids and glycine into central nervous synaptosomes of the rat. *J Neurochem* **21**:1533, 1973.
80. Balcar VJ, Johnston GAR: The structural specificity of the high affinity uptake of L-glutamate and L-aspartate by rat brain slices. *J Neurochem* **19**:2657, 1972.
81. Schwarcz R, Whetsell WO, Mangano RM: Quinolinic acid: An endogenous metabolite that produces axon-sparing lesions in rat brain. *Science* **219**:316, 1983.
82. McGeer EG, Singh E: Neurotoxic effects of endogenous materials: Quinolinic acid, L-pyroglutamic acid and TRH. *Exp Neurol* **86**:410, 1984.
83. Heyes MP: Hypothesis: A role for quinolinic acid in the neuropathology of glutaric aciduria type I. *Can J Neurol Sci* **14**:441, 1987.
84. Monyer H, Burnashev N, Laurie DJ, Sakmann B, Seeburg PH: Developmental and regional expression in the rat brain and functional properties of four NMDA receptors. *Neuron* **12**:529, 1994.
85. Kang ES, Gerald PS: Hyperammonemia and Reye's syndrome. *N Engl J Med* **286**:1216, 1972.
86. Shih VE, Glick TH, Bercu BB: Lysine metabolism in Reye's syndrome. *Lancet* **2**:163, 1974.
87. Goodman SI, Kohlhoff JG: Glutaric aciduria: Inherited deficiency of glutaryl-CoA dehydrogenase activity. *Biochem Med* **13**:138, 1975.
88. Christensen E, Brandt NJ: Studies on glutaryl-CoA dehydrogenase in leucocytes, fibroblasts and amniotic fluid cells: The normal enzyme and the mutant form in patients with glutaric aciduria. *Clin Chim Acta* **88**:267, 1978.
89. Naylor E, Chace D: Unpublished observations.
90. Kyllerman M, Steen G: Glutaric aciduria: A "common" metabolic disorder? *Arch Fr Pediatr* **37**:279, 1980.
91. Bennett MJ, Pollitt RJ, Goodman SI, Hale DE, Vamecq J: Atypical riboflavin-responsive glutaric aciduria, and deficient peroxisomal glutaryl-CoA oxidase activity: A new peroxisomal disorder. *J Inher Metab Dis* **14**:165, 1991.
92. McCabe ERB, Goodman SI, Fennessey PV, Miles BS, Wall M, Silverman A: Glutaric, 3-hydroxypropionic and lactic aciduria with metabolic acidemia, following extensive small bowel resection. *Biochem Med* **28**:229, 1982.
93. Wendel U, Bakkeren J, de Jong J, Bongaerts G: Glutaric aciduria mediated by gut bacteria. *J Inher Metab Dis* **18**:358, 1995.
94. Goodman SI, Braverman N, Valle D: Unpublished observations.
95. Goodman SI, Gallegos DA, Pullin CJ, Halpern B, Truscott RJW, Wise G, Wilcken B, et al.: Antenatal diagnosis of glutaric acidemia. *Am J Hum Genet* **32**:695, 1980.
96. Christensen E: Prenatal diagnosis of glutaryl-CoA dehydrogenase deficiency: Experience using first-trimester chorionic villus sampling. *Prenat Diagn* **14**:333, 1994.
97. Morton DH: Unpublished observations.
98. Davidoff RA, Sear ES: The effects of lioresal on synaptic activity in the isolated spinal cord. *Neurology* **24**:957, 1974.
99. Fukuda H, Kudo Y, Ono H: Effect of β-(p-chlorophenyl)-GABA (baclofen) on spinal synaptic activity. *Eur J Pharmacol* **44**:17, 1977.
100. Brandt NJ, Gregersen N, Christensen E, Gron IH, Rasmussen K: Treatment of glutaryl-CoA dehydrogenase deficiency (glutaric aciduria). *J Pediatr* **94**:669, 1979.
101. Francois B, Jaeken J, Gillia P: Vigabatrin in the treatment of glutaric aciduria type I. *J Inher Metab Dis* **13**:352, 1990.

CHAPTER 96

Glutathione Synthetase Deficiency and Other Disorders of the γ-Glutamyl Cycle

Agne Larsson ■ Mary E. Anderson

Hereditary defects have been described for four of the six enzymes of the γ-glutamyl cycle:

1. **Generalized glutathione synthetase deficiency (MIM 266130) is associated with decreased cellular levels of glutathione, massive urinary excretion of 5-oxoproline, elevated levels of 5-oxoproline in the blood and cerebrospinal fluid, severe metabolic acidosis, increased rate of hemolysis, central nervous system symptoms, and defective granulocyte function. Glutathione normally regulates its own biosynthesis by inhibiting γ-glutamylcysteine synthetase, the enzyme that catalyzes the first step in the γ-glutamyl cycle. Therefore, marked reduction of glutathione levels caused by glutathione synthetase deficiency leads to a modified γ-glutamyl cycle, and γ-glutamylcysteine is formed in increased amounts. This dipeptide is converted to 5-oxoproline and cysteine by the action of γ-glutamyl cyclotransferase. The overproduction of 5-oxoproline exceeds the capacity of 5-oxoprolinase to convert this substrate to glutamate, and some of the 5-oxoproline formed is therefore excreted in the urine. Forty patients in 35 families have been described with generalized glutathione synthetase deficiency. Several mutations in the glutathione synthetase gene (MIM 601002) have been identified.**
   Glutathione synthetase is a homodimer with a subunit with a molecular mass of 52 kDa consisting of 474 amino acids. The gene has been localized to the human chromosome 20 q 11.2. A milder form of glutathione synthetase deficiency (MIM 231900) is associated with decreased erythrocyte glutathione levels and well-compensated hemolytic disease. This disorder, expressed in erythrocytes, has been identified in four families and seems to be less prevalent than the generalized (severe form) of glutathione synthetase deficiency and does not lead to 5-oxoprolinuria. This inborn error is associated with synthesis of an unstable glutathione synthetase. Turnover of the defective but active enzyme is sufficiently rapid in most tissues to compensate for the defect; however, this is not true for erythrocytes in which protein synthesis does not take place.
2. **Deficiency of γ-glutamylcysteine synthetase (MIM 230450) has been described in six patients in five different families. A consistent clinical finding is an increased rate of hemolysis. In addition, two sibs also had spinocerebellar degeneration, peripheral neuropathy, myopathy, and aminoaciduria. The patients had generalized glutathione deficiency and marked deficiency in the synthesis of γ-glutamylcysteine.**
3. **Five patients with hereditary deficiency of γ-glutamyl transpeptidase (MIM 231950) have been reported. They exhibit central nervous system involvement, glutathionemia, and urinary excretion of substantial amounts of glutathione, as well as of γ-glutamylcysteine and cysteine moieties. An animal model indicates that this enzyme deficiency is associated with central nervous system dysfunction and growth retardation.**
4. **Eight individuals with inborn deficiency of 5-oxoprolinase (MIM 260005) have been reported. They excrete increased amounts of 5-oxoproline in their urine and also have elevated plasma levels of 5-oxoproline. The patients do not have chronic acidosis or other symptoms clearly related to the biochemical defect.**

GLUTATHIONE BIOCHEMISTRY AND PHYSIOLOGY

Glutathione, L-γ-glutamyl-L-cysteinylglycine, is found in most cells in high concentration (0.1 to 10 mM). It has an unusual γ-peptide bond that prevents its hydrolysis by all but one peptidase and a thiol moiety that is key to its physiological and biochemical functions. Glutathione participates as a coenzyme in several reactions and is involved in maintaining thiol/disulfide balance. Additionally, it plays a key role in the protection against toxic compounds through nonenzymatic reactions and those catalyzed by GSH S-transferases and GSH peroxidase. A product of the peroxidase reaction, glutathione disulfide (GSSG), is normally reduced by glutathione disulfide reductase using NADPH. Normally there is little cellular GSSG, and the ratio of GSH to GSSG is high. Glutathione has many cellular functions, and the

A list of standard abbreviations is located immediately preceding the index in each volume. Additional abbreviations used in this chapter include: AP = activator protein; ARE = antioxidant response element; BCNU = 1,3-bis (2-chloroethyl)-1-nitrosourea; BSO = buthionine sulfoximine; EpRE = electrophile response element; GCS = γ-glutamylcysteine synthetase; GCT = γ-glutamyl cyclotransferase; GS = glutathione synthetase; GST = glutathione S-transferase; GSH = reduced glutathione; GSSG = glutathione disulfide; GT = γ-glutamyltranspeptidase; MDR = multidrug-resistant protein; MSO = methionine sulfoximine; NAC = *N*-acetylcysteine; NTP = nucleoside triphosphate; OP = 5-oxoprolinase; OTC = oxothiazolidine-4-carboxylate.

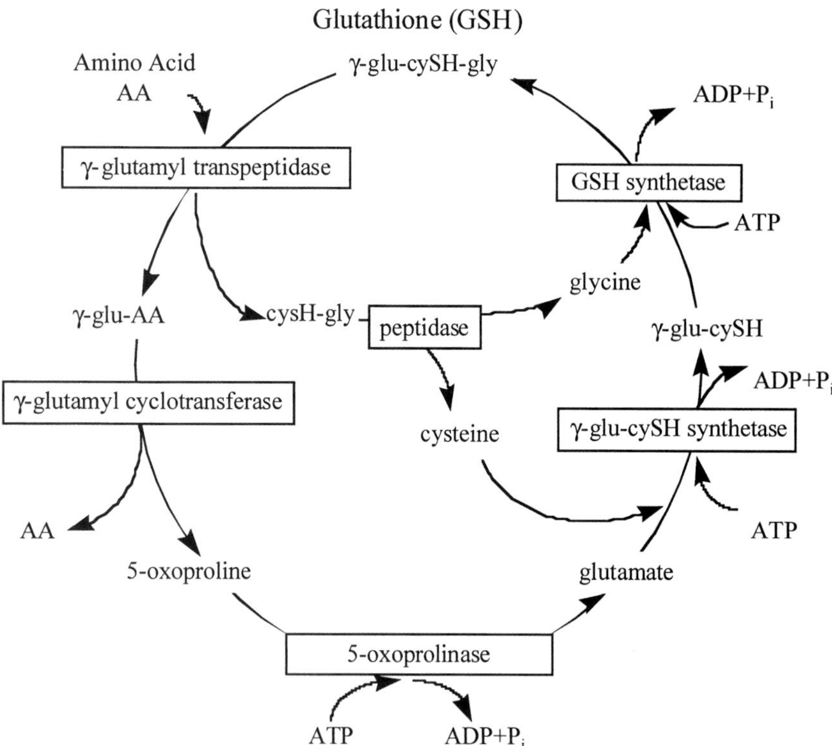

Fig. 96-1 The γ-glutamyl cycle.

study of these has been aided by genetic mutants of enzymes involved in GSH metabolism and by the use of inhibitors of GSH metabolism.[1–5]

The γ-Glutamyl Cycle

Six enzymes form the γ-glutamyl cycle, which catalyzes the synthesis and degradation of GSH (Fig. 96-1). The γ-glutamyl cycle was identified by Meister and coworkers in 1970.[6] Since then, a large body of experimental evidence supports its function *in vivo*.[3,7] Although many tissues and cells have all of the γ-glutamyl cycle enzymes, some cells, such as the erythrocytes, lack γ-glutamyl transpeptidase and 5-oxoprolinase. Glutathione is synthesized intracellularly and exported from most cells. Tissues have very different rates of GSH turnover. For example, rat kidney, liver, lymphocyte, lung, and skeletal muscle have GSH half-times of about 20 min, 60 min, 25 min, 45 min, and 16 h, respectively; the reasons for such differences in GSH turnover are not known. If the γ-glutamyl cycle plays a role in amino acid transport, it is likely that it has an important role in the salvaging of cysteine and GSH moieties and for maintaining cellular thiol and GSH status.

Glutathione Biosynthesis. With the exception of most gram-positive bacteria,[8] GSH is synthesized in all cells from glutamate, cysteine, and glycine by the sequential actions of γ-glutamylcysteine synthetase (GCS) and glutathione synthetase (GS). Both enzymes are cytosolic and use ATP, which is hydrolyzed to ADP and Pi.

γ-Glutamylcysteine Synthetase (GCS). GCS catalyzes the first and rate-limiting step in the biosynthesis of GSH, the formation of γ-glutamylcysteine:

$$\text{L-Glu} + \text{L-Cys} + \text{ATP} \rightarrow \text{L-}\gamma\text{-Glu-Cys} + \text{ADP} + \text{Pi}$$

The enzyme has been partially purified from several sources, including porcine liver, *Xenopus laevis* liver, *E. coli, Proteus mirabilis*, wheat germ, rat kidney, liver and erythrocytes, bovine lens and erythrocytes, sheep erythrocytes, and human erythrocytes.[3]

Rat kidney is the source of the most highly purified and characterized GCS.[9,10] The enzyme is active toward several L-glutamate and L-cysteine analogs. Because of spontaneous oxidation, which causes problems in *in vitro* assays, L-α-aminobutyrate is often used instead of cysteine as the acceptor amino acid. Rat GCS is a heterodimer of separately encoded subunits (molecular weight 73 kDa and 31 kDa).[9,10] Human GCS is highly homologous to rat GCS.[11] The heavy subunit has catalytic activity, but low affinity for glutamate. The light subunit, which by itself is not catalytically active, increases the affinity of the heavy subunit for glutamate and is thus regulatory. The light subunit has 6 cysteine residues and the heavy subunit has 14, one of which is needed for activity. The two subunits are associated by strong hydrophobic interactions. They can also interact through disulfide bond formation, which increases the affinity of the enzyme for glutamate.[10] The disulfide form of the enzyme is likely to be present when GSH levels are low and there is oxidative stress. Thus, GCS activity is controlled by cellular needs for GSH. Also GCS is feedback inhibited, that is, non-allosterically, by GSH at physiological concentrations suggesting that *in vivo* the enzyme is not fully active but can respond rapidly to changing cellular needs for GSH.[9,12] In addition to regulation of GCS activity by GSH and by disulfide formation between the heavy and light subunits, GCS activity may be inhibited by phosphorylation.[13]

The enzyme GCS is inhibited by a number of compounds, which are reactive with thiols.[2] Such inhibitors are cystamine, L-2-amino-4-oxo-5-chloropentanoic acid, and L- and D-3-amino-1-chloro-2-pentanone, all of which interact with a thiol near the active site. D-γ-Methylene glutamate irreversibly inhibits the enzyme by addition to an enzyme thiol moiety. The enzyme is also inactivated by both L- and D- isomers of S-sulfocysteine and S-sulfohomocysteine, which bind tightly to the enzyme and are stabilized by a thiol near the active site. L-Glutamate protects against inactivation by all of these compounds, which suggests that there is an essential thiol at or near the active site.[9,10,14]

Methionine sulfoximine (MSO) inhibits both GCS and glutamine synthetase.[15] Meister and colleagues showed that glutamine synthetase is inhibited by L-methionine-S-sulfoximine phosphate, a transition state inhibitor. Glutamine synthetase is selectively inhibited by α-ethyl MSO, whereas GCS is inhibited by longer amino acid sulfoximines, such as prothionine sulfoximine and buthionine sulfoximine (BSO). These studies suggest that like glutamine synthetase, GCS functions by forming an enzyme-bound γ-glutamyl phosphate intermediate.[16,17]

The mRNA for the heavy subunit of GCS (hGCS) is overexpressed in a number of drug-resistant human tumor cell lines.[18] GCS mRNA levels are increased by cisplatin, insulin, hydrocortisone, hydrogen peroxide, tumor necrosis factor transforming growth factor-$\beta 1$, and β-naphthoflavone.[19–22] The 5′ flanking sequence of the hGCS gene has AP-1 (activator protein 1) and AP-2 binding-site consensus sequences, as well as consensus sequences for ARE4 (antioxidant response element 4) and EpRE (electrophile response element).[19,23–25] The transcription of the light (regulatory) subunit of GCS is increased in response to oxidative stress and cisplatin, but not to insulin[21,26,27] in cultured cell lines. The levels of hGCS and MDR (multidrug-resistant protein) mRNA increase in drug-resistant tumor cell lines.[28,29] The two subunits seem to be induced by oxidative stress and to play a role in certain types of chemotherapeutic drug resistance.

Glutathione Synthetase. Glutathione synthetase (GS) (MIM 601002) is widely distributed in mammalian tissues and catalyzes the formation of GSH.[30] The enzyme has been purified from a number of sources including *E. coli,* yeast pigeon liver, plants, rat kidney, human brain, and erythrocytes. Studies on yeast GS, using pulse labeling and chemical intermediate synthesis, showed that GS catalyzes the formation of an acyl phosphate intermediate, γ-glutamyl-α-aminobutyryl phosphate.[30] Thus, GS, like GCS, proceeds via an acyl phosphate intermediate:

$$\gamma\text{-Glu-Cys} + \text{Gly} + \text{ATP} \rightarrow \text{GSH} + \text{ADP} + \text{Pi}$$

The most studied and first cloned mammalian GS is the rat kidney enzyme.[31] This enzyme is a homodimer with subunits of 52 kDa. It has about 2 percent carbohydrate content,[32] but its expression in *E. coli* yields a fully active enzyme, which suggests that the carbohydrate moiety is not required for enzyme activity. The human enzyme[33] has 88 percent amino acid identity and 98 percent amino acid similarity to the rat enzyme.

Recent studies on human GS have shown that mutations altering Cys-422 lead to decreased enzyme activity.[34] Comparison of human and rat GS shows that there is a highly conserved domain of 13 amino acids that may be important in substrate binding.[35] Furthermore, mutations altering some residues in this domain lead to dramatic loss of enzyme activity. The enzyme exhibits negative cooperativity for both γ-glutamylcysteine and γ-glutamyl-α-aminobutyrate, that is, the binding of the first molecule of γ-glutamyl substrate diminishes the affinity for the second molecule.[35] It is not yet known whether human GS exhibits negative cooperativity.

There is only GS structural gene in the human genome and it maps to chromosome 20.q 11.2.[36] Studies on drug resistant human tumor cells show that GS is not induced, even when GCS transcription is strongly induced,[18] suggesting that there are different response elements in the promotors of GCS and GS, and that there is sufficient GS activity to form GSH. The murine GS gene encodes six transcripts each with different 5′ ends.[37] Mouse GS is reported to be induced by the metal chelator 1,10-phenanthroline.[38]

Glutathione Degradation

Four enzymes catalyze the degradative reactions of the γ-glutamyl cycle (Fig. 96-1). The activity of each of these enzymes varies in different tissues. For instance, erythrocytes lack γ-glutamyl transpeptidase (GT) and OP, and thus GSH turnover in erythrocytes depends on export of GSH to other tissues with a complete set of degrading enzymes.

γ-Glutamyl Transpeptidase. GT is a membrane-bound enzyme whose active site faces the external side of a cell (ectoenzyme), and it is the only enzyme that cleaves the γ-glutamyl bond of GSH. The GT activity is found in many plants and microorganisms, as well as in mammals.[1] In mammals, it is found in cells that have secretory or absorptive functions. The highest levels are found in kidney, pancreas, and intestine, but it is also found in spleen, liver, epididymis, lymphoid cells, choroid plexus, and ciliary body.[1] A soluble form of GT is found in bile and plasma, and its levels in plasma are used clinically as a marker of liver function. The enzyme is localized to microvilli of epithelial cells in the kidney proximal tubules, and to the jejunum, bile duct, retinal pigment epithelium, bronchioles, thyroid follicles, pancreas acinar and ductile epithelial cells, the canalicular portions of hepatocytes, and seminal vesicles.[39]

γ-Glutamyl transpeptidase catalyzes the coupled hydrolysis of the γ-glutamyl bond of GSH (and other γ-glutamyl compounds) with the transfer of the γ-glutamyl moiety to acceptor molecules:

$$\text{GSH} + \text{acceptor} \Leftrightarrow \gamma\text{-glutamyl acceptor} + \text{cysteinylglycine}$$

The acceptor is usually an amino acid, yielding a γ-glutamyl amino acid, but it may also be water or GSH. When the acceptor is water, GSH is hydrolyzed to glutamate and cysteinylglycine. Maleate and hippurate increase the hydrolysis activity of GT.[39] Bile acids and conjugated bile acids also modulate the hydrolysis and γ-glutamyl transfer activity of GT.[1] When GSH is the acceptor, γ-glutamyl GSH is formed.[40] The enzyme has a γ-glutamyl intermediate and a ping-pong mechanism.[1]

γ-Glutamyl transpeptidase is a highly glycosylated heterodimer with subunits of 21 kDa and 38 kDa, which are formed by cleavage of a single, inactive glycopropeptide chain.[41] The heavy subunit has an N-terminal membrane anchor and it is noncovalently linked to the light subunit. The human GT gene is a multigenic family composed of at least seven different loci,[42] five of which are located on chromosome 22.[43] In addition, GT-related sequences have been identified on chromosomes 18, 19, and 20;[44] thus, there are multiple copies of the human GT gene.[45] In contrast, rodent GT is encoded by a single copy gene with multiple promotors, some of which are regulated by oxidative stress.[46–48] Both the human and the rat GT mRNAs are differentially expressed in tissues and during development.[47,49–54] One rat promotor has a negative regulatory region that is similar to the silencer element in the GSH S-transferase gene.[55]

The active site of GT faces the outside of the cell and has three active subsites. The γ-glutamyl donor site has a broad specificity using L- and D- γ-glutamyl donors.[1,39] The cysteinylglycine site binds amino acids and dipeptides (in the L-configuration or glycine) and has two subsites. The best acceptor amino acids are the neutral amino acids, whereas branched chain amino acids are weak acceptors, and D-amino acids and L-proline are inactive.[39] The glycine subsite prefers dipeptides with glycine in the C-terminal position.[3]

γ-Glutamyl transpeptidase is inhibited by L- or D-serine and borate, which forms a transition state inhibitor-complex with an enzyme hydroxyl group.[56] The enzyme is also inhibited by a variety of compounds, such as γ-glutamyl derivatives and glutamine antagonists, and such inhibition is decreased by γ-glutamyl compounds, such as GSH and glutamine.[39] Site-specific mutagenesis and inhibitor-binding studies suggest that several amino acid hydroxyl groups and charged amino acids are important for GT catalysis. These studies[45,57–59] suggest that the active site of the enzyme is at an interface between the heavy and light subunits.

γ-Glutamylcyclotransferase. γ-Glutamylcyclotransferase (GCT) catalyzes the hydrolysis of the γ-glutamyl bond of certain γ-glutamyl compounds to form free amino acid and 5-oxoproline, a cyclic form of glutamate:

$$\text{L-}\gamma\text{-glu-amino acid} \rightarrow \text{5-oxoproline} + \text{amino acid}$$

GCT activity is present in many tissues, including kidney, liver, testes, spleen, brain, lung, heart, thymus, thyroid, skeletal muscle, skin, and adrenal gland.[1] The GCT peptide is 27 kDa and contains 7 half cystines.[1]

Although GCT catalyzes the hydrolysis of L-γ-glutamyl amino acids, it does not catalyze the hydrolysis of the γ-glutamyl bond of GSH or GSSG.[1] It has a broad specificity toward L-γ-glutamyl amino acids; most L-γ-glutamyl amino acids are substrates except for the aromatic, branched chain, and proline L-γ-glutamyl derivatives. The enzyme is not active toward D-γ-glutamyl derivatives. The substrate specificity of GCT parallels that of γ-glutamyl transpeptidase.

Dipeptidase. The enzyme activity that cleaves the GT product cysteinylglycine has been called dipeptidase or cysteinylglycinase. The activity has been found in the cytosol and associated with membranes.[1] A mouse has at least four distinct membrane dipeptidase mRNA transcripts that result from the use of two promoters and two different poly(A) addition sites.[60]

5-Oxoprolinase. 5-Oxoprolinase (OP) catalyzes ATP-dependent ring-opening of 5-oxo-L-proline (pyroglutamic acid; pyrrolidone carboxylate) to yield glutamate.[1]

$$\text{5-Oxoproline} + \text{ATP} \rightarrow \text{L-Glu} + \text{ADP} + \text{Pi}$$

5-Oxoproline can be formed by the action of GCT on γ-glutamyl compounds, enzymatic degradation of proteins with N-terminal 5-oxoprolyl residues, nonenzymatic formation from glutamine, as well as from dietary sources, such as tomato juice and some processed foods, and intestinal microorganism flora.[60]

The enzyme is found in microorganisms, plants, and in most mammalian tissues, except erythrocytes.[1] The activity of OP in cells is low relative to most of the other enzymes of the γ-glutamyl cycle, but normally little 5-oxoproline is found in tissues or urine. The mammalian enzyme is not well studied, but it is composed of two apparently identical subunits, each with several thiol moieties. A putative clone has been reported from rat kidney.[62] Studies on the bacterial enzyme suggest that the enzyme forms a 5-oxoproline phosphate intermediate that couples the hydrolysis of the "internal peptide bond" of 5-oxoproline to the hydrolysis of ATP.[63]

The substrate specificity of OP is narrow.[1] 5-Oxo-D-proline is neither a substrate nor an inhibitor of OP. While ATP is the preferred nucleotide, OP will use dATP and other nucleoside triphosphates (NTPs) to a lesser extent. The enzyme requires both K^+ and Mg^{2+} for activity. An interesting substrate is L-2-oxothiazolidine-4-carboxylate (see below, Cysteine Delivery), which is opened to form intracellular cysteine. The best competitive inhibitor of OP is L-2-imidazolidone-4-carboxylate.

Experimental Deficiency of γ-Glutamyl Cycle Enzymes

A number of methods have been used to study the roles of the individual enzymes of the γ-glutamyl cycle, from cultured cells and tissue slices to rodent models.[1,15] These studies have given insights into the functions of GSH and provided models for testing potential therapies for deficiency of GSH and GSH-related enzymes.

Experimental γ-Glutamylcysteine Synthetase Deficiency. Several compounds have been used to decrease cellular GSH levels; however, many of these compounds are nonspecific. As discussed above, GCS and glutamine synthetase are both inhibited by MSO. Administration of MSO to rodents leads to decreased tissue levels of GSH and glutamine. In addition, BSO, a specific inhibitor of GCS, is transported into many tissues, except across the blood-brain and blood-testis barriers. Glutathione levels decrease in tissues as GSH is used for cellular functions and exported in the absence of GSH synthesis.[1] The levels of GSH decreases in rodent tissues after a few doses of BSO to 10 to 20 percent of control. A series of experiments showed that most of the remaining GSH is present in mitochondria. Mitochondria do not synthesize GSH, but take it up from the cytosol.[64] After long-term administration of BSO to rodents, even mitochondrial GSH is depleted primarily because the electron transport system leaks free radicals, and, eventually, the mitochondria swell and lyse.[2] Long-term BSO administration leads to damage of several organs, including lung, muscle, cerebral cortex, liver, jejunum, colon, and proximal renal tubule, but not heart and stomach; also plasma levels of triglycerides and cholesterol are elevated.[2] Long-term BSO treatment provides a model of endogenous oxidative stress.[65] Guinea pigs and newborn rodents, like humans, cannot synthesize vitamin C, and thus may be useful models for understanding human endogenous oxidative stress. Studies show that administration of vitamin C to rodents can prevent mitochondrial GSH deficiency caused by BSO treatment and that elevating cellular GSH can delay scurvy in vitamin C-deficient rodents.[66–69] Thus, GSH "spares" vitamin C and vitamin C "spares" GSH.

Administration of BSO to rodents increases the toxicity of melphalan, BCNU (1.3-bis(2-chloroethyl)-1-nitrosourea), cisplatin, cadmium ions, mercury ions, and monocrotaline, as well as of radiation. Furthermore, BSO treatment blocks the activation of human T lymphocytes.[4] Such studies emphasize the importance of GSH in protection mechanisms. In addition, BSO is being tested in clinical trials for cancer therapy.[70]

Experimental Glutathione Synthetase Deficiency. No selective inhibitor of mammalian GS is available. Accordingly, there is no pharmacologic model of human GS deficiency. This is unfortunate because such a model would facilitate the testing of therapies for patients with GS deficiency.

Experimental γ-Glutamyl Transpeptidase Deficiency. Administration to mice of acceptor amino acids, such as glycylglycine, stimulate transpeptidation and lead to decreased cellular levels of GSH. When an inhibitor of GT is given prior to the amino acid, GSH levels do not decrease.[15] Administration of effective inhibitors of GT to mice leads to glutathionuria and glutathionemia. After acivicin treatment, urinary thiols (GSH, γ-glutamylcysteine, cysteine) increased; these same thiols were found in the urine of a GT-deficient patient.[71]

γ-Glutamyl transpeptidase knockout mice have been made.[72] Recent studies using these mice showed that GT deficiency leads to glutathionuria, glutathionemia, growth failure, decreased life span, and infertility.[73]

Experimental γ-Glutamylcyclotransferase Deficiency. The best inhibitor of GCT is β-aminoglutaryl-L-α-aminobutyrate with a Ki of 0.6 mM, and it is competitive. When administered to mice, 5-oxoproline levels decrease substantially, suggesting that GCT activity is important *in vivo* for the formation of 5-oxoproline and also that the γ-glutamyl cycle functions *in vivo*.[74]

Experimental 5-Oxoprolinase Deficiency. Administration to mice of competitive inhibitors of OP, such as L-2-imidazolidone-4-carboxylate or D,L-3-methyl-5-oxoproline, showed that the metabolism of 5-oxoproline is significantly decreased and 5-oxoproline may be found in urine.[1]

Experimental Dipeptidase Deficiency. Recent studies[60] using mice, which are deficient in membrane-bound dipeptidase, show that mice still retain the ability to convert leukotriene D4 to E4, but had a slight elevation of urinary cystinyl bisglycine, suggesting that there is more than one enzyme activity with cysteinylglycinase activity.

Elevation of GSH Levels — Potential Therapies

Deficiency of GSH results from inborn errors in the GSH synthetic pathway. Other diseases have also been associated with GSH deficiency, such as HIV infection,[75–79] hepatitis C infection,[78] diabetes,[79] ulcerative colitis,[80] idiopathic pulmonary fibrosis,[81] and adult respiratory distress syndrome.[82] Various toxic compounds can be rendered less harmful by reaction with GSH; such reactions can be nonenzymatic or via the GSH S-transferase family of enzymes. Superoxide dismutase and reactions involving GSH detoxify reactive oxygen species. Glutathione can react through glutathione peroxidase to detoxify hydrogen peroxide and organic peroxides. Reactive oxygen species have been associated with various diseases involving ischemia-reperfusion, namely stroke and myocardial infarction, cancer, AIDS, arthritis, atherosclerosis, adult respiratory distress syndrome, and Parkinson disease.[83,84] It is not clear for any of these pathologic conditions whether the synthesis of GSH is affected or whether the metabolism of GSH is increased. Increasing cellular GSH levels may be beneficial for treating GSH deficiency caused by reactive oxygen species and by deficiency of GSH-related enzymes.

Cysteine Delivery. Administration of GSH is only effective as a cysteine delivery compound. GSH is not readily taken up by cells; it is broken down and its component amino acids used to resynthesize GSH.[15] Administration of cysteine supplies what is usually the limiting substrate for GSH synthesis; however, it is readily oxidized to cystine, which has limited solubility and is reported to be toxic.[85] *N*-Acetyl cysteine (NAC) is commonly used to treat patients who are exposed to paracetamol in overdose. It is transported into cells and deacetylated to form cysteine for GSH synthesis. Two reports of treatment of GS-deficient patients with NAC suggested that NAC has little or no effect.[86] NAC may serve as a reducing agent and liberate GSH from GSSG and other disulfide forms thereby supplying cysteine for GSH synthesis. This would restore cysteine supplies in GS-deficient patients. Alternatively, NAC may provide beneficial reducing power to cells. 2-Oxothiazolidine-4-carboxylate (OTC; procysteine) is a substrate for OP and is opened to form intracellular cysteine.[5,87] It is well transported and increases cellular GSH levels in many cells;[85] however, both GCS and GS activities are required. Administration of OTC has been reported to raise cellular GSH levels in HIV patients.[88–90] In rats, OTC promotes growth and protects against ischemia.[91,92]

γ-Glutamylcysteine Delivery. The cellular level of γ-glutamylcysteine is low and normally it is the rate-limiting substrate for GS. Administration of this dipeptide can increase GSH in cells that can transport γ-glutamyl amino acids, such as those of the kidney.[93] Administration of γ-glutamylcysteine bypasses GCS, the feedback inhibited and rate-limiting step of GSH synthesis. The use of γ-glutamylcysteine for GSH biosynthesis is part of the salvage or alternative pathway of GSH synthesis. In this pathway, GSH is exported, reacts via GT with cystine to form γ-glutamylcystine, which is transported and reduced to γ-glutamylcysteine and used directly by GS for GSH synthesis; the extent to which this pathway functions *in vivo* is not known.

γ-Glutamylcysteine has been shown to increase brain GSH levels after intraventricular injection.[94] γ-Glutamylcysteine ester has been used to transport γ-glutamylcysteine into cells for the synthesis of GSH.[95,96]

GSH Esters. Because GSH is not readily taken up by cells, GSH mono- and diesters were developed.[5,97–99] These esters are transported into cells in many tissues, except brain, and are hydrolyzed to yield free GSH.[100,101] The other product of the reaction is the corresponding alcohol, usually ethanol. Treatment of rodents and cell lines with GSH monoester protects against the toxicity listed above for experimental GSH deficiency produced by BSO treatment. It is also effective in the endogenous oxidative stress model involving newborn rodents (see above, "Experimental GCS Deficiency"). Thus, administration of GSH monoester to rodents prevents cataract formation and mitochondrial damage, and protects against the effects of vitamin C deficiency. Esters of GSH have potential in the therapy of patients with GSH deficiency.

Antioxidants — Vitamin C. Vitamin C and GSH can spare each other in rodent models (see above, "Experimental GCS Deficiency"). Short-term treatment of GS-deficient patients with vitamin C has been reported to increase lymphocyte GSH levels.[86] It is not known whether long-term vitamin C treatment is beneficial, but because vitamin C and GSH are not able to carry out the same functions, it is likely that vitamin C treatment is only partially effective. Treatment with other antioxidants, such as vitamin E, may have effects similar to treatment with vitamin C, but further studies are needed.

INBORN ERRORS OF GLUTATHIONE METABOLISM

In man, hereditary deficiency is described in four of the six enzymes in the γ-glutamyl cycle (Fig. 96-1), namely GCS, GS, GT, and OP. More detailed descriptions of individual patients were published earlier.[102,103] Patients with hereditary defects in γ-glutamyl cyclotransferase and the dipeptidase are still to be detected.

In diagnostic work, it is important to remember that erythrocytes have an incomplete γ-glutamyl cycle — they lack both GT and OP. These enzymes must, therefore, be analyzed in other types of cells, such as leukocytes and fibroblasts.

γ-Glutamylcysteine Synthetase Deficiency

Five patients with GCS deficiency (MIM 230450) have been reported. Two German sibs were originally described in 1972;[104] subsequently, one Polish woman[105] and two Japanese patients have been described.[106] A sixth patient, a woman from the Netherlands, is currently under investigation. This wide geographical distribution of patients suggests allelic heterogeneity.

A common clinical finding among patients with GCS deficiency is hemolytic anemia, which is usually rather mild. The patients exhibit low levels of GCS, γ-glutamylcysteine, and GSH in their erythrocytes. Their GS activity is normal. There is evidence for generalized enzyme deficiency because the patients have decreased levels of γ-glutamylcysteine and GSH in leukocytes, skeletal muscle, and cultured fibroblasts. The deficiency of GCS is postulated as inherited as an autosomal recessive trait.

A remarkable clinical history was found in the first two patients described, a brother and sister 25 to 30 years old.[104,107] Initially their only symptom was hemolytic anemia with erythrocyte GSH deficiency (<5 percent of normal). The female sib required transfusions during pregnancy, but otherwise the increased rate of hemolysis was well compensated in both. Subsequently, in their 30s, they exhibited progressive spinocerebellar degeneration and neuromuscular symptoms with peripheral neuropathy and myopathy. Several years later, the woman became psychotic after treatment with sulfonamide for a urinary tract infection and developed ataxia and dysmetria. Her brother also developed myopathy and ataxia. Generalized aminoaciduria was found in both these patients with especially marked excretion of dibasic and monobasic-monocarboxylic amino acids. Because the levels of amino acids in plasma were essentially normal, a renal transport defect was indicated. This finding is consistent with the involvement in the kidney of the γ-glutamyl cycle in the active transport of amino acids.[6]

The third patient described with GCS deficiency was the child of consanguineous parents.[105] She had a history of transient jaundice during an unspecified viral infection at 10 years of age. At age 21, she presented with anemia and reticulocytosis while pregnant and she received blood transfusions. After the delivery, she continued to be anemic with increased reticulocyte counts. She had GSH deficiency in her erythrocytes (10 percent of normal mean) and markedly diminished activity of GCS (6 percent of normal mean); GS activity was normal.

Two unrelated Japanese patients with GCS deficiency were recently described.[106] A 15-year-old boy had a history of anemia at birth and required a blood transfusion at 1 month of age. Afterward, he was asymptomatic until 10 years of age when he had an episode of anemia, reticulocytosis, jaundice, and hepatosplenomegaly. At 15 years of age, he still had mild hemolytic anemia. He was found to have GSH deficiency in his erythrocytes (0.4 percent of normal mean) and markedly diminished activity of GCS (0.6 percent of normal mean) and GST (16 percent of normal mean). His mother had decreased activity of GCS (56 percent of normal mean) and GST (61 percent of normal mean). His growth and development were normal.[106] The other patient was a 17-year-old girl whose parents were first cousins. She had had anemia and reticulocytosis from childhood. Her erythrocytes had markedly decreased survival with a half-life that was 10 to 20 percent of normal.[106] She had low GSH levels in her erythrocytes (13 percent of normal mean) and her erythrocyte GCS activity was decreased (23 percent of normal mean), as was her GST activity (29 percent of normal mean). Her mother also had a mild deficiency of GCS (75 percent of normal mean) and her father and brother had slightly decreased GST activity (62 percent and 79 percent of normal mean, respectively). Neither of these two Japanese patients with GCS deficiency had signs of central nervous system involvement.

The sixth patient, currently under investigation, is a 66-year-old Dutch women. She was originally reported more than 30 years ago.[108] She had a history of transient jaundice, hemolytic anemia, and very low erythrocyte GSH (3 percent of normal mean) and erythrocyte γ-glutamylcysteine (<2 percent of normal mean). She has markedly diminished GCS activity, but normal GS activity in erythrocytes and leukocytes. She does not have hepatosplenomegaly. The patient has normal levels of amino acids in blood and urine and she did not excrete 5-oxoproline in urine. Several of her family members were found to have transient jaundice and marked erythrocyte GSH deficiency, and some of them also had mild hepatosplenomegaly.

Among the six patients with GCS deficiency so far described, two have had generalized aminoaciduria, three patients have not been investigated with respect to urinary amino acids, and one patient had normal amino acid excretion. This phenotypic variation may have several explanations. If the γ-glutamyl cycle serves an important function in amino acid transport,[6] the absence of aminoaciduria in at least one of the patients could be explained by the residual GCS activity being able to maintain low, but adequate, levels of GSH in the renal tubules to permit amino acid transport via the γ-glutamyl cycle. Alternatively, the aminoaciduria found in the two sibs with GCS deficiency, but so far not in any of the other patients, may reflect a more indirect involvement of GSH in renal amino acid transport. It may, in fact, be analogous to the decreased level of GST[109] or to the decreased hepatic activity of succinylacetoacetase found in a patient with GS deficiency.[110] A third possibility is that alternative mechanisms for renal amino acid transport exist and that the generalized aminoaciduria found in two of the six patients is merely coincidental.

GCS consists of two nonidentical subunits encoded by two separate genes.[111,112] Thus, the clinical heterogeneity may reflect mutations in the genes encoding the heavy and light subunits, respectively. It will be interesting to characterize the molecular basis of GCS deficiency in these patients.

The prognosis, treatment, and genetics in GCS deficiency remain to be established. The partial reduction in GCS activity in first-degree relatives is consistent with autosomal recessive inheritance.

The observation that symptoms worsened in one GCS deficient patient after treatment with sulfonamide[104,107] indicates that patients with this disorder should avoid drugs that are known to precipitate hemolytic crises in patients with G6PD deficiency (see Chap. 179). The postulated mechanism is that increased oxidative stress caused by sulfonamide in a G6PD deficient individual is poorly tolerated by erythrocytes of patients who are unable to keep GSH in the reduced state. In the absence of G6PD, the erythrocytes cannot convert NADP to NADPH, and thus lack an essential substrate for glutathione reductase.

Glutathione Synthetase Deficiency

Clinically, two forms of GS deficiency can be distinguished: one is expressed only in erythrocytes (MIM 231900) and the other is expressed in multiple tissues (MIM 266130). The erythrocyte form of GS deficiency was postulated to be due to a mutation that primarily affected the stability of the enzyme, whereas the generalized form was postulated to be due to mutations affecting the catalytic properties of the enzyme.[113] Glutathione synthetase deficiency results in low levels of GSH in erythrocytes, and in the generalized form, there are also low levels of GSH in leukocytes, fibroblasts, and other tissues. The distinction between the two forms of GS deficiency is clinically useful. The human genome contains only a single GS gene, so it is likely that these two phenotypes reflect allelic heterogeneity.[33]

Generalized Glutathione Synthetase Deficiency

Clinical Signs and Symptoms. The first patient with generalized GS deficiency was a 19-year-old Norwegian boy of normal height and weight who had been mentally retarded since childhood.[114] He showed signs of cerebral damage with spastic tetraparesis and cerebellar disturbances with intentional tremor and ataxic gait. Abnormalities included increased resistance to passive movement, predominantly of the pyramidal type, retarded voluntary movements, pronounced tremor, and impaired coordination. His speech was simple, childlike, and dysarthric. His IQ was about 60. At age 17, the patient was treated surgically for a diaphragmatic hernia, and postoperatively life-threatening acidosis developed, which was corrected by daily infusions of sodium bicarbonate solution. Later, he was maintained on sodium bicarbonate orally (10 to 20 g daily).

A remarkable biochemical finding was excretion in the urine of about 30 g (0.23 mol) of 5-L-oxoproline (L-pyroglutamic acid) per day. His urinary excretion of urea was considered to be only 40 percent of that normally expected; consequently, it was initially postulated that he suffered from a defect in the urea cycle and that his 5-oxoprolinuria was secondary to an enzyme deficiency in the urea cycle. Thin-layer chromatography and gas-liquid chromatography/mass spectrometry identified 5-oxoprolinuria. Elevated levels of serum 5-oxoproline were also demonstrated.

The history of the patient revealed that he became jaundiced and seriously ill immediately after birth, but recovered spontaneously. During childhood, he exhibited various progressive neurologic symptoms. In retrospect, it appears that he had chronic metabolic acidosis, which was compensated for until he underwent surgery for diaphragmatic hernia. His nonconsanguineous parents, an elder brother, and other relatives were healthy.

Forty patients in 35 families with generalized GS deficiency are now known. They originate in all continents of the world. Most patients with generalized GS deficiency show symptoms within the first few days of life, namely metabolic acidosis, hemolytic anemia, jaundice, and 5-oxoprolinuria. After the neonatal period, their condition is usually stabilized, especially if the acidosis is corrected. During episodes of gastroenteritis and other infections, however, the patients may become critically ill due to severe acidosis and electrolyte imbalance. Five of 35 patients have died from infections and severe acidosis in the neonatal period; another died during childhood.

Twelve of 33 patients have had progressive central nervous system damage, including mental retardation, ataxia, spasticity, and seizures. One patient died at the age of 28 years and autopsy revealed atrophy of the granular cell layer of the cerebellum as well as focal lesions of the cortex.[115] The neurologic symptoms in his case were progressive. It is, however, essential to remember that generalized GS deficiency has a variable phenotype and that it is difficult to predict the outcome for individual patients. Some may even escape central nervous system damage. The clinical picture is presumably correlated to the extent of the enzyme deficiency, which, in turn, depends, in part, on the specific mutation. In addition, the degree of environmental challenge on

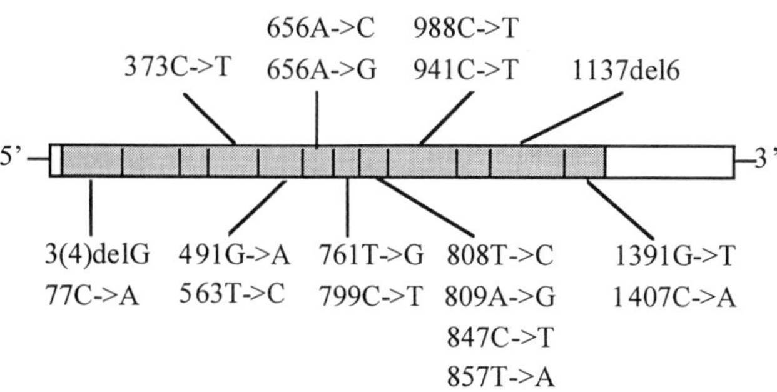

Fig. 96-2 The human glutathione synthetase cDNA and mutations identified. The message is 1.4 kb and composed of 11 exons. Twenty mutations identified in families with glutathione synthetase deficiency are indicated.

the γ-glutamyl cycle might also modify the phenotype of the patients. Two patients have had increased susceptibility to bacterial infections due to defective granulocyte function.[116] GS deficiency also leads to impaired synthesis of leukotrienes,[117–119] other prostaglandins, steroid hormones, and melanin.[1] The clinical consequences of this remain to be established.

It can be speculated that because of reduced antioxidant protection the patients with GS deficiency might be at risk of additional symptoms, such as presenile cataract, increased risk of cancer, atherosclerosis, and immunodeficiency. So far, however, there are no reports of any of these complications.

Diagnosis. The diagnosis is usually considered in a newborn infant with severe metabolic acidosis and hemolytic anemia. In urine, there is massive excretion of L-5-oxoproline (up to 1 g [or 8 mM]/kg body weight/day). Decreased activity of GS can be demonstrated in erythrocytes, leukocytes, or cultured skin fibroblasts. Cellular levels of GSH are usually decreased. Parents show intermediate levels of GS.

Twelve unrelated patients with GS deficiency were analyzed at the cDNA level.[120,121] Splice-site mutations, deletions, and missense mutations have been identified. The mutations are distributed over the whole mRNA but with a tendency to clustering in the central part of the message (Fig. 96-2). All patients found so far have residual GS activity. This may indicate that complete loss of GS activity in critical tissues is lethal.

One patient with generalized GS deficiency was found to have decreased activity of fumarylacetoacetate lyase in liver tissue obtained at autopsy.[110] The authors concluded that most likely GSH is needed to maintain fumarylacetoacetate lyase activity. This suggests that fumarylacetoacetate lyase activity in the absence of GSH may be low. On this basis, assessment of patients with tyrosinemia should include studies of their GSH status. GS deficiency has been observed in a patient with hereditary hepatorenal tyrosinemia.[122] The mechanism for this double deficiency is presumed to be similar to the decreased activity of GSH S-transferase in erythrocytes of a patient with erythrocyte GS deficiency.[109]

Mechanism of 5-Oxoprolinuria. Glutathione normally inhibits GCS. In GS deficiency, there is reduced GSH, lack of feedback inhibition of GCS, and overproduction of γ-glutamyl cysteine (Fig. 96-3). GCT then converts this dipeptide into 5-oxoproline and cysteine. 5-Oxoproline is hydrolyzed to glutamate by OP, the enzyme in the γ-glutamyl cycle with the lowest activity in many tissues. The excessive formation of 5-oxoproline exceeds the capacity of OP. Therefore, 5-oxoproline accumulates in the body fluids, causing metabolic acidosis and 5-oxoprolinuria.

An understanding of the mechanism by which a block of GS produces 5-oxoprolinuria requires consideration of the γ-glutamyl cycle and of the properties of the enzymes involved. Glutathione is not a substrate of GCT; thus, this tripeptide may accumulate in cells in substantial concentrations, as it does under normal conditions. In contrast, γ-glutamylcysteine is an excellent substrate of GCT, as well as of GT and GS (Fig. 96-3). The normal tissue concentration of γ-glutamylcysteine is very low, perhaps less than 1 percent of that of GSH. It is possible that γ-glutamylcysteine is normally protected from the action of GCT by close linkage between the two synthetases or by compartmentalization within the cell. The affinity of GS for γ-glutamylcysteine may be greater than the affinities of the other enzymes that act on this substrate. γ-Glutamylcysteine might replace GSH as a γ-glutamyl donor in transpeptidation reactions with amino acids. However,

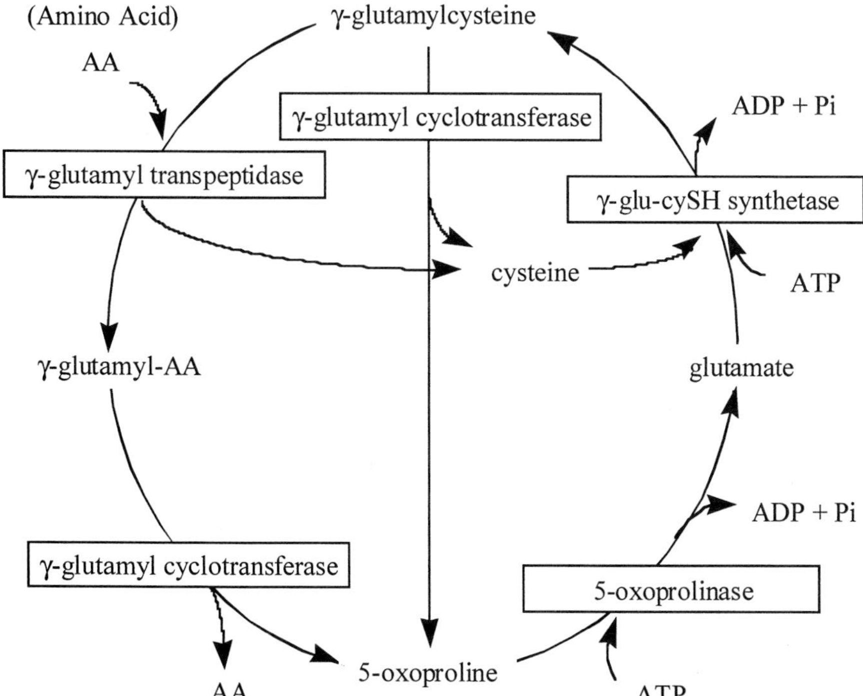

Fig. 96-3 Modified γ-glutamyl cycle in generalized glutathione synthetase deficiency.

γ-glutamylcysteine that is not used for GSH synthesis or in transpeptidation reactions is converted to 5-oxoproline and cysteine. A block in GSH synthesis leads to 5-oxoprolinuria if more than normal amounts of γ-glutamylcysteine are formed and converted to 5-oxoproline by the action of GCT, and if the overproduction of 5-oxoproline exceeds the capacity of OP to convert this substrate to glutamate. This, indeed, seems to be the mechanism of 5-oxoprolinuria. It appears that GCS normally functions at substantially less than its maximal capacity because of feedback inhibition of GSH. In the absence or marked reduction in the cellular level of GSH, there is increased formation of γ-glutamylcysteine, which is efficiently converted to 5-oxoproline.

This is an interesting example of an inborn error that prevents the synthesis of a compound that normally functions as a feedback inhibitor. The compound that accumulates as a result of the block is derived from the immediate precursor of the feedback inhibitor. The metabolic defect in this disease therefore leads to a modified γ-glutamyl cycle (Fig. 96-3) in which γ-glutamylcysteine synthesis is followed by its conversion to 5-oxoproline and cysteine. In the modified cycle, γ-glutamyl-cysteine replaces GSH as a γ-glutamyl donor in transpeptidation reactions and cysteine is recycled. This modified γ-glutamyl cycle is mediated by the action of only four enzymes; neither dipeptidase nor GS activity is involved.

The endogenous production of 5-oxoproline was estimated in tracer studies with ^{14}C-5-oxoproline[123,124] to be 60 to 80 g (or about 0.5 M)/day, or more than twice the amount excreted in the urine. Similarly, studies in which another patient with GS deficiency was given radioactive 5-oxoproline showed a daily synthesis of about 200 mM of 5-oxoproline of which 50 mM were excreted in the urine, indicating an endogenous utilization of 5-oxoproline of about 75 percent.[125] These results are in accord with the explanation for 5-oxoprolinuria given above. Accumulation of 5-oxoproline exceeds the capacity of OP to convert this compound to glutamate.

Treatment. Treatment of patients with GS deficiency involves correction of acidosis using parenteral administration of sodium bicarbonate initially followed by oral maintenance doses of sodium bicarbonate or citrate. During episodes of acute infections, higher doses may be required. Patients with generalized GS deficiency have been postulated to have increased sensitivity to oxidative stress. Therefore, free radical scavengers have been administered. Vitamin E has been claimed to correct the defective granulocyte function[126,127] and is, therefore, usually given in a dose of 10 mg/kg body weight/day. Likewise, vitamin C is also given in high doses — 100 mg/kg body weight/day. Drugs which precipitate hemolytic crises in patients with G6PD deficiency should be avoided in order to prevent hemolytic crises in patients with GS deficiency. Different therapeutic trials have been made in order to substitute for the lack of GSH. Oral administration of GSH analogues, NAC and GSH esters, have been tested. It has been possible to increase GSH levels significantly in certain tissues such as leukocytes. So far, no decrease in 5-oxoproline excretion has been reported. NAC given orally increased the GSH concentration in leukocytes by 20 to 30 percent,[128] in lymphocytes (3.5-fold) and in plasma (sixfold).[86] It has also been shown that GSH esters spare ascorbate and vice versa.[66] Oral administration of GSH monoethyl ester increases GSH concentration in erythrocytes up to sixfold and in leukocytes up to threefold.[129] This therapeutic approach, however, is limited by its expense and high doses of GSH esters required (4 to 10 mM/kg body weight/day). Studies using dietary manipulations, including adjustment of the protein intake, have not decreased the excretion of 5-oxoproline.

During the neonatal period it is essential to correct the metabolic acidosis and to prevent excessive hyperbilirubinemia in order to avoid brain damage caused by bilirubin. Anemia often needs to be treated with transfusions and electrolyte imbalance should be avoided. Additional, long-term trials are required to identify treatments to prevent CNS damage.

Prognosis. The prognosis of patients with generalized GS deficiency is difficult to predict. It likely depends on several factors, including the type of mutation, the extent of the acidosis, and other supportive treatment given, as well as early and intense treatment of invasive bacterial infections with antibiotics. In the families with more than one child affected with generalized GS deficiency, the clinical picture tends to be repeated.

Prenatal Diagnosis. Prenatal diagnosis for GS deficiency has been performed by analysis of 5-oxoproline in amniotic fluid, or by enzyme analysis in cultured amniocytes or chorion villus samples.[130,131] In an affected fetus, the 5-oxoproline level in amniotic fluid was more than fifteenfold elevated.[131] In the future, linkage analysis with suitable markers on chromosome 20 can be used. If the specific mutation(s) in the family is known, the method of choice will be direct analysis of the GS gene in DNA from a chorion villus sample obtained around the twelfth week of gestation.

The first pregnancy known in a woman with generalized GS deficiency recently resulted in the birth of a normal child at term. The pregnancy was uneventful and the urinary excretion of 5-oxoproline was constant during the gestation.

Erythrocyte Glutathione Synthetase Deficiency. Erythrocyte GS deficiency has been reported in at least four unrelated families. The first patients ever reported with an inborn error of GSH metabolism had GS deficiency in erythrocytes.[108,132] Subsequently, three additional families with the same enzyme defect were described.[109,133] The defect is most likely due to mutations that affect enzyme stability and this is supported by experimental evidence.[113] It appears that, in the erythrocyte form of GS deficiency, the genetic lesion leads to synthesis of an unstable GS molecule. The rate of replacement of an unstable but active enzyme appears to be sufficiently great in most tissues to compensate for the defect. However, such a compensatory mechanism is not possible in the erythrocyte in which protein synthesis does not take place. One mutation in the GS gene leading to erythrocyte GS deficiency has been reported.[120] The mode of inheritance is autosomal recessive.

A few of these patients had mild hemolytic anemia. Three patients also had splenomegaly. There was no indication of neurologic defects in any of the patients. No additional symptoms have been reported to be common to all patients.

All these patients had decreased activities of GS and low levels of GSH in erythrocytes. The only patient who has been studied had normal — or near normal — levels of GS and GSH in fibroblasts and leukocytes.[113] All patients had normal urinary levels of 5-oxoproline.

Decreased activity of erythrocyte GSHS-transferase has been found in two patients with erythrocyte GS deficiency.[109] This suggests that under normal conditions the transferase is protected by GSH. This finding has recently been confirmed in patients with GS and GCS deficiency.[106]

γ-Glutamyl Transpeptidase Deficiency

Five patients with GT deficiency have been reported.[134–137] These patients have increased GSH concentrations in plasma and urine but the cellular levels are normal. In addition to glutathionuria, the patients have increased urinary levels of γ-glutamylcysteine and cysteine, which emphasizes the role of GT in the degradation of GSH under normal conditions.

Three of the five patients with GT deficiency were described as having central nervous system involvement, but two sibs apparently had no signs of brain damage. Whether these symptoms are part of the clinical picture remains to be established. The presence of cerebral damage may simply reflect that the first three patients were identified by urinary screening for amino acid defects in populations of mentally retarded individuals, which revealed glutathionuria (up to 1 g per day; controls < 10 mg).[135,138]

Decreased activity of GT can be demonstrated in leukocytes or cultured skin fibroblasts, but not in erythrocytes which lack this enzyme also under normal conditions. No specific treatment has been proposed or tried.

The prognosis should be considered serious if the patient presents with psychiatric or neurologic symptoms. On the other hand, two sibs, aged 20 and 21 years, have so far shown no signs of central nervous system involvement.[137] γ-Glutamyl deficiency is transmitted as an autosomal recessive trait. The human GT gene family is composed of at least seven different loci[42] and five of them are located on chromosome 22.[43]

Recently, Harding *et al.*[73] described a mouse mutant with renal GT deficiency and glutathionuria. These mice exhibited lethargy, severe growth failure, shortened life span, and infertility. This mutant strain offers a useful model for further studies of human GT deficiency. It is interesting that the GT-deficient mice exhibited neurologic abnormalities, agitation, and tremor when stimulated. Furthermore, the mutant mice had impaired renal reabsorption of amino acids, which is in agreement with the γ-glutamyl cycle hypothesis for active transport of amino acids proposed by Orlowski and Meister.[6]

5-Oxoprolinase Deficiency

Eight patients with OP deficiency have been described.[139–144] They were identified because of 5-oxoprolinuria; they excreted 4 to 10 g of L-5-oxoproline per day. All have normal cellular levels of GSH and normal acid-base balance. The clinical symptoms that led to the discovery of these patients are not necessarily related to their metabolic defect. They usually do not have signs of hemolytic anemia.

Two brothers were investigated because of renal stone formation and enterocolitis.[138] The third patient was a woman with mild mental retardation who had given birth to a child with congenital malformations and hyperprolinemia.[140] Additional cases of OP deficiency have been reported. Two brothers — a younger brother who presented neonatally with self-limiting hypoglycemia and his healthy brother[141] — had normal psychomotor development at 4 and 8 years of age, respectively. The sixth patient reported was a 3-year-old child with severe developmental delay, failure to thrive, microcytic anemia, and microcephaly.[142] An 8-year old girl with developmental delay in language skills and gross motor function was found to have OP deficiency.[144] Another patient was recently investigated, a 5.5-year-old girl with markedly delayed psychomotor development.[143]

Thus, two of eight reported patients with OP deficiency have shown some degree of mental retardation. Whether this is coincidental remains to be established. One additional patient with possible OP deficiency has been described[145] — a 36-year-old man who participated as a volunteer in a study of urinary metabolite excretion profiles. His urine was found to contain 6 g of 5-oxoproline per day. He had no clinical signs and symptoms. The enzyme defect in this patient has not yet been established.

5-Oxoprolinase is not present in erythrocytes and therefore leukocytes or other tissues must be used for diagnosis. No specific treatment of patients with OP deficiency has been proposed, and the prognosis remains to be established. The mode of inheritance is autosomal recessive.

5-Oxoprolinuria Without Enzyme Defect in the γ-Glutamyl Cycle

Increased urinary 5-oxoproline has been observed in patients with severe burns and in patients who have Stevens-Johnson syndrome.[146] Possibly in these conditions there is increased metabolism of collagen, fibrinogen, or other proteins that contain substantial amounts of N-terminal 5-oxoproline. 5-Oxoproline can also have a dietary origin. Certain infant formulas and tomato juice may contain proteins modified by preparation that have increased 5-oxoproline content.[147] Patients with homocystinuria have been reported to have increased urinary excretion of 5-oxoproline.[148] The mechanism underlying increased excretion of 5-oxoproline is thought to be related to the ability of GCS to use homocysteine as a substrate. The γ-glutamyl homocysteine formed is a substrate for GCT, thus leading to 5-oxoproline formation. 5-Oxoproline excretion appears to occur when plasma level of homocystine is above 0.2 mM. Normal human urine contains variable amounts of 5-oxo-D-proline formed by enzymatic cyclization of D-glutamate, which probably arises from dietary or bacterial sources,[149] which may complicate the interpretation of analyses of urine for 5-oxoproline. Normal human skin contains large amounts of 5-oxoproline.[1] Somewhat elevated levels of 5-oxo-L-proline and 5-oxo-D-proline have been found in plasma of patients with renal insufficiency.[150] 5-Oxoprolinuria has been described after administration of vigabatrin (DL-γ-vinyl-γ-aminobutyric acid) and antibiotics, indicating that these drugs interfere with the γ-glutamyl cycle.[151] However, conversion of the D-isomer of vigabatrin to D-glutamate, followed by cyclization of the latter to 5-oxo-D-proline might also account for the findings.[1] Transient 5-oxoprolinuria has been described in a preterm infant;[152] the cause of this abnormality is not known.

Mutations in Organisms Other than Humans

Several mutant microorganisms with blocks in the biosynthesis of GSH have been reported and GSH-related mutants of sheep are also known;[102] one mutation involves decreased erythrocyte GCS and another involves decreased transport of cysteine to the erythrocyte.[1]

An interesting mouse mutant with genetic GT deficiency was recently identified.[73] This mutant suffers from glutathionuria, postnatal growth failure, lethargy, and reduced life span.

REFERENCES

1. Meister A, Anderson ME: Glutathione. *Ann Rev Biochem* **52**:711, 1983.
2. Meister A: Glutathione deficiency produced by inhibition of its synthesis and its reversal; Applications in research and therapy. *Pharmacol Ther* **51**:155, 1991.
3. Meister A: A brief history of glutathione and a survey of its metabolism and functions, in Dolphin D, Poulson R, Avramovic O (eds): *Glutathione: Chemical, Biochemical and Medical Aspects*. New York, John Wiley, 1989, p 1.
4. Anderson ME: Glutathione and glutathione delivery compounds. *Adv Pharmacol* **38**:65, 1997.
5. Anderson ME: Modulation of glutathione, in Packer L, Cadenas E (eds): *Handbook of Synthetic Antioixdants*. New York, Marcel Dekker, 1997, p 321.
6. Orlowski M, Meister A: The γ-glutamyl cycle: A possible transport system for amino acids. *Proc Natl Acad Sci U S A* **67**:1248, 1970.
7. Meister A: A trail of research: From glutamine synthetase to selective inhibition of glutathione synthesis. *Chem Tracts-Biochem Mol Biol* **3**:75, 1992.
8. Sherrill C, Fahey RC: Import and metabolism of glutathione by *Streptococcus* mutants. *J Bacteriol* **180**:1454, 1998.
9. Huang CS, Chang LS, Anderson ME, Meister A: Amino acid sequence and function of the light subunit of rat kidney γ-glutamylcysteine synthetase. *J Biol Chem* **268**:20578, 1993.
10. Huang CS, Chang LS, Anderson ME, Meister A: Catalytic and regulatory properties of the heavy subunit of rat kidney gamma-glutamylcysteine synthetase. *J Biol Chem* **268**:19675, 1993.
11. Gipp JJ, Chang C, Mulcahy RT: Cloning and nucleotide sequence of a full-length cDNA for human liver gamma-glutamylcysteine synthetase. *Biochem Biophys Res Commun* **185**:29, 1992.
12. Richman P, Meister A: Regulation of γ-glutamyl cysteine synthetase by nonallosteric feedback inhibition by glutathione. *J Biol Chem* **250**:1422, 1975.
13. Cai J, Sun WM, Lu SC: Hormonal and cell density regulation of hepatic γ-glutamylcysteine synthetase gene expression. *Mol Pharmacol* **48**:212, 1995.
14. Huang CS, Moore W, Meister A: On the active site thiol of γ-glutamylcysteine synthetase: Relationships to catalysis, inhibition and regulation. *Proc Natl Acad Sci U S A* **85**:2464, 1988.
15. Meister A: Glutathione deficiency produced by inhibition of its synthesis and its reversal; Applications in research and therapy. *Pharmacol Ther* **51**(2):155, 1991.

16. Meister A: A trail of research from glutamine synthetase to selective inhibition of glutathione synthesis. *Chem Tracts-Biochem Mol Biol* **3**:75, 1992.
17. Purich DL: Advances in the enzymology of glutamine synthesis. *Adv Enzymol Relat Areas Mol Biol* **72**:9, 1998.
18. Godwin AK, Meister A, O'Dwyer PJ, Hamilton TC, Huang DS, Anderson ME: High resistance to cisplatin in human ovarian cancer cell lines is associated with marked increase of glutathione synthesis. *Proc Natl Acad Sci U S A* **89**:3070, 1992.
19. Wild AC, Gipp JJ, Mulcahy T: Overlapping antioxidant response element and PMA response element sequences mediate basal and β-naphthoflavone-induced expression of the human γ-glutamylcysteine synthetase catalytic subunit gene. *Biochem J* **332**:373, 1998.
20. Arsalane K, Dubois CM, Muanza T, Begin R, Boudreau F, Asselin C, Cantin AM: Transforming growth factor βl is a potent inhibitor of glutathione synthesis in the lung epithelial cell line A549: Transcriptional effect on the GSH rate-limiting enzyme γ-glutamylcysteine synthetase. *Am J Respir Cell Mol Biol* **17**:599, 1997.
21. Cai J, Huang ZZ, Lu SC: Differential regulation of γ-glutamylcysteine synthetase heavy and light subunit gene expression. *Biochem J* **326**:167, 1997.
22. Morales A, Garcia-Ruiz C, Miranda M, Mari M, Cotell A, Ardite E, Fernandez Checa JC: Tumor necrosis factor increases hepatocellular glutathione by transcriptional regulation of the heavy subunit chain of γ-glutamylcysteine synthetase. *J Biol Chem* **272**:30371, 1997.
23. Mulcahy RT, Gipp JJ: Identification of a putative antioxidant response element in the 5′-flanking region of the human γ-glutamylcysteine synthetase heave subunit gene. *Biochem Biophys Res Commun* **209**:227, 1995.
24. Moinova HR, Mulcahyl RT: An electrophile responsive element (EpRE) regulates β-naphthoflavone induction of the human γ-glutamylcysteine synthetase regulatory subunit gene. Constitutive expression is mediated by an adjacent ap-1-site. *J Biol Chem* **273**:14683, 1998.
25. Yao KS, Godwin AK, Johnson SW, Ozols RF, O'Dwyer PJ, Hamilton TC: Evidence for altered regulation of gamma-glutamylcysteine gene expression among cisplatin-sensitive and cisplatin-resistant human ovarian cancer cell lines. *Cancer Res* **55**:4367, 1995.
26. Tian L, Shi MM, Forman H: Increased transcription of the regulatory subunit of γ-glutamylcysteine synthetase in rat lung epithelial L2 cells exposed to oxidative stress or glutathione depletion. *Arch Biochem Biophys* **342**:126, 1997.
27. Oguri T, Fujiwara Y, Isobe T, Katoh O, Watanabe H, Yamakido M: Expression of γ-glutamylcysteine synthetase (γGCS) and multidrug-resistance associated protein/MRP) but not human canicular multi-specific organic anion transporter (cMOAT) genes correlate with exposure of human lung cancer to platinum drugs. *Br J Cancer* **77**:1089, 1998.
28. Kuo MT, Bao J, Furuichi M, Yamane Y, Gomi A, Savaraj N, Masuzawa T, Ishikawa T: Frequent coexpression of MRP/GS-X pump and γ-glutamylcysteine synthetase mRNA in drug resistant cells, untreated tumor cells and normal mouse tissues. *Biochem Pharmacol* **55**:605, 1998.
29. Ogretmen B, Bahadori HR, McCanley MD, Boylan A, Green MR, Safa AR: Co-ordinate over-expression of the MRP and γ-glutamylcysteine synthetase genes, but not MDRI, correlates with doxorubicin resistance in human malignant mesothelioma cell lines. *Int J Cancer* **75**:757, 1998.
30. Meister A: Glutathione synthesis. *Enzymes* **10**:671, 1974.
31. Huang CS, He W, Meister A, Anderson ME: Amino acid sequence of rat kidney glutathione synthetase. *Proc Natl Acad Sci U S A* **92**:1232, 1995.
32. Oppenheimer L, Wellner VP, Griffith OW, Meister A: Glutathione synthetase; Purification from rat kidney and mapping of the substrate binding sites. *J Biol Chem* **254**:5184, 1979.
33. Gali RR, Board PG: Identification of an essential cysteine residue in human glutathione synthetase. *Biochem J* **321**:207, 1997.
34. Gali RR, Board PG: Identification of an essential cysteine residue in human glutathione synthetase. *Biochem J* **321**: 207, 1997.
35. Huang CS, He W, Meister A, Anderson ME: Amino acid sequence of rat kidney glutathione synthetase. *Proc Natl Acad Sci U S A* **92**: 1232, 1995.
36. Webb GC, Vaska VL, Gali RR, Ford JH, Board PG: The gene encoding human glutathione synthetase (GSS) maps to the long arm of chromosome 20 at band 11.2. *Genomics* **30**:617, 1995.
37. Shi ZZ, Carter BZ, Habib GM, He X, Sazer S, Lebovitz RM, Lieberman MW: A single mouse glutathione synthetase gene encodes six mRNAs with different 5′ ends. *Arch Biochem Biophys* **331**:215, 1996.
38. Sun WM, Huang ZZ, LU SC: Regulation of gamma-glutamyl cysteine synthetase by protein phosphorylation. *Biochem J* **320**:321, 1996.
39. Tate SS, Meister A: γ-Glutamyl transpeptidase from kidney. *Method Enzymol* **113**:400, 1985.
40. Abbott WA, Griffith OW, Meister A: γ-Glutamyl-glutathione; Natural occurrence and enzymology. *J Biol Chem* **261**:657, 661, 1986.
41. Nash B, Tate SS: In vitro translation and processing of rat kidney γ-glutamyl transpeptidase. *J Biol Chem* **239**:2553, 1984.
42. Courtay C, Heisterkamp N, Siest G, Groffen J: Expression of multiple γ-glutamyltransferase genes in man. *Biochem J* **297**:503, 1994.
43. Bulle F, Mattei MG, Siegrist S, Pawlak A, Passage E, Chobert MN, Laperche Y, Guellaen G: Assignment of the human γ-glutamyl transferase gene to the long arm of chromosome 22. *Hum Genet* **76**:283, 1987.
44. Figlewicz DA, Delattre O, Guellaen G, Krizus A, Thomas G, Zucman J, Rouleau GA: Mapping of human gamma-glutamyl transpeptidase genes on chromosome 22 and other human autosomes. *Genomics* **17**:299, 1993.
45. Taniguchi N, Ikeda Y: Gamma-glutamyl transpeptidase: Catalytic mechanism and gene expression. *Adv Enzymol Relat Areas Mol Biol* **72**:239, 1998.
46. Markey CM, Rudolph DB, Labus JC, Hinton BT: Oxidative stress differentially regulates the expression of γ-glutamyl transpeptidase mRNAs in the initial segment of the rat epididymis. *J Androl* **19**:92, 1998.
47. Brouillet A, Holic N, Chobert MN, Laperche Y: The γ-glutamyl transpeptidase gene is transcribed from a different promoter in rat hepatocytes and biliary cells. *Am J Pathol* **152**:1039, 1998.
48. Sepulveda AR, Huang SL, Lebovitz RM, Lieberman MW: A 346-base pair region of the mouse γ-glutamyl transpeptidase type II promoter contains sufficient *cis*-acting elements for kidney-restricted expression in transgenic mice. *J Biol Chem* **272**:11959, 1997.
49. Griffiths SA, Manson MM: Rat liver γ-glutamyl transpeptidase mRNA differs from the 5′ untranslated sequence from the corresponding kidney mRNA. *Cancer Lett* **46**:69, 1989.
50. Chobert MN, Lahuna O, Lebargy F, Kurauchi O, Darbony M, Bernaudin JF, Guellaen G, Barouki R, Laperache Y: Tissue-specific expression of two γ-glutamyl transpeptidase mRNAs with alternative 5′ ends encoded by a single copy gene in the rat. *J Biol Chem* **265**:2352, 1990.
51. Coloma J, Garcia-Jimeno A: Tissue-specific methylation in the 5′ flanking region of the γ-glutamyl transpeptidase gene. *Biochem Biophys Res Commun* **177**:229, 1991.
52. Baik JH, Siegrist S, Giuili G, Lahuna O, Bulle F, Guellaen G: Tissue- and developmental stage-specific methylation in the two kidney promoters of the rat γ-glutamyl transpeptidase gene. *Biochem J* **287**:691, 1992.
53. Lahuna O, Brouillet A, Chobert MN, Darbony M, Okamoto T, Laperche Y: Identification of γ-glutamyl transpeptidase in rat kidney and epididymis. *Biochemistry* **31**:9190, 1992.
54. Pawlak A, Cohen EH, Octave JN, Schweickhardt R, Wu SJ, Bulle F, Chikhi N, Baik JH, Siegrist S, Guellaen G: An alternatively processed mRNA specific for γ-glutamyl transpeptidase in human tissue. *J Biol Chem* **265**:3256, 1990.
55. Hudson EA, Munks RJ, Manson MM: Characterization of transcriptional regulation of γ-glutamyl transpeptidase in rat liver involving both positive and negative regulatory elements. *Mol Carcinog* **20**:376, 1997.
56. Tate SS, Meister A: Serine-borate complex as a transition-state inhibitor of γ-glutamyl transpeptidase. *Proc Natl Acad Sci U S A* **75**:4806, 1978.
57. Smith TK, Meister A: Chemical modification of active site residues in γ-glutamyl transpeptidase, aspartate-422 and cysteine-453. *J Biol Chem* **270**:12476, 1995.
58. Ikeda Y, Fujii J, Taniguchi N, Meister A: Human γ-glutamyl transpeptidase mutants involving conserved aspartate residues and the unique cysteine residue of the light subunit. *J Biol Chem* **270**:12471, 1995.
59. Ikeda Y, Fujii J, Anderson EM, Taniguchi N, Meister A: Involvement of Ser-451 and Ser-452 in the catalysis of human γ-glutamyl transpeptidase. *J Biol Chem* **270**:22223, 1995.
60. Habib GM, Barrios RZZS, Lieberman MW: Four distinct membrane-bound dipeptidase RNAs are differentially expressed and show discordant regulation with γ-glutamyl transpeptidase. *J Biol Chem* **271**:16273, 1996.

61. Van Der Werf P, Meister A: The metabolic formation and utilization of 5-oxo-l-proline (L-pyroglutamate, L-pyrrolidone carboxylate). *Adv Enzymol* **43**:519, 1975.
62. Ye GJ, Breslow EB, Meister A: The amino acid sequence of rat kidney 5-oxo-l-prolinase determined by cDNA cloning. *J Biol Chem* **271**:32293, 1996.
63. Li LY, Seddon AP, Meister A: Interaction of the protein components of 5-oxoprolinase: Substrate-dependent enzyme complex formation. *J Biol Chem* **263**:6495, 1988.
64. Griffith OW, Meister A: Origin and turnover of mitochondrial glutathione. *Proc Natl Acad Sci U S A* **82**:4668, 1985.
65. Måartensson J, Jain A, Stole E, Frayer W, Auld PAM, Meister A: Inhibition of glutathione synthesis in the newborn rat: A model for endogenously produced oxidative stress. *Proc Natl Acad Sci U S A* **88**:9360, 1991.
66. Måartensson J, Meister A: Glutathione deficiency decreases tissue ascorbate levels in newborn rats: Ascorbate spares glutathione and protects. *Proc Natl Acad Sci U S A* **88**:4656, 1991.
67. Meister A: On the antioxidant effects of ascorbic acid and glutathione. *Biochem Pharmacol* **44**:1905, 1992.
68. Meister A: Glutathione ascorbic acid antioxidant system in animals. *J Biol Chem* **269**:9397, 1994.
69. Meister A: Mitochondrial changes associated with glutathione deficiency. *Biochim Biophys Acta* **1271**:35, 1995.
70. Meister A: Depletion of glutathione in normal and malignant human cells in vivo by l-buthionine sulfoximine: Possible interaction with ascorbate. *J Natl Cancer Inst* **84**:1601, 1992.
71. Griffith OW, Meister A: Excretion of cysteine and gamma-glutamyl transpeptidase deficiency. *Proc Natl Acad Sci U S A* **77**:3384, 1980.
72. Lieberman MW, Wiseman AL, Shi ZZ, Carter BZ, Barrios R, Ou CN, Chevez-Barrios P, Wang Y, Habib GM, Goodman JC, Huang SL, Lebowitz RM, Matzuk MM: Growth retardation and cysteine deficiency in γ-glutamyl transpepti dase deficient mice. *Proc Natl Acad Sci U S A* **93**:7923, 1996.
73. Harding CO, Williams P, Wagner E, Chang DS, Wild K, Colwell RE, Wolff JA: Mice with genetic γ-glutamyl transpeptidase deficiency exhibit glutathionuria, severe growth failure, reduced life span and infertility. *J Biol Chem* **272**:12560, 1997.
74. Bridges RJ, Griffith OW, Meister A: L-γ-(Threo-β-methyl) glutamyl-L-α-aminobutyrate, a selective substrate of γ-glutamyl cyclotransferase; Inhibition of enzymic activity by β-aminoglutaryl-L-α-aminobutyrate. *J Biol Chem* **255**:10787, 1980.
75. Eck H-P, Gmuender H, Hartmann M, Petzoldt D, Daniel V, Droege W: Low concentrations of acid soluble thios (cysteine) in the blood plasma of HIV-1 infected patients. *Biol Chem Hoppe Seyler* **370**:101, 1989.
76. Buhl R, Holroyd, KJ, Mastrangeli A, Cantin AM, Jaffe HA, Wells FBCS, Crystal RG: Systemic glutathione deficiency in symptom-free HIV-seropositive individuals. *Lancet* **2**:1294, 1989.
77. Pace GW, Leaf CD: The role of oxidative stress in HIV disease. *Free Rad Biol Med* **19**:523, 1995.
78. Suarez M, Beloqui O, Ferrer JV, Fil B, Qian C, Garcia N, Civeira P, Prieto J: Glutathione depletion in chronic hepatitis C. *Int Hepatol Commun* **1**:215, 1993.
79. Forrester TE, Badaloo V, Bennett FI, Jackson AA: Excessive excretion of 5-oxoproline and decreased levels of blood glutathione in type II diabetes mellitus. *Eur J Clin Nutr* **44**:847, 1990.
80. Fields JA, Keshavarzian A, Eiznhamer D, Frommel T, Winship D, Holmes EW: Low levels of blood and colonic glutathione in ulcerative colitis. *Gastroenterology* **106**:A680, 1994.
81. Cantin AM, Hubbard RC, Crystal RG: Glutathione deficiency in the epithelial lining fluid of the lower respiratory tract in idiopathic pulmonary fibrosis. *Am Rev Respir Dis* **139**:370, 1989.
82. Pacht ER, Timmerman AP, Lykens MG, Merola AJ: Deficiency of alveolar fluid glutathione in patients with sepsis and the adult respiratory distress syndrome. *Chest* **100**:1397, 1991.
83. Martinez-Cayuela M: Oxygen free radicals and human disease. *Biochimie* **77**:147, 1998.
84. Meister A: Strategies for increasing cellular glutathione, in Packer L, Cadenas E (eds): *Biothiols*. New York, Marcel Dekker, 1994, pp 165–188.
85. Anderson ME, Meister A: Intracellular delivery of cysteine. *Method Enzymol* **143**:313, 1987.
86. Jain A, Buist NR, Kennaway NG, Powell BR, Auld PAM, Måartensson J: Effect of ascorbate or *N*-acetylcysteine treatment in a patient with hereditary glutathione synthetase deficiency. *J Pediatr* **124**:229, 1994.
87. Williamson JM, Meister A: Stimulation of hepatic glutathione formation by administration of L-2-oxothiazolidine-4-carboxylate, a 5-oxo-L-prolinase substrate. *Proc Natl Acad Sci U S A* **78**:936, 1981.
88. Kalayjian RC, Skowron G, Emgushov R-T, Chance M, Spell SA, Borum PR, Webb LS, Mayer KH, Jackson JB, Yen-Liberman B, Sory KO, Rowe WB, Thompson K, Godlberg D, Trimbo S, Lederman MM: A phase I/II trial of intravenous L-2-oxothiazolidine-4 carboxylic acid (procysteine) in asymptomatic HIV-infected subjects. *J Acq Immune Def Syndr* **7**:369, 1994.
89. Lederman MM, Georger D, Dando S, Schmelzer R, Averill L, Goldberg D: L-2-Oxothiazolidine-4-carboxylic acid (procystein) inhibits expression of the human immunodeficiency virus and expression of the interleukin-2 receptor alpha chain. *J Acq Immune Def Syndr* **8**:107, 1995.
90. Porta P, Aebi S, Summer K, Lauterburg BH: L-2-Oxothiazolidine-4-carboxylic acid, a cysteine prodrug: Pharmacokinetics and effects on thiols in plasma and lymphocytes in human. *J Pharmacol Exp Ther* **257**:331, 1991.
91. Jain A, Madsen DC, Auld PAM, Frayer WW, Schwantz MK, Meister A, Måartensson J: L-2-Oxothiazolidine-4-carboxylate, a cysteine precursor, stimulates growth and normalizes tissue glutathione concentration in rats fed a sulfur amino acid-deficient diet. *J Nutr* **125**:851, 1995.
92. Shug AL, Madsen DC: Protection of the ischemic rat heart by procysteine and amino acids. *J Nutr Biochem* **5**:356, 1994.
93. Anderson ME, Meister A: Transport and direct utilization of γ-glutamylcysteine for glutathione synthesis. *Proc Natl Acad Sci U S A* **80**:707, 1983.
94. Pileblad E, Magnusson T: Increase in rat brain glutathione following intracerebroventricular administration of γ-glutamylcysteine. *Biochem Pharmacol* **44**:895, 1992.
95. Nishida K, Ohta Y, Ishiguro I: Glycine facilates γ-glutamylcysteine ethyl ester-mediated increase in liver glutathione level. *Eur J Pharmacol* **333**:289, 1997.
96. Nishida K, Ohta Y, Ishiguro I: γ-Glutamylcysteine ethyl ester attenuates progression of carbon tetrachloride induced acute liver injury in mice. *Toxicology* **126**:55, 1998.
97. Puri RN, Meister A: Transport of glutathione, as gammα-glutamylcysteinylglycyl ester, into liver and kidney. *Proc Natl Acad Sci U S A* **80**:5258, 1983.
98. Levy EJ, Anderson ME, Meister A: Preparation and use of glutathione diethyl ester. *Method Enzymol* **234**:499, 1994.
99. Minhas H, Thornalley PJ: Comparison of the delivery of reduced glutathione into P388D cells by reduced glutathione and its mono- and diethyl ester derivatives. *Biochem Pharmacol* **49**:1475, 1995.
100. Anderson ME, Powrie F, Puri RN, Meister A: Glutathione monoethyl ester: Preparation, uptake by tissues and conversion to glutathione. *Arch Biochem Biophys* **239**:538, 1985.
101. Anderson ME, Levy EJ, Meister A: Preparation and use of glutathione monoesters. *Method Enzymol* **234**:492, 1994.
102. Larsson A: Hereditary disorders relating to glutathione deficiency, in Dolphin D, Poulson R, Avramovic O (eds): *Coenzymes and Cofactors, part B*. New York, John Wiley, 1989, p 198.
103. Meister A, Larsson A: Glutathione synthetase deficiency and other disorders of the γ-glutamyl cycle, in Scriver CF, Beaudet AL, Sly WS, Valle D, (eds): *The Metabolic and Molecular Bases of Inherited Disease 7th ed*. New York, McGraw Hill, 1995, p 1461.
104. Konrad PN, Richards II F, Valentine WN, Paglia DE: γ-Glutamylcysteine synthetase deficiency. A cause of hereditary hemolytic anemia. *N Engl J Med* **286**:557, 1972.
105. Beutler E, Moroose R, Kramer L, Gelbart T, Forman L: Gamma-glutamylcysteine synthetase deficiency and hemolytic anemia. *Blood* **75**:271, 1990.
106. Hirono A, Lyori H, Sekine I, Ueyama J, Chiba H, Kanno H, Fujii H, Miwa S: Three cases of hereditary nonspherocytic hemolytic anemia associated with red blood cell glutathione deficiency. *Blood* **87**:2071, 1996.
107. Richards II F, Cooper MR, Pearce LA, Cowan RJ, Spurr CL: Familial spinocerebellar degeneration, hemolytic anemia, and glutathione deficiency. *Arch Intern Med* **134**:534, 1974.
108. Prins HK, Oort M, Loos JA, Zürcher C, Beckers T: Congenital nonspherocytic hemolytic anemia, associated with glutathione deficiency of the erythrocytes. *Blood* **27**:145, 1966.
109. Beutler E, Gelbart T, Pegelow C: Erythrocyte glutathione synthetase deficiency leads not only to glutathione but also to glutathione-S-transferase deficiency. *J Clin Invest* **77**:38, 1986.

110. Lloyd AJ, Gray RGF, Green A: Tyrosinemia type I and glutathione synthetase deficiency: Two disorders with reduced hepatic thiol group concentration and a liver 4-fumarylacetoacetate hydrolase deficiency. *J Inherit Metab Dis* **18**(1):48, 1995.
111. Sierra-Rivera E, Summar ML, Dasouki M, Krishnamani MRS, Phillips JA, Freeman ML: Assignment of the human gene (GLCLC) that encodes the heavy subunit of γ-glutamylcysteine synthetase to human chromosome 6. *Cytogenet Cell Genet* **70**:278, 1995.
112. Sierra-Rivera E, Dasouki M, Summar ML, Krishnamani MRS, Meredith M, Rao PN, Phillips III JA, Freeman ML: Assignment of the human gene (GLCLR) that encodes the regulatory subunit of γ-glutamyl-cysteine synthetase to chromosome 1p21. *Cytogenet Cell Genet* **72**:252, 1996.
113. Spielberg SP, Garrick MD, Corash LM, Butler JD, Tietze F, Gorgers LV, Schulman JD: Biochemical heterogeneity in glutathione synthetase deficiency. *J Clin Invest* **61**:1417, 1978.
114. Jellum E, Kluge T, Börresen HC, Stokke O, Eldjarn L: Pyroglutamic aciduria — A new inborn error of metabolism. *Scand J Clin Lab Invest* **26**:327, 1970.
115. Skullerud K, Marstein S, Schrader H, Brundelet PJ, Jellum E: The cerebral lesions in a patient with generalized glutathione synthetase deficiency and pyroglutamic aciduria (5-oxoprolinuria). *Acta Neuropathol* **52**:235, 1980.
116. Mayatepek E, Hoffman GF, Carlsson B, Larsson A, Becker K: Impaired synthesis of lipoxygenase products in glutathione synthetase deficiency. *Pediatr Res* **35**:307, 1994.
117. Mayatepek E, Becker K, Carlsson B, Larsson A, Hoffman GF: Deficient synthesis of cysteinyl leukotrienes in glutathione synthetase deficiency. *Int J Tiss Reac* **15**(6):245, 1993.
118. Mayatepek E, Hoffman GF: Impaired Metabolism of leukotrienes in inherited metabolic disorder. *J Inherit Metab Dis* **17**:263, 1994.
119. Mayatepek E, Hoffman GF: Leukotrienes: Biosynthesis, metabolism, and pathophysiologic significance. *Pediatr Res* **37**:1, 1995.
120. Shi ZZ, Habib GM, Rhead WJ, Gahl WA, He X, Sazer S, Lieberman MW: Mutations in the glutathione synthetase gene cause 5-oxoprolinuria. *Nat Genet* **14**:361, 1996.
121. Dahl N, Pigg M, Ristoff E, Gali RR, Carlsson B, Mannervik B, Larsson A, Board PG: Missense mutations in human glutathione synthetase gene result in severe metabolic acidosis, 5-oxoprolinuria, hemolytic anemia and neurological dysfunction. *Hum Mol Genet* **6**:1147, 1997.
122. Stoner E, Starkman H, Wellner D, Wellner VP, Sassa S, Rifkind AB, Grenier A, Steinhertz PG, Meister A, New MI, Levine LS: Biochemical studies of a patient with hereditary hepatorenal tyrosinemia: Evidence of glutathione deficiency. *Pediatr Res* **18**:1332, 1984.
123. Eldjarn L, Jellum E, Stokke O: Pyroglutamic aciduria: Studies on the enzymic block and on the metabolic origin of pyroglutamic acid. *Clin Chim Acta* **40**:461, 1972.
124. Eldjarn L, Jellum E, Stokke O: Pyroglutamic aciduria, in Hommes FA, Van Den Bern CJ (eds): *Inborn Errors of Metabolism*. New York, Academic, 1973, p 255.
125. Hagenfeldt L, Larsson A, Zetterström R: Pyroglutamic aciduria. Studies of an infant with chronic metabolic acidosis. *Acta Pediatr Scand* **63**:1, 1974.
126. Boxer LA, Oliver JM, Spielberg SP, Allen JM, Schulman JD: Protection of granulocytes by vitamin E in glutathione synthetase deficiency. *N Engl J Med* **301**:901, 1979.
127. Pejaver RK, Watson AH: High-dose vitamin E therapy in glutathione synthetase deficiency. *J Inherit Metab Dis* **17**:749, 1994.
128. Måartensson J, Gustafsson J, Larsson A: A therapeutic trial with *N*-acetylcysteine in subjects with hereditary glutathione synthetase deficiency (5-oxoprolinuria). *J Inherit Metab Dis* **12**:120, 1989.
129. Rhead W: Personal communication, 1998.
130. Manning NJ, Davies NP, Olpin SE, Carpenter KH, Smith MF, Pollitt RJ, Duncan SL, Larsson A, Carlsson B: Prenatal diagnosis of glutathione synthetase deficiency. *Prenat Diagn* **14**(6):475, 1994.
131. Erasmus E, Mienie LJ, de Vries WN, de Wet WJ, Carlsson B, Larsson A: Prenatal analysis in two suspected cases of glutathione synthetase deficiency. *J Inherit Metab Dis* **16**(5):837, 1993.
132. Oort M, Loos JA, Prins HR: Hereditary absence of reduced glutathione in erythrocytes — A new clinical and biochemical entity? *Vox Sang* **6**:370, 1961.
133. Mohler DN, Majerus PW, Minnich V, Hess CE, Garrick MD: Glutathione synthetase deficiency as a cause of hereditary hemolytic disease. *N Engl J Med* **283**:1253, 1970.
134. O'Daly S: An abnormal sulphydryl compound in urine. *Ir J Med Sci* 578, 1968.
135. Goodman SI, Mace JW, and Pollack S: Serum γ-glutamyl transpeptidase deficiency. *Lancet* **1**(692):234, 1971.
136. Wright EC, Stern J, Ersser R and Patrick AD: Glutathionuria: γ-Glutamyl transpeptidase deficiency. *J Inherit Metab Dis* **2**:3, 1980.
137. Hammond J, Potter M, Wilcken B, Truscott R: Siblings with γ-glutamyl transferase deficiency. *J Inherit Metab Dis* **18**:83, 1995.
138. Schulman JD, Goodman SI, Mace JW, Patrick AD, Tietze F, Butler EJ: Glutathionuria: Inborn error of metabolism due to tissue deficiency of γ-glutamyl transpeptidase. *Biochem Biophys Res Commun* **65**:68, 1975.
139. Larsson A, Mattsson B, Wauters EAK, Van Gool JD, Duran M, Wadman SK: 5-Oxoprolinuria due to hereditary 5-oxoprolinase deficiency in two brothers — A new inborn error of the γ-glutamyl cycle. *Acta Paediatr Scand* **70**:301, 1981.
140. Roesel RA, Hommes FA, Samper L: Pyroglutamic acid uria (5-oxoprolinuria) without glutathione synthetase deficiency and with decreased pyroglutamate hydrolase activity. *J Inherit Metab Dis* **4**:89, 1981.
141. Henderson MJ, Larsson A, Carlsson B, Dear PRF: 5-Oxoprolinuria associated with 5-oxoprolinase deficiency; A benign disorder? *J Inherit Metab Dis* **16**:1051, 1993.
142. Mayatepek E, Hoffmann GF, Larsson A, Becker K, Bremer HJ: 5-Oxoprolinase deficiency associated with severe psychomotor developmental delay, failure to thrive, microcephaly and microcytic anemia. *J Inherit Metab Dis* **18**:83, 1995.
143. Cohen LHF, Vamos E, Heinrichs C, Toppet M, Courtens W, Kumps A, Mardens Y, Carlsson B, Grillner L, Larsson A: Growth failure, encephalopathy, and endocrine dysfunction in two siblings, one with 5-oxoprolinase deficiency. *Eur J Pediatr* **156**:935, 1997.
144. Bernier FP, Snyder FF, McLeod DR: Deficiency of 5-oxoprolinase in an 8-year-old with developmental delay. *J Inherit Metab Dis* **19**:367, 1996.
145. Ghauri FYK, Parkes HG, Nicholson JK: Asymptomatic 5-oxoprolinuria detected by proton magnetic resonance spectroscopy. *Clin Chem* **39**:1341, 1993.
146. Tham R, Nyström I, Holmstedt B: Identification by mass spectrometry of pyroglutamide acid as a peak in the gas chromatography of human urine. *Biochem Pharmacol* **17**:1735, 1968.
147. Oberholtzer VG, Wood CBS, Palmer T, Harrison BM: Increased pyroglutamic acid levels in patients on artificial ducts. *Clin Chim Acta* **62**:299, 1975.
148. Jellum E, Marstein S, Skullerud K, Munthe E: Glutathione in pyroglutamic aciduria (5-oxoprolinuria) and rheumatoid arthritis, in Larsson A, Orrenius S, Holmgren A, Mannervik B (eds): *Functions of Glutathione — Biochemical, Physiological Toxicological and Clinical Aspects*. New York, Academic, 1983, p 347.
149. Meister A, Bukenberger MW, Strassburer M: The optically specific enzymatic cyclization of d-glutamate. *Biochem Z* **338**:217, 1963.
150. Palekar AG, Tate SS, Sullivan J, Meister A: Accumulation of 5-oxo-L-proline and 5-oxo-D proline in the blood plasma in end stage renal disease. *Biochem Med* **14**:339, 1975.
151. Bonham JR, Rattenbury JM, Meeks A, Pollitt RJ: Pyroglutamicaciduria from vigabatrin. *Lancet* **1**:1452, 1989.
152. Goto A, Ishida A, Goto R, Hayaaka K, Nanso K, Yamashita A, Yamaguchi S, Takada G: Transient 5-oxoprolinuria in a very low-birthweight infant. *J Inherit Metab Dis* **15**:284, 1992.

CHAPTER 97

Disorders of Glycerol Metabolism

Edward R. B. McCabe

1. **Glycerol kinase (GK) deficiency (MIM 307030) is an X-linked inborn error of metabolism characterized by hyperglycerolemia and glyceroluria. These individuals may evidence "pseudohypertriglyceridemia" if the laboratory measures triglycerides by quantitation of glycerol released after lipolysis. Glycerol kinase deficiency has been subdivided into three clinical forms according to phenotype: (1) complex glycerol kinase deficiency, which is an Xp21 contiguous gene syndrome involving the *GK* locus together with the adrenal hypoplasia congenita (*AHC*) and/or Duchenne muscular dystrophy (*DMD*) loci; (2) the juvenile form, associated with episodic vomiting, acidemia, and central nervous system depression, as well as hypotonia and a Reye-like illness in certain patients, presenting in the first several years of life; and (3) the benign, or adult, form, detected incidentally with pseudohypertriglyceridemia. The juvenile and benign forms result from isolated GK deficiency.**
2. **The diagnosis of GK deficiency may be confirmed by a decrease in GK enzymatic activity and/or identification of a GK gene mutation or deletion. The enzyme activity may be determined in leukocytes, fibroblasts, liver, and/or transformed lymphoblastoid cell lines. Kidney, small intestine, and adrenal gland are also deficient in GK activity among affected individuals.**
3. **Because of the relatively high frequency of interstitial deletions in this chromosomal region, all patients with DMD and developmental delay should be evaluated for adrenal hypoplasia and insufficiency and for GK deficiency.**
4. **Treatment is most critical for patients with adrenal hypoplasia and insufficiency, since all the deaths seem to have resulted from Addisonian crises. These patients require glucocorticoid and mineralocorticoid treatment. Patients with vomiting, acidemia, and stupor associated with GK deficiency or the glycerol intolerance syndrome may be placed on a low-fat (i.e., glycerol-restricted) diet, but most important is the avoidance of prolonged fasts.**
5. **The gene order surrounding the GK locus is: Xpter–*AHC-GK-DMD-OTC*–cen. Human GK cDNAs have been isolated from testis, brain, liver, and adrenal gland, and the deduced amino acid sequences show striking similarities to prokaryotic sequences.**
6. **Patients with the glycerol intolerance syndrome have episodes of sweating, irritability, confusion, marked lethargy, and coma. Hypoglycemia and seizures are variably observed. Episodes can be precipitated by glycerol ingestion or infusion. The patients may outgrow these episodes. Each of the three individuals investigated has a history of prematurity. Measurements of GK activity have been normal. Diminished hepatic fructose 1,6-bisphosphatase activity and increased sensitivity of this enzyme to inhibition by glycerol 3-phosphate have been reported. These observations have prompted speculation that this syndrome may represent an unusual sensitivity to the hypoglycemic effects of glycerol 3-phosphate, possibly due to delayed maturation of enzymes of the glycerol metabolic pathway. Similarity of symptoms to those of the juvenile form of GK deficiency has suggested alternative hypotheses that include abnormal compartmentation of a mutant GK gene with normal enzyme activity or a mutation in the glycerol facilitator gene involved in uptake of glycerol across the cell membrane.**

INTRODUCTION AND HISTORICAL PERSPECTIVE

Glycerol ($C_3H_8O_3$; molecular weight 92.09), also known as glycerin or 1,2,3-propanetriol, is a hygroscopic, clear, colorless, syrupy liquid. The term glycerol is derived, via the French *glycerine,* from the Greek *glykeros* (sweet), reflecting its taste.

Glyceroluria was described originally in 1967 in four mentally retarded patients among a group of 900 screened for polyhydric alcohol excretion.[1] The serum glycerol concentrations of these patients were similar to those of controls.[1,2] The glycerol intolerance syndrome was described in 1975 in a 3-year-old boy with episodic confusion, drowsiness, nausea, vomiting, and loss of consciousness associated with glycerol ingestion or infusion; this patient did not have hyperglycerolemia or glyceroluria and had normal leukocyte GK activity.[3]

Deficiency of the glycerol kinase enzyme (Fig. 97-1) was reported in 1977[4] in two brothers with hyperglycerolemia, glyceroluria, psychomotor retardation, spasticity, osteoporosis, Duchenne-type dystrophic myopathy, and adrenal hypoplasia.[4,5] Glycerol kinase deficiency was documented independently in 1978[6] in a pedigree that included a 70-year-old proband, his clinically normal brother, and his 21-year-old asymptomatic grandson. Subsequent pedigrees confirmed the X-linked inheritance. Glycerol kinase maps to the Xp21 region, and patients with the phenotype that includes AHC, GK deficiency, and dystrophic myopathy are now recognized to represent a contiguous gene syndrome.[8–55]

Glycerol is a neutral compound, and therefore GK deficiency is not an organic acidemia. However, this disorder is frequently

A list of standard abbreviations is located immediately preceding the index in each volume. Nonstandard abbreviations used in this chapter include: AHC = adrenal hypoplasia congenita; CGKD = complex glycerol kinase deficiency; cGPDH:NAD = cytoplasmic NAD-linked glycerol 3-phosphate dehydrogenase; DMD = Duchenne muscular dystrophy; GK = glycerol kinase; GKD = glycerol kinase deficiency; HH = hypogonadotropic hypogonadism; mGPDH:FAD = mitochondrial FAD-linked glycerol 3-phosphate dehydrogenase; mGPDH:NAD = mitochondrial NAD-linked glycerol 3-phosphate dehydrogenase; MIP = major intrinsic protein; OTC = ornithine transcarbamylase; pGPDH:NAD = peroxisomal NAD-linked glycerol 3-phosphate dehydrogenase. See text and tables for genotype and phenotype designations.

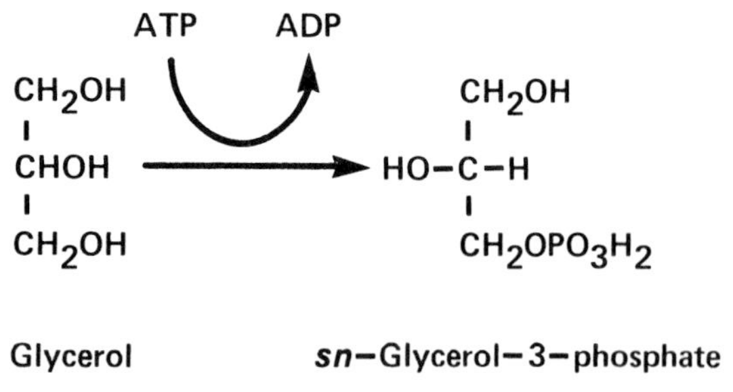

Fig. 97-1 The glycerol kinase reaction.

considered with the organic acidemias, because the diagnosis often is made following urine organic acid analysis by GC/MS performed for evaluation of acute deterioration with shock and acidemia from AHC, as part of a general metabolic evaluation, or during workup for "pseudohypertriglyceridemia."[4,5,7,56–59] Pseudohypertriglyceridemia results from elevation of free glycerol in the blood of these patients, which interferes with the routine measurement of triglycerides based on quantitation of glycerol liberated by lipolysis.[58]

BIOCHEMISTRY AND PHYSIOLOGY OF GLYCEROL METABOLISM

Sources and Fates of Glycerol

The metabolism of glycerol is shown in Fig. 97-2. The sources of glycerol include endogenous breakdown of triglycerides and other glycerolipids and production from glucose, protein, lactate, or pyruvate (a process termed "glyceroneogenesis"); the exogenous source is uptake of glycerol from dietary fats after release during digestion.[60–69] Glycerol supports glycogenesis and gluconeogenesis in various systems.[2,70–92] Glycerol serves as a precursor for synthesis of glycerolipids, which include the acyl-glyceride derivatives, phosphatidic acid, and other glycerol phospholipids, such as phosphatidylinositide and the polyphosphoinositides.[68,93–100] Glycerol is a source for dihydroxyacetone phosphate, which is the immediate precursor for ether lipid synthesis in the peroxisome.[101–104] Glycerol may also be metabolized to lactate,[74,105,106] oxalate,[106] formaldehyde,[107] protein,[108] or carbon dioxide.[66,68]

Pathway of Glycerol Metabolism

The three principal enzymes in the glycerol pathway that will be discussed in this section include glycerol kinase (ATP:glycerol-3-phosphotransferase, EC 2.7.1.30), cytoplasmic NAD-dependent glycerol 3-phosphate dehydrogenase (*sn*-glycerol 3-phosphate: NAD^+ 2-oxidoreductase, EC 1.1.1.8), and mitochondrial FAD-linked glycerol 3-phosphate dehydrogenase (*sn*-glycerol 3-phosphate: (acceptor) 2-oxidoreductase, EC 1.1.99.5). The literature is confusing with respect to cytoplasmic glycerol 3-phosphate dehydrogenase, using the designations EC 1.1.1.8 and EC 1.1.1.94 arbitrarily. These Enzyme Commission numbers refer to *sn*-glycerol 3-phosphate:NAD^+ 2-oxidoreductase (EC 1.1.1.8) and *sn*-glycerol 3-phosphate:$NAD(P)^+$ 2-oxidoreductase (EC 1.1.1.94).[109] Most workers have assayed with NAD+ or NADH and have not attempted to distinguish between these two enzymes. The following convention will be used in this chapter in order to discriminate between the cytoplasmic and mitochondrial enzymes: cGPDH:NAD will specify the cytoplasmic NAD-linked enzyme, and mGPDH:FAD will specify the mitochondrial FAD-linked

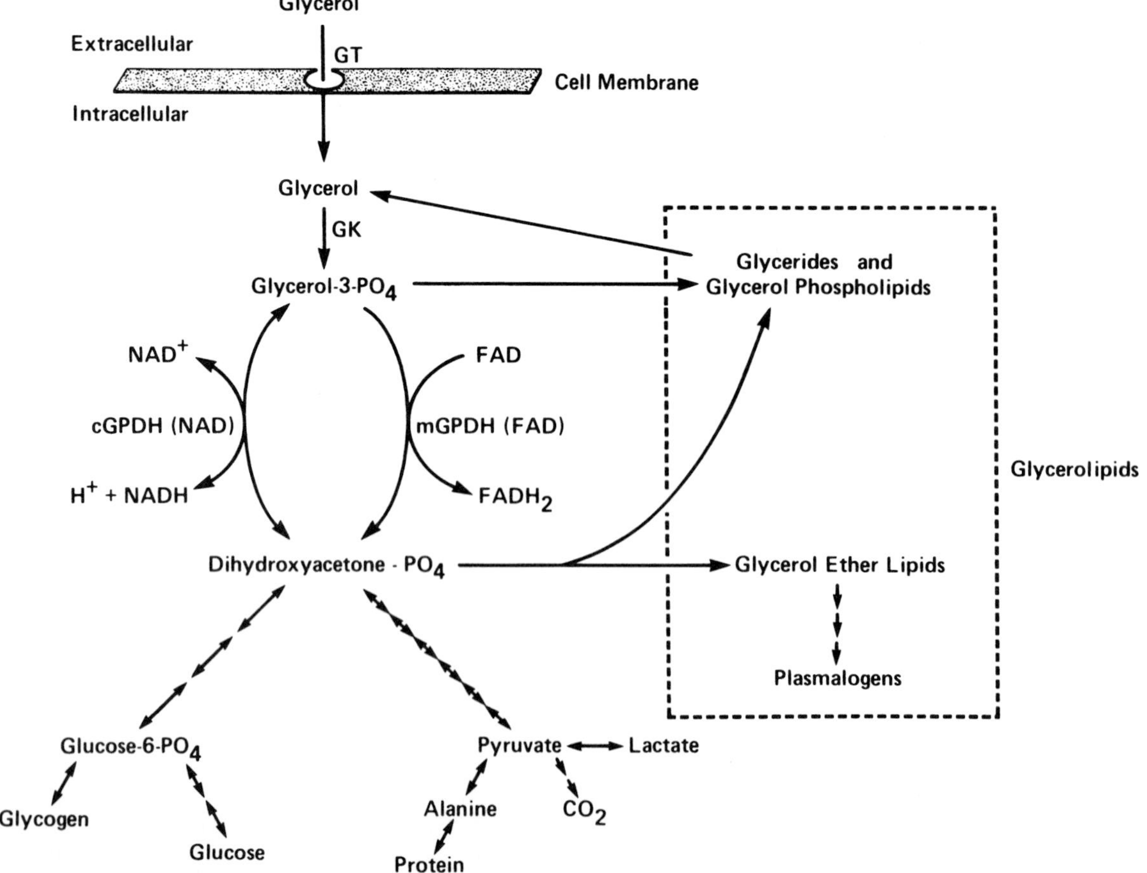

Fig. 97-2 Pathway of glycerol metabolism. GT = glycerol transporter; GK = glycerol kinase; cGPDH:NAD = cytoplasmic NAD-linked glycerol 3-phosphate dehydrogenase; mGPDH:FAD = mitochondrial FAD-linked glycerol 3-phosphate dehydrogenase.

enzyme. Additional enzyme activities will be indicated as follows: mitochondrial NAD-linked activity as mGPDH:NAD and peroxisomal NAD-linked enzyme activity as pGPDH:NAD (see below).

Glycerol Kinase. Glycerol kinase catalyzes the phosphorylation of glycerol by ATP to yield the products glycerol 3-phosphate and ADP.[110] This enzymatic reaction has been demonstrated in a number of tissues and cells, including liver,[95,96,111–129] kidney,[130–134] circulating leukocytes,[4,6,107] intestinal mucosa,[135] brain,[136–138] adrenal gland,[139,140] adipose tissue,[141–159] thyroid gland,[160] cardiac and skeletal muscle,[161–163] lung,[164] mammary gland,[165] spermatozoa,[166–168] and fibroblasts.[5,107,126] GK activity has also been demonstrated in Epstein-Barr-virus transformed lymphoblastoid cell lines,[21] in rat hepatomas and cultured Novikoff rat hepatoma cells,[169,170] and in adenoma alveolar type II cells.[171] Although rat islets and the insulinoma cell line INS-1 contain negligible GK activity and do not respond to glycerol with insulin secretion, transfection with an adenoviral GK construct resulted in insulin release in response to glycerol.[172] The Rous sarcoma virus transforming gene pp60src, a 60-kDa phosphoprotein that phosphorylates protein substrates on tyrosine residues using GTP or ATP, shows ATP-dependent GK activity.[173] A 54-kDa related protein, pp54src, shows similar GK activity, as does the catalytic subunit of cAMP-dependent protein kinase.[174,175] The physiological significance of the GK activity of these protein kinases remains in question because of the relatively high K_m for glycerol.[173,174]

Human *GK* cDNAs were isolated from testis, brain, and liver[176–178] and mouse *Gyk* cDNAs from liver.[179] These mammalian deduced amino acid sequences had remarkable similarities with the prokaryotic and *Caenorhabditis elegans* sequences.[176–179] The rat liver ATP-stimulated glucocorticoid receptor translocation promoter was cloned,[180] and its deduced amino acid sequence was 99 percent identical with the murine Gyk and 95 percent identical with the human GK sequences.[179] There are at least six human genomic loci that make up the human *GK* gene family.[181] The four expressed sequences are encoded on chromosomes 1, 4, Xp, and Xq. The Xp21.3 locus extends over more than 50 kb and is made up of 19 exons. The other members of this human gene family are intronless and map to chromosomes 1, 4, and Xq. Two different testis transcripts have been identified, and both mapped to chromosome 4. Sequence analysis of the GK proteins identified additional, previously unrecognized, members of a carbohydrate-kinase gene family.[182] GK has also been investigated in bacteria,[110,183] including *Escherichia coli*, [184–198] *Bacillus subtilis*, [199,200] *B. stearothermophilus*,[201–204] and *Pseudomonas aeruginosa*.[205]

The bacterial phosphoenolpyruvate-dependent phosphotransferase system appears to be involved in the regulation of GK activity,[206] with studies indicating that the enzyme can be activated by histidyl phosphorylation mediated by the phosphotransferase system[207] and that one of the proteins in this group, enzyme III specific for glucose (III^{Glc}), allosterically inhibits GK.[208] GK has been investigated in *Mycoplasma mycoides;*[209] in fungi,[110,210,211] in particular *Candida,*[115,212–215] *Neurospora,*[216] *Aspergillus,*[217,218] *Microsporum,*[219] and *Fusarium;*[220] and in protozoa, with investigations in *Tetrahymena,*[221] *Leishmania,*[222] and *Trypanosoma brucei,*[223–226] in which it is localized to the peroxisome-like glycosomes.

The properties of GK vary considerably depending on its source and the assay conditions used. While not reproducibly observed by all investigators, dihydroxyacetone and UTP may serve as alternative substrates and glycerol 3-phosphate, AMP, and ADP as inhibitors of GK in liver.[110,112,115,116,227,228] Additional inhibitors of GK activity include D,L-1-chloro-2,3-propanediol (α-chlorhydrin),[229] ($\pm$)-2,3-dihydroxypropyl dichloroacetate,[230] and 1-thioglycerol.[231] Glycerol kinase activity is increased in liver and adipose tissue in response to hyperinsulinemia produced by insulin injection[119,146] or by a hypothalamic lesion,[232] and this may be etiologically related to the elevated enzyme activity observed in homozygous genetically obese (*ob*/*ob*) mice.[69] Castration in rats leads to decreased hepatic GK activity, which is reversed by testosterone injection.[233]

The understanding of the relationship between the structure of the GK protein and its functional properties has been improved dramatically by the report of the solved crystal structure of the *E. coli* enzyme.[234] Key amino acid residues were identified that interacted with the regulatory protein, III^{Glc}, and with the substrates. Structural analyses of related proteins and comparison with the GK structure indicate that GK contains an actin fold made up of two α/β domains flanking a putative hinge region containing an ATP-binding site.[235]

NAD-Linked Glycerol 3-Phosphate Dehydrogenases. cGPDH: NAD catalyzes the reversible oxidation of glycerol 3-phosphate to dihydroxyacetone phosphate with reduction of NAD^+ to NADH + H^+. This enzyme was originally described in muscle extracts[236,237] and was crystallized from muscle.[238] Nearly 90 percent of the total activity in rats is found in skeletal muscle, but cGPDH:NAD has also been described in liver, kidney, smooth muscle, cardiac muscle, and adipose tissue.[69,239] Glucocorticoids induce increased synthesis of the enzyme in cultured glial cells[240] and stimulate cGPDH:NAD activity in cultured rat heart cells;[241] however, T_3 results in decreased enzyme activity in rat heart cells in culture.[242] Forskolin and dibutyryl cAMP induce cGPDH:NAD activity individually in rat glioma C6 cells, and when each of these agents is combined with dexamethasone, the level of induction is greater than observed with either agent individually.[243] Investigations with C6 cells and oligodendrocytes indicate that regulation by glucocorticoids takes place at the transcriptional level.[244,245] Interferon-α/β inhibited the induced expression of the mRNA for this enzyme in C6 cells and oligodendrocytes.[246] Phorbol 12-retinoate 13-acetate and mezerein, two second-stage tumor promoters, also inhibit the induction of cGPDH:NAD activity by glucocorticoids.[247] Stress increases rat hippocampal cGPDH:NAD mRNA, a response presumably mediated by endogenous release of corticosteroids from the adrenal glands.[248] The cDNA for cGPDH:NAD hybridized to 4.7-kb mRNA from rat muscle, rat brain, mouse liver, and C6 cells.[244] A mouse genomic clone for this enzyme also was isolated.[249] The human liver cGPDH:NAD cDNA has been cloned.[250]

In rat liver mitochondria, an NAD-linked glycerol phosphate dehydrogenase (mGPDH:NAD) was described, with properties very similar to those of the cytosolic enzyme.[251] In contrast to the cytosolic enzyme, mGPDH:NAD responded to thyroid status in a manner similar to the way mGPDH:FAD does (see below, FAD-linked glycerol 3-phosphate dehydrogenase.)—that is, thyroidectomy decreased the activity of the mitochondrial oxidoreductase, and T_3 treatment restored it.[251]

An NAD-linked peroxisomal glycerol phosphate dehydrogenase (pGPDH:NAD), with properties differing from those of the cytosolic enzyme, has also been described.[252,253] The activity of pGPDH:NAD increased under conditions associated with increased peroxisomal fatty acid β-oxidation.[253] Peroxisomal oxidoreduction was proposed to play a role in a glycerol 3-phosphate shuttle involving the movement of reducing equivalents between peroxisomes, cytoplasm, and mitochondria (Fig. 97-3).[252,253]

FAD-Linked Glycerol 3-Phosphate Dehydrogenase. The mitochondrial FAD-linked enzyme catalyzes the irreversible oxidation of glycerol 3-phosphate to dihydroxyacetone phosphate. Phenazine methosulfate can serve directly as an artificial electron acceptor.[254] mGPDH:FAD was originally described in frog muscle[255] and has a broad tissue distribution in mammals.[69] In rats, the highest specific activity is in testicular mitochondria,[256] although the activity of this enzyme is quite low in human testis.[257] Other tissues with mGPDH:FAD activity include skeletal muscle, lung, spleen, intestine, brain, placenta, adipose tissue, aorta, and leukocytes.[69,258,259] mGPDH:FAD activity is elevated in

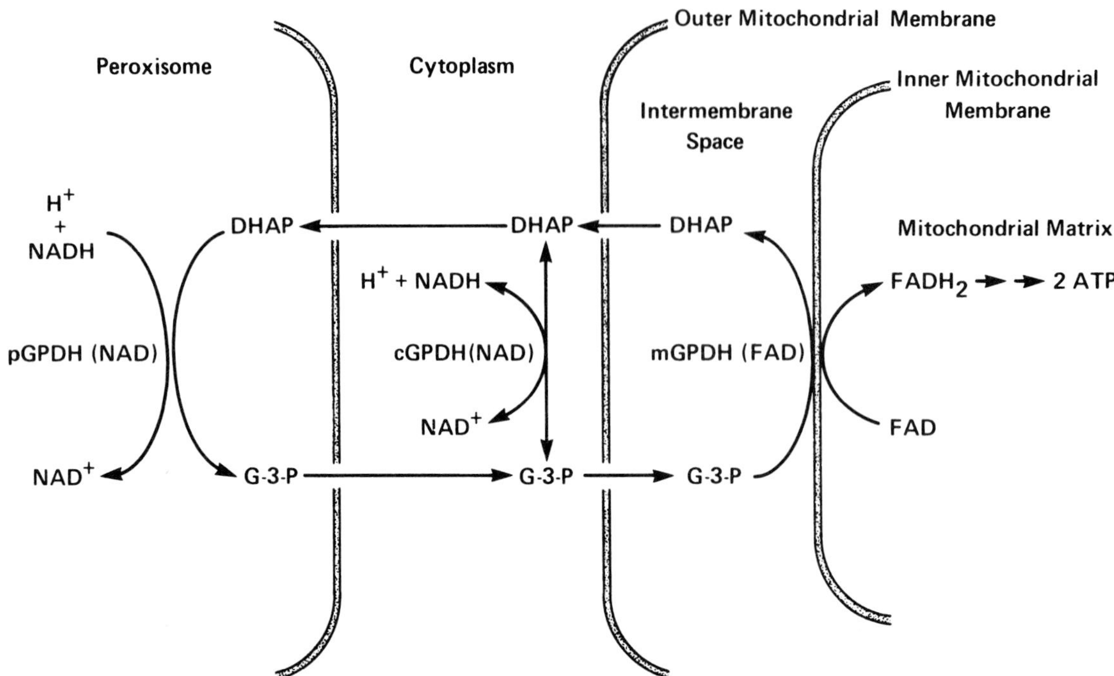

Fig. 97-3 Glycerol phosphate shuttle, showing potential communications between peroxisomes, cytoplasm, and mitochondria. (*Adapted from Tolbert*[252] *and Newsholme and Start.*[297])

most insulinomas and carcinoid tumors, as well as other tumors of the amine precursor uptake decarboxylation system.[260] This enzyme is considered to be localized to the outer surface of the inner mitochondrial membrane.[69,261] The activity of mGPDH:FAD responds to glucocorticoids and thyroid hormone in a manner inversely related to that of cGPDH:NAD. Activity of mGPDH:FAD increases after adrenalectomy[262] or administration of thyroid hormone.[263–266] The rat FAD-dependent mitochondrial glycerol 3-phosphate dehydrogenase cDNA has been cloned and sequenced[267,268] and the genomic organization determined.[269] The deduced amino acid sequence indicates a mitochondrial leader peptide, an FAD-binding domain, a glycerol phosphate-binding domain, and two EF-hand calcium-binding domains with similarity to those in calmodulin.[267] Structure-function analysis suggests that cytoplasmic calcium may play a role in regulation of this enzyme.[270] Human pancreatic islet cell mitochondrial cDNAs have also been cloned and characterized.[271]

Glycerol Transport. Glycerol transport in red blood cells occurs by facilitated diffusion, presumably mediated by a specific carrier that is sensitive to inhibition by Cu^{2+} and other heavy metal ions.[69,272,273] Ethylene glycol acts as a competitive inhibitor for this transport process.[274–276] Transport of glycerol was also investigated in normal hepatocytes[128] and tumor cells, including Novikoff rat hepatoma, HeLa, and Hep-2 cells.[170] The transport process for glycerol was distinct from that for glucose.[128,170] Glycerol uptake was measured in perfused rat liver under steady state conditions, and it was concluded that uptake across the hepatic cell membrane was an important factor in the regulation of glycerol metabolism.[277]

Movement of glycerol across the cell membrane of bacteria and fungi also proceeds by facilitated diffusion.[220,278] The glycerol facilitator (*glpF*) has been cloned and characterized in *E. coli* and *P. aeruginosa* and is in an operon that also includes glycerol kinase (*glpK*).[205,278–280] Based on sequence similarities, a membrane protein family has been described that includes: *glpF;* MIP, involved in lens fiber gap junctions and mutated in mice with congenital cataracts; the aquaporins; and homologues in a variety of organisms, including yeast, plants, and *Drosophila.*[279,281–284] This is referred to as the MIP family of integral membrane transport proteins.[282] These proteins have six putative transmembrane domains[282] and may have arisen by gene duplication.[285] In contrast to the other aquaporins, AQP3 and AQP7 mediate glycerol movement across membranes.[284,286–290] The yeast gene product, FPS1, also serves as a glycerol facilitator.[291] Phylogenetic characterization of more than 50 MIP family members suggests that these proteins derive from two bacterial paralogues, one an aquaporin and the other a glycerol facilitator.[292] It remains to be determined whether AQP3, AQP7, or both are the human glycerol facilitator(s), but they are definite candidates.

Compartmentation of Glycerol Metabolism

Glycerol Phosphate Shuttle. Reducing equivalents serve as energy currency to the cell, since they provide the mitochondria with substrate for oxidative phosphorylation. However, mitochondria are impermeable to the pyridine nucleotides,[293] and indirect pathways, or "shuttles," are used for the transfer of these reducing equivalents from the cytoplasm to the mitochondrial electron transfer chain.[294] One such mechanism is the glycerol phosphate shuttle[294–296] (see Fig. 97-3). Glycerol 3-phosphate moves from the cytoplasm through the outer mitochondrial membrane to the intermembrane space, where it serves as a substrate for mGPDH:FAD on the outer surface of the inner mitochondrial membrane.[69,261] Dihydroxyacetone phosphate formed by mGPDH:FAD exits the intermembrane space, where cGPDH:NAD completes the cycle with production of glycerol 3-phosphate. The directionality of this cycle is ensured by the nonequilibrium reaction catalyzed by the mitochondrial dehydrogenase: The NADH-equivalent of the cytoplasm, with a potential P/O ratio (number of moles of ATP formed per atom of oxygen consumed) of 3, is utilized by mGPDH:FAD, yielding a P/O ratio of only 2, with the additional energy presumably lost as heat.[294,297] Additional options such as glycolysis, gluconeogenesis, and glycerolipid synthesis are available to the intermediates of this shuttle, and, as in any cyclic pathway, the intermediates withdrawn for these metabolic alternatives must be replenished in order for the cycle to continue.

The glycerol phosphate shuttle is clearly important in supplying energy to insect flight muscles.[298,299] Mutations in *Drosophila melanogaster* leading to mGPDH:FAD deficiency result in loss of ability to fly.[300] Glycerol phosphate can serve as a mitochondrial respiratory substrate for a number of tissues, including brain, liver, adipose tissue, intestine, skeletal muscle, aorta, and placenta.[258,301–309] In one study in liver, the glycerol phosphate shuttle accounted for 40 percent of the reducing equivalent flux from the cytoplasm to the mitochondria,[305] and this shuttle appears to play a role in managing the increased reducing equivalents associated with ethanol oxidation.[310–312] It has been suggested that the increased mGPDH:FAD activity observed in tumors involving the amine precursor uptake decarboxylation system, including insulinomas and carcinoids, may facilitate oxidation of the NADH formed by rapid cytosolic metabolism of glucose.[260] In Ehrlich ascites tumor cells, the use of the glycerol phosphate shuttle, which accounts for 80 percent of maximum total reducing equivalent transfer, appears to be dependent on the availability of glycolytic intermediates to provide shuttle substrates.[313] The breast cancer cell line MDA-MB-453 also has an active shuttle.[314] The glycerol phosphate shuttle appears to be important in normal pancreatic islet cells for mitochondrial transfer of reducing equivalents generated by the cytosolic catabolism of glucose.[315–321] The presence of peroxisomal glycerol phosphate dehydrogenase (see above, "Pathway of Glycerol Metabolism") has led to the proposal that there may be a peroxisomal glycerol phosphate shuttle, which would move reducing equivalents generated by fatty acid oxidation out of the peroxisome as glycerol phosphate, and that this might be continuous with the cytoplasmic-mitochondrial shuttle, with reoxidation of glycerol phosphate generated in the peroxisome.[252] The functional role of the mitochondrial glycerol phosphate shuttle in mammals has been questioned, primarily because of studies indicating its limited capacity in a number of tissues.[69,294,322,323]

Direct interactions of cGPDH:NAD with other glycolytic enzymes have been suggested and could influence the activity of the glycerol phosphate shuttle. Interaction of this enzyme with aldolase can be promoted by the addition of polyethylene glycol.[324] The aldolase-cGPDH:NAD complex, representing sequential enzymatic steps, evidences an increased K_m for fructose 1,6-bisphosphate with no change in $V_{\max}$, while the $V_{\max}$ for fructose 1-phosphate increased with no change in K_m. There is a tenfold decrease in K_i for the aldolase-dehydrogenase complex in the presence of fructose 1,6-bisphosphate, but no influence of fructose 1-phosphate or dihydroxyacetone phosphate on K_i. Interaction of cGPDH:NAD with lactate dehydrogenase (LDH) to form a complex for direct transfer of NADH has been discussed[325,326] but remains controversial.[327]

Glycerol Kinase Binding to Porin on the Outer Mitochondrial Membrane. The term "ambiquitous" (meaning both places, by analogy with ubiquitous, or all places) was coined to refer to enzymes with rapid and reversible changes in intracellular distribution.[328] Enzymes considered in this category have included hexokinase,[328,329] aldolase,[330] glyceraldehyde 3-phosphate dehydrogenase,[330] and glycerol kinase.[127,140,331–336] GK may be found in either the cytosolic or the particulate fraction, with differences in subcellular distribution dependent on the tissue, developmental stage, and metabolic state.[126,127,139,140,331–334,337] In the particulate fraction, GK is present in microsomes and mitochondria, and the mitochondrial-bound activity varies with the metabolic state of the animal.[127,333] The mitochondrial receptor for GK is porin, the pore-forming protein of the outer mitochondrial membrane[127,331,333,335,336,338–340] (Fig. 97-4). Porin is identical to the hexokinase binding protein,[331,341,342] and this voltage-dependent anion channel (VDAC)[343,344] is important for movement of adenine nucleotides across the outer mitochondrial membrane.[345,346] ATP flux is controlled by a voltage-gated channel from this membrane.[346] These features explain the competition between mitochondrially bound hexokinase and added GK for

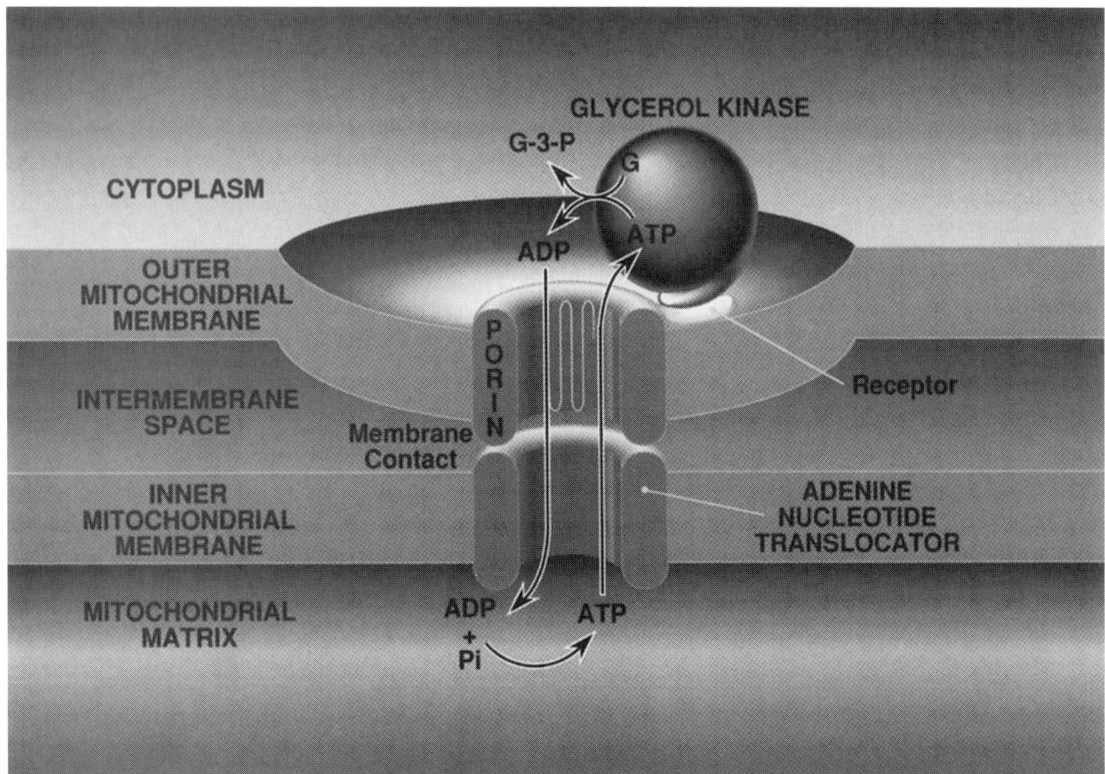

Fig. 97-4 Model for functional compartmentation of glycerol kinase. This model proposes that glycerol kinase binds to its outer mitochondrial membrane receptor protein, porin, at the contact points between the inner and outer mitochondrial membranes. The juxtaposition of porin and the adenine nucleotide translocator, within the outer and inner mitochondrial membranes, respectively, would provide the physical structure that would afford the bound glycerol kinase with preferential access to ATP generated within the mitochondrial matrix. G = glycerol; G-3-P = glycerol 3-phosphate. (*Model adapted from that described by Adams et al.*[336])

mitochondrially generated ATP.[332,341,347,348] The activity of mitochondrially bound GK is stimulated by the respiratory substrates, ADP and succinate, and is inhibited by atractyloside, which blocks the adenine nucleotide carrier of the inner mitochondrial membrane (i.e., GK bound to the outer mitochondrial membrane appears to utilize ATP generated within the mitochondrion).[127,140,334] The reaction product, glycerol 3-phosphate, promotes release of bound GK from porin in liver and adrenal,[127,140,334] and apparent K_m for ATP and for glycerol are lower for the bound enzyme than for that in the supernatant.[140,334] Similarly, mitochondrial hexokinase is specifically solubilized by its product, glucose 6-phosphate,[329,349] utilizes mitochondrially generated ATP,[347,350,351] and has a K_m for ATP that is lower than that for the soluble enzyme.[329] Therefore, GK, like hexokinase, meets the criteria for an ambiquitous enzyme, with rapid and reversible changes in intracellular distribution dependent on cellular energy status and metabolite levels and with distinct kinetic properties dependent on this distribution.[334,336]

The reversible and regulable juxtaposition of an ADP-producing kinase with an ADP-permeable pore suggested the possibility of concerted formation and transport of ADP into the intermembrane space through this pore, allowing ADP to continue to the mitochondrial matrix through the adenine nucleotide carrier of the inner membrane.[332] It was suggested that contact sites between the inner and outer mitochondrial membranes might delimit microcompartments within the intermembrane space.[333,339] The binding of these kinases to the outer mitochondrial membrane and the formation of intermembrane microcompartments become processes that control communication between cytoplasmic and mitochondrial energy production and regulate availability of substrates for alternative metabolic processing.[332–334,336,352] It is known that mammalian mitochondria are capable of synthesizing glycerophospholipids from glycerol and ATP, and the involvement of bound GK in a microcompartmented system has been proposed.[353]

Eukaryotic porin genes have been cloned from *Saccharomyces cerevisiae*,[354] *N. crassa*,[355] *Drosophila melanogaster*,[356] humans,[357] and mice.[358–360] Porin was originally shown to be present in human myocardial particulate material by immunologic cross-reactivity with polyclonal antibodies to bovine myocardial and rat liver porins.[361] The complete amino acid sequence of human porin has been determined by protein sequencing of B-lymphocyte and skeletal muscle porins purified from the tissue plasma membranes.[362–364] These lymphocyte and skeletal muscle plasmalemma porins showed 90 percent sequence identity with partial sequence information from rat kidney and beef heart.[363] Analyses of porin structure suggest that it is a β-barrel consisting of an N-terminal amphipathic α-helix followed by either 13 or 16 membrane-spanning β-strands.[365–368] The presence of porin in the plasma membrane, as well as in the outer mitochondrial membrane, raises interesting questions about the respective roles of this protein in these locations, as well as about the mechanism for controlling solute flow through pores that have relatively low anion selectivity and pass molecules up to 6 to 8 kDa in size.[338,369]

Physiology of Glycerol Metabolism

It is generally recognized that the splanchnic region, and in particular the liver and kidney, represent the principal sites of glycerol metabolism in mammals.[61,69] However, it has been asserted that circulating leukocytes and thrombocytes contribute significantly to the metabolism of glycerol in humans.[370] It is not coincidental that these tissues represent the bulk of the GK activity in the body. The best evidence that GK represents the primary entry of glycerol into metabolism is finding glyceroluria and hyperglycerolemia in patients with GK deficiency (see "Glycerol Kinase Deficiency").

Studies in lean and obese subjects showed that there was a direct correlation between plasma glycerol concentration and glycerol turnover and that both were increased in obese subjects compared with lean individuals.[66] The free fatty acid/glycerol turnover ratio in lean individuals was 4.7:1, differing from the theoretical ratio of 3:1 and indicating incomplete hydrolysis of triglycerides;[66] alternatively, this could be explained by intracellular reutilization of a portion of the glycerol released by hydrolysis. Glycerol did not contribute more than 10 percent of the total respiratory CO_2.[66] Glycerol contribution to gluconeogenesis became substantial under conditions of starvation,[66,371] with glycerol providing 38 percent of the new glucose from protein or glycerol in lean individuals and 79 percent in obese individuals. Increases in the hepatic activities of GK and glycerol 3-phosphate dehydrogenase during starvation were considered to be important for the increased utilization of glycerol released by lipolysis for gluconeogenesis.[372]

During pregnancy there is decreased utilization of glycerol by maternal extrahepatic tissues, associated with a decreased half-life of tracer glycerol and increased gluconeogenesis from this substrate by the maternal liver.[373,374] The fetus is able to respond to maternal fasting and to fetal norepinephrine injection with mobilization of glycerol.[375] The mother is able to supply glycerol to the fetus across the placenta, and the fetus is able to utilize circulating glycerol for gluconeogenesis and glycogen synthesis.[92] The blood glycerol concentration rises rapidly in the postnatal period in premature and term infants.[376,377] The effect of intrauterine asphyxiation on the concentration of blood glycerol is unclear from differing studies.[378,379] In the postnatal period, stress (such as a series of heel pricks or cold exposure) results in elevated blood glycerol.[380,381] Intravenously administered glycerol was eliminated more rapidly in the first day of life in small-for-gestational-age as compared with appropriate-for-gestational-age infants and was eliminated most rapidly at 3 to 5 weeks of age, with term and premature infants showing similar rates of elimination at that age.[85] Malnutrition during lactation results in a decrease in the offspring of the hepatic activities of GK, cGPDH:NAD, and mGPDH:FAD, suggesting that nutritional deprivation might limit the capacity of the liver to use glycerol in the offspring.[382] Animals malnourished after weaning showed striking deficits in gluconeogenic capacity compared with control animals, and these differences were attributed to hepatic accumulation of phosphorylated glycerol metabolites and their inhibiting effects on the pathway of gluconeogenesis.[383]

Studies in rats and hamsters showed a dramatic rise in hepatic GK activity during the neonatal period, but these studies measured the activity of this enzyme only in the supernatant.[384–387] Investigations in human fetuses and newborns did not show similar developmental changes in GK when activity was examined in the whole homogenate.[337,388] There was a marked change in the particulate bound fraction of this enzyme, from 91 percent bound in fetuses to 7 percent bound in infants, the latter being similar to values observed in adults.[139,337] Activity of hepatic cGPDH:NAD paralleled the increase in supernatant GK activity in rats, and both enzyme activities increased in response to hydrocortisone and thyroxine, although the oxidoreductase response to thyroxine was smaller.[386] A second, chromatographically distinct hepatic form of cGPDH:NAD was reported in neonatal mice.[389] Glycerol oxidation to CO_2 by whole rat brain homogenates is lower in the neonate, increasing approximately 30 percent in the suckling period to the higher adult rate.[390] Although discrete areas of the brain differ in glycerol oxidation rates, in general the rates increase with age in hypothalamus, cerebral cortex, hippocampus, and cerebellum. Brain stem is an exception, with maximal glycerol oxidation observed at 4 to 6 days of age, followed by a reduced rate of oxidation.

Diagnostic and Therapeutic Uses of Glycerol

Glycerol is used as an osmotic agent for treatment of increased intraocular and intracerebral pressure[89,391,392] and for diagnosis of endolymphatic hydrops in the differential diagnosis of low frequency hearing loss,[393] as a substrate for the evaluation of disorders of carbohydrate metabolism,[83,90,91] and as a component of emollient solutions, ointments, purgatives, suppositories, and other medications.[60] Our experience indicates that exogenous glycerol is a frequent explanation of glyceroluria.

GLYCEROL KINASE DEFICIENCY

Introduction

Hyperglycerolemia (MIM 307030) is also known as glycerol kinase deficiency (GKD) and GK1 deficiency.[394] GKD can be subdivided into three clinical forms by phenotype. Complex glycerol kinase deficiency (CGKD), or the infantile form,[13,59,332,394,395] is a contiguous gene[8–55] syndrome (see Chap. 65) involving not only the GK locus but also the AHC (see Chap. 167) and/or the DMD (see Chap. 216) locus in the Xp21 region. Two phenotypes have isolated involvement of the GK locus—the juvenile form,[59,395–399] associated with metabolic and central nervous system instability and deterioration, and the benign, or adult, form,[6,59,332,395,400–403] detected incidentally with pseudohypertriglyceridemia.[58]

It is now clear that DMD, GKD, and AHC are caused by mutations in distinct loci, since the cDNAs for the genes responsible for each of these disorders have been cloned.[176–178,394,404,405] The existence of individual genes for the CGKD phenotypes had been previously hypothesized[5,7] and was confirmed by observation of patients with phenotypes including isolated forms of GKD without DMD or AHC, isolated AHC without GKD or DMD, and forms with breakpoints between AHC and GK or between GK and DMD.

Clinical Aspects

Contiguous Gene Syndrome Involving AHC, GKD, and DMD. Two brothers with this phenotype were originally described with GKD in 1977,[4] although the association with AHC was not recognized until later.[5] To date, the largest group of individuals with CGKD have been described with AHC, GKD, and DMD, and others who died prior to the recognition of this syndrome are suspected to have had this diagnosis.[4,5,7,8,11–18,20,21,23–25,27–31,35,37,39,41,42,44,47–55] All but one of the patients were male.[7] One additional male, who died in the neonatal period, also had ornithine transcarbamylase deficiency (OTCD) associated with a deletion extending centromerically beyond the DMD locus.[9,10]

A summary was compiled of the clinical findings in 17 patients with CGKD, of whom 15 had AHC, GKD, and DMD.[27] Among these 15 patients, the following features were observed, with frequencies determined from the number of clinical descriptions in which a comment was made about the particular feature: psychomotor retardation (12/12); short stature (10/12); abnormal genitalia (6/13); osteoporosis (6/13); and characteristic facies with strabismus (6/13), wide-set eyes and drooping mouth (4/13), or dysmorphic facies (1/13, the individual who had AHC, GKD, DMD, and OTCD). The abnormal genitalia included anorchia and cryptorchidism, features of gonadotropin deficiency associated with X-linked cytomegalic AHC.[8,27,406]

The dysmorphic features observed in patients with CGKD, while mild, are characteristic.[53] Facial features include the conformation of the lower forehead, eyebrows, and root and bridge of the nose, with hypertelorism and rounded palpebral fissures, described as an "hourglass" midface appearance. Additional facial features typically seen in these boys are esotropia, a down-turned mouth, and flattened ear lobes. Agenesis of the corpus callosum has been reported in a patient with AHC, GKD, and DMD.[55]

Additional patients have been described with a phenotype involving the AHC and DMD loci without measurement of GK activity or documentation of a *GK* mutation. A Japanese boy presented with vomiting, weight loss, hyponatremia (116 mEq/liter), and hyperkalemia (7.5 mEq/liter) at 23 days of age.[407] Adrenal insufficiency was documented and treated, and an adrenal scintigram showed bilateral absence of the adrenal glands. Serum creatine kinase (CK) was elevated, a muscle biopsy was consistent with DMD, and his clinical course was characteristic of this disorder. Generalized seizures, unconsciousness, and apnea developed after 1 week of insufficient medication, and the patient died at 3 years 5 months of age. Autopsy findings confirmed the adrenal hypoplasia. Two brothers were reported who had adrenal insufficiency and hypoplasia, dystrophic myopathy and elevated serum CK, severe psychomotor retardation, failure to thrive, and megalocornea.[408] Family history included an institutionalized older sister with seizures and mental retardation, a brother with encopresis, and a normal sister. GK activity was not measured in these three patients with AHC and dystrophic myopathy, but they would be expected to have GKD, since the gene loci are ordered AHC, GK, DMD.

There is an extremely high frequency of neonatal and early childhood deaths from unrecognized adrenal insufficiency in these families. Since all the documented patients with AHC, GKD, and DMD living beyond the neonatal period have been developmentally delayed, this would suggest that any patient with DMD and developmental delay should have an evaluation of adrenal function. If this phenotype is ascertained in one family member, then collateral relatives should also be pursued and evaluated. Biochemical or cytogenetic evaluation of 30 patients with DMD identified two patients with deletions extending telomeric of the dystrophin locus.[15]

Contiguous Gene Syndrome Involving AHC and GKD. The second largest group of patients with CGKD have AHC and GKD without DMD.[7,11,14,18,19,21,22,26,29,32–34,36,46,48–50,409] Characteristic features include adrenocortical insufficiency, hyperglycerolemia, and glyceroluria without myopathy. Some patients have had normal genitalia and others have had hypogonadism. Where there is a comment regarding developmental progress, delay is frequently noted, although psychomotor development was reported to be normal in three.[21,34,36] Dysmorphic features were described in one boy, including slightly abnormal pinnae, short palpebral fissures, underdeveloped lower jaw, and decreased hip abduction.[32] Two patients have presented with wheezing, initially attributed to asthma but subsequently considered a mild form of Addisonian crisis.[46] The family histories of these patients and the high frequency of unexplained early deaths indicate that any patient with evidence of GKD, whether or not developmentally delayed, should have an evaluation of adrenal function.

Contiguous Gene Syndrome Involving GKD and DMD. Two brothers have been described with CGKD involving GKD and DMD without AHC, indicating a breakpoint between the AHC and GK loci.[30] Both boys had initial recognition of muscle weakness at 1 year of age. Progressive muscle weakness, elevated serum CK and aldolase activity, and characteristic muscle histology led to the diagnosis of DMD in the older brother. The younger boy also had elevated serum CK values. Both experienced multiple recurring episodes of vomiting beginning at 11 to 12 years of age. The younger boy required hospitalization for intractable vomiting on several occasions, and dehydration, severe metabolic acidemia (arterial pH 7.01, total CO_2 2–3 millimolars), and ketonuria were documented. Both boys showed hyperglycerolemia, glyceroluria, and GKD. Both were developmentally delayed, and normal adrenal function and reserve were documented in them by fasting cortisol and ACTH levels and cosyntropin challenges (Sloan HR: personal communication). They were placed on a low-fat, low-glycerol diet and had no subsequent episodes of vomiting or acidemia during the ensuing 9 months (Sloan HR: personal communication). These episodes and the response to dietary restriction of glycerol are similar to the observations in patients with the juvenile form of isolated GKD. The episodic vomiting and acidemia of these patients with GKD and DMD is particularly interesting, since they have normal adrenal function. Patients with CGKD that includes AHC may have similar episodes, and although these may appear to occur at times of adequate adrenocortical replacement therapy, it may be difficult to determine whether these metabolic abnormalities are truly independent of the AHC. However, the similarity of these episodes to those experienced by children with the isolated symptomatic, or juvenile, form of GKD suggests that the episodes are attributable to deletion of the GK locus in patients with complex GKD.

Isolated Glycerol Kinase Deficiency. There are two clinical subtypes of isolated GKD, referred to previously as the juvenile and the benign, or adult, forms of GKD.[59,332,395]

Symptomatic Juvenile Form. The original two unrelated boys with hyperglycerolemia, glyceroluria, and GKD reported with the juvenile form each presented with an initial episode of vomiting, acidemia, and somnolence or stupor, which on occasion progressed to unconsciousness.[59,396] The patient reported by Eriksson et al.[396] was hospitalized at ages 4, 6, 7, 8.5, and 9 years with fever, vomiting, and diarrhea interpreted as viral gastroenteritis. These episodes were associated with metabolic acidemia: pH 7.2 to 7.31, standard bicarbonate 13.9 to 17.1 mEq/liter, and base deficit 10.5 to 12.9 mEq/liter. On a separate occasion, at 8 years of age, he experienced two grand mal seizures not associated with one of these episodes, for which he was placed on phenytoin. EEG at that time showed rolandic spikes in the central and parietal right hemisphere. Normal studies included serum CK and IV corticotropin stimulation test. Growth and mental development were considered normal. A maternal granduncle had epilepsy. Organic acid analysis revealed glyceroluria.

The second patient[59] presented at 4 years 2 months of age with vomiting, acidemia, hypotonia, fever, and unresponsiveness after ingestion of mouthwash. This episode and those at 4 years 10 months and at 5 years were associated with pH 7.01 to 7.32 and bicarbonate 3.0 to 3.5 mEq/liter. Ketonuria was documented during one episode. Physical and neurologic exams were normal at 6 years 4 months. EEG was normal at 6 years 4 months and at 8 years, except for a single 1-s burst of diffuse bilateral polyspike and wave discharge. A muscle biopsy examined by light and electron microscopy was remarkable only for increased numbers of morphologically normal mitochondria. Serum CK, cortisol, and ACTH were normal. Intelligence was above average at age 7 years, with IQ of 145 and 122 by two different tests. Pseudohypertriglyceridemia led to his diagnosis. A low-fat diet (< 30 percent of total calories) was associated with an absence of further episodes at the time of the report, but subsequent episodes apparently were associated with dietary indiscretions (unpublished), suggesting that the episodes might be related to glycerol ingestion. Family history included hypertriglyceridemia.

A third patient was diagnosed with isolated GKD at 2 years of age but in retrospect had presented initially with episodic hypothermia and lethargy beginning in the first week of life.[397] Temperatures were as low as 94°F, and at 18 months of age an episode was preceded by vomiting and diarrhea beginning 2 days before lethargy and hypothermia. He was developmentally delayed, with a development quotient (DQ) of 69 at 26.5 months of age. He was placed on a low-fat diet and experienced no subsequent episodes. His development was reported to be improving, and at 3.5 years his IQ was 94. His overall performance was considered to be within normal limits, but he did exhibit mild attention problems and slightly delayed fine motor coordination, attributed to mild ataxia.

Bonham and Crawford briefly described a fourth patient who presented at 6 years of age with a Reye syndrome-like illness and hypoglycemia to 0.6 millimolar.[398] They argued that the hypoglycemia resulted from disruption of glucose homeostasis by interruption of glycerol metabolism. In addition, they proposed that the distinction between the symptomatic juvenile and benign adult forms of GKD may be only that those patients with the benign clinical course have not been challenged metabolically[398] (and Bonham JR: personal communication). According to this hypothesis one might expect pedigrees containing individuals with acute episodes as well as those with benign courses. Observations have been extremely limited, and family members with benign courses could be underascertained. Alternatively, the phenotypic distinction between the symptomatic and benign forms of GKD may not be so discrete, as will be discussed below in the section "Genetics."

A fifth patient presented as a neonate with hypotonia, and at age 5 weeks he had apnea and cyanosis requiring stimulation.[399] After another apnea episode at age 5 months and an examination showing persistent truncal hypotonia and symmetrically increased lower extremity deep tendon reflexes, brain imaging revealed mild communicating hydrocephalus, EEG was normal, and the boy exhibited glyceroluria and hyperglycerolemia. His dietary fat was reduced to approximately 20 percent of energy intake until he was 15 months old. By 2 years of age clinical signs had resolved, and repeat MRI at age 2 years 5 months revealed normalization of the earlier abnormalities, with only mild prominence of the lateral ventricles. The authors suggested that the dietary change was unrelated to the resolution of the structural CNS abnormalities and urged consideration of GKD in patients with apnea, hypotonia, mild developmental delay, and/or brain imaging abnormalities.

The resemblance of the acute episodes experienced by patients with the symptomatic, isolated form of GKD (particularly the original two patients[59,396]) and by those with glycerol intolerance (see "Glycerol Intolerance Syndrome" below) is intriguing. These episodes appear to be reduced by restricted fat, and hence glycerol, intake. Patients are susceptible to these acute spells at times of intercurrent illnesses, presumably as a consequence of catabolism and breakdown of fat, with liberation of glycerol. IV glucose during fasting and catabolism imposed by intercurrent illness may prevent these spells. These observations indicate that acute episodes of vomiting, acidemia, and progressive lethargy, at times associated with hypothermia and ketosis, are a feature of symptomatic GKD, whether isolated or part of a contiguous gene syndrome.

Benign Adult Form. Families with the benign, or adult, GKD phenotype are typically ascertained incidentally when a male proband undergoes blood lipid screening that reveals pseudohypertriglyceridemia.[6,58,400–403] Hyperglycerolemia was noted in a mother of three GK-deficient sons in one of these families,[401] and the daughter of one of the men had intermediate GK activity.[58] Hyperglycerolemia is subsequently recognized, because the apparent hypertriglyceridemia is not consistent with the rest of the workup for hyperlipidemia or because the individual does not respond as expected to hyperlipidemia management. The men with this biochemical abnormality ranged in age up to 76 years.

Associated medical problems among those with benign GKD included mild diabetes mellitus,[6,401] myocardial infarctions,[6] laryngeal carcinoma *in situ,*[6] osteoarthritis,[6] herpes zoster ophthalmicus,[6] diarrhea,[401] and a positive family history of diabetes mellitus.[6] Two probands were discovered during routine medical evaluation and were in good health.[58,400] This was in an older population, and while workup of these patients for myopathy and adrenal function was not described, there was no clinical evidence of these features.

Treatment

Patients with adrenal insufficiency consequent to contiguous gene deletion must be treated in the same way as those with isolated AHC (see Chap. 167). This requires replacement doses of a glucocorticoid, such as hydrocortisone, and therapeutic doses of a mineralocorticoid, such as fludrocortisone (Florinef). Patients who have died with these AHC-associated phenotypes died prior to diagnosis or at times when steroid doses had been reduced to subtherapeutic ranges. HH has been treated with testosterone to promote development of secondary sexual characteristics.[33]

Patients with dystrophic myopathy require supportive treatment. It must be noted that not all these patients have the classic

DMD phenotype; early counseling and treatment must recognize that the course of the myopathy is variable and may be mild.

Individuals with GKD, either isolated or part of a contiguous gene syndrome, who have been placed on a low-fat (i.e., low-glycerol) diet have had elimination or reduction of subsequent episodes. Therefore, dietary restriction of glycerol should be considered in patients with GKD and episodic vomiting and acidemia, but it must be recognized that these symptoms may also be attributable to adrenal insufficiency. IV glucose during fasting and catabolism associated with intercurrent illnesses can prevent episodes at these times.

The key to the treatment of these patients is careful documentation of the phenotype. Individuals with the benign form of isolated GKD have required no intervention, although the question has been raised whether metabolic stress might precipitate symptoms in them as well.[398] To date, however, no observations of symptomatic episodes have been reported in individuals or pedigrees with benign isolated GKD.

Diagnosis

All patients with GKD have shown evidence of hyperglycerolemia and glyceroluria. The glyceroluria frequently comes to attention during a general metabolic evaluation, which includes urine organic acid analysis by GC/MS. The glyceroluria is substantial in these patients, leading to contamination of the organic acid fraction by the neutral compound, glycerol, when a solvent extraction procedure is used.[4,56] If ion exchange chromatography is used in preparation of the specimen for GC/MS,[56,57] glycerol may not be seen with the organic acids but will be present in the neutral fraction.[4] Even using solvent extraction procedures, at least two individuals with GKD have been reported with negative initial urine screens for glycerol.[25,396] If glyceroluria is suspected, it is preferable for the GC/MS screen to be performed in a laboratory that has had previous experience in the evaluation of such patients. Quantitation of the urinary concentrations of glycerol in these patients has resulted in values of 41 to 345 millimolars (normal, ≤0.2 millimolars),[7,8,14–16,26–28,34,396,399,410] 90 to 193 mmol/mmol creatinine[55] (normal, not detectable),[25,411] or 11 to 360 mmol/24 h (normal, < 1 mmol/24 h).[6,32,58,400,401]

Hyperglycerolemia may come to attention during evaluation of pseudohypertriglyceridemia,[58] which in fact represents elevated free glycerol in the blood (see "Introduction and Historical Perspective"). Different methods of serum triglyceride measurement may give discrepant results, depending on the method used. The routine clinical laboratory method measures glycerol released after lipolysis; an alternative method relying on solvent extraction and colorimetry does not show interference by water-soluble compounds such as free glycerol.[6] The hyperglycerolemia in individuals with pseudohypertriglyceridemia has been measured in plasma and serum and has ranged from 1.8 to 8.3 millimolars (normal, 0.02 to 0.27 millimolars).[4,7,8,15,16,23,26–28,30,34,55,58,59,396,399–401,410] No differences in degree of glyceroluria or hyperglycerolemia were noted between the different phenotypes described above ("Clinical Aspects"), and the values may vary considerably even within the same individual.

Deficiency of GK activity has been documented in a number of tissues, including intact and disrupted leukocytes,[4,6,8,22,23,27,28,31,33,58,107,396,401] liver,[5,31,107,400] kidney,[5,107] small intestine,[5] adrenal gland,[31] intact and disrupted fibroblasts,[5,7,8,14,16,21,22,25,27,30,33,59,98,107,396] Epstein-Barr-virus-transformed lymphoblastoid cell lines,[21] and cultured amniotic fluid cells.[19,32] These have been assayed using radiochemical or spectrophotometric methods to measure glycerol conversion to glycerol 3-phosphate, to CO_2, to protein, or to phosphoglycerides and triacylglycerols. The radiochemical assay of glycerol GK activity[4,5,21,107] has been superior to the spectrophotometric assay in our hands. Because of the variability of this assay, some may find it helpful to measure the incorporation of labeled glycerol into trichloroacetic acid precipitable counts *in situ* in intact cells[21,25,27,59,107] in parallel with the *in vitro* assay. Incorporation of labeled glycerol into glycerolipids also distinguishes patients from controls.[98] Biochemical methods should be supplemented with molecular genetic diagnostic studies (see "Genetics" below).

Prenatal diagnosis has been successfully performed for GKD. One patient with a deletion resulting in AHC and GKD was diagnosed in utero using maternal estriol measurements before GKD was recognized in his family,[412] and two pregnancies at risk for CGKD with AHC, GKD, and DMD were diagnosed as normal using this approach.[413] GK activity is present in amniocytes.[413] A 26-year-old woman with a son who had died at 12 months of age with the CGKD phenotype, including AHC, GKD, and DMD, underwent amniocentesis at 18 weeks of pregnancy.[19,32] Radiochemical assay of GK activity in homogenates of cultured amniocytes revealed the enzyme deficiency. Total amniotic fluid glycerol (free and triglyceride bound) was 1.740±0.037 millimolar, which was 9.0 SD above the control mean and twice the highest control concentration. Analysis of DNA from cultured amniotic fluid cells and the aborted fetus confirmed the diagnosis of an affected fetus. Prenatal diagnosis performed in another pregnancy at risk for CGKD with AHC and GKD relied on amniotic fluid glycerol and maternal plasma estriol concentrations.[34] The limited genetic probes done in this region at that time did not detect a deletion or an informative polymorphism.[34] Exclusion of the CGKD in a fetus at risk for AHC, GKD, DMD, and OTC was performed using molecular genetic techniques.[10] These studies show that there are several different and complementary approaches to prenatal diagnosis of GKD.

Genetics

The *GK* gene maps to the Xp21 region, where the locus order is Xpter–*AHC-GKD-DMD*–cen (Fig. 97-5). See GenBank X78211 for genomic DNA and pseudogenes. This gene order was initially based on the clinical observation that if only two of these loci are involved, the patients have either AHC and GKD or GKD and DMD, but no patient has been described with AHC and DMD without GKD. Where sublocalization has been possible cytogenetically, it would appear that these deletions involve Xp21.3-p21.2.

An approximate scale for the genomic map in this region was developed by estimation of patient deletion sizes using bivariate flow karyotyping and correlating these results with clinical and molecular genetic data (Fig. 97-6).[49] Data derived from PFGE,[40,414] YACs,[50,415,416] and subsequent identification of

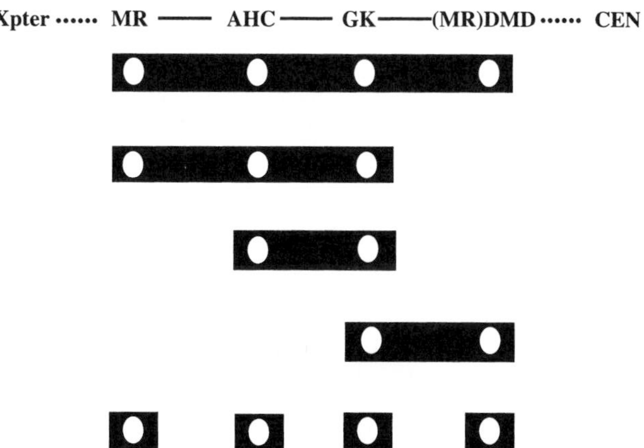

Fig. 97-5 Summary of clinical phenotypes involving the loci surrounding *GK*. The patients' phenotypes allowed ordering of the loci as shown. MR represents a separate locus causing mental retardation, while (MR)DMD represents the mental retardation sometimes seen in DMD patients. Some patients have MR, AHC, GK, and DMD. Some patients have MR, AHC, and GK. Others have AHC and GK, or GK and DMD. Still others have isolated MR, isolated AHC, isolated GK, or isolated DMD. Some DMD patients have associated MR.

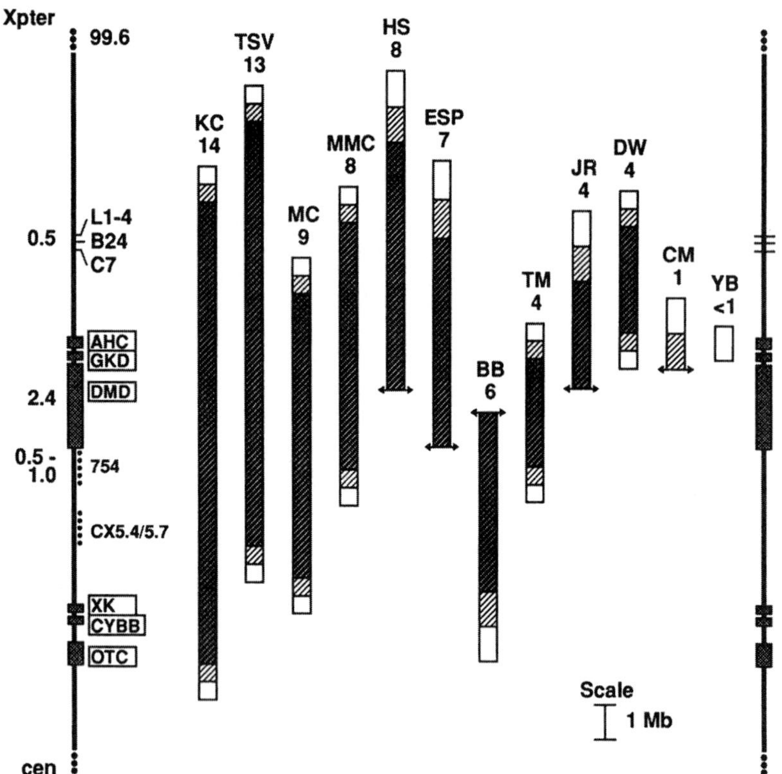

Fig. 97-6 Estimates of deletion sizes among patients with Xp21 contiguous gene syndromes correlated with clinical and molecular genetic data. The sizes of the patients' deletions were estimated using bivariate flow karyotyping and are represented by the vertical bars with the boundary between the open and lighter hatched sections indicating the mean estimate. The sizes of the mean estimates in megabases are shown above the bars and below the letter designations for the patients. The variance was considered to be ± 1 Mb. Breakpoints "anchored" within the DMD locus are shown by double-headed arrows. Loci appear on the left, with numbers to the left of this axis indicating estimates of physical sizes within the specified regions. (*From McCabe et al.*[49] *Used by permission of the publisher.*)

additional genes and markers in this region are consistent with this map (Fig. 97-7). These results indicate that AHC and GK are quite close physically, since the YB deletion affecting both loci was undetectable by these methods, implying it was 1 Mb or less in size. The results also show that AHC and GK are within 1 to 2 Mb of the telomeric end of DMD. These distance estimates are consistent with the observations that patients with CGKD are most likely to have the phenotype of AHC, GKD, and DMD, with deletion of all three loci, and that they are least likely to have the GKD and DMD phenotype, with the telomeric breakpoint between the AHC and GK loci.

Molecular genetic information on the deletions seen in patients with CGKD was crucial to characterization of GK cDNAs by three independent groups (GenBank L13943).[176–178] Partial human GK cDNAs from testis, brain, and liver were identified by sequencing of random clones[176] and by exon trapping,[177] and the complete human hepatic GK coding region was identified by a genomic scanning method.[178] The positional cloning strategies[177,178] relied on cosmids that mapped to the GK critical region defined by CGKD patients. Characterization of the clones isolated by all three of these methods included appropriate mapping in patient deletion panels. Analysis of the deduced amino acid sequence for human liver GK shows a striking similarity with the prokaryotic GK sequence: 50 percent identity and 65 percent similarity with the *E. coli* and 47 percent identity and 63 percent similarity with the *B. subtilis* enzymes[178,198,200] (Fig. 97-8). Human GK activity can be expressed in GK-deficient bacteria.[178] In addition, the three-dimensional crystal structure for *E. coli* GK has been solved, and comparison with the human GK structure indicates strong conservation of amino acid residues involved in substrate interaction.[178,234]

Correlation of human GK mutations with the structural features of the protein may provide insight into structure-function relationships for this protein. Four missense mutations have been

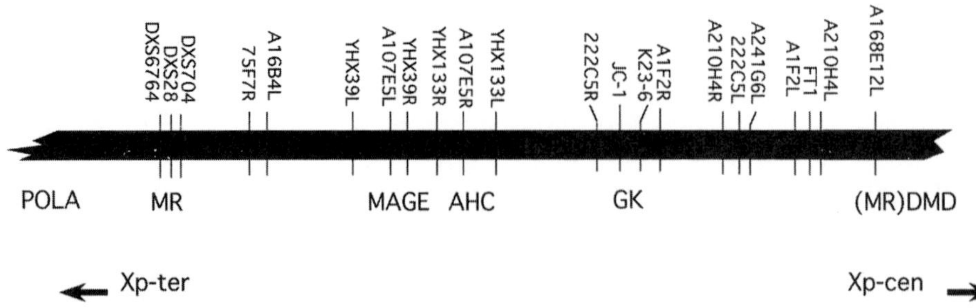

Fig. 97-7 Map of the region surrounding the AHC and GK loci. The Xp21 region, not drawn to scale, is shown, with markers above the chromosome (horizontal black bar) and gene locations below the chromosome. The positions of the cloned MAGE (MIM 300097), AHC (MIM 300200), GK (MIM 307030), and DMD (MIM 310200) loci are accurately localized. However, the positions of the two MR phenotypes observed among patients with deletions in this region, one of which may be due to disturbance of the CNS expression of dystrophin, are given only generally. The DNA polymerase alpha gene (*POLA*; MIM 312040) is telomeric to this region. (*This figure was drawn by W. Guo.*)

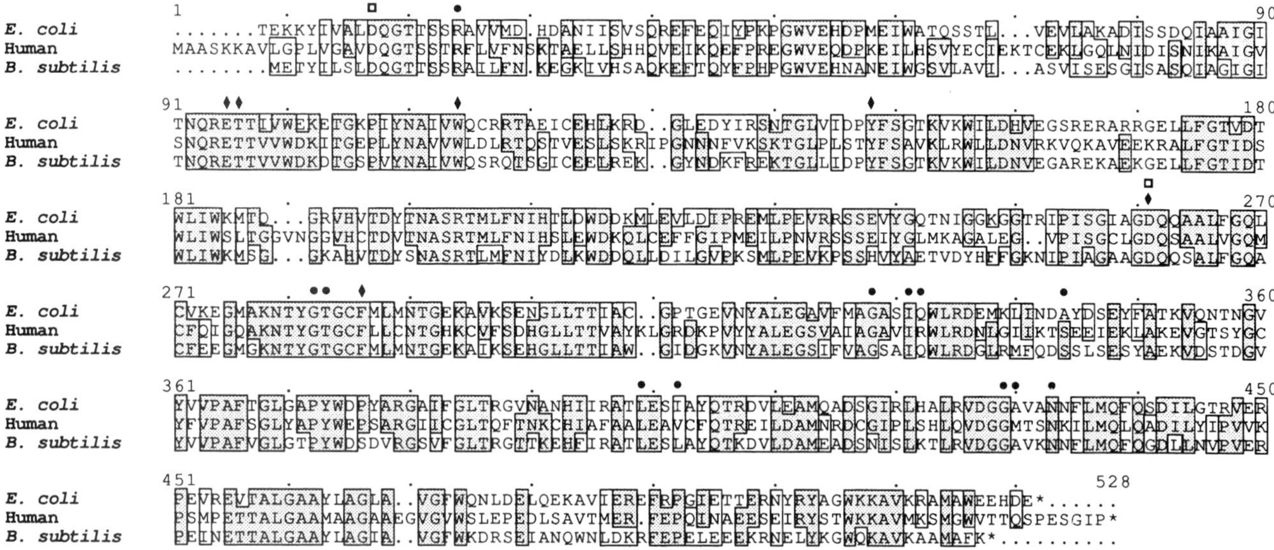

Fig. 97-8 Comparison of the deduced amino acid sequence for human hepatic GK with those for *E. coli* and *B. subtilis.* Amino acids in the prokaryotic sequences that are identical with (shaded) or similar to (open) those in human GK are shown in boxes. Symbols above the *E. coli* sequence show residues identified as interacting with the GK substrates:[234] open squares indicate interactions with Mg^{2+}; closed circles show interactions with ADP; and closed diamonds indicate interactions with glycerol. (*From Guo et al.*[178] *Used by the permission of the publisher.*)

described: two in symptomatic adult males with hyperglycerolemia noted incidentally (862A > G/N288D and 1313A > G/Q438R);[402] one in an infant boy with neonatal asphyxia but no subsequent problems (1823T > C/M428T);[402] and another in a 14-year-old male with mental retardation and no family history of mental retardation (1319A > T/D440V).[403] Knowledge of the crystal structure of prokaryotic GK[234] and its similarity with that of the human protein show that these mutations occur in a residue (M428) corresponding to an alanine in *E. coli* GK that is one member of a cluster of three amino acids interacting with ADP; near this cluster and involving absolutely conserved amino acids in *E. coli, B. subtilis,* and human (Q438 and D440); or in a residue (N288) that is identical in these three organisms and is near a conserved block of amino acids involved in glycerol and ADP binding. Therefore, each of these missense mutations alters an amino acid that has a defined function or is highly conserved.[402]

Understanding of the two additional intragenic mutations in GK relies on a knowledge of the genomic organization of this gene.[181,403] One was a 61-year-old male referred because of "refractory hypertriglyceridemia" due to hyperglycerolemia, who had chronic pancreatitis in the absence of alcohol abuse, gallstones, or hypertriglyceridemia. This man's genomic mutation involved a single base change, G > C, in the 3′ splice site of intron 6 (IVS6-1G > C), resulting in a 2-bp frameshift deletion of the first two nucleotides of exon 7, AG 553 and 554. Two brothers[410] had a genomic deletion resulting in loss of the 81-bp exon 17. Despite the same degree of enzyme deficiency in the two boys, the 7-year-old brother had severe mental retardation, seizures, bone dysplasia, fractures from minor trauma and abnormal teeth, and the 3-year-old brother was clinically normal. The authors speculated that their results might indicate ascertainment bias in identification of patients with signs and symptoms that are unrelated to the GKD; a role for precipitating factors, such as metabolic or environmental stress, in revealing the predisposition to symptoms among those with GKD, as has been suggested by others[398] (Bonham, personal communication); and/or possible interactions between *GK* mutations and other genetic polymorphisms in the individual.[403]

Investigation of the relationship between genotype and phenotype is required in additional patients, including those with the "classic" symptomatic, or juvenile, form of isolated GKD. If no obvious relationship can be determined between the *GK* genotype and phenotype, this may suggest the involvement of environmental/metabolic insult and/or modifying genes[398,403] (Bonham, personal communication). As more patients are ascertained and carefully characterized at the molecular genetic level, the results may either confirm the discrete clinical classification presented above or suggest that the spectrum of phenotypes is broader than previously recognized, with the distinctions between the "classic" clinical delineations less distinct.

Additional possible loci in this region have been suggested by the phenotypes of patients with deletions, including loci for mental retardation, Oregon eye disease (OED), and HH. All patients with the CGKD characterized by AHC, GKD, and DMD have been developmentally delayed, but three with AHC and GKD without myopathy have been reported to be normal developmentally,[21,34,36,417] suggesting the possibility of a mental retardation locus between GK and DMD or perhaps involving the DMD locus and affecting the brain expression of dystrophin or a related Xp21-encoded protein (Fig. 97-5).[418–423] There also appears to be one or more mental retardation loci telomeric to AHC, since patients with isolated AHC and DNA deletions have been mentally retarded[48,50,424] and a patient with an interstitial deletion distal to that involved in AHC had isolated mental retardation (Fig. 97-5).[425] A patient with AHC, GKD, DMD, and a visible Xp21 deletion was also noted to have typical ophthalmologic features of Åland Island eye disease (AIED).[39,42,43] However, since AIED[426,427] maps to Xp11.4-p11.23,[428] the nonallelic Xp21 locus for this phenotypically similar disorder was designated Oregon eye disease.[429] This retinal abnormality is now recognized to be due to loss or malfunction of dystrophin in patients with Becker or Duchenne muscular dystrophy.[430,431] An HH locus was proposed by two groups to be localized telomeric to AHC, based on deletions in patients.[31,33] But, as shown for OED, if a single gene product has pleiotropic effects, then deletion mapping will indicate that these characteristics appear to map adjacently. Individuals with isolated AHC had been reported with gonadotropin deficiency and cryptorchidism,[406,432] and the initial papers identifying *DAX1* as the gene responsible for AHC showed that individuals with intragenic mutations in *DAX1* had both AHC and

HH[404,405,433] (see Chap. 167). Therefore, among the phenotypes suggested by patients' deletions, to date there is clear evidence only for a distinct mental retardation (MR) locus telomeric to *DAX1*.

Pathogenesis

The possibility that the association between GKD and the other phenotypic features was not causal but rather coincidental was considered early in the description of this disorder, and it was hypothesized that these features might represent distinct but closely linked loci on the X chromosome.[7,332] It is now quite clear that this is a contiguous gene syndrome with involvement of discrete AHC, GK, and DMD loci. The size of the genomic region involved in complex GKD is variable but can be quite large[49] (Fig. 97-6), and undoubtedly additional genes that influence the patients' phenotypes will be identified in this region.

Patients with complex GKD and the juvenile form of GKD have episodic vomiting and acidemia, which responds to dietary limitation of glycerol, as noted previously. One could speculate that episodic vomiting and acidosis are associated with more significant mutations in the GK locus than those that cause the benign form of individuals with isolated GKD, but it has been suggested that those with the clinical appearance of the benign form of GKD have not been stressed metabolically.[398] Additional clinical experience and molecular genetic detail will be required to resolve this point. The similarity of these episodes with those observed among patients with glycerol intolerance is intriguing, as is the possibility that disrupted compartmentation of brain GK may play a role.

A mouse model of GKD has been generated by targeted disruption of the murine *Gyk* gene, and all of the hemizygous mutant males die by day 3 or 4 of life with no obvious cause of death.[434] The mutant males have striking hyperglycerolemia (>80-fold normal), indicating a very large flux of glycerol through glycerolipid metabolism, which is phosphorylated by Gyk for reutilization in normal animals. Elevation of plasma free fatty acid levels to approximately three times normal in mutant compared with wild type animals is consistent with a quantitatively important role for Gyk in free fatty acid reesterification, although increased free fatty acid synthesis in the *Gyk* knockout mice cannot be excluded as an alternative explanation. The potential involvement of these metabolic perturbations in the pathogenesis of Gyk deficiency in the mutant mice has yet to be determined. The Gyk protein shows near identity to the ATP-stimulated glucocorticoid receptor translocating promoter (ASTP), a rat liver histone-binding protein that increases the nuclear binding of the activated glucocorticoid receptor complex in the presence of ATP.[180] This sequence similarity has suggested that Gyk deficiency may result not only in hyperglycerolemia and glyceroluria but also in end-organ resistance to glucocorticoid action.[434] The neonatal lethality of the *Gyk* knockout mice has limited its utility in helping us understand the pathogenesis of symptomatic GKD.

Other Causes of Glyceroluria or Hyperglycerolemia

Glyceroluria was observed in four mentally retarded individuals among a group of 900 surveyed.[1] One of these had Down syndrome, and three were reported to have cerebral palsy. Subsequently, glyceroluria was recognized in a normal female.[2] Plasma glycerol concentrations were not elevated (patients, 0.06 to 0.10 millimolar; controls, 0.02 to 0.08 millimolar),[1] suggesting that these patients did not have generalized GKD.[5] Twenty boys with DMD were screened for glyceroluria, and one boy was positive.[15] His urinary glycerol ranged from 3.2 to 10 millimolar with a mean of 7.7 millimolar, which was 40 times the upper limit of normal (≤ 0.2 millimolar) but was less than the concentration in the GK-deficient patient (300 millimolar) examined by the same authors and was less than the values reported for other patients (see "Diagnosis"). Serum glycerol was normal (0.15 millimolar; normal, (≤ 0.2 millimolar), and fibroblast GK activity was above the control range for the authors' laboratory. This patient had no evidence of MR, adrenal hypoplasia, or cytogenetic or molecular deletions.

A series of 3450 urine specimens from healthy workers, adult psychiatric patients, and children selected for metabolic screening were evaluated for glyceroluria.[411] Only two were considered to have "major glyceroluria" (defined as 80 to 120 millimolar), and both of these patients had GKD.[21,25] Four adults and five children had "minor glyceroluria" (defined as 2 to 10 millimolar). Three healthy workers were not investigated further; the fourth was a 33-year-old woman with developmental delay and normal blood glycerol. Two of the children were sibs, a male and a female, with an unknown, familial progressive neurodegenerative disease, mild glyceroluria, and normal blood glycerol and fibroblast GK activity. A 2-year-old boy had mild congenital myopathy and persistent low-level glyceroluria. The fourth was a female infant with infantile spasms, and the fifth was a male, but no further information was available.

Hyperglycerolemia may be seen in patients with diabetes mellitus and hyperthyroidism.[5] The reported values are only severalfold higher than those in controls, and in our experience, even in patients with poorly controlled diabetes mellitus, hyperglycerolemia has not been similar to that in GKD patients. Therapeutic doses of glycerol may result in substantial hyperglycerolemia and glyceroluria,[5,391] as may diagnostic doses of glycerol[435] used for detection of endolymphatic hydrops in the differential diagnosis of low frequency hearing loss.[393]

Our experience in a metabolic screening laboratory indicates that the most common cause of glyceroluria not associated with GKD is contamination of the specimen by exogenous glycerol. Sources of contamination, especially in a "bagged" specimen collected from an infant, include glycerol-containing perineal lotions and glycerin suppositories. Other exogenous sources of glycerol include blood sampling tubes with glycerol-lubricated stoppers, detergents in the laboratory, filters used for sterilization of solutions, and moisturizing lotions used by laboratory personnel.[435]

GLYCEROL INTOLERANCE SYNDROME

Glycerol intolerance was initially described in a 3-year-old boy who presented at 11 months of age with the first of a series of episodes of pallor, sweating, and inability to be aroused.[3] His blood glucose level was 1.6 millimolar, and he improved with glucose administration; he was ketonuric. Subsequent episodes occurring in the fasting and nonfasting state included sweating, confusion, irritability, and marked lethargy. He weighed 2722 g at birth and was 3 weeks premature. There was a possible history of hypoglycemia in two of four paternal uncles. Intelligence and muscle tone were both normal. Oral glycerol tolerance tests were associated with similar episodes and, variably, with hypoglycemia. Hyperglycerolemia was seen only with glycerol loading, and only 1 percent of the glycerol was excreted in the urine. A more pronounced decrease was observed in the patient's serum dopamine β-hydroxylase after oral glycerol compared with control individuals, and prompted speculation regarding altered response of this patient's sympathetic nervous system to glycerol.[436] IV glycerol tolerance testing was associated with rapid loss of consciousness within 4 minutes of the start of the infusion. A generalized convulsive jerk was followed by coma, unreactive constricted pupils, pallor, sweating, and decreased response to pain, but no hypoglycemia. After 1 hour the patient returned to normal. Similar doses of glycerol were not associated with these problems in other children or adults. In the patient's leukocytes, accumulation of phosphorylated products of glycerol, oxidation of glycerol 3-phosphate, and fructose 1,6-bisphosphatase activity were normal. The boy was placed on a low-fat diet and improved, although episodes continued with increased fat intake, infection, or emotional crisis.

Two other patients, one male and one female, have subsequently been reported with the glycerol intolerance syndrome.[437,438] Both were premature–2300 g at 36 weeks and 1850 g at 34 weeks, respectively. The boy had an episode of hypoglycemia at 16 h of age, then had consistent morning irritability relieved by food; at 4.5 years he was hypoglycemic with vomiting and seizures following milk ingestion after an overnight fast.[437] A similar episode with coma was observed 1 month later after a 12-h fast. A liver biopsy revealed mitochondrial swelling and occasional mitochondrial inclusions. On a low-fat diet with frequent snacks, he remained well over the ensuing 2 years. The girl had the first of her recurring hypoglycemic episodes at 5 months of age.[438] Seizures were not observed with all these episodes, and no food intolerances were appreciated. She had a positive family history for chronic seizure disorder and a mentally retarded second cousin. At 5 years 9 months she was begun on a regimen of frequent feedings and avoidance of fatty foods or long fasts and a brief regimen of folic acid administration. She had improved tolerance to fasting and to glycerol after 6 weeks on folic acid therapy. She developed normally and at 15 years 4 months had an improved response to a glycerol tolerance test.

Hepatic activity levels of fructose 1,6-bisphosphatase were less than one-third of control values in both of the last two patients.[437,438] Hepatic cGDPH:NAD and mGPDH:FAD were also measured and found to be decreased in the boy; GK was among the enzymes with normal activity levels in this patient.[437] His hepatic fructose 1,6-bisphosphatase was more sensitive to inhibition by glycerol 3-phosphate than those of controls.[437] The girl's leukocyte fructose 1,6-bisphosphatase activity improved after folic acid treatment and was normal at 15 years 4 months.

It has been suggested that the glycerol intolerance syndrome represents a sensitivity to the hypoglycemic effects of glycerol 3-phosphate, possibly due to delayed maturation of enzymes of the pathway of glycerol metabolism.[383,437,438] The exaggerated hypoglycemic response of malnourished weanling rats to glycerol 3-phosphate[383] and the suggestion that the glycerol intolerance syndrome may represent delayed maturation of glycerol metabolism are interesting in view of the fact that the three reported patients were all born prematurely. Improvement of the patients with age might reflect the decreasing metabolic demands of the liver with age.[438] The clinical similarity between the patients with glycerol intolerance and some of those with symptomatic GKD is quite striking (see "Clinical Aspects" above). This prompted speculation that although GK activity was normal in the glycerol-intolerant patients, compartmentation of this enzyme could be disrupted.[332,334] An alternative hypothesis is that the glycerol intolerance syndrome represents a block in glycerol uptake due to a mutation in the carrier protein that mediates the facilitated diffusion of glycerol across the plasma membrane.[69]

The glycerol intolerance syndrome should be considered in the differential diagnosis of the child with fasting or nonfasting hypoglycemia or with an unusual clinical or metabolic response to glycerol, medium-chain triglycerides, or dietary fat.

REFERENCES

1. Pitkanen E, Palo J: Increased excretion of glycerol in four patients with mental retardation. *Ann Med Exp Fenn* **45**:90, 1967.
2. Palo J, Servo C, Pitkanen E, Tammisto P: Increased urinary excretion of glycerol: Metabolic studies on a patient. *Clin Chim Acta* **80**:391, 1977.
3. Maclaren NK, Cowles C, Ozand PT, Shuttee R, Cornblath M: Glycerol intolerance in a child with intermittent hypoglycemia. *J Pediatr* **86**:43, 1975.
4. McCabe ERB, Fennessey PV, Guggenheim MA, Miles BS, Bullen WW, Sceats DJ, Goodman SI: Human glycerol kinase deficiency with hyperglycerolemia and glyceroluria. *Biochem Biophys Res Commun* **78**:1327, 1977.
5. Guggenheim MA, McCabe ERB, Roig M, Goodman SI, Lum GM, Bullen WW, Ringel SP: Glycerol kinase deficiency with neuromuscular, skeletal and adrenal abnormalities. *Ann Neurol* **7**:441, 1980.
6. Rose CI, Haines DSM: Familial hyperglycerolemia. *J Clin Invest* **61**:163, 1978.
7. Bartley JA, Miller DK, Hayford JT, McCabe ERB: The concordance of X-linked glycerol kinase deficiency with X-linked adrenal hypoplasia in two families. *Lancet* **2**:733, 1982.
8. Renier WO, Nabbe FAE, Hustinx TWJ, Veerkamp JH, Otten BJ, Ter Laak HJ, Ter Haar BGA, et al: Congenital adrenal hypoplasia, progressive muscular dystrophy, and severe mental retardation, in association with glycerol kinase deficiency, in male sibs. *Clin Genet* **24**:243, 1983.
9. Hammond J, Howard NJ, Brookwell R, Purvis-Smith S, Wilcken B, Hoogenraad N: Proposed assignment of loci for X-linked adrenal hypoplasia and glycerol kinase genes. *Lancet* **1**:54, 1985.
10. Old JM, Briand PL, Purvis-Smith S, Howard NJ, Wilcken B, Hammond J, Pearson P, et al: Prenatal exclusion of ornithine transcarbamylase deficiency by direct gene analysis. *Lancet* **1**:73, 1985.
11. Patil SR, Bartley JA, Murray JC, Ionasescu VV, Pearson PL: X-linked glycerol kinase, adrenal hypoplasia and myopathy map at Xp21. *Cytogenet Cell Genet* **40**:720, 1985.
12. Wieringa B, Hustinx T, Scheres J, Hofker M, Ropers HH, ter Haar B: Glycerol kinase deficiency syndrome explained as X-chromosomal deletion. *Cytogenet Cell Genet* **40**:777, 1985.
13. Wieringa B, Hustinx T, Scheres J, Renier W, ter Haar B: Complex glycerol kinase deficiency syndrome explained as X-chromosomal deletion. *Clin Genet* **27**:522, 1985.
14. Bartley JA, Patil S, Davenport S, Goldstein D, Pickens J: Duchenne muscular dystrophy, glycerol kinase deficiency, and adrenal insufficiency associated with Xp21 interstitial deletion. *J Pediatr* **108**:189, 1986.
15. Clarke A, Roberts SH, Thomas NST, Whitfield A, Williams J, Harper PS: Duchenne muscular dystrophy with adrenal insufficiency and glycerol kinase deficiency: High resolution cytogenetic analysis with molecular, biochemical and clinical studies. *J Med Genet* **23**:501, 1986.
16. Dunger DB, Davies KE, Pembrey M, Lake B, Pearson P, Williams D, Whitfield A, et al: Deletion of the X chromosome detected by direct DNA analysis in one of two unrelated boys with glycerol kinase deficiency, adrenal hypoplasia, and Duchenne muscular dystrophy. *Lancet* **1**:585, 1986.
17. Saito F, Goto J, Kakinuma H, Nakamura F, Murayama S, Nakano I, Tonomura A: Inherited Xp21 deletion in a boy with complex glycerol kinase deficiency syndrome. *Clin Genet* **29**:92, 1986.
18. van Ommen GJB, Verkerk JMH, Hofker MH, Monaco AP, Kunkel LM, Ray P, Worton R, et al: A physical map of 4 million bp around the Duchenne muscular dystrophy gene on the human X-chromosome. *Cell* **47**:499, 1986.
19. Borresen A-L, Hellerud C, Moller P, Sovik O, Berg K: Prenatal diagnosis associated with a DNA deletion on the short arm of the X-chromosome. *Clin Genet* **32**:254, 1987.
20. Chelly J, Marlhens F, van Ommen GJB, Dutrillaux B, Harpey JP, Fardeau M, Kaplan JC: Mapping of glycerol kinase (GK) and congenital adrenal hypoplasia (AHC) between J66-H1 (in DMD locus) and L1 (DXS68). *Cytogenet Cell Genet* **46**:592, 1987.
21. Francke U, Harper JF, Darras BT, Cowan JM, McCabe ERB, Kohlschutter A, Seltzer WK, et al: Congenital adrenal hypoplasia, myopathy and glycerol kinase deficiency: Molecular genetic evidence for deletions. *Am J Hum Genet* **40**:212, 1987.
22. Goonewardena P, Dahl N, Ritzen M, Pettersson U: Deletion in Xp associated with glycerol kinase deficiency, adrenal aplasia and hypogonadotropic hypogonadism. *Cytogenet Cell Genet* **46**:621, 1987.
23. Kakinuma H, Nakamura F, Murayama S, Goto J, Nakano I, Saito F, Ohtake A, et al: A case with the infantile type of glycerol kinase deficiency. *Acta Paediatr Jpn* **29**:465, 1987.
24. Kenwrick S, Patterson M, Speer A, Fischbeck K, Davies K: Molecular analysis of the Duchenne muscular dystrophy region using pulsed field gel electrophoresis. *Cell* **48**:351, 1987.
25. Kohlschutter A, Willig RP, Schlamp D, Kruse K, McCabe ERB, Schafer HJ, Beckenkamp G, et al: Infantile glycerol kinase deficiency–A condition requiring prompt identification–Clinical, biochemical and morphological findings in two cases. *Eur J Pediatr* **146**:575, 1987.
26. Marlhens F, Chelly J, Kaplan JC, Lefrancois D, Harpey JP, Dutrillaux B: Familial deletion of Xp21.2 with glycerol kinase deficiency and congenital adrenal hypoplasia. *Hum Genet* **77**:379, 1987.
27. Wise JE, Matalon R, Morgan AM, McCabe ERB: Phenotypic features of patients with congenital adrenal hypoplasia and glycerol kinase deficiency. *Am J Dis Child* **141**:744, 1987.

28. Chelly J, Marlhens F, Dutrillaux B, van Ommen GJ, Lambert M, Haioun B, Boissinot G, et al: Deletion proximal to DXS 68 locus (L1 probe site) in a boy with Duchenne muscular dystrophy, glycerol kinase deficiency, and adrenal hypoplasia. *Hum Genet* **78**:222, 1988.
29. Darras BT, Francke U: Myopathy in complex glycerol kinase deficiency patients is due to 3′ deletions of the dystrophin gene. *Am J Hum Genet* **43**:126, 1988.
30. Davies KE, Patterson M, Kenwrick SM, Bell M, Sloan HR, Westman JA, Elsas LJ, et al: Fine mapping of glycerol kinase deficiency and adrenal hypoplasia within Xp21 on the short arm of the human X chromosome. *Am J Med Genet* **29**:557, 1988.
31. Matsumoto T, Kondoh T, Yoshimoto M, Fujieda K, Matsuura N, Matsuda I, Miike T, et al: Complex glycerol kinase deficiency: Molecular genetic, cytogenetic, and clinical studies of five Japanese patients. *Am J Med Genet* **31**:603, 1988.
32. Sovik O, Jellum E, Madsen B: Glyceroluria with adrenocortical insufficiency, developmental delay and early death. *J Inher Metab Dis* **11**:304, 1988.
33. Goonewardena P, Dahl N, Ritzen M, van Ommen GJ, Pettersson U: Molecular Xp deletion in a male: Suggestion of a locus for hypogonadotropic hypogonadism distal to the glycerol kinase and adrenal hypoplasia loci. *Clin Genet* **35**:5, 1989.
34. Malpuech G, Dastugue B, Giraud G, Jouanel P, Vanlieferinghen P, Carla H: Prenatal diagnosis of X-linked adrenal hypoplasia associated with glycerol kinase deficiency. *J Genet Hum* **37**:155, 1989.
35. McCabe ERB, Towbin J, Chamberlain J, Baumbach L, Witkowski J, van Ommen GJB, Koenig M, et al: Complementary DNA probes for the Duchenne muscular dystrophy locus demonstrate a previously undetectable deletion in a patient with dystrophic myopathy, glycerol kinase deficiency and congenital adrenal hypoplasia. *J Clin Invest* **83**:95, 1989.
36. Oleesky DA, Hakeem V: Congenital adrenal hypoplasia and glycerol kinase deficiency. *Acta Paediatr Scand* **78**:893, 1989.
37. Seltzer WK, McCabe ERB: Glycerol kinase deficiency: Association with Duchenne muscular dystrophy, adrenal insufficiency and mental retardation, in Rowland LP (ed): *Molecular Genetics and Clinical Neurology.* New York, Oxford, 1989, p 380.
38. Towbin JA, Wu D, Chamberlain J, Larsen PD, Seltzer WK, McCabe ERB: Characterization of patients with glycerol kinase deficiency utilizing cDNA probes for the Duchenne muscular dystrophy locus. *Hum Genet* **83**:122, 1989.
39. Weleber RG, Pillers DM, Hanna CE, Powell B, Magenis RE, Buist NRM: Åland island eye disease (Forsius-Eriksson syndrome) associated with contiguous gene syndrome at Xp21: Similarity to incomplete congenital stationary night blindness. *Arch Ophthalmol* **107**:1170, 1989.
40. Love DR, Bloomfield JF, Kenwrick SJ, Yates JRW, Davies KE: Physical mapping distal to the DMD locus. *Genomics* **8**:106, 1990.
41. Love DR, Flint TJ, Marsden RF, Bloomfield JF, Daniels RJ, Forrest SM, Gabrielli O, et al: Characterization of deletions in the dystrophin gene giving mild phenotypes. *Am J Med Genet* **37**:136, 1990.
42. Pillers DM, Towbin JA, Chamberlain JS, Wu D, Ranier J, Powell BR, McCabe ERB: Deletion mapping of Åland island eye disease to Xp21 between DXS67 (B24) and Duchenne muscular dystrophy. *Am J Hum Genet* **47**:795, 1990.
43. Pillers DM, Weleber RG, Powell B, Hanna CE, Magenis RE, Buist NRM: Åland island eye disease (Forsius-Eriksson ocular albinism) and an Xp21 deletion in a patient with Duchenne muscular dystrophy, glycerol kinase deficiency, and congenital adrenal hypoplasia. *Am J Med Genet* **36**:23, 1990.
44. Tonoki H, Fujieda K, Kajii N, Ozutsumi K, Nagano S, Niikawa N: Negative dystrophin staining in muscles of patients with complex glycerol kinase deficiency. *J Pediatr* **117**:268, 1990.
45. Towbin JA, Chamberlain JS, Wu D, Pillers DM, Seltzer WK, McCabe ERB: DXS28 maps centromeric to DXS68 and DXS67 by deletion analysis. *Genomics* **7**:442, 1990.
46. Sakura N, Nishimura S, Kawahara N, Komazawa Y, Yamaguchi S: Asthma as the first presenting symptom of complex glycerol kinase deficiency. *Acta Paediatr Scand* **80**:723, 1991.
47. Stuhrmann M, Heilbronner H, Reis A, Wegner RD, Fischer P, Schmidtke J: Characterization of a Xp21 microdeletion syndrome in a 2-year-old boy with muscular dystrophy, glycerol kinase deficiency and adrenal hypoplasia congenita. *Hum Genet* **86**:414, 1991.
48. Worley KC, Towbin JA, Zhu XM, Barker DF, Ballabio A, Chamberlain J, Biesecker LG, et al: Identification of three new markers in Xp21 between DXS28 (C7) and DMD. *Genomics* **13**:957, 1992.
49. McCabe ERB, Towbin JA, van den Engh GJ, Trask BJ: Xp21 contiguous gene syndromes: Deletion quantitation with bivariate flow karyotyping allows mapping of patient breakpoints. *Am J Hum Genet* **51**:1277, 1992.
50. Worley KC, Ellison KA, Zhang Y-H, Wang D-F, Mason J, Roth EJ, Adams V, et al: Yeast artificial chromosome cloning in the glycerol kinase and adrenal hypoplasia congenita region of Xp21. *Genomics* **16**:407, 1993.
51. Hofker MH, Bergen AAB, Skraastad MI, Bakker E, Francke U, Wieringa B, Bartley J, et al: Isolation of a random cosmid clone, which defines a new polymorphic locus DXS148 near the locus for Duchenne muscular dystrophy. *Hum Genet* **74**:275, 1986.
52. Vogiatzi MG, Gunn SK, Scheuerle A, McCabe ERB, Copeland KC: Adrenal crisis in the newborn: Details leading to correct diagnosis. *J Clin Endo Metab* **80**:1079, 1995.
53. Scheuerle A, Greenberg F, McCabe ERB: Dysmorphic features in patients with complex glycerol kinase deficiency. *J Pediatr* **126**:764, 1995.
54. Worley KC, Lindsay EA, Bailey W, Wise J, McCabe ERB, Baldini A: Rapid molecular cytogenetic analysis of X-chromosomal microdeletions: Fluorescence in situ hybridization (FISH) for complex glycerol kinase deficiency. *Am J Med Genet* **57**:615, 1995.
55. Baranzini SE, del Rey G, Nigro N, Szijan I, Chamoles N, Cresto JC: Patient with an Xp21 contiguous gene deletion syndrome in association with agenesis of the corpus callosum. *Am J Med Genet* **70**:216, 1997.
56. Goodman SI, Markey SP: *Diagnosis of Organic Acidemias by Gas Chromatography—Mass Spectrometry.* New York, Liss, 1981.
57. Chalmers RA, Lawson AM: *Organic Acids in Man–Analytical Chemistry, Biochemistry and Diagnosis of the Organic Acidurias.* New York, Chapman & Hall, 1982.
58. Goussault Y, Turpin E, Neel D, Dreux C, Chann B, Bakir R, Rouffy J: "Pseudohypertriglyceridemia" caused by hyperglycerolemia due to congenital enzyme deficiency. *Clin Chim Acta* **123**:269, 1982.
59. Ginns EI, Barranger JA, McClean SW, Schaefer E, Brady RO, Young R, Goodman SI, et al: Juvenile form of glycerol kinase deficiency with episodic vomiting, acidemia and stupor. *J Pediatr* **104**:736, 1984.
60. Hanke ME: The physiological action of glycerol, in Miner CS, Dalton NN (eds): *Glycerol.* New York, Reinhold, 1953 p 402.
61. Borchgrevink CF, Havel RJ: Transport of glycerol in human blood. *Proc Soc Exp Biol Med* **113**:946, 1963.
62. Shafrir E, Gorin E: Release of glycerol in conditions of fat mobilization and deposition. *Metabolism* **12**:58, 1963.
63. Havel RJ: Some influences of the sympathetic nervous system and insulin in mobilization of fat from adipose tissue: Studies of the turnover rates of free fatty acids and glycerol. *Ann NY Acad Sci* **131**:91, 1965.
64. Ballard FJ, Hanson RW, Leveille GA: Phosphoenolpyruvate carboxykinase and the synthesis of glyceride-glycerol from pyruvate in adipose tissue. *J Biol Chem* **242**:2746, 1967.
65. Bjorntorp P, Bergman H, Varnauskas E, Lindholm B: Lipid mobilization in relation to body composition in man. *Metabolism* **18**:840, 1969.
66. Bortz WM, Paul P, Haff AC, Holmes WL: Glycerol turnover and oxidation in man. *J Clin Invest* **51**:1537, 1972.
67. Reshef L, Meyuhas O, Boshwitz CH, Hanson RW, Ballard FJ: Physiological role and regulation of glyceroneogenesis in rat adipose tissue. *Isr J Med Sci* **8**:372, 1972.
68. Shreeve WW: *Physiological Chemistry of Carbohydrates in Mammals.* Philadelphia, Saunders, 1974.
69. Lin ECC: Glycerol utilization and its regulation in mammals. *Annu Rev Biochem* **46**:765, 1977.
70. Catron LF, Lewis HB: The formation of glycogen in the liver of the young white rat after the oral administration of glycerol. *J Biol Chem* **84**:553, 1929.
71. Shapiro I: Studies on ketosis. V. The comparative glycogenetic and ketolytic action of glucose and some carbohydrate intermediates. *J Biol Chem* **108**:373, 1935.
72. Doerschuk AP: Some studies on the metabolism of glycerol-1-^{14}C. *J Biol Chem* **193**:39, 1951.
73. Ashmore J, Renold AE, Nesbett FB, Hastings AB: Studies on carbohydrate in rat liver slices. V. Glycerol metabolism in relation to substrates in normal and diabetic tissue. *J Biol Chem* **215**:153, 1955.
74. Noble EP, Stjernholm RL, Weisberger AS: Carbohydrate metabolism in the leukocytes. I. The pathway of two- and three-carbon compounds in the rabbit polymorphonuclear leukocyte. *J Biol Chem* **235**:1261, 1960.

75. Jans AW, Willem R: ^{13}C-NMR study of glycerol metabolism in rabbit renal cells of proximal convoluted tubules. *Eur J Biochem* **174**:67, 1988.
76. Voegtlin C, Thompson JW, Dunn ER: Hyperglycemia produced by glycerol. *J Biol Chem* **64**:639, 1925.
77. Chambers WH, Deuel HJ: Animal calorimetry. XXX. The metabolism of glycerol in phlorizen diabetes. *J Biol Chem* **65**:21, 1925.
78. Nikkila EA, Ojala K: Gluconeogenesis from glycerol in fasting rats. *Life Sci* **3**:243, 1964.
79. Bergman EN: Glycerol turnover in the nonpregnant and ketotic pregnant sheep. *Am J Physiol* **215**:865, 1968.
80. Robinson JA, Newsholme EA: The effects of dietary conditions on glycerol uptake by rat liver and kidney-cortex slices. *Biochem J* **112**:449, 1969.
81. Winkler B, Rathgeb I, Steele R, Altszuler N: Conversion of glycerol to glucose in the normal dog. *Am J Physiol* **219**:497, 1970.
82. Wishnofsky M, Kane AP, Spitz WC, Michalover S, Byron CS: Influence of glycerol on glycemia in normal and diabetic individuals. *J Lab Clin Med* **26**:526, 1940.
83. Senior B, Loridan L: Studies of liver glycogenoses with particular reference to the metabolism of intravenously administered glycerol. *N Engl J Med* **279**:958, 1968.
84. Vidnes J, Sovik O: Gluconeogenesis in infancy and childhood. *Acta Paediatr Scand* **65**:297, 1976.
85. Wolf H, Melichar V, Michaelis R: Elimination of intravenously administered glycerol from the blood of newborns. *Biol Neonate* **12**:162, 1968.
86. Ferber J, Rabinowitsch S: Increase in blood sugar following the ingestion of glycerol. *Am J Med Sci* **177**:827, 1929.
87. D'Alena P, Ferguson W: Adverse effects after glycerol orally and parenterally. *Arch Ophthalmol* **75**:201, 1966.
88. Pelkonen R, Nikkila EA, Kekki M: Metabolism of glycerol in diabetes mellitus. *Diabetologia* **3**:1, 1967.
89. Sears ES: Nonketotic hyperosmolar hyperglycemia during glycerol therapy for cerebral edema. *Neurology* **26**:89, 1976.
90. Senior B, Loridan L: Gluconeogenesis and insulin in the ketotic variety of childhood hypoglycemia and in control children. *J Pediatr* **74**:529, 1969.
91. Senior B, Loridan L: Functional differentiation of glycogenoses of the liver with respect to the use of glycerol. *N Engl J Med* **279**:965, 1968.
92. Gilbert M: Origin and metabolic fate of plasma glycerol in the rat and rabbit fetus. *Pediatr Res* **11**:95, 1977.
93. Marinetti GV: Biosynthesis of triglycerides, in Dawson RMC, Rhodes DN (eds): *Comprehensive Biochemistry* vol 18. *Lipid Metabolism*, New York, Wiley, 1964, p 71.
94. Rognstad R, Clark DG, Katz J: Pathways of glyceride glycerol synthesis. *Biochem J* **140**:249, 1974.
95. Lamb RG, Wood CK, Landa BM, Guzelian PS, Fallon HJ: Studies of the formation and release of glycerolipids by primary monolayer cultures of adult rat hepatocytes. *Biochim Biophys Acta* **489**:318, 1977.
96. Wood CK, Lamb RG: The effect of ethanol on glycerolipid biosynthesis by primary monolayer cultures of adult rat hepatocytes. *Biochim Biophys Acta* **572**:121, 1979.
97. Farese RV: Phosphoinositide metabolism and hormone action. *Endocr Rev* **4**:78, 1983.
98. Bartley JA, Ward R: Glycerol kinase deficiency inhibits glycerol utilization in phosphoglyceride and triacylglycerol biosynthesis. *Pediatr Res* **19**:313, 1985.
99. Rasmussen H: The calcium messenger system. *N Engl J Med* **314**:1094, 1986.
100. Uhal BD, Longmore WJ: Glycerol metabolism in type II pneumocytes isolated from streptozotocin-diabetic rats. *Biochim Biophys Acta* **958**:279, 1988.
101. Hajra AK, Agranoff BW: Acyl dihydroxyacetone phosphate–Characterization of a ^{32}P-labeled lipid from guinea pig liver mitochondria. *J Biol Chem* **243**:1617, 1968.
102. Hajra AK: Biosynthesis of glycerolipids via acyldihydroxyacetone phosphate. *Biochem Soc Trans* **5**:34, 1977.
103. Hajra AK, Bishop JE: Glycerolipid biosynthesis in peroxisomes via the acyl dihydroxyacetone phosphate pathway. *Ann NY Acad Sci* **386**:170, 1982.
104. Ballas LM, Lazarow PB, Bell RM: Glycerolipid synthetic capacity of rat liver peroxisomes. *Biochim Biophys Acta* **795**:297, 1984.
105. Esmann V: Dihydroxyacetone as an intermediate during the metabolism of glycerol and glyceraldehyde in leukocytes from rat. *Acta Chem Scand* **22**:2281, 1968.
106. Rofe AM, James HM, Bais R, Edwards JB, Conyers RA: The production of (^{14}C)-oxalate during the metabolism of (^{14}C)-carbohydrates in isolated rat hepatocytes. *Aust J Exp Biol Med Sci* **58**:103, 1980.
107. Winters DK, Cederbaum AI: Oxidation of glycerol to formaldehyde by rat liver microsomes. Effects of cytochrome P-450 inducing agents. *Biochem Pharmacol* **39**:697, 1990.
108. McCabe ERB, Sadava D, Bullen WW, Seltzer WK, McKelvey HA, Rose CI: Human glycerol kinase deficiency: Enzyme kinetics and fibroblast hybridization. *J Inher Metab Dis* **5**:177, 1982.
109. International Union of Biochemistry: *Enzyme Nomenclature 1984*. Orlando, Academic, 1984.
110. Thorner JW, Paulus H: Glycerol and glycerate kinases, in Boyer D (ed): *The Enzymes* vol 8, New York, Academic, 1973 p 487.
111. Kennedy EP: Synthesis of phosphatides in isolated mitochondria. *J Biol Chem* **201**:399, 1953.
112. Bublitz C, Kennedy EP: Synthesis of phosphatides in isolated mitochondria. III. The enzymatic phosphorylation of glycerol. *J Biol Chem* **211**:951, 1954.
113. Bublitz C, Kennedy EP: A note on the asymmetrical metabolism of glycerol. *J Biol Chem* **211**:963, 1954.
114. Bublitz C, Wieland O: Glycerokinase. *Meth Enzymol* **5**:354, 1962.
115. Grunnet N, Lundquist F: Kinetics of glycerol kinases from mammalian liver and *Candida mycoderma*. *Eur J Biochem* **3**:78, 1967.
116. Robinson J, Newsholme EA: Inhibition of liver glycerol kinase by adenosine monophosphate and L-alpha-glycerophosphate. *Biochem J* **104**:70P, 1967.
117. Tepperman HM, Tepperman J: Adaptive changes in alpha-glycerophosphate-generating enzymes in rat liver. *Am J Physiol* **214**:67, 1968.
118. Robinson J, Newsholme EA: Some properties of hepatic glycerol kinase and their relation to the control of glycerol utilization. *Biochem J* **112**:455, 1969.
119. Kampf SC, Seitz HJ, Tarnowski W: Regulation of glycerol metabolism. I. Hormonal and metabolic control of rat liver glycerol kinase activity. *Hoppe-Seyler's Z Physiol Chem* **351**:32, 1970.
120. Lech JJ: Glycerol kinase and glycerol utilization in trout (*Salmo gairdneri*) liver. *Comp Biochem Physiol* **34**:117, 1970.
121. Krause R, Wolf H: Glyzerokinase der schweineleber. I. Allgemeine und kinetische eigenschaften des enzymes. *Acta Biol Med Ger* **33**:385, 1974.
122. Krause R, Wolf H: Glyzerokinase der schweineleber. II. Postnatale entwicklung und intrazellulare verteilung des enzymes. *Acta Biol Med Ger* **33**:393, 1974.
123. Schneider PB: Activation of bovine liver glycerol kinase by ethanol. *Biochim Biophys Acta* **397**:110, 1975.
124. Gardner LB, Reiser S: Serum glycerol and hepatic glycerokinase activity in the carbohydrate-sensitive BHE strain of rat. *Proc Soc Exp Biol Med* **153**:158, 1976.
125. Divakaran P: Regulation of liver lipogenic enzymes by dietary fats. *Experientia* **32**:1128, 1976.
126. Seltzer WK, Bullen WW, McCabe ERB: Human glycerol kinase: Comparison of properties from fibroblasts and liver. *Life Sci* **32**:1721, 1983.
127. Ostlund AK, Gohring U, Krause J, Brdiczka D: The binding of glycerol kinase to the outer membrane of rat liver mitochondria: Its importance in metabolic regulation. *Biochem Med* **30**:231, 1983.
128. Li CC, Lin ECC: Glycerol transport and phosphorylation by rat hepatocytes. *J Cell Physiol* **117**:230, 1983.
129. Pittner RA, Fears R, Brindley DN: Effects of cyclic AMP, glucocorticoids and insulin on the activities of phosphatidate phosphohydrolase, tyrosine aminotransferase and glycerol kinase in isolated rat hepatocytes in relation to the control of triacylglycerol synthesis and gluconeogenesis. *Biochem J* **225**:455, 1985.
130. Kalckar H: Phosphorylation in kidney tissue. *Enzymologia* **2**:47, 1937.
131. Kalckar H: LXXVIII. The nature of phosphoric esters formed in kidney extracts. *Biochem J* **33**:631, 1939.
132. Ackerman RH: Auswirkungen parenteraler glycerinzufuhr auf die glycerokinase-aktivitat und den adenosintriphosphatspiegel in der niere von ratten. *Res Exp Med (Berl)* **166**:251, 1975.
133. Wirthensohn G, Vandewalle A, Guder WG: Renal glycerol metabolism and the distribution of glycerol kinase in rabbit nephron. *Biochem J* **198**:543, 1981.
134. Burch HB, Hays AE, McCreary MD, Cole BR, Chi MM, Dence CN, Lowry OH: Relationships in different parts of the nephron between enzymes of glycerol metabolism and the metabolite changes which result from large glycerol loads. *J Biol Chem* **257**:3676, 1982.

135. Haessler HA, Isslebacher KJ: The metabolism of glycerol by intestinal mucosa. *Biochim Biophys Acta* **73**:427, 1963.
136. Jenkins BT, Hajra AK: Glycerol kinase and dihydroxyacetone kinase in rat brain. *J Neurochem* **26**:377, 1976.
137. Tildon JT, Stevenson JH, Ozand PT: Mitochondrial glycerol kinase activity in rat brain. *Biochem J* **157**:513, 1976.
138. Kaneko M, Kurokawa M, Ishibashi S: Binding and function of mitochondrial glycerol kinase in comparison with those of mitochondrial hexokinase. *Arch Biochem Biophys* **237**:135, 1985.
139. Seltzer WK, McCabe ERB: Human and rat adrenal glycerol kinase: Subcellular distribution and bisubstrate kinetics. *Mol Cell Biochem* **62**:43, 1984.
140. Seltzer WK, McCabe ERB: Subcellular distribution and kinetic properties of soluble and particulate-associated bovine adrenal glycerol kinase. *Mol Cell Biochem* **64**:51, 1984.
141. Koschinsky T, Gries FA, Herberg L: Glycerol kinase activity in isolated fat cells of BHob mice. *Horm Metab Res* **2**:185, 1970.
142. Koschinsky T, Gries FA: Glycerin-kinase und lipolyse des menschlichen fettgewebes in abhangigkeit vom relativen korpergewicht. *Hoppe-Seyler's Z Physiol Chem* **352**:430, 1971.
143. Koschinsky T, Gries FA, Herberg L: Regulation of glycerol kinase by insulin in isolated fat cells and liver of Bar Harbor obese mice. *Diabetologia* **7**:316, 1971.
144. Thenen SW, Mayer J: Adipose tissue glycerokinase activity in genetic and acquired obesity in rats and mice. *Proc Soc Exp Biol Med* **148**:953, 1975.
145. Martin RJ, Lamprey PM: Early development of adipose cell lipogenesis and glycerol utilization in Zucker obese rats. *Proc Soc Exp Biol Med* **149**:35, 1975.
146. Persico PA, Cerchio M, Jeffay H: Glycerokinase in mammalian adipose tissue: Stimulation by lipogenic substances. *Am J Physiol* **228**:1868, 1975.
147. Thenen SW, Mayer J: Hyperinsulinemia and fat cell glycerokinase activity in obese (ob/ob) and diabetic (db/db) mice. *Horm Metab Res* **8**:80, 1976.
148. Bertin R: Glycerokinase activity and lipolysis regulation in brown adipose tissue of cold acclimated rats. *Biochimie* **58**:431, 1976.
149. Ryall RL, Goldrick RB: Glycerokinase in mammalian adipose tissue. *Lipids* **12**:272, 1977.
150. O'Flaherty EJ, McCarty CP: Alteration of rat adipose tissue metabolism associated with dietary chromium supplementation. *J Nutr* **108**:321, 1978.
151. Barrera LA, Ho R: Adipose glycerol kinase: Low molecular weight protein has two Michaelis constants for glycerol. *Biochem Biophys Res Commun* **86**:145, 1979.
152. Taylor WM, Goldrick RB, Ishikawa T: Glycerokinase in rat and human adipose tissue: Response to hormonal and dietary stimuli. *Horm Metab Res* **11**:280, 1979.
153. Ho RJ, Fan C-C, Barrera LA: Comparison of adipose glycerol kinase of hyperglycemic obese mice and lean litter-mates. *Mol Cell Biochem* **27**:89, 1979.
154. Bernfeld P: Glycerokinase levels in adipose tissues of obese hamsters. *Prog Exp Tumor Res* **24**:139, 1979.
155. Kaplan M, Leveille GA: Development of lipogenesis and insulin sensitivity in tissues of the ob/ob mouse. *Am J Physiol* **240**:E101, 1981.
156. Stern JS, Hirsch J, Drewnowski A, Sullivan AC, Johnson PR, Cohn CK: Glycerol kinase activity in adipose tissue of obese rats and mice: Effects of diet composition. *J Nutr* **113**:714, 1983.
157. Chakrabarty K, Chaudhuri B, Jeffay H: Glycerokinase activity in human brown adipose tissue. *J Lipid Res* **24**:381, 1983.
158. Bertin R, Andriamihaja M, Portet R: Glycerokinase activity in brown and white adipose tissues of cold-adapted obese Zucker rats. *Biochimie* **66**:569, 1984.
159. Chakrabarty K, Tauber JW, Sigel B, Bombeck CT, Jeffay H: Glycerokinase activity in human adipose tissue as related to obesity. *Int J Obes* **8**:609, 1984.
160. Schneider PB: Thyroidal glycerol kinase. *Endocrinology* **86**:687, 1970.
161. Robinson J, Newsholme EA: Glycerol kinase activities in rat heart and adipose tissue. *Biochem J* **104**:2C, 1967.
162. Newsholme EA, Taylor K: Glycerol kinase activities in muscles from vertebrates and invertebrates. *Biochem J* **112**:465, 1969.
163. Seltzer WK, Angelini C, Dhariwal G, Ringel SP, McCabe ERB: Muscle glycerol kinase in Duchenne dystrophy and glycerol kinase deficiency. *Muscle Nerve* **12**:307, 1989.
164. Fisher A, Chander A: Glycerol kinase activity and glycerol metabolism of rat granular pneumocytes in primary culture. *Biochim Biophys Acta* **711**:128, 1982.
165. McBride OW, Korn E: Presence of glycerokinase in guinea pig mammary gland and the incorporation of glycerol into glycerides. *J Lipid Res* **5**:442, 1964.
166. Mohri H, Mohri T, Ernster L: Isolation and enzyme properties of the midpiece of bull spermatozoa. *Exp Cell Res* **38**:217, 1965.
167. Mohri H, Masaki J: Glycerokinase and its possible role in glycerol metabolism of bull spermatozoa. *J Reprod Fertil* **14**:179, 1967.
168. Mohri H, Hasegawa S, Masaki J: Seasonal changes in glycerol kinase activity of goat spermatozoa. *Biol Reprod* **2**:352, 1970.
169. Harding JW, Pyeritz EA, Morris HP, White HB: Proportional activities of glycerol kinase and glycerol 3-phosphate dehydrogenase in rat hepatomas. *Biochem J* **148**:545, 1975.
170. Li CC, Lin ECC: Uptake of glycerol by tumor cells and its control by glucose. *Biochem Biophys Res Commun* **67**:677, 1975.
171. Wykle RL, Kraemer WF: Glycerol kinase activity in adenoma alveolar type II cells. *FEBS Lett* **78**:83, 1977.
172. Noel RJ, Antinozzi PA, McGarry JD, Newgard CB: Engineering of glycerol-stimulated insulin secretion in islet beta cells. Differential metabolic fates of glucose and glycerol provide insight into mechanisms of stimulus-secretion coupling. *J Biol Chem* **272**:18621, 1997.
173. Graziani Y, Erikson E, Erikson RL: Evidence that the Rous sarcoma virus transforming gene product is associated with glycerol kinase activity. *J Biol Chem* **258**:2126, 1983.
174. Richert ND, Blithe DL, Pastan I: Properties of the *src* kinase purified from Rous sarcoma virus-induced rat tumors. *J Biol Chem* **257**:7143, 1982.
175. Richert ND: Phosphorylation of glycerol by cAMP-dependent protein kinase: Comparison with *src* kinase. *Biochem Int* **6**:63, 1983.
176. Sargent CA, Affara NA, Bentley E, Pelmear A, Bailey DMD, Davey P, Dow D, et al: Cloning of the X-linked glycerol kinase deficiency gene and its identification by sequence comparison to the *Bacillus subtilis* homologue. *Hum Mol Genet* **2**:97, 1993.
177. Walker AP, Muscatelli F, Monaco AP: Isolation of the human Xp21 glycerol kinase gene by positional cloning. *Hum Mol Genet* **2**:107, 1993.
178. Guo W, Worley K, Adams V, Mason J, Sylvester-Jackson D, Zhang Y-H, Towbin JA, et al: Genomic scanning for expressed sequences in Xp21 identifies the glycerol kinase gene. *Nat Genet* **4**:367, 1993.
179. Huq AH, Lovell RS, Sampson MJ, Decker WK, Dinulos MB, Disteche CM, Craigen WJ: Isolation, mapping, and functional expression of the mouse X chromosome glycerol kinase gene. *Genomics* **36**:530, 1996.
180. Okamoto K, Hirano H, Isohashi F: Molecular cloning of rat liver glucocorticoid-receptor translocation promoter. *Biochem Biophys Res Commun* **193**:848, 1993.
181. Sargent CA, Young C, Marsh S, Ferguson-Smith MA, Affara NA: The glycerol kinase gene family: Structure of the Xp gene, and related intronless retroposons. *Hum Mol Genet* **3**:1317, 1994.
182. Worley KC, King KY, Chau S, McCabe ERB, Smith RF: Identification of new members of a carbohydrate kinase encoding gene family. *J Comput Biol* **2**:451, 1995.
183. Hayashi S, Lin ECC: Capture of glycerol by cells of *Escherichia coli*. *Biochim Biophys Acta* **94**:479, 1965.
184. Hayashi S, Lin ECC: Product induction of glycerol kinase in *Escherichia coli*. *J Mol Biol* **14**:515, 1965.
185. Lin ECC: Glycerol dissimilation and its regulation in bacteria. *Annu Rev Microbiol* **30**:535, 1976.
186. Hayashi S-I, Lin ECC: Purification and properties of glycerol kinase from *Escherichia coli*. *J Biol Chem* **242**:1030, 1967.
187. Zwaig N, Kistler WS, Lin ECC: Glycerol kinase, the pacemaker for the dissimilation of glycerol in *Escherichia coli*. *J Bacteriol* **102**:753, 1970.
188. Thorner JW, Paulus H: Composition and subunit structure of glycerol kinase from *Escherichia coli*. *J Biol Chem* **246**:3885, 1971.
189. de Riel JK, Paulus H: Subunit dissociation in the allosteric regulation of glycerol kinase from *Escherichia coli*. 1. Kinetic evidence. *Biochemistry* **17**:5134, 1978.
190. de Riel JK, Paulus H: Subunit dissociation in the allosteric regulation of glycerol kinase from *Escherichia coli*. 2. Physical evidence. *Biochemistry* **17**:5141, 1978.
191. de Riel JK, Paulus H: Subunit dissociation in the allosteric regulation of glycerol kinase from *Escherichia coli*. 3. Role in desensitization. *Biochemistry* **17**:5146, 1978.
192. Orr GA, Simon J, Jones SR, Chin GJ, Knowles JR: Adenosine 5′-*O*-([γ-^{18}O]γ-thio) triphosphate chiral at the γ-phosphorus: Stereochemical consequences of reactions catalyzed by pyruvate kinase, glycerol kinase, and hexokinase. *Proc Natl Acad Sci USA* **75**:2230, 1978.

193. Blattler WA, Knowles JR: Stereochemical course of the phosphokinases: The use of adenosine [γ-(S)-^{16}O,^{17}O,^{18}O]triphosphate and mechanistic consequences for the reactions catalyzed by glycerol kinase, hexokinase, pyruvate kinase, and acetate kinase. *Biochemistry* **18**:3927, 1979.
194. Pliura DH, Schomburg D, Richard JP, Frey PA, Knowles JR: Stereochemical course of a phosphokinase using a chiral [^{18}O]phosphorothioate: Comparison with the transfer of a chiral [^{16}O,^{17}O,^{18}O]-phosphoryl group. *Biochemistry* **19**:325, 1980.
195. Bethell RC, Lowe G: The stereochemical course of D-glyceraldehyde-induced ATPase activity of glycerokinase from *Escherichia coli*. *Eur J Biochem* **174**:387, 1988.
196. Conrad CA, Stearns GW, Prater WE, Rheiner JA, Johnson JR: Characterization of a *glpK* transducing phage. *Mol Gen Genet* **193**:376, 1984.
197. Pettigrew DW: Inactivation of *Escherichia coli* glycerol kinase by 5,5′-dithiobis(2-nitrobenzoic acid) and N-ethylmaleimide: Evidence for nucleotide regulatory binding sites. *Biochemistry* **25**:4711, 1986.
198. Pettigrew DW, Ma D-P, Conrad CA, Johnson JR: *Escherichia coli* glycerol kinase: Cloning and sequencing of the *glpK* gene and the primary structure of the enzyme. *J Biol Chem* **263**:135, 1988.
199. Holmberg C, Rutberg B: Cloning of the glycerol kinase gene of *Bacillus subtilis*. *FEMS Microbiol Lett* **49**:151, 1989.
200. Holmberg C, Beijer L, Rutberg B, Rutberg L: Glycerol catabolism in *Bacillus subtilis:* Nucleotide sequence of the genes encoding glycerol kinase (glpK) and glycerol-3-phosphate dehydrogenase (glpD). *J Gen Microbiol* **136**:2367, 1990.
201. Scawen MD, Hammond PM, Comer MJ, Atkinson T: The application of triazine dye affinity chromatography to the large-scale purification of glycerokinase from *Bacillus stearothermophilus*. *Anal Biochem* **132**:413, 1983.
202. Goward CR, Atkinson T, Scawen MD: Rapid purification of glucokinase and glycerokinase from *Bacillus stearothermophilus* by hydrophobic interaction chromatography. *J Chromatogr* **369**:235, 1986.
203. Goward CR, Scawen MD, Atkinson T: The inhibition of glucokinase and glycerokinase from *Bacillus stearothermophilus* by the triazine dye Procion Blue MX-3G. *Biochem J* **246**:83, 1987.
204. Burke RM, Tempest DW: Growth of *Bacillus stearothermophilus* on glycerol in chemostat culture: Expression of an unusual phenotype. *J Gen Microbiol* **136**:1381, 1990.
205. Schweizer HP, Jump R, Po C: Structure and gene-polypeptide relationships of the region encoding glycerol diffusion facilitator (glpF) and glycerol kinase (glpK) of *Pseudomonas aeruginosa*. *Microbiology* **143**:1287, 1997.
206. Deutscher J, Sessna G, Gonzy-Treboul G: Regulatory functions of the phosphocarrier protein HPr of the phosphoenol pyruvate-dependent phosphotransferase system in gram-positive bacteria. *FEMS Microbiol Rev* **5**:167, 1989.
207. Romano AH, Saier MH, Jr., Harriott OT, Reizer J: Physiological studies on regulation of glycerol utilization by the phosphoenolpyruvate:sugar phosphotransferase system in *Enterococcus faecalis*. *J Bacteriol* **172**:6741, 1990.
208. Saier MH, Jr. Protein phosphorylation and allosteric control of inducer exclusion and catabolite repression by the bacterial phosphoenolpyruvate:sugar phosphotransferase system. *Microbiol Rev* **53**:109, 1989.
209. Wadher BJ, Henderson CL, Miles RJ, Varsani H: A mutant of *Mycoplasma mycoides* subsp *mycoides* lacking the H_2O_2-producing enzyme L-alpha-glycerophosphate oxidase. *FEMS Microbiol Lett* **60**:127, 1990.
210. Jennings DH: Polyol metabolism in fungi. *Adv Microb Physiol* **25**:149, 1984.
211. Chopra A, Khuller GK: Lipid metabolism in fungi. *CRC Crit Rev Microbiol* **11**:209, 1984.
212. Bergmeyer HU, Holz G, Kauder EM, Molling H, Wieland O: Kristallisierte glycerokinase aus *Candida mycoderma*. *Biochem Z* **333**:471, 1961.
213. Eisenthal R, Harrison R, Lloyd WJ: Specificity of glycerol kinase. *Biochem J* **141**:305, 1974.
214. Knight WB, Cleland WW: Thiol and amino analogues as alternate substrates for glycerokinase from *Candida mycoderma*. *Biochemistry* **28**:5728, 1989.
215. Mago N, Khuller GK: Subcellular localization of the enzymes of phospholipid metabolism in *Candida albicans*. *J Med Vet Mycol* **28**:355, 1990.
216. Pyle JE, Howe HB: Uptake and dissimilation of glycerol by wild type and glycerol nonutilizing strains of *Neurospora crassa*. *Mol Gen Genet* **189**:166, 1983.
217. Witteveen CF, van de Vondervoort P, Dijkema C, Swart K, Visser J: Characterization of a glycerol kinase mutant of *Aspergillus niger*. *J Gen Microbiol* **136**:1299, 1990.
218. Hondemann DH, Busink R, Witteveen CF, Visser J: Glycerol catabolism in *Aspergillus nidulans*. *J Gen Microbiol* **137**:629, 1991.
219. Vaidya S, Khuller GK: Effect of dibutyryl cyclic AMP on lipid synthesis in *Microsporum gypsaeum*. *Biochim Biophys Acta* **960**:435, 1988.
220. Castro IM, Loureiro-Dias MC: Glycerol utilization in *Fusarium oxysporum* var *lini:* Regulation of transport and metabolism. *J Gen Microbiol* **137**:1497, 1991.
221. Lavine JE, Roberts CT, Morse DE: Glucose regulation of specific gene expression is altered in a glucokinase-deficient mutant of *Tetrahymena*. *Mol Cell Biochem* **48**:45, 1982.
222. Hart DT, Opperdoes FR: The occurrence of glycosomes (microbodies) in the promastigote stage of four major *Leishmania* species. *Mol Biochem Parasitol* **13**:159, 1984.
223. Hammond DJ, Aman RA, Wang CC: The role of compartmentation and glycerol kinase in the synthesis of ATP within the glycosome of *Trypanosoma brucei*. *J Biol Chem* **260**:15646, 1985.
224. Misset O, Bos OJM, Opperdoes FR: Glycolytic enzymes of *Trypanosoma brucei*. *Eur J Biochem* **157**:441, 1986.
225. Kiaira JK, Njogu RM: Evidence for glycerol 3-phosphate:glucose transphosphorylase activity in bloodstream *Trypanosoma brucei*. *Int J Biochem* **21**:839, 1989.
226. Krakow JL, Wang CC: Purification and characterization of glycerol kinase from *Trypanosoma brucei*. *Mol Biochem Parasitol* **43**:17, 1990.
227. Barman TE: *Enzyme Handbook* vol 1. New York, Springer-Verlag, 1969.
228. Grunnet N: Inhibition of glycerol kinase by α-glycerophosphate. *Biochem J* **119**:927, 1970.
229. Brooks DE: The interaction of α-chlorohydrin with glycerol kinase. *J Reprod Fertil* **56**:593, 1979.
230. Tisdale MJ, Threadgill MD: ($\pm$)-2,3-Dihydroxypropyl dichloroacetate, an inhibitor of glycerol kinase. *Cancer Biochem Biophys* **7**:253, 1984.
231. Seltzer WK, Dhariwal G, McKelvey HA, McCabe ERB: 1-Thioglycerol: Inhibitor of glycerol kinase activity in vitro and in situ. *Life Sci* **39**:1417, 1986.
232. Kasemsri S, Bernardis LL, Chlouverakis C, Schnatz JD: The incorporation of ^{14}C-glycerol into adipose tissue lipids of weanling rats with hypothalamic obesity. *Proc Soc Exp Biol Med* **141**:38, 1972.
233. Fathipour A, Pridham JB: Control of glycerokinase activity by sex hormones. *Biochem Soc Trans* **2**:1116, 1974.
234. Hurley JH, Faber HR, Worthylake D, Meadow ND, Roseman S, Pettigrew DW, Remington SJ: Structure of the regulatory complex of *Escherichia coli* III^{Glc} with glycerol kinase. *Science* **259**:673, 1993.
235. Kabsch W, Holmes KC: The actin fold. *FASEB J* **9**:167, 1995.
236. Von Euler H, Adler E, Gunther G: Über die komponenten der dehydrasesysteme. XV. Zur kenntnis der dehydrierung von alpha-glycerin-phosphor säure in tierkorpern. *Hoppe-Seyler's Z Physiol Chem* **249**:1, 1937.
237. Adler E, Von Euler H, Hughes W: Uber die komponenten der dehydrasesysteme; glycerophosphat-dehydrase: Oxydoreduction in muskel. *Hoppe-Seyler's Z Physiol Chem* **252**:1, 1938.
238. Baranowski T: Crystalline glycerophosphate dehydrogenase from rabbit muscle. *J Biol Chem* **180**:535, 1949.
239. McGinnis JF, de Vellis J: Glycerol-3-phosphate dehydrogenase isoenzymes in human tissues: Evidence for a heart specific form. *J Mol Cell Cardiol* **11**:795, 1979.
240. McGinnis JF, de Vellis J: Glucocorticoid regulation in rat brain cell cultures–Hydrocortisone increases the rate of synthesis of glycerol phosphate dehydrogenase in C6 glioma cells. *J Biol Chem* **253**:8483, 1978.
241. Freerksen DL, Hartzell CR: Glucocorticoid stimulation of metabolism and glycerol-3-phosphate dehydrogenase activity in cultured heart cells. *J Cell Physiol* **126**:206, 1986.
242. Freerksen DL, Schroedl NA, Hartzell CR: Triiodothyronine depresses NAD-linked glycerol-3-phosphate dehydrogenase activity of cultured neonatal rat heart cells. *Arch Biochem Biophys* **228**:474, 1984.
243. Montiel F, Aranda A, Villa A, Pascual A: Regulation of glycerol phosphate dehydrogenase and lactate dehydrogenase activity by forskolin and dibutyryl cyclic AMP in the C6 glial cells. *J Neurochem* **47**:1336, 1986.
244. Kumar S, Sachar K, Huber J, Weingarten DP, de Vellis J: Glucocorticoids regulate the transcription of glycerol phosphate dehydrogenase in cultured glial cells. *J Biol Chem* **260**:14743, 1985.

245. Kumar S, Cole R, Chiappelli F, de Vellis J: Differential regulation of oligodendrocyte markers by glucocorticoids: Post-transcriptional regulation of both proteolipid protein and myelin basic protein and transcriptional regulation of glycerol phosphate dehydrogenase. *Proc Natl Acad Sci USA* **86**:6807, 1989.
246. Passaquin AC, Coupin G, Schreier WA, Poindron P, Cole RA, de Vellis J: Interferon inhibits the accumulation of glycerol phosphate dehydrogenase mRNA in oligodendrocytes and C6 cells. *Neurochem Res* **14**:987, 1989.
247. Leach KL, Frost MM, Blumberg PM, Bressler JP: Second stage tumor promoters: Differences in biological potency and phorbol ester receptor affinity in C6 cells. *Cancer Lett* **36**:139, 1987.
248. Nichols NR, Masters JN, Finch CE: Changes in gene expression in hippocampus in response to glucocorticoids and stress. *Brain Res Bull* **24**:659, 1990.
249. Ireland RC, Kotarski MA, Johnston LA, Stadler U, Birkenmeier E, Kozak LP: Primary structure of the mouse glycerol-3-phosphate dehydrogenase gene. *J Biol Chem* **261**:11779, 1986.
250. Menaya J, Gonzalez-Manchon C, Parrilla R, Ayuso MS: Molecular cloning, sequencing and expression of a cDNA encoding a human liver NAD-dependent α-glycerol-3-phosphate dehydrogenase. *Biochim Biophys Acta* **1262**:91, 1995.
251. Notsu Y, Omura S, Yoshimoto A, Tomita K: An NAD-linked alpha-glycerophosphate dehydrogenase in rat liver mitochondria and its response to thyroid hormone. *J Biochem* **72**:447, 1972.
252. Tolbert NE: Metabolic pathways in peroxisomes and glyoxysomes. *Annu Rev Biochem* **50**:133, 1981.
253. Gee R, Tolbert NE: Glycerol phosphate dehydrogenase in rat and mouse liver peroxisomes. *Ann NY Acad Sci* **386**:417, 1982.
254. Ringler RL, Singer TP: α-L-glycerophosphate dehydrogenase from pig brain. *Methods Enzymol* **5**:432, 1962.
255. Meyerhof O: Uber die Atmung der froschmuskulatur. *Pfluegers Arch.* **175**:20, 1919.
256. Lee Y-P, Lardy HA: Influence of thyroid hormones on L-α-glycerophosphate dehydrogenase and other dehydrogenases in various organs of the rat. *J Biol Chem* **240**:1427, 1965.
257. Schenkman JB, Richert DA, Westerfeld WW: α-Glycerophosphate dehydrogenase activity in rat spermatozoa. *Endocrinology* **76**:1055, 1965.
258. Kalra VK, Brodie AF: The presence of the glycerol phosphate shuttle and energy dependent transhydrogenase in aortic mitochondria. *Biochem Biophys Res Commun* **51**:414, 1973.
259. Jemelin M, Frei J: Leukocyte energy metabolism. III. Anaerobic and aerobic ATP production and related enzymes. *Enzym Biol Clin* **11**:289, 1970.
260. MacDonald MJ, Warner TF, Mertz RJ: High activity of mitochondrial glycerol phosphate dehydrogenase in insulinomas and carcinoid and other tumors of the amine precursor uptake decarboxylation system. *Cancer Res* **50**:7203, 1990.
261. Klingenberg M: Localization of the glycerol-phosphate dehydrogenase in the outer phase of the mitochondrial inner membrane. *Eur J Biochem* **13**:247, 1970.
262. Henley KS, Kawata H, Pino ME: Effect of adrenalectomy on rat liver mitochondria. *Endocrinology* **73**:366, 1963.
263. Sellinger OZ, Lee K-L: The induction of mitochondrial α-glycerophosphate dehydrogenase by thyroid hormone: Evidence for enzyme synthesis. *Biochim Biophys Acta* **91**:183, 1964.
264. Lee Y-P, Takemori AE, Lardy HA: Enhanced oxidation of α-glycerophosphate by mitochondria of thyroid-fed rats. *J Biol Chem* **234**:3051, 1959.
265. Lardy HA, Lee Y-P, Takemori A: Enzyme responses to thyroid hormones. *Ann NY Acad Sci* **86**:506, 1960.
266. Dummler K, Muller S, Seitz HJ: Regulation of adenine nucleotide translocase and glycerol 3-phosphate dehydrogenase expression by thyroid hormones in different rat tissues. *Biochem J* **317**:913, 1996.
267. Brown LJ, MacDonald MJ, Lehn DA, Moran SM: Sequence of rat mitochondrial glycerol-3-phosphate dehydrogense cDNA: Evidence for EF-hand calcium-binding domains. *J Biol Chem* **269**:14363, 1994.
268. Muller S, Seitz HJ: Cloning of a cDNA for the FAD-linked glycerol-3-phosphate dehydrogenase from rat liver and its regulation by thyroid hormones. *Proc Natl Acad Sci USA* **91**:10581, 1994.
269. Brown LJ, Stoffel M, Moran SM, Fernald AA, Lehn DA, LeBeau MM, MacDonald MJ: Structural organization and mapping of the human mitochondrial glycerol phosphate dehydrogenase-encoding gene and pseudogene. *Gene* **172**:309, 1996.
270. MacDonald MJ, Brown LJ: Calcium activation of mitochondrial glycerol phosphate dehydrogenase restudied. *Arch Biochem Biophys* **326**:79, 1996.
271. Ferrer J, Aoki M, Behn P, Nestorowicz A, Riggs A, Permutt MA: Mitochondrial glycerol-3-phosphate dehydrogenase: Cloning of an alternatively spliced human islet-cell cDNA, tissue distribution, physical mapping, and identification of a polymorphic genetic marker. *Diabetes* **45**:262, 1996.
272. Carlsen A, Wieth JO: Glycerol transport in human red cells. *Acta Physiol Scand* **97**:501, 1976.
273. Yaeger Y, Nathan I, Dvilansky A, Meyerstein N: Permeability of fresh and stored human erythrocytes to glycerol and its acylated derivatives. *Experientia* **35**:1673, 1979.
274. Jacobs MH: A case of apparent physiological competition between ethylene glycol and glycerol. *Biol Bull* **107**:314, 1954.
275. Hunter FR: Facilitated diffusion in human erythrocytes. *Biochim Biophys Acta* **211**:216, 1970.
276. Cainelli SR, Chui A, McClure JD, Hunter FR: Facilitated diffusion in erythrocytes of mammals. *Comp Biochem Physiol* **48A**:815, 1974.
277. Sestoft L, Fleron P: Kinetics of glycerol uptake by the perfused rat liver: Membrane transport, phosphorylation and effect on NAD redox level. *Biochim Biophys Acta* **375**:462, 1975.
278. Sweet G, Gandor C, Voegele R, Wittekindt N, Beuerle J, Truniger V, Lin EC, et al.: Glycerol facilitator of *Escherichia coli:* Cloning of *glpF* and identification of the *glpF* product. *J Bacteriol* **172**:424, 1990.
279. Lupski JR, Zhang Y-H, Rieger M, Minter M, Hsu B, Ooi BG, Koeuth T, et al.: Mutational analysis of the *Escherichia coli glpFK* region with Tn5 mutagenesis and the polymerase chain reaction. *J Bacteriol* **172**:6129, 1990.
280. Maurel C, Reizer J, Schroeder JI, Chrispeels MJ, Saier MH Jr.: Functional characterization of the *Escherichia coli* glycerol facilitator, GlpF, in *Xenopus* oocytes. *J Biol Chem* **269**:11869, 1994.
281. Baker ME, Saier MH: A common ancestor for bovine lens fiber major intrinsic protein, soybean modulin-26 protein and *E. coli* glycerol facilitator. *Cell* **60**:185, 1990.
282. Pao GM, Wu L-F, Johnson KD, Hofte H, Chrispeels MJ, Sweet G, Sandal NN, et al: Evolution of the MIP family of integral membrane transport proteins. *Molec Microbiol* **5**:33, 1991.
283. Van Aelst L, Hohmann S, Zimmermann FK, Jans AW, Thevelein JM: A yeast homologue of the bovine lens fibre MIP gene family complements the growth defect of a *Saccharomyces cerevisiae* mutant on fermentable sugars but not its defect in glucose-induced RAS-mediated cAMP signalling. *EMBO J* **10**:2095, 1991.
284. Lee MD, King LS, Agre P: The aquaporin family of water channel proteins in clinical medicine. *Medicine* **76**:141, 1997.
285. Wistow GJ, Pisano MM, Chepelinsky AB: Tandem sequence repeats in transmembrane channel proteins. *Trends Biochem Sci* **16**:170, 1991.
286. Echevarria M, Windhager EE, Tate SS, Frindt G: Cloning and expression of AQP3, a water channel from the medullary collecting duct of rat kidney. *Proc Natl Acad Sci USA* **91**:10997, 1994.
287. van Lieburg AF, Knoers NV, Deen PM: Discovery of aquaporins: A breakthrough in research on renal water transport. *Pediatr Nephr* **9**:228, 1995.
288. Inase N, Fushimi K, Ishibashi K, Uchida S, Ichioka M, Sasaki S, Marumo F: Isolation of human aquaporin 3 gene. *J Biol Chem* **270**:17913, 1995.
289. Ishibashi K, Kuwahara M, Gu Y, Kageyama Y, Tohsaka A, Suzuki F, Marumo F, et al: Cloning and functional expression of a new water channel abundantly expressed in the testis permeable to water, glycerol, and urea. *J Biol Chem* **272**:20782, 1997.
290. Roudier N, Verbavatz JM, Maurel C, Ripoche P, Tacnet F: Evidence for the presence of aquaporin-3 in human red blood cells. *J Biol Chem* **273**:8407, 1998.
291. Luyten K, Albertyn J, Skibbe F, Prior BA, Ramos J, Thevelein JM, Hohmann S: The FPS1 gene product functions as a glycerol facilitator in the yeast *Saccharomyces cerevisiae*. *Folia Microbiol (Praha)* **39**:534, 1994.
292. Park JH, Saier MH Jr.: Phylogenetic characterization of the MIP family of transmembrane channel proteins. *J Membr Biol* **153**:171, 1996.
293. Lehninger AL: Phosphorylation coupled to oxidation of dihydrodiphosphopyridine nucleotide. *J Biol Chem* **190**:345, 1951.
294. Newsholme EA, Leech AR: *Biochemistry for the Medical Sciences.* New York, Wiley, 1983.
295. Bucher T, Klingenberg M: Wege des wasserstoffs in der lebendigen organisation. *Angew Chem* **245**:552, 1958.
296. Estabrook RW, Sacktor B: α-Glycerophosphate oxidase of flight muscle mitochondria. *J Biol Chem* **233**:1014, 1958.

297. Newsholme EA, Start C: *Regulation in Metabolism*. New York, Wiley, 1973.
298. Sacktor B: The role of mitochondria in respiratory metabolism of flight muscle. *Annu Rev Entomol* **6**:103, 1961.
299. Sacktor B: Regulation of intermediary metabolism with special reference to control mechanisms in insect flight muscle. *Adv Insect Physiol* **7**:267, 1970.
300. Bewley GC, Lucchesi JC: Origin of α-glycerophosphate dehydrogenase isozymes in *Drosophila melanogaster* and their functional relationship in the α-glycerophosphate cycle. *Biochem Genet* **15**:235, 1977.
301. Sacktor B, Packer L, Estabrook RW: Respiratory activity of brain mitochondria. *Arch Biochem Biophys* **80**:68, 1959.
302. Suranyi EM, Hedman R, Luft R, Ernster L: Reconstruction of the glycerol-1-phosphate cycle with subcellular fractions from rat skeletal muscle. *Acta Chem Scand* **17**:877, 1963.
303. Kleitke B, Wollenberger A: Reconstruction of the glycerophosphate cycle in suspensions of rat brain mitochondria. *J Neurochem* **16**:1629, 1969.
304. Galton DJ: Regulation of supply of glycerol phosphate for lipogenesis in human adipose tissue. *Clin Sci* **36**:505, 1969.
305. Berry MN, Kun E, Werner HV: Regulatory role of reducing-equivalent transfer from substrate to oxygen in the hepatic metabolism of glycerol and sorbitol. *Eur J Biochem* **33**:407, 1973.
306. Lamartiniere CA, Weiss G: The role of the glycerolphosphate shuttle in heterogenous liver mitochondria. *Hoppe-Seyler's Z Physiol Chem* **355**:1549, 1974.
307. Swierczynski J, Scislowski P, Aleksandrowicz Z: Regulation of α-glycerophosphate dehydrogenase activity in human term placental mitochondria. *Biochim Biophys Acta* **452**:310, 1976.
308. Schiller CM: Flow of reducing equivalents into intestinal mitochondria. *Metabolism* **28**:105, 1979.
309. Gregory RB, Berry MN: The influence of thyroid state on hepatic glycolysis. *Eur J Biochem* **229**:344, 1995.
310. Curstedt T: Deuterium labeling of glycerol-3-phosphate during metabolism of [1-$^2H_2$]-ethanol in rats. *Eur J Biochem* **49**:355, 1974.
311. Williamson JR, Ohkawa K, Meijer AJ: Regulation of ethanol oxidation in isolated rat liver cells, in Thurman RG, Yonetani T, Williamson JR, Chance B (eds): *Alcohol and Aldehyde Metabolizing Systems*. New York, Academic, 1974 p 365.
312. Poso AR: Influence of the activity of mitochondrial α-glycerophosphate oxidase on the L-alpha-glycerophosphate shuttle during ethanol oxidation. *FEBS Lett* **83**:285, 1977.
313. Grivell AR, Korpelainen EI, Williams CJ, Berry MN: Substrate-dependent utilization of the glycerol 3-phosphate or malate/aspartate redox shuttles by Ehrlich ascites cells. *Biochem J* **310**:665, 1995.
314. Mazurek S, Michel A, Eigenbrodt E: Effect of extracellular AMP on cell proliferation and metabolism of breast cancer cell lines with high and low glycolytic rates. *J Biol Chem* **272**:4941, 1997.
315. Sener A, Malaisse WJ: Stimulation by D-glucose of mitochondrial oxidative events in islet cells. *Biochem J* **246**:89, 1987.
316. Sener A, Rasschaert J, Zahner D, Malaisse WJ: Hexose metabolism in pancreatic islets stimulation by D-glucose of '2-3H:glycerol detritiation. *Int J Biochem* **20**:595, 1988.
317. Giroix MH, Rasschaert J, Bailbe D, Leclercq-Meyer V, Sener A, Portha B, Malaisse WJ: Impairment of glycerol phosphate shuttle in islets from rats with diabetes induced by neonatal streptozocin. *Diabetes* **40**:227, 1991.
318. Rasschaert J, Malaisse WJ: Hexose metabolism in pancreatic islets: Glucose-induced and Ca(2+)-dependent activation of FAD-glycerophosphate dehydrogenase. *Biochem J* **278**:335, 1991.
319. Gerbitz KD, Gempel K, Brdiczka D: Mitochondria and diabetes: Genetic, biochemical, and clinical implications of the cellular energy circuit. *Diabetes* **45**:113, 1996.
320. Ishihara H, Nakazaki M, Kanegae Y, Inukai K, Asano T, Katagiri H, Yazaki Y, et al: Effect of mitochondrial and/or cytosolic glycerol 3-phosphate dehydrogenase overexpression on glucose-stimulated insulin secretion from MIN6 and HIT cells. *Diabetes* **45**:1238, 1996.
321. Sener A, Reusens B, Remacle C, Hoet JJ, Malaisse WJ: Nutrient metabolism in pancreatic islets from protein malnourished rats. *Biochem Molec Med* **59**:62, 1996.
322. Wu BC, Argus MF, Arcos JC: Differential decrease of "shuttle" enzymes of extramitochondrial $NADH_2$ oxidation of heart muscle during progressive thiamine deficiency. *Proc Soc Exp Biol Med* **133**:808, 1970.
323. Carnicero HH, Moor CL, Hoberman HD: Oxidation of glycerol 3-phosphate by the perfused rat liver. *J Biol Chem* **247**:418, 1972.
324. Vertessy BG, Orosz F, Ovadi J: Modulation of the interaction between aldolase and glycerol phosphate dehydrogenase by fructose phosphates. *Biochim Biophys Acta* **178**:236, 1991.
325. Vertessy B, Ovadi J: A simple approach to detect active-site-directed enzyme-enzyme interactions: The aldolase/glycerol-phosphate-dehydrogenase enzyme system. *Eur J Biochem* **164**:655, 1987.
326. Srivastava DK, Smolen P, Betts GF, Fukushima T, Spivey HO, Bernhard SA: Direct transfer of NADH between alpha-glycerol phosphate dehydrogenase and lactate dehydrogenase: Fact or misinterpretation? *Proc Natl Acad Sci USA* **86**:6464, 1989.
327. Wu XM, Gutfreund H, Lakatos S, Chock PB: Substrate channeling in glycolysis: A phantom phenomenon. *Proc Natl Acad Sci USA* **88**:497, 1991.
328. Wilson JE: Ambiquitous enzymes: Variation in intracellular distribution as a regulatory mechanism. *Trends Biochem Sci* **3**:124, 1978.
329. Wilson JE: Brain hexokinase, the prototype ambiquitous enzyme. *Curr Top Cell Regul* **16**:1, 1980.
330. Winzor DJ, Ward LD, Nichol LW: Quantitative considerations of the consequences of an interplay between ligand binding and reversible adsorption of a macromolecular solute. *J Theor Biol* **98**:171, 1982.
331. Fiek C, Benz R, Roos N, Brdiczka D: Evidence for identity between the hexokinase-binding protein and the mitochondrial porin in the outer membrane of rat liver mitochondria. *Biochim Biophys Acta* **688**:429, 1982.
332. McCabe ERB: Glycerol kinase deficiency: An inborn error of compartmental metabolism. *Biochem Med* **30**:215, 1983.
333. Brdiczka D, Knoll G, Riesinger I, Weiler U, Klug G, Benz R, Krause J: Microcompartmentation at the mitochondrial surface: Its function in metabolic regulation, in Brautbar N (ed): *Myocardial and Skeletal Muscle Bioenergetics: Proceedings of 2nd International Congress on Myocardial and Cellular Bioenergetics and Compartmentation*. New York, Plenum, 1986, p 55.
334. McCabe ERB, Seltzer WK: Glycerol kinase deficiency: Compartmental considerations regarding pathogenesis and clinical heterogeneity, in Brautbar N (ed): *Myocardial and Skeletal Muscle Bioenergetics: Proceedings of 2nd International Congress on Myocardial and Cellular Bioenergetics and Compartmentation*. New York, Plenum, 1986, p 481.
335. Brdiczka D: Interaction of mitochondrial porin with cytosolic proteins. *Experientia* **46**:161, 1990.
336. Adams V, Griffin L, Towbin J, Gelb B, Worley K, McCabe ERB: Porin interaction with hexokinase and glycerol kinase: Metabolic microcompartmentation at the outer mitochondrial membrane. *Biochem Med Metab Biol* **45**:271, 1991.
337. Sadava D, Depper M, Gilbert M, Bernard B, McCabe ERB: Development of enzymes of glycerol metabolism in human fetal liver. *Biol Neonate* **52**:26, 1987.
338. Benz R: Porin from bacterial and mitochondrial outer membranes. *CRC Crit Rev Biochem* **19**:145, 1985.
339. Ohlendieck K, Riesinger I, Adams V, Krause J, Brdiczka D: Enrichment and biochemical characterization of boundary membrane contact sites from rat liver mitochondria. *Biochim Biophys Acta* **860**:672, 1986.
340. Krause J, Hay R, Kowollik C, Brdiczka D: Cross-linking analysis of yeast mitochondrial outer membrane. *Biochim Biophys Acta* **860**:690, 1986.
341. Felgner PL: Studies on the physiological raison d'être of mitochondrial hexokinase. *Fed Proc* **32**:488, 1973.
342. Linden M, Gellerfors P, Nelson BD: Pore protein and the hexokinase-binding protein from the outer membrane of rat liver mitochondria are identical. *FEBS Lett* **141**:189, 1982.
343. Colombini M: A candidate for the permeability pathway of the outer mitochondrial membrane. *Nature* **279**:643, 1979.
344. Colombini M: Structure and function of the VDAC ion channel, in Forte M, Colombini M (eds): *Molecular Biology of Mitochondrial Transport Systems*. Berlin, Springer-Verlag, 1994, p 281.
345. Roos N, Benz R, Brdiczka D: Identification and characterization of the pore forming protein in the outer membrane of rat liver mitochondria. *Biochim Biophys Acta* **685**:204, 1982.
346. Rostovtseva T, Colombini M: ATP flux is controlled by a voltage-gated channel from the mitochondrial outer membrane. *J Biol Chem* **271**:28006, 1996.
347. BeltrandelRio H, Wilson JE: Hexokinase of rat brain mitochondria: Relative importance of adenylate kinase and oxidative phosphorylation as sources of substrate ATP, and interaction with intramitochondrial compartments of ATP and ADP. *Arch Biochem Biophys* **286**:183, 1991.

348. Rose IA, Warms JVB: Mitochondrial hexokinase–Release, rebinding and location. *J Biol Chem* **242**:1635, 1967.
349. Chou AS, Wilson JE: Purification and properties of rat brain hexokinase. *Arch Biochem Biophys* **151**:48, 1972.
350. Gots RE, Gorin FA, Bessman SP: Kinetic enhancement of bound hexokinase activity by mitochondrial respiration. *Biochem Biophys Res Commun* **49**:1249, 1972.
351. Bessman SP, Geiger PJ: Compartmentation of hexokinase and creatine phosphokinase, cellular regulation, and insulin action. *Curr Top Cell Regul* **16**:55, 1980.
352. McCabe ERB: Microcompartmentation of energy metabolism at the outer mitochondrial membrane: Role in diabetes mellitus and other diseases. *J Bioenerget Biomemb* **26**:317, 1994.
353. Seltzer WK, Firminger H, Klein J, Pike A, Fennessey P, McCabe ERB: Adrenal dysfunction in glycerol kinase deficiency. *Biochem Med* **33**:189, 1985.
354. Mihara K, Sato R: Molecular cloning and sequencing of cDNA for yeast porin, an outer mitochondrial membrane protein: A search for targeting signal in primary structure. *EMBO J* **4**:769, 1985.
355. Kleene R, Pfanner N, Pfaller R, Link TA, Sebald W, Neupert W, Tropschug M: Mitochondrial porin of *Neurospora crassa:* cDNA cloning, in vitro expression and import into mitochondria. *EMBO J* **6**:2627, 1987.
356. Ryerse J, Blachly-Dyson E, Forte M, Nagel B: Cloning and molecular characterization of a voltage-dependent anion-selective channel (VDAC) from *Drosophila melanogaster. Biochim Biophys Acta* **1327**:204, 1997.
357. Blachly-Dyson E, Zambronicz EB, Yu WH, Adams V, McCabe ERB, Adelman J, Colombini M, et al: Cloning and functional expression in yeast of two human isoforms of the outer mitochondrial membrane channel, VDAC. *J Biol Chem* **268**:1835, 1993.
358. Sampson MJ, Lovell RS, Craigen WJ: Isolation, characterization, and mapping of two mouse mitochondrial voltage-dependent anion channel isoforms. *Genomics* **33**:283, 1996.
359. Sampson MJ, Lovell RS, Davison DB, Craigen WJ: A novel mouse mitochondrial voltage-dependent anion channel gene localizes to chromosome 8. *Genomics* **36**:192, 1996.
360. Sampson MJ, Lovell RS, Craigen WJ: The murine voltage-dependent anion channel gene family: Conserved structure and function. *J Biol Chem* **272**:18966, 1997.
361. Towbin JA, Minter M, Brdiczka D, Adams V, De Pinto V, Palmieri F, McCabe ERB: Demonstration and characterization of human cardiac porin: A voltage-dependent channel involved in adenine nucleotide movement across the outer mitochondrial membrane. *Biochem Med Metab Biol* **42**:161, 1989.
362. Thinnes FP, Goetz H, Kayser H, Benz R, Schmidt WE, Kratzin HD, Hilschmann N: Zur Kenntnis der Porine des Menschen. I. Reinigung eines Porins aus menschlichen B-Lymphozyten (Porin 31HL) und sein topochemischer Nachweis auf dem Plasmalemm der Herkunftszelle. *Biol Chem Hoppe-Seyler* **370**:1253, 1989.
363. Kayser H, Kratzin HD, Thinnes FP, Goetz H, Schmidt WE, Eckart K, Hilschmann N: Zur Kenntnis der Porine des Menschen. II. Charactersierung und Primärstruktur eines 31kDa-Porins aus menschlichen b-Lymphozyten (Porin 31 HL). *Biol Chem Hoppe-Seyler* **370**:1265, 1989.
364. Jurgens L, Ilsemann P, Kratzin HD, Hesse D, Eckart K, Thinnes FP, Hilschmann N: Studies on human porin. IV. The primary structures of "porin 31HM" purified from human skeletal muscle membranes and of "porin 31HL" derived from human B lymphocyte membranes are identical. *Biol Chem Hoppe-Seyler* **372**:455, 1991.
365. DePinto V, Prezioso G, Thinnes F, Link TA, Palmieri F: Peptide-specific antibodies and proteases as probes of the transmembrane topology of the bovine heart mitochondrial porin. *Biochemistry* **30**:10191, 1991.
366. McCabe KM, Wheeler DA, Adams V, McCabe ERB: Comparison of human VDAC1 with streptococcal streptokinase and bovine bactericidal permeability increasing protein: Role of structural information in identifying functionally significant domains. *Biochem Molec Med* **56**:176, 1995.
367. Mannella CA: Minireview: On the structure and gating mechanism of the mitochondrial channel, VDAC. *J Bioenerg Biomemb* **29**:525, 1997.
368. Song J, Colombini M: Indications of a common folding pattern for VDAC channels from all sources. *J Bioenerg Biomemb* **28**:153, 1996.
369. Adams V, McCabe ERB: Role of porin-kinase interactions in disease, in Forte M, Colombini M (eds): *Molecular Biology of Mitochondrial Transport Systems*. Berlin, Springer-Verlag, 1994, p 357.
370. Tibbling G: Glycerol uptake in leukocytes and thrombocytes. *Scand J Clin Lab Invest* **26**:185, 1970.
371. Owen DE, Felig P, Morgan AP, Wahren J, Cahill GF: Liver and kidney metabolism during prolonged starvation. *J Clin Invest* **48**:574, 1969.
372. Harding JW, Pyeritz EA, Copeland ES, White HB: Role of glycerol 3-phosphate dehydrogenase in glyceride metabolism. *Biochem J* **146**:223, 1975.
373. Gilbert M, Ricquier D: Glycerol metabolism in the pregnant and virgin rat. *Biol Neonate* **31**:36, 1977.
374. Chaves JM, Herrera E: In vivo glycerol metabolism in the pregnant rat. *Biol Neonate* **37**:172, 1980.
375. James E, Meschia G, Battaglia FC: A-V differences of free fatty acids and glycerol in the ovine umbilical circulation. *Proc Soc Exp Biol Med* **138**:823, 1971.
376. Persson B, Gentz J: The pattern of blood lipids, glycerol and ketone bodies during the neonatal period, infancy and childhood. *Acta Paediatr Scand* **55**:353, 1966.
377. Melichar V, Wolf H: Postnatal changes in the blood serum content of glycerol and free fatty acids in premature infants–Influence of hypothermia and of respiratory distress. *Biol Neonate* **11**:50, 1967.
378. Sabata V, Wolf H, Lausmann S: Glycerol levels in the maternal and umbilical cord blood under various conditions. *Biol Neonate* **15**:123, 1970.
379. Christensen NC: Concentrations of triglycerides, free fatty acids and glycerol in cord blood of newborn infants with a birthweight of ≤2700 grams. *Acta Paediatr Scand* **66**:43, 1977.
380. Stubbe P, Wolf H: The effect of stress on growth hormone, glucose and glycerol levels in newborn infants. *Horm Metab Res* **3**:175, 1971.
381. Pribylova H, Rylander E: Free fatty acids, glycerol, glucose and β-hydroxybutyrate of plasma of infants protected from cooling and exposed to cold at various times after birth. *Biol Neonate* **20**:425, 1972.
382. Wapnir RA, Mancusi VJ: Glycerol metabolism in experimental malnutrition during lactation. *Biochem Med* **27**:374, 1982.
383. Wapnir RA, Stiel L: Regulation of gluconeogenesis by glycerol and its phosphorylated derivatives. *Biochem Med* **33**:141, 1985.
384. Hahn P, Greenber R: The development of pyruvate kinase, glycerol kinase and phosphoenolpyruvate carboxykinase activities in liver and adipose tissue of the rat. *Experientia* **24**:428, 1968.
385. Vernon RG, Walker DG: Glycerol metabolism in the neonatal rat. *Biochem J* **118**:531, 1970.
386. Ward CJ, Walker DG: Regulation of enzyme development for glycerol utilization by neonatal rat liver. *Biol Neonate* **23**:403, 1973.
387. Seitz HJ, Porsche E, Tarnowski W: Glycerol kinase–A regulatory enzyme of gluconeogenesis? *Acta Biol Med Ger* **35**:141, 1976.
388. Melichar V, Razova M: Glycerokinase in brain and liver of low birthweight newborns. *Acta Paediatr Scand* **65**:10, 1976.
389. Chan AK, Thompson EA: Appearance of a second form of hepatic glycerol-3-phosphate dehydrogenase during neonatal development in the mouse. *Arch Biochem Biophys* **207**:96, 1981.
390. McKenna MC, Tildon JT, Bezold LI: Glycerol oxidation in discrete areas of rat brain from young, adolescent, and adult rats. *J Neurosci Res* **20**:224, 1988.
391. Frank MSB, Nahata MC, Hilty MD: Glycerol: A review of its pharmacology, pharmacokinetics, adverse reactions, and clinical use. *Pharmacotherapy* **1**:147, 1981.
392. Bayer AJ, Pathy MS, Newcombe R: Double-blind randomised trial of intravenous glycerol in acute stroke. *Lancet* **1**:405, 1987.
393. Klockhoff I, Lindblom U: Endolymphatic hydrops revealed by glycerol test. *Acta Otolaryngol* **61**:459, 1966.
394. Online Mendelian Inheritance in Man (OMIM)^{TM}. Center for Medical Genetics, Johns Hopkins University (Baltimore, MD) and National Center for Biotechnology Information, National Library of Medicine (Bethesda, MD). World Wide Web URL: *http://www.ncbi. nim.nih.-gov/Omim.* 1996.
395. McCabe ERB: Glycerol kinase deficiency, in Buyse ML (ed): *Birth Defects Encyclopedia*. Dover, MA, Birth Defects Information Services, 1990, p 791.
396. Eriksson A, Lindstedt S, Ransnas L, von Wendt L: Deficiency of glycerol kinase (EC2.7.1.30). *Clin Chem* **29**:718, 1983.
397. Howell RR, Grier R, Dominguez B, Draehn DK: Neurological manifestations of juvenile glycerol kinase deficiency: Improvement with nutritional therapy. *Brain Dysfunct* **2**:126, 1989.
398. Bonham JR, Crawford M: The effect of isolated glycerol kinase (EC2.7.1.30) deficiency on glucose homeostasis–A cause for concern in affected patients. *Abst Fifth Internat Cong Inborn Errors Metab* OC8.5, 1990.

399. Lewis B, Harbord M, Keenan R, Carey W, Harrison R, Robertson E: Isolated glycerol kinase deficiency in a neonate. *J Child Neurol* **9**:70, 1994.
400. Pometta D, Suenram A, von der Weid N, Widmann JJ: Liver glycerokinase deficiency in man with hyperglycerolaemia and hypertriglyceridaemia. *Eur J Clin Invest* **14**:103, 1984.
401. Wirth A, Heuck CC, Bieger W, Schlierf G: Pseudo-hypertriglyceridamie bei glycerokinase-mangel. *Dtsch Med Wochenschr* **110**: 843, 1985.
402. Zhang Y-H, Huang B-L, Guo W, McCabe LL, Dallongevilla J, Kimura M, Marx H, et al: Glycerol kinase missense mutations provide structure-function but not genotype-phenotype insights. *Pediatr Res* **41**:109A, 1997.
403. Walker AP, Muscatelli F, Stafford AN, Chelly J, Dahl N, Blomquist HK, Delanghe J, et al: Mutations and phenotype in isolated glycerol kinase deficiency. *Am J Hum Genet* **58**:1205, 1996.
404. Zanaria E, Muscatelli F, Bardoni B, Strom TM, Guioli S, Guo W, Lalli E, et al: A novel and unusual member of the nuclear hormone receptor superfamily is responsible for X-linked adrenal hypoplasia congenita. *Nature* **372**:635, 1994.
405. Guo W, Mason JS, Stone CG, Morgan SA, Madu SI, Baldini A, Lindsay EA, et al: Diagnosis of X-linked adrenal hypoplasia congenita by mutation analysis of the DAX-1 gene. *JAMA* **274**:324, 1995.
406. Zachmann M, Illig R, Prader A: Gonadotropin deficiency and cryptorchidism in three prepubertal brothers with congenital adrenal hypoplasia. *J Pediatr* **97**:255, 1980.
407. Toyofuku T, Takashima S, Nagafuji H, Watanabe T: An autopsy case of Duchenne muscular dystrophy with congenital adrenal hypoplasia. *Brain Dev* **3**:241, 1981.
408. Petrykowski WV, Beckmann R, Bohm N, Ketelsen U-P, Ropers HH, Sauer M: Adrenal insufficiency, myopathic hypotonia, severe psychomotor retardation, failure to thrive, constipation and bladder ectasia in 2 brothers: Adrenomyodystrophy. *Helv Paediatr Acta* **37**:387, 1982.
409. Clarke RA, Howard N, O'Sullivan WJ, Svirklys LG, Mackinlay AG: Glycerol kinase deficiency and adrenal hypoplasia congenita. *J Inher Metab Dis* **20**:609, 1997.
410. Blomquist HK, Dahl N, Gustafsson L, Hellerud C, Holme E, Holmgren G, Matsson L, et al: Glycerol kinase deficiency in two brothers with and without clinical manifestations. *Clin Genet* **50**:375, 1996.
411. Kohlschutter A, Seitz HJ, Feldmann B, Lehnert W, Langenbeck U: Glyceroluria in healthy adults, mentally ill adults and children selected for metabolic screening. *Clin Chim Acta* **198**:203, 1991.
412. Hensleigh PA, Moore WV, Wilson K, Tulchinsky D: Congenital X-linked adrenal hypoplasia. *Obstet Gynecol* **52**:228, 1978.
413. Williamson R, Patil S, Bartley J, Greenberg F: Prenatal evaluation for glycerol kinase deficiency (GKD) associated with congenital adrenal hypoplasia. *Am J Hum Genet* **36**:200S, 1984.
414. Burmeister M, Monaco AP, Gillard EF, van Ommen GJB, Affara NA, Ferguson-Smith MA, Kunkel LM, et al: A 10-megabase physical map of human Xp21, including the Duchenne muscular dystrophy gene. *Genomics* **2**:189, 1988.
415. Ellison KA, Roth EJ, McCabe ERB, Chinault AC, Zoghbi HY: Isolation of a yeast artificial chromosome contig spanning the X chromosomal breakpoint in a patient with Rett syndrome. *Am J Med Genet* **47**:1124, 1993.
416. Walker AP, Chelly J, Love DR, Brush YI, Récan D, Chaussain J-L, Oley Ca, et al: A YAC contig in Xp21 containing the adrenal hypoplasia congenita and glycerol kinase deficiency genes. *Hum Mol Genet* **1**:579, 1992.
417. Matfin G, Sheaves R, Muscatelli F, Walker A, Monaco A, Grant D, Nwose O, et al: Gene deletion causing adrenal hypoplasia congenita and hypogonadotropic hypogonadism. *Clin Endocrinol* **40**:807, 1994.
418. Hoffman EP, Brown RH, Kunkel LM: Dystrophin: The protein product of the Duchenne muscular dystrophy locus. *Cell* **51**:919, 1987.
419. Chamberlain JS, Pearlman JA, Muzny DM, Gibbs RA, Ranier JE, Reeves AA, Caskey CT: Expression of the murine Duchenne muscular dystrophy gene in muscle and brain. *Science* **239**:1416, 1988.
420. Nudel U, Robzyk K, Yaffe D: Expression of the putative Duchenne muscular dystrophy gene in differentiated myogenic cell cultures and in the brain. *Nature* **331**:635, 1988.
421. Nudel U, Zuk D, Einat P, Zeelon E, Levy Z, Neuman S, Yaffe D: Duchenne muscular dystrophy gene product is not identical in muscle and brain. *Nature* **337**:76, 1989.
422. Boyce FM, Beggs AH, Feener C, Kunkel LM: Dystrophin is transcribed in brain from a distant upstream promoter. *Proc Natl Acad Sci USA* **88**:1276, 1991.
423. Lederfein D, Levy Z, Augier N, Mornet D, Morris G, Fuchs O, Yaffe D, et al: A 71-kilodalton protein is a major product of the Duchenne muscular dystrophy gene in brain and other nonmuscle tissues. *Proc Natl Acad Sci USA* **89**:5346, 1992.
424. Yates JRW, Gillard EF, Cooke A, Colgan JM, Evans TJ, Ferguson-Smith MA: A deletion of Xp21 maps congenital adrenal hypoplasia distal to glycerol kinase deficiency. *Cytogenet Cell Genet* **46**:723, 1987.
425. Billuart P, Vinet MC, des Portes V, Llense S, Richard L, Moutard ML, Recan D, et al: Identification by STS PCR screening of a microdeletion in Xp21.3–22.1 associated with non-specific mental retardation. *Hum Mol Genet* **5**:977, 1996.
426. Alitalo T, Kruse TA, Forsius H, Eriksson AW, de la Chapelle A: Localization of the Åland island eye disease locus to the pericentromeric region of the X chromosome by linkage analysis. *Am J Hum Genet* **48**:31, 1991.
427. Schwartz M, Rosenberg T: Åland eye disease: Linkage data. *Genomics* **10**:327, 1991.
428. Glass IA, Good P, Coleman MP, Fullwood P, Giles MG, Lindsay S, Nemeth AH, et al: Genetic mapping of a cone and rod dysfunction (Åland Island eye disease) to the proximal short arm of the human X chromosome. *J Med Genet* **30**:1044, 1993.
429. Davies KE, Mandel J-L, Monaco AP, Nussbaum RL, Willard HF: Report of the committee on the genetic constitution of the X chromosome. *Cytogenet Cell Genet* **58**:853, 1991.
430. Pillers DM, Bulman DE, Weleber RG, Sigesmund DA, Musarella MA, Powell BR, Murphey WH, et al: Dystrophin expression in the human retina is required for normal function as defined by electroretinography. *Nat Genet* **4**:82, 1993.
431. Pillers DM, Weleber RG, Woodward WR, Green DG, Chapman VM, Ray PN: mdxCv3 mouse is a model for electroretinography of Duchenne/Becker muscular dystrophy. *Invest Ophthalmol Vis Sci* **36**:462, 1995.
432. Martin MM, Martin ALA: The syndrome of congenital hereditary adrenal hypoplasia and hypogonadotropic hypogonadism. *Int J Adol Med Hlth* **1**:119, 1985.
433. Muscatelli F, Strom TM, Walker AP, Zanaria E, Recan D, Meindl A, Bardoni B, et al: Mutations in the DAX-1 gene give rise to both X-linked adrenal hypoplasia congenita and hypogonadotropic hypogonadism. *Nature* **372**:672, 1994.
434. Huq AH, Lovell RS, Ou C-N, Beaudet AL, Craigen WJ: X-linked glycerol kinase deficiency in the mouse leads to growth retardation, altered fat metabolism, autonomous glucocorticoid secretion and neonatal death. *Hum Mol Genet* **6**:1803, 1997.
435. Nauck M, Winkler K, Siekmeier R, Marangos N, Richter B, Marz W, Wieland H: Pseudohypertriglyceridemia: A case of increased free glycerol without evidence for glycerol kinase deficiency. *Clin Chem* **41**:619, 1995.
436. Karahasanoglu AM, Tildon JT, Ozand PT, Maclaren NK: Glycerol-induced changes in human serum dopamine beta-hydroxylase activity. *Biochem Pharmacol* **27**:2369, 1978.
437. Wapnir RA, Lifshitz F, Sekaran C, Teichberg S, Moak SA: Glycerol-induced hypoglycemia: A syndrome associated with multiple liver enzyme deficiencies: Clinical in vitro studies. *Metabolism* **31**:1057, 1982.
438. Fort P, Wapnir RA, De Rosas F, Lifshitz F: Long-term evolution of glycerol intolerance syndrome. *J Pediatr* **106**:453, 1985.

CHAPTER 98

Sjögren-Larsson Syndrome: Fatty Aldehyde Dehydrogenase Deficiency

William B. Rizzo

1. **Sjögren-Larsson syndrome (SLS; MIM 270200) is an autosomal recessive disorder characterized by ichthyosis, mental retardation, and spastic diplegia or tetraplegia. The disorder is caused by mutations in the gene for fatty aldehyde dehydrogenase (FALDH) that result in deficient enzyme activity and impaired oxidation of long-chain aliphatic aldehydes derived from fatty alcohol metabolism.**
2. **The clinical features of SLS become evident at birth or within the first 2 years of life. Most patients show generalized ichthyosis, mild to moderate mental retardation, and spastic diplegia that often prevents or impedes walking. The presence of glistening white dots on the perifoveal region of the retina is pathognomonic for SLS, but only one-third of patients exhibit this sign. Brain neuroimaging reveals white matter disease in most patients, and seizures are frequently seen. Because other diseases share many of its clinical features, the phenotype of SLS is not sufficiently distinct to permit unambiguous clinical diagnosis without biochemical confirmation.**
3. **Pedigree analyses indicate that SLS is inherited as an autosomal recessive trait, with males and females equally affected. The prevalence of SLS in Sweden, where the largest group of patients has been identified, is 0.4 per 100,000. The disease is seen worldwide, but the incidence is unknown.**
4. **Pathologic changes in the skin of SLS patients include hyperkeratosis, papillomatosis, acanthosis, and a mildly thickened granular layer. Electron microscopy of the skin reveals electron-lucent clefts and membranous inclusions in the stratum corneum and deeper layers. The major pathologic change in the brain involves loss of myelin.**
5. **Long-chain aliphatic aldehydes arise from metabolism of several lipids, including fatty alcohol, ether glycerolipids, sphingolipids, and phytanic acid, a dietary branched chain fatty acid. Of these potential lipid substrates, FALDH has been implicated in the oxidation of aldehydes derived from fatty alcohol and phytanic acid. It remains to be determined whether this enzyme is necessary for oxidation of aldehydes derived from ether glycerolipids and sphingolipids, which are prominent in the brain and skin. Aldehyde-generating lipids are present in the diet, but their contribution to the total body substrate pool is not defined.**
6. **FALDH is a microsomal enzyme that catalyzes the NAD-dependent oxidation of straight- and branched chain aliphatic aldehydes to their corresponding fatty acids. Fatty aldehyde substrates range from 6 to 24-carbons long. The catalytic mechanism involves formation of a covalently bound intermediate consisting of the aldehyde in a thioester linkage with an active site cysteine residue. FALDH is widely expressed in tissues. The active enzyme is probably a homodimer of identical 54-kDa subunits and shows amino acid sequence similarity to several other human aldehyde dehydrogenase isozymes. The 35 C-terminal amino acids of FALDH, missing from related isozymes, are necessary for targeting and anchoring the enzyme to the microsomal membrane.**
7. **The primary biochemical defect in SLS is impaired fatty aldehyde oxidation due to deficient FALDH activity. Owing to FALDH's involvement as a component of fatty alcohol:NAD$^+$ oxidoreductase (FAO), its deficiency is associated with impaired oxidation of fatty alcohol, which results in fatty alcohol accumulation in plasma. A secondary effect of the FALDH defect is a reduction in certain serum polyunsaturated fatty acids in SLS patients.**
8. **The FALDH gene has been mapped to chromosome 17p11.2 and consists of 11 exons. Northern blot analysis shows three transcripts that vary in length due to differences in polyadenylation sites. In addition, splicing of the gene at alternative sites results in two transcripts that encode proteins differing in the C-terminal region.**
9. **A variety of mutations in the FALDH gene cause SLS. Two common mutations in European patients account for about one-half of the mutant alleles in that region of the world.**
10. **The pathogenesis of SLS is hypothesized to arise from accumulation of fatty aldehydes, which form covalent adducts with phosphatidylethanolamine and membrane proteins. The pathogenic effects of fatty alcohol accumulation and polyunsaturated fatty acid deficiency are unclear. Altered lipid composition of multilamellar membranes in the stratum corneum may disrupt the epidermal water barrier, leading to ichthyosis. Lipid alterations in myelin membranes are thought to be responsible for the white matter disease.**
11. **The diagnosis of SLS is readily made by demonstrating deficiency of FALDH or FAO activity in cultured skin fibroblasts, leukocytes, and other tissues. SLS heterozygotes tend to show a partial reduction in enzyme activity.**

A list of standard abbreviations is located immediately preceding the index in each volume. Nonstandard abbreviations used in this chapter include: ALDH = aldehyde dehydrogenase; DHAP = dihydroxyacetone phosphate; FALDH = fatty aldehyde dehydrogenase; FAO = fatty alcohol:NAD$^+$ oxidoreductase; 5-HIAA = 5-hydroxyindoleacetic acid; MRS = magnetic resonance spectroscopy; N-alkyl PE = N-alkylphosphatidylethanolamine; PE = phosphatidylethanolamine; SLS = Sjögren-Larsson syndrome

SLS can now be diagnosed by mutation analysis in targeted populations or select kindreds. Prenatal diagnosis may be performed using enzymatic and DNA-based methods.

12. **Therapy for SLS is largely symptomatic. Ichthyosis improves with topical keratolytic agents or systemic retinoids, and seizures, if present, respond to anticonvulsants. A fat-modified diet with supplemental medium-chain fatty acids has been used in several patients, with inconsistent results.**

INTRODUCTION AND HISTORICAL PERSPECTIVE

In 1956, Sjögren[1] reported a cohort of Swedish patients with a distinctive triad of symptoms: congenital ichthyosis, mental retardation, and spastic diplegia or tetraplegia. The next year, Sjögren and Larsson[2] greatly expanded the clinical description of their 28 patients in a landmark monograph on the disease. Söderhjelm and Enell[3] independently reported on three of the same patients. In most cases, a familial presentation was noted and the disorder could be traced back through several generations to a small number of ancestors living in northern Sweden during the 1700s. The inheritance pattern appeared to be autosomal recessive. This disorder, now known as the Sjögren-Larsson syndrome, constitutes a major neuroichthyotic disorder that has subsequently been recognized in more than 200 patients from all over the world.

Over the next three decades, as additional affected patients were reported, the clinical description of SLS broadened with the inclusion of ancillary symptoms in some patients. Theile[4] summarized the clinical phenotypes of 111 SLS patients reported through 1974, and during the early 1980s Jagell and colleagues[5–8] greatly expanded the description of the clinical findings in the Swedish patients. As often occurs in clinical syndromes lacking objective genetic markers, the diagnosis of SLS in some patients with atypical features gave rise to suspicions concerning genetic heterogeneity.[4,5]

The report by Rizzo and colleagues in 1988[9] that SLS patients had defective fatty alcohol metabolism due to deficient activity of fatty alcohol :NAD^+ oxidoreductase provided the first metabolic insights into SLS. This biochemical marker permitted the reliable diagnosis of SLS and opened up new avenues for understanding the pathogenesis of the disease. Subsequent studies established that the primary enzymatic defect in SLS involved fatty aldehyde dehydrogenase, which is a necessary component of the FAO enzyme complex.[10] Measurement of FALDH or FAO activity allowed the identification of genetic carriers for SLS[10,11] and afforded a safe and convenient means of prenatal diagnosis.[12]

More recently, Pigg *et al.*[13] mapped the SLS gene to chromosome 17 using linkage analysis. In 1996, De Laurenzi *et al.*[14] cloned the FALDH cDNA and found that SLS patients harbored various mutations in the gene, thereby establishing that the FALDH and SLS genes were one and the same. Descriptions of the organization and expression of the FALDH gene quickly followed.[15,16]

These biochemical and genetic advances, occurring largely over the past decade, have transformed the understanding of SLS from a purely clinical syndrome to a molecular genetic disease that disrupts the metabolism of fatty aldehyde and alcohol. Future investigations promise to define the genetic defects in SLS and provide the framework for DNA-based diagnosis. Biochemical and molecular studies on the pathogenic mechanisms responsible for the development of clinical symptoms should hopefully lead to effective therapy.

CLINICAL FEATURES

The three most salient clinical features of SLS are ichthyosis, mental retardation, and spastic diplegia or tetraplegia.[2] For many years, the diagnosis of SLS was based on these clinical criteria alone. With the exception of the Swedish cohort,[2,5] most patients reported in the literature were from isolated kindreds with no known genetic relation to other affected families, and the overwhelming majority of these patients did not receive enzymatic or genetic testing to confirm the diagnosis of FALDH deficiency. Thus, the clinical spectrum of SLS drawn from published cases may be contaminated to some extent by those patients with similar non-SLS disorders. In addition, the phenotype of the Swedish patients, who certainly possess the enzyme defect, may fail to show the diversity of clinical expression seen in other patients because of consanguinity and a more homogeneous genetic background. To provide a more faithful description of the phenotype associated with FALDH deficiency, the clinical features of enzymatically proven SLS patients of non-Swedish origin (see Table 98-1) will be merged with those of SLS patients from the literature who appear more clinically typical. The reader is referred to several excellent reviews that have outlined the clinical features of SLS patients diagnosed prior to discovery of the genetic defect[2,4,5,17–20] and afterward.[21–23]

With rare exception, ichthyosis is seen in all patients with SLS.[2,8,24,25] The ichthyosis is usually apparent at the time of birth or develops in the neonatal period. Although a collodion membrane is usually lacking at birth,[8,25] a membrane was seen in 18 percent of enzymatically confirmed SLS cases (Table 98-1). A small number of SLS patients (14 percent) first developed ichthyosis after the neonatal period in the first year of life, and in a similar percentage (16 percent) of the patients the ichthyosis became apparent between 1 and 2 years of age. None developed ichthyosis after 2 years of age. Erythema may be present at birth and in early infancy, but it usually lessens with age.[8] The ichthyosis is generalized in distribution and typically affects the flexures, trunk, abdomen, back, extremities, nape of the neck, and dorsal areas of the hands and feet (Fig. 98-1). The face tends to be less involved or spared entirely. In more than two-thirds of the patients, hyperkeratosis of the palms and/or soles is seen (Table 98-1). The ichthyosis is usually mild to moderate in severity. Scales can be fine and dandruff-like, larger and more lamellar-like, or even thick and dark brown in appearance,[8,24,25] often resulting in an initial misdiagnosis of lamellar ichthyosis or congenital ichthyosiform erythroderma. Platelike lamellar scales, if present, are usually found on the lower legs;[19] Some patients show prominent hyperkeratosis with accentuated skin markings rather than frank scaling. Alopecia and abnormalities of the hair or nails are not associated with SLS. Diminished sweating rarely occurs,[8,24] but pruritis is a frequent complaint.

The neurologic symptoms of SLS show considerable variation but become evident within the first 3 years of life.[4,6] Spasticity is a constant finding (Table 98-1). Spastic diplegia is much more common than tetraplegia.[6] In some mildly affected patients, the spasticity is evident only as hyperreflexia or a positive Babinski sign. Many patients never gain the ability to walk, and those who do walk often require leg braces or other assisting devices. Developmental delay, particularly in achieving motor and speech milestones, is usually noted prior to 1 year of age. The degree of mental retardation tends to correlate with the severity of spasticity.[6] In a study of the Swedish SLS population, two-thirds of the patients had IQs less than 50.[6] Among enzymatically confirmed cases from around the world, five SLS patients (13 percent) showed no mental retardation (Table 98-1). Four of these five patients were from families with a variant clinical expression[26,27] (see "Atypical SLS"). Of those with mental retardation, 36 percent were mildly retarded and one-third were moderately retarded. Most patients have speech deficits of various types, including delayed speech and dysarthria, that are beyond what might be expected from their degree of mental deficiency.[2,6,28] Two-fifths of the patients have an associated seizure disorder (Table 98-1). Unlike patients with some other lipid storage disorders, those with SLS generally do not show neurologic regression. A loss of ambulation, once achieved, can occur with age, but it is usually due to progressive contractures. Cognitive

Table 98-1 Clinical Features of Enzymatically Confirmed SLS Patients from Throughout the World

Clinical Feature or Symptom	Number of Patients for Whom Data Are Available	Number of Patients with Symptom	Percentage of Patients with Symptom
Ichthyosis	45	44	98
Onset of ichthyosis:			
Congenital or neonatal	44	31	70
1 mo–1 yr	44	6	14
1 yr–2 yr	44	7	16
>2 yr	44	0	0
Collodion membrane	38	7	18
Distribution of ichthyosis:			
Generalized	44	44*	100
Including palms/soles	33	23	70
Including face	28	16	57
Spasticity	45	45	100
Mental retardation	38	33	87
Mild	33	12	36
Moderate	33	11	33
Profound	33	10	30
Retinal glistening white dots	27	8	30
Seizures	41	16	39
White matter disease on brain MRI	19	11	58

* Includes patients with atypical SLS showing patchy but generalized distribution of ichthyosis.

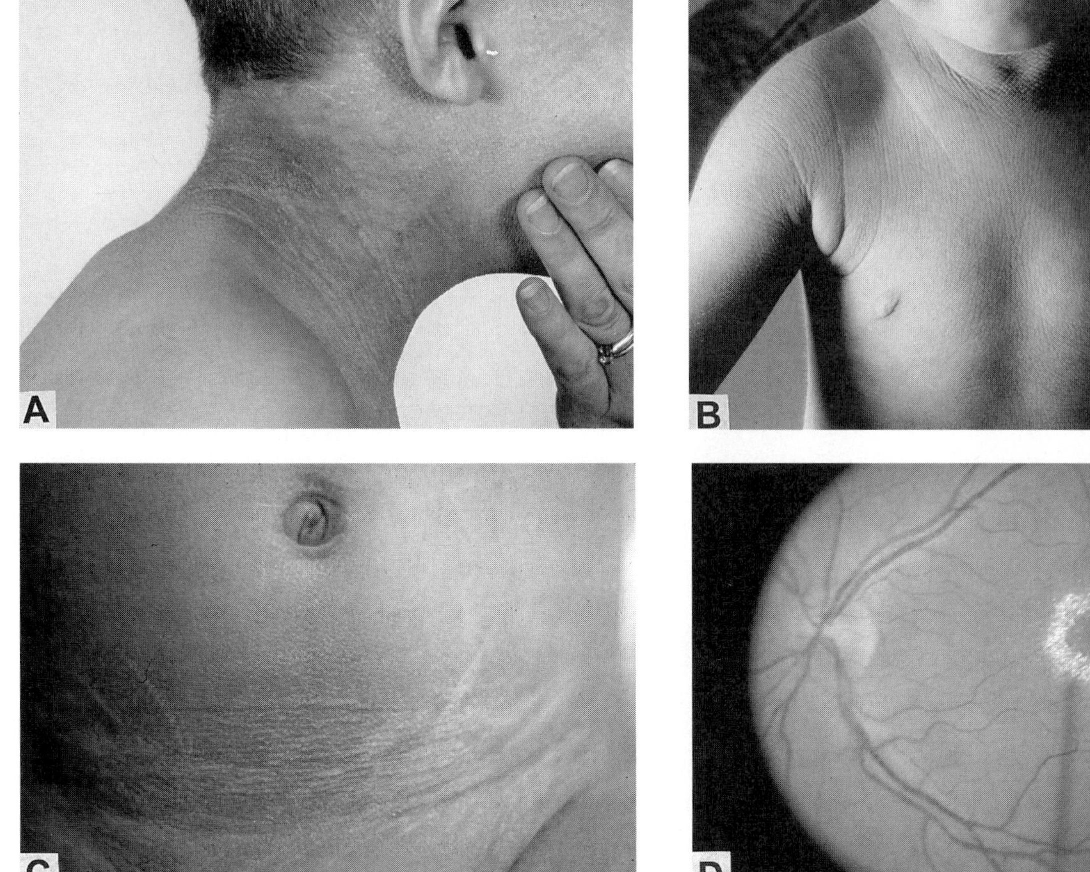

Figure 98-1. Clinical features of SLS. A. Prominent ichthyosis involving the neck. B. Generalized hyperkeratosis of the trunk and shoulders in a 4-year-old patient. (*Photograph provided by Dr. Sherri J. Bale, NIAMS, National Institutes of Health.*) C. Lower abdomen showing hyperkeratosis and excoriations due to pruritus. D. Glistening white dots surrounding the macula of the retina. (*Photograph provided by Dr. Jack A. Cohen, Department of Ophthalmology, Rush-Presbyterian-St. Luke's Medical Center, Chicago, IL.*)

function typically does not worsen over time.[6] It is a notable point that the severity of neurologic disease does not correlate with the cutaneous symptoms.

Abnormalities of the retina are often seen in SLS.[2,4,7,28,29] The most consistent finding is the presence of glistening white dots on the fundus, usually present in the foveal and perifoveal areas (Fig. 98-1). These retinal glistening white dots are pathognomonic for SLS,[7] but they are not a constant feature.[4] The glistening white dots were observed in all 35 Swedish patients who could be examined, including young children,[7] but they were seen in only 30 percent of enzymatically confirmed non-Swedish patients (Table 98-1). The number of glistening white dots is not related to the severity of mental retardation or spasticity.[7] Retinal pigmentary changes and macular degeneration have also been reported in some patients.[2,4,29] Unlike the case in several other forms of ichthyosis, cataracts are not associated with SLS. Visual acuity, however, is sometimes reduced, and photophobia is common.[7]

A variety of other clinical features have been seen in SLS. Most patients with SLS have short stature, due to leg contractures and decreased leg growth rather than to general growth delay.[6] Kyphoscoliosis is not rare, particularly in severely spastic patients. Dental enamel hypoplasia is seen in a minority of patients,[30] and widely spaced teeth have been reported in several patients.[28] Hypertelorism is occasionally present.[28] The disease is not fatal, and most SLS patients who are not institutionalized survive well into adulthood.[5]

Brain neuroimaging exams using either CT[31–33] or MRI[34–37] have ranged from normal to grossly abnormal. The most consistent abnormality in SLS patients has been the presence of white matter disease, most readily detected on T2-weighted images using MRI[34–37] (Fig. 98-2). The areas in the brain most commonly affected include the periventricular regions, centrum semiovale, corpus callosum, and frontal and parietal lobes. The subcortical U-fibers tend to be spared. Among enzymatically confirmed cases, 58 percent showed evidence of white matter disease on brain MRI (Table 98-1). The MRI may be normal during the first year of life and then show evidence of white matter disease several years later, suggesting progressive brain involvement. Electrophysiologic evidence of abnormal myelin includes aberrant somatosensory evoked potentials and brainstem auditory-evoked potentials in some patients.[22] Peripheral nerve conduction studies, however, are normal in SLS.[6]

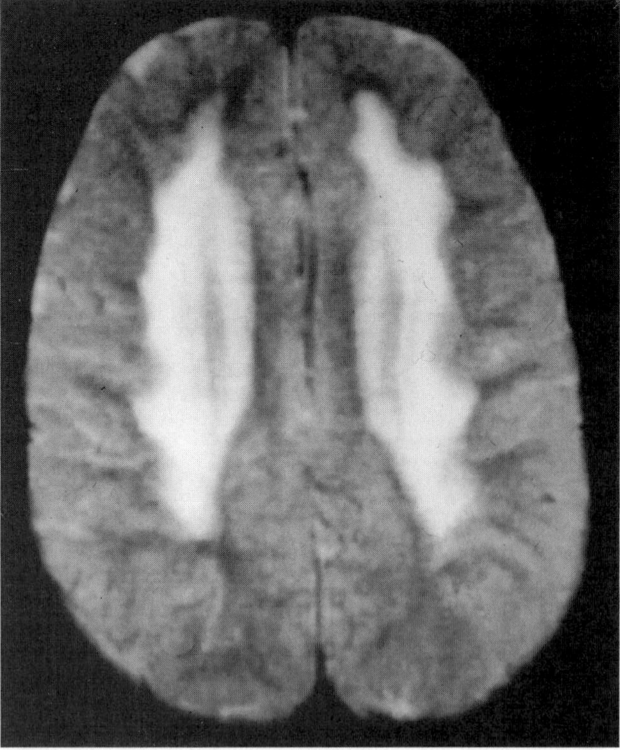

Figure 98-2. Brain MRI of a 4-year-old SLS patient. This T2-weighted image shows widespread white matter disease involving the periventricular and frontal regions. (*Reprinted with permission of the* Journal of Inherited Metabolic Disease.[34])

Atypical SLS

Rarely, SLS patients with documented FALDH deficiency have shown rather atypical clinical features. One Japanese patient[26,38] and two American SLS sibs of mixed European ancestry[27] exhibited patchy and well-demarcated regions of ichthyosis unlike the more usual confluent distribution. The Japanese patient had an IQ of 83 and showed normal development and speech but had mild spasticity with positive Babinski reflexes and hyperreflexia. The two American SLS sibs had a third sib with severe FALDH deficiency, but this child was free of epidermal disease. Surprisingly, a fourth sib who had partial FALDH deficiency consistent with heterozygous status exhibited mild ichthyosis of a more general distribution. All three homozygous SLS children in this family had normal intelligence, although two of them displayed a learning disability that prompted their placement in remedial classes. Like the Japanese patient, the homozygous sibs exhibited spasticity, but the extent of their symptoms was unusually diverse, ranging from mild toe walking to an inability to ambulate. The remarkable clinical variation in this family raises questions concerning its biologic basis. All the homozygous SLS sibs expressed a similar profound enzyme deficiency in their cultured skin fibroblasts. The lack of ichthyosis in one of the sibs suggests greater clinical variation in SLS than previously thought.

SLS-like Diseases (Pseudo-SLS)

A number of patients have been described over the years with clinical features that resembled SLS. Comparing the clinical findings in published cases of SLS with those in the Swedish patients, Jagell *et al.*[5] speculated that more than one-fourth of the patients diagnosed with SLS in the literature actually had genetically distinct diseases. Indeed, the availability of enzymatic testing has clearly distinguished SLS from "SLS-like disorders," or "pseudo-SLS."

In many cases, the clinical phenotype of patients with these "SLS-like" diseases differs from that of typical SLS patients. Three Swedish patients included by Sjögren and Larsson in their original series were later recognized to have a clinically distinct syndrome with severe congenital ichthyosis, mental retardation, alopecia, eclabium, and ectropion but lacking spasticity.[39] Scalais *et al.*[40] reported two sibs with congenital ichthyosis that improved spontaneously over several weeks but did not completely resolve. They developed moderate mental retardation, mild pyramidal involvement, telecanthus, flat facies, stubby long bones, and coxa valga. The bones showed enlarged metaphyses and vertebral dysplasia. FAO and steroid sulfatase activities were normal.

Other patients appear more typical of SLS on physical examination, but biochemical studies rule out the diagnosis. Koone *et al.*[41] described a 19-year-old woman with ichthyosis, mental retardation, and mild spasticity. A skin biopsy showed ultrastructurally abnormal lamellar bodies and membrane-bound lipid vacuoles unlike those seen in SLS. Fibroblast FAO activity was normal.

These pseudo-SLS patients undoubtedly compose a genetically heterogeneous group with ichthyosis, mental retardation, and spasticity. They illustrate the pitfalls of trying to diagnose SLS using clinical criteria alone.

INHERITANCE AND EPIDEMIOLOGY

Pedigree analyses consistently show SLS to be inherited as an autosomal recessive trait.[1,2,4,5] Males and females are equally affected.

Patients with SLS have been diagnosed worldwide and in all ethnic and racial groups.[4] The largest population of patients with SLS resides in northern Sweden, in the counties of Vasterbotten and Norbotten.[5] The prevalence of the disease in Vasterbotten is 8.3 per 100,000, whereas in the whole country of Sweden the prevalence is 0.4 per 100,000. This high prevalence of SLS in northern Sweden is probably due to founder effects and inbreeding. Sjögren and Larsson[2] were able to trace the lineage of most of their patients back to several ancestors living in the 1700s, and haplotype analysis confirms that most Swedish SLS patients are genetically related.[13] It has been hypothesized that the Swedish SLS gene either arose in a founder around the thirteenth century or was brought into this isolated geographic region during a migration of settlers from southern Sweden in the fourteenth century.[42] Mutation and haplotype analysis indicates that many Swedish and northern European SLS patients have a common ancestor.[43] It is speculated that Vikings who established settlements in northern Europe during the ninth and tenth centuries carried this SLS gene from Sweden.

The prevalence or incidence of SLS in other parts of the world is not known. However, the second largest number of patients has been diagnosed from the Mideast, where consanguinity is commonly seen.

PATHOLOGY

In general, the pathologic changes in SLS are poorly defined. Except for the histopathology of the skin, relatively few pathologic studies have been published and most of these involved case reports of patients diagnosed by clinical criteria alone. Without enzymatic or genetic confirmation of the diagnosis, there exists some uncertainty whether some published cases are truly SLS, even when they appear clinically typical. This problem in clinical diagnosis is compounded by the phenotypic variability of patients with SLS.

Skin

The pathologic changes in the skin in SLS are well described.[25,26,44,45] The histologic findings seen on light microscopy, however, are common to other forms of ichthyosis and are not specific for SLS. Skin biopsies show hyperkeratosis, papillomatous changes, and acanthosis (Fig. 98-3). In regions with pronounced hyperkeratosis, the stratum corneum displays a basket-weave appearance. Some patients show prominent follicular hyperkeratosis or occasional parakeratosis. The granular layer tends to be mildly thickened, but it can also be normal or even thinned. Some patients show slight mononuclear cell infiltration in the upper dermis.

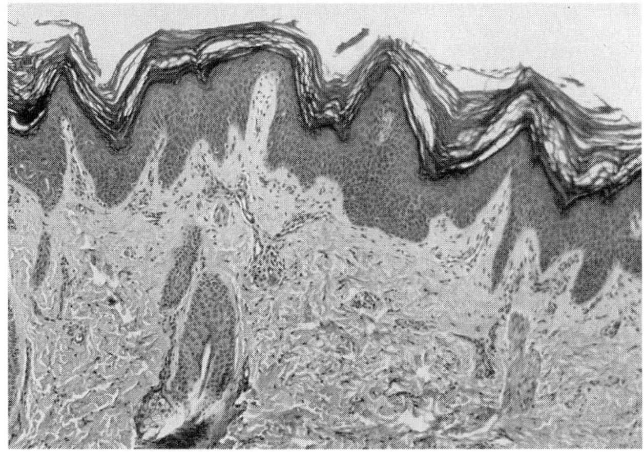

Figure 98-3. Light microscopy of the skin from an SLS patient showing hyperkeratosis and papillomatosis. (*Photo provided by Dr. John DiGiovanna, NIAMS, National Institutes of Health.*)

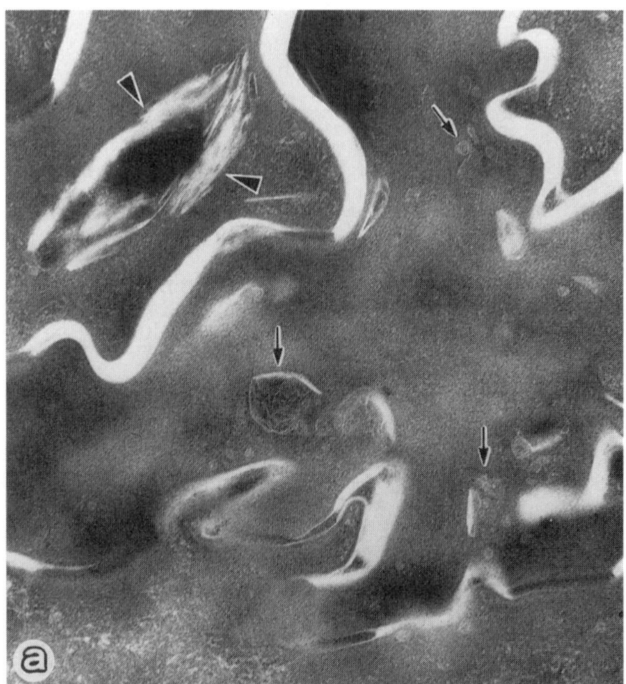

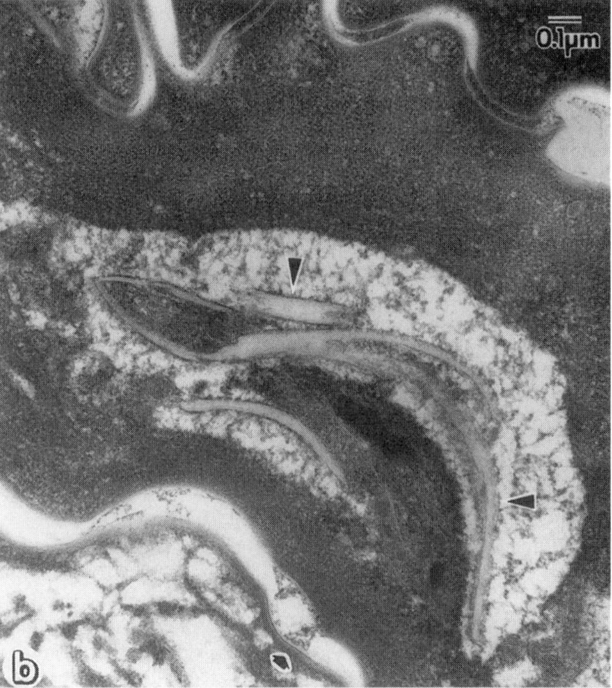

Figure 98-4. Ultrastructure of the stratum corneum of the skin from an SLS patient. a, b. Lamellar membranous inclusions (arrowheads) and small linear or irregularly shaped membranous inclusions (thin arrows) are seen in the cytoplasm. (*Photograph provided by Dr. Masaaki Ito, Department of Dermatology, Niigata University, Niigata, Japan, and reprinted with permission of the* Archives of Dermatologic Research.[26])

At the ultrastructural level, electron-lucent clefts and membranous inclusions are present in the cornified layer.[45] Ito *et al.*[26] found membranous lamellar inclusions in the cytoplasm of granular, spinous, and horny cells of a Japanese SLS patient who was later confirmed to be enzyme-deficient. Two types of inclusions were seen (Fig. 98-4). Larger spindle-shaped inclusions were up to 2 µm in length, and smaller linear membranous ones were up to 0.4 µm long. These membranous inclusions were present in both affected and unaffected skin, suggesting that they

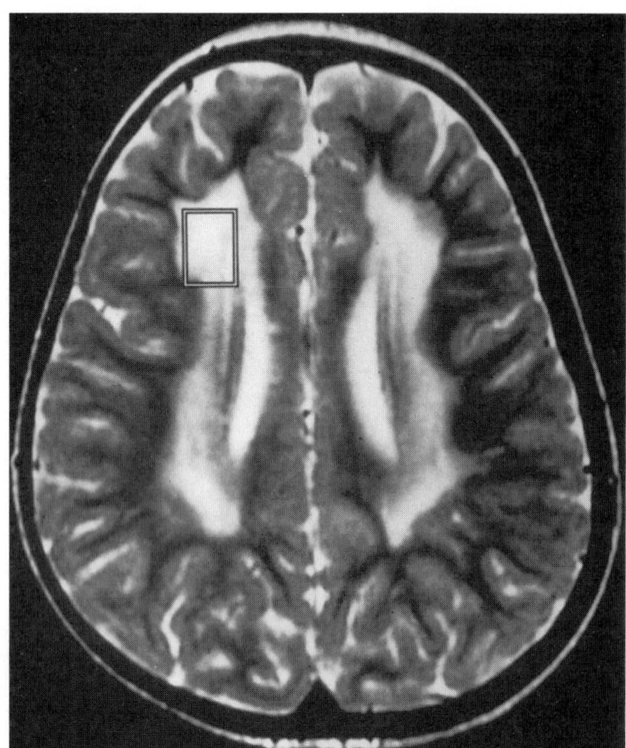

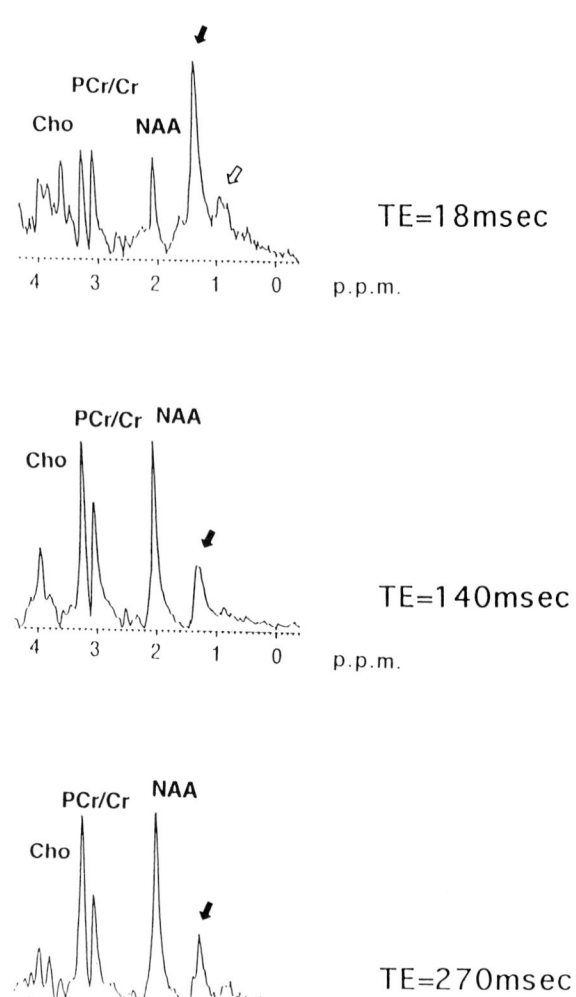

Figure 98-5. Proton magnetic resonance spectroscopy of the brain of a 5-year-old Japanese boy with SLS. Left panel is T2-weighted MRI showing periventricular white matter disease. Right panel is proton magnetic resonance spectrum image of the region of the frontal lobe indicated by a rectangle in the left panel. The filled arrows point to an abnormal peak at 1.3 ppm corresponding to an unidentified lipid. The open arrow identifies a second unidentified lipid at 0.9 ppm. Cho = choline, PCr = phosphocreatine, Cr = creatine, NAA = N-acetyl aspartate. (*This figure is provided by Dr. Toshiyuki Mano, Department of Pediatrics, Osaka University, Osaka, Japan, and reprinted by permission of the* American Journal of Neuroradiology.[55])

are a fundamental pathologic feature and not simply a secondary response to the skin disease. In addition, the keratinocytes and basal cells showed mitochondrial proliferation, and the Golgi apparatus appeared prominent. Within keratinocytes, some lamellar bodies appeared normal, whereas others were elongated or discoid. Nevertheless, the lamellar bodies appeared to fuse normally with the upper cell membrane of the keratinocyte and extrude their contents into the intercellular space at the junction with the stratum corneum. Sweat glands, sebaceous glands, and hair follicles are usually normal in SLS.

The hyperkeratosis in SLS is associated with a hyperproliferative state. In a group of Swedish patients, thymidine-labeling studies of skin punch biopsies demonstrated that SLS skin had 2.7 times more labeled cells than normal.[8] By staining the stratum corneum and measuring the disappearance of fluorescence over time, Jagell and Lidén[8] found that SLS patients have a threefold increased rate of production of the horny layer. In contrast, other investigators used flow cytometry to measure proliferating cells obtained from 0.2-mm shave biopsies of the skin and found a normal proportion of proliferating cells.[46] This method, however, may have underestimated the proliferation rate due to selective sampling of more superficial cells.

The biochemical changes in the skin of SLS patients are not well defined, and a complete analysis of the lipid composition of the skin has not been reported. By analyzing cutaneous scales that reflect the lipid content of the stratum corneum, Paige *et al.*[47] found that the content of ceramide-1 and ceramide-6 were low in SLS, although the total ceramide content was not diminished. Judge *et al.*[48] found the alkane content of SLS scales to be normal.

Nervous System

No extensive neuropathologic report of an enzymatically confirmed SLS patient has been published. Nevertheless, several patients with the typical clinical phenotype of SLS have been studied,[49–52] and the brain neuropathology in two Swedish patients, who assuredly were enzyme-deficient, has been summarized.[53] The patients ranged in age from 5 years to 73 years. The neuropathologic changes were not identical in all of them, and it is unclear whether this represents genetic variation, heterogeneity in the diagnosis, or age-dependent progression of disease.

A consistent neuropathologic finding in all autopsied cases was loss of myelin, either widely distributed or particularly prominent in the centrum semiovale, pyramidal tracts, and frontal lobes.[49–51,53] There was considerable variation, however, in the degree of myelin deficiency and in the sites affected. Two Swedish patients, ages 68 and 73 years, showed widespread loss of myelin.[53] A 24-year-old female with the unusual clinical finding of nystagmus had almost total loss of myelin in the central nervous system, including the optic nerves and tracts.[51] In contrast, a 5-year-old boy, who died of neuroblastoma, showed no myelin loss in the cerebral cortex, internal capsules, basal ganglia, or pons but had marked demyelination of the corticospinal tracts in the medulla and spinal cord.[52] It may be concluded that the distribution of white matter disease in SLS is as variable as indicated by MRI.

The myelin loss is associated with histologic changes in the brain, but there is no pathognomonic alteration specific to SLS. In most cases, the white matter disease is accompanied by a significant degree of gliosis and astrocyte proliferation. Ballooning of myelin sheaths has been noted in areas of myelin loss and near blood vessels throughout the white matter.[50] There is accumulation of sudanophilic fat droplets throughout the gray matter and in the cytoplasm of microglia scattered throughout gray and white matter. The 73-year-old Swedish patient had macrophages containing myelin breakdown products.[53] No inflammatory response has been seen in the brains or spinal cords of SLS patients.

In general, gray matter is much less affected than white matter in SLS. The loss of neurons and axons tends to occur where myelin loss has become extensive, and in most cases it appears to be secondary to the myelin loss. Some regions of the brain may be more susceptible to neuronal loss. Both Swedish patients, one of whom developed Parkinsonian signs at 54 years of age, showed degeneration of the substantia nigra. The 24-year-old patient also had a decreased number of neurons in the substantia nigra.[51]

In three of the cases in which the spinal cord was examined, myelin loss was also extensive.[50–52] At the cervical level of the cord, the demyelination affected the anterior and lateral corticospinal tracts and the vestibulospinal tracts. At the thoracic level, myelin loss was prominent in the anterior and lateral columns and the spinocerebellar tracts. The lumbar spinal cord showed demyelination of the fasciculus gracilis and the dorsal and ventral spinocerebellar tracts. Anterior horn cells were unaffected.[50,51]

Detailed postmortem neuropathologic studies were performed in one Japanese child with the atypical clinical findings of severe growth retardation, micrognathia, protruding forehead, bilateral cryptorchidism, and ichthyosis restricted to the lower legs and the auricles.[54] This patient showed a striking accumulation of peculiar lipoid substances that stained with PAS in the subpial, subependymal, and perivascular glial layers; in the subpial and perivascular spaces; and in the white matter of the cerebrum and brainstem. He also had reduction of myelinated nerve fibers in the cerebral and cerebellar white matter and showed a random arrangement of pyramidal neurons in the insula. Since he was not tested enzymatically, it is unclear whether this patient truly had SLS rather than an SLS-like disorder.

As noted previously for skin, no extensive analysis of the lipid composition of the brain in SLS, particularly with respect to fatty alcohol and aldehyde, has been reported. The lipid composition of the brain of one SLS patient who had widespread loss of myelin on postmortem exam showed global reduction in cerebrosides in the white matter and cortex, along with a decrease in total phospholipids in the cortex but not in the white matter.[50] The patient also accumulated cholesterol esters in the brain, a nonspecific abnormality seen in other white matter diseases.

Indirect evidence, however, suggests that SLS patients have abnormal accumulation of lipid in the brain. Miyanomae *et al.*[35] subjected one FALDH-deficient SLS patient to proton magnetic resonance spectroscopy (MRS). In an area of the brain with white matter disease, they found a strikingly abnormal peak in a region of the spectrum corresponding to a lipid. The spectral peak for N-acetyl aspartate, which is a marker for neuronal metabolism, was low. As shown in Fig. 98-5, this abnormal proton MRS spectrum has been seen in other SLS patients, who showed a second abnormal lipid peak.[55] The MRS abnormality has even been noted in regions of the brain that have a normal T2-weighted signal, suggesting that the lipid accumulation precedes the onset of white matter disease. This abnormal MRS finding is not seen in most other forms of white matter disease. The nature of the lipid(s) is unknown.

A neurotransmitter abnormality was seen in the brains of the two Swedish SLS patients examined at autopsy.[53] The putamen in these patients had a severely reduced dopamine content along with deficient levels of metabolites of homovanillic acid and 3-methoxytyramine. The noradrenaline content was also lower than normal, whereas the contents of serotonin and 5-hydroxyindoleacetic acid (5-HIAA) were elevated. These findings suggest that the patients had a specific monoaminergic dysfunction that might have contributed to their extrapyramidal symptoms of spasticity.

Eye

McLennan *et al.*[51] examined the eyes from a 24-year-old SLS patient who had exhibited nystagmus and optic pallor prior to death but did not have macular degeneration or glistening white dots on the retina. On histologic exam, they found a marked reduction of ganglion cells in the perimacular region. The number of axons in the retinal and optic nerve was reduced, especially at the margins of the optic disc, and myelin was missing from the optic nerve. The retinal pigment epithelium appeared normal.

The histopathologic correlate of the glistening white dots on the retina is still not established. Nilsson and Jagell[56] found evidence of an increased number of lipofuscin granules and a low number of pigment granules in the retinal pigment epithelium of the macula of a 23-year-old SLS patient. Many of the pigment epithelial cells were enlarged, with rounded apical parts. The authors speculated that more extensive accumulation of the lipofuscin granules might lead to clinically apparent glistening white dots.

Other Organs

No consistent pathologic changes are seen in other organs in SLS. On autopsy, the thymus was atrophied in one SLS patient[51] but appeared hypertrophic in another patient.[50] The liver of one 51-year-old patient showed mild centrilobular congestion and fatty metamorphosis, and the kidneys of this patient had groups of fibrotic glomeruli and calcium deposits in the tubules.[49] These findings were not reported in two other patients.[50,51]

BIOCHEMISTRY

Metabolism of Fatty Aldehydes and Alcohols

The fundamental biochemical defect in SLS is an inability to oxidize fatty aldehyde, which is derived from the metabolism of fatty alcohol and related lipids. Since fatty aldehydes are intermediates in the synthesis and oxidation of fatty alcohols, it is relevant to review both fatty alcohol and aldehyde metabolism as a framework for understanding SLS.

Fatty aldehydes and alcohols are aliphatic lipids that exist as free molecules or as components of other lipids (Fig. 98-6). They tend to be saturated or monounsaturated straight chain molecules that range from 14 to 24 carbons.[57,58] Most fatty aldehyde in mammalian tissues is derived from the metabolism of aldehydogenic lipids such as ether glycerolipids and sphingolipids. Free fatty aldehydes appear to be short-lived metabolites that generally do not accumulate in mammalian tissues to any appreciable extent. Fatty alcohols, on the other hand, serve as precursors for biosynthesis of wax esters and ether lipids and are found in most tissues at very low concentrations.[58–60]

As shown in Fig. 98-6, wax esters are composed of fatty alcohols esterified to long-chain fatty acids. Variation in the chain length and degree of unsaturation of the aliphatic components typically results in structural heterogeneity of wax esters. Ether lipids possess even greater diversity than wax esters. These lipids are almost exclusively glycerolipids in which a fatty alcohol is incorporated in an ether linkage at the 1-position of the glycerol backbone (1-O-alkylglycerol)[61] (Fig. 98-6). In most cases, the

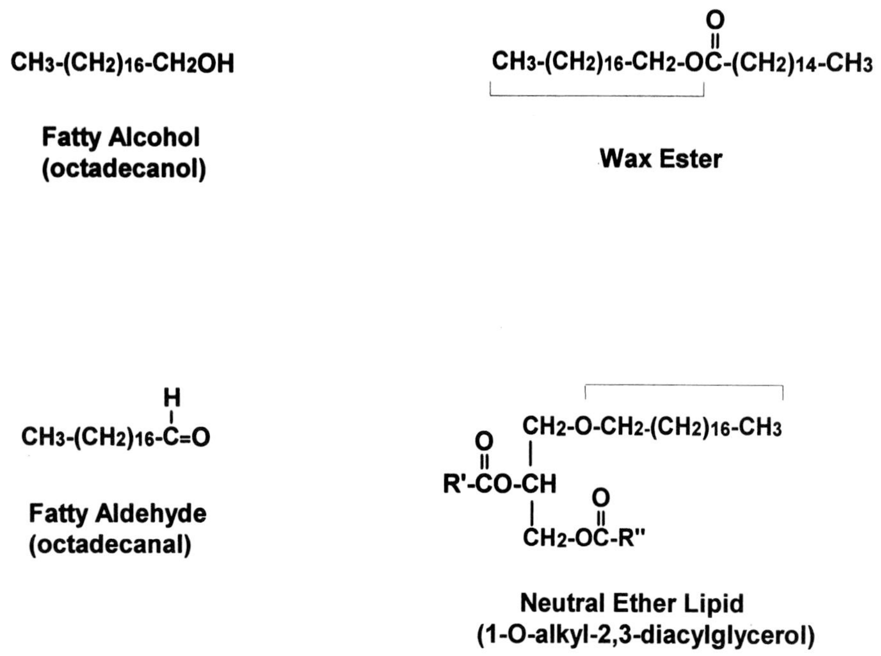

Figure 98-6. Chemical structures of fatty alcohol, fatty aldehyde, wax ester, and neutral ether glycerolipid. The brackets outline the portions of wax ester and ether glycerolipid derived from fatty alcohol incorporation.

2-position of glycerol is esterified with fatty acid. In mammalian tissues, most ether glycerolipids have a 1-O-alkyl chain that is unsaturated at the 1,2 position (alk-1-enyl ether); these are commonly known as plasmalogens. These plasmalogens are usually found as phospholipids, in which the 3-position of the glycerol backbone is occupied by a phosphatidyl diester with ethanolamine, choline, or serine.

It is noteworthy that fatty alcohol-derived lipids are particularly abundant in the skin and brain. Wax esters and alkyldiacylglycerol, which are primarily synthesized by the sebaceous glands, compose up to 24 percent[62] and 15 percent,[63] respectively, of skin surface lipids. In human brain myelin, phosphatidylethanolamine (PE) accounts for 11–14 percent of the total lipids, and almost all of it is in the ether plasmalogen form.[64]

The metabolic pathways for fatty alcohol and fatty aldehyde are shown in Fig. 98-7. The pathways leading to the synthesis and oxidation of fatty alcohol seem to operate as a biochemical cycle.[65] The concept of a "fatty alcohol cycle" is supported by evidence that 1) fatty alcohol is simultaneously synthesized from fatty acid and recycled back to fatty acid by distinct enzymes within the intact cell and 2) the rates at which these two reactions occur far exceed the cell's biosynthetic requirements for fatty alcohol. Studies on mutant Chinese hamster ovary cells[66] and on cells from patients who are genetically deficient in specific steps in fatty alcohol metabolism[9,67,68] have been instrumental in providing experimental evidence for the cycle. It is not known whether the fatty alcohol cycle has an ancillary function besides supplying precursors for lipid biosynthesis or recycling fatty alcohol. In cells that have a low biosynthetic capacity for synthesizing alcohol-derived lipids, fatty alcohol metabolism resembles a "futile cycle"[69] that may function to exchange reducing equivalents between NADPH and NADH for other biosynthetic reactions.[67]

Fatty alcohols are predominantly synthesized from fatty acids by reduction of their corresponding acyl-CoA esters.[70] The initial activation of free fatty acids requires ATP and is catalyzed by acyl-CoA synthetase. The subsequent reduction of acyl CoA to fatty alcohol is catalyzed by acyl-CoA reductase and appears to proceed via an aldehyde intermediate.[71] This enzyme is membrane-bound, utilizes NADPH as nucleotide cofactor, and has a relatively narrow chain-length specificity that determines the profile of alcohols made.[72–74] A cytosolic protein that binds its acyl CoA substrate stimulates the activity of the enzyme.[75] Acyl CoA-reductase is not subject to product inhibition,[71] and studies on intact human fibroblasts indicate that the addition of exogenous fatty alcohol does not decrease endogenous alcohol synthesis.[65] The acyl-CoA reductase enzyme responsible for fatty alcohol synthesis has not been purified from mammalian tissue, and it may consist of more than one protein. Evidence suggests that the reduction of the fatty aldehyde intermediate requires NADPH-cytochrome-*c* reductase or a closely related protein.[76] A distinct cytosolic acyl-CoA reductase that produces hexadecanal and uses NADH as cofactor has been identified in bovine heart,[77] but the role of this enzyme in fatty alcohol metabolism is not known. Fatty alcohol may also be derived from hydroxylation of environmental alkanes;[78] this pathway is undoubtedly minor and may contribute only a minuscule amount of fatty alcohol to the metabolic pool.

The primary function of fatty alcohol in intermediary metabolism is to provide a substrate for the synthesis of wax esters and ether glycerolipids. Wax ester synthesis requires long-chain acyl CoA[73,79] or an acyl chain derived from phosphatidylcholine as a cosubstrate.[80] The incorporation of fatty alcohol into ether glycerolipids is catalyzed by alkyl dihydroxyacetone phosphate (DHAP) synthase.[81] This reaction exchanges the acyl group of 1-acyl-DHAP for fatty alcohol and results in the formation of 1-O-alkyl-DHAP, which is a necessary substrate for subsequent reactions in ether phospholipid synthesis.[82]

Fatty alcohol is oxidized back to fatty acid by fatty alcohol:NAD^+ oxidoreductase (FAO),[65,83] a complex enzyme consisting of at least two separate proteins that catalyze the sequential oxidation of fatty alcohol to fatty aldehyde and fatty acid.[84] This reaction resembles the more widely known oxidation of ethanol, but the enzymes composing FAO are clearly distinct from those involved in short-chain alcohol oxidation. The initial oxidative step is catalyzed by an NAD-dependent alcohol dehydrogenase[83,84] and is probably rate-limiting,[10] but the alcohol dehydrogenase isozyme responsible for this reaction has not yet been identified. The subsequent oxidation of fatty aldehyde to fatty acid is catalyzed by FALDH.[84–86] This enzyme acts on medium- and long-chain aliphatic aldehydes, including branched chain substrates.[86] Although FAO has not yet been purified as an intact protein complex, *in vitro* studies suggest that its two components are in physical contact, since the aldehyde intermediate is not freely accessible.[83] Purified FALDH from rabbit intestine has been reconstituted with partially purified fatty alcohol dehydrogenase to restore the complete oxidation of fatty alcohol to fatty acid.[87] In

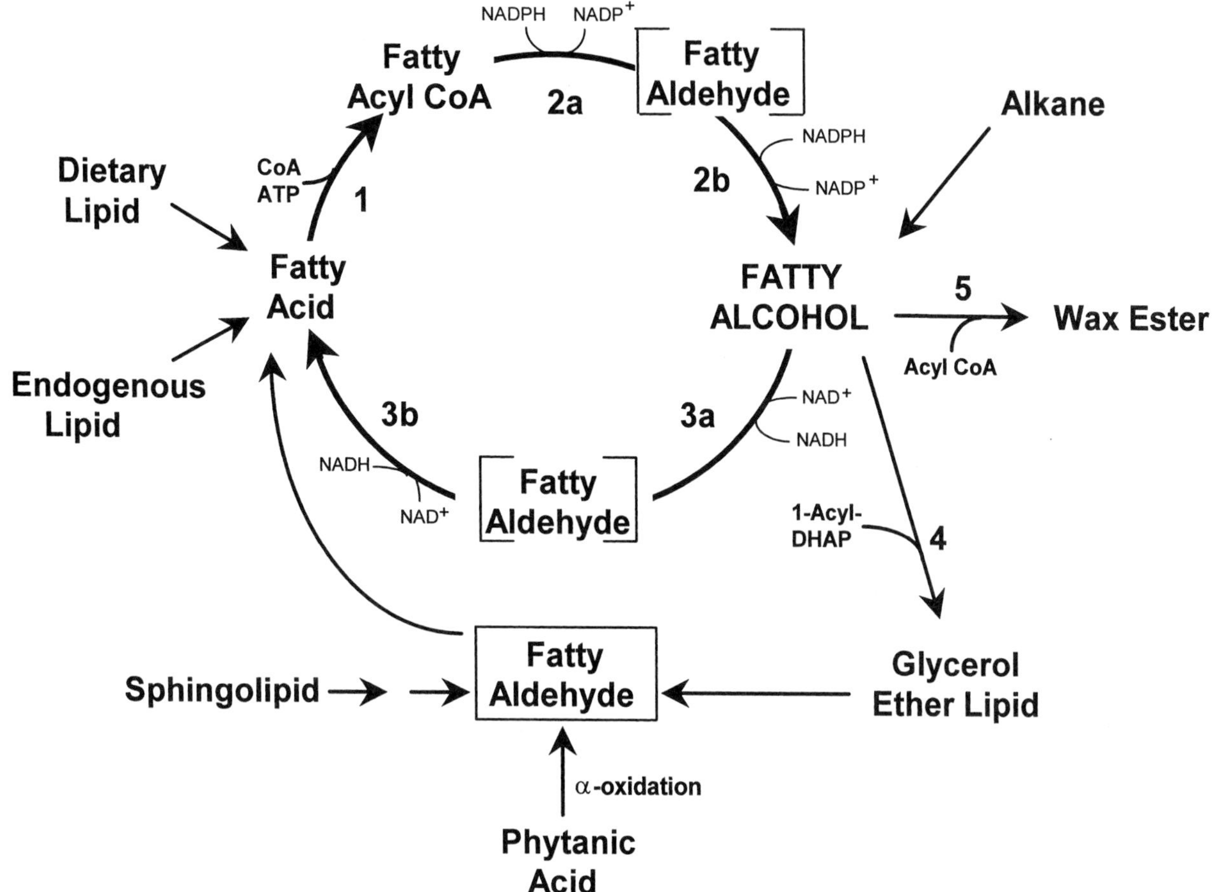

Figure 98-7. Metabolic pathways for fatty aldehyde and fatty alcohol. Brackets surrounding fatty aldehyde indicate enzyme-bound intermediates, whereas a rectangle surrounding fatty aldehyde indicates free fatty aldehyde. 1. Acyl-CoA synthetase. 2. Acyl-CoA reductase. 3. Fatty alcohol:NAD$^+$ oxidoreductase. 3a. Fatty alcohol dehydrogenase. 3b. Fatty aldehyde dehydrogenase. 4. Alkyl-DHAP synthase. 5. Acyl-CoA:fatty alcohol acyl transferase. Figure modified from Rizzo.[67]

addition to its role in fatty alcohol oxidation, FALDH is capable of oxidizing free fatty aldehydes.

Apart from fatty alcohol metabolism, fatty aldehyde is also generated by the catabolism of ether lipids[88,89] and sphingolipids.[90,91] The ether bond of 1-O-alkyl glycerolipids is cleaved by the action of alkylglycerol monooxygenase, a microsomal enzyme that requires molecular oxygen and tetrahydropteridine.[88,89] The product of this reaction is a fatty aldehyde corresponding to the alkyl chain length of the ether lipid substrate. This fatty aldehyde is oxidized to fatty acid via an NAD(P)-dependent enzyme(s).[88] Sphingolipid catabolism generates dihydrosphingosine, which is further cleaved in a pyridoxal-dependent reaction to yield ethanolamine and a fatty aldehyde (hexadecanal) that is 2 carbons shorter.[90,91] The hexadecanal is either oxidized to fatty acid or reduced to fatty alcohol and preferentially channeled into ether lipid biosynthesis.[92] In the catabolic pathways for both ether lipids and sphingolipids, the enzyme(s) responsible for oxidation of the fatty aldehydes—FALDH, another aldehyde dehydrogenase isozyme, or perhaps aldehyde oxidase—has not been positively identified.

It has been shown that the α-oxidation of phytanic acid (3,7,11,15-tetramethylhexadecanoic acid), a branched chain fatty acid of dietary origin, produces a fatty aldehyde product (pristanal) that is one carbon shorter.[93,94] Pristanal is subsequently oxidized to fatty acid by FALDH prior to further β-oxidation.[95] This raises the possibility that the α-oxidation of other fatty acids, perhaps of endogenous origin, may also be a source of fatty aldehydes.

In cultured cells, the flow of fatty alcohol into biosynthetic reactions occurs simultaneously with its oxidative metabolism. The relative flux of fatty alcohol through these pathways is undoubtedly dependent on the wax ester and ether lipid synthetic rates, which may vary between tissues. Cultured human fibroblasts oxidize most fatty alcohol to fatty acid and incorporate only 1–2 percent of the fatty alcohol into the 1-O-alkyl ether bond of plasmalogen PE, the major ether lipid in these cells.[65] In contrast, cultured human AB589 breast cancer cells incorporate about 20 percent of octadecanol into ether lipids, and the remaining fatty alcohol is largely oxidized to fatty acid.[96] Furthermore, the flow of fatty alcohol through its metabolic pathways may be subject to regulation. The addition of fatty acid to the medium of cultured fibroblasts decreases fatty alcohol oxidation, a process that may be mediated in part by long-chain acyl CoA, which inhibits FAO activity.[65] In the presence of 20 μM palmitate in the medium, the turnover rate of the hexadecanol pool in cultured human fibroblasts is estimated to be about 1 hour.

Enzymes involved in the metabolism of fatty alcohol and ether lipids appear to be coordinately regulated to modulate fatty alcohol availability for tissue ether lipid synthesis. In cells or tissues that have a high ether lipid content, the activities of acyl-CoA reductase and alkyl DHAP synthase are increased,[83,97,98] whereas FAO activity is low.[83,98] Cells or tissues with a low ether lipid content show the opposite trend in enzyme activities. Interestingly, alkyl-DHAP synthase, the key enzyme responsible for incorporation of fatty alcohol into ether lipids, is not considered an inducible enzyme,[81] and it may not determine the rate of ether lipid synthesis alone. The tissue ether lipid content may be regulated in part by activity of alkylglycerol monooxygenase.[82]

Fatty alcohol is a substrate for ether lipid synthesis, but it is not clear whether an elevated fatty alcohol concentration results in more ether lipid synthesis. In cultured cells, the addition of increasing amounts of fatty alcohol does not seem to cause elevation of cellular ether lipids, since the excess fatty alcohol is preferentially oxidized to fatty acid.[65,99] However, *in vivo* studies indicate that animals fed large amounts of fatty alcohol accumulate ether phospholipids in liver.[100]

Several enzymatic steps in fatty alcohol metabolism occur within specific subcellular compartments, which may be important for regulating substrate for biosynthetic needs. Activation of fatty acid to acyl CoA occurs in several subcellular locations, including microsomes, mitochondria, and peroxisomes.[101] Acyl-CoA reductase, previously thought to be a microsomal enzyme,[71,73,74,79,102] has now been shown to reside on the outer peroxisomal membrane in guinea pig intestine.[103] This location ensures ready availability of fatty alcohol for entry into the peroxisome, where two key enzymes for ether lipid synthesis reside: alkyl-DHAP synthase, which incorporates fatty alcohol into the ether bond, and DHAP-acyl transferase, which catalyzes the formation of its cosubstrate (1-acyl DHAP).[104–106] The other biosynthetic pathway for fatty alcohol, wax ester synthesis, is reported to be active in microsomes,[73,79] but rigorous subcellular fractionation studies using density gradient separations have not been done to confirm this localization. In contrast to the biosynthetic enzymes, FAO and FALDH in human liver have a microsomal localization,[86] which ensures that fatty alcohol inside peroxisomes is protected from oxidation. Similarly, alkylglycerol monooxygenase is a microsomal enzyme[88,89] and therefore separated from the peroxisomal location where ether lipids are made.

There is evidence that fatty alcohol metabolism may be modified by clofibrate, a drug that induces peroxisome proliferation in rodents. Rats treated with clofibrate have been reported to develop peroxisomal FAO activity in liver.[107] In clofibrate-treated rats, *de novo* synthesis of hexadecanol from acetate appears to occur in liver peroxisomes.[108,109] Whether clofibrate has a similar effect in humans is not known, but clofibrate and other related drugs are generally ineffective in inducing peroxisome proliferation in humans.

Dietary Origin of Fatty Alcohols and Aldehydes

Fatty alcohols and fatty aldehydes may also be derived from dietary lipids, either directly or indirectly, from the metabolism of wax esters and ether lipids. The major dietary sources of free fatty alcohols and aldehydes are probably fruits and vegetables. Fatty alcohols and wax esters are abundant lipids in the cell walls of leafy plants.[110] Free aliphatic aldehydes 8–11 carbons in length are particularly abundant in the peels of oranges, limes, and tangerines,[111] but it is not known to what extent longer-chain aldehydes are present in fruits. Ether lipids and wax esters are major lipid components of certain marine microorganisms and the fish that consume them.[112] Certain cartilaginous fish have a high content of ether lipids, particularly alkyldiacylglycerol, in their oils. A survey of dietary meats, poultry, and fish found that ether phospholipids were present in significant amounts.[113] Among mammals, ether phospholipids are relatively abundant in brain and heart muscle and less so in most other organs, including skeletal muscle.[82] Despite these dietary sources, the consumption and digestibility of aldehydogenic lipids by humans is not well established.

Studies in animals, however, clearly indicate that fatty alcohols,[100,114–116] wax esters,[117] and neutral ether glycerolipids[118–120] are absorbed from the diet. Rats fed fatty alcohol have been shown to incorporate it into 1-O-alkyl ether lipids and wax esters in the small intestine[116] and the liver[100] but showed no change in brain lipids.[100] This suggests that fatty alcohol does not readily cross the blood-brain barrier. Octadecanol is absorbed via the lymphatic system, but most of it is oxidized to fatty acid prior to entry.[121] In addition, dietary phytol (3,7,11,15-tetramethyl-2-hexadecen-1-ol), a plant-derived branched chain fatty alcohol, is absorbed by humans and rodents.[122]

Dietary wax esters may be less digestible than fatty alcohol, in part due to their purgative effect. Evidence suggests that rats fed the wax oleoyl palmitate hydrolyzed much of it in the intestine and reutilized the fatty alcohol for wax ester synthesis.[117]

Neutral ether glycerolipids are also absorbed from the diet. In rodents, dietary neutral alkylglycerol lipids are digested with the 1-O-alkyl bond intact and subsequently incorporated into the ether phospholipids of various tissues.[118–120] Humans show a similar capacity for utilizing dietary ether lipids for biosynthesis. The oral administration of 1-O-alkylglycerol to patients with Zellweger syndrome, who are genetically deficient in alkyl-DHAP synthase and have impaired ether lipid synthesis, caused an increase in erythrocyte plasmalogen levels.[120,123]

In summary, aldehydogenic lipids are absorbed from the diet and are metabolized or incorporated into new lipids. It seems reasonable to conclude that dietary lipids are an indirect source of fatty aldehyde that is subject to oxidation by FALDH. Nevertheless, it is not known to what extent the diet contributes to the total fatty aldehyde pool in humans.

THE FALDH PROTEIN

FALDH (also known as microsomal ALDH) is a member of the aldehyde dehydrogenase (ALDH) family of enzymes.[124] In humans, at least 12 different ALDHs have been purified or their genes cloned.[125] The individual isozymes vary in their substrate specificities, subcellular localizations, and amino acid sequences, which permits their classification into three major subgroups (classes 1, 2, and 3). FALDH is considered a class 3 enzyme.

The ALDHs catalyze the NAD(P)-dependent oxidation of aldehyde substrates to their corresponding carboxylic acids.[126] The reaction is essentially irreversible. Although FALDH has not been studied, other isozymes seem to share an ordered catalytic mechanism characterized by initial binding of NAD^+ to the enzyme, after which the aldehyde substrate binds with the sulfhydryl group of an active-site catalytic cysteine residue to form a thiohemiacetal bond. Hydride ion extraction results in a covalent thioester bond and formation of NADH. Nucleophilic attack by water and hydrolysis of the thioester bond releases the carboxylic acid, after which NADH dissociates. The rate-limiting step in this mechanism appears to be deacylation of the enzyme.

The activity of FALDH has been directly or indirectly demonstrated in several human tissues, including mixed leukocytes,[127,128] skin,[128] liver,[86] cultured skin fibroblasts,[10,65,127,128] intestine,[128] fetal-derived amniocytes,[12] cultured chorionic villi cells,[12] and cultured keratinocytes (Rizzo, unpublished observations). Northern blot analysis of the human FALDH mRNA shows that the gene is widely expressed in tissues, including liver, lung, skeletal muscle, heart, brain, skin, pancreas, and kidney.[15,16] The liver has the highest enzyme activity of any tissue examined. Mature erythrocytes, peripheral blood mononuclear cells, and lymphoblasts have exceedingly low FALDH activity.

The cellular location of FALDH within tissues has been indirectly demonstrated by using a histochemical staining method for fatty alcohol oxidizing activity,[128,129] which is a measure of FAO level. Within the skin, histochemical staining for FAO shows abundant activity in the keratinocytes of the basal, spinous, and granular layers and in the hair follicles and faint activity in fibroblasts[128,129] (Fig. 98-8). No activity is detected in the stratum corneum. The enzyme activity in the intestinal jejunum is largely restricted to the superficial mucosal cells lining the villi.[128]

Xenobiotic agents may induce FALDH activity. Studies on mouse hepatoma cell lines indicate that FALDH mRNA levels are increased threefold by treatment with dioxin (2,3,7,8-tetrachlorodibenzo-*p*-dioxin).[130] In addition, the peroxisome-proliferating drug clofibrate increased mouse FALDH mRNA in cultured hepatoma cells and in mouse liver twofold and eightfold, respectively.

Human FALDH has been purified from normal liver.[86] The enzyme has an apparent subunit molecular weight of 54 kDa. Like other class 3 isozymes, the native FALDH protein probably exists as a homodimer, although the purified enzyme forms polymeric aggregates, which has precluded the unambiguous demonstration

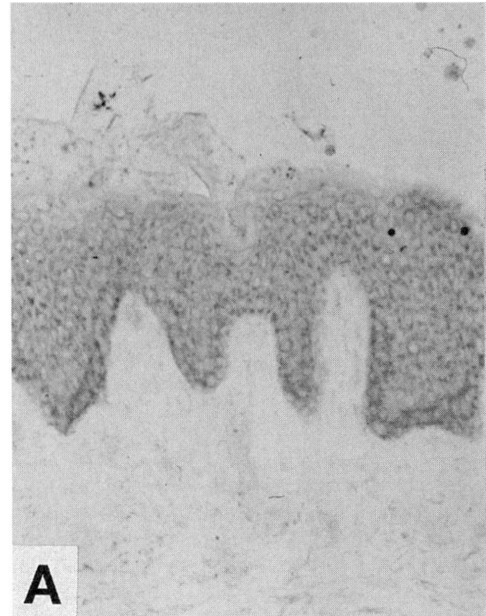

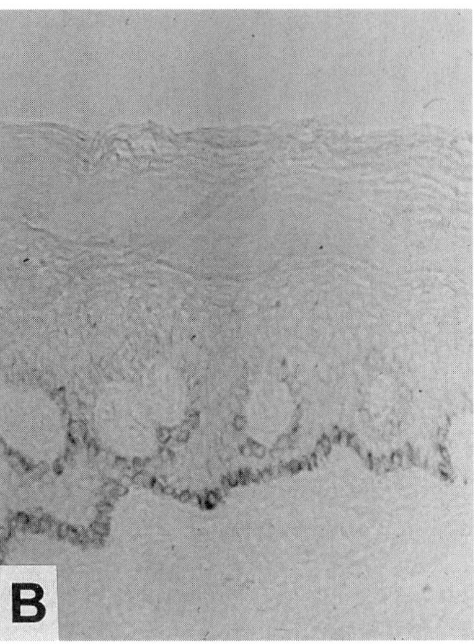

Figure 98-8. Histochemical stain of skin biopsies showing fatty alcohol oxidizing activity using hexanol as substrate. A. The staining pattern of a control patient with nonbullous congenital ichthyosis, showing abundant enzyme activity in the basal, spinous, and granular layers. B. Staining pattern of an SLS patient, showing a striking reduction of activity in the spinous and granular layers. Note that some activity is still detectable in the most basal cells, perhaps arising from an alcohol-oxidizing enzyme(s) that is not deficient in SLS. ***(Dr. Brian Lake, Department of Histopathology, Great Ormond Street Hospital, London, provided this figure.)***

of its native size. The enzyme acts on saturated and unsaturated aliphatic substrates ranging from six to at least 24 carbons long but seems to be most active with aldehydes consisting of eight to 20 carbons. FALDH is also active against 2-methyl[95] and 3-methyl[86] chain aliphatic aldehydes, but it shows no ability to oxidize retinal. By a large margin, purified FALDH prefers NAD^+ to $NADP^+$ as nucleotide cofactor. The enzyme is subject to inhibition by sulfhydryl reagents and disulfiram, which probably interact with the catalytic site.

The FALDH cDNAs from human,[14] rat,[131] and mouse[130] have been cloned. The deduced amino acid sequences of the proteins indicate that they are closely related. Human FALDH shares 84 percent amino acid identity with the rat enzyme and 94 percent amino acid similarity when conservative amino acid substitutions are considered. Human FALDH is comprised of 485 amino acids, whereas the two rodent proteins are 484 amino acids long and each lacks the C-terminal amino acid of the human protein. The human FALDH sequence also shows significant amino acid identity with other class 3 human aldehyde dehydrogenases, particularly the stomach ALDH3 and ALDH7 isozymes, which share 61 percent and 51 percent identity with FALDH, respectively.[14] Because of the sequence similarity between FALDH and ALDH3 and their close gene colocalization on human chromosome 17,[15,132] it is likely that the FALDH and ALDH3 arose from gene duplication and divergent evolution. Both enzymes act on aliphatic substrates, although the ALDH3 isozyme appears to have greater activity with aromatic substrates than does FALDH and has a more restricted tissue distribution.[133] The two enzymes also differ in their subcellular location, ALDH3 being a cytosolic enzyme and FALDH having a microsomal localization. FALDH has considerably less amino acid identity (20–22 percent) with human class 1 and class 2 isozymes (ALDH1, ALDH2, ALDH5, ALDH6).

Comparison of the primary amino acid sequences of 16 aldehyde dehydrogenase isozymes has revealed conserved regions that undoubtedly serve critical catalytic and structural functions.[134] Based on its invariant conservation and studies of other isozymes, Cys-241 of FALDH has been identified as the catalytic cysteine.[14] Like the rodent FALDH homologues, and in contrast to all other aldehyde dehydrogenase isozymes, FALDH contains an extended C-terminal region composed of 35 amino acids. This "tail" consists of amino acids that confer a hydrophobic nature. Site-directed mutagenesis studies on the C-terminal domain of the rat FALDH protein indicate that this domain is essential for binding and anchoring the FALDH enzyme to the microsomal membrane.[135]

The three-dimensional structure of FALDH is expected to resemble that of other aldehyde dehydrogenases. In this regard, the primary sequence of human FALDH, ignoring the C-terminal domain, is 65 percent identical to that of a rat class 3 cytosolic enzyme, the crystalline structure of which has recently been solved.[136] This rat aldehyde dehydrogenase is a homodimer consisting of two asymmetric subunits. The protein is composed of three major functional domains—NAD binding, catalytic, and bridging—and various α and β subdomains. The catalytic site is located at the bottom of a deep funnel-shaped passage and is composed of residues from all three major domains. The catalytic thiol, Cys-243 (corresponding to the FALDH Cys-241), is positioned near the bottom of the passage, which is blocked by the nicotinamide ring. A number of highly conserved residues are found along the catalytic pocket. The protein has a novel NAD-binding domain with a Rossmann fold that contains five rather then the usual six β-strands. Residues involved in hydrogen binding or van der Waals interactions with NAD are scattered throughout amino acid positions 110 to 342. The bridging domain, which extends from and loops back to the central structure, helps stabilize the protein dimer and forms part of the mouth of the catalytic passage. This rat protein affords a model from which basic structural/functional correlations for the human FALDH may be inferred.

ENZYME DEFECT

In 1988, Rizzo *et al.*[9] reported that cultured skin fibroblasts from SLS patients have impaired fatty alcohol oxidation caused by deficient FAO activity. Subsequent studies confirmed this enzyme deficiency in fibroblasts, leukocytes, and cultured keratinocytes from SLS patients.[10,11,127,128] Because FAO is a complex enzyme that consists of at least two separate proteins (fatty alcohol dehydrogenase and FALDH), Rizzo and Craft[10] measured each activity separately and demonstrated that SLS patients were selectively deficient in the FALDH component. No patient was found to be deficient in fatty alcohol dehydrogenase. Using a histochemical staining technique, Judge *et al.*[128] demonstrated impaired hexanol oxidation directly in skin and jejunal biopsies from SLS patients (Fig. 98-8).

As a consequence of the FALDH defect, SLS patients are deficient in both FALDH and FAO activities (Fig. 98-9). To date, FAO and/or FALDH deficiency has been documented in more than 75 SLS patients from around the world. The enzyme defect is specific for SLS and is not seen in other cutaneous or neurologic diseases.[9,21]

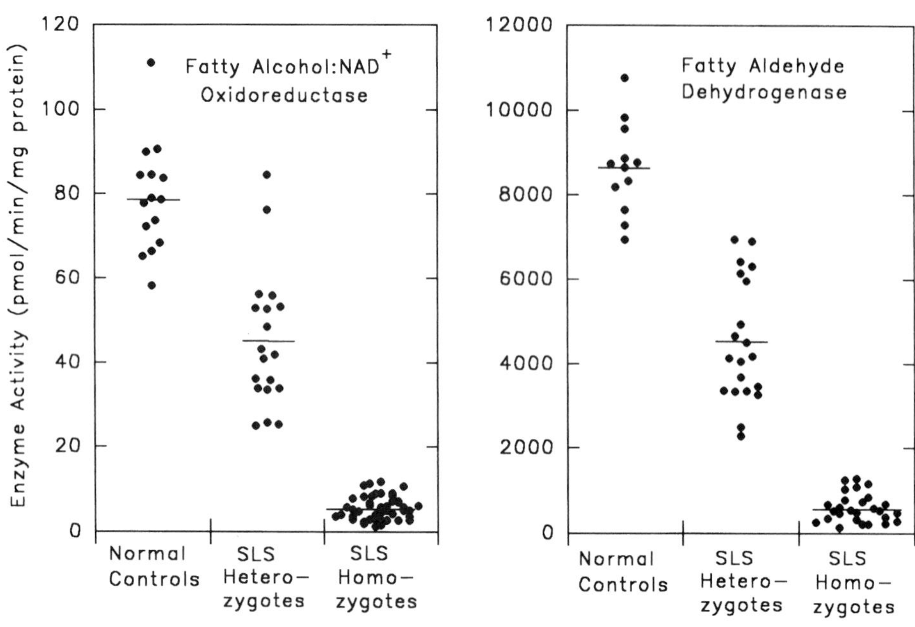

Figure 98-9. Activities of fatty alcohol:NAD$^+$ oxidoreductase and fatty aldehyde dehydrogenase in cultured skin fibroblasts from normal controls, SLS heterozygotes, and SLS homozygotes. (*Reprinted with permission from the* Handbook of Clinical Neurology, *Elsevier.*[22])

All SLS patients exhibit some residual enzyme activity in cultured fibroblasts. The extent of FAO and FALDH deficiency is distinctly more profound when enzyme activities are measured with longer-chain substrates than with shorter-chain ones.[10] As seen in Fig. 98-10, mean FALDH activity in crude homogenates of SLS cells ranged from 27 percent of mean normal activity using dodecanal (12-carbon aldehyde) as substrate to 8 percent of normal using octadecanal (18-carbon aldehyde). An even more severe deficiency of FAO, ranging from 1 percent to 3 percent, is seen when dihydrophytol (a 20-carbon, branched chain alcohol) is used as substrate.[12] Moreover, the extent of FAO or FALDH deficiency in SLS fibroblast is more profound (1–2 percent of normal) when 120,000 x g membrane fractions are tested than when crude homogenates are used (6–8 percent of normal).[10,11] This suggests that the residual FAO and FALDH activities measured with crude cell homogenates arise in part from cytosolic enzymes that are not affected in SLS. These enzymes may include other ALDHs that prefer shorter substrates but possess some minor overlapping activity against long-chain aldehydes. The finding of 6 percent residual FALDH activity in crude homogenates from one patient who was shown to have two mutations leading to severely truncated enzyme supports this conclusion.[14]

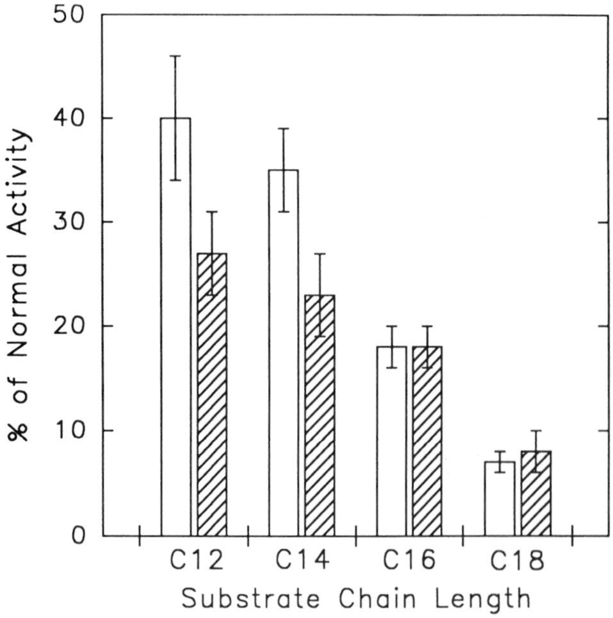

Figure 98-10. Residual enzyme activities measured in cultured skin fibroblasts from SLS patients using substrates with different chain lengths. Open columns, fatty alcohol:NAD$^+$ oxidoreductase. Cross-hatched columns, fatty aldehyde dehydrogenase. Error bars show ± SD. (*Reproduced from* The Journal of Clinical Investigation, *1991, 88:1643–1648, by copyright permission of The American Society for Clinical Investigation.*[10])

As a consequence of deficient FAO activity, cultured skin fibroblasts from SLS patients accumulate fatty alcohol in vitro.[9] Similarly, SLS patients tend to accumulate fatty alcohol in plasma[21,127] (Fig. 98-11). The plasma total octadecanol concentrations, which include both esterified and free alcohol, are increased about two- to three-fold, and hexadecanol levels are about twice the normal concentration. When plasma free fatty alcohols are selectively measured in SLS patients, octadecanol shows a much greater relative accumulation (twenty-five-fold) over normal (Rizzo, unpublished observations).

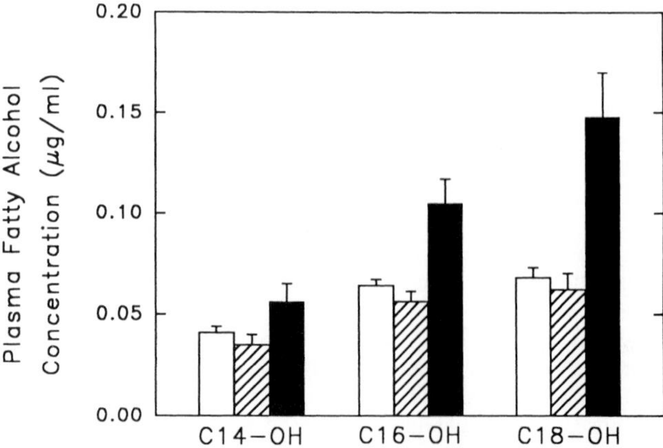

Figure 98-11. Plasma total fatty alcohol concentrations in SLS. Open columns, normal controls. Cross-hatched columns, obligate SLS heterozygotes. Black columns, SLS homozygotes. Error bars show ± SD. (*Reprinted from* Seminars in Dermatology[21] *by permission of WB Saunders Co.*)

In SLS, it is not known whether excess fatty alcohol is diverted into the synthesis of ether lipids and wax esters. Ether lipids are abundant in myelin and skin, but the ether lipid content of these tissues in SLS has not been reported. In erythrocytes from SLS patients, ether lipid content is either normal or only marginally elevated.[127] Even less is known about regulation of wax ester synthesis, and there are no reports of wax ester measurements in SLS tissues.

SLS patients have other biochemical abnormalities, which probably reflect secondary metabolic changes. SLS patients are deficient in polyunsaturated fatty acids in the serum that normally arise from δ-6 desaturation.[137] Their cultured skin fibroblasts, however, possess normal δ-6 desaturase activity,[138] indicating that the fatty acid abnormality occurs only in SLS patients in vivo.

GENETICS

Pigg *et al.*[13] first reported genetic linkage of the SLS gene to chromosome 17 by studying Swedish families. They showed that the microsatellite marker *D17S805* was tightly linked to the SLS gene. Two additional linkage studies in families of diverse ethnic origins confirmed this localization and thereby provided evidence that SLS was a genetically homogeneous disorder.[139,140] Refinement in the mapping of *D17S805* led to the sublocalization of the SLS gene to 17p11.2.[139,141] The FALDH gene was localized to the same chromosome region by finding its DNA sequence on YACs that also contained *D17S805*.[14] The identification of the FALDH gene as the SLS gene was established when De Laurenzi *et al.*[14] cloned the human FALDH cDNA and demonstrated mutations in SLS patients.

As shown in Fig. 98-12, the human FALDH gene (also referred to as ALDH10) consists of 11 exons and spans about 30 kb[15,16] (GenBank NM000382, U75286-U75297). The organization of the FALDH gene resembles that of several other ALDH genes.[125] The sites of intron-exon boundaries within the coding portion of the gene are identical to those noted for the human ALDH3 gene, except for exon 9, which diverges in the two genes, and exons 9′ and 10, which are missing in ALDH3. Both genes are located on chromosome 17p11.2, within 50–85 kb of each other.[15]

Northern blot analysis of FALDH RNA indicates the presence of three mRNA species, 2 kb, 3.8 kb, and 4.0 kb in length, which originate from multiple polyadenylation signals in the 3′ untranslated region.[15,16] All three RNA transcripts are present in a variety of human tissues, but the relative abundance of the mRNA species varies. The two longer transcripts are most abundant in heart, brain, skeletal muscle, and pancreas. All are equally expressed in epidermis, whereas the liver shows an excess of the 2-kb transcript. FALDH mRNA is virtually undetectable in lymphocyte-derived cancer cell lines.

The FALDH promoter lacks a TATA box,[15,16] but the region includes multiple CpG islands, as is characteristic of other TATA-less promoters.[142] Primer extension and RNase protection experiments have identified the transcription initiation site at position — 258 relative to the initiating codon.[15] Using gel-shift analysis with recombinant Spl and nuclear extracts from HeLa cells in which FALDH is actively transcribed, an Spl DNA binding motif at position — 51 was identified as a site of protein-DNA interaction.[15] In addition, a putative initiator sequence 13 nucleotides downstream from the transcription initiation site conforms to the 5′-YYCAYYYYY-3′ (Y = pyrimidine) consensus and interacts with nuclear proteins in gel-shift experiments.

In striking contrast to other aldehyde dehydrogenase genes, alternate splicing of FALDH mRNA produces two distinct transcripts.[15] The major transcript is composed of exons 1–10 and encodes the primary protein, containing 485 amino acids (Fig. 98-12). The alternate transcript contains exon 9′ spliced between exons 9 and 10. This alternately spliced transcript is present in various tissues, including liver, brain, keratinocytes, and fibroblasts, and accounts for less than 10 percent of the major transcript. Exon 9′ contains an in-frame termination codon, and translation of this alternate transcript produces a protein containing 27 amino acids in place of the four C-terminal residues of the more abundant FALDH protein (Fig. 98-12). Thirteen of these amino acids are hydrophobic and are commonly found in transmembrane domains, whereas nine are basic residues. Since the C-terminal region of FALDH is involved in membrane binding, it is possible that the protein encoded by the alternately spliced transcript may have modified membrane-binding properties.

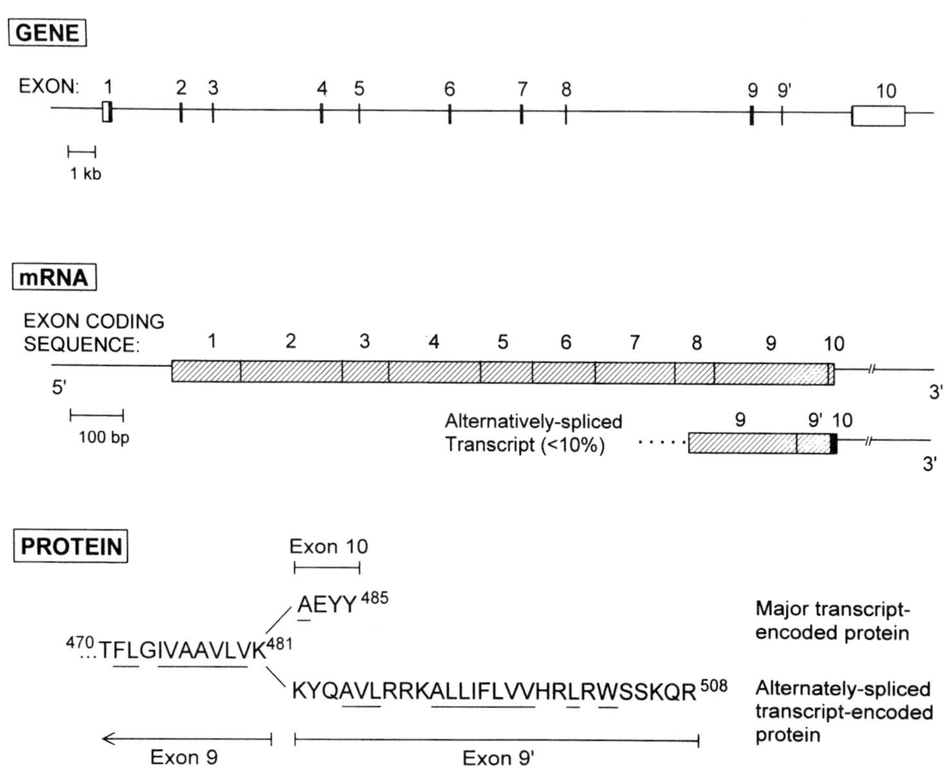

Figure 98-12. Organization of the FALDH gene, mRNA, and protein. The gene map shows the location of the exons, with coding portions as filled rectangles and noncoding portions of exons 1 and 10 as open rectangles. The mRNA consists of two alternately spliced transcripts that encode proteins containing different C-terminal domains. The C-terminal sequences of the alternate FALDH proteins are depicted. Underlined amino acid residues are hydrophobic.

Table 98-2 Mutations in the FALDH Gene Detected in SLS Patients

Type of Mutation	Exon	Nucleotide Change	Protein Change	Ethnic Origin of Patients with Mutation	Reference
Missense	4	641G > A	C214Y	Egyptian	14
	7	943C > T	P315S	Northern European, Swedish	43,144
Deletion	4	521delT	Frameshift and premature termination	Japanese	14
	6	808delG	Frameshift and premature termination	Japanese	14
	9	1297–1298delGA	Frameshift and premature termination	European	143, 145
Insertion	9	1311–1312insACAAA	Frameshift and premature termination	European	143
Deletion + Insertion	7	941–943del and ins21bp	A314G + insert 6 amino acids + P315A	Lebanese/Greek/mixed European	14

FALDH MUTATIONS IN SLS

SLS patients were first reported to have mutations in the FALDH gene by De Laurenzi *et al.*[14] These investigators found four mutations in three unrelated patients. Subsequent studies have identified several additional mutations in the FALDH gene,[43,143–145] including amino acid substitutions, deletions, insertions, and complex deletion/insertion rearrangements (Table 98-2). To date, seven different mutations in the FALDH gene have been reported among SLS patients from around the world.

The 943C > T mutation causes a substitution of Ser for Pro at codon 315 (P315S).[43,144] The Pro-315 residue is highly conserved among aldehyde dehydrogenase proteins.[134] In the structure of the rat class 3 protein,[136] the homologous Pro residue initiates a fold in the protein at the beginning of a short β-domain; it probably serves a similar function in human FALDH. This protein fold is critical for catalytic function, since baculovirus-induced expression of the P315S mutation resulted in a complete loss of enzyme activity.[43] Interestingly, Pro-315 is also altered in another mutation, which is a complex deletion/insertion that changes Pro-315 to Ala and Ala-314 to Gly, and results in the insertion of six additional amino acids into the protein[14] (Table 98-2).

Although most SLS patients have unique mutations, two mutations have been found at a higher frequency among patients of European ancestry, probably as a result of founder effects and/or inbreeding. The P315S mutation is present at a high frequency among kindreds from Sweden and northern Europe.[43,144] Seven SLS probands, not previously known to be genetically related, shared a common haplotype for this mutant allele, suggesting that these patients were distantly related. A second mutation (1297–1298delGA)[143,145] was found in 10 of 21 SLS probands of European origin and accounted for 26 percent of the SLS alleles. Among these 21 European probands, the P315S and 1297–1298delGA mutations together accounted for 48 percent of the SLS alleles, and 66 percent of the probands possessed at least one of them.[145] The existence of these common mutations raises the possibility of DNA-based diagnosis of SLS among this select population.[16]

In addition to mutations listed in Table 98-2, at least two polymorphisms are present within the FALDH gene. One of these is a polymorphic CA repeat in intron 8 that was previously identified as a microsatellite marker (AFMa126yd5).[43] The second is a silent polymorphism within the coding region of exon 10 that involves a change (1446T > A) in the third nucleotide of the codon for Ala482.[16]

PATHOGENESIS

The pathogenic mechanisms originating from mutation in the FALDH gene and culminating in the clinical symptoms of SLS are undoubtedly complex. Unfortunately, our understanding of the pathogenesis is sketchy at best, due to our ignorance of the most basic biochemical changes that occur in the nervous system and skin. Given the biochemical defect in SLS, it must be assumed that the pathogenesis is initiated with altered metabolism of fatty aldehyde and/or fatty alcohol, which results in modification of the lipid composition of tissues. It is not necessary, however, that the critical steps in the development of symptoms involve lipid metabolism. The primary lipid defect may have biochemical effects far removed from the initial abnormality and may cause alterations in structural proteins, enzymes, or even carbohydrates. Since the severity of cutaneous and neurologic symptoms do not correlate well with each other,[6] the pathogenic mechanisms probably differ in the nervous system and the skin. This dichotomy may arise from differences in the susceptibility of two tissues to identical biochemical derangements or may reflect variation between tissues in the biochemical abnormality. Finally, it is likely that these mechanisms are subject to influence from other genetic or environmental factors, because some patients with the same mutation in FALDH do not have identical severity of symptoms.

Based on current knowledge, it may be hypothesized that the initial steps in the pathogenesis of SLS involve 1) accumulation of fatty aldehyde or its metabolites, 2) accumulation of fatty alcohol or its metabolites, or 3) deficiency of polyunsaturated fatty acids.

Accumulation of Fatty Aldehyde or its Metabolites

Free fatty aldehydes have not been detected in intact SLS cells or patients, although they do accumulate in vitro when cell homogenates are incubated with fatty alcohol under optimal assay conditions (pH 9.8).[10,11] The lack of free aldehyde accumulation in intact cells may be caused by the highly reactive nature of aldehyde groups, which form stable and unstable adducts with molecules containing amino and thiol groups. Formation of covalent aldehyde-protein adducts is thought to be responsible for development of alcoholic cirrhosis, in which ethanol-derived acetaldehyde reacts with liver proteins.[146] Although fatty aldehydes were hypothesized to form covalent adducts with proteins or other molecules in SLS,[10,21] James and Zoeller[147] made the important observation that FALDH-deficient Chinese hamster ovary cells and SLS fibroblasts accumulated aldehyde-modified PE when fatty aldehydes were added to the culture medium. N-Alkyl-phosphatidylethanolamine (N-alkyl-PE) is generated when fatty aldehyde forms a Schiff base with the amino group of the ethanolamine moiety of the phospholipid (Fig. 98-13). The unstable Schiff base can become reduced over time to generate stable N-alkyl-PE adducts.

Aldehyde substrates that cannot be metabolized due to FALDH deficiency might be expected to react with PE and form N-alkyl-PE. One such fatty aldehyde is pristanal, which originates from decarboxylation, via α-oxidation, of phytanic acid.[93,94] Verhoeven *et al.*[95] showed that pristanal was a substrate for FALDH and that SLS fibroblasts were deficient in its oxidation. When intact SLS fibroblasts were incubated with radioactive phytanic acid in vitro, the cells accumulated radioactive N-alkyl-PE. SLS patients were found to have normal levels of phytanic acid in their plasma,

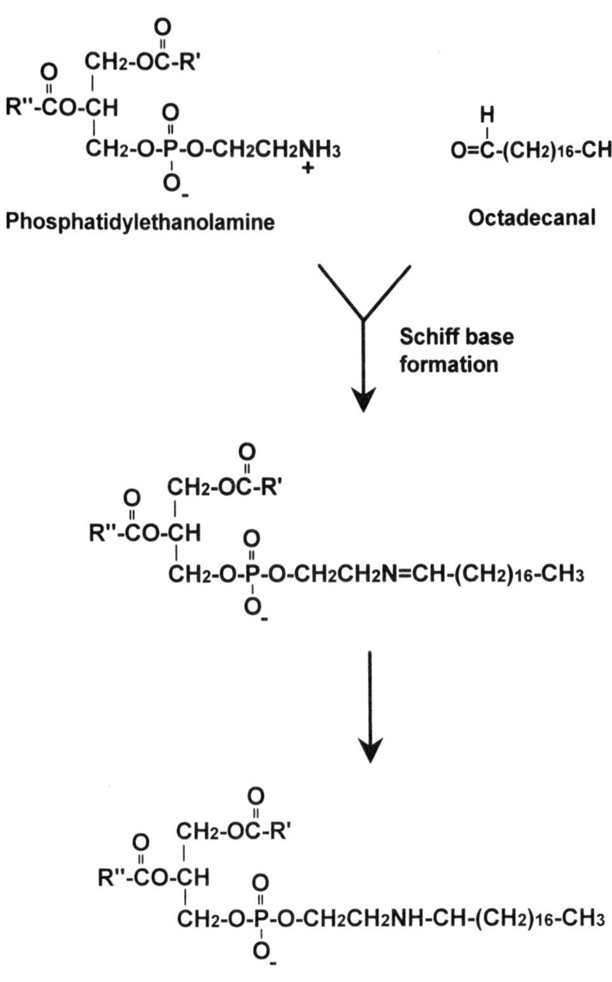

Figure 98-13. Formation of N-alkyl-phosphatidylethanolamine from fatty aldehyde (octadecanal) and phosphatidylethanolamine.

indicating that the block in pristanal oxidation does not prevent the decarboxylation step from occurring. Although the presence of pristanal-modified PE has not yet been demonstrated in vivo, the fibroblast results suggest that N-alkyl-PE may be derived from metabolism of pristanic acid and other fatty acids subjected to α-oxidation.

Formation of N-alkyl-PE would neutralize the positively charged amino group and eliminate its hydrophilic property by replacing it with a hydrophobic alkyl side chain. This dramatic alteration in the structure of PE is expected to have deleterious effects on membrane formation and/or function. It is noteworthy that the cutaneous water barrier within the stratum corneum and the function of myelin are both critically dependent on proper multilamellar membrane assembly. Since PE is a particularly prominent lipid in myelin, accumulation of N-alkyl-PE might be expected to have a profound effect on myelin stability and the function of myelin-associated proteins. The potential formation of fatty aldehyde-mediated Schiff base reactions with amino groups in proteins, carbohydrates, and other lipids raises the possibility of widespread disruption of a variety of biochemical pathways.

Accumulation of Fatty Alcohol or Its Metabolites

The contribution of fatty alcohol to the pathogenesis of SLS is unclear. In SLS, fatty alcohol accumulation appears to be restricted to those aliphatic alcohols that are 16 to 18 carbons long[21,127] (Fig. 98-11). Long-chain alcohols have a high partition coefficient for biologic membranes and would be expected to intercalate into intracellular membranes rather than exist free in solution.[148,149]

Fatty alcohols have been found to exert several potentially detrimental neurologic effects. Saturated alcohols less than 14 carbons long interfere with nerve transmission and have anesthetic properties, but alcohols longer than 14 carbons are virtually devoid of this effect.[150] *In vitro* studies indicate that long-chain alcohols become incorporated into synaptic vesicles.[149] Medium- and long-chain alcohols up to 12 carbons long potentiate $GABA_A$ receptor function and interfere with the righting reflex in mice.[151] With respect to SLS, the effect of longer-chain alcohols with 16–18 carbons on $GABA_A$ receptor function or the righting reflex is not known.

It is possible, however, that fatty alcohol accumulation is responsible for the cutaneous symptoms in SLS. The lipid composition of the skin is important for maintaining the cutaneous water barrier, which is largely derived from the membrane-rich stratum corneum.[152] The intercellular, multilamellar membranes in the stratum corneum are formed when lamellar bodies in the granular cells fuse with the apical plasma membrane and extrude their membrane-rich contents into the junction of the granular and stratum corneum layers. Several inborn errors of metabolism disrupt epidermal lipid composition and are associated with ichthyosis.[153] These include disorders that affect metabolism of cholesterol sulfate (steroid sulfatase deficiency, Chap. 166), phytanic acid (adult Refsum disease, Chap. 132, and rhizomelic chondrodysplasia punctata, Chap. 130), glucocerebrosides (type II Gaucher disease, Chap. 146), and triglycerides (neutral lipid storage disease, (OMIM 275630). Hexadecanol has been found to inhibit lipase activity *in vitro*[154] and could potentially cause triglyceride accumulation in the epidermis. The altered ceramide content of the scales in SLS may be one marker for abnormal stratum corneum lipids.[47] In SLS, it is hypothesized that fatty alcohol storage or diversion of fatty alcohol into the synthetic pathways for wax esters or ether lipids leads to an altered epidermal lipid composition that disrupts the water barrier and induces a hyperproliferative state.[21] The increased transepidermal water loss would cause the skin to dry out and might result in hyperkeratosis and ichthyosis.

Balancing the indirect data suggesting that fatty alcohol is important in SLS pathogenesis is the lack of evidence that straight chain fatty alcohols are toxic to normal animals. Short-term feeding studies in rats revealed no harmful effects of octadecanol,[155] and rats fed a diet containing up to 10 percent (wt/wt) octadecanol for 6 weeks showed no cutaneous or neurologic symptoms.[67] These results in normal animals possessing abundant FALDH activity do not rule out the possibility that patients with SLS are selectively susceptible to fatty alcohol toxicity.

Unlike straight chain fatty alcohols, certain branched chain alcohols may be toxic when fed in large quantities to rodents.[156] One of these is phytol, the metabolic precursor to phytanic acid. Mice fed large amounts of phytol develop cutaneous and neurologic symptoms after several days.[157] This toxic effect, however, may be mediated solely or in part by the metabolism of the phytol to phytanic acid.

In summary, fatty alcohol-induced alterations in the lipid composition of SLS tissues may impair nerve and epidermal function in ways that are not well understood, but direct experimental evidence for such a pathogenic mechanism is still lacking.

Deficiency of Polyunsaturated Fatty Acids

There is convincing evidence that SLS patients are deficient in certain polyunsaturated fatty acids. Hernell *et al.*[137] found that the serum phospholipids from SLS patients had reduced levels of several polyunsaturated fatty acids that are derived from δ-6 desaturation of the essential fatty acid linoleic acid (18:2). The levels of linoleic acid itself were normal, indicating that the patients were not nutritionally deficient in this fatty acid. The polyunsaturated fatty acid deficiencies observed are probably secondary biochemical changes, since cultured skin fibroblasts from SLS patients grown in vitro have a normal fatty acid composition and readily perform delta-6 desaturation.[138] Nevertheless, the fatty acid deficiencies observed in the blood of SLS patients probably also occur in other tissues, including the skin, and may contribute to the cutaneous disease. Essential fatty acid deficiency causes epidermal symptoms of desquamation, probably mediated by alteration in the epidermal lipid composition and disruption of the cutaneous water barrier.[153] Alone, the polyunsaturated fatty acid deficiencies in SLS may not be sufficient to cause frank ichthyosis, but they may contribute to the hyperkeratosis, especially in combination with other lipid changes.

DIAGNOSIS

The diagnosis of SLS should be entertained in any patient with ichthyosis and neurologic symptoms. The cutaneous disease usually brings the patient to medical attention in the neonatal period. At that time, the differential diagnosis includes many other forms of ichthyosis. After the onset of developmental delay and spasticity in infancy or childhood, however, the diagnostic considerations narrow to SLS and several other neuro-ichthyotic disorders, such as neutral lipid storage disease, multiple sulfatase deficiency, Refsum disease, trichothiodystrophy, Rud syndrome, Netherton syndrome, keratitis-ichthyosis-deafness syndrome, and the SLS-like disorders.

Enzymatic testing provides a definitive diagnosis for patients suspected to have SLS. Deficiency of FALDH or FAO is readily demonstrated in cultured skin fibroblasts.[9–11,127,128] The use of 18-carbon aliphatic substrates in the enzymatic assay adds reliability to the results by minimizing the residual activity measured in affected patients.[10] In cultured skin fibroblasts, activity of FAO ranges from 2 percent to 16 percent of mean normal activity using octadecanol as substrate.[21] FALDH deficiency is reduced to a similar extent using octadecanal as substrate. There is no overlap between enzyme activity levels measured in SLS heterozygotes and affected homozygotes using 18-carbon substrates in the assays (Fig. 98-9). The FALDH assay has an advantage over that for FAO because it is less time-consuming, but it must be run on freshly prepared cell homogenates. In contrast, FAO activity can be measured on cell pellets frozen at $-70°C$ for several days, but the method uses a radioactive substrate and is more time-consuming. SLS patients also have deficient FAO and FALDH activity in mixed leukocytes prepared by the dextran sedimentation technique,[127,128] but mononuclear cells prepared by density gradient methods are not a reliable enzyme source. Demonstration of deficient alcohol-oxidizing activity in frozen biopsies of skin and jejunum using a histochemical staining technique affords an alternative method for diagnosing SLS[128,129] (Fig. 98-8). Measurement of plasma fatty alcohols is not recommended as a diagnostic test, because it is technically difficult and not specific for SLS. Elevated plasma fatty alcohols are also seen in rhizomelic chondrodysplasia punctata and possibly in other peroxisomal disorders that disrupt incorporation of fatty alcohol into ether lipids.[67,68]

The enzymatic test is useful for the detection of SLS heterozygotes, who generally show a partial reduction in FALDH activity[10,11] (Fig. 98-10). However, there is overlap between the enzyme activity levels measured in some obligate SLS heterozygotes and those found in normal controls, which precludes the test from being completely reliable for diagnosing at-risk carriers. In at-risk heterozygotes with low-normal FALDH activity, measurement of FAO may demonstrate activity below the normal range.[11] If a mutation has been identified in a family, DNA testing should prove to be the most reliable method for carrier detection.

DNA-based diagnosis of SLS is feasible for families in which the mutation is known and for targeted populations that have a limited number of mutant alleles. Direct sequencing of exons to search for mutations is straightforward but time-consuming. More rapid methods using restriction enzyme digestion or allele-specific PCR amplification have been developed to screen DNA for several of the mutations common in patients of European origin.[43,144,145] For patients with mixed ethnic background or families for which a FALDH mutation has not been identified, the enzymatic method remains the diagnostic test of choice. Linkage analysis using microsatellite markers is potentially useful for family studies when the mutation is not known, but mutation analysis is more direct and eliminates the possibility of misdiagnosis arising from recombination events.

Prenatal diagnosis of SLS was first accomplished by histologic examination of a fetal skin biopsy obtained at 23 weeks' gestation.[158] The biopsy revealed the characteristic hyperkeratosis. However, this method carries a relatively high risk of complications, and the diagnosis of an affected fetus may be missed if fetal skin biopsies are taken before the end of the second trimester, prior to the onset of fetal skin keratinization.[159] Furthermore, newer, less invasive enzymatic and DNA methods have replaced fetal skin biopsy as a diagnostic tool.

Prenatal diagnosis may be performed earlier in gestation by measuring FALDH and FAO activities in cultured amniocytes obtained at 16 weeks and cultured chorionic villus cells collected at 9–11 weeks.[12] To date, our lab has enzymatically diagnosed 12 at-risk fetuses with complete reliability in outcome.

DNA-based prenatal diagnosis has been accomplished in several instances. In the first reported case, mutation analysis of an at-risk fetus revealed a homozygous 943C>T mutation on DNA from chorionic villus tissue.[160] In four other pregnancies involving different mutations, DNA analysis was performed together with enzymatic testing, and results were concordant (Rizzo *et al.*, unpublished data).

THERAPY

The therapy of SLS is largely symptomatic. Although not as serious as the neurologic symptoms, the daily management of the cutaneous disease in SLS is often considered to be a more immediate problem for patients and their families. The main principle for treatment of the ichthyosis is to keep the skin hydrated and remove excessive scales. Daily water baths are often useful, and moisturizing lotions are important for maintaining skin hydration. Topical keratolytic agents, such as urea and lactic acid, help eliminate scales. An initial report of topical administration of the vitamin D_3 calcipotriol in SLS is promising.[161] Systemic retinoids, particularly etretinate[162,163] and the newer short-acting derivative acitretin,[164] are quite effective in improving the skin. Although concern about potential bone toxicity as a side effect of systemic retinoid therapy has limited its use in children, Lacour *et al.*[164] recently found that acitretin was safe and effective in treating the cutaneous disease in three children with SLS.

Treatment of the neurologic disease is limited to supportive measures. Seizures, if present, usually respond well to standard anticonvulsant therapy. Spasticity and contractures are often managed by surgical procedures, such as tendon lengthening and dorsal rhizotomy. Medications to treat the spasticity seem to have limited benefit.

Several patients with SLS have been treated with fat-modified diets. In 1967, Hooft *et al.*[165] reported an SLS patient with exudative enteropathy, peripheral edema, hypoalbuminemia, hypocalcemia, hypolipidemia, and chronic steatorrhea. To improve the fat malabsorption, the patient was placed on a diet in which long-chain fatty acids were replaced with medium-chain fatty acids. Along with correction of his serum abnormalities, the boy showed remarkable resolution of the ichthyosis. Guilleminault *et al.*[166] later placed twin sisters with SLS on a diet containing 13 percent of fat derived from meat and supplemented with an unspecified amount of medium-chain triglycerides. These patients were reported to show improvement in their ichthyosis and neurologic function after 13 months. Chaves-Carballo *et al.*[167]

treated an 8-year-old boy, later confirmed to have FALDH deficiency, with a diet containing 20–40 percent of calories from medium-chain triglycerides. Over a 12-month period, the ichthyosis improved but there was no change in the neurologic symptoms. More recently, Maaswinkel-Mooij *et al.*[168] treated five enzymatically confirmed SLS patients with a diet that reduced fat intake to 15–20 percent of total calories and added medium-chain fatty acids to raise total fat consumption to 45 percent of calories. Plasma octadecanol concentrations did not become normal after 13 months on this diet, and no clinical benefit was observed.

Based on these limited studies, the efficacy of dietary therapy for SLS is still unsettled. In all reports with a favorable response, the diets were poorly described and there was no mention of specific foods that were actually consumed.[165–167] It is possible that the clinical improvement resulted from removing foods that contained fatty alcohols or other lipids that are metabolized into fatty aldehyde. In this regard, the diet used by Maaswinkel-Mooij *et al.* did not restrict vegetables and fruits that might be rich in fatty alcohols and wax esters.

On the assumption that serum polyunsaturated fatty acid deficiency contributed to the symptoms, fatty acid therapy was attempted in several SLS patients.[18,168] Jagell *et al.*[18] summarized their experience feeding evening primrose oil, which provides polyunsaturated fatty acids that bypass the presumed defect in delta-6 desaturation, to nine Swedish patients for 3 months and found no clinical benefit. Maaswinkel-Mooij *et al.*[168] treated two young SLS patients with 3–5 g/kg/day of dietary evening primrose oil. After 16 months, the patients showed no clinical improvement. Surprisingly, they exhibited no increase in serum levels of the δ-6 desaturation products, perhaps due to impaired absorption of the fatty acids.

ADDENDUM

Since completion of this chapter, molecular genetic studies on SLS have advanced considerably. Mutation analyses of the FALDH gene in SLS patients have increased the number of known mutations to 58.[169–172] Three additional single nucleotide polymorphisms were found within introns 1, 3, and 6 of the FALDH gene, raising the total number of intragenic polymorphisms to five.[172] Haplotype analyses using these polymorphic markers showed that several SLS patients, who shared one of four common mutations, had different haplotypes, which suggests that these mutations each recurred independently on different genetic backgrounds. In contrast, haplotype analyses of European patients carrying 1297–1298delGA and 943C > T are consistent with a founder effect and common ancestor.

Progress in sequencing the human genome has resulted in identification of the complete sequence of the FALDH gene along with its neighboring ALDH3 gene on a 190-kb contig from chromosome 17p11.2 (GenBank AC005722). The two genes are located 62 kb apart and are oriented in opposite directions on the chromosome.

Willemsen et al.[173] reported that patients with SLS accumulated the ω-hydroxy oxidation product of leukotriene B_4, a proinflammatory aliphatic lipid mediator, whereas the ω-carboxy metabolite was not detectable. Since leukotriene B is degraded by ω-oxidation, these findings strongly suggest that FALDH is necessary for the complete ω-oxidation of leukotriene B_4. Accumulation of ω-hydroxy-leukotriene B_4 or the corresponding ω-aldehyde derivative, which was not measured in this study, may be involved in the pathogenesis of SLS.

Van Domburg et al.[174] described the clinical and neuroradiographic findings in 11 SLS patients ranging in age from 4 years to 42 years. Most of the patients were born prematurely and all had retinal glistening white dots. The patients showed considerable variation in severity of neurologic symptoms. Each of six patients tested had an abnormal lipid peak on MR spectroscopy of the brain.

REFERENCES

1. Sjögren T: Oligophrenia combined with congenital ichthyosiform erythroderma, spastic syndrome and macular-retinal degeneration. *Acta Genet* **6**:80, 1956.
2. Sjögren T, Larsson T: Oligophrenia in combination with congenital ichthyosis and spastic disorders. *Acta Psychiatr Neurol Scand* **32**(suppl 113):1, 1957.
3. Söderhjelm AL, Enell H: Iktyos, spastisk diplegi i nedre extremiteterna och oligofreni–ett sarskelt syndrom. *Nord Med* **17**:624, 1957.
4. Theile U: Sjögren-Larsson syndrome: Oligophrenia-ichthyosis-di/tetraplegia. *Humangenetik* **22**:91, 1974.
5. Jagell S, Gustavson K-H, Holmgren G: Sjögren-Larsson syndrome in Sweden: A clinical, genetic and epidemiological study. *Clin Genet* **19**:233, 1981.
6. Jagell S, Heijbel J: Sjögren-Larsson syndrome: Physical and neurological features. *Helv Paediat Acta* **37**:519, 1982.
7. Jagell S, Polland W, Sandgren O: Specific changes in the fundus typical for the Sjögren-Larsson syndrome: An ophthalmological study of 35 patients. *Acta Ophthalmol* **58**:321, 1980.
8. Jagell S, Lidén S: Ichthyosis in the Sjögren-Larsson syndrome. *Clin Genet* **21**:243, 1982.
9. Rizzo WB, Dammann AL, Craft DA: Sjögren-Larsson syndrome: Impaired fatty alcohol oxidation in cultured fibroblasts due to deficient fatty alcohol:nicotinamide adenine dinucleotide oxidoreductase activity. *J Clin Invest* **81**:738, 1988.
10. Rizzo WB, Craft DA: Sjögren-Larsson syndrome: Deficient activity of the fatty aldehyde dehydrogenase component of fatty alcohol:NAD oxidoreductase in cultured fibroblasts. *J Clin Invest* **88**:1643, 1991.
11. Kelson TL, Craft DA, Rizzo WB: Carrier detection for Sjögren-Larsson syndrome. *J Inher Metab Dis* **15**:105, 1992.
12. Rizzo WB, Craft DA, Kelson TL, Bonnefont J-P, Saudubray J-M, Schulman JD, Black SH, Tabsh K, Di Rocco M, McKinlay Gardner RJ: Prenatal diagnosis of Sjögren-Larsson syndrome using enzymatic methods. *Prenat Diagn* **14**:577, 1994.
13. Pigg M, Jagell S, Sillen A, Weissenbach J, Gustavson K-H, Wadelius C: The Sjögren-Larsson syndrome gene is close to D17S805 as determined by linkage analysis and allelic association. *Nature* **8**:361, 1994.
14. De Laurenzi V, Rogers GR, Hamrock DJ, Marekov LN, Steinert PM, Compton JG, Markova N, Rizzo WB: Sjögren-Larsson syndrome is caused by mutations in the fatty aldehyde dehydrogenase gene. *Nat Genet* **12**:52, 1996.
15. Rogers GR, Markova NG, De Laurenzi V, Rizzo WB, Compton JG: Genomic organization and expression of the human fatty aldehyde dehydrogenase gene (FALDH). *Genomics* **39**:127, 1997.
16. Chang C, Yoshida A: Human fatty aldehyde dehydrogenase gene (ALDH10): Organization and tissue-dependent expression. *Genomics* **40**:80, 1997.
17. Richards BW: Sjögren-Larsson syndrome, in Winken PJ, Bruyn GW (eds): *Handbook of Clinical Neurology* vol 13. Amsterdam, North-Holland, 1972, p 468.
18. Jagell S, Gustavson K-H, Holmgren G: Sjögren-Larsson syndrome: Update of a clinical, genetic, and epidemiological study, in Berg JM (ed): *Perspectives and Progress in Mental Retardation* vol 2: *Biomedical Aspects*. Baltimore, I.A.S.S.M.D., 1984, p 73.
19. Lidén S, Jagell S: The Sjögren-Larsson syndrome. *Int J Dermatol* **23**:247, 1984.
20. Chaves-Carballo E: Sjögren-Larsson syndrome, in Gomez MR (ed): *Neurocutaneous Diseases*. Boston, Butterworths, 1987, p 219.
21. Rizzo WB: Sjögren-Larsson syndrome. *Semin Dermatol* **12**:210, 1993.
22. Rizzo WB: Sjögren-Larsson syndrome, in Moser HW (ed): *Handbook of Clinical Neurology: Neurodystrophies and Neurolipidoses* vol 22(66). Amsterdam, Elsevier, 1996, p 615.
23. Lacour M: Update on Sjögren-Larsson syndrome. *Dermatology* **193**:77, 1996.
24. Heijer A, Reed WB: Sjögren-Larsson syndrome: Congenital ichthyosis, spastic paralysis, and oligophrenia. *Arch Dermatol* **92**:545, 1965.
25. Goldsmith LA, Baden HP, Canty TG: Sjögren-Larsson syndrome: Diversity of cutaneous manifestations. *Acta Dermatovener* (Stockholm) **51**:374, 1971.
26. Ito M, Oguro K, Sato Y: Ultrastructural study of the skin in Sjögren-Larsson syndrome. *Arch Dermatol Res* **283**:141, 1991.
27. Nigro JF, Rizzo WB, Esterly NB: Redefining the Sjögren-Larsson syndrome: Atypical findings in three siblings and implications regarding diagnosis. *J Am Acad Dermatol* **35**:678, 1996.
28. Selmanowitz VJ, Porter MJ: The Sjögren-Larsson syndrome. *Am J Med* **42**:412, 1967.

29. Gilbert WR, Smith JL, Nyhan WL: The Sjögren-Larsson syndrome. *Arch Ophthalmol* **80**:308, 1968.
30. Forsberg H, Jagell S, Reuterving C-O: Oral conditions in Sjögren-Larsson syndrome. *Swed Dent J* **7**:141, 1983.
31. Probst FP, Jagell S, Heijbel J: Cranial CT in the Sjögren-Larsson syndrome. *Neuroradiology* **21**:101, 1981.
32. Mulder LJMM, Oranje AP, Loonen MCB: Cranial CT in the Sjögren-Larsson syndrome. *Neuroradiology* **29**:560, 1987.
33. Gomori JM, Leibovici V, Zlotogorski A, Wirguin I, Haham-Zadeh S: Computed tomography in Sjögren-Larsson syndrome. *Neuroradiology* **29**:557, 1987.
34. Di Rocco M, Filocamo M, Tortori-Donati P, Veneselli E, Borrone C, Rizzo WB: Sjögren-Larsson syndrome: Nuclear magnetic resonance imaging of the brain in a 4-year-old boy. *J Inher Metab Dis* **17**:112, 1994.
35. Miyanomae Y, Ochi M, Yoshioka H, Takaya K, Kizaki Z, Inoue F, Furuya S, Naruse S: Cerebral MRI and spectroscopy in Sjögren-Larsson syndrome: Case report. *Neuroradiology* **37**:225, 1995.
36. Hussain MZ, Aihara M, Oba H, Ohtomo K, Uchiyama G, Hayashibe H, Nakazawa S: MRI of white matter changes in the Sjögren-Larsson syndrome. *Neuroradiology* **37**:576, 1995.
37. Van Mieghem F, Van Goethem JWM, Parizel PM, Cras P, van den Hauwe L, De Meirleire J, De Schepper AM: MR of the brain in Sjögren-Larsson syndrome. *Am J Neuroradiol* **18**:1561, 1997.
38. Ikarashi M, Morishita M, Ito M, Suzuki M, Sato Y: Sjögren-Larsson syndrome. *Rinsho Hifuka* (Tokyo) **39**:339, 1985.
39. Jagell SF, Holmgren G, Hofer PÅ: Congenital ichthyosis with alopecia, eclabion, ectropion and mental retardation — A new genetic syndrome. *Clin Genet* **31**:102, 1987.
40. Scalais E, Verloes A, Sacre J-P, Pierard GE, Rizzo WB: Sjögren-Larsson-like syndrome with bone dysplasia and normal fatty alcohol NAD^+ oxidoreductase activity. *Pediatr Neurol* **8**:459, 1992.
41. Koone MD, Rizzo WB, Elias PM, Williams ML, Lightner V, Pinnell SR: Ichthyosis, mental retardation, and asymptomatic spasticity: A new neurocutaneous syndrome with normal fatty alcohol:NAD^+ oxidoreductase activity. *Arch Dermatol* **126**:1485, 1990.
42. Iselius L, Jagell S: Sjögren-Larsson syndrome in Sweden: Distribution of the gene. *Clin Genet* **35**:272, 1989.
43. De Laurenzi V, Rogers GR, Tarcsa E, Carney G, Marekov L, Bale SJ, Compton JG, Markova N, Steinert PM, Rizzo WB: Sjögren-Larsson syndrome is caused by a common mutation in northern European and Swedish patients. *J Invest Dermatol* 1997.
44. Hofer P-A, Jagell S: Sjögren-Larsson syndrome: A dermato-histopathological study. *J Cutan Pathol* **9**:360, 1982.
45. Matsuoka LY, Kousseff BG, Hashimoto K: Studies of the skin in Sjögren-Larsson syndrome by electron microscopy. *Am J Dermatopathol* **4**:295, 1982.
46. Lucker GPH, Steijlen PM, Suykerbuyk EJA, Kragballe K, Brandrup F, van de Kerkhof CM: Flow-cytometric investigation of epidermal cell characteristics in monogenic disorders of keratinization and their modulation by topical calcipotriol treatment. *Acta Derm Venereol* (Stockholm) **76**:97, 1996.
47. Paige DG, Morse-Fisher N, Harper JI: Quantification of stratum corneum ceramides and lipid envelope ceramides in the hereditary ichthyoses. *Br J Dermatol* **131**:23, 1994.
48. Judge MR, Morse-Fisher N, Manku M, Harper JI: Quantification of n-alkanes in stratum corneum in the hereditary ichthyoses. *Br J Dermatol* **127**:91, 1992.
49. Baar HS, Galindo J: Pathology of the Sjögren-Larsson syndrome. *J Maine Med Assoc* **56**:223, 1965.
50. Sylvester PE: Pathological findings in Sjögren-Larsson syndrome. *J Mental Defic Res* **13**:267, 1969.
51. McLennan JE, Gilles FH, Robb RM: Neuropathological correlation in Sjögren-Larsson syndrome: Oligophrenia, ichthyosis and spasticity. *Brain* **97**:693, 1974.
52. Silva CA, Saraiva A, Goncalves V, de Sousa G, Martins R, Cruz C: Pathological findings in one of two siblings with Sjögren-Larsson syndrome. *Eur Neurol* **19**:166, 1980.
53. Wester P, Bergström U, Brun A, Jagell S, Karlsson B, Eriksson A: Monoaminergic dysfunction in Sjögren-Larsson syndrome. *Mol Chem Neuropathol* **15**:13, 1991.
54. Yamaguchi K, Handa T: Sjögren-Larsson syndrome: Postmortem brain abnormalities. *Pediatr Neurol* **18**:338, 1998.
55. Mano T, Ono J, Kaminaga T, Imai K, Sakurai K, Harada K, Nagai T, Rizzo WB, Okada S: Proton MR spectroscopy of Sjögren-Larsson's syndrome. *Am J Neuroradiol* **20**:1671, 1999.
56. Nilsson SEG, Jagell S: Lipofuscin and melanin content of the retinal pigment epithelium in a case of Sjögren-Larsson syndrome. *Br J Ophthalmol* **71**:224, 1986.
57. Mahadevan V: Chemistry and metabolism of fatty aldehydes. *Prog Chem Fats Other Lipids* **11**:83, 1971.
58. Mahadevan V: Fatty alcohols: Chemistry and metabolism. *Prog Chem Fats Other Lipids* **15**:255, 1978.
59. Takahashi T, Schmid HHO: Long-chain alcohols in mammalian tissues. *Chem Phys Lipids* **4**:243, 1970.
60. Natarajan V, Schmid HHO: 1-Docosanol and other long chain primary alcohols in developing rat brain. *Lipids* **12**:128, 1977.
61. Hanahan DJ: Ether-linked lipids: Chemistry and methods of measurement, in Snyder F (ed): *Ether Lipids: Chemistry and Biology*. New York, Academic Press, 1972, p 25.
62. Nicolaides N: The monoene and other wax alcohols of human skin surface lipid and their relation to the fatty acids of this lipid. *Lipids* **2**:266, 1967.
63. Oku H, Shudo J, Mimura K, Haratake A, Nagata J, Chinen I: 1-O-Alkyl-2,3-diacylglycerols in the skin surface lipids of the hairless mouse. *Lipids* **30**:169, 1995.
64. O'Brien JS, Sampson EL: Lipid composition of the normal human brain: Gray matter, white matter, and myelin. *J Lipid Res* **6**:537, 1965.
65. Rizzo WB, Dammann AL, Craft DA, Phillips MW: Fatty alcohol metabolism in cultured human fibroblasts: Evidence for a fatty alcohol cycle. *J Biol Chem* **262**:17412, 1987.
66. James PF, Rizzo WB, Lee J, Zoeller RA: Isolation and characterization of a Chinese hamster ovary cell line deficient in fatty alcohol:NAD^+ oxidoreductase activity. *Proc Natl Acad Sci USA* **87**:6102, 1990.
67. Rizzo WB: Inherited disorders of fatty alcohol metabolism. *Mol Genet Metab* **65**:63, 1998.
68. Rizzo WB, Craft DA, Judd LL, Moser HW, Moser AB: Fatty alcohol accumulation in the autosomal recessive form of rhizomelic chondrodysplasia punctata. *Biochem Mol Med* **50**:93, 1993.
69. Hue L: Futile cycles and regulation of metabolism, in Sies H (ed): *Metabolic Compartmentation*. London, Academic Press, 1982, p 71.
70. Riendeau D, Meighen E: Enzymatic reduction of fatty acids and acyl-CoAs to long chain aldehydes and alcohols. *Experientia* **41**:707, 1985.
71. Bishop JE, Hajra AK: Mechanism and specificity of formation of long chain alcohols by developing rat brain. *J Biol Chem* **256**:9542, 1981.
72. Bishop JE, Hajra AK: Specificity of reduction of fatty acids to long chain alcohols by rat brain microsomes. *J Neurochem* **30**:643, 1978.
73. Wykle RL, Malone B, Snyder F: Acyl-CoA reductase specificity and synthesis of wax esters in mouse preputial gland tumors. *J Lipid Res* **20**:890, 1979.
74. Skjeldal OH, Stokke O, Refsum S, Norseth J, Petit H: Clinical and biochemical heterogeneity in conditions with phytanic acid accumulation. *J Neurol Sci* **77**:87, 1987.
75. Moore C, Snyder F: Regulation of acyl coenzyme A reductase by a heat-stable cytosolic protein during preputial gland development. *Arch Biochem Biophys* **214**:500, 1982.
76. Takahashi N, Saito T, Goda Y, Tomita K: Participation of microsomal aldehyde reductase in long-chain fatty alcohol synthesis in the rat brain. *Biochim Biophys Acta* **963**:243, 1988.
77. Johnson RC, Gilbertson JR: Isolation, characterization, and partial purification of a fatty acyl coenzyme A reductase from bovine cardiac muscle. *J Biol Chem* **247**:6991, 1972.
78. Ichihara K, Ishihara K, Kusunose E, Kusunose M: Some properties of a hexadecane hydroxylation system in rabbit intestinal mucosa microsomes. *J Biochem* **89**:1821, 1981.
79. Kolattukudy PE, Rogers L: Acyl-CoA reductase and acyl-CoA: Fatty alcohol acyl transferase in the microsomal preparation from the bovine meibomian gland. *J Lipid Res* **27**:404, 1986.
80. Furuyoshi S, Shi Y-Q, Rando RP: Acyl group transfer from the sn-1 position of phospholipids in the biosynthesis of n-dodecyl palmitate. *Biochemistry* **32**:5425, 1993.
81. van den Bosch H, de Vet ECJM: Alkyl-dihydroxyacetonephosphate synthase. *Biochim Biophys Acta* **1348**:35, 1997.
82. Horrocks LA, Sharma M: Plasmalogens and O-alkyl glycerophospholipids, in Hawthorne, Ansell (eds): *Phospholipids*. New York, Elsevier, 1982, p 51.
83. Lee T-C: Characterization of fatty alcohol: NAD^+ oxidoreductase from rat liver. *J Biol Chem* **254**:2892, 1979.
84. Ichihara K, Kusunose E, Noda Y, Kusunose M: Some properties of the fatty alcohol oxidation system and reconstitution of microsomal oxidation activity in intestinal mucosa. *Biochim Biophys Acta* **878**:412, 1986.

85. Nakayasu H, Mihara K, Sato R: Purification and properties of a membrane-bound aldehyde dehydrogenase from rat liver microsomes. *Biochem Biophys Res Commun* **83**:697, 1978.
86. Kelson TL, Secor McVoy JR, Rizzo WB: Human liver fatty aldehyde dehydrogenase: Microsomal localization, purification, and biochemical characterization. *Biochim Biophys Acta* **1335**:99, 1997.
87. Ichihara K, Noda Y, Tanaka C, Kusunose M: Purification of aldehyde dehydrogenase reconstitutively active in fatty alcohol oxidation from rabbit intestinal microsomes. *Biochim Biophys Acta* **878**:419, 1986.
88. Teitz A, Lindberg M, Kennedy EP: A new pteridine-requiring enzyme system for the oxidation of glyceryl ethers. *J Biol Chem* **239**:4081, 1964.
89. Soodsma JF, Piantadosi C, Snyder F: Partial characterization of the alkylglycerol cleavage enzyme system of rat liver. *J Biol Chem* **247**:3923, 1972.
90. Stoffel W, Sticht G, LeKim D: Degradation in vitro of dihydrosphingosine and dihydrosphingosine phosphate to palmitaldehdye and ethanolamine phosphate. *Hoppe-Seyler's Z Physiol Chem* **349**:1745, 1968.
91. Keenan RW, Maxam A: The in vitro degradation of dihydrosphingosine. *Biochim Biophys Acta* **176**:348, 1969.
92. Stoffel W, LeKim D, Heyn G: Sphinganine (dihydrosphingosine), an effective donor of the alk-1′-enyl chain of plasmalogens. *Hoppe-Seyler's Z Physiol Chem* **351**:875, 1970.
93. Croes K, Casteels M, Asselberghs S, Herdewijn P, Mannaerts GP, Van Veldhoven PP: Formation of a 2-methyl-branched fatty aldehyde during peroxisomal α-oxidation. *FEBS Letters* **412**:643, 1997.
94. Verhoeven NM, Schor DSM, ten Brink HJ, Wanders RJA, Jakobs C: Resolution of the phytanic acid α-oxidation pathway: Identification of pristanal as product of the decarboxylation of 2-hydroxyphytanoyl-CoA. *Biochem Biophys Res Commun* **237**:33, 1997.
95. Verhoeven NM, Jakobs C, Carney G, Somers MP, Wanders RJA, Rizzo WB: Involvement of microsomal fatty aldehyde dehydrogenase in the α-oxidation of phytanic acid. *FEBS Lett* **429**:225, 1998.
96. Welsh CJ, Robinson M, Warne TR, Pierce JH, Yeh GC, Phang JM: Accumulation of fatty alcohol in MCF-7 breast cancer cells. *Arch Biochem Biophys* **315**:41, 1994.
97. Bourre J-M, Daudu O: Stearyl-alcohol biosynthesis from stearyl-CoA in mouse brain microsomes in normal and dysmyelinating mutants (quaking and jimpy). *Neurosci Lett* **7**:225, 1978.
98. Lee T-C, Fitzgerald V, Stephens N, Snyder F: Activities of enzymes involved in the metabolism of ether-linked lipids in normal and neoplastic tissues of rat. *Biochim Biophys Acta* **619**:420, 1980.
99. Cabot MC, Snyder F: Manipulation of alkylglycerolipid levels in cultured cells. Fatty alcohol versus alkylglycerol supplements. *Biochim Biophys Acta* **617**:410, 1980.
100. Gelman RA, Gilbertson JR: Permeability of the blood-brain barrier to long-chain alcohols from plasma. *Nutr Metabol* **18**:169, 1975.
101. Krisans SK, Mortensen RM, Lazarow PB: Acyl-CoA synthetase in rat liver peroxisomes. *J Biol Chem* **255**:9599, 1980.
102. Natarajan V, Schmid HHO: Biosynthesis and utilization of long-chain alcohols in rat brain: Aspects of chain length specificity. *Arch Biochem Biophys* **187**:215, 1978.
103. Burdett K, Larkins LK, Das AK, Hajra AK: Peroxisomal localization of acyl-coenzyme A reductase (long chain alcohol forming) in guinea pig intestine mucosal cells. *J Biol Chem* **266**:12201, 1991.
104. Hajra AK, Burke CL, Jones CL: Subcellular localization of acyl coenzyme A: Dihydroxyacetone phosphate acyltransferase in rat liver peroxisomes (microbodies). *J Biol Chem* **254**:10896, 1979.
105. Hajra AK, Bishop JE: Glycerolipid biosynthesis in peroxisomes via the acyl dihydroxyacetone phosphate pathway. *Ann NY Acad Sci* **386**:170, 1982.
106. Singh H, Beckman K, Poulos A: Exclusive localization in peroxisomes of dihydroxyacetone phosphate acyltransferase and alkyl-dihydroxyacetone phosphate synthase in rat liver. *J Lipid Res* **34**:467, 1993.
107. Sakuraba H, Noguchi T: Alcohol:NAD$^+$ oxidoreductase is present in rat liver peroxisomes. *J Biol Chem* **270**:37, 1995.
108. Hayashi H, Sato A: Fatty alcohol synthesis accompanied with chain elongation in liver peroxisomes. *Biochim Biophys Acta* **1346**:38, 1997.
109. Hayashi H, Hara M: 1-Alkenyl group of ethanolamine plasmalogen derives mainly from de novo-synthesized fatty alcohol within peroxisomes, but not extraperoxisomal fatty alcohol or fatty acid. *J Biochem* **121**:978, 1997.
110. Kolattukudy PE: Plant waxes. *Lipids* **5**:259, 1970.
111. Feron VJ, Til HP, de Vrijer F, Woutersen RA, Cassee FR, van Bladeren PJ: Aldehydes: Occurrence, carcinogenic potential, mechanism of action and risk assessment. *Mutat Res* **259**:363, 1991.
112. Malins DC, Wekell JC: The lipid biochemistry of marine organisms. *Prog Chem Fats Other Lipids* **10**:337, 1969.
113. Blank ML, Cress EA, Smith ZL, Snyder F: Meats and fish consumed in the American diet contain substantial amounts of ether-linked phospholipids. *J Nutr* **122**:1656, 1992.
114. Stetten D, Schoenheimer R: The biological relations of the higher aliphatic alcohols to fatty acids. *J Biol Chem* **133**:347, 1940.
115. Blomstrand R, Rumpf JA: The conversion of [1-^{14}C] cetyl alcohol into palmitic acid in the intestinal mucosa of the rat. *Acta Physiol Scand* **32**:374, 1954.
116. Bandi ZL, Aaes-Jorgensen E, Mangold HK: Metabolism of unusual lipids in the rat. I. Formation of unsaturated alkyl and alk-1-enyl chains from orally administered alcohols. *Biochim Biophys Acta* **239**:357, 1971.
117. Hansen IA, Mead JF: The fate of dietary wax esters in the rat. *Proc Soc Exp Biol Med* **120**:527, 1965.
118. Weber N: Metabolism of orally administered rac-1-O-[1′-^{14}C]dodecylglycerol and nutritional effects of dietary rac-1-O-dodecylglycerol in mice. *J Lipid Res* **26**:1412, 1985.
119. Blank ML, Cress EA, Smith ZL, Snyder F: Dietary supplementation of ether-linked lipids and tissue lipid composition. *Lipids* **26**:166, 1991.
120. Das AK, Holmes RD, Wilson GN, Hajra AK: Dietary ether lipid incorporation into tissue plasmalogens of humans and rodents. *Lipids* **27**:401, 1992.
121. Sieber SM, Cohn VH, Wynn WT: The entry of foreign compounds into the thoracic duct lymph of the rat. *Xenobiotica* **4**:265, 1974.
122. Steinberg D: Refsum disease, in Scriver CR, Beaudet AL, Sly WS, Valle D (eds): *The Metabolic and Molecular Bases of Inherited Disease* vol 2. New York, McGraw-Hill, 1995, p 2351.
123. Holmes RD, Wilson GN, Hajra A: Oral ether lipid therapy in patients with peroxisomal disorders. *J Inher Metab Dis* **10**:239, 1987.
124. Lindahl R: Aldehyde dehydrogenases and their role in carcinogenesis. *Crit Rev Biochem Mol Biol* **27**:283, 1992.
125. Yoshida A, Rzhetsky A, Hsu LC, Chang C: Human aldehyde dehydrogenase gene family. *Eur J Biochem* **251**:549, 1998.
126. Pederson J, Lindahl RG: Aldehyde dehydrogenases, in Guengerich FP (ed): *Comprehensive Toxicology* vol 3, *Biotransformation*. Oxford, Elsevier, 1997.
127. Rizzo WB, Dammann AL, Craft DA, Black SH, Henderson Tilton A, Africk D, Chaves-Carballo E, Holmgren G, Jagell S: Sjögren-Larsson syndrome: Inherited defect in the fatty alcohol cycle. *J Pediatr* **115**:228, 1989.
128. Judge MR, Lake BD, Smith VV, Besley GTN, Harper JI: Depletion of alcohol (hexanol) dehydrogenase activity in the epidermis and jejunal mucosa in Sjögren-Larsson syndrome. *J Invest Dermatol* **95**:632, 1990.
129. Lake BD, Smith VV, Judge MR, Harper JI, Besley GTN: Hexanol dehydrogenase activity shown by enzyme histochemistry on skin biopsies allows differentiation of Sjögren-Larsson syndrome from other ichthyoses. *J Inher Metab Dis* **14**:338, 1991.
130. Vasiliou V, Kozak CA, Lindahl R, Nebert DW: Mouse microsomal class 3 aldehyde dehydrogenase: AHD3 cDNA sequence, inducibility by dioxin and clofibrate, and genetic mapping. *DNA Cell Biol* **15**:235, 1996.
131. Miyauchi K, Masaki R, Taketani S, Yamamoto A, Akayama M, Tashiro Y: Molecular cloning, sequencing, and expression of cDNA for rat liver microsomal aldehyde dehydrogenase. *J Biol Chem* **266**:19536, 1991.
132. Hiraoka LR, Hsu L, Hsieh C-L: Assignment of ALDH3 to human chromosome 17p11.2 and ALDH5 to human chromosome 9p13. *Genomics* **25**:323, 1995.
133. Santisteban I, Povey S, West LF, Parrington JM, Hopkinson DA: Chromosome assignment, biochemical and immunological studies on a human aldehyde dehydrogenase, ALDH3. *Ann Hum Genet* **49**:87, 1985.
134. Hempel J, Nicholas H, Lindahl R: Aldehyde dehydrogenases: Widespread structural and functional diversity within a shared framework. *Protein Sci* **2**:1890, 1993.
135. Masaki R, Yamamoto A, Tashiro Y: Microsomal aldehyde dehydrogenase is localized to the endoplasmic reticulum via its carboxy-terminal 35 amino acids. *J Cell Biol* **126**:1407, 1994.
136. Liu Z-J, Sun Y-J, Rose J, Chung Y-J, Hsiao C-D, Chang W-R, Kuo I, Perozich J, Lindahl R, Hempel J, Wang B-C: The first structure of an aldehyde dehydrogenase reveals novel interactions between NAD and the Rossmann fold. *Nat Struct Biol* **4**:317, 1997.

137. Hernell O, Holmgren G, Jagell SF, Johnson SB, Holman RT: Suspected faulty essential fatty acid metabolism in Sjögren-Larsson syndrome. *Pediatr Res* **16**:45, 1982.
138. Avigan J, Campbell BD, Yost DA, Hernell O, Holmgren G, Jagell SF: Sjögren-Larsson syndrome: Delta 5-and delta 6-fatty acid desaturases in skin fibroblasts. *Neurology* **35**:401, 1985.
139. Rogers GR, Rizzo WB, Zlotogorski A, Hashem N, Lee M, Compton JG, Bale SJ: Genetic homogeneity in Sjögren-Larsson syndrome: Linkage to chromosome 17p in families of different non-Swedish ethnic origins. *Am J Hum Genet* **57**:1123, 1995.
140. Lacour M, Middleton-Price R, Harper JI: Confirmation of linkage of Sjögren-Larsson syndrome to chromosome 17 in families of different ethnic origins. *J Med Genet* **33**:258, 1996.
141. Sillén A, Alderborn A, Pigg M, Jagell S, Wadelius C: Detailed genetic and physical mapping in the Sjögren-Larsson syndrome gene region in 17p11.2. *Hereditas* **128**:245, 1998.
142. Azizkhan JC, Jensen DE, Pierce AJ, Wade M: Transcription from TATA-less promoters: Dihydrofolate reductase as a model. *Crit Rev Eukaryot Gene Expr* **3**:229, 1993.
143. Tsukamoto N, Chang C, Yoshida A: Mutations associated with Sjögren-Larsson syndrome. *Ann Hum Genet* **61**:235, 1997.
144. Sillén A, Jagell S, Wadelius C: A missense mutation in the FALDH gene identified in Sjögren-Larsson syndrome patients originating from the northern part of Sweden. *Hum Genet* **100**:201, 1997.
145. Rizzo WB, Carney G, De Laurenzi V: A common deletion mutation in European patients with Sjögren-Larsson syndrome. *Biochem Mol Med* **62**:178, 1997.
146. Nicholls R, de Jersey J, Worrall S, Wilce P: Modification of proteins and other biological molecules by acetaldehyde: Adduct structure and functional significance. *Int J Biochem* **24**:1899, 1992.
147. James PF, Zoeller RA: Isolation of animal cell mutants defective in long-chain fatty aldehyde dehydrogenase: Sensitivity to fatty aldehydes and Schiff's base modification of phospholipids: Implications for Sjögren-Larsson syndrome. *J Biol Chem* **272**:23532, 1997.
148. Franks NP, Lieb WR: Partitioning of long-chain alcohols into lipid bilayers: Implications for mechanisms of general anesthesia. *Proc Natl Acad Sci USA* **83**:5116, 1986.
149. Miller KW, Firestone LL, Alifimoff JK, Streicher P: Nonanesthetic alcohols dissolve in synaptic membranes without perturbing their lipids. *Proc Natl Acad Sci USA* **86**:1084, 1989.
150. Pringle MJ, Brown KB, Miller KW: Can the lipid theories of anesthesia account for the cutoff in anesthetic potency in homologous series of alcohols? *Mol Pharmacol* **19**:49, 1981.
151. Didly-Mayfield JE, Mihic SJ, Liu Y, Deitrich RA, Harris RA: Actions of long chain alcohols on $GABA_A$ and glutamate receptors: Relation to in vivo effects. *Br J Pharmacol* **118**:378, 1996.
152. Elias PM: Epidermal lipids, barrier function, and desquamation. *J Invest Dermatol* **80**:44, 1983.
153. Williams ML: Lipids in normal and pathological desquamation, in Elias PM, Havel RJ, Small DM (eds): *Advances in Lipid Research* vol 24. San Diego, Academic Press, 1991, p 211.
154. Ferreira GC, Patton JS: Inhibition of lipolysis by hydrocarbons and fatty alcohols. *J Lipid Res* **31**:889, 1990.
155. Elder RL: Final report on the safety assessment of stearyl alcohol, oleyl alcohol, and octyl dodecanol. *J Am Coll Toxicol* **4**:1, 1985.
156. Steinberg D, Avigan J, Mize CE, Baxter JH, Cammermeyer J, Fales HM, Highet PF: Effects of dietary phytol and phytanic acid in animals. *J Lipid Res* **7**:684, 1966.
157. Van den Branden C, Vamecq J, Wybo I, Roels F: Phytol and peroxisomal proliferation. *Pediatr Res* **20**:411, 1986.
158. Kousseff BG, Matsuoka LY, Stenn KS, Hobbins JC, Mahoney MJ, Hashimoto K: Prenatal diagnosis of Sjögren-Larsson syndrome. *J Pediatr* **101**:998, 1982.
159. Tabsh K, Rizzo WB, Holbrook K, Theroux N: Sjögren-Larsson syndrome: Technique and timing of prenatal diagnosis. *Obstet Gynecol* **82**:700, 1993.
160. Sillén A, Holmgren G, Wadelius C: First prenatal diagnosis by mutation analysis in a family with Sjögren-Larsson syndrome. *Prenat Diagn* **17**:1147, 1997.
161. Lucker GPH, van de Kerkhof PCM, Cruysberg JRM, der Kinderen DJ, Steijlen PM: Topical treatment of Sjögren-Larsson syndrome with calcipotriol. *Dermatology* **190**:292, 1995.
162. Jagell S, Lidén S: Treatment of the ichthyosis of the Sjögren-Larsson syndrome with etretinate (Tegison). *Acta Dermatovener* (Stockholm) **63**:89, 1983.
163. Traupe H, Happle R: Etretinate therapy in children with severe keratinization defects. *Eur J Pediatr* **143**:166, 1985.
164. Lacour M, Mehta-Nikhar B, Atherton DJ, Harper JI: An appraisal of acitretin therapy in children with inherited disorders of keratinization. *Br J Dermatol* **134**:1023, 1996.
165. Hooft C, Kriekemans J, van Acker K, Devos E, Traen S, Verdonk G: Sjögren-Larsson syndrome with exudative enteropathy: Influence of medium-chain triglycerides on the symptomatology. *Helv Paediat Acta* **22**:447, 1967.
166. Guilleminault C, Harpey JP, Lafourcade J: Sjögren-Larsson syndrome: Report of two cases in twins. *Neurology* **23**:367, 1973.
167. Chaves-Carballo E, Frank LM, Bason WM: Treatment of Sjögren-Larsson syndrome with medium-chain triglycerides. *Ann Neurol* **10**:294, 1981.
168. Maaswinkel-Mooij PD, Brouwer OF, Rizzo WB: Unsuccessful dietary treatment of Sjögren-Larsson syndrome. *J Pediatr* **124**:748, 1994.
169. Sillén A, Anton-Lamprecht I, Braun-Quentin C, Kraus CS, Sayli BS, Ayuso C, Jagell S, Köster W, Wadelius C: Spectrum of mutations and sequence variants in the FALDH gene in patients with Sjögren-Larsson syndrome. *Hum Mutat* **12**:377, 1998.
170. Willemsen MAAP, Steijlen PM, de Jong JGN, Rotteveel JJ, IJlst L, van Werkhoven MA, Wanders RJA: A novel 4 bp deletion mutation in the FALDH gene segregating in a Turkish family with Sjögren-Larsson syndrome. *J Invest Dermatol* **112**:827, 1999.
171. IJlst L, Oostheim W, van Werkhoven M, Willemsen MAAP, Wanders RJA: Molecular basis of Sjögren-Larsson syndrome: frequency of the 1297–1298 del GA and 943C→T mutation in 29 patients. *J Inher Metab Dis* **22**:319, 1999.
172. Rizzo WB, Carney G, Lin Z: The molecular basis of Sjögren-Larsson syndrome: mutation analysis of the fatty aldehyde dehydrogenase gene. *Am J Hum Genet* **65**:1547, 1999.
173. Willemsen MAAP, de Jong JGN, van Domburg PHMF, Rotteveel JJ, Wanders RJA, Mayatepek E: Defective inactivation of leukotriene B_4 in patients with Sjögren-Larsson syndrome. *J Pediatr* **136**:258, 2000.
174. Van Domburg PHMF,Willemsen MAAP, Rotteveel JJ, de Jong JGN, Thijssen HOM, Heerschap A, Cruysberg JRM, Wanders RJA, Gabrels FJM, Steijlen PM: Sjögren-Larsson syndrome. Clinical and MRI/MRS findings in FALDH-deficient patients. *Neurology* **52**:1345, 1999.

PART 10

DISORDERS OF MITOCHONDRIAL FUNCTION

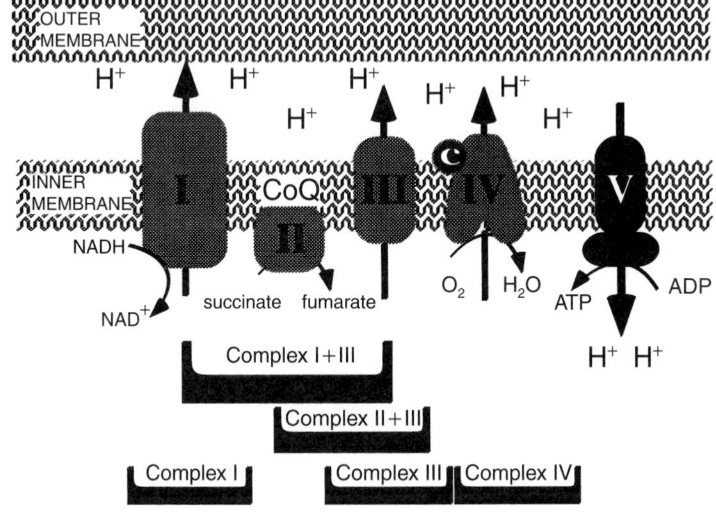

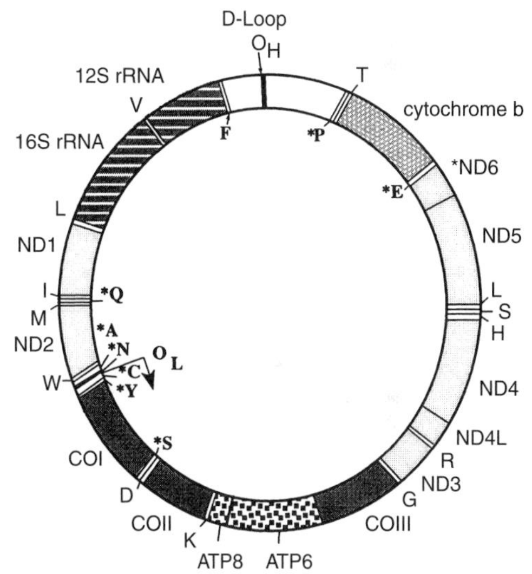

CHAPTER 99

Clinical Presentation of Respiratory Chain Deficiency

Arnold Munnich ▪ Agnès Rötig
Valérie Cormier-Daire ▪ Pierre Rustin

THE METABOLIC DYSFUNCTION

Oxidative phosphorylation, i.e., ATP synthesis by the respiratory chain, is a ubiquitous metabolic pathway that supplies most organs and tissues with energy. Consequently, respiratory chain deficiency can theoretically give rise to any symptom, in any organ or tissue, at any age, with any mode of inheritance, due to the twofold genetic origin of respiratory enzymes (nuclear DNA and mitochondrial DNA).

In the last few years, it has become increasingly clear that genetic defects of oxidative phosphorylation account for a large variety of clinical symptoms in childhood. Among 160 respiratory enzyme chain-deficient patients identified in our center, 40 percent were referred for a neuromuscular symptom and 60 percent presented with a nonneuromuscular disease.[1] Overall, the diagnosis of respiratory chain deficiency is difficult to consider when the first symptom occurs. The diagnosis becomes easier when two seemingly unrelated symptoms are observed.

The mitochondrial respiratory chain catalyzes the oxidation of fuel molecules by oxygen and the concomitant energy transduction into ATP via five complexes, embedded in the inner mitochondrial membrane[2] (Fig. 99-1). Complex I (NADH-coenzyme Q reductase) carries reducing equivalents from NADH to coenzyme Q (CoQ, ubiquinone) and consists of more than 40 different polypeptides, seven of which are encoded by mitochondrial DNA (mtDNA). Complex II (succinate-CoQ reductase) carries reducing equivalents from $FADH_2$ to CoQ and contains four polypeptides, including the FAD-dependent succinate dehydrogenase and three iron-sulfur centers. This is the only complex that does not contain any mtDNA-encoded protein. Complex III (reduced CoQ-cytochrome *c* reductase) carries electrons from CoQ to cytochrome *c*. It contains 11 subunits, one of which (cytochrome *b*) is encoded by mtDNA. Complex IV (cytochrome *c* oxidase, COX), the terminal oxidase of the respiratory chain, catalyzes the transfer of reducing equivalents from cytochrome *c* to molecular oxygen. It is composed of two cytochromes (*a* and a_3), two copper atoms, and 13 different protein subunits, three of which are encoded by mtDNA.[2]

During the oxidation process, electrons are transferred to oxygen via the energy-transducing complexes of the respiratory chain: complexes I, III, and IV for NADH-producing substrates; complexes II, III, and IV for succinate; and complexes III and IV for $FADH_2$, derived from the β-oxidation pathway via the electron transfer flavoprotein (ETF) and the ETF-CoQ oxidoreductase system (Fig. 99-1). CoQ, a highly hydrophobic quinone, and cytochrome *c*, a low-molecular-weight hemoprotein, act as "shuttles" between complexes. The free energy generated from the redox reactions is converted into a transmembrane proton gradient. Protons are pumped through complexes I, III, and IV of the respiratory chain, creating a charge differential. Complex V (ATP synthase) allows protons to flow back into the mitochondrial matrix and uses the released energy to synthesize ATP. Three ATP molecules are made for each NADH molecule oxidized.

Since the respiratory chain transfers NADH to oxygen, a disorder of oxidative phosphorylation should result in 1) an increase of reducing equivalents in both mitochondria and cytoplasm and 2) the functional impairment of the citric acid cycle, due to the excess of NADH and the lack of NAD. Therefore, an increase of ketone body (β-OH butyrate/acetoacetate) and lactate/pyruvate (L/P) molar ratios with secondary elevation of blood lactate might be found in the plasma of affected individuals.[3] This is particularly true in the postabsorptive period, when more NAD is required to adequately oxidize glycolytic substrates. Similarly, as a consequence of the functional impairment of the citric acid cycle, ketone body synthesis increases after meals due to the channeling of acetyl-CoA toward ketogenesis. The elevation of total ketone bodies in a fed individual is paradoxical, as it should normally decrease after meals, due to insulin release (paradoxical hyperketonemia).[4]

CLINICAL PRESENTATIONS

Due to the ubiquitous nature of oxidative phosphorylation, a defect of the mitochondrial respiratory chain should be considered in patients presenting with an unexplained combination of neuromuscular and/or nonneuromuscular symptoms, with a progressive course, involving seemingly unrelated organs or tissues. Table 99-1 lists the clinical symptoms currently observed in respiratory chain deficiency and their frequency in our series of 160 patients.[1] These features, either isolated or in combination, may occur at any stage, but the major feature is the increasing number of organs involved over the course of the disease (Fig. 99-2). This progressive organ involvement occurs regardless of age at onset and clinical presentation. Yet, while the initial symptoms usually

A list of standard abbreviations is located immediately preceding the index in each volume. Nonstandard abbreviations used in this chapter include: CHARGE = coloboma-heart-choanal atresia-mental retardation-genitourinary syndrome; CoQ = coenzyme Q_{10}; DCPIP = dichlorophenol indophenol; FAS = fetal alcohol syndrome; FRDA = Friedreich ataxia; GH = growth hormone; HSP = hereditary spastic paraplegia; KSS = Kearns-Sayre syndrome; L/P : lactate/pyruvate; LHON = Leber hereditary optic neuropathy; MELAS = mitochondrial encephalomyopathy with lactic acidosis and stroke-like episodes; MERRF = myoclonus epilepsy with ragged red fibers; MNGIE = mitochondrial myopathy, peripheral neuropathy, encephalopathy, and gastrointestinal disease; MRS = magnetic resonance spectroscopy; NARP = neurogenic ataxia and retinitis pigmentosa; PCr = phosphocreatine; PEO = progressive external ophthalmoplegia; PPK = palmoplantar keratoderma; RRF = ragged red fiber; SQDR = succinate quinone DCPIP reductase; SSCR = succinate cytochrome *c* reductase; VATER = vertebral-anal-tracheo-esophageal-renal syndrome.

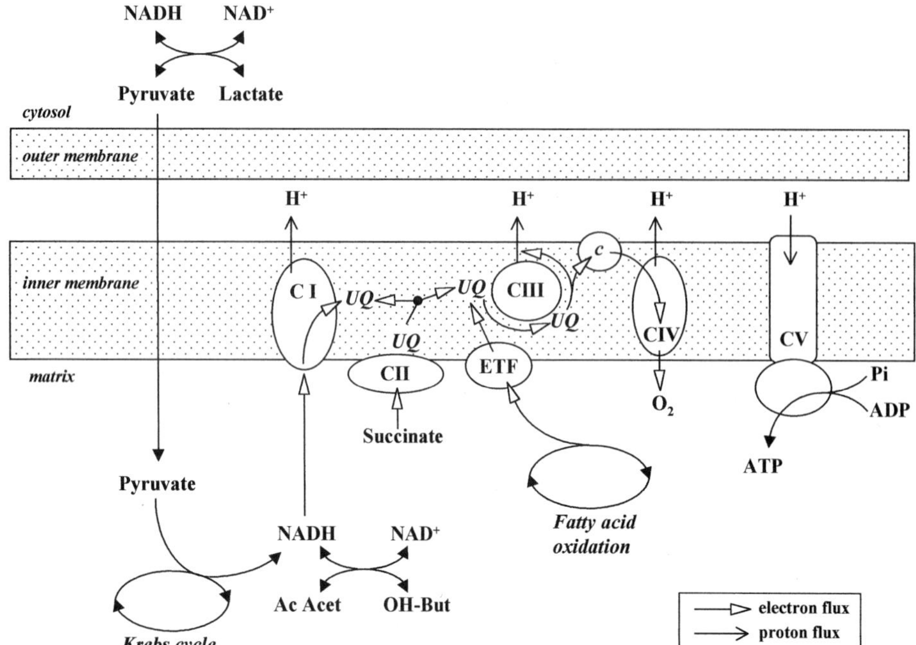

Fig. 99-1. The mitochondrial respiratory chain. ETF = electron transfer flavoprotein; UQ = quinone.

persist and gradually worsen, they occasionally improve or even disappear as other organs become involved.

Neurological presentation

The central and/or peripheral nervous system involvement is frequent at the beginning and almost constant at the late stages of the disease. The disease may start in the neonatal period with drowsiness, poor sucking, severe hypotonia, abnormal movements, seizures, respiratory distress, and fatal ketoacidotic coma with major lactic acidosis. Severe encephalopathy may start later in childhood after a period of apparently normal development. Frequently, the first cause of concern is poor head control, inability to roll over, or delay in ability to sit without support or walk unaided. Later, the clinical profile results from the variable combination of the following neurologic symptoms: trunk hypotonia, cranial nerve and brainstem involvement (e.g., abnormal eye movements, ophthalmoplegia, recurrent apneas), cerebellar ataxia, myoclonia, seizures, pyramidal syndrome, peripheral neuropathy, poliodystrophy, and leukodystrophy (Table 99-1). Patients who follow such a course often present with bouts of drowsiness and frequently get worse following intercurrent infections.[5,6]

Leukodystrophy, i.e., the diffuse impairment of the cerebral white matter, predominantly results in motor disturbance with slow mental retardation and low incidence of seizures. Several syndromes of respiratory chain deficiency involve the white matter, including MELAS, Kearns-Sayre, and Leigh syndromes[7] (see below). However, diffuse involvement of the central white matter can also occur as the major or even unique manifestation of the disease, and respiratory chain deficiency should therefore be regarded as a possible cause of isolated leukodystrophy in childhood.[7]

Muscular presentation

Various degrees of muscle involvement are observed, ranging in severity from fatal infantile myopathy to progressive muscle weakness in childhood and adulthood. Fatal infantile myopathy presents with severe progressive and generalized weakness, respiratory distress, and lactic acidosis. Patients with the fatal form die before 1 year of age of respiratory failure and multiple organ involvement.[5,8] Yet spontaneous remissions have been observed despite severe initial weakness.[9]

The myopathic form is characterized by hypotonia and progressive weakness of the limbs, with intolerance of exertion and muscle atrophy. Symptoms may appear within the first 2 years of life or later in childhood or adulthood. Myopathy may remain isolated or become associated with various additional symptoms, such as retinal dystrophies, ophthalmoplegia, or other organ involvement. Plasma lactate level at rest is normal or mildly elevated, but exercise can trigger a significant elevation of lactic acid.

Other muscular symptoms are occasionally observed, such as myalgias or myoglobinuria. While dystrophinopathies and inborn errors of metabolism (glycolysis, glycogenolysis, and fatty acid oxidation) are known to cause rhabdomyolysis, mitochondrial disorders are not currently regarded as a cause of myoglobinuria. Recently, several children have been reported with recurrent attacks of trunk and limb hypotonia, myalgias, muscle stiffness, lethargy, and repeated episodes of myoglobinuria, ascribed to respiratory chain deficiency.[10,11] Surprisingly, all patients had generalized hyporeflexia during attacks, subnormal plasma lactate levels, and inconstant enzyme deficiency in muscle. Expression of the enzyme deficiency in cultured fibroblasts helps to diagnose this condition, especially when rhabdomyolysis precludes skeletal muscle biopsy during and/or after acute episodes. The pathogenesis of the disease is unknown, but the reduced ATP availability is likely to trigger muscle cell lysis, possibly through the release of respiratory chain components (such as cytochrome *c*) that are known to activate the apoptotic program and worsen muscle injury.[12,13]

Cardiac presentation

Genetic defects of oxidative phosphorylation represent a major cause of cardiomyopathy in children. Cardiomyopathy frequently appears as the onset symptom or as part of multiorgan involvement.[14] In the neonatal period, recurrent apnea, dyspnea, cyanosis, or bronchitis may be the only presenting symptoms of a rapidly fatal mitochondrial cardiomyopathy, whereas delayed-onset forms are frequently diagnosed in patients with unexplained heart failure.[15] The redox status in plasma is consistently disturbed in the neonatal onset form and frequently normal in the delayed onset form. Most patients have concentric hypertrophic and hypokinetic cardiomyopathy; the question of whether the dilated forms are primarily or secondarily dilated is still debated.

Table 99-1 Clinical Symptoms in Respiratory Chain Deficiency

Organ/System	Symptom/Sign	%
Central nervous system	Trunk hypotonica, poor head control	36
	Psychomotor regression, mental retardation	8
	Cranial nerve involvement	18
	Limb spasticity	11
	Peripheral neuropathy	3
	Cerebellar ataxia	8
	Subacute brainstem necrosis	–
	Diffuse white matter involvement (leukodystrophy)	3
	Grey matter involvement (poliodystrophy)	3
	Myoclonus, generalized seizures	–
	Hemicranial headache, migraine	–
	"Stroke-like" episodes	–
	Recurrent apneas, lethargy, drowsiness	–
Body mass	Postnatal growth failure	31
	Intrauterine growth retardation	20
Muscle	Muscle weakness, myopathy	13
	Myalgia, muscle stiffness, exercise intolerance	2
	Recurrent myoglobinuria	2
Liver	Progressive liver enlargement	
	Hepatocellular dysfunction	20
	Hepatic failure (valproate-induced)	
Heart	Cardiomyopathy (hypertrophic +++, dilated	
	Complete heart block	24
	Intraventricular conduction block	
	Right bundle branch block	
Kidney	Proximal tubulopathy (De Toni–Debŕe–Fanconi syndrome)	
	Tubulointerstitial nephritis (mimicking nephrophthisis)	8
	Nephrotic syndrome	
	Renal failure	
	Hemolytic uremic syndrome	
Gut	Chronic diarrhea, villous atrophy	
	Recurrent vomiting, anorexia +++	
	Chronic intestinal pseudoobstruction	
	Exocrine pancreatic dysfunction	8
	Duodenal atresia	
	Failure to thrive	
Bone marrow	Anemia (with ring sideroblasts)	
	Neutropenia (with vacuoles)	
	Thrombopenia	8
	Myelodysplastic syndrome	
	Dyserythropoiesis	
Endocrine	Short stature, delayed bone age	
	GH-unresponsive IgF1 deficiency	
	Recurrent hypoglycemia	–
	Diabetes mellitus, insulin dependent or independent	3
	Hypothyroidism	–
	Hypoparathyroidism	–
	ACTH deficiency	–
	Cryptorchidism	–

Table 99-1 (Continued)

Organ/System	Symptom/Sign	%
Ear	Hearing impairment	
	Sensorineural deafness (brainstem or cochlear)	
	Ototoxicity (aminoside-induced)	
Eye	Lid ptosis	
	Diplopia	
	Progressive external opthalmoplegia (PEO)	
	Limitation of eye movements (all directions, upgaze +++)	8
	Cataract, corneal opacities	
	Optic atrophy	
	Pigmentary retinal degeneration	
Craniofacial/limb malformations	Microcephaly	
	Round face	
	High forehead	
	Flat philtrum	
	Low-set ears	
	Short neck	8
	Short hands, hypoplastic nails	
	Hypoplasia of the distal/ middle phalanges	
	VACTERL association	
Skin	Fatty infiltration of skin	
	Mottled pigmentation (photo-exposed areas)	
	Trichothiodystrophy	5
	Dry, thick, brittle hair	
	Palmoplantar keratoderma	
Metabolic features	Ketoacidotic coma	3
	Metabolic acidosis	
	Hypoglycemia	
	Hyperlactatemia (hyper α-alaninemia)	
	Hypermethioninemia	1
	Hypocitrullinemia	3

The percentages refer to the frequency of the symptoms in a personal series of 160 respiratory enzyme chain–deficient children.[1]

Endomyocardial biopsy is a reliable diagnostic tool in cardiomyopathy.[16] Heart morphology is frequently abnormal (interstitial fibrosis, fibroelastosis). All types of respiratory chain enzyme deficiency have been observed, but complex I deficiency is significantly more frequent.[1] Point mutations as well as multiple mtDNA deletions have been described in several families.[17] Barth syndrome is an important subtype of syndromic cardiomyopathy,[18,19] as this X-linked condition may account for the excess of boys in our series (sex ratio 1.7:1). It is an (ante- or) neonatal-onset cardiomyopathy with cyclic neutropenia and rapidly fatal outcome. It is therefore important to look carefully for neutropenia in boys with neonatal-onset cardiomyopathy, as the recent identification of the disease gene on chromosome Xq28 helps to diagnose this condition.[20] In addition, the endomyocardial biopsy is particularly valuable in the significant fraction of cases that are not expressed in other tissues. Indeed, while multiorgan involvement is usually regarded as a contraindication to organ transplantation, it is reasonable to consider heart transplantation in slowly progressive forms limited to the myocardium.

Renal presentation

Renal involvement is a frequent manifestation of respiratory chain deficiency. The first symptoms develop in the neonatal period or before the age of 2 years. The most common manifestation is a

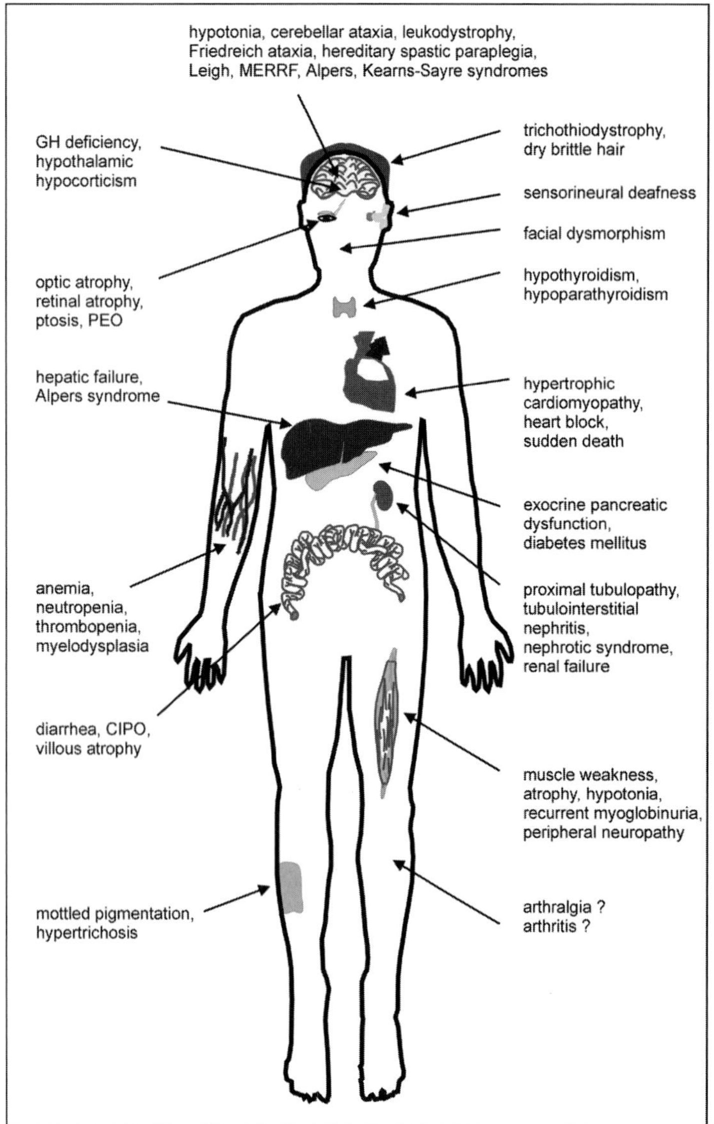

Fig. 99-2. The diversity of organ involvement in respiratory chain deficiency.

proximal tubulopathy with de Toni-Debré-Fanconi syndrome.[21–23] Other renal presentations have been reported, including glomerular disease with a nephrotic syndrome and chronic tubulointerstitial nephropathy.[21,22,24,25] Plasma lactate and L/P ratios are consistently normal, but interestingly, abnormal urinary lactate and Krebs cycle intermediates point toward respiratory chain deficiency. Fanconi syndrome is characterized by impairment of proximal tubular reabsorption, leading to urinary loss of amino acids, glucose, proteins, ions, and water. In respiratory chain deficiency, it is frequently limited to mild aminoaciduria and occasionally responsible for metabolic acidosis. When available, the renal biopsy shows unspecific anomalies of the tubular epithelium with dilations or obliteration by casts, dedifferentiation or atrophy, and occasionally giant mitochondria. Glomerular disease with nephrotic syndrome has been reported in patients with pathologic evidence of focal and segmental glomerular sclerosis.[22] In addition, tubulointerstitial nephritis has occasionally been reported in patients with chronic renal insufficiency. Renal biopsy showed diffuse interstitial fibrosis with tubular atrophy and sclerosed glomeruli in these cases. Finally, the MELAS mutation has been described in several families with cardiomyopathy, diabetes mellitus, sensorineural deafness, and renal failure unrelated to diabetes mellitus.[17,26–28]

Nutritional presentation

A significant fraction of affected neonates are small for gestational age, a feature that illustrates the frequently antenatal expression of the disease.[1,29] Indeed, intrauterine growth retardation was present in 20 percent of cases in our series[1,4,15] (Table 99-1). Alternatively, growth failure may occur postnatally, at any age, after several months of apparently normal development (31 percent of cases in our series). Unexplained inflection of the weight/height curve may long be the unique manifestation of the disease. Severe anorexia, recurrent vomiting, chronic diarrhea with villous atrophy, and/or exocrine pancreatic dysfunction occasionally occur.[30,31] These features are often ascribed to gluten or cow-milk protein intolerance, but they do not resolve with change of diet. These clinical forms are consistently associated with disturbed redox status in plasma and frequently with mtDNA rearrangements in various tissues. Interestingly, while the gastrointestinal symptoms usually persist and gradually worsen, they may occasionally improve or even disappear as other organs become involved. Indeed, remarkable remissions of watery diarrhea have been reported in infants who later developed other organ involvement.[30] In adulthood, chronic intestinal pseudoobstruction has been occasionally ascribed to respiratory chain deficiency.[8,32]

Hepatic presentation

Genetic defects of oxidative phosphorylation have been recognized as possible causes of hepatic failure. Two forms have been identified on the bases of clinical course and severity: a severe neonatal form (40 percent) and a delayed onset form (60 percent).[33] The neonatal form has an early onset (before 1 week), a rapidly fatal course, and frequent neurologic involvement, including severe hypotonia, myoclonic epilepsy, and psychomotor retardation.[34,35] The other type has a delayed onset (from 2 to 18 months), a milder clinical course, inconstant neurologic involvement, and occasionally a fatal outcome.[33] The delayed onset form deserves intensive efforts, because in several cases spontaneous marked improvement after ursodeoxycholic therapy and liver transplantation has occurred. Yet two children developed severe psychomotor retardation and microcephaly following liver transplantation in our series. It is reasonable to limit liver transplantation to patients with severe hepatic failure but no neurologic symptoms or evidence of extrahepatic involvement.

Abnormal histology (steatosis, micro- and macronodular cirrhosis) and elevated plasma or CSF lactate are consistent features of the disease, regardless of the clinical subtype. Deficiency of complexes I and IV and multiple enzyme deficiency have been observed, but no correlation could be made between the enzyme deficiency and the clinical course of the disease. With regard to the extent of the disease, the brain was the most severely affected organ but other organs could occasionally be involved. While mitochondrial DNA depletion has occasionally been observed in severe hepatic failure,[35] the molecular bases of the disease remain largely unknown.[36] The high rate of parental consanguinity in complex IV and I + IV deficiency suggests that autosomal recessive genes are involved,[1] but systematic sequencing of liver-specific nuclear COX subunits (VIA and VIIA) has hitherto failed to identify the disease-causing mutations.

Endocrine presentation

Endocrine presentation includes dwarfism,[29] diabetes mellitus,[37,38] hypoparathyroidism,[39] and rarely, hypothyroidism and ACTH deficiency. Major growth retardation (−4 to −6 SDs) with normal basal and stimulated plasma growth hormone (GH) but markedly reduced plasma IgF1 has been occasionally reported.[15] The redox status in plasma is consistently disturbed, and fatal multiorgan involvement, probably precipitated by exogenous GH administration, eventually occurs.

Diabetes mellitus (either insulin dependent or non-insulin dependent) is seldom the first symptom and rather appears as a complication of the disease. Yet it is important to be aware that diabetes mellitus can occur at very early stages of the disease. Recently, rare cases of neonatal-onset diabetes mellitus have been ascribed to respiratory chain deficiency.[15] The neonates had major hyperglycemia, lacticacidemia, ketosis, and widespread respiratory enzyme deficiency. The main clinical feature of mitochondrial diabetes is its nearly constant association with other symptoms: deafness and heart and renal failure. It is either sporadic[40–44] or maternally inherited.[45–49] The former usually results from mtDNA rearrangements as part of specific syndromes (KSS,[42] Pearson,[41–44] Wolfram syndrome,[40] see below); the latter is the result of either mtDNA mutations[47,49] or deletions/duplications.[45,46,48] The mtDNA mutation that most commonly causes mitochondrial diabetes is the $tRNA^{Leu}$ mutation,[17,47] which is also known to cause MELAS, but other mtDNA point mutations have been also reported.[17,50–53] Several reported patients (aged 20–40 years) had maternally inherited diabetes mellitus and sensorineural hearing loss but usually none of the other MELAS symptoms and no anti-β-islet antibodies.[47] Occasionally, however, diabetes mellitus and deafness have been shown to segregate with the complete MELAS syndrome or even multiple organ involvement in the same pedigree.[38] In Japan, the prevalence of the $tRNA^{Leu}$ mutation is 6 percent and 0 percent in familial and sporadic type I diabetes mellitus, respectively, and 2 percent in familial type II diabetes.[49] In France, the prevalence of the mutation in familial type I diabetes is below 2 percent, but this rate averages 60 percent in patients with combined diabetes mellitus and deafness.[54]

Hematologic presentation

Childhood myelodysplasia occasionally occurs as the initial symptom of a respiratory chain deficiency.[55] Refractory anemia with ring sideroblasts and vacuolization of marrow precursors is usually associated with variable degrees of neutropenia and thrombopenia, as observed in the Pearson syndrome[44,56] (see "Pearson Syndrome" below). The absence of cytogenetic abnormalities and the polyclonal pattern of peripheral neutrophiles and lymphocytes support the view that mitochondrial myelodysplasia should not be regarded as a malignant condition. This clinical presentation emphasizes the difficulty in recognizing the mitochondrial origin of the disease in patients with only hematologic symptoms.

Sensorineural hearing loss

Variable degrees of nonsyndromic sensorineural hearing loss following aminoglycoside exposure have been described in individuals carrying a homoplasmic mitochondrial $tRNA^{Ser}$ (T7445C)[57] or 12S RNA mutation (A1555G).[58–61] This mutation is believed to make the rRNA more similar to the bacterial RNA involved in aminoglycoside-induced bactericidal activity and to alter translation activity. Yet several inbred pedigrees have been reported with family members who are deaf without drug exposure.[59] For this reason, a two-hit model of development has been proposed. The incompletely penetrant heteroplasmic rRNA 12S mutation is maternally transmitted and represents the first hit, the second hit consisting of either aminoglycoside exposure (at nontoxic doses) or homozygosity for an autosomal recessive mutation, altering a putative cochlear-specific rRNA subunit.[62] The major clinical relevance of this is the prevention of antibiotic-induced hearing loss, especially since the A1555G mutation accounts for 15 percent of all cases of aminoglycoside-induced deafness in the USA.[62] Physicians should inquire about a family history of antibiotic-induced hearing loss prior to local or general aminoglycoside administration, and conversely, individuals with aminoglycoside-induced hearing loss should be screened for this mutation, as its detection will allow counseling of maternal relatives to avoid aminoglycosides. More generally, it might be reasonable and cost-effective to screen individuals with nonsyndromic hearing loss for the mutation unless maternal inheritance has been excluded.[62]

Ophthalmologic symptoms

The ophthalmologic manifestations of respiratory chain deficiency are numerous. They frequently occur in the course of the disease, occasionally as part of well-identified syndromes.[63] They involve the retina (pigmentary degeneration, KSS), optic nerve (optic atrophy, Leber disease), anterior chamber (cataract, corneal opacities), and also extraocular muscles (limitation of eye movements, ophthalmoplegia, diplopia, and lid ptosis, in progressive external ophthalmoplegia and KSS).

Dermatologic symptoms

When present, hair and skin anomalies are delayed and consistently associated with other symptoms. They include mottled pigmentation of photo-exposed areas, acrocyanosis, hypertrichosis, alopecia, and abnormal hairs.[40,45,64] Hair anomalies consist of dry, thick, and brittle hair shafts. Amino acid analysis of the hair is largely normal. Electron microscopy shows transverse fractures across the hair shafts through the cuticle and hairs displaying twists (pili torti), longitudinal grooving, cuticle loss, and trichorrhexis nodosa.[64]

Palmoplantar keratoderma (PPK) affecting the plantar surfaces has been reported in association with deafness in large pedigrees segregating the mitochondrial A7445G mutation.[65] Biopsy revealed marked hyperkeratosis, increased thickness of the granular layer, and moderate acanthosis of the epidermis. Less frequent features included epidermal nevus, ichthyosis, and cholesteatoma. While interactions between mitochondria and cytokeratins are known to occur, the link between the A7445G mutation and PPK remains unclear.

Facial dysmorphism

Mitochondrial disorders are not commonly regarded as causes of malformations. Yet respiratory chain deficiency has been observed in several patients with evolutive facial anomalies, microcephaly, and ante- and postnatal growth retardation.[66] Facial features included round face, high forehead, small nose, and long flat philtrum, reminiscent of the fetal alcohol syndrome (FAS). Low-set, posteriorly angulated ears with deficient helix and hypoplastic lobules suggestive of a CHARGE association were occasionally observed. Limb and trunk involvements included short hands, brachydactyly, hypoplasia of the distal and middle phalanges, hypoplastic nails, and the VACTERL association.[66,67] The pathogenesis of these malformations is unknown, but the combination of facial anomalies with prenatal growth failure and skeletal malformations is suggestive of an antenatal expression of the disease. Some of these anomalies common to FAS and metabolic diseases have been described in pyruvate dehydrogenase (PDH) deficiency (Chap. 100).[68] It has been proposed that in FAS, a product of alcohol oxidation, acetaldehyde, inhibits the PDH complex and is responsible for secondary PDH deficiency *in utero*. Whether facial dysmorphism in respiratory chain deficiency is related to this mechanism only or to an intoxication of the fetus by abnormal intermediates as well is presently unknown.

THE SYNDROMES OF RESPIRATORY CHAIN DEFICIENCY

Attempts to delineate tight boundaries between syndromes are questionable, especially as the nature, clinical course, and severity of recruited symptoms vary among (and even within) affected individuals. The overlaps in clinical features account for the difficulties in classifying patients. However, some specific clinical associations are more frequent and have occasionally been recognized as distinct syndromes. Molecular genetic studies have demonstrated that these associations are not fortuitous. The most frequent syndromic forms of respiratory chain deficiency are, in alphabetical order:

Alpers progressive sclerosing poliodystrophy. Respiratory chain deficiency has been found in the livers of children meeting the criteria of Alpers poliodystrophy. Children suffered myoclonic epilepsy, related to the gradual involvement of the gray matter, and developed delayed onset hepatic involvement, frequently triggered by valproate intake. Liver enlargement with mild cytolysis and steatosis were noted, and the children frequently died shortly thereafter.[33,69] Plasma and CSF lactate was normal, and expression of the enzyme deficiency was usually restricted to the liver. Considering the severe prognosis and the expected recurrence risk (25 percent), children with unexplained myoclonic epilepsy in early infancy should be screened for respiratory enzyme deficiency with a needle liver biopsy.

Barth syndrome. This X-linked dilated cardiomyopathy, with cyclic neutropenia, skeletal myopathy, and abnormal mitochondria,[18] has been mapped to chromosome Xq28[19] and ascribed to mutations of the tafazzin gene (G4.5).[20] The same gene might account for nonsyndromic forms of X-linked cardiomyopathy and isolated noncompaction of the left ventricular myocardium.[70]

Friedreich ataxia (FRDA). A common autosomal recessive degenerative disease characterized by cerebellar ataxia with progressive gait and limb ataxia, dysarthria, lack of tendon reflexes, pyramidal weakness of the inferior limbs, and hypertrophic cardiomyopathy,[71] FRDA is caused primarily by a GAA repeat expression in the first intron of the frataxin gene on chromosome 9q13.[72,73] The function of the protein is unknown, but mutated frataxin triggers iron-sulphur (Fe-S) cluster-containing mitochondrial respiratory enzyme deficiency (complexes I-II-III) and aconitase deficiency in heart (and possibly brain) in FRDA patients. The Fe-S-dependent enzyme deficiency in FRDA should be related to the increased mitochondrial iron content reported in heart in the patients, especially since Fe-S proteins are remarkably sensitive to oxygen free radicals. FRDA should therefore be regarded as a frequent nuclearly encoded mitochondrial disorder.[74]

Hereditary spastic paraplegia (HSP). This disorder is characterized by progressive weakness and spasticity of the lower limbs due to degeneration of the corticospinal axons. An autosomal recessive form has been mapped to chromosome 16q24.3. The gene, SPG7, encodes paraplegin, a protein that localizes to mitochondria and is highly homologous to the yeast metalloproteases, with proteolytic and chaperon-like activities at the inner mitochondrial membrane. The exact function of the protein is unknown, but mutated paraplegin results in respiratory chain defects, suggesting that this form of HSP should be regarded as a mitochondrial disorder.[75]

Kearns-Sayre syndrome (KSS). This multisystem disorder is characterized by the unvariant triad of onset before age 20, progressive external ophthalmoplegia, and pigmentary retinal degeneration, plus at least one of the following: complete heart block, CSF protein above 100 mg/dl, and cerebellar ataxia.[8] Large-scale heteroplasmic mitochondrial DNA deletions are frequently detected in skeletal muscle (rarely in other tissues).[17,76,77]

Leber hereditary optic neuroretinopathy (LHON). In this syndrome, rapid bilateral central vision loss is due to optic nerve death.[63] Cardiac dysrhythmia is frequently associated with the disease, but no evidence of skeletal muscle pathology or gross structural mitochondrial abnormality has been documented. The median age of vision loss is 20–24 years, but it can occur at any age between adolescence and late adulthood. Expression among maternally related individuals is variable, and there is a bias toward males' being affected. To date, the disease has been associated with 18 missense mutations in the mtDNA, which can act autonomously or in association with each other to cause the disease.[17,78]

Leigh subacute necrotizing encephalomyopathy. The Leigh syndrome is a devastating encephalopathy characterized by recurrent attacks of psychomotor regression with pyramidal and extrapyramidal symptoms, leukodystrophy, and brainstem dysfunction.[7] The pathologic hallmark consists of focal, symmetric, and necrotic lesions in the thalamus, the brainstem, and the posterior columns of the spinal cord. Microscopically, these spongiform lesions show demyelination, vascular proliferation, and astrocytosis. Various respiratory enzyme deficiencies have been reported (complexes I, II, IV),[79,80] and the T8993G mtDNA mutation has been described in the Leigh syndrome.[17,81] The first nuclear gene mutation reported involved the flavoprotein subunit of complex II and caused Leigh disease.[80] Since then, a significant fraction of cases of complex IV deficiency presenting as Leigh disease has been ascribed to mutations in a mitochondrial assembly protein gene (SURF1).[82]

Mitochondrial encephalomyopathy with lactic acidosis and strokelike episodes (MELAS). Characterized by onset in childhood, MELAS includes intermittent hemicranial headache, vomiting, proximal limb weakness, recurrent neurologic deficit resembling strokes (hemiparesis, cortical blindness, hemianopsia), lactic acidosis, and occasionally ragged red fibers in the muscle biopsy.[7] CT brain scan shows low-density areas (usually posterior) that may affect both white and gray matter, but the findings do not always correlate with clinical symptoms or vascular territories. The pathogenesis of strokelike episodes in MELAS has been ascribed to either cerebral blood flow disruption or acute metabolic decompensation in biochemically deficient areas of the brain. The disease is most frequently caused by a mutation in the $tRNA^{Leu}$ gene (A3243G).[83]

Mitochondrial myopathy, peripheral neuropathy, gastrointestinal, and encephalopathy disease (MNGIE). This autosomal recessive syndrome manifests as intermittent diarrhea and intestinal pseudoobstruction (myoneurogastrointestinal encephalopathy),[32] and has been recently ascribed to mutations of the thymidine phosphorylase gene, with multiple mtDNA deletions in affected tissues.[84]

Mohr-Tranebjaerg syndrome (DFN1). This syndrome is characterized by deafness, visual disability leading to cortical blindness, dystonia, fractures, and mental deficiency. The disease causing this syndrome, DDP (deafness/dystonia peptide), maps to chromosome Xq22[85] and is homologous to yeast Tim8p, a protein involved in the import from the cytoplasm to the mitochondria.[86]

Myoclonic epilepsy with ragged red fibers (MERRF). An encephalomyopathy with myoclonus, ataxia, hearing loss, muscle weakness, and generalized seizures,[87] MERRF is caused by a missense mutation in the mt $tRNA^{Lys}$ gene (A8344G) in 80 percent of cases.[17,88]

Neurogenic muscle weakness, ataxia, retinitis pigmentosa (NARP). This disorder, which causes variable sensory neuropathy, seizures, and mental retardation, is due to an amino acid change in the ATPase6 gene (T8993G) also known occasionally to cause Leigh disease.[17,89]

Pearson syndrome. This is a syndrome of refractory sideroblastic anemia, with variable neutropenia and thrombocytopenia, vacuolization of marrow precursors, and exocrine pancreatic dysfunction. Half of the patients have anemia and half have diarrhea as the initial symptom, but all have impaired redox status in plasma. Both sexes are affected. Severe transfusion-dependent macrocytic anemia begins in early infancy (before 1 year), and the disease is fatal before 3 years in 62 percent of cases.[31,44] Patients who survive spontaneously recover from their myelodysplasia but usually develop KSS. Interestingly, several KSS patients whose disease apparently started in childhood or adulthood were retrospectively shown to have experienced transient sideroblastic anemia, neutropenia, chronic watery diarrhea, or failure to thrive of unexplained origin in early infancy.[90] Large-scale heteroplasmic deletions/duplications of mtDNA are constantly observed in affected and nonaffected organs. Directly repeated sequences are consistently found at the boundaries of the rearrangements, suggesting that these repeats might have triggered molecular mtDNA recombinations.[17]

Progressive external ophthalmoplegia (PEO). A mitochondrial myopathy, PEO causes progressive muscle weakness and external ophthalmoplegia. Ataxia, episodic ketoacidotic coma, and early death have been reported. Single[77] or multiple[91] mtDNA deletions triggered by an unknown nuclear gene mapping to chromosome 3p[92] have been reported in PEO.

Syndromic forms of sensorineural hearing loss. Loss of hearing is not exceptional in respiratory chain deficiency syndromes. The diabetes mellitus and deafness association is frequently accounted for by the A3243G mutation in the $tRNA^{Leu}$ gene, also known to account for MELAS.[47] Hearing loss usually develops after the onset of diabetes. The deafness-ataxia-myoclonus syndrome is caused by a single nucleotide insertion in the $tRNA^{Ser}$ gene (C7472).[93] The deafness-palmoplantar keratoderma association is a recently identified syndrome, ascribed to a maternally inherited mutation altering the $tRNA^{Ser}$ stability.[65] Indeed, the 7445 mutation is adjacent to the 3′ end of the $tRNA^{Ser}$ gene on the light strand and a silent change in the stop codon of the COXI gene on the heavy strand.

Wolfram syndrome. This is a syndrome of diabetes insipidus and diabetes mellitus with optic atrophy and deafness (DIDMOAD). While most cases have been ascribed to an autosomal recessive gene mapping to chromosome 4p16,[94] some cases of early onset DIDMOAD might result from mtDNA mutations[53] or deletions.[40]

METABOLIC SCREENING IN VIVO

Current screening for respiratory chain deficiency includes the determination of plasma lactate, pyruvate, and ketone body levels and molar ratios, as indexes of oxidation/reduction status in cytoplasm and mitochondria, respectively (Table 99-2). Determinations should be made in fasted and 1-hour-fed individuals and repeated (after breakfast, lunch, and dinner). In order to avoid artifactual elevation of lactic acid, blood samples should be taken from a patient at rest through a heparinized venous catheter and immediatly deproteinized with perchloric acid.[95] Samples should be either forwarded in ice to the laboratory or immediately frozen ($-20°C$ or below). Blood glucose and nonesterified fatty acids should be monitored simultaneously.

The observation of a persistent hyperlactatemia (>2.5 μm) with elevated L:P (>20) and ketone body molar ratios is highly suggestive of a respiratory chain deficiency (particularly in the postabsorptive period).[3,4,15] In addition, investigation of the redox status in plasma can help discriminate between the different forms of congenital lactic acidosis, based on L:P and ketone body molar ratios *in vivo*. Indeed, an impairment of oxidative phosphorylation usually results in L:P ratios above 20 and ketone body ratios above 2, whereas a defect of the pyruvate dehydrogenase (PDH) complex results in low L:P ratios ($<$ 10). When basal screening tests are inconclusive, other tests should be carried out (Table 99-2):

- Glucose loading test (2 g/kg, orally) to unmask latent hyperlactatemia and/or paradoxical hyperketonemia;[96]
- Screening for urinary lactate and citric acid cycle intermediates, using GC/MS. Urinary excretion of Krebs cycle intermediates and/or 3-methylglutaconic aciduria has good diagnostic value but is nonspecific, as it is frequently encountered in a variety of respiratory enzyme chain deficiency syndromes;[97]
- Determination of the redox status in the CSF, to detect elective increase of CSF lactate or L:P ratios (This determination is useless when the redox status in plasma is altered.);
- Amino acid chromatography to show indirect evidence of hyperlactatemia (i.e., elevated plasma α-alanine and proline) and occasionally hypermethioninemia. Interestingly, plasma citrulline is low in complex V deficiency caused by the NARP mutation. More generally, hypocitrullinemia might be a nonspecific hallmark of impaired oxidative phosphorylation in vivo. In respiratory chain deficiency, the synthesis of circulating citrulline by enterocytes might be limited by the reduced availability of mitochondrial ATP, required for carbamyl phosphate synthase I activity.

Yet pitfalls in metabolic screening are numerous, and the above diagnostic tests may fail to detect impaired redox status in plasma for several reasons:

- Proximal tubulopathy may lower blood lactate and increase urinary lactate;

Table 99-2 In Vivo Screening or Respiratory Chain Deficiency

Standard screening tests* (at least four determinations overday in fasted and 1-hr-fed individuals)

1) Plasma lactate
2) Lactate/pyruvate molar ratio = redox status in cytoplasm
3) Ketonemia ("paradoxical" elevation in fed individuals)
4) β-OH butyrate/acetoacetate molar ratio = redox status in mitochondria
5) Blood glucose and free fatty acids
6) Urinary organic acids (GC-MS) = lactate, ketone bodies, citric acid cycle intermediates

Provocative tests (when standard tests are inconclusive)

1) Glucose test (2 g/kg orally) in fasted individuals with determination of blood glucose, lactate, pyruvate, ketone bodies, and their molar ratios at 15 min, 30 min, 45 min, 60 min, and 90 min
2) Lactate/pyruvate molar ratios in the CSF (only when no elevation of plasma lactate is observed)
3) Redox status in plasma following exercise

Screening for multiple organ involvement

- Liver = hepatocellular dysfunction?
- Kidney = proximal tubulopathy, distal tubulopathy, proteinuria, renal failure?
- Heart = hypertrophic cardiomyopathy, heart block? (ultrasound, EKG)
- Muscle = myopathic features? (CK, ALAT, ASAT, histologic anomalies, RRF)
- Brain = leukodystrophy; poliodystrophy; hypodensity of the cerebrum, cerebellum, and brainstem; multifocal areas of hyperintense signal (MELAS); bilateral symmetric lesions of the basal ganglia and brainstem (Leigh)? (EEG, NMR, CT scan)
- Peripheral nerve: distal sensory loss, hypo- or areflexia, distal muscle wasting (usually subclinical), reduced motor nerve conduction velocity (NCV) and denervation features? (NCV, EMG, peripheral nerve biopsy showing axonal degeneration and myelinated fiber loss)
- Pancreas = exocrine pancreatic dysfunction?
- Gut = villous atrophy?
- Endocrine = hypoglycemia, hypocalcemia, hypoparathyroidism, growth hormone deficiency? (stimulation tests)
- Bone marrow = anemia, neutropenia, thrombopenia, pancytopenia, vacuolization of marrow precursors?
- Eye = PEO, ptosis, optic atrophy, retinal degeneration? (fundus, electroretinogram, visual evoked potentials)
- Ear = sensorineural deafness? (auditory evoked potentials, brainstem evoked response)
- Skin = trichothiodystrophy, mottled pigmentation of photo-exposed areas?

*See text for critical sampling protocols.

- Diabetes mellitus may hamper entry of pyruvate into the citric acid cycle;
- Tissue-specific isoforms may be selectively impaired, barely altering the redox status in plasma;
- The defect may be generalized but partial: The more those tissues with higher dependence on oxidative metabolism (such as brain and muscle) suffer, the more the oxidation-reduction status in plasma is impaired;

When screening tests are negative, respiratory chain deficiency may be misdiagnosed. For this reason, the investigation of patients at risk of respiratory chain deficiency should include the systematic screening of all possible target organs and tissues, regardless of the onset symptom, as multiple organ involvement is an important diagnostic clue in respiratory chain deficiency.

DIAGNOSTIC TESTS

Diagnostic tests include polarographic and spectrophotometric studies, each providing an independent clue to the diagnosis of respiratory chain deficiency.

Polarographic studies consist of the measurement of oxygen consumption by mitochondria-enriched fractions using a Clarke electrode in the presence of various oxidative substrates (malate + pyruvate, malate + glutamate, succinate, palmitate, etc.).[98,99] In the case of complex I deficiency, polarographic studies show impaired respiration with NADH-producing substrates, while respiration and phosphorylation are normal with $FADH_2$-producing substrates (e.g., succinate). The opposite is observed in the case of complex II deficiency, whereas a block at the level of complex III or IV impairs oxidation of both NADH- and $FADH_2$-producing substrates. In complex V deficiency, there is impaired respiration with various substrates, but adding the uncoupling agent 2,4-dinitrophenol or calcium ions returns the respiratory rate to normal, suggesting that the limiting step involves phosphorylation rather than the respiratory chain. Polarographic studies may also detect PDH deficiency, citric acid cycle enzyme deficiency, and defects of coenzymes, carriers, and shuttles (including cytochrome *c*, quinones, cations, and adenylate), as these conditions also impair the production of reducing equivalents in the mitochondrion. In these cases, however, independent enzyme activities are expected to be normal.

While previous techniques required gram amounts of muscle tissue, the scaled-down procedures now available allow the rapid recovery of mitochondria-enriched fractions (400–500 µg proteins) from small skeletal muscle biopsies (100–200 mg, obtained under local anesthesia) and make polarographic studies feasible in infants and children. Measurement of oxygen consumption by intact or detergent-permeabilized circulating lymphocytes (isolated from 10 ml of blood on a Percoll cushion) and cultured cells (lymphoblastoid cell lines, skin fibroblasts) are also feasible and represent a noninvasive and easily reproducible diagnostic test. The only limitation of these techniques is the absolute requirement of fresh material: polarographic studies are not possible on frozen material.

Spectrophotometric studies consist of isolated or combined respiratory enzyme assays, using specific electron donors and acceptors. They do not require isolation of mitochondrial fractions and can be carried out on tissue homogenates. For this reason, the amount of material required for enzyme assays is very small (1–20 mg) and can be easily derived from liver, kidney, and endomyocardial needle biopsy sample or from a pellet of lymphocytes or cultured skin fibroblasts. Samples should be immediately frozen and kept dry in liquid nitrogen (or at −80°C).[98–103]

The question of what tissue should be investigated deserves particular attention. In principle, the relevant tissue is the one that clinically expresses the disease. In the case of muscle weakness, the appropriate working material is a skeletal muscle (deltoid) microbiopsy sample. When the hematopoietic system expresses the disease (i.e., Pearson syndrome),[31] tests should be carried out on circulating lymphocytes, polymorphonuclear cells, or bone marrow. In liver disease or cardiomyopathy, a needle biopsy of the liver[33] or an endomyocardial biopsy[16] is usually feasible. When the disease is essentially expressed in a barely accessible organ (brain, retina, endocrine gland, smooth muscle), peripheral tissues should be extensively tested (including skeletal muscle, cultured skin fibroblasts, and circulating lymphocytes). Whatever organ is affected, it is mandatory to take skin biopsies for subsequent investigations on cultured fibroblasts (even post mortem).

It should be borne in mind, however, that the *in vitro* investigation of oxidative phosphorylation remains difficult; several pitfalls should be kept in mind:

- Normal respiratory enzyme activities can be found in an organ or tissue that does not clinically express the disease. One might be dealing with a tissue-specific organ deficiency, as observed in Friedreich ataxia.[74]

- Normal respiratory enzyme activity does not preclude mitochondrial dysfunction, even if the tissue tested clinically expresses the disease. One might be dealing with a kinetic mutant, tissular heterogeneity, or cellular mosaicism (heteroplasmy). In this case, one should pay particular attention to histoenzymatic investigations, carry out extensive molecular genetic analyses, test other tissues, and possibly repeat investigations.
- The apparent discrepancy between normal complex I, II, and III activities and impaired combined complex I-III or II-III activities is indicative of a deficient quinone pool. Inborn errors of quinone synthesis remain largely unknown but worth recognizing, as these rare forms of respiratory chain deficiency respond to quinone administration *in vitro* and *in vivo*.[104,105] On the other hand, incorrect freezing may result in a rapid loss of quinone-dependent activities, probably due to peroxidation of membrane lipids. Tissue samples fixed for morphologic studies are inadequate for respiratory enzyme assays.[98]
- The scattering of control activities occasionally hampers the recognition of enzyme deficiencies, as normal values frequently overlap those found in the patients. It is helpful to express results as ratios, especially since normal oxidative phosphorylation requires balanced ratios of respiratory chain enzyme activities. Using activity ratios, patients whose absolute activities are in the low normal range can be unambiguously diagnosed as enzyme deficient.[103] Yet this way of expressing results may fail to identify generalized defects.
- No reliable method is presently available for measurement of complex I activity in circulating or cultured cells, due to the rotenone-resistant cellular NADH-cytochrome *c* reductase activity.
- The phenotypic expression of respiratory enzyme deficiencies in cultured cells is unstable, and activities tend to return to normal values when cells are grown in a standard medium. Adding uridine (200 micromolars) and pyruvate (10 micromolars) to the culture medium prevents counterselection of respiratory enzyme-deficient cells, thereby stabilizing the mutant phenotype (the availability of uridine, required for nucleic acid synthesis, is reduced by the secondary deficiency of the respiratory chain-dependent dihydroorotate dehydrogenase activity).[106,107]
- Discrepancies between control values may indicate faulty experimental conditions. Relative activities should be consistent when tested under non-rate-limiting conditions. For example, normal succinate-cytochrome *c* reductase (SCCR) activity should be twice as high as normal succinate-quinone DCPIP reductase (SQDR) activity (because one e^- is required to reduce cytochrome *c* while two e^- are required to reduce DCPIP).

Histopathologic studies

The muscle specimen taken under local anesthesia must be immediately frozen in liquid nitrogen-cooled isopentane. The histologic hallmark of mitochondrial myopathy is the ragged red fibers (RRF) demonstrated with the modified Gomori trichrome stain, containing peripheral and intermyofibrillar accumulations of abnormal mitochondria.[108] Although the diagnostic importance of RRF is undisputed, it is now clear that absence of RRF does not rule out the diagnosis of mitochondrial disorder. Various histochemical stains specific for oxidative enzymes are used to analyze the distribution of mitochondria in individual fibers and assess enzymatic activities. Histochemical staining helps in estimating severity and detecting heterogeneity of enzyme deficiency in a given muscle section. Myofibrillar integrity, muscle-type fiber predominance, and distribution can be evaluated with the myofibrillar ATPase stain, and studies using antibodies directed against specific subunits are routinely performed in reference centers.

Magnetic resonance spectroscopy of muscle and brain

Phosphorus magnetic resonance spectroscopy (MRS) allows study of muscle and brain energy metabolism *in vivo*. Inorganic phosphate (P_i), phosphocreatine (PCr), AMP, ADP, or ATP, and intracellular pH may be measured. The P_i/PCr ratio is the most useful parameter and may be measured at rest, during exercise, and after recovery. An increased ratio is found in most patients, and MRS is becoming a useful tool for both diagnosing mitochondrial diseases and monitoring therapeutic trials. Yet the observed anomalies are not specific to respiratory enzyme deficiencies, and no correlation between MRS findings and the respiratory enzyme defect can be made.[109]

Molecular genetics studies

The genetic investigation of a mitochondrial disorder requires an extensive pedigree reporting on minor signs in relatives. Such information is of particular importance for deciding what molecular studies should be carried out first. For example, maternal inheritance points toward mtDNA mutations, autosomal dominant inheritance points toward multiple mtDNA deletions, and sporadic cases should be tested for mtDNA deletion/duplications and cases consistent with autosomal recessive inheritance (consanguineous parents) for mtDNA depletions. It should be borne in mind, however, that the molecular genetic investigation of mtDNA is not a routine procedure and that several pitfalls exist:

- A twofold population of mtDNA molecules does not always correspond to deletions and may result from mtDNA polymorphisms.
- The distribution of mutated mtDNA molecules may differ widely among tissues (heteroplasmy), possibly accounting for variable clinical expression. The tissue to be investigated is the one that actually expresses the disease. (mtDNA deletion is frequently absent in circulating lymphocytes of KSS patients.)
- mtDNA deletions may be occasionally associated with duplications. Due to the symmetry of several rearrangements, detection of duplication requires enzymatic cleavage of the mtDNA at sites located within the deletion.[44,110,111]
- mtDNA rearrangements are unstable and gradually disappear in cultured cells unless uridine is included in the culture medium. No conclusion can be drawn from molecular studies based on cell cultures grown in standard conditions.[106,107]
- The detection of mtDNA depletion requires systematic rehybridization of Southern blots using a control nuclear DNA probe for densitometric determination of the mtDNA/nuclear DNA ratio.[112,113]
- Finally, while a positive test supports the mitochondrial nature of the disease, a negative result does not rule out an mtDNA mutation, nor does it represent a clue that a nuclear mutation is involved.

TREATMENT

No satisfactory therapy is presently available for respiratory chain deficiency. Treatment remains largely symptomatic and does not significantly alter the course of the disease. It includes avoidance of drugs and procedures known to have detrimental effects. In particular, it is reasonable to avoid sodium valproate[114] and barbiturates, which inhibit the respiratory chain and have occasionally been shown to precipitate hepatic failure in respiratory enzyme-deficient children. Tetracyclines and chloramphenicol should be avoided as well, as they inhibit mitochondrial protein synthesis. Iron chelators and antioxidant drugs likely to reduce iron are particularly harmful for the respiratory chain in case of mitochondrial iron overload (as in Friedreich ataxia). Due to the increasing number of tissues affected in the course of the disease, it is recommended that organ transplantation (bone marrow, liver, heart) be carefully discussed.

Symptomatic treatments include slow infusion of sodium bicarbonate during acute attacks of lactic acidosis, pancreatic extract administration in instances of exocrine pancreatic dysfunction, and repeated transfusions in cases of anemia or thrombopenia.

Coenzyme Q_{10} administration (5–10 mg/kg/day) has had spectacular effects in rare patients with inborn errors of quinone synthesis.[104,105] Quinone could also play an important protective role against iron-induced injury in various conditions, including FRDA.[74] Carnitine is suggested in patients with secondary carnitine deficiency. Dichloroacetate or 2-chloropropionate administration has been proposed to stimulate PDH activity; each has occasionally reduced the level of lactic acid, but detrimental effects of dichloroacetate have recently been reported (reversible peripheral neuropathy).[8,115]

Dietary recommendations include a high-lipid, low-carbohydrate diet in patients with complex I deficiency. Indeed, a high-glucose diet is a metabolic challenge for patients with impaired oxidative phosphorylation, especially because glucose oxidation is largely aerobic in the liver. Based on our experience, we suggest avoiding a hypercaloric diet and parenteral nutrition and recommend a low-carbohydrate diet in addition to the symptomatic treatment.

GENETIC COUNSELING AND PRENATAL DIAGNOSIS

Any mode of inheritance can be observed in mitochondrial diseases: sporadic, autosomal recessive, dominant, X-linked, or maternal. Indeed, among the numerous genes encoding the respiratory chain proteins, most are located in the nucleus and undergo classic Mendelian inheritance. On the other hand, each human cell contains thousands of molecules of mtDNA,[116] which is a maternally inherited intronless 16,569-bp circular genome encoding genes for a large and a small rRNA, 22 tRNAs, and 13 key subunits of the respiratory enzymes, including seven subunits of complex I, one subunit of complex III, three subunits of complex IV, and two subunits of complex V. The mtDNA has a number of unique genetic features:

- mtDNA is maternally inherited, as it is predominantly transmitted through the egg cytoplasm. The mother transmits her mtDNA to all her progeny, and her daughters transmit their mtDNA to the next generation. Males never transmit their mtDNA. This feature accounts for the maternal inheritance of mtDNA mutations.[8]
- mtDNA has a very high mutation rate, involving both nucleotide substitutions and deletion/insertion mutations.[78]
- mtDNA can switch genotypes completely in two or three generations, as the number of mtDNA molecules is greatly reduced at some points in oogenesis and there is uneven transmission to progeny. This switch appears not to occur as rapidly when mtDNA mutations are harmful, presumably because of selection in favor of wild-type mtDNA.
- In cells with a mixture of mutant and wild-type mtDNAs (heteroplasmy), the mtDNA genotype can shift during cellular replication (replicative segregation). This feature results from the random allotment of mitochondria into daughter cells during cell division.[8] Consequently, some lineages drift toward pure mutant mtDNAs (homoplasmy), others toward pure wild-type mtDNAs, while still others remain heteroplasmic. In cells harboring mutant and wild-type molecules, the phenotype is a reflection of the proportion of mutant mtDNA molecules and the extent to which the cell type relies on mitochondrial function.

Mitochondrial DNA mutations

Pathologic alterations of mtDNA fall into three major classes: point mutations, deletions/duplications, and copy number mutations (depletions).

Point mutations include amino acid substitutions and protein synthesis mutations (tRNA, rRNA). Most of these are maternally inherited and heteroplasmic, but they are associated with a striking variety of clinical phenotypes depending on the proportion of mutant mtDNAs inherited by the different maternal relatives.[17] Indeed, within one particular pedigree, clinical presentations may range from migraines and attention deficit disorders to the full MELAS syndrome. Maternal relatives of patients are generally healthy as long as they have no more than 85 percent mutant mtDNA. Once the percentage of mutant mtDNA rises above this level, there are increasingly serious consequences in the clinical phenotype, illustrating the sharp threshold of protein synthesis mutants.

It is worth noting that there is no strict genotype-phenotype correlation in mtDNA mutations, as a given base substitution can be associated with markedly different clinical profiles. While MERRF,[88] MELAS,[83] NARP,[89] and Leigh[81] syndrome mutations are frequently heteroplasmic, Leber optic neuroretinopathy mutations are usually homoplasmic,[17,117–120] at least in circulating leukocytes. Moreover, several families with such mutations harbor distinct mtDNA base substitutions that may act synergistically to increase the probability of blindness. (Likelihood of blindness might be increased in individuals who have more severe mutations or combinations of base substitutions.[8])

The second class of mtDNA diseases are deletions/duplications of the mitochondrial genome. Although the size and the position of the deletion markedly differ among patients, they usually encompass several coding genes and tRNA genes. They are usually sporadic, heteroplasmic, and unique, and frequently occur between directly repeated sequences, suggesting that they are caused by *de novo* rearrangements that arose during oogenesis or early development.[17,24,25,30,31,40–44,76,77,90] It is worth noting that the most common deletion (4997 bp), found in 30 percent of patients harboring a unique deletion and flanked by a 13-bp direct repeat, has been simultaneously described in Pearson syndrome[44] and KSS[77] and subsequently reported in PEO. Similarly, identical mtDNA duplications have been reported in strikingly different conditions, such as Pearson syndrome[44] and villous atrophy.[30] Thus, no correlation is found between clinical presentation and the nature or extent of rearrangements. The observation of progressive organ involvement should prompt one to consider the diagnosis of mtDNA rearrangement and carry out Southern blot analysis of total DNA. Indeed, unlike mtDNA point mutations, deletions/duplications increase in proportion over the course of the disease, suggesting that they have a replicative advantage over normal molecules. While the vast majority of mtDNA rearrangements are sporadic, occasional pedigrees have been reported in which mtDNA deletions-duplications are present in close maternal relatives.[45–49] This indicates that maternal transmission of rearranged molecules may occur, although germ line transmission is limited. Rare cases are associated with autosomal dominant[87,121] or recessive[122] multiple mtDNA deletions that are flanked by direct repeats. This feature suggests that a mutation occurred in a nuclear gene essential for replication or maintenance of the mitochondrial genome.

The last class of mtDNA diseases are *mtDNA depletions* due to copy number mutations. Rare cases of lethal infantile respiratory, muscle, liver, or kidney failure have been ascribed to mtDNA depletions, and are consistent with autosomal recessive inheritance.[112,113] In these patients, there is a marked (sometimes tissue-specific) deficiency in mtDNA level but not in nuclear gene levels. Yet, it is worth bearing in mind that mtDNA deletions and mutations account for no more than 5 percent of patients, suggesting that in most cases, nuclear gene defects are responsible for respiratory chain deficiency.

Nuclear DNA mutations

Disease-causing nuclear gene mutations are in two categories: 1) mutations in nuclear-encoded respiratory chain subunits, and

2) mutations affecting assembly and maintenance protein genes. While the chromosomal location and cDNA sequence of most respiratory chain subunit genes are known, only a small number of catalytic subunit gene mutations have been reported, namely a mutation in the gene for complex II flavoprotein[80] and mutations in nuclear-encoded complex I genes, including NDUFS,[123] NDUFS7,[124] NDUFS8,[125] and NDUFV1[126] in Leigh syndrome. Yet, mutations are found in the most conserved nuclear-encoded complex I subunit genes and account for only one third of patients with isolated complex I deficiency. Moreover, systematic sequence analysis of nuclear-encoded subunits of complex IV has failed to detect any mutation in their coding sequences.[27] Taken together, these data support the view that mitochondrial assembly and maintenance are primarily altered in respiratory chain deficiency. The discovery of deleterious mutations in the genes encoding three proteins that are essential for the proper assembly of functional complex IV, namely SURF1,[82,128] heme A:farnesyl transferase (COX10),[129] and SCO2[84] in Leigh disease, de Toni-Debré-Fanconi syndrome, and cardioencephalomyopathy, respectively, gives strong support to this view. Along the same lines, it is worth remembering that two nonrespiratory chain subunit genes, thymidine phosphorylase[130] and tafazzin,[20] account for MNGIE and Barth syndrome, respectively. Family studies in dominantly inherited mtDNA deletions[92,131] and autosomal recessive informative families will help to elucidate the genetic heterogeneity of respiratory chain deficiency.

Prenatal diagnosis

Knowledge concerning the mutant genotypes currently associated with clinical presentations sometimes helps predict the heritability of mitochondrial disorders: maternal transmission of base substitutions in LHON,[17,117-120] MERRF,[17,84] MELAS,[17,83] or NARP;[17,89] sporadic occurrence of deletions-duplications in Pearson syndrome[17,44,86] and KSS[17,76,77] (unless germline mosaicism is involved); autosomal recessive transmission of depletions[113,114] in multiorgan failure, autosomal dominant[91,121] or recessive[122] transmission of multiple deletions in PEO. In the case of maternal inheritance of an mtDNA mutation (or deletion), there is no risk for the progeny of an affected male. The risk is high, however, for the progeny of a carrier female. In this case, prenatal diagnosis based on testing of chorionic villi or amniotic cells represents a rational approach to the prevention of these severe diseases. In fact, both diagnosis and prevention are currently hampered by our incomplete knowledge regarding the actual proportion of mutant mtDNA, its relationship to disease severity, its random tissue distribution, and selection against the mutant population during development, possibly related to variable metabolic activities. A percentage of mutant mtDNA below 30 percent or above 80 percent should predict a reasonable chance of good or bad prognosis, respectively.[132] Intermediate results would have an even less certain predictive value. Whatever the results, studies aimed at delivering prenatal diagnosis or predictive genetic advice require careful validation, as proportions of mutant mtDNA may change both between fetal life and infancy and also during adult life.[133]

In the majority of cases, however, the heritability of an mtDNA rearrangement remains unknown and no reliable genetic counseling can be given. Indeed, when dealing with an isolated mtDNA deletion, it is impossible to predict whether a *de novo* event occurred or a heritable mutation is involved (germ line mosaicism). Ongoing systematic screening for disease-causing mtDNA and nuclear gene mutations will hopefully contribute to improvement of genetic counseling. When no mutant genotype is detected, measurement of respiratory enzyme activities in cultured amniocytes or choriocytes represents the unique possibility of prenatal diagnosis.[133,134] Unfortunately, a fraction of enzyme deficiencies are expressed in cultured fibroblasts of probands (even when grown in the presence of uridine).[129]

REFERENCES

1. von Kleist-Retzow JC, Cormier-Daire V, de Lonlay P, Parfait B, Chrétien D, Rustin P, Feingold J, Rötig A, Munnich A: A high rate of parental consanguinity (20–30%) in cytochrome oxidase deficiency. *Am J Hum Genet* **63**:428, 1998.
2. Hatefi Y: The mitochondrial electron transport and oxidative phosphorylation system. *Annu Rev Biochem* **54**:1015, 1985.
3. Robinson BH: Lactic acidemia (disorders of pyruvate carboxylase, pyruvate dehydrogenase), in Scriver CR, Beaudet AL, Sly WS, Valle D (eds): *The Metabolic and Molecular Bases of Inherited Disease* 7th ed. New York, McGraw-Hill, 1995; p 14789.
4. Munnich A, Rötig A, Chretien D, Saudubray JM, Cormier V, Rustin P: Clinical presentations and laboratory investigations in respiratory chain deficiency. *Eur J Pediatr* **155**:262, 1996.
5. Ogier H, Aicardi J: Metabolic diseases, in Aicardi J (ed): *Diseases of the Nervous System in Childhood.* London, MacKeith Press, 1992, p 379.
6. DiMauro S, Bonilla E: Mitochondrial encephalomyopathies. In Rosenberg RN, Prasiner SB, DiMauro S, Barchi RL (eds): *The Molecular and Genetic Basis of Neurological Disease*, Boston, Butterworth-Heinemann, 1997, p 201.
7. de Lonlay-Debeney P, von Kleist-Retzow JC, Hertz-Pannier L, Peudenier S, Cormier-Daire V, Berquin P, Chrétien D, Rötig A, Saudubray JM, Baraton J, Brunelle F, Rustin P, Van Der Knaap M, Munnich A: Cerebral white matter disease in children may be caused by mitochondrial respiratory chain deficiency. *J Pediatr* **136**:209, 2000.
8. Shoffner JM, Wallace DC: Oxidative phosphorylation diseases, in Scriver CR, Beaudet AL, Sly WS, Valle D (eds): *The Metabolic and Molecular Bases of Inherited Disease 7th ed.* New York, McGraw-Hill, 1995, p 1535.
9. DiMauro S, Nicholson JF, Hays AP, Eastwood AB, Papadimitriou A, Koeningsberger R, Devivo DC: Benign infantile mitochondrial myopathy due to reversible cytochrome c oxidase deficiency. *Ann Neurol* **14**:226, 1983.
10. de Lonlay-Debeney P, Edery P, Cormier-Daire V, Parfait B, Chrétien D, Rötig A, Romero N, Saudubray JM, Munnich A, Rustin P: Respiratory chain deficiency presenting as recurrent myoglobinuria in childhood. *Neuropediatrics* **30**:42, 1999.
11. Keightley JA, Hoffbuhr KC, Burton MD, Salas VM, Johnston WSW, Penn AMW, Buist NRM, et al.: A microdeletion in cytochrome c oxidase (COX) subunit III associated with COX deficiency and recurrent myoglobinuria. *Nat Genet* **12**:410, 1996.
12. Kluck RM, Bossy-Wetzel E, Green DR, Newmeyer DD: The release of cytochrome c from mitochondria: A primary site for Bcl-2 regulation of apoptosis. *Science* **275**:1132, 1997.
13. Yang J, Liu X, Bhalla K, Kim CN, Ibrado AM, Cai J, Peng TI, Jones DP, Wang X: Prevention of apoptosis by Bcl-2: Release of cytochrome c from mitochondria blocked. *Science* **275**:1129, 1997.
14. Marin-Garcia J, Goldenthal MJ: Mitochondrial cardiomyopathy: Molecular and biochemical analysis. *Pediatr Cardiol* **18**:251, 1997.
15. Munnich A, Rötig A, Chretien D, Cormier V, Bourgeron T, Bonnefont JP, Saudubray JM, et al: Clinical presentation of mitochondrial disorders in childhood. *J Inher Metab Dis* **19**:521, 1996.
16. Rustin P, Lebidois J, Chretien D, Bourgeron T, Piechaud JF, Rötig A, Munnich A, et al: Endomyocardial biopsies for early detection of mitochondrial disorders in hypertrophic cardiomyopathies. *J Pediatr* **124**:224, 1994.
17. Kogelnik AM, Lott MT, Brown MD, Navathe SB, Wallace DC: MITOMAP: A human mitochondrial genome database (http://www.gen.emory.edu/mitomap.html). Atlanta, Center for Molecular Medicine, Emory University School of Medicine.
18. Barth PG, Scholte HR, Berden JA, Van Der Klei-Van Moorsel JM, Luyt-Houwen IEM, Van't Veer-Korthof ET, Van Der Harten JJ, et al: An X-linked mitochondrial disease affecting cardiac muscle, skeletal muscle, and neutrophil leucocytes. *J Neurol Sci* **62**:327, 1983.
19. Bolhuis PA, Hensels GW, Hulsebos TJM, Baas F, Barth PG: Mapping of the locus for X-linked cardioskeletal myopathy with neutropenia and abnormal mitochondria (Barth syndrome) to Xq28. *Am J Hum Genet* **48**:481, 1991.
20. Bione S, D'adamo P, Maestrini E, Gedeon AK, Bolhuis PA, Toniolo D: A novel X-linked gene, G4.5. is responsible for Barth syndrome. *Nature Genet* **12**:385, 1996.
21. Niaudet P, Rötig A: Renal involvement in mitochondrial cytopathies. *Pediatr Nephrol* **10**:368, 1996.

22. Rötig A, Lehnert A, Rustin P, Chretien D, Bourgeron T, Niaudet P, Munnich A: Renal involvement in the mitochondrial disorders. *Adv Nephrol* **25**:367, 1994.
23. Wendel U, Ruitenbeek W, Bentlage HA, Sengers RC, Trijbels JM: Neonatal de Toni-Debré-Fanconi syndrome due to a defect in complex III of the respiratory chain. *Eur J Pediatr* **154**:915, 1995.
24. Szabolcs MJ, Seigle R, Shanske S, Bonilla E, DiMauro S, D'agati V: Mitochondrial DNA deletion: A cause of chronic tubulointerstitial nephropathy. *Kidney Int* **45**:1388, 1994.
25. Rötig A, Goutières F, Niaudet P, Rustin P, Chretien D, Guest G, Mikol J, et al: Deletion of mitochondrial DNA in patient with chronic tubulointerstitial nephritis. *J Pediatr* **126**:597, 1995.
26. Damian MS, Seibel P, Reichmann H, Schachenmayr W, Laube H, Bachmann G, Wassill KH, et al: Clinical spectrum of the MELAS mutation in a large pedigree. *Acta Neurol Scand* **92**:409, 1995.
27. Hsieh F, Gohh R, Dworkin L: Acute renal failure and the MELAS syndrome, a mitochondrial encephalomyopathy. *J Am Soc Nephrol* **7**:647, 1996.
28. Jansen JJ, Maasen A, Van Der Woude FJ, Lemminck HAJ, Van Den Ouweland JMW, Hart LMT, Smeets HJM, et al: Mutation in mitochondrial tRNALeu (UUR) gene associated with progressive kidney disease. *J Am Soc Nephrol* **8**:1118, 1997.
29. Tulinius MH, Oldfors A, Holme E, Larsson NG, Houshmand M, Fahleson P, Sigstrom L, et al: Atypical presentation of multisystem disorders in two girls with mitochondrial DNA deletions. *Eur J Pediatr* **154**:35, 1995.
30. Cormier-Daire V, Bonnefont JP, Rustin P, Maurage C, Ogier H, Schmitz J, Ricour C, et al: Deletion-duplication of the mitochondrial DNA presenting as chronic diarrhea with villous atrophy. *J Pediatr* **124**:63, 1994.
31. Rötig A, Cormier V, Blanche S, Bonnefont JP, Ledeist F, Romero N, Schmitz J, et al: Pearson's marrow-pancreas syndrome: A multisystem mitochondrial disorder in infancy. *J Clin Invest* **86**:1601, 1990.
32. Hirano M, Silvestri G, Blake DM, Lombès A, Minetti C, Bonilla E, Hays AP, et al: Mitochondrial neurogastrointestinal encephalomyopathy (MNGIE): Clinical, biochemical, and genetic features of an autosomal recessive mitochondrial disorder. *Neurology* **44**:721, 1994.
33. Cormier-Daire V, Chretien D, Rustin P, Rötig A, Dubuisson C, Jacquemin E, Hadchouel M, et al: Neonatal and delayed onset hepatic failure in disorders of oxidative phosphorylation. *J Pediatr* **130**:817, 1997.
34. Edery P, Gérard B, Chrétien D, Rötig A, Cerrone R, Rabier D, Rambaud C, et al: Liver cytochrome c oxidase deficiency in a case of neonatal-onset hepatic failure. *Eur J Pediatr* **153**:190, 1994.
35. Bakker HD, Scholte HR, Dingemans KP, Spelbrink JN, Wijburg FA, Van Den Bogert C: Depletion of mitochondrial deoxyribonucleic acid in a family with fatal neonatal liver disease. *J Pediatr* **128**:683, 1996.
36. Spelbrink JN, Van Galen MJ, Zwart R, Bakker HD, Rovio A, Jacobs HT, Van Den Bogert C: Familial mitochondrial DNA depletion in liver: Haplotype analysis of candidate genes. *Hum Genet* **102**:327, 1998.
37. Rötig A, Bonnefont JP, Munnich A: Mitochondrial diabetes mellitus. *Diab Metab* **22**:291, 1996.
38. Gerbitz KD, Van Den Ouweland JM, Maassen JA, Jaksch M: Mitochondrial diabetes mellitus: A review. *Biochim Biophys Acta* **1271**:253, 1995.
39. Tengan CH, Kiyomoto BH, Rocha MS, Tavares VL, Gabbai AA, Moraes CT: Mitochondrial encephalomyopathy and hypoparathyroidism associated with a duplication and a deletion of mitochondrial deoxyribonucleic acid. *J Clin Endocrinol Metab* **83**:125, 1998.
40. Rötig A, Cormier V, Chatelain P, François R, Saudubray JM, Rustin P, Munnich A: Deletion of the mitochondrial genome in a case of early-onset diabetes mellitus, optic atrophy, and deafness (Wolfram syndrome, MIM 222300). *J Clin Invest* **91**:1095, 1993.
41. Superti-Furga A, Schoenle E, Tuchschmid P, Caduff R, Sabato V, De Mattia D, Gitzelman R, et al: Pearson bone marrow-pancreas syndrome with insulin-dependent diabetes, progressive renal tubulopathy, organic aciduria and elevated fetal haemoglobin caused by a deletion and duplication of mitochondrial DNA. *Eur J Pediatr* **152**:44, 1993.
42. Poulton J, O'Rahilly S, Morten KJ, Clark A: Mitochondrial DNA, diabetes and pancreatic pathology in Kearns-Sayre syndrome. *Diabetologia* **38**:868, 1995.
43. Souied EH, Sales MJ, Soubrane G, Coscas G, Bigorie B, Kaplan J, Munnich A, et al: Macular dystrophy, diabetes, and deafness associated with a large mitochondrial DNA deletion. *Am J Ophthalmol* **125**:100, 1998.
44. Rötig A, Bourgeron T, Chretien D, Rustin P, Munnich A: Spectrum of mitochondrial DNA rearrangements in the Pearson marrow-pancreas syndrome. *Hum Mol Genet* **4**:1327, 1995.
45. Rötig A, Bessis JL, Romero N, Cormier V, Saudubray JM, Narcy P, Lenoir G, et al: Maternally inherited duplication of the mitochondrial genome in a syndrome of proximal tubulopathy, diabetes mellitus, and cerebellar ataxia. *Am J Hum Genet* **50**:364, 1992.
46. Ballinger SW, Shoffner JM, Hedaya EV, Trounce I, Polak AM, Koontz DA, Wallace DC: Maternally transmitted diabetes and deafness associated with a 10.4 kb mitochondrial DNA deletion. *Nature Genet* **1**:11, 1992.
47. Van Den Ouweland JMW, Lemkes HHPJ, Ruitenbeek W, Sandkuijl LA, De Vijlder MF, Struyvenberg PAA, Van De Kamp JJP, et al: Mutation in mitochondrial tRNAleu(UUR) gene in a large pedigree with maternally transmitted type II diabetes mellitus and deafness. *Nature Genet* **1**:368, 1992.
48. Dunbar DR, Moonie PA, Swingler RJ, Davidson D, Roberts R, Holt IJ: Maternally transmitted partial direct tandem duplication of mitochondrial DNA associated with diabetes mellitus. *Hum Mol Genet* **2**:1619, 1993.
49. Kadowaki T, Kadowaki H, Mori Y, Tobe K, Sakuta R, Suzuki Y, Tanabe Y, et al: A subtype of diabetes mellitus associated with a mutation of mitochondrial DNA. *N Engl J Med* **330**:962, 1994.
50. Morten KJ, Cooper JM, Brown GK, Lake BD, Pike D, Poulton J: A new point mutation associated with mitochondrial encephalomyopathy. *Hum Mol Genet* **2**:2081, 1993.
51. Zeviani M, Gellera C, Antozzi C, Rimoldi M, Morandi L, Villani F, Tiranti V, et al: Maternally inherited myopathy and cardiomyopathy: Association with mutation in mitochondrial DNA tRNA(Leu)(UUR). *Lancet* **338**:143, 1991.
52. Moraes CT, Ciacci F, Bonilla E, Jansen C, Hirano M, Rao N, Lovelace RE, et al: Two novel pathogenic mitochondrial DNA mutations affecting organelle number and protein synthesis: Is the tRNA-(Leu(UUR)) gene an etiologic hot spot? *J Clin Invest* **92**:2906, 1993.
53. Pilz D, Quarrell OW, Jones EW: Mitochondrial mutation commonly associated with Leber's hereditary optic neuropathy observed in a patient with Wolfram syndrome (DIDMOAD). *J Med Genet* **31**:328, 1994.
54. Vionnet N, Passa P, Froguel P: Prevalence of mitochondrial gene mutations in families with diabetes mellitus. *Lancet* **342**:1429, 1993.
55. Bader-Meunier B, Rötig A, Mielot F, Lavergne JM, Croisille L, Rustin P, Landrieu P, et al: Refractory anaemia and mitochondrial cytopathy in childhood. *Br J Hematol* **87**:381, 1994.
56. Smith OP, Hann IM, Woodward CE, Brockington M: Pearson's marrow pancreas syndrome: Haematological features associated with deletion and duplication of mitochondrial DNA. *Br J Haematol* **90**:469, 1995.
57. Reid FM, Vernham GA, Jacobs HT: A novel mitochondrial point mutation in a maternal pedigree with sensorineural deafness. *Hum Mutat* **3**:243, 1994.
58. Prezant TR, Agapian JV, Bohlman MC, Bu X, (tm)ztas S, Qiu WQ, Arnos KS, et al: Mitochondrial ribosomal RNA mutation associated with both antibiotic-induced and non-syndromic deafness. *Nature Genet* **4**:289, 1993.
59. Matthijs G, Claes S, Longo-Mbenza B, Cassiman JJ: Non-syndromic deafness associated with a mutation and a polymorphism in the mitochondrial 12S ribosomal RNA gene in a large Zairean pedigree. *Eur J Hum Genet* **4**:46, 1996.
60. El-Schóahawi M, López De Munain A, Sarrazin AM, Shanske AL, Basirico M, Shanske S, DiMauro S: Two large Spanish pedigrees with nonsyndromic sensorineural deafness and the mtDNA mutation at nt 1555 in the 12S rRNA gene: Evidence of heteroplasmy. *Neurol* **48**:453, 1997.
61. Estivill X, Govea N, Barcelo E, Badenas C, Romero E, Moral L, Scozzari R, et al: Familial progressive sensorineural deafness is mainly due to the mtDNA A1555G mutation and is enhanced by treatment with aminoglycosides. *Am J Hum Genet* **62**:27, 1998.
62. Fischel-Ghodsian N: Mitochondrial mutations and hearing loss: Paradigm for mitochondrial genetics. *Am J Hum Genet* **62**:15, 1998.
63. Johns DR: mtDNA mutations and ophthalmological disease, in Wiggs JL (ed): *Molecular Genetics of Ocular Disease*. New York, Wiley-Liss, 1995, p 201.
64. Bodemer C, Rötig A, Rustin P, Cormier V, Niaudet P, Saudubray JM, Rabier D, Munnich A, de Prost Y: Hair and skin disorders as signs of mitochondrial disease. *Pediatrics* **103**:428, 1999.
65. Sevior KB, Hatamochi A, Stewart IA, Bykhovskaya Y, Allen-Powell DR, Fischel-Ghodsian N, Maw MA: Mitochondrial A7445G mutation

in two pedigrees with palmoplantar keratoderma and deafness. *Am J Med Genet* **75**:179, 1998.
66. Cormier-Daire V, Rustin P, Rötig A, Chretien D, Le Merrer M, Belli D, Le Goff A, et al: Craniofacial anomalies and malformations in respiratory chain deficiency. *Am J Med Genet* **66**:457, 1996.
67. Damian MS, Seibel P, Schachenmayr W, Reichmann H, Dorndorf W: VACTERL with the mitochondrial np 3243 point mutation. *Am J Med Genet* **62**:398, 1996.
68. Robinson BH, Macmillan H, Petrova-Benedict R, Sherwood WG: Variable clinical presentation in patients with defective E1 component of pyruvate dehydrogenase complex. *J Pediatr* **111**:525, 1987.
69. DiMauro S, Lombes A, Nakase H, Mita S, Fabrizi GM, Tritschler HJ, Bonilla E, et al: Cytochrome c oxidase deficiency. *Pediatr Res* **28**:536, 1990.
70. Bleyl SB, Mumford BR, Thompson V, Carey JC, Pysher TJ, Chin TK, Ward K: Neonatal, lethal noncompaction of the left ventricular myocardium is allelic with Barth syndrome. *Am J Hum Genet* **61**:868, 1997.
71. Dürr A, Cossée M, Agid Y, Campuzano V, Mignard C, Penet C, Mandel JL, et al: Clinical and genetic abnormalities in patients with Friedreich's ataxia. *N Engl J Med* **335**:1169, 1996.
72. Chamberlain S, Shaw J, Wallis J, Rowland A, Chow L, Farrall M, Keats B, et al: Genetic homogeneity at the Friedreich ataxia locus on chromosome 9. *Am J Hum Genet* **44**:518, 1989.
73. Campuzano V, Montermini L, Molto MD, Pianese L, Cossee M, Cavalcanti F, Monros E, et al: Friedreich's ataxia: Autosomal recessive disease caused by an intronic GAA triplet repeat expansion. *Science* **271**:1423, 1996.
74. Rötig A, De Lonlay P, Chretien D, Foury F, Koenig M, Sidi D, Munnich A, et al: Frataxin expansion causes aconitase and mitochondrial iron-sulfur protein deficiency in Friedreich ataxia. *Nature Genet* **17**:215, 1997.
75. Casari G, De Fusco M, Ciarmatori S, Zeviani M, Mora M, Fernández P, De Michele G, et al: Spastic paraplegia and OXPHOS impairment caused by mutations in paraplegin, a nuclear-encoded mitochondrial metalloprotease. *Cell* **93**:973, 1998.
76. Lestienne P, Ponsot G: Kearns-Sayre syndrome with muscle mitochondrial DNA deletion. *Lancet* **1**:885, 1988.
77. Moraes CT, DiMauro S, Zeviani M, Lombes A, Shanske S, Miranda AF, Nakase H, et al: Mitochondrial DNA deletions in progressive external ophthalmoplegia and Kearns-Sayre syndrome. *N Engl J Med* **320**:1293, 1989.
78. Wallace DC: Mitochondrial DNA sequence variation in human evolution and disease. *Proc Natl Acad Sci U S A* **91**:8739, 1994.
79. Morris AA, Leonard JV, Brown GK, Bidouki SK, Bindoff LA, Woodward CE, Harding AE, et al: Deficiency of respiratory chain complex I is a common cause of Leigh disease. *Ann Neurol* **40**:25, 1996.
80. Bourgeron T, Rustin P, Chretien D, Birch-Machin M, Bourgeois M, Munnich A, Rötig A: Mutation of a nuclear succinate dehydrogenase gene results in mitochondrial respiratory chain deficiency. *Nature Genet* **11**:144, 1995.
81. Tatuch Y, Christodoulou J, Feigenbaum A, Clarke JTR, Wherret J, Smith C, Rudd N, et al: Heteroplasmic mtDNA mutation (T > G) at 8993 can cause Leigh disease when the percentage of abnormal mtDNA is high. *Am J Hum Genet* **50**:852, 1992.
82. Lee N, Morin C, Mitchell G, Robinson BH: Saguenay Lac Saint Jean cytochrome oxidase deficiency: Sequence analysis of nuclear encoded COX subunits, chromosomal localization and a sequence anomaly in subunit VIc. *Biochim Biophys Acta* **1406**:1, 1998.
83. Goto Y, Nonaka I, Horai S: A mutation in the tRNA(Leu)(UUR) gene associated with the MELAS subgroup of mitochondrial encephalomyopathies. *Nature* **348**:651, 1990.
84. Valnot I, von Kleist-Retzow JC, Barrientos A, Gorbatyuk M, Taanman JW, Mehaye B, Rustin P, Tzagoloff A, Munnich A, Rötig A: A mutation in the human heme A:farnesyltransferase gene (COX10) causes cytochrome c oxidase deficiency. *Hum Mol Genet* **9**:1245, 2000.
85. Jin H, May M, Tranebjaerg L, Kendall E, Fontan G, Jackson J, Subramony SH, Arena F, Lubs H, Smith S, Stevenson R, Schwartz C, Vetrie D: A novel X-linked gene, DDP, shows mutations in families with deafness (DFN-1), dystonia, mental deficiency and blindness. *Nature Genet* **14**:177, 1996.
86. Koehler CM, Leuenberger D, Merchant S, Renold A, Junne T, Schatz G: Human deafness dystonia syndrome is a mitochondrial disease. *Proc Nat Acad Sci* **96**:2141, 1999.
87. Wallace DC, Zheng XX, Lott MT, Shoffner JM, Hodge JA, Kelley RI, Epstein CM, et al: Familial mitochondrial encephalomyopathy (MERRF): Genetic, pathophysiological, and biochemical characterization of a mitochondrial DNA disease. *Cell* **55**:601, 1988.
88. Shoffner JM, Lott MT, Lezza AM, Seibel P, Ballinger SW, Wallace DC: Myoclonic epilepsy and ragged-red fiber disease (MERRF) is associated with a mitochondrial DNA tRNA(Lys) mutation. *Cell* **61**:931, 1990.
89. Holt IJ, Harding AE, Petty RKH, Morgan-Hughes JA: A new mitochondrial disease associated with mitochondrial DNA heteroplasmy. *Am J Hum Genet* **46**:428, 1990.
90. Macshane MA, Hammans SR, Sweeney M, Holt IJ, Beattie TJ, Brett EM, Harding AE: Pearson syndrome and mitochondrial encephalomyopathy in a patient with a deletion of mtDNA. *Am J Hum Genet* **48**:39, 1991.
91. Zeviani M, Servidei S, Gellera C, Bertini E, DiMauro S, Didonato S: An autosomal dominant disorder with multiple deletions of mitochondrial DNA starting at the D-loop region. *Nature* **339**:309, 1989.
92. Kaukonen JA, Amati P, Suomalainen A, Rötig A, Piscaglia MG, Salvi F, Weissenbach J, et al: An autosomal locus predisposing to multiple deletions of mtDNA on chromosome 3p. *Am J Hum Genet* **58**:763, 1996.
93. Tiranti V, Chariot P, Carella F, Toscano A, Soliveri P, Girlanda P, Carrara F, et al: Maternally inherited hearing loss, ataxia and myoclonus associated with a novel point mutation in mitochondrial tRNASer(UCN) gene. *Hum Mol Genet* **4**:1421, 1995.
94. Polymeropoulos MH, Swift RG, Swift M: Linkage of the gene for Wolfram syndrome to markers on the short arm of chromosome 4. *Nature Genet* **8**:95, 1994.
95. Trijbels JM, Scholte HR, Ruitenbeek W, Sengers RC, Janssen AJ, Busch HF: Problems with the biochemical diagnosis in mitochondrial (encephalo-)myopathies. *Eur J Pediatr* **152**:178, 1993.
96. Touati G, Rigal O, Lombès A, Frachon P, Giraud M, Ogier De Baulny H: In vivo functional investigations of lactic acid in patients with respiratory chain disorders. *Arch Dis Child* **76**:16, 1997.
97. Gibson KM, Elpeleg ON, Jakobs C, Costeff H, Kelley RI: Multiple syndromes of 3-methylglutaconic aciduria. *Pediatr Neurol* **9**:120, 1993.
98. Rustin P, Chretien D, Bourgeron T, Gerard B, Rötig A, Saudubray JM, Munnich A: Biochemical and molecular investigations in respiratory chain deficiencies. *Clin Chim Acta* **228**:35, 1994.
99. Chretien D, Rustin P, Bourgeron T, Rötig A, Saudubray JM, Munnich A: Reference charts for respiratory chain activities in human tissues. *Clin Chim Acta* **228**:53, 1994.
100. Taylor RW, Birch-Machin MA, Bartlett K, Turnbull DM: Succinate-cytochrome c reductase: Assessment of its value in the investigation of defects of the respiratory chain. *Biochim Biophys Acta* **1181**:261, 1993.
101. Birch-Machin MA, Briggs HL, Saborido AA, Bindoff LA, Turnbull DM: An evaluation of the measurement of the activities of complexes I-IV in the respiratory chain of human skeletal muscle mitochondria. *Biochem Med Metab Biol* **51**:35, 1994.
102. Miró O, Cardellach F, Barrientos A, Casademont J, Rötig A, Rustin P: Cytochrome c oxidase assay in minute amount of human skeletal muscle using simple wavelength spectrophotometers. *J Neurosci Meth* **80**:107, 1997.
103. Chretien D, Gallego J, Barrientos A, Casademont J, Cardellach F, Munnich A, Rötig A, et al: The biochemical parameters for the diagnosis of respiratory chain deficiency in man and their lack of age-related changes. *Biochem J* **329**:249, 1998.
104. Ogasahara S, Engel AG, Frens D, Mack D: Muscle coenzyme Q deficiency in familial mitochondrial encephalomyopathy. *Proc Natl Acad Sci USA* **86**:2379, 1989.
105. Rötig A, Appelkvist EL, Geromel V, Chretien D, Parfait B, Kadhom N, Edery P, Lebideau M, Dallner G, Ernster L, Munnich A, Rustin P: Quinone-responsive mitochondrial encephalomyopathy due to a coenzyme Q10 biosynthesis defect. *Lancet* 2000 (in press).
106. Gérard B, Bourgeron T, Chretien D, Rötig A, Munnich A, Rustin P: Uridine preserves the expression of respiratory enzyme deficiencies in cultured fibroblasts. *Eur J Pediatr* **152**:270, 1992.
107. Bourgeron T, Chretien D, Rötig A, Munnich A, Rustin P: Fate and expression of the deleted mitochondrial DNA differ between heteroplasmic skin fibroblast and Epstein-Barr virus-transformed lymphocyte cultures. *J Biol Chem* **268**:19369, 1993.
108. Romero NB, Lombes A, Touati G, Rigal O, Frachon P, Cheval MA, Giraud M, et al: Morphological studies of skeletal muscle in lactic acidosis. *J Inher Metab Dis* **19**:528, 1996.
109. Radda GK, Odoom J, Kemp G, Taylor DJ, Thompson C, Styles P: Assessment of mitochondrial function and control in normal and diseased states. *Biochim Biophys Acta* **1271**:15, 1995.

110. Poulton J, Morten KJ, Weber K, Brown GK, Bindoff L: Are duplications of mitochondrial DNA characteristic of Kearns-Sayre syndrome? *Hum Mol Genet* **3**:947, 1994.

111. Ballinger SW, Shoffner JM, Gebhart S, Koontz DA, Wallace DC: Mitochondrial diabetes revisited. *Nature Genet* **7**:458, 1994.

112. Moraes CT, Shanske S, Tritschler HJ, Aprile JR, Andreetta F, Bonilla E, Schon EA, et al: mtDNA depletion with variable tissue expression–A novel genetic abnormality in mitochondrial diseases. *Am J Hum Genet* **48**:492, 1991.

113. Poulton J, Holt IJ: Mitochondrial DNA: Does more lead to less? *Nature Genet* 8:313, 1994.

114. Chabrol B, Mancini J, Chretien D, Rustin P, Munnich A, Pinsard N: Valproate-induced hepatic failure in a case of cytochrome c oxidase deficiency. *Eur J Pediatr* **153**:133, 1994.

115. Walker UA, Byrne E: The therapy of respiratory chain encephalomyopathy: A critical review of the past and current perspective. *Acta Neurol Scand* **92**:273, 1995.

116. Anderson S, Bankier AT, Barrell BG, De Bruijn MH, Coulson AR, Drouin J, Eperon IC, et al: Sequence and organization of the human mitochondrial genome. *Nature* **290**:457, 1981.

117. Wallace DC, Singh G, Lott MT, Hodge JA, Schurr TG, Lezza AM, Elsas LJ, et al: Mitochondrial DNA mutation associated with Leber's hereditary optic neuropathy. *Science* **242**:1427, 1988.

118. Howell N, Bindoff LA, McCullough DA, Kubacka I, Poulton J, Mackey D, Taylor L, et al: Leber hereditary optic neuropathy: Identification of the same mitochondrial ND1 mutation in six pedigrees. *Am J Hum Genet* **49**:939, 1991.

119. Brown MD, Voljavec AS, Lott MT, Macdonald I, Wallace DC: Leber's hereditary optic neuropathy: A model for mitochondrial neurodegenerative diseases. *FASEB Journal* **6**:2791, 1992.

120. Brown MD, Voljavec AS, Lott MT, Torroni A, Yang CC, Wallace DC: Mitochondrial DNA complex I and III mutations associated with Leber's hereditary optic neuropathy. *Genetics* **130**:163, 1992.

121. Suomalainen A, Paetau A, Laeinonen H, Majander A, Peltonen L, Somer H: Inherited idiopathic dilated cardiomyopathy with multiple deletions of mitochondrial DNA. *Lancet* **340**:1319, 1992.

122. Bohlega S, Tanji K, Santorelli FM, Hirano M, Al-Jishi A, DiMauro S: Multiple mitochondrial DNA deletions associated with autosomal recessive ophthalmoplegia and severe cardiomyopathy. *Neurology* **46**:1329, 1996.

123. van den Heuvel L, Ruitenbeek W, Smeets R, Gelman-Kohan Z, Elpeleg O, Loeffen J, Trijbels F, Mariman E, de Bruijn D, Smeitink J: Demonstration of a new pathogenic mutation in human complex I deficiency: A 5-bp duplication in the nuclear gene encoding the 18-kD (AQDQ) subunit. *Am J Hum Genet* **62**:262, 1998.

124. Triepels RH, van den Heuvel LP, Loeffen JL, Buskens CA, Smeets RJ, Rubio Gozalbo ME, Budde SM, Mariman EC, Wijburg FA, Barth PG, Trijbels JM, Smeitink JA: Leigh syndrome associated with a mutation in the NDUFS7 (PSST) nuclear encoded subunit of complex I. *Ann Neurol* **45**:787, 1999.

125. Loeffen J, Smeitink J, Triepels R, Smeets R, Schuelke M, Sengers R, Trijbels F, Hamel B, Mullaart R, van den Heuvel L: The first nuclear-encoded complex I mutation in a patient with Leigh syndrome. *Am J Hum Genet* **63**:1598, 1998.

126. Schuelke M, Smeitink J, Mariman E, Loeffen J, Plecko B, Trijbels F, Stockler-Ipsiroglu S, van den Heuvel L: Mutant NDUFV1 subunit of mitochondrial complex I causes leukodystrophy and myoclonic epilepsy. *Nat Genet* **21**:260, 1999.

127. Adams PL, Lightowlers RN, Turnbull DM: Molecular analysis of cytochrome c oxidase deficiency in Leigh's syndrome. *Ann Neurol* **41**:268, 1997.

128. Zhu Z, Yao J, Johns T, Fu K, De Bie I, Macmillan C, Cuthbert AP, Newbold RF, Wang J, Chevrette M, Brown GK, Brown RM, Shoubridge EA: SURF1, encoding a factor involved in the biogenesis of cytochrome c oxidase, is mutated in Leigh syndrome. *Nat Genet* **20**:337, 1998.

129. Tiranti V, Hoertnagel K, Carrozzo R, Galimberti C, Munaro M, Granatiero M, Zelante L, Gasparini P, Marzella R, Rocchi M, Bayona-Bafaluy MP, Enriquez JA, Uziel G, Bertini E, Dionisi-Vici C, Franco B, Meitinger T, Zeviani M: Mutations of SURF-1 in Leigh disease associated with cytochrome c oxidase deficiency. *Am J Hum Genet* **63**:1609, 1998.

130. Papadopoulou LC, Sue CM, Davidson MM, Tanji K, Nishino I, Sadlock JE, Krishna S, Walker W, Selby J, Glerum DM, Coster RV, Lyon G, Scalais E, Lebel R, Kaplan P, Shanske S, De Vivo DC, Bonilla E, Hirano M, DiMauro S, Schon EA: Fatal infantile cardioencephalomyopathy with COX deficiency and mutations in SCO2, a COX assembly gene. *Nat Genet* **23**:333, 1999.

131. Nishino I, Spinazzola A, Hirano M: Thymidine phosphorylase gene mutations in MNGIE, a human mitochondrial disorder. *Science* **283**:689, 1999.

132. Harding AE, Holt IJ, Sweeney MG, Brockington M, Davis MB: Prenatal diagnosis of mitochondrial DNA 8893 T > G disease. *Am J Hum Genet* **50**:629, 1992.

133. Poulton J, Marchington DR: Propects for DNA-based prenatal diagnosis of mitochondrial disorders. *Prenat Diagnosis* **16**:1247, 1996.

134. Faivre L, Cormier-Daire V, Chretien D, von Kleist-Retzow JC, Amiel J, Dommergues M, Dumez Y, Rötig A, Rustin P, Munnich A: Determination of enzyme activities for prenatal diagnosis of respiratory chain deficiency. In press.

CHAPTER

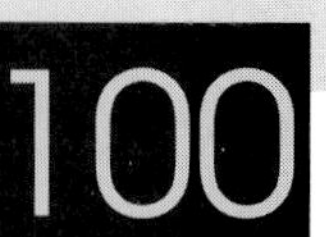

Lactic Acidemia: Disorders of Pyruvate Carboxylase and Pyruvate Dehydrogenase

Brian H. Robinson

1. **The lactic acid that circulates in the human body is the product of the anaerobic metabolism of glucose, which takes place primarily in red cells, skin, kidney medulla, and white skeletal muscle. Some of it is oxidized by red muscle and kidney cortex, but the bulk of it is taken up by the liver and made into glucose. Lactate is always produced by reduction of pyruvate through lactate dehydrogenase and is always removed by a reversal of this process. Deficiency of both the H and the M subunit forms of lactate dehydrogenase are known, but they are relatively benign conditions. The oxidative metabolism of pyruvate proceeds through pyruvate dehydrogenase, the Krebs cycle, and the respiratory chain, whereas anabolic utilization proceeds primarily through pyruvate carboxylase. A defect in any of these pathways may lead to inadequate removal of pyruvate and lactate from the circulation, resulting in a condition of lactic acidemia.**
2. **Deficiency of the pyruvate dehydrogenase complex is the most common of the disorders leading to lactic acidemia. It may be due to a defect in the E_1 (OMIM 312170), E_2 (OMIM 246348), E_3 (OMIM 246900), X-lipoate (OMIM 245349), or pyruvate dehydrogenase phosphatase component of the complex. The most common of these is the defect in the E_1 component. This particular defect can present in three possible ways with a graded spectrum from the most severe to the least. In its most severe form, it presents with overwhelming lactic acidosis at birth, with death in the neonatal period. In a second form of presentation, the lactic acidemia is moderate, but there is profound psychomotor retardation with increasing age and, in many cases, concomitant damage to the brain stem and basal ganglia lead to death in infancy. In the third form of presentation, which is found only in males, there is carbohydrate-induced episodic ataxia, very often coupled with mild developmental delay.**
3. **The E_1 defects are caused by mutations in the $E_1\alpha$ gene which is X-linked (OMIM 312170). Because of its central importance in central nervous system metabolism, pyruvate dehydrogenase deficiency is a problem both in males and in females even though only one $E_1\alpha$ allele in the females carries a mutation. For this reason, this form of pyruvate dehydrogenase complex deficiency should be classified as X-linked dominant. Most defects in the $E_1\alpha$ gene are *de novo* mutations and are not carried somatically by either parent. In males, the defects are either missense mutations or mutations that affect only the 3′ end of the coding sequence. In females, deletions and insertions that completely nullify one allele are more common. The E_2 (OMIM 245348) and protein X-lipoate (OMIM 245349) defects are rare and result in severe psychomotor retardation. A group of X-deficient patients has been characterized at the molecular level.**
4. **The E_3 lipoamide dehydrogenase defect (MIM 246900) leads to deficient activity not only in the pyruvate dehydrogenase complex, but also in the α-ketoglutarate and branched chain ketoacid dehydrogenase complexes. Pyruvate dehydrogenase phosphatase deficiency has been documented in four patients, three of them presenting with Leigh disease and the fourth with unremitting lactic acidemia. The most common pathologic feature of deficiency of the pyruvate dehydrogenase complex is the development of cystic lesions in the cerebral cortex, basal ganglia, and brain stem. More recently, a milder version of E_3 lipoamide dehydrogenase deficiency was described.**
5. **Pyruvate carboxylase deficiency (OMIM 266150) presents in three ways. In the simple (A) form of the disease, the patient presents in the first few months of life with a mild-to-moderate lactic acidemia and delayed development. In the more complex (B) form of the disease, the patient presents soon after birth with a severe lactic acidemia accompanied by hyperammonemia, citrullinemia, and hyperlysinemia. The patients of this latter group rarely survive to 3 months of age. In a single case (C), the presentation is mild and consists only of episodic acidosis with no psychomotor retardation. There is good evidence to suggest that patients in group A have some residual pyruvate carboxylase activity while those in group B have no activity at all. Some patients in group B have absence of both mRNA and pyruvate carboxylase protein in cultured skin fibroblasts. Group A patients who survive are severely mentally retarded and missense mutations have been described for this group. This seems to be due to loss of cerebral neurons, despite the fact that in normal individuals there is pyruvate carboxylase activity in astrocytes but not**

A list of standard abbreviations is located immediately preceding the index in each volume. Additional abbreviations used in this chapter include: HCM = hypertrophic cardiomyopathy; LDH = lactate dehydrogenase; LHON = Lebers hereditary optic neuropathy; MELAS = mitochondrial myopathy, encephalopathy, lactic acidosis, and stroke-like episodes; MERRF = myoclonic epilepsy with ragged red fibers; Protein X = the second lipoate-containing protein other than dihydrolipoamide transacetylase in the pyruvate dehydrogenase complex; NARP = neurodegeneration with ataxia and retinitis pigmentosa; PDH = pyruvate dehydrogenase; PEPCK = phosphoenolpyruvate carboxykinase; PFK = phosphofructokinase; and TPP = thiamine pyrophosphate.

in neurons. This suggests that pyruvate carboxylase has an essential anaplerotic (Greek derivation meaning "filling up") role in astrocytes and that its absence deprives the neuron of an obligatory nutrient normally supplied by astrocyte metabolism.

Several inborn errors of metabolism present with a metabolic acidosis in which the major anionic contributing species is lactate. In others where acidosis is not a problem, the blood lactate level is elevated above normal either on a chronic or an acute basis. For the most part, these elevations of lactic acid are secondary, such as is seen in propionic acidemia, methylmalonic acidemia, hydroxymethylglutaric aciduria, and the fatty acid oxidation defects[1] (see Chaps. 94, 95, and 101), occurring because of interference with coenzyme A (CoA) metabolism in relation to its important function in the pyruvate dehydrogenase complex. Fortunately, these secondary lactic acidemias are easily distinguishable by the presence of unusual organic acids in the urine. Excessive lactic acid production also occurs in many other nongenetic conditions associated with blood vessel occlusion, asphyxia, liver disease, and other pathologic conditions that are not always easy to distinguish from the inborn errors, which are primary causes of lactic acidemia. To understand how lactic acid accumulation occurs, it is necessary to understand the dynamics of lactate production and utilization in the human body.

THE NORMAL METABOLISM OF PYRUVATE AND LACTATE

The Fed State

In the fed state, the average (70-kg) male adult ingests 300 g of carbohydrates per day. Of this 300 g, perhaps 50 g is utilized by the liver for a variety of purposes (glycogen synthesis, energy provision, lipogenesis, etc.) leaving 250 g to be utilized in the periphery (Fig. 100-1). Another 125 g is used by the brain and 125 g by muscle. Additional output of 75 g of glucose from the liver occurs as a result of gluconeogenesis from lactate. This output of 75 g of glucose from the liver is not oxidized to CO_2 and H_2O but is converted in glycolytic tissues to lactate and released into the circulation. Small amounts of lactic acid are also released from brain and white muscle, and much of this lactate is reconverted to glucose in the liver, a small amount being oxidized by red muscle. This conversion of glucose to lactate in the periphery and reconversion of lactate to glucose in the liver is known as the Cori cycle. It is this cycle that is responsible for the turnover of the pool of lactate in the body fluids.[2,3] The major difference that must be appreciated between the adult considered above and the pediatric patient is that the higher brain-to-body weight ratio in a child causes a higher proportion of hepatic glucose output to be used by the brain (Fig. 100-2). The above models for carbohydrate metabolism in the fed state are oversimplified summaries of the average disposition of carbon atoms in a 24-h period, but they do help us put in perspective the relative importance of carbon flow, especially in relation to flux through gluconeogenesis and through oxidative metabolism.

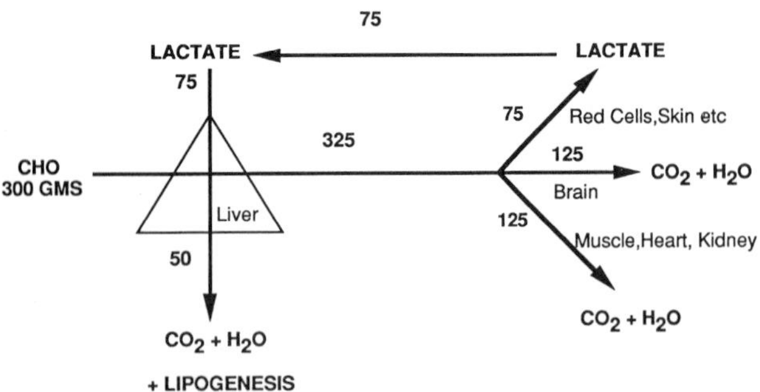

Fig. 100-1 Disposition of ingested carbohydrate (CHO) in an average 70-kg adult in a 24-h period. Values for different branches of metabolic activity are given in grams per 24 h. See text for details.

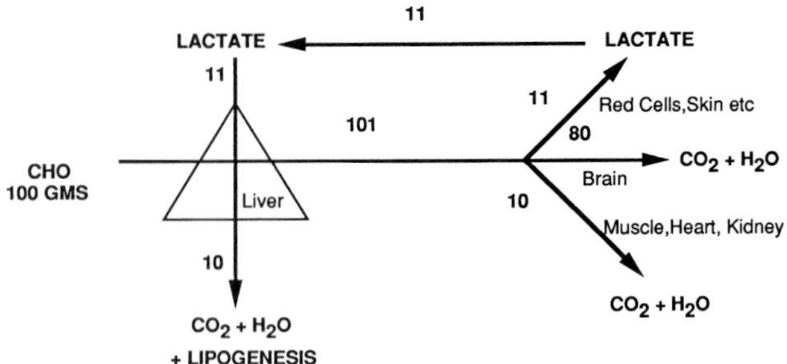

Fig. 100-2 Disposition of ingested carbohydrate (CHO) in a 24-h period in a 10-kg infant. Values for different branches of metabolic activity are given in grams per 24 h. See text for details.

The Fasted State

In the fasted state, major changes occur: (a) fatty acids are substituted as the major fuel for muscle and liver, (b) a major new carbohydrate source from muscle breakdown is available in the form of amino acid as gluconeogenic precursors (mostly alanine), and (c) glycerol derived from triglyceride breakdown contributes to gluconeogenesis (Fig. 100-3). The activity of the Cori cycle and oxidation of glucose remain unchanged in the early stages of fasting.[2,3] As fasting continues, the reliance of the brain on carbohydrate fuels diminishes as ketone body oxidation is substituted as an energy source.[4] This enables the rate of muscle breakdown, which is rapid in the early stages of fasting, to slow, thus conserving lean body mass. Again, this situation is somewhat different for pediatric subjects. Their relatively large brain weight and relatively small lean body mass mean that children are much more prone than adults to the development of hypoglycemia in the fasting situation.[5] The above considerations should lead us to the following series of conclusions about the metabolism of pyruvate and lactate, which are summarized below with reference to Fig. 100-4:

1. In the fed state, the brain utilizes 50 to 90 percent of the ingested carbohydrate that gets oxidized to CO_2 and H_2O, the proportion being high in infants and low in adults.
2. In the fasted state, the brain is the major site of oxidation of glucose produced by the liver.
3. As a result of items 1 and 2, the activity of the pyruvate dehydrogenase complex, the citric acid cycle, and the respiratory chain are essential to the normal working of the human central nervous system.
4. Normal liver pyruvate carboxylase and phosphoenolpyruvate carboxykinase functions are essential for the maintenance of glucose output in the fasting state.

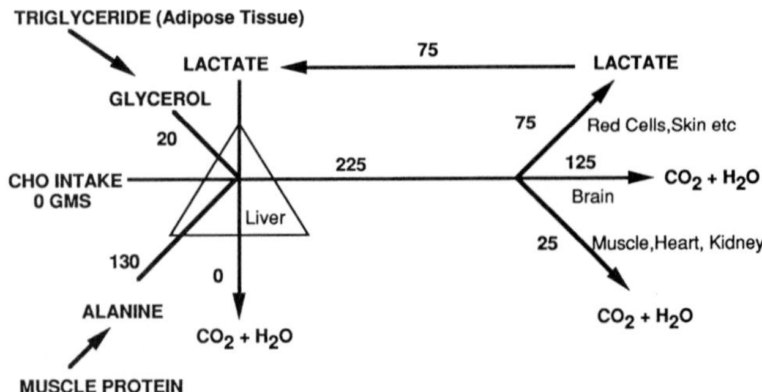

Fig. 100-3 Sources and disposition of carbohydrate (CHO) after 24-h fasting in a 70-kg adult. Carbohydrate is derived from triglyceride glycerol, from muscle protein breakdown, or from lactate, and is utilized primarily by brain. Values are given for different branches of metabolic activity in grams of carbohydrate per 24 h.

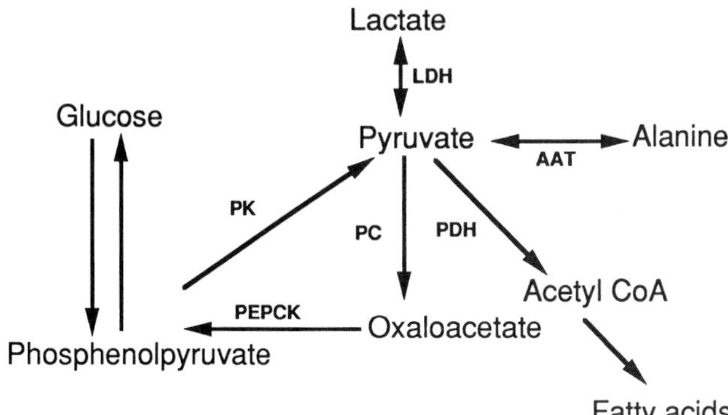

Fig. 100-4 The metabolic fates of pyruvate. Pyruvate can be converted to phosphoenolpyruvate (PEP), oxaloacetate (OAA), acetyl coenzyme A (AcCoA), alanine, or lactate. The enzymes involved are pyruvate kinase (PK), phosphoenolpyruvate carboxykinase (PEPCK), pyruvate dehydrogenase (PDH), pyruvate carboxylase (PC), alanine aminotransferase (AAT), and lactate dehydrogenase (LDH).

Anaerobic Production of Pyruvate and Lactate

For most cell types, providing the oxygen supply is adequate, the bulk of ATP requirements are generated by oxidation of pyruvate, fatty acids, or ketone bodies through the oxidation of acetyl CoA in the tricarboxylic acid cycle. However, as mentioned above, there are some cell types that preferentially derive their energy supply from glycolytic activity, with oxidative metabolism playing a minor role. In such tissues, the end products of metabolism are pyruvic and lactic acids. Some tissues, such as blood, have either very few (white cells) or no (red cells) mitochondria, and thus a glycolytic mode of metabolism is obligatory. Other tissues have such a high glycolytic capacity that oxidative metabolism is suppressed, a phenomenon known as the Crabtree effect (Fig. 100-5).

In the oxidative cell types such as liver, red muscle, and kidney cortex, the products of mitochondrial oxidative phosphorylation (ATP and citrate) act to curtail the activity of the glycolytic pathway by bringing about allosteric inhibition of phosphofructokinase. There are two species of phosphofructokinase (PFK) present in these cell types in varying proportions: an L type, which predominates in liver, and an M type, which predominates in muscle. Both of these species are controlled tightly by the allosteric activators 5′ AMP and fructose 2,6-biphosphate, and by the allosteric inhibitors ATP and citrate, so that glycolytic flow is highly regulated.[6] In skin fibroblasts, platelets, lymphocytes, brain, and kidney medulla, a distinct form of phosphofructokinase (PFK-F) occurs, which has no allosteric activators and is weakly inhibited by ATP and citrate.[7] In cell types where PFK-F predominates, glycolysis is a very important factor in ATP generation, and in these cells lactate production occurs in the presence of adequate supplies of both respiratory substrate and oxygen. This unregulated PFK-F also is present in significant amounts in fetal tissues and in tumor cells, where glycolysis is again a prominent mode of energy production.[7,8]

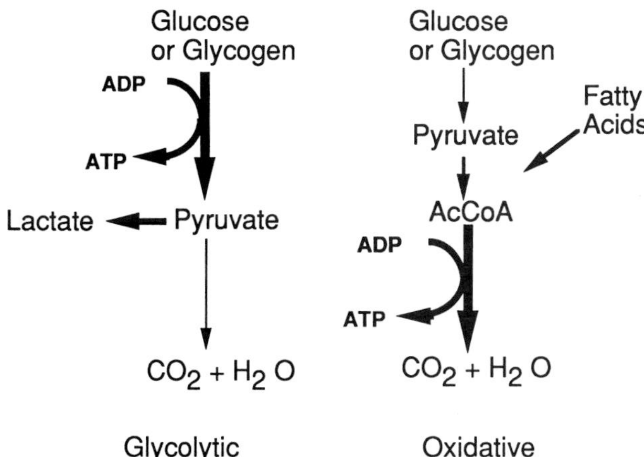

Fig. 100-5 The two modes of cellular energy metabolism. On the left, the glycolytic mode generates the majority of cellular ATP requirements by metabolizing glucose or glycogen to lactate. On the right, the oxidative mode generates the majority of cellular ATP requirements by oxidation of pyruvate, fatty acids, and ketone bodies in the mitochondria.

In the normal individual, who is well-oxygenated and well-perfused, the blood lactate is between 1 and 2 mM and does not change appreciably with fasting, feeding, or any of the simple infectious diseases. CSF lactate levels are similar, with an upper limit of normal of 2.2 mM. The normal range of blood and CSF pyruvate levels vary between 40 and 150 μM in blood and CSF with the lactate to pyruvate ratio being between 10 and 25 to 1. We have already seen that hepatic removal of 75 g lactic acid per 24 h[9] occurs out of a daily lactic acid production of 115 g per day.[10] Of this, 29 g is produced by red cells, 20 g by skin, 17 g by brain, 16 g by skeletal muscle (white), 8 g by intestinal mucosa, and 15 g by renal medulla.[9,10] Thus, about 40 g of lactic acid is removed extrahepatically, mostly by oxidation in red muscle and kidney cortex. The contribution of white skeletal muscle to lactic acid production over and above the normal daily total lactic acid production may be considerable when the subject is involved in explosive exercise, such as sprinting. Hermansen et al.[11] showed in a group of athletes that three bouts of sprinting to exhaustion in a 12-min period generated a mean blood lactic acid level of 22 mM at the end of the third bout of exercise. If the athletes then rested, 6 to 8 h was required to remove the lactic acid load and return the blood lactate to normal, but if the subjects followed the explosive exercise with a period of jogging, then the lactic acid load was removed more rapidly. This experiment illustrates that the normal route for the removal of a lactic acid load via the liver is rather slow,[12] and that the alternative route of removal by direct oxidation in muscle is very efficient,[11] but requires work.

A variety of problems associated with circulatory failure, shock, blood vessel occlusion, and asphyxia, result in an ensuing transient or chronic lactic acidemia.[12] This arises because of lack of sufficient oxygenation of the tissues, a situation in which production of ATP by oxidative phosphorylation is curtailed, and rising intracellular levels of 5′ AMP, ADP, NH^{4+}, and inorganic phosphate trigger a rapid degradation of glycogen to form lactate.[2] In this situation, there is usually a much increased blood lactate-to-pyruvate ratio, indicative of the more reduced intracellular conditions prevailing in hypoxia.[12]

THE ENZYMES OF PYRUVATE METABOLISM

Pyruvate is metabolized through four main enzyme systems in the human body: lactate dehydrogenase, alanine aminotransferase, pyruvate carboxylase, and the pyruvate dehydrogenase complex (Fig. 100-4). Alanine aminotransferase is not discussed in detail here because deficiency of this enzyme in humans has not been reported. Its main functions in overall metabolism are to provide the catalytic function in the fed state, whereby nitrogen derived from branched chain amino acid oxidation can be donated to pyruvate and returned to the liver for fixation, and the catalytic function in fasting, whereby 3-carbon units derived from muscle protein breakdown to amino acids can be aminated and directed to the liver for gluconeogenesis.[13]

Lactate Dehydrogenase

Lactate dehydrogenase exists in two subunit forms: an H form, which predominates in heart, and an M form, which predominates in skeletal muscle. The active form of the enzyme is a tetramer such that in most tissues a spectrum of isoenzymic forms appear to include H_4, H_3M, H_2M_2, H_1M_3, and M_4.[14] Separate deficiencies have been described for the two subunit forms of this enzyme. In one case report, four sibs were totally lacking detectable activity of the M subunit form of the enzyme, and all activity detected in red cells, white cells, and muscle was of the H_4 form.[15] One sib had pigmenturia and easy fatigue on exercise. Ischemic exercise of the forearm led to an exaggerated pyruvic acidemia and to a muted elevation of blood lactic acid. Because muscle damage was evident in this patient, we must conclude that the residual H_4 isoenzyme of lactic dehydrogenase (LDH) present in exercising muscle must have had less than adequate activity to sustain NADH reoxidation rates, thus leading to an early curtailment of glycolysis and loss of intramuscular ATP. This defect is most commonly described in Japanese patients, and Maekawa et al.[16] have demonstrated a 20-bp deletion in exon 6 of the LDH-M isoform gene in 18 individuals from 4 families.

Deficiency of the H subunit was described in a 64-year-old man with moderately impaired glucose tolerance and slight elevation of cholesterol.[17]

Pyruvate Dehydrogenase

Composition of the α-Keto Acid Dehydrogenase Complexes. The three α-keto acid dehydrogenase complexes are made up of three basic functional types of catalytic protein: E_1, an α-keto acid decarboxylase that forms hydroxyalkyl thiamine pyrophosphate (TTP)-E_1 and CO_2; E_2, an acyl transferase that forms acyl CoA; and E_3, dihydrolipoyl dehydrogenase, a flavin-requiring enzyme that forms NADH. In the pyruvate dehydrogenase complex, a further lipoyl-containing functional catalytic protein is present, named protein X, which is also capable of performing an acyl transfer function[18,19] (Fig. 100-6). Lipoyl groups covalently attached through lysine to the E_2 or X backbone act to transfer both hydrogen and acetyl groups between the different component enzymes of the complex.[20,21] In addition to serving a role in acylation reactions, protein X seems to play an essential role in the binding of E_3 to the PDH complex.[22] Recent cDNA cloning of the human X protein demonstrated that it has only one lipoyl domain and both E_2 and E_3 binding domains by homology with other ketoacid dehydrogenase complexes.[23–25]

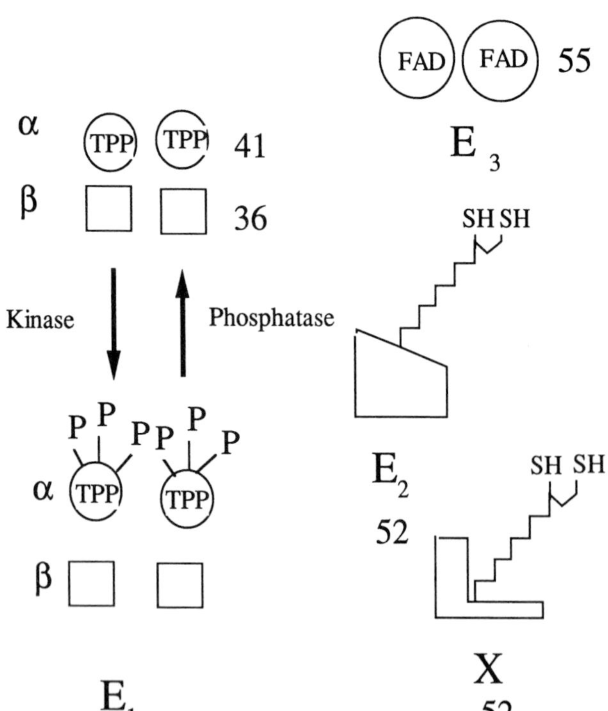

Fig. 100-6 Composition of the pyruvate dehydrogenase complex. See text for details.

Each functional component of a complex is present in multiples in a working undissociated complex such that the actual molecular weight is several million. Thus, the molecular weight of the bovine heart pyruvate dehydrogenase (PDH) complex is 8.5 million, made up of 30 units of E_1, 60 units of E_2, and 6 units each of E_3 and X. The E_1 unit is an $\alpha_2\beta_2$ tetramer with subunits of 41,000 and 36,000 daltons for α and β, respectively. The E_2 is a monomer which gives an apparent M_r of 74,000 on SDS polyacrylamide gel electrophoresis, although its true molecular weight is closer to 52,000.[18] Protein X is also a monomer of $M_r = 51,000$.[20,21]

The E_3 dihydrolipoyl dehydrogenase or lipoamide dehydrogenase is a dimer whose subunit molecular weight is 55,000. In contrast, the E_1 component of the α-ketoglutarate dehydrogenase complex is a dimer of subunit molecular weight 118,000; the E_2 transuccinylase is 48,000; and the E_3 subunit is again 55,000. The branched chain α-keto acid dehydrogenase complex bears a striking resemblance to the PDH complex. Its E_1 component is an $\alpha_2\beta_2$ tetrameric structure with molecular weights of 47,000 and 38,000 for α and β subunits, respectively. The E_2 component is 51,000, and the E_3 is, again, 55,000.[26] The E_3 component of each of the complexes is almost certainly identical, being encoded by the same gene in prokaryotic cells.[27]

The branched chain α-keto acid dehydrogenase complex also resembles the pyruvate dehydrogenase complex in that both can radically change their overall catalytic activity in response to the phosphorylation and dephosphorylation of the $E_1\alpha$ subunit.[19,28,29] Pyruvate dehydrogenase kinase is a dimer of two dissimilar subunits of $M_r = 45,000$ and 48,000,[18] which catalyzes phosphorylation of serine residues in at least two positions on the $E_1\alpha$ protein, rendering the complex inactive. The kinase is strongly inhibited by pyruvate and by ADP, so that the complex tends to stay more active either when rates of ATP turnover are high, or when pyruvate concentrations are high.[18,19] Four isoenzymes of pyruvate dehydrogenase kinase are known to phosphorylate the $E_1\alpha$ subunit of the PDH complex, thereby reducing the activity of the complex.[30–33]

All the PDH kinase isoenzymes (PK1, PK2, PK3, PK4) are inhibited by pyruvate, whereas the PK2 isoenzyme alone is influenced by changes in the NAD/NADH ratio and AcCoA/CoA ratio.[30] These isoenzymes are expressed in most tissues with the exception of PK3, which is present in heart and skeletal muscle only.[30,31]

The same groups are dephosphorylated by the action of PDH phosphatase, a dimer ($M_r = 50,000$ and 98,000) that is weakly bound to the complex.[18,19] This phosphatase requires Mg^{2+} ($K_{0.5} = 1$ mM) and Ca^{2+} ($K_{0.5} = 1$ μM) for full activity, and this activation by Ca^{2+} ions is thought to be physiologically important in muscle and heart under conditions of increased workload (Fig. 100-7). Both the catalytic and regulatory subunit cDNAs of the bovine PDH-complex phosphatase have been determined.[34,35] The catalytic subunit bears a resemblance to the protein phosphatase

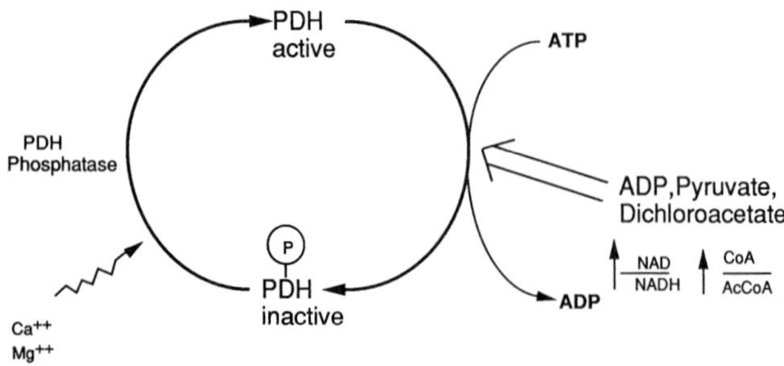

Fig. 100-7 Control of activity in the pyruvate dehydrogenase (PDH) complex. The complex exists in a nonphosphorylated active form or in a phosphorylated inactive form. The phosphorylation is catalyzed by a kinase, which is inhibited by ADP, pyruvate, dichloroacetate-increased mitochondrial NAD^+/NADH and CoA/AcCoA. The dephosphorylation is catalyzed by a phosphatase, which is activated by Ca^{2+} and Mg^{2+}.

2C family, whereas the regulatory subunit shows strong protein sequence similarity to the dimethylglycine dehydrogenase family of proteins.[34,35] Although both α subunits are identical in each PDH-E_1 tetramer, phosphorylation of only one seems to be sufficient to obtain 99 percent inactivation of the complex. Phosphorylation can and does take place to the extent of three serine sites per α subunit, but the physiological significance of this process is not clear.[18,19] The amount of PDH complex present in the active nonphosphorylated form in vivo is known for laboratory animals but not for humans. These figures do change depending on the physiological state. In starvation and diabetes, the percentage activity falls to one-half or one-third of that in the fed state, depending on the length of exposure to the catabolic state.[3] The percentage activity of heart and skeletal muscle PDH complex may rise three- to fourfold after the commencement of heavy exercise.[3,19,36] In the former case, the increasing oxidation of fats brought about by a catabolic hormonal milieu leads to high intramitochondrial NADH/NAD and acetyl CoA/CoA ratios, which have a stimulating effect on the PDH kinase and lead to a decrease in overall activity of the complex. In the case of heavy exercise, increasing concentrations of ADP, pyruvate, and Ca^{2+} has the dual effect of activating the phosphatase and inhibiting the kinase, thus leading to an increase in the overall activity of the complex. The percentage of the pyruvate dehydrogenase complex in the active form can also be increased by the use of dichloroacetate, a pyruvate analogue, and an effective inhibitor of PDH kinase.[37]

DISORDERS OF THE PYRUVATE DEHYDROGENASE COMPLEX

There are now five components in which defects leading to deficiency of the pyruvate dehydrogenase complex have been documented. Individual enzymatic reactions can be documented for each of the components E_1, E_2, and E_3, and for any patient showing deficiency of the pyruvate dehydrogenase complex a profile of activity can be developed using either tissue samples or cultured skin fibroblasts. Thus, PDHC-deficient patients have been described with defects in the E_1 pyruvate dehydrogenase, the E_2 transacetylase, and the E_3 lipoyl dehydrogenase. In addition, patients have been described with defects in the X-component and in PDH-phosphatase.

Pyruvate Decarboxylase Deficiency (OMIM *312170)

There are technical difficulties associated with the measurement of the activity of the pyruvate dehydrogenase complex and its subcomponents in tissue taken at postmortem because of the lability of the complex unless tissue is frozen in liquid N_2 and stored at $-70°C$ or below. The measurement of these activities in fibroblasts, which was pioneered by Blass,[38,40] allowed for the unequivocal documentation of pyruvate dehydrogenase deficiency as an entity. The first cases described were deficient in pyruvate decarboxylase, the first component of the complex.[38–42]

We have carried out reviews of both the patients in the literature and the patients we have collected information from in our lactic acidemia screening program.[43,44] Although we can go some way toward categorizing them in terms of useful symptomatic groupings, it is evident that there is overlap between the groups and the reality is that we are faced with a spectrum of disease severity in which it is difficult to find many patients exactly alike. To demonstrate this point, Fig. 100-8 shows the variation in clinical presentation with residual activity of the complex in cultured fibroblasts measured for a series of 50 patients with PDH-E_1 deficiency.

In general, the severity of the disease is a function of the severity of the lactic acidemia. The most severely affected infants die before 6 months of age, and have low residual activity of the PDH complex and chronic severe lactic acidemia.[44–48] Eleven of 46 PDH-E_1 deficiency cases that we analyzed were of this fatal severe type with a mean activity of 14.6 percent for the total PDH complex[44] (Table 100-1). The second group, although they had lactic acidemia of a mild-to-moderate nature, did not suffer from a major acid-base disturbance except for short periods, usually concurrent with infections.[49–55] Many of these cases did not come to medical attention until it was recognized that they were developmentally delayed. This group with psychomotor retardation is the major group of patients and within this group, there is a wide spectrum. Of 28 cases that we dealt with in this category, 7 died before 3 years of age and 21 were still living. Five of the children that died had cystic lesions in the basal ganglia and brain stems typical of Leigh disease at postmortem,[43,44] a finding reported for many cases in the literature.[49,51,52,54,55] The other two had cerebral atrophy and cysts in the cerebral hemispheres. Of the

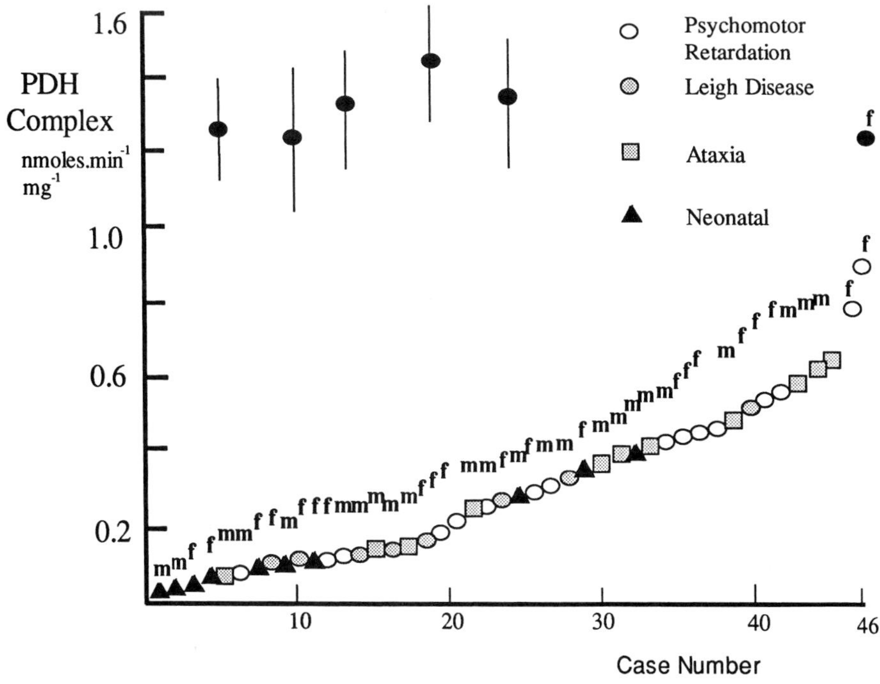

Fig. 100-8 Variation in the clinical presentation and activity of the pyruvate dehydrogenase complex in 46 cases compared to control activities. The clinical presentation is designated by the symbol used and the letters f (female) and m (male) designate the patient's sex.

Table 100-1 Clinical Presentation of PDH-Complex E_1 Deficiency

	Psychomotor Retardation		
Neonatal/Infant Death	**Dead**	**Still Living**	**Ataxic Episodes**
11 Cases	7 Cases	21 Cases	7 Cases
14.6% Activity	21.9% Activity	27.9% Activity	29.8% Activity
5 Males	3 Males	7 Males	7 Males
6 Females	4 Females	14 Females	0 Females
Severe lactic acidemia	Moderate lactic acidemia	Mild lactic acidemia	Mild CHO-sensitive lactic acidemia
7 with cystic lesions in cerebral hemispheres or cerebral atrophy	5 with autopsy-proven Leigh's disease	16 with cortical atrophy and ventricular enlargement	No neuropathology or slow development of lesions in the basal ganglia
2 with cystic lesions in basal ganglia	2 with cerebral atrophy and cysts	5 with hypodensities in basal ganglia by CT scanning	

cases in the neonatal group that came to autopsy, seven also had cystic lesions in the cerebral hemispheres and cerebral atrophy,[43,44] and four had agenesis of the corpus callosum. Two of these children in the neonatal group had cystic lesions in the basal ganglia. In the psychomotor retarded group still living, there was a 2:1 preponderance of females in 21 cases.[44] Sixteen of these had cortical atrophy and ventricular enlargement, while five had hypodensities in the basal ganglia as seen by MRI or CT. The two groups with psychomotor retardation tended to have higher residual PDHC in fibroblasts, 21.9 percent and 27.9 percent, respectively, for the two groups, but overall there was not good correlation between residual activity and survival.[44,56,57]

The final group of patients has a milder form of the disease in which there was either chronic or episodic ataxia.[58–62] Often the ataxia or ataxic episodes are carbohydrate-induced and these children do well on ketogenic diets.[60,61] These patients, who are all males, have blood lactates that are not greatly elevated.[44] Some of them have normal IQ, while others are mentally retarded to varying extents. In many cases, including all those with normal IQ, development is normal and no neuropathology is detectable. In others, there is a slow development of lesions in the brain stem typical of Leigh disease. Leigh disease is a neurodegenerative disease in which bilateral symmetric foci of necrosis, spongiform degeneration, vascular proliferation, and gliosis occur in the thalami, midbrain, pons, medulla, and spinal cord. The mammillary bodies are spared. Brown et al.[57,63] proposed that the condition of the patients not suffering from a systemic acidosis might be referred to as "cerebral" lactic acidosis because the CSF lactate in these patients is usually higher than the blood lactate. This presumably would encompass all the patients outside of the neonatal lactic acidosis patients. In fact, because the pyruvate dehydrogenase complex activity is a rate-limiting step in the aerobic oxidation of glucose by the brain, any deficiency is likely to create an increased CSF lactic acid level over that in the blood.[64] We calculated that there is enough PDH in the human brain to oxidize 180 g of glucose per day when fully activated. Because the actual rate of glucose oxidation by the brain is 125 g per day, there is little reserve capacity in the system to counteract any genetic deficiency.[64]

Facial dysmorphism is a feature in about 35 percent of cases of pyruvate dehydrogenase complex deficiency,[43,63,64] and its features resemble those of fetal alcohol syndrome. Typically, this facial appearance is one of a narrowed head with frontal bossing, wide nasal bridge, an upturned nose, long philtrum, and flared nostrils.[43,63–67] We have suggested that the reason for this parallel between fetal alcohol syndrome dysmorphism and the dysmorphism found in patients with PDH-complex deficiency may be that a common mechanism is involved. In fetal alcohol syndrome, acetaldehyde from the maternal circulation inhibits pyruvate dehydrogenase in the fetus, thus causing malformation. In PDH-complex deficiency, the endogenous low activity of the complex in the fetus causes the same facial malformations.[43]

Partial or total agenesis of the corpus callosum also is a feature of some cases of PDH-complex deficiency, the incidence being particularly high in the neonatal group.[43,44,64,66] This also has a parallel to chronic alcoholism in the Marchiafava-Bignami syndrome, a condition that develops after years of alcohol abuse in which there is a thinning or degeneration of the corpus callosum.[68]

The damage sustained in thiamine deficiency (Wernicke encephalopathy), and in some cases of PDH-complex deficiency, is located in the areas of the greatest metabolic activity of the brain, the brain stem, and basal ganglia.[69] Because Wernicke encephalopathy is invariably associated with alcohol abuse leading to thiamine deficiency, there is probably a reduction in effective PDH-complex activity due to a combination of lack of thiamine pyrophosphate and inhibition by acetaldehyde ($K_i = 50\ \mu M$) (Fig. 100-9).

A partial deficit in PDH complex, in terms of high energy demand, would have to be compensated for by excess glycolysis and excess lactic acid production. Chronic situations arising from this problem may lead to neuronal cell death because of either localized lactic acidosis, or intracellular ATP depletion, or both. Thus, necrotic lesions develop in areas where there is heavy energy demand, or perhaps poor vascularization available to remove the lactic acid produced. Alternatively, neuronal death from this situation may be more generalized, leading to cerebral atrophy and apparent dilation of the ventricles. Several patients with PDH-complex deficiency have shown clinical improvement, or at least have demonstrated more stability on a high fat, low carbohydrate diet which is ketogenic.[43,58,60,61] The provision of ketone bodies as an alternative oxidative substrate to pyruvate for brain mitochondria appears to compensate at least in part for the PDH-complex deficit. Wexler et al.[70] compared groups of patients with the R263G and R378H mutations who had received ketogenic diets at different periods after birth. The earlier the initiation of diet and the greater the carbohydrate restriction, the better was the mental development and longevity. Some patients also seem to benefit from thiamine administration, although, with the exception of one case,[45] the effect does not seem to be due to a direct thiamine or thiamine pyrophosphate dependency of the PDH-complex defect.[43] The response is more likely to result from the elevated levels of thiamine pyrophosphate causing activation of the residual PDH-complex activity.[71] Dichloroacetate administration also has been shown to be useful in patients, especially in an acidotic crisis, again because activation of the residual PDH complex takes place.[72] The variable clinical presentation of patients with similar percentage deficits in the PDH complex is at first sight disconcerting and has led to the expression of difficulty in attempts to make a rational approach to this defect.[56,63,66] The

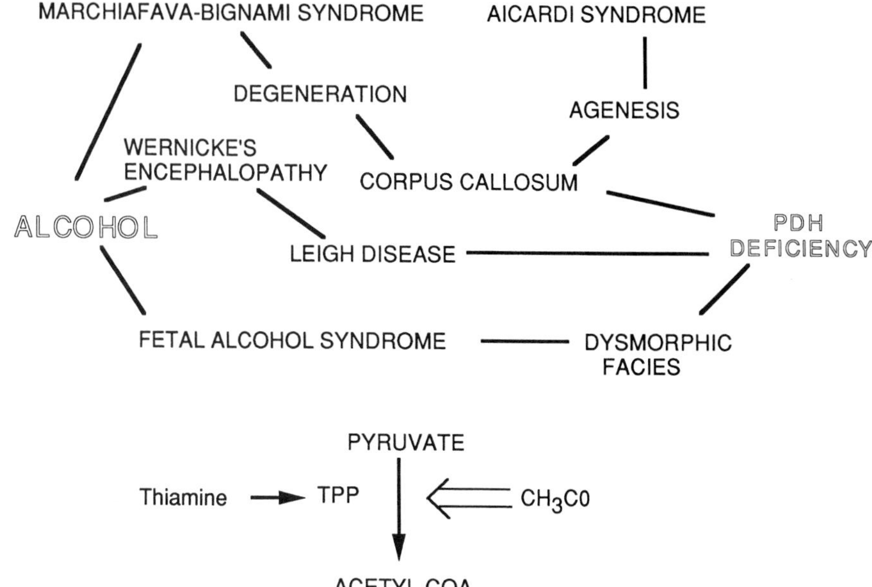

Fig. 100-9 The relationship between defects due to deficiency of the PDH complex and those due to excessive alcohol consumption. Alcohol abuse in adults leads to Wernicke encephalopathy and Marchiafava-Bignami syndrome. It also leads to fetal alcohol syndrome in children of adult female alcohol abusers. The same three areas affected in deficiency of the PDH complex are the corpus callosum, the basal ganglia, and a facial dysmorphic appearance very similar to that seen in fetal alcohol syndrome. The unifying factor is probably acetaldehyde, a potent inhibitor of the PDH complex, which is elevated in chronic alcohol abuse.

basic problem is the lack of correlation of *in vitro* enzymatic data with the clinical spectrum.

PDHC Genes* and Chromosomal Allocation

The isolation of cDNAs for the four PDH-complex catalytic subunits and their chromosomal allocation changed considerably the thinking about the etiology of the clinical spectrum. cDNA isolation for the human PDH-$E_1\alpha$ subunit,[73–77] the $E_1\beta$ subunit,[77–79] the E_2 subunit,[80,81] and the E_3 dihydrolipoyl dehydrogenase have been successful in a number of laboratories. Subsequently, the $E_1\alpha$ subunit was allocated to the X-chromosome at Xp22.1-22.244,[82–84] and the $E_1\beta$ subunit to chromosome 3 at X3p13-q23.[44,79,83] The E_3 lipoamide dehydrogenase was allocated to chromosome 7 at 7q31-q32.[83,85,86] Isolation of cDNAs for the X-protein and allocation to chromosome 11p13 was recently reported.[23–25] A second PDH-$E_1\alpha$ gene, believed to be actively transcribed in testis, was allocated to 4q22.[82]

In terms of gene structure, the $E_1\alpha$ gene consists of 11 exons spanning 17 kb,[87] the $E_1\beta$ gene consists of 10 exons spanning 18 kb,[88] and the E_3 gene consists of 14 exons spanning 20 kb.[89]

The Function of the α and β Subunits of PDH-E_1

Although it has long been known that the E_1 of the mammalian complex acts as a decarboxylase and catalyzes the acetylation of thiamine pyrophosphate, the exact functions of α and β subunits have, until recently, been obscure. It has been pointed out that the α subunit carries the thiamine pyrophosphate-binding motif GDG X26/27 NN[90] common to all TPP-utilizing enzymes. The resolution of the TPP requiring transketolase from yeast at 2.3 Å[91] has recently thrown some light on the likely configurations of the α and β PDH-E_1 subunits. In the transketolase, which is a dimer of a 689 amino acid subunit, the subunits are anteposed in a configuration to bind two TPP molecules.[91] The surprise of this analysis was that the pyrophosphate binding site of the TPP incorporated a lone calcium ion, which implies that all TPP-binding molecules with the GDG X26/27 NN configuration have such a divalent cation enclosed in their operating structure. By aligning an $\alpha\beta$ sequence with the transketolase structure, we observed that in the β subunit of PDH-E_1, there is a motif FMTFNF in an almost identical sequence position to the FFMFYLY hydrophobic pocket of the transketolase that serves to bind the thiazoline ring of thiamine pyrophosphate[92] (Fig. 100-10). The histidine residues 69, 263, and 481 of the transketolase that surround the active site also have their counterparts at His 84 and 263 of α and His 128 of β. Because one of our fatal neonatal cases had an H292L missense mutation (H263L in the mature protein), it is not surprising that there was only 2.5 percent residual activity in the complex, as such a mutation would change the TPP binding site. The conserved residues β I/L 57 and E 59 present in both PDH and branched chain keto acid dehydrogenase β subunits are the counterparts of I416 and E418 in transketolase. They, together with His 481 (128β), are essential to the catalytic mechanism of the PDH-E_1. Perhaps the essentiality of the β subunit residues to the catalytic site accounts for the fact that no patients with β subunit defects have been found.

Thus the overall picture of PDH-E_1 suggests that the $\alpha_2\beta_2$ tetramer is arranged much as are the dimers of transketolase, so that two molecules of TPP are bound per tetramer. This model also provides a clue as to how the phosphorylation of $E_1\alpha$ causes inactivation, because His 263 of $E_1\alpha$, which is involved in the active site, is next to one of the serine phosphorylation sites, serine 264.[92]

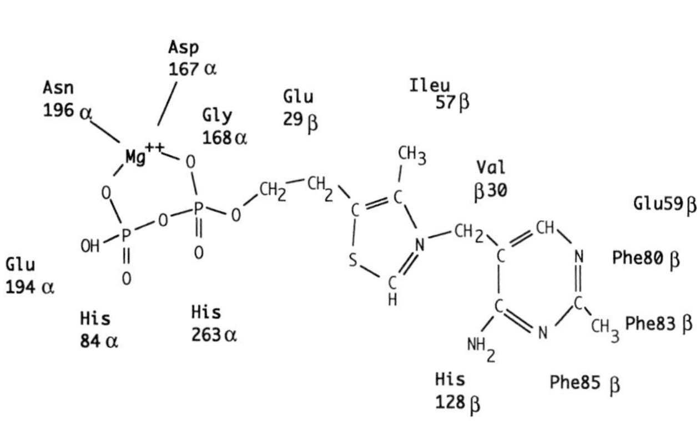

Fig. 100-10 Model of the thiamine pyrophosphate binding site of human pyruvate dehydrogenase E_1. This model is based on sequence alignment of transketolase between human and yeast PDH-E_1,[92] subunits, and the published X-ray crystal structure of transketolase.[91] Residues belonging to the PDH-$E_1\alpha$ subunit are designated α, and residues belonging to the $E_1\beta$ subunit are designated β.

*GenBank accession numbers: PDH-$E_1\alpha$ g1051096; PDH-E_2 g35359; PDH-E_3 g187207; PDH-X (E_3 binding) g297624.

Table 100-2 Observations on the Protein Electrophoresis Mobility of the $E_1\alpha$ Components of the PDH Complex in Patients with PDH-Complex Deficiency

Authors	Classification	Sex	Fibroblast % Activity	Observation on Electrophoresis
MacKay et al.[67]	Neonatal	F	6.7%	Two $E_1\alpha$ bands, one lower M_r
	Psychomotor retardation	F	6.3%	Two $E_1\alpha$ bands, one lower M_r
	Psychomotor retardation	F	18.1%	Two $E_1\alpha$ bands, one lower M_r
Wexler et al.[70]	Ataxia	M	22.8%	No $E_1\alpha$ bands, one lower M_r
	Ataxia	M	18.1%	No $E_1\alpha$ bands, one lower M_r
	Ataxia	M	29.5%	No $E_1\alpha$ protein
	Psychomotor retardation	M	27.9%	No $E_1\alpha$
Kitano et al.[96]	Psychomotor retardation	M	37.3%	2D gels show increased phosphorylated $E_1\alpha$
	Psychomotor retardation	M	38.2%	
Old and DeVivo[93]	Leigh's disease	M	20.2%	$E_1\alpha$ increased M_r
	Ataxia	M	35.5%	$E_1\alpha$ increased M_r
	Neonatal>Sibs	M	14.1%	$E_1\alpha$ decreased protein
	Neonatal>	M	20.4%	$E_1\alpha$ decreased protein
	Psychomotor retardation (Leigh's)	M	16.2%	$E_1\alpha$ decreased protein
Wicking et al.[47]	Neonatal	M	10.2%	No $E_1\alpha$
	Psychomotor retardation	F	40.0%	Increased phosphorylated $E_1\alpha$
Endo et al.[94]	Ataxia, exercise intolerance	M	27.4%	$E_1\alpha$ increased M_r
Robinson et al.[44]	Neonatal	F	2.5%	$E_1\alpha$ normal
Chun et al.[95]	Neonatal	F	3.6%	No $E_1\alpha$
	Neonatal	F	5.5%	No $E_1\alpha$
	Ataxia	M	13.7%	Decreased $E_1\alpha$, two bands one increased M_r
	Psychomotor retardation	F	16.0%	$E_1\alpha$ one band decreased M_r
	Psychomotor retardation	F	20.0%	Reduced $E_1\alpha$

The activity of the PDH complex is expressed as a percentage of the control values given in the reference.

Protein Electrophoretic Abnormalities in PDH-Complex-Deficient Patients

Visualization of the proteins of the PDH complex from deficient patients can be achieved by electrophoresis/immunoprecipitation or electrophoresis/immunoblotting techniques. In patients with PDH-E_1 deficiency, a number of abnormalities have been reported, most of them being associated with the $E_1\alpha$ subunit (Table 100-2). The observations are of four basic types: decreased or absent $E_1\alpha$ protein,[44,47,54,93] increased M_r for $E_1\alpha$,[44,67,93,94] decreased M_r for $E_1\alpha$,[95] and increased amounts of the phosphorylated forms of $E_1\alpha$.[47,96] However, there is no strict linkage between clinical phenotype and the abnormalities seen in the $E_1\alpha$ protein. When the $E_1\alpha$ is decreased, the $E_1\beta$ is always decreased proportionately by the same amount, suggesting that neither $E_1\alpha$ nor $E_1\beta$ subunits can have a prolonged separate existence without each other. At the same time, however, E_2, X, and E_3 proteins appear to be quite normal in the absence of $E_1\alpha$ and $E_1\beta$. Absent $E_1\alpha$ and $E_1\beta$ have been observed in males and females with fatal neonatal lactic acidosis[44,47] and in males with psychomotor retardation and ataxia.[54]

PDH-Complex $E_1\alpha$ Defects and the Effects of Lyonization

Unequivocal allocation of the $E_1\alpha$ gene to the X chromosome coupled with the protein electrophoresis data above strongly suggested that this gene was responsible for the majority of the PDH-complex E_1 deficiency cases. However, because in large surveys of PDH-complex E_1 deficiency[43,44,64] there were equal numbers of males and females affected with the disease, the $E_1\alpha$ defects were designated "X-linked dominant" in genetic terminology. Two observations added credibility to the notion that the $E_1\alpha$ gene was responsible for PDH-E_1 deficiency. First, it was shown by Brown et al.[82] that in a female with PDH-E_1 deficiency, the fibroblast cell culture was a mosaic for the expression of the $E_1\alpha$ protein. Second, it was demonstrated by the same group,[97] using the DXS255 probe for X-inactivation,[98] that in the tissues of this patient, the enzyme activity of the PDH complex and the immunochemically detectable $E_1\alpha$ protein level was directly related to the extent of methylation of the DXS255 site. In this particular case, the female inherited one X chromosome from her father, which chromosome had a normal $E_1\alpha$ gene and an X chromosome from her mother that contained a germ line mutation (GTTAC duplication at nucleotide 903).[99] Random inactivation in different tissues gave rise to low expression of normal protein in kidney and fibroblasts, but close to the expected 50 percent in brain and liver.[97] Despite extensive searches in patients with PDH-E_1 deficiency, no defects have been observed in the $E_1\beta$ gene. Thus the explanation for the equal numbers of affected males and females in this X-linked disease lies with the phenomenon of X inactivation working on a gene coding for a catalytic component of an enzyme that is rate limiting for carbohydrate metabolism in human brain.

Mutations Present in the $E_1\alpha$ Coding Sequence

There are more than 50 families in which the mutation in the $E_1\alpha$ coding sequence has been characterized at the molecular level, 38 of which involve missense mutations and the rest various DNA rearrangements (see URL on HSC Web site at www.sickkids.on.-ca). The majority of the mutations so far discovered are located in the latter half of the coding sequence, in exons 5 to 11. This region of the $E_1\alpha$ protein has a number of features that are important to the functioning of the PDH complex as a whole. The region from aa 130 to 150 is believed to play a part in the binding of pyruvate,[100] that from 195 to 226 has the consensus configuration for a TPP binding site that is found in all TPP-binding proteins,[90] and the region from 231 to 291 contains the serine phosphorylation sites that modulate the activity of the whole complex. Serine residues at positions 293, 300, and 232 of the protein (264, 271, and 203 of the mature protein) are designated as phosphorylation sites 1, 2, and 3, respectively.[18,19] Although there is still disagreement over which of these sites is the most important for inactivation, it seems that there is agreement that once one site is phosphorylated the enzymatic activity of the complex is severely curtailed.[19] The region between the TPP binding site and the phosphorylation sites, residues 249 to 289, is thought to be an important area in the mutual binding of α and β subunits.[101]

As predicted from the consideration of X inactivation of the $E_1\alpha$ gene, the females with PDH-E_1 deficiency have one normal $E_1\alpha$ gene and one bearing a mutation (refer to the HSC Web site at www.sickkids.on.ca). Deletions and insertions accounted for 21 females:11 males while missense/nonsense mutations accounted for 14 females:27 males giving a final ratio of 35 females:38 males in this table. A valine to methionine mutation in the segment that is believed to be involved in pyruvate binding resulted in extremely low activity in the fibroblasts of two sisters who survived to 10 and 11 years of age but with psychomotor retardation.[100] Mutations in the TPP binding zone A198T and F205L produced rather different effects in two males,[99,100] the former producing a slow neurodegeneration and ataxia leading to Leigh disease at the age of 5 years. The latter patient had quite severe lactic acidosis and died at 18 months despite having a higher residual activity (65 percent) in fibroblasts. A threonine for alanine substitution at 231 in front of site 3 for serine phosphorylation at 232, resulted in activity of 1.7 percent in the fibroblasts of a male who died at 7 days of neonatal lactic acidosis.[100] Another mutation, H292L, occurs directly in front of the serine phosphorylation site 1 at 293 giving residual PDH-complex activity of 2.5 percent in a female. This histidine residue is conserved in both the branched chain keto-acid dehydrogenase $E_1\alpha$ and the pyruvate dehydrogenase $E_1\alpha$ in species from bacteria to man,[101] and is quite likely catalytically active. There are 10 patients from 7 families with mutations involving the R263 codon, 8 with R263G and 2 with R263Q. Male patients reported by a number of investigators with the R263G mutation showed symptoms of variable presentation, with ataxia, mild mental retardation, and development of basal ganglia lesions, initially in the caudate and putamen.[100–106] The onset of more severe symptoms associated with Leigh disease was variable. Some were not diagnosed until 8 or 9 years of age. In five of the seven families with R263G, the mother was a carrier — in three instances asymptomatic, but in two instances, with mental retardation or epilepsy. In two families, the mother had siblings with neonatal fatalities. The R263Q mutation also produces Leigh disease, and in one family the mother was a carrier.[107] An R302C mutation has been reported in four females from three families with 10 to 50 percent residual activity of the PDH complex.[106,108,109] These patients had seizures and cerebral atrophy. The mother of one of these individuals, who carried the mutation, had normal PDH-complex activity in fibroblasts; she was mildly mentally retarded and suffered from epilepsy.[110] In another family, the R20P mutation in the leader sequence, which affects the mitochondrial import of the protein and causes Leigh disease, also showed a carrier mother.[111] Finally, an R378H mutation was found in separate males who died at 13 and 18 months with brain atrophy;[110,112] this residue is close to the N-terminus of the sequence.

Deletions and Insertions

All the deletions and insertions found in the $E_1\alpha$ gene so far occur in exons 10 and 11. An insertion of GTTAC at 903 was found in a female who died at 4 weeks of age after suffering from a combination of lactic acidosis and hyperammonemia;[113] this insertion created a GTTAC repeat. In the middle of a GAAGAA repeat at 915 a 21-bp insertion was found again in a male who died at 17 days of age of lactic acidosis.[114] Unlike the first patient whose mutation produced a shortened $E_1\alpha$ protein, the predicted protein length in this case is +7 amino acids. A 7-bp deletion at 927 has been reported twice from separate families. Both cases were females, one dying at 1 month of age with 25 to 30 percent residual activity,[99,115] and the other dying at 3 years of age with 18 percent activity.[99] Enlarged ventricles and agenesis of the corpus callosum were featured in both patients. This 7-bp deletion occurred within an AGTAAGA tandem repeat sequence and would produce a shortened $E_1\alpha$ protein. A deletion of GAA within this same repeat at nucleotide 937 was found in a female who died at 17 years after prolonged psychomotor retardation from birth.[110] This simply deletes lysine 284 from the $E_1\alpha$ sequence. Deletion of a TA within a TATTAT tandem repeat at 948 produced lactic acidosis and death at 7 days in an affected female with only 1.3 percent residual activity of the PDH complex.[99] A 20-bp deletion at nucleotide 1072 in a female with 16.4 percent residual activity produced psychomotor retardation, seizures, optic atrophy, and death at 3.5 years.[99,115] While this mutation again produced a shortened protein, a female with a TT insertion at 1126 is predicted to produce an $E_1\alpha$ protein extended by 35 amino acids.[99] This child is alive at 5 years with psychomotor retardation, blindness, and agenesis of the corpus callosum. ATCA insertions at 1154 have been observed in two nonrelated females with fibroblast PDH-complex activity of 6.372 and 16.7 percent of normal, respectively.[94] They died at 2 and 1 years of age, were psychomotor retarded, and had dilated ventricles. Within the next to last codon, a CAGT deletion within a tandem repeat at 1167 produces an extended $E_1\alpha$ protein of +33 amino acids.[77] Remarkably, this male had only exercise intolerance,[77] although his reported PDH-complex activity in fibroblasts was 24.6 percent.

A number of males with insertions in the last exon have survived quite well — one is now 33 years old with a university degree.[116] Four-bp insertions at 1154 in three female patients was fatal before 2 years of age, while a 4-bp insertion at 1163 in two males produced ataxia and mental retardation.[100,103]

Thus, the X-linked dominant nature of the PDH-E_1 deficiency can be explained by $E_1\alpha$ mutations carried on one X-chromosome of the affected females being expressed as mutant protein. In cells where the normal gene for $E_1\alpha$ is turned off by X inactivation in these individuals, the mutant protein is exclusively expressed, giving rise to a totally or partially blocked entry of pyruvate into the citric acid cycle. Lactate and pyruvate produced in the adversely affected cells may diffuse into neighboring cells whose normal X-$E_1\alpha$ gene has escaped inactivation and may there be oxidized, but this is an inefficient process that may result in the death of cells bearing the inactivated normal gene. This may account for the cortical atrophy so prominent in surviving females. In the affected males, the defects in a single $E_1\alpha$ gene generally seem to allow for some residual activity. In both females and males, the mutations seen so far have been extremely heterogenous confirming the observations on PDH-complex activity and protein electrophoretic mobility.[193–206] This is a good example of the molecular basis of dominance exerted through flux control as proposed by Kacser and Burns in 1981.[117]

CORRELATION BETWEEN $E_1\alpha$ MUTATION, ACTIVITY IN FIBROBLASTS, AND CLINICAL PRESENTATIONS

The new insight that molecular genetics has cast on the subject of PDH-E_1 deficiency, is enabling us to begin resolving some of the associated thorny problems. Knowing about the X linkage of the $E_1\alpha$ has allowed us to put into perspective the equal number of females with PDH-E_1 deficiency. Affected females have one normal $E_1\alpha$ gene and one that carries the mutation, but even random lyonization, giving 50 percent overall activity, where the mutant allele gives no activity may produce an adversely affected individual. In the central nervous system, it is likely that such affected females will lose cells that have low viability because they express a null allele. With affected males, the situation is not quite as clear. Here the activity in skin fibroblasts of the PDH complex might be expected to represent that found in the brain, the organ where most pathology is experienced. For instance, we had two males, one with 1.6 percent residual activity and the other with 10 percent activity (refer to the HSC Web site www.sickkids.on.ca) who died of neonatal lactic acidosis. On the other hand, we have two surviving males with ataxia at 17 percent and 39 percent, while we had one with 30 percent who died at 13 months with psychomotor retardation and brain atrophy. Another male at 27 percent residual activity of the PDH complex merely suffered from exercise intolerance. Clearly some of these activities show little correlation between clinical phenotype and residual activity. In an affected male, we documented activities of 0.8, 4.5, 5.2, 13.2, 18.8, and 22.4 percent of normal activity of the PDH complex for kidney, liver, brain, heart, skeletal muscle, and skin fibroblasts, respectively. As we accumulate data, we begin to see that there is a differential turnover of the PDH complex in different tissues, which accounts for much of the loss of activity.[116] In some males with defects affecting the C-terminus, the CRM+ve material correlates with residual activity, suggesting that if the complex could be stabilized in such cases, it would have close to normal activity. Clearly there is much to learn about the expression of normal and mutant forms of the $E_1\alpha$ protein in tissues.

Defects in the E_2 (OMIM *245348) and X (OMIM *245349) Components of the Pyruvate Dehydrogenase Complex

Seven patients have been described in whom there is good evidence of a defect in protein X or the E_2 dihydrolipoyl transacetylase. In a patient with 24 percent PDH complex residual activity, who presented at 2 weeks of age with hyperammonemia and lactic acidosis, and who eventually died at 3.5 years of age with profound psychomotor retardation, there was only 32 percent of measurable transacetylase while E_1 and E_3 activities were normal.[118] This patient had a normal amount of $E_1\alpha$, $E_1\alpha$, and E_3 proteins, absent E_2, and reduced amounts of protein X. Six patients with an absent protein X on fibroblast Western blots have been described.[23,118–121] These patients had residual PDH complex activities of 12 to 20 percent in skin fibroblasts, and presented with psychomotor retardation usually accompanied by Leigh disease and development of spastic quadriplegia.[23,118–121] Three of these patients were shown to possess homozygous deletions of 4 bp, 59 bp, and 85 bp, respectively, in the cDNA for X-protein.[23,24] These results support the observations that in the bovine PDH complex, when the X protein is removed, only 15 percent residual activity is retained.[123] Further evidence defines a definitive role for the X protein in the binding of the E_3 subunit to the complex.[25,123]

A male born to nonconsanguineous Japanese parents presented at 3 years of age with an ataxic gait but normal mental development. By 5.5 years of age he was significantly worse with loss of fine and gross motor coordination and lesions observable in the putamen and basal ganglia. His lactic acid was elevated between 2.5 and 9 mM, although his residual fibroblast activity was 55 percent.[118] An extra band just below protein X was consistently observed in immunoblots of his skin fibroblasts with anti-PDH antibody; E_2, E_3, $E\alpha$, and $E\beta$ seemed to be present in normal amounts. It was concluded that this extra band was a mutant form of protein X, but subsequent analysis showed it to be an E_2 band.

Lipoamide Dehydrogenase Deficiency (OMIM *246900): Combined α-Keto Acid Dehydrogenase Complex Deficiency

Combined deficiency of the α-keto acid dehydrogenase complexes is a comparatively rare entity, there being few well-documented cases in the world literature.[124–129,134–136,194] Surprisingly, none of the affected children presented at birth, but they developed lactic acidemia that became troublesome at a few months of age. Because the data indicate that the α-keto acid dehydrogenase complexes include only the E_3 component in common,[27] it is appropriate that the E_3 component, otherwise known as lipoamide dehydrogenase, be deficient in most cases of the combined defect. That all complexes are deficient is consistent with the observation of elevated pyruvate, lactate, α-ketoglutarate, and branched chain amino acids levels in blood samples from these patients.[124,125,127,129] The branched chain amino acids are not elevated to the extent seen in classic maple syrup urine disease. Urine organic acids typically show elevated lactate, pyruvate, α-hydroxybutyrate, α-hydroxyisovalerate, and α-ketoglutarate.[126,127,130] In one case, α-ketoisocaproic acid was present in addition to these other acids.[129] When postmortem examination of the brain was carried out,[124–126] myelin loss and cavitation were found in discrete areas of the basal ganglia, thalamus, and brain stem; the cerebral cortex appeared to be free of pathology.

The diagnosis was made initially by measuring activity of the α-keto acid dehydrogenase complexes in tissues or in fibroblasts.[124–126] In seven of nine known cases, the combined defect in the complexes is definitely the result of a defect in lipoamide dehydrogenase,[124–126,128,134–136] which was between 0 and 20 percent of the activity found in controls. In another two cases, despite the α-keto acid dehydrogenases being deficient to the extent of 25 percent of normal, lipoamide dehydrogenase activity was 59 and 63 percent of normal.[127,131] This anomalous situation could be explained if it is postulated that the abnormal protein can carry out the lipoamide dehydrogenase reaction, but the ability of these E_3 proteins to interact with the E_2 transacetylases is affected by the mutation.[127]

Hinman et al.[132] described two patients who died of Leigh disease in which abnormalities were described in the ability of their lipoamide dehydrogenase to restore activity to E_3-depleted PDH-complex preparations. The fibroblasts from these patients had 60 percent of normal PDH complex, even when activated with dichloroacetate.[132] Two mutations in the lipoamide dehydrogenase cDNA, K37E and P453L, were described in a patient with 6 percent E_3 activity but 10 to 30 percent of PDH-complex activity, who died after a ketoacidotic episode at 12 months of age.[133] Two further patients were characterized at the molecular level by the same group. A patient who had a combination of A1173G/del455-457 died at 5 years with microcephaly and psychomotor retardation. Enzyme activity for lipoamide dehydrogenase was 3 percent and PDH complex was 31 percent in fibroblasts.[134] A second patient who died at 28 months with delayed development, hypotonia, and Leigh disease had a combination of insA105/G1533A resulting in one transcript with R460G and one null allele due to the frameshift in the mitochondrial leader sequence.[135] A milder version of the disease has been described with normal cognitive function but some motor impairment at 5 years of age.[136] InsA105 has also been described in two patients with a similar presentation.[137] A patient with prominent hepatocellular disease was also described by the same group with 12 percent residual lipoamide dehydrogenase activity and normal cognitive function.[138]

Pyruvate Dehydrogenase Phosphatase Deficiency

In a small number of cases with congenital lactic acidemia, a defect was demonstrated in the enzyme which activated the PDH complex by removing phosphate groups from $E_1\alpha$ serine residues. Three cases, two reported by Sorbi and Blass[139] and one by De Vivo et al.,[140] had a clinical picture typical of Leigh disease, while a fourth patient described by Robinson and Sherwood[141] died at age 6 months after a course of unremitting lactic acidosis. Two of the cases[140] showed poor reactivation of the PDH complex after inactivation by incubation with ATP in postmortem tissues. The other cases[139] showed a normal activity of the complex in fibroblasts in the native state, but no activation could be demonstrated after incubation of the fibroblasts with dichloroacetate. None of the methods used in these studies was a direct assay of the activity of pyruvate dehydrogenase phosphatase activity. A method was described by Wicking et al.[48] for measuring PDH phosphatase activity in fibroblast by the release of ^{32}P from added ^{32}P-labeled PDH phosphate. This is a more direct method of measurement that should be capable of detecting abnormal activity of this enzyme.

Pyruvate Carboxylase†

Enzymology. Pyruvate carboxylase is a biotin-containing protein of subunit molecular weight $Mr = 125{,}000$, each active enzyme molecule consisting of four tightly bound identical subunits. Each

†GenBank accession number PC g458235.

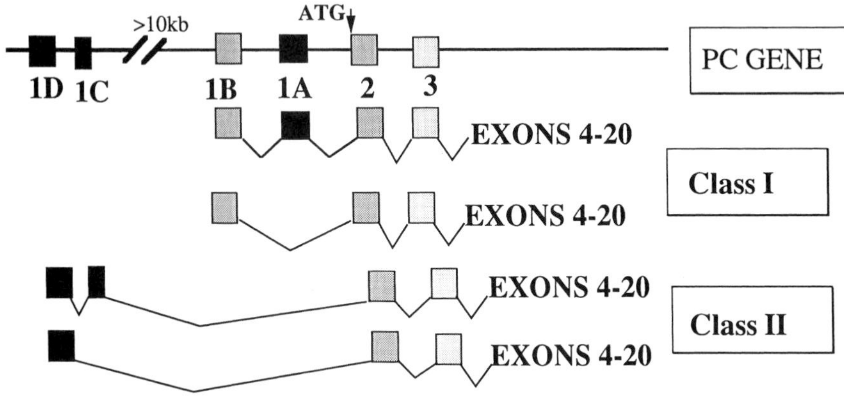

Fig. 100-11 The generation of alternative transcripts from the pyruvate carboxylase gene. Two types of transcript are generated: Class I starting at exon 1D and Class II starting at 1B in a tissue-specific fashion.

subunit has one molecule of covalently bound biotin and possesses binding sites for pyruvate, ATP, HCO_3, and acetyl CoA.[142–144] The enzyme is almost totally dependent on the presence of acetyl CoA as an allosteric activator for activity. As the first enzyme in the gluconeogenic pathway, it is activated in conditions where fatty acids are mobilized and acetyl-CoA is generated.[145]

Pyruvate carboxylase is widely viewed as the major regulatory enzyme and the flux-generating step in the pathway of gluconeogenesis,[145] being regulated by the relative acetyl-CoA/CoA and ATP/ADP ratios in liver mitochondria.[146] This enzyme is always intramitochondrial and has its highest activity in liver and kidney, where its role in gluconeogenesis is important. It is found in lesser amounts in other tissues such as brain, muscle, adipocytes, and fibroblasts where its function is believed to be anaplerotic.[147–149] In these tissues, it plays a role in the maintenance of 4-carbon intermediates in the citric acid cycle.[150]

The full-length cDNA has now been elucidated for both the yeast[151] and mammalian[152,153] pyruvate carboxylase. The partial human gene has been mapped to the long arm of chromosome 11 at 11q13[154], and the coding region of the human gene consists of 19 exons covering 16 kb of sequence.[156] The rat gene structure has been elucidated and found to have 19 exons in the coding sequence, with two alternative 5′ untranslated sequences in front of the initial ATG. The two alternative 5′UTRs are generated from different promoters in such a way that heavy expression of PC takes place in liver and kidney, while a lower level of expression is maintained in other tissues[157] (Fig. 100-11).

Human Deficiency (OMIM 266150). The known instability of pyruvate carboxylase in suboptimal conditions of preservation and storage plagued the early attempts to define the nature of human pyruvate carboxylase deficiency.[155] Many reports were based on measurements of enzyme activity in liver biopsy or postmortem liver specimens, and although some of these cases were undoubtedly bona fide cases of pyruvate carboxylase deficiency, some almost certainly were not. Early reports associated pyruvate carboxylase deficiency with subacute necrotizing encephalomyelopathy (Leigh disease).[158] In a series of nine patients with Leigh disease, skin fibroblast pyruvate carboxylase was examined and found to be normal.[158] In five patients, the diagnosis of Leigh disease was confirmed at autopsy, and in eight the urine inhibitor of thiamine triphosphate synthesis was present. Hommes et al.[155] reviewed a number of cases where diagnosis of pyruvate carboxylase deficiency was made on liver tissue obtained by biopsy or at postmortem. The majority of these determinations are reported as single measurements and many of them have low or undetectable activity. In one case,[159] detailed measurements of the kinetics of pyruvate carboxylase activity were made; it was found that a low K_m component of the enzyme was missing. In the partially purified human enzyme, there are two kinetic components, one with a low K^m and one with a high K^m for pyruvate.[144] This type of defect is difficult to test for and may not be detected in single-measurement assay systems for enzyme activity.

The demonstration that pyruvate carboxylase activity could be measured in cultured skin fibroblasts led to the accurate definition of the clinical sequelae of pyruvate carboxylase deficiency.[148,149,160] There appear to be three distinct groups of patients who have been identified using the highly reproducible cultured skin fibroblast assay (Table 100-3). This initially became evident because the patients presenting with pyruvate carboxylase deficiency in North America (Group A) had a simple presentation of lactic acidemia and psychomotor retardation,[161,162] while the patients presenting in France and the United Kingdom (Group B) had a more complex biochemical presentation with lactic acidemia, hyperammonemia, citrullinemia, and hyperlysinemia.[161,163–165] Those in Group B all presented in the neonatal period and died before 3 months of age as compared with the longer survival of Group A. Group B patients also demonstrated a redox disturbance, the cytosolic compartment being more reduced, as evidenced from an increased ratio of blood lactate to pyruvate, and the mitochondrial compartment being more oxidized, as judged by a higher ratio of blood acetoacetate to β-hydroxybutyrate. In later reports, there are some Group A patients who have a blood lactate to pyruvate ratio above the normal range. Both Group A and Group B patients exhibit hyperalaninemia and hyperprolinemia and have less than 5 percent pyruvate carboxylase activity in their fibroblasts as compared to controls.[160–173] Proximal renal tubular acidosis was present in 3 Group A cases, and 12 of 18 Group A cases were full-blooded North American Indian children, 8 were from either the Manitoba or Ontario Ojibwa, 2 were from the Saskatchewan Cree, and 2 were from the Micmac in Nova Scotia.[174] The one unifying factor about these tribal communities is that they belong to the same linguistic group of Algonquian-speaking Indians.[174] Thus, there was strong epidemiologic and anthropologic evidence for a founder effect in relation to pyruvate carboxylase deficiency in these Amerindian populations.

A third distinct variety of pyruvate carboxylase deficiency was described by Van Coster et al.[175] This child frequently presented with metabolic acidosis as an infant, but between these episodes seemed to be well. Her skin fibroblast pyruvate carboxylase level

Table 100-3 The Presentation of Human Pyruvate Carboxylase (PC) Deficiency

	Group A (18 Cases)	Group B (11 Cases)	Group C
Origin	12 Amerindian, 1 Canadian with Italian parents, 4 U.S. Caucasian, 1 Japanese	2 Canadian (1 with Egyptian parents), 4 French, 2 U.K., 1 West German, 1 Saudi Arabian, 1 Swede	1 U.S. Caucasian
Presentation	Metabolic acidosis Delayed neurologic development	Metabolic acidosis Hepatomegaly	Acute metabolic acidosis
Age of presentation	Birth to 5 months	Neonatal	14 months
Survival	2 survive to 5 years; severe mental retardation	All dead within 3 months	7 years survival with normal development
Biochemical	α-Ketoglutarate in urine Lactic acidosis mild with severe attacks on infection	α-Ketoglutarate in urine Lactic acidosis chronically severe	α-Ketoglutarate in urine
Pyruvate carboxylase activity	$<5\%$ control	$<5\%$ control	$<5\%$ control
Lactate/pyruvate ratio	Normal	Elevated (x5)	—
Acetoacetate/3HOB ratio	Normal?	Elevated (x5)	—
Blood ammonia	Normal	Elevated (x5)	Normal
Alanine	Elevated	Elevated	Elevated
Citrulline	Normal	Elevated (x5)	Normal
Lysine	Normal	Elevated	Elevated
Proline	Elevated	Elevated	Elevated
PC[^{3}H] biotin protein (125 kDa)	Present	Absent in 6/10 cases	—
PC immunoreactive protein	Present	Absent in 6/10 cases	Yes
PC mRNA	Present	Absent in 4/10 cases	Present
	Refs. 159–165 +5 unpublished cases*	Refs. 167–172 +3 unpublished cases*	Ref. 174

Studied by the author (BHR).

was measured at 1.8 percent of control values, which could account for her increased levels of blood lactate. Although many of her blood parameters were the same as the Group A cases of pyruvate carboxylase deficiency, she developed normally and did not become psychomotor retarded. At 7 years she may have a learning deficit in mathematics and slight dysarthria but is otherwise healthy. She is a large child (>95 percentile) for height and weight, who is treated with oral fluids and bicarbonate at the onset of febrile illness.[175]

The biotin-containing enzymes present in cultured skin fibroblasts can be visualized either by [^{3}H]biotin labeling (Fig. 100-12) or by [^{35}S]streptavidin blotting. In both cases, the cell proteins are separated by sodium dodecylsulfate (SDS) polyacrylamide gel electrophoresis.[163,164,166] When this was done with

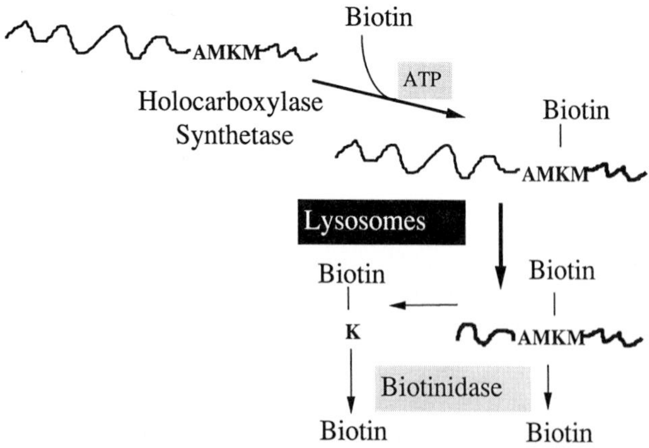

Fig. 100-12 Incorporation of biotin into carboxylase protein. The mRNA for carboxylase produces a translated apocarboxylase, which must incorporate activated biotin in the form of biotinyl-AMP with the release of 5′ AMP. The resulting holocarboxylase protein has biotin covalently attached at a lysine residue.

fibroblasts from patients with pyruvate carboxylase deficiency, it was found that the patients with Group A or C presentation showed the same 125-kDa band corresponding to the subunit of pyruvate carboxylase. However, many of the patients in Group B showed no band for pyruvate carboxylase, but did show normal bands for the α subunit of propionyl CoA carboxylase (73 kDa) and the α subunit of methyl crotonyl CoA carboxylase (75 kDa).[161,164] Immunoprecipitation of labeled protein from cells preincubated with [^{35}S]methionine also showed absence of the 125-kDa protein in some of the Group B patients when antipyruvate carboxylase antiserum was used.[161,164] Finally, Northern blotting with a cloned cDNA probe for pyruvate carboxylase showed absent mRNA in four of six Group B patients who lacked a demonstrable pyruvate carboxylase protein.[164]

In trying to correlate the biochemical symptoms of those patients with the physical and molecular facts about pyruvate carboxylase that arise from the study of the patient's skin fibroblasts, it is evident that in patient Groups A and C, all patients produce a biotin-containing 125-kDa pyruvate carboxylase protein that has little activity. In Group B, there are two groups of patients who are different in molecular terms: those who produce a 125-kDa biotin-containing pyruvate carboxylase protein and those who do not. However, all Group B patients are more severely affected, with death in infancy, and they have a complex biochemical disturbance affecting pyruvate metabolism, the urea cycle, and intracellular redox states.[174] What then determines whether pyruvate carboxylase deficiency presents with the simple phenotype of lactic acidemia or with the complex phenotype of lactic acidemia, citrullinemia, and hyperammonemia? Because we know that the pyruvate carboxylase gene is not expressed in all cases in which the presentation is the complex Group B phenotype, we can associate this phenotype with total absence of activity. Thus, we can hypothesize that the other patients in Group B who have expression of pyruvate carboxylase protein must also have total absence of activity to attain this phenotype. Where there is expression of the enzyme with the milder Groups A and C phenotypes, we must assume that there is enough residual activity

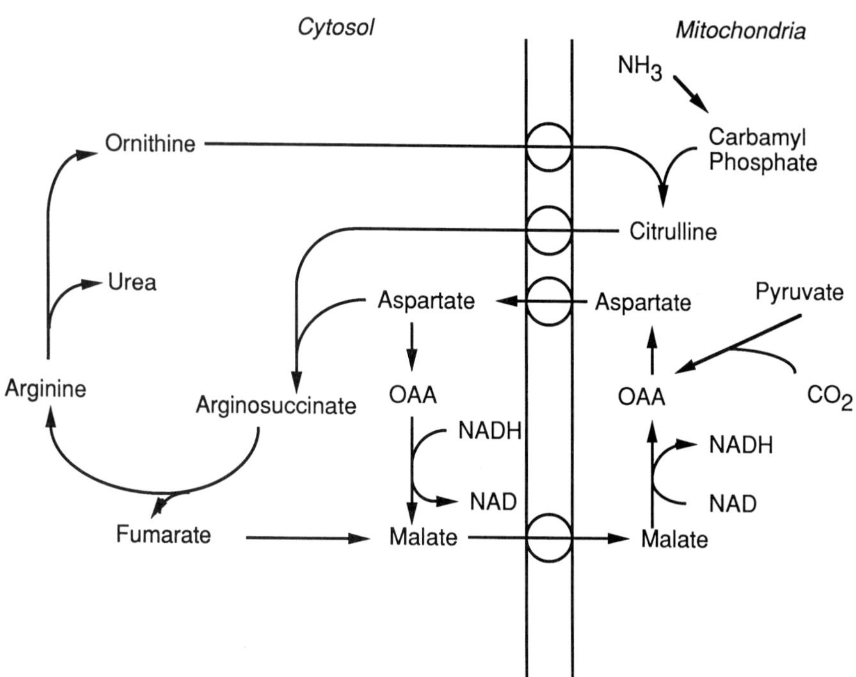

Fig. 100-13 The role of pyruvate carboxylase in the generation of aspartate for use in the urea cycle and the reoxidation of NADH. See text for explanation.

in the mutant pyruvate carboxylase to ameliorate the most severe symptoms of the deficiency, but in the case of Group A, not enough to prevent lactic acidemia and psychomotor retardation.

That all patients with pyruvate carboxylase deficiency develop lactic acidemia is almost certainly due to a failure of the Cori cycle and, in times of starvation, also to a failure of gluconeogenesis itself. Patients in both groups have been documented with hypoglycemic episodes, although this is not a major problem.[164] The Group B patients with the complex presentation show features that are suggestive of depletion of intracellular aspartate and oxaloacetate.[168–170] In the urea cycle, aspartate is the second nitrogen donor, and low levels would cause the accumulation of both citrulline and ammonia (Fig. 100-13). Aspartate is also an essential component of the shuttle system that is responsible for the transport of reducing equivalents from the cytosol to the mitochondria.[176] Electrogenic ejection of aspartate from mitochondria is necessary to maintain the typically very oxidized NAD^+/NADH ratio in the cytosol as opposed to the very reduced NAD>$^+$/NADH ratio in the mitochondrial compartment. A lack of aspartate would result in the cytosol being more reduced and the mitochondria being more oxidized, exactly the situation seen in the Group B patients with the complex phenotype. Thus, it would seem that pyruvate carboxylase activity in the Group B patients is so low that it cannot sustain oxaloacetate and aspartate levels. The few tissue measurements of pyruvate carboxylase activity that have been done in liver have yielded 6.2, 17.2, and 0.0 percent of control values for three Group A patients and 0.3 and 0.3 percent for two Group B patients.[149,158,160,168]

Pathology. The pathology of pyruvate carboxylase deficiency has been documented in one Group A and two Group B cases, and is primarily present in liver and brain. Hepatomegaly, which is seen frequently in this defect, seems to be due to lipid droplet accumulation in hepatocytes.[148,158,160,174] In one Group A case, hyperplasia of hepatocyte endoplasmic reticulum was seen,[148] and the architecture of liver mitochondria had an abnormal appearance with increased matrix density, increased matrix granule size, and dilatation of intracrystal space.[173] The central nervous system pathology common to both Group A and B patients consists of very poor myelination and paucity of neurons in the cerebral cortex, gliosis, ventricular enlargement, thinning of the corpus callosum, and proliferation of astrocytes.[149,168,173] In both Group B patients that came to autopsy, there was additional damage in the form of cavitated infarcts or cysts present in the cerebral cortex.[168,173] In one case, microscopic examination of the kidney showed diffuse vacuolation of the kidney tubules.[148] The appearance of cerebral cortex in pyruvate carboxylase deficiency suggests that myelination is not taking place, that neuronal death is occurring, and that a virtual developmental arrest of the brain is the net result. Thus, pyruvate carboxylase is obviously essential for normal brain development, and this is related to its anaplerotic role in metabolism. It has been documented that pyruvate carboxylase activity is plentiful in astrocytes but is low or absent in neurons.[177] Current evidence suggests that neurotransmitter pools are replenished in part by de novo synthesis within the presynaptic terminals and that glutamine derived metabolically from astrocytes appears to be a major metabolic precursor of the transmitter pools for both glutamate and γ-aminobutyric acid (GABA). The anaplerotic formation of glutamine is thought to occur using pyruvate carboxylation as the initial step, and this can only take place in astrocytes. Thus, in an individual lacking pyruvate carboxylase activity, the neurons lose their ability to be replenished with glutamine from astrocytes, and depletion of 4- and 5-carbon intermediates in the neuron may result in neuronal death. To compound this problem, the lack of the anaplerotic function of pyruvate carboxylase in myelin lipid synthesis at the same time leads to poor or absent myelin formation. The absence of these two essential roles of pyruvate carboxylase in the anaplerotic processes of brain metabolism undoubtedly is a major contributor to the pathology seen in the central nervous system in this disorder. Group A children who survive with this defect are grossly mentally retarded and often have accompanying seizure activity. This lack of a key anaplerotic enzyme may also be the cause of abnormalities seen in kidney and of accumulation of lipid in Type 1 skeletal muscle fibers, in addition to the urea cycle and redox abnormalities previously mentioned. Presumably, the patient placed in Group C has enough activity to maintain normal neurologic function.[175]

Mutations Present in the Pyruvate Carboxylase Gene. Investigation of the Amerindian form of pyruvate carboxylase deficiency has shown that in 13 patients tested, a c.1828G$\rightarrow$A missense mutation was homozygous, these individuals all being either Ojibwa or Cree in origin.[156] A c.2229G→T transversion was present in two Micmac brothers, showing that the deficiency in this group was not due to a founding effect.[156] In some communities of the Ojibwa, the carrier rate for this mutation was as high as 1 in 10 individuals.[156] The two mutations caused an Ala to Thr change at residue 610 and a Met to Ile change at residue 743 respectively, both of these being in conserved regions possibly involved in pyruvate binding.[156]

Heterozygote Detection and Prenatal Diagnosis. The activity of pyruvate carboxylase in the cultured skin fibroblasts from normal individuals varies over quite a wide range. For this reason, although it may be possible to identify heterozygotes for this defect within a family, it is not possible to do this in the general population.[162,178] To add to the confusion, there is a report of a patient with a 50 percent deficiency of pyruvate carboxylase in skin fibroblasts, who had severe chronic lactic acidemia.[179] This patient had a kinetic defect in the enzyme that was perhaps similar to a case described earlier.[159] This type of defect awaits a clearer definition in both enzymatic and clinical terms.

Prenatal diagnosis of an affected child with pyruvate carboxylase deficiency was reported on two occasions. Both families had already had a child who died with the Group B complex presentation of the defect.[180,181] In one case, the absence of [^{3}H]biotin-labeled protein was demonstrated in amniocytes.[181]

Phosphoenolpyruvate Carboxykinase Deficiency

A defect in this enzyme is rarely reported as a cause of lactic acidemia in childhood. The enzyme exists in two compartments in two distinct isoenzymic forms, and for this reason, the diagnosis of a suspected deficiency of either one of the two isoenzymes is difficult.

Recently, the human enzyme cDNA sequence was established for both isoforms, which have 78 percent identity at the amino acid level.[182] Three cases of phosphoenolpyruvate carboxykinase (PEPCK) deficiency have been documented in which the assay of activity was carried out with a liver homogenate.[183,184] In another group of cases, the cytosolic PEPCK in liver was measured and found to be deficient[185] (OMIM 261680). In two cases, the defect was defined by measurement of PEPCK in cultured skin fibroblasts.[74,149] Because it has been shown that the majority of PEPCK present in fibroblasts is mitochondrial in origin, the detection of 15 and 16 percent[74,149] of normal activity in these cases was suggestive of deficiency of mitochondrial PEPCK (MIM 261650). This was confirmed by the demonstration of 6 percent of normal activity in the mitochondria from fibroblasts of one patient.[74]

Both of the children described with mitochondrial PEPCK deficiency had lactic acidemia, hypoglycemia, hypotonia, hepatomegaly, and failure to thrive.[72,186,187] One patient had more severe symptoms, and, in addition, had peripheral edema, disordered liver function, and episodes of unexplained pyrexia; she died at age 6 months.[187] The other patient with mitochondrial PEPCK deficiency had survived to age 10 years with some continuing muscular weakness and hypotonia. These latter symptoms are most likely due to a lack of mitochondrial PEPCK in muscle, where it is thought to play an essential role in the regulation of the pool size of 4-carbon intermediates.[150] A later publication described the sib of one of these PEPCK-deficient cases who had the same clinical presentation but normal PEPCK activity in leukocytes and fibroblasts.[188] This obviously makes it unlikely that PEPCK was the primary deficiency in this family.[188]

The cytosolic form of PEPCK is subject to induction and repression, being induced by catabolic states and repressed by anabolic states.[189] There is a strong suggestion in the cases described by Vidnes and Sovik[185] that the hypoglycemia and low cystolic PEPCK seen in this group of neonates was a result of hyperinsulinism, a condition that would repress cytosolic PEPCK expression in the liver. Hepatomegaly and hypoglycemia were present in two infants described by Hommes et al.[184] with 5 and 10 percent of control PEPCK activity. Localization of the site of the PEPCK was not attempted in postmortem liver samples from these children, both having succumbed to uncontrollable hypoglycemic episodes. Interestingly, one of these children had the inexplicable hypertriglyceridemia and hypercholesterolemia that was evident in the child we described.[72,186,187]

THE DIFFERENTIAL DIAGNOSIS OF LACTIC ACIDEMIA

The patient with lactic acidemia presents one of the more difficult diagnostic problems in the area of genetic metabolic diseases. It is important to assemble as much biochemical and pathologic information as possible on the patient, which, together with the clinical signs and symptoms, will help pinpoint the diagnosis. The basic measurements required are: blood lactate, pyruvate, 3-hydroxybutyrate, acetoacetate; quantitative serum amino acids; urine organic acids done by gas chromatography/mass spectrometry; fasting blood glucose, lactate, and 3-hydroxybutyrate; and, in some cases, muscle biopsy. Measurement of the redox state of cultured fibroblasts using lactate/pyruvate ratio may be helpful, but this is obviously not available at the time of initial diagnosis. A flow chart for diagnosis is shown in Fig. 100-14.

The actual route for establishing a definitive diagnosis by biochemical assay of enzymes in skin fibroblasts, lymphoblasts, tissue biopsies, or by DNA analysis at the level of the gene, is also a complex process. The number and nature of the tests done to establish the diagnosis can be streamlined if the algorithm is used to predict or narrow the possible etiologies. In addition, because testing procedures in many cases are a difficult and lengthy process, treatment regimens may be instituted on the basis of the clinical observations providing caution is exercised by monitoring for adverse reactions.

As an addendum to the biochemical algorithm, there are useful clinical findings (see Chaps. 66 and 99). No one clinical feature is found in all patients with defects in energy metabolism. While this diagnostic treatise concentrates on patients who have a proven increase in blood or CSF lactate there is a wide spectrum of findings in patients with defects in energy metabolism, ranging from those who have quite normal lactate levels to those who have overwhelming lactic acidosis. There are hallmarks of disease severity in the disorders of energy metabolism forming patterns that are compelling. For instance, there are four disorders which follow the pattern of severity: fatal infantile lactic acidosis > Leigh disease > psychomotor retardation > ataxia > muscular weakness/retinal degeneration (Fig. 100-15). These are deficiency of the pyruvate dehydrogenase complex, deficiency of NADH-ubiquinone oxidoreductase (Complex I), deficiency of cytochrome c oxidase (Complex IV), all of which are nuclear encoded, and the mtDNA-encoded ATP6 defects in the oligomycin-sensitive ATPase (Complex V). The variation in severity in any one defect is caused by a variety of factors to include the nature of the mutation, effect on oxygen free radical generation, and the extent of mtDNA heteroplasmy. In all of these defects, a significant proportion of affected children have evidence of midline facial dysplasia, and in both PDH and Complex I deficiency, agenesis of the corpus callosum is common, indicating effects in utero to be involved.

Another constellation of symptoms that are often found associated with lactic acidemia is that of sensorineural hearing loss, muscular weakness, dementia, and strokelike episodes. This constellation of symptoms often point to a mtDNA defect involving tRNA mutation, especially when associated with maternal inheritance. External ophthalmoplegia, ptosis, and exercise intolerance often point to the presence of a mtDNA deletion or mutation, and when combined with either cardiomyopathy or myoclonus epilepsy, they can be a compelling reason to obtain mtDNA sequence information. Most of these

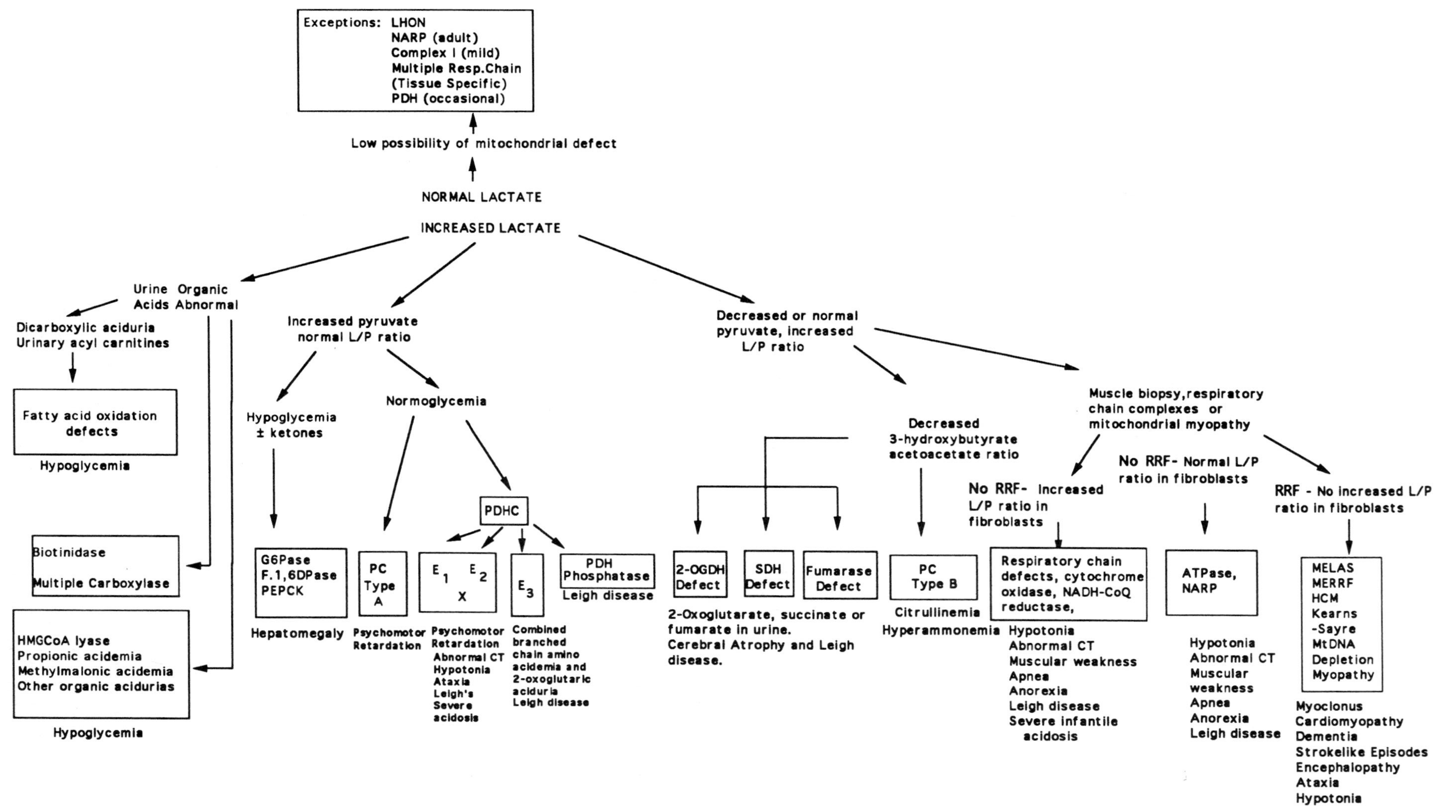

Fig. 100-14 Algorithm for diagnosis of patients with lactic acidemia. See text for detailed explanation. Diagram starts with the observation of increased blood lactic acid with the possibility of mitochondrial defects demonstrating normal blood lactic acid shown in the box above. The differential diagnosis is assisted by observations on urine organic acids, on the status of blood or fibroblast lactate:pyruvate ratio, and the presence of ragged red fibers in muscle. Disease entities or categories are highlighted in boxes.

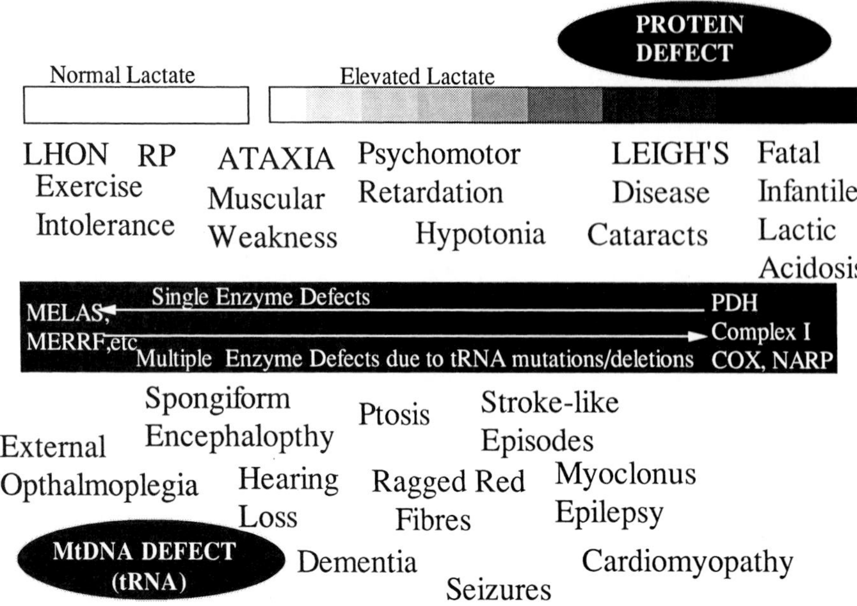

Fig. 100-15 Symptoms of mitochondrial disease grouped above or below the double arrows, depending on the likelihood of being caused by a protein coding defect (either nuclear or mtDNA), or a tRNA coding defect (mtDNA).

mtDNA-encoded tRNA defects have associated ragged red fibers in muscle.

Oxidative Defects with Normal Blood Lactate

It is now known that there are a small number of mitochondrial defects that can be present with a normal blood lactate. These cases are for the most part a rarity, or a small number of cases within a defined defect, which have a normal lactate. The best known of the defined mitochondrial defects with normal blood lactate is Leber hereditary optic neuropathy (LHON), while neurodegeneration with ataxia and retinitis pigmentosa (NARP) caused by a mtDNA mutation at 8993 can also present with no lactic acidemia in its milder and later forms of onset. A small number of cases of NADH-CoQ reductase deficiency have also presented with minimally raised blood lactate levels at 2 to 3 mM. There are also cases with multiple respiratory chain defects present on a tissue-specific basis where lactic acidemia in the neonatal period subsequently settles to present with a normal blood lactate.[190] Finally, in pyruvate dehydrogenase complex deficiency there are a small number of patients with defects in the $E_1\alpha$ gene who have either normal or close to normal lactic acid levels in blood. These patients are mostly females where, because of X inactivation, some cells express the normal $E_1\alpha$ allele, while others express a null or deficient allele. In these cases, the CSF lactate is usually increased above normal because of the cerebral dependence on glucose for ATP generation.

Increased Blood Lactate with Abnormal Organic Acids

Because lactic acid elevation occurs in many of the organic acidurias, these diagnoses should be ruled out in the early stages of investigation by gas chromatography/mass spectrometry analysis of the urine organic acids. Almost any of the organic acidurias can present with an increased blood lactate because of interference with CoA metabolism at the levels of pyruvate dehydrogenase and pyruvate carboxylase. Formation of large amounts of acyl-CoA intermediates due to blocked reactions deprives the PDH complex of CoASH for its reaction and pyruvate carboxylase of its activator acetyl-CoA. Fatty acid oxidation defects have a similar effect and produce a combination of lactic acidemia, hypoglycemia, and dicarboxylic aciduria. Most cases of biotinidase and multiple carboxylase deficiency are detected at this stage by the presence of unusual organic acids, because both defects can present with lactic acid accumulation. The presence of alopecia, dermatitis, and persistent Candida infections should also pinpoint most, but not all, biotinidase and multiple carboxylase deficiency cases. Occasionally, severe Complex I (NADH-CoQ reductase) deficiency can present with dicarboxylic aciduria and mild hypoglycemia, but the accompanying lactic acidosis, which is severe, distinguishes this from fatty acid oxidation defects. Lactic aciduria without lactic acidemia is a common finding, which by itself does not indicate the presence of a mitochondrial defect.

Increased Blood Lactate with Normal L/P Ratio

The ratio of lactate to pyruvate in the blood is one of the most helpful indicators of the underlying problem and may determine the directions of further investigation. A lactate:pyruvate ratio below 25, which we consider to be in the normal range, points to a defect either in pyruvate dehydrogenase or in one of the gluconeogenic enzymes, while a consistently raised lactate:pyruvate ratio, especially of 30 and above, is indicative of either pyruvate carboxylase (Type A) deficiency, a respiratory chain defect, of either nuclear or mtDNA origin, or a Krebs cycle defect.[191,192]

Taking the normal lactate:pyruvate ratio group first, a further differential can be obtained using the response to fasting. A defect in any of the enzymes of the gluconeogenic pathway results in a tendency toward fasting hypoglycemia accompanied by a blood lactate that is higher than in the fed state. The severity of the hypoglycemia experienced is in the order glucose-6-phosphatase > fructose-1,6-biphosphatase > phosphoenolpyruvate carboxykinase > pyruvate carboxylase. Hepatomegaly usually accompanies the gluconeogenic defects, the severity being in the same order as above. Occasionally, neither fasting hypoglycemia nor hepatomegaly is observed in pyruvate carboxylase deficiency (Type A). Muscular hypotonia is present in phosphoenolpyruvate carboxykinase deficiency and pyruvate carboxylase deficiency, but not in glucose-6-phosphatase or fructose-1,6-bisphosphatase deficiency. Psychomotor retardation is present in all pyruvate carboxylase (Type A)-deficient patients, and in most cases of PDH-complex deficiency. Ataxic episodes are a common occurrence, and hypotonia is present in nearly all cases of PDH-complex deficiency. Many patients with PDH-complex deficiency manifest a neurodegenerative course with loss of acquired milestones. Ketone bodies are below normal, even in the fasting state, in most cases of PDH-complex deficiency. CT scanning and MR imaging can be helpful because a significant number of both males and females with PDH-complex deficiency exhibit lesions in the brain stem and basal ganglia, and sometimes also in the cerebral cortex. Cortical atrophy with dilation of the ventricles is very common in female patients with PDH-complex E_1 deficiency. Differential diagnosis between the E_1, E_2, and protein X deficient subtypes of PDH-complex deficiency can only be made by enzyme assay, immunoblotting, and cDNA sequencing. The E_3 subtype of the PDH complex may be distinguished by observing the presence of elevated plasma branched chain amino acids in plasma or branched chain organic acid metabolites in urine.

Increased Blood Lactate with Increased Lactate:Pyruvate Ratio

With Low 3HOB/AcAc Ratio. An increased ratio of blood lactate to pyruvate, which is accompanied by a decreased ratio of 3-hydroxybutyrate to acetoacetate, can be indicative of Type B pyruvate carboxylase deficiency. The presentation will be in infancy and should not be considered in an older child. It can be confirmed by the presence of elevated plasma citrulline and lysine, which is accompanied by hyperammonemia. Mild elevations of ammonia have also been observed in PDH-complex (E_1 type) deficiency. It also appears that infants with defects in the Krebs cycle, including oxoglutarate dehydrogenase, succinate dehydrogenase, and fumarase deficiency, also present with elevated L/P ratio and decreased 3-hydroxybutyrate/acetoacetate ratio.[192,193] This is no doubt a reflection of the lack of intracellular aspartate experienced in functional Krebs cycle defects as oxaloacetate becomes depleted, as happens in Type B pyruvate carboxylase deficiency.

With Increased 3HOB/AcAc Ratio. An increased ratio of blood lactate to pyruvate, which is accompanied by an increased ratio of 3-hydroxybutyrate to acetoacetate ($>2{:}1$), is indicative of a defect somewhere in oxidative phosphorylation. Because this can be due to either nuclear- or mtDNA-encoded defects, the next step is to perform a muscle biopsy. The presence of ragged red fibers in the muscle is typical of a mitochondrial mtDNA defect involving loss of tRNA gene function. This picture is prominent in cases where a mtDNA-encoded tRNA has been affected by mutation or by deletion. This would place the patient in the MELAS, MERRF, Kearns-Sayre group of disorders, especially if this is accompanied by dementia, short stature, and sensorineural hearing loss. Hypertrophic cardiomyopathy (HCM), strokelike episodes, or seizures often appear in isolation, or accompany such mtDNA defects with ragged red fibers. This group of patients is typically older, many of them being in the second or third decade of life. With both nuclear-encoded mitochondrial respiratory chain defects and mtDNA protein-coding defects, mitochondrial proliferation is also seen, but not to the extent of producing ragged red fibers. A useful discriminator between the nuclear- and mitochondrially-encoded defects is measurement of L/P ratio in fibroblasts. Only nuclear-encoded defects appear to have an increased L/P ratio. These patients also have muscular weakness, hypotonia, failure to thrive, and anorexia. Many present as infants or neonates with lactic acidosis, but other reported cases have an adult onset. CT scanning or nuclear magnetic resonance imaging can be helpful. In cytochrome oxidase deficiency, Complex I deficiency, and the mtDNA 8993 mutation (NARP), the cystic lesions and areas of necrosis that develop in the brain stem and basal ganglia may be detectable. A postmortem diagnosis of Leigh disease is often made in these cases. The more severe cases of cytochrome oxidase and Complex I deficiency present with neonatal lactic acidosis, which is overwhelming and fatal.

This outline provides the clinician an overview of the approximate diagnosis of the patient concerned. The final diagnosis must, of course, be confirmed by measurement of enzyme activity where possible in leukocytes, cultured skin fibroblasts, or muscle or liver biopsy, depending on the identity of the suspected defect. Because this is often a lengthy process, some simple attempts at therapy may be instituted (Table 100-4).

Table 100-4 Therapeutic Regimens for Treatment of Lactic Acidemia Syndromes

Defect	Treatment
Glucone 6-phosphatase Fructose 1,6-diphosphatase	High, carbohydrate diet
PEPCK Pyruvate carboxylase Pyruvate dehydrogenase complex	Low CHO or ketogenic diet (excluding E_3 and phosphatase) Dichloroacetate, thiamine, carnitine
Biotinidase	Biotin
Multiple carboxylase	Biotin
NADH-CoQ reductase	Nicotinamide, riboflavin, carnitine, succinate, dimethylglycine
Cytochrome oxidase	Dichloroacetate, carnitine
MELAS, MERRF, Kearns-Sayre	Nicotinamide, riboflavin, dichloroacetate, carnitine
Fatty acid oxidation defects	Carnitine

See Reference 195 for more details and recommended doses.

REFERENCES

1. Tanaka K, Rosenberg LE: Disorders of branched chain-amino acid and organic acid metabolism, in Stanbury JB, Wyngaarden JB, Frederickson DS, Goldstein JL, Brown MS (eds): *The Metabolic Basis of Inherited Disease,* 5th ed. New York: McGraw-Hill, 1983, p 440.
2. Newsholme EA, Leech AR: *Biochemistry for the Medical Sciences.* New York: John Wiley, 1983.
3. Randle PJ, Sugden PH, Kerbey AL, Radcliffe PM, Hutson NJ: Regulation of pyruvate oxidation and the conservation of glucose. *Biochem Soc Symp* **43**:47, 1978.
4. Ahlborg O, Felig P: Lactate and glucose exchange across the forearm, legs and splanchnic bed during and after prolonged leg exercise. *J Clin Invest* **69**:45, 1982.
5. Chaussain JL, Georges P, Olive G, Job JC: Glycemic response to 24-hour fast in normal children and children with ketotic hypoglycemia. *J Pediatr* **85**:776, 1974.
6. Kahn A, Meienhofer MC, Cottreau D, Lagrange JC, Dreyfus JC: Phosphofructokinase (PFK) isozymes in man. *Hum Genet* **48**:93, 1979.
7. Meienhofer MC, Cottreau D, Dreyfus JC, Kahn A: The kinetic properties of human F4 phosphofructokinase. *FEBS Lett* **110**:219, 1980.
8. Davidson M, Collins M, Byrne J, Vora S: Alterations in phosphofructokinase isoenzymes during early human development. *Biochem J* **214**:703, 1983.
9. Kreisberg RA: Glucose-lactate interrelations in man. *N Engl J Med* **287**:132, 1973.
10. Kreisberg RA, Pennington LF, Boshell BR: Lactate turnover and gluconeogenesis in normal and obese humans. *Diabetes* **19**:53, 1970.
11. Hermansen L, Machlum S, Pruett EDR, Vagi O, Waldum H, Wesselaas T: Lactate removal at rest and during exercise, in Howald H, Poortman JR (eds): *Metabolic Adaptation to Prolonged Physical Exercise.* Basel: Birkhauser Verlag, 1975, p 101.
12. Krebs HA, Woods HF, Alberti KGMM: Hyperlactataemia and lactic acidosis, in Marks V, Hales CN (eds): *Essays in Medical Biochemistry.* London: William Clowes, 1975, p 81.
13. Felig P: Amino acid metabolism in man. *Ann Rev Biochem* **44**:993, 1975.
14. Kaplan NO, Everse J: Regulatory characteristics of lactate dehydrogenases. *Adv Enzyme Regul* **10**:323, 1972.
15. Kanno T, Sudo K, Takeuchi I, Kanda S, Honda N, Nishimura Y, Oyama K: Hereditary deficiency of lactate dehydrogenase M-subunit. *Clin Chim Acta* **108**:267, 1980.
16. Maekawa M, Sudo K, Li SS, Kanno T: Analysis of genetic mutations in human lactate dehydrogenase-A (M) deficiency using DNA conformation polymorphism in combination with polyacrylamide gradient gel and silver staining. *Biochem Biophys Res Commun* **180**:1083, 1991.
17. Kitamura M, Hjima N, Hashimoto F, Hiratsuka A: Hereditary deficiency of the subunit H of lactate dehydrogenase. *Clin Chim Acta* **34**:419, 1971.

18. Reed LJ: Regulation of mammalian pyruvate dehydrogenase complex by a phosphorylation-dephosphorylation cycle. *Curr Top Cell Regul* **18**:95, 1981.
19. Randle PJ: Mitochondrial 2-oxoacid dehydrogenase complexes of animal tissues. *Philos Trans* **302**:47, 1983. (Abstract)
20. DeMarcucci GL, Hodgson JA, Lindsay G: The Mr 50,000 polypeptide of mammalian pyruvate dehydrogenase complex participates in acetylation reactions. *Eur J Biochem* **158**:587, 1986.
21. Powers-Greenwood SL, Rahmatullah M, Radke GA, Roche TE: Separation of protein X from the dihydrolipoyl transacetylase component of the mammalian pyruvate dehydrogenase complex and function of protein X. *J Biol Chem* **264**:3655, 1989.
22. Neagle JC, Lindsay JG: Selective proteolysis of the protein X subunit of the bovine heart pyruvate dehydrogenase complex. *Biochem J* **278**:423, 1991.
23. Ling M, McEachern G, Seyda A, MacKay N, Scherer SW, Bratinova S, Beatty B, et al: Detection of a homozygous four base pair deletion in the protein X gene in a case of pyruvate dehydrogenase complex deficiency. *Hum Mol Genet* **7**:501, 1998.
24. Aral B, Benelli C, Ait-Ghezala G, Amessou M, Fouque F, Manoury C, Créau N, et al: Mutations in PDX1, the human lipoyl-containing component X of the pyruvate dehydrogenase-complex gene on chromosome 11p1, in congenital lactic acidosis. *Am J Hum Genet* **61**:1318, 1997.
25. Harris RA, Bowker-Kinley MM, Wu P, Jeng J, Popov KM: Dihydrolipoamide dehydrogenase-binding protein of the human pyruvate dehydrogenase complex. DNA-derived amino acid sequence, expression, and reconstitution of the pyruvate dehydrogenase complex. *J Biol Chem* **272**:19746, 1997.
26. Paxton R, Harris RA: Isolation of rabbit liver branched-chain alpha-ketoacid dehydrogenase and regulation by phosphorylation. *J Biol Chem* **257**:14433, 1982.
27. Guest RJ: Gene-protein relationships of the alpha-keto-acid dehydrogenase complexes of *Escherichia coli* K12: Chromosomal location of the lipoamide dehydrogenase gene. *J Gen Microbiol* **80**:523, 1974.
28. Linn TE, Pettit FH, Hucho F, Reed LJ: Keto acid dehydrogenase complexes. Comparative studies of the regulatory properties of the pyruvate dehydrogenase complexes from kidney, heart and liver mitochondria. *Proc Natl Acad Sci U S A* **64**:227, 1969.
29. McAllister A, Allison SP, Randle PJ: Effects of dichloroacetate on the metabolism of glucose, pyruvate, acetate, 3-hydroxybutyrate and palmitate. *Biochem J* **134**:1067, 1973.
30. Popov KM, Kedishvili NY, Zhao Y, Shimomura Y, Crabb DW, Harris RA: Primary structure of pyruvate dehydrogenase kinase establishes a new family of eukaryotic protein kinases. *J Biol Chem* **35**:26602, 1993.
31. Popov KM, Kedishvili NY, Zhao Y, Gudi R, Harris RA: Molecular cloning of the p45 subunit of pyruvate dehydrogenase kinase. *J Biol Chem* **269**:29720, 1994.
32. Gudi R, Bowker-Kinley MM, Kedishvili NY, Zhao Y, Popov KM: Diversity of the pyruvate dehydrogenase kinase gene family in humans. *J Biol Chem* **270**:28989, 1995.
33. Rowles JC, Scherer SW, Xi T, Majer M, Nickle DC, Popov K, Harris RA, et al: Cloning and characterization of PDK4 on 7q21.3 encoding a fourth human pyruvate dehydrogenase kinase isoenzyme. *J Biol Chem* **271**:22376-22382, 1996.
34. Lawson JE, Niu X-D, Browning KS, Trong HL, Yan J, Reed LJ: Molecular cloning and expression of the catalytic subunit of bovine pyruvate dehydrogenase phosphatase and sequence similarity with protein phosphatase 2C. *Biochem* **32**:8987, 1993.
35. Lawson JE, Park SH, Mattison AR, Yan J, Reed LJ: Cloning, expression, and properties of the regulatory subunit of bovine pyruvate dehydrogenase phosphatase. *J Biol Chem* **272**:31625, 1997.
36. Hogg SA, Taylor SI, Ruderman NB: Pyruvate dehydrogenase activity in starvation, diabetes and exercise. *Biochem J* **158**:203, 1976.
37. Whitehouse S, Cooper RH, Randle PJ: Mechanism of activation of pyruvate dehydrogenase by dichloroacetate and other halogenated carboxylic acids. *Biochem J* **141**:761, 1974.
38. Blass JP, Avigan J, Uhlendorf BW: A defect of pyruvate decarboxylase in a child with an intermittent movement disorder. *J Clin Invest* **49**:423, 1970.
39. Blass JP, Kark RAP, Engel WK: Clinical studies of a patient with pyruvate decarboxylase deficiency. *Arch Neurol* **25**:449, 1971.
40. Blass JP, Lonsdale D, Uhlendorf BW, Ham E: Intermittent ataxia with pyruvate decarboxylase activity. *Lancet* **1**:1302, 1971.
41. Farmer TW, Veath L, Miller AL, O'Brien J, Rosenberg RN: Pyruvate decarboxylase deficiency in a patient with subacute necrotizing encephalomyelopathy. *Neurology* **23**:429, 1973.
42. Farrel DF, Clark AF, Scott CR, Wennberg RP: Absence of pyruvate decarboxylase activity in man. A cause of congenital lactic acidosis. *Science* **187**:1082, 1975.
43. Robinson BH, MacMillan H, Petrova-Benedict R, Sherwood WG: Variable clinical presentation in patients with deficiency of the pyruvate dehydrogenase complex. A review of 30 cases with a defect in the E_1 component of the complex. *J Pediatr* **111**:525, 1987.
44. Robinson BH, Chun K, MacKay N, Otulakowski G, Petrova-Benedict R, Willard H: Isolated and combined deficiencies of the α-keto acid dehydrogenase complexes. *Ann N Y Acad Sci* **573**:337, 1989.
45. Wick H, Schweizerk K, Baumgartner R: Thiamine dependency in a patient with congenital lactic acidemia due to pyruvate dehydrogenase deficiency. *Agents Actions* **7**:405, 1977.
46. Stromme JH, Borud O, Moe PJ: Fatal lactic acidosis in a newborn attributable to a congenital defect of pyruvate dehydrogenase. *Pediatr Res* **10**:60, 1976.
47. Wicking CA, Scholem RD, Hunt SM, Brown GK: Immunochemical analysis of normal and mutant forms of human pyruvate dehydrogenase. *Biochem J* **239**:89, 1986.
48. Matsuo M, Ookita K, Takemine H, Koike K, Koike M: Fatal case of pyruvate dehydrogenase deficiency. *Acta Paediatr Scand* **74**:140, 1985.
49. Evans OB: Pyruvate decarboxylase deficiency in subacute necrotizing encephalomyelopathy. *Arch Neurol* **38**:515, 1981.
50. Papanastasiou D, Lehnert W, Schuchmann L, Hommes FA: Chronic lactic acidosis in an infant. *Helv Paediatr Acta* **35**:253, 1980.
51. Hansen TL, Christensen E, Brandt NJ: Studies on pyruvate carboxylase, pyruvate decarboxylase and lipoamide dehydrogenase in subacute necrotizing encephalomyelopathy. *Acta Paediatr Scand* **71**:263, 1982.
52. Toshima K, Kuroda Y, Hashimoto T, Ito M, Watanabe T, Miyao M, Kunio II: Enzymologic studies and therapy of Leigh's disease associated with pyruvate decarboxylase deficiency. *Pediatr Res* **16**:430, 1982.
53. Miyabayashi S, Ito T, Narisawa K, Iinuma K, Tada K: Biochemical studies in 28 children with lactic acidosis in relation to Leigh's encephalomyelopathy. *Eur J Pediatr* **143**:278, 1985.
54. Ho L, Hu CWC, Packman S, Patel MS: Deficiency of the pyruvate dehydrogenase component in pyruvate dehydrogenase complex-deficient human fibroblasts. Immunological identification. *J Clin Invest* **78**:844, 1986.
55. Ohtake M, Takada G, Miyabayashi S, Arai N, Tada K, Monnada S: Pyruvate decarboxylase deficiency in a patient with Leigh's encephalomyelopathy. *Tohoku J Exp Med* **137**:379, 1982.
56. Wexler ID, Kerr DS, Ho L, Lusk MM, Pepin RA, Javed AA, Mole JE, et al: Heterogenous expression of protein and mRNA in pyruvate dehydrogenase deficiency. *Proc Natl Acad Sci U S A* **85**:7336, 1988.
57. Brown GK, Brown RM, Scholem RD, Kirby DM, Dahl H-HM: The clinical and biochemical spectrum of human pyruvate dehydrogenase complex deficiency. *Ann N Y Acad Sci* **573**:360, 1989.
58. Cederbaum SD, Blass JP, Minkoff N, Brown WJ, Cotton ME, Harris SH: Sensitivity to carbohydrate in a patient with familial intermittent lactic acidosis and pyruvate dehydrogenase deficiency. *Pediatr Res* **10**:713, 1976.
59. Blass JP, Schulman JD, Young DS, Hom E: An inherited defect affecting the tricarboxylic acid cycle in a patient with congenital lactic acidosis. *J Clin Invest* **51**:1845, 1972.
60. Falk RE, Cederbaum SD, Blass JP, Gibson GE, Kark RAP, Carrel RE: Ketonic diet in the management of pyruvate dehydrogenase deficiency. *Pediatrics* **58**:713, 1976.
61. Evans O: Episodic weakness in pyruvate decarboxylase deficiency. *J Pediatr* **105**:961, 1984.
62. Kodama S, Yas R, Ninomiya M, Goji K, Takahashi T, Monshita Y, Matsuo T: The effect of high-fat diet on pyruvate decarboxylase deficiency without involvement of the central nervous system. *Brain Dev* **5**:381, 1983.
63. Brown GK, Haan EA, Kirby DM, Scholem RD, Wrailk JE, Rogers JG, Danks DM: "Cerebral" lactic acidosis: Defects in pyruvate metabolism with profound brain damage and minimal systemic acidosis. *Eur J Pediatr* **147**:10, 1988.
64. Robinson BH, Sherwood WG: Lactic acidemia, the prevalence of pyruvate decarboxylase deficiency. *J Inherit Metab Dis* **7**:69, 1984.
65. Stansbie D, Wallace SJ, Marsac C: Disorders of the pyruvate dehydrogenase complex. *J Inherit Metab Dis* **9**:105, 1986.
66. Robinson BH: The lactic acidemias, in Lloyd JK, Scriver CR (eds): *Genetic and Metabolic Disease in Pediatrics*. London: Butterworth, 1985, p 111.

67. MacKay N, Petrova-Benedict R, Thoene J, Bergen B, Wilson W, Robinson B: Three cases of lactic acidemia due to pyruvate decarboxylase (E_1) deficiency with evidence of protein polymorphism in the α subunit of the enzyme. *Eur J Pediatr* **144**:445, 1986.
68. Marchiafava E, Bignami A: Sopra un alterazione del copo calloso osservata in saggelti alcooliati. *Rev Patol Nerv* **8**:544, 1903.
69. Reynolds SF, Blass JP: A possible mechanism for selective cerebellar damage in partial pyruvate dehydrogenase deficiency. *Neurology* **26**:625, 1976.
70. Wexler ID, Hemalatha SG, McConnell J, Buist NR, Dahl H-H, Berry SA, Cederbaum SD, et al: Outcome of pyruvate dehydrogenase deficiency treated with ketogenic diets. Studies in patients with identical mutations. *Neurology* **49**:1655, 1997.
71. Hommes FA, Berger R, Lutt-DeHann G: The effect of thiamine treatment on the activity of pyruvate dehydrogenase. Relation to the treatment of Leigh's encephalomyelopathy. *Pediatr Res* **7**:616, 1973.
72. McCormick K, Viscardi RM, Robinson BH, Heininger J: Partial pyruvate decarboxylase deficiency with profound lactic acidosis and hyperammonemia: Responses to dichloroacetate and benzoate. *Am J Med Genet* **22**:291, 1985.
73. Kuroda Y, Ito M, Toshima K, Takeda E, Naito E, Hwang TJ, Hashimoto T, et al: Treatment of chronic congenital lactic acidosis by oral administration of dichloroacetate. *J Inherit Metab Dis* **9**:244, 1986.
74. Robinson BH, Taylor J, Sherwood WG: The genetic heterogeneity of lactic acidosis: Occurrence of recognizable inborn errors of metabolism in a pediatric population with lactic acidemia. *Pediatr Res* **14**:956, 1980.
75. Ho L, Wexler ID, Liu T-C, Thekkumkara TJ, Patel MS: Characterization of cDNAs encoding human pyruvate dehydrogenase α subunit. *Proc Natl Acad Sci U S A* **86**:5330, 1989.
76. Koike K, Ohta S, Urata Y, Koike M: Molecular cloning and sequencing of cDNAs encoding α and β subunits of human pyruvate dehydrogenase. *Proc Natl Acad Sci U S A* **85**:41, 1988.
77. Endo H, Hasegawa K, Narisawa K, Tada K, Kagawa Y, Ohta S: Defective gene in lactic acidosis: Abnormal pyruvate dehydrogenase $E_1\alpha$-subunit caused by a frameshift. *Am J Hum Genet* **44**:358, 1989.
78. Ho L, Patel MS: Cloning and cDNA sequence of the β-subunit component of human pyruvate dehydrogenase complex. *Gene* **86**:297, 1990.
79. Chun K, MacKay N, Willard HF, Robinson BH: Isolation, characterization and chromosomal localization of cDNA clones for the $E_1\beta$ subunit of the pyruvate dehydrogenase complex. *Eur J Biochem* **194**:587, 1990.
80. Gershwin E, MacKay IR, Sturgess A, Coppel RL: Identification and specificity of a cDNA encoding the 70Kd mitochondrial antigen recognized in primary biliary cirrhosis. *J Immunol* **183**:3525, 1987.
81. Thekkumkara TJ, Ho L, Wexler ID, Pons G, Liu TC, Patel MS: Nucleotide sequence of a cDNA for dihydrolipoamide acetyltransferase component of human pyruvate dehydrogenase complex. *FEBS Lett* **240**:45, 1988.
82. Brown RM, Dahl H-HM, Brown GK: X chromosome localization of the functional gene for the $E_1\alpha$ subunit of the human pyruvate dehydrogenase complex. *Genome* **7**:215, 1989.
83. Olson S, Song BJ, Hueh TL, Chi YT, Veech RL, McBride OW: Three genes for enzymes of the pyruvate dehydrogenase complex map to human chromosomes 3,7 and X. *Am J Hum Genet* **46**:340, 1990.
84. Szabo P, Sheu KFR, Robinson RM, Grzeschik K-H, Blass JB: The gene for the α polypeptide of pyruvate dehydrogenase is X-linked in humans. *Am J Hum Genet* **46**:874, 1990.
85. Otulakowski G, Robinson BH, Willard HF: Gene for lipoamide dehydrogenase maps to human chromosome 7. *Somat Cell Mol Genet* **14**:411, 1988.
86. Scherer SW, Otulakowski G, Robinson BH, Tsui L-C: Localization of the human dihydrolipoamide dehydrogenase gene (DLD) to 7q31-q32. *Cytogenet Cell Genet* **56**:176, 1991.
87. Maragos C, Hutchison W, Haysaka K, Brown GK, Dahl H-HM: Structural organization of the gene for the $E_1\alpha$ subunit of the human pyruvate dehydrogenase complex. *J Biol Chem* **264**:12294, 1989.
88. Koike K, Urata Y, Koike M: Molecular cloning and characterization of human pyruvate dehydrogenase β subunit gene. *Proc Natl Acad Sci U S A* **87**:5594, 1990.
89. Feigenbaum AS, Robinson BH: The structure of the human dihydrolipoamide dehydrogenase gene (DLD) and its upstream elements. *Genome* **17**:376, 1993.
90. Hawkins CF, Borges A, Perham RN: A common structural motif in thiamine pyrophosphate-binding enzymes. *FEBS Lett* **255**:77, 1989.
91. Lindqvist Y, Schneider G, Erlmer V, Sundstrom M: Three dimensional structure of transketolase, a thiamine diphosphate dependent enzyme, at 2.5 Å resolution. *EMBO J* **11**:2373, 1992.
92. Robinson BH, Chun K: The relationships between transketolase, yeast pyruvate decarboxylase and pyruvate dehydrogenase of the pyruvate dehydrogenase complex. *FEBS Lett* **328**:99, 1993.
93. Old SE, DeVivo DC: Pyruvate dehydrogenase complex deficiency: Biochemical and immunoblot analysis of cultured skin fibroblasts. *Ann Neurol* **26**:746, 1989.
94. Endo H, Miyabayashi S, Toda K, Narisawa K: A four-nucleotide insertion at the $E_1\alpha$ gene in a patient with pyruvate dehydrogenase deficiency. *J Inherit Metab Dis* **14**:793, 1991.
95. Chun K, MacKay N, Petrova-Benedict R, Robinson BH: Pyruvate dehydrogenase deficiency due to a 20bp deletion in exon 11 of the pyruvate dehydrogenase (PDH) $E_1\alpha$ gene. *Am J Hum Genet* **49**:414, 1991.
96. Kitano A, Endo F, Matsuda I: Immunochemical analysis of pyruvate dehydrogenase complex in two boys with primary lactic acidemia. *Neurology* **40**:1312, 1990.
97. Brown RM, Fraser NJ, Brown GK: Differential methylation of the hypervariable locus DXS255 on active and inactive X chromosomes correlates with the expression of a human X-linked gene. *Genome* **7**:215, 1990.
98. Boyd Y, Fraser NJ: Methylation patterns at the hypervariable X-chromosome locus DXS255 (M27β): Correlation with X-inactivation status. *Genome* **7**:182, 1990.
99. Dahl H-HM, Brown GK, Brown RM, Hansen LL, Kerr DS, Wexler ID, Patel MS, et al: Mutations and polymorphisms in the pyruvate dehydrogenase $E_1\alpha$ gene. *Hum Mutat* **1**:97, 1992.
100. Chun K, MacKay N, Petrova-Benedict R, Robinson BH: Mutations in the X-linked $E_1\alpha$ subunit of pyruvate dehydrogenase leading to deficiency of the pyruvate dehydrogenase complex. *Hum Mol Genet* **2**:449, 1993.
101. Wexler ID, Hemalatha SG, Patel MS: Sequence conservation in the α and β subunits of pyruvate dehydrogenase and its similarity to branched-chain α-keto acid dehydrogenase. *FEBS Lett* **282**:209, 1991.
102. Federico A, Doti MT, Fabrizi GM, Palmeri S, Massimo L, Robinson BH, Malandrini A, et al: Congenital lactic acidosis due to a defect of pyruvate dehydrogenase complex (E_1). *Eur Neurol* **30**:123, 1990.
103. Chun K, MacKay N, Petrova-Benedict R, Federico A, Fois A, Cole DEC, Robertson E, et al: Mutations in the X-linked $E_1\alpha$ subunit of pyruvate dehydrogenase; Exon skipping, insertion of duplicate sequence, and missense mutations leading to the deficiency of the pyruvate dehydrogenase complex. *Am J Hum Genet* **56**:558, 1995.
104. Naito E, Ito M, Yokota I, Saijo T, Matsuda J, Osaka H, Kimura S, et al: Biochemical and molecular analysis of an X-linked case of Leigh syndrome associated with thiamin-responsive pyruvate dehydrogenase deficiency. *J Inherit Metab Dis* **20**:539, 1997.
105. Briones P, Lóez MJ, De Meirleir L, Ribes A, Rodés M, Martinez-Costa C, Peris M, et al: Leigh syndrome due to pyruvate dehydrogenase $E_1\alpha$ deficiency (point mutation R263G) in a Spanish boy. *J Inherit Metab Dis* **19**:795, 1996.
106. Lissens W, De Meirleir L, Seneca S, Benelli C, Marsac C, Poll-The BT, Briones P, et al: Mutation analysis of the pyruvate dehydrogenase $E_1\alpha$ gene in eight patients with a pyruvate dehydrogenase complex deficiency. *Hum Mutat* **7**:46, 1996.
107. Awata H, Endo F, Tanoue A, Kitano A, Matsuda I: Characterization of a point mutation in the pyruvate dehydrogenase $E_1\alpha$ gene from two boys with primary lactic acidemia. *J Inherit Metab Dis* **17**:189, 1994.
108. Fujii T, Garcia Alvarez MB, Sheu K-FR, Kranz-Eble PJ, De Vivo DC: Pyruvate dehydrogenase deficiency: The relation of the $E_1\alpha$ mutation to the $E_1\beta$ subunit deficiency. *Pediatr Neurol* **14**:328, 1996.
109. Dahl H-HM, Hansen LL, Brown RM, Danks DM, Rogers JG, Brown GK: X-linked pyruvate dehydrogenase $E_1\alpha$ subunit deficiency in heterozygous females: Variable manifestation of the same mutation. *J Inherit Metab Dis* **15**:835, 1992.
110. Hansen LL, Brown GK, Kirby DM, Dahl H-HM: Characterization of the mutations in three patients with pyruvate dehydrogenase $E_1\alpha$ deficiency. *J Inherit Metab Dis* **14**:140, 1991.
111. Takakubo F, Cartwright P, Hoogenraad N, Thorburn DR, Collins F, Lithgow T, Dahl H-HM: An amino acid substitution in the pyruvate dehydrogenase $E_1\alpha$ gene, affecting mitochondrial import of the precursor protein. *Am J Hum Genet* **57**:772, 1995.
112. Matthews PM, Brown RM, Otero LJ, Marchington DR, LeGris M, Howes R, Meadows LS, et al: Pyruvate dehydrogenase deficiency. Clinical presentation and molecular genetic characterization of five new patients. *Brain* **117**:435, 1994.

113. Brown GK, Scholem RD, Hunt SM, Harrison JR, Pollard AC: Hyperammonemia and lactic acidosis in a patient with pyruvate dehydrogenase deficiency. *J Inherit Metab Dis* **10**:359, 1987.
114. DeMeirleir L, Lissens W, Vamos E, Liebaers I: Pyruvate dehydrogenase deficiency due to mutation of the $E_1\alpha$ subunit. *J Inherit Metab Dis* **14**:301, 1991.
115. Dahl H-HM, Maragos C, Brown RM, Hansen LL, Brown GK: Pyruvate dehydrogenase deficiency caused by deletion of a 7bp repeat sequence in the $E_1\alpha$ gene. *Am J Hum Genet* **47**:286, 1990.
116. Seyda A, MacKay N, Robinson BH: Stability of mutant $E_1\alpha$ enzyme subunit in human pyruvate dehydrogenase complex deficiency. In preparation, 1998.
117. Kacser H, Burns JA: The molecular basis of dominance. *Genetics* **97**:639, 1981.
118. Robinson BH, MacKay N, Petrova-Benedict R, Ozalp I, Coskun T, Stacpoole PW: Defects in the E_2 lipoyl transacetylase and the X-lipoyl-containing component of the pyruvate dehydrogenase complex in patients with lactic acidemia. *J Clin Invest* **85**:1821, 1990.
119. Geoffroy V, Fouque F, Benelli C, et al: Defect in the X-lipoyl-containing component of the pyruvate dehydrogenase complex in a patient with neonatal lactic acidemia. *Pediatrics* **97**:267, 1996.
120. Marsac C, Stansbie D, Bonne G, et al: Defect in the lipoyl-bearing protein X subunit of the pyruvate dehydrogenase complex in two patients with encephalomyelopathy. *J Pediatr* **123**:915, 1993.
121. De Meirleir L, Lissens W, Benelli C, Marsac C, De Klerk J, Scholte J, van Diggelen O, et al: Pyruvate dehydrogenase complex deficiency and absence of subunit X. *J Inherit Metab Dis* **21**:9, 1998.
122. Patel MS, Roche TE: Molecular biology and biochemistry of pyruvate dehydrogenase complexes. *FASEB J* **4**:3224, 1990.
123. Lawson JE, Behal RH, Reed LJ: Disruption and mutagenesis of the saccharomyces cerevisiae PDX1 gene encoding the protein X component of the pyruvate dehydrogenase complex. *Biochem* **30**:2834, 1991.
124. Robinson BH, Taylor J, Sherwood WG: Deficiency of dihydrolipoyl dehydrogenase. A cause of congenital lactic acidosis in infancy. *Pediatr Res* **11**:1198, 1978.
125. Taylor J, Robinson BH, Sherwood WG: A defect in branched-chain amino acid metabolism in a patient with congenital lactic acidosis due to dihydrolipoyl dehydrogenase deficiency. *Pediatr Res* **12**:60, 1978.
126. Robinson BH, Taylor J, Kahler SG, Kirkman HN: Lactic acidemia, neurologic deterioration and carbohydrate dependence in a girl with dihydrolipoyl dehydrogenase deficiency. *Eur J Pediatr* **136**:35, 1981.
127. Munnich A, Saudubray JM, Taylor J, Charpentier C, Marsac C, Rocchiccioli F, Amedee-Manesme O, et al: Congenital lactic acidosis, α-ketoglutaric aciduria and variant form of maple syrup urine disease due to a single enzyme defect. Dihydrolipoyl dehydrogenase deficiency. *Acta Paediatr Scand* **71**:167, 1982.
128. Matalon R, Stumpf DA, Michals K, Hart RD, Parks JK, Goodman SI: Lipoamide dehydrogenase deficiency with primary lactic acidosis: Favorable response to treatment with oral lipoic acid. *J Pediatr* **104**:65, 1984.
129. Kuhara T, Shinka T, Inque Y, Matsumoto M, Yoshino M, Sakaguchi Y, Matsumoto I: Studies of urinary organic acid profiles of a patient with dihydrolipoyl dehydrogenase deficiency. *Clin Chim Acta* **133**:133, 1983.
130. Sweetman L, Nyhan W: Personal communication re patient documented in reference 65. Personal Communication 1985, 1993.
131. Otulakowski G, Nyhan W, Sweetman L, Robinson BH: Immunoextraction of lipoamide dehydrogenase from cultured skin fibroblasts in patients with combined α-ketoacid dehydrogenase deficiency. *Clin Chim Acta* **152**:27, 1985.
132. Hinman LM, Sheu KFR, Baker AC, Kim YT, Blass JP: Deficiency of pyruvate dehydrogenase complex in Leigh's disease fibroblasts—An abnormality in lipoamide dehydrogenase affecting PDHC activation. *Neurology* **39**:70, 1989.
133. Liu T-C, Kim H, Arijmendi C, Kitano A, Patel MS: Identification of two missense mutations in a dihydrolipoamide dehydrogenase deficient patient. *Proc Natl Acad Sci U S A* **90**:5186, 1993.
134. Soo Hong Y, Kerr DS, Liu T-C, Lusk M, Powell BR, Patel MS: Deficiency of dihydrolipoamide dehydrogenase due to two mutant alleles (E340K and G101del). Analysis of a family and prenatal testing. *Biochim Biophys Acta* **1362**:160, 1997.
135. Soo Hong Y, Kerr DS, Craigen WJ, Tan J, Pan Y, Lusk M, Patel MS: Identification of two mutations in a compound heterozygous child with dihydrolipoamide dehydrogenase deficiency. *Hum Mol Genet* **5**:1925, 1996.
136. Elpeleg O, Ruitenbeek W, Jakobs C, Barash V, De Vivo DC, Amir N: Congenital lactic acidemia caused by lipoamide dehydrogenase deficiency with favorable outcome. *J Pediatr* **126**:72, 1995.
137. Elpeleg ON, Shaag A, Glustein JZ, Anikster Y, Joseph A, Saada A: Lipoamide dehydrogenase deficiency in Ashkenazi Jews: An insertion mutation in the mitochondrial leader sequence. *Hum Mutat* **10**:256, 1997.
138. Aptowitzer I, Saada A, Faber J, Kleid D, Elpeleg ON: Liver disease in the Ashkenazi-Jewish lipoamide dehydrogenase deficiency. *J Pediatr Gastroenterol Nutr* **24**:599, 1997.
139. Sorbi S, Blass JP: Abnormal activation of pyruvate dehydrogenase in Leigh disease fibroblasts. *Neurology* **32**:555, 1982.
140. DeVivo DC, Haymond MW, Obert KA, Nelson JS, Pagliara AS: Defective activation of the pyruvate dehydrogenase complex in subacute necrotizing encephalomyelopathy (Leigh disease). *Ann Neurol* **6**:483, 1979.
141. Robinson BH, Sherwood WG: Pyruvate dehydrogenase phosphatase deficiency: A cause of chronic congenital lactic acidosis in infancy. *Pediatr Res* **9**:935, 1975.
142. Bardin RE, Taylor BL, Osohashi I: Structural properties of pyruvate carboxylase from chicken liver and other sources. *Proc Natl Acad Sci U S A* **72**:4308, 1975.
143. Wallace JC, Easterbrook-Smith SB: Substrate binding to pyruvate carboxylase subunits, in Keech DB, Wallace JC (eds): *Pyruvate Carboxylase*. Boca Raton, FL, CRC, 1985, p 65.
144. Scrutton MC, White MD: Purification and properties of human liver pyruvate carboxylase. *Biochem Med* **9**:271, 1974.
145. Barrit GJ: Resolution of gluconeogenic flux by pyruvate carboxylase, in Keech DB, Wallace JC (eds): *Pyruvate Carboxylase*. Boca Raton, FL, CRC, 1985, p 141.
146. Von Glutz G, Walter P: Regulation of pyruvate carboxylation by acetyl-CoA in rat liver mitochondria. *FEBS Lett* **72**:299, 1976.
147. Crabtree B, Higgins SJ, Newsholme EA: The activities of pyruvate carboxylase, phosphoenolpyruvate carboxykinase and fructose 1,6, diphosphatase in muscles from vertebrates and invertebrates. *Biochem J* **130**:391, 1972.
148. Atkin BM, Buist NRM, Utter M, Leiter AB, Banker BQ: Pyruvate carboxylase deficiency and lactic acidosis in a retarded child without Leigh's disease. *Pediatr Res* **13**:109, 1979.
149. Atkin BM, Utter MF, Weinberg MB: Pyruvate carboxylase and phosphoenolpyruvate carboxykinase activity in leucocytes and fibroblasts from a patient with pyruvate carboxylase deficiency. *Pediatr Res* **13**:38, 1979.
150. Lee SH, Davis JE: Carboxylase and decarboxylation reactions anaplerotic flux and removal of citric acid cycle intermediates in skeletal muscle. *J Biol Chem* **254**:420, 1979.
151. Lim F, Morris CP, Occhiodoro F, Wallace JC: Sequence and domain structure of yeast pyruvate carboxylase. *J Biol Chem* **263**:11493, 1988.
152. MacKay N, Rigat B, Douglas C, Chen HS, Robinson BH: cDNA cloning of human kidney pyruvate carboxylase. *Biochem Biophys Res Comm* **202**:1009, 1994.
153. Wexler ID, Du Y, Lisgaris M, Mandel KM, Freytag SO, Yang B-S, Liu T-C, et al: Primary amino acid sequence and structure of human pyruvate carboxylase. *B B Acta* **1227**:46, 1994.
154. Freytag SO, Collier KJ: Molecular cloning of a cDNA for human pyruvate carboxylase. *J Biol Chem* **259**:12831, 1984.
155. Hommes FA, Schrijver J, Dias TH: Pyruvate carboxylase deficiency, studies on patients and on an animal model system, in Burman D, Holton JB, Pennock CA (eds): *Inherited Disorders of Carbohydrate Metabolism*. University Park: Press, 1979, p 239.
156. Carbone MA, MacKay N, Ling M, Cole DEC, Douglas C, Rigat B, Feigenbaum A, et al: Amerindian pyruvate carboxylase deficiency is associated with two distinct missense mutations. *Am J Hum Genet* **62: 1998.**
157. Jitrapakdee S, Booker GW, Cassady AI, Wallace JC: The rat pyruvate carboxylase gene structure. Alternate promoters generate multiple transcripts with the 5′-end heterogeneity. *J Biol Chem* **272**:20522, 1997.
158. Murphy JV, Isohashi F, Weinberg MB, Utter MT: Pyruvate carboxylase deficiency—An alleged biochemical cause of Leigh's disease. *Pediatrics* **88**:401, 1981.
159. Brunette MG, Delvin E, Hazel B, Scriver CR: Thiamine-responsive lactic acidosis in a patient with deficient low K_m pyruvate carboxylase activity in liver. *Pediatrics* **50**:702, 1972.
160. DeVivo D, Haymond MW, Leckie MP, Bussmann YL, McDougal DB, Pagliara AS: Clinical and biochemical implications of pyruvate carboxylase deficiency. *J Clin Endo Metab* **45**:1281, 1977.

161. Robinson BH, Oei J, Sherwood WG, Applegarth D, Wong L, Haworth J, Goodyer P, et al: The molecular basis for the two different clinical presentations of classical pyruvate carboxylase deficiency. *Am J Hum Genet* **36**:283, 1984.
162. Haworth JC, Robinson BH, Perry TL: Lactic acidosis due to pyruvate carboxylase deficiency. *J Inherit Metab Dis* **4**:57, 1981.
163. Gravel RA, Robinson BH: Biotin-dependent carboxylase deficiencies (propionyl-CoA and pyruvate carboxylases). *Ann N Y Acad Sci* **447**:225, 1985.
164. Robinson BH, Oei J, Saudubray JM, Marsac C, Bartlett K, Quan F, Gravel RA: The French and North American phenotypes of pyruvate carboxylase deficiency. Correlation with biotin containing protein by ^{3}H-biotin incorporation, ^{35}S-streptavidin labeling, and Northern blotting with a cloned cDNA probe. *Am J Hum Genet* **40**:50, 1987.
165. Tsuchiyama A, Oyanagi K, Hirano S, Tachi N, Sogawa H, Wagatsuma K, Nakao T, et al: A case of pyruvate carboxylase deficiency with later prenatal diagnosis of an unaffected sibling. *J Inherit Metab Dis* **6**:85, 1983.
166. Robinson BH, Oei J, Saunders M, Gravel R: [^{3}H] biotin-labeled proteins in cultured human skin fibroblasts from patients with pyruvate carboxylase deficiency. *J Biol Chem* **258**:6660, 1983.
167. Oizumi J, Donnel GN, Ng WG, Mulivor PR, Greene AE, Coriell LL: Congenital lactic acidosis associated with pyruvate carboxylase deficiency. Repository identification No. GM 6056. *Cytogenet Cell Genet* **38**:80, 1984.
168. Saudubray JM, Marsac C, Charpentier C, Cathelineau L, Besson LM, Leroux JP: Neonatal congenital lactic acidosis with pyruvate carboxylase deficiency in two siblings. *Acta Paediatr Scand* **65**:717, 1976.
169. Coude FX, Ogier H, Marsac C, Munnich A, Charpentier C, Saudubray JM: Secondary citrullinemia with hyperammonemia in four neonatal cases of pyruvate carboxylase deficiency. *Pediatrics* **68**:914, 1981.
170. Charpentier C, Tetau JM, Ogier H, Saudubray JM, Coude FX, Lemonnier A: Amino acid profile in pyruvate carboxylase deficiency: Comparison with some other metabolic disorders. *J Inherit Metab Dis* **5**:11, 1982.
171. Bartlett K, Ghneim HK, Stirk JH, Dale G, Alberti KGMM: Pyruvate carboxylase deficiency. *J Inherit Metab Dis* **7**:74, 1984.
172. Greter J, Gustafsson J, Holme E: Pyruvate carboxylase deficiency with urea cycle impairment. *Acta Paediatr Scand* **74**:982, 1985.
173. Wong LKT, Davidson GF, Applegarth DA, Dimmick JE, Norman MG, Toone JR, Pirie G, et al: Biochemical and histologic pathology in an infant with cross-reacting material (negative) pyruvate carboxylase deficiency. *Pediatr Res* **20**:274, 1986.
174. Robinson BH: Lactic Acidemia: Biochemical, clinical and genetic considerations, in Harris H, Hirschhorn K (eds): *Advances in Human Genetics*. New York: Plenum Press, 1989, p 151.
175. Van Coster RN, Fernhoff PM, DeVivo DC: Pyruvate carboxylase deficiency: A benign variant with normal development. *Pediatr Res* **30**:1, 1991.
176. Robinson BH, Halperin ML: Transport of reduced nicotinamide adenine dinucleotide into mitochondria of white adipose tissue. *Biochem J* **116**:229, 1970.
177. Shank RP, Bennett GS, Freytag SO, Campbell GL: Pyruvate carboxylase: An astrocyte-specific enzyme implicated in the replenishment of amino acid neurotransmitter pools. *Brain Res* **329**:364, 1985.
178. Atkin B: Carrier detection of pyruvate carboxylase deficiency in fibroblasts and lymphocytes. *Pediatr Res* **13**:1101, 1979.
179. Hansen TL, Christensen E, Willems JL, Trijbels JMF: A mutation of pyruvate carboxylase in fibroblasts from a patient with severe, chronic lactic acidemia. *Clin Chim Acta* **131**:39, 131.
180. Marsac C, Augerau GL, Feldman G, Wolf B, Hansen TL, Berger R: Prenatal diagnosis of pyruvate carboxylase deficiency. *Clin Chim Acta* **119**:121, 1982.
181. Robinson BH, Toone JR, Petrova-Benedict R, Dimmick JE, Oei J, Applegarth DA: Prenatal diagnosis of pyruvate carboxylase deficiency. *Prenat Diagn* **5**:67, 1985.
182. Modaressi S, Christ B, Bratke J, Zahn S, Heise T, Jungermann K: Molecular cloning, sequencing and expression of the cDNA of the mitochondrial form of phosphoenolpyruvate carboxykinase from human liver. *Biochem J* **315**:807, 1996.
183. Fiser RHJR, Melsher HL, Fisher DA: Hepatic phosphoenolpyruvate carboxylase (PEPCK) deficiency. A new cause of hypoglycemia in childhood. *Pediatr Res* **10**:60, 1974.
184. Hommes FA, Bendien K, Elema JD, Bremer HJ, Lombeck I: Two cases of phosphoenolpyruvate carboxykinase deficiency. *Acta Paediatr Scand* **65**:233, 1976.
185. Vidnes J, Sovik O: Gluconeogenesis in infancy and childhood. III. Deficiency of the extramitochondrial form of hepatic phosphoenolpyruvate carboxykinase in a case of persistent neonatal hypoglycemia. *Acta Paediatr Scand* **65**:307, 1976.
186. Robinson BH, Taylor J, Kahler S: Mitochondrial phosphoenolpyruvate carboxykinase deficiency in a child with lactic acidemia, hypotonia and failure to thrive. *Am J Hum Genet* **31**:60, 1979.
187. Clayton PT, Hyland K, Brand M, Leonard JV: Mitochondrial phosphoenolpyruvate carboxykinase deficiency. *Eur J Pediatr* **145**:46, 1986.
188. Leonard JV, Hyland K, Furukawa N, Clayton PT: Mitochondrial phosphoenolpyruvate carboxykinase deficiency. *Eur J Pediatr* **150**:198, 1991.
189. Hanson R, Garber AJ: Phosphoenolpyruvate carboxykinase, its role in gluconeogenesis. *Am J Clin Nutr* **25**:1010, 1972.
190. Robinson BH, Chow W, Petrova-Benedict R, Clarke JTR, Van Allen MI Becker LE, Boulton JE, et al: Fatal combined defects in mitochondrial multienzyme complexes in two siblings. *Eur J Pediatr* **151**:347, 1992.
191. Robinson BH: Mitochondrial defects: An overview of inborn errors associated with lacticacidemia. *Int Pediatr* **10**:82, 1995.
192. Poggi-Travert F, Martin D, Billette De Villemeur T, Bonnefont JP, Vassault A, Rabier D, Charpentier C, et al: Metabolic intermediates in lactic acidosis: Compounds, samples and interpretation. *J Inherit Metab Dis* **19**:478, 1996.
193. Rustin P, Bourgeron T, Parfait B, Chretien D, Munnich A, Rötig A: Inborn errors of the Krebs cycle: A group of unusual mitochondrial diseases in human. *Biochim Biophys Acta* **1361**:185, 1997.
194. Craigen WJ: Leigh disease with deficiency of lipoamide dehydrogenase: Treatment failure with dichloroacetate. *Pediatr Neurol* **14**:69, 1996.
195. Przyrembel H: Therapy of mitochondrial disorders. *J Inher Metab Dis* **10**:129, 1987.

CHAPTER 101

Mitochondrial Fatty Acid Oxidation Disorders

Charles R. Roe ■ Jiahuan Ding

1. Mitochondrial β-oxidation plays a major role in energy production, especially during periods of fasting. The pathway is complex and includes as many as 20 individual steps: cellular uptake of fatty acids; their activation to acyl-CoA esters; transesterification to acylcarnitines; translocation across the mitochondrial membrane; re-esterification to acyl-CoA esters; and the intramitochondrial β-oxidation spiral, generating electrons that are transferred to electron transfer flavoprotein, and acetyl-CoA, which is converted to ketone bodies in the liver. Within the spiral, each step is catalyzed by enzymes with overlapping chain-length specificities. There is also a series of enzymes specifically required for the oxidation of unsaturated fatty acids.

2. Inherited defects of 11 proteins directly involved in this process have been identified in humans. These include defects of plasma membrane carnitine transport (MIM 212140); carnitine palmitoyltransferase (CPT) I (MIM 255120) and CPT II (MIM 255110); carnitine/acylcarnitine translocase (MIM 212138); very long-chain, medium-chain, and short-chain acyl-CoA dehydrogenases [VLCAD (MIM 201475), MCAD (MIM 201450), and SCAD (MIM 201470), respectively]; 2,4-dienoyl-CoA reductase (MIM 222745); and long- and short-chain 3-hydroxyacyl-CoA dehydrogenase [LCHAD (MIM 143450), SCHAD (MIM 601609)]; and mitochondrial trifunctional protein (MIM 600890).

3. MCAD deficiency is the most common defect in the pathway and highlights many of the features that characterize patients with disorders of β-oxidation. It has been described in patients worldwide, most of whom are of northwestern European origin. MCAD deficiency is a disease primarily of hepatic fatty acid oxidation. The most frequent presentation is episodic hypoketotic hypoglycemia provoked by fasting and beginning in the first 2 years of life. Accumulation of fatty acid intermediates results in plasma and urinary metabolites, some of which are general indicators of impaired function of the β-oxidation pathway (e.g., dicarboxylic acids), while others are unique and characteristic of MCAD deficiency (e.g., octanoylcarnitine). Although the first episode may be fatal, resembling sudden infant death syndrome (SIDS), patients with MCAD deficiency are normal between episodes. Therapy includes avoidance of fasting and treatment of acute episodes with IV glucose. Diagnosis can be made by analysis of blood acylcarnitines or, in many cases, by molecular analysis because a single MCAD missense allele accounts for nearly 90 percent of the mutant MCAD genes causing this disorder.

4. Other disorders of the β-oxidation pathway are characterized by skeletal and/or cardiac muscle weakness. These include deficiencies of VLCAD, LCHAD, trifunctional protein, CPT II, SCAD, and carnitine/acylcarnitine translocase deficiencies, as well as a carnitine transport defect. In some of these disorders unique metabolites can be identified in blood or urine; the exceptions are CPT I deficiency and the carnitine transport defect, in which no abnormal metabolites are excreted. In addition, hypoketotic hypoglycemia with increased blood carnitine levels occurs in CPT I deficiency.

5. VLCAD deficiency has two distinct clinical phenotypes: hypertrophic cardiomyopathy (VLCAD-C) and a milder form manifesting recurrent hypoglycemia (VLCAD-H). They can be distinguished biochemically by different acylcarnitine profiles following incubation of fibroblasts or amniocytes with 16-$^2H_3$-palmitate.

6. Carnitine deficiency is a primary manifestation of the carnitine transport defect; patients with this defect respond dramatically to carnitine therapy. Carnitine deficiency is a secondary feature of all other β-oxidation disorders, except CPT I deficiency which is characterized by increased plasma carnitine levels.

7. Syndromes of severe maternal illness (HELLP syndrome and AFLP) have been associated with pregnancies carrying a fetus affected by LCHAD, trifunctional protein, and CPT I deficiencies. These may require emergency delivery in the last trimester. The 1528G > C mutation observed in LCHAD deficiency can often identify a mother at risk for that disease.

Disorders of fatty acid oxidation are relative newcomers to the arena of inborn errors of metabolism. The first well-documented disorders were described in the early 1970s in patients with skeletal muscle weakness or exercise-induced rhabdomyolysis and abnormalities in muscle fatty acid metabolism associated with decreased muscle carnitine[1] or carnitine palmitoyltransferase (CPT).[2] Shortly thereafter, the syndrome of "systemic carnitine deficiency" was identified; in this disorder, plasma, muscle, and liver carnitine levels were low and fatty acid oxidation in both muscle and liver was impaired.[3] Characterization of another group of inborn errors of mitochondrial fatty acid oxidation began in 1982–1983 with the description of medium-chain acyl-CoA dehydrogenase (MCAD) deficiency in patients with a disorder of fasting adaptation by several groups of investigators.[4–7] Altogether, 10 disorders affecting mitochondrial fatty acid

A list of standard abbreviations is located immediately preceding the index in each volume. Additional abbreviations used in this chapter include: CPT = carnitine palmitoyltransferase; EMG = electromyography, electromyogram; ETF = electron transfer flavoprotein; ETF:QO = electron transfer flavoprotein:ubiquinone oxidoreductase; LCAD = matrix long chain acyl coenzyme A dehydrogenase; LCHAD = long chain 3-hydroxyacyl coenzyme A dehydrogenase; MCAD = medium-chain acyl coenzyme A dehydrogenase; MCT = medium-chain triglycerides; MS/MS = tandem mass spectrometry; MTP = mitochondrial trifunctional protein; SCAD = short chain acyl coenzyme A dehydrogenase; SCHAD = short chain L-3-hydroxyacyl coenzyme A dehydrogenase; TCA = tricarboxylic acid; and VLCAD = very long chain acyl coenzyme A dehydrogenase.

oxidation and ketogenesis have been defined.[8] MCAD deficiency in particular, is a common metabolic disease, implicated in some cases of sudden infant death syndrome (SIDS) and Reye syndrome.

Fatty acid oxidation disorders may have escaped attention, in part because the pathway does not play a major role in energy production under nonfasting conditions.[9] Thus, defects in fatty acid oxidation may be clinically silent until relatively late in fasting. Another factor contributing to the delay in their recognition is that routine laboratory tests, other than qualitative urinary ketone analysis, often do not provide clues about potential defects in the fatty acid oxidation pathway. Methods to identify abnormal metabolites of fatty acids using gas chromatography coupled to mass spectrometry (GC-MS) have been available only since the mid-1970s; it is in large measure the availability of these analytic techniques, and others (tandem mass spectrometry) that have evolved more recently, that have permitted the identification of patients with fatty acid oxidation defects, even when they are well.

In this chapter, we describe the pathway of mitochondrial β-oxidation and its constituent enzymes. We then review the clinical, laboratory, pathologic metabolic, and molecular findings in patients with disorders of fatty acid oxidation resulting from deficiency of the four steps of the carnitine cycle—plasma membrane carnitine uptake, CPT I, mitochondrial membrane carnitine/acylcarnitine translocase, and CPT II; deficiency of each of the three acyl-CoA dehydrogenases—very long chain acyl-CoA dehydrogenase (VLCAD), MCAD, and short chain acyl-CoA dehydrogenase (SCAD); deficiency of three other enzymes of the β-oxidation spiral—long chain 3-hydroxyacyl-CoA dehydrogenase (LCHAD), trifunctional protein deficiency and possible short chain 3-hydroxyacyl-CoA dehydrogenase (SCHAD); and deficiency of an enzyme required for unsaturated fatty acid oxidation—2,4-dienoyl-CoA reductase. Details of inherited defects in electron transfer (electron transfer flavoprotein [ETF] and ETF:ubiquinone oxidoreductase [ETF:QO] deficiencies) and ketogenesis (3-hydroxy-3-methylglutaryl [HMG]-CoA lyase deficiency) are given in Chaps. 102 and 103, respectively.

FATTY ACID OXIDATION

Fatty acid oxidation and ketogenesis have been reviewed extensively elsewhere.[10–12] In this section, we outline the major steps in these pathways (Fig. 101-1) including uptake and activation of fatty acids by cells; the carnitine cycle, required for mitochondrial entry of fatty acids; the β-oxidation spiral; and enzymes required for the oxidation of unsaturated fatty acids.

Mobilization, Tissue Uptake, and Activation

Long chain length fatty acids are mobilized from adipose tissue stores and transported in the circulation primarily bound to albumin. During periods of fasting, fatty acids become the predominant substrate for energy production via oxidation in liver, cardiac muscle, and skeletal muscle. During prolonged aerobic exercise, fatty acid oxidation accounts for 60 percent of muscle oxygen consumption.[13] The brain does not directly utilize fatty acids for oxidative metabolism, but readily oxidizes ketone bodies derived from the acetyl-CoA and acetoacetyl-CoA produced by β-oxidation of fatty acids in the liver. Fatty acids are taken up by the liver and other tissues by concentration-dependent mechanisms; these remain poorly understood, but apparently include both saturable carrier-mediated uptake and nonsaturable diffusion.[12] A 40-kDa plasma membrane fatty acid binding protein has been characterized in rat liver, which may function in the sodium-linked ATP-dependent uptake of fatty acids.[14] Long chain fatty acid uptake is inhibited by an antibody raised against the plasma membrane fatty acid binding protein.[15] Inside the cell, fatty acids may become associated with low-molecular-weight cytosolic fatty acid binding proteins. These have been extensively characterized in intestine, liver, heart, skeletal muscle, and other tissues,[16] but their role in mediating fatty acid transfer from the cell membrane to mitochondria remains uncertain. The gene for human-skeletal-muscle-soluble 15-kDa fatty acid binding protein is on chromosome 1 pter-q31.[17] Fatty acids are activated to form CoA thioesters through the action of a series of acyl-CoA synthetases. While long chain acyl-CoA synthetase activities have been characterized in endoplasmic reticulum, peroxisomes, and mitochondria, they are believed to be products of the same gene, which in humans has been localized to chromosome 4.[18] The acyl-CoA esters can serve as substrates for triglyceride, phospholipid, and cholesteryl ester synthesis, and can also be directed to peroxisomes for β-oxidation (Chap. 130). Under fasting conditions, however, they are channeled primarily toward mitochondria for β-oxidation.

The Carnitine Cycle

The carnitine cycle is required for the transport of long chain fatty acids into the mitochondrial matrix, and includes four steps: a plasma membrane carnitine transporter which maintains the intracellular supply of carnitine; an outer mitochondrial membrane

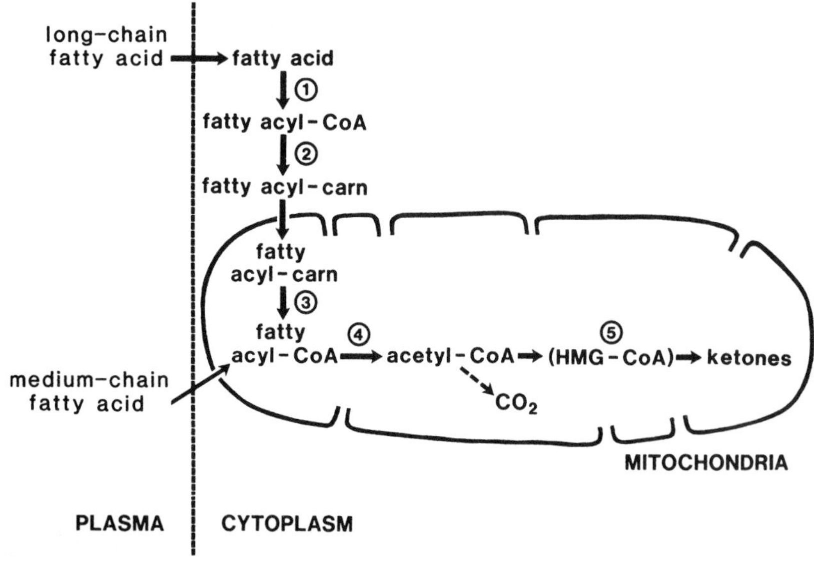

Fig. 101-1 Pathway of fatty acid entry, activation, mitochondrial uptake, β-oxidation, and ketogenesis in liver. The vertical dashed line denotes the liver-cell membrane. Numbers indicate the sequence of reactions: (1) fatty acid activation by acyl-CoA synthetase to form acyl-CoA esters; (2) transesterification of acyl-CoA by CPT I prior to mitochondrial translocation by carnitine/acylcarnitine translocase; (3) reesterification of acylcarnitine to acyl-CoA by CPT II; (4) β-oxidation spiral, each turn of which yields acetyl-CoA, which can be oxidized in the tricarboxylic acid (TCA) cycle to Co2 (broken line with arrow) or can become available for the reactions depicted by 5, the hydroxymethylglutaryl HMG-CoA pathway to form ketone bodies. Medium chain fatty acids can traverse the mitochondrial membrane without the need for carnitine-mediated transport. (*Courtesy of C.A. Stanley, M.D.*)

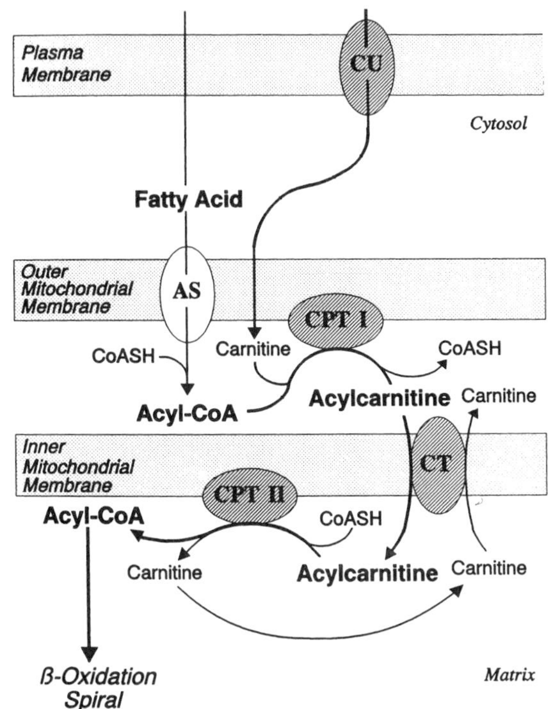

Fig. 101-2 The carnitine cycle. See text for details. AS = acyl-CoA synthetase; CoASH = coenzyme A; CPT = carnitine palmitoyltransferase; CT = carnitine/acylcarnitine translocase; CU = carnitine uptake.

CPT I that converts acyl-CoA compounds to their acylcarnitine analogues; the transmembrane transfer of acylcarnitines, mediated by carnitine/acylcarnitine translocase; and the reesterification of acylcarnitines to form acyl-CoA esters by CPT II within the mitochondrial matrix (Fig. 101-2). Fatty acids <8 carbons in length are believed to traverse the mitochondrial membrane as free acids without the need for carnitine esterification, and then are activated to form acyl-CoA esters within the matrix by the medium chain acyl-CoA synthetase.

Plasma Membrane Carnitine Uptake

There appear to be two distinct plasma membrane carnitine uptake mechanisms. In most tissues, a carnitine transporter has been identified which has a K_m for free carnitine that ranges from 2 to 10 mM in isolated cells and 20 to 200 mM in whole organs.[19] In the liver, by contrast, there is a low-affinity high-capacity transporter with a K_m for carnitine of 2 to 4 mM.[20] The liver, therefore, is dependent on the plasma level of carnitine to maintain normal tissue concentrations. There may be another low-affinity carnitine uptake system present in muscle cells,[21] which gradually develops during muscle maturation, at least in tissue culture, and which operates at carnitine concentrations between 25 and 200 mM.

Carnitine Palmitoyltransferase Activities

CPT I and CPT II are genetically and functionally distinct enzymes.[22]

CPT I is embedded in the outer mitochondrial membrane. In the liver, it is inhibited by malonyl-CoA, thereby providing the site for regulation of fatty acid oxidation and ketogenesis. By contrast, CPT II on the inner mitochondrial membrane is unaffected by malonyl-CoA. Both rat and human liver CPT II cDNAs have been cloned and sequenced, and they have remarkable similarities.[23,24] The gene in humans is on chromosome 1[24] and encodes a precursor polypeptide of 658 amino acids, including a leader peptide of 25 amino acids. The mature CPT II subunit has 633 amino acids, with a molecular weight of 66; the fully active enzyme is a homotetramer.[25] The development of specific antibodies against the individual CPT I and II proteins in rat liver[26–28] has elucidated the structural and functional relationships among the CPT proteins. Anti-CPT I antibody recognizes CPT I, but not CPT II, in rat liver. It recognizes CPT I only in liver and kidney, but not CPT I in muscle or heart. It therefore appears that CPT II is the same enzyme in all tissues of the rat, while CPT I has tissue-specific isoforms. It is likely that these results can be extrapolated to humans, given what we know about the human CPT deficiency states, described below.

Carnitine/Acylcarnitine Translocase

This enzyme facilitates the exchange of carnitine and acylcarnitines across the inner mitochondrial membrane; it also facilitates the unidirectional transport of both free carnitine and acylcarnitine across the membrane so that carnitine concentrations are the same in both cytosolic and mitochondrial matrix spaces. The translocase has been isolated from rat liver mitochondria as a 32.5-kDa protein.[29] It has highest affinity for 12- to 16-carbon acylcarnitines, lower affinity for short chain acylcarnitines, and little or no affinity for free carnitine in reconstituted liposomes.[30]

Mitochondrial β-Oxidation Spiral and Electron Transfer

It is the acyl-CoA ester that enters the pathway of mitochondrial β-oxidation. With each turn of the β-oxidation spiral, the chain length of a saturated acyl-CoA is shortened by two carbon atoms as an acetyl-CoA moiety is released. In most tissues, such as muscle and heart, acetyl-CoA is completely oxidized in the tricarboxylic acid (TCA) cycle, ultimately to carbon dioxide and water. In liver, and to a much smaller extent in kidney, acetyl-CoA produced from β-oxidation is largely converted to the ketone bodies β-hydroxybutyrate and acetoacetate via the HMG-CoA pathway (see "Hepatic Ketogenesis" below). These are then exported for final oxidation by other tissues such as brain and muscle.

Acyl-CoA compounds cycle through β-oxidation as many times as it is possible to generate two-carbon acetyl-CoA fragments; for example, palmitoyl (C16)-CoA makes seven cycles through β-oxidation. Each turn of the β-oxidation spiral is mediated by a sequence of enzymes, all of which exhibit some degree of specificity for the chain length of the acyl-CoA moiety. For a typical saturated acyl-CoA such as palmitoyl-CoA, the sequence of four enzyme steps is (a) acyl-CoA dehydrogenase, (b) 2-enoyl-CoA hydratase, (c) L-3-hydroxyacyl-CoA dehydrogenase, and (d) 3-ketoacyl-CoA (or 3-oxoacyl-CoA) thiolase.

Acyl-CoA Dehydrogenases

Acyl-CoA dehydrogenases mediate the reaction:

$$\mathrm{R-CH_2-CH_2-\underset{\displaystyle O}{\underset{\|}{C}}-SCoA+FAD \longrightarrow R-CH=CH-\underset{\displaystyle O}{\underset{\|}{C}}-SCoA+FADH_2}$$

These enzymes contain noncovalently bound FAD. In the process of inserting a double bond between the α and β (i.e., the second and third) carbons of the acyl-CoA, and forming the corresponding 2-trans-enoyl-CoA, the electrons generated by dehydrogenation are transferred from the FAD of the acyl-CoA dehydrogenase to the FAD of ETF.[31] In turn, reduced ETF is oxidized by ETF:QO and coenzyme Q, with the ultimate transfer of electrons to the electron transport chain.[32] For details of the reactions involving ETF and ETF:QO, see Chap. 103.

The acyl-CoA dehydrogenases represent the best example of the chain-length specificity of β-oxidation enzymes. Except for VLCAD, LCAD, MCAD, and SCAD and the related enzymes, isovaleryl-CoA dehydrogenase and 2-methyl branched-chain acyl-CoA dehydrogenase, are members of a family of enzymes that share many common features. They have been purified and characterized in several laboratories,[33–43] and their substrate specificities have been extensively studied.[33,37,39,40,43,44] They are homotetramers containing one molecule of FAD per subunit;[33] attachment of the FAD ligand occurs after mitochondrial import.[45] ETF is their physiological electron acceptor. In liver, VLCAD in the inner mitochondrial membrane catalyzes the first reaction in β-oxidation of acyl-CoA moieties ranging in length from 20 carbons down to 14 carbons.[46] LCAD was purified and characterized in rat liver mitochondria; it also catalyzes the dehydrogenation of acyl-CoA compounds from 12 to 18 carbons in length. MCAD acts on a broad range of acyl-CoA compounds from 12 carbons down to 4 carbons. SCAD acts only on 6- and 4-carbon compounds.

Although VLCAD also requires ETF as electron acceptor, it is structurally distinct from the other members of this family; it is a heterodimer, and it does not cross-react with antibodies raised against the other acyl-CoA dehydrogenases. The purified VLCAD enzyme has greatest activity toward palmitoyl (C16)-CoA, which overlaps with matrix LCAD. VLCAD has also been termed membrane LCAD, to distinguish it from the previously described matrix LCAD enzyme.[47]

Rat and human cDNAs for LCAD, MCAD, and SCAD have been cloned and sequenced.[48–54] Within the same species, LCAD, MCAD, and SCAD share 30 to 40 percent sequence identity, indicating that they evolved from a common ancestral gene, although they do not cross-react immunologically. This is in contrast to the same enzyme from different mammalian species, which share 87 to 90 percent sequence identity and which generally cross-react immunologically. This family of enzymes also shares similarities with the acyl-CoA oxidases that initiate peroxisomal β-oxidation.[55] The structure-function relationships of these enzymes have become increasingly understood as a result of the x-ray crystallographic detail now available with high resolution.[56] The MCAD monomer, for example, is folded into three domains: N-terminal, middle, and C-terminal. Both N- and C-terminal domains consist mainly of α-helixes; the middle domain is composed of β-sheets. FAD and substrate lay in a crevice between the N-terminal and middle domains, with the reactive side of the flavin ring buried in the crevice. The C-terminal domain forms the core of the tetramer.

2-Enoyl-CoA Hydratases

The second reaction is hydration of the 2-trans-enoyl-CoA catalyzed by 2-enoyl-CoA hydratases:

$$\mathrm{R{-}CH{=}CH{-}\underset{\underset{\displaystyle O}{\|}}{C}{-}SCoA + H_2O \longrightarrow R{-}\underset{\underset{\displaystyle OH}{|}}{CH}{-}CH_2{-}\underset{\underset{\displaystyle O}{\|}}{C}{-}SCoA}$$

This is a reversible reaction, with equilibrium favoring the product, an L-3-hydroxyacyl-CoA. There is evidence for two different 2-enoyl-CoA hydratases in mammalian tissues, a short chain enzyme commonly known as crotonase, and a long chain enzyme.[57,58] Rat crotonase cDNA has been cloned and sequenced; it encodes a 290-amino-acid precursor that is subsequently processed to a 261-amino-acid mature subunit with a molecular weight of 28.3. The fully active crotonase enzyme is a homohexamer and shares considerable sequence similarity with the enoyl-CoA hydratase component of the peroxisomal multifunctional enzyme.[59] It acts on enoyl-CoA substrates with chain lengths of four or more carbons, although enzyme activity decreases with increasing chain length. Long chain 2-enoyl-CoA hydratase, partially purified from pig heart mitochondria,[58] is inactive toward crotonyl-CoA, but is active with all longer-chain substrates (see "Trifunctional Protein," below).

L-3-Hydroxyacyl CoA Dehydrogenases

The freely reversible dehydrogenation of the hydroxy group to a keto group is catalyzed by L-3-hydroxyacyl-CoA dehydrogenases in an (NAD^+)-dependent reaction:

$$\mathrm{R-\underset{\underset{\displaystyle OH}{|}}{CH}-CH_2-\underset{\underset{\displaystyle O}{\|}}{C}-SCoA + NAD \longrightarrow R-\underset{\underset{\displaystyle O}{\|}}{C}-CH_2-\underset{\underset{\displaystyle O}{\|}}{C}-SCoA + NADH_2}$$

Two different L-3-hydroxyacyl-CoA dehydrogenases have been identified in mammalian tissues.[60] Short chain L-3-hydroxyacyl-CoA dehydrogenase (SCHAD) from pig heart is a soluble matrix enzyme with a molecular weight of 65 and is composed of two identical subunits.[61] The rat cDNA has been cloned.[62] It encodes a 34-kDa precursor that is processed to a 31-kDa mature subunit. It is active toward 3-hydroxyacyl-CoA esters from C4 to C16, but its activity declines with increasing chain length. Given its broad substrate specificity, the designation "short-chain" is misleading. Long chain L-3-hydroxyacyl-CoA dehydrogenase (LCHAD) has been partially purified and characterized in the rat liver inner mitochondrial membrane, with a native molecular weight of 230 kDa,[63] which is most active with long chain ester substrates (see "Trifunctional Protein," below).

3-Ketoacyl-CoA Thiolases

The final reaction is thiolytic cleavage of the a,b bond, catalyzed by 3-ketoacyl-CoA thiolases, in the presence of CoA:

$$\mathrm{R{-}\underset{\underset{\displaystyle O}{\|}}{C}{-}CH_2{-}\underset{\underset{\displaystyle O}{\|}}{C}{-}SCoA{+}CoASH \longrightarrow R{-}\underset{\underset{\displaystyle O}{\|}}{C}{-}SCoA{+}CoASAc}$$

where CoASH denotes coenzyme A and CoASAc acetyl coenzyme A. Although this is a reversible reaction, equilibrium considerably favors the products, acetyl-CoA and an acyl-CoA two carbons shorter than the original substrate (e.g., palmitoyl-CoA, a 16-carbon acyl-CoA, yields acetyl-CoA and myristoyl-CoA, with 14 carbons). Mitochondria contain at least two distinct 3-ketoacyl-CoA thiolases, one with a broad chain-length specificity and one specific for acetoacetyl-CoA.[64,65] Acetoacetyl-CoA thiolase is the enzyme involved in β-ketothiolase deficiency.[66] The molecular properties of the broad-specificity 3-ketoacyl-CoA thiolase are unknown (see "Trifunctional Protein" below).

Trifunctional Protein

A trifunctional protein bearing long-chain 2-enoyl-CoA hydratase, LCHAD, and long chain 3-ketoacyl-CoA thiolase activities has been purified from the inner mitochondrial membrane in both rat and human liver.[67,68] In rat liver mitochondria, the native enzyme is an octamer of 46 kDa that consists of α subunits (79 kDa) and two β-subunits called β_1 (51 kDa) and β_2 (49 kDa). The subunits are immunologically distinct. The trifunctional protein exhibits highest enoyl-CoA hydratase activity toward C10 and longer chain substrates. Its activity toward 3-hydroxyacyl-CoA compounds also differs from that of the corresponding short chain hydroxyacyl-CoA dehydrogenase: optimal activity is found with C12 to C16 compounds, in contrast to SCHAD, which has its optimum around C6. Similarly, ketoacyl-CoA thiolase activity of the trifunctional protein is considerably higher with C12 to C16 substrates than is the acetoacetyl-CoA thiolase. Thus, the membrane-bound trifunctional protein contains all three of the enzyme activities with long chain specificity that had been previously purified from various sources. It has been demonstrated that the LCHAD activity previously purified from human liver mitochondria[63] likewise resides in a trifunctional protein.[68]

Unsaturated Fatty Acid Oxidation

Unsaturated acyl-CoA compounds, such as the CoA esters of oleic (C18:1), linoleic (C18:2), and linolenic (C18:3) acids, are also oxidized by the same series of reactions, until the double bond is

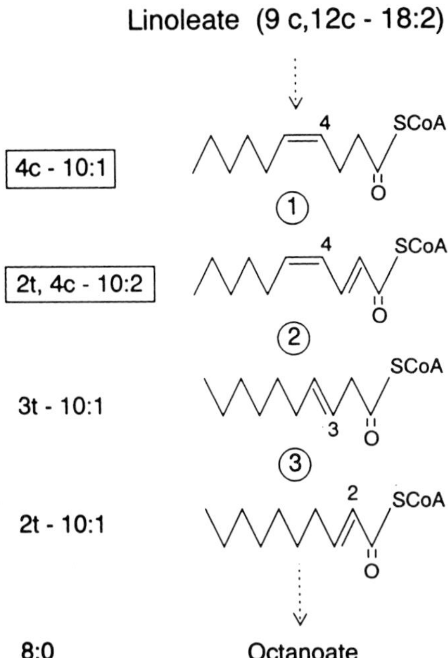

Fig. 101-3 Mitochondrial β-oxidation of linoleic acid. See text for details. Step 1: MCAD inserts a double bond in the C2 position of 4-*cis*-C10:1. Step 2: 2,4-Dienoyl-CoA reductase reduces the series of double bonds, producing the 3-*trans* intermediate. Step 3: D3, D2-Enoyl-CoA isomerase converts this to 2-*trans*-enoyl-CoA for further β-oxidation.

reached (Fig. 101-3).[12] The double bonds in these compounds are usually in the *cis* configuration and extend either from an even-numbered carbon (e.g., the 12-*cis* double bond of linoleic and linolenic acids) or an odd-numbered carbon (e.g., the 9-*cis* double bond of oleic, linoleic, and linolenic acids). Linoleic acid, with its double bonds in the 9- and 12-carbon positions, undergoes three cycles of β-oxidation until 3-*cis*,6-*cis*-dodecadienoyl (C12:2)-CoA is formed.

Δ^3, Δ^2-Enoyl-CoA isomerase converts it to 2-*trans*,6-*cis* -C12:2-CoA. One round of β-oxidation yields 4-*cis*-decenoyl (C10:1)-CoA, which is dehydrogenated by MCAD to 2-*trans*, 4-*cis*-decadienoyl (C10:2)-CoA. Then, the second auxiliary enzyme, 2-4-dienoyl-CoA reductase, catalyzes its reduced nicotinamide adenine dinucleotide phosphate (NADPH)-dependent reduction to 3-*trans*-C10:1-CoA. Isomerization of this compound by the Δ^3, Δ^2-enoyl-CoA isomerase yields an intermediate, 2-*trans*-C10:1-CoA, that reenters the β-oxidation spiral for complete degradation.

The degradation of fatty acids with odd-numbered double bonds, such as oleate (9-*cis*-C18:1), was thought to proceed via β-oxidation to 5-*cis*-tetradecenoyl (C14:1)-CoA, and then to 3-*cis*-dodecenoyl (C12:1)-CoA, with isomerization to 2-*trans*-C12:1-CoA and further oxidation to decanoate. In vitro studies with VLCAD deficient fibroblast lines incubated with oleate or linoleate reveal that all oxidation ceases at the level of 5-*cis*-tetradecenoyl (C14:1)-CoA and 5-*cis*-8-*cis*-tetradecadienoyl (C14:2)-CoA, respectively indicating that in human cells VLCAD is the enzyme responsible for dehydrogenation of substrates with the 5-*cis* double bond. It has also been suggested[69] that the 5-*cis* intermediate is directly reduced by an NADPH-dependent reductase; however, the "5-*cis* reductase" has not been purified or characterized. There appears to be another possible explanation, involving a newly identified NADPH-dependent dienoyl-CoA isomerase.[70] 2-*trans*,5-*cis*-C8:2-CoA produced by dehydrogenation of 5-*cis*-C8:1 is isomerized by enoyl-CoA isomerase to the 3-*trans*,5-*cis*-C8:2 intermediate. This is a substrate for dienoyl-CoA isomerase, producing 2-*trans*,4-*trans*-C8:2. The NADPH-dependent dienoyl-CoA reductase converts this to a 3-*trans* product that is isomerized by Δ^3, Δ^2-enoyl-CoA isomerase to the 2-*trans* intermediate for reentry into the β-oxidation spiral. These other possibilities do not seem to be operational in VLCAD deficient cell lines. Δ^3, Δ^2-Enoyl-CoA isomerase activity is found in two distinct mitochondrial proteins,[71,72] which differ in structure and in their relative activities toward substrates of different chain length. One is an enzyme with its greatest activity toward the 6-carbon 3-enoyl-CoA; it is a homodimer with a subunit molecular weight of 29.3 and has sequence similarities to the amino terminal half of the peroxisomal multifunctional enzyme. The other is a 200-kDa protein with a preference for 10- and 12-carbon substrates;[71] it does not cross-react with antibodies against the short chain enzyme. 2,4-Dienoyl-CoA reductase has been purified from a number of sources, including beef liver,[73] rat liver,[74] and *Escherichia coli*.[73] The gene encodes a monomer of 32 kDa.[74]

Odd-Chain Fatty Acid Oxidation. These acyl-CoA compounds are oxidized by the same series of reactions described above, until the 3-carbon moiety, propionyl-CoA, is formed. This is then degraded by the biotin-dependent enzyme, propionyl-CoA carboxylase.[11]

Hepatic Ketogenesis. Liver is virtually the only tissue which can channel the product of fatty acid β-oxidation, acetyl-CoA, into ketone body formation.[10,11] Especially under conditions of fasting, when carbohydrate stores are depleted, the rate of hepatic ketogenesis is increased. This provides an auxiliary source of substrate for brain oxidative metabolism, sparing glucose oxidation and preventing proteolysis. Acetoacetyl-CoA derived from the last turn of the β-oxidation spiral combines with acetyl-CoA to form HMG-CoA, catalyzed by HMG-CoA synthase. HMG-CoA lyase cleaves HMG-CoA to form acetyl-CoA and acetoacetate, which is reduced to D-3-hydroxybutyrate by the NAD^+-linked D-3-hydroxybutyrate dehydrogenase within mitochondria.

Peroxisomal and Microsomal Fatty Acid Oxidation

Peroxisomal β-oxidation closely parallels the mitochondrial process. It differs from mitochondrial oxidation, however, in some key features: transport of long chain acyl-CoA compounds into peroxisomes does not require carnitine; the first step is catalyzed by a long chain acyl-CoA oxidase (not a dehydrogenase), which does not use ETF as its electron acceptor; the 2-enoyl-CoA hydratase and 3-hydroxyacyl-CoA dehydrogenase steps are carried out by a multifunctional enzyme which also has Δ^3, Δ^2-enoyl-CoA isomerase activity; and peroxisomal β-oxidation apparently proceeds only to the medium-chain acyl-CoA level. Methyl-branched fatty acids such as phytanate and pristanate are sequentially degraded first in the peroxisome down to the level of 2,4-dimethylnonanoyl-CoA, which is converted to an acylcarnitine that is exported. This compound requires carnitine acylcarnitine translocase and CPT II for further oxidation in the mitochondrion.[75] For details of peroxisomal metabolic pathways and the clinical disorders associated with peroxisomal dysfunction, see Chaps. 129 to 132.

Microsomal ω-oxidation of fatty acids is mediated by a cytochrome P450-linked mixed function oxygenase, which catalyzes ω-hydroxylation in the presence of molecular oxygen and NADPH.[76] An NAD^+-dependent oxidation subsequently converts the ω-hydroxy fatty acid into a dicarboxylic acid. The resulting dicarboxylic acid can be transported to the mitochondrial matrix or to peroxisomes for β-oxidation.[77] Dicarboxylic acids may be formed because mitochondrial β-oxidation is overloaded or genetically impaired, and are rapidly and quantitatively excreted in urine. They are also present in the urine of patients fed a diet high in medium-chain triglycerides (MCT).[78] A similar hydroxylation reaction occurs at the ω-1 position, probably using the same microsomal oxygenase pathway.[76] Microsomal α-oxidation degrades fatty acids one carbon at a time; 3-methyl-branched chain fatty acids (e.g., phytanic acid) require an α-oxidation step which uses NADPH and molecular oxygen.[11] For further details, see Chap. 130.

Regulation of Fatty Acid Oxidation

The regulation of fatty acid oxidation in mammals by hormones, competing substrates, cofactors, and diet has been reviewed extensively.[10] Numerous studies have related rates of fatty acid oxidation to the concentrations of free fatty acids mobilized from adipose tissue which are then available for oxidative metabolism. In the transition from the fed to the fasted state, the liver converts from glucose uptake and fatty acid synthesis to glucose production, fatty acid synthesis to glucose production, fatty acid oxidation, and ketogenesis.

Hormonal control of fatty acid oxidation is exerted at the level of substrate mobilization from adipose tissue and at the level of CPT I. Insulin inhibits lipolysis in adipose tissue, decreasing the level of free fatty acids available for oxidative metabolism; it also stimulates lipogenesis and synthesis of malonyl-CoA, an inhibitor of CPT I, and therefore inhibits fatty acid oxidation. Glucagon stimulates hepatic fatty acid oxidation indirectly, by inhibiting acetyl-CoA carboxylase and thereby reducing tissue levels of malonyl-CoA, which results in enhanced activity of CPT I. Therefore, in the fed state, in which the glucagon:insulin ratio is low, the liver directs fatty acid metabolism toward synthesis. In the fasting state, the elevated glucagon:insulin ratio directs fatty acids toward mitochondria for oxidation.

GENETIC DEFECTS OF MITOCHONDRIAL β-OXIDATION

The inherited disorders of mitochondrial β-oxidation are detailed in this section, with emphasis on the clinical, biochemical, and metabolic derangements associated with each of them, their pathogenesis, and when known, their molecular basis. The concluding section describes a general approach to patients in whom a fatty acid oxidation defect is suspected.

Defects of the Carnitine Cycle

Carnitine Transport Defect

Clinical Presentations. An inherited defect in the plasma membrane transport of carnitine was first described in 1988.[79–87] In one review,[82] the ethnic distribution included Caucasian, African-American, North African Arab, Asian Indian, Mexican, and Chinese; the parents were consanguineous in five families. There are two general types of clinical presentation associated with this defect, illustrated by the following case reports.

Case 1. A 3.5-month-old girl,[79] the first child of unrelated parents, previously had been in good health. Four weeks before her initial episode, she had been switched from a cow's-milk formula containing carnitine to a carnitine-free soy-protein formula. She was found limp, unresponsive, and apneic after an overnight fast. Blood glucose was 0.4 mM (7 mg%); amino acid and electrolyte levels were normal. Urine contained only trace ketones and no dicarboxylic acids. Her liver was enlarged, and liver function tests were abnormal [aspartate aminotransferase (AST), 248 IU/L alanine aminotransferase (ALT), 149 IU/liter]. Plasma carnitine was < 1 μM (normal, 40 to 60), and muscle and liver carnitine concentrations were < 5 percent of those found in comparably aged controls. Cardiac evaluation included a normal chest film, sinus tachycardia by ECG, and increased wall thickness of the left ventricle and septum; she had a normal shortening fraction. Her response to IV glucose therapy was rapid. She was treated with long-term oral L-carnitine (100 to 120 mg/kg day) and supplemental nasogastric feeding. Her parents were advised to prevent her from fasting. She had no further episodes of fasting hypoglycemia, but had myoclonic seizures, hypotonia, and delayed mental development. She died from complications of intestinal adhesions after placement of a feeding gastrostomy. There was no family history of SIDS, Reye syndrome, or unexplained cardiac, muscle, or neurologic disease. An unaffected sib had normal plasma carnitine levels.

Case 2. A boy, the second child of distantly related parents, presented at 3.5 years with cardiomegaly and a grade 2 systolic murmur.[85] The ECG was abnormal, and echocardiogram showed left ventricular hypertrophy and dilatation, with greatly reduced left ventricular ejection fraction. He had modest hepatomegaly. Muscle strength and tone were normal. Cardiomegaly increased over the next year and symptoms of congestive heart failure developed. He had muscle weakness; muscle biopsy showed lipid deposition in type 1 fibers with atrophy of type 2 fibers; electromyography (EMG) and nerve conduction studies were normal. He was anemic (hemoglobin [Hb], 10 g/dl) and had modest elevation of AST (31 IU/L) and CPK (138 IU/L). There were no episodes of hypoglycemia. Plasma carnitine was < 5 uM. He began to experience severe dyspnea, and had two episodes of cardiac decompensation with respiratory distress. L-Carnitine therapy (174 mg/kg/day) resulted in rapid and dramatic clinical improvement. His cardiothoracic ratio declined, physical activity increased, and exercise tolerance normalized. A previous male sib died at 2 years with cardiomegaly and anemia; postmortem examination showed fatty infiltration of liver and heart.

Half of the reported patients presented early (3 months to 2.5 years) with episodes characterized by hypoketotic hypoglycemia, hyperammonemia, and elevated transaminases, some with cardiomyopathy and/or skeletal muscle weakness. Cardiomyopathy alone was the presenting sign in the other half of cases; this was frequently of later onset (1 to 7 years), progressive, and associated with skeletal muscle weakness, but without evidence of hypoglycemia. These differences in presentation most likely reflect the occurrence of a period of fasting long enough to result in hypoglycemia (and hence early recognition) before the cardiac and skeletal muscle weakness became apparent. In one family, an affected sib presented early with hypoglycemia, while another presented later with cardiomyopathy and weakness.[82] Several patients were noted to have mild to moderate anemia which responded poorly to iron therapy.[81] The very low plasma carnitine level (< 10 μM) in patients with these clinical findings, especially in the absence of a significant dicarboxylic aciduria, is virtually pathognomonic of the carnitine transport defect. With the exception of one case,[81] pretreatment plasma carnitine levels have been < 10 μM.

Diagnosis. The defect in plasma membrane carnitine transport is expressed in muscle, kidney, leukocytes, and fibroblasts, and presumably in heart, although this has not been measured. Carnitine uptake by fibroblasts and leukocytes from patients is < 10 percent of control rates.[81–84,86,87] Fibroblasts from parents have intermediate rates of carnitine uptake, consistent with heterozygosity. The carnitine transporter is able to maintain a positive gradient across the plasma membrane at low (< 5 μM) extracellular carnitine concentrations in both controls and heterozygotes; above this concentration, there is a linear increase in carnitine uptake by cells, reflecting passive diffusion. Patient fibroblasts cannot maintain a gradient, so the intracellular carnitine level passively follows the extracellular concentration. The failure to transport carnitine into these cells means that intracellular carnitine concentrations are considerably reduced.[17,100] The carnitine transport system in fibroblasts is potently inhibited by medium and long chain acylcarnitines.[82] This may provide an explanation for the secondary carnitine deficiency noted in other β-oxidation defects; the acylcarnitines which accumulate in those disorders may induce a defect in the tissue uptake of free carnitine similar to but less severe than that found in patients with the genetic transport defect.

The oxidation of long chain fatty acids is reported to be low[83] or normal[86] in fibroblasts from a few patients. Addition of carnitine to the medium enhances fatty acid oxidation in all cases studied; under the same conditions there is little or no effect of exogenous carnitine on fatty acid oxidation in control cells.

Pathogenesis. This disorder is a true primary systemic carnitine deficiency for several reasons: It results in extremely low plasma and tissue carnitine levels; it is not secondary to a mitochondrial defect of organic acid oxidation; and patients with this disorder respond dramatically to carnitine therapy. It results from a failure of high-affinity carnitine uptake into several tissues, including muscle, heart, and kidney, but not liver. The failure to concentrate carnitine in cardiac and skeletal muscle means that there is insufficient carnitine to support fatty acid oxidation. The defect in renal transport is evident by studies of carnitine withdrawal. In normal individuals, efficient renal conservation of carnitine permits plasma levels to remain normal even in the face of extended periods of carnitine withdrawal. By contrast, levels of plasma carnitine in affected patients fall to near zero within a few days of stopping carnitine supplementation. During this time, carnitine excretion in urine remains high; even at low plasma levels, the fractional excretion of free carnitine remains at 100 percent of the filtered load (normal, <5 percent). Failure to reabsorb carnitine in the kidney results in very low plasma carnitine levels, which, in turn, diminish the hepatic uptake of carnitine by passive diffusion. Hence, ketogenesis is impaired; it is restored to normal on carnitine supplementation. The accumulated acyl-CoA compounds become substrates for other cellular processes, including peroxisomal β-oxidation and triglyceride synthesis. Peroxisomal β-oxidation produces intermediates such as medium chain fatty acids and dicarboxylic acids, which do not require carnitine for entry into mitochondria. Their complete oxidation in mitochondria explains the lack of dicarboxylic aciduria in patients with this disorder.

Treatment with L-carnitine restores plasma carnitine levels to nearly normal, but muscle carnitine levels rise very slightly, consistent with a failure of carnitine transport into this tissue. It is remarkable that muscle function can be nearly normalized in these patients when their muscle carnitine levels remain less than 10 percent of control levels. This suggests that the normal muscle carnitine level greatly exceeds that necessary to support fatty acid oxidation. While heart carnitine levels have not been measured, there was objective clinical improvement in cardiac ventricular function in one patient, although this remained subnormal even after months of therapy.[81] Therefore, the possibility of later recurrence of cardiomyopathy cannot be ruled out.

Molecular Aspects. Physiological studies suggested the participation of multiple sodium ion-dependent transporters in carnitine movement across cell plasma membranes.[11,79,88,89] Recently, a cDNA of a second member of the human organic cation transporter (OCTN) family, *OCTN2* (GenBank AB015050), has been cloned which has a high similarity (78.5 percent) to human *OCTN1*.[90,91] The full-length *OCTN2* cDNA encodes a polypeptide of 557 amino acids that has many of the characteristics of a high-affinity, sodium ion-dependent carnitine transporter.[91] Furthermore, the *OCTN2* structural gene mapped to 5q31.2-32, the same region shown to harbor the gene for systemic carnitine deficiency in a large Japanese pedigree.[92]

These results focused attention on *OCTN2* as a candidate gene for systemic carnitine. Subsequently, Tsuji and colleagues[309] and others[310,311] identified *OCTN2* mutations in patients with systemic carnitine deficiency including deletions and nonsense mutations. Additionally Tsuji and colleagues surveyed plasma carnitine levels in 973 unrelated Japanese white-collar workers. Fourteen consistently had values <5 percentile, and among these, *OCTN2* mutations were identified in nine. These included W132X (three individuals); S467C (four individuals); W283C (one individual); and M179L (one individual). All but M179L had functional significance when expressed in HEK cells. These results suggest a carrier frequency of about 1 percent in the Japanese population. Furthermore, echocardiographic studies suggested that these heterozygotes were predisposed to asymptomatic cardiac hypertrophy.[312]

Carnitine Palmitoyltransferase I (CPT I) Deficiency. Despite the existence of two isoforms of this enzyme, muscle and liver, mainly the hepatic form of the disease has been documented. This could be due, in part, to the fact that the muscle isoform is not expressed in fibroblasts or amniocytes making a direct muscle biopsy necessary to detect a form of the disease expressed only in heart, muscle, or both. Ten patients (five male, five female) with CPT I deficiency in eight families have been reported. The ethnic origins of patients with the hepatic form of the disease include Caucasian, Middle Eastern, Central American Indian, Inuit, and Asian Indian.[93,94–102]

Clinical Presentation. The first presenting illness is stereotypical and is usually associated with fasting (viral infection, diarrhea). Coma, seizures, hepatomegaly, and hypoketotic hypoglycemia dominate the picture. Elevated CPK, attributable to the MM isozyme, has been seen in acute episodes in two sibs,[99] but without myoglobinuria, and not in other patients. There is no evidence of chronic muscle weakness and cardiomyopathy has not been noted in any patients with CPT I deficiency. Initial illness has occurred between 8 and 18 months, except for one patient who presented as a newborn. In the absence of urinary ketones, there is little or no dicarboxylic aciduria. Plasma carnitine levels are normal to elevated (total, 55 to 141 μM; free, 45 to 93 μM). All but one patient is alive. Renal tubular acidosis was noted in one patient.[100] Persistent neurologic deficit, probably resulting from the initial insult, is common. Recurrent episodes are common and generally have been successfully treated with glucose infusion. They have been avoided by preventing fasting. Frequent feeding and replacement of dietary long chain fat with MCT have been beneficial.

The classical findings of hypoketotic hypoglycemia without dicarboxylic aciduria and with a high plasma carnitine level (both total and free) distinguish CPT I deficiency from the other known defects of the pathway. Acylcarnitines in urine have been examined in only one patient; only acetylcarnitine, the normal species, was excreted.[99] The plasma acylcarnitine profile was normal.

Recently, as with LCHAD deficiency (see below), an Inuit mother was reported to have acute fatty liver of pregnancy (AFLP) while delivering a fetus affected with the hepatic form of CPT I deficiency.[103]

Diagnosis. The definitive diagnosis of CPT I deficiency is made by measuring enzyme activity in fibroblasts, leukocytes, or solid tissues. CPT I activity is measured as palmitoyl-L-[methyl-^{14}C]-carnitine formed from L-[methyl-^{14}C]-carnitine and palmitoyl-CoA in the presence of albumin and carnitine. CPT I, unlike CPT II, is inhibited by malonyl-CoA. Among eight patients, CPT I activity in fibroblasts was 9 to 16 percent of control values. All patients had normal levels of CPT II activity in their fibroblasts. The parents of two sibs with CPT I deficiency had intermediate levels of CPT I activity in their fibroblasts, consistent with heterozygosity. CPT I deficiency has been demonstrated in liver, but not in muscle,[94] of several patients. This supports the hypothesis that CPT I is different in liver and muscle,[96] as in the rat.[28] Fibroblasts from patients with CPT I deficiency oxidize long chain fatty acids poorly, at 5 to 26 percent of control rates.[94,95,99,100,104]

Pathogenesis. CPT I is the enzyme that converts long chain acyl-CoA substrates to their respective acylcarnitines for transport into mitochondria. Deficiency of the enzyme in liver results in a failure of acylcarnitine formation and hence little or no entry of long chain substrates into mitochondria for oxidative metabolism. As is the case with the carnitine transport defect, accumulated long chain acyl-CoA compounds undergo alternative metabolism, producing medium chain intermediates that are fully oxidized by mitochondria. This also provides the rationale for treatment of CPT I-deficient patients with diets containing MCT. The lack of significant muscle findings in most patients with CPT I deficiency is consistent with the normal activity of this enzyme in muscle. It is not easy to explain the striking CPK elevations in the two sibs with hepatic CPT I deficiency whose skeletal muscle CPT I activity was entirely normal.

Molecular Aspects. Two different isoforms of CPT I have been described with distinct tissue distributions.[105,106,109] The hepatic isoform (CPT IA) is expressed in liver, kidney, fibroblasts, and heart; the muscle form (CPT IB) is expressed in skeletal muscle, heart, brown and white adipocytes, and testes. These two forms, the CPT IA and the CPT IB, are encoded by different genes localized on chromosome 11q13.1-13.5 and 22q13.31-13.32, respectively.[107,108] The CPT IA mRNA (GenBank L39211) is approximately 4.7 kb and encodes a protein of 773 amino acids;[109] the CPT IB mRNA (GenBank Y08683) is approximately 3.1 kb and encodes a protein of 772 amino acids.[108,110,111]

Molecular analysis of CPT IA cDNA from one patient with CPT I deficiency revealed a homozygous 1361A > G nucleotide substitution resulting in the missense mutation D454G. The D454G CPT IA cDNA displayed only 2 percent of the activity of expressed wild-type CPT IA.[112] So far, no information is available regarding mutations in CPT IB.

The primary structure of CPT IA and CPT IB have also been established in rat. The nucleotide sequence of the rat CPT IA cDNA and the predicted amino acid sequence of the protein are very similar to those of the human CPT IA (82 percent and 88 percent identity, respectively).[109] The rat CPT IB gene (GenBank AF029875) has 19 exons.[113] The nucleotide sequence of the coding region show 85 percent homology to the human CPT IB cDNA. Interestingly, mutant rat CPT IA protein lacking the first 18 N-terminal amino acid residues still had activity and kinetic properties similar to wild-type of the CPT IA but was insensitive to malonyl-CoA inhibition due to a marked reduction in affinity for malonyl CoA compared to the wild-type liver isoform.[114]

Recently, Yu et al.[115] hypothesized the existence of additional isoforms in heart to account for unique kinetic characteristics of enzyme activity. Hybridization and PCR screening of a human cardiac cDNA library revealed the expression of two novel CPT I isoforms, generated by alternative splicing of the CPT IB transcript. These are present in heart, skeletal muscle, and liver, in differing relative concentrations. The novel isoforms of CPT IB could exhibit unique features with respect to outer mitochondrial membrane topology and response to physiological and pharmacologic inhibitors.

Carnitine/Acylcarnitine Translocase Deficiency

Clinical Presentation. Stanley et al. described the first patient with this defect in mitochondrial acylcarnitine transport.[116] There are two phenotypes for this disorder: severe neonatal onset with cardiomyopathy (no survivors)[117–120] and a milder phenotype with hypoglycemia but no cardiomyopathy.[121,122]

Case Reports: Neonatal Onset. A Caucasian male infant presented with acute cardiorespiratory collapse at 36 h of age associated with fasting stress and ventricular arrhythmias for several days. Over the next 2 years, he had occasional episodes of hypoglycemic coma, recurrent vomiting, gastroesophageal reflux, and mild chronic hyperammonemia. He had severe, chronic muscle weakness and mild hypertrophic cardiomyopathy. Continuous nasogastric feeding of a low-fat, high-carbohydrate diet failed to normalize his muscle strength, although his mental development was normal. At 2.5 years of age, he deteriorated rapidly, with increasing weakness and liver failure; he died following aspiration pneumonia. His total plasma carnitine was low (30 μM), most of which (22 μM) was in the long chain esterified fraction. During treatment with carnitine and a high-carbohydrate diet, his total plasma carnitine level was within normal limits, but it was almost all esterified, including not only long chain acylcarnitines (C16:0, C18:1, C18:2), but also the corresponding dicarboxylic species as acylcarnitines. An older brother died in the newborn period with a similar episode of ventricular arrhythmias and cardiorespiratory arrest; his defect was not documented.[116]

Mild Phenotype. First-cousin Pakistani parents had seven children, four of whom were healthy. One died at 3 months of age without explanation; another died at 48 h of age with undetectable blood glucose and developed ventricular tachycardia and seizures. Autopsy revealed severe steatosis involving myocardium, liver, and kidneys. The seventh child was diagnosed with carnitine acylcarnitine translocase deficiency by analysis of fibroblasts and was found to have a residual activity of 3.0 to 6.8 percent of controls. (The severe neonatal form has no detectable activity.) This child had recurrent hypoglycemia but no cardiac involvement and had normal growth and development at 3 years of age.[122]

Diagnosis. Translocase deficiency was first demonstrated in fibroblasts.[116] The patient's cells had less than 1 percent of control enzyme activity, while cells from his parents had half-normal levels, suggesting autosomal recessive inheritance. Long chain fatty acid oxidation (< 5 percent of control rates with palmitic and oleic acids) was profoundly reduced in fibroblasts. Analysis of blood acylcarnitines by tandem mass spectrometry is also a rapid and simple test to identify the presence of this disease although the profile of acylcarnitines observed is identical for translocase deficiency and CPT II deficiency requiring direct assay of fibroblasts for the definitive diagnosis.

Pathogenesis. A failure to transport long chain (C10 to C18) acylcarnitines formed by CPT I leads to their accumulation along with long chain acyl-CoA intermediates and free long chain fatty acids outside of the mitochondrion. It is not clear which of these intermediates is responsible for the pathogenesis of this deficiency. It is of interest that despite the translocase deficiency, short chain acylcarnitines are excreted in urine and are present in plasma. These include propionylcarnitine, butyryl-/isobutyryl-carnitine, and isovaleryl-/2-methylbutyryl-carnitine. These are produced in the mitochondrial matrix and are derived from the branched-chain amino acid pathways. Incubation of cells from children with the severe neonatal phenotype with $^{2}H_{3}$-L-carnitine reveals that there is a normal exchange of both labeled and unlabeled short chain acylcarnitines across the mitochondrial membrane even when the classical translocase is absent. These results suggest the presence of another translocating system serving the short chain (C3 to C5) intermediates of branched-chain amino acid degradation (Roe DS, Roe CR, et al., unpublished observations).

Treatment of translocase deficiency focuses on the need to control endogenous lipolysis due to fasting or infection as well as attempting to maintain normal glucose homeostasis through frequent feeding. Diets (formulas) containing medium chain triglycerides also form the primary treatment strategy. Aggressive intervention during the neonatal period appears to be vital to survival.[122]

Molecular Aspects. A human carnitine/acylcarnitine translocase cDNA has been cloned[123] and disease-causing mutations have been identified. A C insertion in the cytosine-rich region of bp 955 to 959, the first mutation identified in a patient with mild translocase symptoms, results in a frameshift extending the length of the protein from 301 to 322 amino acids.[123] In other patients, deletions in the coding segment of the transcript suggesting abnormal splicing have been observed.[124,125] Sequencing the intron of the translocase gene from these patients should elucidate the primary mutation that leads to aberrant splicing. Very recently, a 558C > T mutation leading to a premature stop codon has been identified.[126] This nonsense mutation results in a truncated protein of 166 amino acids in a translocase patient with the severe phenotype. The family history was notable for the death of seven siblings in the neonatal period. The parents were first cousins. In another severe translocase patient, a 241G > A substitution producing a G81R missense mutation was reported.[127] This mutation is located in the second membrane-spanning region of the translocase. In addition, a 459C > T substitution producing the missense mutation R133W has been detected in a compound heterozygous patient with severe translocase deficiency. The second mutation has not yet been identified.[125] These results indicate significant genetic heterogeneity in translocase deficiency.

Carnitine Palmitoyltransferase II (CPT II) Deficiency (MIM 600650)

Clinical Presentations. There are three distinct clinical forms of CPT II deficiency. The most common is the "classical" muscular form of CPT II deficiency, described originally in 1973.[2] Patients with this defect generally present in adulthood with episodic myoglobinuria and muscle weakness prompted by prolonged exercise.[128] Occasionally, these episodes have been prompted by fasting, mild infections, emotional stress, or cold exposure. Most patients present with their first episode between 15 and 30 years of age. Most affected patients are males, although the disorder is inherited in an autosomal recessive manner. Between episodes, serum CPK levels are usually normal. Fasting ketogenesis is decreased in some patients, although they rarely show the acute decompensation common in other defects of β-oxidation. Carnitine levels are usually normal in plasma and in tissues. Cardiac dysfunction is rarely seen. Renal failure, as a result of episodes of myoglobinuria, is found in 25 percent of patients. Permanent muscle weakness is rare. Lipid storage in muscle is found in 20 percent of patients; hepatic lipid storage is rare.

An often fatal infantile form of CPT II deficiency has been recognized in six patients.[129–135] The first complete report[129] described a 3-month-old boy with coma, seizures, hypoketotic hypoglycemia without dicarboxylic aciduria, hepatomegaly, cardiomegaly, cardiac arrhythmia, and low plasma and tissue carnitine levels associated with an increase in the long chain acylcarnitine fraction. He died at 17 months of age. Another patient presented at 2 years with fasting hypoglycemia and cardiomyopathy and is still alive.[132] One diagnosis was made prenatally.[133]

The remaining patients reported with CPT II deficiency have presented in the newborn period and died.[130,131,134,135] Hypoketotic hypoglycemia and cardiomyopathy, as well as skeletal muscle involvement point to the defect in these patients affecting multiple tissues. Renal dysgenesis was noted in three patients,[131,133] a feature not observed in other fatty acid oxidation defects although it has been described in some patients with glutaric acidemia type II (see Chap. 103).

Diagnosis. The specific enzyme defect, CPT II deficiency, has been demonstrated in skeletal muscle mitochondria from patients with the adult-onset disease. In spite of the primarily muscular presentation, their enzyme defect is not restricted to muscle, but is expressed in other tissues, such as liver, fibroblasts, and leukocytes. At least some of the phenotypic heterogeneity can be explained by the degree of enzyme deficit. Generally, patients with the late onset form have a partial deficiency of CPT II in fibroblasts, approximately 25 percent of control levels, while those with the more severe neonatal and infantile forms generally have < 10 percent of control activity.[135] Normal rates of long chain fatty acid oxidation have been found in fibroblasts from most, but not all, patients with adult onset CPT II deficiency,[94,135] while cells from patients with the severe infantile form[129,135] have had < 15 percent of control rates. Although not distinguishable from the profile of carnitine-acylcarnitine translocase deficiency, the blood acylcarnitine profile is consistently abnormal in both of these defects with elevations of palmitoylcarnitine, oleoylcarnitine and linoleoylcarnitine reflecting the absence or reduced levels (adult onset) of either translocase or CPT II.

Pathogenesis. In this disorder, long-chain acylcarnitines are translocated across the inner mitochondrial membrane, but are not efficiently converted to their corresponding acyl-CoAs. Hence, there is accumulation of long chain acylcarnitines in the mitochondrial matrix. These must be transported out of mitochondria, as suggested by the prominent long chain acylcarnitine species seen in plasma. It has been speculated[129,130,132] that increased concentrations of long chain acylcarnitines in patients with the severe form of CPT II deficiency, as in the case of translocase deficiency,[116] may promote cardiac arrhythmia. This has been described in a cat heart model,[136] but has not been proven in humans. The absence of arrhythmia in children with the cardiomyopathic form of VLCAD deficiency while receiving oral or intravenous carnitine during illness makes this suggestion seem unlikely in humans (Slonim A, unpublished results).

Molecular Aspects. The human *CPT II* gene, spanning about 20 kb is located at 1p32.[24,137] Its five exons encode a 658 amino acid protein including a 25-residue N-terminal leader peptide.[24,138] The cloning of the *CPT II* gene has enabled the identification of mutations in CPT II patients, and the correlation of mutant genotype to clinical phenotype. In 1992, the first mutation, R631C, was identified in an infant presenting with hypoketotic hypoglycemia and cardiomyopathy.[139] Several *CPT II* mutations have recently been detected (Fig. 101-4). The common mutation in adult CPT II deficiency is S113L,[140,141] while most other mutations have been described only in a single patient.[142–146] In addition, three apparently normal variants, F352C, V368I and M647V, have been identified.[139,146,147] Some of the functionally significant missense mutations have occurred on one of these polymorphic variants. For example, the disease-producing mutation, P227L, occurs on an allele with V368L. The association of P227L with V368L in several patients. In contrast, one patient carrying the S113L mutation presented with the polymorphism M647V, while in another patient, the S113L allele had no such polymorphism. The divergent haplotypes probably reflect the occurrence of independent mutations.

Defects of the β-Oxidation Spiral

Very Long Chain Acyl-CoA Dehydrogenase (VLCAD) Deficiency (MIM 201475)

Clinical Presentations. Until the discovery of VLCFAD, these patients were originally thought to have a deficiency of mitochondrial matrix LCAD.[148–152] The two cases described

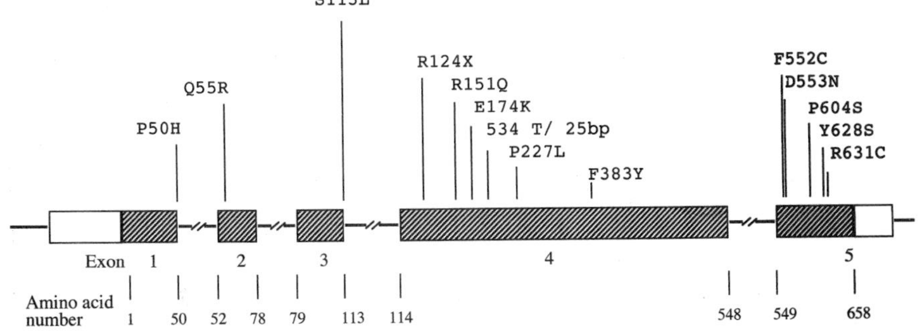

Fig. 101-4 The human CPT II gene and mutations. Boxes indicate exons. The hatched areas are coding regions with mutation positions; open boxes indicate either 5′ or 3′ UTRs. Below the exons, each vertical line indicates the amino acid number in the CPT II protein.

below reflect the distinct clinical phenotypes for this disease: hypertrophic cardiomyopathy with hypoglycemia and skeletal myopathy; or hypoketotic hypoglycemia without cardiac manifestations.

Case 1. Of four children from unrelated parents, two were affected.[153] The first male infant was the 3.3 kg product of a full-term uncomplicated pregnancy and delivery. During the first 24 h, he became tachypneic and intermittently lethargic, which was associated with metabolic acidosis (pH 7.23) and hypoglycemia (0.78 mM or 14 mg%). Urine organic acid analysis revealed dicarboxylic aciduria along with increased blood uric acid (13.3 mg/dl). Negative studies included plasma amino acids, very -long chain fatty acids, ammonia, lactate, pyruvate, and urine acylglycines. He responded to intravenous fluid and glucose therapy and was discharged at 2 weeks of age. At 10 weeks of age, he was readmitted due to poor feeding, irritability, and lethargy associated with metabolic acidosis, hypoglycemia, hepatomegaly, and hyperammonemia (1176 μM). He died following cardiorespiratory arrest. Autopsy revealed cardiac biventricular hypertrophy (weight 83 g; controls 26 g) and hepatomegaly (weight 510 g; controls 160 g) with extensive steatosis and cholestasis.

The fourth child, a female, was the 4.0 kg product of a full-term uncomplicated pregnancy and delivery. At 29 h of age, she became tachypneic, hypotonic, and increasingly lethargic with blood glucose of 0.6 mM (11 mg%). Urine revealed persistent proteinuria and hematuria in the absence of red cells. Liver enzymes were significantly elevated, but CPK was not measured. She responded to intravenous glucose for this event and a similar one at 5 days of age. At 4 months of age, she was admitted for lethargy following 4 days of diarrhea. Abnormal findings included marked hepatomegaly and hypertrophic cardiomyopathy with pericardial effusion by echocardiogram. She had hypoglycemia with an elevated CPK (2255 U/L) and uric acid (13.1 mg/dl), metabolic acidosis, and increased AST and ALT. Blood acylcarnitine analysis revealed dominance of the profile by *cis*-5-tetradecenoylcarnitine (C14:1). Assay of VLCAD activity in fibroblasts revealed an activity of 0.02 nM ETF red/min/mg protein (controls: 1.57 ± 0.31). Unlike most children with the "cardiomyopathic" form of VLCAD deficiency, she recovered and, at 5 years of age, still survives following treatment with a medium chain triglyceride-containing formula (Portagen) and carnitine supplementation.

Case 2. A 32-year-old white female (patient HC in Hale et al.[148] and Naylor et al.[151]) had several unexplained episodes of lethargy and coma associated with fasting, hypoketotic hypoglycemia, and dicarboxylic aciduria early in life. The oldest of six siblings born to healthy unrelated parents, she began at 18 months to experience frequent episodes of lethargy and unresponsiveness, invariably precipitated by an upper respiratory infection. While hospitalized at 2 years for such an episode, hepatomegaly was noted, and liver biopsy showed marked fatty infiltration, moderate lymphocytic infiltration, and perilobular fibrosis. At 5 years, she was hospitalized when she became lethargic, then comatose and unresponsive. Blood glucose was 1.1 mM (20 mg%), blood ammonia was 62 μM, blood urea nitrogen was 31 mg/dl, total CO_2 was 14.8 mM, pH was 7.37, and urine was negative for ketones. She recovered promptly after receiving IV glucose. Glucose infusion was discontinued and the next morning she again became lethargic, although her blood glucose was 3.8 mM (68 mg%). On a high-fat ketogenic diet, she became hypoglycemic and vomited, but no ketones were found in her urine. She had a normal electroencephalogram. She had episodes of hypoglycemia and lethargy over the next few years, which were aggravated by a low-carbohydrate diet. Further investigation was prompted by recurrent episodes of fatigue and muscle soreness, beginning in the second decade. At 20 years, when clinically well, her blood glucose and electrolytes were normal while organic acids revealed dicarboxylic aciduria. Total plasma carnitine was 10.6 μM, of which 4.4 μM was free carnitine, 0.4 μM was short chain acylcarnitine, and 5.8 μM was long chain acylcarnitine. The plasma acylcarnitine profile by tandem MS was dominated by tetradecenoylcarnitine (C14:1). Urinary carnitine excretion (mM/kg/day) was 1.2 total, 0.1 free, and 1.1 acyl (controls 5.4, 3.0, and 2.4, respectively). Unlike plasma, the major urinary species was acetylcarnitine. Her serum CPK was 374 IU/L (controls, < 130). ECG and chest x-ray films were normal. Echocardiography was normal, with no evidence of left ventricular dysfunction. Radionuclide angiogram showed a normal ejection fraction, with normal wall motion at rest or on exercise. She experienced further episodes of fatigue and muscle soreness, usually following either emotional stress or periods of decreased dietary intake, during which CPK levels ranged from 6400 to 32,200 IU/L; only the highest level was associated with frank myoglobinuria. While none of these episodes was associated with obvious hypoglycemia, treatment with 10 percent IV glucose and pain medication has led to a reduction in the CPK level, resolution of dicarboxylic aciduria, and cessation of muscle discomfort. At 25 years of age, she became pregnant. Although the first 16 weeks were uneventful, she had five hospitalizations from 17 to 36 weeks of gestation, all of which were precipitated by muscle tenderness and pain; two were associated with pharyngitis. Peak CPK levels during these admissions ranged from 5600 to 20,580 IU/L, but there was no hypoglycemia. Long-term treatment included a low-fat diet and supplementation with cornstarch at bedtime, fructose, and low-dose carnitine (330 mg four times daily) to normalize plasma carnitine levels, because the implications of her profound carnitine deficiency relative to the fetus were unknown. Short-term treatment included oral starch supplementation, IV glucose, and IV pain medication. She underwent cesarean section at 37 weeks and delivered a normal male infant who was unaffected and was developmentally normal at 8 years of age.

Diagnosis. Most patients with VLCAD deficiency, regardless of phenotype, are at initial risk in the neonatal period often presenting with hypoglycemia, irritability, and lethargy precipitating evaluation for sepsis. Because they often respond rapidly to glucose infusion, they can be discharged without knowledge of the diagnosis until a more severe event occurs. Children with the "cardiomyopathic" form of this disease may also have had transient neonatal hypoglycemia, but then present with hypertrophic cardiomyopathy and pericardial effusion between 2 and 5 months of age, and usually die. Initial studies should include glucose, lactate, ammonia, CPK, electrolytes, and urine organic acid analysis. Urine organic acid analysis, which reveals both saturated and unsaturated dicarboxylic aciduria, is direct evidence for some problem with mitochondrial fat oxidation. Simultaneously, blood acylcarnitine profile analysis should be obtained (usually <72 h for result).The abnormal acylcarnitine profile is identical for both phenotypes of VLCAD deficiency and is dominated by the oleate metabolite, 5-*cis*-tetradecenoylcarnitine (C14:1).[153] Acylglycine analysis will not reveal any diagnostic abnormalities. Skin biopsy should be obtained for direct enzyme assay and in vitro studies using deuterated palmitate to determine which clinical course can be anticipated.[154] Figure 101-5 illustrates the distinctive profiles of acylcarnitines observed with the two phenotypes of VLCAD deficiency when fibroblasts are incubated with 16-$^2H_3$-palmitate. Sixteen cases of VLCAD deficiency (10 cardiomyopathic cases and 6 hypoglycemic forms), documented by direct enzyme assay, were compared to 6 controls. The ratio of $^2H_3$-palmitoylcarnitine (δ3-C16) to $^2H_3$-dodecanoylcarnitine (δ3-C12) was 4.0 in the cardiomyopathic cases, as compared to 1.0 in the children with the milder hypoglycemic phenotype ($P < 0.0005$). Unfortunately, unlike MCAD and LCHAD deficiencies, there is no mutation, sufficiently common, to assist in the acute diagnostic work-up. Similarly, measuring the oxidation rates with various substrates in

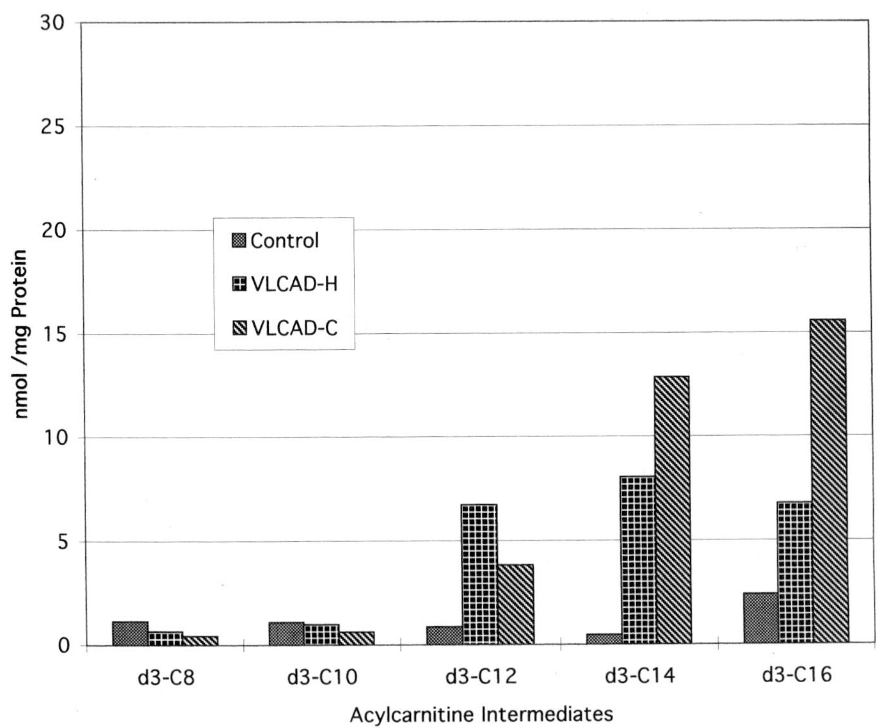

Fig. 101-5 VLCAD phenotypes. Quantitative acylcarnitine intermediates following incubation of fibroblasts from the two clinical phenotypes of VLCAD deficiency with 16-$^2H_3$-palmitate. VLCAD-C = cardiomyopathic phenotype; VLCAD-H = hypoglycemic phenotype. (The differences between these two phenotypes for d3-C16, d3-C14, and d3-C12 were significant: P-values of < 0.002, < 0.02, and < 0.02 respectively.)

fibroblasts will only indicate a problem might be present but will not be definitive as is direct enzyme assay or other more specific in vitro studies.

Families affected by VLCAD deficiency or other mitochondrial fat oxidation defects may have a history of a previous child who died without a specific diagnosis. Often an original newborn screening card or blood obtained by the medical examiner for toxicology studies may still be available for investigation. The diagnosis can often be obtained from these materials by acylcarnitine analysis. When a subsequent pregnancy occurs, direct enzyme assay and in vitro studies with labeled palmitate can provide the specific diagnosis and the anticipated phenotype for an affected fetus.[155]

Management includes avoiding fasting, maintaining high-carbohydrate intake, frequent feeding, maintaining a diet with both high-carbohydrate and medium chain triglyceride, and treating episodes of illness with IV glucose and carnitine. Intravenous and oral carnitine have been used in both phenotypes of this disease without any apparent cardiac side effects despite high plasma levels (45 μM) of long chain acylcarnitines (Slonim A, Roe CR, unpublished observations). MCT replacement of long-chain fatty acids in the diet even during severe episodes involving hypertrophic cardiomyopathy with pericardial effusion appears to be effective for management of these patients.[153,156] Clearly, this approach should only be used after ruling out MCAD deficiency or glutaric acidemia type II.

Pathogenesis. A defect in mitochondrial long chain fatty acid oxidation such as VLCAD deficiency would have far-reaching effects on other metabolic pathways, including impaired energy production during periods of fasting stress, and toxic effects of the long chain acyl-CoA intermediates, which accumulate within mitochondria. The adenine nucleotide translocase, for example, an important site for regulation of oxidative phosphorylation, is sensitive to inhibition by long chain acyl-CoA esters.[157] That peroxisomal β-oxidation and microsomal ω-oxidation play a role in disposing of accumulated acyl-CoA intermediates in VLCAD deficiency is reflected by the significant medium chain dicarboxylic aciduria.

Hepatic light microscopic changes include panlobular steatosis, with both macrovesicular and microvesicular droplets, portal fibrosis, and inflammation usually without necrosis or cholestasis. Electron microscopic findings can reveal increased mitochondrial matrix density and widening of intracristal spaces, giving the mitochondria a condensed appearance.[158] Steatosis is also observed in skeletal and cardiac muscle. In the cardiomyopathic phenotype, heart weight is increased and there is obvious hypertrophy of the ventricular walls.

Molecular Aspects. Sequence analysis of the cloned human VLCAD cDNA (GenBank L46590) isolated from a human heart cDNA library using a rat VLCAD cDNA[159] as a probe revealed a 5′ untranslated sequence of 88 bp, an open reading frame of 1965 bp encoding the entire protein of 655 amino acids, and a 3′ untranslated sequence of 171 bp followed by a short poly A tract.[160] Human heart and liver VLCAD cDNAs have identical coding regions.[161] The human *VLCAD* gene is comprised of 20 exons and is located at 17p13.[160,162,163,166]

The human VLCAD protein has an N-terminal 40 amino acid mitochondrial leader peptide 68 percent identical to the rat VLCAD. This cleavable leader peptide directing the precursor to mitochondria contains basic residues which are similar to other mitochondrial signal peptides. Mature VLCAD is a homodimer of a 70-kDa protein associated with the mitochondrial membrane. MCAD and SCAD, the other acyl-CoA dehydrogenases, are mitochondrial matrix proteins and are homotetramers of approximately 40-kDa polypeptides. The N-terminal region of mature VLCAD shows significant sequence homology to MCAD and SCAD, but the C-terminal 180 amino acid sequence, is not homologous to the other acyl-CoA dehydrogenases.[159,161]

A total of 19 VLCAD mutations have been characterized. These are summarized in Table 101-1. Interestingly, for dimer formation of mature VLCAD, the association of VLCAD protein with the mitochondrial inner membrane is necessary. An S583W mutation identified from a patient with VLCAD deficiency prevents association with the inner membrane after import into the mitochondria. The mutant protein mostly remains in the mitochondrial matrix. However, for VLCHA mutations altering

Table 101-1 Summary of Mutations identified in the Human VLCAD Gene

Mutation	Exon	Amino acid change	References
1-bp g deletion (intron-exon 6 boundary)	6	Frameshift	160
135-bp deletion (343–477)	6	Loss of 45 amino acids	164
3-bp deletion 388–390	6	E130del	164
C 779 T	9	T220M	166
C842A	9	A241D	166
T848C	9	V243A	166
3-bp deletion 895–897	10	K299del	164
T950C	10	V277A	166
105-bp deletion (g + 1 to a) 1078–1182 (exon 11 skipping)	11	Loss of 35 amino acids	160,161
C1096T	11	R326C	166
3-bp deletion 1141–1143	11	E341del	166
A1144C	11	K382Q	164
G1322A	13	G401D	166
G1349A	14	R410H	167
T1372C	14	F458L	156
4-bp insertion (ACAG1679)	18	Frameshift	156,166
C1748G	18	S583W	165
C 1804 A	19	L562I	166,167
C 1837 T	20	R613W	164

the N-terminal region, such as E130del, K299del, and K382Q, the mutant proteins showed some degree of dimer formation.[164,165] The correlation of mutant genotypes to clinical phenotypes is still unclear.

Defects Affecting the Mitochondrial Trifunctional Protein

The mitochondrial trifunctional protein is a heterooctomeric ($\alpha_4\beta_4$) enzyme complex associated with the inner mitochondrial membrane. The complex has been purified and characterized in both rat and human liver.[168,169] It has L-3-hydroxyacyl-CoA dehydrogenase, 2-enoyl-CoA hydratase, and 3-oxoacyl-CoA thiolase activities for the degradation of long chain acyl-CoA thioesters. From a molecular point of view, disorders of this complex can be divided into those patients whose molecular defect is in the gene encoding the α-subunit (*HADH-A*) and those with defects in the gene encoding the β-subunit of the protein (*HADH-B*). However, from a functional viewpoint, these disorders can be considered according to the specific enzyme activities that are affected, for example, L-3-hydroxyacyl-CoA dehydrogenase (LCHAD), 2-enoyl-CoA hydratase, and 3-oxoacyl-CoA thiolase (thiolase). Functional considerations are necessary for the formulation of dietary treatment strategies for these patients. Thus, there are two inherited disorders of this complex that have been described: isolated long chain L-3-hydroxyacyl-CoA dehydrogenase deficiency (LCHAD) and a deficiency affecting the activities of all three enzymatic components—mitochondrial trifunctional protein (MTP) deficiency. MTP deficiency can result from mutations that affect the assembly of and/or degradation of the heterooctomeric holoenzyme. In either case, both the amount of enzyme protein is reduced as is all three enzymatic activities. Unfortunately, the cases reported in the literature often have only enzymatic information related to the impact on LCHAD (α subunit) and thiolase (β subunit) activities but, rarely, information on the status of the long chain enoyl-CoA hydratase.

Long Chain L-3-Hydroxyacyl-CoA Dehydrogenase (LCHAD) Deficiency

Clinical Presentations. This disorder has been documented in many patients,[170–184] and is common among the fatty acid oxidation disorders. There is considerable clinical heterogeneity in LCHAD deficiency, with phenotypes including fulminant hepatic disease, hypertrophic cardiomyopathy, rhabdomyolysis, and in some patients, unusual features such as sensorimotor neuropathy and pigmentary retinopathy.

Case Reports. The first patient in whom LCHAD deficiency was confirmed was initially described clinically by Glasgow et al. in 1983.[170] A boy, one of fraternal twins, presented at 9 months of age with the first of many episodes of fasting-induced vomiting and hypoketotic hypoglycemia resembling Reye syndrome. He had significant hypotonia, cardiomyopathy, and liver dysfunction with low plasma and tissue carnitine levels and dicarboxylic and hydroxydicarboxylic aciduria. Liver biopsy showed mild fibrosis and severe fatty infiltration. He died in cardiorespiratory arrest at 19 months. At autopsy, the liver showed extensive fibrosis, massive necrosis, and steatosis.

His twin sister had a series of similar but less dramatic episodes, also beginning at 9 months. She had cardiomegaly and myopathy early in life, and her episodes were characterized by elevated blood CPK. Treatment with an MCT supplement to her diet appeared to be protective; despite several clinical episodes early in life, her cardiac function and muscle strength normalized.

Of the reported LCHAD-deficient patients, the age of onset of first symptoms has ranged from 1 day to 39 months. Most present with signs of fasting-induced hypoketotic hypoglycemia, although a few have presented with cardiomyopathy (usually hypertrophic) and muscle weakness. Episodes of illness are sometimes associated with striking elevations of serum CPK, occasionally accompanied by myoglobinuria. In a few cases, sensorimotor neuropathy or pigmentary retinopathy has been described. About half the patients died, either from the first episode or with progressive disease ending in cardiorespiratory failure.

Excretion of large quantities of 3-hydroxydicarboxylic acids of 6 to 14 carbons in length, as well as medium chain (C6 to C10) dicarboxylic acids, in urine has most often been the clue to the diagnosis of LCHAD deficiency. Acylcarnitine species corresponding to the 3-hydroxy C16:0, C18:1, and C18:2 monocarboxylic acids have been observed routinely by tandem-MS of blood or plasma from patients with LCHAD deficiency. There are a number of clinical and biochemical features of this disorder that distinguish it from other fatty acid oxidation defects. The degree of liver damage found in some patients with this defect is remarkable. The peripheral neuropathy[172,175] and the pigmentary retinopathy[172,177,178] found in many patients are not characteristic of mitochondrial fatty acid oxidation defects; the latter has been observed in some of the disorders of peroxisomal β-oxidation.

Tyni et al.[185] recently reviewed the most homogeneous population of LCHAD-deficient patients, all 13 of whom were homozygous for the 1528G > C mutation, which affects the L-3-hyroxyacyl-CoA dehydrogenase coding part of the α-subunit of the trifunctional protein producing isolated LCHAD deficiency.[186] The age of onset of symptoms ranged from 2 days to 21 months. The primary symptoms included hypoglycemia, hypotonia, hepatomegaly, and cardiomyopathy. Six of 11 patients examined had pigmentary retinopathy, first detected between 4 and 17 months of age. Jaundice was observed in only two patients who died of hepatic failure within a month of that observation. Most patients were categorized as having hepatopathy but without jaundice. Hypotonia was consistently observed in all patients who were examined. CPK elevation was reported in 6 of 10 patients examined. Neurologically, early psychomotor development was normal but they tended to lose skills with episodes of metabolic illness. Carnitine deficiency was usually observed in these patients. Interestingly, 6 of 10 examined had anemia and thrombocytopenia. Although hypertension was not reported, elevated liver enzymes and low platelets were frequent (see "HELLP Syndrome" below). The cause of death was usually cardiac or respiratory failure, but two died from hepatic failure.

Treatment of patients with LCHAD deficiency has usually involved reducing the long chain fatty acid content of the diet, with frequent carbohydrate-enriched feedings or supplementation with uncooked cornstarch. MCT supplementation has also been used with some success and probably should be a part of the nutritional therapy. Carnitine and riboflavin have also been tried, although without obvious benefit.

Pathologic Findings. Fat accumulation has been found in liver, skeletal muscle, and heart. In the few cases in which electron microscopic study of liver was performed, there were alterations of mitochondrial ultrastructure similar to those seen in MCAD and VLCAD deficiencies, including condensed mitochondrial matrixes and widened cristal spaces.[173,182] In a few cases, the liver was reported to be fibrotic or frankly cirrhotic, which is not a typical feature of fatty acid oxidation disorders.

Diagnosis. Because neonatal hypoglycemia is often the earliest symptom and may respond to therapy, it should not be ignored because the major symptoms of LCHAD deficiency appear shortly thereafter. Blood acylcarnitine analysis at the time of hypoglycemia can often reveal the presence of this disorder permitting early dietary intervention. Similarly, analysis of a blood spot for the 1528G > C mutation can also be helpful. This mutation is present in homozygous form in about 70 percent of affected individuals. For that reason, the combination of acylcarnitine analysis and mutation analysis from blood spots will identify those affected compound heterozygotes compared to true heterozygotes for that mutation.

LCHAD activity in fibroblasts is usually assayed in the reverse of the physiological direction, using 3-ketoacyl-CoA compounds such as 3-ketopalmitoyl-CoA as substrate. Because of the overlapping substrate specificities of LCHAD and SCHAD, however, most patients with LCHAD deficiency have demonstrated 15 to 35 percent of control levels of activity with 3-ketopalmitoyl-CoA as substrate. The specific LCHAD defect is more clearly revealed using an antibody directed against SCHAD to remove this activity. Under these assay conditions, parents' cells have intermediate levels of LCHAD activity, consistent with heterozygosity. As illustrated below, it is best to assay for all three enzyme activities to identify the trifunctional protein deficiency.[185] Prenatal diagnosis can also be accomplished by direct enzyme assay of amniocytes or by probing the β oxidative pathway as previously described.[155]

Obstetrical Complications and LCHAD Deficiency. The association between acute fatty liver of pregnancy and LCHAD deficiency, was first pointed out in 1991 by Wilcken's group.[187] That same year, in an editorial, several kindred were reviewed, which illustrated that this complication of pregnancy, as well as the HELLP syndrome (*h*emolysis, *e*levated *l*iver enzymes, and *l*ow *p*latelets), and/or hyperemesis was observed, and was indeed frequent. Of six pregnancies in which the fetus was affected with LCHAD deficiency, these complications were observed.[188] Subsequently, the evidence for this association with LCHAD deficiency has increased such that it is now prudent to consider determining if the mother with a history of such pregnancy complications or with the initial onset of these problems is heterozygous for 1528G > C.[189–192] With prior history of AFLP or HELLP syndrome and demonstration of this common LCHAD mutation in the mother, amniocentesis should be considered to determine whether the fetus is affected with LCHAD deficiency in order to preserve mother and child and provide opportunity for early therapy of the affected infant.

The study by Tyni et al.[185] revealed that many of the LCHAD-deficient cases they reviewed had anemia (hemolysis), elevated liver enzymes, and low platelets raising the question of HELLP syndrome in the affected children. More detailed investigation of affected children may clarify this issue and might relate to the pathogenesis of the obstetrical complications in mothers of affected fetuses. To date, there has been no clear correlation of obstetrical complications in mothers whose fetus is not affected with LCHAD deficiency.

There has also been a report of acute fatty liver of pregnancy in a mother at risk for having a fetus with carnitine palmitoyltransferase I deficiency (hepatic form).[193] These obstetrical complications have, as yet, not been associated with other disorders of fat oxidation.

The demonstration that both rat[41] and human[90] liver LCHAD activities reside in a trifunctional protein bound to the inner mitochondrial membrane, along with 2-enoyl-CoA hydratase and 3-ketoacyl-CoA thiolase activities, has a bearing on the interpretation of this enzyme defect. Jackson et al.[22] were the first to report a combined defect of these three activities. Most patients with LCHAD deficiency have not been evaluated for the other enzyme activities of the trifunctional protein, but in a few patients in whom they have been measured, long-chain 2-enoyl-CoA hydratase[22,140,147] and long chain 3-ketoacyl-CoA thiolase[22,140,146,147] activities also were reduced. Residual thiolase and hydratase activities were not zero, suggesting that either more than one enzyme contributes to each reaction or that the mutation(s) may have more severe effects on LCHAD than on the other activities of the trifunctional protein.

Mitochondrial Trifunctional Protein Deficiency. Using HPLC techniques and enzyme assays of activities associated with the purified trifunctional enzyme, a combined deficiency of LCHAD long chain oxoacyl-CoA thiolase and long chain 2-enoyl-CoA hydratase has been documented.[181,194] Even though these studies have shown reduction of all three activities, some patients excrete 3-hydroxy monocarboxylic and 3-hydroxy dicarboxylic acids. This observation suggests trifunctional enzyme deficiency in some of those patients previously identified as long chain 3-hydroxyacyl-CoA dehydrogenase deficiency.

Clinical Presentations: Case 1. Of three children in the family, one was normal and two died. The first, a boy, presented at 6 months of age after a period of refusing feeds. He was lethargic, severely hypotonic, areflexic and unresponsive to pain. Serum CPK was 3859 U/liter. He recovered but 6 weeks later was still areflexic and hypotonic. Muscle biopsy when well revealed type 1 fiber predominance and an excess of type 2c fibers. Muscle and serum carnitine concentrations were low. He remained areflexic and hypotonic and by 2 years he had developed plantiflexion contractures and was not walking. Following a 2-week respiratory illness at age 2.5 years, he presented with cardiac failure, an enlarged dilated heart, and generalized weakness. He died and autopsy was refused.

His sister was noted to be areflexic at 3 months of age. A mild equinus deformity and toe walking were noted at 20 months. She had two episodes of anorexia, hypotonia, and weakness by age 3 years without serious consequence. Following a 3-day illness, she was admitted with generalized muscle weakness and areflexia. The weakness progressed rapidly and she died on the third day with severe hyponatremia. Her serum CPK was 33,000 U/liter, glucose levels were normal, lactate was 4.92 mM, and urine organic acids showed small amounts of ethylmalonate, adipic, and suberic acids. A rapid postmortem was performed. In muscle, there was necrosis of 5 to 10 percent of fibers, the 95 percent of which were type II. There was very little lipid storage in muscle fibers, none in heart, and marked steatosis (microvesicular and macrovesicular) in the liver. Direct enzyme assay in isolated mitochondria was consistent with trifunctional protein deficiency with decreased levels of enoyl-CoA hydratase, LCHAD, and thiolase in muscle. Liver and heart mitochondria were assayed for the LCHAD and thiolase (but not the hydratase), and these activities were significantly reduced.[181]

Case 2. This child was the product of a normal uncomplicated pregnancy and delivery. The parents were consanguineous. At 48 h of age, the baby became hypoglycemic and developed hypotonia, which persisted despite normalization of blood glucose. Respiratory failure occurred on the eighth day requiring assisted ventilation. Cardiac failure occurred on the twenty-eighth day due to a hypokinetic-dilated cardiomyopathy. Death occurred on day 30 and autopsy was refused. Serum CPK was not determined. Urine organic acids showed saturated and unsaturated dicarboxylic and 3-hydroxydicarboxylic acids with the longest chain length being 12 carbons. Direct enzyme assay of the trifunctional protein in fibroblasts revealed significant decrease in all three activities.[194]

Pathologic Findings of LCHAD Deficiency. The information on the pathology of LCHAD deficiency is relatively limited. Skeletal muscle seems altered in that there is a predominance of type II fibers (slow oxidative) and necrosis associated with elevated CPK levels consistent with a rhabdomyolytic process. Dilated cardiomyopathy and hepatic steatosis are also prominent, but interestingly, lipid storage in skeletal and cardiac muscle was not impressive.

Diagnosis. Deficiency of the mitochondrial trifunctional protein is difficult to recognize and identify by the usual methods for diagnosis of fatty acid oxidation disorders. Urine organic acid analysis may or may not show dicarboxylic and 3-hydroxydicarboxylic aciduria. Unlike isolated LCHAD deficiency, there is no common mutant allele. The α subunit 1528G > C mutation is not observed in complete trifunctional protein deficiency. The disorder should be considered whenever there is hypoglycemia associated with hypotonia with or without dilated cardiomyopathy, especially when serum CPK and blood lactate levels are increased and hydroxydicarboxylic aciduria is present without the 1528G > C mutation and with a normal blood acylcarnitine profile. The trifunctional protein deficiency seems to be the only fatty acid oxidation disorder in which blood lactate is consistently elevated even when the patient is asymptomatic. Currently, there is no simple direct means to rapidly validate the presence of this defect. Skin biopsy and fibroblast studies are required. Oxidation rates in fibroblasts are reduced with palmitate, but that is not specific for the defect. Direct assay of the three enzyme activities is required to make the diagnosis.

Molecular Aspects. The human mitochondrial trifunctional protein (MTP) is a heteromer of four α and four β subunits. The α and β subunits are encoded by two nuclear genes,[168,195] and in humans, the MTP-α and MTP-β genes are located in the same region of chromosome 2p23.[196,197] The α-subunit (GenBank D16480) has two different activities: long chain enoyl-CoA hydratase and LCHAD; while the β-subunit (GenBank D16481) has the long chain 3-ketoacyl-CoA thiolase activity.

Recently, a G to C mutation at position 1528 (1528G > C) causing the missense mutation E510Q in the MTP α-subunit was reported.[186,190,198] This mutation is frequent in patients with LCHAD deficiency[186] and normal or near normal activities of long chain enoyl-CoA hydratase and long chain 3-ketoacyl-CoA thiolase.

Interestingly, exon skipping or point mutations that result in frameshifts or nonsense mutations in the α subunit cDNA apparently cause complete trifunctional protein deficiency with decreased activity of the three enzyme activities. For example, a patient with neonatal MTP deficiency was a compound heterozygote with two alleles each with mutations in the intron 3 donor splice site: a G to A transversion at the invariant position +1; and, an A to G transversion at position +3. Both alleles caused exon 3 (71 bp) skipping with a resulting frameshift, premature translational termination and undetectable levels of α-subunit protein and complete loss of MTP activity.[199]

Mutations in the β-subunit apparently cause MTP deficiency instead of LCHAD deficiency. Ushikubo et al. first reported disease-causing mutations in the MTP β gene.[200] Two nucleotide substitutions, 182G > A and 740G > A, were identified in a Japanese patient with MTP deficiency and an 788A > G mutation was found in the MTP β-subunit cDNA in another MTP deficiency patient. Aoyama et al. identified two Japanese patients with MTP deficiency.[201] One was homozygous for a 1331G > A transition (R411K) in MTP-β while a second was a compound heterozygote with an exonic insertion of a T which activates a new cryptic 5′ splice site and a 1331G > A transition (R411K). All three enzyme activities of MTP were undetectable in fibroblasts from these patients.[200,201] Mutation and cDNA expression data suggested that MTP activity depends on forming the $\alpha_4\beta_4$ heterooctamer.

Two patients with the unique and infrequent presentation of chronic progressive polyneuropathy and myopathy (with recurrent rhabdomyolysis) but no hepatic or cardiac symptoms were recently described. The mutations were identified only in exon 9 of the MTP α-gene. One child was homozygous for 845T > A while the other was a compound heterozygote for 914T > A (I-N) and 871C > T causing premature termination at residue 255.[202] It is not clear how these mutations produced this specific phenotype. Another study of 46 patients with LCHAD deficiency revealed 12 who were compound heterozygotes for the common mutation (1528G > C). In two of these, the second mutation was a 2129C insertion that changed the α-subunit reading frame and created a premature stop. In a third, a 1025T > C mutation was identified in the α-subunit, resulting in an L342P substitution.[203]

Currently, there are no obvious explanations correlating genotype with the multiple phenotypes associated with defects involving the MTP. Only a few laboratories provide reliable assays of all three enzymatic activities involved in this complex protein. This has impeded the development of a clear picture of the functional impact of the observed mutations on mitochondrial fatty acid oxidation.

2,4-Dienoyl-CoA Reductase Deficiency. *Clinical Presentation.* A single patient[204] has been described with this enzyme deficiency affecting the degradation of unsaturated fatty acids with even-numbered double bonds, such as linoleate (9-*cis*,12-*cis*-C18:2).

Case Report. This 2.2-kg black girl was the product of an uncomplicated pregnancy, born to unrelated parents. Hypotonia, intact deep tendon reflexes, microcephaly, a small ventricular septal defect, short trunk, arms and fingers, small feet, and a large face were noted. Her karyotype was 46XX. Although she was discharged from the hospital at 2 days, she was readmitted a few hours later with sepsis. Despite therapy, she remained hypotonic, with poor feeding, inadequate weight gain, and intermittent vomiting. Gastrostomy and fundoplication were required. Unresponsive respiratory acidosis developed, and she died at 4 months of age. Organic acid analysis of many urine samples was normal, with no evidence of dicarboxylic acids or acylglycines. Plasma amino acid analysis revealed an unexplained hyperlysinemia. Plasma carnitine was low (total, 16 μM; esterified, 6 μM).

Clarification of the phenotype of this disorder must await the identification of other patients. Their recognition appears possible only if hypotonic infants are evaluated for the presence of decadienoyl (C10:2)-carnitine in plasma (see below). Preliminary management of this disorder probably should include avoidance of fasting, reduction of long chain unsaturated fat in the diet and nutritional supplementation with MCT and perhaps carnitine.

Diagnosis. Analysis of acylcarnitines in plasma and urine by tandem mass spectrometry demonstrated a C10:2-acylcarnitine species identified as 2-*trans*,4-*cis*-C10:2, an intermediate in the degradation of linoleic acid and a substrate for 2,4-dienoyl-CoA reductase. Assay of this enzyme in postmortem muscle and liver revealed 17 percent and 40 percent of control activities, respectively. Fibroblasts were not available for analysis. Using a more sensitive assay, enzyme activity in lymphoblastoid cells from the father was 52 percent of controls. It is assumed, therefore, that the defect is inherited as an autosomal recessive trait. A sib born subsequently appears normal, without hypotonia, and with no evidence for the defect, either by enzyme assay or acylcarnitine analysis.

Pathologic Findings. Autopsy revealed only pulmonary vascular congestion and bilateral ventricular hypertrophy, in addition to the congenital abnormalities described above. There was no evidence of steatosis; no ultrastructural studies were performed.

Medium Chain Acyl-CoA Dehydrogenase (MCAD) Deficiency

Clinical Presentations. Since the first children with MCAD deficiency were described in 1982-1983,[4–7] it has become recognized as one of the most common inherited disorders of fatty acid oxidation mainly affecting Caucasians of northern European origin. The family in the following case report illustrates the marked phenotypic heterogeneity associated with MCAD deficiency even in the same family.

Case Report. The parents were unrelated and of English-Irish origin. They had three sons, the youngest of whom had an apparently minor respiratory illness at 18 months of age and was found dead in bed the following morning. Despite his age, the autopsy findings were considered consistent with SIDS. Subsequently, his 23-month-old brother had gastroenteritis and vomiting, which progressed to lethargy and seizures. He was hospitalized and noted to be hypoglycemic and hyperammonemic. He became comatose and died 4 days later. Autopsy revealed marked hepatic steatosis and cerebral edema, and it was concluded that he died of Reye syndrome. An older brother was asymptomatic. At the time of the second child's death, the mother gave birth to her first daughter. A combination of studies—organic acids, enzyme assays, acylcarnitine profiling, and molecular analysis—confirmed that all four siblings had MCAD deficiency; in the two autopsy cases, molecular analysis was performed on paraffin-embedded liver. The oldest male, now 10 years old, has never had an episode of illness related to his MCAD deficiency. He and his sister have been treated with frequent feeding, avoidance of fasting, and long-term carnitine supplementation. His sister had multiple episodes of illness requiring hospitalization during the first 2 years of life, for which she was treated in the short-term with IV glucose and oral carnitine supplementation. Now aged 15 years, she has been free of episodes for over 10 years. Both sibs had varicella with no significant metabolic imbalance during that time.[205] This family exemplifies the considerable phenotypic heterogeneity of MCAD deficiency: sudden death in infancy, Reye syndrome, and asymptomatic and presymptomatic detection with subsequent illness treated with appropriate intervention. It also emphasizes the absolute necessity for evaluating sibs of affected children.

While there is no typical presentation of MCAD deficiency, some common features of the disease should be noted.[8,9] The child with MCAD deficiency often presents with an episode of vomiting and lethargy following a period of fasting. There may have been a prior viral infection (gastrointestinal, upper respiratory), associated with decreased oral intake. There is occasionally a history of previous similar episodes. On presentation, the child may be comatose; blood glucose may be low and often there are no or only low to moderate levels of ketones in the urine. Blood ammonia levels and liver function tests may be abnormally high. Intravenous infusion with 10 percent glucose results in some improvement but even after correction of hypoglycemia, the child may remain obtunded for several hours. These patients are asymptomatic between episodes and can be prevented from having additional episodes by avoidance of fasting and provision of carbohydrate calories as intravenous glucose during intercurrent infections.

With the exception of a few reports in which a parent and several children all had MCAD deficiency,[206] the parents in all other families tested have half-normal levels of MCAD activity and normal plasma carnitine levels; they do not excrete unusual organic acids in urine and are clinically asymptomatic. These data are consistent with heterozygosity for an autosomal recessive disease.

The case report above documents that there is significant phenotypic heterogeneity in MCAD deficiency, even within the same family. There is little doubt that the first episode can be devastating, resulting in sudden death. The children may have only one episode of illness or multiple recurrences; in some cases, they appear to be asymptomatic.

One clinical review[207] showed that of 94 families with MCAD deficiency, 19 (20 percent) had one or more unexplained childhood deaths. In all of these, the diagnosis of MCAD deficiency was made postmortem. Of the 104 affected children in these families, there were 25 deaths. The earliest onset of symptoms and sudden death was in the neonatal period, although this is rare. The latest onset of the first episode, to our knowledge, was at 14 years of age in a girl who enrolled in a weight loss program and became comatose after losing 20 kg of weight (Marsden D, personal communication). To date, there have been a few known MCAD-deficient women who have tolerated pregnancy and delivery without significant problems.

Most children present with acute illness between 3 and 15 months of age. There are few reports of first symptoms after age 4 years, there are fewer recurrent episodes after 4 years, and symptoms requiring repeated hospitalization in the second decade are unusual. In the first year of life, 12 of 63 children (19 percent) died with their first episode. After 12 months of age, 9 of 41 children (22 percent) died with their first episode. Four children died with a later episode. Children with MCAD deficiency clearly are at significant risk of death with either the initial or a later episode. At the time of death, the diagnosis of MCAD deficiency had not been established in 25 children.[207] In contrast, the diagnosis had been established in all 79 survivors. There were no deaths due to MCAD deficiency following diagnosis, suggesting that early diagnosis, possibly by neonatal screening, before onset of symptoms, may be associated with a striking reduction in mortality.

The risk of death in these children is not the only consequence of MCAD deficiency. It was previously assumed, erroneously, that survivors were normal and had few long-term sequelae. A follow-up survey of 78 MCAD-deficient survivors (all $>$ 2 years of age) revealed a number of unexpected problems[207,208] (Table 101-2).

Table 101-2 Consequences of Illness in 78 Surviving MCAD-Deficient Patients

Clinical Finding	No. (%) of Patients*
Developmental disability	16 (21)
Speech and language delay	16 (21)
Behavioral problems	12 (15)
Attention deficit disorder	9 (12)
Proximal muscle weakness	13 (17)
Chronic seizure disorder	13 (17)
Cerebral palsy	8 (10)
Failure to thrive	10 (13)

*These total more than 100 percent because some patients had more than one finding.

Routine developmental assessment was abnormal in 29 patients (37 percent) and showed global developmental disability in 16 (21 percent), speech and language delay in 16 (21 percent), behavioral problems in 12 (15 percent), and attention deficit disorder in 9 (12 percent), 8 of whom were females, in contrast to the usual male preponderance of this disorder in the general population. Complete aphasia followed an episode of illness in four (5 percent). Chronic somatic complaints included proximal muscle weakness in 13 (17 percent), seizure disorder in 13 (17 percent), cerebral palsy in 8 (10 percent), and failure to thrive in 10 (13 percent). The development of muscle weakness was strongly correlated with the length of time between symptomatic presentation and the institution of appropriate measures to prevent further episodes of illness. Therefore, seemingly minor delays in recognizing this disease and initiating appropriate therapy may place these patients at high risk of long-term disability.

Information was also gathered on the sibs of 55 probands with MCAD deficiency.[206] Of 109 sibs, 15 died, 8 of whom were shown to have MCAD deficiency by DNA and acylcarnitine analysis. In all, 64 surviving sibs were investigated: 15 (24 percent) were MCAD-deficient, 29 (46 percent) were carriers, and 20 (32 percent) were normal, close to the expected numbers for an autosomal recessive disorder. These data emphasize the importance of investigating any apparently normal sibs following identification of a new proband with MCAD deficiency. The younger sibs, in particular, are at risk for a fatal first episode. The parents also should be investigated; it is possible, given the frequency of the mutant gene in the population, that an apparently unaffected parent is MCAD-deficient.[206] When unexplained deaths occur in families known to be segregating MCAD deficiency, an effort should be made to establish a postmortem diagnosis, by analysis of postmortem blood or the original newborn screening card. Techniques for these studies are described below.

Diagnosis. The clinical findings of recurrent vomiting leading to obtundation or coma in a child or neonate should immediately raise the possibility of this and other diseases of fatty acid oxidation. Failure to consider the diagnosis of MCAD deficiency in children with this phenotype and to initiate appropriate therapy immediately can have fatal consequences. Even the interval between presentation and receipt of results of diagnosis laboratory results is critical. During the interval of 1 to 2 h required to receive results of such tests, many children with MCAD deficiency have died. In some instances intravenous therapy was instituted but with normal saline rather than a high carbohydrate solution. Although the reflex of administering normal saline may be valid for adults with diabetes mellitus, it is not appropriate for children with these symptoms. Once the blood has been drawn and a blood glucose has been determined at the bedside, a solution of 10 percent glucose, $\frac{1}{4}$ normal saline should be given intravenously at a rate of 1.5 to 2 times maintenance while waiting for the results of early diagnostic tests. It is critical to be aware that the hypoglycemia in this disease follows obtundation. A child with MCAD deficiency may be obtunded due to toxic effects of accumulated metabolites (medium chain fats, ammonium) before hypoglycemia becomes apparent. Correction of hypoglycemia and provision of adequate amounts of fluids and electrolytes is the initial step towards correction of metabolic imbalance and elimination of toxic metabolites.

The diagnosis of MCAD deficiency can be determined in 24 to 48 h by any specialized laboratory using tandem MS of blood spots for acylcarnitine species. The profile of acylcarnitines is unique and specific for MCAD deficiency.[209,210] It includes C6:0-, 4-*cis*- and 5-*cis*-C8:1-, C8:0, and 4-*cis*-C10:1 acylcarnitine species. These can be quantitated by stable isotope dilution mass spectrometry, but the plasma acylcarnitine profile is so specific for MCAD deficiency that quantitation is generally not necessary. With this technique of plasma analysis, there is no longer any requirement for oral carnitine loading as a diagnostic test. Unlike the urinary organic acid profile, the plasma acylcarnitine profile is diagnostic in both sick and well children with MCAD deficiency and can be analyzed with high sensitivity using blood spotted onto a newborn screening (Guthrie) card.[211] Affected infants can therefore be detected prior to the onset of symptoms. Postmortem blood obtained for other reasons (e.g., toxicologic analysis) in cases of sudden death can be analyzed in the same manner.[210–212] Analysis of the same blood spot for the 985G mutation commonly found in MCAD deficiency is also helpful with the caveat that $\approx$10 percent of patients are compound heterozygotes. Urine organic acids during acute illness will show the characteristic acylglycine elevations (hexanoyl- and suberyl-glycine), which are also elevated in children with multiple acyl-CoA dehydrogenase deficiency (glutaric aciduria type II).

In view of the specificity and sensitivity of acylcarnitine analysis, it is not necessary to wait for establishment of a skin fibroblast culture to analyze fatty acid oxidation or to measure MCAD activity directly. The 8- to 10-week delay incurred by these tests is a deterrent to appropriate intervention for the affected child and further delays assessment of potentially affected sibs. In many children with MCAD deficiency, absolute carnitine excretion (μM/kg day) is decreased, paralleling the reduced concentration of carnitine in tissues. Six untreated cases of MCAD deficiency had tissue carnitine levels 16 to 42 percent of normal in liver and 16 to 25 percent of normal in muscle.[7,213,214] Prior to onset of symptoms an affected, breast-fed infant may have normal plasma carnitine levels. However, plasma carnitine levels are not diagnostic and should not precede the analysis of the acylcarnitines by tandem MS for a rapid and specific diagnosis.

The preferred enzymatic method for measuring MCAD and other acyl-CoA dehydrogenase activities is the ETF-based assay.[215,216] The specific enzyme defect has been demonstrated in fibroblasts, peripheral mononuclear leukocytes, liver, heart, skeletal muscle, and amniocytes.[8] There has been no obvious association between the residual MCAD activity and the severity of clinical disease in these patients. Nor has there been any association between measured enzyme activity and genotype, as determined by molecular analysis (described below).

Prenatal diagnosis of MCAD deficiency is an option for early detection of an affected fetus. It is likely, however, that prenatal diagnosis will rarely be sought for the purpose of pregnancy termination, because appropriate management and intervention seem to be effective. At the very least, prenatal diagnosis offers the earliest possible detection of an affected child, so that treatment can be instituted. An alternative to direct enzyme assay for prenatal diagnosis, which is especially useful in pregnancies following the death of a proband not specifically diagnosed, is the incubation of amniocytes with radiolabeled palmitate followed by acylcarnitine analysis of the culture media. This assay permits identification of most fatty acid oxidation defects including MCAD deficiency.[155] It is not reliable for prenatal diagnosis of CPT I and SCAD deficiencies.

Treatment of MCAD deficiency continues to emphasize avoidance of fasting, mild reduction of dietary fat intake (≈20 percent of total calories), and carnitine supplementation which is especially helpful during illness for conjugation of the toxic acyl-CoA intermediates which are then readily excreted as non-toxic acylcarnitines. Considering the high occurrence of sudden death in children under 2 years of age, and our inability to predict episodes, it is wise to provide this supplement from early in life. The family and the personal physician should be educated to understand that an intercurrent viral illness well tolerated by a normal child can produce a fatal episode in a child with MCAD deficiency. Anticipatory treatment with intravenous $D_{10}W$ plus $\frac{1}{4}$ normal saline at 1.5 to 2 times maintenance can prevent these episodes.

Pathologic Findings. The primary pathologic findings in MCAD-deficient patients include light microscopic and ultrastructural changes mainly in liver, but alterations have been observed in other tissues. Cerebral edema is noted postmortem in most cases.[7] Hepatic light microscopic alterations in specimens taken during acute illness are usually limited to steatosis,[158,214] although this is not a universal finding,[217] and may be either macrovesicular or microvesicular in nature.[158] Generally, the steatosis disappears on recovery. In some cases, the microvesicular fat accumulation has been similar to that seen in Reye syndrome. In those instances, however, ultrastructural studies[158,218] clearly demonstrate that the generalized mitochondrial changes characteristic of Reye syndrome are not present. Specifically, the matrix swelling and rarefaction commonly seen in hepatic mitochondria of patients with Reye syndrome have not been observed in MCAD deficiency.[158] Instead, increased matrix density and intracristal widening give the mitochondria a condensed appearance. In a few patients, there are so-called crystalloids in the matrix, associated with an increased number of cristae and with enlargement and abnormal shape of the mitochondria, although some have normal mitochondrial ultrastructure. Condensed mitochondria have been described in other disease states, and crystalloids have been noted in mitochondria from patients with other fatty acid oxidation defects (see above), carnitine-deficient myopathy, and other myopathies,[219] so these findings are not diagnostic.

Molecular Aspects. Within the past few years, a single, highly prevalent mutation within the coding region of MCAD cDNA has been identified among patients with documented MCAD deficiency.[220–230] This nucleotide substitution (985A > G) results in missense mutation (K329E) which alters the amino acid sequence in an α-helical region in the C-terminal half of the peptide.

Figure 101-6 illustrates the structure of the MCAD gene and the location of mutations associated with MCAD deficiency. Among 172 patients with confirmed MCAD deficiency,[229] 138 (80.2 percent) were homozygous for 985A > G, a further 30 (17.4 percent) were compound heterozygotes for this allele and 4 (2.3 percent) did not have the 985A > G change on either allele. Of the 344 mutant MCAD genes, 306 (88.9 percent) were 985A > G. Among the remaining 38, the mutations in 11 were identified: 3 were a 13-bp repeat from nt 999;[227,231,232] 2 were a 4-bp deletion from nt 1100;[233,234] 2 were a 799G > A transition;[227] and 4 were nucleotide substitutions, 157C > T,[232] 447G > A, 730T > C, and 1124T > C,[227] identified in single alleles. Hence, none of the mutations other than 985A > G accounted for more than 1 percent of variant alleles. A total of 27 MCAD mutations remained unidentified in this series of patients, but in many cases, the above-mentioned mutations were excluded. The 985A > G allele, therefore, accounts for most of the mutant MCAD genes characterized in this large series of MCAD deficient patients. The approximate frequency of MCAD deficiency among Caucasians, based on several studies,[235,236] is between 1 in 6400 and 1 in 46,000, with a heterozygote frequency of 1 to 2 percent. That a single mutation accounts for approximately 90 percent of the disease-causing mutant genes in an outbred population is unusual. Furthermore, it is striking that MCAD deficiency is found almost exclusively among Caucasians, particularly those of northwestern European origin.[225,227,232,237] The few patients identified in other populations include one Pakistani patient (homozygous for 985A > G,[223] one African-American (Roe CR, unpublished observation), and isolated cases of southern European and North African origin. No patients have been identified in the Far East, nor were any carriers found by newborn screening in Japan.[236]

The human MCAD gene is highly polymorphic,[238–240] and with the use of three restriction enzymes, *Sac*I (or *Ban*II), *Taq*I and *Pst*I, several restriction fragment-polymorphism (RFLP) haplotypes have been identified.[231,241,242] One haplotype, resistant to all three enzymes (designated − − −), occurred in 23 percent[241] and 35 percent[227] of control alleles, but was found in virtually all of the 985A > G alleles in all three studies. This result suggests that the 985A > G mutation arose on the background of a − − − allele and gradually spread in the population. Two studies have demonstrated the particularly high frequency of the allele in patients of northwestern European origin, particularly among MCAD-deficient patients in the United Kingdom and Germany. These observations suggest that the 985A > G mutation occurred in a historical population occupying one of these regions and spread throughout northwestern Europe.[227,232]

Even before the discovery of the 985A > G allele (K329E), studies aimed at understanding the molecular basis of MCAD deficiency were performed.[243] By pulse-labeling of nascent MCAD in cultured fibroblasts with [^{35}S] methionine, the synthesis of the precursor MCAD subunit and its proteolytic processing to a mature subunit within the mitochondrial matrix were shown to be normal in cells from patients with MCAD deficiency. All but one of these patients were later found to be homozygous for the 985A > G mutation; the exception was a compound heterozygote[231] for 985A > G and the 13-bp insertion beginning at base 999. Immunoblot analysis of MCAD in fibroblasts from all of these patients,[244] as well as from other homozygotes for 985A > G,[245,246] have shown little or no immunoreactive MCAD. These results demonstrate that, despite normal translation and immediate posttranslational processing of the K329E-MCAD subunit, virtually none of the variant protein is detectable in the steady state. This suggests that the K329E-MCAD protein is unstable in the mitochondria. This conclusion is supported by

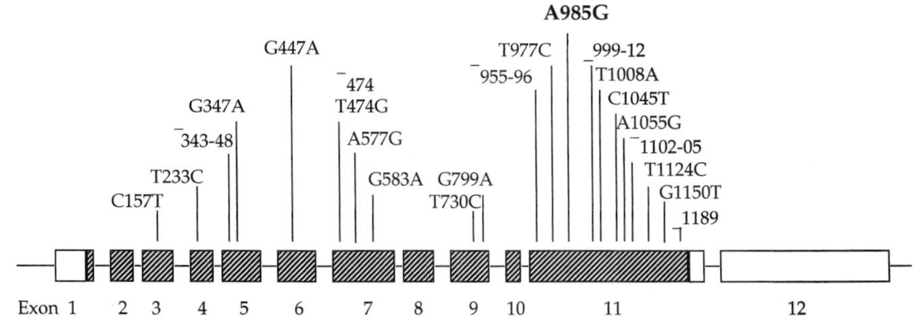

Fig. 101-6 The human MCAD gene and mutations. Boxes indicate exons; hatched areas are coding regions with mutation positions; open boxes indicate either 5′ or 3′ UTRs.

pulse-chase metabolic-labeling experiments using [^{35}S]-methionine, showing that the K329E MCAD protein, in contrast to wild-type MCAD, disappears almost completely over 24 h of incubation in unlabeled methionine.[244] However, these data do not agree with those of Kelly et al.[224] whose immunoblot studies demonstrated that fibroblasts from 985A > G homozygotes had detectable MCAD. There is, as yet, no obvious explanation for the discrepancy between these findings.

Several mechanisms could explain the apparent instability of the K329E MCAD subunit. These mechanisms include inherent instability of the mutant protein, inhibition of tetramer formation or disruption of normal tetramer structure. Computer analysis predicts that the K329E substitution would not cause drastic changes in MCAD secondary structure.[221] K329E is not involved in FAD binding or in substrate binding,[247] but, instead, contributes to the interface between subunits in the tetramer structure.[56,248] Replacement of a basic residue in this region by an acidic one may hinder tetramer formation or disrupt normal tetramer structure. Site-directed mutagenesis showed that a basic residue at position 329 is important for tetramer stability and/or assembly.[249,250]

Transfection of an 985A > G MCAD cDNA into bacteria,[225,251,252] green monkey kidney (COS-7) cells,[251] and Chinese hamster ovary cells[253] demonstrated that the K329E substitution significantly impairs MCAD activity. A normal amount of mRNA was produced but most of the variant protein recovered was in insoluble aggregates (bacteria) or partially degraded (COS-7 cells). By contrast, normal MCAD was soluble.[251,252]

Curiously, the 985A > G mutation, which occurs in exon 11, appears to be associated with a high degree of missplicing of MCAD mRNA; 30 to 40 percent of the mature 985A > G transcripts have exon deletions (particularly exon 2 or 5) and/or intron retention.[54,224,225] In some transcripts, the splicing apparatus utilizes a cryptic acceptor splice site in exon 11 downstream from the site of the nucleotide substitution, with the result that the sequence encoded in the 5′ half of exon 11 is deleted from the mature transcript. The molecular explanation(s) for the association of the aberrant splicing with the nucleotide substitution at position 985 is not known; however, even the transcripts derived from the normal MCAD gene exhibit a high degree of aberrant splicing (5 to 10 percent of the total cDNA clones isolated from various tissues).[54]

Studies of the molecular pathology of some of the other MCAD mutations have been reported. The 4-bp deletion (nt 1100 to 1103) described in two compound heterozygous patients[233,234] predicts a frameshift beginning at codon 369, leading to an MCAD precursor with 16 altered residues and truncated at residue 385, 36 residues shorter than normal. By immunoblot analysis, a variant MCAD precursor 4 to 5 kDa smaller than normal was identified in liver from a patient with this allele[234] and in *E. coli* transfected with mutant cDNA.[233] The 13-bp repeat insertion described in heterozygous form in three patients[231,232] predicts a truncated protein, although none was found in cell labeling[243] or immunoblot[244] experiments. This result suggests that the RNA produced from this allele or its protein product is unstable.[227]

Implications for Diagnosis and Screening. The molecular characterization of MCAD deficiency has made it possible to assess the various methods employed in the diagnosis of this disease. For this purpose, data were gathered on acylcarnitine profiles and DNA analysis in samples from members of 25 families with MCAD deficiency. Of the 62 children analyzed, 36 had MCAD deficiency, 28 were homozygous for 985A > G, and 8 were compound heterozygotes for this mutation and a rarer allele (4-bp deletion from nt 1100, 799A > G, 157C > T). Blood acylcarnitine profiles were diagnostic of MCAD deficiency in all cases. A further 18 children were heterozygotes for A985G and a normal allele, 1 was a carrier for a rare mutation (799A > G), and 5 were normal; acylcarnitine profiles were normal in all 62 of these children. They were also normal in blood from all 46 of their parents. Thus, blood acylcarnitine profile appears to identify all patients with MCAD deficiency and is normal in heterozygotes. Mutation analysis clearly distinguishes 985A > G homozygotes and carriers from normals but cannot distinguish compound heterozygotes for 985A > G and some other rare alleles. The combination of molecular analysis plus acylcarnitine profile provides the most information.

Direct assay of MCAD activity does not always discriminate between affected, carrier, and normal individuals. It can occasionally miss affected individuals, and is not absolutely reliable for carrier detection. Given that other biochemical and molecular methods have been developed which are reliable and rapid, enzyme assay would not have a role in screening.

MCAD deficiency satisfies all the major criteria for newborn screening.[228] It is a common inherited disease, with a frequency approaching that of phenylketonuria. The disorder can result in significant clinical disease that may be fatal. Relatively simple dietary means and anticipatory management can avert the clinical phenotype of MCAD deficiency. Affected individuals are for the most part asymptomatic in the newborn period, but the molecular defect which underlies most mutant alleles, as well as some of the key abnormal metabolites, can be detected with high accuracy and specificity in blood samples spotted onto newborn screening cards.[210,232,235,236,254,255] For these reasons, the screening of all newborns for MCAD deficiency appears to be justified. Similarly, screening of at-risk populations, either retrospectively (e.g., by analysis of postmortem specimens[222,256,257] from patients dying with SIDS) or prospectively (e.g., sibs of patients with confirmed MCAD deficiency) can be done.

Management and Treatment. The primary goals for management of MCAD-deficient patients include provision of adequate caloric intake, avoidance of fasting, and aggressive support during infectious episodes. The anorexia that often accompanies infection and fever predisposes to mobilization of endogenous lipid stores, producing toxic intermediates (see "Pathogenesis of MCAD Deficiency" below) which can lead to vomiting, lethargy, coma, and even death. Although some children with MCAD deficiency appear to have good fasting tolerance in the absence of infection, they usually do not do well with infection and may require IV glucose to halt the process. The risk of death and the frequency of other residual abnormalities (see Table 101-2) leave little doubt about the urgency of early diagnosis and appropriate treatment.

L-Carnitine supplementation has been advocated in the management of MCAD deficiency, as well as other causes of secondary carnitine deficiency. Its use in this setting represents a useful conjugation pathway for the removal of potentially toxic intermediates that accumulate under conditions of fasting stress or infection in these patients.[204] For example,[258] an asymptomatic MCAD-deficient patient receiving oral carnitine supplementation (100 mg/kg day) excreted 7 mM total carnitine per milligram of creatinine, of which only 0.4 mM was octanoylcarnitine. The same patient when acutely ill and treated with IV carnitine (30 mg/kg day) excreted 13 mM octanoylcarnitine/mg creatinine; when she had recovered and was receiving the same IV dose of carnitine, she excreted only 0.6 mM octanoylcarnitine/mg creatinine. Thus, on IV therapy octanoylcarnitine excretion during illness was 21 times greater than that observed when well. The enhanced production and excretion of octanoylcarnitine in the sick child suggests that carnitine supplementation is useful for conjugation and excretion of toxic metabolites during illness, but may serve little purpose during periods of good health.

Carnitine supplementation in MCAD deficiency is analogous to the provision of glycine to patients with isovaleric acidemia (see Chap. 87). Glycine supplementation augments the excretion of toxic intermediates (isovalerate) from tissues while restoring CoA levels. Carnitine supplementation does not correct the underlying defect in MCAD deficiency,[259,260] but neither is it associated with enhanced turnover of fat in this disorder,[261] a theoretical concern that arises because carnitine mediates the mitochondrial uptake of fatty acids. There are apparently no toxic effects from carnitine supplementation other than occasional loose stools and a dose-dependent fishlike body odor in children receiving very high doses. This odor results from bacterial degradation of L-carnitine in the gastrointestinal tract producing trimethylamine, and is not apparent with the usual doses utilized in therapy.

Pathogenesis of MCAD Deficiency. There is substantial information available from controlled fasting studies[9,262] and from the analysis of urinary metabolite excretion profiles[204,263–265] to allow speculation on the sequence of metabolic events in MCAD deficiency and their potential consequences. While the following discussion refers to MCAD deficiency, much of it is relevant to the pathogenesis of all fatty acid oxidation defects.

One major consequence of MCAD deficiency is the failure to make ketone bodies in quantities sufficient to meet tissue energy demands under conditions of fasting stress. During the initial stages of fasting, patients remain well and their glucose levels are normal. As plasma free fatty acids rise with continued fasting, there is no attendant increase in plasma ketones. Hypoglycemia develops presumably as a result of the exhaustion of glucose production, because ketones and fatty acids are unavailable to substitute for glucose as metabolic fuels.

A further consequence is the accumulation of medium chain (C8-C12) acyl-CoA intermediates in mitochondria at the expense of acetyl-CoA. Free CoA, which does not exchange between the mitochondrial and cytosolic compartments, is also compromised. Thus, increased acyl-CoA production results in decreased CoA availability for other mitochondrial reactions. The acyl-CoA:CoA ratio in mitochondria exerts regulatory control over pyruvate dehydrogenase[266] and α-ketoglutarate dehydrogenase.[267] When this ratio is elevated, both enzymes are inhibited, resulting in reduced conversion of pyruvate to acetyl-CoA and reduced flux through the tricarboxylic acid cycle, because citrate synthesis and flux from α-ketoglutarate to succinyl-CoA are impeded. Succinyl-CoA ligase is also inhibited by octanoate,[268] as well as by other acyl-CoA intermediates. When these intermediates accumulate, mitochondrial β-oxidation is inhibited;[11] the expected result is fatty acid incorporation into triglycerides, consistent with the marked accumulation of fat in liver during acute episodes.[158]

Inadequate acetyl-CoA production has significant secondary effects on flux through the tricarboxylic acid cycle, on regulation of fatty acid oxidation in mitochondria, and on the efficiency of gluconeogenesis. Acetyl-CoA is a substrate, along with oxaloacetate, for the citrate synthase reaction. Inadequate amounts of either substrate result in diminished citrate synthesis. Inhibition of α-ketoglutarate dehydrogenase by the elevated acyl-CoA:CoA ratio reduces flux through the tricarboxylic acid cycle and impairs oxaloacetate synthesis. Furthermore, because citrate serves as a means to transport acetyl-CoA to the cytosol, decreased availability of citrate influences the regulation of both fatty acid oxidation and gluconeogenesis. When there is a sufficient quantity of citrate, it is transported to the cytosol and converted by citrate lyase into acetyl-CoA and oxaloacetate. The latter may be converted to malate or to phosphoenolpyruvate and ultimately glucose. Thus, both the redox state and gluconeogenesis are affected. Acetyl-CoA produced from citrate by citrate lyase in the cytoplasm is a substrate for acetyl-CoA carboxylase and synthesis of malonyl-CoA, the primary regulator of CPT I. Citrate not only is the source of substrate for acetyl-CoA carboxylase, but also is its primary activator. Decreased mitochondrial acetyl-CoA limits the amount of cytoplasmic citrate available to both activate and provide substrate for acetyl-CoA carboxylase. Reduced malonyl-CoA levels allow unregulated entry of fatty acids into mitochondria and, in MCAD deficiency, increased production of medium chain acyl-CoA intermediates.

Inadequate mitochondrial acetyl-CoA also affects pyruvate carboxylase. Acetyl-CoA is the primary activator of this biotin-dependent enzyme, which converts pyruvate to oxaloacetate and is critical for gluconeogenesis. Propionyl-CoA also activates pyruvate carboxylase, but longer chain compounds such as octanoyl-CoA do not. Compromise of this pathway in MCAD deficiency may account for the hypoglycemia.

The clinical presentation and many of the routine laboratory observations in MCAD-deficient patients are indistinguishable from those in Reye syndrome.[269] Octanoate infused into rabbits produces many of the pathologic findings of Reye syndrome.[270] The encephalopathy and cerebral edema observed in MCAD deficiency may result from similar mechanisms.[270,271] Acyl compounds with three or more carbons have significant encephalopathic properties;[272] the greater the chain length of the compounds, the more rapidly coma occurs. Furthermore, acyl compounds such as propionate, octanoate, and palmitate enter the central nervous system at rates increasing with longer carbon-chain length. There is potential, therefore, for rapid accumulation of fatty acids within the central nervous system. This may be exacerbated by octanoate-induced inhibition of the choroid plexus organic anion uptake system largely responsible for egress of these compounds from the central nervous system.[273] Experimentally induced octanoic acidemia damages neuronal mitochondria with distension and separation of mitochondrial cristae, and loss of matrix integrity.[271] Cultured astrocytes exposed to octanoate fail to maintain volume control.[274] These structural abnormalities together with depression of energy metabolism and the resultant decreased availability of high-energy phosphate compounds,[275] may lead to cerebral edema. Although hypoglycemia is a common finding in MCAD deficiency, coma in these patients is not due entirely to low blood glucose levels, since they may be encephalopathic despite correction of hypoglycemia.[4,7] Coma is more likely the result of toxic effect of fatty acids or their metabolites.

Short Chain Acyl CoA Dehydrogenase (SCAD) Deficiency

Clinical Presentations. SCAD deficiency has been identified in only a few patients[276–278] with highly variable clinical and laboratory findings, as demonstrated by the following cases.

Case 1. A female infant of unrelated parents (neonate II[277]) was delivered normally and began cow's milk formula on day 2. On day 3, she fed poorly, began to vomit, and became lethargic and hypertonic. She was hypoglycemic, acidotic (pH 7.28), and hyperammonemic (399 μM). In spite of IV glucose therapy, she became more lethargic, unresponsive, and hypotonic, with increasing respiratory effort. Organic acid analysis showed lactic acidosis, ketosis, and increased excretion of butyrate, ethylmalonate, and adipate. She died on day 6. Postmortem examination revealed cerebral edema, hepatosplenomegaly with fatty changes, cholestasis, and focal hepatocellular necrosis.

Case 2. A female infant[278] of unrelated parents presented in early postnatal life with poor feeding and frequent emesis. She exhibited poor weight gain, developmental delay, progressive skeletal muscle weakness, hypotonia, and microcephaly. Skeletal muscle biopsy showed minor generalized lipid accumulation in type I fibers. She never had episodes of hypoglycemia, rarely had organic aciduria, and had low-normal plasma carnitine levels. Her muscle carnitine level was 50 percent of control with 75 percent esterified. She responded poorly to a fat-restricted diet supplemented with L-carnitine. At 21 months, she had significant developmental delay. Increasing difficulty with poor oral intake required a gastrostomy tube at 23 months. At 32 months, she showed significant weight gain and overall improvement in strength.

Case 3. A 46-year-old woman[276] with no previous neuromuscular disorder presented with persistent weakness in one arm and both legs, exacerbated by mild exertion. Neurologic examination revealed a proximal myopathy, which was confirmed by electromyography. Serum CPK was normal. There was excess neutral lipid in type I skeletal muscle fibers, with no other abnormalities. Muscle carnitine levels were low (25 percent of control) with an increased proportion of acyl to free carnitine. Plasma carnitine levels were low-normal. The major urinary metabolite was ethylmalonate, fasting was not associated with hypoglycemia, and blood ketone body levels were elevated. Her weakness did not respond either to carnitine or prednisolone.

Case 4. A female infant born to related Hispanic parents was severely developmentally delayed and extremely hypotonic. She excreted large quantities of ethylmalonate along with methylsuccinate. Her plasma butyrylcarnitine was consistently elevated. Her plasma lactate was normal. When these same parents had another pregnancy, an amniocentesis with enzyme assay in amniocytes yielded equivocal results suggesting partial decrease in SCAD activity. The family elected to terminate the pregnancy. Direct enzyme assay for SCAD with and without anti-MCAD antibody revealed normal activity in fetal liver but severe deficiency in fetal muscle (Kobori J, Vianey-Saban C, Roe CR, unpublished data).

Pathologic Findings. Pathologic findings in Case 3 were limited to muscle and included lipid vacuolization, especially in type I fibers.[276] Despite Case 2's clinical phenotype being primarily muscular,[278] her liver showed ultrastructural evidence of both microvesicular and macrovesicular steatosis, and mitochondrial changes reminiscent of those seen in MCAD deficiency, namely, increased matrix density and crystalloids (Douglas SD, Coates PM, unpublished observation). Case 1 had hepatic steatosis at autopsy.

Organic Acid Analysis. Patients with generalized SCAD deficiency excrete short chain organic acids (ethylmalonate, methylsuccinate, butyrylglycine) and butyrylcarnitine in urine. Although these metabolites are also excreted by patients with multiple acyl-CoA dehydrogenation defects,[279–281] the latter may be recognized by the presence of acylcarnitines[210] and other metabolites[279] derived from defective amino acid oxidation.

Diagnosis. The diagnosis of SCAD deficiency is made by measuring acyl-CoA dehydrogenase activities in available tissues. Because MCAD has broad substrate specificity with some activity towards short chain acyl-CoAs, the most direct measurements of SCAD are made in extracts in which MCAD activity has been eliminated by incubation with anti-MCAD antibody. With butyryl-CoA as substrate, fibroblasts from Cases 1 and 2 and another patient (neonate I)[277] had 50 percent of control SCAD activity, all of which was inhibited by incubation of the cells with anti-MCAD antibody.[277,278] Activity toward palmitoyl-CoA and octanoyl-CoA was normal. Cells from the parents of Case 2 had intermediate SCAD activity, consistent with heterozygosity for an autosomal trait.

Skeletal muscle SCAD activity in Case 3, measured with butyryl-CoA as substrate,[276] was 25 percent of control levels, and was associated with reduced immunoreactive SCAD;[282] dehydrogenase activities toward longer-chain acyl-CoA substrates (C8 or longer) were well within normal limits. SCAD activity in fibroblasts was normal.[277,278] While careful study of SCAD in other tissues from Case 3 could not be performed, the data suggested that this patient had an isolated deficiency of muscle SCAD, although a variant multiple acyl-CoA dehydrogenation defect could not be ruled out. The results with case 4, a severely affected infant, and analysis of an at risk pregnancy in the same family, suggest that there is a form of SCAD deficiency which is limited to muscle, without involvement of liver, which may manifest severe symptoms in infancy. Unfortunately, no direct assays have been performed on muscle or liver from the affected child, so this hypothesis cannot be tested directly. If the hypothesis is correct, prenatal diagnosis of such cases by enzyme assay of amniocyte extracts could be misleading.

In this context, there are a few patients with lipid storage myopathy in whom muscle SCAD (and sometimes MCAD) activity and antigen are substantially reduced,[283,284] who show clinical and biochemical improvement on treatment with pharmacologic doses of riboflavin; furthermore, SCAD activity and antigen are restored. These data are similar to those found in the riboflavin-deficient rat,[285–287] and suggest that patients such as these may have a form of riboflavin-responsive multiple acyl-CoA dehydrogenation defect.[288–295]

Butyryl-CoA dehydrogenase (SCAD) is known to be very labile and easily affected secondarily. Because some patients thought to have SCAD deficiency due to increased ethylmalonate excretion have also had persistent elevations of lactate, the possibility of a primary lesion in the respiratory chain should also be considered.

Pathogenesis. The pathogenesis of disease associated with SCAD deficiency presents some puzzling aspects, because there is no common thread among the patients who have been reported with this defect. Cases 3 and 4 appear to have an isolated muscle SCAD deficiency appearing either in infancy or adulthood, while other patients[277,278] have an enzyme defect expressed in fibroblasts. Because of its position in the β-oxidation pathway, it is unlikely that a defect in SCAD would have a major effect on the yield of energy from fatty acid oxidation, because at least three-fourths of a long chain fatty acid can be oxidized before SCAD activity is required. This prediction is supported by the finding that under conditions of fasting stress, SCAD-deficient patients were capable of mounting a ketogenic response. That some SCAD-deficient patients are profoundly affected suggests that the pathophysiology involves more than simple energy deficit.

Molecular Aspects. SCAD is a homotetrameric mitochondrial flavoenzyme that catalyzes the initial reaction in short chain fatty acid β-oxidation. The human *SCAD* structural gene is approximately 13 kb in length and is located at 12q22-qter.[296,297] Its 10 exons encode the entire 412 amino acid precursor SCAD (44.3 kDa) (GenBank M26393) including the 24-amino acid mitochondrial leader peptide and a 388-amino-acid mature protein (41.7 kDa).[52,297] Comparison of SCAD and MCAD sequences reveals a high degree of similarity, suggesting that these enzymes evolved from a common ancestral gene.[52]

Four *SCAD* gene polymorphisms have been reported. Three are synonymous variants (321T > C, 990C > T, 1260G > C), while one (625G > A) results in a glycine to serine substitution (G209S) that has not been associated with SCAD deficiency but that has been associated with ethylmalonic aciduria.[297]

136C > T (R22W) and 319C > T (R83C) mutations were first reported in a compound heterozygous patient with SCAD deficiency.[298] Four additional mutations, 274G > T, 529T > C, 1147C > T, and 511C > T, have also been identified.[299]

Elevated urinary excretion of ethylmalonic acid (EMA) is a common biochemical finding in patients with SCAD deficiency. When butyryl-CoA oxidation is reduced, as in SCAD deficiency, it is alternatively metabolized by propionyl-CoA carboxylase to EMA. Among 135 individuals with abnormal EMA excretion ranging from 18 to 1185 μmol/mol of creatinine (controls < 18 μmol/mol of creatinine) a significant overrepresentation of a variant allele was found.[300] Eighty-one individuals (60 percent) were homozygous for the 625G > A allele, 40 (30 percent) were heterozygous, and only 14 (10 percent) were homozygous for the wild-type allele. Corydon et al. believe that the 625G > A allele, as well as a recently identified 511C > T mutation,[299] are associated with the development of ethylmalonic aciduria.[297,300] The extent to which these mutations reduce SCAD activity, as determined by direct enzyme assay, has not yet been determined.

The BALB/cBy mouse strain is a model for SCAD deficiency. In this inbred line, a 278-bp deletion was identified in the 3′ end of the structural SCAD gene. This deletion results in missplicing of mRNA. The abnormal transcripts have aberrant stop codons and reduced steady state levels of SCAD mRNA.[301] Although the biochemical markers of the disease are present, there are no comparable symptoms as seen in affected humans.

Short Chain L-3-Hydroxyacyl-CoA Dehydrogenase (SCHAD) Deficiency

Clinical presentations: Case 1. A 16-year-old girl presented with recurrent episodes of myoglobinuria, hypoketotic hypoglycemia, encephalopathy, and hypertrophic cardiomyopathy. Enzyme assays of a skeletal muscle homogenate had normal LCHAD activity with 3-ketopalmitoyl-CoA as substrate, but markedly reduced SCHAD activity with acetoacetyl-CoA as substrate; the defect was not expressed in fibroblasts. SCHAD activity was not measured in liver.[302]

Case 2. This boy was normal at birth and developed normally for the first year of life. At age 13 months, he had an episode of vomiting, lethargy, and dehydration. He also had three seizures associated with hyponatremia. A high-carbohydrate diet was not effective and he had continued to have episodes up to 3.5 years of age. Laboratory studies including glucose, electrolytes, bicarbonate, calcium, bilirubin, liver enzymes, ammonia, lactate/pyruvate, plasma amino acids, carnitine, and acylcarnitine analyses were normal. Urine organic acids revealed to reveal massive ketosis (β-hydroxybutyrate and acetoacetate) associated with long chain saturated and unsaturated dicarboxylic and monocarboxylic acids. Enzyme assays for LCHAD, SCHAD, and short chain 3-ketoacyl-CoA thiolase (SKAT) were performed on fibroblast extracts and on an isolated mitochondrial fraction. These enzyme activities were decreased from 34 to 41 percent in fibroblast extracts, and in mitochondrial fraction, LCHAD was reduced by 29 percent and SKAT by 43 percent, while there was a 95 percent decrease in SCHAD activity.[303]

Case 3. This female was diagnosed with DiGeorge syndrome (MIM 188400) with a microdeletion in 22q11. At 3 months of age, 1 month following cytomegalovirus septicemia, hepatomegaly was noted and electron microscopy of a liver biopsy showed lipid droplets and enlarged mitochondria. At 15 months, she had an episode of mild hypoglycemia associated with ketonuria. MRI of her head revealed bilateral demyelinating lesions of the periventricular white matter. Plasma carnitine was reduced at 22 mM and only C4 (butyryl-isobutyryl-) acylcarnitine was elevated on tandem MS analysis. Skin fibroblasts enzyme assays for LCHAD, SCHAD, and SKAT were not performed on disrupted cells but isolated mitochondria were assayed for SCHAD which was reduced to 6.6 percent of mean values and for SKAT, which was also reduced by 43 percent.[303]

These three cases reflect three very different phenotypes. Many more well-documented cases will have to be studied to determine optimal diagnostic tests, treatment, and pathogenesis.

Molecular Aspects. The human short chain L-3-hydroxyacyl-CoA dehydrogenase (*HADHSC*; EC1.1.1.35) structural gene (GenBank AF026853) is comprised of at least eight exons and is located at 4q22-26.[304,305] A cloned human liver SCHAD cDNA (GenBank X96752) has a 5′ untranslated sequence of 87 bases, an open reading frame of 942 nucleotides encoding a precursor protein of 314 amino acids and a 3′ untranslated sequence of 845 bases including the poly (A) tail.[305] The precursor protein (34.3 kDa) has a mitochondrial import signal peptide of 12 amino acids and a 302-amino-acid mature protein, which has 92 percent identity with the porcine enzyme. The human gene is expressed in skeletal and cardiac muscle, liver, kidney, and pancreas,[305] but not in fibroblasts, which raises a conflict with one of the case reports.[204,303]

A putative SCHAD pseudogene has also been identified and linked to marker D15S1324, located at Chr 15q17-21.[304]

Interestingly, a novel L-3-hydroxyacyl-CoA dehydrogenase from human brain has also been cloned, which is identical to an endoplasmic reticulum amyloid β-peptide-binding protein (ERAB) involved in Alzheimer's disease.[306] This human short chain L-3-hydroxyacyl-CoA dehydrogenase gene is organized into six exons and five introns and maps to chromosome Xp11.2.

No information is available about the mutations in short-chain L-3-hydroxyacyl-CoA dehydrogenase deficiency.

GENERAL APPROACH TO THE PATIENT WITH A SUSPECTED FATTY ACID OXIDATION DISORDER

Individual defects and their various (often multiple) clinical phenotypes have been described above. This concluding section provides a summary of clinical and laboratory considerations for patients in whom a disorder of fatty acid oxidation is suspected.

When the possibility of a mitochondrial fat oxidation disorder is considered, certain routine and specialized tests should be obtained. These include (especially during the acute illness) blood glucose, electrolytes, urea, ammonia, uric acid, CPK, lactate, transaminases (AST/ALT), and complete blood count, including platelets. From routine urinalysis, examine results for "blood" from the dipstick and compare with the presence or absence of red blood cells detected in the microscopic analysis to see if myoglobinuria is present. More specialized tests include plasma carnitine levels (increase suggests CPT I) and an acylcarnitine profile (useful for the diagnosis of translocase, CPT II, VLCAD, LCHAD, MCAD, and possibly SCAD and trifunctional protein deficiencies) along with quantitative urinary organic acid analysis by GC-MS (includes acylglycine quantification-MCAD and MADD only). Skin biopsy to establish a fibroblast culture should be done for direct enzyme assay or for probing the metabolic pathway with 16-$^2H_3$-palmitate as a substrate, in vitro. It is important to recognize that fibroblast fatty acid oxidation studies with labeled myristate or palmitate can only suggest a problem exists without necessarily providing specific information unlike direct enzyme assay or probing the β oxidation pathway using 16-$^2H_3$-palmitate as substrate and tandem-MS analysis of the acylcarnitines as the assay. If deficiency of the muscle-kidney plasma membrane carnitine transporter or hepatic CPT I is prominent on the differential list, then specific direct assays should be sought.

Although there is overlap of presenting symptoms and organ involvement, these disorders generally fall into three major groups dominated by the organ system most involved. These include the hepatic-, cardiac-, and muscle-dominant phenotypes.[307,308]

The hepatic group is mainly characterized by recurrent Reye-like illness involving hypoketotic hypoglycemia leading to obtundation and coma. Metabolic acidosis is unusual unless terminal lactic acidosis has developed. Hyperammonemia, hyperuricemia, and increased levels of serum transaminases are usually observed. Plasma carnitine levels are usually decreased secondarily although they are characteristically increased in the hepatic form of CPT I deficiency. Liver biopsy, acutely or at postmortem, will reveal micro- and/or macrovesicular steatosis. These observations have been reported commonly in MCAD deficiency, and in the hypoglycemic form of VLCAD deficiency, LCHAD, infantile CPT II, mild translocase, and CPT I deficiencies. The cardiac form of VLCAD deficiency often presents with neonatal hypoketotic hypoglycemia responsive to fluid therapy in the neonatal period, but returns between 2 and 5 months of age with severe hypertrophic cardiomyopathy that is usually fatal. Any neonatal hypoglycemia should be evaluated with an acylcarnitine profile to identify this disorder.

When cardiac abnormalities dominate the presentation, there is often an acute or chronic hypertrophic or dilated cardiomyopathy. Pericardial effusion often accompanies the hypertrophic cardiomyopathy and is often responsible for death in the cardiac form of VLCAD deficiency. Isolated transient arrhythmia should not be considered as a major cardiac finding in these diseases. The first case of VLCAD reported had a transient arrhythmia but the real problem was hypoglycemia and the patient never had any other cardiac manifestations. Cardiac abnormalities have been prominent with the muscle-kidney carnitine transporter defect, LCHAD, trifunctional protein deficiency, neonatal CPT II deficiency, as well as the cardiac phenotype of VLCAD deficiency.

A muscle phenotype usually includes moderate to severe hypotonia or recurrent rhabdomyolysis. Hypotonia, developmental delay, with or without seizures, should suggest the muscle phenotype of SCAD deficiency. Hypotonia can be observed during illness in many of these disorders but other organ system involvement often leads to consideration of the other categories. Recurrent rhabdomyolysis is characteristic of the adult form of CPT II deficiency and is often associated with deficiency of LCHAD, trifunctional protein, VLCAD, and in at least one case of SCHAD. It is important to realize that gross myoglobinuria ("burgundy"-colored urine) is often not observed until the serum CPK level is in excess of 30,000 IU/liter. Therefore dark or concentrated-appearing urine can represent myoglobinuria, which is confirmed by a positive urine dipstick test for blood in the absence of red cells in the urinary sediment. Serum CPK should routinely be measured when considering these diseases.

Family history is also important to determine if prior sibs have died—often categorized as SIDS or sudden unexplained death. Many families with these disorders of fat oxidation have already suffered the loss of at least one child. Similarly, prior pregnancies may have been associated with life-threatening acute fatty liver of pregnancy (AFLP) or HELLP syndrome (hemolysis, elevated liver enzymes, and low platelets). These third trimester maternal syndromes have been associated both with fetuses with either LCHAD or CPT I deficiency.

Investigation of sibling deaths is also often extremely helpful. These children are frequently medical examiner cases and extensive information may be obtained from review of the postmortem examination. Steatosis and/or cerebral edema are often observed but the absence of these abnormalities does not, by itself, rule out fatty acid oxidation disorders. The original neonatal screening card may still be available and can be utilized for acylcarnitine assay or molecular analysis. Similarly, blood samples taken for toxicology analysis are frequently stored for up to 1 year and have proved very useful in detecting MCAD, VLCAD, CPT II, translocase, and LCHAD deficiencies. Molecular analysis of these samples, as well as from amplified DNA obtained from either formalin-fixed or paraffin embedded tissues, has been useful in screening for MCAD and LCHAD mutations. Molecular screening for other disorders of fat oxidation has been less useful due to the lack of a frequent disease-causing mutation.

In the past, prenatal diagnosis was traditionally done by direct enzyme assay of amniocytes or chorionic villous samples (CVS). Analysis of cell-free amniotic fluid for metabolites is not a useful alternative for the diagnosis of fat oxidation disorders as diagnostic metabolites are usually undetectable, even in MCAD deficiency. Because the various disorders have overlapping phenotypes, direct enzyme assays are only useful if the disorder segregation in a family has already been identified. An alternative for simultaneous analysis for many of these disorders is the incubation of amniocytes with stable isotope-labeled precursors for the β oxidative pathway such as 16-$^2H_3$-palmitate followed by acylcarnitine analysis of the labeled intermediates by tandem-MS. These quantified, labeled intermediate profiles have been successfully utilized for prenatal diagnosis of deficiency of translocase, CPT II, VLCAD, LCHAD, and MCAD. Complete trifunctional protein deficiency has not yet been studied with this method. Because there are no characteristic acylcarnitines for CPT I deficiency and the muscle-kidney carnitine transporter defect, other methods are needed to diagnosis these disorders. Although SCAD deficiency should be easily detected, in the muscle form of this disease, neither incubation of amniocytes with 16-$^2H_3$-palmitate nor direct enzyme assay with butyryl-CoA and ETF were able to identify an affected fetus (later proven by direct enzyme assay of fetal muscle tissue). Despite these limitations, when the specific defect is not known, the incubation with 16-$^2H_3$-palmitate has proven to be very useful. Given the complexity of the β-oxidation spiral, the fact that all the enzymes in the pathway-acyl-CoA dehydrogenases, 2-enoyl-CoA hydratases, 3-hydroxyacyl-CoA dehydrogenases, and 3-ketoacyl-CoA thiolases have been found to exist in multiple forms with overlapping chain-length specificity, and the fact that the complete oxidation of unsaturated fatty acids requires additional enzyme-mediated steps, it is likely that additional defects in fatty acid oxidation will be identified. They represent ongoing challenges for the study of inherited disorders of mitochondrial fatty acid oxidation.

REFERENCES

1. Engel AG, Angelini C: Carnitine deficiency of human skeletal muscle with associated lipid storage myopathy: A new syndrome. *Science* **179**:899, 1973.
2. DiMauro S, DiMauro PMM: Muscle carnitine palmityltransferase deficiency and myoglobinuria. *Science* **182**:929, 1973.
3. Karpati G, Carpenter S, Engel AG, Watters G, Allen J, Rothman S, Klassen G, Mamer OA: The syndrome of systemic carnitine deficiency: Clinical, morphologic, biochemical, and pathophysiologic features. *Neurology* **25**:16, 1975.
4. Kolvraa S, Gregersen N, Christensen E, Hobolth N: In vitro fibroblast studies in a patient with C6-C10-dicarboxylic aciduria: Evidence for a defect in general acyl-CoA dehydrogenase. *Clin Chim Acta* **126**:53, 1982.
5. Divry P, David M, Gregersen N, Kolvraa S, Christensen E, Collet JP, Dellamonica D, Cotte J: Dicarboxylic aciduria due to medium chain acyl CoA dehydrogenase defect. A cause of hypoglycemia in childhood. *Acta Paediatr Scand* **72**:943, 1983.
6. Rhead WJ, Amendt BA, Fritchman KS, Felts SJ: Dicarboxylic aciduria: Deficient [1-14C] octanoate oxidation and medium-chain acyl-CoA dehydrogenase in fibroblasts. *Science* **221**:73, 1983.
7. Stanley CA, Hale DE, Coates PM, Hall CL, Corkey BE, Yang W, Kelley RI, Gonzales EL, Williamson JR, Baker L: Medium-chain acyl-CoA dehydrogenase deficiency in children with non-ketotic hypoglycemia and low carnitine levels. *Pediatr Res* **17**:877, 1983.
8. Roe CR, Coates PM: Acyl-CoA dehydrogenase deficiencies, in Scriver CR, Beaudet AL, Sly WS, Valle D (eds): *The Metabolic Basis of Inherited Disease*, 7th ed. New York, McGraw-Hill, 1995, Vol I, p 1501.
9. Stanley CA: New genetic defects in mitochondrial fatty acid oxidation and carnitine deficiency. *Adv Pediatr* **34**:59, 1987.
10. McGarry JD, Foster DW: Regulation of hepatic fatty acid oxidation and ketone body production. *Annu Rev Biochem* **49**:395, 1980.
11. Bremer J, Osmundsen H: Fatty acid oxidation and its regulation, in Numa S (ed): *Fatty Acid Metabolism and Its Regulation*. Amsterdam, Elsevier, 1984, p 113.
12. Schulz H: Oxidation of fatty acids, in Vance DE, Vance J (eds): *Biochemistry of Lipids, Lipoproteins and Membranes*. Amsterdam, Elsevier, 1991, p 87.
13. Ahlborg G, Felig P, Hagenfeldt L, Hendler R, Wahren J: Substrate turnover during prolonged exercise in man. Splanchnic and leg metabolism of glucose, free fatty acids, and amino acids. *J Clin Invest* **53**:1080, 1974.
14. Stremmel W, Strohmeyer G, Borchard F, Kochwa S, Berk PD: Isolation and partial characterization of a fatty acid binding protein in rat liver plasma membranes. *Proc Natl Acad Sci U S A* **82**:4, 1985.
15. Stremmel W, Strohmeyer G, Berk PD: Hepatocellular uptake of oleate is energy dependent, sodium linked, and inhibited by an antibody to a hepatocyte plasma membrane fatty acid binding protein. *Proc Natl Acad Sci U S A* **83**:3584, 1986.
16. Ockner RK, Kaikaus RM, Bass NM: Fatty acid binding proteins: Recent concepts of regulation and function, in Coates PM, Tanaka K (eds): *New Developments in Fatty Acid Oxidation*. New York, Wiley-Liss, 1992, p 189.
17. Peeters R, Veerkamp J, Kanda T, Ono T, Geurts van Kessel A: The gene encoding skeletal muscle fatty acid binding protein resides on human chromosome 1, region pter-q31. *Cytogenet Cell Genet* **58**:1861, 1991.
18. Abe T, Fujino T, Fukuyama R, Minoshima S, Shimizu N, Toh H, Suzuki H, Yamamoto T: Human long-chain acyl-CoA synthetase: Structure and chromosomal location. *J Biochem* **111**:123, 1992.
19. Bremer J: Carnitine-metabolism and functions. *Physiol Rev* **63**:1420, 1983.
20. Sandor A, Kispal G, Melegh B, Alkonyi I: Release of carnitine from the perfused rat liver. *Biochim Biophys Acta* **835**:83, 1985.
21. Martinuzzi A, Vergani L, Rosa M, Angelini C: L-Carnitine uptake in differentiating human cultured muscle. *Biochim Biophys Acta* **1095**:217, 1991.

22. Zammit VA, Corstorphine CG, Kelliher MG: Evidence for distinct functional molecular sizes of carnitine palmitoyltransferases I and II in rat liver mitochondria. *Biochem J* **250**:415, 1988.
23. Woeltje KF, Esser V, Weis BC, Sen A, Cox WF, McPhaul MJ, Slaughter CA, Foster DW, McGarry JD: Cloning, sequencing, and expression of a cDNA encoding rat liver mitochondrial carnitine palmitoyltransferase II. *J Biol Chem* **265**:10720, 1990.
24. Finocchiaro G, Taroni F, Rocchi M, Liras Martin A, Colombo I, Torri Tarelli G, DiDonato S: cDNA cloning, sequence analysis, and chromosomal localization of the gene for human carnitine palmitoyltransferase. *Proc Natl Acad Sci U S A* **88**:661, 1991.
25. Finocchiaro G, Colombo I, DiDonato S: Purification, characterization and partial amino acid sequences of carnitine palmitoyl-transferase from human liver. *FEBS Lett* **274**:163, 1990.
26. Woeltje KF, Esser V, Weis BC, Cox WF, Schroeder JG, Liao S-T, Foster DW, McGarry JD: Inter-tissue and inter-species characteristics of the mitochondrial carnitine palmitoyltransferase enzyme system. *J Biol Chem* **265**:10714, 1990.
27. Woeltje KF, Kuwajima M, Foster DW, McGarry JD: Characterization of the mitochondrial carnitine palmitoyltransferase enzyme system. II. Use of detergents and antibodies. *J Biol Chem* **262**:9822, 1987.
28. Kolodziej MP, Crilly PJ, Corstorphine CG, Zammit VA: Development and characterization of a polyclonal antibody against rat liver mitochondrial overt carnitine palmitoyltransferase (CPT I). Distinction of CPT I from CPT II and of isoforms of CPT I in different tissues. *Biochem J* **282**:415, 1992.
29. Indiveri C, Tonazzi A, Palmieri F: Identification and purification of the carnitine carrier from rat liver mitochondria. *Biochim Biophys Acta* **1020**:81, 1990.
30. Indiveri C, Tonazzi A, Prezioso G, Palmieri F: Kinetic characterization of the reconstituted carnitine carrier from rat liver mitochondria. *Biochim Biophys Acta* **1065**:231, 1991.
31. Crane FL, Beinert H: On the mechanism of dehydrogenation of fatty acyl derivatives of coenzyme A. II. The electron-transferring flavoprotein. *J Biol Chem* **218**:717, 1956.
32. Frerman FE: Acyl-CoA dehydrogenases, electron transfer flavoprotein and electron transfer flavoprotein dehydrogenase. *Biochem Soc Trans* **16**:416, 1988.
33. Ikeda Y, Okamura-Ikeda K, Tanaka K: Purification and characterization of short-chain, medium-chain, and long-chain acyl-CoA dehydrogenases from rat liver mitochondria. Isolation of the holo- and apoenzymes and conversion of the apoenzyme to the holoenzyme. *J Biol Chem* **260**:1311, 1985.
34. Finocchiaro G, Ito M, Tanaka K: Purification and properties of short chain acyl-CoA, medium chain acyl-CoA, and isovaleryl-CoA dehydrogenases from human liver. *J Biol Chem* **262**:7982, 1987.
35. Crane FL, Mii S, Hauge JG, Green DE, Beinert H: On the mechanism of dehydrogenation of fatty acyl derivatives of coenzyme A. I. The general fatty acylcoenzyme A dehydrogenase. *J Biol Chem* **218**:701, 1956.
36. Hauge JG, Crane FL, Beinert H: On the mechanism of dehydrogenation of fatty acyl derivatives of coenzyme A. III. Palmitoyl CoA dehydrogenase. *J Biol Chem* **219**:727, 1956.
37. Hall CL, Kamin H: The purification and some properties of electron transfer flavoprotein and general fatty acyl coenzyme A dehydrogenase from pig liver mitochondria. *J Biol Chem* **250**:3476, 1975.
38. Thorpe C, Matthews RG, Williams CH: Acyl-coenzyme A dehydrogenase from pig kidney. Purification and properties. *Biochemistry* **18**:331, 1979.
39. Davidson B, Schulz H: Separation, properties, and regulation of acyl coenzyme A dehydrogenases from bovine heart and liver. *Arch Biochem Biophys* **213**:155, 1982.
40. Dommes V, Kunau W-H: Purification and properties of acyl coenzyme A dehydrogenases from bovine liver. Formation of 2-*trans*, 4-*cis*-decadienoyl coenzyme A. *J Biol Chem* **259**:1789, 1984.
41. Shaw L, Engel PC: The purification and properties of ox liver short-chain acyl-CoA dehydrogenase. *Biochem J* **218**:511, 1984.
42. Ikeda Y, Dabrowski C, Tanaka K: Separation and properties of five distinct acyl-CoA dehydrogenases from rat liver mitochondria. Identification of a new 2-methyl branched-chain acyl-CoA dehydrogenase. *J Biol Chem* **258**:1066, 1983.
43. Furuta S, Miyazawa S, Hashimoto T: Purification and properties of rat liver acyl-CoA dehydrogenases and electron transfer flavoprotein. *J Biochem* **90**:1739, 1981.
44. Engel PC: Acyl-coenzyme A dehydrogenases, in Muller F (ed): *Chemistry and Biochemistry of Flavoenzymes*. Boca Raton, FL: CRC Press, 1992, vol III, p 597.
45. Nagao M, Tanaka K: FAD-dependent regulation of transcription, translation, post-translational processing and post-translational stability of various acyl-CoA dehydrogenase and of electron transfer flavoprotein, and the site of holoenzyme formation. *J Biol Chem* **267**:3052, 1992.
46. Izai K, Uchida Y, Oril T, Yamamoto S, Hashimoto T: Novel fatty acid β-oxidation enzymes in rat liver mitochondria. I. Purification and properties of very long-chain acyl-coenzyme A dehydrogenase. *J Biol Chem* **267**:1027, 1992.
47. Kelley RI: Beta-oxidation of long-chain fatty acids by human fibroblasts: Evidence for a novel long-chain acyl-coenzyme A dehydrogenase. *Biochem Biophys Res Commun* **182**:1002, 1992.
48. Indo Y, Yang-Feng T, Glassberg R, Tanaka K: Molecular cloning and nucleotide sequence of cDNAs encoding human long-chain acyl-CoA dehydrogenase and assignment of the location of its gene (ACADL) to chromosome 2. *Genomics* **11**:609, 1991.
49. Matsubara Y, Indo Y, Naito E, Ozasa H, Glassberg R, Vockley J, Ikeda Y, Kraus J, Tanaka K: Molecular cloning and nucleotide sequence of cDNAs encoding the precursors of rat long chain acyl-coenzyme A, short chain acyl-coenzyme A, and isovaleryl-coenzyme A dehydrogenases. Sequence homology of four enzymes of the acyl-CoA dehydrogenase family. *J Biol Chem* **264**:16321, 1989.
50. Kelly DP, Kim J-J, Billadello JJ, Hainline BE, Chu TW, Strauss AW: Nucleotide sequence of medium-chain acyl-CoA dehydrogenase mRNA and its expression in enzyme-deficient human tissue. *Proc Natl Acad Sci U S A* **84**:4068, 1987.
51. Matsubara Y, Kraus JP, Ozasa H, Glassberg R, Finocchiaro G, Ikeda Y, Mole J, Rosenberg LE, Tanaka K: Molecular cloning and nucleotide sequence of cDNA encoding the entire precursor of rat liver medium chain acyl coenzyme A dehydrogenase. *J Biol Chem* **262**:10104, 1987.
52. Naito E, Ozasa H, Ikeda Y, Tanaka K: Molecular cloning and nucleotide sequence of complementary DNAs encoding human short chain acyl-coenzyme A dehydrogenase and the study of the molecular basis of short chain acyl-coenzyme A dehydrogenase deficiency. *J Clin Invest* **83**:1605, 1989.
53. Matsubara Y, Kraus JP, Yang-Feng TL, Francke U, Rosenberg LE, Tanaka K: Molecular cloning of cDNAs encoding rat and human medium-chain acyl-CoA dehydrogenase and assignment of the gene to human chromosome 1. *Proc Natl Acad Sci U S A* **83**:6543, 1986.
54. Zhang Z, Kelly DP, Kim J-J, Zhou Y, Ogden ML, Whelan AJ, Strauss AW: Structural organization and regulatory regions of the human medium-chain acyl-CoA dehydrogenase gene. *Biochemistry* **31**:81, 1992.
55. Tanaka K, Indo Y: Evolution of the acyl-CoA dehydrogenase/oxidase superfamily, in Coates PM, Tanaka K (eds): *New Developments in Fatty Acid Oxidation*. New York, Wiley-Liss, 1992, p 95.
56. Kim JJP: Crystallographic studies of medium chain acyl-CoA dehydrogenase from pig liver mitochondria, in Curti B, Ronchi S, Zanetti G (eds): *Flavins and Flavoproteins 1990*. Berlin, W. deGruyter, 1991, p 291.
57. Stern JR, del Campillo A: Enzymes of fatty acid metabolism. II. Properties of crystalline crotonase. *J Biol Chem* **218**:985, 1956.
58. Schulz H: Long chain enoyl coenzyme A hydratase from pig heart. *J Biol Chem* **249**:2704, 1974.
59. Minami-Ishii N, Taketani S, Osumi T, Hashimoto T: Molecular cloning and sequence analysis of the cDNA for rat mitochondrial enoyl-CoA hydratase. Structural and evolutionary relationships linked to the bifunctional enzyme of the peroxisomal β-oxidation system. *Eur J Biochem* **185**:73, 1989.
60. El-Fakhri M, Middleton B: The existence of two different l-3-hydroxyacyl-coenzyme A dehydrogenases in rat tissues. *Biochem Soc Trans* **7**:392, 1979.
61. Noyes BE, Bradshaw RA: l-3-Hydroxyacyl coenzyme A dehydrogenase from pig heart muscle. I. Purification and properties. *J Biol Chem* **248**:3052, 1973.
62. Amaya Y, Takiguchi M, Hashimoto T, Mori M: Molecular cloning of cDNA for rat mitochondrial 3-hydroxyacyl-CoA dehydrogenase. *Eur J Biochem* **156**:9, 1986.
63. El-Fakhri M, Middleton B: The existence of an inner-membrane bound, long acyl-chain-specific 3-hydroxyacyl-CoA dehydrogenase in mammalian mitochondria. *Biochim Biophys Acta* **713**:270, 1982.
64. Middleton B: The oxoacyl-coenzyme A thiolases of animal tissues. *Biochem J* **132**:717, 1973.
65. Staack H, Binstock JF, Schulz H: Purification and properties of a pig heart thiolase with broad chain length specificity and comparison of thiolases from pig heart and *Escherichia coli*. *J Biol Chem* **253**:1827, 1978.

66. Fukao T, Yamaguchi S, Kano M, Orii T, Fujiki Y, Osumi T, Hashimoto T: Molecular cloning and sequence of the complementary DNA encoding human mitochondrial acetoacetyl-coenzyme A thiolase and study of the variant enzymes in cultured fibroblasts from patients with 3-ketothiolase deficiency. *J Clin Invest* **86**:2086, 1990.
67. Uchida Y, Izai K, Orii T, Hashimoto T: Novel fatty acid β-oxidation enzymes in rat liver mitochondria. II. Purification and properties of enoyl-coenzyme A (CoA) hydratase/3-hydroxyacyl-CoA dehydrogenase/3-ketoacyl-CoA thiolase trifunctional protein. *J Biol Chem* **267**:1034, 1992.
68. Carpenter K, Pollitt RJ, Middleton B: Human liver long-chain 3-hydroxyacyl-coenzyme A dehydrogenase is a multifunctional membrane-bound β-oxidation enzyme of mitochondria. *Biochem Biophys Res Commun* **183**:433, 1992.
69. Tserng K-Y, Jin S-J: NADPH-dependent reductive metabolism of *cis*-5 unsaturated fatty acids. A revised pathway for the β-oxidation of oleic acid. *J Biol Chem* **266**:11614, 1991.
70. Smeland TE, Nada M, Cuebas D, Schulz H: NADPH-dependent β-oxidation of unsaturated fatty acids with double bonds extending from odd-numbered carbon atoms. *Proc Natl Acad Sci U S A* **89**:6673, 1992.
71. Kilponen JM, Palosaari PM, Hiltunen JK: Occurrence of a long-chain 3,2-enoyl-CoA isomerase in rat liver. *Biochem J* **269**:223, 1990.
72. Palosaari PM, Vihinen M, Mantsala PI, Alexson SEH, Pihlajaniemi T, Hiltunen JK: Amino acid sequence similarities of the mitochondrial short-chain 3,2-enoyl-CoA isomerase and peroxisomal multifunctional 3,2-enoyl-CoA isomerase, 2-enoyl-CoA hydratase, 3-hydroxyacyl-CoA dehydrogenase enzyme in rat liver. The proposed occurrence of isomerization and hydration in the same catalytic domain of the multifunctional enzyme. *J Biol Chem* **266**:10750, 1991.
73. Dommes V, Kunau W-H: 2,4-Dienoyl coenzyme A reductases from bovine liver and *Escherichia coli*. Comparison of properties. *J Biol Chem* **259**:1781, 1984.
74. Hirose A, Kamijo K, Osumi T, Hashimoto T, Mizugaki M: cDNA cloning of rat liver 2,4-dienoyl-CoA reductase. *Biochim Biophys Acta* **1049**:346, 1990.
75. Verhoeven, NM, Roe, DS, Kok, RM, Wanders, RJA, Jakobs, C. and Roe, CR: Phytanic acid and pristanic acid are oxidized by sequential peroxisomal and mitochondrial reactions in human fibroblasts. *J Lipid Res* **39**:66, 1998.
76. Bjorkhem I, Danielson H: ω- and (ω-1)-Oxidation of fatty acids by rat liver microsomes. *Eur J Biochem* **17**:450, 1970.
77. Gregersen N, Mortensen PB: C6-C10-dicarboxylic and C6-C10-ω-1-hydroxy monocarboxylic acids in human and rat with acyl-CoA dehydrogenation deficiencies: In vitro studies on the ω-and ω-1-oxidation of medium-chain (C6–C12) fatty acids in human and rat liver. *Pediatr Res* **17**:828, 1983.
78. Whyte RK, Whelan D, Hill R, McClorry S: Excretion of dicarboxylic and ω-1 hydroxy fatty acids by low birth weight infants fed with medium-chain triglycerides. *Pediatr Res* **20**:122, 1986.
79. Treem WR, Stanley CA, Finegold DN, Hale DE, Coates PM: Primary carnitine deficiency due to a failure of carnitine transport in kidney, muscle, and fibroblasts. *N Engl J Med* **319**:1331, 1988.
80. Eriksson BO, Lindstedt S, Nordin I: Hereditary defect in carnitine membrane transport is expressed in skin fibroblasts. *Eur J Pediatr* **147**:662, 1988.
81. Tein I, De Vivo DC, Bierman F, Pulver P, De Meirleir LJ, Cvitanovic-Sojat L, Pagon RA, Bertini E, Dionisi-Vici C, Servidei S, DiMauro S: Impaired skin fibroblast carnitine uptake in primary systemic carnitine deficiency manifested by childhood carnitine-responsive cardiomyopathy. *Pediatr Res* **28**:247, 1990.
82. Stanley CA, DeLeeuw S, Coates PM, Vianey-Liaud C, Divry P, Bonnefont J-P, Saudubray J-M, Haymond M, Trefz FK, Breningstall GN, Wappner RS, Byrd DJ, Sansaricq C, Tein I, Grover W, Valle D, Rutledge SL, Treem WR: Chronic cardiomyopathy and weakness or acute coma in children with a defect in carnitine uptake. *Ann Neurol* **30**:709, 1991.
83. Garavaglia B, Uziel G, Dworzak F, Carrara F, DiDonato S: Primary carnitine deficiency: Heterozygote and intrafamilial phenotypic variation. *Neurology* **41**:1691, 1991.
84. Stanley CA: Plasma and mitochondrial membrane carnitine transport defects, in Coates PM, Tanaka K (eds): *New Developments in Fatty Acid Oxidation*. New York, Wiley-Liss, 1992, p 289.
85. Waber LJ, Valle D, Neill C, DiMauro S, Shug A: Carnitine deficiency presenting as familial cardiomyopathy: A treatable defect in carnitine transport. *J Pediatr* **101**:700, 1982.
86. Stanley CA, Treem WR, Hale DE, Coates PM: A genetic defect in carnitine transport causing primary carnitine deficiency, in Tanaka K, Coates PM (eds): *Fatty Acid Oxidation: Clinical, Biochemical, and Molecular Aspects*. New York, Alan R. Liss, 1990, p 457.
87. Eriksson BO, Gustafson B, Lindstedt S, Nordin I: Transport of carnitine into cells in hereditary carnitine deficiency. *J Inherit Metab Dis* **12**:108, 1989.
88. Hashimoto N, Suzuki F, Tamai I, Nikaido H, Kuwajima M, Hayakawa J, Tsuji A: Gene-dose effect on carnitine transport activity in embryonic fibroblasts of JVS mice as a model of human carnitine transporter deficiency. *Biochem Pharmacol* **55**:1729, 1998.
89. Stieger B, O'Neill B, Knahenbuhl S: Characterization of L-carnitine transport by rat kidney brush-border-membrane vesicles. *Biochem J* **309**:643, 1995.
90. Tamai I, Yabuuchi H, Nezu J, Sai Y, Oku A, Shimane M, Tsuji A: Cloning and characterization of a novel human pH-dependent organic cation transporter, OCTN1. *FEBS Lett* **419(1)**:107, 1997.
91. Tamai I, Ohashi R, Nezu Ji, Yabuuchi H, Oku A, Shimane M, Sai Y, Tsuji A: Molecular and functional identification of sodium ion-dependent, high affinity human carnitine transporter OCTN2. *J Biol Chem* **273**:20378, 1998.
92. Shoji Y, Koizumi A, Kayo T, Ohata T, Takahashi T, Harada K, Takada G: Evidence for linkage of human primary systemic carnitine deficiency with D5S436: a novel gene locus on chromosome 5q. *Am J Hum Genet* **63(1)**:101, 1998.
93. Bougneres P-F, Saudubray J-M, Marsac C, Bernard O, Odievre M, Girard J: Fasting hypoglycemia resulting from hepatic carnitine palmitoyl transferase deficiency. *J Pediatr* **98**:742, 1981.
94. Demaugre F, Bonnefont J-P, Mitchell G, Nguyen-Hoang N, Pelet A, Rimoldi M, DiDonato S, Saudubray J-M: Hepatic and muscular presentations of carnitine palmitoyl transferase deficiency: Two distinct entities. *Pediatr Res* **24**:308, 1988.
95. Bonnefont J-P, Haas R, Wolff J, Thuy LP, Buchta R, Carroll JE, Saudubray J-M, Demaugre F, Nyhan WL: Deficiency of carnitine palmitoyltransferase I. *J Child Neurol* **4**:197, 1989.
96. Tein I, Demaugre F, Bonnefont J-P, Saudubray J-M: Normal muscle CPT1 and CPT2 activities in hepatic presentation patients with CPT1 deficiency in fibroblasts. Tissue-specific isoforms of CPT1? *J Neurol Sci* **92**:229, 1989.
97. Demaugre F, Bonnefont J-P, Cepanec C, Scholte J, Saudubray J-M, Leroux J-P: Immunoquantitative analysis of human carnitine palmitoyltransferase I and II defects. *Pediatr Res* **27**:497, 1990.
98. Stanley CA, Sunaryo F, Hale DE, Bonnefont J-P, Demaugre F, Saudubray J-M: Elevated plasma carnitine in the hepatic form of carnitine palmitoyltransferase-1 deficiency. *J Inherit Metab Dis* **15**:785, 1992.
99. Haworth JC, Demaugre F, Booth FA, Dilling LA, Moroz SP, Seshia SE, Seargeant LE, Coates PM: Atypical features in the hepatic form of carnitine palmitoyltransferase deficiency in 3 patients in a Hutterite family. *J Pediatr* **121**:553, 1992.
100. Falik-Borenstein ZC, Jordan SC, Saudubray J-M, Brivet M, Demaugre F, Edmond J, Cederbaum SD: Renal tubular acidosis in carnitine palmitoyltransferase type I deficiency. *N Engl J Med* **327**:24, 1992.
101. Marandian MH, Soltanabadi A, Rakchan M, Kouchanfar A, Fallah A: Encephalopathie aigue et steatose hepatique recurrentes avec activite normale de l'acyl-CoA dehydrogenase des acides gras a chaine longue et moyenne. *Arch Fr Pediatr* **44**:369, 1987.
102. Layward EM, Hodges S, Swift PGF, Pollitt RJ, Bennett MJ, Bartlett K: Recurrent encephalopathy in a child of normal growth with a defect of long chain fatty acid oxidation. *Abstracts of the 25th Annual Symposium of the Society for the Study of Inborn Errors of Metabolism*, 1987, p 15.
103. Innes AM, Seargeant LE, Balachandra K, Roe CR, Wanders RJA, Casiro O, Grewar D, Greenberg CR: Hepatic carnitine palmitoyltransferase I deficiency. *Pediatr Res.* **47**:43, 2000.
104. Moon A, Rhead WJ: Complementation analysis of fatty acid oxidation disorders. *J Clin Invest* **79**:59, 1987.
105. Weis BC, Esser V, Foster DW, McGarry JD: Rat heart expresses two forms of mitochondrial carnitine palmitoyltransferase I. The minor component is identical to the liver enzyme. *J Biol Chem* **269(29)**:18712,1994.
106. Yamazaki N, Yamanaka Y, Hashimoto Y, Shinohara Y, Shima A, Terada H: Structural features of the gene encoding human muscle type carnitine palmitoyltransferase I. *FEBS Lett* **409(3)**:401, 1997.
107. Britton CH, Mackey DW, Esser V, Foster DW, Burns DK, Yarnall DP, Froguel P, McGarry JD: Fine chromosome mapping of the genes for human liver and muscle carnitine palmitoyltransferase I (CPT1A and CPT1B). *Genomics* **40**:209, 1997.

108. van der Leij FR, Takens J, van der Veen AY, Terpstra P, Kuipers JR: Localization and intron usage analysis of the human CPT1B gene for muscle type carnitine palmitoyltransferase I. *Biochim Biophys Acta* **1352(2)**:123,1997.
109. Britton CH, Schultz RA, Zhang B, Esser V, Foster DW, McGarry JD : Human liver mitochondrial carnitine palmitoyltransferase I: characterization of its cDNA and chromosomal localization and partial analysis of the gene. *Proc Nat Acad Sci U S A* **92**:1984, 1995.
110. Yamazaki N, Shinohara Y, Shima A, Yamanaka Y, Terada H: Isolation and characterization of cDNA and genomic clones encoding human muscle type carnitine palmitoyltransferase I. *Biochim Biophys Acta* **1307(2)**:157, 1996.
111. Zhu H, Shi J, de Vries Y, Arvidson DN, Cregg JM, Woldegiorgis G: Functional studies of yeast-expressed human heart muscle carnitine palmitoyltransferase I. *Arch Biochem Biophys* **347(1)**:53, 1997.
112. Lodewijk IJ, Mandel HW, Oostheim JOS, Ruiter PN, Gutman A, Wanders RJA: Molecular basis of hepatic carnitine palmitoyltransferase I deficiency. *J Clin Invest* **102(3)**:527, 1998.
113. Wang D, Harrison W, Buja LM, Elder FF, McMillin JB: Genomic DNA sequence, promoter expression, and chromosomal mapping of rat muscle carnitine palmitoyltransferase I. *Genomics* **48(3)**:314, 1998.
114. Shi J, Zhu H, Arvidson DN, Cregg JM, Woldegiorgis G: Deletion of the conserved first 18 N-terminal amino acid residues in rat liver carnitine palmitoyltransferase I abolishes malonyl-CoA sensitivity and binding. *Biochemistry* **37(31)**:11033, 1998.
115. Yu GS, Lu YC, Gulick T: Expression of novel isoforms of carnitine palmitoyltransferase I (CPT-1) generated by alternative splicing of the CPT-iβ gene. *Biochem J* **334(Pt 1)**:225, 1998.
116. Stanley CA, Hale DE, Berry GT, DeLeeuw S, Boxer J, Bonnefont J-P: A deficiency of carnitine-acylcarnitine translocase in the inner mitochondrial membrane. *N Engl J Med* **327**:19, 1992.
117. Pande SV, Brivet M, Slama A, Demaugre F, Aufrant C, Saudubray JM: Carnitine-acyl-carnitine translocase deficiency with severe hypoglycemia and auriculoventricular block: translocase assay in permeabilized fibroblasts. *J Clin Invest* **91**:1247, 1993.
118. Ogier de Baulney H, Slama A, Touati G, Turnbull D, Pourfarzam M, Brivet M: Neonatal hyperammonemia caused by a defect of carnitine-acylcarnitine translocase. *J Pediatr* **127**:723, 1995.
119. Niezen-Koning KE, van Spronsen FJ, Ijlst L,Wanders RJ, Brivet M, Duran M, Reijngoud DJ, Heymans HS, Smit GP: A patient with a lethal cardiomyopathy and a carnitine-acylcarnitine translocase deficiency. *J Inherit Metab Dis* **18**:230, 1995.
120. Chalmers RA, Stanley CA, English N, Wigglesworth JS: Mitochondrial carnitine-acylcarnitine translocase deficiency presenting as sudden neonatal death. *J Pediatr* **131**:220, 1997.
121. Dionisi-Vici C, Garavaglia B, Bartuli A, Invemizzi F, DiDonato S, Sabetta G, Kahler SG, Millington DS: Carnitine acylcarnitine translocase deficiency: Benign course without cardiac involvement [Abstract]. *Pediatr Res* **37**:147A, 1995.
122. Morris AAM, Olpin SE, Brivet M, Turnbull DM, Jones RAK, Leonard JV: A patient with carnitine-acylcarnitine translocase deficiency with a mild phenotype. *J Pediatr* **132**:514, 1998.
123. Huizing M, Iacobazzi V, Ijlst L, Savelkoul P, Ruitenbeek W, van den Heuvel L, Indiveri C, Smeitink J, Trijbels F, Wanders R, Palmieri F: Cloning of the human carnitine-acylcarnitine carrier cDNA and identification of the molecular defect in a patient. *Am J Hum Genet* **61**:1239, 1997.
124. Huizing M, Wendel U, Ruitenbeek W, Iacobazzi V, Ijlst L, Veenhuizen P, Savelkoul P,van den Heuvel LP, Smeitink JA, Wanders RJ, Trijbels JM, Palmieri F: Carnitine-acylcarnitine carrier deficiency: Identification of the molecular defect in a patient. *J Inherit Metab Dis* **21(3)**:262, 1998.
125. Invernizzi E, Garavaglia B, Parini R, Dionisi C, Smith M, Huizing M, Palmieri F, Taroni F: Identification of the molecular defect in patients with carnitine-acylcarnitine carrier deficiency. *J Inherit Metab Dis* **21(Suppl 2)**:56, 1998.
126. Costa C, Costa JM, Slama A, Boutron A, Saudubray JM, Brivet M: Identification of the molecular defect in a severe case of Acylcarnitine carrier deficiency [Abstract]. *J Inherit Metab Dis* **21(Suppl 2)**:57, 1998.
127. IJlst L, Ruiter JPN, Huizing M, Ruitenbeek W, Smeitink J, Trijbels F, Niezen-Koning KE, Oostheim W, Palmieri F, Wanders RJA: Molecular basis of carnitine acyl-carnitine deficiency [Abstract]. *J Inherit Metab Dis* **21(Suppl 2)**:56, 1998.
128. DiMauro S, Papadimitriou A: Carnitine palmitoyltransferase deficiency, in Engel AG, Banker BQ (eds): *Myology: Basic and Clinical*. New York, McGraw-Hill, 1986, p 1697.
129. Demaugre F, Bonnefont J-P, Colonna M, Cepanec C, Leroux J-P, Saudubray JM: Infantile form of carnitine palmitoyltransferase II deficiency with hepatomuscular symptoms and sudden death. Physiopathological approach to carnitine palmitoyltransferase II deficiencies. *J Clin Invest* **87**:859, 1991.
130. Hug G, Bove KE, Soukup S: Lethal neonatal multiorgan deficiency of carnitine palmitoyltransferase II. *N Engl J Med* **325**:1862, 1991.
131. Zinn AB, Zurcher VL, Kraus F, Strohl C, Walsh-Sukys MC, Hoppel CL: Carnitine palmitoyltransferase B (CPT B) deficiency: A heritable cause of neonatal cardiomyopathy and dysgenesis of the kidney. *Pediatr Res* **29**:73A, 1991.
132. Taroni F, Verderio E, Garavaglia B, Fiorucci S, Finocchiaro G, Uziel G, DiDonato S: Biochemical and molecular studies of carnitine palmitoyltransferase II deficiency with hepatocardiomyopathic presentation, in Coates PM, Tanaka K (eds): *New Developments in Fatty Acid Oxidation*. New York, Wiley-Liss, 1992, p 521.
133. Witt DR, Theobald M, Santa-Maria M, Packman S, Townsend S, Sweetman L, Goodman S, Rhead W, Hoppel C: Carnitine palmitoyl transferase-type 2 deficiency: Two new cases and successful prenatal diagnosis. *Am J Hum Genet* **49(Suppl)**:109, 1991.
134. Land JM, Mistry S, Squier W, Hope P, Orford M, Saggerson ED: Neonatal carnitine palmitoyltransferase deficiency: A case with a muscular presentation, in Coates PM, Tanaka K (eds): *New Developments in Fatty Acid Oxidation*. New York, Wiley-Liss, 1992, p 309.
135. Demaugre F, Bonnefont J-P, Brivet M, Cepanec C, Pollitt RJ, Priestley BL, Saudubray JM, Leroux JP: Pathophysiological approach to carnitine palmitoyltransferase II deficiencies, in Coates PM, Tanaka K (eds): *New Developments in Fatty Acid Oxidation*. New York, Wiley-Liss, 1992, p 301.
136. Corr PB, Creer MH, Yamada KA, Saffitz JE, Sobel BE: Prophylaxis of early ventricular fibrillation by inhibition of acylcarnitine accumulation. *J Clin Invest* **83**:927, 1989.
137. Gellera C, Verderio E, Floridia G, Finochiaro G, Montermini L, Cavadini P, Zuffardi O, Taroni F: Assignment of the human carnitine palmitoyltransferase II gene (CPT I) to chromosome 1P32. *Genomics* **24**:195, 1994.
138. Verderio E, Cavadini P, Montermini L, Wang H, Lamantea E, Finocchiaro G, DiDonatoS,Gellera C, Taroni F: Carnitine palmitoyltransferase II deficiency: structure of the gene and characterization of two novel disease-causing mutations. *Hum Mol Genet* **4(1)**:19, 1995.
139. Taroni F, Verderio E, Fiorucci S, Cavadini P, Finocchiaro G, Uziel G, Lamantea E, Gellera C, DiDonato S: Molecular characterization of inherited Carnitine palmitoyltransferase(CPT II) deficiency. *Proc Natl Acad Sci U S A* **89**:8429, 1992.
140. Taroni F, Verderio E, Dworzak F, Willems P J, Cavadini P, DiDonato S: Identification of a common mutation in the carnitine palmitoyltransferase II gene in familial recurrent myoglobinuria patients. *Nat Genet* **4**:314, 1993.
141. Handig I, Dams E, Taroni F, Laere SV, Barsy TD: Inheritance of the S113L mutation within an inbred family with carnitine palmitoyltransferase enzyme deficiency. *Hum Genet* **97**:291, 1996.
142. Gellera C, Witt DR, Verderio E, Cavadini P, DiDonato S, Taroni F: Molecular study of lethal neonatal Carnitine palmitoyltransferase (CPT II) deficiency. *Am J Genet* **51**:A168, 1992.
143. Taroni F, Gellera C, Cavadini P, Baratta S, Lamantea E, Dethlefs S, DiDonato S, Reike PJ: Lethal Carnitine palmitoyltransferase (CPT) II deficiency in newborns: A molecular genetic study. *Am J Hum Genet* **55**:A245, 1994.
144. Yamamoto S, Abe H, Kohgo T, Ogawa A, Ohtake A, Hayashibe H, Sakuraba H, Suzuki Y,Aramaki S, Takayanagi M, Hasegawa S, Niimi H: Two novel gene mutations (Glu174 → Lys, Phe383 → Tyr) causing the "hepatic" form of carnitine palmitoyltransferase II deficiency. *Hum Genet* **98**:116, 1996.
145. Yang BZ, Ding JH, Roe D, Dewese T, Day DW, Roe CR: A novel mutation identified in carnitine palmitoyltransferase II deficiency. *Mol Genet Metab* **63(2)**:110, 1998.
146. Yang BZ, Ding JH, Dewese T, Roe D, He G, Wilkinson J, Day DW, Demaugre F, Rabier D, Brivet M, Roe C: Identification of four novel mutations in patients with carnitine palmitoyltransferase II (CPT II) deficiency. *Mol Genet Metab* **64**:229, 1998.
147. Wataya K, Akanuma J, Cavadini P, Aoki Y, Kure S, Invernizzi F, Yoshida I, Kira J, Taroni F, Matsubara Y, Narisawa K: Two CPT2 mutations in three Japanese patients with carnitine palmitoyltransferase II deficiency: functional analysis and association with polymorphic haplotypes and two clinical phenotypes. *Hum Mutat* **11(5)**:377, 1998.

148. Hale DE, Batshaw ML, Coates PM, Frerman FE, Goodman SI, Singh I, Stanley CA: Long-chain acyl-coenzyme A dehydrogenase deficiency: An inherited cause of nonketotic hypoglycemia. *Pediatr Res* **19**:666, 1985.
149. Hale DE, Stanley CA, Coates PM: The long-chain acyl-CoA dehydrogenase deficiency, in Tanaka K, Coates PM (eds): *Fatty Acid Oxidation: Clinical, Biochemical, and Molecular Aspects*. New York, Alan R. Liss, 1990, p 303.
150. Parini R, Garavaglia B, Saudubray J-M, Bardelli P, Melotti D, Zecca G, DiDonato S: Clinical diagnosis of long-chain acyl-coenzyme A-dehydrogenase deficiency: Use of stress and fat-loading tests. *J Pediatr* **119**:77, 1991.
151. Naylor EW, Mosovich LL, Guthrie R, Evans JE, Tieckelmann H: Intermittent non-ketotic dicarboxylic aciduria in two siblings with hypoglycaemia: An apparent defect in β-oxidation of fatty acids. *J Inherit Metab Dis* **3**:19, 1980.
152. Allison F, Bennett MJ, Variend S, Engel PC: Acylcoenzyme A dehydrogenase deficiency in heart tissue from infants who died unexpectedly with fatty change in the liver. *BMJ* **296**:11, 1988.
153. Brown-Harrison MC, Nada MA, Sprecher H, Vianey-Saban C, Farquhar J, Gilladoga AC, Roe CR: Very long chain acyl-CoA dehydrogenase deficiency: Successful treatment of acute cardiomyopathy. *Biochem Mol Med* **58**:59, 1996.
154. Vianey-Saban C, Divry P, Brivet M, Nada M, Zabot MT, Mathieu M, Roe C: Mitochondrial very-long-chain acyl-coenzyme A dehydrogenase deficiency: Clinical characteristics and diagnostic considerations in 30 patients. *Clin Chim Acta* **269**:43, 1998.
155. Nada MA, Vianey-Saban C, Roe CR, Ding JH, Mathieu M, Wappner RS, Bialer MG, McGlynn JA, Mandon G: Prenatal diagnosis of mitochondrial fatty acid oxidation defects. *Prenat Diagn* **16**:117, 1996.
156. Cox GF, Souri M, Aoyama T, Rockenmacher S, Varvogli L, Rohr F, Hashimoto T, Korson MS: Reversal of severe hypertrophic cardiomyopathy and excellent neuropsychologic outcome in very-long-chain acyl-coenzyme A dehydrogenase deficiency. *J Pediatr* **133**:247, 1998.
157. Tager JM, Wanders RJA, Groen AK, Kunz W, Bohnensack R, Kuster U, Letko G, Bohme G, Duszynski J, Wojtczak L: Control of mitochondrial respiration. *FEBS Lett* **151**:1, 1983.
158. Treem WR, Witzleben CA, Piccoli DA, Stanley CA, Hale DE, Coates PM, Watkins JB: Medium-chain and long-chain acyl-CoA dehydrogenase deficiency. Clinical, pathologic, and ultrastructural differentiation from Reye's syndrome. *Hepatology* **6**:1270, 1986.
159. Aoyama T, Ueno I, Kamijo T, Hashimoto T: Rat very-long-chain acyl-CoA dehydrogenase, a novel mitochondrial acyl-CoA dehydrogenase gene product, is a rate-limiting enzyme in long-chain fatty acid β-oxidation system. cDNA and deduced amino acid sequence and distinct specificities of the cDNA-expressed protein. *J Biol Chem* **269(29)**:19088, 1994.
160. Strauss AW, Powell CK, Hale DE, Anderson MM, Ahuja A, Brackett JC, and Sims HF: Molecular basis of human mitochondrial very-long-chain acyl-CoA dehydrogenase deficiency causing cardiomyopathy and sudden death in childhood. *Proc Natl Acad Sci U S A* **92(23)**:10496, 1995.
161. Aoyama T, Souri M, Ueno I, Kamijo T, Yamaguchi S, Rhead WJ, Tanaka K, Hashimoto T: Cloning of human very-long-chain acyl-coenzyme A dehydrogenase and molecular characterization of its deficiency in two patients. *Am J Hum Genet* **57**:273, 1995.
162. Orii K, Aoyama T, Souri M, Orii K, Kondo N, Orii T, Hashimoto T: Genomic DNA organization of human mitochondrial very-long-chain acyl-CoA dehydrogenase and mutation analysis. *Biochem Biophys Res Commun* **217(3)**:987, 1995.
163. Aoyama T, Wakui K, Fukushima Y, Orii KO, Hashimoto T: Assignment of the human mitochondrial very-long-chain acyl-CoA dehydrogenase gene (LCACD) to 17p13 by in situ hybridization. *Genomics* **37**:144, 1996.
164. Souri M, Aoyama T, Orii K, Yamaguchi S, Hashimoto T: Mutation analysis of very-long-chain acyl-coenzyme A dehydrogenase (VLCAD) deficiency: Identification and characterization of mutant VLCAD cDNAs from four patients. *Am J Hum Genet* **58**:97, 1996.
165. Souri M, Aoyama T, Hoganson G, Hashimoto T: Very-long-chain acyl-CoA dehydrogenase subunit assembles to the dimer form on mitochondrial inner membrane. *FEBS Lett* **426**:187, 1998.
166. Andresen BS, Bross P, Vianey-Saban C, Divry P, Zabot MT, Roe CR, Nada MA, Byskoc A, Kruse TA, Neve S, Kristiansen K, Knudsen I, Corydon MJ, Gregersen N: Cloning and characterization of human very-long-chain acyl-CoA dehydrogenase cDNA, chromosomal assignment of the gene and identification in four patients of nine different mutations within the VLCAD gene. *Hum Mol Genet* **5**:461, 1996.
167. Smelt AH, Poorthuis BJ, Onkenhout W, Scholte HR, Andresen BS, van Duinen SG, Gregersen N, Wintzen AR: Very long chain acyl-coenzyme A dehydrogenase deficiency with adult onset. *Ann Neurol* **43**:540, 1998.
168. Uchida Y, Izai K, Orii T, Hashimoto T: Novel fatty acid β-oxidation enzymes in rat liver mitochondria. II. Purification and properties of enoyl-coenzyme A hydratase/3-hydroxyacyl-CoA dehydrogenase/3-ketoacyl-CoA thiolase trifunctional protein. *J Biol Chem* **267**:1034,1992.
169. Carpenter K, Pollitt RJ, Middleton B: Human liver long-chain 3-hydroxyacyl-CoA dehydrogenase is a multifunctional membrane-bound β-oxidation enzyme of mitochondria. *Biochem Biophys Res Commun* **183**:443, 1992.
170. Glasgow AM, Engel AG, Bier DM, Perry LW, Dickie M, Todaro J, Brown BI, Utter MF: Hypoglycemia, hepatic dysfunction, muscle weakness, cardiomyopathy, free carnitine deficiency and long-chain acylcarnitine excess responsive to medium chain triglyceride diet. *Pediatr Res* **17**:319, 1983.
171. Riudor E, Ribes A, Boronat M, Sabado C, Dominguez C, Ballabriga A: A new case of C6-C14 dicarboxylic aciduria with favourable evolution. *J Inherit Metab Dis* **9(Suppl 2)**:297, 1986.
172. Poll-The BT, Bonnefront JP, Ogier H, Charpentier C, Pelet A, Le Fur JM, Jakobs C, Kok RM, Duran M, Divry P, Scotto J, Saudubray JM: Familial hypoketotic hypoglycaemia associated with peripheral neuropathy, pigmentary retinopathy and C6-C14 hydroxydicarboxylic aciduria. A new defect in fatty acid oxidation? *J Inherit Metab Dis* **11**:183, 1988.
173. Rocchiccioli F, Wanders RJA, Aubourg P, Vianey-Liaud C, Ijlst L, Fabre M, Cartier N, Bougneres P-F: Deficiency of long-chain 3-hydroxyacyl-CoA dehydrogenase: A cause of lethal myopathy and cardiomyopathy in early childhood. *Pediatr Res* **28**:657, 1990.
174. Jackson S, Bartlett K, Land J, Moxon ER, Pollitt RJ, Leonard JV, Turnbull DM: Long-chain 3-hydroxyacyl-CoA dehydrogenase deficiency. *Pediatr Res* **29**:406, 1991.
175. Dionisi Vici C, Burlina AB, Bertini E, Bachmann C, Mazziotta MRM, Zacchello F, Sabetta G, Hale DE: Progressive neuropathy and recurrent myoglobinuria in a child with long-chain 3-hydroxyacyl-coenzyme A dehydrogenase deficiency. *J Pediatr* **118**:744, 1991.
176. Duran M, Wanders RJA, de Jager JP, Dorland L, Bruinvis L, Ketting D, Ijlst L, van Sprang FJ: 3-Hydroxydicarboxylic aciduria due to long-chain 3-hydroxyacyl-coenzyme A dehydrogenase deficiency associated with sudden neonatal death: Protective effect of medium-chain triglyceride treatment. *Eur J Pediatr* **150**:190, 1991.
177. Przyrembel H, Jakobs C, Ijlst L, de Klerk JBC, Wanders RJA: Long-chain 3-hydroxyacyl-CoA dehydrogenase deficiency. *J Inherit Metab Dis* **14**:674, 1991.
178. Tserng K-Y, Jin S-J, Kerr DS, Hoppel CL: Urinary 3-hydroxydicarboxylic acids in pathophysiology of metabolic disorders with dicarboxylic aciduria. *Metabolism* **40**:676, 1991.
179. Wanders RJA, Ijlst L, Duran M, Jakobs C, de Klerk JBC, Przyrembel H, Rocchiccioli F, Aubourg P: Long-chain 3-hydroxyacyl-CoA dehydrogenase deficiency: Different clinical expression in three unrelated patients. *J Inherit Metab Dis* **14**:325, 1991.
180. Bertini E, Dionisi-Vici C, Garavaglia B, Burlina AB, Sabatelli M, Rimoldi M, Bartuli A, Sabetta G, DiDonato S: Peripheral sensory-motor polyneuropathy, pigmentary retinopathy, and fatal cardiomyopathy in long-chain 3-hydroxy-acyl-CoA dehydrogenase deficiency. *Eur J Pediatr* **151**:121, 1992.
181. Jackson S, Singh Kler R, Bartlett K, Briggs H, Bindoff LA, Pourfarzam M, Gardner-Medwin D, Turnbull DM: Combined enzyme defect of mitochondrial fatty acid oxidation. *J Clin Invest* **90**:1219, 1992.
182. Kelley RI, Morton DH: 3-Hydroxyoctanoic aciduria: Identification of a new organic acid in the urine of a patient with non-ketotic hypoglycemia. *Clin Chim Acta* **175**:19, 1988.
183. Hagenfeldt L, von Dobeln U, Holme E, Alm J, Brand- berg G, Enocksson E, Lindeberg L: 3-Hydroxydicarboxylic aciduria — A fatty acid oxidation defect with severe prognosis. *J Pediatr* **116**:387, 1990.
184. Ribes A, Riudor E, Navarro C, Boronat M, Marti M, Hale DE: Fatal outcome in a patient with long-chain 3-hydroxyacyl-CoA dehydrogenase deficiency. *J Inherit Metab Dis* **15**:278, 1992.
185. Tyni T, Palotie A, Viinikka L, Valanne L, Salo MK, von Dobeln U, Jackson S, Wanders R, Venizelos N, Pihko H: Long-chain 3-hydroxyacyl-coenzyme A dehydrogenase deficiency with the G1528C mutation: Clinical presentation of thirteen patients. *J Pediatr* **130**:67, 1997.

186. Ijlst L, Wanders RJA, Ushikubo S, Kamijo T, Hashimoto T: Molecular basis of long-chain 3-hydroxyacyl-CoA dehydrogenase deficiency: identification of the major disease-causing mutation in the α subunit of the mitochondrial trifunctional protein. *Biochim Biophys Acta* **1215**:347, 1994.
187. Shoerman MN, Batey RG, Wilcken B: Recurrent acute fatty liver of pregnancy associated with a fatty-acid oxidation defect in the offspring. *Gastroenterology* **100**:544, 1991.
188. Wilcken G, Leung FC, Hammond J, Kamath R, Leonard JV: Pregnancy and fetal long-chain 3-hydroxyacyl coenzyme A dehydrogenase deficiency. *Lancet* **341**:407, 1993.
189. Treem WR, Rinaldo P, Hale DE, Stanley CA, Millington DS, Hyams JS, Jackson S, Turnbull DM: Acute fatty liver of pregnancy and long-chain 3-hydroxyacyl-coenzyme A dehydrogenase deficiency. *Hepatology* **19**:339, 1994.
190. Sims HF, Brackett JC, Powell CK, Treem WR, Hale DE, Bennett MJ, Gibson B, Shapiro S, Strauss AW: The molecular basis of long-chain 3-hydroxyacyl-CoA dehydrogenase deficiency associated with maternal acute fatty liver of pregnancy. *Proc Natl Acad Sci U S A* **92**:841, 1995.
191. Isaacs JD Jr, Sims HF, Powell CK, Bennett MJ, Hale DE, Treem WR, Strauss AW: Maternal acute fatty liver of pregnancy associated with fetal trifunctional protein deficiency: molecular characterization of a novel maternal mutant allele. *Pediatr Res* **40(3)**:393, 1996.
192. Tyni T, Ekholm E, Pihko H: Pregnancy complications are frequent in long-chain 3-hydroxyacyl-coenzyme A dehydrogenase deficiency. *Am J Obstet Gynecol* **178**:603, 1998.
193. Greenberg CR, Wanders RJA, Roe CR, Grewar D, and Sergeant DE: Complete deficiency of CPT I in an infant born to a mother with acute fatty liver of pregnancy. *Seventh International Congress of Inborn Errors of Metabolism*, May 21–25, 1997, Vienna, Austria.
194. Wanders RJA, Ijlst L, Poggi F, Bonnefont JP, Munnich A, Brivet M, Rabier D, Saudubray JM: Human trifunctional protein deficiency: A new disorder of mitochondrial fatty acid β-oxidation. *Biochem Biophys Res Commun* **188**:1139, 1992.
195. Kamijo T, Aoyama T, Komiyama A, Hashimoto T: Structural analysis of cDNAs for subunits of human mitochondrial fatty acid β-oxidation trifunctional protein. *Biochem Biophys Res Commun* **199**:818, 1994.
196. Yang BZ, Heng HHQ, Ding JH, Roe CR: The gene for the α and β subunits of the mitochondrial trifunctional protein are both located in the same region of human chromosome 2P23. *Genomics* **37**:141, 1996.
197. IJlst L, Ruiter JPN, Hoovers JMN, Jakobs ME, Wanders RJA: Common missence mutation G1528C in long-chain 3-hydroxyacyl-CoA dehydrogenase deficiency: Characterization and expression of the mutant protein, mutation analysis on genomic DNA and chromosomal localization of the mitochondrial trifunctional protein a subunit gene. *J Clin Invest* **98**:1028, 1996.
198. Ding JH, Yang BZ, Nada MA, Roe CR: Improved detection of the G1528C mutation in LCHAD deficiency. *Biochem Mol Med* **58**:46, 1996.
199. Brackett JC, Sims HF, Rinaldo P, Shapiro S, Powell CK, Bennett MJ, Strauss AW: Two alpha subunit donor splice site mutations cause human trifunctional protein deficiency. *J Clin Invest* **95(5)**:2076, 1995.
200. Ushikubo S, Aoyama T, Kamijo T, Wanders RJ, Rinaldo P, Vockley J, Hashimoto T: Molecular characterization of mitochondrial trifunctional protein deficiency: formation of the enzyme complex is important for stabilization of both alpha- and β-subunits. *Am J Hum Genet* **58(5)**:979, 1996.
201. Aoyama T, Wakui K, Fukushima Y, Miyajima H, Yamaguchi S, Orii T, Kondo N: Genomic and mutational analysis of the mitochondrial trifunctional protein β-subunit (HADHB) gene in patients with trifunctional protein deficiency. *Hum Mol Genet* **6(8)**:1215, 1997.
202. Ibdah JA, Tein I, Dionisi-Vici C, Bennett MJ, Ijlst L, Gibson B, Wanders RJA, Strauss AW: Mild trifunctional protein deficiency is associated with progressive neuropathy and myopathy and suggests a novel genotype-phenotype correlation. *J Clin Invest* **102**:1193, 1998.
203. Ijlst L, Oostheim W, Ruiter JPN, Wanders RJA: Molecular basis of long-chain 3-hydroxyacyl-CoA dehydrogenase deficiency: Identification of two new mutations. *J Inherit Metab Dis* **20**:420, 1997.
204. Roe CR, Millington DS, Norwood DL, Kodo N, Sprecher H, Mohammed BS, Nada M, Schulz H, McVie R: 2,4-Dienoyl-coenzyme A reductase deficiency: A possible new disorder of fatty acid oxidation. *J Clin Invest* **85**:1703, 1990.
205. Roe CR, Millington DS, Maltby DA, Kinnebrew P: Recognition of medium-chain acyl-CoA dehydrogenase deficiency in asymptomatic siblings of children dying of sudden infant death or Reye-like syndromes. *J Pediatr* **108**:13, 1986.
206. Duran M, Hofkamp M, Rhead WJ, Saudubray J-M, Wadman SK: Sudden child death and "healthy" affected family members with medium-chain acyl-coenzyme A dehydrogenase deficiency. *Pediatrics* **78**:1052, 1986.
207. Iafolla AK, Millington DS, Chen YT, Ding JH, Kahler SG, Roe CR: Natural course of medium chain acyl-CoA dehydrogenase deficiency. *Am J Hum Genet* **49(Suppl)**:99, 1991.
208. Iafolla AK, Thompson RT, Roe CR: Psychodevelopmental outcome in children with medium chain acyl CoA dehydrogenase deficiency. *Am J Hum Genet* **51**:A351, 1992.
209. Millington DS, Kodo N, Terada N, Roe D, Chace DH: The analysis of diagnostic markers in human blood and urine using tandem mass spectrometry with liquid secondary ion mass spectrometry. *Int J Mass Spectrom Ion Proc* **111**:211, 1991.
210. Millington DS, Terada N, Chace DH, Chen Y-T, Ding J-H, Kodo N, Roe CR: The role of tandem mass spectrometry in the diagnosis of fatty acid oxidation disorders, in Coates PM, Tanaka K (eds): *New Developments in Fatty Acid Oxidation*. New York, Wiley-Liss, 1992, p 339.
211. Millington DS, Kodo N, Norwood DL, Roe CR: Tandem mass spectrometry: A new method for acylcarnitine profiling with potential for neonatal screening for inborn errors of metabolism. *J Inherit Metab Dis* **13**:321, 1990.
212. Bennett MJ, Rinaldo P, Millington DS, Tanaka K, Yokota I, Coates PM: Medium-chain acyl-CoA dehydrogenase deficiency: Postmortem diagnosis in a case of sudden infant death and neonatal diagnosis of an affected sibling. *Pediatr Pathol* **11**:889, 1991.
213. Glasgow AM, Eng G, Engel AG: Systemic carnitine deficiency simulating recurrent Reye syndrome. *J Pediatr* **96**:889, 1980.
214. Cruse RP, DiMauro S, Towfighi J, Trevisan C: Familial systemic carnitine deficiency. *Arch Neurol* **41**:301, 1984.
215. Coates RM, Hale DE, Stanley CA, Corkey BE, Cortner JA: Genetic deficiency of medium-chain acyl-coenzyme A dehydrogenase: Studies in cultured skin fibroblasts and peripheral mononuclear leukocytes. *Pediatr Res* **19**:671, 1985.
216. Frerman FE, Goodman SI: Fluorometric assay of acyl-CoA dehydrogenases in normal and mutant human fibroblasts. *Biochem Med* **33**:38, 1985.
217. Losty HC, Lee P, Alfaham M, Gray OP, Leonard JV: Fatty infiltration in the liver in medium-chain acyl-CoA dehydrogenase deficiency. *Arch Dis Child* **66**:727, 1991.
218. Santer R, Schmidt-Sommerfeld E, Leung YK, Fischer JE, Lebenthal E: Medium-chain acyl CoA dehydrogenase deficiency: Electron microscopic differentiation from Reye syndrome. *Eur J Pediatr* **150**:111, 1990.
219. Engel AG, Banker BQ, Eiben RM: Carnitine deficiency: Clinical, morphological, and biochemical observations in a fatal case. *J Neurol Neurosurg Psychiatry* **40**:313, 1977.
220. Matsubara Y, Narisawa K, Miyabashi S, Tada K, Coates PM: Molecular lesion in patients with medium-chain acyl-CoA dehydrogenase deficiency. *Lancet* **335**:1589, 1990.
221. Yokota I, Indo Y, Coates PM, Tanaka K: Molecular basis of medium chain acyl-coenzyme A dehydrogenase deficiency. An A to G transition at position 985 that causes a lysine-304 to glutamate substitution in the mature protein is the single prevalent mutation. *J Clin Invest* **86**:1000, 1990.
222. Ding J-H, Roe CR, Chen Y-T, Matsubara Y, Narisawa K: Mutations in medium chain acyl-CoA dehydrogenase deficiency. *Lancet* **336**:748, 1990.
223. Matsubara Y, Narisawa K, Miyabayashi S, Tada K, Coates PM, Bachmann C, Elsas LJ, Pollitt RJ, Rhead WJ, Roe CR: Identification of a common mutation in patients with medium-chain acyl-CoA dehydrogenase deficiency. *Biochem Biophys Res Commun* **171**:498, 1990.
224. Kelly DP, Whelan AJ, Ogden ML, Alpers R, Zhang Z, Bellus G, Gregersen N, Dorland L, Strauss AW: Molecular characterization of inherited medium-chain acyl-CoA dehydrogenase deficiency. *Proc Natl Acad Sci U S A* **87**:9236, 1990.
225. Gregersen N, Andresen BS, Bross P, Winter V, Rudiger N, Engst S, Christensen E, Kelly D, Strauss AW, Kolvraa S, Bolund L, Ghisla S: Molecular characterization of medium-chain acyl-CoA dehydrogenase (MCAD) deficiency: Identification of a lys329 to glu mutation in the MCAD gene, and expression of inactive mutant enzyme protein in *E. coli*. *Hum Genet* **86**:545, 1991.
226. Curtis D, Blakemore AIF, Engel PC, MacGregor D, Besley G, Kolvraa S, Gregersen N: Heterogeneity for mutations in medium chain acyl-CoA dehydrogenase deficiency in the UK population. *Clin Genet* **40**:283, 1991.

227. Yokota I, Coates PM, Hale DE, Rinaldo P, Tanaka K: Molecular survey of a prevalent mutation, 985A-to-G transition, and identification of five infrequent mutations in the medium-chain acyl-CoA dehydrogenase (MCAD) gene in 55 patients with MCAD deficiency. *Am J Hum Genet* **49**:1280, 1991.
228. Matsubara Y, Narisawa K, Tada K: Medium-chain acyl-CoA dehydrogenase deficiency: Molecular aspects. *Eur J Pediatr* **151**:154, 1992.
229. Workshop on Molecular Aspects of MCAD Deficiency: Mutations causing medium-chain acyl-CoA dehydrogenase deficiency: A collaborative compilation of the data from 172 patients, in Coates PM, Tanaka K (eds): *New Developments in Fatty Acid Oxidation*. New York, Wiley-Liss, 1992, p 499.
230. Coates PM, Tanaka K: Molecular basis of mitochondrial fatty acid oxidation defects. *J Lipid Res* **33**:1099, 1992.
231. Yokota I, Tanaka K, Coates PM, Ugarte M: Mutations in medium-chain acyl-CoA dehydrogenase deficiency. *Lancet* **336**:748, 1990.
232. Gregersen N, Winter V, Kolvraa S, Andresen BS, Bross P, Blakemore A, Curtis D, Bolund L: Molecular analysis of medium-chain acyl-CoA dehydrogenase deficiency: A diagnostic approach, in Coates PM, Tanaka K (eds): *New Developments in Fatty Acid Oxidation*. New York, Wiley-Liss, 1992, p 441.
233. Ding J-H, Yang B-Z, Bao Y, Roe CR, Chen Y-T: Identification of a new mutation in medium-chain acyl-CoA dehydrogenase (MCAD) deficiency. *Am J Hum Genet* **50**:229, 1992.
234. Kelly DP, Hale DE, Rutledge SL, Ogden ML, Whelan AJ, Zhang Z, Strauss AW: Molecular basis of inherited medium-chain acyl-CoA dehydrogenase deficiency causing sudden child death. *J Inherit Metab Dis* **15**:171, 1992.
235. Blakemore AIF, Singleton H, Pollitt RJ, Engel PC, Kolvraa S, Gregersen N, Curtis D: Frequency of the G985 MCAD mutation in the general population. *Lancet* **337**:298, 1991.
236. Matsubara Y, Narisawa K, Tada K, Ikeda H, Ye-Qi Y, Danks DM, Green A, McCabe ERB: Prevalence of K329E mutation in medium-chain acyl-CoA dehydrogenase gene determined from Guthrie cards. *Lancet* **338**:552, 1991.
237. Yokota I, Coates PM, Hale DE, Rinaldo P, Tanaka K: The molecular basis of medium-chain acyl-CoA dehydrogenase deficiency: Survey and evolution of 985A → G transition, and identification of five rare types of mutations within the medium chain acyl-CoA dehydrogenase gene, in Coates PM, Tanaka K (eds): *New Developments in Fatty Acid Oxidation*. New York, Wiley-Liss, 1992, p 425.
238. Kidd JR, Matsubara Y, Castiglione CM, Tanaka K, Kidd KK: The locus for the medium-chain acyl-CoA dehydrogenase gene on chromosome 1 is highly polymorphic. *Genomics* **6**:89, 1990.
239. Blakemore AIF, Kolvraa S, Gregersen N, Engel PC, Curtis D: Localisation of RFLPs of the medium chain acyl-CoA dehydrogenase gene. *Hum Genet* **86**:537, 1991.
240. Blakemore AIF, Engel PC, Curtis D: BamHI and MspI RFLP's in strong linkage disequilibrium at the medium chain acyl-coenzyme A dehydrogenase locus (ACADM chromosome 1). *Nucleic Acids Res* **18**:2838, 1990.
241. Kolvraa S, Gregersen N, Blakemore AIF, Schneidermann AK, Winter V, Andresen BS, Curtis D, Engel PC, Divry P, Rhead W, Bolund L: The most common mutation causing medium-chain acyl-CoA dehydrogenase deficiency is strongly associated with a particular haplotype in the region on the gene. *Hum Genet* **87**:425, 1991.
242. Matsubara Y, Narisawa K, Tada K, Ikeda H, Yeqi Y, Danks DM, Green A, McCabe ERB: Prevalence of K329E mutation in the medium-chain acyl-CoA dehydrogenase gene determined from Guthrie cards, in Coates PM, Tanaka K (eds): *New Developments in Fatty Acid Oxidation*. New York, Wiley-Liss, 1992, p 453.
243. Ikeda Y, Hale DE, Keese SM, Coates PM, Tanaka K: Biosynthesis of variant medium chain acyl-CoA dehydrogenase in cultured fibroblasts from patients with medium-chain acyl-CoA dehydrogenase deficiency. *Pediatr Res* **20**:843, 1986.
244. Coates PM, Indo Y, Young D, Hale DE, Tanaka K: Immunochemical characterization of variant medium-chain acyl-CoA dehydrogenase in fibroblasts from patients with medium-chain acyl-CoA dehydrogenase deficiency. *Pediatr Res* **31**:34, 1992.
245. Inagaki T, Ohishi N, Bachmann C, Ghisla S, Tsukagoshi N, Udaka S, Yagi K: Immunochemical and molecular analysis of medium-chain acyl-CoA dehydrogenase deficiency. *J Clin Biochem Nutr* **8**:1, 1990.
246. Oglivie I, Jackson S, Bartlett K, Turnbull DM: Immunoreactive enzyme protein in medium-chain acyl-CoA dehydrogenase deficiency. *Biochem Med Metab Biol* **46**:373, 1991.
247. Kim J-JP, Wu J: Structure of the medium-chain acyl-CoA dehydrogenase from pig liver mitochondria at 3-Å resolution. *Proc Natl Acad Sci U S A* **85**:6677, 1988.
248. Kim J-JP, Wang M, Djordjevic S, Paschke R: The three dimensional structure of acyl-CoA dehydrogenase, in Coates PM, Tanaka K (eds): *New Developments in Fatty Acid Oxidation*. New York, Wiley-Liss, 1992, p 111.
249. Yokota I, Saijo T, Vockley J, Tanaka K: Tetramer formation and stability of K304E-variant medium chain acyl-CoA dehydrogenase (MCAD): A site-directed mutagenesis study. *Pediatr Res* **31**:136, 1992.
250. Tanaka K, Yokota I, Coates PM, Strauss AW, Kelly DP, Zhang Z, Gregersen N, Andresen BS, Matsubara Y, Curtis D, Chen Y-T: Mutations in the medium chain acyl-CoA dehydrogenase (MCAD) gene. *Hum Mutat* **1**:271, 1992.
251. Bross P, Jensen T, Krautle F, Winter V, Engst S, Bolund L, Kolvraa S, Ghisla S, Rasched I, Gregersen N: Characterization of medium-chain acyl-CoA dehydrogenase (MCAD) with a point mutation associated with MCAD deficiency, in Coates PM, Tanaka K (eds): *New Developments in Fatty Acid Oxidation*. New York, Wiley-Liss, 1992, p 473.
252. Ding JH, Bross P, Yang BZ, Iafolla AK, Millington DS, Roe CR, Gregersen N, Chen YT: Genetic heterogeneity in MCAD deficiency. Frequency of K329E allele and identification of three additional mutant alleles, in Coates PM, Tanaka K (eds): *New Developments in Fatty Acid Oxidation*. New York, Wiley-Liss, 1992, p 479.
253. Kelly DP, Whelan AJ, Hale DE, Rinaldo P, Rutledge SL, Zhang Z, Strauss AW: Molecular characterization of medium-chain acyl-CoA dehydrogenase deficiency causing sudden death, in Coates PM, Tanaka K (eds): *New Developments in Fatty Acid Oxidation*. New York, Wiley-Liss, 1992, p 463.
254. Gregersen N, Blakemore AIF, Winter V, Andresen B, Kolvraa S, Bolund L, Curtis D, Engel PC: Specific diagnosis of medium-chain acyl-CoA dehydrogenase (MCAD) deficiency in dried blood spots by a polymerase chain reaction (PCR) assay detecting a point mutation (G985) in the MCAD gene. *Clin Chim Acta* **202**:23, 1991.
255. Gregersen N, Winter V, Curtis D, Deufel T, Mack M, Willems P, Ponzone A, Parrella T, Ponzone K, Ding J-H, Zhang W, Kahler SG, Chen Y-T, Roe CR, Kolvraa S, Schneidermann K, Andresen BS, Bross P, Bolund L: Medium-chain acyl-CoA dehydrogenase (MCAD) deficiency: The prevalent mutation K304E (G985) is subject to a strong founder effect from northwestern Europe. *Hum Hered* **43**:342, 1993.
256. Bennett MJ, Hale DE, Coates PM, Stanley CA: Postmortem recognition of fatty acid oxidation disorders. *Pediatr Pathol* **11**:361, 1991.
257. Miller ME, Brooks JG, Forbes N, Insel R: Frequency of medium chain acyl-coenzyme A dehydrogenase deficiency G-985 mutation in sudden infant death syndrome. *Pediatr Res* **31**:305, 1992.
258. Roe CR, Millington DS, Kahler SG, Kodo N, Norwood DL: Carnitine homeostasis in the organic acidurias, in Tanaka K, Coates PM (eds): *Fatty Acid Oxidation: Clinical, Biochemical, and Molecular Aspects*. New York, Wiley-Liss, 1990, p 383.
259. Treem WR, Stanley CA, Goodman SI: Medium-chain acyl-CoA dehydrogenase deficiency: Metabolic effects and therapeutic efficacy of long-term L-carnitine supplementation. *J Inherit Metab Dis* **12**:112, 1989.
260. Stanley CA: Disorders of fatty acid oxidation, in Fernandes J, Saudubray J-M, Tada K (eds): *Inborn Metabolic Diseases: Diagnosis and Treatment*. Berlin, Springer-Verlag, 1990, p 395.
261. Van Hove JLK, Kahler SG, Millington DS, Roe DS, Chace DH, Heales SJR, Roe CR: Intravenous L-carnitine in medium-chain acyl-CoA dehydrogenase deficiency and isovaleric acidemia. *Pediatr Res* **35**:96, 1994.
262. Stanley CA, Hale DE, Coates PM: Medium-chain acyl-CoA dehydrogenase deficiency, in Tanaka K, Coates PM (eds): *Fatty Acid Oxidation: Clinical, Biochemical, and Molecular Aspects*. New York, Alan R. Liss, 1990, p 291.
263. Taubman B, Hale DE, Kelley RJ: Familial Reye-like syndrome: A presentation of medium-chain acyl-coenzyme A dehydrogenase deficiency. *Pediatrics* **79**:382, 1987.
264. Gregersen N, Kolvraa S, Rasmussen K, Mortensen PB, Divry P, David M, Hobolth N: General (medium-chain) acyl-CoA dehydrogenase deficiency (non-ketotic dicarboxylic aciduria): Quantitative urinary excretion pattern of 23 biologically significant organic acids in three cases. *Clin Chim Acta* **132**:181, 1983.

265. Duran M, Mitchell G, de Klerk JBC, de Jager JP, Hofkamp M, Bruinvis L, Ketting D, Saudubray JM, Wadman SK: Octanoic acidemia and octanoylcarnitine excretion with dicarboxylic aciduria due to defective oxidation of medium-chain fatty acids. *J Pediatr* **107**:397, 1985.
266. Denton RM, McCormick JG, Oviasu OA: Short-term regulation of pyruvate dehydrogenase activity in the liver, in Hue L, Van de Werve G (eds): *Short-Term Regulation of Liver Metabolism.* Amsterdam, Elsevier, 1981, p 159.
267. Pogson CI, Munoz-Clares RA, Elliott KRF, Kean EA, Lloyd P, Smith SA: Interactions of amino acids with gluconeogenesis, in Hue L, Van de Werve G (eds): *Short-Term Regulation of Liver Metabolism.* Amsterdam, Elsevier, 1981, p 339.
268. Parker WD, Haas R, Stumpf DA, Eguren LA: Effects of octanoate on rat brain and liver mitochondria. *Neurology* **33**:1374, 1983.
269. Mamunes P, Devries GH, Miller CD, David RB: Fatty acid quantitation in Reye's syndrome, in Pollack JD (ed): *Reye's Syndrome*. New York, Grune & Stratton, 1974, p 245.
270. Trauner DA, Adams H: Intracranial pressure elevations during octanoate infusion in rabbits: An experimental model of Reye's syndrome. *Pediatr Res* **15**:1097, 1981.
271. Heubi JE, Partin JC, Partin JS, Schubert WK: Reye's syndrome: Current concepts. *Hepatology* **7**:155, 1987.
272. Samson FE, Dahl N, Dahl DR: A study on the narcotic action of the short chain fatty acids. *J Clin Invest* **35**:1291, 1956.
273. Kim CS, O'Tuama LA, Mann JD, Roe CR: Effect of increasing carbon chain length on organic acid transport by the choroid plexus: A potential factor in Reye's syndrome. *Brain Res* **259**:340, 1983.
274. Olson JE, Holtzman D, Sankar R, Lawson C, Rosenberg R: Octanoic acid inhibits astrocyte volume control: Implications for cerebral edema in Reye's syndrome. *J Neurochem* **52**:1197, 1989.
275. McCandless DW: Octanoic acid-induced coma and reticular formation energy metabolism. *Brain Res* **335**:131, 1985.
276. Turnbull DM, Bartlett K, Stevens DL, Alberti KGMM, Gibson GJ, Johnson MA, McCulloch AJ, Sherratt HSA: Short-chain acyl-CoA dehydrogenase deficiency associated with a lipid-storage myopathy and secondary carnitine deficiency. *N Engl J Med* **311**:1232, 1984.
277. Amendt BA, Greene C, Sweetman L, Cloherty J, Shih V, Moon A, Teel L, Rhead WJ: Short-chain acyl-coenzyme A dehydrogenase deficiency: Clinical and biochemical studies in two patients. *J Clin Invest* **79**:1303, 1987.
278. Coates PM, Hale DE, Finocchiaro G, Tanaka K, Winter SC: Genetic deficiency of short-chain acyl-coenzyme A dehydrogenase in cultured fibroblasts from a patient with muscle carnitine deficiency and severe skeletal muscle weakness. *J Clin Invest* **81**:171, 1988.
279. Gregersen N: The acyl-CoA dehydrogenation deficiencies. *Scand J Clin Lab Invest Suppl* **174**:1, 1985.
280. Vianey-Liaud C, Divry P, Gregersen N, Mathieu M: The inborn errors of mitochondrial fatty acid oxidation. *J Inherit Metab Dis* **10(Suppl 1)**:159, 1987.
281. Bennett MJ: The laboratory diagnosis of inborn errors of mitochondrial fatty acid oxidation. *Ann Clin Biochem* **27**:519, 1990.
282. Farnsworth L, Shepherd IM, Johnson MA, Bindoff LA, Turnbull DM: Absence of immunoreactive enzyme protein in short-chain acylcoenzyme A dehydrogenase deficiency. *Ann Neurol* **28**:717, 1990.
283. Turnbull DM, Shepherd IM, Ashworth B, Bartlett K, Johnson MA, Cullen MJ, Jackson S, Sherratt HSA: Lipid storage myopathy associated with low acyl-CoA dehydrogenase activities. *Brain* **111**:815, 1988.
284. DiDonato S, Gellera C, Peluchetti D, Uziel G, Antonelli A, Lus G, Rimoldi M: Normalization of short-chain acylcoenzyme A dehydrogenase after riboflavin treatment in a girl with multiple acylcoenzyme A dehydrogenase-deficient myopathy. *Ann Neurol* **25**:479, 1989.
285. Hoppel C, DiMarco JP, Tandler B: Riboflavin and rat hepatic cell structure and function. Mitochondrial oxidative metabolism in deficiency states. *J Biol Chem* **254**:4164, 1979.
286. Sakurai T, Miyazawa S, Furuta S, Hashimoto T: Riboflavin deficiency and β-oxidation systems in rat liver. *Lipids* **17**:598, 1982.
287. Ross NS, Hansen TPB: Riboflavin deficiency is associated with selective preservation of critical flavoenzyme-dependent metabolic pathways. *Biofactors* **3**:185, 1992.
288. Green A, Marshall TG, Bennett MJ, Gray RGF, Pollitt RJ: Riboflavin responsive ethylmalonic adipic aciduria. *J Inherit Metab Dis* **8**:67, 1985.
289. Gregersen N, Wintzensen H, C6-C10-Dicarboxylic aciduria: Investigations of a patient with riboflavin responsive multiple acyl-CoA dehydrogenation defects. *Pediatr Res* **16**:861, 1982.
290. Gregersen N, Christensen MF, Christensen E, Kolvraa S: Riboflavin responsive multiple acyl-CoA dehydrogenation deficiency. *Acta Paediatr Scand* **75**:676, 1986.
291. de Visser M, Scholte HR, Schutgens RBH, Bolhuis PA, Luyt-Houwen IEM, Vaandrager-Verduin MHM, Veder HA, Oey PL: Riboflavin-responsive lipid-storage myopathy and glutaric aciduria type II of early adult onset. *Neurology* **36**:367, 1986.
292. Brivet M, Tardieu M, Khellaf A, Boutron A, Rocchiccioli F, Haengeli CA, Lemonnier A: Riboflavin responsive ethylmalonic-adipic aciduria in a 9-month-old boy with liver cirrhosis, myopathy and encephalopathy. *J Inherit Metab Dis* **14**:333, 1991.
293. Peluchetti D, Antozzi C, Roi S, DiDonato S, Cornelio F: Riboflavin responsive multiple acyl-CoA dehydrogenase deficiency: Functional evaluation of recovery after high dose vitamin supplementation. *J Neurol Sci* **105**:93, 1991.
294. Roettger V, Marshall T, Amendt B, Rhead WJ: Multiple acyl-coenzyme A dehydrogenation disorders (MAD) responsive to riboflavin: Biochemical studies in fibroblasts, in Coates PM, Tanaka K (eds): *New Developments in Fatty Acid Oxidation*. New York, Wiley-Liss, 1992, p 317.
295. Rhead WJ: Inborn errors of fatty acid oxidation in man. *Clin Biochem* **24**:319, 1991.
296. Barton DE, Yang-Feng TL, Finocchiaro G, Ozasa H, Tanaka K, Francke U: Short chain acyl-CoA dehydrogenase (ACADS) maps to chromosome 12 (q22-qter) and electron transfer flavoprotein (ETFA) to 15 (q23-q25). *Cytogenet Cell Genet* **46**:577, 1987.
297. Corydon MJ, Andresen BS, Bross P, Kjeldsen M, Andreasen PH, Eiberg H, Kolvraa S, Gregersen N: Structural organization of the human short-chain acyl-CoA dehydrogenase gene. *Mamm Genome* **8(12)**:922, 1997.
298. Naito E, Indo Y, Tanaka K: Identification of two variant short chain acyl-coenzyme A dehydrogenase alleles, each containing a different point mutation in a patient with short chain acyl-coenzyme A dehydrogenase deficiency. *J Clin Invest* **85(5)**:1575, 1990.
299. Gregersen N, Winter VS, Corydon MJ, Corydon TJ, Rinaldo P, Ribes A, Martinez G, Bennett MJ, Vianey-Saban C, Bhala A, Hale DE, Lehnert W, Kmoch S, Roig M, Riudor E, Eiberg H, Andresen BS, Bross P, Bolund LA, Kolvraa S: Identification of four new mutations in the short-chain acyl-CoA dehydrogenase (SCAD) gene in two patients: One of the variant alleles, 511C $\rightarrow$ T, is present at an unexpectedly high frequency in the general population, as was the case for 625G $\rightarrow$ A, together conferring susceptibility to ethylmalonic aciduria. *Hum Mol Genet* **7(4)**:619, 1998.
300. Corydon MJ, Gregersen N, Lehnert W, Ribes A, Rinaldo P, Kmoch S, Christensen E, Kristensen TJ, Andresen BS, Bross P, Winter V, Martinez G, Neve S, Jensen TG, Bolund L, Kolvraa S: Ethylmalonic aciduria is associated with an amino acid variant of short chain acyl-coenzyme A dehydrogenase. *Pediatr Res* **39(6)**:1059, 1996.
301. Hinsdale ME, Kelly CL, Wood PA: Null allele at Bcd-1 locus in BALB/cByJ mice is due to a deletion in the short-chain acyl-CoA dehydrogenase gene and results in missplicing of mRNA. *Genomics* **16(3)**:605,1993.
302. Tein I, De Vivo DC, Hale DE, Clarke JTR, Zinman H, Laxer R, Shore A, DiMauro S: Short-chain l-3-hydroxyacyl-CoA dehydrogenase deficiency in muscle: A new cause for recurrent myoglobinuria and encephalopathy. *Ann Neurol* **30**:415, 1991.
303. Bennett MJ, Weinberger MJ, Kobori JA, Rinaldo P, Burlina AB: Mitochondrial short-chain L-3-hydroxyacyl-coenzyme A dehydrogenase deficiency: A new defect of fatty acid oxidation. *Pediatr Res* **39**:185, 1996.
304. Vredendaal PJ, van den Berg IE, Malingre HE, Stroobants AK, Olde Weghuis DE, Berger R: Human short-chain L-3-hydroxyacyl-CoA dehydrogenase: Cloning and characterization of the coding sequence. *Biochem Biophys Res Commun* **223**:718, 1996.
305. Vredendaal PJ, van den Berg IE, Stroobants AK, van der A DL, Malingre HE, Bergar R: Structural organization of the human short-chain L-3-hydroxyacyl-CoA dehydrogenase gene. *Mamm Genome* **9**:763, 1998.
306. He XY, Schulz H, Yang SY: A human brain L-3-hydroxyacyl-coenzyme A dehydrogenase is identical to an amyloid β-peptide-binding protein involved in Alzheimer's disease. *J Biol Chem* **273(17)**:10741, 1998.
307. Roe CR: Diagnostic approach to disorders of fat oxidation. *Int Pediatr* **11**:23, 1996.
308. Stanley CA: Dissecting the spectrum of fatty acid oxidation disorders. *J Pediatr* **132**:384, 1998.

309. Nezu J, Tamai I, Oku A, Ohashi R, Yabuuchi H, Hashimoto N, et al: Primary systemic carnitine deficiency is caused by mutations in a gene encoding sodium ion-dependent carnitine transporter. *Nat Genet* **21**:91, 1999.
310. Tang NL, Ganapathy V, Wu X, Hui J, Seth P, Yuen PM, Wanders RJ, Fok TF, Hjelm NM: Mutations in OCTN2, an organic cation/carnitine transporter, lead to deficient cellular carnitine uptake in primary carnitine deficiency. *Hum Mol Genet* **8**:655, 1999.
311. Wang Y, Ye J, Ganapathy V, Longo N: Mutations in the organic cation/carnitine transporter OCTN2 in primary carnitine deficiency. *Proc Natl Acad Sci U S A* **96**:2356, 1999.
312. Koizumi A, Nozaki J, Ohura T, Kayo T, Wada Y, Nezu J, et al: Genetic epidemiology of the carnitine transporter OCTN2 gene in a Japanese population and phenotypic characterization in Japanese pedigrees with primary systemic carnitine deficiency. *Hum Mol Genet* **8**:2247, 1999.

CHAPTER 102

Inborn Errors of Ketone Body Metabolism

Grant A. Mitchell ▪ Toshiyuki Fukao

1. **The ketone bodies acetoacetate (AcAc) and R-3-hydroxybutyrate (3HB) are important vectors of energy transport from hepatocyte mitochondria to extrahepatic tissues during fasting and other lipolytic stress. AcAc is the product of ketogenesis and the substrate for ketolysis. 3HB is derived from AcAc. A third compound, acetone, arises from decarboxylation of AcAc and accounts for the distinct odor of ketotic individuals.**
2. **Ketogenesis is fueled by fatty acids or ketogenic amino acids, principally leucine. Two mitochondrial enzymes mediate ketogenesis from fatty acids: mitochondrial HMG-CoA synthase (mHS) and HMG-CoA lyase (HL). Circulating levels of ketone bodies fluctuate greatly with age, nutrition, lipolytic stress, and other factors.**
3. **Ketolysis occurs in mitochondria of extrahepatic tissues, particularly heart, kidney, and brain, via reversible reactions catalyzed by succinyl-CoA: 3-ketoacid CoA transferase (SCOT) and mitochondrial AcAc-CoA thiolase (T2). Ketolytic rate is determined by the circulating concentration of ketone bodies. The ketolytic capacity of tissues is proportional to their level of SCOT activity.**
4. **Inborn errors of ketogenesis (mHS or HL deficiencies) cause episodes of hypoketotic hypoglycemia, often with coma. Ketolytic (T2 or SCOT) deficiencies cause episodes of ketoacidosis. All four disorders are autosomal recessive. Infancy is the period of highest risk for decompensation. Death or neurologic complications can occur, but with early diagnosis and treatment, many patients are clinically normal. The mainstay of treatment in these disorders is suppression of ketogenesis. Enzyme and molecular diagnosis is possible for each of these conditions.**
5. **mHS undergoes intricate transcriptional and posttranscriptional regulation to control the rate of ketogenesis. In mHS deficiency, the urinary organic acid pattern is not diagnostic. Diagnosis depends upon enzyme assay in liver and/or molecular studies.**
6. **HL is located in mitochondria and peroxisomes of all tissues studied to date. HL deficiency is characterized by high levels of 3-hydroxy-3-methylglutaric acid (HMG) and related leucine metabolites in urine. Enzymatic confirmation is recommended, since rare patients excrete these compounds but have normal HL activity. Mental retardation, epilepsy, and white matter changes may occur following hypoglycemic episodes.**
7. **SCOT is extrahepatic in distribution. The ketolytic capacity of tissues is proportional to their levels of SCOT activity. In SCOT deficiency, ketoacidosis develops rapidly on fasting and ketonuria is often present in the fed state. Urine organic acids show only a nonspecific increase of AcAc and 3HB.**
8. **T2 functions in both ketolysis and ketogenesis. T2 deficiency presents as infantile ketoacidosis. Coma and basal ganglia abnormalities may occur. A diagnostic metabolite profile including 2-methyl-3HB, 2-methylAcAc and tiglylglycine is present in most patients.**
9. **3HB dehydrogenase (3HBD) catalyzes the reversible reduction of AcAc to 3HB, functioning in both ketogenesis and ketolysis. 3HBD deficiency has not been described.**
10. **A distinct cytoplasmic AcAc-CoA thiolase (CT) functions in lipogenesis and cholesterol synthesis. It was reportedly deficient in two girls with progressive mental retardation. Enzyme and molecular diagnosis is possible.**

The presence of ketone bodies has been used for 140 years as a sign of uncontrolled diabetes and as a tool for assessing the severity of dehydration. It is less commonly appreciated that ketone bodies are important vectors of energy metabolism and that the demonstration of abnormal levels of ketone bodies is a useful diagnostic sign. The finding of an appropriate increase of ketone bodies during lipolytic stress implies that the entire pathway of lipid energy metabolism is functional.

Ketogenesis is quiescent under most circumstances but can be activated to an extraordinary degree by fasting and other ketogenic stress, especially in infants and children. As a reflection of this, patients with inborn errors of ketone body metabolism are usually asymptomatic but may experience fulminant, potentially fatal decompensations during lipolytic stress. This is particularly likely in infants. Avoiding ketogenic stress can prevent most episodes.

Ketone body metabolism has been addressed in symposia and reviews over the past 20 years.[1–8] Historical references are given in reference 9.

STRUCTURE AND PROPERTIES OF KETONE BODIES

The term "ketone bodies" refers to three molecules, acetoacetate (AcAc), R-3-hydroxybutyrate (3HB), and acetone (Fig. 102-1). Chemically, 3HB is not a ketone, but the nomenclature is entrenched, and we will use it for the rest of the chapter. Acetoacetate is chemically unstable and generates acetone by spontaneous decarboxylation.[11] In contrast, 3HB is stable and nonvolatile. Acetone is volatile and is responsible for the fruity odor of breath and urine during ketoacidosis.

A list of standard abbreviations is located immediately preceding the index in each volume. Nonstandard abbreviations used in this chapter include: 2MeAcAc = 2-methylacetoacetate; 3HB = R-3-hydroxybutyrate; 3HBD = R-3-hydroxybutyrate dehydrogenase; AcAc = acetoacetate; cHS = cytoplasmic HMG-CoA synthase; CT = cytoplasmic AcAc-CoA thiolase; HL = HMG-CoA lyase; HMG = 3-hydroxy-3-methylglutaric acid; mHS = mitochondrial HMG-CoA synthase; PPRE = peroxisome proliferator response element; SCOT = succinyl CoA-3-ketoacid CoA transferase; T2 = mitochondrial AcAc-CoA thiolase; 2Me3HB = 2-methyl-3-hydroxybutyric acid.

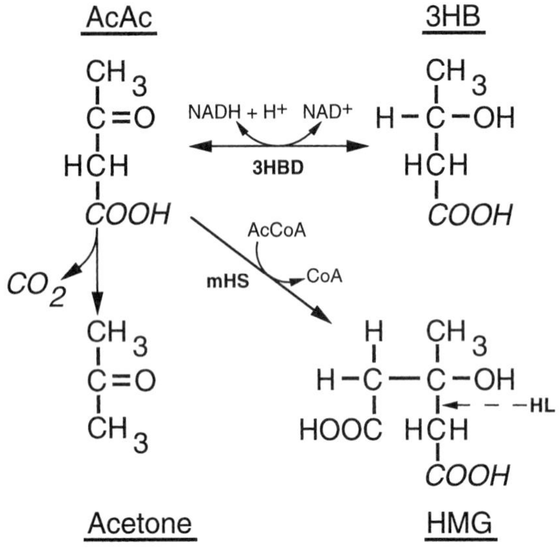

Fig. 102-1 Chemical structures of AcAc-related compounds AcAc, 3HB, and acetone are usually grouped together as "ketone bodies," although chemically this is inexact, since 3HB contains no ketone group. 3HB and acetone are derived from AcAc. HMG-CoA is derived from AcAc-CoA. AcAc and HMG form CoA thioesters at the italicized carbonyl groups. The anatomy of HMG-CoA formation and lysis is shown: an acetyl group derived from Ac-CoA is added to AcAc-CoA at carbon 3 by mHS, then HL liberates free AcAc by cleavage at the bond between carbons 2 and 3, shown by a dashed arrow. Thus, the 4-carbon chain of the AcAc-CoA precursor is cleaved, donating two carbons to the free AcAc.

3HB and AcAc are the 4-carbon analogues of lactic and pyruvic acids, respectively. Their molecular weights and pKa values at 25°C[12] are: AcAc, 102.09, 3.58; 3HB, 104.10, 4.70.

The (R) enantiomorph of 3HB is produced during ketone body metabolism, while the (S) form of 3HB-CoA is produced by beta oxidation.[12] Only the (S) form of HMG-CoA is produced physiologically.[13]

MEASUREMENT OF KETONE BODIES

Urinary Ketone Bodies

Tablet or dipstick tests for urinary ketone bodies are based on the reaction of ketones with nitroprusside in alkaline buffered solution, resulting in a purple color. The lower limit of sensitivity for AcAc is ~0.5 mM.[14] Acetone reacts seven- to tenfold less strongly than AcAc. 3HB is not detected. Phenylketones and N-acetylcysteine can produce false positive results.[15] For screening purposes, urinary ketosis can usually be detected for ≥24 hours in noncontaminated samples at room temperature.[16]

Blood Ketone Body Measurement

AcAc and 3HB are usually measured spectrophotometrically using commercially available 3HB dehydrogenase and following the absorption of the NADH cofactor at 340 nm.[17,19]

Blood AcAc level may be estimated semiquantitatively by testing serial dilutions of plasma using nitroprusside-based reagent sticks or tablets. A strong reaction at dilutions greater than 1:1 is consistent with ketosis.[20]

Blood samples should be processed immediately after sampling. Because AcAc is volatile and unstable, samples should be kept on ice and measurements should be performed soon after sampling. Although arterial levels of ketone bodies can be 20 percent higher than those in venous blood, arterialized venous blood levels do not differ significantly from arterial levels.[21]

OVERVIEW OF KETONE BODY METABOLISM

Ketone bodies transport fat-derived energy from the liver to other organs, particularly the brain. Conceptually, if one defines a metabolic pathway as a series of enzymatic reactions beginning with a rate-determining reaction and ending either with another rate-determining reaction or with terminal metabolites,[12] ketogenesis and ketolysis form a single pathway spanning the liver and an extrahepatic ketolytic tissue.

Ketogenesis

AcAc is synthesized from acetoacetyl-CoA (AcAc-CoA) and acetyl CoA via two enzymatic steps, described by Feodor Lynen and colleagues in 1958:[22] mitochondrial HMG CoA synthase (mHS), a highly regulated enzyme, and HMG CoA lyase (HL) (Fig. 102-2).

A third enzyme, R-3-hydroxybutyrate dehydrogenase (3HBD), catalyzes the reduction of AcAc to 3HB. 3HB synthesis increases the molecule's energy content: Oxidation of one molecule of 3HB can potentially furnish 26 high-energy phosphate bonds, in comparison to 23 for AcAc. 3HB is analogous to lactic acid, in that its only known metabolic role is interconversion with AcAc.

Mitochondrial AcAc-CoA thiolase (T2) equilibrates intramitochondrial pools of CoASAc and of AcAc-CoA, catalyzing the

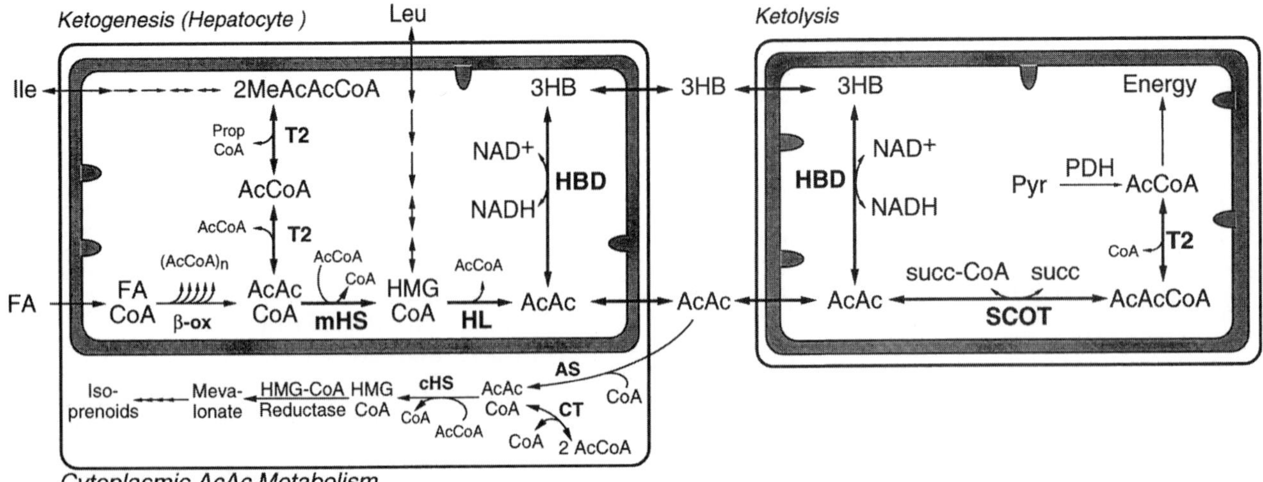

Fig. 102-2 Ketone body metabolism. The pathways of ketogenesis and ketolysis are shown (bold arrows), as are some cytoplasmic reactions of AcAc-CoA and HMG-CoA. Cytosolic pathways are shown only in the hepatocyte. AS = AcAc-CoA synthetase, PDH = pyruvate dehydrogenase, Prop-CoA = propionyl-CoA, Pyr = pyruvate.

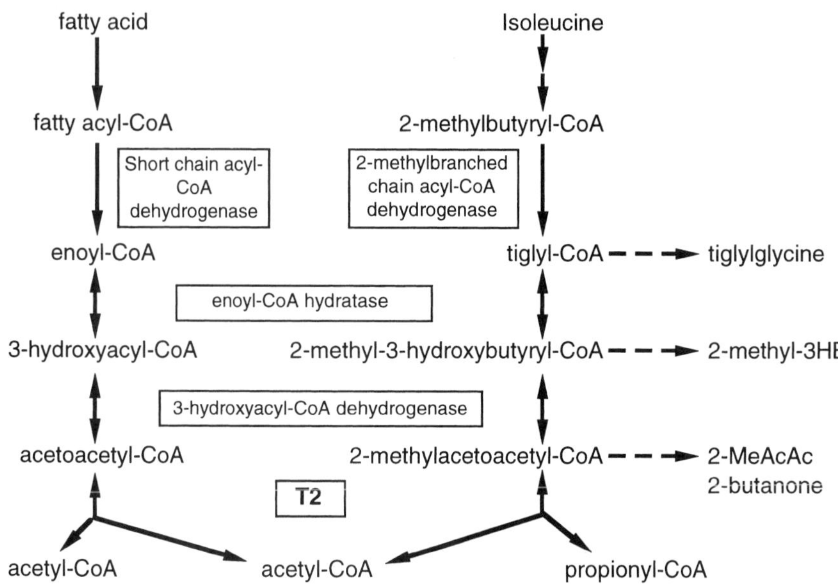

Fig. 102-3 Isoleucine catabolism. The pathway is summarized on the right side, as are the possible origins of abnormal metabolites in T2 deficiency (dotted arrows). Chemically, the final three reactions of isoleucine degradation are analogous to the last steps of short-chain fatty acid oxidation shown on the left. T2 mediates the last reaction of both pathways. The identity of the two preceding enzymes of isoleucine catabolism has not been conclusively established.

reversible transfer of an acetyl group between two CoASAc molecules. If the matrix is rich in acetyl groups from beta oxidation, the *ketogenic threshold* is attained and equilibrium shifts to AcAc-CoA synthesis.

During active ketogenesis in adults, 115–180 g of ketone bodies can be produced daily.[23–25] Since the energy content of ketone bodies is about 4.5 kcal/g,[25] ketogenesis can in theory mobilize the energy equivalent of nearly half of basal energy consumption. This becomes critical at times of glucose scarcity. In comparison, cytoplasmic HMG-CoA metabolism (Fig. 102-2), which leads to the synthesis of isoprenoid compounds, has a capacity of ~2.5 g/day.[26]

Ketogenesis has been evaluated *in vitro* under multiple circumstances. For example, in adult guinea pig liver homogenates, the ketogenic capacity with long-chain substrates is ~30 μmol/h/g, wet weight and is ~1.5-fold greater with medium- and short-chain substrates.[27] In isolated rat hepatocytes incubated with oleate and acetylcarnitine, ketogenesis is ~45 μmol/10^8 cells/h for fed rats and ~110 μmol/10^8 cells/h for fasted rats, ketone bodies accounting for ~90 percent of acid-soluble radioactivity, i.e., the great majority of total fatty acid oxidation.[28]

Lipid and protein sources of ketone bodies. Ketone bodies are derived from fatty acids and from ketogenic amino acids. Ketone bodies are synthesized *conditionally* from fatty acids if CoASAc production by beta oxidation exceeds the use of CoASAc by the hepatocyte. Of note, CoASAc produced by fatty acid oxidation is channeled preferentially to ketogenesis, whereas CoASAc derived from glucose is directed preferentially to the Krebs cycle.[29]

In contrast, the principal ketogenic amino acid, leucine, produces HMG-CoA as an *obligate* intermediate during degradation. Lysine and tryptophan can also produce HMG-CoA but have alternative catabolic pathways. Their quantitative contributions to ketogenesis are less documented than those of leucine. Phenylalanine and tyrosine produce AcAc directly, without an HMG-CoA intermediate (Chap. 79).

A calculation based upon a diet providing 30 percent of energy as fat (palmitate) and 20 percent as protein with a typical amino acid composition shows that, if all possible substrates were converted to ketone bodies, ~1000 mmol of AcAc could be formed from fat and ~115 mmol would be formed from protein via HMG-CoA:leucine (~60 mmol), tryptophan (~10 mmol), lysine (~45 mmol). Phenylalanine plus tyrosine would directly provide an additional ~40 mmol of AcAc, and CoASAc produced from other amino acids could contribute as well. In practice, the relative contributions of each substrate are determined by the intensity of lipolysis and proteolysis as well as by dietary intake. Using isotopic tracers in an HL-deficient child, it was shown that during an infection most HMG-related metabolites in urine were derived from leucine catabolism, whereas during fasting, most were lipid-derived.[30]

In contrast to mHS, HL plays a role in both fat and amino acid catabolism (Fig. 102-2). The same is true for T2, which cleaves a metabolite of isoleucine, 2-methylacetoacetyl CoA (2 MeAcAc-CoA) (Figs. 102-2 and 102-3).

Circulation and transport of ketone bodies. AcAc and 3HB circulate as free molecules. Cell membrane transporters of ketone bodies have not been identified, but 3HB inhibits lactate uptake by liver,[31] suggesting possible interaction with the monocarboxylate transporter MCT2.[32] AcAc enters mitochondria via the monocarboxylic acid transporter.[33]

Ketolysis

In mitochondria of extrahepatic cells, AcAc is activated to AcAcCoA by succinyl CoA: 3-ketoacid ("oxoacid") transferase (SCOT). The ketolytic capacity of tissues varies directly with SCOT activity: heart (assigned as 100 percent) $>$ kidney (~70 percent) $\gg$ brain (~10 percent) $>$ skeletal muscle (~5 percent) $\gg$ liver (undetectable).[6]

The rate of ketone body utilization is proportional to the circulating levels.[5,34–36] However, after 2 weeks of starvation, blood levels of ketone bodies increase despite a constant rate of ketogenesis,[5,24] suggesting that in prolonged fasting ketolysis may be reduced. AcAc concentrations greater than 5 mM inhibit SCOT activity,[37] but it is not proved that this is physiologically relevant.

AcAc-CoA is converted to CoASAc by T2 (Fig. 102-2). T2 can thus be viewed as the first enzyme of ketogenesis[38] and the last enzyme of ketolysis.

Pseudoketogenesis

The 3HBD, SCOT, and T2 reactions are reversible. Although in extrahepatic tissues the net flow of AcAc carbon is in the direction of ketolysis, there is some equilibration between AcAc and cellular CoASAc. The term "pseudoketogenesis" has been applied to this phenomenon, which creates an artifact in isotopic

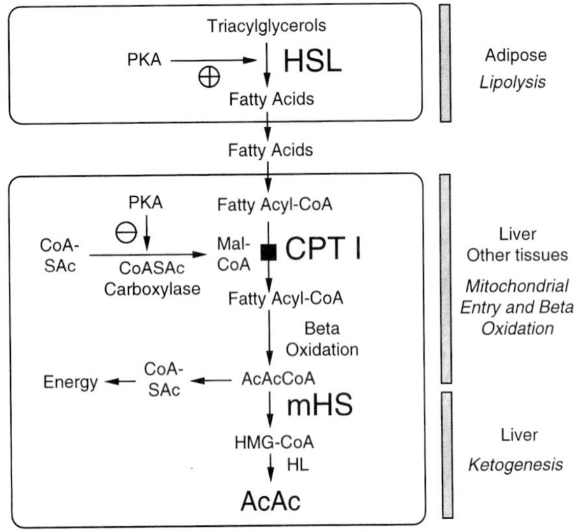

Fig. 102-4 Control of ketogenesis. The three levels of enzymatic control are shown. CPT I = carnitine palmitoyltranferase I, HSL = hormone-sensitive lipase, Mal-CoA = malonyl CoA, PKA = protein kinase A.

tracer studies.[39] Pseudoketogenesis hinders the noninvasive estimation of *in vivo* ketone body flux by stable isotope techniques. Under some experimental conditions, net ketogenesis occurs in heart or kidney.[40,41]

Control of Ketogenesis

Ketogenesis is the final phase of lipid energy metabolism. In the postabsorptive period (3–4 h after eating), lipid energy metabolism is relatively quiescent; it then increases gradually during the period of glycogenolysis (5–24 h).[12] As glycogen stores wane, use of fatty acids as an energy source progressively increases.

Hepatic ketogenesis is regulated at three levels (Fig. 102-4): (1) substrate availability from lipolysis, determined by adipocyte hormone-sensitive lipase; (2) concentration of hepatic malonyl CoA (malonyl CoA inhibits carnitine palmitoyltransferase I, reducing the entry of fatty acids into mitochondria); and (3) mHS. Briefly, the mechanisms of control, reviewed elsewhere,[4,42,43] involve phosphorylation of both hormone-sensitive lipase and acetyl CoA carboxylase (the enzyme that synthesizes malonyl CoA), either by protein kinase A (cyclic AMP-dependent protein kinase) or by AMP-activated protein kinase, at different sites and with opposing effects on enzyme activity.[44] Phosphorylation by protein kinase A, the activity of which is increased by glucagon and reduced by insulin, activates hormone-sensitive lipase[45] and inactivates acetyl CoA carboxylase.[46] The net effect of this is to accelerate lipid catabolism by increasing fatty acid release from adipocytes and by increasing the entry of fatty acids into hepatic mitochondria.

Evidence suggests that mHS exerts some control on ketogenesis and possibly on beta oxidation. Consistent with this are the great fluctuations of mHS activity in response to ketogenic stimuli and the observation that changes in carnitine palmitoyltransferase I cannot completely explain observed rates of ketogenesis.[47–49] Furthermore, in mice transgenic for mHS, with a threefold increase in hepatic mHS activity, basal ketone body levels are twice normal.[50]

Since lipolysis, carnitine palmitoyltransferase I, and mHS are all influenced by the glucagon/insulin ratio, ketogenesis is exquisitely sensitive to carbohydrate ingestion and insulin infusion.[51]

Metabolic Effects of Ketone Bodies

Ketone bodies reduce glucose utilization,[52,53] perhaps by generating citrate that inhibits glycolysis.[54] They can reduce proteolysis,[55] although less effectively than isocaloric amounts of carbohydrate.[56] Ketone bodies can also inhibit lipolysis[57] and reduce gluconeogenesis.[58,59]

Extrahepatic Ketone Body Metabolism

Brain

Brain energy supply. Ketone bodies are an essential link between the body's fat stores and brain mitochondria. The main function of ketone bodies may be to provide the brain with a non-carbohydrate energy source during fasting. The brain cannot use fatty acids as an energy source.[60] In well-nourished individuals, the main energy substrates of brain are glucose and its derivatives (lactic acid, glycerol), but during prolonged fasting, ketone bodies supply nearly two-thirds of brain energy.[61]

Ketone bodies traverse the blood-brain barrier via the monocarboxylate carrier.[60] In cultures from fetal rat brain, neurons have higher levels of SCOT and a greater ketolytic capacity than astrocytes or oligodendroglia.[62]

Brain development. In rodents, ketone bodies are normally used for brain lipid synthesis.[63,64] However, in suckling rats, a carbohydrate-rich diet permits normal brain development.[65] In humans, many HL-deficient patients survive normally for months or years prior to developing symptoms, suggesting that ketone bodies are not necessary for normal human brain development.

Ketone bodies and epilepsy. Ketosis can reduce the severity of some forms of epilepsy, by unknown mechanisms.[66]

Kidney. Experimentally, up to 80 percent of renal cortical energy can be provided by AcAc.[40] Up to 35 percent of fatty acid carbon oxidized in cortex can be released as AcAc,[40] presumably by reversal of ketolysis, since mHS is low in kidney. AcAc and 3HB are filtered but reabsorbed in the proximal tubule.[67–69] Active transport systems are identified, with calculated K_ms of 1.34 (high affinity) and 5.44 mM (low affinity).[70] A high filtered load of ketone bodies reduces uric acid clearance, contributing to hyperuricemia in acidosis,[71] and reduces renal ammoniagenesis, perhaps by reducing the use of glutamine for energy.[72]

Heart. Ketone bodies do not sustain cardiac contractility if provided as the sole energy source for the heart, possibly because CoA sequestration inhibits 2-oxoglutarate dehydrogenase.[73] However, in rat heart perfused with glucose, supplementation of the perfusate with 4 mM 3HB and 1 mM AcAc improves work efficiency by 35 percent.[74]

Gastrointestinal tract. Ketone bodies may provide an important source of energy for adult gut.[75]

Muscle. Because of its large mass, skeletal muscle accounts for substantial ketolysis despite its low SCOT activity.[5]

Hematopoietic tissues. Ketone bodies may share some properties of butyric acid, such as the ability to stimulate fetal hemoglobin synthesis. During a ketoacidotic crisis in a T2-deficient patient, fetal hemoglobin level was 13.5 percent of total hemoglobin,[76] but normalized to 0.5 percent after correction of the ketoacidosis. It will be interesting to test this in other patients.

Placenta and fetus. In contrast to long-chain fatty acids, ketone bodies readily cross the placenta, fetal and maternal ketone body levels being similar.[6,77] In rodent embryos, neural tube defects can be induced by exposure to high levels of 3HB.[78]

Alternative Metabolic Fates of AcAc and AcAc-CoA

Multiple enzymes utilize or produce AcAc.[79] Some reactions are mediated by distinct cytoplasmic enzymes of cholesterol and lipid synthesis. A distinct cytoplasmic HS isozyme (cHS)[80,81] catalyzes an early step of cholesterol synthesis. It is thought that there is

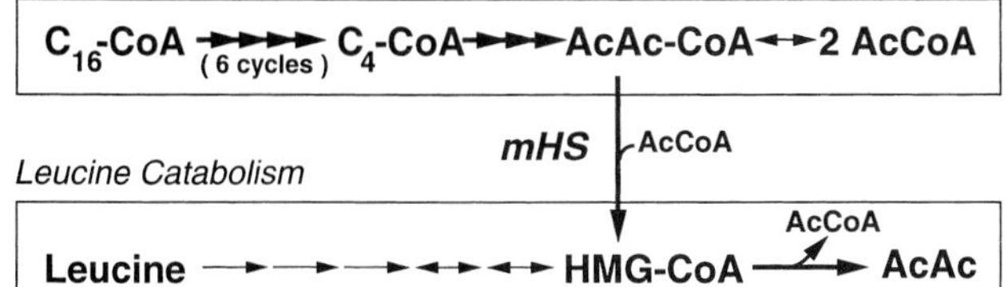

Fig. 102-5 The evolution of ketogenesis, a hypothesis. The mitochondrion prior to invasion by HS is thought to have contained the complete pathways of beta oxidation (top) and leucine catabolism (bottom), in metabolic isolation from one another. The appearance of HS within the mitochondrion linked the two pathways, permitting ketogenesis from fatty acids (bold arrows).

little or no exchange between the cytoplasmic and mitochondrial pools of HMG-CoA,[82] although this has not been formally proven. A cytoplasmic AcAc-CoA synthetase in liver, adipose, and brain[83,84] presumably provides substrate for lipogenesis. In rat liver, ketone bodies account for up to 22 percent of hepatic lipogenesis,[85] showing the hepatic mitochondria and cytoplasm to be metabolically distinct.

Activities of AcAc-CoA hydrolase[86] and acetoacetyl glutathione hydrolase[87] are present in mitochondria. A succinyl-CoA: HMG-CoA transferase has been described.[88] Because the decarboxylation of AcAc proceeds faster in perfused liver than in protein-free solution,[89] an AcAc decarboxylase may exist in mammals, as it does in *Clostridium acetobutylicum*.[90] Acetone may be metabolized to carbohydrate via lactate.[91]

The presence of these enzymes complicates enzymatic diagnosis of some ketone body inborn errors. Their metabolic capacity is insufficient to prevent the clinical manifestations of such inborn errors. Future studies may reveal the extent to which alternative pathways modify the phenotypes of these disorders or perhaps themselves cause as yet undescribed hereditary diseases.

Comparative and Fundamental Aspects of Ketone Body Metabolism

The HMG-CoA pathway in evolution, a hypothesis. Ketogenesis in mammals can be viewed as an "altruistic" pathway by which the liver cell provides energy to other organs. Hence it is useful only to multicellular organisms, which by evolutionary standards arose relatively recently. A primitive form of ketogenesis could be mediated by leakage of ketone bodies from energy-rich tissues via reversal of the ketolytic pathway, but this does not provide the control obtained with the HMG-CoA pathway.

Comparison of the sequences of mHS and cHS suggests that they arose 400–900 million years ago, by gene duplication.[81] The mHS mitochondrial leader, encoded mainly by exon I of the mHS gene,[92] was presumably acquired after the divergence and directed mHS to mitochondria, linking preexisting pathways of beta oxidation and leucine catabolism and creating the HMG-CoA pathway of ketogenesis (Fig. 102-5) to provide fat-derived energy to the brain.

Comparative metabolism. There is great quantitative variation in fat energy metabolism among vertebrates,[93–102] an important consideration in applying results from other species to humans. Discussion of these interesting variants is beyond the scope of this chapter.

Analogies with pyruvate metabolism. The structure and metabolism of AcAc resembles those of pyruvate. These are analogous four- or three-carbon carboxylic acids, penultimate metabolites of major fuels that participate in highly adaptable systems capable of transporting large amounts of energy. The metabolism of both AcAc and pyruvate depends on the supply of their precursor fuels, has complex internal regulation, and is associated with acquired and hereditary metabolic diseases. Similarly, 3HB and lactate are reduced (high-energy) hydroxyacids, whose only metabolic fate is reoxidation to their precursors.

Metabolic paradigms. Ketone body metabolism illustrates metabolic compartmentalization (HMG-CoA and AcAc-CoA)[82,103] and metabolic channeling (AcAc-CoA)[29] and lends itself to metabolic control analysis.[104,105]

THE ENZYMES OF KETONE BODY METABOLISM

The directionality of ketone body flow is due to the combination in liver of high activity of mHS and low activity of SCOT. The substrates and products of the enzymes of ketone body metabolism can be utilized by several other enzymes, which can lead to technical difficulties with their assay.

Mitochondrial HMG-CoA Synthase

Mitochondrial HMG-CoA synthase (mHS, E.C. 4.1.3.5) catalyzes the irreversible rate-limiting reaction of ketogenesis in the mitochondrial matrix (Fig. 102-6):

$$\text{AcAc-CoA} + \text{CoASAc} \rightarrow \text{S-HMG-CoA} + \text{CoA} \qquad (102\text{-}1)$$

The mHS reaction. Schematically, the HS reaction can be divided into three steps:[106,107] (I) reversible acetylation of HS by AcCoA, with release of free CoA; (II) condensation of AcAc-CoA, resulting in covalent bonding of an HMG-CoA molecule to the active site cysteine; and (III) hydrolysis of the enzyme-(HMG-CoA) thioester bond, liberating HMG-CoA. Acetylation of mHS appears to be rate limiting.[108] mHS can also catalyze the hydrolysis of CoA-SAc, although a hundredfold slower than the rate of the full reaction.[107] The HS reaction has ping-pong kinetics.[109] The active site cysteine corresponds to C166 in human mHS.[110]

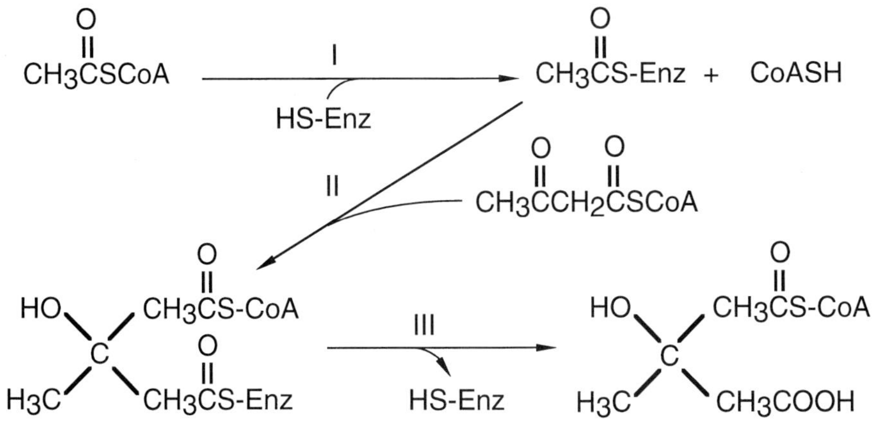

$CH_3C(O)SCoA$ —(I, HS-Enz)→ $CH_3C(O)S\text{-Enz}$ + CoASH

(II) + $CH_3C(O)CH_2C(O)SCoA$ → $HO\!-\!C(CH_3)(CH_2C(O)S\text{-CoA})(CH_2C(O)S\text{-Enz})$

—(III)→ HS-Enz + $HO\!-\!C(CH_3)(CH_2C(O)S\text{-CoA})(CH_2COOH)$

Fig. 102-6 The proposed catalytic mechanism of mHS. See text for details. HS-Enz, mHS enzyme with its catalytic sulfhydryl group.

mHS exhibits both substrate and product inhibition. The kinetic constants for avian[106] and ox[109] liver mHS are: K_m for Ac-CoA, 100 and 51 ± 8 μM; K_m for AcAc-CoA, 0.35 and < 0.5 μM; K_i for AcAc-CoA, 10 and 3.5 ± 0.5 μM; K_i for HMG-CoA in avian mHS, 12 μM. Substrate and product inhibition hinders the determination of V_{max}. The specific activities of purified chicken liver mHS[106] and of recombinant human mHS[111] are 0.7 to 1.0 U/mg.

The mHS protein. The mature human mHS monomer is a 51,350-Da, 471-residue peptide. The N-terminus is inferred to be at Thr38, corresponding to the first residue of the cHS peptide, which lacks a mitochondrial leader.[80] mHS has been purified from chicken[106] and ox[109] liver. We have purified recombinant human mHS from bacterial lysates[111] by a technique similar to that described for recombinant cHS.[112] When studied by gel filtration and by sedimentation, both mHS and cHS migrate as homodimers.[106,109]

The mHS gene and mRNA. The sequences of liver mHS cDNAs from rat[80,113,114] and human[81,115] and of mHS genes of rat[114,116] and human[81,92] have been reported. The mHS locus, *HMGCS2*, maps to human chromosome 1p12–13.[81,117] The human liver mHS mRNA is about 2 kb in length.

The human mHS gene spans 25 kb and contains 10 exons. Exon 1 encodes the translation start site and 33/37 residues of the mitochondrial leader; exon 2, the active site Cys166 residue; and exon 9, the termination codon. Exon 10 is entirely untranslated and contains the polyadenylation signal.[92] A polymorphic short tandem repeat marker is located 23 bp 5′ of the exon 6 acceptor splice site.[117]

The 5′ flanking region of the human mHS gene contains a TATA box 28 bp upstream of the transcription start site plus potential binding sequences for Sp1, nuclear factor 1 (NF1), CAAT-box enhancer binding protein (C/EBP), hepatocyte nuclear factors 1 and 5 (HNF1, HNF5) and activator proteins 1 and 2 (AP1, AP2).[92]

Reported gene studies of the rat mHS gene promoter have demonstrated a peroxisome proliferator-responsive element (PPRE) 104 bp upstream of the start codon.[118] Methylation of the 5′ flanking region is associated with transcriptional inactivation.[119]

Biologic properties. ***Half-life.*** Evidence suggests that mHS has a short half-life, although this has not been measured directly. Near its C-terminal, mHS contains proline-, glutamate-, serine-, and threonine-rich "PEST" sequences[80,81] that are characteristic of short-lived peptides,[120] and on immunoblots, levels of mHS peptide change nearly twofold within 1 h following administration of dibutyryl cyclic AMP (increase) or insulin (decrease).[121]

Tissue distribution. mHS is abundant in liver, accounting for about 0.5 percent of the total protein of ox liver (calculated concentration, > 6 μmol/kg wet weight).[109] Although ketogenesis is reportedly favored in pericentral venous regions of the liver lobule,[122] mHS is distributed throughout the lobule.[123] In male rats, mHS is located in Leydig cells,[124,125] and in females, in proximal oviduct epithelium and theca interna cells of ovarian follicles.[125] In rats, mHS is highly expressed in neonatal intestine[126,127] and to a lesser extent in kidney, brain, and muscle of neonates and adults.[127]

Regulation. mHS activity, protein, and mRNA are highly regulated.[128–131] In rats, liver mHS mRNA is undetectable at fetal day 15 and increases gradually until birth.[132] With suckling, mRNA levels increase threefold, remaining at this level until weaning to a high-carbohydrate diet, at which point they decrease to birth levels within 24 h.[132] This level is maintained in fed adults. Fat feeding, fasting, and diabetes roughly double liver mHS activity,[128] and mHS mRNA increases in liver, intestine, and kidney in response to fat feeding.[132] In rat, the level of liver mHS mRNA is increased tenfold by triiodothyronine administration in thyroidectomized or hypophysectomized rats,[133] is decreased by insulin,[49] and is increased two- to fourfold within 1–2 h after glucagon or dibutyryl cAMP administration[130,132] and twelvefold in streptozocin-induced diabetes.[130] mHS peptide changes in a similar pattern but to a lesser degree than mHS mRNA.[121] Fatty acids upregulate mHS transcription via a the PPRE sequence situated ~104 bp upstream of the transcription start site. Meertens *et al.*[134] have recently described a unique mechanism by which mHS regulates its own transcription: the motif Leu-Ala-Ser-Leu-Leu (residues 390–394) interacts physically with peroxisome proliferator-activated receptor (PPAR)-α, is transported into the nucleus, and stimulates its own transcription by modulating the effect of PPAR-α.

Autosuccinylation and inhibition of mHS occur in the presence of succinyl CoA.[135] In fed rats, mHS is ~40 percent succinylated, diminishing to ~10 percent following treatment with glucagon, which is known to decrease mitochondrial succinyl CoA concentration.[136a] The physiological importance of succinylation is unclear, but it is plausible that it contributes to the reduction of mHS activity in the fed state.[135]

Other roles. A possible role for mHS in cholesterol synthesis is suggested by the interesting observation that expression of an mHS cDNA can correct mevalonate auxotrophy in the cHS-deficient MEV-1 cell line.[137] This challenges current concepts of strict separation between the ketogenic and cholesterologenic pools of HMG-CoA.

mHS and liver metabolism. The mitochondrial matrix is characterized by a high concentration[109] and low specific activity[108,109,111] of mHS and the presence of multiple competing enzymes. The low K_m of mHS for AcAc-CoA (0.35 μM) is suited to the low concentrations of AcAc-CoA (0.2–0.4 μmol/kg wet weight) compared to those of Ac-CoA (50–160 μmol/kg) and free CoA (65–80 μmol/kg).[138] It is unknown whether inhibition by AcAc-CoA, HMG-CoA, or succinyl-CoA has physiological relevance.

HMG-CoA synthase isozymes. The cytoplasmic isozyme of mHS (cHS) is a 57-kDa peptide encoded by a distinct but homologous gene.[139] mHS and cHS have similar kinetic properties and specific activities.[106,112] Antibodies raised to full-length mHS or to cHS peptide cross-react weakly with the other isozyme.[112] The existence of a peroxisomal mHS has been hypothesized[140] but, to our knowledge, remains unproven.

HMG-CoA Lyase

HMG-CoA lyase (HL, EC 4.1.3.4) catalyzes the final step of ketogenesis and of leucine degradation:

$$\text{(S)-HMG-CoA} \rightarrow \text{AcAc} + \text{Ac-CoA} \qquad (102\text{-}2)$$

Structure. Initially, HL was partially purified from pig heart.[141] Many catalytic properties of HL were identified with this preparation, including a requirement for a thiol group and divalent metals such as Mg^{++} or Mn^{++}, an alkaline optimal pH, and the similarity of the HL reaction to that of citrate synthase. Native and recombinant HL has been purified from several sources.[13,82,142] Mature human mitochondrial HL is a homodimer. The 325-residue HL precursor is cleaved to a mature 298-residue 34.4-kDa monomer.[143]

Reaction mechanism. HL mediates a reverse Claisen reaction (Fig. 102-7)[144] proceeding in three steps: (I) abstraction of a proton from the 3-hydroxy group of HMG-CoA by a general base that initiates (II) cleavage of the C2-C3 bond, and then (III) quenching of the resulting Ac-CoA carbanion by a general acid. C266 in human HL is an active site residue, possibly the proton receptor of the earliest step of the reaction after HMG-CoA

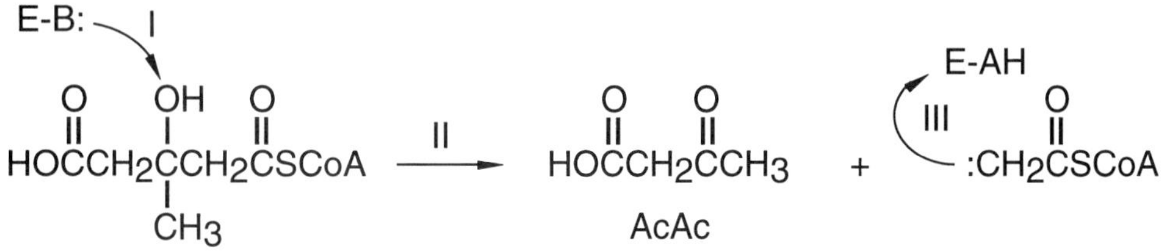

E-B: I

HOCCH$_2$C(OH)(CH$_3$)CH$_2$CSCoA —II→ HOCCH$_2$CCH$_3$ (AcAc) + :CH$_2$CSCoA (III, E-AH)

Fig. 102-7 The proposed catalytic mechanism of HL. The mechanism involves (I) attack on the hydroxyl group of the HMG-CoA by a general base from the active site (E-B:), (II) cleavage of the HMG-CoA molecule to AcAc and a reactive carbanion-CoA species, and (III) quenching by a general acid from the active site (E-AH).

binding.[144] The overall reaction is irreversible, although the final phase, enolization of Ac-CoA, can be reversed to some extent.[145]

Naturally occurring and synthetic HL mutants have demonstrated that H233,[146] R41,[147] and D42[147] are also essential to catalysis. H235 is involved in metal binding.[148] Dimerization is not essential for catalysis.[149]

HL from several sources has been studied. Recombinant human HL is representative:[150] K_m for HMG-CoA, 21.2 μM; V_{max}, 159 units/mg protein; turnover number 158/s at pH 8.2 and 30°C. HL is specific for the (S) diastereomer of HMG-CoA. (R)-HMG-CoA is neither a substrate nor an inhibitor.[151] The HL reaction requires the presence of divalent cations. The K_m for Mg^{++} is 233 μM; that for Mn^{++} is 1.5 μM, with an activation constant (K_a) of 0.5 μM.[142] The high optimal pH (~9.2) of HL presumably enhances its catalytic potential in the mitochondrial matrix, where pH is about 0.5 units higher than in the cytoplasm.[152]

The HL gene and mRNA. HL cDNAs were cloned first from the bacterium *Pseudomonas mevalonii*[153] and subsequently from liver of human,[143] mouse,[154] and rat.[127] All human tissues studied to date contain a ~1.7-kb HL mRNA.

The HL gene has been cloned in humans and mice.[155] The mouse HL gene locus, *Hmgcl*, is on chromosome 4,[154] in a region homologous to that of the human *HMGCL* locus, on human chromosome 1p35.1-36.1.[143] The mouse HL gene has 9 exons and spans ~15–20 kb.[155] The 5′ extremity of the human gene has not been reported, but exons 2–9 are arranged in a similar fashion to those in mouse.[155]

Some functionally important regions of HL are known. The mitochondrial leader spans exons 1 (20 codons of the leader) and 2 (8 codons). A highly conserved region including codons for the catalytically essential R41 and D42 residues is encoded by exon 2. The catalytically essential H233 and cation-binding H235 residues are in exon 7. The active site C266 codon is in exon 8, and the peroxisomal targeting signal (see below) and termination codon are in exon 9.

Biological properties of HL

Control and regulation. HL is expressed in all tissues studied to date. A slight increase in activity occurs in liver of fasting and fat fed rats,[128] and there is a fourfold increase during the fetal-neonatal transition.[156] The mouse HL promoter contains a CpG island and multiple Sp1 binding motifs but neither a TATA nor a CAAT box. It has multiple transcription start sites 9–35 bp upstream of the translational start codon.[155]

Half-life. Metabolic labeling shows a half-life of 13.5–19 h for mitochondrial HL and 12–16 h for peroxisomal HL (see below) in human hepatoma-derived Hep G2 cells, fibroblasts, and lymphoblasts.[157]

Peroxisomal HL. The C-terminal tripeptide of human HL, Cys-Lys-Leu, is a peroxisomal targeting signal 1 motif.[103] About 6 percent of human and mouse liver HL is peroxisomal,[103] as is 16–20 percent of HL in human fibroblasts, lymphoblasts, and HepG2 cells.[157] Compared with mature mitochondrial HL, peroxisomal HL has a greater molecular mass (about 34.5 kDa vs 32 kDa) and more basic pI (7.6 vs 6.2), suggesting that it retains the mitochondrial leader.[103,149] Recombinant HL precursor is enzymatically active, with a K_m for HMG-CoA, V_{max}, and optimal pH similar to those of naturally occurring HL.[149] By gel and ultrafiltration, recombinant precursor HL behaves as a monomer and mature HL as a dimer,[149] suggesting that the presence of the mitochondrial leader inhibits dimerization but does not affect catalytic activity. To our knowledge, HL is the only peptide with dual posttranslational sorting to mitochondria and to peroxisomes under normal conditions. The physiological role of peroxisomal HL, if any, is unknown. A hypothesis is discussed below in the section "HMG-uria with normal HL activity."

R-3-Hydroxybutyrate Dehydrogenase

R-3-Hydroxybutyrate dehydrogenase (3HBD, EC 1.1.1.30) catalyzes the interconversion of AcAc and 3HB in the mitochondrial matrix:

$$\text{AcAc} + \text{NADH} + \text{H}^+ \leftrightarrow \text{3HB} + \text{NAD}^+ \qquad (102\text{-}3)$$

3HBD interacts specifically with phosphatidylcholine, an allosteric activator on the inner mitochondrial membrane.[158] Since apo-3HBD is inactive, purified 3HBD is assayed either with mitochondrial phospholipids or in submitochondrial vesicles. Representative kinetic constants, obtained for bovine heart 3HBD,[159] are: K_m for 3HB, 1.05 ± 0.18 mM (with mitochondrial phospholipids) and 0.84 ± 0.15 mM (with submitochondrial vesicles); K_m for NAD, 0.36 ± 0.05 and 0.29 ± 0.04; K_i for NAD, 0.93 ± 0.24 and 1.16 ± 0.29; V_{max} (μmol/min/mg), 175 ± 5 and 0.85 ± 0.03.[159] A human heart 3HBD cDNA[158] predicts a 33.1-kDa, 297-residue peptide and identifies a 1.3-kb mRNA. 3HBD activity is greatest in liver, about tenfold lower in kidney, heart, and adrenal glands, and twentyfold lower in brain.[34,160] 3HBD is increased in diabetes and decreased by administration of insulin.[161]

Succinyl-CoA: 3-Oxoacid CoA Transferase

Succinyl-CoA:3-oxoacid CoA transferase (SCOT, EC 2.8.3.5) catalyzes the rate-determining step of ketolysis:

$$\text{succinyl-CoA} + \text{AcAc} \leftrightarrow \text{AcAc-CoA} + \text{succinate} \qquad (102\text{-}4)$$

The SCOT reaction. SCOT catalyzes a reversible reaction.[162] In contrast to the physiological direction of ketolysis, AcAc production is favored energetically: In pig heart,[163] the equilibrium constant ([AcAc-CoA][succinate]/[AcAc][succinyl-CoA]) is < 0.1. The energetics of the SCOT reaction have been studied in detail.[164] The mechanism is of the ping-pong type[163,165] and involves a CoA-enzyme thioester intermediate. The determination of kinetic constants is difficult because the K_i is less than the K_m value for succinate, AcAc-CoA, and succinyl-CoA.[163] Approximate K_m values for SCOT are 27–200 μM for AcAc-CoA, 5.6–20 mM for succinate, 0.16–6.5 mM for succinyl-CoA, and 67–100 μM for AcAc.[165,166] SCOT requires succinate or succinyl-CoA as its dicarboxylic acid substrate. The 3-ketoacid moiety may vary from C4 to C6 and may be substituted on the alpha-carbon,[162] but AcAc and AcAc-CoA are the best substrates.

The SCOT peptide. The 520-residue, 56.2-kDa human SCOT precursor is cleaved on mitochondrial entry to a 481-residue, 52.1-kDa mature monomer. In pig heart[163] and sheep kidney,[167] SCOT is a homodimer.

The side-chain carboxyl group of E344 forms the CoA thioester intermediate.[168] The glycine-rich cluster GGFGLCG at human SCOT residues 62–68 is highly conserved among CoA transferases and ADP-binding sites of enzymes that use NAD as a cofactor,[169] suggesting that this region may interact with the adenine moiety of CoA.[170]

Mammalian SCOT can be proteolytically cleaved, with no loss of activity, within a poorly conserved hydrophilic "hinge" region.[171] Integrity of this region does enhance SCOT folding and assembly.[171] Bacterial CoA transferases lack the hinge region and are encoded by two genes (A and B).[172] The crystal structure of another CoA transferase, glutaconate CoA transferase from *Acidaminococcus fermentans*,[173] reveals a A_4B_4 heterooctamer and an active site formed in part by both A and B subunits. The tertiary structure of the A and B subunits is similar, suggesting a distant common origin. By analogy, SCOT is predicted to be a homodimer.

The SCOT gene and RNA. SCOT cDNAs have been cloned from pig heart,[174] rat brain,[175] and human heart.[172] The 3.2-kb human heart SCOT cDNA contains a 1560-bp open reading frame and a long 3′ untranslated tail.[172] The human SCOT locus, *OXCT*, maps to chromosome 5p12-p13.[172] We recently characterized the human SCOT gene,[176] which spans at least 100 Kb and contains 17 exons.[177] The SCOT 5′ flanking region is guanidine- and cytosine-rich and lacks a TATA box.[177]

Biological properties of SCOT. In rats, SCOT is most abundant in kidney and heart and is also high in adrenal gland, stomach, and ileum.[34,178] A similar pattern is seen for humans (heart > kidney, adrenal, and brain).[179] In extrahepatic tissues, the activities of SCOT and T2 correlate well to each other in rats[178] and to a lesser extent in humans.[179] In brain, SCOT and 3HBD are highest in cerebral and cerebellar cortices and thalamus,[180] suggesting that ketolytic capacity varies among brain regions. SCOT activity is not detectable in adult liver. The mechanism of transcriptional suppression of SCOT within hepatocytes is not known.

Mitochondrial AcAc-CoA Thiolase

Mitochondrial AcAc-CoA thiolase (T2, EC 2.3.1.9) is a mitochondrial enzyme that catalyzes the following reversible reactions:

$$\text{AcAc-CoA} + \text{CoA} \leftrightarrow 2\text{Ac-CoA} \qquad (102\text{-}5)$$

$$2\text{MeAcAc-CoA} + \text{CoA} \leftrightarrow \text{Ac-CoA} + \text{propionyl-CoA} \qquad (102\text{-}6)$$

T2 has varied physiological roles. It equilibrates the free CoA and Ac-CoA pools in mitochondria and mediates reactions of ketogenesis and ketolysis (Fig. 102-2) and of isoleucine catabolism (Fig. 102-3).

Nomenclature of 3-oxothiolases. Mammals have at least five distinct 3-oxothiolases ("beta-ketothiolases"), abbreviated "thiolases" in the remainder of this chapter.[178,181,182] They share 34–45 percent amino acid sequence identity.[183] Despite this similarity, antibody to purified T2 is monospecific.[184] Table 102-1 shows the contribution of different thiolases to total AcAc-CoA thiolase activity in fibroblasts.

The designations T1 and T2 were coined in the laboratory of T Hashimoto, referring to the two major mitochondrial AcAc-CoA thiolase activities in rat liver and their order of elution on phosphocellulose column chromatography.

The T2 gene and cDNA. Rat and human T2 cDNAs have been cloned and sequenced.[185,186] The human T2 cDNA is about 1.5 kb long and encodes a precursor peptide of 427 amino acids, including a 33-residue leader. The human T2 gene (*ACAT1*) spans ~27 kb on chromosome 11q22.3-q23.1[187] and contains 12 exons and 11 introns.[188] The 5′ flanking region lacks a conventional TATA box but is GC-rich and has two CAAT boxes, typical of genes with widespread expression. The tissue-specific expression of T2 remains unexplained. Northern blot analysis of human fibroblast RNA reveals a single ~1.7-kb mRNA.

The T2 reaction. T2 has a reversible ping-pong mechanism.[189] Equilibrium favors CoASAc formation: for ox T2, under optimal conditions the rate of AcAc-CoA synthesis is 0.08 times that of AcAc-CoA cleavage.[189] The apparent K_m values for AcAc-CoA and CoA are 7 and 21 μM, respectively, for rat hepatic T2.[178] T2 shows substrate inhibition with >10 μM AcAc-CoA in the direction of CoASAc formation.[178] It also shows product inhibition with both CoA and AcAc-CoA in the direction of AcAc-CoA production.[190] The K_m for CoASAc is 80 μM for ox

Table 102-1 Thiolases in Mammalian Cells

Thiolase[1]	Subcellular Localization	Optimal substrate	Function	Contribution to total AcAc-CoA thiolase activity in human fibroblasts[2]
Mitochondrial acetoacetyl-CoA thiolase[185]	Mitochondrial matrix	C4; 2MeAcAc	Ketogenesis; ketolysis; isoleucine catabolism	50–60%
Mitochondrial medium-chain 3-ketoacyl-CoA thiolase[363]	Mitochondrial matrix	C4–C16; (2MeAcAc)	Beta oxidation (short-medium chain) Beta oxidation (medium chain)	20–24%
Mitochondrial trifunctional protein[364]	Mitochondrial inner membrane	C6–C16<	Beta oxidation (long chain)	0%
Cytosolic acetoacetyl-CoA thiolase[183]	Cytosol	C4	Cholesterol synthesis	13–19%
Peroxisomal 3-ketoacyl-CoA thiolase[365]	Peroxisome	C4–C16<	Peroxisomal beta oxidation	<5%

(1) References refer to human cDNA cloning papers. (2) Data from Fukao et al.[199]
AcAc-CoA thiolase activity was assayed in the direction of thiolysis, with 15 μM AcAc-CoA and 50 μM CoA in the presence of potassium ion.

liver T2.[189] Using purified rat T2, the reaction rate using 2MeAcAc-CoA as substrate is 1.6-fold greater than that with AcAc-CoA, when each are present at 10 μM.[191]

A unique property of T2 that is useful in clinical diagnosis is its activation by potassium ion, an eightfold increase in the case of human T2.[184] The apparent K_a for potassium ion is 1 mM in both rat and human T2.[178,184]

The residue corresponding to C126 in human T2 forms the acyl-S-enzyme intermediate,[192] and C413 mediates deprotonation during AcAc-CoA formation.[193,194]

The T2 peptide

Structure. Human T2 is a homotetramer of 41-kDa subunits.[186] Conserved amino acid residues, presumably essential for function, are distributed along the entire length of mammalian and bacterial thiolase cDNAs.

Although the divergence of the thiolases is ancient, their catalytic mechanism and basic structure are likely conserved. The crystal structure of peroxisomal 3-ketoacyl-CoA thiolase from *Saccharomyces cerevisiae*, reported at 2.8 Å resolution,[195] reveals a homodimer with a five-layered structure constructed from two core domains of identical topology. The active site is a shallow pocket, containing conserved residues corresponding to C126, H385, and C413 in human T2. Based on the yeast peroxisomal thiolase, we proposed a model of human T2, depicted in Fig. 102-8.[196]

CoA modification of T2. Since T2 functions in ketogenesis as well as in ketolysis, the finding of ketoacidosis in T2 deficiency led to speculation that a liver-specific AcAc-CoA thiolase might exist.[178,189] Column chromatography of homogenates variously resolved two or three peaks of T2 activity, termed isozymes A (A1 and A2), found only in liver, and B, found in all tissues.[178] Subsequently, the A isoenzyme was shown to be CoA-modified and the B isoform to be unmodified.[197]

It has now been proven that the A and B isoforms are derived from a single protein. Purified A and B isoforms are indistinguishable by electrophoretic mobility on SDS-PAGE, amino acid composition, or immunoreactivity with polyclonal antibodies raised to the B isozymes of rat or of human.[185,186] Furthermore, molecular cloning of the T2 cDNA and gene[185,186] and chromosomal mapping[187] demonstrate a single T2 gene and mRNA. The apparently paradoxical finding of ketosis in T2 deficiency is discussed below (T2 Deficiency, Pathophysiology).

CoA modification enhances AcAc-CoA formation[189,198] but shortens the half-life of T2.[197] Further studies may reveal a physiological role for CoA-modified T2.

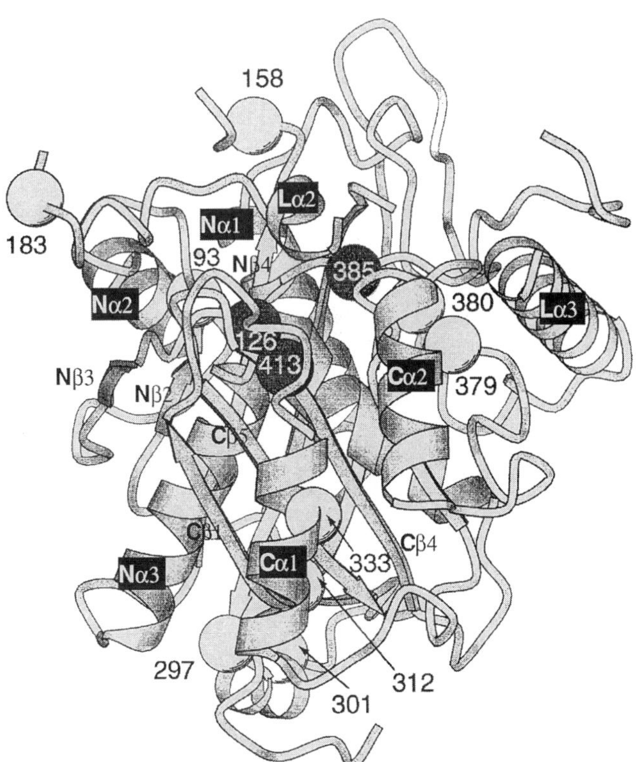

Fig. 102-8 Tertiary structure model of the human T2 monomer. The model shows the active site pocket containing the catalytically essential Cys126, His385, and Cys413 residues (black spheres) and its predicted relationships to the sites of missense mutations in T2 deficiency (white spheres). Alpha helices and beta pleated sheets are shown as helices and arrows, respectively, and numbered as in the peroxisomal thiolase of *S cerevisiae*.[195] (*Produced with assistance from Haruki Nakamura.*)

Biologic characteristics of T2

Redundancy with T1. Mitochondrial medium-chain 3-ketoacyl-CoA thiolase (T1) accounts for 27 percent of the capacity for AcAc-CoA cleavage in rat liver[178] and 20–24 percent of that in human fibroblasts[199] (Table 102-1). Purified rat T1 has some activity towards 2MeAcAc-CoA as well (0.3-fold compared to activity towards AcAc-CoA),[191] accounting for <3 percent of 2MeAcAc-CoA thiolase activity in fibroblasts[191] and ~8 percent of total 2MeAcAc-CoA cleavage capacity in rat liver.

Half-life. The apparent half-life of T2 is 38 h in rat liver[197] and longer in human fibroblasts.[184,200]

Tissue distribution. In the rat, T2 activity is high in liver, kidney, heart, and adrenal gland.[34,178] In immunoblots of human tissues, T2 is abundant in liver, kidney, heart, and adrenal. In extrahepatic tissues, the activities of SCOT and T2 correlate well in rats[178] and to a lesser extent in humans.[179] In rat brain, T2 activity is low at birth, increases fivefold during weaning, then declines to an adult level twofold higher than at birth,[201] a pattern similar to those of 3HBD and SCOT.

Cytosolic Acetoacetyl-CoA Thiolase

Cytosolic acetoacetyl-CoA thiolase (CT, EC 2.3.1.9) catalyzes the same reaction with AcAc-CoA as T2 and shares the same EC number. Cytosolic AcAc-CoA serves as substrate for HMG-CoA synthase, and CT may be viewed as the first enzyme of cholesterol synthesis (Fig. 102-2).

Peptide and reaction. CT has been purified from rat[202] and human[184] liver. Rat CT is a homotetramer.[202] K_m values of rat CT are: for AcAc-CoA, 50 μM and for CoA, 3 μM.[202] Substrate inhibition by CoA is documented.[202]

The CT cDNA and locus. A human hepatic CT cDNA[183] predicts a 397-amino acid, 41.3-kDa CT monomer. A single ~1.7-kb message is present in brain, liver, lung, and kidney.[179] The human CT locus, designated *ACAT2*, maps to chromosome 6q25.3–q26.[203]

Biology of CT. In the adult rat, the distribution of CT activity reflects the capacity of cholesterol synthesis rather than of ketolysis: adrenal and liver > brain > intestine, testis, skeletal muscle, and heart.[178] In newborn rats, brain CT activity is 2.5-fold greater than in adults.[178,201] The tissue distribution in humans is similar to that in rats.[179] Potential substrates for CT include CoASAc (from mitochondrial acetyl groups shuttled via the citrate transporter) and AcAcCoA (provided by cytosolic AcAc-CoA synthetase).

NORMAL KETONE BODY LEVELS

In the clinical setting, the most important variables to consider in interpreting ketone body levels are age and duration of fasting.

Ketosis is particularly common in young children. Numerous other factors, listed below, also influence ketone body levels.

Ketone bodies are the circulating metabolites whose concentrations fluctuate most widely, from < 50 μM in the postprandial state in some individuals to > 25 mM in some ketoacidotic episodes in diabetes or SCOT deficiency. It has been suggested[6] that normal blood concentration of 3HB plus AcAc in the fed state be defined as < 0.2 mM, hyperketonemia as levels > 0.2 mM, and ketoacidosis as levels > 7 mM. In our experience, many patients develop acidosis at lower levels of circulating ketone bodies, perhaps due to dehydration or other associated conditions.

The normal range of ketone body levels is wide even when standardized for age and time of fasting. Presumably, basal metabolic rate, hepatic glycogen stores, and the rates of proteolysis and lipolysis, which together determine the rate of ketolysis, depend upon multiple genetic and nutritional factors. Therefore, *ketone body levels must be interpreted in their clinical context and in relation to the levels of other simultaneously measured metabolites and hormones*. These metabolites include blood glucose, free fatty acids, lactate, pyruvate, amino acids, and urinary organic acid metabolites of fatty acids and branched chain amino acids. Measurement of insulin and, if clinically indicated, cortisol and growth hormone may be useful.

Normal fasting values of blood ketone bodies and other metabolites have been published for children[204–207] and adults[24,208–210] (see Chap. 66). Notably, the lack of ketonuria in a hypoglycemic child is abnormal and is an important diagnostic finding.

The urinary excretion of AcAc and 3HB is 0.1- to 0.4-fold that of inulin.[71] In ketoacidosis, 10–20 percent of ketone body production may be lost in the urine.[24,210] Examples of urinary excretion at different plasma ketone body levels are published,[209,211] but precise correlation is difficult. In cerebrospinal fluid, AcAc and 3HB concentrations are about 50–65 percent of blood levels.[212]

Nutritional Status

Fasting. With growth and aging, the rate of energy utilization per unit body mass slows, and this is reflected in ketone body metabolism. Mild pediatric infections causing anorexia and vomiting are the commonest cause of ketosis. In fasting children under 7 years of age, total ketone body levels $> 1–2$ mM are expected within 24 h (Fig. 102-9).[204] In fasting adults, ketone body levels exceed 1 mM only after 2–3 days, attaining levels of about 5 mM at 1 week[208] and a plateau of 6–8 mM by 3–4 weeks of fasting, with wide variation among individuals.[209,210] During this period the 3HB:AcAc ratio rises steadily from unity to a level of 5–6.[208,209]

Dietary fat content. Ketosis can be induced by high-fat (ketogenic) diets. In comparison to a standard North American diet, which provides 35–40 percent of energy as fat, the 3:1 ketogenic diet (the lipid/carbohydrate ratio being expressed on a weight basis) contains 87 percent of energy as lipid. On this diet, blood ketone levels can, in some children, rise to 4 mM (3HB) and 1.5 mM (AcAc)[213] and urinary ketone bodies are continuously present.

Ketogenic diets form the basis for popular weight-reduction schemes,[214] have recently regained favor as a treatment for epilepsy,[66] and have been used in pyruvate dehydrogenase deficiency[215] and hereditary deficiency of the blood-brain barrier glucose transporter, GLUT-1.[216] However, the therapeutic efficacy of ketogenic diets is limited by several factors. Ketosis is abolished rapidly by glucose administration,[51] and the diets are unpalatable and may lead to obesity and deficiency of certain nutrients.[217] Medium-chain triglycerides induce ketosis more effectively than long-chain triglycerides, and their addition to ketogenic diets may permit a higher nonfat caloric intake.[213,218,219] Ketogenic diets should be supervised by an experienced nutritionist.

Obesity. Obesity is associated with resistance to ketosis, perhaps because of hyperinsulinism and the abundant liver glycogen reserves of obese subjects.[220]

Neonates. Ketone body metabolism is rapidly activated after birth by the high-fat (milk) diet and by the stress of birth. In contrast, in utero metabolism is mainly glycolytic. The metabolic adaptations associated with the fetal-neonatal transition have been extensively documented (reviewed in Girard *et al.*[221]). The neonatal ketogenic response is blunted in premature and small-for-gestational-age infants.[222]

Early reports suggested that neonates develop a physiological ketosis of 0.8–1.2 mM,[223,224] but in infants fed soon after birth in accordance with modern newborn feeding practices, peak 3HB levels of 0.42 ± 0.05 occur at 20 h of life, with AcAc approximately half of this.[225] This mild physiological hyperketonemia does not result in ketonuria detectable by dipstick methods. Ketonuria is unusual in normal newborns and if present, suggests the possibility of a metabolic error (Table 102-2). Ketonuria has been reported in neonates receiving a high concentration of medium-chain triglycerides.

Pregnancy. Pregnancy is associated with slight maternal hyperketonemia and an accelerated increase of blood ketone body levels upon fasting.[226]

Exercise. Mild ketosis (1–2 mM) is observed following prolonged exercise (the Courtice-Douglas effect),[5,227] perhaps attributable to an abrupt decrease in muscular use of fatty acids liberated during exercise that are available to the liver as ketogenic fuel.[12]

Cold exposure. Ketonuria is reportedly increased in cold weather.[211,228] It would be interesting to confirm these classic observations with measurement of blood ketone body levels and under strictly controlled dietary intake.

ABNORMALITIES OF KETONE BODY METABOLISM

There are three principal clinical abnormalities of ketone body metabolism: (1) ketosis and ketoacidosis, (2) hypoketotic hypoglycemia, and (3) abnormal 3HB:AcAc ratio.

Ketosis and Ketoacidosis

The presence of ketosis (Table 102-2) signals two things. First, except in rare patients with ketolytic defects, it is indicative of a substantial lipolytic stress. Second, the presence of ketosis is strong evidence that the pathway of lipid energy metabolism is intact, from lipolysis to ketogenesis (Fig. 102-4). With the possible exception of SCOT deficiency, ketosis is intermittent, and most patients with the following conditions do not have ketonuria or hyperketonemia between episodes.

Differential diagnosis

Ketotic hypoglycemia. This condition[229] is seen primarily in children 1–7 years of age, disappearing around puberty. Patients tend to be short and thin and are normal except for the tendency to develop fasting ketosis and hypoglycemia. Symptoms are variable and include weakness, palpitations, tremulousness, hunger, nausea, sweating, headache, anxiety, personality changes, stupor, seizures, and, in some instances, localized neurologic signs. Ketosis is present. In samples taken during hypoglycemia, levels of insulin and other hormones are appropriate for the degree of hypoglycemia. Plasma amino acids show a low level of alanine,[230] and analysis of urine organic acids is normal aside from ketosis. Symptoms develop during stress, particularly after fasting overnight or longer. The development of cataracts has been associated with recurrent episodes.[231,232] Neurologic sequelae are rare.

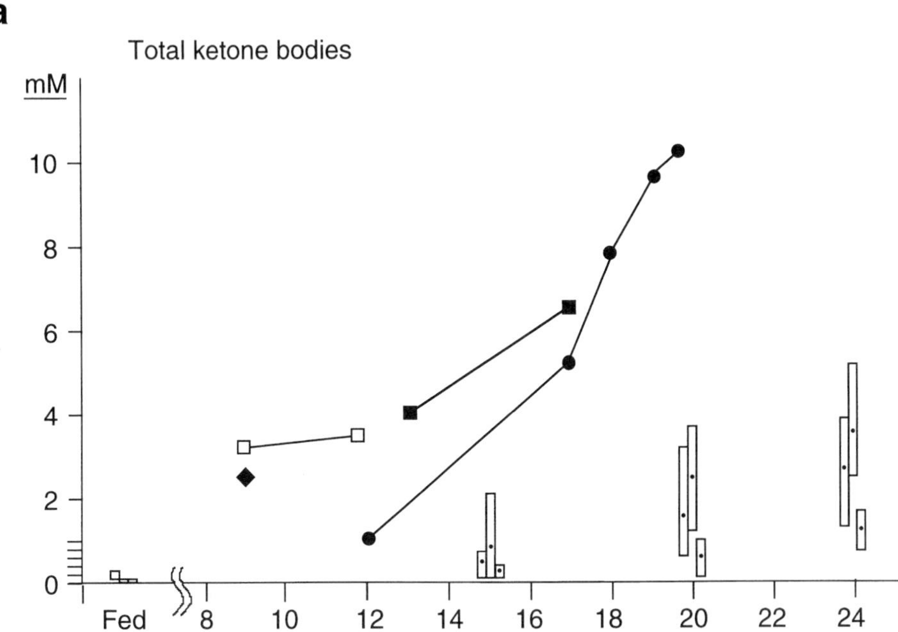

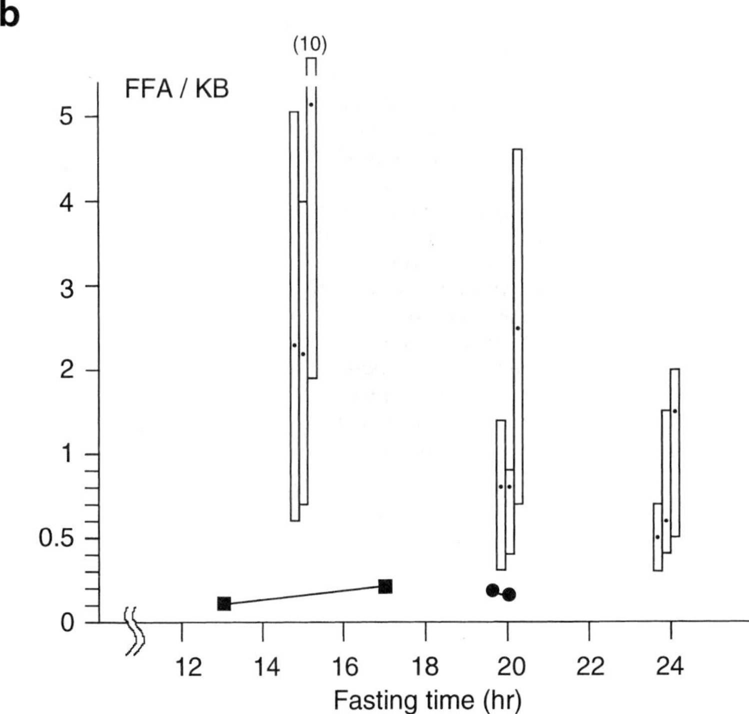

Fig. 102-9 Fasting tests in normal subjects and SCOT-deficient patients. (a) Ketone body levels and (b) free fatty acid/ketone body ratios during controlled fasting. The four SCOT-deficient patients are ◆, a 6-year-old girl;[172,301] □, a 15-month-old-boy;[305] ■, a 12-month-old boy;[304] and ●, a 1-year-old boy (S.C.).[299,300] Normal values are shown by bars, each group of three bars showing, from left to right, values in children aged 1 month to 1 year (n = 12), 1 to 7 years (n = 27), and 7 to 15 years (n = 9), from Bonnefont *et al.*[204] as reproduced in Chap. 66. The bars indicate the range, the internal dot the mean. Note the lower rate of increase in ketone bodies in the older controls. The difference between the SCOT-deficient patients and the controls increases obviously as fasting is prolonged.

Conceptually, ketotic hypoglycemia can be viewed as an imbalance between energy supply and demand in children with reduced stores of hepatic glycogen and muscle protein, the main fuels of gluconeogenesis. Ketogenesis in these children may thus be a normal response to glucopenia, accentuated to the point of ketosis.[233–236] It is important to differentiate ketotic hypoglycemia from adrenocorticoid or growth hormone deficiencies and inborn errors (Table 102-2). Ketotic episodes are treated with intravenous glucose in the acute phase and can usually be prevented by planning frequent meals and bedtime or nighttime snacks during catabolic illness, such as infections.

Recurrent ketosis of childhood. We have adopted this descriptive term for patients whose biochemical and clinical profile resembles that of ketotic hypoglycemia except that hypoglycemia is absent despite the development of ketosis. Patients have a benign course and are normal between episodes. The mechanism(s) underlying this interesting phenomenon, which resembles an exaggerated ketogenic response to stress, with (resulting?) maintenance of blood glucose, has not been studied in detail. Other conditions in Table 102-2 must be considered prior to accepting this diagnosis.

Endocrine ketoses. Diabetic ketoacidosis is the commonest cause of ketoacidosis in childen and adults (Chaps. 67–69) and combines a reduction of insulin effect with a relative excess of glucagon. Ketone body levels above 25 mM can occur.[20] Initial blood glucose levels of < 10 mM (180 mg/dl) are rarely if ever observed.[237]

Table 102-2 Causes of Ketosis

	Blood glucose
Physiologic	**Blood glucose**
Fasting (especially during infancy or pregnancy)	N, D
Prolonged exercise	N, occ D
Ketogenic diet	N, occ D
Hormonal	
Diabetic ketoacidosis	I
Glucocorticoid deficiency	D
Growth hormone deficiency	D
Toxic	
Alcoholic ketoacidosis	Variable
Isopropyl alcohol poisoning	N
Salicylate poisoning	Variable
Inborn errors of metabolism	
Congenital lactic acidoses	Variable
Branched chain organic acidopathies (methylmalonic, propionic, isovaleric acidemias)	Variable
Gluconeogenic and glycogen storage diseases	D
Glycogen synthase deficiency	D
Short-chain hydroxyacyl CoA dehydrogenase deficiency	D
Inborn errors of ketolysis SCOT deficiency	N, rarely D
T2 deficiency	Variable
Cytosolic 3-oxothiolase deficiency (?)	N (?)
Ketotic hypoglycemia	D
Recurrent ketosis of childhood	N

D = decreased; I = increased; N = normal; occ = occasionally.

Other endocrine factors must be considered in patients suspected to have ketotic hypoglycemia, including adrenocortical insufficiency, growth hormone deficiency, and panhypopituitarism.[238] Hyperthyroidism is associated with accelerated ketogenesis.[239] Adrenergic stimulation may increase ketogenesis by increasing lipolysis.[240] Interestingly, in transgenic mice, overexpression of the muscle and fat glucose transporter, GLUT4, results in hyperketonemia,[241] but this condition is not known in humans.

Toxic ketoses. Alcoholic ketoacidosis[20,242] occurs after excessive alcohol consumption and fasting. Gastritis and pancreatitis are frequent. Blood glucose levels are variable but can be elevated. Typical metabolite levels include 3HB, 1.8–20.5 mM; blood pH, 7.2–7.3; lactate, 2.4–4.7 mM (normal <2.2 mM); and plasma free fatty acid levels, ≤ 2.9 mM. The oxidation of ethanol to acetate can create a reduced redox state in the mitochondrial matrix, with a high 3HB:AcAc ratio and low or negative urine tests for ketones.[242] Ethanol is frequently undetectable in blood by the time of presentation.[242] Alcoholic ketosis responds rapidly to intravenous glucose administration.

Poisoning with isopropyl alcohol,[243] found in antifreeze and rubbing alcohol, clinically resembles ethanol intoxication. Isopropyl alcohol is metabolized directly to acetone, producing high levels of acetone but normal AcAc and 3HB levels and minimal acidosis.

Other intoxications, in particular salicylate poisoning,[244,245] can be associated with ketoacidosis. Conversely, ketone bodies can produce a false positive result in some screening tests for salicylates.[246] A toxicology screen should be performed in patients with undiagnosed ketoacidosis.

Infections and ketosis. Mild pediatric infections are the most frequent cause of ketosis, presumably because of their association with fasting and vomiting. In contrast, severe infection is accompanied by hypoketonemia.[247,248]

Inborn errors of metabolism and ketosis. In some congenital lactic acidoses caused by respiratory chain deficiencies, ketoacidosis dominates the clinical picture and hyperlactacidemia is modest. Presumably, ketoacidosis results from mitochondrial engorgement with CoASAc, with activation of ketogenesis in liver and/or reversal of the ketolytic pathway in other tissues. In contrast, in pyruvate dehydrogenase deficiency, ketone body degradation is unaffected (Fig. 102-2) and a ketogenic diet has potential therapeutic value. (See also "Abnormalities of the ketone body ratio," below.) Congenital lactic acidosis should be considered systematically in ketoacidosis of unknown etiology.

Methylmalonic, propionic, and isovaleric acidemias typically present with ketoacidosis and were formerly known as "ketotic hyperglycinemias." The mechanisms of hyperketonemia are unknown. In rat hepatocytes, propionate stimulates ketogenesis.[249] An inhibitory effect on ketolysis has not been excluded in these conditions.

Several inborn errors of glycogen metabolism (Chap. 71) are associated with ketosis, which presumably develops as a response to hypoglycemia. Patients with glycogen synthase deficiency[57,250,251] or glycogen phosphorylase kinase deficiency[252] often experience hyperketotic hypoglycemia with fasting. Glycogen synthase deficiency is not associated with hepatomegaly and should be considered in the differential diagnosis of ketotic hypoglycemia. Although children with glucose-6-phosphatase deficiency are reportedly resistant to ketosis,[253,254] many develop it readily. Interestingly, the ketosis-prone patients seem less susceptible to hypoglycemia.[255]

In general, the presence of ketosis in a hypoglycemic patient militates against disorders of fatty acid oxidation. Surprisingly, a small number of patients with deficiencies of short-chain hydroxyacyl CoA dehydrogenation[256] or, rarely, of medium-chain acyl CoA dehydrogenase [256a] have been reported to have ketotic hypoglycemia. This may reflect the presence of some ketogenic capacity from the unimpeded initial cycles of beta oxidation, disruption of ketolysis in extrahepatic tissues that also oxidize fat, and/or tissue specificity of the deficient enzyme.

Diagnostic approach to the ketotic patient

Acute illness. Pathologic ketosis is present if the degree of ketoacidosis exceeds that expected for the physiological response to stress. It should be suspected if recurrent episodes, coma, organ failure, marked acidosis (systemic pH <7.1), or blood ketone bodies >6 mM are seen. Laboratory evaluation includes blood gases, glucose, ketone bodies, lactate, pyruvate, insulin, free fatty acids, plasma amino acids and carnitine, and urinary organic acids and toxicology screen. One to 2 ml of heparinized plasma and ≥ 10 ml of urine should be obtained during the acute phase and saved for additional measurements.

Between ketoacidotic episodes. If the patient is first seen after an episode, the minimal initial laboratory investigation includes a dipstick test for urinary acetoacetate and urine organic acids determination. Parents should be instructed in urine testing for ketones and test all urines over one 24-h period and first-morning samples for 2 weeks, recording ketonuria, diet, and clinical state.

If suspicion of a ketolytic disorder is strong but definite evidence of permanent ketonuria or the typical organic acid profile of T2 deficiency is lacking, we perform a 24-h metabolite cycle, monitoring ketonuria and measuring blood glucose, ketone bodies, fatty acids, lactate, and pyruvate before and 1 h after each meal.

Functional tests are of limited diagnostic value. Fasting tests have provided confirmatory data in SCOT deficiency (Fig. 102-9) but can be normal with T2 deficiency. Administration of an isoleucine load (L-isoleucine, 100 mg/kg, with collection of urine samples for 4–8 h after loading) may be useful in patients suspected to have T2 deficiency in whom the diagnostic urine organic acid profile is lacking.

Assay of SCOT and T2 is indicated for children with persistent nonfasting ketosis or repeated episodes of severe unexplained ketoacidosis for which no cause is identified, and T2 assay alone for those with a suggestive organic acid profile.

Hypoketotic Hypoglycemia

Usually hypoketonemia is discovered only when it accompanies hypoglycemia, because measurement of ketone body levels is rarely indicated in other circumstances in nonketotic individuals. Hypoketotic hypoglycemia is associated with two groups of diseases: hyperinsulinism (Chaps. 67–69) and inborn errors of fatty acid oxidation (Chap. 101) and of ketogenesis (see mHS deficiency and HL deficiency, below).

Abnormalities of the Ketone Body Ratio

The normal value of the 3HB : AcAc ratio in the postprandial state is approximately unity[24] but rises to 5–6 after 1 week of fasting in adults.[208,209] The 3HB : AcAc ratio reflects the redox state of hepatic mitochondria: the more reduced the matrix, i.e., the higher the NADH : NAD^+ ratio, the higher the 3HB : AcAc ratio. A reduced matrix is frequently associated with inhibition of the respiratory chain as in anoxia or with substrate excess as in uncontrolled diabetes. In interpreting 3HB : AcAc ratios, the clinician must recall that blood levels of 3HB and AcAc reflect both production and consumption of each compound. Ketone body utilization is, in general, related to circulating levels of ketone bodies but differs between AcAc and 3HB and between different organs.[24] These variables have not been exhaustively studied, rendering precise interpretation of 3HB : AcAc ratios difficult.

Technical artefacts may arise if ketosis is measured by nitroprusside-based methods, which detect only AcAc and acetone. In patients with diabetic or alcoholic ketoacidosis, the high 3HB : AcAc ratio nitroprusside-based tests underestimate ketosis. With clinical improvement, decrease of the 3HB : AcAc ratio may cause an increase in AcAc levels despite an overall reduction in ketone bodies, and ketosis may paradoxically appear to worsen. This misinterpretation is avoided if blood levels of both 3HB and AcAc are determined.

The arterial 3HB : AcAc ratio has been used to predict postoperative success in liver transplantation[257] and to assess the fitness of a potential donor livers[258] and the severity of chronic liver disease.[259] High 3HB : AcAc ratios (or low values of the reciprocal AcAc : 3HB ratio, prefered by some investigators) are a poor prognostic factor, suggesting a reduced mitochondrial matrix due to ischemia or other causes.

In congenital lactic acidemias, the 3HB : AcAc ratio is classically low in severe pyruvate carboxylase deficiency,[260] normal in pyruvate dehydrogenase deficiency, and increased in severe defects of the respiratory chain. In our experience, it is an insensitive diagnostic index in mild cases. In 3HBD deficiency, the 3HB:AcAc ratio is predicted to be very low.

DISEASES OF KETONE BODY METABOLISM

HL and mHS deficiencies present as hypoketotic hypoglycemia, whereas SCOT and T2 deficiencies present as ketoacidosis. Patients are often clinically normal between episodes of decompensation, although SCOT-deficient patients may be chronically ketotic.

mHS DEFICIENCY (MIM 600234)

Two mHS-deficient patients are reported (Patients 1[261] and 2[262]). Both presented in childhood with hypoketotic hypoglycemia. Information in this section is taken from the above two references.

Clinical Findings

Both patients presented with hypoketotic hypoglycemia, associated with a convulsion in Patient 1 (at age 6 years) and with coma in Patient 2 (18 months). Patient 2 also had an enlarged, hyperechogenic liver, suggesting fatty infiltration, which resolved with treatment. Neither had further episodes except during provocative testing, and both subsequently had normal mental development.

Pathology

Liver biopsies were studied in both patients. In Patient 1, periportal fatty infiltration was noted, as was moderate variation in the size of mitochondria, many of which contained nonspecific crystalline inclusions. In Patient 2, whose hepatomegaly had resolved at the time of biopsy, fatty infiltration was absent, but electron microscopy showed proliferation and dilatation of the smooth endoplasmic reticulum and a hyperdense matrix in some mitchochondria.

Diagnosis

mHS deficiency should be suspected in patients presenting with hypoketotic hypoglycemia. By extension, it may be a consideration in some cases of Reye syndrome or sudden infant death syndrome.

Diagnostic metabolites and functional testing. In Patient 1, organic acids were normal in urine obtained 2 days after the episode. Following medium-chain triglyceride loading, urinary medium-chain fatty acid derivatives were higher than in controls. Patient 2 had a nonspecific medium-chain dicarboxylic aciduria including unsaturated and 3-hydroxylated derivatives, but ethylmalonate, glutarate, and 3HB were normal, and medium chain glycine conjugates were not detectable. Fasting caused hypoketotic hypoglycemia after 18–22 h. Long-chain triglyceride loading in both patients and medium-chain loading in Patient 1 failed to increase 3HB despite appropriate increases in free fatty acid levels. In contrast, leucine loading (200 mg/kg) in Patient 2 caused an increase in 3HB of 0.45 mM, similar to the result in controls. Functional testing for mHS deficiency should be performed only after the initial screening results have eliminated other inborn errors of fatty acid or amino acid metabolism.

In both patients, tandem mass spectrometry analysis of blood acylcarnitines was normal. In Patient 1, total liver carnitine content was 1278 nmol/g wet weight (normal 900–1800) and free carnitine was 55 percent of total (normal ~70 percent).

Enzymatic diagnosis. Clinical enzymatic diagnosis of mHS deficiency remains challenging for two reasons. First, the substrates and product of mHS are also utilized or synthesized by several other enzymes. For example, in human liver homogenates, less than half of total measured AcAc-CoA disappearance is due to mHS. AcAc-CoA hydrolase activity accounts for 10[111] to 40[140] percent. In our experience, ~15 percent of liver HS activity is cytoplasmic. As for assays that measure HMG-CoA appearance, there is a moderate but not overwhelming excess of HL in liver samples. A second problem in mHS assay is that sampling is not trivial, because mHS is measurable only in liver and gonads.

Methods of mHS assay[106] involve measurement of AcAc-CoA disappearance or of HMG-CoA production. For the first method, T2 activity, which in liver is 20- to 50-fold greater than that of mHS,[128] is assumed to contribute 50 percent of total AcAc-CoA disappearance, stoichiometrically catalyzing the conversion of one AcAc-CoA molecule for each CoASAc liberated by the HS or hydrolase reactions. The assay has been refined by the use of a CoASAc generating system to eliminate the effect of AcAc-CoA hydrolase.[140]

Measurement of HMG-CoA production provides a more specific end point than AcAc-CoA disappearance. Previously, endogenous HL has been used to couple the HS reaction to AcAc synthesis, AcAc being assayed spectrophotometrically as for HL.[27,128] cHS and AcAc-CoA hydrolase activities are also measured by this method.

We have added recombinant HL in the reaction to ensure an excess of HL activity over that of mHS.[111] To increase the specificity of the reaction, an antibody to mHS was added and mHS activity was calculated as the difference between values obtained with and without immunoprecipitation.

Succinylation inactivates purified mHS. An mHS assay in which mHS is desuccinylated has been described.[140] In human liver, desuccinylation reportedly increases mHS activity by ~13 percent (range 1.7 to 30 percent).[140] An abstract has recently appeared[140a] describing a mHS assay that may avoid many of the above problems. In this assay, excess amounts of purified HMG-CoA reductase are added and HMG-CoA production is measured as the conversion of NADPH to NADP.

Despite the above efforts, development of more specific assays in readily available tissues and also molecular analysis are important avenues to explore.

Enzyme results in mHS-deficient patients. With a coupled assay, mean liver mHS activity in Patient 1 was ~10 percent of control (0.035 μmol/min/g wet weight; controls 0.20–0.32). In Patient 2, mHS activity was 50 percent of control levels using the CoASAc regeneration assay, but a complete absence of immunoreactive mHS peptide was reported. Further studies are under way to clarify this observation.

As expected, tests of beta-oxidative flux were normal in cultured lymphoblasts (Patient 1) and fibroblasts (Patient 2). Assays of carnitine palmitoyltransferase and several beta-oxidation enzymes were also normal in patients' cells.

Molecular diagnosis. The human mHS gene[92] and cDNA[81,115] are known. We have recently shown that Patient 1 is homozygous for a phenylalanine-to-leucine substitution at codon 174 (F174L) that yields no detectable activity when expressed, and that Patient 2 is a compound with a premature termination mutation (R424X) and an as-yet uncharacterized mutant allele.[111]

Management

The general principles discussed in the section "General Principles of Management of Inborn Errors of Ketone Body Metabolism" below apply. Avoidance both of fasting and of excessive fat intake and replacement of glucose at times of hypoglycemia or fasting stress are clearly indicated. To date, this has been adequate for normal growth and development.

There is no reason to restrict protein. A high-protein diet may in fact be useful, since ketogenesis from leucine is unimpaired (Fig. 102-2), but no experience with this is available to date.

Asymptomatic sibs are at risk and should be evaluated. Molecular testing by direct mutation detection or with intragenic markers should provide a noninvasive method to assess their status.

Pathophysiology

The occurrence of hypoketotic hypoglycemia coma and susceptibility to medium-chain fatty acid intoxication demonstrates the physiological importance of the HMG-CoA pathway of ketogenesis in humans.

mHS mediates ketogenesis from fatty acids. Ketogenesis from leucine proceeds unimpaired (Fig. 102-2), as demonstrated above in Patient 2. Nothing is known of the precise intracellular events that accompany decompensation in mHS deficiency. AcAc-CoA accumulation is predicted to be the primary intracellular change. Notably, AcAc-CoA is chemically unstable and normally present at low concentration in liver.[138]

mHS-deficient patients are expected to be at risk only when the rate of beta oxidation exceeds the ketogenic threshold. The resulting increase of intramitochondrial Ac-CoA and AcAc-CoA would inhibit beta oxidation, leading to fatty liver, hypoglycemia, and nonspecific dicarboxylic aciduria. Beta oxidation intermediates may accumulate to toxic levels, as suggested by the development of coma in Patient 1 following a medium-chain triglyceride load despite only mild hypoglycemia (2.8 mM [50 mg/dl]).

A critical point is the absence of a specific urinary organic acid pattern. Any AcAc liberated by hydrolysis of AcAc-CoA would be avidly consumed by extrahepatic tissues and not excreted in urine.

mHS is highly expressed in gonads and newborn intestine. To date, no abnormalities have been reported in these tissues in mHS deficiency.

Epidemiology

Why have only two cases of mHS deficiency been described? Perhaps asymptomatic deficient individuals exist. It is also possible that mHS deficiency is underdiagnosed because of the nondiagnostic organic acid pattern, because enzymatic diagnosis requires biopsy specimens, and because many physicians are unaware of the HMG-CoA pathway of ketogenesis.

HL DEFICIENCY (MIM 246450)

HL deficiency, first described in 1971,[263] is usually well tolerated except for episodes of hypoketotic hypoglycemia and acidosis, during which the central nervous system is particularly vulnerable. These may cause severe permanent handicap.

Clinical Findings

HL deficiency has been reviewed previously.[264–267] We have assembled a series of 62 HL-deficient patients from the literature and information from collaborating physicians. Thirty presented in the first week of life. Most of the others presented before 1 year of age, with presentation after 2 years of age being exceptional.

Typically, pregnancy and delivery are normal. Episodes can be precipitated by fasting, infections, protein loading, and the fetal-neonatal transition. Abnormalities of glucose and pH range from mild to severe (e.g., glucose undetectable, pH < 7.0, bicarbonate < 6 mM). Vomiting, lethargy, tachypnea, and moderate hepatomegaly with elevation of serum transaminases are frequent. Hyperammonemia has been reported and may be severe (> 1000 μM).[268] A peculiar odor of the urine has been noted in some patients,[269] perhaps due to accumulation of 3-methylcrotonic acid. Between episodes, children are often normal on physical examination.

The neurologic complications of hypoglycemia may be severe in HL deficiency. The risk of mental retardation and epilepsy exceeds that expected in other conditions for similar lengths of time and severity of hypoglycemia. Several patients have white matter abnormalities located in the deep arcuate fibers,[270–272] hypodense on computerized tomography and hyperintense on T_2-weighted magnetic resonance imaging (Fig. 102-10). Macrocephaly, reported in some HL-deficient patients with marked neurologic complications,[273,274] may be a consequence of the disease; alternatively, perhaps large brain size and high cerebral energy consumption increase the risk of hypoglycemia. Focal neurologic signs can occur.[275]

Single instances of cardiomyopathy,[276] pancreatitis,[277] and nonprogressive deafness and retinitis pigmentosa[278] have been reported in HL deficiency. Because similar findings occur in other organic acidemias (Chaps. 66, 93), these observations cannot be dismissed as coincidental.

Pathology

To date, pathologic changes have been nonspecific. Fatty liver can occur.[279] A brain biopsy in one patient showed gliosis, spongiosis, and an increase in glycogen in astrocytes.[280]

Diagnosis

HL deficiency should be considered in patients with hypoketotic hypoglycemia and acidosis and in children presenting with Reye syndrome or sudden infant death syndrome. Usually urinary organic acid analysis confirms the diagnosis. Because rare children have typical organic aciduria but normal HL activity, the diagnosis should be confirmed enzymatically.

Diagnostic metabolites and functional testing. The diagnosis of HL deficiency usually relies on its distinctive urinary organic acid pattern of leucine metabolites, mainly 3-hydroxy-3-methylglutaric, 3-methylglutaconic, and 3-hydroxyisovaleric acids. This is

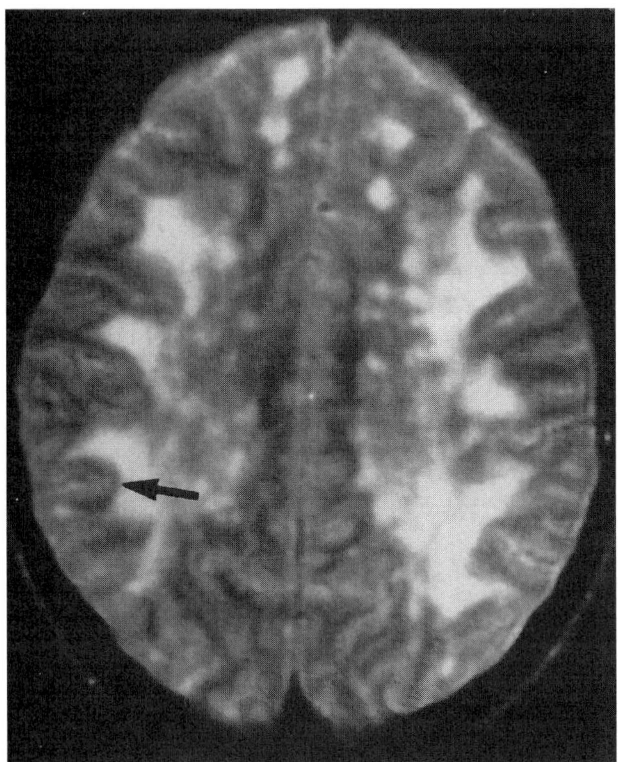

Fig. 102-10 White matter abnormalities in HL deficiency. T_2-weighted image showing disseminated hyperintense regions of the deep arcuate fibers, one area of which is shown by the arrow. In an S69fs(−2) homozygote who had episodes of hypoglycemia. (*From Gordon et al.,*[272] *with permission.*)

discussed in Chap. 93, with other branched chain organic acidemias.

Fasting and leucine loading tests are usually unecessary for diagnosis. They may be useful to determine fasting and protein tolerance, but involve some risk of provoking decompensation and should be performed only under close supervision.

Enzymatic diagnosis. For diagnosis, HL is commonly assayed spectrophotometrically.[281] AcAc produced by HL is reduced to 3HB using commercially available 3HBD and an excess of NADH, and NADH disappearance is followed at 340 nm. Performing the assay at pH 9.25 maximizes HL activity, permitting the use of spectophotometric rather than radioactive techniques.[281] In assays using a [3-^{14}C]HMG-CoA substrate (reviewed in Gibson[282]), [3-^{14}C]AcAc production is quantitated either as volatile radioactivity or with HPLC. Native HL requires the presence of thiol reagents for stability. For study of recombinant mutant and normal HL, it is convenient to use the C323S mutant, which is catalytically indistinguishable from wild-type HL but is more stable in the absence of reducing agents.[142] Published normal ranges for HL activity in nmol/min/mg protein are, for the spectrophotometric assay at pH 9.2, 16–32 in fibroblasts,[281] 15–27 in leukocytes,[283] and 23–35 in platelets,[283] and, for the radioactive assay at pH 7.4, 3.9–5.7 in fibroblasts and ~11.5 in lymphocytes.[284] HL activity is detectable in amniocytes and chorionic villi.[273,285,286]

Molecular diagnosis. We have described our approach to mutation detection, using amplification of exons and screening by single-strand polymorphism analysis followed by expression in bacteria of mutations of biologic interest.[147] cDNA amplification and sequencing is an alternative approach.[143,287] Mutation analysis permits nonambiguous carrier testing for relatives.

Molecular basis of HL deficiency. Eleven mutations have been reported in HL deficiency. The mutations include two large deletions[155] and three frameshift/premature termination mutations (S69fs(−2),[143] N46fs(+1),[273] and F305fs(−2)).[147] Elegant studies of splicing have been carried out for three other premature termination mutations: E37X,[287] IVS8 + 1 G→C,[288] and a 2-bp deletion at cDNA positions 505 and 506,[289] documenting the occurrence of alternately spliced transcripts of these mRNAs containing in-frame stop codons.

To date, publications have concentrated on mutations of biologic or epidemiologic interest. Some naturally occurring point mutations have revealed active site residues in HL.[147] Five mutations in the highly conserved R41 and D42 codons (R41Q, R41X, D42H, D42G, and D42E) accounted for at least 19 out of 82 (23 percent) of the mutant alleles of the 41 probands studied. No explanation to date fully accounts for the clustering in such a small region. When expressed in bacteria and purified, the activity of recombinant HL containing R41Q, D42H, or D42G is reduced 100,000-fold; that of D42E is 4.4 percent of normal. This suggests strongly that R41 and D42 participate in the catalytic mechanism of HL.

Another naturally occurring mutation, H233R, was detected in one of a pair of histidine residues H233 and H235, thought to be important for divalent ion binding.[146] HL peptide containing H233R has a 10,000-fold reduction in activity but little change in either the K_m for HMG-CoA or activation by metal ions,[146] showing H233 to be an active site residue that does not participate in ion binding. In contrast, the mutants H235A and H235E, created by site-directed mutagenesis, both had markedly reduced divalent cation binding. Further study showed that cations normally bind both to HL, presumably at H235, and to substrate.[148]

Other synthetic mutants are C266S and C323S. C266S retains structural integrity and affinity for HMG-CoA, but the reaction rate is reduced 10,000-fold,[150] showing that C266 is an active site residue. Finally, the catalytic properties of one mutant, C323S, are similar to those of wild-type HL.[142] C323S is more stable to oxidative inactivation than is the wild-type HL, a useful property for assays of recombinant HL, but is more vulnerable than wild-type HL to degradation in the absence of glycerol.

Ethnic distribution of mutations. Three mutations have been observed in more than one family: R41Q, F305fs(−2), and E37X. Six of nine Saudi probands are R41Q homozygotes. We also detected R41Q in Turkish and Italian patients. R41Q accounts for 15 out of 82 (18 percent) of mutant alleles in our series of probands. Haplotype analysis has not yet been performed in these patients. Two other Saudi probands were homozygous for F305fs(−2). The final Saudi patient had no detectable abnormality on SSCP analysis. Thus, at least three mutant alleles cause HL deficiency in Saudi patients.

E37X has been reported in two patients,[287] and we have detected it in two others,[111] all of Iberian or Arab descent.

Genotype-phenotype correlations. To date, a strong genotype-phenotype correlation has not emerged in our study of over 40 HL-deficient patients. For instance, a homozygote for D42E, a mutation with 4.4 percent residual activity in purified mutant HL, was diagnosed at 12 months and had had previous feeding difficulties and hypoglycemic convulsions. Conversely, some patients with mutations causing a complete loss of HL activity are thriving, suggesting that residual HL activity alone does not determine clinical phenotype.

Prenatal Diagnosis

Prenatal diagnosis of HL deficiency has been performed using metabolite measurements,[273] enzyme assay,[273,285,286] and molecular techniques.[273] In affected pregnancies, maternal urine may contain elevated HMG-related metabolites,[290] but the diagnostic sensitivity of this method is not known.

Management

With the approach to therapy discussed in the section, "General Principles of Management of Inborn Errors of Ketone Body

Metabolism," we have encountered no symptomatic crises following diagnosis. Some patients' disease may prove more difficult to control, however, and it is important to individualize therapy. Because of frequent white matter changes, it is reasonable to obtain a baseline cerebral MRI evaluation and to carefully follow the neurologic status of patients.

Pathophysiology

The cardinal event in the pathophysiology of HL deficiency is predicted to be the accumulation within mitochondria of HMG-CoA and other acyl CoA derivatives but the cascade by which this leads to clinically identifiable signs is unknown.

Hypoglycemia. Hypoglycemia presumably results both from insufficient glucose production (disruption of gluconeogenesis as a consequence of HMG-CoA accumulation) and from increased glucose consumption (due to the absence of ketone bodies). It is of note that intravenous infusion of 3HB corrected hypoglycemia in one patient.[52]

The brain in HL deficiency. The brain is predicted to be highly sensitive to hypoglycemia in HL deficiency. Because ketone bodies are the only substantial non-glucose-derived fuel for brain in HL deficiency, hypoglycemia in HL deficiency causes a near-complete lack of exogenous energy sources for the brain. The frequent occurrence of white matter lesions and of severe neurologic sequelae in some HL-deficient patients following prolonged crises are consistent with this. The possibility of endogenous HMG-CoA production in brain cannot be excluded as an additional neurotoxic mechanism.

Animal models. In the absence of an appropriate animal model, the intracellular mechanisms of HL deficiency, like those of most inborn errors of CoA metabolism, remain speculative. We created a gene-targeted HL-deficient mouse, but homozygous HL-deficient mouse fetuses die prenatally at $\sim$10.5 days p.c.[291] This observation challenges the clinical notion that prenatal development can be assumed to be normal in inborn errors of CoA ester metabolism.

Epidemiology

HL deficiency has been reported frequently in Saudi Arabia,[267] where for unknown reasons the clinical manifestations are described as neonatal and particularly severe and where in one series it accounts for up to 16 percent of diagnosable neurometabolic disease.[292] A large Bedouin cohort is also described.[293] Most cases have occurred in single families of diverse ethnic origins.

HMG-uria with Normal HL Activity

At least three patients have been reported. Two presented with hyperammonemia,[294,295] one of whom had proven carbamyl phosphate synthetase I deficiency.[294] The third had microcephaly, nerve deafness, and basal ganglia abnormalities.[296] Characteristic HMG-CoA metabolites were modestly increased. If such patients are observed in the future, it will be of interest to document their metabolite excretion in illness and when well, and to examine cells from these individuals to determine the intracellular distribution of HL. It remains to be determined whether these patients have a distinct metabolic condition or whether a mild HL-deficiency-like pattern of urinary organic acids can develop in some individuals in response to stress. As a clinical corollary, the finding of high levels of HMG in a patient with a Reye-syndrome-like presentation does not necessarily exclude the presence of other underlying metabolic abnormalities, including urea cycle diseases and conditions of oxidative stress such as lactic acidoses.[294]

3HBD DEFICIENCY

Deficiency of 3HBD has not, to our knowledge, been reported. Our speculations on the possible phenotype are as follows: 3HB is expected to be absent and AcAc and acetone increased. Urine ketones would quickly become positive with fasting. Since the calculated energy yield of 3HB is only 13 percent greater than that of AcAc, and since both are acids of approximately the same strength, the effects on energy transport and acid-base status are expected to be mild. However, the NADH/NAD$^+$ ratio of the mitochondrial matrix might be increased during active ketogenesis, with secondary metabolic effects in hepatocytes.

SCOT DEFICIENCY (MIM 245050)

SCOT deficiency was described in 1972 by Tildon and Cornblath.[297] All known patients have had ketoacidotic episodes. SCOT deficiency is potentially fatal but is treatable. We know of 14 published[297–305] and unpublished[177] cases.

Clinical Findings

The clinical findings of 14 SCOT-deficient patients are summarized in Table 102-3. About half presented in the first week of life and all before 22 months. Ketoacidosis is frequently precipitated by minor febrile illness and is often severe. When measured, lactate, pyruvate, and ammonia levels have been normal.

Between ketoacidotic episodes, patients are asymptomatic. Available data suggest that persistent hyperketonemia is present in SCOT deficiency even in the fed state. Nonfasting ketonuria is rare and should alert the clinican to possible SCOT deficiency.

Blood glucose is usually normal during ketoacidosis in SCOT deficiency, but hypoglycemia occurred in two severely acidotic newborns. In one[304] a level of 2.1 mM (38 mg/dl) was reported; in the other it was undetectable.[306] In older SCOT-deficient children, blood glucose has been normal. Although the presence of hypoglycemia cannot rule out SCOT deficiency, there was little difficulty differentiating hypoglycemic SCOT-deficient patients from those with ketotic hypoglycemia, based on their young age and severe acidosis of SCOT deficient patients.

Cardiomegaly has been noted in two patients,[297,300] one of whom developed congestive heart failure.[297] The patient with severe hypoglycemia developed convulsions.[306] The full spectrum of SCOT deficiency may not be recognized.

Table 102-3 Clinical Aspects of 14 SCOT-Deficient Patients

Sex	F6, M8	
Consanguinity	5/13	
History of sibling death	3/12	
Survival[1]	12/14	
Onset		
$<$1 wk	6/14	
1 wk–6 mo	3/14	
6–22 mo	5/14	
Neurologic status during ketoacidosis		
Coma	2/9	
Lethargy	4/9	
Normal	3/9	
Number of crises[2]	2.5	(1–6; 8)
Laboratory data during ketoacidosis		
pH	7.08	(6.88–7.29; 11)
Bicarbonate (mM)	5.0	(2.0–12.0; 10)
Ketone bodies (mM)	11.5	(5.1–30; 7)
3HB:AcAc ratio	1.7	(1.5–22.3; 6)
Glucose (mM)	5.0	(UD–10.0; 7)
SCOT activity in fibroblasts (percent of normal)	16.5	(5.0–35.0; 13)

[1]Follow-up of survivors ranges from 15 months to 11 years.
[2]Below this point, the figures in the left column indicate the median value and those in parentheses the range and the number of patients for whom data are available.
UD = undetectable. Ketonuria was present in all acidotic crises.

Pathology

Few data are available except for the succinct description of the first reported case, in which fatty liver, pneumonia, and small brain size were documented.[297]

Diagnosis

SCOT deficiency should be considered in children with severe or recurrent ketoacidosis or nonfasting ketosis. Clinical judgment is essential in comparing the severity and frequency of ketosis with the normal physiological response to stress.

Metabolite Measurement and Functional Testing

As discussed in the section "Diagnostic Approach to the Ketotic Patient" above, SCOT deficiency is suggested by an isolated ketonuria. Because diabetes, congenital lactic acidoses, T2 deficiency, and other branched chain organic acidemias can also produce ketosis, important negative findings include absence of glucose and normal levels of lactate, 2MeAcAc, 2Me3HB, and methylcitrate in urine. Excessive amounts of long- and medium-chain dicarboxylic acids can be present, suggesting deficient short-chain hydroxyacyl CoA oxidation.[256]

Carnitine levels were reported in three cases. They were decreased in one (GS04, free carnitine 8.2 μM; acyl carnitine, 6.8)[304] and normal in two (GS01 and GS08).[177] The blood 3HB:AcAc ratio has been normal except during severe acidosis (Table 102-3).

Between episodes, a simple procedure is repeated testing for ketonuria (see "Diagnostic Approach to the Ketotic Patient" above). There is surprisingly little published documentation of baseline blood ketone body levels SCOT deficiency, but when measured they have been elevated.[298,300] Observations of well-nourished SCOT-deficient patients may be useful in estimating human basal ketogenic rate.

Fasting tests are usually unnecessary for diagnosis but may be useful for assessing fasting tolerance. They demonstrate a rapid increase in blood ketone bodies and a low ratio of free fatty acids to ketone bodies (Fig. 102-9).

Enzymatic Diagnosis

Fibroblast, lymphocyte, and lymphoblast extracts can be used for clinical diagnosis.[302] SCOT is best assayed in the direction of AcAc-CoA degradation, since AcAc-CoA concentration is easily monitored by absorbence at 303 nm and equilibrium favors this direction.[163] It is of technical note that high concentrations of AcAc-CoA increase apparent SCOT activity.

Using an AcAc-CoA concentration of 30 μM, normal SCOT activity values in our lab are 14.7 ± 4.8 nmol/min/mg protein (n = 13); peripheral blood mononuclear cells, 12.0 ± 3.6 (n = 8); and EBV-transformed lymphoblasts, 27.5 ± 11.7 (n = 5).

Interestingly, assay of fibroblasts from SCOT-deficient patients with mutations that completely inactivate SCOT reveals 15–30 percent of control activity.[172,307,308] This apparent residual activity may be due to other acetoacetyl CoA-utilizing enzymes,[79] particularly T2. Although T2 inhibitors are routinely added to the SCOT assay mixture, inhibition is incomplete.[34] Currently available assays in fibroblasts are sufficiently sensitive for clinical diagnosis of SCOT deficiency but not for precise assessment of residual activity.

In our transient expression system, introduction of plasmid encoding wild-type SCOT into SCOT-deficient fibroblasts yields levels ~fifteenfold higher than background levels. This system allows more precise estimation of the residual activity of SCOT mutations.

Immunoblots of all nine SCOT-deficient fibroblast lines tested to date show an absence or marked decrease of SCOT.[177,307]

Molecular Diagnosis

To date, mutation detection in SCOT has been performed with cDNA from patient cells. The recent characterization of the human SCOT gene[176] will be useful for mutation detection. Transient expression is discussed in the preceding section.

Molecular Studies

Five pathogenic SCOT mutations are known. The first to be reported, S283X,[172] is homozygous in the Spanish patient GS01 and causes loss of the essential C-terminus of SCOT and marked reduction of SCOT mRNA level on northern blots. Two Japanese sibs, GS02 and GS03, are genetic compounds: The maternal allele carries the C456F mutation; the paternal, two mutations in *cis*, T58M and V133E. T58M is functionally neutral, but C456F and V133E are immunoblot-negative and possess no detectable SCOT activity.[308] A Dutch patient (GS04) is a genetic compound for G219E and G324E, neither of which yields detectable SCOT activity on transient expression.[177] An unpublished English patient (GS05) is a V221M homozygote. On transient expression, V221M retains about 10 percent residual SCOT activity.[176] Interestingly, GS05 has the mildest phenotype described to date, with onset at 22 months and only two episodes of ketoacidosis by 8 years of age.

Prenatal Diagnosis

Prenatal diagnosis of SCOT deficiency is possible. There are several management options, and genetic counseling should ensure that the couple is aware of the sometimes fatal but usually favorable outcome of the disease. One patient (GS03) had an uneventful neonatal course following predictive prenatal diagnosis and prophylactic intravenous administration of glucose after birth.[177] At-risk neonates could also be followed by enzyme assay and monitoring of ketone body levels after birth, without prenatal diagnosis.

In one affected pregnancy,[309] SCOT activity in cultured amniocytes was < 0.4 nmol/min/mg protein (normal, 5.0 ± 0.5). Amniotic fluid ketone body levels were normal: 3HB was 44.5 μM (normal, 62.3 ± 24.0; n = 5); AcAc was present in trace amounts in both patient and control amniotic fluids.

Enzymatic prenatal diagnosis of SCOT deficiency has also been performed using chorionic villi.[310] Molecular prenatal diagnosis is possible for families in which the causal mutation or mutations are known.

Management

The general approach to treatment is reviewed in the section "General Principles of Management of Inborn Errors of Ketone Body Metabolism," below.

Protein provides a modest amount of ketogenic substrate. Of 13 SCOT-deficient patients for whom information is available, three (33 percent) are on protein-restricted diets. Because ketogenesis decreases with age, protein tolerance may increase and protein tolerance should be reassessed periodically if a low-protein diet is prescribed.

Sodium bicarbonate supplementation can be considered in patients with persistent metabolic acidosis. Its effectiveness should also be periodically evaluated. Of six patients for whom we have information, two are supplemented with bicarbonate.

Monitoring. Blood ketones should be assessed repeatedly to establish the typical baseline of the patient during asymptomatic periods. Home monitoring of ketonuria should be performed on a regular basis and intensified at times of fasting or other lipolytic stress. Periodic cardiac ultrasound and electrocardiographic evaluation, urinalysis for assessment of tubular function, and documentation of development and school performance are reasonable.

Prognosis. Although many recently reported patients are developing normally, SCOT deficiency is potentially fatal (Table 102-3).

Pathophysiology

SCOT deficiency is an exclusively ketolytic defect. Because ketogenesis is normal, hyperketonemia and ketoacidosis occur rapidly with ketogenic stress. In the fed state, asymptomatic hyperketonemia is present. This observation is interesting in relation to normal physiology, suggesting that some ketogenesis occurs even in well-fed humans.

During crises, the main problem is acidosis. Intermediary metabolism is predicted to be otherwise normal, since abnormal CoA esters do not accumulate and free AcAc is thought to have few effects upon metabolism. Because normal liver is devoid of SCOT, gluconeogenesis and other hepatic functions are predicted to be unhindered. Similarly, other organs are able to use glucose and fatty acids as sources of energy, compensating in part for the lack of ketolysis.

Notably, the fibroblasts of the first published patient [311] showed reduced glucose uptake and oxidation, in contrast to the above predictions. It will be interesting to test this in cells from other SCOT-deficient patients.

Clinical severity does not depend solely on genotype. Affected siblings with neonatal and later onset have been observed, and patients with functionally null alleles can have relatively mild phenotypes.[172]

Epidemiology

SCOT deficiency appears to be panethnic, patients originating from North America, Europe (France, England, Spain, Netherlands), Japan, and South Africa. The apparent rarity of SCOT deficiency may be partly due to underdiagnosis, for reasons discussed in the "Epidemiology" section in "mHS Deficiency" above. Perhaps some patients with fatal neonatal acidosis or with mild episodes of ketosis have SCOT deficiency.

T2 DEFICIENCY (MIM 203750)

T2 deficiency (beta-ketothiolase deficiency; 2MeAcAc-CoA thiolase deficiency), first reported in 1971, is a disorder of ketone body and isoleucine metabolism that typically presents as ketoacidotic episodes. A favorable outcome is frequent if the first ketoacidotic crisis is rapidly diagnosed and treated.

Clinical Findings

T2 deficiency usually presents as acute ketoacidosis. Patients are usually asymptomatic between episodes. However, there is great clinical heterogeneity in T2 deficiency.

Ketoacidotic episodes. The first episode usually occurs between 5 and 24 months of age in a previously normal child. The oldest age at which any ketoacidotic episode has been reported in T2 deficiency is 10 years. Episodes typically accompany infections and vomiting. Some patients are initially diagnosed as having encephalitis or aspirin poisoning.[246]

Acidosis is typically severe (pH < 7.1, bicarbonate < 7 mM). Blood glucose is generally normal, but hypoglycemia (0.6 mM, 11 mg/dl)[313] and hyperglycemia (12.7 mM, 229 mg/dl) have been described.[314] Moderate hyperammonemia (up to 307 μM) and hyperglycinemia can occur.[315]

Asymptomatic affected individuals. T2 deficiency has been documented in asymptomatic sibs of probands[316,317] and in GK05, the asymptomatic 36-year-old father of patient GK04.[318]

Neonatal presentation. One atypical patient with probable T2 deficiency[319] presented as a newborn with refractory vomiting, leading to pyloromyotomy at 4 weeks and rehospitalization at 10 weeks of age for dehydration, acidosis (bicarbonate 11 mM), ketonuria, neutropenia (nadir 500/mm^3), thrombocytopenia (nadir 5000/mm^3), and hyperammonemia (220 μM). A protein load (8 g/kg/day) caused ketoacidosis within 12 h. Her condition was well controlled metabolically by a diet providing 1.5 g protein/kg/day but at 8 years of age she developed fatal dilated cardiomyopathy.[320] Her urinary organic acids included metabolites typical of T2 deficiency but also the atypical metabolites hexanone and pentanone.[315] Her fibroblasts showed reduced CO_2 production from isoleucine,[319] but T2 activity was not measured.

Neurologic complications. Some patients have developed severe headaches at 6 or 7 years of age. Clinical descriptions have been succinct but are suggestive of migraine.[321,322] Neurologic and ophthalmologic examination were normal when reported.

Five patients, three of Saudi Arabian origin, had developmental delay prior to their first ketoacidotic attack.[323–325] Brain MRI of the Saudi patients and of a German patient (GK06) revealed basal ganglion abnormalities suggestive of bilateral striatal necrosis (Fig. 102-11). Mental retardation and dystonia can occur. Similar basal ganglion abnormalities are known in other branched chain aminoacidopathies (Chaps. 66, 93).

Other clinical features. Dilated cardiomyopathy,[319,326] prolonged QT interval,[312] neutropenia, and thrombocytopenia[319] have been reported.

Pregnancy in T2 deficiency. Pregnancy and delivery by cesarean section were well tolerated by a T2-deficient woman.[327] She consumed a normal diet throughout her pregnancy and excreted typical urinary organic acids. Low levels of serum carnitine (free 7.9 μM, total 17.2 μM) were corrected by carnitine supplementation. As expected, the baby was a carrier of T2 deficiency and had no detectable clinical symptoms.

Pathology

Data are available for the hearts of three patients,[320,326] in whom T2 was not assayed, but whose urinary metabolite patterns suggested T2 deficiency. All had cardiac hypertrophy (weight 1.5- to 2-fold normal). Fatty infiltration of the liver was present. Neuropathology of two affected brothers[326] revealed neuronal loss, spongiosis, and reactive gliosis in cerebral cortex and basal ganglia.

Diagnostic Metabolites and Functional Testing

The diagnostic metabolites for T2 deficiency are isoleucine derivatives (Fig. 102-3). Other diseases of isoleucine degradation are considered in Chap. 93.

In most cases, the urinary organic acid pattern during or between attacks is diagnostic. However, urine metabolites are highly variable in T2 deficiency, and some (2MeAcAc, 2-butanone) present special challenges for quantitative analysis.[328] For instance, 2MeAcAc decarboxylates to form 2-butanone and both of these compounds are volatile.[321,328] 2Me3HB-CoA and tiglyl-CoA are thought to accumulate due to the reversibility of the 3-hydroxyacyl CoA dehydrogenase and enoyl CoA hydratase reactions and the high mitochondrial NADH : NAD ratio, leading to excretion of 2Me3HB, tiglic acid and tiglylglycine. Elevation of 2Me3HB is the most consistent finding in T2 deficiency. It is difficult to rule out T2 deficiency based only on a normal urinary organic acid pattern in a sample from an asymptomatic period.

Typical values for urinary metabolites are well described in the previous edition of this work.[329] The normal level of 2Me3HB is 1–9 mmol/mol creatinine, which can rise to 200 mmol/mol creatinine with ketosis of any cause. We speculate that the presence of high intracellular concentrations of CoASAc in ketosis may inhibit 2MeAcAc-CoA degradation. In T2 deficiency, typical ranges for 2Me3HB excretion are 200–1000 mmol/mol creatinine when patients are well and 1000–14,400 mmol/mol creatinine during decompensation. 2MeAcAc levels are four- to tenfold less than those of 2Me3HB and may be undetectable during asymptomatic periods. Tiglylglycine levels vary from undetectable to 7000 mmol/mol creatine. In some patients, 2-butanone can be detected in urine. In the only patient with a neonatal presentation, hexanone was detected.[315]

Isoleucine loading (see "Diagnostic Approach to the Ketotic Patient" above) has produced three- to fourfold increases in 2Me3HB and 2MeAcAc[317,324] and the appearance of tiglylglycine in urine of affected individuals.[324]

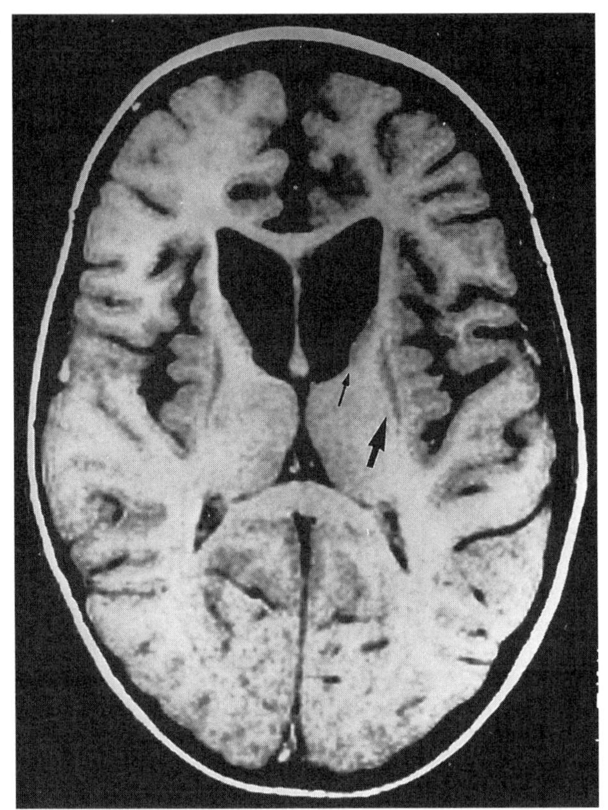

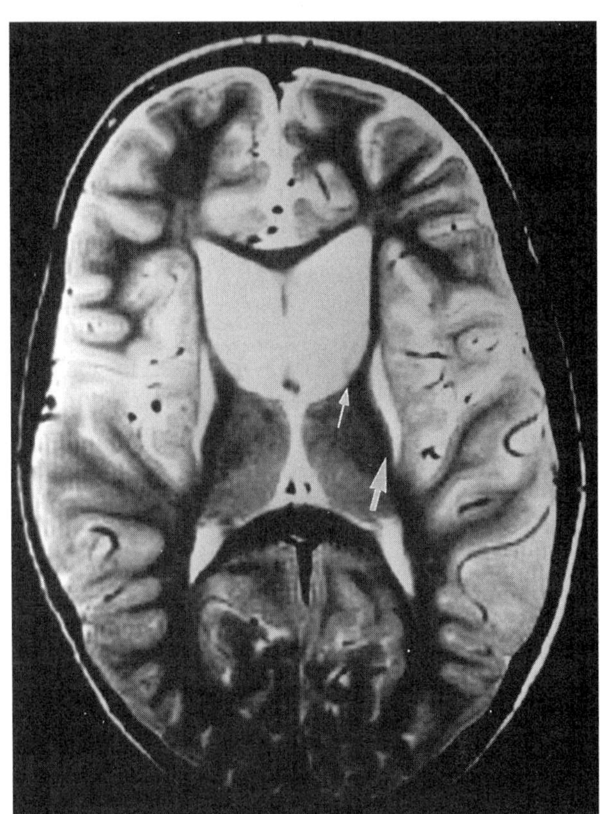

Fig. 102-11 T2 deficiency and striatal necrosis. Cerebral MRI of a T2-deficient patient with extrapyramidal symptoms (see text). (a) T_1- and (b) T_2-weighted images demonstrate atrophy of the caudate nucleus (thin arrow); in (b) T_2 hyperintensity of both the caudate nucleus and the putamen (thick arrow) is consistent with bilateral striatal necrosis. (*Figure courtesy of Georg Fraudienst-Egger.*)

Differential diagnosis by means of metabolites. 2Me3HB and tiglylglycine are also detected in propionic and methylmalonic acidemias. However, these conditions are easily distinguished from T2 deficiency by the prominent occurrence of 3-hydroxypropionic acid, methylcitric acid, and propionylglycine in the blood.

6-Methyluracil. Cromby *et al.*[331] proposed 6-methyluracil as a marker for T2 deficiency, since it was present in two T2-deficient patients and in two children with recurrent infection-related ketoacidemia, but not in patients with fasting ketosis. This finding has not been confirmed,[332] and further studies are needed to clarify its diagnostic usefulness.

Carnitine and acylcarnitines. During ketoacidotic attacks, esterified carnitine level is elevated and the acyl/free carnitine ratio is increased in blood.[314] Tiglylcarnitine is detectable in most patients[314,333] and increases during acute illness.[334] One patient also excreted a tiglylcarnitine isomer, possibly 2-ethylacrylylcarnitine. 3-hydroxyisovalerylcarnitine is a common C5-hydroxycarnitine found in all forms of ketosis.[334] A C5-hydroxycarnitine, suggested to be 2Me3HB carnitine, was proposed as a hallmark of T2 deficiency[323] but has not yet to our knowledge been distinguished from 3-hydroxyisovaleryl carnitine.[334]

Enzyme Diagnosis

Assay for potassium ion-activated acetoacetyl CoA thiolase activity, first reported by Robinson *et al.* in fibroblasts,[246] is a robust diagnostic method for which substrates are commercially available. It is applicable in fibroblasts, peripheral blood lymphocytes, polymorphonuclear cells, and EBV-transformed lymphoblasts.[317,349] Mean values in our laboratory, in nmol/min/mg protein, are: lymphoblasts 26.4 (in the absence of K^+), 48.2 (with K^+), ratio 1.9 ($n = 5$); peripheral blood mononuclear cells 7.6, 14.7, ratio 1.9 ($n = 8$), and fibroblasts 10.1, 18.1, ratio 1.8 ($n = 13$). In cells from carriers of T2 deficiency, T2 activity is stimulated 1.3- to 1.9-fold by potassium ion. Therefore, there is some overlap between the ranges of carriers and of controls.[335] Normal ranges differ among laboratories, so patient results must be compared to control values for the laboratory.

Another assay, using 2MeAcAc-CoA as substrate,[191] is more sensitive and specific than the above method, but 2MeAcAc-CoA is unstable and not commercially available. Using this substrate, fibroblasts from most T2-deficient patients have 0–4 percent of normal activity and the mild T2-deficient patient (GK03) had 7 percent activity. Carriers can be detected using the ratio of thiolase activity levels using 2MeAcAc-CoA vs AcAc-CoA as substrate.[198]

Assays in intact cells. Early publications reported a twofold reduction of CO_2 production from radiolabeled isoleucine in T2-deficient fibroblasts.[246,312,319] Other assays that measure segments of the isoleucine degradation pathway[321,337] have yielded high residual activity in T2-deficient patients with clinically mild presentations.[338] It will be interesting to see whether these findings can be confirmed in other patients.

Immunoblotting. All 26 fibroblasts studied have had either reduced or absent immunoreactive T2 peptide (Table 102-4).[177,335] Carrier detection has been reported by evaluating the ratio of T2 to control proteins.[335] Immunoblotting should not be used as the only diagnostic test, because it would fail to recognize crossreactive material (CRM)-positive mutations.

Molecular Diagnosis

Nineteen T2-deficient patients have been analyzed (Table 102-4); 18 patients are probands; one (GK05) is the asymptomatic T2-deficient father of GK04. Mutations are distributed throughout the T2 gene. Four patients (21 percent) were homozygotes.

Table 102-4 Mutations in T2 Deficiency

Exon/Intron	Mutation	Nucleotide changes	Nucleotide position	CRMT[1]	Activity[2]	Comments[3]	Patient (GK no.)	Ref
E1	M1K	T→A	2	A	–	Init	08	346
E2	83del2	del AT	83	A	nd	FS, PT	14	345
E2	Y33X	T→A	99	A	nd	PT	12	177
E3	149delC	del C	149	A	nd		01	196
E4	delE85	del GAA	253–255	A	–		02	177
E4	N93S	A→G	278	C	10%		19	196
E5	K124R	A→G	371	nd	nd		18	177
I5	435+1G→C	G→C		A	nd	Spl(Ex5), FS, PT	13, 14	345
E6	G152A	G→C	455	B	–		02	177
E6	N158D	A→G	472	E	–	AM	11, 15	340
E6	G183R	G→A	547	C	–		04, 05	366
E7	754ins2	ins CT	754	A	–	FS, PT	13	345
I7–E8	del68	del (Spl −46–752)		A	–	Spl(Ex8)	17	367
E8	Q272X	C→T	816	A	–	Spl(Ex8)	07, 15	342
I8	828+1G→T	G→T		A	–	Spl(Ex8)	05, 16	366
E9	T297M	C→T	890	D	10%		11	340
E9	A301P	G→C	901	F	5%	AM	16	340
E9	I312T	C→T	935	F	10%	AM	17	196
E10	A333P	G→C	997	E	–	AM	01	196
I10	1005−2A→C	A→C		A	–	Spl(Ex11)	04	366
I10	1005−1G→C	G→C		A	–	Spl(Ex11)	10	344
E11	G379V	G→T	1136	B	–		07	342
E11	A380T	G→C	1138	B	7%		06	347
I11	116+2T→C	T→C		A	–	Spl, FS	09, 17	346

[1]CRM subtypes (A to F) are from pulse chase studies: A, no detectable CRM; B, highly unstable, normal electrophoretic mobility; C, moderately unstable, normal electrophoretic mobility; D, stable, normal electrophoretic mobility; E, very unstable, reduced electrophoretic mobility; F, moderately unstable, reduced electrophoretic mobility. In all classes, the amount of CRM is reduced.

[2]Activity as estimated by transient expression of the mutant cDNA, compared to that of a normal cDNA.

[3]AM, altered electrophoretic mobility; FS, frameshift; Init, initiation codon mutation; PT, premature truncation; Spl, abnormal splicing with deletion of the indicated exon; nd, not determined.

Because of allelic heterogeneity,[339] molecular testing is not a first-line diagnostic test in T2 deficiency. We first establish the diagnosis enzymatically, then perform immunoblotting, RT-PCR, and cDNA sequencing. For missense mutations, we perform transient expression using lipofection of the mutant cDNA in T2-null SV40-transformed fibroblasts. For prenatal diagnosis and carrier detection in a family in which a causal mutation or mutations have been identified, molecular analysis is the method of choice.

Protein phenotype. Potassium ion-activated T2 activity is insensitive for detection of residual enzyme activity, having revealed this in only one patient, GK19.[317] Western blot analysis of cells from T2-deficient patients has demonstrated reproducible differences in T2 level among patients (GK19 ≫ GK11, GK16[340] > GK03, GK05[200]). Some point mutations cause abnormal electrophoretic mobility (see Table 102-4).

T2 mRNA phenotype. mRNA expression, examined quantitatively in fibroblasts from patients GK01–GK04 (Table 102-4), was reduced in GK01 and GK03.[186] GK03, who has clinically mild disease and residual T2 activity, has < 10 percent of normal T2 mRNA levels. Detailed study of her T2 cDNA and gene has been normal. We speculate that her causal mutation(s) decrease transcription.

Genotype. In 19 patients, we have identified 24 potential or proven causal mutations on 34 of 38 alleles (89 percent) (Table 102-4).

Polymorphisms. Two single-nucleotide polymorphisms are known. One (A5P) creates an *Msp* I site in the leader. The functional consequences have not been studied in detail, but homozygotes for each variant are clinically normal. A *Taq* I polymorphism is known in intron 9.[341] The frequencies of each of these polymorphisms are about 0.5 in Japanese controls but have not been studied in other populations.

Nonsense, splicing, and frameshift mutations. Two nonsense mutations (Y33X and Q272X) have been identified. Q272X may directly influence splicing,[342] as well as destabilizing its mRNA, as reported for other transcripts containing nonsense mutations.[343] Seven mutations (29 percent) are at splice sites.[339,344,345] 1163 + 2T→C causes a 4-bp extension of exon 11, resulting in a frameshift.[346] Frameshift mutations resulting from small deletions (149delC, 83del2) or an insertion (754ins2) have been identified.[196,345]

Missense mutations. Twelve missense mutations have been identified. M1K reduces T2 mRNA translation to < 5 percent of normal.[346] G379V in GK07 and A380T in GK06 alter residues located in the most conserved region of T2 (residues 378–393),[183] (Fig. 102-8), presumably rendering the mutant T2 unstable.[342]

All missense mutations except K124R have been characterized by transient expression in T2-null SV40-transformed fibroblasts. Residual T2 activity could be detected by transient expression in 5 out of 11 mutations (45 percent): T297M (∼10 percent residual activity), I312T (10 percent), N93S (10 percent), A380T (7 percent), and A301P (5 percent).[196,339]

Dominant negative effects may be active in GK11. This patient is a compound of T298M (10 percent residual activity and CRM when expressed alone) and N158D (no detectable activity or CRM). Cotransfection of both mutant cDNAs resulted in lower levels of activity than expected if each were transfected separately.[340]

We have evaluated some missense mutations in relation to our model of T2 tertiary structure[196] (Fig. 102-8). For example, I312 is predicted to be buried in the hydrophobic region. In I312T, the replacement with threonine may destabilize the enzyme. Consistent with this, in transient expression of I312T, mutant T2 is detected mainly in the pellet, while the fraction of I312T-T2 that is soluble has residual activity but is thermolabile.

Genotype-phenotype correlations. To date, the course of T2 deficiency cannot be predicted from genotype. Some patients are clinically severe despite having mutations with residual activity: GK11 (T297M) presented with severe ketoacidosis and classic organic aciduria, although his development is normal;[340] GK06, who is a genetic compound with one A380T allele, is mentally retarded;[347] and GK16, who was a compound of A301P and a functionally null allele, died during a severe ketoacidotic attack.[340] Conversely, patients with mutations that yield no detectable T2 activity can have a mild clinical course.

Prenatal Diagnosis

T2 is measurable in cultured amniocytes and in chorionic villi.[348] Molecular prenatal diagnosis has been reported.[348] To our knowledge, assay of amniotic fluid metabolites has not been reported for an affected pregnancy.

Management

Ketoacidotic crises. As noted below (see "Principles of Management of Inborn Errors of Ketone Body Metabolism"), acidosis should be treated cautiously because aggressive alkalinization may result in hypernatremia. In patient GK16, hypernatremia (203 mM) was associated with cerebral hemorrhage and death.[340] Plasma ammonia, glucose, and electrolytes should be monitored. Intravenous carnitine supplementation is reasonable although its effect has not been formally demonstrated.

Long-term management. If the patient is febrile or vomits, intravenous glucose should be administered. Carbohydrate-rich snacks should be provided during mild illness, especially if urinary ketones are positive, and medical help should be sought if the urinary ketone body level is moderate. In our experience, frequent feeding has not been necessary to avoid ketonuria when the child is clinically well.

Some patients tolerate normal dietary protein intake.[316–318] Typically, a diet providing $\sim$1.5 g/kg/day of protein is prescribed. This is usually tolerated and is adequate for growth. Protein-rich diets ($>$3g/kg/day) and ketogenic diets should be avoided. Carnitine supplementation can be considered.

Most T2-deficient patients achieve good control with these methods. Because some patients have basal ganglion lesions and cardiopathy, baseline cerebral MRI and periodic cardiology evaluation may be indicated.

Prognosis

This section summarizes a literature review of 40 patients plus an overlapping but more recent series of 26 patients who we diagnosed and whose attending physicians provided clinical data.[177] In the literature series, four patients (10 percent) died.[246,312,319,340] Nine infant deaths in undiagnosed sibs were also reported. Of 36 survivors, 10 (28 percent) showed some degree of mental retardation or ataxia.[312,313,316,323,324,347,349] Poor weight gain was seen in four (11 percent).

Two reports describe long-term follow-up. A 15-year-old girl[322] with four ketoacidotic attacks between 14 months and 4 years of age was subsequently asymptomatic despite normal protein intake. In contrast, a 10-year-old girl[350] who had attacks at 10 months and 2 years of age experienced mild ketosis, vomiting, and migraines during febrile illness despite protein restriction.

In our series, one patient (GK16) died of hypernatremia and cerebral hemorrhage.[340] Among the 25 survivors, two had neurologic abnormalities prior to developing a ketoacidotic crisis. Of these, one remains severely retarded, whereas the other regained normal development. Among the 23 remaining patients with previously normal development, one is slightly retarded but two patients who showed delayed development after a ketoacidotic attack also recuperated and have normal intelligence. The other patients have not developed ketoacidotic episodes while on treatment. Three patients (12 percent) remain asymptomatic without dietary restriction.

Overall, the prognosis for normal development is excellent with therapy, if neurologic damage has not occurred prior to diagnosis.

Pathophysiology

T2 plays several roles. In liver, it equilibrates the mitochondrial pools of CoA, Ac-CoA, and AcAc-CoA. During active beta oxidation in liver, high concentrations of Ac-CoA favor ketogenesis.[189] The reaction in this direction also serves to liberate free CoA. In peripheral tissues, ketolysis is the main function of T2.

If T2 is a ketogenic enzyme, why do T2-deficient patients become ketotic? This question fueled the unsuccessful search for a distinct liver-specific AcAc-CoA thiolase (see the section "CoA modification of T2," above). Clearly, ketogenesis exceeds ketolysis in T2 deficiency. There are at least two mechanisms of T2-independent ketogenesis. First, AcAc-CoA formed at the penultimate step of beta oxidation may be utilized directly for ketogenesis. Thus, at low levels of beta oxidation, T2 is not necessary to supply substrate to mHS. Second, T1 can also mediate AcAc-CoA synthesis[178] and 2MeAcAc-CoA degradation[191] and presumably compensates partially for T2 deficiency in liver. Although AcAc-CoA thiolase activity is not essential for ketogenesis, it is necessary for AcAc-CoA use in ketolytic tissues. We hypothesize that these factors explain the excess of ketogenesis over ketolysis in T2 deficiency, and also the relatively mild hepatic manifestations of T2 deficiency.

Epidemiology

Reports of over 35 patients have been published, and we know of over 20 others. There is no particular ethnic predisposition. Patients have been reported from Europe (the Netherlands, Germany, France, Switzerland, Spain, Italy, the United Kingdom, Norway), the Americas (Canada, USA, Chile, Brazil), the Middle East (Saudi Arabia, Israel, Yemen), and Asia (Laos, Vietnam, Japan).

GENERAL PRINCIPLES OF MANAGEMENT OF INBORN ERRORS OF KETONE BODY METABOLISM

Treatment of Acute Episodes

Suppression of ketogenesis. In all four conditions it is advisable to avoid fasting. Oral or intravenous carbohydrate administration is useful for its antilipolytic effect, and in HL, SCOT, and T2 deficiencies for its antiproteolytic actions as well.

Hypoglycemia. Hypoglycemia can be corrected by administration of 2 ml/kg of 10 percent glucose (1.1 mmol/kg), followed by intravenous perfusion, initially with 10 percent glucose with appropriate electrolytes at a rate equal to the patient's fluid requirements, then adjusted to maintain blood glucose levels in the upper normal range.

Acidosis. Deficiencies of SCOT, T2, and HL are associated with acidotic episodes. Ketoacidosis is the main clinical feature in most cases of SCOT and T2 deficiency. The most important treatment is reduction of ketogenesis by provision of carbohydrates, after which the acidosis improves over several hours.

The treatment of metabolic acidosis is controversial. The complications of acidosis include cardiac depression. At pH 7.10, negative inotropic effects and lack of response to catecholamines can be documented experimentally.[351] Extreme acidosis can also cause hyperventilation, leading to increased energy expenditure and exhaustion. Cerebral vasoconstriction accompanies hyperventilation, with detectable EEG changes occurring at a $P_{CO_2} < 20$ torr.[352]

However, severe systemic acidosis is often well tolerated by the nervous system.[353] In children it is exceptional to encounter clinically important cardiac dysfunction at pH values above 7.0. Therefore, in many instances it is not necessary to correct the acidosis acutely. Aggressive alkalinization may be deleterious[354–356] and can cause hypernatremia, hyperosmolarity, and paradoxical central nervous system acidosis.[353]

As a minimal guideline to initial therapy, in a patient with severe ketoacidosis (pH < 7.1) who is not in circulatory or respiratory failure and is alert neurologically, we recommend a slow bolus of bicarbonate (1 mmol/kg over 10 min) followed by a continuous infusion calculated to increase and maintain pH at > 7.10 and $P_{CO_2} > 20$ over the next 12–18 hours, with rapid tapering of the dose as biochemical improvement begins.

Invasive methods like dialysis are effective in controlling acidosis and metabolite levels, but are rarely necessary. Peritoneal dialysis or hemodialysis has been used in HL deficiency,[268] SCOT deficiency,[301] and T2 deficiency.[246] Consideration of dialysis should not delay the immediate administration of glucose and other supportive treatment designed to suppress ketogenesis.

Preventive measures. Intercurrent illnesses should be identified and treated. After diagnosis, preventive measures like treatment with frequent carbohydrate-rich snacks during mild infections are recommended.[357]

Chronic treatment. ***Fat intake.*** The extremes of dietary fat intake should be avoided. A ketogenic diet is clearly contraindicated. Conversely, we do not support the use of severly fat-restricted diets in patients with inborn errors of ketone body metabolism. Extreme fat restriction is difficult to adhere to, may require synthetic food supplements, and may cause deficiencies of lipid-soluble vitamins. Furthermore, patients with hereditary disorders of ketone body metabolism have normal fat mass, and to our knowledge there is no evidence that chronic dietary fat restriction effectively diminishes lipolysis during stress, which causes the main threat of development of decompensations.

Changes of fat intake within the range of typical North American diets have only modest effects upon the body's choice of energy substrates.[358,359] The "prudent," or step one, diet recommended for mild hypercholesterolemia provides 30 percent of energy as fat and is healthy, palatable, and familiar to dieticians. This level of intake seems reasonable, although its efficacy, if any, in reducing ketogenesis remains unproven. If reduction of dietary fat intake is attempted, it would be useful to document its effect upon metabolite and ketone body levels.

Protein intake. In HL and T2 deficiencies and possibly in SCOT deficiency,[299,300] protein restriction is useful. In contrast, in mHS deficiency, a high protein intake may in theory compensate for the metabolic block and provide a source of ketone bodies, although its long-term deficiency, if any, has not been directly tested. Protein intake should be individualized. In practice, most pediatric patients with HL or T2 deficiencies are stable on intakes of ~ 1.5 g/kg/day.

Other therapy. There are no specific therapeutic agents for these diseases. Carnitine supplementation may be considered, particularly if there is evidence that a child has low levels of carnitine. Long-term follow-up of neurologic and hepatic functions and genetic counseling for the family, including evaluation of asymptomatic sibs, are essential.

CT DEFICIENCY

Two patients, designated Patients 1[360] and 2,[361] have been reported to have cytoplasmic thiolase (CT) deficiency. Both were initially thought to be normal female infants but developed progressive mental retardation. Both had mild hyperketonemia. At the time the patients were described, a specific CT assay was not available. The diagnosis of CT deficiency is therefore considered plausible but unproven in these patients.

Clinical Descriptions

In Patient 1, developmental delay was discovered at 4 months of age. Ataxia, chorea, hypotonia, motor regression, and severe mental retardation were described. Laboratory investigation showed slight elevations of alanine and aspartate aminotransferases, lactate, and pyruvate; a low lactate/pyruvate ratio; and mild metabolic acidosis. She was normoglycemic after a 16-h fast. Three days after she started a ketogenic diet, a blood sample showed pH, 7.09; bicarbonate, 15 mM; 3HB, 4.47 mM; and AcAc, 0.84 mM.

Patient 2 developed normally to age 7 months, when she had an episode of extreme irritability, hypotonia and fever followed by severe developmental delay. Laboratory investigation was normal except for persistent ketonuria. On a normal diet, overnight fasting blood ketone body levels were 3HB, 0.37–1.3 mM; acetoacetate, 0.21–0.38 mM.

Enzyme and Molecular Diagnosis

We have developed two specific CT assays for fibroblasts and lymphocytes. One uses immunoprecipitation with anti-(human CT) antibody;[199] the other, subcellular fractionation with digitonin treatment.[362] Using the first method in fibroblasts, CT accounts for 26–38 percent and 14–22 percent, respectively, of total AcAc-CoA thiolase activities in the absence and in the presence of potassium ion.[199] Therefore, it is difficult to estimate CT activity in assays that do not use immunoprecipitation.

In a liver biopsy from Patient 1, thiolase activity in the cytosolic fraction was in the low-normal range. Increased substrate inhibition was observed with CoA, suggesting a K_m mutant. In fibroblasts from Patient 2, total AcAc-CoA thiolase activity in the presence of potassium ion was about 50 percent of normal, while activity levels of T2 and T1 were normal. Although the decrease in total AcAc-CoA thiolase activity is greater than predicted from our studies of different thiolases, these results are suggestive of CT deficiency. In fibroblasts from Patient 2, cholesterol synthesis was 36–42 percent of normal, a level similar to that seen in cells from patients with mevalonic aciduria (Chap. 93).

Pathophysiology

One can speculate that CT deficiency would decrease the synthesis of cholesterol and other essential isoprenoids like farnesylated protein, heme, ubiquinones, and dolichols, and that complete deficiency may be fatal prenatally. A related disease located on this pathway, mevalonic aciduria (Chap. 93), is associated with mental retardation, failure to thrive, ataxia, cataracts, dysmorphism, and recurrent fever. Similar findings may accompany CT deficiency. Current concepts suggest that CT deficiency should not alter ketone body flux. In any patient with proven CT deficiency, detailed evaluation of both cholesterol and ketone body metabolism would be of great interest.

CONCLUSIONS

Precise diagnosis is now possible for the inborn errors of ketone body metabolism. Their full clinical spectrum remains to be defined. Therapeutic manipulation of ketone body metabolism has potential for treatment of epilepsy and other diseases. Ketone body metabolism illustrates many principles of energy use and coenzyme A metabolism. Several poorly characterized enzymes that mediate other reactions of short-chain acyl-CoA metabolism are potential modifiers of the clinical severity of the inborn errors of ketone body metabolism or may themselves underlie as yet undescribed biochemical diseases.

ACKNOWLEDGMENTS

We thank Seiji Yamaguchi, Shu Pei Wang, Henry Miziorko, K. Michael Gibson, Ronald J. Wanders, and Haruki Nakamura for ongoing collaboration; Jean-Marie Saudubray, France Demaugre, Hélène Ogier, Charles Scriver, and Takashi Hashimoto for their contributions to the early phases of this work; Tadao Orii and Naomi Kondo for their support at Gifu University and the many physicians participating in ongoing molecular and clinical analysis of inborn errors of ketone body metabolism. The following people contributed suggestions or information before publication: G. Berry, G. Besley, J. Dubé, G. Fraudienst-Egger, E. Holme, W. Huth, J. Lacroix, J. Leonard, A. Morris, C. Pérez Cerdá, C. R. Roe, M.-O. Rolland, H. Shintaku, L. Sweetman.

REFERENCES

1. Söling H-D, Seufert C-D: *Biochemical and Clinical Aspects of Ketone Body Metabolism*. Stuttgart, Thieme, 1978.
2. Robinson AM, Williamson DH: Physiological roles of ketone bodies as substrates and signals in mammalian tissues. *Physiol Rev* **60**:143, 1980.
3. McGarry JD, Foster DW: Regulation of hepatic fatty acid oxidation and ketone body production. *Annu Rev Biochem* **49**:395, 1980.
4. McGarry JD, Woeltje KF, Kuwajima M, Foster DW: Regulation of ketogenesis and the renaissance of carnitine palmitoyltransferase. *Diabetes Metab Rev* **5**:271, 1989.
5. Balasse EO, Féry F: Ketone body production and disposal: Effects of fasting, diabetes, and exercise. *Diabetes Metab Rev* **5**:247, 1989.
6. Williamson DH: Ketone body production and metabolism in the fetus and newborn, in Polin RA, Fox WW (eds): *Fetal and Neonatal Physiology*. Philadelphia, Saunders, 1992, p 330.
7. Nosadini R, Avogaro A, Doria A, Fioretto P, Trevisan R, Morocutti A: Ketone body metabolism: A physiological and clinical overview. *Diabetes Metab Rev* **5**:299, 1989.
8. Mitchell GA, Kassovska-Bratinova S, Boukaftane Y, Robert M-F, Wang SP, Ashmarina L, Lambert M, Lapierre P, Potier E: Medical aspects of ketone body metabolism. *Clin Invest Med* **18**:193, 1995.
9. Campbell J, Best CH: Physiologic aspects of ketosis. *Metabolism* **5**:95, 1956.
10. Magnus-Levy A: Die Acetonkörper. *Ergebness der Innerer Med und Kinderheilkeite* **1**:352, 1908.
11. Pedersen KJ: The ketonic decomposition of beta-keto carboxylic acids. *J Am Chem Soc* **51**:2098, 1927.
12. Newsholme EA, Leech AR: *Biochemistry for the Medical Sciences*. New York, Wiley, 1983.
13. Stegink LD, Coon MJ: Stereospecificity and other properties of highly purified beta-hydroxy-beta-methylglutaryl coenzyme A cleavage enzyme from bovine liver. *J Biol Chem* **243**:5272, 1968.
14. Fraser J, Fetter MC, Mast RL, Free AH: Studies with a simplified nitroprusside test for ketone bodies in urine, serum, plasma, and milk. *Clin Chim Acta* **11**:372, 1965.
15. Shih VE, Mandell R, Sheinhait I: General metabolic screening tests, in Hommes FA (ed): *Techniques in Diagnostic Human Biochemical Genetics: A Laboratory Manual*. New York, Wiley-Liss, 1991, p 45.
16. Free AH, Free HM: Nature of nitroprusside reactive material in urine in ketosis. *Am J Clin Pathol* **30**:7, 1958.
17. Williamson DH, Mellanby J, Krebs HA: Enzymic determination of D(−)-β-hydroxybutyric acid and acetoacetic acid in blood. *Biochem J* **82**:90, 1962.
18. Williamson DH, Mellanby J: D-(−)-3-hydroxybutyrate, in Bergmeyer HU (ed): *Methods of Enzymatic Analysis*. New York, Academic Press, 1974, p 1836.
19. Mellanby J, Williamson DH: Acetoacetate, in Bergmeyer HU (ed): *Methods of Enzymatic Analysis*. New York, Academic Press, 1974, p 1840.
20. Foster DW: Diabetes mellitus, in Wilson JD, Braunwald E, Isselbacher KJ, Petersdorf RG, Martin JB, Fauci AS, Root RK (eds): *Harrison's Principles of Internal Medicine* 12th ed. New York, McGraw-Hill, 1991, p 1739.
21. Sonnenberg GE, Keller U: Sampling of arterialized heated-hand venous blood as a noninvasive technique for the study of ketone body kinetics in man. *Metabolism* **31**:1982.
22. Lynen F, Henning UBC, Sörbo B, Kröplin-Rueff L: Der chemische Mechanismus der Acetessigsäurebildung in der Leber. *Biochemische Zeitschrift* **330**:269, 1958.
23. Flatt JP: On the maximal possible rate of ketogenesis. *Diabetes* **21**:50, 1972.
24. Garber AJ, Menzel PH, Boden G, Owen OE: Hepatic ketogenesis and gluconeogenesis in humans. *J Clin Invest* **54**:981, 1974.
25. Reichard GA, Jr., Owen OE, Haff AC, Paul P, Bortz WM: Ketone-body production and oxidation in fasting obese humans. *J Clin Invest* **53**:508, 1974.
26. Goldberg IJ, Holleran S, Ramakrishnan R, Adams M, Palmer RH, Dell RB, Goodman DS: Lack of effect of lovastatin therapy on the parameters of whole body cholesterol metabolism. *J Clin Invest* **86**:801, 1990.
27. Stanley CA, Gonzales E, Baker L: Development of hepatic fatty acid oxidation and ketogenesis in the newborn guinea pig. *Pediatr Res* **17**:224, 1983.
28. Mannaerts GP, Thomas J, Debeer LJ, McGarry JD, Foster DW: Hepatic fatty acid oxidation and ketogenesis after clofibrate treatment. *Biochim Biophys Acta* **529**:201, 1978.
29. Des Rosiers C, David F, Garneau M, Brunengraber H: Nonhomogeneous labeling of liver mitochondrial acetyl-CoA. *J Biol Chem* **266**:1574, 1991.
30. Thompson GN, Chalmers RA, Halliday D: The contribution of protein catabolism to metabolic decompensation in 3-hydroxy-3-methylglutaric aciduria. *Eur J Pediatr* **149**:346, 1990.
31. Metcalfe HK, Monson JP, Welch SG, Cohen RD: Inhibition of lactate removal by ketone bodies in rat liver: Evidence for a quantitatively important role of the plasma membrane lactate transporter in lactate metabolism. *J Clin Invest* **78**:743, 1986.
32. Garcia CK, Brown MS, Pathak RK, Goldstein JL: cDNA cloning of MCT2, a second monocarboxylate transporter expressed in different cells than MCT1. *J Biol Chem* **270**:1843, 1995.
33. Pande SV, Parvin R: Pyruvate and acetoacetate transport in mitochondria. *J Biol Chem* **253**:1565, 1978.
34. Williamson DH, Bates MW, Page MA, Krebs HA: Activities of enzymes involved in acetoacetate utilization in adult mammalian tissues. *Biochem J* **121**:41, 1971.
35. Hawkins RA, Williamson DH, Krebs HA: Ketone-body utilization by adult and suckling rat brain *in vivo*. *Biochem J* **122**:13, 1971.
36. Wick AN, Drury DR: The effect of concentration on the rate of utilization of beta-hydroxybutyric acid by the rabbit. *J Biol Chem* **138**:129, 1941.
37. Fenselau A, Wallis K: Ketone body usage by mammals: Acetoacetate substrate inhibition of CoA transferase from various rat tissues. *Life Sci* **15**:811, 1974.
38. Huth W, Menke R: Regulation of ketogenesis: Mitochondrial acetyl-CoA acetyltransferase from rat liver: Initial-rate kinetics in the presence of the product CoASH reveal intermediary plateau regions. *Eur J Biochem* **128**:413, 1982.
39. Fink G, Desrochers S, Des Rosiers C, Garneau M, David F, Daloze T, Landau BR, et al.: Pseudoketogenesis in the perfused rat heart. *J Biol Chem* **263**:18036, 1988.
40. Weidemann MJ, Krebs HA: The fuel of respiration of rat kidney cortex. *Biochem J* **112**:149, 1969.
41. Williamson JR, Krebs HA: Acetoacetate as fuel of respiration in the perfused rat heart. *Biochem J* **80**:540, 1961.
42. Guzman M, Greelen MJH: Regulation of fatty acid oxidation in mammalian liver. *Biochim Biophys Acta* **1167**:227, 1993.
43. Stralfors P, Olsson H, Belfrage P: Hormone-sensitive lipase, in Boyer PD, Krass EG (eds): *The Enzymes* Vol 18. New York, Academic Press, 1987, p 144.
44. Roach PJ: Multisite and hierarchical protein phosphorylation. *J Biol Chem* **266**:14139, 1991.
45. Holm C, Davis RC, Fredrikson G, Belfrage P, Schotz MC: Expression of biologically active hormone-sensitive lipase in mammalian (COS) cells. *FEBS Lett* **285**:139, 1991.
46. Mabrouk GM, Helmy IM, Thampsy KG, Wakil SJ: Acute hormonal control of acetyl-CoA carboxylase. *J Biol Chem* **265**:6330, 1990.
47. Decaux F-F, Ferré P, Robin D, Robin P, Girard J: Decreased hepatic fatty acid oxidation at weaning in the rat is not linked to a variation of malonyl-CoA concentration. *J Biol Chem* **263**:3284, 1988.
48. Moir AM, Zammit VA: Rapid switch of hepatic fatty acid metabolism from oxidation to esterification during diurnal feeding of meal-fed rats correlates with changes in the properties of acetyl-CoA carboxylase, but not of carnitine palmitoyltransferase I. *Biochem J* **291**:241, 1993.
49. Arias G, Asins G, Hegardt FG, Serra D: The effect of fasting/refeeding and insulin treatment on the expression of the regulatory

genes of ketogenesis in intestine and liver of suckling rats. *Arch Biochem Biophys* **340**:287, 1997.
50. Valera A, Pelegrin M, Asins G, Fillat C, Sabater J, Pujol A, Hegardt FG, et al.: Overexpression of mitochondrial 3-hydroxy-3-methylglutaryl-CoA synthase in transgenic mice causes hepatic hyperketogenesis. *J Biol Chem* **269**:6267, 1994.
51. Page M, Alberti KG, Greenwood R, Gumma KA, Hockaday TD, Lowy C, Nabarro JD, Pyke DA, Sonksen PH, Watkins PJ, West TE: Treatment of diabetic coma with continuous low-dose infusion of insulin. *BMJ* **2**:687, 1974.
52. François B, Bachmann C, Schutgens RBH: Glucose metabolism in a child with 3-hydroxy-3-methylglutaryl-coenzyme A lyase deficiency. *J Inherit Metab Dis* **4**:163, 1981.
53. Randle PJ, Newsholme EA, Garland PB: Regulation of glucose uptake by muscle: Effects of fatty acids, ketone bodies and pyruvate, and of alloxan diabetes and starvation, on the uptake and metabolic fate of glucose in rat heart and diaphragm muscles. *Biochem J* **93**:652, 1964.
54. Randle PJ, England PJ, Denton RM: Control of the tricarboxylate cycle and its interactions with glycolysis during acetate utilization in rat heart. *Biochem J* **117**:677, 1970.
55. Nair KS, Welle SL, Halliday D, Campbell RG: Effect of beta-hydroxybutyrate on whole-body leucine kinetics and fractional mixed skeletal muscle protein synthesis in humans. *J Clin Invest* **82**:198, 1988.
56. Vazquez JA, Adibi SA: Protein sparing during treatment of obesity: Ketogenic versus nonketogenic very low calorie diet. *Metabolism: Clinical & Experimental* **41**:406, 1992.
57. Green A, Newsholme EA: Sensitivity of glucose uptake and lipolysis of white adipocytes of the rat to insulin and effects of some metabolites. *Biochem J* **180**:365, 1979.
58. Henry RR, Brechtel G, Lim K-H: Effects of ketone bodies on carbohydrate metabolism in non-insulin-dependent (type II) diabetes mellitus. *Metabolism: Clinical & Experimental* **39**:853, 1990.
59. Webber J, Simpson E, Parkin H, Macdonald IA: Metabolic effects of acute hyperketonaemia in man before and during an hyperinsulinaemic euglycaemic clamp. *Clin Sci* **86**:677, 1994.
60. Pardridge WM: Blood-brain barrier transport of glucose, free fatty acids, and ketone bodies, in Vranic M, Efendic S, Hollenberg CH (eds): *Fuel Homeostasis and the Nervous System.* New York, Plenum, 1991 p 43.
61. Owen OE, Morgan AP, Kemp HG, Sullivan JM, Herrera MG, Cahill GFJ: Brain metabolism during fasting. *J Clin Invest* **46**:1589, 1967.
62. Edmond J, Robbins RA, Bergstrom JD, Cole RA, de Vellis J: Capacity for substrate utilization in oxidative metabolism by neurons, astrocytes, and oligodendrocytes from developing brain in primary culture. *J Neur Res* **18**:551, 1987.
63. Nehlig A, Pereira de Vasconcelos A: Glucose and ketone body utilization by the brain of neonatal rats. *Prog Neurobiol* **40**:163, 1993.
64. Yeh Y-T, Streuli VL, Zee P: Ketone bodies serve as important precursors of brain lipids in the developing rat. *Lipids* **12**:957, 1977.
65. Auestad N, Fisher R, Chiappelli F, Korsak RA, Edmond J: Growth and development of brain of artificially reared hypoketonemic rat pups. *Proc Soc Exp Biol Med* **195**:335, 1990.
66. Swink TD, Vining EP, Freeman JM: The ketogenic diet. *Adv Pediatr* **44**:297, 1997.
67. Sapir DG, Owen OE: Renal conservation of ketone bodies during starvation. *Metabolism* **24**:23, 1975.
68. Visscher FE: Renal clearance of beta-hydroxybutyric acid in a dog. *Proc Soc Exp Biol Med* **60**:296, 1945.
69. Schwab L, Lotspeich WD: Renal tubular reabsorption of acetoacetate in the dog. *Am J Physiol* **176**:195, 1954.
70. Jorgensen KE, Sheikh MI: Mechanisms of uptake of ketone bodies by luminal-membrane vesicles. *Biochim Biophys Acta* **814**:23, 1985.
71. Goldfinger S, Klinenberg JR, Seegmiller E: Renal retention of uric acid induced by infusion of beta-hydroxybutyrate and acetoacetate. *N Engl J Med* **272**:351, 1965.
72. Lemieux G, Vinay P, Robitaille P, Plante GE, Lussier Y, Martin P: The effect of ketone bodies on renal ammoniagenesis. *J Clin Invest* **50**:1781, 1971.
73. Russell RR III, Taegtmeyer H: Coenzyme A sequestration in rat hearts oxidizing ketone bodies. *J Clin Invest* **89**:968, 1992.
74. Sato K, Kashiwaya Y, Keon CA, Tsuchiya N, King MT, Radda GK, Chance B, et al.: Insulin, ketone bodies, and mitochondrial energy transduction. *FASEB J* **9**:651, 1995.
75. Windmueller HG, Spaeth AE: Identification of ketone bodies and glutamine as the major respiratory fuels *in vivo* for postabsorptive rat small intestine. *J Biol Chem* **253**:69, 1978.
76. Galanello R, Cao A, Olivieri N: Induction of fetal hemoglobin in the presence of increased 3-hydroxybutyric acid associated with beta-ketothiolase deficiency. *N Engl J Med* **331**:746, 1994.
77. Girard JR, Ferré P, Gilbert M, Kervran A, Assan R, Marliss EB: Fetal metabolic response to maternal fasting in the rat. *Am J Physiol* **232**:456, 1977.
78. Moore DCP, Stanisstreet M, Clarke CA: Morphological and physiological effects of beta-hydroxybutyrate on rat embryos grown in vitro at different stages. *Teratology* **40**:237, 1989.
79. Aragon JJ, Lowenstein JM: A survey of enzymes which generate or use acetoacetyl thioesters in rat liver. *J Biol Chem* **258**:4725, 1983.
80. Ayté J, Gil-Gómez G, Haro D, Marrero PF, Hegardt FG: Rat mitochondrial and cytosolic 3-hydroxy-3-methylglutaryl-CoA synthases are encoded by two different genes. *Proc Natl Acad Sci (USA)* **87**:3874, 1990.
81. Boukaftane Y, Duncan A, Wang S, Labuda D, Robert M-F, Sarrazin J, Schappert K, et al: Human mitochondrial HMG CoA synthase (mHS): Liver cDNA and partial genomic cloning, chromosome mapping to 1p12–13 and possible role in vertebrate evolution. *Genomics* **23**:552, 1994.
82. Clinkenbeard KD, Reed WD, Mooney RA, Lane MD: Intracellular localization of the 3-hydroxy-3-methylglutaryl coenzyme A cycle enzymes in liver. *J Biol Chem* **250**:3108, 1975.
83. Buckley BM, Williamson DH: Acetoacetyl-CoA synthetase, a lipogenic enzyme in rat tissues. *FEBS Lett* **60**:7, 1975.
84. Buckley BM, Williamson DH: Acetoacetate and brain lipogenesis: Developmental pattern of acetoacetyl-coenzyme A synthetase in the soluble fraction of rat brain. *Biochem J* **132**:653, 1973.
85. Endemann G, Goetz PG, Edmond J, Brunengraber H: Lipogenesis from ketone bodies in the isolated perfused rat liver. *J Biol Chem* **257**:3434, 1982.
86. Svensson LT, Kilpeläinen SH, Hiltunen JK, Alexson SEH: Characterization and isolation of enzymes that hydrolyze short-chain acyl-CoA in rat-liver mitochondria. *Eur J Biochem* **239**:526, 1996.
87. Sauer F, Erfle JD: On the mechanism of acetoacetate synthesis by guinea pig liver fractions. *J Biol Chem* **241**:30, 1966.
88. Francesconi MA, Donella-Deana A, Furlanetto V, Cavallini L, Palatini P, Deana R: Further purification and characterization of the succinyl-CoA:3-hydroxy-3-methylglutarate coenzyme A transferase from rat-liver mitochondria. *Biochim Biophys Acta* **999**:163, 1989.
89. Gavino VC, Somma J, Philbert L, David F, Garneau M, Bélair J, Brunengraber H: Production of acetone and conversion of acetone to acetate in the perfused rat liver. *J Biol Chem* **262**:6735, 1987.
90. Gerischer U, Dürre P: Cloning, sequencing, and molecular analysis of the acetoacetate decarboxylase gene region from *Clostridium acetobutylicum*. *J Bacteriol* **172**:6907, 1990.
91. Argilás JM: Has acetone a role in the conversion of fat to carbohydrate in mammals? *TIBS* **11**:61, 1998.
92. Boukaftane Y, Mitchell GA: Cloning and characterization of the human mitochondrial 3-hydroxy-3-methylglutaryl CoA synthase gene. *Gene* **195**:121, 1997.
93. Herdt TH, Emery RS: Therapy of diseases of ruminant intermediary metabolism. *Vet Clin North Am* **8**:91, 1992.
94. Nielsen NC, Fleischer S: β-hydroxybutyrate dehydrogenase: Lack in ruminant liver mitochondria. *Science* **166**:1017, 1969.
95. Malcolm A, Dunbrack R, Dunbrack RL: Physiological constraints on life history phenomena: The example of small bear cubs at birth. *Am Naturalist* **127**:735, 1998.
96. Castellini MA, Costa DP: Relationships between plasma ketones and fasting duration in neonatal elephant seals. *Am J Physiol* **259**:R1086, 1998.
97. Phillips JW, Hird FJ: Ketogenesis in vertebrate livers. *Comp Biochem Physiol* **57**:133, 1977.
98. Bailey E, Horne JA: Formation and utilization of acetoacetate and D-3-hydroxybutyrate by various tissues of the adult pigeon (*Columba livia*). *Comp Biochem Physiol* **42B**:659, 1998.
99. Le Maho Y, Vu Van Kha H, Koubi H, Dewasmes G, Girard J, Ferré P, Cagnard M: Body composition, energy expenditure, and plasma metabolites in long-term fasting geese. *Am J Physiol* **241**:E342, 1981.
100. Duée P-H, Pégorier J-P, Quant PA, Herbin C, Kohl C, Girard J: Hepatic ketogenesis in newborn pigs is limited by low mitochondrial 3-hydroxy-3-methylglutaryl-CoA synthase activity. *Biochem J* **298**:207, 1994.

101. Koundakjian PP, Snoswell AM: Ketone body and fatty acid metabolism in sheep tissues: 3-Hydroxybutyrate dehydrogenase, a cytoplasmic enzyme in sheep liver and kidney. *Biochem J* **119**:49, 1970.
102. Crandall LAJ: A comparison of ketosis in man and dog. *J Biol Chem* **138**:123, 1941.
103. Ashmarina LI, Rusnak N, Miziorko HM, Mitchell GA: 3-Hydroxy-3-methylglutaryl-CoA lyase is present in mouse and human liver peroxisomes. *J Biol Chem* **269**:31929, 1994.
104. Quant PA: Experimental application of top-down control analysis to metabolic systems. *Trends Biochem Sci* **18**:26, 1993.
105. Quant PA, Robin D, Robin P, Girard J, Brand MD: A top-down control analysis in isolated rat liver mitochondria: Can the 3-hydroxy-3-methylglutaryl-CoA pathway be rate-controlling for ketogenesis? *Biochim Biophys Acta* **1156**:135, 1993.
106. Miziorko HM: 3-Hydroxy-3-methyglutaryl-CoA synthase from chicken liver. *Methods Enzymol* **110**:19, 1985.
107. Miziorko HM, Clinkenbeard KD, Reed WD, Lane MD: 3-Hydroxy-3-methylglutaryl coenzyme A synthase: Evidence for an acetyl-S-enzyme intermediate and identification of a cysteinyl sulfhydryl as the site of acetylation. *J Biol Chem* **250**:5768, 1975.
108. Miziorko HM, Lane MD: 3-Hydroxy-3-methylglutaryl-CoA synthase: Participation of acetyl-S-enzyme and enzyme-S-hydroxy-methylglutaryl-SCoA intermediates in the reaction. *J Biol Chem* **252**:1414, 1977.
109. Lowe DM, Tubbs PK: 3-hydroxy-3-methylglutaryl-coenzyme A synthase from ox liver. Purification, molecular and catalytic properties. *Biochem J* **227**:591, 1985.
110. Miziorko HM, Behnke CE: Amino acid sequence of an active site peptide of avian liver mitochondrial 3-hydroxy-3-methylglutaryl-CoA synthase. *J Biol Chem* **260**:13513, 1985.
111. Mitchell GA: Unpublished work. 1998.
112. Misra I, Narasimhan C, Miziorko HM: Avian 3-hydroxy-3-methyl-glutaryl-CoA synthase-characterization of a recombinant cholesterogenic isozyme and demonstration of the requirement for a sulfhydryl functionality in formation of the acetyl-enzyme reaction intermediate. *J Biol Chem* **268**:12129, 1993.
113. Ayté J, Gil-Gomez G, Hegardt FG: Nucleotide sequence of a rat liver cDNA encoding the cytosolic 3-hydroxy-3-methylglutaryl coenzyme A synthase. *Nucleic Acids Res* **18**:3642, 1990.
114. Ayté J, Gil-Gomez G, Hegardt FG: Structural characterization of the 3′ noncoding region of the gene encoding rat mitochondrial 3-hydroxy-3-methylglutaryl coenzyme A synthase. *Gene* **123**:267, 1993.
115. Mascaro C, Buesa C, Ortiz JA, Haro D, Hegardt FG: Molecular cloning and tissue expression of human mitochondrial 3-hydroxy-3-methylglutaryl-CoA synthase. *Arch Biochem Biophys* **317**:385, 1995.
116. Gil-Gómez G, Ayté J, Hegardt FG: The rat mitochondrial 3-hydroxy-3-methylglutaryl-coenzyme-A-synthase gene contains elements that mediate its multihormonal regulation and tissue specificity. *Eur J Biochem* **213**:773, 1993.
117. Bouchard L, Boukaftane Y, Bétard C, Hudson TJ, Mitchell GA: The human mitochondrial 3-hydroxy-3-methylglutaryl-CoA synthase gene (HMGCS2): Characterization of an intragenic microsatellite (D1S3752) and gene mapping with radiation hybrids. *Hum Mutat* **12**:291, 1998.
118. Rodriguez JC, Gil-Gómez G, Hegardt FG, Haro D: Peroxisome proliferator-activated receptor mediates induction of the mitochondrial 3-hydroxy-3-methylglutaryl-CoA synthase gene by fatty acids. *J Biol Chem* **269**:18767, 1994.
119. Ayté J, Gil-Gómez G, Hegardt FG: Methylation of the regulatory region of the mitochondrial 3-hydroxy-3-methylglutaryl-CoA synthase gene leads to its transcriptional inactivation. *Biochem J* **295**:807, 1993.
120. Rogers S, Wells R, Rechsteiner M: Amino acid sequences common to rapidly degraded proteins: The PEST hypothesis. *Science* **234**:264, 1986.
121. Serra D, Casals N, Asins G, Royo T, Ciudad CJ, Hegardt FG: Regulation of mitochondrial 3-hydroxy-3-methylglutaryl-coenzyme A synthase protein by starvation, fat feeding, and diabetes. *Arch Biochem Biophys* **307**:40, 1993.
122. Jungermann K, Katz N: Functional specialization of different hepatocyte populations. *Physiol Rev* **69**:708, 1989.
123. Royo T, Pedragosa MJ, Ayté J, Gil-Gómez G, Vilaro S, Hegardt FG: Immunolocalization of mitochondrial 3-hydroxy-3-methylglutaryl CoA synthase in rat liver. *J Cell Physiol* **162**:103, 1995.
124. Pignataro OP, Radicella JP, Calvo JC, Charreau EH: Mitochondrial biosynthesis of cholesterol in Leydig cells from rat testis. *Mol Cell Endocrinol* **33**:53, 1983.
125. Royo T, Pedragosa MJ, Ayté J, Gil-Gómez G, Vilaro S, Hegardt FG: Testis and ovary express the gene for the ketogenic mitochondrial 3-hydroxy-3-methylglutaryl-CoA synthase. *J Lipid Res* **34**:867, 1993.
126. Békési AW, Williamson DH: An explanation for ketogenesis by the intestine of the suckling rat: The presence of an active hydroxymethylglutaryl-coenzyme A pathway. *Biol Neonate* **58**:160, 1990.
127. Cullingford TE, Dolphin CT, Bhakoo KK, Peuchen S, Canevari L, Clark JB: Molecular cloning of rat mitochondrial 3-hydroxy-3-methylglutaryl-CoA lyase and detection of the corresponding mRNA and of those encoding the remaining enzymes comprising the ketogenic 3-hydroxy-3-methylglutaryl-CoA cycle in central nervous system of suckling rat. *Biochem J* **329**(Pt 2):373, 1998.
128. Williamson DH, Bates MW, Krebs HA: Activity and intracellular distribution of enzymes of ketone-body metabolism in rat liver. *Biochem J* **108**:353, 1968.
129. Knight JA, Robertson G, Wu JT: The chemical basis and specificity of the nitrosonaphthol reaction. *Clin Chem* **29**:1969, 1983.
130. Casals N, Roca N, Guerrero M, Gil-Gómez G, Ayté J, Ciudad CJ, Hegardt FG: Regulation of the expression of the mitochondrial 3-hydroxy-3-methylglutaryl-CoA synthase gene: Its role in the control of ketogenesis. *Biochem J* **283**:261, 1992.
131. Hegardt FG: Regulation of mitochondrial 3-hydroxy-3-methylglutaryl-CoA synthase gene expression in liver and intestine from the rat. *Biochem Soc Trans* **23**:486, 1995.
132. Thumelin S, Forestier M, Girard J, Pegorier J-P: Developmental changes in mitochondrial 3-hydroxy-3-methylglutaryl-CoA synthase gene expression in rat liver, intestine and kidney. *Biochem J* **292**:493, 1993.
133. Royo T, Haro D, Hegardt FG: Regulation of cytosolic 3-hydroxy-3-methylglutaryl-CoA synthase mRNA levels by L-tri-iodothyronine. *Biochem J* **289**:557, 1993.
134. Meertens LM, Miyata KS, Cechetto JD, Rachubinski RA, Capone JP: A mitochondrial ketogenic enzyme regulates its gene expression by association with the nuclear hormone receptor PPARα. *EMBO J* **17**: 6972–6978, 1998.
135. Lowe DM, Tubbs PK: Succinylation and inactivation of 3-hydroxy-3-methylglutaryl-CoA synthase by succinyl-CoA and its possible relevance to the control of ketogenesis. *Biochem J* **232**:37, 1985.
136. Quant PA, Tubbs PK, Brand MD: Glucagon activates mitochondrial 3-hydroxy-3-methylglutaryl-CoA synthase in vivo by decreasing the extent of succinylation of the enzyme. *Eur J Biochem* **187**(1):169, 1990.
136a. Siess EA, Fahimi FM, Wieland OH: Decrease by glucagon in hepatic succinyl-CoA. *Biochem Biophys Res Comm* **95**:205, 1980.
137. Ortiz JA, Gil-Gómez G, Casaroli-Marano RP, Vilaro S, Hegardt FG, Haro D: Transfection of the ketogenic mitochondrial 3-hydroxy-3-methylglutaryl-coenzyme A synthase cDNA into Mev-1 cells corrects their auxotrophy for mevalonate. *J Biol Chem* **269**:28523, 1994.
138. Menahan LA, Hron T, Hinkelman DG, Miziorko HM: Interrelationships between 3-hydroxy-3-methylglutaryl-CoA synthase, acetoacetyl-CoA and ketogenesis. *Eur J Biochem* **119**:287, 1981.
139. Mehrabian M, Callaway KA, Clarke CF, Tanaka RD, Greenspan M, Lusis AJ, Sparkes RS, et al: Regulation of rat liver 3-hydroxy-3-methylglutaryl coenzyme A synthase and the chromosomal localization of the human gene. *J Biol Chem* **261**:16249, 1986.
140. Lascelles CV, Quant PA: Investigation of human hepatic mitochondrial 3-hydroxy-3-methylglutaryl-coenzyme A synthase in postmortem or biopsy tissue. *Clin Chim Acta* **260**:85, 1997.
140a. Ijst L, Wanrooij S, Houten S, Waterham HR, Wanders RJA: 3-Hydroxy-3-methyl glutaryl-CoA synthase: Development of a new enzyme assay applicable to liver biopsy specimens. *J Inherit Metab Dis* **23**:107, 2000.
141. Bachhawat BK, Robinson WG, Coon MJ: The enzymatic cleavage of beta-hydroxy-beta-methylglutaryl coenzyme A to aceto-acetate and acetyl coenzyme A. *J Biol Chem* **216**:727, 1955.
142. Roberts JR, Narasimhan C, Hruz PW, Mitchell GA, Miziorko HM: 3-Hydroxy-3-methylglutaryl-CoA lyase: Expression and isolation of the recombinant human enzyme and investigation of a mechanism for regulation of enzyme activity. *J Biol Chem* **269**:17841, 1994.
143. Mitchell GA, Robert M-F, Hruz PW, Fontaine G, Behnke CE, Mende-Mueller LM, Wang S, et al: HMG CoA lyase (HL): Cloning of human and chicken liver HL cDNAs, and characterization of a mutation causing human HL deficiency. *J Biol Chem* **268**:4376, 1993.

144. Hruz PW, Narasimhan C, Miziorko HM: 3-Hydroxy-3-methylglutaryl coenzyme A lyase: Affinity labeling of the *Pseudomonas mevalonii* enzyme and assignment of Cys-237 to the active site. *Biochemistry* **31**:6842, 1992.
145. Kramer PR, Miziorko HM: 3-Hydroxy-3-methylglutaryl-CoA lyase: Catalysis of acetyl coenzyme A enolization. *Biochemistry* **22**:2353, 1983.
146. Roberts JR, Mitchell GA, Miziorko HM: Modeling of a mutation responsible for human 3-hydroxy-3-methylglutaryl-CoA lyase deficiency implicates Histidine-233 as an active-site residue. *J Biol Chem* **271**:24604, 1996.
147. Mitchell GA, Ozand PT, Robert M-F, Ashmarina L, Roberts J, Gibson M, Wanders RJ, et al: HMG CoA lyase deficiency: Identification of five causal point mutations in codons 41 and 42, including a frequent Saudi Arabian mutation, R41Q. *Am J Hum Genet* **62**:295, 1997.
148. Roberts JR, Miziorko HM: Evidence supporting a role for histidine-235 in cation binding to human 3-hydroxy-3-methylglutaryl-CoA lyase. *Biochemistry* **36**:7594, 1997.
149. Ashmarina LI, Robert M-F, Elsliger M-A, Mitchell GA: Characterization of the HMG-CoA lyase precursor, a protein targeted to peroxisomes and mitochondria. *Biochem J* **315**:71, 1996.
150. Roberts JR, Narasimhan C, Miziorko HM: Evaluation of cysteine 266 of human 3-hydroxy-3-methylglutaryl-CoA lyase as a catalytic residue. *J Biol Chem* **270**:17311, 1995.
151. Bischoff KM, Rodwell VW: Biosynthesis and characterization of (*S*)- and (*R*)-3-hydroxy-3-methylglutaryl coenzyme A. *Biochem Med Metab Biol* **48**:149, 1992.
152. Strzelecki T, Thomas JA, Koch CD, LaNoue KF: The effect of hormones on proton compartmentation in hepatocytes. *J Biol Chem* **259**:4122, 1984.
153. Anderson DH, Rodwell VW: Nucleotide sequence and expression in *Escherichia coli* of the 3-hydroxy-3-methylglutaryl coenzyme A lyase gene of *Pseudomonas mevalonii*. *J Bacteriol* **171**:6468, 1989.
154. Wang S, Nadeau JH, Duncan A, Robert M-F, Fontaine G, Schappert K, Johnson KR, et al: 3-Hydroxy-3-methylglutaryl coenzyme A lyase (HL): Cloning and characterization of a mouse liver HL cDNA and subchromosomal mapping of the human and mouse HL genes. *Mamm Genome* **4**:382, 1993.
155. Wang SP, Robert M-F, Gibson KM, Wanders RJA, Mitchell GA: 3-Hydroxy-3-methylglutaryl-CoA lyase (HL): Mouse and human HL gene (HMGCL) cloning and detection of large gene deletions in two unrelated HL-deficient patients. *Genomics* **33**:99, 1996.
156. Hipólito-Reis C, Bailey E, Bartley W: Factors involved in the control of the activity of enzymes of hepatic ketogenesis during development of the rat. *Int J Biochem* **5**:31, 1974.
157. Ashmarina LI, Pshezhetsky AV, Branda SS, Isaya G, Mitchell GA: 3-Hydroxy-3-methylglutaryl coenzyme A lyase: Targeting and processing in peroxisomes and mitochondria. *J Lipid Res* 1998.
158. Marks AR, McIntyre JO, Duncan TM, Erdjument-Bromage H, Tempst P, Fleischer S: Molecular cloning and characterization of (R)-3-hydroxybutyrate dehydrogenase from human heart. *J Biol Chem* **267**:15459, 1992.
159. McIntyre JO, Latruffe N, Brenner SC, Fleischer S: Comparison of 3-hydroxybutyrate dehydrogenase from bovine heart and rat liver mitochondria. *Arch Biochem Biophys* **262**:85, 1988.
160. Lehninger AL, Sudduth HC, Wise JB: D-Beta-hydroxybutyric dehydrogenase of mitochondria. *J Biol Chem* **235**:2450, 1960.
161. Kante A, Malki MC, Coquard C, Latruffe N: Metabolic control of the expression of mitochondrial D-beta-hydroxybutyrate dehydrogenase, a ketone body converting enzyme. *Biochim Biophys Acta* **1033**:291, 1990.
162. Stern JR, Coon MJ, Del Campillo A, Schneider MC: Enzymes of fatty acid metabolism. IV. Preparation and properties of coenzyme A transferase. *J Biol Chem* **221**:15, 1956.
163. Hersh LB, Jencks WP: Coenzyme A transferase: Kinetics and exchange reactions. *J Biol Chem* **242**:3468, 1967.
164. Whitty A, Fierke CA, Jencks WP: Role of binding energy with coenzyme A in catalysis by 3-oxoacid coenzyme A transferase. *Biochemistry* **34**:11678, 1995.
165. Sharp JA, Edwards MR: Initial-velocity kinetics of succinyl-coenzyme A-3-oxo acid coenzyme A-transferase from sheep kidney. *Biochem J* **213**:179, 1983.
166. Moore SA, Jencks WP: Formation of active site thiol esters of CoA transferase and the dependence of catalysis on specific binding interactions. *J Biol Chem* **257**:10893, 1982.
167. Sharp JA, Edwards MR: Purification and properties of succinyl-coenzyme A-3-oxo acid coenzyme A-transferase from sheep kidney. *Biochem J* **173**:759, 1978.
168. Rochet JC, Bridger WA: Identification of glutamate 344 as the catalytic residue in the active site of pig heart CoA transferase. *Protein Sci* **3**:975, 1994.
169. Wierenga RK, Terpstra P, Hol WGJ: Prediction of the occurrence of the ADP-binding beta-alpha-beta fold in proteins, using an amino acid sequence fingerprint. *J Mol Biol* **187**:101, 1986.
170. Williams WA: Structure/function relationships within pig heart CoA transferase. Ph D Thesis. University of Minnesota, Minneapolis, 1990.
171. Rochet J-C, Oikawa K, Hicks LD, Kay CM, Bridger WA, Wolodko WT: Productive interactions between the two domains of pig heart CoA transferase during folding and assembly. *Biochemistry* **36**:8807, 1997.
172. Kassovska-Bratinova S, Fukao T, Song X-Q, Duncan AMV, Chen HS, Robert M-F, Pérez-Cerdá C, et al: Succinyl CoA: 3-oxoacid CoA transferase (SCOT): Human cDNA cloning, human chromosomal mapping to 5p13, and mutation detection in a SCOT-deficient patient. *Am J Hum Genet* **59**:519, 1996.
173. Jacob U, Mack M, Clausen T, Huber R, Buckel W, Messerschmidt A: Glutaconate CoA-transferase from *Acidaminococcus fermentans*: The crystal structure reveals homology with other CoA-transferases. *Structure* **5**:415, 1997.
174. Lin T, Bridger WA: Sequence of a cDNA clone encoding pig heart mitochondrial CoA transferase. *J Biol Chem* **267**:975, 1992.
175. Ganapathi MK, Kwon M, Haney PM, McTiernan C, Javed AA, Pepin RA, Samols D, et al.: Cloning of rat brain succinyl-CoA3-oxoacid CoA-transferase cDNA. *Biochem J* **248**:853, 1987.
176. Fukao T, Mitchell GA, Song X-Q, Nakamura H, Wraith JE, Besley G, Wanders RJA, Niezen-Koning KE, Berry GT, Palmieri M, Kassovska-Bratinova S, Oriil KE, Kondo N: Succinyl-CoA:3-ketoacid CoA transferase (SCOT): Cloning of the human SCOT gene, tertiary structural modelling of the human SCOT monomer and characterization of three pathogenic mutations. *Genomics* 2000 In press.
177. Fukao T: Unpublished work. 1998.
178. Middleton B: The oxoacyl-coenzyme A thiolases of animal tissues. *Biochem J* **132**:717, 1973.
179. Fukao T, Song X-Q, Mitchell GA, Yamaguchi S, Sukegawa K, Hashimoto T, Orii T, et al: Enzymes of ketone body utilization in humans: Protein levels and gene expression in multiple tissues of succinyl-CoA:3-ketoacid CoA transferase and mitochondrial and cytosolic acetoacetyl-CoA thiolases. *Pediatr Res* **42**:498, 1997.
180. Page MA, Williamson DH: Enzymes of ketone-body utilisation in human brain. *Lancet* **66**, 1971.
181. Miyazawa S, Osumi T, Hashimoto T: The presence of a new 3-oxoacyl-CoA thiolase in rat liver peroxisomes. *Eur J Biochem* **103**:589, 1980.
182. Uchida Y, Izai K, Orii T, Hashimoto T: Novel fatty acid beta-oxidation enzymes in rat liver mitochondria. II. Purification and properties of enoyl-coenzyme A (CoA) hydratase/3-hydroxyacyl-CoA dehydrogenase/3-ketoacyl-CoA thiolase trifunctional protein. *J Biol Chem* **267**:1034, 1992.
183. Song XQ, Fukao T, Yamaguchi S, Miyazawa S, Hashimoto T, Orii T: Molecular cloning and nucleotide sequence of complementary DNA for human hepatic cytosolic acetoacetyl-coenzyme A thiolase. *Biochem Biophys Res Commun* **201**:478, 1994.
184. Yamaguchi S, Orii T, Sakura N, Miyazawa S, Hashimoto T: Defect in biosynthesis of mitochondrial acetoacetyl-coenzyme A thiolase in cultured fibroblasts from a boy with 3-ketothiolase deficiency. *J Clin Invest* **81**:813, 1988.
185. Fukao T, Kamijo K, Osumi T, Fujiki Y, Yamaguchi S, Orii T, Hashimoto T: Molecular cloning and nucleotide sequence of cDNA encoding the entire precursor of rat mitochondrial acetoacetyl-CoA thiolase. *J Biochem* **106**:197, 1989.
186. Fukao T, Yamaguchi S, Kano M, Orii T, Fujiki Y, Osumi T, Hashimoto T: Molecular cloning and sequence of the complementary DNA encoding human mitochondrial acetoacetyl-coenzyme A thiolase and study of the variant enzymes in cultured fibroblasts from patients with 3-ketothiolase deficiency. *J Clin Invest* **86**:2086, 1990.
187. Masuno M, Kano M, Fukao T, Yamaguchi S, Soumi T, Hashimoto T, Takahashi E, et al: Chromosome mapping of the human mitochondrial acetoacetyl-coenzyme A thiolase gene to 11q22.3–q23.1 by fluorescence in situ hybridization. *Cytogenet Cell Genet* **60**:121, 1992.

188. Kano M, Fukao T, Yamaguchi S, Orii T, Osumi T, Hashimoto T: Structure and expression of the human mitochondrial acetoacetyl-CoA thiolase-encoding gene. *Gene* **109**:285, 1991.
189. Huth W, Jonas R, Wunderlich I, Seubert W: On the mechanism of ketogenesis and its control: Purification, kinetic mechanism and regulation of different forms of mitochondrial acetoacetyl-CoA thiolases from ox liver. *Eur J Pediatr* **59**:475, 1975.
190. Huth W: The charge heterogeneity of the mitochondrial acetyl-CoA acetyltransferase from rat liver. *Eur J Biochem* **120**:475, 1975.
191. Middleton B, Bartlett K: The synthesis and characterisation of 2-methylacetoacetyl coenzyme A and its use in the identification of the site of the defect in 2-methylacetoacetic and 2-methyl-3-hydroxybutyric aciduria. *Clin Chim Acta* **128**:291, 1983.
192. Gehring H, Harris JI: The active site cysteines of thiolase. *Eur J Biochem* **16**:492, 1970.
193. Masamune S, Walsh CT, Sinskey AJ, Peoples OP: Poly(R)-3-hydroxybutyrate (PHB) biosynthesis: Mechanistic studies on the biological Claisen condensation catalyzed by beta-ketoacyl thiolase. *Pure Appl Chem* **61**:303, 1989.
194. Masamune S, Palmar MAJ, Gambani R, Thompson S, Davies JT, Williams SF, Peoples OP: Bio-Claisen condensation catalyzed by thiolase from *Zoogloea ramigera*: Active site cysteine residues. *J Am Chem Soc* **111**:1879, 1986.
195. Mathieu M, Zeelen JPH, Pauptit RA, Erdmann R, Kunau WH, Wierenga RK: The 2.8 Å crystal structure of peroxisomal 3-ketoacyl-CoA thiolase of *Saccharomyces cerivisiae*: A five layered alpha-beta-alpha-beta-alpha structure constructed from two core domains of identical topology. *Structure* **15**:797, 1994.
196. Fukao T, Nakamura H, Song XQ, Nakamura K, Orii K, Kohno Y, Kano M, et al.: Characterization of N93S, I312T and A333P missense mutations in two Japanese families with mitochondrial acetoacetyl-CoA thiolase deficiency. *Hum Mutat* **12**:245, 1998.
197. Schwerdt G, Huth W: Turnover and transformation of mitochondrial acetyl-CoA acetyltransferase into CoA-modified forms. *Biochem J* **292**:915, 1993.
198. Middleton B: Identification of heterozygotes for the defect of mitochondrial 3-ketothiolase causing 2-methyl-3-hydroxybutyric aciduria. *J Inherit Metab Dis* **10**(Suppl 2):270, 1987.
199. Fukao T, Song XQ, Yamaguchi S, Hashimoto T, Orii T, Kondo N: Immunotitration analysis of cytosolic acetoacetyl-CoA thiolase activity in human fibroblasts. *Pediatr Res* **39**:1055, 1996.
200. Nagasawa H, Yamaguchi S, Orii T, Schutgens RBH, Sweetman L, Hashimoto T: Heterogeneity of defects in mitochondrial acetoacetyl-CoA thiolase biosynthesis in fibroblasts from four patients with 3-ketothiolase deficiency. *Pediatr Res* **26**:145, 1989.
201. Middleton B: The acetoacetyl-coenzyme A thiolases of rat brain and their relative activities during postnatal development. *Biochem J* **132**:731, 1973.
202. Middleton B: The kinetic mechanism and properties of the cytoplasmic acetoacetyl-coenzyme A thiolase from rat liver. *Biochem J* **139**:109, 1974.
203. Masuno M, Fukao T, Song XQ, Orii T, Kondo N, Imaizumi K, Kurozumi Y: Assignment of the human cytosolic acetoacetyl-coenzyme A thiolase (ACAT2) gene to chromosome 6q25.3–q26. *Genomics* **36**:217, 1996.
204. Bonnefont JP, Specola NB, Vassault A, Lombes A, Ogier H, de Klerk JBC, Munnich A, et al: The fasting test in paediatrics: Application to the diagnosis of pathological hypo- and hyperketotic states. *Eur J Pediatr* **150**:80, 1990.
205. Wolsdorf JI, Sadeghi-Nejad A, Senior B: Fat-derived fuels during a 24-hour fast in children. *Eur J Pediatr* **138**:141, 1982.
206. Saudubray JM, Marsac C, Limal JM, Dumurgier E, Charpentier C, Ogier H, Coudé FX: Variation in plasma ketone bodies during a 24-hour fast in normal and in hypoglycemic children: Relationship to age. *J Pediatr* **98**:904, 1981.
207. Morris AA, Thekekara AG, Wilks Z, Clayton PT, Leonard JV, Aynsley-Green A: Evaluation of fasts for investigating hypoglycaemia or suspected metabolic disease. *Arch Dis Child* **75**:115, 1996.
208. Cahill GF, Herrera MG, Morgan AP, Soeldner JS, Steinke J, Levy PL, Reichard GA, et al: Hormone-fuel interrelationships during fasting. *J Clin Invest* **45**:1751, 1966.
209. Marliss EB, Murray FT, Nakhooda AF: The metabolic response to hypocaloric protein diets in obese man. *J Clin Invest* **21**:468, 1978.
210. Owen OE, Felig P, Morgan AP, Wahren J, Cahill GF Jr: Liver and kidney metabolism during prolonged starvation. *J Clin Invest* **48**:574, 1969.
211. Johnson RE, Sargent IF, Passmore R: Normal variations in total ketone bodies in serum and urine of healthy young men. *J Exp Physiol* **43**:339, 1958.
212. Owen OE, Reichard GA, Jr, Boden G, Shuman C: Comparative measurements of glucose, beta-hydroxybutyrate, acetoacetate, and insulin in blood and cerebrospinal fluid during starvation. *Metabolism* **23**:7, 1974.
213. Huttenlocher PR: Ketonemia and seizures: Metabolic and anti-convulsant effects of two ketogenic diets in childhood epilepsy. *Pediatr Res* **10**:536, 1976.
214. Atkins RC: *Dr. Atkins's Diet Revolution.* New York, Bantam, 1973.
215. Falk RE, Cederbaum SD, Blass JP, Gibson GE, Kark R, Carrel RE: Ketogenic diet in the management of pyruvate dehydrogenase deficiency. *Pediatrics* **58**:713, 1976.
216. Seidner G, Garcia Alvarez M, Yeh J-I, O'Driscoll KR, Kelpper J, Stump TS, Wang D, et al: GLUT-1 deficiency syndrome caused by haploinsufficiency of the blood-brain barrier hexose carrier. *Nat Genet* **18**:188, 1998.
217. Dodson WE, Prensky AL, DeVivo DC, Goldring S, Dodge PR: Management of seizure disorders: Selected aspects. *J Pediatr* **89**:695, 1976.
218. Huttenlocher PR, Wilbourn AJ, Signore JM: Medium-chain triglycerides as a therapy for intractable childhood epilepsy. *Neurology* **21**:1097, 1971.
219. Sills MA, Forsythe WI, Haidukewych D, Macdonald A, Robinson M: The medium chain triglyceride diet and intractable epilepsy. *Arch Dis Child* **61**:1168, 1986.
220. Kerwick A, Pawan GLS, Chalmers TM: Resistance to ketosis in obese subjects. *Lancet* **2**:1157, 1959.
221. Girard J, Ferré P, Pégorier J-P, Duée P-H: Adaptations of glucose and fatty acid metabolism during perinatal period and suckling-weaning transition. *Physiol Rev* **72**:507, 1992.
222. Hawdon JM, Ward Platt MP: Metabolic adaptation in small for gestational age infants. *Arch Dis Child* **68**:262, 1993.
223. Persson B, Gentz J: The pattern of blood lipids, glycerol and ketone bodies during the neonatal period, infancy and childhood. *Acta Paediatr Scand* **55**:353, 1966.
224. Melichar V, Drahota Z, Hahn P: Ketone bodies in the blood of full term newborns, premature and dysmature infants and infants of diabetic mothers. *Biol Neonate* **11**:23, 1967.
225. Anday EK, Stanley CA, Baker L, Delivoria-Papadopoulos M: Plasma ketones in newborn infants: Absence of suckling ketosis. *J Pediatr* **98**:628, 1981.
226. Paterson P, Sheath J, Taft P, Wood C: Maternal and foetal ketone concentrations in plasma and urine. *Lancet* **1**:862, 1967.
227. Koeslag JH, Noakes TD, Sloan AW: Post-exercise ketosis. *J Physiol* **301**:79, 1980.
228. Johnson RE, Passmore R, Sargent F: Multiple factors in experimental human ketosis. *Arch Intern Med* **107**:43, 1961.
229. Colle E, Ulstrom RA: Ketotic hypoglycemia. *J Pediatr* **64**:632, 1964, abstract.
230. Pagliara AS, Karl IE, De Vivo DC, Feigin RD, Kipnis DM: Hypoalaninemia: A concomitant of ketotic hypoglycemia. *J Clin Invest* **51**:1440, 1972.
231. Merin S, Crawford JS: Hypoglycemia and infantile cataract. *Arch Ophthalmol* **86**:495, 1971.
232. Wets B, Milot JA, Polomeno RC, Letarte J: Cataracts and ketotic hypoglycemia. *Ophthalmology* **89**:999, 1982.
233. Dahlquist G, Gentz J, Hagenfeldt L, Larsson A, Löw H, Persson B, Zetterström R: Ketotic hypoglycemia of childhood-A clinical trial of several unifying etiological hypotheses. *Acta Paediatr Scand* **68**:649, 1979.
234. Chaussain JL: Glycemic response to 24 hour fast in normal children and children with ketotic hypoglycemia. *J Pediatr* **82**:438, 1973.
235. Chaussain JL, Georges P, Olive G, Job JC: Glycemic response to 24-hour fast in normal children and children with ketotic hypoglycemia: II. Hormonal and metabolic changes. *J Pediatr* **85**:776, 1974.
236. Haymond MW, Karl IE, Pagliara AS, Ketotic hypoglycemia: An amino acid substrate limited disorder. *J Clin Endocrinol Metab* **38**, 521, 1974, abstract.
237. Jenkins D, Close CF, Krentz AJ, Nattrass M, Wright AD: Euglycaemic diabetic ketoacidosis: Does it exist? *Acta Diabetol* **30**:251, 1993.
238. Aynsley-Green A, McGann A, Deshpande S: Control of intermediary metabolism in childhood with special reference to hypoglycaemia and growth hormone. *Acta Paediatr Scand* **377**:43, 1991.

239. Singh I, Srivastava MC: Hyperglycemia: Keto-acidosis and coma in a nondiabetic hyperthyroid patient. *Metabolism* **17**:893, 1968.
240. Avogaro A, Cryer PE, Bier DM: Epinephrine's ketogenic effect in humans is mediated principally by lipolysis. *Am J Physiol* **263**:E250, 1992.
241. Ren J-M, Marshall BA, Mueckler MM, McCaleb M, Amatruda JM, Shulman GI: Overexpression of Glut4 protein in muscle increases basal and insulin-stimulated whole body glucose disposal in conscious mice. *J Clin Invest* **95**:429, 1995.
242. Fulop M: Alcoholic ketoacidosis. *Endocrinol Metab Clin North Am* **22**:209, 1993.
243. Ellenhorn MJ, Barceloux DG: Isopropyl alcohol, in Ellenhorn MJ, Barceloux DG (eds): *Medical Toxicology*. New York, Elsevier, 1988, p 798.
244. Anderson RJ, Potts DE, Gabow PA, Rumack BH, Schrier RW: Unrecognized adult salicylate intoxication. *Ann Intern Med* **85**:745, 1976.
245. Bartels PD, Lund-Jacobsen H: Blood lactate and ketone body concentrations in salicylate intoxication. *Hum Toxicol* **5**:363, 1986.
246. Robinson BH, Sherwood WG, Taylor J, Balfe JW; Mamer OA: Acetoacetyl CoA thiolase deficiency: A cause of severe ketoacidosis in infancy simulating salicylism. *J Pediatr* **95**:228, 1979.
247. De Vasconcelos PRL, Kettlewell MGW, Williamson DH: Time course of changes in hepatic metabolism in response to sepsis in the rat: Impairment of gluconeogenesis and ketogenesis *in vitro*. *Clin Sci* **72**:683, 1987.
248. Lanza-Jacoby S, Rosato E, Braccia G, Tabares A: Altered ketone body metabolism during gram-negative sepsis in the rat. *Metabolism* **39**:1151, 1990.
249. Rosario P, Medina JM: Stimulation of ketogenesis by propionate in isolated rat hepatocytes: An explanation for ketosis associated with propionic acidaemia and methylmalonic acidaemia. *J Inherit Metab Dis* **5**:59, 1982.
250. Lewis GM, Spencer-Peet J, Stewart KM: Infantile hypoglycaemia due to inherited deficiency of glycogen synthetase in liver. *Arch Dis Child* **38**:40, 1963.
251. Aynsley-Green A, Williamson DH, Gitzelmann R: Hepatic glycogen synthetase deficiency: Definition of syndrome from metabolic and enzyme studies on a 9-year-old girl. *Arch Dis Child* **52**:573, 1977.
252. Willems PJ, Gerver WJM, Berger R, Fernandes J: The natural history of liver glycogenosis due to phosphorylase kinase deficiency: A longitudinal study of 41 patients. *Eur J Pediatr* **149**:268, 1990.
253. Binkiewicz A, Senior B: Decreased ketogenesis in von Gierke's disease (type I glycogenosis). *J Pediatr* **83**:973, 1973.
254. Fernandes J, Pikaar NA: Ketosis in hepatic glycogenosis. *Arch Dis Child* **47**:41, 1972.
255. Labrune P, Chalas J, Baussan C, Odièvre M: Tolerance to prolonged fasting in two children with type I glycogen storage disease. *J Inherit Metab Dis* **16**:1044, 1993.
256. Bennett MJ, Weinberger MJ, Kobori JA, Rinaldo P, Burlina AB: Mitochondrial short-chain L-3-hydroxyacyl-coenzyme A dehydrogenase deficiency: A new defect of fatty acid oxidation. *Pediatr Res* **39**:185, 1996.
256a. Patel JS, Leonard JV: Ketonuria and medium-chain-acyl-CoA dehydrogenase deficiency. *J Inherit Metab Dis* **18**(1):98, 1995.
257. Ozaki N, Ringe B, Gubernatis G, Takada Y, Yamaguchi T, Yamaoka Y, Oellerich M, et al: Changes in energy substrates in relation to arterial ketone body ratio after human orthotopic liver transplantation. *Surgery* **113**:403, 1993.
258. Yamaoka Y, Taki Y, Gubernatis G, Nakatani T, Okamoto R, Yamamoto Y, Ishikawa Y, et al: Evaluation of the liver graft before procurement: Significance of arterial ketone body ratio in brain-dead patients. *Transplant Int* **3**:78, 1990.
259. Iwata S, Ozawa Z, Shimahara Y, Mori K, Kobayashi N, Kumada K, Yamaoka Y: Diurnal fluctuations of arterial ketone body ratio in normal subjects and patients with liver dysfunction. *Gastroenterology* **100**:1371, 1991.
260. Saudubray JM, Marsac C, Cathelineau CL, Besson-Leaud M, Leroux JP: Neonatal congenital lactic acidosis with pyruvate carboxylase deficiency in two siblings. *Acta Paediatr Scand* **65**:717, 1998.
261. Thompson GN, Hsu BYL, Pitt JJ, Treacy E, Stanley CA: Fasting hypoketotic coma in a child with deficiency of mitochondrial 3-hydroxy-3-methylglutaryl-CoA synthase. *N Engl J Med* **337**:1203, 1997.
262. Morris AAM, Lascelles CV, Olpin SE, Lake BD, Leonard JV, Quant PA: Hepatic mitochondrial 3-hydroxy-3-methylglutaryl-CoA synthase deficiency. *Pediatr Res* **44**:392, 1998.
263. Faull K, Bolton P, Halpern B, Hammond J, Danks DM, Wilkinson SP, Wysocki SJ, et al: Patient with defect in leucine metabolism. *N Engl J Med* **294**:1013, 1971.
264. Wysocki SJ, Hähnel R: 3-Hydroxy-3-methylglutaryl-coenzyme A lyase deficiency: A review. *J Inherit Metab Dis* **9**:225, 1986.
265. Gibson KM, Breuer J, Kaiser K, Nyhan WL, McCoy EE, Ferreira P, Greene CL, et al: 3-Hydroxy-3-methylglutaryl-coenzyme A lyase deficiency: Report of five new patients. *J Inherit Metab Dis* **11**:76, 1988.
266. Gibson KM, Breuer J, Nyhan WL: 3-Hydroxy-3-methylglutaryl-coenzyme A lyase deficiency: Review of 18 reported patients. *Eur J Pediatr* **148**:180, 1988.
267. Ozand PT, Aqeel A, Gascon G, Brismar J, Thomas E: 3-Hydroxy-3-methylglutaryl-coenzyme A (HMG-CoA) lyase deficiency in Saudi Arabia. *J Inherit Metab Dis* **14**:174, 1991.
268. Stacey TE, de Sousa C, Tracey BM, Whitelaw A, Mistry J, Timbrell P, Chalmers RA: Dizygotic twins with 3-hydroxy-3-methylglutaric aciduria: Unusual presentation, family studies and dietary management. *Eur J Pediatr* **144**:177, 1985.
269. Schutgens RBH, Heymans H, Ketel A, Veder HA: Lethal hypoglycemia in a child with a deficiency of 3-hydroxy-3-methylglutarylcoenzyme A lyase. *J Pediatr* **94**:89, 1979.
270. Ferris NJ, Tien RD: Cerebral MRI in 3-hydroxy-3-methylglutaryl-coenzyme A lyase deficiency: Case report. *Neuroradiology* **35**:559, 1993.
271. Lisson G, Leupold D, Bechinger D, Wallesch C: CT finding in a case of deficiency of 3-hydroxy-3-methylglutaryl-CoA lyase. *Neuroradiology* **22**:99, 1981.
272. Gordon K, Riding M, Camfield P, Bawden H, Ludman M, Bagnell P: CT and MR of 3-hydroxy-3-methylglutaryl-coenzyme A lyase deficiency. *AJNR* **15**:1474, 1994.
273. Mitchell GA, Jakobs C, Gibson KM, Robert M-F, Burlina A, Dionisi-Vici C, Dallaire L: Molecular prenatal diagnosis of 3-hydroxy-3-methylglutaryl CoA lyase deficiency. *Prenat Diagn* **15**:725, 1995.
274. Leupold D, Bojasch M, Jakobs C: 3-Hydroxy-3-methylglutaryl-CoA lyase deficiency in an infant with macrocephaly and mild metabolic acidosis. *Eur J Pediatr* **138**:73, 1982.
275. Leonard JV, Seakins JWT, Griffin NK: Beta-hydroxy-beta-methylglutaricaciduria presenting as Reye's syndrome. *Lancet* **1**:680, 1979.
276. Gibson KM, Cassidy SB, Seaver LH, Wanders RJ, Kennaway NG, Mitchell GA, Spark RP: Fatal cardiomyopathy associated with 3-hydroxy-3-methylglutaryl-CoA lyase deficiency. *J Inherit Metab Dis* **17**:291, 1994.
277. Wilson WG, Cass MB, Sovik O, Gibson KM, Sweetman L: A child with acute pancreatitis and recurrent hypoglycemia due to 3-hydroxy-3-methylglutaryl-CoA lyase deficiency. *Eur J Pediatr* **142**:289, 1984.
278. Jones KJ, Wilcken B, Kilham H: The long-term evolution of a case of 3-hydroxy-3-methylglutaryl-coenzyme A lyase deficiency associated with deafness and retinitis pigmentosa. *J Inherit Metab Dis* **20**:833, 1997.
279. Robinson BH, Oei J, Sherwood WG, Slyper AH, Heininger J, Mamer OA: Hydroxymethylglutaryl CoA lyase deficiency: Features resembling Reye syndrome. *Neurology* **30**:714, 1980.
280. Zoghbi HY, Spence JE, Beaudet AL, O'Brien WE, Goodman CJ, Gibson KM: Atypical presentation and neuropathological studies in 3-hydroxy-3-methylglutaryl-CoA lyase deficiency. *Ann Neurol* **20**:367, 1986.
281. Wanders R, Schutgens R, Zoeters P: 3-Hydroxy-3-methylglutaryl-CoA lyase in human skin fibroblasts: Study of its properties and deficient activity in 3-hydroxy-3-methylglutaric aciduria patients using a simple spectrophotometric method. *Clin Chim Acta* **171**:95, 1988.
282. Gibson KM: Assay of 3-hydroxy-3-methylglutaryl-CoA lyase. *Methods Enzymol* **166**:219, 1988.
283. Wanders RJA, Zoeters PHM, Schutgens RBH, de Klerk JBC, Duran M, Wadman SK, van Sprang FJ, et al: Rapid diagnosis of 3-hydroxy-3-methylglutaryl-coenzyme A lyase deficiency via enzyme activity measurements in leukocytes or platelets using a simple spectrophotometric method. *Clin Chim Acta* **189**:327, 1990.
284. Gibson KM, Lee CF, Kamali V, Johnston K, Beaudet AL, Craigen WJ, Powell BR, et al: 3-Hydroxy-3-methylglutaryl-CoA lyase deficiency as detected by radiochemical assay in cell extracts by thin-layer chromatography, and identification of three new cases. *Clin Chem* **36**:297, 1990.
285. Wanders RJA, Schutgens RBH, Zoeters BHM: Prenatal diagnosis of 3-hydroxy-3-methylglutaric aciduria via enzyme activity measurements in chorionic villi, chorionic villous fibroblasts or amniocytes

using a simple spectrophotometric method. *J Inherit Metab Dis* **11**:430, 1988.

286. Barash V, Elpeleg O, Sheffer R, Mandel H, Wanders RJA: Measurement of 3-hydroxy-3-methylglutaryl-CoA lyase activity in amniotic cells and in chorionic villi. *Prenat Diagn* **8**:691, 1988.
287. Buesa C, Pie J, Barcelo A, Casals N, Mascaro C, Casale CH, Haro D, et al: Aberrantly spliced mRNAs of the 3-hydroxy-3-methylglutaryl coenzyme A lyase (HL) gene with a donor splice-site point mutation produce hereditary HL deficiency. *J Lipid Res* **37**:2420, 1996.
288. Pie J, Casals N, Casale CH, Buesa C, Mascaro C, Barcelo A, Rolland MO, et al: A nonsense mutation in the 3-hydroxy-3-methylglutaryl-CoA lyase gene produces exon skipping in two patients of different origin with 3-hydroxy-3-methylglutaryl-CoA lyase deficiency. *Biochem J* **323**(Pt 2):329, 1997.
289. Casals N, Pié J, Casale CH, Zapater N, Ribes A, Castro-Gago M, Rodriguez-Segade S, et al.: A two-base deletion in exon 6 of the 3-hydroxy-3-methylglutaryl coenzyme A lyase (HL) gene producing the skipping of exons 5 and 6 determines 3-hydroxy-3-methylglutaric aciduria. *J Lipid Res* **38**:2303, 1997.
290. Duran M, Schutgens RBH, Ketel A, Heymans H, Berntssen MWJ, Ketting D, Wadman SK: 3-hydroxy-3-methylglutaryl coenzyme A lyase deficiency: Postnatal management following prenatal diagnosis by analysis of maternal urine. *J Pediatr* **95**:1004, 1979.
291. Wang SP, Marth JD, Oligny L, Vachon M, Robert M-F, Ashmarina L, Mitchell GA: 3-hydroxy-3-methylglutaryl-CoA lyase (HL): Gene targeting causes prenatal lethality in HL-deficient mice. *Hum Mol Genet* **17**:2057, 1998.
292. Ozand PT, Devol EB, Gascon GG: Neurometabolic diseases at a national referral center: Five years experience at the King Faisal specialist hospital and research centre. *J Child Neurol* **7**:(Suppl4), 1992.
293. Barash V, Mandel H, Sella S, Geiger R: 3-Hydroxy-3-methylglutaryl-coenzym A lyase deficiency: Biochemical studies and family investigation of four generations. *J Inherit Metab Dis* **13**:156, 1990.
294. Applegarth DA, Macleod Toone JR, Kirby LT, Maclean JR, Mamer OA, Montgomery JA: Organic acids and Reye's syndrome. *Lancet* **1**:1147, 1979.
295. Truscott RJW, Halpern B, Wysocki SJ, Hahnel R, Wilcken B: Studies on a child suspected of having a deficiency in 3-hydroxy-3-methylglutaryl-CoA lyase. *Clin Chim Acta* **95**:11, 1979.
296. Hammond J, Wilcken B: 3-Hydroxy-3-methylglutaric, 3-methylglutaconic and 3-methylglutaric acids can be non-specific indicators of metabolic disease. *J Inherit Metab Dis* **7**(Suppl 2):117, 1984.
296a. Melov S, Coskun P, Patel M, Tuinstra R, Cottrell B, Jun AS, Zastawny TH, Dizdaroglu M, Goodman SI, Huang TT, Miziorko H, Epstein CJ, Wallace DC: Mitochondrial disease in superoxide dismutase 2 mutant mice. *Proc Natl Acad Sci USA* **96**:846, 1999.
297. Tildon JT, Cornblath M: Succinyl-CoA:3-ketoacid CoA-transferase deficiency: A cause for ketoacidosis in infancy. *J Clin Invest* **51**:493, 1972.
298. Spence MW, Murphy MG, Cook HW, Ripley BA, Embil JA: Succinyl-CoA:3-ketoacid CoA-transferase deficiency: A "new" phenotype? *Pediatr Res* **7**:394, 1973.
299. Middleton B, Day R, Lombes A, Saudubray JM: Infantile ketoacidosis associated with decreased activity of succinyl-CoA:3-ketoacid CoA-transferase. *J Inherit Metab Dis* **10**:273, 1987.
300. Saudubray JM, Specola N, Middleton B, Lombes A, Bonnefont JP, Jakobs C, Vassault A, Charpentier C, Day R: Hyperketotic states due to inherited defects of ketolysis. *Enzyme* **38**:80, 1987.
301. Pérez-Cerdá C, Merinero B, Sanz P, Jiménez A, Hernández C, García MJ, Ugarte M: A new case of succinyl-CoA:acetoacetate transferase deficiency. *J Inherit Metab Dis* **15**:371, 1992.
302. Sakazaki H, Hirayama K, Murakami S, Yonezawa S, Shintaku H, Sawada Y, Fukao T, et al: A new Japanese case of succinyl-CoA:3-ketoacid CoA-transferase deficiency. *J Inherit Metab Dis* **18**:323, 1995.
303. Pretorius CJ, Loy Son GG, Bonnici F, Harley EH: Two siblings with episodic ketoacidosis and decreased activity of succinyl-CoA:3-ketoacid CoA-transferase in cultured fibroblasts. *J Inherit Metab Dis* **19**:296, 1996.
304. Niezen-Koning KE, Wanders RJ, Ruiter JP, Ijlst L, Visser G, Reitsma-Bierens WC, Heymans HS, et al: Succinyl-CoA: acetoacetate transferase deficiency: Identification of a new patient with a neonatal onset and review of the literature. *Eur J Pediatr* **156**:870, 1997.
305. Snyderman SE, Sansaricq C, Middleton B: Succinyl-CoA:3-ketoacid CoA-transferase deficiency. *Pediatrics* **101**:709, 1998.
306. Berry G: Unpublished work, 1998.
307. Song X-Q, Fukao T, Mitchell GA, Kassovska-Bratinova S, Ugarte M, Wanders RJA, Kirayama K, et al: Succinyl-CoA:3-ketoacid coenzyme A transferase (SCOT): Development of an antibody to human SCOT and diagnostic use in hereditary SCOT deficiency. *Biochim Biophys Acta* **1360**:151, 1997.
308. Song X-Q, Fukao T, Watanabe H, Shintaku H, Hirayama K, Kassovska-Bratinova S, Kondo N, et al: Succinyl-CoA: 3-ketoacid CoA transferase (SCOT) deficiency: Two pathogenic mutations, V133E and C456F, in Japanese siblings. *Hum Mutat* **12**:83, 1998.
309. Fukao T, Song XQ, Watanabe H, Hirayama K, Sakazaki H, Shintaku H, Imanaka M, Orii T, Kondo N: Prenatal diagnosis of succinyl-coenzyme A: 3-ketoacid coenzyme A transferase deficiency. *Prenat Diagn* **16**:471, 1996.
310. Rolland MO, Guffon N, Mandon G, Divry P: Succinyl-CoA:aceto-acetate transferase deficiency: Identification of a new case; prenatal exclusion in three further pregnancies. *J Inherit Metab Dis* **21**:687, 1998.
311. Tildon JT, Leffler AT, Cornblath M, Stevenson J: Abnormal glucose metabolism in skin fibroblasts cultured from a patient with a new syndrome of ketoacidemia. *Pediatr Res* **5**:518, 1972.
312. Daum RS, Scriver CR, Mamer OA, Delvin E, Lamm P, Goldman H: An inherited disorder of isoleucine catabolism causing accumulation of alpha-methylacetoacetate and alpha-methyl-beta-hydroxybutyrate, and intermittent metabolic acidosis. *Pediatr Res* **7**:149, 1973.
313. Leonard JV, Middleton B, Seakins JWT: Acetoacetyl CoA thiolase deficiency presenting as ketotic hypoglycemia. *Pediatr Res* **21**:211, 1987.
314. Fontaine M, Briand G, Ser N, Armelin I, Rolland MO, Degand P, Vamecq J: Metabolic studies in twin brothers with 2-methylacetoacetyl-CoA thiolase. *Clin Chim Acta* **255**:67, 1996.
315. Hillman RE, Keating JP: Beta-ketothiolase deficiency as a cause of the "ketotic hyperglycinemia syndrome." *Pediatrics* **53**:221, 1974.
316. Merinero B, Pérez-Cerdá C, García MJ, Carrasco S, Lama R, Ugarte M, Middleton B: Beta-ketothiolase deficiency: Two siblings with different clinical conditions. *J Inherit Metab Dis* **10**:276, 1987.
317. Fukao T, Kodama A, Aoyanagi N, Tsukino R, Uemura S, Song XQ, Kondo N: Mild form of beta-ketothiolase deficiency (mitochondrial acetoacetyl-CoA thiolase deficiency) in two Japanese siblings: Identification of detectable residual activity and cross-reactive material in EB-transformed lymphocytes. *Clin Genet* **50**:263, 1996.
318. Schutgens RB, Middleton B, Blij JF, Oorthuys JW, Veder HA, Vulsma T, Tegelaers WH: Beta-ketothiolase deficiency in a family confirmed by in vitro enzymatic assays in fibroblasts. *Eur J Pediatr* **139**:39, 1982.
319. Keating JP, Feigin RD, Tenenbaum SM, Hillman RE: Hyperglycinemia with ketosis due to a defect in isoleucine metabolism: A preliminary report. *Pediatrics* **50**:890, 1972.
320. Henry CG, Strauss AW, Keating JP, Hillman RE: Congestive cardiomyopathy associated with beta-ketothiolase deficiency. *J Pediatr* **99**:754, 1981.
321. Gompertz D, Saudubray JM, Charpentier C, Bartlett K, Goodey PA, Draffan GH: A defect in L-isoleucine metabolism associated with 2-methyl-beta-hydroxybutyric and 2-methylacetoacetic aciduria: Quantitative *in vivo* and *in vitro* studies. *Clin Chim Acta* **57**:269, 1974.
322. Halvorsen S, Stokke O, Jellum E: A variant form of 2-methyl-3-hydroxybutyric and 2-methylacetoacetic aciduria. *Acta Paediatr Scand* **68**:123, 1979.
323. Ozand PT, Rashed M, Gascon GG, Odaib AA, Shums A, Nester M, Brismar J: 3-Ketothiolase deficiency: A review and four new patients with neurologic symptoms. *Brain Dev* **16**(suppl):38, 1994.
324. Middleton B, Bartlett K, Romanos A, Vazquez JG, Conde C, Cannon RA, Lipson M, Sweetman L, Nyhan WL: Beta-ketothiolase deficiency in a family confirmed by in vitro enzymatic assays in fibroblasts. *Eur J Pediatr* **144**:586, 1986.
325. Wajner M, Sanseverino MT, Giugliani R, Sweetman L, Yamaguchi S, Fukao T, Shih VE: Biochemical investigation of a Brazilian patient with a defect in mitochondrial acetoacetyl-coenzyme A thiolase. *Clin Genet* **42**:202, 1992.
326. Jänisch W, Hesse V, Fiedler B, Förster H, Böhles H: Pathomorphologische befunde bei ketothiolasemangel. *Zentralbl Pathol* **139**:245, 1993.
327. Sewell AC, Herwig J, Wiegratz I, Lehnert W, Niederhoff N, Song XQ, Kondo N, Fukao T Mitochondrial acetoacetyl-CoA thiolase (beta-ketothiolase) deficiency and pregnancy. *J Inherit Metab Dis* **21**:441, 1998.
328. Aramaki S, Lehotay D, Sweetman L, Nyhan WL, Winter SC, Middleton B: Urinary excretion of 2-methylacetoacetate, 2-methyl-3-

hydroxybutyrate and tiglylglycine after isoleucine loading in the diagnosis of 2-methylacetoacetyl-CoA thiolase deficiency. *J Inherit Metab Dis* **14**:63, 1991.

329. Sweetman L, Williams JC: Branched chain organic acidurias, in Scriver CR, Beaudet AL, Sly WS, Valle D (eds): *The Metabolic and Molecular Bases of Inherited Disease* 7th ed. New York, McGraw-Hill, 1995, p 1387.
330. Daum RS, Lamm PH, Mamer OA, Scriver CR: A "new" disorder of isoleucine catabolism. *Lancet* **2**:1289, 1971.
331. Cromby CH, Manning NJ, Pollitt RJ, Powell S, Bennet MJ: 6-Methyluracil excretion in 2-methylacetoacetyl-CoA thiolase deficiency and in two children with an unexplained recurrent ketoacidemia. *J Inherit Metab Dis* **17**:81, 1994.
332. Riudor E, Ribes A, Pérez-Cerdá C, Arranz JA, Mora J, Yeste D, Castello R, et al: Metabolic coma with ketoacidosis and hyperglycaemia in 2-methylacetoacetyl-CoA thiolase deficiency. *J Inherit Metab Dis* **18**:748, 1995.
333. Millington DS, Roe CR, Maltby DA: Characterization of new diagnostic acylcarnitines in patients with beta-ketothiolase deficiency and glutaric aciduria type I using mass spectrometry. *Biomed Envir Mass Spectrometry* **14**:711, 1987.
334. Roe C: Unpublished work. 1998.
335. Yamaguchi S, Sakai A, Fukao T, Wakazo, Kuwahara T, Orii T, Hashimoto T: Biochemical and immunochemical study of seven families with 3-ketothiolase deficiency: Diagnosis of heterozygotes using immunochemical determination of the ratio of mitochondrial acetoacetyl-CoA thiolase and 3-ketoacyl-CoA thiolase proteins. *Pediatr Res* **33**:429, 1993.
336. Daum RS, Lamm PH, Mamer OA, Scriver CR: A "new" disorder of isoleucine catabolism. *Lancet* **2**:1289, 1971.
337. Gibson KM, Lee CF, Kamali V, Sovik O: A coupled assay detecting defects in fibroblast isoleucine degradation distal to enoyl-CoA hydratase: Application to 3-oxothiolase deficiency. *Clin Chim Acta* **205**:127, 1992.
338. Iden P, Middleton B, Robinson BH, Sherwood WG, Gibson KM, Sweetman L, Sovik O: 3-Oxothiolase activities and [1-^{14}C]2-methylbutanoic acid incorporation in cultured fibroblasts from 13 cases of suspected 3-oxothiolase deficiency. *Pediatr Res* **28**:518, 1990.
339. Fukao T, Yamaguchi S, Orii T, Hashimoto T: Molecular basis of beta-ketothiolase deficiency: Mutations and polymorphisms in the human mitochondrial acetoacetyl-coenzyme A thiolase gene. *Hum Mutat* **5**:113, 1995.
340. Wakazono A, Fukao T, Yamaguchi S, Hori T, Orii T, Lambert M, Mitchell GA, Lee GW, Hashimoto T: Molecular, biochemical, and clinical characterization of mitochondrial acetoacetyl coenzyme A thiolase deficiency in two further patients. *Hum Mutat* **5**:34, 1995.
341. Kuwahara T, Fukao T, Kano M, Yamaguchi S, Orii T, Hashimoto T: Identification of Taq I polymorphism in the mitochondrial acetoacetyl-CoA thiolase gene and familial analysis of 3-ketothiolase deficiency. *Hum Genet* **90**:208, 1992.
342. Fukao T, Yamaguchi S, Wakazono A, Orii T, Hoganson G, Hashimoto T: Identification of a novel exonic mutation at −13 from the 5′ splice site causing exon skipping in a girl with mitochondrial acetoacetyl-coenzyme A thiolase deficiency. *J Clin Invest* **93**:1034, 1994.
343. Dietz HC, Valle D, François B, Kendzior RJJ, Pyeritz RE, Cutting GR: The skipping of constitutive exons in vivo induced by nonsense mutations. *Science* **259**:680, 1993.
344. Fukao T, Yamaguchi S, Orii T, Osumi T, Hashimoto T: Molecular basis of 3-ketothiolase deficiency: Identification of an AG to AC substitution at the splice acceptor site of intron 10 causing exon 11 skipping. *Biochim Biophys Acta* **1139**:184, 1992.
345. Fukao T, Song XQ, Yamaguchi S, Kondo N, Matthieu JM, Bachmann C, Orii T: Identification of three novel frameshift mutations (83delAT, 754indCT and 435+1G to A) of mitochondrial acetoacetyl-coenzyme A thiolase gene in two Swiss patients with CRM-negative beta-ketothiolase deficiency. *Hum Mutat* **9**:277, 1997.
346. Fukao T, Yamaguchi S, Scriver CR, Dunbar G, Wakazono A, Kano M, Orii T, Hashimoto T: Molecular studies of mitochondrial acetoacetyl-coenzyme A thiolase in two original families. *Hum Mutat* **2**:214, 1993.
347. Fukao T, Yamaguchi S, Tomatsu S, Orii T, Frauendienst-Egger G, Schrod L, Osumi T, Hashimoto T: Evidence for a structural mutation (^{347}Ala to Thr) in a German family with 3-ketothiolase deficiency. *Biochem Biophys Res Commun* **179**:124, 1991.
348. Fukao T, Wakazono A, Song XQ, Yamaguchi S, Zacharias R, Donlan MA, Orii T: Prenatal diagnosis in a family with mitochondrial acetoacetyl-CoA thiolase deficiency with the use of the polymerase chain reaction followed by the heteroduplex detection method. *Prenat Diagn* **15**:363, 1995.
349. Hiyama K, Sakura N, Matsumoto T, Kuhara T: Deficient beta-ketothiolase activity in leukocytes from a patient with 2-methylacetoacetic aciduria. *Clin Chim Acta* **155**:189, 1986.
350. Sebetta G, Bachmann C, Giardini O, Castro M, Gambarara M, Dionisi-Vici C, Bartlett K, Middleton B: Beta-ketothiolase deficiency with favorable evolution. *J Inherit Metab Dis* **10**:405, 1987.
351. Wildenthal K, Mierzwiak DS, Mysers RW, Mitchell JH: Effects of acute lactic acidosis on left ventricular performance. *Am J Physiol* **214**:1352, 1968.
352. Morgan P, Ward B: Hyperventilation and changes in the electroencephalogram and electroretinogram. *Neurology* **20**:1009, 1970.
353. Posner JB, Plum F: Spinal-fluid pH and neurologic symptoms in systemic acidosis. *N Engl J Med* **277**:605, 1967.
354. Okuda Y, Adrogue HJ, Field JB, Nohara H, Yamashita K: Counterproductive effects of sodium bicarbonate in diabetic ketoacidosis. *J Clin Endocrinol Metab* **81**:314, 1996.
355. Graf H, Leach W, Arieff AI: Evidence for a detrimental effect of bicarbonate therapy in hypoxic lactic acidosis. *Science* **227**:754, 1984.
356. Arieff AI, Leach W, Park R, Lazarowitz VC: Systemic effects of $NaHCO_3$ in experimental lactic acidosis in dogs. *Am J Physiol* **242**:F586, 1982.
357. Dixon MA, Leonard JV: Intercurrent illness in inborn errors of metabolism. *Arch Dis Child* **67**:1387, 1992.
358. Flatt JP, Ravussin E, Acheson KJ, Jéquier E: Effects of dietary fat on postprandial substrate oxidation and on carbohydrate and fat balances. *J Clin Invest* **76**:1019, 1985.
359. Binnert C, Pachiaudi C, Beylot M, Croset M, Cohen R, Riou JP, Laville M: Metabolic fate of an oral long-chain triglyceride load in humans. *Am J Physiol* **270**:E445, 1996.
360. De Groot CJ, Luit-De Haan G, Hulstaert CE, Hoomes FA: A patient with severe neurologic symptoms and acetoacetyl-CoA thiolase deficiency. *Pediatr Res* **11**:1112, 1977.
361. Bennett MJ, Hosking GP, Smith MF, Gray RGF, Middleton B: Biochemical investigations on a patient with a defect in cytosolic acetoacetyl-CoA thiolase, associated with mental retardation. *J Inherit Metab Dis* **7**:125, 1984.
362. Watanabe H, Yamaguchi S, Kimura M, Wakazono A, Song XQ, Fukao T, Orii T: Practical assay method of cytosolic acetoacetyl-CoA thiolase by rapid release of cytosolic enzymes from cultured lymphocytes using digitonin. *Tohoku J Exp Med* **184**:29, 1998.
363. Abe H, Ohtake A, Yamamoto S, Satoh Y, Takayanagi M, Amaya Y, Takiguchi M, Sakuraba H, Suzuki Y, Mori M, Niimi H: Cloning and sequence analysis of a full length cDNA encoding human mitochondrial 3-oxoacyl-CoA thiolase. *Biochim Biophys Acta* **1216**:304, 1993.
364. Kamijo T, Aoyama T, Miyazaki J-I, Hashimoto T: Molecular cloning of the cDNAs for the subunits of rat mitochondrial fatty acid beta-oxidation multienzyme complex. *J Biol Chem* **268**:26452, 1993.
365. Fairbairn LJ, Tanner MJA: Complete cDNA sequence of human foetal liver peroxisomal 3-oxoacyl-CoA thiolase. *Nucleic Acids Res* **17**:3588, 1989.
366. Fukao T, Yamaguchi S, Orii T, Schutgens RB, Osumi T, Hashimoto T: Identification of three mutant alleles of the gene for mitochondrial acetoacetyl-coenzyme A thiolase: A complete analysis of two generations of a family with 3-ketothiolase deficiency. *J Clin Invest* **89**:474, 1992.
367. Fukao T, Song XQ, Yamaguchi S, Orii T, Wanders RJ, Poll-The BT, Hashimoto T: Mitochondrial acetoacetyl-coenzyme A thiolase gene: A novel 68-bp deletion involving a 3′ splice site of intron 7, causing exon 8 skipping in a Caucasian patient with beta-ketothiolase deficiency. *Hum Mutat* **5**:94, 1995.

CHAPTER 103

Defects of Electron Transfer Flavoprotein and Electron Transfer Flavoprotein-Ubiquinone Oxidoreductase: Glutaric Acidemia Type II

Frank E. Frerman ▪ Stephen I. Goodman

1. **Electron transfer flavoprotein (ETF) and ETF-ubiquinone oxidoreductase (ETF-QO) are nuclear encoded proteins through which electrons from flavoprotein acyl CoA dehydrogenases, dimethylglycine dehydrogenase, and sarcosine dehydrogenase enter ubiquinone in the respiratory chain. Inherited defects of either protein cause glutaric acidemia type II.**
2. **Glutaric acidemia type II is characterized clinically by hypoketotic hypoglycemia and metabolic acidosis; pathologically by fatty infiltration of the liver, heart, and kidneys; and biochemically by a diagnostic organic aciduria. Complete enzyme defects, especially of ETF-QO, are often associated with multiple congenital anomalies, including renal cystic dysplasia, and death in infancy.**
3. **Primary defects of ETF-QO and those of either ETF subunit are inherited as autosomal recessive traits. Several pathogenic mutations have been identified in the genes for ETF-QO and the α-ETF subunit. No single ETF-QO mutation is common, but of six that have been identified in the α-ETF gene, αT266M may account for about 40 percent of mutant alleles.**
4. **Prenatal diagnosis of glutaric acidemia type II is possible in some cases by demonstrating increased concentrations of glutaric acid in amniotic fluid, acylcarnitine esters in maternal urine, or impaired substrate oxidation by cultured amniocytes.**
5. **There is no effective treatment for glutaric acidemia type II patients who present in early infancy. Treatment with riboflavin, glycine, and L-carnitine and diets restricted in fat and protein may be effective in less severely affected patients.**

A list of standard abbreviations is located immediately preceding the index in each volume. Nonstandard abbreviations used in this chapter include: DMGDH = dimethylglycine dehydrogenase; ETF = electron transfer flavoprotein; ETF_{ox} = oxidized ETF; ETF_{1e-} = ETF semiquinone; ETF_{2e-} = ETF hydroquinone; ETF-QO = ETF-ubiquinone oxidoreductase; GA2 = glutaric acidemia type II; MADD = multiple acyl CoA dehydrogenation deficiency; MCAD = medium-chain acyl CoA dehydrogenase; and SDH = sarcosine dehydrogenase.

BIOCHEMISTRY OF ELECTRON TRANSFER FLAVOPROTEIN (ETF) AND ETF-UBIQUINONE OXIDOREDUCTASE (ETF-QO)

Electron transfer flavoproteins (ETFs) in mammalian mitochondria and some bacteria act as intermediary electron carriers between primary flavoprotein dehydrogenases and terminal respiratory chains.[1–3] In mammals, ETF in the mitochondrial matrix serves as the electron acceptor for at least nine flavoprotein dehydrogenases and is reoxidized by ETF-ubiquinone oxidoreductase (ETF-QO) in the inner mitochondrial membrane.[4–6] ETF-QO in turn reduces ubiquinone, which communicates with the ubiquinone pool of the main respiratory chain.[7] The ETF/ETF-QO system may thus be viewed as a branch of the electron transport system, with separate input sites for seven acyl CoA dehydrogenases and two N-methyl dehydrogenases.[8–14]

Electron transfer flavoprotein

Mammalian ETFs exist in the mitochondrial matrix as heterodimers of alpha- (30-kDa) and beta- (28-kDa) subunits.[15–19] The heterodimer contains a noncovalently bound flavin adenine dinucleotide (FAD) redox cofactor and an equivalent of noncovalently bound adenosine 5′-monophosphate. The latter is associated with the β-subunit and is apparently required for protein folding and/or dimerization.[20–23]

The cDNAs encoding both human subunits have been cloned[24,25] and co-expressed (from a single vector) in *Escherichia coli* to yield active human ETF.[18] The expressed human protein has been crystallized, and its structure has been resolved to 2.1 Å.[26,27] The α-subunit (GenBank accession number J04058) is synthesized as a 35-kDa precursor that is imported into mitochondria and processed to yield the mature 30-kDa subunit.[28] The β-subunit (GenBank accession number X71129) has no cleavable presequence but contains a sequence in the N-terminal region that is homologous to one in β-ketothiolase,[29] another mitochondrial protein, which is not proteolytically processed after import. Crystal structure[26,27] shows that the FAD is bound entirely within domain II of the α-subunit. This domain, which contains the C-terminal half of the subunit, is highly conserved, even in ETF-like proteins involved in nitrogen fixation and trimethylamine oxidation in bacteria.[2,3,30,31] The xylene subnucleus of the flavin ring is exposed to solvent in the region of the C(8) methyl group, the site that was originally proposed to be the location of electron transfer to ETF from medium-chain acyl CoA dehydrogenase (MCAD).[32]

Although the α-subunit side chains in contact with the flavin are conserved in other ETFs,[26,31,33] the oxidation-reduction (redox) potentials of the FAD extend from near zero for human and porcine ETFs[19,34] to +0.219 V for ETF from methylotrophic bacteria.[35] The redox potentials of FAD in ETF are thus determined not only by amino acids in its immediate vicinity but also by amino acid side chains some distance away. In bacterial flavodoxin, for example, mutations that affect protein charge dipoles can alter the redox potential even when they are not in the immediate vicinity of the flavin.[36,37]

The amino acid residues that form hydrogen bonds to the FAD of human ETF are αT266 [with N(5) and C(4)O], αQ262, and αV263 [with N(3)], and αH286 [with C(2)O]. The 4′ hydroxyl of the ribityl side chain is hydrogen-bonded to the flavin at N(1). The one-electron (semiquinone) and two-electron (hydroquinone) reduced forms of ETF are anions in which charge is delocalized in the region of N(1) and C(2)O, so hydrogen bonding at these positions may help stabilize the anionic reduced species. The αR249 that lies immediately behind the flavin may participate in electron transfer from primary dehydrogenases[27] and may also overcome charge repulsion between ETF-QO and the anionic reduced ETF species in the oxidative half-reaction. Y16 and F41 of the β-subunit are within van der Waals contact distance of the C(8) and C(7) methyl groups of the xylene ring of FAD, but their role in ETF function is not known. Site-directed mutations of βY16 to leucine and alanine cause a tenfold increase in flavin fluorescence but have no effect on the reaction of ETF with MCAD.[38]

A model for the binary complex between ETF and MCAD based on crystal structures[26,27] proposes that the two flavins, which are separated by 19 Å in the static complex, can be brought to within 17 Å of each other by conformational flexibility of the ETF. The model proposes that the polypeptide chains act as a wire to effect electron transfer between the two flavins and that amino acid residues participating in this transfer include E253 and R249 of α-ETF and W166, E212, and R210 of MCAD. It is of interest that W166 is highly conserved among acyl CoA dehydrogenases.

The model is also consistent with crosslinking experiments that indicate that the β-ETF subunit is involved in the association of ETF with MCAD and ETF-QO,[39,40] and with experiments using a human ETF in which residues 1–83 of the β-chain had been replaced by β-chain sequence from *Paracoccus denitrificans*.[18] Sequence identity in the exchanged region was about 70 percent, but the net difference in charge was −6, and k_{cat}/K_m of ETF-QO with the chimeric ETF was 150-fold less than with human ETF. Mutating βK61 and βK58 back to the normal human residues reversed these results, showing that these residues are important in the interaction of ETF with ETF-QO.[41]

The redox potentials of human ETF are slightly more positive than those of porcine ETF; the potential for the first electron transfer to human ETF flavin is about +0.037 V, and the potential for the second electron transfer has been calculated to be about +0.025 V.[19] Pre–steady-state and steady-state kinetic studies of enzymatic reduction and oxidation have been done only with porcine ETF.[42,43] Two molecules of ETF are reduced to the semiquinone oxidation state by the complex of MCAD/2,3-enoyl CoA according to equations 103-1 to 103-3.

$$\mathrm{DH_{2e-}} \cdot \text{2,3-enoyl-CoA} + \mathrm{ETF_{ox}} \leftrightarrows \mathrm{DH_{1e-}} \cdot \text{2,3-enoyl-CoA} + \mathrm{ETF_{1e-}} \qquad (103\text{-}1)$$

$$\mathrm{DH_{1e-}} \cdot \text{2,3-enoyl-CoA} + \mathrm{ETF_{ox}} \leftrightarrows \mathrm{DH_{ox}} \cdot \text{2,3-enoyl-CoA} + \mathrm{ETF_{1e-}} \qquad (103\text{-}2)$$

$$\mathrm{DH_{ox}} \cdot \text{2,3-enoyl-CoA} \leftrightarrows \mathrm{DH_{ox}} + \text{2,3-enoyl-CoA} \qquad (103\text{-}3)$$

How reduced ETF is reoxidized by ETF-QO remains unclear, because there is evidence that the reductant of ETF-QO is ETF hydroquinone (ETF_{2e-}), which is apparently produced from ETF_{ox} by primary dehydrogenases too slowly to be physiologically significant.[43,44] However, the necessary ETF_{2e-} may be produced by disproportionation of ETF_{1e-} by ETF-QO (equation 103-4), and studies on expressed human ETF containing the αT266M mutation support the notion that this reaction is indeed significant physiologically.[19]

$$2\mathrm{ETF_{1e-}} \leftrightarrows \mathrm{ETF_{ox}} + \mathrm{ETF_{2e-}} \qquad (103\text{-}4)$$

Two spectrophotometric assays have been used to assay ETF in crude extracts of tissues and fibroblasts. The first involves determining the rate of electron transfer from a suitable primary dehydrogenase, such as MCAD, and its acyl CoA substrate to 2,6-dichlorophenolindophenol. This assay has been used with soluble extracts of fibroblast mitochondria but gives very high background rates with crude extracts.[45] A second method follows reduction of water soluble analogs of ubiquinone, e.g., Q_1, in a system containing an acyl CoA ester, MCAD, and purified ETF-QO. This assay has a relatively low background rate even with crude extracts of whole fibroblasts or tissue.[46] Both assays require purified primary dehydrogenase, and the second also requires a purified preparation of ETF-QO.

Electron transfer flavoprotein-ubiquinone oxidoreductase (ETF dehydrogenase)

Identical preparations of ETF-QO have been isolated from beef heart mitochondria and pig liver submitochondrial particles,[4,6] and human cDNA has been cloned (GenBank accession number S69232) and expressed in *Saccharomyces cerevisiae*.[47] Mature ETF-QO is a 64-kDa monomer, which is synthesized as a 67-kDa precursor and processed to the mature form in the course of translocation into the mitochondrion, insertion of prosthetic groups, and localization in the inner mitochondrial membrane.[47] The mature protein contains one equivalent of FAD and one 4Fe4S cluster as redox prosthetic groups. One sequence found in most FAD-containing proteins and another found in succinic dehydrogenases and fumarate reductases bind the ADP moiety of the flavin. A region near the C-terminus contains a C-X_n-C-XX-C-XX-C ($n = 23$ residues) sequence, which is found in proteins with 4Fe4S clusters and through which the four cysteine residues act as ligands for the iron atoms of the cluster.

The potentials of the FAD in porcine ETF-QO are +0.028 V and −0.006 V for the first and second electrons, and the potential of the iron sulfur cluster, an obligatory one-electron carrier, is +0.047 V.[48] Enzymatic reduction yields an ETF-QO species containing the flavin semiquinone and the reduced cluster, but reduction with sodium dithionite, a low-potential reductant, is required to reduce the flavin to the hydroquinone.[49] The redox potentials suggest that electrons (from ETF) enter through the flavin center and exit via the iron sulfur cluster to ubiquinone. This pathway of electron transfer is consistent with results obtained by expressing human ETF-QO in which the 5′-most cysteine residue in the cluster binding domain (C561) was replaced by alanine, yielding an ETF-QO that could accept electrons from ETF but could not reduce ubiquinone.[50]

ETF-QO solubilized from mitochondrial membranes can be assayed in several ways. It can be assayed spectrophotometrically by following reduction of Q_1 in a system containing an acyl CoA substrate, MCAD, and ETF.[44] ETF-QO also catalyzes the equilibration of ETF redox states under anaerobic conditions according to equation 4.[4,5,44] Disproportionation of ETF semiquinone (to ETF_{ox} and ETF_{2e-}) can be assayed spectrophotometrically, and comproportionation of oxidized ETF and ETF hydroquinone (to ETF_{1e-}) can be assayed fluorometrically. Both of these assays must be performed under anaerobic conditions. All three assays may be used with crude extracts as well as with purified ETF-QO and require a source of purified ETF. ETF-QO has also been assayed in submitochondrial particles and in the particulate fraction of human fibroblasts as an NADH-ETF reductase.[7,51] Under anaerobic conditions (and in the presence of antimycin or myxothiazole to inhibit ubiquinol-cytochrome *c* reductase [Complex III]), NADH or succinate reduces ETF to the semiquinone. Reduction of ETF is assayed fluorometrically.

GLUTARIC ACIDEMIA TYPE II

Introduction

Glutaric acidemia type II (GA2), or multiple acyl CoA dehydrogenation deficiency, MIM 231680, is an inborn error characterized clinically by hypo- or nonketotic hypoglycemia and metabolic acidosis; pathologically by fatty degeneration of liver parenchymal cells, renal tubular epithelium, and myocardium; and biochemically by the accumulation of metabolites of compounds oxidized by enzymes that transfer electrons to ETF. In most cases the disorder is due to deficiency of either ETF or ETF-QO, but in some it may be due to an as yet undefined abnormality in flavin metabolism or transport. Complete deficiency of ETF-QO is often associated with congenital anomalies, the most frequent and characteristic being cysts and dysplasia of the kidneys. All forms of the disease are transmitted as autosomal recessive traits. Most patients with severe disease do not survive the first few weeks of life.

Clinical phenotype

Patients with glutaric acidemia type II, which was first reported in 1976,[52] fall into one of three groups, each consistent within a family. These have been designated (1) neonatal onset with congenital anomalies, (2) neonatal onset without anomalies, and (3) mild and/or later onset.[53] The first two groups are sometimes said to have multiple acyl CoA dehydrogenation deficiency–severe (MADD:S) and the third to have multiple acyl CoA dehydrogenation deficiency–mild (MADD:M), or ethylmalonic-adipic aciduria.

Neonatal-onset patients with congenital anomalies are often premature and present during the first 24–48 hours of life with hypotonia, hepatomegaly, severe hypoglycemia and metabolic acidosis, and (often) an odor similar to that present in isovaleric acidemia (Chap. 93), i.e., the odor of sweaty feet. In some patients the kidneys are palpably enlarged, and there may be facial dysmorphism (high forehead and low-set ears, hypertelorism, hypoplastic midface, etc.), rocker-bottom feet, muscular defects of the anterior abdominal wall, and anomalies of the external genitalia, including hypospadias and chordee. Most such patients die within the first week of life.[54–58] In other patients, congenital anomalies are not noted on physical examination, and renal cysts are discovered only at autopsy.[59–61]

Infants without congenital anomalies usually develop hypotonia, tachypnea and metabolic acidosis, hepatomegaly, hypoglycemia, and a "sweaty feet" odor within the first few days of life, many of them within the first 24 hours. The few patients with this form of the disease who have survived beyond the first week of life because of prompt diagnosis and treatment have died within a few months, usually with severe cardiomyopathy. A few other infants have been hypoglycemic in the newborn period and only later developed typical episodes of Reye syndrome-like illnesses; these patients have survived somewhat longer.[52,54,62–66]

The course and age at presentation of later-onset glutaric acidemia type II is extremely variable. The first patient to be described with this form of the condition had intermittent episodes of vomiting, hypoglycemia, and acidosis beginning at 7 weeks of age,[67,68] and another was totally symptom free during childhood, presenting in adult life with episodic vomiting, hypoglycemia, hepatomegaly, and proximal myopathy.[69] Several other patients with episodic disease beginning during the first few years of life have been described,[70–72] as well as two others with progressive lipid storage myopathy and carnitine deficiency.[51,73,74] A few

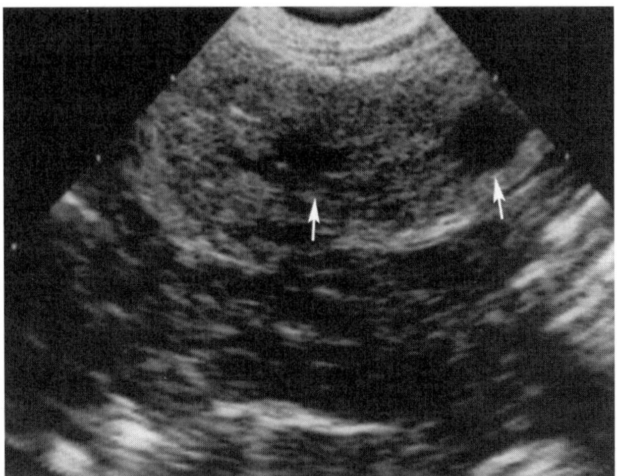

Fig. 103-1 Abdominal ultrasound showing renal cysts in a 2-day-old infant with glutaric acidemia type II due to ETF-QO deficiency. (*Courtesy of Dr. C. Greenberg.*)

patients have had a progressive extrapyramidal movement disorder much more typical of glutaryl CoA dehydrogenase deficiency.[75]

Routine laboratory evaluation shows severe metabolic acidosis, often with an anion gap, mild or moderate hyperammonemia (usually <300 μg/dl), and severe hypoglycemia without ketonuria or ketonemia. Serum transaminases may be elevated, and prothrombin and partial thromboplastin times may be prolonged. Lactic acid in serum is usually elevated. Chest x-ray may show cardiac enlargement, and echocardiography may show evidence of hypertrophic cardiomyopathy. MRI scans of two patients with macrocephaly during the first months of life showed the same symmetric hypoplasia of the temporal lobes seen in glutaryl CoA dehydrogenase deficiency.[76,77] Abdominal ultrasound or CT scan may show renal cysts (Fig. 103-1).

Urine organic acid analysis often shows various combinations of short-chain volatile acids (e.g., isovaleric, isobutyric, 2-methylbutyric); glutaric, ethylmalonic, 3-hydroxyisovaleric, 2-hydroxyglutaric, 5-hydroxyhexanoic, adipic, suberic, sebacic, and dodecanedioic acids: and isovalerylglycine, isobutyrylglycine, and 2-methylbutyrylglycine (Fig. 103-2). 3-Hydroxybutyric and acetoacetic acids are either not seen or not prominent. Organic

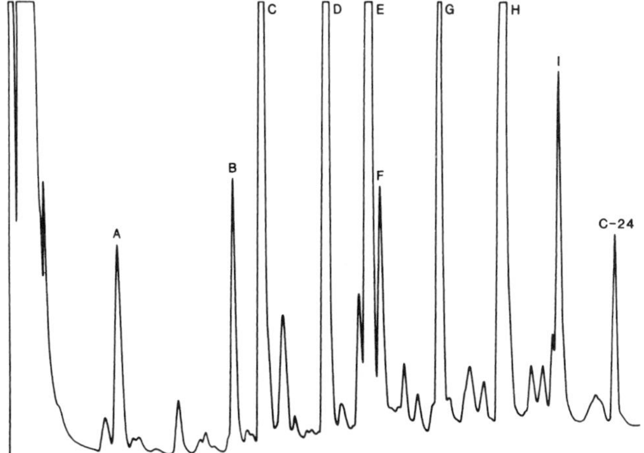

Fig. 103-2 Urine organic acids in an infant with glutaric acidemia type II. A = lactic, B = malonic (internal standard), C = ethylmalonic, D = glutaric, E = adipic, F = 2-hydroxyglutaric, G = suberic, H = sebacic, I = dodecanedioic. (*From SI Goodman and SP Markey, Diagnosis of Organic Acidemias by Gas Chromatography-Mass Spectrometry, Alan R Liss Inc., New York, 1981. Used by permission.*)

acids are also significantly elevated in serum and CSF. In some patients, especially those with episodic disease, urine organic acids are abnormal only during acute episodes.

Generalized aminoacidemia and aminoaciduria, often with marked increases in proline and hydroxyproline, are common in neonatal-onset patients, and elevations of sarcosine in serum and urine are especially frequent in those with later onset.

Carnitine concentrations in serum may be normal or low, but acylcarnitine esters in urine may be significantly increased.[78,79] Treatment of one patient with oral carnitine produced a large increase in several acylcarnitine esters in urine, including acetylcarnitine, isobutyrylcarnitine, isovalerylcarnitine, hexanoylcarnitine, butyrylcarnitine, and propionylcarnitine.[51]

Pathology

All patients autopsied to date have shown severe microvesicular fatty changes in liver parenchymal cells, cells of the proximal renal tubule, and myocardium, but these changes are not diagnostic. Renal anomalies, when present, may be dramatic. The kidneys may be so large that they fill the abdomen, and cysts may occupy all of the cortex and medulla.[57,80,81] Dysplastic changes are present in some cases, but not all (Fig. 103-3).

Brain has been examined in several patients. In two cases there was focal dysplasia of the cerebral cortex with bilateral reduction in the number of gyri in the frontal, parietal, and temporal lobes, with numerous warty protrusions on the temporoparietal cortex, and microscopic evidence of abnormal neuronal migration.[81] Abnormal neuronal migration was observed in three additional patients[82,83] but not in a fourth,[57] in whom the sole finding on routine examination was a reduced number of Purkinje cells in the cerebellar cortex. Electron microscopy in this patient showed moderately electron-dense, membrane-limited, cytoplasmic bodies, and it was suggested that these might be characteristic, if not pathognomonic. One patient with progressive neurologic disease, intermittent dystonic posturing, and ETF deficiency showed only neuronal loss and gliosis in the caudate nucleus and putamen,[75] findings much more typical of glutaryl CoA dehydrogenase deficiency (Chap. 95).

Concentrations of glutaric acid are increased in several tissues, including liver and kidney, and detection of this compound in postmortem tissue has established the diagnosis in several cases, one of them an infant with fatty changes in the liver that were prominent enough to suggest a diagnosis of Wolman's disease (Chap. 142).

Biochemical and Molecular Basis of Disease

In some patients glutaric acidemia type II is due to inherited deficiency of ETF-QO, and in others it is due to inherited deficiency of ETF. While all three clinical forms of the disease can be caused by a defect in either protein, patients with renal cystic dysplasia and other anomalies are much more likely to have ETF-QO deficiency. No single study has correlated the clinical phenotype with ETF and ETF-QO activity and mutations.

Deficiency of ETF-QO antigen was first demonstrated in membranes of liver mitochondria obtained from a female infant with polycystic kidneys and multiple congenital anomalies[53] and then confirmed in fibroblasts from this child and several other infants with and without anomalies.[46,84] Less complete deficiency of ETF-QO antigen and activity has now been demonstrated in patients with less severe and/or later-onset forms of the disease.[46,51,85]

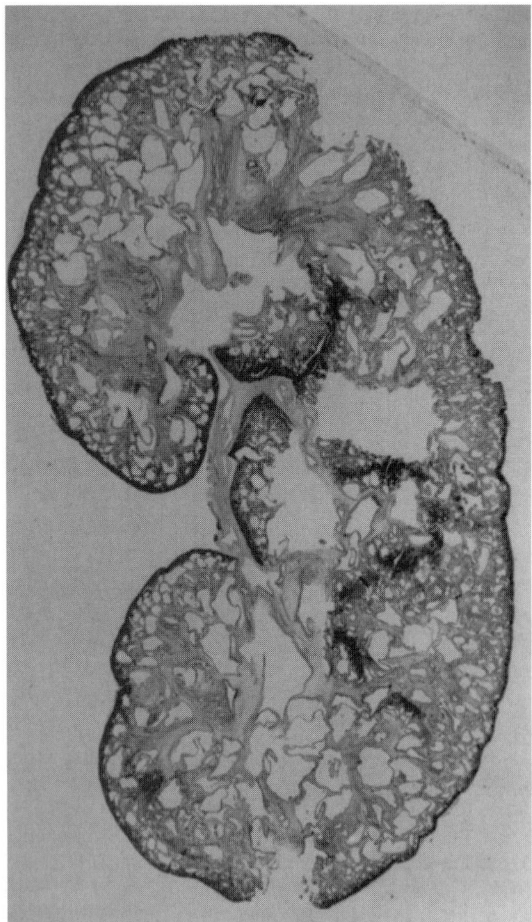

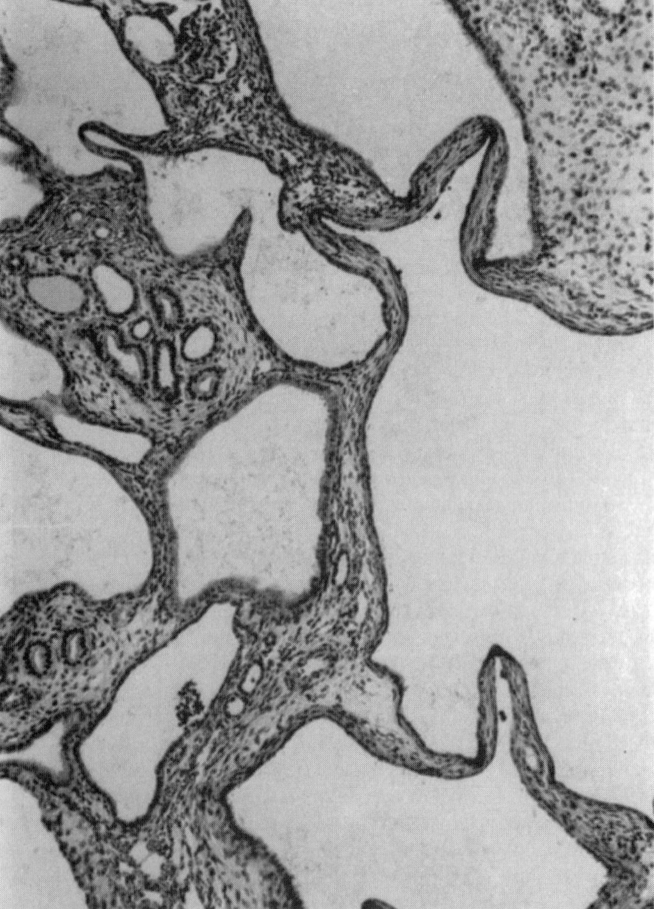

Fig. 103-3 Kidney of a 19-week fetus with glutaric acidemia type II due to ETF-QO deficiency. Left: Not magnified. Right: Cysts derived from Bowman's capsule and renal tubules, with interstitial tissue resembling primitive mesenchyme. Both kidneys showed the same features. H & E; original magnification x50. (*Courtesy of Dr Y. E. Hsia.*)

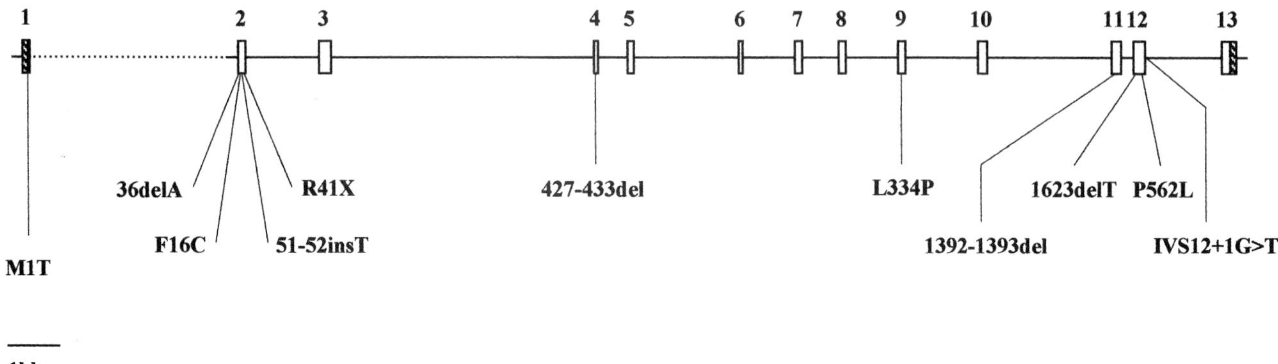

Fig. 103-4 Schematic of the ETF-QO gene, showing nature and location of all mutations detected to date.[84]

cDNA encoding human ETF-QO has been isolated and expressed in *S cerevisiae*;[47] the gene is on chromosome 4q32 → ter and contains 13 exons.[86] Two ETF-QO mutations, i.e., IVS12 +1g → t (c.1810 + 1g → t) and c.427-433del, have been described,[50] and nine others are known to us. Of the mutations shown in Fig. 103-4, only c.427-433del, L334P, 1623delT, and P562L have been found in more than one patient. The genotypes of four patients *with* renal cystic dysplasia[46,53,55] are c.427-433del/L334P, 36delA/36delA, c.427-433del/IVS12 + 1g → t, and L334P/L334P.

IVS12 + 1g → t causes skipping of exon 12, which encodes the 5′-most cysteine residue (C561) of the iron sulfur cluster-binding domain at its 3′ end. When ETF-QO cDNA missing exon 12 is expressed in *S. cerevisiae*, the mutant protein can be reduced by ETF but can no longer reduce ubiquinone.[50] It should be noted that P562 is one residue downstream of C561 and that proline in this position is conserved among 4Fe4S cluster-binding domains.[47]

Deficiency of ETF antigens was first noted in fibroblast lines from two affected infants without congenital anomalies[84] and has now been confirmed by immunoblots or immunoprecipitation and pulse chase on several other patients;[28,45,46,87,88] most of these did *not* have renal cystic dysplasia. Some cells are deficient in only one subunit, but in some lines there is rapid degradation of both, perhaps because the heterodimer is unstable. Pulse chase studies suggest that the primary defect in most of the latter lines, including one from an infant with renal cystic disease,[87] is in the α-subunit. A primary defect of the β-subunit has been found only in two siblings.[87,88] An almost total lack of ETF activity has been demonstrated in cells from patients with neonatal-onset disease, and partial deficiency has been noted in patients with late-onset disease.[45,46]

cDNAs encoding the α- and β-subunits of ETF have been isolated and expressed in *E. coli.*[18,24,25] The α- and β-ETF genes are on human chromosomes 15q23-25 and 19q13.3, respectively;[89,90] gene structure has not been reported. α-ETF mutations delineated to date include 3-, 18-, and 66-bp deletions and V157G, G116R, and T266M.[91,92] The last is common and in one study accounted for five mutant alleles in six patients.[92] Only two β-ETF mutations, R164Q and an IVS12 + 1g → c mutation, have been described.[93] The genotypes of five infants *without* renal cystic dysplasia[46,64,70,87,92] are αT266M/G116R, αV157G/c.453-470del, αT266M/T266M, βR164Q/IVS12 + 1g → c, and αT266M/c.808-810del, respectively.

The αG116R and αT266M mutations have been expressed in *E. coli.* ETF containing the αG116R mutation is unstable and, even when forced to dimerize in the presence of the chaperonins GroEL and GroES, produces an inactive and abnormally folded protein.[19] The hydroxyl group of αT266 is normally hydrogen bonded to the N(5) position of ETF FAD, and the backbone amide hydrogen is hydrogen bonded to C(4)O.[26] ETF containing the αT266M mutation is stable in fibroblasts[92] and *E. coli*,[19] but the redox potentials of the oxidized/semiquinone and semiquinone/hydroquinone flavin couples is lowered to such a point that while the ETF can be reduced by MCAD, disproportionation of the semiquinone to ETF_{2e-}, the putative reductant of ETF-QO, is energetically unfavorable.[19] The activity of purified αT266M ETF in the reaction with ETF-QO is about 8 percent of normal, which is in agreement with the 18 percent found in fibroblasts from a patient homozygous for this mutation.

Fibroblasts from some patients with clinical and biochemical features of GA2 have normal ETF and ETF:QO activities,[94] and since severe riboflavin deficiency can produce a quite similar organic aciduria in rats,[95] the disease in such patients might be due to a defect in FAD biosynthesis or transport. There are, however, no instances in which such defects have been conclusively demonstrated. The central role of flavoproteins in cytosolic, microsomal, mitochondrial, and peroxisomal function suggests that early or complete blocks in FAD biosynthesis would be lethal, but the effects of a less severe block in FAD biosynthesis, or those of an as yet undescribed transport system that might move FAD from the cytoplasm into mitochondria, are more difficult to predict. A defect in cytoplasmic FAD biosynthesis could lead to FAD deficiency in both peroxisomes and mitochondria and might explain why certain patients with glutaric acidemia type II resemble those with Zellweger syndrome,[94] in which peroxisomal assembly is defective (Chap. 129). Defects of this type should affect only mitochondrial (and peroxisomal) processes that are flavoprotein dependent and should especially affect proteins that have low affinity for FAD or, like ETF and glutaryl CoA dehydrogenase, are unstable in its absence.

Pathogenesis

Deficiency of ETF or ETF-QO in severely affected patients is virtually complete, resulting in functional deficiency of several enzymes and accumulation of their substrates and metabolites. Some metabolites, like glutaric acid, derive from simple hydrolysis of the accumulated coenzyme A ester, but most have a more complex origin that involves carboxylation, ω- or (ω-1)-oxidation in microsomes, β-oxidation in peroxisomes, or glycine conjugation, either alone or in combination. For example, microsomal ω-oxidation of accumulated long-chain acyl CoAs probably creates long-chain dicarboxylic esters, with subsequent β-oxidation in peroxisomes generating the C_{12} (dodecanedioic), C_{10} (sebacic), C_8 (suberic), and C_6 (adipic) acids.

The origin of 2-hydroxyglutaric acid, which is now confirmed to be the D-isomer,[63,96] is not clear but suggests that there is yet another flavin dehydrogenase that acts on 2- or 4-D-hydroxyglutaryl CoA and transfers electrons to the respiratory chain via ETF and ETF-QO. A primary defect of this dehydrogenase might cause isolated D-2-hydroxyglutaric acidemia.[97–99]

Sarcosine is frequently found in serum and urine of less severely affected patients but not in patients with acute neonatal onset, perhaps for the following reason. Sarcosine is synthesized by dimethylglycine dehydrogenase (DMGDH) and metabolized by sarcosine dehydrogenase (SDH). Both enzymes transfer flavin-bound electrons to ETF, and sarcosine biosynthesis might be blocked in complete ETF (or ETF-QO) deficiency. With less severe deficiency of ETF or ETF-QO, sarcosine would accumulate if its rate of oxidation were slower than its rate of biosynthesis. The apparent K_m values of DMGDH and SDH for their substrates are 0.5 and 1.0 mM, respectively,[100] which would favor sarcosine accumulation if the enzyme turnover numbers were similar.

Limited availability of acetyl CoA from β-oxidation of fatty acids, with decreased synthesis of N-acetylglutamate (Chap. 85) and reduced allosteric activation of pyruvate carboxylase (Chap. 100), may be important in causing hyperammonemia and hypoglycemia. Decreased generation of NADH could also limit gluconeogenesis by decreasing glyceraldehyde phosphate dehydrogenase activity. Hyperammonemia may contribute to the encephalopathy that occurs during acute episodes, but high circulating levels of toxic short-chain fatty acids and reduced levels of ketone bodies may also play a role. The heart's inability to oxidize long-chain fatty acids and the decreased availability of ketone bodies deprive it of preferred energy sources, perhaps causing cardiomyopathy.

While loss of carnitine esters of organic acids in the urine might cause depletion of carnitine stores and hypocarnitinemia, its role in pathogenesis is not clear. In severely affected infants, for example, complete deficiency of ETF or ETF-QO would preclude mitochondrial β oxidation of fatty acids, even in the presence of normal carnitine stores. Carnitine deficiency is more likely to be of significance in patients with milder disease. In these patients, who presumably have marginally adequate rates of β oxidation, carnitine depletion could further impair β oxidation by impairing uptake of long-chain fatty acids into skeletal muscle mitochondria, leading to fat accumulation and myopathy.

The cause of abnormal fetal development in some patients with ETF or ETF-QO deficiency is not known, but the presence of congenital anomalies suggests a specific toxic effect of one of the accumulated metabolites or the need for this part of the electron transport chain in certain developmental processes. The similarity of the renal lesions to those seen in riboflavin deficiency, Zellweger syndrome, and neonatal carnitine palmitoyltransferase II deficiency has been noted[82,101] but remains unexplained.

Genetics

Many of the first glutaric acidemia type II patients described were males, prompting speculation that the disorder was inherited as an X-linked trait,[60] but additional pedigree data and gene localization studies make it clear that all forms of the disease are transmitted as autosomal recessive traits. Deficiency of ETF-QO in patient fibroblasts, with enzyme activity values in parents intermediate between patient and control values,[46,84] establishes inheritance of ETF-QO deficiency as an autosomal recessive trait, and the gene for ETF-QO is on chromosome 4q32 $\rightarrow$ ter.[86]

The occurrence of defects in α-ETF biosynthesis in males and females, even in the same family, suggests that α-subunit deficiency is also inherited as an autosomal recessive trait, in accord with data indicating that the gene for the β-subunit is on human chromosome 15q23-25.[89] The two siblings with primary defects in the β-ETF subunit are male, but the gene encoding the β-subunit is on chromosome 19q13.3,[90] establishing inheritance as an autosomal trait.

Incidence

The disorder is not screened for in the newborn period, and there are no accurate figures on its incidence. Many reports of the condition have appeared since its first description in 1976,[52] and it is probably one of the more common inborn errors. It is certainly not rare.

Diagnosis

The presence of the characteristic organic acid pattern in urine from a newborn with nonketotic hypoglycemia and metabolic acidosis, with or without congenital anomalies, establishes the diagnosis as glutaric acidemia type II. A very similar organic aciduria occurs in Jamaican vomiting sickness,[102] which occurs after ingestion of unripe ackees — and thus only in areas of the world in which the fruit is eaten — and (probably) also in severe riboflavin deficiency.[95]

Diagnosis in late-onset cases may be considerably more difficult, because metabolic acidosis, the usual indication for examining urine organic acids, may not be present. Further, the organic aciduria in such patients is considerably less pronounced and often intermittent, being present only during acute episodes. The finding of 2-hydroxyglutaric aciduria in such patients is a useful diagnostic point, serving to distinguish the condition from glutaric acidemia (glutaryl CoA dehydrogenase deficiency), in which 3-hydroxyglutaric acid is excreted. Some patients with mild glutaric acidemia type II bear a strong phenotypic resemblance to children with von Gierke's disease (Chap. 71), and liver biopsy will be avoided only if the absence of ketonemia and ketonuria is recognized.

Whole fibroblast metabolism of a variety of radiolabeled compounds may be examined in an attempt to solidify the diagnosis, and this can be done by measuring either oxidation of various ^{14}C-compounds, e.g., [1-^{14}C]palmitate, [1-^{14}C]octanoate, [1-^{14}C]butyrate, [1,5-^{14}C]glutarate, 2-^{14}C]lysine, [2-^{14}C]leucine to $^{14}CO_2$ or incorporation of ^{14}C from appropriate labeled precursors into lipid or protein. Another published method assays oxidation of [1,5-^{14}C]glutaryl CoA to $^{14}CO_2$ in the absence of artificial electron acceptor, when oxidation is totally dependent on the presence of endogenous ETF and ETF-QO.[103,104] However, since there is more than one cause of glutaric acidemia type II, the specific diagnosis can be established only by demonstrating deficiency of ETF or ETF-QO in fibroblasts or other appropriate tissues, e.g., liver, or by showing that cells from a particular patient do not complement those of patients with a known biochemical defect.

In some cases the specific defect can be demonstrated by showing deficient ETF or ETF-QO antigen in appropriate tissues, either by Western blot analysis[46] or by radiolabeling of cells followed by immunoprecipitation.[28] In other cases, usually those with mild disease or late onset, direct assay of ETF or ETF-QO activity is necessary.

Glutaric acidemia type II fibroblasts also show a defect in the ability to release tritium from [9,10(n)-^{3}H]-palmitic acid into cell water, and mutant fibroblasts may be assigned to complementation groups based on their ability to correct the defect in another cell line after polyethylene glycol-induced cell fusion.[105] Such procedures can quickly and accurately identify the enzyme defect in a cell line without growing the large number of cells needed to assay ETF or ETF-QO. An added advantage is that if there are forms of glutaric acidemia type II due to mutations of proteins other than ETF and ETF-QO, cells with such defects can be identified as such without identifying the defective protein.

Prenatal diagnosis

Prenatal diagnosis of glutaric acidemia type II has been established on several occasions by demonstrating increased glutaric acid in amniotic fluid, acylcarnitine esters in maternal urine, and/or impaired substrate oxidation by whole cultured amniocytes.[64,65,106–109] Confirmation of predictions that the fetus would be affected has been obtained by showing deficient substrate oxidation in whole fetal fibroblasts, the presence of large cystic kidneys in ETF-QO-deficient fetuses (Fig. 103-1), or, in other instances, by showing that fetuses that had been allowed to proceed to term indeed had the disease.

Analysis of organic acids in amniotic fluid and substrate oxidation in amniocytes might not clearly indicate fetal status when the proband had mild disease or slight or intermittent organic aciduria. Further, methods of measuring ETF or ETF-QO antigen or activity require amounts of tissue that are not easily obtained by amniocentesis or CVS. It is thus possible that in utero diagnosis of patients with mild and variant forms of this condition will increasingly rely on mutation identification in the probands.

Treatment

Most patients who present within a few days of birth, even those without multiple anomalies, die within the first few months of life. Diets low in fat and protein, with supplementation of carnitine and riboflavin, have been tried without success. Intravenous administration of methylene blue (2 mg/kg per dose) has been tried in one instance, with apparent clinical improvement and almost total clearing of organic aciduria, but the child died soon after the therapeutic trial was terminated.[108] Such treatment assumes that the artificial electron acceptor will enter mitochondria, remove flavin-bound electrons from acyl CoA dehydrogenases, and lessen substrate accumulation behind the metabolic block.

Treatment with riboflavin, carnitine, and diets low in protein and fat have been somewhat more successful when applied to patients with milder or later-onset disease. Treatment with oral riboflavin (100–300 mg/day) has been particularly effective in a few patients, including a woman who developed organic aciduria and sarcosinuria only during pregnancy and intercurrent infection and who without treatment had had six consecutive offspring die by 3 months of age.[71–73,110] With riboflavin treatment during pregnancy, she delivered two normal offspring.[110] The primary defects in these patients have not been identified. Patients with defects in flavin metabolism or transport should be excellent candidates for such treatment, but there may also be patients whose defects in ETF and ETF-QO, both of which contain ionically bound FAD, might respond to higher intramitochondrial FAD concentrations. This might overcome a defect in coenzyme binding, or the FAD might stabilize the mutant electron transferase just enough to increase its activity above a required threshold.

REFERENCES

1. Thorpe C: Electron transferring flavoproteins, in Muller F (ed): *Chemistry and Biochemistry of Flavoenzymes* vol 2. Boca Raton, CRC Press, 1992, p 471.
2. Arigoni F, Kaminski PA, Hennecke H, Elmerich C: Nucleotide sequence of the fix ABC region of *Azorhizobium caulinudans* ORS571: Similarity of the fixB product with eukaryotic flavoproteins, characterization of fixX and identification of nifW. *Mol Gen Genet* **225**:514, 1991.
3. Weidenhaupt M, Rossi P, Beck C, Fischer HM, Hennecke H: Two discrete sets of electron transfer flavoprotein genes: fixA, fixB, etfS and etfL. *Archiv Microbiol* **165**:169, 1996.
4. Ruzicka FJ, Beinert H: A new iron-sulfur flavoprotein of the respiratory chain: A component of the fatty acid βoxidation pathway. *J Biol Chem* **252**:8440, 1977.
5. Beckmann JD, Frerman FE: Electron transfer flavoprotein-ubiquinone oxidoreductase from pig liver: Molecular, catalytic and redox properties. *Biochemistry* **24**:3913, 1985.
6. Beckmann JD, Frerman FE: Interaction of electron transfer flavoprotein and electron transfer flavoprotein ubiquinone oxidoreductase. *Biochemistry* **24**:3922, 1985.
7. Frerman FE: Reaction of electron transfer flavoprotein ubiquinone oxidoreductase with the mitochondrial respiratory chain. *Biochim Biophys Acta* **893**:161, 1987.
8. Hauge J: On the mechanism of dehydrogenation of fatty acyl derivatives of coenzyme A. *J Am Chem Soc* **78**:5266, 1956.
9. Izai K, Uchida Y, Yamamoto S, Hashimoto T: Novel fatty acid beta oxidation enzymes in rat liver mitochondria: Purification and properties of a very long chain acyl-CoA dehydrogenase. *J Biol Chem* **267**:1027, 1992.
10. Ikeda Y, Tanaka K: Purification and characterization of isovaleryl coenzyme. A dehydrogenase from rat liver mitochondria. *J Biol Chem* **258**:1077, 1983.
11. Ikeda Y, Tanaka K: Purification and characterization of 2-methyl-branched chain acyl-coenzyme A dehydrogenase, an enzyme involved in isoleucine and valine metabolism, from rat liver mitochondria. *J Biol Chem* **258**:9477, 1983.
12. Lenich A, Goodman SI: Purification and characterization of glutaryl-CoA dehydrogenase from porcine and human liver. *J Biol Chem* **261**:4090, 1986.
13. Beinert H, Frisell WR: The functional identity of the electron-transferring flavoproteins of the fatty acyl coenzyme A and sarcosine dehydrogenase systems. *J Biol Chem* **237**:2988, 1962.
14. Wittwer AJ, Wagner C: Identification of the folate-binding proteins of rat liver mitochondria as methylglycine dehydrogenase and sarcosine dehydrogenase. *J Biol Chem* **256**:4109, 1981.
15. Gorelick RJ, Mizzer JP, Thorpe C: Purification and properties of electron transferring flavoprotein from pig kidney. *Biochemistry* **21**:6936, 1982.
16. McKean MC, Beckmann JD, Frerman FE: Subunit structure of electron transfer flavoprotein. *J Biol Chem* **258**:1866, 1983.
17. Husain M, Steenkamp DJ: Electron transfer flavoprotein from pig liver mitochondria: A simple purification and re-evaluation of some of the molecular properties. *Biochem J* **209**:541, 1983.
18. Herrick KR, Salazar D, Goodman SI, Finocchiaro G, Bedzyk LA, Frerman FE: Expression and characterization of human and chimeric human-*Paracoccus denitrificans* electron transfer flavoprotein. *J Biol Chem* **269**:32239, 1994.
19. Salazar D, Zhang L, deGala GD, Frerman FE: Expression and characterization of two pathogenic mutations in human electron transfer flavoprotein. *J Biol Chem* **272**:26425, 1997.
20. Sato K, Nichina Y, Shiga K: Anion-induced conformational change of apo-electron transfer flavoprotein. *J Biochem* **111**:359, 1992.
21. Sato K, Nishina Y, Shiga K: Electron transferring flavoprotein has an AMP-binding site in addition to the FAD-binding site. *J Biochem* **114**:215, 1993.
22. Griffin KJ, Dwyer TM, Manning MC, Meyer JD, Carpenter JF, Frerman FE: αT244M mutation affects the redox, kinetic and in vitro folding properties of *Paracoccus denitrificans* electron transfer flavoprotein. *Biochemistry* **36**:4194, 1997.
23. DuPlessis EE, Rohlfs RJ, Hille R, Thorpe C: Electron transferring flavoprotein from pig and the methylotrophic bacterium W3A1 contains AMP as well as FAD. *Biochem Mol Biol Int* **195**:195, 1994.
24. Finocchiaro G, Ito M, Ikeda Y, Tanaka K: Molecular cloning and nucleotide sequence of cDNAs encoding the α-subunit of human electron transfer flavoprotein. *J Biol Chem* **263**:15773, 1988.
25. Finocchiaro G, Colombo I, Garavaglia B, Gallera C, Valdameria G, Garbuglio N, DiDonato S: cDNA cloning and mitochondrial import of the β-subunit of the human electron transfer flavoprotein. *Eur J Biochem* **213**:1003, 1993.
26. Roberts DL, Frerman FE, Kim JJP: Three dimensional structure of human electron transfer flavoprotein to 2.1 Å resolution. *Proc Natl Acad Sci USA* **93**:14355, 1996.
27. Roberts DL, Frerman FE, Kim JJP: Human electron transfer flavoprotein: Three dimensional structure and a possible complex with medium chain acyl-CoA dehydrogenase, In Stevenson KJ, Massey V, Williamson CH, Jr. (eds): *Flavins and Flavoproteins*. Calgary, University of Calgary Press, 1997, p 523.
28. Ikeda Y, Keese SM, Tanaka K: Biosynthesis of electron transfer flavoprotein in a cell free system and in cultured human fibroblasts: Defect in the alpha subunit synthesis is a primary lesion in glutaric aciduria type II. *J Clin Invest* **78**:997, 1986.
29. Arakawa H, Takiguchi M, Amaya Y, Hayashi H, Mori M: cDNA derived amino acid sequence of rat 3-oxoacyl-CoA thiolase with no transit peptide: Structural relationships with the peroxisomal enzyme. *EMBO J* **6**:1361, 1987.
30. Davidson VL, Husain M, Neher JW: Electron transfer flavoprotein from *Methylophilus methylotrophus:* Properties, comparison with other electron transferring flavoproteins, and control of expression by carbon source. *J Bacteriol* **166**:812, 1986.
31. Chen D, Swenson RP: Cloning, sequence analysis, and expresson of the genes ecoding the two subunits of the methylotrophic bacterium W3A1 electron transfer flavoprotein. *J Biol Chem* **269**:32120, 1994.
32. Gorelick RJ, Thorpe C: Electron transferring flavoprotein from pig liver: Flavin analog studies. *Biochemistry* **25**:7092, 1986.
33. Roberts DL, Salazar D, Frerman FE, Fulmer J, Kim JJP: Crystal structure of *Paracoccus denitrificans* electron transfer flavoprotein: Structural and electrostatic analysis of a conserved flavin binding domain *Biochemistry.* **38**:1977, 1999
34. Husain M, Stankovich MT, Fox BG: Measurement of the oxidation-reduction potentials for one-electron and two-electron reduction of electron transfer flavoprotein from pig liver. *Biochem J* **219**:1043, 1984.

35. Byron CM, Stankovich MT, Husain M, Davidson VL: Unusual redox properties of electron transfer flavoprotein from *Methylophilus methylotrophus*. *Biochemistry* **28**:8582, 1989.
36. Zhou JS, Swenson RP: The cumulative effects of aromatic stacking interactions and negative electrostatic environment of the flavin mononucleotide binding site is a major determinant of the reduction potential of the flavodoxin from *Desulfovibrio vulgaris* [Hildenborough]. *Biochemistry* **35**:15980, 1996.
37. Zhou JS, Swenson RP: Evaluation of the electrostatic effect of the 5′ phosphate of flavin mononucleotide cofactor on the oxidation-reduction potential of the flavodoxin from *Desulfovibrio vulgaris* [Hildenborough]. *Biochemistry* **35**:12443, 1996.
38. Dwyer TM, Zhang L, Mueller M, Marrugo F, Frerman FE: The functions of flavin contact residues, αArg249 and βTyr16, in human electron transfer flavoprotein. *Biochem Biophys Acta* **1433**:139, 1999.
39. Steenkamp DJ: Preferential cross-linking of the small subunit of the electron-transfer flavoprotein to general acyl-CoA dehydrogenase. *Biochem J* **243**:519, 1987.
40. Steenkamp DJ: Cross-linking of electron-transfer flavoprotein to electron-transfer flavoprotein-ubiquinone oxidoreductase with hetero-bifunctional reagents. *Biochem J* **255**:869, 1988.
41. Salazar D, Frerman FE: Unpublished.
42. McKean MC, Frerman FE, Mielke DM: General acyl-CoA dehydrogenase from pig liver: Kinetic and binding studies. *J Biol Chem* **254**:2730, 1979.
43. Gorelick RJ, Schopfer LM, Ballou DP, Massey V, Thorpe C: Interflavin oxidation-reduction between pig kidney general acyl-CoA dehydrogenase and electron transfer flavoprotein. *Biochemistry* **24**:6830, 1985.
44. Ramsay RR, Steenkamp DJ, Husain M: Reactions of electron transfer flavoprotein and electron transfer flavoprotein-ubiquinone oxidoreductase. *Biochem J* **241**:883, 1987.
45. Amendt BA, Rhead WJ: The multiple acyl-coenzyme A dehydrogenation disorders, glutaric aciduria type II and ethylmalonic-adipic aciduria: Mitochondrial fatty acid oxidation, acyl-coenzyme A dehydrogenase, and electron transfer flavoprotein activities in fibroblasts. *J Clin Invest* **78**:205, 1986.
46. Loehr JP, Goodman SI, Frerman FE: Glutaric acidemia type II: Heterogeneity of clinical and biochemical phenotypes. *Pediatr Res* **27**:311, 1990.
47. Goodman SI, Axtell KM, Bindoff LA, Beard SE, Gill RE, Frerman FE: Molecular cloning and expression of a cDNA encoding human electron transfer flavoprotein-ubiquinone oxidoreductase. *Eur J Biochem* **219**:277, 1994.
48. Paulsen KE, Orville AM, Frerman FE, Lipscomb JD, Stankovich MT: Redox properties of electron transfer flavoprotein-ubiquinone oxidoreductase as determined by EPR-spectroelectrochemistry. *Biochemistry* **31**:11755, 1992.
49. Johnson MK, Morningstar JE, Oliver M, Frerman FE: Electron paramagnetic resonance and magnetic circular dichroism studies of electron transfer flavoprotein-ubiquinone oxidoreductase from pig liver. *FEBS Lett* **226**:129, 1987.
50. Beard SE, Goodman SI, Bemelen K, Frerman FE: Characterization of a mutation that abolishes quinone reduction by electron transfer flavoprotein-ubiquinone oxidoreductase. *Hum Mol Genet* **4**:157, 1995.
51. Di Donato S, Frerman FE, Rimoldi M, Rinaldo P, Taroni F, Weismann UN: Systemic carnitine deficiency due to lack of electron transfer flavoprotein:ubiquinone oxidoreductase. *Neurology* **36**:957, 1986.
52. Przymembel H, Wendel U, Becker K, Bremer HJ, Bruinvis L, Ketting D, Wadman SK: Glutaric aciduria type II: Report on a previously undescribed metabolic disorder. *Clin Chim Acta* **66**:227, 1976.
53. Goodman SI, Frerman FE: Glutaric acidaemia type II (multiple acyl-CoA dehydrogenation deficiency). *J Inherit Metab Dis* **7**(Suppl 1):33, 1984.
54. Sweetman L, Nyhan WL, Trauner DA, Merritt TA, Singh M: Glutaric aciduria type II. *J Pediatr* **96**:1020, 1980.
55. Lehnert W, Wendel U, Lindenmaier S, Böhm N: Multiple acyl-CoA dehydrogenation deficiency (glutaric aciduria type II), congenital polycystic kidneys, and symmetric warty dysplasia of the cerebral cortex in two brothers: I. Clinical, metabolical, and biochemical findings. *Eur J Pediatr* **139**:56, 1982.
56. Goodman SI, Reale M, Berlow S: Glutaric acidemia type II: A form with deleterious intrauterine effects. *J Pediatr* **102**:411, 1983.
57. Harkin JC, Gill WL, Shapira E: Glutaric acidemia type II: Phenotypic findings and ultrastructural studies of brain and kidney. *Arch Pathol Lab Med* **110**:399, 1986.
58. Whitfield J, Hurst D, Bennett MJ, Sherwood WG, Hogg R, Gonsoulin W: Fetal polycystic kidney disease associated with glutaric aciduria type II: An inborn error of energy metabolism. *Am J Perinatol* **13**:131, 1996.
59. Gregersen N, Kølvraa S, Rasmussen K, Christensen E, Brandt NJ, Ebbesen F, Hansen FH: Biochemical studies in a patient with defects in the metabolism of acyl-CoA and sarcosine: Another possible case of glutaric aciduria type II. *J Inherit Metab Dis* **3**:67, 1980.
60. Coudé FX, Ogier H, Charpentier C, Thomassin G, Checoury A, Amedee-Manesme O, Saudubray JM, Frezal J: Neonatal glutaric aciduria type II: An X-linked recessive inherited disorder. *Hum Genet* **59**:263, 1981.
61. Mitchell G, Saudubray JM, Gubler MC, Habib R, Ogier H, Frezal J, Boué J: Congenital anomalies in glutaric aciduria type 2. *J Pediatr* **104**:961, 1984.
62. Goodman SI, McCabe ERB, Fennessey PV, Mace JW: Multiple acyl-CoA dehydrogenase deficiency (glutaric aciduria type II) with transient hypersarcosinemia and sarcosinuria: Possible inherited deficiency of an electron transfer flavoprotein. *Pediatr Res* **14**:12, 1980.
63. Goodman SI, Stene DO, McCabe ERB, Norenberg MD, Shikes RH, Stumpf DA, Blackburn GK: Glutaric acidemia type II: Clinical, biochemical, and morphologic considerations. *J Pediatr* **100**:946, 1982.
64. Niederwieser A, Steinmann B, Exner U, Neuheiser F, Redweik U, Wang M, Rampini S, et al: Multiple acyl-CoA dehydrogenation deficiency (MADD) in a boy with nonketotic hypoglycemia, hepatomegaly, muscle hypotonia and cardiomyopathy: Detection of N-isovalerylglutamic acid and its monoamide. *Helv Paediatr Acta* **38**:9, 1983.
65. Bennett MJ, Curnock DA, Engel PC, Shaw L, Gray RGF, Hull D, Patrick AD, et al: Glutaric aciduria type II: Biochemical investigation and treatment of a child diagnosed prenatally. *J Inherit Metab Dis* **7**:57, 1984.
66. Mooy PD, Przymembel H, Giesberts MAH, Scholte HR, Blöm W, van Gelderen HH: Glutaric aciduria type II: Treatment with riboflavine, carnitine and insulin. *Eur J Pediatr* **143**:92, 1984.
67. Tanaka K, Mantagos S, Genel M, Seashore MR, Billings BA, Baretz BH: New defect in fatty-acid metabolism with hypoglycemia and organic aciduria. *Lancet* **2**:986, 1977.
68. Mantagos S, Genel M, Tanaka K: Ethylmalonic-adipic aciduria: In vivo and in vitro studies indicating deficiency of activities of multiple acyl-CoA dehydrogenases. *J Clin Invest* **64**:1580, 1979.
69. Dusheiko G, Kew MC, Joffe BI, Lewin JR, Mantagos S, Tanaka K: Recurrent hypoglycemia associated with glutaric aciduria type II in an adult. *N Engl J Med* **301**:1405, 1979.
70. Vergee ZH, Sherwood WG: Multiple acyl-CoA dehydrogenase deficiency: A neonatal onset case responsive to treatment. *J Inherit Metab Dis* **8**(Suppl 2):137, 1985.
71. Green A, Marshall TG, Bennett MJ, Gray RGF, Pollitt RJ: Riboflavin responsive ethylmalonic-adipic aciduria. *J Inherit Metab Dis* **8**:67, 1985.
72. Gregersen G, Wintzensen H, Kølvraa S, Christensen E, Christensen MF, Brandt NJ, Rasmussen K: C_6-C_{10}-Dicarboxylic aciduria: Investigations of a patient with riboflavin responsive multiple acyl-CoA dehydrogenation defects. *Pediatr Res* **16**:861, 1982.
73. de Visser M, Scholte HR, Schutgens RBH, Bolhuis PA, Luyt-Houwen IEM, Vaandrager-Verduin MHM, Veder HA, et al: Riboflavin-responsive lipid-storage myopathy and glutaric aciduria type II of early adult onset. *Neurology* **36**:367, 1986.
74. Cornelio F, Di Donato S, Peluchetti D, Bizzi A, Bentagnolio B, d'Angelo A, Wiesmann U: Fatal cases of lipid storage myopathy with carnitine deficiency. *J Neurol Neurosurg Psychiatr* **40**:170, 1977.
75. Chow CW, Frerman FE, Goodman SI, Brown GK, Pitt JJ, Danks DM: Striatal degeneration in glutaric acidaemia type II. *Acta Neuropathol* **77**:554, 1989.
76. Støckler S, Radner H, Felizitas K, Hauer A, Ebner F: Symmetric hypoplasia of the temporal cerebral lobes in an infant with glutaric aciduria type II (multiple acyl-CoA dehydrogenase deficency). *J Pediatr* **24**:601, 1994.
77. Shevell MI, Didomenicantonio G, Sylvain M, Arnold DL, O'Gorman AM, Scriver CR: Glutaric acidemia type II: Neuroimaging and spectroscopy evidence for a developmental encephalomyopathy. *Pediatr Neurol* **12**:350, 1995.
78. Chalmers RA, Roe CR, Stacey TE, Hoppel CL: Urinary excretion of L-carnitine and acylcarnitines by patients with disorders of organic acid metabolism: Evidence for secondary insufficiency of L-carnitine. *Pediatr Res* **18**:1325, 1984.

79. Mandel H, Africk D, Blitzer M, Shapira E: The importance of recognizing secondary carnitine deficiency in organic acidaemias: Case report in glutaric acidaemia type II. *J Inherit Metab Dis* **11**:397, 1988.
80. Chalmers RA, Tracy BM, King GS, Pettit B, Rocchiccioli F, Saudubray JM, Gray RGF, et al: The prenatal diagnosis of glutaric aciduria type II, using quantitative GC-MS. *J Inherit Metab Dis* **8**(Suppl 2):145, 1985.
81. Böhm N, Uy J, Kießling M, Lehnert W: Multiple acyl CoA dehydrogenation deficiency (glutaric aciduria type II), congenital polycystic kidneys, and symmetric warty degeneration of the cerebral cortex in two newborn brothers: II. Morphology and pathogenesis. *Eur J Pediatr* **139**:60, 1982.
82. Hoganson G, Berlow S, Gilbert EF, Frerman F, Goodman S, Schweitzer L: Glutaric acidemia type II and flavin-dependent enzymes in morphogenesis, in EF Gilbert, JM Opitz (eds): *Genetic Aspects of Developmental Pathology,* Birth Defects: Original Article Series vol 23. New York, Liss, 1987, p 65.
83. Greenberg, C: Personal communication.
84. Frerman FE, Goodman SI: Deficiency of electron transfer flavoprotein or electron transfer flavoprotein ubiquinone oxidoreductase in glutaric acidemia type II fibroblasts. *Proc Natl Acad Sci USA* **82**:4517, 1985.
85. Bell RB, Brownell AKW, Roe CR, Engel AG, Goodman SI, Frerman FE, Seccombe DW, et al: Electron transfer flavoprotein:ubiquinone oxidoreductase (ETF:QO) deficiency in an adult. *Neurology* **40**:1779, 1990.
86. Goodman SI. Unpublished data.
87. Yamaguchi S, Orii T, Suzuki Y, Maeda K, Oshima M, Hashimoto T: Newly identified forms of electron transfer flavoprotein deficiency in two patients with glutaric aciduria type II. *Pediatr Res* **29**:60, 1991.
88. Yamaguchi S, Shimizu N, Orii T, Fukao T, Suzuki Y, Maeda K, Hashimoto T, et al: Prenatal diagnosis and neonatal monitoring of a fetus with glutaric aciduria type II due to electron transfer flavoprotein (β-subunit) deficiency. *Pediatr Res* **30**:439, 1991.
89. Barton DE, Yang-Feng TL, Finocchiaro G, Ozasa H, Tanaka K, Francke U: Short chain acyl-CoA dehydrogenase (ACADS) maps to chromosomes 12 (q22-ter) and electron transfer flavoprotein (ETFA) to 15 (q23-q25). *Cytogenet Cell Genet* **46**:577, 1987.
90. Antonacci R, Colombo I, Archidiacono N, Volta M, Di Donato S, Finocchiaro G, Rocchi M: Assignment of the gene encoding the beta-subunit of the electron-transfer flavoprotein (ETFB) to human chromosome 19q13.3. *Genomics* **19**:177, 1994.
91. Indo Y, Glassberg R, Yokota I, Tanaka K: Molecular characterization of variant alpha-subunit of electron transfer flavoprotein in three patients with glutaric acidemia type II–and identification of glycine substitution for valine-157 in the sequence of the precursor, producing an unstable mature protein in a patient. *Am J Hum Genet* **49**:575, 1991.
92. Freneaux E, Sheffield VC, Molin L, Shires A, Rhead WJ: Glutaric acidemia type II: Heterogeneity in β-oxidation flux, polypeptide synthesis, and complementary DNA mutations in the α subunit of electron transfer flavoprotein in eight patients. *J Clin Invest* **90**:1679, 1992.
93. Colombo I, Finocchiaro G, Garavaglia B, Garbuglio N, Yamaguchi S, Frerman FE, Berra B, et al: Mutations and polymorphisms of the gene encoding the β-subunit of the electron transfer flavoprotein in three patients with glutaric acidemia type II. *Hum Mol Gen* **3**:429, 1994.
94. Loehr J, Frerman FE, Goodman SI: A new form of glutaric acidemia type II (GA2). *Pediatr Res* **21**:291A, 1987 (abstract).
95. Goodman SI: Organic aciduria in the riboflavin-deficient rat. *Am J Clin Nutr* **34**:2434, 1981.
96. Watanabe H, Yamaguchi S, Saiki K, Shimizu N, Fukao T, Kondo N, Orii T: Identification of the D-enantiomer of 2-hydroxyglutaric acid in glutaric aciduria type II. *Clin Chim Acta* **238**:115, 1995.
97. Craigen WJ, Jakobs C, Sekul EA, Levy ML, Gibson KM, Butler IJ, Herman GE: D-2-Hydroxyglutaric aciduria in neonate with seizures and CNS dysfunction. *Pediatr Neurol* **10**:49, 1994.
98. Nyhan ML, Shelton GD, Jakobs C, Holmes B, Bowe C, Curry CJR, Vance C, et al: D-2-Hydroxyglutaric aciduria. *J Child Neurol* **10**:137, 1995.
99. Baker NS, Sarnat HB, Jack RM, Patterson K, Shaw DW, Herndon SP: D-2-Hydroxyglutaric aciduria: Hypotonia, cortical blindness, seizures, cardiomyopathy, and cylindrical spirals in skeletal muscle. *J Child Neurol* **12**:31, 1997.
100. Frisell WR, Mackenzie CG: Separation and purification of sarcosine dehydrogenase and dimethylglycine dehydrogenase. *J Biol Chem* **237**:94, 1962.
101. North KN, Hoppel CL, De Girolami U, Kozakewich HP, Korson MS: Lethal neonatal deficiency of carnitine palmitoyltransferase II associated with dysgenesis of the brain and kidneys. *J Pediatr* **127**:414, 1995.
102. Tanaka K, Kean EA, Johnson B: Jamaican vomiting sickness: Biochemical investigation of two cases. *N Engl J Med* **295**:461, 1976.
103. Christensen E, Kølvraa S, Gregersen N: Glutaric aciduria type II: Evidence for a defect related to the electron transfer flavoprotein or its dehydrogenase. *Pediatr Res* **18**:663, 1984.
104. Christensen E: Glutaryl-CoA dehydrogenase activity determined with intact electron-transport chain: Application to glutaric aciduria type II. *J Inher Metab Dis* **7**(Suppl 2):103, 1984.
105. Moon A, Rhead WJ: Complementation analysis of fatty acid oxidation disorders. *J Clin Invest* **79**:59, 1987.
106. Mitchell G, Saudubray JM, Benoit Y, Rocchiccioli F, Charpentier C, Ogier H, Boué J: Antenatal diagnosis of glutaricaciduria type II. *Lancet* **1**:1099, 1983.
107. Jacobs C, Sweetman L, Wadman SK, Duran M, Saudubray JM, Nyhan WL: Prenatal diagnosis of glutaric aciduria type II by direct chemical analysis of dicarboxylic acids in amniotic fluid. *Eur J Pediatr* **141**:153, 1984.
108. Harpey JP, Charpentier C, Coude M: Methylene-blue for riboflavin-unresponsive glutaricaciduria type II. *Lancet* **1**:391, 1986.
109. Sakuma T, Sugiyama N, Ichiki T, Kobayashi M, Wada Y, Nohara D: Analysis of acylcarnitines in maternal urine for prenatal diagnosis of glutaric aciduria type 2. *Prenat Diagn* **11**:77, 1991.
110. Harpey JP, Charpentier C, Goodman SI, Darbois Y, Lefebvre G, Sebbah J: Multiple acyl-CoA dehydrogenase deficiency occurring in pregnancy and caused by a defect in riboflavin metabolism in the mother. *J Pediatr* **103**:394, 1983.

CHAPTER 104

Oxidative Phosphorylation Diseases

John M. Shoffner

1. Oxidative phosphorylation (OXPHOS) is composed of five intramitochondrial enzyme complexes (complexes I to V) that are responsible for producing the majority of the ATP required for normal cellular function. Assembly and maintenance of OXPHOS requires the coordinate regulation of nuclear DNA and mitochondrial DNA (mtDNA) genes. The mtDNA encodes 12 OXPHOS subunits, 22 tRNAs, and 2 rRNAs, which provide the core elements for OXPHOS function and mitochondrial protein synthesis. The nuclear DNA is responsible for synthesizing approximately 70 OXPHOS subunits, transporting them to the mitochondria via chaperone proteins, ensuring their passage across the mitochondrial inner membrane, and coordinating their proper processing and assembly. OXPHOS is regulated by a wide variety of factors and processes that include hormone levels, oxygen supply, ion gradients, membrane transporters such as the adenine nucleotide translocase that supplies ADP for conversion to ATP, transcription factors that alter the levels of nuclear gene transcription, tissue-specific isoforms, developmental-specific isoforms, mitochondrial replication, mitochondrial transcription, and mitochondrial translation. Defects in any of these processes may produce an OXPHOS disease.

2. The cytoplasmic location of the mtDNA creates a unique genetics. Mitochondrial genetics is defined by these principles: maternal inheritance, replicative segregation, threshold expression, a high mtDNA mutation rate, and a propensity to accumulate somatic mutations with age. The age-related accumulation of mtDNA mutations may contribute to the decline of cellular OXPHOS function with age and to the progression of a variety of degenerative diseases. Increases in somatic mtDNA mutations are associated with increased generation of free radicals that permanently damage the mtDNA. The paucity of mtDNA repair mechanisms means that once mtDNA damage occurs, the mutated mtDNA can persist in the cell and clonally proliferate over time. After sufficient levels of mutant mtDNA are reached, OXPHOS function begins to decline.

3. mtDNA mutations are classified as deletions, duplications, or point mutations. These mutations produce defective OXPHOS subunits or abnormalities in mitochondrial protein synthesis. Mutations in nuclear OXPHOS genes are the most important causes for OXPHOS diseases. These mutations have diverse effects that include increases in the mtDNA mutation rate, decreases in the mtDNA copy number, impaired OXPHOS enzyme assembly, and abnormal function of an OXPHOS enzyme subunit.

4. OXPHOS diseases are a complex family of disorders with a vast array of clinical manifestations that can be caused by mutations in the nuclear DNA or the mtDNA. OXPHOS mutations produce diseases that can affect a variety of developmental stages, tissues, or systems, resulting in a diversity of clinical phenotypes encountered in virtually all age groups. Hence, OXPHOS diseases should be considered in the differential diagnosis of many familial diseases. The evaluation of patients for OXPHOS diseases is complex and should be performed at centers that are experienced with the clinical, biochemical, and genetic characteristics of these disorders. The principles of mitochondrial genetics, as well as of Mendelian genetics, must be considered when interpreting the results of this analysis. This approach permits developing an appropriate management plan, addressing genetic counseling issues for the family, focusing on anxieties associated with the complexities of these diseases processes, providing patient education, and minimizing the need for further complex and expensive diagnostic evaluations.

Oxidative phosphorylation (OXPHOS) is responsible for producing much of the ATP that cells require. The OXPHOS pathway incorporates over 100 polypeptides, whose genes are located in either the nuclear DNA or the mitochondrial DNA (mtDNA). The expression of these genes and the assembly of the five OXPHOS enzyme complexes (complexes I to V) are highly ordered and coordinated processes. A broad array of human diseases result from mutations in either the nuclear or mtDNA genes or even in the systems that coordinate their interactions. Consequently, OXPHOS diseases can have complex inheritance patterns and a broad spectrum of clinical presentations.

The concept of an OXPHOS disease was first formulated in 1962 when a young Swedish woman was found to have a hypermetabolic state, structurally abnormal mitochondria, and abnormalities of OXPHOS function,[1] a rare disorder now known as Luft disease. Over the next two decades, investigations of OXPHOS diseases focused on neuromuscular disorders that were associated with ragged-red muscle fibers (RRF) identified by staining patient muscle sections with the modified Gomori-trichrome,[2] abnormal mitochondrial ultrastructure,[3,4] and various abnormalities in OXPHOS enzyme activity.

The mtDNA was first discovered in 1963,[5,6] but it was not until the late 1970s and early 1980s that the relevance of mtDNA mutations to human disease began to be seriously considered. During that time, the basic principles of mitochondrial genetics, including maternal inheritance of the mtDNA, were elucidated, and the complete mtDNA sequence was determined.[7] Based on these advances, the first pathogenic mtDNA mutations were reported in 1988. Large mtDNA deletions that removed several thousand base pairs (bp) were found in patients who had chronic progressive external ophthalmoplegia, structurally abnormal mitochondria, and abnormal OXPHOS biochemistry.[8] Shortly after this study was published, an mtDNA point mutation in the ND4 gene was shown to be a major cause of a type of maternally inherited blindness called Leber hereditary optic neuropathy.[9] Within 2 years, the major classes of pathogenic mtDNA mutations were identified. Deletions, duplications, and point mutations in the mtDNA were recognized as causes of OXPHOS diseases.

Shortly after the discovery of pathogenic mtDNA mutations, the clinical, biochemical, and molecular features of families with autosomal dominant OXPHOS diseases were described.[10] Individuals from these families had ophthalmoparesis and mitochondrial myopathies caused by the accumulation of a heterogeneous array of mtDNA deletions as a consequence of a nuclear gene mutation. Since the description of these patients, it has become clear that nuclear gene mutations are the major causes of pediatric and adult OXPHOS diseases.

Due to the large number of nuclear genes involved in the assembly and regulation of OXPHOS, the term OXPHOS disease now encompasses an enormous array of clinical disorders whose onset can occur at any time from birth to old age. Clinical diseases are no longer confined to rare neuromuscular disorders with ragged-red fibers and structurally abnormal mitochondria. Disease expression is complex and depends on interactions between nuclear genes and the mtDNA. The catalogue of pediatric and adult phenotypes is expanding at a rate suggesting that OXPHOS diseases may be one of the most commonly encountered classes of degenerative diseases. Current estimates suggest that OXPHOS diseases occur at an incidence of at least 1 in 10,000.[11] Most OXPHOS diseases appear to be transmitted in an autosomal recessive fashion.[12] This chapter reviews the clinical, biochemical, metabolic, and genetic features of OXPHOS diseases. The last time that this chapter was written, diseases were classified according to their molecular defect. However, this classification scheme is limited by the large amount of overlap in the clinical manifestations of nuclear DNA and mtDNA gene mutations, and is difficult for clinicians to use. This chapter organizes OXPHOS diseases according to the major clinical presentations that clinicians encounter (Tables 104-1 and 104-2), thus providing a clinical basis for diagnosis, management, and genetic counseling. Leber hereditary optic neuropathy is reviewed in Chap. 105.

OXIDATIVE PHOSPHORYLATION BIOCHEMISTRY AND GENETICS

Mitochondria are generally about 0.1 to 0.5 μm in diameter and in adult human muscle account for about 4 percent of the total fiber volume.[13] These are cytoplasmic structures with an inner and outer membrane separated by an intermembrane space. The outer membrane is permeable to most small molecules and ions and contains a variety of enzymes, such as monoamine oxidase, long-chain acyl-CoA synthetase, carnitine palmitoyl transferase 1 (CPT1), receptors, and mitochondrial protein import proteins. The inner mitochondrial membrane is impermeable to most metabolites. It has a convoluted structure with multiple folds called cristae. The inner membrane has a high content of protein and cardiolipin. It contains the enzymes of oxidative phosphorylation as well as multiple classes of translocases. The space surrounded by the inner mitochondrial membrane, called the mitochondrial matrix, contains a broad array of enzymes, including those for the Krebs cycle (tricarboxylic acid cycle), the pyruvate dehydrogenase complex, β-oxidation of fatty acids, urea cycle, ketone metabolism, amino acid metabolism, heme metabolism, nucleotide metabolism, and the peptidases, plus chaperonins necessary for mitochondrial protein import and OXPHOS enzyme assembly. The mitochondrial matrix also contains the mitochondrial DNA. The mtDNA is a 16,569-nucleotide pair, double-stranded, circular molecule that codes for 2 ribosomal RNAs (rRNA), 22 transfer RNAs (tRNA), and 13 polypeptides that, together with polypeptides coded by the nuclear DNA, form complexes I, III, IV, and V (Fig. 104-1).

OXPHOS uses about 95 percent of the oxygen delivered to tissues for producing most of the ATP that is required by cells. It produces about 18 times more ATP than glycolysis. The expression of these genes and the assembly of the five OXPHOS enzyme complexes (complexes I to V) into the inner mitochondrial membrane are highly ordered and coordinated processes that depend on gene expression from the mitochondrial DNA as well as the nuclear DNA. Although the mtDNA encodes only 13 polypeptide subunits of the OXPHOS enzymes, approximately 1000 proteins are estimated to be necessary for proper OXPHOS function. OXPHOS enzymes are located in the mitochondrial inner membrane and are designated complex I (NADH:ubiquinone oxidoreductase, EC 1.6.5.3), complex II (succinate:ubiquinone oxidoreductase, EC 1.3.5.1), complex III (ubiquinol:ferrocytochrome c oxidoreductase, EC 1.10.2.2), complex IV (ferrocytochrome c:oxygen oxidoreductase or cytochrome c oxidase, EC 1.9.3.1), and complex V (ATP synthase, EC 3.6.1.34). Complex I transfers electrons to ubiquinone (coenzyme Q_{10}) through a long series of redox groups that include flavin mononucleotide (FMN) and six iron-sulfur clusters. This large and fragile enzyme is composed of approximately 42 subunits, 7 encoded by the mtDNA and the remainder by the nuclear DNA. Complex II performs a key step in the citric acid cycle in which succinate is dehydrogenated to fumarate and the electrons are donated to ubiquinone in the mitochondrial inner membrane. Complex II is localized to the matrix side of the mitochondrial inner membrane and is the only OXPHOS enzyme where the nuclear DNA codes all subunits. Complex III catalyzes electron transfer between two mobile electron carriers, ubiquinol and cytochrome c, and translocates protons across the mitochondrial inner membrane. This enzyme is composed of 11 polypeptides, only 1 of which is encoded by the mtDNA. Complex IV or cytochrome c oxidase is the terminal enzyme complex for electron transport that collects electrons that are transferred from reduced cytochrome c and donates them to oxygen, which is then reduced to water. In conjunction with this process, protons are pumped across the mitochondrial inner membrane into the intermembrane space. Mammalian complex IV is composed of 13 polypeptide subunits, 3 of which the mtDNA encodes. Complex V uses the electrochemical gradient created by complexes I, III, and IV as a source of energy for synthesizing ATP from ADP + P_i. This enzyme is composed of two parts, the F_1 segment that catalyzes ATP synthesis, and the F_o segment that translocates protons into the mitochondrial matrix. It is composed of 12 to 13 subunits: 2 coded by the mtDNA (ATPase 6 and 8 genes) and 11 to 12 subunits coded by the nuclear DNA. The synthesis of ATP by complex V is functionally coupled to electron transport through complexes I, III, IV, and the reduction of oxygen. In coupled mitochondria, electron transport and oxygen consumption increase when ADP is available, and decline to a minimum constant level when ADP is limiting.

The cytoplasmic location of the mtDNA within the mitochondria is associated with a unique inheritance pattern called maternal inheritance. This inheritance pattern refers to the exclusive transmission of mtDNAs from a mother to her children. The mtDNA of the mother is transmitted to all of her children through the egg cytoplasm, which contains approximately 200,000 to 300,000 mtDNAs. Each human cell contains hundreds of pleomorphic mitochondria[14] and thousands of mtDNAs packaged as 2 to 10 mtDNAs per mitochondrion.[15–18] Although sperm (paternal) mitochondrial DNA does enter the oocyte at fertilization, it is actively eliminated.[19] Even with intracytoplasmic injection of the entire sperm into the oocyte, no paternal mtDNA is detectable in the offspring after delivery.[20] During oogenesis and embryogenesis, the density of mitochondria and the mtDNA copy number appear to be independently regulated, but highly coordinated. During oogenesis, the number of mitochondria increases approximately one hundredfold while the mtDNA copy number per mitochondrion decreases from 2–10 to 1–2 mtDNAs.[21,22] Following fertilization, the embryo undergoes rapid nuclear DNA replication and cell cleavage to yield a blastocyst without a significant increase in the number of mitochondria or mtDNAs. After the blastocyst is formed, oxygen consumption increases[23] in association with increased cytochrome c oxidase staining[24] and biogenesis of mitochondria and mtDNAs.[25–27]

When a pathogenic mtDNA mutation is present, the consequences of maternal transmission are influenced by whether the mtDNA is *homoplasmic* or *heteroplasmic*. The mtDNAs within a

Table 104-1 Nuclear DNA Mutations

Multiple mtDNA deletions	Phenotype
438, 676–682, 10, 439– 441, 682–687	Autosomal dominant progressive external ophthalmoplegia
456	Autosomal dominant progressive external ophthalmoplegia, rhabdomyolysis
688	Autosomal dominant progressive external ophthalmoplegia, hypogonadism, anticipation
439	Autosomal dominant ataxia, ketoacidotic coma
689	Autosomal recessive chronic progressive external ophthalmoplegia, oligoasthenospermia
417	Autosomal recessive cardiomyopathy and ophthalmoplegia
483	Autosomal recessive Wolfram syndrome
690	Myoclonic epilepsy and ragged-red fiber disease (MERRF)
166, 167	Multiple symmetrical lipomatosis
691, 692	Chronic progressive ophthalmoplegia
693	Chronic progressive ophthalmoplegia, demyelinating neuropathy, leukoencephalopathy, myopathy, gastrointestinal dysfunction
444	Myopathy, neuropathy
694	Sensory ataxia neuropathy
695	Inherited dilated cardiomyopathy
696	Male infertility
697	Essential hyperCPKemia
697	Subacute onset flaccid tetraplegia
697	Parkinsonism
698	Pigmentary retinopathy, L-dopa responsive tremor, rigidity, micrographia, peripheral neuropathy
699	Brachmann-de Lange syndrome, hyperthermia, mitochondrial myopathy
700	Chronic fatigue syndrome
701	Polymyalgia rheumatica, ragged-red fiber myopathy
281	Diabetes mellitus
702	Multiple sclerosis, mitochondrial myopathy
703	Periodic paralysis
455	Rhabdomyolysis, alcohol intolerance
Multiple mtDNA deletions (thymidine phosphorylase, Chr. 22q13.32-qter)	
446, 451, 453, 454, 676, 704–708	Myo-neuro-gastrointestinal encephalopathy (autosomal recessive)
mtDNA depletion (autosomal recessive)	
709, 403, 404, 710	Mitochondrial myopathy
403	Mitochondrial myopathy, nephropathy
403, 711–714	Hepatopathy (liver failure)
715	Liver disease, lactic acidemia, hypoketotic hypoglycemia
711	Liver failure, Leigh disease, cataracts
430, 431	Hypertrophic cardiomyopathy
716	Weakness, fatigability, post-exercise pain
717	Psychomotor delay, hypotonia, muscle weakness, areflexia, spasticity, ragged-red fiber and COX-negative fiber myopathy, lactic acidemia
405	Fatal cytochrome c oxidase deficient myopathy
718	Infantile fatal encephalomyopathy, lactic acidemia
719, 405, 720	Fatal infantile mitochondrial myopathy
481	Alpers disease, gamma polymerase deficiency
721	Spinal muscular atrophy phenocopy
722	Sideroblastic anemia, mild pancreatic insufficiency, mitochondrial myopathy (Pearson syndrome); multiple deletions present in asymptomatic mother
Succinate dehydrogenase, flavoprotein subunit	
11	Autosomal recessive Leigh disease
Complex I (18-kDa subunit, NDUFS4, AQDQ)	
460	Autosomal recessive Leigh disease
Complex I (NDUSF8 subunit, TYKY)	
461	Autosomal recessive Leigh disease

(Continued on next page)

Table 104-1 (Continued)

Multiple mtDNA deletions	Phenotype
Complex I (51-kDa subunit, NDUFV1, UQOR1)	
462	Autosomal recessive Leigh disease
462	Autosomal recessive Alexander disease
SURF1	
465	Autosomal recessive Leigh disease, cytochrome c oxidase deficiency
Frataxin	
487	Friedreich ataxia (autosomal recessive)
Paraplegin	
485	Autosomal recessive spastic paraplegia with ragged-red fibers
Tafazzin (G4.5)	
498–503	Barth syndrome (X-linked)

cell or tissue are referred to as homoplasmic when all the mtDNAs share the same sequence, and are referred to as heteroplasmic when mtDNAs with different sequences coexist. Individuals who do not have OXPHOS diseases are generally homoplasmic. The exception to this condition is the rare, neutral polymorphism, which is heteroplasmic. Pathogenic mtDNA mutations can be either homoplasmic or heteroplasmic, whereas neutral polymorphisms are usually homoplasmic. When heteroplasmy exists, the normal and mutant mtDNAs segregate randomly during cytokinesis to the daughter cells.[28,29] Once the mutant mtDNAs reach a critical level, cellular phenotype changes rapidly from normal to abnormal. The phenotypic consequences of an mtDNA mutation are a function of the severity of the mtDNA mutation, the percentage of mutant mtDNAs, and the differing energetic requirements of human organs and tissues. Each tissue requires a different minimum level (threshold) of mitochondrial ATP production to sustain normal cellular functions. In families with heteroplasmic mtDNA mutations, the severity of the OXPHOS defect varies with the percentage of normal mtDNAs. Therefore, different family members can inherit different percentages of mutant mtDNAs and can present with different clinical manifestations. The relationship between genotype and phenotype is more complex for pathogenic mtDNA mutations that are homoplasmic. Disease expression appears to be influenced by poorly understood genetic and environmental interactions.

PATIENT DIAGNOSIS ALGORITHM

OXPHOS diseases can result from mutations in mitochondrial genes or in nuclear OXPHOS genes. Because genes for OXPHOS are located in two distinct genomes, the inheritance of OXPHOS diseases may occur by maternal or Mendelian patterns (autosomal dominant, autosomal recessive, X-linked). Sporadic mutations in either the mtDNA or the nuclear DNA may also produce OXPHOS diseases. The basic elements of the algorithm are (a) phenotype recognition, (b) metabolic testing, (c) skeletal muscle pathology, (d) OXPHOS biochemistry, and (e) genetic testing of the mtDNA or nuclear DNA (Fig. 104-2). Due to rapid advances in genetic testing, the entire mtDNA can be screened using single-strand conformation polymorphism (SSCP) analysis and direct sequencing of SSCP variants. This approach to patient evaluation permits assignment of the patient's phenotype to the nuclear DNA or to the mtDNA, which is important for genetic counseling of families.

Phenotype Recognition

Due to the large number of phenotypes that are described, phenotype recognition can be difficult. Tables 104-1 and 104-2 outline major classes of phenotype-genotype associations in patients with OXPHOS diseases. Leber hereditary optic neuropathy is covered in Chap. 105.

Neuroradiology

The neuroradiologic examination is important in patients suspected of having an OXPHOS disease. Since lesions that are important for the diagnosis may be either symptomatic or asymptomatic, brain MRI is frequently indicated. Lesions appear over time. Thus, patients with new or persistent symptoms may require follow-up brain MRI assessment, even if a prior scan was interpreted as normal. When assessing patients for an OXPHOS disease, MR imaging and proton spectroscopy can detect asymptomatic lesions, as well as increases in brain lactate.[30] Neuroradiologic abnormalities include basal ganglia lesions (increased T2-weighted signal), strokes (large or small vessel), cerebellar atrophy or cerebellar lesions (increased T2-weighted signal), cerebral atrophy, and white matter or pyramidal tract lesions (increased T2-weighted signal).[31,32]

Metabolic Testing in OXPHOS Diseases

Abnormalities in oxidative phosphorylation can produce identifiable defects in related metabolic pathways such as glycolysis, pyruvate metabolism, the tricarboxylic acid cycle, protein catabolism, and fatty acid oxidation. Although the quantitation of organic acids and amino acids in blood, urine, and cerebrospinal fluid can provide useful diagnostic information, normal values for metabolic tests do not exclude the diagnosis. Metabolic acidosis as well as elevations of lactate, pyruvate, lactate/pyruvate ratio (>20), alanine, tricarboxylic acid cycle intermediates, dicarboxylic acids, and/or a generalized amino aciduria can be important diagnostic clues to the presence of an OXPHOS disease. Other metabolites that may also be increased are tiglylglycine, ethylmalonic acid,[33] 3-methylglutaconic acid plus 3-hydroxy-3-methylglutaric acid,[34,35] 2-ethylhydracrylic acid,[36] 2-methylsuccinate, butyrylglycine, isovaleryl glycine, and ammonia. Excretion

Table 104-2 mtDNA Genotype and Phenotype Associations

mtDNA deletions/duplications (sporadic, clonal)	
29, 39, 45, 55, 57, 65, 74, 77, 78, 81, 87–90, 92, 96–103, 237, 411, 412, 478, 479, 601, 686, 708, 723–833	Kearns-Sayre and chronic progressive external ophthalmoplegia syndromes
83	Kearns-Sayre syndrome, mitochondrial encephalomyopathy, lactic acidosis, stroke-like episodes (MELAS), hypoparathyroidism, diabetes mellitus
544, 834	Kearns-Sayre syndrome (delivery of healthy children)
835, 836	Kearns-Sayre syndrome, hypoparathyroidism
837	Kearns-Sayre syndrome, hypoparathyroidism, diabetes mellitus
838	Kearns-Sayre syndrome, pernicious anemia, hypoparathyroidism
839	Kearns-Sayre syndrome, pituitary hypothyroidism, periventricular white matter abnormalities
840	Kearns-Sayre syndrome, corneal decompensation
841	Kearns-Sayre syndrome, choroideremia-like fundus
842	Kearns-Sayre syndrome, dilated cardiomyopathy with successful cardiac transplantation
85	Kearns-Sayre syndrome, choroideremia-like fundus
843	Kearns-Sayre syndrome, oculocerebrorenal syndrome (Lowe syndrome)
844	Kearns-Sayre syndrome, anhidrosis, de Toni-Debré-Fanconi syndrome
845	Kearns-Sayre syndrome, Bartter syndrome
	Kearns-Sayre syndrome, onset as renal tubular acidosis + tetany
846	Chronic progressive external ophthalmoplegia presenting with unilateral ptosis
545	Chronic progressive external ophthalmoplegia, pregnancy complicated by preterm labor, hypertension
847	Chronic progressive external ophthalmoplegia plus, stroke, epilepsy
839	Chronic progressive external ophthalmoplegia, periventricular white matter lesions, pituitary hypothyroidism
848	Ptosis, pigmentary retinopathy, normal ocular motility, no ragged-red fibers
842	Chronic progressive external ophthalmoplegia, deafness, cardiomyopathy with successful cardiac transplantation
849	Chronic progressive external ophthalmoplegia, familial hypercholesterolemia
710	Chronic progressive external ophthalmoplegia, abnormal markers of oxidative stress
850	Chronic progressive external ophthalmoplegia, Marfanoid appearance, cytoplasmic bodies in muscle
851	Adult-onset mitochondrial myopathy
110–115, 727, 774, 852–873	Pearson syndrome
874	Pearson syndrome, Kearns-Sayre syndrome
875	Pearson syndrome with neonatal death
876	Pearson syndrome, multiple renal cysts
877, 878	Pearson syndrome, Leigh disease
879	Pearson syndrome, de Toni-Debré-Fanconi syndrome
880	Pearson syndrome variant: sideroblastic anemia with vacuolization of hematopoietic precursors
881	Pearson syndrome, zonular cataract, secondary strabismus
882	Pearson syndrome variant: exocrine pancreas dysfunction, mitochondrial myopathy
883	Pearson syndrome variant: Congenital hypoplastic anemia, diabetes mellitus, exocrine pancreas insufficiency, renal tubule dysfunction, cerebral atrophy
884	Pearson syndrome variant: altered tricarboxylic acid and urea cycle metabolites, adrenal insufficiency, corneal opacities
35	Pearson syndrome, 3-methylglutaconic aciduria
885	Cerebellar ataxia, hypogonadotropic hypogonadism, chorioretinal dystrophy
886	Cerebral palsy and growth hormone deficiency
887	Developmental delay, regression, brainstem dysfunction, lactic acidosis, pancytopenia, failure to thrive, absence of ragged-red and COX-negative fibers
888	Adrenal insufficiency
889	Adrenal insufficiency, growth retardation, deafness, leukodystrophy
890	Diabetes mellitus, optic atrophy, deafness (DIDMOAD, Wolfram phenotype)
891	Diabetes mellitus, cataracts, deafness, macular dystrophy
889	Diabetes mellitus, mitochondrial myopathy, leukodystrophy
892	Diabetes mellitus, diabetic amyotrophy, diabetic myoatrophy, diabetic fatty liver
893	Diabetes mellitus, Fanconi syndrome
894	Mitochondrial myopathy, axonal neuropathy
168	Mitochondrial myopathy, multiple symmetric lipomatosis
895	MELAS, Fanconi syndrome
330	Leigh disease
896	Infantile cardioencephalomyopathy with decreased carnitine acetyltransferase

(*Continued on next page*)

Table 104-2 (Continued)

897, 898	Cluster headache
899	Migrainous strokes (complicated migraines); ragged-red fibers
900	Leukodystrophy, chronic renal failure, tubulointerstitial nephritis
901	Hypoparathyroidism, ataxia, spastic paraparesis, myopathy, deafness, short stature, vitiligo, hirsutism, anemia, diabetes, exocrine pancreas dysfunction
901	Renal tubule dysfunction (polydipsia, polyuria), fatigue, ataxia, deafness
902	Leukodystrophy, ataxia, bulbar palsy, ragged-red fiber myopathy
903	Chronic tubulointerstitial nephropathy, megaloblastic anemia, growth retardation, partial renal Fanconi syndrome
455, 775	Recurrent myoglobinuria
904	Chronic diarrhea, villous atrophy
52	Inclusion body myositis
905	Affective disorder
mtDNA deletion (sporadic, clonal) plus maternally transmitted tRNA$^{Leucine(UUR)}$ A3243G mutation	
906	Kearns-Sayre syndrome, autoimmune polyglandular syndrome (Addison disease, autoimmune insulin-dependent diabetes mellitus, Hashimoto thyroiditis, primary ovarian failure)
mtDNA deletion/duplication (maternally transmitted)	
907	Kearns-Sayre syndrome
263, 908–910	Diabetes, deafness
482, 890	Wolfram syndrome (optic atrophy, diabetes mellitus, diabetes insipidus, deafness, urinary tract abnormalities, neurologic dysfunction)
911, 912	Chronic progressive external ophthalmoplegia
913	Chronic progressive external ophthalmoplegia in mother and Pearson syndrome in son
94	Chronic progressive external ophthalmoplegia in mother and daughters with proximal tubulopathy, diabetes mellitus, cerebellar ataxia
909	Chronic progressive external ophthalmoplegia, diabetes mellitus
Focal mtDNA deletion accumulation	
914, 915	Late-onset mitochondrial myopathy
mtDNA microdeletion	
916	Transient lactic acidosis, newborn
mtDNA microdeletion (15 bp, COX III)	
917	Recurrent myoglobinuria
mtDNA duplication/triplication	
918	Asymptomatic (10–12% muscle levels)
mtDNA duplication/triplication (260 bp, D-Loop)	
919	Mitochondrial myopathy
920	Chronic progressive ophthalmoplegia syndrome patients and asymptomatic mothers
mtDNA point mutations	
tRNA^{Phenylalanine} T618C	
921	Mitochondrial myopathy
12S rRNA 961 (cytosine deletion)	
922	Non-syndromic deafness, aminoglycoside-induced deafness
12S rRNA A1555G	
371–373, 922–938	Non-syndromic deafness, aminoglycoside-induced deafness
939	Maternally inherited cardiomyopathy
tRNA^{Valine} G1606A	
940	Ataxia, seizures, dementia, myopathy, deafness
941	MELAS
tRNA^{Valine} G1642A	
942	MELAS
tRNA^{Valine} G1644A	
943	Adult-onset Leigh disease
16S rRNA C2835T	
944, 945	Rett syndrome
16s rRNA G3196A	
946	Alzheimer and Parkinson disease
tRNA$^{Leucine(UUR)}$ A3243G	
43, 44, 46, 55, 58, 65, 104, 107, 108, 195, 196, 198, 199, 201, 202, 211, 230, 245, 255, 258, 275, 279, 299, 301, 305, 324, 411, 412, 478, 479, 708, 756, 761, 772, 777, 800, 801, 871, 947–1000	MELAS (maternally inherited, sporadic)

Table 104-2 (Continued)

1001	MELAS, cataracts
1002	MELAS, laminar cortical necrosis, severe cortical atrophy
1003	MELAS, cardiomyopathy
1004, 1005	MELAS, diabetes mellitus, hyperthyroidism
1006	MELAS, chronic renal failure
961	MELAS with ophthalmoplegia, developmental delay, pigmentary retinopathy, or intestinal pseudo-obstruction
1007	MELAS, ophthalmoplegia, pigmentary retinopathy
1008	MELAS without ragged-red fiber myopathy, normal lactate level (rest and post-exercise)
1009, 1010	Late onset MELAS ($>$50 years)
1011	Myopathy, seizures
1011	Myopathy, leukoencephalopathy
365	Myopathy, cardiomyopathy
954	Variable combinations of deafness, mitochondrial myopathy, diabetes mellitus, mental retardation
234	Variable intrafamilial combinations of deafness, retinal pigmentary degeneration, migraine headaches, hypothalamic hypogonadism, mitochondrial myopathy
961	Encephalopathy, deafness, ataxia, dementia
964	Chronic mild encephalopathy, short stature, hearing loss
251, 275, 993, 994, 1012	MERRF
169	MERRF, basal ganglia calcifications
1013	MERRF/MELAS overlap
973, 1003, 1014	Hypertrophic cardiomyopathy
994	Kearns-Sayre syndrome
275, 788, 957, 961, 969, 970, 993, 995, 1015–1017	Chronic progressive external ophthalmoplegia syndromes (variable expression of deafness, diabetes mellitus, pigmentary retinopathy)
970, 1018	Chronic progressive external ophthalmoplegia, MELAS
993	Chronic progressive external ophthalmoplegia, MELAS, MERRF features
1019	Chronic progressive external ophthalmoplegia, MELAS, carnitine deficiency
237	Juvenile cataract + retinal pigmentary degeneration
239	Renal failure
239, 1020, 1021	Cardiomyopathy
246, 275, 279, 961, 1022	Mitochondrial myopathy
970, 994	Deafness
224, 229, 230, 235–303	Diabetes mellitus $\pm$ deafness, $\pm$ islet cell antibodies
1023	Diabetes mellitus, pancreatic exocrine dysfunction
1024	Diabetes mellitus, cardiomyopathy, sick sinus syndrome (1st degree AV block, incomplete right bundle branch block) progressing to sinus arrest
300, 1025	Diabetes mellitus, hearing loss, cardiomyopathy
1026	Diabetes mellitus, pregnancy, spontaneous abortion
1027–1030	Diabetes mellitus, hypertrophic cardiomyopathy
1031	Diabetes mellitus, hyperechogenic cardiomyopathy
1032	Diabetes mellitus, decreased cerebral blood perfusion
1033	Diabetes mellitus, pigmentary retinopathy
1034	Diabetes mellitus, deafness, cerebellar ataxia
30	Diabetes mellitus, deafness, Leigh disease variant with asymptomatic basal ganglia and subcortical increase of T2 MRI signal (adult)
1035	Diabetes mellitus, mental retardation, growth hormone deficiency, nephropathy
1036	Diabetes mellitus, psychiatric symptoms
891	Diabetes mellitus, deafness, macular dystrophy, retinal branch vein occlusion
1037–1040	Diabetes mellitus, deafness, macular pattern retinal dystrophy
1041	Diabetes mellitus, deafness, progressive non-diabetic kidney disease (Alport-like phenotype)
258	Diabetic embryopathy (anal atresia, caudal dysgenesis, multicystic dysplastic kidneys)
234	Diabetes mellitus, retinitis pigmentosa, hypothalamic hypogonadism, mitochondrial myopathy (variable manifestations within a pedigree)
255	Gestational diabetes
1042	MERRF, chronic progressive external ophthalmoplegia overlap
1013, 1043	MERRF/MELAS overlap
1044	Leigh disease
1045	Psychosis, mitochondrial myopathy, Alzheimer-like neuropathology
258	Infantile intractable seizures, developmental delay
967	Cardiac and gastrointestinal abnormalities
1046	Recurrent respiratory failure
1047	Depressive disorder
1048	Cluster headache
1049	*No association with larger populations of cluster headache patients
1050	VACTERL (vertebral, anal, cardiovascular, tracheoesophageal, renal, limb defects)

(*Continued on next page*)

Table 104-2 (Continued)

58	Failure to thrive, developmental delay
1051	Failure to thrive, developmental delay, microcephaly, seizures, lactic acidosis, pancreatitis
62, 1052	Demyelinating polyneuropathy
66	Peripheral neuropathy, rhabdomyolysis, severe lactic acidosis
1053	Subacute dementia, cerebral atrophy, myoclonus, periodic synchronous discharge (EEG) (Creutzfeldt-Jakob-like presentation)
1054	Parkinsonism, dementia, vertical supranuclear ophthalmoplegia, deafness
1054	Ataxia, vertical supranuclear ophthalmoplegia, deafness
1055	Asymptomatic retinal abnormalities
1056	Chronic asthma, depression
973	Analysis of fetus
$tRNA^{Leucine(UUR)}$ A3243T	
1057	Mitochondrial encephalomyopathy
$tRNA^{Leucine(UUR)}$ T3250C	
632	Mitochondrial myopathy, riboflavin-responsive
368	Mitochondrial myopathy
$tRNA^{Leucine(UUR)}$ A3251G	
1058	Fatal mitochondrial myopathy, lactic acidosis
1059	Mitochondrial myopathy, psychiatric features, sudden death
$tRNA^{Leucine(UUR)}$ A3252G	
1060	Mitochondrial encephalomyopathy, pigmentary retinopathy, dementia, hypoparathyroidism, and diabetes mellitus
$tRNA^{Leucine(UUR)}$ C3254G	
1061	Mitochondrial myopathy, cardiomyopathy
$tRNA^{Leucine(UUR)}$ C3256T	
1062, 1063	Diabetes mellitus
1064, 1065	MERRF, optic atrophy, retinitis pigmentosa, diabetes mellitus
$tRNA^{Leucine(UUR)}$ A3260G	
1066	MELAS
365, 1067–1070	Cardiomyopathy, myopathy
$tRNA^{Leucine(UUR)}$ T3264C	
1071	Diabetes mellitus
1072	Diabetes mellitus, cervical lipoma, ataxia, deafness, ophthalmoplegia, bilateral facial nerve palsy, olfactory dysfunction
$tRNA^{Leucine(UUR)}$ A3271C	
105, 202, 978, 985, 1073–1075	MELAS
240	Diabetes mellitus
$tRNA^{Leucine(UUR)}$ 3271 thymidine deletion	
1076	Mitochondrial encephalomyopathy with severe intracerebral calcifications (Fahr disease variant)
$tRNA^{Leucine(UUR)}$ T3290C	
1077	Diabetes mellitus
$tRNA^{Leucine(UUR)}$ T3291G	
1078	MELAS
$tRNA^{Leucine(UUR)}$ A3302G	
1079	Mitochondrial myopathy
$tRNA^{Leucine(UUR)}$ C3303T	
1080	Fatal infantile cardiomyopathy
1080	Cardiomyopathy, myopathy
1080	Sudden cardiac death
ND1 T3308C (methionine to threonine)	
1081	MELAS, Leigh variant (bilateral striatal necrosis)
ND1 G3316A (alanine to threonine)	
1077, 1082–1084	Diabetes mellitus, noninsulin-dependent
ND1 T3394C (tyrosine to histidine)	
1085	Japanese noninsulin-dependent diabetes mellitus
ND1 A3397G (methionine to valine)	
1086	Alzheimer and Parkinson disease
ND1 G3460A (alanine to threonine)	
297, 1087–1106	Leber hereditary optic neuropathy
1107	Spastic dystonia
1108	Multiple sclerosis-like phenotype in females

Table 104-2 (Continued)

ND1 T4160C (leucine to proline) plus T14484C (ND6, methionine to valine)	
1095	Juvenile encephalopathy and peripheral neurologic signs
tRNA^{Isoleucine} A4269G	
1109, 1110	Dilated cardiomyopathy, short stature, deafness, epilepsy, focal glomerulosclerosis, mitochondrial myopathy
tRNA^{Isoleucine} T4285C	
1111	Chronic progressive external ophthalmoplegia
tRNA^{Isoleucine} G4295A	
1112	Hypertrophic cardiomyopathy, successful cardiac transplantation
tRNA^{Isoleucine} G4298A	
1113	Chronic progressive external ophthalmoplegia, multiple sclerosis
tRNA^{Isoleucine} A4300G	
1114	Hypertrophic cardiomyopathy, mitochondrial myopathy
tRNA^{Isoleucine} A4317G	
364	Fatal infantile cardiomyopathy
tRNA^{Isoleucine} C4320T	
1115	Infantile encephalopathy, hypotonia, seizures, spastic tetraparesis, hyporeflexia, increased CSF protein, cerebral atrophy, intractable cardiomyopathy
tRNA^{Glutamine} T4336C	
946	Alzheimer and Parkinson disease
tRNA^{Methionine} T4409C	
1116	Mitochondrial myopathy, exercise intolerance
tRNA^{Tryptophan} G5521A	
1117	Mitochondrial myopathy
tRNA^{Tryptophan} T5537 insertion	
1118	Mitochondrial encephalomyopathy
1118	Leigh disease
tRNA^{Tryptophan} G5549A	
1119	Dementia, chorea, cerebellar ataxia, deafness, peripheral neuropathy, ragged-red fiber myopathy
tRNA^{Alanine} A5601G	
991	MELAS
Nucleotide separating tRNA^{Alanine} and tRNA^{Asparagine} A5656G	
1120	Severe mitochondrial encephalomyopathy (intracellular triplasmy, see tRNA^{Glycine} T10010C)
1121	Familial progressive tubulointerstitial nephritis
tRNA^{Asparagine} A5692G	
976, 1122	Chronic progressive external ophthalmoplegia
tRNA^{Asparagine} G5703A	
1065	Chronic progressive external ophthalmoplegia syndromes
tRNA^{Cysterine} A5814G	
1123	Chronic progressive external ophthalmoplegia plus
1124	Mitochondrial encephalomyopathy
tRNA^{Tyrosine} G5877A	
1125	CPEO
COXI, 5-bp deletion	
1126	Motor neuron disease (isolated) with increased CSF protein
COXI T6721C (isoleucine to threonine)	
1127	Acquired sideroblastic anemia
COXI T6742C (methionine to threonine)	
1127	Acquired sideroblastic anemia
RNA$^{Serine(UCN)}$ /COXI A7445G	
1128–1131	Non-syndromic deafness
1132	Non-syndromic deafness ± palmoplantar keratosis
tRNA$^{Serine(UCN)}$ 7472 cytosine insertion	
1133	Deafness, ataxia, myoclonus
1133, 1134	Deafness
577	Deafness, ataxia, dementia
tRNA$^{Serine(UCN)}$ G7497A	
577	Mitochondrial myopathy, exercise intolerance, lactic acidosis, complex I and IV deficiency
tRNA$^{Serine(UCN)}$ T7512C	
1135	MERRF/MELAS
577	Deafness, ataxia, dementia
9-bp insertion: noncoding region COXII/tRNA^{Lysine}	
1136	Mitochondrial encephalomyopathy

(*Continued on next page*)

Table 104-2 (Continued)

1136	Leigh disease
1137	9-bp insertion in population control (eastern Tharu)
tRNA^{Lysine} A8296G	
304	Diabetes mellitus ± sensorineural deafness
tRNA^{Lysine} A8296G	
1138	MERRF (triplasmy: A8296G plus G8363A)
tRNA^{Lysine} G8313A	
1139	Gastrointestinal symptoms, seizures, deafness, peripheral neuropathy, ragged-red fiber myopathy, progressive encephalopathy
tRNA^{Lysine} A8344G	
44, 107, 117, 145–151, 155, 156, 161, 165, 171, 411, 412, 478, 479, 686, 708, 761, 800, 801, 960, 1140–1167	MERRF
237	MERRF, pigmentary retinal degeneration
1168	MERRF, bilateral optic atrophy
1169	MERRF, overwhelming lactic acidosis
163	MERRF, multiple symmetrical lipomatosis with clonal chromosome 6 deletion in lipomas
1170	MERRF, dizygotic twins
1150	Late-onset MERRF (63 years)
165, 1147	Mitochondrial myopathy
1147	Mitochondrial myopathy, sensory neuropathy
1140	Cardiomyopathy
1140	Rapid onset dementia
160, 162	Ekbom syndrome (photomyoclonus, cerebellar ataxia, cervical lipoma)
161, 164, 167	Multiple symmetric lipomatosis
165	Truncal lipomas, myopathy
1171	Leigh disease, dystonia
165, 330, 1044, 1154, 1172–1174	Leigh disease
1154	MELAS
1154	Chronic progressive external ophthalmoplegia
1164	Chronic progressive external ophthalmoplegia, lipoma, mitochondrial myopathy
1172	Spinocerebellar degeneration
1172	Atypical Charcot-Marie-Tooth disease
281, 1175	Diabetes mellitus
1150	Late-onset dementia, seizures, myopathy
tRNA^{Lysine} T8356G	
152, 153, 1176, 1177	MERRF/MELAS overlap
1178	MERRF
tRNA^{Lysine} G8363A	
1179, 1180	MERRF
1138	MERRF (triplasmy: A8296G plus G8363A)
ATP6 T8851C (tryptophan to arginine)	
1181	Leigh disease
ATP6 T8993G (leucine to arginine)	
330–332, 334, 335, 352, 479, 542, 960, 1044, 1182–1194	Leigh disease (sporadic or maternally transmitted)
1195	Leigh disease, hypertrophic cardiomyopathy
1196	Leigh disease, ragged-red fibers
336, 1183, 1190, 1197–1199	Neuropathy, ataxia, retinitis pigmentosa (NARP)
1200	Neuropathy, ataxia, retinitis pigmentosa (NARP), prenatal diagnosis
1201	Retinitis pigmentosa, ataxia, mental retardation
1202	Severe infantile lactic acidosis, encephalopathy
1197	Kearns-Sayre syndrome
1203	Mental retardation, ataxia
1201	Mental retardation, ataxia, retinitis pigmentosa
1204	Non-specific developmental delay
1204	Cerebral palsy
1205	Lactic acidosis
ATP6 T8993C (leucine to proline)	
330, 1206–1208	Leigh disease
ATP6 T9101C (isoleucine to threonine)	
1209	Leber hereditary optic neuropathy

Table 104-2 (Continued)

ATP6 T9176C (leucine to proline)	
1210	Leigh disease, sudden death
1211, 1212	Leigh disease
1211	Ataxia
COXIII, G9952A (stop codon, 13-amino-acid loss)	
1213	Episodic encephalopathy, lactic acidemia, exercise intolerance, proximal myopathy, COX-deficient myofibers
COXIII, T9957C (phenylalanine to leucine)	
1214	MELAS
$tRNA^{Glycine}$ T9997C	
1215, 1216	Infantile hypertrophic cardiomyopathy, fatal ventricular arrhythmia
$tRNA^{Glycine}$ 10006	
976	Chronic intestinal pseudo-obstruction
$tRNA^{Glycine}$ T10010C	
1120	Ataxia, dystonia, increased CSF protein, hepatopathy, seizures, spasticity, mitochondrial myopathy (intracellular triplasmy, see A5656G)
$tRNA^{Glycine}$ A10044G	
1217	Severe encephalopathy, sudden death
ND4 A11696G (valine to isoleucine)	
362	Spastic dystonia, Leber hereditary optic neuropathy
ND4 G11778A (arginine to histidine)	
1088, 1089, 1091–1094, 1096–1101, 1218–1242, 1243, 1102, 1244, 1245, 1246, 1247, 1248, 1249, 1250, 1251, 1252, 1253, 1254, 757, 1255, 9, 76, 757, 776, 1104, 1105, 1251, 1256–1291	Leber hereditary optic neuropathy (± Wolff-Parkinson-White syndrome); maternally inherited and singleton cases
1292	Stargardt type maculopathy
1293	Leber hereditary optic neuropathy, discordant phenotype in twins
1294, 1295	Leber hereditary optic neuropathy, cerebellar ataxia
1296	Leber hereditary optic neuropathy, multiple sclerosis-like syndrome
1297	Absence of association in larger multiple sclerosis populations
1107	Spastic dystonia
1298	Abnormal brain and muscle 31-PNMR
1299	Diabetes mellitus, optic atrophy, generalized seizures, hearing loss (DIDMOAD-like syndrome)
1108, 1300	Multiple sclerosis-like syndrome (females)
1301, 1302	Leber hereditary optic neuropathy, demyelinating disease
1302	Leber hereditary optic neuropathy, oculopalatal myoclonus, Parinaud syndrome
ND4 A12026G (isoleucine to valine)	
1303	Diabetes mellitus
$tRNA^{Serine(GCU)}$ C12246G	
976	Chronic intestinal pseudo-obstruction
$tRNA^{Serine(GCU)}$ C12258A	
1304	Retinitis pigmentosa, deafness
$tRNA^{Leucine(CUN)}$ G12301A	
1305	Acquired sideroblastic anemia
$tRNA^{Leucine(CUN)}$ T12311C	
1306	Chronic progressive external ophthalmoplegia
$tRNA^{Leucine(CUN)}$ G12315A	
1307	Chronic progressive external ophthalmoplegia, ptosis, mitochondrial myopathy, deafness, pigmentary retinopathy
$tRNA^{Leucine(CUN)}$ A12320G	
1308	Mitochondrial myopathy (isolated)
ND5 G13513A	
1309	MELAS
ND6 14484	
1088, 1089, 1091–1093, 1219, 1310–1312, 1095, 1097, 1098, 1104, 1105, 1313, 1314	Leber hereditary optic neuropathy
1315	Leber hereditary optic neuropathy, brainstem involvement

(*Continued on next page*)

Table 104-2 (Continued)

ND6 G14459A (alanine to valine)	
1316–1318	Leber hereditary optic neuropathy, dystonia
ND6 T14498C (tyrosine to cysteine)	
1319	Leber hereditary optic neuropathy
tRNA^{Glutamate} T14709C	
1320	Diabetes mellitus, deafness, mitochondrial myopathy, pigmentary retinal degeneration
1321	Congenital myopathy, mental retardation, ataxia
1321	Adult-onset diabetes mellitus
1321, 1322	Adult-onset diabetes mellitus and ragged-red fiber myopathy
Cytochrome b 14787, 4-base pair deletion	
1323	Parkinsonism, MELAS overlap
Cytochrome b, G15059A (glycine to stop codon; 244-amino-acid loss)	
1324	Exercise intolerance, myoglobinuria
Cytochrome b, C15452A (leucine to isoleucine)	
1325	Ischemic cardiomyopathy
Cytochrome b, G15615A (glycine to aspartate)	
1326, 1327	Progressive exercise intolerance, myopathy, complex III deficiency with antimycin resistance
Cytochrome b, G15762A (glycine to glutamate)	
1328	Mitochondrial myopathy
tRNA^{Threonine} G15915A	
1329, 1330	Deafness, basal ganglia calcifications, cataracts, mental retardation, hypogonadotropic-hypogonadism, short stature, myoclonus, lactic acidemia
tRNA^{Threonine} A15923G	
406, 407, 1331	Lethal infantile mitochondrial disease (newborn, hypoglycemia, lactic acidosis, multisystem failure, cardiac arrest; similarly affected brother, multiple miscarriages in the mother and her sister)
tRNA^{Threonine} A15924G	
406	Lethal infantile mitochondrial disease
tRNA^{Threonine} 15940, thymidine deletion	
	Mitochondrial myopathy
tRNA^{Proline} G15990A	
1332, 1333	Mitochondrial myopathy
tRNA^{Proline} C15990T	
1333	Mitochondrial myopathy

of carnitine esters may be associated with reduced blood and tissue carnitine levels. A 24-h urine collection is useful because it can provide an integrated evaluation of organic and amino acids, as well as insight into the function of the highly OXPHOS-dependent proximal renal tubules. Although this is easily accomplished in adults, a 24-h urine collection is difficult in pediatric patients, and spot urine collection is used.[37] Analysis of organic and amino acids in venous blood can be complicated by technical factors such as duration of tourniquet application, activity such as recent seizures or vigorous crying and struggling that occurs in some children during venipuncture, delays in sample processing, and inconsistencies in the extraction of organic acids from blood samples. To enhance the accuracy of lactate and pyruvate determinations and amino acid analysis, as well as our ability to reliably compare serial determinations, the blood is collected as a morning sample after an overnight fast. CSF lactate and pyruvate testing can be an important aspect of the evaluation. In some patients, an increase in CSF lactate is the only metabolic abnormality found.

Skeletal Muscle Pathology in OXPHOS Diseases

Most patients who are suspected of having an OXPHOS disease require a muscle biopsy. Muscle biopsy is a safe procedure that is performed under general anesthesia in children and under local anesthesia in adults. It is unclear whether children with OXPHOS diseases have a higher risk of anesthetic complications than do children with other types of neurologic diseases. Anesthetic complications are best minimized by close attention to cardiac status (cardiomyopathies and arrhythmias), respiratory muscle weakness, airway protection in patients with oropharyngeal dysfunction, blood glucose control in diabetic patients, and the patient's propensity to develop lactic acidosis. Although it is unclear whether patients with OXPHOS diseases are at increased risk for developing malignant hyperthermia, these precautions are taken in patients with OXPHOS diseases who receive general anesthesia at our institution.

Most patients with OXPHOS diseases will have identifiable biochemical or pathologic manifestations. The primary goals of the muscle biopsy are (a) to assess the muscle for other diseases; (b) to isolate mitochondria for biochemical testing; (c) to isolate DNA for testing; (d) to look for pathologic changes in the muscle such as fibrosis and inflammation that would produce secondary abnormalities in the muscle biochemistry; and (e) to search for those histochemical, immunohistochemical, or ultrastructural changes that support the presence of an OXPHOS disease.

Only a few histochemical changes are predictive of the presence of an OXPHOS disease: (a) ragged-red fibers; (b) abnormal increases in succinate dehydrogenase reactions; and (3)

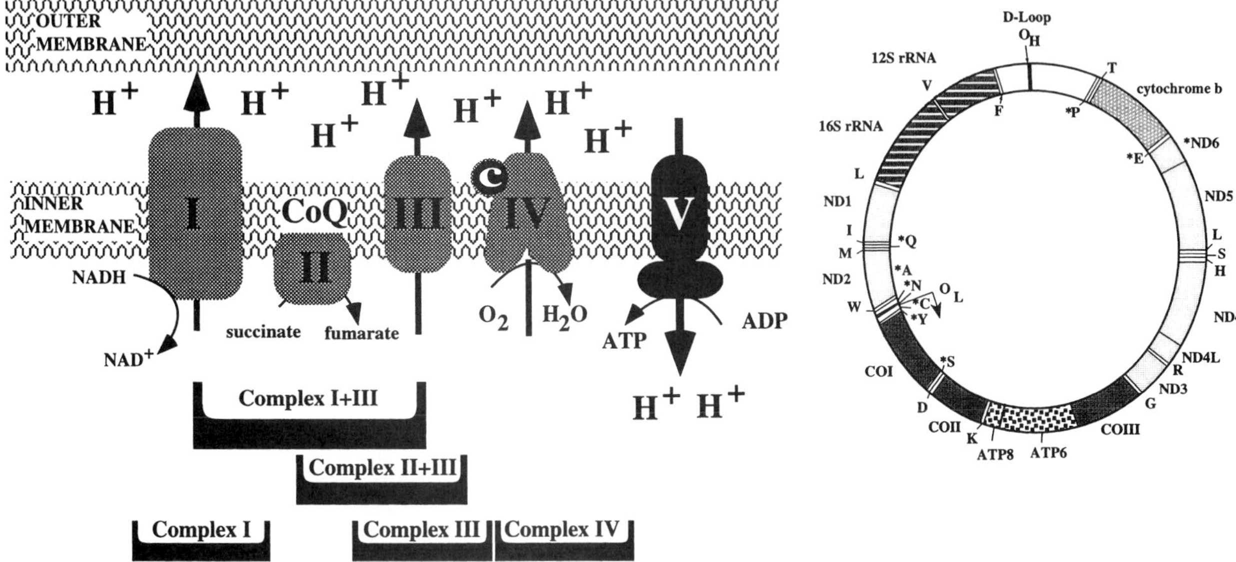

Fig. 104-1 Oxidative phosphorylation and mitochondrial DNA. Complexes I to V are located in the inner mitochondrial membrane. OXPHOS enzyme assays used in our laboratory for patient assessment are listed under the pathway. The assays measuring electron flow across single OXPHOS enzymes are the complex I assay in which the specific activity is measured by following the reduction of the coenzyme Q analog, n-decyl-coenzyme Q, after the addition of NADH; the complex III assay in which the specific activity is measured by following the reduction of cytochrome c with the addition of reduced n-decyl-coenzyme Q; and the complex IV assay in which the specific activity is measured by following the reduction of ferrocytochrome c by oxygen. Two assays assess the movement of electrons between complexes and are the complex I + III assay which follows the reduction of cytochrome c after the addition of NADH. Rotenone, a specific respiratory inhibitor of complex I, is used to determine the proportion of the activity that is specific to OXPHOS. The complex II + III assay measures the reduction of cytochrome c following the addition of succinate. Refer to references 7 and 15 for a description of the assays. Human mtDNA is shown with the locations of polypeptide genes encoding complex I subunits (ND1, ND2, ND3, ND4, ND4L, ND5, ND6), the complex III subunit (cytochrome b), the complex IV subunits (COI, COII, COIII), and the complex V subunits (ATP6, ATP8), the intervening transfer RNAs, and the ribosomal RNA genes (12S rRNA and 16S rRNA). Abbreviations: c = cytochrome c; CoQ = coenzyme Q10; H^+ = protons; O_L = origin of light strand replication; O_H = origin of heavy strand replication. Transfer RNAs: A = alanine; R = arginine; N = asparagine; D = aspartate; C = cysteine; E = glutamate; Q = glutamine; G = glycine; H = histidine; I = isoleucine; L = leucine; K = lysine; M = methionine; F = phenylalanine; P = proline; S = serine; T = threonine; W = tryptophan; Y = tyrosine; V = valine.

cytochrome c oxidase-deficient fibers. Proliferation of subsarcolemmal mitochondria with degeneration of the muscle fibers is called ragged-red fibers. This abnormality can be detected by Gomori-trichrome staining,[2] as well as by succinate dehydrogenase histochemistry. The percentage of ragged-red fibers shows large interindividual variability, ranging from approximately 2 percent to 70 percent of the total fibers. Ragged-red fibers also have mild accumulations of glycogen and neutral lipid. Pathologic alterations are segmental and do not extend the length of the myofiber, thus emphasizing the heterogeneous nature of the skeletal muscle manifestations.[38,39] The abnormal myofiber segments can have sharp boundaries, as in Kearns-Sayre and

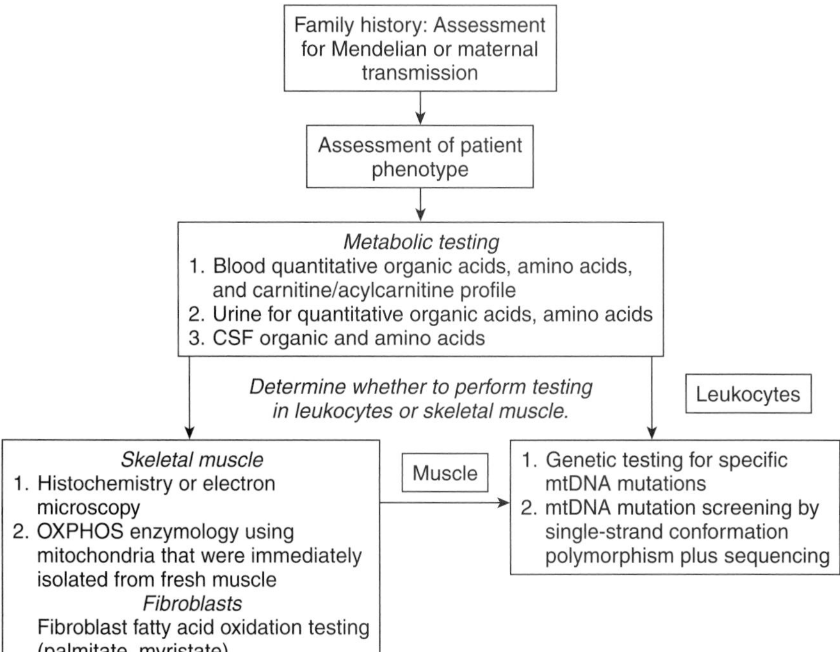

Fig. 104-2 Patient diagnosis algorithm. The basic clinical and laboratory steps important for patient diagnosis are listed in this flow chart.

chronic progressive external ophthalmoplegia syndromes, or they can be somewhat diffuse. Most ragged-red fibers also show an increased succinate dehydrogenase reaction and a decreased cytochrome c oxidase (COX) reaction (COX-negative or COX-deficient fibers). Frequently, the number of COX-negative or COX-deficient fibers is larger than the number of ragged-red fibers. These changes are observed in a variety of oxidative phosphorylation diseases, which include mtDNA-depletion diseases, mtDNA deletions, and mitochondrial transfer RNA mutations. Although COX-deficient fibers provide important evidence for an OXPHOS disease, mutations in COX subunits encoded by the mtDNA or nuclear DNA genes are rare.[40,41] The mitochondrial transfer RNA A3243G mutation in the $tRNA^{Leucine(UUR)}$ gene is an important exception to this pattern of histopathologic observations. This mutation is the most common cause for mitochondrial myopathy, encephalopathy, lactic acidosis, and stroke-like episodes (MELAS). The ragged-red fibers may be either COX-deficient or show a positive COX reaction.[42–46] In addition, the blood vessels characteristically show an increased succinate dehydrogenase reaction.[42–46] It is important to note that COX-deficient fibers, increased succinate dehydrogenase reaction, and ragged-red fibers may be observed in a variety of conditions including normal aging, zidovudine myopathy, myotonic dystrophy, limb-girdle dystrophy, inclusion body myositis, inflammatory myopathies, and nemaline myopathy.[47–55]

Ultrastructural analysis of the muscle may reveal structurally abnormal mitochondria with paracrystalline inclusions that are intermembranous condensations of mitochondrial creatine kinase.[56] A careful search for paracrystalline inclusions is important. When this ultrastructural abnormality is found in conjunction with ragged-red fibers, increases in succinate dehydrogenase reactivity, and cytochrome c oxidase-deficient fibers, the presence of an mtDNA mutation that impairs mitochondrial protein synthesis, such as an mtDNA deletion, mtDNA depletion, or a mitochondrial transfer RNA point mutation, is suggested. This can be important in focusing the genetic testing.

Unfortunately, most patients with OXPHOS diseases do not show any of the above characteristic muscle changes. The muscle pathology may show neurogenic changes, internal nuclei, fiber splitting, myofiber hypertrophy, or hypotrophy involving either type I or type II fibers, accumulations of lipid, or mild increases in glycogen.[57,58] In some individuals, the muscle histology may even be normal. Immunohistochemical approaches that assess levels of proteins such as neurotropin-4, a neuronal signaling molecule, may be able to improve patient detection.[59] Patients with OXPHOS defects (mtDNA or nuclear DNA) do not usually display dystrophic changes in muscle such as increased connective tissue or significant myonecrosis. However, rare exceptions to this rule do exist.[60] This observation can be important in distinguishing patients with OXPHOS diseases from those with other classes of neuromuscular diseases.

Nerve biopsy may be helpful in the investigation of some patients with OXPHOS diseases who present with significant neuropathies. Clinical, as well as subclinical, impairment of central and peripheral myelin is common. Interestingly, the pathology of some cases was consistent with inflammatory demyelination.[61,62] Axonal neuropathies affecting sensory and motor nerves are also frequent findings.[63–65] Although the neuropathy in most patients progresses slowly over a long period of time, acute presentations may occur.[66]

OXPHOS Biochemistry

Biochemical and genetic testing can confirm the presence of an OXPHOS disease. When specific mutations are not implicated by the clinical examination, OXPHOS enzyme analysis in skeletal muscle mitochondria can be used to classify a disorder as an OXPHOS disease. To perform accurate assessments of this delicate enzyme system, immediate isolation of mitochondria from fresh muscle biopsies can be helpful. This approach avoids artifacts in OXPHOS enzyme analysis that can be associated with freezing the biopsy before mitochondrial isolation. Although it is now possible to achieve a precise diagnosis of certain OXPHOS diseases by DNA analysis alone, OXPHOS enzymology is necessary in the majority of cases. To determine the specific activities of OXPHOS enzymes, the complex I, complex III, and complex IV assays are used to assess electron flow across single OXPHOS complexes and the complex I + III and complex II + III assays assess the movement of electrons between complexes (Fig. 104-1). The specificity of these assays is demonstrated by using specific respiratory inhibitors. The proper functioning of the reagents used in these assays is insured by performing each enzyme assay in mitochondria isolated from mouse or rat skeletal muscle in parallel with the patient assays.

Complex I defects are commonly observed in patient samples. Distinguishing between pathogenic defects and those produced by technical factors can be difficult. To assess complex I function, three assays are used, each employing a different electron acceptor: (a) n-decylCoQ as the electron acceptor; (b) CoQ1 as the electron acceptor; and (c) the traditional complex I + III assay. The first two assays are the most specific for mitochondrial complex I activity, but CoQ reduction probably occurs at different sites due to the more hydrophilic nature of CoQ1 and the more lipophilic nature of n-decylCoQ. The complex I + III assays measure the rate of electron flow between complexes I and III. However, approximately 50 percent of the observed activity is nonmitochondrial and must be accounted for in the interpretation. Due to the complexities associated with oxidative phosphorylation assessment, corroborative data are sought by testing for abnormalities in skin fibroblast β-oxidation. β-Oxidation of substrates such as palmitate (C16:0) and myristate (C14:0) is often reduced, thus providing support for the diagnosis of an OXPHOS defect. We observe β-oxidation defects in conjunction with OXPHOS defects (usually complex I defects) in about 24 percent of our patients.

During the first step of β-oxidation, a double bond is added to the fatty acid, electrons are transferred to the electron transfer flavoprotein via $FADH_2$, and electrons are transferred to complex I via NADH (Fig. 104-1). OXPHOS defects, particularly those involving complex I, reduce the oxidation of palmitate and myristate to levels that are approximately 40 percent to 60 percent of the control mean. This contrasts with diseases such as carnitine palmitoyl transferase deficiency and medium chain acyldehydrogenase deficiency, which reduce the oxidation of these fatty acids to <10 percent and <20 percent of the control means, respectively. Assessment of long chain fatty acid oxidation by the trifunctional protein is normal in patients who harbor OXPHOS defects.

Genetic Testing of OXPHOS Diseases

At the time of muscle biopsy, a small portion of the biopsy is frozen in liquid nitrogen for DNA isolation. In our experience, the integrated clinical-genetic, metabolic, and biochemical-genetic protocol increases the probability of reaching the correct biochemical and genetic diagnosis that is necessary for accurate genetic counseling and effective patient management. In general, the level of mtDNA mutations in skeletal muscle appears to correlate best with clinical features.[67] An interesting feature of skeletal muscle is that mtDNA deletions and tRNA point mutations are generally present at significant levels in myofibers, but are rare or undetectable in muscle satellite cells.[68] Therefore, regenerating myofibers demonstrate higher levels of normal mtDNAs than the surrounding nonregenerating myofibers.[68] mtDNA testing in leukocytes can be important for patient diagnosis. However, mutation levels in blood correlate poorly with patient phenotype.[19,67] Tables 104-1 and 104-2 are designed to assist physicians in recognizing genotype and phenotype associations. It is important to remember that a large array of mtDNA mutations is known. Most mtDNA mutations are private or semiprivate mutations (i.e., occurring in relatively few families). Therefore, in order to exclude an mtDNA mutation as a cause for symptoms in a proband, a comprehensive analysis of the mtDNA by SSCP and sequencing can be helpful. This approach permits assignment of the patient's disease manifestations to the nuclear DNA or to the mtDNA. When small SSCP fragments are used for analysis, mutation detection exceeds 90 percent.[69] Some groups use denaturing gradient-gel electrophoresis to screen for mtDNA mutations.[70,71] Over the next several years, more rapid approaches to mutation detection using high-density DNA arrays (DNA "chip" technology) are likely to emerge as important methods of genetic testing for OXPHOS diseases.[72]

MITOCHONDRIAL DNA MUTATIONS

Three classes of pathogenic mtDNA mutations exist: (a) mtDNA rearrangements in which mtDNA genes are deleted or duplicated; (b) mtDNA point mutations in tRNA or ribosomal RNA genes resulting in defects in mitochondrial protein synthesis; and (c) missense mutations that change an amino acid, thus altering a critical function of an OXPHOS polypeptide. The OXPHOS diseases known to be caused by nuclear DNA mutations are inherited in an autosomal dominant or autosomal recessive pattern (Table 104-1). A synopsis of OXPHOS diseases is given below. Leber hereditary optic neuropathy is reviewed in Chap. 105.

mtDNA DELETIONS AND mtDNA DUPLICATIONS: SPORADIC AND MATERNALLY TRANSMITTED VARIANTS

Kearns-Sayre and Chronic Progressive External Ophthalmoplegia (CPEO) Syndromes

Kearns-Sayre syndrome (KSS) has an onset before 20 years of age and is characterized by ophthalmoplegia, atypical retinitis pigmentosa, mitochondrial myopathy, and one of the following: cardiac conduction defect, cerebellar syndrome, or an elevated CSF protein above 100 mg/dl.[73] Individuals whose symptoms begin after 20 years of age are classified as having the chronic progressive external ophthalmoplegia (CPEO) syndrome, which ranges in severity from isolated extraocular eye muscle involvement (CPEO) to CPEO plus a variety of other clinical manifestations (CPEO PLUS). KSS and CPEO PLUS patients have complex disorders with variable combinations of the following manifestations: pigmentary retinopathy; optic atrophy; hearing loss; dementia; seizures; hypertrophic and dilated cardiomyopathies; cardiac conduction defects; atrial and ventricular arrhythmias including preexcitation syndromes; gastrointestinal mobility disturbances; endocrinopathies such as diabetes mellitus and hypoparathyroidism; renal failure due to glomerulosclerosis; proximal renal tubule dysfunction; respiratory failure; mitochondrial myopathy; lactic acidemia; sensory and motor neuropathies; and ataxias.[74–82] Some patients demonstrate overlap with other OXPHOS diseases, such as individuals who have manifestations of both KSS and MELAS.[83]

Four patterns of retinal degeneration are encountered in KSS/CPEO syndromes: (a) a "salt and pepper" retinopathy characterized by a mottled retina due to regions of hypo- and hyperpigmentation; (b) a retinitis pigmentosa characterized by bone spicule formation, optic atrophy, and attenuated blood vessels; (c) generalized loss of the retinal pigment epithelium, choriocapillaris, and optic nerve; and (d) a pattern that is a phenocopy of choroideremia which is characterized by complete atrophy of the choroid and sclera.[80,84,85] Most individuals with KSS and CPEO do not experience significant diplopia. In those individuals who do develop this problem, extraocular muscle resection rather than recession may provide a better postsurgical outcome.[86]

The most common causes for KSS and CPEO syndromes are mtDNA rearrangements that consist of mtDNA deletion mutations and the mtDNA duplication mutations.[8,87–89] Approximately 80 percent of KSS patients, 70 percent of CPEO PLUS patients, and 40 percent of CPEO patients have mtDNA deletions and mtDNA duplications.[78,81] The mtDNA deletion mutation has the simplest structure and consists of an mtDNA molecule that is missing contiguous tRNA and OXPHOS polypeptide genes, thus yielding an mtDNA molecule that is smaller than the normal 16.6-kb mtDNA. The structurally more complex mtDNA duplication mutation produces an mtDNA molecule that is larger than the normal mtDNA and contains two tandemly arranged mtDNA molecules consisting of a full-length 16.6-kb mtDNA coupled to an mtDNA deletion mutation.[87–89] The deletions appear to increase in the patient's tissues with age, possibly contributing to the progressive degenerative course of the disease.[90] The mtDNA deletions that cause KSS and CPEO are heteroplasmic and can remove between 9 percent and 50 percent of the mtDNA genome.[91] The extent of the somatic variation can be extensive.[92]

In most patients with mtDNA rearrangements, the mutation is not inherited, but appears to be a spontaneous event that occurred after fertilization of the oocyte at an early stage of embryonic development.[93] Due to replicative segregation of mutant and normal mtDNAs, the identification of maternal inheritance of an mtDNA rearrangement by clinical criteria can be difficult and often requires analysis of skeletal muscle mtDNA from maternal lineage relatives of the proband. Of the two classes of mtDNA rearrangements, the mtDNA duplication mutation has the greatest probability of being maternally transmitted.[94] Leukocytes and platelets containing mtDNA rearrangements tend to be lost from the circulation. Assessment for mtDNA deletions in blood samples is probably the most common mistake made by physicians. In most cases, this analysis is uninformative. Skeletal muscle is optimal for detection of mtDNA rearrangements due to its ability to retain mtDNA mutations and its easy accessibility.

mtDNA deletions generally spare the two origins of replication, O_H and O_L, thus defining two arcs in which mtDNA deletions occur. Over 90 percent of deletions occur in the large arc between O_H and O_L, which encompasses two-thirds of the genome and contains the cytochrome b, ND6, ND5, ND4, ND4L, ND3, COIII, ATPase 6 and 8, COII, and COI genes, plus the intervening tRNAs. This region also has a high frequency of direct repeats.[74,75,95] Few patients with deletions in the smaller arc between O_L and O_H are described. This region encompasses one-third of the genome and contains the ND2, ND1, 16S rRNA, and 12S rRNA genes, and associated tRNA genes, and relatively few direct repeats.[77,96,97] One O_L to O_H deletion in the smaller arc of the mtDNA has been reported to remove not only the rRNA genes but also the heavy-strand promoter, interfering with heavy-strand transcription.[96,97] The high frequency of direct repeats in the human mtDNA as well as other species suggest that slip-replication may be an important mechanism that results in mtDNA deletions and duplications.[74,98,99] The most commonly encountered mtDNA deletion is 4977 base pairs and originates between two 13-base pair repeats. In cultured human cells, the mutation rate for this specific deletion is estimated to be 5.95×10^{-8} per mitochondrial genome replication. Another possibility is that homologous recombination is important in mtDNA deletion formation.[99,100]

Detailed genetic and histochemical analyses of skeletal muscle from KSS and CPEO patients showed that the deleted mtDNAs are localized in distinct regions along the muscle fiber, whereas the normal mtDNAs are evenly distributed along the fiber's length.[39] This localization pattern results in a periodic respiratory deficiency along the muscle fiber associated with localized accumulation of the transcripts from the deleted mtDNAs.[39,101,102] Because tRNAs are lost during the deletion process, these observations suggest that the availability of normal tRNAs could be rate limiting in these regions, causing deficits in protein synthesis and OXPHOS defects.[39] This is consistent with the prominent defect in mitochondrial protein synthesis observed in cells from KSS and CPEO patients.[103]

Those patients whose manifestations are not caused by mtDNA deletions are likely to represent either mtDNA point mutations or nuclear DNA mutations. For example, significant clinical overlap occurs between individuals with mtDNA deletions and certain individuals who harbor the A3243G mutation. Both types of mtDNA mutations can produce chronic progressive external ophthalmoplegias with or without stroke-like episodes.[83,104–108] Additional mtDNA point mutations that are associated with Kearns-Sayre and CPEO syndromes plus the broad array of phenotypes associated with mtDNA deletion/duplication mutations are listed in Tables 104-1 and 104-2.

Pearson Syndrome

Pearson syndrome is a systemic disorder of oxidative phosphorylation in infants that predominantly affects the bone marrow. Hematopoietic dysfunction is manifested as a severe, transfusion-dependent, macrocytic anemia with varying degrees of neutropenia and thrombocytopenia.[109] Bone marrow examination shows normal cellularity but extensive vacuolization of erythroid and myeloid precursors, hemosiderosis, and ringed sideroblasts. This disease occurs sporadically within pedigrees with no evidence of hematologic dysfunction in other family members and is caused by spontaneously occurring deletions in the mtDNA.[110–115] Patients with this disorder may die early in the course of this disease due to complications of bone marrow failure and repeated transfusions. Some individuals have spontaneous improvement of the pancytopenia, presumably due to repopulation of the bone marrow with stem cells, which have predominantly normal mtDNAs. However, individuals that show improvement of their pancytopenia later develop symptoms of KSS in other organs from OXPHOS defects caused by the deleted mtDNA. Lactic acidosis, growth restriction, pancreas dysfunction, mitochondrial myopathy, and progressive neurologic dysfunction frequently occur. This syndrome further supports the concept that the phenotypes produced by mtDNA deletions are highly variable and dependent on the chance distribution of the deleted molecules among the tissues through replicative segregation.

mtDNA POINT MUTATIONS

Myoclonic Epilepsy and Ragged-Red Fiber Disease (MERRF)

MERRF is a maternally inherited disease characterized by progressive myoclonic epilepsy, a mitochondrial myopathy with ragged-red fibers, and a slowly progressive dementia.[116–128] Although MERRF patients generally have ragged-red fibers on muscle biopsy, some individuals with progressive myoclonic epilepsy and ataxia without ragged-red fibers harbor the MERRF mutation (unpublished observation).[107] Onset of symptoms ranges from late childhood to adulthood.[116–128] Hearing loss and ataxia are common findings,[117,118,120–123,129,130] although in some cases, hearing is normal.[124,126,127] Neuropathologic analysis of the extraocular eye muscles has shown mild endomysial fibrosis, accumulation of abnormal mitochondria without paracrystalline inclusions, myofibril loss, and Hirano bodies.[131]

Energy metabolism impairment in the central nervous system of MERRF patients can be detected by imaging techniques such as positron emission tomography (PET) and ^{31}P-NMR analyses of brain,[122,132] as well as ^{31}P-NMR analysis of skeletal muscle.[117] Brain MRI abnormalities include cerebral atrophy, cerebellar atrophy, cerebellar hyperintense lesions, basal ganglia hyperintense lesions, and hyperintense white matter or pyramidal tract lesions.[31] Generally, MERRF can be clinically distinguished from MELAS (mitochondrial encephalomyopathy, lactic acidosis, and stroke-like episodes) based on the absence of strokes.[133] However, features of both MERRF and MELAS can be seen during the clinical course of some patients,[134–140] as well as within the same pedigree.[141] Neuropathologic analyses of the brains from patients with MERRF revealed degeneration in the dentatorubral and pallidoluysian systems, substantia nigra, cerebellar cortex, inferior olivary nucleus, locus ceruleus, gracile and cuneate nuclei, and the pontine tegmentum.[119,131,142–144] The pathology in the spinal cord resembled that found in Friedreich ataxia.[131,142]

Approximately 80 percent to 90 percent of MERRF cases are caused by a heteroplasmic G to A point mutation at bp 8344 in the TΨC loop of the $tRNA^{Lysine}$ gene (G8344A mutations).[106,107,145–151] Two additional families have been attributed to a heteroplasmic T to C transition mutation at bp 8356 in the $tRNA^{Lys}$ gene (T8356C mutation).[152,153] The T8356C mutation alters a moderately conserved nucleotide that is predicted to disrupt base pairing in the stem of the TΨC loop. Both the dihydrouridine loop and the TΨC loop appear to be involved in interactions with the ribosome.[154] Although the genetic causes for MERRF are limited, biochemical defects are heterogeneous. Combined defects in complexes I and IV are often observed. This is consistent with the protein synthesis defects observed in MERRF patient cells, because complexes I and IV have the greatest number of mtDNA-encoded subunits and thus may be most sensitive to a protein synthesis defect.[155,156] While other MERRF patients have shown biochemical defects in complex II,[157] cytochrome b of complex III,[120,122] cytochrome c oxidase (complex IV),[130,158] complexes III and IV,[122] and coenzyme Q,[128] the difficulties in correlating OXPHOS biochemistry with the mtDNA mutations suggest that both methodologic differences and secondary effects can affect enzyme-specific activities.

Patients with MERRF often demonstrate a characteristic accumulation of lipomas in the anterior and posterior cervical region.[159] Some patients develop a syndrome of multiple symmetrical lipomatosis, which is characterized by large subcutaneous fat masses around the neck, shoulders, and trunk. The MERRF G8344A mutation is present in some patients.[159–165] However, other classes of mutations can also produce this syndrome (Tables 104-1 and 104-2) including multiple mtDNA deletions,[166,167] single (clonal) mtDNA deletions,[168] and the MELAS A3243G mutation.[169] Most of the patients with multiple symmetrical lipomatosis have ragged-red fiber myopathy plus peripheral neuropathy. Alcohol abuse appears to be frequent in this group of patients. Although multiple symmetrical lipomatosis is an important clinical clue to the presence of an OXPHOS disease, mitochondrial abnormalities are not observed in all patients.[170]

The clinical, biochemical, and genetic characterization of a large MERRF pedigree with the G8344A mutation demonstrated that many of the manifestations of this disease are explained by the principles of mitochondrial genetics. The proband had myoclonic epilepsy, mitochondrial myopathy with ragged-red fibers and paracrystalline inclusions, abnormal visual-evoked response (VER) and electroencephalograph (EEG), bilateral neurosensory hearing loss, cerebellar ataxia, lactic acidosis, dementia, a primary central hypoventilation associated with periodic respiratory arrest, and a mild cardiomyopathy.[117,118] A continuum of clinical and biochemical abnormalities can be observed in other family members, emphasizing the wide range of manifestations associated with heteroplasmic mtDNA mutations. Seven family members had mitochondrial myopathies, while one had only aberrations in her EEG and VER. The mitochondrial ATP-generating capacity of these individuals was quantitated in three ways: ^{31}P-NMR assessment of high-energy phosphate metabolism, anaerobic threshold determination as an estimation of the work capacity of oxidative muscle fibers during exercise stress, and biochemical analysis of OXPHOS in isolated skeletal muscle mitochondria. The ^{31}P-NMR quantitation of the phosphocreatine to phosphate ratio (PCR/P_i) revealed a marked reduction in recovery rate of high energy phosphates following exercise, with the severely affected proband recovering much more slowly than the less affected mother. The anaerobic threshold that quantitates the oxidative (type I) muscle fiber work capacity varied between 409 ml O_2/min for the severely affected proband and 1212 ml O_2/min for the mildly affected family members. The OXPHOS enzyme activities correlated with these anaerobic threshold changes and the clinical phenotype.

Significant variation has been observed in the levels of the mutant mtDNA between tissue types of individual MERRF patients. Skeletal muscle frequently has the highest percentages of the G8344A mutation in severely affected individuals ranging from 80 percent to almost 100 percent,[147,155,171] and correlates best with clinical manifestations.[67] Less severely affected family members have been reported to have percentages of the G8344A mutation ranging from 0 percent to 92 percent.[147,171] Relative to skeletal muscle, fibroblasts frequently have the lowest levels of the G8344A mutation, and lymphocytes have intermediate levels, suggesting that the cells with a higher percentage of normal mtDNAs have a selective advantage, although the extent of this effect may vary between different cell types.[171]

The G8344A mutation in $tRNA^{Lys}$ inhibits mitochondrial protein synthesis.[156] The mitochondrial RNA translation defect can be transferred between cells through the mutant mtDNAs. Patient cells are enucleated and the cytoplasmic fragment containing the mitochondria fused to recipient ρ° cells that lack mtDNAs. Recipient cells that acquire the patient mtDNA can be selected in media lacking uridine and pyruvate.[172–181] The ρ° cells require uridine because their OXPHOS deficiency inhibits the dihydrouridine dehydrogenase activity necessary for *de novo* uridine monophosphate synthesis.[182,183] Acquisition of patient mtDNAs relieves the pyrimidine auxotrophy and permits the cytoplasmic hybrids (cybrids) to grow. Mitochondrial transfer can also be achieved by microinjection of intact mitochondria into ρ° cells.[184] Cybrids that are homoplasmic for the G8344A mutation have a severe impairment of mitochondrial protein synthesis, whereas cybrids that are homoplasmic for the normal mtDNA of the patient have normal mitochondrial protein synthesis. This proves that the G8344A mutation is solely responsible for the translation defect.[156]

Consistent with the higher proportion of G8344A mutation mtDNAs in muscle, explanted myoblast clones are frequently found to be homoplasmic for the mutant mtDNA with only a small number of clones being heteroplasmic or homoplasmic for the normal mtDNA.[155] Heteroplasmic myotubes with varying percentages of the G8344A mutation demonstrated a sharp decline in mitochondrial protein synthesis levels when the intracellular percentage of mutant mtDNAs exceeded 85 percent.[155] At this point, the translation efficiency of COI and the cytochrome c oxidase enzyme activity dramatically declined. This indicates that the G8344A mutation is functionally recessive, which is consistent with clinical observations in MERRF family members. When the mutant mtDNAs exceeded 85 percent, large changes in clinical phenotype occur with only small changes in genotype.[147] This implies that patients born with high percentages of mutant mtDNAs would be acutely sensitive to further inhibition of OXPHOS function. The relatively small reductions in OXPHOS function[48,49,185–187] associated with the age-related accumulation of somatic mtDNA mutations[188–192] could then be sufficient to produce clinical manifestations as the patient matures.

The efficiency of protein synthesis was greater in the myotubes than myoblasts that contained similar quantities of the G8344A mutation.[155] This may be due to the induction of OXPHOS gene expression and a 2.4- to 4-fold increase in mtDNA content following fusion of myoblasts to myotubes. OXPHOS gene mRNA levels for the nuclear-encoded ATP synthase β subunit gene and the mtDNA-encoded 16S rRNA, ATPase 6, and COIII genes are high in myoblasts, but fall during exit from the cell cycle and increase again with cell fusion to form myotubes.[193] Transcripts for the heart and skeletal muscle specific isoform of the adenine nucleotide translocase (ANT1) progressively increase following myotube formation.[193,194] Hence, the increased mitochondrial protein synthesis capacity in myotubes may reflect an overall increase in their biosynthetic capacity.

Mitochondrial Myopathy, Encephalomyopathy, Lactic Acidosis, and Stroke-like Episodes (MELAS)

MELAS is a progressive neurodegenerative disease that is characterized by stroke-like episodes and a mitochondrial myopathy.[133] Approximately 80 percent of individuals with the clinical characteristics of MELAS have a heteroplasmic A to G point mutation in the dihydrouridine loop of the $tRNA^{Leucine(UUR)}$ gene at bp 3243 (A3243G mutation).[195–201] An additional 7.5 percent have a heteroplasmic T to C point mutation at bp 3271 in the terminal nucleotide pair of the anticodon stem of the $tRNA^{Leucine(UUR)}$ gene (T3271C mutation).[105,202] The remaining cases appear to be caused by either nuclear DNA mutations[203] or other as yet unidentified mtDNA mutations. In adult populations, the frequency of the A3243G mutations is approximately 16.3/100,000.[204]

Stroke-like episodes are generally associated with infarcts seen on head CT or MRI and can resolve over a few hours or days along with the neurologic deficits. The infarcts are most commonly observed in the posterior temporal, parietal, and occipital lobes and may be associated with other abnormalities, such as ventricular dilatation, cortical atrophy, and basal ganglia calcifications.[105,134,135,205–210] Originally, it was hypothesized that these infarcts are nonvascular and are due to transient OXPHOS dysfunction within the brain parenchyma.[133,136,206,207,211] The infarcts usually do not produce the classical wedge-shaped lesions of gray and white matter produced by thromboembolic cerebrovascular disease, but instead are localized primarily to cortical regions supplied by several large vessels.[133,205–207,212] However, it is now clear that vascular pathology is important in the pathogenesis of stroke. A mitochondrial angiopathy of small vessels produces contrast enhancement of affected regions[206,212] and mitochondrial abnormalities of endothelial cells and smooth muscle cells of blood vessels.[202,213–217] The mitochondrial angiopathy may even be manifest in the skin as purpura.[213,218] Hence, the multisystem dysfunction in MELAS patients appears to be due to both parenchymal and vascular OXPHOS defects. Increased production of free radicals due to an OXPHOS defect could damage potent vasodilators like nitrous oxide, which are generated by the vascular endothelium,[219] leading to areas of vasoconstriction.

The strokes in MELAS can be ascertained by single photon emission computerized tomography (SPECT) studies using *N*-isopropyl-*p*-[^{123}I]-iodoamphetamine (IMP). It can delineate the extent of the lesion and be used to monitor the course of the disease.[220–224] Regional hypoperfusion can be detected by SPECT, even when CT and MRI are normal. Positron emission tomography (PET) studies on MELAS patients revealed a reduced cerebral metabolic rate for oxygen, increased cerebral blood flow in cortical regions, and preservation of the cerebral metabolic rate for glucose.[225] Neuropathologic analyses of MELAS patients demonstrate infarct-like lesions in both cortical and subcortical structures.[135,208,217,226–228] Areas of neuronal loss, demyelination, and astrocytic proliferation are found in a wide variety of brain regions. Mitochondrial abnormalities in the vascular smooth muscle cells and endothelial cells are characteristic findings in these patients.[137,217]

The A3243G mutation can be associated with a variety of clinical manifestations. Patients harboring this mutation may have different combinations of fatigability; myopathy; myalgias; ophthalmoplegia; pigmentary retinopathy; hypertrophic or dilated cardiomyopathy; cardiac conduction defects including ventricular arrhythmias; preexcitation syndromes; cardiac conduction block; myoclonus; dementia; ataxia; deafness; lactic acidemia; various forms of endocrinopathy; and renal disease, particularly proximal renal tubule dysfunction.[104–106,108] Sensorineural deafness appears to be caused by inner ear damage.[229–232] Cochlear implants have improved hearing in patients with MELAS.[233] Migraine headaches are frequently observed in these patients, as well as in their maternal lineage relatives, and they can precede the development of a focal neurologic deficit and/or focal or generalized seizures.[234] The most common form of clinical expression for the A3243G mutation is type II diabetes mellitus, accounting for about 1 percent of all patients with type II diabetes mellitus.[224,229,230,235–303] A second $tRNA^{Leucine(UUR)}$ gene mutation (A8296G) is also estimated to be present in about 1 percent of diabetics.[304] Individuals with the more severe clinical manifestations generally have over 80 percent mutant mtDNAs in stable tissues such as muscle and brain.[104,197,234,305] In rapidly dividing cells, such as hematopoietic lineages, A3243G mutation may segregate to extremely low levels making genetic diagnosis from blood difficult.[104] These patients require analysis of skeletal muscle mtDNA to confirm the presence or absence of the mutation. The absence of ragged-red muscle fibers does not exclude MELAS because ragged-red fibers are not invariably identified in patients with the disease.[104,234,306]

Patients may present as sporadic cases[129,133,137,206,216,228,307–314] or as members of maternal pedigrees with a wide variety of clinical presentations.[129,207,208,315–318] Patients may be normal until their first stroke-like episode, which usually occurs between 5 and 15 years of age.[104,133,196,206,208,216,228,307–315,319,320] The stroke-like episodes may also have their onset in infants or adults.[104,106,107,196,206,207,316,317] Alternatively, patients may present in infancy[213] with a variety of motor and cognitive developmental abnormalities. In fact, the only clinical manifestation of the disease can be a new cortical or subcortical infarct or even a malignant migraine.[234]

A unique patient with MELAS was reported who had a complex I defect in muscle plus the generation of an autoantibody to a 41-kDa matrix polypeptide.[321] This patient was a 15-year-old male who presented initially with episodes of hypoglycemia and loss of consciousness at 10 months of age. Over the subsequent years, he developed recurrent seizures followed by a right hemiparesis, dementia, hearing loss, short stature, ataxia, a Wolf-Parkinson-White type B dysrhythmia, and a generalized myopathy with easy fatigability. Clinical, metabolic, and pathologic investigations showed cerebral and cerebellar atrophy as well as bilateral basal ganglia calcifications, lactic acidemia, and a ragged-red fiber myopathy. The patient's mother had a remote history of seizures and ragged-red fibers on muscle biopsy. No other affected individuals were recognized in the family history. An immunoblot of complex I showed that all subunits were reduced except for the 24-kDa subunit that was absent. This protein defect is not specific for this clinical presentation because patients with an undetectable 24-kDa subunit by immunoblot have also presented with an isolated myopathy or with the more complex clinical manifestations of a mitochondrial encephalomyopathy.[322,323] Hence, the molecular mechanism for this MELAS patient's OXPHOS defect is unclear. While no deletions or duplications of the mtDNA were observed on Southern blot analysis,[8] these individuals were not tested for the common MELAS mutations such as the A3243G mutation. Other patients with MELAS presentations have also developed autoantibodies such as the rheumatoid factor and antimitochondrial antibodies.[320]

Assessment of the pathophysiology of the A3243G mutation is complicated by the fact that the nucleotide change resides in a region of the mtDNA with dual function. This mutation not only alters the dihydrouridine loop of the $tRNA^{Leu(UUR)}$ gene, but also changes a conserved nucleotide at the binding site for a nuclear DNA-encoded transcription termination factor.[324] The transcription termination factor truncates H-strand transcription after the 16S rRNA gene has been traversed, thus maintaining the high rRNA to mRNA ratio in mitochondria. The A3243G mutation was proposed to reduce the binding affinity of the transcription termination factor and gel-shift analysis, DNase I footprinting, and runoff transcription/termination studies indicated that it reduced the efficacy of transcription termination.[324,325] This point mutation could also interfere with processing of the 16S rRNA and the adjacent $tRNA^{Leu(UUR)}$ or increase the production of the termination factor which could bind to other sites in the D-loop and impair L-strand transcription.[324,326] Alternatively, the A3243G mutation may impair protein synthesis directly by interfering with polypeptide chain elongation and have no effect on termination factor function.[325]

By fusing cytoplasts from MELAS patients with the A3243G mutation to ρ° cells, cybrid cell lines have been generated that contained from 0 percent to 100 percent mutant mtDNAs. In these cell lines, the proportion of mutant mtDNAs correlated with the reduction in protein synthesis, OXPHOS dysfunction, and impaired cell growth.[327] The ratio of 12S and 16S rRNAs to OXPHOS subunit mRNA in cybrids with the A3243G mutation was similar to normal cells, suggesting that this ratio may not be significantly altered by this mutation,[325,327] but in some cases, an abnormal RNA species accumulated consisting of the 16S rRNA + $tRNA^{Leu(UUR)}$ + ND1 transcript.[325,327] The mechanism by which the A3243G mutation interferes with protein synthesis remains unclear, though defects in $tRNA^{Leu(UUR)}$ function, rRNA to mRNA ratio, impaired incorporation of leucine into mitochondrial translation products,[328] and rRNA processing remain viable alternatives. A complicating variable in assessing the pathophysiology of the MELAS A3243G mutation is that suppressor mutations may exist in the $tRNA^{Leucine(CUN)}$ gene that allow decoding of UUR-leucine codons. A heteroplasmic variant at position 12300 in the $tRNA^{Leucine(CUN)}$ gene was observed in a patient who also harbored the A3243G mutation.[329] A suppressor function for this variant in the $tRNA^{Leucine(CUN)}$ gene was postulated.

Leigh Disease, Cerebellar Ataxia Plus Pigmentary Retinopathy Syndromes, and Dystonia

Leigh disease, or subacute necrotizing encephalopathy, is suspected when cranial nerve abnormalities, respiratory dysfunction, and ataxia are observed in conjunction with bilateral hyperintense signals on T2-weighted MRI images in the basal ganglia, cerebellum, or brain stem. The incidence of the disease is estimated to be about 1 in 40,000.[330] The age of onset for disease manifestations is usually during infancy or early childhood. Two mtDNA mutations, a T-to-G[331,332] (T8993G) or a T-to-C[333] mutation in the ATPase 6 gene at position 8993 (T8993C), are important causes of Leigh disease. Additional mutations associated with Leigh disease are listed in Table 104-2. The T8993G mutation is the most frequently encountered of the two mutations and changes an evolutionarily conserved leucine to an arginine of the ATPase 6 polypeptide, thus replacing a neutral amino acid with a basic amino acid within the proton channel of complex V and impairing ATP synthesis.[334,335] The T8993G mutation is the most frequently encountered of these two mutations and was originally identified in patients with neuropathy, ataxia, and retinitis pigmentosa syndromes (NARP).[336] In comparing the effects of the ATP6 gene T8993G mutation that causes NARP with the ATP6 gene T9101C mutation that causes Leber hereditary optic neuropathy, is was concluded that the T9101C mutation produced proton leakage through the proton translocating F_o segment, whereas the T8993G mutation blocked proton translocation.[337]

A variety of clinical manifestations can be observed in patients with Leigh disease. Of 18 Leigh disease cases with OXPHOS dysfunction that were characterized pathologically,[130,338–343] six had a typical clinical course with bilateral basal ganglia lucencies detected by CT scan of the head.[338,339,344,345] The mean age of onset of clinical manifestations in these patients was 1.5 years, with a mean duration of illness until death of 5 years. Clinical manifestations included optic atrophy, ophthalmoplegia, nystagmus, respiratory abnormalities, ataxia, hypotonia, spasticity, and developmental delay or regression. The myopathy usually had nonspecific findings, such as fiber size variation with increased fat. Only two cases had ragged-red fibers and these lacked paracrystalline inclusions.[344–347] Liver and heart show the greatest variability in disease expression. Liver may show clinical and biochemical dysfunction[341,342,344–347] or be unaffected.[341,348] Hypertrophic cardiomyopathy was seen in two patients,[341,342] but not in others. A common feature of the clinical course in Leigh disease is abrupt worsening of the patient's clinical and metabolic status with infections. This may be due to a direct effect of certain bacterial endotoxins and viruses on the underlying OXPHOS defect, causing an increase in dysfunction.[349–351]

The T8993G mutation acts in a recessive manner. Patients generally have no manifestations when the level of the T8993G mutation in tissues is less than approximately 60 percent to 70 percent of the total mtDNA. Patients that harbor between approximately 70 percent and 90 percent mutant mtDNAs in their tissues have highly variable disease manifestations. In mildly affected individuals, a pigmentary retinopathy can be the only clinical manifestation. In more severely affected individuals, cerebellar ataxia and retinitis pigmentosa are commonly observed together. Approximately 7 percent to 20 percent of patients with Leigh disease harbor the T8993G mutation (unpublished results).[331,334,335,352]

Pathologically, Leigh disease exhibits demyelination, gliosis, necrosis, relative neuronal sparing, and capillary proliferation in specific brain regions. In decreasing order of severity, the basal ganglia, brain stem, cerebellum, and cerebral cortex are affected.[353,354] Patients with Leigh encephalopathy may have defects in several enzyme complexes associated with mitochondrial respiratory metabolism. Dysfunction in cytochrome c oxidase (complex IV) is the most commonly reported biochemical abnormality,[130,339–341,343–348,355] followed by NADH dehydrogenase (complex I),[338,342,356] pyruvate dehydrogenase,[357–359] and pyruvate carboxylase.[360]

The heteroplasmic T8993G mutation is readily detected by *Ava*I digestion of patient DNA followed by Southern blot and hybridization with a purified mtDNA probe. By this test, patients with Leigh disease have a very high percentage of mutant mtDNAs, usually exceeding 95 percent. Rapid segregation of this mutation within a family poses a significant difficulty in clinically identifying affected individuals, and emphasizes the difficulties of assigning specific phenotypes to particular mtDNA mutations. Rigid correlations between genotype and phenotype are in many respects contrary to the principles of mitochondrial genetics, which predict clinical heterogeneity. A variety of mtDNA mutations can cause Leigh disease, including the G8344A mutation, which causes MERRF,[122,145] and the A3243G mutation, which causes MELAS. This indicates that the Leigh disease phenotype is a final common pathway for severe defects in ATP production.

Certain Leigh disease cases overlap clinically with Leber hereditary optic neuropathy (LHON). These cases are often referred to as LHON plus infantile bilateral striatal necrosis (IBSN) or Leigh disease plus LHON. One carefully studied pedigree revealed early onset dementia with asymmetric dystonia, bulbar dysfunction, corticospinal tract abnormalities, and short stature.[361] Computerized tomography and magnetic resonance imaging of the brain showed basal ganglia abnormalities leading to the designation "infantile bilateral striatal necrosis." The onset of the striatal necrosis was between 1.5 and 9 years of age. Thus, this pedigree could also be clinically classified as LHON + Leigh disease. There was significant variability in the severity of disease expression among affected individuals. Individuals with the mildest manifestations had adolescent-onset visual loss with optic atrophy, similar to LHON. The most severely affected individual had infantile bilateral striatal necrosis and later developed optic atrophy. Muscle biopsy of one severely affected individual showed excessive variation in fiber size and increased central nuclei but no ragged-red fibers or ultrastructural abnormalities of mitochondria. This phenotype is most commonly observed in conjunction with complex I defects. Heteroplasmic mtDNA mutation in the complex I subunits ND4 (A11696G)[362] and ND6 (G14459A)[363] can cause this disease (Table 104-2).

Hypertrophic Cardiomyopathy and Myopathy

Infantile Onset. Hypertrophic cardiomyopathy and myopathy is occasionally observed in infants. In one such case, an A to G transition at bp 4317 in the mtDNA $tRNA^{Ile}$ gene was proposed to be responsible for the phenotype.[364] In this pedigree, a 1-year-old male died with a severe hypertrophic cardiomyopathy accompanied by a complex I and IV defect in cardiac muscle. On autopsy, the heart was dilated and weighed 142 g (normal = 42 g). The only other organ system that demonstrated primary pathologic changes was the skeletal muscle, which had necrosis and basophilic degeneration. The bp 4317 mutation occurred at the junction of the TΨC stem-loop structure and was proposed to alter the conformation of the TΨC loop by producing a new site for G-C pairing. While this mutation is novel, its pathologic significance remains to be proven because only one affected individual was identified in the study, family members were not assessed to determine whether the point mutation was heteroplasmic or homoplasmic, and only 28 controls were surveyed to determine whether the mutation occurred in the general population.

Adult Onset. Hypertrophic cardiomyopathy is a relatively common finding in children and adults with OXPHOS disease and is typically associated with other manifestations of mitochondrial disease. Hypertrophic cardiomyopathy occurs in conjunction with an A to G transition mutation in the $tRNA^{Leu(UUR)}$ gene at bp 3260 (A3260G mutation)[365] and a C to T transition at bp 3303 in the $tRNA^{Leu(UUR)}$ gene (C3303T mutation).[366] Severely affected maternal relatives with the A3260G mutation began to manifest symptoms of congestive heart failure in their twenties and had no clinical evidence for central nervous system involvement. The heart from the most severely affected individual, who died at 30 years of age, demonstrated myocardial fibrosis, hypertrophy, and structural disarray of cardiomyocytes. Other clinical manifestations in this patient included insulin-dependent diabetes mellitus, bilateral cataracts, and the Wolf-Parkinson-White preexcitation syndrome. Maternal relatives frequently had evidence of a mild proximal myopathy with ragged-red fibers. The A3260G mutation was present throughout the maternal lineage; was heteroplasmic, ranging in concentration from 20 percent to 90 percent in skeletal muscle; and was associated with predominantly complex I and complex IV defects. The percentage of mutant mtDNAs correlated with the complex I-specific activities, the percent maximum oxygen consumption, and the clinical severity of the disease. In a pedigree with the C3303T mutation, the clinical manifestations began in infancy and in two individuals resulted in death at 10 weeks and 9 months of age.[366]

The phenotype of hypertrophic cardiomyopathy and mitochondrial myopathy can also be produced by the G8344A and A3243G mutations. Patients with these clinical manifestations can be screened for the A3260G, the G8344A, and the A3243G mutations in blood. If these mutations are not found, then a muscle biopsy can be performed for more detailed pathologic, biochemical, and genetic analyses.

Mitochondrial Myopathy

Many adults and some children present with muscle weakness and fatigability associated with a ragged-red fiber myopathy and/or abnormal mitochondria. In one such family, a heteroplasmic mtDNA T to C mutation at bp 3250 in the $tRNA^{Leu(UUR)}$ gene was observed (T3250C).[367,368] Five individuals along the maternal lineage of the pedigree were affected and manifested varying degrees of fatigability and ragged-red fiber myopathy. One individual also had respiratory muscle weakness. Serum lactates varied from normal to elevated at rest, but were generally abnormal after exercise. Clinical evidence for involvement of other organs was not found. As commonly occurs in disorders with heteroplasmic mtDNA mutations, OXPHOS enzyme levels in skeletal muscle were variable, with different family members demonstrating normal specific activities, a complex I defect, or defects in both complex I and complex IV. Interestingly, the T at bp 3250 is only modestly conserved, being found in human, cow, and rat, but not in chicken or *Xenopus* sequence. Although the percentages of mutant and normal mtDNA in the patient samples were not quantitated, it was clear that significant quantities of normal mtDNA were present in these patients. Possibly, individuals who inherit higher concentrations of the A3243G mutation than observed in this pedigree may demonstrate disease manifestations in tissues other than skeletal muscle.

Mitochondrial myopathy is frequently the primary presenting clinical manifestation for other tRNA mutations as well. Patients who harbor the G8344A mutation may exhibit fatigability and/or myopathy as their only disease manifestations.[75,117] Comparable presentations are seen in family members with low percentages of the A3243G mutation as well. Because of the variety of mtDNA mutations that can present with primary mitochondrial myopathy, extensive testing may be necessary to identify the mtDNA mutation.

Maternally Inherited Sensorineural Deafness

In general, hereditary deafness occurs in isolation in about 60 percent of cases.[369] Given the large number of causes for hereditary deafness, OXPHOS diseases account for a small percentage of cases. However, in families who harbor OXPHOS diseases, sensorineural hearing loss before 50 years of age is commonly encountered and can occur as an isolated finding or in conjunction with more complex clinical manifestations.[75] Generally, however, deafness is variable among maternal relatives, probably reflecting the heteroplasmic nature of many deleterious mtDNA mutations.

In one large maternal Israeli-Arab kindred in which deafness is the primary manifestation, 55 affected subjects were identified across 5 generations.[370] Female transmission of the disease was common in the pedigree, and 6 deaf or 11 unaffected fathers did not transmit deafness. Disease onset was within the first few years of life in most individuals, with two individuals experiencing the adult onset of symptoms. Audiometric studies indicated severe to profound sensorineural hearing loss. Mitochondrial protein synthesis analysis in Epstein-Barr virus-transformed lymphocytes was normal, as was the sensitivity of protein synthesis to chloramphenicol.[371] OXPHOS enzymology performed on mitochondria-enriched lysates of the lymphoblastoid cells were interpreted to represent an increased OXPHOS activity for complexes III and V.[371] This family harbored an A-to-G mutation in the 12S rRNA gene.[372] An important feature of patients who harbor this mutation is that deafness can be precipitated by aminoglycoside exposure. The A1555G mutation appears to enhance the affinity of aminoglycoside antibiotics for this region of the 12S rRNA [FES9].[373] Hearing loss is a very common clinical finding in patients with OXPHOS diseases. Other mutations associated with hearing loss are listed in Tables 104-1 and 104-2.

NUCLEAR DNA MUTATIONS AND OXPHOS DISEASE

Current estimates place the number of nuclear genes required for proper OXPHOS function at about 1000. Because of this large number of nuclear OXPHOS genes, it is likely that most respiratory deficiency diseases are the result of nuclear OXPHOS gene mutations. The most common inheritance pattern is autosomal recessive. A detailed pedigree analysis is a crucial element of the OXPHOS disease evaluation. Particular care must be exercised during pedigree analysis to avoid overlooking minor clinical manifestations of the disease and mistakenly classifying it as Mendelian when it is in fact maternally inherited. In many cases, the distinction between Mendelian and maternal inheritance patterns can only be made after a detailed genetic assessment as described above. This section reviews selected OXPHOS diseases caused by defects in nuclear genes.

Benign Infantile Mitochondrial Myopathy (BIMM)

BIMM is characterized clinically by weakness at birth, hypotonia, difficulty feeding, respiratory difficulties, mitochondrial myopathy, and lactic acidosis. Only skeletal muscle appears to be affected, and this condition improves spontaneously at 6 to 9 months of age.[374–378] Complex IV histochemistry and cytochrome c oxidase enzyme activity are sharply reduced in skeletal muscle early in the patient's course, but return to normal levels after 1 to 3 years.[374,375] In the cases studied to date, only the extrafusal muscle fibers had abnormal complex IV histochemistry. The intrafusal muscle fibers of muscle spindles and the smooth muscle of blood vessels have stained normally.[158,378–380] Immunohistochemical studies using subunit-specific antibodies have revealed a selective absence of the nuclear-encoded subunits VIIa and VIIb as well as the mitochondrial-encoded subunit II.[378] Because one pedigree had a similarly affected relative,[376] this disease was attributed to autosomal recessive or new autosomal dominant mutations.

The improvement of muscle OXPHOS activity correlates with the increase in brain OXPHOS function that occurs over the first year.[381,382] The functional equivalence of the mtDNA in all cells, the clinical and biochemical improvements over the first year, and the inheritance pattern suggest that these cases may be the result of a nuclear DNA mutation in fetal OXPHOS isoform that is specific for muscle. A developmental switch from the defective fetal isoform to a normal adult isoform could account for the gradual improvement in the mitochondrial myopathy seen in this disorder.

Lethal Infantile Mitochondrial Disease (LIMD) and mtDNA Depletion Diseases. LIMD patients can be relatively normal at birth, with a normal clinical exam and Apgar scores. However, OXPHOS function rapidly declines, resulting in death during the first year of life. In biochemically characterized cases of LIMD, the mean age of onset of symptoms was 3 weeks, with death occurring on the average at 5 months and associated with overwhelming lactic acidosis.[379,380,383–401] While the clinical course was similar in all cases, only a few patients have had a multi-organ pathologic or biochemical evaluation that would define the extent of tissue dysfunction.

Infants with LIMD present with failure to thrive, weakness, hypotonia, and severe lactic acidosis. A myopathy characterized by lipid and glycogen accumulation and by abnormally shaped mitochondria without paracrystalline inclusions is commonly observed. However, true ragged-red fibers are infrequent. Hepatic dysfunction is a prominent finding. Although renal function may be normal,[383,384,393] proximal tubule abnormalities are commonly encountered and include a generalized amino aciduria,[388,394,400] or the de Toni-Debré-Fanconi- syndrome.[379,380,385,397] The OXPHOS defects reported in LIMD include defects of complex I,[386,389,390,396] complex III,[401] complex IV,[380,385,392,398] complex IV, and cytochrome aa_3,[383,384] complex IV + cytochrome aa_3 + cytochrome b,[379,388,393–395,397,399,400] and complexes I + IV.[391]

Recent genetic studies suggest that some cases of LIMD are caused by tissue-specific depletions of the mtDNA.[395,402–405] mtDNA depletion diseases are transmitted in an autosomal recessive fashion. In an example of one family,[395] the patients manifested mitochondrial myopathy, hypotonia, progressive external ophthalmoplegia, and severe lactic acidosis. A second cousin died at 9 months with hepatic failure and mitochondrial abnormalities. Quantitative Southern blot analysis demonstrated that the copy number of the mtDNA was greatly reduced in affected tissues, which correlated with the severity of tissue dysfunction and abnormalities identified in complex IV histochemistry and immunohistochemistry.[403–405] Interestingly, the unaffected tissues of some patients may show normal levels of mtDNA. The disorder is transmitted in an autosomal recessive fashion.

Some cases of LIMD were proposed to result from mtDNA mutations though the prevalence of this mechanism is unclear. In two cases, homoplasmic mtDNA point mutations were observed in the $tRNA^{Thr}$ gene at positions 15,923 and 15,924.[406] Both of these mutations were A to G transitions, one located in the terminal nucleotide of the anticodon stem (bp 15,924) and the other in the anticodon loop (bp 15,923). Both infants had lactic acidosis and OXPHOS defects in skeletal muscle, and died within several days of birth. However, the frequency of these mtDNA mutations in the general population was not determined in the original study.[406] The $tRNA^{Thr}$ bp 15,924 mutation was also observed in one of three LIMD infants with OXPHOS defects and lactic acidosis examined.[407] This male died at 4 months postpartum with severe lactic acidosis, ragged-red fibers, and complex I and IV defects in heart and skeletal muscle.[391] His mother, who had normal histochemistry and electron microscopy on her muscle biopsy and normal OXPHOS enzymology, was also homoplasmic for this point mutation. Screening unaffected controls for the bp 15,924 mutation revealed that 11 percent (11/103) of Caucasians were also homoplasmic for this mutation. Hence, the bp 15,924 mutation appears to be a common polymorphism and not the cause of the disease. None of the patients harbored the bp 15,923 mutation, nor was it found in 91 Caucasians, 35 Africans, and 57 Asians. While it is unlikely that either of these $tRNA^{Thr}$ mutations alone can cause LIMD, it is possible that they are pathogenic in association with specific nuclear gene variants.

Some cases of LIMD appear to be characterized by abnormal expression of specific complex I or complex IV subunits. Four cases of LIMD have been analyzed by immunohistochemical staining of skeletal muscle with complex IV-specific antibodies.[378] Skeletal muscle analyses revealed the absence of the nuclear-encoded subunit VIIa and VIIb in all fiber types, whereas subunits II, IV, Va and b, VIa, VIb and c, and VIII were normal. This pattern of complex IV subunit deficiency was distinct from the one found in BIMM, which involved subunit II along with subunits VIIa and VIIb. The absence of expression of the mtDNA-encoded subunit II was proposed to permit differentiation between these two disorders (see "Benign Infantile Mitochondrial Myopathy" below). Two patients with severe neonatal lactic acidosis demonstrated a complex I deficiency and a reduction of the complex I subunits as determined by western blot.[408] Investigation of the mRNA expression for the 75-kDa iron-sulfur protein subunit of complex I revealed a normal 2.6-kb mRNA.[409]

Benign Infantile Mitochondrial Myopathy and Cardiomyopathy (BIMC) and Adult Cardiomyopathies

BIMC appears to be a more severe variant of BIMM and involves both skeletal and cardiac muscle.[410] In one case, healthy consanguineous parents had seven male children of which two died with "hyperpnea" shortly after birth, four had neonatal lactic acidemia and evidence of cardiomyopathy, and one appeared healthy but also had evidence of cardiomyopathy. Three children with neonatal lactic acidosis improved during their first year of life. Muscle biopsy of one child had swollen mitochondria and lipid droplet accumulation. OXPHOS enzymology showed a complex I defect. Analysis of the mitochondrial polypeptides synthesized by myotubes and myoblasts revealed that ND3 migrated more slowly with an apparent molecular weight of 13.1 in contrast to the normal molecular weight of 13.7.

Cardiomyopathy may occur in a variety of clinical settings in adults and children with OXPHOS diseases caused by nuclear gene abnormalities as well as mtDNA gene abnormalities.[411–433] This group of patients is clinically and genetically heterogeneous. Autosomal dominant as well as autosomal recessive variants are described. Autosomal dominant cases may have complex phenotypes that include ragged-red fibers, COX-deficient fibers, limb girdle myopathy, dilated cardiomyopathy, and dementia.[421]

Kearns-Sayre and Chronic Progressive External Ophthalmoplegia (CPEO) Syndromes

Kearns-Sayre and chronic progressive external ophthalmoplegia syndromes can be transmitted in an autosomal dominant or autosomal recessive fashion.[10,79,434–436] mtDNA analysis of affected individuals in these families revealed that each harbors an array of deleted mtDNAs.[10] Clinical manifestations include ophthalmoplegia, proximal muscle weakness, sensorineural hearing loss and abnormal vestibular responses, tremor, ataxia, and sensorimotor neuropathy.[437,438] Although multiple mtDNA deletions accumulated in various tissues of some patients, clinical manifestations within the same pedigree are often highly variable, ranging from individuals with severe manifestations to individuals who are asymptomatic. In one family with this disorder, the male proband exhibited the manifestations of Kearns-Sayre syndrome and Leigh disease.[439] Elevations in blood lactate, a ragged-red fiber myopathy, and OXPHOS defects primarily affecting complexes I and IV occur. The biochemical abnormalities are typical of mutations that cause defects in mitochondrial protein synthesis. Skeletal muscle is the best tissue for detecting multiple mtDNA deletions.[10] These mutations are generally absent in populations of rapidly dividing cells such as cultured fibroblasts, peripheral blood cells, cultured myoblasts,[440] myotubes, or in vitro innervated muscle cells.[437] Autosomal dominant forms of the disease map to chromosome 10q23.3-24.3 in a Finnish family,[441] and chromosome 3p14.1-21.2 in Italian families.[442]

An autosomal recessive variant of CPEO with multiple mtDNA deletions was proposed.[443,444] Two brothers, ages 46 and 48 years, whose parents were first cousins had a disorder characterized by ptosis, early CPEO, muscle weakness and wasting, optic atrophy, and a sensory neuropathy. Mild elevations in lactate and pyruvate as well as creatine kinase were present. Histochemical and ultrastructural analysis of skeletal muscle revealed typical features of a mitochondrial myopathy with ragged-red fibers, abnormal cytochrome c oxidase staining, and paracrystalline inclusions in the mitochondria. Numerous mtDNA deletions were identified in the same region of the mtDNA as the autosomal dominant form of the disease.[444] Autosomal recessive inheritance was proposed in an individual with KSS who had a defect in complex II function,[445] because all of the complex II subunits are encoded entirely by the nuclear DNA.

Myoneurogastrointestinal Disorder and Encephalopathy (MNGIE)

MNGIE is an autosomal recessive disorder characterized by a progressive external ophthalmoplegia, dementia with a progressive leukodystrophy, mitochondrial myopathy, peripheral neuropathy, and prominent involvement of the gastrointestinal tract.[446–452] The gastrointestinal manifestations are heralded by significant diarrhea, malabsorption, and weight loss with normal pancreatic function. Radiologic investigations may show marked thickening of the small intestines, which reflects the pathologic findings of extensive mural thickening and fibrosis of the submucosa and subserosa. Lactate may be elevated along with other tricarboxylic acid cycle intermediates. This disorder is linked to chromosome 22q13.32-qter.[453] Recent investigations demonstrated that this disorder is caused by loss-of-function mutations in the thymidine phosphorylase gene.[454] Thymidine phosphorylase converts thymidine to 2-deoxy-D-ribose-1-phosphate and may function to regulate thymidine availability for DNA synthesis. Thymidine phosphorylase is widely expressed in human tissues. Interestingly, this enzyme shows little expression in skeletal muscle, even though disease manifestations are identifiable in this tissue. At this time, the mechanism for disease expression in skeletal muscle is unknown.

Inherited Exertional Myoglobinuria and Rhabdomyolysis

Exercise-related myoglobinuria is frequently caused by defects in enzymes involved in glycogenolysis, glycolysis, and fatty acid transport: phosphorylase, phosphofructokinase, phosphoglycerate kinase, phosphoglyceromutase, lactate dehydrogenase, and carnitine palmitoyl transferase (type II). However, a novel clinical disorder associated with mtDNA deletions was described that consists of recurrent episodes of rhabdomyolysis induced by strenuous exercise, heavy alcohol intake, or fasting.[455] Until this report, muscle pain and myoglobinuria were not attributed to OXPHOS dysfunction. Two brothers had the onset of these symptoms at approximately 18 years of age. No other systemic manifestations of OXPHOS disease, such as CPEO, epilepsy, dementia, retinal degeneration, or cardiomyopathy, were reported. Creatine kinase levels varied between approximately 1300 and 12,000 U/liter, depending on the clinical state. Metabolic investigations indicated that resting levels of blood lactate and pyruvate were normal, but even mild exercise provoked significant elevations. Muscle biopsy demonstrated central nuclei, actively degenerating and regenerating fibers, and occasional ragged-red fibers containing abnormal mitochondria with paracrystalline inclusions. OXPHOS enzymology was normal in both individuals. mtDNA analysis revealed heterogeneous populations of deleted mtDNAs. Rhabdomyolysis also can be seen in conjunction with mtDNA point mutations, such as the A3243G mutation that causes MELAS,[66] and in patients who have autosomal dominant variants of chronic progressive external ophthalmoplegia.[456] Autosomal dominant myoglobinuria was observed in a Swiss family with COX-deficient muscle fibers and exertional lactic acidemia.[457] mtDNA deletions were not observed in this family.

Several Swedish families were described with a disorder characterized by lifelong exercise intolerance and episodes of fatigability, weakness, muscle swelling, and myoglobinuria.[458] A complex II defect of OXPHOS in conjunction with abnormal aconitase activity of the tricarboxylic acid cycle was reported in one of these individuals.[459] The complex II defect was confirmed histochemically, biochemically, and by immunoblot analysis.

Leigh Disease

Although Leigh disease can be caused by defects in a variety of metabolic pathways, OXPHOS defects are the most commonly identified abnormality in this group of patients. To date, all nuclear OXPHOS gene mutations discovered were transmitted in an autosomal recessive fashion. Complex I, complex IV, and complex V defects are important causes of Leigh disease.[338,342,356130,339–341,343–348,355]

Four mutations in nuclear-encoded OXPHOS subunits were identified in Leigh disease patients. One is in a nuclear OXPHOS gene mutation in the flavoprotein subunit of complex II.[11] The other three mutations groups involve complex I subunits. One is a mutation in the 18-kDa (AQDQ) complex I subunit which maps to chromosome 5.[460] A second represents mutations in the NDUSF8 (TYKY) subunit of complex I.[461] A third represents mutations in the 51-kDa subunit of complex I (NDUFV1).[462] Each of these mutations is transmitted in an autosomal recessive fashion. The complex I mutation in the 18-kDa subunit showed normal organic and amino acids, skeletal muscle light microscopy, and electron microscopy. The complex I defect was present in both skeletal muscle and in fibroblasts. This patient provides genetic confirmation for the common observation that complex I defects generally do not produce detectable metabolic abnormalities. Additional phenotypic heterogeneity was observed with the 51-kDa subunit mutations. One individual was diagnosed as having Alexander disease, which is characterized by megalencephaly with progressive spasticity and dementia.[462]

Although complex IV defects are frequently observed, mutations affecting mtDNA-encoded or nuclear-encoded subunits of complex IV are rare.[41] Mutations in a highly evolutionarily conserved gene, the SURF1 gene (chromosome 9q34), were recognized as a cause for systemic cytochrome c oxidase (complex IV) deficiency.[463,464] These individuals had Leigh disease with early onset hypotonia, ataxia, brainstem abnormalities, regression, and the characteristic bilateral basal ganglia lesions found in Leigh disease. The SURF1 gene appears to be essential for complex IV assembly. Mutations in the SURF1 gene are heterogeneous, consisting of deletions, nonsense mutations, and donor splice-site mutants. Compound heterozygotes are common. The use of functional complementation to discover this gene defect promises to be a powerful tool in uncovering novel mechanisms for OXPHOS disease pathogenesis.

Leigh disease is a genetically heterogeneous group of OXPHOS diseases. A group of Leigh disease patients referred to as the Saguenay Lac-Saint-Jean type show complex IV deficiency.[465–468] Although phenotypically similar to the patients harboring mutations in the SURF1 gene, this recessively transmitted disorder maps to chromosome 2. Whereas the complex IV defect in the group with SURF1 mutations is systemic, the Saguenay Lac-Saint-Jean group has 50 percent activity in muscle, fibroblasts, and amniocytes, less than 10 percent activity in brain and liver, and normal activity in kidney and heart. Other patients with complex Leigh-like features are reported. An interesting variant with the acronym EPEMA consists of encephalopathy, petechiae, and ethymalonic aciduria.[33] Other features include COX-deficient muscle fibers, hypotonia, orthostatic acrocyanosis, and chronic diarrhea.

Alpers Disease (Progressive Infantile Poliodystrophy)

Alpers disease is associated with characteristic neuropathologic lesions accompanied by spongiform or microcystic cerebral degeneration.[318,469–472] Both Leigh and Alpers disease have central nervous system lesions characterized by gliosis, spongiosis, necrosis, or capillary proliferation.[353,354,473–476] Neuropathologically, the primary point of differentiation between Leigh disease and Alpers disease is the severity of involvement of certain brain regions. In order of decreasing severity, Alpers disease affects the cerebral cortex, cerebellum, basal ganglia, and brain stem, whereas Leigh disease preferentially affects the basal ganglia and brain stem. Like Leigh disease, Alpers has a childhood onset at approximately 1 to 2 years of age, with death occurring in 3 to 4 years. Clinical manifestations include various combinations of developmental retardation and regression, myoclonus, ataxia, spasticity, nystagmus, areflexia, hypotonia, abnormal respiration, liver dysfunction, and clinical worsening during infections. The prominent myoclonus in this disorder emphasizes the extensive cortical involvement. Biochemical abnormalities identified for this disorder include decreased NADH utilization,[472,477] complex I defects,[478,479] pyruvate dehydrogenase deficiency,[480] decreased pyruvate utilization,[472] citric acid cycle dysfunction,[471] gamma polymerase deficiency plus mtDNA depletion,[481] and decreased cytochrome $a + a_3$.[318,472] The mode of transmission of Alpers disease is unclear due to the small size of the pedigrees. However, autosomal recessive inheritance is the most likely inheritance pattern.

Wolfram Syndrome

Wolfram syndrome is characterized by diabetes insipidus, insulin-dependent diabetes mellitus, optic atrophy, and deafness. In a small percentage of cases, multiple mtDNA deletions are observed in tissues of these individuals. Muscle biopsy may reveal cytochrome c oxidase-deficient fibers and ragged-red fibers. This autosomal recessive disorder is linked to chromosome 4p16.[482,483]

Hereditary Spastic Paraplegia with Ragged-Red Fiber Myopathy

An autosomal recessive form of spastic paraparesis was identified at chromosome 16q24.3.[484] Patients experience progressive weakness, spasticity, and mild decreases in vibratory sensation as their major manifestations. Dysphagia, scoliosis, and optic nerve atrophy have also occurred. This unique form of hereditary spastic paraplegia is caused by mutations in the gene called paraplegin that is localized to the mitochondria.[485] Paraplegin has a high degree of homology with a subclass of ATPases called the AAA family. This group of ATPases consists of metalloproteases with proteolytic and chaperonin functions. Patients have ragged-red fibers and cytochrome c oxidase-deficient fibers in their skeletal muscle. As noted above, these observations suggest that paraplegin may in some fashion be important to mitochondrial protein synthesis.

Friedreich Ataxia

Friedreich ataxia was recently discovered to be a mitochondrial disease. Clinical manifestations are systemic and include hypoactive or absent deep tendon reflexes, ataxia, corticospinal tract dysfunction, impaired vibratory and proprioceptive function, hypertrophic cardiomyopathy, and diabetes mellitus. This autosomal recessive disorder was mapped to chromosome 9q13. This disease is caused by a GAA trinucleotide repeat expansion in the first intron of the frataxin gene.[486] Frataxin is a mitochondrial protein[487] that is involved in iron homeostasis. Frataxin gene mutations result in impaired activity of the iron-sulfur containing enzymes within the mitochondria: complex I, complex II, complex III, and aconitase.[488]

Lethal Infantile Cardiomyopathy (LIC)

LIC represents a distinct OXPHOS disorder of infancy where the cardiac myocytes have a reduced number of myofibrils, and accumulate abnormal mitochondria, lipid, and glycogen.[432,489] Clinically, cardiomyopathy and cardiac dysrhythmias including supraventricular preexcitation (Wolf-Parkinson-White) and ventricular arrhythmias are the predominant manifestations.[422] Two OXPHOS defects have been reported for LIC: cytochrome b deficiency[432] and cytochrome c + c_1 deficiency.[489]

The LIC patient with cytochrome b deficiency occurred as an isolated case, a frequent situation for patients with similar clinicopathologic findings.[418,419,422,424,425,490–493] However, two pedigrees have been reported with affected siblings.[493] One hypothesis for the origin of these cases could be a spontaneous mutation in the mtDNA cytochrome b gene which becomes enriched during embryogenesis. Alternatively, a recessive nuclear DNA mutation or a new dominant mutation in a complex III subunit could impair cytochrome b incorporation and cause the disease. However, most reported cases are female, which cannot be explained by these genetic models.

Lethal Infantile Cardiomyopathy (LIC): X-linked Cardioskeletal Myopathy (Barth Syndrome)

X-linked cardioskeletal myopathy (CSM) is characterized by a congenital dilated cardiomyopathy and mitochondrial myopathy with growth retardation.[36,489,494–496] The dilated cardiomyopathy may be associated with endocardial fibroelastosis,[495] and ultrastructural studies of the cardiac muscle show mitochondria with abnormally shaped cristae, but no paracrystalline inclusions. Skeletal muscle shows increased lipid on histochemistry and abnormal mitochondrial cristae.[489] Abnormal mitochondria are also found in bone marrow,[489] liver,[496] and renal tubule epithelial cells.[496] Additional features linked to this disease include decreased plasma free carnitine and muscle carnitine,[489] increased urinary 3-methylglutaconic acid and 2-ethylhydracrylic acid,[36] and reduced levels of cytochromes c + c_1 in skeletal muscle.[489] Although the primary enzymologic defect associated with 3-methylglutaconic aciduria is unknown, this organic aciduria was associated with a defect in complex V in a child with retinitis pigmentosa, optic atrophy, and cataracts.[497] Barth syndrome is localized to Xq28 and is caused by mutations in the tafazzin gene (G4.5 gene).[498–503] The function of this gene and its relationship with mitochondrial abnormalities is unknown.

Idiopathic Dystonia

Adult- and pediatric-onset dystonias represent a complex group of disorders in which patients experience involuntary sustained muscle contractions in a focal, segmental, or generalized distribution. Basal ganglia dysfunction is the most likely cause for these muscle spasms. However, precise neuroanatomic or biochemical localization of the defect has not been possible.[504] Pathologic analyses of brains from patients with idiopathic dystonias have been normal.[505] Although the clinical features are highly variable, the most severe variant of the disease, generalized dystonia, generally has its onset in childhood, whereas the less severe focal and segmental dystonias generally become symptomatic during adult life. The inheritance of idiopathic dystonias has also been unclear. Recent genetic studies suggest that an autosomal dominant gene or genes may cause idiopathic dystonias with variable penetrance.[504,506–511] An alternative explanation for the variable penetrance could be that the phenotypic heterogeneity, in some cases, is the result of heteroplasmic mtDNA mutations.

OXPHOS function has been assessed in platelets from a cohort of patients with focal, segmental, and generalized dystonias.[512] Complex I-specific activity as determined by the NADH-ubiquinone assay was significantly reduced in all patients with dystonia relative to controls. Moreover, the patients with segmental or generalized dystonias had greater reductions in this enzyme activity relative to controls than did patients with focal dystonias. Complex III- and complex IV-specific activities were normal. mtDNA analyses will be important in these patients to assess the contribution of mtDNA mutations to the pathogenesis of this disease.

Mitochondrial Myopathy

Mitochondrial myopathies are usually seen in conjunction with disease manifestations in other tissues that include Wolf-Parkinson-White conduction defect,[513] cardiomyopathy,[413,513,514] hearing loss and vertigo,[515,516] seizures,[515,516] and pigmentary retinopathy.[84] The distribution of the myopathy may be in a facioscapulohumeral dystrophy pattern,[516–518] limb-girdle pattern,[413,514,519] a generalized muscle weakness pattern,[520–526] or even polymyalgia rheumatica.[527,528] Childhood,[514,515,517,518,522–526,529] adolescent,[517–520] and adult-onset[516] forms of the disease occur. Most patients present as singleton cases within a pedigree.[514,516,519–521,523,525,526] The reported OXPHOS defects of mitochondrial myopathy cases are as heterogeneous as their clinical descriptions and include complex I dysfunction,[513,519,520,524] complex II dysfunction,[413,530] complex III dysfunction,[521,525,526,531] and complex IV dysfunction.[516,522,532]

Autosomal dominant and recessive forms of mitochondrial myopathy occur with some cases demonstrating tissue-specific patterns of disease expression. However, careful clinical evaluation often reveals that other organs can also be involved. Hence, classification in this group of disorders is problematic due to the difficulty in defining recognizable syndromes.

Defects in multiple OXPHOS complexes were identified by enzymologic and polarographic studies in a young girl with a progressive mitochondrial myopathy.[533] A specific defect in the 27-kDa subunit of complex II and the Rieske iron-sulfur protein from skeletal muscle was observed by immunohistochemistry. No other organ systems were reported to be involved. As is common to many of the OXPHOS diseases, this patient experienced a worsening of her disease manifestations during episodes of fever. The reduced levels of specific nuclear-encoded subunits for complexes II and III was interpreted as a defect in the transport of these subunits from the cytosol to the mitochondria. Because this patient was the only affected individual in her family and the proteins involved are nuclear encoded, she is likely to harbor a recessive form of mitochondrial myopathy.

More complex clinical presentations are described in other families. In a large pedigree with mitochondrial myopathy, cerebellar ataxia, and diabetes mellitus, the complete syndrome appeared in 11 family members along the maternal lineage.[517,518,534] However, seven asymptomatic family members had elevations in creatine kinase and/or electromyographic abnormalities. Three of these individuals were on the paternal lineage, indicating autosomal dominant inheritance with variable penetrance. An autosomal recessive disorder with congenital muscular dystrophy, mitochondrial depletion in the center of the myofibers, and significant ultrastructural abnormalities in the subsarcolemmal mitochondria is described.[60] Rare patients have a primary coenzyme Q_{10} deficiency.[1334,1335] The triad of CNS involvement, recurrent myoglobinuria, and ragged-red fibers suggests the diagnosis. These patients are important to identify since clinical improvements were noted with CoQ_{10} administration.

Luft Disease

Two spontaneous cases of Luft disease have been reported.[1,535–538] These patients presented with nonthyroid hypermetabolism manifested clinically as elevated basal metabolic rate, increased body temperature, profuse sweating, tachycardia, increased respiratory rate, and a generalized myopathy with onset during childhood. Skeletal muscle appears to be the primary tissue affected and exhibits ragged-red fibers and paracrystalline inclusions. mtDNA deletions have been excluded by Southern blot analysis of patient muscle.[81]

Biochemical analysis of Luft patients has suggested that their skeletal muscle mitochondria are uncoupled, with the electrochemical gradient generated by the electron transport chain being dissipated without a concomitant ATP synthesis. Consistent with this hypothesis, oligomycin, an inhibitor of ATP synthase (complex V), does not inhibit the respiration of Luft mitochondria. One mechanism proposed for dissipation of the electrochemical gradient is an inability of patient mitochondria to retain calcium or magnesium. This would result in a futile cycle in which the proton gradient drives the uptake of the divalent cations, which then leak out.[537] Alternatively, the impairment in coupling could be due to mutations in the nuclear-encoded subunits of the F_o portion of the ATPase (complex V), mitochondrially encoded F_o subunits (ATPase subunits 6 or 8), or in the nuclear-encoded uncoupler protein or inhibitor protein. Investigation of the PMI and CBP inhibitor proteins of complex V in fibroblasts from a patient with Luft disease revealed that PMI was deficient.[539] Hence, as the intracellular calcium increases during excitation-contraction coupling of skeletal muscle, the CBP would be inactivated, leaving no mechanism for regulation of ATP hydrolysis and synthesis.[539] This could lead to the abnormal coupling observed in mitochondria from individuals with Luft disease.

GENETIC COUNSELING, PRENATAL DIAGNOSIS, AND PREGNANCY

Mutations in nuclear OXPHOS genes can be detected by standard genetic testing approaches. At this time, the number of identified mutations in nuclear OXPHOS genes is small. Genetic counseling is difficult in many patients with OXPHOS diseases due to the complex genetics of these disorders.[540] If viewed in aggregate, most OXPHOS diseases are transmitted in an autosomal recessive fashion. mtDNA testing (Southern blot, point mutation analysis, SSCP, sequencing) can be helpful in defining whether the nuclear DNA or the mitochondrial DNA is the most likely cause for the OXPHOS disease. These approaches can greatly enhance the accuracy of genetic counseling. Recommendations are given in Table 104-3.

The ability to perform prenatal diagnostic testing for OXPHOS diseases and perform accurate predictions of phenotype is limited. Levels of heteroplasmic mtDNA mutations in chorionic villi or amniocytes may not accurately reflect the levels in patient tissues. For example, chorionic villi and amniocytes might harbor low levels of mutant mtDNA, whereas tissues such as brain, heart, and muscle may harbor very high levels. Alternatively, when the levels of the mtDNA mutation are very high in chorionic villi or amniocytes, it is more likely that the mutant mtDNA levels will be high in fetal tissues.[541,542] For OXPHOS diseases such as Leigh disease, recurrence risk can be very high, probably greater than 70 percent. In a woman with 50 percent of the T8993G mutation in blood, her oocyte analysis revealed one with 0 percent mutant mtDNA and six with >95 percent mutant mtDNA.[543] Biochemical testing of chorionic villus cells or amniocytes is difficult and awaits further investigation of the efficacy of this approach.

Limited information exists concerning appropriate obstetrical care of women who have OXPHOS diseases. A number of women who harbor mtDNA mutations have had uneventful pregnancies (unpublished observations).[544] Reports are emerging that describe various problems that include preterm labor, hypertension, and pregnancy-induced diabetes mellitus.[545] However, it is unclear whether obstetric complications occur at a frequency higher than the general population. Anecdotally, it does not appear that pregnancy in women with OXPHOS diseases precipitates acute disease progression. More data are needed to assess the validity of these assumptions.

Table 104-3 Genetic Counseling Recommendations for OXPHOS Disease Caused by mtDNA Mutations

I. Maternal inheritance of an mtDNA mutation:

A. *Pedigree testing:* Maternal lineage pedigree members are at risk for inheriting the mtDNA mutation. Due to rapid segregation of mtDNA mutations, genetic confirmation of the mutation should be performed in each individual at risk.

B. *Prognosis:* Predictions based on patient genotype of a single tissue (% mutant versus % normal mtDNAs) are generally unreliable except for individuals who harbor high levels of mtDNA mutations. Periodic clinical screening of commonly involved organs is necessary for early detection and treatment of disease manifestations.

C. *Prenatal testing:* Experience with prenatal testing for mtDNA mutations is limited. Due to the variability in patient phenotype with small shifts in the amount of normal mtDNA, accurate phenotype predictions are not possible. Prognosis has been predicted only if the fetus is essentially homoplasmic for a highly pathogenic mtDNA mutation that is heteroplasmic in the mother.

II. Spontaneous mtDNA mutations:

A. *Pedigree testing:* Due to the high replicative rate of blood cells, a failure to detect the mutation in blood does not exclude the presence of the mutation in other tissues. A tissue with low replicative potential such as skeletal muscle must be tested to confirm absence of transmission of the mtDNA mutation. The best characterized categories of spontaneously occurring mtDNA are the mtDNA deletions and duplications. The mtDNA deletions are generally confined to the somatic cell lineage, preventing germ cell transmission. The spontaneous occurrence of mtDNA point mutations is also possible.

B. *Prognosis:* Same as IB.

MEDICATIONS AND OXIDATIVE PHOSPHORYLATION

Although an exhaustive discussion of medication and toxin interactions with OXPHOS is beyond the scope of this chapter, several adverse interactions are important to mention. Medications designed to inhibit viral replication by acting as nucleoside analogues can have deleterious effects on mitochondrial function. AIDS patients treated with zidovudine (AZT), an inhibitor of the mitochondrial gamma polymerase,[546,547] may experience mtDNA depletion associated with severe mitochondrial myopathy, including ragged-red fiber accumulation[548–550] and ultrastructural abnormalities in mitochondria.[551,552] When the AZT treatment is withdrawn, the normal mtDNA level is rapidly restored.[553]

Fialuridine, an antiviral agent of treatment for hepatitis B, caused severe side effects due to mitochondrial injury.[554–563] Adverse effects included nausea, vomiting, painful paresthesias, hepatic failure, pancreatitis, myopathy, and lactic acidosis. Other nucleoside analogues capable of inducing mitochondrial injury are didanosine and zalcitabine.[557,564–569] Interestingly, mitochondrial injury does not appear to occur with all nucleoside analogs. To date, adverse effects are not reported with lamivudine and famciclovir.[557,562,570]

The understanding of the range of medications adversely affecting mitochondrial function is limited. Fatty acid oxidation or OXPHOS function may occur with aspirin and valproic acid through coenzyme A sequestration, tetracyclines, 2-arylpropionate anti-inflammatory drugs, chloramphenicol, amineptine and tianeptine by beta-oxidation impairment, endogen bile acids, amiodarone, perhexiline, diethyl-aminoethoxyhexestrol by impairment of OXPHOS and beta-oxidation, and with alcohol abuse.[571] Although many patients with OXPHOS diseases and seizures benefit from valproate, selected individuals experienced worsening of their OXPHOS disease symptoms after valproate administration,[572–576] or even a Reye-like syndrome.[577]

OXPHOS DISEASE TREATMENT

Metabolic therapies for OXPHOS diseases attempt to increase mitochondrial ATP production and thus arrest the progression of the clinical manifestations. Metabolic therapies that have been reported to produce a positive therapeutic effect include coenzyme Q_{10}, phylloquinone, menadione, succinate, ascorbate, and riboflavin. However, the assessment of the efficacy of these treatments has been difficult due to the clinical and genetic heterogeneity of these disorders. Treatment for most patients is supportive because therapeutic efficacy of any reported compounds is limited.[578]

Coenzyme Q_{10}

Coenzyme Q_{10} (CoQ_{10}) (2,3-dimethoxy-5-methyl-6-decaprenyl-1,4-benzoquinone) is a fat-soluble quinone that contains a side chain of 10 isoprenoid units. CoQ_{10} functions to transfer electrons from complex I to complex III and from complex II to complex III. This compound may also stabilize the OXPHOS complexes within the inner membrane and serve as a potent antioxidant for oxygen free radicals,[579–584] even at physiological concentrations.[585] In humans, the highest concentrations of coenzyme Q are found in heart, liver, kidney, and pancreas.[586] Studies using rat hepatocytes demonstrated that 25 percent to 30 percent of coenzyme Q is localized in the cell nucleus, 40 percent to 50 percent in the mitochondrion, 15 percent to 20 percent in microsomes, and 5 percent to 10 percent in the cytosol.[587]

Plasma levels in children and adults are 0.79 ± 0.22 μg/ml. Following a single 100 mg oral dose, peak plasma levels occur in approximately 5 to 10 h with a mean plasma level of about 1 μg/ml.[588] The plasma half-life is estimated at 33.9 ± 5.32 h and approximately 90 percent of the steady-state concentration can be achieved after 4 days of treatment. In our experience with administration of CoQ_{10} to children and adults, an oral dose of 4.3 mg/kg/day results in an increase in the plasma level to 3 to 4 μg/ml. Oral doses of CoQ_{10} appear to be taken up by chylomicrons, deposited in the liver, and packaged into very-low-density lipoproteins.[589] Excretion is primarily through the biliary tract.[590] During chronic administration, approximately 62.5 percent of the orally administered CoQ_{10} can be recovered in the feces. To date, no side effects have been reported.

CoQ_{10} has been reported to have a beneficial effect on the clinical manifestations of a number of OXPHOS diseases. Clinical and metabolic improvement with CoQ_{10} administration has been noted in various classes of OXPHOS disease.[74,312,314,591–601] CoQ_{10} doses have ranged from 30 to 300 mg/day with no side effects. In MELAS, doses of 300 mg/day were required for optimal therapeutic effects.[312,314] A trial of CoQ_{10} (60 mg/day), vitamin B_6 (180 mg/day), and ferrous citrate (150 mg/day) in 27 Alzheimer disease patients, 2 of whom harbored a missense mutation in the amyloid β-protein at codon 717 (Val to Ile), was reported to result in an improvement of mental status.[602,603] In a multicenter, double-blind study where the participants had chronic progressive external ophthalmoplegias from a variety of causes (i.e., only a subset had mtDNA deletions), a decrease inpost exercise lactate levels was observed in about 30 percent of individuals and intention tremor improved in about 10 percent of individuals with cerebellar signs.[600] This study employed a relatively low dose of CoQ_{10} (2 mg/kg/day) which resulted in only modest increases in blood CoQ_{10} levels. Positive therapeutic effects have also been reported in patients with angina pectoris,[604,605] congestive heart failure,[423,426,427,604–612] Adriamycin cardiotoxicity,[613–616] and cardiac arrhythmias.[592] Symptoms such as sleep disturbances, leg paresthesias, leg edema, and palpitations are anecdotally reported to be improved with CoQ_{10} administration.[243] In our treatment of OXPHOS diseases, we administer CoQ_{10} at a dose of 4.3 mg/kg/day for both pediatric and adult patients. Due to the complexities of CoQ_{10} absorption, particularly in pediatric groups, analysis of CoQ_{10} blood levels can be helpful in optimizing the dose. For children and adults who are unable to swallow the CoQ_{10}, this hydrophobic compound can be dissolved in vegetable oil. Once this is done, the vegetable oil can be added to food (applesauce, cereal, etc.) to make it more palatable.

Menadione and Phylloquinone

Two vitamin K compounds, menadione (vitamin K_3) and phylloquinone (vitamin K_1 or phytonadione), have been administered in conjunction with ascorbate (vitamin C) to donate electrons directly to cytochrome c.[132,617] Menadione (40 to 80 mg/day) and ascorbate (4 g/day) improved cellular phosphate metabolism of a patient with mitochondrial myopathy and complex III dysfunction as measured by ^{31}P-NMR.[132,617] Menadione has also been reported to decrease complex III inhibition by Adriamycin in yeast.[618–620] Moreover, in a yeast mutant (*S. cerevisiae* W7) with abnormal complex III function due to a glycine to serine substitution at amino acid 131 of the cytochrome b gene, the complex III activity was significantly improved by menadione supplementation.[621] Menadione enhances the rate of fumarate reduction by permitting electron transfer to the S3 iron-sulfur cluster of complex II.[622] It also improves electron transfer after complex I inhibition by rotenone in human fibroblasts[623,624] and rat liver,[625] and by diphenylene iodonium in rats.[626]

The water-soluble menadione must be alkylated to menaquinone-4 to be both lipophilic and biologically active.[627] Phylloquinone, by contrast, is already in a lipid-soluble and biologically active form. Although both vitamin K derivatives, phylloquinone and menadione, have relatively short half-lives, phylloquinone appears to have better tissue retention and appears to reach a greater concentration in the mitochondria.[627,628] No side effects have been reported with phylloquinone use, whereas menadione may produce hemolytic anemia, hyperbilirubinemia, or kernicterus in newborns. It is unclear which form of vitamin K is best for the treatment of OXPHOS diseases.

Succinate

Succinate is a tricarboxylic acid-cycle intermediate that donates electrons directly to complex II. Preliminary evidence for positive therapeutic effect for succinate has been reported for two cases. In one of our KS/CPEO syndrome patients with the 4.9-kb mtDNA deletion (see class III mutations) and an associated defect in complex I, IV, and V, respiratory failure resolved on a regimen of 300 mg/day CoQ_{10} and 6 g/day sodium succinate.[74] However, it is difficult to separate the effects of CoQ_{10} and succinate in this patient. Similarly, a MELAS patient was reported to have a decreased frequency of stroke-like episodes when treated with sodium succinate at 6 g/day.[629] Due to the high sodium content of succinate preparations, careful supervision is needed when administering this compound to patients with cardiomyopathy.

Thiamine, Nicotinamide, and Riboflavin

Thiamine and riboflavin have been given to some OXPHOS disease patients. Thiamine, as a cofactor of pyruvate dehydrogenase, has been used to stimulate NADH production, which can then enter OXPHOS at complex I. A KS/CPEO patient showed improved plasma lactate and pyruvate levels when treated with a thiamine dose of 300 mg/day.[630] Riboflavin (vitamin B_2), after conversion to flavin monophosphate and flavin adenine dinucleotide, functions as a cofactor for electron transport in complex I, complex II, and the electron transfer flavoprotein. A mitochondrial myopathy patient with complex I dysfunction was noted to have improvement in exercise capacity after administering 100 mg/day of riboflavin.[631] A patient who harbored the $tRNA^{Leucine(UUR)}$ T3250C mutation was reported to have an improvement in her myopathy.[632]

Complex I accepts electrons from NADH and ultimately transfers electrons to coenzyme Q_{10}. Oral nicotinamide was used to treat a patient with MELAS who inherited the A3243G mutation.[633] The blood NAD and NADH pool showed a twenty-fourfold increase over a 5-month interval. Blood lactate and pyruvate decreased by 50 percent. As with many OXPHOS disease therapies, responses with these agents are anecdotal. Isolated cases responding to mixtures of compounds are common in the literature. For example, clinical improvement was reported in patients with mitochondrial encephalomyopathies with a mixture of cytochrome c, vitamin B_1, and vitamin B_2.[634] The actual efficacy of these mixtures is unknown.

Corticosteroids

Corticosteroids have been reported to produce positive effects in MELAS,[134,311,313,315,320] MERRF,[120] and mitochondrial myopathy patients.[635,636] For example, muscle strength, serum lactate, and energy metabolism demonstrated improvement with a dose of 0.25 mg/kg in six affected family members.[637] The mechanism for clinical improvement is unclear and may include membrane stabilization, enzyme induction, or inhibition of phospholipase activity.[638,639] In general, the use of corticosteroids in OXPHOS diseases is discouraged. Although some patients respond favorably to their use, these individuals may become dependent on the drugs, developing the sequelae of chronic steroid use and undergoing clinical deterioration when the drug is reduced or withdrawn (unpublished observation).[134,320]

Idebenone

Idebenone is a novel quinone compound that has been used to treat neurologic dysfunction caused by ischemia,[640] to improve impaired long- and short-term memory,[641] alter neurotransmitter levels,[642–645] and inhibit lipid peroxidation.[646] Based on the proposed physiological effects and the structural similarity to CoQ_{10}, this compound has been used at doses of 90 mg/day[647] to treat patients with MELAS[42,597,648] and cerebrovascular dementia.[642] Improvements in clinical and metabolic abnormalities were observed in the patients with MELAS. A single patient with LHON caused by the MTND4*LHON11778 mutation has also been treated with idebenone (90 mg/day) for a year and during that time experienced a mild improvement of visual acuity.[649] While idebenone is not approved for patient use in the United States, further investigation of the efficacy of this compound in OXPHOS diseases is warranted.

Dichloroacetate (DCA)

DCA has been studied for many years for its ability to reduce blood glucose in chemical or surgical models of diabetes.[650–653] The primary effect of DCA is to stimulate pyruvate dehydrogenase (PDH) function[654] by inhibiting pyruvate dehydrogenase kinase, the enzyme that normally phosphorylates and inactivates PDH.[654–656] The drug may also stimulate the glycolytic enzyme phosphofructokinase by suppressing levels of the allosteric inhibitor, citrate, and increasing levels of the activator, fructose-2,6-biphosphate.[651,657,658] Inhibition of glyceraldehyde-3-phosphate[659–661] and pyruvate carboxylase[662,663] may also contribute to the metabolic effects of DCA. Hence, in conditions that result in the accumulation of lactate and alanine (compounds which are in equilibrium with pyruvate), activation of PDH decreases the release of these compounds from peripheral tissues and enhances their oxidative metabolism by liver.[664–668] The Cori and alanine cycles, which allow lactate and alanine to be utilized by the liver for glycogen synthesis, are interrupted.

DCA has been used in pediatric and adult patients for the treatment of lactic acidosis. In infants and children, oral or intravenous doses ranging between 15 and 200 mg/kg/day have been used without adverse effect, and have generally been associated with at least a 20 percent fall in blood lactate. Adults have shown a similar response when doses of 35 or 50 mg/kg were administered.[669–671] However, a large multicenter, placebo-controlled, randomized trial of DCA in adult patients from a critical care unit with various types of shock (septic, cardiogenic, hemorrhagic, multisystem failure, etc.) failed to show any benefit from the use of parenteral DCA at 50 mg/kg/day.[672]

It is unknown whether DCA may benefit patients with heritable forms of lactic acidosis. Anecdotal reports of successful and unsuccessful treatment are present in the literature. For example, a patient with MELAS who had auditory hallucinations experienced a normalization of lactate in the blood and CSF and a resolution of his psychiatric symptoms when DCA was administered orally at doses of 12.5 to 100 mg/kg/day.[673] In contrast, DCA was ineffective in a child with Leigh disease who harbored the T8993G mutation.[674] Currently DCA is only available under research protocols in the United States. Its effect on the morbidity and mortality of OXPHOS diseases has not yet been determined and requires more intensive trials to resolve these issues.

Chloramphenicol

The hypermetabolism of Luft disease has been reduced by inducing hypothyroidism or by inhibiting mtDNA protein synthesis with chloramphenicol.[1,535,537] However, the long-term clinical benefits of these treatments are unclear, and chronic chloramphenicol therapy can induce pancytopenia and, in some instances, aplastic anemia.

Dietary Manipulations

Dicarboxylic aciduria and secondary impairment of long chain fatty acid oxidation occur in patients with OXPHOS diseases. Avoidance of fasting, cornstarch supplementation, and decreased dietary long chain fatty acids may be helpful in selected patients. However, the long-term benefits of dietary manipulations are unknown. In addition, improvements in some patients may simply be related to improved attention to nutritional status and hydration.

Exercise

The effects of mild degrees of aerobic activity are a frequent concern voiced by patients and physicians. In 10 adults with mitochondrial myopathies, moderate treadmill training over 8 weeks resulted in a 30 percent improvement of aerobic capacity, a 30 percent drop in resting lactate and postexercise lactate levels, and a 60 percent improvement in adenosine triphosphate recovery as measured by ^{31}P-NMR testing.[675]

SUMMARY

Physicians in all specialties are becoming increasingly aware of OXPHOS diseases. Although the prevalence of OXPHOS diseases in the general population is unknown, the number of requests for pediatric and adult evaluations is increasing rapidly. A basic awareness of OXPHOS disease phenotypes, as well as of the essential elements of patient evaluation, are important for appropriate patient management and referrals. Centers that specialize in OXPHOS disease evaluations can be instrumental in working with referring physicians to develop a cost-effective diagnostic plan that is individualized to suit the patient's needs. Comprehensive mtDNA analysis by SSCP and sequencing is important in defining whether a family harbors an mtDNA mutation or is likely to harbor a nuclear DNA mutation. After a complete evaluation, genetic counseling based on Mendelian principles or mtDNA principles of inheritance can be applied. Although approaches that assess patients for mtDNA mutations are evolving rapidly, significant ambiguity in patient diagnosis often remains even after detailed testing is complete. Advances in our understanding of mutations in nuclear OXPHOS genes will provide a powerful addition to our ability to diagnose, manage, and counsel patients with these disorders, as well as to understand basic elements of OXPHOS disease pathophysiology.

REFERENCES

1. Luft R, Ikkos D, Palmieri G, Ernster L, Afzelius B: A case of severe hypermetabolism of nonthyroid origin with a defect in the maintenance of mitochondrial respiratory control: A correlated clinical, biochemical, and morphological study. *J Clin Invest* **41**:1776, 1962.
2. Engel WK, Cunningham GG: Rapid examination of muscle tissue. An improved method for fresh-frozen biopsy sections. *Neurology* **13**:919, 1963.

3. Shy GM, Gonatas NK: Human myopathy with giant abnormal mitochondria. *Science* **145**:493, 1964.
4. Shy GM, Gonatas NK, Perez M: Two childhood myopathies with abnormal mitochondria. I. Megaconial myopathy. II. Pleoconial myopathy. *Brain* **89**:133, 1966.
5. Nass MK, Nass S: Intramitochondrial fibers with DNA characteristics. I. Fixation and electron staining reactions. *J Cell Biol* **19**:593, 1963.
6. Nass S, Nass MK: Intramitochondrial fibers with DNA characteristics. II. Enzymatic and other hydrolytic treatments. *J Cell Biol* **19**:613, 1963.
7. Anderson S, Bankier AT, Barrell BG, de Bruijn MHL, Coulson AR, Drouin J, Eperon IC, Nierlich DP, Roe BA, Sanger F, Schreier PH, Smith AJH, Staden R, Young IJ: Sequence and organization of the human mitochondrial DNA genome. *Nature* **290**:457, 1981.
8. Holt IJ, Harding AE, Morgan HJA: Deletions of muscle mitochondrial DNA in patients with mitochondrial myopathies. *Nature* **331**:717, 1988.
9. Wallace DC, Singh G, Lott MT, Hodge JA, Schurr TG, Lezza AM, Elsas LJD, Nikoskelainen EK: Mitochondrial DNA mutation associated with Leber's hereditary optic neuropathy. *Science* **242**:1427, 1988.
10. Zeviani M, Servidei S, Gellera C, Bertini E, DiMauro S, DiDonato S: An autosomal dominant disorder with multiple deletions of mitochondrial DNA starting at the D-loop region. *Nature* **339**:309, 1989.
11. Bourgeron T, Rustin P, Chretien D, Birch-Machin M, Bourgeois M, Viegas-Pequignot E, Munnich A, Rotig A: Mutation of a nuclear succinate dehydrogenase gene results in mitochondrial respiratory chain deficiency. *Nat Genet* **11**:144, 1995.
12. von Kleist-Retzow J-C, Cormier-Daire V, de Lonlay P, Parfait B, Chretien D, Rustin P, Feingold J, Rotig A, Munnich A: A high rate (20%–30%) of parental consanguinity in cytochrome oxidase deficiency. *Am J Hum Genet* **63**:428, 1998.
13. Jerusalem F, Engel AG, Peterson HA: Human muscle fiber fine ultrastructure: Morphometric data on controls. *Neurology* **25**:127, 1975.
14. Johnson LV, Walsh ML, Chen LB: Localization of mitochondria in living cells with rhodamine. *Proc Natl Acad Sci U S A* **77**:990, 1980.
15. Shuster RC, Rubenstein AJ, Wallace DC: Mitochondrial DNA in anucleate human blood cells. *Biochem Biophys Res Commun* **155**:1360, 1988.
16. Shmookler-Reiss RJ, Goldstein S: Mitochondrial DNA in mortal and immortal human cells. *J Biol Chem* **258**:9078, 1983.
17. Bogenhagen D, Clayton DA: The number of mitochondrial deoxyribonucleic acid genomes in mouse L and human HeLa cells. Quantitative isolation of mitochondrial deoxyribonucleic acid. *J Biol Chem* **249**:7991, 1974.
18. Robin ED, Wong R: Mitochondrial DNA molecules and virtual number of mitochondria per cell in mammalian cells. *J Cell Physiol* **136**:507, 1988.
19. Manfredi G, Thyagarajan D, Papadopoulou LC, Pallotti F, Schon EA: The fate of human sperm-derived mtDNA in somatic cells. *Am J Hum Genet* **61**:953, 1997.
20. Houshmand M, Holme E, Hanson C, Wennerholm UB, Hamberger L: Is paternal mitochondrial DNA transferred to the offspring following intracytoplasmic sperm injection? *J Assist Reprod Genet* **14**:223, 1997.
21. Michaels GS, Hauswirth WW, Laipis PJ: Mitochondrial DNA copy number in bovine oocytes and somatic cells. *Dev Biol* **94**:246, 1982.
22. Piko L, Matsumoto L: Number of mitochondria and some properties of mitochondrial DNA in the mouse egg. *Dev Biol* **49**:1, 1976.
23. Magnusson C, Einarsson B, Nilsson BO: Oxygen consumption by the mouse blastocyst at activation for implantation. *Acta Physiol Scand* **127**:215, 1986.
24. Nilsson BO, Magnusson C, Widehn S, Hillensjo T: Correlation between blastocyst oxygen consumption and trophoblast cytochrome oxidase reaction at initiation of implantation of delayed mouse blastocysts. *J Embryol Exp Morphol* **71**:75, 1982.
25. Gyllensten U, Wharton D, Josefsson A, Wilson AC: Paternal inheritance of mitochondrial DNA in mice. *Nature* **352**:255, 1991.
26. Piko L: Synthesis of macromolecules in early mouse embryos cultured in vitro: RNA, DNA, and a polysaccharide component. *Dev Biol* **21**:257, 1970.
27. Cascio S, Wassarman PM: Program of early development in the mammal: Synthesis of mitochondrial proteins during oogenesis and early embryogenesis in the mouse. *Dev Biol* **83**:166, 1981.
28. Wallace DC: Mitotic segregation of mitochondrial DNAs in human cell hybrids and expression of chloramphenicol resistance. *Somat Cell Mol Genet* **12**:41, 1986.
29. Moraes CT, Schon EA, DiMauro S, Miranda AF: Heteroplasmy of mitochondrial genomes in clonal cultures from patients with Kearns-Sayre syndrome. *Biochem Biophys Res Commun* **160**:765, 1989.
30. Bowen J, Richards T, Maravilla K: MR imaging and proton MR spectroscopy in A-to-G substitution at nucleotide position 3243 of leucine transfer RNA. *Am J Neuroradiol* **19**:231, 1998.
31. Lindner A, Hofmann E, Naumann M, Becker G, Reichmann H: Clinical, morphological, biochemical, and neuroradiological features of mitochondrial encephalomyopathies. Presentation of 19 patients. *Mol Cell Biochem* **174**:297, 1997.
32. Valanne L, Ketonen L, Majander A, Suomalainen A, Pihko H: Neuroradiologic findings in children with mitochondrial disorders. *Am J Neuroradiol* **19**:369, 1998.
33. Garcia-Silva MT, Ribes A, Campos Y, Garavaglia B, Arenas J: Syndrome of encephalopathy, petechiae, and ethylmalonic aciduria. *Pediatr Neurol* **17**:165, 1997.
34. Ruesch S, Krahenbuhl S, Kleinle S, Liechti-Gallati S, Schaffner T, Wermuth B, Weber J, Wiesmann UN: Combined 3-methylglutaconic and 3-hydroxy-3-methylglutaric aciduria with endocardial fibroelastosis and dilatative cardiomyopathy in male and female siblings with partial deficiency of complex II/III in fibroblasts. *Enzyme Protein* **49**:321, 1996.
35. Gibson KM, Bennett MJ, Mize CE, Jakobs C, Rotig A, Munnich A, Lichter-Konecki U, Trefz FK: 3-Methylglutaconic aciduria associated with Pearson syndrome. *J Pediatr* **121**:940, 1992.
36. Kelly RI, Clark BJ, Morton DH, Sherwood WG: X-linked cardiomyopathy, neutropenia, and increased urinary levels of 3-methylglutaconic and 2-ethylhydracrylic acids. *Am J Hum Genet* **45(Suppl 1)**:A7, 1989.
37. Touati G, Rigal O, Lombes A, Frachon P, Giraud M, Ogier de Baulny H: In vivo functional investigations of lactic acid in patients with respiratory chain disorders. *Arch Dis Child* **76**:16, 1997.
38. Yamamoto M, Nonaka I: Skeletal muscle pathology in chronic progressive external ophthalmoplegia with ragged-red fibers. *Acta Neuropathol* **76**:558, 1988.
39. Shoubridge EA, Karpati G, Hastings KE: Deletion mutants are functionally dominant over wild type mitochondrial genomes in skeletal muscle fiber segments in mitochondrial disease. *Cell* **62**:43, 1990.
40. Parfait B, Percheron A, Chretien D, Rustin P, Munnich A, Rotig A: No mitochondrial cytochrome oxidase (COX) gene mutations in 18 cases of COX deficiency. *Hum Genet* **101**:247, 1997.
41. Adams PL, Lightowlers RN, Turnbull DM: Molecular analysis of cytochrome c oxidase deficiency in Leigh's syndrome. *Ann Neurol* **41**:268, 1997.
42. Yamazaki M, Igarashi H, Hamamoto M, Miyazaki T, Nonaka I: A case of mitochondrial encephalomyopathy with schizophrenic psychosis, dementia and neuroleptic malignant syndrome. *Rinsho Shinkeigaku* **31**:1219, 1991.
43. Mita S, Tokunaga M, Kumamoto T, Uchino M, Nonaka I, Ando M: Mitochondrial DNA mutation and muscle pathology in mitochondrial myopathy, encephalopathy, lactic acidosis, and strokelike episodes. *Muscle Nerve* **3**:S113, 1995.
44. Hasegawa H, Matsuoka T, Goto Y, Nonaka I: Cytochrome c oxidase activity is deficient in blood vessels of patients with myoclonus epilepsy with ragged-red fibers. *Acta Neuropathol (Berl)* **85**:280, 1993.
45. Hasegawa H, Matsuoka T, Goto Y, Nonaka I: Vascular pathology in chronic progressive external ophthalmoplegia with ragged-red fibers. *Rinsho Shinkeigaku* **32**:155, 1992.
46. Chikama M, Himoto Y, Nonaka I: Mitochondrial myopathy, encephalopathy, lactic acidosis, and stroke-like episodes with delayed and decreased cerebral blood flow on cerebral angiography — A case report. *Rinsho Shinkeigaku* **34**:167, 1994.
47. Yamamoto M, Koga Y, Ohtaki E, Nonaka I: Focal cytochrome c oxidase deficiency in various neuromuscular diseases. *J Neurol Sci* **91**:207, 1989.
48. Muller-Hocker J: Cytochrome c oxidase-deficient fibers in the limb muscle and diaphragm of man without muscular disease: An age-related alteration. *J Neurol Sci* **100**:14, 1990.
49. Muller-Hocker J: Cytochrome c oxidase deficient cardiomyocytes in the human heart. An age-related phenomenon. *Am J Pathol* **134**:1167, 1989.

50. Horvath R, Fu K, Johns T, Genge A, Karpati G, Shoubridge EA: Characterization of the mitochondrial DNA abnormalities in the skeletal muscle of patients with inclusion body myositis. *J Neuropathol Exp Neurol* **57**:396, 1998.
51. Moslemi AR, Lindberg C, Oldfors A: Analysis of multiple mitochondrial DNA deletions in inclusion body myositis. *Hum Mutat* **10**:381, 1997.
52. Oldfors A, Larsson NG, Lindberg C, Holme E: Mitochondrial DNA deletions in inclusion body myositis. *Brain* **116**:325, 1993.
53. Oldfors A, Moslemi AR, Fyhr IM, Holme E, Larsson NG, Lindberg C: Mitochondrial DNA deletions in muscle fibers in inclusion body myositis. *J Neuropathol Exp Neurol* **54**:581, 1995.
54. Santorelli FM, Sciacco M, Tanji K, Shanske S, Vu TH, Golzi V, Griggs RC, Mendell JR, Hays AP, Bertorini TE, Pestronk A, Bonilla E, DiMauro S: Multiple mitochondrial DNA deletions in sporadic inclusion body myositis: a study of 56 patients. *Ann Neurol* **39**:789, 1996.
55. Schroder JM, Molnar M: Mitochondrial abnormalities and peripheral neuropathy in inflammatory myopathy, especially inclusion body myositis. *Mol Cell Biochem* **174**:277, 1997.
56. Stadhouders A, Jap P, Walliman TH: Biochemical nature of mitochondrial crystals. *J Neurol Sci* **98(Suppl)**:304, 1990.
57. Reichmann H, Gold R, Meurers B, Naumann M, Seibel P, Walter U, Klopstock T: Progression of myopathology in Kearns-Sayre syndrome: A morphological follow-up study. *Acta Neuropathol (Berl)* **85**:679, 1993.
58. Koo B, Becker LE, Chuang S, Merante F, Robinson BH, MacGregor D, Tein I, Ho VB, McGreal DA, Wherrett JR, et al: Mitochondrial encephalomyopathy, lactic acidosis, stroke-like episodes (MELAS): Clinical, radiological, pathological, and genetic observations. *Ann Neurol* **34**:25, 1993.
59. Walker UA, Schon EA: Neurotrophin-4 is up-regulated in ragged-red fibers associated with pathogenic mitochondrial DNA mutations. *Ann Neurol* **43**:536, 1998.
60. Nishino I, Kobayashi O, Goto Y, Kurihara M, Kumagai K, Fujita T, Hashimoto K, Horai S, Nonaka I: A new congenital muscular dystrophy with mitochondrial structural abnormalities. *Muscle Nerve* **21**:40, 1998.
61. Kalman B, Lublin FD, Alder H: Impairment of central and peripheral myelin in mitochondrial diseases. *Mult Scler* **2**:267, 1997.
62. Rusanen H, Majamaa K, Tolonen U, Remes AM, Myllyla R, Hassinen IE: Demyelinating polyneuropathy in a patient with the tRNA(Leu)(UUR) mutation at base pair 3243 of the mitochondrial DNA [see Comments]. *Neurology* **45**:1188, 1995.
63. Chu CC, Huang CC, Fang W, Chu NS, Pang CY, Wei YH: Peripheral neuropathy in mitochondrial encephalomyopathies. *Eur Neurol* **37**:110, 1997.
64. Fang W: Polyneuropathy in the mtDNA base pair 3243 point mutation. *Neurology* **46**:1494, 1996.
65. Schroder JM: Neuropathy associated with mitochondrial disorders. *Brain Pathol* **3**:177, 1993.
66. Hara H, Wakayama Y, Kouno Y, Yamada H, Tanaka M, Ozawa T: Acute peripheral neuropathy, rhabdomyolysis, and severe lactic acidosis associated with 3243 A to G mitochondrial DNA mutation [Letter]. *J Neurol Neurosurg Psychiatry* **57**:1545, 1994.
67. Chinnery PF, Howell N, Lightowlers RN, Turnbull DM: Molecular pathology of MELAS and MERRF. The relationship between mutation load and clinical phenotypes. *Brain* **120**:1713, 1997.
68. Shoubridge EA, Johns T, Karpati G: Complete restoration of a wild-type mtDNA genotype in regenerating muscle fibres in a patient with a tRNA point mutation and mitochondrial encephalomyopathy. *Hum Mol Genet* **6**:2239, 1997.
69. Barros F, Lareu MV, Salas A, Carracedo A: Rapid and enhanced detection of mitochondrial DNA variation using single-strand conformation analysis of superposed restriction enzyme fragments from polymerase chain reaction-amplified products. *Electrophoresis* **18**:52, 1997.
70. Michikawa Y, Hofhaus G, Lerman LS, Attardi G: Comprehensive, rapid and sensitive detection of sequence variants of human mitochondrial tRNA genes. *Nucleic Acids Res* **25**:2455, 1997.
71. Sternberg D, Danan C, Lombes A, Laforet P, Girodon E, Goossens M, Amselem S: Exhaustive scanning approach to screen all the mitochondrial tRNA genes for mutations and its application to the investigation of 35 independent patients with mitochondrial disorders. *Hum Mol Genet* **7**:33, 1998.
72. Chee M, Yang R, Hubbell E, Berno A, Huang XC, Stern D, Winkler J, Lockhart DJ, Morris MS, Fodor SP: Accessing genetic information with high-density DNA arrays. *Science* **274**:610, 1996.
73. Rowland LP: Molecular genetics, pseudogenetics, and clinical neurology. *Neurology* **33**:1179, 1983.
74. Shoffner JM, Lott MT, Voljavec AS, Soueidan SA, Costigan DA, Wallace DC: Spontaneous Kearns-Sayre/chronic external ophthalmoplegia plus syndrome associated with a mitochondrial DNA deletion: A slip-replication model and metabolic therapy. *Proc Natl Acad Sci U S A* **86**:7952, 1989.
75. Shoffner JM, Wallace DC: Oxidative phosphorylation diseases. Disorders of two genomes. *Adv Hum Genet* **19**:267, 1990.
76. Holt IJ, Miller DH, Harding AE: Genetic heterogeneity and mitochondrial DNA heteroplasmy in Leber's hereditary optic neuropathy. *J Med Genet* **26**:739, 1989.
77. Holt IJ, Harding AE, Morgan-Hughes JA: Deletions of muscle mitochondrial DNA in mitochondrial myopathies: Sequence analysis and possible mechanisms. *Nucleic Acids Res* **17**:4465, 1989.
78. Holt IJ, Harding AE, Cooper JM, Schapira AH, Toscano A, Clark JB, Morgan-Hughes JA: Mitochondrial myopathies: Clinical and biochemical features of 30 patients with major deletions of muscle mitochondrial DNA. *Ann Neurol* **26**:699, 1989.
79. Berenberg RA, Pellock JM, DiMauro S, Schotland DL, Bonilla E, Eastwood A, Hays A, Vicale CT, Behrens M, Chutorian A, Rowland LP: Lumping or splitting? "Ophthalmoplegiaplus" or "Kearns-Sayre syndrome." *Ann Neurol* **1**:37, 1977.
80. Petty RK, Harding AE, Morgan HJA: The clinical features of mitochondrial myopathy. *Brain* **109**:915, 1986.
81. Moraes CT, DiMauro S, Zeviani M, Lombes A, Shanske S, Miranda AF, Nakase H, Bonilla E, Werneck LC, Servidei S, Nonaka I, Koga Y, Spiro AJ, Brownell AKW, Schmidt B, Schotland DL, Zupanc M, DeVivo DC, Schon EA, Rowland LP: Mitochondrial DNA deletions in progressive external ophthalmoplegia and Kearns-Sayre syndrome. *N Engl J Med* **320**:1293, 1989.
82. Zeviani M, Moraes CT, DiMauro S, Nakase H, Bonilla E, Schon EA, Rowland LP: Deletions of mitochondrial DNA in Kearns-Sayre syndrome [see Comments]. *Neurology* **38**:1339, 1988.
83. Zupanc ML, Moraes CT, Shanske S, Langman CB, Ciafaloni E, DiMauro S: Deletion of mitochondrial DNA in patients with combined features of Kearns-Sayre and MELAS syndromes. *Ann Neurol* **29**:680, 1991.
84. Mullie MA, Harding AE, Petty RK, Ikeda H, Morgan HJA, Sanders MD: The retinal manifestations of mitochondrial myopathy. A study of 22 cases. *Arch Ophthalmol* **103**:1825, 1985.
85. Herzberg NH, van Schooneveld MJ, Bleeker Wagemakers EM, Zwart R, Cremers FP, van der Knaap MS, Bolhuis PA, de Visser M: Kearns-Sayre syndrome with a phenocopy of choroideremia instead of pigmentary retinopathy. *Neurology* **43**:218, 1993.
86. Sorkin JA, Shoffner JM, Grossniklaus HE, Drack AV, Lambert SR: Strabismus and mitochondrial defects in chronic progressive external ophthalmoplegia. *Am J Ophthalmol* **123**:235, 1997.
87. Poulton J, Deadman ME, Gardiner RM: Tandem direct duplications of mitochondrial DNA in mitochondrial myopathy: Analysis of nucleotide sequence and tissue distribution. *Nucleic Acids Res* **17**:10223, 1989.
88. Poulton J, Deadman ME, Gardiner RM: Duplications of mitochondrial DNA in mitochondrial myopathy. *Lancet* **1**:236, 1989.
89. Poulton J, Deadman ME, Bindoff L, Morten K, Land J, Brown G: Families of mtDNA re-arrangements can be detected in patients with mtDNA deletions: Duplications may be a transient intermediate form. *Hum Mol Genet* **2**:23, 1993.
90. Larsson NG, Holme E, Kristiansson B, Oldfors A, Tulinius M: Progressive increase in the mutated mitochondrial DNA fraction in Kearns-Sayre syndrome. *Pediatr Res* **28**:131, 1990.
91. Wallace DC, Lott MT, Torroni A, Brown MD: Report of the committee on human mitochondrial DNA. *Cytogenet Cell Genet* **59**:727, 1992.
92. Obermaier-Kusser B, Muller-Hocker J, Nelson I, Lestienne P, Enter C, Riedele T, Gerbitz KD: Different copy numbers of apparently identically deleted mitochondrial DNA in tissues from a patient with Kearns-Sayre syndrome detected by PCR. *Biochem Biophys Res Commun* **169**:1007, 1990.
93. Marzuki S, Berkovic SF, Saifuddin Noer A, Kapsa RM, Kalnins RM, Byrne E, Sasmono T, Sudoyo H: Developmental genetics of deleted mtDNA in mitochondrial oculomyopathy. *J Neurol Sci* **145**:155, 1997.
94. Rotig A, Bessis JL, Romero N, Cormier V, Saudubray JM, Narcy P, Lenoir G, Rustin P, Munnich A: Maternally inherited duplication of the mitochondrial genome in a syndrome of proximal tubulopathy, diabetes mellitus, and cerebellar ataxia. *Am J Hum Genet* **50**:364, 1992.

95. Wallace DC: Mitochondrial genes and neuromuscular disease, in McHugh PR, McKusick VA (eds): *Genes, Brain, and Behavior*, Research Publications: Association for Research in Nervous and Mental Disease, Volume 69. New York, Raven Press, 1991, p 101.
96. Moraes CT, Andreetta F, Bonilla E, Shanske S, DiMauro S, Schon EA: Replication-competent human mitochondrial DNA lacking the heavy-strand promoter region. *Mol Cell Biol* **11**:1631, 1991.
97. Johns DR, Cornblath DR: Molecular insight into the asymmetric distribution of pathogenetic human mitochondrial DNA deletions. *Biochem Biophys Res Commun* **174**:244, 1991.
98. Degoul F, Nelson I, Lestienne P, Francois D, Romero N, Duboc D, Eymard B, Fardeau M, Ponsot G, Paturneau-Jouas M, et al.: Deletions of mitochondrial DNA in Kearns-Sayre syndrome and ocular myopathies: Genetic, biochemical, and morphologic studies. *J Neurol Sci* **101**:168, 1991.
99. Degoul F, Nelson I, Amselem S, Romero N, Obermaier-Kusser B, Ponsot G, Marsac C, Lestienne P: Different mechanisms inferred from sequences of human mitochondrial DNA deletions in ocular myopathies. *Nucleic Acids Res* **19**:493, 1991.
100. Schon EA, Rizzuto R, Moraes CT, Nakase H, Zeviani M, DiMauro S: A direct repeat is a hotspot for large-scale deletion of human mitochondrial DNA. *Science* **244**:346, 1989.
101. Hammans SR, Sweeney MG, Holt IJ, Cooper JM, Toscano A, Clark JB, Morgan-Hughes JA, Harding AE: Evidence for intramitochondrial complementation between deleted and. *J Neurol Sci* **107**:87, 1992.
102. Mita S, Schmidt B, Schon EA, DiMauro S, Bonilla E: Detection of "deleted" mitochondrial genomes in cytochrome c oxidase-deficient muscle fibers of a patient with Kearns-Sayre syndrome. *Proc Natl Acad Sci U S A* **86**:9509, 1989.
103. Nakase H, Moraes CT, Rizzuto R, Lombes A, DiMauro S, Schon EA: Transcription and translation of deleted mitochondrial genomes in Kearns-Sayre syndrome: Implications for pathogenesis. *Am J Hum Genet* **46**:418, 1990.
104. Ciafaloni E, Ricci E, Shanske S, Moraes CT, Silvestri G, Hirano M, Simonetti S, Angelini C, Donati MA, Garcia C, et al: MELAS: Clinical features, biochemistry, and molecular genetics. *Ann Neurol* **31**:391, 1992.
105. Goto Y, Nonaka I, Horai S: A new mutation in the tRNA-Leu(UUR) gene associated with mitochondrial myopathy, lactic acidosis, and stroke-like episodes. *Biochim Biophys Acta* **1097**:238, 1991.
106. Hammans SR, Harding AE: Mitochondrial disease and mitochondrial DNA. *Br J Hosp Med* **46**:20, 1991.
107. Hammans SR, Sweeney MG, Brockington M, Morgan-Hughes JA, Harding AE: Mitochondrial encephalopathies: Molecular genetic diagnosis from blood samples. *Lancet* **337**:1311, 1991.
108. Goto Y, Horai S, Matsuoka T, Koga Y, Nihei K, Kobayashi M, Nonaka I: Mitochondrial myopathy, encephalopathy, lactic acidosis, and stroke-like episodes (MELAS): A correlative study of the clinical features and the mitochondrial DNA mutation. *Neurology* **42**:545, 1992.
109. Pearson HA, Lobel JS, Kocoshis SA, Naiman JL, Windmiller J, Lammi AT, Hoffman R, Marsh JC: A new syndrome of refractory sideroblastic anemia with vacuolization of marrow precursors and exocrine pancreatic function. *J Pediatr* **95**:976, 1979.
110. Rotig A, Cormier V, Koll F, Mize CE, Saudubray JM, Veerman A, Pearson HA, Munnich A: Site-specific deletions of the mitochondrial genome in the Pearson marrow-pancreas syndrome. *Genomics* **10**:502, 1991.
111. Rotig A, Colonna M, Bonnefont JP, Blanche S, Fischer A, Saudubray JM, Munnich A: Mitochondrial DNA deletion in Pearson's marrow/pancreas syndrome. *Lancet* **1**:902, 1989.
112. Rotig A, Colonna M, Blanche S, Fischer A, Le Deist F, Frezal J, Saudubray JM, Munnich A: Deletion of blood mitochondrial DNA in pancytopenia [Letter]. *Lancet* **2**:567, 1988.
113. Rotig A, Cormier V, Blanche S, Bonnefont JP, Ledeist F, Romero N, Schmitz J, Rustin P, Fischer A, Saudubray JM, et al.: Pearson's marrow-pancreas syndrome. A multisystem mitochondrial disorder in infancy. *J Clin Invest* **86**:1601, 1990.
114. Cormier V, Rotig A, Bonnefont JP, Mechinand F, Berthou C, Goulet O, Schmitz J, Blanche S, Vassaut A, Maier M: Pearson's syndrome. Pancytopenia with exocrine pancreatic insufficiency: new mitochondrial disease in the first year of childhood. *Arch Fr Pediatr* **48**:171, 1991.
115. Blaw ME, Mize CE: Juvenile Pearson syndrome. *J Child Neurol* **5**:187, 1990.
116. Lombes A, Mendell JR, Nakase H, Barohn RJ, Bonilla E, Zeviani M, Yates AJ, Omerza J, Gales TL, Nakahara K, et al.: Myoclonic epilepsy and ragged-red fibers with cytochrome oxidase deficiency. *Ann Neurol* **26**:20, 1989.
117. Wallace DC, Zheng XX, Lott MT, Shoffner JM, Hodge JA, Kelley RI, Epstein CM, Hopkins LC: Familial mitochondrial encephalomyopathy (MERRF): Genetic, pathophysiological, and biochemical characterization of a mitochondrial DNA disease. *Cell* **55**:601, 1988.
118. Rosing HS, Hopkins LC, Wallace DC, Epstein CM, Weidenheim K: Maternally inherited mitochondrial myopathy and myoclonic epilepsy. *Ann Neurol* **17**:228, 1985.
119. Fukuhara N: MERRF: A clinicopathological study. Relationships between myoclonus epilepsies and mitochondrial myopathies. *Rev Neurol (Paris)* **147**:476, 1991.
120. Morgan-Hughes JA, Hayes DJ, Clark JB, Landon DN, Swash M, Stark RJ, Rudge P: Mitochondrial encephalomyopathies: Biochemical studies in two cases revealing defects in the respiratory chain. *Brain* **105**:553, 1982.
121. Holliday PL, Climie AR, Gilroy J, Mahmud MZ: Mitochondrial myopathy and encephalopathy: Three cases—A deficiency of NADH-CoQ dehydrogenase? *Neurology* **33**:1619, 1983.
122. Berkovic SF, Carpenter S, Evans A, Karpati G, Shoubridge EA, Andermann F, Meyer E, Tyler JL, Diksic M, Arnold D, S. WL, Andermann E, Hakim AM: Myoclonus epilepsy and ragged-red fibres (MERRF). I. A clinical, pathological, biochemical, magnetic resonance spectrographic and positron emission tomographic study. *Brain* **112**:1231, 1989.
123. Berkovic SF, Andermann F, Karpati G, Carpenter S, Andermann E, Shoubridge E: Mitochondrial encephalomyopathies: A solution to the enigma of the Ramsay-Hunt syndrome. *Neurology* **37(Suppl 1)**:125, 1987.
124. Byrne E, Dennett X, Trounce I, Burdon J: Mitochondrial myoneuropathy with respiratory failure and myoclonic epilepsy. A case report with biochemical studies. *J Neurol Sci* **71**:273, 1985.
125. Fitzsimons RB, Clifton-Bligh P, Wolfenden WH: Mitochondrial myopathy and lactic acidaemia with myoclonic epilepsy, ataxia, and hypothalamic infertility: A variant of Ramsay-Hunt syndrome. *J Neurol Neurosurg Psychiatry* **44**:79, 1981.
126. Feit H, Kirkpatrick J, Van Woert MH, Pandian G: Myoclonus, ataxia, and hypoventilation: Response to l-5-hydroxytryptophan. *Neurology* **33**:109, 1983.
127. Fukuhara N, Tokiguchi S, Shirakawa K, Tsubaki T: Myoclonus epilepsy associated with ragged-red fibers (mitochondrial abnormalities): Disease entity or a syndrome? Light- and electron-microscopic studies of two cases and review of the literature. *J Neurol Sci* **47**:117, 1980.
128. Ogasahara S, Engel AG, Frens D, Mack D: Muscle coenzyme Q deficiency in familial mitochondrial encephalomyopathy. *Proc Natl Acad Sci U S A* **86**:2379, 1989.
129. Berkovic SF, Andermann E, Caarpenter S, Karpati G, Andermann F, Arnold D, Shoubridge E: Mitochondrial encephalomyopathies: Evidence for maternal transmission. *Am J Hum Genet* **41**:A47, 1987.
130. Berkovic SF, Carpenter S, Karpati G, Andermann F, Andermann E, Shoubridge E, Arnold D: Cytochrome c oxidase deficiency: A remarkable spectrum of clinical and neuropathological findings in a single family. *Neurology* **37(Suppl 1)**:223, 1987.
131. Takeda S, Wakabayashi K, Ohama E, Ikuta F: Neuropathology of myoclonus epilepsy associated with ragged-red fibers (Fukuhara's disease). *Acta Neuropathol (Berl)* **75**:433, 1988.
132. Eleff SM, Barker PB, Blackband SJ, Chatham JC, Lutz NW, Johns DR, Bryan RN, Hurko O: Phosphorus magnetic resonance spectroscopy of patients with mitochondrial cytopathies demonstrates decreased levels of brain phosphocreatine. *Ann Neurol* **27**:626, 1990.
133. Pavlakis SG, Phillips PC, DiMauro S, De Vivo DC, Rowland LP: Mitochondrial myopathy, encephalopathy, lactic acidosis, and stroke-like episodes: A distinctive clinical syndrome. *Ann Neurol* **16**:481, 1984.
134. Shapira Y, Cererbaum SD, Cancilla PA, Nielsen D, Lippe BM: Familial poliodystrophy, mitochondrial myopathy, and lactate acidemia. *Neurology* **25**:614, 1975.
135. Kuriyama M, Umezaki H, Fukuda Y, Osame M, Koike K, Tateishi J, Igata A: Mitochondrial encephalomyopathy with lactate-pyruvate elevation and brain infarctions. *Neurology* **34**:72, 1984.
136. Kuriyama M, Igata A: Mitochondrial encephalopathy, lactic acidosis, and stroke-like syndrome (MELAS). *Ann Neurol* **18**:625, 1985.

137. Mukoyama M, Kazui H, Sunohara N, Yoshida M, Nonaka I, Satoyoshi E: Mitochondrial myopathy, encephalopathy, lactic acidosis, and stroke-like episodes with acanthocytosis. *J Neurol* **233**:228, 1986.
138. Fukuhara N: Stroke-like episodes in MERRF. *Ann Neurol* **18**:368, 1985.
139. Lach B, Preston D, Servidei S, Embree G, DiMauro S, Swierenga S: Maternally inherited mitochondrial encephalomyopathy, a vasculopathy. *Muscle Nerve* **9(5S)**:180, 1986.
140. Byrne E, Trounce I, Dennett X, Gilligan B, Morley JB, Marzuki S: Progression from MERRF to MELAS phenotype in a patient with combined respiratory complex I and IV deficiencies. *J Neurol Sci* **88**:327, 1988.
141. Danks RA, Dorevitch M, Cummins JT, Byrne E: Mitochondrial myopathy, encephalopathy, lactic acidosis and stroke-like episodes (MELAS): Adolescent onset with severe cerebral edema. *Aust N Z J Med* **18**:69, 1988.
142. Sasaki H, Kuzuhara S, Kanazawa I, Nakanishi T, Ogata T: Myoclonus, cerebellar disorder, neuropathy, mitochondrial myopathy, and ACTH deficiency. *Neurology* **33**:1288, 1983.
143. Nakano T, Sakai H, Amano N, Yagishita S, Ito Y: An autopsy case of degenerative type myoclonus epilepsy associated with Friedreich's ataxia and mitochondrial myopathy. *Brain Nerve* **34**:321, 1982.
144. Fukuhara N: Myoclonus epilepsy and mitochondrial myopathy, in Scarlato G, Cerri C (eds): *Mitochondrial Pathology in Muscle Diseases*. Padua, Piccin Medical Books, 1983, p 88.
145. Berkovic SF, Shoubridge EA, Andermann F, Andermann E, Carpenter S, Karpati G: Clinical spectrum of mitochondrial DNA mutation at base pair 8344. *Lancet* **338**:457, 1991.
146. Zeviani M, Amati P, Bresolin N, Antozzi C, Piccolo G, Toscano A, DiDonato S: Rapid detection of the A to G (8344) mutation of mtDNA in Italian families with myoclonus epilepsy and ragged-red fibers (MERRF). *Am J Hum Genet* **48**:203, 1991.
147. Shoffner JM, Lott MT, Lezza AM, Seibel P, Ballinger SW, Wallace DC: Myoclonic epilepsy and ragged-red fiber disease (MERRF) is associated with a mitochondrial DNA tRNA(Lys) mutation. *Cell* **61**:931, 1990.
148. Tanno Y, Yoneda M, Nonaka I, Tanaka K, Miyatake T, Tsuji S: Quantitation of mitochondrial DNA carrying tRNALys mutation in MERRF patients. *Biochem Biophys Res Commun* **179**:880, 1991.
149. Seibel P, Degoul F, Romero N, Marsac C, Kadenbach B: Identification of point mutations by mispairing PCR as exemplified in MERRF disease. *Biochem Biophys Res Commun* **173**:561, 1990.
150. Seibel P, Degoul F, Bonne G, Romero N, Francois D, Paturneau-Jouas M, Ziegler F, Eymard B, Fardeau M, Marsac C, et al.: Genetic biochemical and pathophysiological characterization of a familial mitochondrial encephalomyopathy (MERRF). *J Neurol Sci* **105**:217, 1991.
151. Noer AS, Sudoyo H, Lertrit P, Thyagarajan D, Utthanaphol P, Kapsa R, Byrne E, Marzuki S: A tRNA(Lys) mutation in the mtDNA is the causal genetic lesion underlying myoclonic epilepsy and ragged-red fiber (MERRF) syndrome. *Am J Hum Genet* **49**:715, 1991.
152. Silvestri G, Moraes CT, Shanske S, Oh SJ, DiMauro S: A new mutation in the tRNA-Lys gene associated with myoclonic epilepsy and ragged-red fibers (MERRF). *Am J Hum Genet* **51**:1213, 1992.
153. Zeviani M, Muntoni F, Savarese N, Serra G, Tiranti V, Carrara F, Mariotti C, DiDonato S: A MERRF/MELAS overlap syndrome associated with a new point mutation in the mitochondrial DNA tRNA(Lys) gene [published erratum appears in *Eur J Hum Genet* 1(2):124, 1993]. *Eur J Hum Genet* **1**:80, 1993.
154. Rich A, RajBhandary UL: Transfer RNA: Molecular structure, sequence, and properties. *Ann Rev Biochem* **45**:805, 1976.
155. Boulet L, Karpati G, Shoubridge E: Distribution and threshold expression of the tRNA-Lys mutation in skeletal muscle of patients with myoclonic epilepsy and ragged-red fibers (MERRF). *Am J Hum Genet* **51**:1187, 1992.
156. Chomyn A, Meola G, Bresolin N, Lai ST, Scarlato G, Attardi G: In vitro genetic transfer of protein synthesis and respiration defects to mitochondrial DNA-less cells with myopathy-patient mitochondria. *Mol Cell Biol* **11**:2236, 1991.
157. Riggs JE, Schochet SSJ, Fakadej AV, Papadimitriou A, DiMauro S, Crosby TW, Gutmann L, Moxley RT: Mitochondrial encephalomyopathy with decreased succinate-cytochrome c reductase activity. *Neurology* **34**:48, 1984.
158. Lombes A, Mendell JR, Nakase H, Barohn RJ, Bonilla E, Zeviani M, Yates AJ, Omerza J, Gales TL, Nakahara K, Rizzuto R, Engel WK, DiMauro S: Myoclonic epilepsy and ragged-red fibers with cytochrome oxidase deficiency: neuropathology, biochemistry, and molecular genetics. *Ann Neurol* **26**:20, 1989.
159. Berkovic SF, Andermann F, Shoubridge EA, Carpenter S, Robitaille Y, Andermann E, Melmed C, Karpati G: Mitochondrial dysfunction in multiple symmetrical lipomatosis. *Ann Neurol* **29**:566, 1991.
160. Calabresi PA, Silvestri G, DiMauro S, Griggs RC: Ekbom's syndrome: Lipomas, ataxia, and neuropathy with MERRF. *Muscle Nerve* **17**:943, 1994.
161. Holme E, Larsson NG, Oldfors A, Tulinius M, Sahlin P, Stenman G: Multiple symmetric lipomas with high levels of mtDNA with the tRNA(Lys) A → G(8344) mutation as the only manifestation of disease in a carrier of myoclonus epilepsy and ragged-red fibers (MERRF) syndrome. *Am J Hum Genet* **52**:551, 1993.
162. Traff J, Holme E, Ekbom K, Nilsson BY: Ekbom's syndrome of photomyoclonus, cerebellar ataxia and cervical lipoma is associated with the tRNA(Lys) A8344G mutation in mitochondrial DNA. *Acta Neurol Scand* **92**:394, 1995.
163. Larsson NG, Tulinius MH, Holme E, Oldfors A: Pathogenetic aspects of the A8344G mutation of mitochondrial DNA associated with MERRF syndrome and multiple symmetric lipomas. *Muscle Nerve* **3**:S102, 1995.
164. Naumann M, Kiefer R, Toyka KV, Sommer C, Seibel P, Reichmann H: Mitochondrial dysfunction with myoclonus epilepsy and ragged-red fibers point mutation in nerve, muscle, and adipose tissue of a patient with multiple symmetric lipomatosis. *Muscle Nerve* **20**:833, 1997.
165. Silvestri G, Ciafaloni E, Santorelli FM, Shanske S, Servidei S, Graf WD, Sumi M, DiMauro S: Clinical features associated with the A → G transition at nucleotide 8344 of mtDNA ("MERRF mutation"). *Neurology* **43**:1200, 1993.
166. Klopstock T, Naumann M, Schalke B, Bischof F, Seibel P, Kottlors M, Eckert P, Reiners K, Toyka KV, Reichmann H: Multiple symmetric lipomatosis: Abnormalities in complex IV and multiple deletions in mitochondrial DNA. *Neurology* **44**:862, 1994.
167. Klopstock T, Naumann M, Seibel P, Shalke B, Reiners K, Reichmann H: Mitochondrial DNA mutations in multiple symmetric lipomatosis. *Mol Cell Biochem* **174**:271, 1997.
168. Campos Y, Martin MA, Navarro C, Gordo P, Arenas J: Single large-scale mitochondrial DNA deletion in a patient with mitochondrial myopathy associated with multiple symmetric lipomatosis. *Neurology* **47**:1012, 1996.
169. Fabrizi GM, Cardaioli E, Grieco GS, Cavallaro T, Malandrini A, Manneschi L, Dotti MT, Federico A, Guazzi G: The A to G transition at nt 3243 of the mitochondrial tRNALeu(UUR) may cause an MERRF syndrome. *J Neurol Neurosurg Psychiatry* **61**:47, 1996.
170. Matthews PM, Squier MV, Chalk C, Donaghy M: Mitochondrial abnormalities are not invariably present in neurologic syndromes associated with multiple symmetric lipomatosis. *Neurology* **45**:197, 1995.
171. Larsson N-G, Tulinius MH, Holme E, Oldfors A, Anderson O, Wahlstrom J, Aasly J: Segregation and manifestations of the mtDNA tRNA-lys A to G (8344) mutation of myoclonus epilepsy and ragged-red fibers (MERRF) syndrome. *Am J Hum Genet* **51**:1201, 1992.
172. Goldring ES, Grossman LI, Krupnick D, Cryer DR, Marmur J: The petite mutation in yeast. Loss of mitochondrial deoxyribonucleic acid during induction of petites with ethidium bromide. *J Mol Biol* **52**:323, 1970.
173. Desjardins P, Frost E, Morais R: Ethidium bromide-induced loss of mitochondrial DNA from primary chicken embryo fibroblasts. *Mol Cell Biol* **5**:1163, 1985.
174. Desjardins P, de Muys JM, Morais R: An established avian fibroblast cell line without mitochondrial DNA. *Somat Cell Mol Genet* **12**:133, 1986.
175. King ME, Godman GC, King DW: Respiratory enzymes and mitochondrial morphology of HeLa and L cells treated with chloramphenicol and ethidium bromide. *J Cell Biol* **53**:127, 1972.
176. Morais R, Gregoire M, Jeannotte L, Gravel D: Chick embryo cells rendered respiration-deficient by chloramphenicol and ethidium bromide are auxotrophic for pyrimidines. *Biochem Biophys Res Commun* **94**:71, 1980.
177. Nass MM: Differential effects of ethidium bromide on mitochondrial and nuclear DNA synthesis in vivo in cultured mammalian cells. *Exp Cell Res* **72**:211, 1972.
178. Wiseman A, Attardi G: Reversible tenfold reduction in mitochondria DNA content of human cells treated with ethidium bromide. *Mol Gen Genet* **167**:51, 1978.

179. Slonimski PP, Perrodin G, Croft JH: Ethidium bromide induced mutation of yeast mitochondria: Complete transformation of cells into respiratory deficient non-chromosomal "petites." *Biochem Biophys Res Commun* **30**:232, 1968.
180. Nagley P, Linnane AW: Mitochondrial DNA deficient petite mutants of yeast. *Biochem Biophys Res Commun* **39**:989, 1970.
181. King MP, Attardi G: Human cells lacking mtDNA: Repopulation with exogenous mitochondria by complementation. *Science* **246**:500, 1989.
182. Gregoire M, Morais R, Quilliam MA, Gravel D: On auxotrophy for pyrimidines of respiration-deficient chick embryo cells. *Eur J Biochem* **142**:49, 1984.
183. Chen JJ, Jones ME: The cellular location of dihydroorotate dehydrogenase: Relation to de novo biosynthesis of pyrimidines. *Arch Biochem Biophys* **176**:82, 1976.
184. King MP, Attardi G: Injection of mitochondria into human cells leads to a rapid replacement of the endogenous mitochondrial DNA. *Cell* **52**:811, 1988.
185. Muller-Hocker J, Schneiderbanger K, Stefani FH, Kadenbach B: Progressive loss of cytochrome c oxidase in the human extraocular muscles in ageing-a cytochemical-immunohistochemical study. *Mutat Res* **275**:115, 1992.
186. Trounce I, Byrne E, Marzuki S: Decline in skeletal muscle mitochondrial respiratory chain function: Possible factor in ageing. *Lancet* **1**:637, 1989.
187. Yen TC, Su JH, King KL, Wei YH: Ageing-associated 5-kb deletion in human liver mitochondrial DNA. *Biochem Biophys Res Commun* **178**:124, 1991.
188. Corral-Debrinski M, Stepien G, Shoffner JM, Lott MT, Kanter K, Wallace DC: Hypoxemia is associated with mitochondrial DNA damage and gene induction. Implications for cardiac disease. *JAMA* **266**:1812, 1991.
189. Corral-Debrinski M, Shoffner JM, Lott MT, Wallace DC: Association of mitochondrial DNA damage with aging and coronary atherosclerotic heart disease. *Mutat Res* **275**:169, 1992.
190. Corral-Debrinski M, Horton T, Lott MT, Shoffner JM, Beal MF, Wallace DC: Mitochondrial DNA deletions in human brain: Regional variability and increase with advanced age. *Nat Genet* **2**:324, 1992.
191. Cortopassi GA, Arnheim N: Detection of a specific mitochondrial deletion in tissues of older individuals. *Nucleic Acids Res* **18**:6927, 1990.
192. Hattori K, Tanaka M, Sugiyama S, Obayashi T, Ito T, Satake T, Hanaki Y, Asai J, Nagano M, Ozawa T: Age-dependent increase in deleted mitochondrial DNA in the human. *Am Heart J* **121**:1735, 1991.
193. Webster KA, Gunning P, Hardeman E, Wallace DC, Kedes L: Coordinate reciprocal trends in glycolytic and mitochondrial transcript accumulations during the in vitro differentiation of human myoblasts. *J Cell Physiol* **142**:566, 1990.
194. Stepien G, Torroni A, Chung AB, Hodge JA, Wallace DC: Differential expression of adenine nucleotide translocator isoforms in mammalian tissues and during muscle cell differentiation. *J Biol Chem* **267**:14592, 1992.
195. Enter C, Muller HJ, Zierz S, Kurlemann G, Pongratz D, Forster C, Obermaier KB, Gerbitz KD: A specific point mutation in the mitochondrial genome of Caucasians with MELAS. *Hum Genet* **88**:233, 1991.
196. Goto Y, Nonaka I, Horai S: A mutation in the tRNA(Leu)(UUR) gene associated with the MELAS subgroup of mitochondrial encephalomyopathies. *Nature* **348**:651, 1990.
197. Goto Y, Horai S, Matsuoka T, Koga Y, Nihei K, Kobayashi M, Nonaka I: Mitochondrial myopathy, encephalopathy, lactic acidosis, and stroke-like episodes (MELAS). *Neurology* **42**:545, 1992.
198. Kobayashi Y, Momoi MY, Tominaga K, Momoi T, Nihei K, Yanagisawa M, Kagawa Y, Ohta S: A point mutation in the mitochondrial tRNA(Leu)(UUR) gene in MELAS (mitochondrial myopathy, encephalopathy, lactic acidosis and stroke-like episodes). *Biochem Biophys Res Commun* **173**:816, 1990.
199. Inui K, Tsukamoto H, Fukushima H, Taniike M, Tanaka J, Nishigaki T, Okada S: Detection of the A to G(3243) mutation of mitochondrial DNA in Japanese families with mitochondrial encephalomyopathies. *J Inherit Metab Dis* **15**:311, 1992.
200. Obermaier KB, Paetzke BI, Enter C, Muller HJ, Zierz S, Ruitenbeek W, Gerbitz KD: Respiratory chain activity in tissues from patients (MELAS) with a point mutation of the mitochondrial genome [tRNA(Leu(UUR))]. *FEBS Lett* **286**:67, 1991.
201. Moraes CT, Ricci E, Bonilla E, DiMauro S, Schon EA: The mitochondrial tRNA(Leu(UUR)) mutation in mitochondrial. *Am J Hum Genet* **50**:934, 1992.
202. Tokunaga M, Mita S, Sakuta R, Nonaka I, Araki S: Increased mitochondrial DNA in blood vessels and ragged-red fibers in mitochondrial myopathy, encephalopathy, lactic acidosis, and stroke-like episodes (MELAS). *Ann Neurol* **33**:275, 1993.
203. DeQuick M, Lammens M, Dom R, Carton H: MELAS: A family with paternal inheritance. *Ann Neurol* **29**:456, 1991.
204. Majamaa K, Moilanen JS, Uimonen S, Remes AM, Salmela PI, Karppa M, Majamaa-Voltti KA, Rusanen H, Sorri M, Peuhkurinen KJ, Hassinen IE: Epidemiology of A3243G, the mutation for mitochondrial encephalomyopathy, lactic acidosis, and strokelike episodes: Prevalence of the mutation in an adult population. *Am J Hum Genet* **63**:447, 1998.
205. Matthews PM, Tampieri D, Berkovic SF, Andermann F, Silver K, Chityat D, Arnold DL: Magnetic resonance imaging shows specific abnormalities in the MELAS syndrome. *Neurology* **41**:1043, 1991.
206. Hasuo K, Tamura S, Yasumori K, Uchino A, Goda S, Ishimoto S, Kamikaseda K, Wakuta Y, Kishi M, Masuda K: Computed tomography and angiography in MELAS (mitochondrial myopathy, encephalopathy, lactic acidosis and stroke-like episodes): Report of 3 cases. *Neuroradiology* **29**:393, 1987.
207. Yamamoto T, Beppu H, Tsubaki T: Mitochondrial encephalomyopathy: Fluctuating symptoms and CT. *Neurology* **34**:1456, 1984.
208. Hart AH, Chang CH, Perrin EUD, Neerunjun JS, Ayyar R: Familial poliodystrophy, mitochondrial myopathy, and lactate acidemia. *Arch Neurol* **34**:180, 1977.
209. Abe K, Inui T, Hirono N, Mezaki T, Kobayashi Y, Kameyama M: Fluctuating MR images with mitochondrial encephalopathy, lactic acidosis, stroke-like syndrome (MELAS). *Neuroradiology* **32**:77, 1990.
210. Rosen L, Phillips S, Enzmann D: Magnetic resonance imaging in MELAS syndrome. *Neuroradiology* **32**:168, 1990.
211. Di Trapani G, Gregori B, Servidei S, Ricci E, Sabatelli M, Tonali P: Mitochondrial encephalopathy, lactic acidosis, and stroke-like episodes (MELAS). *Clin Neuropathol* **16**:195, 1997.
212. Allard JC, Tilak S, Carter AP: CT and MR of MELAS syndrome. *Am J Neuroradiol* **9**:1234, 1988.
213. Fujii T, Okuno T, Ito M, Mutoh K, Horiguchi Y, Tashiro H, Mikawa H: MELAS of infantile onset: Mitochondrial angiopathy or cytopathy? *J Neurol Sci* **103**:37, 1991.
214. Sakuta R, Nonaka I: Vascular involvement in mitochondrial myopathy. *Ann Neurol* **25**:594, 1989.
215. Hasegawa H, Matsuoka T, Goto Y, Nonaka I: Strongly succinate dehydrogenase-reactive blood vessels in muscles from patients with mitochondrial myopathy, encephalopathy, lactic acidosis, and stroke-like episodes. *Ann Neurol* **29**:601, 1991.
216. Kobayashi Y, Miyabayashi S, Takada G, Narisawa K, Tada K, Yamamoto TY: Ultrastructural study of the childhood mitochondrial myopathic syndrome associated with lactic acidosis. *Eur J Pediatr* **139**:25, 1982.
217. Ohama E, Ohara S, Ikuta F, Tanaka K, Nishizawa M, Miyatake T: Mitochondrial angiopathy in cerebral blood vessels of mitochondrial encephalomyopathy. *Acta Neuropathol (Berl)* **74**:226, 1987.
218. Horiguchi Y, Fujii T, Imamura S: Purpuric cutaneous manifestations in mitochondrial encephalomyopathy. *J Dermatol* **18**:295, 1991.
219. Rubanyi GM, Vanhoutte PM: Oxygen-derived free radicals, endothelium, and responsiveness of vascular smooth muscle. *Am J Physiol* **250**:H822, 1986.
220. Suzuki T, Koizumi J, Shiraishi H, Ishikawa N, Ofuku K, Sasaki M, Hori T, Ohkoshi N, Anno I: Mitochondrial encephalomyopathy (MELAS) with mental disorder. CT, MRI and SPECT findings. *Neuroradiology* **32**:74, 1990.
221. Grunwald F, Zierz S, Broich K, Schumacher S, Bockisch A, Biersack HJ: HMPAO-SPECT imaging resembling Alzheimer-type dementia in mitochondrial encephalomyopathy with lactic acidosis and stroke-like episodes (MELAS). *J Nucl Med* **31**:1740, 1990.
222. Satoh M, Ishikawa N, Yoshizawa T, Takeda T, Akisada M: *N*-isopropyl-*p*-[^{123}I]iodoamphetamine SPECT in MELAS syndrome: Comparison with CT and MR imaging. *J Comput Assist Tomogr* **15**:77, 1991.
223. Morita K, Ono S, Fukunaga M, Yasuda T, Higashi Y, Terao A, Morita R: Increased accumulation of *N*-isopropyl-*p*-(^{123}I)-iodoamphetamine in two cases with mitochondrial encephalomyopathy with lactic acidosis and stroke-like episodes (MELAS). *Neuroradiology* **31**:358, 1989.

224. Suzuki Y, Hata T, Miyaoka H, Atsumi Y, Kadowaki H, Taniyama M, Kadowaki T, Odawara M, Tanaka Y, Asahina T, Matsuoka K: Diabetes with the 3243 mitochondrial tRNALeu(UUR) mutation. Characteristic neuroimaging findings. *Diabetes Care* **19**:739, 1996.
225. Watahiki Y, Tomiyama M, Nagata K, Shishido F, Kobayashi Y, Komatsu K, Goto A, Takada G: Positron emission tomographic study in patients with MELAS. *No To Hattatsu* **20**:404, 1988.
226. Fujii T, Okuno T, Ito M, Motoh K, Hamazaki S, Okada S, Kusaka H, Mikawa H: CT, MRI, and autopsy findings in brain of a patient with MELAS. *Pediatr Neurol* **6**:253, 1990.
227. Mizukami K, Sasaki M, Suzuki T, Shiraishi H, Koizumi J, Ohkoshi N, Ogata T, Mori N, Ban S, Kosaka K: Central nervous system changes in mitochondrial encephalomyopathy: Light and electron microscopic study. *Acta Neuropathol (Berl)* **83**:449, 1992.
228. Bogousslavsky J, Perentes E, Deruaz JP, Regli F: Mitochondrial myopathy and cardiomyopathy with neurodegenerative features and multiple brain infarcts. *J Neurol Sci* **55**:351, 1982.
229. Tamagawa Y, Tanaka H, Hagiwara H, Ishida T, Kitamura K: Audiologic evaluation in a family showing diabetes mellitus and deafness associated with a mutation in mitochondrial DNA. *Nippon Jibiinkoka Gakkai Kaiho* **98**:1257, 1995.
230. Tamagawa Y, Kitamura K, Hagiwara H, Ishida T, Nishizawa M, Saito T, Iwamoto Y: Audiologic findings in patients with a point mutation at nucleotide 3,243 of mitochondrial DNA. *Ann Otol Rhinol Laryngol* **106**:338, 1997.
231. Sawada S, Takeda T, Kakigi A, Saito H, Suehiro T, Nakauchi Y, Chikamori K: Audiological findings of sensorineural deafness associated with a mutation in the mitochondrial DNA. *Am J Otol* **18**:332, 1997.
232. Sue CM, Lipsett LJ, Crimmins DS, Tsang CS, Boyages SC, Presgrave CM, Gibson WP, Byrne E, Morris JG: Cochlear origin of hearing loss in MELAS syndrome. *Ann Neurol* **43**:350, 1997.
233. Yamaguchi T, Himi T, Harabuchi Y, Hamamoto M, Kataura A: Cochlear implantation in a patient with mitochondrial disease—Kearns-Sayre syndrome: A case report. *Adv Otorhinolaryngol* **52**:321, 1997.
234. Mosewich RK, Donat JR, DiMauro S, Ciafaloni E, Shanske S, Erasmus M, George D: The syndrome of mitochondrial encephalomyopathy, lactic acidosis, and strokelike episodes presenting without stroke. *Arch Neurol* **50**:275, 1993.
235. Oka Y: [Diabetes mellitus caused by an A to G transition at 3243 of the mitochondrial gene.] *Nippon Rinsho* **56(Suppl 3)**:525, 1998.
236. Xiang K, Wang Y, Wu S, Lu H, Zheng T, Sun D, Weng Q, Jia W, Shen W, Pu L, He J: Mitochondrial tRNA(Leu(UUR)) gene mutation diabetes mellitus in Chinese. *Chin Med J (Engl)* **110**:372, 1997.
237. Isashiki Y, Nakagawa M, Ohba N, Kamimura K, Sakoda Y, Higuchi I, Izumo S, Osame M: Retinal manifestations in mitochondrial diseases associated with mitochondrial DNA mutation. *Acta Ophthalmol Scand* **76**:6, 1998.
238. Odawara M, Yamashita K: Mutation at nucleotide position 3243 of the mitochondrial DNA as a cause of IDDM—A meta-analysis [Letter; Comment]. *Diabetologia* **40**:1493, 1997.
239. Damian MS, Hertel A, Seibel P, Reichmann H, Bachmann G, Schachenmayr W, Hoer G, Dorndorf W: Follow-up in carriers of the "MELAS" mutation without strokes. *Eur Neurol* **39**:9, 1998.
240. Tsukuda K, Suzuki Y, Kameoka K, Osawa N, Goto Y, Katagiri H, Asano T, Yazaki Y, Oka Y: Screening of patients with maternally transmitted diabetes for mitochondrial gene mutations in the tRNA[Leu(UUR)] region [see Comments]. *Diabet Med* **14**:1032, 1997.
241. Smith PR, Dronsfield MJ, Mijovic CH, Hattersley AT, Yeung VT, Cockram C, Chan JC, Barnett AH, Bain SC: The mitochondrial tRNA[Leu(UUR)] A to G 3243 mutation is associated with insulin-dependent and non-insulin-dependent diabetes in a Chinese population. *Diabet Med* **14**:1026, 1997.
242. Fukunaga Y, Azuma N, Koshiyama H, Inoue D, Sato H, Yoshimasa Y, Nakao K: Mitochondrial DNA 3243 mutation is infrequent in Japanese diabetic patients with auditory disturbance [Letter; Comment]. *Diabetes Care* **20**:1800, 1997.
243. Suzuki Y, Taniyama M, Muramatsu T, Atsumi Y, Hosokawa K, Asahina T, Shimada A, Murata C, Matsuoka K: Diabetes mellitus associated with 3243 mitochondrial tRNA(Leu(UUR)) mutation: Clinical features and coenzyme Q10 treatment. *Mol Aspects Med* **18(Suppl)**:S181, 1997.
244. Kobayashi T, Nakanishi K, Nakase H, Kajio H, Okubo M, Murase T, Kosaka K: In situ characterization of islets in diabetes with a mitochondrial DNA mutation at nucleotide position 3243. *Diabetes* **46**:1567, 1997.
245. Yamamoto M: Did de novo MELAS common mitochondrial DNA point mutation (mtDNA 3243, A → G transition) occur in the mother of a proband of a Japanese MELAS pedigree? *J Neurol Sci* **135**:81, 1996.
246. Smith ML, Hua XY, Marsden DL, Liu D, Kennaway NG, Ngo KY, Haas RH: Diabetes and mitochondrial encephalomyopathy with lactic acidosis and stroke-like episodes (MELAS): Radiolabeled polymerase chain reaction is necessary for accurate detection of low percentages of mutation. *J Clin Endocrinol Metab* **82**:2826, 1997.
247. Fukui M, Nakano K, Obayashi H, Kitagawa Y, Nakamura N, Mori H, Kajiyama S, Wada S, Fujii M, Yoshimori K, Kanaitsuka T, Shigeta H, Kondo M: High prevalence of mitochondrial diabetes mellitus in Japanese patients with major risk factors. *Metabolism* **46**:793, 1997.
248. Maassen JA, van den Ouweland JM, 't Hart LM, Lemkes HH: Maternally inherited diabetes and deafness: A diabetic subtype associated with a mutation in mitochondrial DNA. *Horm Metab Res* **29**:50, 1997.
249. Suzuki Y, Goto Y, Taniyama M, Nonaka I, Murakami N, Hosokawa K, Asahina T, Atsumi Y, Matsuoka K: Muscle histopathology in diabetes mellitus associated with mitochondrial tRNA(Leu(UUR)) mutation at position 3243. *J Neurol Sci* **145**:49, 1997.
250. Rigoli L, Di Benedetto A, Romano G, Corica F, Cucinotta D: Mitochondrial DNA [tRNA(Leu)(UUR)] mutation in a southern Italian diabetic population [Letter]. *Diabetes Care* **20**:674, 1997.
251. Lee HC, Song YD, Li HR, Park JO, Suh HC, Lee E, Lim S, Kim K, Huh K: Mitochondrial gene transfer ribonucleic acid (tRNA)-Leu(UUR) 3243 and tRNA(Lys) 8344 mutations and diabetes mellitus in Korea. *J Clin Endocrinol Metab* **82**:372, 1997.
252. Suzuki Y, Muramatsu T, Taniyama M, Atsumi Y, Suematsu M, Kawaguchi R, Higuchi S, Asahina T, Murata C, Handa M, Matsuoka K: Mitochondrial aldehyde dehydrogenase in diabetes associated with mitochondrial tRNA(Leu(UUR)) mutation at position 3243. *Diabetes Care* **19**:1423, 1996.
253. Kobayashi T, Oka Y, Katagiri H, Falorni A, Kasuga A, Takei I, Nakanishi K, Murase T, Kosaka K, Lernmark A: Association between HLA and islet cell antibodies in diabetic patients with a mitochondrial DNA mutation at base pair 3243 [see Comments]. *Diabetologia* **39**:1196, 1996.
254. Odawara M, Asano M, Yamashita K: Mitochondrial gene mutations that affect the binding of the termination factor and their prevalence among Japanese diabetes mellitus. *Nucleic Acids Symp Ser* **237,** 1995.
255. Chuang LM, Wu HP, Chiu KC, Lai CS, Tai TY, Lin BJ: Mitochondrial gene mutations in familial non-insulin-dependent diabetes mellitus in Taiwan. *Clin Genet* **48**:251, 1995.
256. Suzuki Y, Kadowaki H, Atsumi Y, Hosokawa K, Katagiri H, Kadowaki T, Oka Y, Uyama K, Mokubo A, Asahina T, et al.: A case of diabetic amyotrophy associated with 3243 mitochondrial tRNA(leu; UUR) mutation and successful therapy with coenzyme Q10. *Endocr J* **42**:141, 1995.
257. Isashiki Y, Ohba N, Hokita N, Sakamoto Y, Uemura A, Nakagawa M, Osame M, Izumo S: Assessment of mitochondrial gene in proliferative vitreoretinal tissues from patients with familial diabetes mellitus. *Jpn J Ophthalmol* **40**:66, 1996.
258. Feigenbaum A, Chitayat D, Robinson B, MacGregor D, Myint T, Arbus G, Nowaczyk MJ: The expanding clinical phenotype of the tRNA(Leu(UUR)) A → G mutation at np 3243 of mitochondrial DNA: Diabetic embryopathy associated with mitochondrial cytopathy. *Am J Med Genet* **62**:404, 1996.
259. Odawara M, Yamashita K: Are MELAS and diabetes mellitus caused solely by the same mutation at np 3243 of the mitochondrial gene [Letter]? *Diabetologia* **38**:1488, 1995.
260. Silvestre-Aillaud P, BenDahan D, Paquis-Fluckinger V, Pouget J, Pelissier JF, Desnuelle C, Cozzone PJ, Vialettes B: Could coenzyme Q_{10} and L-carnitine be a treatment for diabetes secondary to 3243 mutation of mtDNA [Letter]? *Diabetologia* **38**:1485, 1995.
261. Odawara M: Involvement of mitochondrial gene abnormalities in the pathogenesis of diabetes mellitus. *Ann N Y Acad Sci* **786**:72, 1996.
262. Uchigata Y, Mizota M, Yanagisawa K, Nakagawa Y, Otani T, Ikegami H, Yamada H, Miura J, Ogihara T, Matsuura N, Omori Y: Large-scale study of an A-to-G transition at position 3243 of the mitochondrial gene and IDDM in Japanese patients [Letter]. *Diabetologia* **39**:245, 1996.
263. Gebhart SS, Shoffner JM, Koontz D, Kaufman A, Wallace D: Insulin resistance associated with maternally inherited diabetes and deafness. *Metabolism* 45:526, 1996.

264. Iwanishi M, Obata T, Yamada S, Maegawa H, Tachikawa-Ide R, Ugi S, Hasegawa M, Kojima H, Oguni T, Toudo R, et al.: Clinical and laboratory characteristics in the families with diabetes and a mitochondrial tRNA(LEU(UUR)) gene mutation. *Diabetes Res Clin Pract* **29**:75, 1995.
265. Malaisse WJ, Pueyo ME, Nadi AB, Malaisse-Lagae F, Froguel P, Velho G: D-glucose metabolism in lymphocytes of patients with mitochondrial point mutation of the tRNALeu(UUR) gene. *Biochem Mol Med* **54**:91, 1995.
266. Yamasoba T, Oka Y, Tsukuda K, Nakamura M, Kaga K: Auditory findings in patients with maternally inherited diabetes and deafness harboring a point mutation in the mitochondrial transfer RNA(Leu) (UUR) gene. *Laryngoscope* **106**:49, 1996.
267. Oshima T, Ueda N, Ikeda K, Abe K, Takasaka T: Bilateral sensorineural hearing loss associated with the point mutation in mitochondrial genome. *Laryngoscope* **106**:43, 1996.
268. Tamagawa Y, Tanaka H, Hagiwara H, Ishida T, Kitamura K, Nishizawa M: [Detection of a mutation in mitochondrial DNA in a family with sensorineural deafness and diabetes mellitus as the predominant clinical features.] *Nippon Jibiinkoka Gakkai Kaiho* **98**:1104, 1995.
269. Iwasaki N, Ohgawara H, Nagahara H, Kawamura M, Bell GI, Omori Y: Characterization of Japanese families with early-onset type 2 (non-insulin dependent) diabetes mellitus and screening for mutations in the glucokinase and mitochondrial tRNA(Leu(UUR)) genes. *Acta Diabetol* **32**:17, 1995.
270. Odawara M, Sasaki K, Tachi Y, Yamashita K: Selection of primers for detection of A to G mutation at nucleotide 3243 of the mitochondrial gene [Letter; Comment]. *Diabetologia* **38**:377, 1995.
271. Thomas AW, Morgan R, Majid A, Rees A, Alcolado JC: Detection of mitochondrial DNA mutations in patients with diabetes mellitus [Letter; Comment]. *Diabetologia* **38**:376, 1995.
272. Kadowaki T, Sakura H, Otabe S, Yasuda K, Kadowaki H, Mori Y, Hagura R, Akanuma Y, Yazaki Y: A subtype of diabetes mellitus associated with a mutation in the mitochondrial gene. *Muscle Nerve* **3**:S137, 1995.
273. Oka Y, Katagiri H, Ishihara H, Asano T, Kikuchi M, Kobayashi T: Mitochondrial diabetes mellitus — Glucose-induced signaling defects and beta-cell loss. *Muscle Nerve* **3**:S131, 1995.
274. van den Ouweland JM, Lemkes HH, Gerbitz KD, Maassen JA: Maternally inherited diabetes and deafness (MIDD): A distinct subtype of diabetes associated with a mitochondrial tRNA(Leu)(UUR) gene point mutation. *Muscle Nerve* **3**:S124, 1995.
275. Hammans SR, Sweeney MG, Hanna MG, Brockington M, Morgan-Hughes JA, Harding AE: The mitochondrial DNA transfer RNA-Leu(UUR) A → G(3243) mutation. A clinical and genetic study. *Brain* **118**:721, 1995.
276. Gerbitz KD, van den Ouweland JM, Maassen JA, Jaksch M: Mitochondrial diabetes mellitus: A review. *Biochim Biophys Acta* **1271**:253, 1995.
277. Odawara M, Asakura Y, Tada K, Tsurushima Y, Yamashita K: Mitochondrial gene mutation as a cause of insulin resistance [Letter; Comment]. *Diabetes Care* **18**:275, 1995.
278. Alcolado JC, Thomas AW: Maternally inherited diabetes mellitus: The role of mitochondrial DNA defects. *Diabet Med* **12**:102, 1995.
279. Campos Y, Bautista J, Gutierrez-Rivas E, Chinchon D, Cabello A, Segura D, Arenas J: Clinical heterogeneity in two pedigrees with the 3243 bp tRNA(Leu(UUR)) mutation of mitochondrial DNA. *Acta Neurol Scand* **91**:62, 1995.
280. Alcolado JC, Majid A, Brockington M, Sweeney MG, Morgan R, Rees A, Harding AE, Barnett AH: Mitochondrial gene defects in patients with NIDDM [see Comments]. *Diabetologia* **37**:372, 1994.
281. Suzuki S: [Clinical characterization of diabetes mellitus in the families with mitochondrial encephalomyopathies.] *Nippon Rinsho* **52**:2606, 1994.
282. 't Hart LM, Lemkes HH, Heine RJ, Stolk RP, Feskens EJ, Jansen JJ, van der Does FE, Grobbee DE, Kromhout D, van den Ouweland JM, et al.: Prevalence of maternally inherited diabetes and deafness in diabetic populations in The Netherlands [Letter]. *Diabetologia* **37**:1169, 1994.
283. Oka Y, Katagiri H, Yazaki Y, Murase T, Kobayashi T: Mitochondrial gene mutation in islet-cell-antibody-positive patients. *Lancet* **342**:527, 1993.
284. Oka Y: NIDDM — Genetic marker, glucose transporter, glucokinase, and mitochondria gene. *Diabetes Res Clin Pract* **24(Suppl)**:S117, 1994.
285. Blanche H, Froguel P, Dausset J, Cohen D, Cohen N: Non-isotopic and sensitive method for diagnosis of maternally-inherited diabetes and deafness [Letter; see Comments]. *Diabetologia* **37**:842, 1994.
286. Suzuki S, Hinokio Y, Hirai S, Onoda M, Matsumoto M, Ohtomo M, Kawasaki H, Satoh Y, Akai H, Abe K, et al.: Pancreatic beta-cell secretory defect associated with mitochondrial point mutation of the tRNA(LEU(UUR)) gene: A study in seven families with mitochondrial encephalomyopathy, lactic acidosis and stroke-like episodes (MELAS). *Diabetologia* **37**:818, 1994.
287. Kanamori A, Tanaka K, Umezawa S, Matoba K, Fujita Y, Iizuka T, Yajima Y: Insulin resistance in mitochondrial gene mutation [Letter; see Comments]. *Diabetes Care* **17**:778, 1994.
288. Suzuki Y, Kadowaki H, Katagiri H, Suematsu M, Atsumi Y, Hosokawa K, Kadowaki T, Oka Y, Yazaki Y, Matsuoka K: Posttreatment neuropathy in diabetic subjects with mitochondrial tRNA (Leu) mutation [Letter]. *Diabetes Care* **17**:777, 1994.
289. van den Ouweland JM, Lemkes HH, Trembath RC, Ross R, Velho G, Cohen D, Froguel P, Maassen JA: Maternally inherited diabetes and deafness is a distinct subtype of diabetes and associates with a single point mutation in the mitochondrial tRNA(Leu(UUR)) gene. *Diabetes* **43**:746, 1994.
290. Otabe S, Sakura H, Shimokawa K, Mori Y, Kadowaki H, Yasuda K, Nonaka K, Hagura R, Akanuma Y, Yazaki Y, et al.: The high prevalence of the diabetic patients with a mutation in the mitochondrial gene in Japan. *J Clin Endocrinol Metab* **79**:768, 1994.
291. Katagiri H, Asano T, Ishihara H, Inukai K, Anai M, Yamanouchi T, Tsukuda K, Kikuchi M, Kitaoka H, Ohsawa N, et al.: Mitochondrial diabetes mellitus: Prevalence and clinical characterization of diabetes due to mitochondrial tRNA(Leu(UUR)) gene mutation in Japanese patients. *Diabetologia* **37**:504, 1994.
292. Kadowaki T, Kadowaki H, Mori Y, Tobe K, Sakuta R, Suzuki Y, Tanabe Y, Sakura H, Awata T, Goto Y, et al.: A subtype of diabetes mellitus associated with a mutation of mitochondrial DNA. *N Engl J Med* **330**:962, 1994.
293. Vionnet N, Passa P, Froguel P: Prevalence of mitochondrial gene mutations in families with diabetes mellitus [Letter]. *Lancet* **342**:1429, 1993.
294. Awata T, Matsumoto T, Iwamoto Y, Matsuda A, Kuzuya T, Saito T: Japanese case of diabetes mellitus and deafness with mutation in mitochondrial tRNA(Leu(UUR)) gene [Letter; Comment]. *Lancet* **341**:1291, 1993.
295. Kadowaki H, Tobe K, Mori Y, Sakura H, Sakuta R, Nonaka I, Hagura R, Yazaki Y, Akanuma Y, Kadowaki T: Mitochondrial gene mutation and insulin-deficient type of diabetes mellitus [Letter]. *Lancet* **341**:893, 1993.
296. Sasagasako N, Shida N, Yoshimura T, Kobayashi T, Goto I: [A family with MELAS whose main manifestations are maternally transmitted deafness and diabetes mellitus.] *Rinsho Shinkeigaku* **33**:657, 1993.
297. Norby S: Screening for the two most frequent mutations in Leber's hereditary optic neuropathy by duplex PCR based on allele-specific amplification. *Hum Mutat* **2**:309, 1993.
298. Alcolado JC: Mitochondrial DNA defects in diabetes mellitus [Letter; Comment]. *Diabetologia* **36**:578, 1993.
299. Remes AM, Majamaa K, Herva R, Hassinen IE: Adult-onset diabetes mellitus and neurosensory hearing loss in maternal relatives of MELAS patients in a family with the tRNA(Leu(UUR)) mutation. *Neurology* **43**:1015, 1993.
300. Gerbitz KD, Paprotta A, Jaksch M, Zierz S, Drechsel J: Diabetes mellitus is one of the heterogeneous phenotypic features of a mitochondrial DNA point mutation within the tRNALeu(UUR) gene. *FEBS Lett* **321**:194, 1993.
301. Onishi H, Inoue K, Osaka H, Kimura S, Nagatomo H, Hanihara T, Kawamoto S, Okuda K, Yamada Y, Kosaka K: Mitochondrial myopathy, encephalopathy, lactic acidosis and stroke-like episodes (MELAS) and diabetes mellitus: Molecular genetic analysis and family study. *J Neurol Sci* **114**:205, 1993.
302. Reardon W, Ross RJM, Sweeney MG, Luxon LM, Pembrey ME, Harding AE, Trembath RC: Diabetes mellitus associated with a pathogenic point mutation in mitochondrial DNA. *Lancet* **340**:1376, 1992.
303. van den Ouweland JM, Lemkes HH, Ruitenbeek W, Sandkuijl LA, de Vijlder MF, Struyvenberg PA, van de Kamp JJ, Maassen JA: Mutation in mitochondrial tRNA(Leu)(UUR) gene in a large pedigree with. *Nat Genet* **1**:368, 1992.

304. Kameoka K, Isotani H, Tanaka K, Azukari K, Fujimura Y, Shiota Y, Sasaki E, Majima M, Furukawa K, Haginomori S, Kitaoka H, Ohsawa N: Novel mitochondrial DNA mutation in tRNA(Lys) (8296A → G) associated with diabetes. *Biochem Biophys Res Commun* **245**:523, 1998.
305. Ciafaloni E, Ricci E, Servidei S, Shanske S, Silvestri G, Manfredi G, Schon EA, DiMauro S: Widespread tissue distribution of a tRNALeu(UUR) mutation in the mitochondrial DNA of a patient with MELAS syndrome. *Neurology* **41**:1663, 1991.
306. Melberg A, Akerlund P, Raininko R, Silander HC, Wibom R, Khaled A, Nennesmo I, Lundberg PO, Olsson Y: Monozygotic twins with MELAS-like syndrome lacking ragged red fibers and lactic acidaemia. *Acta Neurol Scand* **94**:233, 1996.
307. Ichiki T, Tanaka M, Nishikimi M, Suzuki H, Ozawa T, Kobayashi M, Wada Y: Deficiency of subunits of complex I and mitochondrial encephalomyopathy. *Ann Neurol* **23**:287, 1988.
308. Yoda S, Terauchi A, Kitahara F, Akabane T: Neurologic deterioration with progressive CT changes in a child with Kearns-Shy syndrome. *Brain Dev* **6**:323, 1984.
309. Kobayashi M, Morishita H, Sugiyama N, Yokochi K, Nakano M, Wada Y, Hotta Y, Terauchi A, Nonaka I: Mitochondrial myopathy, encephalopathy, lactic acidosis and stroke-like episodes syndrome and NADH-CoQ reductase deficiency. *J Inherit Metab Dis* **9**:301, 1986.
310. Kobayashi M, Morishita H, Sugiyama N, Yokochi K, Nakano M, Wada Y, Hotta Y, Terauchi A, Nonaka I: Two cases of NADH-coenzyme Q reductase deficiency: Relationship to MELAS syndrome. *J Pediatr* **110**:223, 1987.
311. Goda S, Ishimoto S, Goto I, Kuroiwa Y, Koike K, Koike M, Nakagawa M, Reichmann H, DiMauro S: Biochemical studies in mitochondrial encephalomyopathy. *J Neurol Neurosurg Psychiatry* **50**:1348, 1987.
312. Goda S, Hamada T, Ishimoto S, Kobayashi T, Goto I, Kuroiwa Y: Clinical improvement after administration of coenzyme Q10 in a patient with mitochondrial encephalomyopathy. *J Neurol* **234**:62, 1987.
313. Hayes DJ, Hilton-Jones D, Arnold DL, Galloway G, Styles P, Duncan J, Radda GK: A mitochondrial encephalomyopathy: A combined 31P magnetic resonance and biochemical investigation. *J Neurol Sci* **71**:105, 1985.
314. Yamamoto M, Sato T, Anno M, Ujike H, Takemoto M: Mitochondrial myopathy, encephalopathy, lactic acidosis, and strokelike episodes with recurrent abdominal symptoms and coenzyme Q10 administration. *J Neurol Neurosurg Psychiatry* **50**:1475, 1987.
315. Montagna P, Gallassi R, Medori R, Govoni E, Zeviani M, DiMauro S, Lugaresi E, Andermann F: MELAS syndrome: Characteristic migrainous and epileptic features and maternal transmission. *Neurology* **38**:751, 1988.
316. Ishitsu T, Miike T, Kitano A, Haraguchi Y, Ohtani Y, Matsuda I, Shimoji A, Kimura H: Heterogeneous phenotypes of mitochondrial encephalomyopathy in a single kindred. *Neurology* **37**:1867, 1987.
317. Driscoll PF, Larsen PD, Gruber AB: MELAS syndrome involving a mother and two children. *Arch Neurol* **44**:971, 1987.
318. Prick MJJ, Gabreels FJM, Trijbels JMF, Janssen AJM, le Coultre R, van Dam K, Jaspar HHJ, Ebels EJ, Op de Coul AAW: Progressive poliodystrophy (Alpers' disease) with a defect in cytochrome aa_3 in muscle: A report of two unrelated patients. *Clin Neurol Neurosurg* **85**:57, 1983.
319. Rouslin W: Mitochondrial complexes I, II, III, IV, and V in myocardial ischemia and autolysis. *Am J Physiol* **244**:H743, 1983.
320. Skoglund RR: Reversible alexia, mitochondrial myopathy, and lactic acidemia. *Neurology* **29**:717, 1979.
321. Schapira AHV, Cooper JM, Manneschi L, Vital C, Morgan-Hughes JA, Clark JB: A mitochondrial encephalomyopathy with specific deficiencies of two respiratory chain polypeptides and a circulating autoantibody to a mitochondrial matrix protein. *Brain* **113**:419, 1990.
322. Schapira AHV, Cooper JM, Morgan-Hughes JA, Patel SD, Cleeter MJW, Ragan CI, Clark JB: Molecular basis of mitochondrial myopathies: Polypeptide analysis in complex I deficiency. *Lancet* **i**:500, 1988.
323. Morgan-Hughes JA, Schapira AHV, Cooper JM, Clark JB: Molecular defects of NADH-ubiquinone oxidoreductase (complex I) in mitochondrial diseases. *J Bioenerg Biomembr* **20**:365, 1988.
324. Hess JF, Parisi MA, Bennett JL, Clayton DA: Impairment of mitochondrial transcription termination by a point mutation associated with the MELAS subgroup of mitochondrial encephalomyopathies. *Nature* **351**:236, 1991.
325. Chomyn A, Martinuzzi A, Yoneda M, Daga A, Hurko O, Johns D, Lai ST, Nonaka I, Angelini C, Attardi G: MELAS mutation in mtDNA binding site for transcription termination factor causes defects in protein synthesis and in respiration but no change in levels of upstream and downstream mature transcripts. *Proc Natl Acad Sci U S A* **89**:4221, 1992.
326. Christianson TW, Clayton DA: In vitro transcription of human mitochondrial DNA: accurate termination requires a region of DNA sequence that can function bidirectionally. *Proc Natl Acad Sci U S A* **83**:6277, 1986.
327. King MP, Koga Y, Davidson M, Schon EA: Defects in mitochondrial protein synthesis and respiratory chain activity segregate with the tRNA(Leu(UUR)) mutation associated with mitochondrial myopathy, encephalopathy, lactic acidosis, and strokelike episodes. *Mol Cell Biol* **12**:480, 1992.
328. Flierl A, Reichmann H, Seibel P: Pathophysiology of the MELAS 3243 transition mutation. *J Biol Chem* **272**:27189, 1997.
329. El Meziane A, Lehtinen SK, Hance N, Nijtmans LG, Dunbar D, Holt IJ, Jacobs HT: A tRNA suppressor mutation in human mitochondria. *Nat Genet* **18**:350, 1998.
330. Rahman S, Blok RB, Dahl HH, Danks DM, Kirby DM, Chow CW, Christodoulou J, Thorburn DR: Leigh syndrome: Clinical features and biochemical and DNA abnormalities. *Ann Neurol* **39**:343, 1996.
331. Shoffner JM, Fernhoff PM, Krawiecki NS, Caplan DB, Holt PJ, Koontz DA, Takei Y, Newman NJ, Ortiz RG, Polak M, et al.: Subacute necrotizing encephalopathy: oxidative phosphorylation defects. *Neurology* **42**:2168, 1992.
332. Tatuch Y, Christodoulou J, Feigenbaum A, Clarke JT, Wherret J, Smith C, Rudd N, Petrova-Benedict R, Robinson BH: Heteroplasmic mitochondrial DNA mutation (T to G) at 8993 can cause Leigh disease when the percentage of abnormal mtDNA is high. *Am J Hum Genet* **50**:852, 1992.
333. Santorelli FM, Shanske S, Jain KD, Tick D, Schon EA, DiMauro S: A T to C mutation at nt 8993 of mitochondrial DNA in a child with Leigh syndrome. *Neurology* **44**:972, 1994.
334. Tatuch Y, Pagon RA, Vlcek B, Roberts R, Korson M, Robinson BH: The 8993 mtDNA mutation: Heteroplasmy and clinical presentation in three families. *Eur J Hum Genet* **2**:35, 1994.
335. Trounce I, Neill S, Wallace DC: Cytoplasmic transfer of the mtDNA nt 8993 T → G (ATP6) point mutation associated with Leigh syndrome into mtDNA-less cells demonstrates cosegregation with a decrease in state III respiration and ADP/O ratio. *Proc Natl Acad Sci U S A* **91**:8334, 1994.
336. Holt IJ, Harding AE, Petty RK, Morgan-Hughes JA: A new mitochondrial disease associated with mitochondrial DNA heteroplasmy. *Am J Hum Genet* **46**:428, 1990.
337. Majander A, Lamminen T, Juvonen V, Aula P, Nikoskelainen E, Savontaus ML, Wikstrom M: Mutations in subunit 6 of the F1F0-ATP synthase cause two entirely different diseases. *FEBS Lett* **412**:351, 1997.
338. Van Erven PMM, Gabreels FJM, Wevers RA, Doesvurg WH, Ruitenbeek W, Renier WO, Lamers KJB: Intravenous pyruvate loading test in Leigh syndrome. *J Neurol Sci* **77**:217, 1987.
339. Miyabayashi S, Ito T, Abukawa D, Narisawa K, Tada K, Tanaka M, Ozawa T, Droste M, Kadenbach B: Immunochemical study in three patients with cytochrome c oxidase deficiency presenting as Leigh's encephalomyopathy. *J Inherit Metab Dis* **10**:289, 1987.
340. Hoganson GE, Paulson DJ, Chun R, Sufit RL, Shug AL: Deficiency of muscle cytochrome c oxidase in Leigh's disease. *Pediatr Res* **18**:222A, 1984.
341. DiMauro S, Servidei S, Zeviani M, DiRocco M, DeVivo DC, DiDonato S, Uziel G, Berry K, Hoganson G, Johnsen SD, Johnson PC: Cytochrome c oxidase deficiency in Leigh syndrome. *Ann Neurol* **22**:498, 1987.
342. Hoppel CL, Kerr DS, Dahms B, Roessmann U: Deficiency of the reduced nicotinamide adenine dinucleotide dehydrogenase component of complex I of mitochondrial electron transport: Fatal infantile lactic acidosis and hypermetabolism with skeletal-cardiac myopathy and encephalopathy. *J Clin Invest* **80**:71, 1987.
343. Miranda DF, Ishii S, DiMauro S, Shay JW: Cytochrome c oxidase (COX) deficiency in Leigh's syndrome: Genetic evidence for a nuclear DNA-encoded mutation. *Neurology* **39**:697, 1989.
344. Arts WF, Scholte HR, Loonen MC, Przyrembel H, Fernandes J, Trijbels JM, Luyt HIE: Cytochrome c oxidase deficiency in subacute necrotizing encephalomyelopathy. *J Neurol Sci* **77**:103, 1987.
345. Miyabayashi S, Narisawa K, Iinuma K, Tada K, Sakai K, Kobayashi K, Kobayashi Y, Morinaga S: Cytochrome c oxidase deficiency in two siblings with Leigh encephalomyelopathy. *Brain Dev* **6**:362, 1984.

346. Miyabayashi S, Ito T, Narisawa K, Iinuma K, Tada K: Biochemical study in 28 children with lactic acidosis, in relation to Leigh's encephalopathy. *Eur J Pediatr* **143**:278, 1985.
347. Miyabayashi S, Narisawa K, Tada K, Sakai K, Kobayashi K, Kobayashi Y: Two siblings with cytochrome c oxidase deficiency. *J Inherit Metab Dis* **6**:121, 1983.
348. Willems JL, Monnens LAH, Trijbels LMF, Veerkamp JH, Meyer AEFH, van Dam K, van Haelst U: Leigh's encephalomyelopathy in a patient with cytochrome c oxidase deficiency in muscle tissue. *Pediatrics* **60**:850, 1977.
349. Mela L, Bacalzo LV, Miller LD: Defective oxidative metabolism of rat liver mitochondria in hemorrhagic and endotoxin shock. *Am J Physiol* **220**:571, 1971.
350. Schumer W, Das Gupta TK, Moss GS, Nyhus LM: Effect of endotoxemia on liver cell mitochondria in man. *Ann Surg* **171**:875, 1970.
351. Trauner DA, Horvath E, Davis LE: Inhibition of fatty acid beta oxidation by influenza B virus and salicylic acid in mice: Implications for Reye's syndrome. *Neurology* **38**:239, 1988.
352. Santorelli FM, Shanske S, Macaya A, DeVivo DC, DiMauro S: The mutation at nt 8993 of mitochondrial DNA is a common cause of Leigh's syndrome. *Ann Neurol* **34**:827, 1993.
353. Pincus JH: Subacute necrotizing encephalomyelopathy (Leigh's disease): A consideration of clinical features and etiology. *Dev Med Child Neurol* **14**:87, 1972.
354. Montpetit VJA, Andermann F, Carpenter S, Fawcett JS, Zborowska-Sluis D, Gibersun HR: Subacute necrotizing encephalomyelopathy: A review and a study of two families. *Brain* **94**:1, 1971.
355. Glerum M, Robinson BH, Spratt C, Wilson J, Patrick D: Abnormal kinetic behavior of cytochrome oxidase in a case of Leigh disease. *Am J Hum Genet* **41**:584, 1987.
356. Robinson BH, De Meirleir L, Glerum M, Sherwood G, Becker L: Clinical presentation of mitochondrial respiratory chain defects in NADH-coenzyme Q reductase and cytochrome oxidase: Clues to pathogenesis of Leigh disease. *J Pediatr* **110**:216, 1987.
357. Stansbie D, Wallace SJ, Marsac C: Disorders of the pyruvate dehydrogenase complex. *J Inherit Metab Dis* **9**:105, 1986.
358. Robinson BH: Cell culture studies on patients with mitochondrial diseases: Molecular defects in pyruvate dehydrogenase. *J Bioenerg Biomembr* **20**:313, 1988.
359. Kretzchmar HA, DeArmond SJ, Koch TK, Patel MS, Newth CJL, Schmidt KA, Packman S: Pyruvate dehydrogenase complex deficiency as a cause of subacute necrotizing encephalopathy (Leigh's disease). *Pediatrics* **79**:370, 1987.
360. Hommes FA, Polman HA, Reerink JD: Leigh's encephalomyelopathy: An inborn error of gluconeogenesis. *Arch Dis Child* **43**:423, 1968.
361. Novotny EJJ, Singh G, Wallace DC, Dorfman LJ, Louis A, Sogg RL, Steinman L: Leber's disease and dystonia: A mitochondrial disease. *Neurology* **36**:1053, 1986.
362. De Vries DD, Went LN, Bruyn GW, Scholte HR, Hofstra RM, Bolhuis PA, van Oost BA: Genetic and biochemical impairment of mitochondrial complex I activity in a family with Leber hereditary optic neuropathy and hereditary spastic dystonia. *Am J Hum Genet* **58**:703, 1996.
363. Jun AS, Brown MD, Wallace DC: A mitochondrial DNA mutation at np 14459 of the ND6 gene associated with maternally inherited Leber's hereditary optic neuropathy and dystonia. *Proc Natl Acad Sci U S A* **91**:6206, 1994.
364. Tanaka M, Ino H, Ohno K, Hattori K, Sato W, Ozawa T, Tanaka T, Itoyama S: Mitochondrial mutation in fatal infantile cardiomyopathy. *Lancet* **336**:1452, 1990.
365. Zeviani M, Gellera C, Antozzi C, Rimoldi M, Morandi L, Villani F, Tiranti V, DiDonato S: Maternally inherited myopathy and cardiomyopathy: association with mutation in mitochondrial DNA tRNA-(Leu)(UUR). *Lancet* **338**:143, 1991.
366. Silvestri G, Shanske S, Whitley CB, Schimmenti LA, Smith SA, DiMauro S: A new mtDNA mutation in the tRNALeu(UUR) gene associated with cardiomyopathy and ragged-red fibers. *Neurology* **43**:A402, 1993.
367. Koga Y, Nonaka I, Kobayashi M, Tojyo M, Nihei K: Findings in muscle in complex I (NADH coenzyme Q reductase) deficiency. *Ann Neurol* **24**:749, 1988.
368. Goto Y, Tojo M, Tohyama J, Horai S, Nonaka I: A novel point mutation in the mitochondrial tRNA(Leu)(UUR) gene in a family with mitochondrial myopathy. *Ann Neurol* **31**:672, 1992.
369. Fischel-Ghodsian N, Falk RE: Deafness, in Rimoin DL, Connor JM, Pyeritz RE (eds): *Emery and Rimoin's Principles and Practice of Medical Genetics*. New York, Churchill Livingstone, 1996, p 1150.
370. Jaber L, Shohat M, Bu X, Fischel-Ghodsian N, Yang H-Y, Wang S-J, Rotter JI: Sensorineural deafness inherited as a tissue specific mitochondrial disorder. *J Med Genet* **29**:86, 1992.
371. Prezant TR, Shohat M, Jaber L, Pressman S, Fischel-Ghodsian N: Biochemical characterization of a pedigree with mitochondrially inherited deafness. *Am J Med Genet* **44**:465, 1992.
372. Prezant TR, Agapian JV, Bohlman MC, Bu X, Oztas S, Qiu WQ, Arnos KS, Cortopassi GA, Jaber L, Rotter JI, et al.: Mitochondrial ribosomal RNA mutation associated with both antibiotic-induced and non-syndromic deafness. *Nat Genet* **4**:289, 1993.
373. Hamasaki K, Rando RR: Specific binding of aminoglycosides to a human rRNA construct based on a DNA polymorphism which causes aminoglycoside-induced deafness. *Biochemistry* **36**:12323, 1997.
374. DiMauro S, Nicholson JF, Hays AP, Eastwood AB, Papadimitriou A, Koenigsberger R, DeVivo DC: Benign infantile mitochondrial myopathy due to reversible cytochrome c oxidase deficiency. *Ann Neurol* **14**:226, 1983.
375. Zeviani M, Peterson P, Servidei S, Bonilla E, DiMauro S: Benign reversible muscle cytochrome c oxidase deficiency: A second case. *Neurology* **37**:64, 1987.
376. Roodhooft AM, Van AKJ, Martin JJ, Ceuterick C, Scholte HR, Luyt HIE: Benign mitochondrial myopathy with deficiency of NADH-CoQ reductase and cytochrome c oxidase. *Neuropediatrics* **17**:221, 1986.
377. Jerusalem F, Angelini C, Engel A, Groover RV: Mitochondria-lipid-glycogen (MLG) disease of muscle: A morphologically regressive congenital myopathy. *Arch Neurol* **29**:162, 1973.
378. Tritschler HJ, Bonilla E, Lombes A, Andreetta F, Servidei S, Schneyder B, Miranda AF, Schon EA, Kadenbach B, DiMauro S: Differential diagnosis of fatal and benign cytochrome c oxidase-deficient myopathies of infancy: An immunohistochemical approach. *Neurology* **41**:300, 1991.
379. DiMauro S, Mendell JR, Sahenk Z, Bachman D, Scarpa A, Scofield RM, Reiner C: Fatal infantile mitochondrial myopathy and renal dysfunction due to cytochrome c oxidase deficiency. *Neurology* **30**:795, 1980.
380. Zeviani M, Nonaka I, Bonilla E, Okino E, Moggio M, Jones S, DiMauro S: Fatal infantile mitochondrial myopathy and renal dysfunction caused by cytochrome c oxidase deficiency: Immunological studies in a new patient. *Ann Neurol* **17**:414, 1985.
381. Diebler MF, Farkas-Bargeton E, Wherle R: Developmental changes of enzymes associated with energy metabolism and the synthesis of some neurotransmitters in discrete areas of human neocortex. *J Neurochem* **32**:429, 1979.
382. Chugani HT, Phelps ME, Mazziotta JC: Positron emission tomography study of human brain development. *Ann Neurol* **22**:487, 1987.
383. Zeviani M, H. Van Dyke DH, Servidei S, Bauserman SC, Bonilla E, Beaumont ET, Sharda J, VanderLaan K, DiMauro S: Myopathy and fatal cardiopathy due to cytochrome c oxidase deficiency. *Arch Neurol* **43**:1198, 1986.
384. Bresolin N, Zeviani M, Bonilla E, Miller RH, Leech RW, Shanske S, Nakagawa M, DiMauro S: Fatal infantile cytochrome c oxidase deficiency: Decrease of immunologically detectable enzyme in muscle. *Neurology* **35**:802, 1985.
385. Heiman PTD, Bonilla E, DiMauro S, Foreman J, Schotland DL: Cytochrome c oxidase deficiency in a floppy infant. *Neurology* **32**:898, 1982.
386. Moreadith RW, Batshaw ML, Ohnishi T, Kerr D, Knox B, Jackson D, Hruban R, Olson J, Reynafarje B, Lehninger AL: Deficiency of the iron-sulfur clusters of mitochondrial reduced nicotinamide-adenine dinucleotide-ubiquinone oxidoreductase (complex I) in an infant with congenital lactic acidosis. *J Clin Invest* **74**:685, 1984.
387. Muller-Hocker J, Ibel H, Paetzke I, Deufel T, Endres W, Kadenbach B, Gokel JM, Hubner G: Fatal infantile mitochondrial cardiomyopathy and myopathy with heterogeneous tissue expression of combined respiratory chain deficiencies. *Virchows Arch A Pathol Anat Histopathol* **419**:355, 1991.
388. Muller-Hocker J, Pongratz D, Deufel T, Trijbels JM, Endres W, Hubner G: Fatal lipid storage myopathy with deficiency of cytochrome-c-oxidase and carnitine. A contribution to the combined cytochemical-fine structural identification of cytochrome c oxidase in long-term frozen muscle. *Virchows Arch A Pathol Anat Histopathol* **399**:11, 1983.
389. Robinson BH, McKay N, Goodyer P, Lancaster G: Defective intramitochondrial NADH oxidation in skin fibroblasts from an infant with fatal neonatal lacticacidemia. *Am J Hum Genet* **37**:938, 1985.

390. Robinson BH, Ward J, Goodyer P, Baudet A: Respiratory chain defects in the mitochondria of cultured skin fibroblasts from three patients with lacticacidemia. *J Clin Invest* **77**:1422, 1986.
391. Zheng X, Shoffner JM, Lott MT, Voljavec AS, Krawiecki NS, Winn K, Wallace DC: Evidence in a lethal infantile mitochondrial disease for a nuclear mutation affecting respiratory complexes I and IV. *Neurology* **39**:1203, 1989.
392. Rimoldi M, Bottachi E, Rossi L, Cornelio F, Uziel G, Di Donato S: Cytochrome c oxidase deficiency in muscles of a floppy infant without mitochondrial myopathy. *J Neurol* **227**:201, 1982.
393. Sengers RC, Trijbels JMF, Bakkeren JAJM, Ruitenbeek W, Fischer JC, Janssen AJM, Stadhouders AM, ter Laak HJ: Deficiency of cytochromes b and aa_3 in muscle from a floppy infant with cytochrome c oxidase deficiency. *Eur J Pediatr* **141**:178, 1984.
394. Aprille JR: Tissue specific cytochrome deficiencies in human infants, in Quagliarello E, Slater EL, Palmieri F, Saccone C, Kroon AM (eds): *Achievements and Perspectives of Mitochondrial Research, Biogenesis*. New York, Elsevier Science, 1985, p 465.
395. Boustany RN, Aprille JR, Halperin J, Levy H, DeLong GR: Mitochondrial cytochrome deficiency presenting as a myopathy with hypotonia, external ophthalmoplegia, and lactic acidosis in an infant and as fatal hepatopathy in a second cousin. *Ann Neurol* **14**:462, 1983.
396. Moreadith RW, Cleeter MW, Ragan CI, Batshaw ML, Lehninger AL: Congenital deficiency of two polypeptide subunits of the iron-protein fragment of mitochondrial Complex I. *J Clin Invest* **79**:463, 1987.
397. Van Biervliet JPGM, Bruinvis L, Ketting D, De Bree PK, Van der Heiden C, Wadman SK, Willems NL, Bookelman H, Van Haelst U, Monnens LAH: Hereditary mitochondrial myopathy with lactic acidemia, a De Toni-Fanconi-Debre syndrome and a defective respiratory chain in voluntary striated muscles. *Pediatr Res* **11**:1088, 1977.
398. Trijbels JMF, Sengers R, Monnens L, Janssen AJM, Willems JL, ter Laak HJ, Stadhouders AM: A patient with lactic acidaemia and cytochrome oxidase deficiency. *J Inherit Metab Dis* **6**:127, 1983.
399. Stansbie D, Dormer RL, Hughes IA, Minchom PE, Hendry GAF, Jones OTG, Cross AR, Sherratt HSA, Turnbull DM, Johnson MA: Mitochondrial myopathy with skeletal muscle cytochrome oxidase deficiency. *J Inherit Metab Dis* **5**:27, 1982.
400. Minchom PE, Dormer RL, Hughes IA, Stansbie D, Cross AR, Hendry GAF, Jones OTG, Johnson MA, Sherratt HSA, Turnbull DM: Fatal infantile mitochondrial myopathy due to cytochrome c oxidase deficiency. *J Neurol Sci* **60**:453, 1983.
401. Birch Machin MA, Shepherd IM, Watmough NJ, Sherratt HS, Bartlett K, Darley Usmar VM, Milligan DW, Welch RJ, Aynsley-Green A, Turnbull DM: Fatal lactic acidosis in infancy with a defect of complex III of the respiratory chain. *Pediatr Res* **25**:553, 1989.
402. Figarella-Branger D, Pellissier JF, Scheiner C, Wernert F, Desnuelle C: Defects of the mitochondrial respiratory chain complexes in three pediatric cases with hypotonia and cardiac involvement. *J Neurol Sci* **108**:105, 1992.
403. Moraes CT, Shanske S, Tritschler HJ, Aprille JR, Andreetta F, Bonilla E, Schon EA, DiMauro S: mtDNA depletion with variable tissue expression: A novel genetic abnormality in mitochondrial diseases. *Am J Hum Genet* **48**:492, 1991.
404. Tritschler HJ, Andreetta F, Moraes CT, Bonilla E, Arnaudo E, Danon MJ, Glass S, Zelaya BM, Vamos E, Telerman-Toppet N: Mitochondrial myopathy of childhood associated with depletion of mitochondrial DNA. *Neurology* **42**:209, 1992.
405. Telerman-Toppet N, Biarent D, Bouton JM, de Meirleir L, Elmer C, Noel S, Vamos E, DiMauro S: Fatal cytochrome c oxidase-deficient myopathy of infancy associated with mtDNA depletion. Differential involvement of skeletal muscle and cultured fibroblasts. *J Inherit Metab Dis* **15**:323, 1992.
406. Yoon KL, Aprille JR, Ernst SG: Mitochondrial tRNA(thr) mutation in fatal infantile respiratory enzyme deficiency. *Biochem Biophys Res Commun* **176**:1112, 1991.
407. Brown MD, Torroni A, Shoffner JM, Wallace DC: Mitochondrial tRNA(Thr) mutations and lethal infantile mitochondrial myopathy. *Am J Hum Genet* **51**:446, 1992.
408. Robinson BH, Glerum DM, Chow W, Petrova-Benedict R, Lightowlers R, Capaldi R: The use of skin fibroblast cultures in the detection of respiratory chain defects in patients with lactic acidemia. *Pediatr Res* **28**:549, 1990.
409. Chow W, Ragan I, Robinson BH: Determination of the cDNA sequence for the human mitochondrial 75-kDa Fe-S protein of NADH-coenzyme Q reductase. *Eur J Biochem* **201**:547, 1991.
410. Bolhuis PA, Barth PG, Wijburg FA, Sinjorgo KMC, Ruttenbeek W: Molecular basis of mitochondrial myopathies. *Lancet* **i**:884, 1988.
411. Anan R: Cardiac involvement in mitochondrial disease: A clinical study of 38 patients. *Igaku Kenkyu* **61**:49, 1991.
412. Anan R, Nakagawa M, Miyata M, Higuchi I, Nakao S, Suehara M, Osame M, Tanaka H: Cardiac involvement in mitochondrial diseases. A study on 17 patients with documented mitochondrial DNA defects [see Comments]. *Circulation* **91**:955, 1995.
413. Angelini C, Micaglio GF, Sforza P, Melacini P, Carrozzo R, Fanin M, Ferrarese A, Rosa N: Familial lipid storage cardiomyopathy with mitochondrial complex II defect. *Neurology* **38(Suppl 1)**:152, 1988.
414. Antozzi C, Zeviani M: Cardiomyopathies in disorders of oxidative metabolism. *Cardiovasc Res* **35**:184, 1997.
415. Bernucci P, D'Amati G, Casali C, De Biase L, Autore C, Fedele F, Gallo P: [Mitochondrial cardiomyopathies: A new entity in cardiology research and diagnosis.] *G Ital Cardiol* **26**:1031, 1996.
416. Besley GT, Lendon M, Broadhead DM, Till J, Heptinstall LE, Phillips B: Mitochondrial complex deficiencies in a male with cardiomyopathy and 3-methylglutaconic aciduria. *J Inherit Metab Dis* **18**:221, 1995.
417. Bohlega S, Tanji K, Santorelli FM, Hirano M, al-Jishi A, DiMauro S: Multiple mitochondrial DNA deletions associated with autosomal recessive ophthalmoplegia and severe cardiomyopathy. *Neurology* **46**:1329, 1996.
418. Bruton D, Herdson PB, Becroft DMO: Histiocytoid cardiomyopathy of infancy: An unexplained myofiber degeneration. *Pathology* **9**:115, 1977.
419. Amini M, Bosman C, Marino B: Histiocytoid cardiomyopathy in infancy: A new hypothesis? *Chest* **77**:556, 1980.
420. Cruysberg JRM, Sengers RCA, Pinckers A, Kibat K, van Haelst UJGM: Features of a syndrome with congenital cataract and hypertrophic cardiomyopathy. *Am J Ophthalmol* **102**:740, 1986.
421. Fabrizi GM, Lodi R, D'Ettorre M, Malandrini A, Cavallaro T, Rimoldi M, Zaniol P, Barbiroli B, Guazzi G: Autosomal dominant limb girdle myopathy with ragged-red fibers and cardiomyopathy. A pedigree study by in vivo 31P-MR spectroscopy indicating a multisystem mitochondrial defect. *J Neurol Sci* **137**:20, 1996.
422. Ferrans VJ, McAllister HAJ, Haese WH: Infantile cardiomyopathy with histiocytoid change in cardiac muscle cells. Report of six patients. *Circulation* **53**:708, 1976.
423. Frustaci A, Schiavoni G, Pennestri F, Mazzari M, Rossi E, Ferri T, Lippa S, Oradei A, Littarru GP, Manzoli U: Coenzyme Q10 in dilated cardiomyopathy: A biochemical approach to the treatment. *Cardiologia* **30**:533, 1985.
424. Hug G, Schubert WK: Idiopathic cardiomyopathy. Mitochondrial and cytoplasmic alterations in heart and liver. *Lab Invest* **22**:541, 1970.
425. Kauffman SL, Chandra N, Peress NS, Rodriguez-Torres R: Idiopathic infantile cardiomyopathy with involvement of the conduction system. *Am J Cardiol* **30**:648, 1972.
426. Langsjoen PH, Langsjoen PH, Folkers K: Long-term efficacy and safety of coenzyme Q10 therapy for idiopathic dilated cardiomyopathy. *Am J Cardiol* **65**:521, 1990.
427. Langsjoen PH, Folkers K, Lyson K, Muratsu K, Lyson T, Langsjoen P: Effective and safe therapy with coenzyme Q10 for cardiomyopathy. *Klin Wochenschr* **66**:583, 1988.
428. Kurabayashi M, Yamaoki K, Yazaki Y: [Familial dilated cardiomyopathy.] *Ryoikibetsu Shokogun Shir* **14**:49, 1996.
429. Marian AJ, Roberts R: Molecular basis of hypertrophic and dilated cardiomyopathy. *Tex Heart Inst J* **21**:6, 1994.
430. Marin-Garcia J, Ananthakrishnan R, Goldenthal MJ, Filiano JJ, Perez-Atayde A: Cardiac mitochondrial dysfunction and DNA depletion in children with hypertrophic cardiomyopathy. *J Inherit Metab Dis* **20**:674, 1997.
431. Marin-Garcia J, Ananthakrishnan R, Goldenthal MJ: Hypertrophic cardiomyopathy with mitochondrial DNA depletion and respiratory enzyme defects. *Pediatr Cardiol* **19**:266, 1998.
432. Papadimitriou A, Neustein HB, DiMauro S, Stanton R, Bresolin N: Histiocytoid cardiomyopathy of infancy: Deficiency of reducible cytochrome b in heart mitochondria. *Pediatr Res* **18**:1023, 1984.
433. Pitkanen S, Merante F, Ross Mcleod D, Applegarth D, Tong T, Robinson B: Familial cardiomyopathy with cataracts and lactic acidosis: A defect in complex I (NADH dehydrogenase) of the mitochondria respiratory chain. *Pediatr Res* **39**:513, 1996.
434. Bastiaensen LA, Jaspar HHJ, Stadhouders AM: Ophthalmoplegia-plus. *Doc Ophthalmol* **46**:365, 1979.
435. Barron SA, Heffner RRJ, Zwirecki R: A familial mitochondrial myopathy with central defect in neural transmission. *Arch Neurol* **36**:553, 1979.

436. McAuley FD: Progressive external ophthalmoplegia. *Br J Ophthalmol* **40**:686, 1956.
437. Zeviani M: Nucleus-driven mutations of human mitochondrial DNA. *J Inherit Metab Dis* **15**:456, 1992.
438. Suomalainen A, Majander A, Wallin M, Setala K, Kontula K, Leinonen H, Salmi T, Paetau A, Haltia M, Valanne L, Lonnqvist J, Peltonen L, Somer H: Autosomal dominant progressive external ophthalmoplegia with multiple deletions of mtDNA: Clinical, biochemical, and molecular genetic features of the 10q-linked disease. *Neurology* **48**:1244, 1997.
439. Cormier V, Rotig A, Tardieu M, Colonna M, Saudubray JM, Munnich A: Autosomal dominant deletions of the mitochondrial genome in a case of progressive encephalomyopathy. *Am J Hum Genet* **48**:643, 1991.
440. Servidei S, Zeviani M, Manfredi G, Ricci E, Silvestri G, Bertini E, Gellera C, DiMauro S, Di Donato S, Tonali P: Dominantly inherited mitochondrial myopathy with multiple deletions of mitochondrial DNA: Clinical, morphologic, and biochemical studies. *Neurology* **41**:1053, 1991.
441. Suomalainen A, Kaukonen J, Amati P, Timonen R, Haltia M, Weissenbach J, Zeviani M, Somer H, Peltonen L: An autosomal locus predisposing to deletions of mitochondrial DNA. *Nat Genet* **9**:146, 1995.
442. Kaukonen JA, Amati P, Suomalainen A, Rotig A, Piscaglia MG, Salvi F, Weissenbach J, Fratta G, Comi G, Peltonen L, Zeviani M: An autosomal locus predisposing to multiple deletions of mtDNA on chromosome 3p. *Am J Hum Genet* **58**:763, 1996.
443. Mizusawa H, Watanabe M, Kanazawa I, Nakanishi T, Kobayashi M, Tanaka M, Suzuki H, Nishikimi M, Ozawa T: Familial mitochondrial myopathy associated with peripheral neuropathy: Partial deficiencies of complex I and complex IV. *J Neurol Sci* **86**:171, 1988.
444. Yuzaki M, Ohkoshi N, Kanazawa I, Kagawa Y, Ohta S: Multiple deletions in mitochondrial DNA at direct repeats of non-D-loop regions in cases of familial mitochondrial myopathy. *Biochem Biophys Res Commun* **164**:1352, 1989.
445. Rivner MH, Shamsnia M, Swift TR, Trefz J, Roesel RA, Carter AL, Yanamura W, Hommes FA: Kearns-Sayre syndrome and complex II deficiency. *Neurology* **39**:693, 1989.
446. Bardosi A, Creutzfeldt W, DiMauro S, Felgenhauer K, Friede RL, Goebel HH, Kohlschutter A, Mayer G, Rahlf G, Servidei S, Van Lessen G, Wetterling T: Myo-, neuro-, gastrointestinal encephalomyopathy (MNGIE syndrome) due to partial deficiency of cytochrome c oxidase. A new mitochondrial multisystem disorder. *Acta Neuropathol* **74**:248, 1987.
447. Ionasescu V, Thompson HS, Aschenbrener C, Anuras S, Risk WS: Late-onset oculogastrointestinal muscular dystrophy. *Am J Med Genet* **18**:781, 1984.
448. Ionasescu V, Thompson SH, Ionasescu R, Searby CH, Anuras S, Christensen J, Mitros F, Hart M, Bosch P: Inherited ophthalmoplegia with intestinal pseudo-obstruction. *J Neurol Sci* **59**:215, 1983.
449. Ionasescu V: Oculogastrointestinal muscular dystrophy. *Am J Med Genet* **15**:103, 1983.
450. Simon LT, Horoupian DS, Dorfman LJ, Marks M, Herrick MK, Wasserstein P, Smith ME: Polyneuropathy, ophthalmoplegia, leukoencephalopathy, and intestinal pseudo-obstruction: POLIP syndrome. *Ann Neurol* **28**:349, 1990.
451. Blake D, Lombes A, Minetti C: MNGIE syndrome: Report of 2 new patients. *Neurology* **40(Suppl 1)**:294, 1990.
452. Rowland LP: Progressive external ophthalmoplegia and ocular myopathies, in Rowland LP, DiMauro S (eds): *Handbook of Clinical Neurology*. Oxford, UK, Elsevier Science, 1992, p 287.
453. Hirano M, Garcia-de-Yebenes J, Jones AC, Nishino I, DiMauro S, Carlo, Jose R., Bender AN, Hahn AF, Salberg LM, Weeks DE, Nygaard TG: Mitochondrial neurogastrointestinal encephalomyopathy syndrome maps to chromosome 22q13.32-qter. *Am J Hum Genet* **63**:526, 1998.
454. Nishino I, Spinazzola A, Hirano M: Thymidine phosphorylase gene mutations in MNGIE, a human mitochondrial disorder. *Science* **283**:689, 1999.
455. Ohno K, Tanaka M, Sahashi K, Ibi T, Sato W, Yamamoto T, Takahashi A, Ozawa T: Mitochondrial DNA deletions in inherited recurrent myoglobinuria. *Ann Neurol* **29**:364, 1991.
456. Melberg A, Holme E, Oldfors A, Lundberg PO: Rhabdomyolysis in autosomal dominant progressive external ophthalmoplegia. *Neurology* **50**:299, 1998.
457. Martin-Du Pan RC, Morris MA, Favre H, Junod A, Pizzolato GP, Bottani A: Mitochondrial anomalies in a Swiss family with autosomal dominant myoglobinuria. *Am J Med Genet* **69**:365, 1997.
458. Linderholm H, Essen-Gustavsson B, Thornell L-E: Low succinate dehydrogenase (SDH) activity in a patient with a hereditary myopathy with paroxysmal myoglobinuria. *J Intern Med* **228**:43, 1990.
459. Haller RG, Henriksson KG, Jorfeldt L, Hultman E, Wibom R, Sahlin K, Areskog N-H, Gunder M, Ayyad K, Blomqvist CG, Hall RE, Thuiller P, Kennaway NG, Lewis SF: Deficiency of skeletal muscle succinate dehydrogenase and aconitase. Pathophysiology of exercise in a novel human muscle oxidative defect. *J Clin Invest* **88**:1197, 1991.
460. van den Heuvel L, Ruitenbeek W, Smeets R, Gelman-Kohan Z, Elpeleg O, Loeffen J, Trijbels F, Mariman E, de Bruijn D, Smeitink J: Demonstration of a new pathogenic mutation in human complex I deficiency: A 5-bp duplication in the nuclear gene encoding the 18-kD (AQDQ) subunit. *Am J Hum Genet* **62**:262, 1998.
461. Loeffen J, Smeitink J, Triepels R, Smeets R, Schuelke M, Sengers R, Trijbels F, Hamel B, Mullaart R, van den Huevel L: The first nuclear-encoded complex I mutation in a patient with Leigh syndrome. *Am J Human Genet* **63**:1598, 1998.
462. Schuelke M, Smeitink J, Mariman E, Loeffen J, Plecko B, Trijbels F, Stockler-Ipsiroglu S, van den Heuvel L: Mutant NDUFV1 subunit of mitochondrial complex I causes leukodystrophy and myoclonic epilepsy. *Nat Genet* **21**:260, 1999.
463. Tiranti V, Hoertnagel K, Carrozzo R, Galimberti C, Munaro M, Granatiero M, Zelante L, Gasparini P, Marzella R, Rocchi M, Bayona-Bafaluy MP, Enriquez J-A, Uziel G, Bertini E, Dionisi-Vici C, Franco B, Meitinger T, Zeviani M: Mutations of SURF-1 in Leigh disease associated with cytochrome c oxidase deficiency. *Am J Hum Genet* **63**:1609, 1998.
464. Zhu Z, Yao J, Johns T, Fu K, De Bie I, Macmillan C, Cuthbert A, Newbold R, Wang J, Chevrette M, Brown G, Brown R, Shoubridge E: SURF1, encoding a factor involved in the biogenesis of cytochrome c oxidase. *Nat Genet* **20**:337, 1998.
465. Merante F, Petrova-Benedict R, MacKay N, Mitchell G, Lambert M, Morin C, De Braekeleer M, Laframboise R, Gagne R, Robinson BH: A biochemically distinct form of cytochrome oxidase (COX) deficiency in the Saguenay-Lac-Saint-Jean region of Quebec. *Am J Hum Genet* **53**:481, 1993.
466. Heyer E: Mitochondrial and nuclear genetic contribution of female founders to a contemporary population in northeast Quebec. *Am J Hum Genet* **56**:1450, 1995.
467. Lee N, Morin C, Mitchell G, Robinson B: Saguenay Lac Saint Jean cytochrome oxidase deficiency: sequence analysis of nuclear encoded COX subunits, chromosomal localization and a sequence anomaly in subunit VIc. *Biochim Biophys Acta* **27**:1, 1998.
468. Morin C, Mitchell G, Larochelle J, Lambert M, Ogier H, Robinson B, De Braekeleer M: Clinical, metabolic, and genetic aspects of cytochrome C oxidase deficiency in Saguenay-Lac-Saint-Jean. *Am J Hum Genet* **53**:488, 1993.
469. Packer L, Smith JR: Extension of the lifespan of cultured normal human cells by vitamin E. *Proc Natl Acad Sci U S A* **71**:4763, 1974.
470. Prick MJ, Gabreels FJ, Renier WO, Trijbels JM, Sengers RC, Slooff JL: Progressive infantile poliodystrophy. Association with disturbed pyruvate oxidation in muscle and liver. *Arch Neurol* **38**:767, 1981.
471. Prick MJ, Gabreels FJ, Renier WO, Trijbels JM, Willems JL, Janssen AJ, Slooff JL, Geelen JA, de Jager JP: Progressive infantile poliodystrophy (Alpers' disease) with a defect in citric acid cycle activity in liver and fibroblasts. *Neuropediatrics* **13**:108, 1982.
472. Gabreels FJ, Prick MJ, Trijbels JM, Renier WO, Jaspar HH, Janssen AJ, Slooff JL: Defects in citric acid cycle and the electron transport chain in progressive poliodystrophy. *Acta Neurol Scand* **70**:145, 1984.
473. Egger J, Harding BN, Boyd SG, Wilson J, Erdohazi M: Progressive neuronal degeneration of childhood (PNDC) with liver disease. *Clin Pediatr* **26**:167, 1987.
474. Greenhouse AH, Neuberger KT: The syndrome of progressive cerebral poliodystrophy. *Arch Neurol* **10**:47, 1964.
475. Jellinger K, Seitelberger F: Spongy glio-neuronal dystrophy in infancy and childhood. *Acta Neuropathol* **16**:125, 1970.
476. Sandbank U, Lerman P: Progressive cerebral poliodystrophy: Alpers' disease. Disorganized giant neuronal mitochondria on electron microscopy. *J Neurol Neurosurg Psychiatry* **35**:749, 1972.
477. Fischer JC, Ruitenbeek W, Gabreels FJ, Janssen AJ, Renier WO, Sengers RC, Stadhouders AM, ter LHJ, Trijbels JM, Veerkamp JH: A mitochondrial encephalomyopathy: The first case with an established defect at the level of coenzyme Q. *Eur J Pediatr* **144**:441, 1986.

478. Tulinius MH, Holme E, Kristiansson B, Larsson NG, Oldfors A: Mitochondrial encephalomyopathies in childhood. I. Biochemical and morphological investigations. *J Pediatr* **119**:242, 1991.
479. Tulinius MH, Holme E, Kristiansson B, Larsson NG, Oldfors A: Mitochondrial encephalomyopathies in childhood. II. Clinical manifestations and syndromes. *J Pediatr* **119**:251, 1991.
480. Prick M, Gabreels F, Renier W, Trijbels F, Jaspar H, Lamers K, Kok J: Pyruvate dehydrogenase deficiency restricted to brain. *Neurology* **31**:398, 1981.
481. Naviaux RK, Nyhan WL, Barshop BA, Poulton J, Markusic D, Karpinski NC, Haas RH: Mitochondrial DNA polymerase γ deficiency and mtDNA depletion in a child with Alpers' syndrome. *Ann Neurol* **45**:54, 1999.
482. Barrientos A, Casademont J, Saiz A, Cardellach F, Volpini V, Solans A, Tolosa E, Urbano-Marquez A, Estivill X, Nunes V: Autosomal recessive Wolfram syndrome associated with an 8.5-kb mtDNA single deletion. *Am J Hum Genet* **58**:963, 1996.
483. Barrientos A, Volpini V, Casademont J, Genis D, Manzanares JM, Ferrer I, Corral J, Cardellach F, Urbano-Marquez A, Estivill X, Nunes V: A nuclear defect in the 4p16 region predisposes to multiple mitochondrial DNA deletions in families with Wolfram syndrome. *J Clin Invest* **97**:1570, 1996.
484. De Michele G, De Fusco M, Cavalcanti F, Filla A, Marconi R, Volpe G, Monticelli A, Ballibio A, Casari G, Cocozza S: A new locus for autosomal recessive hereditary spastic paraplegia maps to chromosome 16q24.3. *Am J Hum Genet* **63**:135, 1998.
485. Casari G, De Fusco M, Ciarmatori S, Zeviani M, Mora M, Fernandez P, De Michele G, Filla A, Cocozza S, Marconi R, Durr A, Fontaine B, Ballabio A: Spastic paraplegia and OXPHOS impairment caused by mutations in paraplegin, a nuclear encoded mitochondrial metalloprotease. *Cell* **93**:973, 1998.
486. Campuzano V, Montermini L, Molto MD, Pianese L, Cossee M, Cavalcanti F, Monros E, et al.: Friedreich's ataxia: Autosomal recessive disease caused by an intronic GAA triplet repeat expansion. *Science* **271**:1423, 1996.
487. Koutnikova H, Campuzano V, Foury F, Dolle P, Cazzalini O, Koenig M: Studies of human, mouse and yeast homologues indicate a mitochondrial function for frataxin. *Nat Genet* **16**:345, 1997.
488. Rotig A, de Lonlay P, Chretien D, Foury F, Koenig M, Sidi D, Munnich A, Rustin P: Aconitase and mitochondrial iron-sulphur protein deficiency in Friedreich ataxia. *Nat Genet* **17**:215, 1997.
489. Barth PG, Scholte HR, Berden JA, Van der Klei Van Moorsel JM, Luyt-Houwen IE, Van t Veer Korthof ET, Van der Harten JJ, Sobotka Plojhar MA: An X-linked mitochondrial disease affecting cardiac muscle, skeletal muscle and neutrophil leucocytes. *J Neurol Sci* **62**:327, 1983.
490. Haese WH, Maron BJ, Mirowski M, Rowe RD, Hutchins GM: Peculiar focal myocardial degeneration and fatal ventricular arrhythmias in a child. *N Engl J Med* **287**:180, 1972.
491. Ross CF, Belton EM: A case of cardiac lipidosis. *Br Heart J* **30**:726, 1968.
492. Witzleben CL, Pinto M: Foamy myocardial transformation of infancy: Lipid or histiocytoid myocardiopathy. *Arch Pathol Lab Med* **102**:306, 1978.
493. Suarez V, Fuggle WJ, Cameron AH, French TA, Hollingworth T: Foamy myocardial transformation of infancy: An inherited disease. *J Clin Pathol* **40**:329, 1987.
494. Ino T, Sherwood WG, Cutz E, Benson LN, Rose V, Freedom RM: Dilated cardiomyopathy with neutropenia, short stature, and abnormal carnitine metabolism. *J Pediatr* **113**:511, 1988.
495. Hodgson S, Child A, Dyson M: Endocardial fibroelastosis: possible X linked inheritance. *J Med Genet* **24**:210, 1987.
496. Neustein HB, Lurie PR, Dahms B, Takahashi M: An X-linked recessive cardiomyopathy with abnormal mitochondria. *Pediatrics* 64:24, 1979.
497. Costeff H, Elpeleg O, Apter N, Divry P, Gadoth N: 3-Methylglutaconic aciduria in "optic atrophy plus." *Ann Neurol* **33**:103, 1993.
498. Bleyl SB, Mumford BR, Brown-Harrison M-C, Pagotto LT, Carey JC, Pysher TJ, Ward K, Chin TK: Xq28-linked noncompaction of the left ventricular myocardium: prenatal diagnosis and pathologic analysis of affected individuals. *Am J Med Genet* **72**:257, 1997.
499. Ades LC, Gedeon AK, Latham M, Partington M, Sillence DO, Mulley JC: Confirmation of localisation of Barth syndrome to distal Xq28. *Cytigenet Cell Genet* **58**:2053, 1991.
500. Bolhuis PA, Hensels GW, Hulsebos TJ, Baas F, Barth PG: Mapping of the locus for X-linked cardioskeletal myopathy with neutropenia and abnormal mitochondria (Barth syndrome) to Xq28. *Am J Hum Genet* **48**:481, 1991.
501. Bionne S, D'Adamo P, Maestrini E, Gedeon AK, Bolhuis PA, Toniolo D: A novel X-linked gene, G4.5 is responsible for Barth syndrome. *Nat Genet* **12**:385, 1996.
502. Bleyl SB, Mumford BR, Thompson V, Carey JC, Pysher TJ, Chin TK, Ward K: Neonatal, lethal noncompaction of the left ventricular myocardium is allelic to Barth syndrome. *Am J Hum Genet* **61**:868, 1997.
503. D'Adamo P, Fassone L, Gedeon A, Janssen EAM, Bione S, Bolhuis PA, Barth PG, Wilson M, Haan E, Orstavik KH, Patton MA, Green AJ, Zammarchi E, Donati MA, Toniolo D: The x-linked gene G4.5 is responsible for different infantile dilated cardiomyopathies. *J Hum Genet* **61**:862, 1997.
504. Hornykiewicz O, Kish SJ, Becker LE, Farley I, Shannak K: Brain neurotransmitters in dystonia musculorum deformans. *N Engl J Med* **315**:347, 1986.
505. Zweig RM, Hedreen JC, Jankel WR, Casanova MF, Whitehouse PJ, Price DL: Pathology in brainstem regions of individuals with primary dystonia. *Neurology* **38**:702, 1988.
506. Bressman SB, De Leon D, Brin M, Risch N, Burke RE, Greene PE, Shale H, Fahn S: Idiopathic dystonia among Ashkenazi Jews: Evidence for autosomal recessive dominant inheritance. *Ann Neurol* **26**:612, 1989.
507. Fletcher NA, Harding AE, Marsden CD: A genetic study of idiopathic torsion dystonia in the United Kingdom. *Brain* **113**:379, 1990.
508. Waddy HM, Fletcher NA, Harding AE, Marsden CD: A genetic study of idiopathic focal dystonias. *Ann Neurol* **29**:320, 1991.
509. Zilber N, Korczyn AD, Kahana E, Fried K, Alter M: Inheritance of idiopathic torsion dystonia among Jews. *J Med Genet* **21**:13, 1984.
510. Bundey S, Harrison MJG, Marsden CD: A genetic study of torsion dystonia. *J Med Genet* **12**:12, 1975.
511. Eldridge R: The torsion dystonias: Literature review and genetic and clinical studies. *Neurology* **20(Suppl 1)**:1, 1970.
512. Benecke R, Strumper P, Weiss H: Electron transfer Complex I defect in idiopathic dystonia. *Ann Neurol* **32**:683, 1992.
513. Bet L, Bresolin N, Moggio M, Meola G, Prelle A, Schapira AH, Binzoni T, Chomyn A, Fortunato F, Cerretelli P, Scarlato G: A case of mitochondrial myopathy, lactic acidosis and complex I deficiency. *J Neurol* **237**:399, 1990.
514. Schotland DL, DiMauro S, Bonilla E, Scarpa A, Lee CP: Neuromuscular disorder associated with a defect in mitochondrial energy supply. *Arch Neurol* **33**:475, 1976.
515. Hackett TNJ, Bray PF, Ziter FA, Nyhan WL, Creer KM: A metabolic myopathy associated with chronic lactic acidemia, growth failure, and nerve deafness. *J Pediatr* **83**:426, 1973.
516. Servidei S, Lazaro RP, Bonilla E, Barron KD, Zeviani M, DiMauro S: Mitochondrial encephalomyopathy and partial cytochrome c oxidase deficiency. *Neurology* **37**:58, 1987.
517. Worsfold M, Park DC, Pennington RJ: Familial "mitochondrial" myopathy. A myopathy associated with disordered oxidative metabolism in muscle fibres. 2. Biochemical findings. *J Neurol Sci* **19**:261, 1973.
518. Hudgson P, Bradley WG, Jenkison M: Familial "mitochondrial" myopathy. A myopathy associated with disordered oxidative metabolism in muscle fibres. 1. Clinical, electrophysiological and pathological findings. *J Neurol Sci* **16**:343, 1972.
519. Land JM, Morgan HJA, Clark JB: Mitochondrial myopathy. Biochemical studies revealing a deficiency of NADH-cytochrome b reductase activity. *J Neurol Sci* **50**:1, 1981.
520. Trockel U, Scholte HR, Toyka KV, Busch HF, Luyt HIE, Berden JA: Myopathy with abnormal mitochondria, transient low electron transport capacity in the respiratory chain, and absence of energy transduction at sites 1 and 2 in vitro. *J Neurol Neurosurg Psychiatry* **49**:645, 1986.
521. Kennaway NG, Buist NR, Darley Usmar VM, Papadimitriou A, Dimauro S, Kelley RI, Capaldi RA, Blank NK, D'Agostino A: Lactic acidosis and mitochondrial myopathy associated with deficiency of several components of complex III of the respiratory chain. *Pediatr Res* **18**:991, 1984.
522. Monnens L, Gabreels F, Willems J: A metabolic myopathy associated with chronic lactic acidemia, growth failure, and nerve deafness. *J Pediatr* **86**:983, 1975.
523. Morgan-Hughes JA, Darveniza P, Kahn SN, Landon DN, Sherratt RM, Land JM, Clark JB: A mitochondrial myopathy characterized by a deficiency in reducible cytochrome b. *Brain* **100**:617, 1977.
524. Morgan-Hughes JA, Darveniza P, Landon DN, Land JM, Clark JB: A mitochondrial myopathy with a deficiency of respiratory chain NADH-CoQ reductase activity. *J Neurol Sci* **43**:27, 1979.

525. Hayes DJ, Lecky BR, Landon DN, Morgan HJA, Clark JB: A new mitochondrial myopathy. Biochemical studies revealing a deficiency in the cytochrome b-c1 complex (complex III) of the respiratory chain. *Brain* **107**:1165, 1984.
526. Reichmann H, Rohkamm R, Zeviani M, Servidei S, Ricker K, DiMauro S: Mitochondrial myopathy due to complex III deficiency with normal reducible cytochrome b concentration. *Arch Neurol* **43**:957, 1986.
527. Harle JR, Pellissier JF, Desnuelle C, Disdier P, Figarella BD, Weiller PJ: Polymyalgia rheumatica and mitochondrial myopathy: Clinicopathologic and biochemical studies in five cases. *Am J Med* **92**:167, 1992.
528. Serratrice G, Daumen LV, Lafforgue P, Perrier H, Acquaviva PC, Pellissier JF, Desnuelle C: Inflammatory myalgic syndrome and muscular mitochondrial abnormalities: 4 cases. *Rev Rhum Mal Osteoartic* **59**:395, 1992.
529. Tarlow MJ, Lake BD, Lloyd JK: Chronic lactic acidosis in association with myopathy. *Arch Dis Child* **48**:489, 1973.
530. Werneck LC, DiMauro S: Myopathy due to succinate cytochrome C oxidoreductase deficiency: Possible defect of complex II of the respiratory chain. *Arq Neuropsiquiatr* **47**:461, 1989.
531. Kim SJ, Lee KO, Takamiya S, Capaldi RA: Mitochondrial myopathy involving ubiquinol-cytochrome c oxidoreductase (complex III) identified by immunoelectron microscopy. *Biochim Biophys Acta* **894**:270, 1987.
532. Bresolin N, Bet L, Moggio M, Mirata P, Prelle A, Pellegrini G, Scarlato G: Low cytochromes content and normal polarographic studies in a familial mitochondrial myopathy. *Neurology* **38(Suppl 1)**:188, 1988.
533. Schapira AHV, Cooper JM, Morgan-Hughes JA, Landon DN, Clark JB: Mitochondrial myopathy with a defect of mitochondrial protein transport. *N Engl J Med* **323**:37, 1990.
534. Mechler F, Fawcett PR, Mastaglia FL, Hudgson P: Mitochondrial myopathy: A study of clinically affected and asymptomatic members of a six generation family. *J Neurol Sci* **50**:191, 1981.
535. Afifi AK, Ibrahim MZM, Bergman RA, Haydar NA, Mire J, Bahuth N, Kaylani F: Morphological features of hypermetabolic mitochondrial disease: A light microscopic, histochemical and electron microscopic study. *J Neurol Sci* **15**:271, 1972.
536. Ernster L, Luft R: Further studies on a population of human skeletal muscle mitochondria lacking respiratory control. *Exp Cell Res* **32**:26, 1963.
537. DiMauro S, Bonilla E, Lee CP, Schotland DL, Scarpa A, Conn HJ, Chance B: Luft's disease. Further biochemical and ultrastructural studies of skeletal muscle in the second case. *J Neurol Sci* **27**:217, 1976.
538. Haydar NA, Conn HL, Afifi A, Wakid N, Ballas S, Fawaz K: Severe hypermetabolism with primary abnormality of skeletal muscle mitochondria. *Ann Intern Med* **74**:548, 1971.
539. Yamada EW, Huzel NJ: Distribution of the ATPase inhibitor proteins of mitochondria in mammalian tissues including fibroblasts from a patient with Luft's disease. *Biochim Biophys Acta* **1139**:143, 1992.
540. Warner TT, Schapira AH: Genetic counselling in mitochondrial diseases. *Curr Opin Neurol* **10**:408, 1997.
541. Poulton J, Marchington DR: Prospects for DNA-based prenatal diagnosis of mitochondrial disorders. *Prenat Diagn* **16**:1247, 1996.
542. Ferlin T, Landrieu P, Rambaud C, Fernandez H, Dumoulin R, Rustin P, Mousson B: Segregation of the G8993 mutant mitochondrial DNA through generations and embryonic tissues in a family at risk of Leigh syndrome. *J Pediatr* **131**:447, 1997.
543. Blok RB, Gook DA, Thorburn DR, Dahl HH: Skewed segregation of the mtDNA nt 8993 (T $\rightarrow$ G) mutation in human oocytes. *Am J Hum Genet* **60**:1495, 1997.
544. Kokot W, Iwaszkiewicz-Bilikiewiczowa B, Lewczuk A, Sworczak K: A case of Kearns-Sayre syndrome. *Klin Oczna* **98**:327, 1996.
545. Ewart RM, Burrows RF: Pregnancy in chronic progressive external ophthalmoplegia: A case report. *Am J Perinatol* **14**:293, 1997.
546. Simpson MV, Chin CD, Keilbaugh SA, Lin TS, Prusoff WH: Studies on the inhibition of mitochondrial DNA replication by 3′-azido-3′-deoxythymidine and other dideoxynucleoside analogs which inhibit HIV-1 replication. *Biochem Pharmacol* **38**:1033, 1989.
547. Izuta S, Saneyoshi M, Sakurai T, Suzuki M, Kojima K, Yoshida S: The 5′-triphosphates of 3′-azido-3′-deoxythymidine and 2′, 3′-dideoxynucleosides inhibit DNA polymerase gamma by different mechanisms. *Biochem Biophys Res Commun* **179**:776, 1991.
548. Pezeshkpour G, Illa I, Dalakas MC: Ultrastructural characteristics and DNA immunocytochemistry in human immunodeficiency virus and zidovudine-associated myopathies. *Hum Pathol* **22**:1281, 1991.
549. Dalakas MC, Illa I, Pezeshkpour GH, Laukaitis JP, Cohen B, Griffin JL: Mitochondrial myopathy caused by long-term zidovudine therapy. *N Engl J Med* **322**:1098, 1990.
550. Mhiri C, Baudrimont M, Bonne G, Geny C, Degoul F, Marsac C, Roullet E, Gherardi R: Zidovudine myopathy: A distinctive disorder associated with mitochondrial dysfunction. *Ann Neurol* **29**:606, 1991.
551. Lewis W, Gonzalez B, Chomyn A, Papoian T: Zidovudine induces molecular, biochemical, and ultrastructural changes in rat skeletal muscle mitochondria. *J Clin Invest* **89**:1354, 1992.
552. Lamperth L, Dalakas MC, Dagani F, Anderson J, Ferrari R: Abnormal skeletal and cardiac muscle mitochondria induced by zidovudine (AZT) in human muscle in vitro and in an animal model. *Lab Invest* **65**:742, 1991.
553. Arnaudo E, Dalakas M, Shanske S, Moraes CT, DiMauro S, Schon EA: Depletion of muscle mitochondrial DNA in AIDS patients with zidovudine-induced myopathy. *Lancet* **337**:508, 1991.
554. Colacino JM: Mechanisms for the anti-hepatitis B virus activity and mitochondrial toxicity of fialuridine (FIAU). *Antiviral Res* **29**:125, 1996.
555. Colacino JM, Malcolm SK, Jaskunas SR: Effect of fialuridine on replication of mitochondrial DNA in CEM cells and in human hepatoblastoma cells in culture. *Antimicrob Agents Chemother* **38**:1997, 1994.
556. Dusheiko GM: Treatment and prevention of chronic viral hepatitis. *Pharmacol Ther* **65**:47, 1995.
557. Honkoop P, Scholte HR, de Man RA, Schalm SW: Mitochondrial injury. Lessons from the fialuridine trial. *Drug Saf* **17**:1, 1997.
558. Kleiner DE, Gaffey MJ, Sallie R, Tsokos M, Nichols L, McKenzie R, Straus SE, Hoofnagle JH: Histopathologic changes associated with fialuridine hepatotoxicity. *Mod Pathol* **10**:192, 1997.
559. Lewis W, Levine ES, Griniuviene B, Tankersley KO, Colacino JM, Sommadossi JP, Watanabe KA, Perrino FW: Fialuridine and its metabolites inhibit DNA polymerase gamma at sites of multiple adjacent analog incorporation, decrease mtDNA abundance, and cause mitochondrial structural defects in cultured hepatoblasts. *Proc Natl Acad Sci U S A* **93**:3592, 1996.
560. Lewis W, Perrino FW: Severe toxicity of fialuridine (FIAU) [Letter; Comment]. *N Engl J Med* **334**:1136; discussion 1137, 1996.
561. McKenzie R, Fried MW, Sallie R, Conjeevaram H, Di Bisceglie AM, Park Y, Savarese B, Kleiner D, Tsokos M, Luciano C, et al.: Hepatic failure and lactic acidosis due to fialuridine (FIAU), an investigational nucleoside analogue for chronic hepatitis B [see Comments]. *N Engl J Med* **333**:1099, 1995.
562. Schalm SW, de Man RA, Heijtink RA, Niesters HG: New nucleoside analogues for chronic hepatitis B. *J Hepatol* **22**:52, 1995.
563. Semino-Mora C, Leon-Monzon M, Dalakas MC: Mitochondrial and cellular toxicity induced by fialuridine in human muscle in vitro. *Lab Invest* **76**:487, 1997.
564. Lewis W, Dalakas MC: Mitochondrial toxicity of antiviral drugs. *Nat Med* **1**:417, 1995.
565. Benbrik E, Chariot P, Bonavaud S, Ammi-Said M, Frisdal E, Rey C, Gherardi R, Barlovatz-Meimon G: Cellular and mitochondrial toxicity of zidovudine (AZT), didanosine (ddI) and zalcitabine (ddC) on cultured human muscle cells. *J Neurol Sci* **149**:19, 1997.
566. Domanski MJ, Sloas MM, Follmann DA, Scalise PPR, Tucker EE, Egan D, Pizzo PA: Effect of zidovudine and didanosine treatment on heart function in children infected with human immunodeficiency virus [see Comments]. *J Pediatr* **127**:137, 1995.
567. Famularo G, Moretti S, Marcellini S, Trinchieri V, Tzantzoglou S, Santini G, Longo A, De Simone C: Acetyl-carnitine deficiency in AIDS patients with neurotoxicity on treatment with antiretroviral nucleoside analogues. *Aids* **11**:185, 1997.
568. Medina DJ, Tsai CH, Hsiung GD, Cheng YC: Comparison of mitochondrial morphology, mitochondrial DNA content, and cell viability in cultured cells treated with three anti-human immunodeficiency virus dideoxynucleosides. *Antimicrob Agents Chemother* **38**:1824, 1994.
569. Pedrol E, Masanes F, Fernandez-Sola J, Cofan M, Casademont J, Grau JM, Urbano-Marquez A: Lack of muscle toxicity with didanosine (ddI). Clinical and experimental studies. *J Neurol Sci* **138**:42, 1996.
570. Honkoop P, de Man RA, Scholte HR, Zondervan PE, Van Den Berg JW, Rademakers LH, Schalm SW: Effect of lamivudine on morphology and function of mitochondria in patients with chronic hepatitis B. *Hepatology* **26**:211, 1997.
571. Fromenty B, Pessayre D: Impaired mitochondrial function in microvesicular steatosis. Effects of drugs, ethanol, hormones and cytokines. *J Hepatol* **26(Suppl 2)**:43, 1997.

572. Lam CW, Lau CH, Williams JC, Chan YW, Wong LJ: Mitochondrial myopathy, encephalopathy, lactic acidosis and stroke-like episodes (MELAS) triggered by valproate therapy. *Eur J Pediatr* **156**:562, 1997.
573. Chabrol B, Mancini J, Chretien D, Rustin P, Munnich A, Pinsard N: Cytochrome c oxidase defect, fatal hepatic failure and valproate: A case report. *Eur J Pediatr* **153**:133, 1994.
574. Munnich A, Rotig A, Chretien D, Saudubray JM, Cormier V, Rustin P: Clinical presentations and laboratory investigations in respiratory chain deficiency. *Eur J Pediatr* **155**:262, 1996.
575. Ponchaut S, Veitch K: Valproate and mitochondria. *Biochem Pharmacology* **46**:199, 1993.
576. Hayasaka K, Takahashi I, Kobayashi Y, Iinuma K, Narisawa K, Taka K: Effects of valproate on biogenesis and function of liver mitochondria. *Neurology* **36**:351, 1986.
577. Jaksch M, Klopstock T, Kurlemann G, Dorner M, Hofmann S, Kleinle S, Hegemann S, Weissert M, Muller-Hocker J, Pongratz D, Gerbitz K-D: Progressive myoclonus epilepsy and mitochondrial myopathy associated with mutations in the tRNA-Serine(UCN) gene. *Ann Neurol* **44**:635, 1998.
578. Taylor RW, Chinnery PF, Clark KM, Lightowlers RN, Turnbull DM: Treatment of mitochondrial disease. *J Bioenerg Biomembr* **29**:195, 1997.
579. Takeshige K, Takayanagi R, Shigeki M: Reduced coenzyme Q10 as an antioxidant of lipid peroxidation in bovine heart mitochondria, in Yamamura Y, Folkers, Ito Y (eds): *Biomedical and Clinical Aspects of Coenzyme Q*. Amsterdam, Elsevier/North-Holland Biomedical, 1980, p 15.
580. Landi L, Cabrini L, Sechi AM, Pasquali P: Antioxidative effect of ubiquinones in mitochondrial membranes. *Biochem J* **222**:463, 1984.
581. Lenaz G, Esposti MD: Physical properties of ubiquinones in model systems and membranes, in Lenaz G (ed): *Coenzyme Q*. New York, Wiley, 1985, p 83.
582. Lenaz G, De Santis A, Bertoli E: A survey of the function and specificity of ubiquinone in the mitochondrial respiratory chain, in Lenaz G (ed): *Coenzyme Q*. New York, Wiley, 1985, p 165.
583. Sugiyama S, Kitazawa M, Ozawa T, Suzuki K, Izawa Y: Antioxidative effect of coenzyme Q10. *Experientia* **36**:1002, 1980.
584. Spisni A, Masotti L, Lenaz G, Bertoli E, Pedulli GF, Zannoni C: Interactions between ubiquinones and phospholipid bilayers. A spin-label study. *Arch Biochem Biophys* **190**:454, 1978.
585. Frei B, Kim MC, Ames BN: Ubiquinol-10 is an effective lipid-soluble antioxidant at physiological concentrations. *Proc Natl Acad Sci U S A* **87**:4879, 1990.
586. Linn BO, Page AC, Wong EL, Gale PH, Shunk CH, Folkers K: Isolation and distribution of coenzyme Q10 in animal tissues. *J Am Chem Soc* **81**:4007, 1959.
587. Sustry PS, Jayaraman J, Ramasarma T: Distribution of coenzyme Q in rat liver cell fractions. *Nature* **189**:577, 1961.
588. Tomono Y, Hasegawa J, Seki T, Motegi K, Morishita N: Pharmacokinetic study of deuterium-labelled coenzyme Q10 in man. *Int J Clin Pharmacol Ther Toxicol* **24**:536, 1986.
589. Yuzuriha T, Takada M, Katayama K: Transport of [14C]coenzyme Q10 from the liver to other tissues after intravenous administration to guinea pigs. *Biochim Biophys Acta* **759**:286, 1983.
590. Lucker PF, Wetzelsberger N, Hennings G, et al.: Pharmakokinetics of coenzyme ubidecarenone in healthy volunteers, in Folkers K, Yamamura Y (eds): *Biomedical and Clinical Aspects of Coenzyme Q*. Amsterdam, Elsevier Science, 1984, p 143.
591. Ogasahara S, Yorifuji S, Nishikawa Y, Takahashi M, Wada K, Hazama T, Nakamura Y, Hashimoto S, Kono N, Tarui S: Improvement of abnormal pyruvate metabolism and cardiac conduction defect with coenzyme Q10 in Kearns-Sayre syndrome. *Neurology* **35**:372, 1985.
592. Ogasahara S, Nishikawa Y, Yorifuji S, Soga F, Nakamura Y, Takahashi M, Hashimoto S, Kono N, Tarui S: Treatment of Kearns-Sayre syndrome with coenzyme Q10. *Neurology* **36**:45, 1986.
593. Bet L, Bresolin N, Binda A, Nador F, Ferrante C, Comi G, Scarlato G: Cardiac improvement after coenzyme Q10 treatment with Kearns-Sayre syndrome. *Neurology* **37(Suppl 1)**:202, 1987.
594. Bresolin N, Bet L, Binda A, Moggio M, Comi G, Nador F, Ferrante C, Carenzi A, Scarlato G: Clinical and biochemical correlations in mitochondrial myopathies treated with coenzyme Q10. *Neurology* **38**:892, 1988.
595. Desnuelle C, Pellisier JF, Serratrice G, Pouget J: Chronic progressive external ophthalmoplegia (CPEO) associated with diaphragm paralysis: Successful treatment with coenzyme Q (CoQ). *Neurology* **38(Suppl 1)**:102, 1988.
596. Nishikawa Y, Takahashi M, Yorifuji S, Nakamura Y, Ueno S, Tarui S, Kozuka T, Nishimura T: Long-term coenzyme Q10 therapy for a mitochondrial encephalomyopathy with cytochrome c oxidase deficiency: A 31P NMR study. *Neurology* **39**:399, 1989.
597. Ihara Y, Namba R, Kuroda S: A case of mitochondrial myopathy, encephalopathy, lactic acidosis and strokelike episodes (MELAS)—Treatment with coenzyme Q10 and idebenone. *Rinsho Shinkeigaku* **28**:62, 1988.
598. Abe K, Fujimura H, Nishikawa Y, Yorifuji S, Mezaki T, Hirono N, Nishitani N, Kameyama M: Marked reduction in CSF lactate and pyruvate levels after CoQ therapy in a patient with mitochondrial myopathy, encephalopathy, lactic acidosis and stroke-like episodes (MELAS). *Acta Neurol Scand* **83**:356, 1991.
599. Bendahan D, Desnuelle C, Vanuxem D, Confort GS, Figarella BD, Pellissier JF, Kozak RG, Pouget J, Serratrice G, Cozzone PJ: ^{31}P NMR spectroscopy and ergometer exercise test as evidence for muscle oxidative performance improvement with coenzyme Q in mitochondrial myopathies. *Neurology* **42**:1203, 1992.
600. Bresolin N, Doriguzzi C, Ponzetto C, Angelini C, Moroni I, Castelli E, Cossutta E, Binda A, Gallanti A, Gabellini S, et al.: Ubidecarenone in the treatment of mitochondrial myopathies: A multi-center double-blind trial. *J Neurol Sci* **100**:70, 1990.
601. Zierz S, Jahns G, Jerusalem F: Coenzyme Q in serum and muscle of 5 patients with Kearns-Sayre syndrome and 12 patients with ophthalmoplegia plus. *J Neurol* **236**:97, 1989.
602. Imagawa M: Therapy with a combination of coenzyme Q10, vitamin B6, and iron for Alzheimer's disease and senile dementia of Alzheimer's type, in Iqbal Kea (ed): *Alzheimer's Disease: Basic Mechanisms, Diagnosis, and Strategies*. New York, Wiley, 1991, p 649.
603. Imagawa M, Naruse S, Tsuji S, Fujioka A, Yamaguchi H: Coenzyme Q10, iron, and vitamin B6 in genetically-confirmed Alzheimer's disease. *Lancet* **340**:671, 1992.
604. Hiasa Y, Ishida T, Maeda T, et al.: Effects of coenzyme Q10 on exercise tolerance in patients with stable angina pectoris, in Folkers K, Yamamura Y (eds): *Biomedical and Clinical Aspects of Coenzyme Q*. Amsterdam, Elsevier Science, 1984, p 269.
605. Karlsson J, Diamant B, Folkers K, Lund B: Muscle fibre types, ubiquinone content and exercise capacity in hypertension and effort angina. *Ann Med* **23**:339, 1991.
606. Langsjoen PH, Vadhanavikit S, Folkers K: Effective treatment with coenzyme Q10 of patients with chronic myocardial disease. *Drugs Exp Clin Res* **11**:577, 1985.
607. Langsjoen PH, Vadhanavikit S, Folkers K: Response of patients in classes III and IV of cardiomyopathy to therapy in a blind and crossover trial with coenzyme Q10. *Proc Natl Acad Sci U S A* **82**:4240, 1985.
608. Littarru GP, Ho L, Folkers K: Deficiency of coenzyme Q 10 in human heart disease. II. *Int J Vitam Nutr Res* **42**:413, 1972.
609. Folkers K, Littarru GP, Ho L, Runge TM, Havanonda S, Cooley D: Evidence for a deficiency of coenzyme Q10 in human heart disease. *Int Z Vitaminforsch* **40**:380, 1970.
610. Folkers K, Vadhanavikit S, Mortensen SA: Biochemical rationale and myocardial tissue data on the effective therapy of cardiomyopathy with coenzyme Q10. *Proc Natl Acad Sci U S A* **82**:901, 1985.
611. Mortensen SA, Vadhanavikit S, Baandrup U, Folkers K: Long-term coenzyme Q10 therapy: A major advance in the management of resistant myocardial failure. *Drugs Exp Clin Res* **11**:581, 1985.
612. Vadhanavikit S, Sakamoto N, Ashida N, Kishi T, Folkers K: Quantitative determination of coenzyme Q10 in human blood for clinical studies. *Anal Biochem* **142**:155, 1984.
613. Cortes EP, Gupta M, Chou C, Amin VC, Folkers K: Adriamycin cardiotoxicity: Early detection by systolic time interval and possible prevention by coenzyme Q10. *Cancer Treat Rep* **62**:887, 1978.
614. Kishi T, Watanabe T, Folkers K: Bioenergetics in clinical medicine: Prevention by forms of coenzyme Q of the inhibition by Adriamycin of coenzyme Q10-enzymes in mitochondria of the myocardium. *Proc Natl Acad Sci U S A* **73**:4653, 1976.
615. Kishi T, Folkers K: Letter: Prevention by coenzyme Q10 (NSC-140865) of the inhibition by Adriamycin (NSC-123127) of coenzyme Q10 enzymes. *Cancer Treat Rep* **60**:223, 1976.
616. Folkers K, Baker L, Richardson PC, Shizukuishi S, Takemura K, Drzewoski J, Lewandowski J, Ellis JM: in Folkers K, Yamamura Y (eds): *Biomedical and Clinical Aspects of Coenzyme Q*. Amsterdam, North-Holland Biomedical Press, 1981, p 399.
617. Argov Z, Bank WJ, Maris J, Eleff S, Kennaway NG, Olson RE, Chance B: Treatment of mitochondrial myopathy due to complex III deficiency with vitamins K3 and C: A ^{31}P-NMR follow-up study. *Ann Neurol* **19**:598, 1986.

618. Warshaw JR, Lam KW, Sanadi DR: Studies on oxidative phosphorylation XI. Energy dependent reduction of diphosphopyridine nucleotide by enediol compounds in the presence of dyes. *Arch Biochem Biophys* **115**:307, 1966.
619. Sanadi DR: On the mechanism of oxidative phosphorylation IX. Energy-dependent reduction of nicotinamide adenine dinucleotide by ascorbate and ubiquinone or menadione. *Biochim Biophys Acta* **89**:367, 1964.
620. Nosoh Y, Kajioka J, Itoh M: Effect of menadione on the electron transport pathway of yeast mitochondria. *Arch Biochem Biophys* **127**:1, 1968.
621. Brivet-Chevillotte P, di Rago JP: Electron-transfer restoration by vitamin K3 in a complex III-deficient mutant of *S. cerevisiae* and sequence of the corresponding cytochrome b mutation. *FEBS Lett* **255**:5, 1989.
622. Kotlyar AB, Gutman M, Ackrell BAC: Interaction of ubiquinone and vitamin K3 with mitochondrial succinate-ubiquinone oxidoreductase. *Biochem Biophys Res Commun* **186**:1656, 1992.
623. Wijburg FA, Feller N, De Groot CJ, Wanders RJA: Menadione partially restores NADH-oxidation and ATP-synthesis in complex I deficient fibroblasts. *Biochem Int* **22**:303, 1990.
624. Wijburg FA, De Groot CJ, Feller N, Wanders JA: Restoration of NADH-oxidation in complex I and complex III deficient fibroblasts by menadione. *J Inherit Metab Dis* **14**:293, 1991.
625. De Groot H, Noll T, Sies H: Oxygen dependence and subcellular partitioning of hepatic menadione mediated oxygen uptake: Studies with isolated hepatocytes, mitochondria, and microsomes from rat liver in an oxystat system. *Arch Biochem Biophys* **243**:556, 1985.
626. Cooper JM, Hayes DJ, Challiss RAJ, Morgan-Hughes JA, Clark JB: Treatment of experimental NADH ubiquinone reductase deficiency with menadione. *Brain* **115**:991, 1992.
627. Suttie JW: Vitamin K, in Diplock AT (ed): *Fat-Soluble Vitamins: Their Biochemistry and Applications.* Lancaster, Technomic, 1985, p 225.
628. Thierry MJ, Hermodson MA, Suttie JW: Vitamin K and warfarin distribution and metabolism in the warfarin-resistant rat. *Am J Physiol* **219**:354, 1970.
629. Kobayashi M, Morishita H, Okajima K, Sugiyama N, Wada Y: Successful treatment with succinate supplement in a patient with a deficiency of Complex I (NADH-CoQ reductase). *The Fourth International Congress of Inborn Errors of Metabolism*, May 23-30, Sendai, Japan, 1987, p 148.
630. Lou HC: Correction of increased plasma pyruvate and plasma lactate levels using large doses of thiamine in patients with Kearns-Sayre syndrome. *Arch Neurol* **38**:469, 1981.
631. Arts WF, Scholte HR, Bogaard JM, Kerrebijn KF, Luyt Houwen IE: NADH-CoQ reductase deficient myopathy: Successful treatment with riboflavin. *Lancet* **2**:581, 1983.
632. Ogle RF, Christodoulou J, Fagan E, Blok RB, Kirby DM, Seller KL, Dahl HH, Thorburn DR: Mitochondrial myopathy with tRNA(-Leu(UUR)) mutation and complex I deficiency responsive to riboflavin. *J Pediatr* **130**:138, 1997.
633. Majamaa K, Rusanen H, Remes A, Hassinen IE: Metabolic interventions against complex I deficiency in MELAS syndrome. *Mol Cell Biochem* **174**:291, 1997.
634. Nagai TJ, Arai H, Inui K, Jamanouchi H, Goto Y, Nonaka I, Okada S: Treatment of mitochondrial encephalomyopathy with a combination of cytochrome c and vitamins B1 and B2. *Brain Dev* **19**:262, 1997.
635. Patten BM, Phillips PC, DiMauro S, De Vivo DC, Rowland LP: Mitochondrial myopathy associated with abnormal lactate metabolism: Response to prednisone in three patients. *Neurology* **26**:370, 1984.
636. Mastaglia FL, Thompson PL, Papadimitriou JM: Mitochondrial myopathy with cardiomyopathy, lactic acidosis and response to prednisone and thiamine. *Aust N Z J Med* **10**:660, 1980.
637. Heiman-Patterson TD, Argov Z, Chavin JM, Kalman B, Alder H, DiMauro S, Bank W, Tahmoush AJ: Biochemical and genetic studies in a family with mitochondrial myopathy. *Muscle Nerve* **20**:1219, 1997.
638. Bachynski BN, Flynn JT, Rodrigues MM, Rosenthal S, Cullen R, Curless RG: Hyperglycemic acidotic coma and death in Kearns-Sayre syndrome. *Ophthalmology* **93**:391, 1986.
639. Peterson PL, Martens M, Lee CP: The treatment of mitochondrial disease. *Neurology* **36(Suppl 1)**:95, 1986.
640. Nagaoka A, Suno M, Shibota M, Kakihana M: Effects of idebenone (CV-2619) on neurological deficits, local cerebral blood flow, and energy metabolism in rats with experimental cerebral ischemia. *Nippon Yakurigaku Zasshi* **84**:303, 1984.
641. Yamazaki N, Take Y, Nagaoka A, Nagawa Y: Beneficial effect of idebenone (CV-2619) on cerebral ischemia-induced amnesia in rats. *Jpn J Pharmacol* **36**:349, 1984.
642. Kawakami M, Itoh T: Effects of idebenone on monoamine metabolites in cerebrospinal fluid of patients with cerebrovascular dementia. *Arch Gerontol Geriatr* **8**:343, 1989.
643. Narumi S, Nagaoka A, Nagawa Y: Effects of idebenone (CV-2619) on endogenous monoamine release and cyclic AMP formation in diencephalon slices from rats. *Jpn J Pharmacol* **37**:218, 1985.
644. Narumi S, Nagai Y, Kakihana M, Yamazaki N, Nagaoka A, Nagawa Y: Effects of idebenone (CV-2619) on metabolism of monoamines, especially serotonin, in the brain of normal rats and rats with cerebral ischemia. *Jpn J Pharmacol* **37**:235, 1985.
645. Kakihana M, Yamazaki N, Nagaoka A: Effects of idebenone (CV-2619) on the concentrations of acetylcholine and choline in various brain regions of rats with cerebral ischemia. *Jpn J Pharmacol* **36**:357, 1984.
646. Suno M, Nagaoka A: Inhibition of lipid peroxidation by a novel compound, idebenone (CV-2619). *Jpn J Pharmacol* **35**:196, 1984.
647. Barkworth MF, Dyde CJ, Johnson KI, Schnelle K: An early phase I study to determine the tolerance, safety and pharmacokinetics of idebenone following multiple oral doses. *Arzneimittelforschung* **35**:1704, 1985.
648. Ihara Y, Namba R, Kuroda S, Sato T, Shirabe T: Mitochondrial encephalomyopathy (MELAS): Pathological study and successful therapy with coenzyme Q10 and idebenone. *J Neurol Sci* **90**:263, 1989.
649. Mashima Y, Hiida Y, Oguchi Y: Remission of Leber's hereditary optic neuropathy with idebenone [Letter]. *Lancet* **340**:368, 1992.
650. Latipaa PM, Hiltunen JK, Peuhkurinen KJ, Hassinen IE: Regulation of fatty acid oxidation in heart muscle. Effects of pyruvate and dichloroacetate. *Biochem Biophys Acta* **752**:162, 1983.
651. Satcpoole PW, Felts JM: Diisopropylammonium dichloroacetate: Regulation of metabolic intermediates in muscle of alloxan diabetic rats. *Metabolism* **20**:830, 1971.
652. McAllister A, Allison SP, Randle PJ: Effects of dichloroacetate on the metabolism of glucose, pyruvate, acetate, 3-hydroxybutyrate and palmitate in rat diaphragm and heart muscle in vitro and on extraction of glucose, lactate, pyruvate, and free fatty acids by dog heart in vivo. *Biochem J* **134**:1067, 1973.
653. Stacpoole PW, Felts JM: Diisopropylammonium dichloroacetate (DIPA) and sodium dichloroacetate (DCA): Effect on glucose and fat metabolism in normal and diabetic tissue. *Metabolism* **19**:71, 1970.
654. Whitehouse S, Randle PJ: Activation of pyruvate dehydrogenase in perfused rat heart by dichloroacetate. *Biochem J* **134**:651, 1973.
655. Pratt ML, Roche TE: Mechanism of pyruvate inhibition of kidney pyruvate dehydrogenase kinase and synergistic inhibition by pyruvate and ADP. *J Biol Chem* **254**:7191, 1979.
656. Whitehouse S, Cooper RH, Randle PJ: Mechanism of activation of pyruvate dehydrogenase by dichloroacetate and other halogenated carboxylic acids. *Biochem J* **141**:761, 1974.
657. Passoneau JV, Lowry OH: Phosphofructokinase and the Pasteur effect. *Biochem BIophys Res Commun* **7**:10, 1962.
658. Sobrino F, Gualberto A, Gonzalez-Rivero J: Regulation of fructose-2,6-biphosphate and glycogen synthesis by dichloroacetate and phenazine methosulphate in rat adipose tissue. *Biochem Intern* **12**:767, 1986.
659. Crabb DW, Harris RA: Mechanism responsible for the hypoglycemic actions of dichloroacetate and 2-chloropropionate. *Arch Biochem Biophys* **198**:145, 1979.
660. Harris RA, Crabb DW: Inhibition of hepatic gluconeogenesis by dichloroacetate. *Arch Biochem Biophys* **189**:364, 1978.
661. Stacpoole PW: Effect of dichloroacetate on gluconeogenesis in isolated rat hepatocytes. *Metabolism* **26**:107, 1976.
662. Lasey JH, Randle PJ: Inhibition of lactate gluconeogenesis in rat kidney by dichloroacetate. *Biochem J* **170**:551, 1978.
663. Demaugre F, Cepanec C, Leroux JP: Characterization of oxalate as a catabolite of dichloroacetate responsible for the inhibition of gluconeogenesis and pyruvate carboxylation in rat liver cells. *Biochem Biophys Res Commun* **85**:1180, 1978.
664. Snell K, Duff DA: Branched-chain amino acid metabolism and alanine formation in rat diaphragm muscle in vitro. *Biochem J* **223**:831, 1984.
665. Goodman ML, Ruderman NB, Aoki TT: Glucose and amino acid metabolism in perfused skeletal muscle. Effect of dichloroacetate. *Diabetes* **27**:1065, 1978.

666. Snell K, Duff DA: The release of alanine by rat diaphragm muscle in vitro. *Biochem J* **162**:399, 1977.
667. Snell K: Alanine release by rat hemidiaphragm muscle in vitro. *Bio Soc Trans* **4**:287, 1976.
668. Searle GL, Felts JM, Shakelford R: Acute effects of dichloroacetate in the depancreatized dog: Glucose synthesis and turnover. *Diabetologia* **23**:45, 1982.
669. Stacpoole PW, Harman EM, Curry SH, Baumgartner TG, Misbin RI: Treatment of lactic acidosis with dichloroacetate. *N Engl J Med* **309**:390, 1983.
670. Stacpoole PW, Lorenz AC, Thomas RG, Harman EM: Dichloroacetate in the treatment of lactic acidosis. *Ann Intern Med* **108**:58, 1988.
671. Blackshear PJ, Fang LST, Axelrod L: Treatment of severe lactic acidosis with dichloroacetate. *Diabetes Care* **5**:391, 1982.
672. Stacpoole PW, Wright EC, Baumgartner TG, Bersin RM, Buchalter S, Curry SH, Duncan CA, Harman EM, Henderson GN, Jenkinson S, Lachin JM, Lorenz A, Schneider SH, Siegel JH, Summer WR, Thompson DT, Wolfe CL, Zorovich B, Group TDS: A controlled clinical trial of dichloroacetate for treatment of lactic acidosis in adults. *N Engl J Med* **327**:1564, 1992.
673. Saijo T, Naito E, Ito M, Takeda E, Hashimoto T, Kuroda Y: Therapeutic effect of sodium dichloroacetate on visual and auditory hallucinations in a patient with MELAS. *Neuropediatrics* **22**:166, 1990.
674. Takanashi J, Sugita K, Tanabe Y, Maemoto T, Niimi H: Dichloroacetate treatment in Leigh syndrome caused by mitochondrial DNA mutation. *J Neurol Sci* **145**:83, 1997.
675. Taivassalo T, De Stefano N, Argov Z, Matthews PM, Chen J, Genge A, Karpati G, Arnold DL: Effects of aerobic training in patients with mitochondrial myopathies. *Neurology* **50**:1055, 1998.
676. Carrozzo R, Hirano M, Fromenty B, Casali C, Santorelli FM, Bonilla E, DiMauro S, Schon EA, Miranda AF: Multiple mtDNA deletions features in autosomal dominant and recessive diseases suggest distinct pathogeneses. *Neurology* **50**:99, 1998.
677. Moslemi AR, Melberg A, Holme E, Oldfors A: Clonal expansion of mitochondrial DNA with multiple deletions in autosomal dominant progressive external ophthalmoplegia [see Comments]. *Ann Neurol* **40**:707, 1996.
678. Shoubridge EA: Autosomal dominant chronic progressive external ophthalmoplegia: a tale of two genomes [Editorial; Comment]. *Ann Neurol* **40**:693, 1996.
679. Kawai H, Akaike M, Yokoi K, Nishida Y, Kunishige M, Mine H, Saito S: Mitochondrial encephalomyopathy with autosomal dominant inheritance: A clinical and genetic entity of mitochondrial diseases. *Muscle Nerve* **18**:753, 1995.
680. Kawashima S, Ohta S, Kagawa Y, Yoshida M, Nishizawa M: Widespread tissue distribution of multiple mitochondrial DNA deletions in familial mitochondrial myopathy. *Muscle Nerve* **17**:741, 1994.
681. Kawashima S, Nishizawa M: [Multiple mitochondrial DNA deletions in chronic progressive external ophthalmoplegia (CPEO).] *Nippon Rinsho* **51**:2391, 1993.
682. Kawai H, Akaike M, Yokoi K, Tamaki Y, Saito S: [Mitochondrial myopathy with autosomal dominant inheritance — Report of a family and review of the literature.] *Rinsho Shinkeigaku* **33**:162, 1993.
683. Suomalainen A, Majander A, Haltia M, Somer H, Lonnqvist J, Savontaus ML, Peltonen L: Multiple deletions of mitochondrial DNA in several tissues of a patient with severe retarded depression and familial progressive external ophthalmoplegia. *J Clin Invest* **90**:61, 1992.
684. Haltia M, Suomalainen A, Majander A, Somer H: Disorders associated with multiple deletions of mitochondrial DNA. *Brain Pathol* **2**:133, 1992.
685. Zeviani M, Bresolin N, Gellera C, Bordoni A, Pannacci M, Amati P, Moggio M, Servidei S, Scarlato G, DiDonato S: Nucleus-driven multiple large-scale deletions of the human mitochondrial genome: A new autosomal dominant disease. *Am J Hum Genet* **47**:904, 1990.
686. Marsac C, Degoul F, Bonne G, Romero N, Nelson I, Fardeau M, Francois D, Ponsot G, Harpey JP, Eymard B: Mitochondrial function and mitochondrial DNA in a series of 64 patients suspected of having mitochondrial myopathy. *Rev Neurol (Paris)* **147**:462, 1991.
687. Otsuka M, Niijima K, Mizuno Y, Yoshida M, Kagawa Y, Ohta S: Marked decrease of mitochondrial DNA with multiple deletions in a patient with familial mitochondrial myopathy. *Biochem Biophys Res Commun* **167**:680, 1990.
688. Melberg A, Arnell H, Dahl N, Stalberg E, Raininko R, Oldfors A, Bakall B, Lundberg PO, Holme E: Anticipation of autosomal dominant progressive external ophthalmoplegia with hypogonadism. *Muscle Nerve* **19**:1561, 1996.
689. Lestienne P, Reynier P, Chretien MF, Penisson-Besnier I, Malthiery Y, Rohmer V: Oligoasthenospermia associated with multiple mitochondrial DNA rearrangements. *Mol Hum Reprod* **3**:811, 1997.
690. Blumenthal DT, Shanske S, Schochet SS, Santorelli FM, DiMauro S, Jaynesm M, Bodensteiner J: Myoclonus epilepsy with ragged red fibers and multiple mtDNA deletions. *Neurology* **50**:524, 1998.
691. Campos Y, Martin MA, Rubio JC, Ricard C, Cabello A, Arenas J: Multiple deletions of mitochondrial DNA in muscle from a patient with benign progressive external ophthalmoplegia. *J Inherit Metab Dis* **19**:366, 1996.
692. Ville-Ferlin T, Dumoulin R, Stepien G, Matha V, Bady B, Flocard F, Carrier H, Mathieu M, Mousson B: Fine mapping of randomly distributed multiple deletions of mitochondrial DNA in a case of chronic progressive external ophthalmoplegia. *Mol Cell Probes* **9**:207, 1995.
693. Uncini A, Servidei S, Silvestri G, Manfredi G, Sabatelli M, Di Muzio A, Ricci E, Mirabella M, DiMauro S, Tonali P: Ophthalmoplegia, demyelinating neuropathy, leukoencephalopathy, myopathy, and gastrointestinal dysfunction with multiple deletions of mitochondrial DNA: A mitochondrial multisystem disorder in search of a name. *Muscle Nerve* **17**:667, 1994.
694. Fadic R, Russell JA, Vedanarayanan VV, Lehar M, Kuncl RW, Johns DR: Sensory ataxic neuropathy as the presenting feature of a novel mitochondrial disease. *Neurology* **49**:239, 1997.
695. Suomalainen A, Paetau A, Leinonen H, Majander A, Peltonen L, Somer H: Inherited idiopathic dilated cardiomyopathy with multiple deletions of. *Lancet* **340**:1319, 1992.
696. Reynier P, Chretien MF, Penisson-Besnier I, Malthiery Y, Rohmer V, Lestienne P: Male infertility associated with multiple mitochondrial DNA rearrangements. *C R Acad Sci III* **320**:629, 1997.
697. Checcarelli N, Prelle A, Moggio M, Comi G, Bresolin N, Papadimitriou A, Fagiolari G, Bordoni A, Scarlato G: Multiple deletions of mitochondrial DNA in sporadic and atypical cases of encephalomyopathy. *J Neurol Sci* **123**:74, 1994.
698. Chalmers RM, Brockington M, Howard RS, Lecky BR, Morgan-Hughes JA, Harding AE: Mitochondrial encephalopathy with multiple mitochondrial DNA deletions: A report of two families and two sporadic cases with unusual clinical and neuropathological features. *J Neurol Sci* **143**:41, 1996.
699. Melegh B, Bock I, Gati I, Mehes K: Multiple mitochondrial DNA deletions and persistent hyperthermia in a patient with Brachmann-de Lange phenotype. *Am J Med Genet* **65**:82, 1996.
700. Zhang C, Baumer A, Mackay IR, Linnane AW, Nagley P: Unusual pattern of mitochondrial DNA deletions in skeletal muscle of an adult human with chronic fatigue syndrome. *Hum Mol Genet* **4**:751, 1995.
701. Reynier P, Pellissier JF, Harle JR, Malthiery Y: Multiple deletions of the mitochondrial DNA in polymyalgia rheumatica. *Biochem Biophys Res Commun* **205**:375, 1994.
702. Bet L, Moggio M, Comi GP, Mariani C, Prelle A, Checcarelli N, Bordoni A, Bresolin N, Scarpini E, Scarlato G: Multiple sclerosis and mitochondrial myopathy: An unusual combination of diseases. *J Neurol* **241**:511, 1994.
703. Prelle A, Moggio M, Checcarelli N, Comi G, Bresolin N, Battistel A, Bordoni A, Scarlato G: Multiple deletions of mitochondrial DNA in a patient with periodic attacks of paralysis. *J Neurol Sci* **117**:24, 1993.
704. Threlkeld AB, Miller NR, Golnik KC, Griffin JW, Kuncl RW, Johns DR, Lehar M, Hurko O: Ophthalmic involvement in myo-neuro-gastrointestinal encephalopathy. *Am J Ophthalmol* **114**:322, 1992.
705. Johns DR, Threlkeld AB, Miller NR, Hurko O: Multiple mitochondrial DNA deletions in myo-neuro-gastrointestinal encephalopathy syndrome [Letter]. *Am J Ophthalmol* **115**:108, 1993.
706. Hirano M, Silvestri G, Blake DM, Lombes A, Minetti C, Bonilla E, Hays AP, Lovelace RE, Butler I, Bertorini TE, et al.: Mitochondrial neurogastrointestinal encephalomyopathy (MNGIE): Clinical, biochemical, and genetic features of an autosomal recessive mitochondrial disorder. *Neurology* **44**:721, 1994.
707. Hamano H, Ohta T, Takekawa Y, Kouda K, Shinohara Y: Mitochondrial neurogastrointestinal encephalomyopathy presenting with protein-losing gastroenteropathy and serum copper deficiency: A case report. *Rinsho Shinkeigaku* **37**:917, 1997.
708. Rowland LP, Blake DM, Hirano M, DiMauro S, Schon EA, Hays AP, Devivo DC: Clinical syndromes associated with ragged red fibers. *Rev Neurol (Paris)* **147**:467, 1991.
709. Macmillan CJ, Shoubridge EA: Mitochondrial DNA depletion: Prevalence in a pediatric population referred for neurologic evaluation. *Pediatr Neurol* **14**:203, 1996.

710. Andreetta F, Tritschler HJ, Schon EA, DiMauro S, Bonilla E: Localization of mitochondrial DNA in normal and pathological muscle using immunological probes: A new approach to the study of mitochondrial myopathies. *J Neurol Sci* **105**:88, 1991.
711. Morris AA, Taanman JW, Blake J, Cooper JM, Lake BD, Malone M, Love S, Clayton PT, Leonard JV, Schapira AH: Liver failure associated with mitochondrial DNA depletion. *J Hepatol* **28**:556, 1998.
712. Spelbrink JN, Van Galen MJ, Zwart R, Bakker HD, Rovio A, Jacobs HT, Van den Bogert C: Familial mitochondrial DNA depletion in liver: Haplotype analysis of candidate genes. *Hum Genet* **102**:327, 1998.
713. Bakker HD, Van den Bogert C, Scholte HR, Zwart R, Wijburg FA, Spelbrink JN: Fatal neonatal liver failure and depletion of mitochondrial DNA in three children of one family. *J Inherit Metab Dis* **19**:112, 1996.
714. Mazziotta MR, Ricci E, Bertini E, Vici CD, Servidei S, Burlina AB, Sabetta G, Bartuli A, Manfredi G, Silvestri G, et al.: Fatal infantile liver failure associated with mitochondrial DNA. *J Pediatr* **121**:896, 1992.
715. Maaswinkel-Mooij PD, Van den Bogert C, Scholte HR, Onkenhout W, Brederoo P, Poorthuis BJ: Depletion of mitochondrial DNA in the liver of a patient with lactic acidemia and hypoketotic hypoglycemia [see Comments]. *J Pediatr* **128**:679, 1996.
716. Genge A, Karpati G, Arnold D, Shoubridge EA, Carpenter S: Familial myopathy with conspicuous depletion of mitochondria in muscle fibers: A morphologically distinct disease. *Neuromuscul Disord* **5**:139, 1995.
717. Mariotti C, Uziel G, Carrara F, Mora M, Prelle A, Tiranti V, DiDonato S, Zeviani M: Early-onset encephalomyopathy associated with tissue-specific mitochondrial DNA depletion: A morphological, biochemical and molecular-genetic study. *J Neurol* **242**:547, 1995.
718. Paquis-Flucklinger V, Pellissier JF, Camboulives J, Chabrol B, Saunieres A, Monfort MF, Giudicelli H, Desnuelle C: Early-onset fatal encephalomyopathy associated with severe mtDNA depletion. *Eur J Pediatr* **154**:557, 1995.
719. Larsson NG, Oldfors A, Holme E, Clayton DA: Low levels of mitochondrial transcription factor A in mitochondrial DNA depletion. *Biochem Biophys Res Commun* **200**:1374, 1994.
720. Bodnar AG, Cooper JM, Holt IJ, Leonard JV, Schapira AH: Nuclear complementation restores mtDNA levels in cultured cells from a patient with mtDNA depletion. *Am J Hum Genet* **53**:663, 1993.
721. Pons R, Andreetta F, Wang CH, Vu TH, Bonilla E, DiMauro S, De Vivo DC: Mitochondrial myopathy simulating spinal muscular atrophy. *Pediatr Neurol* **15**:153, 1996.
722. Casademont J, Barrientos A, Cardellach F, Rotig A, Grau JM, Montoya J, Beltran B, Cervantes F, Rozman C, Estivill X, et al.: Multiple deletions of mtDNA in two brothers with sideroblastic anemia and mitochondrial myopathy and in their asymptomatic mother. *Hum Mol Genet* **3**:1945, 1994.
723. Muller-Hocker J, Jacob U, Seibel P: The common 4977 base pair deletion of mitochondrial DNA preferentially accumulates in the cardiac conduction system of patients with Kearns-Sayre syndrome. *Mod Pathol* **11**:295, 1998.
724. Kim SH, Chi JG: Characterization of a mitochondrial DNA deletion in patients with mitochondrial myopathy. *Mol Cells* **7**:726, 1997.
725. Consalvo D, Villegas F, Villa AM, Kohler G, Molina H, Benchuga E, Chamoles N, Sanz OP, Sica RE: [Severe cardiac failure in Kearns-Sayre syndrome.] *Medicina (B Aires)* **57**:67, 1997.
726. Kiyomoto BH, Tengan CH, Moraes CT, Oliveira AS, Gabbai AA: Mitochondrial DNA defects in Brazilian patients with chronic progressive external ophthalmoplegia. *J Neurol Sci* **152**:160, 1997.
727. Kleinle S, Wiesmann U, Superti-Furga A, Krahenbuhl S, Boltshauser E, Reichen J, Liechti-Gallati S: Detection and characterization of mitochondrial DNA rearrangements in Pearson and Kearns-Sayre syndromes by long PCR. *Hum Genet* **100**:643, 1997.
728. Barrientos A, Casademont J, Nunes V: [Rearrangement of the mitochondrial DNA in Kearns-Sayre syndrome: Is it necessary to differentiate deletions from duplications or polymerization?] *Neurologia* **11**:257, 1996.
729. Fromenty B, Carrozzo R, Shanske S, Schon EA: High proportions of mtDNA duplications in patients with Kearns-Sayre syndrome occur in the heart. *Am J Med Genet* **71**:443, 1997.
730. Lewczuk A, Sworczak K, Falkiewicz B: [Kearns-Sayre syndrome: Encephalomyopathy caused by deletion of mitochondrial DNA.] *Pol Arch Med Wewn* **96**:597, 1996.
731. Hirt L, Magistretti PJ, Hirt L, Bogousslavsky J, Boulat O, Borruat FX: Large deletion (7.2 kb) of mitochondrial DNA with novel boundaries in a case of progressive external ophthalmoplegia [Letter]. *J Neurol Neurosurg Psychiatry* **61**:422, 1996.
732. Brockington M, Alsanjari N, Sweeney MG, Morgan-Hughes JA, Scaravilli F, Harding AE: Kearns-Sayre syndrome associated with mitochondrial DNA deletion or duplication: A molecular genetic and pathological study. *J Neurol Sci* **131**:78, 1995.
733. Klopstock T, Bischof F, Gerok K, Deuschl G, Seibel P, Ketelsen UP, Reichmann H: 3.1-kb deletion of mitochondrial DNA in a patient with Kearns-Sayre syndrome. *Acta Neuropathol (Berl)* **90**:126, 1995.
734. Poulton J, O'Rahilly S, Morten KJ, Clark A: Mitochondrial DNA, diabetes and pancreatic pathology in Kearns-Sayre syndrome. *Diabetologia* **38**:868, 1995.
735. Midro AT, Zalewska R, Skrzypczak-Adamiak G, Wilichowski E: [Retinitis pigmentosa in Kearns-Sayre syndrome resulting from mutation of mitochondrial DNA "de novo."] *Klin Oczna* **97**:203, 1995.
736. Barrientos A, Casademont J, Grau JM, Cardellach F, Montoya J, Estivill X, Urbano-Marquez A, Nunes V: [Progressive external ophthalmoplegia and the Kearns-Sayre syndrome: A clinical and molecular study of 6 cases.] *Med Clin (Barc)* **105**:180, 1995.
737. Vazquez-Acevedo M, Coria R, Gonzalez-Astiazaran A, Medina-Crespo V, Ridaura-Sanz C, Gonzalez-Halphen D: Characterization of a 5025 base pair mitochondrial DNA deletion in Kearns-Sayre syndrome. *Biochim Biophys Acta* **1271**:363, 1995.
738. Poulton J, Morten KJ, Marchington D, Weber K, Brown GK, Rotig A, Bindoff L: Duplications of mitochondrial DNA in Kearns-Sayre syndrome. *Muscle Nerve* **3**:S154, 1995.
739. Moraes CT, Sciacco M, Ricci E, Tengan CH, Hao H, Bonilla E, Schon EA, DiMauro S: Phenotype-genotype correlations in skeletal muscle of patients with mtDNA deletions. *Muscle Nerve* **3**:S150, 1995.
740. Blok RB, Thorburn DR, Thompson GN, Dahl HH: A topoisomerase II cleavage site is associated with a novel mitochondrial DNA deletion. *Hum Genet* **95**:75, 1995.
741. Poulton J, Morten KJ, Weber K, Brown GK, Bindoff L: Are duplications of mitochondrial DNA characteristic of Kearns-Sayre syndrome? *Hum Mol Genet* **3**:947, 1994.
742. Ulicny KS, Jr., Detterbeck FC, Hall CD: Sinus dysrhythmia in Kearns-Sayre syndrome. *Pacing Clin Electrophysiol* **17**:991, 1994.
743. Heddi A, Lestienne P, Wallace DC, Stepien G: Steady state levels of mitochondrial and nuclear oxidative phosphorylation transcripts in Kearns-Sayre syndrome. *Biochim Biophys Acta* **1226**:206, 1994.
744. Ernst BP, Wilichowski E, Wagner M, Hanefeld F: Deletion screening of mitochondrial DNA via multiprimer DNA amplification. *Mol Cell Probes* **8**:45, 1994.
745. Norby S, Lestienne P, Nelson I, Nielsen IM, Schmalbruch H, Sjo O, Warburg M: Juvenile Kearns-Sayre syndrome initially misdiagnosed as a psychosomatic disorder. *J Med Genet* **31**:45, 1994.
746. Crisi G, Ferrari G, Merelli E, Cocconcelli P: MRI in a case of Kearns-Sayre syndrome confirmed by molecular analysis. *Neuroradiology* **36**:37, 1994.
747. Remes AM, Peuhkurinen KJ, Herva R, Majamaa K, Hassinen IE: Kearns-Sayre syndrome case presenting a mitochondrial DNA deletion with unusual direct repeats and a rudimentary RNAase mitochondrial ribonucleotide processing target sequence. *Genomics* **16**:256, 1993.
748. Soga F, Ueno S, Yorifuji S: [Deletions of mitochondrial DNA in Kearns-Sayre syndrome.] *Nippon Rinsho* **51**:2386, 1993.
749. Sudoyo H, Marzuki S, Byrne E, Mastaglia F: Phenotypic expression of mtDNA heteroplasmy in the skeletal muscle of patients with oculomyopathy: Defect in mitochondrial protein synthesis. *J Neurol Sci* **117**:83, 1993.
750. Byrne E, Jean-Francois B, Thyagarajan D, Collins S, Dennett X, Marzuki S: Biochemical and molecular investigation of mitochondrial disease: An illustrative case showing the value of a multifaceted approach. *Aust N Z J Med* **21**:837, 1991.
751. Yamamoto M, Clemens PR, Engel AG: Mitochondrial DNA deletions in mitochondrial cytopathies: Observations in 19 patients. *Neurology* **41**:1822, 1991.
752. Ota Y, Tanaka M, Sato W, Ohno K, Yamamoto T, Maehara M, Negoro T, Watanabe K, Awaya S, Ozawa T: Detection of platelet mitochondrial DNA deletions in Kearns-Sayre syndrome. *Invest Ophthalmol Vis Sci* **32**:2667, 1991.
753. Meola G, Rotondo G, Velicogna M, Toppi R, Sansone V, Bresolin N, Comi G, Bordoni A, Amati P, Ausenda C: Expression of a defect in the respiratory chain in cultured human cells. *Riv Neurol* **61**:122, 1991.

754. Geny C, Cormier V, Meyrignac C, Cesaro P, Degos JD, Gherardi R, Rotig A: Muscle mitochondrial DNA in encephalomyopathy and ragged red fibres: A Southern blot analysis and literature review. *J Neurol* **238**:171, 1991.
755. Poulton J, Deadman ME, Ramacharan S, Gardiner RM: Germ-line deletions of mtDNA in mitochondrial myopathy. *Am J Hum Genet* **48**:649, 1991.
756. McKelvie PA, Morley JB, Byrne E, Marzuki S: Mitochondrial encephalomyopathies: A correlation between neuropathological findings and defects in mitochondrial DNA. *J Neurol Sci* **102**:51, 1991.
757. Kosmorsky G, Johns DR: Neuro-ophthalmologic manifestations of mitochondrial DNA disorders: Chronic progressive external ophthalmoplegia, Kearns-Sayre syndrome, and Leber's hereditary optic neuropathy. *Neurol Clin* **9**:147, 1991.
758. Merelli E, Selleri L, Ferrari S, Sola P, Colombo A, Torelli G: Mitochondrial DNA deletion in oculoskeletal myopathy. *Eur Neurol* **31**:160, 1991.
759. Morgan-Hughes JA, Cooper JM, Schapira AH, Sweeny M, Holt IJ, Harding AE, Clark JB: The molecular pathology of human respiratory chain defects. *Rev Neurol (Paris)* **147**:450, 1991.
760. Miyabayashi S, Hanamizu H, Endo H, Tada K, Horai S: A new type of mitochondrial DNA deletion in patients with encephalomyopathy. *J Inherit Metab Dis* **14**:805, 1991.
761. Sparaco M, Bonilla E, DiMauro S, Powers JM: Neuropathology of mitochondrial encephalomyopathies due to mitochondrial DNA defects. *J Neuropathol Exp Neurol* **52**:1, 1993.
762. Sato W, Tanaka M, Sugiyama S, Hattori K, Ito T, Kawaguchi H, Onozuka H, Yasuda H, Ito K, Takada G, et al.: Deletion of mitochondrial DNA in a patient with conduction block. *Am Heart J* **125**:550, 1993.
763. Johnson MA, Bindoff LA, Turnbull DM: Cytochrome c oxidase activity in single muscle fibers: Assay techniques and diagnostic applications. *Ann Neurol* **33**:28, 1993.
764. Haginoya K, Miyabayashi S, Iinuma K, Tada K: Quantitative evaluation of electron transport system proteins in mitochondrial encephalomyopathy. *Acta Neuropathol (Berl)* **85**:370, 1993.
765. Muller-Hocker J, Seibel P, Schneiderbanger K, Zietz C, Obermaier-Kusser B, Gerbitz KD, Kadenbach B: In situ hybridization of mitochondrial DNA in the heart of a patient. *Hum Pathol* **23**:1431, 1992.
766. Perocchio M, Tomassini B, Biasia R, Belli Valletta M, Cerutti A, Bobba F: [Mitochondrial disease and complete heart block. Kearns-Sayre.] *Minerva Med* **83**:7, 1992.
767. Anan R, Nakagawa M, Higuchi I, Nakao S, Nomoto K, Tanaka H: Deletion of mitochondrial DNA in the endomyocardial biopsy sample from. *Eur Heart J* **13**:1718, 1992.
768. Remes AM, Hassinen IE, Majamaa K, Peuhkurinen KJ: Mitochondrial DNA deletion diagnosed by analysis of an endomyocardial. *Br Heart J* **68**:408, 1992.
769. Oldfors A, Larsson NG, Holme E, Tulinius M, Kadenbach B, Droste M: Mitochondrial DNA deletions and cytochrome c oxidase deficiency in muscle fibers. *J Neurol Sci* **110**:169, 1992.
770. Fischel-Ghodsian N, Bohlman MC, Prezant TR, Graham JM, Jr., Cederbaum SD, Edwards MJ: Deletion in blood mitochondrial DNA in Kearns-Sayre syndrome. *Pediatr Res* **31**:557, 1992.
771. Quade A, Zierz S, Klingmuller D: Endocrine abnormalities in mitochondrial myopathy with external ophthalmoplegia. *Clin Investig* **70**:396, 1992.
772. Hammans SR, Sweeney MG, Wicks DA, Morgan HJA, Harding AE: A molecular genetic study of focal histochemical defects in mitochondrial encephalomyopathies. *Brain* **115**:343, 1992.
773. Poulton J: Duplications of mitochondrial DNA: Implications for pathogenesis. *J Inherit Metab Dis* **15**:487, 1992.
774. Harding AE, Hammans SR: Deletions of the mitochondrial genome. *J Inherit Metab Dis* **15**:480, 1992.
775. Ohno K, Tanaka M, Ino H, Suzuki H, Tashiro M, Ibi T, Sahashi K, Takahashi A, Ozawa T: Direct DNA sequencing from colony: Analysis of multiple deletions of the mitochondrial genome. *Biochim Biophys Acta* **1090**:9, 1991.
776. Phillips CI, Gosden CM: Leber's hereditary optic neuropathy and Kearns-Sayre syndrome: Mitochondrial DNA mutations. *Surv Ophthalmol* **35**:463, 1991.
777. Zammarchi E: Kearns-Sayre and Melas syndromes. *Minerva Pediatr* **43**:111, 1991.
778. Poulton J, Deadman ME, Turnbull DM, Lake B, Gardiner RM: Detection of mitochondrial DNA deletions in blood using the polymerase chain reaction: Non-invasive diagnosis of mitochondrial myopathy. *Clin Genet* **39**:33, 1991.
779. Holt IJ, Harding AE, Morgan-Hughes JA: Deletions of muscle mitochondrial DNA in patients with mitochondrial myopathies. *Nature* **331**:717, 1988.
780. Takeshita K: Mitochondrial myopathy and abnormal mitochondrial DNA. *Tanpakushitsu Kakusan Koso* **33**:834, 1988.
781. Lestienne P, Ponsot G: Kearns-Sayre syndrome with muscle mitochondrial DNA deletion. *Lancet* **1**:885, 1988.
782. Holt IJ, Cooper JM, Morgan-Hughes JA, Harding AE: Deletions of muscle mitochondrial DNA. *Lancet* **1**:1462, 1988.
783. Zeviani M, Moraes CT, DiMauro S, Nakase H, Bonilla E, Schon EA, Rowland LP: Deletions of mitochondrial DNA in Kearns-Sayre syndrome. *Neurology* **38**:1339, 1988.
784. Nelson I, Degoul F, Obermaier-Kusser B, Romero N, Borrone C, Marsac C, Vayssiere JL, Gerbitz K, Fardeau M, Ponsot G, et al.: Mapping of heteroplasmic mitochondrial DNA deletions in Kearns-Sayre. *Nucleic Acids Res* **17**:8117, 1989.
785. Nelson I, d'Auriol L, Galibert F, Ponsot G, Lestienne P: Nucleotide mapping and a kinetic model of a heteroplasmic deletion of 4,666 base pairs from mitochondrial DNA in the Kearns-Sayre syndrome. *C R Acad Sci III* **309**:403, 1989.
786. Poulton J, Gardiner RM: Non-invasive diagnosis of mitochondrial myopathy. *Lancet* **1**:961, 1989.
787. Akaike M, Kawai H, Yokoi K, Kunishige M, Mine H, Nishida Y, Saito S: Cardiac dysfunction in patients with chronic progressive external ophthalmoplegia. *Clin Cardiol* **20**:239, 1997.
788. Drouet A: [Chronic progressive external ophthalmoplegia with mitochondrial anomalies. Clinical, histological, biochemical and genetic analysis (9 cases).] *Rev Med Interne* **17**:200, 1996.
789. Magalhaes PJ, Sjo O, Norby S: Ocular myopathy and mitochondrial DNA deletion. A presentation of seven identified Danish patients. *Acta Ophthalmol Scand Suppl* **219**:29, 1996.
790. Barbiroli B, Medori R, Tritschler HJ, Klopstock T, Seibel P, Reichmann H, Iotti S, Lodi R, Zaniol P: Lipoic (thioctic) acid increases brain energy availability and skeletal muscle performance as shown by in vivo 31P-MRS in a patient with mitochondrial cytopathy. *J Neurol* **242**:472, 1995.
791. Munakata S, Yamazaki H, Sato T: [Progressive external ophthalmoplegia with extensive mitochondrial DNA deletion.] *Nippon Ganka Gakkai Zasshi* **98**:1036, 1994.
792. Fassati A, Bordoni A, Amboni P, Fortunato F, Fagiolari G, Bresolin N, Prelle A, Comi G, Scarlato G: Chronic progressive external ophthalmoplegia: A correlative study of quantitative molecular data and histochemical and biochemical profile. *J Neurol Sci* **123**:140, 1994.
793. Matsuoka T, Goto Y, Nonaka I: "All-or-none" cytochrome c oxidase positivity in mitochondria in chronic progressive external ophthalmoplegia: An ultrastructural-cytochemical study. *Muscle Nerve* **16**:206, 1993.
794. Collins S, Rudduck C, Marzuki S, Dennett X, Byrne E: Mitochondrial genome distribution in histochemically cytochrome c oxidase-negative muscle fibres in patients with a mixture of deleted and wild type mitochondrial DNA. *Biochim Biophys Acta* **1097**:309, 1991.
795. Nakagawa M, Tokimura M, Kuriyama M, Higuchi I, Osame M: Chronic progressive external ophthalmoplegia (CPEO); mitochondrial DNA deletion, brain MRI and electrophysiological studies. *Rinsho Shinkeigaku* **31**:981, 1991.
796. Piccolo G, Banfi P, Azan G, Rizzuto R, Bisson R, Sandona D, Bellomo G: Biological markers of oxidative stress in mitochondrial myopathies with progressive external ophthalmoplegia. *J Neurol Sci* **105**:57, 1991.
797. Trounce I, Byrne E, Marzuki S, Dennett X, Sudoyo H, Mastaglia F, Berkovic SF: Functional respiratory chain studies in subjects with chronic progressive external ophthalmoplegia and large heteroplasmic mitochondrial DNA deletions. *J Neurol Sci* **102**:92, 1991.
798. Lowsky R, Davidson G, Wolman S, Jeejeebhoy KN, Hegele RA: Familial visceral myopathy associated with a mitochondrial myopathy. *Gut* **34**:279, 1993.
799. Matsuoka T, Goto Y, Hasegawa H, Nonaka I: Segmental cytochrome c-oxidase deficiency in CPEO: Teased muscle fiber analysis. *Muscle Nerve* **15**:209, 1992.
800. Goto Y: Clinical application of molecular diagnosis for mitochondrial encephalomyopathies. *Hokkaido Igaku Zasshi* **67**:27, 1992.
801. Thyagarajan D, Byrne E, Dennet X, Marzuki S: The molecular genetics of mitochondrial cytopathies: The Melbourne experience. *Clin Exp Neurol* **29**:172, 1992.

802. Hayashi J, Ohta S, Kikuchi A, Takemitsu M, Goto Y, Nonaka I: Introduction of disease-related mitochondrial DNA deletions into HeLa cells lacking mitochondrial DNA results in mitochondrial dysfunction. *Proc Natl Acad Sci U S A* **88**:10614, 1991.
803. Noer AS, Marzuki S, Trounce I, Byrne E: Mitochondrial DNA deletion in encephalomyopathy [Letter]. *Lancet* **2**:1253, 1988.
804. Johns DR, Drachman DB, Hurko O: Identical mitochondrial DNA deletion in blood and muscle. *Lancet* **1**:393, 1989.
805. Sato W, Tanaka M, Ohno K, Yamamoto T, Takada G, Ozawa T: Multiple populations of deleted mitochondrial DNA detected by a novel gene amplification method. *Biochem Biophys Res Commun* **162**:664, 1989.
806. Johns DR, Hurko O: Preferential amplification and molecular characterization of junction sequences of a pathogenetic deletion in human mitochondrial DNA. *Genomics* **5**:623, 1989.
807. Tanno Y, Yoneda M, Ohnishi Y, Miyatake T, Ozawa T: Chronic progressive external ophthalmoplegia (CPEO) with deleted mitochondrial DNA. *Rinsho Shinkeigaku* **29**:1176, 1989.
808. Johns DR, Rutledge SL, Stine OC, Hurko O: Directly repeated sequences associated with pathogenic mitochondrial DNA deletions. *Proc Natl Acad Sci U S A* **86**:8059, 1989.
809. Tanaka M, Sato W, Ohno K, Yamamoto T, Ozawa T: Direct sequencing of deleted mitochondrial DNA in myopathic patients. *Biochem Biophys Res Commun* **164**:156, 1989.
810. Romero NB, Lestienne P, Marsac C, Paturneau-Jouas M, Nelson I, Francois D, Eymard B, Fardeau M: Immunocytological and histochemical correlation in Kearns-Sayre syndrome with mtDNA deletion and partial cytochrome c oxidase deficiency in skeletal muscle. *J Neurol Sci* **93**:297, 1989.
811. Tanaka-Yamamoto T, Tanaka M, Ohno K, Sato W, Horai S, Ozawa T: Specific amplification of deleted mitochondrial DNA from a myopathic patient and analysis of deleted region with S1 nuclease. *Biochim Biophys Acta* **1009**:151, 1989.
812. Nakamura S, Sato T, Hirawake H, Kobayashi R, Fukuda Y, Kawamura J, Ujike H, Horai S: In situ hybridization of muscle mitochondrial mRNA in mitochondrial myopathies. *Acta Neuropathol (Berl)* **81**:1, 1990.
813. Oldfors A, Fyhr IM, Holme E, Larsson NG, Tulinius M: Neuropathology in Kearns-Sayre syndrome. *Acta Neuropathol (Berl)* **80**:541, 1990.
814. Shanske S, Moraes CT, Lombes A, Miranda AF, Bonilla E, Lewis P, Whelan MA, Ellsworth CA, DiMauro S: Widespread tissue distribution of mitochondrial DNA deletions in Kearns-Sayre syndrome. *Neurology* **40**:24, 1990.
815. Melacini P, Angelini C, Buja G, Micaglio G, Valente ML: Evolution of cardiac involvement in progressive ophthalmoplegia with deleted mitochondrial DNA. *Jpn Heart J* **31**:115, 1990.
816. Gerbitz KD, Obermaier-Kusser B, Zierz S, Pongratz D, Muller-Hocker J, Lestienne P: Mitochondrial myopathies: Divergences of genetic deletions, biochemical defects and the clinical syndromes. *J Neurol* **237**:5, 1990.
817. Mita S, Rizzuto R, Moraes CT, Shanske S, Arnaudo E, Fabrizi GM, Koga Y, DiMauro S, Schon EA: Recombination via flanking direct repeats is a major cause of large-scale deletions of human mitochondrial DNA. *Nucleic Acids Res* **18**:561, 1990.
818. Sensi A, Bonfatti A: Mitochondrial DNA deletions and ophthalmoplegia. *N Engl J Med* **322**:701, 1990.
819. Gerbitz KD, Obermaier-Kusser B, Lestienne P, Zierz S, Muller-Hocker J, Pongratz D, Paetzke-Brunner I, Deufel T: Mutations of the mitochondrial DNA: The contribution of DNA techniques to the diagnosis of mitochondrial encephalomyopathies. *J Clin Chem Clin Biochem* **28**:241, 1990.
820. Luppi M, Marasca R, Sola P, Corradi M, Fancinelli M, Montorsi M, Manfredini R, Selleri L: Mitochondrial DNA deletion in a case of progressive ophthalmoplegia. *Medicina (Firenze)* **10**:166, 1990.
821. Kadenbach B, Muller-Hocker J: Mutations of mitochondrial DNA and human death. *Naturwissenschaften* **77**:221, 1990.
822. Bordarier C, Duyckaerts C, Robain O, Ponsot G, Laplane D: Kearns-Sayre syndrome. Two clinicopathological cases. *Neuropediatrics* **21**:106, 1990.
823. Ponzetto C, Bresolin N, Bordoni A, Moggio M, Meola G, Bet L, Prelle A, Scarlato G: Kearns-Sayre syndrome: Different amounts of deleted mitochondrial DNA are present in several autoptic tissues. *J Neurol Sci* **96**:207, 1990.
824. Zierz S, von Wersebe O, Gerbitz KD, Jerusalem F: Ophthalmoplegia-plus: Clinical variability, biochemical defects of the mitochondria respiratory chain and deletions of the mitochondria genome. *Nervenarzt* **61**:332, 1990.
825. Reichmann H, Gold R, Lestienne P, Meurers B: The mitochondrial genome and its deletions as a cause of disease. *Dtsch Med Wochenschr* **115**:980, 1990.
826. Zeviani M, Gellera C, Pannacci M, Uziel G, Prelle A, Servidei S, DiDonato S: Tissue distribution and transmission of mitochondrial DNA deletions in mitochondrial myopathies. *Ann Neurol* **28**:94, 1990.
827. Scholte HR, Agsteribbe E, Busch HF, Hoogenraad TU, Jennekens FG, van Linge B, Luyt-Houwen IE, Ross JD, Ruiters MH, Verduin MH: Oxidative phosphorylation in human muscle in patients with ocular myopathy and after general anesthesia. *Biochim Biophys Acta* **1018**:211, 1990.
828. Morgan-Hughes JA, Schapira AH, Cooper JM, Holt IJ, Harding AE, Clark JB: The molecular pathology of respiratory-chain dysfunction in human mitochondrial myopathies. *Biochim Biophys Acta* **1018**:217, 1990.
829. Johns DR: mtDNA deletions in Kearns-Sayre. *Neurology* **40**:1322, 1990.
830. Hurko O, Johns DR, Rutledge SL, Stine OC, Peterson PL, Miller NR, Martens ME, Drachman DB, Brown RH, Lee CP: Heteroplasmy in chronic external ophthalmoplegia: Clinical and molecular observations. *Pediatr Res* **28**:542, 1990.
831. Goto Y, Koga Y, Horai S, Nonaka I: Chronic progressive external ophthalmoplegia: a correlative study of mitochondrial DNA deletions and their phenotypic expression in muscle biopsies. *J Neurol Sci* **100**:63, 1990.
832. Reichmann H, Degoul F, Gold R, Meurers B, Ketelsen UP, Hartmann J, Marsac C, Lestienne P: Histological, enzymatic and mitochondrial DNA studies in patients with Kearns-Sayre syndrome and chronic progressive external ophthalmoplegia. *Eur Neurol* **31**:108, 1991.
833. Collins S, Dennett X, Byrne E, Marzuki S: Chronic progressive external ophthalmoplegia in patients with large heteroplasmic mitochondrial DNA deletions: An immunohistochemical study. *Acta Neuropathol (Berl)* **82**:185, 1991.
834. Larsson NG, Eiken HG, Boman H, Holme E, Oldfors A, Tulinius MH: Lack of transmission of deleted mtDNA from a woman with Kearns-Sayre syndrome to her child. *Am J Hum Genet* **50**:360, 1992.
835. Tengan CH, Kiyomoto BH, Rocha MS, Tavares VL, Gabbai AA, Moraes CT: Mitochondrial encephalomyopathy and hypoparathyroidism associated with a duplication and a deletion of mitochondrial deoxyribonucleic acid. *J Clin Endocrinol Metab* **83**:125, 1998.
836. Wilichowski E, Gruters A, Kruse K, Rating D, Beetz R, Korenke GC, Ernst BP, Christen HJ, Hanefeld F: Hypoparathyroidism and deafness associated with pleioplasmic large-scale rearrangements of the mitochondrial DNA: A clinical and molecular genetic study of four children with Kearns-Sayre syndrome. *Pediatr Res* **41**:193, 1997.
837. Isotani H, Fukumoto Y, Kawamura H, Furukawa K, Ohsawa N, Goto Y, Nishino I, Nonaka I: Hypoparathyroidism and insulin-dependent diabetes mellitus in a patient with Kearns-Sayre syndrome harbouring a mitochondrial DNA deletion. *Clin Endocrinol (Oxf)* **45**:637, 1996.
838. Abramowicz MJ, Cochaux P, Cohen LH, Vamos E: Pernicious anaemia and hypoparathyroidism in a patient with Kearns-Sayre syndrome with mitochondrial DNA duplication. *J Inherit Metab Dis* **19**:109, 1996.
839. Yasui M, Kihira T, Ota K, Uematsu Y, Komai N, Oku H, Hashimoto T: [A case of chronic progressive external ophthalmoplegia with pituitary hypothyroidism.] *No To Shinkei* **45**:741, 1993.
840. Chang TS, Johns DR, Stark WJ, Drachman DB, Green WR: Corneal decompensation in mitochondrial ophthalmoplegia plus (Kearns-Sayre) syndrome. A clinicopathologic case report. *Cornea* **13**:269, 1994.
841. Herzberg NH, van Schooneveld MJ, Bleeker-Wagemakers EM, Zwart R, Cremers FP, van der Knaap MS, Bolhuis PA, de Visser M: Kearns-Sayre syndrome with a phenocopy of choroideremia instead of pigmentary retinopathy. *Neurology* **43**:218, 1993.
842. Tranchant C, Mousson B, Mohr M, Dumoulin R, Welsch M, Weess C, Stepien G, Warter JM: Cardiac transplantation in an incomplete Kearns-Sayre syndrome with mitochondrial DNA deletion. *Neuromuscul Disord* **3**:561, 1993.
843. Moraes CT, Zeviani M, Schon EA, Hickman RO, Vicek BW, DiMauro S: Mitochondrial DNA deletion in a girl with manifestations of Kearns-Sayre and Lowe syndromes: An example of phenotypic mimicry? *Am J Hum Genet* **41**:301, 1991.
844. Mori K, Narahara K, Ninomiya S, Goto Y, Nonaka I: Renal and skin involvement in a patient with complete Kearns-Sayre syndrome. *Am J Med Genet* **38**:583, 1991.

845. Goto Y, Itami N, Kajii N, Tochimaru H, Endo M, Horai S: Renal tubular involvement mimicking Bartter syndrome in a patient with Kearns-Sayre syndrome. *J Pediatr* **116**:904, 1990.
846. Rossier J, Hatt M: [Atypical manifestation of progressive external ophthalmoplegia.] *Klin Monatsbl Augenheilkd* **208**:366, 1996.
847. Furuya H, Sugimura T, Yamada T, Hayashi K, Kobayashi T: [A case of incomplete Kearns-Sayre syndrome with a stroke like episode.] *Rinsho Shinkeigaku* **37**:680, 1997.
848. Ota Y, Miyake Y, Awaya S, Kumagai T, Tanaka M, Ozawa T: Early retinal involvement in mitochondrial myopathy with mitochondrial DNA deletion. *Retina* **14**:270, 1994.
849. Orimo S, Arai M, Hiyamuta E, Goto Y: A case of chronic progressive external ophthalmoplegia associated with familial hypercholesterolemia. *Rinsho Shinkeigaku* **32**:37, 1992.
850. Sahashi K, Ohno K, Tanaka M, Ibi T, Yamamoto T, Tashiro M, Sato W, Takahashi A, Ozawa T: Cytoplasmic body and mitochondrial DNA deletion. *J Neurol Sci* **99**:291, 1990.
851. Manfredi G, Vu T, Bonilla E, Schon EA, DiMauro S, Arnaudo E, Zhang L, Rowland LP, Hirano M: Association of myopathy with large-scale mitochondrial DNA duplications and deletions: which is pathogenic? *Ann Neurol* **42**:180, 1997.
852. Muraki K, Nishimura S, Goto Y, Nonaka I, Sakura N, Ueda K: The association between haematological manifestation and mtDNA deletions in Pearson syndrome. *J Inherit Metab Dis* **20**:697, 1997.
853. Seneca S, De Meirleir L, De Schepper J, Balduck N, Jochmans K, Liebaers I, Lissens W: Pearson marrow pancreas syndrome: a molecular study and clinical management. *Clin Genet* **51**:338, 1997.
854. Smith OP, Hann IM, Woodward CE, Brockington M: Pearson's marrow/pancreas syndrome: Haematological features associated with deletion and duplication of mitochondrial DNA. *Br J Haematol* **90**:469, 1995.
855. Rotig A, Bourgeron T, Chretien D, Rustin P, Munnich A: Spectrum of mitochondrial DNA rearrangements in the Pearson marrow-pancreas syndrome. *Hum Mol Genet* **4**:1327, 1995.
856. Rotig A, Bourgeron T, Rustin P, Munnich A: Phenotypic expression of mitochondrial genotypes in cultured skin fibroblasts and in Epstein-Barr virus-transformed lymphocytes in Pearson syndrome. *Muscle Nerve* **3**:S159, 1995.
857. Spelbrink JN, Van Oost BA, Van den Bogert C: The relationship between mitochondrial genotype and mitochondrial phenotype in lymphoblasts with a heteroplasmic mtDNA deletion. *Hum Mol Genet* **3**:1989, 1994.
858. Kapsa R, Thompson GN, Thorburn DR, Dahl HH, Marzuki S, Byrne E, Blok RB: A novel mtDNA deletion in an infant with Pearson syndrome. *J Inherit Metab Dis* **17**:521, 1994.
859. Bader-Meunier B, Rotig A, Mielot F, Lavergne JM, Croisille L, Rustin P, Landrieu P, Dommergues JP, Munnich A, Tchernia G: Refractory anaemia and mitochondrial cytopathy in childhood. *Br J Haematol* **87**:381, 1994.
860. Superti-Furga A, Schoenle E, Tuchschmid P, Caduff R, Sabato V, DeMattia D, Gitzelmann R, Steinmann B: Pearson bone marrow-pancreas syndrome with insulin-dependent diabetes, progressive renal tubulopathy, organic aciduria and elevated fetal haemoglobin caused by deletion and duplication of mitochondrial DNA. *Eur J Pediatr* **152**:44, 1993.
861. Morikawa Y, Matsuura N, Kakudo K, Higuchi R, Koike M, Kobayashi Y: Pearson's marrow/pancreas syndrome: A histological and genetic study. *Virchows Arch A Pathol Anat Histopathol* **423**:227, 1993.
862. Sano T, Ban K, Ichiki T, Kobayashi M, Tanaka M, Ohno K, Ozawa T: Molecular and genetic analyses of two patients with Pearson's marrow-pancreas syndrome. *Pediatr Res* **34**:105, 1993.
863. Baerlocher KE, Feldges A, Weissert M, Simonsz HJ, Rotig A: Mitochondrial DNA deletion in an 8-year-old boy with Pearson syndrome. *J Inherit Metab Dis* **15**:327, 1992.
864. Danse PW, Jakobs C, Rotig A, Munnich A, Veerman AJ: Pearson's syndrome: A multi-system disorder based on an mt-DNA deletion. *Tijdschr Kindergeneeskd* **59**:196, 1991.
865. Jakobs C, Danse P, Veerman AJ: Organic aciduria in Pearson syndrome [Letter]. *Eur J Pediatr* **150**:684, 1991.
866. McShane MA, Hammans SR, Sweeney M, Holt IJ, Beattie TJ, Brett EM, Harding AE: Pearson syndrome and mitochondrial encephalomyopathy in a patient with a deletion of mtDNA. *Am J Hum Genet* **48**:39, 1991.
867. Nelson I, Bonne G, Degoul F, Marsac C, Ponsot G, Lestienne P: Kearns-Sayre syndrome with sideroblastic anemia: molecular. *Neuropediatrics* **23**:199, 1992.
868. Imai T, Kondo M, Ito S, Onishi K, Isobe K, Sotoyama Y: [Magnetic resonance imaging and spectroscopy of Pearson syndrome.] *No To Hattatsu* **24**:393, 1992.
869. Gurgey A, Rotig A, Gumruk F, Cemeroglu P, Sarialioglu F, Altay C: Pearson's marrow-pancreas syndrome in 2 Turkish children. *Acta Haematol* **87**:206, 1992.
870. de Vries DD, Buzing CJ, Ruitenbeek W, van der Wouw MP, Sperl W, Sengers RC, Trijbels JM, van Oost BA: Myopathology and a mitochondrial DNA deletion in the Pearson marrow and pancreas syndrome. *Neuromuscul Disord* **2**:185, 1992.
871. de Vries DD, Ruitenbeek W, van Oost BA: Detection of extremely low levels of wild-type mitochondrial DNA in the liver of a patient with Pearson syndrome by a sensitive PCR assay. *J Inherit Metab Dis* **15**:307, 1992.
872. Cormier V, Rotig A, Quartino AR, Forni GL, Cerone R, Maier M, Saudubray JM, Munnich A: Widespread multi-tissue deletions of the mitochondrial genome in the Pearson marrow-pancreas syndrome. *J Pediatr* **117**:599, 1990.
873. Munnich A, Rotig A: Metabolic, enzymological and molecular assessment of mitochondrial cytopathies. *Pediatrie (Bucur)* **46**:509, 1991.
874. Simonsz HJ, Barlocher K, Rotig A: Kearns-Sayre's syndrome developing in a boy who survived pearson's syndrome caused by mitochondrial DNA deletion. *Doc Ophthalmol* **82**:73, 1992.
875. Muraki K, Goto Y, Nishino I, Hayashidani M, Takeuchi S, Horai S, Sakura N, Ueda K: Severe lactic acidosis and neonatal death in Pearson syndrome. *J Inherit Metab Dis* **20**:43, 1997.
876. Gurgey A, Ozalp I, Rotig A, Coskun T, Tekinalp G, Erdem G, Akeoren Z, Caglar M, Bakkaloglu A: A case of Pearson syndrome associated with multiple renal cysts. *Pediatr Nephrol* **10**:637, 1996.
877. Santorelli FM, Barmada MA, Pons R, Zhang LL, DiMauro S: Leigh-type neuropathology in Pearson syndrome associated with impaired ATP production and a novel mtDNA deletion. *Neurology* **47**:1320, 1996.
878. Yamadori I, Kurose A, Kobayashi S, Ohmori M, Imai T: Brain lesions of the Leigh-type distribution associated with a mitochondriopathy of Pearson's syndrome: Light and electron microscopic study. *Acta Neuropathol (Berl)* **84**:337, 1992.
879. Niaudet P, Heidet L, Munnich A, Schmitz J, Bouissou F, Gubler MC, Rotig A: Deletion of the mitochondrial DNA in a case of de Toni-Debre-Fanconi syndrome and Pearson syndrome. *Pediatr Nephrol* **8**:164, 1994.
880. Mielot F, Bader-Meunier B, Tchernia G, Dommergues JP: [Myelodysplasia in children and mitochondrial cytopathies.] *Pathol Biol (Paris)* **45**:594, 1997.
881. Cursiefen C, Kuchle M, Scheurlen W, Naumann GO: Bilateral zonular cataract associated with the mitochondrial cytopathy of Pearson syndrome. *Am J Ophthalmol* **125**:260, 1998.
882. Morris AA, Lamont PJ, Clayton PT: Pearson's syndrome without marrow involvement. *Arch Dis Child* **77**:56, 1997.
883. Majander A, Suomalainen A, Vettenranta K, Sariola H, Perkkio M, Holmberg C, Pihko H: Congenital hypoplastic anemia, diabetes, and severe renal tubular dysfunction associated with a mitochondrial DNA deletion. *Pediatr Res* **30**:327, 1991.
884. Ribes A, Riudor E, Valcarel R, Salva A, Castello F, Murillo S, Dominguez C, Rotig A, Jakobs C: Pearson syndrome: altered tricarboxylic acid and urea-cycle metabolites, adrenal insufficiency and corneal opacities. *J Inherit Metab Dis* **16**:537, 1993.
885. Barrientos A, Casademont J, Genis D, Cardellach F, Fernandez-Real JM, Grau JM, Urbano-Marquez A, Estivill X, Nunes V: Sporadic heteroplasmic single 5.5 kb mitochondrial DNA deletion associated with cerebellar ataxia, hypogonadotropic hypogonadism, choroidal dystrophy, and mitochondrial respiratory chain complex I deficiency. *Hum Mutat* **10**:212, 1997.
886. Gucuyener K, Seyrantepe V, Topaloglu H, Ozguc: Mitochondrial deletion in a boy with growth hormone deficiency mimicking cerebral palsy. *J Inherit Metab Dis* **21**:173, 1998.
887. Blok RB, Thorburn DR, Danks DM, Dahl HH: mtDNA deletion in a patient with symptoms of mitochondrial cytopathy but without ragged red fibers. *Biochem Mol Med* **56**:26, 1995.
888. Bruno C, Minetti C, Tang Y, Magalhaes PJ, Santorelli FM, Shanske S, Bado M, Cordone G, Gatti R, DiMauro S: Primary adrenal insufficiency in a child with a mitochondrial DNA deletion. *J Inherit Metab Dis* **21**:155, 1998.

889. Nicolino M, Ferlin T, Forest M, Godinot C, Carrier H, David M, Chatelain P, Mousson B: Identification of a large-scale mitochondrial deoxyribonucleic acid deletion in endocrinopathies and deafness: Report of two unrelated cases with diabetes mellitus and adrenal insufficiency, respectively. *J Clin Endocrinol Metab* **82**:3063, 1997.
890. Rotig A, Cormier V, Chatelain P, Francois R, Saudubray JM, Rustin P, Munnich A: Deletion of mitochondrial DNA in a case of early onset diabetes mellitus, optic atrophy and deafness (DIDMOAD, Wolfram syndrome). *J Inherit Metab Dis* **16**:527, 1993.
891. Souied EH, Sales MJ, Soubrane G, Coscas G, Bigorie B, Kaplan J, Munnich A, Rotig A: Macular dystrophy, diabetes, and deafness associated with a large mitochondrial DNA deletion. *Am J Ophthalmol* **125**:100, 1998.
892. Hinokio Y, Suzuki S, Komatu K, Ohtomo M, Onoda M, Matsumoto M, Hirai S, Sato Y, Akai H, Abe K, et al.: A new mitochondrial DNA deletion associated with diabetic amyotrophy, diabetic myoatrophy and diabetic fatty liver. *Muscle Nerve* **3**:S142, 1995.
893. Luder A, Barash V: Complex I deficiency with diabetes, Fanconi syndrome and mtDNA deletion. *J Inherit Metab Dis* **17**:298, 1994.
894. Molnar M, Zanssen S, Buse G, Schroder JM: A large-scale deletion of mitochondrial DNA in a case with pure mitochondrial myopathy and neuropathy. *Acta Neuropathol (Berl)* **91**:654, 1996.
895. Campos Y, Garcia-Silva T, Barrionuevo CR, Cabello A, Muley R, Arenas J: Mitochondrial DNA deletion in a patient with mitochondrial myopathy, lactic acidosis, and stroke-like episodes (MELAS) and Fanconi's syndrome. *Pediatr Neurol* **13**:69, 1995.
896. Melegh B, Seress L, Sumegi B, Trombitas K, Bock I, Kispal G, Olah E, Mehes K: [Mitochondrial DNA deletion in hereditary cardio-encephalo-myopathy.] *Orv Hetil* **136**:1275, 1995.
897. Montagna P, Cortelli P, Barbiroli B: A case of cluster headache associated with mitochondrial DNA deletions [Letter; Comment]. *Muscle Nerve* **21**:127, 1998.
898. Odawara M, Tamaoka A, Mizusawa H, Yamashita K: A case of cluster headache associated with mitochondrial DNA deletions [Letter; see Comments]. *Muscle Nerve* **20**:394, 1997.
899. Bresolin N, Martinelli P, Barbiroli B, Zaniol P, Ausenda C, Montagna P, Gallanti A, Comi GP, Scarlato G, Lugaresi E: Muscle mitochondrial DNA deletion and 31P-NMR spectroscopy alterations in a migraine patient. *J Neurol Sci* **104**:182, 1991.
900. Rotig A, Goutieres F, Niaudet P, Rustin P, Chretien D, Guest G, Mikol J, Gubler MC, Munnich A: Deletion of mitochondrial DNA in patient with chronic tubulointerstitial nephritis. *J Pediatr* **126**:597, 1995.
901. Tulinius MH, Oldfors A, Holme E, Larsson NG, Houshmand M, Fahleson P, Sigstrom L, Kristiansson B: Atypical presentation of multisystem disorders in two girls with mitochondrial DNA deletions. *Eur J Pediatr* **154**:35, 1995.
902. Nakai A, Goto Y, Fujisawa K, Shigematsu Y, Kikawa Y, Konishi Y, Nonaka I, Sudo M: Diffuse leukodystrophy with a large-scale mitochondrial DNA deletion. *Lancet* **343**:1397, 1994.
903. Szabolcs MJ, Seigle R, Shanske S, Bonilla E, DiMauro S, D'Agati V: Mitochondrial DNA deletion: A cause of chronic tubulointerstitial nephropathy. *Kidney Int* **45**:1388, 1994.
904. Cormier-Daire V, Bonnefont JP, Rustin P, Maurage C, Ogler H, Schmitz J, Ricour C, Saudubray JM, Munnich A, Rotig A: Mitochondrial DNA rearrangements with onset as chronic diarrhea with villous atrophy. *J Pediatr* **124**:63, 1994.
905. Stine OC, Luu SU, Zito M, Casanova M: The possible association between affective disorder and partially deleted mitochondrial DNA. *Biol Psychiatry* **33**:141, 1993.
906. Ohno K, Yamamoto M, Engel AG, Harper CM, Roberts LR, Tan GH, Fatourechi V: MELAS- and Kearns-Sayre-type co-mutation [corrected] with myopathy and autoimmune polyendocrinopathy [published erratum appears in *Ann Neurol* 40(3):480, 1996]. *Ann Neurol* **39**:761, 1996.
907. Akaike M, Kawai H, Kashiwagi S, Kunishige M, Saito S: [A case of Kearns-Sayre syndrome whose asymptomatic mother had abnormal mitochondria in skeletal muscle.] *Rinsho Shinkeigaku* **35**:190, 1995.
908. Ballinger SW, Shoffner JM, Gebhart S, Koontz DA, Wallace DC: Mitochondrial diabetes revisited [Letter]. *Nat Genet* **7**:458, 1994.
909. Dunbar DR, Moonie PA, Swingler RJ, Davidson D, Roberts R, Holt IJ: Maternally transmitted partial direct tandem duplication of mitochondrial DNA associated with diabetes mellitus. *Hum Mol Genet* **2**:1619, 1993.
910. Ballinger SW, Shoffner JM, Hedaya EV, Trounce I, Polak MA, Koontz DA, Wallace DC: Maternally transmitted diabetes and deafness associated with a 10.4 kb. *Nat Genet* **1**:11, 1992.
911. Ozawa T, Yoneda M, Tanaka M, Ohno K, Sato W, Suzuki H, Nishikimi M, Yamamoto M, Nonaka I, Horai S: Maternal inheritance of deleted mitochondrial DNA in a family with mitochondrial myopathy. *Biochem Biophys Res Commun* **154**:1240, 1988.
912. Tanaka M, Yoneda M, Ohno K, Sato W, Yamamoto M, Nonaka I, Horai S, Ozawa T: Differently deleted mitochondrial genomes in maternally inherited chronic progressive external ophthalmoplegia. *J Inherit Metab Dis* **12**:359, 1989.
913. Bernes SM, Bacino C, Prezant TR, Pearson MA, Wood TS, Fournier P, Fischel-Ghodsian N: Identical mitochondrial DNA deletion in mother with progressive external ophthalmoplegia and son with Pearson marrow-pancreas syndrome. *J Pediatr* **123**:598, 1993.
914. Johnston W, Karpati G, Carpenter S, Arnold D, Shoubridge EA: Late-onset mitochondrial myopathy [see Comments]. *Ann Neurol* **37**:16, 1995.
915. Mendell JR: Mitochondrial myopathy in the elderly: exaggerated aging in the pathogenesis of disease [Editorial; Comment] [see Comments]. *Ann Neurol* **37**:3, 1995.
916. Seneca S, Abramowicz M, Lissens W, Muller MF, Vamos E, de Meirleir L: A mitochondrial DNA microdeletion in a newborn girl with transient lactic acidosis. *J Inherit Metab Dis* **19**:115, 1996.
917. Keightley JA, Hoffbuhr KC, Burton MD, Salas VM, Johnston WS, Penn AM, Buist NR, Kennaway NG: A microdeletion in cytochrome c oxidase (COX) subunit III associated with COX deficiency and recurrent myoglobinuria. *Nat Genet* **12**:410, 1996.
918. Tengan CH, Moraes CT: Duplication and triplication with staggered breakpoints in human mitochondrial DNA. *Biochim Biophys Acta* **1406**:73, 1998.
919. Manfredi G, Servidei S, Bonilla E, Shanske S, Schon EA, DiMauro S, Moraes CT: High levels of mitochondrial DNA with an unstable 260-bp duplication in a patient with a mitochondrial myopathy. *Neurology* **45**:762, 1995.
920. Brockington M, Sweeney MG, Hammans SR, Morgan-Hughes JA, Harding AE: A tandem duplication in the D-loop of human mitochondrial DNA is associated with deletions in mitochondrial myopathies. *Nat Genet* **4**:67, 1993.
921. Kleinle S, Schneider V, Moosmann P, Brandner S, Krahenbuhl S, Liechti-Gallati S: A novel mitochondrial tRNA(Phe) mutation inhibiting anticodon stem formation associated with a muscle disease. *Biochem Biophys Res Commun* **247**:112, 1998.
922. Bacino C, Prezant TR, Bu X, Fournier P, Fischel-Ghodsian N: Susceptibility mutations in the mitochondrial small ribosomal RNA gene in aminoglycoside induced deafness. *Pharmacogenetics* **5**:165, 1995.
923. Estivill X, Govea N, Barcelo E, Badenas C, Romero E, Moral L, Scozzri R, D'Urbano L, Zeviani M, Torroni A: Familial progressive sensorineural deafness is mainly due to the mtDNA A1555G mutation and is enhanced by treatment of aminoglycosides [see Comments]. *Am J Hum Genet* **62**:27, 1998.
924. Gardner JC, Goliath R, Viljoen D, Sellars S, Cortopassi G, Hutchin T, Greenberg J, Beighton P: Familial streptomycin ototoxicity in a South African family: a mitochondrial disorder. *J Med Genet* 34:904, 1997.
925. Hutchin TP, Cortopassi GA: Multiple origins of a mitochondrial mutation conferring deafness. *Genetics* 145:771, 1997.
926. Matthijs G, Claes S, Longo-Mbenza B, Cassiman JJ: Non-syndromic deafness associated with a mutation and a polymorphism in the mitochondrial 12S ribosomal RNA gene in a large Zairean pedigree. *Eur J Hum Genet* **4**:46, 1996.
927. Fischel-Ghodsian N, Prezant TR, Chaltraw WE, Wendt KA, Nelson RA, Arnos KS, Falk RE: Mitochondrial gene mutation is a significant predisposing factor in aminoglycoside ototoxicity. *Am J Otolaryngol* **18**:173, 1997.
928. Pandya A, Xia X, Radnaabazar J, Batsuuri J, Dangaansuren B, Fischel-Ghodsian N, Nance WE: Mutation in the mitochondrial 12S rRNA gene in two families from Mongolia with matrilineal aminoglycoside ototoxicity. *J Med Genet* **34**:169, 1997.
929. el-Schahawi M, Lopez de Munain A, Sarrazin AM, Shanske AL, Basirico M, Shanske S, DiMauro S: Two large Spanish pedigrees with nonsyndromic sensorineural deafness and the mtDNA mutation at nt 1555 in the 12s rRNA gene: evidence of heteroplasmy. *Neurology* **48**:453, 1997.
930. Tamagawa Y, Kitamura K, Ishida T, Hagiwara H, Abe K, Nishizawa M: Mitochondrial DNA mutation at nucleotide 1555 in a patient with bilateral sensorineural hearing loss of unknown etiology. *Acta Otolaryngol (Stockh)* **116**:796, 1996.

931. Guan MX, Fischel-Ghodsian N, Attardi G: Biochemical evidence for nuclear gene involvement in phenotype of non-syndromic deafness associated with mitochondrial 12S rRNA mutation. *Hum Mol Genet* **5**:963, 1996.
932. Braverman I, Jaber L, Levi H, Adelman C, Arons KS, Fischel-Ghodsian N, Shohat M, Elidan J: Audiovestibular findings in patients with deafness caused by a mitochondrial susceptibility mutation and precipitated by an inherited nuclear mutation or aminoglycosides. *Arch Otolaryngol Head Neck Surg* **122**:1001, 1996.
933. Inoue K, Takai D, Soejima A, Isobe K, Yamasoba T, Oka Y, Goto Y, Hayashi J: Mutant mtDNA at 1555 A to G in 12S rRNA gene and hypersusceptibility of mitochondrial translation to streptomycin can be co-transferred to rho 0 HeLa cells. *Biochem Biophys Res Commun* **223**:496, 1996.
934. Fischel-Ghodsian N, Prezant TR, Bu X, Oztas S: Mitochondrial ribosomal RNA gene mutation in a patient with sporadic aminoglycoside ototoxicity. *Am J Otolaryngol* **14**:399, 1993.
935. Hutchin T, Haworth I, Higashi K, Fischel-Ghodsian N, Stoneking M, Saha N, Arnos C, Cortopassi G: A molecular basis for human hypersensitivity to aminoglycoside antibiotics. *Nucleic Acids Res* **21**:4174, 1993.
936. Hu DN, Qui WQ, Wu BT, Fang LZ, Zhou F, Gu YP, Zhang QH, Yan JH, Ding YQ, Wong H: Genetic aspects of antibiotic induced deafness: mitochondrial inheritance. *J Med Genet* **28**:79, 1991.
937. Gold M, Rapin I, Shanske S: Mitochondrial inheritance of acquired deafness. *Ann N Y Acad Sci* **630**:301, 1991.
938. Bu X, Shohat M, Jaber L, Rotter JI: A form of sensorineural deafness is determined by a mitochondrial and an autosomal locus: Evidence from pedigree segregation analysis. *Genet Epidemiol* **10**:3, 1993.
939. Santorelli FM, Tanji K, Manta P, Casali C, Krishna S, Hays AP, Mancini DM, DiMauro S, Hirano M: Maternally inherited cardiomyopathy: An atypical presentation of the mtDNA 12S rRNA gene A1555G mutation. *Am J Hum Genet* **64**:295, 1999.
940. Tiranti V, D'Agruma L, Pareyson D, Mora M, Carrara F, Zelante L, Gasparini P, Zeviani M: A novel mutation in the mitochondrial tRNA(Val) gene associated with a complex neurological presentation. *Ann Neurol* **43**:98, 1998.
941. Taylor RW, Chinnery PF, Haldane F, Morris AA, Bindoff LA, Wilson J, Turnbull DM: MELAS associated with a mutation in the valine transfer RNA gene of mitochondrial DNA. *Ann Neurol* **40**:459, 1996.
942. de Coo IF, Sistermans EA, de Wijs IJ, Catsman-Berrevoets C, Busch HF, Scholte HR, de Klerk JB, van Oost BA, Smeets HJ: A mitochondrial tRNA(Val) gene mutation (G1642A) in a patient with mitochondrial myopathy, lactic acidosis, and stroke-like episodes. *Neurology* **50**:293, 1998.
943. Chalmers RM, Lamont PJ, Nelson I, Ellison DW, Thomas NH, Harding AE, Hammans SR: A mitochondrial DNA tRNA(Val) point mutation associated with adult-onset Leigh syndrome. *Neurology* **49**:589, 1997.
944. Tang J, Qi Y, Bao XH, Wu XR: Mutational analysis of mitochondrial DNA of children with Rett syndrome. *Pediatr Neurol* **17**:327, 1997.
945. Tang J, Qi Y, Bao X: [Mutation analysis of mitochondrial DNA of children with Rett syndrome.] *Chung Hua I Hsueh Tsa Chih* **76**:684, 1996.
946. Shoffner JM, Brown MD, Torroni A, Lott MT, Cabell MF, Mirra SS, Beal MF, Yang CC, Gearing M, Salvo R, et al.: Mitochondrial DNA variants observed in Alzheimer disease and Parkinson. *Genomics* **17**:171, 1993.
947. McEntagart M, Droogan O, Burke M, Brett F, Murphy S, Farrell M: Mitochondrial encephalopathy with lactic acidosis and stroke-like episodes (MELAS) in a Donegal kindred—Clinical features and molecular genetic analysis. *Ir Med J* **90**:144, 1997.
948. Sano M, Ishii K, Momose Y, Uchigata M, Senda M: Cerebral metabolism of oxygen and glucose in a patient with MELAS syndrome. *Acta Neurol Scand* **92**:497, 1995.
949. Maassen JA, Jansen JJ, Kadowaki T, van den Ouweland JM, t Hart LM, Lemkes HH: The molecular basis and clinical characteristics of Maternally Inherited Diabetes and Deafness (MIDD), a recently recognized diabetic subtype. *Exp Clin Endocrinol Diabetes* **104**:205, 1996.
950. Huang CC, Chen RS, Chu NS, Pang CY, Wei YH: Random mitotic segregation of mitochondrial DNA in MELAS syndrome. *Acta Neurol Scand* **93**:198, 1996.
951. Kaufmann P, Koga Y, Shanske S, Hirano M, DiMauro S, King MP, Schon EA: Mitochondrial DNA and RNA processing in MELAS. *Ann Neurol* **40**:172, 1996.
952. Walker M, Taylor RW, Stewart MW, Bindoff LA, Shearing PA, Anyaoku V, Jackson MJ, Humphriss DB, Johnston DG, Alberti KG: Insulin and proinsulin secretion in subjects with abnormal glucose tolerance and a mitochondrial tRNA(Leu(UUR)) mutation [Letter; see Comments]. *Diabetes Care* **18**:1507, 1995.
953. Kovalenko SA, Tanaka M, Yoneda M, Iakovlev AF, Ozawa T: Accumulation of somatic nucleotide substitutions in mitochondrial DNA associated with the 3243 A-to-G tRNA(leu)(UUR) mutation in encephalomyopathy and cardiomyopathy. *Biochem Biophys Res Commun* **222**:201, 1996.
954. Damian MS, Seibel P, Reichmann H, Schachenmayr W, Laube H, Bachmann G, Wassill KH, Dorndorf W: Clinical spectrum of the MELAS mutation in a large pedigree. *Acta Neurol Scand* **92**:409, 1995.
955. Morten KJ, Poulton J, Sykes B: Multiple independent occurrence of the 3243 mutation in mitochondrial tRNA(leuUUR) in patients with the MELAS phenotype. *Hum Mol Genet* **4**:1689, 1995.
956. Tanno Y, Yoneda M, Tanaka K, Tanaka H, Yamazaki M, Nishizawa M, Wakabayashi K, Ohama E, Tsuji S: Quantitation of heteroplasmy of mitochondrial tRNA(Leu(UUR)) gene using PCR-SSCP. *Muscle Nerve* **18**:1390, 1995.
957. Mariotti C, Savarese N, Suomalainen A, Rimoldi M, Comi G, Prelle A, Antozzi C, Servidei S, Jarre L, DiDonato S, et al.: Genotype to phenotype correlations in mitochondrial encephalomyopathies associated with the A3243G mutation of mitochondrial DNA. *J Neurol* **242**:304, 1995.
958. Chiang LM, Jong YJ, Huang SC, Tsai JL, Pang CY, Lee HC, Wei YH: Heteroplasmic mitochondrial DNA mutation in a patient with mitochondrial myopathy, encephalopathy, lactic acidosis and stroke-like episodes. *J Formos Med Assoc* **94**:42, 1995.
959. Goto Y: Clinical features of MELAS and mitochondrial DNA mutations. *Muscle Nerve* **3**:S107, 1995.
960. Holme E, Tulinius MH, Larsson NG, Oldfors A: Inheritance and expression of mitochondrial DNA point mutations. *Biochim Biophys Acta* **1271**:249, 1995.
961. Morgan-Hughes JA, Sweeney MG, Cooper JM, Hammans SR, Brockington M, Schapira AH, Harding AE, Clark JB: Mitochondrial DNA (mtDNA) diseases: correlation of genotype to phenotype. *Biochim Biophys Acta* **1271**:135, 1995.
962. Erro E, Gomez Moreno I, Gomez Romero L, Lopez A: [MELAS syndrome with peripheral neuropathy.] *Neurologia* **10**:117, 1995.
963. Lee ML, Chaou WT, Yang AD, Jong YJ, Tsai JL, Pang CY, Wei YH: Mitochondrial myopathy, encephalopathy, lactic acidosis and stroke-like episodes (MELAS): Report of a sporadic case and review of the literature. *Chung Hua Min Kuo Hsiao Erh Ko I Hsueh Hui Tsa Chih* **35**:148, 1994.
964. Damian MS, Reichmann H, Seibel P, Bachmann G, Schachenmayr W, Dorndorf W: [MELAS syndrome. Clinical aspects, MRI, biochemistry and molecular genetics.] *Nervenarzt* **65**:258, 1994.
965. Liou CW, Huang CC, Chee EC, Jong YJ, Tsai JL, Pang CY, Lee HC, Wei YH: MELAS syndrome: Correlation between clinical features and molecular genetic analysis. *Acta Neurol Scand* **90**:354, 1994.
966. Campos Y, Bautista J, Gutierrez-Rivas E, Llabres J, Lorenzo G, Arenas J: Variable clinical expression associated with the mutation 3243 np of mitochondrial DNA. *J Inherit Metab Dis* **17**:634, 1994.
967. Dougherty FE, Ernst SG, Aprille JR: Familial recurrence of atypical symptoms in an extended pedigree with the syndrome of mitochondrial encephalomyopathy, lactic acidosis, and stroke-like episodes (MELAS). *J Pediatr* **125**:758, 1994.
968. de Vries D, de Wijs I, Ruitenbeek W, Begeer J, Smit P, Bentlage H, van Oost B: Extreme variability of clinical symptoms among sibs in a MELAS family correlated with heteroplasmy for the mitochondrial A3243G mutation. *J Neurol Sci* **124**:77, 1994.
969. Petruzzella V, Moraes CT, Sano MC, Bonilla E, DiMauro S, Schon EA: Extremely high levels of mutant mtDNAs co-localize with cytochrome c oxidase-negative ragged-red fibers in patients harboring a point mutation at nt 3243. *Hum Mol Genet* **3**:449, 1994.
970. Jean-Francois MJ, Lertrit P, Berkovic SF, Crimmins D, Morris J, Marzuki S, Byrne E: Heterogeneity in the phenotypic expression of the mutation in the mitochondrial tRNA(Leu) (UUR) gene generally associated with the MELAS subset of mitochondrial encephalomyopathies. *Aust N Z J Med* **24**:188, 1994.
971. Huang CC, Chen RS, Chen CM, Wang HS, Lee CC, Pang CY, Hsu HS, Lee HC, Wei YH: MELAS syndrome with mitochondrial tRNA(Leu(UUR)) gene mutation in a Chinese family. *J Neurol Neurosurg Psychiatry* **57**:586, 1994.

972. Tokunaga M, Mita S, Murakami T, Kumamoto T, Uchino M, Nonaka I, Ando M: Single muscle fiber analysis of mitochondrial myopathy, encephalopathy, lactic acidosis, and stroke-like episodes (MELAS). *Ann Neurol* **35**:413, 1994.

973. Matthews PM, Hopkin J, Brown RM, Stephenson JB, Hilton-Jones D, Brown GK: Comparison of the relative levels of the 3243 (A → G) mtDNA mutation in heteroplasmic adult and fetal tissues. *J Med Genet* **31**:41, 1994.

974. Hirano M, Pavlakis SG: Mitochondrial myopathy, encephalopathy, lactic acidosis, and strokelike episodes (MELAS): Current concepts. *J Child Neurol* **9**:4, 1994.

975. Shiraiwa N, Ishii A, Iwamoto H, Mizusawa H, Kagawa Y, Ohta S: Content of mutant mitochondrial DNA and organ dysfunction in a patient with a MELAS subgroup of mitochondrial encephalomyopathies. *J Neurol Sci* **120**:174, 1993.

976. Munscher C, Muller-Hocker J, Kadenbach B: Human aging is associated with various point mutations in tRNA genes of mitochondrial DNA. *Biol Chem Hoppe Seyler* **374**:1099, 1993.

977. Miyabayashi S, Hanamizu H, Nakamura R, Hayashi JI, Tada K: Clinical and biochemical phenotype of the MELAS mutation. *J Inherit Metab Dis* **16**:886, 1993.

978. Goto Y: [MELAS (mitochondrial myopathy, encephalopathy lactic acidosis, and stroke-like episodes): Clinical features and mitochondrial DNA mutations.] *Nippon Rinsho* **51**:2373, 1993.

979. Macmillan C, Lach B, Shoubridge EA: Variable distribution of mutant mitochondrial DNAs (tRNA(Leu[3243])) in tissues of symptomatic relatives with MELAS: the role of mitotic segregation. *Neurology* **43**:1586, 1993.

980. Love S, Nicoll JA, Kinrade E: Sequencing and quantitative assessment of mutant and wild-type mitochondrial DNA in paraffin sections from cases of MELAS. *J Pathol* **170**:9, 1993.

981. Stroh EM, Winterkorn JM, Jalkh AE, Lessell S: MELAS syndrome: A mitochondrially inherited disorder. *Int Ophthalmol Clin* **33**:169, 1993.

982. Suomalainen A, Majander A, Pihko H, Peltonen L, Syvanen AC: Quantification of tRNA3243(Leu) point mutation of mitochondrial DNA in MELAS patients and its effects on mitochondrial transcription. *Hum Mol Genet* **2**:525, 1993.

983. Hamazaki S, Koshiba M, Sugiyama T: Organ distribution of mutant mitochondrial tRNA(leu(UUR)) gene in a MELAS patient. *Acta Pathol Jpn* **43**:187, 1993.

984. Shoji Y, Sato W, Hayasaka K, Takada G: Tissue distribution of mutant mitochondrial DNA in mitochondrial myopathy, encephalopathy, lactic acidosis and stroke-like episodes (MELAS). *J Inherit Metab Dis* **16**:27, 1993.

985. Sakuta R, Goto Y, Horai S, Nonaka I: Mitochondrial DNA mutations at nucleotide positions 3243 and 3271 in mitochondrial myopathy, encephalopathy, lactic acidosis, and stroke-like episodes: a comparative study. *J Neurol Sci* **115**:158, 1993.

986. Kobayashi Y, Ichihashi K, Ohta S, Nihei K, Kagawa Y, Yanagisawa M, Momoi MY: The mutant mitochondrial genes in mitochondrial myopathy, encephalopathy, lactic acidosis and stroke-like episodes (MELAS) were selectively amplified through generations. *J Inherit Metab Dis* **15**:803, 1992.

987. Miyabayashi S, Hanamizu H, Nakamura R, Endo H, Tada K: Defects of mitochondrial respiratory enzymes in cloned cells from MELAS fibroblasts. *J Inherit Metab Dis* **15**:797, 1992.

988. Hirano M, Ricci E, Koenigsberger MR, Defendini R, Pavlakis SG, DeVivo DC, DiMauro S, Rowland LP: Melas: An original case and clinical criteria for diagnosis. *Neuromuscul Disord* **2**:125, 1992.

989. Inui K, Fukushima H, Tsukamoto H, Taniike M, Midorikawa M, Tanaka J, Nishigaki T, Okada S: Mitochondrial encephalomyopathies with the mutation of the mitochondrial tRNA(Leu(UUR)) gene. *J Pediatr* **120**:62, 1992.

990. Kobayashi Y, Momoi MY, Tominaga K, Shimoizumi H, Nihei K, Yanagisawa M, Kagawa Y, Ohta S: Respiration-deficient cells are caused by a single point mutation in the mitochondrial tRNA-Leu(UUR) gene in mitochondrial myopathy, encephalopathy, lactic acidosis, and stroke-like episodes (MELAS). *Am J Hum Genet* **49**:590, 1991.

991. Tanaka M, Ino H, Ohno K, Ohbayashi T, Ikebe S, Sano T, Ichiki T, Kobayashi M, Wada Y, Ozawa T: Mitochondrial DNA mutations in mitochondrial myopathy, encephalopathy, lactic acidosis, and stroke-like episodes (MELAS). *Biochem Biophys Res Commun* **174**:861, 1991.

992. Ino H, Tanaka M, Ohno K, Hattori K, Ikebe S, Sano T, Ozawa T, Ichiki T, Kobayashi M, Wada Y: Mitochondrial leucine tRNA mutation in a mitochondrial encephalomyopathy. *Lancet* **337**:234, 1991.

993. Chang TS, Johns DR, Walker D, de la Cruz Z, Maumence IH, Green WR: Ocular clinicopathologic study of the mitochondrial encephalomyopathy overlap syndromes. *Arch Ophthalmol* **111**:1254, 1993.

994. Crimmins D, Morris JG, Walker GL, Sue CM, Byrne E, Stevens S, Jean-Francis B, Yiannikas C, Pamphlett R: Mitochondrial encephalomyopathy: Variable clinical expression within a single kindred. *J Neurol Neurosurg Psychiatry* **56**:900, 1993.

995. Martinuzzi A, Bartolomei L, Carrozzo R, Mostacciuolo M, Carbonin C, Toso V, Ciafaloni E, Shanske S, DiMauro S, Angelini C: Correlation between clinical and molecular features in two MELAS. *J Neurol Sci* **113**:222, 1992.

996. Yoneda M, Chomyn A, Martinuzzi A, Hurko O, Attardi G: Marked replicative advantage of human mtDNA carrying a point mutation that causes the MELAS encephalomyopathy. *Proc Natl Acad Sci U S A* **89**:11164, 1992.

997. Ito T, Hattori K, Obayashi T, Tanaka M, Sugiyama S, Ozawa T: Mitochondrial DNA mutations in cardiomyopathy. *Jpn Circ J* **56**:1045, 1992.

998. Schon EA, Koga Y, Davidson M, Moraes CT, King MP: The mitochondrial tRNA(Leu)(UUR)) mutation in MELAS: a model for. *Biochim Biophys Acta* **1101**:206, 1992.

999. Onishi H, Inoue K, Osaka H, Nagatomo H, Ando N, Yamada Y, Suzuki K, Hanihara T, Kawamoto S, Okuda K, et al.: [MELAS associated with diabetes mellitus and point mutation in mitochondrial DNA.] *No To Shinkei* **44**:259, 1992.

1000. Sato W, Hayasaka K, Komatsu K, Sawaishi Y, Sakemi K, Shoji Y, Takada G: Genetic analysis of three pedigrees of mitochondrial myopathy. *Am J Hum Genet* **50**:655, 1992.

1001. Terauchi A, Tamagawa K, Morimatsu Y, Kobayashi M, Sano T, Yoda S: An autopsy case of mitochondrial encephalomyopathy, lactic acidosis and stroke-like episodes (MELAS) with a point mutation of mitochondrial DNA. *Brain Dev* **18**:224, 1996.

1002. Valanne L, Paetau A, Suomalainen A, Ketonen L, Pihko H: Laminar cortical necrosis in MELAS syndrome: MR and neuropathological observations. *Neuropediatrics* **27**:154, 1996.

1003. Cristofari M, Bertocchi P, Vigano M: [The MELAS syndrome and dilated-hypertrophic cardiomyopathy: A case report.] *G Ital Cardiol* **25**:69, 1995.

1004. Li JY, Kong KW, Chang MH, Cheung SC, Lee HC, Pang CY, Wei YH: MELAS syndrome associated with a tandem duplication in the D-loop of mitochondrial DNA. *Acta Neurol Scand* **93**:450, 1996.

1005. Yang CY, Lam HC, Lee HC, Wei YH, Lu CC, Han TM, Tsai JL, Chuang YH, Lee JK: MELAS syndrome associated with diabetes mellitus and hyperthyroidism: A case report from Taiwan. *Clin Endocrinol (Oxf)* **43**:235, 1995.

1006. Ihara M, Tanaka H, Yashiro M, Nishimura Y: [Mitochondrial myopathy, encephalopathy, lactic acidosis, and stroke-like episodes (MELAS) with chronic renal failure: Report of mother-child cases.] *Rinsho Shinkeigaku* **36**:1069, 1996.

1007. Rummelt V, Folberg R, Ionasescu V, Yi H, Moore KC: Ocular pathology of MELAS syndrome with mitochondrial DNA nucleotide 3243 point mutation. *Ophthalmology* **100**:1757, 1993.

1008. Ujike H, Wakagi T, Kohira I, Kuroda S, Otsuki S, Sato T: MELAS without ragged red fibers or lactic acidosis diagnosed by. *Jpn J Psychiatry Neurol* **47**:637, 1993.

1009. Kimata KG, Gordan L, Ajax ET, Davis PH, Grabowski T: A case of late-onset MELAS. *Arch Neurol* **55**:722, 1998.

1010. Minamoto H, Kawabata K, Okuda B, Shibuya N, Tachibana H, Sugita M, Goto Y, Nishino I, Nonaka I: Mitochondrial encephalomyopathy with elderly onset of stroke-like episodes [see Comments]. *Intern Med* **35**:991, 1996.

1011. Degoul F, Diry M, Pou-Serradell A, Lloreta J, Marsac C: Myoleukoencephalopathy in twins: Study of 3243-myopathy, encephalopathy, lactic acidosis, and strokelike episodes mitochondrial DNA mutation. *Ann Neurol* **35**:365, 1994.

1012. Folgero T, Torbergsen T, Oian P: The 3243 MELAS mutation in a pedigree with MERRF. *Eur Neurol* **35**:168, 1995.

1013. Chen RS, Huang CC, Lee CC, Wai YY, Hsi MS, Pang CY, Wei YH: Overlapping syndrome of MERRF and MELAS: Molecular and neuroradiological studies. *Acta Neurol Scand* **87**:494, 1993.

1014. Hiruta Y, Chin K, Shitomi K, Ichihara T, Mochizuki M, Adachi K, Obayashi T, Tanaka M, Ozawa T: Mitochondrial encephalomyopathy with A to G transition of mitochondrial transfer RNA(Leu(UUR)) 3,243 presenting hypertrophic cardiomyopathy. *Intern Med* **34**:670, 1995.

1015. Hoshino S, Tamaoka A, Ohkoshi N, Shoji S, Goto Y: [A case of mitochondrial encephalomyopathy showing ophthalmoplegia, diabetes mellitus and hearing loss associated with the A3243G mutation of mitochondrial DNA.] *Rinsho Shinkeigaku* **37**:326, 1997.
1016. Laforet P, Lombes A, Eymard B, Danan C, Chevallay M, Rouche A, Frachon P, Fardeau M: Chronic progressive external ophthalmoplegia with ragged-red fibers: Clinical, morphological and genetic investigations in 43 patients. *Neuromuscul Disord* **5**:399, 1995.
1017. Moraes CT, Ciacci F, Silvestri G, Shanske S, Sciacco M, Hirano M, Schon EA, Bonilla E, DiMauro S: Atypical clinical presentations associated with the MELAS mutation at position 3243 of human mitochondrial DNA. *Neuromuscul Disord* **3**:43, 1993.
1018. Fang W, Huang CC, Lee CC, Cheng SY, Pang CY, Wei YH: Ophthalmologic manifestations in MELAS syndrome. *Arch Neurol* **50**:977, 1993.
1019. Hsu CC, Chuang YH, Tsai JL, Jong HJ, Shen YY, Huang HL, Chen HL, Lee HC, Pang CY, Wei YH, et al.: CPEO and carnitine deficiency overlapping in MELAS syndrome. *Acta Neurol Scand* **92**:252, 1995.
1020. Vilarinho L, Santorelli FM, Rosas MJ, Tavares C, Melo-Pires M, DiMauro S: The mitochondrial A3243G mutation presenting as severe cardiomyopathy. *J Med Genet* **34**:607, 1997.
1021. Silvestri G, Bertini E, Servidei S, Rana M, Zachara E, Ricci E, Tonali P: Maternally inherited cardiomyopathy: A new phenotype associated with the A to G AT nt.3243 of mitochondrial DNA (MELAS mutation). *Muscle Nerve* **20**:221, 1997.
1022. Kawakami Y, Sakuta R, Hashimoto K, Fujino O, Fujita T, Hida M, Horai S, Goto Y, Nonaka I: Mitochondrial myopathy with progressive decrease in mitochondrial tRNA(Leu)(UUR) mutant genomes. *Ann Neurol* **35**:370, 1994.
1023. Onishi H, Hanihara T, Sugiyama N, Kawanishi C, Iseki E, Maruyama Y, Yamada Y, Kosaka K, Yagishita S, Sekihara H, Satoh S: Pancreatic exocrine dysfunction associated with mitochondrial tRNA(-Leu)(UUR) mutation. *J Med Genet* **35**:255, 1998.
1024. Inamori M, Ishigami T, Takahashi N, Hibi K, Ashino K, Sumita S, Tamura K, Ochiai H, Umemura S, Ishii M, Tanaka S, Sekihara H, Inayama Y: [A case of mitochondrial cardiomyopathy with heart failure, sick sinus syndrome and diabetes mellitus: Mitochondrial DNA adenine-to-guanine transition at 3243 of mitochondrial tRNA(LEU)(UUR) gene.] *J Cardiol* **30**:341, 1997.
1025. Shinomiya H, Fukuda N, Takeichi N, Soeki T, Shinohara H, Yui Y, Tamura Y, Fukada Y, Nakamura M, Miyatake K, Yutani C: [Evaluation of cardiac function by various cardiac imaging techniques in mitochondrial cardiomyopathy: a case report.] *J Cardiol* **31**:109, 1998.
1026. Yanagisawa K, Uchigata Y, Sanaka M, Sakura H, Minei S, Shimizu M, Kanamuro R, Kadowaki T, Omori Y: Mutation in the mitochondrial tRNA(leu) at position 3243 and spontaneous abortions in Japanese women attending a clinic for diabetic pregnancies. *Diabetologia* **38**:809, 1995.
1027. Takeda N: Cardiomyopathies and mitochondrial DNA mutations. *Mol Cell Biochem* **176**:287, 1997.
1028. Yoshida R, Ishida Y, Abo K, Hozumi T, Ueno H, Shiotani H, Kishimoto-Hashiramoto M, Hashiramoto M, Matsunaga K, Kasuga M, et al.: Hypertrophic cardiomyopathy in patients with diabetes mellitus associated with mitochondrial tRNA(Leu)(UUR) gene mutation [see Comments]. *Intern Med* **34**:953, 1995.
1029. Takeda N: Mitochondrial DNA mutations in diabetes mellitus and heart disease [Editorial; Comment]. *Intern Med* **34**:931, 1995.
1030. Kitaoka H, Kameoka K, Suzuki Y, Sasaki E, Majima M, Takada K, Katagiri H, Oka Y, Ohsawa N: A patient with diabetes mellitus, cardiomyopathy, and a mitochondrial gene mutation: Confirmation of a gene mutation in cardiac muscle. *Diabetes Res Clin Pract* **28**:207, 1995.
1031. Kuzuya N, Noda M, Fujii M, Kanazawa Y: [A pedigree with maternally transmitted diabetes mellitus, deafness and cardiomyopathy.] *Nippon Rinsho* **52**:2611, 1994.
1032. Odawara M, Tada K, Yamashita K: Decreased cerebral blood perfusion in an NIDDM patient with an A-to-G mutation in the mitochondrial gene: A possible contribution to cognition deficits in diabetes [Comment]. *Diabetologia* **38**:1004, 1995.
1033. Vialettes B, Paquis-Fluckinger V, Silvestre-Aillaud P, Ben Dahan D, Pelissier JF, Etchary-Bouyx F, Raccah D, Gin H, Guillausseau PJ, Vanuxen D, et al.: Extra-pancreatic manifestations in diabetes secondary to mitochondrial DNA point mutation within the tRNALeu(UUR) gene. *Diabetes Care* **18**:1023, 1995.
1034. Arai M, Ohshima S: Maternally inherited diabetes and deafness with cerebellar ataxia: A new clinical phenotype associated with the mitochondrial DNA 3243 mutation [Letter]. *J Neurol* **244**:468, 1997.
1035. Yorifuji T, Kawai M, Momoi T, Sasaki H, Furusho K, Muroi J, Shimizu K, Takahashi Y, Matsumura M, Nambu M, Okuno T: Nephropathy and growth hormone deficiency in a patient with mitochondrial tRNA(Leu(UUR)) mutation. *J Med Genet* **33**:621, 1996.
1036. Inagaki T, Ishino H, Seno H, Ohguni S, Tanaka J, Kato Y: Psychiatric symptoms in a patient with diabetes mellitus associated with point mutation in mitochondrial DNA. *Biol Psychiatry* **42**:1067, 1997.
1037. Harrison TJ, Boles RG, Johnson DR, LeBlond C, Wong LJ: Macular pattern retinal dystrophy, adult-onset diabetes, and deafness: A family study of A3243G mitochondrial heteroplasmy. *Am J Ophthalmol* **124**:217, 1997.
1038. Bonte CA, Matthijs GL, Cassiman JJ, Leys AM: Macular pattern dystrophy in patients with deafness and diabetes. *Retina* **17**:216, 1997.
1039. Bonte C, Leys A, Matthijs G, Missotten L: Fundus changes in patients with the mitochondrial DNA point mutation at position 3243. *Bull Soc Belge Ophtalmol* **261**:9, 1996.
1040. Massin P, Guillausseau PJ, Vialettes B, Paquis V, Orsini F, Grimaldi AD, Gaudric A: Macular pattern dystrophy associated with a mutation of mitochondrial DNA. *Am J Ophthalmol* **120**:247, 1995.
1041. Jansen JJ, Maassen JA, van der Woude FJ, Lemmink HA, van den Ouweland JM, t' Hart LM, Smeets HJ, Bruijn JA, Lemkes HH: Mutation in mitochondrial tRNA(Leu(UUR)) gene associated with progressive kidney disease. *J Am Soc Nephrol* **8**:1118, 1997.
1042. Verma A, Moraes CT, Shebert RT, Bradley WG: A MERRF/PEO overlap syndrome associated with the mitochondrial DNA 3243 mutation. *Neurology* **46**:1334, 1996.
1043. Campos Y, Martin MA, Lorenzo G, Aparicio M, Cabello A, Arenas J: Sporadic MERRF/MELAS overlap syndrome associated with the 3243 tRNA(Leu(UUR)) mutation of mitochondrial DNA. *Muscle Nerve* **19**:187, 1996.
1044. Nakase H: [Leigh's syndrome and mitochondrial myopathy.] *Nippon Rinsho* 51:2403, 1993.
1045. Kaido M, Fujimura H, Soga F, Toyooka K, Yoshikawa H, Nishimura T, Higashi T, Inui K, Imanishi H, Yorifuji S, Yanagihara T: Alzheimer-type pathology in a patient with mitochondrial myopathy, encephalopathy, lactic acidosis and stroke-like episodes (MELAS). *Acta Neuropathol (Berl)* **92**:312, 1996.
1046. Kamakura K, Abe H, Tadano Y, Nakamura R, Kobayashi H, Kawaguchi S, Nagata N, Matsuoka T, Sakuta R, Nonaka I: Recurrent respiratory failure in a patient with 3243 mutation in mitochondrial DNA [Letter]. *J Neurol* **242**:253, 1995.
1047. Onishi H, Kawanishi C, Iwasawa T, Osaka H, Hanihara T, Inoue K, Yamada Y, Kosaka K: Depressive disorder due to mitochondrial transfer RNALeu(UUR) mutation. *Biol Psychiatry* **41**:1137, 1997.
1048. Seibel P, Grunewald T, Gundolla A, Diener HC, Reichmann H: Investigation on the mitochondrial transfer RNA(Leu)(UUR) in blood cells from patients with cluster headache. *J Neurol* **243**:305, 1996.
1049. Cortelli P, Zacchini A, Barboni P, Malpassi P, Carelli V, Montagna P: Lack of association between mitochondrial tRNA(Leu(UUR)) point mutation and cluster headache [Letter; Comment]. *Lancet* **345**:1120, 1995.
1050. Damian MS, Seibel P, Schachenmayr W, Reichmann H, Dorndorf W: VACTERL with the mitochondrial np 3243 point mutation [see Comments]. *Am J Med Genet* **62**:398, 1996.
1051. Kishnani PS, Van Hove JL, Shoffner JS, Kaufman A, Bossen EH, Kahler SG: Acute pancreatitis in an infant with lactic acidosis and a mutation at nucleotide 3243 in the mitochondrial DNA tRNA-Leu(UUR) gene. *Eur J Pediatr* **155**:898, 1996.
1052. King MD, O'Neill G, Poulton J, Moran M, Burke M, Redmond J, Farrell MA: Polyneuropathy in the mtDNA base pain 3243 point mutation [Letter; Comment]. *Neurology* **46**:1495, 1996.
1053. Isozumi K, Fukuuchi Y, Tanaka K, Nogawa S, Ishihara T, Sakuta R: A MELAS (mitochondrial myopathy, encephalopathy, lactic acidosis, and stroke-like episodes) mtDNA mutation that induces subacute dementia which mimics Creutzfeldt-Jakob disease. *Intern Med* **33**:543, 1994.
1054. Hara K, Yamamoto M, Anegawa T, Sakuta R, Nakamura M: [Mitochondrial encephalomyopathy associated with parkinsonism and a point mutation in the mitochondrial tRNA(Leu)(UUR)) gene.] *Rinsho Shinkeigaku* **34**:361, 1994.
1055. Sue CM, Mitchell P, Crimmins DS, Moshegov C, Byrne E, Morris JG: Pigmentary retinopathy associated with the mitochondrial DNA 3243 point mutation. *Neurology* **49**:1013, 1997.
1056. Shanske AL, Shanske S, Silvestri G, Tanji K, Wertheim D, Lipper S: MELAS point mutation with unusual clinical presentation. *Neuromuscul Disord* **3**:191, 1993.

1057. Shaag A, Saada A, Steinberg A, Navon P, Elpeleg ON: Mitochondrial encephalomyopathy associated with a novel mutation in the mitochondrial tRNA(leu)(UUR) gene (A3243T). *Biochem Biophys Res Commun* **233**:637, 1997.

1058. Houshmand M, Larsson NG, Oldfors A, Tulinius M, Holme E: Fatal mitochondrial myopathy, lactic acidosis, and complex I deficiency associated with a heteroplasmic A → G mutation at position 3251 in the mitochondrial tRNALeu(UUR) gne. *Hum Genet* **97**:269, 1996.

1059. Sweeney MG, Bundey S, Brockington M, Poulton KR, Winer JB, Harding AE: Mitochondrial myopathy associated with sudden death in young adults and a novel mutation in the mitochondrial DNA leucine transfer RNA(UUR) gene. *Q J Med* **86**:709, 1993.

1060. Morten KJ, Cooper JM, Brown GK, Lake BD, Pike D, Poulton J: A new point mutation associated with mitochondrial encephalomyopathy. *Hum Molec Genet* **2**:2081, 1993.

1061. Kawarai T, Kawakami H, Kozuka K, Izumi Y, Matsuyama Z, Watanabe C, Kohriyama T, Nakamura S: A new mitochondrial DNA mutation associated with mitochondrial myopathy: tRNA(Leu)(UUR) 3254C-to-G. *Neurology* **49**:598, 1997.

1062. Hirai M, Suzuki S, Onoda M, Hinokio Y, Hirai A, Ohtomo M, Chiba M, Kasuga S, Hirai S, Satoh Y, Akai H, Miyabayashi S, Toyota T: Mitochondrial deoxyribonucleic acid 3256C-T mutation in a Japanese family with noninsulin-dependent diabetes mellitus. *J Clin Endocrinol Metab* **83**:992, 1998.

1063. Hirai M, Suzuki S: [Diabetes mellitus with mitochondrial DNA tRNA(Leu)(UUR) mutation at 3256(C-T).] *Nippon Rinsho* **56(Suppl 3)**:530, 1998.

1064. Hao H, Moraes CT: Functional and molecular mitochondrial abnormalities associated with a C → T transition at position 3256 of the human mitochondrial genome. The effects of a pathogenic mitochondrial tRNA point mutation in organelle translation and RNA processing. *J Biol Chem* **271**:2347, 1996.

1065. Moraes CT, Ciacci F, Bonilla E, Jansen C, Hirano M, Rao N, Lovelace RE, Rowland LP, Schon EA, DiMauro S: Two novel pathogenic mitochondrial DNA mutations affecting organelle number and protein synthesis. Is the tRNA(Leu(UUR)) gene an etiologic hot spot? *J Clin Invest* **92**:2906, 1993.

1066. Nishino I, Komatsu M, Kodama S, Horai S, Nonaka I, Goto Y: The 3260 mutation in mitochondrial DNA can cause mitochondrial myopathy, encephalopathy, lactic acidosis, and strokelike episodes (MELAS). *Muscle Nerve* **19**:1603, 1996.

1067. Zeviani M, Mariotti C, Antozzi C, Fratta GM, Rustin P, Prelle A: OXPHOS defects and mitochondrial DNA mutations in cardiomyopathy. *Muscle Nerve* **3**:S170, 1995.

1068. Mariotti C, Tiranti V, Carrara F, Dallapiccola B, DiDonato S, Zeviani M: Defective respiratory capacity and mitochondrial protein synthesis in transformant cybrids harboring the tRNA(Leu(UUR)) mutation associated with maternally inherited myopathy and cardiomyopathy. *J Clin Invest* **93**:1102, 1994.

1069. Sweeney MG, Brockington M, Weston MJ, Morgan-Hughes JA, Harding AE: Mitochondrial DNA transfer RNA mutation Leu(UUR)A → G 3260: A second family with myopathy and cardiomyopathy. *Q J Med* **86**:435, 1993.

1070. Deleted in proof.

1071. Suzuki Y, Suzuki S: [Diabetes mellitus with mitochondrial DNA tRNA(Leu)(UUR) mutation at 3264(T → C).] *Nippon Rinsho* **56(Suppl 3)**:534, 1998.

1072. Suzuki Y, Suzuki S, Hinokio Y, Chiba M, Atsumi Y, Hosokawa K, Shimada A, Asahina T, Matsuoka K: Diabetes associated with a novel 3264 mitochondrial tRNA(Leu)(UUR) mutation. *Diabetes Care* **20**:1138, 1997.

1073. Tarnopolsky MA, Maguire J, Myint T, Applegarth D, Robinson BH: Clinical, physiological, and histological features in a kindred with the T3271C melas mutation. *Muscle Nerve* **21**:25, 1998.

1074. Marie SK, Goto Y, Passos-Bueno MR, Zatz M, Carvalho AA, Carvalho M, Levy JA, Palou VB, Campiotto S, Horai S, et al.: A Caucasian family with the 3271 mutation in mitochondrial DNA. *Biochem Med Metab Biol* **52**:136, 1994.

1075. Hayashi J, Ohta S, Takai D, Miyabayashi S, Sakuta R, Goto Y, Nonaka I: Accumulation of mtDNA with a mutation at position 3271 in tRNA(Leu)(UUR) gene introduced from a MELAS patient to HeLa cells lacking mtDNA results in progressive inhibition of mitochondrial respiratory function. *Biochem Biophys Res Commun* **197**:1049, 1993.

1076. Shoffner JM, Bialer MG, Pavlakis SG, Lott M, Kaufman A, Dixon J, Teichberg S, Wallace DC: Mitochondrial encephalomyopathy caused by a single nucleotide deletion in the mitochondrial tRNA-leucine(UUR) gene. *Neurology* **45**:286, 1995.

1077. McCarthy M, Cassell P, Tran T, Mathias L, t Hart LM, Maassen JA, Snehalatha C, Ramachandran A, Viswanathan M, Hitman GA: Evaluation of the importance of maternal history of diabetes and of mitochondrial variation in the development of NIDDM. *Diabet Med* **13**:420, 1996.

1078. Goto Y-i, Tsugane K, Tanabe Y, Nonaka I, Horai S: A new point mutation at nucleotide pair 3291 of the mitochondrial tRNA-Leu(UUR) gene in a patient with mitochondrial myopathy, encephalopathy, lactic acidosis, and stroke-like episodes (MELAS). *Biochem Biophys Res Commun* **202**:1624, 1994.

1079. Bindoff LA, Howell N, Poulton J, McCullough DA, Morten KJ, Lightowlers RN, Turnbull DM, Weber K: Abnormal RNA processing associated with a novel tRNA mutation in mitochondrial DNA. A potential disease mechanism. *J Biol Chem* **268**:19559, 1993.

1080. Silvestri G, Santorelli FM, Shanske S, Whitley CB, Schimmenti LA, Smith SA, DiMauro S: A new mtDNA mutation in the tRNA(-Leu(UUR)) gene associated with maternally inherited cardiomyopathy. *Hum Mutat* **3**:37, 1994.

1081. Campos Y, Martin MA, Rubio JC, Gutierrez del Olmo MC, Cabello A, Arenas J: Bilateral striatal necrosis and MELAS associated with a new T3308C mutation in the mitochondrial ND1 gene. *Biochem Biophys Res Commun* **238**:323, 1997.

1082. Odawara M, Sasaki K, Yamashita K: A G-to-A substitution at nucleotide position 3316 in mitochondrial DNA is associated with Japanese non-insulin-dependent diabetes mellitus. *Biochem Biophys Res Commun* **227**:147, 1996.

1083. Kalinin VN, Schmidt W, Poller W, Olek K: [A new point mutation in the mitochondrial gene ND1, detected in a patient with type II diabetes.] *Genetika* **31**:1180, 1995.

1084. Nakagawa Y, Ikegami H, Yamato E, Takekawa K, Fujisawa T, Hamada Y, Ueda H, Uchigata Y, Miki T, Kumahara Y, et al.: A new mitochondrial DNA mutation associated with non-insulin-dependent diabetes mellitus [published erratum appears in *Biochem Biophys Res Commun* 212(2):718, 1995]. *Biochem Biophys Res Commun* **209**:664, 1995.

1085. Hirai M, Suzuki S, Onoda M, Hinokio Y, Ai L, Hirai A, Ohtomo M, Komatsu K, Kasuga S, Satoh Y, Akai H, Toyota T: Mitochondrial DNA 3394 mutation in the NADH dehydrogenase subunit 1 associated with non-insulin-dependent diabetes mellitus. *Biochem Biophys Res Commun* **219**:951, 1996.

1086. Shoffner JM, Brown MD, Torroni A, Lott MT, Cabell MF, Mirra SS, Beal MF, Yang C-C, Gearing M, Salvo R, Watts RL, Juncos JL, Hansen LA, Crain BJ, Fayad M, Reckord CL, Wallace DC: Mitochondrial DNA mutations associated with Alzheimer's and Parkinson's disease. *Genomics* **17**:171, 1993.

1087. Black GC, Craig IW, Oostra RJ, Norby S, Rosenberg T, Morten K, Laborde A, Poulton J: Leber's hereditary optic neuropathy: Implications of the sex ratio for linkage studies in families with the 3460 ND1 mutation. *Eye* **9**:513, 1995.

1088. Howell N, Kubacka I, Halvorson S, Howell B, McCullough DA, Mackey D: Phylogenetic analysis of the mitochondrial genomes from Leber hereditary optic neuropathy pedigrees. *Genetics* **140**:285, 1995.

1089. Harding AE, Sweeney MG, Govan GG, Riordan-Eva P: Pedigree analysis in Leber hereditary optic neuropathy families with a pathogenic mtDNA mutation. *Am J Hum Genet* **57**:77, 1995.

1090. Hiida Y, Mashima Y, Saga M, Shuu M, Akiya S, Kudoh J, Shimizu N, Oguchi Y: [Molecular genetic analysis of Leber's hereditary optic neuropathy with the 3460 mutation in Japanese pedigrees.] *Nippon Ganka Gakkai Zasshi* **99**:728, 1995.

1091. Harding AE, Riordan-Eva P, Govan GG: Mitochondrial DNA diseases: Genotype and phenotype in Leber's hereditary optic neuropathy. *Muscle Nerve* **3**:S82, 1995.

1092. Riordan-Eva P, Sanders MD, Govan GG, Sweeney MG, Da Costa J, Harding AE: The clinical features of Leber's hereditary optic neuropathy defined by the presence of a pathogenic mitochondrial DNA mutation. *Brain* **118**:319, 1995.

1093. Leo-Kottler B, Christ-Adler M, Reck B, Wissinger B, Zrenner E: [Correlation between clinical and molecular genetic findings in Leber's optic atrophy.] *Ophthalmologe* **92**:86, 1995.

1094. Smith PR, Cooper JM, Govan GG, Harding AE, Schapira AH: Platelet mitochondrial function in Leber's hereditary optic neuropathy. *J Neurol Sci* **122**:80, 1994.

1095. Mackey DA: Three subgroups of patients from the United Kingdom with Leber hereditary optic neuropathy. *Eye* **8**:431, 1994.

1096. Nikoskelainen EK, Savontaus ML, Huoponen K, Antila K, Hartiala J: Pre-excitation syndrome in Leber's hereditary optic neuropathy. *Lancet* **344**:857, 1994.

1097. Oostra RJ, Bolhuis PA, Zorn-Ende I, de Kok-Nazaruk MM, Bleeker-Wagemakers EM: Leber's hereditary optic neuropathy: No significant evidence for primary or secondary pathogenicity of the 15257 mutation. *Hum Genet* **94**:265, 1994.

1098. Oostra RJ, Bolhuis PA, Wijburg FA, Zorn-Ende G, Bleeker-Wagemakers EM: Leber's hereditary optic neuropathy: Correlations between mitochondrial genotype and visual outcome. *J Med Genet* **31**:280, 1994.

1099. Borruat FX, Sanders MD: [Atypical presentation of Leber's optic neuropathy.] *Klin Monatsbl Augenheilkd* **204**:400, 1994.

1100. Juvonen V, Huoponen K, Syvanen AC, Nikoskelainen E, Savontaus ML: Quantification of point mutations associated with Leber hereditary optic neuroretinopathy by solid-phase minisequencing. *Hum Genet* **93**:16, 1994.

1101. Huoponen K, Lamminen T, Juvonen V, Aula P, Nikoskelainen E, Savontaus ML: The spectrum of mitochondrial DNA mutations in families with Leber hereditary optic neuroretinopathy. *Hum Genet* **92**:379, 1993.

1102. Majander A, Huoponen K, Savontaus ML, Nikoskelainen E, Wikstrom M: Electron transfer properties of NADH:ubiquinone reductase in the ND1/3460 and the ND4/11778 mutations of the Leber hereditary optic neuroretinopathy (LHON). *FEBS Lett* **292**:289, 1991.

1103. Huoponen K, Vilkki J, Aula P, Nikoskelainen EK, Savontaus ML: A new mtDNA mutation associated with Leber hereditary optic neuroretinopathy. *Am J Hum Genet* **48**:1147, 1991.

1104. Tanno Y, Yoneda M, Tanaka K, Tsuji S: [Molecular genetic analysis for Leber's hereditary optic neuropathy.] *Nippon Rinsho* **51**:2396, 1993.

1105. Newman NJ: Leber's hereditary optic neuropathy. New genetic considerations. *Arch Neurol* **50**:540, 1993.

1106. Johns DR, Smith KH, Miller NR: Leber's hereditary optic neuropathy. Clinical manifestations of the 3460 mutation. *Arch Ophthalmol* **110**:1577, 1992.

1107. Meire FM, Van Coster R, Cochaux P, Obermaier-Kusser B, Candaele C, Martin JJ: Neurological disorders in members of families with Leber's hereditary optic neuropathy (LHON) caused by different mitochondrial mutations. *Ophthalmic Genet* **16**:119, 1995.

1108. Kellar-Wood H, Robertson N, Govan GG, Compston DA, Harding AE: Leber's hereditary optic neuropathy mitochondrial DNA mutations in multiple sclerosis. *Ann Neurol* **36**:109, 1994.

1109. Hayashi J, Ohta S, Kagawa Y, Takai D, Miyabayashi S, Tada K, Fukushima H, Inui K, Okada S, Goto Y, et al.: Functional and morphological abnormalities of mitochondria in human cells containing mitochondrial DNA with pathogenic point mutations in tRNA genes. *J Biol Chem* **269**:19060, 1994.

1110. Taniike M, Fukushima H, Yanagihara I, Tsukamoto H, Tanaka J, Fujimura H, Nagai T, Sano T, Yamaoka K, Inui K, et al.: Mitochondrial tRNA(Ile) mutation in fatal cardiomyopathy. *Biochem Biophys Res Commun* **186**:47, 1992.

1111. Silvestri G, Servidei S, Rana M, Ricci E, Spinazzola A, Paris E, Tonali P: A novel mitochondrial DNA point mutation in the tRNA(Ile) gene is associated with progressive external ophthalmoplegia. *Biochem Biophys Res Commun* **220**:623, 1996.

1112. Merante F, Myint T, Tein I, Benson L, Robinson BH: An additional mitochondrial tRNA(Ile) point mutation (A-to-G at nucleotide 4295) causing hypertrophic cardiomyopathy. *Hum Mutat* **8**:216, 1996.

1113. Taylor RW, Chinnery PF, Bates MJ, Jackson MJ, Johnson MA, Andrews RM, Turnbull DM: A novel mitochondrial DNA point mutation in the tRNA(Ile) gene: Studies in a patient presenting with chronic progressive external ophthalmoplegia and multiple sclerosis. *Biochem Biophys Res Commun* **243**:47, 1998.

1114. Casali C, Santorelli FM, D'Amati G, Bernucci P, DeBiase L, DiMauro S: A novel mtDNA point mutation in maternally inherited cardiomyopathy. *Biochem Biophys Res Commun* **213**:588, 1995.

1115. Santorelli FM, Mak SC, Vazquez-Acevedo M, Gonzalez-Astiazaran A, Ridaura-Sanz C, Gonzalez-Halphen D, DiMauro S: A novel mitochondrial DNA point mutation associated with mitochondrial encephalocardiomyopathy. *Biochem Biophys Res Commun* **216**:835, 1995.

1116. Vissing J, Salamon MB, Arlien-Soborg P, Norby S, Manta P, DiMauro S, Schmalbruch H: A new mitochondrial tRNA(Met) gene mutation in a patient with dystrophic muscle and exercise intolerance. *Neurology* **50**:1875, 1998.

1117. Silvestri G, Rana M, DiMuzio A, Uncini A, Tonali P, Servidei S: A late-onset mitochondrial myopathy is associated with a novel mitochondrial DNA (mtDNA) point mutation in the tRNA(Trp) gene. *Neuromuscul Disord* **8**:291, 1998.

1118. Santorelli FM, Tanji K, Sano M, Shanske S, El-Shahawi M, Kranz-Eble P, DiMauro S, De Vivo DC: Maternally inherited encephalopathy associated with a single-base insertion in the mitochondrial tRNATrp gene. *Ann Neurol* **42**:256, 1997.

1119. Nelson I, Hanna MG, Alsanjari N, Scaravilli F, Morgan-Hughes JA, Harding AE: A new mitochondrial DNA mutation associated with progressive dementia and chorea: a clinical, pathological, and molecular genetic study. *Ann Neurol* **37**:400, 1995.

1120. Bidooki SK, Johnson MA, Chrzanowska-Lightowlers Z, Bindoff LA, Lightowlers RN: Intracellular mitochondrial triplasmy in a patient with two heteroplasmic base changes. *Am J Hum Genet* **60**:1430, 1997.

1121. Zsurka G, Ormos J, Ivanyi B, Turi S, Endreffy E, Magyari M, Sonkodi S, Venetianer P: Mitochondrial mutation as a probable causative factor in familial progressive tubulointerstitial nephritis. *Hum Genet* **99**:484, 1997.

1122. Seibel P, Lauber J, Klopstock T, Marsac C, Kadenbach B, Reichmann H: Chronic progressive external ophthalmoplegia is associated with a novel mutation in the mitochondrial tRNA(Asn) gene. *Biochem Biophys Res Commun* **204**:482, 1994.

1123. Santorelli FM, Siciliano G, Casali C, Basirico MG, Carrozzo R, Calvosa F, Sartucci F, Bonfiglio L, Murri L, DiMauro S: Mitochondrial tRNA(Cys) gene mutation (A5814G): A second family with mitochondrial encephalopathy. *Neuromuscul Disord* **7**:156, 1997.

1124. Manfredi G, Schon EA, Bonilla E, Moraes CT, Shanske S, DiMauro S: Identification of a mutation in the mitochondrial tRNA(Cys) gene associated with mitochondrial encephalopathy. *Hum Mutat* **7**:158, 1996.

1125. Sahashi K, Ibi T, Yoneda M, Tanaka M, Ohno K: [A mitochondrial DNA mutation in the heteroplasmic tRNA-Tyr gene associated with chronic progressive external ophthalmoplegia—Clinical and molecular biological study.] *Nippon Rinsho* **55**:3265, 1997.

1126. Comi GP, Bordoni A, Salani S, Franceschina L, Sciacco M, Prelle A, Fortunato F, Zeviani M, Napoli L, Bresolin N, Moggio M, Ausenda CD, Taanman JW, Scarlato G: Cytochrome c oxidase subunit I microdeletion in a patient with motor neuron disease. *Ann Neurol* **43**:110, 1998.

1127. Gattermann N, Retzlaff S, Wang YL, Hofhaus G, Heinisch J, Aul C, Schneider W: Heteroplasmic point mutations of mitochondrial DNA affecting subunit I of cytochrome c oxidase in two patients with acquired idiopathic sideroblastic anemia. *Blood* **90**:4961, 1997.

1128. Hyslop SJ, James AM, Maw M, Fischel-Ghodsian N, Murphy MP: The effect on mitochondrial function of the tRNA Ser(UCN)/COI A7445G mtDNA point mutation associated with maternally inherited sensorineural deafness. *Biochem Mol Biol Int* **42**:567, 1997.

1129. Fischel-Ghodsian N, Prezant TR, Fournier P, Stewart IA, Maw M: Mitochondrial mutation associated with nonsyndromic deafness. *Am J Otolaryngol* **16**:403, 1995.

1130. Reid FM, Vernham GA, Jacobs HT: A novel mitochondrial point mutation in a maternal pedigree with sensorineural deafness. *Hum Mutat* **3**:243, 1994.

1131. Guan M-X, Enriquez JA, Fischel-Ghodsian N, Puranam RS, Lin CP, Maw MA, Attardi G: The deafness associated mitochondrial DNA mutation at position 7445, which affects tRAN serine(UCN) precursor processing, has long-range effects on NADH dehydrogenase subunit ND6 gene expression. *Mol Cell Biol* **18**:5868, 1998.

1132. Sevior KB, Hatamochi A, Stewart IA, Bykhovskaya Y, Allen-Powell DR, Fischel-Ghodsian N, Maw MA: Mitochondrial A7445G mutation in two pedigrees with palmoplantar keratoderma and deafness. *Am J Med Genet* **75**:179, 1998.

1133. Tiranti V, Chariot P, Carella F, Toscano A, Soliveri P, Girlanda P, Carrara F, Fratta GM, Reid FM, Mariotti C, et al.: Maternally inherited hearing loss, ataxia and myoclonus associated with a novel point mutation in mitochondrial tRNASer(UCN) gene. *Hum Mol Genet* **4**:1421, 1995.

1134. Vernham GA, Reid FM, Rundle PA, Jacobs HT: Bilateral sensorineural hearing loss in members of a maternal lineage with mitochondrial point mutation. *Clin Otolaryngol* **19**:314, 1994.

1135. Nakamura M, Nakano S, Goto Y, Ozawa M, Nagahama Y, Fukuyama H, Akiguchi I, Kaji R, Kimura J: A novel point mutation in the mitochondrial tRNA(Ser(UCN)) gene detected in a family with MERRF/MELAS overlap syndrome. *Biochem Biophys Res Commun* **214**:86, 1995.

1136. Fabrizi GM, Tiranti V, Mariotti C, Guazzi GC, Malandrini A, DiDonato S, Zeviani M: Sequence analysis of mitochondrial DNA in a new maternally inherited encephalomyopathy. *J Neurol* **242**:490, 1995.

1137. Passarino G, Semino O, Modiano G, Santachiara-Benerecetti AS: COII/tRNA(Lys) intergenic 9-bp deletion and other mtDNA markers. *Am J Hum Genet* **53**:609, 1993.
1138. Arenas J, Campos Y, Bornstein B, Ribacoba R, Martin MA, Rubio JC, Santorelli FM, Zeviani M, DiMauro S, Garesse R: A double mutation (A8296G and G8363A) in the mitochondrial DNA tRNA-Lysine gene associated with myoclonus epilepsy with ragged-red fibers. *Neurology* **52**:377, 1999.
1139. Verma A, Piccoli DA, Bonilla E, Berry GT, DiMauro S, Moraes CT: A novel mitochondrial G8313A mutation associated with prominent initial gastrointestinal symptoms and progressive encephaloneuropathy. *Pediatr Res* **42**:448, 1997.
1140. Ozawa M, Goto Y, Sakuta R, Tanno Y, Tsuji S, Nonaka I: The 8,344 mutation in mitochondrial DNA: A comparison between the proportion of mutant DNA and clinicopathologic findings. *Neuromuscul Disord* **5**:483, 1995.
1141. Campos Y, Martin MA, Vaamonde J, Cabello A, Esteban J, Arenas J: Clinical variability associated with the mutation at nucleotide position 8344 of the mitochondrial DNA. *J Inherit Metab Dis* **19**:119, 1996.
1142. Chen RS, Huang CC, Chu NS, Chu CC, Shih KD, Pang CY, Wei YH: Tissue distribution of mutant mitochondrial DNA in a patient with MERRF syndrome. *Muscle Nerve* **19**:519, 1996.
1143. Oldfors A, Holme E, Tulinius M, Larsson NG: Tissue distribution and disease manifestations of the tRNA(Lys) A → G(8344) mitochondrial DNA mutation in a case of myoclonus epilepsy and ragged red fibres. *Acta Neuropathol (Berl)* **90**:328, 1995.
1144. Huang CC, Chu NS, Shih KD, Pang CY, Wei YH: Distribution and clinical expression of the tRNA(Lys) mutation in mitochondrial DNA in MERRF syndrome. *J Formos Med Assoc* **94**:159, 1995.
1145. Thompson PD, Hammans SR, Harding AE: Cortical reflex myoclonus in patients with the mitochondrial DNA transfer RNA(Lys)(8344) (MERRF) mutation. *J Neurol* **241**:335, 1994.
1146. Fang W, Huang CC, Chu NS, Lee CC, Chen RS, Pang CY, Shih KD, Wei YH: Myoclonic epilepsy with ragged-red fibers (MERRF) syndrome: report of a Chinese family with mitochondrial DNA point mutation in tRNA(Lys) gene [see Comments]. *Muscle Nerve* **17**:52, 1994.
1147. Graf WD, Sumi SM, Copass MK, Ojemann LM, Longstreth WT, Jr., Shanske S, Lombes A, DiMauro S: Phenotypic heterogeneity in families with the myoclonic epilepsy and ragged-red fiber disease point mutation in mitochondrial DNA. *Ann Neurol* **33**:640, 1993.
1148. Suomalainen A, Kollmann P, Octave JN, Soderlund H, Syvanen AC: Quantification of mitochondrial DNA carrying the tRNA(8344Lys) point mutation in myoclonus epilepsy and ragged-red-fiber disease. *Eur J Hum Genet* **1**:88, 1993.
1149. Tanno Y, Yoneda M, Tanaka K, Kondo R, Hozumi I, Wakabayashi K, Yamada M, Fukuhara N, Ikuta F, Tsuji S: Uniform tissue distribution of tRNA(Lys) mutation in mitochondrial DNA in MERRF patients. *Neurology* **43**:1198, 1993.
1150. Nomura T, Ota M, Kotake N, Tanaka K: [Two cases of MERRF (myoclonus epilepsy associated with ragged red fibers) showing different clinical features in the same family.] *Rinsho Shinkeigaku* **33**:1198, 1993.
1151. Piccolo G, Focher F, Verri A, Spadari S, Banfi P, Gerosa E, Mazzarello P: Myoclonus epilepsy and ragged-red fibers: Blood mitochondrial DNA heteroplasmy in affected and asymptomatic members of a family. *Acta Neurol Scand* **88**:406, 1993.
1152. Ohtsuka Y, Amano R, Oka E, Ohtahara S: Myoclonus epilepsy with ragged-red fibers: A clinical and electrophysiologic follow-up study on two sibling cases. *J Child Neurol* **8**:366, 1993.
1153. Franceschetti S, Antozzi C, Binelli S, Carrara F, Nardocci N, Zeviani M, Avanzini G: Progressive myoclonus epilepsies: An electroclinical, biochemical, morphological and molecular genetic study of 17 cases. *Acta Neurol Scand* **87**:219, 1993.
1154. Hammans SR, Sweeney MG, Brockington M, Lennox GG, Lawton NF, Kennedy CR, Morgan-Hughes JA, Harding AE: The mitochondrial DNA transfer RNA(Lys)A → G(8344) mutation and the syndrome of myoclonic epilepsy with ragged red fibres (MERRF). Relationship of clinical phenotype to proportion of mutant mitochondrial DNA. *Brain* **116**:617, 1993.
1155. de Vries DD, de Wijs IJ, Wolff G, Ketelsen UP, Ropers HH, van Oost BA: X-linked myoclonus epilepsy explained as a maternally inherited mitochondrial disorder. *Hum Genet* **91**:51, 1993.
1156. Lombes A, Diaz C, Romero NB, Ziegler F, Fardeau M: Analysis of the tissue distribution and inheritance of heteroplasmic mitochondrial DNA point mutation by denaturing gradient gel electrophoresis in MERRF syndrome. *Neuromuscul Disord* **2**:323, 1992.
1157. Matsuoka T, Goto Y, Yoneda M, Nonaka I: Muscle histopathology in myoclonus epilepsy with ragged-red fibers (MERRF). *J Neurol Sci* **106**:193, 1991.
1158. Yoneda M, Tanno Y, Nonaka I, Miyatake T, Tsuji S: Simple detection of tRNA(Lys) mutation in myoclonus epilepsy associated with ragged-red fibers (MERRF) by polymerase chain reaction with a mismatched primer. *Neurology* **41**:1838, 1991.
1159. Bindoff LA, Desnuelle C, Birch-Machin MA, Pellissier JF, Serratrice G, Dravet C, Bureau M, Howell N, Turnbull DM: Multiple defects of the mitochondrial respiratory chain in a mitochondrial encephalopathy (MERRF): A clinical, biochemical and molecular study. *J Neurol Sci* **102**:17, 1991.
1160. Shih KD, Yen TC, Pang CY, Wei YH: Mitochondrial DNA mutation in a Chinese family with myoclonic epilepsy and ragged-red fiber disease. *Biochem Biophys Res Commun* **174**:1109, 1991.
1161. Shoffner JM, Lott MT, Wallace DC: MERRF: A model disease for understanding the principles of mitochondrial genetics. *Rev Neurol (Paris)* **147**:431, 1991.
1162. Byrne E, Trounce I, Marzuki S, Dennett X, Berkovic SF, Davis S, Tanaka M, Ozawa T: Functional respiratory chain studies in mitochondrial cytopathies. Support for mitochondrial DNA heteroplasmy in myoclonus epilepsy and ragged red fibers (MERRF) syndrome. *Acta Neuropathol (Berl)* **81**:318, 1991.
1163. Lertrit P, Noer AS, Byrne E, Marzuki S: Tissue segregation of a heteroplasmic mtDNA mutation in MERRF. *Hum Genet* **90**:251, 1992.
1164. Suomalainen A, Ciafaloni E, Koga Y, Peltonen L, DiMauro S, Schon EA: Use of single strand conformation polymorphism analysis to detect. *J Neurol Sci* **111**:222, 1992.
1165. Iwanga K, Mori K, Inoue M, Yoshimura T, Tanno Y: [Myoclonus epilepsy associated with ragged-red fibers—Report of a patient with negative myoclonus.] *Rinsho Shinkeigaku* **32**:870, 1992.
1166. Yoneda M, Tanno Y, Horai S, Ozawa T, Miyatake T, Tsuji S: A common mitochondrial DNA mutation in the t-RNA(Lys) of patients with myoclonus epilepsy associated with ragged-red fibers. *Biochem Int* **21**:789, 1990.
1167. Tanno Y, Yoneda M, Tanaka K, Tsuji S: Molecular genetic analysis for myoclonus epilepsy associated with ragged-red fibers (MERRF). *Nippon Rinsho* **51**:2379, 1993.
1168. Isashiki Y, Nakagawa M, Yamada H, Miyata M: [Ocular manifestations in mitochondrial DNA abnormalities.] *Nippon Ganka Gakkai Zasshi* **98**:3, 1994.
1169. Sanger TD, Jain KD: MERRF syndrome with overwhelming lactic acidosis. *Pediatr Neurol* **14**:57, 1996.
1170. Penisson-Besnier I, Degoul F, Desnuelle C, Dubas F, Josi K, Emile J, Lestienne P: Uneven distribution of mitochondrial DNA mutation in MERRF dizygotic. *J Neurol Sci* **110**:144, 1992.
1171. Huang WY, Chi CS, Mak SC, Wu HM, Yang MT: Leigh syndrome presenting with dystonia: Report of one case. *Chung Hua Min Kuo Hsiao Erh Ko I Hsueh Hui Tsa Chih* **36**:378, 1995.
1172. Howell N, Kubacka I, Smith R, Frerman F, Parks JK, Parker WD Jr: Association of the mitochondrial 8344 MERRF mutation with maternally inherited spinocerebellar degeneration and Leigh disease. *Neurology* **46**:219, 1996.
1173. Sweeney MG, Hammans SR, Duchen LW, Cooper JM, Schapira AH, Kennedy CR, Jacobs JM, Youl BD, Morgan-Hughes JA, Harding AE: Mitochondrial DNA mutation underlying Leigh's syndrome: Clinical, pathological, biochemical, and genetic studies of a patient presenting with progressive myoclonic epilepsy. *J Neurol Sci* **121**:57, 1994.
1174. Santorelli FM, Tanji K, Shanske S, Krishna S, Schmidt RE, Greenwood RS, DiMauro S, De Vivo DC: The mitochondrial DNA A8344G mutation in Leigh syndrome revealed by analysis in paraffin embedded sections: Revisiting the past. *Ann Neurol* **44**:962, 1998.
1175. Suzuki S, Hinokio Y, Hirai S, Onoda M, Matsumoto M, Ohtomo M, Kawasaki H, Satoh Y, Akai H, Abe K, et al.: Diabetes with mitochondrial gene tRNALYS mutation. *Diabetes Care* **17**:1428, 1994.
1176. Sano M, Ozawa M, Shiota S, Momose Y, Uchigata M, Goto Y: The T-C(8356) mitochondrial DNA mutation in a Japanese family. *J Neurol* **243**:441, 1996.
1177. Serra G, Piccinnu R, Tondi M, Muntoni F, Zeviani M, Mastropaolo C: Clinical and EEG findings in eleven patients affected by mitochondrial encephalomyopathy with MERRF-MELAS overlap. *Brain Dev* **18**:185, 1996.
1178. Masucci JP, Davidson M, Koga Y, Schon EA, King MP: In vitro analysis of mutations causing myoclonus epilepsy with ragged-red fibers in the mitochondrial tRNA(Lys)gene: two genotypes produce similar phenotypes. *Mol Cell Biol* **15**:2872, 1995.

1179. Ozawa M, Nishino I, Horai S, Nonaka I, Goto YI: Myoclonus epilepsy associated with ragged-red fibers: A G-to-A mutation at nucleotide pair 8363 in mitochondrial tRNA(Lys) in two families. *Muscle Nerve* **20**:271, 1997.
1180. Ozawa M, Nishino I, Watanabe A, Yamamoto H, Fujimoto M, Horai S, Nonaka I, Goto Y: A novel point mutation in mitochondrial lysine tRNA in two Japanese families with myoclonic epilepsy and ragged-red fiber disease (MERRF). *Am J Hum Genet* **57(Suppl)**:A223, 1995.
1181. De Meirleir L, Seneca S, Lissens W, Schoentjes E, Desprechins B: Bilateral striatal necrosis with a novel point mutation in the mitochondrial ATPase 6 gene. *Pediatr Neurol* **13**:242, 1995.
1182. Takahashi S, Makita Y, Oki J, Miyamoto A, Yanagawa J, Naito E, Goto Y, Okuno A: De novo mtDNA nt 8993 (T → G) mutation resulting in Leigh syndrome [Letter]. *Am J Hum Genet* **62**:717, 1998.
1183. Uziel G, Moroni I, Lamantea E, Fratta GM, Ciceri E, Carrara F, Zeviani M: Mitochondrial disease associated with the T8993G mutation of the mitochondrial ATPase 6 gene: A clinical, biochemical, and molecular study in six families. *J Neurol Neurosurg Psychiatry* **63**:16, 1997.
1184. Degoul F, Francois D, Diry M, Ponsot G, Desguerre I, Heron B, Marsac C, Moutard ML: A near homoplasmic T8993G mtDNA mutation in a patient with atypic Leigh syndrome not present in the mother's tissues. *J Inherit Metab Dis* **20**:49, 1997.
1185. Seller A, Kennedy CR, Temple IK, Brown GK: Leigh syndrome resulting from de novo mutation at position 8993 of mitochondrial DNA. *J Inherit Metab Dis* **20**:102, 1997.
1186. Naito E, Ito M, Yokota I, Saijo T, Matsuda J, Osaka H, Kimura S, Kuroda Y: [Defects of pyruvate metabolism in cultured lymphoblastoid cells of 20 patients with Leigh syndrome.] *No To Hattatsu* **28**:495, 1996.
1187. Tulinius MH, Houshmand M, Larsson NG, Holme E, Oldfors A, Holmberg E, Wahlstrom J: De novo mutation in the mitochondrial ATP synthase subunit 6 gene (T8993G) with rapid segregation resulting in Leigh syndrome in the offspring. *Hum Genet* **96**:290, 1995.
1188. Marin-Garcia J, Ananthakrishnan R, Korson M, Goldenthal MJ, Perez-Atayde A: Cardiac mitochondrial dysfunction in Leigh syndrome. *Pediatr Cardiol* **17**:387, 1996.
1189. Degoul F, Diry M, Rodriguez D, Robain O, Francois D, Ponsot G, Marsac C, Desguerre I: Clinical, biochemical, and molecular analysis of a maternally inherited case of Leigh syndrome (MILS) associated with the mtDNA T8993G point mutation. *J Inherit Metab Dis* **18**:682, 1995.
1190. Makela-Bengs P, Suomalainen A, Majander A, Rapola J, Kalimo H, Nuutila A, Pihko H: Correlation between the clinical symptoms and the proportion of mitochondrial DNA carrying the 8993 point mutation in the NARP syndrome. *Pediatr Res* **37**:634, 1995.
1191. Ciafaloni E, Santorelli FM, Shanske S, Deonna T, Roulet E, Janzer C, Pescia G, DiMauro S: Maternally inherited Leigh syndrome. *J Pediatr* **122**:419, 1993.
1192. Ortiz RG, Newman NJ, Shoffner JM, Kaufman AE, Koontz DA, Wallace DC: Variable retinal and neurologic manifestations in patients harboring the mitochondrial DNA 8993 mutation. *Arch Ophthalmol* **111**:1525, 1993.
1193. Yoshinaga H, Ogino T, Ohtahara S, Sakuta R, Nonaka I, Horai S: A T-to-G mutation at nucleotide pair 8993 in mitochondrial DNA in a patient with Leigh's syndrome. *J Child Neurol* **8**:129, 1993.
1194. Sakuta R, Goto Y, Horai S, Ogino T, Yoshinaga H, Ohtahara S, Nonaka I: Mitochondrial DNA mutation and Leigh's syndrome [Letter]. *Ann Neurol* **32**:597, 1992.
1195. Pastores GM, Santorelli FM, Shanske S, Gelb BD, Fyfe B, Wolfe D, Willner JP: Leigh syndrome and hypertrophic cardiomyopathy in an infant with a mitochondrial DNA point mutation (T8993G). *Am J Med Genet* **50**:265, 1994.
1196. Mak SC, Chi CS, Liu CY, Pang CY, Wei YH: Leigh syndrome associated with mitochondrial DNA 8993 T → G mutation and ragged-red fibers. *Pediatr Neurol* **15**:72, 1996.
1197. Santorelli FM, Tanji K, Shanske S, DiMauro S: Heterogeneous clinical presentation of the mtDNA NARP/T8993G mutation. *Neurology* **49**:270, 1997.
1198. Lodi R, Montagna P, Iotti S, Zaniol P, Barboni P, Puddu P, Barbiroli B: Brain and muscle energy metabolism studied in vivo by 31P-magnetic resonance spectroscopy in NARP syndrome. *J Neurol Neurosurg Psychiatry* **57**:1492, 1994.
1199. Tatuch Y, Robinson BH: The mitochondrial DNA mutation at 8993 associated with NARP slows the rate of ATP synthesis in isolated lymphoblast mitochondria. *Biochem Biophys Res Commun* **192**:124, 1993.
1200. Harding AE, Holt IJ, Sweeney MG, Brockington M, Davis MB: Prenatal diagnosis of mitochondrial DNA8993 T → G disease. *Am J Hum Genet* **50**:629, 1992.
1201. Puddu P, Barboni P, Mantovani V, Montagna P, Cerullo A, Bragliani M, Molinotti C, Caramazza R: Retinitis pigmentosa, ataxia, and mental retardation associated with mitochondrial DNA mutation in an Italian family. *Br J Ophthalmol* **77**:84, 1993.
1202. Houstek J, Klement P, Hermanska J, Houstkova H, Hansikova H, Van den Bogert C, Zeman J: Altered properties of mitochondrial ATP-synthase in patients with a T → G mutation in the ATPase 6 (subunit a) gene at position 8993 of mtDNA. *Biochim Biophys Acta* **1271**:349, 1995.
1203. de Coo IF, Smeets HJ, Gabreels FJ, Arts N, van Oost BA: Isolated case of mental retardation and ataxia due to a de novo mitochondrial T8993G mutation [Letter]. *Am J Hum Genet* **58**:636, 1996.
1204. Fryer A, Appleton R, Sweeney MG, Rosenbloom L, Harding AE: Mitochondrial DNA 8993 (NARP) mutation presenting with a heterogeneous phenotype including "cerebral palsy." *Arch Dis Child* **71**:419, 1994.
1205. Klement P, Zeman J, Hansikova H, Houstkova H, Baudysova M, Houstek J: Different restriction fragment pattern of mtDNA indicative of generalized 8993 point mutations in a boy with lactic acidosis. *J Inherit Metab Dis* **17**:249, 1994.
1206. Santorelli FM, Mak SC, Vazquez-Memije E, Shanske S, Kranz-Eble P, Jain KD, Bluestone DL, De Vivo DC, DiMauro S: Clinical heterogeneity associated with the mitochondrial DNA T8993C point mutation. *Pediatr Res* **39**:914, 1996.
1207. Santorelli FM, Shanske S, Jain KD, Tick D, Schon EA, DiMauro S: A T → C mutation at nt 8993 of mitochondrial DNA in a child with Leigh syndrome. *Neurology* **44**:972, 1994.
1208. De Vries DD, Van Engelen BG, Gabreels FJ, Ruitenbeek W, Van Oost BA: A second missense mutation in the mitochondrial ATPase 6 gene in Leigh's syndrome. *Ann Neurol* **34**:410, 1993.
1209. Lamminen T, Majander A, Juvonen V, Wikstrom M, Aula P, Nikoskelainen E, Savontous ML: A mitochondrial mutation at nt 9101 in the ATP synthase 6 gene associated with deficient oxidative phosphorylation in a family with Leber hereditary optic neuroretinopathy [Letter]. *Am J Hum Genet* **56**:1238, 1995.
1210. Dionisi-Vici C, Seneca S, Zeviani M, Fariello G, Rimoldi M, Bertini E, De Meirleir L: Fulminant Leigh syndrome and sudden unexpected death in a family with the T9176C mutation of the mitochondrial ATPase 6 gene. *J Inherit Metab Dis* **21**:2, 1998.
1211. Campos Y, Martin MA, Rubio JC, Solana LG, Garcia-Benayas C, Terradas JL, Arenas J: Leigh syndrome associated with the T9176C mutation in the ATPase 6 gene of mitochondrial DNA. *Neurology* **49**:595, 1997.
1212. Thyagarajan D, Shanske S, Vazquez-Memije M, De Vivo D, DiMauro S: A novel mitochondrial ATPase 6 point mutation in familial bilateral striatal necrosis. *Ann Neurol* **38**:468, 1995.
1213. Hanna MG, Nelson IP, Rahman S, Lane RJM, Land J, Heales S, Cooper MJ, Schapira AHV, Morgan-Hughes JA, Wood NW: Cytochrome c oxidase deficiency associated with the first stop-codon point mutation in human mtDNA. *Am J Hum Genet* **63**:29, 1998.
1214. Manfredi G, Schon EA, Moraes CT, Bonilla E, Berry GT, Sladky JT, DiMauro S: A new mutation associated with MELAS is located in a mitochondrial DNA polypeptide-coding gene. *Neuromuscul Disord* **5**:391, 1995.
1215. Merante F, Tein I, Benson L, Robinson BH: A novel T-to-C transition at nucleotide 9997 in the mitochondrial tRNA-Glycine gene giving rise to maternally inherited hypertrophic cardiomyopathy. *Am J Hum Genet* **53(Suppl)**:928, 1993.
1216. Merante F, Tein I, Benson L, Robinson BH: Maternally inherited hypertrophic cardiomyopathy due to a novel T-to-C transition at nucleotide 9997 in the mitochondrial tRNA(glycine) gene. *Am J Hum Genet* **55**:437, 1994.
1217. Santorelli FM, Schlessel JS, Slonim AE, DiMauro S: Novel mutation in the mitochondrial DNA tRNA glycine gene associated with sudden unexpected death. *Pediatr Neurol* **15**:145, 1996.
1218. Hotta Y, Fujiki K, Hayakawa M, Nakajima A, Kanai A, Mashima Y, Hiida Y, Shinoda K, Yamada K, Oguchi Y, et al.: Clinical features of Japanese Leber's hereditary optic neuropathy with 11778 mutation of mitochondrial DNA. *Jpn J Ophthalmol* **39**:96, 1995.
1219. Wakakura M, Yokoe J: Evidence for preserved direct pupillary light response in Leber's hereditary optic neuropathy. *Br J Ophthalmol* **79**:442, 1995.

1220. Mashima Y, Saga M, Hiida Y, Oguchi Y, Wakakura M, Kudoh J, Shimizu N: Quantitative determination of heteroplasmy in Leber's hereditary optic neuropathy by single-strand conformation polymorphism. *Invest Ophthalmol Vis Sci* **36**:1714, 1995.
1221. Mashima Y, Hiida Y, Oguchi Y: Lack of differences among mitochondrial DNA in family members with Leber's hereditary optic neuropathy and differing visual outcomes. *J Neuroophthalmol* **15**:15, 1995.
1222. Mashima Y, Hiida Y, Saga M, Oguchi Y, Kudoh J, Shimizu N: Risk of false-positive molecular genetic diagnosis of Leber's hereditary optic neuropathy. *Am J Ophthalmol* **119**:245, 1995.
1223. Borruat FX, Hirt L, Regli F: [Optic neuropathy caused by alcoholism and smoking: a diagnostic pitfall of Leber's optic neuropathy.] *Rev Neurol (Paris)* **150**:799, 1994.
1224. Zhang LS, Huang Y, Li FY: [Mitochondrial DNA mutation in Leber's hereditary optic neuropathy in China.] *Chung Hua I Hsueh Tsa Chih* **74**:349, 1994.
1225. Degli Esposti M, Carelli V, Ghelli A, Ratta M, Crimi M, Sangiorgi S, Montagna P, Lenaz G, Lugaresi E, Cortelli P: Functional alterations of the mitochondrially encoded ND4 subunit associated with Leber's hereditary optic neuropathy. *FEBS Lett* **352**:375, 1994.
1226. Oostra RJ, Van den Bogert C, Nijtmans LG, van Galen MJ, Zwart R, Bolhuis PA, Bleeker-Wagemakers EM: Simultaneous occurrence of the 11778 (ND4) and the 9438 (COX III) mtDNA mutations in Leber hereditary optic neuropathy: Molecular, biochemical, and clinical findings [Letter]. *Am J Hum Genet* **57**:954, 1995.
1227. Kobayashi Y, Sharpe H, Brown N: Single-cell analysis of intercellular heteroplasmy of mtDNA in Leber hereditary optic neuropathy [Letter]. *Am J Hum Genet* **55**:206, 1994.
1228. Howell N, Xu M, Halvorson S, Bodis-Wollner I, Sherman J: A heteroplasmic LHON family: Tissue distribution and transmission of the 11778 mutation [Letter]. *Am J Hum Genet* **55**:203, 1994.
1229. Nakamura N, Furukawa Y, Fujiki K, Hayakawa M, Mizuno Y: [Leber's hereditary optic neuropathy with onset at the age of 54 years.] *Rinsho Shinkeigaku* **34**:258, 1994.
1230. Nakamura M, Yamamoto M: [Genetic characteristics of Japanese pedigrees with Leber's hereditary optic neuropathy.] *Nippon Ganka Gakkai Zasshi* **98**:319, 1994.
1231. Huoponen K, Juvonen V, Iitia A, Dahlen P, Siitari H, Aula P, Nikoskelainen E, Savontaus ML: Time-resolved fluorometry in the diagnosis of Leber hereditary optic neuroretinopathy. *Hum Mutat* **3**:29, 1994.
1232. Mashima Y, Hiida Y, Oguchi Y, Kudoh J, Shimizu N: High frequency of mutations at position 11778 in mitochondrial ND4 gene in Japanese families with Leber's hereditary optic neuropathy. *Hum Genet* **92**:101, 1993.
1233. Yen MY, Liu JH, Pang CY, Wei YH: Molecular diagnosis of Leber's hereditary optic neuropathy. *J Formos Med Assoc* **92**:42, 1993.
1234. Nakamura M: Genetic analysis of Japanese pedigrees with Leber's hereditary optic neuropathy. *Kobe J Med Sci* **39**:171, 1993.
1235. Smith KH, Johns DR, Heher KL, Miller NR: Heteroplasmy in Leber's hereditary optic neuropathy. *Arch Ophthalmol* **111**:1486, 1993.
1236. Cullom ME, Heher KL, Miller NR, Savino PJ, Johns DR: Leber's hereditary optic neuropathy masquerading as tobacco-alcohol amblyopia. *Arch Ophthalmol* **111**:1482, 1993.
1237. Zhang LS: [A molecular genetic study of Leber's disease.] *Chung Hua Yen Ko Tsa Chih* **29**:103, 1993.
1238. Weiner NC, Newman NJ, Lessell S, Johns DR, Lott MT, Wallace DC: Atypical Leber's hereditary optic neuropathy with molecular confirmation. *Arch Neurol* **50**:470, 1993.
1239. Moorman CM, Elston JS, Matthews P: Leber's hereditary optic neuropathy as a cause of severe visual loss in childhood. *Pediatrics* **91**:988, 1993.
1240. Erickson CE, Castora FJ: PCR amplification using a single cell allows the detection of the mtDNA lesion associated with Leber's hereditary optic neuropathy. *Biochim Biophys Acta* **1181**:77, 1993.
1241. Nakamura M, Fujiwara Y, Yamamoto M: Homoplasmic and exclusive ND4 gene mutation in Japanese pedigrees with Leber's disease. *Invest Ophthalmol Vis Sci* **34**:488, 1993.
1242. Cavelier L, Gyllensten U, Dahl N: Intrafamilial variation in Leber hereditary optic neuropathy revealed by direct mutation analysis. *Clin Genet* **43**:69, 1993.
1243. Van Caelenberghe E, Meire F, Broux C, Vassart G, Cochaux P: Leber's hereditary optic neuropathy: clinical and molecular genetic aspects. Preliminary results in our families. *Bull Soc Belge Ophtalmol* **243**:139, 1992.
1244. Kormann BA, Schuster H, Berninger TA, Leo-Kottler B: Detection of the G to A mitochondrial DNA mutation at position 11778 in German families with Leber's hereditary optic neuropathy. *Hum Genet* **88**:98, 1991.
1245. Poulton J, Deadman ME, Bronte-Stewart J, Foulds WS, Gardiner RM: Analysis of mitochondrial DNA in Leber's hereditary optic neuropathy. *J Med Genet* **28**:765, 1991.
1246. Larsson NG, Andersen O, Holme E, Oldfors A, Wahlstrom J: Leber's hereditary optic neuropathy and complex I deficiency in muscle. *Ann Neurol* **30**:701, 1991.
1247. Carducci C, Leuzzi V, Scuderi M, De Negri AM, Gabrieli CB, Antonozzi I, Pontecorvi A: Mitochondrial DNA mutation in an Italian family with Leber hereditary optic neuropathy. *Hum Genet* **87**:725, 1991.
1248. Jacobson DM, Stone EM: Difficulty differentiating Leber's from dominant optic neuropathy in a patient with remote visual loss. *J Clin Neuroophthalmol* **11**:152, 1991.
1249. Ara F, Hotta Y, Hayakawa M, Yanashima K, Kanai A, Fujiki K: A trial of molecular diagnosis in Leber's optic neuropathy. *Nippon Ganka Gakkai Zasshi* **95**:715, 1991.
1250. Cortelli P, Montagna P, Avoni P, Sangiorgi S, Bresolin N, Moggio M, Zaniol P, Mantovani V, Barboni P, Barbiroli B, et al.: Leber's hereditary optic neuropathy: Genetic, biochemical, and phosphorus magnetic resonance spectroscopy study in an Italian family. *Neurology* **41**:1211, 1991.
1251. Newman NJ, Lott MT, Wallace DC: The clinical characteristics of pedigrees of Leber's hereditary optic neuropathy with the 11,778 mutation. *Am J Ophthalmol* **111**:750, 1991.
1252. Fujiki K, Hotta Y, Hayakawa M, Saito K, Ara F, Ueda S, Goto T, Ishida M, Yanashima K, Shiono T, et al.: A mutation of mitochondrial DNA in Japanese families with Leber's hereditary optic neuropathy. *Jinrui Idengaku Zasshi* **36**:143, 1991.
1253. Norby S, Lestienne P, Nelson I, Rosenberg T: Mutation detection in Leber's hereditary optic neuropathy by PCR with allele specific priming. *Biochem Biophys Res Commun* **175**:631, 1991.
1254. Johns DR, Berman J: Alternative, simultaneous complex I mitochondrial DNA mutations in Leber's hereditary optic neuropathy. *Biochem Biophys Res Commun* **174**:1324, 1991.
1255. Hiida Y, Mashima Y, Oguchi Y, Uemura Y, Kudoh J, Sakai K, Shimizu N: Mitochondrial DNA analysis of Leber's hereditary optic neuropathy. *Jpn J Ophthalmol* **35**:102, 1991.
1256. Isashiki Y, Nakagawa M: Clinical correlation of mitochondrial DNA heteroplasmy and Leber's hereditary optic neuropathy. *Jpn J Ophthalmol* **35**:259, 1991.
1257. Mashima Y, Hiida Y, Kubota R, Oguchi Y, Kudoh J, Shimizu N: DNA diagnosis of Leber's hereditary optic neuropathy by using dried blood specimens [Letter]. *Am J Ophthalmol* **116**:773, 1993.
1258. Oostra RJ, Bolhuis PA, Bleeker-Wagemakers EM: Mitochondrial DNA analysis as a diagnostic tool in singleton cases of Leber's hereditary optic neuropathy [see Comments]. *Ophthalmic Paediatr Genet* **14**:109, 1993.
1259. Mackey DA: Leber's hereditary optic neuropathy. Is it a disease of northern Europe and Asia? [Editorial; Comment]. *Ophthalmic Paediatr Genet* **14**:105, 1993.
1260. Norby S: Mutation-specific PCR: A rapid and inexpensive diagnostic method, as exemplified by mitochondrial DNA analysis in Leber's hereditary optic neuropathy. *DNA Cell Biol* **12**:549, 1993.
1261. Mackey D, Nasioulas S, Forrest S: Finger prick blood testing in Leber hereditary optic neuropathy. *Br J Ophthalmol* **77**:311, 1993.
1262. Gerbitz KD, Paprotta A, Obermaier-Kusser B, Rietschel M, Zerres K: No genetic differences between affected and unaffected members of a German family with Leber's hereditary optic neuropathy (LHON) with respect to ten mtDNA point mutations associated with LHON. *FEBS Lett* **314**:251, 1992.
1263. Barboni P, Mantovani V, Montagna P, Bragliani M, Cortelli P, Lugaresi E, Puddu P, Caramazza R: Mitochondrial DNA analysis in Leber's hereditary optic neuropathy. *Ophthalmic Paediatr Genet* **13**:219, 1992.
1264. Borruat FX, Green WT, Graham EM, Sweeney MG, Morgan-Hughes JA, Sanders MD: Late onset Leber's optic neuropathy: A case confused with ischaemia. *Br J Ophthalmol* **76**:571, 1992.
1265. Mackey DA, Buttery RG: Leber hereditary optic neuropathy in Australia. *Aust N Z J Ophthalmol* **20**:177, 1992.
1266. Yen MY, Yen TC, Pang CY, Liu JH, Wei YH: Mitochondrial DNA mutation in Leber's hereditary optic neuropathy. *Invest Ophthalmol Vis Sci* **33**:2561, 1992.

1267. Dumur V, Lalau G, Boone P, Roussel P, Francois P, Hache JC, Hemery B, Puech B: Rapid diagnosis of mitochondrial mutation at position 11778-associated Leber hereditary optic neuropathy. *Clin Chem* **38**:1390, 1992.
1268. Ortiz RG, Newman NJ, Manoukian SV, Diesenhouse MC, Lott MT, Wallace DC: Optic disk cupping and electrocardiographic abnormalities in an American pedigree with Leber's hereditary optic neuropathy. *Am J Ophthalmol* **113**:561, 1992.
1269. Stone EM, Newman NJ, Miller NR, Johns DR, Lott MT, Wallace DC: Visual recovery in patients with Leber's hereditary optic neuropathy and the 11778 mutation. *J Clin Neuroophthalmol* **12**:10, 1992.
1270. Sudoyo H, Marzuki S, Mastaglia F, Carroll W: Molecular genetics of Leber's hereditary optic neuropathy: Study of a six-generation family from Western Australia. *J Neurol Sci* **108**:7, 1992.
1271. Howell N, McCullough D, Bodis-Wollner I: Molecular genetic analysis of a sporadic case of Leber hereditary optic neuropathy. *Am J Hum Genet* **50**:443, 1992.
1272. Zhu DP, Economou EP, Antonarakis SE, Maumenee IH: Mitochondrial DNA mutation and heteroplasmy in type I Leber hereditary optic neuropathy. *Am J Med Genet* **42**:173, 1992.
1273. Nakamura M, Ara F, Yamada M, Hotta Y, Hayakawa M, Fujiki K, Kanai A, Sakai J, Inoue M, Yamamoto M, et al.: High frequency of mitochondrial ND4 gene mutation in Japanese pedigrees with Leber hereditary optic neuropathy. *Jpn J Ophthalmol* **36**:56, 1992.
1274. Pagot V, Malecaze F, Rotig A, Simorre V, Maillard P, Mathis A, Munnich A: Leber's optic neuropathy: New diagnostic prospects. *J Fr Ophtalmol* **15**:19, 1992.
1275. Isashiki Y, Ohba N, Uto M, Nakagawa M, Nakano T, Kitahara K, Hotta A, Okamura R, Ozaki M, Futami Y, et al.: Nonfamilial and unusual cases of Leber's hereditary optic neuropathy identified by mitochondrial DNA analysis. *Jpn J Ophthalmol* **36**:197, 1992.
1276. Cormier V, Rotig A, Geny C, Cesaro P, Dufier JL, Munnich A: mtDNA heteroplasmy in Leber hereditary optic neuroretinopathy. *Am J Hum Genet* **48**:813, 1991.
1277. Nikoskelainen E, Vilkki J, Huoponen K, Savontaus ML: Recent advances in Leber's hereditary optic neuroretinopathy. *Eye* **5**:291, 1991.
1278. Yoneda M, Tsuji S, Yamauchi T, Inuzuka T, Miyatake T, Horai S, Ozawa T: Mitochondrial DNA mutation in family with Leber's hereditary optic neuropathy. *Lancet* **1**:1076, 1989.
1279. Singh G, Lott MT, Wallace DC: A mitochondrial DNA mutation as a cause of Leber's hereditary optic neuropathy. *N Engl J Med* **320**:1300, 1989.
1280. Vilkki J, Savontaus ML, Nikoskelainen EK: Genetic heterogeneity in Leber hereditary optic neuroretinopathy revealed by mitochondrial DNA polymorphisms. *Am J Hum Genet* **45**:206, 1989.
1281. Hotta Y, Hayakawa M, Saito K, Kanai A, Nakajima A, Fujiki K: Diagnosis of Leber's optic neuropathy by means of polymerase chain reaction amplification. *Am J Ophthalmol* **108**:601, 1989.
1282. Larsson NG, Holme E, Tulinius MH: DNA diagnosis of mitochondrial diseases is now possible. *Lakartidningen* **86**:4235, 1989.
1283. Lott MT, Voljavec AS, Wallace DC: Variable genotype of Leber's hereditary optic neuropathy patients. *Am J Ophthalmol* **109**:625, 1990.
1284. Newman NJ, Wallace DC: Mitochondria and Leber's hereditary optic neuropathy. *Am J Ophthalmol* **109**:726, 1990.
1285. Newman NJ: Leber's hereditary optic neuropathy. *Ophthalmol Clin North Am* **4**:431, 1991.
1286. Vilkki J, Savontaus ML, Nikoskelainen EK: Segregation of mitochondrial genomes in a heteroplasmic lineage with Leber hereditary optic neuroretinopathy. *Am J Hum Genet* **47**:95, 1990.
1287. Mashima Y, Oguchi Y, Uemura Y, Kudoh J, Sakai K, Shimizu N: DNA diagnosis of Leber's hereditary optic neuropathy. *Nippon Ganka Gakkai Zasshi* **94**:683, 1990.
1288. Bolhuis PA, Bleeker-Wagemakers EM, Ponne NJ, Van Schooneveld MJ, Westerveld A, Van den Bogert C, Tabak HF: Rapid shift in genotype of human mitochondrial DNA in a family with Leber's hereditary optic neuropathy. *Biochem Biophys Res Commun* **170**:994, 1990.
1289. Stone EM, Coppinger JM, Kardon RH, Donelson J: Mae III positively detects the mitochondrial mutation associated with Type I Leber hereditary optic neuropathy. *Arch Ophthalmol* **108**:1417, 1990.
1290. Norby S, Rosenberg T: Leber's hereditary optic atrophy. A hereditary disease caused by mitochondrial DNA mutation. *Ugeskr Laeger* **152**:3149, 1990.
1291. Smith JL, Tse DT, Byrne SF, Johns DR, Stone EM: Optic nerve sheath distention in Leber's optic neuropathy and the significance of the "Wallace mutation." *J Clin Neuroophthalmol* **10**:231, 1990.
1292. Yen MY, Wei YH, Liu JH: Stargardt's type maculopathy in a patient with 11778 Leber's optic neuropathy. *J Neuroophthalmol* **16**:120, 1996.
1293. Johns DR, Smith KH, Miller NR, Sulewski ME, Bias WB: Identical twins who are discordant for Leber's hereditary optic neuropathy. *Arch Ophthalmol* **111**:1491, 1993.
1294. Murakami T, Mita S, Tokunaga M, Maeda H, Ueyama H, Kumamoto T, Uchino M, Ando M: Hereditary cerebellar ataxia with Leber's hereditary optic neuropathy mitochondrial DNA 11778 mutation. *J Neurol Sci* **142**:111, 1996.
1295. Funakawa I, Kato H, Terao A, Ichihashi K, Kawashima S, Hayashi T, Mitani K, Miyazaki S: Cerebellar ataxia in patients with Leber's hereditary optic neuropathy. *J Neurol* **242**:75, 1995.
1296. Olsen NK, Hansen AW, Norby S, Edal AL, Jorgensen JR, Rosenberg T: Leber's hereditary optic neuropathy associated with a disorder indistinguishable from multiple sclerosis in a male harbouring the mitochondrial DNA 11778 mutation. *Acta Neurol Scand* **91**:326, 1995.
1297. Nishimura M, Obayashi H, Ohta M, Uchiyama T, Hao Q, Saida T: No association of the 11778 mitochondrial DNA mutation and multiple sclerosis in Japan. *Neurology* **45**:1333, 1995.
1298. Barbiroli B, Montagna P, Cortelli P, Iotti S, Lodi R, Barboni P, Monari L, Lugaresi E, Frassineti C, Zaniol P: Defective brain and muscle energy metabolism shown by in vivo 31P magnetic resonance spectroscopy in nonaffected carriers of 11778 mtDNA mutation. *Neurology* **45**:1364, 1995.
1299. Pilz D, Quarrell OW, Jones EW: Mitochondrial mutation commonly associated with Leber's hereditary optic neuropathy observed in a patient with Wolfram syndrome (DIDMOAD). *J Med Genet* **31**:328, 1994.
1300. Harding AE, Sweeney MG, Miller DH, Mumford CJ, Kellar-Wood H, Menard D, McDonald WI, Compston DA: Occurrence of a multiple sclerosis-like illness in women who have a. *Brain* **115**:979, 1992.
1301. Flanigan KM, Johns DR: Association of the 11778 mitochondrial DNA mutation and demyelinating disease. *Neurology* **43**:2720, 1993.
1302. Paulus W, Straube A, Bauer W, Harding AE: Central nervous system involvement in Leber's optic neuropathy. *J Neurol* **240**:251, 1993.
1303. Tawata M, Ohtaka M, Iwase E, Ikegishi Y, Aida K, Onaya T: New mitochondrial DNA homoplasmic mutations associated with Japanese patients with type 2 diabetes. *Diabetes* **47**:276, 1998.
1304. Mansergh FC, Millington-Ward S, Kennan A, Kiang A-S, Humphries M, Farrar GJ, Humphries P, Kenna PF: Retinitis pigmentosa and progressive sensorineural hearing loss caused by a C12258A mutation in the mitochondrial MTTS2 gene. *Am J Hum Genet* **64**:971, 1999.
1305. Gattermann N, Retzlaff S, Wang YL, Berneburg M, Heinisch J, Wlaschek M, Aul C, Schneider W: A heteroplasmic point mutation of mitochondrial tRNALeu(CUN) in non-lymphoid haemopoietic cell lineages from a patient with acquired idiopathic sideroblastic anaemia. *Br J Haematol* **93**:845, 1996.
1306. Hattori Y, Goto Y-i, Sakuta R, Nonaka I, Mizuno Y, Horai S: Point mutations in mitochondrial tRNA genes: Sequence analysis of chronic progressive external ophthalmoplegia (CPEO). *J Neurol Sci* **125**:50, 1994.
1307. Fu K, Hartlen R, Johns T, Genge A, Karpati G, Shoubridge EA: A novel heteroplasmic tRNAleu(CUN) mtDNA point mutation in a sporadic patient with mitochondrial encephalomyopathy segregates rapidly in skeletal muscle and suggests an approach to therapy. *Hum Mol Genet* **5**:1835, 1996.
1308. Weber K, Wilson JN, Taylor L, Brierley E, Johnson MA, Turnbull DM, Bindoff LA: A new mtDNA mutation showing accumulation with time and restriction to skeletal muscle. *Am J Hum Genet* **60**:373, 1997.
1309. Santorelli FM, Tanji K, Kulikova R, Shanske S, Vilarinho L, Hays AP, DiMauro S: Identification of a novel mutation in the mtDNA ND5 gene associated with MELAS. *Biochem Biophys Res Commun* **238**:326, 1997.
1310. Cock HR, Cooper JM, Schapira AH: The 14484 ND6 mtDNA mutation in Leber hereditary optic neuropathy does not affect fibroblast complex I activity [Letter]. *Am J Hum Genet* **57**:1501, 1995.
1311. Hedges TRr, Sedwick LA, Newman NJ: Two brothers with bilateral optic neuropathy [Clinical Conference]. *Surv Ophthalmol* **39**:417, 1995.
1312. Rizzo JFR: Adenosine triphosphate deficiency: A genre of optic neuropathy. *Neurology* **45**:11, 1995.
1313. Johns DR, Heher KL, Miller NR, Smith KH: Leber's hereditary optic neuropathy. Clinical manifestations of the 14484 mutation. *Arch Ophthalmol* **111**:495, 1993.

1314. Johns DR, Neufeld MJ, Park RD: An ND-6 mitochondrial DNA mutation associated with Leber hereditary. *Biochem Biophys Res Commun* **187**:1551, 1992.
1315. Funalot B, Ranoux D, Mas JL, Garcia C, Bonnefont JP: Brainstem involvement in Leber's hereditary optic neuropathy: Association with the 14,484 mitochondrial DNA mutation [Letter]. *J Neurol Neurosurg Psychiatry* **61**:533, 1996.
1316. Jun AS, Trounce IA, Brown MD, Shoffner JM, Wallace DC: Use of transmitochondrial cybrids to assign a complex I defect to the mitochondrial DNA-encoded NADH dehydrogenase subunit 6 gene mutation at nucleotide pair 14459 that causes Leber hereditary optic neuropathy and dystonia. *Mol Cell Biol* **16**:771, 1996.
1317. Shoffner JM, Brown MD, Stugard C, Jun AS, Pollock S, Haas RH, Kaufman A, Koontz D, Kim Y, Graham JR, et al.: Leber's hereditary optic neuropathy plus dystonia is caused by a mitochondrial DNA point mutation. *Ann Neurol* **38**:163, 1995.
1318. Jun AS, Brown MD, Wallace DC: A mitochondrial DNA mutation at nucleotide pair 14459 of the NADH dehydrogenase subunit 6 gene associated with maternally inherited Leber hereditary optic neuropathy and dystonia. *Proc Natl Acad Sci U S A* **91**:6206, 1994.
1319. Leo-Kottler B, Christ-Adler M, Baumann B, Zrenner E, Wissinger B: Leber's hereditary optic neuropathy: clinical and molecular genetic results obtained in a family with a new point mutation at nucleotide position 14498 in the ND 6 gene. *Ger J Ophthalmol* **5**:233, 1996.
1320. Vialettes BH, Paquis-Flucklinger V, Pelissier JF, Bendahan D, Narbonne H, Silvestre-Aillaud P, Montfort MF, Righini-Chossegros M, Pouget J, Cozzone PJ, Desnuelle C: Phenotypic expression of diabetes secondary to a T14709C mutation of mitochondrial DNA. Comparison with MIDD syndrome (A3243G mutation): A case report. *Diabetes Care* **20**:1731, 1997.
1321. Hanna MG, Nelson I, Sweeney MG, Cooper JM, Watkins PJ, Morgan-Hughes JA, Harding AE: Congenital encephalomyopathy and adult-onset myopathy and diabetes mellitus: Different phenotypic associations of a new heteroplasmic mtDNA tRNA glutamic acid mutation. *Am J Hum Genet* **56**:1026, 1995.
1322. Hao H, Bonilla E, Manfredi G, DiMauro S, Moraes CT: Segregation patterns of a novel mutation in the mitochondrial tRNA glutamic acid gene associated with myopathy and diabetes mellitus. *Am J Hum Genet* **56**:1017, 1995.
1323. De Coo IFM, Renier WO, Ruitenbeek W, Ter Laak HJ, Bakker M, Schagger H, Van Oost BA, Smeets HJM: A 4-base pair deletion in the mitochondrial cytochrome b gene associated with Parkinsonism/MELAS overlap syndrome. *Ann Neurol* **45**:130, 1999.
1324. Andreu AL, Bruno C, Dunne TC, Tanji K, Shanske S, Sue CM, Krishna S, Hadjogeorgiou GM, Shtilbans A, Bonillan E, DiMauro S: A nonsense mutation (G15059A) in the cytochrome b gene in a patient with exercise intolerance and myoglobinuria. *Ann Neurol* **45**:127, 1999.
1325. Marin-Garcia J, Hu Y, Ananthakrishnan R, Pierpont ME, Pierpont GL, Goldenthal MJ: A point mutation in the cytb gene of cardiac mtDNA associated with complex III deficiency in ischemic cardiomyopathy. *Biochem Mol Biol Int* **40**:487, 1996.
1326. Dumoulin R, Sagnol I, Ferlin T, Bozon D, Stepien G, Mousson B: A novel gly290asp mitochondrial cytochrome b mutation linked to a complex III deficiency in progressive exercise intolerance. *Mol Cell Probes* **10**:389, 1996.
1327. Bouzidi MF, Carrier H, Godinot C: Antimycin resistance and ubiquinol cytochrome c reductase instability associated with a human cytochrome b mutation. *Biochim Biophys Acta* **1317**:199, 1996.
1328. Andreu AL, Bruno C, Shanske S, Shtilbans A, Hirano M, Krishna S, Hayward L, Systrom DS, Brown RH, Jr., DiMauro S: Missense mutation in the mtDNA cytochrome b gene in a patient with myopathy. *Neurology* **51**:1444, 1998.
1329. Seki A, Nishino I, Goto Y-i, Maekagi Y, Koeda T: Mitochondrial encephalomyopathy with 15915 mutation: Clinical report. *Pediatr Neurol* **17**:161, 1997.
1330. Nishino I, Seki A, Maegaki Y, Takeshita K, Horai S, Nonaka I, Goto Y: A novel mutation in the mitochondrial tRNA(Thr) gene associated with a mitochondrial encephalomyopathy. *Biochem Biophys Res Commun* **225**:180, 1996.
1331. Yoon KL, Ernst SG, Rasmussen C, Dooling EC, Aprille JR: Mitochondrial disorders associated with newborn cardiopulmonary arrest. *Pediatr Res* **33**:433, 1993.
1332. Ionasescu VV, Hart M, DiMauro S, Moraes CT: Clinical and morphologic features of a myopathy associated with a point mutation in the mitochondrial tRNA(Pro) gene. *Neurology* **44**:975, 1994.
1333. Moraes CT, Ciacci F, Bonilla E, Ionasescu V, Schon EA, DiMauro S: A mitochondrial tRNA anticodon swap associated with a muscle disease. *Nat Genet* **4**:284, 1993.
1334. Ogasahara S, Engel AG, Frens D, Mack D: Muscle coenzyme Q deficiency in familial mitochondrial encephalomyopathy. *Proc Natl Acad Sci U S A* **86**:2379, 1989.
1335. Sobreira C, Hirano M, Shanske S, Keller RK, Haller RG, Davidson E, Santorelli FM, et al.: Mitochondrial encephalomyopathy with coenzyme Q_{10} deficiency. *Neurology* **48**:1238, 1997.

CHAPTER 105

Mitochondria and Neuro-ophthalmologic Diseases

Douglas C. Wallace ▪ Marie T. Lott
Michael D. Brown ▪ Keith Kerstann

1. **Defects in mitochondrial oxidative phosphorylation (OXPHOS) frequently manifest with neuro-ophthalmologic symptoms. Acute-onset, bilateral, optic atrophy is the primary clinical sign of Leber hereditary optic neuropathy (LHON), which is caused by missense mutations in the mitochondrial DNA (mtDNA). Retinitis pigmentosa, frequently in association with Leigh syndrome, can be caused by mtDNA base substitutions, as well as by nuclear DNA (nDNA) OXPHOS gene mutations. Ophthalmoplegia and ptosis, together with mitochondrial myopathy, are associated with chronic progressive external ophthalmoplegia (CPEO) and the Kearns-Sayre syndrome (KSS), and can be caused by mtDNA rearrangements, nDNA mutations that destabilize the mtDNA, or mtDNA base substitutions. To understand the biochemical and molecular bases of mitochondrial neuro-ophthalmologic disease, it is necessary to understand the biochemistry and genetics of the mitochondrion, and the association between mitochondrial gene mutations and clinical symptoms.**
2. **Mitochondrial OXPHOS participates in three major cellular functions relevant to the pathophysiology of mitochondrial disease. First, the mitochondria generate much of the energy of the cell and this process regulates cellular redox potential, mitochondrial membrane potential, ATP production, and Ca^{++} uptake. Second, the mitochondria generate most of the endogenous reactive oxygen species (ROS) as a toxic byproduct of OXPHOS. Third, the mitochondria integrate many of the signals for initiating apoptosis through regulating the opening of the mitochondrial permeability transition pore (mtPTP). Opening of the mtPTP results in the release of cytochrome c and apoptotic enzymes from the mitochondrial intermembrane space, precipitating programmed cell death. All three of these processes use common OXPHOS polypeptides and functions.**

   The OXPHOS complexes are composed of multiple polypeptides distributed between the mtDNA and nDNA. Complex I has 43 polypeptides, 7 (ND1, 2, 3, 4, 4L, 5, 6) from the mtDNA. Complex II has four nDNA subunits. Complex III has 11 subunits, 1 (CYTB) from the mtDNA. Complex IV has 13 polypeptides, 3 (COI, COII, COIII) from the mtDNA; and complex V has 16 polypeptides, 2 (ATP6, 8) from the mtDNA. In addition, the mtDNA encodes the 12S and 16S rRNAs and the 22 RNAs necessary for mitochondrial protein synthesis. The nDNA codes for all of the remaining OXPHOS complex subunits as well as the proteins necessary for their expression and assembly. The nDNA also codes for the mitochondrial inner membrane anion carriers, including the adenine nucleotide translocator (ANT), which exchanges mitochondrial ATP for cytosolic ADP; the mitochondrial Mn superoxide dismutase (MnSOD) and glutathione peroxidase (GPx1), which are involved in detoxifying mitochondrial ROS; and for proteins that constitute the mtPTP, including the ANT, the voltage-dependent anion channels (VDAC), the pro-apoptotic BAX family, the antiapoptotic BCL2 family, and cyclophilin D. The mechanisms for electron transport and proton pumping of each of the OXPHOS complexes are rapidly being elucidated, and this is permitting a detailed physiological understanding of some of the mitochondrial disease mutants. For example, the ATP synthases (complex V) are composed of a fixed component, the stator, which projects from the membrane into the matrix and is composed of the barrel of 3 α and 3 β subunits anchored to the inner membrane ATP6 polypeptide by an arm composed of two "b" subunits and a δ subunit. This stator interacts with a rotor composed of a wheel of about 12 ATP9 subunits attached to an axle of ε and γ subunits, which projects up into the 3 α and 3 β barrel. The outer rim of the ATP9 wheel has a negative amino acid Glu,[58] located in the middle of the membrane. This interacts with the adjacent ATP6 subunit to form a pair of half proton channels, such that the flow of protons through the ATP6 channels causes the rotor to rotate. The spinning of the asymmetric γ subunit axle inside the 3 α and 3 β barrel causes the β subunit to move through three conformational states: binding ADP + P_i, condensing it to ATP, and releasing the ATP. Mutations distort the interaction between ATP6 and ATP9, inhibiting the rotation of the rotor and limiting ATP synthesis in the mtDNA MTATP6 gene causing retinitis pigmentosa and Leigh syndrome.

   Inhibition of OXPHOS lowers mitochondrial energy output and redirects mitochondrial electrons to ROS production. Reduced energy and increased ROS, in turn, impinge on the mtPTP, stimulating it to open and initiate apoptosis. Hence, mitochondrial energy production, ROS generation, and apoptosis are all intimately interrelated in the processes of cell and tissue decline and failure.
3. **The genetics of mitochondrial disease are particularly complex because they involve the interaction of two very different genomes, the mtDNA and nDNA. The mtDNA is maternally inherited, present in thousands of copies per cell, has a high mutation rate, and can exist within the cell as a mixture of mutant and normal mtDNAs (heteroplasmy). Heteroplasmic cells and maternal lineages can segregate the mutant and normal mtDNAs during mitosis and meiosis to give different ratios, creating variable bioenergetic defects and symptoms. The nDNA-encoded mitochondrial genes are dispersed across all of the chromosomes. Their proteins are synthesized on cytosolic**

ribosomes, and their polypeptides transported into the mitochondrial matrix or inner membrane by an outer (Tom) and either of two inner (Tim) membrane transport systems.

The high mtDNA mutation rate has created a large number of neutral or near-neutral population-specific polymorphisms, which have accumulated as sequential mutations on radiating maternal lineages as women migrated out of Africa and occupied Europe, Asia, and the Americas. It is essential to have a detailed understanding of natural mtDNA variation in order to discriminate pathogenic mutations from nonpathogenic polymorphisms. To this end, the analysis of mtDNA polymorphisms has allowed the reconstruction of the origin and radiation of *Homo sapiens*. According to the mtDNA, humans originated in Africa about 150,000 years before present (YBP). Currently about two-thirds of all African mtDNAs belong to an ancient African-specific group of mtDNA haplotypes, designated macrohaplogroups L1 + L2. About one-third of African mtDNAs are distinctive and designated L3. A subset of the people with the L3 mtDNAs left Africa and migrated to Asia and later to Europe. European populations developed nine distinctive mtDNA lineages distributed between two macrohaplogroups (+/−, −/−) defined by the presence or absence of a *Dde*I restriction site at np 10394 and an *Alu*I site at np 10397. The +/− haplogroups are I, J, and K, while the −/− haplogroups are H, T, U, V, W, and X. The age of European mtDNAs is about 40,000 to 50,000 YBP. Asian mtDNA haplogroups also fall into two similar macrohaplogroups: −/− and +/+. The −/− macrohaplogroup encompasses Asian haplogroups like A, B, and F, while the +/+ macrohaplogroup encompasses other haplogroups such as C, D, E, and G. Asia was occupied about 60,000 to 70,000 YBP. From Asia, haplogroups A, B, C, and D migrated either through Siberia or along the Siberian coast to populate the Americas in two to four migrations starting 20,000 to 30,000 YBP. It also appears that a small group of individuals came to America from Europe, carrying haplogroup X and arriving in central North America about 15,000 to 30,000 YBP.

4. The high mtDNA mutation rate also generates many nonneutral mutations that disrupt essential mitochondrial gene functions, resulting in mitochondrial disease. Mitochondrial genetic disease can also result from nDNA mutations, because both genomes code for genes essential for the assembly and maintenance of the mitochondria as well as OXPHOS.

mtDNA mutations can either be base substitution mutations or rearrangement mutations. Base substitution mutations can, in turn, either be missense mutations affecting polypeptides or protein synthesis mutations affecting the tRNA or rRNA genes. mtDNA missense mutations have been associated with a number of clinical phenotypes, the most common of which are LHON and NARP (neurogenic muscle weakness, ataxia, and retinitis pigmentosa), which can also present as Leigh syndrome.

LHON is a maternally inherited, late-onset, acute, optic atrophy. While most LHON families manifest only optic atrophy, some patients present with additional or alternative clinical symptoms including pediatric-onset dystonia associated with bilateral striatal necrosis. Some LHON family members can also manifest a multiple sclerosis-like optic neuritis. More than 90 percent of European and Asian LHON cases result from three mtDNA missense mutations. These include a G to A mutation in the MTND4 gene at nucleotide 11778 (MTND4*LHON11778A), which converts the highly conserved arginine at codon 340 of the ND4 gene to a histidine. This mutation accounts for about 50 percent of European cases and about 95 percent of Asian LHON patients. In addition, the MTND1*LHON3460A (ND1 Ala52Thr) and MTND6*LHON14484C (ND6 Met64Val) mutations each account for about 15 percent of European cases. A number of rare mutations also appear to cause LHON. These include MTND6*LHON14482G, which changes the same codon as MTND6*LHON14484C; MTND6*14498T; MTND2*LHON5244A; MTND5*LHON13730A; and MTATP6*LHON9101C.

In addition to these LHON mutations, additional mutations can cause both LHON and dystonia (LDYT). The best characterized of these is the MTND6*LDYT14459A mutation, which changes a highly conserved alanine at codon 72 of ND6 to a valine. Rarer mutations associated with LDYT include MTND6*LDYT14596A and MTND4*LDYT11696G.

Analysis of the background haplotypes of patients with LHON and LDYT mutations has shown that the common mutations have arisen repeatedly in the population, consistent with the high rate of mtDNA mutation. In three independent MTND6*LDYT14459A families, the mutation was associated with Native American haplogroup D, African haplogroup L, and European haplogroup I mtDNAs. Similarly, in a study of European LHON patients, with the MTND1*LHON3460A and MTND4*LHON11778A mutations, both mutations were found to be associated with a variety of different European haplogroups, although 37 percent of the MTND4*LHON11778A cases were found on a haplogroup J background. By contrast, when the MTND6*LHON14484C cases were examined, 80 percent were found to be associated with European haplogroup J. This latter association was not due to common descent because haplogroup J LHON patients and controls are randomly interspersed in the haplogroup J lineage. Hence, it appears that the European haplogroup J mtDNA increases the probability that the MTND6*LHON14484C, and to a lesser extent the MTND4*LHON11778A, mutations will cause clinical blindness. This might be due to one or more of the three amino acid substitutions associated with haplogroup J: MTND1*LHON4216G, MTND5*LHON13708A, and MTCYB*LHON15257A.

Biochemical analysis has revealed that the MTND6*LDYT14459A mutation is associated with a 55 percent reduction in complex I-specific activity, but only a minor reduction in the respiration rate on complex I substrates. This biochemical defect has been correlated with an altered binding of the complex I electron acceptor, coenzyme Q_{10} (CoQ_{10}). A similar biochemical defect is found in the MTND1*LHON3460A mutation, and ND1 has also been proposed to be involved in CoQ_{10} binding. The MTND4*LHON11778A mutation has no significant reduction in complex I enzyme activity, although it is associated with a 30 percent to 50 percent reduction in complex I respiration rates, as well as altered rotenone binding, which implicates CoQ_{10} interactions. Finally, the MTND6*LDYT14459A mutation exhibits only a mild inhibition of respiration, but it is located in the same gene as the MTND6*LHON14484C mutation, in a region between codons 26 and 72, encompassing six LHON and LDYT mutations. Hence, it is likely that all of these mutations affect electron transfer from complex I to CoQ_{10}. The mechanism by which inhibition of CoQ_{10} reduction by complex I could cause optic atrophy is still unclear. The pathophysiology could be the simple result of energy deficiency. Alternatively, the inhibition of the electron transport chain could direct more electrons into ROS production, increasing the tendency for retinal ganglion cell apoptosis or, alternatively, promoting the destruction of nitric oxide (NO) from retinal vessels causing spasm and ischemia.

Retinitis pigmentosa and Leigh syndrome are most frequently associated with three missense mutations: MTND6*NARP8993G, MTND6*NARP8993C, and MTATP6*FBSN9176C. However, these phenotypes can also result from the more severe mtDNA protein synthesis mutations such as MTTK*MERRF8344G and MTTL1*MELAS3243G.

The MTATP6*NARP8993G/C mutations are the best characterized. These mutations are invariably heteroplasmic, with the mutant and normal mtDNAs segregating along the maternal lineage. This random genotypic variation results in striking clinical variation among maternal relatives, with symptoms ranging from unaffected, to mild salt-and-pepper retinitis pigmentosa, to macular degeneration and olivopontocerebellar atrophy, to lethal Leigh syndrome.

The biochemical defect of the MTATP6*NARP8993G mutation has been extensively analyzed and found to be associated with a 24 percent to 53 percent reduction in ADP-stimulated respiration and a 30 percent reduction in ADP/O ratios. Correlation of these data with current information on the mechanism of the ATP synthase (complex V) indicates that the MTATP6*NARP8993G mutation adds an additional positive charge to the ATP6 stator subunit, increasing its attraction to the Glu^{58} in the ATP9 rotor subunit, inhibiting the rotation of the rotor. Other potentially pathogenic ATP6 mutations may impinge on these same interactions. The inhibition of the ATP synthase would limit ATP production, but also inhibit the electron transport chain. This could stimulate ROS production and increase damage due to oxidative stress.

Leigh syndrome, frequently with retinitis pigmentosa and ophthalmoplegia, has also been shown to result from nDNA mutations. This syndrome, as well as other more severe mitochondrial diseases, is associated with the degeneration of the basal ganglia of the brain. Nuclear gene variants identified in Leigh syndrome patients include mutations in the structural genes of the pyruvate dehydrogenase (E1α gene), various complex I subunit genes, the complex II flavoprotein gene, and the putative complex IV assembly gene, SURF-1. Nuclear DNA mutations affecting mitochondrial functions have also been associated with pediatric encephalomyopathy including basal ganglia degeneration, dystonia and deafness, hereditary spastic paraplegia, and Friedreich ataxia.

Ophthalmoplegia and ptosis, with mitochondrial myopathy, have been associated with mtDNA rearrangements in 83 percent of KSS and 47 percent of CPEO cases, and with autosomal dominant PEO in about 6 percent of cases; mtDNA tRNA mutations occur in at least 4 percent of KSS and 14 percent of CPEO. Mitochondrial myopathy is a distinctive muscle pathology involving ragged-red muscle fibers (RRFs) resulting from the degeneration of muscle fibers accompanied by the proliferation of abnormal muscle mitochondria.

The KSS and CPEO cases resulting from rearrangements are generally spontaneous, isolated cases. The severity of the disease, and hence the age of onset and number of organs involved, appears to depend on the number and distribution of rearranged mtDNAs at conception, and the relentless, preferential propagation of the rearranged mtDNAs. Once the mutant mtDNAs exceed expression thresholds, symptoms appear and progress. High proportions of deleted mtDNAs inhibit cell replication. Consequently, most bone marrow stem cells with high proportions of mutant mtDNAs stop replicating, and only normal bone marrow cells grow. As a result, most CPEO and KSS patients lack rearranged mtDNAs in their blood cells, requiring that definitive diagnostics involving mtDNA rearrangements be done on a postmitotic tissue such as muscle.

If all bone marrow cells contain rearranged mtDNAs, then all the stem cells stop growing, resulting in children with pancytopenia, a condition known as Pearson marrow syndrome. These children have rearranged mtDNAs in their circulating blood cells, and often die unless they have repeated transfusions. In rare cases, the pancytopenia spontaneously reverts, but the children subsequently develop KSS.

A milder mtDNA rearrangement syndrome manifests only as maternally inherited diabetes mellitus and deafness, with occasional individuals experiencing stroke-like episodes. The reason for the mildness of these symptoms is less clear.

mtDNA rearrangements can include deletions, duplications, or both. The deletions most commonly occur in the two-thirds of the mtDNA between the origins of replication, O_H and O_L. Duplications generally occur in association with deletions and are reciprocal to the deletion, sharing a common breakpoint. This suggests that the duplications might give rise to deletions. The duplicated molecules appear to have a replicative advantage in cultured cells and hence may have a higher predilection for maternal transmission. Indeed, the maternally inherited diabetes and deafness syndrome family harbored a reciprocal 10.4-kb deletion and 6.1-kb duplication.

Mitochondrial myopathy, frequently with ophthalmoplegia and ptosis, can also result from nDNA mutations that destabilize the mtDNA. Mutations in the thymidine phosphorylase gene result in mitochondrial neurogastrointestinal encephalomyopathy (MNGIE). Defects in at least two nDNA loci result in the multiple deletion syndrome, AD-PEO, and nDNA defects have been implicated in the lethal mtDNA depletion syndrome.

Finally, ophthalmoplegia, ptosis, and mitochondrial myopathy can also be the presenting clinical symptoms in patients harboring mtDNA tRNA mutations. The most common of these is the MELAS mutation, MTTL1*MELAS3243C. However, multiple additional tRNA mutations have also been associated with CPEO, including MTTN*CPEO5692G, MTTN*CPEO5703G, MTTI*CPEO4298A, MTTL2*CPEO12308G, MTTL2* CPEO12311G, and so on.

The association between mtDNA tRNA mutations and ophthalmoplegia, ptosis, and mitochondrial myopathy may provide some insights into the pathophysiology of these symptoms. Because essentially all mtDNA rearrangements remove at least one tRNA or rRNA gene, then it seems that ophthalmoplegia, ptosis, and mitochondrial myopathy are most commonly caused by defects in mitochondrial protein synthesis. This has been supported by biochemical analysis of cybrids containing mtDNA deletions and the MTTL*MELAS3243G and MTTK*MERRF8344G tRNA mutations, which reveal a severe defect in mitochondrial protein synthesis.

Mitochondrial diseases generally have a delayed onset and progress with age. This has been correlated with the age-related decline in mitochondrial function in association with the accumulation of somatic mtDNA mutations. It has

been hypothesized that the accumulation of these somatic mtDNA mutations is the result of ROS damage, and that the damaged mtDNAs are selectively amplified. Experimental data continue to support this hypothesis, both as it relates to mitochondrial disease and aging.

5. **While identification of the mtDNA mutations associated with neuro-ophthalmologic disease has defined this field, efforts to understand the pathophysiology of these diseases and to develop effective metabolic therapies have been hampered by an inadequate understanding of mitochondrial physiology, the variability in clinical presentations, difficulty in studying the affected tissues, and concerns about experimental drug toxicity to patients. These limitations are being overcome by the application of transgenic mouse technology for the development of mouse models of mitochondrial disease. Three targeted nuclear gene mutations have created animals that have been informative. The first of these was the inactivation of the heart/muscle isoform of the ANT (ANT1). These mice develop classical hypertrophic cardiomyopathy and a mitochondrial myopathy with RRFs and the massive proliferation of giant mitochondria. Because elimination of the ANT would limit ADP/ATP exchanged across the mitochondrial inner membrane, this would limit the availability of ADP to the ATP synthase. Inhibition of the ATP synthase would result in hyperpolarization of the electrochemical gradient ($\Delta\Psi$), which would inhibit the electron transfer chain, redirecting a greater percentage of mitochondrial electrons into generating ROS. The increased ROS would damage mitochondrial membranes, proteins, and mtDNA. These predictions have been confirmed by demonstrating that the hydrogen peroxide production rates of mitochondria from ANT1-deficient mice were maximal in heart and muscle. Moreover, the antioxidant enzyme GPx1 was induced threefold in the mitochondria of both tissues and MnSOD was induced fifteenfold in muscle, but not in heart. The high ROS production in heart coupled with the lack of compensating MnSOD induction would be expected to create imbalance between pro-oxidants and antioxidants, resulting in oxidative stress. Consistent with this expectation, the level of heart mtDNA rearrangement mutations was greatly elevated. Hence, inherited OXPHOS defects can also increase oxidative stress and stimulate the accumulation of somatic mtDNA mutants.**

   The importance of mitochondrial ROS in the pathophysiology of mitochondrial disease was further confirmed in mice lacking the mitochondrial MnSOD. These animals die at about 8 days of age of dilated cardiomyopathy and the massive accumulation of fat in the liver. Biochemical analysis has shown that this results from the inactivation of the iron-sulfur centers in respiratory complexes I, II, and III, as well as in the tricarboxylic acid (TCA) cycle enzyme aconitase. Hence, acute ROS toxicity shuts down the electron transport chain and the TCA cycle, starving the cell of energy and resulting in cardiac failure. This same model has been evoked to explain the pathophysiology of Friedreich ataxia.

   This interpretation has been confirmed by treating the MnSOD-deficient mice with the catalytic antioxidant drug, MnTBAP. This drug completely rescued the cardiomyopathy and fatty liver of the mutant mice. However, MnTBAP does not cross the blood-brain barrier, and the animals developed a movement disorder reminiscent of dystonia and Parkinson disease in association with a spongiform encephalopathy. Clearly, the pathophysiology of mitochondrial encephalomyopathy must involve both inhibited energy generation and increased ROS production.

   A third knockout mouse involves the inactivation of the gene for the mitochondrial transcription factor Tfam. Animals with a systemic defect in Tfam died *in utero* of severe mtDNA depletion. In mice where the mutation is confined to heart, the animals die at about 20 days of age of a cardiomyopathy. Hence, defects in mitochondrial biogenesis also can cause mitochondrial myopathy.

   While these nuclear mutations are proving useful in understanding the pathophysiology of mitochondrial disease, they lack the stochastic element of pathogenic mtDNA mutations. To create models of mtDNA disease, efforts are being made to introduce mtDNA mutations isolated in cultured cells into mouse female embryonic stem cells by mitochondrial cybrid transfer. These mutant female stem cells are then being used to create mouse maternal lineages harboring the mutant mtDNAs. Using the mtDNA mutation imparting resistance to the mitochondrial ribosome inhibitor chloramphenicol (CAP), chimeric mice have been established in which up to 50 percent of the kidney mtDNAs harbor the mutant mtDNAs. Efforts are now underway to achieve female germ line transmission of the mutant mtDNAs. Because the CAP^R mutation causes a partial reduction in complexes I and IV, a heteroplasmic CAP^R mouse may be a good model for human heteroplasmic mtDNA protein synthesis mutation diseases.

6. **These various studies have led to a mitochondrial hypothesis for degenerative diseases and aging. Each individual is envisioned as born with a bioenergetic genotype. If the individual inherits primarily functional mitochondrial genes, then the individual starts with a high bioenergetic capacity. However, if the individual inherits one or more defective mitochondrial genes (either nuclear or cytoplasmic), then the individual starts with a lower energetic capacity. With aging the individual begins to accumulate somatic mtDNA mutations, presumably as a result of chronic ROS damage. These somatic mtDNA rearrangements, together with any systemic mtDNA rearrangement mutations, are subsequently selectively replicated in postmitotic tissues. Therefore, with aging the individual's bioenergetic capacity declines. Ultimately, the energetic capacity of the individual's cells and tissues drops below the minimum necessary for normal function, resulting in dysfunction, induction of apoptosis, and tissue and organ failure. The lower the initial bioenergetic state, the earlier the bioenergetic threshold is traversed and the sooner symptoms appear.**

Ophthalmologic symptoms are among the most conspicuous clinical features of mitochondrial disease. Indeed, acute-onset optic neuropathy and ophthalmoplegia are the most prominent features for the first two mitochondrial diseases to be shown to result from mitochondrial DNA (mtDNA) mutations. Acute-onset optic atrophy is the primary symptom of Leber hereditary optic neuropathy (LHON), a disease caused by a missense mutation in the mtND4 subunit of NADH dehydrogenase, the first enzyme of the oxidative phosphorylation pathway (OXPHOS).[1] Ophthalmoplegia, or paralysis of the extraocular eye muscles, ptosis, and droopy eyelids are the most obvious features of chronic progressive external ophthalmoplegia (CPEO) and Kearns-Sayre syndrome (KSS), both of which are commonly caused by mtDNA deletions.[2] Since the discovery of these mutations in 1988, over 50 pathogenic base substitutions have been identified in the mtDNA and over 100 mtDNA rearrangement mutations have been characterized, many of these having ophthalmologic sequelae.

This raises the question: what are the genetic and pathophysiological features of mitochondrial disease that so frequently affect the eye? New insights into this question are being obtained through studies of mitochondrial physiology, biogenesis, and genetics in both human mitochondrial disease, and in mice with genetically engineered defects in mitochondrial function.

MITOCHONDRIAL BIOLOGY AND BIOENERGETICS

Over the past 5 years, a number of seemingly disparate lines of biomedical research into the causes of degenerative diseases and aging have all converged upon the mitochondrion. This has spawned a new paradigm for the pathophysiology of degenerative disease that integrates mitochondrial energy deficiency, oxygen radical production, and regulation of apoptosis to explain tissue decline and failure.

It is now clear that the mitochondria make three major contributions to cellular biology: (a) they provide most of the energy of the cell, thus generating most of the cellular ATP, regulating cellular redox state, and modulating cytosolic Ca^{++} levels; (b) they produce most of the endogenous cellular oxygen radicals, also known as reactive oxygen species (ROS); and (c) they integrate a variety of signals that can initiate programmed cell death or apoptosis, via the opening of the mitochondrial permeability transition pore (mtPTP). Because a decline in energy production would inhibit cellular metabolism and a rise in mitochondrial ROS production would damage mitochondrial structure and function, these factors could contribute to cell and tissue decline over time. Furthermore, a decline in mitochondrial energy production and an increase in mitochondrial ROS production and oxidative stress can both act on the mtPTP to initiate pore opening and apoptosis. Hence, defects in any of the critical functions of the mitochondria can initiate a progressive program ultimately leading to cell death and tissue and organ failure.

Mitochondrial Structure and Function

Mitochondrial Morphology. The mitochondria are highly pleomorphic, double-membrane structures. The inner mitochondrial membrane is highly involved, forming cristae that create an enormous surface area on which OXPHOS can take place. The outer membrane surrounds the enfolded inner membrane, with the whole structure resulting in four compartments: the central mitochondrial matrix where the tricarboxylic acid (TCA) cycle and β-oxidation take place, the inner membrane that contains the OXPHOS complexes, the intermembrane space that stores key proteins, and the outer membrane that medicates the interaction between the mitochondria and the cytosol. The inner membrane is rich in cardiolipin (22 percent), relative to the outer membrane (3 percent), with the outer membrane lipid composition being more similar to the other cellular membranes.[3]

The overall shape and distribution of the mitochondria vary from one cell to another. The pleomorphic nature of the mitochondrial structure can be readily determined by staining the cells with the heterocyclic action dye rhodamine 124 (Fig. 105-1). This and related cationic compounds are selectively transported into the mitochondrial matrix because of the electrostatic difference across the mitochondrial inner membrane, which is negatively charged and alkaline on the inside and positively charged and acid on the outside. In a cultured mammalian cell, the mitochondria can vary from spherical dots, to long branched structures, to an interconnected network.

The mitochondrial shapes and distribution within the cell are beginning to be understood as the product of the interaction of the mitochondria with each other through regular fusion and fission, and between the mitochondria and the cytoskeleton. Proteins that are involved in mitochondrial fusion and fission include the large membrane-bound GTP-binding protein, *fuzzy onion*, first described in *Drosophila,*[4] and its yeast homologue Fzo1p. Mutations in Fzo1p cause fragmentation of the mitochondria.[5,6]

Mitochondrial mobility within the cell has been shown to be associated with movement along the microtubules and intermediate filaments of the cytoskeleton. Movement along microtubules is mediated by the microtubular motor proteins dynein and kinesin. Several members of the kinesin family have been localized to the mitochondria. These include KIF1B, KLP67B, and KIF5B. Disruption of the KIF5B gene in mice results in an embryonic lethal, but in cells derived from mutant embryos, the mitochondrial distribution is shifted from dispersed around the cell to clustered near the nucleus. Because KIF5B cofractionates with the mitochondria, it follows that it assists in the radial movement of the mitochondria along the cytoskeleton of the cell.[7] Maintenance of mitochondrial morphology and distribution also involves the dynamin superfamily of GTP-binding proteins, including Drp1.[8] These and other genes are required for regulating mitochondrial morphology, interaction, mobility, fission, fusion, and transmission.[6] Thus, the biology of the mitochondrion involves many levels of complexity that are just beginning to be perceived.

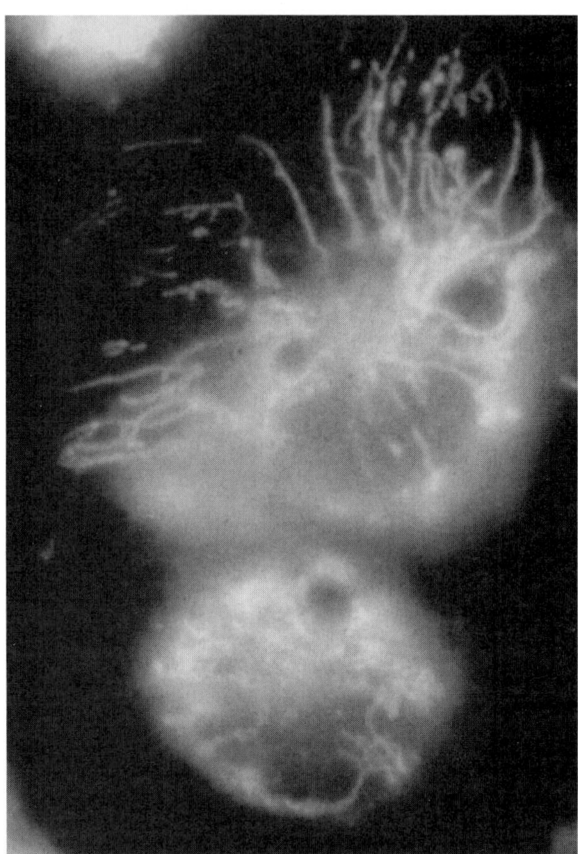

Fig. 105-1 Human HT1080C fibrosarcoma cells stained with the mitochondria-specific vital dye rhodamine 123. The mitochondria are seen to be broadly distributed throughout the cell and to have a variety of sizes and shapes. This is now understood to be the product of the action of a variety of genes involving fusion of the mitochondria and the interaction of mitochondria with the cytoskeleton. (*Reproduced from Wallace.*[824] *Used with permission.*)

Mitochondrial OXPHOS: Energy, ROS, and Apoptosis. Mitochondrial energy production, ROS generation, and apoptosis regulation all involve the enzymes of OXPHOS located within the mitochondrial inner membrane.

OXPHOS is composed of five multipolypeptide enzyme complexes. Complexes I, II, III, and IV make up the electron transport chain (ETC), while complex V is the ATP synthase (Fig. 105-2). Carbohydrates and fats from our diet are transported to the mitochondria where they are oxidized by the tricarboxylic acid (TCA) cycle and the β-oxidation pathways, respectively (Fig. 105-2). This liberates CO_2 and hydrogen atoms, the latter carried on soluble NAD^+ as $NADH + H^+$ or on enzyme-bound FAD as $FADH_2$. $NADH + H^+$ is oxidized by complex I (NADH:

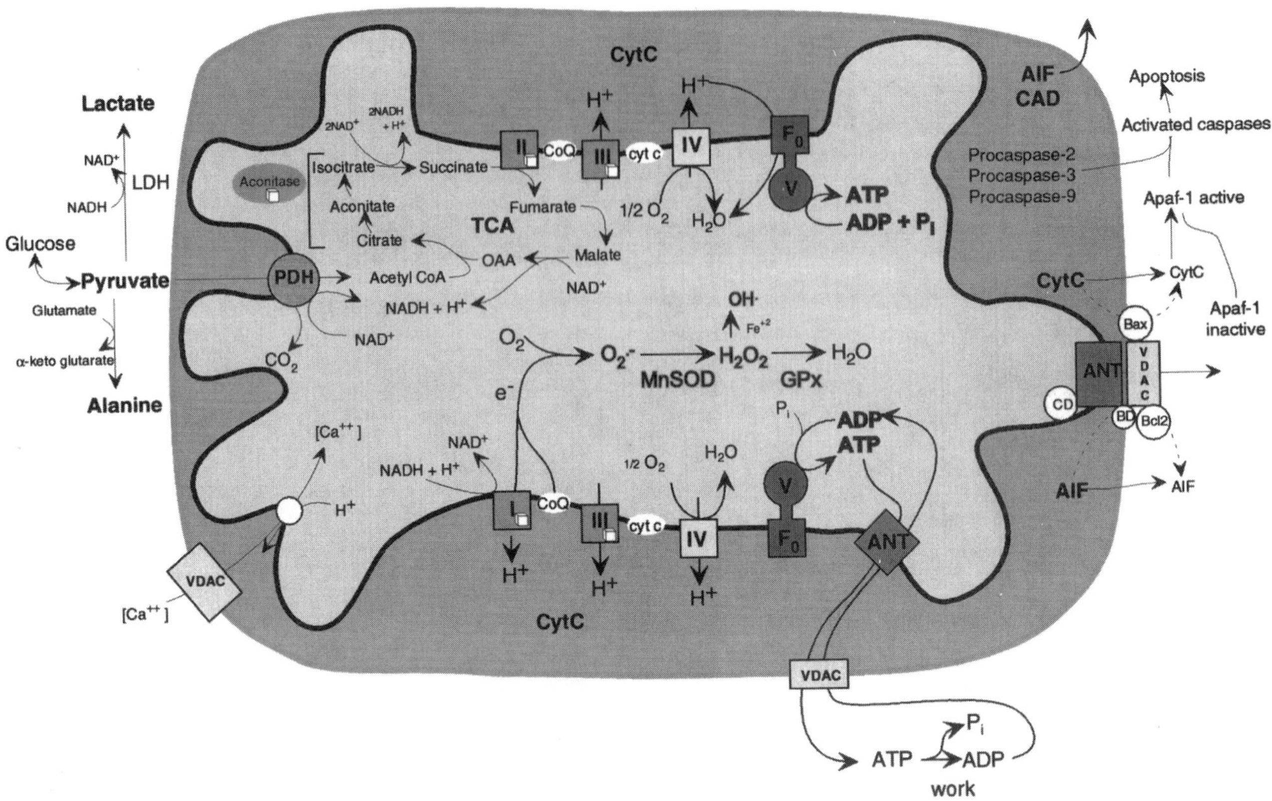

Fig. 105-2 Diagram of a mitochondrion, illustrating the relationships between mitochondrial oxidative phosphorylation and (a) the production of energy (ATP), (b) the generation of reactive oxygen species (ROS), and (c) the initiation of apoptosis through activation of the mitochondrial permeability transition pore (mtPTP). The respiratory enzyme complexes involved in OXPHOS are complex I [NADH:ubiquinone oxidoreductase], complex II [succinate:ubiquinone oxidoreductase], complex III [ubiquinol:cytochrome c oxidoreductase], complex IV [cytochrome c oxidase], and complex V [H^+-translocating ATP synthase]. Pyruvate from glucose enters the mitochondria via pyruvate dehydrogenase (PDH), generating acetyl CoA, which enters the tricarboxylic acid (TCA) cycle by combining with oxaloacetate (OOA). *cis*-Aconitase converts citrate to isocitrate. All enzymes containing an iron-sulfur cluster are designated with a cube. Lactate dehydrogenase (LDH) converts excess pyruvate plus NADH to lactate. Small molecules diffuse through the outer membrane via the voltage-dependent anion channels (VDAC) or porin. VDACs together with the adenine nucleotide translocator (ANT), Bax, and cyclophilin D (CD) are thought to come together at the mitochondrial inner and outer membrane contact points to create the mtPTP. Bax is pro-apoptotic and is thought to interact with the antiapoptotic protein BCL-2 and the benzodiazepine receptor (BD). The opening of the mtPTP is associated with the release of cytochrome c, AIF (apoptosis initiating factor), CAD (caspase-activated DNAase), and the procaspase-2, -3, and -9. In the cytosol, cytochrome c activates Apaf-1, which actives procaspase-2 and -9. The activated caspases activate caspase-3, -6, -7, and CAD. The caspases degrade the cytoplasm, while AIF and CAD migrate to the nucleus and degrade the chromatin. (*Modified from Koehler et al.*[825] *Used with permission.*)

ubiquinone oxidoreductase, EC 1.6.5.3) and the electrons transported through flavin mononucleotide (FMN) and multiple iron-sulfur centers until they are transferred to ubiquinone (CoQ_{10}). CoQ_{10} is sequentially reduced to ubisemiquinone ($CoQ_{10}H\cdot$) and then to ubiquinol ($CoQ_{10}H_2$). $CoQ_{10}H_2$ is also generated by complex II (succinate: ubiquinone oxidoreductase, EC 1.3.5.1) and by the electron transfer flavoprotein together with the ETF dehydrogenase (EC 1.5.5.1). Complex II collects electrons from the oxidation of succinate to fumarate in the TCA cycle, while ETF and ETF dehydrogenase collect electrons from fatty acid β-oxidation. Both enzymes contain an FAD and one or more iron sulfur centers. $CoQ_{10}H_2$ ferries the electrons through the inner membrane from complexes I, II, and ETF dehydrogenase to complex III (ubiquinol: ferrocytochrome c oxidoreductase, EC 1.10.2.2), also known as the cytochrome bc1 complex. Within this complex, the electrons move through the Q cycle, cytochrome b, the Rieske iron-sulfur, and cytochrome c1. The electrons are then transferred to cytochrome c, which is loosely associated with the exterior of the inner membrane. Cytochrome c transfers the electrons from complex III to complex IV (ferrocytochrome c: oxygen oxidoreductase, EC 1.9.3.3.1), also known as cytochrome c oxidase or COX. Within this complex the electrons are transferred through the CuA and CuB centers and cytochromes a and a_3, and ultimately combine with $\frac{1}{2}$ O_2 to give H_2O. The energy that is released in this controlled oxidation of the electrons is used to pump protons from inside the mitochondrial matrix out across the inner membrane to the intermembrane space through complexes I, III, and IV. The resulting electrochemical gradient [$\Delta p = \Delta\psi + \Delta\mu^{H+}$] involves both pH ($\Delta\mu^{H+}$) and electrostatic ($\Delta\psi$) differences, and serves as a source of potential energy for synthesizing adenosine triphosphate (ATP) from adenosine diphosphate (ADP) and inorganic phosphate (Pi). ATP is synthesized by complex V (ATP phosphohydrolase [$-H^+$-transporting], or ATP synthase, EC 3.6.1.34) which contains three distinctive components: the base, F_0; the stalk; and the spherical head, F_1. As protons move back through F_0, they cause the central core of F_0 and the stalk to rotate within the hexagonal array of 3 α and 3 β subunits of the F_1. This causes each β subunit to sequentially change its conformation, first binding ADP + Pi, condensing them to ATP, and releasing the ATP. The matrix ATP is then exchanged for spent cytosolic ADP by the adenine nucleotide translocator (ANT)[9–11] (Fig. 105-2).

Because OXPHOS oxidizes reduced NADH and $FADH_2$, it is central to maintaining the redox balance of the cell. The $\Delta\psi$ is also utilized as a source of potential energy for the uptake of cytosolic Ca^{++} into the mitochondria (Fig. 105-2). Finally, expression of uncoupler proteins in the mitochondrial inner membrane results in an increased proton leak back into the matrix. This increases the rate of mitochondrial oxidation of hydrogen generating heat, a process central to mammalian thermal regulation.

As a toxic byproduct of mitochondrial energy generation by OXPHOS, the mitochondria generate most of the cellular ROS ($O_2^{\cdot-}$, H_2O_2, and OH·) (Fig. 105-2). This is because when the ETC is inhibited, the electrons accumulate in the early stages of the ETC, complex I, II, and III, all of which generate $CoQ_{10}H\cdot$. $CoQ_{10}H\cdot$ is electronegative enough to donate electrons directly to molecular oxygen (O_2) to give superoxide anion ($O_2^{\cdot-}$). Superoxide anion is detoxified by the mitochondrial manganese superoxide dismutase (MnSOD) (EC 1.15.1.1) to give hydrogen peroxide (H_2O_2) and H_2O_2 is converted to H_2O by glutathione peroxidase (GPx) (EC 1.11.1.9). H_2O_2, in the presence of reduced transition metals, can also be converted to the highly reactive hydroxyl radical (·OH) by the Fenton reaction. Chronic ROS exposure can result in oxidative damage to the mitochondrial and cellular proteins, lipids, and nucleic acids; acute ROS exposure can inactivate the iron-sulfur (Fe-S) centers of ETC complexes I, II, and III, and TCA cycle enzyme aconitase, shutting down mitochondrial energy metabolism.[12,13]

The mitochondria also have the capacity to integrate a number of factors associated with the initiation of apoptosis. This is thought to occur via the opening of a nonspecific mitochondrial inner membrane channel, the mitochondrial permeability transition pore (mtPTP). The mtPTP is thought to be composed of the ANT, porin (voltage-dependent anion channel), Bax, Bcl2, cyclophilin D and the benzodiazepine receptor (Fig. 105-2).[14–16] The mitochondrial inner membrane space contains a number of cell death-promoting factors including cytochrome c, apoptosis initiating factor (AIF, a flavoprotein), latent forms of caspases (procaspase-2, procaspase-3, and procaspase-4), as well as the caspase-activated DNAse (CAD). Current evidence suggests that the opening of the mtPTP results in the collapse of $\Delta\Psi$, the swelling of the mitochondrial inner membrane, and the rupture of the mitochondrial outer membrane. This releases cytochrome c, AIF, the procaspases, and CAD into the cytosol.[17–21] The released cytochrome c activates the cytosolic Apaf-1, which activates procaspase-9 and procaspase-2. Caspase-9 and -2 activate caspase-3, -6, and -7, and these destroy the cell. The AIF, which has a nuclear targeting sequence, is transported to the nucleus where it initiates chromatin condensation and degradation. CAD also participates in nDNA degradation.

The opening of the mtPTP can be initiated by the mitochondrion's excessive uptake of Ca^{++}, increased exposure to ROS, or a decline in energetic capacity such as a drop in $\Delta\Psi$.[15,18] Thus, disease states which lead to an increase in mitochondrial uptake of Ca^{++}, a decline in OXPHOS bioenergetics capacity, or an increase in ROS production could all activate the mtPTP and precipitate apoptosis-mediated cell death.[15,22,23]

Mitochondrial OXPHOS Complexes

Complex I. OXPHOS complex I is composed of approximately 42 polypeptides, 7 (MTND1, 2, 3, 4, 4L, 5, and 6) of which are encoded by the mtDNA (Fig. 105-3). These encompass 3 flavoproteins (FPs), 7 iron-sulfur proteins (ISPs), and over 24 hydrophobic proteins (Fig. 105-4*A*).[24–36] The complex I proteins, cDNAs, gene structures, and chromosomal locations are given in Table 105-1.

Complex I oxidizes NADH, reduces CoQ_{10}, and uses the energy released to pump protons across the mitochondrial inner membrane. Electrons from NADH are transferred through FMN and up to nine iron-sulfur centers, including N-1a, N-1b, N-2, N-3, N-4, and N-5.[37,38] The overall structure of complex I is slipper-shaped, with the foot lying in the membrane and the ankle extending into the mitochondrial matrix (Fig. 105-4).[39,40]

The bovine complex I consists of a globular hydrophilic region containing the NADH binding site, FMN, and all ISPs; a 30-Å diameter stalk, and a hydrophobic membrane component (Fig. 105-4*A*). The overall molecular mass is 890 kDa. The hydrophilic globular component and stalk are 175 Å and have a mass of about 520 kDa. The hydrophobic component is 200 Å long and has a mass of about 370 kDa.[40] The complex can be split into two major components, Iα and Iβ, by the detergent lauryl-dimethylamine oxide (LDAO). The Iα component is an active NADH dehydrogenase, and contains the NADH binding site, FMN, and all of the known Fe-S centers. It can oxidize NADH and reduce ubiquinone, and represents the ankle. The Iβ component has no enzymatic activity, is hydrophobic, and probably represents the membrane-bound component. The Iα component has a mass of about 540 kDa. It consists of 23 polypeptides including polypeptides 75 kDa, 51 kDa, 24 kDa, TYKY, PSST, and PGIV, which bind the redox centers.[34] The 75-kDa protein contains two iron-sulfur centers and the human gene is located on chromosome 2q33-34.[41–43] The 51-kDa polypeptide forms the NADH and FMN binding sites and also binds a tetranuclear iron-sulfur center. The 24-kDa subunit contains a binuclear iron-sulfur center and the gene is located on chromosome 18p11.2-p11.13.[42,44–49] A subfraction of Iα, Iλ, has a mass of 360 kDa and can be obtained by treatment with LDAO in high salt. It is able to transfer electrons from NADH to the synthetic electron acceptor ferricyanide, but not to quinones. The Iλ encompasses 15 polypeptides including 75 kDa, 51 kDa, 24 kDa, TYKY, and PSST. The Iβ fragment is 200 Å long and has a mass of about 266 kDa. It contains 17 polypeptides, 13 of which contain at least one membrane-spanning segment and two of which are ND4 and ND5.[34,50,51] During the biosynthesis of the *Neurospora crassa* complex I, a transient intermediate occurs with molecular mass of 350 kDa. This contains all of the mitochondrial-synthesized subunits (same as mammals) and is thought to encompass most of the membrane domain.[40,52] Thus, most of the mtDNA-encoded polypeptides probably reside in the foot-shaped membrane component IB (Fig. 105-4*A*).

Two of the subunits of complex I may be involved in specialized means for respiration. These include an acyl carrier protein with a phosphopantetheine group and a member of a family of NAD(P)H-dependent reductases/isomerases.[39]

Respiratory complex I can also be subfractionated by treatment with the chaotropic anion perchlorate into three fragments: the flavoprotein fragment, the iron-protein fragment, and the hydrophobic fragment.[38] The flavoprotein fragment encompasses FMN, six iron atoms, and the 51-kDa, the 24-kDa, and the 10-kDa polypeptides. The function of the 10-kDa polypeptide is unknown.[34,53] The iron-protein fragment contains 9 or 10 iron atoms,[54,55] and a 15-kDa protein that may be a ubiquinone-binding protein.[56] The mtDNA ND6 polypeptide may also be located in this fragment[29] and involved in CoQ_{10} binding.[57] The hydrophobic fragment probably contains the majority of the mtDNA-encoded polypeptides including MTND1, MTND3, and MTND4L,[29,38] and may also contain MTND2, MTND4, and MTND5. The hydrophobic fragment may also encompass the iron-sulfur centers that donate electrons to CoQ_{10}. MTND1 is thought to interact with the CoQ_{10} binding site and may be involved in electron transfer to CoQ_{10}. It also binds rotenone and rotenone analogues,[38,58] although the rotenone and CoQ_{10} binding sites may not be the same.[59] MTND6 may also occupy the CoQ_{10} binding site, because mutations in the MTND6 gene associated with optic atrophy and dystonia[60] also alter the efficiency of electron transfer to CoQ_{10}.[57]

Respiratory-deficient mutants lacking complex I have been isolated in cultured human VA_2 B cells. Two of these mutants, C4T and C5T, had an insertion of a single C within a stretch of six Cs at nps 10947 to 10952 toward the N-terminus of ND4. This created a frameshift in the ND4 protein, generating a stop codon about 150 nucleotides downstream, and a truncated protein of about 13 kDa. Two other mutants, C8T and C9T, had a single A insertion in a stretch of eight As encompassing np 12417 to 12424 at the N-terminal end of ND5. This also created a frameshift and a truncated protein of about 6.9 kDa. Both types of mutants had severely reduced mitochondrial oxygen consumption using NADH-linked substrates and NADH:CoQ oxidoreductase activities. However, both retained their NADH:Fe $(CN)_6$

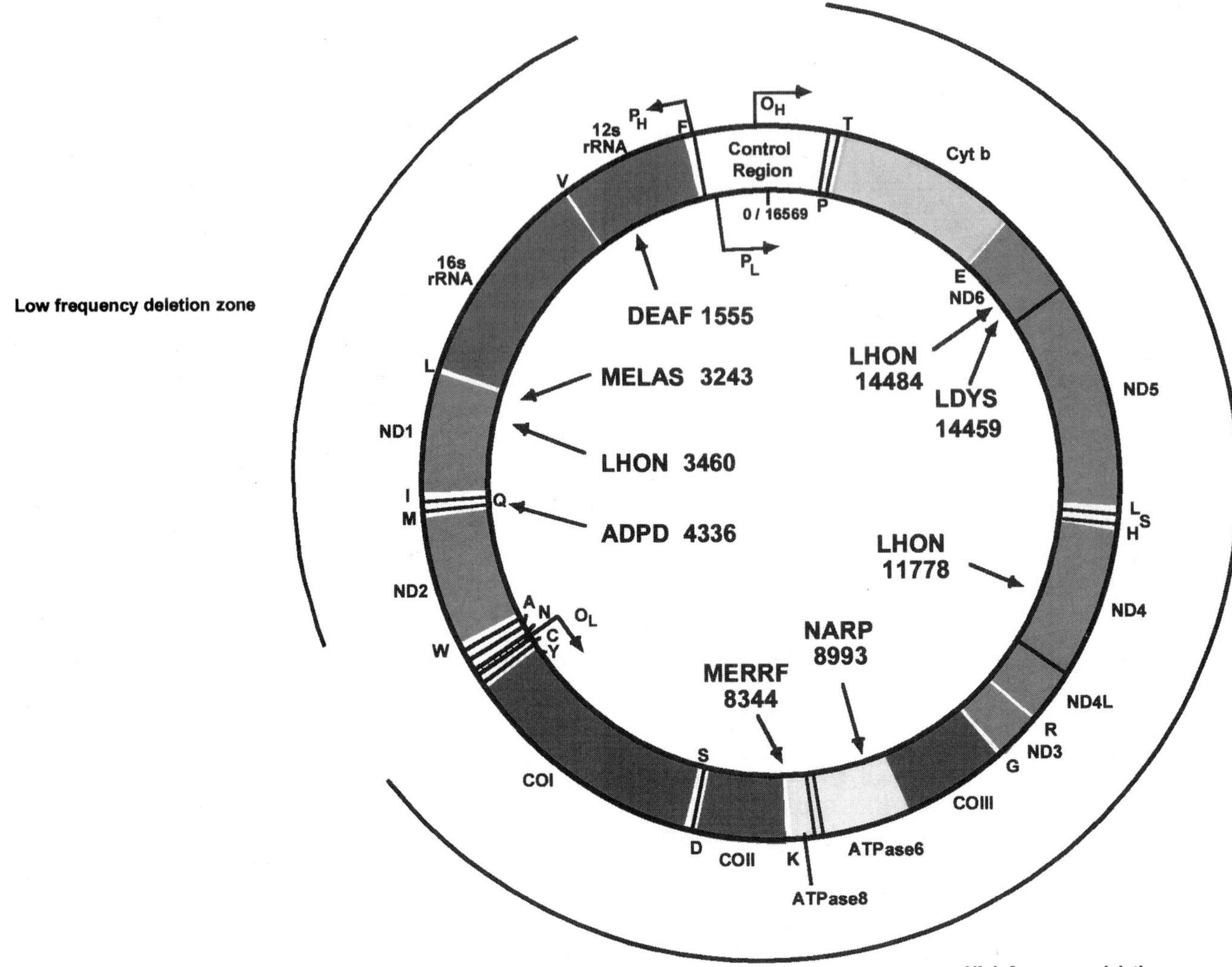

Fig. 105-3 The human mtDNA map, showing the location of selected pathogenic mutations. The human mtDNA is a 16,569-base-pair circular molecule which codes for seven (ND1, 2, 3, 4L, 5, and 6) of the 43 subunits of complex I; one (cytochrome b, cyt b) of the 11 subunits of complex III; three (COI, II, and III) of the 13 subunits of complex IV; and two (ATPase 6 and 8) of 16 subunits of complex V. It also codes for the small and large rRNAs, and 22 tRNAs, with the adjacent letters indicating the cognate amino acids. The heavy (H)-strand origin of replication (O_H) and the H-strand and light (L)-strand promoters, P_H and P_L, are indicated in the control region. The mitochondrial transcription factor Tfam binds between the promoters. Tfam is important in initiating transcription and in generating the primer from the L-strand transcripts to initiate H-strand DNA replication at O_H. The L-strand origin of replication (O_L) is located two-thirds of the way around the genome. The positions of representative pathogenic point mutations are shown on the inside of the circle, with the nucleotide position and disease acronym. The regions of the mtDNA that can be deleted in various diseases are shown by the external arcs. The most common deletion zone is between O_H and O_L on the right side of the molecule. (*Adapted from Koehler et al.*[825] *Used with permission.*)

oxidoreductase activities, suggesting retention of a functional Iα component. Immunoprecipitation of complex I using antibodies to the nuclear-encoded 49-kDa iron-sulfur protein revealed that the ND4 mutants lacked the mtDNA-encoded subunits, suggesting a failure to assemble the membrane Iβ component. The ND5 mutants contained the other mtDNA subunits, implying a more normal assemble. This suggests that ND4 but not ND5 is essential for assembly of the Iβ component of complex I.[61,62]

The actual mechanism of electron transfer and protein pumping for complex I is unknown. The redox differential across complex I is from -320 mV for NADH to $+60$ mV for CoQ_{10}. The approximate redox potentials for selected iron-sulfur centers are N-1 (≈ -305 mV), N-4 (≈ -245 mV), N-2 (≈ -20 mV). Hence, N-1 and N-4 are closest to NADH/FMN and N-2 is closest to CoQ_{10}. The ratios of protons pumped to electrons transported is also unknown, although one determination suggests $3H^+/2e^-$. The model presented in Fig. 105-4*B* is the synthesis of several current proposals. In this model, the FMN oxidation-reduction by NADH + H^+ is coupled to the transport of two protons across the membrane and the sequential transfer of two electrons to the iron-sulfur center N-1, and then on to the isopotential iron-sulfur N-3 and N-4. The electrons are then transferred to N-2, where two successive electrons reduce two ubiquinones (CoQ_{10} or "Q"), one bound to the "B" site on the cytosolic side ("o" or out) and the other to the "A" site on the matrix side ("i" or in). Each electron reduction is accompanied by acquisition of a matrix proton to create a ubisemiquinone. The ubisemiquinone at site B transfers its electron to the ubisemiquinone at site A and releases its proton on the cytosolic side. The fully reduced ubiquinone acquires another matrix proton to create bound ubiquinol on the matrix side (QH_2 bi). This ubiquinol then moves into the C site and is released into the membrane. The CoQ_{10} bound to the B site is then ready to acquire another electron from N-2 (Fig. 105-4*B*).[3,63–66]

Complex I is affected by a wide variety of inhibitors. One notable example is the activated form of 1-methyl-4-phenyl-1,2,3,4-tetrahydropyridine (MPTP), 1-methyl-4-phenylpyridinium

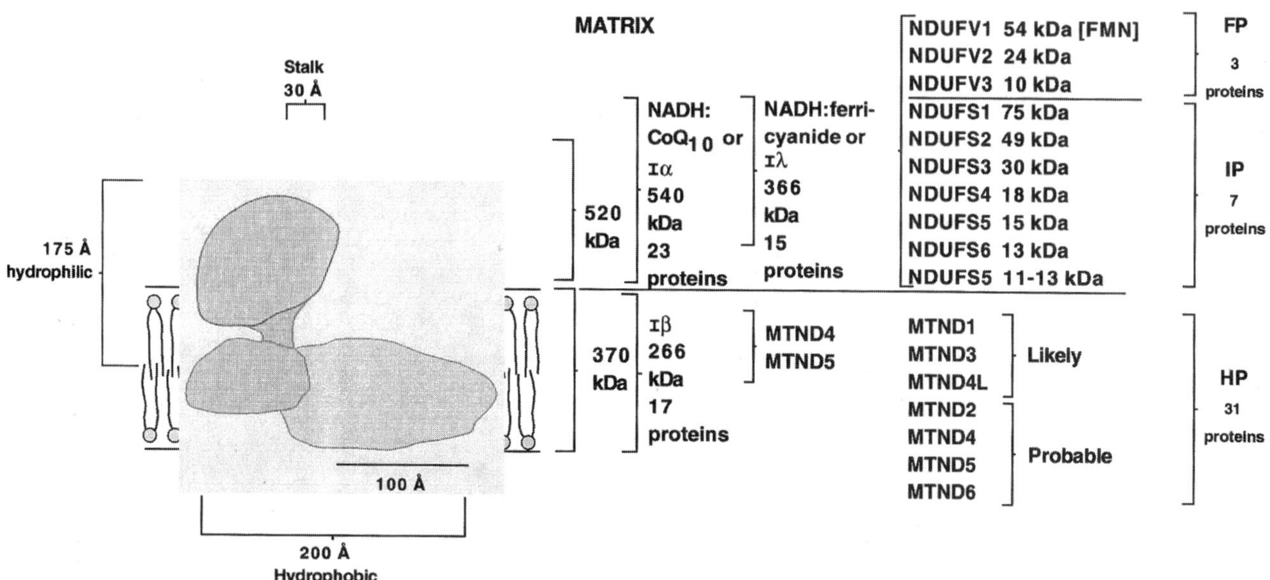

A

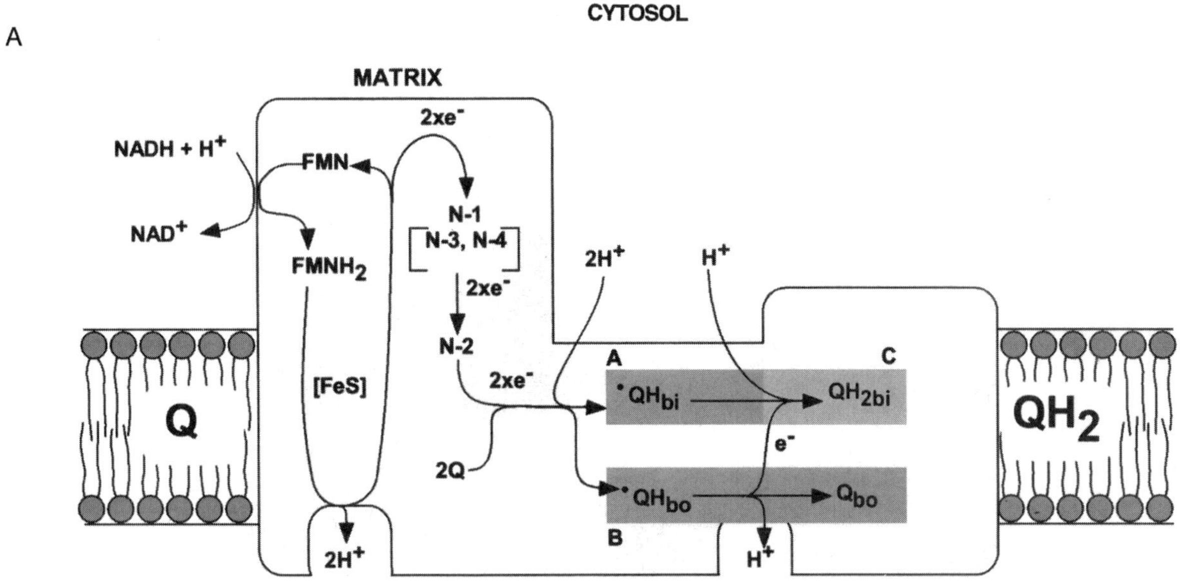

B

Fig. 105-4 Structure and function of complex I. *Panel A:* The structure of complex I is shown, determined at 22-Å resolution using electron microscopy of frozen specimens.[40] The L-shaped structure involves a hydrophilic globular component projecting into the matrix, attached by a 30-Å diameter stalk to a foot-shaped hydrophobic membrane component.[39,40] The hydrophilic component is estimated to be about 520 kDa, and to roughly correspond to the catalytic fraction of the enzyme Iα. Iα is capable of the complete NADH:ubiquinone oxidoreductase (OR) reaction, is composed of 23 polypeptides, and encompasses all the flavoprotein (Fs) and iron-sulfur proteins (ISP). These same catalytic sites are found in the Iλ subfraction capable of the NADH:ferricyanide oxidoreductase (OR) reaction.[34,50] This same region of the enzyme can be subdivided into an Fp component of three polypeptides and an ISP (IP) component of seven polypeptides.[53] The hydrophobic membrane component encompasses the Iβ fraction of the enzyme involving 17 polypeptides[34,35,50] and is probably virtually encompassed by the hydrophobic (HP) fraction of the enzyme encompassing 31 polypeptides.[53] All of the mtDNA-encoded subunits are likely located in the hydrophobic membrane component.[29] *Panel B:* Hypothetical model of electron transport and proton pumping for complex I. Model adapted from conjectures by authors in references 46, 64, 65, 67, and 404. This proposal gives a ratio of $3H^+/2e^-$, involves elements of the bcl Q cycle, and hypothesizes two proton channels on the cytosolic, high H^+ side. The first set of protons is proposed to be transported during the oxidation-reduction of FMN, in conjunction with certain of the Fe-S centers. Electrons then flow through an array of Fe-S centers including N-1 and the isopotential N-3 and N-4, and are then donated to the most positive center, N-2. N-2 then donates sequentially two electrons to two ubiquinones (Q), each of which picks up a proton, to create two bound (b) ubisemiquinones: one on the outside ("o" or site B) and one on the inside ("i" or site A). These dismutate with the ubisemiquinone bound to the "o/B" site gives up its proton to the cytosolic side and transmits its electron to the ubisemiquinone bound to the "i/A" site. The reduced ubisemiquinone at the "i/A" picks up another proton from the matrix to give ubiquinol (QH_2 bi) which then occupies the "C" site and is released into the lipid bilayer. The ubiquinone bound to the "o/B" site is then ready to pick up the next electron from N-2.

Table 105-1 **Complex I: Proteins, cDNAs, and Genes**

A. Hydrophobic Proteins

Gene	Description	Accession #	Chr. location	Sequence	Leader	Gene Characterization	Comments
MTND1	NADH dehydrogenase (ubiquinone), subunit ND1	M10546, J01415, V00662	mtDNA[25]	mDNA[25]	N/A	Polypeptide = 318 aa, encoded by 954 bp, nucleotide position 3307–4262	Mutations include: Leber optic atrophy (MTND1*LHON3460A, MTND1*LHON4160C, MTND1*LHON4216C, MTND1*LHON3394C, MTND1*LHON4136G), Alzheimer[690] disease and Parkinson disease (MTND1*ADPD3397G)
MTND2	NADH dehydrogenase (ubiquinone), subunit ND2	J01415, V00662	mtDNA[25]	mDNA[25]	N/A	Polypeptide = 347 aa, encoded by 1041 bp, nucleotide position 4470–5511	Mutations include: Leber optic atrophy (MTND2*LHON4917G, MTND2*LHON5244A)
MTND3	NADH dehydrogenase (ubiquinone), subunit ND3	J01415, V00662	mtDNA[25]	mDNA[25]	N/A	Polypeptide = 115 aa, 345 bp, nucleotide position 10,059–10,404	
MTND4	NADH dehydrogenase (ubiquinone), subunit ND4	J01415, V00662	mtDNA[25]	mDNA[25]	N/A	Polypeptide = 459 aa, encoded by 1377 bp, nucleotide position 10,760–12,137	Mutations include: Leber optic atrophy (MTND4*LHON11778A), MELAS sydrome (MTND4*MELAS11084G), and Leber optic atrophy and spastic dystonia (MTND4, 11696A-G, VAL312ILE)
MTND4L	NADH dehydrogenase (ubiquinone), subunit ND4L	J01415, V00662	mtDNA[25]	mDNA[25]	N/A	Polypeptide = 98 aa, encoded by 294 bp, nucleotide position 10,470–10,766	
MTND5	NADH dehydrogenase (ubiquinone), subunit ND5	J01415, V00662	mtDNA[25]	mDNA[25]	N/A	Polypeptide = 603 aa, encoded by 1809 bp, nucleotide position 12,337–14,148	Mutations include: Leber optic atrophy (MTND5*LHON13708A, MTND5*LHON13730A)
MTND6	NADH dehydrogenase (ubiquinone), subunit ND6	J01415, V00662	mtDNA[25]	mDNA[25]	N/A	Polypeptide = 174 aa, encoded by 522 bp, nucleotide position 14,149–14,673	Mutations include: Leber optic atrophy (MTND6*LHON14484A), and Leber optic atrophy and dystonin (MTND6*LDYT14459A, MTND6*LDYT14596A)
NDUFA1	NADH dehydrogenase (ubiquinone) 7.5K chain	U54993	Xq24[584]	gDNA, cDNA[584]	–	Gene has 3 exons, polypeptide = 70 aa, coded by 210 bp	
NDUFA2	NADH dehydrogenase (ubiquinone) 8K chain	AF047185	5q31.2[585]	cDNA[586]	–	Polypeptide = 99 aa, encoded by 297 bp	Limb girdle muscular dystrophy-1 A maps to 5q22.3-q31.3, implicating NDUFA2 as a candidate gene.[587]
NDUFA3	NADH dehydrogenase (ubiquinone) 9K chain	AF044955		cDNA[588]	–	Polypeptide = 84 aa, encoded by 252 bp	

NDUFA4	NADH dehydrogenase (ubiquinone) 9K chain	U94586		cDNA[589]		Polypeptide = 81 aa, encoded by 243 bp	
NDUFA6	NADH dehydrogenase (ubiquinone) 14K chain	NM_002490	21q13.1[590]	cDNA[586]		Polypeptide = 128 aa, encoded by 384 bp	
NDUFA7	NADH dehydrogenase (ubiquinone) 14.5K chain	AF050637	19p13.2[590]	cDNA[588]	–	Polypeptide = 113 aa, encoded by 339 bp	
NDUFA8	NADH dehydrogenase (ubiquinone) 19K chain	AA338496	9q33.2-34.11[591]	cDNA[592]		Polypeptide = 172 aa, encoded by 516 bp	
NDUFA9	NADH dehydrogenase (ubiquinone) 39K chain	L04490	12p13[593]	cDNA[593]	+ (35 aa)	Polypeptide = 377 aa, encoded by 1131 bp	A pseudogene has been localized to 22q12-qter.[593]
NDUFA10	NADH dehydrogenase (ubiquinone) 42K chain	AF087661		cDNA[588]	+	Polypeptide = 355 aa, encoded by 1065 bp	
NDUFAB1	NADH dehydrogenase (ubiquinone) 8K chain	AF087660	16p12.3-12.1[591]	cDNA[588]		Polypeptide = 156 aa, encoded by 468 bp	
NDUFB1	NADH dehydrogenase (ubiquinone) 7K chain	AF054181	14q31.3[591]	cDNA[594]		Polypeptide = 58 aa, encoded by 174 bp	
NDUFB2	NADH dehydrogenase (ubiquinone) 8K chain	AF050639	7q34-35[591]	cDNA[588]	+	Polypeptide = 105 aa, encoded by 315 bp	
NDUFB3	NADH dehydrogenase (ubiquinone) 12K chain	AF047183		cDNA[586]			
NDUFB4	NADH dehydrogenase (ubiquinone) 15K chain	AF044957		cDNA[588]	–	Polypeptide = 129 aa, encoded by 387 bp	
NDUFB5	NADH dehydrogenase (ubiquinone) 16K chain	NM_002492		cDNA[586]	+(46 aa)	Polypeptide = 189 aa, encoded by 567 bp	
NDUFB6	NADH dehydrogenase (ubiquinone) 17K chain	NM_002493	9p13.2[591]	cDNA[595]		Polypeptide = 128 aa, encoded by 384 bp	
NDUFB7	NADH dehydrogenase (ubiquinone) 18K chain	NM_004146	19p13.12-13.11[591]	cDNA[596]	–	Polypeptide = 135 aa, encoded by 405 bp	
NDUFB8	NADH dehydrogenase (ubiquinone) 19K chain	AF044958	10q23.2-23.33[590]	cDNA[588]	+(28 aa)	Polypeptide = 186 aa, encoded by 558 bp	
NDUFB9	NADH dehydrogenase (ubiquinone) 22K chain	S82655	8p13.3[591,597]	gDNA,[598] cDNA[597]	–	Gene has 4 exons, polypeptide = 179* aa, encoded by 537 bp	Branchio-oto-renal syndrome maps to this region, to date, no patients have shown mutations in NDUFB9.[597] *The N-terminus is acetylated in bovine NDUFB9.[598]
NDUFB10	NADH dehydrogenase (ubiquinone) 22K chain	AF044954	16p13.3[591]	cDNA[588]	–	Polypeptide = 172 aa, encoded by 516 bp	
NDUFC1	NADH dehydrogenase (ubiquinone) 6K chain	NM_002494	4q28-q31.1[591]	cDNA[586]	+(27 aa)	Polypeptide = 76 aa, encoded by 228 bp	

(Continued on next page)

Table 105-1 (Continued)

A. Hydrophobic Proteins

Gene	Description	Accession #	Chr. location	Sequence	Leader	Gene Characterization	Comments
NDUFC2	NADH dehydrogenase (ubiquinone) 14.5K chain	AF087659		cDNA[588]	–	Polypeptide = 119 aa, encoded by 357 bp	
NDUFS7	NADH dehydrogenase (ubiquinone) 20K chain		19p13[599]	cDNA[599]	+(38 aa)	Polypeptide = 213 aa, encoded by 639 bp	
NDUFS8	NADH dehydrogenase (ubiquinone) 23K chain	U65579, AF038406	11q13.1-Q13.3[590,600]	gDNA,[601] cDNA[600]	+ (34 aa)	Gene has 7 exons, polypeptide = 210 aa, encoded by 630 bp	Mutations include: Leigh syndrome (NDUFS8, PRO79LEU and NDUFS8, ARG102HIS)[419]
B. Iron-Sulfur Proteins							
NDUFS1	NADH dehydrogenase (ubiquinone) 75K chain	X61100	2q33–34[41]	cDNA[43]	+(23 aa)	Polypeptide = 727 aa encoded by 2181 bp	Contains 2 Fe-S centers
NDUFS2	NADH dehydrogenase (ubiquinone) 49K chain	AF050640	1q23[602,603]	cDNA[602,603]	+(33 aa)	Polypeptide = 463 aa, encoded by 1389 bp	
NDUFS3	NADH dehydrogenase (ubiquinone) 30K chain	NM_004551	11p11.11[591]	cDNA[603]	+(36 aa)	Polypeptide = 264 aa, encoded by 792 bp	
NDUFS4	NADH dehydrogenase (ubiquinone) 18K chain	AF020351	5q11.1[591]	cDNA[437]	+(42 aa)	Polypeptide = 175 aa, encoded by 525 bp	Mutations include: 5-bp deletion[437]
NDUFS5	NADH dehydrogenase (ubiquinone) 15K chain	AF020352	1p34.2-p33[591]	cDNA[594]		Polypeptide = 106 aa, encoded by 318 bp	
NDUFS6	NADH dehydrogenase (ubiquinone) 13K chain	AF044959	5pter-5p15.33[591]	cDNA[603]	+(28 aa)	Polypeptide = 124 aa, encoded by 372 bp	A pseudogene has been localized to chromosome 5 or 6.[591]
NDUFA5	NADH dehydrogenase (ubiquinone) 13K chain	U53468	7q32[604]	cDNA[604,605]	*	Polypeptide = 116*aa, encoded by 348 bp	A pseudogene has been localized to 11p15.5.[604] *One aa is removed post translationally.[606]
C. Flavoprotein Proteins							
NDUFV1	NADH dehydrogenase (ubiquinone) 51K chain	AF053069, AF053070	11q13.1–13.3[44]	gDNA[45,607]	+(20 aa)	Gene has 10 exons, polypeptide = 464 aa, encoded by 1392 bp	The 3′ UTR of NDUFV 1 mRNA is homologous to 5′ UTR for IP-30.[607] Mutations include Leigh syndrome, leukodystrophy and/or myoclonic epilepsy (NDUFV1, THR423MET; NDUFV1, 175T-C; NDUFV1, ALA341VAL)[608]
NDUFV2	NADH dehydrogenase (ubiquinone) 24K chain	M22538	18p11.2-p11.31[48,49]	gDNA[48,49], cDNA[46,47]	+(32 aa)	Gene has 8 exons, polypeptide = 249 aa, encoded by 747 bp	This protein contains the binuclear iron-sulfur cluster. A pseudogene has been localized to 19q13.3-qter.[49]
NDUFV3	NADH dehydrogenase (ubiquinone) 10K chain	X99728, X99727, X99726, X59048	21q22.3[609]	gDNA, cDNA[609]	+34 aa	Gene has 3 exons, polypeptide = 74 aa, encoded by 324 bp	

Table 105-2 Complex II: Proteins, cDNAs, and Genes

Gene	Description	Accession	Chr. location	Sequence	Leader	Characterization	Comments
SDH1	Succinate dehydrogenase (ubiquinone) 27K iron-sulfur protein	U17248	1p35-36.1[76]	gDNA[75], cDNA[74]	+	Gene has 8 exons, polypeptide = 280 aa, encoded by 840 bp	
SDH2	Succinate dehydrogenase (ubiquinone) 70K flavoprotein	L21936, X53943	5p15[77]	cDNA[77,78]	+(43 aa)	Polypeptide = 664 aa, encoded by 1992 bp	Mutations include Leigh syndrome R554W mutation (see Table 105-14).
SDHC	Succinate dehydrogenase (ubiquinone) cytochrome b large subunit	D49737	1q21[80]	cDNA[80]		Polypeptide = 140 aa, encoded by 420 bp	
SDHD	Succinate dehydrogenase (ubiquinone) cytochrome b small subunit	AB006202	11q23[80]	cDNA[80]		Polypeptide = 103 aa, encoded by 309 bp	

(MPP^+). Exposure to MPTP in both humans and other mammals results in the selective destruction of basal ganglia neurons and induction of parkinsonism.[12,67]

It has been proposed that complex I inhibitors interrupt the CoQ_{10} reduction cycle of complex I at the three CoQ_{10} binding sites, A, B, and C (Fig. 105-9*B*). Site B antagonists include MPP^+, rotenone, piericidin B, and Amytal. Site A antagonists include piericidin A and idebenone; and site C antagonists include quinol products like meperidine (Demerol).[67] Hence, inhibitors of complex I are both vital to biomedical science and also to characterizing biochemical defects in disease patients.

Complex II. Complex II oxidizes succinate to fumarate and transfers the electrons to CoQ_{10}. The enzyme is composed of four subunits: a 70-kDa flavoprotein (FP), a 27-kDa iron-sulfur protein (ISP), a 15-kDa membrane polypeptide, and a 5- to 7-kDa membrane polypeptide (Table 105-2).

All four complex II subunits are nuclear encoded. Their chromosomal locations are given in Table 105-2. The 70-kDa flavoprotein contains the succinate binding site and a covalently bound FAD moiety; the 27-kDa iron-sulfur protein contains three iron-sulfur clusters (center 1 $[2Fe\text{-}2S]^{2+,1+}$, center 2 $[4Fe\text{-}4S]^{2+,1+}$, and center 3 $[3Fe\text{-}4S]^{1+,0}$), which transport electrons to CoQ_{10}. CoQ_{10} is presumably bound to the two membrane-intrinsic subunits CII-3 and CII-4. A b_{560} -type heme is also associated with to CII-3 and CII-4, but its function is unclear.[68–72] However, the *C. elegans mev*-1 mutant is the result of a mutation in the CII-3 subunit which increases ROS and decreases life span, suggesting that the cytochrome b_{560} may function to stabilize or dismutate ubisemiquinone (CoQ_{10} H·).[73]

The cDNA[74] and genomic clones[75] for the iron-sulfur protein have been reported. The iron-sulfur protein gene has eight exons[75] and is located on chromosome 1p35-36.1.[76] The cDNA for the flavoprotein has also been cloned,[77,78] and the gene found to be duplicated in the genome on chromosomes 3q29 and 5p15, with the chromosome 5 gene being expressed.[79] The bovine CII-3 cDNA has been isolated and characterized,[69] and the succinate dehydrogenase (ubiquinone) cytochrome b large and small subunits have been cloned and mapped to chromosome 1q 21 and 11q23, respectively.[80]

Complex III. Complex III is composed of 11 polypeptides, 1 (cytochrome b, MTCYB) encoded by the mtDNA (Figs. 105-2 and 105-5).[81,82] The proteins, cDNAs, and gene structure and chromosome locations of six of the subunits is given in Table 105-3.

The crystal structure of complex III has been determined (Fig. 105-6). This revealed that it functions as a dimer with a monomer mass of 240 kDa.[83,84] This enzyme oxidizes ubiquinol (CoQ_{10} H_2), reduces ferricytochrome c to ferrocytochrome c, and uses the energy released to pump protons across the mitochondrial inner membrane via the Q cycle (Fig. 105-5). The polypeptides of complex III include two core proteins (subunit I on chromosome 3q21.3 and subunit II on chromosome 16q 12.3), MTCYB (subunit III), cytochrome c1 (subunit IV on chromosome 8q 24.3), the "Rieske" iron-sulfur protein (ISP) (subunit V on chromosome 19q12), and seven smaller polypeptides, subunits 6 to 11.

The complex can be roughly subdivided into three major domains, parallel to the plane of the membrane. The intermembrane space domain includes cytochrome c1, the Rieske ISP, and subunit 8. The intermembrane domain includes cytochrome b and subunits 7, 10, and 11. The matrix side domain includes the two core proteins 1 and 2, and subunits 6 and 9. Cytochrome b, cytochrome c1, and the Rieske ISP provide the major redox centers of the enzyme[83].

The Rieske ISP and cytochrome c1, on the intermembrane side of the enzyme, both contain one membrane-spanning domain. Cytochrome c1 is primarily an α-helix protein composed of seven helices, one of which enters the membrane. The heme is covalently bound to Cys[37] and Cys[40] and its ligands are His[41] and Met[160].[81,85,86] Subunit 8, or the "acidic/hinge protein," lies above cytochrome c1 and the two form the docking site for cytochrome c, possibly involving the 14 NH_2-terminal amino acids of subunit 8, together with helix $\alpha 1^1$ and loop $\alpha 3$-$\beta 1$ of cytochrome b. The Rieske ISP encompasses a single 2Fe-2S iron-sulfur center and changes conformation, switching from intermediate (int), to b, to c1 forms. In this process, its relationship to the adjacent cytochromes c1 and b changes, facilitating directional electron flow. In the c1 state, the iron-sulfur center is adjacent to the heme of cytochrome c1; in the int state, the iron-sulfur center is displaced from both cytochromes c1 and b; and in the b state, it interacts with cytochrome b.

The central core of the transmembrane domain is composed of cytochrome b. Cytochrome b has eight transmembrane α helices (αA through αH) and four horizontal helices on the intermembrane side (αab, αcd1, αcd2, and αef). The high-potential heme b_L (b_{566}) and the low-potential heme b_H (b_{560}) are in the center of a four α-helix bundle formed by αA, αB, αC, and αD. Heme b_L is close to the intermembrane side, while heme b_H is on the matrix side. The inhibitor myxothiazol binds in the ubiquinol binding site (Qp) close to heme b_L, while the inhibitor antimycin A binds to the ubiquinone binding site (Qn) close to heme b_H on the matrix side of cytochrome b.[83,85,87–89]

Subunits 10 and 11 of the transmembrane region each have a single transmembrane helix with the NH_3 end on the matrix side. They interact with cytochrome b in the membrane and cytochrome c1 and the iron-sulfur protein on the intermembrane side.

The core of the matrix side of the enzyme is composed of the core 1 and core 2 proteins, together with subunits 6 and 9. Subunit 6 lies at the interface between cytochrome b and core 1, with core

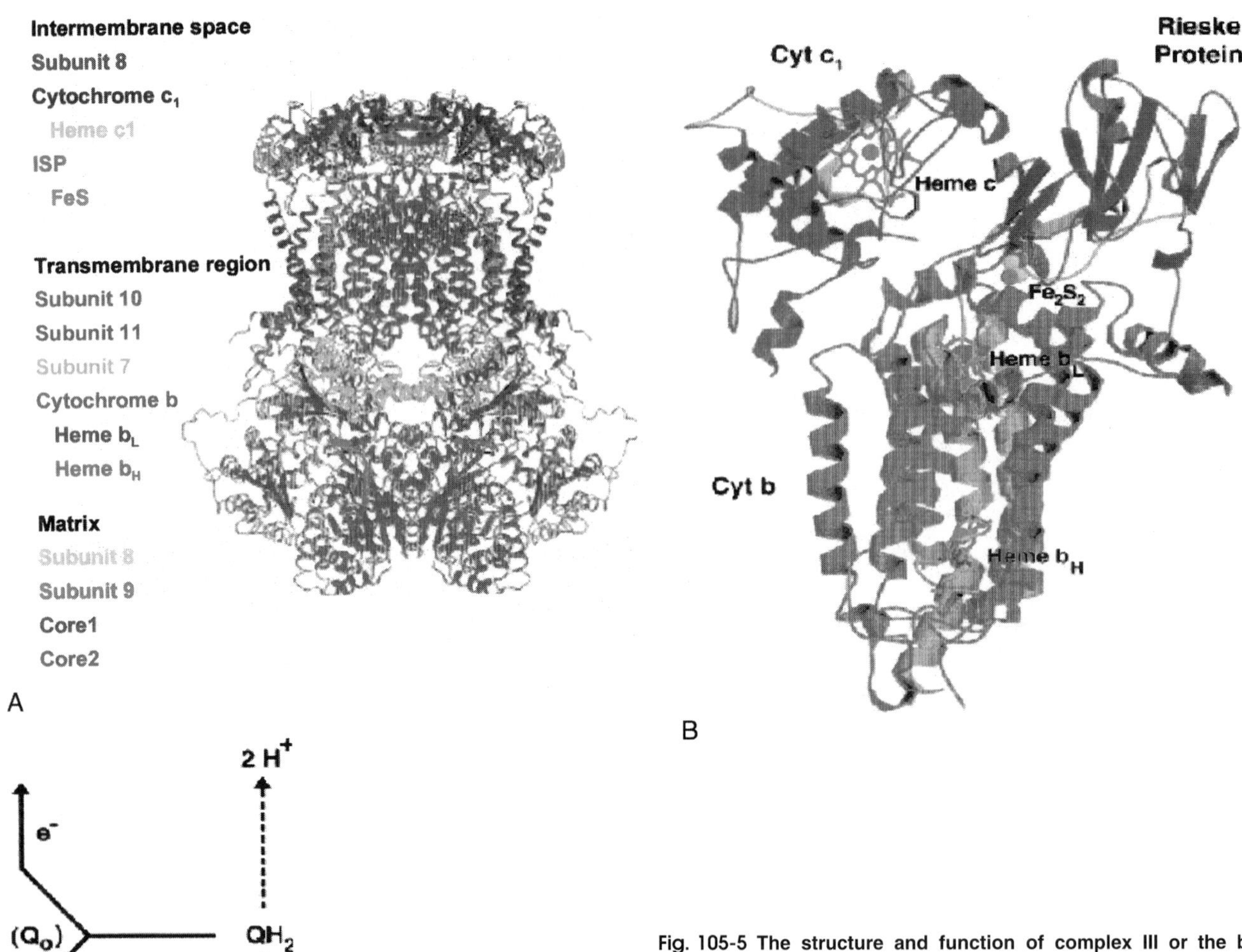

Fig. 105-5 The structure and function of complex III or the bc1 complex. ***Panel A:*** **The structure of the dimeric enzyme showing the relative positions of all 11 subunits. The cytochrome c1 and Rieske ISP are located on the cytoplasmic side of the membrane, while cytochrome b lies below them and within the membrane. The two core proteins 1 and 2 are located at the matrix end of the protein. (*Panel A is reprinted from Iwata et al.*[83] *Used with permission.*)** ***Panel B:*** **The relative positions of the catalytic bc1 complex subunits [cytochrome b, Rieske ISP, and cytochrome c1] showing the location of their prosthetic groups. The Rieske ISP changes conformation permitting its Fe-S cluster to interact alternatively with the heme b_L and heme c of cytochromes b and c1, respectively.** ***Panel C:*** **The electron transfer and proton pumping associated with the Q cycle of the bc1 complex. (*Panels B and C reprinted from Saraste.*[84] *Used with permission.*)**

2 binding beneath core 1. Surprisingly, subunit 9 is derived from the NH_2-terminal 78 amino acids of the nascent Rieske ISP, and this is cleaved from the intact protein precursor by metalloprotease activity built into the core 1 and 2 proteins. Core 1 shows sequence homology to the mitochondrial processing protease β-MPP and core 2 to α-MPP. Core 2 has an inverse zinc-binding motif (HXXEH), suggesting that it might bind Zn and be the actual protease.

Proton translocation of complex III is linked to electron transport through the intermediates of CoQ_{10} oxidation-reduction in the proton-motive Q cycle.[42,85,90,91] Complex III has two CoQ_{10} binding sites, one on the cytoplasmic side (Q_o or Q_p site) and one on the matrix side (Q_i or Q_N site) of the inner membrane. $CoQ_{10}H_2$ binds to the Q_o site and transfers one electron to the Rieske ISP, which passes it on to cytochrome c1. The resulting ubisemiquinone donates the other electron to the adjacent b_L heme located on the cytoplasmic side of the membrane. The transfer of the two electrons from $CoQ_{10}H_2$ releases the two ubiquinol protons to the outside of the mitochondrial membrane. The electron at the b_L heme is then transported to the more matrix b_H heme where it is transferred to CoQ_{10} at the Q_i site to generate ubisemiquinone. A second molecule of $CoQ_{10}H_2$ is oxidized as above, and the resulting b_H electron is donated to the ubisemiquinone at the Q_i site. This reduced quinone then combines with two protons from the matrix to generate ubiquinone, $CoQ_{10}H_2$. Hence two protons are transported through the membrane for each pair of electrons that exits complex III (Fig. 105-5).[92]

The Q cycle is driven by the conformational changes of the Rieske ISP. When complex III is oxidized, the Rieske ISP is in the int state. When $CoQ_{10}H_2$ binds to the Q_o site in cytochrome b at helices αC and acdl plus the ef loop, the $CoQ_{10}H_2$ is deproteinated to $CoQ_{10}H\cdot$, which overcomes the activation barrier. This pulls the ISP to the b position. An electron is transferred to the Rieske ISP while it is adjacent to the $CoQ_{10}H\cdot$ (ubisemiquinone) in the b conformation. The second electron from $CoQ_{10}H\cdot$ is then transferred to heme b_L, weakening the interaction between the quinone and the Rieske ISP, permitting the ISP to move to the c1 state. Here it transfers the electron to cytochrome c1, and the ISP moves to the int state. The cytochrome c1 electron moves on to cytochrome c and the heme b_L electron moves on to the heme b_H site.[83]

Table 105-3 Complex III: Proteins, cDNAs, and Genes

Gene	Description	Accession #	Chr. location	Sequence	Leader	Characterization	Comments
CYC1	Ubiquinol—cytochrome c reductase subunit IV: cytochrome cl	X06994, J04444	8q24.3[610]	cDNA[95] gDNA[94]	+(84 aa)	Gene has 7 exons, polypeptide = 325 aa, encoded by 975 bp	
MTCYB	Ubiquinol—cytochrome c reductase subunit III: cytochrome b	V00662	mtDNA[25]	mDNA[25]	N/A	Polypeptide = 380 aa, encoded by 1140 bp, nucleotide position 14747-15887	Mutations include: Leber optic atrophy (MTCYTB*LHON15257, MTCYB*LHON15812).
UQCRB	Ubiquinone-binding protein QP-C	X13585, M35761, M26706, M26707		cDNA[611], gDNA[612]	–	Gene has 4 exons, polypeptide = 111 aa, encoded by 333 bp	Two pseudogenes have been identified for this gene.[612]
UQCRC1	Ubiquinol—cytochrome c reductase subunit I: core I protein	L16842	3p21.3–3p21.3[613]	cDNA, gDNA[613]	+(34 aa)	Gene has 13 exons, polypeptide = 480 aa, encoded by 1440 bp	
UQCRC2	Ubiquinol—cytochrome c reductase subunit II: core protein II	J04973	16p12.3-16p12.3[614]	cDNA[615]	+(14 aa)	Polypeptide = 453 aa, encoded by 1359 bp	11 potential pseudogenes have been identified for this gene.[615]
UQCRFS1	Ubiquinol—cytochrome c reductase subunit V: iron-sulfur subunit	L32977	19q12[616,93]	cDNA[617]	+(78 aa)	Polypeptide = 274 aa, encoded by 822 bp	This protein is the Rieske Fe-S redox-active subunit.[618] A potential pseudogene has been localized to 22q13.[93,616]
UQCRH	Ubiquinol—cytochrome c reductase 11K hinge protein	Y00764		cDNA[619]	+(13 aa)	Polypeptide = 91 aa encoded by 273 bp	

The proteins, cDNAs, gene structures, and chromosome locations for complex III are described in Table 105-3. The Rieske ISP is located on chromosome 19p12[93] and the cytochrome c1 gene is located on chromosome 8q24. It contains seven exons with exon III encompassing the heme binding sites and exons IV and V the cytochrome c interaction site.[94–96]

Cytochrome c. Cytochrome c ferries electrons along the outside of the inner mitochondrial membrane from complex III to complex IV (Fig. 105-2). It contains a single covalently bound heme and is encoded by two isoform genes, a systemic cytochrome c and a testis cytochrome c.[97,98] The systemic cytochrome c is located on chromosome 8q24.3 and encompasses 2 exons.[99,100]

Complex IV. Complex IV is composed of 13 polypeptides, three (COI, COII, and COIII) encoded by the mtDNA. The remaining nuclear polypeptides have been designated IV, Va, Vb, VIa, VIb, VIc, VIIa, VIIb, VIIc, and VIII (Fig. 105-6).[101] The proteins, cDNAs, gene structures, and chromosomal locations of the complex IV genes are given in Table 105-4.

The crystal structure of complex IV has been determined (Fig. 105-7).[84,102] It is a functional dimer with a minimal monomer molecular weight of 204 kDa. Complex IV collects electrons from reduced cytochrome c (ferrocytochrome c), transfers them to CuA, then to cytochrome a, then to the bimetallic cytochrome a3/CuB active site, and then to oxygen to give water, concurrently pumping 4 protons across the mitochondrial inner membrane (Fig. 105-2 and 105-6).

Comparisons of the data from the crystal structure of beef heart complex IV[102] and the molecular genetic studies of *Rhodobacter sphaeroides* cytochrome c oxidase (cytochrome aa_3) and *Escherichia coli* ubiquinol oxidase (cytochrome b_O) have provided important insights into the structure and function of cytochrome c oxidase.[103] Such comparisons have been possible because of the high homology between the mammalian and bacterial enzymes. *R. sphaeroides* subunit I is 62.1 kDa and 52 percent identical and 76 percent similar to beef-heart COI; subunit II is 32.9 kDa and 39 percent identical and 63 percent similar to bovine COII; and subunit III is 30.1 kDa and 49 percent identical and 71 percent similar to bovine COIII. The spectra and extinction coefficients are similar between the two enzymes.[92,104,105]

Complex IV encompasses two hemes a ($a + a_3$), three coppers (two for CuA and one for CuB), one magnesium, and one zinc. The two coppers forming the binuclear center CuA are associated with mtDNA subunit II (COII), while the two hemes and CuB (heme a and heme a_3 − CuB) form a trinuclear center associated with mtDNA subunit I (COI). Electron flow is from cytochrome c to CuA, then to heme a, and then to the heme a_3 − CuB binuclear center where oxygen is reduced to water.[102,103,106] Molecular oxygen (O_2) binds to the a_3 − CuB binuclear center and electron transfer to O_2 is probably linked to proton transport. Complex IV uses four electrons to reduce O_2 and four protons from the matrix

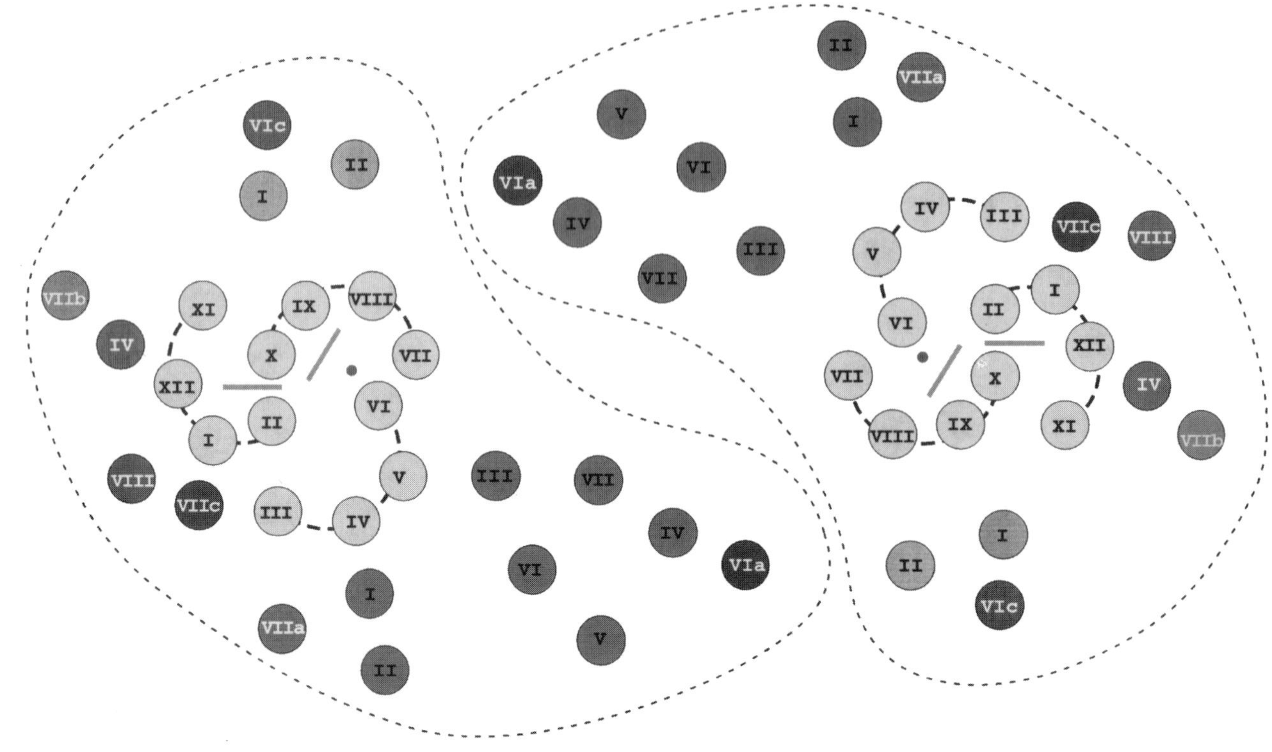

A

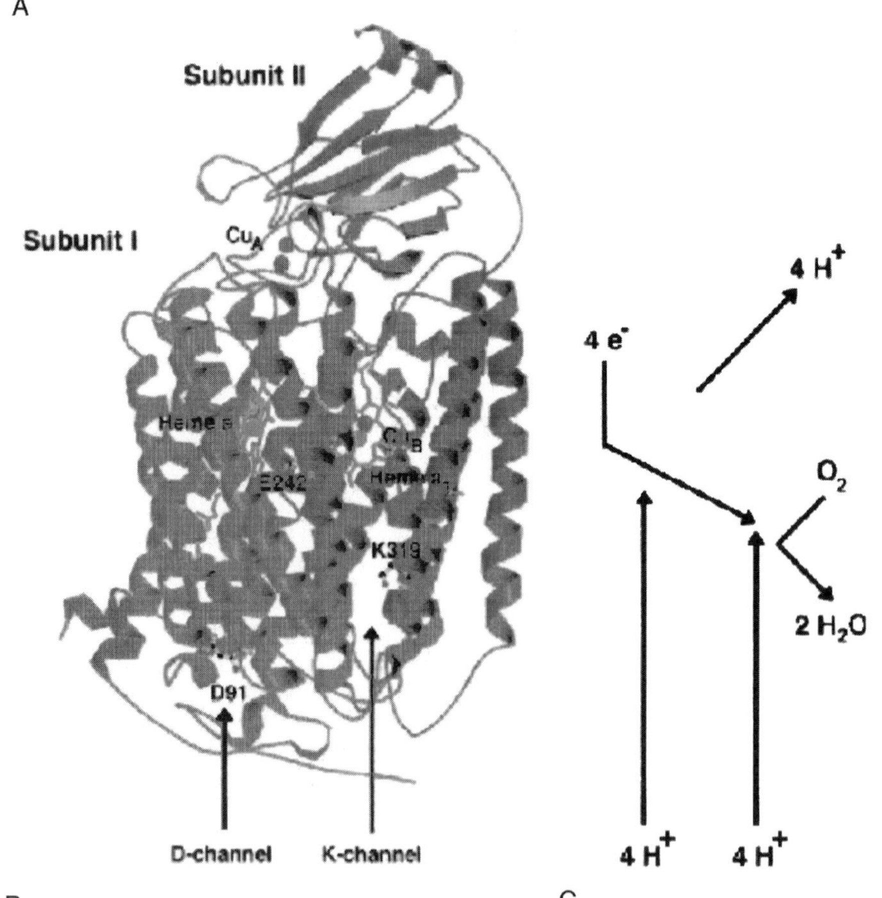

B C

Fig. 105-6 The structure and function of complex IV (cytochrome c oxidase). ***Panel A:*** **This diagram shows the relative location of the transmembrane α-helixes that are derived from the mtDNA- and nDNA-encoded subunits, as they are arranged in the functional dimer. This is the arrangement that would be seen from the top of the membrane on the cytoplasmic side. The 12 α-helixes of the mtDNA COI subunit and their associated hemes a and a_3 and CuB form spiral arrays at the center of each monomer. The two mtDNA COII α-helixes lie on one side of COI, adjacent to helixes IX and VIII, while the seven helixes of mtDNA COIII lie on the other side of COI, adjacent to helixes III, IV, and V. The individual membrane-spanning α-helixes of nuclear subunits IV, VIa, VIc, VIIa, VIIb, VIIc, and VIII surround the central mtDNA encoded subunits. (*Panel A is reproduced from Tsukihara et al.*[102] *Used with permission.*)** ***Panel B:*** **This shows the relative locations of the catalytic sites of the mtDNA-encoded subunits COI and COII, as viewed from the plane of the membrane. The cytochrome c binding site is located in subunit II, adjacent to the CuA site. Electrons flow from CuA to heme a, then to heme a_3 + CuB, where they react with O_2. Protons move into the complex along the D and K channels.** ***Panel C:*** **The movement of electrons, protons and oxygen during COX catalysis. (*Panels B and C reprinted from Saraste.*[84] *Used with permission.*)**

to generate two H_2O. Four additional protons are transferred from the matrix, across the mitochondrial membrane, possibly in the proximity of heme a_3[107] (Fig. 105-6).

The three mtDNA-encoded subunits form the core of the monomer, with the nuclear-encoded subunits surrounding it. COI has 12 membrane-spanning domains (I to XII). These form three sets of four transmembrane helices forming a "spiral galaxy"-like array of three comma-shaped spokes radiating out from the center (Fig. 105-6*A*). One comma-shaped spoke includes helices II-I-XII-X, listed from inside out; the second, helices

Table 105-4 Complex IV: Proteins, cDNAs, and Genes

Gene	Description	Accession #	Chr. location	Sequence	Leader	Characterization	Comments
MTCOI	Cytochrome c oxidase subunit I	V006622, J01415	mtDNA[25]	mDNA[25]	N/A	Polypeptide = 513 aa, encoded by 1539 bp, nucleotide position 5904 to 7444	This protein contains the CuB and hemes a and a_3 that form redox centers for electron transfer. Mutations include: Leber optic atrophy (MTCO1*LHON7444A), acquired idiopathic sideroblastic anemia (MTCO1*AISA6742C, MTCO1*AISA6721C), and mitochondrial syndromic encephalopathy with COX deficiency (MTCO1*COX6480A).
MTCOII	Cytochrome c oxidase subunit II	V00662, X15759	mtDNA[25]	mDNA[25]	N/A	Polypeptide = 227 aa, encoded by 681 bp, nucleotide position 7586 to 8294	This protein contains the CuA. Mutations include: COX II deficiency (MTCO2, 7587T-C).
MTCOIII	Cytochrome c oxidase subunit III	V00662, J01415	mtDNA[25]	mDNA[25]	N/A	Polypeptide = 261 aa, encoded by 783 bp, nucleotide position 9207 to 9990	Mutations include: Leber optic atrophy (MTCO3*LHON9438A, MTCO3*LHON9804A), COX deficiency with recurrent myoglobinuria (MTCO3, 15-bp deletion), and COX deficiency (MTCO3, 9952G-A).
COX4	Cytochrome c oxidase chain IV	X54802	16q22-qter[128,127]	cDNA[115]	+(22 aa)	Polypeptide = 169 aa, encoded by 507 bp	A pseudogene has been mapped to 14q21-qter.[127,128]
COX5A	Cytochrome c oxidase chain Va	M22760	15q25[129]	cDNA[116]	+(41 aa)	Polypeptide = 150 aa, encoded by 450 bp	
COX5B	Cytochrome c oxidase chain Vb	M19961, M59250	2cen-2q13[125]	cDNA, gDNA[117]	+(31 aa)	Gene has 5 exons, polypeptide = 129 aa, encoded by 387 bp	7 pseudogenes have been mapped to 4cen-q31, 6, 7, 11q, 12, 13, 22.[125]
COX6A1	Cytochrome c oxidase chain VIa, hepatic	X15341	6p21[620]	cDNA[118]	–	Polypeptide = 86 aa, encoded by 258 bp	
COX6A2	Cytochrome c oxidase chain VIa, cardiac and skeletal muscle	M83308	16p[130]	cDNA[621]	+ (11aa)	Polypeptide = 96 aa, encoded by 288 bp	
COX6B	Cytochrome c oxidase chain VIb	X13923	19q13.1[131]	cDNA[119,622]	*	Polypeptide = 86 aa*, encoded by 258 bp	*This protein potentially undergoes N-terminal posttranslational methionine removal and alanine acetylation.[622] Multiple potential pseudogenes have been identified.[623]
COX6C	Cytochrome c oxidase chain VIc	X13238	8q22-q23[129]	cDNA[120]		Polypeptide = 75 aa, encoded by 225 bp	

(Continued to next page)

Table 105-4 (Continued)

Gene	Description	Accession #	Chr. location	Sequence	Leader	Characterization	Comments
COX7A1	Cytochrome c oxidase chain VIIa, cardiac and skeletal muscle	M83186	19q13.1–19q13.1[121]	cDNA[121]	+(21 aa)	Polypeptide = 79 aa, encoded by 237 bp	
COX7A2	Cytochrome c oxidase chain VIIa, liver	X15822	4q31–35[121]	cDNA[624]	+(23 aa)	Polypeptide = 83 aa, encoded by 249 bp	
COX7B	Cytochrome c oxidase chain VIIb	Z14244	14q21-qter	cDNA[122]	+(24 aa)	Polypeptide = 80 aa, encoded by 240 bp	This gene has potential pseudogenes.[122]
COX7C	Cytochrome c oxidase chain VIIc	X16560	5q14[129]	cDNA[123]	+(16 aa)	Polypeptide = 63 aa, encoded by 189 bp	
COX8	Cytochrome c oxidase chain VIII	J04823	11q12-q13[124]	cDNA[124]	+(25 aa)	Polypeptide = 69 aa, encoded by 207 bp	

X-IX-VIII-VII; and the third, helices VI-V-IV-III. COII has two transmembrane domains that lie adjacent to COI helices IX and VIII. COIII has seven transmembrane domains that lie on the opposite site of COI from COII. Finally, 7 of the 10 nDNA subunits (IV, VIa, VIc, VIIb, VIIc, and VIII) have one membrane-spanning domain that surrounds the core COI, COII, and COIII subunits in the membrane. The remaining three nDNA subunits, Va, Vb, and VIb, do not have transmembrane domains. Subunits Va and Vb lie on the matrix side and subunit VIb on the cytosolic side of complex IV.

Subunits II, VIa, and VIb appear to form the 25-Å diameter cytochrome c binding site composed of acidic residues that interact with the basic residues of cytochrome c.[102] The CuA coppers are separated by 2.7 Å, suggesting a Cu–Cu bond, and are associated with two cysteine residues (Cys^{196} and Cys^{200}) of subunit II. The CuA center lies near the outside of the membrane, at the interface of COII and COI. The heme a and heme a_3 – CuB centers are located 13 Å into the membrane. Heme a is bound to two histidines located on the adjacent transmembrane helices II (His^{61}) and X (His^{378}). Heme a_3 is also ligated to a histidine in helix X (His^{376}), putting the two hemes close together, perpendicular to the membrane, and at a 104° angle relative to each other, possibly permitting rapid electron transfer along the heme edges. The CuB is coordinated by three histidines, His^{240} in helix VI, and His^{290} and His^{291} in the nonhelical region between helixes VII and VIII. The heme a_3 – CuB distance is 4.5 Å. The Mg atom is located close to the trinuclear center, at the interface between COII and COI and ligated to both, directly between CuA and heme a_3. The Zn is associated with the nuclear encoded subunit Vb on the matrix side of the enzyme bound to cysteine residues.[92,103,106,108]

Molecular genetic studies on *R. sphaeroides* cytochrome aa_3 and *Escherichia coli* cytochrome b_0 have provided support for the highly conserved functional groups of human and bovine COI.[25,92,108,109] The *R. sphaeroides* cytochrome aa_3 COI subunit has been found to interact with the complex IV prosthetic groups at evolutionarily conserved amino acids. The heme a is located between helix II and X, bound to invariant histidines at amino acid 102 (human and bovine COI His^{61}) of helix II and at 421 (human and bovine His^{378}) of helix X. Hemes a and a_3 are on opposite sides of helix X, with heme a_3 bound to the invariant histidine 419 (human and bovine COI His^{376}). CuB and heme a_3 make up a binuclear center and are adjacent to each other, with CuB ligated to helix VI at histidine 284 (human and bovine His^{240}) and helix VII at histidines 333 and 334 (human and bovine His^{290} and His^{291}).[110]

Complex IV has two hydrophobic proton-conducting channels, D (Asp^{91}) and K (Lys^{319}), named after conserved amino acids that form the matrix sides of the channels (Fig. 105-6). Channel D is delineated by Asp^{91}, Asn^{80}, Asn^{98}, Ser^{156}, Ser^{157}, and ends at the conserved Glu^{242} in the middle of the membrane. Glu^{242} resides in a hydrophobic cavity extending towards the binuclear heme-copper center and is required for proton translocation. The K channel encompasses Ser^{255}, Lys^{319}, Thr^{316}, and Tyr^{244}, and ends at the binuclear center. Protons for both water formation and proton pumping move through these channels, presumably along a chain of water molecules.

Proton pumping involves reduction of both metals (a3 and CμB) at the active site with two electrons and two protons taken up. Oxygen then reacts, initially forming an oxygen intermediate. An additional electron is acquired, creating the peroxy state. Then three protons are acquired, generating the ferryl intermediate and creating an H_2O and translocating two protons. A fourth electron is then accepted, resulting in a second water and transport of two additional protons. The overall reaction involves oxidation of four e^-, generation of two H_2O, and translocation of four H^+.[84,111]

While COIII is a universal component of all cytochrome c oxidase enzymes, its function is unclear. It does bind dicyclohexylcarbodiimide (DCCD).[112]

The functions of the 10 nuclear-encoded subunits are still unclear. Two of the human subunits (VIa and VIIa) have two isoenzymes, one systemic and the other heart- and muscle-specific,[108,113] which can be regulated at both the transcriptional and posttranscriptional levels.[114] Complementary cDNAs have been cloned for all of the human COX genes including IV systemic/liver;[115] Va muscle;[116] Vb muscle;[117] VIa liver;[118] VIb muscle;[119] VIc fibroblast;[120] VIIa liver;[121] VIIa muscle;[121] VIIb heart;[122] VIIc muscle;[123] and VIII liver/heart.[124] Genomic clones have been isolated for subunit Vb[125] and VIb.[126] Chromosomal locations have been determined for subunit IV at 16q22-ter;[127,128] subunit Va at 15q25;[129] subunit Vb at 2cen-q13;[125] subunit VIa muscle at 16p;[130] subunit VIb at 19q13.1;[131] subunit VIIa muscle at 19q13.1; subunit VIIa liver on 4q31-35 and 14q21-qter;[121] and subunit VIII at 11q12-13.[124]

A number of adenosine nucleotide binding sites have been identified in complex IV, at least some of which can alter the kinetics of the enzyme. Equilibrium dialysis has revealed seven high-affinity binding sites for ATP in bovine heart mitochondrial

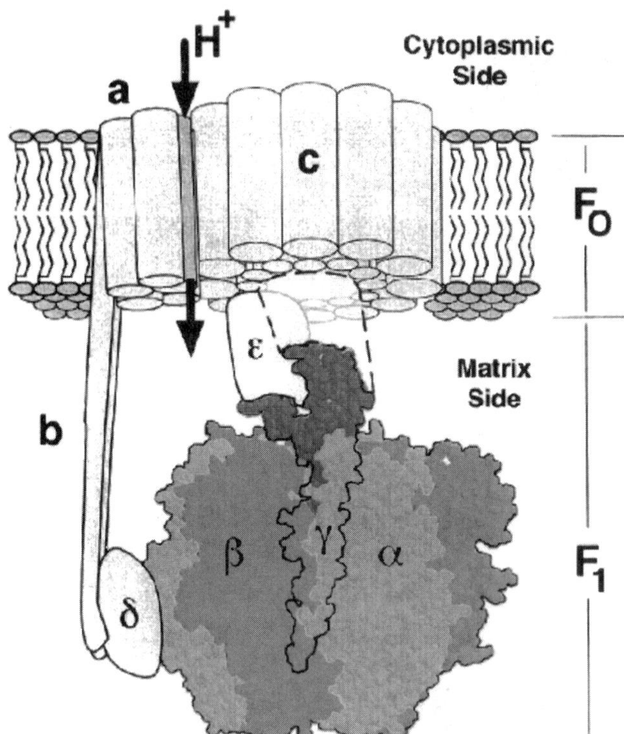

Fig. 105-7 The structure and function of complex V (H^+-translocating ATP synthase). The structure of the α, β and γ subunit interaction in F_1, is derived from the crystal structure.[141] The model for the remaining subunits, using *E. coli* nomenclature, is from the proposals of Wang and Oster[142] and Elster, Wang, and Oster.[144] The two-stalk structure of the model is supported by the electron microscopic data by Ogilvie et al.[143] The complex is proposed to function in two parts, a "stator" and a "rotor." The stator is anchored in the membrane by subunit a, the mtDNA-encoded subunit ATP6. From subunit a, subunit b extends into the matrix. At the opposite end of b from the membrane is bound the δ subunit. Subunit δ is disulfide bonded to one of the α subunits of the hexagonal barrel of 3α and 3β subunits, thus anchoring the barrel "statically" to membrane subunit a (ATP6). The rotor is a wheel of presumably 12 (10 to 12) spokes composed of the two α helices of subunit c. The wheel rotates in the plane of the membrane with the axle perpendicular to the membrane and pointing out into the matrix. The outer edge of the wheel is composed of subunit c (ATP9) helix 2 faces, which rotate past the subunit a helical 4 face. Between the faces of subunit a and c is the proton channel. The axle of the rotor is composed of the ε and γ subunits. The γ subunit projects into the lumen of the 3α:3β barrel, and is asymmetrically shaped. As the rotor spins, driven by the flux of protons through the subunit a/subunit c channel, the comma-shaped γ subunit interacts sequentially with each of the three β subunits, causing them to change conformation. Three different conformational states occur. These states are sequentially the O (open) or E (empty) state in which the β subunit is in the β_E conformation and does not bind adenine nucleotides; the L (loose) state in which the β subunit is in the β_{DP} conformation and binds ADP + Pi; and the T (tight) state in which the β subunit is in the β_{TP} conformation that condenses the ADP + Pi to ATP. The β subunit then cycles back to the β_E state and releases the ATP. The γ subunit interacts with the β subunit using two different "catches" that drive the conformational changes. The ATP synthase functions at nearly 100 percent efficiency. Using 4 H^+ to make 1 ATP or 12 H^+ per turn of the wheel to make three ATPs, one for each β subunit. (*Reproduced from Wang and Oster.*[142] *Used with permission.*)

complex IV and six in bovine liver complex IV. In addition, three lower-affinity binding sites have been detected for ADP. A variety of studies have localized five nucleotide binding sites: one between subunits I and III on the cytosolic side of the enzyme, two in subunit IV, one each on the cytosolic and matrix ends of the molecule, and two in subunit IVa, again cytosolic and matrix.[132] Two of these sites have been localized from cholate binding within the crystal structure. Cholate is used in complex IV isolation and mimics the structure of adenine nucleotides. One cholate binding site was found on the cytosolic side between subunit I, helix III, Tyr^{304} and subunit III, helix III, His^{103} and Trp^{99}. The other binding site was on the matrix end of the subunit VIa interacting with Arg^{14} and Arg^{17}.[102] Cytosolic nucleotide binding sites for subunit VIa have been identified in bovine heart complex IV by inhibition of nucleotide binding by monoclonal antibody reaction[133] and in yeast complex IV by subunit mutagenesis.[134] Matrix nucleotide binding sites for subunit VIa have been identified in bovine heart, but not bovine liver complex IV.[133] Cytosolic and matrix interactions of nucleotides to subunit IV have also been detected using monoclonal antibodies. Nucleotide binding to the matrix side of subunit VIa changes the H^+/e^- stoichiometry, while nucleotide binding to the cytosolic domain of subunit IV affects the affinity of cytochrome c.[132,133,135–137]

Complex IV is sensitive to a variety of common toxic chemicals. These include cyanide and azide, which form a bridge between cytochrome a_3 and CuB, and thiocyanate and formate, which bind other locations in the binuclear center.[138]

The complex structure of the respiratory complexes suggests that the assembly of active complexes requires the action of additional gene products. This has been shown to be the case for complex IV, where an additional protein, SURF-1, is required for generating normal human complex IV (COX) activity. Mutations in the SURF-1 gene have been found to be the primary cause of COX-deficient Leigh syndrome.[139,140] The SURF-1 gene is located at chromosome 9q34. It consists of nine exons spanning 5 kb of genomic sequence. It is embedded in a cluster of six housekeeping genes (SURF-1 to -6) spanning approximately 36 kb of sequence, with SURF-1 and SURF-2 sharing a bidirectional promoter, transcribed in opposite directions. SURF-1 is 25.6 percent homologous to the yeast gene SHY-1, with SURF-1 being 300 amino acids and SHY-1 being 389 amino acids. Both proteins have a mitochondrial-targeting peptide, two membrane-spanning domains, and are targeted to the mitochondria, presumably residing in the mitochondrial inner membrane. While the human SURF-1 mutation gives a specific COX defect, the yeast SHY-1 mutation is more pleiotropic. Hence, it has been suggested that SURF-1 may function in the assembly or maintenance of an active holoenzyme COX complex.[139,140]

Complex V. Complex V encompasses 16 polypeptides, including 2 (ATPase6 and ATPase8) that are encoded by the mtDNA (Fig. 105-3).[34] The available information on the proteins, cDNAs, and genes of the complex V is provided in Table 105-5. This H^+-translocating ATP synthase utilizes the electrochemical gradient ($\Delta\rho = \Delta\psi + \Delta\mu^{pH}$) generated by complexes I, III, and IV to catalyze the condensation of ATP and Pi to make ATP. This enzyme uses a rotary catalytic mechanism which is close to 100 percent efficient.

The F_0 component of the enzyme is based in the mitochondrial inner membrane, with the enzyme projecting into the matrix in a lollipop involving a 45-Å long stalk, and a 90- to 100-Å diameter barrel (F_1) (Fig. 105-7). The approximate subunit composition of these three domains for the mitochondrial (bovine) and bacterial (*E. coli*) enzymes is given in Table 105-6. The F_1, as isolated, is composed of five subunits α, β, γ, δ, and ε, with amino acid lengths in cow of 510, 482, 272, 146, and 50 amino acids, respectively. The ratio of these subunits in the F_1 particle is 3:3:1:1:1, with a total mass of about 370 kDa.[42] The α and β subunits are highly homologous, 20 percent identical, and form a hexagonal array of alternating α and β subunits. While both α and β subunits bind nucleotides, only the β subunits are catalytic. The crystal structure for the F_1 has been solved, and resolved the α, β, and γ subunits. The α and β subunits form a hollow barrel into which the γ subunit projects up from the stalk to form an axle.[141]

Based on the concept of rotary catalysis, complex V has been divided into two functional components: a "rotor" and a "stator" (Fig. 105-7).[142–144] The rotor consists of a hydrophobic wheel of

Table 105-5 **Complex V: Proteins, cDNAs, and Genes**

Gene	Description	Accession #	Chr. location	Sequence	Leader	Characterization	Comments
ATP5A1	H^+-transporting ATP synthase, F_1 complex, alpha subunit	X59066, X65460	18q12-q21[625]	gDNA[163], cDNA[150,152]	+(43 aa)	Genes has 12 exons, polypeptide = 553 aa, encoded by 1659 bp	Pseudogenes have been mapped to 9p12, chromosomes 2 and 16[625] and chromosmes 9 and 18.[164]
ATP5B	H^+-transporting ATP synthase, F_1 complex, beta subunit	M27132, M19482, M19483	12p13-qter[164,166]	gDNA[167], cDNA[153,154]	+ (59 aa)	Gene has 10 exons, polypeptide = 539 aa, encoded by 1617 bp	This subunit contains the catalytic site. Pseudogenes (ATPMBL1 and ATPMBL2) have been mapped to chromosome 2 and 17, respectively.[164]
ATP5C1	H^+-transporting ATP synthase, F_1 complex, gamma subunit—liver-specific	D16561, D16562	c10, c14[164]	gDNA, cDNA[168]	+(25 aa)	Gene has 10 exons, polypeptide = 298 aa, encoded by 894 bp	Tissue specificity produced by alternative RNA splicing of exon 9, exact chromosomal location still undetermined.[164,168]
ATP5C2	H^+-transporting ATP synthase, F_1 complex, gamma subunit—heart specific	D16561, S16563	c10, c14[164]	gDNA, cDNA[168]	+ (25 aa)	Gene has 10 exons, polypeptide = 297 aa, encoded by 891 bp	Tissue specificity produced by alternative RNA splicing of exon 9; exact chromosomal location still undetermined.[164]
ATP5D	H^+-transporting ATP synthase, F_1 complex, delta chain	X63422		CDNA[155]	+(22 aa)	Polypeptide = 168 aa, encoded by 504 bp	
ATP5F1	H^+-transporting ATP synthase, F_0 complex, subunit b	X60221		CDNA[156]	+(42 aa)	Polypeptide = 256 aa, encoded by 768 bp	
ATP5G1	ATP synthase, F_0 complex, chain 9 (subunit c), isoform 1	X69907	c17[158]	gDNA, cDNA[158]	+(61 aa)	Gene has 5 exons, polypeptide = 136 aa, encoded by 408 bp	This is the gene product from the P1 gene. All three ATP5G genes encode the same polypeptide with three different leader peptides.
ATP5G2	ATP synthase, F_0 complex, chain 9 (subunit c), isoform 2	X69908	c12[158]	GDNA, cDNA[158]	+(66 aa)	Gene has 5 exons, polypeptide = 141 aa, encoded by 423 bp	This is the gene product from the P2 gene. A pseudogene has been isolated for the P2 gene. See ATP5G1.
ATP5G3	ATP synthase, F_0 complex, chain 9 (subunit c), isoform 3	U09813	c2[162]	CDNA[162]	+(67 aa)	Polypeptide = 142 aa, encoded by 426 bp	This is the gene product from the P3 gene. See ATP5G1.
ATP5J	ATP synthase, F_0 complex, subunit F6	M37104		CDNA[156,157]	+(32 aa)	Polypeptide = 108 aa, encoded by 324 bp	
MTATP6	H^+-transporting ATP synthase, F_0 complex, protein 6 (subunit A)	J01415, V00662	mtDNA[25]	MDNA[25]	N/A	Polypeptide = 226 aa, encoded by 678 bp, nucleotide position 8527-9207	Mutations include: NARP syndrome, Leigh disease, hypertrophic cardiomyopathy (MTATP6*8993T-G).
ATP50	ATP synthase oligomycin sensitivity conferral protein precursor (OSCP), mitochondrial H^+-transporting ATP synthase, subunit 8—mitochondrial	X83218	21q22.1–q22.2[626]	CDNA[626]	+(23 aa)	Polypeptide = 213 aa, encoded by 639 bp	
MTATP8	H^+-transporting ATP synthase, subunit 8	J01415, V00662	mtDNA[25]	MDNA[25]	N/A	Polypeptide = 68 aa, encoded by 204 bp, nucleotide positions 8366–8572	

Table 105-6 Complex V: Subunit Structure in Mitochondria and Bacteria[627–631]

	MITOCHONDRIAL (Bovine)				BACTERIAL (*E. coli*)	
COMPONENT	**SUBUNIT**	**STOICHIOMETRY**	**M.WT.**	**AA**	**SUBUNIT**	**STOICHIOMETRY**
F_0	α	3		510	α	3
	β	3		482	β	3
	γ	1		272	γ	1
	δ	1		146	δ	1
	ϵ	1		50	ϵ	1
Stalk	OSCP	1	20,967	190		
	F6	2	8958	76		
	b	2	24,670	256	b	2
	d	1	18,603			
	A (ATP6)	1	24,815	226	a	1
F_0	c (ATP9)	−12	7608	75	c	10–12
	A6L (ATP8)	1	7964	68		
	c		8189			
	f		10,209	87		
	g		11,328	102		
	IF1		9578	84		

12 c (ATP9) subunits lying in the plane of the inner membrane, which rotates with its axle extending into the matrix (Fig. 105-7). The axle is composed of the ε subunit at the base and the γ projecting up into the F_1 barrel. The stator is composed of a base made by the a subunit (ATP6) embedded in the membrane. This is adjacent to the c subunit wheel. The a (ATP6) subunit anchors a pair of b subunits, which project out of the membrane and end with the δ subunit. The δ subunit binds to the α subunit of the α-β barrel. Thus, the F_0 subunit a (ATP6) is linked to the 3α:3β barrel in a static structure through the b subunits and δ. As the rotor spins, the wheel of c (ATP6) subunits rotate past the stators a (ATP6) subunit, and the rotor's axle, ending in the γ subunit, rotates within the α and β barrel. The γ subunit makes two contacts with the β subunit, thus mediating the two components of the catalytic cycle.

The subunit a (ATP6)/subunit c (ATP9) interface mediates the proton flux from the intermembrane space to the matrix, thus driving the rotor's rotation and causing the γ axle to spin within the α and β subunit barrel. This generates sequential conformational changes in the β subunit nucleotide binding sites that bind ADP + Pi, condense it to ATP, and release the ATP into the matrix.[142,144]

The mechanism by which the proton motive force drives rotor rotation has been proposed to be electrostatic (Fig. 105-8). In Fig. 105-8, the F_0 is viewed from the plane of the membrane, with the subunit a (ATP6) of the stator in the center, and the wheel of about 12 subunit c (ATP9) subunits behind. All functional ATP subunits have a key negative charge in the c subunit in the middle of the membrane. For the bacterial enzyme, this is the Asp^{61} of subunit c, helix 2. For the mammalian enzyme this is the Glu^{58}. This carboxylate group faces outward from the wheel adjacent to the opposing face of the stator subunit a (ATP6) and also the hydrophobic core of the membrane's lipid bilayer. The stator subunit a (ATP6) has an opposing positive charge, Arg^{210} for the bacterial subunit c helix 4 and Arg^{159} for the mammalian subunit ATP6. This positive charge is offset 0.52 nm from the plane, such that it exerts electrostatic attraction without being capable of forming a salt bridge to stop rotation. The stator subunit c has two half-proton channels that penetrate halfway into the membrane from opposite sides, but are offset from each other. One half channel is open to the intermembrane space, and the other to the matrix (Fig. 105-8). In the presence of an electrochemical gradient, the half channel open to the intermembrane space has a high concentration of positively charged protons, while the half well open to the matrix space has very few protons. The intermembrane space well permits the protons to protonate the subunit c (ATP9) carboxyl group (Asp^{61}, Glu^{58}), neutralizing its charge and permitting the subunit to rotate into the hydrophobic lipid bilayer without energetic inhibition. The protonated subunit c will rotate all of the way around the wheel until it returns to the subunit a (ATP6) of the stator where it encounters the other half well. In this environment, the proton leaves subunit c (Asp^{61}, Glu^{58}) and enters into the negatively charged and alkaline matrix. The exposed negative charge of Asp^{61} (Glu^{58}) is then attracted to the displaced positive charge Arg^{210} (Arg^{159}) causing the Asp^{61} (Glu^{58}) carboxyl group to rotate until it reenters the environment of the proton-rich intermembrane space channel, where it can be reprotonated.[142,144–146] The stoichiometry of proton translocation to ATP synthesis is $4H^+$/ATP. Given that there are 3 β subunit active sites, 3 ATPs are synthesized per rotation of the rotor. Hence, 12 H^+ must be bound for each complete turn of the wheel. Given that each subunit c (ATP9) has only one carboxylate group, the wheel must have 12 spokes provided by 12 c (ATP9) subunits.

The coupling of rotor rotation to ATP synthesis is mediated by the asymmetric interaction of the γ subunit of the wheel axle with the inside surface of the β subunits of the F_1 barrel. This coupling is now understood at the molecular level due to the solution of the F_1 crystal structure.[141] The three α and three β subunits are capped by β-pleated sheets. Just below this cap is a hydrophobic ring forming a bearing in which the C-terminal end of the γ subunit rotates. The γ subunit consists of two long α-helixes folded in the middle so that both the N- and C-terminal ends extend into the 3α:3β barrel, with the C-terminal end extending furthermost. The C-terminal residues of γ, amino acids 253 to 272, are hydrophobic, such that the bearing is lubricated by hydrophobic surfaces.

Below the β sheet, and in the middle of the α and β subunits, are the nucleotide binding sites. The conformation and nucleotide binding sites of the α subunits are relatively static, while those of the β subunits are dynamic. According to the Boyer hypothesis of rational catalysis[147] and the F_1 crystal structure, the three β subunits sequentially go through three states: "O" or open with very low affinity for ligands and catalytically inactive; "L" or loose with the capacity to binding the ligands ADP and Pi, but catalytically inactive; and "T" or tight, with the ligands tightly bound associated with catalysis. These three states are generated as the asymmetric γ subunit interacts with the interior side of the β subunits.

The nucleotide binding site of the β subunit is centered around the phosphate-binding amino acids, or P-loop, with the motif G(X)nGKT/S and including Gly^{159}, Lys^{162}, and Thr^{163}. Additional interactions occur through the positively charged β subunit Arg^{189} and Arg^{260} amino acids as well as the adjacent α subunit

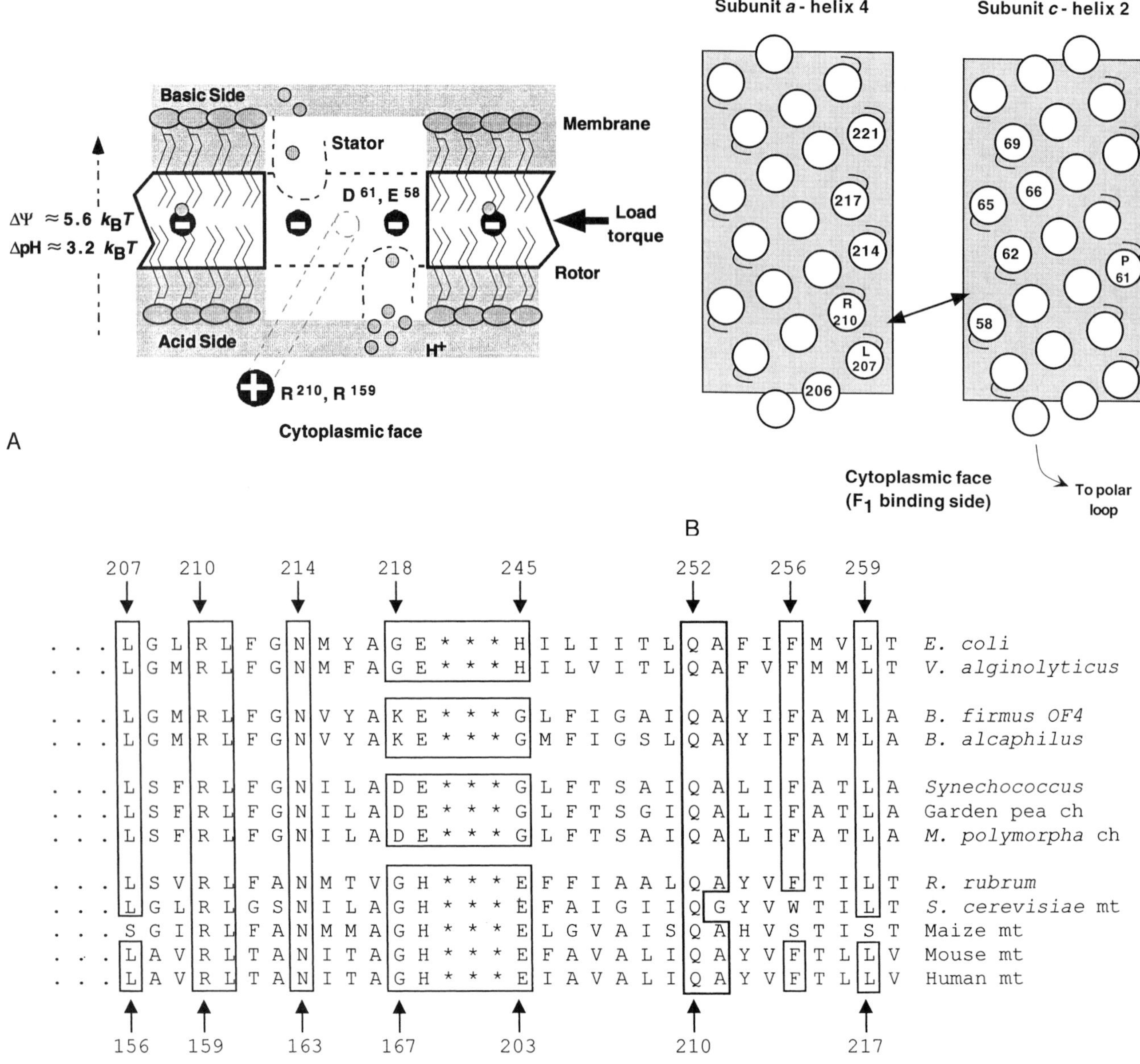

Fig. 105-8 Proposed models for the interaction of the ATP synthase subunit a (ATP6) and subunit c (ATP9) polypeptides in creation of the proton channel. *Panel A:* The interface between subunits a and c as viewed along the plane of the membrane. In this drawing, the cytoplasmic side (intermembrane space) is at the bottom and the mitochondrial matrix side is on top. The outer edge of the 12-spoke subunit c wheel is shown in the plane of the membrane with the face of subunit a in front. Subunit a is proposed to form two half-proton channels, offset from each other. At the center of helix 2 of subunit c is the critical negatively charged amino acid, Asp,^{61} in bacterial subunit c, and Glu^{58} in mitochondria subunit ATP6. As the wheel spins, the negative charge of Asp^{61}/Glu^{58} encounters the high-proton half-channel on the right where the carboxyl group becomes protonated. The neutralized amino acid can then rotate to the right and into the lipid belayer. It moves through the membrane one complete turn of the wheel and reenters the subunit "a" interface on the left where it encounters the low proton half channel. Here Asp^{61}/Glu^{58} is deprotonated, again acquiring a negative charge. An offset arginine, Arg^{210} for bacterial subunit a and Arg^{159} for mitochondrial subunit ATP6, attracting the negative charge and pulling it toward the high-proton half-channel where it will be reprotonated. (*Panel A is reproduced from Elston, Wang, and Oster.*[144] *Used with permission.*) *Panel B:* Proposed structure of the interaction between bacterial subunit a helix 4 (mitochondrial ATP6) and subunit c helix 2 (mitochondrial ATP9). The amino acid numbering is that of *E. coli*; however, subunit c D61 (Asp^{61}) is equivalent to ATP6 Glu^{58} and subunit a R210 (Arg^{210}) is equivalent to ATP6 Arg^{159}. Subunit a amino acid L207 (Leu^{207}) is equivalent to the mitochondrial ATP6 Leu^{156}, which is mutated to an arginine in the MTATP6*NARP8993G Leigh disease. (*Panel B is adapted from Fillingame et al.*[145] *Used with permission.*) *Panel C:* The alignment of subunit a and ATP6

amino acids Arg^{373} and Ser^{344}. In addition the γ phosphate of ATP interacts with the β subunits Glu^{188} in association with a bound water. The ribonucleotide binding pocket involves the β subunit Ala^{421} and the phenylalanines Phe^{418} and Phe^{424}. The binding site also uses the α subunit Tyr^{345}.

The binding affinity for this site for adenine nucleotides is modified by sequential changes in the β subunit conformation. In the βE (empty or [O] open) conformation the interaction between strands 3 and 7 is disrupted, rotating part of the nucleotide binding site 30° from the βTP (triphosphate or [T] tight) and βDP (diphosphate or [L] loose) forms. This rotation is accomplished by a major "catch," which is a loop following strand 7 that protrudes into the interior of the 3α:3β barrel. In the βEO form the β subunit amino acids Asp^{316}, Thr^{318}, and Asp^{319} hydrogen bond with γ subunits Arg^{254} and Glu^{255}, and the α subunit Asp^{333} forms a salt bridge with Arg^{252}. A second minor catch separates βTP (triphosphate, tight) from βDP (diphosphate, loose) and βE (empty, open). This involves the interaction of γ subunit amino acids Lys^{87}, Lys^{90}, and Ala^{80} with the β subunit amino acids Asp^{394} and Glu^{398} in the sequence DELSEED (β 394 to 400),[141] which forms part of the binding site for amphipathic cationic inhibitors.[148,149]

These molecular interactions create a catalytic engine driven by elastic forces rather than thermal effects, which permits the near 100 percent efficiency.[142] This has been envisioned as involving a passive and an active spring that opens and closes the nucleotide binding site in the β subunit as the asymmetric γ subunit rotates, hitting the two alternative catches. Studying the reverse reaction of the F_1, ATP hydrolysis, these conformational changes can be defined as having four energetic intermediates: E (empty), T (ATP bound), DP (ADP and Pi bound following hydrolysis), D (ADP bound, Pi released), and E (ADP released). The major energetic transitions occur going from E to T, when ATP is bound (or released), and from DP to D, when phosphate is released (or bound). These major energetic changes correspond to the switches in β conformation, S1 and S2, respectively. Switch 1 (S1) is located at γ subunit Gln^{269} and β subunit Thr^{304}, while switch 2 (S2) occurs between γ Arg^{242} and β Glu^{381} in the DELSEED sequence of the β subunit. In the direction of hydrolysis, the primary power stroke is PSI or ATP binding, which drives the bending of the β subunit, creating an elastic stress that turns γ and compresses the passive elastic element. The secondary power stroke (PS2), triggered by the release of the phosphate, causes the elastic energy stored from the primary power stroke to be liberated during the first power stroke of the next site in the sequence. This motor rotates in steps of $2\Pi/3$, generating up to 45 pNnm of torque and consuming one ATP per step.[84,142]

A number of the nuclear-encoded complex V subunit cDNA and genomic clones have been reported (Table 105-5). Complementary DNAs have been reported for the ATPsynthase (ATPsyn) α subunit, including systemic and heart-skeletal muscle isoforms,[150–152] ATPsynβ,[153,154] ATPsynδ,[155] F_0 subunit b,[156] F_0 subunit F6,[157] and F_0 subunit 9 or c, which has three isoforms, two with the same mature polypeptide but different N-terminal targeting sequences and one with an 80 percent identical polypeptide that maps to chromosome 2.[158–162] Genomic clones have been reported for the ATPsynα gene, which is a single copy gene encompassing 12 exons with no evidence of isoforms[163] and with homologous sequences on chromosomes 9 and 18.[164] The ATPsynβ gene, which encompasses 10 exons, has a complex promoter including the novel OXBOX/REBOX element, and is located on chromosome 12p13-qter.[165–167] The ATPsynγ gene also has 10 exons and maps to chromosome 14.[99,164,168] The ATPsynγ gene generates two alternative mRNAs, liver and heart, by alternate splicing. The heart isoform lacks exon 9 and is the only isoform expressed in heart and skeletal muscle. The liver isoform predominates in brain, liver, pancreas, kidney, and testes, and both mRNAs are found in stomach, intestine, and skin.[168] The exclusion of exon 9 involves synthesis of a *trans*-acting factor that is inducible by high extracellular pH through a protein kinase C signaling mechanism.[169]

Adenine Nucleotide Translocator and Uncoupling Protein. The mitochondrial anion carrier protein family functions to transport solutes through the mitochondrial inner membrane. This group of related proteins has a tripartite repeating domain, each domain of about 100 amino acids. This family includes two classes of carriers of particular relevance to bioenergetics, the ADP/ATP carriers (AAC) or adenine nucleotide translocators (ANT) and the uncoupling proteins (UCP) (Tables 105-7 and 105-8). ANT exchanges mitochondrial ATP for cytosolic ADP across the mitochondrial inner membrane. Three distinct human ANT cDNAs have been cloned: a heart-muscle-specific isoform ANT1,[170–172] an inducible isoform ANT2,[171,173] and a generally systemic isoform ANT3.[171,172] ANT1 is expressed almost exclusively in heart and muscle,[174] has four exons, and has a promoter with classical TATA and CCAAT elements,[175,176] as well as the novel OXBOX/REBOX elements that it shares with the ATPsynβ gene and certain other bioenergetic genes.[165,177,178] The gene maps to 4q35-qter, close to the facioscapulohumeral muscular dystrophy locus.[179–181] ANT2 is expressed at low levels in mature tissues, but is inducible in situations of metabolic stress.[172,174,182–184] ANT2 has been mapped to Xq24-q24, has the same four-exon structure as ANT1, a promoter with a canonical TATA and five potential Sp1 sites, but no CCAAT box, and multiple pseudogenes.[185–187] In addition, ANT2 contains an element about 1.2 kb from the transcriptional start site, termed the GRBOX (glycolysis regulated box). This binds a negative regulator in normal cells, coinciding with the shut-off of the gene. This factor is lost in glycolytic and transformed cells in association with the induction of ANT2.[172] ANT3 is expressed in most mature tissues, as well as in skin fibroblasts.[174,182] It also has the classical four-exon structure, but its promoter lacks TATA and CCAAT elements, although it has potential Sp1 sites.[175] This gene maps to Xp22.3, 1.3 Mb from the telomere within the pseudoautosomal region. The ANT3 gene escapes X inactivation and is transcribed from both X and Y chromosomes. It has one pseudogene on chromosome 9.[188,189]

In contrast to humans, the mouse has only two ANT genes (Ant1 and Ant2). The deduced proteins are homologous to the human ANT1 and ANT2 proteins. The mouse Ant1 maps to chromosome 8, with no recombinants to the mouse D8Mit5 locus and only one recombinant to the D8Mit6 and Klk3 loci.[190,191] This region is syntenic with human chromosome 4q35, the chromosomal location of ANT1. Mouse Ant2 has been mapped to regions A-D of the mouse X chromosome. This excludes the pseudoautosomal region, suggesting the mouse Ant2 may be syntenic to human ANT2.[192] No mouse homologue to the human ANT3 gene could be isolated.[190,192] Southern blots from a variety of mammalian species suggest that the pseudoautosomal Ant3 may have been lost from the entire rodent lineage.[192] The structure of the mouse Ant1 gene is identical to that of the human ANT1, having four exons and three introns.[190]

The uncoupling proteins form a proton channel through the inner membrane, thus depolarizing the electrochemical gradient. This uncouples electron transport from the ATP synthase and ADP phosphorylation. The uncoupler protein-1 (UCP1) was initially identified in brown adipose tissue (BAT), where it functions in thermal regulation. Acute exposure of rodents to cold results in the tenfold induction of UCP1 mRNA, and an associated rapid oxidation of the fats in BAT to generate heat. UCP1 maps to human chromosome 4q31.[193–196] In addition to UPC1, two additional uncoupler protein genes have been cloned. Uncoupler protein-2 (UCP2) has 59 percent amino acid identity to UCP1 and is widely expressed in adult human tissues with mRNA levels being highest in skeletal muscle. It is also up-regulated in white fat in response to an increased fat diet. The gene is located on human chromosome 11q13 and on mouse chromosome 7 where it is linked to a quantitative trait locus for hyperinsulinemia and obesity.[196] A third uncoupler protein-3 (UCP3) gene has been identified; it is 57 percent identical to UCP1 and 73 percent identical to UCP2. UCP3 is also widely expressed in adult tissues, and at particularly high levels in skeletal muscle. Moreover, it is hormonally regulated, being induced in skeletal muscle by thyroid hormone, in white fat by β3-adrenergic agonists, and also regulated by dexamethasone, leptin, and starvation. UCP3 is located adjacent to UCP2 in human chromosome 11q13 and mouse chromosome 7.[197–200]

Mitochondrial Protein Import Apparatus. Because the vast majority of mitochondrial proteins are encoded by nuclear genes and translated on cytosolic ribosomes, a highly efficient procedure has evolved for selectively transporting these proteins into the mitochondria and assembling them into functional complexes. This is accomplished by a set of outer and inner mitochondrial

Table 105-7 OXPHOS-Associated Functions: Proteins, cDNAs, and Genes

Gene	Description	Accession #	Chr. location	Sequence	Leader	Characterization	Comments
ETFQO	Electron transfer flavoprotein ubiquinone oxidoreductase	S69232	4q32-qter[632]	cDNA[632]	+(33 aa)	Polypeptide = 617 aa, encoded by 1851 bp	Mutations include: T-C change in initiator methionine, one- and seven-bp deletions, skipping of the 136-bp exon, and skipping of the 222-bp exon all causing glutaric acidemia type II.[633]
IDH3A	NAD(H)-specific isocitrate dehydrogenase alpha chain	U07681		cDNA[634]	+(27 aa)	Polypeptide = 366 aa, encoded by 1098 bp	
ETFB	Electron transfer flavoprotein beta chain	X71129	19q13.3[635]	cDNA[635]		Polypeptide = 255 aa, encoded by 765 bp	Mutations include: glutaricaciduria IIB (ETFB, bp ARG164GLN and a G-C transversion at the first nucleotide of the intron donor site, causing a deletion of 159 bp, spanning nt 466 to 624, leading to the removal of 53 aa.[636]
PDHA1	Pyruvate dehydrogenase (lipoamide) alpha chain precursor (E1)	J03575	Xp22.1	gDNA, cDNA[637]	+(29 aa)	Gene has 11 exons, polypeptide = 361 aa, encoded by 1170 bp	Many mutations have been isolated in PDHA1 causing pyruvate dehydrogenase deficiency.
PDHB(1)	Pyruvate dehydrogenase (lipoamide) beta chain precursor (El)	J03576, D90086	3p13-q23	gDNA,[638] cDNA[637]	+(30 aa)	Gene has 10 exons, polypeptide = 359 aa, encoded by 1077 bp	This gene was cloned from a human foreskin fibroblast cDNA library. The sequence has been contested by Chun et al., see PDHB(2).
PDHB(2)	Pyruvate dehydrogenase (lipoamide) beta chain precursor (E1)	X57778 (Chun)	3p13-q23	cDNA[639]	+	Polypeptide = 358 aa, encoded by 1074 bp	This gene was cloned from a human foreskin fibroblast cDNA library. This sequence differs from Koike et al. by 19 aa.
PDHA2	Pyruvate dehydrogenase (lipoamide) alpha chain precursor, testis-specific (E1)	M86808	4q22-q23[640]	gDNA, cDNA[640]		Polypeptide = 388 aa, encoded by 1164 bp	This gene lacks introns and possesses characteristics of a functional processed gene.
DLAT	Dihydrolipoamide S-acetyltransferase (E2)	Y00978; HSPDCE2		cDNA[641,642]	+(54 aa)	Polypeptide = 561 aa, encoded by 1686 bp	
CCHU	Cytochrome c	M22877	8q24.3[99]	cDNA[100]		Polypeptide = 105 aa, encoded by 315 aa	
DLD	Dihydrolipoamide dehydrogenase (E3)	J03620, J03490		cDNA[643,644]	+35 aa	Polypeptide = 509 aa, encoded by 1527 bp	
ACO2	Mitochondrial aconitate hydratase, (citrate hydrolyase) (aconitase)	AH006514, U80040	22q13[645]	gDNA, cDNA[645]		Gene has 18 exons, polypeptide = 780 aa, encoded by 2340 bp	

Table 105-8 Inner Membrane Carrier Proteins: Proteins, cDNAs, and Genes

Gene	Description	Accession	Chr. location	Sequence	Leader	Characterization	Comments
ANT1	ADP, ATP carrier protein T1	J04982, J02966	4q35[176]	gDNA[175,176], cDNA[170]		Gene has 4 exons, polypeptide = 297 aa, encoded by 891 bp	
ANT2	ADP ATP carrier protein T3	J02683	Xq24-q26[185]	gDNA[186], cDNA[173]		Gene has 4 exons, polypeptide = 298 aa, encoded by 894 bp	7 pseudogenes were isolated.[185]
ANT3	ADP, ATP carrier protein T2	J03591, J03592, J03593	Xp22.32[189]	gDNA, cDNA[171,175]		Gene has 4 exons, polypeptide = 297 aa, encoded by 894 bp	The partial cDNA clones isolated by Houldsworth et al. are from the 3′ end of the gene. These clones contain some sequence differences from the sequence reported by Cozens et al. A pseudogene has been localized to chromosome 9.[188,189]
PCP	Phosphate carrier protein, from B	X60036		gDNA[646], cDNA[647]	+(49 aa)	Gene has 9 exons, polypeptide = 361 aa, encoded by 1083 bp	An alternatively spliced form of the protein has been observed in which the normal exon IIIB is spliced out and replaced with exon IIIA resulting in a polypeptide that is 1 aa longer.[646,647]
UCP1	Uncoupling protein, mitochondrial	X51952, X51953, X51954, X51955	4q31[193]	gDNA, cDNA[193]	–	Gene has 6 exons, polypeptide = 307 aa, encoded by 921 pp	
UCP2	Uncoupling protein 2, mitochondrial	U76367, AJ223479, AJ223478, AJ223477	11q13[196]	gDNA, cDNA[196]		Gene has 6 exons, polypeptide = 309 aa, encoded by 930 bp	
UCP3L	Uncoupling protein 3—large, mitochondrial	U84763	11q13[648]	cDNA[199,200]	–	Polypeptide = 312 aa, encoded by 936 bp	
UCP3S	Uncoupling protein 3—short, mitochondrial	U82818	11q13[648]	cDNA[199]	–	Polypeptide = 275 aa, encoded by 825 bp	This polypeptide is an isoform of UCP3L that lacks a portion of the 3′ end.
SLC25A12	Solute carrier family 25, member 12-mitochondrial carrier protein aralar1	Y14494		cDNA[649]	–	Polypeptide = 678 aa, encoded by 2034 bp	
SLC20A3	Solute carrier family 20, member 3-tricarboxylate transport protein precursor (citrate transport protein) (CTP)	U25147	22q11[650]	gDNA[651], cDNA[652]	+(13 aa)	Gene has 8 exons, Polypeptide = 311 aa, encoded by 933 bp	
GT	Mitochondrial solute carrier protein homolog	M31659	c10[653]	cDNA[653]	–	Polypeptide = 348 aa, encoded by 1044 bp	

complexes: the Tom complexes for transport across the outer membrane and the Tim complexes for transport across the inner membrane. These systems have been most extensively studied in yeast[201,202] and *Neurospora.*[203] A diagram of the major membrane components is presented in Fig. 105-9.

Proteins to be imported into the mitochondrion have embedded into their structure specific amino acid sequences that target them to the mitochondrion and to specific regions of the organelle. Most proteins to be imported into the mitochondrial matrix have an amino-terminal targeting peptide that is amphiphilic and basic

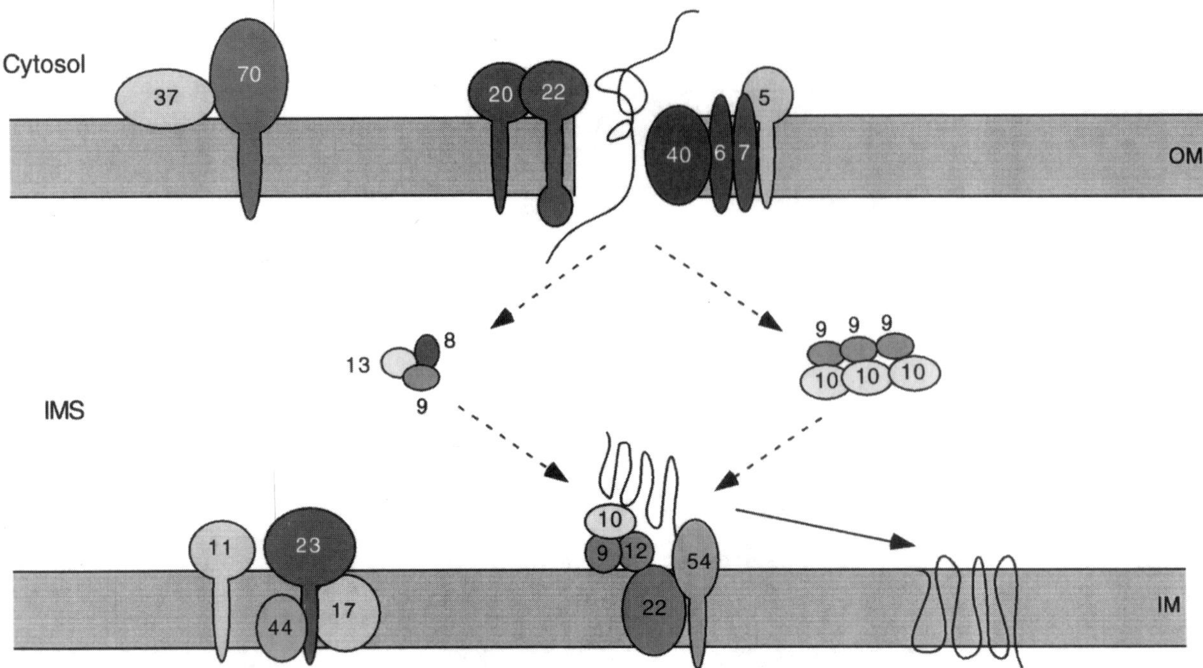

Fig. 105-9 Proteins thought to be involved in the import of cytosolically synthesized polypeptides through the outer and inner mitochondrial membranes. The outer membrane Tom (transport across the outer membrane) complexes consist of two main receptor complexes and the general insertion pore (GIP) complex. Receptor complex Tom20 + Tom22 binds proteins with amino-terminal targeting peptides and feeds them through the GIP, of which Tom22 is thought to be a component. Tom37 + Tom70 are thought to bind proteins with internal targeting sequences and to transfer them to Tom20 + Tom22. The central channel protein of the GIP is thought to be Tom40, with Tom5, Tom6, and Tom7 also being important components. Proteins with amino-terminal targeting peptides destined for the matrix are transferred from the intermembrane space domain of Tom22 to the Tim complex. Tim23 is the central channel protein, and Tim44 binds to the preprotein as it emerges from the Tim23 channel on the matrix side. Anion carrier proteins destined for integration into the mitochondrial inner membrane, such as the ANT, follow a different pathway. As they emerge into the intermembrane space they interact with either of two soluble complexes (Tim8 + - Tim9 + Tim13) or (3 Tim9 + 3 Tim10). These soluble complexes transport the protein through the intermembrane space to the other Tim complex, which is composed of Tim9 + Tim10 + Tim12+ Tim22 + Tim54. ***(Reprinted from Wallace and Murdock,[214] which was adapted from Koehler et al.[211,826] Used with permission.)***

(positively charged), usually due to an excess of arginine residues. These amino-terminal targeting peptides are cleaved from the protein on import. Other proteins can have internal targeting sequences.

While in the cytosol, proteins destined for mitochondrial import interact with cytosolic chaperones. These include members of the cytosolic 70-kDa heat-shock protein (hsp70) family, which bind to nonnative proteins. In addition, there is at least one cytosolic chaperone specific for mitochondrial proteins. This is the heterochimeric mitochondrial import-stimulating factor (MSF) that specifically binds matrix-targeting signals. Both Hsp70 and MSF are ATPases.[201–203]

The mitochondrial proteins, presumably maintained in a random conformation by the chaperone proteins, then interact with the receptor complexes on the mitochondrial outer membrane. Two receptor complexes have been identified: Tom20 + Tom22 and Tom37 + Tom70. Current thinking is that Tom20 + Tom22 binds to proteins with amino-terminal targeting peptides because this complex has "acid bristles" on the cytosolic domains that can interact with the basic targeting peptides. The Tom37 + Tom70 complex is thought to interact with proteins with internal targeting sequences such as the inner membrane carrier proteins ANT and UCP. This complex then transfers the protein to the Tom20 + - Tom22 complex which then moves on to the general insertion pore (GIP). The Tom37 + Tom70 complex and Tom20 + Tom22 complex are known to interact through 34 amino acid "tetra-trico-peptide" motifs.[201–203]

The outer membrane GIP is thought to be composed of Tom40, Tom22, Tom5, Tom6, and Tom7.[204] Tom40 is deeply embedded in the outer membrane and forms a 22-Å hydrophilic transmembrane channel.[205] The smaller polypeptides, Tom5 and Tom6, are also components of the channel, while Tom7 functions as an assembly factor.[204] Tom22 functions both as a key component of the receptor complex and as an integral part of the GIP channel.[201–204]

Once the protein traverses the outer membrane, it can go two different directions. It can either proceed through the inner membrane to the matrix or be inserted directly into the inner membrane. Proteins destined for transport through the inner membrane generally carry an amino-terminal targeting sequence. These targeting sequences are electrostatically attracted to the inner membrane import complex consisting of Tim23, Tim11, Tim14, and Tim17. Tim33 might also be a component. Most of these proteins are embedded in the inner membrane and together constitute the protein-conducting channel. The Tim23 protein is central to this channel and it dimerizes in the presence of $\Delta\Psi$, possibly providing a gating mechanism for the channel. Proteins with basic targeting peptides have been shown to move down an "acid chain" gradient of increasing affinities. This includes the external acidic domain of Tom20, followed by the intermembrane domain of Tom22, followed by the inner membrane pore protein Tim23.

The Tim23, Tim11, Tim14, and Tim17 inner membrane pore complex interacts with a second complex on the matrix side of the inner membrane consisting of Tim44, mtHsp70, and MGE. Tim44 interacts with the preprotein as it emerges from the Tim23 pore. Tim44 also binds mtHsp70, which, in turn, interacts with the preprotein and promotes its import, in conjunction with the hydrolysis of ATP.

The interaction of Tim44 and mtHsp70 is regulated by adenine nucleotides and also by the nucleotide exchange factor (MGE) which regulates Tim44–mtHsp70 dissociation.[201–203]

Table 105-9 Mitochondrial Channels and Apoptosis Functions: Proteins, cDNAS, and Genes

Gene	Description	Accession #	Chr. location	Sequence	Leader	Characterization	Comments
VDAC1	Voltage-dependent anion channel 1	L06132	Xq13-q21[654]	cDNA[655]	–	Polypeptide = 283 aa, encoded by 849 bp	
VDAC2	Voltage-dependent anion channel 2	L06328	21pter-21qter[654]	cDNA[655]	–	Polypeptide = 294 aa, encoded by 882 bp	
VDAC3	Voltage-dependent anion channel 3	S75494	c12[654]	cDNA			VDAC3 and 4 have only partial cDNAs recorded
VDAC4	Voltage-dependent anion channel 4	S75651	1q24-q25[654]	cDNA			see VDAC3
SOD2	Superoxide dismutase (Mn)	Y00472	6q25.3[656]	cDNA[657]	+(24 aa)	Polypeptide = 222 aa, encoded by 666 bp	
GPX1	Human glutathione peroxidase 1	Y00433, M21304	3p21.3[658]	cDNA[659,660]		Polypeptide = 201 aa, encoded by 603 bp	Complications in determining chromosomal location of this gene are due to presence of pseudogenes
BAXA	BCL2-associated X protein-apoptosis regulator BAX, alpha isoform	L22473, L22474, L22475, U19599	19q13.3-q13.4	cDNA[661]		Polypeptide = 192 aa, encoded by 576 bp	Each isoform is transcribed from the same gene and alternately spliced to form each variant. Mutations include 1-bp insertions, 1-bp deletions involved in colorectal cancer, BAX GLY67 ARG and BAX7-bp deletion 114-121G involved in T-cell acute lymphoblastic leukemia.[662,663]
BAXB	BCL2-associated X protein-apoptosis regulator BAX, beta isoform	L22474	19q13.3-q13.4[664]	cDNA[661]		Polypeptide = 218 aa, encoded by 654 bp	see BAXA
BAXG	BCL2-associated X protein-apoptosis regulator BAX, gamma isoform	L22475	19q13.3-q13.4[664]	cDNA[661]		Polypeptide = 41 aa, encoded by 123 bp	see BAXA
BAXD	BCL2-associated X protein-apoptosis regulator BAX delta isoform	U19599	19q13.3-q13.4[664]	cDNA[664]		Polypeptide = 143 aa, encoded by 429 bp	see BAXA
BCL2	Transforming protein (bcl-2-beta)	M13995	18q21.3[665]	cDNA[665]		Polypeptide = 205 aa, encoded by 615 bp	
BCL2	Transforming protein (bcl-2-alpha)	M13994	18q21.3[665]	cDNA[665]		Polypeptide = 239 aa, encoded by 717 bp	
BZRP	Peripheral benzodiazepine receptor	M36035, L21951, L21952, L21953, L21954	22q13.3[666]	gDNA, cDNA[666]		Gene has 4 exons, Polypeptide = 169 aa, encoded by 507 bp	

(Continued on next page)

Table 105-9 (Continued)

Gene	Description	Accession #	Chr. location	Sequence	Leader	Characterization	Comments
—	Peripheral benzodiazepine receptor-related protein	L21950	22q13.3[666]	gDNA, cDNA[667]	–	Gene has 4 exons, polypeptide = 102 aa*, encoded by 306 bp	*This protein is a result of alternative splicing of BZRP that excludes exon 2.
PRAX-1	Peripheral benzodiazepine receptor-associated protein 1—human	AF039571	17q22-q23[668]	cDNA[668]		Polypeptide = 1857 aa, encoded by 5571 bp	
AIF	Apoptosis-including factor	AF100928	Xq25-q26[20]	CDNA[20]	+(31 aa, 27 aa)	Polypeptide = 613 aa*, encoded by 1839 bp	*The mature protein is 510 aa after processing. The sequence also contains two nuclear localization sequences that are utilized after apoptosis is induced.[20]
LON-PEN	Lon proteinase homolog	X76040, X74215		cDNA[669]		Polypeptide = 937 aa (845 aa)*, encoded by 2811 bp (2535 bp)	*Two putative start codons were identified, the second is more likely due to homology to eubacteria.[669]
MPP	Mitochondrial processing peptidase alpha subunit precursor (alpha-MPP) (P-55)	D50913		cDNA[670]		Polypeptide = 528 aa, encoded by 1584 bp	This cDNA was identified by homology to rat MPP.
TOM20	Mitochondrial import receptor subunit TOM20 homolog (translocase on the mitochondrial outer membrane)	D13641	1q42[671]	cDNA[671]		Polypeptide = 145 aa, encoded by 435 bp	Two pseudogenes have been isolated, Ψ1Tom20 and Ψ2Tom20.[671,672]
SPA9B	Mitochondrial heat-shock 70-kDa protein 9B (mortalin-2)	L15189, NM_004134	5q31.1[673]	cDNA[674]	+(51 aa)	Polypeptide = 679 aa, encoded by 2037 bp	Also known as mthsp 75, mthsp70.
HSPD1	heat-shock protein 60	M34664		cDNA[675]	+(26 aa)	Polypeptide = 573 aa, encoded by 1719 bp	

Once in the matrix, the targeting peptides are cleaved off by the mitochondrial processing peptidase (MPP). MPP consists of two subunits, α-MPP of about 55 kDa and β-MPP of about 25 kDa. The β-MPP has the catalytic activity, containing the HXXEH sequence motif characteristic of metal-binding enzyme. A subset of preproteins has a second processing step, mediated by the mitochondrial intermediate peptidase (MIP). Proteins in the matrix also need to be folded, a process mediated by several chaperones. The mtHsp70 plays an important role, as do the cochaperones MD5 and MGE. In addition, the chaperone system involving Hsp60 and Hsp10 plays an essential role in processing proteins into functional forms. Finally, mitochondrial cyclophilins, which are sensitive to cyclosporin A, can act as folding catalysts.[201–203]

Mitochondrial inner membrane transport proteins such as the ANTs and UCPs follow a different pathway. Once they enter the intermembrane space via the Tom complex, they interact with one of two soluble complexes. One complex involves three Tim9 and three Tim10 subunits (Fig. 105-9), while the other involves one each of Tim8, Tim9, and Tim13 polypeptides. These complexes deliver the carrier protein to a 300-kDa complex composed of Tim54, Tim22, Tim12, Tim10, and Tim9, bound to the outer face of the inner membrane. The polypeptides Tim8, Tim9, Tim10, Tim12, and Tim13 all belong to the same gene family, which contains a distinctive duplicated C(N3)C motif reminiscent of a Zn finger.[211–214] The known genes involved in protein import are listed in Table 105-9. For example, mtHsp70 is located on chromosome 5q311.

The Mitochondrial Permeability Transition Pore (mtPTP). The mtPTP complex spans the mitochondrial inner and outer membranes and is thought to be a major mediator for the initiation of apoptosis. Under normal physiological conditions, the pore is closed. However, in response to a variety of signals, including increased mitochondrial Ca^{++}, decreased $\Delta\Psi$, or increased oxidative stress, the pore opens, creating a channel that allows molecules up to 1500 daltons to freely diffuse in or out of the mitochondria. This disrupts the integrity of the mitochondrial inner membrane, causes the collapse of $\Delta\Psi$, and permits water to rush into the mitochondria, causing the mitochondria to swell and rupture.

The core elements of the mtPTP (Fig. 105-2) are thought to be the voltage-dependent anion channel (VDAC) or porin in the outer membrane, and the ANT in the inner membrane. Associated with the outer membrane, VDAC is associated with the benzodiazepine receptor, and with the ANT on the matrix side is cyclophilin D. The involvement of cyclophilin D impacts the cyclosporin A sensitivity which is diagnostic of phenomena associated with the mtPTP.[15,16,22,23,215] In addition to these components, and central to the function and regulation of the mtPTP, is the BCL-2 gene family. This family possesses both proapoptotic and antiapoptotic family members. The proapoptotic proteins are BAX, BAD, BID, BAK, BCL-Xs, Blk, BIM, and HRK. The antiapoptotic members are BCL-2, BCL-X_l, BCL-W, MCL-1, and A1. BAX, together with the ANT, have been shown by both genetic and biochemical reconstitution experiments to be essential to permeabilize the mitochondrial membranes.[23] Most of the BCL-2 is consistently mitochondria bound. By contrast, BAX is found in two states: soluble in the cytosol or bound to the mitochondrial membranes. This transition is modulated by signals that initiate apoptosis. In the absence of apoptotic signals, BAX is soluble as a monomer in the cytosol. However, when the cell is exposed to an apoptotic signal, BAX migrates to the mitochondria where it binds as a homodimer. The binding of this homodimer induces apoptosis in cells, which is inhibited if BCL-2 is also up-regulated. In the absence of high BCL-2, the cells experience a decrease in $\Delta\Psi$ and an increase in ROS production, although cytochrome c is not released.[216] This corresponds to the capacity of BAX to form a channel in the membrane, which is inhibited by the presence of BCL-2.[217,218] Taken together, these data indicate that the core components of the mtPTP are the ANT, BAX, cyclophilin D, and probably also the VDAC and benzodiazepine receptor (Fig. 105-2).

Signals that are known to activate mtPTP opening include high matrix Ca^{++}; oxidizing agents such as H_2O_2, t-butylhydroperoxide, NO (peroxynitrite), menadione, and alloxan; $\Delta\Psi$ reduction; disulfide bridge formation by diamide; thio-derivatization; and the ANT ligands atractyloside and pyridoxal-5-phosphate. Signals or agents that inhibit the opening of the mtPTP include Ca^{++} chelators, certain divalent actions such as Mg^{++} and Zn^{++}, high $\Delta\psi$; ADP and ATP, free radical scavengers such as N-acetylcysteine; reducing agents such as dithiothreitol; the ANT ligand bongkrekic acid; polyamines such as spermine; carnitine and acylcarnitine; and cytosporin A.[16,215]

A number of the genes involved in the mtPTP have been cloned and mapped. These included the three ANTs, four VDACs, BAX on chromosome 19q1.3; BCL-2 α and β on chromosome 8q21.33; the benzodiazepine receptor on 22q13.31-22qter; and AIF on Xq2-Xq26 (Table 105-9).

MITOCHONDRIAL GENES AND GENETICS

Mitochondrial Genes

mtDNA. mtDNA is a 16,569-nucleotide-pair (np), closed circular molecule, located within the mitochondrial matrix and present in thousands of copies per cell. It codes for the structural RNAs of mitochondrial protein synthesis including the small (12S, MTRNR1) and large (16S, MTRNR2) rRNAs as well as 22 tRNAs (Fig. 105-3). These 22 tRNAs can interpret the entire mtDNA genetic code through the use of modified wobble codon rules. Certain tRNAs also have differences in their anticodons that impart a modified genetic code to the mtDNA. In particular, the anticodon of the tryptophan tRNA is modified so that it reads both the normal tryptophan codon (UGG) as well as the opal stop codon (UGA). Similarly, the methionine tRNA recognizes both AUG and AUA as methionine. Finally, the tRNA for recognizing the arginine codons AGA and AGG is absent such that these are now stop codons.[219]

In addition to the rRNAs and tRNAs, the mtDNA also encodes 13 polypeptides (Fig. 105-4). Twelve of these polypeptides, as well as the rRNAs and 13 tRNAs, are encoded by the guanine (G)-rich heavy (H)-strand of the mtDNA, while 1 polypeptide and 9 tRNAs are encoded by the cytosine (C)-rich light (L)-strand. The H-strand polypeptides are the MTND1, 2, 3, 4, 4L, and 5 subunits of complex I; cytochrome b (MTCYB) of complex III; the COI, COII, and COIII (MTCO1, MTCO2, MTCO3) polypeptides of complex IV; and the ATPase6 and 8 (MTATP6, MTATP8) polypeptides of complex V. The only L-strand polypeptide is the complex I subunit MTND6 (Fig. 105-3).[36]

The mtDNA has two origins of replication. The H-strand origin (O_H) is located in the 1121 np, noncoding control region. DNA replication initiates at O_H using an RNA primer generated from the L-strand transcript. The L-strand transcript initiates at the adjacent L-strand promoter (P_L) and is cleaved by the nuclear-encoded mitochondrial RNA processing endonuclease (RNase MRP) located at chromosome 9p12-9p21 (GenBank HSMRP). RNase MRP cleaves at runs of G nucleotides in the conserved sequence blocks CSBIII, CSBII, and CSBI, primarily after CSBI[220–223]. The resulting 3′-OH is utilized by DNA polymerase γ as a primer. The polymerase γ gene is located on chromosome 15q24-15q25 (GenBank DPOG HUMAN), and initially synthesizes a 7S DNA which ends at the termination-associated sequence (TAS) at the end of the control region. The TAS binds to a specific factor that may regulate this replication pause site.[224] This newly synthesized region of the H-strand displaces the parental H-strand to create the displacement-loop (D-loop).[224,225] The 7S DNA is subsequently utilized as a primer to synthesize a new H-strand. From the 7S DNA, H-strand synthesis proceeds two-thirds of the way around the mtDNA, displacing the parental H-strand until it reaches the light strand origin (O_L), situated in a cluster of five tRNA genes (WANCY). Once exposed by the displaced H-strand, O_L folds into a stem-loop structure and L-strand synthesis initiates and proceeds back along the H-strand template. Consequently, mtDNA replication is bidirectional but asynchronous.[226]

mtDNA transcription initiates from two promoters in the control region, one for each strand: P_L and P_H. Both promoters are associated with a nuclear-encoded mitochondrial transcription factor (mtTF1 or Tfam) binding site. Tfam is a high-mobility group DNA-binding protein with two DNA-binding domains and a C-terminal tail essential for transcription.[227–229] It binds with higher affinity to P_L than P_H, consistent with their relative transcription frequencies.[230,231] Tfam also binds with a 40- to 50-base periodicity throughout the D-loop, with CSBII and CSBIII being unbound and CSBI being strongly bound. The mtTF1 phasing downstream from CSBI on the H-strand DNA corresponds to DNA synthesis initiation sites, suggesting that mtTF1 may help define the transitions between RNA and DNA.[232] Transcription from both promoters proceeds around the mtDNA circle creating a polycistronic RNA. The tRNA genes that punctuate the larger rRNA and mRNA sequences then fold within the transcript and are cleaved out by an RNaseP-like activity. The freed mRNAs and rRNAs are post-transcriptionally polyadenylated and the tRNAs are modified and the 3′ terminal CCA added.[233–235]

The rRNAs are present in about a 50:1 ratio with the mRNAs. This differential transcription is accomplished in part by a transcriptional terminator (5′-TGGCAGAGCCCGG-3′) located within the $tRNA^{Leu(UUR)}$ gene, immediately downstream from the 16S rRNAs in the direction of H-strand transcription from P_H. This terminator is bidirectional, thus accounting for the reduction in read-through of the H-strand promoter as well as the termination of the L-strand transcripts prior to its reaching the rRNA genes.[231,236,237]

The mtDNA mRNAs are translated on mitochondrial 55S ribosomes (mitoribosomes) composed of a large 39S and small 28S subunit. These ribosomes have a smaller amount of rRNA than bacterial or eukaryotic ribosomes but a larger number of ribosomal proteins.[238–240] mtDNA mRNAs lack the traditional Shine-Dalgarno sequence for ribosome binding and generally start with the initiation codon at the 5′ end. Translation is thought to initiate with the binding of the small subunit to a 40-base region of the mRNA. The ribosome then moves back to the 5′ end to initiate translation. The mRNA has been proposed to wrap around the ribosome, thus limiting polysome formation.[241,242]

The mitoribosomes are sensitive to the bacterial ribosome inhibitor chloramphenicol (CAP), but resistant to the cytosolic 80S ribosome inhibitors cycloheximide and emetine. They are also relatively insensitive to the aminoglycoside antibodies such as streptomycin and gentamycin.[243]

nDNA. In addition to the 13 mtDNA-encoded polypeptides, the mitochondrion is assembled from a large number of nuclear-encoded polypeptides. These polypeptides are synthesized on cytosolic 80S ribosomes and vectorially transported into the mitochondria via receptor binding to the outer membrane and transfer through the mitochondrial outer and inner membrane import channels.

The exact number of nuclear genes necessary to assemble a mitochondrion is not known. However, the analysis of various eukaryotic genomes suggests that on the order of 1000 nuclear genes may be required to assemble the human mitochondrion. The sequence of the entire yeast genome has provided one data set for estimating the number of genes necessary to assemble a mitochondrion. According to the MITOP database, 437 yeast genes have been identified as functioning in the mitochondria. This is presumably an underestimate because many relevant genes probably have not yet been recognized, suggesting the actual number may be somewhat higher. However, because the central functions of the mitochondria have remained the same throughout eukaryotic evolution, it is unlikely that the number of nuclear genes for mitochondrial functions could have doubled. Thus, we can estimate that the number of nuclear genes necessary for assembling the human mitochondrion is probably on the order of 1000.

Data on the genes involved in mitochondrial biogenesis in humans have been compiled in Tables 105-1 to 105-8. A larger list of nDNA mitochondrial genes is available at the Web site MITOP Mitochondrial Project at (www.mips.biochem.mpg.de/proj/medgen/mitop).[244] Currently, MITOP lists 334 human mitochondrial genes.

While determination of the proteins that make up mitochondrial structures has permitted the cloning of many of the structural polypeptides of the mitochondrion, many mitochondrial functions are currently unknown. To obtain a more complete catalogue of nDNA-encoded mitochondrial genes, a more general method was needed for cloning genes involved in mitochondrial biogenesis. Our laboratory developed such a method based on our observation that mice harboring severe mitochondrial OXPHOS defects attempt to compensate for the energetic defect by the synthesis of more mitochondria. This involves the coordinate up-regulation of both nDNA and mtDNA mitochondria gene transcripts. For example, in mice in which the heart/skeletal muscle ANT1 gene has been knocked out, the mutant mice muscle accumulates about four times more mitochondria than normal animals.[190] In concert with this increase in mitochondria, many of the mitochondrial gene transcripts are increased. Thus, by comparing the mRNA levels of the ANT1 −/− muscle with those of the ANT1 +/+ muscle, we cloned a variety of previously unknown proteins involved in mitochondrial biogenesis.

Transcripts that are up-regulated in the ANT1 −/− mice have been identified using differential display (DD) of ANT1 −/− versus ANT1 +/+ muscle mRNA. Our first set of differential display experiments identified 38 up-regulated transcripts. Seventeen of these mRNA/cDNAs were sufficiently abundant that their transcriptional induction could be confirmed by filter hybridization. Of these 17, 7 were mtDNA transcripts, including 4 of the mtDNA genes for complex I (MTND1, MTND4, MTND5, MTND6), 1 of the mtDNA subunits of complex IV (COI), the mtDNA 16S rRNA, and a cluster of mtDNA tRNAs. The nine up-regulated nDNA transcripts identified included several known energy metabolism proteins. There were the mitochondrial malate dehydrogenase, glycogen phosphorylase, two subunits of complex I (subunits 18 kDa and B8), and two subunits of complex IV (COXVa and COXVb). In addition, three novel cDNAs were found: Mcl-1, the muscle homologue of Bcl-2; WS-3; and Skd3.[245]

The Skd3 protein is particularly intriguing. This protein had been previously identified based on its ability to suppress a yeast K^+ transporter mutant, which could also be complemented by two other genes, both encoding members of the NSF family of proteins known to be involved in membrane fusion and organelle biogenesis.[246] The Skd3 protein is a 76-kDa protein with the C-terminal domain having homology to the Clp/HSP104 family of proteins. This family includes Hsp78 of *S. cerevisiae* that appears to cooperate with the mitochondrial matrix protein Hsp70 in mitochondrial maintenance. Skd3 also contains four ankyrin-like domains and a putative amino-terminal mitochondrial-targeting domain.[245] Hence, this protein might function to link the cellular cytoskeleton via the ankyrin domains with mitochondrial protein assembly through the Clp/HSP104 domain.

The cloning of novel proteins for mitochondrial assembly is valuable not only for increasing our understanding of the biology of the mitochondria, but also for providing candidate genes for determining the role of mitochondrial defects in degenerative disease. This was dramatically demonstrated when the DD products cloned from the ANT1 −/− skeletal muscle were compared to the predicted proteins of various movement disorder genes. The Skd3 protein was found to have significant similarity to the early-onset torsion dystonia gene (DYT1) product torsinA. This is the most severe and common form of hereditary dystonia, and is inherited in an autosomal dominant fashion with almost all cases resulting from a 3-np deletion (GAG) that removes one glutamate codon.[247]

The association between dystonia and up-regulated nDNA-encoded, mitochondrial genes was further extended by comparison of the lower abundance transcripts identified by differential display. Homology was found between one low abundance DD product, DD14p, and the DRN-1 protein responsible for the Mohr-Tranebjaerg syndrome, an X-linked dystonia and deafness disease.[212,245] This association between mitochondrial defects and dystonia is discussed further later.

Mitochondrial DNA Genetics

Each human cell contains hundreds of cytoplasmic mitochondria and thousands of mtDNAs. While the nDNA genes encoding mitochondrial functions follow traditional patterns of Mendelian inheritance, the cytoplasmic mitochondria and mtDNAs do not. Hence, to understand mitochondrial disease, we must understand the genetics of the mtDNA.

Mitochondria are Semiautonomous. Because the mitochondria retain their own self-replicating genome and associated replication, transcription, and translation systems, they behave as semiautonomous organisms within the human cell cytoplasm. This was first demonstrated through studies of cultured mammalian cells selected for resistance to the mitochondrial ribosome inhibitor, chloramphenicol (CAP) (Fig. 105-10). CAP-resistant (CAP^R) cells were enucleated by treatment with cytochalasin B to disaggregate the cytoskeleton and suspension in a centrifugal field, generally created using a density gradient. Under these conditions, the dense nucleus bands lower in the gradient than the cytoplasm. Consequently, the nucleus is pulled out of the cell on a long

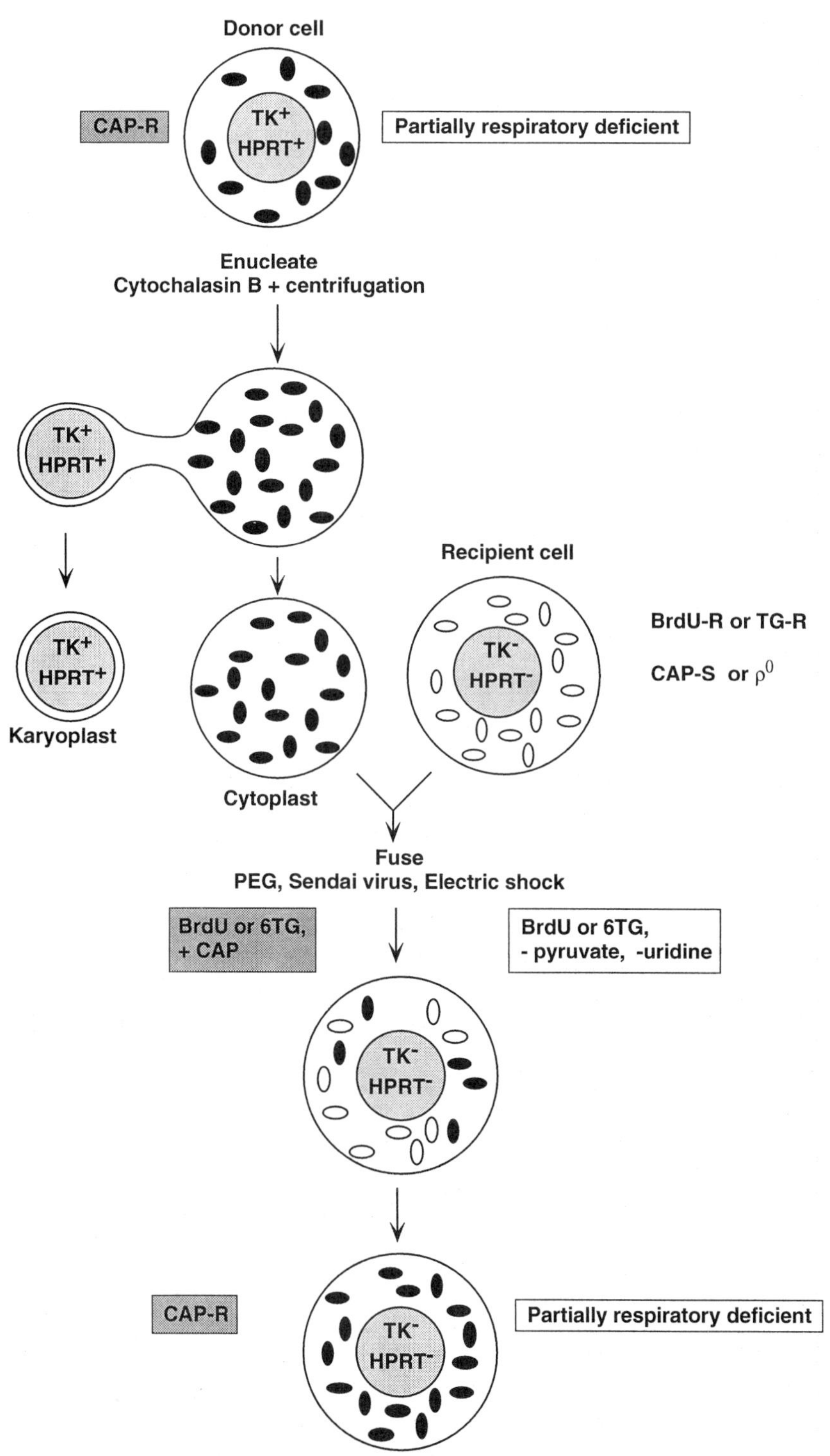

Fig. 105-10 Cybrid-transfer procedure for identifying mtDNA mutations. Cybrid transfer has been used for demonstrating the cytoplasmic inheritance of CAP resistance and for linking clinically important mtDNA mutations to mitochondrial OXPHOS defects. This drawing shows the successive stages of cybrid fusion. The mtDNA donor cell is enucleated and fused to the recipient cell. The cybrids are isolated by selecting for the recipient cell nucleus and for the donor cell mtDNAs. For transfer of CAP resistance (shaded boxes on left of cells), the CAP-R cytoplasts are fused to recipient cells containing CAP-S mtDNAs, and the cybrids are selected in BrdU or 6TG plus CAP. For transfer of disease-associated mtDNA mutations, the patient cytoplasts are fused to cells that have been cured of their mtDNAs (ρ^0). The cybrids are selected in BrdU or 6TG plus media deficient in uridine and/or pyruvate. Since ρ^0 cells die without these two metabolites, only the cybrids with partially functional respiratory chains will grow. (*Reprinted from Wallace.*[11] *Used with permission.*)

cytoplasmic thread that ultimately breaks, leaving a plasma membrane-bound nuclear fragment (karyoplast) and a plasma membrane-encapsulated cytoplasm containing the mitochondria and mtDNAs (cytoplast). The cytoplasts from CAP^R cells can then be fused to whole CAP-sensitive (CAP^S) cells. The resulting cytoplasmic hybrids or "cybrids" are selected by growth in an inhibitor, which selectively kills nonenucleated cytoplasmic donor cells, and in CAP, which kills unfused CAP^S recipient cells. Only those CAP^S cells that fused to CAP^R cytoplasms become doubly resistant and survive.[248,249] By this cybrid transfer procedure, CAP resistance was transferred from cell to cell and shown to be linked to restriction fragment length polymorphisms (RFLPs) of the mtDNA,[250] as well as to mtDNA-encoded protein polymorphisms.[33]

Subsequent molecular analysis of the CAP^R mtDNAs revealed that CAP resistance was due to single nucleotide changes in the peptidyl transferase region near the 3′ end of the 16S rRNA (MTRNR1). In CAP^R human cells the mutation was either a T to C transition at np 2991 or a C to A transversion at np 2939.[251] In CAP^R mouse cells, the mutation is a T to C transition at np 2433 in the 16S rRNA.[252,253] Subsequent studies have shown that CAP^R mtDNAs can be transferred to cells of a variety of differentiated states within the same species and function normally.[254] This process can be facilitated by removing the resident mtDNAs of the recipient cell prior to fusion using various techniques. One technique is to enucleate the recipient cell and fuse the resulting karyoplast with the cytoplast to yield a reconstituted cell.[255] A second technique was to cure the recipient cell of its resident mitochondria and mtDNAs by treatment with the ATP synthase inhibitory dye rhodamine-6G.[256] This eliminates the resident mitochondria mtDNAs.[257] The final approach has been to cure the recipient cell of its resident mtDNAs by growth in the mtDNA replication-inhibitor, ethidium bromide (EtBr). EtBr was first shown to be capable of eliminating the mtDNAs from cultured chicken cells, rendering them auxotrophic for uridine.[258] More recently, this same approach has been used to generate human cells that lack mtDNA (ρ^0 cells) and require pyruvate and uridine for growth.[259] Such ρ^0 recipient cells have provided a powerful tool for studying the biochemical basis of mtDNA disease mutations by permitting demonstration that a specific biochemical defect in a patient cell line can be transferred along with the patient mtDNAs to a ρ^0 cell having a different set of nuclear genes.[57,259–261]

Maternal Inheritance. The human mtDNA is strictly maternally inherited.[262,263] This is due in large measure to the fact that the mammalian egg contains about 100,000 mitochondria and mtDNAs, whereas the sperm contains on the order of 100 mtDNAs.[264,265] The sperm mtDNAs are contributed to the zygote at fertilization and will persist in interspecific crosses.[266] However, in intraspecific crosses the sperm mitochondria are selectively eliminated.[267] This has recently been correlated with the observation that the mitochondria in the sperm mid-piece are ubiquinated[268] and hence may be labeled for immediate destruction within the oocyte cytoplasm.

Replicative Segregation and Heteroplasmy. When a mutation arises in a cellular mtDNA, it creates a mixed intracellular population of mutant and normal molecules known as heteroplasmy. When a cell divides, it is a matter of chance whether the mutant mtDNAs are partitioned into one daughter cell or another. Thus, over time the percentage of mutant mtDNAs in different cell lineages can drift toward either pure mutant or normal (homoplasmy), a process known as replicative segregation. In somatic cell hybrids between transformed human cell lines, the direction of segregation appears to be random.[269] However, in crosses between HeLa cells and either diploid fibroblasts[270–272] or lymphoblastoid cell lines,[254] the HeLa mtDNAs are preferentially lost, even when selected for using CAP resistance. The reason for this directional replicative segregation is unknown. However, it may have clinical significance because it has been reported that in five of seven ρ^0 cybrids heteroplasmic for the pathogenic tRNA mutation MTTL1*MELAS3243G,[273] the wild-type mtDNAs were selectively lost and the mutant mtDNAs preferentially retained.[274] This directional segregation may also involve nuclear genes. In a another study, using the same osteosarcoma 143B TK$^-$ ρ^0 recipient cell above, one of 14 heteroplasmic cybrids segregated toward mutant mtDNAs, while the others remained stable. By contrast, using a different ρ^0 recipient cell (A549, B2), 5 of 25 heteroplasmic cybrids segregated to wild-type mtDNAs.[275] Preferential growth of cells with wild-type mtDNAs has also been observed during cybrid clone isolation[276] and in propagation of heteroplasmic fibroblasts.[277] Hence, the rules governing the directionality of mtDNA segregation and the factors that influence it still remain to be elucidated.

Threshold Expression. Different tissues and organs rely on mitochondrial energy generation to different extents. This has been well established through studies of respiratory inhibitor toxicity in mammals including primates. Acute respiratory toxicity can result in unconsciousness, while chronic toxicity can result in optic atrophy, basal ganglia degeneration, and cardiac and renal failure.[278] Studies on maternal pedigrees harboring heteroplasmic mtDNA mutations indicate that as the percentage of mutant mtDNAs increases, energy production declines. Ultimately, energy output falls below the minimum necessary for normal tissue function, and clinical manifestations result. Observations from many cases now indicate that the bioenergetic expression thresholds for human organs are, in decreasing order, the central nervous system, heart and skeletal muscle, the renal system, the endocrine system, and the liver.[11,279–281]

In somatic cell hybrids between CAP^R and CAP^S cells, as little as 10 percent of the mtDNAs need to be CAP^R for the cell to survive and grow in CAP.[269] By contrast, in diseases resulting from mtDNA tRNA mutations, the percentage of mutant mtDNAs must be high before the biochemical and clinical expression threshold is exceeded. In families harboring the MTTK*MERRF8344G mutation,[279] it has been observed that individuals in the 20- to 40-year-old range require at least 85 percent mutant mtDNAs for symptoms to appear.[279,281,282] This is consistent with data from cultured somatic cells in which the percentage of MTTK*MERRF8344G or MTTLI*MELAS 3243G mutant mtDNAs must exceed 90 percent before both protein synthesis and O_2 consumption decline.[283]

Mitochondrial DNA Complementation. The mitochondria and mtDNAs within a cell also appear to fuse, permitting the mtDNA genomes to complement each other in *trans*. This was first demonstrated by fusing two human cells together to form hybrids, one cell carrying the CAP^R mutation linked to an MTND3 protein polymorphism (MV-1) and the other carrying a CAP^S mtDNA linked to the other MTND3 allele (MV-2). When the mitochondrial translation products of the hybrids were selectively labeled by growth in ^{35}S-methionine together with emetine to block cytosolic protein synthesis, both MV-1 and MV-2 were synthesized in proportion to the percentage of the two mtDNAs. Moreover, when the mitochondrial proteins were labeled in the presence of both emetine and CAP, both proteins were still labeled in proportion to the parental genomes. This implies that in these hybrids the CAP^R mtDNA ribosomes were able to translate the MTND3 mRNAs from the CAP^S mtDNAs, thus suggesting that the CAP^R and CAP^S mtDNA genomes occupied the same mitochondrial structures.[33]

Intracellular mtDNA complementation has also been demonstrated in cells heteroplasmic for the pathogenic tRNA mutations MTTL1*MERRF 8344G. In cybrids derived from heteroplasmic cells, as little as 10 percent of normal mtDNAs was able to restore oxygen consumption and mitochondrial protein synthesis. However, when essentially homoplasmic MTTL1*MELAS3243G genomes were mixed with homoplasmic MTTK*MERRF8344G genomes by two-step cybrid selection, complementation was not observed for either oxygen consumption or mitochondrial translation.[283] This result contrasts with recent studies in which complementation was observed in fusions between cells harboring nonoverlapping mtDNA deletions.[284] Hence, the majority of evidence supports intracellular mitochondrial fusion and mtDNA complementation.

Mitochondrial DNA Recombination. The strict maternal inheritance of the mtDNA means that independent mtDNA lineages rarely become mixed in the same cytoplasm, and hence rarely, if ever, recombine.[285,286] While recombination in cultured mammalian cells is infrequent,[287] evidence for the interconversion of duplicated and deleted mtDNA molecules with the same breakpoint junction within patient cells has suggested that intramolecular recombination may be relatively frequent.[288] This has been confirmed by showing that somatic cell hybrids between two cells, each homoplasmic for a different nonoverlapping mtDNA deletion, will not only complement each other, but in rare circumstances, actually coalesce to form a recombinant molecule containing the two genomes in a tandem array.[284]

High Mutation Rate. The mtDNA mutation rate is much higher than that of nuclear genes.[289] Assessment of the rate of accumulation of sequence polymorphisms between nuclear and mtDNA genes which function in the same enzymes indicates that the mtDNA nucleotide sequence evolves about 10 to 17 times faster than the nuclear DNA sequence.[154,170] This high sequence evolution rate has resulted in the accumulation of a broad spectrum of mtDNA sequence polymorphisms in human populations, but also may be a common source of hereditary disease mutations.

mtDNA VARIATION IN HUMAN POPULATIONS

The high mtDNA mutation rate is reflected by extensive mtDNA sequence variation between populations. Polymorphisms that arise in the various human populations and subsequently reach polymorphic frequencies must be selectively neutral or near-neutral to avoid being eliminated by selection and to become prevalent through genetic drift. Hence these population-specific polymorphisms represent only a fraction of the actual mtDNA mutations that occur in the mtDNA.

The majority of mtDNA mutations are deleterious and are rapidly eliminated by selection. These deleterious mutations can be either base substitutions or rearrangement mutations, and the resulting respiratory phenotype is manifested in the individual as a genetic disease.[290]

When analyzing the mtDNA of an individual from a possible mtDNA disease, it is generally not immediately apparent which of the multiple sequence differences present in the patient's mtDNA, relative to the "Cambridge" reference sequence,[25] is the pathogenic mutation. Hence, it is necessary to know the nature and extent of "normal" mtDNA variation in populations before it is possible to effectively identify disease mutations.

Therefore, there are two major clinical reasons for characterizing the nature and extent of population-specific mtDNA polymorphism. First, by knowing which mtDNA variants are normal, these can be ignored when analyzing a patient's mtDNA. Second, not all population variants are completely neutral. As a result, the mtDNA background can affect the expression and clinical symptoms associated with certain deleterious mtDNA mutations.

World mtDNA Phylogeny and the Origin of Women

Because the mtDNA is strictly maternally inherited, the mtDNA sequence has evolved by the sequential accumulation of base substitutions along radiating maternal lineages. Thus, as women migrated out of Africa into the different continents about 130,000 YBP they accumulated mtDNA mutations that today are seen as high-frequency, continent-specific mtDNA sequence polymorphisms. These polymorphisms are associated with specific mtDNA haplotypes, and groups of related haplotypes (haplogroups).[11,291]

The first clear evidence that mtDNA variation correlated with the ethnic and geographic origin of the individual came from our survey of *Hpa*I RFLPs in African, Asian, and European-American mtDNAs. This revealed that in Africans, 96 percent of Pygmies, 93 percent of San Bushmen, and 71 percent of Bantus harbored an *Hpa*I restriction site at np 3592 not seen in Asians or Europeans. By convention, all polymorphic restriction sites, including the *Hpa*I np 3592 site, are defined by the 5′ end of the recognition sequence, but the polymorphic nucleotide may be different. For example, the *Hpa*I np 3592 site change is caused by a C-to-T transition at np 3594. In contrast to African mtDNAs, about 13 percent of Asians lacked an *Hpa*I restriction site at np 12406 (G to A at np 12406), which was present in all other mtDNAs.[292] A further survey of the mtDNA variation detected using six highly informative restriction enzymes (*Hpa*I, *Bam*HI, *Hae*II, *Msp*I, and *Ava*II) and Southern blotting confirmed that mtDNA variation was high and correlated strongly with the geographic origin of the individual. It also showed that all mtDNAs were part of a single phylogenetic tree, that the greatest variation was in Africa, and that the tree was about 100,000 years old.[293] Extensive studies by our group, as well as by others, ultimately led to the characterization of 3065 mtDNAs from 62 geographic samples using these 6 enzymes. This revealed 149 haplotypes and 81 polymorphic sites. This analysis confirmed (a) that the mtDNA polymorphisms within each mtDNA were virtually in total linkage disequilibrium, consistent with a low frequency of recombination; (b) that mtDNA variation correlated highly with the ethnic and geographic origin of the individual; (c) that there was a single mtDNA tree; (d) and that the greatest variation and deepest root of the tree was in Africa, consistent with an African origin of humans. The extent of mtDNA sequence differences between continental populations was estimated from this data by calculating the GST statistic. For the mtDNA, the GST was 0.35 +/− 0.025, implying that about 35 percent of the mtDNA variation was continent-specific. By contrast, the comparable nDNA value was 0.12. Hence, the mtDNA encompasses much greater continent-specific sequence diversity than the nDNA.[285]

A recent African origin of human mtDNAs was also demonstrated by the investigations of Wilson, Cann, Stoneking, and coworkers.[294] These investigators purified the individual mtDNAs from cells or tissues, digested the DNA with 12 restriction endonucleases (*Hpa*I, *Ava*II, *Fnu*DII, *Hha*I, *Hpa*II, *Mbo*I, *Taq*I, *Rsa*I, *Hin*fI, *Hae*III, *Alu*I, and *Dde*I), end-labeled the fragments, and resolved the fragments using polyacrylamide gels and autoradiography.[295] A survey of 147 mtDNAs, including 34 Asians, 21 aboriginal Australians, 26 aboriginal New Guineans, 46 Caucasians, and 20 Africans (18 of whom were African-Americans), also revealed that there was a single mtDNA tree, that the deepest root occurred in Africa, and that Africa harbored the greatest sequence diversity. Hence, Africa is the origin of *Homo sapiens*. Using an estimated sequence evolution rate of 2 percent to 4 percent per million years (MYR), the human mtDNA tree was calculated to be about 200,000 years old.[294]

This analysis was extended to include 62 Japanese[296] and 119 Papua New Guineans.[297] The Papua New Guineans were sampled from 25 localities, and significant differences in mtDNA variation were found between the highland and coastal populations. Combining the Papua New Guinea data with the previous European, Asian, and African data permitted calculation of a global GST of 0.31,[297] a value similar to that found for the six-enzyme analysis discussed above.

The African origin of mtDNA variation was also supported through sequence analyses of the 1121-np noncoding control region of the mtDNA. This region has a three- to fourfold greater sequence diversity than the coding region. Analysis of the control-region sequences from 189 individuals, 121 of whom were native African, once again confirmed that the greatest sequence diversity was in Africans, that the deepest root was between Africans, and that the coalescence time of the mtDNA tree (phylogeny) was between 166,000 and 249,000 YBP.[298] The African root of this phylogeny was subsequently challenged on the basis that multiple equally probable parsimony trees could be generated from the data.[299] However, other phylogenetic analysis procedures, such as neighbor-joining trees, have reaffirmed the cohesiveness of the deepest African associations and thus support the African origin of the mtDNA phylogeny.[300]

Analysis of the control-region sequence of 95 individuals, including 61 Japanese, confirmed that the greatest diversity and deepest root occurred in Africa and revealed that "Mongoloid" mtDNAs were subdivided into two distinct groups.[301] Analysis of 117 Caucasian mtDNAs confirmed the distinctive nature of many European mtDNAs and revealed that the various mtDNA lineages were widely disseminated throughout Europe.[302]

Finally, comparison of the original European mtDNA sequence[25] with that from an African, a Japanese, and four African apes (common and pygmy chimpanzees, gorilla, and orangutan) revealed that the European and Japanese mtDNAs were most similar, that the African mtDNA was more divergent, and that the nearest ape relatives, the chimpanzees, were 10 times more divergent from humans than Africans are from Asians and Europeans. Using the orangutan-African ape divergence time of 13 million YBP as reference, this study gave an age for human mtDNA radiation of 143,000 ± 18,000 YBP and a time for European and Japanese radiation of 70,000 ± 13,000 YBP.[303]

All of these studies lead to the same conclusion. The human mtDNA tree appears to have originated in Africa about ≈150,000 YBP. As women migrated from Africa to colonize new lands, additional mtDNA mutations arose and became established by genetic drift, resulting in continent-specific mtDNA variation. Today, these population-specific polymorphisms constitute the background on which potentially pathogenic mtDNA mutations must be identified.

Cataloging Continent-Specific mtDNA Variation

While the above methods permitted elucidation of the general features of human mtDNA evolution, a more detailed analysis of mtDNA variation was necessary for clinical studies and for addressing additional anthropologic questions on the age and origin of Africans, Europeans, Asians, and Native Americans. To increase the sensitivity of our analyses, we developed a new mtDNA analysis procedure — high-resolution RFLP analysis — in which the mtDNAs from a variety of human samples could be amplified by using PCR in nine overlapping fragments. Each fragment was then digested with 14 restriction endonucleases (*Alu*I, *Ava*II, *Bam*HII, *Dde*I, *Hae*II, *Hha*I, *Hinf*I, *Hinc*II, *Hpa*I, *Hpa*I, *Msp*I, *Mbo*I, *Rsa*I, and *Taq*I), and the fragments resolved on agarose gels and detected by ethidium bromide staining and UV fluorescence. This procedure surveys >20 percent of the mtDNA sequence, and the aggregate of the restriction-site polymorphisms for each mtDNA is used to define the mtDNA haplotype.[304,305] The regional PCR fragments can also be sequenced, permitting extension of the analysis to areas of interest such as the hypervariable control region.[306,307] The sequence differences between mtDNAs can then be compared by using various phylogenetic procedures including parsimony, neighbor-joining, and unweighed pair-group analyses. These phylogenetic trees reveal the relatedness of the mtDNAs, with the more similar mtDNAs clustering together. The extent of sequence diversity within or between groups of related haplotypes (haplogroups) can also be calculated.[308–311]

African mtDNA Variation

To better characterize African mtDNA variation, we surveyed, using high-resolution RFLP analysis, the mtDNAs from 214 Africans, including 101 from Senegal (60 Mandenkalu, 20 Wolof, 8 Pular, and 13 others from eight tribes); 22 Mbuti (Eastern) Pygmies from Zaire and 17 Biaka (Western) Pygmies from Central African Republic; and 74 South Africans including 43 Kung and 31 Khwe.[312,313] This survey revealed 105 haplotypes defined by greater than 157 polymorphic sites. Phylogenetic analysis revealed that 75 of the haplotypes formed a single, coherent, African-specific haplogroup designated "L" (Fig. 105-11), which is defined by the African-specific *Hpa*I site at np 3592 together with the *Dde*I site at np 10394 (A to G at np 10398). This lineage is subdivided into two sublineages, Ll and L2. Ll encompasses 52 percent of the L haplotypes and 29 percent of all African mtDNAs and is defined by an additional *Hinf*I site at np 10806 (T to C at np 10810). L2 encompasses 48 percent of the L haplotypes and 34 percent of the African mtDNAs and is defined by an additional combined *Hinf*I site gain at np 16389 and *Ava*II site loss at np 16390 (G to A at np 16390). All *Hpa*I np 3592-positive haplotypes are of African origin, with the only exceptions occurring in populations known from historical evidence to have had Africa contact.

Several other features of haplogroup L are of interest. Two length mutations were observed in L1: a 9-np COII/tRNA^{Lys} deletion between nps 8272 and 8289[314,315] found in two African haplotypes, AFR 60 (representing 27 percent of Mbuti Pygmies) and AFR 61 (representing 24 percent of Biaka Pygmies); and a 10- to 12-bp insertion of cytosines (Cs) between the tRNA^{Tyr} and COI gene (nps 5895 to 5899) in Biaka Pygmies with the ARF66 haplotype (Fig. 105-11).

The remaining African mtDNAs form a heterogeneous array of four lineages, which is designated haplogroup L3, each defined by specific restriction-site gains or losses.[316] One of these lineages is defined by loss of the *Dde*I site at np 10394. This lineage represents only a few percent of the African mtDNAs, yet it appears to be the progenitor of roughly half of all European, Asian, and Native American mtDNAs. Within this lineage are mtDNAs that also lack a *Hinf*I site at np 12308. This mtDNA haplotype is closely related to the European-specific haplogroup H.

Analysis of African mtDNA control region sequences reveals many of the same population subdivisions. However, in some cases the control region sequences subdivide haplotypes and in others haplotype markers subdivide control region sequence groups.[313]

Analyses of the population distribution of the African haplotypes revealed that each of the four primary populations studied (the Senegalese of West Africa, the Mbuti Pygmies, the Biaka Pygmies, and the Vasekela Kung) has a distinctive set of related core haplotypes that are specific for that population (Fig. 105-11). The core haplotypes of the Vasekela Kung of South Africa, designated "α," occur in haplogroup L1 and are defined by *Msp*I site losses at np 8112 and 8150, and *Ava*II site gain at np 8249, and an *Hae*III site loss at np 8250. This cluster of Vasekela Kung haplotypes is at the deepest root of the African phylogeny, suggesting that the Kung are one of the oldest populations. The Biaka Pygmy core haplotypes, designated β, also reside in haplogroup L1 and are defined by an *Alu*I site gain at np 10319. The Mbuti Pygmies, designated γ, reside in haplogroup L2 and are delineated by a *Dde*I site loss at np 13065, and an *Rsa*I site gain at np 11776. Finally, the Bantu-derived Senegalese core haplotypes also belong to haplogroup L2 and are defined by an *Hae*III site loss at np 322, A *Dde*I site loss at np 679, and an *Hae*III site loss at np 13957. Calculation of the sequence divergence of the core haplotypes for each population reveals that the Vasekela Kung α lineage and Biaka Pygmy β lineages are the oldest, while the Mbuti Pygmy and Senegalese lineages are much younger. Hence, the Kung and Biaka Pygmies are more representative of the proto-Africans and the Biaka and Mbuti Pygmies may have had independent origins.

Calculation of the accumulated sequence diversity of the African-specific haplogroup L and its subhaplogroups L1 and L2 gave values of 0.356 percent, 0.328 percent, and 0.171 percent, respectively. The total African mtDNA sequence diversity was 0.364 percent. This means that haplogroup L has the highest sequence diversity of any continent-specific haplogroup and that Africa encompasses the greatest diversity of any continent. Using our estimate of the mtDNA sequence evolution rate of 2.2 percent-2.9 percent/million years (Myr),[317] the L haplogroup is between 123,000 and 162,000 years old, and the total African mtDNA lineage is between 126,000 and 166,000 years old (Fig. 105-4).

Calculation of the intragroup and intergroup sequence variation of the various African groups strengthen these observations. The Biaka Pygmies and the Vasekela Kung had the greatest intragroup sequence variation: 0.342 percent and 0.320 percent, respectively, comparable to that of Africa as a whole. This further supports the conclusion that these are among the oldest populations. The Mbuti Pygmies and Senegalese have intragroup sequence diversities in the range of 0.241 to 0.277, confirming that these populations are younger. A neighbor-joining tree analysis clearly separates the Biaka Pygmies from the Mbuti Pygmies, and places the Mbuti Pygmies on the same side of the tree as the Bantu-derived populations. Hence, the Mbuti and Biaka pygmies probably are distinct populations.[313]

Overall, the mtDNA data show that African mtDNAs are distinct, that they are the oldest with the greatest diversity and deepest root, that the Vasekela Kung and Biaka Pygmies are among the original populations of Africa, and that the "Pygmy" morphology arose two independent times in Africa.

European mtDNA Variation

European mtDNA sequence variation has been defined by the analysis of 259 samples from individuals of European ancestry living in the United States, Canada, Finland, Italy, and

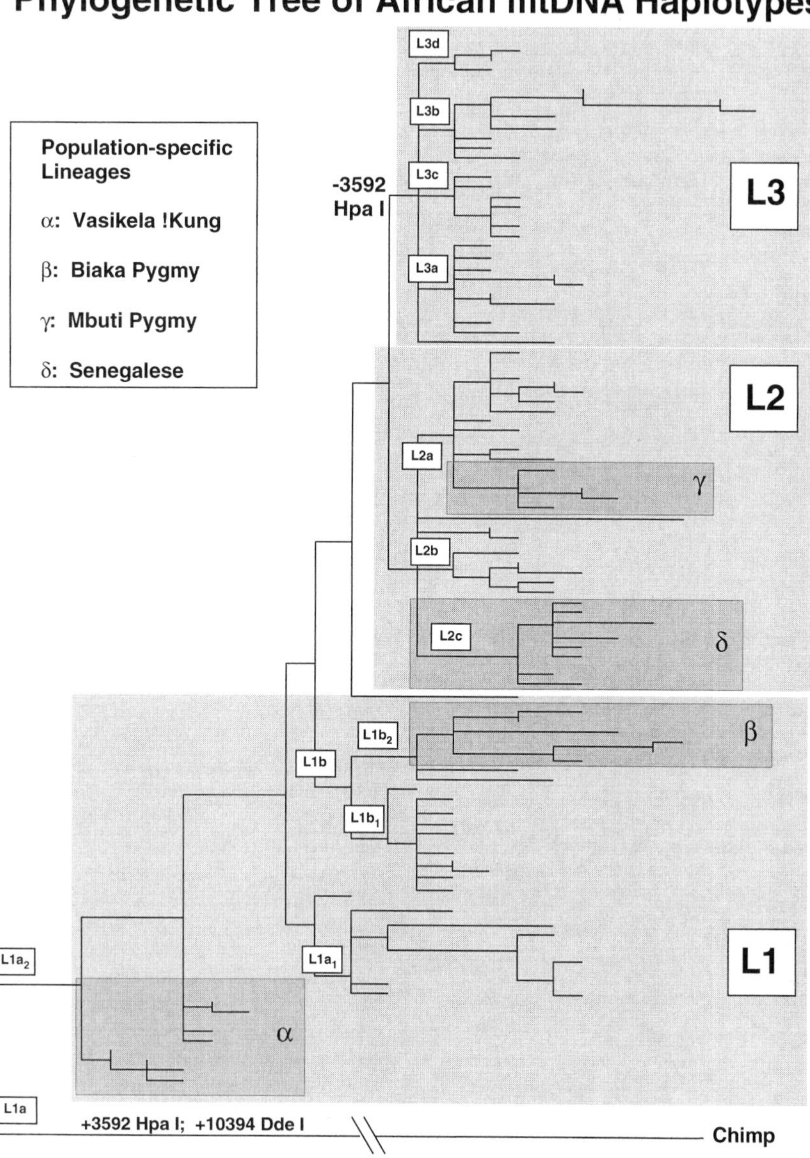

Fig. 105-11 **Phylogeny of African mtDNA haplotypes. This tree summarizes the results from 214 from Africans including 101 Senegalese, 22 Mbuti Pygmies, 17 Biaka Pygmies, 43 Kung, and 31 Khwe, encompassing 105 haplotypes. Each haplotype is positioned relative to the others based on number of genetic similarities or differences. The closer together two haplotypes are in the tree, the more similar is their sequence. mtDNA polymorphisms that arose recently are present in only one or a few mtDNAs and define the terminal twigs of the tree. By contrast, polymorphisms that arose early in human mtDNA evolution are shared by larger groups of related mtDNAs and define major branches of the tree. These groups of related mtDNA haplotypes are called haplogroups. To identify the oldest mtDNA haplogroups, the human mtDNA haplotypes are compared to that of a more distantly related mtDNA, the outgroup, in this case chimpanzee mtDNA. This permits the "rooting" of the tree. For African mtDNAs, one of the oldest and most significant polymorphisms is the *Hpa*I site at np 3592. This site is African-specific with the oldest two-thirds of the tree having the *Hpa*I 3592 site (+3592 *Hpa*I) and being defined as macro-haplogroup L, with haplogroup subdivisions L1 and L2. The absence of this site is defined as haplogroup L3. Haplogroup L3 forms the bridge between African mtDNAs and European and Asian mtDNAs. Within the L1, L2, and L3 divisions are multiple haplogroups and subhaplogroups, some of which correlate highly with the population sampled. Thus a core block of related haplotypes in Lla, designated α, are specific for the Kung; a second block in Llb2, labeled β, are specific for the Biaka Pygmies; a third block in L2a, designated γ, are specific for Mbuti Pygmies; while a fourth block in L2c, labeled δ, are specific for the Senegalese. This implies that these core haplotypes arose with these populations. The fact that the α block of the Kung and the β block the Biaka Pygmies are closest to the root of the tree implies that these are among the oldest African populations. While the deep branches of this tree are very robust, the most distal twigs are subject to greater interpretive fluctuation. Hence, this tree is one of the thousands that could be drawn in which the major branches are retained but the precise branching order of the individual haplotypes can vary. This is standard. (*Reproduced from Chen et al.*[313] *Used with permission.*)**

Sweden.[318,319] Restriction analysis revealed 178 polymorphic sites that define approximately 170 haplotypes.[318,319] Phylogenetic analysis showed that all European mtDNAs could be subdivided into two groups by the presence (1/4) or absence (3/4) of the *Dde*I site at np 10394 (Fig. 105-12). Thus, Europeans exhibit a marked increase in the proportion of −10394 *Dde*I mtDNAs over the 4 percent seen in Africans.

In addition to the macro subdivision of European mtDNAs by the *Dde*I site at np 10394, nine distinct European mtDNA haplogroups have also been observed. Those lacking the *Dde*I site at np 10394 are haplogroups H, T, U, V, W, and X, while those retaining the *Dde*I np 10394 site are I, J, and K.

Of the haplogroups that lack the *DdeI* np 10394 site, haplogroup H also lacks an *Alu*I site at np 7025 (C to T at np

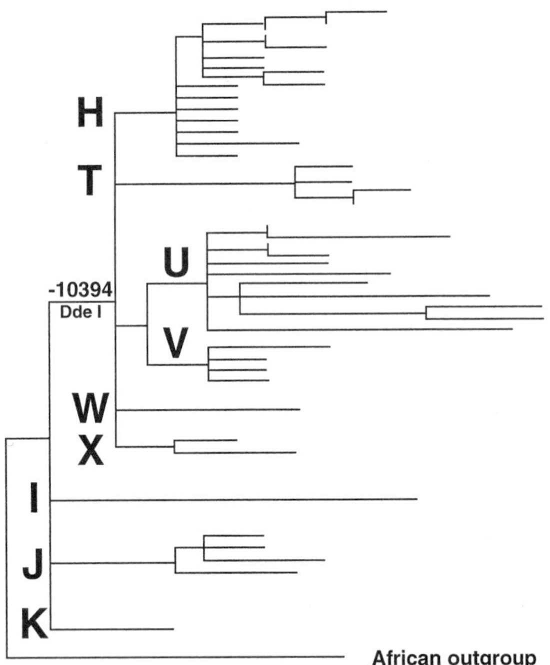

Fig. 105-12 Phylogeny of European mtDNA haplotypes. This representative tree encompasses the analysis of 86 samples from individuals of European ancestry. The tree is bifurcated by the presence or absence of an ancient polymorphism, the *DdeI* site at np 10394. European mtDNAs lacking the 10394 site fall into six distinct haplogroups: H, T, U, V, W, and X; while those retaining the site fall into three major haplogroups: I, J, and K. Each haplogroup is defined by distinctive polymorphisms (see text). These nine European-specific haplogroups account for over 98 percent of all mtDNAs found in Europe.[318,319] As for all parsimony trees, there are many alternative European mtDNA phylogenies, but the central branches are quite robust.

7028). This haplogroup encompasses 40.5 percent of European mtDNAs. Haplogroup T is defined by the presence of a *Bam*HI site at np 13366 and an *Alu*I site at np 15606 and accounts for 15.2 percent of European mtDNAs. Haplogroup U is defined by the presence of a *Hin*fI site at np 12308 and accounts for 14.7 percent of European mtDNAs. Haplogroup V is delineated by the loss of and *Nla*III site at np 4577 and is found in 4.8 percent of Europeans, while haplogroup X is in part defined by the loss of a *Dde*I site at np 1715 and is found in about 6.9 percent of European mtDNAs. Of the haplotypes that retain the *Dde*I site, haplogroup I is defined by the loss of the *Dde*I np 1715 site, and the gain of an *Ava*II site at 8249 and an *Alu*I site at np 10028 and represents 6.7 percent of European mtDNAs. Haplogroup J is identified by the loss of a *Bst*NI site at np 13708 and is found in about 11.3 percent of European mtDNAs; haplogroup K is delineated by the loss of an *Hae*II site at np 9052 and the gain of a *Hin*fI site at np 12308 and is found in 9.1 percent of Europeans. The sequence diversity of haplogroup H is 0.065 percent, giving an age of this lineage of 22,000 to 30,000 YBP. However, the sequence divergence of haplogroup U, which is shared between Europeans and African Bantu, is 0.148 percent, giving an age of 51,000 to 67,000 YBP. Hence, haplogroup U may represent one of the founder lineages of Europe.[319] The overall sequence divergence between the two major branches of the European phylogeny is 0.113 percent, giving an age for the colonization of Europe of between 39,000 and 51,000 YBP.[318]

Analysis of the control regions of the European mtDNAs revealed additional continent-specific markers.[302] However, one control-region mutation in haplogroup I proved to be totally novel, with potential implications for the evolution of the human mtDNAs. All haplogroup I mtDNAs had a homoplasmic insertion of two to six Cs within a cluster of Cs in the sequence ACCCCCC (box 2), where the A is located at np 567. This germ line mutation increases the homology between this sequence and the nearby control-region sequence ACGCCCCCTCCCCCGCT (box 1), where the A is located at np 302. Because of this homology, every individual who inherits the box 2 germ line insertion mutation becomes prone to undergo a somatic mutation during development. In this somatic mutation, the region between boxes 1 and 2 is duplicated as a 270-np direct repeat, possibly through slipped misreplication.[318] The somatic 270-bp duplication duplicates the H-strand promoter (nps 545 to 567), the L-strand promoter (nps 392 to 445), the two intervening mitochondrial transcription factor binding sites (nps 418 to 445 and nps 523 to 550), CSBIII (nps 346 to 363), part of CSBII (nps 299 to 315), and the putative replication primer processing site (nps 317 to 321).[318,320] This raises the possibility that the duplicated molecules are transcribed twice as frequently and may be preferentially replicated, providing selective advantage for this mutation. This may explain why the unstable box 2 insertion has been maintained throughout the 34,000-year history of haplogroup I.[318]

Asian mtDNA Variation

To further define Asian mtDNA sequence variation, we analyzed the mtDNAs from 153 central and Southeast Asians, including aboriginal Malays and Orang Ash, aboriginal Borneans, Han Chinese, Vietnamese, Koreans, and Malaysian Indians,[304] as well as 54 Tibetans[321] and 758 Siberians from 11 aboriginal populations, including the Chukchi and Koryaks from northeastern-most Siberia.[307,322,323] A representative Asian phylogenetic tree encompassing 42 Tibetan haplotypes, 106 Asian haplotypes, and 34 Siberian haplotypes is presented in Fig. 105-13. This phylogeny shows that all Asian mtDNAs can be subdivided into two macro-haplogroups defined by the presence or absence of the polymorphic site at *Dde*I at np 10394, which also bifurcates the European mtDNA lineages. Moreover, every Asian mtDNA that harbors the *Dde*I site at np 10394 also has an adjacent *Alu*I site at np 10397 (C to T at np 10400). The macro-haplogroup defined by the presence of the *Dde*I np 10394 and the *Alu*I np 10397 sites has been designated macro-haplogroup M (or also as "(+/+)"). The constant association of the *Dde*I np 10394 and *Alu*I np 10394 in Asians, but not in Africans or Europeans, implies that the *Alu*I np 10397 mutation must have arisen on an mtDNA carrying the *Dde*I np 10394 mutation as women migrated out of Africa and into Asia.

In addition to this major bifurcation of Asian mtDNAs, there are a number of distinctive sublineages of relevance to Asian and Native American prehistory. Haplogroups A, B, C, and D have proved to be the progenitors of virtually all Native American mtDNAs. Haplogroups A and B lack both the *Dde*I site at np 10394 and the *Alu*I site at np 10397, while haplogroups C and D have these sites. In addition, haplogroup A is defined by an *Hae*III site at np 663 (A to G at np 663), haplogroup B by an independent occurrence of the 9-np deletion between the COII and $tRNA^{Lys}$ genes, haplogroup C by the simultaneous *Hin*cII site loss at np 13259 and an *Alu*I site gain at np 13262 (A to G at np 13262), and haplogroup D by the loss of an *Alu*I site at np 5176 (C to A at np 5178). These haplogroups are further delineated in most Asians and Native Americans by specific control-region variants. For haplogroup A, these include variants at nps 16362 (T to C), 16319 (G to A), 16290 (C to T), and 16223 (C to T); for haplogroup B, variants at nps 16217 (T to C) and 16189 (T to C); for haplogroup C, variants at nps 16327 (C to T), 16298 (T to C), and 16223 (C to T); and, for haplogroup D, variants at nps 16362 (T to C) and 16223 (C to T).[306]

Three other prominent Asian haplogroups are E, F, and G. Haplogroups E and G have the combined *Dde*I and *Alu*I sites at nps 10394 and 10397; haplogroup F lacks these sites. Haplogroup E is further defined by an *Hpa*I site loss at np 7598, haplogroup G by the presence of an *Hae*III site at np 4830 and an *Hpa*I site at np 4831, and haplogroup F is delineated by the combined

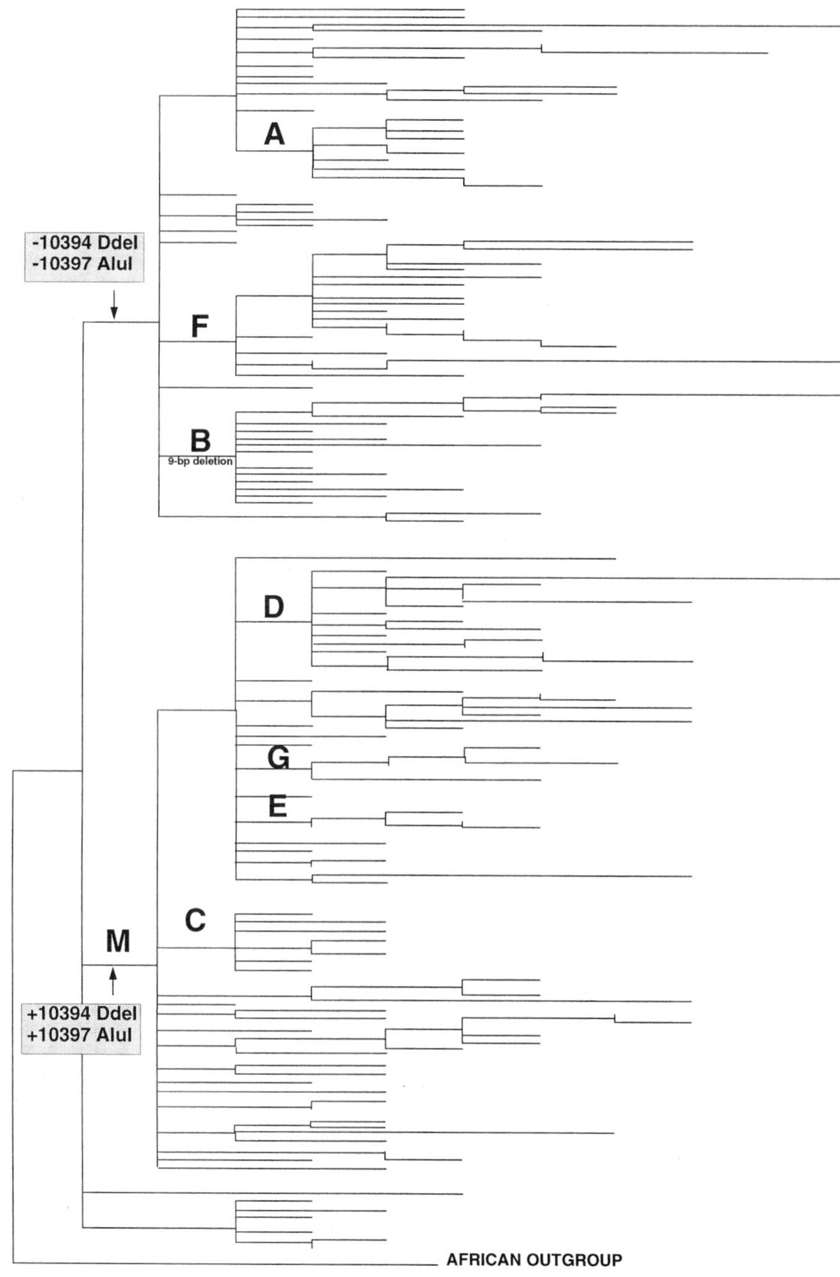

Fig. 105-13 Phylogeny of Asian mtDNA Haplotypes. This representative tree is based on data from 153 central and southeast Asians, 54 Tibetans, and 758 aboriginal Siberians. The Asian mtDNA phylogeny is bifurcated into two macro-haplogroups. One macro-haplogroup lacks the *DdeI* site at np 10394 as well as an *AluI* site at np 10397, and thus is designated (−/−), while the other macro-haplogroup has these restriction sites and is thus designated (+/+). The latter group is called macro-haplogroup M. Within these two major Asian mtDNA lineages are multiple important haplogroups. Haplogroup F is (−/−) and is found at high frequency in Southeast Asia but declines toward the northeast. Haplogroups A and B are −/− while haplogroups C and D are (+/+). These four mtDNAs lineages are at a low frequency in southern Asia but rise to high frequencies in northeast Asia, where they participated in the peopling of the Americas. (*Reprinted from Torroni et al.*[321] *Used with permission.*)

HpaI/HincII site loss at np 12406, the first Asian-specific polymorphism observed.[292,324] All of these haplogroups show marked frequency variation throughout Asia. Haplogroup F is prominent in southern Asian populations, being found in 32 percent of Vietnamese mtDNAs and 21 percent of Malay mtDNAs. It is present in about 15 percent of Koreans and Tibetans but is virtually absent in Siberia. By contrast, haplogroups A, C, D, E, and G are absent in southern Asian populations, including Vietnamese, Malays, Sabah, Malay aboriginals, and New Guineans, but are found at significant frequencies in Tibetans, Koreans, and Han Chinese. This north-south distinction supports the dichotomization of Asians into the Sinodont (northern) and Sundadont (southern) Asian populations.[325,326] Furthermore, haplogroups A, C, and D extend into Siberia populations analyzed, reaching maximum frequencies of 68 percent, 84 percent, and 28 percent, respectively. Haplogroup A reaches its highest frequencies in the Chukchi and Koryaks, the northeastern most populations of Siberia and likely progenitors of Native Americans. The haplogroup frequencies of the Koryaks are 5 percent A, 36 percent C, 1 percent D, and 42 percent G, 10 percent Y, and 6 percent other, while those of the Chukchi are 68 percent A, 11 percent C, 12 percent D, and 9 percent G.[307,322,323]

Haplogroup B, defined by the 9-np COII-tRNA^{Lys} deletion, displays a markedly different distribution. It is common throughout central and southern Asia and is prominent in coastal Asian populations, approaching fixation (100 percent) in certain Pacific island populations.[297,304,327] It is virtually absent from all nine Siberian populations analyzed, yet reappears throughout North, Central, and South American Native American populations.[286,306,307] The high frequency of this haplogroup among coastal Asian and Pacific island populations and its striking absence in Siberians relative to Central Asians and Native Americans raises the possibility that haplogroup B mtDNAs did not come to the Americas via a trans-Siberian migration, but rather may have crossed from Asia to the Americas by migration along the Siberian coast. This deduction has been questioned, however, based on mathematical analysis of control-region sequence diversity.[328]

The co-occurrence of the *Alu*I site at np 10397 and the *Dde*I site at np 10394 in macro-haplogroup M mtDNAs throughout Asia indicates that the *Alu*I site gain occurred at the beginning of Asian habitation. This hypothesis has been supported by the discovery of macro-haplogroup M mtDNAs in east African Ethiopians. Either the haplogroup M mtDNA entered east Africa through relatively recent migrations from Asia, or they originated in east Africa. If the latter is true, this would place the origin of M close to the time of the migration of proto-Asians out of Africa and into Asia.[329,330] Consequently, the sequence diversity that has accumulated in the *Dde*I np 10394 + *Alu*I np 10397 lineage should be indicative of the age of the Asian population. The overall sequence diversity in this lineage is 0.161 percent. This gives an age for the Asian population of 56,000 to 73,000 YBP.

Native American mtDNA Variation

To learn more about the origin of Native Americans, we analyzed 743 Native American mtDNAs. Multiple hypotheses have been put forward to explain the origin and radiation of Native Americans. One hypothesis is based on the classification of Native American languages by Greenberg et al.[331] These authors divided all Native American languages into three major groups: Amerind, which encompasses the great diversity of languages spoken by the Paleo-Indian peoples occupying most of North America and all of Central and South America; Na-Déné, which is spoken by the Athapaskans of the northwestern United States, Canada, and Alaska, as well as the Navajo and Apache who migrated south through the great plains around 1000 AD; and the Eskaleut languages, which are spoken by the Eskimos and Aleuts of the Arctic region. Greenberg hypothesized that each of these language groups corresponded to a different migration, arising in a different geographic homeland. Using glottochronology dating based on the divergence rate of languages, they estimated that these migrations occurred at about 11,000 YBP, 9000 YBP, and 5000 YBP, respectively.

In our first studies on Native American mtDNA variation, we focused on the Pima and the Papago, Paleo-Indians of the southwestern United States. Using Southern blot analysis and our initial six informative restriction endonucleases, we discovered that about 40 percent of these Native American mtDNAs lacked the *Hinc*II site at np 13259,[332] while only 1.8 percent of central Asian mtDNAs lacked this site.[324] This led to the hypothesis that Native American mtDNAs were derived from a limited number of founding mtDNA haplotypes present in people who crossed the Bering land bridge in distinct migrations.[286,332,333] This hypothesis was subsequently confirmed by our more extensive analysis encompassing 563 Paleo-Indians from 24 tribes, 130 Na-Déné representing 5 tribes, and 50 Eskimos.[305,306,317,334]

Our analysis of mtDNA variation in Paleo-Indians revealed a dramatic result. Virtually all of the mtDNAs fell into one of the four Asian haplogroups: A (*Hae*III site at np 663), B (9-np deletion between COII/$tRNA^{Lys}$), C (*Hinc*II site loss at np 13259 and *Alu*I site gain at np 13262), and D (*Alu*I site loss at np 5176), with haplogroups C and D also belonging to macro-haplogroup M and thus harboring the *Dde*I np 10394 and *Alu*I np 10397 site gains found in their Asian progenitors[286,305,334] (Fig. 105-14). Each of the four primary Native American haplogroups traces back to a single nodal mtDNA haplotype that is shared by Asia and the Americas and that initiated the mtDNA radiation in the Americas. However, none of the derived haplotypes are shared by Asians and Americans, as demonstrated by analyzing haplogroup C and D mtDNAs from Siberians and Native Americans.[307] Hence, it appears that primarily these four mtDNA haplotypes crossed from Siberia into the Americas. All four of these haplogroups are distributed throughout the Paleo-Indians of North, Central, and South America, although individual tribes may have lost one or more of the haplogroups through genetic drift. The broad distribution of all four mtDNA haplogroups suggests that they either came together or were subsequently thoroughly mixed.

The calculation of the mtDNA sequence diversity that has accumulated within each haplogroup revealed that haplogroups A, C, and D had relatively similar values: A = 0.075 percent, C = 0.096 percent, and D = 0.053 percent, with a mean value of 0.075 percent. By contrast, haplogroup B had a much lower value, 0.034 percent, suggesting that haplogroup B arrived in the Americas much more recently than A, C, and D.[322] This difference is consistent with the absence of haplogroup B in Siberia, even though haplogroups A, C, and D are prevalent. These two results imply that the Paleo-Indians of the Amerind linguistic group may have been derived from two migrations. The first migration moved up from central Asia through Siberia, during which it became progressively enriched for the founder haplotypes of haplogroups A, C, and D. Ultimately, only people carrying these haplotypes crossed the Bering land bridge to found the Paleo-Indians. The second migration came much later, bearing the founder haplotype of haplogroup B. This migration bypassed Siberia, possibly moving along the Siberian and Alaskan coasts, and entered the Americas, where it interspersed with the already present haplogroups A, C, and D.[286,305,306] An independent analysis of the number of Native American migrations based on mtDNA control region sequence data concluded that all Paleo-Indians (Amerinds) were derived from a single migration. That is, B came with A, C, and D.[328]

To further investigate the Paleo-Indian tribalization process, we examined the mtDNAs from isolated groups of Aztec descendants in central Mexico: the Mixtec of Alta and Baja, the Zapotecs, and the adjacent Mixe. These tribes were compared with the Pima of Arizona, the Maya of Yucatan, the Chibchan-speakers of Panama, the Bella Coola and the Nuu-Chah-Nulth of North America, and the Yanomama and Wapishana of South America. In aggregate, the Aztec-derived Mixtec and Zapotecs harbored three haplogroups: 66 percent A, 18 percent B, and 16 percent C. The linguistically related Pima of Arizona harbored the same haplogroups, as did the Mixe, suggesting a common ancestry. The Maya were more similar to the North American Paleo-Indians, while the Chibchans and South American tribes differed from the more northern tribes and from each other. These results suggest that the Maya and Aztecs may have been derived from different populations.[334]

The prevalence of haplogroup A, B, C, and D mtDNAs in Native American populations has now been confirmed by multiple investigators.[335–338] These same four haplogroups have also been found in the Native American skeletons excavated from a pre-Columbian burial site in Central North America.[339] While some Native American mtDNAs have been found not to exhibit one of the four primary mtDNA restriction site markers,[305,306,340] most of these mtDNAs can be shown to result from either recent genetic admixture with European or African immigrants or the secondary gain or loss of informative restriction sites.[341] The major exception to this is found in the Native Americans of Central North America. These populations have been discovered to harbor a fifth ancient founding mtDNA lineage, designated haplogroup X (Fig. 105-14). Analysis of the mtDNA of 42 Ojibwa of the Great Lakes region revealed 11 (26 percent) that were not from haplogroups A, B, C, or D. Similarly, of the Nuu-Chah-Nulth and the Bella Coola of the Pacific northwest, 13.3 percent and 4 percent, respectively, were non-A–D. Extensive analysis of these mtDNAs revealed that they had some features in common with the rare European haplogroup, haplogroup X. The shared markers included restriction site polymorphisms for an *Acc*I site at np 14465; the absence of *Dde*I sites at np 1715 and at np 10394; and the presence of the *Hae*III site at np 16517. Control region sequence analysis further revealed that both the Native American and European haplogroup X mtDNAs shared additional nucleotide variants, located at 16189C, 16223T, 16278T, 73G, 153G, 195G, 225A, and 263G. However, comparison of the European and Native American control region sequences also revealed clear differences, indicating that the last common ancestor of the European and Native American haplogroup X mtDNAs lived long ago. Moreover, while the above-mentioned survey of the pre-Columbian burial site

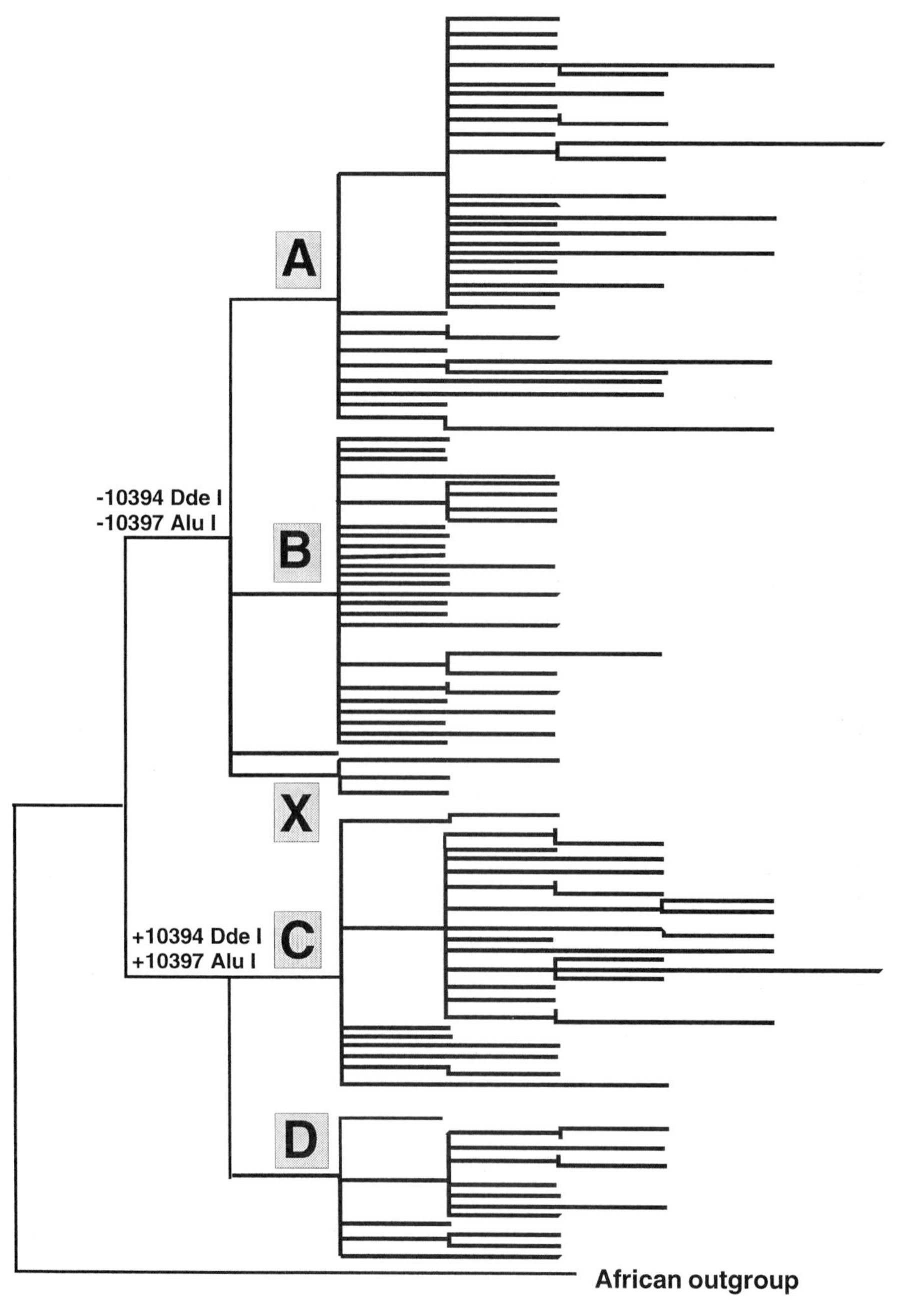

Fig. 105-14 Phylogeny of Native American mtDNAs. This representative tree was derived from the haplotype data obtained from approximately 563 Paleo-Indians, 130 Na-Déné, and 50 Eskimos, and reveals a dramatic point—all Native American mtDNAs were derived from only five founder mtDNAs. These founders originated from haplogroups A, B, C, and D found in Asia and, from haplogroup X, found only in Europe. The Amerind-speaking Paleo-Indians of North, Central, and South America encompass haplogroups A, B, C, and D. The Paleo-Indians of north-central North America also encompass haplogroup X. The Na-Déné of the Pacific Northwest and Southwest (Apache and Navajo) are primarily A with one-third having the Na-Déné-specific marker, an *Rsa*I site loss at np 16329. The Eskimos of the subarctic are primarily haplogroups A and D. This phylogeny is derived from data reported in references 286, 305, 306, 317, 322, 323, 332, 334, 341, and 342.

revealed mostly mtDNAs of haplogroups A, B, C, or D, two skeletons were found to be different and to have the same control region sequence as a subset of the Ojibwa haplogroup X mtDNAs.[342] Hence, the central North American haplogroup X mtDNAs are not the result of recent European admixture with Native Americans, but arrived in an ancient, pre-Columbian, migration.[342] A survey of the distribution of haplogroup X throughout Asia including 411 Siberians[307] and 207 Asians[304,321] failed to reveal a single haplogroup X mtDNA. This implies that the Native American haplogroup X may not be of Asian ancestry, which raises the possibility that haplogroup X came to the Americas in a separate migration originating in Europe. Analysis of the haplogroup X restriction and control region sequence data has permitted us to estimate the divergence time of the American and European haplogroup X mtDNAs, which proved to be in the range of 15,000 to 30,000 YBP. Thus, haplogroup X must have come to the Americas with the original Native American migrations and represents a novel founder lineage of possibly European origin.[342]

Analysis of mtDNA variation of the Na-Déné has confirmed that they are distinct from the Paleo-Indians. Analysis of northern Na-Déné including Dogrib, Tlingit, and Haida, indicates that these people harbor mtDNAs from only one of the founding mtDNA haplogroups, haplogroup A.[305,306] This is substantiated by the southern Na-Déné, including the Apache and Navajo, who are >60 percent haplogroup A. The remaining Apache and Navajo mtDNAs are from haplogroups B, C, and D and probably represent recent admixture with adjacent Paleo-Indian tribes. The distinctive nature of the Na-Déné mtDNAs is confirmed by the fact that about a third of all Na-Déné haplogroup A mtDNAs carry a novel variant, an *Rsa*I site loss at np 16329 (A to G at 16331). Interestingly, this variant is found in all Na-Déné but the Haida. This may suggest that the *Rsa*I site loss occurred in the original Beringian populations that gave rise to the Na-Déné in the Americans.

Analyses of the sequence diversity of the Na-Déné haplogroup A mtDNAs gave a value of 0.021 percent. This is substantially lower than the diversity of the Paleo-Indian haplogroups

A + C + D, and also different from the Paleo-Indian haplogroup B. Hence, the Na-Déné do appear to have arrived as a single independent migration, which occurred more recently than the Paleo-Indians migration.[305,306] This conclusion has been confirmed by analysis of control region sequence data.[328]

Analysis of the mtDNA variation in Eskimos has been more difficult, because of the limited availability of samples and their recent divergence from ancestral populations. However, a survey of 129 Siberian Yupik Eskimos, who represent Eskimo peoples inhabiting both sides of the Bering Strait, revealed only haplogroups A and D. Hence, the Eskimos may also be distinct from the Na-Déné and Paleo-Indians, as predicted from linguistic associations.[307,323]

Times of the Native American migrations, as in the cases of the African, European, and Asian populations, were calculated using the haplogroup-specific mtDNA sequence diversity and the mtDNA sequence evolution rate of 2.2 percent to 2.9 percent/Myr. This rate was calculated using the Chibcha-speaking peoples of Central America, who are estimated from anthropological and nuclear genetic data to have originated about 8000 to 10,000 YBP. Analyzing the mtDNA variation of 110 Chibchans representing five tribes revealed that all but one of the Chibchan mtDNAs were from haplogroups A or B, the exception being a single haplogroup D. Moreover, 62 percent of the Chibchan haplogroup A mtDNAs showed a distinctive private polymorphism, the loss of an *Msp*I site at np 104, the result of a small deletion in the 3′ end of the D-loop hypervariable region II.[317,337] Averaging the sequence diversity of the haplogroup A and B mtDNAs and dividing by the putative age of the population gave the sequence evolution rate of 2.2 percent to 2.9 percent/Myr.[317]

Using this Native American sequence evolution rate, we calculated that the first Paleo-Indian migration carrying haplogroups A, C, and D (sequence diversity of 0.075 percent) arrived 26,000 to 34,000 YBP and that the second Paleo-Indian migration bringing haplogroup B (0.034 percent) arrived 12,000 to 15,000 YBP. The Na-Déné migration with a sequence diversity of 0.021 percent was estimated to have arrived 7200 to 9000 YBP, a value strikingly similar to the 9500 YBP value estimated by glottochronology[317] (Fig. 105-4).

Comparable estimates from control region sequence data have suggested an initial major expansion out of northeastern Siberia into the Americas to generate the Paleo-Indians (Amerind) occurring about 20,000 to 25,000 YBP, followed by a second rapid expansion out of Beringia about 11,300 YBP, giving rise to the Na-Déné and Eskimos.[328]

Siberian Antecedents to Native American Migrations

With the Siberian origin of Native Americans established, it was of interest to determine which Siberian populations are the most likely progenitors of the various Native American migrations. To address this question, we have performed an extensive analysis of the mtDNAs of the Siberian Eskimos and Chukchi of the Chukotka peninsula, and of the Koryaks and Itel'men of the Kamchatka peninsula. The Chukotka peninsula is the region of northeastern Siberia closest to Alaska, while the Kamchatka peninsula extends south from the Chukotka peninsula forming the eastern border of the Sea of Okhotsk. Analysis of 79 Siberian Eskimos revealed an mtDNA haplogroup distribution of 77.2 percent A, 2.5 percent C, and 20.3 percent D. Similarly, the haplotype distribution of the Chukchi was 68.2 percent A, 10.6 percent C, 12.1 percent D, and 9.1 percent G. Control region sequence analysis of the Chukotka haplogroup A mtDNAs, and comparison with those of Native American Na-Déné and northwestern Amerinds, revealed a 16111 C to T transition which appears to delineate an "American" enclave of northeastern Siberian mtDNAs. Furthermore, derivatives of this sublineage were found to include some of the progenitors of the coastal Amerinds, some bearing an additional 16129A variant; the Haida and Bella Coola who bear an additional 16355T variant; and some Eskimos who bear an additional 16265G variant. The 16111T lineage of haplogroup A is further subdivided by the additional 16192T variant. In addition to being found in Chukotka, this 16111T + 16192T lineage is the progenitor of the Na-Déné lineage, which bears the variants 16233G and 16331G, the latter site generating the characteristic Na-Déné *Rsa*I site loss at np 16329 (16331 A to G). Hence Chukotka seems to harbor some remnants of the progenitors of a Beringia expansion which gave rise to the Na-Déné and Eskimo populations.[323]

Analysis of the Koryaks and Itel'men of the Kamchatka peninsula revealed a very different haplogroup distribution. The Koryaks proved to be 5.2 percent A; 36.1 percent C, 1.3 percent D, 41.9 percent G, 9.7 percent Y, and 5.8 percent Z. The Itel'men were 6.4 percent A, 14.9 percent C, 68.1 percent G, 4.3 percent Y, and 6.4 percent Z. Thus, even though the Chukotka and Kamchatka populations are proximate and the Chukchi and Koryaks have related languages, the mtDNAs of these are strikingly distinct. Indeed, in a neighbor-joining tree analysis, the Eskimos and Chukchi were located at one end of the tree with the Amerinds and Na-Déné, while the Koryaks and Itel'men were at the other end of the tree with the Ainu, Japanese, Koreans, and other Siberians.[322]

The predominance of haplogroup C in the Paleo-Indians (Amerind) is most similar to the haplogroup distribution seen in the central Siberian, where the Evenks and Udegeys are 84.3 percent and 17.8 percent C, respectively. This raises the possibility that the progenitors of the Paleo-Indians may currently reside in central Siberia.[322,323]

MITOCHONDRIAL MUTATIONS IN NEURO-OPHTHALMOLOGIC DISEASE

Mitochondrial Gene Mutations and Disease

While some germ line mtDNA mutations are neutral and become established in the human populations by genetic drift, most mtDNA mutations alter essential cellular functions and are eliminated by selection. In humans, this process of selection manifests as genetic disease. Because of the high mtDNA mutation rate, deleterious mtDNA mutations, and hence mitochondrial disease, may be relatively common. Pathogenic mtDNA mutations can include either base substitutions or rearrangement mutations. The mtDNA base substitution mutations can be subdivided into missense mutations affecting the mtDNA proteins (Table 105-10) or protein synthesis mutations affecting the rRNA or tRNA genes (Table 105-11).

mtDNA missense mutations can be associated with two common ophthalmologic manifestations, optic atrophy and retinitis pigmentosa (RP). Optic atrophy is the predominant clinical manifestation of LHON. Retinitis pigmentosa can be associated with a variety of other neurodegenerative symptoms, including neurogenic muscle weakness, ataxia, and retinitis pigmentosa (NARP), and Leigh syndrome. Leigh syndrome with retinitis pigmentosa can either be caused by mtDNA missense mutations or by mutations in nuclear genes necessary for OXPHOS assembly.

A common neuro-ophthalmologic presentation for mtDNA protein-synthesis base-substitution mutations and mtDNA rearrangements is ophthalmoplegia and ptosis, together with mitochondrial myopathy. Ophthalmoplegia and ptosis result from the paralysis of the extraocular eye muscles, which are highly reliant on mitochondria for energy, resulting in an inability to move the eyes (ophthalmoplegia) and droopy eye lids (ptosis) (Fig. 105-15). Mitochondrial myopathy involves the degeneration of the type I oxidative muscle fibers and the accumulation of aggregates of abnormal mitochondria. On staining with Gomori modified trichrome stain, this gives ragged-red muscle fibers (RRFs) (Fig. 105-16). mtDNA rearrangements can either be spontaneous mtDNA mutations or result from nuclear mutations which destabilize the mtDNA.

Table 105-10 Reported Mitochondrial DNA Missense Diseases

Locus	Disease	Allele	np	Nucleotide Change	AA Change	Ho	He	Status	References
MTND1	MELAS	3308C	3308	T-C	M-T	−	+	Prov	676
MTND1	NDDM	3316A	3316	G-A	A-T	+	−	Prov	677
MTND1	LHON	3394C	3394	T-C	Y-H	+	−	Prov	951, 353, 355, 363, 678
MTND1	NIDDM	3394C	3394	T-C	Y-H	+	−	P.M.	679
MTND1	ADPD	3397G	3397	A-G	M-V	+	−	Prov	680, 681
MTND1	LHON	3460A	3460	G-A	A-T	+	+	Cfrm	348–350, 363, 395, 403, 682–685
MTND1	LHON	4136G	4136	A-G	Y-C	+	−	Prov	355, 370, 377, 686
MTND1	LHON	4160C	4160	T-C	L-P	+	−	Prov	356, 377, 387, 686, 687
MTND1	LHON	4216C	4216	T-C	Y-H	+	−	Cfrm	352, 353, 356, 369, 370, 373, 387, 688, 689
MTND2	LHON	4917G	4917	A-G	D-N	+	−	Cfrm	353, 356, 369, 370, 387, 683, 688
MTND2	LHON	5244A	5244	G-A	G-S	−	+	Prov	353, 373, 387, 686
MTND2	AD	5460A	5460	G-A	A-T	+	+	P.M.	690–692
MTND2	AD	5460T	5460	G-T	A-S	+	+	Prov	690–692
MTCO1	LHON	7444A	7444	G-A	Term-K	+	−	Prov	350, 353, 363, 365, 374, 387, 693, 694
MTATP6	NARP	8993G	8993	T-G	L-R	−	+	Cfrm	422–426, 435, 678, 695–697
MTATP6	NARP/ Leigh Disease	8993C	8993	T-C	L-P	−	+	Cfrm	427, 428, 698, 699
MTATP6	LHON	9101C	9101	T-C	I-T	+	−	Prov	366
MTATP6	FBSN	9176C	9176	T-C	L-P	+	+	Prov	429
MTCO3	LHON	9438A	9438	G-A	G-S	+	−	Prov	366, 375, 376, 694, 700–703
MTCO3	LHON	9738T	9738	G-T	A-T	+	−	Prov	702
MTCO3	LHON PEM;	9804A	9804	G-A	A-T	+	−	Prov	365, 694
MTCO3	MELAS	9957C	9957	T-C	F-L	−	+	Prov	704, 705
MTND4	MELAS	11084G	11084	A-G	T-A	+	+	P.M.	706, 707
MTND4	LHON	11778A	11778	G-A	R-H	+	+	Cfrm	1,708–716
MTND4	DM	12026G	12026	A-G	I-V	+	−	Prov	717
MTND5	LHON	13708A	13708	G-A	A-T	+	−	Prov	351, 352, 363, 372, 373, 387, 683, 684, 688, 718
MTND5	LHON	13730A	13730	G-A	G-E	−	+	Prov	364, 686
MTND6	LDYT	14459A	14459	G-A	A-V	+	+	Cfrm	57, 60, 347, 353, 686
MTND6	LHON	14484C	14484	T-C	M-V	+	+	Cfrm	351, 352, 365, 369, 371, 387, 686, 687, 719
MTCYB	PD/MELAS	14787del4	14787	CTCC-del	I-frameshift	−	+	Prov	720
MTCYB	MM	15059A	15059	G-A	G-Term	−	+	Prov	721
MTCYB	LHON	15257A	15257	G-A	D-N	+	−	Prov	350, 352, 372, 373, 387, 684, 718, 722–724
MTCYB	MM	15762A	15762	G-A	G-E	−	+	Prov	725
MTCYB	LHON	15812A	15812	G-A	V-M	+	−	Prov	352, 353, 356, 370, 372, 373, 387, 736

NOTE: In the "Status" column Prov=provisional, Cfrm=confirmed, and P.M.=polymorphism (originally thought by some groups to be a pathogenic mutation).

Leber Hereditary Optic Neuropathy

LHON classically manifests as acute-onset, bilateral, central vision loss associated with the degeneration of the retinal ganglion cell layer and optic nerve. Typically, the onset and progression of blindness is relatively rapid, with both eyes developing vision loss within a year of each other and with blindness usually the only clinical sign. However, in some LHON cases other neurologic abnormalities are also observed.

The inheritance pattern of LHON was ambiguous for many years for three reasons. First, the expressivity of optic atrophy and blindness in families is highly variable, and many families are only singleton cases. Second, blindness is much more common in males than females. Third, penetrance can be quite variable between LHON families and populations.[343–346] A key factor in clarifying the genetic complexity of LHON was the discovery that LHON is caused by missense mutations in the mtDNA.[1] A current paradigm for the clinical evaluation of LHON is provided in Fig. 105-17. A typical pedigree for the most common mtDNA mutation MTND4*LHON11778A is shown in Fig. 105-18.

mtDNA Mutations and LHON. Twenty-three mtDNA missense mutations have been associated with LHON patients (Table 105-12). However, detailed genetic analysis has revealed that only a few "primary" mutations contribute in a major way to the development of blindness. The remaining "secondary" mutations may contribute to LHON by increasing the probability of expressing the phenotype or may simply be linked to other clinically important variants in the same mtDNA haplotype.

The four "primary" LHON mutations are MTND6*LDY-T14459A,[60,347] MTND4*LHON11778A,[1] MTND1*LHON3460 A,[348–350] and MTND6*LHON14484C[351,352] (Table 105-12). Primary mutations, considered individually, represent strong risk factors for maternally inherited LHON expression; have been observed in a number of unrelated LHON families; rarely co-occur with each other; and have not been detected in a large number of control mtDNAs.[353–356] Together these four mutations account for roughly 90 percent of Caucasian patients, with MTND4*LHO-N11778A encompassing about 50 percent of cases and the MTND1*LHON3460A and MTND6*LHON14484C mutations encompassing roughly 15 percent each (Table 105-13). In Asia, the MTND4*LHON11778A mutation accounts for 95 percent of patients.[357]

The MTND6*LDYT14459A mutation is relatively rare, having been reported in three independent pedigrees.[60,347] This mutation changes the highly conserved alanine at codon 72 in the ND6 polypeptide to a valine and can manifest as two very different phenotypes: LHON and/or generalized dystonia (Fig. 105-19). This mutation has been found to be heteroplasmic in at least some family members in every pedigree studied (Table 105-13).[60,347]

Table 105-11 Reported Mitochondrial DNA Protein Synthesis Disease

Locus	Disease	Allele	np	RNA	Ho	He	Status	References
MTTF	MM	618C	618	tRNA Phe	−	+	Prov	727
MTRNR1	DM	1310T	1310	12S	+	−	Prov	717
MTRNR1	DM	1438G	1438	12S	+	−	Prov	717
MTRNR1	DEAF	1555G	1555	rRNA 12S	+	−	Cfrm	434, 728–734
MTTV	AMDF	1606A	1606	tRNA Val	−	+	Prov	735
MTTV	MELAS	1642A	1642	rRNA Val	−	+	Prov	736
MTRNR2	ADPD	3196A	3196	rRNA 16S	+	+	Prov	680, 681
MTTL1	MELAS	3243G	3243	rRNA Leu (UUR)	−	+	Cfrm	273, 451, 547, 737–743
MTTL1	DM/DMDF	3243G	3243	tRNA Leu (UUR)	−	+	Cfrm	532, 539, 744–751
MTTL1	MM	3243T	3243	tRNA Leu(UUR)	−	+	Prov	752
MTTL1	MM	3250C	3250	tRNA Leu (UUR)	−	+	Prov	753
MTTL1	MM	3251G	3251	tRNA Leu (UUR)	−	+	Prov	754
MTTL1	MELAS	3252G	3252	tRNA Leu (UUR)	−	+	Prov	450, 755
MTTL1	MM	3254G	3254	tRNA Leu (UUR)	−	+	Prov	756
MTTL1	MELAS	3256T	3256	tRNA Leu (UUR)	−	+	Cfrm	534, 757
MTTL1	MMC	3260G	3260	tRNA Leu (UUR)	−	+	Cfrm	758–760
MTTL1	DM	3264C	3264	tRNA Leu (UUR)	−	+	Prov	761
MTTL1	MELAS	3271C	3271	tRNA Leu (UUR)	−	+	Conf	450, 545, 550, 762–765
MTTL1	PEM	3271delT	3271	tRNA Leu (UUR)	−	+	Prov	766
MTTL1	DM	3271C	3271	tRNA Leu (UUR)	−	+	Prov	767
MTTL1	MELAS	3291C	3291	tRNA Leu (UUR)	−	+	Prov	450, 768
MTTL1	MM	3302G	3302	tRNA Leu (UUR)	−	+	Cfrm	356, 769, 770
MTTL1	MMC	3303T	3303	tRNA Leu (UUR)	+	+	Prov	771
MTTI	FICP	4269G	4269	tRNA Ile	−	+	Prov	772, 773
MTTI	CPEO/MS	4298A	4298	tRNA Ile	−	+	Prov	535
MTTI	MICM	4300G	4300	tRNA Ile	−	+	Prov	774
MTTI	FICP	4317G	4317	tRNA Ile	nd	nd	Prov	775, 776
MTTQ	ADPD	4336C	4336	tRNA Gln	+	−	Cfrm	680, 681, 777–779
MTTM	MM	4409C	4409	tRNA Met	−	+	Prov	780
MMTW	MM	5521A	5521	tRNA Trp	−	+	Prov	781
MTTW	DEMCHO	5549A	5549	tRNA Trp	−	+	Prov	782
MTTN	CPEO	5692G	5692	tRNA Asn	−	+	Prov	453, 783
MTTN	CPEO, MM	5703G	5703	tRNA Asn	−	+	Prov	534, 784
MTTS1	DEAF	7445G	7445	tRNA Ser (UCN)	+	+	Prov	785–788
MTTS1	PEM/AMDF	7472insC	7472	tRNA Ser (UCN)	+	+	Cfrm	789–792
MTTS1	MM	7497A	7497	tRNA Ser (UCN)	+	+	Prov	750
MTTS1	PEM/MERME	7512C	7512	tRNA Ser (UCN)	+	+	Prov	790, 791, 793
MTTK	DMDF	8296G	8296	tRNA Lys	−	+	Prov	794, 795
MTTK	MNGIE	8313A	8313	tRNA Lys	−	+	Prov	796
MTTK	MERRF	8344G	8344	tRNA Lys	−	+	Cfrm	279, 287, 431, 536, 551, 554, 742, 797–799
MTTK	MERRF	8356C	8356	tRNA Lys	−	+	Cfrm	555, 800, 801
MTTK	MERRF	8363A	8363	tRNA Lys	−	+	Prov	802
MTTG	MHCM	9997C	9997	tRNA Gly	nd	+	Prov	803
MTTG	CIPO	10006G	10006	tRNA Gly	nd	nd	Prov	536, 783
MTTG	PEM	10010C	10010	tRNA Gly	−	+	Prov	804
MTTS1	CIPO	12246G	12246	tRNA Ser (AGY)	nd	nd	Prov	536, 783
MTTS2	DMDF	12258A	12258	tRNA Ser (AGY)		+	Prov	805
MTTL2	CPEO	12308G	12308	tRNA Leu (CUN)	nd	nd	P.M.	534, 536, 551, 803, 806–808
MTTL2	CPEO	12311C	12311	tRNA Leu (CUN)	+	+	Prov	537, 757
MTTL2	CPEO	12315A	12315	tRNA Leu (CUN)	−	+	Prov	538
MTTL2	MM	12320G	12320	tRNA Leu (CUN)	−	+	Prov	809
MTTE	MM+DM	14709C	14709	tRNA Glu	−	+	Conf	810–812
MTATT	MM	15915A	15915	tRNA Thr	−	+	Prov	813, 814
MTTT	LIMM	15923G	15923	tRNA Thr	nd	−	Prov	815–817
MTTT	LIMM	15924G	15924	tRNA Thr	nd	−	P.M.	815, 816, 818
MTTT	MM	15940delT	15940	tRNA Thr	+	−	Prov	819
MTTP	MM	15990T	15990	tRNA Pro	−	+	Prov	820, 821

NOTE: In the "Status" column, Prov = provisional, Cfrm = confirmed, and P.M. = polymorphism (originally thought by some groups to be a pathogenic mutation).

The MTND4*LHON11778A mutation converts the highly conserved ND4 codon 340 from an arginine to a histidine.[1] This mutation typically displays variable expression in families, with males being predominantly affected (Fig. 105-18), and is heteroplasmic in about 14 percent of cases.[358] The MTND1*LHON3460A mutation changes a moderately conserved alanine at codon 52 in the ND1 gene to a threonine and has been observed to be heteroplasmic in a number of families.[348–350] Finally, the MTND6*LHON14484C mutation changes the weakly conserved methionine at codon 64 in the ND6 protein to a valine. This

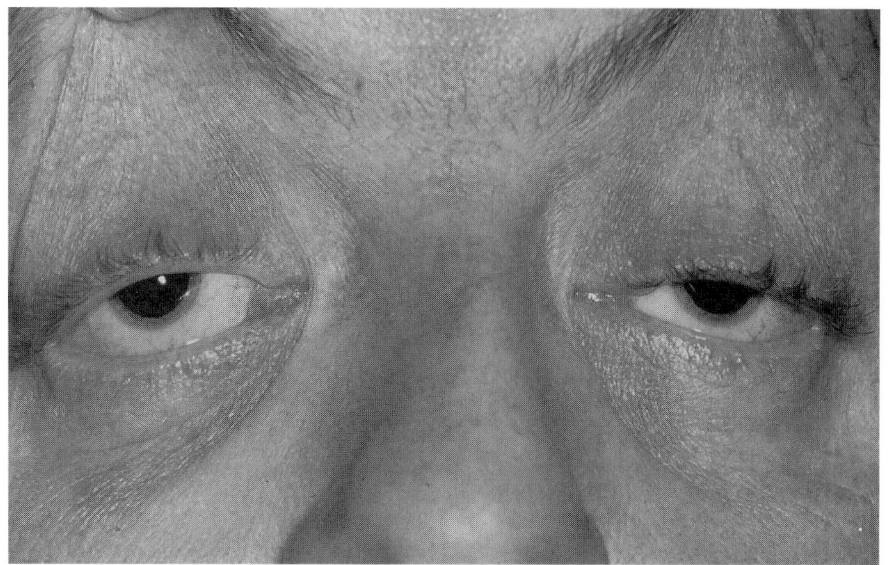

A

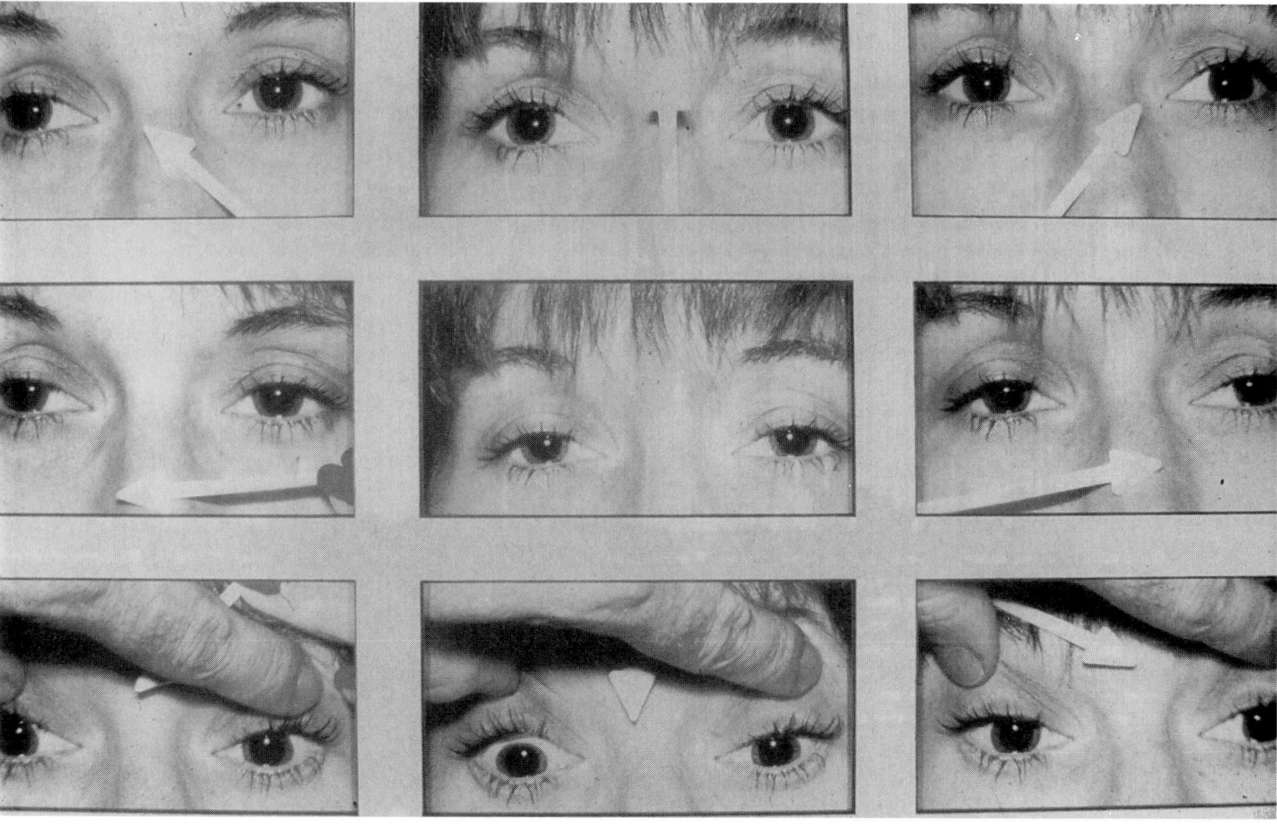

B

Fig. 105-15 ***Panel A:*** **Severe ptosis in a patient with CPEO. In this photograph, the patient was asked to look directly upward while eyelids were manually lifted by the examiner.** ***Panel B:*** **Ophthalmoplegia in a 37-year-old woman with CPEO and mitochondrial myopathy. Ocular motility is shown in nine cardinal positions, arrows indicating the requested direction of gaze. Note mild bilateral ptosis and omnidirectional ophthalmoparesis (*Courtesy of Nancy J. Newman, M.D., Emory University School of Medicine. Reprinted from Wallace, Brown, and Lott.*[13] *Used with permission.*)**

mutation is frequently homoplasmic in LHON families,[351,352] having been reported to be heteroplasmic in only a few pedigrees (Table 105-13).[359]

Analysis of the background mtDNA haplotypes in LHON families harboring the various primary mutations has shown that most families are new mutations and revealed some interesting genetic associations. For example, the MTND6*LDYT14459A mutation was first identified in a large Hispanic family (Fig. 105-19), which proved to harbor a Native American mtDNA from haplogroup D[60] (Fig. 105-20). Subsequently, the same mutation was found in an African-American family encompassing a mother and daughter with LHON in which the daughter also had unilateral striatal degeneration and in a European child with generalized dystonia. The background haplogroups for these families were the sub-Saharan haplogroup L and the European haplogroup I, respectively (Fig. 105-20).[60,347] Because mtDNA haplotypes of

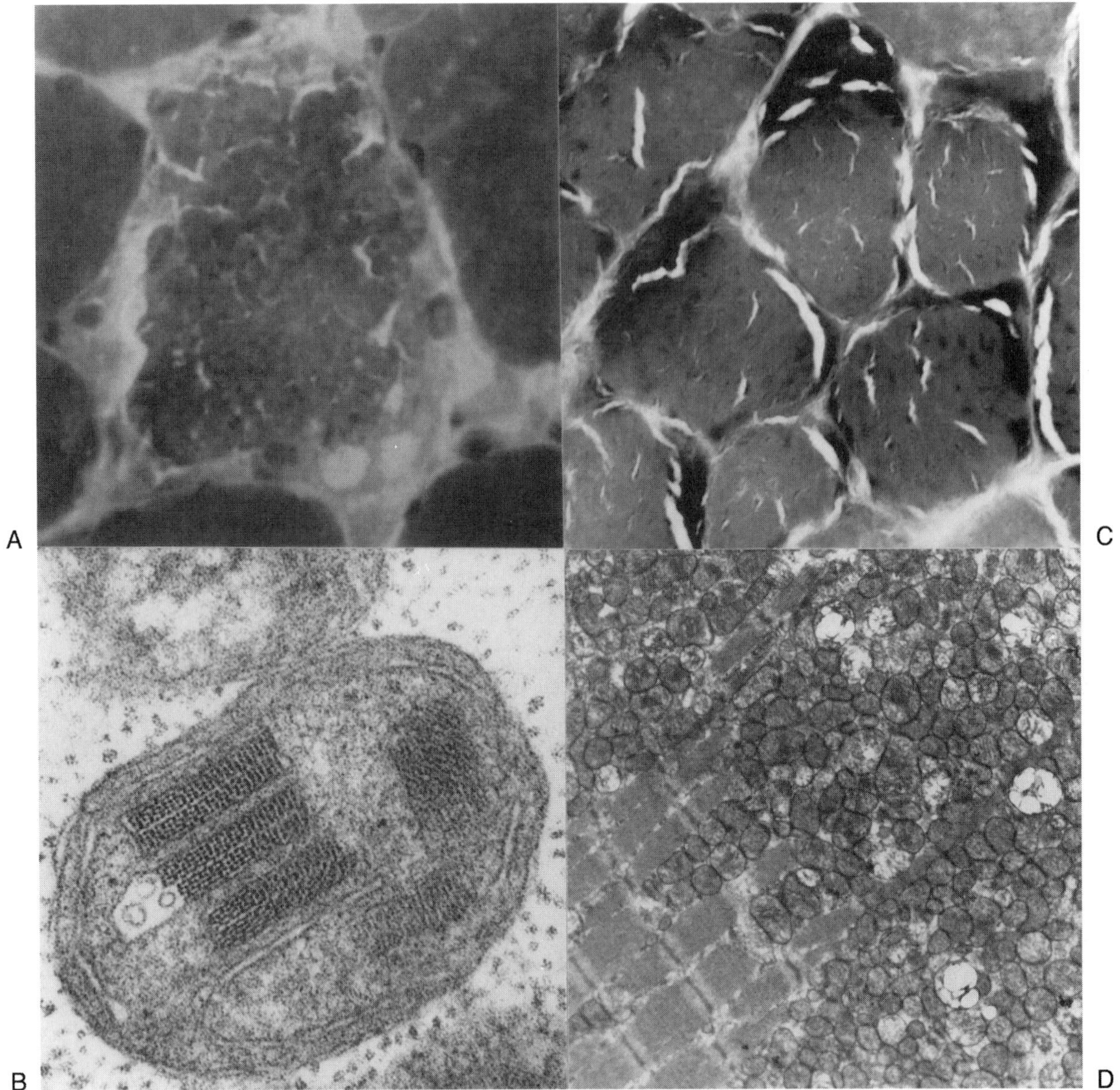

Fig. 105-16 Mitochondrial myopathy in man and mouse. ***Panel A*** **and** ***Panel C*** **are skeletal muscle samples from a patient with myoclonic epilepsy and ragged-red fiber disease (MERRF), which is caused by a mutation in the mitochondrially encoded $tRNA^{Lys}$ gene.[279,281]** ***Panel B*** **and** ***Panel D*** **are skeletal muscle samples from a mouse with mitochondrial myopathy and hypertrophic cardiomyopathy resulting from the targeted inactivation of the gene encoding the heart-muscle isoform of the adenine nucleotide translocator (ANT1).[190] Frozen sections showing a single fiber (A) or several fibers (B) were stained with Gomori modified trichrome to show the ragged-red muscle fibers (RRFs). Electron micrographs show (C) an abnormal mitochondrion with paracrystalline arrays in a human RRF, and (D) the abnormal proliferation of mitochondria and degeneration of the contractile elements in a mouse RRF. (*Reproduced from Wallace.[825] Used with permission.*) See Color Plate 3.**

these three families encompass most of the world's mtDNA sequence diversity, it is not possible that the MTND6*LDY-T14459A mutations are related by descent through a common ancestor. Rather, all three MTND6*LDYT14459A mutations must have arisen recently and independently. This conclusion is supported by the fact that all three families were heteroplasmic. Because all three families had similar disease, this mutation must be the cause of this disease.[60,347]

A similar haplotype analysis has been performed on 47 LHON patients of European descent harboring the three common "primary" mutations: MTND4*LHON11778A, MTND1*LHO-N3460A, and MTND6*LHON14484C (Fig. 105-21).[353] This revealed that patients harboring the MTND4*LHON11778A and MTND1*LHON3460A mutations had a variety of different mtDNA background haplotypes which were dispersed throughout the European mtDNA haplogroups, thus demonstrating that many LHON families with these mutations are due to independent mutational events. On the other hand, most patients harboring the MTND6*LHON14484C mutation clustered together on a single mtDNA lineage, haplogroup J (Fig. 105-21). However, the MTND6*LHON14484C patients were still dispersed throughout haplogroup J, and interspersed with control haplogroup J mtDNAs, which did not harbor the MTND6*LHON14484C mutation (Fig. 105-21).[353] This implies that most, if not all, MTND6*LHON14484C mutation families are also independent mutational events, but that the haplogroup J mtDNA background in some way contributes to the MTND6*LHON14484C mutation's propensity to cause blindness.

The conclusion that mtDNA haplogroup J contributes to the expression of LHON is supported by the fact that haplogroup J is present in only about 9 percent of the general European population, but is present in 37 percent of LHON patients harboring the MTND4*LHON11778A mutation and 80 percent of LHON patients harboring the MTND6*LHON14484C mutation.[360] Indeed, only rarely have European patients with the MTND6*LHON14484C mutation been found on a nonhaplogroup

Leber Hereditary Optic Neuropathy Diagnostic Paradigm

Clinical Presentations:

1. Age: Typically between 15 and 35 years of age with mean of approximately 27 years.
2. Primary clinical signs: Primarily bilateral, painless, progressive loss of central vision. Visual acuity usually decreases to less than 20/200. May be associated with headache, dizziness, Uthoff symptom, photopsia, limb paresthesias, or eye discomfort. [go to 1st testing phase]
   Progression: Simultaneous bilateral vision loss in 20-50% of reported cases. In sequential visual loss, typically 2-3 months between first eye and second eye involvement. In an affected eye, visual acuity progressively worsens, usually over an approximately 2-month period. Spontaneous recovery of some vision does occur, with frequency linked to age of onset and mtDNA mutation.
3. Alternative clinical signs: In some instances the proband or one or more family members may present with neurodegenerative disease, age of onset childhood to young adult. The most common clinical manifestation is dystonia (rigidity of lower and later upper extremities and gait disturbance) frequently with pseudo-bulbar syndrome, impaired intelligence, short stature, and myopathic signs. [include both 1st and 2nd testing phase]
   Progression: Early onset, relatively rapid progression, followed by slower more steady decline.
4. Occasional clinical signs: Cardiac conduction defects, skeletal abnormalities, hearing loss, tremor, sensory neuropathy, mild cerebellar ataxia, extrapyramidal signs, or multiple sclerosis-like presentation.
5. Neuro-ophthalmologic findings: Typical fundus appearance includes circumpapillary telangiectatic microangiopathy, nerve fiber layer swelling and no disc leakage upon fluorescein angiography. Visual fields indicate central or cecocentral scotomas. VEPs and BAEPs may be abnormal. Neuroradiological findings: In cases of dystonia, bilateral striatal necrosis seen on CT and MRI.
6. Family history: Transmission along maternal lineage in many cases, although singleton cases are common. Penetrance is incomplete in LHON and dystonia, and for LHON males can be three or four times more likely to be affected than females.

Diagnostic Testing:

There are no reliable metabolic, neuroradiological, or biochemical tests available for LHON. However, greater than 90% of cases are due to mtDNA missense mutations, which can be readily detected in white blood cells. Hence, direct mutational screening of blood cell DNA is the diagnostic method of choice. Because of the relative frequency of the various mutations this can most efficiently be done in phases.

1st phase testing: accounting for more than 90% of cases of European and Asian descent, and many cases of African descent
MTND4*LHON11778A
MTND1*LHON3460A
MTND6*LHON14484C

2nd phase testing: especially if additional neurodegenerative disease symptoms such as dystonia are observed
MTND6*LDYT14459A
MTND6*LDYT14596A
MTND4*LDYT11696G

3rd phase testing: testing for haplogroup J association, which can be suggestive of mtDNA defect
MTND1*LHON4216C
MTND5*LHON13708A
MTND2*LHON4917G
MTCYB*LHON15259A

4th phase testing: testing for rare pathogenic mutations
MTND2*LHON5244A
MTND5*LHON13730A
MTCO3*LHON9804A
MTND3*LHON10663C
MTATP6*LHON9101C
MTND6*LHON14498T
MTND6*LHON14568T

Fig. 105-17 Diagnostic paradigm for LHON.

J mtDNA,[359] and in only one case has the MTND6*LHON14484C mutation be reported to be associated with the African haplogroup L mtDNA.[361] Hence, haplogroup J appears to augment the pathogenicity of certain primary LHON mutations. The possible cause of this is discussed later in relationship to the "secondary" LHON mutations.

In addition to the four recurrent "primary" LHON mutations, an additional 10 mutations have a number of features characteristic of primary mutations. However, most of these have only been reported in one paper or family, and their status remains to be confirmed (Table 105-13).

One of the rare mutations nicely legitimates the pathogenicity of the MTND6*LHON14484C mutation. This MTND6*-LHON14482G mutation alters the same codon as the MTND6*-LHON14484C mutation, but converts the methione at codon 64 to an isoleucine instead of a valine.[362]

Two of the rare mutations, MTND2*LHON5244A[363] and MTND5*LHON13730A,[364] altered conserved amino acids and were heteroplasmic. Hence, they are likely to be pathogenic mutations. Three other mutations, MTCO3*LHON9804A,[365] MTND4L*LHON10663C,[353] and MTATP6*LHON 9101C,[366] were homoplasmic. Hence the pathogenicity of these mutants remains unclear. The MTCO3*LHON9804 mutation changed the conserved alanine at codon 200 to a threonine in the COIII polypeptide. It was reported in 1.5 percent of LHON patients without other known primary mutations, but not in any of the controls surveyed.[365] The MTND4L*LHON10663C mutation was found to change a poorly conserved valine to an alanine at amino acid 65 in the ND4L polypeptide. However, this mutation was found in two independent LHON patients, and was not detected in a large number of racial group or haplotype-matched controls. The two MTND4L*LHON10663C-positive patients had similar haplogroup J mtDNA haplotypes, incorporating the MTND1*LHON4216C, MTND5*LHON13708A, and MTCYB*LHON15257A secondary variants. One of the patients also harbored the heteroplasmic, primary MTND2*LHON5244A mutation. Determination of the complete mtDNA sequence for the other patient, the proband of a three-generation LHON pedigree, revealed no other candidate mutations.[353] This would imply that either the MTND4L*LHON10663C mutation or the MTND1*LHON4216C + MTND5*LHON13708A + MTCYB*LHON15257A haplotype causes LHON, or alternatively that they act together to precipitate the clinical phenotype. Finally, the MTATP6*LHON9101C mutation converts the poorly conserved isoleucine at amino acid 192 in the MTATP6 polypeptide to a threonine. This mutation was not found in 100 geographically matched controls and was associated with a complex V biochemical defect.[366]

Of the four remaining primary mutations, the MTND4*-LDYT11696G and MTND6*LDYT14596A mutations were identified in the mtDNA of a large maternal pedigree with LHON and dystonia, with the MTND6*LDYT14596A mutation being heteroplasmic.[367] The MTND6*LHON14498T[368] and MTND6*-LHON14568T[368] mutations were both found in individual LHON pedigrees.

The MTCYB*LHON15257A mutation converts the highly conserved aspartate at codon 171 in the cytochrome b gene to an asparagine.[363] However, this variant clearly arose on a single sublineage of haplogroup J (Fig. 105-21). Therefore, it is possible that most, if not all, of its contribution to the LHON phenotype may be due to other sequence variants in the haplogroup J mtDNA, specifically the MTND1*LHON4216C and MTND5*LHON13708A mutations.

The eight remaining LHON mutations have been classified as secondary because their pathogenic role in LHON is particularly unclear (Table 105-13). Like the MTCYB*LHON15257A variant, several are associated with haplogroup J. These include the two variants that define the main haplogroup J lineage: MTND5*LHON13708A and MTND1*LHON4216C.[346,351,353,356,369–371] The MTND5*LHON13708A mutation converts a moderately con-

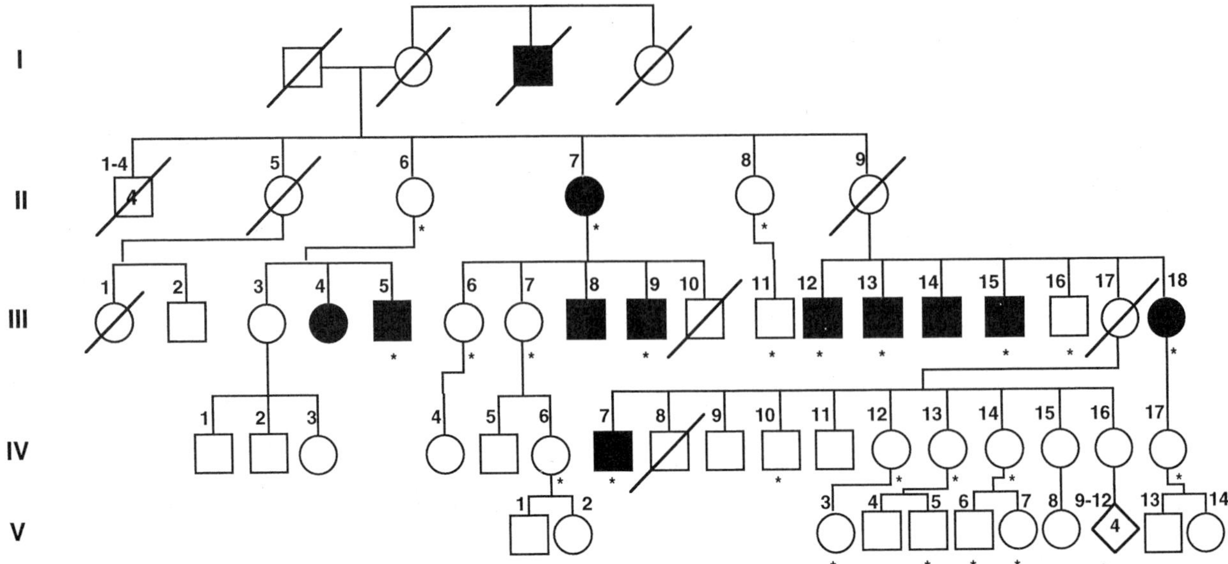

Fig. 105-18 Maternally inherited pedigree of LHON due to the MTND4*LHON11778A mutation. Affected individuals (filled symbols) experience acute-onset optic atrophy and central vision loss, generally as young adults. Even though the mutation is essentially homoplasmic, penetrance among maternal relatives is highly variable. Moreover, males are about three to four times more likely to lose their vision than females.[1,358]

served alanine at codon 458 in the ND5 protein to a threonine,[363,372] while the MTND1*LHON4216C mutation converts a weakly conserved tyrosine at codon 304 in the ND1 protein to histidine.[363,372] The sequencing of multiple haplogroup J mtDNAs has failed to reveal any other obvious sequence variants which could account for this mtDNA lineage's predilection toward increased expression of LHON.[373] Sub-branches of haplogroup J are delineated by the MTCYB*LHON15257A variant, described above, and by the MTND1*LHON3394C variant, which changes the highly conserved tyrosine at codon 30 in the ND1 protein to histidine (Fig. 105-21). The MTND1*LHON3394C variant is prevalent in French Canadians, but like other patients harboring haplogroup J mtDNAs with this mutation, the LHON patients generally also harbor the MTND6*LHON14484C primary mutation.[363,373] The MTCYB*LHON15257A haplogroup J lineage is further subdivided by the MTCYB*LHON15812A variant.[363] Hence, the MTCYB*LHON15812A variant is unlikely to contribute to LHON.

All haplogroup J mtDNAs harbor the MTND1*LHON4216C variant along with the MTND5*LHON13708A variant. However, MTND1*LHON4216C can also be associated with MTND2*LHON4917G. The MTND2*LHON4917G variant changes a highly conserved aspartate at codon 150 in the ND2 protein to an asparagine.[353] The sharing of the MTND1*LHON4216C between these two lineages raises the possibility that the two lineages may be sub-branches of a common single large haplogroup which predisposes individuals to LHON.[356] If so, then the pathogenic significance of the MTND1*-LHON4216C variant might be greater than the mild amino acid substitution might suggest. Alternatively, the predisposition to LHON might be caused by MTND5*LHON13708A on the one lineage and MTND2*LHON4917 on the other.

The MTCO1*LHON7444A mutation changes the termination codon of the COI polypeptide, extending the polypeptide by three charged amino acids.[374] However, the pathogenicity of this mutation is unclear because both reported cases harboring this mutation were also found to harbor a primary mutation, either the MTND6*LHON14484C or the MTND1*LHON3460A mutation.[353] The MTCO3*LHON9438A variant was reported in about 2.5 percent of European patients and to change a highly conserved glycine to a serine.[365] However, the MTCO3*LHON9438A variant is always homoplasmic, has also been found in a low frequency in African and African-American controls,[375] and has been found to co-occur with the MTND4*LHON11778A mutation.[376] Hence, it is unlikely to contribute substantially to the pathophysiology of LHON.

The MTND1*LHON4160 mutation was found together with the MTND6*LHON14484C mutation in the mtDNA of a large pedigree with acute-onset optic atrophy as well as other neurologic symptoms.[377] Hence, this mutation may augment the pathogenicity of the MTND6*LHON14484C mutation. The pathogenicity of the MTND6*LHON14484C mutation has also been underscored by its co-occurrence with the MTND4*LHON11778A mutation.[346]

Clinical Features of the Primary LHON Mutations. LHON is remarkable in that the predominant clinical manifestation is acute onset of central vision loss, even though in most patients the pathogenic mutation is homoplasmic in blood, and thus, presumably, is present in all tissues of the body. This stands in stark contrast to most mtDNA-based diseases, which show a spectrum of neurologic, cardiac, and/or endocrinologic symptoms, often associated with the segregation of heteroplasmic mtDNA mutations among maternal relatives and between the tissues in

Table 105-12 mtDNA Missense Mutation Diseases: Leigh Syndrome

		Amino Acid				
No.	Mutation	Change	Cons	% Controls	Heteroplasmy	Reference
1	MTATP6*NARP8993G	L156R	H	0	+	422, 425, 426
2	MTATP*NARP8993C	L156P	H	0	+	427, 428
3	MTATP6*FBSN9176C	L217P	H	0	+	429

Table 105-13 Leber Hereditary Optic Neuropathy (LHON) Disease Mutations

No.[a]	Mutation	Class[b]	Other Neurol. Disease	Amino Acids[c] Change	Cons	Approx, % European Patients	% Controls	Het.[e]	Penetrance[f] % Relatives	% Males	% Recovery[g]	References
1	MTND6*LDYT14459A	Primary	+/−	A72V	M	Rare	0	+	61	58	Low	60, 347
2	MTND4*LHON11778A	Primary	+/−	R340H	H	50	0	+/−	33–60	82	4	1, 357, 358
3	MTND1*LHON3460A	Primary	+/−	A52T	M	15	0	+/−	14–75	40–80	22	348, 349
4	MTND6*LHON14484C	Primary	−	M64V	L	15	0	+/−	27–80	68	37–50	351, 373, 377
5	MTND2*LHON5244A	Primary	−	G2595	H	Rare	0	+	NA	NA	UN	353
6	MTND5*LHON13730A	Primary	−	G465E	M	Rare	0	+	NA	NA	Yes	364
7	MTCO3*LHON9804A	Primary ?	−	A200T	H	1.5	0	−	UN	UN	UN	365
8	MTND3*LHON10663C	Primary ?	−	V65A	L	Rare	0	−	56	60	UN	353
9	MTATP6*LHON9101C	Primary ?	−	I192T	L	Rare	0	−	NA	NA	UN	353
10	MTND4*LDYT11696G	Primary ?	+/−	V3121	L	Rare	0	−	UN	UN	UN	367
11	MTND6*LHON14482G	Primary ?	−	M64I	L	Rare	0	−	UN	89	UN	822
12	MTND6*LHON14498T	Primary ?	−	Y59C	M	Rare	0	+	31	50	UN	368
13	MTND6*LHON14568T	Primary ?	−	G36S	L	Rare	0	−	NA	NA	UN	368
14	MTND6*LDYT14596A	Primary ?	+/−	I26M	M	Rare	0	+	UN	UN	UN	367
15	MTCYB*LHON15257A	Intermediate	−	D171N	H	9	0.4	−	NA	NA	NA	353, 363, 372
16	MTND5*LHON13708A	Secondary	−	A458T	M	30	6	−	NA	NA	NA	363, 688
17	MTND1*LHON3394C	Secondary	−	Y30H	H	Rare	0.9	−	NA	NA	NA	373
18	MTND1*LHON4160C	Secondary	++	L285P	H	Rare	0	−	76	54	0	377
19	MTND1*LHON4216C	Secondary	−	Y304H	L	−40	13	−	NA	NA	NA	363, 688
20	MTND2*LHON4917G	Secondary	−	D150N	H	3	3	−	NA	NA	NA	688
21	MTCO1*LHON7444A	Secondary	−	Ter→K	NA	5	1	−	NA	NA	UN	374
22	MTCO3*LHON9438A	Secondary	−	G78S	H	2.5	4.6	−	NA	UN	NA	365
23	MTCYB*LHON15812A	Secondary	−	V357M	M	4	0.1	−	NA	NA	NA	363

[a]The first 10 LHON-associated mtDNA mutations are listed in order of estimated severity (see text).
[b]C = confirmed; NC = not confirmed; A = ambiguous. A question mark in classification indicates transient assignment pending more data.
[c]H = high amino acid conservation, M = moderate; L = low; NA = not applicable; Ter = termination codon.
[d]M = multiple background haplotypes; F = few; UN = unknown; 1* = one reported case or family. Mutant association numbers refer to numbers in column one of this table.
[e]Het = Heteroplasmy
[f]NA = not applicable; UN = unknown; penetrance estimate for the 10663 mutation is from a single LHON family which does not harbor a common primary LHON mutation by complete mtDNA sequence analysis.
[g]Low = anecdotal low degree of vision recovery; UN = unknown; NA = not applicable

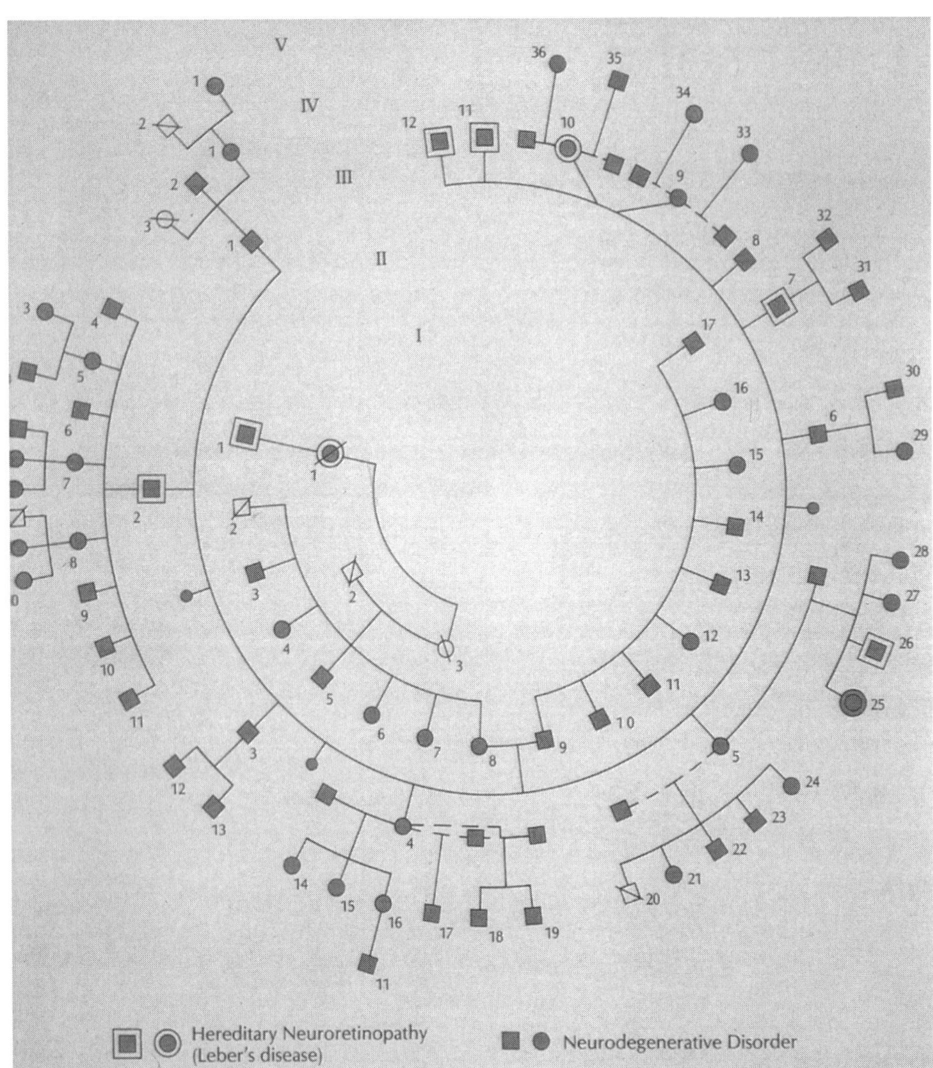

Fig. 105-19 Hispanic family with maternally inherited LHON and/or dystonia due to the heteroplasmic mtDNA mutation at MTND6*LDYT14459A. Individuals with LHON experience acute onset optic atrophy and central vision loss, generally as young adults. Individuals with neurodegenerative disease have a much earlier age of onset and experience gait disturbance, rigidity, pseudobulbar syndrome, impaired intelligence, short stature, and frequently infantile bilateral striatal necrosis (IBSN)[60,378]. *(Reprinted from Wallace.[824] Used with permission.)*

each individual.[13] Moreover, many individuals that inherit mtDNA mutations never manifest symptoms (Fig. 105-18), while others may develop other neurologic, cardiac, and skeletal problems. Hence, the etiology of LHON must be multifactorial.

The relative pathogenicity of the common primary LHON mutations can be assessed by: (a) the potential for co-occurrence of additional clinical signs; (b) the frequency with which independent pedigrees represent new mutations; (c) the frequency of heteroplasmy; (d) the frequency of the mutation in the unaffected population; (e) the penetrance of the mutation in apparently homoplasmic pedigrees; (f) the proportion of affected individuals that is male; (g) the propensity for visual recovery in patients harboring the mutation; and (h) the severity of an OXPHOS biochemical defect.

Applying these criteria, the MTND6*LDYT14459A mutation is the most pathogenic of the LHON mutations. This mutation can cause isolated LHON, but in many patients can also cause the generalized movement disorder, dystonia, as well as other neurologic symptoms. In one large five-generation pedigree, among 42 maternal relatives, 19 percent had LHON, 31 percent had dystonia and bilateral striatal necrosis, and 2 percent had both (Fig. 105-19).[378] The mean age of onset of dystonia was 4 years, with a range of 1.5 to 9 years. The motor system was primarily involved and resulted in gait disturbance and rigidity of the lower extremities that advanced with age to include the upper extremities. Patients also developed pseudobulbar syndrome (swallowing and speech problems), impaired intelligence, short stature, and myopathic features. These symptoms were often associated with bilateral striatal necrosis[378] and the loss of cells in the striatum, putamen, and caudate. Among the three MTND6*-LDYT 14459A-positive families (each with a different mtDNA background), the symptoms differed. The family with the African haplogroup L mtDNA presented with primarily optic atrophy, the family with a Native American haplogroup D mtDNA manifested optic atrophy and/or dystonia, and the individual with European haplogroup I mtDNA developed only dystonia.[60,347] Currently, it is unclear whether the background haplotype modulates the expression of the MTND6*LDYT14459A mutation.

The MTND6*LDYT14459A mutation must be sufficiently severe that it is rapidly eliminated from the population.[290] This conclusion is supported by the fact that it is consistently heteroplasmic, suggesting new mutations, and has not been observed in the normal population including 108 Asian, 103 Caucasian, and 99 African control mtDNAs, nor was it observed in 38 mtDNA haplotype D-matched Native American controls.[60] Its penetrance among maternal relatives is about 61 percent, with 58 percent of the affected individuals being male, and there is no record of an affected individual recovering (Table 105-12).

The MTND4*LHON11778A mutation is the most common cause of LHON. It has a highly variable penetrance, such that many individuals who harbor this mutation are phenotypically normal (Fig. 105-21). Of the affected individuals, the mean age of onset is 27.6 years, with a range of onset from 8 to 60 years. About 58 percent of patients show additional ophthalmologic features, including peripapillary telangiectasias, microangiopathy, disk pseudoedema, and vascular tortuosity. Fifty-five percent of

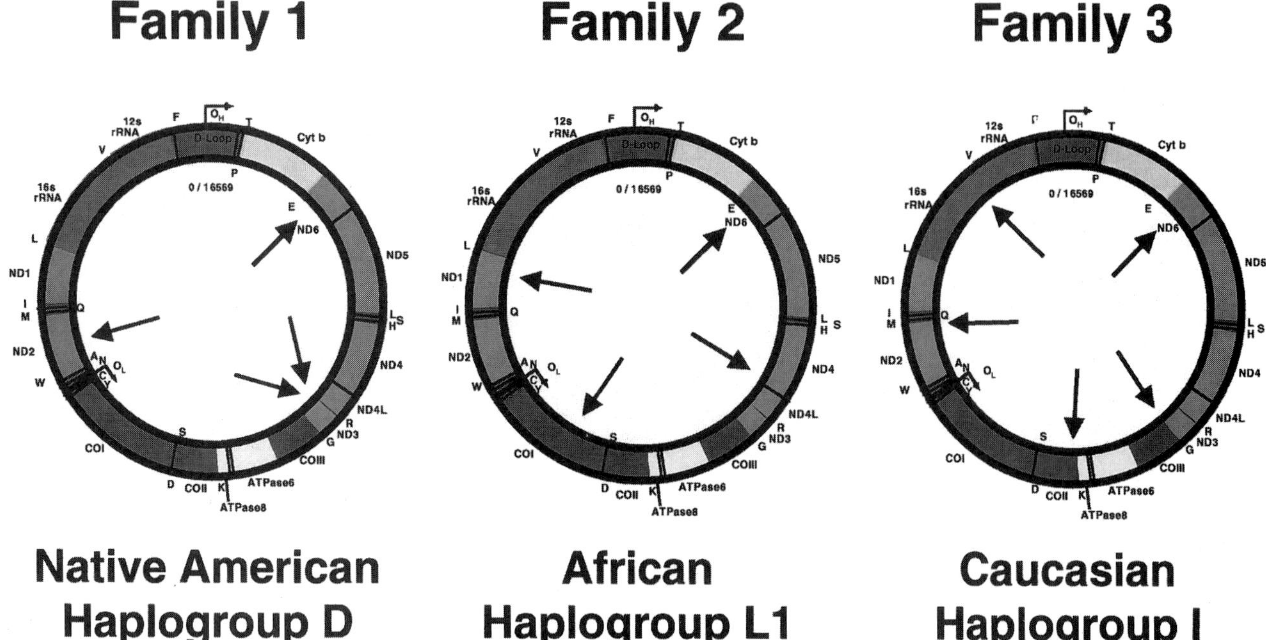

Fig. 105-20 Background haplotypes of three independent families harboring the MTND6*LDY14459A mutation. The family on the left is the Hispanic family presented in Fig. 105-19. This family had a Native American mtDNA from haplogroup D. The center family was an African-American mother and daughter, both of which manifested LHON, with the daughter also having unilateral striatal necrosis. This pedigree harbored an African mtDNA from haplogroup L. The third patient on the right had generalized dystonia. He had a European-derived mtDNA from haplogroup I. Thus, each family must be the result of an independent MTND6*LDYT14459A mutation.[60,347]

patients have a simultaneous onset of vision loss in both eyes, while the overall mean interocular interval is 1.8 months, and the maximum interval is about 9 months. Once vision loss begins, it can progress rapidly or slowly. The mean length of progression for the MTND4*LHON11778A mutation is 3.7 months, with a range of 0 to 24 months. In about 98 percent of cases, the final visual acuity is 20/200 or worse, while only 2 percent are better than 20/200.[358] Most cases are limited to optic atrophy, although a variety of other mild abnormalities have been associated with this mutation. These include cardiac conduction defects such as abnormal QT interval,[379] skeletal abnormalities, and other neurologic signs.[345] One individual, who lost his vision at 37, developed cerebellar-extrapyramidal tremor and left-side rigidity associated with bilateral basal ganglia lesions at age 38.[380] A second MTND4*LHON11778A patient suffered visual loss at 23, showed pyramidal signs including spastic paraparesis, inexhaustible patellar and ankle clonus, diffuse muscle weakness and multiple periventricular and subcortical hyperintensities on MRI compatible with demyelinating disease.[381] A third family (mother and son) exhibited ataxia associated with cerebellar and pontine atrophy.[382] Thus, in unusual cases, the MTND4*LHON11778A mutations can be associated with the same motor disturbances that are a common presentation for the MTND6*LDYT14459A mutation. In LHON pedigrees with the MTND4*LHON11778A mutation, about 1 to 2 percent of female patients also have a diagnosis of multiple sclerosis-like demyelination disease.[358,383–387] Eight females with the MTND4*LHON11778A mutation have been described with LHON who subsequently developed the clinical and/or neuroradiologic signs consistent with multiple sclerosis.[384] A number of similar reports have appeared of females harboring the MTND4*LHON11778A mutation and exhibiting signs of multiple sclerosis,[383,388] and this phenomenon has also been seen in males.[385,388] Although the MTND4*LHON11778A mutation accounts for greater than 90 percent of Japanese LHON cases, no association has been found between this mutation and multiple sclerosis in the Japanese population.[389] LHON mutational associations with multiple sclerosis have been evident only when patients are ascertained through presentation with LHON (with or without family history) or through multiple sclerosis patients with early and prominent optic nerve involvement.[383] Given the rare population frequency of both diseases, it is unlikely, therefore, that the frequent coincidence of LHON and multiple sclerosis occurs by chance. The mechanism by which LHON mtDNA mutations could cause multiple sclerosis remains undefined. However, it is possible that neuronal cell lysis resulting from the mitochondrial defect releases cellular proteins which initiate an autoimmune response.[385,390]

In one patient, the MTND4*LHON11778A mutation was associated with Wolfram syndrome, which included diabetes mellitus, optic atrophy, and sensorineural deafness.[391]

As mentioned, most pedigrees harboring the MTND4*LHON11778A mutation represent independent mutational events.[353,392] Consistent with this conclusion, approximately 14 percent of MTND4*LHON11778A families are heteroplasmic.[358] Moreover, this mutation has not been detected in over 250 controls.[393] Hence, the MTND4*LHON11778A mutation, like the MTND6*LDYT14459A mutation, must be relatively rapidly removed from the population by selection.

Among MTND4*LHON11778A families, approximately 33 to 60 percent of maternal relatives are affected, with 82 percent of the affected individuals being male and 18 percent female.[358,393] Furthermore, only about 4 percent of affected individuals experience visual recovery. Hence, the MTND4*LHON11778A mutation has a slightly lower penetrance than the MTND6*LDYT14459A mutation, and a much greater bias towards males being affected.

The MTND1*LHON3460A mutation is the next most severe primary mutation. Generally, the clinical manifestations of this mutation are confined to LHON, with features quite similar to MTND4*LHON11778A. Only occasionally is the MTND1*LHON3460A mutation associated with other neurologic signs (Table 105-12), although patients harboring this mutation can manifest multiple sclerosis.[383,388] Virtually every MTND1*LHON3460A family is due to an independent mutation,[353] a small percentage of the families are heteroplasmic, and the mutation has not been detected in over 400 normal controls.[393] The number of affected

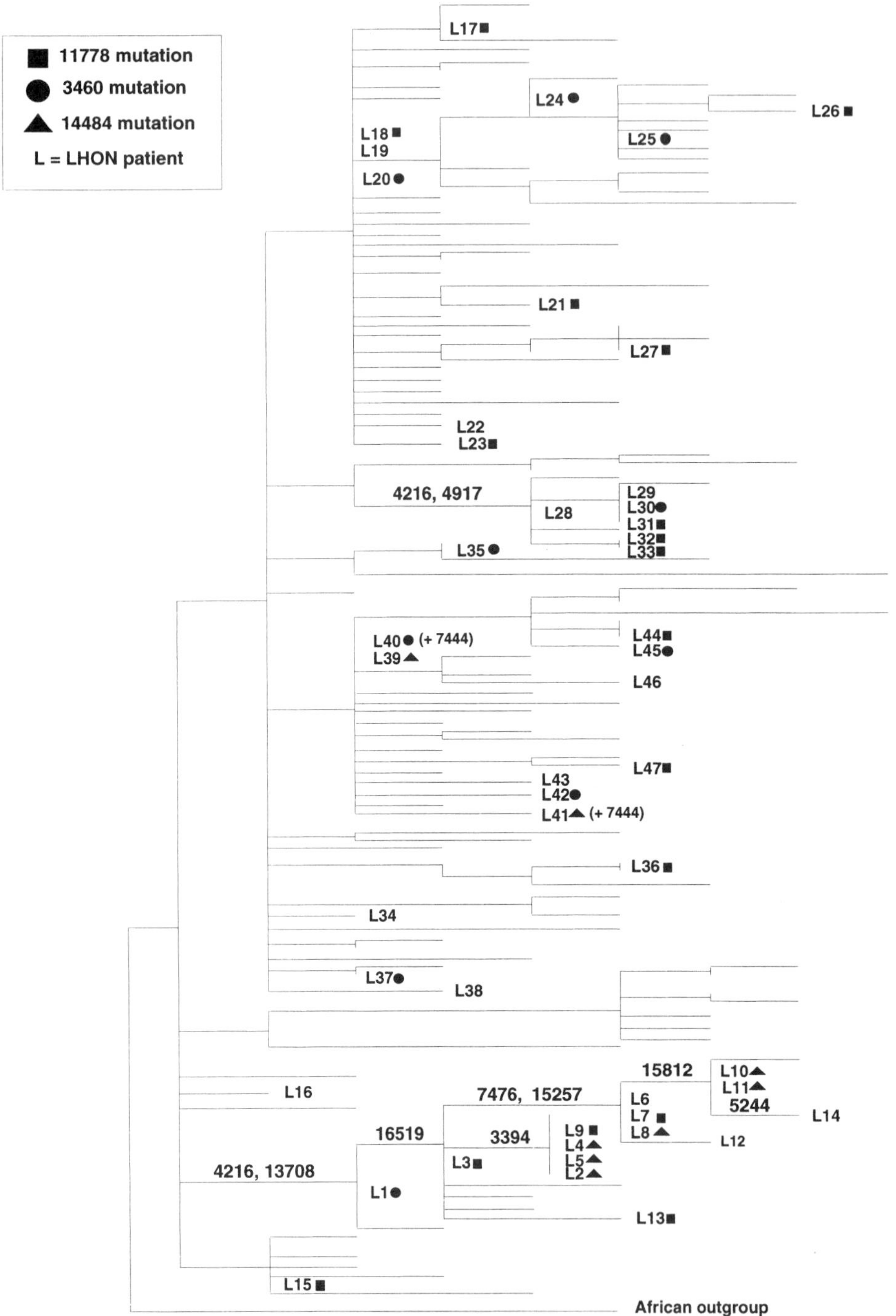

Fig. 105-21 Phylogenetic tree of Caucasian mtDNAs from 47 LHON patients (L1-L47, bold) and 175 Caucasian controls obtained from the United States and Canada. Haplotypes were determined by RFLP analysis using the entire mtDNA. For the patients, all mtDNA haplotypes are shown and the presence of a common primary mutation is indicated (see key). Additional mutations of interest are noted in parentheses. Multiple occurrences of the three common primary LHON mutations are indicated by their presence in independent mtDNA lineages, and, when occurring within the same large mtDNA lineage, by the presence of intermediate haplotypes lacking LHON mutations. The numbers in large, bold characters on branches indicate mutations that define specific groups of mtDNAs but are not necessarily the mutational steps used to create the phylogeny. The horizontal branch lengths are proportional to the number of mutational events that separate haplotypes. (*From Brown et al.*[353] *Used with permission.*)

maternal relatives has varied widely in different studies, but can approach 75 percent,[394,395] with between 40 percent and 80 percent of all affected individuals being male. In contrast to the MTND4*LHON11778A mutation, however, approximately 22 percent of affected individuals with the MDND1*LHON3460A have been reported to experience visual recovery.[371] Hence, in some respects the MTND1*LHON3460A mutation may be considered less deleterious than the MTND4*LHON11778A mutation.

The MTND6*LHON14484C mutation is the mildest of the common primary mutations. Clinically, this mutation is rarely associated with a complex neurologic phenotype. The penetrance of the MTND6*LHON14484C mutation is comparable to that of the other primary LHON mutations, resulting in symptoms in 27 to 80 percent of maternal relatives. Also, the male-to-female ratio of affected individuals is high when compared to that for the MTND4*LHON11778A and MTND1*LHON3460A mutations.[346,371,394] While most MTND6*LHON14484C families are likely to be independent mutations, the strong association with haplogroup J perhaps indicates that the MTND6*LHON14484C is less capable of causing LHON alone than are the MTND4*LHON11778A and MTND1*LHON3460A mutations.[360,396] Moreover, the MTND6*LHON14484C mutation is only rarely heteroplasmic,[359] suggesting that the great majority of mtDNAs in a patient must be mutant to cause a sufficient biochemical defect to result in optic atrophy.

The MTND6*LHON14484C mutation is additionally noteworthy for the tendency of patients to experience visual recovery. Fully 37 to 50 percent of patients with this mutation report visual improvement (Table 105-12).[346,371] Thus, the MTND6*-LHON14484C mutation has the lowest pathogenicity of the primary LHON mutations and may be pathogenic only when present in certain mtDNA contexts. Clearly, the MTND6*-LHON14484C mutation is at the transition between primary causal and secondary enhancing mutations.

While the MTND6*LHON14484C mutation by itself is relatively mild, its phenotype can be severe when paired with certain other mtDNA mutations. In one large pedigree encompassing LHON and severe neurodegenerative disease, the MTND6*LHON14484C mutation was combined with the MTND1*LHON4160C mutation.[377] This latter mutation changed a highly conserved leucine at codon 285 of the ND1 polypeptide to a proline. Both mutations were homoplasmic (Table 105-12). The clinical presentations included sudden onset optic atrophy with an approximately twofold excess of affected males. In addition to the optic atrophy, there were two neurologic presentations. The first had an onset in the first or second decade of life, starting as a gait abnormality and progressing to include ataxia, spasticity, tremor, dysarthria, posterior column signs, and skeletal deformities. The second had a childhood-onset (5 to 10 years) severe encephalitic disease, occasionally resulting in death. Initial signs include headache, convulsions, and abnormal respiration. A novel feature of this later presentation was that some individuals appeared to recover fully.[397] One branch of the pedigree had less severe symptoms and was found to have a second homoplasmic mutation, MTND1*LHON4136G, which was hypothesized to be protective.[377] Biochemical analysis of platelet-derived mitochondria from four subjects revealed an 80 percent reduction in rotenone-sensitive NADH-CoQ oxidoreductase specific activity.[398] Thus, the combination of the MTND6*LHON14484C + MTND1*LHON4160C mutation appears to have the same effect on complex I activity as the MTND6*LDYT14459A mutation does.

OXPHOS Dysfunction and LHON. Multiple studies have been conducted on the biochemical defects associated with each LHON mutation. Virtually all of the primary LHON mutations alter mtDNA-encoded, inner membrane proteins that contribute to NADH:ubiquinone oxidoreductase or complex I. Therefore, it would seem logical that all of the primary mutations would have a common, deleterious effect on complex I, which, in turn, would result in a bioenergetic defect sufficient to precipitate the disease. However, extensive biochemical analysis has not substantiated this contention. Rather, all of the primary LHON mutations have been found to have quite different effects on complex I.

Bioenergetic capacity of mitochondrial mutants is typically determined using respiration and/or enzymologic studies. For LHON, respiration experiments typically measure oxygen consumption rates and ADP phosphorylation efficiency when complex I (NADH)-linked substrates are provided to patient cells or intact mitochondria. OXPHOS enzyme assays measure the specific activity of OXPHOS enzymes in mitochondrial membrane fragments (submitochondrial particles). Both types of experiments are technically complicated, such that variation exists among laboratories with respect to materials assayed (cells versus isolated mitochondria), methods for mitochondrial isolation, assay conditions, and so on. For example, biochemical analysis of LHON mutations has been performed on cells and/or mitochondria from leukocytes, platelets, skeletal muscle, lymphoblasts, and fibroblasts. Even with this methodologic variability, a number of common observations have been made and substantiated.

Analysis of MTND6*LDYT14459A patient skeletal muscle mitochondria has revealed that complex I activity is essentially eliminated.[347] In contrast, biochemical analysis of OXPHOS enzymes and respiration in mitochondria isolated from Epstein-Barr virus (EBV)-transformed lymphoblastoid cell lines of MTND6*LDYT14459A patients revealed a 55 percent reduction in complex I-specific activity when normalized to citrate synthase or mitochondrial protein.[57] This defect could be transferred along with the mutant mtDNAs to ρ^0 lymphoblastoid cells in cybrid experiments.[57] In contrast to the greater than 50 percent reduction in complex I-specific activity, the overall mitochondrial respiration rate using complex I substrates was not significantly reduced. This implies that the complex I defect alone is not sufficient to be rate limiting, consistent with respiratory control theory.[399,400]

Kinetic analysis of the MTND6*LDYT14459A complex I defect revealed that the V_{max} for NADH is reduced, but the K_m is not.[57] Furthermore, the enzyme activity with increased decylubiquinone (DB), a CoQ_{10} analogue, showed a maximum activity at 5 mM and then declined as DB was increased to 10 mM, a result in marked contrast to the steady increase in activity seen in the control enzyme over this same concentration range. Finally, there was a marked product inhibition of the enzyme by 5 mM DBH_2 with the specific activity being inhibited 71 percent. These data suggest that the MTND6*LDYT14459A mutation may alter the CoQ_{10} binding site of complex I.[57] Hence, the MTND6*LDYT14459A mutation places MTND6 near the CoQ_{10} binding site.

Some studies on the MTND4*LHON11778A mutation have reported complex I enzymatic defects ranging from 0 to 50 percent relative to control complex I activity. However, most studies have found no statistically significant reduction in complex I activity.[380,401–405] By contrast, most studies have observed a reduction in mitochondrial respiration using complex I-linked substrates of 30 to 50 percent, while respiration rates using succinate are normal.[380,401,403,406] When the MTND4*LHON11778A mtDNAs are transferred to a different nuclear background by cybrid transfer, the respiration defect is transferred, indicating that the respiration defect is linked to the mtDNA mutation.[381,401,407] The MTND4*LHON11778A mutation has also been reported to have an increased resistance to rotenone, a complex I inhibitor which acts as a ubiquinone antagonist. The mutant enzyme also has an altered affinity for ubiquinone analogs, though other groups have not detected this alteration in rotenone sensitivity.[402,404,406] These observations have led to the postulation that the MTND4*LHON11778A mutation alters the complex I interaction with ubiquinone. Alternatively, the amino acid change has been hypothesized to compromise the enzyme's energy conserving (proton translocation) function, or to destabilize ubisemiquinone intermediates promoting the production of ROS. The absence of an enzymologic defect in the presence of a clear respiration defect might be due to a defect in proton translocation or to an alternation of coenzyme Q affinity that is masked in the enzyme assays by the use of coenzyme Q analogues at nonphysiological concentrations as electron acceptors.

In striking contrast to the MTND4*LHON11778A mutation, the MTND1*LHON3460A mutation is associated with markedly reduced complex I activity, but a less severe reduction in respiration. In multiple studies of patient cells, the MTND1*LHON3460A mutation has been found to be associated with a 60 to 80 percent reduction in the complex I-specific activity.[349,401–403,405] Despite the pronounced reduction in complex I activity, ATP synthesis in MTND1*LHON3460A mitochondria is not compromised.[408] Respiration studies have shown a roughly 30 percent reduction in maximal respiration rates using complex I-linked substrates—slightly less than the reduced rate found associated with the MTND4*LHON11778A mutation.[401,406] In cybrid transfer experiments, the complex I defect transfers faithfully,[401] although nuclear genetic backgrounds may alter the magnitude of the functional defect found in cybrids.[409] When complex I activity was titrated with ubiquinone analogues/derivatives, a substrate inhibition pattern was observed.[409] This is very similar to the functional defect associated with the MTND6*LDYT14459A mutation.[57] The parallel observations for the MTND1*LHON3460A and the MTND6*LDYT14459A mutations are consistent with altered ubiquinone binding affinity, which would be in line with the proposal that both the ND1 and ND6 polypeptides are components of the ubiquinone binding site. Given the similarity in biochemical defect between the two mutations, it is surprising that the two mutations can give quite different phenotypes, LHON for the MTND1*LHON3460A mutation and LHON and dystonia for the MTND6*LDYT14459A mutation.

The biochemical defect of the MTND6*LHON14484C mutation has proven very difficult to detect. Thus, the functional defects associated with this mutation may match the milder genetic and clinical signature of this mutation. In our enzyme and respiration analysis on patient lymphoblasts and cybrids, we found that the specific activity of complex I was essentially normal, even though maximal respiration rates were reduced 15 to 20 percent with complex I-linked substrates.[401] Similarly, in separate, independent studies, no reduction in complex I activity in was found in MTND6*LHON14484C-positive patient fibroblasts,[410,411] although another study reported a severe (65 percent) reduction in complex I activity and an associated 20 percent reduction in complex I-linked ATP synthesis in its patients.[412] One recent report implicates this mutation in complex I-ubiquinone interactions as platelet mitochondria containing the MTND6*LHON14484C mutation were found to have increased sensitivity to the complex I product inhibitors mixothiazol and $NBQH_2$.[411] While additional studies will be needed to reach a consensus concerning the functional defects of this mutation, it is apparent that the biochemical defect of the MTND6*LHON14484C mutation is milder than that of the MTND1*LHON3460A, MTND4*LHON11778A, and MTND6*LDYT14459A mutations.

Potential Pathophysiological Mechanisms of LHON. The pathophysiology of the acute or subacute vision loss of LHON is unknown. The LHON mutations do not appear to alter the amount, assembly, or stability of complex I. However, various mutations have been found to alter the electron transport capacity, respiration rate, and ATP production of complex I. Consequently, it seems possible that all LHON mutations may have a common respiratory defect, and that they differ primarily in the magnitude of this defect.

One respiratory defect that might tie many LHON mutations together is an inhibition in the transfer of electrons from complex I to CoQ_{10}. A faulty interaction between CoQ_{10} and complex I has been documented for the MTND6*LDYT14459A mutation,[57] and suggested for the MTND6*LHON14484C mutation,[411] implying that the region of ND6 around codons 64 to 72 may be involved in CoQ_{10} interaction with complex I. Furthermore, four other pathogenic missense mutations have been found in this same region of ND6, which encompasses the most evolutionarily conserved transmembrane helix (helix c) as well as a region similar to the ubiquinone-reacting domain of cytochrome b in complex III.[411] These are the MTND6*LHON14482C mutation that alters codon 64, the MTND6*LHON14498T mutation that alters codon 59, the MTND6*LHON14568T mutation that affects codon 36, and the MTND6*LDYT14596A mutation that changes codon 26 (Table 105-13). Moreover, the biochemical defects of the MTND6*LDYT14459A and MTND1*LHON3460A mutations are similar, suggesting a common mechanism, and ND1 is also thought to be important in electron transfer to CoQ_{10}. Finally, the MTND4*LHON11778A mutation has been associated with altered rotenone binding and thus of transfer to CoQ_{10}.[402,404,406] Thus, all of the primary LHON mutations have been implicated in problems with CoQ_{10} interaction with complex I. Such a defect might be difficult to evaluate accurately given the difficulties with assaying complex I with the physiological substrate, CoQ_{10}, necessitating the use of the CoQ_{10} analogues such as DB. The possibility that all of these mutations impair electron transfer to CoQ_{10} is supported by the observation that all of the primary LHON and LDYT mutations that have been studied (MTND6*LDYT14459A, MTND4*LHON11778A, MTND1*LHON3460A, and MTND6*LHON14484C) show at least a partial defect in complex I-linked respiration, with reductions in maximal respiration rates for the various mutations ranging from 15 to 40 percent. Given metabolic threshold studies that show that complex I must be reduced by more than 70 percent before oxygen consumption or ATP production are perturbed,[399] it is possible that even the small reduction in respiration observed for the MTND6*LHON14484C mutation might reflect a significant defect in electron transfer within the mitochondria under physiological conditions.

Assuming that the primary defect of most LHON and LDYT mutations is an inhibition of the electron transport chain, then the pathophysiological basis of the disease might either be chronic energy deficiency or increased ROS generation due to the redirection of electrons from complex I and CoQ_{10} to molecular oxygen. If increased ROS production and oxidative stress have a role in LHON, then this might contribute to the pathology of LHON in two ways. It is possible that chronic oxidative stress to the retinal ganglion cells and optic nerve might damage the mtDNA and degrade mitochondrial function to such an extent that ultimately the neuronal mtPTP is activated and the cells undergo a wave of programmed cell death. Such a model is attractive because it explains how a chronic disease could result in a sudden onset of symptoms with a precipitous course. Indeed, this hypothesis could be generalized into a common mechanism for a variety of neurodegenerative diseases, including amyotrophic lateral sclerosis (ALS). ALS patients appear normal until middle age, when they precipitously begin to manifest symptoms of motor weakness due to motor neuron loss, rapidly leading to paralysis and death. Some cases of familial ALS have been associated with mutations in the cytosolic Cu/ZnSOD. These mutations appear to be gain-of-function mutations that increase oxidative stress. A primary target of this increased oxidative stress may be the mitochondria, which show marked changes in mitochondrial morphology and OXPHOS enzyme activities in transgenic mice carrying the human Gly93Ala mutation, preceding the onset of motor decline.[413]

Alternatively, the increased mitochondrial production of ROS might inactivate the vasodilator NO, resulting in chronic vasoconstriction, ischemia, and death of the retinal ganglion cells. A common set of preclinical findings in LHON families includes microangiopathy, retinal vessel telangiectasias, and tortuous vessels, consistent with LHON being due to a retinal vasculopathy. NO is a natural vasodilator, and it is acutely sensitive to inactivation by ROS.[414] If the LHON mutations inhibit the electron transport chain and increase mitochondrial ROS production, then it is possible that these ROS chronically deplete the retinal vascular NO, causing vasoconstriction and ultimately resulting in the spasmodic constriction of the retinal blood vessels, depriving the retinal ganglia cells of oxygen and nutrients. This would lead to ischemia and neuronal death. Thus sudden onset of vision loss would be envisioned as a form of a retinal stroke.

While it will be difficult to define the pathophysiology of mitochondrial ophthalmologic disease in human studies, it is likely that more progress will be made using mouse models for mitochondrial disease. If LHON is the result of increased oxidative stress, then mice lacking mitochondrial antioxidant defenses should be more prone to ophthalmologic decline.

Diagnostic Paradigm for LHON. Because the MTND4*LHON11778A, MTND1*LHON3460A, MTND6*LHON14484C and MTND6*LDYT14459A account for 90 percent of all LHON, molecular testing for the primary LHON mutations is justified to confirm the LHON diagnosis. Simple PCR-based restriction endonuclease assays are available for the common LHON mutations (Fig. 105-17).

In the event that a patient does not harbor one of the above primary mutations, but LHON is strongly suspected, then additional tiers of genetic tests can be applied, including

LEIGH SYNDROME DIAGNOSTIC PARADIGM

Clinical Presentations:

1. Age: generally pediatric onset involving children of 1 to 5 years.
2. Primary clinical signs: can include hypotonia, weakness, ataxia, tremor, respiratory distress (dyspnea), apnea, Cheyne-Stokes breathing.
3. Occasional clinical signs: hypertrophic cardiomyopathy and liver involvement.
4. Neuro-ophthalmologic findings: ophthalmoplegia, sluggish pupils, optic atrophy, retinitis pigmentosa (RP).
5. Family history: possible (a) maternal history of Leigh, RP, ataxia, etc.; (b) X-linked with affected males; (c) autosomal recessive with possible consanguinity.

Diagnostic Testing:

1. Metabolic: (a) possible elevated urine and/or serum lactate and pyruvate as well as other TCA cycle intermediates (e.g., α-ketoglutarate, citrate, succinate etc.). (b) possible elevated alanine and other TCA cycle associated amino acids (e.g., glutamate)
2. Neuroradiological: possible increased bilateral basal ganglia lucencies on MRI; possible cortical and cerebellar atrophy
3. Muscle biopsy:
   a. histochemical analysis: possible altered fiber type size, rarely ragged-red fibers (RRFs), occasionally abnormal mitochondrial ultrastructure.
   b. OXPHOS enzymology: frequently highly significant deficiencies in one or more enzyme complexes.
   c. cultured cell enzymology (lymphocytes and/or fibroblasts): frequently specific defects in pyruvate dehydrogenase, pyruvate carboxylase, complex I, complex IV, or complex V.
4. Genetic: mtDNA mutations for sporadic and maternally inherited cases; nDNA mutations in complex I, II, and IV genes, as well as E1α subunit gene of pyruvate dehydrogenase.

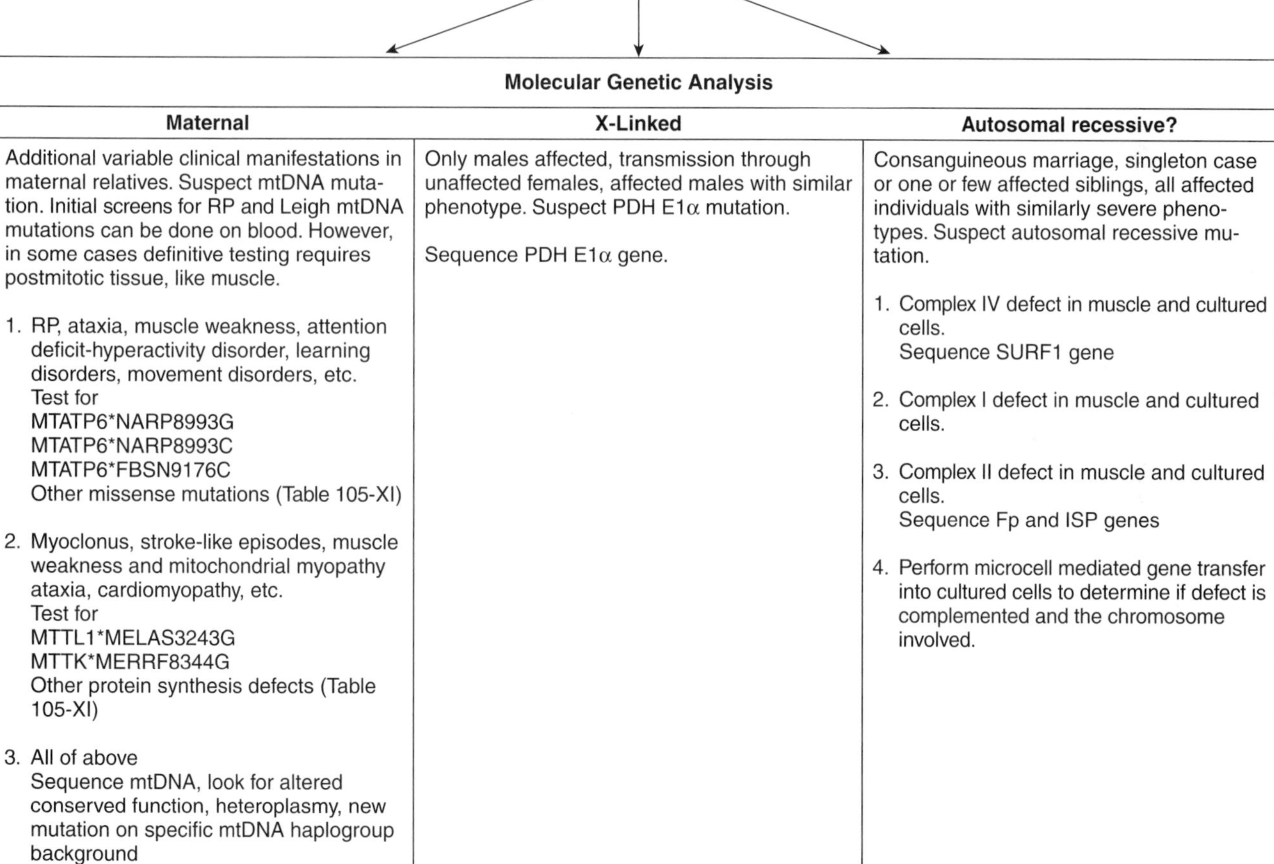

Molecular Genetic Analysis

Maternal	X-Linked	Autosomal recessive?
Additional variable clinical manifestations in maternal relatives. Suspect mtDNA mutation. Initial screens for RP and Leigh mtDNA mutations can be done on blood. However, in some cases definitive testing requires postmitotic tissue, like muscle. 1. RP, ataxia, muscle weakness, attention deficit-hyperactivity disorder, learning disorders, movement disorders, etc. Test for MTATP6*NARP8993G MTATP6*NARP8993C MTATP6*FBSN9176C Other missense mutations (Table 105-XI) 2. Myoclonus, stroke-like episodes, muscle weakness and mitochondrial myopathy ataxia, cardiomyopathy, etc. Test for MTTL1*MELAS3243G MTTK*MERRF8344G Other protein synthesis defects (Table 105-XI) 3. All of above Sequence mtDNA, look for altered conserved function, heteroplasmy, new mutation on specific mtDNA haplogroup background	Only males affected, transmission through unaffected females, affected males with similar phenotype. Suspect PDH E1α mutation. Sequence PDH E1α gene.	Consanguineous marriage, singleton case or one or few affected siblings, all affected individuals with similarly severe phenotypes. Suspect autosomal recessive mutation. 1. Complex IV defect in muscle and cultured cells. Sequence SURF1 gene 2. Complex I defect in muscle and cultured cells. 3. Complex II defect in muscle and cultured cells. Sequence Fp and ISP genes 4. Perform microcell mediated gene transfer into cultured cells to determine if defect is complemented and the chromosome involved.

Fig. 105-22 Diagnostic paradigm for Leigh syndrome.

low-frequency primary mutations (MTND6*LHON14482G, MTND2*LHON5244A, MTCO3*LHON9804A, MTATP6*LHON9101C, MTND3*LHON10663C, MTND5*LHON13730A, and possibly MTND*11696G, MTND6*LHON14489T, MTND6*LHON14568T, and MTND6*LDYT14596A), as well as the high-frequency secondary mutations associated with haplogroup J (MTND1*LHON4216C, MTND2*LHON4917C, MTND5*LHON13708A, and MTCYB*LHON15257A). Maternally inherited cases of optic neuropathy that do not harbor any of the above mutations might be the result of new mtDNA mutations. In this case, further investigations might require sequencing of the mtDNA, preferably from a postmitotic tissue such as muscle (Fig. 105-17).

Retinitis Pigmentosa and Leigh Syndrome

Pigmentary retinopathy, neurodegeneration, and Leigh syndrome have been associated with mutations in the mtDNA MTATP6 gene, as well as with mutation in several nDNA genes involved in the assembly of the respiratory complexes. A diagnostic paradigm for Leigh syndrome and retinitis pigmentosa is given in Fig. 105-22.

Leigh syndrome (subacute necrotizing encephalomyopathy) has an average age of onset of about 1.5 years, with a mean duration of illness until death of about 5 years. Clinical manifestations include ataxia, hypotonia, spasticity, developmental delay and regression, optic atrophy, nystagmus, respiratory abnormalities, and ophthalmoplegia. The myopathy is generally nonspecific and includes fat accumulations. Occasional patients can show liver involvement, cardiomyopathy and mitochondrial myopathy including ragged-red muscle fibers (RRFs), and mitochondria with paracrystalline inclusions, although most patients have normal muscle fiber and mitochondria morphology. A common observation is the abrupt worsening of the patient's clinical and metabolic status with infections or febrile episodes. A common neuroradiologic finding of end-stage patients is the bilateral degeneration of the basal ganglion, readily observed by CT and MRI analysis. Brain pathology classically reveals basal ganglia necrosis associated with marked vascular proliferation in the brain stem.[242]

Current estimates of the proportion of cases resulting from the known biochemical and molecular defects[415] include: (a) about 18 percent mtDNA mutations; (b) about 10 percent pyruvate dehydrogenase defects;[416–418] (c) about 19 percent complex I defects;[417,419] (d) about 18 percent complex IV defects including SURF-1 mutations;[139,140,271,420] and (e) about 35 percent other causes including complex II[79] and pyruvate carboxylase defects.[421] That so many different mitochondrial bioenergetic defects can cause the same lethal phenotype, Leigh syndrome, indicates that the clinical manifestations of Leigh syndrome represent the common clinical endpoint for the most severe mitochondrial OXPHOS defects.

While the clinical presentation for Leigh syndrome is relatively constant, regardless of the molecular defect, the clinical manifestations of other family members can be greatly affected by the nature of the genetic defect. Generally, in families in which disease results from a nuclear gene mutation, the clinical presentation of affected family members is similar to that of the proband. Thus, for X-linked Leigh syndrome due to PDH E1α mutations, males are primary affected and should have a similarly severe phenotype. Likewise, Leigh patients with recessive mutations in nuclear genes will have similar phenotypes in affected family members, with consanguineous marriages being more common. By contrast, Leigh syndrome resulting from a heteroplasmic mtDNA mutation will be associated with highly variable clinical presentations among maternal relatives, with symptoms including retinitis pigmentosa, ophthalmoplegia, optic atrophy, cerebellar ataxia, stroke-like episodes, epilepsy, short stature, behavior disorders, movement disorders, and so on (Fig. 105-22).

mtDNA Mutations Associated with Retinitis Pigmentosa and Leigh Syndrome. The three main mtDNA mutations associated with retinitis pigmentosa and Leigh syndrome are MTATP6*NARP8993G,[422–426] MTATP6*NARP8993C,[427,428] and MTATP6*FBSN9176C[429] (Table 105-12). Leigh syndrome has also been seen in individuals harboring the protein synthesis mutations MTTK*MERRF8344G[430,431] and MTTL1*MELAS3243G[242] (Fig. 105-22).

The first description of maternally inherited retinitis pigmentosa came with the report of the MTATP6*NARP8993G mutation. MTATP6*NARP8993G pedigrees are invariably maternally inherited and heteroplasmic.[422] The initial three-generation pedigree included individuals who presented with neurogenic muscle weakness, ataxia, and retinitis pigmentosa, hence the acronym NARP. The severity of the symptoms varied markedly between individuals and generally correlated with the percentage of mutant mtDNAs harbored by the individual. Neurodegenerative symptoms included generalized seizures, axonal sensory neuropathy, dementia, corticospinal tract degeneration, and cerebellar and brain stem atrophy.[422] This last-mentioned clinical feature can manifest as olivopontocerebellar atrophy on MRI, as seen in subject I-1 of the pedigree in Fig. 105-23. This individual exhibited mental retardation, macular degeneration, and spicular

OPCA + RP and Leigh syndrome associated with mtATP6*8993

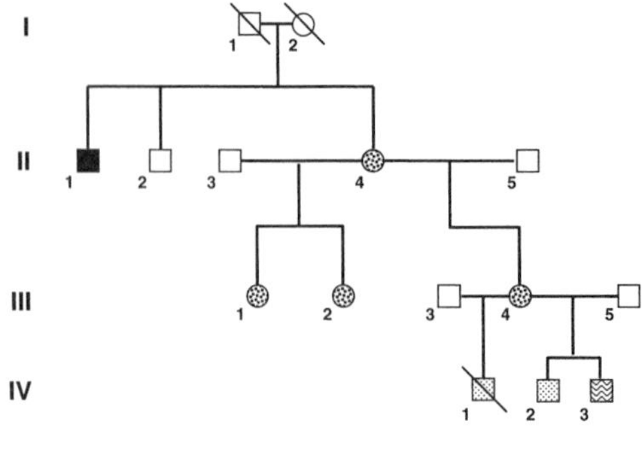

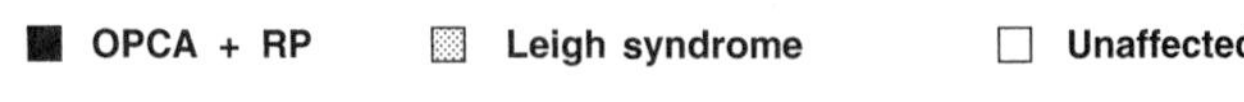

Fig. 105-23 Maternal pedigree segregating retinitis pigmentosa and Leigh syndrome due to the heteroplasmic MTATP6*NARP8993G mutation. The clinical phenotypes of the different maternal relatives ranged from mild salt and pepper retinitis pigmentosa in individuals II4, III1, III2, and III4; to mental retardation, macular degeneration, spicular retinitis pigmentosa, and massive olivopontocerebellar atrophy in individual II-1, to cerebellar ataxia in individual IV-3, to severe childhood-onset Leigh disease in individuals IV-1 and IV-2. This clinical variability is a reflection, at least in part, of the replicative segregation of the heteroplasmic MTATP6*NARP8993G mutation. (*Adapted from Ortiz et al.*[423] *Used with permission.*)

retinitis pigmentosa.[423] Subsequently, families harboring the MTATP6*NARP8993G mutation were found to include individuals presenting with Leigh syndrome.[425,426,432–434]

The variability in clinical presentation of the MTATP6*NARP8993G and C mutations is primarily due to the replicative segregation of the heteroplasmic mutation among maternal relatives. This is demonstrated in the pedigree in Fig. 105-23 in which the symptoms ranged from family members with mild salt-and-pepper retinitis pigmentosa, to an individual with olivopontocerebellar atrophy, to a child with cerebellar ataxia, and to two children with Leigh syndrome. Generally, adults with retinitis pigmentosa harbor about 75 percent mutant mtDNAs, while children with lethal Leigh syndrome have in excess of 90 percent mutant mtDNAs.[423]

The pathophysiology of the MTATP6*NARP8993G and C mutations has been elucidated through the biochemical analysis of patient mitochondria isolated from cultured cells, and through studies of the mechanism of ATP synthesis by the ATP synthase. The MTTP6*NARP8993G and C mutations change the highly conserved leucine 156 in the ATP6 polypeptide to an arginine or proline, respectively. Biochemical analysis of the MTATP6*NARP8993G mutation in patient lymphoblasts or fibroblasts has revealed a 30 percent to 50 percent reduction in the rate of ATP synthesis.[432,433,435] Moreover, in patient lymphoblasts and in their *trans*-mitochondrial cybrids, there was a 30 percent to 40 percent reduction in the rate of maximal (state III) respiration and a comparable reduction in ADP/O ratios.[261] Thus, the MTATP6*NARP8993G mutation results in a significant bioenergetic defect in ATP synthesis.

Correlating the position and nature of the amino acid changes caused by the MTATP6*NARP8993G and C mutations with recent data on the rotor–stator mechanism of the ATP synthase (Figs. 105-7 and 105-8) indicates that the MTATP6*NARP8993 G and C mutations must compromise the ATP synthase proton channel. The highly conserved leucine at ATP6 amino acid 156 is analogous to the *E. coli* amino acid 207 (Fig. 105-8). This forms the base of α-helix 4 in the bacterial protein a, the homologue of ATP6. As is clear from Fig. 105-8*B*, leucine 156 (bacterial 207) is on the same face of the helix as arginine 159 (bacterial 210). Arginine 159 (bacterial 210) is thought to provide the positive charge which pulls the negatively charged, deprotonized glutamate 58 (bacterial aspartate 61) from the matrix-space half proton channel around to the intermembrane-space half-proton channel. Arginine 159 (bacterial 210) is displaced from the glutamate 58 (aspartate 61) so as to provide attraction without forming a salt bridge and blocking rotation of the ATP9 (subunit c) protein wheel. However, conversion of leucine 156 to arginine adds a second positive charge on the ATP6 (a)/ATP9 (c) interface, and conversion of leucine 156 to proline disrupts the α-helix and presumably the interface between ATP6 (a) and ATP9 (c). Hence, both mutations would stall the rotor, block the proton channel, and inhibit ATP synthesis.

Two other pathogenic missense mutations have also been localized in the MTATP6 gene. These are MTATP6*FBSN9176C (Table 105-12) and MTATP6*LHON9101C (Table 105-13) mutations. The MTATP6*FBSN9176C variant changes the highly conserved leucine at codon 217 to a proline, while the MTATP6*LHON9101C changes the weakly conserved leucine at amino acid 192 to a threonine. These mutations are 61 and 36 codons away from the MTATP6*NARP8993G and C mutations, respectively. In *E. coli*, mutations in the c subunit (ATP9) which change aspartate 61 to glycine can be suppressed by mutations in the a subunit (ATP6) at Ala217, Ile221, and Leu224. Moreover, mutations at Gly218 and His214 of protein a (ATP6) result in uncoupling proton translocation from ATP synthesis, while the double mutant Gly218 to Lys plus His245 to Gly restores activity.[146] This implies that the region of human ATP6 around amino acid 197 (bacteria 245) may also be important in coupling the proton gradient to ATP synthesis. Thus, the MTATP6*LHON9101C mutation affecting ATP6 amino acid 192 (approximately bacterial 240) and the MTATP6*FBSN9176C mutation affecting ATP6 amino acid 217 (bacterial 256) flank the bacterial His 245, and hence might also alter the integrity of the ATP synthase proton channel. Hence, all of the pathogenic ATP6 missense mutations appear to affect the ATP synthase proton channel and thus inhibit the coupling of the proton gradient to the synthesis of ATP.

The observation that the MTATP6*LHON9101C mutation causes LHON and not retinitis pigmentosa and Leigh syndrome, like the other ATP6 mutations, may provide further insight into the pathophysiology of LHON. Mice in which the heart/muscle isoform of ANT (ANT1) has been genetically inactivated cannot import adequate ADP into the heart and skeletal muscle mitochondria to provide substrate for the ATP synthase. This inhibits the use of the ATP synthase proton channel, which blocks the depolarization ΔΨ. Hyperpolarization of ΔΨ then inhibits the electron transport chain and diverts the excess electrons into ROS production.[190,436] Assuming that the ATP6 mutations also block the ATP synthase proton channel, then the MTATP6*LHON9101C mutation might also increase ROS production and oxidative stress. This would support the hypothesis that LHON is the product of chronic oxidative stress acting on the retinal ganglia cells or the vascular endothelial cell-generated NO.

nDNA Mutations Associated with Retinitis Pigmentosa, Leigh Syndrome, and Related Neurodegenerative Disease. Mutations in a number of nuclear genes can also cause Leigh syndrome in association with retinitis pigmentosa (Tables 105-14, 105-15, and 105-16). These include mutations in the X-linked E1α subunit of pyruvate dehydrogenase,[418] in the autosomal NDUFS8 N-2 iron-sulfur center protein and the NDUFS7 protein of complex I,[24,419] in the autosomal flavoprotein subunit of complex II,[79] and in the autosomal SURF-1 gene associated with complex IV defects.[139,140]

The best described Leigh patient with a complex I gene mutation was the product of a compound heterozygote for mutations in the complex I subunit NDUFS8 (TYKY). NDUFS8 (TYKY) contains two 4Fe-4S ferredoxin consensus motifs, potentially forming the binding site for the N-2 iron-sulfur cluster. The missense mutations in the two alleles were Pro79Leu and Arg102His (Table 105-14).[419] The other two Leigh syndrome

Table 105-14 Nuclear OXPHOS Gene Disease Mutations

Phenotype	Gene funtion	Mutation	Chromosome	Reference
Leigh syndrome	Complex I–NDUFS8 N-2 FeS	P79L, R102H	9q33.2-34.11	24, 419
Leigh syndrome	Complex I–NDUFS7	V122M	11q13.1-13.3	24
Leigh syndrome	Complex I–NDUFS7	V122M	11q13.1-13.3	24
Leigh syndrome	Complex II–Fp subunit	R554W	5p16	79
Leigh syndrome	Complex IV–SURF-1	Multiple*	9q34	139, 140
Leigh syndrome	PDH–E1α	Multiple	X	418
Pediatric hypotonia, retardation, convulsions, brain and basal ganglia atrophy	Complex I–NDUFS4 18kDa protein	5-bp duplication	5	437
Pediatric hypotonia, vomiting, strabismus, myoclonus, CNS atrophy	Complex I–NDUFVI	R59X, T423M	11q13	24
Pediatric hypotonia, vomiting, strabismus, myoclonus, CNS atrophy	Complex I–NDUFVI	R59X, T423X	11q13	24
Pediatric myoclonic epilepsy, CNS atrophy	Complex I–NDUFVI	A341V	11q13	24
Spastic paraplegia	ATPase protease	Δ gene, 784del2 2228insA	16q24.3	438
Mohr-Tranebjaerg syndrome, deafness and dystonia	DFN-1, mitochondrial import	Δ gene, 183del10, 151delT	X21-22	212, 214, 439
Friedreich ataxia, neuropathy, cardiomyopathy, diabetes	frataxin mito. Fe transport, ROS toxicity	Trinuc.* repeat, structural	9q13	140, 823
MNGIE†	Thymidine phosphorylase	Multiple* missense	22q13.32-qter	522
AP-PEO	mtDNA stability	Unknown	3p14.2-21.2	512, 518
MtDNA Depletion	MtDNA copy control (?)	Unknown	Unknown	523, 524–531

*trinucleotide repeat
†MNGIE=Mitochondrial neurogastrointestinal encephalomyopathy

Table 105-15 Leigh Disease SURF-1 Mutations

Patient	Mutation	Exons	Type(s) mutation	Reference
A	37ins17/37in17	1/1	Frame/Frame	139
B	516+2T→G/550delAG	5/6	Splice/Frame	139
C	868insT/868insT	9/9	Frame/Frame	139
D	312del10, insAT/—	4/—	Frame	139
E	845delCT/845delCT	9/9	Frame/Frame	139
F	312del10, insAT/845delCT	4/9	Frame/Frame	139
G	751C→T (Q251X)/751C→T (Q251X)	7/7	Stop/Stop	139
H	845delCT/—	9/—	Frame/-	139
I	772delCC/—	8/—	Frame/-	139
W	C76ST/337+2T→C	7/4	Stop/del Frame	140
C	326insATdel10/855delCT	4/9	Frame/Frame	140
D	882insT	9/9	Frame/Frame	140

complex I cases had the same genotype. This was a homozygous missense mutation in the NDUFS7 gene causing a Val122Met substitution (Table 105-14).[24]

The Leigh syndrome complex II mutation altered the flavoprotein gene on chromosome 5p15 and was observed in two siblings. The proband had isolated complex II deficiency in skeletal muscle, cultured skin fibroblasts, and circulating lymphocytes, with the enzyme showing a heightened sensitivity to oxaloacetate, the physiological inhibitor. The causal mutation was a C to T transition at nucleotide 1684 in the cDNA resulting in an Arg544Trp substitution in a highly conserved domain of the protein. Both siblings were homozygous mutant, while the two parents were heterozygotes[79] (Table 105-14).

Multiple Leigh syndrome families with complex IV deficiency have been found to harbor mutations in the SURF-1 gene on chromosome 9q34. The SURF-1 protein appears to be involved in the assembly or maintenance of an active complex IV. The reported SURF-1 mutations have included nonsense mutations, missense mutations, and frameshift mutations resulting from small insertions and deletions, and are listed in Table 105-15.[139,140]

Four additional pathogenic mutations have been reported in nDNA complex I subunits in children with progressive degenerative disease. These children had a variety of symptoms, many reminiscent of Leigh syndrome, including hypotonia, feeding problems, vomiting, strabismus, myoclonic epilepsy, and MRI findings including basal ganglia abnormalities and atrophy. The complex I genes affected are for the NDUFS4 18-kDa protein (5-bp duplication),[437] the NDUFV1 protein (two compound heterozygotes for Arg59Stop + Thr423Met), and the NDUFV1 protein (Ala341Val).[24]

Table 105-16 MNGIE TP Gene Disease Mutations[522]

Patient	Mutations	Exons/Introns
1	E289A/E289A	E7/E7
2	E289A/t1504C, E4 skip	I4/E7
3	G145R/G145R	E4/E4
4	K222S/ins4196C	E6/E10
5	G145R/G145R	E4/E4
6	G145R/G145R	E4/E4
7	E289A/g3867c E9 Skip	E7/I8
8	G145R/—	E4/I7
9	Del6bp/q4090a	E9/I9
10	G153S/E289A	E4/E7
11	G153S/E289A	E4/E7
12	G153S/G153S	E4/E4

MNGIE = Mitochondrial neurogastrointestinal encephalomyopathy

The most detailed report of an nDNA complex I mutation patient involved the 18-kDa NDUFS4 mutation resulting from a 5-bp duplication. This child presented with hypotonia, mental retardation, convulsions, and brain and basal ganglia degeneration. The patient was found to be homozygous for a 5-bp duplication, which resulted in a frameshift at codon Lys158, causing a change in the amino acid sequence of the protein from amino acid 178 to the end. This frameshift destroyed a consensus phosphorylation site and extended the protein 14 amino acids. The 18-kDa complex I gene was mapped to chromosome 5.[437]

Nuclear DNA mutations in other mitochondrial genes have also been shown to cause other neurodegenerative diseases including hereditary spastic paraplegia (HSP) and dystonia. HSP, in the "pure" form, presents primarily with progressive weakness and spasticity of the lower limbs. However, in the "complicated" form, symptoms can include mental retardation, peripheral neuropathy, amyotrophy, ataxia, retinitis pigmentosa, optic atrophy, deafness, and ichthyosis. Muscle histology of patients in one mutant family revealed RRFs, which were SDH hyperreactive and contained packed abnormal mitochondria. HSP was initially found to be linked to the paraplegin gene on chromosome 16q24.3 in a large Italian family. The paraplegin gene consists of 5 exons extending over 10.8 kb of genomic sequence. The index family was found to harbor a complex rearrangement in the gene, possibly associated with the interactions of multiple Alu repeat elements. Paraplegin mutations have also been observed in two additional families: a homozygous 2-bp deletion that caused a frameshift that abolished 60 percent of the protein and a single A insertion that created a frameshift and stop codon, two amino acids downstream, thus removing the C-terminal 57 amino acids. The paraplegin protein is an 88-kDa polypeptide with a 40- to 45-amino-acid targeting peptide. It shows homology to a subfamily of adenosine triphosphatases (AAA proteins) that are yeast mitochondrial metalloproteases. In yeast, such proteins have both protease and chaperon-like activities.[438]

Dystonia, associated with the MTND6*LDYT14459A mutation, is also associated with basal ganglia degeneration, and the demonstration that complex I defects can cause dystonia has spurred interest in the possibility that nDNA mutations in mitochondrial genes may also cause movement disorders. This has been dramatically confirmed for the Mohr-Tranebjaerg syndrome, which presents in early childhood with sensorineural hearing loss that can progress to dystonia, spasticity, mental deterioration, paranoia, and cortical blindness. Those patients who develop the movement disorder characteristically exhibit progressive degeneration of the basal ganglia, corticospinal tract, and brain stem. The gene responsible for Mohr-Tranebjaerg syndrome was identified through a patient with a deletion of the locus. The identity of the gene was confirmed in two additional families, one harboring a 10-np deletion in exon 2 and the second resulting from

Tim8 Alignment

```
                        10         20         30         40         50

hDDP1p      1 MDSSS--SSS AAGLGAVD-P QLQHFIEVET QKQRFQQLVH QMT---EL--   50
mDDP1p      1 MESST--SSS GSALGAVD-P QLQHFIEVET QKQRFQQLVH QMT---EL--   50
hDDP2       1 -------MRQ QWRLGEADEA ELQRLVAAEQ QKAQFTAQVH ---HFMEL--   50
DD14p       1 -------MA- --ELGEADEA ELQRLVAAEQ QKAQFTAQVH ---HFMEL--   50
Tim8p       1 MGLSSIFGG- ----GAPSQQ KEAATTAKTT PNPIAKELKN QIAQELAVAN   50

                        60         70         80         90        100
hDDP1p     51 ---CWEKCMD KPGPKLDSRA EACFVNCVER FIDTSQFILN RLEQTQKSKP  100
mDDP1p     51 ---CWEKCMD KPGPKLDSRA EACFVNCVER FIDTSQFILN RLEQTQKSKP  100
hDDP2      51 ---CWDKCVE KPGNRLDSRT ENCLSSCVDR FIDTTLAITS RFAQ------  100
DD14p      51 ---CWDKCVE KPGSRLDSRT ENCLSSCVDR FIDTTLAITG RFAQ------  100
Tim8p      51 ATECFEKCLT SP---YATRN DACIDQCLAK YMRSWNVISK AYISRIQNAS  100
                 *   *                *   *

                       110        120        130        140        150
hDDP1p    101 VFSESLSD.. .......... .......... .......... ..........  150
mDDP1p    101 VFSESLSD.. .......... .......... .......... ..........  150
hDDP2     101 -IVQKGGQ.. .......... .......... .......... ..........  150
DD14p     101 -IVQQGGQ.. .......... .......... .......... ..........  150
Tim8p     101 A---SGEI.. .......... .......... .......... ..........  150
```

Fig. 105-24 Demonstration that the Mohr-Tranebjaerg deafness and dystonia syndrome is due to a defect in the mitochondrial protein import system. The human Mohr-Tranebjaerg syndrome protein (hDDP1)[439] is aligned with the homologous mouse expressed sequence tag (EST) (mDDP2p), the hDDP2 protein, which is closely linked to hDDP1,[439] the mouse DD14P, which was isolated by differential display[245] because it was up-regulated in the skeletal muscle of mice with mitochondrial myopathy (Figs. 105-15 and 105-16),[190] and the yeast homologue to hDDP1, which has been shown to be involved in the import of carrier proteins such as the ANT into the mitochondrial inner membrane (Fig. 105-9).[212] (*Adapted from Wallace and Murdock.*[214] *Used with permission.*)

a 1-np deletion in exon 1. This gene, designated DFN-1, generates a 1,167-np cDNA encoding a 97-amino acid, 11-kDa polypeptide, designated DDP1p. The predicted polypeptide has a high homology to a *Schizosaccharomyces pombe* gene of unknown function.[439]

The mouse homologue of the DDP1 cDNA was first isolated by applying differential display to the skeletal muscle mRNAs of ANT1 −/− knockout mice. Because a variety of energy genes had been found to be induced in this system, the discovery that a homology of DDP1 is unregulated in ANT1 −/− muscle provided preliminary evidence that this gene was involved in mitochondrial biogenesis and assembly (Fig. 105-24). The role of DDP1 in mitochondrial protein import was demonstrated in concurrent studies of the yeast mitochondrial import proteins. While studying the *Saccharomyces cerevisiae* import pathway for mitochondrial inner-membrane carrier proteins such as the ANT (yeast ACC), the Tim8p family of proteins was discovered to be located in the mitochondrial intermembrane space.[212] This family includes Tim8p, Tim9p, Tim10p, Tim12p, and Tim13p, all of which are similar in size and contain a distinctive duplicated $C(N)_3$ C motif, reminiscent of a Zn finger protein. Surprisingly, the DDP1 protein of the Mohr-Tranebjaerg syndrome was found to have the same duplicated $C(N)_3$ C motif as the Tim8p family protein. Moreover, synthetic DDP1 is incorporated into the mitochondrial intermembrane space in yeast and haptin-tagged DDP1 is specifically localized to yeast and mammalian mitochondria. Hence, it appears that the deafness and dystonia associated with Mohr-Tranebjaerg syndrome is due to a defect in the import of carrier proteins into the mitochondria and insertion into the mitochondrial inner membrane.[212]

The demonstration that the DDP1 protein is probably involved in the import of the mitochondrial proteins implies that the underlying defect of the Mohr-Tranebjaerg syndrome is a defect in mitochondrial OXPHOS, specifically due to deficiencies in carrier proteins such as ANT/ACC. This is particularly satisfying because the phenotypes associated with the systemic OXPHOS defects resulting from mutations in the mtDNA give an array of clinical symptoms that nicely overlap with those of the Mohr-Tranebjaerg syndrome. Hence, deafness and dystonia associated with basal ganglia degeneration can now be linked to mitochondrial defects resulting from nDNA as well as mtDNA mutations.

Nuclear gene mutations associated with neurologic symptoms such as cerebellar ataxia can also exert their phenotypic effects by increasing mitochondrial ROS production and inactivating the OXPHOS enzymes. One example is Friedreich ataxia, an autosomal recessive disease that results in cerebellar ataxia, peripheral neuropathy, hypertrophic cardiomyopathy, and diabetes. This disease has been linked to mutations in the frataxin gene on chromosome 9q3. It is autosomal recessive and inactivation of frataxin can either result from the expansion of an intron 1 trinucleotide repeat or from specific structural mutations. The mutant frataxin protein is targeted to the mitochondrial inner membrane and is thought to transport excess iron out of the mitochondrion. With the loss of this protein, iron accumulates in the matrix, stimulating the conversion of H_2O_2 to ·OH by the Fenton reaction. This inactivates the mitochondrial Fe-S center enzymes (complexes I, II, III, and aconitase), reducing mitochondrial energy production.[440–442]

Ophthalmoplegia and Ptosis Associated with Mitochondrial Myopathy

Ophthalmoplegia and ptosis are other prominent neuro-ophthalmologic presentation of mitochondrial disorders. When associated with mitochondrial myopathy, these clinical manifestations are reliable indicators of severe mitochondrial myopathy. Mitochondrial patients with ophthalmoplegia, ptosis, and mitochondrial myopathy can have a wide range of additional symptoms. Patients with milder disorders may manifest only ophthalmoplegia, ptosis, and mitochondrial myopathy, with an age of onset ranging from the late twenties up to late adulthood and a relatively mild course. Such patients are said to have "chronic progressive external ophthalmoplegia" (CPEO). By contrast, other patients can manifest ophthalmoplegia, ptosis, and mitochondrial myopathy prior to age 20 and experience multiple additional symptoms including retinitis pigmentosa and at least one of the following: cardiac conduction defects, cerebellar ataxia, or elevated cerebral spinal fluid protein above 100 mg/dl.[443,444] These patients are said to have the Kearns-Sayre syndrome (KSS). Other symptoms that may be observed in KSS or CPEO patients can include optic atrophy, hearing loss, seizures, dementia, cardiomyopathy, cardiac dysrhythmias, renal failure, endocrine disorders including diabetes mellitus, respiratory failure, lactic acidosis,[242,445] chronic diarrhea, and villous atrophy in early childhood.[446]

Approximately 83 percent of KSS and 47 percent of CPEO patients are the product of mtDNA rearrangements.[447] The great majority of these cases are new spontaneous mutations derived from a single clonal event such that all of the affected tissues of the patient are heteroplasmic for normal mtDNAs plus rearranged mtDNAs with a common unique breakpoint junction. Most of these cases are confined to a single individual in the family and presumably are due to mutations that arose in the oocyte or early in development. A few cases, however, involve rearrangements that can also be detected at low levels in the mother and/or other maternal relatives.[448] A small percentage of patients with progressive external ophthalmoplegia (PEO) harbor multiple rearrangements, caused by the inheritance of an autosomal dominant nuclear mutation that predisposes the mtDNAs to rearrangements.[449] Still other cases of the KSS/CPEO result from a variety of tRNA mutations, including the tRNA mutations MTTL1*MELAS3243G[273,450–452] and MTTN*CPEO5692G.[453] A diagnostic paradigm for ophthalmoplegia and ptosis is provided in Fig. 105-25.

Ophthalmoplegia Associated with mtDNA Rearrangements. The most common causes of CPEO and KSS are mtDNA rearrangements, which can include deletions, insertions, or a combination of the two.[288] The first mtDNA rearrangements were recognized in skeletal muscle of patients with mitochondrial myopathy.[2] Subsequent analysis of a large number of patients revealed that mtDNA rearrangements could be associated with four interrelated phenotypes: KSS, CPEO, Pearson marrow/pancreas syndrome, and maternally inherited diabetes mellitus and deafness.

CPEO and KSS Associated with mtDNA Rearrangements. In addition to ophthalmoplegia and ptosis, patients with CPEO and KSS due to mtDNA rearrangements have a progressive severe mitochondrial myopathy (Fig. 105-16). Additional histologic analysis of CPEO and KSS muscle revealed bands of COX-deficient (COX^-) and SDH-hyper-reactive (SDH^+) activity along the muscle fibers. These COX^- and SDH^+ fibers generally correspond to regions of mitochondrial proliferation and RRFs, high levels of mutant mtDNA, and induction of nDNA and mtDNA OXPHOS gene expression.[183,184,454–456]

The great majority of KSS and CPEO cases are due to spontaneous mtDNA rearrangements.[452,457] Of the 89 different breakpoints which have been reported, 80 percent were flanked by direct repeats of 4 to 16 nucleotides, 7 percent involved direct repeats of 4 to 6 nucleotides, and 12 percent did not involve a direct repeat.[457] Hence, the majority of rearrangements involve a region of homology suggesting some type of sequence-associated rearrangement mechanism. Many KSS patients harbor an interrelated family of rearranged molecules, all of which share a common breakpoint junction. These frequently include, in addition to normal mtDNAs, a duplicated mtDNA, a deletion monomer that retains only the duplicated region, and a deletion dimer containing two copies of the inserted sequence.[444,458]

Duplications may predispose individuals to the more severe disease, because in one survey 10 of 10 KSS patients were found to have duplications as well as deletions, while 8 of 8 CPEO patients harbored only deletion monomers.[459] Furthermore, the amount of the duplicated molecule in the KSS patients appears to correlate with the duplication size. The larger the duplication, the lower the level of duplicated molecules. Moreover, the patients with the smallest duplications (largest deletions) were the only patients with deletion dimers. In skeletal muscle, as the disease progresses, the normal and duplicated mtDNAs decline while the deletion dimers increase, and the patients harboring duplications are more likely to develop diabetes mellitus than those with only deletions.[444] These observations have led to the speculation that duplicated molecules are propagated more readily than deleted molecules and thus are more widely distributed among the tissues. Hence, patients harboring duplications have more organ systems affected and more severe disease.[444,460]

While a wide variety of rearrangement breakpoints have been mapped, the great majority of deletions tend to fall into two areas defined by the O_H and O_L origins of replication.[9] Moreover, deletions are not uniformly distributed. Approximately one-third to one-half of all deletion events occur at the common deletion breakpoint between nps 8469 and 13447 joining the mtDNA genes MTND5 and MTATP8, and removing 4977 nps. This "common" 5-kb deletion occurs between two 13-base pair direct repeats at 8470 to 8482 and 13447 to 13459, one repeat of which is lost and the other retained.[461–463] Two other frequently observed rearrangements bring together nps 7841 and 13905 in the MTCO2 and MTND5 genes, removing 6063 np at a 6- to 8-base direct repeat, and between nps 8648 and 16085 in gene MTATP6 and MTTP, removing 7436 np at a 12-np direct repeat.[457] The increased frequency of deletions at these breakpoints suggests a predominant rearrangement mechanism. In one case of the common 4977-np deletion, the break occurred 1 nucleotide outside the direct repeat. This permitted a demonstration that the upstream 13447 to 13459 repeat was retained, while the downstream 8470 to 8482 repeat was lost. Because this corresponds to the direction of H-strand replication, it was proposed that one mechanism for mtDNA rearrangement was slip-mispairing. Specifically, as the new H-strand is synthesized along the L-strand template starting from O_H and moving down in nucleotide numbers from 16,569 np, the parental H-stand is displaced. As replication proceeds, direct repeats in the parental H-strand are exposed and can base pair with downstream homologous repeats exposed on the L-strand by the replicating fork. Breakage of the single-stranded H-strand on the downstream side of the repeat would create at 3′-OH which would permit reinitiation of replication continuing along the template after the downstream repeat and skipping the intervening mtDNA.[462,464]

Slip-mispairing has been confirmed as an important mutational mechanism in the mtDNA through studies of a spontaneous mtDNA mutation that occurs in the D-loop of a specific European mtDNA lineage. This lineage, designated haplogroup I, is defined by multiple novel restriction site polymorphisms including an *Hae*II site loss at np 4529, an *Ava*II site gain at np 8249, an *Alu*I site gain at np 10028, and a *Bam*HI site gain at np 16389.[318] In studies of KSS patients that happened to harbor this mtDNA haplotype, it was discovered that these patients were heteroplasmic for a 270-np duplication in the D-loop between np 302 and np 567. This tandem duplication duplicates P_H (np 545 to 567), P_L (np 392 to 445), CSBIII (np 346 to 363), and part of CSBII (np 299 to 315).[320] While the original report proposed that this duplication predisposed mtDNAs to subsequent large-scale deletions,[320] this has not been confirmed.[318,444,465] Subsequent analysis revealed that the somatic generation of the duplication was always linked to the Caucasian mtDNA haplogroup I, and that the flanking ends of the 270-bp duplication in these mtDNAs harbored a

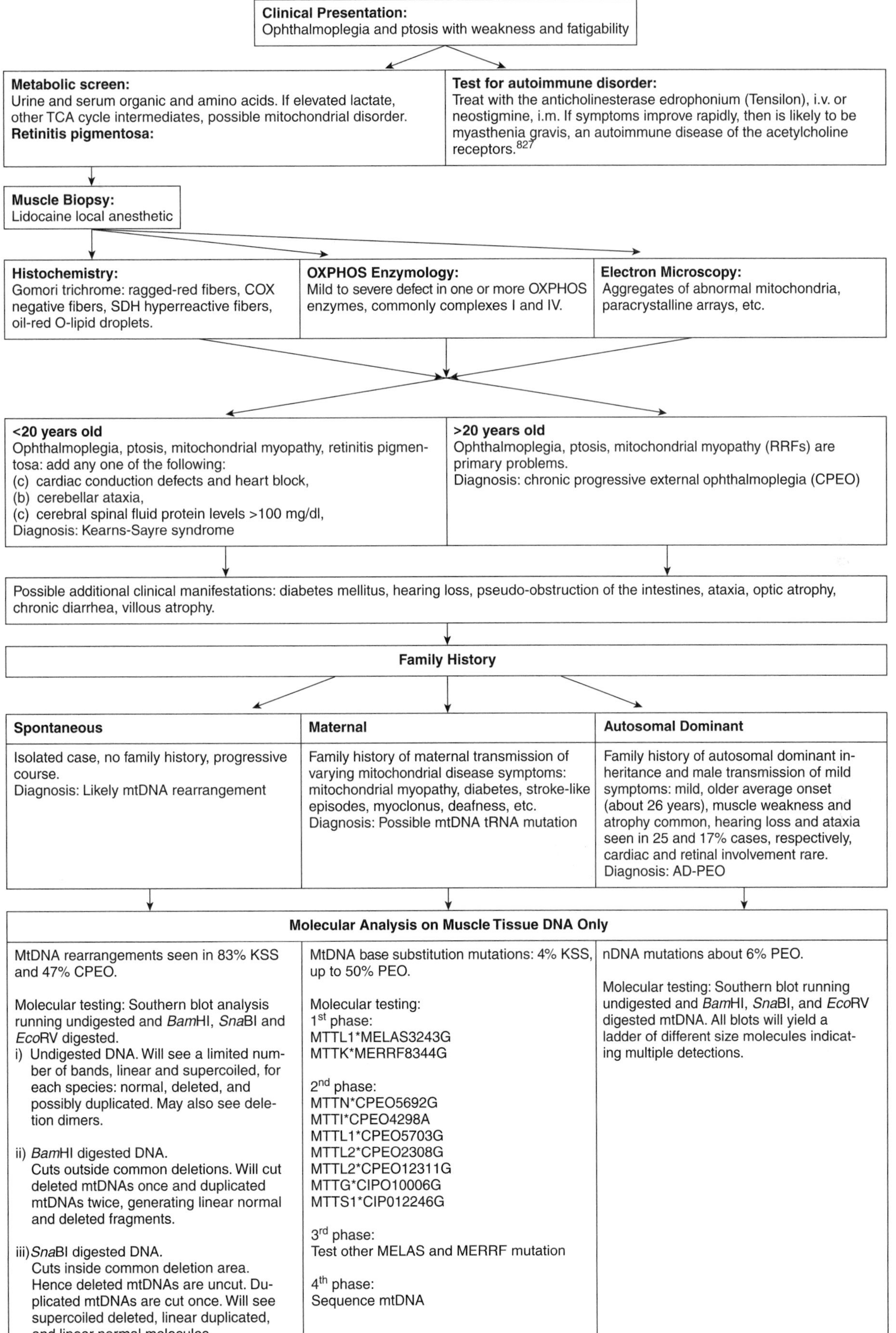

OPHTHALMOPLEGIA DIAGNOSTIC PARADIGM
Clinical Presentation:
Ophthalmoplegia and ptosis with weakness and fatigability
Metabolic screen:
Urine and serum organic and amino acids. If elevated lactate, other TCA cycle intermediates, possible mitochondrial disorder.
Retinitis pigmentosa:
Test for autoimmune disorder:
Treat with the anticholinesterase edrophonium (Tensilon), i.v. or neostigmine, i.m. If symptoms improve rapidly, then is likely to be myasthenia gravis, an autoimmune disease of the acetylcholine receptors.[827]
Muscle Biopsy:
Lidocaine local anesthetic
Histochemistry:
Gomori trichrome: ragged-red fibers, COX negative fibers, SDH hyperreactive fibers, oil-red O-lipid droplets.
OXPHOS Enzymology:
Mild to severe defect in one or more OXPHOS enzymes, commonly complexes I and IV.
Electron Microscopy:
Aggregates of abnormal mitochondria, paracrystalline arrays, etc.
<20 years old
Ophthalmoplegia, ptosis, mitochondrial myopathy, retinitis pigmentosa: add any one of the following:
(c) cardiac conduction defects and heart block,
(b) cerebellar ataxia,
(c) cerebral spinal fluid protein levels >100 mg/dl,
Diagnosis: Kearns-Sayre syndrome
>20 years old
Ophthalmoplegia, ptosis, mitochondrial myopathy (RRFs) are primary problems.
Diagnosis: chronic progressive external ophthalmoplegia (CPEO)
Possible additional clinical manifestations: diabetes mellitus, hearing loss, pseudo-obstruction of the intestines, ataxia, optic atrophy, chronic diarrhea, villous atrophy.
Family History
Spontaneous
Isolated case, no family history, progressive course.
Diagnosis: Likely mtDNA rearrangement
Maternal
Family history of maternal transmission of varying mitochondrial disease symptoms: mitochondrial myopathy, diabetes, stroke-like episodes, myoclonus, deafness, etc.
Diagnosis: Possible mtDNA tRNA mutation
Autosomal Dominant
Family history of autosomal dominant inheritance and male transmission of mild symptoms: mild, older average onset (about 26 years), muscle weakness and atrophy common, hearing loss and ataxia seen in 25 and 17% cases, respectively, cardiac and retinal involvement rare.
Diagnosis: AD-PEO
Molecular Analysis on Muscle Tissue DNA Only
MtDNA rearrangements seen in 83% KSS and 47% CPEO.
Molecular testing: Southern blot analysis running undigested and *Bam*HI, *Sna*BI and *Eco*RV digested.
i) Undigested DNA. Will see a limited number of bands, linear and supercoiled, for each species: normal, deleted, and possibly duplicated. May also see deletion dimers.
ii) *Bam*HI digested DNA.
Cuts outside common deletions. Will cut deleted mtDNAs once and duplicated mtDNAs twice, generating linear normal and deleted fragments.
iii) *Sna*BI digested DNA.
Cuts inside common deletion area. Hence deleted mtDNAs are uncut. Duplicated mtDNAs are cut once. Will see supercoiled deleted, linear duplicated, and linear normal molecules.
MtDNA base substitution mutations: 4% KSS, up to 50% PEO.
Molecular testing:
1st phase:
MTTL1*MELAS3243G
MTTK*MERRF8344G
2nd phase:
MTTN*CPEO5692G
MTTI*CPEO4298A
MTTL1*CPEO5703G
MTTL2*CPEO2308G
MTTL2*CPEO12311G
MTTG*CIPO10006G
MTTS1*CIPO12246G
3rd phase:
Test other MELAS and MERRF mutation
4th phase:
Sequence mtDNA
nDNA mutations about 6% PEO.
Molecular testing: Southern blot running undigested and *Bam*HI, *Sna*BI, and *Eco*RV digested mtDNA. All blots will yield a ladder of different size molecules indicating multiple detections.

Fig. 105-25 Diagnostic paradigm for ophthalmoplegia.

germline mutation which inserted a run of C nucleotides at np 568 to 573. This created a tandem repeat of the sequence 5′-ACCCCCCCC...CCCC-3′ on each side of duplicated region. Every individual harboring this germ line mutation was found to be heteroplasmic for the duplication in all somatic tissues tested. Because the duplicated regions are tandemly arrayed, the simplest explanation for this self-generating D-loop duplication is slip-mispairing.[318] While predisposition to this duplication does not appear to be pathogenic per se, it has been found to be present at relatively high levels (32 percent) in one patient with mitochondrial myopathy including RRFs and partial COX deficiency. This patient also had a small percentage of mtDNAs with this region triplicated.[465] This observation could suggest that either the duplication can be toxic at high levels or, alternatively, that the duplicated mtDNA is preferentially amplified in mitochondrial myopathy due to the presence of the additional promoters and O_H.

Proposed alternative deletion mechanisms include topoisomerase II cleavage[464] and homologous recombination. Putative topoisomerase II recognition sequences have been observed in the vicinity of certain mtDNA deletions and proposed to play a role in removal of sequences.[466,467] Recombination is likely to play an important role because it is now established that many rearrangement patients harbor a complex array of related molecules including duplication molecules, deletion monomers, and deletion dimers, suggesting that they may be interconverted by a recombinational process.[288,458,459] mtDNA recombination has now been confirmed in somatic cell hybrids between two cell lines harboring nonoverlapping CPEO deletions, both of which retained O_H and O_L. In the hybrids, the mtDNAs complemented each other to give respiratory competence and a few cell lines were found to contain recombinant molecules involving the coalescence of the two deleted molecules.[284] Hence, mtDNA recombination does occur in cultured human cells, although in this experiment its frequency was very low.

The pathophysiology of KSS and CPEO resulting from spontaneous mtDNA rearrangements appears to be the result of a protein synthesis defect combined with the stochastic distribution of the mutant molecules during development. All KSS- and CPEO-associated deletions studied to date remove at least one structural RNA (tRNA or rRNA) essential for mitochondrial protein synthesis. Cytoplasmic transfer of deleted molecules from patient cells to ρ^0 HeLa cells confirmed that the deleted molecules caused a defect in mitochondrial protein synthesis. In cybrids with up to 60 percent deleted mtDNAs, the normal mtDNAs complemented in *trans*, permitting high respiration and synthesis of the mtDNA-encoded polypeptides. However, above the 60 percent mutant mtDNA threshold, mitochondrial respiration, protein synthesis, and the level of the individual mitochondrial polypeptides declined precipitously, ultimately falling to zero.[468] This threshold effect on protein synthesis for deletion mutations explains why KSS and CPEO, like the pathogenic tRNA mutations, are frequently associated with mitochondrial myopathy and RRFs. Analysis of the tissue distribution of mtDNA deletions in KSS and CPEO patients at autopsy has revealed that the rearranged molecules are broadly distributed throughout the tissues of the body.[460,469,470] The interesting exception is blood, which is commonly devoid of the mtDNA deletions,[2,460,462,470] although duplications have been found.[444] Hence, molecular diagnosis of KSS and CPEO generally requires a muscle biopsy.

The time in development when pathogenic mtDNA deletions arise is not yet known. However, their broad tissue distribution would imply a mutation in the oocyte or very early in development. This is supported by surveys of the mtDNAs of human oocytes left over from in vitro fertilization clinics that have revealed that many oocytes do harbor deletions. Eight of 15 oocytes harbored the common 4977-np deletion, confirming that deletions must occur early in development.[265,471] The maximum number of molecules containing the 5-kb deletion was 171 molecules, or about 0.1 percent.[265] Moreover, a survey of oocytes from women of different ages revealed that of women less than 38 years, 28 percent of the oocytes had the common deletion while for women older than 38, 93 percent of the oocytes had this deletion. Consequently, the mean age of women without oocyte deletions was 31.4 years, while that of women with deletions was 37.7 years.[471] This correlates with a marked increase in ovarian mtDNA deletions at menopause, about age 45.[472] Thus, it appears that mtDNA rearrangements may arise in the oocyte or early in development, and the frequency of mtDNA rearrangement syndromes may increase with maternal age at conception.

Molecular histologic analysis of the distribution of deleted mtDNAs in skeletal muscle of KSS and CPEO patients has revealed that the levels of mtDNA deletions increase with age,[444,473,474] and that the deleted molecules are not uniformly distributed along the length of the muscle fiber. Staining muscle fibers for COX and SDH has revealed that the COX levels vary from normal to absent and that the SDH staining is normal where COX is normal, but greatly increased in COX-negative regions.[475] *In situ* hybridization and regional PCR amplification show that regions that are COX-negative have increased levels of the deleted mtDNAs and a coordinate induction of mtDNA transcripts from the undeleted genes. By contrast, the COX-positive regions have predominantly normal mtDNAs.[454,455,476] These observations imply that the deleted mtDNAs are initially scattered along the muscle fiber, but that as the individual ages, there is a selective amplification of the deleted molecules, ultimately reaching a high enough concentration to inhibit mitochondrial protein synthesis and cause COX deficiency.

The mechanism by which the deleted mtDNAs are selectively amplified remains unknown, although two hypotheses have been proposed. The first hypothesis is that the deleted molecules are shorter and thus have a replicative advantage.[9] Mitochondrial proteins and mtDNAs are known to be continuously, albeit slowly, turned over in postmitotic tissues.[477–480] Hence, repeated replication cycles might favor shorter deleted mtDNAs or duplicated molecules with extra origins. The alternative hypothesis is that the nuclei adjacent to mutant mtDNAs and mitochondria sense the OXPHOS defect of the mutant mitochondria and attempt to compensate by inducing mtDNA replication and mitochondrial biogenesis in the surrounding mitochondria. Coordinate induction of nuclear and mtDNA OXPHOS gene expression has been documented in skeletal muscle of patients with both mtDNA rearrangement and tRNA mutations,[183,184,456] and because skeletal muscles are syncytia, each nucleus controls a particular cytosolic domain.[481] If nDNA OXPHOS gene expression is modulated by a mitochondrial substrate such as NADH, then inhibition of the ETC by an mtDNA mutation would cause a local rise in NADH and concomitant increase in mitochondrial gene expression in the adjacent nucleus. Such a process could be a mediated via a nuclear transcription factor that activates OXPHOS gene expression. Such a factor has been identified which binds to the REBOX sequence element located 5′ to a variety of nuclear bioenergetic genes and possibly also in the D-loop of the mtDNA. The binding of the REBOX-binding factor (RBF) is stimulated by a reducing environment.[165,177] Thus, in cells with partial respiratory deficiency, increased NADH could activate RBF to bind to the REBOX element and thus stimulate the nucleus to induce the biogenesis of the surrounding mitochondria, including the associated mutant mtDNA. The resulting increase in number of mutant mtDNAs would further increase the NADH and stimulate the nuclear gene expression, creating a self-perpetuating feedback loop that would preferentially amplify the mutant mtDNAs.[482,483] Whatever the mechanism, it would appear that it is the regional bioenergetic defect caused by the selective amplification of the mutant mtDNAs that causes the progressive decline in muscle function in KSS and CPEO.

Pearson Syndrome and mtDNA Rearrangements. A more severe form of the CPEO/KSS mtDNA rearrangement syndrome presents in the first 5 years of life with pancytopenia (loss of all blood cells). This condition is known as the Pearson marrow/pancreas syndrome. Pearson patients develop a severe transfusion-dependent, macrocytic anemia with varying degrees of neutropenia and thrombocytopenia. The bone marrow of Pearson patients shows extensive vacuolization of erythroid and myeloid precursors, hemosiderosis, and ringed sideroblasts. Pearson patients generally die due to complications of the bone marrow dysfunction or transfusions. In addition to pancytopenia, many Pearson patients develop exocrine pancreatic insufficiency, hepatic failure, renal failure, and other neuromuscular problems.[242,484–488] Analysis of circulating white blood cells has revealed a generalized respiratory defect in association with mtDNA rearrangements, both deletions and duplications. As with most CPEO and KSS patients, Pearson patients are generally isolated cases, suggesting mutational events early in development.[489–492] Moreover, autopsy analysis of Pearson patients has revealed that the mtDNA rearrangements are not simply localized to the bone marrow, but are systemic,[493,494] and the rare Pearson patients who spontaneously recover the ability to make blood cells and survive, ultimately progress to a KSS-like phenotype.[444,485,495] These observations suggest that the Pearson marrow/pancreas syndrome and CPEO-KSS are the same disease, with the phenotypic differences resulting from the distribution of the rearranged molecules in the different tissues. This interpretation is supported by the observation that some Pearson patients, including patients who have progressed to KSS, harbor duplications as well as deletions.[444,459] One explanation for the difference between Pearson syndrome and KSS/CPEO is that in Pearson syndrome the rearranged mtDNAs are widely distributed and include all of the bone marrow precursor cells. As the bone marrow stem cells replicate, the rearranged mtDNAs accumulate until there is insufficient energy for further proliferation and/or maturation. At this point the rearranged molecules are prevalent in the peripheral blood and blood cell production declines, leading to pancytopenia. By contrast, in KSS/CPEO patients or in Pearson syndrome patients who survive and progress to KSS, the rearranged molecules may be distributed such that a portion of the bone marrow precursor cells are free of mutant mtDNAs. As the stem cells containing rearranged molecules decline in their replicative potential, the cells having only normal mtDNAs continue to proliferate and ultimately supplant the mutant cells and repopulate the bone marrow. At this point, the patient loses the rearranged mtDNAs in the circulating white blood cells, but still retains rearranged mtDNAs in other organs. These mutant mtDNAs would exert their effects later in life, leading to the multisystem diseases of KSS and CPEO.

Maternally Inherited Diabetes Mellitus and Deafness Due to mtDNA Rearrangements. The mildest clinical presentation of CPEO/KSS mtDNA rearrangement syndrome presents as maternally inherited diabetes mellitus and deafness. Diabetes mellitus is a common clinical manifestation in patients with mtDNA duplications, generally in association with KSS.[444,470] However, in one large African-American family, type 2 diabetes mellitus together with sensorineural hearing loss was maternally inherited along with an mtDNA duplication-deletion rearrangement.[496,497] In this pedigree, maternal relatives developed hearing loss in their twenties and thirties and type 2 diabetes mellitus in their thirties and forties. Occasional individuals in the rearrangement pedigree experienced stroke-like episodes associated with cortical and brain stem lucencies on MRI examination. None of the patients had ophthalmoplegia or ptosis, nor did they have mitochondrial myopathy as detected by muscle histology. However, detailed biochemical analysis of several family members revealed a generalized OXPHOS defect in the skeletal muscle. Physiological analysis indicated that all maternal relatives developed an insulin-dependent diabetes mellitus, with some individuals developing diabetic ketoacidosis. Glucose tolerance tests revealed that severely affected individuals were unable to respond to hyperglycemia with increase insulin production from β cells or decreased glycogen production from α cells.[497] This defect in the "glucose sensor" is similar to that seen in maturity onset diabetes of the young (MODY), which results from mutations in the pancreatic islet cell glucokinase gene. The K_m of the islet cell glucokinase is higher than that of other cellular hexokinases; hence, glucokinase is only active during hyperglycemia.[498–502] Because most glucokinase is attached to the mitochondrial outer membrane by porin, and porin interacts with the ANT of the inner membrane,[503,504] it is possible that glucose sensing involves the linkage between glucokinase and OXPHOS through this *trans*-mitochondrial membrane macromolecular complex. Hence, mutations in either the glucokinase gene that binds glucose during hyperglycemia or mitochondrial OXPHOS that provides the ATP for glucose phosphorylation could affect the ability of the pancreas to respond to hyperglycemia.[483,505]

The mtDNA in this maternally inherited pedigree consisted of three main types of mtDNA molecules: (a) normal mtDNAs; (b) duplicated mtDNAs containing an insertion of 6.1 kb of the mtDNA encompassing from np 4389 in the $tRNA^{Gln}$ gene to np 14,822 in the MTCYB gene and including the ND1, 16S rRNA, 12S rRNA, and part of the MTCYB genes, as well as the $tRNA^{Ile}$, $tRNA^{Leu(UUR)}$, $tRNA^{Val}$, $tRNA^{Phe}$, $tRNA^{Pro}$, and $tRNA^{Thr}$ genes, and the D-loop including O_H ; and (c) deleted mtDNAs which lack 10.4 kb of mtDNA including 11 of the 13 OXPHOS genes; 15 of 22 tRNAs, $-O_L$, and 75 bp of the 5′ end of the MTCYB gene. The deleted molecules appear to be present as a dimer of about 12 kb, and the rearrangement is encompassed by a 10-bp direct repeat (5′-CACCCCATCC-3′). Lymphoblastoid cell lines carrying this rearrangement exhibit a partial protein synthesis defect. Extended propagation results in the selective enrichment for the duplicated molecules and loss of the deleted and normal mtDNAs. Moreover, white blood cells from patients have an excess of duplicated molecules while the postmitotic muscle had a higher proportion of deleted than duplicated mtDNAs. These results suggest that the duplicated molecules with the extra O_H are preferentially replicated and hence transmitted through the germ line, and that the deleted molecules are generated from the duplicated molecules through a recombinational process in postmitotic tissues. While the deleted molecules have only one origin O_H, it is possible that they could also replicate. If the two components of the dimers were arrayed in a head-to-tail position, then there would be an O_H for each strand.[496,497]

This pedigree is remarkable in that it harbored the same type of duplication and deletion dimer molecular defect that has been documented for diabetes mellitus in association with KSS patients and Pearson syndrome patients who progress to KSS,[444,458,459,470,506] yet none of the patients exhibited evidence of ptosis, ophthalmoplegia, or mitochondrial myopathy. In another family, a patient was described with dystonia, external ophthalmoplegia, slowly progressive proximal muscle weakness, no RRFs on muscle biopsy even though showing mitochondrial hyperplasia, and diabetes mellitus that developed at age 36 and was treated with insulin. This individual also had normal and duplicated mtDNAs with the duplication encompassing nucleotides 13445 to 3318 and flanked by imperfect direct repeats at nps 3318 to 3337 and 13445 to 13462. This duplication duplicated the 12S and 16S rRNAs, ND6 and MTCYB genes, O_H and the encompassed tRNAs, and was found in 15 percent of the proband's muscle mtDNA, 80 percent of his blood mtDNA, and 40 percent of his mother's blood mtDNA.[507] In a second family, the child presented at age 8 years with diabetes mellitus and occasional episodes of ketoacidosis, which progressed on to CPEO and mitochondrial myopathy, with the individual dying at age 20 of cardiac dysrhythmia. The patient harbored a family of mtDNA molecules including normal, duplicated, deleted, and deletion dimers that were widely distributed among her tissues, including her pancreas.[470] Thus, these two families have duplications similar to the maternally inherited diabetes mellitus and deafness family and also had diabetes without or without RRFs, but the patients did have ophthalmoplegia. This implies that mtDNA rearrangement syndromes represent a phenotypic continuum with isolated diabetes mellitus and deafness being the mildest presentation, CPEO and KSS intermediate, and Pearson marrow/pancreas syndrome the most severe.

Diabetes mellitus and deafness can also be associated with mtDNA base substitutions in protein synthesis genes. However, in the phenotypes produced by the mtDNA rearrangements and the MTLL1*MELAS3243G mutation patients are more frequently insulin-requiring diabetics.[470,496,497] In one case, this was associated with the loss of pancreatic β cells.[470]

Because of the clinical variability of the mtDNA rearrangement syndromes, diabetes mellitus together with mtDNA rearrangements can be associated with a spectrum of other clinical symptoms. A 5-kb deletion has been identified in an infant with diabetic ketoacidosis, rickets, and de Toni-Debré-Fanconi syndrome.[508] A 5778-np deletion was detected by PCR in patients with diabetic amyotrophy, diabetic myoatrophy and nephropathy, and diabetic fatty liver, although this deletion was not confirmed by Southern blot and the same deletion was found at lower levels in controls.[509] Finally, one patient has been reported with Wolfram syndrome including early-onset diabetes mellitus, optic atrophy, and deafness in association with a 7.6-kb mtDNA deletion,[492] although analysis of another Wolfram patient failed to reveal an mtDNA defect.[510]

Ophthalmoplegia Associated with nDNA Mutations that Destabilized the mtDNA. While most ophthalmoplegia, ptosis, and mitochondrial myopathy patients are the result of spontaneous mtDNA rearrangement mutations and thus have no family history,[462,511] approximately 6 percent of PEO cases harbor multiple deletions and show a clear autosomal dominant inheritance pattern. Such families are known as autosomal dominant-PEO (AD-PEO) (Fig. 105-25).[449,512–514]

In AD-PEO, each affected individual has a different array of mtDNA deletions. This demonstrates that it is a nuclear mutation which increases the tendency toward deletion that is inherited, not the deletion itself (Table 105-14).[449,512,513] Clinically, the mean age of onset of AD-PEO is 26 years, which is older than the average spontaneous CPEO case. In addition to PEO, these patients experience proximal muscle atrophy and weakness in about 62 percent of cases, hearing loss in 25 percent, and ataxia in 17 percent of cases. Cardiac and retinal involvement are rare, and the most common cause of death is respiratory failure.[515] Multiple deletions have also been found in four patients with RRFs but atypical neurologic symptoms. Two individuals presented with Parkinsonism, one with ptosis, a third with exercise intolerance and limb weakness, and a fourth with elevated blood creatine phosphokinase.[516] The nature of the deletions in multiple-deletion syndrome is similar to that found in spontaneous deletion patients. Among the 81 deletions reported from multiple-deletion syndrome patients, 96 percent are encompassed by direct repeats of 4 to 13 nucleotides, while 4 percent involve indirect repeats of 4 base pairs.[457] Moreover, patients show multiple deletions in tissues throughout the body.[517] Efforts to localize the nuclear gene mutations responsible for multiple-deletion syndrome have employed extended families and linkage analysis. At least three loci are currently known. One Finnish locus has been linked to chromosome 10q23.3-24.3,[518,519] and a second Italian locus to chromosome 3p14.2-21.1, with a few families remaining unlinked (Table 105-13).[520,521] The nature of the mutant genes is unknown, although the structural genes for mtTFA and mtSSB have been excluded.[519]

Two other nDNA diseases are known which also result in the destabilization or loss of the mtDNA: the mitochondrial neurogastrointestinal encephalomyopathy (MNGIE) syndrome and the mtDNA depletion syndrome. MNGIE is associated with mitochondrial myopathy, including RRFs and abnormal mitochondria; decreased respiratory chain activity; and multiple mtDNA deletions, mtDNA depletion, or both. This autosomal recessive disease has been linked to multiple mutations in the nuclear thymidine phosphorylase (TP) gene. The published mutant alleles are listed in Table 105-16. While the disease is caused by TP mutations, the clinical symptoms are probably the result of the destruction of the mtDNA. Hence, it has been hypothesized that inactivation of TP alters cellular thymidine pools that are important in mtDNA maintenance.[522]

The mtDNA depletion syndrome results in severe reductions in the mtDNA levels of various organs (muscle, liver, or kidney), resulting in organ failure and death. This is probably the result of a nuclear mutation that disrupts the regulation of the mtDNA copy number during development, resulting in the chance loss of the mtDNA (105-14).[523–531]

Ophthalmoplegia Associated with mtDNA Base Substitution Mutations. A variety of mtDNA tRNA base substitution mutations have also been found to cause ophthalmoplegia, ptosis, and mitochondrial myopathy (Fig. 105-25). The tRNA mutation that is the most common cause of ophthalmoplegia is the MELAS mutation, MTL1*MELAS3243G.[450–452,532,533] In a survey of 28 KSS and 109 PEO patients, 28 KSS patients had deletions and one harbored the MTTL1*MELAS3243G mutation, while of the PEO patients 46 (42 percent) harbored mtDNA deletions while 15 (14 percent) harbored the MTTL1*MELAS3243G mutation. One additional PEO patient had the MTTK*MERRF8344G mutation. KSS and CPEO patients who harbor mtDNA tRNA mutations are generally members of larger maternal pedigrees with several variously affected family members.[514]

In addition to the MTTLI*MELAS3243G mutation, other tRNA base substitution mutations that present with CPEO are the $tRNA^{Asn}$ mutations MTTN*CPEO5692G[453] and MTTN*CPEO5703G;[534] the $tRNA^{Ile}$ mutation MTTI*CPEO4298A;[535] and the $tRNA^{Leu(CUN)}$ mutations MTTL2*CPEO12308G,[536] and MTTL2*CPEO12311G,[537] and MTTL2*CPEO12315A.[538] Ophthalmoplegia is also a major clinical feature of the $tRNA^{Glu}$ mutation at MTTG*CIP01000GG,[536] and the $tRNA^{Ser(AGY)}$ mutation at MTTS1*CIP012246G.[536] Ophthalmoplegia is also a major clinical feature of the $tRNA^{Glu}$ mutation at MTTG*CIPO10006G[536] and the $tRNA^{Ser(AGY)}$ mutation at MTTS1*CIPO12246G.[536] Ophthalmoplegia is also an occasional symptom for a variety of other deleterious mtDNA tRNA mutations, including the MTTK*MERRF8344G mutation[514] and potentially others of the $tRNA^{Leu(UUR)}$ MELAS mutations.[450] As is the case for mtDNA rearrangement mutations, milder renditions of the CPEO mutations can also cause diabetes mellitus and deafness. This phenotype is a common presentation of patients harboring 5 to 30 percent of the MTTL1*MELAS3243G mutation.[450,539]

The occurrence of ophthalmoplegia in the mtDNA tRNA mutations indicates that the pathophysiology of these symptoms might be further understood through studies of the biochemical defects of the tRNA mutations. The best studied of these mutations are MTTL1*MELAS3243G and MTTK*MERRF8344G. Both the MERRF mutation, MTTK*MERRF8344G, and two MELAS mutations, MTTL1*MELAS3243G and MTTL1*MELAS3271C, have been shown to result in a marked defect in mitochondrial protein synthesis. The mtDNA-encoded polypeptides have been found to be reduced by histologic and immunohistochemical analysis in patient skeletal muscle harboring the MTTL1*MELAS3243G mutation.[540] Because the translation of the larger mtDNA proteins would be the most severely compromised, this should preferentially affect complexes I and IV, which has been observed by several groups in assays on skeletal muscle mitochondria.[533,541–543] In cybrid prepared from MTTL1*MELAS3243G and MTTL1*MELAS3271C patient cell lines, oxygen consumption rates can be reduced by up to 70 percent, when the mutant mtDNAs exceed 94 percent.[544–546] A lesser inhibition of respiration was seen in the cybrids prepared with the MTTL1*MELAS3271C mutation.[546]

The actual pathophysiological mechanism by which the MTTL1*MELAS3243G mutation results in MELAS remains unclear. Because the 3243 nucleotide lies within the transcriptional terminator sequence for the rRNA genes, it is possible that this mutation perturbs the transcriptional processes. In in vitro experiments, diminished affinity for the partially purified mitochondrial transcription terminator protein (mTERM) for the mutant terminator sequence has been reported.[547] This was related to an impairment of transcript termination for the 16S rRNA gene and suggested that MELAS may be related to a perturbation in the type and amount of mRNAs relative to rRNAs. Subsequent studies have confirmed a reduced affinity of mTERM for the mutant termination sequence[544] and, in some cases, reduced transcriptional termination.[548] However, others have found no evidence of abnormal termination, altered rRNA production, or a MELAS-specific perturbation in rRNA to mRNA ratios.[540,544,548–550] Moreover, the MTTL1*MELAS3271C mutation is not found within the transcription termination sequence, yet still results in MELAS. This suggests that alteration of the mTERM-associated transcriptional termination may not be the primary causal factor in MELAS. Alternatively, the MELAS mutations may cause an RNA processing defect. One group has shown in MTTL1*MELAS3243G and MTTL1*MELAS3271C cybrids an accumulation of steady state levels of precursor RNA 19, which corresponds to a transcript containing the contiguous 16S rRNA + $tRNA^{Leu(UUR)}$ + ND1 genes,[545,546] and a decreased 5′ and 3′ processing of $tRNA^{Leu(UUR)}$ has been observed in MTTL1*MELAS3243G patient -cybrids.[545]

Similarly, a severe mitochondrial protein synthesis defect has been found to be associated with the MTTK*MERRF8344G mutation in patient skeletal muscle,[551] myoblasts/myotubes,[552,553] and fibroblasts.[554] The translation defect is manifested as a general reduction in the overall rate of protein synthesis, with the larger mitochondrial polypeptides preferentially affected, and in the generation of abnormal translation products. Accompanying the translation defect is a reduction in mitochondrial O_2 consumption and electron transport chain enzyme activity.[281,554] The protein synthesis abnormalities and OXPHOS defects have been unambiguously assigned to both the MTTK*MERRF8344G and MTTK*MERRF8356C mutations by cybrid transfer using both patient myoblasts (MTTK*MERRF8344G only[552]) and fibroblasts.[555] It is postulated that the reduction of mitochondria protein synthesis results in a lowering of the steady state levels of OXPHOS enzyme complexes, perhaps due to premature termination of translation at lysine codons secondary to a 50 to 60 percent decrease in $tRNA^{Lys}$ aminoacylation.[556]

The clear demonstration that both the MELAS and MERRF tRNA mutations inhibit mitochondrial protein synthesis indicates that this is the underlying mechanism that causes ophthalmoplegia, ptosis, and mitochondrial myopathy. This would also explain the origin of the symptoms in the CPEO and KSS patients with mtDNA rearrangements, because every pathogenic rearrangement that has been studied to date alters or removes one or more tRNA genes.[36] Hence, the rearrangement mutations would also cause protein synthesis defects, a result confirmed by cybrid studies of CPEO patient deletion cell lines. Hence, ophthalmoplegia, ptosis, and mitochondrial myopathy must result from primary defects in mitochondrial protein synthesis. Because the mtDNA encodes seven complex I subunits and three complex IV subunits, these would be the OXPHOS enzymes likely to be most affected. This is observed. Hence, ophthalmoplegia, ptosis, and mitochondrial myopathy probably reflect severe defects in mitochondrial energy production.

Somatic mtDNA Mutations in Degenerative Disease and Aging

While inherited mtDNA mutations generally define the nature and extent of patient symptoms, they do not explain why mitochondrial diseases frequently have a delayed onset and progression course. This suggests that a second factor must be required for the pathogenesis of mitochondrial disease, a factor that is age-related and that initiates the onset and progression of the disease. This aging factor correlates with the age-related decline of mitochondrial OXPHOS enzyme activities, which has been documented in primate skeletal muscle, liver, and brain.[12,557] This OXPHOS decline is associated with the age-related accumulation of somatic mtDNA rearrangements in these same postmitotic tissues. For example, in human skeletal muscle, the activities of mitochondrial complexes I, I + II, and II + III decline with age from 20 to 80 years. Analysis of the mtDNAs of those subjects under age 40, by amplification of full-length mtDNAs using the long extension-PCR (LX-PCR) method, revealed primarily full-length mtDNAs, with only an occasional mtDNA rearrangement. By contrast, the skeletal muscle mtDNAs of individuals over the age of 50 have been found to accumulate a wide array of mtDNA rearrangements, the nature of which is specific to each individual muscle sample.[558] The skeletal muscle of elderly subjects has been found to contain RRFs, with each COX^- and SDH^+ fiber containing a different mtDNA mutation.[12,559] This implies that each of these somatic mtDNA mutations arose *de novo* and was selectively amplified within the cell to create the regional respiratory defects.

Somatic mtDNA mutations also occur in the brain. Analysis of mtDNA rearrangements by LX-PCR in human brains has revealed very few rearrangements in young individuals, but a wide spectrum of rearrangements in older individuals.[560] This has been correlated with the quantitation of the common 5-kb mtDNA deletion, which revealed that mtDNA deletions accumulated in all regions of the cortex and basal ganglia after age 75, with the levels being highest in the basal ganglia and reaching a plateau at age 80.[561,562]

An analogous accumulation of somatic mtDNA rearrangements has also been found in chimpanzee tissues,[560] mouse tissues,[563] and *C. elegans.*[560] Thus, mtDNA rearrangements appear to accumulate with age in postmitotic tissues of all multicellular animals, with the level of rearrangements being proportional to life span rather than absolute time.

The cause of the somatic mtDNA mutations is likely to be oxidative damage. Oxidative damage, quantitated using 8-hydroxy-deoxyguanosine (8 OH-dG), increases in the mtDNA with age in both man and mouse.[12,564,565] Moreover, patients with chronic ischemic heart disease, which is associated with cyclic bursts of mitochondrial ROS during ischemia and reperfusion,[566] have been found to harbor 8- to 2000-fold more mtDNA deletions in the heart than age-matched controls.[567]

The hypothesis that OXPHOS decline is a major factor in aging has been supported by the genetic and physiological analysis of *C. elegans* mutants with altered life spans. The *mev-1 (kn1)* mutation imparts a phenotype of rapid aging in the presence of hyperbaric oxygen. Animals exposed to high oxygen not only age more rapidly, but also prematurely accumulate biomarkers for aging such as fluorescent materials and protein carbonyls. The *mev-1* mutation is a glycine to glutamate missense mutation in the succinate dehydrogenase (complex II) cytochrome b560 gene. This mutation might act to destabilize the ubisemiquinone intermediate of CoQ_{10} generated by complex II, thus promoting donation of electrons directly to O_2 to give O_2^{-}.[73]

Metabolic analysis of the increased longevity mutants *age-1*, *daf-2*, and the *clk-1 (e2519)* and *daf-2 (e1370)* double mutant has revealed that all three have metabolic rates significantly less than the wild type (N2). When controlled for size and developmental age, the *daf-2* and *clk-1* + *daf-2* mutants have metabolic rates that are 60 percent less than the metabolic rate of the wild type. For *daf-2* mutants, which also harbor the complementing *daf-16* mutation that restores normal life span, the metabolic rate is restored to normal.[568] These observations are consistent with the hypothesis that *C. elegans* longevity is inversely proportional to mitochondrial respiration rate and hence mitochondrial oxygen radical production. This conclusion is further substantiated by the genetic analyses of the *clk-1* mutation.

The CLK-1 protein is a 187-residue polypeptide with two tandemly repeated core domains of 82 amino acids. The protein is highly conserved and has been found in all eukaryotic cells examined, as well as in *Rickettsia prowazekii*, which is thought to be close to the bacterial progenitor of the mitochondrion. Three mutations in the *clk-1* gene have been characterized—qm30, which is due to a 590-base pair deletion, qm51, which alters the splice site of intron 2, and e2519, which is a glutamate to lysine missense mutation in amino acid 148. In the yeast mutation of the *clk-1* homologue *(Coq7p)*, CoQ_{10} production is lost, resulting in respiratory deficiency.[569] In *C. elegans*, the *clk-1* protein has been found to be present in all cells and targeted to the mitochondria. The *clk-1* mutants have reduced mitochondrial capacity to retain rhodamine 6G and a partial reduction in succinate:cytochrome c oxidoreductase, a reaction that links complexes II and III through CoQ_{10}.[570] Thus, the extended life span of the *clk-1* mutants may be the product of a reduction in the ubisemiquinone available for ROS production. Taken together, most of the current data on the genetic control of longevity in *C. elegans* can be explained by alterations in the mitochondrial production of energy and ROS.

These observations provide strong support for the hypothesis that aging in multicellular animals is associated with an increase in mitochondrial ROS production, which results in damage to mitochondrial function and the generation of somatic mtDNA mutations. The resulting age-related accumulation of mitochondrial damage causes a decline in OXPHOS, ultimately degrading the tissue's energy capacity to below its bioenergetic threshold, resulting in symptoms and senescence.

THE PATHOPHYSIOLOGY OF MITOCHONDRIAL DISEASE EXPLORED USING MOUSE MODELS

While patient studies have revealed much about the genetics of mitochondrial disease, the physiological causes of the observed symptoms have been difficult to study in humans. The creation and analysis of mouse models for mitochondrial disease are overcoming this limitation. Three nuclear gene mutations in the mouse have provided new insight into the pathophysiology of mitochondrial disease. These mutations alter (a) the heart/muscle ANT isoform gene (Ant1), (b) the mitochondrial MnSOD gene, and (c) the mitochondrial transcription factor (Tfam) gene. Mutant mtDNAs are also being introduced into the mouse female germ line, with both naturally occurring polymorphisms as well as the CAP^R mutation transferred into mice. These model systems are permitting the analysis of the combined effects of genotype variation due to mitotic segregation and physiological variation due to changes in energy production, ROS generation, and apoptosis.

Ant1-Deficient Mice

The genetic inactivation of the nDNA-encoded Ant1 gene has provided an excellent model for demonstrating the pathophysiological effects of chronic ATP deficiency. Surprisingly, ANT1-deficient [$Ant1^{tm2Mgr}$ (−/−)] animals are viable, although they developed classical mitochondrial myopathy and hypertrophic cardiomyopathy (Fig. 105-15).[190]

Unlike human Ant gene, the mouse only has two ANTs. Mouse Ant1 gene is expressed at high levels in skeletal muscle and heart and at lower levels in brain, while mouse Ant2 is expressed in all tissues but skeletal muscle.[190] Consequently, mice mutant in Ant1 have a virtually complete deficiency of ANT in skeletal muscle where only ANT1 is expressed, a partial deficiency in heart where both ANT1 and ANT2 are expressed, but normal ANT levels in liver where only ANT2 is expressed.

The skeletal muscle of Ant1 −/− animals exhibits classic RRFs and increased SDH and COX staining in the type I oxidative muscle fibers. These elevated OXPHOS enzyme activities correlate with a massive proliferation of giant mitochondria in the skeletal muscle fibers, degeneration of the contractile fibers, and marked exercise fatigability. The hearts of the ANT1-deficient mice also exhibited a striking hypertrophic cardiomyopathy, associated with a significant proliferation of cardiomyocyte mitochondria. The proliferation of mitochondria in the ANT1-deficient mouse skeletal muscle and heart is associated with the coordinate up-regulation of both nDNA and mtDNA OXPHOS genes. Up-regulated transcripts identified in skeletal muscle by differential display include the nDNA complex I 18-kDa polypeptide mRNA and the complex IV COXVa and COXVb mRNAs, various mtDNA transcripts, and the transcripts of several novel genes including Mcl-1, the muscle Bcl-2 homologue (Fig. 105-2).[245] This implies that ANT1-deficiency affects mitochondrial bioenergetics, as well as oxidative stress and possibly predisposition to mitochondrial permeability transition.

The ANT1-deficient mice also have an elevated serum lactate, alanine, succinate, and citrate, consistent with inhibition of the respiratory chain and TCA cycle. The inhibition of mitochondrial ADP/ATP exchange and of ADP-coupled respiration was confirmed in the skeletal muscle mitochondria of the Ant1 −/− mice by showing their complete resistance to stimulation of oxygen consumption by exogenous ADP. The heart mitochondrial respiration rate was only partially stimulated by ADP, while liver mitochondrial respiration was fully stimulated by ADP. This is consistent with the complete lack of ANT and ADP/ATP exchange in skeletal muscle mitochondria and a partial reduction in heart, but no reduction in liver. Hence, the ANT1 mouse provides direct proof that inhibition of the cell's access to mitochondrial energy production can result in the symptoms of mitochondrial myopathy and cardiomyopathy.[190]

The inhibition of ADP/ATP exchange in heart and skeletal muscle would be expected to limit the availability of matrix ADP for the ATP synthase, thus reducing proton flux through the ATP synthase proton channel. This would result in the hyperpolarization of the mitochondrial inner membrane, $\Delta\Psi$, which would inhibit the ETC and cause the redirection of electrons from the ETC into the ROS-generating pathway.

Consistent with this expectation, the mitochondrial production rate of H_2O_2 was increased six- to eightfold in the ANT1-deficient skeletal muscle and heart mitochondria, levels comparable to those obtained for control mitochondria when the ETC was inhibited by the complex III inhibitor antimycin A. ANT1-deficient brain cortex and cerebellum mitochondria also had elevated H_2O_2 production, but less than that produced in control mitochondria by antimycin A. Finally, the liver mitochondrial H_2O_2 production was the same for mutant and normal animals. Thus, the increased ROS production was proportional to the reduction in mitochondrial ANT levels and associated inhibition of the respiratory chain.

The increased oxidative stress caused by the ANT1 deficiency was paralleled by an induction of the ROS-detoxifying enzymes MnSOD and GPx. In ANT1-deficient skeletal muscle, MnSOD protein was increased about fifteenfold in tissue and sixfold in isolated mitochondria. The GPx levels in skeletal muscle tissue and mitochondria were increased about threefold. In ANT1-deficient heart, the MnSOD level was increased about twofold in tissue, but not at all in isolated mitochondria. The GPx levels in heart tissue and mitochondria were also increased about threefold. Hence, the increased oxidative stress resulting from inhibition of OXPHOS is associated with the induction of the mitochondrial ROS defense systems in skeletal muscle, though less so in heart.[436]

The increased ROS production in heart and muscle would be expected to increase mitochondrial macromolecular damage, unless countered by a comparable induction of antioxidant defenses. Analyses of the heart and skeletal muscle mtDNAs of 16- to 20-month-old ANT1-deficient mice confirmed this. These mutant animals had much higher levels of mtDNA rearrangements in their hearts than did age-matched controls. In fact, the level of mtDNA rearrangements in the 16- to 20-month-old Ant1 −/− heart was comparable to that seen in the heart of very old (30-month) normal mice. By contrast, while the level of mtDNA rearrangements was also increased in skeletal muscle, it was not to the extent of that of heart mtDNA. Because both heart and muscle mitochondria produced maximal levels of ROS, but the skeletal muscle, although not heart mitochondria, compensated by induction of the antioxidant enzyme MnSOD, it would follow that the heart would be exposed to greater residual oxidative stress than skeletal muscle. This can then explain the differential level of mtDNA damage in ANT1 −/− heart over skeletal muscle. Hence, inhibition of OXPHOS not only reduced energy output but increases ROS production and secondarily mitochondrial macromolecular damage, including mtDNA mutations.[436]

MnSOD-Deficient Mice

The origins and consequences of increased mitochondrial ROS production were further clarified by studying mice deficient in the mitochondrial MnSOD. Two mouse lines lacking MnSOD (Sod2) have also been reported: *Sod2*^{tm1Cje} and *Sod2*^{tm1Leb}.[571,572] The *Sod2*^{tm1Cje} mutation was originally studied on the CD1 background and resulted in neonatal death due to dilated cardiomyopathy.[571] The *Sod2*^{tm1Cje} mutation was studied on the C57BL/6 background and resulted in death after about 18 days. It was associated with degenerative injury to the large neurons, particularly in the basal ganglia and brain stem, and injury to the neuronal mitochondria.[572]

The *Sod2*^{tm1Cje} mutation on the CD1 background has been extensively characterized. In addition to death due to dilated cardiomyopathy at about 8 days of age,[571,573] histochemical analysis has revealed striking deposits of lipid in the liver and marked deficiency in SDH (complex II) in the hearts.[571] The complex II defect was confirmed by enzymologic analysis of complex II + complex III activity, which revealed a 65 percent reduction in skeletal muscle and a 76 percent reduction in heart. Heart complex I activity was also reduced 41 percent, and mitochondrial aconitase was almost entirely inactivated in heart (89 percent) and in brain (67 to 76 percent). Finally, urine organic acid analysis of the *Sod2* −/− animals revealed large quantities of 3-methylglutaconic, 2-hydroxyglutaric, 3-hydroxy-3 methylglutaric, and 3-hydroxyisovaleric acids. This is characteristic of human HMG-CoA lyase deficiency, and this enzyme was found to be reduced 36 percent in the mutant mouse livers.[574]

Testing for DNA oxidation revealed that the mutant hearts had large (215 percent to 300 percent) increases in 8-hydroxy-guanine, 8-hydroxy-adenine, and 5-hydroxy-cytosine. The brain also had increased levels of 5-hydroxy-cytosine.[574]

These observations indicate that the high levels of mitochondrial superoxide anion resulting from the MnSOD deficiency can cause the inhibition of the ETC (complexes I and II) and the TCA cycle (aconitase), probably due to the inactivation of the Fe-S centers in these enzymes. This conclusion was confirmed by demonstrating that the cardiac defect can be rescued by treating the Sod2 −/− animals with the exogenous antioxidant MnTBAP (manganese 5,10,15,20-tetrakis (4-benzoic acid) porphyrin), which catalytically converts O_2^- to H_2O_2. Peritoneal injection of the Sod2 −/− mice with MnTBAP eliminated the dilated cardiomyopathy, reduced the liver lipid deposition, and extended the mean life span of the animals to about 16 days of age. Unfortunately, the MnTBAP does not cross the blood-brain barrier, and by 12 days of age the MnTBAP-treated animals began to exhibit gait disturbances that progressed to ataxia, dystonia, repetitive movements, tremor, and immobility by 21 days of age. Histologic analysis of the brains of these mice revealed a symmetric spongiform encephalopathy, together with glial fibrillary acid protein deposition, in regions of the cortex and brain stem. This suggests that the increased mitochondrial ROS production is extremely toxic to the brain, possibly causing neuronal cell apoptosis.[573]

While that acute pathology observed in the Sod2 −/− animals confirms the importance of mitochondrial ROS toxicity in causing mitochondrial dysfunction, many clinical syndromes such as Friedreich ataxia are associated with chronic ROS exposure. Consequently, the analysis of heterozygous Sod2 +/− mice, with a 50 percent reduction in MnSOD, may provide a better model for chronic mitochondrial disease. The liver mitochondria of Sod2 +/− mice have been found to have a 30 percent reduction in mitochondrial glutathione levels, although normal levels of GPx. The mitochondrial aconitase activity was reduced 30 percent, but could be reactivated to control levels by exposure to iron and a reducing agent, confirming the inactivation of the Fe-S centers. Mitochondrial complex I was reduced 30 percent, mitochondrial protein carbonyl groups (aldehydes and ketones) were increased, and the mtDNA had a 30 percent increase in 8-OHdG. Respiration studies revealed a reduction in ADP-stimulated respiration, indicating partial uncoupling of the mitochondria, and the mitochondria had increased sensitivity to the calcium and oxidative stress-induced opening of the of the mtPTP, implying a predilection to apoptosis.[575] Thus, chronic exposure to mitochondrial ROS does impair mitochondrial function, confirming that increased mitochondrial ROS production can play a significant role in the pathophysiology of mitochondrial induction of apoptosis.

Tfam-Deficient Mice

Genetic inactivation of the nDNA-encoded mitochondrial transcription factor Tfam has provided a model for the mtDNA deletion and depletion syndromes. The Tfam gene was inactivated by bracketing the terminal two exons (exons 6 and 7) with loxP sites, and eliminating these exons by crossing the Tfam +/− animals with animals bearing the *Cre* recombinase.

Systemic mtDNA defects were obtained by transcribing the *Cre* recombinase from a constitutive β-actin promoter. The resulting heterozygous Tfam +/− animals were viable and reproductively competent, while the homozygous Tfam −/− animals were embryonic lethals.[576] The Tfam heterozygous animals had a 50 percent reduction in Tfam transcripts and protein, and a partial reduction in mtDNA copy number mitochondrial transcripts, and COXI protein in heart, but not in liver. The homozygous Tfam −/− mutant animals died between embryonic days E8.5 and E10.5, with a complete absence of Tfam protein, and either a severely reduced or a complete absence of mtDNA. The mitochondria in the Tfam −/− animals were enlarged with abnormal cristae and were deficient in COX but not SDH.[576]

Heart- and muscle-specific mtDNA defects were obtained by combining the homozygous Tfam^{loxP} allele with the *Cre* recombinase gene driven by the muscle creatine kinase promoter. This resulted in the selective destruction of heart and skeletal muscle Tfam genes. While the hearts of 18.5 day embryos had reduced levels of Tfam, they appeared to be otherwise morphologically and biochemically normal. By contrast, these mutant animals proved to be postnatal lethals, dying of dilated cardiomyopathy at a mean age of 20 days. The animals also developed cardiac conduction defects. This was associated with a reduction in Tfam protein and mtDNA transcript levels in heart and muscle, a reduction in heart mtDNA by three quarters and in skeletal muscle mtDNA by 40 percent, and a reduction of respiratory complexes I and IV, but not of complex II. Finally, histochemical analysis of the hearts revealed a mosaic-staining pattern with some of the cardiomyocyte being COX$^-$ and SDH$^+$, comparable to the mosaic OXPHOS deficiencies seen in human mitochondrial myopathy patient.[577] Hence, these animals exhibit many of the features seen in the mtDNA deletion and depletion syndromes.

CAP^R Mice

While mice with the nDNA-encoded ANT1, MnSOD, and Tfam-deficiency mutations have provided important new insights into the pathophysiology of mitochondrial disease, they do not reflect the genetic complexity of mtDNA diseases. To create a more accurate mouse model for mtDNA disease, efforts are being made to introduce deleterious mtDNA mutations into the mouse female germ line.

Several approaches have been used to introduce genetically distinctive mtDNAs into the mice. Heteroplasmic mice have been obtained by fusion of cytoplasts collected from mouse oocytes harboring one mtDNA type (e.g., NZB/B1NJ) with oocytes harboring a different mtDNA type (e.g., C57BL/6 or BALB/c).[578–580] Alternatively, membrane-bound karyoplasts containing a zygote nucleus and a portion of the oocyte cytoplasm have been fused to enucleated eggs.[580,581] In both cases, heteroplasmic mice have been obtained and used to study the kinetics of replicative segregation. While neither of these techniques permits the introduction of deleterious mtDNA mutations, they did reveal that certain tissues show directional mtDNA segregation with age, with the BALB mtDNA coming to predominate in blood and spleen but the NZB mtDNA predominating in liver and kidney.[579]

Two approaches have been attempted for introducing exogenous mitochondria and mtDNAs into the mouse female germ line. In the first, mitochondria have been isolated from the livers of *Mus spretus* mice and microinjected into *Mus musculus domesticus* oocytes. Of the 23 surviving blastocysts that were analyzed, all had detectable levels of *M. spretus* mtDNA by PCR analysis.[582]

In the second, the cybrid transfer technique has been used to introduce the CAP^R mtDNA mutation into mouse female embryonic stem (ES) cells. The mtDNA mutant ES cells were then injected into blastocysts and chimeric females generated. Introduction of CAP^R mtDNAs into the mouse should produce a good model of the human mtDNA protein synthesis diseases because this mutation alters the mitochondrial ribosome, resulting in the reduction of the complex I and complex IV activities.

The first attempt to introduce CAP^R mutant mtDNA mutation into the mouse employed CAP^R B16 melanoma cells. These were enucleated, fused to the teratocarcinoma cell line OTT6050, and the teratocarcinoma cybrids injected into blastocysts. Five of the six chimeric animals were found by isoenzyme analysis to have 10 to 15 percent chimerism in various organs. However, no direct evidence was obtained that the CAP^R mtDNA was present in the transgenic mice.[583]

In the second attempt, CAP^R mtDNAs from mouse 501-1 cells were transferred into the mouse female ES line AK11.1. The 501-1 CAP^R mutation is due to a single T to C transition at np 2433 in the 16S rRNA gene,[252] which creates an *Mae*III site. In some cases, the ES cells were cured of their resident CAP^S mitochondria, prior to fusion with the CAP^R cytoplasts, by treatment with the mitochondrial toxin rhodamine 6-G. Using the resulting nearly homoplasmic CAP^R ES cells, chimerism was obtained in 20 animals, ranging from 10 to 30 percent. Three of five chimeric animals were analyzed for the CAP^R mtDNA and were positive. The highest percentage of CAP^R mtDNAs was found in the kidneys, where it ranged from 20 to 50 percent of the total mtDNA. Mutant mtDNA of 15 percent or less was also found in the hearts of two mice and the brain and liver of two additional mice.[253]

These results suggest that it may soon be possible to introduce pathogenic mtDNA mutations, isolated in cultured cells, into the mouse germline via female ES cells. If so, this should permit a direct investigation of the interplay between the stochastic fluctuation of heteroplasmic mtDNA mutations and the variation in mitochondrial energy production, oxidative stress, and apoptosis. Such mouse models promise to recapitulate the full range of genetic and physiological variation seen in mitochondrial diseases and thus to provide important new insights into the role of mitochondrial defects in a spectrum of progressive diseases, possibly including aging and cancer.

MITOCHONDRIAL PARADIGM FOR DEGENERATIVE DISEASES AND AGING

The genetics of mitochondrial disease can now be envisioned as the product of two factors, the inheritance of a deleterious mtDNA or nDNA mutation on a mitochondria gene and the age-related accumulation of mtDNA damage and decline in mitochondria, which exacerbates the inherited defect, pushing the individual over tissue and organ bioenergetic thresholds and resulting in the delayed onset and progressive course of mitochondrial diseases (Fig. 105-26). It is hypothesized that each individual is born with

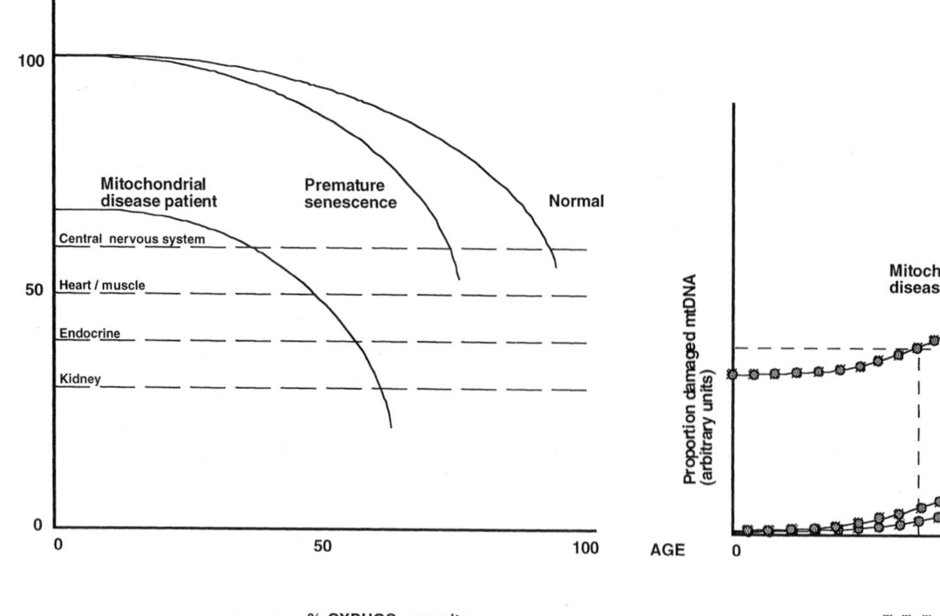

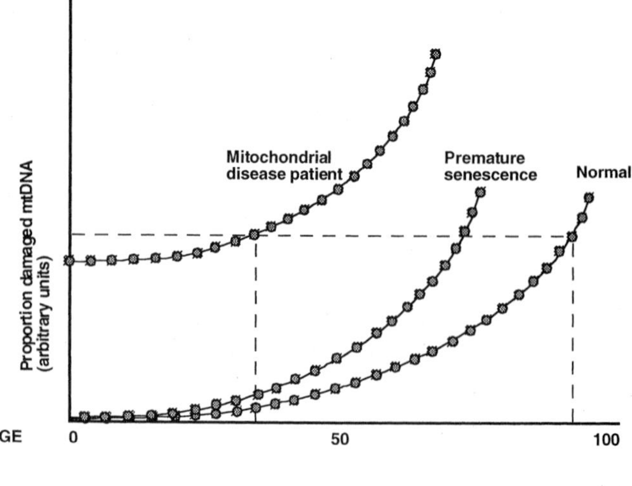

Fig. 105-26 Hypothesis relating the acquisition of mtDNA mutations (inherited and somatic) to the age-related decline of OXPHOS and the progression of OXPHOS diseases and of senescence. The dashed horizontal lines in both panels represent different tissue-specific expression thresholds. The left panel shows the age-related decline of OXPHOS in individuals born with a normal OXPHOS genotype, a mutant OXPHOS gene, and an increased mtDNA somatic mutation rate. The right panel shows the relative levels of defective mtDNA with age for each of these individuals.

an array of nDNA and mtDNA alleles that determines the individual's initial bioenergetic capacity. An individual who inherits a strong genotype will have a high initial energy capacity, well above the minimum energetic thresholds required by his or her tissues. However, if the individual inherits a deleterious mutation, then his or her initial energetic capacity will be lower. Somatic mtDNA mutations in postmitotic cells, which further erode an individual's tissues' energy capacities, accumulate as the individual ages. Ultimately, the combined effects of the inherited and somatic mitochondrial defects push the tissues' energy capacity below bioenergetic thresholds, resulting in symptoms and ultimately failures. By this hypothesis, the more deleterious the inherited mitochondrial gene defects, the sooner tissue thresholds will be traversed and symptoms ensue. Thus, for very mild mutations, such as the mtDNA Alzheimer disease MTTQ*ADPD4336C mutation, symptoms may not occur until late in life. By contrast, for severe mutations, such as the nDNA complex I subunit or SURF-1 gene mutations, the defect is sufficiently severe that expression thresholds are crossed early in life, causing the lethal childhood Leigh disease (Fig. 105-26).

The pathophysiological mechanism that leads to tissue failure can now be understood as the interplay between the decline of mitochondrial energetic capacity, a rise in mitochondrial ROS production, and the impinging of these two processes on the mtPTP, ultimately resulting in the opening of the mtPTP, disruption of the mitochondria, and destruction of the cell. Given this framework, it is now possible to envision several new therapeutic approaches to mitochondrial disease including augmentation of energy production, removal of toxic ROS with drugs such as MnTBAP, and/or inhibition of the activation of the mtPTP. In the future, such approaches might improve the clinical status of mitochondrial disease patients, but also retard disease progression.

REFERENCES

1. Wallace DC, Singh G, Lott MT, Hodge JA, Schurr TG, Lezza AM, Elsas LJ, et al.: Mitochondrial DNA mutation associated with Leber's hereditary optic neuropathy. *Science* **242:**1427, 1988.
2. Holt IJ, Harding AE, Morgan-Hughes JA: Deletions of muscle mitochondrial DNA in patients with mitochondrial myopathies. *Nature* **331:**717, 1988.
3. Tzagoloff A: *Mitochondria*. New York, Plenum Press, 1982.
4. Hales KG, Fuller MT: Developmentally regulated mitochondrial fusion mediated by a conserved, novel, predicted GTPase. *Cell* **90:**121, 1997.
5. Hermann GJ, Thatcher JW, Mills JP, Hales KG, Fuller MT, Nunnari J, Shaw JM: Mitochondrial fusion in yeast requires the transmembrane GTPase Fzo1p. *J Cell Biol* **143:**359, 1998.
6. Yaffe MP: The machinery of mitochondrial inheritance and behavior. *Science* **283:**1493, 1999.
7. Tanaka Y, Kanai Y, Okada Y, Nonaka S, Takeda S, Harada A, Hirokawa N: Targeted disruption of mouse conventional kinesin heavy chain, kif5B, results in abnormal perinuclear clustering of mitochondria. *Cell* **93:**1147, 1998.
8. Smirnova E, Shurland DL, Ryazantsev SN, van der Bliek AM: A human dynamin-related protein controls the distribution of mitochondria. *J Cell Biol* **143:**351, 1998.
9. Wallace DC: Diseases of the mitochondrial DNA. *Annu Rev Biochem* **61:**1175, 1992.
10. Wallace DC: Mitochondrial genetics: a paradigm for aging and degenerative diseases? *Science* **256:**628, 1992.
11. Wallace DC: 1994 William Allan Award Address. Mitochondrial DNA variation in human evolution, degenerative disease, and aging. *Am J Hum Genet* **57:**201, 1995.
12. Wallace DC: Mitochondrial DNA mutations and bioenergetic defects in aging and degenerative diseases, in Rosenberg RN, Prusiner SB, DiMauro S, Barchi RL (eds): *The Molecular and Genetic Basis of Neurological Disease*, 2nd ed. Boston, Butterworth-Heinemann, 1997, p 237.
13. Wallace DC, Brown MD, Lott MT: Mitochondrial Genetics, in Rimoin DL, Connor JM, Pyeritz RE, Emery AEH (eds): *Emery and Rimoin's Principles and Practice of Medical Genetics*, 3rd ed, vol 1. London, Churchill Livingstone, 1996, p 277.
14. Petit PX, Susin SA, Zamzami N, Mignotte B, Kroemer G: Mitochondria and programmed cell death: Back to the future. *FEBS Lett* **396:**7, 1996.
15. Green DR, Reed JC: Mitochondria and apoptosis. *Science* **281:**1309, 1998.
16. Zoratti M, Szabo I: The mitochondrial permeability transition. *Biochim Biophys Acta* **1241:**139, 1995.
17. Mancini M, Nicholson DW, Roy S, Thornberry NA, Peterson EP, Casciola-Rosen LA, Rosen A: The caspase-3 precursor has a cytosolic and mitochondrial distribution: Implications for apoptotic signaling. *J Cell Biol* **140:**1485, 1998.
18. Liu X, Kim CN, Yang J, Jemmerson R, Wang X: Induction of apoptotic program in cell-free extracts: requirement for dATP and cytochrome c. *Cell* **86:**147, 1996.
19. Earnshaw WC: Apoptosis. A cellular poison cupboard [News]. *Nature* **397:**387, 1999.
20. Susin SA, Lorenzo HK, Zamzami N, Marzo I, Snow BE, Brothers GM, Mangion J, et al.: Molecular characterization of mitochondrial apoptosis-inducing factor. *Nature* **397:**441, 1999.
21. Susin SA, Lorenzo HK, Zamzami N, Marzo I, Brenner C, Larochette N, Prevost MC, et al.: Mitochondrial release of caspase-2 and -9 during the apoptotic process. *J Exp Med* **189:**381, 1999.
22. Brustovetsky N, Klingenberg M: Mitochondrial ADP/ATP carrier can be reversibly converted into a large channel by Ca^{2+}. *Biochemistry* **35:**8483, 1996.
23. Marzo I, Brenner C, Zamzami N, Jurgensmeier JM, Susin SA, Vieira HL, Prevost MC, et al.: Bax and adenine nucleotide translocator cooperate in the mitochondrial control of apoptosis. *Science* **281:**2027, 1998.
24. Smeitink J, van den Heuvel L: Protein biosynthesis '99. Human mitochondrial complex I in health and disease. *Am J Hum Genet* **4:**1505, 1999.
25. Anderson S, Bankier AT, Barrell BG, de Bruijn MH, Coulson AR, Drouin J, Eperon IC, et al.: Sequence and organization of the human mitochondrial genome. *Nature* **290:**457, 1981.
26. Arizmendi JM, Skehel JM, Runswick MJ, Fearnley IM, Walker JE: Complementary DNA sequences of two 14.5 kDa subunits of NADH:ubiquinone oxidoreductase from bovine heart mitochondria. Complementation of the primary structure of the complex? *FEBS Lett* **313:**80, 1992.
27. Attardi G, Chomyn A, Doolittle RF, Mariottini P, Ragan CI: Seven unidentified reading frames of human mitochondrial DNA encode subunits of the respiratory chain NADH dehydrogenase. *Cold Spring Harb Symp Quant Biol* **1:**103, 1986.
28. Chomyn A, Mariottini P, Cleeter WJ, Ragan CI, Matsuno-Yagi A, Hatefi Y, Doolittle RF, et al.: Six unidentified reading frames of human mitochondrial DNA encode components of the respiratory-chain NADH dehydrogenase. *Nature* **314:**592, 1985.
29. Chomyn A, Cleeter WJ, Ragan CI, Riley M, Doolittle RF, Attardi G: URF6, last unidentified reading frame of human mtDNA, codes for an NADH dehydrogenase subunit. *Science* **234:**614, 1986.
30. Chomyn A, Mariottini P, Gonzalez-Cadavid N, Attardi G, Strong DD, Trovato D, Riley M, et al.: Identification of the polypeptides encoded in the ATPase 6 gene and in the unassigned reading frames 1 and 3 of human mtDNA. *Proc Natl Acad Sci U S A* **80:**5535, 1983.
31. Skehel JM, Fearnley IM, Walker JE: NADH:ubiquinone oxidoreductase from bovine heart mitochondria: sequence of a novel 17.2-kDa subunit. *FEBS Lett* **438:**301, 1998.
32. Galante YM, Hatefi Y: Purification and molecular and enzymic properties of mitochondrial NADH dehydrogenase. *Arch Biochem Biophys* **192:**559, 1979.
33. Oliver NA, Wallace DC: Assignment of two mitochondrially synthesized polypeptides to human mitochondrial DNA and their use in the study of intracellular mitochondrial interaction. *Mol Cell Biol* **2:**30, 1982.
34. Walker JE: Determination of the structures of respiratory enzyme complexes from mammalian mitochondria. *Biochim Biophys Acta* **1271:**221, 1995.
35. Walker JE, Arizmendi JM, Dupuis A, Fearnley IM, Finel M, Medd SM, Pilkington SJ, et al.: Sequences of 20 subunits of NADH:ubiquinone oxidoreductase from bovine heart mitochondria. Application of a novel strategy for sequencing proteins using the polymerase chain reaction. *J Mol Biol* **226:**1051, 1992.
36. MITOMAP: A Human Mitochondrial Genome Database, Center for Molecular Medicine, Emory University (Atlanta, GA), http://www.gen.emory.edu/mitomap.html, 1999.
37. Ohnishi T: *Mitochondrial Iron-Sulfur Flavohydrogenases*. New York, Dekker, 1979.

38. Ragan CI: Structure of NADH-ubiquinone reductase (complex I). *Curr Top Bioenerget* **15:**1, 1987.
39. Guenebaut V, Schlitt A, Weiss H, Leonard K, Friedrich T: Consistent structure between bacterial and mitochondrial NADH:ubiquinone oxidoreductase (complex I). *J Mol Biol* **276:**105, 1998.
40. Grigorieff N: Three-dimensional structure of bovine NADH:ubiquinone oxidoreductase (complex I) at 22 Å in ice. *J Mol Biol* **277:**1033, 1998.
41. Duncan AM, Chow W, Robinson BH: Localization of the human 75-kDal Fe-S protein of NADH-coenzyme Q reductase gene (NDUFS1) to 2q33 → q34. *Cytogenet Cell Genet* **60:**212, 1992.
42. Hatefi Y: The mitochondrial electron transport and oxidative phosphorylation system. *Annu Rev Biochem* **54:**1015, 1985.
43. Chow W, Ragan I, Robinson BH: Determination of the cDNA sequence for the human mitochondrial 75-kDa Fe-S protein of NADH-coenzyme Q reductase. *Eur J Biochem* **201:**547, 1991.
44. Ali ST, Duncan AM, Schappert K, Heng HH, Tsui LC, Chow W, Robinson BH: Chromosomal localization of the human gene encoding the 51-kDa subunit of mitochondrial complex I (NDUFV1) to 11q13. *Genomics* **18:**435, 1993.
45. Spencer SR, Taylor JB, Cowell IG, Xia CL, Pemble SE, Ketterer B: The human mitochondrial NADH:ubiquinone oxidoreductase 51-kDa subunit maps adjacent to the glutathione S-transferase P1-1 gene on chromosome 11q13. *Genomics* **14:**1116, 1992.
46. Pilkington SJ, Walker JE: Mitochondrial NADH-ubiquinone reductase: Complementary DNA sequences of import precursors of the bovine and human 24-kDa subunit. *Biochemistry* **28:**3257, 1989.
47. Toda H, Hosokawa Y, Nishikimi M, Suzuki H, Kato K, Ozawa T: Cloning and sequencing of a cDNA encoding the precursor to the 24-kDa iron-sulfur protein of human mitochondrial NADH dehydrogenase. *Int J Biochem* **21:**1161, 1989.
48. Hattori N, Suzuki H, Wang Y, Minoshima S, Shimizu N, Yoshino H, Kurashima R, et al.: Structural organization and chromosomal localization of the human nuclear gene (NDUFV2) for the 24-kDa iron-sulfur subunit of complex I in mitochondrial respiratory chain. *Biochem Biophys Res Commun* **216:**771, 1995.
49. de Coo R, Buddiger P, Smeets H, van Kessel AG, Morgan-Hughs J, Weghuis DO, Overhauser J, et al.: Molecular cloning and characterization of the active human mitochondrial NADH:ubiquinone oxidoreductase 24-kDa gene (NDUFV2) and its pseudogene. *Genomics* **26:**461, 1995.
50. Fearnley IM, Skehel JM, Walker JE: Electrospray ionization mass spectrometric analysis of subunits of NADH:ubiquinone oxidoreductase (complex I) from bovine heart mitochondria. *Biochem Soc Trans* **22:**551, 1994.
51. Walker JE: The NADH:ubiquinone oxidoreductase (complex I) of respiratory chains. *Q Rev Biophys* **25:**253, 1992.
52. Tuschen G, Sackmann U, Nehls U, Haiker H, Buse G, Weiss H: Assembly of NADH: ubiquinone reductase (complex I) in Neurospora mitochondria. Independent pathways of nuclear-encoded and mitochondrially encoded subunits. *J Mol Biol* **213:**845, 1990.
53. Belogrudov G, Hatefi Y: Catalytic sector of complex I (NADH:ubiquinone oxidoreductase): subunit stoichiometry and substrate-induced conformation changes. *Biochemistry* **33:**4571, 1994.
54. Ragan CI, Galante YM, Hatefi Y: Purification of three iron-sulfur proteins from the iron-protein fragment of mitochondrial NADH-ubiquinone oxidoreductase. *Biochemistry* **21:**2518, 1982.
55. Ragan CI, Galante YM, Hatefi Y, Ohnishi T: Resolution of mitochondrial NADH dehydrogenase and isolation of two iron-sulfur proteins. *Biochemistry* **21:**590, 1982.
56. Suzuki H, Ozawa T: An ubiquinone-binding protein in mitochondrial NADH-ubiquinone reductase (complex I). *Biochem Biophys Res Commun* **138:**1237, 1986.
57. Jun AS, Trounce IA, Brown MD, Shoffner JM, Wallace DC: Use of transmitochondrial cybrids to assign a complex I defect to the mitochondrial DNA-encoded NADH dehydrogenase subunit 6 gene mutation at nucleotide pair 14459 that causes Leber hereditary optic neuropathy and dystonia. *Mol Cell Biol* **16:**771, 1996.
58. Earley FG, Ragan C: Photoaffinity labelling of mitochondrial NADH dehydrogenase with arylazidoamorphigenin, an analogue of rotenone. *Biochem J* **224:**525, 1984.
59. Ahmed I, Krishnamoorthy G: The non-equivalence of binding sites of coenzyme quinone and rotenone in mitochondrial NADH-CoQ reductase. *FEBS Lett* **300:**275, 1992.
60. Jun AS, Brown MD, Wallace DC: A mitochondrial DNA mutation at np 14459 of the ND6 gene associated with maternally inherited Leber's hereditary optic neuropathy and dystonia. *Proc Natl Acad Sci U S A* **91:**6206, 1994.
61. Hofhaus G, Attardi G: Lack of assembly of mitochondrial DNA-encoded subunits of respiratory NADH dehydrogenase and loss of enzyme activity in a human cell mutant lacking the mitochondrial ND4 gene product [published erratum appears in *EMBO J* 13(23):5794, 1994]. *EMBO J* **12:**3043, 1993.
62. Hofhaus G, Attardi G: Efficient selection and characterization of mutants of a human cell line which are defective in mitochondrial DNA-encoded subunits of respiratory NADH dehydrogenase [published erratum appears in *Mol Cell Biol* 15(6):3461, 1995]. *Mol Cell Biol* **15:**964, 1995.
63. Pilkington SJ, Arizmendi JM, Fearnley IM, Runswick MJ, Skehel JM, Walker JE: Structural organization of complex I from bovine mitochondria. *Biochem Soc Trans* **21:**26, 1993.
64. Vinogradov AD: Kinetics, control, and mechanism of ubiquinone reduction by the mammalian respiratory chain-linked NADH-ubiquinone reductase. *J Bioenerg Biomembr* **25:**367, 1993.
65. Weiss H, Friedrich T, Hofhaus G, Preis D: The respiratory-chain NADH dehydrogenase (complex I) of mitochondria. *Eur J Biochem* **197:**563, 1991.
66. Degli Esposti M, Ghelli A: The mechanism of proton and electron transport in mitochondrial complex I. *Biochim Biophys Acta* **1187:**116, 1994.
67. Degli Esposti M: Inhibitors of NADH-ubiquinone reductase: An overview. *Biochim Biophys Acta* **1364:**222, 1998.
68. Clarkson GH, Neagle J, Lindsay JG: Topography of succinate dehydrogenase in the mitochondrial inner membrane. A study using limited proteolysis and immunoblotting. *Biochem J* **273:**719, 1991.
69. Cochran B, Capaldi RA, Ackrell BA: The cDNA sequence of beef heart C_{II-3}, a membrane-intrinsic subunit of succinate-ubiquinone oxidoreductase. *Biochim Biophys Acta* **1188:**162, 1994.
70. Davis KA, Hatefi Y: Succinate dehydrogenase. I. Purification, molecular properties, and substructure. *Biochemistry* **10:**2509, 1971.
71. Davis KA, Hatefi Y: Spectral and reconstitution properties of cytochrome b in complexes II and 3. *Biochem Biophys Res Commun* **44:**1338, 1971.
72. Hatefi Y, Galante YM: Isolation of cytochrome b560 from complex II (succinateubiquinone oxidoreductase) and its reconstitution with succinate dehydrogenase. *J Biol Chem* **255:**5530, 1980.
73. Ishii N, Fujii M, Hartman PS, Tsuda M, Yasuda K, Senoo-Matsuda N, Yanase S, et al.: A mutation in succinate dehydrogenase cytochrome b causes oxidative stress and ageing in nematodes [see Comments]. *Nature* **394:**694, 1998.
74. Kita K, Oya H, Gennis RB, Ackrell BA, Kasahara M: Human complex II (succinate-ubiquinone oxidoreductase): cDNA cloning of iron sulfur (Ip) subunit of liver mitochondria. *Biochem Biophys Res Commun* **166:**101, 1990.
75. Au HC, Ream-Robinson D, Bellew LA, Broomfield PL, Saghbini M, Scheffler IE: Structural organization of the gene encoding the human iron-sulfur subunit of succinate dehydrogenase. *Gene* **159:**249, 1995.
76. Leckschat S, Ream-Robinson D, Scheffler IE: The gene for the iron sulfur protein of succinate dehydrogenase (SDH-IP) maps to human chromosome 1p35-36.1. *Somat Cell Mol Genet* **19:**505, 1993.
77. Hirawake H, Wang H, Kuramochi T, Kojima S, Kita K: Human complex II (succinate-ubiquinone oxidoreductase): cDNA cloning of the flavoprotein (Fp) subunit of liver mitochondria. *J Biochem (Tokyo)* **116:**221, 1994.
78. Morris AA, Farnsworth L, Ackrell BA, Turnbull DM, Birch-Machin MA: The cDNA sequence of the flavoprotein subunit of human heart succinate dehydrogenase. *Biochim Biophys Acta* **1185:**125, 1994.
79. Bourgeron T, Rustin P, Chretien D, Birch-Machin M, Bourgeois M, Viegas-Pequignot E, Munnich A, et al.: Mutation of a nuclear succinate dehydrogenase gene results in mitochondrial respiratory chain deficiency. *Nat Genet* **11:**144, 1995.
80. Hirawake H, Taniwaki M, Tamura A, Kojima S, Kita K: Cytochrome b in human complex II (succinate-ubiquinone oxidoreductase): cDNA cloning of the components in liver mitochondria and chromosome assignment of the genes for the large (SDHC) and small (SDHD) subunits to 1q21 and 11q23. *Cytogenet Cell Genet* **79:**132, 1997.
81. Gonzalez-Halphen D, Lindorfer MA, Capaldi RA: Subunit arrangement in beef heart complex III. *Biochemistry* **27:**7021, 1988.
82. Schagger H, Link TA, Engel WD, von Jagow G: Isolation of the eleven protein subunits of the bc1 complex from beef heart. *Methods Enzymol* **126:**224, 1986.
83. Iwata S, Lee JW, Okada K, Lee JK, Iwata M, Rasmussen B, Link TA, et al.: Complete structure of the 11-subunit bovine mitochondrial cytochrome bc1 complex [see Comments]. *Science* **281:**64, 1998.
84. Saraste M: Oxidative phosphorylation at the fin de siecle. *Science* **283:**1488, 1999.

85. Trumpower BL, Gennis RB: Energy transduction by cytochrome complexes in mitochondrial and bacterial respiration: The enzymology of coupling electron transfer reactions to transmembrane proton translocation. *Annu Rev Biochem* **63:**675, 1994.
86. Weiss H, Linke P, Haiker H, Leonard K: Structure and function of the mitochondrial ubiquinol:cytochrome c reductase and NADH:ubiquinone reductase. *Biochem Soc Trans* **15:**100, 1987.
87. Degli Esposti M, DeVries S, Crimi M, Ghelli A, Patarnello T, Meyer A: Mitochondrial cytohrome b: evolution and structure of the protein. *Biochim Biophys Acta* **1143:**243, 1993.
88. Saraste M: Location of haem-binding sites in the mitochondrial cytochrome b. *FEBS Lett* **166:**367, 1984.
89. Wikstrom M, Krab K, Saraste M: Proton-translocating cytochrome complexes. *Annu Rev Biochem* **50:**623, 1981.
90. Mitchell P: Possible molecular mechanisms of the protonmotive function of cytochrome systems. *J Theor Biol* **62:**327, 1976.
91. Wikstrom M, Krab K: The semiquinone cycle. A hypothesis of electron transfer and proton translocation in cytochrome bc-type complexes. *J Bioenerg Biomembr* **18:**181, 1986.
92. Hosler JP, Ferguson-Miller S, Calhoun MW, Thomas JW, Hill J, Lemieux L, Ma J, et al.: Insight into the active-site structure and function of cytochrome oxidase by analysis of site-directed mutants of bacterial cytochrome *aa3* and cytochrome *bo*. *J Bioenerg Biomembr* **25:**121, 1993.
93. Pennacchio LA, Bergmann A, Fukushima A, Okubo K, Salemi A, Lennon GG: Structure, sequence and location of the UQCRFS1 gene for the human Rieske Fe-S protein. *Gene* **155:**207, 1995.
94. Suzuki H, Hosokawa Y, Nishikimi M, Ozawa T: Structural organization of the human mitochondrial cytochrome c1 gene. *J Biol Chem* **264:**1368, 1989.
95. Nishikimi M, Ohta S, Suzuki H, Tanaka T, Kikkawa F, Tanaka M, Kagawa Y, et al.: Nucleotide sequence of a cDNA encoding the precursor to human cytochrome c1. *Nucleic Acids Res* **16:**3577, 1988.
96. Nishikimi M, Suzuki H, Yamaguchi M, Matsukage A, Yoshida MC, Ozawa T: Assignment of the human cytochrome c1 gene to chromosome 8. *Biochem Int* **16:**655, 1988.
97. Limbach KJ, Wu R: Characterization of a mouse somatic cytochrome c gene and three cytochrome c pseudogenes. *Nucleic Acids Res* **13:**617, 1985.
98. Virbasius JV, Scarpulla RC: Structure and expression of rodent genes encoding the testis-specific cytochrome *c*. Differences in gene structure and evolution between somatic and testicular variants. *J Biol Chem* **263:**6791, 1988.
99. Cuticchia AJ: *Human Gene Mapping 1994: A Compendium*. Baltimore, MD, Johns Hopkins University Press, 1995.
100. Evans MJ, Scarpulla RC: The human somatic cytochrome c gene: Two classes of processed pseudogenes demarcate a period of rapid molecular evolution. *Proc Natl Acad Sci U S A* **85:**9625, 1988.
101. Kadenbach B, Jarausch J, Hartmann R, Merle P: Separation of mammalian cytochrome c oxidase into 13 polypeptides by a sodium dodecyl sulfate-gel electrophoretic procedure. *Anal Biochem* **129:**517, 1983.
102. Tsukihara T, Aoyama H, Yamashita E, Tomizaki T, Yamaguchi H, Shinzawa-Itoh K, Nakashima R, et al.: The whole structure of the 13-subunit oxidized cytochrome c oxidase at 2.8 A [see Comments]. *Science* **272:**1136, 1996.
103. Gennis R, Ferguson-Miller S: Structure of cytochrome *c* oxidase, energy generator of aerobic life. *Science* **269:**1063, 1995.
104. McKusick VA, Antonarakis SE: *Mendelian Inheritance in Man: A Catalog of Human Genes and Genetic Disorders*. Baltimore, Johns Hopkins University Press, 1998.
105. Online Mendelian Inheritance in Man, OMIM, Center for Medical Genetics, Johns Hopkins University (Baltimore, MD) and National Center for Biotechnology Information, National Library of Medicine (Bethesda, MD), www.ncbi.nlm.nih.gov/omim/, 1999.
106. Tsukihara T, Aoyama H, Yamashita E, Tomizaki T, Yamaguchi H, Shinzawa-Itoh K, Nakashima R, et al.: Structures of metal sites of oxidized bovine heart cytochrome c oxidase at 2.8 Å. *Science* **269:**1069, 1995.
107. Rousseau DL, Ching Y, Wang J: Proton translocation in cytochrome c oxidase: redox linkage through proximal ligand exchange on cytochrome a3. *J Bioenerg Biomembr* **25:**165, 1993.
108. Capaldi RA: Structure and function of cytochrome c oxidase. *Annu Rev Biochem* **59:**569, 1990.
109. Anderson S, deBruijn MHL, Coulson AR, Eperon IC, Sanger F, Young IG: Complete sequence of bovine mitochondrial DNA. Conserved features of the mammalian mitochondrial genome. *J Mol Biol* **156:**683, 1982.
110. Fetter JR, Qian J, Shapleigh J, Thomas JW, Garcia-Horsman A, Schmidt E, Hosler J, et al.: Possible proton relay pathways in cytochrome *c* oxidase. *Proc Natl Acad Sci U S A* **92:**1604, 1995.
111. Wikstrom M: Proton translocation by bacteriorhodopsin and heme-copper oxidases. *Curr Opin Struct Biol* **8:**480, 1998.
112. Prochaska LJ, Bisson R, Capaldi RA, Steffens GC, Buse G: Inhibition of cytochrome c oxidase function by dicyclohexylcarbodiimide. *Biochim Biophys Acta* **637:**360, 1981.
113. Lomax MI, Grossman LI: Tissue-specific genes for respiratory proteins. *Trends Biochem Sci* **14:**501, 1989.
114. Preiss T, Lightowlers RN: Post-transcriptional regulation of tissue-specific isoforms. A bovine cytosolic RNA-binding protein, COLBP, associates with messenger RNA encoding the liver-form isopeptides of cytochrome c oxidase. *J Biol Chem* **268:**10659, 1993.
115. Zeviani M, Nakagawa M, Herbert J, Lomax MI, Grossman LI, Sherbany AA, Miranda AF, et al.: Isolation of a cDNA clone encoding subunit IV of human cytochrome *c* oxidase. *Gene* **55:**205, 1987.
116. Rizzuto R, Nakase H, Zeviani M, DiMauro S, Schon EA: Subunit Va of human and bovine cytochrome c oxidase is highly conserved. *Gene* **69:**245, 1988.
117. Zeviani M, Sakoda S, Sherbany AA, Nakase H, Rizzuto R, Samitt CE, DiMauro S, et al.: Sequence of cDNAs encoding subunit Vb of human and bovine cytochrome *c* oxidase. *Gene* **65:**1, 1988.
118. Fabrizi GM, Rizzuto R, Nakase H, Mita S, Kadenbach B, Schon EA: Sequence of a cDNA specifying subunit VIa of human cytochrome c oxidase. *Nucleic Acids Res* **17:**6409, 1989.
119. Taanman JW, Schrage C, Ponne N, Bolhuis P, de Vries H, Agsteribbe E: Nucleotide sequence of cDNA encoding subunit VIb of human cytochrome *c* oxidase. *Nucleic Acids Res* **17:**1766, 1989.
120. Otsuka M, Mizuno Y, Yoshida M, Kagawa Y, Ohta S: Nucleotide sequence of cDNA encoding human cytochrome c oxidase subunit VIc. *Nucleic Acids Res* **16:**10916, 1988.
121. Arnaudo E, Hirano M, Seelan RS, Milatovich A, Hsieh CL, Fabrizi GM, Grossman LI, et al.: Tissue-specific expression and chromosome assignment of genes specifying two isoforms of subunit VIIa of human cytochrome c oxidase. *Gene* **119:**299, 1992.
122. Sadlock JE, Lightowlers RN, Capaldi RA, Schon EA: Isolation of a cDNA specifying subunit VIIb of human cytochrome *c* oxidase. *Biochim Biophys Acta* **1172:**223, 1993.
123. Koga Y, Fabrizi GM, Mita S, Arnaudo E, Lomax MI, Aqua MS, Grossman LI, et al.: Sequence of a cDNA specifying subunit VIIc of human cytochrome c oxidase. *Nucleic Acids Res* **18:**684, 1990.
124. Rizzuto R, Nakase H, Darras B, Francke U, Fabrizi G, M., Mengel T, Walsh F, et al.: A gene specifying subunit VIII of human cytochrome c oxidase is localized to chromosome 11 and is expressed in both muscle and non-muscle tissues. *J Biol Chem* **264:**10595, 1989.
125. Lomax MI, Hsieh CL, Darras BT, Francke U: Structure of the human cytochrome *c* oxidase subunit Vb gene and chromosomal mapping of the coding gene and of seven pseudogenes. *Genomics* **10:**1, 1991.
126. Taanman JW, Schrage C, Bokma E, Reuvekamp P, Agsteribbe E, De Vries H: Nucleotide sequence of the last exon of the gene for human cytochrome *c* oxidase subunit VIb and its flanking regions. *Biochim Biophys Acta* **1089:**283, 1991.
127. Darras BT, Zeviani M, Schone EA, Francke U: Sequences homologous to cytochrome c oxidase subunit IV are located on human chromosome 14q21-qter and 16q22-q24 [Abstract]. *Cytogenet Cell Genet* **46:**603, 1987.
128. Lomax MI, Welch MD, Darras BT, Francke U, Grossman LI: Novel use of a chimpanzee pseudogene for chromosomal mapping of human cytochrome *c* oxidase subunit IV. *Gene* **86:**209, 1990.
129. Hofmann S, Lichtner P, Schuffenhauer S, Gerbitz KD, Meitinger T: Assignment of the human genes coding for cytochrome c oxidase subunits Va (COX5A), VIc (COX6C) and VIIc (COX7C) to chromosome bands 15q25, 8q22 → q23 and 5q14 and of three pseudogenes (COX5AP1, COX6CP1, COX7CP1) to 14q22, 16p12 and 13q14 → q21 by FISH and radiation hybrid mapping. *Cytogenet Cell Genet* **83:**226, 1998.
130. Bachman NJ, Riggs PK, Siddiqui N, Makris GJ, Womack JE, Lomax MI: Structure of the human gene (COX6A2) for the heart/muscle isoform of cytochrome c oxidase subunit VIa and its chromosomal location in humans, mice, and cattle. *Genomics* **42:**146, 1997.
131. Taanman JW, van der Veen AY, Schrage C, de Vries H, Buys CH: Assignment of the gene coding for human cytochrome *c* oxidase subunit VIb to chromosome 19, band q13.1, by fluorescence *in situ* hybridisation. *Hum Genet* **87:**325, 1991.

132. Napiwotzki J, Shinzawa-Itoh K, Yoshikawa S, Kadenbach B: ATP and ADP bind to cytochrome c oxidase and regulate its activity. *Biol Chem* **378:**1013, 1997.
133. Anthony G, Reimann A, Kadenbach B: Tissue-specific regulation of bovine heart cytochrome-c oxidase activity by ADP via interaction with subunit VIa. *Proc Natl Acad Sci U S A* **90:**1652, 1993.
134. Taanman JW, Turina P, Capaldi RA: Regulation of cytochrome c oxidase by interaction of ATP at two binding sites, one on subunit VIa. *Biochemistry* **33:**11833, 1994.
135. Napiwotzki J, Kadenbach B: Extramitochondrial ATP/ADP-ratios regulate cytochrome c oxidase activity via binding to the cytosolic domain of subunit IV. *Biol Chem* **379:**335, 1998.
136. Arnold S, Kadenbach B: Cell respiration is controlled by ATP, an allosteric inhibitor of cytochrome-c oxidase. *Eur J Biochem* **249:**350, 1997.
137. Arnold S, Kadenbach B: The intramitochondrial ATP/ADP-ratio controls cytochrome c oxidase activity allosterically. *FEBS Lett* **443:**105, 1999.
138. Palmer G: Current issues in the chemistry of cytochrome c oxidase. *J Bioenerg Biomembr* **25:**145, 1993.
139. Tiranti V, Hoertnagel K, Carrozzo R, Galimberti C, Munaro M, Granatiero M, Zelante L, et al.: Mutations of SURF-1 in Leigh Disease associated with cytochrome c oxidase deficiency. *Am J Hum Genet* **63:**1609, 1998.
140. Zhu Z, Yao J, Johns T, Fu K, De Bie I, Macmillan C, Cuthbert AP, et al.: SURF1, encoding a factor involved in the biogenesis of cytochrome c oxidase, is mutated in Leigh syndrome. *Nat Genet* **20:**337, 1998.
141. Abrahams JP, Leslie AG, Lutter R, Walker JE: Structure at 2.8 Å resolution of F_1-ATPase from bovine heart mitochondria [see Comments]. *Nature* **370:**621, 1994.
142. Wang H, Oster G: Energy transduction in the F_1 motor of ATP synthase. *Nature* **396:**279, 1998.
143. Ogilvie I, Wilkens S, Rodgers AJ, Aggeler R, Capaldi RA: The second stalk: The delta-b subunit connection in ECF_1 F_0. *Acta Physiol Scand Suppl* **643:**169, 1998.
144. Elston T, Wang H, Oster G: Energy transduction in ATP synthase. *Nature* **391:**510, 1998.
145. Fillingame RH, Girvin ME, Jiang W, Valiyaveetil F, Hermolin J: Subunit interactions coupling H^+ transport and ATP synthesis in F_1F_0 ATP synthase. *Acta Physiol Scand Suppl* **643:**163, 1998.
146. Hartzog PE, Cain BD: Second-site suppressor mutations at glycine 218 and histidine 245 in the alpha subunit of F_1F_0 ATP synthase in *Escherichia coli*. *J Biol Chem* **269:**32313, 1994.
147. Boyer PD: The binding change mechanism for ATP synthase—Some probabilities and possibilities. *Biochim Biophys Acta* **1140:**215, 1993.
148. Bullough DA, Ceccarelli EA, Roise D, Allison WS: Inhibition of the bovine-heart mitochondrial F_1-ATPase by cationic dyes and amphipathic peptides. *Biochim Biophys Acta* **975:**377, 1989.
149. Zhuo S, Paik SR, Register JA, Allison WS: Photoinactivation of the bovine heart mitochondrial F_1-ATPase by [^{14}C]dequalinium cross-links phenylalanine-403 or phenylalanine-406 of an alpha subunit to a site or sites contained within residues 440–459 of a beta subunit. *Biochemistry* **32:**2219, 1993.
150. Breen GA: Bovine liver cDNA clones encoding a precursor of the alpha-subunit of the mitochondrial ATP synthase complex. *Biochem Biophys Res Commun* **152:**264, 1988.
151. Kataoka H, Biswas C: Nucleotide sequence of a cDNA for the alpha subunit of human mitochondrial ATP synthase. *Biochim Biophys Acta* **1089:**393, 1991.
152. Walker JE, Powell SJ, Vinas O, Runswick MJ: ATP synthase from bovine mitochondria: Complementary DNA sequence of the import precursor of a heart isoform of the alpha subunit. *Biochemistry* **28:**4702, 1989.
153. Ohta S, Kagawa Y: Human F1-ATPase: Molecular cloning of cDNA for the beta subunit. *J Biochem (Tokyo)* **99:**135, 1986.
154. Wallace DC, Ye JH, Neckelmann SN, Singh G, Webster KA, Greenberg BD: Sequence analysis of cDNAs for the human and bovine ATP synthase b-subunit: Mitochondrial DNA genes sustain seventeen times more mutations. *Curr Genet* **12:**81, 1987.
155. Jordan EM, Breen GAM: Molecular cloning of an import precursor of the delta-subunit of the human mitochondrial ATP synthase complex. *Biochim Biophys Acta* **1130:**123, 1992.
156. Higuti T, Tsurumi C, Osaka F, Kawamura Y, Tsujita H, Yoshihara Y, Tani I, et al.: Molecular cloning of cDNA for the import precursor of human subunit B of H(+)-ATP synthase in mitochondria. *Biochem Biophys Res Commun* **178:**1014, 1991.
157. Javed AA, Ogata K, Sanadi DR: Human mitochondrial ATP synthase: cloning cDNA for the nuclear-encoded precursor of coupling factor 6. *Gene* **97:**307, 1991.
158. Dyer MR, Walker JE: Sequences of members of the human gene family for the c subunit of mitochondrial ATP synthase. *Biochem J* **293:**51, 1993.
159. Farrell LB, Nagley P: Human liver cDNA clones encoding proteolipid subunit 9 of the mitochondrial ATPase complex. *Biochem Biophys Res Commun* **144:**1257, 1987.
160. Gay NJ, Walker JE: Two genes encoding the bovine mitochondrial ATP synthase proteolipid specify precursors with different import sequences and are expressed in a tissue-specific manner. *EMBO J* **4:**3519, 1985.
161. Higuti T, Kawamura Y, Kuroiwa K, Miyazaki S, Tsujita H: Molecular cloning and sequence of two cDNAs for human subunit c of H^+-ATP synthase in mitochondria. *Biochim Biophys Acta* **1173:**87, 1993.
162. Yan WL, Lerner TJ, Haines JL, Gusella JF: Sequence analysis and mapping of a novel human mitochondrial ATP synthase subunit 9 cDNA (ATP5G3). *Genomics* **24:**375, 1994.
163. Akiyama S, Endo H, Inohara N, Ohta S, Kagawa Y: Gene structure and cell type-specific expression of the human ATP synthase alpha subunit. *Biochim Biophys Acta* **1219:**129, 1994.
164. Jabs EW, Thomas PJ, Bernstein M, Coss C, Ferreira GC, Pedersen PL: Chromosomal localization of genes required for the terminal steps of oxidative metabolism: Alpha and gamma subunits of ATP synthase and the phosphate carrier. *Hum Genet* **93:**600, 1994.
165. Haraguchi Y, Chung AB, Neill S, Wallace DC: OXBOX and REBOX, overlapping promoter elements of the mitochondrial F_0F_1-ATP synthase beta subunit gene. OXBOX/REBOX in the ATPsyn beta promoter. *J Biol Chem* **269:**9330, 1994.
166. Neckelmann N, Warner C, K., Chung A, Kudoh J, Minoshima S, Fukuyama R, Maekawa M, et al.: The human ATP synthase beta subunit gene: Sequence analysis, chromosome assignment, and differential expression. *Genomics* **5:**829, 1989.
167. Ohta S, Tomura H, Matsuda K, Kagawa Y: Gene structure of the human mitochondrial adenosine triphosphate synthase beta subunit. *J Biol Chem* **263:**11257, 1988.
168. Matsuda C, Endo H, Ohta S, Kagawa Y: Gene structure of human mitochondrial ATP synthase gamma-subunit. Tissue specificity produced by alternative RNA splicing. *J Biol Chem* **268:**24950, 1993.
169. Endo H, Matsuda C, Kagawa Y: Exclusion of an alternatively spliced exon in human ATP synthase gamma-subunit pre-mRNA requires *de novo* protein synthesis. *J Biol Chem* **269:**12488, 1994.
170. Neckelmann N, Li K, Wade RP, Shuster R, Wallace DC: cDNA sequence of a human skeletal muscle ADP/ATP translocator: Lack of a leader peptide, divergence from a fibroblast translocator cDNA, and coevolution with mitochondrial DNA genes. *Proc Natl Acad Sci U S A* **84:**7580, 1987.
171. Houldsworth J, Attardi G: Two distinct genes for ADP/ATP translocase are expressed at the mRNA level in adult human liver. *Proc Natl Acad Sci U S A* **85:**377, 1988.
172. Giraud S, Bonod-Bidaud C, Wesolowski-Louvel M, Stepien G: Expression of human ANT2 gene in highly proliferative cells: GRBOX, a new transcriptional element, is involved in the regulation of glycolytic ATP import into mitochondria. *J Mol Biol* **281:**409, 1998.
173. Battini R, Ferrari S, Kaczmarek L, Calabretta B, Chen ST, Baserga R: Molecular cloning of a cDNA for a human ADP/ATP carrier which is growth-regulated. *J Biol Chem* **262:**4355, 1987.
174. Stepien G, Torroni A, Chung AB, Hodge JA, Wallace DC: Differential expression of adenine nucleotide translocator isoforms in mammalian tissues and during muscle cell differentiation. *J Biol Chem* **267:**14592, 1992.
175. Cozens AL, Runswick MJ, Walker JE: DNA sequences of two expressed nuclear genes for human mitochondrial ADP/ATP translocase. *J Mol Biol* **206:**261, 1989.
176. Li K, Warner CK, Hodge JA, Minoshima S, Kudoh J, Fukuyama R, Maekawa M, et al.: A human muscle adenine nucleotide translocator gene has four exons, is located on chromosome 4, and is differentially expressed. *J Biol Chem* **264:**13998, 1989.
177. Chung AB, Stepien G, Haraguchi Y, Li K, Wallace DC: Transcriptional control of nuclear genes for the mitochondrial muscle ADP/ATP translocator and the ATP synthase beta subunit. Multiple factors interact with the OXBOX/REBOX promoter sequences. *J Biol Chem* **267:**21154, 1992.
178. Li K, Hodge JA, Wallace DC: OXBOX, a positive transcriptional element of the heart-skeletal muscle ADP/ATP translocator gene. *J Biol Chem* **265:**20585, 1990.

179. Wijmenga C, Winokur ST, Padberg GW, Skraastad MI, Altherr MR, Wasmuth JJ, Murray JC, et al.: The human skeletal muscle adenine nucleotide translocator gene maps to chromosome 4q35 in the region of the facioscapulohumeral muscular dystrophy locus. *Hum Genet* **92:**198, 1993.
180. Wijmenga C, Hewitt JE, Sandkuijl LA, Clark LN, Wright TJ, Dauwerse HG, Gruter AM, et al.: Chromosome 4q DNA rearrangements associated with facioscapulohumeral muscular dystrophy. *Nat Genet* **2:**26, 1992.
181. Haraguchi Y, Chung AB, Torroni A, Stepien G, Shoffner JM, Wasmuth JJ, Costigan DA, et al.: Genetic mapping of human heart-skeletal muscle adenine nucleotide translocator and its relationship to the facioscapulohumeral muscular dystrophy locus. *Genomics* **16:**479, 1993.
182. Torroni A, Stepien G, Hodge JA, Wallace DC: Neoplastic transformation is associated with coordinate induction of nuclear and cytoplasmic oxidative phosphorylation genes. *J Biol Chem* **265:**20589, 1990.
183. Heddi A, Lestienne P, Wallace DC, Stepien G: Steady state levels of mitochondrial and nuclear oxidative phosphorylation transcripts in Kearns-Sayre syndrome. *Biochim Biophys Acta* **1226:**206, 1994.
184. Heddi A, Lestienne P, Wallace DC, Stepien G: Mitochondrial DNA expression in mitochondrial myopathies and coordinated expression of nuclear genes involved in ATP production. *J Biol Chem* **268:**12156, 1993.
185. Chen ST, Chang CD, Huebner K, Ku DH, McFarland M, DeRiel JK, Baserga R, et al.: A human ADP/ATP translocase gene has seven pseudogenes and localizes to chromosome X. *Somat Cell Mol Genet* **16:**143, 1990.
186. Ku DH, Kagan J, Chen ST, Chang CD, Baserga R, Wurzel J: The human fibroblast adenine nucleotide translocator gene. Molecular cloning and sequence. *J Biol Chem* **265:**16060, 1990.
187. Schiebel K, Mertz A, Winkelmann M, Nagaraja R, Rappold G: Localization of the adenine nucleotide translocase gene ANT2 to chromosome Xq24-q25 with tight linkage to DXS425. *Genomics* **24:**605, 1994.
188. Schiebel K, Weiss B, Wohrle D, Rappold G: A human pseudoautosomal gene, ADP/ATP translocase, escapes X-inactivation whereas a homologue on Xq is subject to X-inactivation. *Nat Genet* **3:**82, 1993.
189. Slim R, Levilliers J, Ludecke HJ, Claussen U, Nguyen VC, Gough NM, Horsthemke B, et al.: A human pseudoautosomal gene encodes the ANT3 ADP/ATP translocase and escapes X-inactivation. *Genomics* **16:**26, 1993.
190. Graham B, Waymire K, Cottrell B, Trounce IA, MacGregor GR, Wallace DC: A mouse model for mitochondrial myopathy and cardiomyopathy resulting from a deficiency in the heart/skeletal muscle isoform of the adenine nucleotide translocator. *Nat Genet* **16:**226, 1997.
191. Mills KA, Ellison JW, Mathews KD: The Ant1 gene maps near Klk3 on proximal mouse chromosome 8. *Mamm Genome* **7:**707, 1996.
192. Ellison JW, Li X, Francke U, Shapiro LJ: Rapid evolution of human pseudoautosomal genes and their mouse homologs. *Mamm Genome* **7:**25, 1996.
193. Cassard AM, Bouillaud F, Mattei MG, Hentz E, Raimbault S, Thomas M, Ricquier D: Human uncoupling protein gene: Structure, comparison with rat gene, and assignment to the long arm of chromosome 4. *J Cell Biochem* **43:**255, 1990.
194. Kozak LP, Britton JH, Kozak UC, Wells JM: The mitochondrial uncoupling protein gene. Correlation of exon structure to transmembrane domains. *J Biol Chem* **263:**12274, 1988.
195. Jacobsson A, Stadler U, Glotzer MA, Kozak LP: Mitochondrial uncoupling protein from mouse brown fat. Molecular cloning, genetic mapping, and mRNA expression. *J Biol Chem* **260:**16250, 1985.
196. Fleury C, Neverova M, Collins S, Raimbault S, Champigny O, Levi-Meyrueis C, Bouillaud F, et al.: Uncoupling protein-2: A novel gene linked to obesity and hyperinsulinemia [see Comments]. *Nat Genet* **15:**269, 1997.
197. Gong DW, He Y, Karas M, Reitman M: Uncoupling protein-3 is a mediator of thermogenesis regulated by thyroid hormone, beta3-adrenergic agonists, and leptin. *J Biol Chem* **272:**24129, 1997.
198. Solanes G, Vidal-Puig A, Grujic D, Flier JS, Lowell BB: The human uncoupling protein-3 gene. Genomic structure, chromosomal localization, and genetic basis for short and long form transcripts. *J Biol Chem* **272:**25433, 1997.
199. Vidal-Puig A, Solanes G, Grujic D, Flier JS, Lowell BB: UCP3: an uncoupling protein homologue expressed preferentially and abundantly in skeletal muscle and brown adipose tissue. *Biochem Biophys Res Commun* **235:**79, 1997.
200. Boss O, Samec S, Paoloni-Giacobino A, Rossier C, Dulloo A, Seydoux J, Muzzin P, et al.: Uncoupling protein-3: A new member of the mitochondrial carrier family with tissue-specific expression. *FEBS Lett* **408:**39, 1997.
201. Schatz G: The protein import system of mitochondria. *J Biol Chem* **271:**31763, 1996.
202. Schatz G, Dobberstein B: Common principles of protein translocation across membranes. *Science* **271:**1519, 1996.
203. Neupert W: Protein import into mitochondria. *Annu Rev Biochem* **66:**863, 1997.
204. Dekker PJ, Ryan MT, Brix J, Muller H, Honlinger A, Pfanner N: Preprotein translocase of the outer mitochondrial membrane: molecular dissection and assembly of the general import pore complex. *Mol Cell Biol* **18:**6515, 1998.
205. Hill K, Model K, Ryan MT, Dietmeier K, Martin F, Wagner R, Pfanner N: Tom40 forms the hydrophilic channel of the mitochondrial import pore for preproteins [Comment]. *Nature* **395:**516, 1998.
206. Glick B, Schatz G: Import of proteins into mitochondria. *Annu Rev Genet* **25:**21, 1991.
207. Glick BS, Beasley EM, Schatz G: Protein sorting in mitochondria. *Trends Biochem Sci* **17:**453, 1992.
208. Pfanner N, Neupert W: The mitochondrial protein import apparatus. *Annu Rev Biochem* **59:**331, 1990.
209. Pfanner N, Sollner T, Neupert W: Mitochondrial import receptors for precursor proteins. *Trends Biochem Sci* **16:**63, 1991.
210. Roise D: Import of proteins into mitochondria. *Prog Clin Biol Res* **282:**43, 1988.
211. Koehler CM, Jarosch E, Tokatlidis K, Schmid K, Schweyen RJ, Schatz G: Import of mitochondrial carriers mediated by essential proteins of the intermembrane space. *Science* **279:**369, 1998.
212. Koehler CM, Leuenberger D, Merchant S, Renold A, Junne T, Schatz G: Human deafness dystonia sydrome is a mitochondrial disease. *Proc Natl Acad Sci U S A* **96:**2141, 1999.
213. Sirrenberg C, Endres M, Folsch H, Stuart RA, Neupert W, Brunner M: Carrier protein import into mitochondria mediated by the intermembrane proteins Tim10/Mrs11 and Tim12/Mrs5. *Nature* **391:**912, 1998.
214. Wallace DC, Murdock DG: Mitochondria and dystonia: the movement disorder connection? *Proc Natl Acad Sci U S A* **96:**1817, 1999.
215. Kroemer G, Zamzami N, Susin SA: Mitochondrial control of apoptosis. *Immunol Today* **18:**44, 1997.
216. Gross A, Jockel J, Wei MC, Korsmeyer SJ: Enforced dimerization of BAX results in its translocation, mitochondrial dysfunction and apoptosis. *EMBO J* **17:**3878, 1998.
217. Antonsson B, Conti F, Ciavatta A, Montessuit S, Lewis S, Martinou I, Bernasconi L, et al.: Inhibition of Bax channel-forming activity by Bcl-2. *Science* **277:**370, 1997.
218. Schlesinger PH, Gross A, Yin XM, Yamamoto K, Saito M, Waksman G, Korsmeyer SJ: Comparison of the ion channel characteristics of proapoptotic BAX and antiapoptotic BCL-2. *Proc Natl Acad Sci U S A* **94:**11357, 1997.
219. Wallace DC: Structure and evolution of organelle genomes. *Microbiol Rev* **46:**208, 1982.
220. Chang DD, Clayton DA: A mammalian mitochondrial RNA processing activity contains nucleus-encoded RNA. *Science* **235:**1178, 1987.
221. Chang DD, Clayton DA: A novel endoribonuclease cleaves at a priming site of mouse mitochondrial DNA replication. *EMBO J* **6:**409, 1987.
222. Chang DD, Clayton DA: Mouse RNAase MRP RNA is encoded by a nuclear gene and contains a decamer sequence complementary to a conserved region of mitochondrial RNA substrate. *Cell* **56:**131, 1989.
223. Clayton DA: A nuclear function for RNase MRP. *Proc Natl Acad Sci U S A* **91:**4615, 1994.
224. Madsen CS, Ghivizzani SC, Hauswirth WW: Protein binding to a single termination-associated sequence in the mitochondrial DNA D-loop region. *Mol Cell Biol* **13:**2162, 1993.
225. Doda JN, Wright CT, Clayton DA: Elongation of displacement-loop strands in human mouse mitochondrial DNA is arrested near specific template sequences. *Proc Natl Acad Sci U S A* **78:**6116, 1981.
226. Clayton DA: Replication of animal mitochondrial DNA. *Cell* **28:**693, 1982.
227. Dairaghi DJ, Shadel GS, Clayton DA: Addition of a 29-residue carboxyl-terminal tail converts a simple HMG box-containing protein into a transcriptional activator. *J Mol Biol* **249:**11, 1995.
228. Parisi MA, Clayton DA: Similarity of human mitochondrial transcription factor 1 to high mobility group proteins. *Science* **252:**965, 1991.

229. Milatovich A, Parisi MA, Poulton J, Clayton DA, Francke U: Sequences homologous to MTTF1, mitochondrial transcription factor 1, are located on human chromosomes 7 (7pter-cen), 10, and 11 (11cen-qter). *Cytogenet Cell Genet* **58:**1929, 1991.
230. Ikeda S, Sumiyoshi H, Oda T: DNA binding properties of recombinant human mitochondrial transcription factor 1. *Cell Mol Biol* **40:**489, 1994.
231. Ghivizzani SC, Madsen CS, Hauswirth WW: *In organello* footprinting. Analysis of protein binding at regulatory regions in bovine mitochondrial DNA. *J Biol Chem* **268:**8675, 1993.
232. Ghivizzani SC, Madsen CS, Nelen MR, Ammini CV, Hauswirth WW: In organello footprint analysis of human mitochondrial DNA: Human mitochondrial transcription factor A interactions at the origin of replication. *Mol Cell Biol* **14:**7717, 1994.
233. Attardi G, Chomyn A, Montoya J, Ojala D: Identification and mapping of human mitochondrial genes. *Cytogenet Cell Genet* **32:**85, 1982.
234. Attardi G, Montoya J: Analysis of human mitochondrial RNA. *Methods Enzymol* **97:**435, 1983.
235. Clayton DA: Transcription of the mammalian mitochondrial genome. *Annu Rev Biochem* **53:**573, 1984.
236. Christianson TW, Clayton DA: A tridecamer DNA sequence supports human mitochondrial RNA 3′-end formation in vitro. *Mol Cell Biol* **8:**4502, 1988.
237. Christianson TW, Clayton DA: In vitro transcription of human mitochondrial DNA: Accurate termination requires a region of DNA sequence that can function bidirectionally. *Proc Natl Acad Sci U S A* **83:**6277, 1986.
238. Hamilton MG, O'Brien TW: Ultracentrifugal characterization of the mitochondrial ribosome and subribosomal particles of bovine liver: Molecular size and composition. *Biochemistry* **13:**5400, 1974.
239. O'Brien TW, Denslow ND, Anders JC, Courtney BC: The translation system of mammalian mitochondria. *Biochim Biophys Acta* **1050:**174, 1990.
240. Matthews DE, Hessler RA, Denslow ND, Edwards JS, O'Brien TW: Protein composition of the bovine mitochondrial ribosome. *J Biol Chem* **257:**8788, 1982.
241. Liao HX, Spremulli LL: Effects of length and mRNA secondary structure on the interaction of bovine mitochondrial ribosomes with messenger RNA. *J Biol Chem* **265:**11761, 1990.
242. Shoffner JM, Wallace DC: Oxidative phosphorylation diseases, in Scriver CR, Beaudet AL, Sly WS, Valle D (eds): *The Metabolic and Molecular Basis of Inherited Disease*, 7th ed. New York, McGraw-Hill, 1995, p 1535.
243. Wallace DC: Cytoplasmic inheritance of chloramphenicol resistance in mammalian cells, in Shay JW (ed): *Techniques in Somatic Cell Genetics*, vol 12. New York, Plenum Press, 1982, p 159.
244. Scharfe C, Zaccaria P, Hoertnagel K, Jaksch M, Klopstock T, Lill R, Prokisch H, et al.: MITOP: database for mitochondria-related proteins, genes and diseases. *Nucleic Acids Res* **27:**153, 1999.
245. Murdock D, Boone BE, Esposito L, Wallace DC: Up-regulation of nuclear and mitochondrial genes in the skeletal muscle of mice lacking the heart/muscle isoform of the adenine nucleotide translocator. *J Biol Chem* **274:**14429, 1999.
246. Perier F, Radeke CM, Raab-Graham KF, Vandenberg CA: Expression of a putative ATPase suppresses the growth defect of a yeast potassium transport mutant: Identification of a mammalian member of the Clp/HSP104 family. *Gene* **152:**157, 1995.
247. Ozelius LJ, Hewett JW, Page CE, Bressman SB, Kramer PL, Shalish C, de Leon D, et al.: The early-onset torsion dystonia gene (DYT1) encodes an ATP-binding protein. *Nat Genet* **17:**40, 1997.
248. Bunn CL, Wallace DC, Eisenstadt JM: Cytoplasmic inheritance of chlormaphenicol resistance in mouse tissue culture cells. *Proc Natl Acad Sci U S A* **71:**1681, 1974.
249. Wallace DC, Bunn CL, Eisenstadt JM: Cytoplasmic transfer of chloramphenicol resistance in human tissue culture cells. *J Cell Biol* **67:**174, 1975.
250. Wallace DC: Assignment of the chloramphenicol resistance gene to mitochondrial deoxyribonucelic acid and analysis of its expression in cultured human cells. *Mol Cell Biol* **1:**697, 1981.
251. Blanc H, Adams CW, Wallace DC: Different nucleotide changes in the large rRNA gene of the mitochondrial DNA confer chloramphenicol resistance on two human cell lines. *Nucleic Acids Res* **9:**5785, 1981.
252. Blanc H, Wright CT, Bibb MJ, Wallace DC, Clayton DA: Mitochondrial DNA of chloramphenicol-resistant mouse cells contains a single nucleotide change in the region encoding the 3′ end of the large ribosomal RNA. *Proc Natl Acad Sci U S A* **78:**3789, 1981.
253. Levy S, Waymire K, Kim Y, MacGregor G, Wallace DC: Transfer of chloramphenicol-resistant mitochondrial DNA into the chimeric mouse. *Transgenic Res* **8:**137, 1999.
254. Wallace DC, Pollack Y, Bunn CL, Eisenstadt JM: Cytoplasmic inheritance in mammalian tissue culture cells. *In Vitro* **12:**758, 1976.
255. Ege T, Krondahl U, Ringertz NR: Introduction of nuclei and micronuclei into cells and enucleated cytoplasms by Sendai virus induced fusion. *Exp Cell Res* **88:**428, 1974.
256. Ziegler ML, Davidson RL: Elimination of mitochondrial elements and improved viability in hybrid cells. *Somat Cell Mol Genet* **7:**73, 1981.
257. Trounce I, Wallace DC: Production of transmitochondrial mouse cell lines by cybrid rescue of rhodamine-6G pre-treated L-cells. *Somat Cell Mol Genet* 22:81, 1996.
258. Desjardins P, Frost E, Morais R: Ethidium bromide-induced loss of mitochondrial DNA from primary chicken embryo fibroblasts. *Mol Cell Biol* **5:**1163, 1985.
259. King MP, Attardi G: Injection of mitochondria into human cells leads to a rapid replacement of the endogenous mitochondrial DNA. *Cell* **52:**811, 1988.
260. Chomyn A, Lai ST, Shakeley R, Bresolin N, Scarlato G, Attardi G: Platelet-mediated transformation of mtDNA-less human cells: Analysis of phenotypic variability among clones from normal individuals and complementation behavior of the $tRNA^{Lys}$ mutation causing myoclonic epilepsy and ragged red fibers. *Am J Hum Genet* **54:**966, 1994.
261. Trounce I, Neill S, Wallace DC: Cytoplasmic transfer of the mtDNA nt 8993 TG (ATP6) point mutation associated with Leigh syndrome into mtDNA-less cells demonstrates cosegregation with a decrease in state III respiration and ADP/O ratio. *Proc Natl Acad Sci U S A* **91:**8334, 1994.
262. Case JT, Wallace DC: Maternal inheritance of mitochondrial DNA polymorphisms in cultured human fibroblasts. *Somat Cell Mol Genet* **7:**103, 1981.
263. Giles RE, Blanc H, Cann HM, Wallace DC: Maternal inheritance of human mitochondrial DNA. *Proc Natl Acad Sci U S A* **77:**6715, 1980.
264. Michaels GS, Hauswirth WW, Laipis PJ: Mitochondrial DNA copy number in bovine oocytes and somatic cells. *Dev Biol* **94:**246, 1982.
265. Chen X, Prosser R, Simonetti S, Sadlock J, Jagiello G, Schon EA: Rearranged mitochondrial genomes are present in human oocytes. *Am J Hum Genet* **57:**239, 1995.
266. Gyllensten U, Wharton D, Josefsson A, Wilson AC: Paternal inheritance of mitochondrial DNA in mice. *Nature* **352:**255, 1991.
267. Kaneda H, Hayashi J, Takahama S, Taya C, Lindahl KF, Yonekawa H: Elimination of paternal mitochondrial DNA in intraspecific crosses during early mouse embryogenesis. *Proc Natl Acad Sci U S A* **92:**4542, 1995.
268. Hopkin K: Death to sperm mitochondria [News]. *Sci Am* **280:**21, 1999.
269. Wallace DC: Mitotic segregation of mitochondrial DNAs in human cell hybrids and expression of chloramphenicol resistance. *Somat Cell Mol Genet* **12:**41, 1986.
270. Hayashi J, Werbin H, Shay JW: Effects of normal human fibroblast mitochondrial DNA on segregation of HeLaTG Mitochondrial DNA and on tumorigenicity of HeLaTG cells. *Cancer Res* **46:**4001, 1986.
271. Miranda AF, Ishii S, DiMauro S, Shay JW: Cytochrome c oxidase deficiency in Leigh's syndrome: Genetic evidence for a nuclear DNA-encoded mutation. *Neurology* **39:**697, 1989.
272. White FA, Bunn CL: Segregation of mitochondrial DNA in human somatic cell hybrids. *Mol Gen Genet* **197:**453, 1984.
273. Goto Y, Nonaka I, Horai S: A mutation in the $tRNA^{Leu(UUR)}$ gene associated with the MELAS subgroup of mitochondrial encephalomyopathies [Comments]. *Nature* **348:**651, 1990.
274. Yoneda M, Chomyn A, Martinuzzi A, Hurko O, Attardi G: Marked replicative advantage of human mtDNA carrying a point mutation that causes the MELAS encephalomyopathy. *Proc Natl Acad Sci U S A* **89:**11164, 1992.
275. Dunbar DR, Moonie PA, Jacobs HT, Holt IJ: Different cellular backgrounds confer a marked advantage to either mutant or wild-type mitochondrial genomes. *Proc Natl Acad Sci U S A* **92:**6562, 1995.
276. Shoubridge EA: Segregation of mitochondrial DNAs carrying a pathogenic point mutation ($tRNA^{Leu3243}$) in cybrid cells. *Biochem Biophys Res Commun* **213:**189, 1995.
277. Matthews PM, Brown RM, Morten K, Marchington D, Poulton J, Brown G: Intracellular heteroplasmy for disease-associated point mutations in mtDNA: Implications for disease expression and evidence for mitotic segregation of heteroplasmic units of mtDNA. *Hum Genet* **96:**261, 1995.

278. Wallace DC: Maternal genes: mitochondrial diseases, in McKusick VA, Roderick TH, Mori J, Paul MW (eds): *Medical and Experimental Mammalian Genetics: A Perspective*, vol 23. New York, Alan R. Liss for the March of Dimes Foundation, 1987, p 137.
279. Shoffner JM, Lott MT, Lezza AM, Seibel P, Ballinger SW, Wallace DC: Myoclonic epilepsy and ragged-red fiber disease (MERRF) is associated with a mitochondrial DNA $tRNA^{Lys}$ mutation. *Cell* **61:**931, 1990.
280. Wallace DC, Lott MT, Shoffner JM, Ballinger S: Mitochondrial DNA mutations in epilepsy and neurological disease. *Epilepsia* **35:**S43, 1994.
281. Wallace DC, Zheng X, Lott MT, Shoffner JM, Hodge JA, Kelley RI, Epstein CM, et al.: Familial mitochondrial encephalomyopathy (MERRF): Genetic, pathophysiological, and biochemical characterization of a mitochondrial DNA disease. *Cell* **55:**601, 1988.
282. Wallace DC: Mitochondrial diseases: Genotype versus phenotype. *Trends Genet* **9:**128, 1993.
283. Attardi G, Yoneda M, Chomyn A: Complementation and segregation behavior of disease-causing mitochondrial DNA mutations in cellular model systems. *Biochim Biophys Acta* **1271:**241, 1995.
284. Davidson M, King MP, Koga Y, Zhang L, Schon EA: Physical communication between mammalian mitochondria: a genetic approach [Abstract PS111. EUROMIT III]. Chantilly, France, Third International Meeting on Human Mitochondrial Pathology, 1995, p 23.
285. Merriwether DA, Clark AG, Ballinger SW, Schurr TG, Soodyall H, Jenkins T, Sherry ST, et al.: The structure of human mitochondrial DNA variation. *J Mol Evol* **33:**543, 1991.
286. Schurr TG, Ballinger SW, Gan YY, Hodge JA, Merriwether DA, Lawrence DN, Knowler WC, et al.: Amerindian mitochondrial DNAs have rare Asian mutations at high frequencies, suggesting they derived from four primary maternal lineages. *Am J Hum Genet* **46:**613, 1990.
287. Zuckerman SH, Solus JF, Gillespie FP, Eisenstadt JM: Retention of both parental mitochondrial DNA species in mouse-Chinese hamster somatic cell hybrids. *Somat Cell Mol Genet* **1984:**85, 1984.
288. Poulton J, Holt I: Mitochondrial DNA: Does more lead to less? *Nat Genet* **8:**313, 1994.
289. Brown WM, George M, Wilson AC: Rapid evolution of animal mitochondrial DNA. *Proc Natl Acad Sci U S A* **76:**1967, 1979.
290. Wallace DC: Mitochondrial DNA sequence variation in human evolution and disease. *Proc Natl Acad Sci U S A* **91:**8739, 1994.
291. Torroni A, Wallace DC: Mitochondrial DNA variation in human populations and implications for detection of mitochondrial DNA mutations of pathological significance. *J Bioenerg Biomembr* **26:**261, 1994.
292. Denaro M, Blanc H, Johnson MJ, Chen KH, Wilmsen E, Cavalli-Sforza LL, Wallace DC: Ethnic variation in *Hpa*I endonuclease cleavage patterns of human mitochondrial DNA. *Proc Natl Acad Sci U S A* **78:**5768, 1981.
293. Johnson MJ, Wallace DC, Ferris SD, Rattazzi MC, Cavalli-Sforza LL: Radiation of human mitochondria DNA types analyzed by restriction endonuclease cleavage patterns. *J Mol Evol* **19:**255, 1983.
294. Cann RL, Stoneking M, Wilson AC: Mitochondrial DNA and human evolution. *Nature* **325:**31, 1987.
295. Brown WM: Polymorphism in mitochondrial DNA of humans as revealed by restriction endonuclease analysis. *Proc Natl Acad Sci U S A* **77:**3605, 1980.
296. Horai S, Matsunaga E: Mitochondrial DNA polymorphism in Japanese. II. Analysis with restriction enzymes of four or five base pair recognition. *Hum Genet* **72:**105, 1986.
297. Stoneking M, Jorde LB, Bhatia K, Wilson AC: Geographic variation in human mitochondrial DNA from Papua New Guinea. *Genetics* **124:**717, 1990.
298. Vigilant L, Stoneking M, Harpending H, Hawkes K, Wilson AC: African populations and the evolution of human mitochondrial DNA. *Science* **253:**1503, 1991.
299. Templeton AR: Human origins and analysis of mitochondrial DNA sequences [Letter; Comment]. *Science* **255:**737, 1992.
300. Hedges SB, Kumar S, Tamura K: Human origins and analysis of mitochondrial DNA sequences [Letter; Comment]. *Science* **255:**737, 1991.
301. Horai S, Hayasaka K: Intraspecific nucleotide sequence differences in the major noncoding region of human mitochondrial DNA. *Am J Hum Genet* **46:**828, 1990.
302. Di Rienzo A, Wilson AC: Branching pattern in the evolutionary tree for human mitochondrial DNA. *Proc Natl Acad Sci U S A* **88:**1597, 1991.
303. Horai S, Hayasaka K, Kondo R, Tsugane K, Takahata N: Recent African origin of modern humans revealed by complete sequences of hominoid mitochondrial DNAs. *Proc Natl Acad Sci U S A* **92:**532, 1995.
304. Ballinger SW, Schurr TG, Torroni A, Gan YY, Hodge JA, Hassan K, Chen KH, et al.: Southeast Asian mitochondrial DNA analysis reveals genetic continuity of ancient mongoloid migrations [Erratum appears in *Genetics* **130**(4):957, 1992]. *Genetics* **130:**139, 1992.
305. Torroni A, Schurr TG, Yang C-C, Szathmary EJ, Williams RC, Schanfield MS, Troup GA, et al.: Native American mitochondrial DNA analysis indicates that the Amerind and the Nadene populations were founded by two independent migrations. *Genetics* **130:**153, 1992.
306. Torroni A, Schurr TG, Cabell MF, Brown MD, Neel JV, Larsen M, Smith DG, et al.: Asian affinities and continental radiation of the four founding Native American mtDNAs [Comments]. *Am J Hum Genet* **53:**563, 1993.
307. Torroni A, Sukernik RI, Schurr TG, Starikovskaya YB, Cabell MF, Crawford MH, Comuzzie AG, et al.: MtDNA variation of aboriginal Siberians reveals distinct genetic affinities with Native Americans. *Am J Hum Genet* **53:**591, 1993.
308. Tateno Y, Nei M, Tajima F: Accuracy of estimated phylogenetic trees from molecular data. I. Distantly related species. *J Mol Evol* **18:**387, 1982.
309. Nei M, Tajima F: Maximum likelihood estimation of the number of nucleotide substitutions from restriction sites data. *Genetics* **105:**207, 1983.
310. Saitou N, Nei M: The neighbor-joining method: A new method for reconstructing phylogenetic trees. *Mol Biol Evol* **4:**406, 1987.
311. Swofford DL: *Phylogenetic Analysis Using Parsimony (PAUP).* Champaign, IL, University of Illinois, 1993.
312. Chen YS, Torroni A, Excoffier L, Santachiara-Benerecetti AS, Wallace DC: Analysis of mtDNA variation in African populations reveals the most ancient of all human continent-specific haplogroups. *Am J Hum Genet* **57:**133, 1995.
313. Chen YS, Olckers A, Schurr TG, Kogelnik A, Huoponen K, Wallace DC: Mitochondrial DNA variation in the South African !Kung and Khwe and their genetic relationships to other African populations. *Am J Hum Genet* **66:**1362, 2000.
314. Cann RL, Wilson AC: Length mutations in human mitochondrial DNA. *Genetics* **104:**699, 1983.
315. Wrischnik LA, Higuchi RG, Stoneking M, Erlich HA, Arnheim N, Wilson AC: Length mutations in human mitochondrial DNA: Direct sequencing of enzymatically amplified DNA. *Nucleic Acids Res* **15:**529, 1987.
316. Watson E, Bauer K, Aman R, Weiss G, von Haeseler A, Paabo S: mtDNA sequence diversity in Africa [Comments]. *Am J Hum Genet* **59:**437, 1996.
317. Torroni A, Neel JV, Barrantes R, Schurr TG, Wallace DC: A mitochondrial DNA "clock" for the Amerinds and its implication for timing their entry into North America. *Proc Natl Acad Sci U S A* **91:**1158, 1994.
318. Torroni A, Lott MT, Cabell MF, Chen Y, Laverge L, Wallace DC: MtDNA and the origin of Caucasians. Identification of ancient Caucasian-specific haplogroups, one of which is prone to a recurrent somatic duplication in the D-loop region. *Am J Hum Genet* **55:**760, 1994.
319. Torroni A, Huoponen K, Francalacci P, Petrozzi M, Morelli L, Scozzari R, Obinu D, et al.: Classification of European mtDNAs from an analysis of three European populations. *Genetics* **144:**1835, 1996.
320. Brockington M, Sweeney MG, Hammans SR, Morgan-Hughes JA, Harding AE: A tandem duplication in the D-loop of human mitochondrial DNA is associated with deletions in mitochondrial myopathies. *Nat Genet* **4:**67, 1993.
321. Torroni A, Miller JA, Moore LG, Zamudio S, Zhuang J, Droma R, Wallace DC: Mitochondrial DNA analysis in Tibet. Implications for the origin of the Tibetan population and its adaptation to high altitude. *Am J Phys Anthropol* **93:**189, 1994.
322. Schurr TG, Sukernik RI, Starikovskaya YB, Wallace DC: Mitochondrial DNA variation in Koryaks and Itel'men: Population replacement in the Okhotsk Sea–Bering Sea region during the Neolithic. *Am J Phys Anthropol* **108:**1, 1999.
323. Starikovskaya EB, Sukernik RI, Schurr TG, Kogelnik AM, Wallace DC: Mitochondrial DNA diversity in Chukchi and Siberian Eskimos: Implications for genetic history of ancient Beringia and peopling of the New World. *Am J Hum Genet* **63:**1473, 1998.
324. Blanc H, Chen KH, D'Amore MA, Wallace DC: Amino acid change associated with the major polymorphic *Hinc*II site of Oriental and Caucasian mitochondrial DNAs. *Am J Hum Genet* **35:**167, 1983.

325. Turner CG II: Dental evidence for the peopling of the Americas, in Shutler R Jr (ed): *Early Man in the New World.* Beverly Hills, CA, Sage, 1983, p 147.
326. Turner CG, II: Late Pleistocene and Holocene population history of East Asia based on dental variation. *Am J Phys Anthropol* **73:**305, 1987.
327. Hertzberg M, Mickleson KNP, Serjeantson SW, Prior JF, Trent RJ: An Asian specific 9-bp deletion of mitochondrial DNA is frequently found in Polynesians. *Am J Hum Genet* **44:**504, 1989.
328. Forster P, Harding R, Torroni A, Bandelt HJ: Origin and evolution of Native American mtDNA variation: A reappraisal. *Am J Hum Genet* **59:**935, 1996.
329. Passarino G, Semino O, Bernini LF, Santachiara-Benerecetti AS: Pre-Caucasoid and Caucasoid genetic features of the Indian population, revealed by mtDNA polymorphisms. *Am J Hum Genet* **59:**927, 1996.
330. Passarino G, Semino O, Quintana-Murci L, Excoffier L, Hammer M, Santachiara-Benerecetti AS: Different genetic components in the Ethiopian population, identified by mtDNA and Y-chromosome polymorphisms. *Am J Hum Genet* **62:**420, 1998.
331. Greenberg JH, Turner CG, II, Zegura SL: The settlement of the Americas: A comparison of the linguistic, dental, and genetic evidence. *Curr Anthropol* **27:**477,1986.
332. Wallace DC, Garrison K, Knowler WC: Dramatic founder effects in Amerindian mitochondrial DNAs. *Am J Phys Anthropol* **68:**149, 1985.
333. Wallace DC, Torroni A: American Indian prehistory as written in the mitochondrial DNA: A review. *Hum Biol* **64:**403, 1992.
334. Torroni A, Chen Y, Semino O, Santachiara-Beneceretti AS, Scott CR, Lott MT, Winter M, et al.: MtDNA and Y-chromosome polymorphisms in four native American populations from southern Mexico. *Am J Hum Genet* **54:**303, 1994.
335. Ward RH, Redd A, Valencia D, Frazier B, Paabo S: Genetic and linguistic differentiation in the Americas. *Proc Natl Acad Sci U S A* **90:**10663, 1993.
336. Ward RH, Frazier BL, Dew-Jager K, Paabo S: Extensive mitochondrial diversity within a single Amerindian tribe. *Proc Natl Acad Sci U S A* **88:**8720, 1991.
337. Santos M, Barrantes R: D-loop mtDNA deletion as a unique marker of Chibchan Amerindians [Letter; Comment]. *Am J Hum Genet* **55:**413, 1994.
338. Horai S, Kondo R, Nakagawa-Hattori Y, Hayashi S, Sonoda S, Tajima K: Peopling of the Americas, founded by four major lineages of mitochondrial DNA. *Mol Biol Evol* **10:**23, 1993.
339. Stone AC, Stoneking M: Ancient DNA from a pre-Columbian Amerindian population. *Am J Phys Anthropol* **92:**463, 1993.
340. Bailliet G, Rothhammer F, Carnese FR, Bravi CM, Bianchi NO: Founder mitochondrial haplotypes in Amerindian populations. *Am J Hum Genet* **55:**27, 1994.
341. Torroni A, Wallace DC: MtDNA haplogroups in Native Americans [Comment, *Am J Hum Genet* 56:1236, 1995]. *Am J Hum Genet* **56:**1234, 1995.
342. Brown MD, Hosseini SH, Torroni A, Bandelt HJ, Allen JC, Schurr TG, Scozzari R, et al.: mtDNA Haplogroup X: An ancient link between Europe/Western Asia and North America? *Am J Hum Genet* **63:**1852, 1998.
343. Erickson RP: Leber's optic atrophy, a possible example of maternal inheritance. *Am J Hum Genet* **24:**348, 1972.
344. Newman NJ, Wallace DC: Mitochondria and Leber's hereditary optic neuropathy. *Am J Ophthalmol* **109:**726730, 1990.
345. Newman NJ: Leber's hereditary optic neuropathy. New genetic considerations. *Arch Neurol* **50:**540, 1993.
346. Riordan-Eva P, Sanders MD, Govan GG, Sweeney MG, Da Costa J, Harding AE: The clinical features of Leber's hereditary optic neuropathy defined by the presence of a pathogenic mitochondrial DNA mutation. *Brain* **118:**319, 1995.
347. Shoffner JM, Brown MD, Stugard C, Jun AS, Pollok S, Haas RH, Kaufman A, et al.: Leber's hereditary optic neuropathy plus dystonia is caused by a mitochondrial DNA point mutation in a complex I subunit. *Ann Neurol* **38:**163, 1995.
348. Huoponen K, Vilkki J, Aula P, Nikoskelainen EK, Savontaus ML: A new mtDNA mutation associated with Leber hereditary optic neuroretinopathy. *Am J Hum Genet* **48:**1147, 1991.
349. Howell N, Bindoff LA, McCullough DA, Kubacka I, Poulton J, Mackey D, Taylor L, et al.: Leber hereditary optic neuropathy: Identification of the same mitochondrial ND1 mutation in six pedigrees. *Am J Hum Genet* **49:**939, 1991.
350. Huoponen K, Lamminen T, Juvonen V, Aula P, Nikoskelainen E, Savontaus JL: The spectrum of mitochondrial DNA mutations in families with Leber hereditary optic neuroretinopathy. *Hum Genet* **92:**379, 1993.
351. Johns DR, Neufeld MJ, Park RD: An ND-6 mitochondrial DNA mutation associated with Leber hereditary optic neuropathy. *Biochem Biophys Res Commun* **187:**1551, 1992.
352. Mackey D, Howell N: A variant of Leber hereditary optic neuropathy characterized by recovery of vision and by an unusual mitochondrial genetic etiology. *Am J Hum Genet* **51:**1218, 1992.
353. Brown MD, Torroni A, Reckord CL, Wallace DC: Phylogenetic analysis of Leber's hereditary optic neuropathy mitochondrial DNAs indicates multiple independent occurrences of the common mutations. *Hum Mutat* **6:**311, 1995.
354. Brown MD, Wallace DC: Spectrum of mitochondrial DNA mutations in Leber's hereditary optic neuropathy. *Clin Neurosci* **2:**138, 1994.
355. Howell N: Leber hereditary optic neuropathy: How do mitochondrial DNA mutations cause degeneration of the optic nerve? *J Bioenerg Biomembr* **29:**165, 1997.
356. Howell N, Kubacka I, Halvorson S, Howell B, McCullough DA, Mackey D: Phylogenetic analysis of the mitochondrial genomes from Leber hereditary optic neuropathy pedigrees. *Genetics* **140:**285, 1995.
357. Mashima Y, Hiida Y, Oguchi Y, Kudoh J, Shimizu N: High frequency of mutations at position 11778 in mitochondrial ND4 gene in Japanese families with Leber's hereditary optic neuropathy. *Hum Genet* **92:**101, 1993.
358. Newman NJ, Lott MT, Wallace DC: The clinical characteristics of pedigrees of Leber's hereditary optic neuropathy with the 11778 mutation. *Am J Ophthalmol* **111:**750762, 1991.
359. Biousse V, Brown MD, Newman NJ, Allen JC, Rosenfeld J, Meola G, Wallace DC: De novo 14484 mitochondrial DNA mutation in monozygotic twins discordant for Leber's hereditary optic neuropathy. *Neurology* **49:**1136, 1997.
360. Brown MD, Sun F, Wallace DC: Clustering of Caucasian Leber hereditary optic neuropathy patients containing the 11778 or 14484 mutations on an mtDNA lineage. *Am J Hum Genet* **60:**381, 1997.
361. Torroni A, Carelli V, Petrozzi M, Terracina M, Barboni P, Malpassi P, Wallace DC, et al.: Detection of the mtDNA 14484 mutation on an African-specific haplotype: Implications about its role in causing Leber hereditary optic neuropathy. *Am J Hum Genet* **59:**248, 1996.
362. Howell N: Leber hereditary optic neuropathy: respiratory chain dysfunction and degeneration of the optic nerve. *Vision Res* **38:**1495, 1998.
363. Brown MD, Voljavec AS, Lott MT, Torroni A, Yang C-C, Wallace DC: Mitochondrial DNA complex I and III mutations associated with Leber's hereditary optic neuropathy. *Genetics* **130:**163, 1992.
364. Howell N, Halvorson S, Burns J, McCullough DA, Poulton J: When does bilateral optic atrophy become Leber hereditary optic atrophy [Letter]? *Am J Hum Genet* **53:**959, 1993.
365. Johns DR, Neufeld MJ: Cytochrome c oxidase mutations in Leber hereditary optic neuropathy. *Biochem Biophys Res Commun* **196:**810, 1993.
366. Lamminen T, Majander A, Juvonen V, Wikstrom M, Aula P, Nikoskelainen E, Savontous ML: A mitochondrial mutation at nt 9101 in the ATP synthase 6 gene associated with deficient oxidative phosphorylation in a family with Leber hereditary optic neuroretinopathy [Letter]. *Am J Hum Genet* **56:**1238, 1995.
367. De Vries DD, Went LN, Bruyn GW, Scholte HR, Hofstra RM, Bolhuis PA, van Oost BA: Genetic and biochemical impairment of mitochondrial complex I activity in a family with Leber hereditary optic neuropathy and hereditary spastic dystonia. *Am J Hum Genet* **58:**703, 1996.
368. Wissinger B, Besch D, Baumann B, Fauser S, Christ-Adler M, Jurklies B, Zrenner E, et al.: Mutation analysis of the ND6 gene in patients with Leber's hereditary optic neuropathy. *Biochem Biophys Res Commun* **234:**511, 1997.
369. Oostra RJ, Bolhuis PA, Wijburg FA, Zorn-Ende G, Bleeker-Wagemakers EM: Leber's hereditary optic neuropathy: Correlations between mitochondrial genotype and visual outcome. *J Med Genet***31:**280, 1994.
370. Obermaier-Kusser B, Lorenz B, Schubring S, Paprotta A, Zerres K, Meitinger T, Meire F, et al.: Features of mtDNA mutation patterns in European pedigrees and sporadic cases with Leber hereditary optic neuropathy. *Am J Hum Genet* **55:**1063, 1994.
371. Johns DR, Heher KL, Miller NR, Smith KH: Leber's hereditary optic neuropathy. Clinical manifestations of the 14484 mutation. *Arch Ophthalmol* **111:**495, 1993.
372. Johns DR, Neufeld MJ: Cytochrome b mutations in Leber hereditary optic neuropathy. *Biochem Biophys Res Commun* **181:**1358, 1991.

373. Brown MD, Voljavec AS, Lott MT, MacDonald I, Wallace DC: Leber's hereditary optic neuropathy: a model for mitochondrial neurodegenerative diseases. *FASEB J* **6:**2791, 1992.
374. Brown MD, Yang C-C, Trounce I, Torroni A, Lott MT, Wallace DC: A mitochondrial DNA variant, identified in Leber hereditary optic neuropathy patients, which extends the amino acid sequence of cytochrome c oxidase subunit I. *Am J Hum Genet* **51:**378, 1992.
375. Brown MD, Torroni A, Huoponen K, Chen YS, Lott MT, Wallace DC: Pathological significance of the mtDNA COX III mutation at nucleotide pair 9438 in Leber hereditary optic neuropathy [Letter]. *Am J Hum Genet* **55:**410, 1994.
376. Oostra RJ, Van den Bogert C, Nijtmans LG, van Galen MJ, Zwart R, Bolhuis PA, Bleeker-Wagemakers EM: Simultaneous occurrence of the 11778 (ND4) and the 9438 (COX III) mtDNA mutations in Leber hereditary optic neuropathy: molecular, biochemical, and clinical findings [Letter]. *Am J Hum Genet* **57:**954, 1995.
377. Howell N, Kubacka I, Xu M, McCullough DA: Leber hereditary optic neuropathy: Involvement of the mitochondrial ND1 gene and evidence for an intragenic suppressor mutation. *Am J Hum Genet* **48:**935, 1991.
378. Novotny EJ, Singh G, Wallace DC, Dorfman LJ, Louis A, Sogg RL, Steinman L: Leber's disease and dystonia: A mitochondrial disease. *Neurology* **36:**1053, 1986.
379. Ortiz RG, Newman NJ, Manoukian SV, Diesenhouse MC, Lott MT, Wallace DC: Optic disk cupping and electrocardiographic abnormalities in an American pedigree with Leber's hereditary optic neuropathy. *Am J Ophthalmol* **113:**561, 1992.
380. Larsson NG, Andersen O, Holme E, Oldfors A, Wahlstrom J: Leber's hereditary optic neuropathy and complex I deficiency in muscle. *Ann Neurol* **30:**701, 1991.
381. Vergani L, Martinuzzi A, Carelli V, Cortelli P, Montagna P, Schievano G, Carrozzo R, et al.: MtDNA mutations associated with Leber's hereditary optic neuropathy: Studies on cytoplasmic hybrid (cybrid) cells. *Biochem Biophys Res Commun* **210:**880, 1995.
382. Funakawa I, Kato H, Terao A, Ichihashi K, Kawashima S, Hayashi T, Mitani K, et al.: Cerebellar ataxia in patients with Leber's hereditary optic neuropathy. *J Neurol* **242:**75, 1995.
383. Kellar-Wood H, Robertson N, Govan GG, Compston DA, Harding AE: Leber's hereditary optic neuropathy mitochondrial DNA mutations in multiple sclerosis. *Ann Neurol* **36:**109, 1994.
384. Harding AE, Sweeney MG, Miller DH, Mumford CJ, Kellar-Wood H, Menard D, McDonald WI, et al.: Occurrence of a multiple sclerosis-like illness in women who have a Leber's heditary optic neuropathy mitochondrial DNA mutation. *Brain* **115:**979, 1992.
385. Olsen NK, Hansen AW, Norby S, Edal AL, Jorgensen JR, Rosenberg T: Leber's hereditary optic neuropathy associated with a disorder indistinguishable from multiple sclerosis in a male harbouring the mitochondrial DNA 11778 mutation. *Acta Neurol Scand* **91:**326, 1995.
386. Flanigan KM, Johns DR: Association of the 11778 mitochondrial DNA mutation and demyelinating disease. *Neurology* **43:**2720, 1993.
387. Hanefeld FA, Ernst BP, Wilichowski E, Christen HJ: Leber's hereditary optic neuropathy mitochondrial DNA mutations in childhood multiple sclerosis. *Neuropediatrics* **25:**331, 1994.
388. Nikoskelainen EK, Marttila RJ, Huoponen K, Juvonen V, Lamminen T, Sonninen P, Savontaus ML: Leber's "plus": Neurological abnormalities in patients with Leber's hereditary optic neuropathy. *J Neurol Neurosurg Psychiatry* **59:**160, 1995.
389. Nishimura M, Obayashi H, Ohta M, Uchiyama T, Hao Q, Saida T: No association of the 11778 mitochondrial DNA mutation and multiple sclerosis in Japan. *Neurology* **45:**1333, 1995.
390. Chalmers RM, Robertson N, Kellar-Wood H, Compston DA, Harding AE: Sequence of the human homologue of a mitochondrially encoded murine transplantation antigen in patients with multiple sclerosis. *J Neurol* **242:**332, 1995.
391. Pilz D, Quarrell OW, Jones EW: Mitochondrial mutation commonly associated with Leber's hereditary optic neuropathy observed in a patient with Wolfram syndrome (DIDMOAD). *J Med Genet* **31:**328, 1994.
392. Torroni A, Petrozzi M, D'Urbano L, Sellitto D, Zeviani M, Carrara F, Carducci C, et al.: Haplotype and phylogenetic analyses suggest that one European-specific mtDNA background plays a role in the expression of Leber hereditary optic neuropathy by increasing the penetrance of the primary mutations 11778 and 14484. *Am J Hum Genet* **60:**1107, 1997.
393. Brown MD, Wallace DC: Molecular basis of mitochondrial DNA disease. *J Bioenerg Biomembr* **26:**273, 1994.
394. Harding AE, Sweeney MG, Govan GG, Riordan-Eva P: Pedigree analysis in Leber hereditary optic neuropathy families with a pathogenic mtDNA mutation. *Am J Hum Genet* **57:**77, 1995.
395. Johns DR, Smith KH, Miller NR: Leber's Hereditary Optic Neuropathy. Clinical manifestations of the 3460 mutation. *Arch Ophthalmol* **110:**1577, 1992.
396. Torroni A, Semino O, Scozzari R, Sirugo G, Spedini G, Abbas N, Fellous M, et al.: Y chromosome DNA polymorphisms in human populaitons: Differences between Caucasoids and Africans detected by 49a and 49f probes. *Ann Hum Genet* **54:**287, 1990.
397. Wallace DC: A new manifestation of Leber's disease and a new explanation for the agency responsible for its unusual pattern of inheritance. *Brain* **93:**121, 1970.
398. Parker WD Jr, Oley CA, Parks JK: A defect in mitochondrial electron-transport activity (NADH-coenzyme Q oxidoreductase) in Leber's hereditary optic neuropathy. *N Engl J Med* **320:**1331, 1989.
399. Letellier T, Heinrich R, Malgat M, Mazat JP: The kinetic basis of threshold effects observed in mitochondrial diseases:a systemic approach. *Biochem J* **302:**171, 1994.
400. Malgat M, Letellier T, Jouaville SL, Mazat JP: Value of control theory in the study of cellular metabolism — Biomedical implications. *J Biol Sys* **3:**165, 1995, p.
401. Brown MD, Trounce I, Jun AS, Allen JC, Wallace DC: Functional analysis of lymphoblast and cybrid mitochondria containing the 3460, 11778, or 14484 Leber's hereditary optic neuropathy mtDNA mutations. Submitted for publication, 2000.
402. Carelli V, Ghelli A, Ratta M, Bacchilega E, Sangiorgi S, Mancini R, Leuzzi V, et al.: Leber's hereditary optic neuropathy: biochemical effect of 11778/ND4 and 3460/ND1 mutations and correlation with the mitochondrial genotype. *Neurology* **48:**1623, 1997.
403. Majander A, Huoponen K, Savontaus ML, Nikoskelainen E, Wikstrom M: Electron transfer properties of NADH:ubiquinone reductase in the ND1/3460 and the ND4/11778 mutations of the Leber hereditary optic neuroretinopathy (LHON). *FEBS Lett* **292:**289, 1991.
404. Degli Esposti M, Carelli V, Ghelli A, Ratta M, Crimi M, Sangiorgi S, Montagna P, et al.: Functional alterations of the mitochondrially encoded ND4 subunit associated with Leber's hereditary optic neuropathy. *FEBS Lett* **352:**375, 1994.
405. Smith PR, Cooper JM, Govan GG, Harding AE, Schapira AH: Platelet mitochondrial function in Leber's hereditary optic neuropathy. *J Neurol Sci* **122:**80, 1994.
406. Majander A, Finel M, Savontaus ML, Nikoskelainen E, Wikstrom M: Catalytic activity of complex I in cell lines that possess replacement mutations in the ND genes in Leber's hereditary optic neuropathy. *Eur J Biochem* **239:**201, 1996.
407. Hofhaus G, Johns DR, Hurko O, Attardi G, Chomyn A: Respiration and growth defects in transmitochondrial cell lines carrying the 11778 mutation associated with Leber's hereditary optic neuropathy. *J Biol Chem* **271:**13155, 1996.
408. Cock HR, Cooper JM, Shapira AHV: Functional consequences of the 3460-bp mitochondrial DNA mutation associated with Leber's hereditary optic neuropathy. *J Neurol Sci* **165:**10, 1999.
409. Cock HR, Tabrizi SJ, Cooper JM, Schapira AH: The influence of nuclear background on the biochemical expression of 3460 Leber's hereditary optic neuropathy. *Ann Neurol* **44:**187, 1998.
410. Cock HR, Cooper JM, Schapira AH: The 14484 ND6 mtDNA mutation in Leber hereditary optic neuropathy does not affect fibroblast complex I activity [Letter]. *Am J Hum Genet* **57:**1501, 1995.
411. Carelli V, Ghelli A, Bucchi L, Montagna P, De Negri A, Leuzzi V, Carducci C, et al.: Biochemical features of mtDNA 14484 (ND6/M64V) point mutation associated with Leber's hereditary optic neuropathy. *Ann Neurol* **45:**320, 1999.
412. Oostra RJ, Van Galen MJ, Bolhuis PA, Bleeker-Wagemakers EM, Van den Bogert C: The mitochondrial DNA mutation ND6/14484C associated with Leber hereditary optic neuropathy, leads to deficiency of complex I of the respiratory chain. *Biochem Biophys Res Commun* **215:**1001, 1995.
413. Kong J, Xu Z: Massive mitochondrial degeneration in motor neurons triggers the onset of amyotrophic lateral sclerosis in mice expressing a mutant SOD1. *J Neurosci* **18:**3241, 1998.
414. Bandy B, Davison AJ: Mitochondrial mutations may increase oxidative stress: Implications for carcinogenesis and aging? *Free Radic Biol Med* **8:**523, 1990.
415. Dahl HH: Getting to the nucleus of mitochondrial disorders: identification of respiratory chain-enzyme genes causing Leigh syndrome [Editorial; Comment]. *Am J Hum Genet* **63:**1594, 1998.
416. Kretzchmar HA, DeArmond SJ, Koch TK, Patel MS, Newth CJL, Schmidt KA, Packman S: Pyruvate dehydrogenase complex deficiency as a cause of subacute necrotizing encephalopathy (Leigh's disease). *Pediatrics* **79:**370, 1987.

417. Robinson BH, De Meirleir L, Glerum M, Sherwood G, Becker L: Clinical presentation of mitochondrial respiratory chain defects in NADH-coenzyme Q reductase and cytochrome oxidase: Clues to pathogenesis of Leigh disease. *J Pediatr* **110:**216, 1987.
418. Matthews PM, Marchington DR, Squier M, Land J, Brown RM, Brown GK: Molecular genetic characterization of an X-linked form of Leigh's syndrome. *Ann Neurol* **33:**652, 1993.
419. Loeffen J, Smeitink J, Triepels R, Smeets R, Schuelke M, Sengers R, Trijbels F, et al.: The first nuclear-encoded complex I mutation in a patient with Leigh Syndrome. *Am J Hum Genet* **63:**1598, 1998.
420. DiMauro S, Servidei S, Zeviani M, DiRocco M, DeVivo DC, DiDonato S, Uziel G, et al.: Cytochrome c oxidase deficiency in Leigh syndrome. *Ann Neurol* **22:**498, 1987.
421. Hommes FA, Polman HA, Reerink JD: Leigh's encephalomyelopathy: An inborn error of gluconeogenesis. *Arch Dis Child* **43:**423, 1968.
422. Holt IJ, Harding AE, Petty RK, Morgan-Hughes JA: A new mitochondrial disease associated with mitochondrial DNA heteroplasmy. *Am J Hum Genet* **46:**428, 1990.
423. Ortiz RG, Newman NJ, Shoffner JM, Kaufman AE, Koontz DA, Wallace DC: Variable retinal and neurologic manifestations in patients harboring the mitochondrial DNA 8993 mutation. *Arch Ophthalmol* **111:**1525, 1993.
424. Santorelli FM, Shanske S, Macaya A, DeVivo DC, DiMauro S: The mutation at nt 8993 of mitochondrial DNA is a common cause of Leigh's syndrome. *Ann Neurol* **34:**827, 1993.
425. Shoffner JM, Fernhoff MD, Krawiecki NS, Caplan DB, Holt PJ, Koontz DA, Takei Y, et al.: Subacute necrotizing encephalopathy: Oxidative phosphorylation defects and the ATPase 6 point mutation. *Neurology* **42:**2168, 1992.
426. Tatuch Y, Christodoulou J, Feigenbaum A, Clarke JTR, Wherret J, Smith C, Rudd N, et al.: Heteroplasmic mtDNA mutation (T-G) at 8993 can cause Leigh disease when the percentage of abnormal mtDNA is high. *Am J Hum Genet* **50:**852, 1992.
427. De Vries DD, Van Engelen BG, Gabreels FJ, Ruitenbeek W, Van Oost BA: A second missense mutation in the mitochondrial ATPase 6 gene in Leigh's syndrome. *Ann Neurol* **34:**410, 1993.
428. Santorelli FM, Shanske S, Jain KD, Tick D, Schon EA, DiMauro S: A T-C mutation at nt 8993 of mitochondrial DNA in a child with Leigh syndrome. *Neurology* **44:**972, 1994.
429. Thyagarajan D, Shanske S, Vazquez-Memije M, De Vivo D, DiMauro S: A novel mitochondrial ATPase 6 point mutation in familial bilateral striatal necrosis. *Ann Neurol* **38:**468, 1995.
430. Berkovic SF, Carpenter S, Evans A, Karpati G, Shoubridge EA, Andermann F, Meyer E, et al.: Myoclonus epilepsy and ragged-red fibres (MERRF). I. A clinical, pathological, biochemical, magnetic resonance spectrographic and positron emission tomographic study. *Brain* **112:**1231, 1989.
431. Berkovic SF, Shoubridge EA, Andermann F, Andermann E, Carpenter S, Karpati G: Clinical spectrum of mitochondrial DNA mutation at base pair 8344. *Lancet* **338:**457, 1991.
432. Houstek J, Klement P, Hermanska J, Houstkova H, Hansikova H, Van den Bogert C, Zeman J: Altered properties of mitochondrial ATP-synthase in patients with a T $\rightarrow$ G mutation in the ATPase 6 (subunit a) gene at position 8993 of mtDNA. *Biochim Biophys Acta* **1271:**349, 1995.
433. Makela-Bengs P, Suomalainen A, Majander A, Rapola J, Kalimo H, Nuutila A, Pihko H: Correlation between the clinical symptoms and the proportion of mitochondrial DNA carrying the 8993 point mutation in the NARP syndrome. *Pediatr Res* **37:**634, 1995.
434. Tulinius MH, Houshmand M, Larsson NG, Holme E, Oldfors A, Holmberg E, Wahlstrom J: De novo mutation in the mitochondrial ATP synthase subunit 6 gene (T8993G) with rapid segregation resulting in Leigh syndrome in the offspring. *Hum Genet* **96:**290, 1995.
435. Tatuch Y, Robinson BH: The mitochondrial DNA mutation at 8993 associated with NARP slows the rate of ATP synthesis in isolated lymphoblast mitochondria. *Biochem Biophys Res Commun* **192:**124, 1993.
436. Esposito LA, Melov S, Panov A, Cottrell BA, Wallace DC: Mitochondrial disease in mouse results in increased oxidative stress. *Proc Natl Acad Sci U S A* **96:**4820, 1999.
437. van den Heuvel L, Ruitenbeek W, Smeets R, Gelman-Kohan Z, Elpeleg O, Loeffen J, Trijbels F, et al.: Demonstration of a new pathogenic mutation in human complex I deficiency: A 5-bp duplication in the nuclear gene encoding the 18-kD (AQDQ) subunit. *Am J Hum Genet* **62:**262, 1998.
438. Casari G, De Fusco M, Ciarmatori S, Zeviani M, Mora M, Fernandez P, De Michele G, et al.: Spastic paraplegia and OXPHOS impairment caused by mutations in paraplegin, a nuclear-encoded mitochondrial metalloprotease. *Cell* **93:**973, 1998.
439. Jin H, May M, Tranebjaerg L, Kendall E, Fontan G, Jackson J, Subramony SH, et al.: A novel X-linked gene, DDP, shows mutations in families with deafness (DFN-1), dystonia, mental deficiency and blindness. *Nat Genet* **14:**177, 1996.
440. Rotig A, de Lonlay P, Chretien D, Foury F, Koenig M, Sidi D, Munnich A, et al.: Aconitase and mitochondrial iron-sulphur protein deficiency in Friedreich ataxia. *Nat Genet* **17:**215, 1997.
441. Wilson RB, Roof DM: Respiratory deficiency due to loss of mitochondrial DNA in yeast lacking the frataxin homologue. *Nat Genet* **16:**352, 1997.
442. Koutnikova H, Campuzano V, Foury F, Dolle P, Cazzalini O, Koenig M: Studies of human, mouse and yeast homologues indicate a mitochondrial function for frataxin. *Nat Genet* **16:**345, 1997.
443. Rowland LP: Molecular genetics, pseudogenetics, and clinical neurology. *Neurology* **33:**1179, 1983.
444. Poulton J, Morten KJ, Marchington D, Weber K, Brown GK, Rotig A, Bindoff L: Duplications of mitochondrial DNA in Kearns-Sayre syndrome. *Muscle Nerve* **3:**S154, 1995.
445. Ota Y, Miyake Y, Awaya S, Kumagai T, Tanaka M, Ozawa T: Early retinal involvement in mitochondrial myopathy with mitochondrial DNA deletion. *Retina* **14:**270, 1994.
446. Cormier-Daire V, Bonnefont JP, Rustin P, Maurage C, Ogler H, Schmitz J, Ricour C, et al.: Mitochondrial DNA rearrangements with onset as chronic diarrhea with villous atrophy. *J Pediatr* **124:**63, 1994.
447. Moraes CT, DiMauro S, Zeviani M, Lombes A, Shanske S, Miranda AF, Nakase H, et al.: Mitochondrial DNA deletions in progressive external ophthalmoplegia and Kearns-Sayre syndrome. *N Engl J Med* **320:**1293, 1989.
448. Poulton J, Deadman ME, Ramacharan S, Gardiner RM: Germ-line deletions of mtDNA in mitochondrial myopathy. *Am J Hum Genet* **48:**649, 1991.
449. Zeviani M, Servidei S, Gellera C, Bertini E, DiMauro S, DiDonato S: An autosomal dominant disorder with multiple deletions of mitochondrial DNA starting at the D-loop region. *Nature* **339:**309, 1989.
450. Goto Y: Clinical features of MELAS and mitochondrial DNA mutations. *Muscle Nerve* **3:**S107, 1995.
451. Johns DR, Hurko O: Mitochondrial leucine tRNA mutation in neurological diseases [Letter]. *Lancet* **337:**927, 1991.
452. Schon EA, Hirano M, DiMauro S: Mitochondrial encephalomyopathies: clinical and molecular analysis. *J Bioenerg Biomembr* **26:**291, 1994.
453. Seibel P, Lauber J, Klopstock T, Marsac C, Kadenbach B, Reichmann H: Chronic progressive external ophthalmoplegia is associated with a novel mutation in the mitochondrial $tRNA^{Asn}$ gene. *Biochem Biophys Res Commun* **204:**482, 1994.
454. Mita S, Schmidt B, Schon EA, DiMauro S, Bonilla E: Detection of "deleted" mitochondrial genomes in cytochrome-c oxidase-deficient muscle fibers of a patient with Kearns-Sayre syndrome. *Proc Natl Acad Sci U S A* **86:**9509, 1989.
455. Shoubridge EA, Karpati G, Hastings KEM: Deletion mutants are functionally dominant over wild-type mitochondrial genomes in skeletal muscle fiber segments in mitochondrial disease. *Cell* **62:**43, 1990.
456. Heddi A, Stepien G, Benke PJ, Wallace DC: Coordinate induction of energy gene expression in tissues of mitochondrial disease patients. *J Biol Chem* **274:**22968, 1999.
457. Wallace DC, Lott MT, Brown MD, Huoponen K, Torroni A: Report of the committee on human mitochondrial DNA, in Cuticchia AJ (ed): *Human Gene Mapping 1994, A Compendium*. Baltimore, MD, Johns Hopkins University Press, 1995, p 910.
458. Poulton J, Deadman ME, Bindoff L, Morten K, Land J, Brown G: Families of mtDNA re-arrangements can be detected in patients with mtDNA deletions: Duplications may be a transient intermediate form. *Hum Mol Genet* **2:**23, 1993.
459. Poulton J, Morten KJ, Weber K, Brown GK, Bindoff L: Are duplications of mitochondrial DNA characteristic of Kearns-Sayre syndrome? *Hum Mol Genet* **3:**947, 1994.
460. Brockington M, Alsanjari N, Sweeney MG, Morgan-Hughes JA, Scaravilli F, Harding AE: Kearns-Sayre syndrome associated with mitochondrial DNA deletion or duplication: A molecular genetic and pathological study. *J Neurol Sci* **131:**78, 1995.
461. Schon EA, Rizzuto R, Moraes CT, Nakase H, Zeviani M, DiMauro S: A direct repeat is a hotspot for large-scale deletion of human mitochondrial DNA. *Science* **244:**346, 1989.

462. Shoffner JM, Lott MT, Voljavec AS, Soueidan SA, Costigan DA, Wallace DC: Spontaneous Kearns-Sayre/chronic external ophthalmoplegia plus syndrome associated with a mitochondrial DNA deletion: A slip-replication model and metabolic therapy. *Proc Natl Acad Sci U S A* **86:**7952, 1989.
463. Holt IJ, Harding AE, Morgan-Hughes JA: Deletions of muscle mitochondrial DNA in mitochondrial myopathies: Sequence analysis and possible mechanisms. *Nucleic Acids Res* **17:**4465, 1989.
464. Lestienne P, Bataille N, Lucas-Heron B: Role of the mitochondrial DNA and calmitine in myopathies. *Biochim Biophys Acta* **1271:**159, 1995.
465. Manfredi G, Servidei S, Bonilla E, Shanske S, Schon EA, DiMauro S, Moraes CT: High levels of mitochondrial DNA with an unstable 260-bp duplication in a patient with a mitochondrial myopathy. *Neurology* **45:**762, 1995.
466. Mita S, Rizzuto R, Moraes CT, Shanske S, Arnaudo E, Fabrizi GM, Koga Y, et al.: Recombination via flanking direct repeats is a major cause of large-scale deletions of human mitochondrial DNA. *Nucleic Acids Res* **18:**561, 1990.
467. Blok RB, Thorburn DR, Thompson GN, Dahl HH: A topoisomerase II cleavage site is associated with a novel mitochondrial DNA deletion. *Hum Genet* **95:**75, 1995.
468. Hayashi J, Ohta S, Kikuchi A, Takemitsu M, Goto Y, Nonaka I: Introduction of disease-related mitochondrial DNA deletions into HeLa cells lacking mitochondrial DNA results in mitochondrial dysfunction. *Proc Natl Acad Sci U S A* **88:**10614, 1991.
469. Shanske S, Moraes CT, Lombes A, Miranda AF, Bonilla E, Lewis P, Whelan MA, et al.: Widespread tissue distribution of mitochondrial DNA deletions in Kearns-Sayre syndrome. *Neurology* **40:**24, 1990.
470. Poulton J, O'Rahilly S, Morten KJ, Clark A: Mitochondrial DNA, diabetes and pancreatic pathology in Kearns-Sayre syndrome. *Diabetologia* **38:**868, 1995.
471. Keefe DL, Niven-Fairchild T, Powell S, Buradagunta S: Mitochondrial deoxyribonucleic acid deletions in oocytes and reproductive aging in women. *Fertil Steril* **64:**577, 1995.
472. Kitagawa T, Suganuma N, Nawa A, Kikkawa F, Tanaka M, Ozawa T, Tomoda Y: Rapid accumulation of deleted mitochondrial deoxyribonucleic acid in postmenopausal ovaries. *Biol Reprod* **49:**730, 1993.
473. Larsson NG, Holme E, Kristiansson B, Oldfors A, Tulinius M: Progressive increase of the mutated mitochondrial DNA fraction in Kearns-Sayre syndrome. *Pediatr Res* **28:**131, 1990.
474. Fassati A, Bordoni A, Amboni P, Fortunato F, Fagiolari G, Bresolin N, Prelle A, et al.: Chronic progressive external ophthalmoplegia: a correlative study of quantitative molecular data and histochemical and biochemical profile. *J Neurol Sci* **123:**140, 1994.
475. Muller-Hocker J: Cytochrome c oxidase deficient fibres in the limb muscle and diaphragm of man without muscular disease: An age-related alteration. *J Neurol Sci* **100:**14, 1990.
476. Moraes CT, Sciacco M, Ricci E, Tengan CH, Hao H, Bonilla E, Schon EA, et al.: Phenotype-genotype correlations in skeletal muscle of patients with mtDNA deletions. *Muscle Nerve* **3:**S150, 1995.
477. Gross NJ, Getz GS, Rabinowitz M: Apparent turnover of mitochondrial deoxyribonucleic acid and mitochondrial phospholipids in the tissues of the rat. *J Biol Chem* **244:**1552, 1969.
478. Kadenbach B: Half-lives of cytochrome *c* from various organs of the rat. *Biochim Biophys Acta* **186:**399, 1969.
479. Menzies RA, Gold PH: The turnover of mitochondria in a variety of tissues of young adult and aged rats. *J Biol Chem* **246:**2425, 1971.
480. Neubert D, Oberdisse E, Bass R: Biosynthesis and degradation of mammalian mitochondrial DNA, in Slater EC, Tager JM, Papa S, Quagliarello E (eds): *Biochemical Aspects of the Biogenesis of Mitochondria*. Bari, Adriatica Editrice, 1968, p 103.
481. Pavlath GK, Rich K, Webster SG, Blau HM: Localization of muscle gene products in nuclear domains. *Nature* **337:**570, 1989.
482. Wallace DC, Richter C, Bohr VA, Cortopassi G, Kadenbach B, Linn S, Linnane AW, et al.: Group Report: The role of bioenergetics and mitochondrial DNA mutations in aging and age-related diseases, in Esser K, Martin GM (eds): *Molecular Aspects of Aging*. New York, John Wiley & Sons, 1995, p 199.
483. Wallace DC: Mitochondrial DNA mutations in diseases of energy metabolism. *J Bioenerg Biomembr* **26:**241, 1994.
484. Kapsa R, Thompson GN, Thorburn DR, Dahl HH, Marzuki S, Byrne E, Blok RB: A novel mtDNA deletion in an infant with Pearson syndrome. *J Inherit Metab Dis* **17:**521, 1994.
485. Rotig A, Bourgeron T, Chretien D, Rustin P, Munnich A: Spectrum of mitochondrial DNA rearrangements in the Pearson marrow-pancreas syndrome. *Hum Mol Genet* **4:**1327, 1995.
486. Smith OP, Hann IM, Woodward CE, Brockington M: Pearson's marrow/pancreas syndrome: haematological features associated with deletion and duplication of mitochondrial DNA. *Br J Haematol* **90:**469, 1995.
487. Cormier V, Rotig A, Bonnefont JP, Mechinand F, Berthou C, Goulet O, Schmitz J, et al.: Pearson's syndrome. Pancytopenia with exocrine pancreatic insufficiency: New mitochondrial disease in the first year of childhood. *Arch Fr Pediatr* **48:**171, 1991.
488. Pearson HA, Lobel JS, Kocoshis SA, Naiman JL, Windmiller J, Lammi AT, Hoffman R, et al.: A new syndrome of refractory sideroblastic anemia with vacuolization of marrow precursors and exocrine pancreatic function. *J Pediatr* **95:**976, 1979.
489. Rotig A, Cormier V, Koll F, Mize CE, Saudubray J-M, Veerman A, Pearson HA, et al.: Site-specific deletions of the mitochondrial genome in the Pearson marrow-pancreas syndrome. *Genomics* **10:**502, 1991.
490. Rotig A, Colonna M, Blanche S, Fischer A, LeDeist F, Frezal J, Saudubray JM, et al.: Deletion of blood mitochondrial DNA in pancytopenia. *Lancet* **2:**567, 1988.
491. Rotig A, Colonna M, Bonnefont JP, Blanche S, Fischer A, Saudubray JM, Munnich A: Mitochondrial DNA deletion in Pearson's marrow-pancreas syndrome. *Lancet* **1:**902, 1989.
492. Rotig A, Cormier V, Chatelain P, Francois R, Saudubray JM, Rustin P, Munnich A: Deletion of mitochondrial DNA in a case of early-onset diabetes mellitus, optic atrophy, and deafness (Wolfram syndrome, MIM 222300). *J Clin Invest* **91:**1095, 1993.
493. De Vries DD, Buzing CJM, Ruitenbeek W, van de Wouw MPME, Sperl W, Sengers RCA, Trijbels JMF, et al.: Myopathology and a mitochondrial DNA deletion in the Pearson marrow and pancreas syndrome. *Neuromuscul Disord* **2:**185, 1992.
494. Cormier V, Rotig A, Quartino AR, Forni GL, Cerone R, Maier M, Saudubray JM, et al.: Widespread multitissue deletions of the mitochondrial genome in the Pearson marrow-pancreas syndrome. *J Pediatr* **117:**599, 1990.
495. McShane MA, Hammans M, Sweeney I, Holt IJ, Beattie TJ, Brett EM, Harding AE: Pearson Syndrome and mitochondrial encephalomyopathy in patient with a deletion of mtDNA. *Am J Hum Genet* **48:**39, 1991.
496. Ballinger SW, Shoffner JM, Hedaya EV, Trounce I, Polak MA, Koontz DA, Wallace DC: Maternally transmitted diabetes and deafness associated with a 10.4 kb mitochondrial DNA deletion. *Nat Genet* **1:**11, 1992.
497. Ballinger SW, Shoffner JM, Gebhart S, Koontz DA, Wallace DC: Mitochondrial diabetes revisited [Letter]. *Nat Genet* **7:**458, 1994.
498. German MS: Glucose sensing in pancreatic islet beta cells: The key role of glucokinase and the glycolytic intermediates. *Proc Natl Acad Sci U S A* **90:**1781, 1993.
499. Gidh-Jain M, Takeda J, Xu LZ, Lange AJ, Vionnet N, Stoffel M, Froguel P, et al.: Glucokinase mutations associated with non-insulin-dependent (type 2) diabetes mellitus have decreased enzymatic activity: implications for structure/function relationships. *Proc Natl Acad Sci U S A* **90:**1932, 1993.
500. Stoffel M, Froguel P, Takeda J, Zouali H, Vionnet N, Nishi S, Weber IT, et al.: Human glucokinase gene: Isolation, characterization, and identification of two missense mutations linked to early-onset non-insulin-dependent (type 2) diabetes mellitus [Erratum appears in *Proc Natl Acad Sci U S A* 89(21):10562, 1992]. *Proc Natl Acad Sci U S A* **89:**7698, 1992.
501. Stoffel M, Patel P, Lo YM, Hattersley AT, Lucassen AM, Page R, Bell JI, et al.: Missense glucokinase mutation in maturity-onset diabetes of the young and mutation screening in late-onset diabetes. *Nat Genet* **2:**153, 1992.
502. Stoffel M, Bell KL, Blackburn CL, Powell KL, Seo TS, Takeda J, Vionnet N, et al.: Identification of glucokinase mutations in subjects with gestational diabetes mellitus. *Diabetes* **42:**937, 1993.
503. Malaisse-Lagae F, Malaisse WJ: Hexose metabolism in pancreatic islets: Regulation of mitochondrial hexokinase binding. *Biochem Med Metab Biol* **39:**80, 1988.
504. Adams V, Griffin L, Towbin J, Gelb B, Worley K, McCabe ER: Porin interaction with hexokinase and glycerol kinase: Metabolic microcompartmentation at the outer mitochondrial membrane. *Biochem Med Metab Biol* **45:**271, 1991.
505. McCabe ER: Microcompartmentation of energy metabolism at the outer mitochondrial membrane: Role in diabetes mellitus and other diseases. *J Bioenerg Biomembr* **26:**317, 1994.
506. Poulton J, Deadman ME, Gardiner RM: Duplications of mitochondrial DNA in mitochondrial myopathy. *Lancet* **1:**236, 1989.

507. Dunbar DR, Moonie PA, Swingler RJ, Davidson D, Roberts R, Holt IJ: Maternally transmitted partial direct tandem duplication of mitochondrial DNA associated with diabetes mellitus. *Hum Mol Genet* **2**:1619, 1993.
508. Luder A, Barash V: Complex I deficiency with diabetes, Fanconi syndrome and mtDNA deletion. *J Inherit Metab Dis* **17**:298, 1994.
509. Hinokio Y, Suzuki S, Komatu K, Ohtomo M, Onoda M, Matsumoto M, Hirai S, et al.: A new mitochondrial DNA deletion associated with diabetic amyotrophy, diabetic myoatrophy and diabetic fatty liver. *Muscle Nerve* **3**:S142, 1995.
510. Jackson MJ, Bindoff LA, Weber K, Wilson JN, Ince P, Alberti KG, Turnbull DM: Biochemical and molecular studies of mitochondrial function in diabetes insipidus, diabetes mellitus, optic atrophy, and deafness. *Diabetes Care* **17**:728, 1994.
511. Larsson NG, Eiken HG, Boman H, Holme E, Oldfors A, Tulinius MH: Lack of transmission of deleted mtDNA from a woman with Kearns-Sayre Syndrome to her child. *Am J Hum Genet* **50**:360, 1992.
512. Zeviani M, Bresolin N, Gellera C, Bordoni A, Pannacci M, Amati P, Moggio M, et al.: Nucleus-driven multiple large-scale deletions of the human mitochondrial genome: A new autosomal dominant disease. *Am J Hum Genet* **47**:904, 1990.
513. Cormier V, Rotig A, Tardieu M, Colonna M, Saudubray JM, Munnich A: Autosomal dominant deletions of the mitochondrial genome in a case of progressive encephalomyopathy. *Am J Hum Genet* **48**:643, 1991.
514. Moraes CT, Ciacci F, Silverstri G, Shanske S, Sciacco M, Hirano M, Schon EA, et al.: Atypical clinical presentations associated with the MELAS mutation at position 3243 of human mitochondrial DNA. *Neuromuscul Disord* **3**:43, 1993.
515. Kawai H, Akaike M, Yokoi K, Nishida Y, Kunishige M, Mine H, Saito S: Mitochondrial encephalomyopathy with autosomal dominant inheritance: A clinical and genetic entity of mitochondrial diseases. *Muscle Nerve* **18**:753, 1995.
516. Checcarelli N, Prelle A, Moggio M, Comi G, Bresolin N, Papadimitriou A, Fagiolari G, et al.: Multiple deletions of mitochondrial DNA in sporadic and atypical cases of encephalomyopathy. *J Neurol Sci* **123**:74, 1994.
517. Suomalainen A, Majander A, Haltia M, Somer H, Lonnqvist J, Savontaus ML, Peltonen L: Multiple deletions of mitochondrial DNA in several tissues of a patient with severe retarded depression and familial progressive external ophthalmoplegia. *J Clin Invest* **90**:61, 1992.
518. Suomalainen A, Kaukonen J, Amati P, Timonen R, Haltia M, Weissenbach J, Zeviani M, et al.: An autosomal locus predisposing to deletions of mitochondrial DNA. *Nat Genet* **9**:146, 1995.
519. Zeviani M, Amati P, Comi G, Fratta G, Mariotti C, Tiranti V: Searching for genes affecting the structural integrity of the mitochondrial genome. *Biochim Biophys Acta* **1271**:153, 1995.
520. Kaukonen J, Amati P, Suomalainen A, Rotig A, Antozzi C, Salvi F, Weissenbach J, et al.: Identification of a second autosomal locus predisposing to multiple deletions of mitochondrial DNA [Abstract 1246]. *Am J Hum Genet* **57**:A216, 1995.
521. Kaukonen JA, Amati P, Suomalainen A, Rotig A, Piscaglia MG, Salvi F, Weissenbach J, et al.: An autosomal locus predisposing to multiple deletions of mtDNA on chromosome 3p. *Am J Hum Genet* **58**:763, 1996.
522. Nishino I, Spinazzola A, Hirano M: Thymidine phosphorylase gene mutations in MNGIE, a human mitochondrial disorder. *Science* **283**:689, 1999.
523. Bodnar AG, Cooper JM, Holt IJ, Leonard JV, Schapira AH: Nuclear complementation restores mtDNA levels in cultured cells from a patient with mtDNA depletion. *Am J Hum Genet* **53**:663, 1993.
524. Moraes CT, Shanske S, Tritschler HJ, Aprille JR, Andreetta F, Bonilla E, Schon EA, et al.: MtDNA depletion with variable tissue expression: A novel genetic abnormality in mitochondrial diseases. *Am J Hum Genet* **48**:492, 1991.
525. Bodnar AG, Cooper JM, Leonard JV, Schapira AH: Respiratory-deficient human fibroblasts exhibiting defective mitochondrial DNA replication. *Biochem J* **305**:817, 1995.
526. Boustany RN, Aprille JR, Halperin J, Levy H, DeLong GR: Mitochondrial cytochrome deficiency presenting as a myopathy with hypotonia, external ophthalmoplegia, and lactic acidosis in an infant and as fatal hepatopathy in a second cousin. *Ann Neurol* **14**:462, 1983.
527. Figarella-Branger D, Pellissier JF, Scheiner C, Wernert F, Desnuelle C: Defects of the mitochondrial respiratory chain complexes in three pediatric cases with hypotonia and cardiac involvement. *J Neurol Sci* **108**:105, 1992.
528. Mazziotta MR, Ricci E, Bertini E, Vici CD, Servidei S, Burlina AB, Sabetta G, et al.: Fatal infantile liver failure associated with mitochondrial DNA depletion. *J Pediatr* **121**:896, 1992.
529. Poulton J, Sewry C, Potter CG, Bougeron T, Chretien D, Wijburg FA, Morten KJ, et al.: Variation in mitochondrial DNA levels in muscle from normal controls. Is depletion of mtDNA in patients with mitochondrial myopathy a distinct clinical syndrome? *J Inherit Metab Dis* **18**:4, 1995.
530. Telerman-Toppet N, Biarent D, Bouton JM, de Meirleir L, Elmer C, Noel S, Vamos E, et al.: Fatal cytochrome c oxidase-deficient myopathy of infancy associated with mtDNA depletion. Differential involvement of skeletal muscle and cultured fibroblasts. *J Inherit Metab Dis* **15**:323, 1992.
531. Tritschler H-J, Andreetta F, Moraes CT, Bonilla E, Arnaudo E, Danon MJ, Glass S, et al.: Mitochondrial myopathy of childhood associated with depletion of mitochondrial DNA. *Neurology* **42**:209, 1992.
532. Hammans SR, Sweeney MG, Hanna MG, Brockington M, Morgan-Hughes JA, Harding AE: The mitochondrial DNA transfer $RNA^{Leu(UUR)}$ $A \rightarrow G^{3243}$ mutation. A clinical and genetic study. *Brain* **118**:721, 1995.
533. Mariotti C, Savarese N, Suomalainen A, Rimoldi M, Comi G, Prelle A, Antozzi C, et al.: Genotype to phenotype correlations in mitochondrial encephalomyopathies associated with the A3243G mutation of mitochondrial DNA. *J Neurol* **242**:304, 1995.
534. Moraes CT, Ciacci F, Bonilla E, Jansen C, Hirano M, Rao N, Lovelace RE, et al.: Two novel pathogenic mitochondrial DNA mutations affecting organelle number and protein synthesis. Is the $tRNA^{Leu(UUR)}$ gene an etiologic hot spot? *J Clin Invest* **92**:2906, 1993.
535. Taylor RW, Chinnery PF, Bates MJ, Jackson MJ, Johnson MA, Andrews RM, Turnbull DM: A novel mitochondrial DNA point mutation in the tRNA(Ile) gene: Studies in a patient presenting with chronic progressive external ophthalmoplegia and multiple sclerosis. *Biochem Biophys Res Commun* **243**:47, 1998.
536. Lauber J, Marsac C, Kadenbach B, Seibel P: Mutations in mitochondrial tRNA genes: A frequent cause of neuromuscular diseases. *Nucleic Acids Res* **19**:1393, 1991.
537. Hattori Y, Goto Y, Sakuta R, Nonaka I, Mizuna Y, Horai S: Point mutations in mitochondrial tRNA genes: Sequence analysis of chronic progressive external ophthalmoplegia (CPEO) [Comments]. *J Neurol Sci* **125**:50, 1994.
538. Fu K, Hartlen R, Johns T, Genge A, Karpati G, Shoubridge EA: A novel heteroplasmic tRNAleu(CUN) mtDNA point mutation in a sporadic patient with mitochondrial encephalomyopathy segregates rapidly in skeletal muscle and suggests an approach to therapy. *Hum Mol Genet* **5**:1835, 1996.
539. Gerbitz KD, van den Ouweland JM, Maassen JA, Jaksch M: Mitochondrial diabetes mellitus: A review. *Biochim Biophys Acta* **1271**:253, 1995.
540. Moraes CT, Ricci E, Bonilla E, DiMauro S, Schon EA: The mitochondrial $tRNA^{Leu(UUR)}$ mutation in mitochondrial encephalomyopathy, lactic acidosis, and strokelike episodes (MELAS): Genetic, biochemical, and morphological correlations in skeletal muscle. *Am J Hum Genet* **50**:934, 1992.
541. De Vries D, De Wijs I, Ruitenbeek W, Begeer J, Smit P, Bentlage H, van Oost B: Extreme variability of clinical symptoms among sibs in a MELAS family correlated with heteroplasmy for the mitochondrial A3243G mutation. *J Neurol Sci* **124**:77, 1994.
542. Goto Y, Horai S, Matsuoka T, Koga Y, Nihei K, Kobayashi M, Nonaka I: Mitochondrial myopathy, encephalopathy, lactic acidosis, and stroke-like episodes (MELAS): A correlative study of the clinical features and mitochondrial DNA mutation. *Neurology* **42**:545, 1992.
543. Obermaier-Kusser B, Paetzke-Brunner I, Enter C, Muller-Hocker J, Zierz S, Ruitenbeek W, Gerbitz K-D: Respiratory chain activity in tissues from patients (MELAS) with a point mutation of the mitochondrial genome ($tRNA^{Leu(UUR)}$). *FEBS Lett* **286**:67, 1991.
544. Chomyn A, Martinuzzi A, Yoneda M, Daga A, Hurko O, Johns D, Lai ST, et al.: MELAS mutation in mtDNA binding site for transcription termination factor causes defects in protein synthesis and in respiration but no change in levels of upstream and downstream mature transcripts. *Proc Natl Acad Sci U S A* **89**:4221, 1992.
545. King MP, Koga Y, Davidson M, Schon EA: Defects in mitochondrial protein synthesis and respiratory chain activity segregate with the $tRNA^{Leu(UUR)}$ mutation associated with mitochondrial myopathy, encephalopathy, lactic acidosis, and stroke-like episodes. *Mol Cell Biol* **12**:480, 1992.

546. Koga Y, Davidson M, Schon EA, King MP: Analysis of cybrids harboring MELAS mutations in the mitochondrial tRNA$^{Leu(UUR)}$ gene. *Muscle Nerve* **3:**S119, 1995.
547. Hess JF, Parisi MA, Bennett JL, Clayton DA: Impairment of mitochondrial transcription termination by a point mutation associated with the MELAS subgroup of mitochondrial encephalomyopathies. *Nature* **351:**236, 1991.
548. Suomalainen A, Majander A, Pihko H, Peltonen L, Syvanen AC: Quantification of tRNA$^{3243(Leu)}$ point mutation of mitochondrial DNA in MELAS patients and its effects on mitochondrial transcription. *Hum Mol Genet* **2:**525, 1993.
549. Koga Y, Davidson M, Schon EA, King MP: Fine mapping of mitochondrial RNAs derived from the mtDNA region containing a point mutation associated with MELAS. *Nucleic Acids Res* **21:**657, 1993.
550. Tokunaga M, Mita S, Sakuta R, Nonaka I, Araki S: Increased mitochondrial DNA in blood vessels and ragged-red fibers in mitochondrial myopathy, encephalopathy, lactic acidosis, and stroke-like episodes (MELAS). *Ann Neurol* **33:**275, 1993.
551. Noer AS, Sudoya H, Lertrit P, Thyagarajan D, Utthanaphol P, Kapsa R, Byrne E, et al.: A tRNA^{Lys} mutation in the mtDNA is the causal genetic lesion underlying myoclonic epilepsy and ragged-red fiber (MERRF) syndrome. *Am J Hum Genet* **49:**715, 1991.
552. Chomyn A, Meola G, Bresolin N, Lai ST, Scarlato G, Attardi G: *In vitro* genetic transfer of protein synthesis and respiration defects to mitochondrial DNA-less cells with myopathy-patient mitochondria. *Mol Cell Biol* **11:**2236, 1991.
553. Boulet L, Karpati G, Shoubridge EA: Distribution and threshold expression of the tRNA^{Lys} mutation in skeletal muscle of patients with myoclonic epilepsy and ragged-red fibers (MERRF). *Am J Hum Genet* **51:**1187, 1992.
554. Seibel P, Degoul F, Bonne G, Romero N, Francois D, Paturneau-Jouas M, Ziegler F, et al.: Genetic biochemical and pathophysiological characterization of a familial mitochondrial encephalomyopathy (MERRF). *J Neurol Sci* **105:**217, 1991.
555. Masucci JP, Davidson M, Koga Y, Schon EA, King MP: In vitro analysis of mutations causing myoclonus epilepsy with ragged-red fibers in the mitochondrial tRNA^{Lys}gene: Two genotypes produce similar phenotypes. *Mol Cell Biol* **15:**2872, 1995.
556. Enriquez JA, Chomyn A, Attardi G: MtDNA mutation in MERRF syndrome causes defective aminoacylation of tRNA^{Lys} and premature translation termination. *Nat Genet* **10:**47, 1995.
557. Trounce I, Byrne E, Marzuki S: Decline in skeletal muscle mitochondrial respiratory chain function: possible factor in ageing. *Lancet* **1:**637, 1989.
558. Melov S, Shoffner JM, Kaufman A, Wallace DC: Marked increase in the number and variety of mitochondrial DNA rearrangements in aging human skeletal muscle [Erratum *Nucleic Acids Res* **23(23):**4938, 1995]. *Nucleic Acids Res* **23:**4122, 1995.
559. Muller-Hocker J, Schneiderbanger K, Stefani FH, Kadenbach B: Progressive loss of cytochrome c oxidase in the human extraocular muscles in ageing—a cytochemical-immunohistochemical study. *Mutat Res* **275:**115, 1992.
560. Melov S, Coskun EP, Wallace DC: Mouse models of mitochondrial disease, oxidative stress, and senescence. *Mutat Res* **434:**233, 1999.
561. Corral-Debrinski M, Horton T, Lott MT, Shoffner JM, Beal MF, Wallace DC: Mitochondrial DNA deletions in human brain: Regional variability and increase with advanced age. *Nat Genet* **2:**324, 1992.
562. Soong NW, Hinton DR, Cortopassi G, Arnheim N: Mosaicism for a specific somatic mitochondrial DNA mutation in adult human brain. *Nat Genet* **2:**318, 1992.
563. Melov S, Hinerfeld D, Esposito L, Wallace DC: Multi-organ characterization of mitochondrial genomic rearrangements in ad libitum and caloric restricted mice show striking somatic mitochondrial DNA rearrangements with age. *Nucleic Acids Res* **25:**974, 1997.
564. Ames BN, Shigenaga MK, Hagen TM: Oxidants, antioxidants, and the degenerative diseases of aging. *Proc Natl Acad Sci U S A* **90:**7915, 1993.
565. Mecocci P, MacGarvey U, Kaufman AE, Koontz D, Shoffner JM, Wallace DC, Beal MF: Oxidative damage to mitochondrial DNA shows marked age-dependent increases in human brain. *Ann Neurol* **34:**609, 1993.
566. Das DK, George A, Liu XK, Rao PS: Detection of hydroxyl radical in the mitochondria of ischemic-reperfused myocardium by trapping with salicylate. *Biochem Biophys Res Commun* **165:**1004, 1989.
567. Corral-Debrinski M, Shoffner JM, Lott MT, Wallace DC: Association of mitochondrial DNA damage with aging and coronary atherosclerotic heart disease. *Mutat Res* **275:**169, 1992.
568. Van Voorhies WA, Ward S: Genetic and environmental conditions that increase longevity in *Caenorhabditis elegans* decrease metabolic rate. *Proc Natl Acad Sci U S A* **96:**11399, 1999.
569. Jonassen T, Proft M, Randez-Gil F, Schultz JR, Marbois BN, Entian KD, Clarke CF: Yeast Clk-1 homologue (Coq7/Cat5) is a mitochondrial protein in coenzyme Q synthesis. *J Biol Chem* **273:**3351, 1998.
570. Felkai S, Ewbank JJ, Lemieux JJ, Labbe C, Brown GG, Hekimi S: CLK-1 controls respiration, behavior and aging in the nematode *Caenorhabditis elegans. EMBO J* **18:**1783, 1999.
571. Li Y, Huang TT, Carlson EJ, Melov S, Ursell PC, Olson JL, Noble LJ, et al.: Dilated cardiomyopathy and neonatal lethality in mutant mice lacking manganese superoxide dismutase. *Nat Genet* **11:**376, 1995.
572. Lebovitz RM, Zhang H, Vogel H, Cartwright J, Jr., Dionne L, Lu N, Huang S, et al.: Neurodegeneration, myocardial injury, and perinatal death in mitochondrial superoxide dismutase-deficient mice. *Proc Natl Acad Sci U S A* **93:**9782, 1996.
573. Melov S, Schneider JA, Day BJ, Hinerfeld D, Coskun P, Mirra SS, Crapo JD, et al.: A novel neurological phenotype in mice lacking mitochondrial manganese superoxide dismutase [Comments]. *Nat Genet* **18:**159, 1998.
574. Melov S, Coskun P, Patel M, Tunistra R, Cottrell B, Jun AS, Zastawny TH, et al.: Mitochondrial disease in superoxide dismutase 2 mutant mice. *Proc Natl Acad Sci U S A* **96:**846, 1999.
575. Williams MD, Van Remmen H, Conrad CC, Huang TT, Epstein CJ, Richardson A: Increased oxidative damage is correlated to altered mitochondrial function in heterozygous manganese superoxide dismutase knockout mice. *J Biol Chem* **273:**28510, 1998.
576. Larsson NG, Wang J, Wilhelmsson H, Oldfors A, Rustin P, Lewandoski M, Barsh GS, et al.: Mitochondrial transcription factor A is necessary for mtDNA maintenance and embryogenesis in mice [Comments]. *Nat Genet* **18:**231, 1998.
577. Wang J, Wilhelmsson H, Graff C, Li H, Oldfors A, Rustin P, Bruning JC, et al.: Dilated cardiomyopathy and atrioventricular conduction blocks induced by heart-specific inactivation of mitochondrial DNA gene expression. *Nat Genet* **21:**133, 1999.
578. Jenuth JP, Peterson AC, Fu K, Shoubridge EA: Random genetic drift in the female germline explains the rapid segregation of mammalian mitochondrial DNA [Comments]. *Nat Genet* **14:**146, 1996.
579. Jenuth JP, Peterson AC, Shoubridge EA: Tissue-specific selection for different mtDNA genotypes in heteroplasmic mice. *Nat Genet* **16:**93, 1997.
580. Meirelles FV, Smith LC: Mitochondrial genotype segregation during preimplantation development in mouse heteroplasmic embryos. *Genetics* **148:**877, 1998.
581. Meirelles FV, Smith LC: Mitochondrial genotype segregation in a mouse heteroplasmic lineage produced by embryonic karyoplast transplantation. *Genetics* **145:**445, 1997.
582. Pinkert CA, Irwin MH, Johnson LW, Moffatt RJ: Mitochondria transfer into mouse ova by microinjection. *Transgenic Res* **6:**379, 1997.
583. Watanabe T, Dewey MJ, Mintz B: Teratocarcinoma cells as vehicles for introducing specific mutant mitochondrial genes into mice. *Proc Natl Acad Sci U S A* **75:**5113, 1978.
584. Zhuchenko O, Wehnert M, Bailey J, Sun ZS, Lee CC: Isolation, mapping, and genomic structure of an X-linked gene for a subunit of human mitochondrial complex I. *Genomics* **37:**281, 1996.
585. Dunbar DR, Shibasaki Y, Dobbie L, Andersson B, Brookes AJ: In situ hybridisation mapping of genomic clones for five human respiratory chain complex I genes. *Cytogenet Cell Genet* **78:**21, 1997.
586. Ton C, Hwang DM, Dempsey AA, Liew CC: Identification and primary structure of five human NADH-ubiquinone oxidoreductase subunits. *Biochem Biophys Res Commun* **241:**589, 1997.
587. Yamaoka LH, Westbrook CA, Speer MC, Gilchrist JM, Jabs EW, Schweins EG, Stajich JM, et al.: Development of a microsatellite genetic map spanning 5q31-q33 and subsequent placement of the LGMD1A locus between D5S178 and IL9. *Neuromuscul Disord* **4:**471, 1994.
588. Loeffen JL, Triepels RH, van den Heuvel LP, Schuelke M, Buskens CA, Smeets RJ, Trijbels JM, et al.: cDNA of eight nuclear encoded subunits of NADH:ubiquinone oxidoreductase: Human complex I cDNA characterization completed. *Biochem Biophys Res Commun* **253:**415, 1998.
589. Kim JW, Lee Y, Kang HB, Chose YK, Chung TW, Chang SY, Lee KS, et al.: Cloning of the human cDNA sequence encoding the NADH:ubiquinone oxidoreductase MLRQ subunit. *Biochem Mol Biol Int* **43:**669, 1997.

590. Emahazion T, Brookes AJ: Mapping of the NDUFA2, NDUFA6, NDUFA7, NDUFB8, and NDUFS8 electron transport chain genes by intron based radiation hybrid mapping. *Cytogenet Cell Genet* **82:**114, 1998.
591. Emahazion T, Beskow A, Gyllensten U, Brookes AJ: Intron based radiation hybrid mapping of 15 complex I genes of the human electron transport chain. *Cytogenet Cell Genet* **82:**115, 1998.
592. Triepels R, van den Heuvel L, Loeffen J, Smeets R, Trijbels F, Smeitink J: The nuclear-encoded human NADH:ubiquinone oxidoreductase NDUFA8 subunit: cDNA cloning, chromosomal localization, tissue distribution, and mutation detection in complex-I-deficient patients. *Hum Genet* **103:**557, 1998.
593. Baens M, Chaffanet M, Cassiman JJ, van den Berghe H, Marynen P: Construction and evaluation of a hncDNA library of human 12p transcribed sequences derived from a somatic cell hybrid. *Genomics* **16:**214, 1993.
594. Mao M, Fu G, Wu JS, Zhang QH, Zhou J, Kan LX, Huang QH, et al.: Identification of genes expressed in human CD34(+) hematopoietic stem/progenitor cells by expressed sequence tags and efficient full-length cDNA cloning. *Proc Natl Acad Sci U S A* **95:**8175, 1998.
595. Smeitink J, Loeffen J, Smeets R, Triepels R, Ruitenbeek W, Trijbels F, van den Heuvel L: Molecular characterization and mutational analysis of the human B17 subunit of the mitochondrial respiratory chain complex I. *Hum Genet* **103:**245, 1998.
596. Wong YC, Tsao SW, Kakefuda M, Bernal SD: cDNA cloning of a novel cell adhesion protein expressed in human squamous carcinoma cells. *Biochem Biophys Res Commun* **166:**984, 1990.
597. Gu JZ, Lin X, Wells DE: The human B22 subunit of the NADH-ubiquinone oxidoreductase maps to the region of chromosome 8 involved in branchio-oto-renal syndrome. *Genomics* **35:**6, 1996.
598. Lin X, Wells DE, Kimberling WJ, Kumar S: Human NDUFB9 gene: Genomic organization and a possible candidate gene associated with deafness disorder mapped to chromosome 8q13. *Hum Hered* **49:**75, 1999.
599. Hyslop SJ, Duncan AM, Pitkanen S, Robinson BH: Assignment of the PSST subunit gene of human mitochondrial complex I to chromosome 19p13. *Genomics* **37:**375, 1996.
600. Procaccio V, Depetris D, Soularue P, Mattei MG, Lunardi J, Issartel JP: cDNA sequence and chromosomal localization of the NDUFS8 human gene coding for the 23 kDa subunit of the mitochondrial complex I. *Biochim Biophys Acta* **1351:**37, 1997.
601. de Sury R, Martinez P, Procaccio V, Lunardi J, Issartel J-P: Genomic structure of the human NDUFS8 gene coding for the iron-sulfur TYKY subunit of the mitochondrial NADH:ubiquinone oxidoreductase. *Gene* **215:**1, 1998.
602. Procaccio V, de Sury R, Martinez P, Depetris D, Rabilloud T, Soularue P, Lunardi J, et al.: Mapping to 1q23 of the human gene (NDUFS2) encoding the 49-kDa subunit of the mitochondrial respiratory Complex I and immunodetection of the mature protein in mitochondria. *Mamm Genome* **9:**482, 1998.
603. Loeffen J, van den Heuvel L, Smeets R, Triepels R, Sengers R, Trijbels F, Smeitink J: cDNA sequence and chromosomal localization of the remaining three human nuclear encoded iron sulphur protein (IP) subunits of complex I: The human IP fraction is completed. *Biochem Biophys Res Commun* **247:**751, 1998.
604. Russell MW, du Manoir S, Collins FS, Brody LC: Cloning of the human NADH:ubiquinone oxidoreductase subunit B13: Localization to chromosome 7q32 and identification of a pseudogene on 11p15. *Mamm Genome* **8:**60, 1997.
605. Pata I, Tensing K, Metspalu A: A human cDNA encoding the homologue of NADH:ubiquinone oxidoreductase subunit B13. *Biochim Biophys Acta* **1350:**115, 1997.
606. Fearnley IM, Walker JE: Conservation of sequences of subunits of mitochondrial complex I and their relationships with other proteins. *Biochim Biophys Acta* **1140:**105, 1992.
607. Schuelke M, Loeffen J, Mariman E, Smeitink J, van den Heuvel L: Cloning of the human mitochondrial 51 kDa subunit (NDUFV1) reveals a 100% antisense homology of its 3′UTR with the 5′UTR of the gamma-interferon inducible protein (IP-30) precursor: Is this a link between mitochondrial myopathy and inflammation? *Biochem Biophys Res Commun* **245:**599, 1998.
608. Schuelke M, Smeitnik J, Mariman E, Loeffen J, Plecko B, Trijbels F, Stockler-Ipsiroglu S, et al.: Mutant NDUFV1 subunit of mitochondrial complex I causes leukodystrophy and myoclonic epilepsy. *Nat Genet* **21:**260, 1999.
609. de Coo RF, Buddiger P, Smeets HJ, van Oost BA: Molecular cloning and characterization of the human mitochondrial NADH:oxidoreductase 10-kDa gene (NDUFV3). *Genomics* **45:**434, 1997.
610. Duncan AM, Ozawa T, Suzuki H, Rozen R: Assignment of the gene for the cytochrome c1 subunit of the mitochondrial cytochrome bc1 complex (CYC1) to human chromosome 8q24.3. *Genomics* **19:**400, 1994.
611. Suzuki H, Hosokawa Y, Toda H, Nishikimi M, Ozawa T: Cloning and sequencing of a cDNA for human mitochondrial ubiquinone-binding protein of complex III. *Biochem Biophys Res Commun* **156:**987, 1988.
612. Suzuki H, Hosokawa Y, Toda H, Nishikimi M, Ozawa T: Isolation of a single nuclear gene encoding human ubiquinone-binding protein in complex III of mitochondrial respiratory chain. *Biochem Biophys Res Commun* **161:**371, 1989.
613. Hoffman GG, Lee S, Christiano AM, Chung-Honet LC, Cheng W, Katchman S, Uitto J, et al.: Complete coding sequence, intron/exon organization, and chromosomal location of the gene for the core I protein of human ubiquinol-cytochrome c reductase. *J Biol Chem* **268:**21113, 1993.
614. Duncan AM, Ozawa T, Suzuki H, Rozen R: Assignment of the gene for the core protein II (UQCRC2) subunit of the mitochondrial cytochrome bc1 complex to human chromosome 16p12. *Genomics* **18:**455, 1993.
615. Hosokawa Y, Suzuki H, Toda H, Nishikimi M, Ozawa T: Complementary DNA encoding core protein II of human mitochondrial cytochrome bc1 complex. Substantial diversity in deduced primary structure from its yeast counterpart. *J Biol Chem* **264:**13483, 1989.
616. Duncan AM, Anderson L, Duff C, Ozawa T, Suzuki H, Worton R, Rozen R: Assignment of the gene (UQCRFS1) for the Rieske iron-sulfur protein subunit of the mitochondrial cytochrome bc1 complex to the 22q13 and 19q12-q13.1 regions of the human genome. *Genomics* **21:**281, 1994.
617. Nishikimi M, Hosokawa Y, Toda H, Suzuki H, Ozawa T: The primary structure of human Rieske iron-sulfur protein of mitochondrial cytochrome bc1 complex deduced from cDNA analysis. *Biochem Int* **20:**155, 1990.
618. Rieske JS: Composition, structure, and function of complex III of the respiratory chain. *Biochim Biophys Acta* **456:**195, 1976.
619. Ohta S, Goto K, Arai H, Kagawa Y: An extremely acidic amino-terminal presequence of the precursor for the human mitochondrial hinge protein. *FEBS Lett* **226:**171, 1987.
620. Hey Y, Hoggard N, Burt E, James LA, Varley JM: Assignment of COX6A1 to 6p21 and a pseudogene (COX6A1P) to 1p31.1 by in situ hybridization and somatic cell hybrids. *Cytogenet Cell Genet* **77:**167, 1997.
621. Fabrizi GM, Sadlock J, Hirano M, Mita S, Koga Y, Rizzuto R, Zeviani M, et al.: Differential expression of genes specifying two isoforms of subunit VIa of human cytochrome *c* oxidase. *Gene* **119:**307, 1992.
622. Taanman JW, Schrage C, Ponne NJ, Das AT, Bolhuis PA, de Vries H, Agsteribbe E: Isolation of cDNAs encoding subunit VIb of cytochrome c oxidase and steady-state levels of coxVIb mRNA in different tissues. *Gene* **93:**285, 1990.
623. Carrero-Valenzuela RD, Quan F, Lightowlers R, Kennaway NG, Litt M, Forte M: Human cytochrome c oxidase subunit VIb: Characterization and mapping of a multigene family. *Gene* **102:**229, 1991.
624. Fabrizi GM, Rizzuto R, Nakase H, Mita S, Lomax MI, Grossman LI, Schon EA: Sequence of a cDNA specifying subunit VIIa of human cytochrome c oxidase. *Nucleic Acids Res* **17:**7107, 1989.
625. Godbout R, Pandita A, Beatty B, Bie W, Squire JA: Comparative genomic hybridization analysis of Y79 and FISH mapping indicate the amplified human mitochondrial ATP synthase alpha-subunit gene (ATP5A) maps to chromosome 18q12 → q21. *Cytogenet Cell Genet* 77:253, 1997.
626. Chen H, Morris MA, Rossier C, Blouin JL, Antonarakis SE: Cloning of the cDNA for the human ATP synthase OSCP subunit (ATP5O) by exon trapping and mapping to chromosome 21q22.1-q22.2. *Genomics* **28:**470, 1995.
627. Collinson IR, Runswick MJ, Buchanan SK, Fearnley IM, Skehel JM, van Raaij MJ, Griffiths DE, et al.: F_0 membrane domain of ATP synthase from bovine heart mitochondria: Purification, subunit composition, and reconstitution with F_1-ATPase. *Biochemistry* **33:**7971, 1994.
628. Belogrudov GI, Tomich JM, Hatefi Y: ATP synthase complex. Proximities of subunits in bovine submitochondrial particles. *J Biol Chem* **270:**2053, 1995.
629. Walker JE, Collinson IR: The role of the stalk in the coupling mechanism of F_1 F_0-ATPases. *FEBS Lett* **346:**39, 1994.

630. Walker JE, Falk G, Gay NJ, Tybulewicz VL: Genes for bacterial and mitochondrial ATP synthase. *Biochem Soc Trans* **12:**234, 1984.
631. Frangione B, Rosenwasser E, Penefsky HS, Pullman ME: Amino acid sequence of the protein inhibitor of mitochondrial adenosine triphosphatase. *Proc Natl Acad Sci U S A* **78:**7403, 1981.
632. Goodman SI, Axtell KM, Bindoff LA, Beard SE, Gill RE, Frerman FE: Molecular cloning and expression of a cDNA encoding human electron transfer flavoprotein-ubiquinone oxidoreductase. *Eur J Biochem* **219:**277, 1994.
633. Beard SE, Spector EB, Seltzer WK, Frerman FE, Goodman SI: Mutations in electron transfer flavoprotein:ubiquinone oxidoreductase (ETF:QO) in glutaric acidemia type II (GA2). *Clin Res* **41:**271a, 1993.
634. Kim YO, Oh IU, Park HS, Jeng J, Song BJ, Huh TL: Characterization of a cDNA clone for human NAD(+)-specific isocitrate dehydrogenase alpha-subunit and structural comparison with its isoenzymes from different species. *Biochem J* **308:**63, 1995.
635. Finocchiaro G, Archidiacono N, Gellera C, Bloisi W, Colombo I, Valdameri G, Romeo G, et al.: Molecular cloning and chromosomal localization of the beta-subunit of human electron transfer flavoprotein (ETF). *Am J Hum Genet* **45:**A185, 1989.
636. Colombo I, Finocchiaro G, Garavaglia B, Garbuglio N, Yamaguchi S, Frerman FE, Berra B, et al.: Mutations and polymorphisms of the gene encoding the beta-subunit of the electron transfer flavoprotein in three patients with glutaric acidemia type II. *Hum Mol Genet* **3:**429, 1994.
637. Koike K, Ohta S, Urata Y, Kagawa Y, Koike M: Cloning and sequencing of cDNAs encoding alpha and beta subunits of human pyruvate dehydrogenase. *Proc Natl Acad Sci U S A* **85:**41, 1988.
638. Koike K, Urata Y, Koike M: Molecular cloning and characterization of human pyruvate dehydrogenase beta subunit gene. *Proc Natl Acad Sci U S A* **87:**5594, 1990.
639. Chun K, Mackay N, Willard HF, Robinson BH: Isolation, characterization and chromosomal localization of cDNA clones for the E1 beta subunit of the pyruvate dehydrogenase complex. *Eur J Biochem* **194:**587, 1990.
640. Dahl HH, Brown RM, Hutchison WM, Maragos C, Brown GK: A testis-specific form of the human pyruvate dehydrogenase E1 alpha subunit is coded for by an intronless gene on chromosome 4. *Genomics* **8:**225, 1990.
641. Thekkumkara TJ, Ho L, Wexler ID, Pons G, Liu TC, Patel MS: Nucleotide sequence of a cDNA for the dihydrolipoamide acetyltransferase component of human pyruvate dehydrogenase complex. *FEBS Lett* **240:**45, 1988.
642. Coppel RL, McNeilage LJ, Surh CD, Van de Water J, Spithill TW, Whittingham S, Gershwin ME: Primary structure of the human M2 mitochondrial autoantigen of primary biliary cirrhosis: Dihydrolipoamide acetyltransferase. *Proc Natl Acad Sci U S A* **85:**7317, 1988.
643. Pons G, Raefsky-Estrin C, Carothers DJ, Pepin RA, Javed AA, Jesse BW, Ganapathi MK, et al.: Cloning and cDNA sequence of the dihydrolipoamide dehydrogenase component human alpha-ketoacid dehydrogenase complexes. *Proc Natl Acad Sci U S A* **85:**1422, 1988.
644. Otulakowski G, Robinson BH: Isolation and sequence determination of cDNA clones for porcine and human lipoamide dehydrogenase. Homology to other disulfide oxidoreductases. *J Biol Chem* **262:**17313, 1987.
645. Mirel DB, Marder K, Graziano J, Freyer G, Zhao Q, Mayeux R, Wilhelmsen KC: Characterization of the human mitochondrial aconitase gene (ACO2). *Gene* **213:**205, 1998.
646. Dolce V, Iacobazzi V, Palmieri F, Walker JE: The sequences of human and bovine genes of the phosphate carrier from mitochondria contain evidence of alternatively spliced forms. *J Biol Chem* **269:**10451, 1994.
647. Dolce V, Fiermonte G, Messina A, Palmieri F: Nucleotide sequence of a human heart cDNA encoding the mitochondrial phosphate carrier. *DNA Seq* **2:**133, 1991.
648. Walder K, Norman RA, Hanson RL, Schrauwen P, Neverova M, Jenkinson CP, Easlick J, et al.: Association between uncoupling protein polymorphisms (UCP2-UCP3) and energy metabolism/obesity in Pima indians. *Hum Mol Genet* **7:**1431, 1998.
649. del Arco A, Satrustegui J: Molecular cloning of Aralar, a new member of the mitochondrial carrier superfamily that binds calcium and is present in human muscle and brain. *J Biol Chem* **273:**23327, 1998.
650. Stoffel M, Karayiorgou M, Espinosa R, 3rd, Beau MM: The human mitochondrial citrate transporter gene (SLC20A3) maps to chromosome band 22q11 within a region implicated in DiGeorge syndrome, velo-cardio-facial syndrome and schizophrenia. *Hum Genet* **98:**113, 1996.
651. Iacobazzi V, Lauria G, Palmieri F: Organization and sequence of the human gene for the mitochondrial citrate transport protein. *DNA Seq* **7:**127, 1997.
652. Kaplan RS, Mayor JA, Wood DO: The mitochondrial tricarboxylate transport protein. cDNA cloning, primary structure, and comparison with other mitochondrial transport proteins. *J Biol Chem* **268:**13682, 1993.
653. Zarrilli R, Oates EL, McBride OW, Lerman MI, Chan JY, Santisteban P, Ursini MV, et al.: Sequence and chromosomal assignment of a novel cDNA identified by immunoscreening of a thyroid expression library: Similarity to a family of mitochondrial solute carrier proteins. *Mol Endocrinol* **3:**1498, 1989.
654. Blachly-Dyson E, Baldini A, Litt M, McCabe ER, Forte M: Human genes encoding the voltage-dependent anion channel (VDAC) of the outer mitochondrial membrane: mapping and identification of two new isoforms. *Genomics* **20:**62, 1994.
655. Blachly-Dyson E, Zambronicz EB, Yu WH, Adams V, McCabe ER, Adelman J, Colombini M, et al.: Cloning and functional expression in yeast of two human isoforms of the outer mitochondrial membrane channel, the voltage-dependent anion channel. *J Biol Chem* **268:**1835, 1993.
656. Church SL, Grant JW, Meese EU, Trent JM: Sublocalization of the gene encoding manganese superoxide dismutase (MnSOD/SOD2) to 6q25 by fluorescence in situ hybridization and somatic cell hybrid mapping. *Genomics* **14:**823, 1992.
657. Beck Y, Oren R, Amit B, Levanon A, Gorecki M, Hartman JR: Human Mn superoxide dismutase cDNA sequence. *Nucleic Acids Res* **15:**9076, 1987.
658. Kiss C, Li J, Szeles A, Gizatullin RZ, Kashuba VI, Lushnikova T, Protopopov AI, et al.: Assignment of the ARHA and GPX1 genes to human chromosome bands 3p21.3 by in situ hybridization and with somatic cell hybrids. *Cytogenet Cell Genet* **79:**228, 1997.
659. Ishida K, Morino T, Takagi K, Sukenaga Y: Nucleotide sequence of a human gene for glutathione peroxidase. *Nucleic Acids Res* **15:**10051, 1987.
660. Sukenaga Y, Ishida K, Takeda T, Takagi K: cDNA sequence coding for human glutathione peroxidase. *Nucleic Acids Res* **15:**7178, 1987.
661. Oltvai ZN, Milliman CL, Korsmeyer SJ: Bcl-2 heterodimerizes in vivo with a conserved homolog, Bax, that accelerates programmed cell death. *Cell* **74:**609, 1993.
662. Rampino N, Yamamoto H, Ionov Y, Li Y, Sawai H, Reed JC, Perucho M: Somatic frameshift mutations in the BAX gene in colon cancers of the microsatellite mutator phenotype. *Science* **275:**967, 1997.
663. Meijerink JP, Mensink EJ, Wang K, Sedlak TW, Sloetjes AW, de Witte T, Waksman G, et al.: Hematopoietic malignancies demonstrate loss-of-function mutations of BAX. *Blood* **91:**2991, 1998.
664. Apte SS, Mattei MG, Olsen BR: Mapping of the human BAX gene to chromosome 19q13.3-q13.4 and isolation of a novel alternatively spliced transcript, BAX delta. *Genomics* **26:**592, 1995.
665. Tsujimoto Y, Croce CM: Analysis of the structure, transcripts, and protein products of bcl-2, the gene involved in human follicular lymphoma. *Proc Natl Acad Sci U S A* **83:**5214, 1986.
666. Riond J, Mattei MG, Kaghad M, Dumont X, Guillemot JC, Le Fur G, Caput D, et al.: Molecular cloning and chromosomal localization of a human peripheral-type benzodiazepine receptor. *Eur J Biochem* **195:**305, 1991.
667. Lin D, Chang YJ, Strauss JFI, Miller WL: The human peripheral benzodiazepine receptor gene: Cloning and characterization of alternative splicing in normal tissues and in a patient with congenital lipoid adrenal hyperplasia. *Genomics* **18:**643, 1993.
668. Galiegue S, Jbilo O, Combes T, Bribes E, Carayon P, Le Fur G, Casellas P: Cloning and characterization of PRAX-1. A new protein that specifically interacts with the peripheral benzodiazepine receptor. *J Biol Chem* **274:**2938, 1999.
669. Amerik A, Petukhova GV, Grigorenko VG, Lykov IP, Yarovoi SV, Lipkin VM, Gorbalenya AE: Cloning and sequence analysis of cDNA for a human homolog of eubacterial ATP-dependent Lon proteases. *FEBS Lett* **340:**25, 1994.
670. Nagase T, Seki N, Tanaka A, Ishikawa K, Nomura N: Prediction of the coding sequences of unidentified human genes. IV. The coding sequences of 40 new genes (KIAA0121-KIAA0160) deduced by analysis of cDNA clones from human cell line KG-1. *DNA Res* **2:**167, 1995.
671. Hanson B, Nuttal S, Hoogenraad N: A receptor for the import of proteins into human mitochondria. *Eur J Biochem* **235:**750, 1996.
672. Hernandez JM, Blat B, Iruela C, Vila F, Hernandez-Yago J: Identification of two processed psuedogenes of the human Tom20 gene. *Mol Gen Genet* **258:**117, 1998.

673. Kaul SC, Wadhwa R, Matsuda Y, Hensler PJ, Pereira-Smith OM, Komatsu Y, Mitsui Y: Mouse and human chromosomal assignments of mortalin, a novel member of the murine hsp70 family of proteins. *FEBS Lett* **361**:269, 1995.
674. Bhattacharyya T, Karnezis AN, Murphy SP, Hoang T, Freeman BC, Phillips B, Morimoto RI: Cloning and subcellular localization of human mitochondrial hsp70. *J Biol Chem* **270**:1705, 1995.
675. Venner TJ, Singh B, Gupta RS: Nucleotide sequences and novel structural features of human and Chinese hamster hsp60 (chaperonin) gene families. *DNA Cell Biol* **9**:545, 1990.
676. Campos Y, Martin MA, Rubio JC, Gutierrez del Olmo MC, Cabello A, Arenas J: Bilateral striatal necrosis and MELAS associated with a new T3308C mutation in the mitochondrial ND1 gene. *Biochem Biophys Res Commun* **238**:323, 1997.
677. Nakagawa Y, Ikegami H, Yamato E, Takekawa K, Fujisawa T, Hamada Y, Ueda H, et al.: A new mitochondrial DNA mutation associated with non-insulin-dependent diabetes mellitus [Erratum appears in *Biochim Biophys Res Commun* 209:664, 1995]. *Biochem Biophys Res Commun* **209**:664, 1995.
678. Obayashi T, Hattori K, Sugiyama S, Tanaka M, Tanaka T, Itoyama S, Deguchi H, et al.: Point mutations in mitochondrial DNA in patients with hypertrophic cardiomyopathy. *Am Heart J* **124**:1263, 1992.
679. Thomas AW, Edwards A, Sherratt EJ, Majid A, Gagg J, Alcolado JC: Molecular scanning of candidate mitochondrial tRNA genes in type 2 (non-insulin dependent) diabetes mellitus. *J Med Genet* **33**:253, 1996.
680. Wallace DC, Shoffner JM, Brown MD, Torroni A, Lott MT, Cabell M: Mitochondrial DNA mutations associated with Alzheimer's and Parkinson's disease. *Am J Hum Genet* **51**:A30, 1992.
681. Shoffner JM, Brown MD, Torroni A, Lott MT, Cabell MR, Mirra SS, Beal MF, et al.: Mitochondrial DNA variants observed in Alzheimer disease and Parkinson disease patients. *Genomics* **17**:171, 1993.
682. Howell N, McCullough D, Bodis-Wollner I: Molecular genetic analysis of a sporadic case of Leber hereditary optic neuropathy [Letter]. *Am J Hum Genet* **50**:443, 1992.
683. Johns DR: Mitochondrial ND-1 mutation in Leber hereditary optic neuropathy [Letter]. *Am J Hum Genet* **50**:872, 1992.
684. Johns DR, Neufeld M: Pitfalls in the molecular genetic diagnosis of Leber hereditary optic neuropathy (LHON). *Am J Hum Genet* **53**:916, 1993.
685. Norby S: Screening for the two most frequent mutations in Leber's hereditary optic neuropathy by duplex PCR based on allele-specific amplification. *Hum Mutat* **2**:309, 1993.
686. Riordan-Eva P, Harding AE: Leber's hereditary optic neuropathy: the clinical relevance of different mitochondrial DNA mutations. *J Med Genet* **32**:81, 1995.
687. Mackey DA: Three subgroups of patients from the United Kingdom with Leber hereditary optic neuropathy. *Eye* **8**:431, 1994.
688. Johns DR, Berman J: Alternative, simultaneous complex I mitochondrial DNA mutations in Leber's hereditary optic neuropathy. *Biochem Biophys Res Commun* 174:1324, 1991.
689. Salmaggi A, Carrara F, Zeviani M: Remarkable recovery of visual function in a patient with Leber's optic neuropathy and multiple mutations of mitochondrial DNA. *Int J Neurosci* **77**:261, 1994.
690. Lin F, Lin R, Wisniewski HM, Hwang Y, Grundke-Iqbal I, Healy-Louie G, Iqbal K: Detection of point mutations in codon 331 of mitochondrial NADH dehydrogenase subunit 2 in Alzheimer's brains. *Biochem Biophys Res Commun* **182**:238, 1992.
691. Petruzzella V, Chen X, Schon EA: Is a point mutation in the mitochondrial ND2 gene associated with Alzheimer's disease? *Biochem Biophys Res Commun* **186**:491, 1992.
692. Kosel S, Egensperger R, Mehraein P, Graeber MB: No association of mutations at nucleotide 5460 of mitochondrial NADH dehydrogenase with Alzheimer's disease. *Biochem Biophys Res Commun* **203**:745, 1994.
693. Reynier P, Figarella-Branger D, Serratrice G, Charvet B, Malthiery Y: Association of deletion and homoplasmic point mutation of the mitochondrial DNA in an ocular myopathy. *Biochem Biophys Res Commun* **202**:1606, 1994.
694. Newman NJ, Torroni A, Brown MD, Lott MT, Wallace DC, Philen R, Roman GC: Cuban optic neuropathy [Letter; Comment]. *Neurology* **45**:397, 1995.
695. Harding AE, Holt IJ, Sweeney MG, Brockington M, Davis MB: Prenatal diagnosis of mitochondrial DNA8993 T-G disease. *Am J Hum Genet* **50**:629, 1992.
696. Ciafaloni E, Santorelli FM, Shanske S, Deonna T, Roulet E, Janzer C, Pescia G, et al.: Maternally inherited Leigh syndrome. *J Pediatr* **122**:419, 1993.
697. Puddu P, Barboni P, Mantovani V, Montagna P, Cerullo A, Bragliani M, Molinotti C, et al.: Retinitis pigmentosa, ataxia, and mental retardation associated with mitochondrial DNA mutation in an Italian family. *Br J Ophthalmol* **77**:84, 1993.
698. Chakrapani A, Heptinstall L, Walter J: A family with Leigh syndrome caused by the rarer T8993C mutation. *J Inherit Metab Dis* **21**:685, 1998.
699. Mak SC, Chi CS, Tsai CR: Mitochondrial DNA 8993 T > C mutation presenting as juvenile Leigh syndrome with respiratory failure. *J Child Neurol* **13**:349, 1998.
700. Howell N: Mitochondrial gene mutations and human diseases: A prolegomenon [Editorial]. *Am J Hum Genet* **55**:219, 1994.
701. Johns DR: Pathological significance of the mtDNA COX III mutation at nucleotide pair 9438 in Leber hereditary optic neuropathy. [Reply to Brown et al.] *Am J Hum Genet* **55**:410, 1994.
702. Johns DR, Neufeld MJ, Hedges TR: Mitochondrial DNA mutations in Cuban optic and peripheral neuropathy. *J Neuroophthalmol* **14**:135, 1994.
703. Newman NJ, Torroni A, Brown MD, Lott MT, Fernandez MM, Wallace DC, Cuba Neuropathy Field Investigation Team: Epidemic neuropathy in Cuba not associated with mitochondrial DNA mutations found in Leber's hereditary optic neuropathy patients. *Am J Ophthalmol* **118**:158, 1994.
704. Manfredi G, Bonilla E, Schon EA, DiMauro S, Moraes C: A mitochondrial DNA missense mutation in the cytochrome oxidase subunit III gene associated with a progressive encephalopathy. *Miami Short Reports* **4**:17, 1994.
705. Manfredi G, Schon EA, Moraes CT, Bonilla E, Berry GT, Sladky JT, DiMauro S: A new mutation associated with MELAS is located in a mitochondrial DNA polypeptide-coding gene. *Neuromuscul Disord* **5**:391, 1995.
706. Lertrit P, Noer AS, Jean-Francois MJ, Kapsa R, Dennett X, Thyagarajan D, Lethlean K, et al.: A new disease-related mutation for mitochondrial encephalopathy lactic acidosis and strokelike episodes (MELAS) syndrome affects the ND4 subunit of the respiratory complex I [Comments]. *Am J Hum Genet* **51**:457, 1992.
707. Sakuta R, Goto Y, Nonaka I, Horai S: An A-to-G transition at nucleotide pair 11084 in the ND4 gene may be an mtDNA polymorphism [Letter; Comment]. *Am J Hum Genet* **53**:964, 1993.
708. Holt IJ, Miller DH, Harding AE: Genetic heterogeneity and mitochondrial DNA heteroplasmy in Leber's hereditary optic neuropathy. *J Med Genet* **26**:739, 1989.
709. Hotta Y, Hayakawa M, Saito K, Kanai A, Nakajima A, Fujiki K: Diagnosis of Leber's optic neuropathy by means of polymerase chain reaction amplification. *Am J Ophthalmol* **108**:601, 1989.
710. Singh G, Lott MT, Wallace DC: A mitochondrial DNA mutation as a cause of Leber's hereditary optic neuropathy. *N Engl J Med* **320**:1300, 1989.
711. Vilkki J, Savontaus ML, Nikoskelainen EK: Genetic heterogeneity in Leber hereditary optic neuroretinopathy revealed by mitochondrial DNA polymorphism. *Am J Hum Genet* **45**:206, 1989.
712. Yoneda M, Tsuji S, Yamauchi T, Inuzuka T, Miyatake T, Horai S, Ozawa T: Mitochondrial DNA mutation in family with Leber's hereditary optic neuropathy. *Lancet* **1**:1076, 1989.
713. Bolhuis PA, Bleeker-Wagemakers EM, Ponne NJ, Van Schooneveld MJ, Westerveld A, Van den Bogert C, Tabak HF: Rapid shift in genotype of human mitochondrial DNA in a family with Leber's hereditary optic neuropathy. *Biochem Biophys Res Commun* **170**:994, 1990.
714. Huoponen K, Vilkki J, Savontaus ML, Aula P, Nikoskelainen EK: Analysis of mitochondrial ND4 gene DNA sequence in Finnish families with Leber hereditary optic neuroretinopathy. *Genomics* **8**:583, 1990.
715. Johns DR: The molecular genetics of Leber's hereditary optic neuropathy. *Arch Ophthalmol* **108**:1405, 1990.
716. Lott MT, Voljavec AS, Wallace DC: Variable genotype of Leber's hereditary optic neuropathy patients. *Am J Ophthalmol* **109**:625, 1990.
717. Tawata M, Ohtaka M, Iwase E, Ikegishi Y, Aida K, Onaya T: New mitochondrial DNA homoplasmic mutations associated with Japanese patients with type 2 diabetes. *Diabetes* **47**:276, 1998.
718. Haferkamp O, Scheuerle A, Schlenk R, Melzner I, Pavenstadt-Grupp I, Rodel G: Mitochondrial complex I and III mutations and neutral-lipid storage in activated mononuclear macrophages and neutrophils: A case presenting with necrotizing myopathy, poikiloderma atrophicans vasculare, and xanthogranulomatous bursitis. *Hum Pathol* **25**:419, 1994.

719. Govan GG, Smith PR, Kellar-Wood H, Schapira AH, Harding AE: HLA class II genotypes in Leber's hereditary optic neuropathy. *J Neurol Sci* **126:**193, 1994.
720. de Coo IF, Renier WO, Ruitenbeek W, Ter Laak HJ, Bakker M, Schagger H, Van Oost BA, et al.: A 4-base pair deletion in the mitochondrial cytochrome b gene associated with parkinsonism/ MELAS overlap syndrome. *Ann Neurol* **45:**130, 1999.
721. Andreu AL, Bruno C, Dunne TC, Tanji K, Shanske S, Sue CM, Krishna S, et al.: A nonsense mutation (G15059A) in the cytochrome b gene in a patient with exercise intolerance and myoglobinuria. *Ann Neurol* **45:**127, 1999.
722. Heher KL, Johns DR: A maculopathy associated with the 15257 mitochondrial DNA mutation. *Arch Ophthalmol* **111:**1495, 1993.
723. Howell N, Kubacka I, Halvorson S, Mackey D: Leber's hereditary optic neuropathy: the etiological role of a mutation in the mitochondrial cytochrome b gene [Letter]. *Genetics* **133:**133, 1993.
724. Johns DR, Smith KH, Savino PJ, Miller NR: Leber's hereditary optic neuropathy. Clinical manifestations of the 15257 mutation. *Arch Ophthalmol* **100:**981, 1993.
725. Andreu AL, Bruno C, Shanske S, Shtilbans A, Hirano M, Krishna S, Hayward L, et al.: Missense mutation in the mtDNA cytochrome b gene in a patient with myopathy. *Neurology* **51:**1444, 1998.
726. Haferkamp O, Rosenau W, Scheuerle A, Pietrczyk C, Skowronek P, Rodel G: Disseminated neocortical and subcortical encephalopathy (DNSE) with widespread activation of brain macrophages: a new dementia disorder? Autopsy reports of two postmenopausal women from families with mitochondrial DNA mutations. *Clinical Neuropathology* **17:**85, 1998.
727. Kleinle S, Schneider V, Moosmann P, Brandner S, Krahenbuhl S, Liechti-Gallati S: A novel mitochondrial tRNA(Phe) mutation inhibiting anticodon stem formation associated with a muscle disease. *Biochem Biophys Res Commun* **247:**112, 1998.
728. Fischel-Ghodsian N, Prezant TR, Bu X, Oztas S: Mitochondrial ribosomal RNA gene mutation in a patient with sporadic aminoglycoside ototoxicity. *Am J Otolaryngol* **14:**399, 1993.
729. Hutchin T, Haworth I, Higashi K, Fischel-Ghodsian N, Stoneking M, Saha N, Arnos C, et al.: A molecular basis for human hypersensitivity to aminoglycoside antibiotics. *Nucleic Acids Res* **21:**4174, 1993.
730. Prezant TR, Agapian JV, Bohlman MC, Bu X, Oztas S, Qiu WQ, Arnos KS, et al.: Mitochondrial ribosomal RNA mutation associated with both antibiotic-induced and non-syndromic deafness. *Nat Genet* **4:**289, 1993.
731. Matthijs G, Claes S, Longo-Mbenza B, Cassiman JJ: Teenage onset non-syndromic deafness associated with a mutation and a polymorphism in the mitochondrial 12S ribosomal RNA gene in a large Zairese pedigree [Abstract]. *Am J Hum Genet* **55:**A23, 1994.
732. Shoffner JM, Brown M, Huoponen K, Stugard C, Koontz D, Kaufman A, Graham J, et al.: A mitochondrial DNA (mtDNA) mutation associated with maternally inherited Parkinson's disease (PD) and deafness [Abstract 1417]. *Am J Hum Genet* **55:**A242, 1994().
733. Tono T, Ushisako Y, Kiyomizu K, Usami S, Abe S, Shinkawa H, Komune S: Cochlear implantation in a patient with profound hearing loss with the A1555G mitochondrial mutation. *Am J Otol* **19:**754, 1998.
734. Usami S, Abe S, Shinkawa H, Kimberling WJ: Sensorineural hearing loss caused by mitochondrial DNA mutations: Special reference to the A1555G mutation. *J Commun Dis* **31:**423, 1998.
735. Tiranti V, D'Agruma L, Pareyson D, Mora M, Carrara F, Zelante L, Gasparini P, et al.: A novel mutation in the mitochondrial tRNA(Val) gene associated with a complex neurological presentation. *Ann Neurol* **43:**98, 1998.
736. de Coo IF, Sistermans EA, de Wijs IJ, Catsman-Berrevoets C, Busch HF, Scholte HR, de Klerk JB, et al.: A mitochondrial tRNA(Val) gene mutation (G1642A) in a patient with mitochondrial myopathy, lactic acidosis, and stroke-like episodes. *Neurology* **50:**293, 1998.
737. Poulton J, Turnbull DM, Mehta AB, Wilson J, Gardiner RM: Restriction enzyme analysis of the mitochondrial genome in mitochondrial myopathy. *J Med Genet* **25:**600, 1988.
738. Ino H, Tanaka M, Ohno K, Hattori K, Ikebe S, Sano T, Ozawa T, et al.: Mitochondrial leucine tRNA mutation in a mitochondrial encephalomyopathy [Letter; Comment]. *Lancet* **337:**234, 1990.
739. Kobayashi Y, Momoi MY, Tominaga K, Momoi T, Nihei K, Yanagisawa M, Kagawa Y, et al.: A point mutation in the mitochondrial $tRNA^{Leu(UUR)}$ gene in MELAS (mitochondrial myopathy, encephalopathy, lactic acidosis and stroke-like episodes). *Biochem Biophys Res Commun* **173:**816, 1990.
740. Ciafaloni E, Ricci E, Servidei S, Shanske S, Silvestri G, Manfredi G, Schon EA, et al.: Widespread tissue distribution of a $tRNA^{Leu(UUR)}$ mutation in the mitochondrial DNA of a patient with MELAS syndrome. *Neurology* **41:**1663, 1991.
741. Enter C, Muller-Hocker J, Zierz S, Kurlemann G, Pongratz D, Forster C, Obermaier-Kusser B, et al.: A specific point mutation in the mitochondrial genome of Caucasians with MELAS. *Hum Genet* **88:**233, 1991.
742. Hammans SR, Sweeney MG, Brockington M, Morgan-Hughes JA, Harding AE: Mitochondrial encephalopathies: Molecular genetic diagnosis from blood samples. *Lancet* **337:**1311, 1991.
743. Kobayashi Y, Momoi MY, Tominaga K, Shimoizumi H, Nihei K, Yanagisawa M, Kagawa Y, et al.: Respiration-deficient cells are caused by a single point mutation in the mitochondrial $tRNA^{Leu(UUR)}$ gene in mitochondrial myopathy, encephalopathy, lactic acidosis, and stroke-like episodes (MELAS). *Am J Hum Genet* **49:**590, 1991.
744. van den Ouweland JM, Lemkes HHP, Ruitenbeek W, Sandkjujl LA, deVijlder MF, Struyvenberg PAA, van de Kamp JJP, et al.: Mutation in mitochondrial $tRNA^{Leu(UUR)}$ gene in a large pedigree with maternally transmitted type II diabetes mellitus and deafness. *Nat Genet* **1:**368, 1992.
745. Alcolado JC, Majid A, Brockington M, Sweeney MG, Morgan R, Rees A, Harding AE, et al.: Mitochondrial gene defects in patients with NIDDM. *Diabetologia* **37:**372, 1994.
746. van den Ouweland JM, Lemkes HH, Trembath RC, Ross R, Velho G, Cohen D, Froguel P, et al.: Maternally inherited diabetes and deafness is a distinct subtype of diabetes and associates with a single point mutation in the mitochondrial $tRNA^{Leu(UUR)}$ gene. *Diabetes* **43:**746, 1994.
747. Alcolado JC, Thomas AW: Maternally inherited diabetes mellitus: The role of mitochondrial DNA defects. *Diabet Med* **12:**102, 1995.
748. Campos Y, Bautista J, Gutierrez-Rivas E, Chinchon D, Cabello A, Segura D, Arenas J: Clinical heterogeneity in two pedigrees with the 3243 bp $tRNA^{Leu(UUR)}$ mutation of mitochondrial DNA. *Acta Neurol Scand* **91:**62, 1995.
749. Kadowaki T, Sakura H, Otabe S, Yasuda K, Kadowaki H, Mori Y, Hagura R, et al.: A subtype of diabetes mellitus associated with a mutation in the mitochondrial gene. *Muscle Nerve* **3:**S137, 1995.
750. Manouvrier S, Rotig A, Hannebique G, Gheerbrandt JD, Royer-Legrain G, Munnich A, Parent M, et al.: Point mutation of the mitochondrial $tRNA^{Leu}$ gene (A 3243 G) in maternally inherited hypertrophic cardiomyopathy, diabetes mellitus, renal failure, and sensorineural deafness. *J Med Genet* **32:**654, 1995.
751. Massin P, Guillausseau PJ, Vialettes B, Paquis V, Orsini F, Grimaldi AD, Gaudric A: Macular pattern dystrophy associated with a mutation of mitochondrial DNA. *Am J Ophthalmol* **120:**247, 1995.
752. Shaag A, Saada A, Steinberg A, Navon P, Elpeleg ON: Mitochondrial encephalomyopathy associated with a novel mutation in the mitochondrial tRNA(leu)(UUR) gene (A3243T). *Biochem Biophys Res Commun* **233:**637, 1997.
753. Goto Y, Tojo M, Tohyama J, Horai S, Nonaka I: A novel point mutation in the mitochondrial $tRNA^{Leu(UUR)}$ gene in a family with mitochondrial myopathy. *Ann Neurol* **31:**672, 1992.
754. Sweeney MG, Bundey S, Brockington M, Poulton KR, Winer JB, Harding AE: Mitochondrial myopathy associated with sudden death in young adults and a novel mutation in the mitochondrial DNA leucine transfer $RNA^{(UUR)}$ gene. *QJM* **86:**709, 1993.
755. Morten K, Brown G, Lake B, Wilson J, Poulton J: A new point mutation associated with the MELAS phenotype. Second International Congress of Human Mitochondrial Pathology (EUROMIT), 1992, p 39.
756. Kawarai T, Kawakami H, Kozuka K, Izumi Y, Matsuyama Z, Watanabe C, Kohriyama T, et al.: A new mitochondrial DNA mutation associated with mitochondrial myopathy: tRNA(Leu)(UUR) 3254C-to-G. *Neurology* **49:**598, 1997.
757. Sato W, Hayasaka K, Shoji Y, Takahashi T, Takada G, Saito M, Fukawa O, et al.: A mitochondrial tRNA(Leu)(UUR) mutation at 3,256 associated with mitochondrial myopathy, encephalopathy, lactic acidosis, and stroke- like episodes (MELAS). *Biochem Mol Biol Int* **33:**1055, 1994.
758. Zeviani M, Gellera C, Antozzi C, Rimoldi M, Morandi L, Villani F, Tiranti V, et al.: Maternally inherited myopathy and cardiomyopathy: Association with mutation in mitochondrial DNA $tRNA^{Leu(UUR)}$. *Lancet* **338:**143, 1991.
759. Sweeney MG, Brockington M, Weston MJ, Morgan-Hughes JA, Harding AE: Mitochondrial DNA transfer RNA mutation $Leu^{(UUR)}$ A-G 3260: A second family with myopathy and cardiomyopathy. *QJM* **86:**435, 1993.

760. Mariotti C, Tiranti V, Carrara F, Dallapiccola B, DiDonato S, Zeviani M: Defective respiratory capacity and mitochondrial protein synthesis in transformant cybrids harboring the $tRNA^{Leu(UUR)}$ mutation associated with maternally inherited myopathy and cardiomyopathy. *J Clin Invest* **93:**1102, 1994.
761. Suzuki Y, Suzuki S, Hinokio Y, Chiba M, Atsumi Y, Hosokawa K, Shimada A, et al.: Diabetes associated with a novel 3264 mitochondrial tRNA(Leu)(UUR) mutation. *Diabetes Care* **20:**1138, 1997.
762. Goto Y, Nonaka I, Horai S: A new mtDNA mutation associated with mitochondrial myopathy, encephalopathy, lactic acidosis and stroke-like episodes (MELAS). *Biochim Biophys Acta* **1097:**238, 1991.
763. Hayashi J, Ohta S, Takai D, Miyabayashi S, Sakuta R, Goto Y, Nonaka I: Accumulation of mtDNA with a mutation at position 3271 in $tRNA^{Leu(UUR)}$ gene introduced from a MELAS patient to HeLa cells lacking mtDNA results in progressive inhibition of mitochondrial respiratory function. *Biochem Biophys Res Commun* **197:**1049, 1993.
764. Sakuta R, Goto Y, Horai S, Nonaka I: Mitochondrial DNA mutations at nucleotide positions 3243 and 3271 in mitochondrial myopathy, encephalopathy, lactic acidosis, and stroke-like episodes: a comparative study. *J Neurol Sci* **115:**158, 1993.
765. Takeda A, Chiba S, Takaaki I, Tanamura A, Yamaguchi Y, Takeda N: Cell cycle of myocytes of cardiac and skeletal muscle in mitochondrial myopathy. *Jpn Circ J* **62:**695, 1998.
766. Shoffner JM, Bialer MG, Pavlakis SG, Lott MT, Kaufman A, Dixon J, Teichberg S, et al.: Mitochondrial encephalomyopathy associated with a single nucleotide pair deletion in the mitochondrial $tRNA^{Leu(UUR)}$ gene. *Neurology* **45:**286, 1995.
767. Tsukuda K, Suzuki Y, Kameoka K, Osawa N, Goto Y, Katagiri H, Asano T, et al.: Screening of patients with maternally transmitted diabetes for mitochondrial gene mutations in the tRNA[Leu(UUR)] region [Comments]. *Diabet Med* **14:**1032, 1997.
768. Goto Y, Tsugane K, Tanabe Y, Nonaka I, Horai S: A new point mutation at nucelotide pair 3291 of the $tRNA^{Leu(UUR)}$ gene in a patient with mitochondrial myopathy, encephalopathy, lactic acidosis, and stroke-like episodes (MELAS). *Biochem Biophys Res Commun* **202:**1624, 1994.
769. Bindoff LA, Howell N, Poulton J, McCullough DA, Morten KJ, Lightowlers RN, Turnbull DM, et al.: Abnormal RNA processing associated with a novel tRNA mutation in mitochondrial DNA. A potential disease mechanism. *J Biol Chem* **268:**19559, 1993.
770. Shoffner JM, Krawiecki N, Cabell MF, Torroni A, Wallace DC: A novel $tRNA^{Leu(UUR)}$ mutation in childhood mitochondrial myopathy. *Am J Hum Genet* **53(Suppl):** 949, 1993.
771. Silvestri G, Santorelli FM, Shanske S, Whitley CB, Schimmenti LA, Smith SA, DiMauro S: A new mtDNA mutation in the $tRNA^{Leu(UUR)}$ gene associated with maternally inherited cardiomyopathy. *Hum Mutat* **3:**37, 1994.
772. Taniike M, Fukushima H, Yanagihara I, Tsukamoto H, Tanaka J, Fujimura H, Nagai T, et al.: Mitochondrial $tRNA^{Ile}$ mutation in fatal cardiomyopathy. *Biochem Biophys Res Commun* **186:**47, 1992.
773. Hayashi J, Ohta S, Kagawa Y, Takai D, Miyabayashi S, Tada K, Fukushima H, et al.: Functional and morphological abnormalities of mitochondria in human cells containing mitochondrial DNA with pathogenic point mutations in tRNA genes. *J Biol Chem* **269:**19060, 1994.
774. Casali C, Santorelli FM, D'Amati G, Bernucci P, DeBiase L, DiMauro S: A novel mtDNA point mutation in maternally inherited cardiomyopathy. *Biochem Biophys Res Commun* **213:**588, 1995.
775. Tanaka M, Ino H, Ohno K, Hattori K, Sato W, Ozawa T, Tanaka T, et al.: Mitochondrial mutation in fatal infantile cardiomyopathy. *Lancet* **336:**1452, 1990.
776. Ito T, Hattori K, Obayashi T, Tanaka M, Sugiyama S, Ozawa T: Mitochondrial DNA mutations in cardiomyopathy. *Jpn Circ J* **56:**1045, 1992.
777. Cortopassi GA, Hutchin TP: Germline inheritance of a rare mtDNA variant leads to greatly increased risk for Alzheimer's disease [Abstract 857]. *Am J Hum Genet* **55:**A149, 1994 (.
778. Leroy D, Norby S: A new human mtDNA polymorphism: $tRNA^{Gln}$/ 4336 T(C). *Clin Genet* **45:**109, 1994.
779. Hutchin T, Cortopassi G: A mitochondrial DNA clone is associated with increased risk for Alzheimer disease. *Proc Natl Acad Sci U S A* **92:**6892, 1995.
780. Vissing J, Salamon MB, Arlien-Soborg P, Norby S, Manta P, DiMauro S, Schmalbruch H: A new mitochondrial tRNA(Met) gene mutation in a patient with dystrophic muscle and exercise intolerance. *Neurology* **50:**1875, 1998.
781. Silvestri G, Rana M, DiMuzio A, Uncini A, Tonali P, Servidei S: A late-onset mitochondrial myopathy is associated with a novel mitochondrial DNA (mtDNA) point mutation in the tRNA(Trp) gene. *Neuromuscul Disord* **8:**291, 1998.
782. Nelson I, Hanna MG, Alsanjari N, Scaravilli F, Morgan-Hughes JA, Harding AE: A new mitochondrial DNA mutation associated with progressive dementia and chorea: A clinical, pathological, and molecular genetic study. *Ann Neurol* **37:**400, 1995.
783. Munscher C, Muller-Hocker J, Kadenbach B: Human aging is associated with various point mutations in tRNA genes of mitochondrial DNA. *Biol Chem Hoppe-Seyler* **374:**1099, 1993.
784. Hao H, Moraes CT: A disease-associated G5703A mutation in human mitochondrial DNA causes a conformational change and a marked decrease in steady-state levels of mitochondrial tRNA(Asn). *Mol Cell Biol* **17:**6831, 1997.
785. Reid FM, Vernham GA, Jacobs HT: A novel mitochondrial point mutation in a maternal pedigree with sensorineural deafness. *Hum Mutat* **3:**243, 1994.
786. Reid FM, Vernham GA, Jacobs HT: Complete mtDNA sequence of a patient in a maternal pedigree with sensorineural deafness. *Hum Mol Genet* **3:**1435, 1994.
787. Vernham GA, Reid FM, Rundle PA, Jacobs HT: Bilateral sensorineural hearing loss in members of a maternal lineage with mitochondrial point mutation. *Clin Otolaryngol* **19:**314, 1994.
788. Guan MX, Enriquez JA, Fischel-Ghodsian N, Puranam RS, Lin CP, Maw MA, Attardi G: The deafness-associated mitochondrial DNA mutation at position 7445, which affects tRNASer(UCN) precursor processing, has long-range effects on NADH dehydrogenase subunit ND6 gene expression. *Mol Cell Biol* **18:**5868, 1998.
789. Tiranti V, Chariot P, Carella F, Toscano A, Soliveri P, Girlanda P, Carrara F, et al.: Maternally inherited hearing loss, ataxia and myoclonus associated with a novel point mutation in mitochondrial $tRNA^{Ser(UCN)}$ gene. *Hum Mol Genet* **4:**1421, 1995.
790. Jaksch M, Klopstock T, Kurlemann G, Dorner M, Hofmann S, Kleinle S, Hegemann S, et al.: Progressive myoclonus epilepsy and mitochondrial myopathy associated with mutations in the tRNA(Ser(UCN)) gene. *Ann Neurol* **44:**635, 1998.
791. Jaksch M, Hofmann S, Kleinle S, Liechti-Gallati S, Pongratz DE, Muller-Hocker J, Jedele KB, et al.: A systematic mutation screen of 10 nuclear and 25 mitochondrial candidate genes in 21 patients with cytochrome c oxidase (COX) deficiency shows tRNA(Ser)(UCN) mutations in a subgroup with syndromal encephalopathy. *J Med Genet* **35:**895, 1998.
792. Schuelke M, Bakker M, Stoltenburg G, Sperner J, von Moers A: Epilepsia partialis continua associated with a homoplasmic mitochondrial tRNA(Ser(UCN)) mutation. *Ann Neurol* **44:**700, 1998.
793. Nakamura M, Nakano S, Goto Y, Ozawa M, Nagahama Y, Fukuyama H, Akiguchi I, et al.: A novel point mutation in the mitochondrial $tRNA^{Ser(UCN)}$ gene detected in a family with MERRF/MELAS overlap syndrome. *Biochem Biophys Res Commun* **214:**86, 1995.
794. Kameoka K, Isotani H, Tanaka K, Azukari K, Fujimura Y, Shiota Y, Sasaki E, et al.: Novel mitochondrial DNA mutation in tRNA(Lys) (8296A $\rightarrow$ G) associated with diabetes. *Biochem Biophys Res Commun* **245:**523, 1998.
795. Kameoka K, Isotani H, Tanaka K, Kitaoka H, Ohsawa N: Impaired insulin secretion in Japanese diabetic subjects with an A-to-G mutation at nucleotide 8296 of the mitochondrial DNA in tRNA(Lys) [Letter]. *Diabetes Care* **21:**2034, 1998.
796. Verma A, Piccoli DA, Bonilla E, Berry GT, DiMauro S, Moraes CT: A novel mitochondrial G8313A mutation associated with prominent initial gastrointestinal symptoms and progressive encephaloneuropathy. *Pediatr Res* **42:**448, 1997.
797. Yoneda M, Tanno Y, Horai S, Ozawa T, Miyatake T, Tsuji S: A common mitochondrial DNA mutation in the $tRNA^{Lys}$ of patients with myoclonus epilepsy associated with ragged-red fibers. *Biochem Int* **21:**789, 1990.
798. Shoffner JM, Lott MT, Wallace DC: MERRF: A model disease for understanding the principles of mitochondrial genetics. *Rev Neurol (Paris)* **147:**431, 1991.
799. Tanno Y, Yondea M, Nonaka I, Tanaka K, Miyatake T, Tsuji S: Quantitation of mitochondrial DNA carrying $tRNA^{Lys}$ mutation in MERRF patients. *Biochem Biophys Res Commun* **179:**880, 1991.
800. Silvestri G, Moraes CT, Shanske S, Oh SJ, DiMauro S: A new mtDNA mutation in the $tRNA^{Lys}$ gene associated with myoclonic epilepsy and ragged-red fibers (MERRF). *Am J Hum Genet* **51:**1213, 1992.
801. Zeviani M, Muntoni F, Savarese N, Serra G, Tiranti V, Carrara F, Mariotti C, et al.: A MERRF/MELAS overlap syndrome associated with a new point mutation in the mitochondrial DNA $tRNA^{Lys}$ gene. *Eur J Hum Genet* **1:**80, 1993.

802. Ozawa M, Nishino I, Horai S, Nonaka I, Goto YI: Myoclonus epilepsy associated with ragged-red fibers: a G-to-A mutation at nucleotide pair 8363 in mitochondrial tRNA(Lys) in two families [Comments]. *Muscle Nerve* **20:**271, 1997.
803. Merante F, Tein I, Benson L, Robinson BH: Maternally inherited hypertrophic cardiomyopathy due to a novel T-to-C transition at nucleotide 9997 in the mitochondrial tRNA(glycine) gene. *Am J Hum Genet* **55:**437, 1994.
804. Bidooki SK, Johnson MA, Chrzanowska-Lightowlers Z, Bindoff LA, Lightowlers RN: Intracellular mitochondrial triplasmy in a patient with two heteroplasmic base changes. *Am J Hum Genet* **60:**1430, 1997.
805. Lynn S, Wardell T, Johnson MA, Chinnery PF, Daly ME, Walker M, Turnbull DM: Mitochondrial diabetes: investigation and identification of a novel mutation. *Diabetes* **47:**1800, 1998.
806. Marzuki S, Noer AS, Letrit P, Thyagarajan D, Kapsa R, Utthanaphol P, Byrne E: Normal variants of human mitochondrial DNA and translation products: the building of a reference data base. *Hum Genet* **88:**139, 1991.
807. van den Ouweland JM, Bruining GJ, Lindhout D, Wit JM, Veldhuyzen BF, Maassen JA: Mutations in mitochondrial tRNA genes: Non-linkage with syndromes of Wolfram and chronic progressive external ophthalmoplegia. *Nucleic Acids Res* **20:**679, 1992.
808. Houshmand M, Larsson NG, Holme E, Oldfors A, Tulinius MH, Andersen O: Automatic sequencing of mitochondrial tRNA genes in patients with mitochondrial encephalomyopathy. *Biochim Biophys Acta* **1226:**49, 1994.
809. Weber K, Wilson JN, Taylor L, Brierley E, Johnson MA, Turnbull DM, Bindoff LA: A new mtDNA mutation showing accumulation with time and restriction to skeletal muscle. *Am J Hum Genet* **60:**373, 1997.
810. Hanna MG, Nelson I, Sweeney MG, Cooper JM, Watkins PJ, Morgan-Hughes JA, Harding AE: Congenital encephalomyopathy and adult-onset myopathey and diabetes mellitus: Different phenotypic associations of a new heteroplasmic mtDNA tRNA glutamic acid mutation. *Am J Hum Genet* **56:**1026, 1995.
811. Hao H, Bonilla E, Manfredi G, DiMauro S, Moraes CT: Segregation patterns of a novel mutation in the mitochondrial tRNA glutamic acid gene associated with myopathy and diabetes mellitus. *Am J Hum Genet* **56:**1017, 1995.
812. Vialettes BH, Paquis-Flucklinger V, Pelissier JF, Bendahan D, Narbonne H, Silvestre-Aillaud P, Montfort MF, et al.: Phenotypic expression of diabetes secondary to a T14709C mutation of mitochondrial DNA. Comparison with MIDD syndrome (A3243G mutation): A case report. *Diabetes Care* **20:**1731, 1997.
813. Nishino I, Seki A, Maegaki Y, Takeshita K, Horai S, Nonaka I, Goto Y: A novel mutation in the mitochondrial $tRNA^{Thr}$ gene associated with a mitochondrial encephalomyopathy. *Biochem Biophys Res Commun* **225:**180, 1996.
814. Seki A, Nishino I, Goto Y, Maegaki Y, Koeda T: Mitochondrial encephalomyopathy with 15915 mutation: Clinical report. *Pediatr Neurol* **17:**161, 1997.
815. Yoon KL, Aprille JR, Ernst SG: Mitochondrial $tRNA^{Thr}$ mutation in fatal infantile respiratory enzyme deficiency. *Biochem Biophys Res Commun* **176:**1112, 1991.
816. Brown MD, Torroni A, Shoffner JM, Wallace DC: Mitochondrial $tRNA^{Thr}$ mutations and lethal infantile mitochondrial myopathy. *Am J Hum Genet* **51:**446, 1992.
817. Yoon KL, Ernst SG, Rasmussen C, Dooling EC, Aprille JR: Mitochondrial disorder associated with newborn cardiopulmonary arrest. *Pediatr Res* **33:**433, 1993.
818. Ozawa T, Tanaka M, Sugiyama S, Ino H, Ohno K, Hattori K, Ohbayashi T, et al.: Patients with idiopathic cardiomyopathy belong to the same mitochondrial DNA gene family of Parkinson's disease and mitochondrial encephalomyopathy. *Biochem Biophys Res Commun* **177:**518, 1991.
819. Seneca S, Lissens W, Liebaers I, van den Bergh P, Nassogne MC, Benatar A, de Meirleir L: Pitfalls in the diagnosis of mtDNA mutations [Letter]. *J Med Genet* **35:**963, 1998.
820. Moraes CT, Ciacci F, Bonilla E, Ionasescu V, Schon EA, DiMauro S: A mitochondrial tRNA anticodon swap associated with a muscle disease. *Nat Genet* **4:**284, 1993.
821. Ionasescu VV, Hart M, DiMauro S, Moraes CT: Clinical and morphologic features of a myopathy associated with a point mutation in the mitochondrial $tRNA^{Pro}$ gene. *Neurology* **44:**975, 1994.
822. Howell N, Bogolin C, Jamieson R, Marenda DR, Mackey DA: mtDNA mutations that cause optic neuropathy: how do we know? [Letter]. *Am J Hum Genet* **62:**196, 1998.
823. Campuzano V, Montermini L, Molto MD, Pianese L, Cossee M, Cavalcanti F, Monros E, et al.: Friedreich's ataxia: autosomal recessive disease caused by an intronic GAA triplet repeat expansion [Comments]. *Science* **271:**1423, 1996.
824. Wallace DC: Mitochodrial genes and disease. *Hosp Pract (Off Ed)* **21:**77, 1986.
825. Wallace DC: Mitochondrial diseases in man and mouse. *Science* **283:**1482, 1999.
826. Koehler CM, Merchant S, Oppliger W, Schmid K, Jarosch E, Dolfini L, Junne T, et al.: Tim9p, an essential partner subunit of Tim10p for the import of mitochondrial carrier proteins. *EMBO J* **17:**6477, 1998.
827. Simon RP, Aminoff MJ, Greenberg DA: *Clinical Neurology.* Stamford, CT, Appleton & Lange, 1999.

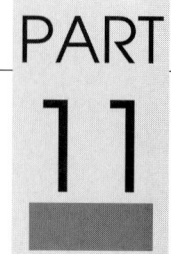

PURINES AND PYRIMIDINES

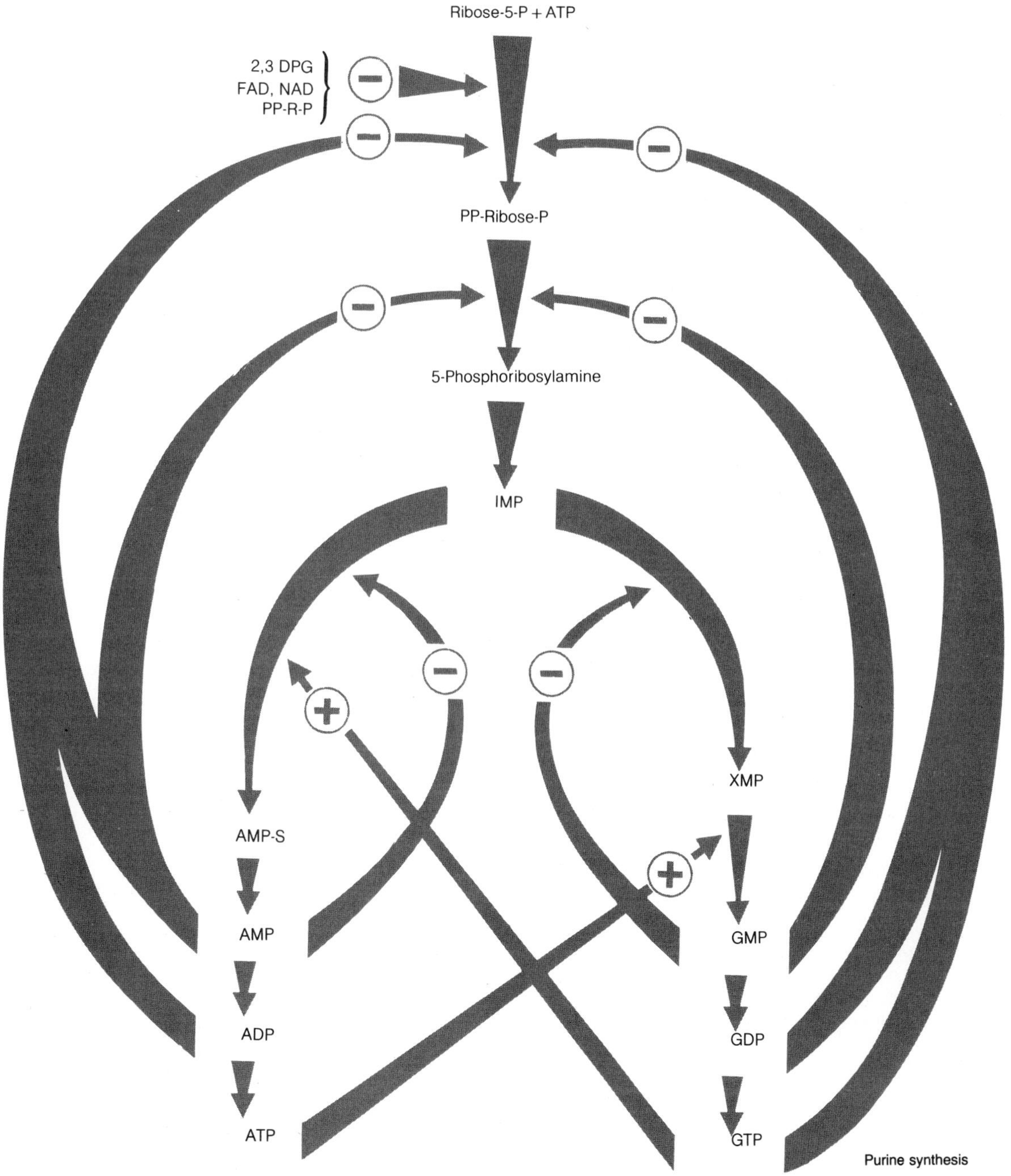

Ribose-5-P + ATP

2,3 DPG
FAD, NAD
PP-R-P

PP-Ribose-P

5-Phosphoribosylamine

IMP

AMP-S

AMP

ADP

ATP

XMP

GMP

GDP

GTP

Purine synthesis

CHAPTER 106

Hyperuricemia and Gout

Michael A. Becker

1. **Gout (urate crystal deposition disease) is characterized by hyperuricemia and manifested by recurrent attacks of acute inflammatory arthritis; accumulation of urate crystals to form tophaceous deposits; uric acid urolithiasis, which may precede arthritis or punctuate the course of gout; and nephropathy, which, although common among patients with gout, is usually due to comorbid causes.**
2. **Hyperuricemia is appropriately defined as serum urate concentrations exceeding 7.0 mg/dl in men and 6.0 mg/dl in women, employing enzyme-based (uricase) methods of measurement. Serum urate concentrations exceeding 7.0 mg/dl are associated with increased risk for gouty arthritis and uric acid urolithiasis, and the prevalence of these manifestations correlates strongly with the magnitude of hyperuricemia in population studies.**
3. **Serum urate values vary considerably among populations sampled and are influenced by many factors, including ethnic background, age, sex, body weight, and body surface area. Renal function, blood pressure, and use of ethanol and a variety of pharmacologic agents are important determinants of urate levels in many individuals.**
4. **Hyperuricemia is a common biochemical aberration and is a necessary but not sufficient precondition for development of the gouty state. The majority of hyperuricemic individuals never manifest the clinical features of gout, and moderate hyperuricemia appears to confer no independent risk for development of functionally significant renal impairment. In addition, there is no evidence that hyperuricemia (or gout) plays a causal role in the important disorders with which it is frequently associated, such as obesity, hyperlipidemia, hypertension, atherosclerosis, and the syndrome of hyperinsulinemia and resistance to insulin action.**
5. **Acute gouty arthritis is triggered when monosodium urate crystals initiate an inflammatory response. Multiple factors regulate both urate crystal deposition and the inflammatory response, but direct urate crystal interactions with neutrophils and with inflammatory mediator pathways that potentiate neutrophil activation and entry into the joint are crucial to the induction and perpetuation of the attack.**
6. **Uric acid is the end product of human purine metabolism, a complex of interacting biochemical pathways whereby (1) purine nucleotides are synthesized either from nonpurine precursors (purine synthesis *de novo*) or from dietary purines or products of purine nucleotide interconversion and degradation reactions (purine salvage); (2) purine nucleotides are interconverted to provide adequate supplies of adenylates and guanylates for nucleic acid synthesis and for the additional essential roles of purine compounds in differentiated cell activation, cellular energy metabolism, and nonpurine biosynthetic and catabolic pathways; and (3) purines are degraded to uric acid in a series of catabolic reactions. These pathways are regulated and integrated at several levels.**
7. **Uric acid production and excretion are balanced processes in which, under normal circumstances, about two thirds of the uric acid turned over daily is excreted by the kidneys and virtually all the rest is eliminated via intestinal bacterial uricolysis. In renal failure and in many hyperuricemic individuals, extrarenal uric acid disposal is increased.**
8. **Serum urate concentration is a function of both synthetic and degradative rates. Hyperuricemia may result from uric acid overproduction or underexcretion or from a combination of both mechanisms. Hyperuricemia may be primary or the secondary result of a concurrent condition. Excessive dietary purine intake is rarely a cause of sustained hyperuricemia.**
9. **Primary gout is a biochemically and genetically heterogeneous category, presumably attributable to inborn metabolic errors altering uric acid homeostasis. The biochemical defects in the majority of patients are not yet defined. In most gouty subjects, there is reduced renal fractional clearance of urate, which is most prominent in individuals with normal or reduced daily urinary uric acid excretion. This defect may be the major or sole basis of hyperuricemia.**
10. **Three different inherited enzyme defects result in early development of marked hyperuricemia and gout. In glucose-6-phosphatase deficiency (glycogen storage disease type I), hyperuricemia results from both excessive uric acid production and impaired uric acid excretion. In severe and partial deficiencies of hypoxanthine-guanine phosphoribosyltransferase (HPRT) and in superactivity of 5-phosphoribosyl-1-pyrophosphate synthetase (PRS), the basis of hyperuricemia is purine nucleotide and uric acid overproduction. Accelerated purine synthesis in these two disorders is a consequence of increased intracellular availability of PP-ribose-P, a critical regulatory intermediate in the pathway of purine synthesis *de novo*. The precise biochemical bases of neurologic manifestations encountered in patients with severe HPRT deficiency or defects in the regulation of PRS activity remain unknown.**
11. **Both genetic and environmental factors contribute to the high prevalence of hyperuricemia in many populations. Cumulative effects of multiple genes are more prominent when heterogeneous populations are studied. Single gene influences, some autosomal dominantly transmitted and some X-linked, are identifiable in studies of less genetically diverse groups. Glucose-6-phosphatase deficiency is an autosomal recessive trait. Both HPRT deficiency and PRS superactivity are X-linked traits.**

A list of standard abbreviations is located immediately preceding the index in each volume. Nonstandard abbreviations used in this chapter include: AmidoPRT = amidophosphoribosyltransferase; GFR = glomerular filtration rate; HPRT = hypoxanthine-guanine phosphoribosyltransferase; PP-ribose-P = 5-phosphoribosyl-1-pyrophosphate; PRS = PP-ribose-P synthetase; Rib-5-P = ribose-5-phosphate.

12. **Although accelerated PP-ribose-P and purine nucleotide synthesis characterize all instances of PRS superactivity, the kinetic mechanisms and genetic defects underlying this disorder are heterogeneous. Point mutations in *PRPS1*, one of two X-linked genes encoding highly homologous PRS isoforms, result in mutant PRS1 enzymes with defective allosteric properties and account for PRS superactivity with resistance to inhibition of enzyme activity by purine nucleotides. In contrast, PRS1 structure and regulation of PRS activity are normal in another form of PRS overactivity ("catalytic superactivity"), but the PRS1 isoform is overexpressed as a consequence of selectively accelerated transcription of *PRPS1*.**
13. **Specific and effective pharmacologic therapy for gout is available. Anti-inflammatory drugs and colchicine are used to treat and prevent acute gouty attacks. Two classes of antihyperuricemic agents are available to lower serum urate levels into the normal range, thus reducing the frequency of acute gouty arthritis, tophus formation, and urolithiasis. Uricosuric agents inhibit renal tubular post-secretory reabsorption of uric acid, promoting renal uric acid excretion. Uric acid production is decreased by administration of allopurinol, a purine base analogue that inhibits xanthine oxidase.**

DEFINITIONS AND BACKGROUND

Deposition of monosodium urate and uric acid crystals in tissues as a result of supersaturation of extracellular fluids with urate, the end product of human purine metabolism, constitutes the fundamental pathophysiologic event defining gout. Because many factors may promote urate supersaturation, gout (urate deposition disease) may be regarded as a clinical syndrome reflecting a heterogeneous group of genetic and acquired metabolic aberrations.[1] The range of clinical manifestations of gout is narrow and includes recurrent attacks of a characteristic acute inflammatory arthritis (acute gouty arthritis); accumulation of potentially destructive and deforming crystalline aggregates (tophi), especially in connective tissue structures; uric acid urolithiasis; and, uncommonly, renal impairment. Virtually all patients with gout show hyperuricemia (urate supersaturation of serum) at some point in the course of their disease; however, only a minority of hyperuricemic individuals ever experience a clinical event resulting from urate deposition.[2] Hyperuricemia is the necessary pathogenetic common denominator predisposing to gout, but this biochemical aberration should be distinguished from the disease state.

The current level of pathogenetic understanding and the effectiveness of contemporary management of gout represent triumphs of biomedical research. Prior to 1950, gout was a major clinical problem despite two millennia of careful and accurate disease descriptions and a century of recognition of the cause-and-effect relationship between urate deposition and gouty inflammation.[1] In the past 50 years, the elucidation of purine biochemistry, the discovery of inborn errors of metabolism leading to hyperuricemia, and the development of effective therapies to reduce serum urate concentration have led to success in controlling the consequences of the gouty state. Although the precise metabolic basis for gout in the majority of affected patients remains uncertain, successful management is nearly always possible. Moreover, the evolution of knowledge of the regulation of purine metabolic pathways, fostered in large part through the study of inherited enzyme defects, provides an important model for the study of inborn errors of metabolism. Few examples better illustrate the classical progression of scientific sophistication from bedside observation to the precise molecular genetic level.

Epidemiology of Hyperuricemia and Gout

Automated enzymatic (uricase) methods that measure production of H_2O_2 generated in the oxidation of urate have provided greater accuracy and reproducibility in the clinical measurement of serum and urinary uric acid than prior colorimetric methods.[3] Automated methods approach in accuracy the uricase-spectrophotometric assay,[4] although the latter remains preferable for research studies. At the concentrations of sodium present in extracellular fluids, the theoretic limit of solubility of monosodium urate in serum at 37°C is about 6.5 mg/dl, providing a physical chemical definition of hyperuricemia.[5] Most population studies utilizing the uricase-spectrophotometric method have defined upper limits of normal serum urate [mean ± 2 standard deviations (SD)] of about 7.0 mg/dl in adult men and 6.0 mg/dl in premenopausal women.[1] The distribution of serum urate values is not symmetrical about the mean; the majority of values falling outside 2 SD are high. Serum urate values in excess of 7.0 mg/dl confer increased risk for gouty arthritis[6,7] and urolithiasis.[7]

Serum urate concentrations vary with age in patterns that are distinctive in men and women. Childhood serum urate concentrations of 3 to 4 mg/dl increase during male puberty[1,8] to adult levels and remain rather constant or increase slightly thereafter.[9] In contrast, women show little change in urate concentrations until the menopause, when values increase to approach those in adult men.[5] Higher urinary fractional excretion of urate in women, due to lower tubular urate postsecretory reabsorption, is most likely related to the action of estrogenic compounds, but the precise mechanism is not well defined.[10,11]

Among the many factors influencing serum urate levels in adults are ethnic background (e.g., indigenous Pacific islanders have significantly higher mean serum urate levels than other population groups),[12–14] anthropomorphic and social factors, and physiologic/pharmacologic determinants such as body weight, fat distribution,[15] blood pressure,[16] drug and alcohol intake, and renal function.[1] The annual incidence of gout is estimated at 0.20 to 0.35 per 1000 persons, and an overall prevalence of 2 to 3 per 1000 has been reported for North America and Europe.[1] Increasing age and serum urate concentration as well as male gender are associated with increased prevalence.[7,17,18] For example, among French men 35 to 44 years of age, the prevalence of gout was 11 per 1000 previously asymptomatic men in the group 35 to 39 years of age and 20 per 1000 in those 40 to 44 years of age.[17] In the New Zealand Maori population, with increased mean serum urate levels, the prevalence of gout in adult males and females is reported to exceed 10 and 4 percent, respectively.[12,13] The overall annual incidence rate of gout is 4.9 percent in individuals with urate levels exceeding 9 mg/dl, 0.5 percent with concentrations between 7.0 and 8.9 mg/dl, and 0.1 percent with urate values less than 7.0 mg/dl.[6] Although the 5-year cumulative incidence of gout among individuals with serum urate values greater than 9 mg/dl is reported to be 22 percent, patients with such levels represent only about 20 percent of most gouty populations.[6,7]

Asymptomatic Hyperuricemia

Asymptomatic hyperuricemia is the state in which urate concentration is abnormally high but symptoms have not occurred. It is common among adult men and elderly women. For example, a prevalence rate of 5 to 8 percent has been estimated for asymptomatic hyperuricemia among American men. Hyperuricemia frequently begins at puberty in men and may persist throughout life. In both prospective and retrospective studies assessing the consequences of hyperuricemia and gout on long-term renal function, these variables impose no substantial independent risk for the development of chronic renal insufficiency.[6,19–23] In fact, in the range of serum urate values for which sufficient information is available (up to 13 mg/dl in men and 10 mg/dl in women), hyperuricemia appears to be of no clinical importance in determining the course of renal function.[20]

CLINICAL DESCRIPTION

Symptomatic manifestations of gout arise in only the minority of hyperuricemic persons, and usually only after 20 or 30 years of sustained hyperuricemia.[1] In the natural history of the untreated disorder, acute gouty arthritis, intercritical gout, and chronic tophaceous gout represent stages in progressive urate crystal deposition disease, with uric acid urolithiasis preceding or punctuating the course. However, antihyperuricemic drug therapies have substantially altered the classic description by reducing the frequency of gouty arthritis, urolithiasis, and tophus formation.

Acute Gouty Arthritis

Numerous vivid descriptions of acute gouty arthritis have been given, such as that of Sydenham:

> **The patient goes to bed and sleeps quietly till about two in the morning when he is awakened by a pain which usually seizes the great toe, but sometimes the heel, ankle, or instep. The pain resembles that of a dislocated bone... and is immediately preceded by a chillness and slight fever in proportion to the pain which is mild at first but grows gradually more violent every hour; sometimes resembling a laceration of ligaments, sometimes the gnawing of a dog, and sometimes a weight and constriction of the parts affected, which becomes so exquisitely painful as not to endure the weight of the clothes nor the shaking of the room from a person walking briskly therein.[24]**

Episodes of painful inflammatory arthritis are the most common manifestation of gout. Initial attacks are self-limited, remitting completely after hours to several weeks and are monoarticular in 80 to 90 percent of instances.[1] About half involve the first metatarsophalangeal joint (podagra)[25] (Fig. 106-1). Polyarticular episodes and accompanying constitutional features (fever, leukocytosis, increased sedimentation rate) are more common during recurrences. The peak incidence of gouty arthritis in men is during the fourth to sixth decades of life,[1,25] which contrasts with the sixth to eighth decade peak onset in women.[26–29] Childhood-, juvenile-, or early adult-onset gout or gout in a premenopausal woman should suggest the possibility of an underlying inherited enzyme defect, a hereditary or toxic renal disorder, or ingestion of an agent affecting uric acid metabolism.[30]

The intensity of inflammation and the usual monoarticular distribution of gouty arthritis always warrant differentiation from septic arthritis (or even cellulitis), calcium pyrophosphate crystal deposition disease (pseudogout), basic calcium phosphate crystal deposition disease,[31,32] and acute trauma. The diagnosis of acute gouty arthritis can be made with certainty only by identification of negatively birefringent monosodium urate crystals in neutrophilic leukocytes by polarizing light microscopic examination of synovial fluid from an affected joint.[1] However, other clinical features of gouty inflammation are often distinctive enough to be helpful diagnostically.[1] Up to 90 percent of affected men have

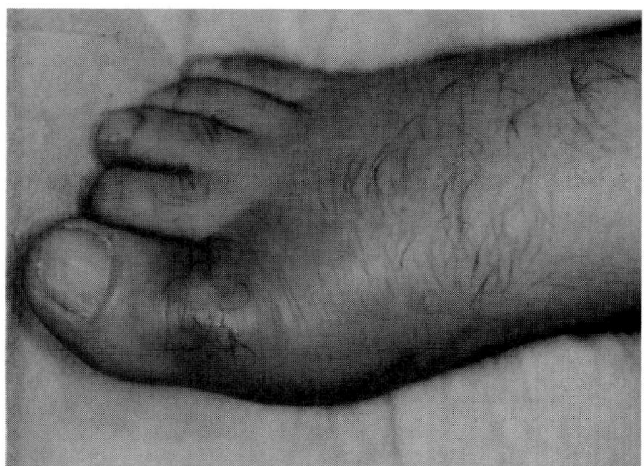

Fig. 106-1 Acute gouty arthritis of the first metatarsophalangeal joint (podagra). Intense swelling and discoloration (redness) spreading well beyond the confines of the joint (periarticular inflammation) are typical of acute gout.

podagra at some point in the disease. Other target joints include mid-tarsal joints, ankles, and knees, with upper extremity involvement more common in wrists, interphalangeal joints, and elbows (olecranon bursa). Gout of the shoulders, hips, spine, and sacroiliac joints is uncommon except in advanced disease. Resolution of acute gouty arthritis is frequently accompanied by desquamation of the overlying skin, and the subsequent period of complete freedom from joint symptoms is an important diagnostic clue.

Circumstances that appear capable of inciting attacks of gouty arthritis include trauma, surgery, excessive ingestion of alcohol or purine-rich foods, starvation, and administration of certain drugs. Each of these circumstances is associated with either hyperuricemia or hypouricemia, but the precise means by which these sometimes abrupt changes in extracellular urate concentrations provoke acute inflammation is uncertain. In fact, serum urate concentrations are normal in up to 40 percent of individuals during episodes of acute gouty arthritis.[33] Alcohol binges, overeating, or starvation can induce hyperuricemia,[1] as can thiazide diuretics[26–30,34] and cyclosporine.[34–38] On the other hand, acute gouty arthritis in the setting of intravenous hyperalimentation,[39] allopurinol or uricosuric agent treatment for hyperuricemia, surgery, or trauma may occur despite hypouricemia.[1]

Acute gout is the prototype for crystal-induced synovitis.[40] Extracellular fluid urate supersaturation is necessary but not sufficient for production of acute gouty inflammation. Among additional factors that may regulate urate crystal deposition in articular tissues are lower temperature,[41] proteoglycan content, changes in pH, trauma, aging, and local increases in urate concentrations resulting from more rapid fluid than urate reabsorption from joint structures.[42]

The pathophysiology of acute gouty inflammation has long centered on the urate crystal–polymorphonuclear leukocyte interaction.[40,43] Protein-coated free urate crystals stimulate the formation of multiple inflammatory mediators from serum proteins (including C5a, bradykinin, and kallikrein) and from synovial lining cells [e.g., cyclooxygenase and lipoxygenase arachidonate metabolites, lysosomal proteases, tumor necrosis factor α (TNF-α), the chemokine KC/GROα,[44] and interleukin 1 (IL-1), IL-6, and IL-8]. Urate crystal induction of cyclooxygenase 2 (COX-2) in human monocytes has recently been described.[45] Neutrophil ingress is promoted by chemotactic properties of these mediators and by a specific glycoprotein crystal-induced chemotactic factor elaborated on neutrophil phagocytosis of urate crystals.[46] This process is enhanced by endothelial cell activation by IL-1 and TNF-α and is accompanied by activation of neutrophils both by the soluble mediators and by direct contact of the cells with urate crystals. Recruitment and activation of neutrophils are ongoing processes, constituting a cycle necessary to perpetuate gouty inflammation because of the limited functional life span of neutrophils.[40] Systemic release of interleukins and TNF-α from the site of gouty inflammation into the circulation is likely responsible for the constitutional accompaniments of some gouty attacks and also may promote inflammation in other joints, as in polyarticular attacks.[43]

Activated neutrophils ingest urate crystals within phagosomes, which ultimately merge with lysosomes. Crystal binding to lysosomal membranes, probably through electrostatic interaction, results in membrane lysis and augmentation of the inflammatory response by released lysosomal hydrolases and mediators and by superoxide anions also generated in the neutrophil-crystal interaction.[40]

The changing nature of the protein components coating urate crystals in the course of gouty inflammation appears to explain experimental observations implicating the proteins adhering to crystals as both promoters and inhibitors of the process. For example, apolipoprotein B (Apo B) and Apo E increasingly replace proinflammatory and complement-activating immunoglobulin G (IgG) and C-reactive protein on crystals during the course of the acute attack and inhibit crystal phagocytosis, superoxide generation, leukotriene elaboration, and neutrophil cytolysis.[40,43,47] Thus, the fact that urate crystals may exist for long periods in joint structures and tophi with no evident inflammatory response may be due in part to the antiphlogistic properties of proteins adhering to crystal surfaces. The details governing the self-limited nature of acute gouty attacks remain under investigation. The roles of additional cytokines and inhibitors, neutrophil modulatory responses, central humoral responses, crystal clearance, and crystal properties have been reviewed.[43]

Intercritical Gout

Intercritical periods are the intervals between gouty attacks. For most untreated patients, the first intercritical period lasts less than a year. In one series, 62 percent of patients had second attacks within the first year and 78 percent within 2 years.[1] Seven percent of patients were free of recurrences for 10 years or more. With repeated recurrences, intercritical periods generally diminish in length. Establishing a diagnosis of gout may be difficult during an intercritical period. Aspiration of a previously inflamed joint can often corroborate the diagnosis, especially in untreated patients. In one study, 36 of 37 aspirates from previously affected joints were positive for urate crystals.[48] Crystals were identified, however, in only 50 percent of aspirates from such joints in patients receiving urate-lowering drugs and in only 22 percent of samples from joints not previously involved. This test is also of limited value in renal failure patients because of occasional false-positive results.

Chronic Tophaceous Gout

After a number of years in which the untreated patient may experience a series of more severe, long-lasting, and polyarticular attacks, pain-free intercritical periods may disappear entirely. This stage of chronic polyarticular gout may be punctuated by acute attacks, occurring in sequence, in a migratory pattern, or in a cluster of adjacent joints.

Accompanying these developments, deposition of solid urate (tophi) often occurs in articular and other connective tissues, with ultimate development of a destructive arthropathy (Fig. 106-2). The identification of tophi with or prior to the initial gouty attack has been reported in 0.5 percent of subjects with gout secondary to myeloproliferative disease[1] and in patients with type 1 glycogen storage disease (see Chap. 71), and with the Lesch-Nyhan syndrome (see Chap. 107). This occurrence was thought to be rare in patients with primary gout[49] (gout occurring in the absence of an identifiable associated disorder) but has been described with increasing frequency in recent years.[50–52] Even in untreated patients, chronic tophaceous gout is usually a late occurrence, visible tophi appearing an average of 11.6 years (range 3–42 years) after the initial attack.[53] In one series, 72 percent of patients had tophi after 20 years, and severe tophaceous involvement was found in 24 percent.[54] With uricosuric agents and allopurinol, reduction in the frequency of chronic tophaceous gout to as low as 3 percent has been documented,[55] but certain patient groups remain at unusual risk: poorly instructed or noncompliant patients; postmenopausal women; elderly patients of both sexes whose osteoarthritic changes mask coexistent gout; and organ transplant patients receiving cyclosporine A.

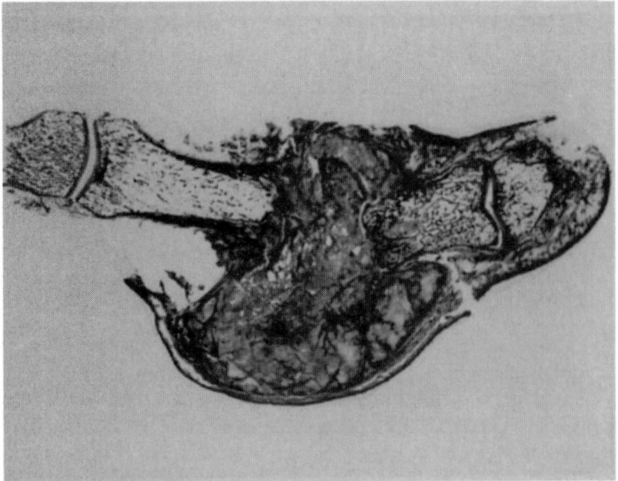

Fig. 106-2 Chronic tophaceous gout. In this sagittal section of a surgical specimen, complete destruction of the first metatarsophalangeal joint is evident. Light microscopy with polarization confirmed replacement of articular and adjacent bony structures as well as the subcutaneous layers by fibrous tissue containing relatively few chronic inflammatory cells but masses of monosodium urate crystals. The tarsometatarsal and interphalangeal joints remain intact. (*Courtesy of Dr. M.A. Simon, University of Chicago.*)

Tophaceous gout is associated with an early age of onset, a long duration of active but untreated disease, frequent attacks, high serum urate values, and a predilection for upper extremity and polyarticular episodes.[54,56,57] Additional factors in this progression are excessive ethanol consumption, diuretic use, and, especially, poor compliance or poor physician-patient communication.[56,57] Elderly patients, particularly women, who are receiving uricoretentive diuretics and anti-inflammatory drugs and who have mild renal insufficiency are another group at high risk for tophus formation and polyarticular gout.[26–29,58] In a particular subset of such individuals, nodal osteoarthritis of distal and proximal interphalageal joints delays the recognition of urate crystal deposition in these damaged joints, often for years.[26–29,59–62] years. Finally, transplant recipients receiving cyclosporine to prevent organ rejection have a substantial risk for gout and early tophus formation.[35–38]

Extraarticular sites of predilection for tophi include the helix of the ear, olecranon and prepatellar bursae, ulnar surfaces of the forearms, Achilles tendons, and finger pads.[63] In some instances, including finger pad tophi, urate crystal deposits may be intradermal rather than subcutaneous in location.[63,64] Tophi have been reported in virtually all parenchymal organs except the brain. Deposits may produce irregular and grotesque deformities on the hands or feet, with accompanying joint destruction and crippling. The atrophic skin overlying tophi may ulcerate and extrude white, chalky material composed of urate crystals. Rarely, ulcerated tophi become secondarily infected.

Radiologic changes early in gout are nonspecific and include periarticular and soft tissue swelling during acute episodes. Normal joint spaces and bone density are usually retained well into the disease. Degenerative changes (bony sclerosis, osteophytes, and subchondral cysts) may be present at onset, especially in bunion joints and in the interphalangeal joints of the hands and may represent prior osteoarthritis on which gout is superimposed.[59] With greater duration of gout, tophi may be seen as nodulated densities in soft tissues or in bone.[56] Bony erosions are frequent in chronic gout and are often seen with overlying tophi (Fig. 106-2). Gouty erosions appear as punched-out oval-shaped defects with sclerotic borders and, sometimes, rather characteristic overhanging edges of bone. Magnetic resonance and computed tomographic imaging have been applied to the identification of urate tophi in a variety of articular and organ structures, but the features of tophi with these imaging techniques do not appear sufficiently specific to allow definitive diagnosis.[65–67]

Renal Disease

Several types of renal disease occur in patients with gout, comprising the most frequent complication of hyperuricemia apart from arthritis and tophus formation.[1] Urate nephropathy is attributed to deposition of monosodium urate crystals in renal interstitial tissue. In contrast, uric acid nephropathy, caused by deposition of uric acid crystals from urine in the collecting tubules, renal pelvis, or ureter, can impair urine flow and be manifested by either acute uric acid nephropathy or uric acid calculi. Calcium oxalate urolithiasis also occurs more commonly in hyperuricemic than in normouricemic individuals.[68]

Urate Nephropathy. Urate nephropathy appears to be a distinct entity but is not believed to be an important contributor to declining renal function in the majority of patients with gout. Mild proteinuria (in 20–40 percent of patients with gout) and inability to generate a maximally concentrated urine are the earliest signs of urate nephropathy, preceding decreases in glomerular filtration rate (GFR).[1] These changes are observed even when the 30 to 40 percent of gouty patients with hypertension are excluded from the study population. Although renal failure accounts for 10 percent of deaths among patients with gout, coexistent hypertension,[16,23,69] ischemic heart disease,[69] chronic lead exposure,[69,70] anti-inflammatory drug use,[71] and prior renal insufficiency[23] rather than hyperuricemia appear to constitute primary renal risk factors in gouty individuals.

Acute Uric Acid Nephropathy. Acute renal failure as a result of precipitation of uric acid crystals in the collecting ducts and ureters most often results from rapid destruction of malignant cells during chemotherapy. Massive amounts of nucleic acids and nucleotides released during cytolysis are rapidly converted to uric acid. The acute tumor lysis syndrome[72] is defined by hyperuricemia, lactic acidosis, hyperphosphatemia, hyperkalemia, and hypocalcemia. Acute renal failure also may result from uric acid overproduction due to inherited enzyme defects, such as hypoxanthine-guanine phosphoribosyltransferase (HPRT) deficiency.

Uric Acid Urolithiasis. Uric acid stones account for nearly 10 percent of all urinary calculi in the United States and for a considerably higher proportion in nations with arid, hot climates.[73] Among patients with primary gout, the 10 to 25 percent incidence of renal stones is more than 1000 times that in the general population.[74] An even higher incidence (42 percent) was reported among patients with secondary gout. The incidence of stones in both instances increases with serum urate concentration[7] and urinary uric acid excretion,[74] reaching 50 percent with serum urate in excess of 13 mg/dl and daily urinary uric acid excretion greater than 1100 mg.[74] The risk for development of uric acid urolithiasis among patients with gouty arthritis is about 1 percent per year and among hyperuricemic persons about 0.27 percent per year.[20] Uric acid stones also occur in patients with no history of gout; in fact, only about 20 percent of these people are hyperuricemic. Lower fasting urinary pH and higher urine specific gravities may predispose these individuals to stone formation.[73]

Gouty patients also have an increased incidence of calcium stones, particularly calcium oxalate. Thirty percent of calcium oxalate stone formers have either hyperuricemia or hyperuricosuria,[68] and allopurinol administration significantly reduces recurrence rates,[75] supporting an etiologic association between formation of uric acid and calcium oxalate stones. Xanthine and oxypurinol calculi also have been reported in patients with Lesch-Nyhan syndrome receiving allopurinol.[76]

Other Nephropathy in Gout

Familial Juvenile Gouty Nephropathy. This term has been applied to families in which hyperuricemia and gout appear in multiple members of both sexes early in life in association with hypertension and progressive renal impairment, leading to death by age 40. Severely impaired renal uric acid excretion is demonstrable in this autosomal dominantly inherited disorder and precedes other overt evidence of renal dysfunction.[77] Affected patients do not exhibit other features suggestive of hereditary renal diseases in which hyperuricemia may precede renal insufficiency, such as polycystic kidney disease,[1] medullary cystic disease,[78] and focal tubulointerstitial nephropathy.[79] Stabilization of progressive renal impairment with allopurinol has been inconstant. It seems likely that a primary disruption of renal hemodynamics marked initially by reduced uric acid excretion underlies this disorder, which, as pointed out by Puig et al.,[80] may better be described as autosomal dominant nephropathy associated with hyperuricemia and gout.

Lead Intoxication. A renal defect in chronic lead intoxication appears to underlie complicating hyperuricemia and gout (saturnine gout), but the precise nature of the defect remains poorly defined. Lead levels in patients with primary gout but no overt lead exposure are higher than those in matched controls, suggesting that lead intoxication may be etiologic in some of these patients.[81] Also, the presence of more mobilizable lead in patients with gout and renal impairment than in gouty persons with normal kidney function implies a potentially important role for lead in the pathogenesis of gouty nephropathy.[70] No correlation was found, however, between the extent of reduced uric acid or creatinine clearance and the amount of lead excreted after ethylenediamine-tetraacetic acide (EDTA) infusion in a study of patients with histories of ingestion of unbonded distilled spirits ("moonshine").[69] The occurrence of gout in chronic renal failure may be a useful marker for lead overload.[82]

Disorders Associated with Hyperuricemia and Gout

Frequent coexistence of gout and hyperuricemia with a number of important disorders has long been recognized. The associated disorders include obesity,[9,83–85] hyperlipidemia,[83,86–88] hypertension,[16,83,89–91] atherosclerosis,[92–96] and ethanol abuse.[1,97,98] With the exception of ethanol abuse—which contributes to hyperuricemia by enhancing purine nucleotide catabolism to uric acid[97,98] and by reducing uric acid excretion through the induction of dehydration,[99] ketonemia,[100] and lactic acidemia—no cause-and-effect relationship of these diseases with gout and hyperuricemia has been established. In fact, the frequent presence of several of these metabolic and degenerative cardiovascular processes in hyperuricemic individuals makes the delineation of primary relationships extremely difficult. Although more extensive discussions of these relationships appear elswhere,[1,83] Emmerson[101] has commented on the complexity of such associations. Emmerson has identified independent or combined roles of obesity,[102–105] alcohol consumption,[106,107] and impaired glucose tolerance and excessive insulin secretion[108–112] in mediating both hypertriglyceridemia and hyperuricemia. With regard to impaired glucose tolerance and excessive insulin secretion, recent evidence supports the view that hyperuricemia resulting from reduced renal clearance of urate constitutes an intrinsic part of the metabolic syndrome of hyperinsulinemia and resistance to insulin action,[113] characterized by increased body mass index, abdominal obesity, hypertriglyceridemia, increased apolipoprotein B and very low density lipoprotein cholesterol, reduced high-density lipoprotein cholesterol, hypertension, and coronary artery disease.[110–113] Thus, hyperuricemic individuals, especially those with abdominal obesity, should be thought of as at risk for the consequences of insulin resistance.[101]

BIOCHEMICAL BASIS

Purine compounds contain the nine-member purine nucleus, consisting of fused pyrimidine and imidazole rings (Fig. 106-3).[1]

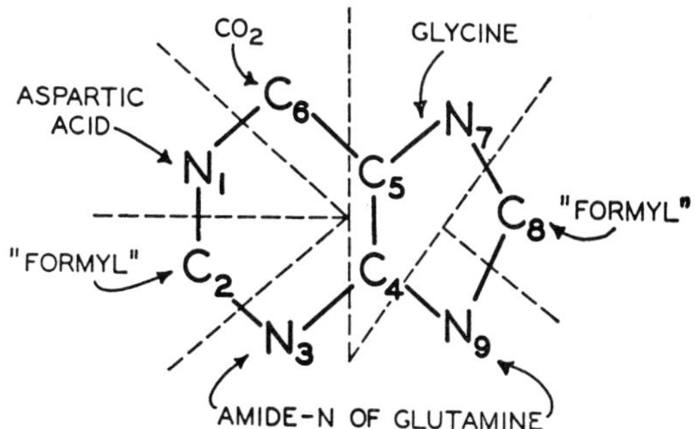

Fig. 106-3 Origins of the atoms of the purine ring.

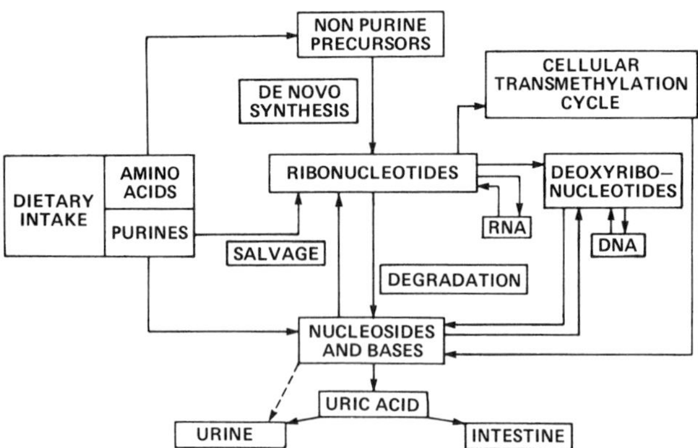

Fig. 106-4 Overview of human purine metabolism. There are two pathways leading to purine ribonucleotide synthesis. One is biosynthesis *de novo*; the second is the purine salvage pathway by which purine bases and nucleosides, including purines contained in the diet, can be resynthesized to ribonucleotides. Purine ribonucleotides can be converted to the diphosphate and triphosphate forms as well as to the cyclic nucleotides. The ribonucleoside diphosphate derivatives are converted to deoxyribonucleoside diphosphate derivatives, substrates for DNA synthesis. ATP is a substrate for the cellular transmethylation cycle to form S-adenosylmethionine. During cellular transmethylation, S-adenosylhomocysteine and adenosine are formed, and adenosine feeds into the pathway of purine nucleotide degradation. Purine ribonucleoside triphosphates are substrates for RNA synthesis, and nucleotides are products of RNA degradation. Purine ribonucleoside monophosphates are the main substrates for the pathway of purine nucleotide degradation, a pathway by which purine nucleotides are converted in humans to uric acid. (*Reprinted with permission from Fox IH: Disorders of purine and pyrimidine metabolism, Spittell JA (ed):* Clinical Medicine. *Vol 9. Philadelphia. Harper & Row, 1986, p 1.*)

The overall scheme of human purine metabolism is depicted in Fig. 106-4.

Pathways of Human Purine Metabolism

Purine Synthesis *De Novo*. Net contributions to body pools of purine compounds are provided only by dietary purine ingestion and endogenous synthesis of purine nucleotides from nonpurine precursors (Figs. 106-4 and 106-5). The pathway of purine synthesis *de novo* encompasses 11 enzymatic reactions by which the purine ring is sequentially constructed from small molecule donors on a ribose 5-phosphate backbone provided by 5-phosphoribosyl-1-pyrophosphate (PP-ribose-P) to form the parent purine compound inosine monophosphate (IMP).[1]

PP-ribose-P is a key regulatory substrate in purine synthesis *de novo*.[1,114,115] The PP-ribose-P synthetase (PRS) reaction in which this compound is produced from MgATP and ribose-5-phosphate (Rib-5-P) may be regarded as the initial step, even though this reaction is not uniquely committed to the pathway, because PP-ribose-P is also used in pyrimidine and pyridine nucleotide synthesis and in purine base salvage synthesis of purine nucleotides.[1,114] PP-ribose-P then condenses irreversibly with L-glutamine to generate 5-β-phosphoribosyl-1-amine in the first committed step, catalyzed by amidophosphoribosyltransferase (AmidoPRT). Alternative reactions resulting in formation of phosphoribosylamine have been described in bacterial, avian, and mammalian cell extracts, but their physiologic importance in human purine synthesis is uncertain.[1,116] The succeeding reactions in the pathway are directed at the stepwise construction and closure of the purine ring[1] and are summarized in Fig. 106-5.

Purine Nucleotide Interconversions and Catabolism. All newly synthesized purine compounds are ultimately derived from IMP, which serves as a branchpoint for alternative biosynthetic pathways leading to production of adenylates and guanylates, the major classes of purine nucleotides involved in RNA and DNA synthesis, or to the purine catabolic pathway, terminating in the irreversible formation of uric acid (Fig. 106-6). Two-step pathways accomplish interconversion of IMP to adenosine monophosphate (AMP) and guanosine monophosphate (GMP), the respective precursors of adenosine diphosphate (ADP) and adenosine triphosphate (ATP) and guanosine diphosphate (GDP) and guanosine triphosphate (GTP).[1] AMP is derived from IMP by way of adenylosuccinic acid (adenylosuccinate synthase [AMPS]), formed in a reaction requiring GTP as the energy source. In the conversion of IMP to GMP through the intermediate xanthosine 5-monophosphate (XMP), ATP provides the energy for transfer of the amido group of glutamine to the C-2 of XMP.[1] Thus, each of these nucleotide interconversion pathways depends on the availability of a product of the other. Deamination of AMP to IMP with the release of ammonia is an additional purine nucleotide interconversion reaction and is catalyzed by AMP deaminase. This reaction together with the two steps to formation of AMP from IMP comprise a purine nucleotide cycle, which is particularly active in muscle and is discussed in Chap. 110.

The purine catabolic pathway (Fig. 106-6) encompasses reactions through which purine nucleoside 5′-monophosphates are eventually degraded to uric acid in humans.[117] Dephosphorylation of AMP, IMP, XMP, and GMP to their corresponding ribonucleosides, with release of P_i, is catalyzed by nonspecific phosphatases and by specific purine 5′-nucleotidases. Both cytoplasmic and plasma membrane-bound (ecto) 5′-nucleotidases have been studied,[117–119] and an important role for cytoplasmic 5′-nucleotidase in the pathogenesis of the immunodeficiency disorders associated with inherited adenosine deaminase and purine nucleoside phosphorylase deficiencies has been proposed[119] (see Chaps. 109 and 185). Purine nucleoside phosphorylase cleaves the nucleosides inosine and guanosine (as well as their corresponding 2′-deoxynucleosides) and, less effectively, xanthosine to the respective purine bases, hypoxanthine, guanine, and xanthine, and ribose (or d-ribose)-1-phosphate.[120] The reaction is reversible and favors nucleoside synthesis under ordinary conditions, but the catabolic reaction is favored under circumstances promoting nucleoside excess. Adenosine, derived from both AMP and S-adenosylhomocystine metabolism, is, however, not a substrate for the human enzyme.[120] Adenine nucleotide and nucleoside catabolism proceed through deamination of AMP to IMP and of adenosine to inosine. The latter reaction is catalyzed by adenosine deaminase, an enzyme that also readily converts deoxyadenosine to deoxyinosine (Chap. 109).

Guanine is converted to xanthine by guanine deaminase. Both of the oxidation steps converting hypoxanthine to xanthine and xanthine to uric acid are catalyzed by xanthine oxidase, an enzyme found in appreciable amounts only in the liver and small intestine, and in trace amounts in endothelial cells.[1,117] Xanthine oxidase is a flavoprotein that contains iron and molybdenum and exists in oxidase (O) and dehydrogenase (D) forms. In the course of catalyzing the oxidation reactions leading to production of uric acid, superoxide anion and H_2O_2 are generated, with further conversion of H_2O_2 to free hydroxyl radicals. Production of these mediators of inflammation and tissue injury in the course of xanthine oxidase activity has led to a proposed role for the enzyme in the events surrounding tissue injury and ischemia,[121] circumstances shown to accelerate adenine nucleotide catabolism and uric acid production.[122] Deficiency of xanthine oxidase is discussed in Chap. 111. In contrast, uric acid is a strong peroxynitrite scavenger, suggesting that the protective role for this end product in murine experimental allergic encephalomyelitis may be explained by this mechanism and, in turn, may explain the rare coexistence of gout and multiple sclerosis in humans.[123]

Purine Reutilization Pathways. The pathway of purine synthesis *de novo* requires 6 moles of ATP for generation of each mole of purine nucleotide product.[1] However, a complex network of reactions, including those of nucleotide interconversion (discussed above) and of nucleoside and base salvage (Fig. 106-6), ensures

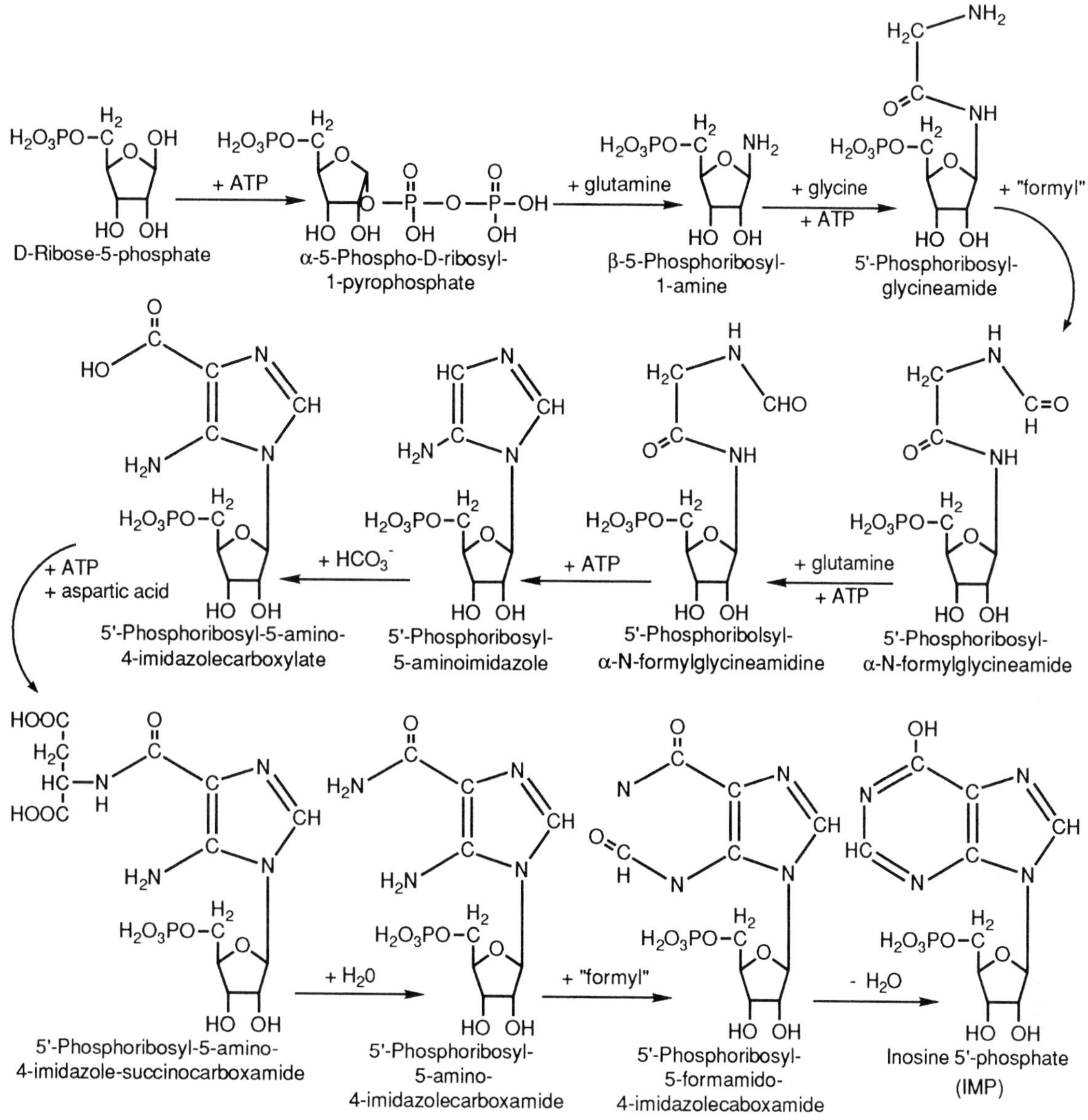

Fig. 106-5 ***De novo*** **biosynthesis of the purine ring.**

efficient reutilization of preformed purines, thus conserving much of the cellular energy that might otherwise be consumed in the synthesis of new purines. Foremost among these are the single-step purine base salvage reactions involving the enzymes HPRT and adenine phosphoribosyltransferase (APRT), which catalyze phosphoribosylation of the respective purine bases directly to the corresponding nucleotides by reaction with PP-ribose-P.[1,124] These enzymes, which also accept alternative purine base and base analogue substrates, are discussed in detail in Chaps. 107 and 108, respectively.

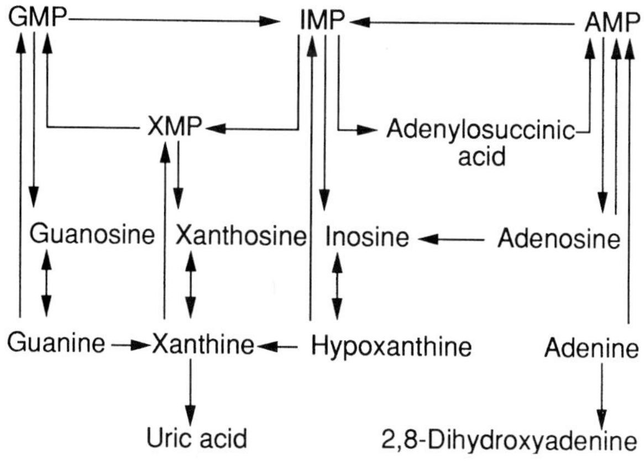

Fig. 106-6 Purine catabolic pathway.

In the apparent absence of inosine and guanosine kinases in human cells, these nucleosides cannot be directly converted to the respective nucleoside 5′-monophosphates. Salvage of inosine and guanosine is thus dependent on HPRT-catalyzed conversion of hypoxanthine and guanine derived from these nucleosides in the purine nucleoside phosphorylase catabolic reaction. In contrast, adenosine can be phosphorylated to AMP by adenosine kinase in a reaction using ATP as the phosphate donor and resulting in generation of ADP.[125] The dephosphorylation of AMP to adenosine by 5′-nucleotidase and the rephosphorylation of adenosine to AMP by adenosine kinase thus forms an adenosine cycle.[126] This cycle may have a role in modulating the availability of adenosine for a variety of cell surface receptor–mediated signaling functions of this nucleoside[126] and in maintaining cellular "energy charge," a proposed composite metabolic regulator of biosynthetic events, defined by intracellular concentrations of adenylates: ATP + 1/2ADP/ATP + ADP + AMP.[127] Finally, reutilization of adenosine in the series of reactions—adenosine → inosine → hypoxanthine → IMP → XMP → GMP—may, in some human cell types, provide the major means for provision of guanylates from the adenine nucleotide pool, particularly under conditions in which guanylate production from purine synthesis *de novo* is otherwise insufficient to permit cell growth and survival.[128]

Regulation of Purine Nucleotide Biosynthesis

Purine nucleotide synthesis *de novo* and purine base salvage reactions provide alternative but concerted means for regulating production of purine nucleotides to meet cellular requirements. Control of purine synthesis *de novo* (Fig. 106-7) is effected in a regulatory domain encompassing the first reaction (AmidoPRT) uniquely committed to the pathway[129,130] and the preceding PRS reaction, in which PP-ribose-P is produced.[115]

The allosteric regulatory and quaternary structural properties of AmidoPRT are consistent with a functionally critical antagonistic interaction between PP-ribose-P and pathway end products at the level of the enzyme.[129–131] Binding of PP-ribose-P to the enzyme induces a conformational change favoring activation.[129] Purine nucleotides (in order of potency—monophosphates, diphosphates, triphosphates) inhibit AmidoPRT, apparently by binding at sites distinct from substrate binding sites.[130,132,133] Inhibition by purine nucleotides shows synergism between nucleotides bearing different (amino and hydroxy) substituents at position 6 of the purine ring, but synergistic mononucleotide inhibition can be overcome by very high concentrations of PP-ribose-P.[130,132,134] However, levels of PP-ribose-P in normal cells[114] are less than the apparent affinity constant of AmidoPRT for this compound,[130] suggesting that availability of PP-ribose-P is the basis for rate limitation of the pathway at the AmidoPRT reaction. Under all but a few experimental conditions, increased intracellular PP-ribose-P concentrations accelerate purine synthesis *de novo*, and depletion of this compound slows the rate of the pathway.[114] Only under unusual conditions of glutamate deprivation is rate limitation by this substrate demonstrable.[135,136]

AmidoPRT can assume two subunit conformations[129] (Fig. 106-8). Active 133-kDa monomers are reversibly converted into

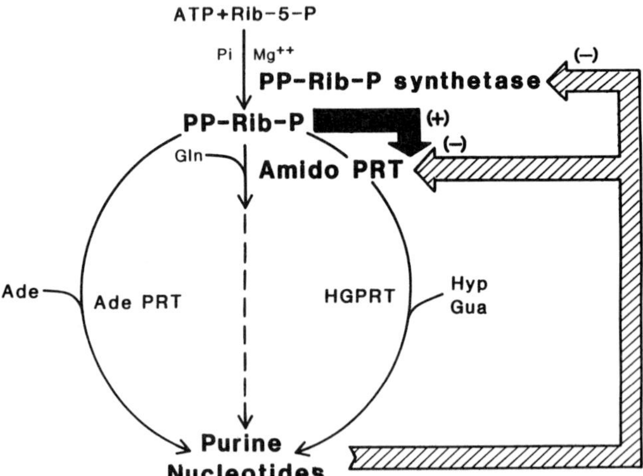

Fig. 106-7 Schematic representation of the pathways of PP-ribose-P and purine nucleotide synthesis and the regulation of rates of purine synthesis *de novo* by PP-ribose-P and purine nucleotide end products. Curved arrows depict single-step purine base salvage pathways of purine nucleotide synthesis, requiring PP-ribose-P and catalyzed by the phosphoribosyltransferase (PRT) enzymes, HPRT and adenine PRT. Purine synthesis *de novo* is shown by a solid arrow (representing the rate-limiting AmidoPRT reaction) and a dashed arrow (depicting the final nine steps in this sequence of reactions). Purine nucleotide inhibition (−) of PP-ribose-P synthetase and AmidoPRT is indicated by the heavy hatched arrow, and allosteric activation (+) of AmidoPRT by PP-ribose-P is shown by the heavy dark arrow. (*Reprinted with permission from Becker MA, Kim M, Husain K, Kang T: Regulation of purine nucleotide synthesis in human B lymphoblasts with both hypoxanthine-guanine phosphoribosyltransferase deficiency and phosphoribosylpyrophosphate synthetase superactivity.* J Biol Chem *267:4317, 1992.*)

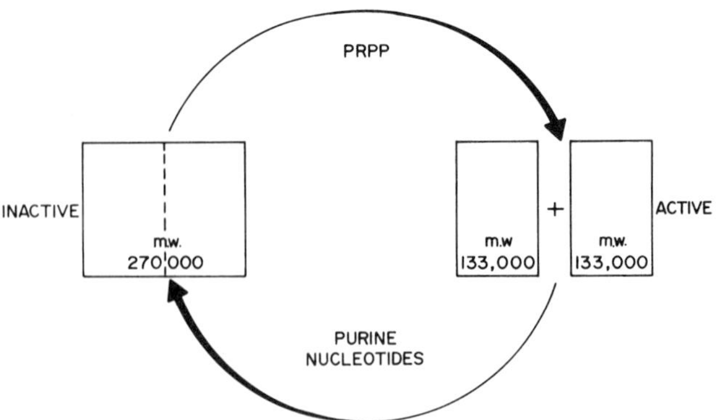

Fig. 106-8 Model of interconversion of small (active) and large (inactive) forms of amidophosphoribosyltransferase. (*Courtesy of Dr. E.W. Holmes, Duke University.*)

inactive 272-kDa dimers by addition of nucleotide inhibitors, and this effect is blocked by increasing concentrations of PP-ribose-P. This potential molecular mechanism for control of AmidoPRT activity has been shown *in vivo* as well as in purified preparations of the enzyme.[131] The molecular cloning of human[137] and avian[138] AmidoPRT complementary DNAs (cDNAs) and the crystallographic analysis of bacteria (*Bacillus subtilis*) AmidoPRT[139] have provided molecular insight into the complicated amidotransferase and glutaminase functions of this important enzyme.

An additional level of inhibitory control of rates of purine synthesis *de novo* is exerted by the action of purine nucleotides on PRS.[115] This enzyme catalyzes synthesis of PP-ribose-P from MgATP and Rib-5-P in a reaction requiring P_i and free Mg^{2+} (Fig. 106-9). The identification in humans of at least three highly homologous PRS cDNAs and isoforms,[140–142] products of separate genes (*PRPS* genes),[140,142,143] has made previous studies of the kinetic and structural properties of this enzyme subject to reinterpretation. Nevertheless, human erythrocyte PRS (largely or entirely the PRS1 isoform) is an allosteric enzyme with at least three potential regulatory sites[144,145] defined by competitive inhibition by ADP with respect to MgATP; competitive inhibition by 2,3-diphosphoglycerate (2,3-DPG) with respect to Rib-5-P; and noncompetitive inhibition with respect to both substrates by many purine, pyrimidine, and pyridine nucleotides, particularly nucleoside diphosphates and triphosphates.[144,146] The subunit of the erythrocyte enzyme has a molecular weight of 34.5 kDa[146,147] and can undergo reversible enzyme concentration- and effector-mediated subunit association to aggregates containing 2, 4, 8, 16, and 32 identical subunits,[147] with enzyme activity residing only in the two largest multimers.[148] As discussed below, overactivity of PRS has been described among some families with gout and uric acid overproduction.

Of importance with regard to the control of purine synthesis *de novo*, PRS is less sensitive to purine nucleotide inhibition than is AmidoPRT.[115,136] Moreover, PRS activity is also inhibited by pyrimidine and pyridine nucleotides, products of pathways that, like purine nucleotide synthesis, require PP-ribose-P. Overall,

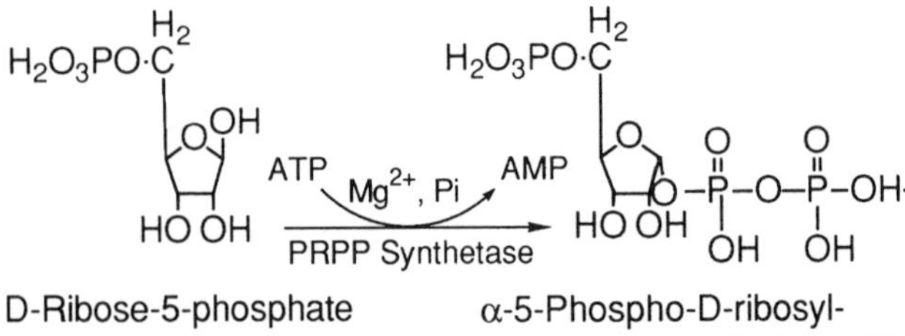

$H_2O_3PO{\cdot}CH_2$ — D-Ribose-5-phosphate $\xrightarrow[\text{PRPP Synthetase}]{\text{ATP} \rightarrow \text{AMP};\ Mg^{2+},\ P_i}$ α-5-Phospho-D-ribosyl-1-pyrophosphate(PP-ribose-P)

Fig. 106-9 The phosphoribosylpyrophosphate synthetase reaction.

regulation of purine synthesis *de novo* at each of two early steps in the pathway (Fig. 106-7) appears well suited to maintenance of both fine and broad control over changes in end-product availability. Fine control is ensured by alterations in AmidoPRT subunit structure and activity in response to small changes in purine concentrations.[115,129,131,136] Broad control is maintained by the addition of changes in PRS activity in response to larger variations in the concentrations of the nucleotide products of several biosynthetic pathways.[115,136,146,149]

Additional Levels of Control of Purine Metabolism. Purine nucleotide interconversion reactions (Fig. 106-6) governing the alternative conversion of IMP to either AMP or GMP in separate two-step pathways are subject to end-product inhibition directed at the first reaction in the respective sequence: AMPS synthetase is inhibited by AMP (as well as GDP), and IMP dehydrogenase is inhibited by GMP.[1] The additional requirements for GTP and ATP, respectively, in the synthesis of AMP and GMP from IMP suggest control over the balance of nucleotide classes produced by interconversion reactions as well as control over the individual classes by means of direct product inhibition.

Ribonucleotide degradation (Fig. 106-6) is also a regulated process of some complexity.[117,150] The critical reactions governing this pathway are catalyzed by AMP deaminase and 5′-nucleotidases. AMP deaminase is activated by ATP and ADP and is inhibited by GTP and P_i. Release of this enzyme from inhibition, as in circumstances requiring rapid phosphorylation of substrates by ATP, results in acceleration of nucleotide degradation to uric acid.[117] The multiplicity of soluble 5′-nucleotidases, each with a different pattern of substrate preference and responsiveness to nucleotides and P_i, has limited understanding of regulation at the level of dephosphorylation. Nevertheless, it appears that nucleotides, especially ATP and ADP, as well as P_i, are key modulators of nucleotide catabolism. Working through activation of AMP deaminase or 5′-nucleotidase or both, different stimuli or even the same stimuli in different tissues may result in catabolic processes distinctive in the dynamics of degradation and in the degree to which uric acid formation or purine reutilization is favored.[117]

URIC ACID HOMEOSTASIS AND MECHANISMS OF HYPERURICEMIA

Humans and great apes are unique among mammals in the requirement to excrete uric acid as the end product of purine metabolism as a result of a lack of the enzyme uricase, which catalyzes degradation of uric acid to the readily excretable compound allantoin.[151] Uric acid, a trioxypurine with oxygen at positions 2, 6, and 8 of the purine ring, is a weak organic acid ionized at position 9 with a pKa of 5.75 and at position 3 with a pKa of 10.3 (Fig. 106-10).[1] The solubility properties of uric acid condition humans to the development of supersaturated body fluids, with the attendant risks of urate crystal deposition and clinical sequelae. The theoretic limit of solubility of the un-ionized acid form of uric acid in aqueous solution is about 6.5 mg/dl. This form predominates in normal acidic urine, where at pH 5.0 saturation occurs at about 15 mg/dl. The solubility of the ionized urate form that constitutes 98 percent of the uric acid at the pH and sodium concentration of other extracellular fluids is comparably limited—only about 6.5 mg/dl. Therefore, in many normal adult male populations at least, mean serum urate concentrations approach the limit of urate solubility in serum. Furthermore, in most individuals, excretion of an acid urine is accompanied by uric acid concentrations considerably in excess of saturation.[1] Despite these considerations, manifestations of urate deposition are relatively uncommon. The factors determining in whom hyperuricemia and gout will develop are diverse and can be appreciated in light of knowledge of the physiologic mechanisms maintaining uric acid homeostasis in normal and hyperuricemic individuals.

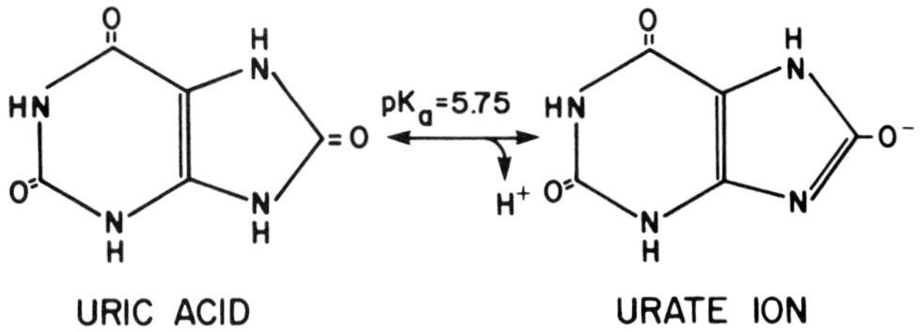

Fig. 106-10 Ionization of uric acid. The weakly acidic nature of uric acid is due to ionization of hydrogen atoms. Ionization at position 9 (pKa = 5.75) is shown above. The ionized forms of uric acid readily form salts. In extracellular fluids in which sodium is the principal cation, about 98 percent of uric acid is in the form of the monosodium salt at pH 7.4. The crystals, which form in the synovial fluid or the tophi of gouty patients when solubility limits are exceeded, are composed of monosodium urate monohydrate.

Uric acid is synthesized mainly in the liver and is released into the circulation. In the absence of significant plasma protein binding (<4 percent under physiologic conditions),[152,153] the vast majority of circulating urate is readily available for filtration at the glomerulus and the subsequent mechanisms of renal uric acid handling. The size and dynamics of the miscible pool of uric acid and the overall contribution of renal excretion to uric acid disposal have been estimated at steady state in normal and gouty individuals by sequential measurements of isotopic enrichment of urinary uric acid following intravenous administration of [^{15}N] or [^{14}C] urate. (Details of the isotopic analyses discussed in this section are reviewed in a previous edition of this chapter[5] and elsewhere.[1]) In normal men, the miscible urate pool averages about 1200 mg (range 866–1587 mg), with a mean rate of turnover of about 700 mg/day (range 513–1108 mg/day). A mean urate pool size of about 600 mg and a turnover rate of about 0.6 pool/day have been found in normal women. Urinary uric acid excretion ordinarily accounts for two thirds to three fourths of daily uric acid disposal. Intestinal uricolysis, degradation by gut bacteria of uric acid secreted into the gut, accounts for nearly all urate disposed of by extrarenal routes.[1]

All untreated patients with gout have enlarged uric acid pools, usually ranging from 2000 to 4000 mg in the absence of evident tophi but reaching 30,000 mg or more in tophaceous gout.[1] Extrarenal uric acid disposal in hyperuricemic or gouty individuals is normal or increased to as much as 50 percent of total daily excretion. Impaired intestinal uricolysis is thus not a mechanism of hyperuricemia.[154] Many patients with gout have rates of turnover of the uric acid pool that overlap the normal range. However, increased rates of turnover have invariably been found in patients who show excessive rates of purine synthesis *de novo* and uric acid overproduction as reflected by increased incorporation of radioactively labeled precursor molecules (such as [^{14}C] glycine) into urinary uric acid[1,155,156] and by daily urinary uric acid excretion clearly exceeding that of normal individuals.[1,154]

These findings provided evidence for heterogeneity in the mechanisms accounting for uric acid accumulation, hyperuricemia, and the consequent predisposition to urate crystal deposition among gouty patients. Additional study has confirmed that excessive production and diminished renal excretion of uric acid, operating singly or in combination, are the major abnormalities demonstrable among hyperuricemic individuals with or without gout.[1] Whether hyperuricemia occurs as a result of hereditary metabolic disease (primary hyperuricemia) or is a consequence of a coexisting acquired condition (secondary hyperuricemia), one or both of these mechanisms underlie the development of hyperuricemia. The known causes of hyperuricemia are listed in Table 106-1.

Distinction in individual patients between uric acid overproduction and impaired renal uric acid excretion as the basis of hyperuricemia has therapeutic and investigative significance and is warranted in most patients with primary gout and, perhaps, all patients with normal renal function.[83] An accurate approach to

Table 106-1 Etiology of Hyperuricemia in Humans

Increased purine biosynthesis or urate poduction

- Inherited enzymatic defects
  - Genetically undefined
  - HPRT deficiency
  - PRS overactivity
  - Glycogen storage diseases (types I, III, V, VIII)
- Disease states leading to purine or urate overproduction
  - Myeloproliferative disorders
  - Malignancies
  - Hemolysis
  - Psoriasis
  - Obesity
  - Tissue hypoxia
  - Down syndrome
- Associated with drugs or dietary habits
  - Cytolytic agents
  - Vitamin B_{12} (pernicious anemia)
  - Warfarin
  - Nicotinic acid
  - 4-Amino-5-imidazole carboxamide riboside
  - Pancreatic extract
  - Fructose
  - Ethanol
  - Excessive dietary purine intake

Decreased renal clearance of urate

- Inherited defects of glomerular or tubular function (undefined)
- Disease states leading to reduced urate clearance
  - Chronic renal insufficiency
  - Polycystic kidney disease
  - Dehydration
  - Starvation
  - Diabetes insipidus
  - Lactic acidosis (tissue hypoxia)
  - Obesity
  - Hyperparathyroidism
  - Hypothyroidism
  - Sarcoidosis
  - Eclampsia
  - Bartter syndrome
  - Lead poisoning
  - Beryllium poisoning
- Associated with drug administration
  - Diuretics
  - Ethanol
  - Salicylates (low dose)
  - Laxative abuse (alkalosis)
  - Cyclosporine
  - Pyrazinamide
  - Ethambutol
  - Levodopa
  - Methoxyflurane

achieving this distinction in persons with normal renal function is measurement of daily urinary uric acid excretion on two consecutive samples obtained 5 days after initiation of an isocaloric purine-free diet.[83,155] Medications affecting uric acid production or excretion and uricosuric radiologic contrast agents should be avoided for at least 10 days prior to measurements. Under these conditions of steady state with regard to uric acid metabolism, urinary excretion of uric acid represents a minimal estimate of the rate of uric acid synthesis (uncorrected for extrarenal uric acid disposal).[155]

In normal white men tested in this manner, daily urinary uric acid excretion averages about 425 mg/day (SD 75–80 mg/day). Values in excess of 600 mg/day (mean ± 2 SD) are indicative of uric acid overproduction.[1,155]

Strict dietary control is necessary to ensure the accuracy of this determination but is often impractical and thus difficult to achieve in ambulatory patients. Measurement of daily urinary uric acid excretion during normal dietary intake is an alternative approach frequently used; excretion of more than 1000 mg/day is regarded as clearly excessive.[22] Values between 800 and 1000 mg/day are deemed equivocal, and retesting under closer dietary control is usually advisable. Standardized normal values are unavailable for women, children, and obese or very large individuals. For such persons, daily urinary uric acid excretion in excess of about 12 mg per kilogram of body weight most likely indicates uric acid overproduction.

Uric Acid Overproduction

Excessive urinary uric acid excretion is demonstrable in 10 to 15 percent of patients with gout and primary hyperuricemia and in most patients in whom hyperuricemia reflects increased cell turnover (e.g., a lymphoproliferative or myeloproliferative disease or psoriasis) or a toxic state or pharmacologic intervention resulting in increased uric acid production (Table 106-1).[1] In such individuals with normal renal function and no evident tophaceous deposits, in vivo isotopic labeling studies almost invariably confirm the presence of increased purine nucleotide and uric acid synthesis (Fig. 106-11),[155] so that it is rarely necessary to use the accurate but costly and cumbersome isotopic procedures. In vivo labeling studies or direct measurement of rates of purine synthesis *de novo* in fibroblasts cultured from skin biopsy material[149,157] may, however, prove useful in confirming a strong suspicion of uric acid overproduction when urinary uric acid

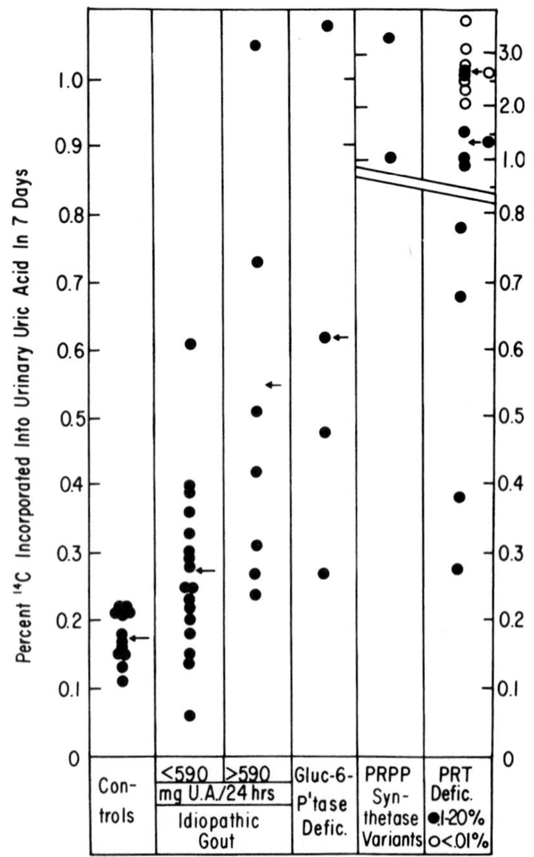

Fig. 106-11 Summary of values of cumulative incorporation of ^{14}C into urinary uric acid in control and gouty subjects reported from 1957 through 1980.

excretion values fail to do so, as in some patients with extensive tophaceous deposits or renal insufficiency, or other circumstances in which there is increased extrarenal uric acid disposal.

Sustained uric acid overproduction in patients with gout and primary hyperuricemia indicates excessive rates of purine synthesis *de novo*, which in the framework of current understanding of the regulation of this pathway should reflect altered interaction between PP-ribose-P and purine nucleotides on AmidoPRT activity[115,131] (Fig. 106-6). In fact, in several circumstances in which inherited or acquired hyperuricemia is associated with uric acid overproduction, alterations in the availability of these small molecule effectors have been demonstrated, with either increased PP-ribose-P availability or decreased purine nucleotide concentrations constituting the apparent basis for excessive purine nucleotide and uric acid synthesis. Structural mutations in AmidoPRT leading to decreased responsiveness to nucleotide inhibition or to increased responsiveness to PP-ribose-P also might result in purine overproduction,[157,158] but defects in this enzyme have yet to be demonstrated among gouty individuals.

Increased PP-ribose-P Availability. The role of PP-ribose-P as a critical component in the regulation of purine nucleotide and uric acid production has been supported by extensive biochemical, pharmacologic, and clinical investigations since first proposed by Wyngaarden and Kelley 30 years ago.[1,115,159] Increased PP-ribose-P availability is the driving force for excessive rates of purine synthesis *de novo* in two X chromosome–linked inborn errors of purine metabolism: PRS superactivity[160,161] and HPRT deficiency[162,163] (discussed below and in Chap. 107). Uric acid overproduction, hyperuricemia, and hyperuricosuria occur in each of these disorders in conjunction with increased intracellular PP-ribose-P concentrations, but no apparent decreases in concentrations of purine nucleotides.[115,149,161,164,165] In PRS superactivity, increased PP-ribose-P levels result from overproduction of this regulatory substrate.[149,166] In contrast, PP-ribose-P accumulates in excess in HPRT deficiency as a consequence of underutilization in this salvage reaction.[128,149] Increased PP-ribose-P availability in both instances results in activation of AmidoPRT and acceleration of purine nucleotide and uric acid synthesis.

PRS superactivity and HPRT deficiency account for only a small proportion (perhaps 10 percent) of patients with primary uric acid overproduction[1] but represent the only states in which excessive PP-ribose-P availability clearly constitutes the sole basis of uric acid overproduction. However, a unique or contributory role for increased PP-ribose-P availability has been suggested in several other proposed or established enzymatic defects or metabolic states in which there is evidence of uric acid overproduction.

In patients with glucose-6-phosphatase deficiency (glycogen storage disease type I; see Chap. 71), hyperuricemia may appear as early as infancy, and gout has been reported by the end of the first decade of life. Patients surviving into adulthood with this autosomal recessive disorder may then suffer tophaceous gout as a major clinical problem.[167,168] Hyperuricemia in these patients is multifactorial, involving both purine nucleotide and uric acid overproduction[167] and impaired renal uric acid excretion, due to lactic acidemia and ketonemia.[168] Two tenable mechanisms through which increased PP-ribose-P production may contribute to hyperuricemia have been proposed and studied in humans and in animal models. First, glucose-6-phosphate accumulation in the liver as a consequence of the inherited enzyme deficiency may stimulate the oxidative branch of the pentose phosphate pathway, resulting in increased Rib-5-P and, ultimately, PP-ribose-P synthesis.[169] Second, reduced hepatic concentrations of inhibitory purine nucleotides during recurrent episodes of hypoglycemia may result in activation of AmidoPRT and PRS by release of these enzymes from nucleotide feedback inhibition.[131]

Excessive PP-ribose-P production resulting from enhanced oxidative pentose phosphate pathway generation of Rib-5-P also may explain hyperuricemia in some primary gout patients with normal glucose 6-phosphatase activity. Increased concentrations and rates of production of Rib-5-P and PP-ribose-P were demonstrated in fibroblasts cultured from two patients with documented purine nucleotide and uric acid overproduction but no identifiable enzyme defect.[158] In addition, a high frequency of overactive, electrophoretically variant forms of glutathione reductase was reported in erythrocyte lysates from patients with gout.[170] Glutathione reductase promotes reduction of glutathione and oxidation of NADPH to NADP, a cofactor in the first two reactions of the oxidative pathway. Because the rate of operation of the pathway depends at least in part on the regulation of glucose-6-phosphatase activity by the ratio NADPH/NADP, increased glutathione reductase activity could provide a tenable mechanism for excessive PP-ribose-P synthesis and purine nucleotide and uric acid overproduction.

These findings suggest that abnormalities in carbohydrate metabolism may manifest themselves in hyperuricemia and gout due to purine overproduction. However, neither purine overproduction nor increased glutathione reductase activity has been confirmed in hemolysates from patients with gout.[171] Moreover, experimental evidence linking rates of the oxidative and nonoxidative pathways of pentose phosphate generation to rates of PP-ribose-P and purine nucleotide synthesis under physiologic conditions has not, to date, been definitive. If confirmed, a link between changes in carbohydrate metabolism and rates of PP-ribose-P production may have significant bearing on observed associations between metabolic abnormalities, such as obesity and hypertriglyceridemia, and hyperuricemia. The presumed mechanism would be that in states of carbohydrate excess and accelerated lipogenesis, metabolic flux through the pentose phosphate shunt is increased with increased Rib-5-P and, potentially, PP-ribose-P production.

Decreased Purine Nucleotide Concentrations. Despite impaired purine base salvage,[172] normal intracellular purine nucleotide concentrations have been found in cells deficient in HPRT.[149,165,173] However, uric acid overproduction due to nucleotide depletion has been identified in a number of circumstances having in common net degradation of ATP as a consequence of either increased ATP consumption or impaired ATP regeneration[174] (Table 106-2). Under conditions in which the supply of P_i, oxygen, glucose, or fatty acids is restricted, ATP synthesis may be impaired, and severe ATP depletion and accompanying hyperuricemia may ensue, particularly if the demands for ATP consumption are increased. Net ATP degradation results in accumulation of ADP and AMP, which are rapidly converted to uric acid through the intermediates inosine, hypoxanthine, and xanthine. Increases in any or all of these intermediates accompanying excessive uric acid levels in serum or urine provide evidence in support of this mechanism of hyperuricemia.[5,97,98,122,175–179]

Table 106-2 Conditions Resulting in Disordered ATP Metabolism

Increased ATP degradation
Fructose infusion
Exercise
Ethanol ingestion
Glucose-6-phosphatase deficiency
Hereditary fructose intolerance
Fructose-1,6-diphosphatase deficiency
Decreased ATP synthesis
Tissue hypoxia
Ischemia
Hypoxemia
Metabolic myopathies
Hypophosphatemia

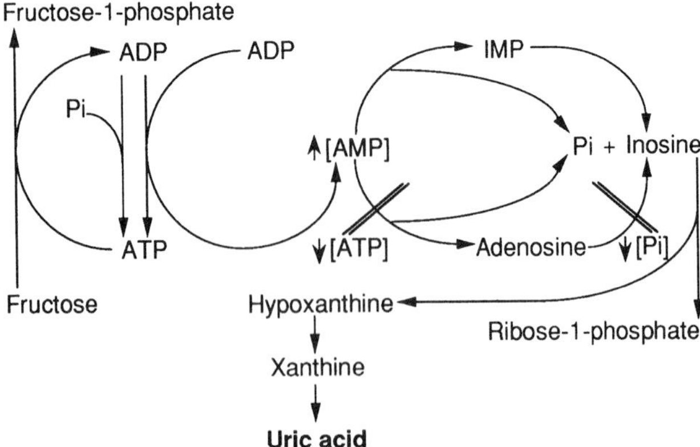

Fig. 106-12 Mechanism of fructose-induced purine nucleotide degradation. Fructose triggers rapid breakdown of purine nucleotides to uric acid in the liver. Phosphorylation of fructose to fructose-1-phosphate causes ATP to be degraded to ADP. Fructose-1-phosphate accumulates and thus traps inorganic phosphate. ADP is converted back to ATP by the mitochondrial electron transport system or glycolysis, which uses inorganic phosphate, or by adenylate kinase. The reaction with adenylate kinase also forms AMP. The net result is a diminution of intracellular ATP and inorganic phosphate and buildup of AMP. Elevated AMP concentrations also lead to increased IMP concentration. Dephosphorylation by 5′-nucleotidase is triggered. If AMP and IMP concentrations are high enough, then the nonspecific phosphatase can be activated. Once dephosphorylation is activated, there is a cascade of nucleotide degradation through catabolic pathways leading to increased synthesis of uric acid. This accounts for the resultant hyperuricemia and elevated urinary excretion of inosine, hypoxanthine, xanthine, and uric acid. Interrupted arrows indicate enzyme inhibition. Bold arrows indicate changes in the levels of ATP, AMP and P_i induced by fructose infusion. (*Adapted with permission from Fox IH: Metabolic basis for disorders of purine nucleotide degradation.* Metabolism *30:616, 1981.*)

The effects of rapid administration of fructose in humans provide an experimental model for the hyperuricemia related to ATP depletion[180] (Fig. 106-12). Fructose is phosphorylated in the liver using ATP, and the accompanying P_i depletion limits regeneration of ATP from ADP, which in turn serves as substrate for the catabolic pathway to uric acid formation.[174] Within minutes after fructose infusion, plasma (and later urinary) inosine, hypoxanthine, xanthine, and uric acid concentrations are increased.[180] In conjunction with purine nucleotide depletion, rates of purine synthesis *de novo* are accelerated, thus potentiating increased uric acid production.[177] The increased purine synthetic rate is also accompanied by increased PP-ribose-P levels, presumably as a result of release of PRS from nucleotide inhibition and by a shift in the apparent molecular weight of hepatic AmidoPRT toward that of the active monomeric form[131] (Fig. 106-8).

Unusual physiologic as well as pathologic states can provoke net ATP degradation and consequent hyperuricemia. Strenuous exercise or prolonged training in otherwise normal individuals may result in muscle hypoxia, leading to muscle adenylate depletion and generation of inosine and hypoxanthine.[174,175] These purine catabolic intermediates are then transported to the liver for conversion to uric acid, ultimately contributing more to the ensuing hyperuricemia than the accompanying lactic acidemia and dehydration. In glycogen storage diseases type III (debrancher deficiency), type V (myophosphorylase deficiency), and type VII (muscle phosphofructokinase deficiency) (see Chap. 71), mild exercise provokes myogenic hyperuricemia and hyperuricosuria as a consequence of impaired glucose availability for generation of ATP from ADP in muscle.[178,179] A similar mechanism has been proposed for hyperuricemia in myoadenylate deaminase deficiency (see Chap. 110). Finally, in glucose-6-phosphatase deficiency, hypoglycemia or glucagon administration results in reduced hepatic ATP concentrations and purine catabolism, contributing to hyperuricemia.[169]

Hyperuricemia, related at least in part to net ATP degradation, is encountered commonly in two additional situations. First, in acutely ill patients with diseases such as adult respiratory distress syndrome, myocardial infarction, or status epilepticus, tissue hypoxia may impair ATP synthesis from ADP in mitochondria, resulting in ADP catabolism and high plasma and urinary concentrations of inosine, hypoxanthine, xanthine, and uric acid.[122] These findings are associated with a poor prognosis in such patients,[181] indicating that significant hypoxia is required for activation of the purine catabolic pathway. Second, alcohol consumption results in accelerated conversion of ATP to AMP and enhanced production of uric acid and its immediate precursors when the rate of ATP utilization in ethanol metabolism via acetate to form acetyl CoA exceeds the capacity for ATP regeneration.[98] This mechanism plays a major role in the hyperuricemia associated with ethanol ingestion,[97] along with renal uric acid retention resulting from dehydration and metabolic acidosis.

Uric Acid Excretion

Renal Handling Mechanisms. Renal excretion of uric acid is a complicated physiologic function (Fig. 106-13); the component mechanisms of urate handling by the kidney have been defined over a number of years as a result of pharmacologic and physiologic studies in experimental animals and in humans. These mechanisms are discussed in detail in Chap. 198, and only a brief review pertinent to hyperuricemia and gout is presented here.

Despite essentially free filtration of urate at the glomerulus, renal clearance of uric acid in normal subjects is only 7 to 10 percent that of creatinine or inulin clearances, implying net reabsorption of at least 90 to 93 percent of filtered urate in the nephron.[182] The proximal renal tubule is the site of a uric acid reabsorption process facilitated by active transport independent of nonionic diffusion or passive forces.[183] The identification of an otherwise healthy man in whom marked hypouricemia was accompanied by a urate clearance far in excess of inulin clearance

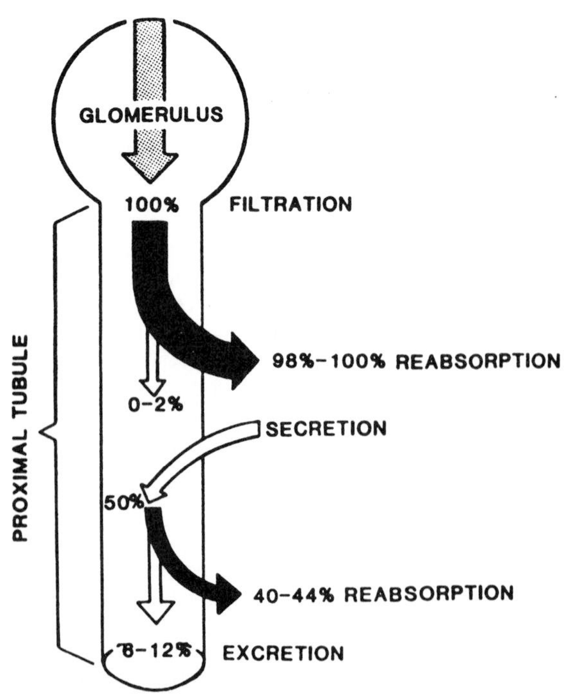

Fig. 106-13 Four-component model illustrating bidirectional urate transport by the kidney. Tubular secretion and reabsorption are shown as a percentage of filtered urate. (*Reprinted with permission from Koopman WJ:* Arthritis and Allied Conditions, *13th ed. Baltimore, Williams & Wilkins, 1997, p 2051.*)

led to the proposal, later confirmed, of tubular urate secretion.[184] The existence of this third mechanism appeared to explain the paradoxical effects of salicylates and probenecid on uric acid excretion. In low doses, these drugs decrease uric acid excretion, but high doses result in uricosuria.[185] These phenomena were best explained by hypothesizing inhibition of tubular secretion at low doses and inhibition of both secretion and reabsorption at higher doses. Urate is secreted in the proximal tubule in humans, apparently by an energy-dependent transport system, shared with and potentially in competition with a lengthy list of endogenously generated and drug-derived organic acids.[182]

Although tubular urate secretion may be the single most important factor in establishing urinary uric acid excretion,[186,187] the relative contributions of reabsorption and secretion to this process in humans remain uncertain. In fact, a variety of seemingly paradoxical drug effects on human uric acid excretion and studies in Cebus monkeys and in individuals and families with apparent defects in renal uric acid handling have led to the proposal of a four-component model (Fig. 106-13) incorporating extensive postsecretory reabsorption of secreted urate at a site either coextensive with or distal to the secretory site.[186–189] As recently stated,[182] however, validation of this model of urate handling and quantitation of the flux of uric acid through the individual transport mechanisms have yet to be achieved, particularly as doubts have emerged with the interpretation of the results of the pyrazinamide suppression test, formerly in wide use to distinguish the relative contributions of secreted and filtered but nonreabsorbed uric acid to urinary uric acid excretion.[186,188]

Decreased Uric Acid Excretion in Hyperuricemia and Gout

In 80 percent or more of individuals with gout, a deficit in renal uric acid excretion is the major mechanism leading to hyperuricemia.[1] Underexcretion of uric acid, rigorously defined as a daily urinary content of less than 250 to 300 mg of uric acid in a hyperuricemic person receiving a purine-free diet, may occur on either a primary or secondary basis. Even among the majority of gout patients who excrete normal amounts of uric acid, however, these amounts are inappropriately low with respect to the corresponding serum urate concentrations. That is, gouty patients with primary underexcretion of uric acid have lower uric acid clearance rates than nongouty subjects.[1,182,190–192] When urinary urate excretion rates (expressed in milligrams per minute per 100 ml of glomerular filtrate) are plotted as a logarithmic function of plasma urate concentration in gouty and nongouty individuals (Fig. 106-14), parallel regression lines are generated, with the line for gouty persons displaced such that these individuals must have a mean plasma urate value nearly 2 mg/dl greater than nongouty controls in order to achieve equivalent excretion rates.[190] From these data, Simkin has found that gouty patients excrete an average of 41 percent less uric acid than normal subjects at any given plasma urate concentration. Similar findings are observed when the curate/cinulin ratio (fractional excretion of urate) is studied.[1,182,190]

Decreased urate clearance in primary gout could be due to reduced uric acid filtration, enhanced tubular uric acid reabsorption, or diminished tubular urate secretion. Increased urate binding to plasma proteins has been reported in conjunction with the hyperuricemia of the Maoris of New Zealand[12,193] and in a few gouty subjects. Excessive plasma protein binding of urate could reduce the filtered load of urate. However, these findings have not been accompanied by urate clearance data. Both increased reabsorption and decreased secretion of uric acid have been proposed as the basis for the lower urate clearances observed in most patients with primary gout, but there is no compelling experimental evidence to affirm enhanced proximal tubular reabsorption of uric acid as a common mechanism.[186,188,194] In contrast, diminished renal urate secretion per nephron has been implicated in the hyperuricemia of primary gout not associated with overproduction of uric acid.[186,187,189,195,196] Studies employing the uricosuric response to benzbromarone, a drug that selectively inhibits reabsorption of secreted urate, to measure minimum tubular secretory rate are also reported to show decreased secretion of uric acid in such patients in comparison with nongouty controls or gouty subjects with overproduction hyperuricemia.[186] To date, no alteration in postsecretory reabsorption has been documented in conjunction with hyperuricemia.

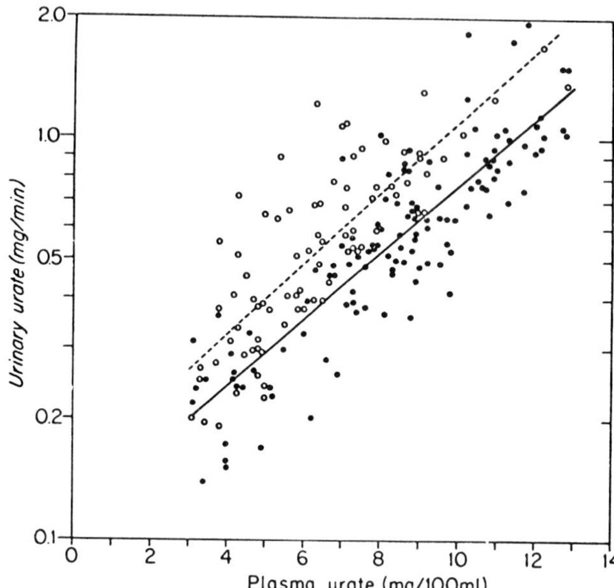

Fig. 106-14 Urate excretion at varying concentrations of plasma urate. Urinary urate is expressed in mg/(min · 100 ml of glomerular filtrate). The slopes of the normal (○—○) and gout (•—•) regressions are not significantly different from each other. The average gouty individual must have a serum urate level 1.7 mg/dl higher than normal in order to equal the normal rate of urate excretion. (*Reprinted with permission from Simkin PA: Urate excretion in normal and gouty men.* Adv Exp Med Biol *76B:41, 1977.*)

In contrast to the limited insight into the individual contributions of uric acid handling mechanisms to renal urate retention in primary gout, mechanisms of secondary hyperuricemia and gout are better understood. For example, advanced chronic renal failure is commonly accompanied by hyperuricemia resulting from the progressive decline in GFR, which obviates the need for compensatory mechanisms that earlier in the course of the disease promote uric acid excretion through enhanced fractional excretion of filtered urate.[197] Similarly, conditions resulting in extracellular volume depletion are associated with hyperuricemia, in part due to reduced GFR. In such conditions as dehydration, diabetes insipidus, and diuretic therapy, however, enhanced reabsorption of uric acid plays an important and perhaps dominant role in inducing hyperuricemia.[99] Diuretic treatment is an important and frequent cause of renal hyperuricemia.[26–29] Finally, decreased tubular secretion as a mechanism for secondary renal hyperuricemia is exemplified by the effects of elevated blood levels of a wide array of endogenous and drug-derived organic acids (such as lactate, β-hydroxybutyrate, acetoacetate, and low-dose salicylates), which inhibit uric acid excretion by competing with urate at tubular secretory sites.[100,185,198]

GENETIC BASIS

Idiopathic Gout and Hyperuricemia

The familial nature of gout was recognized in antiquity, but an ordered approach to the genetics of gout became possible only when the biochemical basis of the disorder was identified as excessive accumulation of uric acid. Gout was included among the inborn errors of metabolism in 1931 by A.E. Garrod, who regarded gout as a dominantly inherited trait.[199]

In the subsequent three decades, several studies established a 25 percent prevalence of hyperuricemia among the relatives of gout patients and a 20 percent incidence of gout in these family members.[1] Overall, familial incidence figures for gout ranged from 6 to 18 percent.[1] These data were interpreted as consistent with the concept of an autosomal-dominant allele as the inherited basis of gout, with greater penetrance in men than women.[200] Further support for this hypothesis was provided by bimodal distributions of serum urate values in studies of racially selected or geographically isolated populations.[1] Reexamination of some of these data failed to confirm such bimodality, however, leading to an alternative hypothesis—that hyperuricemia and the gouty diathesis are influenced by multiple genes.[201,202] Strong polygenic hereditary influences, some suggesting autosomal dominant transmission and some indicating X-linked inheritance, were found for serum urate values in Blackfoot and Pima Indians[203] and were supported by the lack of bimodality of urate concentrations in studies conducted in other large populations.[1,7] Overall, polygenic control is more prominently displayed as the heterogeneity of the population under study increases, and, conversely, expression of a single gene is more likely to be manifested within more genetically homogeneous groups, potentially obscuring gene interactions.

A particularly striking example of hereditary influence is provided by the fact that 71 percent of patients with early adult-onset gout (mean age 28 years), in the setting of nephropathy[77,80] but no identifiable inherited enzyme defect, had a family history of other affected members.[204] Thus, although there is little doubt about the existence of multiple genetic determinants governing serum urate concentration in humans, the impact of many of these on gout remains unclear and will await definition of the accompanying biochemical or physiologic aberrations. In several instances, however, specific genetic defects have been intimately linked with gout.

Gout Associated with Specific Inborn Errors

PP-Ribose-P Synthetase Superactivity. PP-ribose-P is a substrate in the synthesis of virtually all nucleotides[114] and is an important regulator of the *de novo* pathways of purine[115] and pyrimidine[205] nucleotide synthesis. Formation of PP-ribose-P is catalyzed in eukaryotes by a family of PRS isoforms.[140–142,206,207] Synthesis of PP-ribose-P in mammalian cells appears to be regulated in a complex manner that includes, but is not limited to, allosteric control of PRS enzymatic activity.[114,115,208–215] The existence of multiple PRS isoforms with differing kinetic properties,[208,209] apparent alterations in PRS activity in response to mitogens[213] and changes in intracellular divalent cation concentrations,[212] and tissue-specific differences in abundance of PRS transcripts[210] and isoforms suggest additional mechanisms of control of PP-ribose-P production, involving the selective expression of genes encoding PRS[210,211] and perhaps modifications of the structure or functional organization of the gene products by interaction with one another[148] or with specific PRS-associated modifier proteins.[214,215] For example, Tatibana et al. have cloned and characterized cDNAs for two PRS-associated proteins[214,215] that bind PRS isoforms and inhibit enzyme activity. Whether these interactions affect intracellular PP-ribose-P production is unknown, but they raise the possibility of substantial complexity in postranslational regulation of PRS isoform expression.

Multiple isoforms of PRS were first identified by Tatibana and colleagues,[142,207] who cloned and sequenced three distinct PRS cDNAs (numbered 1, 2, and 3) encoding highly homologous polypeptides of identical length. Each human and rodent PRS cDNA is encoded by a separate *PRPS* gene: human *PRPS1* and *PRPS2* map to different regions of the X chromosome (Xq22-q24 and Xp22.2-p22.3, respectively)[140] and are widely expressed.[210] *PRPS3* maps to human chromosome 7 and appears to be transcribed only in the testes.[142,210] X-linked human PRS1 and PRS2 cDNAs show 80 percent nucleotide sequence identity throughout their 954-bp translated regions but show no homology in the corresponding 5′- and 3′-untranslated regions.[140] PRS1 and PRS2 cDNAs hybridize with transcripts of 2.3 and 2.7 kb, respectively.[140] Human organs, tissues, and cell lines contain both PRS1 and PRS2 transcripts[210] and isoforms,[216] but the relative abundances of these gene products vary with the cell source. Studies of tissue-specific expression of *PRPS1* and *PRPS2* genes indicate that *PRPS1* may be a constitutively expressed gene,[208,211,213] whereas *PRPS2* expression may be responsive to mitogenic stimulation or transformation.[213,216] Both X-linked *PRPS* genes exceed 30 kb and contain 7 exons with virtually identical exon-intron borders. However, 5′-promoter regions of the genes are structurally distinct.[211]

Normal human PRS1 and PRS2 cDNAs have been expressed in *Escherichia coli*, and purified recombinant PRS isoforms have been compared.[208] Despite 95 percent amino acid homology, recombinant PRS1 and PRS2 isoforms differ in several physical and kinetic properties, including thermal stability and sensitivity to subunit disaggregation and inactivation in the absence of MgATP and Mg^{2+}; isoelectric points; pH optima; and kinetic constants for substrates, activators, and inhibitors.[208] The difference in isoelectric points of PRS1 and PRS2 has allowed the development of an isoelectric focusing–immunoblotting method for separation and quantitation of the isoforms in tissue and cell samples.[216]

Superactivity of PRS was initially described by Sperling et al. in brothers with early adult-onset uric acid urolithiasis and gout associated with severe hyperuricemia and hyperuricosuria.[160,217] Purine nucleotide overproduction, reflected by daily urinary excretion of 2400 mg of uric acid in the proband, was accompained by an accelerated rate of erythrocyte PP-ribose-P synthesis and a variant form of PRS with normal maximal velocity and dissociation constants for substrates and activators but a defect in allosteric regulation of enzyme activity by purine nucleotide (ADP, GDP) inhibitors.[218] In the nearly two dozen kindreds in which PRS superactivity has been reported in conjunction with uric acid overproduction, heterogeneous kinetic mechanisms leading to excessive enzyme activity have been displayed. These include (1) defective regulation of PRS, involving impaired responsiveness to allosteric effectors of PRS activity;[166,218–222] (2) catalytic overactivity, in which excessive enzyme activity results from an overabundance of the normal PRS1 isoform;[145,216,223–225] (3) combined regulatory defects and catalytic overactivity;[222,226] and (4) increased affinity for the substrate Rib-5-P,[158] which is normally present in cells at concentrations below the apparent dissociation constant of PRS for this substrate. Catalytic superactivity is the most common class of kinetic aberration reported to date.[221]

Despite the variety of functional abnormalities in the enzyme, purine nucleotide and uric acid overproduction in PP-ribose-P superactivity is explainable in all instances as a consequence of increased PP-ribose-P availability, which is, in turn, due to accelerated PP-ribose-P synthesis.[149,166] Increased PP-ribose-P availability activates AmidoPRT, accelerating purine synthesis *de novo*. Affected males with regulatory or combined regulatory defects and catalytic overactivity in the enzyme generally have greater rates of PP-ribose-P production and, ultimately, greater acceleration of purine nucleotide and uric acid synthesis than individuals with isolated overabundance of normal PRS1.[149]

In common with HPRT deficiency, PRS superactivity is inherited as an X-linked trait,[227,228] which is expressed in two clinical phenotypes.[221,225] In families with the more severe phenotype, affected hemizygous males show early childhood symptoms and signs of uric acid overproduction in association with neurodevelopmental impairment, frequently including sensorineural deafness.[221] Gout may develop in heterozygous female carriers in these families during the reproductive period; in two of these families, the women were deaf.[226,229] Six kindreds have been found with these features. In five, affected patients and their cultured cells show regulatory or combined defects in the enzyme,[218,220,221,226] along with severe functional derangements in PP-ribose-P and purine metabolism.[149,222] PRS in the sixth family[230] is catalytically superactive, and overproduction of

PP-ribose-P and purine nucleotides is apparently no more severe than is encountered in the later onset phenotype.[225] Abnormal purine metabolic and neurologic features in this family appeared much later in childhood.[230] Moreover, not all families with nucleotide inhibitor–resistant PRS have neurologic impairment or even childhood presentation, as exemplified by the family initially described.[160] As discussed below, the genetic basis of impaired allosteric regulation of PRS has been identified.[222,231] Nevertheless, the mechanisms relating metabolic and neurologic derangements in PRS superactivity remain unknown.[222]

The late juvenile-onset to early adult-onset variety of PRS superactivity is restricted to males who show gout or uric acid urolithiasis but no neurologic deficits.[221,225] Overabundance of the normal PRS1 isoform is, with the single exception noted above, associated with this clinical pattern. Functional defects in the PP-ribose-P and purine nucleotide metabolism of cells from such patients are less aberrant than is the case with allosteric regulation-impaired forms of the enzyme.[149]

PRS overactivity was reported in association with symmetric lipomatosis in a single patient, but this may have represented a chance occurrence because the patient had a gouty brother without lipomatosis.[232] A severe deficiency of PRS was reported in erythrocytes of a hypouricemic and retarded child with seizures and progressive electroencephalographic abnormalities. PRS activity was partially deficient in each parent,[233] suggesting autosomal-recessive inheritance. However, studies in fibroblasts cultured from this patient did not confirm enzyme deficiency in this tissue.

The genetic heterogeneity suggested by differences in the kinetic abnormalities and phenotypic expressions of inherited PRS superactivity has been confirmed: point mutations in the translated region of *PRPS1* provide the genetic basis for altered allosteric control of PRS activity;[223,231] in contrast, PRS catalytic superactivity reflects altered regulation of the expression of the normal PRS1 isoform.[216]

Reverse-transcriptase polymerase chain reaction (RT-PCR) analysis of patient and normal fibroblast and lymphoblast RNA identified single base substitutions in the PRS1 cDNAs derived from each of six unrelated male patients with superactive, purine nucleotide-resistant PRS (Table 106-3).[222,231] In each instance, the base change in PRS1 cDNA predicted a single amino acid substitution in PRS1, ranging from amino acid residue 51 to 192 of the 317-residue polypeptide. The functional significance of the mutation predicted for each PRS1 was established by demonstrating that each patient's recombinant PRS1 showed the pattern and magnitude of aberrant allosteric responses to purine nucleotide inhibitors and Pi characteristic of PRS in cells from that patient.[222] Thus, the genetic basis of inherited PRS superactivity associated with altered allosteric regulation is a point mutation in the PRS1-coding region of the *PRPS1* gene.

Table 106-3 Mutations in PRS1 in Patients with PRS Superactivity and Purine Nucleotide Inhibitor Resistance

Patient	Base Substitution	Type of Mutation	Deduced Amino Acid Replacement*
O.G.	G154 → C	Transversion	Asp51 → His
N.B.	A341 → G	Transition	Asn113 → Ser
R.D.	C385 → A	Transversion	Leu128 → Ile
S.M.	G547 → C	Transversion	Asp182 → His
A.L.	C569 → T	Transition	Ala89 → Val
V.R.G.	C579 → G	Transversion	Hisl92 → Gln

*In mature PRS1, N-terminal Met has been removed. As a consequence, amino acid residues are numbered relative to the N-terminal Pro residue corresponding to nucleotides through 4 to 6.

Reprinted with permission from Becker MA, Smith PR, Taylor W, Mustafi R, Switzer RL: The genetic and functional basis of purine nucleotide feedback-resistant phosphoribosylpyrophosphate synthetase superactivity. *J Clin Invest* **96**:2133, 1995.

These variant PRS1s provide some insight into the molecular basis of regulation of PRS1 activity. The fact that single-residue substitutions dispersed over a major portion of PRS1 result in diminished responsiveness to inhibition by ADP and GDP suggests that these compounds share an extensive allosteric nucleotide inhibitory mechanism and that most or all of the mutations alter transmission of allosteric effects to the active site of PRS1 rather than the primary structure of nucleotide binding residues in the allosteric site. The MgATP binding properties of the recombinant mutant PRS1s are normal,[222] indicating that the active site is not directly altered. Overall, multiple residues and regions of the PRS1 polypeptide appear involved in determining isoform activity and sensitivity to GDP and ADP inhibition. Concurrent impairment of nucleotide inhibition and enhancement of P_i responsiveness in mutant PRS1s suggest that these effectors share a mechanism in which inhibited conformations favored by nucleotide binding are in equilibrium with more active conformations favored by P_i binding. In such a model, mutant PRS1s are likely altered in residues involved in stabilizing the inhibited conformations, rather than directly in P_i or nucleotide binding.

The kinetics of ADP and GDP inhibition of purified recombinant normal and mutant PRS1s[222] also provide information regarding mechanisms by which inhibition is effected in vivo. ADP inhibition of normal PRS1 involves both noncompetitive and competitive mechanisms, but only a competitive mechanism of ADP inhibition is demonstrable for recombinant mutant PRS1s. Despite retention of this mechanism, however, mutant PRS1s clearly resist inhibition by ADP and the noncompetitive inhibitor GDP in the presence of saturating concentrations of ATP. These findings suggest that point mutations in PRS1 disrupt a major noncompetitive component of the allosteric nucleotide inhibitory mechanism without altering the ATP substrate-binding region and that the competitive mechanism exerts little or no control on PRS1 activity under physiologic conditions in which ATP concentrations are saturating for the enzyme.

When RT-PCR analysis of PRS1 and PRS2 transcripts was applied to 6 patients with X-linked catalytic superactivity of PRS, no alterations in the sequences of the translated regions of PRS1 and PRS2 cDNAs were identified,[216] showing that mutations in the translated region of X-linked *PRPS1* or *PRPS2* genes did not account for this class of PRS superactivity. Rather, this variety of PRS overactivity appeared to involve increased expression of one or both X-linked PRS isoforms with normal primary sequence. Using northern blot analysis and quantitative isoelectric focusing–immunoblotting, levels of X chromosome–linked PRS transcripts and isoforms in cultured fibroblasts from normal and affected individuals were determined and showed that PRS catalytic superactivity was associated with two- to sixfold increased fibroblast concentrations of PRS1 isoform with physical and catalytic properties indistinguishable from those of normal PRS1.[216] Total PRS activities in both normal and patient cells closely correlated with total PRS isoform contents (>80 percent of which is PRS1), so that superactivity was clearly associated with increased PRS1 content. In fact, PRS isoform specific activities (PRS activity per milligram PRS isoform) in cell extracts were comparable in normal and patient cells and close to those of purified recombinant normal PRS isoforms.[208] PRS catalytic superactivity is thus not due to preferential inhibition of normal PRS, such as by specific PRS-associated proteins.[214,215] In addition, relative steady state levels of PRS1 transcripts were increased two- to fivefold in patient cells, and PRS2 isoform and transcript levels were comparable in normal and patient cells.[216] Together, these findings demonstrated that the enzymatic basis of PRS catalytic superactivity is selectively increased concentration of the normal PRS1 isoform and that PRS1 overexpression is determined at least in major part by an altered pretranslational mechanism of control of *PRPS1* gene expression.

Studies aimed at identifying the aberrant pretranslational mechanism of *PRPS1* expression in PRS catalytic superactivity[234] have excluded *PRPS1* gene amplification or altered structure or processing of PRS1 mRNA as likely explanations for the increased *PRPS1* expression.[216,234] In addition, PRS1 mRNA stability in normal and patient cells is nearly identical: half-lives of the PRS1 transcript are 10.8 ± 1.4 and 11.1 ± 0.9 (mean ±1 SD), respectively, in normal and patient cells.[234] In contrast, rates of *PRPS1* transcription (by nuclear runoff analysis) were two- to fourfold greater relative to those of *GAPDH* and *PRPS2* transcription in patient lymphoblasts and fibroblasts than in corresponding normal cells. Taken together, these findings establish that the pretranslational mechanism underlying inherited overexpression of the normal PRS1 isoform involves increased rates of *PRPS1* gene transcription in the cells of affected individuals.[234] Selectively increased *PRPS1* transcription rates could reflect altered structure and/or function of 5′ *PRPS1* promoter region. However, no differences were found in the 850 bp of DNA immediately 5′ to the transcription initiation site of *PRPS1* when the promoter region sequences of patient and normal *PRPS1*s were compared, raising the possibility of altered regulation of structurally normal *PRPS1* promoters in PRS catalytic superactivity. Extended cloning and sequencing of the 5′ DNA flanking *PRPS1* and measurements of *PRPS1* promoter activities by reporter gene analysis may help resolve this question.

Hypoxanthine-guanine Phosphoribosyltransferase Deficiency. Virtually complete deficiency of HPRT or virtually complete absence of catalytically active HPRT[162] is associated with the Lesch-Nyhan syndrome.[235] The clinical manifestations of the syndrome include uric acid overproduction and overexcretion leading to urolithiasis or gout, mental and growth retardation, choreoathetosis, spasticity, and compulsive self-mutilation. Partial deficiency of HPRT (Kelley-Seegmiller syndrome)[163] is typically an early adult-onset disorder of men, characterized by uric acid overproduction, gout, and urolithiasis, with only occasional mild neurologic accompaniments. Both disorders are transmitted in an X-linked manner, reflecting localization of the HPRT gene to the long arm of the X chromosome. Both severe and partial HPRT deficiencies have been studied extensively at the molecular level and have served as useful genetic models for inborn metabolic disorders; they are discussed in detail in Chap. 107.

Glycogen Storage Diseases

Glucose-6-Phosphatase Deficiency (Type 1). Hyperuricemia and gout occur frequently in type 1 glycogen storage disease (see also Chap. 71).[167] Both decreased renal clearance of urate secondary to lactic acidemia and ketonemia[169] and increased production of uric acid[167] contribute to the hyperuricemia, as discussed earlier.

Myogenic Hyperuricemia. In type III, type V, and type VII glycogen storage diseases, hyperuricemia has been noted either in the resting state or after exercise. Each of these enzyme deficiencies involves abnormal muscle glycogen metabolism, and the mechanism of hyperuricemia is related to excessive ATP breakdown in muscle during exercise as a result of decreased formation of carbohydrate substrates needed for ATP synthesis.[178]

TREATMENT

Hyperuricemia is a common biochemical aberration for which consideration of the cause is always required. In the absence of symptomatic events, however, specific treatment aimed at lowering serum urate levels is usually not warranted. Such treatment is appropriate for gout, for renal calculi associated with hyperuricemia, for significant hyperuricosuria, and for prevention of acute uric acid nephropathy.

Asymptomatic Hyperuricemia

Most hyperuricemic persons remain asymptomatic even after many years of modest to moderate increases in serum urate.[1] Moreover, evidence is lacking to support either a significant renal risk resulting from hyperuricemia of such a degree[6,19–23] or a causal or contributory role for hyperuricemia in the major associated disorders[83,101] described earlier. A decision regarding treatment of the asymptomatic hyperuricemic individual should be made primarily by the statistical risk for development of gouty arthritis, tophi, uric acid or calcium oxalate stones, urate nephropathy, or acute uric acid nephropathy.

The magnitude of the risk for articular gout or tophi is related to the degree and duration of hyperuricemia as well as to the sex and age of the individual.[6,7,17,18] Gouty arthritis and tophi are treatable and reversible if they occur and are not life-threatening. It is reasonable to withhold antihyperuricemic therapy until gouty arthritis occurs. Similarly, antihyperuricemic therapy need not be instituted as prophylaxis against stone disease but should be started on discovery of a stone in the hyperuricemic or hyperuricosuric individual.

Three specific clinical circumstances warrant the institution of antihyperuricemic treatment in asymptomatic subjects. First, persistent hyperuricemia with serum urate levels greater than 13 mg/dl in men and 10 mg/dl in women may carry some significant nephrotoxic risk, perhaps related to the likelihood of accompanying uric acid overproduction.[20] Second, excretion of daily urinary uric acid in excess of 1100 mg is associated with a 50 percent risk of uric acid calculi.[74] Finally, patients about to receive radiotherapy or chemotherapy expected to result in extensive tumor cytolysis should be treated with allopurinol to prevent acute uric acid nephropathy.

Gouty Arthritis. The aims of the treatment of gout are to terminate the acute arthritic attack as promptly and safely as possible, to prevent recurrences of acute gouty arthritis, to prevent or reverse complications resulting from urate crystal deposition in joints, kidneys, and other tissues, and to prevent formation or recurrence of renal stones. Reversal of deleterious manifestations of disorders associated with gout, such as obesity, hypertension, ethanol abuse, and hyperlipidemia, is an additional aim requiring action directed to the specific accompanying process rather than the abnormal purine metabolism.[236,237] It is critical for the physician and the patient to distinguish between management of acute inflammatory features and control of hyperuricemia. Drugs effective in reducing acute gouty inflammation are generally of no value in controlling hyperuricemia, and antihyperuricemic agents, while capable of ultimately reducing the frequency of acute attacks, have no value in treatment of ongoing gouty inflammation.

Anti-inflammatory Therapy. Acute gouty arthritis is usually responsive to any of a broad array of anti-inflammatory measures, the most prompt and complete resolution occurring the earlier the therapy is introduced.[238] Virtually any of the available nonsteroidal anti-inflammatory agents (e.g., indomethacin, naproxen, ibuprofen, sulindac, piroxicam) or colchicine can be administered orally with the expectation of a satisfactory response, although frequent nausea, vomiting, and diarrhea often limit the hourly use of the latter agent. Prednisone and parenteral corticosteroids have a definite effect on gouty inflammation[239] but withdrawal may be attended by a rebound attack. In the frequent hospital setting of acute gouty arthritis in the postoperative period, intraarticular corticosteroids are useful, especially if only a single joint or bursa is involved. The use of intravenous colchicine in patients with polyarticular gout or in those unable to take oral medications should be restricted to hospitalized patients and should be supervised by physicians experienced in the use of colchicine by this route of administration, following the required precautions, detailed elsewhere.[238] In brief, leukopenia, hepatic and renal disease, and recent use of oral colchicine should be considered contraindications for use of intravenous colchicine,[238,240–242] which should be given with great care to avoid local infiltration into the extravascular space of this highly sclerotic agent, and never in total doses exceeding 4 mg during any attack.

Prophylactic Therapy. Despite recent contentions to the contrary,[243] therapy with oral colchicine (0.6 mg twice daily) appears valuable in reducing the frequency of recurrent acute gouty arthritis in patients with a prior history of gout, and is an especially important adjunct early in the course of administration of antihyperuricemic agents, when patients are at high risk for gouty attacks.[244] In many elderly patients, reduced dosage mandated by loose stools or diarrhea appears adequate for prophylaxis. Indomethacin (25 mg twice daily) appears to be effective in patients intolerant of low doses of colchicine. In patients with no evident tophi, prophylaxis can be safely discontinued 6 to 12 months after normal serum urate values have been achieved, when urate pools are presumably normalized. Patients with tophi should continue to receive prophylaxis until these lesions resolve. Suppression of chemotactic factor release by synovial lining cells appears to underlie this action of colchicine.[43,238]

Antihyperuricemic Therapy. Dietary purine restriction is not often practical or effective in the management of hyperuricemia and gout in patients with normal dietary habits. Although a severely purine-restricted diet may reduce daily urinary uric acid excretion by 200 to 400 mg, mean serum urate concentrations decrease only by about 1 mg/dl.[1] In some instances, however, unusual dietary habits may benefit from avoidance of specific dietary components. Patients who customarily ingest large quantities of organ-rich foods (liver, sweetbreads), beer, or distilled spirits may benefit greatly from avoiding these stimuli to increasing urate levels, particularly if such ingestion is temporally associated with acute gouty episodes. Patients who have had dysuria, crystalluria, or gouty arthritis associated with hyperuricemia and hyperuricosuria in the course of high-dose pancreatic extract therapy in cystic fibrosis[245,246] may benefit from dose reduction with a return to more normal urate levels. With the advent of effective antihyperuricemic drug therapy, dietary restriction is limited to hyperuricemic individuals with severe renal insufficiency or with intolerance to pharmacologic management. Unfortunately, low-purine diets are rather unpalatable and may in the long run be atherogenic.

Anti-inflammatory and prophylactic drug treatments provide effective means to control and prevent attacks of gouty arthritis but are insufficient to reverse hyperuricemia and thus modify the natural history of the disorder. For this purpose, potent agents are available that can reduce serum urate levels either by enhancing renal excretion of uric acid or by decreasing uric acid synthesis. Antihyperuricemic therapy generally aims at achieving urate concentrations of 5 to 6 mg/dl, well below that at which monosodium urate saturates extracellular fluid (6.5 mg/dl).[236–238]

The uricosuric agents most widely used in the United States are probenecid and sulfinpyrazone, but others, including benzbromarone, are popular elsewhere. Allopurinol, a xanthine oxidase inhibitor, is currently the only available and effective drug for reducing uric acid synthesis. Treatment with an antihyperuricemic agent is usually continued for an indefinite period, and it is thus important for the choice of drug to be made on a rational basis.[236–238]

Although allopurinol is likely to be effective in treating virtually all patients warranting therapy, cost and safety considerations, as well as the demonstrated efficacy of uricosuric drugs over four decades of experience, dictate an important role for these compounds as agents of choice in many patients with gout. Specifically, the majority of patients with gout who excrete less than 700 mg of uric acid per day are potential candidates for uricosuric drug therapy in the absence of other evidence for uric acid overproduction, significant renal insufficiency (creatinine clearance less than 80 ml/min), or a history of urolithiasis.[236–238] Even if age (older than 60 years) and the presence of tophi are considered relative indications for allopurinol (rather than uricosuric) treatment, a high proportion of gouty individuals remain candidates for uricosuric agents. It is important to stress that, in this group of patients, both uricosuric agents and allopurinol have comparable efficacy in establishing normouricemia and, ultimately, in decreasing or abolishing attacks of gouty arthritis and preventing tophi and urolithiasis. In view of the difficulty in relating hyperuricemia and gout to chronic renal insufficiency, however, an effect of either class of antihyperuricemic drugs in preventing functionally significant renal impairment has yet to be established.

Uricosuric Agents. Uricosuric drugs are weak organic acids that increase the renal clearance of uric acid by inhibiting renal tubular reabsorption of uric acid at a postsecretory site.[238] Therapy with uricosuric drugs is started at a low dose to minimize the risk of renal calculi associated with the transient increase in uric acid excretion. The maintenance of adequate urine flow by hydration (2 or more liters of fluids daily) further diminishes the possibility of uric acid stone formation, but alkalinization is unnecessary in most patients. Probenecid is started at a dose of 250 mg twice per day, increasing after several weeks to 500 to 1000 mg two or three times each day; the maximum effective dose is 3 g/day. Sulfinpyrazone is started at a dose of 50 mg twice per day, increasing over several weeks to 100 mg three or four times each day; the maximum effective dose is 800 mg/day.

Probenecid and sulfinpyrazone are effective for most gouty patients. Seventy-five to eighty percent of patients with tophaceous gout have demonstrated improvement. The major side effects of uricosuric drugs include skin rash, precipitation of acute gouty arthritis, gastrointestinal intolerance, and uric acid calculus formation. Probenecid has a calciuric action in gouty patients, reinforcing the contraindication for its use in patients with prior nephrolithiasis.[247] Probenecid should not be used in hyperuricemic cystinuria patients because of increased urinary cystine and decreased cysteine–penicillamine mixed disulfide and penicillamine disulfide metabolites.[248] Uricosuric drugs alter the transport of other organic acids across cell membranes, resulting in many drug interactions. For example, the renal excretion of penicillin and ampicillin is decreased by probenecid, so the half-lives of these antibiotics are prolonged. An autoimmune hemolytic anemia has also been reported with probenecid therapy.[249,250]

Xanthine Oxidase Inhibitors. Allopurinol inhibits uric acid production in major part by virtue of inhibition of xanthine oxidase by the drug and by its major metabolite and oxidation product, oxypurinol.[251] Allopurinol and oxypurinol are structural analogues of hypoxanthine and xanthine, respectively, and the complex metabolism and pharmacodynamics of these compounds have been reviewed in detail in a previous version of this chapter.[5]

Administration of allopurinol results in multiple effects on human purine and pyrimidine metabolism.[1,251] Allopurinol is a competitive inhibitor of xanthine oxidase and, along with oxipurinol, produces pseudoirreversible inactivation of the enzyme. As a result, hypoxanthine and xanthine accumulate in body fluids, producing a pharmacologic xanthinuric state. During allopurinol treatment, total urinary purine excretion diminishes as a result of inhibition of purine synthesis *de novo* either by nucleotide derivatives of allopurinol and oxipurinol[1,251] or by nucleotide products arising from enhanced rates of reutilization of hypoxanthine.[172] The decrement in total urinary purine excretion during allopurinol administration requires HPRT activity and, by potentiating the inhibition of uric acid production, contributes to the antihyperuricemic effect of the drug, except when this enzyme is deficient.[5] Oxypurinol nucleotide derivatives of allopurinol block the pyrimidine pathway enzyme orotidylate decarboxylase, inducing a state of orotidinuria and orotic aciduria in patients receiving the drug.[252,253]

The daily single dose of allopurinol required to achieve control of serum urate concentration varies considerably in individuals with normal renal function, ranging from 100 mg to over 600 mg, with a mean of 300 mg. Because the half-life of oxypurinol is prolonged in renal failure, dose reduction is important in this state.[254–256] Reduction in serum urate levels begins within 2 days of allopurinol administration and reaches a stable level in 1 to 2 weeks. Failure of allopurinol to decrease urate concentrations to therapeutic levels may occur in patients with many tophi early in the course of treatment, but refractoriness to the drug is rare and usually denotes a failure of patient compliance or physician-patient communication.[5,237,238]

Therapeutic effectiveness of this drug has been excellent for over 20 years.[251] Nevertheless, side effects and adverse reactions, some severe, have been encountered.[238,254,255] As with uricosuric agents, allopurinol administration can precipitate acute gouty arthritis, particularly if colchicine prophylaxis has been omitted. Adverse reactions, which occur in 3 to 5 percent of patients,[254] include skin rashes, leukopenia or thrombocytopenia, diarrhea, and drug fever. A life-threatening allopurinol hypersensitivity syndrome,[255,257] consisting of erythematous skin rash, fever, hepatitis, eosinophilia, and renal failure, has been encountered, especially when patients receiving diuretics and with mild renal insufficiency receive standard doses of the drug. Accumulation of oxypurinol in these circumstances has been suggested to play a role in this adverse reaction.[256] The mortality rate in reported cases has been nearly 25 percent, reinforcing caution in restricting allopurinol use to patients with appropriate indications and to the minimum dose necessary to achieve adequate antihyperuricemic effect.[255–257] Additional adverse reactions include gastrointestinal intolerance, vasculitis, and interstitial nephritis. Xanthine urolithiasis or crystalluria has been reported only in patients with HPRT deficiency or those who have received cytolytic cancer chemotherapy.

Among clinically relevant drug interactions involving allopurinol[5] are potentiation of the actions of 6-mercaptopurine and azathioprine, requiring reduction of doses of these agents; bone marrow suppression in patients receiving cyclophosphamide; prolongation of the actions of dicumarol and warfarin; and increased incidence of ampicillin-induced skin rash. Concomitant use of allopurinol and a uricosuric agent has been undertaken in patients incompletely responsive to either class of agent alone. Despite documented pharmacologic interactions between these drugs, combined therapy at standard doses has been efficacious when required.

Urolithiasis

Uric acid stones can generally be managed with alkalinization of the urine to pH 6.0 to 6.5 (with oral potassium bicarbonate or potassium citrate, typically at doses of 60 to 80 meq/day), allopurinol, and fluid intake of 2 to 3 L/day.[73,238] Patients with recurrent calcium oxalate stones and hyperuricosuria frequently benefit from allopuriol,[68,73,258] high fluid intake, and modest reduction in dietary purines.

Acute Uric Acid Nephropathy

Prophylaxis against this serious complication of renal uric acid overload can usually be achieved by measures that decrease uric acid concentrations and increase uric acid solubility in urine: urinary alkalinization, maintenance of high urine flow, and treatment with allopurinol.[73] In the acute tumor lysis syndrome, these measures may not entirely prevent significant increases in urinary uric acid and may still permit sufficient urinary xanthine concentrations to precipitate xanthine nephropathy.[259] An alternative approach to treatment or prevention of acute uric acid nephropathy is degradation of uric acid by administration of recombinant uricase, the enzyme catalyzing oxidation of uric acid to allantoin.[260,261] The need for parenteral administration and the documentation of allergic reactions[262] limit the routine use of this approach in prophylaxis of chemotherapy-induced hyperuricemia, but the production of a longer lasting nonantigenic polyethylene glycol–conjugated uricase preparation[263,264] holds promise for successful use of this approach in this setting and perhaps in the treatment of refractory tophaceous gout.[265]

ACKNOWLEDGMENTS

This work was supported by a grant from the U.S. Public Health Service (DK28554). I wish to thank Danette Shine for excellent preparation of the manuscript.

REFERENCES

1. Wyngaarden JB, Kelley WN: *Gout and Hyperuricemia.* New York, Grune & Stratton, 1976, pp 1–512 (and references therein).
2. Paulus HE, Coutts A, Calabro JJ, Klinenberg JR: Clinical significance of hyperuricemia in routinely screened hospitalized men. *JAMA* **211**:277, 1970.
3. Price CP, James DR: Analytical reviews in biochemistry: The measurement of urate. *Ann Clin Biochem* **25**:484, 1988.
4. Liddle L, Seegmiller JE, Laster L: Automated analysis of uric acid. *J Lab Clin Med* **54**:903, 1959.
5. Palella TD, Fox IH: Hyperuricemia and gout, in Scriver CR, Beaudet AL, Sly WS, Valle D (eds): *The Metabolic Basis of Inherited Disease*, 6th ed. Vol 1. New York, McGraw-Hill, 1989, p 965.
6. Campion EW, Glynn RJ, DeLabry LO: Asymptomatic hyperuricemia. Risks and consequences in the Normative Aging Study. *Am J Med* **82**:421, 1987.
7. Hall AP, Barry PE, Dawber TR, McNamara PM: Epidemiology of gout and hyperuricemia. A long-term population study. *Am J Med* **42**:27, 1967.
8. Cameron JS, Moro F, Simmonds HA: Gout, uric acid and purine metabolism in paediatric nephrology. *Pediatr Nephrol* **7**:105, 1995.
9. Glynn RJ, Campion EW, Silbert JE: Trends in serum uric acid levels 1961–1980. *Arthritis Rheum* **26**:87, 1983.
10. Mateos Anton F, Garcia Puig J, Ramos T, Gonzalez P, Ordas J: Sex differences in uric acid metabolism in adults: Evidence for a lack of influence of estradiol-17 beta (E_2) on the renal handling of urate. *Metabolism* **35**:343, 1986.
11. Marinello E, Riario-Sforza G, Marcolongo R: Plasma follicle-stimulating hormone, luteinizing hormone, and sex hormones in patients with gout. *Arthritis Rheum* **28**:127, 1985.
12. Gibson T, Waterworth R, Hatfield P, Robinson G, Bremner K: Hyperuricaemia, gout and kidney function in New Zealand Maori men. *Br J Rheumatol* **23**:276, 1984.
13. Klemp P, Stansfield SA, Castle B, Robertson MC: Gout is on the increase in New Zealand. *Ann Rheum Dis* **56**:22, 1997.
14. Darmavan J, Valkenburg HA, Muirden KD, Wigley RD: The epidemiology of gout and hyperuricemia in a rural population of Java. *J Rheumatol* **19**:1595, 1992.
15. Takahashi S, Yamamoto T, Tsutsumi Z, Moriwaki Y, Yamakita J, Higashino K: Close correlation between visceral fat accumulation and uric acid metabolism in healthy men. *Metabolism* **46**:1162, 1997.
16. Hochberg MC, Thomas J, Thomas DJ, Mead L, Levine DM, Klag MJ: Racial differences in the incidence of gout: The role of hypertension. *Arthritis Rheum* **38**:628, 1995.
17. Zalokar J, Lellouch J, Claude JR: Serum urate and gout in 4663 young male workers. *Semin Hop Paris* **57**:664, 1981.
18. Nishioka K, Mikanagi K: Hereditary and environmental factors influencing on the serum uric acid throughout ten years population study in Japan. *Adv Exp Med Biol* **122**:155, 1980.
19. Langford HG, Blaufox MD, Borhani NO, Curb JD, Molteni A, Schneider KA, Pressel S: Is thiazide-produced uric acid elevation harmful? Analysis of data from the Hypertension Detection and Follow-up Program. *Arch Intern Med* **147**:645, 1987.
20. Fessel WJ: Renal outcomes of gout and hyperuricemia. *Am J Med* **67**:74,1979.
21. Gibson T, Highton J, Potter C, Simmonds HA: Renal impairment and gout. *Ann Rheum Dis* **39**:417, 1980.
22. Berger L, Yu TF: Renal function in gout. IV. An analysis of 524 gouty subjects including long-term follow-up studies. *Am J Med* **59**:605, 1975.
23. Yu TF, Berger L: Impaired renal function in gout: Its association with hypertensive vascular disease and intrinsic renal disease. *Am J Med* **72**:95, 1982.
24. Copeman WSC: *A Short History of Gout.* Berkeley, University of California Press, 1964.
25. Grahame R, Scott JT: Clinical survey of 354 patients with gout. *Ann Rheum Dis* **29**:461, 1970.
26. Myers OL, Monteagudo FSE: Gout in females: An analysis of 92 patients. *Clin Exp Rheumatol* **3**:105, 1985.
27. Macfarlane DG, Dieppe PA: Diuretic-induced gout in elderly women. *Br J Rheumatol* **24**:155, 1985.

28. Lally EV, Ho G Jr, Kaplan SR: The clinical spectrum of gouty arthritis in women. *Arch Intern Med* **146**:2221, 1986.
29. Puig JG, Michan AD, Jimenez ML, Perez de Ayala C, Mateos FA, Capitan CF, de Miguel E, et al.: Female gout: Clinical spectrum and uric acid metabolism. *Arch Intern Med* **151**:726, 1991.
30. Hayem G, Delahousse M, Meyer O, Palazzo E, Chazerain P, Kahn M-F: Female premenopausal tophaceous gout induced by longterm diuretic abuse. *J Rheumatol* **23**:2166, 1996.
31. Fam AG, Rubenstein J: Hydroxapatite pseudopodagra: A syndrome of young women. *Arthritis Rheum* **32**:741, 1989.
32. Mines D, Abduhl SB: Hydroxyapatite pseudopodagra in a young man: Acute calcific periarthritis of the first metatarsophalangeal joint. *Am J Emerg Med* **14**:180, 1996.
33. Logan JA, Morrison E, McGill P: Serum uric acid in acute gout. *Ann Rheum Dis* **56**:696, 1997.
34. Scott JT: Drug-induced gout. *Ballieres Clin Rheumatol* **5**:39, 1991.
35. Kahl LE, Thompson ME, Griffith BP: Gout in the heart transplant recipient. Physiological puzzle and therapeutic challenge. *Am J Med* **87**:289, 1989.
36. Burack DA, Griffith BP, Thompson ME, Kahl LE: Hyperuricemia and gout among heart transplant recipients receiving cyclosporine. *Am J Med* **92**:141, 1992.
37. Lin HY, Rocher LL, McQuillan MA, Schmaltz S, Palella TD, Fox IH: Cyclosporine-induced hyperuricemia and gout. *N Engl J Med* **321**:287, 1989.
38. Baethge BA, Work J, Landreneau MD, McDonald JC: Tophaceous gout in patients with renal transplants treated with cyclosporine A. *J Rheumatol* **20**:718, 1993.
39. Derus CL, Levinson DJ, Bowman B, Bengoa JM, Sitrin MD: Altered fractional excretion of uric acid during total parenteral nutrition. *J Rheumatol* **14**:978, 1987.
40. Terkeltaub RA, Ginsberg MH: The inflammatory reaction to crystals. *Rheum Dis Clin North Am* **14**:353, 1988.
41. McCarty DJ: Gout without hyperuricemia. *JAMA* **271**:302, 1994.
42. Simkin PA: The pathogenesis of podagra. *Ann Intern Med* **86**:230, 1977.
43. Terkeltaub RA: What stops a gouty attack? *J Rheumatol* **19**:8, 1992.
44. Terkeltaub R, Baird S, Sears P, Santigo R, Boisvert W: The murine homolog of the interleukin-8 receptor CXCR-2 is essential for the occurrence of neutrophilic inflammation in the air pouch model of acute urate crystal-induced gouty synovitis. *Arthritis Rheum* **41**:900, 1998.
45. Pouliot M, James MJ, McColl SR, Naccache PH, Cleland LG: MSU crystals induce COX-2 in human monocytes. *Blood* **91**:1769, 1998.
46. Spilberg I, Mandell B: Crystal-induced chemotactic factor, in Weissman G (ed): *Advances in Inflammation Research*. New York, Raven, 1982, p 57.
47. Terkeltaub RA, Dyer CA, Martin J, Curtiss LK: Apolipoprotein (apo) E inhibits the capacity of monosodium urate crystals to stimulate neutrophils. Characterization of intraarticular apo E and demonstration of apo E binding to urate crystals *in vivo*. *J Clin Invest* **87**:20, 1991.
48. Pascual E: Persistence of monosodium urate crystals and low-grade inflammation in the synovial fluid of patients with untreated gout. *Arthritis Rheum* **34**:141, 1991.
49. Holingworth P, Scott JT, Burry HC: Nonarticular gout: Hyperuricemia and tophus formation without gouty arthritis. *Arthritis Rheum* **26**:98, 1983.
50. Wernick R, Winkler C, Campbell S: Tophi as the initial manifestation of gout. Report of six cases and review of the literature. *Arch Intern Med* **152**:873, 1992.
51. Iglesias A, Londono JC, Saaibi DL, Pena M, Lizarazo H, Gonzalez EB: Gout nodulosis: Widespread subcutaneous deposits without gout. *Arthritis Care Res* **9**:74, 1996.
52. Liu K, Moffatt EJ, Hudson ER, Layfield LJ: Gouty tophus presenting as a soft-tissue mass diagnosed by fine-needle aspiration: A case report. *Diagn Cytopathol* **15**:246, 1996.
53. Hench PS: Diagnosis of gout and gouty arthritis. *J Lab Clin Med* **22**:48, 1936.
54. Gutman AB: The past four decades of progress in the knowledge of gout, with an assessment of the present status. *Arthritis Rheum* **16**:431, 1973.
55. O'Duffy JD, Hunder GG, Kelly PJ: Decreasing prevalence of tophaceous gout. *Mayo Clin Proc* **50**:227, 1975.
56. Nakayama DA, Barthelemy C, Carrera G, Lightfoot RW Jr, Wortmann RL: Tophaceous gout: A clinical and radiographic assessment. *Arthritis Rheum* **27**:468, 1984.
57. Lawry GV II, Fan PT, Bluestone R: Polyarticular versus monoarticular gout: A prospective comparative analysis of clinical features. *Medicine* **67**:335, 1988.
58. Wordsworth BP, Mowat AG: Rapid development of gouty tophi after diuretic therapy. *J Rheumatol* **12**:376, 1985.
59. Lally EV, Zimmermann B, Ho G Jr, Kaplan SR: Urate-mediated inflammation in nodal osteoarthritis: Clinical and roentgenographic correlations. *Arthritis Rheum* **32**:86, 1989.
60. Simkin PA, Campbell PM, Larson EB: Gout in Heberden's nodes. *Arthritis Rheum* **26**:94, 1983.
61. Fam AG, Stein JG, Rubenstein J: Gouty arthritis in nodal osteoarthritis. *J Rheumatol* **23**:684, 1996.
62. Foldes K, Petersilge CA, Weisman MH, Resnick D: Nodal osteoarthritis and gout. *Skel Radiol* **25**:421, 1996.
63. Holland NW, Jost D, Beutler A, Schumacher HR, Agudelo CA: Finger pad tophi in gout. *J Rheumatol* **23**:690, 1996.
64. Fam AG, Assad D: Intradermal urate tophi. *J Rheumatol* **24**:1126, 1997.
65. Popp JD, Bidgood WD Jr, Edwards NL: Magnetic resonance imaging of tophaceous gout in the hands and wrists. *Semin Arthritis Rheum* **25**:282, 1996.
66. Yu JS, Chung C, Recht M, Dailiana T, Jurdi R: MRI imaging of tophaceous gout. *AJR* **168**:523, 1997.
67. Gerster JC, Landry M, Duvoisin B, Rappoport G: Computed tomography of the knee joint as an indicator of intraarticular tophi in gout. *Arthritis Rheum* **39**:1406, 1996.
68. Coe FL, Kavalach AG: Hypercalciuria and hyperuricosuria in patients with calcium nephorolithiasia. *N Engl J Med* **291**:1344, 1974.
69. Reynolds PP, Knapp MJ, Baraf HS, Holmes EW: Moonshine and lead. Relationship to the pathogenesis of hyperuricemia in gout. *Arthritis Rheum* **26**:1057, 1983.
70. Batuman V, Maesaka JK, Haddad B, Tepper E, Landy E, Wedeen RP: The role of lead in gout nephropathy. *N Engl J Med* **304**:520, 1981.
71. Simon LS, Mills JA: Nonsteroidal antiinflammtory drugs. *N Engl J Med* **302**:1179;1237, 1980.
72. Cohen LF, Balow JE, Poplack DG: Acute tumor lysis syndrome: A review of 37 patients with Burkitt's lymphoma. *Am J Med* **68**:486, 1980.
73. Asplin JR: Uric acid stones. *Semin Nephrol* **16**:412, 1996.
74. Yu T, Gutman AB: Uric acid nephrolithiasis in gout. Predisposing factors. *Ann Intern Med* **67**:1133, 1967.
75. Ettinger B, Tang A, Citron JT, Livermore B, Williams T: Randomized trial of allopurinol in the prevention of calcium oxalate calculi. *N Engl J Med* **315**:1386, 1986.
76. Brock WA, Golden J, Kaplan GW: Xanthine calculi in the Lesch-Nyhan syndrome. *J Urol* **130**:157, 1983.
77. Simmonds HA, Cameron JS, Potter CF, Warren D, Gibson T, Farebrother D: Renal failure in young subjects with familial gout. *Adv Exp Med Biol* **122**:15, 1980.
78. Thompson GR, Weiss JJ, Goldman RT, Rigg GA: Familial occurrence of hyperuricemia, gout, and medullary cystic disease. *Arch Intern Med* **138**:1614, 1978.
79. Leumann EP, Wegmann W: Familial nephropathy with hyperuricemia and gout. *Nephron* **34**:51, 1983.
80. Puig JG, Miranda ME, Mateos FA, Picazo ML, Jimenez ML, Calvin TS, Gil AA: Hereditary nephropathy associated with hyperuricemia and gout. *Arch Intern Med* **153**:357, 1993.
81. Campbell BC, Moore MR, Goldberg A, Hernandez LA, Dick WC: Subclinical lead exposure: A possible cause of gout. *BMJ* **2**:1403, 1978.
82. Craswell PW, Price J, Boyle PD, Heazlewood VJ, Baddeley H, Lloyd HM, Thomas BJ, et al.: Chronic renal failure with gout: A marker of chronic lead poisoning. *Kidney Int* **26**:319, 1984.
83. Becker MA: Clinical aspects of monosodium urate monohydrate crystal deposition disease (gout). *Rheum Dis Clin North Am* **14**:377, 1988.
84. Seidell JC, Bakx KC, Deurenberg P, van den Hoogen HJ, Hautvast JG, Stijnen T: Overweight and chronic illness—a retrospective cohort study, with a follow-up of 6–17 years, in men and women of initially 20–50 years of age. *J Chron Dis* **39**:585, 1986.
85. Scott JT: Obesity and hyperuricemia. *Clin Rheum Dis* **3**:25, 1977.
86. Jiao S, Kameda K, Matsuzawa Y, Tarui S: Hyperlipoproteinaemia in primary gout: Hyperlipoproteinaemic phenotype and influence of alcohol intake and obesity in Japan. *Ann Rheum Dis* **45**:308, 1986.
87. Fox IH, John D, DeBruyne S, Dwosh I, Marliss EB: Hyperuricemia and hypertriglyceridemia: Metabolic basis for the association. *Metabolism* **34**:741, 1985.

88. Darlington LG, Slack J, Scott JT: Family study of lipid and purine levels in gout patients. *Ann Rheum Dis* **41**:253, 1982.
89. Messerli FH, Frohlich ED, Dreslinski GR, Suarez DH, Aristimuno GG: Serum uric acid in essential hypertension: An indicator of renal vascular involvement. *Ann Intern Med* **93**:817, 1980.
90. Heyden S, Borhani NO, Tyroler HA, Schneider KA, Langford HG, Hames CG, Hutchinson R, et al.: The relationship of weight change to changes in blood pressure, serum uric acid, cholesterol and glucose in the treatment of hypertension. *J Chron Dis* **38**:281, 1985.
91. The Hypertension Detection and Follow-up Program Cooperative Research Group: Mortality findings for stepped-care and referred-care participants in the hypertension detection and follow-up program, stratified by other risk factors. *Prev Med* **14**:312, 1985.
92. Abbott RD, Brand FN, Kannel WB, Castelli WP: Gout and coronary heart disease: The Framingham Study. *J Clin Epidemiol* **41**:237, 1988.
93. Nishioka K, Mikanagi K: A retrospective study on the cause of death, in Japan, of patients with gout. *Ryumachi* **21**(suppl):29, 1981.
94. Fessel WJ: High uric acid as an indicator of cardiovascular disease. Independence from obesity. *Am J Med* **68**:401, 1980.
95. Macfarlane DG, Slade R, Hopes PA, Hartog MH: A study of platelet aggregation and adhesion in gout. *Clin Exp Rheumatol* **1**:63, 1983.
96. Gelber AC, Klag MJ, Mead LA, Thomas J, Thomas DJ, Pearson TA, Hochberg MC: Gout and risk for subsequent coronary heart disease. The Meharry-Hopkins Study. *Arch Intern Med* **157**:1436, 1997.
97. Faller J, Fox IH: Ethanol-induced hyperuricemia: Evidence for increased urate production by activation of adenine nucleotide turnover. *N Engl J Med* **307**:1598, 1982.
98. Puig JG, Fox IH: Ethanol-induced activation of adenine nucleotide turnover. Evidence for a role of acetate. *J Clin Invest* **74**:936, 1984.
99. Feinstein EI, Quion-Verde H, Kaptein EM, Massry SG: Severe hyperuricemia in patients with volume depletion. *Am J Nephrol* **4**:77, 1984.
100. Goldfinger S, Klinenberg JR, Seegmiller JE: Renal retention of uric acid induced by infusion of beta-hydroxybutyrate and acetoacetate. *N Engl J Med* **272**:351, 1965.
101. Emmerson B: Hyperlipidaemia in hyperuricaemia and gout. *Ann Rheum Dis* **57**:509, 1998.
102. Gibson T, Kilbourn K, Horner I, Simmonds HA: Mechanism and treatment of hypertriglyceridaemia in gout. *Ann Rheum Dis* **38**:31, 1979.
103. Vague J: The degree of masculine differentiation of obesities: A factor determining predisposition to diabetes, atherosclerosis, gout and uric calculous disease. *Am J Clin Nutr* **4**:20, 1956.
104. Carey GDP: Abdominal obesity. *Curr Opin Lipidol* **9**:35, 1998.
105. Roubenoff R, Klag MG, Mead LA, Liang KY, Seidler AJ, Hochberg MC: Incidence and risk factors for gout in white men. *JAMA* **266**:3004, 1991.
106. Ostrander LD, Lamphiear DE, Block WD, Johnson BC, Ravenscroft C, Epstein FH: Relationship of serum lipid concentrations to alcohol consumption. *Arch Intern Med* **134**:451, 1974.
107. Ginsberg H, Olefsky J, Farquhar JW, Reaven GM: Moderate ethanol ingestion and plasma triglyceride levels: A study in normal and hypertriglyceridemic persons. *Ann Intern Med* **80**:143, 1974.
108. Wiedmann E, Rose H, Schwartz E: Plasma lipoproteins, glucose tolerance and insulin response in primary gout. *Am J Med* **53**:299, 1972.
109. Collantes Estevez E, Pineda Priego M, Anon Barbudo J, Sanchez Guijo P: Hyperuricemia–hyperlipidemia association in the absence of obesity and alcohol abuse. *Clin Rheumatol* **9**:28, 1990.
110. Lee J, Sparrow D, Vokonas PS, Landsberg L, Weiss ST: Uric acid and coronary heart disease risk: Evidence for a role of uric acid in the obesity-insulin resistance syndrome. *Am J Epidemiol* **142**:288, 1995.
111. Vuorin-Markkola H, Yki-Jarvonen H: Hyperuricemia and insulin-resistance. *J Clin Endocrinol Metab* **78**:25, 1994.
112. Facchini F, Chen Y-D, Hollenbeck CB, Reaven GM: Relationship between resistance to insulin-mediated glucose uptake, urinary uric acid clearance, and plasma uric acid concentration. *JAMA* **266**:3008, 1991.
113. Reaven GM: Role of insulin-resistance in human disease. *Diabetes* **37**:1595, 1988.
114. Becker MA, Raivio KO, Seegmiller JE: Synthesis of phosphoribosylpyrophosphate in mammalian cells. *Adv Enzymol Relat Areas Mol Biol* **49**:281, 1979.
115. Becker MA, Kim M: Regulation of purine synthesis *de novo* in human fibroblasts by purine nucleotides and phosphoribosylpyrophosphate. *J Biol Chem* **262**:14531, 1987.
116. Holmes EW, King GL, Leyva A, Singer SC: A purine auxotroph deficient in phosphoribosylpyrophosphate amidotransferase and phosphoribosylpyrophosphate aminotransferase activities with normal activity of ribose-5-phosphate aminotransferase. *Proc Natl Acad Sci U S A* **73**:2458, 1976.
117. Fox IH: Degradation of purine nucleotides, in Kelley WN, Weiner IM (eds): *Uric Acid*. New York, Springer-Verlag, 1978, p 93.
118. Fox IH: Metabolic basis for disorders of purine nucleotide degradation. *Metabolism* **30**:616, 1981.
119. Carson DA, Carrera CJ, Wasson DB, Iizasa T: Deoxyadenosine-resistant human T lymphoblasts with elevated 5′-nucleotidase activity. *Biochim Biophys Acta* **1091**:22, 1991.
120. Krenitsky TA, Elion GB, Henderson AM, Hitchings GH: Inhibition of human purine nucleoside phosphorylase. Studies with intact erythrocytes and the purified enzyme. *J Biol Chem* **243**:2876, 1968.
121. McCord JM: Oxygen-derived free radicals in postischemic tissue injury. *N Engl J Med* **312**:159, 1985.
122. Woolliscroft JO, Fox IH: Increased body fluid purine levels during hypotensive events. Evidence for ATP degradation. *Am J Med* **81**:472, 1986.
123. Hooper DC, Spitsin S, Kean RB, Champion JM, Dickson GM, Chaudhry I, Koprowski H: Uric acid, a natural scavenger of peroxynitrite, in experimental allergic encephalomyelitis and multiple sclerosis. *Proc Natl Acad Sci U S A* **95**:675, 1998.
124. Arnold WJ: Purine salvage enzymes, in Kelley WN, Weiner IM (eds): *Uric Acid*. New York, Springer-Verlag, 1978, p 43.
125. Palella TD, Andres CM, Fox IH: Human placental adenosine kinase. Kinetic mechanism and inhibition. *J Biol Chem* **255**:5264, 1980.
126. Fox IH, Kelley WN: The role of adenosine and 2′-deoxyadenosine in mammalian cells. *Annu Rev Biochem* **47**:655, 1978.
127. Atkinson DE: The energy charge of the adenylate pool as a regulatory parameter. Interaction with feedback modifiers. *Biochemistry* **7**:4030, 1968.
128. Becker MA, Kim M, Husain K, Kang T: Regulation of purine nucleotide synthesis in human B lymphoblasts with both hypoxanthine-guanine phosphoribosyltransferase deficiency and phosphoribosylpyrophosphate synthetase superactivity. *J Biol Chem* **267**:4317, 1992.
129. Holmes EW, Wyngaarden JB, Kelley WN: Human glutamine phosphoribosylpyrophosphate amidotransferase. Two molecular forms interconvertible by purine ribonucleotides and phosphoribosylpyrophosphate. *J Biol Chem* **248**:6035, 1973.
130. Holmes EW, McDonald JA, McCord JM, Wyngaarden JB, Kelley WN: Human glutamine phosphoribosylpyrophosphate amidotransferase. Kinetic and regulatory properties. *J Biol Chem* **248**:144, 1973.
131. Itakura M, Sabina RL, Heald PW, Holmes EW: Basis for the control of purine biosynthesis by purine ribonucleotides. *J Clin Invest* **67**:994, 1981.
132. Holmes EW: Kinetic, physical, and regulatory properties of amidophosphoribosyltransferase. *Adv Enzyme Regul* **19**:215, 1980.
133. Averil BA, Dwiredi A, Debrunner P, Vollmer SJ, Wong JY, Switzer RL: Evidence for a tetra-nuclear iron-sulfur center in glutamine phosphoribosylpyrophosphate amidotransferase from *Bacillus subtilis*. *J Biol Chem* **255**:6007, 1980.
134. Grindey GB, Lowe JK, Divekar AY, Hakala MT: Potentiation by guanine nucleosides of the growth-inhibitory effects of adenosine analogs on L1210 and sarcoma 180 cells in culture. *Cancer Res* **36**:379, 1976.
135. Raivio KO, Seegmiller JE: Role of glutamine in purine synthesis and in guanine nucleotide formation in normal fibroblasts and in fibroblasts deficient in hypoxanthine phosphoribosyltransferase activity. *Biochim Biophys Acta* **299**:283, 1973.
136. Yen RC, Raivio KO, Becker MA: Inhibition of phosphoribosylpyrophosphate synthesis in human fibroblasts by 6-methylthioinosinate. *J Biol Chem* **256**:1839, 1981.
137. Iwahana H, Oka J, Mizusawa N, Kudo E, Setsuko I, Yoshimoto K, Holmes EW, et al.: Molecular cloning of human amidophosphoribosyltransferase. *Biochem Biophys Res Commun* **190**:192, 1993.
138. Zhou GC, Dixon JE, Zalkin H: Cloning and expression of avian glutamine phosphoribosylpyrophosphate amidotransferase. Conservation of a bacterial propeptide sequence supports a role for posttranslational processing. *J Biol Chem* **265**:21152, 1990.
139. Smith JL, Zaluzec EJ, Wery J-P, Niu L, Switzer RL, Zalkin H, Satow Y: Structure of the allosteric regulatory enzyme of purine biosynthesis. *Science* **264**:1427, 1994.
140. Becker MA, Heidler SA, Bell GI, Seino S, Le Beau MM, Westbrook CA, Neuman W, et al.: Cloning of cDNAs for human phosphoribosylpyrophosphate synthetases 1 and 2 and X chromosome localization of PRPS1 and PRPS2 genes. *Genomics* **8**:555, 1990.

141. Iizasa T, Taira M, Shimada H, Ishijima S, Tatibana M: Molecular cloning and sequencing of human cDNA for phosphoribosyl pyrophosphate synthetase subunit II. *FEBS Lett* **244**:47, 1989.
142. Taira M, Iizasa T, Shimada H, Kudoh J, Shimizu N, Tatibana M: A human testis-specific mRNA for phosphoribosylpyrophosphate synthetase that initiates from a non-AUG codon. *J Biol Chem* **265**:16491, 1990.
143. Taira M, Kudoh J, Minoshima S, Iizasa T, Shimada H, Shimizu Y, Tatibana M, et al.: Localization of human phosphoribosylpyrophosphate synthetase subunit I and II genes (PRPS1 and PRPS2) to different regions of the X chromosome and assignment of two PRPS1-related genes to autosomes. *Somat Cell Mol Genet* **15**:29, 1989.
144. Fox IH, Kelley WN: Human phosphoribosylpyrophosphate synthetase. Kinetic mechanism and end product inhibition. *J Biol Chem* **247**:2126, 1972.
145. Becker MA, Kostel PJ, Meyer LJ: Human phosphoribosylpyrophosphate synthetase. Comparison of purified normal and mutant enzymes. *J Biol Chem* **250**:6822, 1975.
146. Fox IH, Kelley WN: Human phosphoribosylpyrophosphate synthetase. Distribution, purification, and properties. *J Biol Chem* **246**:5739, 1971.
147. Becker MA, Meyer LJ, Huisman WH, Lazar C, Adams WB: Human erythrocyte phosphoribosylpyrophosphate synthetase. Subunit analysis and states of subunit association. *J Biol Chem* **252**:3911, 1977.
148. Meyer LJ, Becker MA: Human erythrocyte phosphoribosylpyrophosphate synthetase. Dependence of activity on state of subunit association. *J Biol Chem* **252**:3919, 1977.
149. Becker MA, Losman MJ, Kim M: Mechanisms of accelerated purine nucleotide synthesis in human fibroblasts with superactive phosphoribosylpyrophosphate synthetases. *J Biol Chem* **262**:5596, 1987.
150. Lomax CA, Bagnara AS, Henderson JF: Studies of the regulation of purine nucleotide catabolism. *Can J Biochem* **53**:231, 1975.
151. Hitchings GH: Uric acid: Chemistry and synthesis, in Kelley WN, Weiner IM (eds): *Uric Acid*. New York, Springer-Verlag, 1978, p 1.
152. Kovarsky J, Holmes EW, Kelley WN: Absence of significant urate binding to human serum proteins. *J Lab Clin Med* **93**:85, 1979.
153. Holmes EW, Blondet P: Urate binding to serum albumin: Lack of influence on renal clearance of uric acid. *Arthritis Rheum* **22**:737, 1979.
154. Sorensen LB: The pathogenesis of gout. *Arch Intern Med* **109**:379, 1962.
155. Seegmiller JE, Grayzel AI, Laster L, Liddle L: Uric acid production in gout. *J Clin Invest* **40**:1304, 1961.
156. Wyngaarden JB: Overproduction of uric acid as the cause of hyperuricemia in primary gout. *J Clin Invest* **36**:1508, 1957.
157. Henderson JF, Rosenbloom FM, Kelley WN, Seegmiller JE: Variations in purine metabolism of cultured skin fibroblasts from patients with gout. *J Clin Invest* **47**:1511, 1968.
158. Becker MA: Patterns of phosphoribosylpyrophosphate and ribose-5-phosphate concentration and generation in fibroblasts from patients with gout and purine overproduction. *J Clin Invest* **57**:308, 1976.
159. Jones OW Jr, Ashton DM, Wyngaarden JB: Accelerated turnover of phosphoribosylpyrophosphate, a purine nucleotide precursor, in certain gouty subjects. *J Clin Invest* **41**:1805, 1962.
160. Sperling O, Boer P, Persky-Brosh S, Kanarek E, de Vries A: Altered kinetic property of erythrocyte phosphoribosylpyrophosphate synthetase in excessive purine production. *Rev Eur Etud Clin Biol* **17**:703, 1972.
161. Becker MA, Meyer LJ, Wood AW, Seegmiller JE: Purine overproduction in man associated with increased phosphoribosylpyrophosphate synthetase activity. *Science* **179**:1123, 1973.
162. Seegmiller JE, Rosenbloom FM, Kelley WN: Enzyme defect associated with a sex-linked human neurological disorder and excessive purine synthesis. *Science* **155**:1682, 1967.
163. Kelley WN, Rosenbloom FM, Henderson JF, Seegmiller JE: A specific enzyme defect in gout associated with overproduction of uric acid. *Proc Natl Acad Sci U S A* **57**:1735, 1967.
164. Kelley WN, Greene ML, Rosenbloom FM, Henderson JF, Seegmiller JE: Hypoxanthine-guanine phosphoribosyltransferase deficiency in gout. *Ann Intern Med* **70**:155, 1969.
165. Rosenbloom FM, Henderson JF, Caldwell IC, Kelley WN, Seegmiller JE:Biochemical bases of accelerated purine biosynthesis de novo in human fibroblasts lacking hypoxanthine-guanine phosphoribosyltransferase. *J Biol Chem* **243**:1166, 1968.
166. Zoref E, de Vries A, Sperling O: Mutant feedback-resistant phosphoribosylpyrophosphate synthetase associated with purine overproduction and gout. Phosphoribosylpyrophosphate and purine metabolism in cultured fibroblasts. *J Clin Invest* **56**:1093, 1975.
167. Alepa FP, Howell RR, Klineberg JR, Seegmiller JE: Relationships between glycogen storage disease and tophaceous gout. *Am J Med* **42**:58, 1967.
168. Reitsma-Bierens WCC: Renal complications in glycogen storage disease type I. *Eur J Pediatr* **152**:560, 1993.
169. Greene HL, Wilson FA, Hefferan P, Terry AB, Moran JR, Slonim AE, Claus TH, et al.: ATP depletion, a possible role in the pathogenesis of hyperuricemia in glycogen storage disease type I. *J Clin Invest* **62**:321, 1978.
170. Long WK: Glutathione reductase in red blood cells: Variant associated with gout. *Science* **155**:712, 1967.
171. Braven J, Hardwell TR, Hickling P, Whittaker M: Effect of treatment on erythrocyte phosphoribosyl pyrophosphate synthetase and glutathione reductase activity in patients with primary gout. *Ann Rheum Dis* **45**:941, 1986.
172. Edwards NL, Recker D, Fox IH: Overproduction of uric acid in hypoxanthine-guanine phosphoribosyltransferase deficiency. Contribution by impaired purine salvage. *J Clin Invest* **63**:922, 1979.
173. Hershfield MS, Seegmiller JE: Regulation of *de novo* purine synthesis in human lymphoblasts. Similar rates of *de novo* synthesis during growth by normal cells and mutants deficient in hypoxanthine-guanine phosphoribosyltransferase activity. *J Biol Chem* **252**:6002, 1977.
174. Fox IH, Palella TD, Kelley WN: Hyperuricemia: A marker for cell energy crisis [Editorial]. *N Engl J Med* **317**:111, 1987.
175. Yamanaka H, Kawagoe Y, Taneguchi A: Accelerated purine nucleotide degradation by anaerobic but not by aerobic ergometer muscle exercise. *Metabolism* **41**:364, 1992.
176. Fox IH: Adenosine triphosphate degradation in specific disease. *J Lab Clin Med* **106**:101, 1985.
177. Raivio KO, Becker A, Meyer LJ, Greene ML, Nuki G, Seegmiller JE: Stimulation of human purine synthesis *de novo* by fructose infusion. *Metabolism* **24**:861, 1975.
178. Mineo I, Kono N, Hara N, Shimizu T, Yamada Y, Kawachi M, Kiyokawa H, et al.: Myogenic hyperuricemia. A common pathophysiologic feature of glycogenosis types III, V, and VII. *N Engl J Med* **317**:75, 1987.
179. Jinnai K, Kono N, Yamamoto Y: Glycogenosis V (McArdle's disease) with hyperuricemia. A case report and clinical investigation. *Eur Neurol* **33**:204–207, 1993.
180. Fox IH, Kelley WN: Studies on the mechanism of fructose-induced hyperuricemia in man. *Metabolism* **21**:713, 1972.
181. Woolliscroft JO, Colfer H, Fox IH: Hyperuricemia in acute illness: A poor prognostic sign. *Am J Med* **72**:58, 1982.
182. Roch-Ramel F, Diezi J: Renal transport of organic ions and uric acid, in Schrier RW, Gottschalk CW (eds): *Diseases of the Kidney, 6th ed.* Boston, Little, Brown, 1996, p 231.
183. Roch-Ramel F, Weiner IM: Excretion of urate by the kidneys of Cebus monkeys: A micropuncture study. *Am J Physiol* **224**:1369, 1973.
184. Praetorius E, Kirk JE: Hypouricemia: With evidence for tubular elimination of uric acid. *J Lab Clin Med* **35**:865, 1950.
185. Yu T-F, Gutman AB: Study of the paradoxical effects of salicylate in low, intermediate and high dosage on the renal mechanisms for excretion of urate in man. *J Clin Invest* **38**:1298, 1959.
186. Levinson DJ, Sorensen LB: Renal handling of uric acid in normal and gouty subjects: Evidence for a 4-component system. *Ann Rheum Dis* **39**:173, 1980.
187. Puig JG, Anton FM, Jimenez ML, Guitierrez PC: Renal handling of uric acid in gout: Impaired tubular transport of urate is not dependent on serum urate values. *Metabolism* **35**:1147, 1986.
188. Diamond HS, Paolino JS: Evidence for a postsecretory reabsorptive site for uric acid in man. *J Clin Invest* **52**:1491, 1973.
189. Puig JG, Anton MF, Sanz MA, Gaspar G, Lesmes A, Ramos T, Vazquez OJ: Renal handling of uric acid in normal subjects by means of the pyrazinamide and probenecid tests. *Nephron* **35**:183, 1983.
190. Simkin PA: Urate excretion in normal and gouty men. *Adv Exp Med Biol* **76B**:41, 1977.
191. Zollner N, Griebsch A: Diet and gout. *Adv Exp Med Biol* **41B**:435, 1974.
192. Levinson DJ, Decker DE, Sorensen LB: Renal handling of uric acid in man. *Ann Clin Lab Sci* **12**:73, 1982.
193. Campion DW, Olsen RW, Caughey D, Bluestone R, Klinenberg JR: Does increased free serum urate concentration cause gout? [Abstract]. *Clin Res* **23**:261A, 1975.
194. Steele TH: Urate secretion in man: The pyrazinamide suppression test. *Ann Intern Med* **79**:734, 1973.
195. Rieselbach RE, Sorensen LB, Shelp WD, Steele TH: Diminished renal urate secretion per nephron as a basis for primary gout. *Ann Intern Med* **73**:359, 1970.

196. Holmes EW, Kelley WN: The renal pathophysiology of gout, in Kurtzman NA, Martinez-Moldanado M (eds): *Pathophysiology of the Kidney*. Springfield, IL, Charles C Thomas, 1977, p 696.
197. Steele TH, Rieselbach RE: The contribution of residual nephrons within the chronically diseased kidney to urate homeostasis in man. *Am J Med* **43**:876, 1967.
198. Schulman JD, Lustberg TJ, Kennedy JL, Museles M, Seegmiller JE: A new variant of maple syrup urine disease (branched chain ketoaciduria). Clinical and biochemical evaluation. *Am J Med* **49**:118, 1970.
199. Garrod AE: *The Inborn Factors in Disease: An Essay*. Oxford, Clarendon, 1931.
200. Stecher RM, Hersh AH, Solomon WM: The heredity of gout and its relationship to familial hyperuricemia. *Ann Intern Med* **31**:595, 1949.
201. Hauge M, Harvald B: Heredity in gout and hyperuricemia. *Acta Med Scand* **152**:247, 1955.
202. Neel JV, Rakic MT, Davidson RI, Valkenburg HA, Mikkelsen WM: Studies on hyperuricemia. II. A reconsideration of the distribution of serum uric acid values in the families of Smyth, Cotterman, and Freyberg. *Am J Hum Genet* **17**:14, 1965.
203. O'Brien WM, Burch TA, Bunim JJ: Genetics of hyperuricemia in Blackfeet and Pima Indians. *Ann Rheum Dis* **25**:117, 1966.
204. Calabrese G, Simmonds HA, Cameron JS, Davies PM: Precocious familial gout with reduced fractional urate clearance and normal purine enzymes. *Q J Med* **75**:441, 1990.
205. Tatibana M, Shigesada K: Two carbamyl phosphate synthetases of mammals: Specific roles in control of pyrimidine and urea biosynthesis. *Adv Enzyme Regul* **10**:249, 1972.
206. Sonoda T, Taira M, Ishijima S, Ishizuka T, Iizasa T, Tatibana M: Complete nucleotide sequence of human phosphoribosylpyrophosphate synthetase subunit I and a comparison with human and rat *PRPS* gene families. *J Biochem* **109**:36, 1991.
207. Taira M, Ishijima S, Kita K, Yamada K, Iizasa T, Tatibana M: Nucleotide and deduced amino acid sequences of two distinct cDNAs for rat phosphoribosylpyrophosphate synthetase. *J Biol Chem* **262**:14867, 1987.
208. Nosal JM, Switzer RL, Becker MA: Overexpression, purification, and characterization of recombinant human 5-phosphoribosyl-1-pyrophosphate synthetase isozymes I and II. *J Biol Chem* **268**:10168, 1993.
209. Ishijima S, Kita K, Ahmad I, Ishizuka T, Taira M, Tatibana M: Expression of rat phosphoribosylpyrophosphate synthetase subunits I and II in *Escherichia coli*. Isolation and characterization of the recombinant isoforms. *J Biol Chem* **266**:15693, 1992.
210. Taira M, Iizasa T, Yamada K, Shimada H, Tatibana M: Tissue-differential expression of two distinct genes for phosphoribosylpyrophosphate synthetase and existence of the testis-specific transcript. *Biochim Biophys Acta* **1007**:203, 1989.
211. Ishizuka T, Iizasa T, Taira M, Ishijima S, Sonoda T, Shimada H, Nagatake N, et al.: Promoter regions of the human X-linked housekeeping genes PRPS1 and PRPS2 encoding phosphoribosylpyrophosphate synthetase subunit I and II isoforms. *Biochim Biophys Acta* **1130**:139, 1992.
212. Ishijima S, Kita K, Tatibana M: External Mg^{2+}-dependent early stimulation of nucleotide synthesis in Swiss 3T3 cells. *Am J Physiol* **257**:C1113, 1989.
213. Becker MA, Heidler SA, Nosal JM, Switzer RL, LeBeau MM, Shapiro LJ, Palella TD, et al.: Human phosphoribosylpyrophosphate synthetase (PRS)2: An independently active, X-chromosome-linked PRS isoform. *Adv Exp Med Biol* **309B**:129, 1991.
214. Kita K, Ishizuka T, Ishijima S, Sonoda T, Tatibana M: A novel 39-kDa phosphoribosylpyrophosphate synthetase-associated protein of rat liver. *J Biol Chem* **269**:8334, 1997.
215. Sonoda T, Ishizuka T, Kita K, Ishijima S, Tatibana M: Cloning and sequencing of rat cDNA for the 41-kDa phosphoribosylpyrophosphate synthetase–associated protein has a high homology to the catalytic subunits and the 39 kDa associated protein. *Biochim Biophys Acta* **1350**:6, 1997.
216. Becker MA, Taylor W, Smith PR, Ahmed M: Overexpression of the normal phosphoribosylpyrophosphate synthetase isoform 1 underlies catalytic superactivity of human phosphoribosylpyrophosphate synthetase. *J Biol Chem* **271**:19894, 1996.
217. Sperling O, Eilam G, Persky-Brosh S, de Vries A: Accelerated erythrocyte 5-phosphoribosyl-1-pyrophosphate synthesis. A familial abnormality associated with excessive uric acid production and gout. *Biochem Med* **6**:310, 1972.
218. Sperling O, Persky-Brosh S, Boer P, de Vries A: Human erythrocyte phosphoribosylpyrophosphate synthetase mutationally altered in regulatory properties. *Biochem Med* **7**:389, 1973.
219. Lejeune E, Bouvier M, Mousson B, Llorca G, Baltassat P: Phosphoribosylpyrophosphate synthetase anomalies in 2 cases of gout beginning at an early age. *Rev Rhum Mal Osteoartic* **46**:457, 1979.
220. Becker MA, Losman MJ, Wilson J, Simmonds HA: Superactivity of human phosphoribosylpyrophosphate synthetase due to altered regulation by nucleotide inhibitors and inorganic phosphate. *Biochim Biophys Acta* **882**:168, 1986.
221. Becker MA, Puig JG, Mateos FA, Jimenez ML, Kim M, Simmonds HA: Inherited superactivity of phosphoribosylpyrophosphate synthetase: Association of uric acid overproduction and sensorineural deafness. *Am J Med* **85**:383, 1988.
222. Becker MA, Smith PR, Taylor W, Mustafi R, Switzer RL: The genetic and functional basis of purine nucleotide feedback-resistant phosphoribosylpyrophosphate synthetase superactivity. *J Clin Invest* **96**:2133, 1995.
223. Akaoka I, Fujimori S, Kamatani N, Takeuchi F, Yano E, Nishida Y, Hashimoto A, et al.: A gouty family with increased phosphoribosylpyrophosphate synthetase activity: Case reports, familial studies, and kinetic studies of the abnormal enzyme. *J Rheumatol* **8**:563, 1981.
224. Becker MA, Losman MJ, Itkin P, Simkin PA: Gout with superactive phosphoribosylpyrophosphate synthetase due to increased enzyme catalytic rate. *J Lab Clin Med* **99**:495, 1982.
225. Becker MA, Losman MJ, Rosenberg AL, Mehlman I, Levinson DJ, Holmes EW: Phosphoribosylpyrophosphate synthetase superactivity. A study of five patients with catalytic defects in the enzyme. *Arthritis Rheum* **29**:880, 1986.
226. Becker MA, Raivio KO, Bakay B, Adams WB, Nyhan WL: Variant human phosphoribosylpyrophosphate synthetase altered in regulatory and catalytic functions. *J Clin Invest* **65**:109, 1980.
227. Zoref E, de Vries A, Sperling O: Metabolic cooperation between human fibroblasts with normal and with mutant superactive phosphoribosylpyrophosphate synthetase. *Nature* **260**:787, 1976.
228. Yen RCK, Adams WB, Lazar C, Becker MA: Evidence for X-linkage of human phosphoribosylpyrophosphate synthetase. *Proc Natl Acad Sci U S A* **75**:782, 1978.
229. Simmonds HA, Webster DR, Lingham S, Wilson J: An inborn error of purine metabolism, deafness and neurodevelopmental abnormality. *Neuropediatrics* **16**:106, 1985.
230. Rosenberg AL, Bergstrom L, Troost BT, Bartholomew BA: Hyperuricemia and neurologic deficits. A family study. *N Engl J Med* **282**:992, 1970.
231. Roessler BJ, Nosal JM, Smith PR, Heidler SA, Palella TD, Switzer RL, Becker MA: Human X-linked phosphoribosylpyrophosphate synthetase superactivity is associated with distinct point mutations in the *PRPS1* gene. *J Biol Chem* **268**:26476, 1993.
232. Muller MM, Frank O: Lipid and purine metabolism in benign symmetric lipomatosis. *Adv Exp Med Biol* **41B**:509, 1973.
233. Wada Y, Nishimura Y, Tanaba M, Yoshimura Y, Iinuma K, Yoshida T, Arakawa T: Hyperuricemic mentally retarded infant with a defect of phosphoribosy-1-pyrophosphate synthetase of erythrocytes. *Tohuku J Exp Med* **113**:149, 1974.
234. Ahmed M, Taylor W, Smith PR, Becker MA: Acclerated transcription of *PRPS1* in X-linked overactivity of normal human phosphoribosylpyrophosphate synthetase. *J Biol Chem* **274**:7482, 1999.
235. Lesch M, Nyhan WL: A familial disorder of uric acid metabolism and central nervous system function. *Am J Med* **36**:561, 1964.
236. Emmerson BT: The management of gout. *N Engl J Med* **334**:445, 1996.
237. Simkin PA: Gout and hyperuricemia. *Curr Opin Rheumatol* **9**:268, 1997.
238. Wallace SL, Singer JZ: Therapy in gout. *Rheum Dis Clin North Am* **14**:441, 1988.
239. Werlen D, Gabay C, Vischer TL: Corticosteroid therapy for the treatment of acute attacks of crystal induced arthritis: An effective alternative to nonsteroidal antiinflammatory drugs. *Rev Rhum* **63**:248, 1996.
240. Ferrannini E, Pentimone F: Marrow aplasia following colchicine treatment for gouty arthritis. *Clin Exp Rheumatol* **2**:173, 1984.
241. Neuss MN, McCallum RM, Brenckman WD, Silberman HR: Long-term colchicine administration leading to colchicine toxicity and death. *Arthritis Rheum* **29**:448, 1986.
242. Kuncl RW, Duncan G, Watson D, Alderson K, Rogawski MA, Peper M: Colchicine myopathy and neuropathy. *N Engl J Med* **316**:1562, 1987.
243. Fam AG: Should patients with interval gout be treated with urate lowering drugs? *J Rheumatol* **22**:1621, 1995.
244. Yu T-F: The efficacy of colchicine prophylaxis in articular gout. A reappraisal after 20 years. *Arthritis Rheum* **12**:256, 1982.

245. Stapleton FB, Kennedy J, Nousia-Arvanitakis S, Linshaw MA: Hyperuricosuria due to high-dose pancreatic extract therapy in cystic fibrosis. *N Engl J Med* **295**:246, 1976.
246. Sack J, Blau H, Goldfarb D, Ben-Zaray S, Katznelson D: Hyperuricosuria in cystic fibrosis patients treated with pancreatic enzyme supplements. A study of 16 patients in Israel. *Isr J Med Sci* **16**:417, 1980.
247. Weinberger A, Schindel B, Liberman UA, Pinkhas J, Sperling O: Calciuric effect of probenecid in gouty patients. *Isr J Med Sci* **19**:377, 1983.
248. Yu TF, Roboz J, Johnson S, Kaung C: Studies on the metabolism of D-penicillamine and its interaction with probenecid in cystinuria and rheumatoid arthritis. *J Rheumatol* **11**:467, 1984.
249. Sosler SD, Behzad O, Garratty G, Lee CL, Postoway N, Khomo O: Immune hemolytic anemia associated with probenecid. *Am J Clin Pathol* **84**:391, 1985.
250. Kickler TS, Buck S, Ness P, Shirey RS, Sholar PW: Probenecid induced immune hemolytic anemia. *J Rheumatol* **13**:208, 1986.
251. Rundles RW: The development of allopurinol. *Arch Intern Med* **145**:1492, 1985.
252. Fox RM, Royse-Smith D, O'Sullivan WJ: Orotidinuria induced by allopurinol. *Science* **168**:861, 1970.
253. Beardmore TD, Kelley WN: Mechanism of allopurinol-mediated inhibition of pyrimidine biosynthesis. *J Lab Clin Med* **78**:696, 1971.
254. McInnes GT, Lawson DH, Jick H: Acute adverse reactions attributed to allopurinol in hospitalised patients. *Ann Rheum Dis* **40**:245, 1981.
255. Hande KR, Noone RM, Stone WJ: Severe allopurinol toxicity. Description and guidelines for prevention in patients with renal insufficiency. *Am J Med* **76**:47, 1984.
256. Saji M: A study of oxipurinol concentration and renal function in patients administered allopurinol. *Jpn J Nephrol* **38**:640, 1996.
257. Singer JZ, Wallace SL: The allopurinol hypersensitivity syndrome. Unnecessary morbidity and mortality. *Arthritis Rheum* **29**:82, 1986.
258. Pak CY, Peters P, Hurt G, Kadesky M, Fine M, Reisman D, Splann F, Caramela C, Freeman A, Britton F, Sakhaee K, Breslau NA: Is selective therapy of recurrent nephrolithiasis possible? *Am J Med* **71**:615, 1981.
259. Hande KR, Hixson CV, Chabner BA: Postchemotherapy purine excretion in lymphoma patients receiving allopurinol. *Cancer Res* **41**:2273, 1981.
260. Masera G, Jankovic M, Zurlo MG, Locasciulli A, Rossi MR, Uderzo C, Recchia M: Urate-oxidase prophylaxis of uric acid-induced renal damage in childhood leukemia. *J Pediatr* **100**:152, 1982.
261. Louyot P, Montet Y, Roland J, Pourel J: L'urate oxydase dans le traitement de la goutte et de l'hyperuricemie. *Rev Rhum Mal Osteoartic* **37**:795, 1970.
262. Montagnac R, Schillinger F: Accident anaphylactique lie a l'injection intraveinuse d'urate oxydase chez ne dialysee. *Nephrologie* **11**:259, 1990.
263. Davis S, Park YK: Hypouricaemic effect of polyethyleneglycol modified urate oxidase. *Lancet* **1**:281, 1981.
264. Chua CC, Greenberg ML, Viau AT, Nucci M, Brenckman WD Jr, Hershfield MS: Use of polyethylene glycol-modified uricase (PEG-uricase) to treat hyperuricemia in a patient with non-Hodgkins lymphoma. *Ann Intern Med* **114**:1988.
265. Rozenberg S, Koeger A-C, Bourgeois P: Urate-oxydase for gouty arthritis in cardiac transplant recipients. *J Rheumatol* **20**:2171, 1993.
266. Fox IH: Disorders of purine and pyrimidine metabolism, Spittell JA (ed): *Clinical Medicine.* Vol 9. Philadelphia, Harper & Row, 1986, p 1.

CHAPTER 107

Lesch-Nyhan Disease and Its Variants

H. A. Jinnah ▪ Theodore Friedmann

1. **Inherited deficiency of the purine salvage enzyme hypoxanthine-guanine phosphoribosyltransferase (HPRT) causes three overlapping clinical syndromes, depending on the amount of residual enzyme activity. Patients with at least 8 percent of residual enzyme activity demonstrate marked overproduction of uric acid, with associated hyperuricemia, nephrolithiasis, and gout. Patients with 1.5 to 8 percent of residual activity demonstrate uric acid overproduction with neurologic disability that varies from minor clumsiness to debilitating extrapyramidal and pyramidal motor dysfunction. Patients with less than 1.5 percent of residual activity demonstrate overproduction of uric acid, debilitating neurologic disability, varying degrees of cognitive disability, and behavioral abnormalities that include impulsive and self-injurious behaviors. This latter and most severe form of the disease is known as Lesch-Nyhan disease (LND).**
2. **HPRT deficiency is inherited as an X-linked recessive condition, and the HPRT gene has been mapped to Xq26-q27. The entire HPRT gene has been cloned and sequenced and more than 200 mutations responsible for disease have been characterized. These advances at the molecular genetic level have allowed for the development of rapid and convenient methods for diagnosis, carrier identification, and prenatal testing.**
3. **The metabolic basis for the overproduction of uric acid in HPRT deficiency has been determined to result from changes in the regulation of purine synthesis and degradation. The overproduction of uric acid can be blocked by the administration of allopurinol, providing an effective means to reduce the risk of nephrolithiasis and gout in affected patients. Unfortunately, allopurinol has no efficacy against the neurobehavioral features.**
4. **The pathogenesis of the neurologic and behavioral features remains incompletely understood, although growing evidence suggests that these features result from dysfunction of the dopamine transmitter systems of the basal ganglia. Treatments for the neurobehavioral features are limited to protective physical devices and behavior therapy.**
5. **Current research efforts are focused on prevention, elucidating the basis for the central nervous system dysfunction, and developing more effective treatment strategies for the neurobehavioral features.**

A list of standard abbreviations is located immediately preceding the index in each volume. Additional abbreviations used in this chapter include: 5′NT = 5′-nucleotidase; AK = adenosine kinase; AMPRT = amidophosphoribosyltransferase; AS = adenylosuccinate; ASL = adenylosuccinate synthetase-lyase; IDH = isocitrate dehydrogenase; GA = guanase; LND = Lesch-Nyhan disease; PNP = purine nucleoside phosphorylase; XA = xanthylic acid; XO = xanthine oxidase.

HISTORICAL ASPECTS

In 1964, Lesch and Nyhan described two brothers with hyperuricemia and a characteristic neurobehavioral syndrome that included motor dysfunction and self-injurious behavior.[1] Both boys had been diagnosed with cerebral palsy, but the familial occurrence and unusual clinical features suggested that this was a previously unrecognized inherited metabolic disease. Within a few years, multiple additional cases were identified to confirm the existence of a distinct clinical syndrome. In retrospect, the same syndrome may have been described in earlier reports. According to Beck, Jacobus de Voragine described a syndrome of self-injurious behavior, uncontrolled movements, mental deficiency, gout, and renal failure in the twelfth century.[2] Though the syndrome was ascribed as a punishment rendered by God upon the murderers of St. Thomas, the unusual collection of features suggests he may have drawn on personal experience with an individual suffering from the syndrome described by Lesch and Nyhan.

In 1967, Seegmiller and colleagues demonstrated a deficiency of HPRT as the underlying biochemical cause of the syndrome.[3] This discovery facilitated the identification of similar patients with less severe forms of the disease. Catel and Schmidt had already reported a patient with hyperuricemia and neurologic disability but lacking any behavioral abnormalities in 1959.[4] This patient was later shown to have low residual amounts of HPRT,[5] and may be the first case of partial HPRT deficiency described. Kelley and colleagues later reported several additional patients who displayed an incomplete syndrome due to partial HPRT deficiency, including several who had hyperuricemia with no obvious neurologic or behavioral abnormalities.[6] The full spectrum of disease associated with HPRT deficiency is now recognized to range from isolated hyperuricemia to hyperuricemia with profound neurobehavioral dysfunction. In recognition of the careful early clinical descriptions, the full spectrum of clinical abnormalities associated with HPRT deficiency has been designated Lesch-Nyhan disease (LND). Patients who lack the full clinical manifestations as a result of partial HPRT deficiency are designated LND variants.

The isolation of the human HPRT gene was facilitated by the discovery of repetitive interspersed Alu sequences in the human genome. In 1982, Jolly and colleagues used the Alu sequences to identify and clone the human gene in HPRT-deficient murine cells transformed with human genomic DNA.[7,8] Simultaneous with the identification of the human HPRT gene, Konecki, Brennand, and colleagues took advantage of a murine cell line that contained highly amplified HPRT genomic sequences to clone and sequence the mouse HPRT cDNA.[9,10] The ensuing years witnessed the characterization of more than 200 genetic mutations responsible for disease. Detailed historical accounts of the discovery of the syndrome and its causes have been presented.[11,12]

Despite its rarity, a great deal of research has focused on LND and HPRT for a number of reasons. First, observations of patients with LND led to the concept that recognizable patterns of

Table 107-1 Presenting Features of *HPRT* Deficiency*

Presenting Feature	Classic LND (total = 132)	Neurologic Variant (total = 22)	Hyperuricemic Variant (total = 23)
Neurobehavioral	84.8% (112)	36.4% 8	0
Motor delay	78.0% (103)	9.1% (2)	0
Other motor	9.8% (13)	27.3% (6)	0
Uric acid excess	8.3% (1)	63.6% (14)	95.7% (22)
Hyperuricemia	0.8% (1)	0	0.4% (1)
Crystalluria	1.5% (2)	9.1% (2)	8.0% (2)
Nephrolithiasis	0.8% (1)	18.2% (4)	30.4% (7)
Renal failure	3.4% (5)	13.6% (3)	0
Gout	1.5% (2)	22.7% (5)	47.8% (11)
Other	8.3% (11)	0	0.4% (1)
Emesis	5.3% (7)	0	0
Irritability	3.0% (4)	0	4.3% (1)

*Data were collected from cases reported in the prior literature.[1,5,6,26–121] Subgroup percentages may total more than 100%, since some patients presented with more than one feature. The numbers in parentheses indicate the actual number of patients in each group.

abnormal behavior might result from specific genetic insults,[13] analogous to inherited patterns of physical malformation already recognized by dysmorphologists. There continues to be a great deal of interest in the concept of neurobehavioral phenotypes and in elucidating the mechanisms by which a single gene or gene defect can influence complex behavioral patterns. Second, because the HPRT gene was one of the first genes associated with a human disease to be cloned, LND has served as a model for development of the concepts and techniques of gene therapy.[14–16] The development of simple methods to identify[17,18] and amplify[19] single cells with or without HPRT has provided a unique tool for the detection of rare events in studies of gene transfer. These methods have also made the HPRT locus a favorite for studies of X-chromosome inactivation,[20,21] somatic cell mutation,[22–25] and cell hybridization.[19]

CLINICAL FEATURES

Presentation

The clinical features associated with HPRT deficiency have been described in a number of prior reviews and case reports. The clinical features may be broadly divided into three categories, including overproduction of uric acid and its consequences, neurobehavioral manifestations indicative of central nervous system dysfunction, and a miscellaneous category that includes growth retardation and anemia. A summary of the clinical features described for a total of 171 published cases of LND[1,26–107] is described below and summarized in Tables 107-1 and 107-2 and Figs. 107-1 and 107-2. Subsequently, the clinical features resulting from 49 cases of partial HPRT deficiency[5,6,30,84,95,108–121] are described.

The overwhelming majority of patients with LND present between 3 and 12 months of age with motor delay, most commonly hypotonia or failure to reach normal motor milestones (Table 107-1). Others are first identified by the presence of involuntary movements or increased muscle tone. A smaller number of patients may present with complications related to the overproduction of uric acid. Sometimes, there is an early history that diapers contain an "orange sand" that is caused by uric acid crystals and microhematuria.[32,34,77] Other patients may present with renal failure or hematuria as a result of nephrolithiasis.[55,65,66,88,95,104,107] In contrast, patients with partial deficiency of HPRT more often present with consequences related to overproduction of uric acid rather than neurologic or behavioral impairments (Table 107-1).

Uric Acid in LND

Hyperuricemia. Nearly all patients with LND overproduce large quantities of uric acid. Although elevated levels of uric acid can usually be detected in the blood, the degree of hyperuricemia may be sufficiently small that it escapes notice in routine studies (Table 107-2, Fig. 107-1*A*). In addition, some patients have serum uric acid levels that repeatedly fall in the normal range.

Hyperuricosuria. Although all patients with LND overproduce large quantities of uric acid, marked increases in serum levels are apparently prevented by efficient renal clearance. Consequently, urinary measurements provide a more accurate estimate of total uric acid production. Isolated urinary uric acid values are not useful, because there is a broad range of normal values produced by variations in hydration status, diet, age, ethnic background, comorbid diseases, and medications.[122] However, the uric acid to creatinine ratio corrects for much of the variation among urine specimens (Table 107-2, Fig. 107-1*B*) and is usually abnormal among patients with LND.[39,45,52,71,74,78,81,96,97,123,124] Another method to correct for sample variability is to measure 24-h urinary uric acid production.[1,35,36,38,44,46,47,50,55,68,71,73,77,88,96,124,125] This measure is also usually abnormal among patients with LND, particularly when adjusted for the relatively small size of the patients (Table 107-2, Fig. 107-1*C*). Although the urinary uric acid to creatinine ratio and 24-h uric acid excretion values are typically abnormal in LND, neither measure is considered reliable enough to serve as a definitive diagnostic tool.[125]

Nephrolithiasis. In untreated patients, the marked increases in the production and excretion of uric acid frequently lead to the formation of stones in the renal medullae or other portions of the urological system. Before the advent of effective treatment for hyperuricemia, a significant proportion of patients with LND died from complications of nephrolithiasis, such as renal failure or sepsis from urinary tract infection. Even with adequate control of uric acid production with allopurinol, subclinical renal

Table 107-2 Uric Acid in HPRT Deficiency*

Measurement	Normals	Classic LND	Neurologic Variant	Hyperuricemic Variant
Serum (mg/dL)	4.5 ± 1.3	11.7 ± 4.4 (70)	13.1 ± 3.5 (15)	13.4 ± 6.2 (22)
Urine ratio (uric acid/creatinnie)	0.3 ± 0.1	3.0 ± 1.1 (17)	1.3 ± 0.7 (7)	1.0 ± 0.4 (10)
Urine excretion (mg/kg/day)	9.7 ± 3.7	39.6 ± 13.9 (24)	25.5 ± 13.5 (9)	25.4 ± 16.4 (10)

*Average ± SD serum or urinary uric acid values were collected from cases reported in the prior literature.[1,5,6,26–105,107–121] The numbers in parentheses show the number of individual cases for which data were available. Normal ranges for serum uric acid,[581] urine uric acid to creatinine,[123] and urine total excretion[1,5,68] are for adults only.

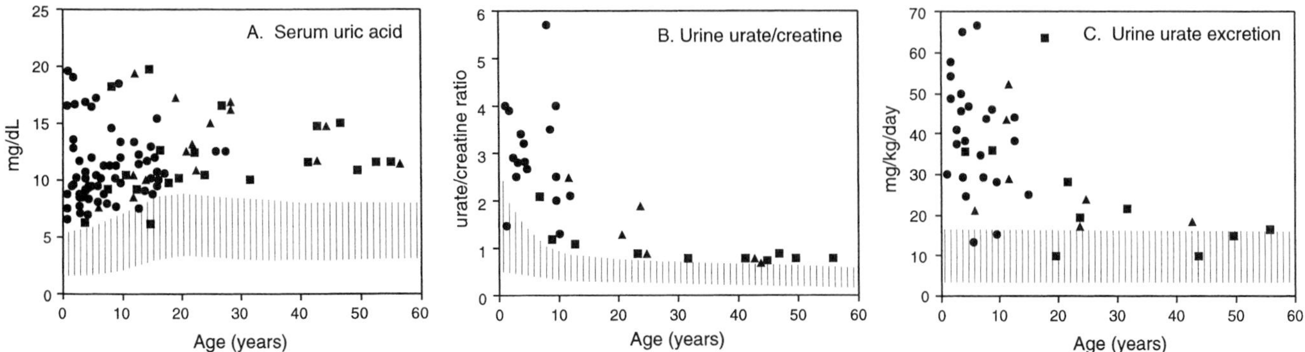

Fig. 107-1 Serum and urine uric acid. Uric acid values were collected from prior case reports and reviews.[1,5,6,26–105,107–121] Each symbol reflects the value reported for an individual with LND (circle), a neurologic variant without self-injurious behavior (triangle), or a hyperuricemic subject with partial HPRT deficiency (square). Serum values are shown in *panel A* in mg/dl, where the shaded area depicts 95 percent confidence intervals for the range of normal values (average ± 2 SD), estimated from data collected by Mikkelsen and colleagues from 2987 males of different ages.[581] Urinary uric acid to creatinine ratios are shown in *panel B*, where the 95 percent confidence intervals for normative data were estimated from data collected by Kaufman and colleagues from more than 1500 subjects of different ages.[123] The total uric acid excreted in the urine over a 24-h period is shown in *panel C*. The confidence limits for normal values were obtained from data collected from 24 normal individuals and are not age-adjusted.[1,6,68]

dysfunction is often evident from calculated creatinine clearance values.[30,31,50,84,101] Nephrolithiasis remains a significant problem even after control of hyperuricemia with allopurinol, and numerous reports have described kidney stones developing among patients already receiving adequate doses of allopurinol.[126–130] The subnormal renal function in treated patients may therefore reflect cumulative damage from chronic unrecognized nephrolithiasis, or a direct deleterious effect of the metabolic defect on kidney function.

Tophi. Untreated hyperuricemia may lead to the development of solid deposits of uric acid tophi in the subcutaneous tissues.[122] Because these tophi do not typically develop for several years, other clinical features typically lead to the diagnosis prior to their development. Though tophi were described in early cases, early recognition of the disease and treatment with allopurinol effectively prevents their occurrence.

Gout. Hyperuricemia due to HPRT deficiency may result in gout, but gout is relatively uncommon in children[32,107] and an unusual presenting feature of LND (Table 107-1). However, gout may develop in patients with LND if hyperuricemia is not treated. As described below, gout is more commonly a presenting feature in cases with partial HPRT deficiency.

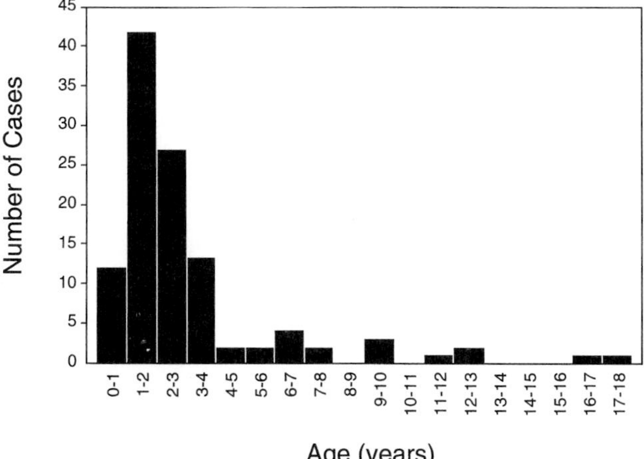

Fig. 107-2 Onset of self-injurious behavior. The age to onset of self-injurious behavior was collected from prior case reports and reviews.[1,26–106,362] The data are presented as a frequency histogram, with 1-year intervals. The onset of self-injurious behavior occurred at an average of 3.3 years and a median of 2 years. The histogram does not include similar data from the 40 patients previously summarized by Anderson and Ernst.[157]

Neurobehavioral Features in LND

Development. All patients with LND exhibit profound motor disability, which is usually first recognized during the first 3 to 9 months of life when the infant fails to develop the ability to hold up the head or sit unsupported and is found to be hypotonic.[26,31,32,53,68,104] In rare cases, hypotonia has been recognized shortly after birth.[31,37,53,61,70,89] Further motor development is delayed, and extrapyramidal and pyramidal signs typically begin to develop between 1 and 2 years of age.[31,38,68] Crawling is difficult or impossible, and patients are eventually confined to a wheelchair because the motor impairments are sufficiently severe that they prevent ambulation. A loss of motor milestones is evident in some cases. Whether this loss reflects a degenerative process or impairment of previously acquired skills because of the emergence of extrapyramidal features is unknown. This sequence of events closely resembles that occurring in dyskinetic cerebral palsy, and many patients are initially suspected of suffering from cerebral palsy until hyperuricemia or self-injury become apparent.[32,34]

Extrapyramidal Features. Extrapyramidal motor features indicative of dysfunction of the basal ganglia are universal among LND patients (Table 107-3). However, the descriptive terminology applied to these features has varied widely among different reports. Two large case series including a total of 29 patients have reported choreoathetosis as a universal feature.[32,34] Only one of these studies described dystonia in a minority of the patients.[32] However, a third study focusing specifically on the neurologic features of eight patients reported that all patients had dystonia rather than choreoathetosis.[31] A fourth study of five patients described a combination of choreoathetosis and dystonia in all patients.[28]

Although the differences described in these studies might represent clinical heterogeneity among patients reported by different groups, it is more likely that they represent variations in the use of descriptive terminology. Variations in the application of terms such as chorea, athetosis, and dystonia have long been recognized in the neurologic literature, and have led to recommendations for a standardized nomenclature by a Task Force on the Classification of Extrapyramidal Disorders.[131] These recommendations were recently applied in a detailed study of motor dysfunction in 12 LND patients.[132] In this study, all patients had a severely disabling action dystonia with excessive cocontraction of agonist and antagonist muscles during voluntary movement, twisting and sometimes sustained postures, overflow of contractions to extraneous muscle groups, and hypertrophy of chronically active muscles. Less than half of the patients also had chorea. In general, the chorea was less severe than dystonia, and it typically emerged only with stress or excitement.

In addition to dystonia and chorea, other extrapyramidal signs may also be apparent. Many reports have described opisthotonus, extensor spasms of the trunk, back arching, and sudden retrocollis.[31,32,36,38,42,44,45,51–53,60,64,66,68,70,74,84,89,90] Flinging or flailing movements of the limbs suggestive of ballismus may also occur.[30–32,51,68,99] These features are all attributable to dysfunction of the basal ganglia or its connections.[133]

Pyramidal Features. Pyramidal features indicative of dysfunction of the corticospinal motor system are also commonly recognized among patients with LND, although the incidence varies widely among different reports (Table 107-3). Three major signs have been assessed as indices of pyramidal dysfunction: spasticity, hyperreflexia, and the extensor plantar reflex. Two large series described spasticity and hyperreflexia among nearly all affected patients.[32,34] However, other studies have considered most patients hypotonic, with spasticity being uncommon.[31,132] In these later studies, only a minority of patients displayed spasticity or hyperreflexia, and these signs were nearly always limited to the legs in a pattern suggestive of a cervical or thoracic myelopathy.

The involvement of the cervical spinal cord may result directly from the metabolic defect or indirectly from the chronic and sometimes forceful involuntary movements of the neck. The development of a cervical myelopathy as a result of involuntary neck movements has been amply documented for several other conditions, including dyskinetic cerebral palsy,[134–139] torticollis,[140] paroxysmal dystonia,[141] and Tourette syndrome.[140,142] In fact, cervical instability leading to myelopathy has been documented by radiographic studies in two patients with LND.[31] Another report described atlantoaxial dislocation as result of violent retrocollis in a patient with LND.[38] A third report described an unexplained high cervical fracture in one patient, and an os odontoideum in another.[43] These orthopedic problems could have resulted from chronic and forceful involuntary neck movements. Because baseline motor disability is severe in these patients, the potential development of a secondary myelopathy may be difficult to identify without neuroimaging studies.

Dorsiflexion of the great toe in response to plantar stimulation has also been observed frequently in LND. This reflex is commonly associated with dysfunction of the pyramidal motor system, and is often termed the Babinski sign. Unfortunately, the Babinski sign is indistinguishable from another sign known as the striatal toe response, which is associated with extrapyramidal diseases.[143] Because LND is associated with prominent extrapyramidal signs, the upgoing toe response does not provide unequivocal evidence for pyramidal tract involvement.[132]

Table 107-3 Neurobehavioral Features of LND*

Feature	Christie et al., 1982 (total = 19)	Watts et al., 1982 (total = 8)	Jinnah et al., 1998 (total = 15)
Self-injury	100% (19)	100% (8)	100% (15)
Dysarthria	100% (19)	100% (8)	100% (15)
Extrapyramidal			
Dystonia	21% (4)	100% (8)	100% (15)
Choreoathetosis	100% (19)	0	40% (6)
Ballismus	0	38% (3)	30% (5)
Pyramidal			
Hyerreflexia	100% (19)	25% (2)	93% (14)
Extensor plantar	100% (19)	25% (2)	30% (5)
Baseline tone			
Hypotonia	0	100% (8)	100% (15)
Spasticity	100% (19)	25% (2)	40% (6)

*Neurologic features reported in three studies of LND.[31,32,132] The numbers in parentheses indicate the actual number of patients in each group.

Other Neurologic Features. Epileptic seizures have been reported for a number of cases.[32,34,37,38,64,68,69,81,87,96,104] However, the true incidence of epilepsy is difficult to determine, because violent and sometimes prolonged opisthotonic spasms or posturing may closely resemble seizures.[45] Epileptiform discharges are rarely seen on electroencephalograms, which most often show normal results[30,31,35,44,46,52,68,72,91,119] or nonspecific changes such as diffuse slowing or disorganization.[68,84,89]

A few LND patients and variants have been described as ataxic or suffering from a condition resembling a spinocerebellar syndrome.[6,69,108] Unfortunately, the term *ataxia* is so widely used that its meaning is difficult to decipher. The term is sometimes used as a general term to describe clumsiness that may result from cerebellar, pyramidal, extrapyramidal, or sensory dysfunction. More properly, it is employed to describe a combination of dysmetria, dysdiadochokinesis, and decomposition of movements that implies dysfunction of the cerebellum and its connections.[144] The occurrence of true cerebellar ataxia in LND and its variants is difficult to ascertain with confidence when considered against the background of the severe extrapyramidal features and is not widely accepted.[31,32,34,132,145,146]

Dysarthria occurs in all patients,[31,32,34,132] and some patients are difficult, if not impossible, to understand. Although the nature of the dysarthria has never been fully characterized, it has been described as an "athetoid dysarthria" typical of disease of the basal ganglia.[146–148] Dysphagia, most likely related to oropharyngeal dystonia, is also common in LND, and may lead to inadequate nutrition. Other patients have recurrent and persistent emesis,[36,41,68,80,90] which can also lead to inadequate nutrition or dehydration. Some patients have required gastrostomy tubes to maintain nutrition.

The cause of death in most reported cases has been pneumonia, most likely related to aspiration. However, there are several reports of sudden and unexplained death in previously well-managed patients.[31,34,35,90] The cause of sudden death could not be determined after autopsy in one case,[34] and in most cases remains uncertain. However, a neurologic basis is often suspected. A potentially related problem has been recurrent episodes of apnea and cyanosis[31,106] or recurrent and unexplained coma.[87] The reasons for these events remain unclear, and may be related to a mechanical cervical myelopathy leading to diaphragmatic paralysis, brainstem ischemia due to compromise of nutrient arteries from the neck, prolonged laryngospasm, or primary failure of brain stem respiratory centers.[31,38,106,146,149] One group has suggested an increased risk of stroke from a hypercoagulable state,[150,151] although this finding has not been confirmed.

Cognition. Many studies have reported moderate to severe mental retardation in LND. Standardized IQ scores for 13 reported cases have ranged from less than 50 to 105, with an average of approximately 71 ± 16.[30,36–38,47,51,68,72,84,87,94,97,105] One systematic study applied a battery of standardized cognitive tests to 7 patients and found an average composite IQ of approximately 60 ± 15.[152] A follow-up study of the same cohort of patients 2 years later indicated little developmental progress, suggesting an upper limit to cognitive development rather than a progressive cognitive decline.[153] A similar study of 12 additional patients again demonstrated an average IQ score of 60 ± 15.[154] The latter study also demonstrated a pattern of cognitive deficits suggestive of predominantly subcortical dysfunction, with relatively severe involvement of attention, working memory, and delayed recall.[154]

Other studies have suggested that LND patients may not be as cognitively impaired as formal test measures indicate because they appear to function at levels much higher than expected from standardized test scores.[155] In addition, some patients with apparently normal intelligence have been reported.[5,54,87] Adequate assessments of cognitive abilities in these patients have been difficult to obtain for several reasons. First, the severe neurologic and behavioral abnormalities restrict the availability of normal educational opportunities. Second, the motor and speech impairments, together with the behavioral abnormalities, may subjectively influence the interpretation of responses to test questions. Third, many patients exhibit reduced attention and oppositional behavior with poor cooperation in formal testing situations. Overall, some degree of cognitive impairment seems apparent when LND patients are considered as a group, although the range of cognitive abilities is broad, with some patients functioning in the normal range.

Behavior. Patients with LND often strike out at those around them, use foul language, or spit toward people.[98,147,156,157] Although these behaviors are often interpreted as a manifestation of aggression, it is important to recognize that the occurrence of these behaviors is not synonymous with aggression because they can have many different underlying causes. The expression of these behaviors may also reflect a failure of impulse control, an uncontrollable compulsion, or a tic analogous to the coprolalia or copropraxia of Tourette syndrome. Although many patients will indeed strike at people, they will often warn those close enough to be hit. They often don't intend to hurt people, and they will frequently apologize afterwards. These behaviors may be triggered by excitement, or by the awareness that the behavior provokes a negative reaction.

Self-Injury. Self-injurious behavior is a striking neurobehavioral feature of LND and is considered a hallmark feature of the disease. In one study of 40 patients, the average age of onset to self-injurious behavior was 3 years, with a range of 1 to 8 years.[157] A review of the literature disclosed 111 cases in which the age of onset was reported. The median to onset was 2 years, the average was 3.3 years, and the range was 6 months to 18 years (Fig. 107-2). Although self-injury is often considered an invariant feature of severe HPRT deficiency, the recognition of rare patients who don't develop self-injury until the late teens suggests the potential existence of other patients who may have severe HPRT deficiency yet never self-injure.

The most common expression of self-injury involves biting.[157] Most patients bite their lips and fingers, although some also bite their tongue, arms, shoulders, or toes.[157] Other forms of injury include banging or snapping the head backward against wheelchair supports, injuring hands or feet on sharp parts of a wheelchair, or poking the eyes with the fingers (Table 107-4). Over time, the behavior may wax and wane, with wide variations in severity. In the most severe cases, self-injurious behavior occurs daily and may lead to major medical complications including partial amputations of lips or fingers, major infections, or near-blindness. Serious tissue loss is common (Fig. 107-3). In other cases, the behavior may disappear for months or even years. It is exacerbated by intercurrent illnesses, such as an upper respiratory infection, a painful joint, or renal colic. It is also exacerbated by psychologic stress such as formal medical evaluation, the presence of a stranger, or changes in environment. The behavior is least severe when patients are actively engaged in a comfortable and familiar environment. With age, the frequency and severity of self-injurious behaviors may decline, and may rarely even disappear.[34]

Table 107-4 Self-Injurious Behavior in LND*

Type of Self-Injury	Number (total = 40)
Biting	
Lips	33
Fingers	29
Arms	16
Tongue	14
Other	
Limb extension at doorway	35
Head snapping	34
Head banging	30
Feet under wheelchair	23
Fingers in wheelchair	17
Eye poking	13

*This table was modified from data presented by Anderson and Ernst.[157]

Individuals with LND clearly do not wish to injure themselves, and often learn to call for help when they feel that injury is imminent. Some have learned to sit on their hands as a deterrent, while others wear socks or gloves on their hands to reduce self-injury.[156] A number of neurobehavioral theories have been presented to account for the occurrence of self-injurious behavior in LND. Neurologic models have considered that self-injury might be related to insensitivity to pain,[36] irritating paresthesias from a sensory neuropathy,[158] the manifestation of a complex partial seizure,[159] a stereotypic movement disorder,[160] or a defect in somatotopic recognition analogous to the alien limb phenomenon.[161] Psychologic models have suggested that self-injury is an attention-seeking tool,[98] a form of autoaggression,[39] or an uncontrollable compulsion.[98,148,162–164] The factors responsible for the onset of self-injury may differ from those responsible for the maintenance of the behavior over time.[165] It seems most likely

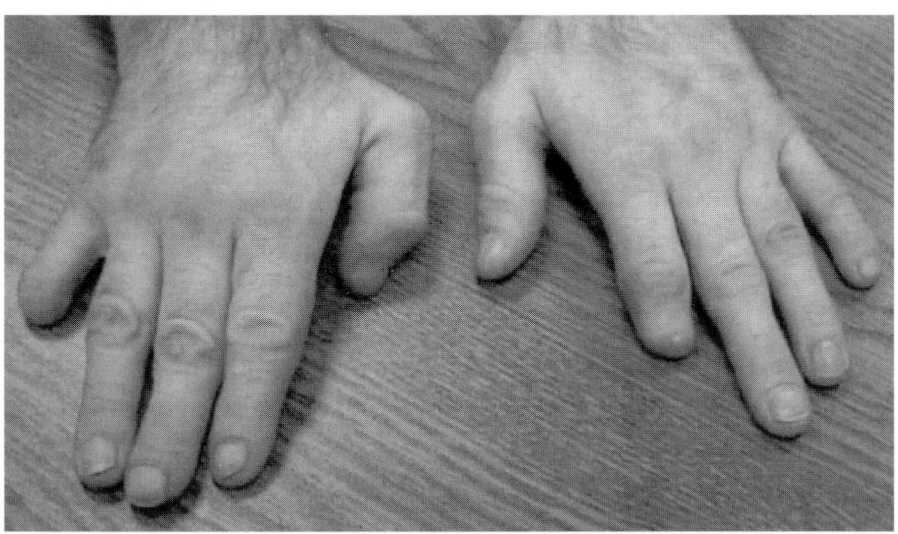

Fig. 107-3 Self-injurious finger biting. The hands of this LND patient demonstrate partial amputation of the fingers caused by prior self-biting.

that self-injurious behavior is a form of obsessive-compulsive disorder analogous to onychophagia or trichotillomania,[133] although formal evidence is lacking.

Other Manifestations in LND

Megaloblastic Anemia. A megaloblastic anemia, sometimes profound, is an occasional, although inconsistent, finding among patients with LND.[31,34,50,146,166,167] One autopsy case revealed extramedullary hematopoiesis in the liver and spleen.[31] In most cases, the cause for anemia is uncertain because serum B_{12}, folate, and thyroid function tests are normal; and folate or B_{12} supplements are not routinely effective in treatment. On the other hand, adenine supplements may be effective in reversing the anemia,[50] suggesting that purine limitation may be the cause of the anemia. It has been suggested that bone marrow stem cells are particularly dependent on HPRT-mediated purine salvage to maintain cell purine levels.[167–170] Unfortunately, adenine therapy is associated with a significantly increased risk for renal failure,[46,77] and is not routinely used for treatment.

Growth Retardation. Somatic growth appears subnormal in LND. Although markedly reduced birth weights are not common, one careful study revealed average birth weights to be significantly reduced in eight LND patients.[103] Serial anthropomorphic measures reveal that these patients grow more slowly than age-matched normal individuals, and height and weight often fall below two standard deviations of age-adjusted normative data.[32,34,103,171] Head circumference during development is also reduced, although often less than somatic growth, and bone age is only slightly delayed.[32,34,103,171]

Testicular atrophy is also common, and puberty is delayed or absent.[103] There are several reports of undescended testes,[31,34,72,103] and testicular tissue could not be identified in one autopsied case.[31] The relatively prominent dysfunction of the testes is thought to be related to the importance of HPRT-mediated purine salvage in this tissue.[103]

Unexplained Fevers. Unexplained hyperpyrexia has been noted in several published cases.[32,55,58,68] Hyperpyrexia is probably not a direct consequence of the metabolic lesion because there are many potential sources of fever in these patients. For example, dysphagia and recurrent emesis predispose to aspiration and bronchopneumonia. The deposition of uric acid crystals in the joints or subcutaneous tissues can produce inflammatory changes with fever. Nephrolithiasis increases the risk for pyelonephritis or infection in other parts of the urogenital system. Therefore, the occurrence of hyperpyrexia must prompt a thorough medical evaluation.

Partial HPRT Deficiency Syndromes

Patients with HPRT deficiency may be categorized into three groups based on the presence and severity of various clinical features. Although initial studies reported a poor correlation between the clinical phenotype and the amount of residual enzyme activity,[6,30,172] a further refinement of methods used to measure HPRT demonstrated a good correlation.[111,173,174] Patients with near-complete deficiency of the enzyme demonstrate overproduction of uric acid and the characteristic neurobehavioral phenotype described above. These patients are considered to have *classic LND*. Patients with 1.5 to 8 percent of residual enzyme activity demonstrate overproduction of uric acid with neurologic abnormalities, but they lack the behavioral abnormalities such as impulsive and self-injurious behaviors. Because of the absence of behavioral abnormalities, these patients are often designated as *LND variants*. Patients with more than 8 percent of residual enzyme activity suffer from overproduction of uric acid, but neurologic and behavioral abnormalities are not evident (Fig. 107-4). This least-severely affected group has only HPRT-related hyperuricemia.

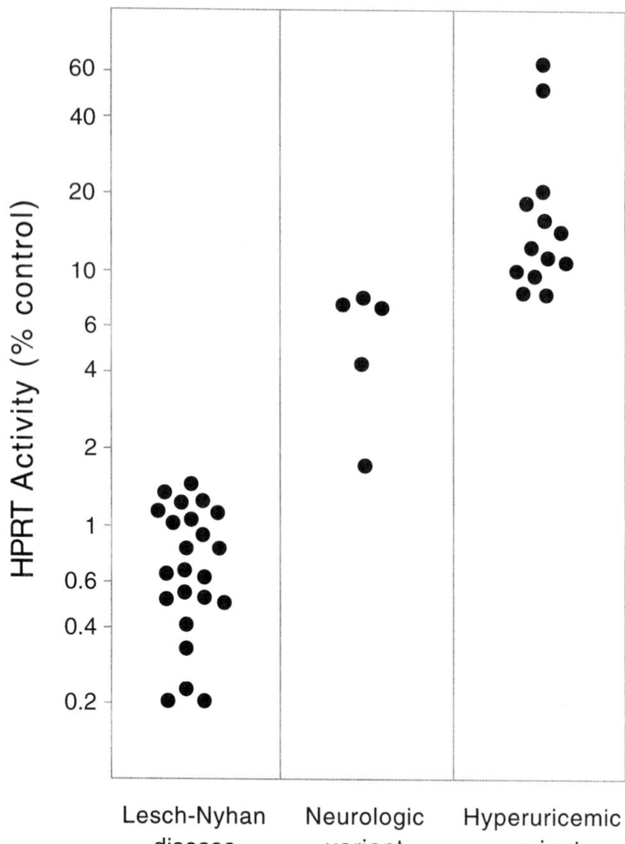

Fig. 107-4 Correlation of disease with residual HPRT function. HPRT activity was assessed by measuring the incorporation of radiolabeled hypoxanthine into purine nucleotides in fibroblasts growing in tissue culture.[111,173,174] Each symbol reflects results obtained from a single patient. Results show HPRT activity as a percentage of normal values, as described by Page and colleagues.[173,174]

LND Variants. This group of patients spans a broad range of severity. The most severe cases are neurologically indistinguishable from the classic patients, with such profound extrapyramidal and pyramidal dysfunction that they are confined to a wheelchair.[5,108,113] On the other hand, the least severe cases may appear grossly normal, with subtle defects emerging only after careful neurologic assessment. For example, some patients have had only mildly clumsy fine motor skills or gait.[6,30,95,109,114] Several have had persistent stuttering or indistinct speech, or merely a history of transient speech impediment during childhood.[6,30,110,111,114]

These patients are distinguished from the classic cases of LND by the absence of prominent self-injurious or other undesirable behaviors. However, this distinction may not be absolute, because abnormal behaviors have been reported in some cases. One patient reported to have only mild choreoathetosis and hyperreflexia compulsively tore out a large patch of his hair at age 18 when hospitalized with a painful kidney stone.[105] Two additional patients with the typical neurologic features of LND but no self-injury began to bite their lips for the first time in their late teenage years when hospitalized for urgent medical care (unpublished observations). Another patient with only mild clumsiness and dysarthria was reported to engage in recurrent high-risk behaviors, such as impulsively jumping from his motorcycle at high speed or a compulsion to insert metal objects into electrical outlets.[110] Other patients have only mild clumsiness and prominent onychophagia,[30,145,175] sometimes with minor bleeding. Although such patients are rare, they suggest the existence of a continuum of neurologic and behavioral abnormalities related to HPRT deficiency, rather than clearly distinct subgroups.

The LND variants may have systemic manifestations similar to those of classic cases. Although neurologic disability may be present during early development, the diagnosis is generally not considered until uric acid overproduction is identified. The overproduction of uric acid may fall in the same range as in the classic cases,[6,124,125] although the average uric acid overproduction is generally less severe (Table 107-2). Megaloblastic anemia,[6] subnormal renal function,[6,30,110] and testicular dysfunction[110,114] have all been reported for the neurologic variants with hyperuricemia.

HPRT-Related Hyperuricemia. This group of patients demonstrates overproduction of uric acid with all of its consequences, but no obvious neurologic or behavioral abnormalities. These patients typically present with gout, nephrolithiasis, or renal failure (Table 107-1). Hyperuricemia is common in adults, and results from a variety of causes.[122] Only 20 percent of patients with hyperuricemia develop gout, a painful inflammatory condition caused by uric acid crystal deposition in the tissues or joints. Attacks of gout commonly occur in the great toe, but other joints may be involved. Although gout is a relatively common disorder, partial deficiency of HPRT is not a common cause. In a large survey of 425 patients with gout, only 7 had HPRT deficiency, and 5 were all from the same family.[176] Another study of 110 gouty patients disclosed only 5 with HPRT deficiency, and 3 were from the same family.[177]

Some patients with HPRT-related hyperuricemia have no obvious neurobehavioral abnormalities, but slight clumsiness or indistinct speech may become evident with careful testing. Thus, the identification of patients with hyperuricemia alone is not always clearcut, suggesting the existence of a continuum of metabolic, neurologic, and behavioral abnormalities associated with HPRT deficiency. The eponym *Kelley-Seegmiller syndrome* has occasionally been applied to patients with partial HPRT deficiency.[117,122,124] Some restrict this term to HPRT-related hyperuricemia without neurologic manifestations,[122,178] while others use it to describe partial HPRT deficiency with or without neurologic manifestations.[124] Unfortunately, either use of the term implies the existence of clearly distinct subgroups of patients with HPRT deficiency, and has little practical value when the full spectrum of disease is considered as a continuum.

Females with LND. LND results from an X-linked and recessive genetic defect, so affected females are rarely encountered because defective expression from both alleles is required to produce a level of HPRT enzyme deficiency severe enough to be symptomatic. The first female case was reported to have all of the typical features seen in affected males, including hyperuricemia, extrapyramidal and pyramidal neurologic disability, and self-injurious behavior.[179] This case was subsequently shown to have a microdeletion of the maternally derived HPRT gene and nonrandom inactivation of the paternally derived X chromosome.[180] Four additional cases have been reported,[181–184] and two of these were determined to have a point mutation in one allele and markedly reduced mRNA expression from the other allele.[181,185] Thus LND may occur in females, although the mode of inheritance makes this quite rare.

MOLECULAR BASIS

Normal HPRT Gene

LND is inherited as an X-linked recessive disease with an approximate incidence of 1:380,000.[186,187] The mode of inheritance dictates that the disease occur nearly exclusively in males, although affected females do occur rarely.[180–185] The disease results from mutation of the HPRT gene, which spans approximately 45 kb on the distal end of the long arm of the X chromosome at Xq26-q27.[188–190] There is only one functional copy of the HPRT gene in the human genome, but four pseudogenes have been identified. One of these is located on chromosome 3, another on chromosome 5, and two are located on chromosome 11.[191] These additional sequences are nonfunctional because they do not appear to be transcribed.

The structure of the human HPRT gene has been studied in great detail.[20,22,192,193] There are nine exons as shown schematically in Fig. 107-5. The entire gene, including all introns, has been subject to sequence analysis.[194] Approximately 30 percent of the noncoding sequences consist of short repeat sequences, including 49 Alu repeats,[195] but the functional significance of these repeat structures in not yet known. To date, a single restriction fragment-length polymorphism with three alleles has been identified in the human HPRT gene.[196,197] The restriction endonuclease *Bam*HI generates a 22/25 kb pair, a 12/25 kb pair, and a 18/22 kb pair.[196] The frequency of heterozygote females varies from 29 to 38 percent in Americans to 45 to 49 percent in Orientals.[196,198–200] A screening study for low blood HPRT among 1000 normal volunteers has also identified one asymptomatic individual with 37 to 46 percent residual HPRT activity resulting from a point mutation changing histidine to arginine at codon 60.[201] Whether this case should be considered as a rare polymorphism or an asymptomatic mutant is not clear.

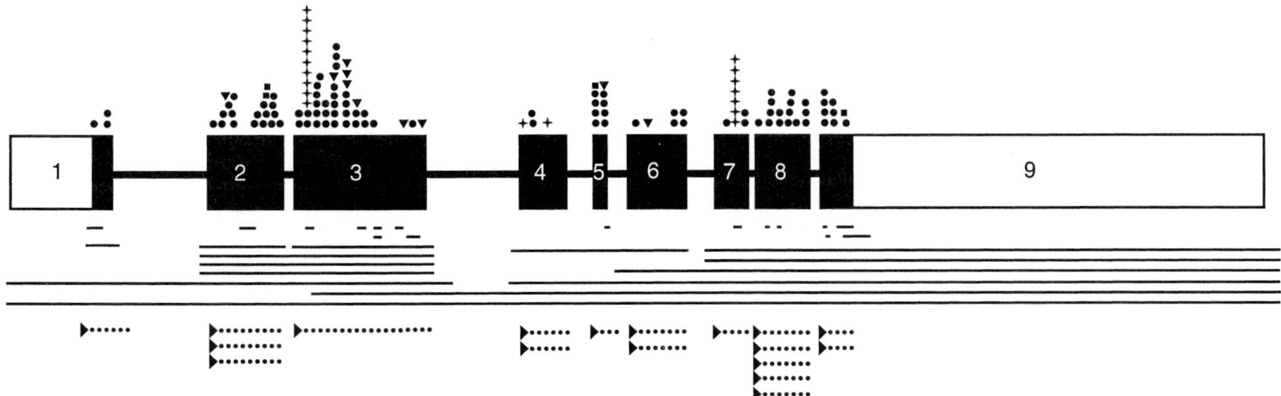

Fig. 107-5 Schematic of the HPRT gene and known mutations. The nine exons of the HPRT gene are depicted as boxes connected by intronic sequences represented by narrow lines. The coding region is shown in black, with noncoding sequences in white. Each symbol above the gene shows the approximate location of a single base alteration described for a patient with HPRT deficiency. Types of mutations shown include amino acid substitutions (circles), stop mutations (stars), single base insertions (triangles), and single base deletions (squares). The solid lines below the gene show deletion mutations characterized for individual patients, and the dotted lines headed by a triangle show splice mutations leading to exon skipping. Insertions of more than one base, duplications, and substitutions are not shown.

The coding sequence of the HPRT gene has been determined for a variety of species from bacteria to man, including *Rhodobacter capsulatus*,[202] *Vibrio harvei*,[203] *Plasmodium falciparum*,[204] *Schistosoma mansoni*,[205] *Trypanosoma cruzi*,[206] mouse,[9,207] rat,[208] and Chinese hamster.[9,209] Sequence homology among the mammalian species is greater than 95 percent in the coding regions. The structures of the mouse[9,207] and Chinese hamster[9,209] HPRT genes have also been elucidated, and their exon/intron arrangements appear similar to those of the human gene. The Australian wallaroo apparently has a functional HPRT minigene expressed only in the liver, in addition to a normal copy of the gene that is ubiquitously expressed.[210,211]

HPRT Gene Expression

Factors regulating the expression of the HPRT gene have been carefully studied by a number of investigators and previously summarized.[20,21] The promoter region of the gene lacks conventional CAAT-like and TATA-like sequences typically found within 80 base pairs of the 5′-end of many genes transcribed by RNA polymerase II.[20,21] Instead, the promoter region has several GC-rich regions characteristic of other mammalian housekeeping genes and some viral genes associated with the SP1 transcription factor complex.[20,21] The first exon of the gene is flanked by four copies of the 5′-GGGCGG-3′ sequence on the 5′ side and three more copies on the 3′ side.[192,193] RNase protection and primer extension studies have demonstrated multiple transcriptional start sites for the human HPRT gene.[192,193]

A region spanning approximately 600 base pairs upstream of the 5′ start site of the gene harbors both positive and negative influences on HPRT gene expression. A segment from positions −219 to −122 relative to the translational start point encompasses all of the 5′ GC-rich regions and functions as a core promoter with partial bidirectionality.[212,213] A second segment from positions −570 to −388 contains repressor elements.[212] Additional regulatory elements are present within the first two introns of the HPRT gene. Sequences in intron 1 act as enhancer elements, and sequences in intron 2 appear necessary for permitting expression of the gene in embryonic stem cells.[214]

Expression of the HPRT gene also appears to be related to the extent of methylation of cytosine residues in CpG clusters. Though females have two copies of the HPRT gene, the one on the inactivated X-chromosome is transcriptionally silent. The silent copy has the majority of its CpG clusters methylated, while the active copy of the gene is largely unmethylated.[215–220]

The majority of studies on relative HPRT expression patterns in mammals have employed biochemical assays for enzyme activity, which are likely to reflect the net combination of differences in gene transcription, mRNA translation, protein turnover, and enzyme activity. Because tissue differences in HPRT enzyme stability have been recognized,[221] enzyme activity does not provide a reliable index of differences in gene expression. A smaller number of studies have looked at relative differences in mRNA levels, which are likely to reflect differences in gene expression more accurately.

The relative expression of HPRT mRNA has not been systematically compared for different human tissues or brain regions. In the mouse, HPRT mRNA expression has been studied in different tissues and brain regions with conflicting results. *In situ* hybridization has revealed significant variations among different regions and cell types of the mouse brain. Two different mouse strains expressed HPRT mRNA at higher levels in neurons in comparison with glia, with relatively high levels in cortex, hippocampus, cerebellum, and motor nuclei.[222] Notably, the basal ganglia expressed particularly low levels.[222] In contrast, semi-quantitative measures involving reverse transcription of mRNA followed by amplification with the polymerase chain reaction have suggested that the basal ganglia have abundant HPRT mRNA.[223] Transgenic mice harboring a human HPRT minigene driven by the metallothionein promoter were reported to express particularly high levels of both the endogenous mouse and the human transcript in the basal ganglia, suggesting that regional variations in HPRT expression might be controlled by elements within the coding region of the human HPRT gene.[224] Another study of transgenic mice expressing β-galactosidase from various fragments of 5′ noncoding regions from the HPRT gene also reported high levels of expression in specific brain regions, suggesting important control elements in the promotor region.[223] However, a subsequent report using the same strategy revealed remarkably distinct temporal and spatial patterns of expression of the transgene that were thought to reflect control by the transgene insertion site rather than the promoter or transgene sequences.[225] These highly specific expression profiles displayed stable patterns of inheritance in five transgenic strains, with only one of the strains showing significant expression in the basal ganglia. Although it is often stated that HPRT mRNA expression is higher in the basal ganglia than most other brain regions and tissues, systematic studies are lacking; and the available evidence does not provide consistent results.

Mutations Causing Disease

Advances in molecular techniques have led to progressive refinements in the characterization of gene mutations responsible for disease among patients. The initial genetic mutations were predicted after purification and sequencing of aberrant HPRT protein from affected patients.[226] These methods were limited to cases where residual HPRT proteins could be detected and purified. Once the HPRT gene was cloned, mutations could be identified more directly. Major structural abnormalities of the HPRT gene were detected in only 15 to 20 percent of cases by Southern or northern analysis, suggesting that the majority of cases had point mutations.[227–232] Some of these point mutations could be detected by RNase protection assays.[231,233,234] Subsequent methods relied on direct gene sequencing of cDNA transcripts amplified by reverse transcription from mRNA isolated from patients. These methods depend on the expression of mRNA and cannot distinguish splice-site mutations from deletions. The most precise methods use direct amplification of genomic DNA by the polymerase chain reaction with primers for each of the exons.[233,235–238] A review of the literature through August 1999 discloses 202 defined mutations reported for patients with HPRT deficiency.[53,61,95,112,113,116,121,180,181,226–228,231,233,235,236,238–274] These mutations are summarized in Table 107-5 and shown schematically in Fig. 107-5. Mutations determined from analysis of mRNA only were not included in this summary, because it is not possible to distinguish point mutations leading to splicing errors from genomic deletions without genomic DNA analysis.

Overall, mutations causing disease appear throughout the HPRT gene. The recognition of potential hot spots for mutation is complicated by the occasional repeated publication of results for the same patient or family, sometimes by the same authors. However, a few mutations have appeared several times in apparently unrelated patients. For example, a C to T substitution changing arginine to stop at codon 51 has emerged multiple times at a CpG motif.[226,233,238,240,251,252,262,269] A similar C-to-T mutation has been identified at another CpG motif at codon 169.[61,233,238,242,251,272] The mechanism for this type of mutation is thought to be related to the frequent methylation of cytosines at CpG motifs, with subsequent deamination of 5-methylcytosine to produce thymine.[251]

Several authors have proposed that clinically relevant mutations might cluster in regions of the gene that encode important functional domains of the HPRT enzyme, such as the putative PP-ribose-P binding site.[233,238,244,249,275] This site was initially inferred by comparing sequence homologies among different phosphoribosyltransferases[244,276] and subsequently confirmed by x-ray crystallography.[277–279] However, most of the kinetic mutations associated with an altered affinity for PP-ribose-P are actually located outside this site.[226,235,247,248,250,254] Evidently, mutations distant from the active site may have a significant influence on enzyme function as a result of conformational

Table 107-5 Molecular Basis of HPRT Deficiency

Mutation	LND (n=200)	Variant (n=63)	NA (n=8)	Total (n=271)
Point				
Substitution	63	48	4	225
Early	23	1	1	25
Splice error	25	6	0	31
Deletion				
Coding	56	2	3	61
Splice error	4	0	0	4
Insertion				
Coding	18	1	0	19
Splice error	1	0	0	1
Other				
Duplication	3	3	0	6
Substitution	2	0	0	6
Double mutant	0	2	0	2
Females	5	0	0	5

Data for this were obtained from published mutations described for patients with varying degrees of HPRT deficiency.[53,61,95,112,113,118,121,180,181,226–228,231,233,235,236,238–274] Clinical information was not available for 8 cases (NA).

changes that indirectly alter the active site, or change mRNA or protein stability.

A consideration of the known mutations in the context of differences in phenotypic expression leads to some important concepts. First, most of the patients with variant forms of the disease resulting from partial enzyme deficiency have point mutations leading to amino acid substitutions rather than nonsense mutations or complex mutations disrupting major portions of the coding sequence. This is to be expected if the phenotypic severity depends on residual enzyme activity encoded by the mutant gene. Some of the variants that have mutations predicting complete absence of HPRT activity appear to represent exceptions to this concept, but careful analysis of several of these patients has provided an explanation for the discrepancy. For example, one patient with an early nonsense mutation was reported as a variant because of the absence of self-injury by age 10,[272] although the emergence of self-injury at a later age would require that he be reclassified as having classic LND. In addition, some variants with deletion mutations may permit some residual HPRT enzyme function. One of these has an early deletion, but a functional mRNA is transcribed from an alternate GUG start codon.[260] Another has a 51-base pair deletion that is predicted to produce an HPRT protein missing only the last 2 amino acids.[271] Three variants have partial gene duplications predicting complete loss of HPRT expression, but two of these mutations are unstable *in vitro*, with high rates of reversion leading to the expression of residual HPRT enzyme activity.[239,240,257] These duplications may undergo a similar reversion *in vivo*, resulting in significant residual HPRT activity depending on the extent of somatic mosaicism, and might explain the relatively mild symptoms in these patients. Another variant with a 3 base pair insertion might have significant residual enzyme activity because the resultant HPRT protein is predicted to include only one additional amino acid without disturbing the normal reading frame.[240]

Another lesson learned from genotype-phenotype correlations is that the same mutation may have somewhat different phenotypic consequences among different patients. For example, a C-to-T mutation at nucleotide position 508 that changed an arginine residue to a stop at codon 170 has been reported for several patients. Two of these patients were reported to have the full spectrum of the disease with self-injury,[233,242] while the last was considered a variant because of the absence of self-injury.[272] Other authors have remarked on significant differences in disease severity among different patients with the same mutation[233] or even among multiple affected members of the same kindred.[53,109] These observations suggest that the molecular mutation cannot always be used to reliably predict disease severity, because the expression of the disease may be modified to some degree by other genetic or environmental factors.

Somatic Mutation

The HPRT gene has provided a uniquely powerful tool to investigate the frequency and type of acquired mutations in cultured cells or circulating lymphocytes.[23,25,178] The purine analog 6-thioguanine is not toxic to normal cells unless it is first converted by HPRT into its nucleotide form. Cells that have acquired a mutation in the HPRT gene can be grown *in vitro* and readily identified by their resistance to this analog. The differential growth of normal and HPRT-deficient cells provides a rapid method for the determination of mutation frequencies. The HPRT gene can then be sequenced to determine the type of mutations incurred.

The frequency of HPRT mutants identified in this way in circulating lymphocytes ranges from 0.4 to 27.8 per 10^6 cells in healthy adults.[25] Elevated mutation frequencies are observed in normal aging, in tobacco smokers, in radiotherapists, in oncology patients treated with radiation or chemotherapy, in patients with defects of DNA repair such as ataxia telangiectasia and xeroderma pigmentosum, and in survivors of atomic bomb explosions.[25]

BIOCHEMICAL BASIS

Purine Metabolism

Synthesis. The purines form a class of molecules with diverse functions in cell physiology.[280] They play an essential role in energy-requiring reactions, nucleic acid synthesis, cofactor reactions, and inter- and intracellular signaling. The pathways for synthesis, metabolism, and degradation of the purines are shown in Fig. 107-6. In general, cellular purines are obtained through three different processes. These processes include *de novo* synthesis from smaller organic molecules, salvage of preformed purine bases, and uptake from the extracellular environment.

The *de novo* synthesis of purines occurs through a multistep process that is regulated at several points.[122,281] The first and rate-limiting step in the synthesis of purines is mediated by the enzyme amidophosphoribosyltransferase. This step is stimulated by increased concentrations of the substrate PP-ribose-P, and is

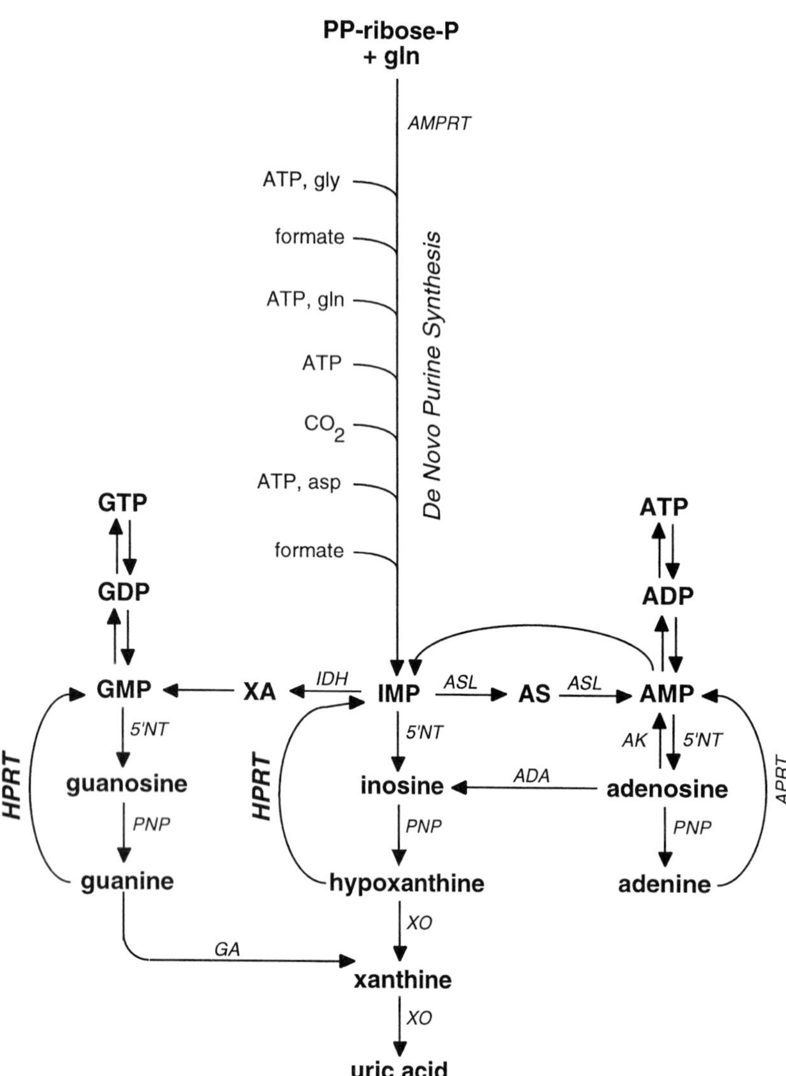

Fig. 107-6 Role of HPRT in purine metabolism. Abbreviations used are: 5′NT, 5′-nucleotidase; ADA, adenosine deaminase; ADP, adenosine diphosphate; AK, adenosine kinase; AMP, adenosine monophosphate; AMPRT, amidophosphoribosyltransferase; APRT, adenine phosphoribosyltransferase; AS, adenylosuccinate; ASL, adenine succinate-synthase/lyase; ATP, adenosine triphosphate; GA, guanase; GDP, guanosine diphosphate; gln, glutamine; gly, glycine; GMP, guanosine monophosphate; GTP, guanosine triphosphate; HPRT, hypoxanthine-guanine phosphoribosyltransferase; IDH, IMP dehydrogenase; IMP, inosine monophosphate; PNP, purine nucleoside phosphorylase; PP-ribose-P, phosphoribosylpyrophosphate; XA, xanthylic acid; XO, xanthine oxidase.

subject to feedback inhibition by IMP, AMP, and GMP. The branch point, which involves the conversion of IMP into either the guanine or adenine nucleotide pool, is also under feedback control. The conversion of IMP to xanthylic acid by the enzyme IMP dehydrogenase is the first step along the pathway leading to the production of guanine nucleotides and is inhibited by GTP. Similarly, the conversion of IMP to adenylosuccinate by adenylosuccinate synthase-lyase is the first step along the pathway leading to the production of adenine nucleotides and is inhibited by AMP. GTP also regulates the activity of adenylosuccinate synthase-lyase because it serves as a substrate for this enzyme. Although most cells have the machinery to synthesize purines *de novo*, it is important to note that this pathway is metabolically expensive. The synthesis of one molecule of IMP, for example, involves multiple steps and requires contributions from four amino acids, two folates, one PP-ribose-P, and three ATP.

Salvage. Purine recycling in humans is mediated by three different enzymes: HPRT, APRT, and adenosine kinase. In humans, it is estimated that 90 percent of free purines generated during intracellular metabolism are recycled rather than degraded or excreted.[280] HPRT serves to recycle free hypoxanthine and guanine into IMP and GMP, respectively. APRT, which is structurally and functionally very similar to HPRT, serves to recycle free adenine into AMP. Adenosine kinase, although not strictly considered as one of the salvage pathway enzymes, prevents the diffusion of free adenosine from the cell by phosphorylating it to produce AMP. In this way, free adenosine that would otherwise be lost to the extracellular environment through diffusion is salvaged. Like HPRT and APRT, adenosine kinase helps to maintain the purine nucleotide pools by recycling a preformed purine moiety into the cellular purine pools. Although none of these salvage enzymes is essential for cell survival, their presence allows for more economical functioning with regard to the metabolism of purines.[280]

The final mechanism contributing to the maintenance of cellular purines involves the incorporation of free purine bases and nucleosides produced from extracellular sources. For example, digestion of dietary plant and animal matter produces purines through the degradation of DNA and RNA. A portion of these compounds is then taken up from the gut into the bloodstream and incorporated into utilizable purines by the liver.[280] The liver then produces purine bases and exports them into the bloodstream for use by other tissues.[282] The incorporation of these preformed purines into cellular purine pools is mediated by the salvage enzymes described above. Therefore, the absence of the purine salvage enzymes results not only in an inability to salvage purines produced through intracellular metabolism, but an inability to incorporate purines derived from extracellular sources.

Degradation. The degradation of purines occurs through the action of 5′-nucleotidase, adenosine deaminase, purine nucleoside phosphorylase, guanase, and xanthine oxidase as shown in Fig. 107-6. In general, the activity of each of these enzymes is regulated by substrate availability. In primates, the final degradation product is uric acid; but in other animals, uric acid is further degraded to allantoin by the action of the enzyme uricase.

HPRT Biochemistry

Structure. The mature HPRT mRNA of approximately 1.3 kb is initially translated into a protein of 218 amino acids with a mass of 25 kDa. The initial methionine at the N-terminus is cleaved from the protein, and the newly exposed alanine is acetylated.[226] Cross-linking studies and isoelectric focussing experiments have suggested that four identical subunits aggregate to form a dimer of dimers, or a tetramer, depending on ionic strength and pH.[283–285] Several other modifications occur in a time-dependent manner. The asparagine at position 106 is partially deamidated,[286,287] resulting in multiple distinct bands on isoelectric focusing gels. In addition, the cysteine at position 23 is partially oxidized, leading to a progressive loss of specific activity due to a decrease in the affinity of the enzyme for PP-ribose-P.[288]

A three-dimensional structure for HPRT was initially predicted from analysis of amino acid sequences.[226,289] The sequence of 12 amino acids from positions 129 through 140 has been proposed to comprise the PP-ribose-P binding site of the enzyme, because this area was noted to be highly conserved among different phosphoribosyltransferases isolated from several species.[226,289,290] The three-dimensional structure of human HPRT with bound GMP,[277] IMP,[291] or a nonmetabolizable hypoxanthine substrate[279] has been resolved by x-ray crystallography (Fig. 107-7). The crystal structure suggests that the human enzyme has a core α/β structure similar to other dehydrogenases and a cleft in which the PP-ribose-P and purine bases bind. The results from crystallography have confirmed earlier predictions regarding a central role for amino acids 129 to 140 at the active site.

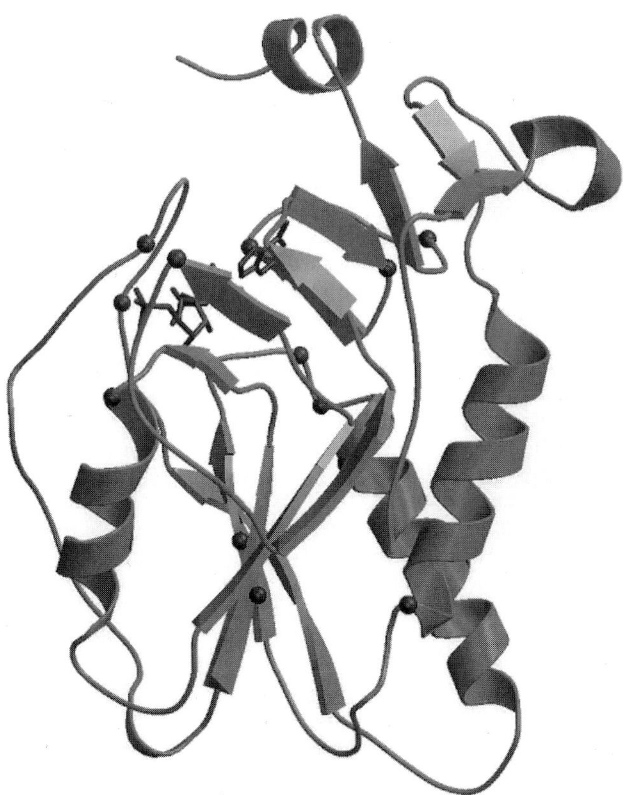

Fig. 107-7 **Structure of human HPRT. The three-dimensional structure of human HPRT with PP-ribose-P and a nonmetabolizable analog of hypoxanthine (7-hydroxy [4,3-d]pyrazolo pyrimidine) was determined by x-ray crystallography.[277–279] The enlarged arrows show the locations of beta strands, and the coils represent alpha helices. The round balls depict some of the known mutations affecting the kinetic properties of the enzyme. (*The graphical depiction was kindly provided by Drs. G.K. Balendiron and J.C. Sacchettini.*)**

Function. HPRT is one of a family of 10 enzymes that use the high-energy phosphodiester bonds of PP-ribose-P rather than ATP for catalysis.[290,292] These enzymes are involved in the metabolism of the amino acids histidine and tryptophan, as well as in the metabolism of purine, pyrimidine, and pyridine nucleotides. More specifically, HPRT catalyzes the transfer of the 5-phosphoribosyl group from PP-ribose-P to the 9 position of hypoxanthine or guanine in the presence of magnesium to form the respective nucleotide and pyrophosphate. The molecular mechanism of the reaction has been studied in great detail.[278,291,293,294] The forward reaction begins with the binding of the magnesium salt of PP-ribose-P to the active site of the enzyme. The purine base binds next and forms a short-lived ternary complex before the transfer reaction. After the transfer reaction, the pyrophosphate product is released first, followed by release of either IMP or GMP.

The K_m values reported for human HPRT from various sources range from 220 to 250 μM for PP-ribose-P, 9.9 to 17 μM for hypoxanthine, and 4.0 to 21 μM for guanine.[278,291,293,294] The equilibrium of the reaction lies far toward the nucleotide products, with an approximate K_{eq} constant of 1.6×10^{-5}. Alterations in the kinetic properties of the enzyme have been identified in several patients. These alterations have included reduced affinities for PP-ribose-P, the purine base, or reduced maximal enzyme velocity.[89,115,247–249,254,288,295–297] The kinetic properties of the rodent enzyme are similar to those of the human.[283,298]

Expression. HPRT enzyme activity is widely expressed in many species throughout phylogeny from bacteria through mammals. In mammals, activity is measurable in essentially all tissues throughout development. It exists chiefly in the cytosolic fraction, though subcellular fractionation studies with rat brain have suggested that it may be somewhat enriched in synaptosomal preparations.[298] Though expression of HPRT is ubiquitous among mammalian tissues, there are significant quantitative variations in relative amounts measured in different tissues at different developmental stages.

The tissue distribution of HPRT enzyme activity has been studied in a variety of organisms, including humans. Early studies led to the concept that the human brain expressed particularly high levels of HPRT activity, with marked variations in different regions of the brain. The earliest study comparing HPRT enzyme activities among different tissues of one case demonstrated the brain to have markedly higher levels than eight other tissues tested, with the basal ganglia showing the highest activity among four brain regions examined.[6,172] Early studies in the rhesus monkey seemed to confirm that the brain had high levels of HPRT activity.[299] These studies contributed to the concept that the brain, and in particular the basal ganglia, was particularly dependent upon HPRT-mediated salvage to maintain purine levels.

However, later studies of human tissues revealed two factors that have forced a revision of these early concepts. First, HPRT activity varies markedly among different tissues during development. Second, different tissues express varying amounts of several competing enzymes may artifactually alter apparent HPRT enzyme activities with standard in vitro assays. During early human development, HPRT enzyme activity is present even in the preimplantation oocyte and generally increases during embryogenesis.[300] In the developing fetus, HPRT activity differs little among several tissues.[258,301–303] In one neonate, HPRT activity varied twofold among different tissues and brain regions, with the basal ganglia expressing midrange values.[301] The amount and distribution of HPRT activity varies considerably between children and adults. In one thorough study employing special precautions to minimize artifactual changes in apparent HPRT activity due to competing enzymes, HPRT activity was assessed in eight tissues of multiple subjects of different ages.[304] In adults, the testis expressed higher levels than the brain. Within the brain, cortical tissue had slightly higher HPRT activity than the basal ganglia. Measurements of HPRT activity among 12 brain regions from another adult human brain specimen revealed a twofold variation in activity, with the basal ganglia in the high to middle range of recorded values.[31] Another study of four adult brain specimens revealed little variation in HPRT activity among the caudate, putamen, thalamus, and cortex.[27]

More systematic studies of differences in HPRT expression have been conducted with rodent tissues. In mice, HPRT enzyme activity increases three- to fivefold in several tissues during early postnatal development before reaching stable adult values.[305] Comparisons among different mouse tissues have generally suggested that the brain has higher HPRT activity than most other tissues, although in many cases the differences appear minor.[221,305,306] Only one study reported the mouse brain to have markedly elevated HPRT enzyme levels in comparison with other tissues.[224] Within the mouse brain, HPRT activity varies less than twofold among different regions.[307] In the rat, HPRT expression also increases during early postnatal development,[298,304,305,308–311] although there is very little variation in HPRT enzyme activity among different tissues[298,304,306,308] or different regions of the brain.[304,310,312]

HPRT activity also appears to vary during different growth cycles of the cell. Activity is often higher in rapidly dividing cells in comparison to quiescent cells.[306,313,314] A similar situation occurs in vivo, where HPRT activity increases in regenerating liver after partial hepatectomy.[306] It has been suggested that the increased activity is important for the maintenance of purines for nucleic acid synthesis in the dividing cells. However, the high levels of HPRT activity in the adult brain and other postmitotic tissues, suggests processes other than nucleic acid synthesis also depend heavily on purine salvage.[310]

HPRT Deficiency

Accumulation of Oxypurines. The absence of HPRT results in the accumulation of its substrates, hypoxanthine and guanine. Because there is no other pathway for reincorporating hypoxanthine and guanine into utilizable purines, they are eventually degraded or excreted. In the blood, hypoxanthine and xanthine are converted primarily to uric acid and excreted in the urine. Concentrations of xanthine and hypoxanthine remain elevated in the blood and urine of LND patients, reflecting incomplete metabolism of these purines to uric acid.[315–319]

Because brain tissue has relatively high levels of guanase, the majority of guanine produced in the brain is degraded to xanthine. LND patients excrete into their cerebrospinal fluid four to five times the normal concentration of hypoxanthine, but relatively normal levels of xanthine.[172,316,320] However, brain tissue has relatively low levels of xanthine oxidase,[321] so the generation of uric acid from xanthine and hypoxanthine is limited. Cerebrospinal fluid uric acid is either normal[172] or slightly elevated.[89]

Increased Intracellular PP-Ribose-P. Although direct measurements of PP-ribose-P levels in tissue samples from LND patients have not been possible for technical reasons, several studies have demonstrated increased PP-ribose-P levels in HPRT-deficient erythrocytes or cultured cells. Approximately two- to tenfold increases in PP-ribose-P levels have been demonstrated in HPRT-deficient human erythrocytes,[322–324] human lymphoblasts,[325–327] human fibroblasts,[328–332] and rat C6 glioma cells[333] in culture. The increased PP-ribose-P levels appear to result from at least two separate processes. First, the absence of HPRT results in underuse and therefore increased availability of PP-ribose-P. Second, PP-ribose-P synthetase activity is enhanced in HPRT-deficient cells including human fibroblasts,[89,329,334] human lymphocytes,[335] and rat hepatoma cells[336] in culture.

Care must be taken in interpreting results from *in vitro* experiments, because intracellular PP-ribose-P concentrations have been shown to vary significantly depending on cellular growth rates or the availability of carbohydrates and amino acids in the tissue culture medium.[325,334,337] Currently, no direct deleterious effects are known to result from the elevated PP-ribose-P levels in HPRT-deficient cells. However, several studies have suggested that the elevated levels of PP-ribose-P are indirectly responsible for increasing the rates of reactions of other enzymes that use PP-ribose-P as a substrate. For example, APRT activity, which is dependent on the availability of PP-ribose-P, is typically elevated by twofold in HPRT-deficient erythrocytes[51,75,105,322,338–340] and cultured cells.[71,89,341] Amidophosphoribosyltransferase and orotidine phosphoribosyltransferase activities are also increased.[323] The increase in the activity of other enzymes dependent upon PP-ribose-P is thought to result from the phenomenon of substrate stabilization.[322,338–340]

Purine Depletion. Given the role of HPRT in purine recycling, it seems likely that the absence of HPRT would be associated with continual loss of purines leading to an intracellular purine deficit.[45,167,342–344] The severity of the deficit in different tissues is likely to depend on the proportion of purines derived from synthesis versus salvage. Technical limitations have precluded the direct measurement of purine pools in tissue samples from LND patients, so most attempts to measure purines have focused on blood cells obtained from LND patients, HPRT-deficient cells grown in culture, and an HPRT-deficient knockout mouse.

Two reports have described an approximately 30 percent reduction in guanine nucleotides with normal levels of adenine nucleotides in erythrocytes obtained from LND patients.[345,346] On the other hand, another study of HPRT-deficient erythrocytes described a 30 percent reduction in adenine nucleotides with normal guanine nucleotides.[347] A small reduction in ATP together with normal ADP and guanine nucleotides has also been reported for LND platelets.[348] These conflicting results are difficult to interpret. In addition, erythrocytes and platelets are anucleate and lack a complete pathway for *de novo* purine synthesis, so results obtained with these preparations may not apply to most other tissues.

A purine deficit has also been sought for HPRT-deficient cells grown in culture. Studies including HPRT-deficient human fibroblasts,[328] human lymphoblasts,[349] rat neuroma cells,[350] and mouse neuroblastoma cells,[351] have consistently failed to produce any evidence for purine depletion. The major limitation of these studies is that cells grown *in vitro* typically have unlimited access to cellular nutrients supplied in the tissue culture medium which may be limiting *in vivo*. In fact, HPRT-deficient human lymphoblasts grown in tissue culture under conditions of limited nutrition have lower levels of adenine and guanine nucleotides when compared to normal cells grown under similar conditions.[352] Unfortunately, the biologic relevance of purine deficits occurring only with nutrient starvation *in vitro* are unclear. Therefore, conclusions derived from the *in vitro* studies cannot be readily extrapolated to the *in vivo* situation.

Purines have also been measured in the brains of HPRT-deficient mice.[307] Although there was no evidence for purine depletion in whole-brain tissue or any of six different subregions examined, purine synthesis was accelerated four- to fivefold. These results are also difficult to extrapolate to the human condition, because the mice do not suffer from any obvious neurobehavioral deficits. In summary, although purine depletion seems a likely consequence of impaired purine salvage, no definite loss of purines has been demonstrated in studies of blood cells from patients, HPRT-deficient cells in vitro, or an HPRT-deficient mouse model.

Accelerated Purine Synthesis. In addition to the buildup in HPRT substrates and potential depletion of purine nucleotide products, several studies have documented that HPRT-deficiency is associated with a pronounced activation of *de novo* purine synthesis. *De novo* purine synthesis has most commonly been studied by monitoring the incorporation of radiolabeled glycine or formic acid into the purine pools. In LND patients, radiolabeled glycine or formic acid administered intravenously is incorporated into urinary uric acid at least 10 times faster than in normal individuals.[1,3,55,68,186] Although never directly demonstrated, it is assumed that a similar increase in *de novo* purine synthesis occurs in the LND brain. Increased incorporation of radiolabeled glycine or formic acid into purines has also been observed in HPRT-deficient human fibroblasts,[328] human lymphoblasts,[325–327] rat C6 glioma cells,[333] and rat neuroma cells[350] in culture. It has also been demonstrated in the HPRT-deficient mouse.[307]

The increased synthesis of purines appears to result from two separate processes.[122] First, an increase in the availability of PP-ribose-P may accelerate purine synthesis *de novo* because it is one of the substrates of the rate-limiting step. Second, a decrease in intracellular purine nucleotides may result in decreased feedback inhibition on purine synthesis. It is the combination of increased purine synthesis together with the failure of purine recycling that is responsible for the marked overproduction of uric acid associated with HPRT deficiency.

PATHOLOGIC BASIS

Renal Dysfunction

The subnormal renal function among patients with HPRT deficiency may be related to uric acid nephropathy, a direct deleterious effect of the enzyme deficiency on renal function, or both. Stones composed of uric acid, xanthine, hypoxanthine, and oxypurinol are all radiolucent. As a result, plain films and CT images of the kidneys are often unrevealing. Stones are more readily detected with ultrasound[63–65,88,353,354] or intravenous pyelograms.[126,128,355] Another common finding on ultrasound has been a diffuse hyperechoic signal from the renal medulla.[64,65,88,353,354]

Several gross abnormalities have been described in the kidneys at autopsy, including stones[37,67,81] and diffuse atrophy.[33,37] At the microscopic level, there are often inflammatory changes consisting of interstitial nephritis and fibrosis, focal glomerulosclerosis, giant cells, and granuloma.[33,42,73,106,107,120] These findings are thought to be due to the ability of uric acid crystals to induce a marked inflammatory response.

Neurobehavioral Features

Neuroimaging. There are few detailed neuroimaging studies of LND, in part due to the rarity of the disease and in part to the difficulty of obtaining adequate images without general anesthesia. Normal CT images of the brain were reported in seven case reports,[31,57,78,87,119] while diffuse atrophy was reported in another.[356] A review of brain CT images from 12 patients revealed mild to moderate atrophy in many, but not all, of these cases.[357]

The first study involving MRI in LND included four patients.[28] One patient had moderate cerebral atrophy, another had decreased T2 signal in the basal ganglia, and the remaining two were considered normal. MR images were considered normal for 1 case report[87] and for all 12 patients in a PET study.[358] The most detailed MRI study included seven patients.[359] Brain atrophy was evident in most cases, as judged by enlargement of the cerebrospinal fluid spaces. The application of quantitative methods confirmed brain atrophy, with apparent preferential involvement of the basal ganglia. In comparison to a group of age-matched controls, total brain volumes in the patients were decreased by 17 percent, and caudate volumes were decreased by 34 percent.[359] A concurrent enlargement of the cranial sinuses suggested that the volume loss reflected poor brain development rather than a degenerative process, so the term dystrophy might be preferable to atrophy, which implies a degenerative process.[359]

Neuropathology. Neuropathologic studies have been reported for 15 LND patients at autopsy.[31,33–35,37,38,42,70,360,361] Brain size was considered small in 4 of these cases.[33,35,37,361] Focal softenings,[34,37,38] areas of gliosis,[34,37,42,106,362] and loss of cerebellar cells[34,37,42] have each reported in several cases. Less commonly noted findings included a thin cortex,[70] demyelinative lesions,[37] cerebral edema,[35] severe hydrocephalus,[42] and PAS-positive inclusions in the olives.[361] Two patients had increased dopamine receptor immunoreactivity in the basal ganglia, with normal numbers of midbrain neurons immunopositive for tyrosine hydroxylase.[362] Although many different abnormalities have been described, the lack of any consistent findings suggests that they do not play a central role in pathogenesis. In fact, some of the reported abnormalities may be related to chronic renal failure in untreated patients or from ischemia among patients dying from aspiration pneumonia. It is therefore noteworthy that neuropathologic examination was completely normal in three cases.[33,35,360]

The histopathologic appearance of peripheral nerves has been described for five patients. The sural nerve of a 31-year-old who died of pneumonia showed a decrease in the number of large myelinated fibers and lipid-like inclusions in Schwann cells.[48] Sural nerve biopsies were normal in four additional cases, except for mild increased mitochondrial density in three.[158]

In summary, routine neuroimaging and autopsy studies do not provide diagnostic information. Brain atrophy is evident in many cases, but the degree of atrophy may be sufficiently small to escape detection in routine studies.

Monoamine Neurochemistry. Multiple studies employing different methodologies have demonstrated that HPRT deficiency is associated with abnormalities of the neurochemistry of monoamines, and in particular dopamine. The prominent neurobehavioral features suggesting dysfunction of the basal ganglia in LND led to a neurochemical assessment of the major neurotransmitter systems of this region in three cases at autopsy.[27] This study showed 60 to 90 percent reductions of dopamine and its metabolite homovanillic acid in all subregions of the basal ganglia including the caudate, putamen, globus pallidus, and nucleus accumbens. Two enzymes involved in dopamine synthesis, tyrosine hydroxylase and aromatic amino acid decarboxylase, were similarly affected. However, dopamine was not significantly reduced in the midbrains of these patients, leading to the proposal that the midbrain dopamine neurons were intact but their fiber projections to the basal ganglia were reduced.[27]

Profound dopamine loss in the basal ganglia was confirmed in two additional cases.[362] Measures of monoamine metabolites in cerebrospinal fluid specimens from affected patients have generally confirmed a slight reduction in the dopamine metabolite, homovanillic acid.[28,29,41,363] However, the interpretation of these results is confounded by significant changes in normative data during development.[29] PET has also been used to assess basal ganglia dopamine systems *in vivo*. In one study that included 7 patients, the binding of the ligand WIN 35,428 to dopamine uptake transporters was reduced by an average of 73 percent in the putamen and 56 percent in the caudate.[364] Another study of 12 patients demonstrated average reductions in fluorodopa uptake of 69 percent in the putamen and 61 percent in the caudate.[358] Both of these studies provide indirect evidence for a reduction in dopamine fiber density in the basal ganglia of patients with LND.

Dopamine deficiency also occurs in an HPRT-deficient mouse[365–369] and in HPRT-deficient subclones of the rat PC12 pheochromocytoma cell line *in vitro*.[177,370] Taken together, the data from clinical and basic research studies have provided strong support that HPRT deficiency causes significant dysfunction of neuronal systems that use dopamine as a neurotransmitter. The mechanisms by which HPRT deficiency affects dopamine systems remain enigmatic, because no direct relationship between the biochemical functions of HPRT and dopamine metabolism is currently known.

Norepinephrine and the enzyme most directly responsible for its synthesis, dopamine β-hydroxylase, were not altered in the human autopsy study.[27] However, average serum dopamine β-hydroxylase activity was abnormally high in one study of 10 LND patients[371] and abnormally low in a subsequent study of 14 additional patients.[372] Both studies revealed abnormal sympathetic responses to cold stress or postural changes. Abnormalities of the sympathetic nervous system are perhaps not surprising given the chronic physical and psychologic stressors experienced by these patients. In the autopsy study, serotonin levels were elevated by 24 percent and the serotonin metabolite 5-hydroxyindoleacetic acid was increased by 92 percent.[27] In cerebrospinal fluid, 5-hydroxyindole acetic acid has been reported to be slightly reduced[29,41,363] or unchanged.[28,316]

Monoamine oxidase, an enzyme responsible for the degradation of monoamines, was increased up to twofold in the autopsy study.[27] However, *in vitro* studies repeatedly demonstrated abnormally low levels of this enzyme among HPRT-deficient cells grown in culture. Monoamine oxidase activity was reduced by 60 to 90 percent in HPRT-deficient human fibroblasts,[373–375] mouse neuroblastoma cells,[373] rat C6 glioma cells,[376] and rat PC12 pheochromocytoma cells.[177]

Amino Acid Neurochemistry. In brain tissue obtained from 5 LND patients at autopsy, almost all amino acids were significantly reduced in the cortex, cerebellum, hippocampus, and putamen.[377] One exception was glutamine, which appeared to be elevated in most regions. These findings were interpreted to reflect a poor nutritional status of the subjects. In another study, the amino acid concentrations in brain and serum were reported for one LND patient.[316] Significant reductions were found in almost all amino acids in brain, but amino acid levels were normal in the serum. These results suggested that poor nutritional status was not the only explanation for the abnormally low brain amino acid concentrations. In the cerebrospinal fluid, amino acid levels have been reported to be normal, increased, or decreased.[41,316,378]

In tissue culture, amino acid levels in HPRT-deficient mouse neuroblastoma[379] and rat C6 glioma cells[380] were reported to be normal, with the exception of glycine, which was elevated approximately twofold in both cell types. In these studies, the presence of a full complement of essential amino acids in the tissue culture medium probably precluded the finding of any amino acid deficits. However, the consistent elevation of glycine suggests the occurrence of an intrinsic abnormality of amino acid metabolism in HPRT-deficient cells. The significance of the reported abnormalities of amino acid content, and their relationship to HPRT deficiency, remain to be elucidated.

Neuropathogenesis. A large number of hypotheses have been presented to explain the mechanisms by which HPRT deficiency might cause the neurobehavioral abnormalities observed in LND.[381] In general, these hypotheses can be grouped into two categories (Table 107-6). The first category postulates the accumulation of excess quantities of a metabolite that exerts neurotoxic effects, and the second category postulates dysfunction or maldevelopment related to deficiency of a metabolite. Because the pathogenesis of the neurobehavioral features is one of the least-well understood areas in HPRT deficiency, these hypotheses and associated data are reviewed in detail below.

Table 107-6 Theories for Neuropathogenesis in LND

Theories
Toxicity hypotheses
Uric acid
Oxypurines
Phosphoribosylpyrophosphate
Z-nucleotides
Oxidant stress
Glutamate
Deficiency hypotheses
Adenine nucleotides
ATP (energy)
Cofactors
Adenosine
Guanine nucleotides
Tetrahydrobiopterin
G-proteins

Uric Acid Toxicity. The demonstration of gross increases in plasma and urinary uric acid in LND led to early proposals that the accumulation of this compound might result in a toxic effect on the developing nervous system.[45,55,342] Uric acid toxicity is perhaps one of the most often proposed hypotheses for neuropathogenesis in LND, but current evidence suggests that this is an inadequate explanation. If high levels of uric acid have a toxic effect on the nervous system, then suppression of uric acid production in LND patients should suppress the subsequent development of neurobehavioral abnormalities. To the contrary, treatment of LND patients from birth with allopurinol has no influence on the development of neurobehavioral defects.[26] If uric acid toxicity is responsible for neuropathogenesis in LND, one might expect LND-like neurobehavioral disturbances in other clinical situations involving the overproduction of uric acid. This is not the case; patients with partial HPRT deficiency and overactivity of PP-ribose-P synthetase have plasma and urinary uric acid levels that fall in the same range as those of LND patients, but these patients have little or no neurologic impairment.[122] Taken together, these observations indicate that uric acid toxicity is not responsible for the neurobehavioral impairments observed in LND.

Oxypurine Toxicity. The accumulation of excessive concentrations of hypoxanthine or xanthine might also cause pathologic effects in the LND brain.[172,344,382–385] These oxypurines bind to benzodiazepine receptors in brain tissue, and could potentially interfere with the normal functions of these receptors.[382,384,386] Despite the low affinity of the oxypurines for the benzodiazepine receptor, these bases may reach sufficiently high concentrations to have a physiologically relevant effect on receptor function. In addition, implantation of solid hypoxanthine crystals into the basal ganglia of rats has been reported to produce self-injurious behavior.[385]

Although hypoxanthine and xanthine accumulate in HPRT-deficient cells and appear to be elevated in the cerebrospinal fluid of patients with LND,[172,316] there is so far no direct evidence that these bases are neurotoxic in the Lesch-Nyhan brain. Furthermore, several additional observations argue against the oxypurine toxicity hypothesis. First, the administration of allopurinol to patients with LND results in large increases in serum oxypurines, but does not exacerbate the neurobehavioral features.[172,316] In addition, if elevated hypoxanthine or xanthine concentrations are responsible for neuropathophysiology in LND, one might expect LND-like neurobehavioral abnormalities in other clinical situations where these bases are found at elevated levels. This is not the case; patients with extremely high levels of plasma and urinary hypoxanthine and xanthine resulting from congenital deficiency of xanthine oxidase do not exhibit any of the neurobehavioral abnormalities observed in LND.

PP-Ribose-P Toxicity. PP-ribose-P accumulates to supranormal levels in HPRT-deficient cells[326–328,333,335] and may accumulate in the LND brain. It is therefore possible that this compound interferes with specific cellular functions or is directly cytotoxic. However, there is currently no direct evidence to support a role for PP-ribose-P toxicity in LND. Further evidence arguing against a pathogenic role for PP-ribose-P comes from observations among patients with elevated PP-ribose-P levels due to a superactive PP-ribose-P synthetase.[122] Overproduction of PP-ribose-P in these patients is associated with hyperuricemia and toxicity to the auditory nerve, but neurobehavioral abnormalities similar to those occurring in LND are not observed.

Z-Nucleotide Toxicity. The accelerated rate of *de novo* purine synthesis among patients with HPRT deficiency results in increased concentrations of some purine intermediates which are normally present only at very low concentrations. These intermediates, nucleotide derivatives of 5-amino-4-imidazolecarboxamide riboside, are collectively known as Z-nucleotides and have been proposed as potential mediators of neuropathogenesis in LND.[345] Currently, evidence is insufficient to support the involvement of Z-nucleotide toxicity in LND, and increases in these compounds have been noted in other metabolic disorders that are not associated with the neurobehavioral abnormalities of LND.[345]

Oxidant Stress. The mechanisms responsible for pathogenesis in Parkinson disease are relevant to HPRT deficiency in so far as both diseases are associated with relatively selective pathology in the basal ganglia dopamine systems. A progressive loss of nigrostriatal dopamine neurons in Parkinson disease has been proposed to result from oxidant stress in the form of excessive production of superoxide radicals, hydrogen peroxide, and hydroxyl radicals.[387,388] Several factors may contribute to the selective vulnerability of the nigrostriatal dopamine neurons in this disease. First, the enzymatic metabolism of dopamine via monoamine oxidase results in the stoichiometric production of hydrogen peroxide as a by-product. Second, the substantia nigra dopamine neurons contain high amounts of iron that accelerate the production of oxidant molecules. Third, dopamine and other catecholamines undergo spontaneous autoxidation, resulting in the production of superoxide radicals. Multiple studies have repeatedly demonstrated that dopamine and other catecholamines are directly toxic to many cell types, both *in vitro* and *in vivo*.[389–392] The mechanism of toxicity is thought to involve the spontaneous and metal-catalyzed oxidation of dopamine to produce reactive quinones and oxidant species.

The association between HPRT-deficiency and brain dopamine loss could be explained by an increased susceptibility to dopamine-associated oxidant toxicity. At least three potential mechanisms could account for the increased vulnerability of HPRT-deficient cells to this mode of toxicity. First, xanthine oxidase produces superoxide anions during the normal metabolism of oxypurines,[393] and the pronounced hyperuricemia observed in LND implies increased activity of xanthine oxidase. Patients with LND may therefore be exposed to an added burden of superoxide anions because of increased xanthine oxidase activity. Second, the marked increase in purine synthesis associated with HPRT deficiency may increase demands for energy production by mitochondria, a major intracellular source for oxidant species.[394] Finally, HPRT deficiency may be associated with ATP depletion, resulting in impaired metabolic defenses against oxidant stress. The oxidant stress hypothesis of LND provides an attractive explanation for selective vulnerability of the basal ganglia dopamine systems, although experimental evidence is currently lacking.

Purine Depletion. A failure of purine salvage could lead to purine depletion if an increase in purine synthesis cannot compensate for purine wasting. Early studies indicating high levels of purine salvage with low levels of *de novo* purine synthesis in the normal human basal ganglia suggested that this region might be particularly susceptible to purine depletion and provided an attractive explanation for selective vulnerability of this region. However, this explanation is likely to be oversimplified for a number of reasons. As reviewed above, marked regional differences in purine metabolism in the human brain may be more apparent than real. In addition, a selective vulnerability of basal ganglia dopamine systems is evident in the HPRT-deficient mouse model of LND,[365–369] yet regional differences in purine metabolism are not significant.[307] These results indicate that the presumed differences in tissue HPRT expression are insufficient to account for selective brain dysfunction in LND.

Many neurogenetic diseases exhibit a selective vulnerability of specific cell populations that is not directly related to differential expression of the associated gene. For example, Huntington disease is associated with early degeneration of intrinsic neurons of the basal ganglia[395] despite expression of the associated *IT15* gene in all cells of the body and brain.[396] Similarly, superoxide dismutase is expressed in many cells of the brain and body, yet genetic mutations lead to selective degeneration of spinal cord motor neurons in familial amyotrophic lateral sclerosis.[397] Thus, selective vulnerability of basal ganglia dopamine systems does not require preferential expression of HPRT in this brain region. Although regional differences in HPRT expression or purine synthesis cannot account for the selective vulnerability of basal ganglia dopamine neurons, it seems likely that purine deficiency may contribute to the process.

Brain dysfunction could result from global purine depletion, or from depletion of more specific purine molecules. Some authors have emphasized the potential importance of adenine nucleotide depletion,[6,45,47,149,167,170,342,398] while others have stressed the importance of guanine nucleotide depletion.[6,45,310,342,399] One group has reported empirical evidence that the severity of neurobehavioral features among the partial variants correlates better with residual hypoxanthine salvage rather than guanine salvage, suggesting that depletion of adenine nucleotides might be more relevant than depletion of guanine nucleotides.[111,173,174] However, mathematical models of the changes in purine metabolism associated with varying degrees of HPRT deficiency have led to the suggestion that depletion of guanine nucleotides was the more significant pathogenic process.[400]

ATP Depletion. ATP depletion may cause brain dysfunction by interfering with energy-dependent processes, brain development, or cofactor-dependent reactions. HPRT-deficient cells derived from the bone marrow often grow poorly in tissue culture, presumably because they rely heavily on HPRT-mediated purine salvage to maintain purine levels.[167,170,398] A similar dependence of the brain on HPRT-mediated purine salvage could account for poor brain growth during development.[167,170,398] ATP depletion could also slow the activity of poly ADP-ribose polymerase, resulting in inadequate DNA repair.[149] ATP depletion could also interfere with the packaging of neurotransmitters such as dopamine into storage vesicles, with the result that they may diffuse into the cytosol where their toxic properties become difficult to control.[177,370]

GTP and Tetrahydrobiopterin Depletion. GTP depletion has been proposed to result in deficiency of the cofactor tetrahydrobiopterin, because GTP is utilized in the first and rate-limiting step in its synthesis.[399,401] A deficit in tetrahydrobiopterin levels might then impair the activities of specific enzymes that require it, including tyrosine hydroxylase, tryptophan hydroxylase, and phenylalanine hydroxylase. These enzymes are involved in the synthesis of catecholamines, serotonin, and tyrosine, respectively. This hypothesis is attractive because it specifies a biochemical explanation for the abnormalities of monoamine systems observed among patients with LND. However, this hypothesis is not consistent with several observations.

First, urinary tetrahydrobiopterin metabolites have been reported to be normal or increased in three LND patients.[90,363,402] Second, a depletion of tetrahydrobiopterin would be expected to cause reductions in all tetrahydrobiopterin-dependent enzyme reactions, with a consequent reduction in the levels of all monoamine neurotransmitters. Although the levels of dopamine are clearly reduced in the brains of patients with LND, the levels of norepinephrine are not; and serotonin values appear to be elevated.[403] Tetrahydrobiopterin is also a required cofactor for phenylalanine hydroxylase, the enzyme that converts phenylalanine to tyrosine. A deficiency of phenylalanine hydroxylation might be predicted to produce hyperphenylalaninemia and phenylketonuria similar to that occurs in classic phenylalanine hydroxylase deficiency, but hyperphenylalaninemia is not observed in LND. Third, the consequences of tetrahydrobiopterin deficiency, as observed in deficiency of GTP-cyclohydrolase or dihydropterin reductase are not identical with those observed in LND.[404] These disorders can be effectively managed by the administration of tetrahydrobiopterin or a combination of levodopa and 5-hydroxytryptophan. Patients with LND have been treated with tetrahydrobiopterin, levodopa, and 5-hydroxy-tryptophan with little long-term benefit.[28,363]

GTP Depletion and G-Proteins. Many neurotransmitter, neuro-peptide, and hormone receptors use G-proteins for signal transduction.[405,406] To date, multiple different G-proteins have been identified with different tissue distributions and pharmacologic properties.[405,406] One common feature of these proteins is that their activation requires the binding of GTP. After signal transduction occurs, spontaneous hydrolysis of the bound GTP to GDP returns the G-protein to its inactive state. GTP depletion as a result of HPRT deficiency has been proposed to impair G-protein-mediated signal transduction.[310,399] However, given the wide-spread function of G-proteins in neural and hormonal signal transduction throughout the brain and body, it seems unlikely that any process that globally compromised G-protein function would be compatible with life. Such a mechanism also fails to account for selective dysfunction of basal ganglia dopamine systems.

Adenosine Depletion. Several purines are now recognized as neurotransmitters or neuromodulators in different brain regions.[407,408] Adenosine is particularly attractive in view of several studies documenting important regulatory and trophic influences of this purine on basal ganglia dopamine systems.[409–411] A number of investigators have suggested that the neurobehavioral abnormalities observed in LND might be due to a deficit in adenosine-mediated neural transmission.[222,412–416] Although HPRT is not directly involved in the metabolism of adenosine, a mechanism whereby HPRT deficiency could influence adenosine metabolism is well-recognized.[222] Adenosine released as a neurotransmitter can be metabolized via three different pathways (Fig. 107-6). The degradation of adenosine to adenine by purine nucleoside phosphorylase is quantitatively unimportant in most tissues. The main pathway of adenosine metabolism involves the reuptake and phosphorylation of adenosine into adenine nucleotides by adenosine kinase, while the other pathway involves enzymatic degradation of adenosine by adenosine deaminase and/or purine nucleoside phosphorylase to inosine and hypoxanthine. The metabolism of adenosine by the latter route requires HPRT for reincorporating hypoxanthine into the utilizable purine pools. The absence of HPRT may therefore cause a continual depletion of purines from cells that depend heavily this route of metabolism, such as neuronal systems that use adenosine as a neuromodulator.

Accelerated* De Novo *Purine Synthesis. As previously noted, *de novo* purine synthesis is markedly accelerated in HPRT-deficient cells and tissues. The acceleration of purine synthesis has usually been interpreted to play a protective role, preventing purine depletion in the presence of reduced purine salvage.[307,317,350] However, the acceleration of *de novo* purine synthesis may also be deleterious, by causing a depletion of intermediary molecules that are required for other neural functions[342,343] Alternatively, the generation of free radicals by enhanced flux through the purine metabolic pathways may have neurotoxic effects as previously described. Currently, insufficient information exists to determine what role, if any, the acceleration of *de novo* purine synthesis plays in the generation of the neurobehavioral abnormalities in LND.

ANIMAL MODELS

Surrogate models have been particularly valuable for investigating the pathogenesis of LND for two reasons. First, LND is relatively rare, so there are few patients available for study. Second, the types of rigorously controlled studies that are required to address pathophysiology in LND cannot be performed in human subjects. Many investigators disagree on the minimum criteria that define a model for a disease, but it is unrealistic to expect a disease model to mimic all features of its human counterpart. Incomplete models may nevertheless be quite useful, because the value of a model of a human disease lies not in how much it can be made to resemble its human counterpart, but in how it can be used to answer questions regarding the disease process and operations of the normal organism.[381,417]

HPRT-Deficient Mice

The application of molecular genetic techniques to murine development has made it possible to produce genetic animal models for specific human disorders. One strain of HPRT-deficient mice has been produced by retroviral interruption of the HPRT gene in pluripotent embryonic stem cells,[418] and another was produced by selecting stem cells for spontaneous mutations in the HPRT gene.[419] Because these mice carry mutations in the same gene responsible for producing LND in humans, they represent true genetic models for the disease. The mouse strain carrying the HPRT deletion mutation has been studied in most detail. Southern analysis has revealed that the mutation encompasses the first two exons of the gene, as well as several kb of upstream sequences.[222] Because the mutation spans the promotor region of the gene, transcription of HPRT mRNA does not occur. These mice have no residual HPRT antigenic material on western blots and no residual enzyme activity in the brain.[307] These mice also display several of the metabolic and neurochemical features of LND, so the mice can be studied as metabolic models as well. Although there is no obvious depletion of purines in the brains of the HPRT-deficient mice, *de novo* purine synthesis is accelerated approximately four-to fivefold.[307]

In addition to the changes in purine metabolism, the HPRT-deficient mice have significantly reduced brain dopamine levels, particularly in the basal ganglia.[365–369,420] Five different mouse strains carrying one of two mutations in the HPRT gene each displayed a 50 to 60 percent loss of dopamine in the basal ganglia.[369] Brain dopamine is normal shortly after birth, but does not show the normal increases during the first 4 to 6 weeks of postnatal development.[368,369] This period coincides with the development and maturation of basal ganglia dopamine systems, suggesting an abnormal developmental process or an early degenerative process. Other markers associated with the dopamine systems, including homovanillic acid, tyrosine hydroxylase, and aromatic amino acid decarboxylase, are also significantly reduced.[368,369]

In contrast to the marked reductions in basal ganglia dopamine in the mutants, other transmitter systems appear normal. Norepinephrine, serotonin, tryptophan hydroxylase, and glutamic acid decarboxylase were normal in all brain regions examined.[368] Choline acetyltransferase was slightly though consistently reduced in the basal ganglia.[368,369] The neuroanatomically and neuro-chemically selective deficits of basal ganglia dopamine in the HPRT-deficient mice confirm an important relationship between HPRT and brain dopamine systems initially described for patients with LND.

Despite the molecular and biochemical derangements, the HPRT-deficient mice do not exhibit any overt neurobehavioral abnormalities.[365,367,421] There are several potential explanations for the absence of an obvious neurobehavioral phenotype in these mice. For example, there may be important species differences in purine metabolism between mice and humans that attenuate or prevent the neuropathologic consequences of HPRT deficiency in mice. It has been proposed that uricase, which occurs in normal mice but not in humans, may prevent the accumulation of neurotoxic levels of uric acid.[422] However, as noted above, hyperuricemia is not likely to contribute to the neurobehavioral aspects of LND. In addition, uricase-deficient knockout mice, and HPRT/uricase double mutants do not develop any obvious neurobehavioral deficits.[422] Others have suggested that APRT may play a more important role than HPRT for purine salvage in the normal mouse.[423] This proposal was initially supported by observations that the putative APRT inhibitor 9-ethyladenine produced self-injurious grooming behavior in the HPRT-deficient mice,[423] but others have been unable to confirm these effects of the drug.[424] In addition, APRT-deficient knockout mice and APRT/HPRT double mutants do not display any significant neurobehavioral deficits.[425,426] Yet a third possibility is that the enhanced brain purine synthesis seen in HPRT-deficient mice may not occur in the LND brain, leading to more severe purine depletion in the human.[307]

Despite the absence of gross neurobehavioral abnormalities in the HPRT-deficient mice, their behaviors cannot be considered entirely normal. They display exaggerated behavioral responses to dopamine-releasing drugs such as amphetamine, methylphenidate, and nomifensine.[367,421] However, they appear to have normal densities of postsynaptic dopamine receptors[420] and normal behavioral responses to direct-acting dopamine receptor agonists such as apomorphine and SKF-38393.[365,367] These abnormal behavioral responses are likely to reflect the underlying dysfunction of the basal ganglia dopamine systems. Though the behavioral differences so far described for these mice are subtle, they raise the possibility of provoking more obvious abnormalities by appropriate pharmacologic interventions. Despite the absence of an obvious neurobehavioral phenotype in this model, it is particularly valuable for exploring the mechanisms by which HPRT deficiency causes disruption of basal ganglia dopamine systems.

Neonatal Dopamine Depletion in Rats

The relevance of brain dopamine depletion to the neurobehavioral phenotype of LND has been carefully assessed in studies involving the pharmacologic manipulation of dopamine systems in rats during early development. Brain dopamine neurons can be destroyed by the administration of the neurotoxin 6-hydroxydopamine.[427,428] The destruction of brain dopamine systems in adult rats or primates results in a hypokinetic neurobehavioral phenotype characterized by a slowness and paucity of movements. This behavior can be reversed by the administration of dopamine agonists or levodopa, the metabolic precursor to dopamine. The hypokinetic behavioral phenotype is similar to that occurring in Parkinson disease, and these animals have therefore served as models for this disorder. However, the same lesion in a developing animal produces a very different neurobehavioral phenotype. Rats treated with 6-hydroxydopamine within the first few days of birth develop spontaneous hyperactivity as they grow to adults, rather than the typical hypokinetic phenotype observed in rats treated as adults.[427–436] In addition, treatment of neonatally lesioned animals with levodopa does not restore their behavior to normal; rather, it exacerbates their hyperactivity and induces the emergence of self-biting.[427,437] These studies have demonstrated that the age at which dopamine lesions occur has a profound influence on behavioral outcome.

The neurobiologic basis for the self-biting in this model has been thoroughly investigated. Self-biting appears to be mediated by the pharmacologically defined D_1 dopamine receptor, because either nonselective dopamine receptor agonists or agonists selective for this receptor can reproduce the behavior.[438] In contrast, selective D_2 dopamine receptor agonists do not produce self-biting. These studies have led to the suggestion that self-biting results from overstimulation of supersensitized D_1 dopamine receptors.[439] Regional microinjection studies with this model have shown that the caudoputamen complex is the anatomic locus responsible for the generation of self-biting, and the accumbens is responsible for the motor hyperactivity.[440]

Although these studies provide strong support for the involvement of brain dopamine systems in the generation of self-biting, it is unlikely that dopaminergic dysfunction alone is sufficient to cause this behavior. Self-injurious behavior is not observed in other human metabolic disorders associated with brain dopamine loss, such as deficiency of tyrosine hydroxylase,[441] aromatic amino acid decarboxylase,[442] or tetrahydrobiopterin synthesis.[443] In view of these observations, it seems likely that early dopamine loss contributes to the expression of the neurobehavioral phenotype in LND along with additional influences.

Neurotransmitter systems other than the dopamine system also appear to contribute to self-biting after neonatal destruction of dopamine neurons. Early destruction of the dopamine projections to the basal ganglia leads to a massive secondary overgrowth of serotonergic fibers to this region,[429,444–451] and recent studies have suggested that aberrant serotonergic influences may contribute to the expression of self-biting.[452] These observations in rodents may be relevant to the increased levels of serotonin and 5-hydroxyindole acetic acid in the LND basal ganglia,[27] and the transient reductions in self-injury reported for the serotonin precursor 5-hydroxytryphtophan in LND.[39–41,49,53,97,148,363,453–456] The involvement of serotonin systems is also supported by recent proposals that self-injurious behaviors in LND and other disorders may reflect an obsessive-compulsive phenomenon related to serotonergic dysfunction.[133,162,163,457]

In addition to the potential influences of serotonin neurotransmitter systems, levodopa-induced self-biting in rats with neonatal lesions of brain dopamine systems can be attenuated with adenosine receptor agonists and exacerbated by adenosine antagonists.[416] Extrapolation of these results to the human condition has led to the proposal that self-biting in LND results from the activation of supersensitive dopamine receptors in the presence of impaired neuromodulatory functions of adenosine. Self-biting in this model can also be reduced by treatment of the animals with the glutamate receptor antagonist MK-801.[458]

The neonatal 6-hydroxydopamine model for LND has been particularly useful for elucidating the biologic substrates of self-injurious behavior associated with early damage to basal ganglia dopamine systems. The observation that dysfunction of the dopamine systems mediates the expression of self-injury in this model is intriguing when considering that the major neurochemical abnormality detected in the LND brain also involves the dopamine systems. The main limitation of this model is that it is not possible to investigate initial steps in the pathogenic process resulting from HPRT deficiency, such as changes in purine metabolism. It is also not possible to study the mechanisms by which HPRT deficiency causes dysfunction of the basal ganglia dopamine systems to begin with.

Pharmacologic Models

Dopamine Stimulation. Several pharmacologic models have also been developed for studies of LND. Under certain conditions, administration of amphetamine and related psychostimulants can cause self-biting in a variety of species. Self-biting has been demonstrated in rodents after systemic administration of a single high dose of amphetamine, methamphetamine, or pemoline.[459–462] Self-biting also emerges with chronic administration of low doses of these drugs[463–466] or chronic administration of the dopamine reuptake inhibitor GBR-12909.[467] Direct microinjection of amphetamine[468,469] or the D_1 dopamine receptor agonist SKF-38393[470] into the brain may also cause self-biting in rodents. The behavioral actions of these drugs are thought to be mediated by direct or indirect stimulation of brain dopamine systems, providing further evidence to support the concept that self-injurious behavior in LND may result from dysfunction of basal ganglia dopamine systems.

Methylxanthines. Chronic administration of the methylxanthines caffeine and theophylline cause self-biting in rats and rabbits.[360,403,471–474] Animals are typically given more than 100 mg/kg caffeine or theophylline per day for several days, and self-biting appears in 10 to 80 percent of the animals over several days. The percentage of animals exhibiting self-biting appears to depend on several variables, including the strain of rat[403] and nutritional status.[403,471] The mechanisms by which caffeine and theophylline cause self-biting remain unclear. Pharmacologically, these drugs are thought to exert their behavioral effects by acting as antagonists at adenosine receptors in the brain,[475] although the high doses required may influence other neural processes as well.

Clonidine. Under very specific conditions, clonidine has been reported to provoke self-biting in mice. In the presence of other animals, mice treated with high doses of clonidine exhibit aggressiveness and attack behavior.[476–478] When isolated, the drug induces compulsive gnawing on any available objects, such as bedding, cage bars, or food pellets.[479] However, when tested in isolation in a smooth-walled container with nothing to bite, the biting is directed towards the animal's own body.[477,479–482] The ability of clonidine to provoke self-biting appears to be somewhat species specific, because rats and rabbits are resistant to this effect of the drug.[481] Pharmacologically, clonidine is often used as an agonist for α-noradrenergic receptors.[483] However, clonidine-induced self-biting is not blocked, but rather potentiated, by noradrenergic antagonists, suggesting that activation of these receptors is not responsible for clonidine's ability to produce the behavior.[477,478] Clonidine, like the methylxanthines, also appears to antagonize adenosine receptors.[484–487] In fact, the ability of clonidine to provoke self-biting seems to be related to blockade of adenosine receptors, because the behavior can be inhibited by coadministration of adenosine agonists and potentiated by adenosine antagonists.[477,478,480]

The pharmacologic models have been useful to identify neurotransmitter and neurochemical mechanisms mediating self-injurious behaviors. They have provided additional indirect evidence that dysfunction of basal ganglia dopamine systems can cause self-injurious behavior in a normal animal with normal HPRT levels. The results from the methylxanthine and clonidine models also suggest a potential role for dysfunction of purinergic neurotransmitter systems as well. These studies are valuable because they may guide pharmacologic interventions for self-injury in affected patients. However, they have been of limited value in understanding the role of HPRT deficiency in the generation of these behaviors.

DIAGNOSIS AND PREVENTION

Differential Diagnosis

Self-Injurious Behavior. The occurrence of self-injurious behavior often leads to the suspicion for LND. However, self-injury may occur in many different clinical populations, most commonly profound mental retardation or autism.[162,488,489] Self-injury is also seen in several genetic conditions, including Rett syndrome,[163] Cornelia de Lange syndrome,[490] Prader-Willi syndrome,[491] neuroacanthocytosis,[163,492] and congenital insensitivity to pain.[156] Self-injurious behavior has also been reported after encephalitis and in a significant proportion of patients with Tourette syndrome.[493,494] Patients with dementia or psychiatric diseases may also develop thought or mood-congruent behaviors that lead to self-injury.[457,495]

The self-injury of LND can often be distinguished from that appearing in these other diseases. In LND, self-injury is always accompanied by profound motor impairment. In contrast, self-injurious behavior associated with other diseases often occurs on a background of normal or near-normal motor function. In addition, self-injury in LND often appears to result from a frequent and irrepressible urge to inflict pain and injury, while in other diseases it may be an indirect result of a highly stereotyped behavior such as hand-wringing in Rett syndrome or mostly accidental as in the congenital neuropathies. LND should be suspected chiefly when self-injurious behavior is associated with the typical motor dysfunction, especially if it also associated with evidence for excessive production of uric acid.

Developmental Delay with Extrapyramidal Signs. The most common presenting feature for LND is developmental delay, followed by the appearance of extrapyramidal and sometimes pyramidal signs. The differential diagnosis for developmental delay is broad,[496] and few features point specifically towards LND. However, LND should be suspected if delayed development is accompanied by self-injurious behavior or evidence for excessive production of uric acid.

LND variants often present with a history of developmental delay without self-injurious behavior. These patients may develop moderate to severe neurologic disability, with dysarthria, cognitive disability, and extrapyramidal and pyramidal signs. Other patients may have such mild neurologic disability that they readily go undetected. The diagnosis of such patients is challenging, and HPRT deficiency is generally not suspected until hyperuricemia, nephrolithiasis, or gout become apparent.[81]

Several cases have been reported where neurobehavioral abnormalities are combined with hyperuricemia, although most cases are readily distinguished from LND. Rosenberg and colleagues described a family with progressive ataxia, deafness, and hyperuricemia.[497] Confusion with LND is unlikely because the neurologic phenotype was not typical of LND and symptoms began after 10 years of age. Mavrikakis and colleagues described a family with tremor, ataxia, cognitive disability, mild self-biting of the lips and fingers, and hyperuricemia leading to gout and renal insufficiency.[498] These patients could be distinguished from LND by their atypical neurologic phenotype, the presence of early cardiomyopathy, and sensorineural deafness. Laszlo and colleagues reported a boy with severe retardation, dysarthria, hypotonia, pyramidal signs, finger and lip biting, aggressive behavior, and hyperuricemia in association with an 18q deletion.[499] He could be distinguished from typical LND by facial dysmorphism and his comparatively mild motor impairments.

Hyperuricemia. Rare patients with LND present with hyperuricemia leading to renal failure or gout during the first year of life, sometimes before neurobehavioral abnormalities are apparent.[55,55,65,66,88,95,104] Patients with less severe HPRT deficiency present with nephrolithiasis or gout, with no obvious neurobehavioral defects. The differential diagnosis of hyperuricemia in pediatric cases includes superactivity of PP-ribose-P synthase, disorders of carbohydrate metabolism, iatrogenic causes such as treatment of leukemia, and other medications.[122,500] Although hyperuricemia is common in adults, HPRT-deficiency is an uncommon cause of gout, and many cases likely go undetected without rigorous screening methods.

Confirmatory Testing

Uric Acid. As previously noted, the majority of patients with LND have elevated serum uric acid levels. However, hyperuricemia is neither sufficiently sensitive nor specific to serve as a reliable diagnostic test. Some increase in sensitivity and specificity can be obtained by measuring 24-h urinary uric acid to creatinine ratios or total uric acid excretion, especially when adjusted for patient weight; but adequate specimens are notoriously difficult to collect. Uric acid measures may provide important clues to the diagnosis, but are not considered sufficient for definitive diagnosis.

HPRT Enzyme Activity. The measurement of HPRT enzyme activity using *in vitro* methods is the most commonly used confirmatory test for LND. The assays can be conducted with lysates from any conveniently obtained tissue, such as peripheral blood cells. However, the use of cell lysates has been reported to provide misleading results in rare cases. For example, several cases with classic LND have been reported with near-normal HPRT enzyme activity in cell lysates.[78,89,501] These discrepancies are related to kinetic mutations of the HPRT enzyme. A patient may express a mutant HPRT enzyme with a markedly decreased affinity for the cosubstrate PP-ribose-P, so that enzyme activity is essentially absent with the PP-ribose-P concentrations normally present in intact cells, but much higher with concentrations used for the *in vitro* assays. Other patients may have absent HPRT activity in cell lysates, with significant residual activity in intact cells, presumably as a result of an HPRT mutant with reduced stability outside the normal cellular environment.[5,109,310,501] Nevertheless, the measurement of HPRT enzyme activity in cell lysates may provide diagnostic information when appropriate precautions are applied.

A more accurate method involves the measurement of HPRT enzyme activity in intact cells in tissue culture. Fibroblasts[111,173,174] or lymphocytes[502,503] may be cultured, and HPRT activity is assessed in the growing cells by monitoring the incorporation of isotopically labeled hypoxanthine into the purine pools. Although this method is both technically demanding and time-consuming, it avoids the pitfalls associated with measurement of the enzyme in cell lysates by simulating the *in vivo* situation more precisely. The results also provide some predictive value concerning severity of disease (Fig. 107-4). Patients with more than 1.5 percent of residual HPRT enzyme activity may have the neurologic features without self-injury or other behavioral problems. Patients with more than 8 percent activity may have hyperuricemia with few obvious neurobehavioral impairments. Care must be taken to avoid contamination of long-term cultures with bacterial L-forms[504] or mycoplasma[505] because these organisms produce endogenous HPRT leading to misleading results.

Molecular Genetic Tests. Because rapid and reliable methods have been developed for the identification of HPRT gene mutations, diagnostic confirmation can also be obtained with molecular genetic methods.[233,235,238,240,241] The identification of a large deletion, early nonsense mutation, or mutation identified in a prior patient is likely to be a good predictor of disease severity. However, small duplications, in-frame deletions, and some point mutations may not predict disease severity because the influence of these mutations on the resultant enzyme activity is difficult to determine. A single point mutation may cause classic LND or a less-severe variant depending on its effect on residual enzyme activity. Nevertheless, the characterization of a genetic mutation in an affected index patient facilitates the subsequent identification of at-risk carriers or pregnancies.

Prevention

Carrier Testing. Because there are currently no effective therapies for the devastating neurobehavioral features of LND, prevention remains the cornerstone of effective medical intervention. Genetic counseling plays an important role in identifying other potentially affected family members. The patient's mother must be screened to determine whether she is a carrier and at risk for producing more affected children. The patient's sisters and other female family members should also be evaluated to determine their risk.

Many methods have been employed for the identification of carrier females. Because one copy of the HPRT gene is silenced during X-chromosome inactivation in the female, carrier females are functional mosaics with varying proportions of normal and HPRT-deficient cells. These two populations of cells can be distinguished by autoradiographic methods after exposing them to isotopically labeled hypoxanthine in tissue culture.[506–508] Because X-chromosome inactivation is a random process, approximately half of a carrier's cells should be normal, and half HPRT-deficient. However, different cell types from known carriers often do not show the expected equal proportions of normal and mutant cells, suggesting a selective growth advantage to the X chromosome carrying the normal HPRT allele or nonrandom inactivation of the X chromosome carrying the mutant allele. Cultured fibroblasts come closest to demonstrating equal proportions, with one study of 7627 individual clones from 41 heterozygous carriers being 59 percent normal and 41 percent HPRT-deficient.[509] Circulating lymphocytes and erythrocytes demonstrate even greater deviations from equal proportions, with fewer than 5 percent of the cells being HPRT-deficient.[170,508,510] A similar selection against HPRT-deficient cells occurs among intestinal cells.[508] Thus blood and other tissues representing pooled cell populations do not yield intermediate HPRT enzyme levels that allow prediction of gene dosage. The extent of deviation from the expected equal proportions among various cell types is thought to reflect the dependence of the particular cell type on HPRT-mediated purine salvage for normal growth and function.

Differential growth of cultured cells exposed to media capable of discriminating between normal and HPRT-deficient cells has also been employed for carrier detection.[169,511–517] Another popular technique has relied on HPRT assays of single hair follicles.[61,508,518–523] This technique relies on the observation that human hair follicles are each derived from only a small number primordial cells.[518,524] Because APRT activity is typically increased in HPRT-deficient cells, simultaneous measurements of APRT and calculation of HPRT/APRT ratios provides even greater sensitivity.[519–522] Although serum hypoxanthine and xanthine are not elevated in heterozygote carriers, urinary excretion is sufficiently increased that it may provide a useful screening test.[525] Today, the most convenient and accurate method for carrier detection involves molecular genetic techniques. If a mutation can first be characterized in an affected LND patient, methods can be devised to rapidly identify the same mutation in any potential carriers.[526]

Mothers of documented cases of LND are not necessarily obligate carriers because many cases result from *de novo* mutation during gametogenesis or early development. Conversely, if a mother is screened and determined not to be a carrier, subsequent pregnancies may still be at risk as a result of gonadal mosaicism.[526] It is therefore prudent to monitor all pregnancies from a mother who has given birth to a child with LND, whether or not she is determined to be a carrier.

Prenatal Diagnosis. The identification of a carrier mandates the monitoring of all subsequent pregnancies if the family wishes to consider termination of affected pregnancies. Again, several methods have been used to identify affected fetuses. The earliest efforts relied on assessments of amniotic fluid cells. These cells can be assessed by microassay of HPRT activity,[302,303,527,528] HPRT/APRT activity ratios,[18,529,530] autoradiographic identification cells cultured with isotopically labeled hypoxanthine,[17,301,530–532] or growth in selective media.[530] These methods provide a diagnosis relatively late in a pregnancy because amniocentesis is not practical until at least 3 months after conception, and assessment of HPRT activity requires an additional 1 to 3 weeks.

Subsequent efforts focused on the measurement of HPRT/APRT ratios in chorionic villus samples, because they can be obtained as early at 2 months after conception.[533,534] Nevertheless, at least one failure has been reported with this method.[535] It is important to exclude contamination of the sample with maternal tissues by microscopy in the operating theater.[535,536] In addition, special precautions must be taken to inhibit the high levels of 5′-nucleotidase activity in chorionic villus samples that can interfere with the proper measurement of HPRT activity.[537]

Currently, the most rapid and accurate method for prenatal diagnosis involves molecular genetic methods.[526] If a proband's mutation can be positively characterized, a rapid method can be devised for identifying the mutation in potential carriers, amniotic fluid cells, or chorionic villus samples. These methods can often provide a result in only a few days, and provide the earliest opportunity for therapeutic abortion if desired.

TREATMENT

Physical Methods

Protective Devices. A properly designed wheelchair is a critical element of supportive management.[538] Care must be taken to remove or cover any hard or sharp surfaces that a patient may reach to injure himself (Fig. 107-8). Behaviors such as thrusting

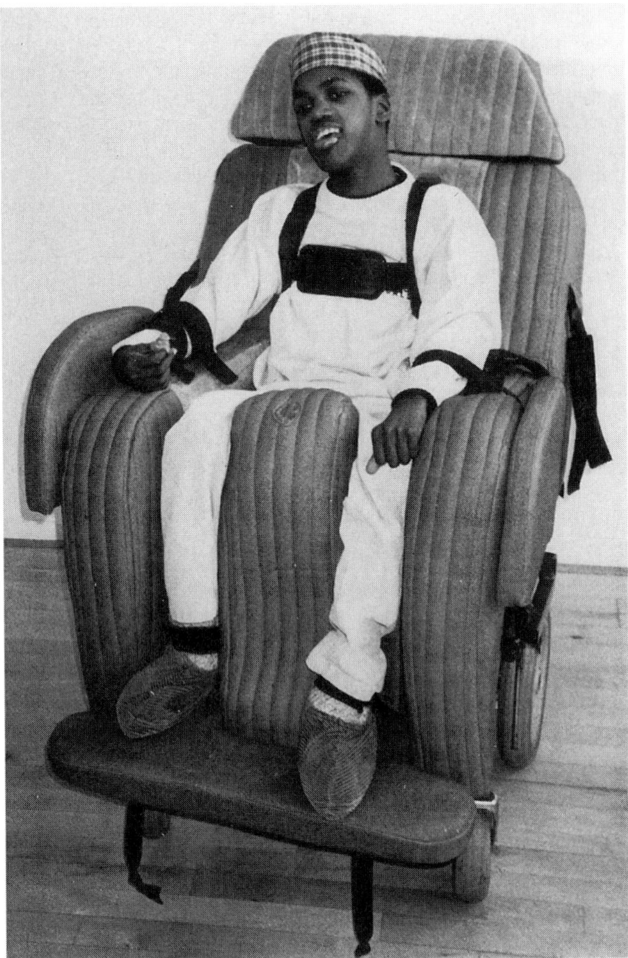

Fig. 107-8 Special devices to prevent self-injury. This boy with LND had a wheelchair specifically designed to prevent self-injury. All sharp surfaces within reach are covered by soft material. Protective straps for the chest and limbs allow mobility while preventing potentially harmful movements. He wears a headband tethered to the back of the chair to assist him in preventing his habit of lacerating his lip on his shoulder. (*The photograph was kindly provided by Dr. J.E. Visser.*)

fingers into the spokes of a wheelchair or abrading the ankles on the sides of foot supports necessitates that these be properly covered. In addition, a soft but firm support should be attached behind the head, because frequent opisthotonic spasms and extreme backward head thrusts may lead to cervical spine injury.[31]

Protective trunk harnesses and limb straps are often attached to the wheelchairs and beds to prevent self-injury. Flexible arm splints[94] or helmets with retractable mouth barriers[93] may provide an alternative to protective straps. Other patients find that covering their hands with gloves or socks provides an adequate deterrent to prevent self-injury.[156]

Dental Care. Although biting of the fingers can be prevented by appropriate hand and arm protection, biting of the lips and tongue is much more difficult to manage. Extraction of the permanent teeth, though drastic, is a reliable means to prevent this behavior when it occurs. The prevention of self-inflicted tissue damage with a permanently disfiguring procedure seems paradoxical, but delays in tooth extraction often result in an individual who is both edentulous and disfigured. Any tooth causing damage should be extracted without delay when behavior therapy and other conservative measures fail.[57,82,86,539] Patients are often quite relieved once the procedure is completed.

A variety of dental devices have been constructed with the goal of preserving the teeth while preventing self-biting. These have included flexible appliances inserted in the mouth[540] or over the lips,[85] and rigid dental splints retained with cement,[541] wire,[58] or head straps.[56] Unfortunately, several problems have been identified with these devices. These include an impediment to adequate dental hygiene, uncontrolled drooling, the need for multiple revisions with age, and excoriation and inflammation of the lips or gums. In addition, the risk of the device breaking or becoming dislodged may result in the patient injuring himself with it. In a short time, these patients can produce significant tissue damage with permanent disfigurement if the device fails. They are perhaps most appropriate for sparing the dentition in a patient with only mild or predictably intermittent self-biting.[539]

Pharmacotherapy

Hyperuricemia. The marked overproduction of uric acid in LND and its variants leads to hyperuricemia with the associated risk of nephrolithiasis, renal failure, gouty arthritis, and tophi. Allopurinol, which inhibits the catabolism of xanthine and hypoxanthine into uric acid by the enzyme xanthine oxidase,[542] effectively reduces serum uric acid levels to normal among patients with LND.[45,315,318,543] Doses are titrated to maintain uric acid levels within the high-normal range. Doses generally range from 50 to 600 mg per day, and must be adjusted for renal insufficiency. The drug is generally well tolerated, although a severe allergic reaction known as the allopurinol hypersensitivity syndrome may occur.[544]

The normalization of serum uric acid values reduces the complications of hyperuricemia, but may not entirely protect against the formation of kidney stones. For example, inadequate doses of allopurinol may allow the continued propagation of uric acid stones. The use of allopurinol is also associated with a corresponding increase in serum and urinary xanthine and hypoxanthine concentrations.[45,315,318,543] As a result, stones comprised of these purine bases may form.[126–130] Xanthine is particularly insoluble, and unlike urate stones, xanthine stones do not readily dissolve at a urine pH achieved by typical alkalinization procedures.[126] It has been proposed that xanthine stones might be managed by increasing the dose of allopurinol, which promotes solubility by reducing the ratio of xanthine to hypoxanthine.[62,126] However, allopurinol itself is metabolized by xanthine oxidase to oxypurinol, a relatively insoluble compound that may also contribute to stone formation.[126,127] In some cases, stones consist of mixtures of urate, hypoxanthine, xanthine, and oxypurinol.[127] The formation of stones is best prevented by allopurinol in combination with generous hydration at all times.

Renal stones are often identified after the development of renal colic or urinary obstruction. However, patients may develop extensive nephrolithiasis without overt symptoms, so regular ultrasound evaluations have been recommended to avert the development of long-term renal complications.[130,355] Stones composed of urate, xanthine, hypoxanthine, and oxypurinol are all radiolucent unless they calcify, so renal ultrasound is the preferred modality for diagnosis. Small urate stones can often be managed by increasing fluid intake and alkalinization of the urine, while large stones may require lithotripsy or surgery. Stones composed of the oxypurines may be managed with lithotripsy and hydration, although they can be much more difficult to eliminate.[130]

Behavioral Manifestations. A variety of agents has been tested for controlling the neurobehavioral abnormalities in LND. No agent has consistently demonstrated effectiveness in managing this aspect of the disease. The identification of useful drugs has been hampered by several factors. First, the collection of large cohorts of patients for conclusive studies is limited by the rarity of the condition. Second, a rational approach for the selection of candidate drugs is hindered by our limited understanding of the pathogenesis of the neurobehavioral features. Finally, the severity of the neurobehavioral features varies from patient to patient over time, and reliable quantitative measures are lacking. Most patients are admitted to specialized clinical research centers for evaluation, and the stress of this change in environment can be associated with a transient increase in both behavioral and neurologic impairments that confounds assessment of short-term therapeutic trials.[455] Despite these caveats, several trials have provided useful information, and these are reviewed below. Most of these studies focused on a reduction in self-injury as the primary outcome measure, with secondary assessment of the neurologic dysfunction.

The early discovery of hyperuricemia in LND led to proposals that nervous system damage results from high circulating levels of uric acid.[342] Although therapy with allopurinol is very effective in reducing hyperuricemia and the associated nephrotoxicity and arthropathy, it appears to have no beneficial effect on the neurobehavioral aspects.[44] Two patients have been treated from birth with allopurinol with the hope that prevention of possible early toxicity would block the emergence of neurobehavioral abnormalities.[26,148] Unfortunately, both patients developed the full neurobehavioral phenotype with no obvious benefit from the prior therapy.

The role of HPRT in purine recycling has also led to proposals that HPRT deficiency results in purine deficiency.[149,170,342] Because many purine compounds are interconvertible through reversible enzymatic reactions, the introduction of purine precursors into a common cellular pool may correct any potential deficit. Early studies focussed on the application of adenine, which can be incorporated into the purine pools by the salvage enzyme APRT. Multiple patients have been treated with adenine, including several neonates.[45–47,50,52,77,545,546] The efficacy of adenine therapy has been demonstrated by its ability to restore deficient ATP levels and reduce elevated PP-ribose-P levels in circulating erythrocytes,[46,347] and to correct the anemia often associated with LND.[50] Although some investigators have reported modest improvements in neurobehavioral abnormalities, no consistent benefit has been observed. In addition, the administration of high doses of adenine is associated with a significant risk for 2,8-dihydroxyadenine nephrolithiasis and renal failure.[46,77] Because of the unfavorable risk/benefit ratio, adenine therapy is no longer used. Recent studies have addressed the possibility of using other purine precursors, such as 5-aminoimidazole-4-carboxamide riboside.[547] Further clinical trials with these purine precursors will require detailed studies on their bioavailability and toxicity.

The marked increase in *de novo* purine synthesis has also been proposed to consume exaggerated quantities of intermediates such as folate or glutamine, and deficiencies of these intermediates may be responsible for nervous system dysfunction.[44,45,342,343] In tissue culture, HPRT-deficient cells grow poorly in medium with low levels of glutamine or folate. Based on these considerations, some patients with LND have been treated with folate and/or monosodium glutamate, which is readily metabolized to glutamine. An early study reported significant improvement of the neurobehavioral abnormalities in a single patient with LND,[44] but subsequent studies were not encouraging.[39,47] Emerging evidence for glutamate neurotoxicity, especially in the developing nervous system, has discouraged further attempts with large glutamate supplements.[548]

In cases in which there is a small amount of residual HPRT activity resulting from a mutation affecting enzyme kinetics, there may be some therapeutic value in supplying artificially large amounts of substrates or cofactors to drive maximal activity. This strategy has been attempted in LND with the substrate hypoxanthine[363] and the cofactor magnesium.[549] Although this is a logical approach toward therapy, it has not been effective in the few patients with whom it has been tried. The success of this strategy depends on a number of variables including the amount of residual activity, absorption of substrate or cofactor from the site of administration, uptake of hypoxanthine or magnesium into the nervous system, metabolism through other routes, timing of therapy, and toxicity. This approach is not likely to benefit the majority of patients who do not have kinetic mutations.

The marked depletion of basal ganglia dopamine in LND patients and evidence from animal models has led to the hypothesis that self-injury results from dopamine receptor supersensitivity.[438,550–553] As a result, several dopamine receptor antagonists have been examined. Fluphenazine suppressed self-injury in only one of two patients,[551] and chlorpromazine[52] or pimozide[31] had little effect in one patient each. It is likely that any apparent benefits observed with these neuroleptics are a side effect of their potent sedating properties. Because improvements have not been consistent and the chronic administration of these agents is associated with the risk for development of tardive dyskinesia, classic neuroleptics are now only rarely used. However, atypical agents such as Risperdal may have a lower incidence of adverse long-term side effects and might prove useful in the future. One patient was reported to demonstrate a sustained reduction in self-injurious behavior with this drug,[554] but more experience with this agent is required before it can be recommended for routine therapy.

Several investigators have also focused on the manipulation of brain serotonin systems, in view of psychologic theories that self-injurious behavior is a form of autoaggression mediated by brain serotonin systems.[39,555] In particular, efforts have been directed at increasing brain serotonin levels by the administration of the serotonin precursor 5-hydroxytryptophan. In initial studies, the administration of this agent abolished self-injury in four patients; and the behavior recurred when the agent was discontinued.[39,453] Subsequent studies revealed that the drug had only transient effects lasting a few days or weeks, even when given with a peripheral decarboxylase inhibitor to augment brain levels.[40,41,49,53,97,148,363,454–456] This drug is no longer widely used. Other attempts to manipulate brain serotonin metabolism with the precursor tryptophan were not successful.[39,453] The serotonin reuptake inhibitors clomipramine and fluoxetine had no effect in one patient each,[31] though paroxetine and sertraline were recently reported to be effective in a single case report.[556]

The hypothesis that self-biting in LND may result from peripheral dysesthesias due to an underlying neuropathy has led to a trial of carbamazepine.[158] Although sural nerve biopsies provided no evidence for neuropathy, self-injury was suppressed by carbamazepine in three patients, and modestly reduced in a fourth. Because there is little evidence for neuropathy in LND, carbamazepine presumably works via some other mechanism. It should be noted that this drug has complex mechanisms of action and proven effectiveness in a number of neurologic and psychiatric conditions, including neuropathic dysesthesias, epilepsy, and disorders of mood and impulse control. Although the theoretic basis for the effectiveness of carbamazepine is uncertain, its potential benefits deserve further attention.

A deleterious effect of elevated hypoxanthine levels on benzodiazepine levels has led to the proposal that benzodiazepines might be useful in LND.[382,384,529] However, a specific beneficial effect of these drugs is difficult to separate from their anxiolytic and sedating properties. Nevertheless, because stress and anxiety exacerbate self-injury, the anxiolytic properties of these drugs may be useful on a temporary basis. Limited trials of other agents have also been reported, including AMP,[557] GMP,[557] inosine,[45] diaminopurine,[45] nicotinamide,[187] chlordiazepoxide,[39] tetrahydrobiopterin,[363] and gabapentin.[274]

Neurologic Manifestations. Most drug trials have focused on behavioral measures, but a few have focused primarily on the neurologic abnormalities. As noted above, the neurologic manifestations are a combination of extrapyramidal and pyramidal features. These features must be distinguished and evaluated separately, since they are likely to respond to different approaches.

Dystonia occurs in a number of neurologic conditions, and it is often quite resistant to most therapies.[558] The marked depletion of basal ganglia dopamine in LND has led to attempts to restore the levels of this neurotransmitter with its precursor, levodopa with or without a peripheral decarboxylase inhibitor. The motor disorder was reported to improve modestly in two patients,[363,453] worsen in four patients,[28,31] and remain unchanged in two patients.[53,363] The dopamine agonist bromocriptine improved motor function in one patient and worsened it in another.[28]

Choreiform and ballismic movements also occur in a number of neurologic disorders, and typically respond to dopamine receptor antagonists or drugs that deplete dopamine stores. It is therefore surprising that fluphenazine, pimozide, and tetrabenazine do not consistently benefit patients with LND.[28,31,52,551] It is possible that beneficial responses to these agents are obscured by the superimposed dystonia, which often does not respond to these agents.

Pyramidal manifestations such as spasticity can be managed with baclofen or benzodiazepines. Benzodiazepines have the added advantage of reducing anxiety, which can often exacerbate the extrapyramidal and behavioral features of the disease. Often, baclofen and benzodiazepines are used concurrently.

Behavior Therapy

Psychologically based techniques have been used to manage self-injury and other unwanted behaviors in LND. Some of the first reports involved extinction methods,[59] which consist of actively ignoring an unwanted behavior, so that the patient receives no positive reinforcement in terms of added attention. Eventually, the patient learns other behavior patterns that replace the unwanted behavior. This method is quite difficult to apply in LND, because attempts at self-injury may lead quickly to permanent tissue damage and must be physically terminated. In addition, self-injurious behaviors invoke an almost immediate emotional reaction of horror and empathy among any witnesses, and this reaction may unintentionally reinforce the behavior. Nevertheless, appropriately trained therapists who can summarily terminate attempts at self-injury while avoiding any explicit or implicit acknowledgment that the behavior occurred may have a major impact in reducing self-injury in some patients.[92,99,559] Unfortunately, patients treated in this manner may rapidly revert when returned to the home situation,[102] unless parents or other caretakers are properly trained.

Other learning-based techniques are also useful. In most conditions associated with undesirable behaviors, a combination of negative reinforcement for unwanted behaviors and positive reinforcement for alternate behaviors leads to the desired behavioral modification. However, negative reinforcement in LND is ineffective and may even increase undesirable behavior.[92,99,559–561] The failure of negative reinforcement to suppress an unwanted behavior is not due to an inability to learn, because positive reinforcement appears to be effective. Overall, the most effective management involves engaging the patient in an active environment, providing positive reinforcement for desired behaviors, and actively ignoring undesirable behaviors.

Experimental Approaches

Thalamotomy. Two LND patients with prominent extrapyramidal features were treated with thalamotomy, with no obvious benefit.[68,84] The refinement of surgical techniques in recent years for the treatment of patients with extrapyramidal syndromes including dystonia may provide a viable option in the near future.[562]

Bone Marrow Transplantation. In cases in which disease results from deficiency of a single protein product, an obvious approach to therapy is to attempt to replace the missing product from exogenous sources. This approach has been reported to be partially successful for several of the lysosomal and peroxisomal storage diseases, including adrenoleukodystrophy, metachromatic leukodystrophy, globoid cell leukodystrophy, and Hurler syndrome.[563] Evidence has been presented that the therapeutic effect is mediated by marrow-derived microglia.[564]

Based on observations that patients with only 5 percent of residual HPRT enzyme activity have a much less severe phenotype, restoration of even small amounts of active enzyme may have therapeutic potential. Active HPRT has been administered to two LND patients by repeated exchange transfusions of blood cells containing HPRT, with restoration of blood enzyme activity to near-normal levels.[52,504] Unfortunately, patients derived no obvious benefit.

Blood HPRT has also been restored chronically in affected patients by bone marrow transplantation.[565,566] Once again, no obvious benefit was observed. Bone marrow transplantation also failed to correct the neurochemical and neuropharmacologic abnormalities observed in the HPRT-deficient mouse model of LND.[567] Enthusiasm for further development of these methods has waned because morbidity is significant and because the majority of LND patients died shortly after marrow transplantation.[565–567] Patients with LND may be particularly sensitive to toxicity from the immunosuppressants required for successful bone marrow because many of these drugs interfere with purine metabolism (azathioprine, methotrexate) or impair renal function (cyclosporin, FK-506).

There are two potential reasons why restoration of blood HPRT fails to correct the neurobehavioral abnormalities. First, HPRT restored in the blood may not gain access to relevant diseased sites in the nervous system. Unlike lysosomal storage enzymes that may be released from donor cells and taken up by diseased cells, there is little evidence that HPRT can be transferred. The second potential reason for the failure of enzyme replacement is that HPRT deficiency may lead to irreversible brain pathology early in development, and enzyme replacement after this has occurred does not help. These methods should probably be restricted to carefully monitored research protocols until there is more compelling evidence that enzyme replacement has therapeutic potential and until issues related to safety are more thoroughly addressed for this patient population.

Gene Therapy. LND was one of the first diseases proposed as a candidate for gene therapy,[14] and continues to serve as a model for its development.[15,16] Currently, two different strategies for gene therapy are used. The indirect "*ex vivo* approach" involves the genetic modification of appropriate surrogate cells in culture, followed by the engraftment of these cells into an affected organism. Alternatively, the "*in vivo* approach" involves the introduction of a transgene directly into tissues *in vivo*, usually with the aid of a viral vector.

LND has been studied as a model for both strategies.[15,16] The earliest work focused on the *ex vivo* approach to gene therapy, and numerous studies have demonstrated that functional HPRT can be introduced into HPRT-deficient cells *in vitro*.[568–572] Expression of HPRT in these cells has also been shown to correct some of the metabolic abnormalities associated with HPRT deficiency. Other studies have shown that human HPRT can be expressed in vitro in bone marrow stem cells[568,572] or fibroblasts[573] and detected after transplantation of the cells into rats or mice. Exogenous HPRT has also been introduced directly into the mouse, rat, or Macaque brain with vectors derived from human herpes virus type 1[574] or adenoviral vectors.[575,576] However, the functional consequences of gene transfer have not yet been examined.

Recent advances in gene transfer technology have provided new avenues for the potential correction of defects affecting the nervous system. Particularly helpful has been the development of viral vectors that allow for long-term stable expression of a transgene in postmitotic cells such as neurons. Vectors based on the herpes simplex virus can transduce neurons and other cells, but may produce cytopathic effects.[574,577] Vectors derived from adenoviruses have also been successful in introducing genes into postmitotic cells such as neurons, but host immune responses have made application challenging.[575] More recently, vectors based on the adeno-associated virus[578] and on lentiviruses, such as the human immunodeficiency virus,[579,580] have been developed and may prove useful for gene therapy.

CONCLUSIONS

Inherited deficiency of the purine salvage enzyme HPRT results in a spectrum of clinical dysfunction. The least severe manifestation of HPRT deficiency is expressed only as overproduction of uric acid, with hyperuricemia, nephrolithiasis, and gout. The most severe manifestation is LND, which is characterized by overproduction of uric acid, severe neurologic disability, and self-injurious behavior. Between these two extremes are patients with evidence of overproduction of uric acid with varying degrees of neurobehavioral abnormality.

HPRT deficiency results from mutations in the HPRT gene, which has been mapped, cloned, and characterized in detail. Multiple mutations responsible for disease have been identified, facilitating the development of rapid and reliable diagnostic tools. Extensive biochemical and metabolic studies have also delineated the basis for hyperuricemia, and allopurinol is very useful for controlling the overproduction of uric acid. However, the pathogenesis of the neurologic and behavioral aspects associated with HPRT deficiency remains incompletely understood, although increasing evidence has implicated dysfunction of dopamine systems of the basal ganglia.

Current and future efforts must be devoted towards prevention and elucidating the biologic basis for the neurobehavioral disturbances. The development of new pharmacologic, surgical, or genetic strategies for treating the devastating neurobehavioral features must assume a high priority.

ACKNOWLEDGMENTS

We would like to thank Drs. T. Page, B.K. Balendiron, J.C. Sacchettini, and J.E. Visser for their assistance with some of the figures; Dr. J.P. O'Neill for his assistance with the summary of genetic mutations; and Dr. J.E. Visser for reviewing the manuscript. This work was supported in part by NINDS NS01985 and the Lesch-Nyhan Syndrome Children's Research Foundation, 210 South Green Bay Road, Lake Forest, IL 60045.

REFERENCES

1. Lesch M, Nyhan WL: A familial disorder of uric acid metabolism and central nervous system function. *Am J Med* **36**:561, 1964.
2. Beck ChTh: Jacobus de Voragine (1230–1298): First to describe a Lesch-Nyhan syndrome? *Eur J Pediatr Surg* **2**:355, 1991.
3. Seegmiller JE, Rosenbloom FM, Kelley WN: Enzyme defect associated with a sex-linked human neurological disorder and excessive purine synthesis. *Science* **155**:1682, 1967.
4. Catel W, Schmidt J: Uber familiare gichtische Diathese in Verbindung mit zerebralen und renalen Symptomen bei einem Kleinkind. *Dtsch Med Wschr* **84**:2145, 1959.
5. Bakay B, Nissinen E, Sweetman L, Francke U, Nyhan WL: Utilization of purines by an HPRT variant in an intelligent, nonmutilative patient with features of the Lesch-Nyhan syndrome. *Pediatr Res* **13**:1365, 1979.
6. Kelley WN, Greene ML, Rosenbloom FM, Henderson JF, Seegmiller JE: Hypoxanthine-guanine phosphoribosyltransferase deficiency in gout. *Ann Intern Med* **70**:155, 1969.
7. Jolly DJ, Okayama H, Berg P, Esty AC, Filpula D, Bohlen P, Johnson GG, Shively JE, Hunkapillar T, Friedmann T: Isolation and characterization of a full-length expressible cDNA for human hypoxanthine phosphoribosyltransferase. *Proc Natl Acad Sci U S A* **80**:477, 1983.
8. Jolly DJ, Esty AC, Bernard HU, Friedmann T: Isolation of a genomic clone partially encoding human hypoxanthine phosphoribosyltransferase. *Proc Natl Acad Sci U S A* **79**:5038, 1982.
9. Konecki DS, Brennand J, Fuscoe JC, Caskey CT, Chinault AC: Hypoxanthine-guanine phosphoribosyltransferase genes of mouse and Chinese hamster: Construction and sequence analysis of cDNA recombinants. *Nucleic Acids Res* **10**:6763, 1982.
10. Brennand J, Chinault AC, Konecki DS, Melton DW, Caskey CT: Cloned cDNA sequences of the hypoxanthine/guanine phosphoribosyltransferase gene from a mouse neuroblastoma cell line found to have amplified genomic sequences. *Proc Natl Acad Sci U S A* **79**:1950, 1982.
11. Nyhan WL: The recognition of Lesch-Nyhan syndrome as an inborn error of purine metabolism. *J Inherit Metab Dis* **20**:171, 1997.
12. Seegmiller JE: Contributions of Lesch-Nyhan syndrome to the understanding of purine metabolism. *J Inherit Metab Dis* **12**:184, 1989.
13. Nyhan WL: Behavioral phenotypes in organic genetic disease: Presidential address to the Society for Pediatric Research. *Pediatr Res* **6**:1, 1972.
14. Friedmann T, Roblin R: Gene therapy for human genetic disease? *Science* **175**:949, 1972.
15. Jinnah HA, Friedmann T: Gene therapy and the brain. *Br Med Bull* **51**:138, 1995.
16. Lowenstein PR, Southgate TD, Smith-Arica JR, Smith J, Castro MG: Gene therapy for inherited neurological disorders: Towards therapeutic intervention in the Lesch-Nyhan syndrome. *Prog Brain Res* **117**:485, 1998.
17. DeMars R, Sarto G, Felix JS, Benke P: Lesch-Nyhan mutation: Prenatal detection with amniotic fluid cells. *Science* **164**:1303, 1969.
18. Berman PH, Balis ME, Dancis J: A method for the prenatal diagnosis of the Lesch-Nyhan syndrome using fresh amniotic cells. *Trans Am Neurol Assoc* **94**:222, 1969.
19. Szybalski W: Use of the HPRT gene and the HAT selection technique in DNA-mediated transformation of mammalian cells: First steps towards developing hybridoma techniques and gene therapy. *Bioessays* **14**:495, 1992.
20. Melton DW: HPRT gene organization and expression. *Oxf Surv Euk Genes* **4**:35, 1987.
21. Jiralerspong S, Patel PI: Regulation of the hypoxanthine phosphoribosyltransferase gene: In vitro and in vivo approaches. *Proc Soc Exp Biol Med* **212**:116, 1996.
22. Stout JT, Caskey CT: HPRT: Gene structure, expression, and mutation. *Ann Rev Genet* **19**:127, 1985.
23. Lambert B, Andersson B, He SM, Marcus S, Steen AM: Molecular analysis of mutation in the human gene for hypoxanthine phosphoribosyltransferase. *Mol Genet Med* **2**:161, 1992.
24. Albertini RJ: Drug-resistant lymphocytes in man as indicators of somatic cell mutation. *Teratog Carcinog Mutagen* **1**:25, 1980.
25. Cariello NF, Skopek TR: In vivo mutation at the human HPRT locus. *Trends Genet* **9**:322, 1993.
26. Marks JF, Baum J, Keele DK, Kay JL, MacFarlen A: Lesch-Nyhan syndrome treated from the early neonatal period. *Pediatrics* **42**:357, 1968.
27. Lloyd KG, Hornykiewicz O, Davidson L, Shannak K, Farley I, Goldstein M, Shibuya M, Kelley WN, Fox IH: Biochemical evidence of dysfunction of brain neurotransmitters in the Lesch-Nyhan syndrome. *N Engl J Med* **305**:1106, 1981.
28. Jankovic J, Caskey CT, Stout JT, Butler IJ: Lesch-Nyhan syndrome: A study of motor behavior and cerebrospinal fluid neurotransmitters. *Ann Neurol* **23**:466, 1988.
29. Silverstein FS, Johnston MV, Hutchinson RJ, Edwards NL: Lesch-Nyhan syndrome: CSF neurotransmitter abnormalities. *Neurology* **35**:907, 1985.
30. Emmerson BT, Thompson L: The spectrum of hypoxanthine-guanine phosphoribosyltransferase deficiency. *QJM* **166**:423, 1973.
31. Watts RWE, Spellacy E, Gibbs DA, Allsop J, McKeran RO, Slavin GE: Clinical, post-mortem, biochemical and therapeutic observations on the Lesch-Nyhan syndrome with particular reference to the neurological manifestations. *QJM* **201**:43, 1982.
32. Christie R, Bay C, Kaufman IA, Bakay B, Borden M, Nyhan WL: Lesch-Nyhan disease: Clinical experience with nineteen patients. *Devel Med Child Neurol* **24**:293, 1982.
33. Crussi FG, Robertson DM, Hiscox JL: The pathological condition of the Lesch-Nyhan syndrome. *Am J Dis Child* **118**:501, 1969.
34. Mizuno T: Long-term follow-up of ten patients with Lesch-Nyhan syndrome. *Neuropediatrics* **17**:158, 1986.
35. Bassermann R, Gutensohn W, Jahn H, Springmann JS: Pathological and immunological observations in a case of Lesch-Nyhan syndrome. *Eur J Pediatr* **132**:93, 1979.
36. Partington MW, Hennen BKE: The Lesch-Nyhan syndrome: Self-destructive biting, mental retardation, neurological disorder and hyperuricemia. *Devel Med Child Neurol* **9**:563, 1967.
37. Sass JK, Itabashi HH, Dexter RA: Juvenile gout with brain involvement. *Arch Neurol* **13**:639, 1965.
38. Hoefnagel D, Andrew ED, Mireault NG, Berndt WO: Hereditary choreoathetosis, self-mutilation, and hyperuricemia in young males. *N Engl J Med* **273**:130, 1965.

39. Mizuno T, Yugary Y: Prophylactic effect of L-5-hydroxytryptophan on self-mutilation in the Lesch-Nyhan syndrome. *Neuropediatrics* **6**:13, 1975.
40. Anders TF, Cann HM, Ciaranello RD, Barchas JD, Berger PA: Further observations on the use of 5-hydroxytryptophan in a child with Lesch-Nyhan syndrome. *Neuropediatrics* **9**:157, 1978.
41. Castells S, Chakrabarti C, Winsberg BG, Hurwic M, Perel JM, Nyhan WL: Effect of L-5-hydroxytryptophan on monoamine and amino acids turnover in the Lesch-Nyhan syndrome. *J Autism Dev Disord* **9**:95, 1979.
42. Wada Y, Arakawa T, Loizumi K: Lesch-Nyhan syndrome: Autopsy findings and in vitro study of incorporation of 14C-8-inosine into uric acid, guanosine-monophosphate and adenosine-monophosphate in the liver. *Tohoku J Exp Med* **95**:253, 1968.
43. Shewell PC, Thompson AG: Atlantoaxial instability in Lesch-Nyhan syndrome. *Spine* **21**:757, 1996.
44. Ghadimi H, Bhalla CK, Kirchenbaum DM: The significance of the deficiency state in Lesch-Nyhan syndrome. *Acta Pediatr Scand* **59**:233, 1970.
45. Berman PH, Balis ME, Dancis J: Congenital hyperuricemia: An inborn error of purine metabolism associated with psychomotor retardation, athetosis, and self-mutilation. *Arch Neurol* **20**:44, 1969.
46. Schulman JD, Greene ML, Fujimoto WY, Seegmiller JE: Adenine therapy for Lesch-Nyhan syndrome. *Pediatr Res* **5**:77, 1971.
47. Benke PJ, Herrick N, Smitten L, Aradine C, Laessig R, Wolcott GJ: Adenine and folic acid in the Lesch-Nyhan syndrome. *Pediatr Res* **7**:729, 1973.
48. Origuchi Y, Miyoshino S, Mishima K, Mine K: Quantitative histologic study of the sural nerve in Lesch-Nyhan syndrome. *Pediatr Neurol* **6**:353, 1990.
49. Ciaranello RD, Anders TF, Barchas JD, Berger JD, Berger PA: The use of 5-hydroxytryptophan in a child with Lesch-Nyhan syndrome. *Child Psychiatry Hum Devel* **7**:127, 1976.
50. Van Der Zee SPM, Lommen EJP, Trijbels JMF, Schretland EDAM: The influence of adenine on the clinical features and purine metabolism in the Lesch-Nyhan syndrome. *Acta Pediatr Scand* **59**:259, 1970.
51. Wood MH, Fox RM, Vincent L, Reye C, O'Sullivan WJ: The Lesch-Nyhan syndrome: Report of three cases. *Aust N Z J Med* **1**:57, 1972.
52. Watts RWE, McKeran RO, Brown E, Andrews TM, Griffiths MI: Clinical and biochemical studies on treatment of Lesch-Nyhan syndrome. *Arch Dis Child* **49**:693, 1974.
53. Hunter TC, Melancon SB, Dallaire L, Taft S, Skopek TR, Albertini RJ, O'Neill JP: Germinal HPRT splice donor site mutation results in multiple RNA splicing products in T-lymphocyte cultures. *Somat Cell Mol Genet* **22**:145, 1996.
54. Scherzer AL, Ilson JB: Normal intelligence in the Lesch-Nyhan syndrome. *Pediatrics* **44**:116, 1969.
55. Nyhan WL, Oliver WJ, Lesch M: A familial disorder of uric acid metabolism and central nervous system function II. *J Pediatr* **67**:257, 1965.
56. Chen LR, Liu JF: Successful treatment of self-inflicted oral mutilation using an acrylic splint retained by a headgear. *Am Acad Pediatr Dent* **18**:408, 1996.
57. Salman RA, Glickman RS, Super S: Lesch-Nyhan syndrome: Report of two cases. *J Oral Med* **42**:10, 1987.
58. Shapira J, Zilberman Y, Becker A: Lesch-Nyhan syndrome: A non-extracting approach to prevent mutilation. *Dent Health* **25**:6, 1987.
59. Duker P: Behaviour control of self-biting in a Lesch-Nyhan patient. *J Ment Defic Res* **19**:11, 1975.
60. Riley ID: Gout and cerebral palsy in a three-year-old boy. *Arch Dis Child* **35**:293, 1960.
61. Marcus S, Steen AM, Andersson B, Lambert B, Kristoffersson U, Francke U: Mutation analysis and prenatal diagnosis in a Lesch-Nyhan family showing non-random X-inactivation interfering with carrier detection tests. *Hum Genet* **89**:395, 1992.
62. Hiraishi K, Nakamura S, Yamamoto S, Kurokawa K: Prevention of xanthine stone formation by augmented dose of allopurinol in the Lesch-Nyhan syndrome. *Br J Urol* **59**:362, 1987.
63. Stevens SK, Parker BR: Renal oxypurine deposition in Lesch-Nyhan syndrome: Sonographic evaluation. *Pediatr Radiol* **19**:479, 1989.
64. Kenney IJ: Renal sonography in long-standing Lesch-Nyhan syndrome. *Clin Radiol* **43**:39, 1991.
65. Ludman CN, Dicks-Mireaux C, Saunders AJ: Renal ultrasonographic appearances at presentation in an infant with Lesch-Nyhan syndrome. *Br J Radiol* **65**:724, 1992.
66. Jenkins EA, Hallett RJ, Hull RG: Lesch-Nyhan syndrome presenting with renal insufficiency in infancy and transient neonatal hypothyroidism. *Br J Rheumatol* **33**:392, 1994.
67. Mizuno T, Endoh H, Konishi Y, Miyachi Y, Akoaka I: An autopsy case of the Lesch-Nyhan syndrome: Normal HGPRT activity in liver and xanthine calculi in various tissues. *Neuropaediatrie* **7**:351, 1976.
68. Michener WM: Hyperuricemia and mental retardation. *Am J Dis Child* **113**:195, 1967.
69. Pullon DH, Ballantyne GH, Webster D, Becroft DM: The Lesch-Nyhan syndrome: A family study. *N Z Med J* **86**:518, 1977.
70. Storey B: The Lesch-Nyhan syndrome. *Med J Aust* **2**:696, 1969.
71. Shaltiel A, Katzuni E, Boer P, Zoref-Shani E, Sperling O: Lesch-Nyhan syndrome in an Arab family. Detection and biochemical manifestation of heterozygosity. *Isr J Med Sci* **17**:1169, 1981.
72. Reed WB, Fish CH: Hyperuricemia with self-mutilation and choreoathetosis: Lesch-Nyhan syndrome. *Arch Dermatol* **94**:194, 1966.
73. Mahnovski V, Dozic S, Vulovic D, Marjanovic B, Tasic G: Necropsy findings in a case of Lesch-Nyhan syndrome. *Arch Dis Child* **50**:666, 1975.
74. Steadman RH, McIntosh G, Gross BD: Lesch-Nyhan syndrome. *J Oral Maxillofac Surg* **40**:750, 1982.
75. Itiaba K, Banfalvi M, Crawhall JC, Mongeau JG: Family studies of a Lesch-Nyhan patient from an isolated Canadian community. *Am J Hum Genet* **25**:134, 1973.
76. Mangano M, Azzia N, Russo A, Romeo MA: Lesch-Nyhan syndrome in two brothers: Why early diagnosis is essential. *Clin Pediatr* **33**:125, 1994.
77. Ceccarelli M, Ciompi ML, Pasero G: Acute renal failure during adenine therapy in Lesch-Nyhan syndrome. *Adv Exp Med Biol* **41**:671, 1974.
78. Fattal A, Spirer Z, Zoref-Shani E, Sperling O: Lesch-Nyhan syndrome: Biochemical characterization of a case with attenuated behavioral manifestation. *Enzyme* **31**:55, 1984.
79. Kulkarni ML, Sureshkumar C, George VG: Lesch-Nyhan syndrome. *Indian Pediatr* **30**:537, 1993.
80. Gilbert RD, Wiggelinkhuizen J, Harley EH, Marinaki A: The Lesch-Nyhan syndrome — An under-recognised condition in South Africa? A case report. *S Afr Med J* **81**:375, 1992.
81. Mitchell G, McInnes RR: Differential diagnosis of cerebral palsy: Lesch-Nyhan syndrome without self-mutilation. *Can Med Assoc J* **130**:1323, 1984.
82. LaBanc J, Epker BN: Lesch-Nyhan syndrome: Surgical treatment in a case with lip chewing: A case report. *J Maxillofac Surg* **9**:64, 1981.
83. Shnier MH, Sims F, Zail S: The Lesch-Nyhan syndrome: First case description in a South African family. *S Afr Med J* **46**:947, 1972.
84. Bunn DN, Moss IK, Nicholls A, Scott JT, Snaith ML, Watson MR: Clinical and biochemical observations on three cases of hypoxanthine-guanine phosphoribosyltransferase deficiency. *Ann Rheum Dis* **34**:249, 1975.
85. Evans J, Sirikumara M, Gregory M: Lesch-Nyhan syndrome and the lower lip guard. *Oral Surg Oral Med Oral Pathol* **76**:437, 1993.
86. Smith BM, Cutilli BJ, Fedele M: Lesch-Nyhan syndrome: A case report. *Oral Surg Oral Med Oral Pathol* **78**:317, 1994.
87. Lynch BJ, Noetzel MJ: Recurrent coma and Lesch-Nyhan syndrome. *Pediatr Neurol* **7**:389, 1991.
88. Erhard U, Herkenrath P, Benz-Bohm G, Querfeld U: Lesch-Nyhan syndrome: Clinical diagnosis and confirmation by biochemical and genetic methods. *Pediatr Nephrol* **11**:124, 1997.
89. Rijksen G, Staal GEJ, van der Vlist MJM, Beemer FA, Troost J, Gutensohn W, van Laarhoven JPRM, De Bruyn CHMM: Partial hypoxanthine-guanine phosphoribosyl transferase deficiency with full expression of the Lesch-Nyhan syndrome. *Hum Genet* **57**:39, 1981.
90. Singh S, Willers I, Ullrich K, Gustmann H, Niederwieser A, Goedde HW: A case of Lesch-Nyhan syndrome with delayed onset of self-mutilation: Search for abnormal biochemical, immunological and cell growth characteristic in fibroblasts and neurotransmitters in urine. *Adv Exp Med Biol* **195A**:205, 1986.
91. Hatanaka T, Higashino H, Woo M, Yasuhara A, Sugimoto T, Kobayashi Y: Lesch-Nyhan syndrome with delayed onset of self-mutilation: Hyperactivity of interneurons at the brainstem and blink reflex. *Acta Neurol Scand* **81**:184, 1990.
92. McGreevy P, Arthur M: Effective behavioral treatment of self-biting by a child with Lesch- Nyhan syndrome. *Dev Med Child Neurol* **29**:536, 1987.
93. Eguchi S, Tokioka T, Motoyoshi A, Wakamura S: A self-controllable mask with helmet to prevent self finger-mutilation in the Lesch-Nyhan syndrome. *Arch Phys Med Rehabil* **75**:709, 1994.
94. Ball TS, Datta PC, Rios M, Constantine C: Flexible arm splints in the control of a Lesch-Nyhan victim's finger biting and a profoundly retarded client's finger sucking. *J Autism Dev Disord* **15**:177, 1985.

95. Marcus S, Christensen E, Malm G: Molecular analysis of the mutations in five unrelated patients with the Lesch Nyhan syndrome. *Hum Mutat* **2**:473, 1993.
96. Puliyel JM, Kumar M: Lesch Nyhan syndrome. *Indian Pediatr* **21**:251, 1984.
97. Barry RG, Buckley BM, Tully ER: Clinical and biochemical observations on a patient with the Lesch-Nyhan syndrome. *Ir J Med Sci* **147**:213, 1978.
98. Dizmang LH, Cheatham CF: The Lesch-Nyhan syndrome. *Am J Psychiatry* **127**:671, 1970.
99. Bull M, LaVecchio F: Behavior therapy for a child with Lesch-Nyhan syndrome. *Dev Med Child Neurol* **20**:368, 1978.
100. Itiaba K, Melancon SB, Dallaire L, Crawhall JC: Adenine phosphoribosyl transferase deficiency in association with sub-normal hypoxanthine phosphoribosyl transferase in families of Lesch-Nyhan patients. *Biochem Med* **19**:252, 1978.
101. Larson LO, Wilkins RG: Anesthesia and the Lesch-Nyhan syndrome. *Anesthesiology* **63**:197, 1985.
102. Gilbert S, Spellacy E, Watts RW: Problems in the behavioural treatment of self-injury in the Lesch-Nyhan syndrome. *Dev Med Child Neurol* **21**:795, 1979.
103. Watts RW, Harkness RA, Spellacy E, Taylor NF: Lesch-Nyhan syndrome: Growth delay, testicular atrophy and a partial failure of the 11 beta-hydroxylation of steroids. *J Inherit Metab Dis* **10**:210, 1987.
104. Roscioni G, Farnetani MA, Pagani R, Pizzichini M, Marinello E, Porcelli B: Plasma and urinary oxypurines in Lesch-Nyhan patient after allopurinol treatment. *Adv Exp Med Biol* **370**:357, 1994.
105. Benke PJ, Herrick N: Azaguanine-resistance as a manifestation of a new form of metabolic overproduction of uric acid. *Am J Med* **52**:547, 1972.
106. Saito Y, Hanaoka S, Fukumizu M, Morita H, Ogawa T, Takahasi K, Ito M, Hashimoto T: Polysomnographic studies of Lesch-Nyhan syndrome. *Brain Dev* **20**:579, 1998.
107. Holland PC, Dillon MJ, Pincott J, Simmonds HA, Barratt TM: Hypoxanthine guanine phosphoribosyltransferase deficiency presenting as gout and renal failure in infancy. *Arch Dis Child* **58**:831, 1983.
108. Adler CH, Wrabetz L: Lesch-Nyhan variant: Dystonia, ataxia, near-normal intelligence, and no self-mutilation. *Mov Disord* **11**:583, 1996.
109. Dancis J, Yip LC, Cox RP, Piomelli S, Balis ME: Disparate enzyme activity in erythrocytes and leukocytes: A variant of hypoxanthine phosphoribosyl-transferase deficiency with an unstable enzyme. *J Clin Invest* **52**:2068, 1973.
110. Geerdink RA, De Vries WHM, Willemse J, Oei TL, De Bruyn CHMM: An atypical case of hypoxanthine-guanine phosphoribosyltransferase deficiency (Lesch-Nyhan syndrome). I. Clinical studies. *Clin Genet* **4**:348, 1973.
111. Hersh JH, Page T, Hand ME, Seegmiller JE, Nyhan WL, Weisskopf B: Clinical correlations in partial hypoxanthine guanine phosphoribosyltransferase deficiency. *Pediatr Neurol* **2**:302, 1986.
112. Marcus S, Hellgren D, Lambert B, Fallstrom SP, Wahlstrom J: Duplication in the hypoxanthine phosphoribosyl-transferase gene caused by Alu-Alu recombination in a patient with Lesch-Nyhan syndrome. *Hum Genet* **90**:477, 1993.
113. Skopek TR, Recio L, Simpson D, Dellaire L, Melancon SB, Ogier H, O'Neill JP, Falta MT, Nicklas JA, Albertini RJ: Molecular analyses of a Lesch-Nyhan syndrome mutation ($hprt_{\mathrm{Montreal}}$) by use of T-lymphocyte cultures. *Hum Genet* **85**:111, 1990.
114. Snyder FF, Chudley AE, MacLeod PM, Carter RJ, Fung E, Lowe JK: Partial deficiency of hypoxanthine-guanine phosphoribosyltransferase with reduced affinity for PP-ribose-P in four related males with gout. *Hum Genet* **67**:18, 1984.
115. Zanic T, Gamulin V, Lipovac K: A case of severe hypoxanthine-guanine phosphoribosyl transferase deficiency. *J Inherit Metab Dis* **8**:79, 1985.
116. Choi Y, Koo JW, Ha IS, Yamada Y, Goto H, Ogasawara N: Partial hypoxanthine-guanine phosphoribosyl transferase deficiency in two Korean siblings — A new mutation. *Pediatr Nephrol* **7**:739,1993.
117. Khattak FH, Morris IM, Harris K: Kelley-Seegmiller syndrome: A case report and review of the literature. *Brit J Rheumatol* **37**:580, 1998.
118. Toyo-Oka T, Hanaoka F, Akaoka I, Yamada MA: X-linked hypoxanthine-guanine phosphoribosyltransferase deficiency without neurological disorders: A report of a family. *Clin Genet* **7**:181, 1975.
119. Andres A, Praga M, Ruilope LM, Martinez JM, Millet VG, Bellow I, Rocicio JL: Partial deficit of hypoxanthine guanine phosphoribosyl transferase presenting as acute renal failure. *Nephron* **46**:179, 1987.
120. Lorentz WB, Burton BK, Trillo A, Browning MC: Failure to thrive, hyperuricemia, and renal insufficiency in early infancy secondary to partial hypoxanthine-guanine phosphoribosyl transferase deficiency. *J Pediatr* **104**:94, 1984.
121. Hikita M, Hosoya T, Ichida K, Okabe H, Saji M, Ohno I, Kuriyama S, Tomonari H, Hayashi F, Onouchi K, Fujimori S, Yamaoka N, Sakuma R: Partial deficiency of hypoxanthine-guanine-phosphoribosyltransferase manifesting as acute renal damage. *Intern Med* **37**:945, 1998.
122. Becker MA, Roessler BJ: Hyperuricemia and gout, in Scriver CR, Beaudet AL, Sly WS, Valle D (eds): *The Metabolic and Molecular Basis of Inherited Disease*, 7th ed. New York, McGraw-Hill, 1995, p 1192.
123. Kaufman JM, Greene ML, Seedmiller JE: Urine uric acid to creatinine ratio — A screening test for inherited disorders of purine metabolism. *J Pediatr* **73**:583, 1968.
124. Mateos EA, Puig JG: Purine metabolism in Lesch-Nyhan syndrome versus Kelley-Seegmiller syndrome. *J Inherit Metab Dis* **17**:138, 1994.
125. Wortmann RL, Fox IH: Limited value of uric acid to creatinine ratios in estimating uric acid excretion. *Ann Intern Med* **93**:822, 1980.
126. Brock WA, Golden J, Kaplan GW: Xanthine calculi in the Lesch-Nyhan syndrome. *J Urol* **130**:157, 1983.
127. Kranen S, Keough D, Gordon RB, Emmerson BT: Xanthine-containing calculi during allopurinol therapy. *J Urol* **133**:658, 1985.
128. Ogawa A, Watanabe K, Minejima N: Renal xanthine stone in Lesch-Nyhan syndrome treated with allopurinol. *Urol* **26**:56, 1985.
129. Oka T, Utsunomiya M, Ichikawa Y, Koide T, Takaha M, Mimaki T, Sonoda T: Xanthine calculi in the patient with the Lesch-Nyhan syndrome associated with urinary tract infection. *Urol Int* **40**:138, 1985.
130. Morino M, Shiigai N, Kusuyama H, Okada K: Extracorporeal shock wave lithotripsy and xanthine calculi in Lesch-Nyhan syndrome. *Pediatr Radiol* **22**:304, 1992.
131. Ad hoc committee on extrapyramidal disorders: Classification of extrapyramidal disorders. *J Neurol Sci* **51**:311, 1981.
132. Jinnah HA, Harris JC, Reich SG, Visser JE, Garabas G, Eddey GE: The motor disorder of Lesch-Nyhan disease. *Mov Disord* **13(Suppl 2)**:98, 1998.
133. Visser JE, Baer P, Jinnah HA: Lesch-Nyhan syndrome and the basal ganglia. *Brain Res Rev* **32**:449, 2000.
134. Anderson WW, Wise BL, Itabashi HH, Jones M: Cervical spondylosis in patients with athetosis. *Neurology* **12**:410, 1962.
135. Levine RA, Rosenbaum AE, Waltz JM, Scheinberg LC: Cervical spondylosis and dyskinesias. *Neurology* **20**:1194, 1970.
136. Hirose G, Kadoya S: Cervical spondylotic radiculomyelopathy in patients with athetoid-dystonic cerebral palsy: Clinical evaluation and surgical treatment. *J Neurol Neurosurg Psychiatry* **47**:775, 1984.
137. Ebara S, Harada T, Yamazaki Y: Unstable cervical spine in athetoid cerebral palsy. *Spine* **14**:1154, 1989.
138. El-Mallakh RS, Rao K, Barwick M: Cervical myelopathy secondary to movement disorders: case report. *Neurosurg* **24**:902, 1989.
139. Harada T, Ebara S, ANwar MM: The cervical spine in athetoid cerebral palsy: A radiological study of 180 patients. *J Bone Joint Surg* **78**:613, 1996.
140. Adler CH, Zimmerman RS, Lyons MK, Simeone F, Brin MF: Perioperative use of botulinum toxin for movement disorder-induced cervical spine disease. *Mov Disord* **11**:79, 1996.
141. Rosenfeld M, Friedman JH: Cervical stenosis and dystonic cerebral palsy. *Mov Disord* **14**:194, 1999.
142. Krauss JK, Jankovic J: Severe motor tics causing cervical myelopathy in Tourette's syndrome. *Mov Disord* **11**:563, 1996.
143. Nausieda PA, Weiner WJ, Klawans HL: Dystonic foot response of Parkinsonism. *Arch Neurol* **37**:132, 1980.
144. Massaquoi SG, Hallet M: Ataxia and other cerebellar syndromes, in Jankovic J, Tolosa E (eds): *Parkinson's Disease and Movement Disorders*. Baltimore, Williams and Wilkins, 1998, p 623.
145. Nyhan WL: Ataxia and disorders of purine metabolism: Defects in hypoxanthine guanine phosphoribosyl transferase and clinical ataxia. *Adv Neurol* **21**:279, 1978.
146. Nyhan WL: Lesch-Nyhan syndrome: Summary of clinical features. *Fed Proc* **27**:1034, 1968.
147. Nyhan WL: The Lesch-Nyhan syndrome. *Hand Clin Neurol* **29**:263, 1977.
148. Nyhan WL: Clinical features of the Lesch-Nyhan syndrome. *Arch Intern Med* **130**:186, 1972.
149. McCreanor GM, Harkness RA: Lesch-Nyhan syndrome and its pathogenesis: Normal nicotinamide-adenine dinucleotide but reduced ATP concentrations that correlate with reduced poly(ADP-ribose) synthetase activity in HPRT-deficient lymphoblasts. *J Inherit Metab Dis* **18**:737, 1995.

150. Imamura A, Yamanouchi H, Kurokawa T, Arima M: Elevated fibrinopeptide A (FPA) in patients with Lesch-Nyhan syndrome. *Brain Dev* **14**:424, 1992.
151. Imamura A, Yamanouchi H, Arima M: Decreased 6-keto prostaglandin F1 alpha (6-keto PGF1 alpha) in patients with Lesch-Nyhan syndrome. *Brain Dev* **15**:381, 1993.
152. Matthews WS, Solan A, Barabas G: Cognitive functioning in Lesch-Nyhan syndrome. *Dev Med Child Neurol* **37**:715, 1995.
153. Solan A, Matthews W, Barabas G, Robey K: Cognition in LND: A two-year follow-up study. *Dev Med Child Neurol* **39**:492, 1997.
154. Schretlen DJ, Harris JC, Park KS, Jinnah HA, Ojeda del Pozo N: Neurocognitive functioning in Lesch-Nyhan disease and partial hypoxanthine-guanine phosphoribosyltransferase dificiency. *J Int Neuropsychol Soc*, in press.
155. Anderson LT, Ernst M, Davis SV: Cognitive abilities of patients with Lesch-Nyhan disease. *J Autism Dev Disord* **22**:189, 1992.
156. Nyhan WL: Behavior in the Lesch-Nyhan syndrome. *J Autism Child Schizophren* **6**:235, 1976.
157. Anderson LT, Ernst M: Self-injury in Lesch-Nyhan disease. *J Autism Dev Disord* **24**:67, 1994.
158. Roach ES, Delgado M, Anderson L, Iannoccone ST, Burns DK: Carbamazepine trial for Lesch-Nyhan self-mutilation. *J Child Neurol* **11**:476, 1996.
159. Gedye A: Serotonin-GABA treatment is hypothesized for self-injury in Lesch-Nyhan syndrome. *Med Hypoth* **38**:325, 1992.
160. Hanna GL: Stereotypic movement disorder and disorder of infancy, childhood, or adolescence NOS, in Kaplan HI, Sadock BJ (eds): *Comprehensive Textbook of Psychiatry*. Baltimore, Williams and Wilkins, 1995, p 2359.
161. Pellicer F, Buendia-Roldan I, Pallares-Trujillo VC: Self-mutilation in the Lesch-Nyhan syndrome: A corporal consciousness problem? A new hypothesis. *Med Hypoth* **50**:43, 1998.
162. King BH: Self-injury by people with mental retardation: A compulsive behavior hypothesis. *Am J Ment Retard* **98**:93, 1993.
163. Jankovic J: Orofacial and other self-mutilations. *Adv Neurol* **49**:365, 1988.
164. Van Woert MH, Yip LC, Balis ME: Purine phosphoribosyltransferase in Gilles de la Tourette syndrome. *N Engl J Med* **296**:210, 1977.
165. Guess G, Carr E: Emergence and maintenance of stereotypy and self-injury. *Am J Ment Retard* **96**:299, 1991.
166. Van Der Zee SPM, Schretlen EDAM, Monnens LAH: Megaloblastic anemia in the Lesch-Nyhan syndrome. *Lancet* **1**:1427, 1968.
167. McKeran RO: Factors in the pathogenesis of the brain damage and anaemia in the Lesch-Nyhan syndrome. *CIBA Found Symp* **48**:83, 1977.
168. Ansell JD, Samuel K, Whittingham DG, Patek CE, Hardy K, Handyside AH, Jones KW, Muggleton-Harris AL, Taylor AH, Hooper ML: Hypoxanthine phosphoribosyl transferase deficiency, haematopoiesis and fertility in the mouse. *Development* **112**:489, 1991.
169. Hakoda M, Hirai Y, Akiyama M, Yamanaka H, Terai C, Kamatani N, Kashiwazaki S: Selection against blood cells deficient in hypoxanthine phosphoribosyltransferase (HPRT) in Lesch-Nyhan heterozygotes occurs at the level of multipotent stem cells. *Hum Genet* **96**:674, 1995.
170. McKeran RO, Howell A, Andrews TM, Watts RWE, Arlett CF: Observations on the growth in vitro of myeloid progenitor cells and fibroblasts from hemizygotes and heterozygotes for "complete" and "partial" hypoxanthine-guanine phosphoribosyltransferase (HGPRT) deficiency, and their relevance to the pathogenesis of brain damage in the Lesch-Nyhan syndrome. *J Neurol Sci* **22**:183, 1974.
171. Skyler JS, Neelon FA, Arnold WJ, Kelly WN, Lebovitz HE: Growth retardation in the Lesch-Nyhan syndrome. *Acta Endocrinol* **75**:3, 1974.
172. Rosenbloom FM, Kelley WN, Miller J, Henderson JF, Seegmiller JE: Inherited disorder of purine metabolism. *JAMA* **202**:175, 1967.
173. Page T, Nyhan WL: The spectrum of HPRT deficiency: An update. *Adv Exp Med Biol* **253A**:129, 1989.
174. Page T, Bakay B, Nissinen E, Nyhan WL: Hypoxanthine-guanine phosphoribosyltransferase variants: Correlation of clinical phenotype with enzyme activity. *J Inherit Metab Dis* **4**:203, 1981.
175. Kogut MD, Donnell GN, Nyhan WL, Sweetman L: Disorder of purine metabolism due to partial deficiency of hypoxanthine-guanine phosphoribosyltransferase. *Am J Med* **48**:148, 1970.
176. Yu TF, Balis ME, Krenitsky TA, Dancis J, Silvers DN, Elion GB, Gutman AB: Rarity of X-linked partial hypoxanthine-guanine phosphoribosyltransferase deficiency in a large gouty population. *Ann Int Med* **76**:255, 1972.
177. Bitler CM, Howard BD: Dopamine metabolism in hypoxanthine-guanine phosphoribosyltransferase-deficient variants of PC12 cells. *J Neurochem* **47**:107, 1986.
178. O'Neill JP, Rogan PK, Cariello N, Nicklas JA: Mutations that alter RNA splicing of the human HPRT gene: A review of the spectrum. *Mutat Res* **411**:179, 1998.
179. Hara K, Kashiwamata S, Ogasawara N, Ohishi H, Natsume R, Yamanaka T, Hakamada S, Miyazaki S, Watanabe K: A female case of the Lesch-Nyhan syndrome. *Tohoku J Exp Med* **137**:275, 1982.
180. Ogasawara N, Stout JT, Goto H, Sonta SI, Matsumoto A, Caskey CT: Molecular analysis of a female Lesch-Nyhan patient. *J Clin Invest* **4**:1024, 1989.
181. Aral B, de Saint B, Al-Garawi S, Kamoun P, Ceballos-Picot I: Novel nonsense mutation in the hypoxanthine guanine phosphoribosyltransferase gene and nonrandom X-inactivation causing Lesch-Nyhan syndrome in a female patient. *Hum Mutat* **7**:52, 1996.
182. Hooft C, Van Nevel C, De Schaepdryver AF: Hyperuricosuric encephalopathy without hyperuricaemia. *Arch Dis Child* **43**:734, 1968.
183. van Bogaert P, Ceballos I, Desguerre I, Telvi L, Kamoun P, Ponsot G: Lesch-Nyhan syndrome in a girl. *J Inherit Metab Dis* **15**:790, 1992.
184. Yukawa T, Akazawa H, Miyake Y, Takahashi Y, Nagao H, Takeda E: A female patient with Lesch-Nyhan syndrome. *Dev Med Child Neurol* **34**:543, 1992.
185. Yamada Y, Goto H, Yukawa T, Akazawa H, Ogasawara N: Molecular mechanisms of the second female Lesch-Nyhan patient. *Adv Exp Med Biol* **370**:337, 1994.
186. Nyhan WL, Pesek J, Sweetman L, Carpenter DG, Carter CH: Genetics of an X-linked disorder of uric acid metabolism and cerebral function. *Pediatr Res* **1**:5, 1967.
187. Crawhall JC, Henderson JF, Kelley WN: Diagnosis and treatment of the Lesch-Nyhan syndrome. *Pediatr Res* **6**:504, 1972.
188. Shows TB, Brown JA: Localization of genes coding for PGK, HPRT, and G6PD on the long arm of the X chromosome in somatic cell hybrids. *Cytogenet Cell Genet* **14**:426, 1975.
189. Pai GS, Sprenkle JA, Do TT, Mareni CE, Migeon BR: Localization of loci for hypoxanthine phosphoribosyltransferase and glucoe-6-phosphate dehydrogenase and biochemical evidence of nonrandom X chromosome expression from studies of a human X-autosome translocation. *Proc Natl Acad Sci U S A* **77**:2810, 1980.
190. Franke U, Taggart RT: Comparative gene mapping: Order of loci on the X chromosome is different in mice and humans. *Proc Natl Acad Sci U S A* **77**:3595, 1980.
191. Patel PE, Nussbaum RL, Framson PE, Ledbetter DH, Caskey CT, Chinault AC: Organization of the HPRT gene and related sequences in the human genome. *Somat Cell Mol Genet* **10**:483, 1984.
192. Patel PI, Framson PE, Caskey CT, Chinault AC: Fine structure of the human hypoxanthine phosphoribosyltransferase gene. *Mol Cell Biol* **6**:393, 1986.
193. Kim SH, Mores JC, Respess JG, Jolly DJ, Friedmann T: The organization of the human *HPRT* gene. *Nucleic Acids Res* **14**:3103, 1986.
194. Edwards A, Voss H, Rice P, Civitello A, Stegemann J, Schwager C, Zimmermann J, Erfle H, Caskey CT, Ansorge W: Automated DNA sequencing of the human HPRT locus. *Genomics* **6**:593, 1990.
195. Renwick PJ, Birley AJ, Hulten MA: Study of Alu sequences at the hypoxanthine phosphoribosyltransferase (hprt) encoding region of man. *Gene* **184**:155, 1997.
196. Nussbaum RL, Crowder WE, Nyhan WL, Caskey CT: A three-allele restriction-fragment-length polymorphism at the hypoxanthine phosphoribosyltransferase locus in man. *Proc Natl Acad Sci U S A* **80**:4035, 1983.
197. Gibbs DA, Headhouse-Benson CM, Watts RW: Family studies of the Lesch-Nyhan syndrome: The use of a restriction fragment length polymorphism (RFLP) closely linked to the disease gene for carrier state and prenatal diagnosis. *J Inherit Metab Dis* **9**:45, 1986.
198. Ogasawara N, Goto H: Restriction fragment length polymorphisms of HPRT and APRT gene in Japanese population. *Adv Exp Med Biol* **253A**:461, 1989.
199. Igarishi T, Ikegami H, Yamazaki H, Minami M: Bam HI restriction fragment length polymorphisms for hypoxanthine-guanine phosphoribosyltransferase (HPRT) gene of carrier and controls of HPRT deficiency in Japan. *Acta Paediatr Jpn* **32**:12, 1990.
200. Chan LC, Tse E, Pittaluga S: X-linked polymorphism of hypoxanthine phosphoribosyl transferase gene (HPRT) in Chinese females. *Cancer Genet Cytogenet* **64**:192, 1992.
201. Fujimori S, Sakuma R, Yamaoka N, Hakoda M, Yamanaka H, Kamatani N: An asymptomatic germline missense base substitution in the hypoxanthine phosphoribosyltransferase (HPRT) gene that reduces the amount of enzyme in humans. *Hum Genet* **99**:8, 1997.

202. Beckman DL, Kranz RG: A bacterial homolog to HPRT. *Biochem Biophys Acta* **1129**:112, 1991.
203. Showalter RE, Silverman MR: Nucleotide sequence of a gene, *hpt*, for hypoxanthine phosphoribosyltransferase from *Vibrio harveyi*. *Nucleic Acids Res* **18**:4621, 1990.
204. King A, Melton DW: Characterisation of cDNA clones for hypoxanthine-guanine phosphoribosyltransferase from the human malarial parasite, *Plasmodium falciparum*: comparison to the mammalian gene and protein. *Nucleic Acids Res* **15**:10469, 1987.
205. Craig SPI, McKerrow JH, Newport GR, Wang CC: Analysis of cDNA encoding the hypoxanthine-guanine phosphoribosyltransferase (HGPRTase) of *Schistosoma mansoni*: A putative target for chemotherapy. *Nucleic Acids Res* **16**:7087, 1988.
206. Focia PJ, Craig SPI, Nieves-Alicea R, Fletterick RJ, Eakin AE: A 1.4 Å crystal structure of the hypoxanthine phosphoribosyltransferase of *Trypanosoma cruzi*. *Biochem* **37**:15066, 1998.
207. Melton DW, Konecki DS, Brennand J, Caskey CT: Structure, expression, and mutation of the hypoxanthine phosphoribosyltransferase gene. *Proc Natl Acad Sci U S A* **81**:2147, 1984.
208. Chiaverotti TA, Battula N, Monnat RJ: Rat hypoxanthine phosphoribosyltransferase cDNA cloning and sequence analysis. *Genomics* **11**:1158, 1991.
209. Rossiter BJ, Fuscoe JC, Muzny DM, Fox M, Caskey CT: Chinese hamster HPRT gene: Restriction map, sequence analysis, and multiplex PCR deletion screen. *Genomics* **9**:247, 1991.
210. Conaty J, Piper AA: Full-length cDNA sequence of the X-linked HPRT gene of an Australian marsupial, the wallaroo (*Macropus robustus*). *Mamm Genome* **7**:74, 1996.
211. Noyce L, Conaty J, Piper AA: Identification of a novel tissue-specific processed HPRT gene and comparison with X-linked gene transcription in the Australian marsupial *Macropus robustus*. *Gene* **186**:87, 1997.
212. Rincon-Limas DE, Drueger DA, Patel PI: Functional characterization of the human hypoxanthine phosphoribosyltransferase gene promoter: Evidence for a negative regulatory element. *Mol Cell Biol* **11**:4157, 1991.
213. Johnson P, Friedmann T: Limited bidirectional activity of two housekeeping gene promotors: Human *HPRT* and *PGK*. *Gene* **88**:207, 1990.
214. Reid LH, Gregg RG, Smithies O, Koller BH: Regulatory elements in the introns of the human HPRT gene are necessary for its expression in embryonic stem cells. *Proc Natl Acad Sci U S A* **87**:4299, 1990.
215. Wolf SF, Jolly DJ, Lunnen KD, Friedmann TF, Migeon BR: Methylation of the hypoxanthine phosphoribosyltransferase locus on the human X chromosome: Implications for X-chromosome inactivation. *Proc Natl Acad Sci U S A* **81**:2806, 1984.
216. Yen PH, Patel P, Chinault AC, Mohandas T, Shapiro LJ: Differential methylation of hypoxanthine phosphoribosyltransferase genes on active and inactive human X chromosomes. *Proc Natl Acad Sci U S A* **81**:1759, 1984.
217. Lock LF, Melton DW, Caskey CT, Martin GR: Methylation of the mouse hprt gene differs on the active and inactive X chromosomes. *Mol Cell Biol* **6**:914, 1986.
218. Lock LF, Takagi N, Martin GR: Methylation of the hprt gene on the inactive X occurs after chromosome inactivation. *Cell* **48**:39, 1987.
219. Hornstra IK, Yang TP: High-resolution methylation analysis of the human hypoxanthine-phosphoribosyltransferase gene 5′ region on the active and inactive X-chromosomes: Correlation with binding sites for transcription factors. *Mol Cell Biol* **14**:1419, 1994.
220. Subramanian PS, Chinault AC: Replication timing properties of the human HPRT locus on active, inactive, and reactivated X chromosomes. *Somat Cell Mol Genet* **23**:97, 1997.
221. Lo YV, Palmour M: Developmental expression of murine HPRT. I. Activities, heat stabilities, and electrophoretic mobilities in adult tissues. *Biochem J* **17**:737, 1979.
222. Jinnah HA, Hess EJ, Wilson MC, Gage FH, Friedmann T: Localization of hypoxanthine-guanine phosphoribosyltransferase mRNA in the mouse brain by *in situ* hybridization. *Mol Cell Neurosci* **3**:64, 1992.
223. Rincon-Limas DE, Geske RS, Xue JJ, Hsu CY, Overbeek PA, Patel PI: 5′-Flanking sequences of the human HPRT gene direct neuronal expression in the brain of transgenic mice. *J Neurosci Res* **38**:259, 1994.
224. Stout JT, Chen JY, Brennand J, Caskey CT, Brinster RL: Expression of human HPRT in the central nervous system of transgenic mice. *Nature* **317**:250, 1985.
225. Bonnerot C, Grimber G, Briand P, Nicolas JF: Patterns of expression of position-dependent integrated transgenes in mouse embryo. *Proc Natl Acad Sci U S A* **87**:6331, 1990.
226. Wilson JM, Young AB, Kelley WN: Hypoxanthine-guanine phosphoribosyltransferase deficiency. The molecular basis of the clinical syndromes. *N Engl J Med* **309**:900, 1983.
227. Yang TP, Patel PI, Chinault AC, Stout JT, Jackson LG, Hildebrand BM, Caskey CT: Molecular evidence for new mutation at the hprt locus in Lesch-Nyhan patients. *Nature* **310**:412, 1984.
228. Wilson JM, Stout JT, Palella TD, Davidson BL, Kelley WN, Caskey CT: A molecular survey of hypoxanthine-guanine phosphoribosyltransferase deficiency in man. *J Clin Invest* **77**:188, 1986.
229. Gordon RB, Keough DT, Sculley DG, de Jersey J, Emmerson BT, Beacham IR: Characterization of genomic DNA, mRNA and enzyme protein in cases of HPRT-deficiency. *Adv Exp Med Biol* **253A**:151, 1989.
230. Lambert B, Andersson B, He SM, Hellgren D, Marcus S, Steen AM: Molecular analysis of mutation at the human hprt locus. *Acta Physiol Scand Suppl* **592**:85, 1990.
231. Singh S, Willers I, Held K, Goedde W: Lesch-Nyhan syndrome and HPRT variants: Study of heterogeneity at the gene level. *Adv Exp Med Biol* **253A**:145, 1989.
232. Sinnett D, Lavergne L, Melancon SB, Dallaire L, Potier M, Labuda D: Lesch-Nyhan syndrome: Molecular investigation of three French Canadian families using a hypoxanthine-guanine phosphoribosyltransferase cDNA probe. *Hum Genet* **81**:4, 1988.
233. Davidson BL, Tarle SA, Van Antwerp M, Gibbs DA, Watts RWE, Kelley WN, Palella TD: Identification of 17 independent mutations responsible for human hypoxanthine-guanine phosphoribosyltransferase (HPRT) deficiency. *Am J Hum Genet* **48**:951, 1991.
234. Gibbs RA, Caskey CT: Identification and localization of mutations at the Lesch-Nyhan locus by ribonuclease A cleavage. *Science* **236**:303, 1987.
235. Gibbs RA, Nguyen PN, Edwards A, Civitello AB, Caskey CT: Multiplex DNA deletion detection and exon sequencing of the hypoxanthine phosphoribosyltransferase gene in Lesch-Nyhan families. *Genomics* **7**:235, 1990.
236. Sculley DG, Dawson PA, Emmerson BT, Gordon RB: A review of the molecular basis of hypoxanthine-guanine phosphoribosyltransferase (HPRT) deficiency. *Hum Genet* **90**:195, 1992.
237. Sege-Peterson K, Nyhan WL, Page T: Lesch-Nyhan disease and HPRT deficiency, in Rosenberg RN, Prusiner SB, DiMauro S, Barchi RL, Kunkel LM (eds): *The Molecular and Genetic Basis of Neurological Disease*. Boston, Butterworth-Heinemann, 1992, p 241.
238. Tarle SA, Davidson BL, Wu VC, Zidar FJ, Seegmiller JE, Kelley WN, Palella TD: Determination of the mutations responsible for the Lesch-Nyhan syndrome in 17 subjects. *Genomics* **10**:499, 1991.
239. Yang TP, Stout JT, Konecki DS, Patel PI, Alford RL, Caskey CT: Spontaneous reversion of novel Lesch-Nyhan mutation by HPRT gene rearrangement. *Somat Cell Mol Genet* **14**:293, 1988.
240. Sege-Peterson K, Chambers J, Page T, Jones OW, Nyhan WL: Characterization of mutations in phenotypic variants of hypoxanthine phosphoribosyltransferase deficiency. *Hum Mol Genet* **1**:427, 1992.
241. Davidson BL, Tarle SA, Palella TD, Kelley WN: Molecular basis of hypoxanthine-guanine phosphoribosyltransferase deficiency in ten subjects determined by direct sequencing of amplified transcripts. *J Clin Invest* **84**:342, 1989.
242. Gibbs RA, Nguyen PN, McBride LJ, Koepf SM, Caskey CT: Identification of mutations leading to the Lesch-Nyhan syndrome by automated direct DNA sequencing of in vitro amplified cDNA. *Proc Natl Acad Sci U S A* **86**:1919, 1989.
243. Davidson BL, Pashmforoush M, Kelley WN, Palella TD: Genetic basis of hypoxanthine guanine phosphoribosyltransferase deficiency in a patient with the Lesch-Nyhan syndrome (HPRT Flint). *Gene* **63**:331, 1988.
244. Davidson BL, Palella TD, Kelley WN: Human hypoxanthine-guanine phosphoribosyltransferase: A single nucleotide substitution in cDNA clones isolated from a patient with Lesch-Nyhan syndrome (HPRT Midland). *Gene* **68**:85, 1988.
245. Kim KJ, Yamada Y, Suzumori K, Choi Y, Yang SW, Cheong HI, Hwang YS, Goto H, Ogasawara N: Molecular analysis of hypoxanthine guanine phosphoribosyltransferase (HPRT) gene in five Korean families with Lesch-Nyhan syndrome. *J Korean Med Sci* **12**:332, 1997.
246. Wehnert M, Herrmann FH: Characterization of three new deletions at the 5′ end of the HPRT structural gene. *J Inherit Metab Dis* **13**:178, 1990.
247. Lightfoot T, Lewkonia RM, Snyder FF: Sequence, expression, and characterization of $\text{HPRT}_{\text{Moose Jaw}}$: A point mutation resulting in cooperativity and decreased substrate affinities. *Hum Mol Genet* **3**:1377, 1994.

248. Davidson BL, Pashmforoush M, Kelley WN, Palella TD: Human hypoxanthine-guanine phosphoribosyltransferase deficiency: The molecular defect in a patient with gout ($HPRT_{Ashville}$). *J Biol Chem* **264**:520, 1989.
249. Fujimori S, Hidaka Y, Davidson BL, Palella TD, Kelley WN: Identification of a single nucleotide change in a mutant gene for hypoxanthine-guanine phosphoribosyltransferase ($HPRT_{Ann\ Arbor}$). *Hum Genet* **79**:39, 1988.
250. Gordon RB: Identification of a single nucleotide substitution in the coding sequence of in vitro amplified cDNA from a patient with partial HPRT deficiency ($HPRT_{Brisbane}$). *J Inherit Metab Dis* **13**:692, 1990.
251. O'Neill JP, Finette BA: Transition mutations at CpG dinucleotides are the most frequent in vivo spontaneous single-base substitution mutation in the human HPRT gene. *Environ Molec Mutagen* **32**:188, 1998.
252. Jinnah HA, DeGregorio L, Harris JC, Nyhan WL, O'Neill JP: The spectrum of inherited mutations causing HPRT deficiency: 75 new cases and a review of 196 previously reported cases. *Mutat Res* **463**:309, 2000.
253. Tvrdik T, Marcus S, Hou SM, Falt S, Noori P, Podlutskaja N, Hanefeld F, Stromme P, Lambert B: Molecular characterization of two deletion events involving *Alu*-sequences, one novel base substitution and two tentative hotspot mutations in the hypoxanthine-phosphoribosyltransferase (HPRT) gene in five patients with Lesch-Nyhan syndrome. *Hum Genet* **103**:311, 1998.
254. Wilson JM, Kelley WN: Molecular basis of hypoxanthine-guanine phosphoribosyltransferase deficiency in a patient with the Lesch-Nyhan syndrome. *J Clin Invest* **71**:1331, 1983.
255. Fujimori S, Davidson BL, Kelley WN, Palella TD: Identification of a single nucleotide change in the hypoxanthine-guanine phosphoribosyltransferase gene ($HPRT_{Yale}$) responsible for Lesch-Nyhan syndrome. *J Clin Invest* **83**:11, 1989.
256. Gordon RB, Dawson PA, Sculley DG, Emmerson BT, Caskey CT, Gibbs RA: The molecular characterisation of $HPRT_{Chermside}$ and $HPRT_{Coorparoo}$: Two Lesch-Nyhan patients with reduced amounts of mRNA. *Gene* **108**:299, 1991.
257. Monnat RJ Jr, Chiaverotti TA, Hackmann AF, Maresh GA: Molecular structure and genetic stability of human hypoxanthine phosphoribosyltransferase (HPRT) gene duplications. *Genomics* **13**:788, 1992.
258. Bouwens-Rombouts AG, van den Boogaard MJ, Puig JG, Mateos FA, Hennekam RC, Tilanus MG: Identification of two new nucleotide mutations ($HPRT_{Utrecht}$ and $HPRT_{Madrid}$) in exon 3 of the human hypoxanthine-guanine phosphoribosyltransferase (HPRT) gene. *Hum Genet* **91**:451, 1993.
259. Yamada Y, Goto H, Tamura S, Ogasawara N: Molecular genetic study of a Japanese family with Lesch-Nyhan syndrome: A point mutation at the consensus region of RNA splicing ($HPRT_{Keio}$). *Jpn J Hum Genet* **38**:413, 1993.
260. Davidson BL, Golovoy N, Roessler BJ: A 13 base pair deletion in exon 1 of $HPRT_{Illinois}$ forms a functional GUG initiation codon. *Hum Genet* **93**:300, 1994.
261. Renwick PJ, Birley AJ, McKeown CM, Hulten M: Southern analysis reveals a large deletion at the hypoxanthine phosphoribosyltransferase locus in a patient with Lesch-Nyhan syndrome. *Clin Genet* **48**:80, 1995.
262. Yamada Y, Suzumori K, Tanemura M, Goto H, Ogasawara N: Molecular analysis of a Japanese family with Lesch-Nyhan syndrome: Identification of mutation and prenatal diagnosis. *Clin Genet* **50**:164, 1996.
263. Tohyama J, Nanba E, Ohno K: Hypoxanthine-guanine phosphoribosyltransferase (HPRT) deficiency: Identification of point mutations in Japanese patients with Lesch-Nyhan syndrome and hereditary gout and their permanent expression in an HPRT-deficient mouse cell line. *Hum Genet* **93**:175, 1994.
264. Boyd M, Lanyon WG, Connor JM: Screening for molecular pathologies in Lesch-Nyhan syndrome. *Hum Mutat* **2**:127, 1993.
265. Fuscoe JC, Nelsen AJ: Molecular description of a hypoxanthine phosphoribosyltransferase gene deletion in Lesch-Nyhan syndrome. *Hum Mol Genet* **3**:199, 1994.
266. Sculley DG, Dawson PA, Beacham IR, Emmerson BT, Gordon RB: Hypoxanthine-guanine phosphoribosyltransferase deficiency: Analysis of HPRT mutations by direct sequencing and allele-specific amplification. *Hum Genet* **87**:688, 1991.
267. Yamada Y, Goto H, Suzumori K, Adachi R, Ogasawara N: Molecular analysis of five independent Japanese mutant genes responsible for hypoxanthine guanine phosphoribosyltransferase (HPRT) deficiency. *Hum Genet* **90**:379, 1992.
268. Yamada Y, Goto H, Ogasawara N: Identification of two independent Japanese mutant HPRT genes using the PCR technique. *Adv Exp Med Biol* **309B**:121, 1991.
269. Fujimori S, Tagaya T, Yamaoka N, Saito H, Kamatani N, Akaoka I: Direct evidence for a hot spot of germline mutation at HPRT locus. *Adv Exp Med Biol* **370**:679, 1994.
270. Hidalgo-Laos RI, Kedar A, Williams CA, Neiberger RE: A new point mutation in a hypoxanthine phosphoribosyltransferase-deficient patient. *Pediatr Nephrol* **11**:645, 1997.
271. Igarishi T, Minami M, Nishida Y: Molecular analysis of hypoxanthine-guanine phosphoribosyltransferase mutation in five unrelated Japanese patients. *Acta Paediatr Jpn* **31**:303, 1989.
272. Burgemeister R, Gutensohn W, Van den Berghe G, Jaeken J: Genetic and clinical heterogeneity in hypoxanthine phosphoribosyltransferase deficiencies. *Adv Exp Med Biol* **370**:331, 1994.
273. Torres RJ, Mateos FA, Molano J, Gathoff BS, O'Neill JP, Fundel RM, Trombley L, Puig JG: Molecular basis of hypoxanthine-guanine phosphoribosyltransferase deficiency in thirteen Spanish families. *Hum Mutat* (Online) **15**:383, 2000.
274. Chang SJ, Chang JG, Chen CJ, Wang JC, Ou TT, Chang KL, Ko YC: Identification of a new single nucleotide substitution on the hypoxanthine-guanine phosphoribosyltransferase gene ($HPRT_{Tsou}$) from a Taiwanese aboriginal family with severe gout. *J Rheumatol* **26**:1802, 1999.
275. Fujimori S, Tagaya T, Kamatani N, Akaoka I: A germ line mutation within the coding sequence for the putative 5-phosphoribosyl-1-pyrophosphate binding site of hypoxanthine-guanine phosphoribosyltransferase (HPRT) in a Lesch-Nyhan patient: Missense mutations within a functionally important region probably cause disease. *Hum Genet* **90**:385, 1992.
276. Hershey HV, Taylor MW: Nucleotide sequence and deduced amino acid sequence of *Escherichia coli* adenine phosphoribosyltransferase and comparison with other analogous enzymes. *Gene* **43**:287, 1986.
277. Eads JC, Scapin G, Xu Y, Grubmeyer C, Sacchettini JC: The crystal structure of human hypoxanthine-guanine phosphoribosyltransferase with bound GMP. *Cell* **78**:325, 1994.
278. Giacomello A, Salerno C: Human hypoxanthine-guanine phosphoribosyltransferase: Steady state kinetics of the forward and reverse reactions. *J Biol Chem* **253**:6038, 1978.
279. Balendiran GK, Molina JA, Xu Y, Torres-Martinez J, Stevens R, Focia PJ, Eakin AE, Sacchettini JC, Craig SP: Ternary complex structure of human HGPRTase, PRPP, Mg^{2+}, and the inhibitor HPP reveals the involvement of the flexible loop in substrate binding. *Protein Sci* **8**:1023, 1999.
280. Murray AW: The biological significance of purine salvage. *Ann Rev Biochem* **40**:811, 1971.
281. Patterson D: De novo purine and pyrimidine biosynthesis, in Bottesman MM (ed): *Molecular Cell Genetics*. New York, John Wiley, 1985, p 267.
282. Pritchard JB, Chavez-Peon F, Berlin RD: Purines: Supply by liver to tissues. *Am J Physiol* **219**:1263, 1970.
283. Johnson GG, Eisenberg LR, Migeon BR: Human and mouse hypoxanthine-guanine phosphoribosyltransferase: Dimers and tetramers. *Science* **203**:174, 1979.
284. Holden JA, Kelley WN: Human HPRT: Evidence for tetrameric structure. *J Biol Chem* **253**:4459, 1978.
285. Arnold WJ, Kelley WN: Human hypoxanthine-guanine phosphoribosyltransferase: Purification and subunit structure. *J Biol Chem* **246**:7398, 1971.
286. Wilson JM, Landa LE, Kobayashi R, Kelley WN: Human hypoxanthine-guanine phosphoribosyltransferase: Tryptic peptides and post-translational modification of the erythrocyte enzyme. *J Biol Chem* **257**:14830, 1982.
287. Johnson GG, Ramage AL, Littlefield JW, Kazazian HHJr: Hypoxathine-guanine phosphoribosyltransferase in human erythroid cells: Posttranslational modification. *Biochem* **21**:960, 1982.
288. Keough DT, Emmerson BT, de Jersey J: Localization of the 5-phospho-α-D-ribosyl-1-pyrophosphate binding site of human hypoxanthine-guanine phosphoribosyltransferase. *Biochim Biophys Acta* **1096**:95, 1991.
289. Argos P, Hanei M, Wilson JM, Kelley WN: A possible nucleotide-binding domain in the tertiary fold of phosphoribosyltransferases. *J Biol Chem* **258**:6450, 1983.
290. Musick WDL: Structural features of the phosphoribosyltransferases and their relationship to the human deficiency disorders of purine and pyrimidine metabolism. *Crit Rev Biochem* **11**:1, 1981.

291. Xu Y, Eads J, Sacchettini JC, Grubmeyer C: Kinetic mechanism of human hypoxanthine-guanine phosphoribosyltransferase: Rapid phosphoribosyl transfer chemistry. *Biochem* **36**:3700, 1997.
292. Fox IH, Kelley WN: Phosphoribosylpyrophosphate in man: Biochemical and clinical significance. *Ann Intern Med* **74**:424, 1971.
293. Salerno C, Giacomello A: Human hypoxanthine-guanine phosphoribosyltransferase: IMP-GMP exchange stoichiometry and steady state kinetics of the reaction. *J Biol Chem* **254**:10232, 1979.
294. Salerno C, Giacomello A: Human hypoxanthine guanine phosphoribosyltransferase: the role of magnesium ion in a phosphoribosylpyrophosphate-utilizing enzyme. *J Biol Chem* **256**:3671, 1981.
295. Richardson BJ, Ryckman DL, Komarnicki LM, Hamerton JL: Heterogeneity in the biochemical characteristics of red blood cell hypoxanthine-guanine phosphoribosyl transferase from two unrelated patients with the Lesch-Nyhan syndrome. *Biochem Genet* **9**:197, 1973.
296. Benke PJ, Herrick N, Hebert A: Hypoxanthine-guanine phosphoribosyltransferase variant associated with accelerated purine synthesis. *J Clin Invest* **52**:2234, 1973.
297. Keough DT, Gordon RB, de Jersey J, Emmerson BT: Biochemical basis of hypoxanthine-guanine phosphoribosyltransferase deficiency in nine families. *J Inherit Metab Dis* **11**:229, 1988.
298. Gutensohn W, Guroff G: Hypoxanthine-guanine-phosphoribosyltransferase from rat brain (purification, kinetic properties, development and distribution). *J Neurochem* **19**:2139, 1972.
299. Krenitsky RA: Tissue distribution of purine ribosyl- and phosphoribosyltransferases in the rhesus monkey. *Biochem Biophys Acta* **179**:506, 1969.
300. Braude PR, Monk M, Pickering SJ, Cant A, Johnson MH: Measurement of HPRT activity in the human unfertilized oocyte and pre-embryo. *Prenat Diagn* **9**:839, 1989.
301. Boyle JA, Raivio KO, Astrin KH, Schulman JD, Graf ML, Seegmiller JE, Jacobsen CB: Lesch-Nyhan syndrome: Preventive control by prenatal diagnosis. *Science* **169**:688, 1970.
302. Van Heeswijk PJ, Blank CH, Seegmiller JE, Jacobson CB: Preventive control of the Lesch-Nyhan syndrome. *Obstet Gynecol* **40**:109, 1972.
303. Shin-Buehring YS, Osang M, Wirtz A, Haas B, Rahm P, Schaub J: Prenatal diagnosis of Lesch-Nyhan syndrome and some characteristics of hypoxanthine-guanine phosphoribosyltransferase and adenine phosphoribosyltransferase in human tissues and cultivated cells. *Pediatr Res* **14**:825, 1980.
304. Adams A, Harkness RA: Developmental changes in purine phosphoribosyltransferases in human and rat tissues. *Biochem J* **160**:565, 1976.
305. Planet G, Willemot J: Changes in purine phosphoribosyltransferase activities in mouse brain, liver and muscle with age. *Biochem Biophys Acta* **364**:236, 1974.
306. Murray AW: Purine-phosphoribosyltransferase activities in rat and mouse tissues and in Ehrlich ascites-tumor cells. *Biochem J* **100**:664, 1966.
307. Jinnah HA, Page T, Friedmann T: Brain purines in a genetic mouse model of Lesch-Nyhan disease. *J Neurochem* **60**:2036, 1993.
308. Allsop J, Watts RWE: Activities of amidophosphoribosyltransferase and purine phosphoribosyltransferases in developing rat brain. *Adv Exp Med Biol* **122A**:361, 1979.
309. Ikeda K, Iida T, Nakagawa S: Postnatal expression of hypoxanthine-guanine phosphoribosyltransferase in the mouse brain. *Enz Prot* **47**:65, 1993.
310. Allsop J, Watts RW: Activities of amidophosphoribosyltransferase (EC2.4.2.14) and the purine phosphoribosyltransferases (EC2.4.2.7 and 2.4.2.8), and the phosphoribosylpyrophosphate content of rat central nervous system at different stages of development-their possible relationship to the neurological dysfunction in the Lesch-Nyhan syndrome. *J Neurol Sci* **46**:221, 1980.
311. Brosh S, Sperling O, Bromberg Y, Sidi Y: Developmental changes in the activity of enzymes of purine metabolism in rat neuronal cells in culture and in whole brain. *J Neurochem* **54**:1776, 1990.
312. Shaw G, Thomas SE: Purine nucleotide de novo biosynthesis in the brain. *J Neurochem* **27**:637, 1976.
313. Itiaba K, Banfalvi M, Crawhall JC: Variations in purine phosphoribosyl transferase enzymes during growth of fibroblast cell cultures. *Biochem Med* **6**:495, 1972.
314. Wood S, Pinsky L: Lesch-Nyhan mutation: The influence of population density on purine phosphoribosyltransferase activities and exogenous purine utilization in monolayer cultures of skin fibroblasts. *J Cell Physiol* **80**:33, 1972.
315. Balis ME, Krakoff IH, Berman PH, Dancis J: Urinary metabolites in congenital hyperuricosuria. *Science* **156**:1122, 1967.
316. Harkness RA, McCreanor GM, Watts RWE: Lesch-Nyhan syndrome and its pathogenesis: Purine concentrations in plasma and urine with metabolite profiles in CSF. *J Inherit Metab Dis* **11**:239, 1988.
317. Puig JG, Jimenez ML, Mateos FA, Fox IH: Adenine nucleotide turnover in hypoxanthine-guanine phosphoribosyl-transferase deficiency: Evidence for an increased contribution of purine biosynthesis de novo. *Metabolism* **38**:410, 1989.
318. Sweetman L, Nyhan WL: Excretion of hypoxanthine and xanthine in a genetic disease of purine metabolism. *Nature* **215**:859, 1967.
319. Sweetman L, Nyhan WL: Detailed comparison of the urinary excretion of purines in a patient with the Lesch-Nyhan syndrome and a control subject. *Biochem Med* **4**:121, 1970.
320. Sweetman L: Urinary and cerebrospinal fluid oxypurine levels and allopurinol metabolism in the Lesch-Nyhan syndrome. *Fed Proc* **27**:1055, 1968.
321. Schultz V, Lowenstein JM: Purine nucleotide cycle: Evidence for the occurrence of the cycle in the brain. *J Biol Chem* **251**:485, 1974.
322. Greene ML, Boyle JA, Seegmiller JE: Substrate stabilization: Genetically controlled reciprocal relationship of two human enzymes. *Science* **167**:887, 1970.
323. Beardmore TD, Meade JC, Kelley WN: Increased activity of two enzymes of pyrimidine biosynthesis de novo in erythrocytes from patients with the Lesch-Nyhan syndrome. *J Lab Clin Med* **81**:43, 1973.
324. Fairbanks LD, Simmonds HA, Webster DR: Use of intact erythrocytes in the diagnosis of inherited purine and pyrimidine disorders. *J Inherit Metab Dis* **10**:174, 1987.
325. Hershfield MS, Seegmiller JE: Regulation of de novo purine synthesis in human lymphoblasts. *J Biol Chem* **252**:6002, 1977.
326. Nuki G, Lever J, Seegmiller JE: Biochemical characteristics of 8-azaguanine resistant human lymphoblast mutants selected in vitro. *Adv Exp Med Biol* **41A**:255, 1973.
327. Wood AW, Becker MA, Seegmiller JE: Purine nucleotide synthesis in lymphoblasts cultured from normal subjects and a patient with Lesch-Nyhan syndrome. *Biochem Genet* **9**:261, 1973.
328. Rosenbloom FM, Henderson JF, Caldwell IC, Kelley WN, Seegmiller JE: Biochemical bases of accelerated purine biosynthesis de novo in human fibroblasts lacking hypoxanthine-guanine phosphoribosyltransferase. *J Biol Chem* **243**:1166, 1968.
329. Torrelio BM, Paz MA: Increased phosphoribosylpyrophosphate synthetase activity in fibroblasts of hypoxanthine-guanine phosphoribosyl transferase deficient patients. *Biochem Biophys Res Comm* **87**:380, 1979.
330. Benke PJ, Dittmar D: Phosphoribosylpyrophosphate synthesis in cultured human cells. *Science* **198**:1171, 1977.
331. Becker MA: Regulation of purine nucleotide synthesis. Effects of inosine on normal and hypoxanthine-guanine phosphoribosyltransferase-deficient fibroblasts. *Biochim Biophys Acta* **435**:132, 1976.
332. Boyle JA, Raivio KO, Becker MA, Seegmiller JE: Effects of nicotinic acid on human fibroblast purine biosynthesis. *Biochim Biophys Acta* **269**:179, 1972.
333. Skaper SD, Seegmiller JE: Purine metabolism in thioguanine-resistant glioma cells. *Exp Cell Res* **100**:415, 1976.
334. Martin DW, Maler BA: Phosphoribosylpyrophosphate synthetase is elevated in fibroblasts from patients with the Lesch-Nyhan syndrome. *Science* **193**:408, 1976.
335. Reem GH: Phosphoribosylpyrophosphate overproduction, a new metabolic abnormality in the Lesch-Nyhan syndrome. *Science* **190**:1098, 1975.
336. Graf LH, McRoberts JA, Harrison TM, Martin DW: Increased PRPP synthetase activity in cultured rat hepatoma cells containing mutations in the hypoxanthine-guanine phosphoribosyltransferase gene. *J Cell Physiol* **88**:331, 1976.
337. Henderson JF, Khoo MK: Synthesis of 5-phosphoribosyl 1-pyrophosphate from glucose in Ehrlich ascites tumor cells in vitro. *J Biol Chem* **240**:2349, 1965.
338. Rubin CS, Balis ME, Piomelli S, Berman PH, Dancis J: Elevated AMP pyrophosphorylase activity in congenital IMP pyrophosphorylase deficiency (Lesch-Nyhan disease). *J Lab Clin Med* **74**:732, 1969.
339. Bashkin P, Sperling O, Schmidt R, Szeinberg A: Erythrocyte adenine phosphoribosyltransferase in the Lesch-Nyhan syndrome. *Isr J Med Sci* **9**:1553, 1973.
340. Zoref E, Sperling O, Vries Ad: Abnormal property of human mutant hypoxanthine-guanine phosphoribosyltransferase: Insensitivity of fibroblast enzyme to stabilization against freezing and thawing by 5-phosphoribosyl-1- pyrophosphate. *Eur J Clin Invest* **4**:43, 1974.

341. De Bruyn CHMM, Oei TL, Geerdink RA, Lommen EJP: An atypical case of hypoxanthine-guanine phosphoribosyltransferase deficiency (Lesch-Nyhan syndrome). II. Genetic studies. *Clin Genet* **4**:353, 1973.
342. Henderson JF: Possible functions of hypoxanthine-guanine phosphoribosyltransferase and their relation to the biochemical pathology of the Lesch-Nyhan syndrome. *Fed Proc* **27**:1075, 1968.
343. Raivio KO, Seegmiller JE: Role of glutamine in purine synthesis and in guanine nucleotide formation in normal fibroblasts and in fibroblasts deficient in hypoxanthine phosphoribosyltransferase activity. *Biochim Biophys Acta* **299**:283, 1973.
344. Thorpe WP: The Lesch-Nyhan syndrome. *Enzyme* **12**:129, 1971.
345. Sidi Y, Mitchell BS: Z-nucleotide accumulation in erythrocytes from Lesch-Nyhan patients. *J Clin Invest* **76**:2416, 1985.
346. Simmonds HA, Fairbanks LD, Morris GS, Morgan G, Watson AR, Timms P, Singh B: Central nervous system dysfunction and erythrocyte guanosine triphosphate depletion in purine nucleoside phosphorylase deficiency. *Arch Dis Child* **62**:385, 1987.
347. Lommen EJP, Vogels GD, Van Der Zee SPM, Trijbels JMF, Schretlen EDAM: Concentrations of purine nucleotides in erythrocytes of patients with the Lesch-Nyhan syndrome before and during oral administration of adenine. *Acta Pediatr Scand* **60**:642, 1971.
348. Rivard GE, Izadi P, Lazerson J, McLaren JD, Parker C, Fish CH: Functional and metabolic studies of platelets from patients with Lesch-Nyhan syndrome. *Br J Haematol* **31**:245, 1975.
349. Brenton DP, Astrin KH, Cruikshank MK, Seegmiller JE: Measurement of free nucleotides in cultured human lymphoid cells using high pressure liquid chromatography. *Biochem Med* **17**:231, 1977.
350. Zoref-Shani E, Bromberg Y, Brosh S, Sidi Y, Sperling O: Characterization of alterations in purine nucleotide metabolism in hypoxanthine-guanine phosphoribosyltransferase-deficient rat neuroma cell line. *J Neurochem* **61**:457, 1993.
351. Snyder FF, Cruikshank MK, Seegmiller JE: A comparison of purine metabolism and nucleotide pools in normal and hypoxanthine-guanine phosphoribosyltransferase-deficient neuroblastoma cells. *Biochem Biophys Acta* **543**:556, 1978.
352. Skaper SD, Willis RC, Seegmiller JE: Intracellular 5-phosphoribosyl-1-pyrophosphate: Decreased availability during glutamine limitation. *Science* **193**:587, 1976.
353. Toyoda K, Miyamoto Y, Ida M, Tada S, Utsunomiya M: Hyperechoic medulla of the kidneys. *Radiology* **173**:431, 1989.
354. Rosenfeld DL, Preston MP, Salvaggi-Fadden K: Serial renal sonographic evaluation of patients with Lesch-Nyhan syndrome. *Pediatr Radiol* **24**:509, 1994.
355. Morton WJ: Lesch-Nyhan syndrome. *Urol* **20**:506, 1982.
356. Holdeigel M: Craniales Computertomogramm bei inkomplettem Lesch-Nyhan-Syndrom. *Radiologe* **27**:127, 1987.
357. Wong CJ: Radiology of Lesch-Nyhan disease. School of Medicine Thesis, University of California, San Diego 1988.
358. Ernst M, Zametkin AJ, Matochik JA, Pascualvaca D, Jons PH, Hardy K, Hankerson JG, Doudet DJ, Cohen RM: Presynaptic dopaminergic deficits in Lesch-Nyhan disease. *N Engl J Med* **334**:1568, 1996.
359. Harris JC, Lee RR, Jinnah HA, Wong DF, Yaster M, Bryan N: Craniocerebral magnetic resonance imaging measurement and findings in Lesch-Nyhan syndrome. *Arch Neurol* **55**:547, 1998.
360. Hoefnagel D: Summary: Pathology and pathologic physiology. *Fed Proc* **27**:1042, 1968.
361. Warzok R, Schwesinger G, Knapp A, Seidlitz F: Neuropathologische befunde beim Lesch-Nyhan Syndrom. *Zbl Allg Pathol U Pathol Anat* **126**:95, 1982.
362. Saito Y, Ito M, Hanaoka S, Ohama E, Akaboshi S, Takashima S: Dopamine receptor upregulation in Lesch-Nyhan syndrome: A postmortem study. *Neuropediatrics* **30**:66, 1999.
363. Manzke H, Gustmann H, Koke HB, Nyhan WL: Hypoxanthine and tetrahydrobiopterin treatment of a patient with features of the Lesch-Nyhan syndrome. **195A**:197, 1986.
364. Wong DF, Harris JC, Naidu S, Yokoi F, Marenco S, Dannals RF, Ravert HT, Yaster M, Evans A, Rousset O, Bryan RN, Gjedde A, Kuhar MJ, Breese GR: Dopamine transporters are markedly reduced in Lesch-Nyhan disease in vivo. *Proc Natl Acad Sci U S A* **93**:5539, 1996.
365. Finger S, Heavens RP, Sirinathsinghji DJS, Kuehn MR, Dunnett SB: Behavioral and neurochemical evaluation of a transgenic mouse model of Lesch-Nyhan syndrome. *J Neurol Sci* **86**:203, 1988.
366. Dunnett SB, Sirinathsinghji DJS, Heavens R, Rogers DC, Kuehn MR: Monoamine deficiency in a transgenic (Hprt−) mouse model of Lesch-Nyhan syndrome. *Brain Res* **501**:401, 1989.
367. Jinnah HA, Langlais PJ, Friedmann T: Functional analysis of brain dopamine systems in a genetic mouse model of Lesch-Nyhan syndrome. *J Pharmacol Exp Ther* **263**:596, 1992.
368. Jinnah HA, Wojcik BE, Hunt MA, Narang N, Lee KY, Goldstein M, Wamsley JK, Langlais PJ, Friedmann T: Dopamine deficiency in a genetic mouse model of Lesch-Nyhan disease. *J Neurosci* **14**:1164, 1994.
369. Jinnah HA, Jones MD, Wojcik BE, Rothstein JD, Hess EJ, Friedman T, Breese GR: Influence of age and strain on striatal dopamine loss in a genetic mouse model of Lesch-Nyhan disease. *J Neurochem* **72**:225, 1999.
370. Yeh J, Zheng S, Howard BD: Impaired differentiation of HPRT-deficient dopaminergic neurons: a possible mechanism underlying neuronal dysfunction in Lesch-Nyhan syndrome. *J Neurosci Res* **53**:78, 1998.
371. Rockson S, Stone R, Van der Weyden M, Kelley WN: Lesch-Nyhan syndrome: Evidence for abnormal adrenergic function. *Science* **186**:934, 1974.
372. Lake CR, Ziegler MG: Lesch-Nyhan syndrome: Low dopamine-β-hydroxylase activity and diminished sympathetic response to stress and posture. *Science* **196**:905, 1977.
373. Breakefield XO, Castiglione CM, Edelstein SB: Monoamine oxidase activity decreased in cells lacking hypoxanthine phosphoribosyltransferase activity. *Science* **192**:1018, 1976.
374. Singh S, Willers I, Kluss EM, Goedde HW: Monoamine oxidase and catechol-O-methyltransferase activity in cultured fibroblasts from patients with maple syrup urine disease, Lesch-Nyhan syndrome and healthy controls. *Clin Genet* **15**:153, 1979.
375. Skaper SD, Schafer IA: Monoamino oxidase activity reduced in cultured human fetal cells deficient in hypoxanthine-guanine phosphoribosyltransferase activity. *Biochem Genet* **16**:1135, 1978.
376. Skaper SD, Seegmiller JE: Hypoxanthine-guanine phosphoribosyltransferase mutant glioma cells: Diminished monoamine oxidase activity. *Science* **194**:1171, 1976.
377. Rassin DK, Lloyd KG, Kelley WN, Fox I: Decreased amino acids in various brain areas of patients with Lesch-Nyhan syndrome. *Neuropediatrics* **13**:130, 1982.
378. Harkness RA: Lesch-Nyhan syndrome: Reduced amino acid concentrations in CSF and brain. *Adv Exp Med Biol* **253A**:159, 1989.
379. Skaper SD, Seegmiller JE: Increased concentrations of glycine in hypoxanthine-guanine phosphoribosyltransferase-deficient mouse neuroblastoma cells. *J Neurochem* **26**:689, 1976.
380. Skaper SD, Seegmiller JE: Elevated intracellular glycine associated with hypoxanthine-guanine phosphoribosyltransferase deficiency in glioma cells. *J Neurochem* **29**:83, 1977.
381. Jinnah HA, Breese GR: Animal models for Lesch-Nyhan disease, in Iannocconne PM, Scarpelli DG (eds): *Biological Aspects of Disease: Contributions from Animal Models*. Amsterdam, Harwood Academic, 1997, p 93.
382. Dasheiff RM: Benzodiazepine treatment for Lesch-Nyhan syndrome? *Dev Med Child Neurol* **22**:101, 1980.
383. Norstrand IF: Lesch-Nyhan syndrome. *N Engl J Med* **306**:1368, 1982.
384. Kish SJ, Fox IH, Kapur BM, Lloyd KG, Hornykiewicz O: Brain benzodiazepine receptor binding and purine concentration in Lesch-Nyhan syndrome. *Brain Res* **336**:117, 1985.
385. Palmour RM: Animal models for Lesch-Nyhan disease, in Boulton A, Baker G, Butterworth R (eds): *Animal Models of Neurological Disease, I*. Totowa, NJ Humana Press, 1992, p 295.
386. Skolnick P, Marangos PJ, Goodwin FK, Edwards M, Paul SM: Identification of inosine and hypoxanthine as endogenous inhibitors of [^{3}H] diazepam binding in the central nervous system. *Life Sci* **23**:1473, 1978.
387. Fahn S, Cohen G: The oxidant stress hypothesis in Parkinson's disease: Evidence supporting it. *Ann Neurol* **32**:804, 1992.
388. Coyle JT, Puttfarcken P: Oxidative stress, glutamate, and neurodegenerative disorders. *Science* **262**:689, 1993.
389. Ben-Shachar D, Zuk R, Glinka Y: Dopamine neurotoxicity: Inhibition of mitochondrial respiration. *J Neurochem* **64**:718, 1995.
390. Filloux F, Townsend JJ: Pre- and postsynaptic neurotoxic effect of dopamine demonstrated by intrastriatal injection. *Exp Neurol* **119**:79, 1993.
391. Hasting TG, Lewis DA, Zigmond MJ: Role of oxidation in the neurotoxic effects of intrastriatal dopamine injections. *Proc Natl Acad Sci U S A* **93**:1956, 1996.
392. Michel PP, Hefti F: Toxicity of 6-hydroxydopamine and dopamine for dopaminergic neurons in culture. *J Neurosci Res* **26**:428, 1990.

393. Parks DA, Granger DN: Xanthine oxidase: Biochemistry, distribution and physiology. *Acta Physiol Scand Suppl* **548**:87, 1986.
394. Beal MF: Aging, energy, and oxidative stress in neurodegenerative disease. *Ann Neurol* **38**:357, 1995.
395. Hersch SM, Ferrante RJ: Neuropathology and pathophysiology of Huntington's disease, in Watts RL, Koller WC (eds): *Movement Disorders: Neurological Principles and Practice*. New York, McGraw-Hill, 1997, p 503.
396. Sharp AH, Loev SJ, Schilling B, Li SH, Li XJ, Bao J, Wagster MV, Kotzuk JA, Steiner JP, Lo A, Hedreen H, Sisodia S, Snyder SH, Dawson TM, Ryugo DK, Ross CA: Widespread expression of Huntington's disease gene (IT15) protein product. *Neuron* **14**:1065, 1995.
397. Brown RH: Amyotrophic lateral sclerosis: Recent insights from genetics and transgenic mice. *Cell* **80**:687, 1995.
398. McKeran RO, Watts RW: Use of phytohaemagglutinin stimulated lymphocytes to study effects of hypoxanthine-guanine phosphoribosyltransferase (HGPRT) deficiency on polynucleotide and protein synthesis in the Lesch-Nyhan syndrome. *J Med Genet* **13**:91, 1976.
399. Watts RWE: Defects of tetrahydrobiopterin synthesis and their possible relationship to a disorder of purine metabolism (the Lesch-Nyhan Syndrome). *Adv Enz Regul* **23**:25, 1985.
400. Curto R, Voit EO, Cascante M: Analysis of abnormalities in purine metabolism leading to gout and to neurological dysfunctions in man. *Biochem J* **329**:477, 1998.
401. Goldstein M: Dopaminergic mechanisms in self-inflicting biting behavior. *Psychopharmacol Bull* **25**:349, 1989.
402. Sebesta I, Krijt J, Kmoch S, Hyanek J: Urinary pterins in Lesch-Nyhan syndrome. *Adv Exp Med Biol* **309B**:261, 1991.
403. Lloyd HGE, Stone TW: Chronic methylxanthine treatment in rats: A comparison of Wistar and Fisher 344 strains. *Pharmacol Biochem Behav* **14**:827, 1981.
404. Scriver CR, Eisensmith RC: The hyperphenylalaninemias, in Scriver CR, Beaudet AL, Sly WS, Valle D (eds): *The Metabolic and Molecular Basis of Inherited Disease* 5th ed. New York, McGraw-Hill, 1983, p 270.
405. Birnbaumer L: G-proteins in signal transduction. *Ann Rev Pharmacol Toxicol* **30**:675, 1990.
406. Gilman AG: G proteins: Transducers of receptor-generated signals. *Ann Rev Biochem* **56**:615, 1987.
407. Dunwiddie TV: The physiological role of adenosine in the central nervous system. *Int Rev Neurobiol* **27**:63, 1985.
408. Snyder SH: Adenosine as a neuromodulator. *Ann Rev Neurosci* **8**:103, 1985.
409. Jarvis MF, Williams M: Adenosine and dopamine function in the CNS. *Trends Pharmacol Sci* **8**:330, 1987.
410. Ferre S, Fuxe K, Von Euler G, Johansson B, Fredholm BB: Adenosine-dopamine interactions in the brain. *Neuroscience* **51**:501, 1992.
411. Ferre S, Fredholm BB, Morelli M, Popoli P, Fuxe K: Adenosine-dopamine receptor-receptor interactions as an integrative mechanism in the basal ganglia. *Trends Neurosci* **20**:482, 1997.
412. Pritchard JB, O'Connor N, Oliver JM, Berlin RD: Uptake and supply of purine compounds by the liver. *Am J Physiol* **229**:967, 1975.
413. Stone TW: Physiological roles for adenosine and adenosine 5′-triphosphate in the nervous system. *Neuroscience* **6**:523, 1981.
414. Kopin IJ: Neurotransmitters and the Lesch-Nyhan syndrome. *N Engl J Med* **305**:1148, 1981.
415. Green RD, Proudfit JK, Yeung SH: Modulation of striatal dopaminergic function by local injection of 5′-N-ethylcarboxamide adenosine. *Science* **218**:58, 1982.
416. Criswell H, Mueller RA, Breese GR: Assessment of purine-dopamine interaction in 6-hydroxydopamine-lesioned rats: Evidence for pre- and postsynaptic influences by adenosine. *J Pharmacol Exp Ther* **244**:493, 1988.
417. Jinnah HA, Gage FH, Friedmann T: Animal models of Lesch-Nyhan syndrome. *Brain Res Bull* **25**:467, 1990.
418. Kuehn MR, Bradley A, Robertson EJ, Evans MJ: A potential animal model for Lesch-Nyhan syndrome through introduction of HPRT mutations into mice. *Nature* **326**:295, 1987.
419. Hooper M, Hardy K, Handyside A, Hunter S, Monk M: HPRT-deficient (Lesch-Nyhan) mouse embryos derived from germline colonization by cultured cells. *Nature* **326**:292, 1987.
420. Williamson DJ, Sharkey J, Clarke AR, Jamieson A, Arbuthnott GW, Kelly PAT, Melton DW, Hooper ML: Analysis of forebrain dopaminergic pathways in HPRT− mice. *Adv Exp Med Biol* **309B**:269, 1991.
421. Jinnah HA, Gage FH, Friedmann T: Amphetamine-induced behavioral phenotype in a hypoxanthine-guanine phosphoribosyltransferase-deficient mouse model of Lesch-Nyhan syndrome. *Behav Neurosci* **105**:1004, 1991.
422. Wu X, Wakamiya M, Vaishnav S, Geske R, Montgomery C Jr, Jones P, Bradley A, Caskey CT: Hyperuricemia and urate nephropathy in urate oxidase-deficient mice. *Proc Natl Acad Sci U S A* **91**:742, 1994.
423. Wu CL, Melton DW: Production of a model for Lesch-Nyhan syndrome in hypoxanthine phosphoribosyltransferase-deficient mice. *Nature Genet* **3**:235, 1993.
424. Edamuar K, Sasai H: No self-injurious behavior was found in HPRT-deficient mice treated with 9-ethyladenine. *Pharmacol Biochem Behav* **61**:175, 1998.
425. Redhead NJ, Selfridge J, Wu ChL, Melton DW: Mice with adenine phosphoribosyltransferase deficiency develop fatal 2,8-dihydroxyadenine lithiasis. *Hum Gene Ther* **1**:1491, 1996.
426. Engle SJ, Womer DE, Davies PM, Boivin G, Sahota A, Simmonds HA, Stambrook PJ, Tischfield JA: HPRT-APRT deficient mice are not a model for Lesch-Nyhan syndrome. *Hum Mol Genet* **5**:1607, 1996.
427. Breese GR, Baumeister AA, McCown TJ, Emerick SG, Frye GD, Crotty K, Mueller RA: Behavioral differences between neonatal and adult 6-hydroxydopamine-treated rats to dopamine agonists: Relevance to neurological symptoms in clinical syndromes with reduced brain dopamine. *J Pharmacol Exp Ther* **231**:343, 1984.
428. Breese GR, Duncan GE, Napier TC, Bondy SC, Iorio LC, Mueller RA: 6-hydroxydopamine treatments enhance behavioral responses to intracerebral microinjection of D1- and D2-dopamine agonists into nucleus accumbens and striatum without changing dopamine antagonist binding. *J Pharmacol Exp Ther* **240**:167, 1987.
429. Erinoff L, Snodgrass SR: Effects of adult or neonatal treatment with 6-hydroxydopamine or 5,7-dihydroxytryptamine on locomotor activity, monoamine levels, and response to caffeine. *Pharmacol Biochem Behav* **24**:1039, 1986.
430. Archer T, Danysz W, Fredriksson A, Jonsson G, Luthman J, Sundstrom E, Teiling A: Neonatal 6-hydroxydopamine-induced dopamine depletions: Motor activity and performance in maze learning. *Pharmacol Biochem Behav* **31**:357, 1988.
431. Miller FE, Heffner TG, Kotake C, Seiden LS: Magnitude and duration of hyperactivity following neonatal 6-hydroxydopamine is related to the extent of brain dopamine depletion. *Brain Res* **229**:123, 1981.
432. Pappas BA, Peters DAV, Sobrian SK, Blouin A, Drew B: Early behavioral and catecholaminergic effects of 6-hydroxydopamine and guanethidine in the neonatal rat. *Pharmacol Biochem Behav* **3**:681, 1974.
433. Shaywitz BA, Klopper JH, Yager RD, Gordon JW: Paradoxical response to amphetamine in developing rats treated with 6-hydroxydopamine. *Nature* **261**:153, 1976.
434. Castenada E, Whishaw IQ, Lermer L, Robinson TE: Dopamine depletion in neonatal rats: Effects on behavior and striatal dopamine release assessed by intracerebral microdialysis during adulthood. *Brain Res* **508**:30, 1990.
435. Shaywitz BA, Yager RD, Klopper JH: Selective brain dopamine depletion in developing rats: An experimental model of minimal brain dysfunction. *Science* **191**:305, 1976.
436. Pappas BA, Gallivan JV, Dugas T, Saari M, Ings R: Intraventricular 6-hydroxydopamine in the newborn rat and locomotor responses to drugs in infancy: No support for the dopamine depletion model of minimal brain dysfunction. *Psychopharmacol* **70**:41, 1980.
437. Breese GR, Baumeister AA, McCown TJ, Emerick SG, Frye GD, Mueller RA: Neonatal-6-hydroxydopamine treatment: Model of susceptibility for self-mutilation in the Lesch-Nyhan syndrome. *Pharmacol Biochem Behav* **21**:459, 1984.
438. Breese GR, Baumeister A, Napier TC, Frye GD, Mueller RA: Evidence that D-1 dopamine receptors contribute to the supersensitive behavioral responses induced by L-dihydroxyphenylalanine in rats treated neonatally with 6-hydroxydopamine. *J Pharmacol Exp Ther* **235**:287, 1985.
439. Breese GR, Criswell HE, Mueller RA: Evidence that lack of brain dopamine during development can increase the susceptibility for aggression and self-injurious behavior by influencing D1-dopamine receptor function. *Prog Neuro-Psychopharmacol Biol Psychiat* **14**:S65, 1990.
440. Breese GR, Napier TC, Mueller RA: Dopamine agonist-induced locomotor activity in rats treated with 6-hydroxydopamine at differing ages: Functional supersensitivity of D-1 dopamine receptors in neonatally lesioned rats. *J Pharmacol Exp Ther* **234**:447, 1985.
441. Brautigam C, Wevers RA, Jansen RJT, Smeitink JAM, De Rijk-Van Andel JF, Gabreels FJM, Hoffmann GF: Biochemical hallmarks of tyrosine hydroxylase deficiency. *Clin Chem* **44**:1897, 1998.

442. Hyland K, Surtees RAH, Rodeck C, Clayton PT: Aromatic L-amino acid decarboxylase deficiency: Clinical features, diagnosis, and treatment of a new inborn error of neurotransmitter amine synthesis. *Neurology* **42**:1980, 1992.
443. Rajput AH, Gibb WRG, Zhong XH, Shannak KS, Kish S, Chang LG, Hornykiewicz O: Dopa-responsive dystonia: Pathological and biochemical observations in a case. *Ann Neurol* **35**:396, 1994.
444. Blue ME, Molliver ME: 6-hydroxydopamine induces serotonergic axon sprouting in cerebral cortex of newborn rat. *Dev Brain Res* **32**:255, 1987.
445. Sivam SP, Krause JE, Breese GR, Hong JS: Dopamine-dependent postnatal development of enkephalin and tachykinin neurons of rat basal ganglia. *J Neurochem* **56**:1499, 1991.
446. Dewar KM, Soghomonian JJ, Bruno JP, Descarries L, Reader TA: Elevation of dopamine D2 but not D1 receptors in adult rat neostriatum after neonatal 6-hydroxydopamine denervation. *Brain Res* **536**:287, 1990.
447. Berger TW, Kaul S, Stricker EM, Zigmond MJ: Hyperinnervation of the striatum by dorsal raphe afferents after dopamine-depleting brain lesions in neonatal rats. *Brain Res* **336**:354, 1985.
448. Towle AC, Criswell HE, Maynard EH, Lauder JM, Joh TH, Mueller RA, Breese GR: Serotonergic innervation of the rat caudate following a neonatal 6-hydroxydopamine lesion: An anatomical, biochemical and pharmacological study. *Pharmacol Biochem Behav* **34**:367, 1989.
449. Stachowiak MK, Bruno JP, Snyder AM, Stricker EM, Zigmond MJ: Apparent sprouting of striatal serotonergic terminals after dopamine-depleting brain lesions in neonatal rats. *Brain Res* **291**:164, 1984.
450. Luthman J, Bolioli B, Tsutsumi T, Verhofstad A, Jonsson G: Sprouting of striatal serotonin nerve terminals following selective lesions of nigro-striatal dopamine neurons in neonatal rat. *Brain Res Bull* **19**:269, 1987.
451. Snyder AM, Zigmond MJ, Lund RD: Sprouting of serotoninergic afferents into striatum after dopamine-depleting lesions in infant rats: A retrograde transport and immunocytochemical study. *J Comp Neurol* **245**:274, 1986.
452. Allen SM, Freeman JN, Davis WM: Evaluation of risperidone in the neonatal 6-hydroxydopamine model of Lesch-Nyhan syndrome. *Pharmacol Biochem Behav* **59**:327, 1998.
453. Mizuno T, Yugari Y: Self-mutilation in Lesch-Nyhan syndrome. *Lancet* **1**:761, 1974.
454. Anderson LT, Herrmann L, Dancis J: The effect of L-5-hydroxytryptophan on self-mutilation in Lesch-Nyhan disease: A negative report. *Neuropediatrics* **7**:439, 1976.
455. Frith CD, Johnstone EC, Joseph MH, Powell RJ, Watts RWE: Double-blind clinical trial of 5-hydroxytryptophan in a case of Lesch-Nyhan syndrome. *J Neurol Neurosurg Psychiatry* **39**:656, 1976.
456. Sweetman L, Borden M, Kulovich S, Kaufman I, Nyhan WL: Altered excretion of 5-hydroxyindoleacetic acid and glycine in patients with the Lesch-Nyhan disease. *Adv Exp Med Biol* **76A**:398, 1977.
457. Primeau F, Fontaine R: Obsessive disorder with self-mutilation: A subgroup responsive to pharmacotherapy. *Can J Psychiat* **32**:699, 1987.
458. Criswell HE, Johnson KB, Mueller RA, Breese GR: Evidence for involvement of brain dopamine and other mechanisms in the behavioral action of the *N*-methyl-D-aspartic acid antagonist MK-801 in control and 6-hydroxydopamine-lesioned rats. *J Pharmacol Exp Ther* **265**:1001, 1993.
459. Genovese E, Napoli PA, Bolego-Zonta N: Self-aggressiveness: A new type of behavioral change induced by pemoline. *Life Sci* **8**:513, 1969.
460. Mueller K, Hsiao S: Pemoline-induced self-biting in rats and self-mutilation in the de Lange syndrome. *Pharmacol Biochem Behav* **13**:627, 1980.
461. Mueller K, Nyhan WL: Pharmacologic control of pemoline induced self-injurious behavior in rats. *Pharmacol Biochem Behav* **16**:957, 1982.
462. King BH, Au D, Poland RE: Pretreatment with MK-801 inhibits pemoline-induced self-biting behavior in prepubertal rats. *Dev Neurosci* **17**:47, 1995.
463. Huberman HS, Eison MS, Bryan KS, Ellison G: A slow-release silicone pellet for chronic amphetamine administration. *Eur J Pharmacol* **45**:237, 1977.
464. Mueller K, Saboda S, Palmour R, Nyhan WL: Self-injurious behavior produced in rats by daily caffeine and continuous amphetamine. *Pharmacol Biochem Behav* **17**:613, 1982.
465. Brien JF, Peachy JE, Rogers BJ, Kitney JC: Amphetamine-induced stereotyped behaviour and brain concentrations of amphetamine and its hydroxylated metabolites in mice. *J Pharm Pharmacol* **29**:49, 1977.
466. Mueller K, Hollingsworth E, Pettit H: Repeated pemoline produces self-injurious behavior in adult and weanling rats. *Pharmacol Biochem Behav* **25**:933, 1986.
467. Sivam SP: GBR-12909-induced self-injurious behavior: Role of dopamine. *Brain Res* **690**:259, 1995.
468. Kelley AE, Lang CG, Gauthier AM: Induction of oral stereotypy following amphetamine microinjection into a discrete subregion of the striatum. *Psychopharmacol* **95**:556, 1988.
469. Kelley AE, Gauthier AM, Lang CG: Amphetamine microinjections into distinct striatal subregions cause dissociable effects on motor and ingestive behavior. *Behav Brain Res* **35**:24, 1989.
470. Delfs JM, Kelley AE: The role of D1 and D2 dopamine receptors in oral stereotypy induced by dopaminergic stimulation of the ventrolateral striatum. *Neuroscience* **39**:59, 1990.
471. Peters JM: Caffeine-induced hemorrhagic automutilation. *Arch Intern Pharmacodyn* **169**:139, 1967.
472. Morgan LL, Schneiderman N, Nyhan WL: Theophylline: Induction of self-biting in rabbits. *Psychon Sci* **19**:37, 1970.
473. Sakata T, Fuchimoto H: Stereotyped and aggressive behavior induced by sustained high dose of theophylline in rats. *Jpn J Pharmacol* **23**:781, 1973.
474. Ferrer I, Costell M, Grisolia S: Lesch-Nyhan syndrome-like behavior in rats from caffeine ingestion. *FEBS Lett* **141**:275, 1982.
475. Daly JW, Bruns RF, Snyder SH: Adenosine receptors in the central nervous system: relationship to the central actions of methylxanthines. *Life Sci* **28**:2083, 1981.
476. Morpurgo C: Aggressive behavior induced by large doses of 2-(2,6-dichlorphenylamino)-2-imidazoline hydrochloride (ST 155) in mice. *Eur J Pharmacol* **3**:374, 1968.
477. Katsuragi T, Ushijima I, Furukawa T: The clonidine-induced self-injurious behavior of mice involves purinergic mechanisms. *Pharmacol Biochem Behav* **20**:943, 1984.
478. Ushijima I, Katsuragi T, Furukawa T: Involvement of adenosine receptor activities in aggressive responses produced by clonidine in mice. *Psychopharmacol* **83**:335, 1984.
479. Razzak A, Fujiwara M, Ueki S: Automutilation induced by clonidine in mice. *Eur J Pharmacol* **30**:356, 1975.
480. Razzak A, Fujiwara M, Oishi R, Ueki S: Possible involvement of a central noradrenergic system in automutilation induced by clonidine in mice. *Jpn J Pharmacol* **27**:145, 1977.
481. Mueller K, Nyhan WL: Clonidine potentiates drug induced self-injurious behavior in rats. *Pharmacol Biochem Behav* **18**:891, 1983.
482. De Feo G, Lisciani R, Pavan L, Samarelli M, Valeri P: Possible dopaminergic involvement in biting compulsion induced by large doses of clonidine. *Pharmacol Res Commun* **15**:613, 1983.
483. Hoffman BB, Lefkowitz RJ: Catecholamines, sympathomimetic drugs, and adrenergic receptor antagonists, in Hardman JG, Limbird LE, Molinoff PB, Ruddon RW, Gilman AG (eds): *The Pharmacological Basis of Therapeutics*. New York, McGraw-Hill, 1985, p 199.
484. Kulkarni SK, Mehta AK: P1-purinoceptor antagonism by clonidine in the rat caecum. *Life Sci* **34**:2273, 1984.
485. Stone TW, Taylor DA: Clonidine as an adenosine antagonist. *J Pharm Pharmacol* **30**:792, 1978.
486. Stone TW, Taylor DA: Antagonism by clonidine of neuronal depressant responses to adenosine and adenosine-5′-monophosphate and adenosine triphosphate. *Br J Pharmacol* **64**:369, 1978.
487. Katsuragi T, Su C: Facilitation by clonidine of purine release induced by high KCl from the rabbit pulmonary artery. *Br J Pharmacol* **74**:709, 1981.
488. Baumeister AA, Rollings JP: Self-injurious behavior. *Int Rev Res Mental Retard* **8**:1, 1976.
489. Winchel RM, Stanley M: Self-injurious behavior: A review of the behavior and biology of self-mutilation. *Am J Psychiatry* **148**:306, 1991.
490. Shear CS, Nyhan WL, Kirman BH, Stern J: Self-mutilative behavior as a feature of the de Lange syndrome. *J Pediatr* **78**:506, 1971.
491. Warnock JK, Kestenbaum T: Pharmacologic treatment of severe skin-picking behaviors in Prader-Willi syndrome. *Arch Dermatol* **128**:1623, 1992.
492. Hardie RJ: Acanthocytosis and neurological impairment — A review. *QJM* **71**:291, 1989.
493. Moldofsky H, Tullis C, Lamon R: Multiple tic syndrome (Gilles de la Tourette's syndrome). *J Nerv Ment Dis* **159**:282, 1974.
494. Comings DE, Comings BG: Tourette syndrome: Clinical and psychological aspects of 250 cases. *Am J Hum Genet* **37**:435, 1985.
495. Shua-Haim JR, Gross JS: Lesch-Nyhan syndrome in an Alzheimer's disease patient: A case report. *J Am Geriatr Soc* **45**:1034, 1997.

496. Fenichel GM: *Clinical Pediatric Neurology: A Signs and Symptoms Approach*. Philadelphia, WB Saunders, 1997.
497. Rosenberg AL, Bergstrom L, Troost T, Bartholomew BA: Hyperuricemia and neurological deficits. *N Engl J Med* **282**:992, 1970.
498. Mavrikakis ME, Sfikakis PP, Kontoyannis DA, Antoniades LG, Tsaknikas C: Gout and neurological abnormalities associated with cardiomyopathy in a young man. *Ann Rheum Dis* **49**:942, 1990.
499. Laszlo A, Osztovics M, Dallmann L, Mattyus A: Hyperuricaemia associated with 18q deletion. Atypical Lesch-Nyhan syndrome? *Ann Genet* **24**:17, 1981.
500. Cameron JS, Moro F, Simmonds HA: Gout, uric acid and purine metabolism in paediatric nephrology. *Pediatr Nephrol* **7**:105, 1993.
501. Holland MJ, DiLorenzo AM, Dancis J, Balis ME, Yu TF, Cox RP: Hypoxanthine phosphoribosyltransferase activity in intact fibroblasts from patients with X-linked hyperuricemia. *J Clin Invest* **57**:1600, 1976.
502. Cox RP, Krauss MR, Balis ME, Yip LC, Jansen V, Dancis J: Incorporation of hypoxanthine by PHA-stimulated HPRT-deficient lymphocytes. *Exp Cell Res* **88**:289, 1974.
503. Gordon RB, Keough DT, Emmerson BT: HPRT-deficiency associated with normal PRPP concentration and APRT activity. *J Inherit Metab Dis* **10**:82, 1987.
504. Willers I, Singh S, Held KR, Goedde HW: High HPRT activity in fibroblasts from patients with Lesch-Nyhan syndrome due to bacterial "L-form" contamination. *Adv Exp Med Biol* **122A**:327, 1980.
505. Stanbridge EJ, Tischfield JA, Schneider EL: Appearance of hypoxanthine guanine phosphoribosyltransferase activity as a consequence of mycoplasma contamination. *Nature* **256**:329, 1975.
506. Salzmann J, DeMars R, Benke P: Single-allele expression at an X-linked hyperuricemia locus in heterozygous human cells. *Proc Natl Acad Sci U S A* **60**:545, 1968.
507. Johnson LA, Gordon RB, Emmerson BT: Two populations of heterozygote erythrocytes in moderate hypoxanthine guanine phosphoribosyltransferase deficiency. *Nature* **264**:172, 1976.
508. McKeran RO, Andrews TM, Howell A, Gibbs DA, Chinn S, Watts WE: The diagnosis of the carrier state for the Lesch-Nyhan syndrome. *QJM* **44**:189, 1975.
509. Migeon BR, Axelman J, Beggs AH: Effect of ageing on reactivation of the human X-linked HPRT locus. *Nature* **335**:93, 1988.
510. Nyhan WL, Bakay B, Connor JD, Marks JF, Keele DK: Hemizygous expression of glucose-6-phosphate dehydrogenase in erythrocytes of heterozygotes for the Lesch-Nyhan syndrome. *Proc Natl Acad Sci U S A* **65**:214, 1970.
511. Migeon BR: Studies of skin fibroblasts from 10 families with HGPRT deficiency, with reference to X-chromosomal inactivation. *Am J Hum Genet* **23**:199, 1971.
512. Dancis J, Cox RP, Berman PH, Jansen V, Balis ME: Cell population density and phenotypic expression of tissue culture fibroblasts from heterozygotes of Lesch-Nyhan's disease (inosinate pyrophosphorylase deficiency). *Biochem Genet* **3**:609, 1969.
513. Albertini RJ, DeMars R: Mosaicism of peripheral blood lymphocyte populations in females heterozygous for the Lesch-Nyhan mutation. *Biochem Genet* **11**:397, 1974.
514. Migeon BR: X-linked hypoxanthine-guanine phosphoribosyltransferase deficiency: Detection of heterozygotes by selective medium. *Biochem Genet* **4**:377, 1970.
515. Felix JS, DeMars R: Detection of females heterozygous for the Lesch-Nyhan mutation by 8-azaguanine-resistant growth of cultured fibroblasts. *J Lab Clin Med* **77**:596, 1971.
516. Kamatani N, Yamanaka H, Nishioka K, Nakamura T, Nakano K, Tanimoto K, Mizuno T, Nishida Y: A new method for the detection of Lesch-Nyhan heterozygotes by peripheral blood T cell culture using T cell growth factor. *Blood* **63**:912, 1984.
517. Dempsey JL, Morley AA, Seshadri RS, Emmerson BT, Gordon R, Bhagat CI: Detection of the carrier state for an X-linked disorder, the Lesch-Nyhan syndrome, by the use of lymphocyte cloning. *Hum Genet* **64**:288, 1983.
518. Dancis J, Silvers DN, Balis ME, Cox RP, Schwartz MS: Evidence for the derivation of individual hair roots from three progenitor cells. *Hum Genet* **58**:414, 1981.
519. Bruyn CH, Oei TL, Haar BG: Studies on hair roots for carrier detection in hypoxanthine-guanine phosphoribosyl transferase deficiency. *Clin Genet* **5**:449, 1974.
520. Silvers DN, Cox RP, Balis ME, Dancis J: Detection of heterozygote in Lesch-Nyhan disease by hair-root analysis. *N Engl J Med* **286**:390, 1972.
521. Francke U, Bakay B, Nyhan WL: Detection of heterozygous carriers of the Lesch-Nyhan syndrome by electrophoresis of hair root lysates. *J Pediatr* **82**:472, 1973.
522. Bakay B, Tucker-Pian C, Seegmiller JE: Detection of Lesch-Nyhan syndrome carriers: Analysis of hair roots for HPRT by agarose gel electrophoresis and autoradiography. *Clin Genet* **17**:369, 1980.
523. Page T, Bakay B, Nyhan WL: An improved procedure for detection of hypoxanthine-guanine phosphoribosyl transferase heterozygotes. *Clin Chem* **28**:1181, 1982.
524. Gartler SM, Scott RC, Goldstein JL, Campbell B: Lesch-Nyhan syndrome: Rapid detection of heterozygotes by use of hair follicles. *Science* **172**:572, 1971.
525. Puig JG, Mateos FA, Torres RJ, Buno AS: Purine metabolism in female heterozygotes for hypoxanthine-guanine phosphoribosyltransferase deficiency. *Eur J Clin Invest* **28**:950, 1998.
526. Alford RL, Redman JB, O'Brien WE, Caskey CT: Lesch-Nyhan syndrome: carrier and prenatal diagnosis. *Prenat Diagn* **15**:329, 1995.
527. Singh S, Willers I, Goedde HW: A rapid micromethod for prenatal diagnosis of Lesch-Nyhan syndrome. *Clin Genet* **10**:12, 1976.
528. Hosli P, de Bruyn CH, Oerlemans FJ, Verjaal M, Nobrega RE: Rapid prenatal diagnosis of HG-PRT deficiency using ultra-microchemical methods. *Hum Genet* **37**:195, 1977.
529. Richardson BJ, Cox DM: Rapid tissue culture and microbiochemical methods for analyzing colonially grown fibroblasts from normal, Lesch-Nyhan and Tay-Sachs patients and amniotic fluid cells. *Clin Genet* **4**:376, 1973.
530. Zoref-Shani E, Bromberg Y, Goldman B, Shaki R, Barkai G, Legum C, Sperling O: Prenatal diagnosis of Lesch-Nyhan syndrome: Experience with three fetuses at risk. *Prenat Diagn* **9**:657, 1989.
531. Burkhardt WC Jr, Jackson JF, Clement EG, Sherline DM: Prenatal diagnosis of the Lesch-Nyhan syndrome. *J Reprod Med* **21**:169, 1978.
532. Halley D, Heukels-Dully MJ: Rapid prenatal diagnosis of the Lesch-Nyhan syndrome. *J Med Genet* **14**:100, 1977.
533. Stout JT, Jackson LG, Caskey CT: First trimester diagnosis of Lesch-Nyhan syndrome: Applications to other disorders of purine metabolism. *Prenat Diagn* **5**:183, 1985.
534. Graham GW, Aitken DA, Connor JM: Prenatal diagnosis by enzyme analysis in 15 pregnancies at risk for the Lesch-Nyhan syndrome. *Prenat Diagn* **16**:647, 1996.
535. Gruber A, Zeitune M, Fejgin M: Failure to diagnose Lesch-Nyhan syndrome by first trimester chorionic villus sampling. *Prenat Diagn* **9**:452, 1989.
536. Gibbs DA, McFadyen IR, Crawfurd MD, De Muinck K, Headhouse-Benson CM, Wilson TM, Farrant PH: First-trimester diagnosis of Lesch-Nyhan syndrome. *Lancet* **2**:1180, 1984.
537. Page T, Broock RL: A pitfall in the prenatal diagnosis of Lesch-Nyhan syndrome by chorionic villus sampling. *Prenat Diagn* **10**:153, 1990.
538. Letts RM, Hobson DA: Special devices as aids in the management of child self-mutilation in the Lesch-Nyhan syndrome. *Pediatr* **55**:852, 1975.
539. Dicks JL: Lesch-Nyhan syndrome: A treatment planning dilemma. *Pediatr Dent* **4**:127, 1982.
540. Sugahar T, Mishim K, Mori Y: Lesch-Nyhan syndrome: Successful prevention of lower lip ulceration caused by self-mutilation by use of mouth guard. *Int J Maxillofac Surg* **23**:37, 1994.
541. Budnick J: The Lesch-Nyhan syndrome. *J Dent Child* **36**:277, 1969.
542. Smith GW, Wright V: Allopurinol. *Br J Clin Practice* **41**:710, 1987.
543. Edwards NL, Puig JG, Mateos FA: The effect of allopurinol on cerebral spinal fluid (CSF) purines in hypoxanthine-guanine phosphoribosyltransferase (HPRT) deficiency syndromes. *Adv Exp Med Biol* **204**:465, 1986.
544. Arellano F, Sacristan JA: Allopurinol hypersensitivity syndrome: A review. *Ann Pharmacother* **27**:337, 1993.
545. Demus A, Kaiser W, Schaub J: Metabolic studies during administration of adenine. *Z Kinderheildk* **114**:119, 1973.
546. Nissim S, Ciopi ML, Barzan L, Pasero G: Behavioral changes during adenine therapy in Lesch-Nyhan syndrome. *Adv Exp Med Biol* **41**:677, 1974.
547. Page T, Barshop B, Yu AL, Nyhan WL: Treatment of Lesch-Nyhan syndrome with AICAR. *Adv Exp Med Biol* **370**:353, 1995.
548. Choi DW: Glutamate neurotoxicity and diseases of the nervous system. *Neuron* **1**:623, 1988.
549. Benke PJ, Hebert A, Herrick N: In vitro effects of magnesium ions on mutant cells from patients with the Lesch-Nyhan syndrome. *N Engl J Med* **289**:446, 1973.

550. Casas-Bruge M, Almenar C, Grau IM, Jane J, Herrera-Marschitz M, Ungerstedt U: Dopaminergic receptor supersensitivity in self-mutilatory behaviour of Lesch-Nyhan disease. *Lancet* **1**:991, 1985.
551. Goldstein M, Anderson LT, Reuben R, Dancis J: Self-mutilation in Lesch-Nyhan disease is caused by dopaminergic denervation. *Lancet* **1**:338, 1985.
552. Baumeister AA, Frye GD: The biochemical basis of the behavioral disorder in the Lesch-Nyhan syndrome. *Neurosci Biobehav Rev* **9**:169, 1985.
553. Breese GR, Criswell HE, Johnson KB, O'Callaghan JP, Duncan GE, Jensen KF, Simson PE, Mueller RA: Neonatal destruction of dopaminergic neurons. *Neurotoxicology* **15**:149, 1994.
554. Allen SM, Rice SN: Risperidone antagonism of self-mutilation in a Lesch-Nyhan patient. *Prog Neuropsychopharmacol Biol Psychiat* **20**:793, 1996.
555. Van Praag HM, Plutchik R, Conte H: The serotonin hypothesis of (auto)aggression: Critical appraisal of the evidence. *Ann N Y Acad Sci* **487**:150, 1986.
556. Kirkpatrick-Sanchez S, Williams DE, Gualtieri CT, Raichman JA: Case report: the effects of selective serotonergic reuptake inhibitors combined with behavioral treatment on self-injury associated with Lesch-Nyhan syndrome. *J Dev Phys Disabil* **10**:283, 1998.
557. Rosenberg D, Monnet P, Mamelle JC, Colombel M, Salle B, Bovier-LaPierre M: Encephalopathie avec troubles du metabolisme des purines. *Presse Med* **76**:2333, 1968.
558. Jankovic J, Fahn S: Dystonic disorders, in Jankovic J, Tolosa E (eds): *Parkinson's Disease and Movement Disorders.* Baltimore, Williams and Wilkins, 1998, p 513.
559. Anderson L, Dancis J, Alpert M: Behavioral contingencies and self-mutilation in Lesch-Nyhan disease. *J Consult Clin Psychol* **46**:529, 1978.
560. Anderson LT, Dancis J, Alpert M, Herrmann L: Punishment learning and self-mutilation in Lesch-Nyhan disease. *Nature* **265**:461, 1977.
561. Anderson LT, David R, Bonnet K, Dancis J: Passive avoidance learning in Lesch-Nyhan disease: Effect of 1-desamino-8-arginine-vasopressin. *Life Sci* **24**:905, 1979.
562. Andrew J, Fowler CJ, Harrison MJG: Stereotaxic thalamotomy in 55 cases of dystonia. *Brain* **106**:981, 1983.
563. Krivit W, Lockman LA, Watkins PA, Hirsh J, Shapiro EG: The future for treatment by bone marrow transplantation for adrenoleukodystrophy, metachromatic leukodystrophy/globoid cell leukodystrophy and Hurler syndrome. *J Inherit Metab Dis* **18**:398, 1995.
564. Krivit W, Sung JH, Shapiro EG, Lockman LA: Microglia: The effector cell for reconstitution of the central nervous system following bone marrow transplantation for lysosomal and peroxisomal storage diseases. *Cell Transplant* **4**:385, 1995.
565. Nyhan WL, Parkman R, Page T, Gruber HE, Pyati J, Jolly D, Friedmann T: Bone marrow transplantation in Lesch-Nyhan disease. *Adv Exp Med Biol* **195A**:167, 1986.
566. Endres W, Helmig M, Shin YS, Albert E, Wank R, Ibel H, Weiss M, Hadorn HB, Hass R: Bone marrow transplantation in Lesch-Nyhan disease. *J Inherit Metab Dis* **14**:270, 1991.
567. Wojcik BE, Jinnah HA, Muller-Sieburg CE, Friedmann T: Bone marrow transplantation does not ameliorate the neurologic symptoms in mice deficient in hypoxanthine guanine phosphoribosyl transferase (HPRT). *Metab Brain Dis* **14**:57, 1999.
568. Miller AD, Eckner RJ, Jolly DJ, Friedmann T, Verma IM: Expression of a retrovirus encoding human HPRT in mice. *Science* **225**:630, 1984.
569. Palella TD, Silverman LJ, Schroll CT, Homa FL, Levine M, Kelley WN: Herpes simplex virus-mediated human hypoxanthine-guanine phosphoribosyltransferase gene transfer into neuronal cells. *Mol Cell Biol* **8**:457, 1988.
570. Miller AD, Jolly DJ, Friedmann T, Verma IM: A transmissible retrovirus expressing human hypoxanthine phosphoribosyltransferase (HPRT): Gene transfer into cells obtained from humans deficient in HPRT. *Proc Natl Acad Sci U S A* **80**:4709, 1983.
571. Willis RC, Jolly DJ, Miller AD, Plent MM, Esty AC, Anderson PJ, Chang HC, Jones OW, Seegmiller JE, Friedmann T: Partial phenotypic correction of human Lesch-Nyhan (hypoxanthine-guanine phosphoribosyltransferase-deficient) lymphoblasts with a transmissible retroviral vector. *J Biol Chem* **259**:7842, 1984.
572. Chang SMW, Wager-Smith K, Tsao TY, Henkel-Tigges J, Vaishnav S, Caskey CR: Construction of a defective retrovirus containing the human hypoxanthine phosphoribosyltransferase cDNA and its expression in cultured cells and mouse bone marrow. *Mol Cell Biol* **7**:854, 1991.
573. Gage FH, Wolff JA, Rosenberg MB, Xu L, Yee YK, Shultz C, Friedmann T: Grafting genetically modified cells to the brain: Possibilities for the future. *Neurosci* **23**:795, 1987.
574. Palella TD, Hidaka Y, Silverman LJ, Levine M, Glorioso J, Kelley WN: Expression of human HPRT mRNA in brains of mice infected with a recombinant herpes simplex virus-1 vector. *Gene* **80**:137, 1989.
575. Davidson BL, Doran SE, Shewach DS, Latta JM, Hartman JW, Roessler BJ: Expression of Escherichia coli beta-galactosidase and rat HPRT in the CNS of Macaca mulatta following adenoviral-mediated gene transfer. *Exp Neurol* **125**:258, 1994.
576. Plumb TJ, Bosch A, Roessler BJ, Shewach DS, Davidson BL: Hypoxanthine-guanine phosphoribosyltransferase (HPRT) expression in the central nervous system of HPRT-deficient mice following adenoviral-mediated gene transfer. *Neurosci Lett* **214**:159, 1996.
577. Johnson PA, Miyanohara A, Levine F, Cahill T, Friedmann T: Cytotoxicity of a replication-defective mutant of herpes simplex virus type 1. *J Virol* **66**:2952, 1992.
578. Xiao X, McCown TJ, Samulski RJ: Gene transfer by adeno-associated virus vectors into the central nervous system. *Exp Neurol* **144**:113, 1997.
579. Naldini L, Blomer U, Gallay P, Ory D, Mulligan R, Gage FH, Verma IM, Trono D: In vivo gene delivery and stable transduction of nondividing cells by a lentiviral vector. *Science* **272**:263, 1996.
580. Peoschla E, Corbeau P, Wong-Staal F: Development of HIV vectors for anti-HIV gene therapy. *Proc Natl Acad Sci U S A* **93**:11395, 1996.
581. Mikkelsen WM, Dodge HJ, Valkenburg H: The distribution of serum uric acid values in a population unselected as to gout or hyperuricemia. *Am J Med* **39**:242, 1965.

CHAPTER 108

Adenine Phosphoribosyltransferase Deficiency and 2,8-Dihydroxyadenine Lithiasis

Amrik S. Sahota ▪ Jay A. Tischfield
Naoyuki Kamatani ▪ H. Anne Simmonds

1. **Adenine phosphoribosyltransferase (APRT) catalyzes the synthesis of AMP from adenine and 5-phosphoribosyl-1-pyrophosphate (PP-ribose-P). An inherited deficiency of this enzyme (MIM 1026000) results in inability to utilize adenine, which, in the absence of any other significant pathway of metabolism in humans, is oxidized by xanthine dehydrogenase (XDH) via the 8-hydroxy intermediate to 2,8-dihydroxyadenine (2,8-DHA). 2,8-DHA is extremely insoluble, and its accumulation in the kidney can lead to crystalluria and the formation of urinary stones. Adenine and 2,8-DHA are secreted by the human kidney, and 2,8-DHA is protein-bound in the circulation. Both these factors tend to minimize toxicity in tissues other than the kidney. Administration of exogenous adenine itself has produced 2,8-DHA nephrotoxicity in a variety of animal systems and also in humans with normal APRT activity given massive transfusions of adenine-containing blood.**
2. **Clinical symptoms, which include renal colic, hematuria, urinary tract infection, and dysuria, are due to 2,8-DHA stone formation or crystalluria and may be present from birth. Age at diagnosis has ranged from 5 months to 74 years, and approximately 60 percent of patients have been male. As many as 50 percent of APRT-deficient individuals may be asymptomatic. Acute renal failure may occur as the presenting symptom and can be reversible. Some patients have developed chronic renal failure, requiring dialysis or transplantation, and in a subset of these, 2,8-DHA crystals were first detected during biopsy analysis of the native or the transplanted kidney. Homozygotes do not show any evidence of immunodeficiency.**
3. **Except for the excretion of adenine and its metabolites, no biochemical abnormalities have been recorded. Purine production and excretion are normal, indicating that, unlike the companion enzyme hypoxanthine-guanine phosphoribosyltransferase, APRT is not vital for the overall control of purine metabolism in humans. Adenine metabolites in the urine account for 20–30 percent of total purine excretion, even on a low-purine diet. The main source of endogenous adenine is probably polyamine synthesis, of which adenine is a metabolic byproduct. Adenine-rich foods may be a contributing factor in precipitating urolithiasis.**
4. **Two types of APRT deficiency have been recognized, based on the level of residual enzyme activity in erythrocyte lysates. Patients with type I deficiency have no detectable activity in erythrocyte lysates. Approximately 140 such patients have been identified in many countries, including 45 in Japan. These patients are homozygotes or compound heterozygotes for null alleles. Patients with type II deficiency have significant enzyme activity (5–25 percent of wild-type in hemolysates) and have been found only in Japan to date (138 cases). Approximately 75 percent of the patients in Japan have the type II defect. The type II enzyme has reduced affinity for PP-ribose-P compared with the wild-type enzyme. In both types of deficiency, APRT activity is neither demonstrable in intact cells nor functional in vivo. Intact cells are resistant to the toxic effects of 2,6-diaminopurine (DAP) and other adenine analogues that depend on APRT for their metabolism.**
5. **APRT deficiency is inherited in an autosomal recessive manner. The frequency of heterozygosity is quite high (0.4–1.2 per 100), but the number of identified cases is smaller than expected, especially in non-Japanese populations. This may be due to the wide variability in the clinical expression of the defect, coupled with problems of diagnosis.**
6. **Heterozygotes for the type I or type II defect do not appear to have any clinical or biochemical abnormalities. Intact cells from both types of heterozygote incorporate significant amounts of adenine into nucleotides and are sensitive to DAP, and APRT activity is detectable in hemolysates. Thus, the two types of heterozygote cannot readily be distinguished from each other by assays in intact cells or in cell extracts. The distinction can be made by culturing peripheral blood lymphocytes from these individuals in DAP, isolating DAP-resistant colonies, and**

A list of standard abbreviations is located immediately preceding the index in each volume. Nonstandard abbreviations used in this chapter include: AAA = azaserine-alanosine-adenine; DAP = 2,6-diaminopurine; 2,8-DHA = 2,8-dihydroxyadenine; ES cells = embryonic stem cells; GALNS = N-acetylgalactosamine-6-sulfate sulfatase; 8-HA = 8-hydroxyadenine; LOH = loss of heterozygosity; MTA = 5′-methylthioadenosine; PNP = purine nucleoside phosphorylase; SAHH = S-adenosylhomocysteine hydrolase; SSCP = single-strand conformational polymorphism; XDH = xanthine dehydrogenase.

carrying out APRT assay in cell extracts. Both types of heterozygote give rise to DAP-resistant colonies, but only colonies from type II heterozygotes have enzyme activity. Type I and type II heterozygotes can also be distinguished by starch gel electrophoresis.

7. **APRT is a dimer with 179 amino acid residues per subunit and a subunit molecular weight of 19,481. The *APRT* gene is located on chromosome 16q24.3 and encompasses 2.8 kb of genomic DNA. The gene is similar in size and intron-exon arrangement to the rodent genes and has five exons and four introns. Fourteen polymorphisms have been identified in the immediate 5′ and 3′ flanking regions of the gene. Other polymorphisms include two *Taq*I sites and a *Bgl*II site within the gene and an *Sph*I site upstream. Most of the polymorphisms have been detected in both Japanese and non-Japanese subjects.**
8. **The molecular basis of APRT deficiency has been determined in many patients by sequence analysis of genomic DNA amplified by the polymerase chain reaction (PCR). Fifteen mutations have been identified in non-Japanese patients. Nine of these were single base substitutions, two were single base-pair insertions, three were small deletions (2–7 bp), and one was a complex mutation. At least three mutations appeared to have common ancestral origins. Three mutations accounted for 95 percent of the mutant alleles identified in Japanese patients. These were the M136T missense mutation (67 percent), observed exclusively in type II patients, and the W98X nonsense mutation (21 percent) and a 4-bp duplication in exon 3 (7 percent), each found in both type I and type II patients. Approximately 79 percent of type II patients are homozygous for the M136T mutation, the remainder being compound heterozygotes with an M136T/null genotype.**
9. **The nature of spontaneous somatic mutations ("second hits") affecting the normal allele in APRT heterozygotes has been determined by studying DAP-resistant T cell clones. In approximately 75 percent of the DAP-resistant clones, there was loss of the wild-type allele and flanking markers (loss of heterozygosity) due to mitotic recombination. The remaining clones contained point mutations or other minor structural changes within the wild-type alleles, and the nature of these mutations was similar to those observed in the germline.**
10. **In the past, 2,8-DHA stones were generally confused with uric acid stones, because of their identical chemical reactivity. Correct identification requires UV, IR, MS, x-ray crystallography, HPLC, or capillary electrophoresis. The presence of brownish spots on the diaper or of yellow-brown, round crystals in the urine in both symptomatic and asymptomatic individuals is suggestive of APRT deficiency. The diagnosis may be confirmed by the identification of adenine and 2,8-DHA in the urine, together with the absence of functional APRT activity in intact erythrocytes. The latter will be impossible to establish if a recent transfusion has formed an essential part of the therapy.**
11. **Treatment has included dietary purine restriction and high fluid intake. Allopurinol administration has prevented further 2,8-DHA excretion and stone formation. The use of alkali should be avoided. Renal transplantation has been successful in several patients. Shock-wave lithotripsy has been beneficial in a small number of patients.**
12. **Homozygous APRT-deficient mice have been produced by targeted homologous recombination in embryonic stem cells. The APRT knockout mice appear to be a faithful model for human APRT deficiency. These mice excrete adenine and 2,8-DHA crystals in the urine, and renal histopathology shows extensive tubular dilatation, inflammation, necrosis, and fibrosis that varies in severity with the mouse background.**

INTRODUCTION

Adenine phosphoribosyltransferase (APRT, EC 2.4.2.7) catalyzes the synthesis of AMP from adenine and 5-phosphoribosyl-1-pyrophosphate (PP-ribose-P) in the presence of Mg^{2++}. In the absence of APRT, adenine is oxidized, via 8-hydroxyadenine (8-HA), to 2,8-dihydroxyadenine (2,8-DHA) by xanthine dehydrogenase (XDH). The chief clinical manifestation directly related to the enzyme defect is 2,8-DHA urolithiasis (Fig. 108-1). This is not an invariable finding, but when present, it can lead to serious complications.[1–3] 2,8-DHA stones sometimes have been mistaken for uric acid stones. Patients with no detectable APRT activity in cell extracts or in intact cells have been identified in many countries, including Japan (type I APRT deficiency).[2,3] Patients with measurable activity in cell extracts but no activity in intact cells have been identified only in Japan so far (type II APRT deficiency).[2,3] Approximately 140 cases of the type I defect and 138 cases of the type II defect have been diagnosed or reported in the literature. The type II defect accounts for approximately 75 percent of known cases in Japan.

Brief case histories representing the most extreme forms of expression of the disease, and results from enzymatic, metabolic, and genetic analyses have been recorded in previous editions of this chapter.[1,2] The main characteristics of APRT deficiency, and the more recent studies since the seventh edition of this text,[3] are presented here. References from 1991 onwards only are listed; references to the earlier literature may be found in the previous editions.

CLINICAL FEATURES OF APRT DEFICIENCY

Clinical symptoms of APRT deficiency occur only when 2,8-DHA stones or crystals are formed as a consequence of the enzyme defect.[1–22] The clinical situation among patients may vary from benign to life-threatening. In patients with 2,8-DHA lithiasis, the whole range of symptoms associated with stone formation has been observed, including fever from urinary tract infection, macroscopic hematuria, dysuria, urinary retention, and abdominal colic. APRT deficiency was reported initially in children, but adults now make up 60–75 percent of cases.[3,23] Age at diagnosis has ranged from 5 months to 74 years, and approximately 60 percent of symptomatic patients have been male.[3]

In many cases it took 20–50 years before the exact nature of the stones was recognized following the initial presentation with urolithiasis.[24–26] In six cases, acute, reversible anuric renal failure first drew attention to the underlying lithiasis.[3,19,21] Twenty-eight patients, including 16 from Japan, have developed chronic renal failure,[3,6,8,10,18,20] and some have died. Several of these patients have been on dialysis, and 14 have subsequently had renal transplants, 10 of which are known to have been successful. In several cases, the defect was first identified from the 2,8-DHA crystals in renal biopsies, performed at the stage of terminal renal insufficiency or after episodes of acute allograft rejection.[10,18,20] Hypoplastic kidneys or other renal developmental abnormalities have been observed in 17 Japanese patients, but this figure is likely to be an underestimate, as kidney shape and size have not been examined in all patients.[12]

2,8-DHA crystalluria can occur without clinical symptoms; the abnormality is then detected only during family investigations. Initial studies suggested that approximately 15 percent of APRT homozygotes may be asymptomatic[3,14,19,27,28] (see "Types of APRT Deficiency" below). Severe neurologic abnormalities in a number of recently described cases have been attributed to the coexistence of mucopolysaccharidosis type IVA (see "APRT

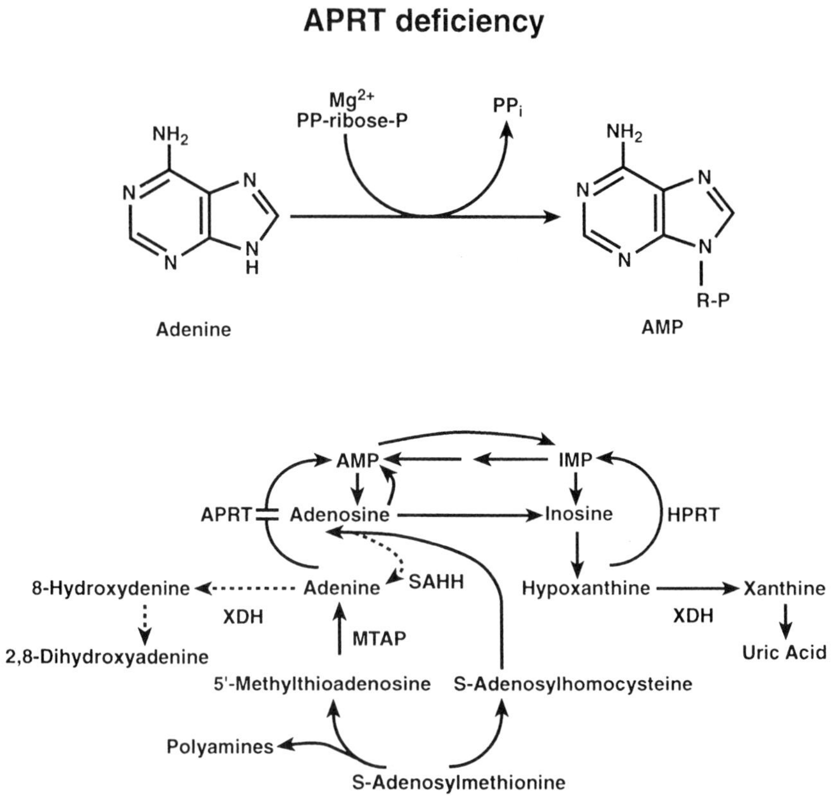

Fig. 108-1 Metabolic pathways for the formation and disposal of adenine and adenosine in humans, compared with those for hypoxanthine. Adenine phosphoribosyltransferase (APRT) catalyzes the synthesis of AMP from adenine and 5-phosphoribosyl-1-pyrophosphate (PP-ribose-P) in the presence of Mg^{2++}. In APRT deficiency, adenine is oxidized, via 8-hydroxyadenine (8-HA), to 2,8-dihydroxyadenine (2,8-DHA) by XDH. Adenine is formed, as a by-product of polyamine synthesis, from 5′-methylthioadenosine by the action of 5′-methylthioadenosine phosphorylase (MTAP). This is probably the principal route of adenine formation in vivo. A novel route of adenine formation involving S-adenosylhomocysteine hydrolase (SAHH) is indicated by the dotted line.

Activity in Other Disorders" below).[16,29] APRT deficiency is not associated with immunodeficiency.[3]

BIOCHEMICAL FEATURES OF APRT DEFICIENCY

Adenine and its derivatives, 8-HA and 2,8-DHA, are excreted in the urine in the approximate ratio 1.0:0.03:1.5.[3] The excretion of 8-HA in APRT deficiency confirms that adenine, unlike hypoxanthine, is oxidized by XDH via the 8- and not the 2-hydroxy intermediate (Fig. 108-1). Subjects with APRT deficiency generally have normal levels of uric acid in plasma and urine. The total urinary purine excretion (uric acid + precursor oxypurines + adenine derivatives) is also normal (0.05–0.1 mmol/kg/24 h), but adenine metabolites compose 20–30 percent of this total. No other abnormal purines or pyrimidines have been detected in plasma or urine. All other biochemical and hematologic parameters studied have been normal, including lymphocyte function. Erythrocytes from homozygotes for APRT deficiency have normal levels of ATP and PP-ribose-P. The former observation confirms that the erythrocyte must maintain its ATP pool through the action of adenosine kinase. The latter, together with the normal PP-ribose-P synthetase activity and purine production, suggests that APRT, unlike its companion salvage enzyme hypoxanthine-guanine phosphoribosyltransferase (HPRT), is not vital for the overall control of purine metabolism in humans.

TYPES OF APRT DEFICIENCY

As indicated above, two types of APRT deficiency have been identified.[3] These are type I deficiency (demonstrated by complete enzyme deficiency in intact cells or in cell extracts) and type II deficiency (demonstrated by complete enzyme deficiency in intact cells but only a partial deficiency in cell extracts). Homozygotes for the type II defect have been found only in Japan,[23] but two heterozygotes have been identified in Korea recently[30] (see "Molecular Bases of APRT Deficiency" below). In both types of deficiency, APRT is not functional in vivo. Cultured cells from type I and type II patients are resistant to the toxic effects of 2,6-diaminopurine (DAP) and other adenine analogues that depend on APRT for their metabolism. Patients with type I deficiency are homozygotes or compound heterozygotes for a variety of null alleles (see "Molecular Bases of APRT Deficiency" below). Seventy-nine percent of patients with the type II defect are homozygous for the M136T allele, the remainder being compound heterozygotes with the genotypes M136T/null.[23,30] In the last two editions of this chapter,[2,3] null alleles have been designated *APRT*Q0* and the M136T mutant allele has been designated *APRT*J*.

Type I Deficiency

Approximately 140 patients with type I APRT deficiency have been identified in 19 countries, including 45 in Japan, 31 in France, and 17 in Iceland.[3,13–15,19,24] Iceland, with a population of 267,000, has the largest proportion of homozygotes in a population. About 60 percent of patients have been adults.[3] Approximately 15 percent of APRT homozygotes appear to be asymptomatic,[3,14,19,27,28] but this figure is likely to be an underestimate, as family data are not available for all cases (see "APRT Deficiency Among the Japanese" below). APRT activity in erythrocyte lysates was extremely low to undetectable in type I homozygotes, but the majority of heterozygotes had erythrocyte enzyme levels of about 25 percent of the normal mean.[3,16,27] Lymphocytes and fibroblasts from type I patients also lacked APRT activity, and heterozygotes had approximately 50 percent of normal levels (see "Properties of the Mutant Enzymes" below). Intact erythrocytes from homozygotes showed no conversion of adenine into nucleotides under any incubation conditions. At physiological levels of adenine and phosphate (approximately 1 μM and 1 mM, respectively), nucleotide synthesis in intact erythrocytes from heterozygotes was indistinguishable from that in controls, but at higher adenine concentrations (10 μM) nucleotide synthesis was reduced to 40–60 percent of normal.[3] Cultured cells from homozygotes were killed in azaserine-alanosine-adenine (AAA) medium but grew normally in DAP medium.[3,31,32] Conversely, cells from heterozygotes grew in AAA but were killed in DAP.[3,31] These observations confirm that the enzyme from type I homozygotes is not functional in vivo or in vitro.

Type II Deficiency

2,8-DHA urolithiasis associated with type II APRT deficiency has been found only in Japan so far. M136T homozygotes had up to 25 percent of normal APRT activity in hemolysates and about 50 percent of normal activity in T-lymphocyte extracts. M136T heterozygotes had 50–70 percent of normal activity in hemolysates. Patients with the M136T/null genotype had approximately 5 percent and 25 percent of normal APRT activity in erythrocyte and lymphocyte extracts, respectively.[3] As with type I patients, cultured cells from type II patients did not grow in AAA medium and were resistant to the adenine analogues 6-methylpurine and DAP.[33–36] Furthermore, intact erythrocytes from these patients incorporated very little or no radioactive adenine into nucleotides.[3] These observations indicate that although the enzyme from type II patients can be detected in cell extracts, it is not functional in intact cells or in vivo.

APRT Deficiency Among the Japanese

Since the largest number of patients with APRT deficiency has been identified in Japan, it is instructive to examine the nature of the defect in this population in more detail. The data presented here are based on 200 patients from 173 families described in the literature or seen at the Tokyo Women's Medical University.[23,30] Forty-five of these patients (from 39 families) had type I (~ 25 percent) and 138 (from 118 families) had type II (~ 75 percent) disease. The nature of the defect was not identified in the remaining 17 patients. Of the 200 patients, 177 were symptomatic (urolithiasis or renal failure), 19 were asymptomatic, and four had an unclear clinical picture. This suggests that approximately 10 percent of Japanese patients are asymptomatic. However, 27 of the 200 subjects with APRT deficiency were identified because they were family members of symptomatic patients. Twelve of them were symptomatic, 12 were asymptomatic, and the clinical picture was not clear in three. Thus, as many as 50 percent of APRT-deficient individuals among the Japanese may be asymptomatic.

Among 169 symptomatic individuals whose sex was recorded, 104 (62 percent) were male and 65 (38 percent) were female. In contrast, among 19 asymptomatic individuals, 7 (37 percent) were male and 12 (63 percent) were female. Among 16 renal failure patients, 12 were male and 4 were female. Among 152 symptomatic individuals whose ages at diagnosis were known, the mean age at diagnosis for males ($n = 93$) was 25.1 ± 18.9 years (range 5 months to 74 years), whereas for females ($n = 59$) it was 28.1 ± 18.6 years (range 10 months to 72 years). These data suggest that males may be more prone to urolithiasis than females. Among 140 symptomatic individuals, the mean age at diagnosis for type I patients was 23.2 ± 18.7 years and for type II patients 27.0 ± 19.2 years, suggesting that type I patients may be more susceptible to urolithiasis. Approximately 75 percent of Japanese patients have been adults at diagnosis.

Distinction Between Type I Heterozygotes and Type II Patients

As indicated above, type I heterozygotes and type II patients have comparable levels of APRT activity in hemolysates. Thus, these two groups cannot be reliably distinguished from each other on the basis of hemolysate assay alone. However, cells from type II patients do not grow in AAA, are resistant to adenine analogues, and do not incorporate significant amounts of radioactive adenine, whereas cells from type I heterozygotes show the reverse phenomena.[3,31,34–36] These properties can be used to differentiate type II patients from type I heterozygotes.

Distinction Between Type I and Type II Heterozygotes

Intact cells from type I and type II heterozygotes incorporate significant amounts of adenine into nucleotides, are sensitive to adenine analogs, and have variable levels of hemolysate activity. Thus, the two types of heterozygote cannot be readily distinguished from each other, or from normal subjects, by assays in intact cells or in cell extracts. The distinction can be made by culturing peripheral blood T lymphocytes from these individuals in DAP, isolating DAP-resistant clones, and carrying out APRT assay in cell extracts. Both type I and type II heterozygotes give rise to DAP-resistant clones at high frequency, but only clones from type II heterozygotes have enzyme activity.[34–36] The occurrence of DAP-resistant clones from normal subjects was extremely low and undetectable by standard methods.

PROPERTIES OF THE NORMAL ENZYME

Biochemical Properties

In humans and higher animals, APRT appears to provide the only mechanism by which free adenine is converted to the nucleotide form. In some prokaryotes and lower eukaryotes, adenine can be deaminated to hypoxanthine by adenine aminohydrolase, which can then enter the nucleotide pool via HPRT. The properties of APRT from human and other mammalian sources have been reviewed previously;[3] only a summary is given here. APRT is widely distributed in human tissues. Enzyme activity in erythrocyte lysates from healthy subjects is in the range of 16–32 nmol/h per milligram of hemoglobin. This is about one third of the corresponding HPRT activity. Both enzyme's activity levels are of the same order of magnitude in leukocytes, platelets, and fibroblasts, APRT activity being five- to tenfold higher in these cells than in erythrocytes. The highest APRT activity level is found in liver, where it is three times that of HPRT. It is similarly in excess over HPRT in muscle, but here activity levels of both are extremely low. APRT activity in brain is about one tenth of that of HPRT. It is generally assumed that APRT is a soluble, cytoplasmic enzyme.

The K_m for adenine for the human erythrocyte enzyme is in the range of 1.1 to 2.7 μM. The K_m for PP-ribose-P is Mg^{2++}-dependent and is in the range of 6–29 μM. APRT is strongly inhibited by both products of the reaction. The enzyme is a dimer with 179 amino acid residues per subunit, and this is in agreement with the cDNA sequence data. The calculated subunit molecular weight is 19,481.

Adenine Analogues as Substrates for APRT

In addition to adenine, many adenine analogues are substrates for APRT. Adenine, however, has a much higher affinity for APRT than any of the analogues, which include DAP, 4-amino-5-imidazolecarboxamide, 4-aminopyrazolo (3,4-d)pyrimidine (pyrazoloadenine), 8-azaadenine, 4-carbamoylimidazolium-5-olate, 2-fluoroadenine, 6-methylaminopurine, and 6-methylpurine.[3] Once converted into nucleotides, these analogues are often toxic to cells. Analogue metabolites may also inhibit other enzymes of purine metabolism, as in the inhibition of inosine monophosphate (IMP) dehydrogenase by the nucleotide of 4-carbamoylimidazolium-5-olate. DAP and 8-azaadenine are the most widely used analogues for selecting drug-resistant cells. Cells resistant to one analogue are usually cross-resistant to the others, and resistant cells are generally defective in APRT activity, although some DAP-resistant cells have been shown to have APRT activity.[37,38]

PROPERTIES OF THE MUTANT ENZYMES

Type I Deficiency

Detailed immunochemical and electrophoretic analyses of APRT have been carried out in hemolysates and B lymphoblast extracts from families with the type I defect.[3] APRT activity and immunoreactive protein in both cell types from patients was less than 1 percent of control values. Hemolysate APRT activity in the heterozygotes was approximately 25 percent of normal, but the levels of immunoreactive protein ranged from 22 percent to normal. The corresponding values in lymphoblasts were 46 and 41 percent of normal, respectively. These studies suggest that in patients with the type I defect, either very little enzyme is synthesized or the enzyme is degraded very rapidly. Immunoreactive protein also has not been detected in B lymphoblast extracts from type I Japanese patients.

The above differences between erythrocytes and other cell types may relate to the fact that APRT is a dimer. It has been assumed that of all the possible dimer combinations, only the dimer consisting of the wild-type subunits is active in erythrocyte lysates from heterozygotes, whereas the wild-type dimer and the hybrid dimer (consisting of wild-type and mutant subunits) may be active in fibroblast and lymphoblast extracts. Alternatively, the expression of the normal allele may be increased in these cells, while either the mutant allele is not expressed or its product is labile.

Type II Deficiency

APRT from patients with type II deficiency had reduced affinity for PP-ribose-P compared with the wild-type enzyme, but affinity for adenine was unchanged.[3] The mutant enzyme showed sigmoidal rather than hyperbolic kinetics with respect to PP-ribose-P. The $S_{0.5}$ value for PP-ribose-P for the normal enzyme was 2.9 μM, but it was in the 47–82 μM range for the mutant enzyme. The concentration of PP-ribose-P was normal in erythrocytes from patients and heterozygotes for type II deficiency. The amount of immunoreactive APRT protein was decreased in hemolysates from type II patients, probably because of the lability of the enzyme.

No differences in the isoelectric point between wild-type APRT and the type II mutant enzyme have been reported. However, the two enzymes can be distinguished by starch-gel electrophoresis, and the increased K_m for PP-ribose-P for the type II enzyme can also be demonstrated by this technique.[31] Since the wild-type and type II enzymes have the same molecular weight, it is likely that small differences in charge are responsible for the starch-gel separation. The migration of the mutant enzyme was more anodal than that of the wild-type enzyme. Heterozygotes for the type II defect displayed a three-band pattern (wild-type, hybrid, and type II), consistent with the fact that APRT is a dimer. Thus, starch-gel electrophoresis can be used for the detection of type II heterozygotes.

APRT ACTIVITY IN OTHER DISORDERS

Partial APRT Deficiency and Hyperuricemia

Partial APRT deficiency was discovered prior to the recognition of the complete deficiency, during screening for HPRT deficiency in gouty subjects. Initial observations linking partial APRT deficiency with hyperuricemia and gout and with disturbances in lipid metabolism have not been substantiated. However, investigations are currently under way in families with an unusual combination of heterozygote levels of APRT activity and familiar juvenile hyperuricemic nephropathy, an autosomal dominant disorder affecting young females and males equally.[3,39–41]

Elevated APRT Activity in Purine, Pyrimidine, and Other Disorders

Erythrocyte APRT activity is elevated in most patients with HPRT deficiency, and this has been attributed to the increased levels of PP-ribose-P in this defect.[3] PP-ribose-P is considered to stabilize APRT in vivo, resulting in a diminished rate of degradation or an increase in specific activity. Elevated APRT activity has also been found in brain and liver, but not in cultured fibroblasts or lymphoblasts from HPRT-deficient patients, despite the fact that the intracellular concentration of PP-ribose-P is raised in all these cell types. APRT activity and PP-ribose-P levels are also increased in erythrocytes from patients with purine nucleoside phosphorylase (PNP) deficiency, but PP-ribose-P levels are normal in fibroblasts. PP-ribose-P levels in erythrocytes are also normal in hereditary orotic aciduria, but APRT activity is raised. This may be related to increased APRT synthesis rather than to diminished degradation.

Elevated erythrocyte APRT levels have been noted in newborns, in patients with megaloblastic anemia and reticulocytosis, and in patients with renal failure, confirming the general pattern of increased enzyme activity in young erythrocytes.[3] An increase in APRT activity has been observed in partial trisomy of chromosome 16q22.2–qter and in a patient with a duplication of 16q and a deletion of 15q, reflecting increased gene dosage.

Combined APRT and GALNS Deficiency

Two unrelated patients with combined APRT and N-acetylgalactosamine-6-sulfate sulfatase (GALNS) deficiency (mucopolysaccharidosis type IVA, or Morquio syndrome A) have been described recently.[16,29] The phenotype in these patients was consistent with a deletion involving both genes. *GALNS* and *APRT* are both located on chromosome 16q24.3 (see "The *APRT* Gene" below). These observations suggest that patients with GALNS deficiency who have unexplained renal problems should be examined for APRT deficiency.

GENETICS OF APRT DEFICIENCY

Mode of Inheritance

The mode of inheritance of APRT deficiency is autosomal recessive (Fig. 108-2). The majority of patients with type I deficiency have been Caucasian, but the defect has been found in Arab, Asian, African-American, and Japanese families, confirming that it is not restricted to certain ethnic groups.[3] Patients with type II deficiency, on the other hand, have been found only in Japan. Consanguinity has been observed in a number of families. In three Japanese families both a parent and a child were affected, and this is most likely to be due to a homozygote's marrying a heterozygote, given the high frequency of heterozygosity in the Japanese population[42] (see "Frequency of Heterozygosity" below). As mentioned previously, in the non-Japanese population the genotype null/null (type 1) is associated with 2,8-DHA urolithiasis or crystalluria, whereas three genotypes are found among Japanese patients with these problems. The relative proportions of these genotypes among 136 Japanese individuals were 62 percent M136T/M136T (type II), 17 percent M136T/null (type II), and 21 percent null/null (type 1).

Frequency of Heterozygosity

The frequency of heterozygosity for APRT deficiency in different Caucasian populations has been estimated to be 0.4–1.1 percent.[3] The most recent figures for the Japanese population indicate an estimated heterozygote frequency of 0.73 percent for the M136T mutation and a calculated heterozygote frequency of 1.1 percent for the entire APRT deficiency.[23,30] This is a relatively high frequency and would suggest that 1 in 250,000 to 1 in 33,000 individuals would be affected with this disorder. These figures are similar in magnitude to those for some of the more common autosomal recessive disorders, but the number of observed cases in Caucasian populations is much lower than expected.

The potentially lethal nature of the defect when unrecognized or misdiagnosed in homozygotes, the asymptomatic status in other cases, death in utero (rare as in Fig. 108-2), and the difficulties of diagnosis may be contributory factors for the observed discrepancy in Caucasian populations.[3] It is also possible that a common but as yet unidentified mutation in Caucasians, even when present in double dose, does not completely abolish APRT activity. Two hundred homozygotes have been reported in Japan, but many more have been diagnosed and not reported. In addition, the proportion of homozygotes who are asymptomatic is approximately 50 percent. Thus, there is little discrepancy between the

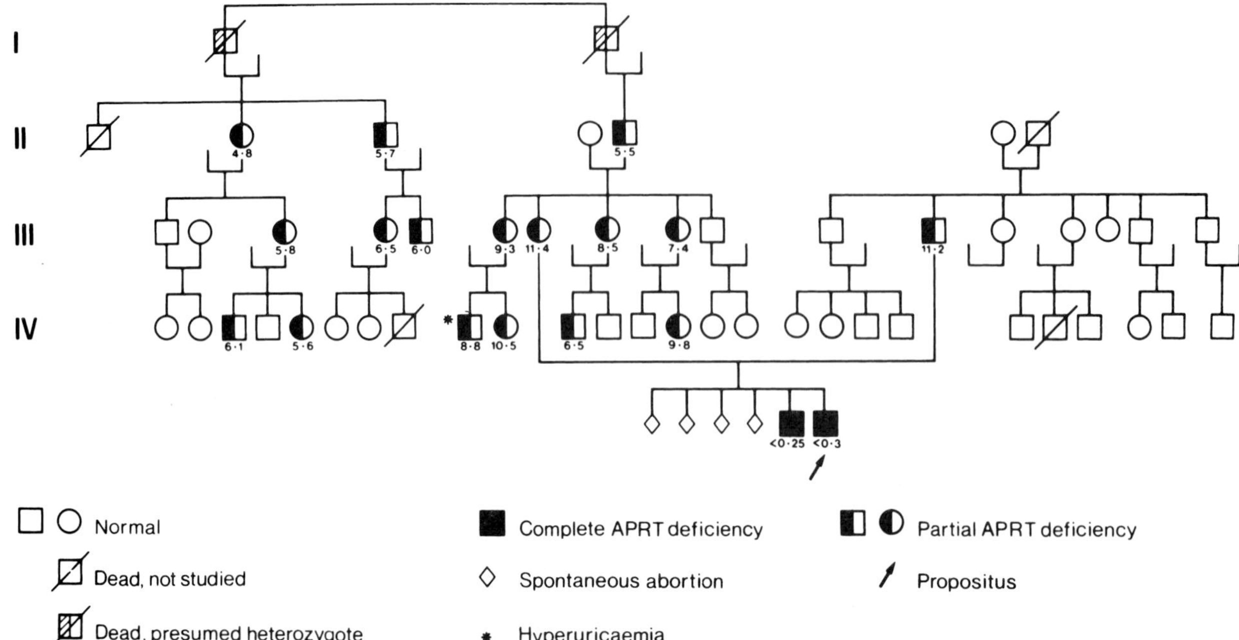

Fig. 108-2 Pedigree of a Belgian patient and his asymptomatic sib showing the recessive mode of inheritance. The absence of any other heterozygotes in the father's kindred suggests a new mutation. The numbers refer to the levels of APRT activity in erythrocyte lysates from the heterozygotes. The high proportion of members with enzyme levels approximately 25 percent of the control mean (24.4 ± 4.8 nmol/h per milligram of hemoglobin) was also a feature in other kindreds.

heterozygote frequency and the number of DHA lithiasis patients in Japan.[30]

THE *APRT* GENE

Structure

The human *APRT* gene has been mapped to chromosome 16q24.3 and is the most telomeric gene on 16q so far identified;[3,43] (see GenBank M16446 and Y00486). The fully functional gene is contained within a 2.8-kb *Bgl*II-*Cla*I fragment, including the 5′ flanking region and the 3′ untranslated region. The gene contains five exons and four introns (Fig. 108-3). There are 2202 base pairs from the start to the stop codon, and the protein-encoding region spans 540 base pairs.[3,44] The amino acid sequence deduced from the cDNA is in full agreement with that obtained from peptide mapping (see "Properties of the Normal Enzyme" above).

Comparative studies of APRT from different organisms reveal a high degree of conservation. The mouse and human enzymes are identical at 80 percent of their amino acids, with most substitutions having no effect on charge, whereas the human and *Escherichia coli* enzymes are 42 percent identical. There is, however, no significant homology in the 5′ flanking, the 3′ untranslated, or the intron sequences between the human and the rodent genes. The introns are located at the same positions in the human and the rodent genes, although they vary somewhat in size.[3,45,46] Like a number of other housekeeping genes, the promoter region of human *APRT* lacks TATA and CCAAT sequences.

The human gene contains five GC-rich boxes in the promoter region, and the mouse gene contains three such boxes. These boxes probably are the binding sites for Sp1 and other transcriptional factors that facilitate the binding of RNA polymerase to DNA.[3,47] A striking feature of the human and mouse genes is the way CpG dinucleotides are distributed within the gene. The frequency of occurrence of these dinucleotides is lower than expected and is nonrandom. They are overrepresented at the 5′ end but underrepresented at the 3′ end. By comparison, the distribution of GpC dinucleotides is relatively constant over the length of both genes.

Polymorphisms

A *Taq*I restriction-fragment-length polymorphism (RFLP) site is located within intron 2 of human *APRT*, and an *Sph*I RFLP site lies outside the gene (2.8 kb upstream of the *Taq*I site in intron 2).[3] Fourteen additional polymorphisms have recently been identified by heteroduplex analysis, single-strand conformational polymorphism (SSCP) analysis, and DNA sequence analysis of PCR-amplified DNA from obligate heterozygotes.[48] Two regions

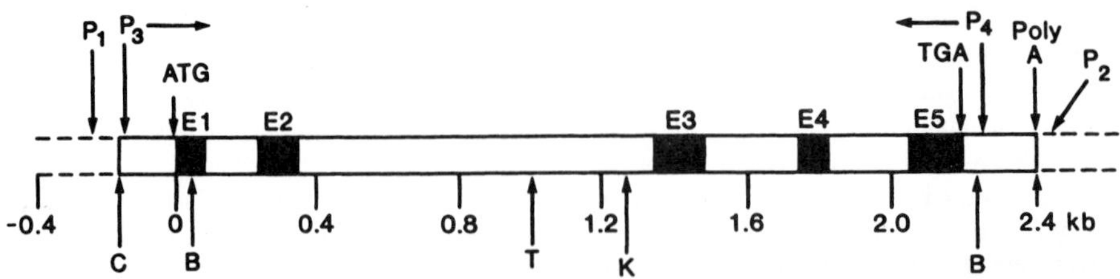

Fig. 108-3 Diagram showing the coding region and flanking sequences of *APRT*. E1 through E5 are the five exons; B = *Bam*HI; C = *Cla*I; K = *Kpn*I; T = polymorphic *Taq*I. The start and stop codons and the polyadenylation site are also shown. P1 and P2 are the primer pairs that were used for PCR amplification of *APRT*, and P3 and P4 are the other. The polymorphic *Sph*I site is upstream of the gene (not shown). (*From Chen et al.,[44] with the permission of the publisher.*)

flanking *APRT* were examined, one 1.2 kb upstream of the initiation codon and the other 1.8 kb downstream of the termination codon. Six of these polymorphisms were observed in the upstream and eight in the downstream region. The polymorphisms occurred with an average frequency of 1 in 212, consistent with the notion that the flanking regions of *APRT* contain noncoding rather than coding sequences. Most of the polymorphisms were observed in both Caucasian and Japanese heterozygotes. PCR amplification and SSCP analysis of a fragment spanning nucleotides 2344 and 2750 of *APRT* in 955 blood samples from random Japanese, Korean, and Taiwanese nationals identified five variant sequences in addition to the M136T mutation.[30] Sequence analysis of one of the variants revealed a base substitution in intron 4, suggesting that this and the other variants are neutral substitutions.

MOLECULAR BASES OF APRT DEFICIENCY

Non-Japanese Patients

The molecular bases of type I APRT deficiency have been determined by PCR amplification and DNA sequence analysis of the *APRT* gene[3,23,30,49–51] (Fig. 108-3). Fifteen different mutant alleles have been identified in the above families (Table 108-1). A T insertion at the intron 4 splice donor site was found in five families, four from Middle Europe and one from the United States, but in the last case the mutation was found in a heterozygote only. The mutation results in the replacement of an A by a T at the third base downstream from the splice site. A purine at this position appears to be essential for normal splicing. The mutation leads to deletion of exon 4 from the mRNA because of aberrant splicing. In three of the European families (one each from Belgium, Germany, and Austria), the patients were homozygous or compound heterozygous for the T insertion mutation and also for a 2.1-kb *Taq*I RFLP (restriction site present). Twins from Germany with these mutations were also homozygous for an 8-kb *Sph*I RFLP. These data suggest that the T insertion mutation in these families may have a common origin.[3] However, the fourth case (from Austria) was a compound heterozygote, with a T insertion in one allele and a complex mutation in the other (Table 108-1). Furthermore, this T insertion was not associated with the above-mentioned *Taq*I RFLP, possibly suggesting more than one origin for this mutation.[51] The T insertion creates an *Mse*I site that can be used for diagnostic or screening purposes.[52,53] Pedigree analysis of the Belgian family (Fig. 108-2) indicated that one of the mutant alleles was already present in the early 1800s. A G-to-T transversion at the intron 4 splice donor site was identified in a patient from Iraq, and this is also believed to disrupt normal splicing.

A total of 17 patients have been identified in Iceland, but they have been shown to have the previously identified D65V mutation (Table 108-1). The same mutation was identified in a British patient. All patients were homozygous for the 2.1-kb *Taq*I RFLP. The Icelandic patients were also homozygous for the 8-kb *Sph*I RFLP, whereas the British patient was heterozygous at this site. These studies support the concept that a founder effect is responsible for APRT deficiency in the Icelandic population and that the mutation may have originated in mainland Europe.[54] Common ancestors dating back to the early 1700s have been identified for several of the APRT-deficient Icelandic families.[13]

A 7-bp deletion in *APRT* exon 3 was found in both alleles from a patient of Turkish origin.[27] Her older sister was also deficient in APRT activity but is so far asymptomatic. This mutation has been identified previously in an unrelated APRT-deficient patient from Hungary[55] (Table 108-1). The Ottoman Turks invaded Hungary a number of times from the 15th to the 17th centuries, suggesting that the mutant allele may be of Turkish origin.

An insertion of a T nucleotide in exon 2 was found in two patients and probably leads to a frameshift after Ile at position 61. The other non-Japanese patients had a variety of mutations, mainly single base changes and small deletions (Table 108-1). None of the patients had gross alterations in *APRT,* and no polymorphic amino acid substitutions were detected. The largest number of patients has been described in France, but with one exception (Table 108-1), no mutation data are available for these patients,[24] or for those from Spain[14] or Italy.[15]

We have not been able to find a mutation in one APRT-deficient patient after completely sequencing the 2.4-kb genomic region. This patient, from Quebec, first presented with chronic renal

Table 108-1 Mutations at the *APRT* Locus in Non-Japanese Patients

No.	Country of Origin	Base Change	Amino Acid Change	Location	Allele No.	Mutation
1.	Hungary	A→G	MIV	Exon 1	1	Initiation codon
		GGCCCCA deletion		Exon 3	2	Frameshift after P93
2.	Turkey	GGCCCCA deletion		Exon 3	Both	Frameshift after P93
3.	Greece	T insertion		Exon 2	Both	Frameshift after I61
4.	USA	T insertion		Exon 2	1	Frameshift after I61
		G→A	R67Q	Exon 3	2	Missense
5.	Iceland	A→T	D65V	Exon 3	Both	Missense
6.	Britain	A→T	D65V	Exon 3	Both	Missense
7.	Pakistan	C→T	R87X	Exon 3	Both	Nonsense
8.	France	AC deletion		Exon 3	Both	Frameshift after P95
9.	Canada	T→C	L110P	Exon 4	Both	Missense
10.	Bermuda	A→T	I112F	Exon 4	1	Missense
		T→C	C153R	Exon 5	2	Missense
11.	Iraq	G→T		Intron 4	Both	Splice donor
12.	Belgium	TTC deletion	ΔF173	Exon 5	1	Triplet deletion
		T insertion		Intron 4	2	Splice donor
13.	Germany	T insertion		Intron 4	Both	Splice donor
14.	Austria	T insertion		Intron 4	Both	Splice donor
15.	Austria	T insertion		Intron 4	1	Splice donor
		Insertion/deletion			2	Complex mutation
16.	USA	T insertion		Intron 4	1	Splice donor; heterozygote
17.	Ausralia	G→A	R89Q	Exon 3	1	Missense; heterozygote

SOURCE: Adapted from Sahota et al.,[50] with permission of the publisher.

Table 108-2 Mutations at the *APRT* Locus in Japanese Patients

No.	Base Change	Amino Acid Change	Location	Mutation	No. of Alleles	Percentage
1.	T→C	M136T	Exon 5	Missense	96	67
2.	G→A	W98X	Exon 3	Nonsense	30	21
3.	CCGA insertion		Exon 3	Frameshift after I86	10	7
4.	G→C	X1816S	Stop codon	Termination failure	2	1
5.	Major deletion				2	1
6.	Undefined				4	3
	TOTAL				144	100

failure, and the diagnosis of APRT deficiency was made following the identification of microcrystalline deposits of 2,8-DHA in a kidney allograft biopsy specimen.[10] Whether APRT deficiency in this patient derives from mutations outside the 2.4-kb genomic fragment or from epigenetic phenomena (e.g., methylation)[56,57] has not been investigated. Neither has a mutation been found in a subject with reduced APRT activity in hemolysates. We have previously identified a missense mutation (R89Q, Table 108-1) in one allele in a number of families with reduced APRT activity in hemolysates, but not in 500 random samples.[58]

Japanese Patients

One hundred forty-four mutant *APRT* alleles have been analyzed from 74 different Japanese families (70 affected and four heterozygotes), and a total of five mutations have been identified[23,30] (Table 108-2). Among these, the three main mutations were the missense mutation (M136T) observed exclusively in type II patients, a nonsense mutation (W98X), and a 4-bp duplication (CCGA, codon 87) observed in both type I and type II patients. These three mutations account for 95 percent (67 percent, 21 percent, and 7 percent, respectively) of the *APRT* mutant alleles in Japanese patients. One type I patient was homozygous for X181S, a G-to-C transition at the physiological termination codon (TGA to TCA, Ter to Ser),[59] and two heterozygotes had a major deletion. The deleted region appeared to contain a gene necessary for cell survival and would have been expected to be lethal in homozygotes. Mutations have not been identified in four alleles (3 percent). PCR amplification and sequence analysis of all five exons and the exon-intron junctions from three of these patients did not reveal any abnormalities,[30] suggesting that, as with the non-Japanese patient from Quebec mentioned above, the mutations may occur in the sequences upstream or downstream of the coding region.[60] All patients with the W98X mutation had a silent base substitution at codon 99 (GCC to GCT, Ala).[3,50,61] The M136T mutation lies within the putative PP-ribose-P binding region and may be responsible for the increased K_m for PP-ribose-P in type II deficiency.[3]

There is strong linkage disequilibrium between the M136T mutation and the *Taq*I polymorphic site in intron 2, and there is evidence for a crossover event between the M136T mutation site and the *Sph*I site.[3,23,30] These data strongly suggest that a single ancestral mutation is responsible for type II APRT deficiency and that this mutation probably has a long evolutionary history.[23] A recent study of the geographic distribution of *APRT* mutations showed that the codon M136T mutation was distributed uniformly in all four islands of Japan and in Okinawa and also found two heterozygotes with this mutation in 356 Korean blood samples but none in 231 samples from Taiwan.[30] Based on crossover data mentioned above, the age of this mutation was estimated to be between 4,340 and 43,360 years. The recent finding of this mutation in Korean heterozygotes indicates that the mutation originated at least 2,300 years ago, since the Koreans and Okinawans are believed to share ancestors only before the Yayoi era (3rd century BC to 3rd century AD).[30]

APRT Deficiency in Somatic Cells In Vivo

For comparison with germline mutations and to gain insight into the mechanisms of loss of heterozygosity (LOH) in somatic cells, we have investigated in vivo somatic mutations in normal human T cells.[32–36] Because of the autosomal nature of *APRT*, these mutations are best studied in heterozygotes. T cells from the heterozygotes were cultured in medium containing DAP to select for APRT-deficient clones. These clones were observed at a frequency of 10^{-4} to 10^{-5}. DAP-resistant clones from transformed B cells have been selected at a similar frequency.[35] About 20 percent of the DAP-resistant clones retained both *APRT* alleles, and 19 different mutations have been detected in previously wild-type *APRT* allele (the allele that did not bear the germline mutation) from these clones.[32,33] These mutations tended to cluster at two positions within the gene (at the intron 4 splice donor site and around codon 87). These regions appear to be mutational hot spots in both T cells and germline cells. Further, the types of mutations in somatic and germline cells were quite similar, suggesting that they were a consequence of similar mechanisms.[33] In vitro somatic mutations in human *APRT* do not appear to show this clustering.

About 80 percent of the DAP-resistant clones exhibited LOH of linked microsatellite markers on chromosome 16q.[32] Ten of these clones were examined further, and nine of them showed a normal diploid karyotype by conventional cytogenetics and two copies of *APRT* by fluorescence in situ hybridization. One clone was hemizygous for *APRT*, and it had the smallest region of LOH. These results indicate that mitotic recombination and, to a much lesser extent, interstitial deletion may be the primary mechanism for the relatively high frequency of in vivo LOH in human T cells. Similar results have been reported in T and B cells from Japanese heterozygotes.[35,36]

ADENINE METABOLISM IN HUMANS

Adenine Metabolism

The ubiquitous distribution of APRT in human tissues had long been puzzling in view of the presence of extremely low levels of adenine in blood (reported range 0.07–1.13 μM) and almost undetectable levels (less than 1.5 mg [11 μmol]/24 h) in the urine of normal humans.[3,62] The finding of homozygotes for APRT deficiency, eliminating up to 100 mg (740 μmol) of adenine and its oxidation products per 24 h, indicates the presence of a significant source of adenine production in vivo. Although hypoxanthine and guanine are readily formed from the corresponding nucleosides (Fig. 108-1), no significant formation of adenine from adenosine (or vice versa) via PNP has been demonstrated in mammalian cells, as distinct from bacterial and other cells.[3]

The alternative possibility that the adenine metabolites excreted in APRT deficiency were derived from the diet was excluded when dietary purine restriction yielded only a slight reduction in total adenine metabolites. Nevertheless, diet may be an important precipitating factor in the clinical expression of the defect. This is suggested by the larger number of patients identified in France than in the United Kingdom or United States and underscored by the permanent renal damage suffered by a child from a commune whose members consumed diets rich in adenine-containing compounds.[3]

Origin of Adenine in APRT Deficiency

The polyamine pathway has been identified as the main source of endogenous adenine in humans (Fig. 108-1). This pathway is active in dividing and regenerating cells and tissues, and adenine is derived from 5′-methylthioadenosine (MTA), the end product of this pathway, by the action of MTA phosphorylase.[3] Studies in two APRT-deficient patients over 23 years have demonstrated a remarkable constancy in the levels of adenine metabolites (20–30 percent of total daily purine excretion on a low-purine diet), which has tended to parallel the increase in body weight during childhood.[5] Increased excretion of MTA and adenine has been noted in patients with neoplastic diseases, consequent to increased polyamine synthesis.[63]

Studies in intact erythrocytes from normal subjects, from patients with complete adenosine deaminase (ADA) and PNP deficiencies, and from APRT-deficient subjects (forming an effective adenine trap) have established the existence of a novel route of adenine formation from deoxyadenosine/adenosine and adenosine analogues in human erythrocytes.[3,64,65]

These studies were stimulated by the unexpected incorporation of the radiolabeled adenine moiety from [^{14}C]2′-deoxyadenosine into ATP by erythrocytes from ADA- and PNP-deficient subjects, which could not be explained by the operation of any known pathway. The incorporation of labeled adenine into ATP was not observed in erythrocytes from APRT-deficient patients, but free adenine accumulated. This implicated APRT, with free adenine as an obligatory intermediate. The involvement of S-adenosylhomocysteine hydrolase (SAHH) was postulated to explain these in vitro findings, but the significance of this pathway in vivo is difficult to assess. Although under normal circumstances little adenine is likely to be produced this way, such a pathway (if present in cells other than the erythrocyte) offers a potential new route not only for ATP generation but also for the conversion to nucleotides of nucleoside analogues used in chemotherapy.

2,8-DHA NEPHROTOXICITY AND STONE FORMATION

2,8-DHA Solubility

The chief clinical manifestation in APRT deficiency relates to the nephrotoxicity of 2,8-DHA. A similar pathology can occur following adenine overload in animals or humans with normal APRT activity. The nephrotoxicity of 2,8-DHA is due to its poor solubility, which does not vary significantly within the normal physiological pH range, solubility in vitro being 2.68 ± 0.84 mg/liter at pH 5.0 and 4.97 ± 1.49 mg/liter at pH 7.8. Human urine at 37°C apparently exhibits an enhanced capacity for solubilizing 2,8-DHA, which may remain supersaturated in vitro at levels up to 40.4 ± 3.3 mg/liter for 16 h; while values as high as 96 mg/liter have been noted in the urine of patients receiving oral adenine. Concentrations up to 0.5 mM (80 mg/liter) were noted in a growing asymptomatic patient, confirming in vivo supersaturation of 2,8-DHA in APRT deficiency. Varying ability to supersaturate the urine may thus explain the existence of affected and asymptomatic sibs in several families. The apparent lack of in vivo toxicity to tissues other than the kidney may be related to the high degree of protein binding in the circulation, coupled with the active secretion of 2,8-DHA by the human kidney.[3]

2,8-DHA and Adenine Toxicity

The potential nephrotoxicity of adenine, via 2,8-DHA, was first noted as early as 1898 during the feeding of adenine to animals. Since then, 2,8-DHA nephrotoxicity has been demonstrated in most mammalian species, the severity varying with the species and the route and duration of adenine administration.[3] In all species, little 2,8-DHA was formed below 10 mg/kg of adenine, but with increasing dosages, yellowish spheres of 2,8-DHA appeared in the urine and tubular lumens. Higher doses produced extensive deposits within the interstitium as well, followed by progressive renal failure and death. A similar pathology has been reported in liver, kidney, and lymph nodes of cattle.[66] It is curious that tissues in addition to the kidney appear to be affected in cattle. The renal pathology in animals corresponded closely with the findings in a patient described earlier (Fig. 108-4 and detailed in ref. 1) and confirmed acute intratubular crystal deposition as the primary event.

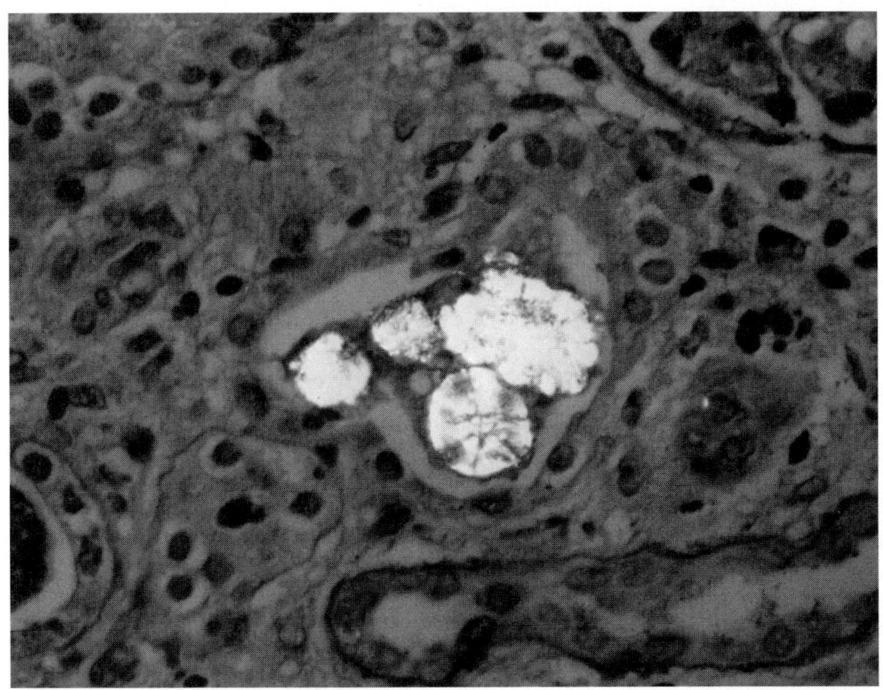

Fig. 108-4 Photomicrograph of renal biopsy X800 (original magnification) from a previously described patient,[1] stained with the periodic acid-Schiff technique and photographed in semipolarized light. Several large crystals are seen within the lumen of a distended, atrophied cortical tubule (center). There is a greatly increased amount of interstitial connective tissue with lymphocytes; within this tissue is a reactive multinucleate giant cell (right), which has formed around a further small crystal.

The addition of adenine to blood to prolong its shelf life is a common practice. It is considered that 10–15 mg/kg of adenine does not normally produce 2,8-DHA crystals in humans, but a fatal incidence has been reported in a patient receiving massive amounts of adenine-containing blood. Thus, it should be recognized that heterozygotes as well as homozygotes for APRT deficiency may be at increased risk from transfusion of adenine-containing blood.[3]

There is no evidence for any long-term toxicity or immunodeficiency due to adenine accumulation, as evidenced by follow-up studies over 19 years in a patient who presented at age 4 with severe renal damage requiring dialysis and then transplantation.[3] The normal clinical and immunologic status over 23 years of two APRT-deficient sibs, one of whom was on allopurinol therapy (during which adenine accumulated and was excreted in quantity), also argues against significant adenine toxicity in vivo.[5] Several homozygotes identified in their 40s have had healthy children, indicating a lack of toxicity of adenine and its metabolites to the reproductive system (unpublished observations).

DIAGNOSIS

2,8-DHA Crystalluria and Urolithiasis

APRT deficiency in a symptomatic or asymptomatic child may be suspected initially by an astute parent or clinician from the brownish spots on a diaper.[13,19] The appearance of round, brownish crystals in urine deposits under a light microscope also suggests the presence of 2,8-DHA[3,13,17] (Fig. 108-5). These findings are highly suggestive of APRT deficiency, but they should be confirmed by specific techniques. In a review of 15 Japanese patients who had no DHA lithiasis but whose urine contained round crystals indistinguishable from 2,8-DHA by light microscopy, only seven were later found to be APRT homozygotes. 2,8-DHA crystals have Maltese cross birefringence under polarized light.

2,8-DHA stones are detectable by ultrasonography, but there must be a large degree of deposition in the kidney (as with nephrocalcinosis) before crystals can be detected this way. Accidental discovery during routine abdominal ultrasound led to the first case of 2,8-DHA nephrolithiasis identified in twins.[3] Scanning electron microscopy has also been used for analysis of 2,8-DHA stones.[67] The stones are generally 95–98 percent 2,8-DHA, the remainder being predominantly uric acid.

2,8-DHA is an analogue of uric acid and is indistinguishable from it by routine chemical and thermogravimetric analyses. The two compounds may also be confused if only the alkaline ultraviolet spectrum is examined. Both kinds of stones are radiolucent, although in three Japanese patients the stones also contained calcium phosphate and thus were radiopaque. Some or all of these factors may be responsible for the frequent misdiagnosis of 2,8-DHA stones as "uric acid" stones.[3]

Simple guidelines for correct stone identification include noting the macroscopic appearance of the stones. 2,8-DHA stones are whitish to pale gray, rough, and friable, whereas uric acid stones are generally yellowish, smooth, hard, and difficult to crush. 2,8-DHA can also be distinguished from uric acid by wet chemistry or by its intense phosphorescence on a filter paper strip

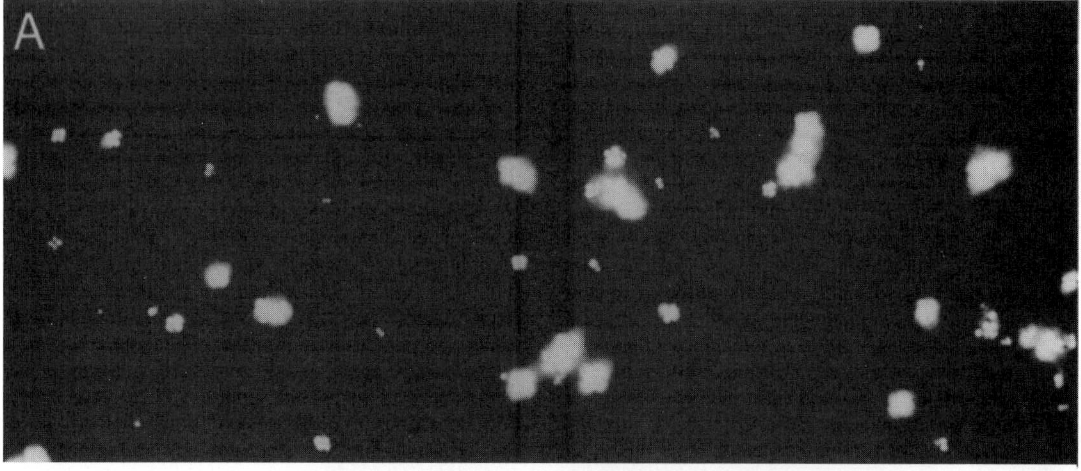

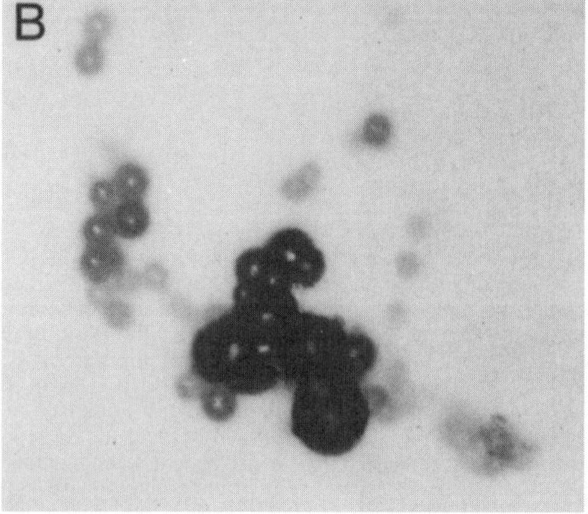

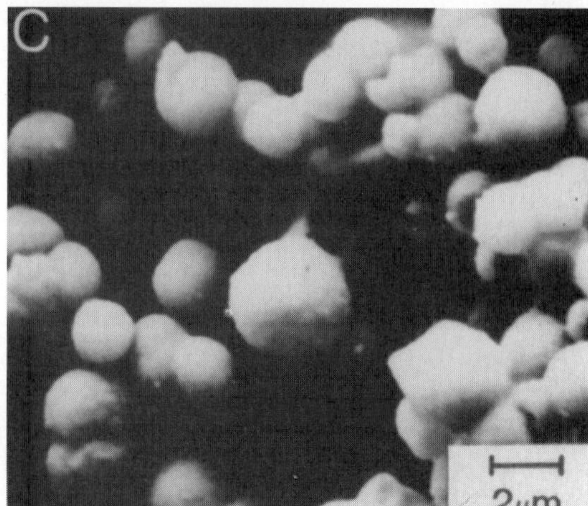

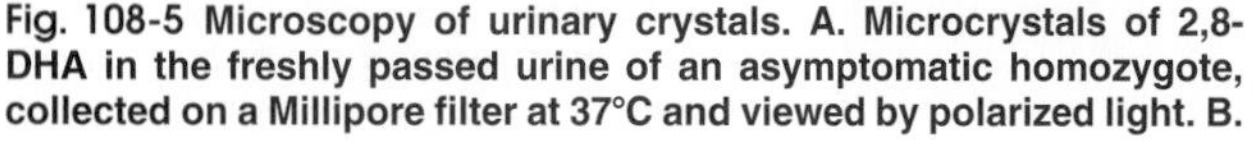

Fig. 108-5 Microscopy of urinary crystals. A. Microcrystals of 2,8-DHA in the freshly passed urine of an asymptomatic homozygote, collected on a Millipore filter at 37°C and viewed by polarized light. B. Round brown crystals in urine of a boy with 2,8-DHA stones. C. Scanning electron micrograph of the crystals. (*Panels B and C courtesy of the publishers of* Urology.)

dipped in liquid nitrogen and then exposed to ultraviolet light. Final confirmation may be obtained from the ultraviolet spectrum in both acid and alkali, the infrared spectrum, MS, X-ray crystallography, HPLC, or electrophoretic analyses.[3,62,68] 2,8-DHA, unlike uric acid, is resistant to the action of uricase. The diagnosis of uric acid stones should always be suspect, especially in children who are otherwise normal.

The three adenine metabolites excreted in the urine by both symptomatic and asymptomatic subjects can be detected and quantitated by HPLC, TLC, or capillary electrophoresis.[3,62,68] Co-elution problems with methylated xanthine derivatives in subjects not on caffeine-free diets or with metabolites with the same retention times in those taking acetaminophen, may lead to a false "adenine" peak when using HPLC without in-line diode-array detection. Therefore, confirmation by measurement of APRT activity is essential.

Confirmation of APRT Deficiency

APRT deficiency can be confirmed by a combination of studies in intact cells and cell extracts.[3,69] Assays in erythrocyte lysates alone will not distinguish the various mutant forms of the enzyme and can be misleading when a recent transfusion has formed part of the treatment protocol. Patients and heterozygotes for type I or type II deficiency can be distinguished based on (i) APRT activity in intact cells and in cell extracts; (ii) adenine uptake by intact cells; (iii) sensitivity of cultured cells to adenine analogues; and (iv) analysis of urine for adenine and its oxidation products by HPLC or other analytic techniques. The most reliable method for establishing homozygosity for the type II defect is to determine whether proliferating T cells are resistant to DAP or 6-methylpurine.[34–36] Compound heterozygotes with the M136T/null genotype also have the type II phenotype and can be detected only in this way.

Molecular Diagnostics

Given the small size of the *APRT* gene (genomic region 2.8 kb, coding region 0.54 kb), APRT deficiency can be identified readily in new patients by PCR amplification, subcloning, and DNA sequencing of a 2.4-kb genomic fragment.[44] A number of assays for the detection of existing mutations have been described. These include: (i) *Mse*I digestion of PCR-amplified DNA for the detection of the T insertion mutation common in Caucasian populations;[52,53] (ii) oligonucleotide probe or SSCP analysis of the M136T mutation in the Japanese;[17,70–72] and (iii) allele-specific oligonucleotide probe hybridization for the R89Q mutation detected in some heterozygotes.[58] Reverse-transcription PCR has also been used to examine *APRT* mutations, especially in cases involving nonsense mutations that can result in shorter transcripts through exon skipping.[73]

TREATMENT AND PROGNOSIS

Allopurinol Therapy

2,8-DHA formation has been controlled by allopurinol treatment, but some is still excreted. Allopurinol therapy did not reduce the total levels of adenine compounds excreted (still 20–30 percent of total purine excretion on a low-purine diet) but rearranged the proportion so that adenine became the major urinary component.[3] Allopurinol at 10 mg/kg/day (child) or 300 mg/day (adult) has almost eliminated 2,8-DHA from the urine in most cases. In subjects with acute or chronic renal failure, the dose should be reduced to 5 mg/kg/day in children and 100 mg/day in adults, because of the well-documented retention of oxypurinol (the active metabolite of allopurinol) in renal failure, with the associated risk of bone marrow depression and other undesirable side effects. When possible, plasma oxypurinol levels should be monitored and dosage adjusted accordingly. A careful watch should be kept on all hematologic parameters. Allopurinol was discontinued after 14 years in the longest-studied case without recurrence of symptoms,[5] indicating that withdrawal may be possible after puberty.

Importance of Diet

A high fluid intake is encouraged and the use of allopurinol without alkali advised, since the solubility of 2,8-DHA is not altered within the physiological pH range. A low-purine/low-adenine diet is recommended, since dietary adenine, as well as dietary-derived uric acid, can contribute to the severity of the clinical manifestations. A child presenting with acute or chronic renal failure was from a commune whose members consumed diets rich in lentils, grains, and vegetable extracts–all foods with a reputedly high adenine content.[3]

Shock Wave Lithotripsy

As with stones of other origins, therapy using shock-wave lithotripsy with sonograph stone localization has proven beneficial in the treatment of 2,8-DHA stones,[74] with the exception of one case, where the treatment was effective in only one of the affected kidneys.[20] In Japan, the use of lithotripsy has contributed to an increase in the number of patients diagnosed correctly. In Europe, this is generally not the case, except possibly in France; and patients successfully treated for radiolucent or radiopaque stones are not tested for the underlying cause, which may thus remain unrecognized. The significance of this is underlined by a recently identified family with two sibs (now both dead) with a long history of recurrent nephrolithiasis requiring dialysis whose cause was not recognized (H. Gault, personal communication).

Prognosis

The prognosis clearly depends on renal function at the time of diagnosis.[3,6,8,10,18,20,24] At least 14 patients with terminal renal failure have had replacement of renal function by transplantation, which is known to have been successful in 10 of them. A number of patients have died. One patient, undiagnosed at the time of transplantation, suffered recurrent stones after transplantation until APRT deficiency was recognized and allopurinol therapy commenced. In four cases the defect was first identified from the 2,8-DHA crystals in renal biopsies, performed in two at the stage of terminal renal insufficiency and in the other two after renal allograft rejection. Therefore, the importance of early diagnosis and treatment must again be stressed.

Studies over more than 20 years have allayed doubts about the possibility of any long-term adverse effects of adenine toxicity or of allopurinol therapy in growing children with APRT deficiency.[5] The defect itself does not appear to have any adverse effects on physical or intellectual development. A child who developed terminal renal failure and had a successful transplant 14 years ago at the age of 12 has shown normal growth and development.[3]

KNOCKOUT MOUSE MODEL FOR APRT DEFICIENCY

Production of APRT- and HPRT-deficient Mice

Two groups have recently described the production of APRT-deficient mice using targeted homologous recombination in embryonic stem (ES) cells and subsequent breeding of heterozygous offspring. In one case the positive/negative targeting vector was created by inserting a neomycin resistance cassette into the middle of *Aprt* exon 3[75] and in the other by replacing exons 1 and 2 of *Aprt* with this cassette.[76] In both cases, a herpes simplex virus thymidine kinase gene fragment was introduced at the 3′ end of the gene. Both vectors contained sufficient regions of homology at the 5′ and 3′ ends to promote homologous recombination in ES cells. The linearized targeting vector was electroporated into ES cells, and colonies were selected in G418 (positive selection) followed by ganciclovir (negative slection). DNA from the G418- and ganciclovir-resistant colonies was screened by Southern blotting or PCR to identify clones containing one wild-type and one mutant (null) copy of *Aprt*. Correctly targeted ES cells were microinjected into blastocysts, which were then re-implanted into pseudopregnant mice. The offspring were genotyped to identify heterozygous mice, which were then interbred to produce homozygous deficient animals. The mutant *Aprt* allele has been bred into mice of several different strains (Shao et al., unpublished data), and we have also produced mice that are HPRT- and APRT-deficient by breeding appropriate strains.[77] Unlike a number of other knockout mouse models of purine metabolic disease that have been described (e.g., HPRT deficiency),[78,79] the APRT knockout mouse appears to be a faithful model for human APRT deficiency.

Metabolic and Other Studies in APRT- and HPRT-deficient Mice

The availability of *Aprt* knockout mice has allowed study of several aspects of APRT deficiency that cannot be tested in human subjects. These include: (i) changes in kidney structure and function during the progression from 2,8-DHA crystalluria to urolithiasis, (ii) activation of genes during the early stages of the disease process, (iii) the role of XDH in stone formation among different mouse strains, (iv) sex differences in the frequency or severity of 2,8-DHA-associated renal failure, (v) the contribution of diet to the disease process, (vi) possible effects on organs and tissues other than kidney, and (vii) the suggested involvement of APRT in a mouse model for Lesch-Nyhan syndrome.

APRT-deficient male mice excreted adenine and 2,8-DHA crystals in the urine, and renal histopathology showed extensive tubular dilatation, inflammation, necrosis, and fibrosis. Both intracellular and intratubular 2,8-DHA crystal formation was noted.[75,76] As in human APRT deficiency, the severity of symptoms varied widely among APRT-deficient mice. By 12 weeks of age, APRT-deficient males showed extensive renal damage and had elevated blood urea nitrogen; their glomerular filtration rate was approximately half that of animals with the wild-type gene.[80] The most severely affected males died by about 6 months of age, but this appeared to be strain-specific. The consequences of APRT deficiency appeared to be less severe in females. As in humans, allopurinol treatment prevented the accumulation of 2,8-DHA and much of the resultant renal damage in APRT-deficient mice.[75,76] Experiments to confirm and extend these early findings are in progress. It has been hypothesized that inactivation of both *Aprt* and *Hprt* is essential to generate a mouse model for the Lesch-Nyhan syndrome.[81] Preliminary biochemical and behavior studies in APRT- and HPRT-deficient mice showed that they excreted adenine and 2,8-DHA in the urine but showed no evidence for any of the features associated with Lesch-Nyhan syndrome.[77] Thus, APRT deficiency is not essential for generating a mouse model for Lesch-Nyhan syndrome.

ACKNOWLEDGMENTS

This work was supported by NIH grant DK38185, and update of European data was facilitated by EC grant BMH4-CT98-3079. AS and HAS would like to thank Karel J. Van Acker for his contributions to the previous editions of this chapter.

REFERENCES

1. Simmonds HA, Van Acker KJ: Adenine phosphoribosyltransferase deficiency: 2,8-Dihydroxyadenine lithiasis, in Stanbury JB, Wyngaarden JB, Fredrickson DS, Goldstein JL, Brown MS (eds): *The Metabolic Basis of Inherited Disease* 5th ed. New York, McGraw-Hill, 1983, p 1144.
2. Simmonds HA, Sahota AS, Van Acker KJ: Adenine phosphoribosyltransferase deficiency and 2,8-dihydroxyadenine lithiasis, in Scriver CR, Beaudet AL, Sly WS, Valle D (eds): *The Metabolic Basis of Inherited Disease* 6th ed. New York, McGraw-Hill, 1989, p 1029.
3. Simmonds HA, Sahota AS, Van Acker KJ: Adenine phosphoribosyltransferase deficiency and 2,8-dihydroxyadenine lithiasis, in Scriver CR, Beaudet AL, Sly WS, Valle D (eds): *The Metabolic and Molecular Bases of Inherited Disease* 7th ed. New York, McGraw-Hill, 1995, p 1707.
4. Osawa O, Ohara T, Komatz Y: Two cases of 2,8-dihydroxyadenine stone with a partial deficiency of adenine phosphoribosyltransferase [Japanese]. *Hinyokika Kiyo* **37**:1535, 1991.
5. Van Acker KJ, Simmonds HA: Long-term evolution of type I adenine phosphoribosyltransferase (APRT) deficiency. *Adv Exp Med Biol* **309B**:91, 1991.
6. Gelb AB, Fye KH, Tischfield JA, Sahota AS, Sparks JW, Hancock DC, Sibley RK: Renal insufficiency secondary to 2,8-dihydroxyadenine urolithiasis. *Hum Path* **23**:1081, 1992.
7. Katsuoka Y, Miyakita H, Shiramizu M, Iwagaki H, Ikeda T: 2,8-Dihydroxyadenine urolithiasis due to partial deficit in adenine phosphoribosyltransferase: A case report [Japanese]. *Hinyokika Kiyo* **38**:573, 1992.
8. Fye KH, Sahota A, Hancock DC, Gelb AB, Chen J, Sparks JW, Sibley RK, Tischfield JA: Adenine phosphoribosyltransferase deficiency with renal deposition of 2,8-dihydroxyadenine leading to nephrolithiasis and chronic renal failure. *Arch Inter Med* **153**:767, 1993.
9. Takeuchi H, Kaneko Y, Fujita J, Yoshida O: A case of a compound heterozygote for adenine phosphoribosyltransferase deficiency *(APRT*J/APRT*Q0)* leading to 2,8-dihydroxyadenine urolithiasis: Review of the reported cases with 2,8-dihydroxyadenine stones in Japan. *J Urol* **149**:824, 1993.
10. Gagne ER, Deland E, Daudon M, Noel LH, Nawar T: Chronic renal failure secondary to 2,8-dihydroxyadenine deposition: The first report of recurrence in a kidney transplant. *Am J Kid Dis* **24**:104, 1994.
11. Kambayashi T, Nakanishi T, Suzuki K, Fujita K, Tajima A, Kawabe K: Two siblings with 2,8-dihydroxyadenine urolithiasis [Japanese]. *Hinyokika Kiyo* **40**:1097, 1994.
12. Konishi N, Takeshita K, Yasui H: A case of adenine phosphoribosyltransferase (APRT) deficiency discovered by urine examination [Japanese]. *Nippon Jinzo Gakkai Shi* **31**:1191, 1994.
13. Laxdal T: 2,8-Dihydroxyadeninuria [Icelandic]. *Laeknabladid* **80**:141, 1994.
14. Wuhl O, Vila R, Barcelo P, Laguna P, Rousaud A: 2,8 dihydroxyadenine (2,8 DHA) lithiasis: Report of 3 cases [Spanish]. *Acta Urol Espanol* **18**:43, 1994.
15. Malfi B, Rotunno M, Mazzucco G, et al: Depositi di cristalli di 2,8-diidrossi-adenini su rene transplanto. *G Ital di Nefrol* **12**:63, 1995.
16. Sebesta I, Krijt J, Hrebiček M, et al: Adenine phosphoribosyltransferase deficiency with suspected mucopolysaccharidosis Type IVA. *Pharm World Sci* **17**:K15, 1995.
17. Terai C, Hakoda M, Yamanaka H, Kamatani N, Okai M, Takahashi F, Kashiwazaki S: Adenine phosphoribosyltransferase deficiency identified by urinary sediment analysis: Cellular and molecular confirmation. *Clin Genet* **48**:246, 1995.
18. de Jong DJ, Assmann KJ, De Abreu RA, Monnens LA, van Liebergen FJ, Dijkman HB, Huysmans FT: 2,8-Dihydroxyadenine stone formation in a renal transplant recipient due to adenine phosphoribosyltransferase deficiency. *J Urol* **156**:1754, 1996.
19. Laxdal T: 2,8-Dihydroxyadeninuria in Iceland. *Klin Kemi I Norden* **8**:53, 1996.
20. Thomas J, Conort P, Fompeydie D, Bellin J, Rechke JP, Arvis G: A case of lithiasis caused by 2,8 dihydroxyadenine: Evolutive characteristics: Therapeutic problems [French]. *J d'Urol* **102**:161, 1996.
21. Arnadottir M, Laxdal T, Hardarson S, Asmundsson P: Acute renal failure in a middle-aged woman with 2,8-dihydroxyadeninuria. *Nephrol Dialysis Transplant* **12**:1985, 1997.
22. Suzuki K, Kobayashi S, Kawamura K, Kuhara T, Tsugawa R: Family study of 2,8-dihydroxyadenine stone formation: Report of two cases of a compound heterozygote for adenine phosphoribosyltransferase deficiency *(APRT*J/APRT*Q0)*. *Int J Urol* **4**:304, 1997.
23. Kamatani N, Hakoda M, Otsuka S, Yoshikawa H, Kashiwazaki S: Only three mutations account for almost all defective alleles causing adenine phosphoribosyltransferase deficiency in Japanese patients. *J Clin Invest* **90**:130, 1992.
24. Ceballos-Picot I, Perignon JL, Hamet M, Daudon M, Kamoun P: 2,8-Dihydroxyadenine urolithiasis, an underdiagnosed disease. *Lancet* **339**:1050, 1992.
25. Laxdal T: 2,8-Dihydroxyadenine crystalluria vs urolithiasis. *Lancet* **340**:184, 1992.
26. Simmonds HA, Van Acker KJ, Sahota AS: 2,8-Dihydroxyadenine urolithiasis. *Lancet* **339**:1295, 1992.
27. Bye S, Mallmann R, Duley J, Simmonds HA, Chen J, Tischfield JA, Sahota A: Identification of a 7-basepair deletion in the adenine

phosphoribosyltransferase gene as a cause of 2,8-dihydroxyadenine urolithiasis. *Clin Invest* **72**:550, 1994.

28. Sahota A, Chen J, Boyadjiev SA, Gault MH, Tischfield JA: Missense mutation in the adenine phosphoribosyltransferase gene causing 2,8-dihydroxyadenine urolithiasis. *Hum Mol Genet* **3**: 817, 1994.
29. Fukuda S, Tomatsu S, Masuno M, et al: Mucopolysaccharidosis IVA: Submicroscopic deletion of 16q24.3 and a novel R386C mutation of N-acetylgalactosamine-6-sulfate sulfatase gene in a classical case of Morquio disease. *Hum Mutat* **7**:123, 1996.
30. Kamatani N, Terai C, Kim SY, et al: The origin of the most common mutation of adenine phosphoribosyltransferase among Japanese goes back to a prehistoric era. *Hum Genet* **98**:596, 1996.
31. Sahota A, Chen J, Behzadian MA, Ravindra R, Takeuchi H, Stambrook PJ, Tischfield JA: 2,8-Dihydroxyadenine lithiasis in a Japanese patient heterozygous at the adenine phosphoribosyltransferase locus. *Am J Hum Genet* **48**:983, 1991.
32. Gupta PK, Sahota A, Boyadjiev SA, et al: High frequency in vivo loss of heterozygosity is primarily a consequence of mitotic recombination. *Cancer Res* **57**:1188, 1997.
33. Chen J, Sahota A, Martin GF, Hakoda M, Kamatani N, Stambrook PJ, Tischfield JA: Analysis of germline and in vivo somatic mutations in the human adenine phosphoribosyltransferase genes: Mutational hotspots at the intron 4 splice donor site and at codon 87. *Mutat Res* **287**:217, 1993.
34. Hakoda M, Yamanaka H, Kamatani N, Kamatani N: Diagnosis of heterozygote states for adenine phosphoribosyltransferase deficiency based on detection of in vivo somatic mutants in blood T cells: Application to screening of heterozygotes. *Am J Hum Genet* **48**:552, 1991.
35. Hakoda M, Kamatani N, Terai C, Yamanaka H, Taniguchi A, Ueda H, Kashiwazaki S: Similarity of *in vivo* somatic mutations at an autosomal adenine phosphoribosyltransferase locus between T- and B-cells in human peripheral blood. *Mutat Res* **98**:107, 1996.
36. Hakoda M, Kamatani N, Kurumada S: Intervention of somatic mutational events *in vivo* by a germline defect at adenine phosphoribosyltransferase locus. *Hum Genet* **99**:164, 1997.
37. Khattar NH, Cooper GE, DiMartino DL, Bishop PL, Turker MS: Molecular and biochemical elucidation of a cellular phenotype characterized by adenine analogue resistance in the presence of high levels of adenine phosphoribosyltransferase activity. *Biochem Genet* **30**:635, 1992.
38. Khattar NH, Turker MS: A role for certain mouse *Aprt* sequences in resistance to toxic adenine analogs. *Somat Cell Molec Genet* **23**:51, 1997.
39. Moro F, Ogg CS, Simmonds HA, et al: Familial juvenile gouty nephropathy with renal urate hypoexcretion preceding renal disease. *Clin Nephrol* **35**:263, 1991.
40. Mateos FA, Puig JG: Renal hemodynamics in familial nephropathy associated with hyperuricemia (FNAH). *Adv Exp Med Biol* **370**:31, 1994.
41. McBride MB, Simmonds HA, Hatfield PJ, Graham R, McCaskey J, Jackson M: Renal urate hypoexcretion in Polynesian women is not as severe as in United Kingdom (UK) women with familial juvenile hyperuricemic nephropathy (FJHN). *Adv Exp Med Biol* **370**:35, 1994.
42. Ishidate T, Igarashi S, Kamatani N: Pseudodominant transmission of an autosomal recessive disease, adenine phosphoribosyltransferase deficiency. *J Pediatr* **118**:90, 1991.
43. Richards RI, Holman K, Lane S, Sutherland GR, Callen DF: Chromosome 16 physical map: Mapping of somatic cell hybrids using multiplex PCR deletion analysis of sequence tagged sites. *Genomics* **10**:1047, 1991.
44. Chen J, Sahota A, Stambrook PJ, Tischfield JA: Polymerase chain reaction amplification and sequence analysis of human mutant adenine phosphoribosyltransferase genes: The nature and frequency of errors caused by *Taq* DNA polymerase. *Mutat Res* **249**:169, 1991.
45. Fieldhouse D, Golding GB: The rat adenine phosphoribosyltransferase sequence shows evolutionary rate variation among exons in rodents. *Genome* **36**:1107, 1993.
46. Fieldhouse D, Yazdani F, Golding GB: Substitution rate variation in closely related rodent species. *Heredity* **78**:21, 1997.
47. Frank D, Keshet I, Shani M, Levine A, Razin A, Cedar H: Demethylation of CpG islands in embryonic cells. *Nature* **351**:239, 1991.
48. Boyadjiev SA, Sahota A, Tischfield JA: Identification and application of polymorphisms flanking the human adenine phosphoribosyltransferase gene. *Hum Mutat* **8**:214, 1996.
49. Sahota A, Chen J, Stambrook PJ, Tischfield JA: Mutational basis of adenine phosphoribosyltransferase deficiency. *Adv Exp Med Biol* **309B**:73, 1991.
50. Sahota A, Chen J, Stambrook PJ, Tischfield JA: Genetic basis of adenine phosphoribosyltransferase deficiency, in Gresser U (ed): *Molecular Genetics, Biochemistry and Clinical Aspects of Disorders of Purine and Pyrimidine Metabolism*. Heidelberg, Springer-Verlag, 1993, p 54.
51. Menardi C, Schneider R, Neuschmid-Kaspar F: et al: Human APRT deficiency: Indication for multiple origins of the most common Caucasian mutation and detection of a novel type of mutation involving intrastrand-templated repair. *Hum Mutat* **10**:251, 1997.
52. Gathof BS, Sahota A, Gresser U, Chen J, Stambrook PJ, Tischfield JA, Zollner N: A splice mutation at the adenine phosphoribosyltransferase locus in a German family. *Adv Exp Med Biol* **309B**:83, 1991.
53. Gathof BS, Zollner N: The restriction enzyme *MseI* applied for the detection of a possibly common mutation of the *APRT* locus. *Clin Invest* **70**:535, 1992.
54. Chen J, Sahota A, Laxdal T, Scrine M, Bowman S, Cui C, Stambrook PJ, Tischfield JA: Identification of a single missense mutation in the adenine phosphoribosyltransferase gene from five Icelandic patients and a British patient. *Am J Hum Genet* **49**:251, 1991.
55. Sahota A, Chen J, Bye S, Jaing J, Berenyi M, Fekete G, Tischfield JA: Occurrence of a missense mutation in one allele and a seven basepair deletion in the other allele in a patient with adenine phosphoribosyltransferase deficiency. *Hum Mutat* **3**:315, 1994.
56. Mummaneni P, Bishop PL, Turker MS: A *cis*-acting element accounts for a conserved methylation pattern upstream of the mouse adenine phosphoribosyltransferase gene. *J Biol Chem* **268**:552, 1993.
57. Mummaneni P, Walker KA, Bishop PL, Turker MS: Epigenetic gene inactivation induced by a *cis*-acting methylation center. *J Biol Chem* **270**:788, 1995.
58. Sahota A, Bye S, Chen J, Khattar NH, Turker MS, Moro F, Simmonds HA, Emmerson BT, Gordon RB, Tischfield JA: Molecular characterization of a novel mutation in APRT heterozygotes. *Adv Exp Med Biol* **370**:675, 1994.
59. Taniguchi A, Hakoda M, Yamanaka H, Terai C, Hikiji K, Kawaguchi R, Konishi N, Kashiwazaki S, Kamatani N: A germline mutation abolishing the original stop codon of the human adenine phosphoribosyltransferase (APRT) gene leads to complete loss of the enzyme protein. *Hum Genet* **102**:197, 1998.
60. Higashimoto H, Ouchi A, Kawaguchi R: Detection of the three common mutations of adenine phosphoribosyltransferase deficiency among Japanese. *Clin Chim Acta* **234**:1, 1995.
61. Mimori A, Hidaka Y, Wu VC, Tarle SA, Kamatani N, Kelley WN, Palella TD: A mutant allele common to the type I adenine phosphoribosyltransferase deficiency in Japanese subjects. *Am J Hum Genet* **48**:102, 1991.
62. Simmonds HA, Duley JA, Davies PM: Analysis of purines and pyrimidines in blood, urine, and other physiological fluids, in Hommes F (ed): *Techniques in Diagnostic Human Biochemical Genetics: A Laboratory Manual*. New York, Wiley-Liss, 1991, p 397.
63. Kaneko K, Fujimori S, Kumakawa T, Kamatani N, Akaoka I: Disturbance in the metabolism of 5′-methylthioadenosine in patients with neoplastic diseases and those with a deficiency of adenine phosphoribosyltransferase. *Metabolism* **40**:918, 1991.
64. Smolenski RT, Montero C, Duley JA, Simmonds HA: Effects of adenosine analogues on ATP concentration: Further evidence for a route independent of adenosine kinase. *Biochem Pharmacol* **42**:1767, 1991.
65. Smolenski RT, Fabianowska-Majewska K, Montero C, Duley JA, Fairbanks LD, Marlewski M, Simmonds HA: A novel route of ATP synthesis. *Biochem Pharmacol* **43**:2053, 1992.
66. McCaskey PC, Ribsby WE, Hinton DM, Friedlander L, Hurst VJ: Accumulation of 2,8-dihydroxyadenine in bovine liver, kidneys and lymph nodes. *Vet Pathol* **28**:99, 1991.
67. Winter P, Hesse A, Klocke K, Schaefer RM: Scanning electron microscopy of 2,8-dihydroxyadenine crystals and stones. *Scanning Microsc* **7**:1075, 1993.
68. Terai C, Hakoda M, Yamanaka H, Kamatani N, Okai M, Takahashi F, Kashiwazaki S: A fast and simple screening method for detection of 2,8-dihydroxyadenine urolithiasis. *Clin Chim Acta* **93**:85, 1996.
69. Adam T, Sevick J, Fairbanks LD, Bartak P: Determination of purine enzyme activities in human erythrocytes by capillary electrophoresis. *Adv Exp Med Biol* **431**:759, 1998.
70. Kawaguchi R, Higashimoto H, Hikiji K, Hakoda M, Kamatani N: Detection of the most common mutation of adenine phosphoribosyltransferase deficiency among Japanese by a non-radioactive method. *Clin Chim Acta* **203**:183, 1991.
71. Higashimoto H, Kawaguchi R, Hikiji K: Detection of the mutation responsible for adenine phosphoribosyltransferase deficiency among Japanese patients [Japanese]. *Jap J Clin Path* **40**:1067, 1992.

72. Kaneko Y, Takeuchi H, Takenawa J, Yoshida O, Takano S, Fujita JL: Detection of mutant adenine phosphoribosyltransferase genes by polymerase chain reaction-single strand conformation polymorphism analysis [Japanese]. *Hinyokika Kiyo* **38**:641, 1992.
73. Bye S, Sahota A, Chen J, Tischfield JA: Analysis of *APRT* mutations by reverse transcription PCR. *Adv Exp Med Biol* **370**:671, 1994.
74. Frick J, Sarica K, Kohle R, Kunit G: Long-term follow-up after extracorporeal shock wave lithotripsy in children. *Eur Urol* **19**:225, 1991.
75. Engle SJ, Stockelman MG, Chen J, et al: Adenine phosphoribosyltransferase deficient mice develop 2,8-dihydroxyadenine nephrolithiasis. *Proc Natl Acad Sci USA* **93**:5307, 1996.
76. Redhead NJ, Selfridge J, Wu CL, Melton DW: Mice with adenine phosphoribosyltransferase deficiency develop fatal 2,8-dihydroxyadenine lithiasis. *Hum Gene Therapy* **7**:1491, 1996.
77. Engle SJ, Womer DE, Davies PM, et al: HPRT-APRT-deficient mice are not a model for Lesch-Nyhan syndrome. *Hum Molec Genet* **5**:1607, 1996.
78. Hooper M, Hardey K, Handyside A, Hunter S, Monk M: HPRT-deficient (Lesch-Nyhan) mouse embryos derived from germline colonization by cultured cells. *Nature* **326**:292, 1987.
79. Huehn MR, Bradley A, Robertson EJ, Evans MJ: A potential animal model for Lesch-Nyhan syndrome through introduction of HPRT mutations into mice. *Nature* **326**:295, 1987.
80. Stockelman MG, Lorenz JN, Smith FN et al: Chronic renal failure in a mouse model of human adenine phosphoribosyltransferase deficiency. *Am J Physiol* **275**:F154, 1998.
81. Wu C-L, Melton DW: Production of a model for Lesch-Nyhan syndrome in hypoxanthine phosphoribosyltransferase-deficient mice. *Nat Genet* **3**:235, 1993.

CHAPTER 109

Immunodeficiency Diseases Caused by Adenosine Deaminase Deficiency and Purine Nucleoside Phosphorylase Deficiency

Michael S. Hershfield ▪ Beverly S. Mitchell

1. Adenosine deaminase (ADA) and purine nucleoside phosphorylase (PNP) catalyze sequential steps in the metabolism of purine ribo- and deoxyribonucleosides. They are expressed at very high levels in lymphoid cells. In patients with heritable deficiency of ADA or PNP, actions of their substrates or related metabolites impair lymphocyte differentiation, viability, and function, resulting in lymphopenia and immunodeficiency. Most patients with ADA deficiency lack both cell-mediated (T cell) and humoral (B cell) immunity, resulting in severe combined immunodeficiency disease (SCID). PNP-deficient children have defective cell-mediated immunity but may have normal, hyperactive, or reduced humoral immunity. Most patients with these disorders are severely affected and present during infancy and early childhood with recurrent infections involving pathogens and opportunistic organisms. Autoimmunity and neurologic abnormalities may occur with either enzyme deficiency, and hepatic dysfunction occurs in some patients with ADA deficiency.

2. ADA deficiency (MIM 102700) has been identified in several hundred families, and PNP deficiency in less than 50. Increasingly, enzyme-deficient patients with later onset and milder or atypical clinical presentations are being recognized. These diagnoses should be considered in patients with unexplained T-cell lymphopenia and late manifestations of immunodeficiency, such as chronic pulmonary insufficiency, sometimes with a history of autoimmunity and neurologic abnormalities, during the first two decades of life and even later. Diagnosis is made by finding absent or very low enzyme activity in erythrocytes or in nucleated blood cells. Heterozygotes have normal immune function and approximately half the normal erythrocyte enzyme levels. Prenatal diagnosis can be established by measuring enzyme activity in amniotic cells or chorionic villi.

3. Both conditions are inherited in an autosomal-recessive manner. Structural genes are located on chromosomes 20q13.11 (ADA) and 14q13 (PNP). Over 60 ADA gene mutations have been identified in immune-deficient patients. Several others have been found in a small group of individuals with so-called partial ADA deficiency, who are clinically unaffected owing to significant ADA activity in nucleated cells despite nearly absent levels in erythrocytes. There is a good correlation between the ADA activity expressed *in vitro* by mutant ADA alleles and clinical severity. Fourteen PNP mutations have been identified. The developmental and tissue-specific expression of ADA and PNP genes have been investigated, and the three-dimensional crystal structures of murine ADA and human PNP have been determined.

4. In ADA deficiency, levels of adenosine (Ado) and 2′-deoxyadenosine (dAdo) are elevated in the plasma; dAdo is elevated in the urine. Two major metabolic findings in erythrocytes are markedly elevated deoxyadenosine triphosphate (dATP) and reduced activity of *S*-adenosylhomocysteine (AdoHcy) hydrolase (usually <5 percent of normal), owing to suicide-like inactivation by dAdo; erythrocyte adenosine triphosphate (ATP) is decreased substantially in patients with SCID. The level of dATP in erythrocytes correlates with clinical severity and with the level of ADA activity expressed in *Escherichia coli* by mutant ADA alleles. In PNP deficency, plasma and urinary levels of PNP substrates are elevated, whereas uric acid is markedly decreased. In erythrocytes deoxyguanosine triphosphate (dGTP) may be detectable and guanosine triphosphate (GTP) may be decreased.

5. The primary lymphotoxic substrates of ADA and PNP—dAdo and 2′-deoxyguanosine (dGuo), respectively—are derived largely from the breakdown of DNA associated with cell death. Several effects of dAdo may contribute to lymphopenia and immune dysfunction in ADA deficiency: (a) dATP pool expansion can induce apoptosis in both dividing and nondividing lymphoid cells. This effect may be related to dATP-induced inhibition of ribonucleotide

A list of standard abbreviations is located immediately preceding the index in each volume. Nonstandard abbreviations used in this chapter include: ADA, adenosine deaminase; Ado, adenosine; AdoHcy, *S*-adenosylhomocysteine; AdoMet, *S*-adenosylmethionine; dAdo, 2′-deoxyadenosine; dAXP, dAdo nucleotides; dGuo, 2′-deoxyguanosine; DPP-IV, dipeptidyl peptidase IV; GVHD, graft-versus-host disease; HPRT, hypoxanthine-guanine phosphoribosyltransferase; PEG-ADA, polyethylene glycol–modified ADA; PNP, purine nucleoside phosphorylase; SCID, severe combined immunodeficiency disease.

reductase, blocking DNA replication in dividing cells, and dATP-induced DNA strand breaks in nondividing lymphocytes. dATP directly activates a protease (caspase 9) involved in apoptosis. (b) AdoHcy accumulation can block vital *S*-adenosylmethionine (AdoMet)-mediated transmethylation reactions. (c) Formation of dATP from dAdo activates adenosine monophosphate (AMP) deamination and inosine monophosphate (IMP) dephosphorylation, leading to depletion of cellular ATP. Impaired lymphocyte function also may result from aberrant signal transduction, mediated by Ado acting through G protein–associated receptors, or from altered costimulatory function of T cell–associated ADA complexing protein CD26/dipeptidyl peptidase IV. In PNP deficiency, dGTP accumulation can inhibit ribonucleotide reductase and DNA replication in thymocytes, and can induce apoptosis.

6. **Bone marrow transplantation from a human leukocyte antigen (HLA)-identical donor is the preferred treatment and can result in complete or partial immune reconstitution. Transplantation of T cell–depleted marrow from an HLA-haploidentical donor also has been successful, but is associated with greater morbidity and mortality and is less effective in restoring humoral immune function. For patients with ADA deficiency, an alternative to haploidentical transplantation is replacement therapy by intramuscular injection (once or twice weekly) of bovine ADA modified by attachment of polyethylene glycol (PEG-ADA). The high plasma ADA activity achieved with PEG-ADA, by degrading circulating dAdo, reverses intracellular dATP pool expansion and AdoHcyase inactivation. Immune function improves in most cases, resulting in sustained clinical benefit. Antibody to bovine ADA often becomes detectable with restoration of humoral immunity, but no allergic reactions have occurred and efficacy has usually not been impaired. About a dozen PEG-ADA–treated patients have become subjects for ongoing gene therapy experiments involving *ex vivo* retrovirus-mediated transfer of ADA complementary DNA. Mature blood T cells, as well as $CD34^+$ cells isolated from bone marrow and umbilical cord blood, have been targeted. The efficiency of transducing stem cells has been low, but persistence of vector in myeloid cells and in T-lymphocytes has been demonstrated in several patients. These patients have continued to receive PEG-ADA, making evaluation of the benefit from gene transfer problematic.**

In 1972, Dr. Eloise Giblett reported the association of combined immunodeficiency with the absence of erythrocyte adenosine deaminase (ADA) activity.[1] She made this discovery while analyzing polymorphic genetic markers in a patient being considered for bone marrow transplantation (BMT). "As luck would have it,"[2] an unrelated patient studied a few weeks later was also ADA deficient. Indeed, ADA deficiency had been observed independently in an immunodeficient Danish child, but (as luck would have it) normal activity in a second patient obscured the significance.[3] Within a year a half dozen such patients had been reported.[1,3–5] Giblett and her colleagues then began to screen levels of other enzymes of purine and pyrimidine metabolism in patients with various immune disorders. In 1975, these efforts were rewarded with the discovery of the first case of purine nucleoside phosphorylase (PNP) deficiency, found in a 5-year-old girl with a defect in cellular immunity but with apparently normal humoral immunity.[6] Additional cases were soon reported.[7–11]

Until these assignments of specific molecular defects, heritable immunodeficiency syndromes had been categorized solely by clinical and pathologic criteria. The defining characteristics and means of isolating lymphocyte subpopulations were just being worked out; very little was known about their biochemistry. Inborn errors of hypoxanthine-guanine phosphoribosyltransferase (HPRT) and PP-ribose-P synthase, which cause hyperuricemia and gout, were paradigms for thinking about the consequences of defective purine salvage. Thus, from both an immunologic and metabolic viewpoint, the association of ADA and PNP deficiencies with selective immune dysfunction was entirely unexpected and provided challenging new directions for research.

The original report on ADA deficiency closed by anticipating that "Eventually it may be possible to determine, not only the genetic mechanism involved, but also the biochemical reasons for the immunological defect."[1] These goals have largely been realized during the past three decades. Specific therapies have been developed based on knowledge of the underlying gene defect and understanding of pathogenesis in terms of the abnormal metabolism.

CLINICAL ASPECTS

The major functional arms of the adaptive immune system—*cell-mediated*, effected primarily by T-lymphocytes, and *humoral*, mediated by antibodies produced by B-lymphocytes and plasma cells—are highly interdependent. Nevertheless, heritable (primary) immune defects occur that dramatically affect one arm while leaving the other relatively intact. T-cell disorders are associated mainly with infections caused by viral and opportunistic organisms; immunoglobulin deficiencies result in susceptibility to encapsulated bacteria and certain viruses. Combined immunodeficiency (CID) is a rare disorder, caused by several different genetic defects, in which both forms of immunity are impaired.[12] The simple designation *CID* encompasses patients with variable degrees of cellular or humoral immune dysfunction over time. In milder cases the underlying immune disorder may be masked by supportive therapy, delaying diagnosis for months or years.[13] The most complete form, known as severe combined immunodeficiency disease (SCID), presents in the first weeks to a few months of life, often with the constellation of thrush, pneumonia, diarrhea, and failure to thrive; it is usually fatal by 2 years of age.[14] About half of all cases of SCID are X linked, and the rest have autosomal recessive inheritance.

Immunodeficiency, manifested by profound lymphopenia and recurrent infections, is the most conspicuous manifestation of both ADA and PNP deficiency. Most ADA-deficient patients have CID; impaired cellular immunity usually predominates in PNP-deficient individuals, who may have normal or even hyperactive humoral function. The recognized clinical spectrum of each disease has broadened as patients with atypical or milder immunodeficiency have been found to be enzyme deficient. The diagnoses should be considered in patients presenting with unexplained immunodeficiency during, and even beyond, the first two decades of life.

ADA Deficiency

Historically, 85 to 90 percent of ADA-deficient patients are infants with SCID. The frequency of ADA deficiency among all forms of SCID can be gauged from the experience of two marrow transplant centers in Paris and the United States: among a total of 225 SCID patients treated over a combined period of 53 years, 32 (14%) were ADA deficient.[15,16] The incidence of ADA deficiency has been estimated to be from less than 1 in 1,000,000 births to as high as 1 in 200,000.[17]

SCID Presentation. Although clinically similar to SCID due to other genetic defects, patients with ADA deficiency are over-represented among the most seriously ill, often presenting by 1 month of age with failure to thrive and life-threatening interstitial pneumonitis.[15] Pneumonia may be caused by *Pneumocystis carinii* or viral infection, but an organism frequently is not isolated. The skin and gastrointestinal tract are also common sites of initial infections. A variety of pathogens and opportunistic agents (viral, fungal, bacterial, and protozoan) are encountered. Candidiasis is usually present at some stage, first as "diaper rash," then as a more extensive infection involving skin, oral and esophogeal mucosa, and the vagina. Persistent diarrhea, either viral or secondary to abnormal intestinal flora, is common. Physical findings are related to infection, failure to thrive, and the absence of lymph nodes and pharyngeal lymphoid tissue. Prominent costochondral junctions, similar to a so-called rachitic rosary, may be present.[18]

Various neurologic abnormalities have been reported, including spasticity, head lag, movement disorders, nystagmus, inability to focus, and sensorineural deafness.[19–21] Among 16 French ADA-deficient SCID patients, 6 presented with developmental delay without evidence of central nervous system infection, a higher incidence than was found among non–enzyme-deficient SCID patients.[15] Whether ADA deficiency per se is responsible for these diverse neurologic problems is unclear because they only occur in a minority of patients and infection often cannot be excluded. Central neurologic involvement has been related in some cases to vaccination with live poliovirus, to hypoxia associated with pneumonia or mechanical ventilation, or to an episode of cardiorespiratory arrest.

Adenosine deaminase–deficient SCID is often diagnosed by 1 to 2 months of age, when recurrent infections first prompt evaluation of immune function. The average age for a group of 31 ADA-deficient patients was 4.4 months.[22] This is similar to other forms of SCID[15,16] and reflects an estimated average delay of about 2 months between onset of symptoms and diagnosis of SCID.[15] Longer delays may occur when initial symptoms are related more to failure to thrive than to opportunistic infection. If immunologic function is not restored, SCID is fatal by 1 to 2 years, often due to complications of infection with parainfluenza, cytomegalovirus, varicella, or various other DNA and RNA viruses. Vaccination with live organisms (bacillus Calmette-Guérin, poliovirus), and graft-versus-host disease (GVHD) resulting from transfusion of unirradiated blood, also may be fatal. There is an increased risk of B-cell lymphomas, which may be related to Epstein-Barr virus (EBV). SCID patients who do survive beyond early childhood are subject to pulmonary insufficiency and other chronic consequences of recurrent infections experienced prior to institution of definitive therapy.

Delayed or Late/Adult-Onset Presentation. Ten to fifteen percent of ADA-deficient patients present with a less complete form of CID that is diagnosed beyond the first year of life, but within the first decade,[18,23–27] (and unpublished observations). This clinical phenotype has been referred to as delayed onset. In some of these patients serious infections have not begun until 2 to 3 years of age, but in others, recurrent episodes of otitis, as well as sinus and upper respiratory infections, including bacterial pneumonia, have begun by 6 to 18 months, but because these have not involved opportunistic organisms or required hospitalization, CID has not been considered until 2 to 8 years of age. Prior to reaching the correct diagnosis, these patients have been diagnosed as having asthma, chronic allergy, or isolated defects in regulation of humoral immunity owing to the presence of eosinophilia, increased immunoglobulin E (IgE) or decreased IgG2 subclass levels, or autoimmune phenomena.

Combined immunodeficiency due to ADA deficiency has been diagnosed beyond the first decade (late/adult onset) in several patients who had been symptomatic for long periods.[26,28,29] For example, at diagnosis a 15-year-old boy had *P. carinii* pneumonia and pancytopenia; when hospitalized several years earlier he had been lymphopenic, but lymphocyte response to mitogens and antibody titers to encapsulated organisms were significant (K. Weinberg, unpublished observations).[26] Sisters diagnosed at 34 and 35 years of age in England had progressive pulmonary insufficiency and recurrent warts beginning in their late teens.[28] A 39-year-old Swiss woman was discovered to be ADA deficient during evaluation for recurrent pneumonia.[29] Lymphopenia, frequent respiratory infections, and recurrent hepatitis of unknown etiology had been documented by age 5 years (ADA deficiency was then unknown). She did relatively well until her late twenties, but in her thirties she developed chronic hepatobiliary disease, asthma with markedly elevated serum IgE, recurrent sinopulmonary infections, and pulmonary tuberculosis. At age 40, she died of leukoencephalopathy due to JC papovavirus, a disorder associated with impaired cellular immunity, including acquired immunodeficiency syndrome (AIDS). Prior to appreciation of their underlying immunodeficiency, these adult women had been treated for extended periods with glucocorticoids and immunosuppressive drugs in attempts to control progressive pulmonary insufficiency. Also, each had gone through normal pregnancies. This is of interest in view of embryotoxicity associated with ADA inhibition in mice, and because high levels of ADA are normally expressed in portions of the placenta.[30,31]

These extraordinary adult cases, and some pediatric cases diagnosed late in the first decade, suggest that there may be an underdiagnosed class of ADA-deficient individuals in whom the degree of immunodeficiency is compatible with long survival, albeit with gradual immunologic and clinical deterioration over years. Early diagnosis of ADA deficiency is essential, both to avoid treatment with immunosuppressive agents and because specific therapy may restore immune function sufficiently to prevent this deterioration. It is important to stress that T-cell lymphopenia is the sign that has most often led to consideration of CID and ADA deficiency in patients with delayed/late onset.

Clinical heterogeneity within a family can occur, but it is difficult to evaluate. In most cases awareness of one affected child leads to diagnosis and treatment of subsequent affected sibs at birth, before the clinical condition is full blown. There have been exceptions. Giblett's second patient had been well until 2 years of age, whereas her younger sib, diagnosed with CID at 14 months, had a first episode of pneumonia at 9 months.[1,23,32] In another family,[27] the younger of two sibs presented first with SCID, with persistent diarrhea, respiratory infections, and failure to thrive from 4 months of age; she was diagnosed at 9 months during evaluation for *Pseudomonas sepsis* and *P. carinii* pneumonia. Her 39-month-old "healthy" sib was then tested and found to be ADA deficient; her benign clinical history included an uneventful recovery from varicella at 12 months of age and normal growth. Lymphopenia had been noted at 1 year of age, but at diagnosis she showed some preservation of both cellular and humoral immunity. Clinical and immunologic deterioration over the next several months eventually led to enzyme replacement therapy.[27]

Autoimmunity. Dysregulated humoral immunity has occurred in untreated patients with milder immune dysfunction, and in SCID patients during the initial period of enzyme replacement therapy, when return of B cells precedes that of T cells (see later section on Therapy). Autoimmune thyroid insufficiency was found at presentation in a 14-month-old[32] and was recognized at 9 years of age in a second patient, in whom ADA deficiency was diagnosed at 8 years.[24] Transient immune thrombocytopenia precipitated by a viral syndrome occurred in a 2-year-old girl with delayed onset of CID shortly after starting enzyme replacement therapy.[33] Fatal autoimmune hemolytic anemia has occurred in two SCID patients: in one after a virus infection in the second month of enzyme replacement therapy (A. Junker, unpublished observations), and in the other after 2 years of erythrocyte transfusion therapy.[20,34] ADA deficiency was diagnosed at 2 years of age in a patient with a history of mild infections who presented at 1 year of age with severe atopic dermatitis and insulin-dependent diabetes.[35] Autoimmunity should be considered a consequence of ADA deficiency, but, as with neurologic abnormalities, it is more commonly associated with PNP deficiency.

Clinical Manifestations Unrelated to Immune Function. It is not uncommon for serum transaminases to be elevated, but usually without overt hepatic dysfunction; etiology has rarely been pursued. In one patient in whom persisting neonatal hepatitis was the presenting illness, an extensive search for etiology, including liver biopsy, failed to reveal any known infectious agent or GVHD; hepatic function normalized with enzyme replacement therapy, suggesting that metabolic injury per se was responsible for hepatitis.[36] We are aware of other patients in whom overt hepatobiliary dysfunction was a presenting or a major finding[29] (and unpublished observations), or in whom an increase in serum transaminases followed interruption of ADA replacement therapy to evaluate gene therapy,[37] or prior to BMT (unpublished observations) (hepatic injury in ADA-deficient mice is discussed in the section on Pathogenesis). Fine, sparse hair, anatomic malformations of the urinary tract, and transient renal tubular acidosis have been reported,[18] but it is unclear whether these are secondary to chronic infection or if their association with ADA deficiency is only coincidental.

Radiographic Features. As in other forms of SCID, x-rays show absence of a thymic shadow and suggest diminution or lack of adenoids. Cupping and flaring of the anterior rib ends has been described in ADA-deficient patients with a rachitic rosary.[38] Other x-ray abnormalities include pelvic dysplasia, shortening of the vertebral transverse processes with flattening or convexity of their ends, platyspondyly, and unusually thick growth arrest lines.[38] None of these changes are pathognomonic, and they have been construed as nonspecific reactions to metabolic insult. Nevertheless, rib abnormalities on chest x-ray have come to be associated with ADA deficiency.

Pathology. An early report suggested a difference in thymic histopathology between ADA-deficient patients and SCID patients with normal ADA levels.[39] No consistent differences were found in later studies.[18,40] In most autopsy specimens the thymus is hypoplastic, without corticomedullary demarcation; lymphocytes are absent and Hassall bodies cannot be identified. This was found in thymic tissue obtained from an affected fetus at 18 weeks of gestation.[41] In some cases areas of differentiated thymic epithelium and Hassall bodies are seen, and in one case normal thymic architecture and cellularity were present when the thymus was examined via biopsy at 6 months of age.[42] Few or no lymphocytes are found in lymph nodes and spleen.[40]

A number of cartilaginous growth plate abnormalities have been noted, which differ from those seen in other metaphyseal chondrodysplasias and correspond to the x-ray abnormalities described above.[43,44] Mesangial sclerosis in renal glomeruli and adrenal cortical sclerosis also have been noted.[44] It is not clear whether the latter findings have significant clinical correlates.

Laboratory Findings Related to Combined Immunodeficiency. Among all patients with SCID, those with ADA deficiency have the most profound lymphopenia, affecting T, B, and natural killer (NK) cells.[16] The total lymphocyte count is usually less than 500 per μl. Skin tests for delayed hypersensitivity to *Candida*, streptokinase, and other antigens are negative. *In vitro* lymphocyte responses to lectins (phytohemagglutinin, pokeweed mitogen, concanavalin A), allogeneic cells, and specific antigens are attenuated or absent. Total immunoglobulin levels may be only slightly depressed at birth owing to the maternal contribution of IgG, but IgM and IgA, which ordinarily do not cross the placenta, are often absent. IgG levels decline as maternal antibodies are cleared, and by 1 to 2 months of age pronounced hypogammaglobulinemia signals the lack of humoral immunity. Antibody responses to specific antigens such as tetanus toxoid and ϕX174 bacteriophage usually cannot be elicited; blood group isoagglutinins are absent in patients with SCID. Other laboratory abnormalities that may be present and are possibly related to chronic infection or to immunodeficiency include mild to moderate anemia and eosinophilia. Abnormal platelet function *in vitro* has been described.[45,46]

Diagnosis of ADA Deficiency. ADA activity is very low or undetectable in all tissues. The diagnosis is most easily made by measuring ADA activity in hemolysates by any of several modifications of spectrophotometric or radiochemical methods. The former measure the ADA-dependent conversion of adenosine (Ado) or deoxyadenosine (dAdo) to inosine or deoxyinosine,[47] or to uric acid in a coupled assay in which excess PNP and xanthine oxidase are added.[48] Spectrophotometric determination of ammonia has been used but is considered less reliable. Radiochemical assays measure conversion of labeled nucleoside substrate to nucleoside product, employing thin-layer, high-performance liquid chromatography (HPLC), or paper chromatographic separation. In radiochemical assays, phosphate-containing buffers must be avoided to prevent destruction of the product by PNP, which is present at high levels relative to ADA in hemolysates and in extracts of some nucleated cells. Fractionation of cell extracts over G-25 Sephadex spun columns equilibrated in Tris buffer has been used to remove phosphate and nucleotides that might generate phosphate.[49]

It is not uncommon that very ill patients have been transfused before the possibility of ADA deficiency has been considered. In this situation, measuring ADA in plasma is of no help because plasma ADA activity is normally very low and due in large part to a nonspecific aminohydrolase rather than to the ADA gene product. As discussed below, one of the metabolic hallmarks of ADA deficiency is a markedly increased concentration of dAdo nucleotides [dAXP, >90 percent deoxyadenosine triphosphate (dATP)] in red blood cells (RBCs). Because dAXP are almost undetectable in normal erythrocytes, the finding of appreciable dATP (dAXP) may be useful in pointing to ADA deficiency following transfusion. The diagnosis can then be confirmed by assaying ADA activity in erythrocyte-free preparations of blood mononuclear cells. Alternatively, if the patient is too lymphopenic, sufficient nucleated cells may be obtained from 1 to 2 ml of heparinized bone marrow. Analysis of DNA can be used for diagnosis if previous studies have identified the mutant ADA allele(s) in the family.

Prenatal Diagnosis and Heterozygote Detection. ADA deficiency has been diagnosed in the first trimester by direct enzyme assay of chorionic villi.[50,51] Second trimester diagnosis has usually been based on absence of ADA activity in cultured amniotic cells.[52–55] We have found two to four times higher ADA activity in fibroblasts cultured from chorionic villi than in the fresh tissue, and in cultured amniocytes compared with uncultured cells from amniotic fluid (M.S.H., unpublished observations). Therefore, we prefer to analyze the cultured cells, although this entails a delay of about 2 weeks. ADA deficiency also has been detected by assay of fetal erythrocytes.[56] T-cell lymphopenia and increased levels of erthrocyte dATP have been demonstrated in blood obtained from affected fetuses.[41] ADA and metabolite levels in amniotic fluid have not been useful for diagnosis.

Most obligate heterozygotes have approximately half-normal erythrocyte ADA activity. Because of overlap between about 10 percent of normal individuals and some obligate heterozygotes, erythrocyte ADA activity is not entirely reliable for carrier identification.[57] ADA levels in cultured skin fibroblasts, as well as in cultured amniocytes and chorionic villus fibroblasts, are also too variable to be useful in heterozygote detection.[58] Occasionally ADA polymorphisms have been used to identify carriers of a mutant or null gene.[59–61] In families where genotype has previously been determined, we have used DNA analysis to both confirm and to exclude the prenatal diagnosis of ADA deficiency, as well as for heterozygote detection (M.S.H. and colleagues, unpublished observations).

Partial ADA Deficiency. Shortly after the first description of ADA deficiency in SCID, a report appeared of a 10-year-old !Kung tribesman in Southwest Africa, who lacked erythrocyte ADA while retaining normal immune function.[62] This individual, who appears to be homozygous for a mutant ADA allele common among the !Kung (gene frequency 0.11),[63] had aproximately 2, 10, and 26 percent of normal ADA activity in his erythrocytes, leukocytes, and cultured fibroblasts, respectively.[64] Immune function was still normal at 18 years of age.[65] About a dozen other immunocompetent individuals have been found, with erythrocyte ADA ranging from about 20 percent of normal to undetectable, but about 4 to 70 percent of normal activity in lymphocytes or fibroblasts, a condition referred to as partial ADA deficiency.[42,66–71] Most "partials" have been ascertained through a newborn screening program in New York State.[72] The absence of erythrocyte ADA is believed to be due to the time-dependent inactivation of a relatively unstable mutant enzyme in cells that cannot synthesize new protein. ADA activity in nucleated cells of these individuals is sufficient to prevent the metabolic consequences of ADA deficiency, preserving immune function.[34,66,70,73]

Hereditary Elevation of Erythrocyte ADA Activity (MIM 102730). An inherited form of hemolytic anemia with erythrocyte ADA levels 40 to 85 times normal has been reported in three unrelated families.[74–76] Lymphocyte ADA levels and immune function were normal. Erythrocytes from patients in all three families contained an increased amount of catalytically and immunologically normal ADA.[74,76–78] The nonspherocytic, Coombs'-negative anemia was attributed to diminished erythrocyte adenosine triphosphate (ATP), resulting from increased adenosine monophosphate (AMP) catabolism and decreased adenine nucleotide synthesis from Ado.[76]

The molecular basis of this disorder is not known. A pedigree analysis of one family suggested autosomal dominant inheritance.[74] The erythroid-specific overproduction of ADA in one family was associated with increased levels of ADA messenger RNA (mRNA) in reticulocytes; the sequence of ADA complementary DNA (cDNA) cloned from reticulocytes was normal.[79,80] Analysis of a highly polymorphic region 2 kb upstream of the ADA transcriptional start site indicated that a single ADA allele was inherited concordantly with the overproduction phenotype in nine family members and was not present in eight unaffected individuals.[81] These data strongly suggest that enhanced ADA transcription in reticulocytes is due to a *cis*-acting mutation in an ADA gene regulatory element. Attempts to locate a specific mutation in the 5′ flanking region and first intron that confers ADA overexpression in transgenic mice have been unsuccessful.[82]

PNP Deficiency

This rare autosomal recessive disorder has been reported in fewer than 50 patients. The finding of a very low serum uric acid (see later section on Purine Nucleoside Metabolism) distinguishes PNP deficiency from other primary immunodeficiency disorders. Hypouricemia in association with T-cell lymphopenia in a child with recurrent infections, who also may have a neurologic or autoimmune disorder, should raise suspicion of PNP deficiency.

Presentation. The age of onset of clinical manifestations has ranged from 4 months to 6 years.[83] Presentations have included recurrent otitis, pharyngitis, sinus infections, pneumonia, disseminated varicella, diarrhea, and urinary tract infections.[84] A broad spectrum of organisms has been encountered, but viral pathogens are common, including cytomegalovirus, parainfluenza type 3, herpes, EBV, and ECHO meningoencephalitis. Routine bacterial pathogens such as *Hemophilus influenzae*, *Pseudomonas*, and *Streptococcus pneumoniae* have been found, as have opportunistic infections with *Candida albicans* and *P. carinii*. Most patients have received childhood immunizations without difficulty, but death due to generalized vaccinia has occurred.[9] Although PNP deficiency has been described as primarily a disorder of cellular immunity, the clinical profile of many cases suggests an associated humoral defect.

Neurologic abnormalities have been reported in more than half of PNP-deficient children, including spastic diplegia or tetraparesis, retarded motor development, ataxia, tremor, hyper- or hypotonia, behavioral difficulties, and varying degrees of mental retardation.[7,11,83,85,86] Five children were described with a syndrome of dysequilibrium characterized by hypotonia and difficulty in maintaining posture associated with spastic diplegia and deficient cellular immunity[87–89]; PNP deficiency was documented in each of the three children who were tested. Neurologic disease has preceded the presentation of immunodeficiency in at least seven patients. Although the neurologic manifestations are variable, the concurrence of immunodeficiency and neurologic problems strongly suggests PNP deficiency.

As with milder forms of ADA deficiency, autoimmune disorders are also common: hemolytic anemia (seven cases), idiopathic thrombocytopenic purpura, and autoimmune neutropenia have been reported, as have single cases of systemic lupus and central nervous system vasculitis.[10,11,83] The association of these disorders with PNP deficiency has been felt to reflect B-lymphocyte hyperactivity resulting from a loss of T-cell regulation. B-cell lymphomas, in one case associated with EBV infection, also occur and have been ascribed to primary T-cell dysfunction.[86,90]

Physical findings are compatible with a history of recurrent infections and may include mild hepatomegaly, splenomegaly, and developmental retardation. The thymus is absent on chest x-ray and tonsils are reduced in size or absent. The total lymphocyte count is frequently less than 500/μl. T-cell counts have decreased with age in several patients, although fluctuations and occasional spontaneous amelioration also have been noted.[83,91] T-cell function, as assessed by mitogenic responsiveness and by the mixed lymphocyte reaction, is reduced.[7,92] The number and function of B-lymphocytes have been normal in most cases, although increased serum immunoglobulins, monoclonal gammopathies, and specific autoantibodies reflecting aberrant B-lymphocyte regulation have been found with some frequency. In a review of 33 patients, 9 had some degree of B-cell dysfunction, such as low antibody or serum immunoglobulin levels.[91] These findings indicate that PNP deficiency may cause a SCID-like syndrome, and underscore the importance of measuring the activities of both ADA and PNP in all patients presenting with SCID.

Laboratory Diagnosis. PNP deficiency is usually diagnosed by finding extremely low or undetectable enzymatic activity in RBC lysates. In radiochemical assays, nucleoside substrates labeled in the purine ring are separated from the purine base product by HPLC, thin-layer chromatography, or paper chromatography. Spectrophotometric assays monitor the conversion of inosine to uric acid in the presence of excess xanthine oxidase; this assay has been optimized to yield a mean normal erythryocyte PNP activity of 18.6 U/ml packed cells at 37°C.[93] A colorimetric assay dependent on the oxidation of a chromogenic substrate in the presence of peroxidase,[94] as well as an isotopic assay based on the release of tritium from [2-^{3}H]inosine in the presence of xanthine oxidase,[93] also have been reported. The presence of 13 to 50 mM phosphate at a pH of 7.5 results in optimal enzymatic activity.

Purine nucleoside phosphorylase deficiency results in low serum (usually <1 mg/dl) and urinary levels of uric acid. Increased serum inosine and guanosine levels, and elevated levels of inosine, 2′-deoxyinosine, guanosine, and 2′-deoxyguanosine in urine, are pathognomonic (see later section on Purine Nucleoside Metabolism). Elevated deoxyguanosine triphosphate (dGTP) and decreased *S*-adenosylhomocysteinase (AdoHcyase) activity have been reported in RBCs, but to far lesser degrees than the dATP and AdoHcyase abnormalities found in ADA deficiency. Therefore, in patients who have been transfused, PNP deficiency can, for practical purposes (i.e., when PNP mutations in the family are unknown), only be diagnosed by assaying PNP activity in cleanly isolated blood mononuclear cells or in fibroblasts. In most cases, erythrocyte PNP activity is half-normal in obligate heterozygotes. PNP deficiency has been correctly excluded in a fetus at risk by assay of cultured amniotic cells[95]; measuring PNP in cultured chorionic villus fibroblasts is feasible[51] (and M.S.H., unpublished observations).

Table 109-1 Purine Compounds in Plasma or Serum: ADA and PNP Deficiency

Compound	Controls (μM)	ADA Deficiency (μM)	PNP Deficiency (μM)	References
Adenosine	<0.05–0.4	<0.1–10		73, 96, 104, 107, 632
Deoxyadenosine	Undetected	<0.1–7		96, 104, 107
Inosine	Undetected		14–115	6, 7, 11, 96, 116, 633–635
Guanosine	Undetected		6–29	7, 85, 633, 635
Deoxyinosine	Undetected		2–19	85
Deoxyguanosine	Undetected		2–14	85
Urate	220 ± 60	80–260	Trace to 150	6, 11, 85, 96, 116, 634, 635

Some data have been recalculated to allow comparison in common units.

Metabolic Abnormalities in Plasma, Erythrocytes, and Urine of ADA- and PNP-Deficient Patients

Data from several metabolic studies of ADA- and PNP-deficient patients are summarized in Tables 109-1 to 109-3. In ADA deficiency, uric acid levels are in the normal range.[96] Plasma Ado and dAdo are variably elevated to between 0.5 and 10 μM. Urinary excretion of dAdo is invariably elevated, and much greater than excretion of Ado, reflecting the more efficient reutilization (i.e., phosphorylation) of Ado than dAdo by cells. Urine also contains elevated levels of methylated and incompletely characterized derivatives of Ado.[97–100]

In ADA deficiency two pathognomonic consequences of impaired catabolism of dAdo are found in erythrocytes: (a) markedly elevated dATP and total dAdo nucleotides (dAXP, usually >90 percent dATP)[73,101]; and (b) decreased activity of the enzyme AdoHcyase, which is inactivated by dAdo, to less than 10 percent, and often to less than 5 percent of normal.[26,33,102–105] The magnitude of these abnormalities is related to clinical severity. This is most evident for dAXP, which are normally less than 2 nmol/ml packed RBCs, but range from about 300 to 2000 nmol/ml in early onset SCID, 30 to 300 nmol/ml in delayed /late onset SCID, and less than 30 nmol/ml in healthy individuals with partial ADA deficiency.[22,26,66,69,70,73,96,106] dATP accumulation has been found in the RBCs of ADA-deficient fetuses at 16 to 17 weeks of gestation[41,96] and in cord blood at birth.[96,107,108] Erythrocyte dAXP levels increase substantially after birth (M.S.H., unpublished observations). For example, in dizygotic ADA-deficient twin boys, dAXP increased from 253 and 289 nmol/ml in cord blood erythrocytes to 725 and 630 nmol/ml in venous erythrocytes at 10 days of age. In the most severely ADA-deficient patients, dAXP in erythrocytes may equal or exceed the level of AXP. In these cases, the absolute content of AXP is decreased, and may be half the normal level or less[102,103,109,110] (and M.S.H., unpublished observations).

Table 109-2 Purine Compounds in Urine: ADA Deficiency

Compound	Control	ADA Deficiency	References
Adenosine			
μmol/24h	<2	<2–5.6	113, 636
mmol/mmol creatine	<1	10.3 ± 20.4	96
μmol/g creatinine	<1	29.4 ± 5.7	100
Deoxyadenosine			
μmol/24h	Undetected	60–124	113, 636
mmol/mmol creatine	<1	140 ± 74	96
μmol/g creatinine	<0.1	582 ± 363	100
Uric acid			
mmol/mmol creatine	400–600	400–1600	96

Some data have been recalculated to allow comparison in common units.

In PNP deficiency, serum urate is usually less than 1 mg/dl and urinary excretion of uric acid is decreased. These low levels are due to the block in forming hypoxanthine and guanine, the substrates for xanthine oxidase, from PNP substrates. Plasma inosine is often greater than 20 μM and may exceed 100 μM; plasma guanosine, deoxyinosine, and 2′-deoxyguanosine (dGuo) range from 1 to 30 μM (Tables 109-1 and 109-3). Normally undetectable in RBCs, dGTP in the range of 2 to 11 nmol/ml packed cells (much less than the increase in dATP in ADA deficiency) has been found in patients with PNP deficiency.[85,110,111] Depletion of GTP to about 10 percent of normal in RBCs also has been observed.[85,110,112]

Aside from erythrocytes, there are limited data on dATP levels in other hematopoietic cells of ADA-deficient patients; dGTP pool expansion has only been demonstrated in erythrocytes of PNP-deficient patients. Marked dATP pool expansion (770 and 1760 pmol/10^6 cells; normal 2–4 pmol/10^6 cells) was found on two occasions in blood mononuclear cells of one ADA-deficient patient who had been receiving RBC transfusions for over a year.[113] In a later study of this patient over a 40-month period, mononuclear cell dATP was barely elevated (10 ± 3.9 pmol/10^6 cells, vs. 5.3 ± 1.3 in controls).[114] Interestingly, dATP was elevated (40–80 pmol/10^6 cells) in lymphocytes of donor origin isolated from an ADA-deficient patient who had undergone successful transplantation.[115] Blood mononuclear cell dATP levels of 5.4 and 14.4 pmol/10^6 cells were found in two other successfully transplanted patients.[105] dATP was about 2 percent of the ATP pool in nucleated cells, representing mostly immature nonlymphoid hematopoietic cells, from the bone marrow of one ADA-deficient patient, whereas in RBCs from the same marrow sample dATP was 70 percent of the ATP level.[102]

Purine Overexcretion in PNP Deficiency. By blocking the formation of hypoxanthine and guanine, PNP deficiency not only causes hypouricemia, but also interrupts a major salvage pathway for purine nucleotide synthesis via the HPRT reaction. As in primary HPRT deficiency (see Chapter 107), this results in overproduction of purines *de novo*. This is evident by the finding that total urinary excretion of the nucleoside substrates for PNP, the end products of purine catabolism in this setting, exceeds the normal excretion of uric acid.[97,116] For example, a 10-kg PNP-deficient child excreted in 24 h 0.08 mmol of uric acid, and 1.78, 0.71, 0.40, and 0.53 mmol each of inosine, guanosine, deoxyinosine, and dGuo, for a total purine excretion of 3.59 mmol. A 12.8-kg control child excreted 0.92 mmol of total purines, 95 percent as uric acid.[97] No clinical consequences of this purine overproduction have been noted. This reflects the greater solubility of nucleosides than uric acid, and the distribution among four rather than one compound.

In HPRT deficiency, two mechanisms contribute to purine overproduction *de novo*: (a) decreased synthesis of feedback-inhibitory nucleotides via the salvage pathway, and (b) increased intracellular PP-ribose-P (see Chapter 107). The PP-ribose-P

Table 109-3 Purine Compounds in Urine: PNP Deficiency

Compound	Controls*	PNP Deficiency*	References
Inosine	Undetected	1.3–4.3 (4.5–17)	6, 11, 85, 97, 116, 634–636
Guanosine	Undetected	0.61–2.3 (1.4–7.7)	6, 11, 85, 97, 116, 634–636
Deoxyinosine	Undetected	1.7, 0.4 (2.8–4.7)	85, 97, 116, 636
Deoxyguanosine	Undetected	0.82, 0.53 (2.3–3.6)	85, 97, 116, 636
Uric acid	(2.9–5.2)†	0.01–1.19 (0.16–3.13)	6, 11, 85, 97, 116, 634–636
Urate equivalents	(2.9–5.2)†	(11.3–30.3)	6, 11, 97, 116, 634–636

Some data have been recalculated to allow comparison in common units.
*Units = mmol/24 h (mmol/g creatinine).
†Data for children from Balis et al., *Science* **156**:1122 1967.

concentration is markedly elevated in cultured fibroblasts of patients with HPRT deficiency, but the level was normal in fibroblasts from a PNP-deficient patient.[116] This has been explained by the different ways in which HPRT and PNP deficiency interrupt an inosinate cycle[117]:

$$\begin{array}{c} \quad\quad PNP \quad\quad\quad\quad\quad\quad HPRT \\ \text{IMP} \rightarrow \text{Ino} \rightarrow \text{Hx} + \text{rib-PO}_4\ [\rightarrow \text{PP-rib-P}] \rightarrow \text{IMP} \end{array}$$

HPRT deficiency prevents reutilization of hypoxanthine (Hx) (and guanine), but salvage of the other PNP product, ribose-1-PO_4, after conversion to PP-ribose-P, can still occur, resulting in an increased steady-state concentration of PP-ribose-P. PNP deficiency blocks equally the salvage of the base and ribosyl moieties of PNP substrates, preventing excess PP-ribose-P formation. Thus, reduced salvage synthesis of feedback inhibitory nucleotides alone accounts for increased *de novo* purine production.[117]

PURINE NUCLEOSIDE METABOLISM

Adenosine deaminase catalyzes the irreversible, hydrolytic deamination of Ado and 2′-deoxyadenosine (dAdo) to inosine and 2′-deoxyinosine, respectively, and ammonia (Fig. 109-1). ADA also can hydrolyze six-position substituents of some purine nucleoside analogues. The reported Michaelis constant (K_m) values for Ado and dAdo are similar, 7 to 40 μM; the maximal rate for dAdo is about 30 percent that for Ado.[118–120] PNP catalyzes the reversible phosphorolysis of inosine and 2′-deoxyinosine (the ADA products), and of guanosine and dGuo, yielding hypoxanthine or guanine and the appropriate pentose-1-phosphate (Fig. 109-1). K_m values of 44 to 60 μM have been reported for the nucleoside substrates of PNP.[121,122] Although nucleoside formation is favored ($K_{eq} = 54$ for inosine and 2′-deoxyinosine formation[123,124]), phosphorolysis occurs readily, probably because the inorganic phosphate concentration in cells exceeds those of ribose- or 2-deoxyribose-1-phosphate, and because the subsequent metabolism of hypoxanthine and guanine is efficient. These bases may be reutilized by conversion to nucleoside monophosphates by the enzyme HPRT (see Chapter 107), or catabolized to xanthine and uric acid by the actions of guanase and xanthine oxidase (see Chapter 111).

The normal concentration of Ado in plasma has been reported as 82 ± 14 nM.[125] Other ADA and PNP substrates are usually reported as undetectable or negligible in plasma and in urine (Tables 109-1 to 109-3). By comparison, the plasma urate level is 0.2 to 0.45 mM, and 2 to 4 mMol of uric acid are excreted daily in urine. In cells, purines exist almost exclusively as nucleotides and nucleic acids, or in other forms such as AdoMet and AdoHcy, in which the substituent on the 5′ carbon of the pentose moiety is an amino acid. Purine nucleosides are generated as transient intermediates in the catabolism, interconversion, and normal metabolic turnover of these entities. Despite the low level of free nucleosides, the flux of Ado[125] and possibly other purine nucleosides through the circulation is very high. Their low steady state levels in normal plasma and urine reflect rapid uptake and efficient metabolism by cells. The discussion below summarizes aspects of metabolism relevant to understanding the consequences of ADA and PNP deficiencies, and some forms of therapy.

Extracellular Nucleoside Production and Transport

High levels of 5′-nucleotidase, alkaline phosphatase, ADA, PNP, xanthine oxidase, and guanase are coexpressed in epithelial cells lining some regions of the gastrointestinal tract.[126–128] *In situ* studies indicate that these enzymes constitute an efficient pathway of nucleotide catabolism to urate.[127] This probably accounts for the finding that dietary purine nucleotides and nucleosides are largely catabolized in the gut before gaining access to the circulation.[129–133] ADA or PNP deficiency would disrupt this degradative pathway, potentially increasing absorption of ADA or PNP substrates derived from diet; this possibility has not been studied.

Nucleosides can enter and leave all cells via a facilitated diffusion transporter with broad specificity and high capacity, which functions to equilibrate intra- and extracellular nucleoside concentrations.[134] cDNAs have been cloned for two equilibrative

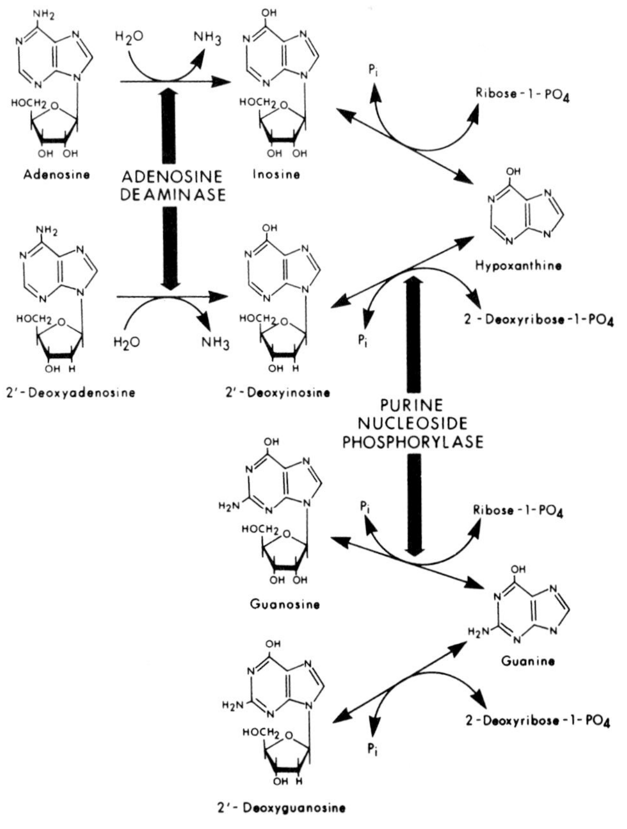

Fig. 109-1 Reactions catalyzed by ADA and PNP.

(e-type) transporters, distinguishable by their sensitivity or insenstivity (es or ei) to the nucleoside analogue nitrobenzylthioinosine.[135–137] Some specialized tissues and cell types also possess concentrative (c-type), sodium-dependent nucleoside transporters, which function mainly in the direction of cellular uptake. At least two types have been identified—one selective for purine and the other for pyrimidine nucleosides—although Ado and uridine are substrates for both.[134] There is no evidence that nucleoside transport is altered as a consequence of ADA or PNP deficiency.

Ecto-ATPases, as well as an ecto-5′-nucleotidase with broad specificity for 5′ nucleoside monophosphates but a preference for AMP, are associated with the external surfaces of endothelial and other cell types, including subsets of T- and B-lymphocytes, follicular dendritic cells, and thymic medullary epithelial cells.[138,139] These ecto-enzymes can generate Ado from adenine nucleotides released under certain conditions from platelets, neutrophils, neurons, and possibly other cell types, and thus may modulate the signaling and neurotransmitter actions of extracellular adenine nucleotides and Ado.[140–143] A tight coupling between ecto-nucleotidase activity and Ado uptake via sodium-dependent nucleoside transporters also has been suggested.[144]

Ecto-5′-nucleotidase is a homodimer of 61-kDa subunits linked to the cell membrane via a C-terminal glycosylphosphatidylinositol anchor.[145] A low K_m soluble nucleotidase with a preference for AMP has been isolated from many sources, including serum and human B- and T-lymphoblastoid cell lines.[146] This may be an easily solubilized form of ecto-5′-nucleotidase. Participation of ecto-nucleotidase in the metabolism of intracellular nucleotides has been questioned.[147]

Intracellular Metabolism of Purine Ribonucleosides

Several cytosolic 5′-nucleotidases have been characterized.[148–150] These appear to be involved, along with nucleoside kinases and in some cases ADA and PNP, in purine nucleoside-nucleotide substrate cycles that help to maintain ribo- and deoxyribonucleotide pools.[151–154] Deficiency of ADA or PNP would interrupt cycles in which they participate, potentially elevating levels of their substrates and altering some nucleotide pools.

In neutrophils and lymphoid cells, the major route of AMP catabolism appears to be deamination to IMP, rather than dephosphorylation to Ado, both under normal metabolic conditions[117,155–157] and conditions that increase ATP breakdown.[155,158–160] A cytosolic nucleotidase with nucleoside phosphotransferase activity, which prefers IMP and GMP to AMP, occurs in lymphoid cells and other tissues.[150,161] This enzyme is strongly activated by purine nucleoside triphosphates, including dATP.[149,157,162,163] In cultured lymphoblasts and fibroblasts, AMP deamination initiates an inosinate (IMP) cycle, involving this nucleotidase and PNP, but not ADA.[117,164,165] In contracting skeletal muscle, AMP deamination initiates a purine nucleotide cycle, which involves neither nucleotidase nor ADA or PNP (see Chapter 106).

In some tissues Ado can be derived from intracellular AMP by the action of a cytoplasmic 5′-nucleotidase.[151,154,166,167] A soluble nucleotidase in cardiac muscle, which may not occur in other tissues, prefers AMP to IMP and is activated by ADP.[149,168,169] Ado is also formed in all cells from the hydrolysis of AdoHcy, a by-product of AdoMet-dependent methylation. Metabolic balance studies, in which the intake and excretion of methylated compounds were determined in normal adults, indicate that 14 to 23 mmol of Ado are generated from AdoHcy daily.[170] Hepatic methylation of guanidinoacetic acid to form creatine alone accounts for about 85 percent of this total. In liver and other tissues, methylation of nucleic acids, proteins, phospholipids, biogenic amines, and various other acceptors accounts for the remainder of the Ado derived from this route.

In mammalian cells, Ado can either be rephosphorylated by Ado kinase or deaminated by ADA (cleavage to adenine is negligible). The K_m for Ado of human Ado kinase is 0.4 to 3 μM[171–173] versus 25 to 74 μM for human ADA.[119,120,174] In human lymphocytes[175] and B-lymphoblastoid cells[156] phosphorylation exceeded deamination at 0.5 to 5 μM Ado, even though total ADA activity far exceeds Ado kinase activity in these cells. Continuous cycling between AMP and Ado via cytosolic 5′-nucleotidase and Ado kinase has been demonstrated in normoxic liver and heart.[151,167] Thus, at Ado levels that exist under normal physiologic conditions, rephosphorylation is the major route of Ado metabolism. ADA plays a greater role under conditions that increase adenine nucleotide breakdown and AMP dephosphorylation.

Because of the high capacity for intracellular metabolism, the level of free Ado in cytoplasm is lower than in extracellular fluid, and net Ado movement is into cells via the nonconcentrative nucleoside transporter. When conditions (e.g., anoxia) favor adenine nucleotide catabolism to Ado, Ado kinase becomes saturated and is also subject to both substrate and product inhibition; Ado is then released from anoxic tissues with relatively low ADA activity, such as myocardium or liver.[154,171,176–180] Treating neuronal tissues with neurotransmitters increases extracellular Ado, which appears to be derived from release of adenine nucleotides that are then degraded by ectonucleotidases.[181,182]

Kinases for inosine, guanosine, and deoxyinosine do not occur in mammalian cells, and significant phosphorylation of dGuo probably occurs only in PNP deficiency. These nucleosides are normally metabolized exclusively by phosphorolysis (PNP) to purine bases, which may either be reconverted to nucleotides by HPRT or oxidized via xanthine oxidase to uric acid.

Purine Deoxynucleosides and Deoxynucleotides

With sensitive methods, and using ADA inhibitors or mutants lacking ADA or nucleoside kinases, it is possible to detect the release of only small amounts of dAdo from cultured lymphoblastoid cell lines.[183–185] *In vivo*, purine deoxynucleosides are largely derived from the degradation of DNA of senescent cells, the nuclei of erythroid progenitors, and various cell populations undergoing apoptosis. Cell turnover and apoptosis, and hence the generation of dAdo and dGuo, are particularly active in bone marrow, during stages of thymopoiesis, and in lymph nodes after antigenic stimulation.[186,186a,187]

2′-Deoxyadenosine and dGuo are normally acted on by ADA and PNP, either before release from macrophages involved in DNA degradation[186,187] or after uptake from the circulation or extracellular space by viable cells. Deficiency of ADA or PNP exposes these bystander cells to elevated levels of dAdo or dGuo, which may result in toxic effects, particulary resulting from expansion of intracellular dATP and dGTP pools (see later section on Pathogenesis). The degree of pool expansion is a function of the relative levels of deoxynucleoside kinase and deoxynucleotidase activities in target cells.[188,189]

Routes of purine deoxynucleotide catabolism are more limited than for their ribonucleotide counterparts. dAMP is a poor substrate for AMP deaminase; dAMP catabolism in T-lymphoblasts was shown to proceed almost exclusively via dephosphorylation to produce dAdo (in contrast to the efficient metabolism of AMP to IMP rather than to Ado).[157,159,190] In mouse T-lymphoblasts, GMP could be degraded either by deamination or dephosphorylation, but dGMP was exclusively converted to dGuo.[191]

The properties of kinases capable of phosphorylating purine deoxynucleosides have been reviewed.[192] dAdo can be phosphorylated by Ado kinase, but for the human enzyme the Km for dAdo is 135 to 540 μM, versus 0.3 to 3 μM for Ado.[171–173,193] A mitochondrial purine deoxynucleoside kinase with a preference for dGuo and a Km in the low micromolar range has been cloned.[194] The role of this enzyme in mediating dGuo cytotoxicity is uncertain. Most dAdo and dGuo phosphorylating activity in cell extracts is associated with deoxycytidine (dCyd) kinase.[195,196] This substrate specificity and its high level of expression in lymphoid cells have strongly implicated dCyd kinase in the development of lymphopenia of ADA and PNP deficiency (see section on Pathogenesis).

Human dCyd kinase is a 60-kDa homodimer encoded by a seven-exon gene on chromosome 4.[197–201] Although usually considered to be cytoplasmic, overexpressed human dCyd kinase localized to the nucleus.[202] Several purified preparations of dCyd kinase have been characterized.[192] The affinity for dCyd is much greater than for the purine substrates. For example, with enzyme from human T-lymphoblasts, apparent K_m values for dCyd, dAdo, and dGuo were, respectively, 0.8, 500, and 430 μM,[203] and 1, 120, and 150 μM for the enzyme from leukemic spleen.[197] The enzyme can use either ATP or uridine triphosphate (UTP) as phosphate donor, and it is feedback inhibited by deoxycytidine triphosphate (dCTP); dCyd strongly inhibits phosphorylation of both purine substrates.[192,195,197,198,203,204]

Mature RBCs lack dCyd kinase activity. This probably explains the lack of dGTP accumulation in erythrocytes of patients with PNP deficiency (Tables 109-1 to 109-3). The extraordinary accumulation dATP found in the RBCs of patients with ADA-deficient SCID can therefore be attributed to the action of Ado kinase. The relative contributions of Ado kinase and dCyd kinase to the phosphorylation of dAdo and dGuo have been evaluated in intact lymphoblastoid cells, which contain substantial levels of both activities. With S49 mouse T-lymphoma cells[205] and the human B-cell line WI-L2,[173,206] loss of Ado kinase diminished the toxicity of dAdo and eliminated the ability of dAdo to cause dATP pool expansion; loss of dCyd kinase had little effect on either dAdo toxicity or dATP accumulation. In the CEM human T-cell line, both dCyd kinase and Ado kinase were active in phosphorylating dAdo, with dCyd kinase predominating at low concentrations of dAdo, and Ado kinase at higher concentrations.[207–209] Mutational loss of dCyd kinase eliminated[209,210] and exogenous dCyd blocked[207,211–214] dGTP accumulation from dGuo in T-cell lines. With human thymocytes, dCyd was able to completely block accumulation of dATP and dGTP from their deoxynucleoside precursors.[215]

Consistent with the relative activities of ADA, Ado kinase, and dCyd kinase, deamination was by far the major route of dAdo metabolism in several mouse tissues and human erythrocytes.[216] Using kinetic constants determined in extracts of rat thymocytes, it was caclulated that the ratio of deamination to phosphorylation would be greater than 2000:1 at 0.1 μM dAdo, and greater than 200:1 even at 1 mM; analogous ratios for Ado were 3:1 and 80:1.[120] The major route of dGuo metabolism by cultured T- and B-lymphoblasts was via PNP.[217,218] The K_m for dGuo of human erythrocyte PNP, 44 μM,[219] is much lower than the K_m for dCyd kinase, and in lymphoid cells PNP activity far exceeds that of dCyd kinase.[220–222] Taken together, available data indicate that in normal cells dAdo and dGuo are metabolized almost entirely by deamination and phosphorolysis, respectively. Phosphorylation only plays a significant role in their metabolism in ADA and PNP deficiency.

GENETIC ASPECTS

ADA Enzyme and Gene

Distribution of ADA. The enzyme is found in all tissues, but levels vary over a 10^3- to 10^4-fold range.[223,224] In humans the highest ADA activity is found in thymus (~800 IU per mg protein) and other lymphoid tissues; the lowest is in erythrocytes (~1 IU/mg).[127,220,224–228] Among nonlymphoid tissues, ADA is relatively high in the villi of epithelial cells lining the duodenum (570 IU/mg), but lower in other regions of the gastrointestinal tract.[127,228] In mice, ADA levels are more than 10-fold higher in epithelial cells lining the proximal alimentary tract than in the thymus.[126,127,228–230] ADA was estimated to account for 5 to 20 percent of total soluble protein in the murine tongue, esophagus, forestomach, and proximal small intestine. Maternal-derived decidual cells of the placenta are also rich in ADA in both the mouse[30,127,231] and human.[51] As noted (see earlier section on Purine Nucleoside Metabolism), in the foregut, decidua, and proximal small intestine of mice, ADA and PNP colocalize with other enzymes involved in nucleotide catabolism to uric acid.[126–128]

In addition to varying widely among tissues, ADA expression is also developmentally regulated. Among human lymphoid cells, expression in immature cortical thymocytes is higher than in medullary thymocytes and mature T-lymphocytes; a decrease in ADA activity with maturation also occurs in B cells.[232–235] In mice, ADA activity and ADA mRNA both increased by approximately 80-fold in the placenta between days 6 and 9 after implantation,[30,127,231] and by 100- to 1000-fold in the alimentary tract during the first weeks after birth.[126,127,228–230,236] ADA protein and mRNA in these tissues is highly localized, being confined in the placenta to maternally derived decidual cells, and in the foregut to the terminal portions of villi of postmitotic epithelial cells.

Structure and Chemistry of ADA. Human ADA is a 40,762-dalton peptide composed of 363 amino acids.[237–242] The N-terminal methionine is removed after translation to give a mature enzyme with 362 residues.[240] The *E. coli* and murine ADA genes respectively encode a 332–amino acid protein (Mr 36,345) with 33 percent and a 352–amino acid protein with 83.1 percent homology to human ADA.[243,244] Due to an earlier translation stop codon, murine ADA lacks the 11 C-terminal amino acids of the human protein.

The 2.4-Å crystal structure of recombinant murine ADA revealed a parallel α/β barrel architecture, with eight central β strands and eight peripheral α helices.[245,246] Each ADA molecule contained one very tightly associated zinc atom situated deep within the active site pocket (Fig. 109-2). A cofactor requirement had not previously been suspected because purified ADA is fully active after prolonged dialysis. However, *in vitro* mutagenesis of three of the residues involved in zinc coordination (H17, H214, D295) eliminated ADA activity,[247] and a naturally occurring mutation of the fourth zinc-binding residue (H15D) was responsible for ADA deficiency in a patient with SCID.[248] The zinc atom also coordinated with the 6-hydroxyl of the enzyme-bound transition state analogue 6-hydroxy-1,6-dihydropurine ribonucleoside.[245] It was suggested that this interaction may account for the extraordinarily high binding affinity of ADA-inhibitory analogues possessing a 6-hydroxyl group in the proper configuration.[249,250] Adenylate (AMP) deaminase, which catalyzes a hydrolytic deamination similar to that of ADA, is also a zinc enzyme. Several short amino acid sequences found in AMP deaminases from several species are conserved among procaryotic and mammalian ADAs, suggesting a common evolution of these two enzymes.[244]

Association with ADA Complexing Protein. Purified, catalytically active ADA from several human tissues is a monomer of 36 to 44 kDa.[174,251–253] However, ADA activity in crude extracts fractionates from about 40 kDa, the only species present in hemolysates, up to about 280 kDa, found in fibroblasts and various organs. These larger forms result from binding of the 41-kDa ADA gene product to a noncatalytic homodimeric glycoprotein, with a subunit of 110 kDa, termed ADA conversion factor, binding protein, or complexing protein (ADA-CP).[224,254–257] ADA-CP is predominantly plasma membrane associated and localizes to secretory or adsorptive surfaces of epithelia of liver, gut, kidney, and exocrine glands; it is also found free in plasma, urine, saliva, and tears.[255,256,258–265]

Dimeric ADA-CP was shown to bind two molecules of catalytic ADA; this interaction did not affect the activity of ADA.[255] The equilibrium constant for binding of human, rabbit, and calf ADA to ADA-CP was estimated at 4 to 20 nM, using rabbit kidney membrane ADA-CP.[265] Genes on chromosomes 2 and 6 were required for ADA-CP expression in somatic cell

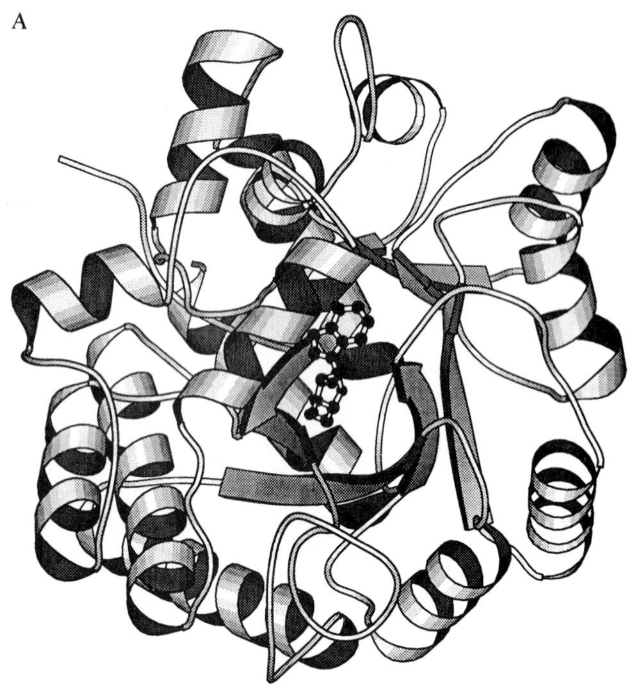

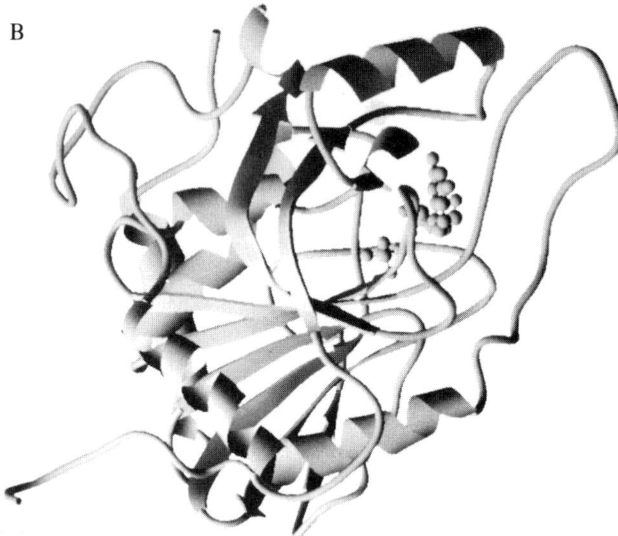

Fig. 109-2 ***A.*** **Structure of recombinant murine ADA (*courtesy of F. Quiocho*).** ***B.*** **Structure of human erythrocyte PNP (*courtesy of S. Ealick*).**

hybrids.[266–268] The function of ADA-CP–associated ADA was unclear, but a role in ADA deficiency was generally not suspected. A low level of surface-bound ADA was detected on blood mononuclear cells,[269,270] but ADA associated with these cells is largely intracellular. It was speculated that a high level of ADA-CP on kidney tubular epithelium mediates the renal clearance of ADA.[256,260,265,271,272] It was also speculated that ADA-CP regulates the level of plasma ADA or of extracellular Ado.[258,259,273]

Recent studies have shown that ADA-CP is identical to a multifunctional protein known as CD26/dipeptidyl peptidase IV (DPP-IV).[274,275] CD26 was initially defined as a surface antigen of activated T cells[276] and was later shown to be identical to DPP-IV, an extensively studied ecto-peptidase with the same tissue distribution as ADA-CP and a structural gene on chromosome 2.[277–279] cDNAs cloned from human T cells and intestine predict a 766-residue polypeptide of 88,300 kDa with 10 potential N-glycosylation sites.[279–281] CD26/DPP-IV is a type II membrane protein; a 34-residue, uncleaved signal peptide anchors it into the plasma membrane, leaving only the six N-terminal residues facing into the cytoplasm.[282,283] The serine protease (DPP-IV) active site is in the extracellular C-terminal domain (residues 628–632 of the human protein). DPP-IV cleaves the N-terminal dipeptide from peptides with proline or alanine as the second amino acid; it may be involved in the absorption or degradation of proline-containing peptides, including several hormones and cytokines.

Although similar in amino acid sequence to the human protein, CD26/DPP-IV from mouse and rat does not bind ADA.[263,284] Replacing small regions of human CD26 with rat sequences identified residues 340 to 343 of the extracellular portion of CD26 as essential for ADA binding.[285] ADA associated with CD26 on human T cells was not derived from intracellular ADA, and only a fraction of cell surface–associated CD26 was occupied by ADA.[286] It was concluded that ADA bound to CD26/DPP-IV/ADA-CP is not transported to the cell surface, but is probably scavenged from the circulation after release from senescent cells.

CD26 is expressed on medullary thymocytes late in differentiation, and in the periphery on activated T-lymphocytes, particularly those with a helper/memory phenotype.[287] CD26 is a costimulator of human T-cell and thymocyte proliferation and of interleukin-2 (IL-2) production, acting apparently through multiple signal transduction pathways, possibly via interaction with the CD45 protein tyrosine phosphatase.[288–290] CD26 is also a costimulator of immature thymocytes and cells of other hematopoietic lineages in the mouse and rat,[291,292] and it has been reported to be essential for thymocyte maturation in the mouse.[293]

With the discovery that ADA-CP is CD26, it has been speculated that in humans binding of ADA is important to the costimulatory function of CD26, that such binding protects lymphocytes from effects of extracellular Ado, and even that immunodeficiency in patients with ADA deficiency is due to absence of CD26-associated ADA.[287] There are several reasons to be skeptical about these hypotheses. Regarding regulation of extracellular Ado, (a) the saturation of human T cell CD26 with ADA is low, and the bound ADA seems to be scavenged from plasma, rather than regulated; (b) plasma Ado and dAdo levels are far below the K_m for ADA; (c) these ADA substrates can enter cells very efficiently; and (d) not only does cytosolic ADA activity far exceed CD26-associated ADA in lymphoid cells, but cytosolic Ado kinase may play a greater role in Ado metabolism than ADA (see earlier section on Purine Nucleoside Metabolism). Regarding the role of CD26-associated ADA in regulating the thymocyte proliferation and lymphocyte function, although the costimulatory function of CD26 on thymocytes and activated T cells seems to be conserved in humans and rodents, as noted above, rodent CD26 does not bind ADA. Moreover, an apparently healthy strain of rats totally lacks cell surface expression of CD26/DPP-IV owing to a destabilizing mutation at the DPP-IV active site.[294,295] We have localized the CD26 binding site of human ADA to the carboxy end of a peripheral helical segment comprising residues 126–143. Mutation of Arg 142 to Gln (found at this position in mouse ADA) largely prevented CD26 binding (E. Richard, FX Arredondo-Vega, I Santisteban, SJ Kelly, DD Patel, MS Hershfield, submitted). We have identified a healthy adult with partial ADA deficiency, whose only expressed ADA allele carries the R142Q mutation (reference 344, cited in Table 109-4). These findings suggest that in humans, as in mice, binding of ADA to CD26 is not essential for the development or maintenance of immune function.

Structure and Regulation of the ADA Gene. The ADA locus has been assigned to the long arm of human chromosome 20,[296,297] region 20q13.11.[298,299] The human ADA gene has been cloned[300,301] and completely sequenced.[301] Spanning 32,040 bp from the transcription start site to polyadenylation site, it consists

Table 109-4 ADA Gene Missense and Nonsense Mutations

Mutation Designation	Site	Nucleotide*	Change	Effect	References
Missense					
H15D	Ex2	43 (138)	CAT → GAT	His15 → Asp	248
G20R	Ex2	58 (153)	GGA → AGA	Gly20 → Arg	364
G74C	Ex4	220 (315)	GGC → TGC	Gly74 → Cys	342
G74V	Ex4	221 (316)	GGC → GTC	Gly74 → Val	36
R76W	Ex4	226 (321)	CGG → TGG	Arg76 → Trp	355
A83D	Ex4	248 (343)	GCC → GAC	Ala83 → Asp	248
Y97C	Ex4	290 (385)	TAT → TGT	Tyr97 → Cys	637
R101W	Ex4	301 (396)	CGG → TGG	Arg101 → Trp	348
R101Q	Ex4	302 (397)	CGG → CAG	Arg101 → Gln	359
R101L	Ex4	302 (397)	CGG → CTG	Arg101 → Leu	26
P104L	Ex4	311 (406)	CCG → CTG	Pro104 → Leu	638
L106V	Ex4	316 (411)	CTG → GTG	Leu106 → Val	637
L107P	Ex4	320 (415)	CTG → CCG	Leu107 → Pro	355
P126Q	Ex5	377 (472)	CCA → CAA	Pro126 → Gln	29
V129M	Ex5	385 (480)	GTG → ATG	Val129 → Met	342
G140E	Ex5	419 (514)	GGG → GAG	Gly140 → Glu	342
R142Q	Ex5	425 (520)	CGA → CAA	Arg142 → Gln	344
R149W	Ex5	445 (540)	CGG → TGG	Arg149 → Trp	342
R149Q	Ex5	446 (541)	CGG → CAG	Arg149 → Gln	355
L152M	Ex5	454 (549)	CTG → ATG	Leu152 → Met	353
R156C	Ex5	466 (561)	CGC → TGC	Arg156 → Cys	365
R156H	Ex5	467 (562)	CGC → CAC	Arg156 → His	26
V177M	Ex6	529 (624)	GTG → ATG	Val177 → Met	26
A179D	Ex6	536 (631)	GCC → GAC	Ala179 → Asp	248
Q199P	Ex6	596 (691)	CAG → CCG	Gln199 → Pro	342
R211C	Ex7	631 (726)	CGT → TGT	Arg211 → Cys	355
R211H	Ex7	632 (727)	CGT → CAT	Arg211 → His	348
A215T	Ex7	643 (738)	GCC → ACC	Arg215 → Thr	29, 355
G216R	Ex7	646 (741)	GGG → AGG	Gly216 → Arg	26, 363
E217K	Ex7	649 (744)	GAG → AAG	Glu217 → Lys	338
T233I	Ex8	698 (793)	ACA → ATA	Thr233 → Ile	353
R253P	Ex8	758 (853)	CGG → CCG	Arg253 → Pro	366
P274L	Ex9	821 (916)	CCG → CTG	Pro274 → Leu	355
S291L	Ex10	872 (967)	TCG → TTG	Ser291 → Leu	26, 365
P297Q	Ex10	890 (985)	CCG → CAG	Pro297 → Gln	354
A329V	Ex11	986 (1081)	GCG → GTG	Ala329 → Val	348
Nonsense					
Q3X	Ex1	7 (102)	CAG → TAG	Gln3 → Term	344
R142X	Ex5	424 (519)	CGA → TGA	Arg142 → Term skip Ex 5	344
Q254X	Ex8	760 (855)	CAG → TAG	Gln254 → Term	340

*cDNA numbering: from start of translation (transcription) (based on method of Wiginton et al.[301])

of 12 exons ranging in size from 62 to 325 bp and 11 introns, the first of which is larger than 15 kb (Fig. 109-3). The major mRNA is 1.5 kb, consisting of 95 nucleotides of 5′- and 311 of 3′-untranslated sequences flanking a 1089-nucleotide open reading frame. Scattered through the gene are 23 Alu repetitive elements, 13 within intron 1. Basal promoter activity was localized to 81 bp of the 5′ flanking sequence. This promoter consists of 82 percent G + C residues, lacks TATA and CCAT sequences, and possesses six functional binding sites for the Sp1 transcriptional activator.[302] The murine ADA gene promoter has similar characteristics.[303,304] Although apparently sufficient to determine constitutive (house-keeping) ADA expression, neither the basal human promoter nor 3.7 kb of upstream sequence conferred specific ADA expression in T-cell lines or in thymus of transgenic mice.[228,300,305]

Widely distributed *cis*-acting sequences appear to control tissue-specific ADA gene expression. A cluster of DNase hypersensitive sites 4.3 to 8.5 kb downstream of the first exon, within the large first intron of the human ADA gene was found to have T cell–specific enhancer activity.[228,306] Constructs bearing this region in addition to the promoter were expressed at very high levels in the thymus of transgenic mice. The active enhancer was a 230-bp element containing functional consensus binding sites for several transcription factors, including AP1, E box, c-Myb, Ets, and LEF-1.[228,306–308] A mouse ADA gene enhancer with similar features has been characterized.[309] Facilitator sequences flanking the human ADA T-cell enhancer had locus control region (LCR) properties, resulting in position-independent transgene expression.[306,307,310] A discrete region in the human ADA gene situated 3′ from the T-cell enhancer has been found to confer high-level expression in the duodenum of transgenic mice.[311] In the case of the murine ADA gene, *cis*-acting sequences and *trans*-acting factors that mediate high-level forestomach and placental expression of mouse ADA have been identified.[312–314]

Other Regulatory Aspects of ADA Gene Expression. As in tissues of mice, ADA levels correlated with steady state levels of ADA mRNA in cultured human T- and B-lymphoblasts, HL-60 promyelocytic cells, and fibroblasts,[238,315,316] suggesting

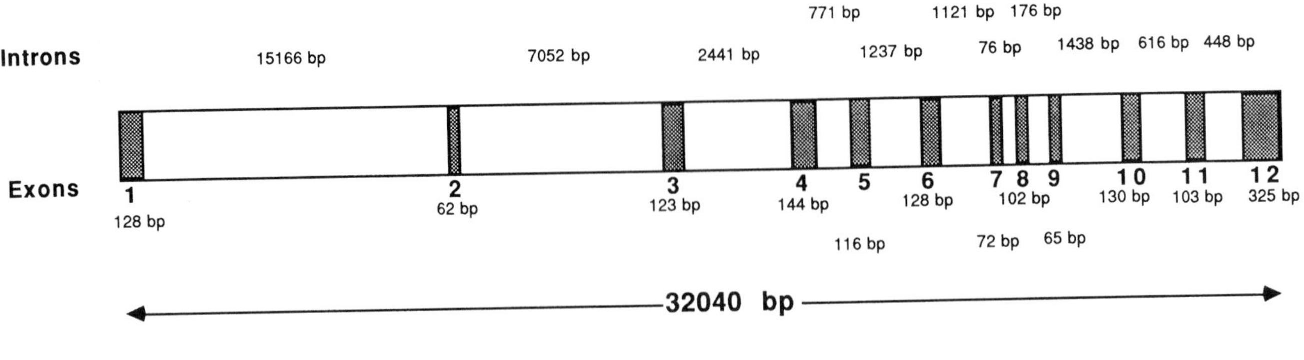

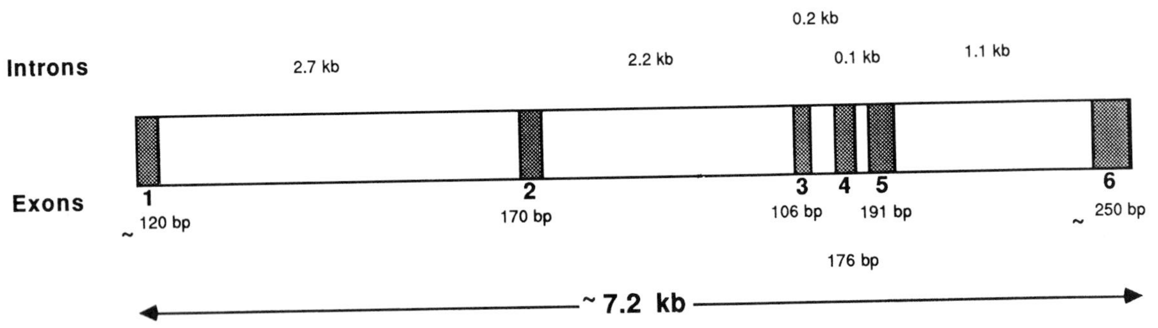

Fig. 109-3 Genes for human ADA and PNP. Exons are shown as *shaded* regions, introns as *open*. The scale is not proportional to nucleotide length. (*From the data of Wiginton et al.*[301] *for the ADA gene and Williams et al.*[371,372] *for the PNP gene.*)

transcriptional control of ADA expression. Human leukocyte antigen (HLA)-60 cells and Molt-4 T-lymphoblasts differing by approximately 17- and 20-fold, respectively, in levels of ADA activity and ADA mRNA showed little difference in rates of initiation of ADA mRNA synthesis or in the stability of the mRNA in cytoplasm. The difference in ADA mRNA levels was attributed to a difference in posttranscriptional processing or in stability of the message in the nucleus.[315] By contrast, steady state levels of ADA mRNA in human T- and B-lymphoblasts and fibroblasts correlated well with rates of ADA mRNA transcription.[316]

Arrest of transcript elongation appears to play a role in determining ADA mRNA levels in murine and human cell lines and murine tissues.[236,303,316,317] Transcription of human and murine ADA gene constructs in frog oocytes gave rise to 105-bp (human) and 96-bp (mouse) properly initiated but prematurely terminated transcripts; the major sites of arrest were, respectively, at 10 and 7 nucleotides distal to the translational start site in exon 1.[317,318] Similar results with murine ADA gene constructs were obtained with an *in vitro* RNA polymerase II–mediated transcription system.[319] Sequences approximately 65 bp downstream from the 3′ end of murine exon 1 were necessary for production of the short transcript.[318]

Differences in rates of ADA protein turnover provide another level of control of cellular ADA activity. A three- to sixfold faster rate of ADA degradation in human B-cell than T-cell lines contributed to the 7- to 12-fold difference in their ADA activity.[320] It was estimated that of the approximately 50-fold higher ADA activity in the Molt-4 T-cell line than in B-lymphoblasts, approximately 10-fold was due to a greater rate of Molt-4 ADA gene transcription and the remainder to more rapid ADA degradation in the B-cell lines.[316]

The Primary Genetic Defect. Early studies found that ADA-deficient patients lacked both the small (41-kDa) erythrocyte and larger tissue ADA isozymes, indicating a defect in a common catalytic component.[321] ADA-complexing protein (CD26/DPP-IV) was normal in fibroblasts, liver, and kidney of patients.[322,323] A minor Ado deaminating activity found in spleen, serum, and lymphoblasts of ADA-deficient and normal individuals was shown to differ from the major enzyme with respect to its size, insensitivity to ADA inhibitors, lack of immunologic cross-reactivity, and a K_m of 2 to 3 mM for Ado[324–326] versus approximately 50 μM for ADA.[174] The minor Ado deaminase appears to be a spurious aminohydrolase activity of some unknown enzyme, and it plays no physiologic role in Ado metabolism.

The residual ADA in extracts of erythrocytes, fibroblasts, and lymphoid cell lines of immunodeficient patients has been characterized with regard to electrophoretic mobility, stability, immunologic cross-reactivity, and, where activity was detectable, kinetic parameters.[322,327–329] Considerable heterogeneity was found, but some early studies did not distinguish residual ADA from the nonspecific aminohydrolase. Concerns also have been raised that cultured fibroblasts can endocytose bovine ADA from fetal calf serum, and that fibroblast ADA-CP–associated ADA may not be quantified accurately in immunoassays developed with purified ADA.[257,328] Lymphoblastoid cell lines from several SCID patients had less than 5 percent (usually <1 percent) of normal ADA activity; ADA protein detected by western blot and radioimmunoassay was less than 12 percent of normal (usually much less).[70,328,330] In most patient cell lines, levels of ADA mRNA were normal or increased.[238,240,329–332] Many of these cell lines were later discovered to have been derived from compound heterozygotes.

Table 109-5 ADA Gene Deletion and Splicing Mutations

Mutation Designation	Site/Nucleotide*	Change	Effect	References
Deletion				
alu 1 → *alu* 3	†g−1491 to †g + 1757 ± 13	del 3.25 kb	del promoter, Ex1	335, 336
alu 1 → *alu* 3	†g − 1533 to †g + 1735 ± 16	del 3.25 kb	del promoter, Ex1	337
>30 kb 5′ gene	>4 kb 5′ to g + 26620	del >30 kb	del promoter, Ex1-5	338
367del1	367 (462)	del **G**	frameshift	342
539del2	539–540 (634–635)	del **TT**	frameshift	639
955del5	955–959 (1050–1054)	del **GAAGA**	frameshift	26, 339, 340
E337del	1009–1011 (1104–1106)	del **AGA**	del Glu337	342
1019del2	1019–1020 (1114–1115)	del **AG**	frameshift	26
Splicing				
33 (128) + 1G → T	IVS1 5′ ss	**GT → TT**	↓mRNA	349
95 (190) + 1G → A	IVS2 5′ ss	**GT → AT**	ins 4 bp, skip Ex2 ↓mRNA	343
219 (314) − 2A → G	IVS3 3′ ss	**AG → GG**	skip Ex 4	348
478 (573) + 1G → A	IVS5 5′ ss	**GT → AT**	skip Ex 5, ↓mRNA	248
478 (573) + 6T → A	IVS5 5′ ss	GTGAGT → GTGAG**A**	skip Ex5, ↓mRNA	26
678 (773) + 1G → A	IVS7 5′ ss	**GT → AT**	skip Ex7	639
781 (876) − 3 → + 1 ins/rearr	IVS8/Ex9 boundary	TC**CAG/AT** → TC**TGGAAGAG CAGATCTGG**T	skip Ex9, ↓mRNA	343
975 (1070) + 1G → A	IVS10 5′ ss	**GT → AG**	ins 4 bp, ↓mRNA	26
976 (1071) − 34 G → A	IVS10 3′ ss	**GG → AG**	ins 32 bp, extend reading frame, add 100 amino acids	26

*cDNA numbering: from start of translation (transcription); "g" preceding a number indicates genomic DNA (cDNA and genomic numbering based on the method of Wiginton et al.[301]).
†Approximate position.

Over 60 different ADA mutations have now been identified (Tables 109-4 and 109-5). Almost two thirds alter single amino acids; deletions and splicing mutations each account for about 15 percent, and three are nonsense mutations. Some aspects of the mutational spectrum are noteworthy.

Homologous recombination between the first and third Alu repeats has resulted in two different deletions of about 3.2 kb that eliminate the promoter and exon 1.[333–337] A third large deletion beginning at an undefined point upstream extends through more than 25 kb of the 5′ end of the ADA gene, eliminating the promoter and exons 1 to 5.[338] Most ADA deletions are short (1–5 bp) and introduce premature translation stop signals, resulting in decreased levels of ADA mRNA. A recurrent 5-bp deletion in exon 10 (955del5)[26,339,340] and a 2-bp deletion in exon 11[26] occur in sequences containing several 2- to 4-bp direct repeats that resemble short deletional hot spots.[341] A 3-bp deletion in exon 11 eliminates the codon for Glu337.[342]

Most ADA splice site mutations are intronic single base pair substitutions that cause exon skipping or activate cryptic splice sites, resulting in premature translation termination and decreased levels of mRNA. Skipping of exon 9 was caused by a complex 17-bp insertion rearrangement, apparently due to template strand switching during replication, which inserts a run of seven purines into the polypyrimidine tract of the 3′splice site of IVS 8.[343] A G → A mutation in IVS 10, at bp −34 from the start of exon 11, activates a strong cryptic 3′ splice site, inserting 32 intronic nucleotides into the mRNA; this had the interesting effect of extending the reading frame through the 3′-untranslated region to add 100 amino acids to the carboxy end of ADA.[26] The homozygous patient in whom this allele was found was diagnosed at age 15 years. Several other splicing mutations also have been identified in patients with later onset phenotypes, suggesting that a low level of correct splicing may provide sufficient wild-type ADA mRNA to modify the phenotype.[26,343]

In addition to exon skipping due to intronic mutations, a nonsense mutation in the middle of exon 5 (R142X), apparently situated in a purine-rich splicing enhancer, caused exon 5 skipping in two homozygous Canadian Mennonite SCID patients.[29,344] Nonsense mutations in exons 1 and 8 did not appear to affect splicing.[340,344] Skipping of exon 7 or inclusion of intron 7 has been found in 10 to 15 percent of ADA cDNAs cloned from normal individuals, and from ADA-deficient patients without mutations in or near exon 7. This has been attributed to the relatively short intron 7 (76 bp) or to a weak 5′ splice site.[332,345] An increased frequency of exon 7 skipping was associated with the A215T missense mutation situated in the middle of the exon.[29] Other exon 7 missense mutations did not appear to have this effect.

Over 35 ADA missense mutations have been identified in immunodeficient patients and in healthy individuals with partial ADA deficiency (Table 109-4). Reduced enzymic activity resulting from these mutations has been demonstrated by expression of cloned cDNA, or by *in vitro* translation of transcripts generated from cDNA. As noted in references cited in Table 109-4, several of these mutations are recurrent, arising from CpG mutational hot spots.[346] Some recurrent mutations have been shown to occur on different haplotypes (e.g., A329V).[347] Among patients undergoing enzyme replacement therapy, we have found R211H in black, white, Hispanic, and Asian (Indian) patients; G216R in black, white, and Asian (Indian) patients; and A329V in black and white patients (I. Santisteban, F.X. Arredondo-Vega, and M.S. Hershfield, unpublished observations). Some mutations are probably recurrent by descent (e.g., L107P and V129M, identified in multiple patients of French and Italian origin, respectively).

The effects of several amino acid substitutions found in patients have been modeled on the crystal structure of murine ADA.[245] Only two directly involve active site residues. Glu217 (changed to Lys338) hydrogen bonds to the N-1 atom of substrate, and His15 (changed to Asp248) coordinates with zinc. Several other mutated residues, including Arg101, Arg211, Gly216, Ser291, and Leu304 are close to the active site, or to peptide segments that deploy active site residues. Several of these residues, as well as Leu107 and Ala179, are highly conserved.[244] It has been postulated that other missense mutations, including several found in individuals with partial ADA deficiency, may cause misalignment of β strands that line the ADA active site pocket.[245] In several cases where it has been examined, levels of immunologically detectable ADA protein have been reduced in erythrocytes and cell lines from patients with SCID[327,328] (and unpublished observations). Thus, the primary effect of many missense mutations may be to interfere with the folding or stability of ADA, predisposing it to proteolysis.

Cultured T cells of one SCID patient surprisingly expressed nearly normal ADA activity, whereas her B cells and other hematopoietic cells expressed less than 1 percent of normal activity.[49] Satellite DNA analysis gave no evidence of mosaicism, and all cDNA clones from her ADA-expressing T cells possessed either the R101W or R211H mutations, which had been identified in an ADA-deficient B-cell line from this patient.[348] It was speculated that one of these mutant alleles could be expressed as catalytically active ADA in cells where stable folding was favored, but in other cells the protein was labile and inactive.[49]

There have been reports of two ADA-deficient patients who presented with immunodeficiency as children, but later had spontaneous clinical remissions sustained until at least ages 12 and 20 years.[349,350] Each patient showed mosaicism in B-lymphoblastoid cell lines, one for an IVS1 splice site mutation, and the other for a maternally inherited missense mutation in exon 5 of the ADA gene, which had apparently undergone reversion. Although this is probably a rare event, these intriguing cases provide *in vivo* evidence for a selective advantage of ADA-expressing lymphoid cells, an effect that may prove important in gene therapy.

Genetic Defect in Partial ADA Deficiency. Compared with cell lines from patients with SCID, those from healthy individuals with partial ADA deficiency have had higher levels of residual ADA activity (about 2–80 percent of normal) and cross-reacting ADA protein, in some cases with altered stability or electrophoretic mobility.[29,66,67,70,344,351–353] A P297Q substitution was shown to cause heat lability.[354] In four cases, reduced levels of ADA protein in B-cell lines were associated with relatively normal levels of ADA mRNA and rates of enzyme synthesis, but 1.5- to 3-fold enhanced rates of ADA degradation.[352]

Most healthy individuals with partial ADA deficiency have been compound heterozygotes, with one allele providing substantially more residual activity than the other. Most of these mild alleles have not been found in patients with SCID. However, R211C, first identified in a healthy child,[355] also has been found in two immunodeficient sisters diagnosed with ADA deficiency as adults.[337] The L152M allele, identified in a healthy homozygous child of Afghanistani descent, may have been associated with immunodeficiency in other family members.[353] Based on these cases, it has been estimated that 2 to 5 percent of residual ADA activity may be the threshhold necessary to sustain protection from metabolic lymphotoxicity.[353,355]

Polymorphisms. Analysis of ADA in hemolysates (which is not complexed with ADA-CP/CD26) by starch gel electrophoresis gives a relatively simple pattern consisting of one major and two minor bands, the latter apparently due to posttranslational modification. This system has been used extensively to study ADA genetic polymorphism.[48,356,357] The most common normal variant, designated ADA 2, has a slightly slower anodal mobility (more basic) than the predominant ADA 1 allozyme, and a gene frequency estimated at approximately 0.06 in Western populations and 0.03 to 0.11 in African and Southeast Asian populations. ADA 2 results from a substitution of asparagine for aspartic acid at codon 8 (D8N).[358] Several other nucleotide differences that result in synonomous codons (silent polymorphisms), and polymorphisms that do not significantly reduce activity, also have been identified.[345,359–361] A highly polymorphic $(TAAA)_n$ repeat in an Alu sequence 1.1 kb 5′ to the ADA transcription initiation site also has been identified and used in analyzing ADA allele inheritance.[337,344,362]

Relationship of Genotype and Metabolic Status to Clinical Phenotype in ADA Deficiency. Erythrocyte ADA activity is low in all phenotypes associated with ADA deficiency; this most likely reflects the low ADA expression and lack of protein turnover in RBCs, which favor loss of unstable mutant enzymes. In contrast to ADA activity, RBC dAXP levels tend to correlate with clinical phenotype, with SCID > delayed/late onset > partial deficiency (see earlier section on Metabolic Abnormalities in Plasma, Erythrocytes, and Urine of ADA- and PNP-Deficient Patients).[22,26,66,69,70,73,96,106] Lacking DNA, erythrocytes neither require dATP nor produce dAdo; thus, dAXP pool expansion results from uptake of circulating dAdo. Assuming no systematic differences among patients in dAdo production, transport, or excretion, phenotype-related differences in RBC dAXP should reflect overall residual capacity of nonerythroid cells to catabolize dAdo (i.e., residual ADA activity), determined mainly by ADA genotype.

Although most mutations have been reported in single cases, a pattern relating ADA genotype to clinical status has emerged. Several SCID patients have been homozygous or functionally hemizygous for deletions or nonsense mutations,[333,335,339,342,344] or for amino acid substitutions at or close to the active site (G20R, R211H, G216R, E217K).[22,338,363,364] Other missense and some splicing mutations are preferentially associated with delayed/late onset phenotypes.[26,342,365,366] For example, R156H, found in three of seven such patients, has not been found in patients with the more common SCID phenotype.[26] Other missense alleles first found in children with partial deficiency also have not been found in SCID.[29,353,355] One of these, R211C, has occurred in functionally hemizygous sisters who developed clinical immunodeficiency as adults.[337] Another, A215T, has been found in a healthy adult with partial ADA deficiency.[29] These observations suggest that SCID results from having two "severe" alleles providing less than some critical level of ADA activity; alleles providing more than this level of activity, either due to a functional mutant protein or to some normal mRNA processing at a mutant splice site,[26,343] could confer a milder phenotype.

More precisely assessing the influence of ADA genotype and defining a critical threshold of ADA activity has been complicated because ADA deficiency is so rare and genetically diverse, and because quantitating the effects of disease-associated mutations has been difficult. As noted, erythrocyte ADA activity is very low in all phenotypes; lymphoid cells, the lineage with highest ADA expression, can rarely be obtained from immunodeficient patients. In defining genotype, missense mutations have been distinguished from polymorphisms by transfecting mammalian cell lines with cDNA, or by translating cDNA-derived transcripts *in vitro*. In these studies, a high background of endogenous ADA activity has precluded quantitation of much lower mutant ADA activity, which has been estimated using a relatively insensitive, nonlinear histochemical procedure.

In an attempt to address these limitations comprehensively, cDNAs for 29 patient-derived alleles (28 missense, 1 single amino acid deletion) were expressed in an *E. coli* strain deleted for the homologous bacterial ADA gene.[22] Mutant ADA activity, quantitated by radiochemical assay, was related to clinical and metabolic status of a diverse group of 52 patients who possessed 43 genotypes derived from 42 different alleles, including 28 of the mutations expressed in *E. coli*. Consistent with estimates that 5 percent of normal ADA activity is sufficient to prevent immunodeficiency, 3 alleles from healthy subjects with partial deficiency expressed 5 to 28 percent of the activity from normal human ADA cDNA; 26 disease-associated alleles expressed 0.001 to 0.6 percent.[22] To simplify correlations, genotypes were ranked according to the potential of their constituent alleles to provide ADA activity: deletion and nonsense alleles formed group 0 (no activity); missense mutations were assigned to groups I to IV, with increasing ADA activity expressed in *E. coli* (Table 109-6); splicing mutations were grouped together, making no assumption about potential for providing some normal ADA mRNA and enzyme.[22]

Using these designations, 28 of 31 SCID patients fell into three genotype categories (0/0, 0/I, I/I) that could express no more than

Table 109-6 Mutant ADA Alleles Grouped by Activity Expressed in *E. coli* Sϕ3834

Group	Mutations	Expressed ADA Activity* (nmol/h/mg protein)	Percentage of Wild Type*
I	H15D, G74V, A83D, R101L, R101Q, R101W, P104L, L107P, G140E, R149W, R156C, R211H, G216R, E217K, S291L, A329V, E337del	30.4 ± 35.8 (3.0–134.2)	0.012 ± 0.014 (0.001–0.051)
II	V129M, R156H, V177M, A179D, Q199P, R253P	280 ± 104 (164–456)	0.11 ± 0.04 (0.06–0.17)
III	G74C, P126Q, R211C	1,093 ± 487 (711–1642)	0.42 ± 0.19 (0.27–0.63)
IV	R142Q, R149Q, A215T	34,253 ± 34,443 (12,492–73,963)	13.0 ± 13.1 (4.8–28.2)
	Wild Type	262,593 ± 21,590	

*Mean ± SD (range).

Wild-type human ADA cDNA and cDNAs for 29 patient-derived mutant alleles that alter single amino acid residues were expressed in *E. coli* Sϕ3834, which has a deletion of the bacterial ADA gene. Based on increasing ADA activity expressed, mutant alleles were assigned to groups to I to IV. In addition, alleles with deletions or nonsense mutations were assigned to Group 0 (no activity), and splicing mutations to a separate group (making no assumption about capacity to provide ADA activity). As discussed, Sϕ3834 Arredondo-Vega et al.[22] these allele group designations can be used to assign patients to genotype categories based on capacity to provide ADA activity. (Adapted with permission from Table 3 of Arredondo-Vega et al.[22])

0.05 percent of normal ADA activity (that expressed by two copies of the normal cDNA). Only 2 of 21 patients with milder phenotypes had one of these severe genotypes.[22] The sum of the expressed ADA activity derived from each patient's alleles correlated well with indices of both metabolic (RBC dAXP) and clinical (age at diagnosis) phenotype (Fig. 109-4). Thus, nearly all SCID patients had RBC dAXP of greater than 350 nmol/ml and total expressed ADA activity of less than 200 nmol/h/mg (0.04% of wild type). In contrast, nearly all patients with delayed, late, or partial phenotypes had RBC dAXP of less than 300 nmol/ml, and total expressed ADA activity of greater than 190 nmol/h/mg.[22] This expression-based classification system provides a quantitative framework for evaluating the implications of gentoype and novel amino acid subsititutions.

PNP Enzyme and Gene

The gene encoding human PNP is located on chromosome 14q13.[367–369] The 1.7-kb cDNA contains a 289-codon open reading frame encoding a 32-kDa peptide.[370] The PNP gene cloned from a normal individual[371] and from a PNP-deficient patient[372] consists of 6 exons extending over 9 kb (Fig. 109-3). A functional promoter contains a TATA box, an inverted CCAAT sequence, and two G/C-rich regions within a 216-bp segment.[373] A 444-bp region in the first intron confers enhancer activity on both the endogenous and heterologous promoters.[374] PNP is considered a housekeeping gene and is expressed in all tissues, but highest levels are found in erythrocytes and kidney.[220] Treating human thymocytes[375] and lymphoid leukemic cell lines[376] with phorbol ester increased the levels of PNP mRNA and PNP activity by severalfold, whereas those of ADA decreased, mimicking changes observed during normal maturation from prothymocytes to mature T cells.[234]

Purified native human PNP, although active as a monomer, appears to be a trimer composed of approximately 32,000-kDa subunits.[377–379] Non–Michaelis-Menten kinetics have been attributed to substrate-induced dissociation of the trimer[380] or to nonequivalent, interacting active sites resulting from the trimeric structure. Fluorescence analysis of calf spleen PNP has shown that guanine and ribose-1-phosphate bind to free enzyme, indicating that nucleoside synthesis proceeds by a random mechanism, whereas phosphorolysis of inosine and guanosine requires the prior binding of phosphate, indicating an ordered reaction.[381] PNP appears to be sensitive to environmental factors. Thus, dissociation of the trimer into more active, but less stable monomers was a function of enzyme concentration and ligand effectors.[380] Oxidation eliminated cooperativity and decreased affinity for inosine.[382]

Crystallographic analysis of erythrocyte PNP has confirmed a trimeric structure (Fig. 109-2).[383] Each subunit contains an eight-stranded and a five-stranded mixed β sheet that forms a distorted β barrel. Seven α helices of 9 to 17 residues flank the β core, giving

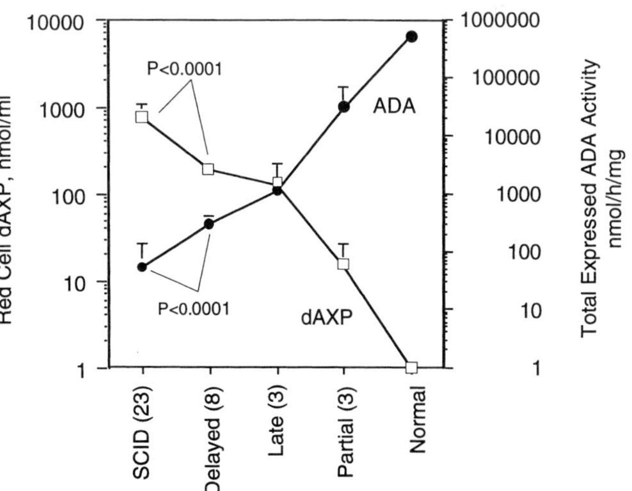

Fig. 109-4 Relationship of expressed ADA activity to clinical and metabolic phenotype. The sum of the ADA activity expressed in *E. coli* strain Sϕ3834 by both mutant ADA alleles (total expressed ADA activity) was determined for each of 34 immunodeficient subjects whose clinical phenotype was defined by age at diagnosis (SCID, first year of life; delayed onset, 1–10 years; late onset, beyond 10 years), and for 3 healthy subjects with partial deficiency. The mean (±SD) of total expressed ADA activity (•) and red cell dAXP level (□) for each of these phenotypes are plotted. ADA expression for a normal individual was taken as twice the ADA activity expressed in Sϕ3834 by wild-type ADA cDNA (plotted from data in Table 5 of Arredondo-Vega et al.[22]).

an α/β structure without apparent homology to other α/β proteins. The active site is located near the interface of two subunits within the trimer, and is formed by seven segments from a single subunit and one from an adjacent subunit. Many of the residues involved in substrate binding occur near the four center strands of the eight-stranded β sheet. The arrangement of hydrogen bond donors and acceptors within the active site predicts specificity for guanine, hypoxanthine, and their analogues, but not for adenine,[383] an observation consonant with the known substrate specificity of the mammalian enzyme.[384] Extensive site-directed mutagenesis studies at the active site have identified Asn243 and Glu201 as the residues largely responsible for substrate specificity and efficient catalysis.[385–387]

Inhibitors of PNP have been sought as potential immunosuppressive agents that might mimic the T-cell deficiency state associated with inherited PNP deficiency. Modeling on the crystalline enzyme with a series of known PNP inhibitors has defined characteristics required for optimal competitive inhibition with respect to inosine.[388] In particular, 50 mM, as opposed to 1 mM, phosphate was shown to decrease the potency of a wide range of substituted guanine analogues by as much as 100-fold, due to displacement of contact between inhibitors and a sulfate ion that occupies a phosphate binding site. Crystallographic data have been used to improve the design of PNP inhibitors and have resulted in the synthesis of a number of compounds with Kis in the low nanomolar range.[389,390] Clinical trials are underway.

Following transfection of *E. coli* PNP cDNA, the broader substrate specificity of the bacterial enzyme has been used as a mechanism for converting nontoxic prodrugs, including 6-methylpurine-2′-deoxyriboside and fludarabine, into toxic metabolites for killing tumor cells, both directly and through a bystander effect, in several experimental models.[391,392] Because *E. coli* PNP can use Ado and dAdo as substrates, it has been theorized that this enzyme may be used as a basis for PEG-enzyme replacement therapy of both PNP and ADA deficiencies.[393] This possibility is being tested in studies with ADA and PNP knockout mice.

Primary Genetic Defect. To date, 10 different mutations have been defined in eight PNP-deficient patients (Table 109-7).[90,372,394–396] These include 6 missense and 2 splice site mutations, a 1-codon deletion, and a 1-bp deletion resulting in a frameshift. Correlations with phenotype are limited by this heterogeneity and small number of patients. However, one patient (patient 7) with a late onset of symptoms had about 3 percent of normal lymphocyte PNP activity.[397] Analysis of a B-cell line suggested that residual activity was due to low levels of normal PNP mRNA derived from an allele carrying an intronic point mutation that created an alternative 3′ splice site, the predominant effect of which was to introduce 16 bp of intron 3 into the majority of transcripts. As in the case of some splicing mutations found in ADA-deficient patients with delayed and late onset, this finding suggests that low levels of PNP activity can ameliorate the clinical course.

PATHOGENESIS

The basis for selective lymphocyte depletion in ADA and PNP deficiency has necessarily been investigated in model systems ranging from cultured cells to mice (discussed separately). Most cell culture studies have used inhibitors of ADA, such as erythro-9-(2-hydroxy-3-nonyl)adenine (EHNA), coformycin, and 2′-deoxycoformycin with a Ki of 10^{-9} to 10^{-12} M, or less potent PNP inhibitors with Ki 10^{-5} to 10^{-7} M, such as 8-aminoguanosine.[398,399] A consistent finding has been that inhibiting ADA or PNP is not particularly toxic, but greatly enhances sensitivity to exogenous Ado and dAdo in the former case, and to dGuo in the latter (guanosine is cytotoxic, but only upon conversion by PNP to guanine). This reflects the limited endogenous production of dAdo and dGuo by cultured cells, and the ability of Ado kinase to detoxify Ado generated metabolically. When ADA/PNP is inhibited, exogenous Ado is usually toxic at 5 to 50 μM, dAdo at 0.2 to 50 μM, and dGuo at 1 to 50 μM (sensitivity varies with cell type, species, and experimental design).

The use of the tight-binding ADA inhibitor 2′-deoxycoformycin (dCF) (Ki 2.5×10^{-12} M) to treat lymphocytic leukemias has provided an *in vivo* model in which the actions of endogenous ADA substrates can be assessed.[400–403] In addition to an antileukemic effect, dCF causes rapid depletion of nonmalignant lymphocytes, which persists for months after therapy.[404] This implies pathogenic mechanisms that act on nondividing mature lymphocytes as well on their replicating precursors (it also raises a question regarding the reversibility of lymphopenia following enzyme replacement or gene therapy). Nonlymphoid toxicity occurs in some patients treated with dCF. This has been attributed to some inhibition of AMP deaminase as well as ADA,[405,406] or to minor phosphorylated derivatives of dCF.[407] A more likely explanation is that massive leukemic cell lysis generates far more dAdo, and hence less selective toxicity, than occurs in SCID patients.[408]

The following section emphasizes those potentially pathogenic mechanisms (Fig. 109-5) for which *in vivo* findings or *in vitro*

Table 109-7 PNP Gene Mutations

Mutation Designation	Site	Nucleotide*	Change	Effect	References
Missense					
E89K	Ex3	265	**G**AA → **A**AA	Glu89 → Lys	372, 375
D128G	Ex4	383	G**A**T → G**G**T	Asp128 → Gly	394
A174P	Ex5	520	**G**CT → **C**CT	Ala174 → Pro	395
G190V	Ex5	569	G**G**C → G**T**C	Gly190 → Val	395
Y192C	Ex5	575	T**A**T → T**G**T	Tyr192 → Cys	90
R234P	Ex6	701	C**G**A → C**C**A	Arg234 → Pro	394, 395
Deletion					
I129del	Ex4	385–387	del **ATC**	del Ile129	395
730del1	Ex6	730	del **A**	frameshift	90
Splicing					
181G → T	Ex2 5′ ss	181	A**G** → A**T**	skip Ex2, ↓mRNA	396
286–18G → A	IVS3 3′ ss	286–18	C**G**G → C**A**G	ins 16 bp, ↓mRNA	395

*cDNA numbering: from start of translation, based on method of Williams et al.[371]

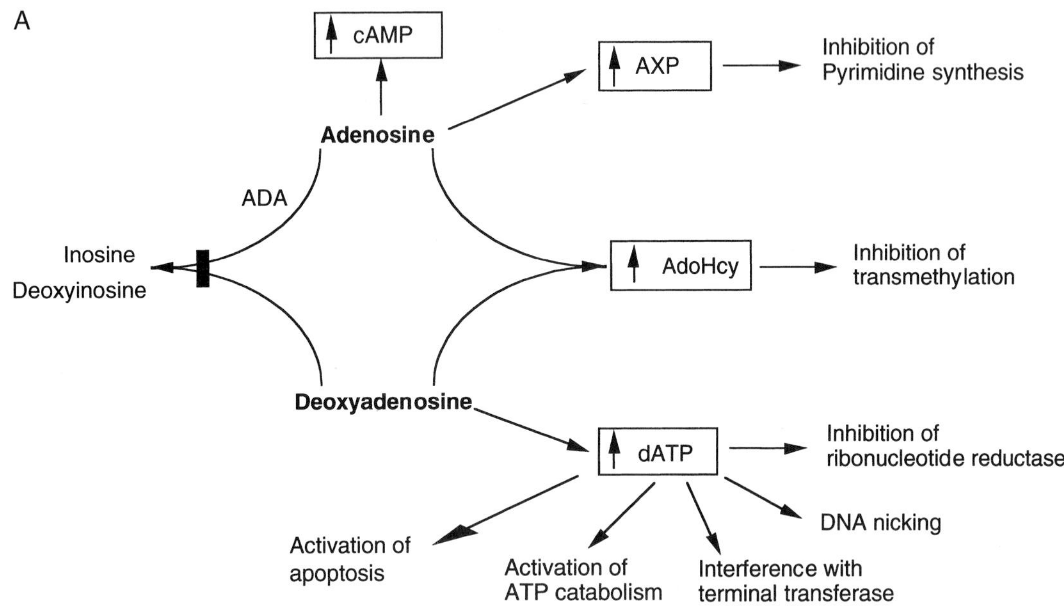

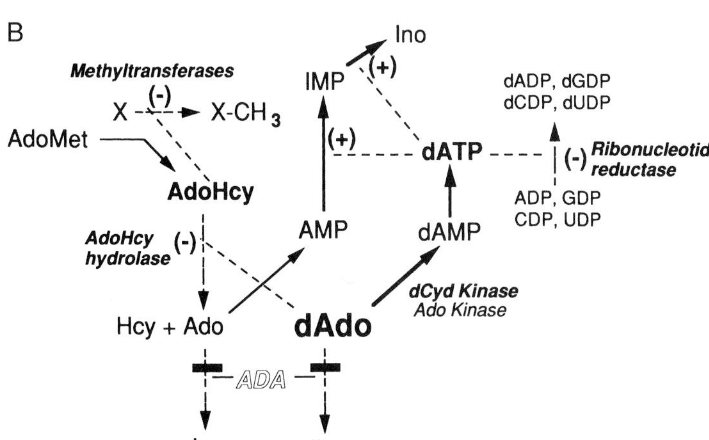

Fig. 109-5 ***A.*** **Effects of adenosine and deoxyadenosine that have been considered as potential causes of immune dysfunction in ADA deficiency. AdoHcy, *S*-adenosylhomocysteine; AXP, adenosylnucleotides.** ***B.*** **Schema showing the effects of dAdo on AdoHcy hydrolysis, adenine ribonucleotide catabolism, and deoxyribonucleotide synthesis in ADA deficiency. dCyd, deoxycytidine; Hcy, homocysteine.**

evidence seem most compelling. However, the basis for purinogenic immunodeficiency remains uncertain. Invoking a common mechanism for ADA and PNP deficiency, such as inhibition of ribonucleotide reductase, seems overly reductionist in view of the multiplicity of mechanisms shown to operate in various models, which could adversely affect lymphoid development from the stem cell to the mature lymphocyte, as well as interfere with function. Some attempt at a unifying theme nevertheless seems in order.

Adenosine triphosphate and GTP act as RNA precursors, phosphate donors, and effectors of signal transduction; their concentrations can modulate the activity of enzymes in all cellular compartments. dATP and dGTP serve much more limited functions, which may all be related to DNA metabolism in the nucleus. Elevated levels of purine deoxyribosyl metabolites could potentially act as structural analogues, interfering with reactions that have evolved with specificity for their ribosyl counterparts. Examples of such effects are the inactivation of AdoHcyase by dAdo and the ability of excessive dATP formation to activate ATP catabolism. The toxic inhibition of ribonucleotide reductase by expanded pools of dATP and dGTP is an accentuation of a physiologic regulatory mechanism. To avoid analogue effects, cells appear to have evolved mechanisms for limiting the size of purine deoxyribonucleoside and deoxyribonucleotide pools (e.g., the stringent regulation of ribonucleotide reductase and the inefficiency of purine deoxynucleoside kinases).

High ADA and PNP expression in lymphoid progenitors may be a lineage-specific adaptation, needed to protect lymphocytes from high levels of dAdo and dGuo generated by physiologic apoptosis associated with intrathymic negative selection or antigen-specific activation. In the absence of ADA or PNP, accumulation of purine 2′-deoxyribonucleoside triphosphate (dNTP) may be harmful in several ways, by inducing apoptosis of positively selected thymocytes destined to make up the mature T-cell repertoire, by interfering with gene rearrangement and somatic mutation necessary for generating antigen receptor diversity, or by interefering with signaling pathways essential to T- and B-cell differentiation and function.

dATP and dGTP Toxicity

Lymphoblast mutants unable to transport or phosphorylate dAdo and dGuo are largely (dAdo) or completely (dGuo) resistant to these nucleosides, evidence that activation, presumably to the triphosphate, is the primary cause of *in vitro* toxicity.[173,205,206,209,210] Early studies found that T-cell lines were more sensitive than B cell lines to dAdo and dGuo. This correlated with the greater ability of T cell lines to accumulate dATP[188,211,222,409–413] and dGTP[111,211,213,409,413–418] Human thymocytes resembled T-lymphoblasts in this respect.[215,419–422] The response of T-lymphoblastic leukemia to dCF, and to the dGuo analogue arabinosyl guanine, correlates with dATP and araGTP accumulation in malignant cells.[400–403,408,423,424] dATP and dGTP accumulation has been related to higher dCyd kinase[207,220,234,419,425] and lower deoxynucleotidase activity[188,189,222,419,426] in T-lymphocyte precursors as compared with other cell types. These observations have led to a hypothesis explaining the predominantly T cell–deficient phenotype of ADA and PNP deficiency in terms of a selective capacity of immature T cells to efficiently trap dAdo and dGuo as toxic intracellular dNTPs.

Although dATP/dGTP accumulation in thymocytes plays a significant pathogenic role, the emphasis on T-cell selectivity based on a unique ability to undergo marked dATP/dGTP pool expansion now appears oversimplified. Some B-cell lines accumulate dATP and dGTP as efficiently as T-cell lines, and this capacity seems related more to the degree of maturity than to lineage.[218,427] Relatively mature indolent T- and B-cell leukemias and hairy cell leukemia with limited ability to accumulate dATP and dGTP readily respond to dCF[428–430] and are sensitive to 2-chlorodeoxyadenosine, the active metabolite of which is 2-chloro-dATP.[431] Compared with T-lymphoblasts, mature T-lymphocytes have small dNTP pools and little ability to accumulate dATP or dGTP.[419,421,422,428,432] ADA-inhibited B-lymphocytes incubated with dAdo accumulated dATP efficiently,[422,433] although they did not accumulate dGTP from dGuo.[419] In a colony assay, ADA-inhibited T and B cells were equally sensitive to dAdo and Ado.[434] Erythrocytes, which contain Ado kinase but virtually no dCyd kinase, accumulate massive amounts of dATP in ADA-deficient patients. Other tissues have not been examined systematically, but elevated dATP has been found in nonlymphoid tissues from an ADA-deficient SCID patient,[435] and in two leukemia patients treated with dCF, dATP levels in kidney and liver exceeded levels in spleen.[403]

Specific Mechanisms of Deoxynucleotide Toxicity

Inhibition of Ribonucleotide Reductase. In dividing cells, *de novo* synthesis of dNTP occurs via reduction of ADP, GDP, CDP, and UDP, all catalyzed by ribonucleotide reductase (EC 1.17.4.1). This stringently regulated process maintains dNTP pools at about 1 percent of the corresponding NTP pools, sufficient to support only a few minutes of DNA replication. The reductase is composed of nonidentical peptides: M1, an effector binding subunit, and M2, which contains nonheme iron and the tyrosyl radical essential for catalytic activity. A balanced production of DNA precursors is achieved by complex allosteric effects of dATP, dGTP, dTTP, and ATP, which bind to M1[436–442] (Fig. 109-6). ATP is a general activator and dATP a general inhibitor of the reduction of all four substrates. dGTP and dTTP inhibit CDP reduction; dGTP also inhibits UDP reduction. Reduction of ADP and GDP is stimulated by dGTP and dTTP, respectively. Ki values for dATP as an inhibitor of the reduction of CDP, UDP, GDP and ADP were 40, 55, 1500, and 4 μM for the enzyme purified from the Molt-4 human T-cell line.[443] Ki values for dGTP as an inhibitor of CDP and UDP reduction were 25 to 47 μM, and 1.5 to 4.3 μM, respectively.

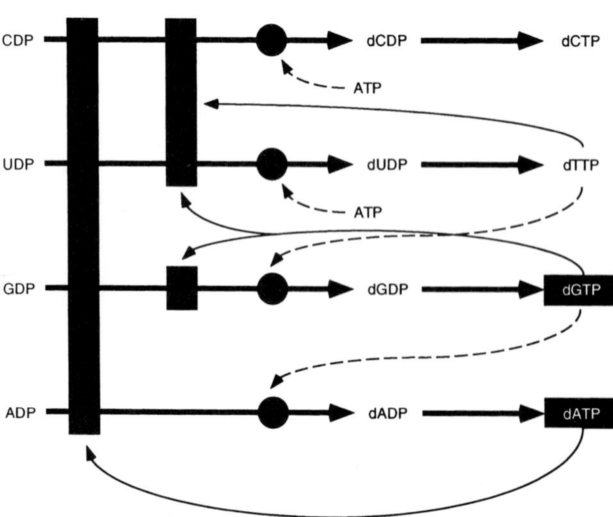

Fig. 109-6 Schema of the regulation of ribonucleotide reductase by nucleotides. Solid lines and bars indicate inhibition. Dotted lines and circles indicate activation. (*Adapted with permission from Thelander and Reichard.*[438])

Studies in nonlymphoid cells identified inhibition of ribonucleotide reductase in general, and of dCTP production in particular, as a primary event in the inhibition of DNA synthesis caused by dAdo, dGuo, or thymidine. After the discovery of dATP accumulation in ADA deficiency, dAdo- and dGuo-induced toxicity to mouse and human lymphoblastoid cell lines was likewise shown to be associated with depletion of dNTP pools, and was often diminished by dCyd.[184,205,210,212,416,444–448] dCyd was presumed to act by restoring dCTP, but may simply have inhibited dAdo and dGuo phosphorylation by dCyd kinase. More convincing evidence was the finding that CEM T-lymphoblast mutants with increased levels of ribonucleotide reductase, or with a reductase resistant to inhibition by dATP or dGTP, showed reduced sensitivity to dAdo and dGuo.[184,210,446,447] These findings led to the hypothesis that T-cell depletion in ADA and PNP deficiency results from inhibition of ribonucleotide reductase by dATP and dGTP, leading to inhibiton of DNA replication.

Several observations have pointed to purine dNTP-induced toxicity unrelated to ribonucleotide reductase. For example, dAdo and dGuo halted growth of CEM cells in the G1, not S, phase of the cell cycle.[445,449] As noted, dCF therapy eliminates nonmalignant, resting lymphocytes; dCF plus micromolar dAdo is lethal to such cells *in vitro*,[420,450] and after mitogen addition dAdo blocked their transition from G0 to G1 within 24 h,[451–453] when ribonucleotide reductase activity is very low.[454,455]

Deoxyribonucleotide-Induced Apoptosis. Immature thymocytes are highly sensitive to apoptosis induced by various stimuli (glucocorticoids, radiation), and during normal thymic ontogeny a majority of these cells are deleted by apoptosis (negatively selected). Human T-lymphoblasts and murine thymocytes treated with dAdo and dGuo,[456–458] as well as nondividing blood lymphocytes treated with dAdo and its ADA-resistant 2-chloro analogue,[431] have been shown to undergo apoptosis. Treating mice with dCF induced apoptosis in cortical thymocytes at the $CD4^+CD8^+$ double-positive stage; this effect was suppressed by overexpression of the antiapoptotic protein Bcl-2, and by elimination of p53 expression.[457]

Both the G0 and G1 blocks induced by dAdo and dGuo, preventing progression to DNA replication, as well as dAdo and dGuo-induced apoptosis, may now be understood as alternative fates determined by p53 protein–regulated cell cycle checkpoints, possibly responding to dATP/dGTP pool expansion as a potential threat to genome stability.[459] Apoptosis results from irreversible cell damage caused by the activation of several aspartate-specific cysteine proteases (caspases).[460] In an early step in an apoptotic program (Fig. 109-7), it has been found that cytochrome c released from mitochondria binds in the presence of dATP to cytoplasmic apoptotic protease–activating factor 1 (Apaf1) to activate Casp9.[461,462] The Apaf-1/activated Casp9 complex then recruits and proteolytically activates other caspases in a cascade that leads to cleavage of many target proteins and activation of a DNase that degrades nuclear DNA.[460,463] *Bcl2*, by blocking the release of cytochrome c from mitochondria, antagonizes this process.[464,465] 2-Chloro-dATP (derived from 2-chlorodeoxyadenosine) acts in a manner similar to dATP in inducing apoptosis.[466] Thus, activation of the caspase cascade in both thymocytes and peripheral blood cells by dATP could account for thymocyte depletion in ADA deficiency and the therapeutic efficacy and immunosuppression of ADA inhibitors and dAdo analogues in lymphoproliferative disorders. T lymphocytes from PNP-deficient mice exhibited

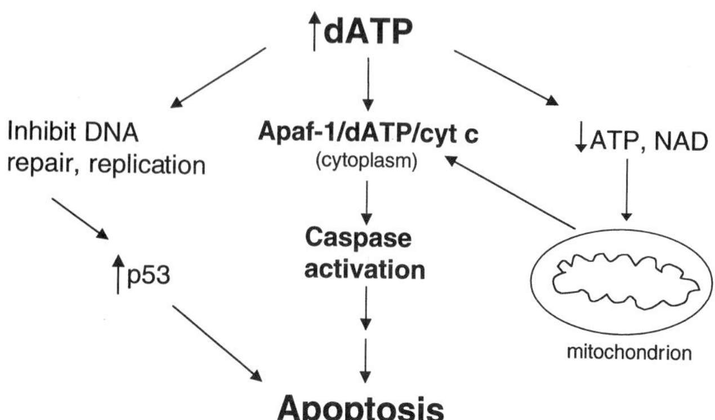

Fig. 109-7 Factors contributing to the induction of apoptosis by 2′-deoxyATP (dATP). dATP and its analogue 2-chloro-2′-dATP directly complex with cytoplasmic cytochrome c and apoptotic protease activating factor-1 (Apaf-1) to activate the caspase pathway, culminating in DNA fragmentation and other events associated with apoptotic cell death. Other effects of dATP pool expansion also may contribute to the induction of apoptosis, including ATP and NAD depletion, which may potentiate cytochrome c leakage from mitochodria, and impaired DNA replication and repair, which may induce the tumor suppressor p53. (*Adapted with permission from Leoni et al.*[466])

increased apoptosis and higher sensitivity to irradiation than lymphocytes from heterozygous littermates. This and other evidence suggested that the immune deficiency in PNP deficiency results from apoptosis induced by inhibition of mitochondrial DNA repair by dGTP (resulting from activation of dGuo by mitochondrial dGuo kinase).[466a]

Deoxyribonucleotide Pool Imbalance and VDJ Recombination. In addition to effects on replicative DNA synthesis and apoptosis, it has been suggested that dATP pool expansion could modify the product of terminal deoxynucleotidyl transferase (TdT).[101] This template-independent DNA polymerase expressed in thymocytes and B-lymphocyte progenitors is thought to play a role in generating immunologic diversity by inserting nucleotides into N regions of rearranging immunoglobulin and T-cell receptor genes at sites of V(D)J recombination.[467,468] In a cell model expressing V(D)J recombination substrates in conjunction with recombinase activating proteins and TdT, elevating dATP concentration markedly increased the proportion of AT as compared with GC residues within N regions, and decreased overall recombination frequency.[469] A similar alteration was found in N regions in B-lymphoblasts from ADA-deficient patients. In contrast, elevation of dGTP pools did not result in alterations in the already high GC content of N regions. Whether or not these alterations play any role in the B-cell defect found in ADA deficiency is presently unclear.

Maintaining balanced levels of dNTPs is also important to the fidelity of DNA replication. Perturbing this balance has been found to increase the mutation rate at several genetic loci.[470–473] It has been proposed that mutations result primarily from misincorporation of the nucleotide in excess,[470,474] although treating cultured T-lymphoblasts with dAdo or dGuo resulted in a variety of mutations at the HPRT locus, including deletions and insertions.[473] Hydroxyurea, an inhibitor of ribonucleotide reductase, is not mutagenic,[473,475] suggesting that reductase inhibition does not underlie the mutagenic effects of dNTP pool perturbations.

NAD Depletion/DNA Nicking in Resting Lymphocytes. This mechanism was proposed to account for the lethality of dAdo to nondividing lymphocytes. Resting lymphocytes normally contain DNA strand breaks that are rapidly rejoined after addition of mitogens[476,477]; dAdo caused single strand breaks to accumulate in DNA of unstimulated human T cells.[478] Seto et al.[431] found that in resting (but not dividing) lymphocytes, dAdo not only induced DNA strand breaks, but also depleted NAD and ATP. This was attributed to activation by DNA strand breaks of the chromatin-associated poly(ADP-ribose) polymerase (PARP), which uses NAD as a substrate.[479,480] NAD depletion and loss of viability, measured by dye exclusion, were diminished by high concentrations of nicotinamide, a precursor of NAD, or 3-aminobenzamide, an inhibitor of PARP. It was proposed that dATP interferes with DNA repair in resting lymphocytes, stimulating NAD utilization by PARP, and exhausting cellular ATP in a failed attempt to maintain NAD pools.[431]

In similar experiments, others have shown that rescue by nicotinamide and 3-aminobenzamide is only apparent: such lymphocytes are "metabolically dead," being unable to synthesize protein or RNA, or to respond to mitogens.[481] As little as 1 μM dAdo, but not Ado or dGuo, inhibited RNA synthesis in unstimulated, ADA-inhibited human lymphocytes.[482] Inhibition occurred within 4 hours and was associated with dATP accumulation but not ATP depletion. Neither DNA strand breaks nor NAD or ATP depletion were observed in dCF-sensitive malignant cells obtained from patients with hairy cell leukemia and T-cell lymphoma.[430,483] Although these findings do not support the DNA nicking/NAD depletion hypothesis, these indolent malignant cells may differ from resting lymphocytes in capacity to synthesize NAD or to repair DNA.

ATP Catabolism. Erythrocyte ATP is reduced in ADA-deficient patients, and in those with early onset SCID (lowest residual ADA activity); ATP is often less than 50 percent of normal and below the level of dATP[22,109,484] (and unpublished observations). A striking decline in erythrocyte ATP also occurs during dCF therapy, and has been associated with hemolysis[402]; a decline in lymphoblast ATP also has been observed.[485] The mechanism of hemolysis during dCF therapy is unclear. *In vitro*, almost complete replacement of ATP with dATP in dCF-treated RBCs had no detectable effect on energy metabolism or various tests of structural integrity.[486] Hemolysis is uncommon in ADA-deficient SCID, but it has been reported in one patient with half normal RBC ATP, in whom several other causes were excluded.[102] Reduced erythrocyte ATP associated with hemolysis occurs in patients with familial elevated erythrocyte ADA activity.

The mechanism of dAdo-induced ATP catabolism has been studied in ADA-inhibited human T-lymphoblasts[157] and erythrocytes.[487] ATP breakdown was dependent on continuous dATP formation (it did not occur in nucleoside kinase–deficient or –inhibited cells), and proceeded via the pathway AMP → IMP → inosine → hypoxanthine. Coformycin, an inhibitor of AMP deaminase as well as ADA, dissociated dATP accumulation and ATP catabolism.[157] Selective deamination of elevated levels of AMP, generated from ATP used to phosphorylate dAdo, could be explained by the findings that dAMP was a poor substrate for AMP deaminase, whereas dATP was as effective as ATP as a potent activator of both AMP deaminase and a cytoplasmic 5′-IMP nucleotidase.

Effects of Adenosine

Adenosine Receptor–Mediated Effects. Extracellular Ado has widespread physiologic effects mediated through plasma membrane–associated Ado receptors, which are coupled via G (GTP-binding) proteins to a growing list of effectors, including adenylylcyclase, potassium and calcium channels, phospholipase C, and phospholipase A2.[488] Four receptor subtypes designated A1, A2a, A2b, and A3 have been identified and their cDNAs cloned. A1 and A3 appear to couple with members of the G_i family, and A2a and A2b with members of the G_s family. Cells may express multiple Ado receptor subtypes, G proteins, and effectors.

Adenosine-induced increase in intracellular cyclic adenosine monophosphate (cAMP) mediated via the A2 Ado receptor was an early mechanism proposed to account for Ado lymphotoxicity. Although inhibiting Ado transport potentiated Ado-induced cAMP elevation, mutational loss of the nucleoside transporter abolished Ado toxicity to S49 murine T-lymphoma cells.[489] Also, S49 mutants with a defective adenylylcyclase remained sensitive to Ado toxicity.[490] Ado-induced apoptosis of murine thymocytes and T-lymphocytes has been attributed to cAMP elevation, but effects due to Ado uptake and metabolism were not evaluated.[456,491,492] Indeed, a transport inhibitor prevented Ado-induced apoptosis of thymocytes and lymphocytes from occurring in irradiated mice.[493] Ado-induced apoptosis of endothelial cells was also prevented by blocking Ado transport, and apoptosis was attributed to metabolic effects, possibly inhibition of AdoHcyase.[494]

It has been speculated that nontoxic Ado receptor–mediated effects of Ado might cause immune dysregulation leading to autoimmunity, possibly by impairing antigen-dependent responses. Brief exposure of human CD4 T-helper cells to Ado induced a rapid expression of CD8 antigen, followed by development of suppressor activity.[495,496] Ado suppressed various T-cell receptor–triggered functions of murine lymphocytes, such as expression of activation antigens and IL-2 receptor; these actions occurred in the presence of an Ado transport inhibitor and were attributed to A2a receptor–mediated stimulation of adenylylcyclase.[492,497] Others have proposed that extracellular ADA bound to ADA-CP/CD26 may modulate Ado signaling through lymphocyte Ado receptors.[287] Exogenous ADA has been shown to cointernalize with the A1 Ado receptor on cultured smooth muscle cells (there was no indication that CD26 was involved).[498] Other effects of Ado, presumed to be via Ado receptors, on neutrophil function have been proposed, including actions that could be both inflammatory and antiinflammatory.[499–501]

There are species differences in Ado receptor ligand binding properties, as well as species and cell line differences in expression of receptor subtypes, G proteins, and downstream effectors of signal transduction.[488] Many pharmacologic studies have been performed not with Ado, but with analogues that are neither transported nor metabolized. These factors complicate extrapolation from animal and cell culture models to the ADA-deficient patient. Ado receptor research has focused heavily on neurophysiologic and cardiovascular consequences of effects of Ado, such as on neurotransmitter release and cardiac and smooth muscle tone; on antiadrenergic effects on lipolysis and heart rate; on platelet aggregation due to effects on ADP release; and on bronchospasm resulting both from effects of Ado on smooth muscle and mast cell degranulation. Clinical correlates of these Ado receptor–related actions do not occur in ADA-deficient patients any more often than in patients with other forms of SCID. Nor has treatment with polyethylene glycol–modified ADA (PEG-ADA; see later section on Therapy), which can elevate extracellular ADA activity to 100-fold over the normal level, had any clinical effects related to Ado receptor signaling.

Inhibition of Pyrimidine Synthesis. Treating a variety of cultured cells with Ado causes depletion of cellular pyrimidine nucleotides; this was one of the first mechanisms proposed for Ado cytotoxicity and lymphopenia in ADA deficiency.[502] Pyrimidine depletion appears to result from Ado nucleotide–induced inhibition of PP-ribose-P–dependent phosphoribosylation of orotic acid.[405] There is evidence that pyrimidine starvation causes a p53-dependent cell cycle arrest in G1 and S phase,[503,504] and that inhibition of orotate synthesis underlies the immunosuppressive actions of the drug leflunomide.[505] In some cell lines, growth inhibition by Ado could be prevented by adding uridine or eliminating Ado kinase. However, uridine did not prevent Ado from inhibiting the response of human lymphocytes to mitogens,[506,507] and Ado toxicity to a human B-cell line was not diminished by loss of Ado kinase or by exogenous uridine.[508] Normal levels of UTP and CTP in blood mononuclear cells and normal excretion of orotic acid were found in studies of an ADA-deficient child.[509,510]

Toxicity Due to Effects of Ado and dAdo on AdoHcy Hydrolase

The AdoHcy product of transmethylation reactions is a competitive inhibitor of all methyltransferases; Ki values for AdoHcy of 10^{-7} to 10^{-5} M are often lower than the K_m for AdoMet (Fig. 109-8).[511] Normal operation of methylation-dependent processes (e.g., gene expression, RNA splicing, protein synthesis, and prenylation) therefore requires efficient elimination of AdoHcy. In mammalian cells this is catalyzed by the highly conserved housekeeping enzyme AdoHcy hydrolase (EC 3.3.1.1).[512,513] AdoHcy is a significant source of Ado, and is the only metabolic precursor of homocysteine. A deletion of the AdoHcyase structural gene is lethal to mouse embryos.[514]

S-adenosylhomocysteine hydrolysis is reversible and thermodynamically unfavorable ($K_{eq} = 1.4 \times 10^{-6}$ M).[512] AdoHcyase also has a high affinity for Ado: for the human enzyme K_m is approximately 1 μM in the AdoHcy synthesis reaction, and K_D is 0.2 to 0.5 μM for Ado binding in the absence of homocysteine.[515,516] Because of these properties, AdoHcy breakdown depends on both adequate AdoHcyase activity and efficient metabolism of Ado and homocysteine. Normal removal of Ado by phosphorylation and deamination, and of homocysteine by transsulfuration and remethylation, maintains the ratio AdoMet/AdoHcy at ≥10 : 1. This ratio, sometimes called the methylation index, is a useful indicator of the capacity of a cell to transmethylate.

In ADA deficiency, two mechanisms interfere with AdoHcy hydrolysis. First, elevated Ado drives the AdoHcyase reaction in the direction of AdoHcy formation.[517] Second, dAdo irreversibly inactivates AdoHcyase with kinetics characteristic of suicide

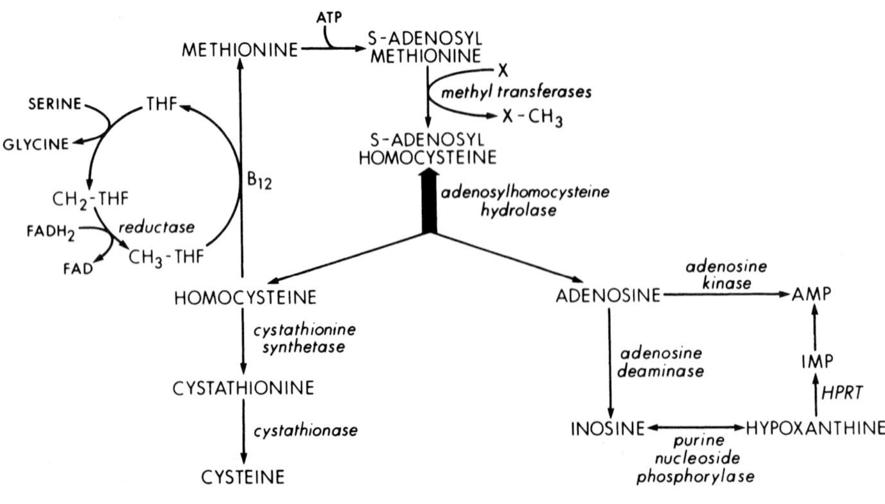

Fig. 109-8 The transmethylation pathway showing the relationships between methionine, homocysteine, and adenosine metabolism. Because of the reversibility of the *S*-adenosylhomocysteine hydrolase reaction, an increase in adenosine concentration, as would occur from a lack of ADA, is accompanied by a higher steady-state level of *S*-adenosylhomocysteine, a potent inhibitor of methyl transfer reactions. THF, tetrahydrofolate.

inactivation; for the human enzyme the inactivation constant (K_I) for dAdo was 66 μM, and V_{max} was 0.12 min^{-1}.[518] The PNP substrate inosine is both a weak substrate and a weak inactivator of AdoHcyase, with K_m and K_I values of 9.3 and 5.9 mM, respectively.[519] Inactivation by dAdo, adenine arabinoside, and other Ado analogues has been shown to involve reduction of the enzyme-bound NAD cofactor, associated with cleavage of the nucleoside inhibitor to release adenine.[520–522] As noted, erythrocyte AdoHcyase activity of ADA-deficient SCID patients is invariably less than 10 percent, and often less than 2 percent of normal[26,33,102–105]; AdoHcyase activity is more modestly decreased in PNP deficiency.[519,523] Nucleated cells from bone marrow of three ADA-deficient patients had normal amounts of immunologically reactive AdoHcyase protein, but specific activity was approximately 15 percent of normal[102,524] (and M.S.H., unpublished observation).

In ADA-inhibited lymphoblasts[517,525] and activated lymphocytes,[526] concentrations of Ado that blocked proliferation (10–50 μM) increased AdoHcy by 3- to 20-fold, reduced the AdoMet/AdoHcy ratio from ≥10 to ≤3, and inhibited DNA and RNA methylation. Homocysteine potentiated AdoHcy accumulation and Ado toxicity. AdoHcyase inhibition accounts for the residual toxicity of adenine, Ado, and dAdo to lymphoblast mutants unable to convert these compounds to nucleotides.[173,508,525] Expanded AdoMet pools and export of AdoHcy may act in some cell types to diminish toxicity due to AdoHcyase inhibition.[527–529]

In patients with acute leukemia, dCF therapy resulted in a decrease in T-lymphoblast AdoHcyase activity by 80 to 95 percent.[400,408,530] AdoHcy increased by 20- to 30-fold, and the AdoMet/AdoHcy ratio decreased from about 40:1 before treatment to 3 to 4:1.[408,530] Methylation of newly synthesized lymphoblast RNA was shown to be inhibited to a degree that correlated with the decrease in methylation index.[408] Accumulation of dATP is probably the primary lymphotoxic effect of dCF in acute leukemia. More mature malignant T and B cells of patients with chronic lymphocytic and hairy cell leukemias accumulate much less dATP, yet respond to relatively low doses of dCF. In one such patient with chronic T-cell leukemia, circulating malignant cells accumulated no detectable dATP and showed minimal change in levels of ATP. However, AdoHcyase activity in these cells decreased by about 70 percent and accumulation of AdoHcy occurred, with a decline in the methylation index from 47:1 to 6:1.[429]

Lymphocyte AdoMet pools increase sharply within 2 hours after mitogen addition, suggesting a need for methylation during activation.[531] A potent AdoHcyase inactivator, (Z)-5′-fluoro-4′,5′-didehydro-5′-deoxyadenosine (MDL 28842), which cannot be deaminated or phosphorylated, inhibited antigen-specific murine and human T-cell proliferation (concomitant with AdoHcy accumulation); in mice MDL 28842 selectively blocked a T cell–dependent immune response and ameliorated collagen-induced arthritis.[532,533] It also blocked murine thymocyte differentiation at the double positive stage, associated with impaired expression of mRNAs for the T-cell receptor and CD4 and CD8 molecules.[534] MDL 28842 did not induce thymocyte apoptosis.

Effects on Lymphocyte Function and Differentiation. Purine deoxynucleosides have been reported to influence lymphocyte function at several levels. As little as 1 μM dAdo inhibited the action of human T cells in a mixed lymphocyte culture assay; higher concentrations blocked IL-2 production and IL-2 receptor expression, although addition of IL-2 did not overcome the antiproliferative effect of dAdo.[535] Micromolar dGuo blocked antigen-induced human T-suppressor cell activity; much higher concentrations blocked nonproliferative T-helper cell function and B-lymphocyte proliferation and differentiation.[413] dGuo abrogated the development of suppressor T cells in mice.[536–538] These immune dysregulatory effects may underlie the autoimmune disorders associated with PNP deficiency.

In the presence of dCF, dAdo equally blocked formation of erythroid, myeloid, and T-lymphoid colonies from committed progenitors from human marrow[539] and blood.[434] In the latter study Ado was only slightly less toxic than dAdo, and both nucleosides inhibited T- and B-cell colony formation equally. Depending on conditions, dAdo was more toxic to T-cell than to myeloid colonies[540] or was equally toxic to T cells and nonlymphoid progenitors; Ado killed nondividing T cells but did not affect the viability or differentiation of hematopoietic progenitors.[541]

Incubation with normal thymic epithelium induced E rossette receptor expression on bone marrow precursor cells from children with ADA-deficient SCID. Such expression was not observed if the thymic epithelium was treated with an ADA inhibitor, but was restored by adding exogenous ADA.[542] This was interpreted as demonstrating a requirement for ADA at the earliest stage of thymocyte differentiation. Treating newborn mice with dCF appeared to interfere with thymocyte differentiation at two points. The first block resulted in depletion of immature cortical thymocytes, and the second in a failure of $CD4^+CD8^+$ medullary thymocytes to mature into single positive, functional T cells.[543]

Direct effects of ADA inhibition on differentiation of pluripotent stem cells have been inferred from observations in two patients with acute stem cell leukemia. In each case an abrupt conversion from a T-lymphoblastoid to a myeloid phenotype occurred in close association with dCF therapy.[530,544] In one of these patients[530] phenotypic conversion occurred within 3 to 4 days of a 3-day infusion of dCF. Cytogenetic evidence showed that pretreatment T-lymphoblasts and postconversion myeloid cells arose from the same clone. Both dATP and AdoHcy accumulated in leukemia cells during treatment. These and other findings suggested that biochemical effects of ADA inhibition had induced a change in the direction of differentiation of a malignantly transformed, pluripotent stem cell from lymphoid to myeloid.[530] A cell line derived from the latter patient was capable of multilineage differentiation.[530,545] Treating the cell line in its undifferentiated state with dAdo, Ado, and nucleoside analogues that selectively inhibit AdoHcyase induced the expression of myeloid properties.

Mouse Models of ADA and PNP Deficiency

Mice show the major effects of ADA deficiency in humans, but the phenotype of complete deficiency in mice is less selective and more severe, reflecting differences in purine metabolism and in lymphoid and organ development. In adult and newborn mice, dCF treatment caused lymphoid depletion, associated with dATP accumulation and AdoHcyase inactivation.[187,543,546–550] Higher doses also produced hemolysis associated with RBC ATP depletion, and caused hepatic and renal tubular injury.[187,547,550] Death occurred within 1 to 3 days following a continuous 5-day infusion of dCF.[547] Besides lymphoid depletion, the only histologic abnormality noted was hepatitis, which was attributed to impaired immunity rather than to direct hepatotoxicity. However, fatal hepatic necrosis occurred in mice treated with dCF and dAdo; this was associated with AdoHcy accumulation, a profound decrease in the AdoMet/AdoHcy ratio, and inhibition of AdoMet-dependent transmethylation in the liver.[551]

Treating pregnant mice with dCF at 7 to 8 days of gestation arrested fetal development within 2 to 4 days, associated with extensive fetal cell death.[31,552] In contrast, homozygous ADA-deficient knockout mice bred from heterozygous (ADA-expressing) mothers survived gestation (19–21 days), but died perinatally with hepatocellular degeneration and failure of lung expansion; unlike human SCID patients, thymic and peripheral lymphoid development was normal at birth.[553,554] Whole fetuses showed increased levels of Ado and dAdo; dATP was increased in blood.[553] In neonates, Ado, dAdo, and dAXP were increased in RBCs, thymus, liver, and spleen.[554] dAXP was only modestly elevated in thymus, representing less than 5 percent of total adenine nucleotides versus greater than 50 percent in T-lymphoblasts of human leukemic patients during dCF therapy. This difference, which might account for normal thymic development, may reflect less efficient dAdo phosphorylation by murine than human dCyd kinase.[555] Fetal murine thymocytes also may be relatively resistant to toxic effects of ADA deficiency. Thus, apoptotic negative selection of thymocytes occurs during fetal development in the human, but begins postnatally in the mouse.[556] dAXP was even less elevated in liver, and it was speculated that hepatic injury in ADA knockout mice is more likely due to impaired AdoHcy hydrolysis. Thus, hepatic AdoHcyase activity was reduced by 85 percent and AdoHcy was increased by four- to sixfold; the AdoMet/AdoHcy ratio was decreased to less than 2 : 1, and AdoMet was increased by twofold, changes consistent with inhibition of AdoMet-dependent transmethylation.[554]

Perinatal death of ADA knockout mice could be prevented by selective placental expression of an ADA transgene.[557] The rescued knockouts survived for 3 weeks before dying from pulmonary failure due to airway thickening and inflammation; bone and cartilage abnormalities of ribs and renal hemorrhage were also noted. Lymphocytes were reduced in the thymus (eightfold) and spleen (threefold). There appeared to be a partial block in thymocyte development at the CD4/CD8 double-negative stage. Treating these mice with PEG-ADA during the first 2 weeks of life reduced metabolic abnormalities in lung tissue, resulting in resolution of pulmonary eosinophilia and other histopathology, and prolonged survival.[557a] At higher doses of PEG-ADA, which produced circulating ADA activity comparable to levels observed in human SCID patients (see Enzyme Replacement with PEG-ADA below), metabolic abnormalities in thymus and spleen were also corrected, and both immunologic and pulmonary status improved.[557b] Ongoing studies are aimed at addressing the hypothesis, posed in these studies, that the dramatic pulmonary injury in ADA-deficient mice results from effects of Ado mediated via Ado receptors.

Purine nucleoside phosphorylase–deficient mice carrying several different missense mutations have been derived from mutagenized males.[558–560] Strains with greater than 5 percent of normal erythrocyte PNP activity overexcreted PNP substrates, but were not immunodeficient. Strains with about 1 percent of normal activity showed a partial block in thymocyte maturation at the double-negative stage. Splenic T-lymphocytes were reduced by 50 percent, and their response to T-cell mitogens was reduced by 80 percent.[560] In the most severely PNP-deficient strain, dGTP in thymocytes was elevated by about fivefold. This limited dGTP accumulation was attributed to an unexplained, separable deficiency of dGuo kinase activity.[559] This model may be relevant to partial PNP deficiency in humans, and it is consistent with a pivotal role of deoxynucleoside kinase activity in mediating immunodeficiency in PNP deficiency. PNP knockout mice have recently been developed.[466a] The metabolic and immunologic findings were similar to those to PNP-deficient mice with severe missense mutations, including the secondary reduction in mitochondrial dGuo kinase activity.

THERAPY

At diagnosis of SCID, aggressive supportive care and therapy for specific infections are essential. Prophylaxis for *P. carinii*, herpes virus, and fungal infections, and appropriate isolation to prevent exposure to common childhood viruses are also required. Live virus vaccines and unirradiated blood products must be avoided. Intravenous immunoglobulin (IVIG) is used in the management of both ADA and PNP deficiencies. Unfortunately, these measures alone do not restore health or prevent an eventually fatal outcome unless immune function is restored. When ADA and PNP deficiencies were discovered, HLA-identical allogeneic BMT was the only means of achieving this. Because most patients lack a histocompatible sib, attempts were soon initiated to develop treatment based on specific etiology and emerging concepts of metabolic pathogenesis.

As reviewed in previous versions of this chapter, treatment with dCyd, which blocks dAdo phosphorylation and might correct a putative deficiency of dCTP due to inhibition of ribonucleotide reductase, has been attempted in four ADA-deficient patients and in two PNP-deficient patients. Persistent increase in plasma dCyd was documented when dCyd was infused continuously along with an inhibitor of dCyd deaminase.[561] Transient improvement in *in vitro* T-cell function was noted in single ADA- and PNP-deficient patients.[561,562] No well-documented clinical benefit resulted from nucleoside administration. Fetal liver and thymus transplantation have been used with limited success in several patients with ADA and one with PNP deficiency. Thymosin and other thymic peptide hormones also have been used, but with little or no long-term efficacy in patients with both ADA and PNP deficiency. As discussed below, erythrocyte transfusion as a form of enzyme replacement benefited some patients with ADA deficiency.

More promising therapy for patients who lack a matched marrow donor has been evolving in three areas: (a) HLA-mismatched BMT; (b) enzyme replacement with PEG-ADA; and (c) somatic cell gene therapy. The first two are now established therapies for ADA deficiency. Each has its limitations so that patient selection remains, in many cases, a difficult matter of judgment. Gene therapy for ADA deficiency is still in an experimental stage, and at the time of this writing has not been applied without simultaneous treatment with PEG-ADA. *In utero* therapy (transplantation, enzyme replacement, or gene transduction) is in theory possible, but has not yet been attempted.

Transplantation of Marrow/Hematopoietic Stem Cells

Adenosine deaminase–deficient patients have successfully undergone transplantation with marrow from HLA-identical siblings, HLA-haploidentical parents, and HLA-matched unrelated donors.[91,563–566] Engraftment is usually characterized by lymphoid chimerism: T cells are exclusively of donor origin, but B cells often arise from host stem cells. Disparity of HLA class I and II antigens on host-derived antigen-presenting cells and donor-derived T cells may account for the frequent persistence of humoral immune dysfunction. Although potentially curative, BMT is an intensive and essentially irreversible procedure. The posttransplantation period can be associated, often unpredictably, with complications that may be fatal or cause chronic morbidity. These include opportunistic infections (reactivated or acquired from the donor), GVHD, graft rejection, interstitial pneumonitits, autoimmunity, and lymphoma. Complications are more frequent with transplants from HLA-nonidentical donors, with patients who have active pulmonary infections, and in older patients who may be chronically ill and who may harbor cytomegalovirus, EBV, or other viruses. Mortality is also greater in first affected children, who are often more seriously ill at diagnosis than are their subsequent affected sibs.

Transplantation with marrow from an HLA-identical sib is considered the treatment of choice for typical cases of SCID (all causes). Engraftment of functional T cells usually begins within a month. At this time, activation of cytolytic donor T cells by minor host alloantigens may initiate acute GVHD in as many as 60 percent of patients, but the risk of severe GVHD is lower.[563,566] Humoral immune function recovers more slowly and is often partial. One review found that greater than 90 percent of second-affected sibs who received an HLA-identical bone marrow graft for SCID had long-term T-cell engraftment; about 30 percent of first-affected children died within 6 months.[563] In a review of the overall European experience from 1983 to 1989, 97 percent of 32 SCID patients, including all 8 with ADA deficiency, who received HLA-identical bone marrow grafts were reported to be cured.[564] Buckley et al. reported 100 percent survival among 12 SCID patients (4 ADA deficient) who received HLA-identical bone marrow grafts between 1982 and 1998.[566]

With HLA-nonidentical BMT (usually from a haploidentical parent), removal of T cells from donor marrow (e.g., by lectin agglutination or with monoclonal antibodies) has greatly reduced the risk of severe GVHD.[563–567] As a result of T-cell depletion, mature donor T cells usually do not appear in blood for 3 to 4 months, and full T-cell function may not develop for 8 to 12 months. B-cell function remains abnormal in the majority of patients, even years after transplantation. Delayed T-cell engraftment, and a higher incidence of graft failure than with HLA-identical BMT, increase the risk of serious posttransplantation viral infections. Infection is largely responsible for the greater early mortality associated with haploidentical than with HLA-identical BMT.

Cytoablative and immunosuppressive preconditioning of the recipient (e.g., with alkylating agents, antimetabolites, antithymocyte globulin) prior to T cell–depleted BMT has been advocated, with the aim of impairing host mechanism(s) that interfere with engraftment of donor T and B cells.[563–565] In an unusual approach, one ADA-deficient patient was conditioned by continuous infusion of dAdo for 3 weeks prior to, and for 17 days after, haploidentical BMT. Despite substantial increases in plasma dAdo and erythrocyte dATP, the patient failed to engraft.[568] This treatment may have been toxic to donor as well as to host lymphoid cells. There is evidence that pretransplantation conditioning is unnecessary and unacceptably increases posttransplantation morbidity.[566,569] Agents that are hepatotoxic or that are metabolized in liver (such as cyclophosphamide) pose an additional risk for patients who manifest hepatotoxic effects of ADA substrates.

The success of haploidentical BMT for SCID (all causes) has varied widely among transplant centers in North America and Europe. A 1989 review reported actuarial probabilities of survival with engraftment and recovery of T-cell function 2 to 3 years posttransplantation ranging from 28 to 67 percent.[563] In some series, ADA-deficient patients have fared worse than patients with other forms of SCID. For example, among a combined 74 patients treated through 1992 at a center in Paris and another in California, overall survival was approximately 55 percent, but none of the 8 ADA-deficient patients survived.[15,570] The largest experience with T cell–depleted HLA-nonidentical BMT for SCID is from a long-term European cooperative trial. Between 1983 and 1989, the overall 2-year survival rate for 100 patients was 56 percent, and 53 percent for the 19 patients with ADA deficiency.[564] In an update through 1993, 48 percent of 193 SCID patients were alive 6 years posttransplantation; of the 20 with ADA deficiency, 60 percent survived with T-cell engraftment 6 months posttransplantation, but only 8 (40%) were still alive after 6 years.[565] The largest series from a single center in the United States has reported that from 1982 to 1998, survival among 77 SCID patients who received haploidentical bone marrow grafts was 78 percent; 6 of 9 (67%) with ADA deficiency engrafted successfully.[566]

Bone marrow transplantation for PNP deficiency has been problematic. Only two of eight patients have engrafted with long-term survival following transplantation of grafts from HLA-identical siblings.[397,571] One patient who failed a first T cell–depleted haploidentical transplant engrafted following a second BMT performed after more intensive conditioning.[572] The remainder of the patients have died as a consequence of infection, graft failure, and GVHD.[83,571]

Metabolic Effects of Marrow Transplantation. Successful HLA-identical BMT substantially corrects RBC dATP content and AdoHcyase activity.[105,573] The effect is greatest when erythroid as well as lymphoid cells are donor derived. Following haploidentical BMT, erythrocytes usually remain of host origin (ADA deficient). In this setting, we have found that erythrocyte dAXP content provides a semiquantitative indicator of the progress and stability of lymphoid engraftment (although not of graft function), which may be useful when low numbers of circulating donor lymphocytes are difficult to quantify. With engraftment, erythrocyte dAXP levels decrease progressively; with unstable engraftment, erythrocyte dAXP increases to pretreatment levels[103,574] (and M.S.H., unpublished observations).

Metabolic effects of engrafted donor cells can reduce systemic nucleoside toxicity (Fig. 109-9). However, ADA activity provided by engrafted T cells is apparently insufficient to rescue ADA-deficient host thymocytes. Thus, following haploidentical BMT performed without preconditioning, circulating T cells are exclusively donor derived. In some patients, B cells are derived from endogenous stem cells, which may reflect the greater sensitivity of ADA-deficient T than B cells to ADA substrates. As discussed below, more effective metabolic correction achieved with PEG-ADA therapy can rescue functional, ADA-deficient T cells.

Enzyme Replacement with PEG-ADA

For many enzyme deficiencies, replacement therapy requires targeting to specific cells in which an abnormal substrate is stored. This is not the case for ADA, and probably PNP, deficiency. dAdo and dGuo derived from DNA degradation in ADA- or PNP-deficient macrophages must traverse the extracellular space before exerting toxic effects on lymphocytes (e.g., by expanding pools of dATP, dGTP, and AdoHcy). These compounds cross cell membranes poorly, but are metabolically interconvertible with ADA and PNP substrates, which rapidly equilibrate with plasma via the nonconcentrative nucleoside transporter. The latter has greater affinity and capacity for dAdo and dGuo than either Ado kinase or deoxycytidine kinase. Thus, maintaining sufficient levels of ectopic ADA or PNP in plasma, or in circulating cells, should prevent macrophage-derived nucleosides from reaching

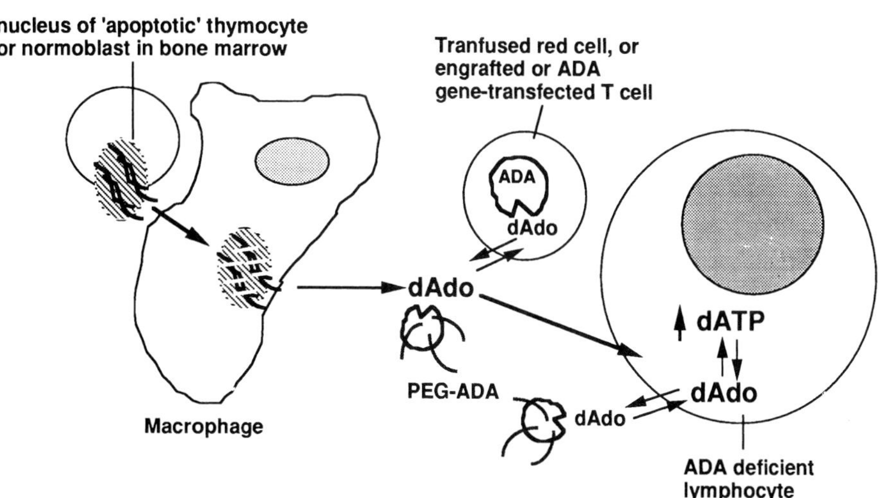

Fig. 109-9 Schema indicating the basis for the efficacy of circulating ADA as therapy for ADA deficiency. 2′-Deoxyadenosine (dAdo) arising from DNA degradation in macrophages (or from dATP turnover in cells) is in equilibrium with plasma. Efficient deamination of extracellular dAdo by PEG-ADA in plasma, or by the ADA-containing transfused erythrocytes, transplanted donor T cells, or ADA gene-transduced autologous T cells, will result in depletion of dAdo and reversal of its metabolic effects in ADA-deficient lymphocytes. (*Data from Hershfield and Chaffee.*[631])

lymphocytes, and also promote nucleoside export from lymphocytes, ultimately depleting them of toxic metabolites (Fig. 109-9).

The finding that exogenous ADA improved the *in vitro* response of lymphocytes from an ADA deficient patient to mitogens[575] first prompted investigation of erythrocyte transfusion therapy.[19] Transfusing twice monthly (with frozen, irradiated RBCs to prevent GVHD) increased blood ADA activity to near normal and reduced plasma levels of Ado,[73] dAdo,[20,576] and urinary dAdo.[20] Erythrocyte dATP decreased by 90 percent or more.[20,73,114,577] Immune function and clinical status improved in some children,[19,20,576,577] but the response was usually transient or inadequate.[114,578–580] Among 10 treated patients, the 5 who had a good response had residual T- and B-cell function prior to treatment, which was absent in 4 nonresponders.[581] Of the 5 who initially responded, 1 subsequently died of varicella pneumonia (U. Sorensen, unpublished observation), and another died of refractory hemolytic anemia (R. Hirschhorn, unpublished observation). The 3 long-term survivors developed iron overload and eventually switched to PEG-ADA therapy at 9 to 12 years of age. Chronic transfusion carries a risk for transmitting serious viral infections. It is traumatic, inconvenient, and in young patients must be carefully monitored to avoid circulatory embarrassment.

In recent years, transfusion has been replaced by intramuscular injection of purified bovine ADA, modified by covalent attachment of the inert polymer monomethoxypoly(ethylene glycol) (PEG-ADA). Attachment of PEG to proteins through lysine residues, which can be achieved by various chemical couplings, was shown in animal studies to prolong circulating life and block cellular uptake, diminish immunogenicity, and prevent antibody binding and proteolytic attack.[582,583] These effects, which have been demonstrated for bovine ADA[584] and *E. coli* PNP,[393] result from increased mass and from steric effects of the flexible, bulky, and hydrophilic PEG strands. On a volume basis, the clinical preparation of PEG-ADA (Adagen®, Enzon, Inc.) has approximately 1800 times the ADA activity of erythrocytes.

The lack of toxicity of free PEG and PEG-ADA in animals, and the potential for achieving much higher levels of circulating ADA activity than is possible by transfusion, led to the first clinical test of PEG-ADA in a critically ill patient who had twice failed haploidentical BMT and had not responded to transfusion therapy.[103] To date, over 85 patients have received PEG-ADA for up to 12.5 years, including 46 for more than 2 years and 33 for more than 5 years (mean for these patients is 8 years). About two thirds of the patients have had SCID and one third a delayed- or late-onset phenotype. The clinical and immunologic responses of several patients have been reported.[25,27,33,35,36,103,574,585–587] The overall experience through 1994 has been reviewed.[588] PEG-ADA (Adagen®) was approved by the U.S. Food and Drug Administration in 1990.

Polyethylene glycol–modified ADA is not appreciably taken up by blood cells, and it does not bind to CD26 (M.S.H., unpublished observations). After intramuscular injection of PEG-ADA, plasma ADA activity peaks in 24 to 48 hours, then declines with a half-life of 3 to greater than 6 days. Clearance is more rapid in some infants and newly diagnosed children who are severely ill[587] (and M.S.H., unpublished observations). Treatment is therefore initiated with twice weekly injections of 30 U/kg (60 U/kg/wk), based on ideal body weight (i.e., 50th percentile for the patient's age). At this schedule, preinjection plasma ADA activity is maintained at 50 to 150 μMol/h/ml (normal plasma ADA activity is <0.4 μMol/h/ml), or approximately 4 to 10 times normal total blood (erythrocyte) ADA activity. After several months, the dose is often reduced to 30 U/kg once a week, which maintains trough plasma ADA activity at approximately 25 to 60 μMol/h/ml. By 2 months of treatment, dAXP in erythrocytes falls to ≤2 to 10 nmol/ml packed RBCs (normal, ≤2 nmol/ml); AdoHcyase activity also normalizes (Fig. 109-10). This metabolic state is similar to that of healthy individuals with partial ADA deficiency.

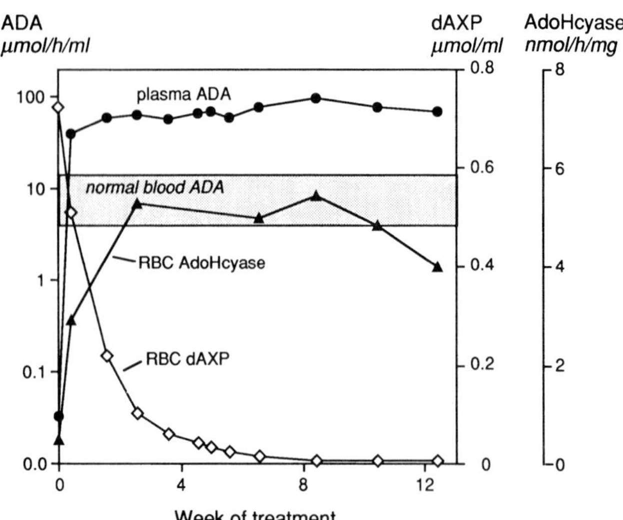

Fig. 109-10 Plasma ADA activity and levels of dAXP and AdoHcy hydrolase activity in erythrocytes of an SCID patient with ADA deficiency during the first 3 months of treatment with PEG-ADA at a dose of 30 U/kg twice a week (M.S.H., unpublished data).

Lymphocyte counts and immune function improve within a few weeks to several months of starting PEG-ADA. Circulating B cells may increase sharply during the first month, whereas an increase in T cells may not occur until 6 to 12 weeks of treatment[36] (Fig. 109-11). The proliferative response of blood lymphocytes to mitogens increases over this period, and a thymic shadow may reappear[33] (Fig. 109-12). Several SCID patients have developed transient thrombocytosis, without clinical consequence, in the first month of treatment (H.M. Rosenblatt and colleagues, unpublished observations). The time course and pattern of T-cell reconstitution, as judged by surface antigen expression and *in vitro* function, resembles that of intrathymic lymphoid ontogeny.[587] Maintaining immune function requires continued treatment with PEG-ADA. Any sustained decrease in plasma ADA activity to below about 10 μMol/h/ml has been associated with an increase in dAXP, a decrease in AdoHcyase activity in RBCs, and a decline in lymphocyte counts and function.[37,589,590]

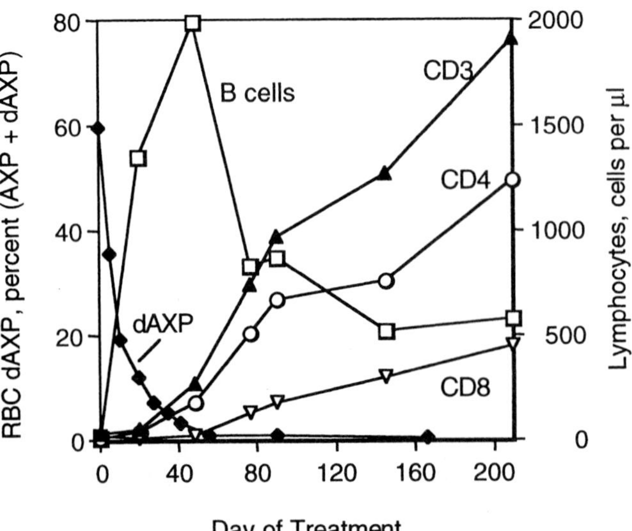

Fig. 109-11 Reappearance of circulating B- and T-lymphocytes in an SCID patient after initiation of PEG-ADA therapy at 2 months of age. (*Reprinted with permission from Bollinger et al.*[36])

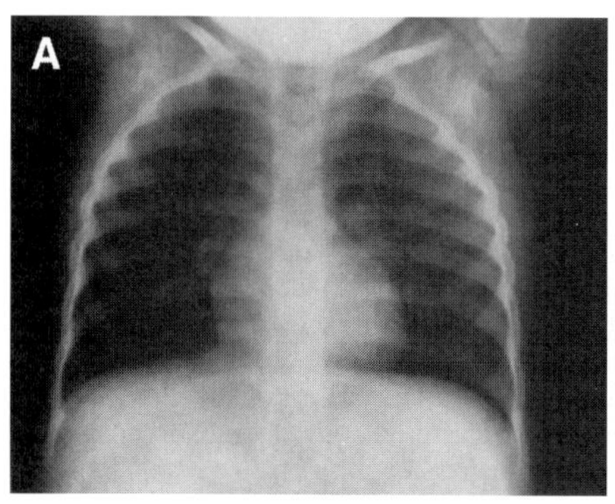

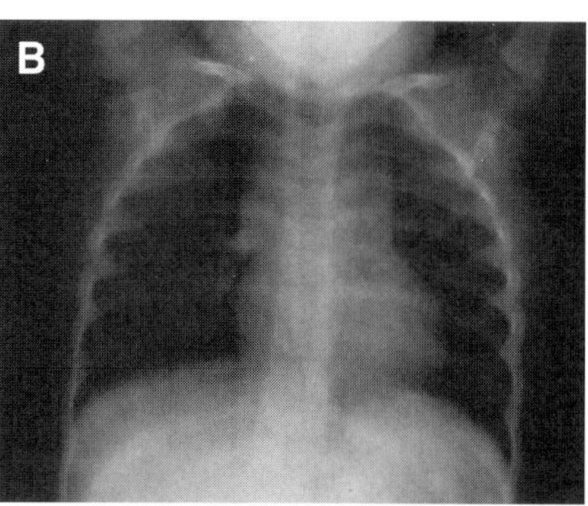

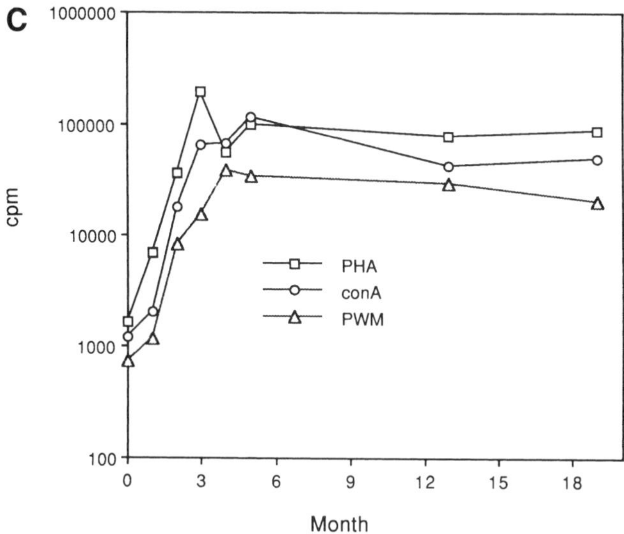

Fig. 109-12 Observations in a patient with delayed-onset phenotype who began treatment at 2 years of age, showing reappearance of thymic shadow on x-ray (*A*, pretreatment; *B*, after 3 months of treatment), and recovery of proliferative response of blood mononuclear cells to mitogens (*C*). (*Reprinted with permission from Hershfield et al.*[33])

Although PEG-ADA consistently corrects metabolic abnormalities, the degree of immune reconstitution varies.[33,588] About 20 percent of patients, mostly with early onset SCID, have shown only slight improvement in *in vitro* lymphocyte response to mitogens, compared with 30 percent to more than 90 percent of normal responses in the majority. Most patients with good clinical responses remain lymphopenic with fluctuating *in vitro* lymphocyte function. Over half of patients tested have developed significant lymphocyte responses to recall antigens. About half have discontinued IVIG, in several cases within 6 months of starting PEG-ADA. In these patients, normal immunoglobulin, isohemagglutinin, and specific antibody levels after immunization and infection have been demonstrated. There is evidence that humoral immunity is more effectively reconstituted in patients who respond to PEG-ADA than in ADA-deficient patients with stable engraftment after BMT.[574]

Clinically, PEG-ADA has been effective even in some patients with little improvement in T-cell counts and *in vitro* function. Acute illnesses are usually controlled in the first 1 to 3 months of treatment. After 6 months, opportunistic infections cease to occur and the frequency and duration of respiratory infections and diarrhea decrease markedly, permitting growth to resume. With long-term treatment, restrictions on social interaction, including school attendance, have been removed or greatly eased. Several patients have had uncomplicated chicken pox and have developed normal and persisting antivaricella antibody titers[33] (MS Hershfield et al., unpublished observations). As in the posttransplantation period,[563] immune dysregulation may occur early in treatment with PEG-ADA. However, this has not been common. Two patients have developed autoimmune phenomena after viral infections in the first 2 to 3 months. One had transient thrombocytopenia that responded to brief treatment with IVIG.[33] The second patient developed hemolytic anemia, which did not respond to aggressive immunosuppression; she died in the fourth month of treatment (A. Junker, unpublished observations).

There have been no toxic or allergic reactions to PEG-ADA. Nor has immunogenicity led to discontinuation of therapy.[589,591] IgG antibody to bovine-specific peptide epitopes of PEG-ADA became detectable by enzyme-linked immunosorbent assay (ELISA), usually after 3 to 8 months of treatment, in 10 of 17 patients treated for 1.1 to 5.5 years.[589] Titers did not correlate with plasma ADA activity, which remained stable in 8 of 10 anti–ADA-positive patients for periods of 24 to 60 months. Two patients developed enhanced enzyme clearance when ADA-inhibitory antibody, apparently directed toward the ADA active site, appeared at 4 to 5 months of treatment. In one case, tolerance was induced, allowing a weekly injection schedule to be resumed (she has now been treated for >10 years).[589,590] The other patient has required twice weekly injections to maintain therapeutic levels of plasma ADA activity. Continued monitoring by ELISA indicates that anti-ADA IgG can be detected in 75 to 80 percent of patients on long-term therapy.[591] Because of the possibility of developing enhanced clearance, regular monitoring of plasma ADA activity is advisable, particularly during the first 12 to 18 months of treatment.

Many patients have received PEG-ADA because they were considered too ill to safely undergo BMT. Nevertheless, the mortality rate among the first 85 PEG-ADA patients is less than 20 percent, which compares favorably with haploidentical BMT. Of 14 deaths related to immunodeficiency, 7 occurred in the first month of treatment, and 4 others within the first 5 months. These deaths occurred among critically ill infants with viral pneumonia or serious central neurologic deficits. Three late deaths have occurred after 3 to 6 years; two of these patients died of severe pulmonary insufficiency that was present when PEG-ADA was started at 9 and 33 years of age. The third had a severe neurologic deficit at the time PEG-ADA was initiated; this did not improve during treatment.

Sixteen patients have initially been treated with PEG-ADA with the intent of performing BMT when clinical status permitted and a suitable donor had been identified. Five of the donors were HLA identical, and 11 were haploidentical or matched unrelated. Twelve patients received PEG-ADA for longer than a month; in these cases enzyme was discontinued from several weeks to 3 months before transplantation. All 11 patients with nonidentical donors received pretransplantation conditioning. Among these 11 patients there have been 4 deaths (36%). One patient died from drug toxicity during conditioning; 3 others died a few weeks to a year posttransplantation, due to infections or GVHD following transplantation of marrow from haploidentical (1 case) or matched-unrelated (2 cases) donors.

Polyethylene glycol–modified ADA is very expensive, primarily because it is used in so few patients (it was one of the first "orphan" drugs[592]). It has been used selectively to treat SCID patients who lacked an HLA-identical marrow donor and were considered at too high a risk to undergo haploidentical BMT, and to treat late onset patients whose residual immune function made graft rejection likely. The deciding factor in both situations is concern with the mortality and morbidity of HLA-mismatched BMT, particularly when cytoablative conditioning is deemed necessary.

Attempts have been made to treat four PNP-deficient patients by RBC transfusion. No improvement was noted in two patients.[593,594] Limited improvement in percentage of T cells and in mitogenic response was seen in the other two.[595,596] In the latter there was marked decrease in urinary excretion of PNP substrates and total purines, an increase in plasma and urinary urate, and reduction in RBC dGTP.[596] Based on these results, the development of PEG-PNP for treating PNP deficiency seems a reasonable goal. Mammalian PNP appears to be too unstable at 37°C to be used for therapy. However, the far more stable *E. coli* PNP has been PEG modified and shown to have markedly prolonged circulating life, but considerable immunogenicity in mice. To reduce immunogenicity, a mutant *E. coli* PNP was prepared in which three Arg residues were replaced with Lys to provide additional potential sites for PEG attachment. The PEG-modified mutant enzyme retained full enzymatic activity and had significantly reduced immunogenicity.[393] Preliminary studies indicate that this PEG-PNP is effective in correcting the phenotype of PNP-knockout mice.[466a]

Somatic Cell Gene Therapy

It has been proposed that correction of specific ADA mutations in genomic DNA of stem cells could be achieved by homologous recombination.[597] Another proposal has been to graft patients with autologous epidermal keratinocytes transduced in culture with an ADA cDNA.[598] However, clinical gene therapy trials for ADA deficiency, now underway for almost a decade, have been based on extensive *in vitro* studies of retrovirus vector-mediated transduction. PNP gene therapy remains at the *in vitro* stage. Retrovirus-mediated transduction of the PNP-deficient NSU-1 subline of murine S49 T-lymphoma cells resulted in substantial expression of both human and murine PNP, as well as resistance to dGuo toxicity.[599] Peripheral blood T cells from a PNP-deficient patient, expanded *in vitro* with IL-2, were transduced with the same vectors, resulting in a fivefold increase in PNP activity to 1.1 percent of normal.[600] Proliferative responses to phytohemagglutinin and allogeneic cells were improved, but sensitivity to dGuo was unaffected. It was postulated that endogenous mutated PNP subunits, by virtue of inclusion in trimeric enzyme, might have a dominant negative effect on overall PNP activity. Work on PNP gene transfer is continuing with modifications of the retroviral vectors to enhance transduction efficiency and level of expression.[601]

Several observations suggest that introducing a functional human ADA gene into lymphohematopoietic stem cells, or into mature T cells, could reverse immunodeficiency, even if normal expression were not achieved: (a) T-cell chimerism achieved by BMT is of long-term benefit; (b) the response to PEG-ADA shows that, if protected from metabolic toxicity, endogenous stem cells retain some capacity to generate functional T- and B-lymphocytes; (c) immune function is normal in individuals with as little as 4 to 5 percent of normal ADA activity; (d) inherited erythroid ADA overexpression does not have severe consequences; and (e) gene-corrected lymphoid cells should have a survival advantage. Selective survival of ADA gene–transduced versus ADA-deficient human T cells has been observed after introduction into immunodeficient mice.[602] More pertinent is the discovery of two ADA-deficient patients who had spontaneous clinical remissions, each associated with mosaicism for ADA expression in B-lymphoblastoid cell lines; in one case, this was due to reversion of a mutant allele, presumably a rare event.[349,350]

Inefficient transduction of stem cells, the major obstacle to *ex vivo* retrovirus-mediated gene therapy, results from several factors: stem cells account for less than 0.1 percent of marrow nucleated cells, and they are largely nondividing, and hence do not permit retroviral integration. Induction of cell division often results in loss of the potential for multilineage differentiation. Other problems have included lack of persistent proviral integration, and clonal fluctuation in functioning stem cells in recipients. Long-term, multilineage expression of human ADA cDNA has been achieved in mice[603–606] owing to improvements in vector design,[605,607–609] as well as in the use of cytokines to induce stem cell replication but not differentiation.[610,611] Unfortunately, conditions used in the murine model have not worked as well in nonhuman primates[612,613] or with cultured human marrow.[614–617]

Despite poor results in primates, human trials of gene therapy for ADA deficiency began in 1990, when a proposal for targeting mature T cells was approved by the National Institutes of Health (NIH) Recombinant DNA Advisory Committee.[618] Because mature T cells are absent in ADA deficiency and have a finite life span, this approach involved repeated cycles of transduction with the aim of stabilizing the T-cell repertoire generated by treatment with PEG-ADA. Two trials targeting marrow stem cells, enriched by immunoselection for CD34 antigen-expression, began in Europe in 1993. In the same year, a U.S.-Canadian trial was conducted in prenatally diagnosed newborns, targeting $CD34^+$ cells isolated from umbilical cord blood. Patients in the stem cell trials also received maintenance therapy with PEG-ADA.

Entry into gene therapy trials required persisting lymphopenia and abnormalities in some tests of immune function, features found in most patients treated with PEG-ADA. A severe phenotype was not required, and all patients involved were clinically stable when they began gene therapy. For example, the first NIH patient had been diagnosed at age 2 years, and had never been hospitalized; the second was well until age 3, and was diagnosed at 5 years.[25,33] They had responded to PEG-ADA, which they had received for 1.7 and 3.5 years, with improved immune function (Fig. 109-12 shows responses of the first patient), restored growth, and sustained clinical benefit; each had discontinued IVIG, and the older patient was attending school.[33] In all, 11 patients have been involved in four trials. They include 3 neonates, who started PEG-ADA at 1 to 4 days of age, and 8 children 0.7 to 9.5 years of age, 7 of whom had received PEG-ADA for 1.8 to 3.7 years prior to gene therapy (one started PEG-ADA within 4 months). All subjects were still receiving PEG-ADA at the time reports based on these trials were published, 1 to 3 years following the last infusion of transduced cells.[108,619–622] PEG-ADA therapy has complicated evaluation of benefit, but it does not enter cells, so vector persistence and the level of ADA expression in target cells have provided objective, semiquantitative end points.

In the NIH trial, leukapheresed blood mononuclear cells were cultured for a few days with a T-cell mitogen (anti-CD3 antibody) and IL-2, then incubated with supernatant containing the LASN amphotropic retroviral vector, in which human ADA cDNA is under control of the Moloney murine leukemia virus long terminal repeat promoter.[608] After expansion for several days, the activated T cells were reinfused (without IL-2 or selection for transduced cells). The two patients received 11 and 12 infusions of treated T cells over about 2 years.[619] Transduction efficiency varied from 1 to 10 percent in the first patient, increasing ADA activity in her circulating T cells to 20 to 25 percent of normal. This level has persisted for more than 4 years since the last treatment. In the second patient, transduction efficiency was only 0.1 to 1 percent; no increase in ADA activity was detectable in blood T cells during or after treatment. In 1995, a 5-year-old who had been receiving PEG-ADA for almost 4 years was treated in Japan using the NIH protocol and vector. Four cycles of treatment resulted in transduction of 10 to 20 percent of T cells, as well as an increase in T-cell ADA activity to almost 50 percent of normal.[622]

Two Italian patients received both blood T cells and $CD34^+$ marrow cells that had been separately treated with retroviral vectors bearing different restriction enzyme sites, allowing the origin of transduced progeny to be identified.[620] One patient received about 7×10^8 transduced T cells and 0.4×10^8 marrow cells in 9 infusions over 24 months; the second received slightly fewer cells in five infusions over 10 months. Sixteen months after their last treatment, blood T cells of the two patients had about 11 percent and 7 percent of control T-cell ADA activity. ADA activity was also detected in granulocytes and erythrocytes, and in multilineage marrow colony-forming cells. Analysis of vector persistence suggested that transduced T cells had a life span of 6 to 12 months (much less than estimated for the first NIH patient). Over longer periods, these were replaced by T cells derived from transduced marrow progenitors. In a second European trial, three patients received single infusions of $CD34^+$ marrow cells, which were isolated and transduced at Leiden University.[621] Transduction of 5 to 12 percent of colony-forming cells was achieved, but after reinfusion, vector was detected only transiently in circulating granulocytes and mononuclear cells. Vector was never detected in T cells, nor was ADA expressed in any hematopoietic cells.

The last trial involved three prenatally diagnosed infants from the United States and Canada, born within a month of one another. Investigators at Childrens Hospital of Los Angeles isolated $CD34^+$ cells from umbilical cord blood of each patient. These cells were cultured for 3 days with IL-3, IL-6, and stem cell factor, and transduced with the LASN vector; the autologous cells were reinfused at 4 days of age.[108] It was estimated that no more than 1 percent of the $CD34^+$ cells had been transduced, and that these represented about 0.01 percent of endogenous marrow mass. When analyzed at age 18 months, 4 to 6 percent of marrow colony-forming cells, but only 0.001 to 0.03 percent of the patients' blood leukocytes contained vector. ADA activity in T cells was not measurably increased.[108] Reverse transcriptase polymerase chain reaction analysis of T cells from one of the patients, who was homozygous for a mutation that caused skipping of ADA exon 5, failed to detect transcripts derived from the transduced normal ADA cDNA.[344]

In an effort to enhance selection for ADA-expressing cells, the dose of PEG-ADA was reduced by half in these three patients. By age 4 years the frequency of vector-bearing T cells had increased to 1 to 10 percent, compared with 0.01 to 0.1 percent of B cells and other hematopoietic cells.[37] At this time PEG-ADA was withheld for 2 months in the patient with the highest levels of gene marking and T-cell numbers. Clearance of PEG-ADA from plasma was accompanied by a 100-fold increase in RBC dAXP and a decrease in RBC AdoHcyase activity to pretreatment levels; serum transaminase activity increased by sixfold to five times the upper limit of normal. During this period, the numbers of circulating B and NK cells decreased sharply; T-cell counts were relatively stable, but the *in vitro* response to tetanus toxoid disappeared. The patient became ill with an upper respiratory infection and sinusitis, and he developed an opportunistic monilial infection. Within a month of restarting PEG-ADA, these biochemical, immunologic, and clinical abnormalities all resolved, and the patient gained 2 kg in weight.[37] It was concluded that ADA gene-transduced cells provided far less ADA activity than PEG-ADA, and that transduced T cells, although they remained viable, were unable, in the absence of PEG-ADA, to sustain immunologic function.

The dose of PEG-ADA has been modestly reduced or held constant in several other gene therapy patients.[619,620,622] It is unclear how much selective pressure this achieves, or that the lower dose PEG-ADA is without benefit. In most of these cases, PEG-ADA still provides, each week, the ADA activity of about 10^{12} normal T cells, and when measured, plasma ADA activity in these patients has remained within the therapeutic range. Some reports have attributed improvement in immune function to gene therapy in patients receiving concomitant enzyme replacement.[619,620,622] However, rapid increases in lymphocyte counts and isoagglutinin titers have been observed when transduction efficiency was $\leq$10 percent, and when minimal gene marking and ADA expression had been achieved.[619] Some of these phenomena may be due to immunomodulatory effects of infusing large numbers of IL-2–activated T cells ($\geq$90% untransduced). An independent evaluation of ADA gene therapy trials by a panel established by the NIH has concluded that attributing benefit to gene therapy is premature, and that efforts should be focused on research to improve stem cell isolation and transduction.[623] Recent encouraging developments, which may be applied in future trials, include the use of fibronectin to increase the interaction between retroviral vectors and human target cells, refinement of vector design, and progress in understanding human stem cell biology.[624–630] Using some of these principles, gene therapy targeting $CD34^+$ bone marrow cells has recently led to the expression in circulating T and NK cells of the transduced cDNA for the normal γc subunit of the IL−2, −4, −7, −9, and −15 cytokine receptors in two patients with the X-linked SCID (due to mutation of γc subunit). Full correction of clinical and immunologic phenotype was achieved.[630a] New trials of gene therapy for SCID due to ADA deficiency are anticipated.

REFERENCES

1. Giblett ER, Anderson JE, Cohen F, Pollara B, Meuwissen HJ: Adenosine deaminase deficiency in two patients with severely impaired cellular immunity. *Lancet* **2**:1067, 1972.
2. Giblett ER: ADA and PNP deficiencies: How it all began. *Ann NY Acad Sci* **451**:1, 1985.
3. Dissing J, Knudsen JB: Adenosine deaminase deficiency and combined immunodeficiency syndrome. *Lancet* **2**:1316, 1972.
4. Ochs HD, Yount JE, Giblett ER, Chen SH, Scott CR, Wedgwood RJ: Adenosine-deaminase deficiency and severe combined immunodeficiency syndrome. *Lancet* **1**:1393, 1973.
5. Pollara B, Pickering RJ, Meuwissen HJ: Combined immunodeficiency disease and adenosine deaminase deficiency, an inborn error of metabolism. *Pediatr Res* **7**:362, 1973.
6. Giblett ER, Ammann AJ, Wara DW, Sandman R, Diamond LK: Nucleoside-phosphorylase deficiency in a child with severely defective T-cell immunity and normal B-cell immunity. *Lancet* **1**:1010, 1975.
7. Stoop JW, Zegers BJM, Hendrickx GFM, Siegenbeek Van Heukelom LH, Staal GEJ, De Bree PK, Wadman SK, et al.: Purine nucleoside phosphorylase deficiency associated with selective cellular immunodeficiency. *N Engl J Med* **296**:651, 1977.
8. Biggar WD, Giblett ER, Ozere RL, Grover BD: A new form of nucleoside phosphorylase deficiency in two borthers with defective T-cell function. *J Pediatr* **92**:354, 1978.
9. Virelizier JL, Hamet M, Ballet JJ, Reinert P, Griscelli C: Impaired defense against vaccinia in a child with T-lymphocyte deficiency associated with inosine phosphorylase defect. *J Pediatr* **92**:358, 1978.
10. Carapella-De Luca E, Aiuti F, Lacarelli P, Bruni L, Baroni CD, Imperato C, Roos D, et al.: A patient with nucleoside phosphorylase deficiency, selective T-cell deficiency, and autoimmune hemolytic anemia. *J Pediatr* **93**:1000, 1978.
11. Rich KC, Arnold WJ, Palella T, Fox IH: Cellular immune deficiency with autoimmune hemolytic anemia in purine nucleoside phosphorylase deficiency. *Am J Med* **67**:172, 1979.

12. Fischer A, Cavazzana-Calvo M, De Saint Basile G, DeVillartay JP, Di Santo JP, Hivroz C, Rieux-Laucat F, et al.: Naturally occurring primary deficiencies of the immune system. *Annu Rev Immunol* **15**:93, 1997.
13. Ammann AJ, Hong RH: Disorders of the T-cell system, in Stiehm ER (ed): *Immunologic Disorders in Infants and Children*. Philadelphia, WB Saunders, 1989, p 257.
14. Primary immunodeficiency diseases. Report of a WHO scientific group. *Clin Exp Immunol* **109**(suppl 1):1, 1997.
15. Stephan JL, Vlekova V, Le Deist F, Blanche S, Donadieu J, De Saint-Basile G, Durandy A, et al.: Severe combined immunodeficiency: A retrospective single center study of clinical presentation and outcome in 117 patients. *J Pediatr* **123**:564, 1993.
16. Buckley RH, Schiff RI, Schiff SE, Markert ML, Williams LW, Harville TO, Roberts JL, et al.: Human severe combined immunodeficiency: Genetic, phenotypic, and functional diversity in one hundred eight infants. *J Pediatr* **130**:378, 1997.
17. Hirschhorn R: Incidence and prenatal detection of adenosine deaminase deficiency and purine nucleoside phosphorylase deficiency, in Pollara B, Pickering RJ, Meuwissen HJ, Porter IH (eds): *Inborn Errors of Specific Immunity*. New York, Academic, 1979, p 5.
18. Hirschhorn R: Clinical delineation of adenosine deaminase deficiency, in Elliot K, Whelan J (eds): *Enzyme Defects and Immune Dysfunction, Ciba Foundation Symposium 68*. New York, Excerpta Medica, 1979, p 35.
19. Polmar SH, Stern RC, Schwartz AL, Wetzler EM, Chase PA, Hirschhorn R: Enzyme replacement therapy for adenosine deaminase deficiency and severe combined immunodeficiency. *N Engl J Med* **295**:1337, 1976.
20. Hirschhorn R, Papageorgiou PS, Kesariwala HH, Taft LT: Amelioration of neurologic abnormalities after "enzyme replacement" in adenosine deaminase deficiency. *N Engl J Med* **303**:377, 1980.
21. Tanaka C, Hara T, Suzaki I, Maegaki Y, Takeshita K: Sensorineural deafness in siblings with adenosine deaminase deficiency. *Brain Dev* **18**:304, 1996.
22. Arredondo-Vega FX, Santisteban I, Daniels S, Toutain S, Hershfield MS: Adenosine deaminase (ADA) deficiency: Genotype-phenotype correlations based on expressed activity of 29 mutant alleles. *Am J Hum Genet* **63**:1049, 1998.
23. Cohen F, Cejka J, Chang CH, Brough AJ, Rowe BJ, Gaines PJ: Adenosine deaminase deficiency and immunodeficiency, in Pollara B, Pickering RJ, Meuwissen HJ, Porter IH (eds): *Inborn Errors of Specific Immunity*. New York, Academic, 1979, p 401.
24. Geffner ME, Stiehm ER, Stephure D, Cowan MJ: Probable autoimmune thyroid disease and combined immunodeficiency disease. *Am J Dis Child* **140**:1194, 1986.
25. Levy Y, Hershfield MS, Fernandez-Mejia C, Polmar SH, Scudiery D, Berger M, Sorensen RU: Adenosine deaminase deficiency with late onset of recurrent infections: Response to treatment with polyethylene glycol-modified adenosine deaminase (PEG-ADA). *J Pediatr* **113**:312, 1988.
26. Santisteban I, Arredondo-Vega FX, Kelly S, Mary A, Fischer A, Hummell DS, Lawton A, et al.: Novel splicing, missense, and deletion mutations in 7 adenosine deaminase deficient patients with late/delayed onset of combined immunodeficiency disease: Contribution of genotype to phenotype. *J Clin Invest* **92**:2291, 1993.
27. Umetsu DT, Schlossman CM, Ochs HD, Hershfield MS: Heterogeneity of phenotype in two siblings with adenosine deaminase deficiency. *J Allergy Clin Immunol* **93**:543, 1994.
28. Shovlin CL, Hughes JMB, Simmonds HA, Fairbanks L, Deacock S, Lechler R, Roberts I, et al.: Adult presentation of adenosine deaminase deficiency. *Lancet* **341**:1471, 1993.
29. Ozsahin H, Arredondo-Vega FX, Santisteban I, Fuhrer H, Tuchschmid P, Jochum W, Aguzzi A, et al.: Adenosine deaminase δ(ADA) deficiency in adults. *Blood* **89**:2849, 1997.
30. Knudsen TB, Green JD, Airhart MJ, Higley HR, Chinsky JM, Kellems RD: Developmental expression of adenosine deaminase in placental tissues of the early postimplantation mouse embryo and uterine stroma. *Biol Reprod* **39**:937, 1988.
31. Knudsen TB, Gray MK, Church JK, Blackburn MR, Airhart MJ, Kellems RE, Skalko RG: Early postimplantation embryolethality in mice following in utero inhibition of adenosine deaminase with 2′-deoxycoformycin. *Teratology* **40**:615, 1989.
32. Hong R, Gatti R, Rathbun JC, Good RA: Thymic hypoplasia and thyroid dysfunction. *N Engl J Med* **282**:470, 1970.
33. Hershfield MS, Chaffee S, Sorensen RU: Enzyme replacement therapy with polyethylene glycol-adenosine deaminase in adenosine deaminase deficiency: Overview and case reports of three patients, including two now receiving gene therapy. *Pediatr Res* **33**(suppl):42, 1993.
34. Hirschhorn R: Adenosine deaminase deficiency, in Rosen FS, Seligmann M (eds): *Immunodeficiency Reviews*. New York, Harwood Academic, 1990, p 175.
35. Notarangelo LD, Stoppoloni G, Toraldo R, Mazzolari E, Coletta A, Airo P, Bordignon C, et al.: Insulin-dependent diabetes mellitus and severe atopic dermatitis in a child with adenosine deaminase deficiency. *Eur J Pediatr* **151**:811, 1992.
36. Bollinger ME, Arredondo-Vega FX, Santisteban I, Schwarz K, Hershfield MS, Lederman HM: Hepatic dysfunction as a complication of adenosine deaminase δ(ADA) deficiency. *N Engl J Med* **334**:1367, 1996.
37. Kohn DB, Hershfield MS, Carbonaro D, Shigeoka A, Brooks J, Smogorzewska EM, Barsky LW, et al.: Selective accumulation of T lymphocytes containing a normal ADA gene four years after transplantation of transduced autologous umbilical cord blood CD34+ cells in ADA-deficient SCID neonates. *Nature Medicine* **4**:775, 1998.
38. Wolfson JJ, Cross VF: The radiographic findings in 49 patients with combined immunodeficiency, in Pollara B, Pickering RJ, Meuwissen HJ, Porter IH (eds): *Combined Immunodeficiency Disease and Adenosine Deaminase Deficiency: A Molecular Defect*. New York, Academic, 1975, p 225.
39. Huber J, Kersey J: Pathologic features, in Pollara B, Pickering RJ, Meuwissen HJ, Porter IH (eds): *Combined Immunodeficiency Disease and Adenosine Deaminase Deficiency: A Molecular Defect*. New York, Academic, 1975, p 279.
40. Ratech H, Hirschhorn R, Greco MA: Pathologic findings in adenosine deaminase deficient-severe combined immunodeficiency. II. Thymus, spleen, lymph node, and gastrointestinal tract lymphoid tissue alterations. *Am J Pathol* **135**:1145, 1989.
41. Linch DC, Levinski RJ, Rodeck CH, Maclennan KA, Simmonds HA: Prenatal diagnosis of three cases of severe combined immunodeficiency severe T cell deficiency—during the first half of gestation in fetuses with adenosine deaminase deficiency. *Clin Exp Immunol* **56**:223, 1984.
42. Schmalstieg FC, Mills GC, Tsuda H, Goldman AS: Severe combined immunodeficiency in a child with a healthy adenosine deaminase deficient mother. *Pediatr Res* **17**:935, 1983.
43. Cederbaum SD, Kaitila I, Rimoin DL, Stiehm ER: The chondro-osseous dysplasia of adenosine deaminase deficiency with severe combined immunodeficiency. *J Pediatr* **89**:737, 1976.
44. Ratech H, Greco MA, Gallo G, Rimoin DL, Kamino H, Hirschhorn R: Pathologic findings in adenosine deaminase–deficient severe combined immunodeficiency. *Am J Pathol* **120**:157, 1985.
45. Schwartz AL, Polmar SH, Stern RC, Cowan DH: Abnormal platelet aggregation in severe combined immunodeficiency disease with adenosine deaminase deficiency. *Br J Haematol* **39**:189, 1978.
46. Lee CH, Evans SP, Rozenberg MC, Bagnara AS, Ziegler JB, Van Der Weyden MB: *In vitro* platelet abnormality in adenosine deaminase deficiency and severe combined immunodeficiency. *Blood* **53**:465, 1979.
47. Cercignani G, Allegrini S: On the validity of continuous spectrophotometric assays for adenosine deaminase activity: A critical reappraisal. *Anal Biochem* **192**:312, 1991.
48. Hopkinson DA, Cook PHL, Harris H: Further data on the adenosine deaminase (ADA) polymorphism and a report of a new phenotype. *Ann Hum Genet* **32**:361, 1969.
49. Arredondo-Vega FX, Kurtzberg J, Chaffee S, Santisteban I, Reisner E, Povey MS, Hershfield MS: Paradoxical expression of adenosine deaminase in T cells cultured from a patient with adenosine deaminase deficiency and combined immunodeficiency. *J Clin Invest* **86**:444, 1990.
50. Aitken DA, Gilmore DH, Frew CA, Ferguson-Smith ME, Carty MJ, Chatfield WR: Early prenatal investigation of a pregnancy at risk of adenosine deaminase deficiency using chorionic villi. *J Med Genet* **23**:52, 1986.
51. Dooley T, Fairbanks LD, Simmonds HA, Rodeck CH, Nicolaides KH, Soothill PW, Stewart P, et al.: First trimester diagnosis of adenosine deaminase deficiency. *Prenat Diagn* **7**:561, 1987.
52. Hirschhorn R, Beratis N, Rosen FS, Parkman R, Stern R, Polmar S: Adenosine-deaminase deficiency in a child diagnosed prenatally. *Lancet* **1**:73, 1975.
53. Hirschhorn R: Prenatal diagnosis and heterozygote detection in adenosine deaminase deficiency, in Guttler F, Seakins JWT, Harkness

RA (eds): *Inborn Errors of Immunity and Phagocytosis*. Lancaster, MTP Press, 1979, p 121.

54. Aitken DA, Kleijer WJ, Niermeijer MF, Herbschleb-Voogt E, Galjaard H: Prenatal detection of a probable heterozygote for ADA deficiency and severe combined immunodeficiency disease using a microradioassay. *Clin Genet* **17**:293, 1980.
55. Ziegler JB, Van der Weyden MB, Lee CH, Daniel A: Prenatal diagnosis for adenosine deaminase deficiency. *J Med Genet* **18**:154, 1981.
56. Simmonds HA, Fairbanks LD, Webster DR, Rodeck CH, Linch DC, Levinsky RJ: Rapid prenatal diagnosis of adenosine deaminase deficiency and other purine disorders using fetal blood. *Biosci Rep* **3**:31, 1983.
57. Scott CR, Chen SH, Giblett ER: Detection of the carrier state in combined immunodeficiency disease associated with adenosine deaminase deficiency. *J Clin Invest* **53**:1194, 1974.
58. Chen SH, Scott CR, Swedberg DR: Heterogeneity for adenosine deaminase deficiency: Expression of the enzyme in cultured skin fibroblasts and amniotic fluid cells. *Am J Hum Genet* **27**:46, 1975.
59. Brinkmann B, Brinkman M, Martin H: A new allele in red cell adenosine deaminase polymorphism: ADAo. *Hum Hered* **23**:603, 1973.
60. Chen SH, Scott CR, Giblett ER: Adenosine deaminase: Demonstration of a "silent" gene associated with combined immunodeficiency disease. *Am J Hum Genet* **26**:103, 1974.
61. Chen SH, Scott CR, Giblett ER, Levin AS: Adenosine deaminase deficiency: Another family with a "silent" ADA allele and normal ADA activity in two heterozygotes. *Am J Hum Genet* **29**:642, 1977.
62. Jenkins T: Red-blood-cell adenosine deaminase deficiency in a "healthy" Kung individual. *Lancet* **2**:736, 1973.
63. Jenkins T, Lane AB, Nurse GT, Hopkinson DA: Red cell adenosine deaminase (ADA) polymorphism in Southern Africa, with special reference to ADA deficiency among the !Kung. *Ann Hum Genet* **42**:425, 1979.
64. Jenkins T, Rabson AR, Nurse GT, Lane AB: Deficiency of adenosine deaminase not associated with severe combined immunodeficiency. *J Pediatr* **89**:732, 1976.
65. Jenkins T, Lane AB: The red cell adenosine deaminase polymorphism in Southern African populations with particular reference to the !Kung of Tsumkwe, Southwest Africa/Nambia, in Pollara B, Pickering RJ, Meuwissen HJ, Porter IH (eds): *Inborn Errors of Specific Immunity*. New York, Academic, 1979, p 73.
66. Hirschhorn R, Roegner V, Jenkins T, Seaman C, Piomelli S, Borkowsky W: Erythrocyte adenosine deaminase deficiency without immunodeficiency. Evidence for an unstable mutant enzyme. *J Clin Invest* **64**:1130, 1979.
67. Hirschhorn R, Ellenbogen A: Genetic heterogeneity in adenosine deaminase (ADA) deficiency: Five different mutations in five new patients with partial ADA deficiency. *Am J Hum Genet* **38**:13, 1986.
68. Perignon JL, Hamet M, Broyer M, Griscelli C, Lenoir G, Cartier P: Primary hyperoxaluria and adenosine deaminase deficiency without immunodeficiency. *Int J Pediatr Nephrol* **1**:26, 1980.
69. Borkowsky W, Gershon AA, Shenkman L, Hirschhorn R: Adenosine deaminase deficiency without immunodeficiency: Clinical and metabolic studies. *Pediatr Res* **14**:885, 1980.
70. Daddona PE, Mitchell BS, Meuwissen HJ, Davidson BL, Wilson JM, Koller CA: Adenosine deaminase deficiency with normal immune function. *J Clin Invest* **72**:483, 1983.
71. Hart SL, Lane AB, Jenkins T: Partial adenosine deaminase deficiency: Another family from southern Africa. *Hum Genet* **74**:307, 1986.
72. Moore EC, Meuwissen HJ: Screening for ADA deficiency. *J Pediatr* **85**:802, 1974.
73. Cohen A, Hirschhorn R, Horowitz SD, Rubinstein A, Polmar SH, Hong R, Martin DWJr: Deoxyadenosine triphosphate as a potentially toxic metabolite in adenosine deaminase deficiency. *Proc Natl Acad Sci U S A* **75**:472, 1978.
74. Valentine WN, Paglia DE, Tartaglia AP, Gilsanz F: Hereditary hemolytic anemia with increased red cell adenosine deaminase (45- to 70-fold) and decreased adenosine triphosphate. *Science* **195**:783, 1977.
75. Miwa S, Fujii H, Matsumoto N, Nakatsuji T, Oda S, Asano H, Asano S: A case of red-cell adenosine deaminase overproduction associated with hereditary hemolytic anemia found in Japan. *Am J Hematol* **5**:107, 1978.
76. Perignon JL, Hamet M, Buc HA, Cartier PH, Derycke M: Biochemical study of a case of hemolytic anemia with increased (85-fold) red cell adenosine deaminase. *Clin Chim Acta* **124**:205, 1982.
77. Fujii H, Miwa S, Tani K, Fujinami N, Asano H: Overproduction of structurally normal enzyme in man: Hereditary haemolytic anaemia with increased red cell adenosine deaminase activity. *Br J Haematol* **51**:427, 1982.
78. Chottiner EG, Cloft HJ, Tartaglia AP, Mitchell BS: Elevated adenosine deaminase activity and hereditary hemolytic anemia: Evidence for abnormal translational control of protein synthesis. *J Clin Invest* **79**:1001, 1987.
79. Chottiner EG, Ginsburg D, Tartaglia AP, Mitchell BS: Erythrocyte adenosine deaminase overproduction in hereditary hemolytic anemia. *Blood* **74**:448, 1989.
80. Chottiner EG, Gribbin TE, Ginsburg D, Mitchell BS: Erythrocyte-specific overproduction of adenosine deaminase: Molecular genetic studies. *Prog Clin Biol Res* **319**:55, 1989.
81. Chen EH, Tartaglia AP, Mitchell BS: Hereditary overexpression of adenosine deaminase in erythrocytes: Evidence for a cis-acting mutation. *Am J Hum Genet* **53**:889, 1993.
82. Chen EH, Mitchell BS: Hereditary overexpression of adenosine deaminase in erythrocytes: Studies in erythroid cell lines and transgenic mice. *Blood* **84**:2346, 1994.
83. Markert ML: Purine nucleoside phosphorylase deficiency. *Immunodeficiency Rev* **3**:45, 1991.
84. Ammann AJ: Immunologic abberations in purine nucleoside phosphorylase deficiencies, in Elliot K, Whelan J (eds): *Enzyme Defects and Immune Dysfunction, Ciba Foundation Symposium 68*. New York, Excerpta Medica, 1979, p 55.
85. Simmonds HA, Fairbanks LD, Morris GS, Morgan G, Watson AR, Timms P, Singh B: Central nervous system dysfunction and erythrocyte guanosine triphosphate depletion in purine nucleoside phosphorylase deficiency. *Arch Dis Child* **62**:385, 1987.
86. Watson AR, Evans DK, Marsden HB, Miller V, Rogers PA: Purine nucleoside phosphorylase deficiency associated with a fatal lymphoproliferative disorder. *Arch Dis Child* **56**:563, 1981.
87. Soutar RL, Day RE: Dysequilibrium/ataxic diplegia with immunodeficiency. *Arch Dis Child* **66**:982, 1991.
88. Hagberg B, Hansson O, Liden S, Nilsson K: Familial ataxic diplegia with deficient cellular immunity. *Acta Pediatr Scand* **59**:545, 1970.
89. Graham-Poole J, Gibson AAM, Stephenson JBP: Familial dysequilibrium-diplegia with T lymphocyte deficiency. *Arch Dis Child* **50**:927, 1975.
90. Pannicke U, Tuchschmid P, Friedrich W, Bartram CR, Schwarz K: Two novel missense and frameshift mutations in exons 5 and 6 of the purine nucleoside phosphorylase (PNP) gene in a severe combined immunodeficiency (SCID) patient. *Hum Genet* **98**:706, 1996.
91. Markert ML, Hershfield MS, Schiff RI, Buckley RH: Adenosine deaminase and purine nucleoside phosphorylase deficiencies: Evaluation of therapeutic interventions in eight patients. *J Clin Immunol* **7**:389, 1987.
92. Rijksen G, Kuis W, Wadman SK, Spaapen L, Duran M, Voorbrood BS, Staal G, et al.: A new case of purine nucleoside phosphorylase deficiency: Enzymologic, clinical and immunologic characteristics. *Pediatr Res* **21**:137, 1987.
93. Chu SY, Cashion P, Jiang M: Purine nucleoside phosphorylase in erythrocytes: Determination of optimum reaction conditions. *Clin Biochem* **22**:3, 1989.
94. Chu SY, Cashion P, Jiang M: A new colorimetric assay for purine nucleoside phosphorylase. *Clin Biochem* **22**:357, 1989.
95. Carapella De Luca E, Stegagno M, Dionisi Vici C, Paesano R, Fairbanks LD, Morris GS, Simmonds HA: Prenatal exclusion of purine nucleoside phosphorylase deficiency. *Eur J Pediatr* **145**:51, 1986.
96. Morgan C, Levinsky RJ, Hugh JK, Fairbanks LD, Morris GS, Simmonds HA: Heterogeneity of biochemical, clinical and immunological parameters in severe combined immunodeficiency due to adenosine deaminase deficiency. *Clin Exp Immunol* **70**:491, 1987.
97. Simmonds HA, Sahota A, Potter CF, Cameron JS, Wadman SK: Purine metabolism and immunodeficiency. Urinary purine excretion as a diagnostic screening test in adenosine deaminase and purine nucleoside phosphorylase deficiency. *Clin Sci Mol Med* **54**:579, 1978.
98. Kuttesch JF, Schmalstieg FC, Nelson JA: Analysis of adenosine and other adenine compounds in patients with immunodeficiency diseases. *J Liquid Chromatogr* **1**:97, 1978.
99. Mills GC, Goldblum RM, Newkirk KE, Schmalstieg FC: Urinary excretion of purines, purine nucleosides, and pseudouridine in adenosine deaminase deficiency. *Biochem Med* **20**:180, 1978.
100. Hirschhorn R, Ratech H, Rubinstein A, Papageorgiou P, Kesarwala H, Gelfand E, Roegner Maniscalco V: Increased excretion of modified

adenine nucleosides by children with adenosine deaminase deficiency. *Pediatr Res* **16**:362, 1982.

101. Coleman MS, Donofrio J, Hutton JJ, Hahn L, Daoud A, Lampkin B, Dyminski J: Identification and quantitation of adenine deoxynucleotides in erythrocytes of a patient with adenosine deaminase deficiency and severe combined immunodeficiency. *J Biol Chem* **253**:1619, 1978.
102. Hershfield MS, Kurtzberg J, Aiyar VN, Suh EJ, Schiff R: Abnormalities in *S*-adenosylhomocysteine hydrolysis, ATP catabolism, and lymphoid differentiation in adenosine deaminase deficiency. *Ann NY Acad Sci* **451**:78, 1985.
103. Hershfield MS, Buckley RH, Greenberg ML, Melton AL, Schiff R, Hatem C, Kurtzberg J, et al.: Treatment of adenosine deaminase deficiency with polyethylene glycol-modified adenosine deaminase. *N Engl J Med* **316**:589, 1987.
104. Hershfield MS, Kredich NM, Ownby DR, Ownby H, Buckley R: *In vivo* inactivation of erythrocyte *S*-adenosylhomocysteine hydrolase by 2′-deoxyadenosine in adenosine deaminase-deficient patients. *J Clin Invest* **63**:807, 1979.
105. Hirschhorn R, Roegner-Maniscalco V, Kuritsky L, Rosen FS: Bone marrow transplantation only partially restores purine metabolites to normal in adenosine deaminase–deficient patients. *J Clin Invest* **68**:1387, 1981.
106. Hirschhorn R: Adenosine deaminase deficiency: Molecular basis and recent developments. *Clin Immunol Immunopathol* **76**(suppl):219, 1995.
107. Hirschhorn R, Roegner V, Rubinstein A, Papageorgiou P: Plasma deoxyadenosine, adenosine, and erythrocyte deoxyATP are elevated at birth in an adenosine deaminase–deficient child. *J Clin Invest* **65**:768, 1980.
108. Kohn DB, Weinberg KI, Nolta JA, Heiss LN, Lenarsky C, Crooks GM, Hanley ME, et al.: Engraftment of gene-modified umbilical cord blood cells in neonates with adenosine deaminase deficiency. *Nat Med* **1**:1017, 1995.
109. Simmonds HA, Sahota A, Potter CF, Perrett D, Hugh-Jones K, Watson JG: Purine metabolism in adenosine deaminase deficiency, in Elliot K, Whelan J (eds): *Enzyme Defects and Immune Dysfunction, Ciba Foundation Symposium*. New York, Excerpta Medica, 1979, p 255.
110. Simmonds HA, Watson AR, Webster DR, Sahota A, Perrett D: GTP depletion and other erythrocyte abnormalities in inherited PNP deficiency. *Biochem Pharmacol* **31**:941, 1982.
111. Cohen A, Gudas LJ, Ammann AJ, Staal GEJ, Martin DW Jr: Deoxyguanosine triphosphate as a possible toxic metabolite in the immunodeficiency associated with purine nucleoside phosphorylase deficiency. *J Clin Invest* **61**:1405, 1978.
112. Sidi Y, Mitchell BS: Z-nucleotide accumulation in erythrocytes from Lesch-Nyhan patients. *J Clin Invest* **76**:2416, 1985.
113. Donofrio J, Coleman MS, Hutton JJ, Daoud A, Lampkin B, Dyminski J: Overproduction of adenine deoxynucleosides and deoxynucleotides in adenosine deaminase deficiency with severe combined immunodeficiency disease. *J Clin Invest* **62**:884, 1978.
114. Hutton JJ, Wiginton DA, Coleman MS, Fuller SA, Limouze S, Lampkin BC: Biochemical and functional abnormalities in lymphocytes from an adenosine deaminase deficient patient during enzyme replacement therapy. *J Clin Invest* **68**:413, 1981.
115. Rich KC, Richman CM, Mejias E, Daddona PA: Immunoreconstitution by peripheral blood leukocytes in adenosine deaminase-deficient severe combined immunodeficiency. *J Clin Invest* **66**:389, 1980.
116. Cohen A, Doyle D, Martin DW Jr, Ammann AJ: Abnormal purine metabolism and purine overproduction in a patient deficient in purine nucleoside phosphorylase. *N Engl J Med* **295**:1449, 1976.
117. Hershfield MS, Seegmiller JE: Regulation of *de novo* purine synthesis in human lymphoblasts. Similar rates of *de novo* synthesis during growth by normal cells and mutants deficient in hypoxanthine-guanine phosphoribosyltransferase activity. *J Biol Chem* **252**:6002, 1977.
118. Akedo H, Nishihara H, Shinkai K, Komatsu K, Ishikawa S: Multiple forms of human adenosine deaminase. I. Purification and characterization of two molecular species. *Biochim Biophys Acta* **276**:257, 1972.
119. Agarwal RP, Sagar SM, Parks REJr: Adenosine deaminase from human erythrocytes. Purification and effects of adenosine analogs. *Biochem Pharmacol* **24**:693, 1975.
120. Snyder FF, Lukey T: Purine ribonucleoside and deoxyribonucleoside metabolism in thymocytes. *Adv Exp Med Biol* **122B**:259, 1980.
121. Kim BK, Cha S, Parks RE Jr: Purine nucleoside phosphorylase from human erythrocytes. I. Purification and properties. *J Biol Chem* **243**:1763, 1968.
122. Lewis AS, Lowy BA: Human erythrocyte purine nucleoside phosphorylase: Molecular weight and physical properties. A Theorell-Chance catalytic mechanism. *J Biol Chem* **254**:9927, 1979.
123. Kalkar HM: The enzymatic synthesis of purine ribosides. *J Biol Chem* **167**:477, 1947.
124. Friedkin M: Desoxyribose-1-phosphate. II. The isolation of crystalline desoxyribose-1-phosphate. *J Biol Chem* **184**:449, 1950.
125. Moser GH, Schrader J, Deussen A: Turnover of adenosine in plasma of human and dog blood. *Am J Physiol* **256**:C799, 1989.
126. Lee PC: Developmental changes of adenosine deaminase, xanthine oxidase and uricase in mouse tissues. *Dev Biol* **31**:227, 1973.
127. Witte DP, Wiginton DA, Hutton JJ, Aronow BJ: Coordinate developmental regulation of purine catabolic enzyme expression in gastrointestinal and postimplantation reproductive tracts. *J Cell Biol* **115**:179, 1991.
128. Mohamedali KA, Guicherit OM, Kellems RE, Rudolph FB: The highest levels of purine catabolic enzymes are present in the proximal small intestine. *J Biol Chem* **268**:23728, 1993.
129. Wilson D, Beyer A, Bishop C, Talbott JH: Urinary uric acid excretion after ingestion of isotopic yeast nucleic acid in the normal and gouty human. *J Biol Chem* **209**:227, 1954.
130. Sonoda T, Tatibana M: Metabolic fate of pyrimidines and purines in dietary nucleic acids ingested by mice. *Biochim Biophys Acta* **521**:55, 1978.
131. Ho CY, Miller KV, Savaiano DA, Crane RT, Ericson KA, Clifford AJ: Absorption and metabolism of orally administered purines in fed and fasted rats. *J Nutr* **109**:1377, 1979.
132. Savaiano DA, Ho CY, Chu V, Clifford AJ: Metabolism of orally and intravenously administered purines in rats. *J Nutr* **110**:1793, 1980.
133. Uauy R: Dietary nucleotides and requirements in early life, in Lebenthal E (ed): *Textbook of Gastroenterology and Nutrition in Infancy*. New York, Raven, 1989, p 265.
134. Griffith DA, Jarvis SM: Nucleoside and nucleobase transport systems of mammalian cells. *Biochim Biophys Acta* **1286**:153, 1996.
135. Griffiths M, Beaumont N, Yao SY, Sundaram M, Boumah CE, Davies A, Kwong FY, et al.: Cloning of a human nucleoside transporter implicated in the cellular uptake of adenosine and chemotherapeutic drugs [Comments]. *Nat Med* **3**:89, 1997.
136. Griffiths M, Yao SY, Abidi F, Phillips SE, Cass CE, Young JD, Baldwin SA: Molecular cloning and characterization of a nitrobenzylthioinosine-insensitive (ei) equilibrative nucleoside transporter from human placenta. *Biochem J* **328**:739, 1997.
137. Crawford CR, Patel DH, Naeve C, Belt JA: Cloning of the human equilibrative, nitrobenzylmercaptopurine riboside (NBMPR)-insensitive nucleoside transporter ei by functional expression in a transport-deficient cell line. *J Biol Chem* **273**:5288, 1998.
138. Plesner L: Ecto-ATPases: Identities and functions. *Int Rev Cytol* **158**:141, 1995.
139. Resta R, Yamashita Y, Thompson LF: Ecto-enzyme and signaling functions of lymphocyte CD73. *Immunol Rev* **161**:95, 1998.
140. Strohmeier GR, Lencer WI, Patapoff TW, Thompson LF, Carlson SL, Moe SJ, Carnes DK, et al.: Surface expression, polarization, and functional significance of CD73 in human intestinal epithelia. *J Clin Invest* **99**:2588, 1997.
141. Burnstock G: The past, present and future of purine nucleotides as signalling molecules. *Neuropharmacology* **36**:1127, 1997.
142. Todorov LD, Mihaylova-Todorova S, Westfall TD, Sneddon P, Kennedy C, Bjur RA, Westfall DP: Neuronal release of soluble nucleotidases and their role in neurotransmitter inactivation. *Nature* **387**:76, 1997.
143. Resta R, Hooker SW, Laurent AB, Jamshedur Rahman SM, Franklin M, Knudsen TB, Nadon NL, et al.: Insights into thymic purine metabolism and adenosine deaminase deficiency revealed by transgenic mice overexpressing ecto-5′-nucleotidase (CD73). *J Clin Invest* **99**:676, 1997.
144. Che M, Nishida T, Gatmaitan Z, Arias IM: A nucleoside transporter is functionally linked to ectonucleotidases in rat liver canalicular membrane. *J Biol Chem* **267**:9684, 1992.
145. Misumi Y, Ogata S, Ohkubo K, Hirose S, Ikehara Y: Primary structure of human placental 5′-nucleotidase and identification of the glycolipid anchor in mature form. *Eur J Biochem* **191**:563, 1990.
146. Madrid-Marina V, Lestan B, Nowak PJ, Fox IH, Spychala J: Altered properties of human T-lymphoblast soluble low K_m 5′-nucleotidase: Comparison with B-lymphoblast enzyme. *Leuk Res* **17**:231, 1993.
147. Newby AC, Worku Y, Meghji G: Critical evaluation of the role of ecto- and cytosolic 5′-nucleotidase in adenosine formation, in Gerlach

E, Becker BF (eds): *Topics and Perspectives in Adenosine Research*. Berlin, Springer-Verlag, 1987, p 155.

148. Hoglund L, Reichard P: Cytoplasmic 5′(3′)-nucleotidase from human placenta. *J Biol Chem* **265**:6589, 1990.
149. Zimmermann H: 5′-Nucleotidase: molecular structure and functional aspects. *Biochem J* **285**:345, 1992.
150. Itoh R: IMP-GMP 5′-nucleotidase. *Comp Biochem Physiol [B]* **105**:13, 1993.
151. Bontemps F, Van den Berghe G, Hers HG: Evidence for a substrate cycle between AMP and adenosine in isolated hepatocytes. *Proc Natl Acad Sci U S A* **80**:2829, 1983.
152. Newsholme EA, Challiss RAJ, Crabtree B: Substrate cycles their role in improving sensitivity in metabolic control. *Trends Biochem Sci* **9**:277, 1984.
153. Nicander B, Reichard P: Evidence for the involvement of substrate cycles in the regulation of deoxyribonucleoside triphosphate pools in 3T6 cells. *J Biol Chem* **260**:9216, 1985.
154. Decking UK, Schlieper G, Kroll K, Schrader J: Hypoxia-induced inhibition of adenosine kinase potentiates cardiac adenosine release. *Circ Res* **81**:154, 1997.
155. Matsumoto SS, Raivio KO, Seegmiller JE: Adenine nucleotide degradation during energy depletion in human lymphoblasts. Adenosine accumulation and adenylate energy charge correlation. *J Biol Chem* **254**:8865, 1979.
156. Snyder FF, Trafzer RJ, Hershfield MS, Seegmiller JE: Elucidation of aberrant purine metabolism. Application of hypoxanthine-guanine phosphoribosyltransferase– and adenosine kinase–deficient mutants, and IMP dehydrogenase– and adenosine deaminase–inhibited human lymphoblasts. *Biochim Biophys Acta* **609**:492, 1980.
157. Bagnara AS, Hershfield MS: Mechanism of deoxyadenosine-induced catabolism of adenine ribonucleotides in adenosine deaminase-inhibited human T lymphoblastoid cells. *Proc Natl Acad Sci U S A* **79**:2673, 1982.
158. Newby AC: Role of adenosine deaminase, ecto-(5′-nucleotidase) and ecto-(non-specific phosphatase) in cyanide-induced adenosine monophosphate catabolism in rat polymorphonuclear leucocytes. *Biochem J* **186**:907, 1980.
159. Barankiewicz J, Cohen A: Evidence for distinct catabolic pathways for adenine ribonucleotides and deoxyribonucleotides in human T lymphoblastoid cells. *J Biol Chem* **259**:15178, 1984.
160. Barankiewicz J, Ronlov G, Jimenez R, Gruber HE: Selective adenosine release from human B but not T lymphoid cell lines. *J Biol Chem* **265**:15738, 1990.
161. Allegrini S, Pesi R, Tozzi MG, Fiol CJ, Johnson RB, Eriksson S: Bovine cytosolic IMP/GMP-specific 5′-nucleotidase: Cloning and expression of active enzyme in *Escherichia coli*. *Biochem J* **328**:483, 1997.
162. Carson DA, Wasson DB: Characterization of an adenosine 5′-triphosphate– and deoxyadenosine 5′-triphosphate–activated nucleotidase from human malignant lymphocytes. *Cancer Res* **42**:4321, 1982.
163. Spychala J, Madrid-Marina V, Fox IH: High K_m soluble 5′-nucleotidase from human placenta: Properties and allosteric regulation by IMP and ATP. *J Biol Chem* **263**:18759, 1988.
164. Barankiewicz J, Gelfand EW, Issekutz A, Cohen A: Evidence for active purine nucleoside cycles in human mononuclear cells and fibroblasts. *J Biol Chem* **257**:11597, 1982.
165. Willis RC, Kaufman AH, Seegmiller JE: Purine nucleotide reutilization by human lymphoblast lines with aberrations of the inosinate cycle. *J Biol Chem* **259**:4157, 1984.
166. Chan TS, Ishii K, Long C, Green H: Purine excretion by mammalian cells deficient in adenosine kinase. *J Cell Physiol* **81**:315, 1973.
167. Schrader J, Deussen A, Decking UKM: Adenosine metabolism and transport in the mammalian heart, in Pelleg A, Belardinelli L (eds): *Effects of Extracellular Adenosine and ATP on Cardiomyocytes*. Austin, TX, RG Landes, 1998, p 39.
168. Truong VL, Collinson AR, Lowenstein JM: 5′-Nucleotidases in rat heart: Evidence for the occurrence of two soluble enzymes with different substrate specificities. *Biochem J* **253**:117, 1988.
169. Yamazaki Y, Truong VL, Lowenstein JM: 5′-Nucleotidase I from rabbit heart. *Biochemistry* **30**:1503, 1991.
170. Mudd HS, Poole JR: Labile methyl balances for normal humans on various dietary regimens. *Metabolism* **24**:721, 1975.
171. Palella TD, Andres CM, Fox IH: Human placental adenosine kinase kinetic mechanism and inhibition. *J Biol Chem* **255**:5264, 1980.
172. Meyskens FL, Williams HE: Adenosine metabolism in human erythrocytes. *Biochim Biophys Acta* **240**:170, 1971.
173. Hershfield MH, Kredich NM: Resistance of an adenosine kinase-deficient human lymphoblastoid cell line to effects of deoxyadenosine on growth, *S*-adenosylhomocysteine hydrolase inactivation, and dATP accumulation. *Proc Natl Acad Sci U S A* **77**:4292, 1980.
174. Daddona PE, Kelley WN: Human adenosine deaminase: Purification and subunit structure. *J Biol Chem* **252**:110, 1977.
175. Snyder FF, Mendelsohn J, Seegmiller JE: Adenosine metabolism in phyto- hemagglutinin-stimulated human lymphocytes. *J Clin Invest* **58**:654, 1976.
176. Plagemann PGW: Transport and metabolism of adenosine in human erythrocytes: Effect of transport inhibitors and regulation by phosphate. *J Cell Physiol* **128**:491, 1986.
177. Henderson JF, Mikoshiba A, Chu SY, Caldwell IC: Kinetic studies of adenosine kinase from Ehrlich ascites tumor cells. *J Biol Chem* **247**:1972, 1972.
178. Hawkins CF, Kyd JM, Bagnara AS: Adenosine metabolism in human erythrocytes A study of some factors which affect the metabolic fate of adenosine in intact red cells *in vitro*. *Arch Biochem Biophys* **202**:380, 1980.
179. Snyder FF, Dyer C, Seegmiller JE, Goldblum RM, Mills GC, Schmalstieg FC: Substrate inhibition of adenosine phosphorylation in adenosine deaminase deficiency and adenosine-mediated inhibition of PP-ribose-P dependent nucleotide synthesis in hypoxanthine phosphoribosyltransferase deficient erythrocytes. *J Inherit Metab Dis* **11**:174, 1988.
180. Bontemps F, Vincent MF, Van den Berghe G: Mechanisms of elevation of adenosine levels in anoxic hepatocytes. *Biochem J* **290**:671, 1993.
181. van Waeg G, Van den Berghe G: Purine catabolism in polymorphonuclear neutrophils. Phorbol myristate acetate-induced accumulation of adenosine owing to inactivation of extracellularly released adenosine deaminase. *J Clin Invest* **87**:305, 1991.
182. Hoehn K, White TD: Glutamate-evoked release of endogenous adenosine from rat cortical synaptosomes is mediated by glutamate uptake and not by receptors. *J Neurochem* **54**:1716, 1990.
183. Iizasa T, Kubota M, Carson DA: Differential production of deoxyadenosine by human T and B lymphoblasts. *J Immunol* **131**:1776, 1983.
184. Kubota M, Carrera CJ, Wasson DB, Carson DA: Deoxynucleoside overproduction in deoxyadenosine-resistant, adenosine deaminase-deficient human histiocytic lymphoma cells. *Biochim Biophys Acta* **804**:804, 1984.
185. Bianchi V, Ferraro P, Borella S, Bonvini P, Reichard P: Effects of mutational loss of nucleoside kinases on deoxyadenosine 5′-phosphate/deoxyadenosine substrate cycle in cultured CEM and V79 cells. *J Biol Chem* **269**:16677, 1994.
186. Chan T-S: Purine excretion by mouse peritoneal macrophages lacking adenosine deaminase activity. *Proc Natl Acad Sci U S A* **76**:925, 1979.
186a. Thompson LF, Van De Wiele CJ, Laurent AB, Hooker SW, Jiang H, Khare K, Kellems RE, et al.: Thymopoiesis is inhibited by metabolites from apoptotic thymocytes in adenosine deaminase deficient murine fetal thymic organ cultures. *J Clin Invest* in Press: 2000.
187. Henderson JF, Smith CM: Mechanisms of deoxycoformycin toxicity *in vivo*, in Tattersal MHN, Fox RM (eds): *Nucleosides in Cancer Treatment*. Sydney, Academic, 1981, p 208.
188. Carson DA, Kaye J, Matsumoto S, Seegmiller JE, Thompson L: Biochemical basis for the enhanced toxicity of deoxyribonucleosides toward malignant human T cell lines. *Proc Natl Acad Sci U S A* **76**:2430, 1979.
189. Carson DA, Kaye J, Wasson DB: The potential importance of soluble deoxynucleotidase activity in mediating deoxyadenosine toxicity in human lymphoblasts. *J Immunol* **126**:348, 1981.
190. Valentine WN, Paglia DE, Clarke S, Morimoto BH, Nakatani M, Brockway R: Adenine ribo- and deoxyribonucleotide metabolism in human erythrocytes, B- and T-lymphocyte cell lines, and monocyte-macrophages. *Proc Natl Acad Sci U S A* **82**:6682, 1985.
191. Barankiewicz J, Cohen A: Evidence for distinct catabolic pathways for deoxy-GTP and GTP in purine nucleoside phosphorylase-deficient mouse T lymphoblasts. *J Biol Chem* **260**:4565, 1985.
192. Arner ES, Eriksson S: Mammalian deoxyribonucleoside kinases. *Pharmacol Ther* **67**:155, 1995.
193. Hurley MC, Lin B, Fox IH: Regulation of deoxyadenosine and nucleoside analog phosphorylation by human placental adenosine kinase. *J Biol Chem* **260**:15675, 1985.
194. Sjoberg AH, Wang L, Eriksson S: Substrate specificity of human recombinant mitochondrial deoxyguanosine kinase with cytostatic

and antiviral purine and pyrimidine analogs. *Mol Pharmacol* **53**:270, 1998.

195. Ives DH, Durham JP: Deoxycytidine kinase kinetics and allosteric regulation of the calf thymus enzyme. *J Biol Chem* **245**:2285, 1970.
196. Krenitsky TA, Tuttle JV, Koszalka GW, Chen IS, Beachman LM, Rideout JL, Elion GB: Deoxycytidine kinase from calf thymus substrate and inhibitor specificity. *J Biol Chem* **251**:4055, 1976.
197. Bohman C, Eriksson S: Deoxycytidine kinase from human leukemic spleen: Preparation and characteristics of homogeneous enzyme. *Biochemistry* **27**:4258, 1988.
198. Datta NS, Shewach DS, Hurley MC, Mitchell BS, Fox IH: Human T-lymphoblast deoxycytidine kinase: Purification and properties. *Biochemistry* **28**:114, 1989.
199. Chottiner EG, Shewach DS, Datta NS, Ashcraft E, Gribbin D, Ginsburg D, Fox IH, et al.: Cloning and expression of human deoxycytidine kinase. *Proc Natl Acad Sci U S A* **88**:1531, 1991.
200. Song JJ, Walker S, Chen E, Johnson EEd, Spychala J, Gribbin T, Mitchell BS: Genomic structure and chromosomal localization of the human deoxycytidine kinase gene. *Proc Natl Acad Sci U S A* **90**:431, 1993.
201. Stegmann AP, Honders MW, Bolk MW, Wessels J, Willemze R, Landegent JE: Assignment of the human deoxycytidine kinase (DCK) gene to chromosome 4 band q13.3-q21.1. *Genomics* **17**:528, 1993.
202. Johansson M, Brismar S, Karlsson A: Human deoxycytidine kinase is located in the cell nucleus. *Proc Natl Acad Sci U S A* **94**:11941, 1997.
203. Datta NS, Shewach DS, Mitchell BS, Fox IH: Kinetic properties and inhibition of human T lymphoblast deoxycytidine kinase. *J Biol Chem* **264**:9359, 1989.
204. Hughes TL, Hahn TM, Reynolds KK, Shewach DS: Kinetic analysis of human deoxycytidine kinase with the true phosphate donor uridine triphosphate. *Biochemistry* **36**:7540, 1997.
205. Ullman B, Gudas LJ, Cohen A, Martin DW Jr: Deoxyadenosine metabolism and cytotoxicity in cultured mouse T lymphoma cells: A model for immunodeficiency disease. *Cell* **14**:365, 1978.
206. Ullman B, Levinson BB, Hershfield MS, Martin DW Jr: A biochemical genetic study of the role of specific nucleoside kinases in deoxyadenosine phosphorylation by cultured human cells. *J Biol Chem* **256**:848, 1981.
207. Carson DA, Kaye J, Wasson DB: Differences in deoxyadenosine metabolism in human and mouse lymphocytes. *J Immunol* **124**:8, 1980.
208. Hershfield MS, Kredich NM: Effects of adenosine deaminase inhibition of transmethylation, in Tattersall MNH, Fox RM (eds): *Nucleosides and Cancer Treatment*. New York, Academic, 1981, p 161.
209. Hershfield MS, Fetter JE, Small WC, Bagnara AS, Williams SR, Ullman B, Martin DW Jr, et al.: Effects of mutational loss of adenosine kinase and deoxycytidine kinase on deoxyATP accumulation and deoxyadenosine toxicity in cultured CEM cells. *J Biol Chem* **257**:6380, 1982.
210. Ullman B, Gudas LJ, Clift SM, Martin DW Jr: Isolation and characterization of purine-nucleoside phosphorylase-deficient T-lymphoma cells and secondary mutants with altered ribonucleotide reductase. Genetic model for immunodeficiency diseasa. *Proc Natl Acad Sci U S A* **76**:1074, 1979.
211. Mitchell BS, Mejias E, Daddona PE, Kelley WN: Purinogenic immunodeficiency diseases Selective toxicity of deoxyribonucleosides for T cells. *Proc Natl Acad Sci U S A* **75**:5011, 1978.
212. Wilson JM, Mitchell BS, Daddona PE, Kelley WN: Purinogenic immuno-deficiency diseases. Differential effects of deoxyadenosine and deoxyguanosine on DNA synthesis in human T lymphoblasts. *J Clin Invest* **64**:1475, 1979.
213. Osborne WRA, Scott CR: The metabolism of deoxyguanosine and guanosine in human B and T lymphoblasts. *Biochem J* **214**:711, 1983.
214. Spaapen LJM, Rijkers GT, Staal GEJ, Rijksen G, Wadman SK, Stoop JW, Zegers BJM: The effect of deoxyguanosine on human lymphoctye function I. Analysis of the interference with lymphocyte proliferation *in vitro*. *J Immunol* **132**:2311, 1984.
215. Cohen A, Barankiewicz J, Lederman HM, Gelfand E: Purine and pyrimidine metabolism in human thymocytes. *J Biol Chem* **258**:12334, 1983.
216. Snyder FF, Henderson JF: Alternative pathways of deoxyadenosine and adenosine metabolism. *J Biol Chem* **248**:5899, 1973.
217. Simmonds HA, Goday A, Morris GS, Brolsma MFJ: Metabolism of deoxynucleosides by lymphocytes in long-term culture deficient in different purine enzymes. *Biochem Pharmacol* **33**:763, 1984.
218. Goday A, Simmonds HA, Morris GS, Fairbanks LD: B cells as well as T cells form deoxynucleotides from either deoxyadenosine or deoxyguanosine. *Clin Exp Immunol* **56**:56, 1984.
219. Stoeckler JD, Cambor C, Parks RE Jr: Human erythrocyte purine nucleoside phosphorylase reaction with sugar modified nucleoside substrates. *Biochemistry* **19**:102, 1980.
220. Carson DA, Kaye J, Seegmiller JE: Lymphospecific toxicity in adenosine deaminase deficiency and purine nucleoside phosphorylase deficiency: Possible role of nucleoside kinase(s). *Proc Natl Acad Sci U S A* **74**:5677, 1977.
221. North ME, Newton CA, Webster ADB: Phosphorylation of deoxyguanosine by B and T lymphocytes evidence against selective trapping of deoxyguanosine by T lymphocytes in purine nucleoside phosphorylase deficiency. *Clin Exp Immunol* **42**:523, 1980.
222. Kurtzberg J, Hershfield MS: Determinants of deoxyadenosine toxicity in hybrids between human T- and B-lymphoblasts as a model for the development of drug resistance in T-cell acute lymphoblastic leukemia. *Cancer Res* **45**:1579, 1985.
223. Brady TG, O'Donovan C: A study of the tissue distribution of adenosine deaminase in 6 species. *Comp Biochem Physiol* **14**:101, 1965.
224. Van Der Weyden MB, Kelley WN: Human adenosine deaminase: Distribution and properties. *J Biol Chem* **251**:5448, 1976.
225. Edwards YH, Hopkinson DA, Harris H: Adenosine deaminase in human tissues. *Ann Hum Genet* **35**:207, 1971.
226. Adams A, Harkness RA: Adenosine deaminase activity in thymus and other human tissues. *Clin Exp Immunol* **26**:647, 1976.
227. Hirschhorn R, Martiniuk F, Rosen FS: Adenosine deaminase activity in normal tissues and tissues from a child with severe combined immunodeficiency and adenosine deaminase deficiency. *Clin Immunol Immunopathol* **9**:287, 1978.
228. Aronow B, Lattier D, Silbiger R, Dusing M, Hutton J, Jones G, Stock J, et al.: Evidence for a complex regulatory array in the first intron of the human adenosine deaminase gene. *Genes Dev* **3**:1384, 1989.
229. Chinsky JM, Ramamurthy V, Fanslow WC, Ingolia DE, Blackburn MR, Shaffer KT, Higley HR, et al.: Developmental expression of adenosine deaminase in the upper alimentary tract of mice. *Differentiation* **42**:172, 1990.
230. Rauth S, Yang KG, Seibold AM, Ingolia DE, Ross SR, Yeung CY: GC-rich murine adenosine deaminase gene promoter supports diverse tissue -specific gene expression. *Somat Cell Mol Genet* **16**:129, 1990.
231. Knudsen TB, Blackburn MR, Chinsky JM, Airhart MJ, Kellems RE: Ontogeny of adenosine deaminase in the mouse decidua and placenta: Immunolocalization and embryo transfer studies. *Biol Reprod* **44**:171, 1991.
232. Barton R, Martiniuk F, Hirschhorn R, Goldschneider I: Inverse relationship between adenosine deaminase and purine nucleoside phosphorylase in rat lymphocyte populations. *Cell Immunol* **49**:208, 1980.
233. Chechik BE, Schrader WP, Minowada J: An immunomorphologic study of adenosine deaminase distribution in human thymus tissue, normal lymphocytes, and hematopoietic cell lines. *J Immunol* **126**:1003, 1981.
234. Ma DDF, Sylwestrowicz TA, Granger S, Massaia M, Franks R, Janossy G, Hoffbrand AV: Distribution of terminal deoxynucleotidyl transferase and purine degradative and synthetic enzymes in subpopulations of human thymocytes. *J Immunol* **129**:1430, 1982.
235. Chechik BE, Schrader WP, Perets A, Fernandes B: Immunohistochemical localization of adenosine deaminase distribution in human benign extrathymic lymphoid tissues and B-cell lymphomas. *Cancer* 53:70, 1984.
236. Chinsky JM, Maa MC, Ramamurthy V, Kellems RE: Adenosine deaminase gene expression. Tissue-dependent regulation of transcriptional elongation. *J Biol Chem* **264**:14561, 1989.
237. Valerio D, Duyvesteyn MGC, Meera Kahn P, van Kessel AG, de Waard A, van der Eb A: Isolation of cDNA clones for human adenosine deaminase. *Gene* **25**:231, 1983.
238. Wiginton DA, Adrian GS, Friedman D, Suttle DP, Hutton JJ: Cloning of cDNA sequences of human adenosine deaminase. *Proc Natl Acad Sci U S A* **80**:7481, 1983.
239. Orkin SH, Dadonna PE, Shewach DS, Markham AF, Bruns GA, Goff SC, Kelley W: Molecular cloning of human adenosine deaminase gene sequences. *J Biol Chem* **258**:12753, 1983.
240. Daddona PE, Shewach DS, Kelley WN, Argos P, Markham AF, Orkin SH: Human adenosine deaminase cDNA and complete primary amino acid sequence. *J Biol Chem* **259**:12101, 1984.
241. Wiginton DA, Adrian GS, Hutton JJ: Sequence of human adenosine deaminase cDNA including the coding region and a small intron. *Nucl Acids Res* **12**:2439, 1984.

242. Dadonna PE, Orkin SH, Shewach DS, Kelley WN: cDNA and amino acid sequence of human adenosine deaminase. *Ann NY Acad Sci* **451**:238, 1985.
243. Yeung C-Y, Ignolia DE, Roth DB, Shoemaker C, Al-Ubaidi AU, Yen J-Y, Ching C, et al.: Identification of functional murine adenosine deaminase cDNA clones by complementation in *Escherichia coli*. *J Biol Chem* **260**:10299, 1985.
244. Chang ZY, Nygaard P, Chinault AC, Kellems RE: Deduced amino acid sequence of *Escherichia coli* adenosine deaminase reveals evolutionarily conserved amino acid residues: Implications for catalytic function. *Biochemistry* **30**:2273, 1991.
245. Wilson DK, Rudolph FB, Quiocho FA: Atomic structure of adenosine deaminase complexed with a transition-state analog: Understanding catalysis and immunodeficiency mutations. *Science* **252**:1278, 1991.
246. Sharff AJ, Wilson DK, Chang Z, Quiocho FA: Refined 2.5 Å structure of murine adenosine deaminase at pH 6.0. *J Mol Biol* **226**:917, 1992.
247. Bhaumik D, Medin J, Gathy K, Coleman MS: Mutational analysis of active site residues of human adenosine deaminase. *J Biol Chem* **268**:5464, 1993.
248. Santisteban I, Arredondo-Vega FX, Kelly S, Debré M, Fischer A, Pérignon JL, Hilman B, et al.: Four new adenosine deaminase mutations, altering a zinc-binding histidine, two conserved alanines, and a 5′ splice site. *Hum Mutat* **5**:243, 1995.
249. Kurz LC, Frieden C: Adenosine deaminase converts purine riboside into an analogue of a reactive intermediate: A ^{13}C NMR and kinetic study. *Biochemistry* **26**:8450, 1987.
250. Kati WM, Wolfenden R: Major enhancement of the affinity of an enzyme for a transition-state analog by a single hydroxyl group. *Science* **243**:1591, 1989.
251. Schrader WP, Stacy AR, Pollara B: Purification of human erythrocyte adenosine deaminase by affinity column chromatography. *J Biol Chem* **251**:4026, 1976.
252. Schrader WP, Stacy AR: Purification and subunit structure of adenosine deaminase from human kidney. *J Biol Chem* **252**:6409, 1977.
253. Wiginton DA, Coleman MS, Hutton JJ: Purification, characterization and radioimmunoassay of adenosine deaminase from human leukemic granulocytes. *Biochem J* **195**:389, 1981.
254. Nishihara H, Ishikawa S, Shinkai K, Akedo H: Multiple forms of human adenosine deaminase. II. Isolation and properties of a conversion factor from human lung. *Biochim Biophys Acta* **302**:429, 1973.
255. Daddona PE, Kelley WN: Human adenosine deaminase binding protein. Assay, purification, and properties. *J Biol Chem* **253**:4617, 1978.
256. Schrader WP, Woodward FJ, Pollara B: Purification of an adenosine deaminase complexing protein from plasma. *J Biol Chem* **254**:11964, 1979.
257. Daddona PE, Kelley WN: Analysis of normal and mutant forms of human adenosine deaminase-a review. *Mol Cell Biochem* **29**:91, 1980.
258. Trotta PP: Identification of a membrane associated adenosine deaminase binding protein from human placenta. *Biochemistry* **21**:4014, 1982.
259. Andy RJ, Kornfeld R: The adenosine deaminase binding protein of human skin fibroblasts is located on the cell surface. *J Biol Chem* **257**:7922, 1982.
260. Schrader WP, Bryer PJ: Characterization of an insoluble adenosine deaminase complexing protein from human kidney. *Arch Biochem Biophys* **215**:107, 1982.
261. Weisman MI, Caiolfa VR, Parola AH: Adenosine deaminase–complexing protein from bovine kidney. *J Biol Chem* **263**:5266, 1988.
262. Schrader WP, West CA, Strominger NL: Localization of adenosine deaminase and adenosine deaminase complexing protein in rabbit brain. *J Histochem Cytochem* **35**:443, 1988.
263. Dinjens WN, ten Kate J, van der Linden E, Wijnen JT, Meera Khan P, Bosman FT: Distribution of adenosine deaminase complexing protein (ADCP) in human tissues. *J Histochem Cytochem* **37**:1869, 1989.
264. Dinjens WN, ten Kate J, Wijnen JT, van der Linden EP, Beek CJ, Lenders MH, Meera Khan P, et al.: Distribution of adenosine deaminase-complexing protein in murine tissues. *J Biol Chem* **264**:19215, 1989.
265. Schrader WP, West CA, Miczek AD, Norton EK: Characterization of the adenosine deaminase–adenosine deaminase complexing protein binding reaction. *J Biol Chem* **265**:19312, 1990.
266. Koch G, Shows TB: A gene on human chromosome 6 functions in assembly of tissue-specific adenosine deaminase isozymes. *Proc Natl Acad Sci U S A* **75**:3876, 1978.
267. Herbschleb-Voogt E, Grzeschik KH, de Wit J, Pearson PL, Meera Khan P: Assignment of a structural gene for adenosine deaminase complexing protein (ADCP) to human chromosome 2 in interspecific somatic cell hybrids. *Cytogenet Cell Genet* **25**:163, 1979.
268. Koch G, Shows TB: Somatic cell genetics of adenosine deaminase expression and severe combined immunodeficiency disease in humans. *Proc Natl Acad Sci U S A* **77**:4211, 1980.
269. SenGupta S, Petsche D, Gelfand E, Chechick BE: A flow cytometric method for the detection of adenosine deaminase in mononuclear cells. *J Immunol Methods* **80**:155, 1985.
270. Aran JM, Colomer D, Matutes E, Vives-Corrons JL, Franco R: Presence of adenosine deaminase on the surface of mononuclear blood cells: immunohistochemical localization using light electron microscopy. *J Histochem Cytochem* **39**:1001, 1991.
271. Schrader WP, Harder CM, Schrader DK, West CA: Metabolism of different molecular forms of adenosine deaminase intravenously infused into the rabbit. *Arch Biochem Biophys* **230**:158, 1984.
272. Schrader WP, Miczek AD, West CA, Samsonhoff WA: Evidence for receptor-mediated uptake of adenosine deaminase in rabbit kidney. *J Histochem Cytochem* **36**:1481, 1988.
273. Porat N, Gill D, Parola AH: Adenosine deaminase in cell transformation. Biophysical manifestation of membrane dynamics. *J Biol Chem* **263**:14608, 1988.
274. Morrison ME, Vijayasaradhi S, Engelstein D, Albino AP, Houghton AN: A marker fo neoplastic progression of human melanocytes is a cell surface ectopeptidase. *J Exp Med* **177**:1135, 1993.
275. Kameoka J, Tanaka T, Nojima Y, Schlossman S, Morimoto C: Direct association of adenosine deaminase with a T cell activation antigen, CD26. *Science* **261**:466, 1993.
276. Fox DA, Hussey RE, Fitzgerald KA, Acuto O, Poole C, Palley L, Daley JF, et al.: TA1, a novel 105kd human T cell activation antigen defined by a monoclonal antibody. *J Immunol* 133:1250, 1984.
277. Hegen M, Niedobitek G, Klein E, Stein H, Fleischer B: The T cell triggering molecule Tp103 is associated with dipeptidyl peptidase IV activity. *J Immunol* **144**:2908, 1990.
278. Ulmer AJ, Mattern T, Feller AC, Heymann E, Flad H-D: CD26 antigen is a surface dipeptidyl peptidase IV (DPPIV) as characterized by monoclonal antibodies clone TII-19-4-7 and 4EL1C7. *Scand J Immunol* **31**:429, 1990.
279. Darmoul D, Lacasa M, Chantret I, Swallow DM, Trugnan G: Isolation of a cDNA for the human intestinal dipeptidylpeptidase IV and assignment of the gene locus DPP4 to chromosome 2. *Ann Hum Genet* **54**:191, 1990.
280. Darmoul D, Lacasa M, Baricault L, Marguet D, Sapin C, Trotot P, Barbat A, et al.: Dipeptidyl peptidase IV (CD26) gene expression in enterocyte-like colon cancer cell lines HT-29 and Caco-2. *J Biol Chem* **267**:4824, 1992.
281. Tanaka T, Camerini D, Seed B, Torimoto Y, Dang NH, Kameoka J, Dahlberg HN, et al.: Cloning and functional expression of the T cell activation antigen CD26. *J Immunol* **149**:481, 1992.
282. Ogata S, Misumi Y, Ikehara Y: Primary structure of rat liver dipeptidyl peptidase IV deduced from its cDNA and identification of the NH_2-terminal signal sequence as the membrane-anchoring domain. *J Biol Chem* 264:3596, 1989.
283. Hong WJ, Doyle D: Molecular dissection of the NH_2-terminal signal/anchor sequence of rat dipeptidyl peptidase IV. *J Cell Biol* 111:323, 1990.
284. Iwaki-Egawa S, Watanabe Y, Fujimoto Y: CD26/dipeptidyl peptidase IV does not work as an adenosine deaminase-binding protein in rat cells. *Cell Immunol* **178**:180, 1997.
285. Dong RP, Tachibana K, Hegen M, Munakata Y, Cho D, Schlossman SF, Morimoto C: Determination of adenosine deaminase binding domain on CD26 and its immunoregulatory effect on T cell activation. *J Immunol* **159**:6070, 1997.
286. Dong RP, Kameoka J, Hegen M, Tanaka T, Xu Y, Schlossman SF, Morimoto C: Characterization of adenosine deaminase binding to human CD26 on T cells and its biological role in immune response. *J Immunol* **156**:1349, 1996.
287. Morimoto C, Schlossman SF: The structure and function of CD26 in the T-cell immune response. *Immunol Rev* **161**:55, 1998.
288. Dang NH, Torimoto Y, Shimamura K, Tanaka T, Daley JF, Schlossman SF, Morimoto C: 1F7 (CD26): A marker of thymic maturation involved in the differential regulation of the CD3 and CD2 pathways of human thymocyte activation. *J Immunol* **147**:2825, 1991.
289. Tanaka T, Kameoka J, Yaron A, Schlossman SF, Morimoto C: The costimulatory activity of the CD26 antigen requires dipeptidyl peptidase IV enzymatic activity. *Proc Natl Acad Sci U S A* **90**:4586, 1993.

290. Torimoto Y, Dang NH, Vivier E, Tanaka T, Schlossman S, Morimoto C: Coassociation of CD26 (dipeptidyl peptidase IV) with CD45 on the surface of human T lymphocytes. *J Immunol* **147**:2514, 1991.
291. Vivier I, Marguet D, Naquet P, Bonicel J, Black D, Li CX, Bernard A, et al.: Evidence that thymocyte activating molecule is mouse CD26 (dipeptidyl peptidase IV). *J Immunol* **147**:447, 1991.
292. Bristol LA, Sakaguchi K, Appella E, Doyle D, Takacs L: Thymocyte costimulating antigen is CD26 (dipeptidyl peptidase IV). Costimulation of granulocyte, macrophage, and T cell lineage cell proliferation via CD26. *J Immunol* **149**:367, 1992.
293. Kishihara K, Penninger J, Wallace VA, Kundig TM, Kawai K, Wakeham A, Timms E, et al.: Normal B Lymphocyte development but impaired T cell maturation in CD45-exon6 protein tyrosine phosphatase-deficient mice. *Cell* **74**:143, 1993.
294. Tsuji E, Misumi Y, Fujiwara T, Takami N, Ogata S, Ikehara Y: An active site mutation (Gly633->Arg) of dipeptidyl peptidase IV causes its retentiona and rapid degradation in the endoplasmic reticulum. *Biochemistry* **31**:11921, 1992.
295. Erickson RH, Suzuki Y, Sedlmayer A, Kim YS: Biosynthesis and degradation of altered immature forms of intestinal dipeptidyl peptidase IV in a rat strain lacking the enzyme. *J Biol Chem* **267**:21623, 1992.
296. Tischfield JA, Creagan RP, Nichols EA, Ruddle FH: Assignment of a gene for adenosine deaminase to human chromosome 20. *Hum Hered* **24**:1, 1974.
297. Mohandas T, Sparkes RS, Passage MB, Sparkes MC, Miles JH, Kaback MM: Regional mapping of ADA and ITP on chromosome 20: Cytogenetic and somatic cell studies in an X/20 translocation. *Cytogenet Cell Genet* **26**:28, 1980.
298. Mohandas T, Sparkes RS, Suh EJ, Hershfield MS: Regional localization of the human genes for *S*-adenosylhomocysteine hydrolase (cen > q131) and adenosine deaminase (q131 > qter) on chromosome 20. *Hum Genet* **66**:292, 1984.
299. Jhanwar SC, Berkvens TM, Breukel C, Van Ormondt H, van der Eb AJ, Meera Kahn P: Localization of human adenosine deaminase (ADA) gene sequences to the q12-q13.11 region of chromosome 20 by *in situ* hybridization. *Cytogenet Cell Genet* **50**:168, 1989.
300. Valerio D, Duyvesteyn MGC, Dekkler BMM, Weeda G, Berkvens TM, van der Voorn L, van Ormondt H, et al.: Adenosine deaminase: Characterization and expression of a gene with a remarkable promoter. *Embo J* **4**:437, 1985.
301. Wiginton DA, Kaplan DJ, States JC, Akeson AL, Perme CM, Bilyk IJ, Vaughn AJ, et al.: Complete sequence and structure of the gene for human adenosine deaminase. *Biochemistry* **25**:8234, 1986.
302. Dusing MR, Wiginton DA: Sp1 is essential for both enhancer-mediated and basal activation of the TATA-less human adenosine deaminase promoter. *Nucleic Acids Res* **22**:669, 1994.
303. Ingolia DE, al-Ubaidi MR, Yeung CY, Bigo HA, Wright DA, Kellems RE: Molecular cloning of the murine adenosine deaminase gene from a genetically enriched source: Identification and characterization of the promoter region. *Mol Cell Biol* **6**:4458, 1986.
304. Innis JW, Moore DJ, Kash SF, Ramamurthy V, Sawadogo M, Kellems RE: The murine adenosine deaminase promoter requires an atypical TATA box which binds transcription factor IID and transcriptional activity is stimulated by multiple upstream Sp1 binding sites. *J Biol Chem* **266**:21765, 1991.
305. Valerio D, van der Putten H, Botteri FM, Hoogerbrugge PM: Activity of the adenosine deaminase promoter in transgenic mice. *Nucleic Acids Res* **16**:10083, 1988.
306. Aronow BJ, Silbiger RN, Dusing MR, Stock JL, Yager KL, Potter S, Hutton JJ, et al.: Functional analysis of the human adenosine deaminase gene thymic regulatory region and its ability to generate position-independent transgene expression. *Mol Cell Biol* **12**:4170, 1992.
307. Ess KC, Whitaker TL, Cost GJ, Witte DP, Hutton JJ, Aronow BJ: A central role for a single c-Myb binding site in a thymic locus control region. *Mol Cell Biol* **15**:5707, 1995.
308. Haynes TL, Thomas MB, Dusing MR, Valerius MT, Potter SS, Wiginton DA: An enhancer LEF-1/TCF-1 site is essential for insertion site- independent transgene expression in thymus. *Nucleic Acids Res* **24**:5034, 1996.
309. Brickner AG, Gossage DL, Dusing MR, Wiginton DA: Identification of a murine homolog of the human adenosine deaminase thymic enhancer. *Gene* **167**:261, 1995.
310. Aronow BJ, Ebert CA, Valerius MT, Potter SS, Wiginton DA, Witte DP, Hutton JJ: Dissecting a locus control region: facilitation of enhancer function by extended enhancer-flanking sequences. *Mol Cell Biol* **15**:1123, 1995.
311. Dusing MR, Brickner AG, Thomas MB, Wiginton DA: Regulation of duodenal specific expression of the human adenosine deaminase gene. *J Biol Chem* **272**:26634, 1997.
312. Winston JH, Hanten GR, Overbeek PA, Kellems RE: 5′ Flanking sequences of the murine adenosine deaminase gene direct expression of a reporter gene to specific prenatal and postnatal tissues in transgenic mice. *J Biol Chem* **267**:13472, 1992.
313. Shi D, Winston JH, Blackburn MR, Datta SK, Hanten G, Kellems RE: Diverse genetic regulatory motifs required for murine adenosine deaminase gene expression in the placenta. *J Biol Chem* **272**:2334, 1997.
314. Shi D, Kellems RE: Transcription factor AP-2gamma regulates murine adenosine deaminase gene expression during placental development. *J Biol Chem* **273**:27331, 1998.
315. Berkvens TM, Schoute F, van Ormondt H, Meera Khan P, van der Eb AJ: Adenosine deaminase gene expression is regulated posttranscriptionally in the nucleus. *Nucleic Acids Res* **16**:3255, 1988.
316. Lattier DL, States JC, Hutton JJ, Wiginton DA: Cell type–specific transcriptional regulation of the human adenosine deaminase gene. *Nucleic Acids Res* **17**:1061, 1989.
317. Chen Z, Harless ML, Wright DA, Kellems RE: Identification and characterization of transcriptional arrest sites in exon 1 of the human adenosine deaminase gene. *Mol Cell Biol* **10**:4555, 1990.
318. Ramamurthy V, Maa MC, Harless ML, Wright DA, Kellems RE: Sequence requirements for transcriptional arrest in exon 1 of the murine adenosine deaminase gene. *Mol Cell Biol* **10**:1484, 1990.
319. Innis JW, Kellems RE: A heat-labile factor promotes premature 3′ end formation in exon 1 of the murine adenosine deaminase gene in a cell-free transcription system. *Mol Cell Biol* **11**:5398, 1991.
320. Daddona PE: Human adenosine deaminase: properties and turnover in cultured T and B lymphoblasts. *J Biol Chem* **256**:12496, 1981.
321. Hirschhorn R, Levytska V, Pollara B, Meuwissen HJ: Evidence for control of several different tissue-specific isozymes of adenosine deaminase by a single genetic locus. *Nature* **246**:200, 1973.
322. Daddona PE, Frohman MA, Kelley WN: Human adenosine deaminase and its binding protein in normal and adenosine deaminase–deficient fibroblast cell strains. *J Biol Chem* **255**:5681, 1980.
323. Hirschhorn R: Conversion of human erythrocyte-adenosine deaminase activity to different tissue specific isozymes. Evidence for a common catalytic unit. *J Clin Invest* **55**:661, 1975.
324. Schrader WP, Pollara B, Meuwissen HJ: Characterization of the residual adenosine deaminating activity in the spleen of a patient with combined immunodeficiency and adenosine deaminase deficiency. *Proc Natl Acad Sci U S A* **75**:446, 1978.
325. Ratech H, Hirschhorn R: Serum adenosine deaminase in normals and in a patient with adenosine deaminase–deficient severe combined immunodeficiency. *Clin Chim Acta* **115**:341, 1981.
326. Daddona PE, Kelley WN: Characterization of an aminohydrolase distinct from adenosine deaminase in cultured human lymphocytes. *Biochim Biophys Acta* **658**:280, 1981.
327. Daddona PE, Frohman MA, Kelley WN: Radioimmunochemical quantitation of human adenosine deaminase. *J Clin Invest* **64**:798, 1979.
328. Wiginton DA, Hutton JJ: Immunoreactive protein in adenosine deaminase deficient human lymphoblast cell lines. *J Biol Chem* **257**:3211, 1982.
329. Valerio D, Duyvesteyn MGC, van Ormondt H, Meera Khan P, van der Eb AJ: Adenosine deaminase (ADA) deficiency in cells derived from humans with severe combined immunodeficiency disease is due to an aberration of the ADA protein. *Nucleic Acids Res* **12**:1015, 1984.
330. Adrian GS, Hutton JJ: Adenosine deaminase messenger RNAs in lymphoblast cell lines derived from leukemic patients and patients with hereditary adenosine deaminase deficiency. *J Clin Invest* **71**:1649, 1983.
331. Adrian GS, Wiginton DA, Hutton JJ: Characterization of normal and mutant adenosine deaminase messenger RNAs by translation and hybridization to a cDNA probe. *Hum Genet* **68**:169, 1984.
332. Adrian GS, Wiginton DA, Hutton JJ: Structure of adenosine deaminase mRNAs from normal and adenosine deaminase-deficient human cell lines. *Mol Cell Biol* **4**:1712, 1984.
333. Berkvens TM, Gerritsen EJ, Oldenburg M, Breukel C, Wijnen JT, van Ormondt H, Vossen JM, et al.: Severe combined immune deficiency due to a homozygous 3.2-kb deletion spanning the promoter and first

exon of the adenosine deaminase gene. *Nucleic Acids Res* **15**:9365, 1987.
334. Markert ML, Hershfield MS, Wiginton DA, States JC, Ward FE, Bigner SH, Buckley RH, et al.: Identification of a deletion in the adenosine deaminase gene in a child with severe combined immunodeficiency. *J Immunol* **138**:3203, 1987.
335. Markert ML, Hutton JJ, Wiginton DA, States JC, Kaufman RE: Adenosine deaminase (ADA) deficiency due to deletion of the ADA gene promoter and first exon by homologous recombination between two Alu elements. *J Clin Invest* **81**:1323, 1988.
336. Berkvens TM, van Ormondt H, Gerritsen EJ, Meera Khan P, van der Eb AJ: Identical 3250-bp deletion between two *AluI* repeats in the ADA genes of unrelated ADA-SCID patients. *Genomics* **7**:486, 1990.
337. Shovlin CL, Simmonds HA, Fairbanks L, Deacock S, Hughes JMB, Lechler R, Webster ADB, et al.: Adult onset immunodeficiency caused by inherited adenosine deaminase deficiency. *J Immunol* **153**:2331, 1994.
338. Hirschhorn R, Nicknam MN, Eng F, Yang DR, Borkowsky W: Novel deletion and a new missense mutation (Glu 217 Lys) at the catalytic site in two adenosine deaminase (ADA) alleles of a patient with neonatal onset ADA–severe combined immunodeficiency. *J Immunol* **149**:3107, 1992.
339. Gossage DL, Norby-Slycord CJ, Hershfield MS, Markert ML: A homozygous five nucleotide deletion in the adenosine deaminase (ADA) mRNA in a child with ADA deficiency and very low levels of ADA mRNA and protein. *Hum Mol Genet* **2**:1493, 1993.
340. Hirschhorn R, Chen AS, Israni A, Yang DR, Huie ML: Two new mutations at the ADA locus (Q254X and del nt955-959) unusual for not being missense mutations. *Hum Mutat* **2**:320, 1993.
341. Krawczak M, Cooper DN: Gene deletions causing human genetic disease: Mechanisms of mutagenesis and the role of the local DNA sequence environment. *Hum Genet* **86**:425, 1991.
342. Arredondo-Vega FX, Santisteban I, Notarangelo LD, El Dahr J, Buckley R, Roifman C, Conley ME, et al.: Seven novel mutations in the adenosine deaminase (ADA) gene in patients with severe and delayed onset combined immunodeficiency: G74C, V129M, G140E, R149W, Q199P, 462delG, and E337del. *Hum Mutat* **11**:482, 1998.
343. Arredondo-Vega FX, Santisteban I, Kelly S, Schlossman C, Umetsu D, Hershfield MS: Correct splicing despite a G → A mutation at the invariant first nucleotide of a 5′ splice site: A possible basis for disparate clinical phenotypes in siblings with adenosine deaminase (ADA) deficiency. *Am J Hum Genet* **54**:820, 1994.
344. Santisteban I, Arredondo-Vega FX, Kelly S, Loubser M, Meydan N, Roifman C, Howell PL, et al.: Three new adenosine deaminase mutations that define a splicing enhancer and cause severe and partial phenotypes: Implications for evolution of a CpG hotspot and expression of a transduced ADA cDNA. *Hum Mol Genet* **4**:2081, 1995.
345. Akeson AL, Wiginton DA, Hutton JJ: Normal and mutant human adenosine deaminase genes. *J Cell Biochem* **39**:217, 1989.
346. Cooper DN, Youssoufian H: The CpG dinucleotide and human genetic disease. *Hum Genet* **78**:151, 1988.
347. Markert ML, Norby SC, Ward FE: A high proportion of ADA point mutations associated with a specific alanine-to-valine substitution. *Am J Hum Genet* **45**:354, 1989.
348. Akeson AL, Wiginton DA, Dusing MR, States JC, Hutton JJ: Mutant human adenosine deaminase alleles and their expression by transfection into fibroblasts. *J Biol Chem* **263**:16291, 1988.
349. Hirschhorn R, Yang DR, Israni A, Huie ML, Ownby DR: Somatic mosaicism for a newly identified splice-site mutation in a patient with adenosine deaminase-deficient immunodeficiency and spontaneous clinical recovery. *Am J Hum Genet* **55**:59, 1994.
350. Hirschhorn R, Yang DR, Puck JM, Huie ML, Jiang C-K, Kurlandsky LE: Spontaneous reversion to normal of an inherited mutation in a patient with adenosine deaminase deficiency. *Nat Genet* **13**:290, 1996.
351. Hirschhorn R, Martiniuk F, Roegner-Maniscalco V, Ellenbogen A, Perignon JL, Jenkins T: Genetic heterogeneity in partial adenosine deaminase deficiency. *J Clin Invest* **71**:1887, 1983.
352. Daddona PE, Davidson BL, Perignon JL, Kelley WN: Genetic expression in partial adenosine deaminase deficiency: mRNA levels and protein turnover for the enzyme variants in human B-lymphoblast cell lines. *J Biol Chem* **260**:3875, 1985.
353. Hirschhorn R, Borkowsky W, Jiang CK, Yang DR, Jenkins T: Two newly identified mutations (Thr233Ile and Leu152Met) in partial adenosine deaminase-deficient (ADA-) individuals that result in differing biochemical and metabolic phenotypes. *Hum Genet* **100**:22, 1997.
354. Hirschhorn R, Tzall S, Ellenbogen A, Orkin SH: Identification of a point mutation resulting in a heat-labile adenosine deaminase (ADA) in two unrelated children with partial ADA deficiency. *J Clin Invest* **83**:497, 1989.
355. Hirschhorn R, Tzall S, Ellenbogen A: Hot spot mutations in adenosine deaminase deficiency. *Proc Natl Acad Sci U S A* **87**:6171, 1990.
356. Spencer N, Hopkinson DA, Harris H: Adenosine deaminase polymorphism in man. *Ann Hum Genet* **32**:9, 1968.
357. Weissmann J, Vollmer M, Pribilla O: Survey of the distribution of adenosine deaminase and superoxide dismutase markers in different populations. *Hum Hered* **32**:344, 1982.
358. Hirschhorn R, Yang DR, Israni A: An Asp8Asn substitution in the adenosine deaminase (ADA) genetic polymorphism (ADA 2 allozyme): Occurrence on different chromosomal backgrounds and apparent intragenic crossover. *Ann Hum Genet* **58**:1, 1994.
359. Bonthron DT, Markham AF, Ginsberg D, Orkin SH: Identification of a point mutation in the adenosine deaminase gene responsible for immunodeficiency. *J Clin Invest* **76**:894, 1985.
360. Valerio D, Dekker BMM, Duyvesteyn MGC, van der Voorn L, Berkvens TM, van Ormondt H, van der Eb AJ: One adenosine deaminase allele in a patient with severe combined immunodeficiency contains a point mutation abolishing enzyme activity. *EMBO J* **5**:113, 1986.
361. Akeson AL, Wiginton DA, States JC, Perme CM, Dusing MR, Hutton JJ: Mutations in the human adenosine deaminase gene that affect protein structure and RNA splicing. *Proc Natl Acad Sci U S A* **84**:5947, 1987.
362. Economou EP, Bergen AW, Warren AC, Antonarakis SE: The polydeoxyadenylate tract of Alu repetitive elements is polymorphic in the human genome. *Proc Natl Acad Sci U S A* **87**:2951, 1990.
363. Hirschhorn R, Chakravarti V, Puck J, Douglas SD: Homozygosity for a newly identified missense mutation in a patient with very severe combined immunodeficiency due to adenosine deaminase deficiency (ADA-SCID). *Am J Hum Genet* **49**:878, 1991.
364. Yang DR, Huie ML, Hirschhorn R: Homozygosity for a missense mutation (G20R) associated with neonatal onset adenosine deaminase-deficient severe combined immunodeficiency disease (ADA-SCID). *Clin Immunol Immunopathol* **70**:171, 1994.
365. Hirschhorn R: Identification of two new missense mutations (R156C and S291L) in two ADA-SCID patients unusual for response to therapy with partial exchange transfusions. *Hum Mutat* **1**:166, 1992.
366. Hirschhorn R, Yang DR, Insel RA, Ballow M: Severe combined immunodeficiency of reduced severity due to homozygosity for an adenosine deaminase missense mutation (Arg253Pro). *Cell Immunol* **152**:383, 1993.
367. Ricciuti F, Ruddle FH: Assignment of nucleoside phosphorylase to D-14 and localization of X-linked loci in man by somatic cell genetics. *Nature* **241**:180, 1973.
368. George DL, Francke U: Gene dose effect: regional mapping of human nucleoside phosphorylase on chromosome 14. *Science* **194**:851, 1976.
369. Aitkin DA, Ferguson-Smith MA: Regional assignment of nucleoside phosphorylase by exclusion to 14q13. *Cytogenet Cell Genet* **22**:490, 1978.
370. Goddard JM, Caput D, Williams SR, Martin DWJr: Cloning of human purine nucleoside phosphorylase cDNA sequences by complementation in *Escherichia coli*. *Proc Natl Acad Sci U S A* **80**:4281, 1983.
371. Williams SR, Goddard JM, Martin DWJr: Human purine nucleoside phosphorylase cDNA sequence and genomic clone characterization. *Nucleic Acids Res* **12**:5779, 1984.
372. Williams SR, Gekeler V, McIvor RS, Martin DWJr: A human purine nucleoside phosphorylase deficiency caused by a single base change. *J Biol Chem* **262**:2332, 1987.
373. Jonsson JJ, Williams SR, McIvor RS: Sequence and functional characterization of the human purine nucleoside phosphorylase promoter. *Nucleic Acids Res* **19**:5015, 1991.
374. Jonsson JJ, Converse A, McIvor RS: An enhancer in the first intron of the human purine nucleoside phosphorylase-encoding gene. *Gene* **140**:187, 1994.
375. Martinez-Valdez H, Cohen A: Coordinate regulation of mRNAs encoding adenosine deaminase, purine nucleoside phosphorylase, and terminal deoxynucleotidyl transferase by phorbol esters in human thymocytes. *Proc NY Acad Sci* **85**:6900, 1988.
376. Madrid-Marina V, Martinez-Valdez H, Cohen A: Phorbol esters induce changes in adenosine deaminase, purine nucleoside phosphorylase, and terminal deoxynucleotidyl transferase messenger RNA levels in human leukemic cell lines. *Cancer Res* **50**:2891, 1990.

377. Zannis V, Doyle D, Martin DWJr: Purification and characterization of human erythrocyte purine nucleoside phosphorylase and its subunits. *J Biol Chem* **253**:504, 1978.
378. Stoeckler JE, Agarwal RP, Agarwal KC, Schmid K, Parks RE Jr: Purine nucleoside phosphorylase from human erythrocytes. Physiochemical properties of the crystalline enzyme. *Biochemistry* **17**:278, 1978.
379. Osborne WR: Human red cell purine nucleoside phosphorylase. Purification by biospecific affinity chromatography and physical properties. *J Biol Chem* **255**:7089, 1980.
380. Ropp PA, Traut TW: Purine nucleoside phosphorylase. Allosteric regulation of a dissociating enzyme. *J Biol Chem* **266**:7682, 1991.
381. Porter DJT: Purine nucleoside phosphorylase. Kinetic mechanism of the enzyme from the calf spleen. *J Biol Chem* **267**:7342, 1992.
382. Ropp PA, Traut TW: Allosteric regulation of purine nucleoside phosphorylase. *Arch Biochem Biophys* **288**:614, 1991.
383. Ealick SE, Rule SA, Carter DC, Greenhough TJ, Babu YS, Cook WJ, Habash J, et al.: Three dimensional structure of human erythrocytic purine nucleoside phosphorylase at 3.2 Å resolution. *J Biol Chem* **265**:1812, 1990.
384. Zimmerman TP, Gersten NB, Ross RF, Miech RP: Adenine as substrate for purine nucleoside phosphorylase. *Can J Biochem* **49**:1050, 1971.
385. Erion MD, Takabayashi K, Smith HB, Kessi J, Wagner S, Honger S, Shames SL, et al.: Purine nucleoside phosphorylase. 1. Structure-function studies. *Biochemistry* **36**:11725, 1997.
386. Erion MD, Stoeckler JD, Guida WC, Walter RL, Ealick SE: Purine nucleoside phosphorylase. 2. Catalytic mechanism. *Biochemistry* **36**:11735, 1997.
387. Stoeckler JD, Poirot AF, Smith RM, Parks RE Jr, Ealick SE, Takabayashi K, Erion MD: Purine nucleoside phosphorylase. 3. Reversal of purine base specificity by site-directed mutagenesis. *Biochemistry* **36**:11749, 1997.
388. Ealick SE, Babu YD, Bugg CE, Erion MD, Guida WC, Montgomery JA, Secrist JA III: Application of crystallographic and modeling methods in the design of purine nucleoside phosphorylase inhibitors. *Proc Natl Acad Sci U S A* **88**:11540, 1991.
389. Erion MD, Niwas S, Rose JD, Ananthan S, Allen M, Secrist JAd, Babu YS, et al.: Structure-based design of inhibitors of purine nucleoside phosphorylase. 3. 9-Arylmethyl derivatives of 9-deazaguanine substituted on the methylene group [erratum *J Med Chem* **37**:1034, 1994]. *J Med Chem* **36**:3771, 1993.
390. Guida WC, Elliott RD, Thomas HJ, Secrist JA 3rd, Babu YS, Bugg CE, Erion MD, et al.: Structure-based design of inhibitors of purine nucleoside phosphorylase. 4. A study of phosphate mimics. *J Med Chem* **37**:1109, 1994.
391. Parker WB, King SA, Allan PW, Bennett LL Jr, Secrist JA 3rd, Montgomery JA, Gilbert KS, et al.: *In vivo* gene therapy of cancer with *E. coli* purine nucleoside phosphorylase. *Hum Gene Ther* **8**:1637, 1997.
392. Da Costa LT, Jen J, He TC, Chan TA, Kinzler KW, Vogelstein B: Converting cancer genes into killer genes. *Proc Natl Acad Sci U S A* **93**:4192, 1996.
393. Hershfield MS, Chaffee S, Koro-Johnson L, Mary A, Smith AA, Short SA: Use of site directed mutagenesis to enhance the epitope shielding effect of covalent modifcation of proteins with polyethylene glycol. *Proc Natl Acad Sci USA* **88**:7185, 1991.
394. Aust MR, Andrews LG, Barrett MJ, Nordby-Sylcord CJ, Markert ML: Molecular analysis of mutations in a patient with purine nucleoside phosphorylase deficiency. *Am J Hum Genet* **51**:763, 1992.
395. Markert ML, Finkel BD, McLaughlin TM, Watson TJ, Collard HR, McMahon CP, Andrews LG, et al.: Mutations in purine nucleoside phosphorylase deficiency. *Hum Mutat* **9**:118, 1997.
396. Andrews LG, Markert ML: Exon skipping in purine nucleoside phosphorylase mRNA processing leading to severe immunodeficiency. *J Biol Chem* **267**:7834, 1992.
397. Broome CB, Graham ML, Saulsbury FT, Hershfield MS, Buckley RH: Correction of purine nucleoside phosphorylase deficiency by transplantation of allogeneic bone marrow from a sibling. *J Pediatr* **128**:373, 1996.
398. Agarwal RP, Spector T, Parks REJr: Tight-binding inhibitors-IV. Inhibition of adenosine deaminases by various inhibitors. *Biochem Pharmacol* **26**:359, 1977.
399. Stoeckler JD, Ealick SE, Bugg CE, Parks REJr: Design of purine nucleoside phosphorylase inhibitors. *Fed Proc* **45**:2773, 1986.
400. Mitchell BS, Koller CA, Heyn R: Inhibition of adenosine deaminase results in cytotoxicity to T lymphoblasts *in vivo*. *Blood* **56**:556, 1980.
401. Smyth JF, Paine RM, Jackman AL, Harrap KR, Chassin MM, Adamson RH, Johns DG: The clinical pharmacology of the adenosine deaminase inhibitor 2′-deoxycoformycin. *Cancer Chemother Pharmacol* **5**:93, 1980.
402. Siaw MFE, Mitchell BS, Koller CA, Coleman MS, Hutton JJ: ATP depletion as a consequence of adenosine deaminase inhibition in man. *Proc Natl Acad Sci U S A* **77**:6157, 1980.
403. Grever MR, Siaw MFE, Jacob WF, Neidhart JA, Miser JS, Coleman MS, Hutton JJ, et al.: The biochemical and clinical consequences of 2′-deoxycoformycin in refractory lymphoproliferative malignancy. *Blood* **57**:406, 1981.
404. Urba WJ, Baseler MW, Kopp WC, Steis RG, Clark JW, Smith JW II, Coggin DL, et al.: Deoxycoformycin-induced immunosuppression in patients with hairy cell leukemia. *Blood* **73**:38, 1989.
405. Debatisse M, Buttin G: The control of cell proliferation by preformed purines A genetic study. II. Pleiotropic manifestations and mechanisms of a control exerted by adenylic purines on PRPP synthesis. *Somatic Cell Genet* **3**:513, 1977.
406. Agarwal RP, Parks RJr: Potent inhibition of muscle 5′-AMP deaminase by the nucleoside antibiotics coformycin and deoxycoformycin. *Biochem Pharmacol* **26**:663, 1977.
407. Siaw MFE, Coleman MS: *In vitro* metabolism of deoxycoformycin in human T lymphoblastoid cells. Phosphorylation of deoxycoformycin and incorporation into cellular DNA. *J Biol Chem* **259**:9426, 1984.
408. Hershfield MS, Kredich NM, Koller CA, Mitchell BS, Kurtzberg J, Kinney TR, Falletta JM: *S*-Adenosylhomocysteine catabolism and basis for acquired resistance during treatment of T-cell acute lymphoblastic leukemia with 2′-deoxycoformycin alone and in combination with 9-β-D-arabinofuranosyladenine. *Cancer Res* **43**:3451, 1983.
409. Ochs UH, Chen SH, Ochs HD, Osborne WRA, Scott CR: Deoxyribonucleoside toxicity on adenosine deaminase and purine nucleoside phosphorylase positive and negative cultured lymphoblastoid cells, in Pollara B, Pickering RJ, Meuwissen HJ, Porter IH (eds): *Inborn Errors of Specific Immunity*. New York, Academic, 1979, p 191.
410. Horibata K, Harris AW: Mouse myelomas and lymphomas in culture. *Exp Cell Res* **60**:61, 1970.
411. Reynolds EC, Harris AW, Finch LR: Deoxyribonucleoside triphosphate pools and differential thymidine sensitivities of cultured mouse lymphoma and myeloma cells. *Biochim Biophys Acta* **561**:110, 1979.
412. Carson DA, Kaye J, Seegmiller JE: Differential sensitivity of human leukemic T cell lines and B cell lines to growth inhibition by deoxyadenosine. *J Immunol* **121**:1726, 1978.
413. Gelfand EW, Lee JJ, Dosch HM: Selective toxicity of purine deoxynucleosides for human lymphocyte growth and function. *Proc Natl Acad Sci U S A* **76**:1998, 1979.
414. Kazmers IS, Mitchell BS, Dadonna PE, Wotring LL, Townsend LB, Kelley WN: Inhibition of purine nucleoside phosphorylase by 8-aminoguanosine: Selective toxicity for T lymphoblasts. *Science* **214**:1137, 1981.
415. Fox RM, Tripp EH, Piddington SK, Tattersall MHN: Sensitivity of leukemic human null lymphocytes to deoxynucleosides. *Cancer Res* **40**:3383, 1980.
416. Chan TS: Deoxyguanosine toxicity on lymphoid cells as a cause for immunosuppression in purine nucleoside phosphorylase deficiency. *Cell* **14**:523, 1978.
417. Ochs UH, Chen SH, Ochs HD, Osborne WRA, Scott CR: Purine nucleoside phosphorylase deficiency: A molecular model for selective loss of T cell function. *J Immunol* **122**:2424, 1979.
418. Gudas LJ, Ullman B, Cohen A, Martin DWJr: Deoxyguanosine toxicity in a mouse T lymphoma relationship to purine nucleoside phosphorylase-associated immune dysfunction. *Cell* **14**:531, 1978.
419. Cohen A, Lee JWW, Dosch HM, Gelfand EW: The expression of deoxyguanosine toxicity in T lymphocytes at different stages of maturation. *J Immunol* **125**:1578, 1980.
420. Kefford RF, Fox RM: Purine deoxyribonucleoside toxicity in nondividing cells. *Cancer Res* **42**:324, 1982.
421. Cohen A, Barankiewicz J, Gelfand E: Roles of alternative synthetic and catabolic purine pathways in T lymphocyte differentiation. *Ann NY Acad Sci* **451**:26, 1985.
422. Goday A, Simmonds HA, Morris GS, Fairbanks LD: Human B lymphocytes and thymocytes but not peripheral blood mononuclear cells accumulate high dATP levels in conditions simulating ADA deficiency. *Biochem Pharmacol* **34**:3561, 1985.
423. Prentice HG, Ganeshaguru K, Bradstock KF, Goldstone AH, Smyth JF, Wonke B, Janossy G, et al.: Remission induction with the adenosine deaminase inhibitor 2′-deoxycoformycin in thy- lymphoblastic leukemia. *Lancet* **2**:170, 1980.

424. Gandhi V, Plunkett W, Rodriguez CO Jr, Nowak BJ, Du M, Ayres M, Kisor DF, et al.: Compound GW506U78 in refractory hematologic malignancies: Relationship between cellular pharmacokinetics and clinical response. *J Clin Oncol* **16**:3607, 1998.
425. Durham JP, Ives DH: Deoxycytidine kinase I. Distribution in normal and neoplastic tissues and interrelationships of deoxycytidine and 1-β-D-arabinofuranosylcytidine phosphorylation. *Mol Pharmacol* **5**:358, 1969.
426. Wortmann RL, Mitchell BS, Edwards NL, Fox IH: Biochemical basis for differential deoxyadenosine toxicity to T and B lymphoblasts: Role for 5′-nucleotidase. *Proc Natl Acad Sci U S A* **76**:2434, 1979.
427. Lee N, Russell N, Ganeshaguru K, Jackson BFA, Piga A, Prentice HG, Foa R, et al.: Mechanisms of deoxyadenosine toxicity in human lymphoid cells *in vitro* relevance to the therapeutic use of inhibitors of adenosine deaminase. *Br J Haematol* **56**:107, 1984.
428. Sidi Y, Edwards NL, Winkler C, Bunn P, Mitchell BS: Differential metabolism of deoxyribonucleosides by leukaemic T cells of immature and mature phenotype. *Br J Haematol* **61**:125, 1985.
429. Mitchell BS, Sidi Y, Hershfield M, Koller CA: Biochemical consequences of adenosine deaminase inhibition *in vivo*. *Ann NY Acad Sci* **451**:129, 1985.
430. Johnston JB, Begleiter A, Pugh L, Leith MK, Wilkins JA, Cavers DJ, Israels LG: Biochemical changes induced in hairy-cell leukemia following treatment with the adenosine deaminase inhibitor 2′-deoxycoformycin. *Cancer Res* **46**:2179, 1986.
431. Seto S, Carrera CJ, Kubota M, Wasson DB, Carson DA: Mechanism of deoxyadenosine and 2-chlorodeoxyadenosine toxicity to nondividing human lymphocytes. *J Clin Invest* **75**:377, 1985.
432. Gruber H, Cohen A, Redelman D, Bluestein H: Levels of dATP in ADA-inhibited human peripheral blood B and T lymphocytes cultured in deoxyadenosine. *Ann NY Acad Sci* **45**:315, 1985.
433. Gruber HE, Cohen A, Firestein GS, Redelman D, Bluestein HG: Deoxy-ATP accumulation in adenosine deaminase-inhibited human T and B lymphocytes. *Adv Exp Med Biol* **195A**:503, 1986.
434. Brox LW, Pollock E, Belch A: Adenosine and deoxyadenosine toxicity in colony assay systems for human T-lymphocytes, B-lymphocytes, and granulocytes. *Cancer Chemother Pharmacol* **9**:49, 1982.
435. Coleman MS, Danton MJ, Phillips A: Adenosine deaminase and immune dysfunction. *Ann NY Acad Sci* **451**:54, 1985.
436. Nordenskjøld BA, Skoog L, Brown NC, Reichard P: Deoxyribonucleotide pools and deoxyribonucleic acid synthesis in cultured mouse embryo cells. *J Biol Chem* **245**:5360, 1970.
437. Reichard P: Control of deoxyribonucleotide synthesis *in vitro* and *in vivo*. *Adv Enz Reg* **10**:3, 1972.
438. Thelander L, Reichard P: Reduction of ribonucleosides. *Ann Rev Biochem* **48**:133, 1979.
439. Eriksson S, Thelander L, Akerman M: Allosteric regulation of calf thymus ribonucleoside diphosphate reductase. *Biochemistry* **18**:2948, 1979.
440. Hunting D, Henderson JF: Models of the regulation of ribonucleotide reductase and their evaluation in intact mammalian cells. *CRC Crit Rev Biochem* **13**:325, 1983.
441. Thelander L, Berg P: Isolation and characterization of expressible subunits of mouse ribonucleotide reductase. *Mol Cell Biol* **6**:3433, 1986.
442. Bjorklund S, Skog S, Tribukait B, Thelander L: S-phase expression of mammalian R1 and R2 subunit mRNAs. *Biochemistry* **29**:5452, 1990.
443. Chang CH, Chen YC: Effects of nucleoside triphosphates on human ribonucleotide reductase from Molt-4F cells. *Cancer Res* **39**:5087, 1979.
444. Henderson JF, Fraser WS, Lowe JK: Toxicity of naturally occurring purine deoxyribonucleosides. *Pharmacol Ther* **8**:573, 1980.
445. Mann GJ, Fox RM: Deoxyadenosine triphosphate as a mediator of deoxyguanosine toxicity in cultured T lymphoblasts. *J Clin Invest* **78**:1261, 1986.
446. Ullman B, Clift SM, Gudas LJ, Levinson BB, Wormsted MA, Martin DWJr: Alterations in deoxyribonucleotide metabolism in cultured cells with ribonucleotide reductase activities refractory to feedback inhibition by 2′-deoxyadenosine triphosphate. *J Biol Chem* **255**:8308, 1980.
447. Waddell D, Ullman B: Characterization of a cultured human T-cell line with genetically altered ribonucleotide reductase activity. *J Biol Chem* **258**:4226, 1983.
448. Albert D, Bluestein HG, Thompson L, Seegmiller JA: The mechanism of inhibition and "reversal" of mitogen-induced lymphocyte activation in a model of adenosine deaminase deficiency. *Cell Immunol* **86**:510, 1984.
449. Fox RM, Kefford RF, Tripp EH, Taylor IW: G1-Phase arrest of cultured human leukemic T-cells induced by deoxyadenosine. *Cancer Res* **41**:5141, 1981.
450. Carson DA, Wasson DB, Lakow E, Kamatani N: Possible metabolic basis for the different immunodeficient states associated with genetic deficiencies of adenosine deaminase and purine nucleoside phosphorylase. *Proc Natl Acad Sci U S A* **79**:3848, 1982.
451. Uberti J, Lightbody JJ, Johnson RM: The effect of nucleosides and deoxycoformycin on adenosine and deoxyadenosine inhibition of human lymphocyte activation. *J Immunol* **123**:189, 1979.
452. Redelman D, Bluestein HG, Cohen AH, Depper JM, Wormsley S: Deoxyadenosine (AdR) inhibition of newly activated lymphocytes: Blockade at the G0-G1 interface. *J Immunol* **132**:2030, 1984.
453. Sato T, Chan T-S: Deoxyadenosine blockade of G0 to G1 transition in lymphocytes: Possible involvement of protein kinases. *J Cell Physiol* **166**:288, 1996.
454. Munch-Petersen B, Tyrsted G, Dupont B: The deoxyribonucleoside 5′-triphosphate (dATP and dTTP) pools in phytohemagglutinin-stimulated and non-stimulated human lymphocytes. *Exp Cell Res* **79**:249, 1973.
455. Tyrsted G, Gamulin V: Cytidine 5′-diphosphate reductase activity in phytohemagglutinin stimulated human lymphocytes. *Nucleic Acids Res* **6**:305, 1979.
456. Kizaki H, Shimada H, Ohsaka F, Sakurada T: Adenosine, deoxyadenosine, and deoxyguanosine induce DNA cleavage in mouse thymocytes. *J Immunol* **141**:1652, 1988.
457. Benveniste P, Cohen A: p53 expression is required for thymocyte apoptosis induced by adenosine deaminase deficiency. *Proc Natl Acad Sci U S A* **92**:8373, 1995.
458. Gao X, Knudsen TB, Ibrahim MM, Haldar S: Bcl-2 relieves deoxyadenylate stress and suppresses apoptosis in pre-B leukemia cells. *Cell Death Differentiation* **2**:69, 1995.
459. Levine AJ: p53, the cellular gatekeeper for growth and division. *Cell* **88**:1997.
460. Salvesen GS, Dixit VM: Caspases: Intracellular signaling by proteolysis. *Cell* **91**:443, 1997.
461. Liu X, Kim CN, Yang J, Jemmerson R, Wang X: Induction of apoptotic program in cell-free extracts: requirement for dATP and cytochrome c. *Cell* **86**:147, 1996.
462. Li P, Nijhawan D, Budihardjo I, Srinivasula SM, Ahmad M, Alnemri ES, Wang X: Cytochrome c and dATP-dependent formation of Apaf-1/caspase-9 complex initiates an apoptotic protease cascade. *Cell* **91**:479, 1997.
463. Enari M, Sakahira H, Yokoyama H, Okawa K, Iwamatsu A, Nagata S: A caspase-activated DNase that degrades DNA during apoptosis, and its inhibitor ICAD. *Nature* **391**:43, 1998.
464. Yang J, Liu X, Bhalla K, Kim CN, Ibrado AM, Cai J, Peng T-I, et al.: Prevention of apoptosis by Bcl-2:Release of cytochrome c from mitochondria blocked. *Science* **275**:1129, 1997.
465. Kluck RM, Bossy-Wetzel E, Green DR, Newmeyer DD: The release of cytochrome c from mitochondria: A primary site for Bcl-2 regulation of apoptosis. *Science* **275**:1132, 1997.
466. Leoni LM, Chao Q, Cottam HB, Genini D, Rosenbach M, Carrera CJ, Budihardjo I, et al.: Induction of an apoptotic program in cell-free extracts by 2-chloro-2′-deoxyadenosine 5′-triphosphate and cytochrome c. *Proc Natl Acad Sci U S A* **95**:9567, 1998.
466a. Arpaia E, Benveniste P, Di Cristofano A, Gu Y, Dalal I, Kelly S, Hershfield M, et al.: Mitochondrial basis for immune deficiency: Evidence from purine nucleoside phosphorylase-deficient mice. *J Exp Med* **191**:2197, 2000.
467. Komori T, Okada A, Stewart V, Alt FW: Lack of N regions in antigen receptor variable region genes of TdT-deficient lymphocytes. *Science* **261**:1171, 1993.
468. Gilfillan S, Dierich A, Lemeur M, Benoist C, Mathis D: Mice lacking TdT: Mature animals with an immature lymphocyte repertoire. *Science* **261**:1175, 1993.
469. Gangi-Peterson L, Sorscher DH, Reynolds JW, Kepler TB, Mitchell BS: Nucleotide pool imbalance and adenosine deaminase deficiency induce alterations in N-region insertions during V(D)J recombination. *J Clin Invest* **103**:833, 1999.
470. Meuth M: Sensitivity of a mutator gene in Chinese hamster ovary cell to deoxynucleoside triphosphate pool alterations. *Mol Cell Biol* **1**:652, 1981.
471. Weinberg G, Ullman B, Martin DWJr: Mutator phenotypes in mammalian cell mutants with distinct biochemical defects and abnormal deoxyribonucleoside triphosphate pools. *Proc Natl Acad Sci U S A* **78**:2447, 1981.

472. Sargent RG, Mathews CK: Imbalanced deoxyribonucleoside triphosphate pools and spontaneous mutation rates determined during dCMP deaminase-defective bacteriophage T4 infections. *J Biol Chem* **262**:5546, 1987.
473. Mattano SS, Palella TD, Mitchell BS: Mutations induced at the hypoxanthine-guanine phosphoribosyltransferase locus of human T-lymphoblasts by perturbations of purine deoxyribonucleoside triphosphate pools. *Cancer Res* **50**:4566, 1990.
474. Phear G, Nalbantoglu J, Meuth M: Next-nucleotide effects in mutations driven by DNA precursor pool imbalances at the aprt locus of Chinese hamster ovary cells. *Proc Natl Acad Sci U S A* **84**:4450, 1987.
475. Rossman TG, Stone-Wolff DS: Inhibition of DNA synthesis is not sufficient to cause mutagenesis in Chinese hamster cells. *Biochimie* **64**:809, 1982.
476. Johnstone AP, Williams GT: Role of DNA breaks and ADP-ribosyl transferase activity in eukaryotic differentiation demonstrated in human lymphocytes. *Nature* **300**:368, 1982.
477. Johnstone AP: Rejoining of DNA strand breaks is an early nuclear event during the stimulation of quiescent lymphocytes. *Eur J Biochem* **140**:401, 1984.
478. Brox L, Ng A, Pollock E, Belch E: DNA strand breaks induced in human T-lymphocytes by the combination of deoxyadenosine and deoxycoformycin. *Cancer Res* **44**:934, 1984.
479. Benjamin RC, Gill DM: ADP-ribosylation in mammalian cell ghosts. Dependence of poly(ADP-ribose) synthesis on strand breakage in DNA. *J Biol Chem* **255**:10493, 1980.
480. Benjamin RC, Gill DM: Poly(ADP-ribose) synthesis *in vitro* programmed by damaged DNA. A comparison of DNA molecules containing different types of strand breaks. *J Biol Chem* **255**:10502, 1980.
481. Ganeshaguru K, Piga A, Latini L, Hoffbrand AV: Inability of poly-ADP-ribosylation inhibitors to protect peripheral blood lymphocytes from the toxic effects of ADA inhibition. *Adv Exp Med Biol* **253B**:251, 1989.
482. Matsumoto SS, Yu J, Yu AL: Inhibition of RNA synthesis by deoxyadenosine plus deoxycoformycin in resting lymphocytes. *J Immunol* **131**:2762, 1983.
483. de Korte D, Haverkort WA, van Leeuwen EF, Roos D, van Gennip AH: Biochemical consequences of 2′-deoxycoformycin treatment in a patient with T-cell lymphoma. *Cancer* **60**:750, 1987.
484. Simmonds HA, Levinsky RJ, Perrett D, Webster DR: Reciprocal relationship between erythrocyte ATP and deoxy-ATP levels in inherited ADA deficiency. *Biochem Pharmacol* **31**:947, 1982.
485. Yu AL, Bakay B, Kung FH, Nyhan WL: Effects of 2′-deoxycoformycin on the metabolism of purines and the survival of malignant cells in a patient with T-cell leukemia. *Cancer Res* **41**:2677, 1981.
486. Nakashima K, Nakashima H, Shimoyama M: Deoxyadenosine triphosphate acting as an energy-transferring molecule in adenosine deaminase inhibited human erythrocytes. *Biochim Biophys Acta* **1094**:257, 1991.
487. Bontemps F, Van den Berghe G: Mechanism of ATP catabolism induced by deoxyadenosine and other nucleosides in adenosine deaminase-inhibited human erythrocytes. *Adv Exp Med Biol* **253B**:267, 1989.
488. Olah ME, Stiles GL: Adenosine receptor-mediated signal transduction, in Pelleg A, Belardinelli L (eds): *Effects of Extracellular Adenosine and ATP on Cardiomyocytes*. Austin, TX, RG Landes, 1998, p 1.
489. Cohen A, Ullman B, Martin DWJr: Characterization of a mutant mouse lymphoma cell with deficient transport of purine and pyrimidine nucleosides. *J Biol Chem* **254**:112, 1979.
490. Ullman B, Cohen A, Martin DW: Characterization of a cell culture model for the study of adenosine deaminase– and purine nucleoside phosphorylase–deficient immunologic disease. *Cell* **9**:205, 1976.
491. Kizaki H, Suzuki K, Tadakuma T, Ishimura Y: Adenosine receptor-mediated accumulation of cyclic AMP-induced T-lymphocyte death through internucleosomal DNA cleavage. *J Biol Chem* **265**:5280, 1990.
492. Apasov SG, Koshiba M, Chused TM, Sitkovsky MV: Effects of extracellular ATP and adenosine on different thymocyte subsets: Possible role of ATP-gated channels and G protein-coupled purinergic receptor. *J Immunol* **158**:5095, 1997.
493. Bohacek J, Hosek B, Pospisil M: Postirradiation administration of adenosine monophosphate combined with dipyridamole reduces early cellular damage in mice. *Life Sci* **53**:1317, 1993.
494. Dawicki DD, Chatterjee D, Wyche J, Rounds S: Extracellular ATP and adenosine cause apoptosis of pulmonary artery cells. *Am J Physiol* **273**:L485, 1997.
495. Birch RE, Polmar SH: Pharmacologic modification of immunoregulatory T-lymphocytes I. Effect of adenosine, H1 and H2 histamine agonists upon T-lymphocyte regulation of B-lymphocyte differentiation in vitro. *Clin Exp Immunol* **48**:218, 1982.
496. Birch RE, Rosenthal AK, Polmar SH: Pharmacologic modification of immunoregulatory T-lymphocytes II. Modulation of T-lymphocyte cell surface characteristics. *Clin Exp Immunol* **48**:231, 1982.
497. Koshiba M, Kojima H, Huang S, Apasov S, Sitkovsky MV: Memory of extracellular adenosine A2A purinergic receptor-mediated signaling in murine T cells. *J Biol Chem* **272**:25881, 1997.
498. Saura CA, Mallol J, Canela EI, Lluis C, Franco R: Adenosine deaminase and A1 adenosine receptors internalize together following agonist-induced receptor desensitization. *J Biol Chem* **273**:17610, 1998.
499. Cronstein BN, Daguma L, Nichols D, Hutchison AJ, Williams M: The adenosine/neutrophil paradox resolved: Human neutrophils possess both A1 and A2 receptors that promote chemotaxis and inhibit O_2 generation, respectively. *J Clin Invest* **85**:1150, 1990.
500. Salmon JE, Cronstein BN: Fc gamma receptor-mediated functions in neutrophils are modulated by adenosine receptor occupancy. A1 receptors are stimulatory and A2 receptors are inhibitory. *J Immunol* **145**:2235, 1990.
501. Cronstein BN, Levin RI, Philips M, Hirschhorn R, Abramson SB, Weissmann G: Neutrophil adherence to endothelium is enhanced via adenosine A2 receptors. *J Immunol* **148**:2201, 1992.
502. Green H, Chan TS: Pyrimidine starvation induced by adenosine in fibroblasts and lymphoid cells. Role of adenosine deaminase. *Science* **182**:836, 1973.
503. Wahl GM, Linke SP, Paulson TG, Huang LC: Maintaining genetic stability through TP53 mediated checkpoint control. *Cancer Surv* **29**:183, 1997.
504. Agarwal ML, Agarwal A, Taylor WR, Chernova O, Sharma Y, Stark GR: A p53-dependent S-phase checkpoint helps to protect cells from DNA damage in response to starvation for pyrimidine nucleotides. *Proc Natl Acad Sci U S A* **95**:14775, 1998.
505. Linke SP, Clarkin KC, Di Leonardo A, Tsou A, Wahl GM: A reversible, p53-dependent G0/G1 cell cycle arrest induced by ribonucleotide depletion in the absence of detectable DNA damage. *Genes Dev* **10**:934, 1996.
506. Harrap KR, Paine RM: Adenosine metabolism in cultured lymphoid cells. *Adv Enzyme Regul* **15**:169, 1977.
507. Carson DA, Seegmiller JE: Effect of adenosine deaminase inhibition upon human lymphocyte blastogenesis. *J Clin Invest* **57**:274, 1976.
508. Hershfield MS, Snyder FF, Seegmiller JE: Adenine and adenosine are toxic to human lymphoblast mutants defective in purine salvage enzymes. *Science* **197**:1284, 1977.
509. Schmalstieg FC, Nelson JA, Mills GC, Monahan TM, Goldman AS, Goldblum RM: Increased purine nucleotides in adenosine deaminase-deficient lymphocytes. *J Pediatr* **91**:48, 1977.
510. Mills GC, Schmalstieg FC, Newkirk KE, Goldblum RM: Cytosine and orotic acid in urine of immunodeficient children. *Clin Chem* **25**:419, 1979.
511. Borchardt RT, Creveling CR, Ueland PM: *Biological Methylation and Drug Design*. Clifton, NJ, Humana,, 1986.
512. De La Haba G, Cantoni GL: The enzymatic synthesis of *S*-adenosyl-L-homocysteine from adenosine and homocysteine. *J Biol Chem* **234**:603, 1959.
513. Turner MA, Yuan CS, Borchardt RT, Hershfield MS, Smith GD, Howell PL: Structure determination of selenomethionyl *S*-adenosylhomocysteine hydrolase using data at a single wavelength. *Nat Struct Biol* **5**:369, 1998.
514. Miller MW, Duhl DMJ, Winkes BM, Arredondo-Vega F, Saxon PJ, Wolff GL, Epstein CJ, et al.: The mouse lethal nonagouti (Ax) mutation deletes the *S*-adenosylhomocysteine hydrolase (*Ahcy*) gene. *EMBO J* **13**:1806, 1994.
515. Hershfield MS, Kredich NM: *S*-Adenosylhomocysteine hydrolase is an adenosine-binding protein A target for adenosine toxicity. *Science* **202**:757, 1978.
516. Hershfield MS, Aiyar VN, Premakumar R, Small WC: *S*-adenosylhomocysteine hydrolase from human placenta. *Biochem J* **230**:43, 1985.
517. Kredich NM, Martin DWJr: Role of *S*-adenosylhomocysteine in adenosine- mediated toxicity in cultured moust T-lymphoma cells. *Cell* **12**:931, 1977.
518. Hershfield MS: Apparent suicide inactivation of human lymphoblast *S*-adenosylhomocysteine hydrolase by 2′-deoxyadenosine and adenine arabinoside. A basis for direct toxic effects of analogs of adenosine. *J Biol Chem* **254**:22, 1979.

519. Hershfield MS: Proposed explanation for *S*-adenosylhomocysteine hydrolase deficiency in purine nucleoside phosphorylase and hypoxanthine guanine phosphoribosyltransferase-deficient patients. *J Clin Invest* **67**:696, 1981.
520. Abeles RH, Fish S, Lapinskas B: *S*-adenosylhomocysteinase—Mechanism of inactivation by 2′-deoxyadenosine and interaction with other nucleosides. *Biochemistry* **21**:5557, 1982.
521. Helland S, Ueland PM: Inactivation of *S*-adenosylhomocysteine hydrolase by 9-β-D-arabinofuranosyladenine in intact cells. *Cancer Res* **42**:1130, 1982.
522. Hershfield MS, Small WC, Premakumar R, Bagnara AS, Fetter JE: Inactivation of *S*-adenosylhomocysteine hydrolase. Mechanism and occurrence *in vivo* in disorders of purine nucleoside catabolism, in Borchardt RT, Usdin E, Creveling CR (eds): *Biochemistry of S-Adenosylmethionine and Related Compounds*. London, Macmillan, 1982, p 657.
523. Kaminska JE, Fox IH: Decreased *S*-adenosylhomocysteine hydrolase in inborn errors of purine metabolism. *J Lab Clin Med* **96**:141, 1980.
524. Hershfield MS, Aiyar VN, Chaffee S, Curtis S, Greenberg ML: Probes for examining the structure and function of human *S*-adenosylhomocysteine hydrolase, and for isolation of cDNA, in Borchardt RT, Creveling CR, Ueland PM (eds): *Biological Methylation and Drug Design*. Clifton, NJ, Humana, 1986, p 253.
525. Kredich NM, Hershfield MS: *S*-Adenosylhomocysteine toxicity in normal and adenosine kinase-deficient lymphoblasts of human origin. *Proc Natl Acad Sci U S A* **76**:2450, 1979.
526. Johnston JM, Kredich NM: Inhibition of methylation by adenosine in adenosine deaminase-inhibited, phytohemagglutinin-stimulated human lymphocytes. *J Immunol* **123**:97, 1979.
527. Kajander EO, Kubota M, Carrera CJ, Montgomery JA, Carson DA: Resistance to multiple adenine nucleosides and methionine analogues in murine lymphoma cells with enlarged *S*-adenosylmethionine pools. *Cancer Res* **46**:2866, 1986.
528. Ueland PM, Svardal A, Refsum H, Lillehaug JR, Schance J-S, Helland S: Disposition of endogenous *S*-adenosylhomocysteine and homocysteine following exposure to nucleoside analogues and methotrexate, in Borchardt RT, Creveling CR, Ueland PM (eds): *Biological Methylation and Drug Design. Experimental and Clinical Roles of S-Adenosylmethionine*. Clifton, NJ, Humana, 1986, p 263.
529. Greenberg ML, Chaffee S, Hershfield MS: Basis for resistance to 3-deazaaristeromycin, an inhibitor of *S*-adenosylhomocysteine hydrolase, in human B-lymphoblasts. *J Biol Chem* **264**:795, 1989.
530. Hershfield MS, Kurtzberg J, Moore JO, Whang Peng J, Haynes BF: Conversion of a stem cell leukemia from T-lymphoid to a myeloid phenotype by the adenosine deaminase inhibitor 2′-deoxycoformycin. *Proc Natl Acad Sci U S A* **81**:253, 1984.
531. German DC, Bloch CA, Kredich NM: Measurements of *S*-adenosylmethionine and L-homocysteine metabolism in cultured human lymphoid cells. *J Biol Chem* **258**:10997, 1983.
532. Wolos JA, Frondorf KA, Davis GF, Jarvi ET, McCarthy JR, Bowlin TL: Selective inhibition of T cell activation by an inhibitor of *S*-adenosyl-L-homocysteine hydrolase. *J Immunol* **150**:3264, 1993.
533. Wolos JA, Frondorf KA, Esser RE: Immunosuppression mediated by an inhibitor of *S*-adenosyl-L-homocysteine hydrolase. *J Immunol* **151**:526, 1993.
534. Benveniste P, Zhu W, Cohen A: Interference with thymocyte differentiation by an inhibitor of *S*-adenosylhomocysteine hydrolase. *J Immunol* **155**:536, 1995.
535. Ruers TJM, Buurman WA, Van Der Linden CJ: 2′-Deoxycoformycin and deoxyadenosine affect IL 2 production and IL 2 receptor expression of human T cells. *J Immunol* **138**:116, 1987.
536. Dosch HM, Mansour A, Cohen A, Shore A, Gelfand EW: Inhibition of suppressor T-cell development following deoxyguanosine administration. *Nature* **285**:494, 1980.
537. Bril H, Van Den Akker TW, Molendijk Lok BD, Bianchi ATJ, Brenner R: Influence of 2′-deoxyguanosine upon the development of DTH effector T cells and suppressor T cells *in vivo*. *J Immunol* **132**:599, 1984.
538. Lelchuk R, Cooke A, Playfair JHL: Differential sensitivity to 2′-deoxyguanosine of antigen-specific and nonspecific suppressor T cells in delayed hypersensitivity. *Cell Immunol* **72**:202, 1982.
539. Aye MT, Dunn JV, Yang WC: Studies on the effect of deoxyadenosine on deoxycoformycin-treated myeloid and lymphoid stem cells. *Blood* **60**:872, 1982.
540. Russell NH, Carron J, Hoffbrand AV, Bellingham AJ: The relative sensitivity of peripheral blood T-lymphocyte colony forming cells and bone marrow CFU-GM to deoxyadenosine and 2′-deoxycoformycin. *Leuk Res* **9**:315, 1985.
541. Fabian I, Williams Z: The effect of deoxycoformycin on bone marrow cells treated with adenosine and deoxyadenosine and hematopoietic growth factors. *Hum Immunol* **21**:181, 1988.
542. Shore A, Dosch HM, Gelfand EW: Role of adenosine deaminase in the early stages of precursor T cell maturation. *Clin Exp Immunol* **44**:152, 1981.
543. Doherty PJ, Pan S, Mulloy JC, Thompson E, Thorner P, Barankiewiecz J, Roifman CM, et al.: Adenosine deaminase and thymocyte maturation. *Scand J Immunol* **33**:405, 1991.
544. Murphy SB, Stass S, Kalwinsky D, Rivera G: Phenotypic conversion of acute leukemia from T-lymphoblastic to myeloblastic induced by therapy with 2′-deoxycoformycin. *Br J Haematol* **55**:285, 1983.
545. Kurtzberg J, Bigner SH, Hershfield MS: Establishment of the DU.528 human lymphohematopoietic stem cell line. *J Exp Med* **162**:1561, 1985.
546. Tedde A, Balis ME, Ikehara S, Pahwa R, Good RA, Trotta PP: Animal model for immune dysfunction associated with adenosine deaminase deficiency. *Proc Natl Acad Sci U S A* **77**:4899, 1980.
547. Trotta PP, Tedde A, Ikehara S, Pahwa R, Good RA, Balis ME: Specific immunosuppressive effects of constant infusion of 2′-deoxycoformycin. *Cancer Res* **41**:2189, 1981.
548. Ratech H, Thorbecke GJ, Hirschhorn R: Metabolic abnormalities of human adenosine deaminase deficiency reproduced in the mouse by 2′-deoxycoformycin, and adenosine deaminase inhibitor. *Clin Immunol Immunopathol* **21**:119, 1981.
549. Helland S, Ueland PM: Effect of 2′-deoxycoformycin infusion on *S*-adenosylhomocysteine hydrolase and the amount of *S*-adenosylhomocysteine and related compounds in tissues of mice. *Cancer Res* **43**:4142, 1983.
550. Ratech H, Hirschhorn R, Thorbecke GJ: Effects of deoxycoformycin in mice. III. A murine model reproducing multisystem pathology of human adenosine deaminase deficiency. *Am J Pathol* **119**:65, 1985.
551. Renshaw J, Harrap KR: *In vivo* inhibition of mouse liver methyltransferase enzymes following treatment with 2′-deoxycoformycin and 2′-deoxyadenosine. *Adv Exp Med Biol* **195B**:673, 1986.
552. Gao X, Blackburn MR, Knudsen TB: Activation of apoptosis in early mouse embryos by 2′-deoxyadenosine exposure. *Teratology* **49**:1, 1994.
553. Wakamiya M, Blackburn MR, Jurecic R, McArthur MJ, Geske RS, Cartwright JJr, Mitani K, et al.: Disruption of the adenosine deaminase gene causes hepatocellular impairment and perinatal lethality in mice. *Proc Natl Acad Sci U S A* **92**:3673, 1995.
554. Migchielsen AAJ, Breuer ML, van Roon MA, te Riele H, Zurcher C, Ossendorp F, Toutain S, et al.: Adenosine deaminase-deficient mice die perinatally, exhibiting liver-cell degeneration, small intestinal cell death, and lung atelectasis. *Nat Genet* **10**:279, 1995.
555. Johansson M, Karlsson A: Differences in kinetic properties of pure recombinant human and mouse deoxycytidine kinase. *Biochem Pharmacol* **50**:163, 1995.
556. Surh CD, Sprent J: T-cell apoptosis detected *in situ* during positive and negative selection in the thymus. *Nature* **372**:100, 1994.
557. Blackburn MR, Datta SK, Kellems RE: Adenosine deaminase–deficient mice generated using a two-stage genetic engineering strategy exhibit a combined immunodeficiency. *J Biol Chem* **273**:5093, 1998.
557a. Blackburn MR, Volmer JB, Thrasher JL, Zhong H, Crosby JR, Lee JJ, Kellems RE: Metabolic consequences of adenosine deaminase deficiency in mice are associated with defects in alveogenesis, pulmonary inflammation, and airway obstruction. *J Exp Med* **192**:159, 2000.
557b. Blackburn MR, Aldrich M, Volmer JB, Chen W, Zhong H, Kelly S, Hershfield M, et al.: The use of enzyme therapy to regulate the metabolic and phenotypic consequences of adenosine deaminase deficiency in mice: Differential impact on pulmonary and immunologic abnormalities. *J Biol Chem* In press: 2000.
558. Mably ER, Fung E, Snyder FF: Genetic deficiency of purine nucleoside phosphorylase in the mouse. Characterization of partially and severely enzyme deficient mutants. *Genome* **32**:1026, 1989.
559. Snyder FF, Jena P, Dilay JE, Fung E, Lightfoot T, Mably ER: Secondary loss of deoxyguanosine kinase activity in purine nucleoside phosphorylase deficient mice. *Biochim Biophys Acta* **33**:1227, 1994.
560. Snyder FF, Jenuth JP, Mably ER, Mangat RK: Point mutations at the purine nucleoside phosphorylase locus impair thymocyte differentiation in the mouse. *Proc Natl Acad Sci U S A* **94**:2522, 1997.

561. Cowan MJ, Wara DW, Ammann AJ: Deoxycytidine therapy in two patients with adenosine deaminase deficiency and severe immunodeficiency disease. *Clin Immunol Immunopathol* **37**:30, 1985.
562. Stoop JW, Zegers BJM, Spaapen LJM, Kuis W, Roord JJ, Rijkers GT, Staal GEJ, et al.: The effect of deoxycytidine and tetrahydrouridine in purine nucleoside phosphorylase deficiency. *Adv Exp Med Biol* **165A**:61, 1984.
563. O'Reilly RJ, Keever CA, Small TN, Brochstein J: The use of HLA–non-identical T-cell–depleted marrow for transplants for correction of severe combined immunodeficiency disease. *Immunodeficiency Rev* **1**:273, 1989.
564. Fischer A, Landais P, Friedrich W, Morgan G, Gerritsen B, Fasth A, Porta F, et al.: European experience of bone marrow transplantation for severe combined immunodeficiency. *Lancet* **336**:850, 1990.
565. Haddad E, Landais P, Friedrich W, Gerritsen B, Cavazzana-Calvo M, Morgan G, Bertrand Y, et al.: Long-term immune reconstitution and outcome after HLA-nonidentical T-cell-depleted bone marrow transplantation for severe combined immunodeficiency: A European retrospective study of 116 patients. *Blood* **91**:3646, 1998.
566. Buckley RH, Schiff SE, Schiff RI, Markert ML, Williams LW, Roberts JL, Myers LA, et al.: Hematopoietic stem-cell transplantation for the treatment of severe combined immunodeficiency. *N Engl J Med* **340**:508, 1999.
567. Buckley RH, Schiff SE, Sampson HA, Schiff RI, Markert ML, Knutsen AP, Hershfield MS, et al.: Development of immunity in human severe primary T cell deficiency following haploidentical bone marrow stem cell transplantation. *J Immunol* **136**:2398, 1986.
568. Cowan MJ, Shannon KM, Wara DM, Ammann AJ: Rejection of bone marrow transplant and resistance of alloantigen reactive cells to *in vivo* deoxyadenosine in adenosine deaminase deficiency. *Clin Immunol Immunopathol* **49**:242, 1988.
569. Buckley RH, Schiff SE, Schiff RI, Roberts JL, Markert ML, Peters W, Williams LW, et al.: Haploidentical bone marrow stem cell transplantation in human severe combined immunodeficiency. *Semin Hematol* **30**:92, 1993.
570. Dror Y, Gallagher R, Wara DW, Colombe BW, Merino A, Benkerrou M, Cowan MJ: Immune reconstitution in severe combined immunodeficiency disease after lectin-treated, T-cell-depleted haplocompatible bone marrow transplantation. *Blood* **81**:2021, 1993.
571. Carpenter PA, Ziegler JB, Vowels MR: Late diagnosis and correction of purine nucleoside phosphorylase deficiency with allogeneic bone marrow transplantation. *Bone Marrow Transplant* **17**:121, 1996.
572. Fischer A, Landais P, Friedrich W, Gerritsen B, Fasth A, Porta F, Vellodi A, et al.: Bone marrow transplantation (BMT) in Europe for primary immunodeficiencies other than severe combined immunodeficiency: A report from the European Group for BMT and the European Group for Immunodeficiency. *Blood* 83:1149, 1994.
573. Chen SH, Ochs HD, Scott CR, Giblett ER, Tingle AJ: Adenosine deaminase deficiency. Disappearance of adenine deoxynucleotides from a patient's erythrocytes after successful marrow transplantation. *J Clin Invest* **62**:1386, 1978.
574. Ochs HD, Buckley RH, Kobayashi RH, Kobayashi AL, Sorensen RU, Douglas SD, Hamilton BL, et al.: Antibody responses to bacteriophage 0X174 in patients with adenosine deaminase deficiency. *Blood* **80**:1163, 1992.
575. Polmar SH, Wetzler EM, Stern RC, Hirschhorn R: Restoration of *in vitro* lymphocyte responses with exogenous ADA in a patient with severe combined immunodeficiency. *Lancet* **2**:743, 1975.
576. Rubinstein A, Hirschhorn R, Sicklick M, Murphy RA: *In vivo* and *in vitro* effects of thymosin and adenosine deaminase on adenosine-deaminase–deficient lymphocytes. *N Engl J Med* **300**:387, 1979.
577. Dyminski JW, Daoud A, Lampkin BC, Limouze S, Donofrio J, Coleman MS, Hutton JJ: Immunological and biochemical profiles in response to transfusion therapy in an adenosine deaminase–deficient patient with severe combined immunodeficiency disease. *Clin Immunol Immunopathol* **14**:307, 1979.
578. Davies EG, Levinski RJ, Webster DR, Simmonds HA, Perrett D: Effect of red cell transfusions, thymic hormone and deoxycytidine in severe combined immunodeficiency due to adenosine deaminase deficiency. *Clin Exp Immunol* **50**:303, 1982.
579. Schmalsteig FC, Mills GC, Nelson JA, May LT, Goldman AS, Goldblum RM: Limited effect of erythrocyte and plasma infusions in adenosine deaminase deficiency. *J Pediatr* **93**:597, 1978.
580. Ziegler JB, Lee CL, Van der Weyden MB, Bagnara AS, Beveridge J: Severe combined immunodeficiency and adenosine deaminase deficiency failure of enzyme replacement therapy. *Arch Dis Child* **55**:452, 1980.
581. Polmar SH: Enzyme replacement and other biochemical approaches to the therapy of adenosine deaminase deficiency, in Elliot K, Whelan J (eds): *Enzyme Defects and Immune Dysfunction, Ciba Foundation Symposium*. New York, Excerpta Medica, 1979, p 213.
582. Abuchowski A, Van Es T, Palczuk NC, Davis FF: Alteration of immunological properties of bovine serum albumin by covalent attachment of polyethylene glycol. *J Biol Chem* **252**:3578, 1977.
583. Davis FF, Kazo GM, Nucci ML, Abuchowski A: Reduction of immunogenicity and extension of circulating life of peptides and proteins, in Lee VHL (eds): *Peptide and Protein Drug Delivery*. New York, Marcel Dekker, 1991, p 831.
584. Davis S, Abuchowski A, Park YK, Davis FF: Alteration of the circulating life and antigenic properties of bovine adenosine deaminase in mice by attachment of polyethylene glycol. *Clin Exp Immunol* **46**:649, 1981.
585. Bory C, Boulieu R, Souillet G, Chantin C, Rolland MO, Mathieu M, Hershfield MS: Comparison of red cell transfusion and polyethylene glycol-modified adenosine deaminase therapy in an adenosine deaminase–deficient child. *Pediatr Res* **28**:127, 1990.
586. Girault D, Le Deist F, Debré M, Pérignon JL, Herbelin C, Griscelli C, Scudiery D, et al.: Traitement du deficit en adenosine desaminase par l'adenosine desaminase couplee au polyethylene glycol (PEG-ADA). *Arch Fr Pediatr* **49**:339, 1992.
587. Weinberg K, Hershfield MS, Bastian J, Kohn D, Sender L, Parkman R, Lenarsky C: T lymphocyte ontogeny in adenosine deaminase deficient severe combined immune deficiency following treatment with polyethylene glycol modified adenosine deaminase. *J Clin Invest* **92**:596, 1993.
588. Hershfield MS: PEG-ADA replacement therapy for adenosine deaminase deficiency: An update after 8.5 years. *Clin Immunol Immunopathol* **76**(suppl):228, 1995.
589. Chaffee S, Mary A, Stiehm ER, Girault D, Fischer A, Hershfield MS: IgG antibody response to polyethylene glycol-modified adenosine deaminase (PEG-ADA) in patients with adenosine deaminase deficiency. *J Clin Invest* **89**:1643, 1992.
590. Chun JD, Lee N, Kobayashi RH, Chaffee S, Hershfield MS, Stiehm ER: Suppression of an antibody to adenosine deaminase (ADA) in an ADA deficient severe combined immunodeficiency patient receiving polyethylene glycol modified adenosine deaminase (PEG-ADA). *Ann Allergy* **70**:462, 1993.
591. Hershfield M, S.: Biochemistry and immunology of poly(ethylene glycol)-modified adenosine deaminase (PEG-ADA), in Harris JM, Zalipsky S (eds): *Poly(ethylene glycol) Chemistry and Biological Applications*. Washington, DC, ACS, 1997, p 145.
592. Hershfield MS: The role of PEG-ADA in the evolution of therapy for adenosine deaminase deficiency, in Gupta S, Griscelli C (eds): *New Concepts in Immunodeficiency Diseases*. Chichester, England, Wiley, 1993, p 417.
593. Sandman R, Ammann AJ, Grose C, Wara DW: Cellular immunodeficiency associated with nucleoside phosphorylase deficiency. *Clin Immunol Immunopathol* **8**:247, 1977.
594. Gelfand EW, Dosch HM, Biggar WD, Fox IH: Partial purine nucleoside phosphorylase deficiency Studies of lymphocyte function. *J Clin Invest* **61**:1071, 1978.
595. Zegers BJM, Stoop JW, Staal GEJ, Wadman SK: An approach to the restoration of T cell function in a purine nucleoside phosphorylase deficient patient, in Elliot K, Whelan J (eds): *Enzyme Defects and Immune Dysfunction*. New York, Excerpta Medica, 1979, p 231.
596. Rich KC, Mejias E, Fox IH: Purine nucleoside phosphorylase deficiency: Improved metabolic and immunologic function with erythrocyte transfusions. *N Engl J Med* **303**:973, 1980.
597. Vega MA: Adenosine deaminase deficiency: a model for human somatic cell gene correction. *Biochim Biophys Acta* **1138**:253, 1992.
598. Fenjves ES, Schwartz PM, Blaese RM, Taichman LB: Keratinocyte gene therapy for adenosine deaminase deficiency: A model approach for inherited metabolic disorders. *Hum Gene Ther* **8**:911, 1997.
599. Foresman MD, Nelson DM, McIvor RS: Correction of purine nucleoside phosphorylase deficiency by retroviral-mediated gene transfer in mouse S49 T cell lymphoma: A model for gene therapy of T cell immunodeficiency. *Hum Gene Ther* **3**:625, 1992.
600. Nelson DM, Butters KA, Markert ML, Reinsmoen NL, McIvor RS: Correction of proliferative response in purine nucleoside phosphorylase (PNP)-deficient T lymphocytes by retroviral-mediated PNP gene transfer and expression. *J Immunol* **154**:3006, 1995.
601. Jonsson JJ, Habel DE, McIvor RS: Retrovirus-mediated transduction of an engineered intron-containing purine nucleoside phosphorylase gene. *Hum Gene Ther* **6**:611, 1995.

602. Ferrari G, Rossini S, Giavazzi R, Maggioni D, Nobili N, Soldati M, Ungers G, et al.: An *in vivo* model of somatic cell gene therapy for human severe combined immunodeficiency. *Science* **251**:1363, 1991.
603. Osborne WR, Hock RA, Kaleko M, Miller AD: Long-term expression of human adenosine deaminase in mice after transplantation of bone marrow infected with amphotropic retroviral vectors. *Hum Gene Ther* **1**:31, 1990.
604. Moore KA, Fletcher FA, Villalon DK, Utter AE, Belmont JW: Human adenosine deaminase expression in mice. *Blood* **75**:2085, 1990.
605. Van Beusechem VW, Kukler A, Einerhand MPW, Bakx TA, van der Eb AJ, van Bekkum DW, Valerio D: Expression of human adenosine deaminase in mice transplanted with hemopoietic stem cells infected with amphotropic retroviruses. *J Exp Med* **172**:729, 1990.
606. Apperley JF, Luskey BD, Williams DA: Retroviral gene transfer of human adenosine deaminase in murine hematopoietic cells: Effect of selectable marker sequences on long-term expression. *Blood* **78**:310, 1991.
607. Hantzopoulos PA, Sullenger BA, Ungers G, Gilboa E: Improved gene expression upon transfer of the adenosine deaminase minigene outside the transcriptional unit of a retroviral vector. *Proc Natl Acad Sci U S A* **86**:3519, 1989.
608. Hock RA, Miller AD, Osborne WR: Expression of human adenosine deaminase from various strong promoters after gene transfer into human hematopoietic cell lines. *Blood* **74**:876, 1989.
609. Armentano D, Yu S-F, Kantoff PW, von Ruden T, Anderson WF, Gilboa E: Effect of internal viral sequences on the utility of retroviral vectors. *J Virol* **61**:1647, 1987.
610. Bodine DM, Karlsson S, Nienhuis AW: Combinations of interleukins 3 and 6 preserves stem cell function in culture and enhances retrovirus-mediated gene transfer into hematopoietic stem cells. *Proc Natl Acad Sci U S A* **86**:8897, 1989.
611. Fletcher FA, Moore KA, Ashkenazi M, De Vries P, Overbeek PA, Williams DE, Belmont JW: Leukemia inhibitory factor improves survival of retroviral vector-infected hematopoietic stem cells *in vitro*, allowing efficient long-term expression of vector-encoded human adenosine deaminase in vivo. *J Exp Med* **174**:837, 1991.
612. Kantoff PW, Gillio A, McLachlin JR, Bordignon C, Eglitis MA, Kernan NA, Moen RC, et al.: Expression of human adenosine deaminase in non-human primates after retroviral mediated gene transfer. *J Exp Med* **166**:219, 1987.
613. Van Beusechem VW, Kukler A, Heidt PJ, Valerio D: Long-term expression of human adenosine deaminase in rhesus monkeys transplanted with retrovirus-infected bone-marrow cells. *Proc Natl Acad Sci U S A* **89**:7640, 1992.
614. Bordignon C, Yu SF, Smith CA, Hantzopoulos P, Ungers GE, Keever CA, O'Reilly RJ, et al.: Retroviral vector-mediated high-efficiency expression of adenosine deaminase (ADA) in hematopoietic long-term cultures of ADA-deficient marrow cells. *Proc Natl Acad Sci U S A* **86**:6748, 1989.
615. Hughes PDF, Eaves CJ, Hogge DE, Humphries RK: High-efficiency gene transfer to human hematopoietic cells maintained in long-term marrow culture. *Blood* **74**:1915, 1989.
616. Nolta JA, Kohn DB: Comparison of the effects of growth factors on retroviral vector-mediated gene transfer and the proliferative status of human hematopoietic progenitor cells. *Hum Gene Ther* **1**:257, 1990.
617. Cournoyer D, Scarpa M, Mitani K, Moore KA, Markowitz D, Bank A, Belmont JW, et al.: Gene transfer of adenosine deaminase into primitive human hematopoietic progenitor cells. *Hum Gene Ther* **2**:203, 1991.
618. Blaese RM: Development of gene therapy for immunodeficiency: Adenosine deaminase deficiency. *Pediatr Res* **33**(suppl):49, 1993.
619. Blaese RM, Culver KW, Miller AD, Carter CS, Fleisher T, Clerici M, Shearer G, et al.: T lymphocyte-directed gene therapy for ADA-SCID: Initial trial results after 4 years. *Science* **270**:475, 1995.
620. Bordignon C, Notarangelo L, Nobili N, Ferrari G, Casorati G, Panina P, Mazzolari E, et al.: Gene therapy in peripheral blood lymphocytes and bone marrow for ADA-immunodeficient patients. *Science* **270**:470, 1995.
621. Hoogerbrugge PM, van Beusechem VW, Fischer A, Debree M, le Deist F, Perignon JL, Morgan G, et al.: Bone marrow gene transfer in three patients with adenosine deaminase deficiency. *Gene Ther* **3**:179, 1996.
622. Onodera M, Ariga T, Kawamura N, Kobayashi I, Ohtsu M, Yamada M, Tame A, et al.: Successful peripheral T-lymphocyte–directed gene transfer for a patient with severe combined immune deficiency caused by adenosine deaminase deficiency. *Blood* **91**:30, 1998.
623. Orkin S, Motulsky A: Report and recommendations of the panel to assess the NIH investment in research on gene therapy. *World Wide Web* http://www.nih.gov/news/panelrep.html:1995.
624. Larochelle A, Vormoor J, Hanenberg H, Wang JC, Bhatia M, Lapidot T, Moritz T, et al.: Identification of primitive human hematopoietic cells capable of repopulating NOD/SCID mouse bone marrow: Implications for gene therapy. *Nat Med* **2**:1329, 1996.
625. Hanenberg H, Xiao XL, Dilloo D, Hashino K, Kato I, Williams DA: Colocalization of retrovirus and target cells on specific fibronectin fragments increases genetic transduction of mammalian cells. *Nat Med* **2**:876, 1996.
626. Veena P, Traycoff CM, Williams DA, McMahel J, Rice S, Cornetta K, Srour EF: Delayed targeting of cytokine-nonresponsive human bone marrow CD34(+) cells with retrovirus-mediated gene transfer enhances transduction efficiency and long-term expression of transduced genes. *Blood* **91**:3693, 1998.
627. Wildner O, Candotti F, Krecko EG, Xanthopoulos KG, Ramsey WJ, Blaese RM: Generation of a conditionally neo(r)-containing retroviral producer cell line: Effects of neo(r) on retroviral titer and transgene expression. *Gene Ther* **5**:684, 1998.
628. Onodera M, Nelson DM, Yachie A, Jagadeesh GJ, Bunnell BA, Morgan RA, Blaese RM: Development of improved adenosine deaminase retroviral vectors. *J Virol* **72**:1769, 1998.
629. Pollok KE, Hanenberg H, Noblitt TW, Schroeder WL, Kato I, Emanuel D, Williams DA: High-efficiency gene transfer into normal and adenosine deaminase–deficient T lymphocytes is mediated by transduction on recombinant fibronectin fragments. *J Virol* **72**:4882, 1998.
630. Miyoshi H, Smith KA, Mosier DE, Verma IM, Torbett BE: Transduction of human $CD34^+$ cells that mediate long-term engraftment of NOD/SCID mice by HIV vectors. *Science* **283**:682, 1999.
630a. Cavazzana-Calvo M, Hacein-Bey S, de Saint Basile G, Gross F, Yvon E, Nusbaum P, Selz F, et al.: Gene Therapy of human severe combined immunodeficiency (SCID)-X1 disease. *Science* **288**:669, 2000.
631. Hershfield MS, Chaffee S: PEG-enzyme replacement therapy for adenosine deaminase deficiency, in Desnick RJ (ed): *Treatment of Genetic Diseases*. New York, Churchill Livingstone, 1991, p 169.
632. Mills GC, Schmalstieg FC, Trimmer KB, Foldman AS, Goldblum RS: Purine metabolism in adenosine deaminase deficiency. *Proc Natl Acad Sci U S A* **73**:2867, 1976.
633. Osborne WR, Chen SH, Giblett ER, Biggar WD, Ammann AA, Scott CR: Purine nucleoside phosphorylase deficiency. Evidence for molecular heterogeneity in two families with enzyme-deficient members. *J Clin Invest* **60**:741, 1977.
634. Edwards NL, Gelfand EW, Biggar D, Fox IH: Partial deficiency of purine nucleoside phosphorylase: Studies of purine and pyrimidine metabolsim. *J Lab Clin Med* **91**:736, 1978.
635. Siegenbeek Van Heukelom LH, Akermann JWN, Staal JEJ, De Bruyn CHMM, Stoop JW, Zegers BJM, De Bree PK, et al.: A patient with purine nucleoside phosphorylase deficiency enzymological and metabolic aspects. *Clin Chim Acta* **74**:271, 1977.
636. Simmonds HA, Watson JG, Hugh JK, Perret D, Sahota A, Potter CF: Deoxynucleoside excretion in adenosine deaminase deficiency and purine nucleoside phosphorylase deficiency, in Pollara B, Pickering RJ, Meuwissen HJ, Porter IH (eds): *Inborn Errors of Specific Immunity*. New York, Academic, 1979, p 377.
637. Jiang C, Hong R, Horowitz SD, Kong X, Hirschhorn R: An adenosine deaminase (ADA) allele contains two newly identified deleterious mutations (Y97C and L106V) that interact to abolish enzyme activity. *Hum Mol Genet* **6**:2271, 1997.
638. Atasoy U, Norby-Slycord CJ, Markert ML: A missense mutation in exon 4 of the human adenosine deaminase gene causes severe combined immunodeficiency. *Hum Mol Genet* **2**:1307, 1993.
639. Kawamoto H, Ito K, Kashii S, Monden S, Fujita M, Norioka M, Sasai Y, et al.: A point mutation in the 5′ splice region of intron 7 causes a deletion of exon 7 in adenosine deaminase mRNA. *J Cell Biochem* **51**:322, 1993.

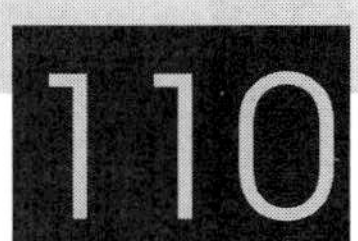

CHAPTER 110

Myoadenylate Deaminase Deficiency

Richard L. Sabina ▪ Edward W. Holmes

1. **Myoadenylate deaminase is the muscle-specific isoenzyme of AMP deaminase (EC 3.5.4.6). Deficiency of myoadenylate deaminase is heterogeneous in etiology and results in derangement of purine nucleotide catabolism and interconversion. More than 200 patients with this disorder have been reported, and reduced myoadenylate deaminase has been demonstrated in approximately 2 percent of muscle biopsy specimens submitted for pathologic examination for a wide array of indications.**
2. **Two distinct forms of myoadenylate deaminase deficiency are recognized. Inherited (primary) deficiency is either asymptomatic or associated with exercise-related cramps and myalgias. Acquired (secondary) deficiency is associated with a wide array of other neuromuscular or rheumatologic disorders. Because of the high frequency of one mutant myoadenylate deaminase allele, many patients with myopathy due to any of a variety of etiologies have a "coincidental" inherited deficiency of myoadenylate deaminase. In most patients with associated disorders, it is difficult to determine the contribution, if any, of the myoadenylate deaminase deficiency to the clinical phenotype. However, a coincidental inherited myoadenylate deaminase deficiency may be synergistic when associated with a second metabolic myopathy.**
3. **Recent evidence indicates that those individuals carrying at least one mutant myoadenylate deaminase allele have an improved clinical outcome should they develop congestive heart failure.**
4. **Inherited deficiency of myoadenylate deaminase is transmitted as an autosomal recessive trait. A single mutant allele harboring a nonsense mutation that results in the production of a severely truncated myoadenylate deaminase peptide is responsible for all cases of inherited myoadenylate deaminase deficiency characterized to date. The acquired disorder may result from a limitation in myoadenylate deaminase transcript availability, perhaps as a consequence of pathologic abnormalities caused by the associated disease. Genetic testing can be used to determine whether these latter individuals actually harbor a coincidental inherited myoadenylate deaminase deficiency.**
5. **Despite the relatively low incidence of the clinical phenotype associated with inherited deficiency of muscle AMP deaminase, the frequencies of the mutant allele are high, for example, 0.10 to 0.14 in several Caucasian sample populations.**
6. **When patients with myoadenylate deaminase deficiency exercise, their skeletal muscle does not accumulate NH_3 and IMP, as occurs in normal subjects.**
7. **The myopathy in patients with inherited myoadenylate deaminase deficiency indicates that this enzyme and the purine nucleotide cycle, of which it is one component, play an important role in skeletal muscle metabolism during exercise.**

The purine nucleotide cycle (Fig. 110-1), of which the adenylate deaminase (AMP deaminase) reaction is one component, is thought to play an important role in skeletal muscle function for several reasons. The activities of all three enzymes in the purine nucleotide cycle are several-fold greater in skeletal muscle than in other tissues, and the activity of AMP deaminase is approximately 100 times greater than that of the other two enzymes.[1–3] During exercise, NH_3 production and inosine monophosphate (IMP) content of skeletal muscle increase in proportion to the work performed by the muscle,[1–8] indicating increased AMP deaminase activity under these conditions. Activation of myoadenylate deaminase and increased flux through the purine nucleotide cycle during exercise lead to an increase in energy production through the generation of intermediates for the citric acid cycle from amino acids and through stimulation of glycolysis.[1–7] Thus, one might anticipate that deficiency of myoadenylate deaminase activity and disruption of the purine nucleotide cycle would lead to skeletal muscle dysfunction.

In 1978, Fishbein et al. described five patients with skeletal muscle dysfunction following mild to moderate exercise.[9] In these patients, myoadenylate deaminase activity was virtually absent. To date, over 200 additional patients with myoadenylate deaminase deficiency have been described.[9–47] Data from several institutions demonstrate that this myopathy is relatively common; about 2 percent of all biopsies submitted for pathologic evaluation are found deficient in myoadenylate deaminase activity.[9,11,20,38]

CLINICAL FEATURES

The clinical features and laboratory abnormalities associated with myoadenylate deaminase deficiency in over 200 reported cases are summarized in Table 110-1. As detailed below (see "Clinical Spectrum and Variability"), myoadenylate deaminase-deficient individuals can be separated clinically into two groups: one with postexercise symptoms as the only manifestations and one with a wide array of other neuromuscular and rheumatologic complications. In the latter group, the characteristics of the associated disorder dominate the clinical picture. Of the former group, 62 percent of patients are male and 93 percent develop fatigue, cramps, or myalgias following moderate to vigorous exercise. Myoglobinuria following strenuous exercise has been reported in three patients. The median age at the time of diagnosis is 37 years, with a range of 4 to 76 years (also see Table 110-1). In 79 percent of patients, the onset of symptoms occurred between childhood and the early adult years. Increased serum creatine kinase has been found in 48 percent. In many patients, however, serum creatine kinase activity was normal at rest and increased into the abnormal range only following exercise. Electromyogram (EMG) findings may be normal, although minor abnormalities have been described in some patients. Results of muscle biopsy examined by routine

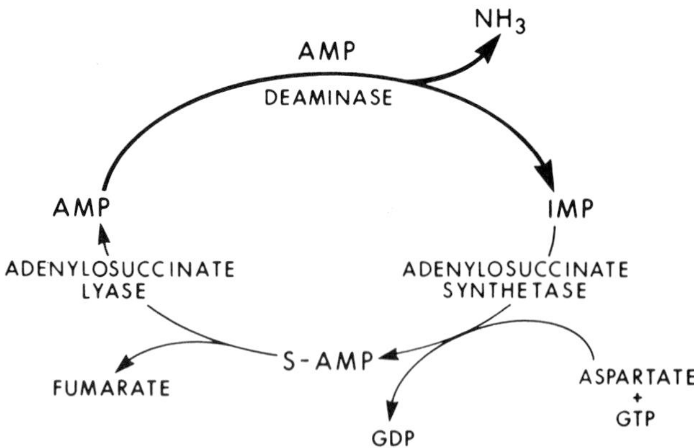

Fig. 110-1 Purine nucleotide cycle. S-AMP refers to adenylosuccinate.

histochemical stains and electron microscopy have varied from no pathologic findings to mild abnormalities in distribution of fiber size.

Histochemical stain for myoadenylate deaminase activity has produced negative results in all patients tested. By extending the incubation time to 3 h, however, it may be possible to distinguish between patients with acquired and inherited deficiencies of myoadenylate deaminase.[31] Residual activity varies from virtually absent (< 0.2) to 15.7 percent of the control mean. The percentage of residual activity may also be helpful in distinguishing an inherited from an acquired deficiency, but it should not be used as the sole criterion (Table 110-2 and References 27 and 45). In all patients with myoadenylate deaminase deficiency, no NH_3 is produced following ischemic forearm exercise. A test measuring NH_3 production has been used to screen patients for this enzyme deficiency. The test is not specific for myoadenylate deaminase deficiency, but it does appear to be a sensitive screening procedure.[9,33,35]

Table 110-1 Clinical Features and Laboratory Abnormalities

Clinical features of inherited AMP deaminase deficiency
Sex: 59 Male, 95 total
Age at time of diagnosis
Mean: 37 years
Median: 37 years
Range:: 4–76 years
Post-exercise symptoms
Easy fatigue, cramps, myalgias; 94 of 101 (93%)
Age at time of onset of symptoms
Infancy (< 2 years): 0 of 34 (0%)
Childhood (2–12 years): 9 of 34 (26%)
Teenage (13–19 years): 7 of 34 (21%)
Young adult (20–40 years): 11 of 34 (32%)
Older adult (> 40 years): 7 of 34 (21%)
Laboratory abnormalities in patients with inherited AMP deaminase deficiency
Elevated serum CPK*: 22 of 45 (48%)
Failure to produce NH_3 on ischemic testing: 57 of 57 (100%)
Negative histochemical stain for AMP deaminase: 62 of 62 (100%)
Diminished (< 0.2 – 15.7% of normal) AMP deaminase activity on direct assay: 95 of 95 (100%)
Other clinical diagnoses in patients with acquired AMP deaminase deficiency (105 cases in the literature)†
Neurogenic disorders: 44
Myopathies: 37
Miscellaneous disorders: 10
Collagen vascular disease: 9
Other metabolic disorders: 5

*CPK = creatine phosphokinase.

†Patients with an acquried deficiency also fail to produce NH_3 on ischemic testing and show negative results of histochemical stain.

CLINICAL SPECTRUM AND VARIABILITY

Myoadenylate deaminase deficiency presents a heterogeneous clinical picture. Although in nearly 50 percent of all reported cases the patients exhibit exercise-related symptoms only, many other associated clinical presentations have been described. For example, the first patient reported to have myoadenylate deaminase deficiency was also diagnosed as having primary hypokalemic periodic paralysis.[10] To date, myoadenylate deaminase deficiency has been reported in association with numerous neurogenic disorders, myopathies, collagen vascular diseases, other metabolic disorders, and several miscellaneous derangements, such as cardiomyopathy and chronic licorice ingestion. In addition, many asymptomatic individuals have been reported.[20,35,39,46,48,49] Therefore, some clinicians have labeled myoadenylate deaminase deficiency a "harmless genetic variant."[11,14,21] It still is not clear what relationship, if any, the deficiency of myoadenylate deaminase activity has to the neuromuscular and rheumatologic disorders exhibited in more than 50 percent of all reported cases. Several key advances, however, have provided critical information that may explain the clinical variability associated with this deficiency.

In 1985, Fishbein presented clinical, biochemical, and immunologic data on numerous patients and proposed two forms of myoadenylate deaminase deficiency.[27] As summarized in Table 110-2, patients can be classified as either inherited, acquired, or coincidental inherited, on the basis of their clinical presentation, amount and immunoreactivity of residual activity, relative activities of other muscle-specific enzymes and AMPD1 genotype. Others have presented data supporting these classifications.[45,50–55] Advances in the molecular biology of AMP deaminase expression have provided additional information that may be used to explain the basis of these two forms of myoadenylate deaminase deficiency (see "Molecular Basis of Myoadenylate Deaminase Deficiency," below). As discussed in subsequent sections of this chapter, the postexercise symptoms experienced by inherited myoadenylate deaminase-deficient patients may be explained by homozygosity for a mutant allele with resultant lack of enzymatic activity and disruption of the purine nucleotide cycle. On the other hand, the depression of myoadenylate deaminase and other muscle-specific enzymatic activities in patients with an acquired deficiency appears to be a limitation in transcript availability. Reduction of myoadenylate deaminase mRNA may reflect a regulatory derangement in muscle-specific gene expression as a consequence of other pathologic neuromuscular and rheumatologic abnormalities. Regardless of the explanation for the molecular abnormalities in an acquired deficiency, the clinical presentation in these patients is dominated by symptoms of the associated disorder. Because the frequency of the nonfunctional myoadenylate deaminase allele is high (e.g., 0.10 to 0.14 in several Caucasian sample populations),[46,48,49] a third class of myoadenylate deaminase-deficient patients has been identified that is comprised of individuals with other neuromuscular and rheumatologic diseases in whom muscle biopsy is performed as part of their diagnostic evaluation and who demonstrate a coincidental inherited deficiency of myoadenylate deaminase.[51–54] The contribution of the enzyme deficiency to the clinical phenotype of these patients is uncertain, but may be synergistic in combination with other disorders of energy metabolism.

The reactions catalyzed by AMP deaminase and other enzymes in the purine nucleotide cycle (see Fig. 110-1) play an important role in the metabolism of the fast-twitch glycolytic fiber following vigorous exercise (see "Purine Nucleotide Cycle," below). This series of reactions also appears to play a role in the metabolism of slow-twitch oxidative fibers.[56] Some of the variability in postexercise symptoms associated with myoadenylate deaminase deficiency may be related to individual differences in the

Table 110-2 Characteristics of Different Forms of Myoadenylate Deaminase Deficiency

	Inherited Myoadenylate Deaminase Deficiency	Acquired Myoadenylate Deaminase Deficiency	Coincidental Inherited Myoadenylate Deaminase Deficiency
Clinical presentation	Exercise-related aches, cramps, and pains	Other neuromuscular manifestations	Other neuromuscular manifestations (can be more severe than either condition alone)
Residual activity	$<2\%$ of control	$>2\%$ of control	$<2\%$ of control
Immunoreactivity of residual activity	Variably precipitated by muscle-specific antiserum	Precipiatated by muscle-specific antiserum	Variably precipitated by muscle-specific antiserum
Other muscle-specific enzymatic activities	Unaffected	Reduced; dependent on severity of associated disorder	Reduced; dependent on severity of associated disorder
Molecular basis	Inherited defect in the AMPD1 gene	Heterozygous for inherited defect combined with limitation in AMPD1 transcript	Inherited defect in the AMPD1 gene

proportion of fast-twitch glycolytic versus slow-twitch oxidative fibers in a given muscle group and the extent to which the purine nucleotide cycle contributes to energy production in each fiber type. Individual differences in the developmental and fiber-type regulated alternative splicing event (see "AMP Deaminase Genes and Transcripts," below), which would remove the mutation responsible for the inherited deficiency (see "Molecular Basis of Myoadenylate Deaminase Deficiency," below), may also contribute to variations in postexercise symptoms. In addition, inherited deficiency of myoadenylate deaminase may be associated with adaptive changes in the expression of another AMP deaminase gene expressed in skeletal myocytes (see "AMP Deaminase Genes and Transcripts," below) or in other metabolic pathways, which may moderate the clinical picture.

Pedigree analyses of inherited myoadenylate deaminase-deficient families indicate autosomal recessive inheritance.[39] The localization of the myoadenylate deaminase gene (AMPD1) to the short arm of human chromosome 1[57] provides physical evidence that the gene is autosomal. Moreover, combined biochemical and genetic characterizations of a healthy population sample have revealed high, intermediate, and low skeletal muscle enzyme activities that correlate with homozygous normal, heterozygous, and homozygous mutant genotypes, respectively.[49]

Recent studies suggest there may be a physiological consequence in heterozygotes for the C34T transition in the AMPD1 gene (see "Molecular Basis of Myoadenylate Deaminase Deficiency," below). These individuals have a striking improvement in clinical outcome should they develop congestive heart failure.[58] The odds ratio of surviving without cardiac transplantation for greater than 5 years following hospitalization for heart failure symptoms is 8.6 times greater (95 percent CI 3.05, 23.87) for those individuals carrying at least one mutant AMPD1 allele. The physiological basis for this striking survival advantage in heterozygotes who develop heart failure remains to be determined, but may be related to metabolic changes that occur in tissues, such as skeletal muscle, that exhibit reduced AMP deaminase activity. The high prevalence of this mutant allele in Caucasian populations with nearly one in four individuals heterozygous for this mutant allele, indicates that it arose early in the course of human evolution and may have conferred some unknown selective advantage on their ancestors.

PURINE NUCLEOTIDE CYCLE

Three enzymes participate in the purine nucleotide cycle (see Fig. 110-1): AMP deaminase (AMP aminohydrolase) (EC 3.5.4.6), adenylosuccinate synthetase (EC 6.3.4.4), and adenylosuccinate lyase (EC 4.3.2.2). At first glance this series of reactions might appear to be a futile cycle; that is, AMP $\rightarrow$ IMP $\rightarrow\rightarrow$ AMP. However, each turn of the cycle results in the utilization of one molecule of aspartate and guanosine triphosphate (GTP) and the production of one molecule of guanosine diphosphate (GDP), fumarate, and NH_3. Before discussing the potential role(s) this cycle plays in muscle function, it may be helpful to review the data that establish that flux through the cycle increases in skeletal muscle during exercise.

Several laboratories have shown that the purine nucleotide cycle is operative in vivo.[2–7,24,56,59] Biopsies obtained from the hindlimbs of rodents following nerve stimulation or treadmill running demonstrate the following sequence of biochemical changes: (a) In fast-twitch glycolytic muscle, the ATP concentration falls when the capacity for energy production by substrate oxidation is exceeded. (b) The resultant increases in AMP and adenosine diphosphate (ADP) production coupled with the decrease in adenosine triphosphate (ATP) concentration lead to an increase in AMP deaminase activity (see "AMP Deaminase Isoforms," below). (c) IMP accumulates in an amount that is almost stoichiometric with the decrease in adenine nucleotides. (d) NH_3 content of the muscle increases stoichiometrically with IMP, and spillover of additional NH_3 into the blood leads to an increase in plasma NH_3 concentration. (e) Aspartate concentration in the muscle falls while the concentrations of fumarate, malate, and citrate increase. This sequence of events demonstrates that myoadenylate deaminase activity increases in muscle following vigorous exercise, and activation of this enzyme in turn leads to increased flux through the purine nucleotide cycle. These experiments establish a central role for myoadenylate deaminase in the control of flux through this cycle.

It has been difficult to quantify flux through the purine nucleotide cycle and, consequently, to estimate the extent to which flux is increased during exercise. Several studies indicate that flux through the cycle is substantially increased during exercise. Meyer et al.[7] showed that blood NH_3 concentration increases 5.5 times in rats following vigorous exercise. The magnitude of increase in blood NH_3 cannot be accounted for by the stoichiometric conversion of ATP to IMP, which suggests that a substantial proportion of the NH_3 released into the blood is derived from aspartate through the purine nucleotide cycle. Aragon and Lowenstein[3] demonstrated that citrate, isocitrate, and succinate concentrations in muscle increase following exercise and that almost three-quarters of this expansion of the pool of citric acid cycle intermediates is derived from aspartate via the purine nucleotide cycle. These studies demonstrate that the IMP that accumulates in skeletal muscle during exercise is continuously recycled to AMP and back to IMP. Reconstitution experiments with muscle extracts have documented simultaneous flux through both "arms"—that is, AMP $\rightarrow$ IMP + NH_3 and IMP + aspartate + GTP $\rightarrow\rightarrow$ AMP + fumarate + GDP—of the purine nucleotide cycle, and flux through the cycle is controlled by adenylate energy charge.[60] These results, taken together, support the conclusion that flux through both arms of the purine nucleotide cycle increases during exercise.

During the rest period following vigorous muscle contraction, IMP is converted first to adenylosuccinate and then to AMP.[3,5–7] Because the capacity for ATP synthesis is greater than the rate of ATP utilization in resting muscle, any AMP formed from IMP is rapidly rephosphorylated to ATP. Thus, the IMP that accumulates during exercise is used to restore the ATP pool during rest. In most studies, the ATP pool is fully replenished by 15 to 30 min postexercise.[3,5–7,61,62]

Sequential muscle biopsies have also been obtained in human subjects at rest, following exercise, and during recovery.[61] Changes in IMP and adenine nucleotide content of human skeletal muscle are similar to those reported in animal experiments.[3,5–7] Blood NH_3 concentration rises following vigorous exercise, and the increase in NH_3 concentration is proportional to the work load.[63–66] Ischemic forearm exercise also leads to NH_3 production by human skeletal muscle.[9,13,15,31,32,34,35,37] Studies in which subjects performed dynamic knee extension exercises to exhaustion demonstrate that net NH_3 production exceeds IMP accumulation. These results suggest flux through both arms of the purine nucleotide cycle during this exercise regimen.[59] These combined results indicate that AMP deaminase activity and flux through the purine nucleotide cycle are increased in human skeletal muscle, much as in rodent skeletal muscle, during exercise.

Several mechanisms have been proposed to explain the role of the purine nucleotide cycle in muscle function. One hypothesis is that the increase in flux through the purine nucleotide cycle during exercise maintains the adenylate energy charge of the myocyte under these conditions.[2,67,68] The adenylate energy charge would be maintained through the following mechanism: The increase in AMP deaminase activity that occurs during exercise would prevent AMP accumulation following ATP catabolism, and this, in turn, would displace the adenylate kinase (myokinase) reaction toward ATP formation. A second hypothesis is that local production of NH_3 acts in conjunction with the decrease in ATP to stimulate the activity of phosphofructokinase and enhance the rate of glycolysis.[68] It has also been suggested that the increase in IMP concentration may contribute to the activation of glycogen phosphorylase and further enhance glycolysis.[69] However, reports of normal lactate accumulation in exercising AMP deaminase-deficient skeletal muscle[9,29,31,32,35,37] document that a disruption of the purine nucleotide cycle does not lead to any significant changes in flux through the glycolytic pathway. Still another hypothesis is that the generation of fumarate, malate, and citrate from aspartate provides a mechanism by which intermediates of the citric acid cycle could be replenished during a time of increased demand for ATP production.[3,70] Finally, the accumulation of IMP may provide a mechanism for preserving the pool of purine nucleotides during exercise, and this reservoir of IMP may be used to replenish the ATP pool rapidly during recovery.[15] These proposed mechanisms are not mutually exclusive, and more than one, or all, may have validity.

It is not clear which fiber type—glycolytic or oxidative—is more dependent on the purine nucleotide cycle for maintenance of energy production. In fast-twitch glycolytic fibers, ATP depletion and flux through the purine nucleotide cycle are readily evident following anaerobic exercise protocols.[5–7] One might postulate that AMP deaminase plays a role in maintaining energy charge in these fibers by preventing AMP accumulation and by producing any positive effects that NH_3 and IMP accumulation have on energy metabolism. In slow-twitch oxidative fibers, ATP levels are usually maintained during aerobic exercise protocols,[5–7] which suggests that the purine nucleotide cycle is of little importance in these types of fibers. However, inhibition of adenylosuccinate lyase activity is associated with rapid onset of fatigue in stimulation protocols that simulate aerobic exercise.[56,71] We might conclude from these studies that the purine nucleotide cycle is important for production of citric acid cycle intermediates for enhanced oxidative metabolism during aerobic exercise, even when ATP levels are not markedly reduced. Thus, it is not unexpected that AMP deaminase deficiency might lead to dysfunction of both glycolytic and oxidative muscle fibers. What is unexpected, however, is how mild and variable the symptoms are in many patients with AMP deaminase deficiency. Although currently there is no definitive explanation for this finding, recent advances in the molecular biology of AMP deaminase (see "Molecular Basis of Myoadenylate Deaminase Deficiency," below) suggest an incomplete block in myoadenylate deaminase expression. Alternatively, the contribution of other AMP deaminase isoforms present in the skeletal myocyte may be sufficient for low-level functioning of the purine nucleotide cycle to such a degree that severe symptoms are alleviated. Abrupt interruption of flux through the purine nucleotide cycle with pharmacologic agents, on the other hand, is likely to be complete and result in a phenotype with more severe symptoms.

EXERCISE-RELATED METABOLIC AND FUNCTIONAL ABNORMALITIES IN PATIENTS WITH MYOADENYLATE DEAMINASE DEFICIENCY

Although numerous reports document biochemical abnormalities in patients with myoadenylate deaminase deficiency,[15,22,24,26,33,34,36,43] relatively few address skeletal muscle function in these individuals.[24,34,36] Among the latter studies, different exercise protocols and subjects, both with inherited and with acquired forms of myoadenylate deaminase deficiency, were employed.

Relative to controls, patients with myoadenylate deaminase deficiency exhibit a number of exercise-related derangements in metabolism (Table 110-3). Many of these are predicted effects of a block in purine catabolic flow as the result of a deficiency in AMP deamination and confirm a biochemical disruption of the purine nucleotide cycle.

Functional data generated from studies employing myoadenylate deaminase-deficient subjects are limited and variable owing to the use of different exercise protocols and patients who have inherited and acquired forms of the disease. Functional abnormalities (i.e., diminished endurance and enhanced depletion of high-energy phosphate pools per unit of work) have been reported in patients with inherited myoadenylate deaminase deficiency during vigorous aerobic exercise,[24] whereas no significant differences from control subjects were observed in a similar patient cohort after a less-intense protocol employing ischemic forearm exercise.[36] An additional study examined a single patient with a combined deficiency of myoadenylate deaminase and myophosphorylase (McArdle Disease).[34] Cycle ergometry failed to show quantitative or qualitative differences between the patient with the

Table 110-3 Exercise-Related Metabolic Abnormalities Associated with Myoadenylate Deaminase Deficiency

Observation	Reference
Anaerobic exercise	
Impaired increase in plasma NH_4 and plasma purines	22, 33
↓ Adenylate catabolism (intracellular)	36
↓ IMP accumulation (intracellular)	36
Aerobic exercise	
↓ Adenylate catabolism	24
↓ IMP accumulation	24
↑ Adenosine production	24
↑ Energy substrate (i.e., ATP, CP)* depletion per unit work	24

*CP = creatine phosphate.

combined defect and individuals with McArdle Disease alone, although all were significantly different from controls in maximal work rate, maximum oxygen consumption, and pH at the end of exercise.

AMP DEAMINASE ISOFORMS

There are several isoenzymes of AMP deaminase in mammalian tissues. Different tissues contain varying proportions of these isoenzymes, and the kinetic, physical, and immunologic properties of these isoenzymes are distinct. In humans, four isoenzymes of AMP deaminase are known.[72] Isoenzyme M, or myoadenylate deaminase, is found only in skeletal muscle; isoenzyme L is the predominant form in liver and brain; isoenzymes E_1 and E_2 are found in erythrocytes. Tissues such as heart, kidney, and spleen contain isoenzymes L, E_1, and E_2. Consequently, skeletal muscle is the only affected tissue in myoadenylate deaminase-deficient patients.[9,13,73] At least three isoenzymes of AMP deaminase have been identified in the rat[74,75] and, as in humans, one is found exclusively in skeletal muscle. Molecular studies have demonstrated that all the mammalian myoadenylate deaminase isoenzymes are encoded by transcripts produced from different genes (see "AMP Deaminase Genes and Transcripts," below).

During the course of development, the total amount of AMP deaminase activity in a given tissue may vary, as may the relative distribution of isoenzyme types.[76–83] Human skeletal muscle exhibits a greater than fivefold increase in total AMP deaminase activity from the 11-week-old fetus to the adult.[81] In rat skeletal muscle, the observed increase from birth is greater than eightfold.[82] In both cases, there is a switch in AMP deaminase isoforms produced in skeletal muscle at different stages of development. Moreover, adult skeletal muscle fiber types exhibit differential AMP deaminase activities and patterns of isoenzyme expression. For example, rat skeletal muscles composed predominantly of fast-twitch white (type IIb) fibers contain three- to tenfold more AMP deaminase activity[84] than do those with a majority of slow-twitch red (type I) fibers. Adult human skeletal muscle exhibits predominant anti-isoform M and anti-isoform E sera reactivity in type II and type I fibers, respectively.[85] In exercising human skeletal muscle, calculated AMP deaminase activity[86] and NH_3 production[87] are directly related to the percentage of fast-twitch fibers in postexercise biopsy. A shift in isoenzyme type has also been observed in human,[88] rat,[83] and chick[77] skeletal myocytes grown in culture, which appears to explain the findings of AMP deaminase activity in primary myoblasts grown in culture from muscle biopsy specimens of patients with well-documented myoadenylate deaminase deficiency.[13,88]

Myoadenylate deaminase (isoform M) has been purified to homogeneity from many mammalian sources, including humans.[72,89–91] The native molecular mass of the enzyme from human skeletal muscle is approximately 300 kDa,[72,91] and following treatment with denaturing agents, such as guanidine hydrochloride or sodium dodecylsulfate, the enzyme dissociates into a single polypeptide with a reported molecular mass of 71 to 72 kDa.[72,91] However, these and many other purifications of mammalian skeletal muscle AMP deaminase were performed in the absence of protease inhibitors that can yield proteolyzed polypeptides lacking up to nearly 100 N-terminal amino acid residues.[92] Purification of rat skeletal muscle AMP deaminase performed in the presence of protease inhibitors yielded a subunit molecular mass of 80 kDa.[93] This latter estimation is closer to the calculated molecular mass of 86 to 87 kDa as predicted from available rat[94] and human[45] myoadenylate deaminase cDNA sequences. Nevertheless, all data are consistent with the conclusion that AMP deaminase from skeletal muscle is composed of four polypeptide chains, and tryptic maps suggest that these subunits are identical. Protein kinase C-mediated phosphorylation of rat skeletal muscle myoadenylate deaminase has been reported.[95] Other post-translational modifications, such as glycosylation or fatty acylation of skeletal muscle myoadenylate deaminase, have not been investigated.

Myoadenylate deaminase is closely associated with the contractile apparatus in skeletal myocytes. Histochemical studies have demonstrated that myoadenylate deaminase is bound to the myofibril in the region of the A band[96] and that 2 mol of native enzyme bind to 1 mol of myosin.[97] Myoadenylate deaminase binds to a specific region of rabbit myosin heavy chain, that is, heavy meromyosin or subfragment 2, and an association between myoadenylate deaminase and myosin appears to have a functional significance in controlling this enzymatic activity (see below). In vitro, the rat 80-kDa muscle myoadenylate deaminase peptide binds much more tightly to myosin than does the 66-kDa proteolyzed fragment.[93]

In vitro and *in vivo* studies suggest that myoadenylate deaminase exhibits a striking increase in activity in skeletal muscle during exercise (see "Purine Nucleotide Cycle," above). Reconstitution experiments that attempt to mimic conditions found in resting muscle *in vivo* suggest that myoadenylate deaminase is inhibited by as much as 80 to 90 percent under these conditions, whereas conditions that mimic contracting muscle are associated with marked increases in activity and flux through the purine nucleotide cycle.[60] Many factors that affect myoadenylate deaminase activity *in vitro* have been identified: adenylate energy charge; ratio of purine nucleoside triphosphates to diphosphates to monophosphates; concentration of K^+, H^+, P_i, and creatine phosphate; and binding to myosin.[60,97–100] Changes in one or more of these variables are thought to lead to the release of inhibition of myoadenylate deaminase and the increase in activity of this enzyme during exercise.

It is not established how each of the above factors influences myoadenylate deaminase activity, but the data obtained by Ashby and Frieden[99] from kinetic and binding studies led them to propose a model that explains many of the regulatory properties of this enzyme. They suggest that the enzyme has three distinct types of purine nucleotide binding sites: a catalytic site that binds AMP, an inhibitory site that binds purine nucleoside triphosphates, and a stimulatory site that binds all types of purine nucleotides, but diphosphates in preference to monophosphates, and monophosphates in preference to triphosphates. K^+ ions affect the activity of the enzyme through cooperative effects on the catalytic site.

Nucleoside triphosphates (ATP and GTP) bind avidly to the inhibitory site and produce effects on cooperativity at the catalytic site. Nucleoside diphosphates and monophosphates (ADP, GDP, AMP, and GMP) bind avidly to the stimulatory site and indirectly decrease the affinity of the inhibitory site for nucleoside triphosphates. IMP, a product of the reaction, also binds to the stimulatory site and may, under some conditions, lead to enzyme activation. In resting muscle, purine nucleoside triphosphates are present in considerable excess relative to diphosphates and monophosphates. Nucleoside triphosphate content decreases following vigorous work, producing a lower concentration of ligands for binding at the inhibitory site. Nucleoside diphosphate and monophosphate content increases, leading to higher ligand concentrations for binding at the stimulatory site and secondarily decreasing the affinity of the inhibitory site for nucleoside triphosphates. AMP content increases, providing more substrate, and probably enhanced enzyme activity, by binding of this monophosphate at the stimulatory site.

This model accommodates a close correlation between the increase in myoadenylate deaminase activity and the drop in adenylate energy charge that occurs with exercise.[61,101] The drop in myocyte pH that follows exercise also contributes to the increase in myoadenylate deaminase activity, especially in fast-twitch glycolytic fibers.[102] The pH optimum of myoadenylate deaminase (i.e., pH 6.5) reflects the role of metabolic acidosis in AMP deaminase activation.[103] Changes in creatine phosphate concentration probably do not play a role in controlling the activity of this enzyme.[104] The association of myoadenylate deaminase with myosin, on the other hand, represents a physical interaction with potential physiological significance. In vitro binding studies indicate an association of the myosin components with the nucleoside triphosphate, or inhibitory site, of AMP deaminase.[97]

Studies performed with rat skeletal muscle have provided *in vivo* evidence for the significance of the myofibrillar binding of myoadenylate deaminase. In resting muscle or during contractions, when energy balance is well maintained, nearly all AMP deaminase is found in the cytosol. During intense contraction, however, conditions favor binding, which increases in a first-order manner and precedes initiation of IMP formation.[105] Furthermore, myosin-bound AMP deaminase exhibits bimodal kinetics, including a component that allows for a higher rate of AMP deamination at the low [AMP] found physiologically.[106] Together, these data imply that the myofibrillar association of myoadenylate deaminase is critical to defining its role in skeletal muscle function. Studies performed with human skeletal muscle, however, have observed higher percentages of bound AMP deaminase in resting skeletal muscle that do not increase during high-intensity exercise.[107,108]

Isoenzyme L of AMP deaminase has been purified to apparent homogeneity from platelets[109] and autopsy liver.[72] The native molecular mass, determined on the latter, is also approximately 300 kDa. Under denaturing conditions, however, the preparation from platelets exhibited a subunit molecular mass of 83 to 85 kDa, whereas that from liver was 68 kDa. Isoenzyme L cDNA sequence[110] would predict that the former estimation is the more accurate and that the latter may reflect proteolysis during preparation. Among all the human AMP deaminase variants, isoenzyme L exhibits the unique property of allosteric activation by ATP in the presence of 150 mM KCl.[72]

Isoenzymes E_1 and E_2 display similar kinetic and immunologic characteristics. Deficiency of AMP deaminase activity restricted to erythrocytes has been described in several asymptomatic families in Japan[111,112] and is characterized by a lack of both E_1 and E_2.[111] The combined information about the E isoenzymes has been used to hypothesize that both are the product of the same gene and that the relatively less abundant E_2 is merely a proteolytic, or otherwise modified, derivative of E_1.[111] Accordingly, an AMPD3 mutant allele has now been identified in Japanese individuals who have a deficiency of erythrocyte AMP deaminase.[113] Anti-isoenzyme E_1 serum reactivity in adult human skeletal muscle sections appears confined primarily to type I fibers,[85] and a similarly reactive component is the major residual activity in extracts prepared from skeletal muscle of patients with inherited myoadenylate deaminase deficiency.[114] Isoenzyme E_1, purified to apparent homogeneity from human erythrocytes, also exhibits a native molecular mass of approximately 300 kDa, which is converted to 80 kDa under denaturing conditions.[72,115] Available cDNA sequence predicts subunit molecular masses ranging from 88 to 90 kDa for alternative forms of isoenzyme E_1.[116]

Availability of cDNA sequences for three of the human AMP deaminase isoenzymes[45,110,116] allows for alignments of their predicted primary amino acid sequences.[110,116] The C-terminal domains, encompassing approximately two-thirds of the polypeptide chains, exhibit 62 to 73 percent amino acid identity. Included in this region is the AMP deaminase signature sequence found in all AMP deaminases in organisms ranging from yeast to humans, SLSTDDP.[45,94,110,116–120] This motif also is highly conserved (i.e., S[I/L]NTDDP) in adenosine deaminases in organisms ranging from bacteria to humans.[121] Significantly, x-ray crystallographic analysis of murine adenosine deaminase has revealed that the consecutive aspartate residues in this motif are involved in the catalytic site of the enzyme.[122] By analogy, a catalytic role has been proposed for the conserved aspartate residues in AMP deaminase,[121] and site-directed mutagenesis that replaces an aspartate residue leads to complete loss of enzymatic activity.[123] Unlike C-terminal domains, the N-terminal third of different human isoenzymes of AMP deaminase exhibits divergent sequences. Several gaps must be inserted into these alignments to generate any similarities.[110,116] However, alignments between rat and human sequences reveal high identities along the entire AMPD1[45] and AMPD3[120] predicted polypeptides, respectively. These data suggest a functional significance for isoenzyme-specific N-terminal sequences of AMP deaminase. Identified roles for divergent N-terminal domains include contributions to isoform-specific kinetic properties,[124] protein-protein interaction,[92] and post-translational modification (unpublished data).

AMP DEAMINASE GENES AND TRANSCRIPTS

Advances in the molecular biology of AMP deaminase expression in mammalian tissues contribute to an understanding of normal and deficient states. Three AMP deaminase genes exist in humans and rats: AMPD1 produces isoenzyme M (myoadenylate deaminase) transcripts; AMPD2 produces isoenzyme L transcripts; and AMPD3 produces the E isoenzyme transcripts. Each of these genes produces multiple transcripts through the regulated use of multiple promoters and/or alternative splicing events resulting in alternative mRNAs that differ at, or near, their 5′ ends. Although the functional significance of alternative AMP deaminase transcripts is unknown, most are predicted to encode small differences at, or near, the N-terminus of their respective AMP deaminase polypeptide.

AMPD1

The human and rat AMPD1 genes have been cloned and exhibit similar sizes and exon distributions.[57] AMPD1 is composed of 16 exons asymmetrically distributed across approximately 23 kb of human and 21 kb of rat genomic DNA. Exons containing the coding information for the C-terminal domain of the myoadenylate deaminase polypeptide are clustered in the 3′ end of the gene. The human AMPD1 gene is on the short arm of chromosome 1 in the region p13-p21. Four highly conserved regions of nucleotide sequence are observed immediately upstream of the transcription start site of the human and rat AMPD1 genes,[57] two of which contain *cis*-acting elements required for skeletal muscle-specific expression.[125] One element (−100 to −79) appears to behave like an enhancer and has an A/T-rich core similar to the MEF2-binding motif. The other element (−60 to −40) has properties of a skeletal muscle-specific promoter element.

The AMPD1 gene produces two ~2.5-kb transcripts as the result of alternative splicing of the small (12-bp) second exon (Fig. 110-2). This alternative splicing event, which exhibits developmental[83] and fiber-type[126] differences in expression, is determined by two sequential reactions: exon recognition and nucleocytoplasmic partitioning.[127] Alternative splicing of the AMPD1 primary transcript occurs at much higher levels (30 to 50 percent) in rat, as compared to human (0.6 to 2 percent), adult skeletal muscle.[126,128] This alternative splicing event is proposed to have a clinical significance (see "Molecular Basis of Myoadenylate Deaminase Deficiency," below) and produces a polypeptide in which the sequence beginning at residue 8 (−AEEKQ−) is replaced by a single −E− with resultant reduction in the overall length of the polypeptide from 747 to 743 residues (Fig. 110-3). Alternative AMPD1 isoforms exhibit different myosin-binding capacities,[129] a potentially important regulatory interaction (see "AMP Deaminase Isoforms," above).

The human AMPD1 gene is expressed at high levels only in adult skeletal muscle[110] and at low levels, predominantly as the exon 2 minus transcript, in other tissues.[128] Immunocytochemical analysis of adult human skeletal muscle[85] and molecular analyses of adult rat skeletal muscle[94,126] demonstrate relative higher AMPD1 expression in type II (glycolytic) fibers.

AMPD2

Human AMPD2 cDNAs[110,130] and genomic DNA[131] have been cloned and partially characterized. A portion of the rat AMPD2 cDNA, representing unprocessed mRNA, has also been isolated.[118] The human AMPD2 gene is comprised of 19 exons asymmetrically distributed across nearly 14 kb of genomic DNA,

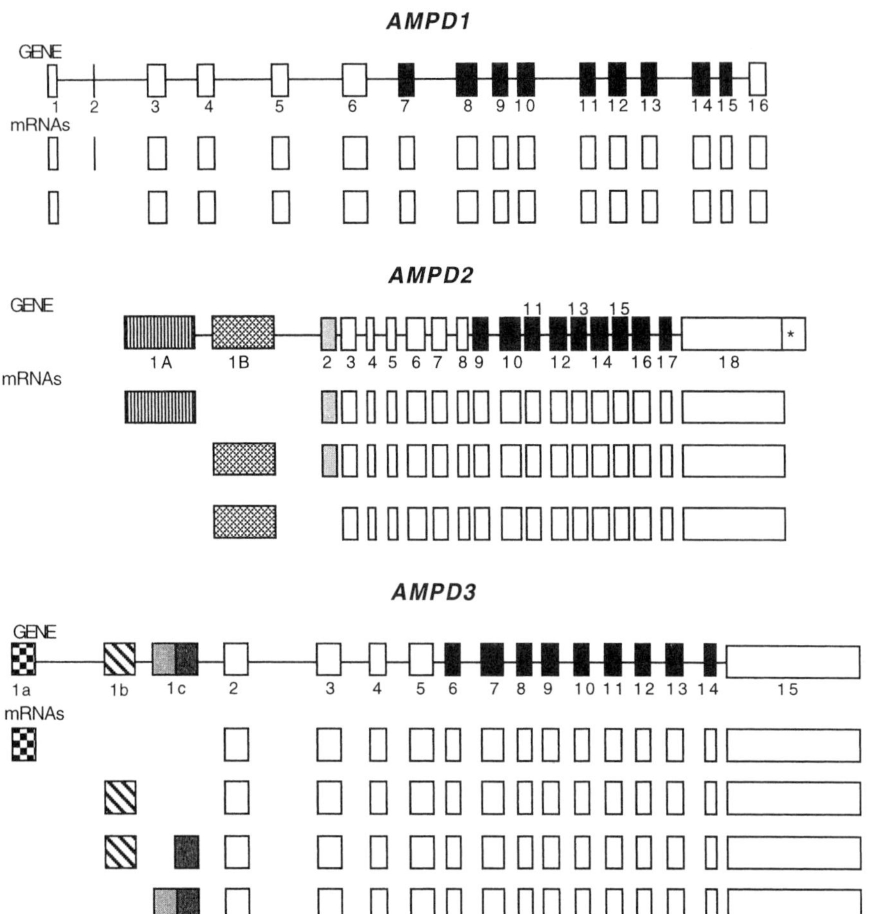

Fig. 110-2 Molecular diversity across the human AMP deaminase multigene family. Alternative mRNAs are produced from each gene as the result of 5′ exon shuffling involving the use of multiple promoters and/or alternative splicing events. Relative gene structures are depicted above alternative mRNAs. Exons (numbered boxes) and introns (horizontal lines) are drawn proportionately, but not to each other. Black boxes denote those exons containing coding information for the conserved C-terminal region of each AMP deaminase polypeptide. Alternative exons are highlighted with other shading patterns. Alternative transcriptional termination events in the AMPD2 gene are indicated by the asterisked extension of exon 18.

and is located on the short arm of chromosome 1 near the p13.3 boundary. Whereas 17 exons are clustered in the 3′-terminal half of the gene, two alternative 5′ exons are remotely located upstream and have associated promoter activities. Both AMPD2 promoter regions lack readily identifiable TATA boxes and are G+C-rich.

The human AMPD2 gene produces three ~4 kb transcripts (Fig. 110-2) through the regulated expression of two closely spaced promoters and an alternative splicing event involving exon 2.[131] Although the functional significance of alternative AMPD2 transcripts is unknown, they are predicted to encode variable

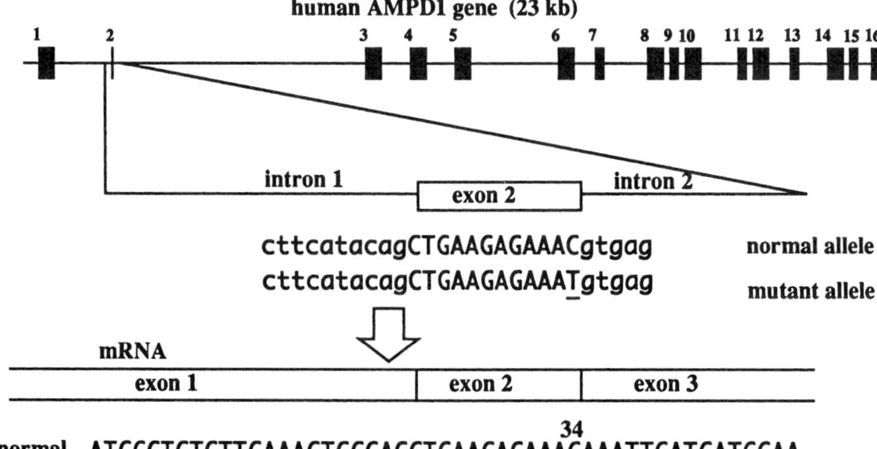

Fig. 110-3 Molecular basis for an inherited myoadenylate deaminase deficiency. The C→T transition at nucleotide +34 in the mutant allele results in a Q12X nonsense mutation in AMPD1 mRNA. This mutation would be predicted to result in a severely truncated myoadenylate polypeptide. An alternative splicing event that removes the exon 2 sequence from mature AMPD1 transcripts would eliminate the mutation, thereby enabling catalytically active protein to be produced from all alleles. This splicing event occurs in 0.6 to 2 percent of mature AMPD1 transcripts.

N-terminal extensions of 47 to 128 amino acid residues on the isoform L polypeptide.[130]

The human AMPD2 gene is widely expressed in nonmuscle tissues, but only at low levels in adult skeletal muscle[110] where it is most likely confined to nonmyocyte elements of this tissue.[85]

AMPD3

Human[116,132] and rat[120] AMPD3 cDNAs and the human gene[132] have been cloned and partially characterized. The human AMPD3 gene is comprised of 17 exons asymmetrically distributed across approximately 60 kb of genomic DNA and is located on the short arm of chromosome 11 in the p13-pter region. Each of three 5′-terminal exons (1a, 1b, and 1c) have associated promoter activities and exhibit multiple transcription initiation sites. Helix-loop-helix/E-box interactions are proposed to mediate exon 1b promoter activity in skeletal myocytes.

The human AMPD3 gene produces at least four transcripts (Fig. 110-2) through the regulated expression of three tandem promoters and an alternative splicing event involving an internal splice acceptor site in exon 1c.[132] The functional significance of alternative AMPD3 transcripts is unknown. Three of the four alternative transcripts are predicted to encode small (7 to 9 amino acid residues) N-terminal extensions on the core isoform E polypeptide, which initiates from exon 2-encoded sequence.

The human AMPD3 gene is also widely expressed, but relative mRNA abundance is greatest in adult skeletal muscle.[132] Immunocytochemical analysis of adult human skeletal muscle[85] and RNase protection analysis of adult rat skeletal muscle groups[120] demonstrate that AMPD3 expression is confined primarily to type I (oxidative) fibers. However, AMPD1 expression is relatively greater than AMPD3 expression in both human and rat skeletal muscle.

MOLECULAR BASIS OF MYOADENYLATE DEAMINASE DEFICIENCY

Availability of immunologic reagents and molecular probes for myoadenylate deaminase has resulted in elucidation of the underlying molecular derangement in patients with the inherited disorder. Although not as extensively studied, an understanding of the acquired deficiency of myoadenylate deaminase is beginning to emerge. Finally, combined molecular and population studies now indicate a third class of myoadenylate deaminase deficiency: a coincidental inherited defect in the AMPD1 gene in patients with other documented neuromuscular and rheumatologic disorders.

Inherited Myoadenylate Deaminase Deficiency

Initial molecular analyses in skeletal muscle of patients with the inherited deficiency reveal no immunoreactive polypeptide, although they do show normal (or even elevated) levels of apparently normal-sized AMPD1 transcript.[45,46] Southern blot analyses of genomic DNA, furthermore, reveal no differences between patients and controls.[41] These observations indicate that an inherited deficiency of myoadenylate deaminase results from a nucleotide substitution, or small deletion, duplication, or rearrangement, in the AMPD1 gene. In agreement with this, 11 unrelated individuals with inherited myoadenylate deaminase deficiency were shown to be homozygous for a mutant allele containing C → T transitions at nucleotide 34 in exon 2 and at nucleotide 143 in exon 3.[46] The C → T transition at nucleotide 143 results in a missense mutation (P48L). Expression of myoadenylate deaminase containing the P48L mutation in a prokaryotic expression system yielded enzymatic activity quantitatively indistinguishable from that of the wild-type allele.[46] This result suggests that the P48L mutation does not affect catalytic function and is not responsible for the severe reduction in enzyme activity observed in the muscle of patients with inherited myoadenylate deaminase deficiency. In contrast, the nucleotide substitution at position 34 produces a nonsense mutation, Q12X, which severely truncates the myoadenylate deaminase peptide and accounts for the lack of enzymatic function (see Fig. 110-3).

Nucleotide 34, positioned at the 3′ end of exon 2, is normally part of a *Mae*II restriction endonuclease site (ACGT) in genomic DNA (see Fig. 110-3). The C → T transition at this position destroys this recognition site (ATGT), allowing development of simple diagnostic tests for identifying the mutant allele.[46,49,133,134] These diagnostic tests have been used to estimate mutant allele frequencies of 0.10 to 0.14 in several randomly selected Caucasian sample populations.[46,48,49] This mutant allele has also been found in the African-American population, but not in the Japanese population.[46] These frequencies are sufficient to account for the reported 2 percent incidence of myoadenylate deaminase deficiency in muscle biopsies. Together, these data imply that one mutant allele is responsible for the vast majority of inherited deficiency of myoadenylate deaminase. Rare mutant alleles are likely, however, based on a report of an asymptomatic, deficient subject who is only a carrier of the C → T transition.[49]

While providing a molecular explanation for the common metabolic myopathy associated with an inherited deficiency of myoadenylate deaminase, these studies also have identified a much larger group of individuals with the same defect in the AMPD1 gene who are relatively asymptomatic. The disparity in frequency of the mutant allele and the prevalence of myopathic symptoms may be explained in a number of ways: that the defect is not the primary cause of the muscle dysfunction seen in individuals with this inherited defect; that some compensating mechanism protects some individuals from the harmful effects of this mutation; or that there is another unidentified factor that, together with the inherited defect in the AMPD1 gene, causes myopathic symptoms. Although it has been referred to as simply a "harmless genetic variant,"[11,14,21] there is a wealth of information supporting a cause and effect relationship between an inherited deficiency of myoadenylate deaminase and myopathic symptoms. Furthermore, amelioration of symptoms caused by the nonsense mutation in the AMPD1 gene may have a demonstrable molecular basis. For example, exon 2 of the AMPD1 gene is alternatively spliced (see "AMP Deaminase Genes and Transcripts," above); excision of exon 2 removes the C → T transition at nucleotide 34. As demonstrated in the rat,[46] the resulting exon 2 minus AMPD1 transcript encodes a catalytically active polypeptide. Thus, if a sufficient fraction of AMPD1 transcripts have exon 2 deleted, deleterious clinical consequences of this mutation may be partially or completely corrected. Furthermore, skeletal myocyte expression of other members of the AMP deaminase multigene family (i.e., AMPD3) may also affect the clinical picture of inherited myoadenylate deaminase deficiency. Molecular and cytochemical analyses have demonstrated AMPD3 expression in adult human skeletal muscle, predominantly in type I (oxidative) fibers.[85,116] Finally, assembly of hybrid AMPD1/AMPD3 tetrameric enzymes[92] may serve to maximize myoadenylate deaminase expression in deficient individuals, particularly in type I fibers. A definitive test of these hypotheses will require careful study of a number of patients and asymptomatic individuals to establish correlations between relative AMP deaminase expression and the presence and absence of clinical symptoms.

Acquired Myoadenylate Deaminase Deficiency

Molecular analyses of acquired myoadenylate deaminase deficiency remain limited. This form of the disease is proposed to have both genetic and pathologic components; that is, carriers of the AMPD1 mutant allele in whom pathological changes related to associated primary neuromuscular or rheumatologic disorders result in further reductions of enzyme activity into the deficient range.[27] Available information is consistent with this hypothesis. For example, two individuals classified as having an acquired form of the disease (i.e., secondary to inflammatory myopathy with relatively high residual AMP deaminase activity that is reactive with antimyoadenylate deaminase serum and reduced creatine kinase activity) displayed reduced levels of AMPD1 transcript as compared to controls and to patients with inherited myoadenylate deaminase deficiency.[45] Furthermore, several studies have presented data linking progressive pathologic change in numerous primary disorders of muscle with declining AMP deaminase activity[135–137] and AMPD1 transcript abundance.[137] Finally, genetic testing revealed the carrier state for the AMPD1 mutant allele in a 53-year-old woman with diagnosed fibromyalgia, type II muscle fiber atrophy, and abnormal forearm ammonia production.[55]

Coincidental Inherited Myoadenylate Deaminase Deficiency

The high frequency of the mutant allele in several populations suggests that some cases of "acquired" myoadenylate deaminase deficiency with myopathy as part of a multisystem disorder would also have a coincidental inherited deficiency of myoadenylate deaminase. This scenario has now been documented in 13 patients with a variety of associated disorders.[51–54] Notably, three of these individuals have an inherited glycolytic defect and exhibit clinical features that are more severe than expected for either condition alone.[51–53] These observations suggest that myoadenylate deaminase deficiency may have a synergistic effect in association with other metabolic disorders.

TREATMENT

No therapies are unequivocally documented to be effective in treating myoadenylate deaminase deficiency. On the basis of an initial study of muscle biopsies obtained from a single patient,[15] it was hypothesized that therapeutic programs aimed at enhancing the rate of replenishment of the ATP pool might benefit myoadenylate deaminase-deficient individuals. One approach, which was successful in increasing the rate of ATP synthesis in myocardium of the rat, is administration of ribose.[138] Ribose increases the rate of synthesis of PP-ribose-P by increasing the availability of ribose-5-phosphate. The increases in PP-ribose-P content of the cell could enhance salvage and *de novo* synthesis of purine nucleotides. Oral ribose has been administered to patients deficient in myoadenylate deaminase, reportedly leading to enhanced stamina[139] and diminished exercise-related symptoms in some[32] while being ineffective in others.[23] Although the biochemical basis for the therapeutic effect of ribose is unclear, it appears to be almost completely absorbed when administered orally[140] and to be without side effects in doses under 200 mg/kg/h.[32,140] Xylitol, which can be metabolically converted to ribose, was reportedly also beneficial when administered orally at 15 to 20 g/day to a single patient with myoadenylate deaminase deficiency.[141]

Another aspect of treatment is related to the different forms of myoadenylate deaminase deficiency. A genetic approach for managing an inherited deficiency of myoadenylate deaminase might be feasible through a clearer understanding of factors that control the alternative splicing event involving exon 2 of the AMPD1 gene. By enhancing the rate at which exon 2 is removed from the primary transcript, one could rescue individuals homozygous for the mutant allele from their clinical complications. Determining which factors control AMPD3 gene expression may also have an impact on treatment of these patients. For an acquired myoadenylate deaminase deficiency, the overwhelming nature of the associated primary neuromuscular complications will likely dictate courses of treatment of these patients.

REFERENCES

1. Lowenstein JM: Ammonia production in muscle and other tissues: The purine nucleotide cycle. *Physiol Rev* **52**:382, 1972.
2. Lowenstein JM, Goodman MN: The purine nucleotide cycle in skeletal muscle. *Fed Proc* **37**:2308, 1978.
3. Aragon JJ, Lowenstein JM: The purine nucleotide cycle: Comparison of the levels of citric acid cycle intermediates with the operation of the purine nucleotide cycle in rat skeletal muscle during exercise and recovery from exercise. *Eur J Biochem* **110**:371, 1980.
4. Goodman MN, Lowenstein JM: The purine nucleotide cycle: Studies of ammonia production by skeletal muscle in situ and in perfused preparations. *J Biol Chem* **252**:5054, 1977.
5. Meyer RA, Terjung RL: Differences in ammonia and adenylate metabolism in contracting fast and slow muscle. *Am J Physiol* **237**:C111, 1979.
6. Meyer RA, Terjung RL: AMP deamination and IMP reamination in working skeletal muscle. *Am J Physiol* **239**:C32, 1980.
7. Meyer RA, Dudley GA, Terjung RL: Ammonia and IMP in different skeletal muscle fibers after exercise in rats. *J Appl Physiol* **49**:1037, 1980.
8. Brooke MH, Choski R, Kaiser KK: Inosine monophosphate production is proportional to muscle force in vitro. *Neurology* **36**:288, 1986.
9. Fishbein WN, Armbrustmacher VW, Griffin JL: Myoadenylate deaminase deficiency: A new disease of muscle. *Science* **200**:545, 1978.
10. Engel AG, Potter CS, Rosevear JW: Nucleotides and adenosine monophosphate deaminase activity of muscle in primary hypokalaemic periodic paralysis. *Nature* **202**:670, 1964.
11. Schumate JB, Katnik R, Ruiz M, Kaiser K, Frieden C, Brooke MH, Carroll JE: Myoadenylate deaminase deficiency. *Muscle Nerve* **2**:213, 1979.
12. Fishbein WN, Griffin JL, Magarajan K, Winkert JW, Armbrustmacher VW: Myoadenylate deaminase deficiency: Association with collagen disease. *Clin Res* **27**:37A, 1979.
13. DiMauro S, Miranda AF, Hays AP, Franck WA, Hoffman GS, Schoenfeldt RS, Singh N: Myoadenylate deaminase deficiency: Muscle biopsy and muscle culture in a patient with gout. *J Neurol Sci* **47**:191, 1980.
14. Schumate JB, Kaiser KK, Carroll JE, Brooke MH: Adenylate deaminase deficiency in a hypotonic infant. *J Pediatr* **96**:885, 1980.
15. Sabina RL, Swain JL, Patten BM, Ashizawa T, O'Brien WE, Holmes EW: Disruption of the purine nucleotide cycle: A potential explanation for muscle dysfunction in myoadenylate deaminase deficiency. *J Clin Invest* **66**:1419, 1980.
16. Heffner RR: Myoadenylate deaminase deficiency. *J Neuropathol Exper Neurol* **39**:360, 1980.
17. Merceles R, Martin JJ, DeHaene I, DeBarsy TH, Van den Berghe G: Myoadenylate deaminase deficiency in a patient with facial and limb girdle myopathy. *J Neurol* **225**:157, 1981.
18. Scholte HR, Busch HFM, Luyt-Houwen IEM: Familial AMP deaminase deficiency with skeletal muscle type I atrophy and fatal cardiomyopathy. *J Inherit Metab Dis* **4**:169, 1981.
19. Kar NC, Pearson CM: Muscle adenylate deaminase deficiency: Report of six new cases. *Arch Neurol* **38**:279, 1981.
20. Keleman J, Rice DR, Bradley WG, Munsat TL, DiMauro S, Hogan EL: Familial myoadenylate deaminase deficiency and exertional myalgia. *Neurology* **32**:857, 1982.
21. Hayes DI, Summers BA, Morgan-Hughes JA: Myoadenylate deaminase deficiency or not? Observations on two brothers with exercise-induced muscle pain. *J Neurol Sci* **53**:125, 1982.
22. Patterson VH, Kaiser KK, Brooke MH: Exercising muscle does not produce hypoxanthine in adenylate deaminase deficiency. *Neurology* **33**:784, 1983.
23. Lecky BRF: Failure of D-ribose in myoadenylate deaminase deficiency. *Lancet* **1**:193, 1983.
24. Sabina RL, Swain JL, Olanow CW, Bradley WG, Fishbein WN, DiMauro S, Holmes EW: Myoadenylate deaminase deficiency: Functional and metabolic abnormalities associated with disruption of the purine nucleotide cycle. *J Clin Invest* **73**:720, 1984.
25. Gertler PA, Jacobs RP: Myoadenylate deaminase deficiency in a patient with progressive systemic sclerosis. *Arthritis Rheum* **27**:586, 1984.
26. Raivio KO, Santavuori P, Somer H: Metabolism of AMP in muscle extracts from patients with deficient activity of myoadenylate deaminase. *Adv Exp Med Biol* **165**:431, 1984.
27. Fishbein WN: Myoadenylate deaminase deficiency: Inherited and acquired forms. *Biochem Med* **33**:158, 1985.
28. Fishbein WN, Muldoon SM, Deuster PA, Armbrustmacher VW: Myoadenylate deaminase deficiency and malignant hypothermia susceptibility: Is there a relationship? *Biochem Med* **34**:344, 1985.
29. Lally EV, Friedman JH, Kaplan SR: Progressive myalgias and polyarthralgias in a patient with myoadenylate deaminase deficiency. *Arthritis Rheum* **28**:1298, 1985.
30. Ashwal S, Peckham N: Myoadenylate deaminase deficiency in children. *Pediatr Neurol* **1**:185, 1985.

31. Goebel HH, Bardosi A, Conrad B, Kuhlendahl HD, DiMauro S, Rumpf KW: Myoadenylate deaminase deficiency. *Klin Wochenschr* **64**:342, 1986.
32. Zollner N, Reiter S, Gross M, Pongratz D, Reimers CD, Gerbitz K, Paetzke I, Deufel T, Hubner G: Myoadenylate deaminase deficiency: Successful symptomatic therapy by high-dose oral administration of ribose. *Klin Wochenschr* **64**:1281, 1986.
33. Sinkeler SPT, Joosten EMG, Wevers RA, Binkhorst RA, Oerlemans FT, van Bennekom CA, Coerwinkel MM, Oei TL: Ischaemic exercise test in myoadenylate deaminase deficiency and McArdle's disease: Measurement of plasma adenosine, inosine and hypoxanthine. *Clin Sci* **70**:399, 1986.
34. Heller SL, Kaiser KK, Planer GJ, Hagberg JM, Brooke MH: McArdle's disease with myoadenylate deaminase deficiency: Observations in a combined enzyme deficiency. *Neurology* **37**:1039, 1987.
35. Sinkeler SPT: Myoadenylate deaminase deficiency: A study of its clinical significance. Dissertation, University of Nijmegen, The Netherlands, 1987.
36. Sinkeler SPT, Binkhorst RA, Joosten EMG, Wevers RA, Coerwinkel MM, Oei TL: AMP deaminase deficiency: Study of the human skeletal muscle purine metabolism during ischaemic isometric exercise. *Clin Sci* **72**:475, 1987.
37. Valen PA, Nakayama DA, Veum J, Sulaiman AR, Wortmann RL: Myoadenylate deaminase deficiency and forearm ischemic exercise testing. *Arthritis Rheum* **30**:661, 1987.
38. Mercelis R, Martin J-J, de Barsy T, Van den Berghe G: Myoadenylate deaminase deficiency: Absence of correlation with exercise intolerance in 452 muscle biopsies. *J Neurol* **234**:385, 1987.
39. Sinkeler SPT, Joosten EMG, Wevers RA, Oei TL, Jacobs AEM, Veerkamp JH, Hamel BCJ: Myoadenylate deaminase deficiency: A clinical, genetic, and biochemical study in nine families. *Muscle Nerve* **11**:312, 1988.
40. Tonin P, Lewis P, Servidei S, DiMauro S: Metabolic causes of myoglobinuria. *Ann Neurol* **27**:181, 1990.
41. Gross M, Morisaki T, Pongratz D, Holmes EW, Zollner N: Normal restriction pattern (*Hin*dIII) of the myoadenylate deaminase gene in enzyme deficient patients. *Klin Wochenschr* **68**:1084, 1990.
42. Kaletha K, Nowak G: Myoadenylate deaminase deficiency: Studies on normal and deaminase-deficient skeletal muscle. *Clin Chim Acta* **190**:147, 1990.
43. Wagner DR, Felbel J, Gresser U, Zollner N: Muscle metabolism and red cell ATP/ADP concentration during bicycle ergometer in patients with AMPD-deficiency. *Klin Wochenschr* **69**:251, 1991.
44. Zimmer C, Altenkirch H, Dorfmuller-Kuchlin S, Pongratz D, Paetzke I, Gosztonyi G: Type 2a fibre rhabdomyolysis in myoadenylate deaminase deficiency. *J Neurol* **238**:31, 1991.
45. Sabina RL, Fishbein WN, Pezeshkpour G, Clarke PRH, Holmes EW: Molecular analysis of the myoadenylate deaminase deficiencies. *Neurology* **42**:170, 1992.
46. Morisaki T, Gross M, Morisaki H, Pongratz D, Zollner N, Holmes EW: Molecular basis of AMP deaminase deficiency in skeletal muscle. *Proc Natl Acad Sci U S A* **89**:6457, 1992.
47. Caradonna P, Gentiloni N, Servidei S, Perrone GA, Greco AV, Russo MA: Acute myopathy associated with chronic licorice ingestion: Reversible loss of myoadenylate deaminase activity. *Ultrastruct Pathol* **16**:529, 1992.
48. Gross M: Clinical heterogeneity and molecular mechanisms in inborn muscle AMP deaminase deficiency. *J Inherit Metab Dis* **20**:186, 1997.
49. Norman B, Mahnke-Zizelman DK, Vallis A, Sabina RL: Genetic and other determinants of AMP deaminase activity in healthy adult skeletal muscle. *J Appl Physiol* **85**:1273, 1998.
50. Sabina RL: Myoadenylate deaminase deficiency, in Rosenberg RN, Prusiner SB, DiMauro S, Barchi RL, Kunkel LM (eds): *The Molecular and Genetic Basis of Neurological Disease*. Boston, London, Butterworth-Heinemann, 1993, p 261.
51. Tsujino S, Shanske S, Carroll JE, Sabina RL, DiMauro S: Double trouble: Combined myophosphorylase and AMP deaminase deficiency in a child homozygous for nonsense mutations at both loci. *Neuromusc Disord* **5**:263, 1995.
52. Rubio JC, Martin MA, Bautista J, Campos Y, Segura D, Arenas J: Association of genetically proven deficiencies of myophosphorylase and AMP deaminase: A second case of double trouble. *Neuromusc Disord* **7**:387, 1997.
53. Bruno C, Minetti C, Shanske S, Morreale G, Bado M, Cordone G, DiMauro S: Combined defects of muscle phosphofructokinase and AMP deaminase in a child with myoglobinuria. *Neurology* **50**:296, 1998.
54. Verzijl HTFM, van Engelen BGM, Luyten JAFM, Steenbergen GCH, van den Heuvel LPWJ, ter Laak HJ, Padberg GW, Wevers RA: Genetic characteristics of myoadenylate deaminase deficiency. *Ann Neurol* **44**:140, 1998.
55. Marin R, Connick E: Tension myalgia versus myoadenylate deaminase deficiency: A case report. *Arch Phys Med Rehabil* **78**:95, 1997.
56. Flanagan WF, Holmes EW, Sabina RL, Swain JL: Importance of the purine nucleotide cycle to energy production in skeletal muscle. *Am J Physiol* **251**:C795, 1986.
57. Sabina RL, Morisaki T, Clarke P, Eddy R, Shows TB, Morton CC, Holmes EW: Characterization of the human and rat myoadenylate deaminase genes. *J Biol Chem* **265**:9423, 1990.
58. Loh E, Rebbeck TR, Mahoney PD, DeNofrio D, Swain JL, Holmes EW: A common variant in the AMPD1 gene predicts prolonged survival in patients with heart failure. *Circulation* **29**:1422, 1999.
59. Bangsbo J, Graham T, Johansen L, Strange S, Christensen C, Saltin B: Elevated muscle acidity and energy production during exhaustive exercise in humans. *Am J Physiol* **263:R891, 1992.**
60. Manfredi JP, Holmes EW: Control of the purine nucleotide cycle in extracts of rat skeletal muscle: Effects of energy state and concentrations of cycle intermediates. *Arch Biochem Biophys* **233**:515, 1984.
61. Sahlin K, Palmskog G, Hultman E: Adenine nucleotide and IMP content of the quadriceps muscle in man after exercise. *Pflugers Arch* **374**:193, 1978.
62. Hettleman BD, Sabina RL, Drezner MK, Holmes EW, Swain JL: Defective adenosine triphosphate synthesis: An explanation for skeletal muscle dysfunction in phosphate-deficient mice. *J Clin Invest* **72**:582, 1983.
63. Wilkerson JE, Batterton DL, Horvath SM: Exercise-induced changes in blood ammonia levels in humans. *Eur J Appl Physiol* **37**:255, 1977.
64. Babij P, Matthews SM, Rennie MJ: Changes in blood ammonia, lactate, and amino acids in relation to workload during bicycle ergometer exercise in man. *Eur J Appl Physiol* **50**:405, 1983.
65. Banister EW, Allen ME, Mekjavic IB, Singh AK, Legge B, Mutch BJC: The time course of ammonia and lactate accumulation in blood during bicycle exercise. *Eur J Appl Physiol* **51**:195, 1983.
66. Katz A, Broberg S, Sahlin K, Wahren J: Muscle ammonia and amino acid metabolism during dynamic exercise in man. *Clin Physiol* **6**:365, 1986.
67. Tornheim K, Lowenstein JM: The purine nucleotide cycle: Interactions with oscillations of the glycolytic pathway in muscle extracts. *J Biol Chem* **249**:3241, 1974.
68. Tornheim K, Lowenstein JM: The purine nucleotide cycle: Control of phosphofructokinase and glycolytic oscillations in muscle extracts. *J Biol Chem* **250**:6304, 1975.
69. Aragon JJ, Tornheim K, Lowenstein JM: On a possible role of IMP in the regulation of phosphorylase activity in skeletal muscle. *FEBS Lett* **117**:suppl K56, 1980.
70. Scislowski PWD, Aleksandrowicz Z, Swierczynski J: Purine nucleotide cycle as a possible anaplerotic process in rat skeletal muscle. *Experientia* **38**:1035, 1982.
71. Swain JL, Hines JJ, Sabina RL, Harbury OL, Holmes EW: Disruption of the purine nucleotide cycle by inhibition of adenylosuccinate lyase produces skeletal muscle dysfunction. *J Clin Invest* **74**:1422, 1984.
72. Ogasawara N, Goto H, Yamada Y, Watanabe T, Asano T: AMP deaminase isozymes in human tissues. *Biochim Biophys Acta* **714**:298, 1982.
73. Fishbein WN, David JI, Nagarajon K, Winkert JW, Foellmer JW: Immunologic distinction of human muscle adenylate deaminase from the isozyme in human peripheral blood cells: Implications for myoadenylate deaminase deficiency. *Arch Biochem Biophys* **205**:360, 1980.
74. Ogasawara N, Goto H, Watanabe T: Isozymes of rat AMP deaminase. *Biochim Biophys Acta* **403**:530, 1975.
75. Ogasawara N, Goto H, Yasukazu Y, Watanabe T: Distribution of AMP-deaminase isozymes in rat tissue. *Eur J Biochem* **87**:297, 1978.
76. Kendrick-Jones J, Perry SV: The enzymes of adenine nucleotide metabolism in developing skeletal muscle. *Biochem J* **103**:207, 1967.
77. Sammons DW, Chilson OP: AMP deaminase: Stage-specific isoenzymes in differentiating chick muscle. *Arch Biochem Biophys* **191**:561, 1978.
78. Kaletha K: Regulatory properties of 14-day embryo and adult hen skeletal muscle AMP deaminase. *Biochim Biophys Acta* **759**:99, 1983.
79. Kaletha K, Skladanowski A: Regulatory properties of 14-day embryo and adult hen heart AMP deaminase. *Int J Biochem* **16**:75, 1984.
80. Spychala J, Kaletha K, Makarewicz W: Developmental changes of chicken liver AMP deaminase. *Biochem J* **231**:329, 1985.

81. Kaletha K, Spychala J, Nowak G: Developmental forms of human skeletal muscle AMP-deaminase. *Experientia* **43**:440, 1987.
82. Marquetant R, Desai NM, Sabina RL, Holmes EW: Evidence for sequential expression of multiple AMP deaminase isoforms during skeletal muscle development. *Proc Natl Acad Sci U S A* **84**:2345, 1987.
83. Sabina RL, Ogasawara N, Holmes EW: Expression of three stage-specific transcripts of AMP deaminase during myogenesis. *Mol Cell Biol* **9**:2244, 1989.
84. Winder WW, Terjung RL, Baldwin KM, Holloszy JO: Effect of exercise on AMP deaminase and adenylosuccinase in rat skeletal muscle. *Am J Physiol* **227**:1411, 1974.
85. van Kuppevelt THv, Veerkamp JH, Fishbein WN, Ogasawara N, Sabina RL: Immunolocalization of AMP-deaminase isozymes in human skeletal muscle and cultured muscle cells: Concentration of isoform M at the neuromuscular junction. *J Histochem Cytochem* **42**:861, 1994.
86. Katz A, Sahlin K, Henriksson J: Muscle ammonia metabolism during isometric contraction in humans. *Am J Physiol* **250**:C834, 1986.
87. Dudley GA, Staron RS, Murray TF, Hagerman FC, Luginbuhl A: Muscle fiber composition and blood ammonia levels after intense exercise in humans. *J Appl Physiol* **54**:582, 1983.
88. Jacobs AEM, Oosterhof A, Benders AAGM, Veerkamp JH: Expression of different isoenzymes of adenylate deaminase in cultured human muscle cells. Relation to myoadenylate deaminase deficiency. *Biochim Biophys Acta* **1139**:91, 1992.
89. Coffee CJ, Kofke WA: Rat muscle 5′-adenylic acid aminohydrolase. I. Purification and subunit structure. *J Biol Chem* **250**:6653, 1975.
90. Boosman A, Chilson OP: Subunit structure of AMP-deaminase from chicken and rabbit skeletal muscle. *J Biol Chem* **251**:1847, 1976.
91. Stankiewicz A: AMP-deaminase from human skeletal muscle: Subunit structure, amino acid composition, and metal content of the homogeneous enzyme. *Int J Biochem* **13**:1177, 1981.
92. Mahnke-Zizelman DK, Tullson PC, Sabina RL: Novel aspects of tetramer assembly and N-terminal domain structure and function are revealed by recombinant expression of human AMP deaminase isoforms. *J Biol Chem* **273**:35118, 1998.
93. Marquetant R, Sabina RL, Holmes EW: Identification of a noncatalytic domain in AMP deaminase that influences binding to myosin. *Biochemistry* **28**:8744, 1989.
94. Sabina RL, Marquetant R, Desai NM, Kaletha K, Holmes EW: Cloning and sequence of rat myoadenylate deaminase cDNA: Evidence for tissue-specific and developmental regulation. *J Biol Chem* **262**:12397, 1987.
95. Tovmasian EK, Hairapetian RL, Bykova EV, Severin SE, Haroutunian AV: Phosphorylation of the skeletal muscle AMP-deaminase by protein kinase C. *FEBS Lett* **259**:321, 1990.
96. Ashby B, Frieden C, Bischoff R: Immunofluorescent and histochemical localization of AMP deaminase in skeletal muscle. *J Cell Biol* **81**:361, 1979.
97. Ashby B, Frieden C: Interaction of AMP aminohydrolase with myosin and its subfragments. *J Biol Chem* **252**:1869, 1977.
98. Solano C, Coffee CJ: Differential response of AMP deaminase isoenzymes to changes in the adenylate energy charge. *Biochem Biophys Res Commun* **85**:564, 1978.
99. Ashby B, Frieden C: Adenylate deaminase. Kinetic and binding studies on the rabbit muscle enzyme. *J Biol Chem* **253**:8728, 1978.
100. Wheeler TJ, Lowenstein JM: Adenylate deaminase from rat muscle: Regulation by purine nucleotides and orthophosphate in the presence of 150 mM KCl. *J Biol Chem* **254**:8994, 1979.
101. Sutton JR, Toews CJ, Ward GR, Fox IH: Purine metabolism during strenuous muscle exercise in man. *Metabolism* **29**:254, 1980.
102. Dudley GA, Terjung RL: Influence of acidosis on AMP deaminase activity in contracting fast-twitch muscle. *Am J Physiol* **248**: C43, 1985.
103. Solano C, Coffee CJ: Comparison of AMP deaminase from skeletal muscle of acidotic and normal rats. *Biochim Biophys Acta* **582**:369, 1979.
104. Wheeler TJ, Lowenstein JM: Creatine phosphate inhibition of adenylate deaminase is mainly due to pyrophosphate. *J Biol Chem* **254**:1484, 1979.
105. Rundell KW, Tullson PC, Terjung RL: AMP deaminase binding in contracting rat skeletal muscle. *Am J Physiol* **263**:C287, 1992.
106. Rundell KW, Tullson PC, Terjung RL: Altered kinetics of AMP deaminase by myosin binding. *Am J Physiol* **263**:C294, 1992.
107. Tullson PC, Bangsbo J, Hellsten Y, Richter EA: IMP metabolism in human skeletal muscle after exhaustive exercise. *J Appl Physiol* **78**:146, 1995.
108. Rush JWE, MacLean DA, Hultman E, Graham TE: Exercise causes branched-chain oxoacid dehydrogenase dephosphorylation but not AMP deaminase binding. *J Appl Physiol* **78**:2193, 1995.
109. Ashby B, Holmsen H: Platelet AMP deaminase: Purification and kinetic studies. *J Biol Chem* **256**:10519, 1981.
110. Bausch-Jurken MT, Mahnke-Zizelman DK, Morisaki T, Sabina RL: Molecular cloning of AMP deaminase isoform L: Sequence and bacterial expression of human AMPD2 cDNA. *J Biol Chem* **267**:22407, 1992.
111. Ogasawara N, Goto H, Yamada Y, Nishigaki I, Itoh T, Hasegawa I: Complete deficiency of AMP deaminase in human erythrocytes. *Biochem Biophys Res Commun* **122**:1344, 1984.
112. Ogasawara N, Goto H, Yamada Y, Nishigaki I, Itoh T, Hasegawa I, Park KS: Deficiency of AMP deaminase in erythrocytes. *Hum Genet* **75**:15, 1987.
113. Yamada Y, Goto H, Ogasawara N: A point mutation responsible for human erythrocyte AMPD deaminase deficiency. *Hum Mol Genet* **3**:331, 1994.
114. Fishbein WN, Sabina RL, Ogasawara N, Holmes EW: Immunologic evidence for three isoforms of AMP deaminase (AMPD) in mature skeletal muscle. *Biochim Biophys Acta* **1163**:97, 1993.
115. Yun S-L, Suelter CH: Human erythrocyte 5′-AMP aminohydrolase: Purification and characterization. *J Biol Chem* **253**:404, 1978.
116. Mahnke-Zizelman DK, Sabina RL: Cloning of human AMP deaminase isoform E cDNAs: Evidence for a third AMPD gene exhibiting alternatively spliced 5′-exons. *J Biol Chem* **267**:20866, 1992.
117. Meyer SL, Kvalnes-Krick KL, Schramm VL: Characterization of AMD, the AMP deaminase gene in yeast. Production of AMP strain, cloning, nucleotide sequence, and properties of the protein. *Biochemistry* **28**:8734, 1989.
118. Morisaki T, Sabina RL, Holmes EW: Adenylate deaminase: A multigene family in humans and rats. *J Biol Chem* **265**:11482, 1990.
119. Wang X, Morisaki H, Sermsuvitayawong K, Mineo I, Toyama K, Ogasawara N, Mukai T, Morisaki T: Cloning and expression of cDNA encoding heart-type isoform of AMP deaminase. *Gene* **188**:285, 1997.
120. Mahnke-Zizelman DK, D'Cunha J, Wojnar JM, Brogley MA, Sabina RL: Regulation of rat AMP deaminase 3 (isoform C) by development and skeletal muscle fibre type. *Biochem J* **326**:521, 1997.
121. Chang Z, Nygaard P, Chinault AC, Kellems RE: Deduced amino acid sequence of *Escherichia coli* adenosine deaminase reveals evolutionarily conserved amino acid residues: Implications for catalytic function. *Biochemistry* **30**:2273, 1991.
122. Wilson DK, Rudolph FB, Quiocho FA: Atomic structure of adenosine deaminase complexed with a transition-state analog: Understanding catalysis and immunodeficiency mutations. *Science* **252**:1278, 1991.
123. Gross M, Morisaki H, Morisaki T, Holmes EW: Identification of functional domains in AMPD1 by mutational analysis. *Biochem Biophys Res Comm* **205**:1010, 1995.
124. Bausch-Jurken MT, Sabina RL: Divergent N-terminal regions of AMP deaminase and isoform-specific properties of the enzyme. *Arch Biochem Biophys* **321**:372, 1994.
125. Morisaki T, Holmes EW: Functionally distinct elements are required for expression of the AMPD1 gene in myocytes. *Mol Cell Biol* **13**:5853, 1993.
126. Mineo I, Clarke PRH, Sabina RL, Holmes EW: A novel pathway for alternative splicing: Identification of an RNA intermediate that generates an alternative 5′ splice donor site not present in the primary transcript of AMPD1. *Mol Cell Biol* **10**:5271, 1990.
127. Mineo I, Holmes EW: Exon recognition and nucleocytoplasmic partitioning determine AMPD1 alternative transcript production. *Mol Cell Biol* **11**:5356, 1991.
128. Morisaki H, Morisaki T, Newby LK, Holmes EW: Alternative splicing: A mechanism for phenotypic rescue of a common inherited defect. *J Clin Invest* **91**:2275, 1993.
129. Hisatome I, Morisaki T, Kamma H, Sugama T, Morisaki H, Ohtahara A, Holmes EW: Control of AMP deaminase 1 binding to myosin heavy chain. *Am J Physiol* **275**:C870, 1998.
130. Van den Bergh F, Sabina RL: Characterization of human AMP deaminase 2 (AMPD2) gene expression reveals alternative transcripts encoding variable N-terminal extensions of isoform L. *Biochem J* **312**:401, 1995.
131. Mahnke-Zizelman DK, Van den Bergh F, Bausch-Jurken MT, Eddy R, Sait S, Shows TB, Sabina RL: Cloning, sequence and characterization of the human AMPD2 gene: Evidence for transcriptional

regulation by two closely spaced promoters. *Biochim Biophys Acta* **1308**:122, 1996.

132. Mahnke-Zizelman DK, Eddy R, Shows TB, Sabina RL: Characterization of the human AMPD3 gene reveals that 5′ exon usage is subject to transcriptional control by three tandem promoters and alternative splicing. *Biochim Biophys Acta* **1306**:75, 1996.
133. Gross M: New method for detection of C34-T mutation in the AMPD1 gene causing myoadenylate deaminase deficiency. *Ann Rheum Dis* **53**:353, 1994.
134. Fishbein WN, Davis JI, Foellmer JW, Nieves S, Merezhinskaya N: A competitive allele-specific oligomers polymerase chain reaction assay for the *cis* double mutation in AMPD1 that is the major cause of myoadenylate deaminase deficiency. *Mol Diagn* **2**:121, 1997.
135. Kar NC, Pearson CM: Muscle adenylic acid deaminase activity: Selective decrease in early-onset Duchenne muscular dystrophy. *Neurology* **23**:478, 1973.
136. Nagao H, Habara S, Morimoto T, Sano N, Takahashi M, Kida K, Matsuda H, Nonaka I: AMP deaminase activity of skeletal muscle in neuromuscular disorders in childhood. *Neuropediatrics* **17**:193, 1986.
137. Sabina RL, Sulaiman AR, Wortmann RL: Molecular analysis of acquired myoadenylate deaminase deficiency in polymyositis (idiopathic inflammatory myopathy). *Adv Exp Med Biol* **309B**:203, 1991.
138. Zimmer HG, Gerlach E: Stimulation of myocardial adenine nucleotide biosynthesis by pentoses and pentitols. *Pflugers Arch* **376**:223, 1978.
139. Patten BM: Beneficial effect of D-ribose in a patient with myoadenylate deaminase deficiency. *Lancet* **1**:1071, 1982.
140. Gross M, Reiter S, Zollner N: Metabolism of D-ribose administered continuously to healthy persons and to patients with myoadenylate deaminase deficiency. *Klin Wochenschr* **67**:1205, 1989.
141. Bruyland M, Ebinger G: Beneficial treatment with xylitol in a patient with myoadenylate deaminase deficiency. *Clin Neuropharm* **17**:492, 1994.

CHAPTER 111

Xanthine Oxidoreductase—Role in Human Pathophysiology and in Hereditary Xanthinuria

Kari O. Raivio ▪ Mika Saksela ▪ Risto Lapatto

1. **Xanthine oxidoreductase (XOR) catalyzes the final reactions of the purine catabolic pathway, oxidizing hypoxanthine to xanthine and xanthine to uric acid. Inherited deficiency of the enzyme results in xanthinuria (MIM 278300), which is usually clinically mild or asymptomatic. Precipitation of xanthine in the urinary tract or muscle may give rise to the most common symptoms, urolithiasis (with secondary renal damage) and muscle pain. Biochemically the disease is characterized by low uric acid and elevated xanthine in plasma and urine. Xanthinuria is an autosomal recessive disease.**
2. **In addition to hypoxanthine and xanthine, XOR oxidizes adenine, 6-mercaptopurine, and allopurinol; a number of pyrimidines, aldehydes, and pterins are also substrates. Under physiological conditions, XOR functions mainly as a dehydrogenase, with NAD^+ as the cosubstrate, but it can be converted into an oxidase, which utilizes molecular oxygen as the cosubstrate and produces hydrogen peroxide and superoxide. The enzyme may also form nitric oxide by reducing nitrite or by cleaving nitrosothiols. The K_m values of both the dehydrogenase and the oxidase for the purine substrates are in the range of 10^{-6}–10^{-5} M.**
3. **Reversible conversion of xanthine dehydrogenase into oxidase occurs by sulfhydryl group oxidation, which results in loss of the NAD^+ binding site. Irreversible proteolytic conversion into oxidase occurs upon enzyme purification, tissue ischemia, or treatment with proteolytic enzymes. In cell and tissue extracts, 7–35 percent of total enzyme activity is accounted for by the oxidase. Inactive enzyme forms include desulfo-XOR and demolybdo-XOR.**
4. **The human XOR gene is located on chromosome 2p22, spans at least 60 kb, and consists of 36 exons and 35 introns. The cDNA for human xanthine dehydrogenase corresponds to a polypeptide of 1333 amino acids, with a predicted molecular weight of ~146 kDa. Purified human XOR is a dimer of two identical subunits of ~150 kDa. Each subunit consists of three domains, cleavable by proteolysis but remaining associated under nondenaturing conditions. The N-terminal 20-kDa domain contains two nonidentical Fe-S centers, the middle 40-kDa domain contains an FAD center, and the C-terminal 85-kDa domain contains molybdenum bound to a cofactor. Catalysis is initiated by the transfer of two electrons to the Mo(VI) atom, followed by intramolecular electron transfer to the Fe-S centers and finally to FAD, which is then oxidized by either NAD^+ or oxygen. Allopurinol inhibits the enzyme after being converted into oxypurinol, which binds tightly to the molybdenum center.**
5. **Enzyme activity, immunoreactive protein, and mRNA of XOR are abundantly expressed in human proximal small intestine and liver; low activity is inconsistently present in kidney and lung. Immunohistochemistry shows expression in intestinal epithelial cells and hepatocytes, faintly in other organs' capillary endothelial cells. Resting mammary epithelium contains enzyme protein, which increases during lactation. No activity, protein, or mRNA can be detected in human myocardium or brain. Basal expression is increased during hypoxia by posttranslational mechanisms. Hyperoxia suppresses enzyme activity by inactivation of the enzyme protein and by inhibition of transcription. Several cytokines (e.g., γ-interferon) activate transcription. Nitric oxide donors and NO itself suppress XOR activity.**
6. **Xanthine oxidase has been ascribed a role in ischemia-reperfusion damage. Hypoxanthine and xanthine accumulate during ischemia, and a burst of oxidants is produced upon reperfusion. This phenomenon, and the attendant tissue injury, can be alleviated by allopurinol or inactivation of XOR by tungsten pretreatment. Clinical trials giving allopurinol to patients undergoing coronary bypass surgery support the role of XOR in reperfusion injury, but it is unlikely that conversion of dehydrogenase to oxidase is required. The product of XOR, uric acid, has been proposed to be a physiological antioxidant.**
7. **Human aldehyde oxidase is closely related to XOR but functions only as an oxidase. The predicted amino acid sequences are 49 percent homologous; both enzymes contain similar molybdenum, FAD, and Fe-S centers; and the intron-exon structures are almost identical, but the regulatory 5′-flanking regions are different. The substrate specificity of the two enzymes overlap widely, N^1-methylnicotinamide being relatively specific for aldehyde oxidase and hypoxanthine or xanthine for XOR. Aldehyde oxidase is expressed at a high level in the liver and lung but at a low level in the intestine.**
8. **Hereditary xanthinuria (MIM 278300) results from a genetic deficiency of XOR (type I) or both XOR and aldehyde oxidase (type II). The two types are clinically similar, but whereas type I patients can metabolize allopurinol, type II patients cannot. Over 100 cases have**

A list of standard abbreviations is located immediately preceding the index in each volume. Nonstandard abbreviations used in this chapter include: AR = adenosine; EPR = electron paramagnetic resonance; GR = guanosine; HXR = inosine; TNF- = tumor necrosis factor ; XMP = xanthosine monophosphate; XOR = xanthine oxidoreductase; XR = xanthosine.

been reported, roughly equally divided between type I and type II. Less than half of the patients have symptoms, which are caused by deposition of xanthine in the urinary tract, resulting in hematuria or renal colic and rarely in acute renal failure or chronic complications related to urolithiasis. Muscle pains due to xanthine deposition occur in a minority of cases. Plasma uric acid is below 5 μM and plasma xanthine over 10 μM. The urinary excretion of uric acid is low or unmeasurable and that of xanthine is elevated. Treatment consists of a low-purine diet and high fluid intake.

9. **Xanthinuria is inherited in an autosomal recessive manner. A single-nucleotide mutation responsible for type I disease has been characterized in four Japanese patients and results in a nonsense mutation. In type II xanthinuria, the mutation may be not in the structural gene of either XOR or aldehyde oxidase but possibly in the mechanism responsible for inserting the essential sulfur atom into the active centers of both enzymes.**

Hereditary xanthinuria was originally described as a benign disorder of purine metabolism caused by a genetic defect in the enzyme xanthine oxidoreductase (XOR). Subsequent studies have revealed that XOR deficiency may either be isolated or occur in combination with defects in two other molybdoenzymes, aldehyde oxidase and sulfite oxidase. A combined loss of xanthine and aldehyde oxidases results in a clinical disease that is similar to isolated XOR deficiency and is known as xanthinuria type II. In contrast, combined deficiency of all three molybdoenzymes is associated with a devastating disease that leads to death in infancy or early childhood. This disease is clinically similar to isolated sulfite oxidase deficiency and is caused by failure to synthesize the molybdenum cofactor common to all three oxidases. It is described in Chap. 128.

Both types of xanthinuria are rare and thus do not represent a public health problem. The disease is usually asymptomatic or benign and rarely causes severe problems for the individual. Nevertheless, XOR is the subject of considerable interest and active research because, on one hand, it is a potential source of reactive oxygen metabolites and thus a cause of cell and tissue damage. On the other hand, it produces uric acid, which is an antioxidant and thus potentially protects the organism against the adverse effects of free radicals.

CATABOLISM OF PURINES

The main physiological substrates of XOR, hypoxanthine and xanthine, are derived from the breakdown of the major purine compounds in the cell: adenine and guanine ribo- and deoxyribonucleotides and nucleic acids (Fig. 111-1). Because the energy cost of synthesizing a purine nucleotide *de novo* is six times higher, in ATP equivalents, than that of reutilizing an intact purine ring, cells have efficient mechanisms for the salvage of degraded purines. This occurs either from the nucleoside (adenosine) or from the purine base (hypoxanthine, guanine, adenine) level. Hypoxanthine is quantitatively the most important purine catabolic product formed in the cell, mainly from adenine nucleotide turnover, and it also readily diffuses out of the cell. Its main metabolic fate is phosphoribosylation to inosine 5′-monophosphate (IMP) through hypoxanthine-guanine phosphoribosyltransferase (HPRT), not oxidation to xanthine through XOR. Guanine nucleotides are catabolized to guanine, which is also effectively salvaged by HPRT. However, many cells also contain an active guanase, which deaminates guanine to xanthine. Since xanthine is not well reutilized, this pathway of guanine nucleotide catabolism appears to be the main source of substrate for XOR.

Under a number of conditions the production of purine catabolites, and hence of substrates for XOR, is greatly increased. Cellular hypoxia prevents resynthesis of ATP and salvage of

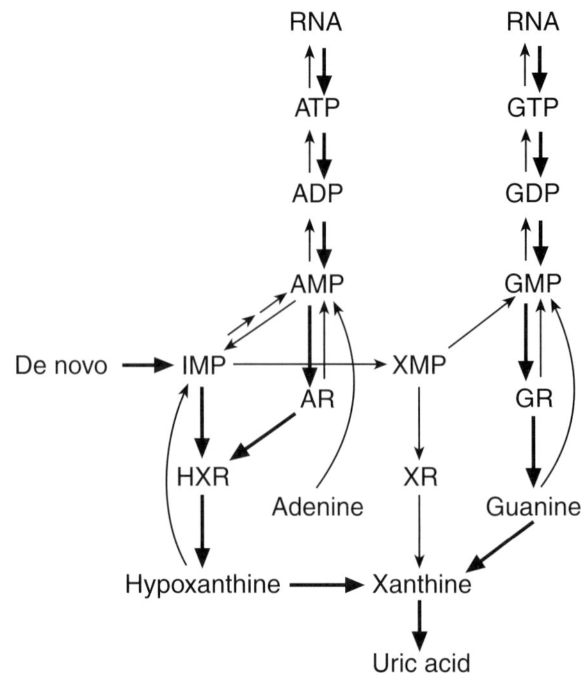

Fig. 111-1 Interconversions of purine compounds synthetized through the de novo pathway. The main catabolic routes leading to the substrates of xanthine oxidoreductase and its end product, uric acid, are indicated by thick arrows. Deoxyribose derivatives are not shown because of their minor role in purine base production. XMP = xanthosine monophosphate, XR = xanthosine, AR = adenosine, HXR = inosine, GR = guanosine.

adenosine and hypoxanthine, which are both energy-dependent processes, resulting in increased production of hypoxanthine.[1] The nucleic acids and nucleotides in dying cells are catabolized, and induction of massive cell death (e.g., at the start of intensive chemotherapy for cancer) causes a massive increase in purine catabolic products.[2] At the level of the whole organism, strenuous exercise increases adenine nucleotide turnover and hypoxanthine production. Dietary nucleic acids and other purines are degraded prior to reutilization and thus contribute to the production of hypoxanthine and xanthine.

In view of the importance of animal models for the study of genetic diseases and their pathophysiology, it must be pointed out that only in humans and higher apes is XOR the last enzyme in the purine catabolic chain and uric acid the end product. In other animals, uricase converts uric acid to allantoin and urate concentrations in the extracellular compartment are low. Although the XOR protein from mammalian sources appears quite similar to the human enzyme, its expression in cells and organs, as well as its regulation, shows marked differences between species.[3] Therefore, the role of XOR in human physiology and pathophysiology cannot be extrapolated from animal data. Neither can the potential role of uric acid as an antioxidant be deduced from animal experiments. For these reasons, this review will focus mainly on the biology and pathology of human XOR. However, since in many respects human studies are incomplete or impossible, reference will also be made to animal experiments, which must be interpreted with caution.

NORMAL HUMAN XANTHINE OXIDOREDUCTASE

Basic Reaction and Substrate Specificity

Depending on the state of the XOR protein and the availability of electron acceptors, the oxidation of hypoxanthine to xanthine

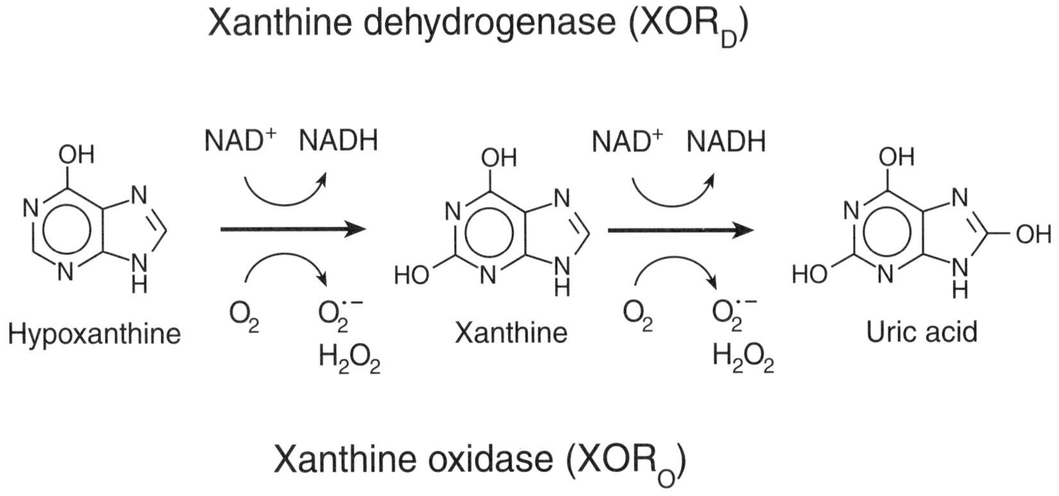

Xanthine dehydrogenase (XOR_D)

Hypoxanthine → Xanthine → Uric acid

(NAD^+ → NADH; O_2 → $O_2^{\cdot -}$, H_2O_2)

Xanthine oxidase (XOR_O)

Fig. 111-2 Basic reactions catalyzed by the dehydrogenase and oxidase forms of xanthine oxidoreductase (XOR).

and of xanthine to uric acid occurs by one of two reactions (Fig. 111-2).[4] Under physiological conditions the enzyme exists as xanthine dehydrogenase [EC 1.1.1.204] and uses NAD^+ as the electron acceptor; the reaction products are oxidized substrate and NADH.[5] Both in vivo and in vitro, the dehydrogenase can be converted into xanthine oxidase [EC 1.2.3.22], which utilizes molecular oxygen as the electron acceptor and yields, in addition to oxidized substrate, superoxide (O_2^-) and hydrogen peroxide (H_2O_2).[5]

Of the naturally occurring purine compounds, XOR oxidizes not only hypoxanthine and xanthine but also adenine (see Chap. 108). Many synthetic purine derivatives, some of which are used as drugs, bind with very low affinity to XOR and thus lack practical significance as substrates.[6] The exceptions are 6-mercaptopurine, which is the active compound derived from azathioprine, and allopurinol, which is effectively converted by the enzyme to oxypurinol, a tight-binding and virtually irreversible inhibitor of XOR.[7] Purine ribonucleosides are extremely poor substrates, 2′-deoxyribonucleosides only slightly better. In addition to purine derivatives, XOR oxidizes a variety of pyrimidines, aldehydes, and pterins. These compounds have been studied mainly by using enzyme preparations from animal sources,[8] but the substrate specificity of human XOR is generally similar to that of the enzyme from animals.[6]

NAD^+ is the physiological electron acceptor for xanthine dehydrogenase. Although this enzyme form is also able to utilize molecular oxygen,[4,9] the reaction has little importance under physiological conditions, because it is effectively inhibited by NAD^+[10] and the K_m for O_2 is fivefold higher than that of the oxidase.[11] The oxidase form is unable to use NAD^+ as the cosubstrate. Nitrosocysteine may also act as an electron acceptor, being itself decomposed to cysteine and NO in the process.[12] Another mechanism of NO formation is reduction of nitrite by xanthine oxidase, in which NADH is required as the electron donor.[13] Both enzyme forms are able to use a number of synthetic electron acceptors, including methylene blue, ferricyanide, and phenazine metho- or ethosulfate.

cDNA and Protein Structure

Crystallographic data on XOR itself are not available, but the active-site structure seems to be quite similar to that of a crystallized molybdoenzyme, aldehyde oxidoreductase from *Desulfovibrio gigas*.[14] Conventional protein studies and cloning of the cDNA[15–17] (GenBank D11456) have provided information about the structure of human XOR and allow basic conclusions concerning functional properties.

The polypeptide chain of human XOR consists of 1333 amino acids, compared with 1331 in rat,[18] 1335 in mouse,[19] and 1358 in chicken[20] liver enzymes. All the mammalian enzymes are highly homologous at the amino acid level. For example, human and rat enzymes are 90 percent and mouse and rat enzymes 94 percent homologous, whereas human and *Drosophila* enzymes are only 52 percent homologous.

The purified protein is a homodimer, consisting of identical subunits of ~150 kDa as estimated by SDS-PAGE.[6,21] The amino acid composition deduced from the cDNA sequence corresponds to a molecular mass of 146 kDa. The protein is not glycosylated.

Each subunit contains a molybdenum center, an FAD center, and two Fe-S centers.[4] Limited proteolysis of the polypeptide chain of the rat liver enzyme by trypsin, which results in conversion of dehydrogenase to active oxidase, cuts the polypeptide chain at two sites (Lys184 and Lys551). This initially produces three fragments, of 20 kDa, 40 kDa, and 85 kDa, which are not dissociated under nonreducing conditions.[18,22] A similar pattern of XOR proteolytic fragments can be seen by treatment of purified xanthine dehydrogenase in vitro with a number of proteolytic enzymes, (e.g., trypsin, chymotrypsin, subtilisin, or papain[5,18,22,23]) or spontaneously in human liver homogenates, with initial proteolysis close to the N-terminus followed by cleavage at a site further downstream.[21] However, it is likely that in most cases the degradation of the 150-kDa polypeptide represents a purification artifact.[6,24] Sequence comparisons with proteins containing similar functional groups have indicated that the N-terminal 20-kDa fragment contains the two Fe-S centers, the middle 40-kDa fragment contains the FAD center with the associated NAD^+ binding site, and the C-terminal 85-kDa fragment contains the molybdenum center.[4,16] Electron microscopy suggests that the three proteolytic fragments correspond to distinct globular structures[25] that may represent functional domains (Fig. 111-3). Although the size of the N-terminal fragment, 20 kDa, corresponds to the size of the fragment cleaved during irreversible conversion in vitro and in vivo, the relationship between nicking of the polypeptide chain at this point and modification of the NAD^+ binding site in the middle fragment is unclear.

The molybdenum is present in the form of a molybdenum cofactor, similar in structure to that in several other molybdoenzymes (see Chap. 128), and is covalently linked to two essential cysteines. The N-terminal part of the XOR molecule is rich in cystine residues, which are essential for binding the Fe atoms in the two nonidentical Fe-S centers.

Kinetics and Reaction Mechanism

Detailed kinetic studies of human XOR have not been published. However, the virtually identical primary structures and active-site conformations of the mammalian enzymes studied allow extrapolations from animal experiments.

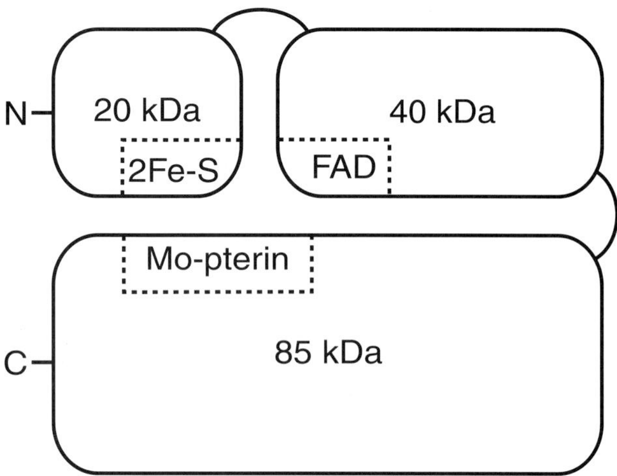

Fig. 111-3 The three structural and functional domains of xanthine oxidoreductase.

In a purified preparation from human liver, in which 90 percent of the enzyme was in the oxidase form, the estimated K_m values were 9 μM for hypoxanthine, 7 μM for xanthine, and 5 μM for adenine.[6] Approximately similar values for hypoxanthine and xanthine have been found for XOR from other sources, including an oxidase preparation from bovine milk. When the bovine milk enzyme was purified in the dehydrogenase form, the K_m for xanthine was clearly lower, at < 1 μM. The K_m for NAD^+ of the latter preparation was 7 μM, and the K_m of the oxidase form for oxygen was 53 μM.[11] This means that at normal atmospheric pressure the oxidase may not be fully saturated with its cosubstrate, which may partly account for the findings of higher activity of the oxidase form with artificial electron acceptors than with O_2. When reduced rat liver xanthine oxidase reacts with molecular oxygen, hydrogen peroxide and superoxide are produced at a molar ratio of approximately 4:1, similar to the ratio found for the human liver enzyme.[6] Xanthine dehydrogenase also reacts with O_2 and produces reactive oxygen metabolites, but its K_m is fivefold that of the oxidase (260 μM), and the reaction is strongly inhibited by NAD^+.[4,26] The dehydrogenase form is also able to oxidize NADH, with a K_m of 1.2 μM, by oxygen and yield superoxide as a by-product. This reaction occurs at the FAD site and thus is not inhibited by allopurinol or oxypurinol.[27] On the other hand, reduction of nitrite occurs at the molybdenum site, the electron donor NADH being bound at the FAD site.[13] Despite some controversial reports, inhibition of XOR by excess purine substrate or product does not seem physiologically relevant.

A large number of inhibitors of XOR have been developed, mainly to treat hyperuricemia. Allopurinol, the prime example, is readily oxidized by XOR, with a K_m of 2 μM.[7] The product, oxypurinol, has a high affinity for the reduced molybdenum site, resulting in essentially irreversible inhibition, with an overall K_i of 85 nM.[7] Diphenyliodonium acts at the flavin site, inhibiting dehydrogenase and NADH oxidizing activity.

Studies on the mechanism of the enzymatic reaction have indicated that the purine substrate is bound to the molybdenum center and donates two electrons, reducing Mo(VI) to Mo(IV). The oxygen incorporated into the oxidized substrate is derived not from the essential oxo group bound to the Mo center but from a water ligand at the molybdenum site.[28,29] After the initial reduction of the molybdenum, there is a rapid intramolecular transfer of electrons via the Fe-S clusters to the flavin center, the latter then being reoxidized by either NAD^+ or O_2. In both cases, first a bivalent and then a univalent reduction of oxygen produces H_2O_2 and superoxide[4].

Enzyme Forms and Their Interconversion

Depending on the experimental conditions, purification of mammalian xanthine oxidoreductases yields one of two interconvertible enzyme forms.[5] By rapid purification, avoidance of proteolysis, and use of dithiothreitol, the enzyme from rat liver[26] or bovine milk[11] remains in the dehydrogenase form, which is its physiological state in intact cells. Xanthine dehydrogenase can be converted into oxidase by sulfhydryl (SH) group oxidation (Fig. 111-4). Titration of bovine milk dehydrogenase with the disulfide-forming reagent 4,4′-dithiopyridine suggests that complete conversion is associated with the generation of four new disulfide bridges.[11] This alters the conformation of the enzyme protein and results in loss of the NAD^+ binding site. The process can be reversed by the SH-reducing agents dithiothreitol or β-mercaptoethanol. In the reversible conversion of rat liver xanthine dehydrogenase to oxidase, Cys535 and Cys992 are implicated.[30]

Conditions favoring reversible oxidase formation include glutathione depletion,[11,31,32] ischemia without or with reperfusion, and presence of oxidants such as hydrogen peroxide and peroxynitrite.[33] Preparation of tissue extracts for enzyme assay or purification also leads to conversion, if thiol reagents are not included in the homogenization medium. If proper precautions are taken, the proportion of the enzyme in the oxidase form in tissues from a number of animal species, including humans, varies between 7 and 35 percent. The possibility that even this residual oxidase activity is an artifact cannot be excluded.

Irreversible conversion of dehydrogenase into oxidase occurs through proteolytic cleavage of a fragment of ~20 kDa from each subunit of the dimeric enzyme,[34] followed by proteolysis further downstream, yielding additional fragments of 40 and 85 kDa.[24] This conversion may occur during extraction and purification of the enzyme as well as in cells and tissues under various pathophysiological conditions, in which irreversible conversion is preceded by an increase in reversible oxidase.[35,36] The protease responsible for the conversion in vivo has not been identified,[37–39] but a mitochondrial protease has been implicated.[24]

Although proteolysis is the basis for the irreversible dehydrogenase-to-oxidase conversion, fragments are dissociated only under reducing conditions, otherwise remaining associated with the enzyme molecule.[18] In the in vivo irreversible conversion, that is, without exogenous proteases, the fragment is cleaved from the N-terminus of the dehydrogenase molecule, between Gln183 and Lys184,[24] and subsequently further downstream, possibly at Gln550 (Fig 111-5). Although XOR, as well as other molybdoenzymes, has been relatively well conserved in evolution, both the reversible and the irreversible conversion of dehydrogenase to oxidase occur only in mammalian species. The reason may be that Cys992, which is involved in the reversible conversion, is conserved only in mammalian XORs.[30]

Cyanide treatment converts xanthine dehydrogenase into an inactive form by removing an essential sulfur atom from the molybdenum center (Fig. 111-4). This desulfo-enzyme can be partly reactivated in vitro in the presence of rhodanese plus thiosulfate and a sulfhydryl reagent[40] or of mercaptopyruvate sulfotransferase plus mercaptopyruvate. Since substantial amounts of desulfo-XOR have been found in homogenates of rat liver[41] and purified preparations from cow's milk, the desulfo-sulfo

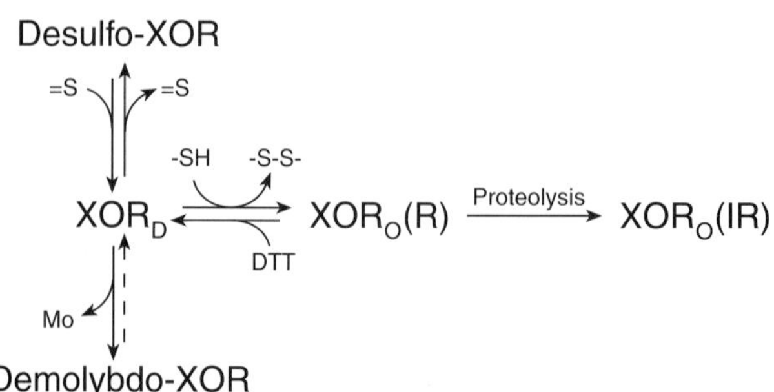

Fig. 111-4 Molecular forms of xanthine oxidoreductase (XOR). XOR_D = dehydrogenase, XOR_O(R) = reversible oxidase, XOR_O(IR) = irreversible oxidase.

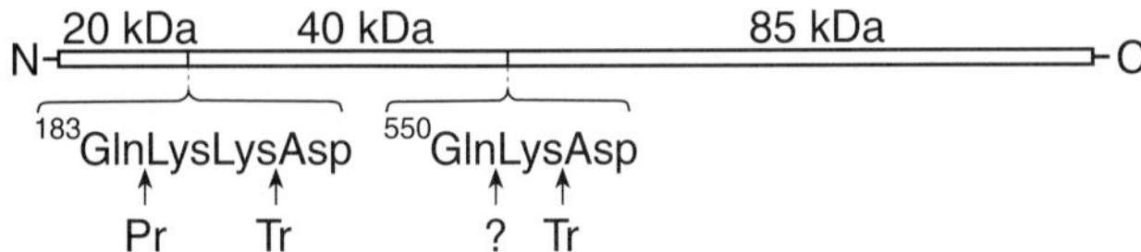

Fig. 111-5 Primary proteolytic sites of xanthine oxidoreductase. Tr = tryptic cleavage sites, Pr = cleavage site of mitochondrial protease, ? = putative cleavage site of mitochondrial protease.

interconversion may have physiological significance. In samples of human liver and intestine, specific activity is 2.7–3.0 nmol/min per milligram XOR protein, whereas in human milk, specific activity is only 20 percent of that.[21] This indicates that milk contains the enzyme mostly in inactive form. In another preparation from human milk, less than 2 percent of the enzyme was active, and a fivefold increase in activity was obtained by a resulfuration procedure.[42] XOR protein may also be inactivated by the loss of molybdenum. This may be due to a mutation (see Chap. 128) or to experimental tungsten supplementation, which results in reversible replacement of the molybdenum atom by tungsten.[43] Enzyme forms from bovine milk have been characterized that lack either just the molybdenum atom or the molybdopterin cofactor.[44] The demolybdo-enzyme is not known to have physiological significance.

The Xanthine Oxidoreductase Gene

Xanthine oxidoreductase is coded for by a single gene, located on human chromosome 2p22[45–47] and in a homologous region on mouse chromosome 21.[48] The gene has been cloned and sequenced from mouse[48] and human,[49] and data are also available on the 5′-untranslated region and the 5′-end of the rat gene.[50–51] The completely characterized mammalian genes show a complex but highly similar structure, consisting of 36 exons and 35 introns, with well-conserved splice sites, the main difference being in the length of the second intron. The genes are quite large, spanning at least 60 kb. Although the cDNA and protein sequences of mammalian and insect (*Drosophila melanogaster*,[52] *D. pseudoobscura*,[53] and *Calliphora vicina*[54]) xanthine dehydrogenases are more than 50 percent homologous, the insect genes consist of only four or five exons, with well-conserved splice sites compared with those in the mammalian genes.

The 5′-flanking region of the human XOR gene contains a number of consensus sequences of potential regulatory interest. These include binding motifs for C/EBP, NF-κB, AP-1, AP-2, ETS-1, ATF, GATA, and homeobox transcription factors, as well as responsive elements for IL-1, IL-6, TNF-α, interferon-γ, glucocorticoids, and thyroid hormones.[49] Which of these actually participate in the regulation of enzyme activity in vivo remains to be established. It should be pointed out, however, that despite the remarkable similarity in the structure of the respective genes themselves, the 5′-untranslated regions in human, rat, and mouse show a number of differences. These may account for the known differences in organ-specific expression and regulation of XOR activity between species.

Enzyme Assay

Many different assay methods for XOR activity have been described, usually to obtain an estimate of quantities of both the oxidase and the dehydrogenase forms. The significant issues concerning the assay method include preparation of samples from biologic sources, choice of substrate (natural or artificial), incubation conditions, and measurement of product. Since the effect of these variables is tissue specific, the assay should be optimized for each application.

Xanthine oxidoreductase is cytosolic and thus can be measured in high-speed supernatants of homogenized or sonicated tissues or cells. To prevent reversible conversion of dehydrogenase to oxidase, dithiothreitol should be included in the sample preparation buffer. Protease inhibitors (e.g., phenylmethylsulfonylfluoride and leupeptin) have been recommended to prevent irreversible conversion and EDTA to avoid heavy metal inhibition. Removal of low-molecular-weight inhibitors (e.g., endogenous purines) by dialysis or gel filtration may be desirable, and necessary if activity is to be measured in human plasma with a high uric acid content. The optimal pH varies between 5.6, with pterin as substrate, and 8.4, with xanthine as substrate, but the actual pH chosen will depend on whether maximal sensitivity or physiological relevance is the prime consideration.

The classic method for assaying xanthine oxidoreductase activity is spectrophotometric, using xanthine as the substrate and measuring uric acid formation at 295 nm ($\varepsilon = 1.1 \times 10^{-4}\ M^{-1}\ cm^{-1}$) in the absence (for oxidase) and presence (for dehydrogenase plus oxidase) of NAD^+. To avoid possible NADH inhibition, pyruvate and LDH can be added. Hypoxanthine, although more soluble, is not as suitable a substrate because of its two-stage oxidation and potential underestimation of enzyme activity by measurement of uric acid alone.

Since XOR activity in most human tissues is low, the sensitivity of the assay becomes an issue. By using [^{14}C]-xanthine as the substrate and separating the radioactive uric acid by HPLC for measurement, sensitivity can be substantially increased.[55]

A fluorometric enzyme assay has been developed using pterin as substrate and measuring the product isoxanthopterin.[56] Its sensitivity is about two orders of magnitude greater than that of the spectrophotometric method. In this assay, methylene blue must be used as the electron acceptor, but, at least in human liver and rat tissues, it gives results similar to those obtained with NAD^+. However, in quantitative terms, the activity levels are not comparable with those obtained with the natural substrate. Although pterin appears to be a poor substrate for aldehyde oxidase, the overlapping specificities of the molybdoenzymes make the use of physiological substrates preferable.

Cell and Organ Distribution

Marked species differences in activity of XOR, as well as in expression of its mRNA, in various organs and cells have been documented.[3] In human tissues, conflicting data have been presented, reflecting (at least in part) differences in assay methodology and specificities of antibodies or hybridization probes. Although animal data are relevant in interpreting disease models using animals, we will mainly review human studies on enzyme localization.

In human autopsy samples, substantial activity is present only in liver and small intestine.[21] In kidney and lung, low or undetectable activity is found, whereas in other organs (e.g., brain, myocardium, skeletal muscle), activity measurements are consistently negative. These findings do not rule out expression of enzyme activity in a small subpopulation of cells in these organs. Levels of immunoreactive XOR protein correlate well with enzyme activity, which suggests that substantial amounts of inactive enzyme forms are not present.[21] Enzyme activity is present in human milk, although at about two orders of magnitude lower than that in cow's milk, but most of the enzyme protein in milk from either source is inactive, presumably in the desulfo form. Normal human plasma does not contain either enzyme activity or protein.

Northern hybridization or ribonuclease protection assay of mRNA extracted from human organs detects expression of XOR only in intestine and liver.[57,58] In autopsy samples from human newborn infants, quantitative RT-PCR analysis indicated the presence of mRNA in heart, brain, lung, kidney, liver, and intestine, in increasing order, but the relative amount in liver and intestine was several orders of magnitude larger than that in heart.[58]

The cellular localization of human XOR has been studied using immunohistochemistry.[59,60] We found most of the intestinal enzyme in duodenal and jejunal epithelium, with little or no protein detectable in large intestine and rectum.[60] Capillary endothelium in the gut showed slight antibody staining, but the enzyme is clearly not localized exclusively in these cells, as suggested in bovine studies.[61] In human liver, hepatocytes are most strongly stained, with some antigen present in the endothelium and less in Kupffer cells. In hepatocytes the enzyme appears to be located in the cytoplasm, analogous to the case with rat liver, in which the cytoplasmic location was confirmed by immunoelectron microscopy.[62] In other organs, immunologically detectable xanthine oxidoreductase has been shown in capillary endothelium and vascular smooth muscle cells from the heart and skeletal muscle,[63] as well as in retina, which also showed staining of the cones.[64] Resting mammary epithelium contains detectable enzyme protein,[65] which becomes much more abundant during lactation.[60] Malignant cells from human breast tumors are negative for the protein.[65]

Cell lines of human origin generally express very low levels of active XOR under normal culture conditions. An exception seems to be endothelial cells from aorta,[66] whereas umbilical vein endothelial cells have either low or unmeasurable activity.[67] An explanation may be loss of enzyme activity upon adaptation of the cells to culture, which has been demonstrated in rat pulmonary epithelial cells.[68]

Regulation of Xanthine Oxidoreductase Expression

Animal and cell culture experiments have indicated that the activity of XOR is regulated at least at the transcriptional and posttranslational levels by a number of effectors. These responses appear to be not only species but also cell type specific.

Changes in oxygen tension have an inverse effect on enzyme activity in many cells, hypoxia causing induction[67,69–72] and hyperoxia suppression of activity.[67,73] The effect of hypoxia seems to be both transcriptional and posttranslational[67,69,70] Hypoxia in cell culture does not convert xanthine dehydrogenase into oxidase.[67,71,74] In whole lung from rats exposed to hypoxia, XOR activity and mRNA levels are doubled.[75]

Hyperoxia causes rapid loss of enzyme activity, partly through inactivation by reactive oxygen metabolites,[76,77] and partly through a decrease in mRNA levels[67,78].

Nitric oxide may participate in the regulation of XOR; on the other hand, the product of the enzyme, superoxide, reacts with NO to form peroxynitrite. Enzyme activity in bovine endothelial cells appears to be rapidly and reversibly inhibited by NO itself and by NO donors, e.g., nitrosoglutathione.[72] Elevation of NO levels by L-arginine supplementation suppresses enzyme activity in normoxic and hypoxic rat endothelial cells as well as in rat lung[79] but has no effect on mRNA levels. On the other hand, inhibitors of NO synthesis induce enzyme activity in normoxic and especially hypoxic cells.[79] However, some of the effects of NO may be only apparent, accounted for by oxidation of uric acid by peroxynitrite, while true inhibition of the enzyme under physiological conditions, in the presence of purine substrates, may be minimal.[80]

The effects of inflammatory mediators and cytokines on XOR activity are well documented in experimental animals but again vary depending on the cell and species. For example, TNF-α and interferon-γ, as well as interleukins 1 and 6, induce enzyme activity in bovine renal epithelial cells,[81] but of these mediators only interferon-γ is active in rat pulmonary endothelial cells.[82] The mechanism of the increase seems to be transcriptional activation, since mRNA levels are elevated.[81,82] Lipopolysaccharide induces enzyme activity and mRNA production in most mouse tissues except those of the gastrointestinal tract and heart[19,83] and doubles enzyme activity and mRNA quantities in rat lung.[75] Strong induction can also be seen in the alveolar epithelium of the lactating mouse mammary gland. In rat macrophages, interferon-γ has a paradoxical effect, since XOR mRNA is increased but enzyme activity disappears. The explanation seems to be inactivation of the enzyme by nitric oxide, the production of which is rapidly induced by the cytokine in macrophages.[84] Inflammatory mediators may also convert xanthine dehydrogenase to oxidase without altering total enzyme activity.[85]

Examples of hormonal regulation of XOR include glucocorticoid induction of activity in bovine renal[81] and mouse breast[83] epithelial cells; in the latter, prolactin has a synergistic effect.

The molecular basis for regulation of human XOR activity has not been elucidated. However, with the recent cloning of the 5′-untranslated region, it will be possible to analyze which of the several consensus recognition sites for transcriptional regulators have physiological significance.

PHYSIOLOGICAL AND PATHOPHYSIOLOGICAL FUNCTIONS

Since XOR is the terminal enzyme in purine degradation in humans but not in most other animals, its physiological role may also be different. In humans, the extracellular concentrations of its substrates, hypoxanthine and xanthine, are low, but the concentration of its product, uric acid, is two orders of magnitude higher. Thus, the enzyme cannot be considered rate-limiting for purine catabolism under normal conditions.

Uric acid has been ascribed a role as an antioxidant, because it is able to scavenge singlet oxygen, peroxyl radical, hydroxyl radical, ozone, and hypochlorous acid. High extracellular urate levels have been hypothesized to explain the low cancer rates and long life span of humans in comparison to those of lower mammals.[86] *Drosophila* mutants, which are deficient in xanthine dehydrogenase, have a reduced life span, as well as increased sensitivity to hyperoxia, paraquat, and ionizing radiation,[87] which has been interpreted to support the antioxidant role of uric acid. Measurable quantities of allantoin, the oxidation product of uric acid, can be found in serum and urine from patients presumably subjected to oxidative stress (e.g., adults with rheumatoid arthritis[88] or preterm infants treated with oxygen[89]).

The other products of XOR, superoxide radicals and hydrogen peroxide, may have physiological as well as pathophysiological functions. Superoxide, like other free radicals, has microbicidal activity, and xanthine oxidase, as well as nitric oxide synthesis, has been implicated in host defense against *Salmonella*[90] and influenza virus[91] infection in mice. In both instances, allopurinol and NO synthase inhibitors increase mortality. Superoxide reacts readily with NO to produce peroxynitrite.[92] Xanthine oxidase activity may thus modulate the physiological effects of NO in the vascular wall, with ensuing increase of vascular tone,[93] or expose tissues to the strong oxidant action of peroxynitrite. Inactivation of the enzyme by tungsten feeding or inhibition of enzyme activity has a hypotensive effect in spontaneously hypertensive rats.[94] A similar effect has been obtained with endothelium-targeted recombinant superoxide dismutase.[95] However, hypotension is not a significant side effect of allopurinol in humans.

The main role of XOR in human pathology has been connected with its ability to produce substantial quantities of reactive oxygen metabolites under a number of conditions, mainly associated with ischemia-reperfusion injury and inflammation. On the basis of animal studies on the intestine, the following hypothesis has been proposed:[96–98] During ischemia, ATP is broken down to hypoxanthine and xanthines, and XOR is converted from dehydrogenase into oxidase. Upon reperfusion, when oxygen is reintroduced, the enzyme has excess substrates present and produces, in addition to uric acid, hydrogen peroxide and superoxide (Fig. 111-6). These, as well as hydroxyl radicals produced in the Fe^{2+}-catalyzed Fenton reaction, are responsible for the ensuing cellular damage.

Both indirect and direct evidence for each of these propositions has been presented in several animal models of reperfusion after ischemia of intestine, liver, heart, brain, kidney, skeletal muscle, and skin. Breakdown of ATP and other high-energy phosphates does occur, and hypoxanthine and xanthine accumulate rapidly both in hypoxic cells[99,100] and ischemic organs[101,102] and in blood.[98,103] Conversion of dehydrogenase into oxidase occurs in some animal models[35,104] but not in others,[105] and the time course of the conversion varies depending on the animal, the organ, and even the cell type. For example, in Kupffer cells isolated from rat liver, hypoxia caused a faster conversion of dehydrogenase into oxidase than it did in hepatocytes or endothelial cells.[106] Clear

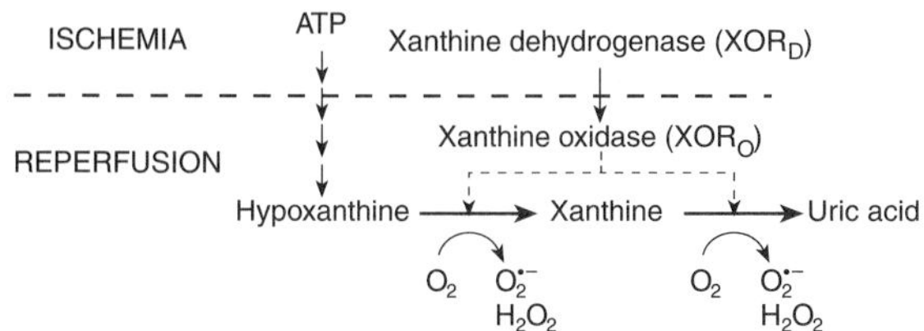

Fig. 111-6 Hypothesis of oxidant production in ischemia-reperfusion injury. During ischemia, ATP is catabolized to hypoxanthine and xanthine dehydrogenase is converted into oxidase. During reperfusion, oxygen becomes available and xanthine oxidase produces hydrogen peroxide and superoxide.

signs of cell damage may appear before significant conversion has taken place.[36,107] Nutritional status also may affect the conversion, at least in the liver, since fasted rats are more susceptible to reperfusion damage and show more rapid conversion than fed animals.[35,105]

Electron paramagnetic resonance (EPR) spectrometry as well as chemiluminescence studies have shown that reperfusion of ischemic rat heart is followed by a burst of reactive oxygen metabolites, which lasts no more than five minutes.[108,109] XOR has been implicated because this burst can be suppressed by allopurinol or oxypurinol.[108] However, the time course of oxidant production coincides with that of accumulation of XOR substrates but not of the increase in the proportion of the oxidase form,[110] again calling into question the significance of the conversion.

A large number of publications have documented alleviation of cellular damage upon reperfusion by inhibitors of XOR, allopurinol, or oxypurinol. For such experiments, oxypurinol is superior, because the oxidation of allopurinol into its active form, oxypurinol, produces superoxide, and allopurinol inhibition can be counteracted by the presence of hypoxanthine or xanthine.[111] That the effect of these inhibitors is due to decreased reactive oxygen metabolite production rather than scavenging of free radicals or accelerated resynthesis of adenine nucleotides is supported by two considerations. First, damage prevention can be obtained with low concentrations of the inhibitors, sufficient to inhibit the enzyme but not to scavenge oxidants.[112] Second, ischemia-reperfusion damage can also be alleviated by pretreatment of the animal with tungsten, which inactivates the enzyme.[43]

Despite ample evidence for the role of XOR in reperfusion damage in animal models, doubt remains concerning its role in human pathology. Important examples of relevant clinical situations include myocardial infarction, stroke, organ transplantation, acute tubular necrosis, and recovery from global ischemia (e.g., circulatory shock, perinatal asphyxia). Accumulation of nucleotide catabolic products has been documented in many of these situations, but the crucial questions are the following: Is XOR expressed in the relevant organ or cell? If present, is it converted from dehydrogenase into oxidase? If it is, by what mechanism and over what time course? Regardless of conversion, is the enzyme capable of generating oxygen radicals under the conditions prevailing in ischemic tissue upon reperfusion? If so, what are the relative contributions of dehydrogenase and oxidase, and what is the role of NO production, favored in ischemic tissue by accumulation of nitrite and NADH?[13] Obviously, other potential sources of oxidants, such as the mitochondria, microsomal oxidases, and cyclooxygenases, have to be taken into consideration.

The only clinical situation in which the hypothesis on the role of XOR in reperfusion injury has been directly tested in randomized clinical trials is allopurinol treatment in connection with coronary bypass surgery. Although the time of drug administration has been variable and the trial end points less than satisfactory, in most published trials a beneficial effect has been claimed.[113–129] Allopurinol is also frequently added to organ preservation solutions in transplantation surgery, even though rigorous scientific evidence for its effectiveness is lacking.

Xanthine oxidoreductase, mostly in the oxidase form, may be released into the circulation from ischemic organs both in animals[105,130,131] and in humans.[132–136] Constitutive release of the oxidase has also been demonstrated in cultured bovine endothelial cells under normal culture conditions.[74] Both bovine and porcine endothelial cells bind anti-XOR antibodies and also hybridoma cells producing monoclonal anti-XOR antibodies onto their surfaces, suggesting that at least a part of the enzyme produced by these cells is localized on the outer surface.[137] In animal experiments, ischemia-reperfusion of the liver[138] or the intestine[130] leads to leakage of fluid into pulmonary alveoli and to respiratory distress that can be alleviated with tungsten pretreatment or XOR inhibitors. In human patients with adult respiratory distress syndrome, xanthine oxidase can be detected in plasma and may contribute to pulmonary damage.[139] Substantial amounts of the enzyme, all in oxidase form, are released from transplanted human liver after restoration of blood flow, in connection with release of nonspecific markers of cell damage.[136]

Extracellular enzyme may be removed from the circulation by endothelial cells, which bind XOR on their surfaces.[140–143] The enzyme is bound with high affinity to glycosaminoglycans, preferably heparin, and remains active, albeit with somewhat altered kinetic characteristics. For example, the K_m for xanthine increases fivefold, to 15 μM; the proportion of superoxide to hydrogen peroxide production is altered;[140] and reduction of nitrite to NO seems to be facilitated.[13] In hypercholesterolemic rabbits, xanthine oxidase bound to endothelial cell surface impairs vasorelaxation due to NO.[144]

As reviewed above, information on the expression of XOR in human tissues and cells is still incomplete. Although activity in most organs is undetectable, there is suggestive evidence of localization of enzyme activity in vascular endothelial cells. Damage to these cells would account for the microvascular injury that is an essential component of reperfusion damage. It would then compromise neighboring cells because of secondary circulatory disturbances. Thus, despite low overall activity in an organ, the enzyme could still be significant. In human aortic endothelial cells reoxygenated after anoxia, EPR measurements showed production of reactive oxygen metabolites that was suppressed by oxypurinol, which also prevented cell death.[145]

Evidence for the conversion of dehydrogenase to oxidase is less convincing. The time course of irreversible oxidase formation appears much slower than that of radical generation. The protease catalyzing the conversion has been assumed to be Ca^2-dependent, but a role for calpains has been ruled out.[38] Our recent data, using labeled recombinant human xanthine dehydrogenase as substrate, indicate that the protease is located in the intermembrane space of mitochondria, from where it may be released under conditions inducing mitochondrial permeability transition, including Ca^{2+}-overload, freezing and thawing, and ischemia-reperfusion.[24] The cleavage occurs between Gln183 and Lys184, which differs from the cleavage sites of known proteases, including the caspase family; none of the protease inhibitors tested was able to prevent conversion of xanthine dehydrogenase by the mitochondrial enzyme. The larger (130 kDa) fragment is subsequently degraded further, first to 85 kDa and then to smaller fragments, possibly by other intracellular proteases.

The possibility remains that XOR is able to produce reactive oxygen metabolites upon reperfusion without increased conversion into oxidase. This may be accounted for by the small amount of basal oxidase in the presence of excess substrate, or by the dehydrogenase under the conditions prevailing after ischemia (i.e., acid pH, low NAD^+, high NADH).

HUMAN ALDEHYDE OXIDASE

Because in some patients with a genetic deficiency of XOR (xanthinuria) the activity of aldehyde oxidase is also deficient, the properties of this enzyme will be briefly reviewed.

Aldehyde oxidase catalyzes the oxidation of a large number of N-oxides, nitrosamines, hydroxamic acids, azo dyes, nitropolycyclic aromatic hydrocarbons, sulfoxides, and cancer chemotherapeutic agents containing the purine ring.[146,147] Its substrate specificity overlaps widely with that of XOR,[8] which makes evaluation of the specific physiological role of each enzyme somewhat difficult. N^1-methylnicotinamide, 6-methylpurine, and 6-phenantridone have been employed as relatively specific substrates for aldehyde oxidase, which, on the other hand, does not react with hypoxanthine or xanthine.

Aldehyde oxidase uses only molecular oxygen as its physiological electron acceptor, and attempts to convert the enzyme into a dehydrogenase, to react with NAD^+ as xanthine dehydrogenase does, have been unsuccessful.[148] Notably, aldehyde oxidase also produces superoxide radicals and H_2O_2. The enzyme can oxidize NADH in a reaction that produces NAD^+ and superoxide.[149] The active-site molybdenum contains an essential sulfido ligand, which may be lost in the process of extracting the enzyme from tissue; resulfuration under aerobic conditions is very slow.[148]

Aldehyde oxidase has been purified and characterized from a number of mammalian sources. Its cDNA has been cloned from bovine,[150] mouse,[151] rat,[152] and human[57,153] (GenBank L11005) liver. The bovine and human cDNAs predict 86 percent identity of their translation products. Comparison of the structures of XOR and aldehyde oxidase reveals a large degree of similarity. Both enzymes are dimers of ~150 kDa, and both contain one molybdopterin, one FAD, and two Fe-S centers per subunit. EPR spectroscopy indicates very similar structures of the Fe-S, flavin, and molybdenum centers.[148] Sequence comparisons of the reported cDNAs of human XOR and aldehyde oxidase reveal 49 percent similarity at the protein level. A considerably higher degree of identity is found in the cysteine-rich N-terminal domain, containing the two Fe-S centers, as well as in the C-terminal domain, where the molybdenum center is located. However, aldehyde oxidase lacks the consensus sequence coding for an NAD^+ binding site.[150]

Human aldehyde oxidase is coded for by a single gene, located on chromosome 2q33[57,153] and in a homologous region on chromosome 1 in the mouse.[154] The gene is ~85 kb long and has a great degree of similarity with the XOR gene. Each has a highly complex intron/exon structure. However, except for suppression of one intron in aldehyde oxidase, which thus contains 35 instead of 36 exons, the locations and types of intron/exon junctions in the two genes are identical.[153] This strongly supports the hypothesis that they have a common evolutionary origin by gene duplication. However, the 5′-flanking region of the human aldehyde oxidase gene is totally different from that of the XOR gene, which indicates that the transcriptional regulation and organ distribution of the gene products are different.

In all species studied, the highest aldehyde oxidase activity is found in the liver, with substantial activity also in the lung. In a survey of bovine organs, liver, lung, and spleen contained the largest amounts of immunoreactive protein and mRNA, as detected by western and northern blotting, respectively.[150] Many organs showed lower levels of expression, and in mouse, a highly selective localization in the choroid plexus and motor neurons has been demonstrated.[151] In human organs, aldehyde oxidase mRNA was found to be expressed in liver, kidney, lung, pancreas, prostate, testis, and ovary, whereas expression in the intestine was low.[57,155]

Because of its substrate specificity and organ distribution, aldehyde oxidase has been proposed to have an important function in the metabolism of xenobiotics.[150] Its physiological substrates include retinaldehyde,[156] which suggests a potential function in the eye, and dihydroxymandelaldehyde, which is involved in the breakdown of adrenaline and noradrenaline. The gene for aldehyde oxidase is closely linked with the locus for recessively inherited amyotropic lateral sclerosis and has been proposed as a candidate gene for it,[57,157] but a credible hypothesis on a pathophysiological mechanism, or any data on gene or protein abnormality in diseased patients, has not been presented. The potential role of aldehyde oxidase as a source of reactive oxygen metabolites in other human diseases has not received nearly as much attention as that of XOR. However, it has been implicated in ethanol-induced hepatotoxicity.[158]

HEREDITARY XANTHINURIA

Definition and Subtypes

A genetic deficiency of XOR was first recognized clinically in a girl, aged $4\frac{1}{2}$ years, presenting with hematuria and a renal stone.[159] Hypouricemia and accumulation of hypoxanthine and xanthine in body fluids was then demonstrated,[160] and the enzyme defect was documented.[161] In later studies, two types of patients with xanthinuria were characterized on the basis of their ability to oxidize allopurinol to oxypurinol.[162] In type I, allopurinol metabolism is quantitatively normal, since it is metabolized by aldehyde oxidase, whereas patients with type II disease are unable to convert allopurinol to oxypurinol. The former patients have isolated deficiency of XOR, whereas the latter have a combined deficiency of aldehyde oxidase and XOR[163]

Cases of isolated aldehyde oxidase deficiency have not been reported. Patients with combined deficiency are clinically indistinguishable from those with a deficiency of XOR alone, thus giving no clues to the physiological function of aldehyde oxidase. On the other hand, molybdenum cofactor deficiency, in which sulfite oxidase activity is missing in addition to aldehyde oxidase and XOR, is clinically much more severe. The symptomatology is similar to that of isolated sulfite oxidase deficiency, which illustrates the important but largely unknown physiological function of this enzyme (see Chap. 128).

More than 100 cases of hereditary xanthinuria have been described, from a variety of population groups. Incidence estimates vary between 1 in 6000 and 1 in 69,000.[164,165] This large spread may reflect the rarity of the disease as well as epidemiological differences. In those clinical studies that report on the subtypes, type I and type II appear to be roughly equal in incidence. Xanthine stones are rarely identified as a cause of urolithiasis, and published surveys suggest an incidence of less than 1 per 1000 cases. There are some indications that xanthine stones, and possibly hereditary xanthinuria, are more common in Mediterranean countries than in the rest of the world.[166]

Clinical Features

Less than one-half of patients with xanthinuria present with symptoms attributable to the disease. An equal number are detected on the basis of very low serum uric acid concentrations, measured in population studies or as part of a workup for an unrelated disease. One-fifth have been diagnosed in family studies after an index case was found.

The clinical symptoms of hereditary xanthinuria can be accounted for by the accumulation in body fluids of the highly insoluble xanthine. The most common presentation is urinary tract calculi due to precipitation of xanthine, which may cause a variety of symptoms, including hematuria, crystalluria, renal colic, or even acute renal failure.[167–170] Repeated episodes of stone formation predispose to recurrent urinary tract infections and may lead to hydronephrosis, chronic renal failure, and even death from uremia. Infants may present with nonspecific symptoms, including irritability and poor feeding. About one-half of the reported cases that included renal symptoms have been diagnosed by the age of 10 years.

Another consequence of xanthine deposition is muscle pain and cramps, which have been documented in at least eight cases.[171,172] Increased concentrations of xanthine and hypoxanthine in muscle tissue have been measured.[173] The symptoms may be precipitated by strenuous exercise, which increases muscle nucleotide turnover. Recurrent joint pains have been experienced by some patients, but in contrast with the finding of urate crystals in synovial fluid in patients with gout, crystal-induced arthropathy has not been documented in hereditary xanthinuria.

Duodenal ulcers have been diagnosed in approximately one-tenth of patients, which is somewhat more than expected by a chance association. However, the relevance to the genetic disease of this feature, as well as of other fortuitous clinical associations, is doubtful.

Biochemical Features

Hereditary xanthinuria is characterized by typical alterations in plasma and urine oxypurine concentrations, which can with good reliability be used as the basis for diagnosis. While in normal individuals plasma uric acid levels range from 250 to 400 μM (see Chap. 106), the levels in xanthinurics are usually less than 5 μM. Plasma xanthine levels, which normally are below 1 μM, may rise to 10–40 μM in patients with xanthinuria.[174–176] Hypoxanthine concentrations are below 5 μM in plasma of normal individuals, and they are usually not elevated in xanthinuric patients.

The renal handling of oxypurines in normal individuals is complex, and at least with uric acid and xanthine, there is a tubular secretion component. For this reason the renal clearance of xanthine exceeds, while that of hypoxanthine approximates, the glomerular filtration rate. The urinary excretion of oxypurines varies with the purine content of the diet, and to a lesser extent with sex and age.[164,174,177] On a low-purine diet, total oxypurine excretion normally amounts to 2–3 mmol/24 h, of which over 90 percent is uric acid and the rest hypoxanthine and xanthine at a ratio of approximately 1.4:1. In xanthinuric individuals, total oxypurine excretion is somewhat reduced, to 1–2 mmol/24 h; uric acid is usually below the limit of detection; and the ratio of hypoxanthine to xanthine is reversed, to ca. 1:4.[164,174,177,178]

The high renal clearance of xanthine accounts for the modest elevation in plasma levels and the high urinary concentrations in relation to the solubility of xanthine. The solubility is approximately 0.5 mM at pH 5.0 and is increased only to 0.9 mM upon alkalinization to pH 7.0, which contrasts with the greatly enhanced solubility of uric acid with a rise in pH.

Hypoxanthine is the main purine base formed in the catabolism of adenine nucleotides, but it is normally very efficiently reutilized by HPRT (see Chap. 107). The pattern of plasma and urinary oxypurines in xanthinuria indicates that in this condition the salvage of hypoxanthine is at least as effective as in normal individuals. One study of adenine nucleotide turnover suggests that hypoxanthine salvage may actually be enhanced in xanthinuria.[179] Although guanine, which is the primary purine base formed upon degradation of guanine nucleotides, is also salvaged by HPRT, it is partly deaminated to xanthine by guanase, which is present and active in many organs both in animals and humans. Isotope studies both in pigs[180] and in xanthinuric humans[179] have indicated that guanine nucleotides are the main source of xanthine.

Oxypurine levels have been measured in muscle tissue from several patients with xanthinuria. While in normal individuals muscle hypoxanthine and xanthine concentrations are below 30 ng/mg and below 50 ng/mg dry weight, respectively, the levels in patients were found to be in the range of 240 to 350 and 315 to 450 ng/mg dry weight, respectively.[173] Vigorous exercise increases plasma hypoxanthine in both normal and xanthinuric subjects,[164,172] a fact accounted for by increased adenine nucleotide turnover. However, the relevance of this elevation is unclear, since hypoxanthine is much more soluble than urate or xanthine. Whether increased amounts of xanthine are formed depends on whether guanine nucleotide turnover is also enhanced by exercise, which has not been documented.

The differential diagnosis of isolated XOR deficiency (type I) from that combined with aldehyde oxidase deficiency (type II) was originally based on the ability of the patient to oxidize allopurinol.[162] The substrate specificities of the two enzymes overlap, and both oxidize allopurinol to oxypurinol, thiopurinol to oxythiopurinol, and pyrazinamide to 5-hydroxypyrazinamide.[181] Each of these oxidation products can be measured in plasma or urine of type I xanthinuric patients after a loading dose of the substrate.[182] On the other hand, hypoxanthine, xanthine, pterin, and pyrazinoic acid are not substrates for aldehyde oxidase, and these compounds are not metabolized in either type of xanthinuria. Substrates relatively specific for aldehyde oxidase, (e.g., N^1-methylnicotinamide or 6-methylpurine)[6] could also be used for distinguishing the two types of xanthinuria.

Diagnosis

Because of the nonspecificity, and frequently the total absence, of symptoms, the clinical picture can lead the way to a proper diagnostic workup, but except in familial cases, only rarely does it provide a solid suspicion of the disease. Hematuria, especially if associated with crystalluria and not explained by more common causes, is an indication to rule out xanthinuria. Acute renal failure, especially with a history of hematuria and/or crystalluria and without a prerenal or parenchymal cause, may also be a manifestation of the disease.

Xanthine stones are a specific manifestation of hereditary xanthinuria, except in the obvious iatrogenic cases associated with allopurinol therapy of massive uric acid overproduction. Such cases include the Lesch-Nyhan syndrome (see Chap. 107) and malignant diseases with a large mass of tumor cells, which are lysed by aggressive chemotherapy started concomitantly with allopurinol and may give rise to xanthine concentrations of nearly 1 mM in plasma and urine.[2] Pure xanthine stones are not radiopaque, but particularly in young children, they frequently contain calcium salts because of the associated hypercalciuria and may be detectable by ultrasound or X-ray studies. The chemical nature of renal stones must be established by specific studies, and xanthine is readily identified by several standard methods, including spectrophotometry, thin-layer or liquid chromatography, infrared or mass spectroscopy, and X-ray crystallography.

For practical purposes, the diagnosis can be established by documenting markedly low uric acid concentrations and elevated hypoxanthine and xanthine levels in plasma and urine. Uric acid assay is usually based on the uricase method (see Chap. 106). To measure the other oxypurines, HPLC methods are currently recommended because of their sensitivity, rapidity, and specificity, which is based on the characteristic ultraviolet absorption spectra of the purine bases.[183]

The ratio of urinary pterin to isoxanthopterin after an oral dose of tetrahydrobiopterin allows an estimation of the in vivo activity of xanthine dehydrogenase and a clear distinction among patients with xanthinuria, molybdenum cofactor deficiency, and controls.[184] In order to distinguish between the two types of hereditary xanthinuria, an allopurinol loading test is the most practical.[182] A plasma sample for oxypurinol determination is taken 90 min after an oral dose of 300 mg allopurinol, and a measurable level of oxypurinol indicates the presence of aldehyde oxidase activity, identifying xanthinuria type I.

For direct demonstration of deficient activity of XOR, a needle biopsy of the liver or a mucosal biopsy of the intestine is necessary. These procedures are seldom indicated for clinical purposes. DNA diagnosis is discussed below.

Treatment and Prognosis

There is no specific treatment to compensate for the deficient enzyme activity. Since the predominance of xanthine over hypoxanthine in body fluids is not due to residual XOR activity but to generation of xanthine from guanine nucleotides, allopurinol cannot reverse the ratio of the two oxypurines in favor of the more soluble hypoxanthine.[162,163,182,186] A low-purine diet and high fluid intake are indicated to decrease oxypurine production and prevent precipitation of xanthine in the urine.

The treatment of xanthine stones follows the general therapeutic guidelines for urinary calculi. In persistent cases of renal colic or acute renal failure, shock-wave lithotripsy has replaced lithotomy. If these potentially grave complications are treated adequately, the prognosis of hereditary xanthinuria is excellent.

Because of the rarity of the disease, it is not possible to conclude whether the patients actually benefit from their inability to generate reactive oxygen metabolites through the XOR reaction. This might conceivably be reflected in the outcome of ischemia-reperfusion damage in clinical situations such as myocardial infarction or stroke. Likewise, there are not sufficient epidemiologic grounds for assessing the potentially harmful effects of deficiency of the antioxidant activity of uric acid.

GENETICS OF HEREDITARY XANTHINURIA

Mode of Inheritance

Family studies had already established the autosomal recessive mode of inheritance of xanthinuria before the era of molecular genetic studies.[166,187] This was later borne out by the localization of the single XOR gene in human chromosome 2p22.[45–47]

Obligate heterozygotes carrying the hereditary xanthinuria defect are asymptomatic, and their plasma oxypurine concentrations are normal. Some heterozygotes have a relatively low uric acid-to-oxypurine excretion ratio, accounted for by elevated hypoxanthine and xanthine excretion,[187,188] but this pattern of oxypurine excretion is too inconsistent to be useful for heterozygote detection. Enzyme activity in the duodenal mucosa of obligate heterozygotes has been reported to be approximately 50 percent of normal.[188]

The Mutation and Its Effects

Despite unmeasurably low XOR activity, immunoreactive protein was detectable by double immunodiffusion in an extract from the duodenal mucosa of a patient with type II xanthinuria[189] but not by western blotting in the duodenal mucosa of a patient with type I disease.[190]

The mutation responsible for hereditary xanthinuria has been documented in four Japanese patients on the basis of analysis of cDNA generated by RT-PCR, which was feasible because in two of the cases XOR mRNA was present at normal levels.[190] Two of the patients were siblings and had type I xanthinuria, as did a third patient, but in the fourth patient the type was not established. The last patient and both the siblings had a C-to-G base change at nucleotide position 682, predicted to generate a nonsense substitution from CGA (Arg) to TGA (Ter) at codon 228. The siblings were homozygous for the mutation, but the unrelated patient was a compound heterozygote with an unidentified second mutation. The fourth case involved a different mutation, a deletion of C at nucleotide 2567, predicted to generate a termination codon from nucleotide 2783. Analysis of genomic DNA confirmed a homozygous mutation at the locus indicated by the cDNA studies.

The cause of type I hereditary xanthinuria thus clearly seems to be a mutation or mutations in the XOR gene. In type II xanthinuria, mutations in the genes coding for XOR and for aldehyde oxidase are unlikely, since these genes are located far apart, albeit both on chromosome 2. A possible explanation has been proposed by analogy to a mutation characterized in *D. melanogaster* that results in failure to incorporate a sulfur atom into the molybdenum center of desulfo xanthine and aldehyde oxidases.[191] This sulfur atom is essential for the function of these two molybdenum hydroxylases but not of sulfite oxidase. The finding of immunoreactive protein but no enzyme activity in a type II patient[189] is in line with this explanation.

Since the cDNA and genomic structure of XOR have been characterized, it is now possible to identify mutations in additional patients with hereditary xanthinuria. Such studies will indicate whether the C-to-T substitution at nucleotide 682, detected in two unrelated Japanese patients, is explained by a mutational hotspot at this locus or by an ancestral mutation. Carrier detection and prenatal diagnosis will also become reliable. However, given the benign nature of the disease and the lack of an effective method of treatment, such diagnostic possibilities can be justified only for scientific purposes, not for clinical needs.

REFERENCES

1. Saugstad OD: Hypoxanthine as an indicator of hypoxia: Its role in health and disease through free radical production. *Pediatr Res* **23**: 143, 1988.
2. Simmonds HA, Cameron JS, Morris GS, Davies PM: Allopurinol in renal failure and the tumour lysis syndrome. *Clin Chim Acta* **160**: 189, 1986.
3. Parks DA, Granger DN: Xanthine oxidase: Biochemistry, distribution and physiology. *Acta Physiol Scand Suppl* **548**: 87, 1986.
4. Hille R, Nishino T: Xanthine oxidase and xanthine dehydrogenase. *FASEB J* **9**: 995, 1995.
5. Stirpe F, DellaCorte E: The regulation of rat liver xanthine oxidase: Conversion *in vitro* of the enzyme activity from dehydrogenase (type D) to oxidase (type O). *J Biol Chem* **244**: 3855, 1969.
6. Krenitsky TA, Spector T, Hall WW: Xanthine oxidase from human liver: Purification and characterization. *Arch Biochem Biophys* **247**: 108, 1986.
7. Spector T, Hall WW, Krenitsky TA: Human and bovine xanthine oxidases: Inhibition studies with oxypurinol. *Biochem Pharmacol* **35**: 3109, 1986.
8. Krenitsky TA, Neil SM, Elion GB, Hitchings GH: A comparison of the specificities of xanthine oxidase and aldehyde oxidase. *Arch Biochem Biophys* **150**: 585, 1972.
9. Nishino T: The conversion of xanthine dehydrogenase to xanthine oxidase and the role of the enzyme in reperfusion injury. *J Biochem* **(Tokyo) 116**: 1, 1994.
10. Nishino T, Nishino T: The nicotinamide adenine dinucleotide-binding site of chicken liver xanthine dehydrogenase: Evidence for alteration of the redox potential of the flavin by NAD binding or modification of the NAD-binding site and isolation of a modified peptide. *J Biol Chem* **264**: 5468, 1989.
11. Hunt J, Massey V: Purification and properties of milk xanthine dehydrogenase. *J Biol Chem* **267**: 21479, 1992.
12. Trujillo M, Alvarez MN, Peluffo G, Freeman BA, Radi R: Xanthine oxidase-mediated decomposition of S-nitrosothiols. *J Biol Chem* **273**: 7828, 1998.
13. Zhang Z, Naughton D, Winyard PG, Benjamin N, Blake DR, Symons MC: Generation of nitric oxide by a nitrite reductase activity of xanthine oxidase: A potential pathway for nitric oxide formation in the absence of nitric oxide synthase activity. *Biochem Biophys Res Comm* **249**: 767, 1998.
14. Romão MJ, Archer M, Moura I, Moura JJG, LeGall J, Engh R, Schneider M, et al.: Crystal structure of the xanthine oxidase-related aldehyde oxido-reductase from *D. gigas*. *Science* **270**: 1170, 1995.
15. Saksela M, Raivio KO: Cloning and expression *in vitro* of human xanthine dehydrogenase/oxidase. *Biochem J* **315**: 235, 1996.
16. Ichida K, Amaya Y, Noda K, Minoshima S, Hosoya T, Sakai O, Shimizu N, Nishino T: Cloning of the cDNA encoding human xanthine dehydrogenase (oxidase)–structural analysis of the protein and chromosomal location of the gene. *Gene* **133**: 279, 1993.
17. Xu P, Huecksteadt TP, Harrison R, Hoidal JR: Molecular cloning, tissue expression of human xanthine dehydrogenase. *Biochem Biophys Res Commun* **199**: 998, 1994.
18. Amaya Y, Yamazaki K, Sato M, Noda K, Nishino T, Nishino T: Proteolytic conversion of xanthine dehydrogenase from the NAD-dependent type to the O_2-dependent type: Amino acid sequence of rat liver xanthine dehydrogenase and identification of the cleavage sites of the enzyme protein during irreversible conversion by trypsin. *J Biol Chem* **265**: 14170, 1990.
19. Terao M, Cazzaniga G, Ghezzi P, Bianchi M, Falciani F, Perani P, Garattini E: Molecular cloning of a cDNA coding for mouse liver xanthine dehydrogenase: Regulation of its transcript by interferons *in vivo*. *Biochem J* **283**: 863, 1992.
20. Sato A, Nishino T, Noda K, Amaya Y, Nishino T: The structure of chicken liver xanthine dehydrogenase–cDNA cloning and the domain structure. *J Biol Chem* **270**: 2818, 1995.
21. Sarnesto A, Linder N, Raivio KO: Organ distribution and molecular forms of human xanthine dehydrogenase/xanthine oxidase protein. *Lab Invest* **74**: 48, 1996.
22. Coughlan MP, Betcher LS, Rajagopalan KV: Isolation of the domain containing the molybdenum, iron-sulfur I, and iron-sulfur II centers of chicken liver xanthine dehydrogenase. *J Biol Chem* **254**: 10694, 1979.

23. Nagler LG, Vartanyan LS: Subunit structure of bovine milk xanthine oxidase: Effect of limited cleavage by proteolytic enzymes on activity and structure. *Biochim Biophys Acta* **427**:78, 1976.
24. Saksela M, Lapatto R, Raivio KO: Irreversible conversion of xanthine dehydrogenase into xanthine oxidase by a mitochondrial protease. *FEBS Lett* **443**:117, 1999.
25. Coughlan M, Ljungdahl LG, Mayer F: Aspects of the macromolecular organization of bovine milk xanthine oxidase as revealed by electron microscopy. *IRCS J Med Sci* **14**:736, 1986.
26. Saito T, Nishino T: Differences in redox and kinetic properties between NAD-dependent and O_2-dependent types of rat liver xanthine dehydrogenase. *J Biol Chem* **264**:10015, 1989.
27. Sanders SA, Eisenthal R, Harrison R: NADH oxidase activity of human xanthine oxidoreductase--generation of superoxide anion. *Eur J Biochem* **245**:541, 1997.
28. Huber R, Hof P, Duarte RO, Moura JJG, Moura I, Liu MY, Legall J, et al.: A structure-based catalytic mechanism for the xanthine oxidase family of molybdenum enzymes. *Proc Natl Acad Sci U S A* **93**:8846, 1996.
29. Kisker C, Schindelin H, Rees DC: Molybdenum-cofactor-containing enzymes: Structure and mechanism. *Annu Rev Biochem* **66**:233, 1997.
30. Nishino T, Nishino T: The conversion from the dehydrogenase type to the oxidase type of rat liver xanthine dehydrogenase by modification of cysteine residues with fluorodinitrobenzene. *J Biol Chem* **272**:29859, 1997.
31. Bindoli A, Cavallini L, Rigobello MP, Coassin M, Di Lisa F: Modification of the xanthine-converting enzyme of perfused rat heart during ischemia and oxidative stress. *Free Radic Biol Med* **4**:163, 1988.
32. Cighetti G, Debiasi S, Paroni R: Effect of glutathione depletion on the conversion of xanthine dehydrogenase to oxidase in rat liver. *Biochem Pharmacol* **45**:2359, 1993.
33. Sakuma S, Fujimoto Y, Sakamoto Y, Uchiyama T, Yoshioka K, Nishida H, Fujita T: Peroxynitrite induces the conversion of xanthine dehydrogenase to oxidase in rabbit liver. *Biochem Biophys Res Commun* **230**:476, 1997.
34. Waud WR, Rajagopalan KV: The mechanism of conversion of rat liver xanthine dehydrogenase from an NAD^+-dependent form (type D) to an O_2-dependent form (type O). *Arch Biochem Biophys* **172**:365, 1976.
35. Brass CA, Narciso J, Gollan JL: Enhanced activity of the free radical producing enzyme xanthine oxidase in hypoxic rat liver: Regulation and pathophysiologic significance. *J Clin Invest* **87**:424, 1991.
36. McKelvey TG, Hollwarth ME, Granger DN, Engerson TD, Landler U, Jones HP: Mechanisms of conversion of xanthine dehydrogenase to xanthine oxidase in ischemic rat liver and kidney. *Am J Physiol* **254**:G753, 1988.
37. Phan SH, Gannon DE, Ward PA, Karmiol S: Mechanism of neutrophil-induced xanthine dehydrogenase to xanthine oxidase conversion in endothelial cells: Evidence of a role for elastase. *Am J Respir Cell Mol Biol* **6**:270, 1992.
38. Stark K, Seubert P, Lynch G, Baudry M: Proteolytic conversion of xanthine dehydrogenase to xanthine oxidase: Evidence against a role for calcium-activated protease (calpain). *Biochem Biophys Res Commun* **165**:858, 1989.
39. Wakabayashi Y, Fujita H, Morita I, Kawaguchi H, Murota S: Conversion of xanthine dehydrogenase to xanthine oxidase in bovine carotid artery endothelial cells induced by activated neutrophils: Involvement of adhesion molecules. *Biochim Biophys Acta* **1265**:103, 1995.
40. Nishino T, Usami C, Tsushima K: Reversible interconversion between sulfo and desulfo xanthine oxidase in a system containing rhodanese, thiosulfate, and sulfhydryl reagent. *Proc Natl Acad Sci U S A* **80**:1826, 1983.
41. Ikegami T, Nishino T: The presence of desulfo xanthine dehydrogenase in purified and crude enzyme preparations from rat liver. *Arch Biochem Biophys* **247**:254, 1986.
42. Abadeh S, Killacky J, Benboubetra M, Harrison R: Purification and partial characterization of xanthine oxidase from human milk. *Biochim Biophys Acta* **1117**:25, 1992.
43. Johnson JL, Rajagopalan KV, Cohen HJ: Molecular basis of the biological function of molybdenum: Effect of tungsten on xanthine oxidase and sulfite oxidase in the rat. *J Biol Chem* **249**:859, 1974.
44. Gardlik S, Barber MJ, Rajagopalan KV: A molybdopterin-free form of xanthine oxidase. *Arch Biochem Biophys* **259**:363, 1987.
45. Xu P, Zhu XL, Huecksteadt TP, Brothman AR, Hoidal JR: Assignment of human xanthine dehydrogenase gene to chromosome 2p22. *Genomics* **23**:289, 1994.
46. Rytkönen EMK, Halila R, Laan M, Saksela M, Kallioniemi O-M Palotie A, Raivio KO: The human gene for xanthine dehydrogenase is localized on chromosome 2p22. *Cytogenet Cell Genet* **68**:61, 1995.
47. Minoshima S, Wang Y, Ichida K, Nishino T, Shimizu N: Mapping of the gene for human xanthine dehydrogenase (oxidase) (XDH) to band p23 of chromosome 2. *Cytogenet Cell Genet* **68**:52, 1995.
48. Cazzaniga G, Terao M, Lo Schiavo P, Galbiati F, Segalla F, Seldin MF, Garattini E: Chromosomal mapping, isolation, and characterization of the mouse xanthine dehydrogenase gene. *Genomics* **23**:390, 1994.
49. Xu P, Huecksteadt TP, Hoidal JR: Molecular cloning and characterization of the human xanthine dehydrogenase gene (XDH). *Genomics* **34**:173, 1996.
50. Chow C-W, Clark MP, Rinaldo JE, Chalkley R: Identification of the rat xanthine dehydrogenase/oxidase promoter. *Nucleic Acids Res* **22**:1846, 1994.
51. Chow C-W, Clark MP, Rinaldo JE, Chalkley R: Multiple initiators and C/EBP binding sites are involved in transcription from the TATA-less rat XDH/XO basal promoter. *Nucleic Acids Res* **23**:3132, 1995.
52. Keith TP, Riley MA, Kreitman M, Lewontin RC, Curtis D, Chambers G: Sequence of the structural gene for xanthine dehydrogenase (rosy locus) in *Drosophila melanogaster*. *Genetics* **116**:67, 1987.
53. Riley MA: Nucleotide sequence of the *Xdh* region in *Drosophila pseudoobscura* and an analysis of the evolution of synonymous codons. *Mol Biol Evol* **6**:33, 1989.
54. Houde M, Tiveron MC, Bregegere F: Divergence of the nucleotide sequences encoding xanthine dehydrogenase in *Calliphora vicina* and *Drosophila melanogaster*. *Gene* **85**:391, 1989.
55. Dougherty TM: A sensitive assay for xanthine oxidase using commercially available [^{14}C]xanthine. *Anal Biochem* **74**:604, 1976.
56. Beckman JS, Parks DA, Pearson JD, Marshall PA, Freeman BA: A sensitive fluorometric assay for measuring xanthine dehydrogenase and oxidase in tissues. *Free Radic Biol Med* **6**:607, 1989.
57. Wright RM, Vaitaitis GM, Weigel LK, Repine TB, McManaman JL, Repine JE: Identification of the candidate ALS2 gene at chromosome 2q33 as a human aldehyde oxidase gene. *Redox Rep* **1**:313, 1995.
58. Saksela M, Lapatto R, Raivio KO: Xanthine oxidoreductase gene expression and enzyme activity in developing human tissues. *Biol Neonate* **74**:274, 1998.
59. Moriwaki Y, Yamamoto T, Yamaguchi K, Suda M, Yamakita J, Takahashi S, Higashino K: Immunohistochemical localization of xanthine oxidase in human tissues. *Acta Histochem Cytochem* **29**:153, 1996.
60. Linder N, Rapola J, Raivio KO: Cellular expression of xanthine oxidoreductase protein in normal human tissues. *Lab Invest* **79**:967, 1999.
61. Jarasch ED, Grund C, Bruder G, Heid HW, Keenan TW, Franke WW: Localization of xanthine oxidase in mammary-gland epithelium and capillary endothelium. *Cell* **25**:67, 1981.
62. Ichikawa M, Nishino T, Nishino T, Ichikawa A: Subcellular localization of xanthine oxidase in rat hepatocytes: High-resolution immunoelectron microscopic study combined with biochemical analysis. *J Histochem Cytochem* **40**:1097, 1992.
63. Hellsten-Westing Y: Immunohistochemical localization of xanthine oxidase in human cardiac and skeletal muscle. *Histochemistry* **100**:215, 1993.
64. Fox NE, van Kuijk FJGM: Immunohistochemical localization of xanthine oxidase in human retina. *Free Radic Biol Med* **24**:900, 1998.
65. Cook WS, Chu RY, Saksela M, Raivio KO, Yeldandi AV: Differential immunohistochemical localization of xanthine oxidase in normal and neoplastic human breast epithelium. *Int J Oncol* **11**:1013, 1997.
66. Zweier JL, Kuppusamy P, Lutty GA: Measurement of endothelial cell free radical generation: Evidence for a central mechanism of free radical injury in postischemic tissues. *Proc Natl Acad Sci U S A* **85**:4046, 1988.
67. Hassoun PM, Yu FS, Shedd AL, Zulueta JJ, Thannickal VJ, Lanzillo JJ, Fanburg BL: Regulation of endothelial cell xanthine dehydrogenase/xanthine oxidase gene expression by oxygen tension. *Am J Physiol* **266**:L163, 1994.
68. Panus PC, Burgess B, Freeman BA: Characterization of cultured alveolar epithelial cell xanthine dehydrogenase/oxidase. *Biochim Biophys Acta* **1091**:303, 1991.
69. Poss WB, Huecksteadt TP, Panus PC, Freeman BA, Hoidal JR: Regulation of xanthine dehydrogenase and xanthine oxidase activity by hypoxia. *Am J Physiol* **270**:L941, 1996.
70. Terada LS, Piermattei D, Shibao GN, McManaman JL, Wright RM: Hypoxia regulates xanthine dehydrogenase activity at pre- and posttranslational levels. *Arch Biochem Biophys* **348**:163, 1997.

71. Terada LS, Guidot DM, Leff JA, Willingham IR, Hanley ME, Piermattei D, Repine JE: Hypoxia injures endothelial cells by increasing endogenous xanthine oxidase activity. *Proc Natl Acad Sci U S A* **89**:3362, 1992.
72. Hassoun PM, Yu FS, Zulueta JJ, White AC, Lanzillo JJ: Effect of nitric oxide and cell redox status on the regulation of endothelial cell xanthine dehydrogenase. *Am J Physiol* **268**:L809, 1995.
73. Panus PC, Wright SA, Chumley PH, Radi R, Freeman BA: The contribution of vascular endothelial xanthine dehydrogenase/oxidase to oxygen-mediated cell injury. *Arch Biochem Biophys* **294**:695, 1992.
74. Partridge CA, Blumenstock FA, Malik AB: Pulmonary microvascular endothelial cells constitutively release xanthine oxidase. *Arch Biochem Biophys* **294**:184, 1992.
75. Hassoun PM, Yu FS, Cote CG, Zulueta JJ, Sawhney R, Skinner KA, Skinner HB, et al.: Upregulation of xanthine oxidase by lipopolysaccharide, interleukin-1, and hypoxia–role in acute lung injury. *Am J Respir Crit Care Med* **158**:299, 1998.
76. Terada LS, Leff JA, Guidot DM, Willingham IR, Repine JE: Inactivation of xanthine oxidase by hydrogen peroxide involves site-directed hydroxyl radical formation. *Free Radic Biol Med* **10**:61, 1991.
77. Terada LS, Beehler CJ, Banerjee A, Brown JM, Grosso MA, Harken AH, McCord JM, et al.: Hyperoxia and self- or neutrophil-generated O_2 metabolites inactivate xanthine oxidase. *J Appl Physiol* **65**:2349, 1988.
78. Lanzillo JJ, Yu FS, Stevens J, Hassoun PM: Determination of xanthine dehydrogenase mRNA by a reverse transcription-coupled competitive quantitative polymerase chain reaction assay: Regulation in rat endothelial cells by hypoxia and hyperoxia. *Arch Biochem Biophys* **335**:377, 1996.
79. Cote CG, Yu FS, Zulueta JJ, Vosatka RJ, Hassoun PM: Regulation of intracellular xanthine oxidase by endothelial-derived nitric oxide. *Am J Physiol* **271**:L869, 1996.
80. Houston M, Chumley P, Radi R, Rubbo H, Freeman BA: Xanthine oxidase reaction with nitric oxide and peroxynitrite. *Arch Biochem Biophys* **355**:1, 1998.
81. Pfeffer KD, Huecksteadt TP, Hoidal JR: Xanthine dehydrogenase and xanthine oxidase activity and gene expression in renal epithelial cells–cytokine and steroid regulation. *J Immunol* **153**:1789, 1994.
82. Dupont GP, Huecksteadt TP, Marshall BC, Ryan US, Michael JR, Hoidal JR: Regulation of xanthine dehydrogenase and xanthine oxidase activity and gene expression in cultured rat pulmonary endothelial cells. *J Clin Invest* **89**:197, 1992.
83. Kurosaki M, Zanotta S, Li Calzi M, Garattini E, Terao M: Expression of xanthine oxidoreductase in mouse mammary epithelium during pregnancy and lactation: Regulation of gene expression by glucocorticoids and prolactin. *Biochem J* **319**:801, 1996.
84. Rinaldo JE, Clark M, Parinello J, Shepherd VL: Nitric oxide inactivates xanthine dehydrogenase and xanthine oxidase in interferon-gamma-stimulated macrophages. *Am J Respir Cell Mol Biol* **11**:625, 1994.
85. Friedl HP, Till GO, Ryan US, Ward PA: Mediator-induced activation of xanthine oxidase in endothelial cells. *FASEB J* **3**:2512, 1989.
86. Ames BN, Cathcart R, Schwiers E, Hochstein P: Uric acid provides an antioxidant defense in humans against oxidant- and radical-caused aging and cancer: A hypothesis. *Proc Natl Acad Sci U S A* **78**:6858, 1981.
87. Hilliker AJ, Duyf B, Evans D, Phillips JP: Urate-null rosy mutants of *Drosophila melanogaster* are hypersensitive to oxygen stress. *Proc Natl Acad Sci U S A* **89**:4343, 1992.
88. Grootveld M, Halliwell B: Measurement of allantoin and uric acid in human body fluids: A potential index of free-radical reactions *in vivo*? *Biochem J* **243**:803, 1987.
89. Ogihara T, Okamoto R, Kim HS, Nagai A, Morinobu T, Moji H, Kamegai H, et al.: New evidence for the involvement of oxygen radicals in triggering neonatal chronic lung disease. *Pediatr Res* **39**:117, 1996.
90. Umezawa K, Akaike T, Fujii S, Suga M, Setoguchi K, Ozawa A, Maeda H: Induction of nitric oxide synthesis and xanthine oxidase and their roles in the antimicrobial mechanism against Salmonella typhimurium infection in mice. *Infect Immun* **65**:2932, 1997.
91. Akaike T, Ando M, Oda T, Doi T, Ijiri S, Araki S, Maeda H: Dependence on O_2- generation by xanthine oxidase of pathogenesis of influenza virus infection in mice. *J Clin Invest* **85**:739, 1990.
92. Beckman JS, Beckman TW, Chen J, Marshall PA, Freeman BA: Apparent hydroxyl radical production by peroxynitrite: Implications for endothelial injury from nitric oxide and superoxide. *Proc Natl Acad Sci U S A* **87**:1620, 1990.
93. Ellis A, Li CG, Rand MJ: Effect of xanthine oxidase inhibition on endothelium-dependent and nitrergic relaxations. *Eur J Pharmacol* **356**:41, 1998.
94. Suzuki H, DeLano FA, Parks DA, Jamshidi N, Granger DN, Ishii H, Suematsu M, et al.: Xanthine oxidase activity associated with arterial blood pressure in spontaneously hypertensive rats. *Proc Natl Acad Sci U S A* **95**:4754, 1998.
95. Nakazono K, Watanabe N, Matsuno K, Sasaki J, Sato T, Inoue M: Does superoxide underlie the pathogenesis of hypertension? *Proc Natl Acad Sci U S A* **88**:10045, 1991.
96. McCord JM: Oxygen-derived free radicals in postischemic tissue injury. *N Engl J Med* **312**:159, 1985.
97. Granger DN: Role of xanthine oxidase and granulocytes in ischemia-reperfusion injury. *Am J Physiol* **255**:H1269, 1988.
98. Saugstad OD, Aasen AO: Plasma hypoxanthine levels in pigs: A prognostic aid in hypoxia. *Eur J Surg Res* **12**:123, 1980.
99. Hassoun PM, Shedd AL, Lanzillo JJ, Thappa V, Landman MJ, Fanburg BL: Inhibition of pulmonary artery smooth muscle cell growth by hypoxanthine, xanthine, and uric acid. *Am J Respir Cell Mol Biol* **6**:617, 1992.
100. Zweier JL, Broderick R, Kuppusamy P, Thompson-Gorman S, Lutty GA: Determination of the mechanism of free radical generation in human aortic endothelial cells exposed to anoxia and reoxygenation. *J Biol Chem* **269**:24156, 1994.
101. Mentzer RMJ, Rubio R, Berne RM: Release of adenosine by hypoxic canine lung tissue and its possible role in pulmonary circulation. *Am J Physiol* **229**:1625, 1975.
102. Buhl MR, Jorgensen S: Breakdown of 5′-adenine nucleotides in ischaemic renal cortex estimated by oxypurine excretion during perfusion. *Scand J Clin Lab Invest* **35**:211, 1975.
103. Saugstad O-D: Hypoxanthine as a measurement of hypoxia. *Pediatr Res* **9**:158, 1975.
104. Engerson TD, McKelvey TG, Rhyne DB, Boggio EB, Snyder SJ, Jones HP: Conversion of xanthine dehydrogenase to oxidase in ischemic rat tissues. *J Clin Invest* **79**:1564, 1987.
105. Kooij A, Schiller HJ, Schijns M, Van Noorden CJF, Frederiks WM: Conversion of xanthine dehydrogenase into xanthine oxidase in rat liver and plasma at the onset of reperfusion after ischemia. *Hepatology* **19**:1488, 1994.
106. Wiezorek JS, Brown DH, Kupperman DE, Brass CA: Rapid conversion to high xanthine oxidase activity in viable Kupffer cells during hypoxia. *J Clin Invest* **94**:2224, 1994.
107. de Groot H, Littauer A: Reoxygenation injury in isolated hepatocytes: Cell death precedes conversion of xanthine dehydrogenase to xanthine oxidase. *Biochem Biophys Res Commun* **155**:278, 1988.
108. Thompson-Gorman SL, Zweier JL: Evaluation of the role of xanthine oxidase in myocardial reperfusion injury. *J Biol Chem* **265**:6656, 1990.
109. Xia Y, Khatchikian G, Zweier JL: Adenosine deaminase inhibition prevents free radical-mediated injury in the postischemic heart. *J Biol Chem* **271**:10096, 1996.
110. Xia Y, Zweier JL: Substrate control of free radical generation from xanthine oxidase in the postischemic heart. *J Biol Chem* **270**:18797, 1995.
111. Spector T: Oxypurinol as an inhibitor of xanthine oxidase-catalyzed production of superoxide radical. *Biochem Pharmacol* **37**:349, 1988.
112. Klein AS, Joh JW, Rangan U, Wang D, Bulkley GB: Allopurinol: Discrimination of antioxidant from enzyme inhibitory activities. *Free Radic Biol Med* **21**:713, 1996.
113. Adachi H, Motomatsu K, Yara I: Effect of allopurinol (Zyloric) on patients undergoing open heart surgery. *Jpn Circ J* **43**:395, 1979.
114. Bochenek A, Religa Z, Spyt TJ, Mistarz K, Bochenek A, Zembala M, Gryzbek H: Protective influence of pretreatment with allopurinol on myocardial function in patients undergoing coronary artery surgery. *Eur J Cardiothorac Surg* **4**:538, 1990.
115. Castelli P, Condemi AM, Brambillasca C, Fundaro P, Botta M, Lemma M, Vanelli P, et al.: Improvement of cardiac function by allopurinol in patients undergoing cardiac surgery. *J Cardiovasc Pharmacol* **25**:119, 1995.
116. Coetzee A, Roussouw G, Macgregor L: Failure of allopurinol to improve left ventricular stroke work after cardiopulmonary bypass surgery. *J Cardiothorac Vasc Anesth* **10**:627, 1996.
117. Coghlan JG, Flitter WD, Clutton SM, Panda R, Daly R, Wright G, Ilsley CD, Slater TF: Allopurinol pretreatment improves postoperative recovery and reduces lipid peroxidation in patients undergoing coronary artery bypass grafting. *J Thorac Cardiovasc Surg* **107**:248, 1994.

118. Emerit I, Fabiani JN, Ponzio O, Murday A, Lunel F, Carpentier A: Clastogenic factor in ischemia-reperfusion injury during open-heart surgery: Protective effect of allopurinol. *Ann Thorac Surg* **46**:619, 1988.
119. England MD, Cavarocchi NC, O'Brien JF, Solis E, Pluth JR, Orszulak TA, Kaye MP, Schaff HV: Influence of antioxidants (mannitol and allopurinol) on oxygen free radical generation during and after cardiopulmonary bypass. *Circulation* **74**:III134, 1986.
120. Gimpel JA, Lahpor JR, van der Molen AJ, Damen J, Hitchcock JF: Reduction of reperfusion injury of human myocardium by allopurinol: A clinical study. *Free Radic Biol Med* **19**:251, 1995.
121. Johnson WD, Kayser KL, Brenowitz JB, Saedi SF: A randomized controlled trial of allopurinol in coronary bypass surgery. *Am Heart J* **121**:20, 1991.
122. Lindsay WG Toledo-Pereyra LH, Foker JE, Varco RL: Metabolic myocardial protection with allopurinol during cardiopulmonary bypass and aortic cross-clamping. *Surg Forum* **26**:259, 1975.
123. MacGowan SW, Regan MC, Malone C, Sharkey O, Young L, Gorey TF, Wood AE: Superoxide radical and xanthine oxidoreductase activity in the human heart during cardiac operations. *Ann Thorac Surg* **60**:1289, 1995.
124. Movahed A, Nair KG, Ashavaid TF, Kumar P: Free radical generation and the role of allopurinol as a cardioprotective agent during coronary artery bypass grafting surgery. *Can J Cardiol* **12**:138, 1996.
125. Rashid MA, William-Olsson G: Influence of allopurinol on cardiac complications in open heart operations. *Ann Thorac Surg* **52**:127, 1991.
126. Sisto T, Paajanen H, Metsä-Ketelä T, Harmoinen A, Nordback I, Tarkka M: Pretreatment with antioxidants and allopurinol diminishes cardiac onset events in coronary artery bypass grafting. *Ann Thorac Surg* **59**:1519, 1995.
127. Tabayashi K, Suzuki Y, Nagamine S, Ito Y, Sekino Y, Mohri H: A clinical trial of allopurinol (Zyloric) for myocardial protection. *J Thorac Cardiovasc Surg* **101**:713, 1991.
128. Taggart DP, Young V, Hooper J, Kemp M, Walesby R, Magee P, Wright JE: Lack of cardioprotective efficacy of allopurinol in coronary artery surgery. *Br Heart J* **71**:177, 1994.
129. Zoran P, Juraj F, Ivana D, Reik H, Dusan N, Mihailo V: Effects of allopurinol on oxygen stress status during open heart surgery. *Int J Cardiol* **44**:123, 1994.
130. Terada LS, Dormish JJ, Shanley PF, Leff JA, Anderson BA, Repine JE: Circulating xanthine oxidase mediates lung neutrophil sequestration after intestinal ischemia-reperfusion. *Am J Physiol* **263**:L394, 1992.
131. Yokoyama Y, Beckman JS, Beckman TK, Wheat JK, Cash TG, Freeman BA, Parks DA: Circulating xanthine oxidase: Potential mediator of ischemic injury. *Am J Physiol* **258**:G564, 1990.
132. Tan S, Gelman S, Wheat JK, Parks DA: Circulating xanthine oxidase in human ischemia reperfusion. *South Med J* **88**:479, 1995.
133. Trewick AL, el Hassan K, Round JM, Adiseshiah M: Xanthine oxidase in critically ischaemic and claudicant limbs: Profile of activity during early reperfusion. *Br J Surg* **83**:798, 1996.
134. Supnet MC, David CR, Walther FJ: Plasma xanthine oxidase activity and lipid hydroperoxide levels in preterm infants. *Pediatr Res* **36**:283, 1994.
135. Friedl HP, Smith DJ, Till GO, Thomson PD, Louis DS, Ward PA: Ischemia-reperfusion in humans: Appearance of xanthine oxidase activity. *Am J Pathol* **136**:491, 1990.
136. Pesonen EJ, Linder N, Raivio KO, Sarnesto A, Lapatto R, Höckerstedt K, Mäkisalo H, Andersson S: Circulating xanthine oxidase and neutrophil activation during human liver transplantation. *Gastroenterology* **114**:1009, 1998.
137. Vickers S, Schiller HJ, Hildreth JEK, Bulkley GB: Immunoaffinity localization of the enzyme xanthine oxidase on the outside of the endothelial cell plasma membrane. *Surgery* **124**:551, 1998.
138. Nielsen VG, Tan S, Weinbroum A, McCammon AT, Samuelson PN, Gelman S, Parks DA: Lung injury after hepatoenteric ischemia-reperfusion: Role of xanthine oxidase. *Am J Respir Crit Care Med* **154**:1364, 1996.
139. Grum CM, Ragsdale RA, Ketai LH, Simon RH: Plasma xanthine oxidase activity in patients with sepsis and adult respiratory distress syndrome. *J Crit Care* **2**:223, 1987.
140. Radi R, Rubbo H, Bush K, Freeman BA: Xanthine oxidase binding to glycosaminoglycans: Kinetics and superoxide dismutase interactions of immobilized xanthine oxidase-heparin complexes. *Arch Biochem Biophys* **339**:125, 1997.
141. Tan S, Yokoyama Y, Dickens E, Cash TG, Freeman BA, Parks DA: Xanthine oxidase activity in the circulation of rats following hemorrhagic shock. *Free Radic Biol Med* **15**:407, 1993.
142. Adachi T, Fukushima T, Usami Y, Hirano K: Binding of human xanthine oxidase to sulphated glycosaminoglycans on the endothelial-cell surface. *Biochem J* **289**:523, 1993.
143. Fukushima T, Adachi T, Hirano K: The heparin-binding site of human xanthine oxidase. *Biol Pharm Bull* **18**:156, 1995.
144. White CR, Darley-Usmar V, Berrington WR, McAdams M, Gore JZ, Thompson JA, Parks DA, et al.: Circulating plasma xanthine oxidase contributes to vascular dysfunction in hypercholesterolemic rabbits. *Proc Natl Acad Sci U S A* **93**:8745, 1996.
145. Zweier JL, Kuppusamy P, Thompson-Gorman S, Klunk D, Lutty GA: Measurement and characterization of free radical generation in reoxygenated human endothelial cells. *Am J Physiol* **266**:C700, 1994.
146. Yoshihara S, Tatsumi K: Guinea pig liver aldehyde oxidase as a sulfoxide reductase: Its purification and characterization. *Arch Biochem Biophys* **242**:213, 1985.
147. Yoshihara S, Tatsumi K: Sulfoxide reduction catalyzed by guinea pig liver aldehyde oxidase in combination with one-electron reducing flavoenzymes. *J Pharmacobiodyn* **8**:996, 1985.
148. Turner NA, Doyle WA, Ventom AM, Bray RC: Properties of rabbit liver aldehyde oxidase and the relationship of the enzyme to xanthine oxidase and dehydrogenase. *Eur J Biochem* **232**:646, 1995.
149. Mira L, Maia L, Barreira L, Manso CF: Evidence for free radical generation due to NADH oxidation by aldehyde oxidase during ethanol metabolism. *Arch Biochem Biophys* **318**:53, 1995.
150. Li Calzi M, Raviolo C, Ghibaudi E, de Gioia L, Salmona M, Cazzaniga G, Kurosaki M, et al.: Purification, cDNA cloning, and tissue distribution of bovine liver aldehyde oxidase. *J Biol Chem* **270**:31037, 1995.
151. Bendotti C, Prosperini E, Kurosaki M, Garattini E, Terao M: Selective localization of mouse aldehyde oxidase mRNA in the choroid plexus and motor neurons. *Neuroreport* **8**:2343, 1997.
152. Wright RM, Clayton DA, Riley MG, McManaman JL, Repine JE: cDNA cloning, sequencing, and characterization of male and female rat liver aldehyde oxidase (rAOX1). Differences in redox status may distinguish male and female forms of hepatic APX. *J Biol Chem* **274**:3878, 1999.
153. Terao M, Kurosaki M, Demontis S, Zanotta S, Garattini E: Isolation and characterization of the human aldehyde oxidase gene–conservation of intron/exon boundaries with the xanthine oxidoreductase gene indicates a common origin. *Biochem J* **332**:383, 1998.
154. Holmes RS: Genetics, ontogeny, and testosterone inducibility of aldehyde oxidase isozymes in the mouse: Evidence for two genetic loci (Aox-I and Aox-2) closely linked on chromosome 1. *Biochem Genet* **17**:517, 1979.
155. Wright RM, Vaitaitis GM, Wilson CM, Repine TB, Terada LS, Repine JE: cDNA cloning, characterization, and tissue-specific expression of human xanthine dehydrogenase/xanthine oxidase. *Proc Natl Acad Sci U S A* **90**:10690, 1993.
156. Huang DY, Ichikawa Y: Two different enzymes are primarily responsible for retinoic acid synthesis in rabbit liver cytosol. *Biochem Biophys Res Commun* **205**:1278, 1994.
157. Berger R, Mezey E, Clancy KP, Harta G, Wright RM, Repine JE, Brown RH, et al.: Analysis of aldehyde oxidase and xanthine dehydrogenase/oxidase as possible candidate genes for autosomal recessive familial amyotrophic lateral sclerosis. *Somat Cell Mol Genet* **21**:121, 1995.
158. Shaw S, Jayatilleke E: The role of aldehyde oxidase in ethanol-induced hepatic lipid peroxidation in the rat. *Biochem J* **268**:579, 1990.
159. Dent CE, Philpot GR: Xanthinuria: An inborn error of metabolism. *Lancet* **1**:182, 1954.
160. Dickinson CJ, Smellie JM: Xanthinuria. *Br Med J* **2**:1217, 1959.
161. Engelman, K, Watts RWE, Klinenberg JR, Sjoerdsma A, Seegmiller JE: Clinical, physiological and biochemical studies of a patient with xanthinuria and pheochromocytoma. *Am J Med* **37**:839, 1964.
162. Simmonds HA, Levin B, Cameron JS: Variations in allopurinol metabolism by xanthinuric subjects. *Clin Sci Mol Med* **47**:173, 1974.
163. Reiter S, Simmonds HA, Zollner N, Braun SL, Knedel M: Demonstration of a combined deficiency of xanthine oxidase and aldehyde oxidase in xanthinuric patients not forming oxypurinol. *Clin Chim Acta* **187**:221, 1990.
164. Harkness RA, Coade SB, Walton KR, Wright D: Xanthine oxidase deficiency and 'Dalmatian' hypouricaemia: Incidence and effect of exercise. *J Inherit Metab Dis* **6**:114, 1983.
165. Harkness RA, McCreanor GM, Simpson D, MacFadyen IR: Pregnancy in and incidence of xanthine oxidase deficiency. *J Inherit Metab Dis* **9**:407, 1986.

166. Frayha RA, Salti IS, Arnaout A, Khatchadurian A, Uthman SM: Hereditary xanthinuria: Report on three patients and short review of the literature. *Nephron* **19**:328, 1977.
167. Bradbury MG, Henderson M, Brocklebank JT, Simmonds HA: Acute renal failure due to xanthine stones. *Pediatr Nephrol* **9**:476, 1995.
168. Carpenter TO, Lebowitz RL, Nelson D, Bauer S: Hereditary xanthinuria presenting in infancy with nephrolithiasis. *J Pediatr* **109**:307, 1986.
169. Bradbury MS, Henderson M, Brocklebank JT, Simmonds HA: Acute renal failure due to xanthine stones. *Pediatr Nephrol* **9**:476, 1995.
170. Simmonds HA, Cameron JS, Barratt TM, Dillon MJ Meadow SR, Trompeter RS: Purine enzyme defects as a cause of acute renal failure in childhood. *Pediatr Nephrol* **3**:433, 1989.
171. Chalmers RA, Watts RW, Bitensky L, Chayen J: Microscopic studies on crystals in skeletal muscle from two cases of xanthinuria. *J Pathol* **99**:45, 1969.
172. Landaas S, Borch K, Aagaard E: A new case with hereditary xanthinuria: Response to exercise. *Clin Chim Acta* **181**:119, 1989.
173. Parker R, Snedden W, Watts RW: The quantitative determination of hypoxanthine and xanthine ("oxypurines") in skeletal muscle from two patients with congenital xanthine oxidase deficiency (xanthinuria). *Biochem J* **116**:317, 1970.
174. Kojima T, Nishina T, Kitamura M, Hosoya T, Nishioka K: Biochemical studies on the purine metabolism of four cases with hereditary xanthinuria. *Clin Chim Acta* **137**:189, 1984.
175. Boulieu R, Bory C, Baltassat P, Divry P: Hypoxanthine and xanthine concentrations determined by high performance liquid chromatography in biological fluids from patients with xanthinuria. *Clin Chim Acta* **142**:83, 1984.
176. Bennett MJ, Carpenter KH, Hill PG: Asymptomatic xanthinuria detected as a result of routine analysis of serum for urate. *Clin Chem* **31**:492, 1985.
177. Simmonds HA, Stutchbury JH, Webster DR, Spencer RE, Fisher RA, Wooder M, Buckley BM: Pregnancy in xanthinuria: Demonstration of fetal uric acid production? *J Inherit Metab Dis* **7**:77, 1984.
178. van Gennip AH, van Noordenburg-Huistra DY, de Bree PK, Wadman SK: Two-dimensional thin-layer chromatography for the screening of disorders of purine and pyrimidine metabolism. *Clin Chim Acta* **86**:7, 1978.
179. Mateos FA, Puig JG, Jimenez ML, Fox IH: Hereditary xanthinuria: Evidence for enhanced hypoxanthine salvage. *J Clin Invest* **79**:847, 1987.
180. Simmonds HA, Rising TJ, Cadenhead A, Hatfield PJ, Jones AS, Cameron JS: Radioisotope studies of purine metabolism during administration of guanine and allopurinol in the pig. *Biochem Pharmacol* **22**:2553, 1973.
181. Moriwaki Y, Yamamoto T, Nasako Y, Takahashi S, Suda M, Hiroishi K, Hada T, Higashino K: *In vitro* oxidation of pyrazinamide and allopurinol by rat liver aldehyde oxidase. *Biochem Pharmacol* **46**:975, 1993.
182. Yamamoto T, Higashino K, Kono N, Kawachi M, Nanahoshi M, Takahashi S, Suda M, Hada T: Metabolism of pyrazinamide and allopurinol in hereditary xanthine oxidase deficiency. *Clin Chim Acta* **180**:169, 1989.
183. Bory C, Chantin C, Boulieu R: Comparison of capillary electrophoretic and liquid chromatographic determination of hypoxanthine and xanthine for the diagnosis of xanthinuria. *J Chromatogr A* **730**:329, 1996.
184. Blau N, de Klerk KJ, Thony B, Heizmann CW, Kierat L, Smeitink JA, Duran M: Tetrahydrobiopterin loading test in xanthine dehydrogenase and molybdenum cofactor deficiencies. *Biochem Mol Med* **58**:199, 1996.
185. Ichida K, Yoshida M, Sakuma R, Hosoya T: Two siblings with classical xanthinuria type 1: Significance of allopurinol loading test. *Intern Med* **37**:77, 1998.
186. Salti IS, Kattuah N, Alam S, Wehby V, Frayha R: The effect of allopurinol on oxypurine excretion in xanthinuria. *J Rheumatol* **3**:201, 1976.
187. Wilson DM, Tapia HR: Xanthinuria in a large kindred. *Adv Exp Med Biol* **41**:343, 1973.
188. Kawachi M, Kono N, Mineo I, Yamada Y, Tarui S: Decreased xanthine oxidase activities and increased urinary oxypurines in heterozygotes for hereditary xanthinuria. *Clin Chim Acta* **188**:137, 1990.
189. Yamamoto T, Moriwaki Y, Suda M, Takahashi S, Hada T, Nanahoshi M, Agbedana EO, Higashino K: An immunoreactive xanthine oxidase protein-possessing xanthinuria and her family. *Clin Chim Acta* **208**:93, 1992.
190. Ichida K, Amaya Y, Kamatani N, Nishino T, Hosoya T, Sakai O: Identification of two mutations in human xanthine dehydrogenase gene responsible for classical type I xanthinuria. *J Clin Invest* **99**:2391, 1997.
191. Wahl RC, Warner CK, Finnerty V, Rajagopalan KV: *Drosophila melanogaster ma-l* mutants are defective in the sulfuration of desulfo Mo hydroxylases. *J Biol Chem* **257**:3958, 1982.

CHAPTER 112

Adenylosuccinate Lyase Deficiency

Georges Van den Berghe ▪ Jaak Jaeken

1. The deficiency of adenylosuccinate lyase (ADSL) (OMIM 103050) causes variable degrees of psychomotor retardation, often accompanied by epileptic seizures and/or autistic features. About half of patients display moderate to severe retardation and epilepsy after the first years, occasionally associated with growth retardation and muscular wasting. Others present with convulsions within the first days to weeks of life. Rare patients display only mild psychomotor retardation or profound muscle hypotonia.

2. ADSL deficiency is characterized by the appearance in cerebrospinal fluid and urine, and to a much smaller extent in plasma, of succinylaminoimidazolecarboxamide riboside (SAICAriboside) and succinyladenosine (S-Ado). These succinylpurines are the dephosphorylated derivatives of, respectively, SAICAribotide (SAICAR) and adenylosuccinate (S-AMP), the two substrates of ADSL. This enzyme intervenes twice in the synthesis of purine nucleotides: it catalyzes the eighth step of their *de novo* synthesis, and the second step of the conversion of IMP into AMP.

3. To date, about 40 patients have been identified. Most of them have been diagnosed in the low countries, Belgium and The Netherlands, and in the Czech Republic. Other patients have been identified in Australia, France, Germany, Italy, Morocco, Spain, Turkey, and the USA. The marked clinical heterogeneity of ADSL deficiency justifies systematic screening for the disorder in patients with unexplained psychomotor retardation and/or neurologic disease.

4. ADSL deficiency is inherited in an autosomal recessive manner. The ADSL gene is located on chromosome 22q. Nineteen ADSL gene mutations have been identified to date. Most seem to lead to structural instability of the enzyme, without modifications of its kinetic properties.

5. Although ADSL intervenes twice in purine biosynthesis, decreased concentrations of purine nucleotides could not be evidenced in various tissues of ADSL-deficient patients. This can be explained by residual activity of ADSL, and by supply of purines via the purine salvage pathway. The symptoms of ADSL deficiency are most likely caused by neurotoxic effects of the accumulating succinylpurines. In most patients, S-Ado/SAICAriboside ratios are around 1. The observation of generally less severe mental retardation in patients with similar SAICAriboside levels but S-Ado/SAICAriboside ratios above 2, suggests that SAICAriboside is the offending compound, and that S-Ado could protect against its toxic effects.

6. The prognosis of ADSL-deficient subjects is generally poor. Several patients, particularly those presenting with early epilepsy, have died in early infancy. Nevertheless, some patients, particularly those with higher S-Ado/SAICAriboside ratios, fare relatively well. With the aim to replenish hypothetically decreased concentrations of purine nucleotides in ADSL-deficient tissues, some patients have been treated with oral supplements of adenine and allopurinol, the latter to avoid conversion of adenine into minimally soluble 2,8-dihydroxyadenine. No clinical or biochemical improvement was recorded, with the exception of some acceleration of growth.

A list of standard abbreviations is located immediately preceding the index in each volume. Additional abbreviations used in this chapter include: AICAR = aminoimidazolecarboxamide ribotide; ADSL = adenylosuccinate lyase (adenylosuccinase); CAIR = carboxylateaminoimidazole ribotide; FAICAR = formylaminoimidazolecarboxamide ribotide; FGAR = formylglycineamide ribotide; GAR = glycineamide ribotide; S-Ado = succinyladenosine; S-AMP = adenylosuccinate; SAICAR = succinylaminoimidazolecarboxamide ribotide; SAICAriboside = succinylaminoimidazolecarboxamide riboside; ZMP = aminoimidazolecarboxamide riboside monophosphate (AICAR); and ZTP = aminoimidazolecarboxamide riboside triphosphate.

INTRODUCTION AND HISTORY

Adenylosuccinase deficiency, the first enzyme deficiency reported on the *de novo* pathway of purine synthesis in man, was discovered in the course of a systematic study of the influence of strong acid hydrolysis on amino acid chromatograms of deproteinized samples of cerebrospinal fluid.[1] This procedure elevates, probably by hydrolysis of small, nonprecipitated peptides, the concentration of several amino acids. Among these, aspartic acid and glycine increase from approximately 1 and 7 μM, respectively, to maximally 40 μM in control samples. In the cerebrospinal fluid of three children with severe psychomotor retardation and autistic features, acid hydrolysis provoked a much larger, equimolar increase of the concentration of both amino acids, to 200 to 300 μM. The elevation of both amino acids originated from one or more ninhydrin-negative compounds because no abnormality was noted on the amino acid chromatograms performed before hydrolysis. Thin-layer chromatography of sugars[2] in the three patients' cerebrospinal fluid before hydrolysis revealed an abnormal spot located between sucrose and galactose; after mild acid hydrolysis it disappeared and was replaced by a spot that coincided with ribose. Quantification by gas chromatography showed that the concentration of ribose was roughly equimolar with that of aspartate and glycine. This led to a search for purine compounds. Anion-exchange HPLC of deproteinized but otherwise untreated cerebrospinal fluid of the three patients revealed the presence of two UV absorbing compounds that were undetectable in control samples (Fig. 112-1). Both peaks were similarly prominent in urine, and two small peaks were also visible in the patients' plasma. The retention times of the two abnormal compounds indicated that both carried two negative charges, and spectral scanning showed that both displayed a maximum extinction at 268 nm. Comparison with standard solutions led to the identification of peak I as succinyladenosine (S-Ado), and of peak II as succinylaminoimidazolecarboxamide riboside (SAICAriboside). These succinylpurines are the dephosphorylated

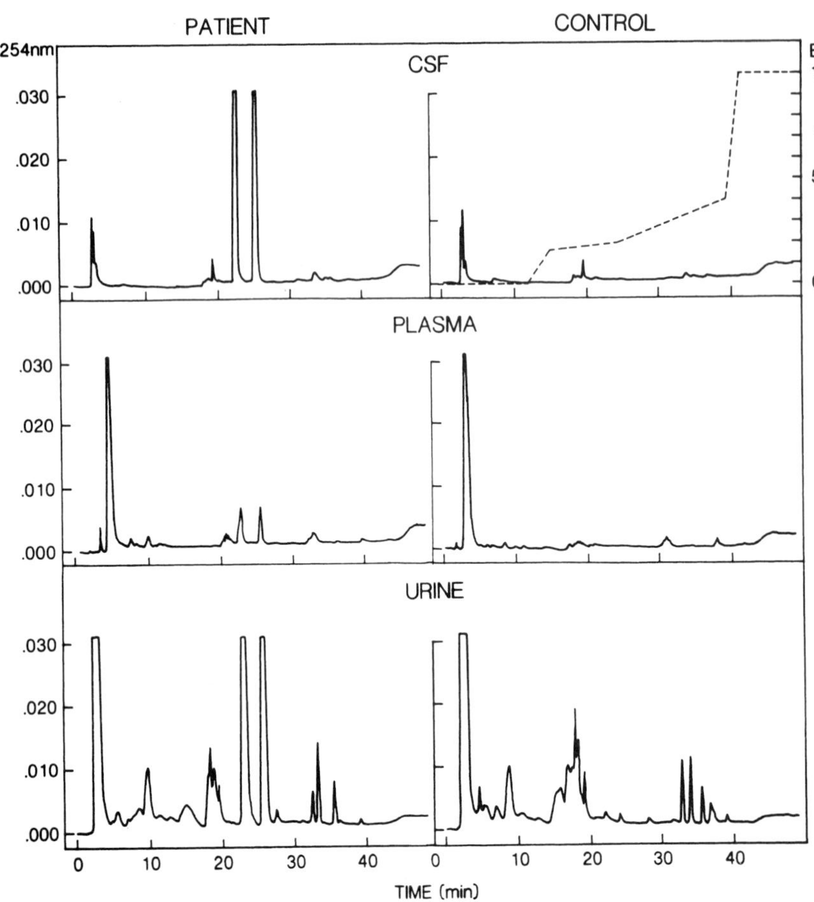

Fig. 112-1 High-pressure liquid chromatography of deproteinized cerebrospinal fluid (CSF), plasma, and urine of an ADSL-deficient patient (left panels) and of a control child (right panels). Samples equivalent to 50 μl were injected into an anion exchange column. The first of the twin peaks in the patient sample is S-Ado; the second is SAICAriboside. Dotted line shows percentage of high concentration eluate (B) in gradient. 254 nm: absorbance at 254 nm. (*From Jaeken & Van den Berghe.*[1] *Used by permission of The Lancet Ltd.*)

counterparts of adenylosuccinate (S-AMP), and SAICAribotide (SAICAR), respectively, the two substrates of adenylosuccinate lyase. This enzyme, also termed adenylosuccinase (ADSL), catalyzes two steps in the synthesis of purine nucleotides (Fig. 112-2): the conversion of SAICAR into aminoimidazole carboxamide ribotide (AICAR), the eighth step of the *de novo* pathway, and the formation of AMP from S-AMP, the second step in the conversion of IMP into AMP.

Enzyme assays in the patients' liver and kidney[1] confirmed that the accumulation of succinylpurines resulted from a deficiency of ADSL. Since then, approximately 40 patients with the disorder have been identified, and reports on 20 of them have been published.[3–11] The 20 reported patients belong to 17 families and 8 nationalities: American,[9] Belgian,[1,3,4] Czech,[5,7] Dutch,[3,8,10] German,[11] Italian,[6] Moroccan,[1,3] and Turkish.[3] In addition, unpublished patients have been identified in Australia, France, and Spain.

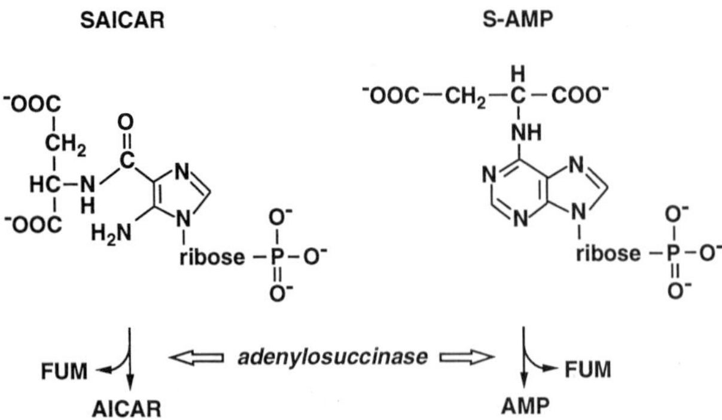

Fig. 112-2 The reactions catalyzed by ADSL (adenylosuccinase). SAICAR, succinylaminoimidazolecarboxamide ribotide; S-AMP, adenylosuccinate; FUM, fumarate; AICAR, aminoimidazolecarboxamide ribotide.

CLINICAL SPECTRUM AND VARIABILITY OF ADSL DEFICIENCY

As a rule, patients with ADSL deficiency reported hitherto presented with a pure encephalopathy comprising variable associations of these symptoms: psychomotor retardation; autistic features (failure to make eye-to-eye contact, repetitive behavior, agitation, temper tantrums, autoaggressivity); epilepsy; hypotonia (axial or generalized); peripheral hypertonia; and secondary feeding problems. Dysmorphic features are absent. Somewhat arbitrarily, patients can be categorized into four main clinical presentations. In the first reported presentation, sometimes referred to as type I,[12] and observed in eight families, patients displayed moderate to severe psychomotor retardation, epilepsy after the first years, and variable behavior disturbances.[1,3–7] In one of these families, represented by two published,[3] and two unpublished sibs, severe growth retardation associated with muscular wasting starting between 1 and 2 years of age was also recorded. A second clinical presentation, observed in seven families, is characterized by early epilepsy, with convulsions starting within the first days to weeks of life.[5,7,8,10,11] A third clinical picture, which has been referred to as type II,[12] comprises one patient, a girl, presenting with strikingly mild psychomotor retardation as compared to the other cases, and only transient contact disturbances.[3] Finally, another girl displayed only delayed motor development and profound muscle hypotonia.[9]

The following technical investigations yielded normal results in the patients in whom they were performed: fundoscopy,[3,9,11] auditory and visual evoked responses,[3,10,11] electroretinography,[11] and nerve conduction velocities.[3] Electromyography and skeletal muscle biopsy were normal in the patients with muscular wasting,[3] and in the girl with profound muscle hypotonia.[9] Somatosensory-evoked potentials were either normal[3] or abnormal without cortical responses.[10] Electroencephalography varied from normal to severely epileptic, with hypsarhythmia in one patient,[3] and a burst-suppression pattern in two patients.[10,11] CT scan of the brain showed cerebellar hypoplasia mainly of the vermis, and cortical and subcortical hypotrophy.[3] MRI of the brain was normal,[3] or revealed myelin disturbances ranging from areas of increased T2 signal in white matter,[9] to severe leukodystrophy.[8,11]

BIOCHEMICAL FEATURES OF ADSL DEFICIENCY

In subjects with ADSL deficiency, concentrations of SAICAriboside and S-Ado in cerebrospinal fluid are between 100 and 500 μM.[1,3,4,5,13] The levels of both succinylpurines are twenty- to one hundredfold higher in cerebrospinal fluid than in plasma, in which their concentrations vary from 2 to 12 μM.[1,3,5,6,13] This concentration gradient indicates that the succinylpurines are produced in the central nervous system and do not cross the blood-brain barrier readily. In urine, the concentrations of both succinylpurines vary from 25 to 700 mmol/mol of creatinine.[1,3,5,6,8,11,13] Calculation shows that the urinary clearance of both succinylpurines reaches two- to threefold that of creatinine, indicating that both compounds are not only filtered but also secreted by the kidney. In a series of seven ADSL-deficient children, the output of both succinylpurines together was found to reach between 50 and 130 percent of that of uric acid.[3] The latter was in the normal range for the age of the children, both when expressed as a uric acid to creatinine ratio[14] and, in the children from whom 24-h urine outputs were available, as mg/kg body weight per 24 h.

In most patients, concentrations of S-Ado are in the same range as those of SAICAriboside, and the S-Ado/SAICAriboside ratios are around 1. Ratios in plasma and urine reflect those in cerebrospinal fluid.[3] Noteworthy, in some patients, body fluid concentrations of S-Ado are distinctly higher than those of SAICAriboside. Presently available evidence suggests that the more severe clinical presentations of ADSL deficiency tend to be associated with higher SAICAriboside levels and lower S-Ado/SAICAriboside ratios, whereas milder clinical pictures are found in association with lower SAICAriboside levels and higher S-Ado/SAICAriboside ratios. In a strikingly less retarded ADSL-deficient girl, cerebrospinal fluid S-Ado reached 475 μM and the S-Ado/SAICAriboside ratio was 3.7.[3] In another mildly affected girl, the urinary S-Ado/SAICA-riboside ratio was about 2.5.[9] In a patient with intermediate symptomatology, cerebrospinal fluid S-Ado was 379 μM and the S-Ado/SAICAriboside ratio reached 1.8.[4] In two siblings with intermediate symptomatology, cerebrospinal fluid S-Ado levels were 283 and 260 μM, and S-Ado/SAICAriboside ratios were 2.2 and 2.1.[5] In five severely affected cases, cerebrospinal fluid S-Ado was 134 to 166 μM, with S-Ado/SAICAriboside ratios around 1.[3,5] Taken together, these findings suggest that SAICAriboside is the most deleterious compound for neural function, and that S-Ado could protect against its toxic effects.

Apart from the accumulation and excretion of the normally undetectable succinylpurines, all routine biochemical analyses of cerebrospinal fluid, plasma, and urine are within normal limits.

PROPERTIES OF THE NORMAL ENZYME

Adenylosuccinate lyase (adenylosuccinate adenosine 5′-monophosphate lyase, EC 4.3.2.2) was discovered in yeast and chick liver by Carter and Cohen,[15] and by Buchanan's group.[16] The enzyme is found in nearly all organisms and tissues examined.[17–22] A brief review of its properties is mostly restricted to the mammalian enzyme.

Enzymology

The two reactions catalyzed by ADSL involve the nonhydrolytic cleavage of the C-N bond linking the succinate moiety to the nucleotide part of the substrate, to yield fumarate (Fig. 112-2). Both eliminations are similar to that catalyzed by the urea cycle enzyme, argininosuccinate lyase.[19] The conclusion that both SAICAR and S-AMP are cleaved by the same enzyme is based on the following evidence (reviewed in reference 19): (a) the ratio of activities with both substrates remains the same along all purification procedures of the enzyme; (b) both substrates exhibit mutual competitive inhibition; and (c) mutant lower organisms which lack S-AMP cleavage activity are also unable to cleave SAICAR. ADSL displays hyperbolic kinetics. K_m of both SAICAR and S-AMP is 1 to 10 μM for the enzyme of human erythrocytes,[23] rat muscle,[24] human cultured fibroblasts,[25] and for human recombinant enzyme.[26] The product of the two reactions, which it catalyzes, inhibits ADSL. K_i is 5 to 10 μM for AICAR and AMP, and 0.2 to 2.8 mM for fumarate.[23,26,27] Competitive inhibition by AICAR and AMP, and noncompetitive inhibition by fumarate, indicate that ADSL from various sources, including yeast,[28] murine cells,[29] human erythrocytes,[23] and the human recombinant enzyme,[26] follows a simple, ordered, sequential reaction mechanism in which fumarate is the first product released, followed by the nucleotide. Intraperitoneal administration of AICAriboside, which is phosphorylated into AICAR by adenosine kinase,[30] has been used to inhibit ADSL in skeletal muscle of rats *in vivo*.[31,32]

ADSL is also capable of efficiently cleaving a variety of purine and nonpurine analogues, among which 6-mercaptopurinoadenylosuccinate,[33] 2′-deoxyadenylosuccinate, β-D-arabinosyladenylosuccinate,[34] 8-aza-adenylosuccinate and succino-4-aminopyrazolo(3,4-*d*)pyrimidine ribonucleotide, an allopurinol derivative,[21] and 2′-3′-dideoxyadenylosuccinate.[35] The latter is an intermediate in the conversion of the anti-HIV compounds 2′,3′-dideoxyadenosine and 2′,3′-dideoxyinosine into their active triphosphate derivatives.[36] Other adenylosuccinate analogues are inhibitory of ADSL and have been investigated as potential antimetabolites (see below).

Structure

Studies of purified ADSL from human erythrocytes,[23] rat liver,[37] and muscle[24] have shown that the native enzyme has a molecular weight of ≈200,000 and is composed of 4 subunits. Nucleotide-predicted amino acid sequences of ADSL have been reported for a number of tissues, including chicken liver,[38] human liver,[39] and mouse kidney.[40] From open cDNA reading frames of 1377 nucleotides, a sequence of 459 amino acids was deduced for both the chicken and human enzyme. However, the high degree of identity of the nucleotide sequence upstream of the originally reported initiation codon of the cDNAs cloned from both sources with the mouse sequence,[40] and correction from C to A of the third nucleotide of the human sequence,[41] have revealed a first ATG, 75 nucleotides 5′ of the originally reported initiation codon. The open reading frame thus comprises 1452 nucleotides and encodes a protein that is 25 amino acids longer at the N-terminus, containing 484 amino acids. At the amino acid level, human ADSL was found 85 percent identical to the chicken enzyme,[39] and 94 percent identical to the murine enzyme.[40]

ADSL also bears sequence homology to a group of enzymes that generate fumarate from different substrates, namely argininosuccinate lyase, aspartase, and class II fumarases. Moreover, it displays sequence similarity with δ-crystallin, the major structural component of the lenses of most birds and reptiles.[42–44] This transparent protein is considered to have evolved from argininosuccinate lyase by gene sharing,[45] because it has retained its enzymic activity. Most highly conserved among the similar regions of the enzymes cited above is an 11-amino acid span (amino acids 288 to 298; GSSAMPYKRNP in the corrected sequence of human ADSL), which is considered the "fumarate lyase" signature.[38] (See also Chap. 85.)

The catalytic mechanism of ADSL has been shown to involve a general base catalyst, removing a proton from the succinyl group of the substrate, acting in concert with a general acid catalyst that protonates the amino group left on AICAR or AMP.[46,47] Several phylogenetically conserved amino acid residues have been proposed to perform these functions.[26,38] Affinity labeling of *Bacillus subtilis* ADSL with 4-bromo-2,3-dioxobutyl thio derivatives of AMP has led to the suggestion that a highly conserved Arg112 is involved in the binding of the substrate by the enzyme, and that another highly conserved residue, His141, corresponding to His134 in human ADSL, may be the general base catalyst.[48–50]

Crystal structures of two enzymes of this superfamily of lyases have been solved, namely those of turkey δ-crystallin,[43] and *E. coli* fumarase.[44] Both reveal a putative active-site cleft, located on the boundary between three subunits of the tetramer, in which the highly conserved histidine is located, which is proposed to serve as general base catalyst. In this structure, the general acid function is attributed to a closely positioned glutamate. Crystallization of *Bacillus subtilis* ADSL was recently reported,[51] but its structure has not yet been determined.

Tissue Distribution and Isozymes

In man, ADSL activity has been measured in erythrocytes,[1,23,52] granulocytes, lymphocytes, liver, kidney, and muscle.[3,53] ADSL remains active in cultured mammalian cells, including fibroblasts[3,25,53–55] and lymphoblasts.[56] A number of observations indicate that isoforms of ADSL exist. Whereas starvation induced a profound decrease of the activity of ADSL in rat liver and spleen, it had no effect on the activity of the enzyme in muscle, brain, and kidney.[20] Isoelectric focusing of rat muscle ADSL showed the existence of three isomeric forms present in similar amounts.[57] Expression of cDNA clones in an epidermoid carcinoma and two colon carcinoma cell lines revealed two ADSL mRNAs with different sizes: 1.8 and 2.5 kb.[58] Northern blots of mouse tissues,[40] revealed only a single predominant 1.9-kb message, but in chicken liver,[38] an abundant mRNA of approximately 1.7 kb was accompanied by two minor messages of 1.2 and 3.0 kb. Finally, studies in patients with ADSL deficiency (see below) show that the activity of the enzyme is lost to a different extent in various tissues, and is normal in others. Further characterization of the isozymes of ADSL has, however, not yet been accomplished.

Adenylosuccinate Lyase in Cancer Cells

Up to threefold elevated activities of ADSL as compared to normal are found in a variety of tumor cells, particularly those derived from liver and kidney.[59,60] These increases appear specific for neoplasia insofar as they are not seen in regenerating liver. Kinetic properties of the enzyme of a rapidly growing hepatoma were similar to those of normal ADSL.[60] Increases in liver ADSL activity were also noted as early as 48 to 72 h following the administration of hepatocarcinogens such as 3′-methyl-4-dimethylaminobenzene and thioacetamide.[61] In experimentally induced rat tumor models, elevation of ADSL activity was a reliable early indicator of the presence of hepatic or breast tumor.[62] In human breast and prostate tumors, a high activity of ADSL was also an indicator of malignancy.[63] On the other hand, differentiation of colon carcinoma cells has been shown to be accompanied by downregulation of the expression of ADSL.[58]

Because enhancement of the *de novo* synthesis of purines is one of the main characteristics of tumor cells, and because ADSL intervenes twice in this process, the potential exists for use of inhibitors of ADSL as antimetabolites. Adenylophosphonopropionate, in which the aspartate moiety of S-AMP is replaced by 3-phosphoalanine, is the most potent inhibitor ($K_i \approx 0.02$ μM) of the enzyme reported sofar.[64] Yet, owing to their multiple negative charges, both adenylophosphonopropionate and its nucleoside fail to penetrate cells.[65] The fluorinated derivatives of aspartate, *threo*-β-fluoroaspartate and *erythro*-β-fluoroaspartate, also potently inhibit ADSL after their conversion into adenylosuccinate and SAICAR derivatives by adenylosuccinate synthetase and SAICAR synthetase, respectively.[24,66] However, both compounds are highly toxic because fluoroaspartate can substitute for aspartate in other pathways, most notably protein synthesis.[67] Alanosine, an investigational anticancer drug, can substitute for aspartate in the SAICAR synthetase reaction, forming alanosyl-carboxylateaminoimidazole ribotide (alanosyl-CAIR), which acts mainly as an inhibitor of adenylosuccinate synthetase, but which also exerts an inhibitory effect on ADSL.[68]

PROPERTIES OF THE MUTANT ENZYMES

Residual Activities

Initially, the activity of ADSL was only measured with S-AMP as substrate in ADSL-deficient patients.[1,3] In the liver of five cases, enzymatic activity was reduced to 15 to 25 percent of normal; in the liver of two other patients it was undetectable. In three patients in whom a kidney biopsy was performed, similar results were found; in one patient, ADSL activity was undetectable, whereas in a brother and sister pair it was reduced to less than 20 percent of normal. In muscle, the activity of ADSL was within the normal range in three patients; in three others, it was reduced to 10 to 20 percent of the mean control value. In two of the latter subjects, severe growth retardation in weight and length and muscle wasting were observed. In the third case, a slow weight-velocity curve was recorded. In peripheral blood lymphocytes, ADSL activity was about 40 percent of normal.[7,53] Diminished activity of ADSL was also measured in lymphoblasts derived from patients' lymphocytes.[56] In some patients, normal activities of ADSL were found in erythrocytes.[53] However, in four other patients, decreased erythrocyte activity has since been reported.[6,7] A partial deficiency of ADSL with S-AMP as substrate was also measured in cultured skin fibroblasts of several patients.[3,9,53]

Later on, measurements of the activity of ADSL with both S-AMP and SAICAR as substrates, showed that both activities were decreased in parallel in liver[69] and in fibroblasts[25] of a number of profoundly retarded patients. In fibroblasts of a mildly retarded patient, however, activity with S-AMP was reduced to 3 percent of normal, whereas that with SAICAR was 30 percent of control.[25] This nonparallel loss of both activities of ADSL, if also present in other tissues, provides an explanation for the higher S-Ado/SAICAriboside ratio, reaching approximately 4, in the body fluids of this mildly retarded patient. Taken together, the enzyme data indicate genetic heterogeneity of the defect, and corroborate the presumed existence of isoforms of ADSL.

Information concerning the activity of ADSL in brain tissue of affected patients is not available. The twenty- to one hundredfold higher concentration of the succinylpurines in the cerebrospinal fluid of the patients, as compared to those in plasma,[1,3,13] provides, nevertheless, a strong indication that cerebral ADSL is also deficient.

Characterization

Heat denaturation studies show that mutant ADSL is substantially more labile than normal in fibroblasts,[55] lymphoblasts,[56] and erythrocytes.[6] Decreased thermal stability of a recombinant mutant human enzyme has also been documented.[39] The apparent K_m of S-AMP for fibroblast ADSL from profoundly retarded, type I patients (≈10 μM) was not modified as compared to control cells.[25] Similar results were obtained with ADSL from cultured lymphoblasts derived from these patients.[56] Owing to the very low residual activity with S-AMP in the fibroblasts from a mildly retarded, type II patient, K_m of S-AMP could not be measured. In both mutant cell types, precise determinations of K_m of SAICAR were also hampered by low enzyme activities.[25] Yet, detailed studies of a recombinant N-terminus-truncated enzyme expressing the mutation of a profoundly retarded patient, showed that its kinetic constants for both substrates were indistinguishable from those of the truncated normal enzyme.[26] In control fibroblasts, as in cells from type I patients, the activity of ADSL, measured both with S-AMP and SAICAR, was not influenced by the addition of 100 mM KCl.[25] In contrast, KCl markedly inhibited ADSL activity with SAICAR in type II fibroblasts (activity decreased by ≈60 percent with 100 mM KCl). Further studies showed that this inhibition was due to the anion, competitive (K_m with SAICAR increased to 270 μM in the presence of 90 mM KCl), and also exerted by other anions which inhibited in this order: $KH_2PO_4 > K_2SO_4 > KI > KBr > KCl > KF > KCOOH$. In cells from controls and from type I patients, the activity with SAICAR was not inhibited by purine and pyrimidine nucleoside triphosphates. In contrast, the activity of ADSL in cells of a type II patient was markedly (60 to 90 percent) inhibited by 2.5 mM ATP, GTP, ITP, ZTP, UTP, and CTP.[25]

Taken together, the enzyme studies suggest that in profoundly retarded, type I patients, the ADSL defect results in a structural defect, provoking decreased stability of the enzyme, whereas in a mildly retarded, type II patient, a catalytic defect impairs binding of S-AMP to a much more marked extent than binding of SAICAR, possibly as a result of addition of positive charges in the active site.

THE ADSL GENE

The ADSL gene has been mapped to chromosome 22q13.1-q13.2 in humans.[70–72] Using chicken liver cDNA[38] as a hybridization probe, Stone et al.[39] deduced that the cDNA sequence of human liver ADSL comprised 1377 nucleotides (EMBL accession number X65867). As already discussed, comparison of the latter sequence with a mouse cDNA[40] led to the conclusion that the open reading frame is 75 nucleotides longer, containing 1452 nucleotides.[41] The fumarate lyase signature comprises nucleotides 864 to 896 of the corrected sequence, encoding amino acids 288 to 298. The mouse cDNA has 87 percent identity to the human sequence.[40] Characterization of the gene-encoding murine ADSL has shown that it is about 27 kb long and contains 13 exons that vary in size from 45 to 204 bp.[40] Like other constitutively expressed housekeeping genes, the promoter region of the human ADSL gene contains no TATA sequence. It possesses several potential transcription-binding sites and also has a high—66 percent—GC content. Comparison of the exon/intron structure with that of the argininosuccinate lyase gene revealed extensive sequence similarity and the presence of the conserved GSSA and GFTH domains found in the fumarase gene family, but did not suggest that the evolution of the family resulted from gene duplication or exon shuffling.[40]

GENETICS AND MOLECULAR BASES OF ADSL DEFICIENCY

The occurrence of the enzyme defect in more than one child in two families, in patients of both sexes, and in two consanguineous marriages,[1,3] indicates that ADSL deficiency is transmitted as an autosomal recessive trait. In a first-investigated Moroccan family with four affected children,[1,3] the molecular basis of the deficiency was found to be a single T to C substitution, resulting in an amino acid change that was initially labeled S413P when the enzyme was considered to be 459 amino acids long,[39] but is now termed S438P in the 484 amino acid protein. A search for this mutation, which introduces a new *Hph*I restriction site, in a group of 119 patients with autistic features gave negative results.[73] However, in accordance with the variability of the clinical picture, analysis of additional ADSL-deficient patients has revealed a high degree of molecular heterogeneity.[74–77] Through June 1998, 19 different mutant alleles were identified in the ADSL cDNA of 17 families (Table 112-1). All were of the missense type, with the exception of a 39-bp deletion. Ten mutations resulted in the appearance or the

Table 112-1 Mutations of the ADSL Locus

Family No.	Country	Base Change	Amino Acid Change	Exon No.	Restriction Site
1*	Morocco	c.1314T→C	S438P	12	+ Hph I
2†	Belgium	c.1279G→A	R426H	12	none
3†	Netherlands	c.1279G→A	R426H	12	none
4†	Netherlands	c.909C→T	R303C	9	– Mae II
5†	Belgium	c.571G→A	R190Q	5	none
		c.738A→G	K246E	7	none
6†	Belgium	c.216A→G	172V	2	+ Mae II
		c.738A→G	K246E	7	none
7§	Italy	c.300C→G	P100A	2	none
		c.1266G→T	D422Y	12	none
8†	Netherlands	c.1279G→A	R426H	12	none
9¶	Czech Republic	c.342T→C	Y114H	2	+ Nla III
		c.571G→A	R190Q	5	none
10¶	Czech Republic	c.10C→T	A3V	1	– Fnu 4H1
		c.1011C→T	R337X	9	none
11¶	Czech Republic	c.582C→T	R194C	5	– Hha I
		c.804G→A	D268N	8	none
12¶	Czech Republic	c.1279G→A	R426H	12	none
13¶	USA	c.1279G→A	R426H	12	none
		c.1290G→A	D430N	12	+ Mse I
14†	Netherlands	c.7C→T	A2V	1	– Fnu 4HI
		c.1187C→A	S395R	11	– Fnu 4HI
15†	Germany	c.423C→T	R141W	4	none
		c.620C→A**	del 206-18	5	– Hae III
16†	Germany	c.78A→T	M26L	1	none
		c.1279G→A	R426H	12	none
17†	Netherlands	c.1279G→A	R426H	12	none

The nucleotide sequence of the human ADSL cDNA is deposited in the EMBL database under accession number X65867.
*Originally described by Stone et al.[39] as S413P.
†Originally described by Marie et al.[77]
§Originally described by Verginelli et al.[76] as P75A and D397Y.
¶Originally described by Kmoch et al.[75]
**Splice-site mutation resulting in del 618-56 in cDNA.[77]

disappearance of a restriction site. In about half the families, the patients are compound heterozygotes. Seven apparently unrelated patients from five different countries were found to carry a R426H mutation. Five of these patients were homozygotes, and two were compound heterozygotes. With the exceptions of a R190Q and a K346E mutation, each of which was found in the heterozygous form in two apparently unrelated patients, all other mutations were only found in a single family. Further analysis on genomic DNA of the 39-bp deletion in the cDNA of patient 15 revealed that it was caused by a base change in exon 5 (c.620 C → A), creating a GC consensus 5′ donor splice site, namely AG gcaag.[77]

The mutations found in the patients seem to be evenly distributed along the ADSL gene, without suggestion of hotspots for mutation. Most missense-mutated amino acids are absolutely conserved in the murine and chicken ADSL sequences, highlighting their functional importance. Moreover, all mutations are located outside the fumarate lyase signature (amino acids 288 to 298). This suggests that they may lead to structural instability of the enzyme, without modifications of its kinetic properties, as demonstrated for the S438P mutated[56] and recombinant[26] enzyme. Interestingly, in the mildly retarded type II patient belonging to family 4, in whom a catalytic defect is suggested because binding of S-AMP is much more impaired than that of SAICAR,[25] the mutation was found to be located on amino acid 303, five amino acids distal from the fumarate lyase signature.

PATHOGENESIS OF ADSL DEFICIENCY

Two main hypotheses can be put forward to explain the symptoms of ADSL deficiency: impaired synthesis of purine nucleotides and toxic effects of the accumulating succinylpurines. Other mechanisms might also play a role.

Impaired Synthesis of Purine Nucleotides

From the dual function of ADSL in the pathway of purine biosynthesis (Fig. 112-3), one might expect its deficiency to lead to decreased concentrations of purine, particularly adenine nucleotides. However, measurements of the concentrations of adenine and guanine nucleotides in freeze-clamped liver, kidney, and muscle of ADSL-deficient patients[53] revealed normal values. Nevertheless, in an affected girl, muscle ATP levels, as well as those of creatine phosphate, measured by ^{31}P NMR, were reported to be decreased, both at rest and after exercise.[78] In this same patient, fructose loading provoked an elevation of plasma magnesium, which might reflect ATP loss.[6] Assessment of nucleoside phosphates by ^{31}P NMR in the brain of ADSL-deficient patients[79] has given normal results. This suggests that in various tissues the residual activity of ADSL remains sufficient to allow flux through the pathway of purine synthesis. In addition, the ADSL defect could be circumvented by supply of purines from non- or little-affected cell types (erythrocytes, granulocytes), via the purine salvage enzymes, HPRT, APRT, and adenosine kinase (Fig. 112-3). Accordingly, in medium containing undialyzed fetal calf serum, and hence purine bases, growth of fibroblasts from both profoundly retarded type I patients and from a mildly retarded type II patient was similar to that of control cells.[80]

The functional consequences of decreased ADSL activity on the *de novo* synthesis of purines have been assessed by measuring the incorporation of [^{14}C]formate into the latter compounds in fibroblasts.[55,80] This incorporation proceeds at two steps along the pathway (Fig 112-3): the conversion of glycineamide ribotide (GAR) into formylglycineamide ribotide (FGAR, not illustrated), and of AICAR into formylaminoimidazolecarboxamide ribotide (FAICAR). Paradoxically, it was found enhanced in ADSL-deficient cells as compared to control fibroblasts, indicating an increase of the *de novo* synthesis. The mechanism of this increase remains to be determined, but may explain the higher growth rates of ADSL-deficient fibroblasts in medium containing dialyzed fetal calf serum. In type II, but not in type I, cells incubated with [^{14}C]formate, small amounts of labeled SAICAR, SAICAriboside, S-AMP, and S-Ado accumulated.[80] This can be explained by the inhibitory effect of salts and nucleotides on the residual activity of ADSL with SAICAR ($\approx$30 percent of normal) and by the low residual activity of ADSL with S-AMP ($\approx$3 percent of normal) in the type II fibroblasts.[25] Both render conversion of SAICAR into AICAR and of S-AMP into AMP rate-limiting.

Conversion of S-AMP into AMP was also evaluated by following the incorporation via HPRT (Fig. 112-3) of labeled hypoxanthine into fibroblast adenine nucleotides. In fibroblasts of type I patients, fluxes of [^{14}C]hypoxanthine into adenine nucleotides were similar to those measured in control cells, and no accumulation of S-AMP was recorded.[80] This confirms that in these cells the 30 percent decrease in ADSL activity, measured with S-AMP, does not render the enzyme rate-limiting. In contrast,

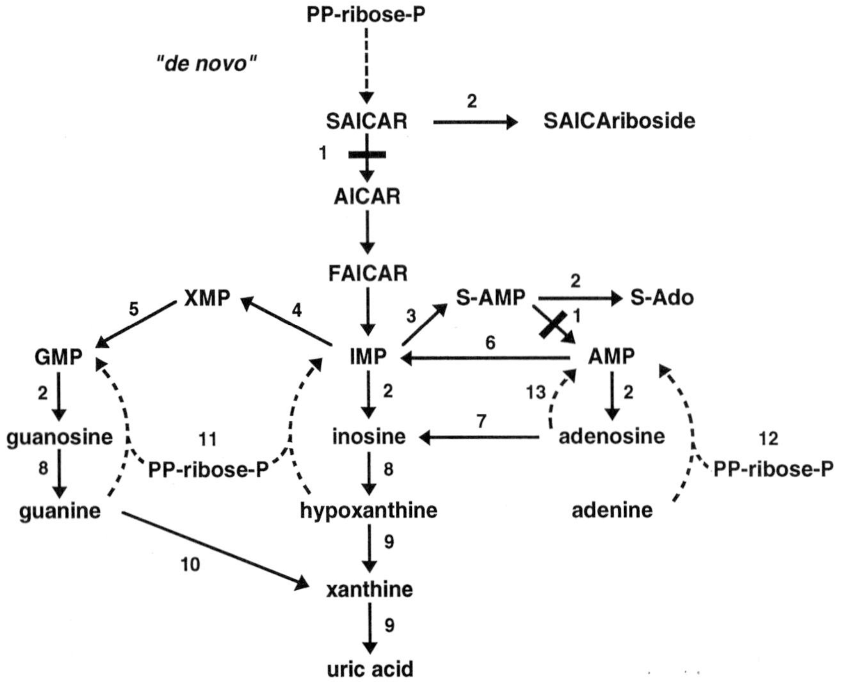

Fig. 112-3 Pathways of purine metabolism. PP-ribose-P, phosphoribosylpyrophosphate; FAICAR, formyl-AICAR; S-Ado, succinyladenosine; other abbreviations as in Fig. 112-2. 1, ADSL; 2, cytosolic 5′-nucleotidase; 3, adenylosuccinate synthetase; 4, IMP dehydrogenase; 5, GMP synthetase; 6, AMP deaminase; 7, adenosine deaminase; 8, purine nucleoside phosphorylase; 9, xanthine dehydrogenase (oxidase); 10, guanine deaminase; 11, hypoxanthine-guanine phosphoribosyltransferase; 12, adenine phosphoribosyl transferase; 13, adenosine kinase. The first seven steps of the *de novo* pathway are represented by a dotted line. The ADSL defect is indicated by solid bars. *(From Van den Berghe et al.[12] Used by permission of Kluwer Academic Publishers, Lancaster, England.)*

in fibroblasts of the type II patient, flux decreased by about 75 percent. There was also a marked accumulation of S-AMP accompanied by formation of S-Ado. This indicates that the pronounced deficiency of ADSL activity with S-AMP, with only 3 percent residual activity, hampers metabolic flux through the enzyme step. Nevertheless, even with this small residual activity, conversion of S-AMP into AMP can still proceed. This provides an explanation for the observation of normal *in vivo* concentrations of adenine and guanine nucleotides in liver, kidney, and muscle of ADSL-deficient patients.[53] Nevertheless, a deficiency of purine nucleotides could occur in some, hitherto unidentified, cell types with profound deficiency of ADSL and low activities of the salvage enzymes.

Toxic Effects of Succinylpurines

Taken together, the data described in the previous paragraph suggest that the symptoms of ADSL deficiency are not caused by purine nucleotide deficiency, but more likely due to toxic effects of the accumulating succinylpurines. Moreover, the observations of generally less severe mental retardation in patients with similar SAICAriboside levels, but with S-Ado/SAICAriboside ratios above 2,[5,9] and of a strikingly mild psychomotor retardation in the type II patient with S-Ado/SAICAriboside ratios around 4,[3] suggest that SAICAriboside is the offending compound, and that S-Ado could protect against its toxic effects. Owing to the resemblance of both succinylpurines with adenosine and to their accumulation to 100 to 500 μM concentrations in the cerebrospinal fluid of the patients, the possibility has been explored that they might interfere with cerebral adenosine receptors, and thereby with the numerous physiological functions of adenosine. In the central nervous system, besides vasodilation, these include sedation and inhibition of neurotransmitter release and of nerve cell firing (reviewed in reference 81). Studies with crude membrane fractions of rat cerebral cortex, however, failed to show interference of SAICAriboside and S-Ado with binding of adenosine.[82] Also, neither of the succinylpurines modified synaptic transmission or the effects of glutamate or adenosine on synaptic potentials in rat hippocampus.[83]

Measurements of the cerebral uptake of [^{18}F]-labeled 2-fluoro-2-deoxyglucose by positron emission tomography have shown that it is markedly reduced in the cortical areas of ADSL-deficient patients,[84] suggesting interference of the succinylpurines with glucose metabolism. However, no effects of SAICAriboside and/or S-Ado were seen on glucose metabolism in isolated hepatocytes (M.F. Vincent and G. Van den Berghe, unpublished data). Recently, infusion of SAICAriboside to rats has been shown to cause neuronal damage in specific regions of the hippocampus.[85]

Other Hypothetical Mechanisms

The deficiency of ADSL could impair the purine nucleotide cycle, composed of adenylosuccinate synthetase, ADSL, and AMP deaminase (Fig. 112-3). This cycle is particularly active in muscle (reviewed in references 86 and 87). Moreover, both inherited and acquired muscular disorders are associated with muscle AMP deaminase deficiency (reviewed in Chap. 110). Decreased activities of ADSL have also been recorded in dystrophic mice,[88] and in subjects with congenital or acquired myopathies.[89] Impairment of the purine nucleotide cycle could thus play a role in the pathogenesis of the muscle wasting and growth retardation of the patients in whom the ADSL defect is expressed in muscle.

AICAR (now often called ZMP), which is the product of the ADSL reaction with SAICAR (Fig. 112-2), can be converted into the corresponding triphosphate ZTP. Accumulation of ZTP has been documented in red blood cells of patients with deficiency of HPRT,[90] and upon addition of AICAriboside to the incubation medium of various cell types.[30,91] Whether small concentrations of ZTP are present in normal cells under physiological conditions, and whether ZTP is an essential cellular constituent, remain open questions. If yes, however, ADSL deficiency could induce a deleterious ZTP depletion.

Accumulation of both substrates of ADSL, S-AMP and SAICAR, was undetectable in liver and muscle, but a slight buildup of S-AMP could be measured in the kidney of two ADSL-deficient patients.[53] This might be explained by less efficient dephosphorylation of S-AMP in kidney as compared to liver and muscle. Nevertheless, the possibility exists that small intracellular accumulations of the substrates of ADSL, remaining below or at the limit of the level of detection of the methods used, may have deleterious effects in some cell types.

DIAGNOSIS

The marked clinical heterogeneity of ADSL deficiency justifies systematic screening for the disorder in the numerous patients with unexplained psychomotor retardation and/or neurologic disease. Diagnosis is based on the presence in urine and cerebrospinal fluid of SAICAriboside and S-Ado, both normally undetectable with routine techniques, although concentrations of S-Ado of about 1 μM have been reported in control cerebrospinal fluid.[92] For systematic screening, a modified Bratton-Marshall test,[93] performed on fresh urine stored at −20°C owing to the instability of SAICAriboside at room temperature and alkaline pH, appears most practical. False positive results are, however, recorded in patients who receive antibiotics, particularly sulfonamides, for the measurement of which the test was initially devised,[94] and/or antiepileptic medications. The succinylpurines can also be detected by other techniques: two-dimensional thin-layer chromatography with staining of imidazole compounds,[13] silica thin-layer chromatography with liquid nitrogen-induced phosphorescence,[95] determination of A270/250 ratio,[96] and capillary electrophoresis,[97,98] HPLC with UV detection being a method of choice for final diagnosis.[1,99] Amino acid analysis before and after strong acid hydrolysis of deproteinized extracts of cerebrospinal fluid, which method was the starting point of the discovery of ADSL deficiency,[1] also remains of interest for the detection of ADSL deficiency, as well as for the search for as yet unknown metabolic disorders.[100] Applied to urine, it can also be used for the diagnosis of inborn errors of pyrimidine catabolism.[101]

Several methods have been described for the assay of ADSL. The activity of the enzyme with S-AMP can be readily measured by a dual-wavelength spectrophotometric method, based on the decrease in absorbance at 282 nm minus that at 320 nm accompanying the conversion of S-AMP into AMP.[102] A similar assay with SAICAR is, however, an order of magnitude less sensitive than with S-AMP, precluding its utilization with patients' biopsies. A coupled assay procedure, involving conversion of fumarate produced by ADSL into L-malate by fumarase, followed by oxidative decarboxylation of L-malate into pyruvate by malic enzyme, and measurement of NADPH produced, has been developed as a gel-staining procedure applicable to purified enzyme.[57] Synthesis of radioactive SAICAR and S-AMP from [2,3-^{14}C]fumarate and, respectively, AICAR and AMP with partially purified ADSL from yeast, has allowed development of a radiochemical assay of ADSL, applicable to small tissue samples.[69] A microassay of ADSL by capillary electrophoresis has also been described.[103] Owing to the instability of ADSL on freezing and thawing,[20] diagnostic assays should be preferentially performed on fresh tissue. Nevertheless, diagnosis of ADSL deficiency is possible in frozen liver and muscle.[69]

ADSL deficiency is a rare disorder, although its frequency is probably higher than that of other inborn errors of purine metabolism, with the exception of muscle AMP deaminase deficiency. Hitherto, most patients have been diagnosed in the low countries, Belgium and The Netherlands, and in the Czech Republic. Cases have also been diagnosed in Australia, France, Germany, Italy, Morocco, Spain, Turkey, and the USA. Strikingly, no subjects with ADSL deficiency have been found yet in the UK, Ireland, or Norway, despite screening of nearly 20,000 "at-risk" patients.[104] This supports genetic data indicating a common ancestry for the latter populations.

TREATMENT AND PROGNOSIS

With the aim to replenish hypothetically decreased concentrations of adenine nucleotides in ADSL-deficient tissues, some patients have been treated for several months with oral supplements of adenine (10 mg/kg per day) and allopurinol (5 to 10 mg/kg per day). Adenine can be incorporated into the adenine nucleotides by way of APRT (Fig. 112-3). Allopurinol is required to avoid conversion of adenine, by xanthine dehydrogenase, into minimally soluble 2,8-dihydroxyadenine, which forms kidney stones. No clinical or biochemical improvement was recorded, with the exception of some acceleration of growth.[3]

The prognosis of ADSL-deficient subjects is generally poor. Several patients, particularly those referred to as type I, and those presenting with early epilepsy have died in early infancy.[7,10,11] Others have died at around 10 years of age. In most cases, further evolution is characterized by absent or minimal progression of psychomotor development and persistence of autistic behavior, except for occasional improvement of eye contact. Nevertheless, some patients, particularly those with higher S-Ado/SAICAriboside ratios, fare relatively well, and as of this writing, the oldest of these patients has reached 31 years of age.[105]

REFERENCES

1. Jaeken J, Van den Berghe G: An infantile autistic syndrome characterised by the presence of succinylpurines in body fluids. *Lancet* **2**:1058, 1984.
2. Kraffczyk F, Helger F, Bremer HJ: Thin-layer chromatographic screening tests for carbohydrate anomalies in plasma, urine and faeces. *Clin Chim Acta* **42**:303, 1972.
3. Jaeken J, Wadman SK, Duran M, van Sprang FJ, Beemer FA, Holl RA, Theunissen PM, De Cock P, Van den Bergh F, Vincent MF, Van den Berghe G: Adenylosuccinase deficiency: An inborn error of purine nucleotide synthesis. *Eur J Pediatr* **148**:126, 1988.
4. Jaeken J, Van den Bergh F, Vincent MF, Casaer P, Van den Berghe G: Adenylosuccinase deficiency: A newly recognized variant. *J Inherit Metab Dis* **15**:416, 1992.
5. Krijt J, Sebesta I, Svehlakova A, Zumrova A, Zeman J: Adenylosuccinate lyase deficiency in a Czech girl and two siblings. *Adv Exp Med Biol* **370**:367, 1995.
6. Salerno C, Crifo C, Giardini O: Adenylosuccinase deficiency: A patient with impaired erythrocyte activity and anomalous response to intravenous fructose. *J Inherit Metab Dis* **18**:602, 1995.
7. Sebesta I, Krijt J, Kmoch S, Hartmannova H, Wojda M, Zeman J: Adenylosuccinase deficiency: Clinical and biochemical findings in 5 Czech patients. *J Inherit Metab Dis* **20**:343, 1997.
8. Maaswinkel-Mooij PD, Laan LAEM, Onkenhout W, Brouwer OF, Jaeken J, Poorthuis BJHM: Adenylosuccinase deficiency presenting with epilepsy in early infancy. *J Inherit Metab Dis* **20**:606, 1997.
9. Valik D, Miner PT, Jones JD: First U.S. case of adenylosuccinate lyase deficiency with severe hypotonia. *Pediatr Neurol* **16**:252, 1997.
10. Van den Bergh FAJTM, Bosschaart AN, Hageman G, Duran M, Poll-The BT: Adenylosuccinase deficiency with neonatal onset severe epileptic seizures and sudden death. *Neuropediatrics* **29**:51, 1998.
11. Köhler M, Assmann B, Bräutigam C, Storm W, Marie S, Vincent MF, Van den Berghe G, Hoffmann GF: Adenylosuccinase deficiency: Possibly underdiagnosed encephalopathy with variable clinical features. *Eur J Pediatr Neurol* **3**:6, 1999.
12. Van den Berghe G, Vincent MF, Jaeken J: Inborn errors of the purine nucleotide cycle: Adenylosuccinase deficiency. *J Inherit Metab Dis* **20**:193, 1997.
13. De Bree PK, Wadman SK, Duran M, Fabery de Jonge H: Diagnosis of inherited adenylosuccinase deficiency by thin-layer chromatography of urinary imidazoles and by automated cation exchange column chromatography of purines. *Clin Chim Acta* **156**:279, 1986.
14. Kaufman JM, Greene ML, Seegmiller JE: Urine uric acid to creatinine ratio: A screening test for inherited disorders of purine metabolism. *J Pediatr* **73**:583, 1968.
15. Carter CE, Cohen LH: Enzymic synthesis of adenylosuccinic acid. *J Am Chem Soc* **77**:499, 1955.
16. Miller RW, Lukens LN, Buchanan JM: The enzymatic cleavage of 5-amino-4-imidazole-N-succinocarboxamide ribotide. *J Am Chem Soc* **79**:1513, 1957.
17. Giles NH, Partridge CWH, Nelson NJ: The genetic control of adenylosuccinase in Neurospora crassa. *Proc Natl Acad Sci U S A* **43**:305, 1957.
18. Gollub EG, Gots JS: Purine metabolism in bacteria. VI. Accumulations by mutants lacking adenylosuccinase. *J Bacteriol* **78**:320, 1959.
19. Ratner S: Argininosuccinases and adenylosuccinases, in Boyer PD (ed): *The Enzymes*. 3rd ed. New York, Academic Press, 1972, p 167.
20. Brand LM, Lowenstein JM: Effect of diet on adenylosuccinase activity in various organs of rat and chicken. *J Biol Chem* **253**:6872, 1978.
21. Spector T, Jones TE, Elion GB: Specificity of adenylosuccinate synthetase and adenylosuccinate lyase from *Leishmania donovani*. Selective amination of an antiprotozoal agent. *J Biol Chem* **254**:8422, 1979.
22. Spector T, Berens RL, Marr JJ: Adenylosuccinate synthetase and adenylosuccinate lyase from *Trypanosoma cruzi*. Specificity studies with potential chemotherapeutic agents. *Biochem Pharmacol* **31**:225, 1982.
23. Barnes LB, Bishop SH: Adenylosuccinate lyase from human erythrocytes. *Int J Biochem* **6**:497, 1975.
24. Casey PJ, Lowenstein JM: Purification of adenylosuccinate lyase from rat skeletal muscle by a novel affinity column. Stabilization of the enzyme, and effects of anions and fluoro analogues of the substrate. *Biochem J* **246**:263, 1987.
25. Van den Bergh F, Vincent MF, Jaeken J, Van den Berghe G: Residual adenylosuccinase activities in fibroblasts of adenylosuccinase-deficient children: Parallel deficiency with adenylosuccinate and succinyl-AICAR in profoundly retarded patients and non-parallel deficiency in a mildly retarded girl. *J Inherit Metab Dis* **16**:415, 1993.
26. Stone RL, Zalkin H, Dixon JE: Expression, purification, and kinetic characterization of recombinant human adenylosuccinate lyase. *J Biol Chem* **268**:19710, 1993.
27. Sabina RL, Kernstine KH, Boyd RL, Holmes EW, Swain JL: Metabolism of 5-amino-4-imidazolecarboxamide riboside in cardiac and skeletal muscle. Effects on purine nucleotide synthesis. *J Biol Chem* **257**:10178, 1982.
28. Bridger WA, Cohen LH: The kinetics of adenylosuccinate lyase. *J Biol Chem* **243**:644, 1968.
29. Brox LW: The cleavage of adenylosuccinate and 5-amino-4-imidazole-*N*-succino-carboxamide ribonucleotide by an adenylosuccinate lyase from Ehrlich ascites tumor cells. *Can J Biochem* **51**:1072, 1973.
30. Sabina RL, Patterson D, Holmes EW: 5-Amino-4-imidazolecarboxamide riboside (Z-riboside) metabolism in eukaryotic cells. *J Biol Chem* **260**:6107, 1985.
31. Swain JL, Hines JJ, Sabina RL, Harbury OL, Holmes, EW: Disruption of the purine nucleotide cycle by inhibition of adenylosuccinate lyase produces skeletal muscle dysfunction. *J Clin Invest* **74**:1422, 1984.
32. Flanagan WF, Holmes EW, Sabina RL, Swain JL: Importance of purine nucleotide cycle to energy production in skeletal muscle. *Am J Physiol* **251**:C795, 1986.
33. Hampton A: Studies of the action of adenylosuccinase with 6-thio analogues of adenylosuccinic acid. *J Biol Chem* **237**:529, 1962.
34. Spector T: Mammalian adenylosuccinate lyase. Participation in the conversion of 2′-dIMP and β-d-arabinosyl-IMP to adenine nucleotides. *Biochim Biophys Acta* **481**:741, 1977.
35. Nair V, Sells TB: Interpretation of the roles of adenylosuccinate lyase and of AMP deaminase in the anti-HIV activity of 2′,3′-dideoxyadenosine and 2′,3′-dideoxyinosine. *Biochim Biophys Acta* **1119**:201, 1992.
36. Johnson MA, Ahluwalia G, Connelly MC, Cooney DA, Broder S, Johns DG, Fridland A: Metabolic pathways for the activation of the antiretroviral agent 2′,3′-dideoxyadenosine in human lymphoid cells. *J Biol Chem* **263**:15354, 1988.
37. Smith LD, Emerson RL, Morrical SW: A comparison of hepatic adenylosuccinate lyase from rats fed either a chow diet or a semisynthetic basal diet low in riboflavin. *Int J Biochem* **14**:875, 1982.
38. Aimi J, Badylak J, Williams J, Chen Z, Zalkin H, Dixon JE: Cloning of a cDNA encoding adenylosuccinate lyase by functional complementation in *Escherichia coli*. *J Biol Chem* **265**:9011, 1990.
39. Stone RL, Aimi J, Barshop BA, Jaeken J, Van den Berghe G, Zalkin H, Dixon JE: A mutation in adenylosuccinate lyase associated with mental retardation and autistic features. *Nat Genet* **1**:59, 1992.
40. Wong L-JC, O'Brien WE: Characterization of the cDNA and the gene encoding murine adenylosuccinate lyase. *Genomics* **28**:341, 1995.
41. Kmoch S: Personal communication, 1997.
42. Wistow GJ, Piatigorsky J: Gene conversion and splice-site slippage in the argininosuccinate lyases/delta-crystallins of the duck lens: Members of an enzyme superfamily. *Gene* **96**:263, 1990.

43. Simpson A, Bateman O, Driessen H, Lindley P, Moss D, Mylvaganam S, Narebor E, Slingsby C: The structure of avian eye lens delta-crystallin reveals a new fold for a superfamily of oligomeric enzymes. *Nat Struct Biol* **1**:724, 1994.
44. Weaver TM, Levitt DG, Donnelly MI, Stevens PP, Banaszak LJ: The multisubunit active site of fumarase C from *Escherichia coli*. *Nat Struct Biol* **2**:654, 1995.
45. Piatigorski J, Wistow GJ: Enzyme/crystallins: Gene sharing as an evolutionary strategy. *Cell* **57**:197, 1989.
46. Cohen LH, Bridger WA: Studies of the mechanism of action of adenylosuccinase. *Can J Biochem* **42**:715, 1964.
47. Hanson KR, Havir EA: The enzymatic elimination of ammonia, in Boyer PD (ed.): *The Enzymes*. 3rd ed. New York, Academic Press, 1992, p 75.
48. Gite SU, Colman RF: Affinity labeling of the active site of rabbit muscle adenylosuccinate lyase by 2-[(4-bromo-2,3-dioxobutyl)thio]-adenosine 5′-monophosphate. *Biochemistry* **35**:2658, 1996.
49. Lee TT, Worby C, Dixon JE, Colman RF: Identification of His[141] in the active site of *Bacillus subtilis* adenylosuccinate lyase by affinity labeling with 6-(4-bromo-2,3-dioxobutyl)thioadenosine 5′-monophosphate. *J Biol Chem* **272**:458, 1997.
50. Colman RF: Chemical arrows for enzymatic targets. *FASEB J* **11**:217, 1997.
51. Redinbo MR, Eide SM, Stone RL, Dixon JE, Yeates TO: Crystallization and preliminary structural analysis of *Bacillus subtilis* adenylosuccinate lyase, an enzyme implicated in infantile autism. *Protein Sci* **5**:786, 1996.
52. Lowy BA, Dorfman B: Adenylosuccinase activity in human and rabbit erythrocyte lysates. *J Biol Chem* **245**:3043, 1970.
53. Van den Berghe G, Jaeken J: Adenylosuccinase deficiency. *Adv Exp Med Biol* **195A**:27, 1986.
54. McFall E, Magasanik B: The control of purine biosynthesis in cultured mammalian cells. *J Biol Chem* **235**:2103, 1960.
55. Laikind PK, Gruber HE, Janssen I, Miller L, Hoffer M, Seegmiller JE, Willis RC, Jaeken J, Van den Berghe G: Purine biosynthesis in Chinese hamster cell mutants and human fibroblasts partially deficient in adenylosuccinate lyase. *Adv Exp Med Biol* **195B**:363, 1986.
56. Barshop BA, Alberts AS, Gruber HE: Kinetic studies of mutant human adenylosuccinase. *Biochim Biophys Acta* **999**:19, 1989.
57. Mack DO, Smith LD: Isoelectrofocusing of rat muscle adenylosuccinase. *Biochem Int* **23**:855, 1991.
58. Van Belzen N, Diesveld MPG, van der Made ACJ, Nozawa Y, Dinjens WNM, Vlietstra R, Trapman J, Bosman FT: Identification of mRNAs that show modulated expression during colon carcinoma cell differentiation. *Eur J Biochem* **234**:843, 1995.
59. Jackson RC, Morris HP, Weber G: Increased adenylosuccinase activity in hepatomas and kidney tumors. *Life Sci* **18**:1043, 1976.
60. Jackson RC, Morris HP, Weber G: Enzymes of the purine ribonucleotide cycle in rat hepatomas and kidney tumors. *Cancer Res* **37**:3057, 1977.
61. Smith LD, Emerson RL, Nixon LK: Effect of hepatocarcinogens on the adenine purine nucleotide cycle during the initiation phase of carcinogenesis. *Cancer Res* **39**:2132, 1979.
62. Mack DO, Lewis EM, Butler EM, Archer WH, Smith LD: A comparison of succinyladenylate lyase activity and serum sialic acid as markers of malignancy. *Biochem Med* **34**:327, 1985.
63. Reed VL, Mack DO, Smith LD: Adenylosuccinate lyase as an indicator of breast and prostate malignancies: A preliminary report. *Clin Biochem* **20**:349, 1987.
64. Brand LM, Lowenstein JM: Inhibition of adenylosuccinase by adenylophosphonopropionate and related compounds. *Biochemistry* **17**:1365, 1978.
65. Casey PJ: Doctoral dissertation, Brandeis University, 1986.
66. Casey PJ, Abeles RH, Lowenstein JM: Metabolism of *threo-β*-fluoroaspartate by H4 cells. Inhibition of adenylosuccinate lyase by fluoro analogs of its substrates. *J Biol Chem* **261**:13637, 1986.
67. Stern AM, Foxman BM, Tashjian AH, Abeles RH: dl-*threo-β*-Fluoroaspartate and dl-*threo-β*-fluoroasparagine: Selective cytotoxic agents for mammalian cells in culture. *J Med Chem* **25**:544, 1982.
68. Casey PJ, Lowenstein JM: Inhibition of adenylosuccinate lyase by l-alanosyl-5-aminoimidazole-4-carboxylic acid ribonucleotide (alanosyl-AICOR). *Biochem Pharmacol* **36**:705, 1987.
69. Van den Bergh F, Vincent MF, Jaeken J, Van den Berghe G: Radiochemical assay of adenylosuccinase: Demonstration of parallel loss of activity toward both adenylosuccinate and succinylaminoimidazole carboxamide ribotide in liver of patients with the enzyme defect. *Anal Biochem* **193**:287, 1991.
70. Van Keuren ML, Hart IM, Kao FT, Neve RL, Bruns GAP, Kurnit DM, Patterson D: A somatic cell hybrid with a single human chromosome 22 corrects the defect in the CHO mutant (Ade-1) lacking adenylosuccinase activity. *Cytogenet Cell Genet* **44**:142, 1987.
71. Delattre O, Azambuja CJ, Aurias A, Zucman J, Peter M, Zhang F, Hors-Cayla MC, Rouleau G, Thomas G: Mapping of human chromosome 22 with a panel of somatic cell hybrids. *Genomics* **9**:721, 1991.
72. Fon EA, Demczuk S, Delattre O, Thomas G, Rouleau GA: Mapping of the human adenylosuccinate lyase (ADSL) gene to chromosome 22q13.1 → q13.2. *Cytogenet Cell Genet* **64**:201, 1993.
73. Fon EA, Sarrazin J, Meunier C, Alarcia J, Shevell MI, Philippe A, Leboyer M, Rouleau GA: Adenylosuccinate lyase (ADSL) and infantile autism: Absence of previously reported point mutation. *Am J Med Genet* **60**:554, 1995.
74. Kmoch S, Hartmannova H, Krijt J, Sebesta I: Adenylosuccinase deficiency — Identification of a new disease causing mutation. *J Inherit Metab Dis* **19(Suppl 1)**:13, 1996.
75. Kmoch S, Hartmannova H, Krijt J, Valik D, Jones JD, Sebesta I: Genetic heterogeneity in adenylosuccinate lyase deficiency. *Clin Biochem* **30**:22, 1997.
76. Verginelli D, Luckow B, Crifo C, Salerno C, Gross M: Identification of new mutations in the adenylosuccinate lyase gene associated with impaired enzyme activity in lymphocytes and red blood cells. *Biochim Biophys Acta* **1406**:81, 1998.
77. Marie S, Cuppens H, Heuterspreute M, Jaspers M, Zambrano Tola E, Gu XX, Legius E, Vincent MF, Jaeken J, Cassimman JJ, Van den Berghe G: Mutation analysis in adenylosuccinate lyase deficiency. Eight novel mutations in the re-evaluated full ADSL coding sequence. *Hum Mut* **13**:197, 1999.
78. Salerno C, Iotti S, Lodi R, Crifo C, Barbiroli B: Failure of muscle energy metabolism in a patient with adenylosuccinate lyase deficiency: An in vivo study by phosphorus NMR spectroscopy. *Biochim Biophys Acta* **1360**:271, 1997.
79. Dorland L, van Sprang FJ, van Echteld CJA, Duran M, Wadman SK, den Hollander JA, Luyten PR: In vivo magnetic resonance spectroscopy and imaging of patients with adenylosuccinase deficiency. *Annual Meeting of SSIEM, Amersfoort, The Netherlands, Abstract book P 150,* 1986.
80. Van den Bergh F, Vincent MF, Jaeken J, Van den Berghe G: Functional studies in fibroblasts of adenylosuccinase-deficient children. *J Inherit Metab Dis* **16**:425, 1993.
81. Dunwiddie TV: The physiological role of adenosine in the central nervous system. *Int Rev Neurobiol* **27**:63, 1985.
82. Vincent MF, Van den Berghe G: Influence of succinylpurines on the binding of adenosine to a particulate fraction of rat cerebral cortex. *Adv Exp Med Biol* **253B**:441, 1989.
83. Stone TW, De Abreu RA, Duley JA, Gross M, Salerno C, Van den Berghe G: Succinylpurines do not modify glutamate or adenosine effects in the cerebrospinal fluid. *Clin Biochem* **30**:42, 1997.
84. De Volder AG, Jaeken J, Van den Berghe G, Bol A, Michel C, Cogneau M, Goffinet AM: Regional brain glucose utilization in adenylosuccinase-deficient patients measured by positron emission tomography. *Pediatr Res* **24**:238, 1988.
85. Stone TW, Roberts LA, Morris BJ, Jones PA, Duley JA, Ogilvy HV: Are succinylpurines neurotoxic? *Clin Biochem* **30**:41, 1997.
86. Lowenstein JM: Ammonia production in muscle and other tissues: The purine nucleotide cycle. *Physiol Rev* **52**:382, 1972.
87. Van den Berghe G, Bontemps F, Vincent MF, Van den Bergh F: The purine nucleotide cycle and its molecular defects. *Progr Neurobiol* **39**:547, 1992.
88. Sanada H, Yamaguchi M: A defect of purine nucleotide cycle in the skeletal muscle of hereditary dystrophic mice. *Biochem Biophys Res Commun* **90**:453, 1979.
89. Operti MG, Vincent MF, Brucher JM, Van den Berghe G: Enzymes of the purine nucleotide cycle in muscle of patients with exercise intolerance. *Muscle Nerve* **21**:401, 1998.
90. Sidi Y, Mitchell BS: Z-nucleotide accumulation in erythrocytes from Lesch-Nyhan patients. *J Clin Invest* **76**:2416, 1985.
91. Vincent MF, Marangos PJ, Gruber HE, Van den Berghe G: Inhibition by AICA riboside of gluconeogenesis in isolated rat hepatocytes. *Diabetes* **40**:1259, 1991.
92. Krijt J, Kmoch S, Hartmannova H, Sebesta I, Havlicek V: Succinyladenosine is a normal component of cerebrospinal fluid. *Clin Biochem* **30**:23, 1997.
93. Laikind PK, Seegmiller JE, Gruber HE: Detection of 5′-phosphoribosyl-4-(*N*-succinylcarboxamide)-5-aminoimidazole in urine by use

of the Bratton-Marshall reaction: Identification of patients deficient in adenylosuccinate lyase activity. *Anal Biochem* **156**:81, 1986.

94. Bratton AC, Marshall AK: A new coupling component for sulfanilamide determination. *J Biol Chem* **128**:537, 1939.
95. Maddocks J, Reed T: Urine test for adenylosuccinase deficiency in autistic children. *Lancet* **1**:158, 1989.
96. Domkin VD, Lazebnik TA, Roudneff AY, Smirnov MN: A new diagnostic technique for adenylosuccinate lyase deficiency. *J Inherit Metab Dis* **18**:291, 1995.
97. Jellum E, Thorsrud AK, Time E: Capillary electrophoresis for diagnosis and studies of human disease, particularly metabolic disorders. *J Chromatogr* **559**:455, 1991.
98. Gross M, Gathof BS, Kölle P, Gresser U: Capillary electrophoresis for screening of adenylosuccinate lyase deficiency. *Electrophoresis* **16**:1927, 1995.
99. Simmonds HA, Duley JA, Davies PM: Analysis of purines and pyrimidines in blood, urine, and other physiological fluids, in Hommes FA (ed.): *Techniques in Diagnostic Human Biochemical Genetics*. New York, Wiley-Liss, 1991, p 397.
100. Jaeken J: Cerebrospinal fluid as a tool in the diagnosis of neurometabolic diseases: amino acid analysis before and after acid hydrolysis. *Eur J Pediatr* **153(Suppl 1)**:S86, 1994.
101. Van Gennip AH, Driedijk PC, Elzinga A, Abeling NGGM: Screening for defects of dihydropyrimidine degradation by analysis of amino acids in urine before and after acid hydrolysis. *J Inherit Metab Dis* **15**:413, 1992.
102. Schultz V, Lowenstein JM: Purine nucleotide cycle. Evidence for the occurrence of the cycle in brain. *J Biol Chem* **251**:485, 1976.
103. Salerno C, Crifo C: Microassay of adenylosuccinase by capillary electrophoresis. *Anal Biochem* **226**:377, 1995.
104. Davies PM, Duley JA, Simmonds HA: Unpublished studies supported by European Community Concerted Action No. BMH1-CT94-1384.
105. Duran M, Huijmans JGM, de Klerk JBC: Personal communication, 1998.

CHAPTER 113

Hereditary Orotic Aciduria and Other Disorders of Pyrimidine Metabolism

Dianne R. Webster ▪ David M. O. Becroft
Albert H. van Gennip ▪ André B. P. Van Kuilenburg

1. Pyrimidines and purines are the building blocks of DNA and RNA and are thus required for the retention and transmission of genetic information. In addition they function in the formation of coenzymes and active intermediates in carbohydrate and phospholipid metabolism. Purines and pyrimidines have two routes for nucleotide formation, the *de novo* pathway, which begins with ribose phosphate, amino acids, CO_2, and ammonia; and the salvage pathway, which takes free bases and nucleosides back to nucleotides. *De novo* and salvage pathways are balanced and connected through the enzymes, which degrade the nucleotides to β-amino acids, CO_2, and ammonia.
2. In contrast to the well-known defects of purine metabolism, most of the seven defects of pyrimidine metabolism are recently discovered: hereditary orotic aciduria (UMP synthase deficiency; MIM 25890, 25892), pyrimidine 5′-nucleotidase deficiency (MIM 26612), dihydropyrimidine dehydrogenase deficiency (MIM 27427), dihydropyrimidinase (dihydropyrimidinuria, MIM), ureidopropionase deficiency, thymidine phosphorylase deficiency, and pyrimidine 5′-superactivity. Purine metabolism has an easily recognizable, easily measurable endpoint in uric acid. There is no equivalent compound in pyrimidine metabolism.
3. The first defect, hereditary orotic aciduria, is in the *de novo* synthetic pathway. This autosomal recessive disorder results from a severe deficiency of the last two activities in the pathway, orotate phosphoribosyltransferase and orotidine-5′-monophosphate decarboxylase. Although orotic aciduria was thought to be unique because of the loss of two enzymes, it is now known that these activities reside in separate domains of a single polypeptide coded by a single gene. This bifunctional protein, uridine-5′-monophosphate synthase, has been purified, the amino acid sequence determined by cDNA sequencing, and the gene localized to chromosome 3q13. Two point mutations resulting in amino acid substitutions and loss of enzyme activity have been identified in one orotic aciduria patient.
4. There are 15 known patients with hereditary orotic aciduria. All have had a macrocytic hypochromic megaloblastic anemia and orotic acid crystalluria. Thirteen have been treated with uridine with good effect in the majority. Five young adults remain well but require continued therapy. One adult has not received uridine therapy and is well despite persisting anemia. Other features have included renal tract obstruction by crystals, cardiac malformations, and strabismus. Infections have been a problem in some, associated with various abnormalities of in vitro tests of immune function. One patient had severe congenital abnormalities. Mild intellectual impairment has been an inconstant feature prior to treatment. The progressive neurologic deterioration in one young adult may be unrelated to the metabolic error.
5. The other disorders involve defects in the pyrimidine degradative pathway. Deficiency of pyrimidine-5′-nucleotidase causes hemolytic anemia, possibly due to accumulation in erythrocytes of pyrimidine nucleotides, mostly uridine triphosphate (UTP) and cytidine triphosphate (CTP). The disorder is transmitted in an autosomal recessive manner, and there is no specific treatment available. Pyrimidine 5′-nucleotidase superactivity has been described in four unrelated patients with developmental delay and neurologic abnormalities. The patients were treated with uridine with good effect. Deficiency of dihydropyrimidine dehydrogenase causes an increase in blood and urine levels of uracil and thymine. This deficiency is detected in a variety of clinical situations including pediatric metabolic screens for neurologic and other problems and adverse reactions to 5-fluorouracil, and is also found in asymptomatic relatives of detected patients. The enzyme deficiency is transmitted in an autosomal recessive manner, and there is some doubt whether there is a causal relationship between the deficiency and the symptoms. Dihydropyrimidinase deficiency (dihydropyrimidinuria) results in a large excretion of dihydrouracil and dihydrothymine. Four Dutch patients have been

A list of standard abbreviations is located immediately preceding the index in each volume. Nonstandard abbreviations used in this chapter include: ALTE = acute life-threatening event; ATC = aspartate transcarbamylase; 5AZOA = 5-azaorotic acid; 6AZUMP = 6-azauridine-5′-monophosphate; 6AZUR = 6-azauridine; BA = barbituric acid; BAIBPAT = β-aminoisobutyrate pyruvate aminotransferase; BAKAT = β-alanine-α-ketoglutarate aminotransferase; BMP = barbituric acid monophosphate; BAPAT = β-alanine pyruvate aminotransferase; CPS = carbamylphosphate synthase; DHO = dihydroorotase; DHODH = dihydroorotate dehydrogenase; DPD = dihydropyrimidine dehydrogenase; DPH = dihydropyrimidine hydrase; DUMPS = deficiency of uridine-5′-monophosphate; ECGF1 = endothelial growth factor 1; HPLC = high performance liquid chromatography; MNGIE = mitochondrial neurogastrointestinal encephalomyopathy; OA = orotic acid; ODC, OMP = orotidine-5′-monophosphate; ODC = orotidine-5′-monophosphate decarboxylase; OPRT = orotate phosphoribosyltransferase; PD-ECGF = platelet-derived endothelial cell growth factor; P5N = pyrimidine-5′-nucleotidase; PF = pyrazofurin; PNMK = pyrimidine nucleoside monophosphate kinase; TMP = thymidine monophosphate; TP = thymidine phosphorylase; UMP = uridine-5′-monophosphate; UP = ureidopropionase.

ascertained following investigation of neurologic and other problems and five asymptomatic Japanese patients by population screening. One patient has been reported with N-carbamyl-β-aminoaciduria due to a deficiency of ureidopropionase. The patient presented with choreoathetosis, hypotonia, and microcephaly. A deficiency of thymidine phosphorylase has been described in patients with juvenile mitochondrial neurogastrointestinal encephalomyopathy (MNGIE).

PYRIMIDINE ENZYMES

The enzymes of pyrimidine metabolism are summarized in Table 113-1, and a diagram of the interrelationship between the enzymes of *de novo* synthesis, interconversion, salvage, and degradation is given in Fig. 113-1. The body's requirement for pyrimidines can be met either by synthesis from small molecules or by reutilization of preformed pyrimidines available from body cell turnover or dietary sources (Figs. 113-1 and 113-2). *De novo* pyrimidine synthesis has been estimated at 4 to 16 mM/day,[1] or 450 or 700 mg/day, approximately equal to the daily purine requirement.[2] There are a number of excellent reviews and sources of information on basic pyrimidine biochemistry.[3,4]

De Novo Synthesis

The six activities of *de novo* pyrimidine biosynthesis in animals are coded by three structural genes. The first gene codes for a large multifunctional protein containing the first three activities of the pathway, carbamyl-phosphate synthetase (CPS, enzyme 1 on Figs. 113-1 and 113-2), aspartate transcarbamylase (ATC, enzyme 2), and dihydroorotase (DHO, enzyme 3). The second gene codes for dihydroorotate dehydrogenase (DHODH, enzyme 4). The third gene codes for the last two activities of the *de novo* pathway, orotate phosphoribosyltransferase (OPRT, enzyme 5) and orotidine-5′-monophosphate decarboxylase (ODC, enzyme 6).

Carbamylphosphate synthase, Aspartate transcarbamylase, and Dihydroorotase are contained in a single polypeptide (CAD, or pyr 1 to 3) with a molecular weight of 220 kDa.[5,6] This cytosolic multifunctional protein appears to be composed of three distinct catalytic domains in the following arrangements:

Table 113-1 Enzymes of Pyrimidine *De Novo* Synthesis, Biosynthesis (Interconversion), Salvage, and Degradation

Enzyme number	Name	Abbreviation	EC Number
***De Novo* synthetic**			
1–3	Multienzyme pyr 1–3 (CPS-ATC-DHO)	CAD	
1	Carbamylphosphate synthetase	CPS	2.7.2.9
2	Aspartate transcarbamylase	ATC	2.1.3.2
3	Dihyroorotase	DHO	3.5.2.3
4	Dihydroorotate dehydrogenase	DHODH	1.3.3.1
5, 6	UMP synthase (multienzyme pyr 5,6) (OPRT-ODC)	UMPS	
5	Orotate phosphorilbosyltransferase	OPRT	2.4.2.10
6	Orotidine 5′-monophosphate decarboxylase	ODC	4.1.1.23
Biosynthetic			
7	Uridine (pyrimidine) monophosphate kinase		2.7.4.14
8	Ribonucleoside diphosphate reductase		1.17.4.1
9	Pyrimidine diphosphate kinase		2.7.4.6
10	Thymidylate synthetase		2.1.1.45
11	Thymidine monophosphate kinase		2.7.4.9
12	Cytidine triphosphate synthetase		6.3.4.2
13	RNA nucleotidyltransferase		2.7.7.6
14	DNA nucleotidyltransferase		2.7.7.7
Salvage			
15	Uridine kinase		2.7.1.48
16	Uridine phosphorylase		2.4.2.3
17	Thymidine kinase		2.7.1.21
18	Thymidine phosphorylase		2.4.2.4
19	Deoxycytidine kinase		2.7.1.74
Catabolic			
20	Cytidine deaminase		3.5.4.5
21	Deoxycytidine monophosphate deaminase		3.5.4.12
22	Dihydropyrimidine dehydrogenase	DPD	1.3.1.2
23	Dihydropyrimidinase	DPH	3.5.2.2
24	β-Ureidopropionase	UP	3.5.1.6
25	Pyrimidine 5′-nucleotidase		3.1.3.5
26	Orotidine-5′-monophosphate phosphohydrolase		
27	R(−)β-aminoisobutyrate-pyruvate aminotransferase	BAIBPAT	2.6.1.40
28	β-alanine-pyruvate aminotransferase	BAPAT	2.6.1.18
29	β-alanine-α-ketoglutarate aminotransferase	BAKAT	2.6.1.19

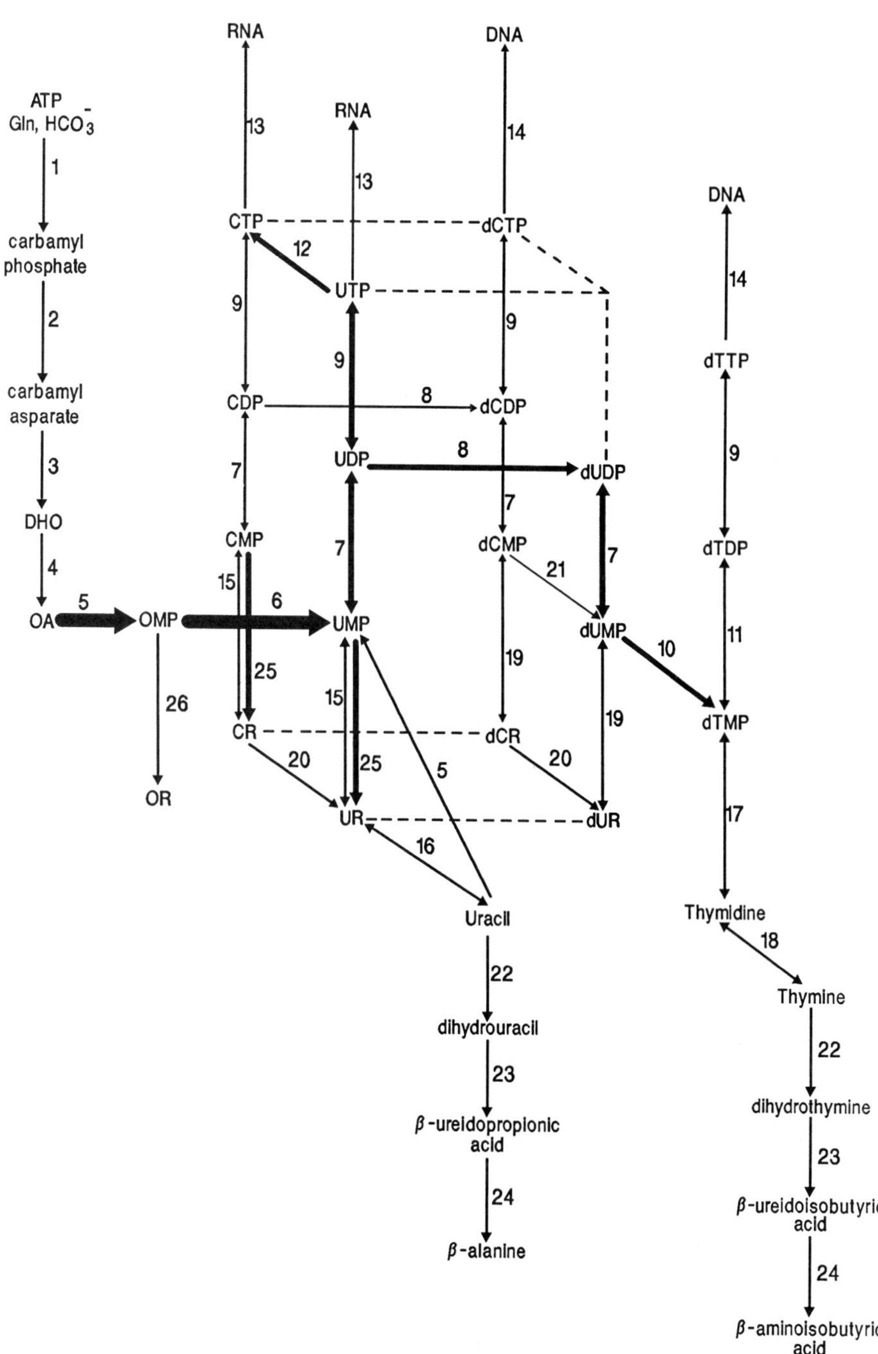

Fig. 113-1 Diagram of the interrelationship of *de novo* pyrimidine synthesis, conversion of UMP to other ribonucleotides and deoxyribonucleotides, salvage from cell turnover or dietary sources, and degradation. The ribonucleosides and ribonucleotides form the left face of the interconversion box. The deoxynucleosides and deoxynucleotides form the right face of the box. Uridine nucleosides and nucleotides form the front face and cytidine nucleosides and nucleotides form the back face of the box. Thymidine nucleotides parallel the deoxy face of the box. Hereditary orotic aciduria (UMP synthase deficiency) is caused by the functional absence of enzymes 5 and 6 (UMPS); pyrimidine-5′-nucleotidase deficiency by the absence of enzyme 25 (P5N); dihydropyrimidine dehydrogenase deficiency by the absence of enzyme 22 (DHPDH), and dihydropyrimidinase deficiency by the absence of enzyme 23 (DHP).

NH_2-DHO-CPS-ATC-COOH.[7,8] Sedimentation analysis and chemical cross-linking studies indicate the native form of the protein consists of stable trimers and hexamers of the basic polypeptide.[5,9,10] The hexamers have an open planar appearance by electron microscopy and can associate to form higher oligomeric forms.[10] Treatment of the CAD protein with staphylococcal proteinase results in cleavage of the protein but no loss in activity. One fragment of 182 kDa contains CPS and DHO. A 42 kDa fragment retains the ATC activity.[11] Similar results were obtained when the CAD protein was digested with elastase,[12] and the ATC domain was shown to self-associate and form well-defined oligomers.

The CAD gene spans a region of more than 25 kb and has over 30 introns.[13] The size of the mRNA coding for the CAD protein is 7.9 kb.[14] The ATC is coded by a 2.2-kb piece from the 3′ end of the total CAD message. Transformation of bacteria defective in ATC activity with this cDNA fragment results in complementation of the defect. Sequence homology is noted between the hamster and *Escherichia coli* ATC at the areas of the protein structure that are critical to catalysis.[8]

The first activity, CPS, produces carbamyl phosphate from glutamine and CO_2, and two molecules of ATP (Fig. 113-2). This activity is referred to as CPS II to distinguish it from CPS I, the mitochondrial enzyme of liver and kidney which produces carbamyl phosphate from ammonia and CO_2 for utilization in the urea cycle. Because of the presence of the next two activities of the complex, almost all the carbamyl phosphate produced by CPS II is used for pyrimidine synthesis. The activity of CPS is the rate-limiting step in the *de novo* synthesis of UMP except when ATP levels are increased at a time when uridine nucleotides and phosphoribosyl pyrophosphate (PP-ribose-P) levels are low. Under these conditions orotic acid (OA) accumulates and OPRT is the rate-limiting reaction.[15] Increased availability of carbamyl phosphate produced by CPS I in various urea cycle deficiencies causes

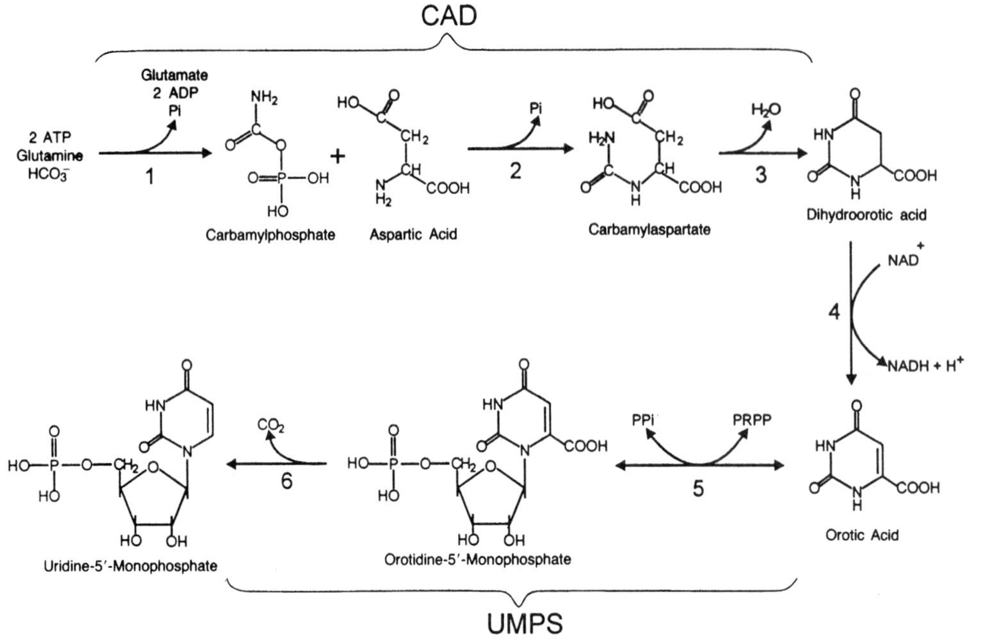

Fig. 113-2 Chemical structure of the intermediaries of *de novo* pyrimidine biosynthesis. Enzyme numbers are from Table 113-1.

vast increases in the rate of *de novo* pyrimidine synthesis.[16] The next activities are aspartate transcarbamylase, which catalyzes the irreversible formation of carbamylaspartate from carbamyl phosphate and aspartate, and dihydroorotase, which effects ring closure to form dihydroorotic acid (Fig. 113-2).

Dihydroorotate dehydrogenase (DHODH) catalyzes the oxidation of dihydroorotic acid to OA. This protein is located on the outer surface of the inner membrane of the mitochondrion. The activity of DHODH is lower when assayed in crude tissue preparations than the activity found with isolated mitochondria. The lower activity appears to be due to the rapid conversion of OA to orotidine-5′-monophosphate (OMP) by UMP synthase when OA is measured as the end point of the reaction.[17]

UMP synthase (UMPS, pyr 5,6) is a bifunctional protein containing the activities OPRT and ODC in a single polypeptide of 52 kDa. OPRT utilizes PP-ribose-P to add the ribose-5′-monophosphate moiety to OA and produce OMP. ODC releases CO_2 from OMP to produce uridine-5′-monophosphate (UMP) (Fig. 113-2). This enzyme will be discussed in detail later in the chapter (see "Enzymology of UMP Synthase").

Interconversion

The pyrimidine nucleus in UMP may be converted to all the other required pyrimidine nucleotides, or these may be salvaged from dietary sources or cell turnover (Table 113-1, Fig. 113-1). Pyrimidine mononucleotides are further phosphorylated by pyrimidine monophosphatase kinase (enzyme 7) and pyrimidine diphosphate kinase (enzyme 9). Cytidine nucleotides are formed by the action of cytidine triphosphate synthetase (enzyme 12) from uridine triphosphate. Reduction of ribonucleotides to deoxyribonucleotides is by the action of ribonucleoside diphosphate reductase (enzyme 8), which forms dUMP and dCDP. The thymidine nucleotides are formed by thymidylate synthetase (enzyme 10), which produces dTMP from dUMP. 5,10-Methylene-5,6,7,8-tetrahydrofolate is a cofactor for the reaction. dTMP may be further phosphorylated by thymidine monophosphate kinase (enzyme 11). Triphosphate nucleotides form DNA and RNA by the action of the appropriate nucleotidyltransferases (enzymes 13 and 14).

Pyrimidine Salvage

De novo synthesis requires 5 mol ATP for each mol of UMP produced, whereas reutilization of uridine from cell turnover or dietary sources costs only 1 mol ATP per mole of UMP. Studies in rate hepatoma and human breast cancer cells have shown that the rate of *de novo* synthesis is substantially reduced when exogenous uridine is supplied,[18,19] and the mechanism of this control may be an alteration of the amount of OPRT enzyme produced.[18] The amount of salvage in the breast cancer cells was controlled by the size of the uridine nucleotide pool.[19] Although *de novo* pyrimidine synthesis has been estimated (4 to 16 mM/day) to be approximately equal to the daily purine requirement,[2] it is possible to supply the greater part of the pyrimidine requirement through the salvage pathway, as is done in the treatment of hereditary orotic aciduria. Uptake studies in human leukemic cells have shown that in these cells (most at G_1 or G_0) the salvage pathway was 100 to 300 times more active than the *de novo* pathway; however, it was calculated that up to 70 percent of the pyrimidine requirement could be met from *de novo* synthesis and that about 30 percent of the requirement in normal bone marrow was from this source.[20] The major enzymes of pyrimidine salvage include uridine kinase (enzyme 15), which phosphorylates both uridine and cytidine; deoxycytidine kinase (enzyme 19); and thymidine kinase (enzyme 17).

Degradation

The pyrimidine mononucleotides are degraded to the corresponding nucleosides by pyrimidine 5′-nucleotidase (P5N, enzyme 25, Fig. 113-1), sometimes called UMP hydrolase. The pyrimidine degradative pathway proceeds in parallel through uridine and thymidine. Cytidine is deaminated to uridine by cytidine deaminase (enzyme 20), and uridine is reduced to uracil by uridine phosphorylase (enzyme 16) (uridine + $P_i \rightarrow$ uracil + ribose-1-phosphate). Although this reaction is reversible in vitro, it appears not to form uridine from uracil in vivo in humans, as evidenced by the unsuccessful use of uracil in the treatment of hereditary orotic aciduria.[21] Recent studies indicate that lymphoblasts are unable to salvage pyrimidine bases. While lymphocytes can synthesize deoxyuridine and thymidine from bases, it is only at high and nonphysiological concentrations, and neither cell can form uridine from uracil.[22] Thymidine phosphorylase is a separate enzyme (enzyme 18), which also catabolizes deoxyuridine nucleotides via dTMP. Following the formation of uracil and thymine, dihydropyrimidine dehydrogenase (DPD, enzyme 22) reduces them to dihydrouracil and dihydrothymine, whence dihydropyrimidine hydrase (DPH, enzyme 23) converts dihydrouracil to N-carbamyl-β-alanine and dihydrothymine-b N-carbamyl-β-aminoisobutyric acid. Urerdopropionase (UP, enzyme 24) converts N carbamyl-β-alanine to β-alanine and N-carbamyl-β-aminoisobutyric acid-b β-aminoisobutyric acid. The fourth step of the two degradation pathways is catalyzed by different enzymes: the reaction of R-β-aminoisobutyric acid into R-methylmalonic acid semialdehyde is catalyzed by BAIBPAT, the reaction of β-alanine into malonic acid semialdehyde is catalyzed by BAPAT or BAKAT. β-Alanine can also be converted into carnosine, the reaction being catalyzed by carnosine synthetase.

It has been suggested that a potential degradative pathway exists as a reversal of the steps of *de novo* synthesis, but this is not quantitatively important in humans.[16,23]

HEREDITARY OROTIC ACIDURIA

Enzymology of UMP Synthase

Purification and Characterization. The early attempts to isolate either OPRT or ODC from mammalian sources resulted in the coordinated purification of both activities, with OPRT more labile and sometimes lost in the later stages.[24,25] It was therefore postulated that the two activities form a complex, but there were reports that the activities could be separated. Kasbekar and colleagues reported separation of the activities by starch gel electrophoresis.[26] Brown and O'Sullivan reported the separation of a 62 kDa complex into two 20 kDa subunits with ODC activity and two 13 kDa subunits with OPRT activity following treatment of the complex with guanidine hydrochloride.[27] Formation of higher molecular weight complexes was associated with increased thermal stability and was induced by OA and competitive inhibitors. An early observation that the activity of ODC in fibroblasts was an exponential function of the amount of protein suggested that there may be an equilibrium between subunits and enzyme aggregate.[28]

The association of the two activities throughout all the purification procedures and the coordinate increase in both activities in the presence of competitive inhibitors caused speculation that the complex was a multifunctional protein that contained two domain centers.[16] Evidence to confirm the bifunctional nature came from: 1) the purification of a single peptide that retained both activities; 2) the characterization of cells resistant to inhibitors of ODC that had coordinately increased levels of OPRT and overproduction of a single protein; and 3) the isolation, sequencing and expression of a single cDNA that contains sequences from both OPRT and ODC domains.

The UMPS protein was first purified to apparent homogeneity from mouse Ehrlich ascites cells.[29] The protein recovered from columns gave a single band in polyacrylamide gel electrophoresis with a molecular weight of about 51.5 kDa and contained both OPRT and ODC activities. The ratio of ODC to OPRT was increased about fivefold in the purified preparation due to loss of OPRT activity. The more stable ODC activity was purified 2300-fold by this procedure. The activities cosedimented in sucrose density gradients at 3.7 S. Two-dimensional electrophoresis revealed two bands with isoelectric points of 5.85 and 5.65, with both bands containing both activities. The pI of the protein is 7.17. The physiological significance of the isoenzyme forms has not been determined.

More recently the UMPS protein has been purified from human placenta.[30] Following two affinity chromatography steps (Dye Matrix green A and phosphocellulose), the enzyme is more than 99 percent pure. The human enzyme has a similar molecular weight and isoenzyme pattern to the murine enzyme.

Substantiating evidence that the two activities, OPRT and ODC, reside within a single polypeptide chain came from enzyme studies in pyrazofurin (PF, 3,β-D-ribofuranosyl-4-hydroxypyrazole-5-carboxamide) and 6-azauridine (6AZUR)-resistant cells that had coordinate increases in both OPRT and ODC activities.[31–33] The increases are most likely caused by monophosphate metabolites of the inhibitors, which are specific inhibitors of ODC. In rat hepatoma cell lines grown in the absence of PF, there was a gradual loss of both activities until their levels were only three- to fourfold above wild-type cells. Analysis of cell extracts by SDS-PAGE revealed only a single band of approximately 55 kDa that was increased in the PF-resistant cells and subsequently decreased in the revertant cells.[33] Two-dimensional gel electrophoresis of extracts from sensitive and resistant cells showed overproduction of two spots in the resistant cells with the same molecular weight of 55 kDa but different isoelectric points.[34] These two overproduced proteins correspond to the two isoenzyme forms found in the mouse ascites enzyme.[29] Antibodies prepared against the affinity-purified mouse ascites UMPS protein were used in Western blot analysis to conclusively demonstrate that this band is UMPS. The overproduction of the UMPS protein is the result of an amplification of the UMPS gene.[35]

Conformation. In studies of mouse Ehrlich ascites cells, it has been demonstrated that UMPS protein exists in three different species or conformations as determined by sucrose density gradient sedimentation and gel filtration chromatography.[36,37] Conformation states with $S_{20,w}$ values of 3.5 S, 5.1 S, and 5.6 S are found depending on the effector molecules in the environment. Since distinct peaks can be distinguished on sucrose gradients, the different forms of the protein are not in rapid equilibrium. The monomer form of the protein has an $S_{20,w}$ value of 3.6 S. In the presence of substrates, products, or their analogs, a 5.1 S dimer is formed. A third species of 5.6 S is formed in the presence of nucleotide monophosphates or their analogs, OMP being the most efficient. The formation of the dimer appears to be the result of binding of the ligand molecule to the ODC catalytic site.[37] The stronger this binding, the lower the amount required to convert the monomer to the dimer form. In the presence of dithiothreitol and the absence of either substrates or products, the larger conformations are converted back to the 3.6 S monomer. The predicted interactions of the monomer units of UMPS are illustrated diagrammatically in Fig. 113-3.

Kinetic studies of UMPS have shown that ODC activity is predominantly associated with the 5.6 S dimer.[38] The OPRT activity is found in all three forms of the protein. The 5.1 and 5.6 S dimers are probably conformationally different. The data could be explained by the presence of a regulatory site separate from the two catalytic sites. The function of the monomer-dimer system could be to control enzyme activity or to enhance stability of the protein. Regulation of the monomer-dimer transitions may therefore by physiologically significant.

Domain Structure. The tertiary structure of multifunctional proteins is now generally accepted to consist of autonomous globular domains connected by peptide bridges.[39,40] The globular structural domains are relatively protease-resistant, compared to the polypeptide linker that is often protease-sensitive. With limited proteolytic digestion it is often possible to separate the structural domains of the multifunctional protein and study individual catalytic steps.

Limited proteolysis of partially purified murine UMPS with elastase produces separate peaks of OPRT and ODC activity in sucrose gradient analysis.[41] The recovery of ODC activity was approximately 70 percent, but only about 7 percent of OPRT activity was recovered. Digestion of purified human UMPS resulted in only a slight decrease in ODC activity, but OPRT activity was no longer detectable.[42] Analysis of the digest on SDS-PAGE showed only a single band of 28.5 kDa. This size is similar to the yeast ODC protein that has an apparent molecular weight of 27.5 kDa.[43] The ODC domain was isolated from digest using immobilized trypsin,[42] and found to be much less stable than the ODC activity of the undigested UMPS protein. This may reflect an inherent stability in the conformation of UMPS as a bifunctional protein. This increased instability in the isolated domains has also been observed in the multifunctional CAD protein.[12]

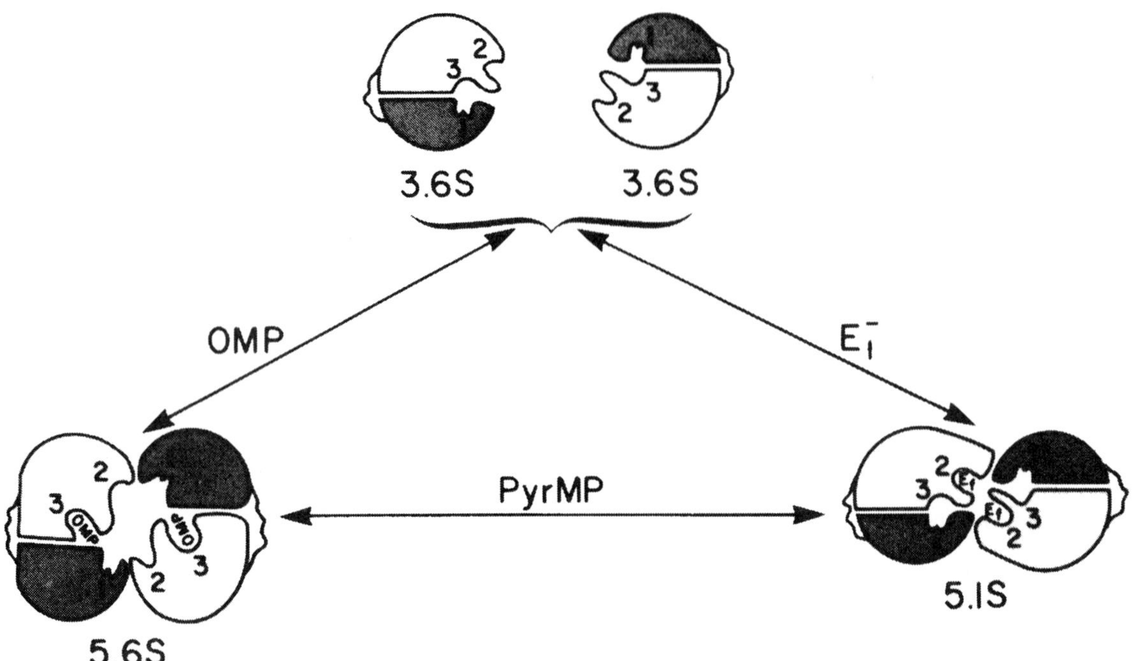

Fig. 113-3 Representation of the three conformational states of UMP synthase. Dimerization and conformational alterations of the UMPS monomer unit are shown. Each monomer is composed of an OPRT (gray) and an ODC (white) domain joined by a linker peptide: (1) OPRT catalytic site; (2) ODC catalytic site; (3) pyrimidine binding-regulatory site; E_i, anionic effector molecules other than OMP; PyrMP, pyrimidine ribonucleoside monophosphate. (*Reproduced from Floyd and Jones.*[42] *Used with permission.*)

The domain structure of the UMPS protein was also demonstrated by the expression of a murine UMPS cDNA in ODC-deficient bacteria.[44] The cDNA was selected from a murine cDNA library by hybridization with a rat UMPS probe. A fragment of 1600 bp was inserted into an expression vector (pUC12) and used to transform strains of bacteria that were deficient in ODC activity. Bacterial colonies that grew in the absence of uracil were shown to express the murine ODC domain by immunotitration assays and by immunoblot analysis. The expressed ODC protein had a molecular weight of 26 to 27.3 kDa.

In further studies, the cDNA encoding the ODC domain was inserted into a yeast expression vector and used to transform ODC-deficient yeast.[45] Selected yeast transformants expressed the ODC domain and had a high specific activity for ODC. Compared to intact UMPS or the ODC domain isolated by proteolytic digestion, the ODC domain expressed in yeast has a lower affinity for the substrate OMP and the inhibitor 6AZUMP. The expressed ODC domains contain a dimerization surface but there was no evidence for the formation of an altered dimer comparable to the 5.6 S species associated with intact UMPS. Thus the expressed ODC domain does not appear to contain the regulatory site predicted from the studies of purified UMPS protein.[45]

Production and Activity of the Monofunctional Domains.

Activity in Bacterial Systems. As described below ("Analysis of mRNA and Gene Sequence"), the UMP synthase amino acid sequence shows a very high degree of homology with the monofunctional OPRT and ODC proteins of yeast and bacteria. Lin and Suttle used PCR techniques to produce the separate cDNA fragments proposed to encode the independent OPRT and ODC independent domains.[46,47] Following cloning into bacterial expression vectors and transfection into uridine auxotrophic bacteria strains (pyr e or pyr f), they demonstrated that the bacteria could grow in media without uridine supplement and that they contained OPRT or ODC enzyme activity. The level of OPRT activity was only 9 percent of that found in normal bacteria, but ODC activity was up to 20 times greater than the normal level in bacteria. These levels could not be normalized for the number of plasmid copies in the bacteria, and the activity of the purified monofunctional proteins has not been determined. The proteins produced in the bacteria are of the size predicted for the separate domains as demonstrated by western blotting with antibody to UMP synthase. These studies convincingly demonstrate that both the OPRT and the ODC domains can produce a catalytically active monofunctional protein, and that these proteins can complement the uridine auxotrophic bacteria.

Activity in Mammalian Systems. Lin and Suttle have also demonstrated that the two separated monofunctional domains of UMP synthase can complement a UMP synthase-deficient hamster cell line.[47] The same cDNA fragments that produced the OPRT and ODC domains in bacteria were inserted into mammalian expression vectors and co-transfected into the deficient hamster cells. Colonies were selected in media without uridine and characterized for catalytic activity and protein production. Both OPRT and ODC activities were detected in cell extracts. The level of each activity was dependent on the number of copies of the respective vector that was integrated into the genome of the deficient hamster cells. In some cell lines the level of OPRT and ODC activity was 8 and 12 times increased respectively above that of the normal Chinese hamster cell. Western blots showed the presence of proteins of the predicted size for the independent domains that hybridized with polyclonal UMP synthase antiserum.[47]

These studies demonstrate convincingly that the bifunctional nature of UMPS is not necessary in mammalian cells for enzyme activity and cell growth. Although the production of the two independent domains does complement the UMP synthase hamster cells, the advantage of the bifunctional protein may be the result of increased protein stability. In tests of the stability of activity of the monofunctional proteins to incubation at increased temperatures, it is apparent that the OPRT domain is more heat-labile than the ODC domain and that both domains are much less stable that the bifunctional protein.[47]

OPRT Reaction Mechanism. Studies of yeast OPRT have demonstrated that the involvement of metal ions in the reaction may be at more than one site.[48,49] It has also been postulated that the reaction may proceed through a BiBi ping-pong kinetic mechanism. The first half of the reaction may be formation of an active ribosylphosphate-enzyme intermediate from PP-ribose-P with release of pyrophosphate from the α position. The second half would involve formation of a β_1'-glycosidic bond between orotate and the ribose-phosphate moiety on the enzyme to form OMP. The reaction mechanism must be more complex than double displacement, because stereochemical inversion occurs.[50]

ODC Characterization and Mechanism. Most studies of the reaction mechanism of ODC have been conducted using the yeast enzyme. The yeast enzyme can be produced in relatively large amounts using yeast expression vectors carrying the URA3 gene and has been purified to homogeneity.[51] Because of the high degree of amino acid conservation among the known sequences for ODC proteins (see discussion below, "Analysis of mRNA and Gene Sequence") studies of the mechanism of the yeast enzyme should be applicable to the mammalian enzyme as well. The yeast ODC enzyme has been crystallized with the transition state analog barbituric acid monophosphate (BMP).[51]

Two alternative mechanisms have been proposed for the decarboxylation reaction. The first mechanism involves the formation of a nitrogen ylide following protonation by the enzyme to form a zwitterion transition state.[52] The second mechanism requires formation of a covalent enzyme-substrate intermediate by attack of an enzymic nucleophile at C-5 of the substrate.[53] Data from NMR studies using [^{13}C]BMP and kinetic isotope effect studies with [^{2}H]OMP suggest that C-5 does not undergo significant changes in geometry during the rate-limiting step of the catalytic process,[54,55] and thus argue against formation of a covalent intermediate between ODC and its ligands. These results and the previous studies of the relative binding affinities of inhibitors of ODC[56] are consistent with a nitrogen ylide mechanism in which the enzyme protonates OMP at either the 2- or 4- keto group yielding a zwitterion with the positive charge on N-1. The positively charged N-1 could momentarily stabilize the C-6 carbanion formed on decarboxylation of OMP until a proton is acquired by C-6 to form the product UMP.[57]

In the conserved regions of the ODC enzyme the most likely proton donor to the 2-keto group of the orotate ring is the lysine at position 93 in yeast or position 97 in the mouse protein. Using the mouse ODC domain in a bacterial expression vector, K97 was changed to 15 alternative amino acids and the expressed proteins tested for active.[58] All of the substitutions were inactive indicating that this lysine is essential for the proposed reaction mechanism.

Channeling of OMP. In the metabolism of OA to UMP the possibility exists that the intermediate product, OMP, would be "channeled" from the OPRT catalytic site to the ODC site. Channeling would mean that no OMP would diffuse away from UMPS to form a free pool of OMP.[59] To determine if channeling was occurring, Traut and Jones[60] measured the amount of UMP formed from OA in the presence of exogenous OMP. Although strict channeling of OMP was found not to occur at high concentrations of exogenous OMP, the results were interpreted as showing partial channeling at all concentrations of OMP studied. One purpose of the channeling could be to protect the OMP from degradation by nucleotidases.[61] The presence of OMP channeling by UMPS has been disputed by McClard and Shokat,[62] who used a computer modeling analysis of the Traut and Jones data to show that the experimentally observed amounts of UMP produced from exogenous OMP were as predicted. The question of channeling of OMP in UMPS is presently unresolved.

Molecular Biology of UMP Synthase

cDNA Selection. The first isolate of a UMPS cDNA was from rat hepatoma cells (3924A) selected in multiple steps for resistance to PF.[33,63] These cells had levels of UMPS activity approximately fortyfold that of sensitive cells. Comparison of cell extracts on SDS-PAGE showed overproduction of a protein of approximately 55.2 kDa, which was confirmed as UMPS using antibody prepared to the mouse Ehrlich ascites UMPS. In vitro translation of mRNA from the PF-resistant cells showed that the UMPS mRNA was present at increased levels. It was then determined that the UMPS gene is amplified approximately fourteenfold in the PF-resistant cells.[63]

The increased level of UMPS mRNA in the PF-resistant rat cells provided a significant advantage in the selection of a cDNA clone for UMPS.[63] Poly(A)+ mRNA from these cells was further enriched for UMPS mRNA by size fractionation on sucrose density gradients. The partially purified mRNA fraction was used to produce a cDNA library that was inserted into the plasmid vector pBR322 using the G-C tailing technique. Recombinant plasmids with inserts complementary to UMPS sequences were selected by differential hybridization to single-stranded cDNA prepared from wild-type and resistant cell poly(A)+ mRNA. Recombinants that demonstrated increased hybridization to the PF-resistant cell cDNA were then tested further for hybrid selection of UMPS mRNA.[63]

cDNA clones for the human UMPS mRNA were selected from a library generated with mRNA from a T-cell leukemic cell line, HPB-ALL.[64] The human UMPS clone was selected by cross-hybridization with the rat sequence described above.[35] A fragment of this rat UMPS probe was also used to select a murine cDNA encompassing the ODC domain of UMPS from Ehrlich ascites cells.[44]

Analysis of mRNA and Gene Sequence. The size of the mRNA for human UMPS was determined by Northern blot analysis of mRNA from HeLa cells and a PF-resistant HeLa cell line to be approximately 2.0 kb.[35] The UMPS mRNA in the PF-resistant rat hepatoma cell line was estimated to be about 1.8 kb.[33] The minimum size of the human UMPS gene containing the coding region can be estimated to be a minimum of 15 kb, based on the size of genomic fragments that contain sequences for the 5′ and 3′ ends of the coding region of the mRNA.[34]

The sequence of 2420 base pairs 5′ of the AUG translation start site has been determined for the UMPS gene. This region contains no consensus TATA or CAAT box at the predicted positions for a RNA polymerase II transcribed gene.[34] This is characteristic of the promoter region of "housekeeping" genes. Similar to other constitutively expressed genes, the region around and immediately 5′ of the AUG translation start site is very CpG rich.

The transcription initiation start site for UMPS has been determined by mRNA primer extension and S1 nuclease mapping techniques. The major transcription start site is 18 nucleotides 5′ of the AUG translation start codon, with a secondary initiation site located 44 base pairs 5′ of the start codon.

Sequence of UMP Synthase and Homology with OPRT and ODC Proteins. The complete coding region of the human UMPS mRNA has been determined by sequencing of cDNAs and a 5′-genomic fragment containing the ATG initiation codon.[65] The UMPS protein is composed of 480 amino acids with a molecular weight of 52 kDa. The bifunctional nature of the UMPS protein is clearly apparent by comparison of its amino acid sequence with that of the monofunctional OPRT and ODC proteins from other species, both prokaryotic[66,67] and eukaryotic.[43,44,67]

Homology with ODC Proteins. Alignment of ODC proteins or domains from 20 species reveals 4 short regions of sequence homology common to all.[67] In the human sequence the amino acids that comprise these regions of sequence similarity are residues 267 to 287, 295 to 323, 411 to 419, and 443 to 454. Region two is the most noticeably conserved, containing six strictly conserved residues within the consensus sequence: DxKxxDI(P/G)(S/T/N)T.[67] Six other residues are strictly conserved within the eukaryotic species. Region three consists of the consensus sequence (D/E)(F/W)hhhT(T/P)Gh, where h is an hydrophobic amino acid with a bulky side chain (L, M, I, V, F, or W).[67]

Between the murine ODC domain and the yeast ODC sequence, 52 percent of the amino acid residues are identical. If amino acids that have similar hydration potential are considered equivalent, these sequences are 75 percent homologous.[44] The amino acid sequence of the murine ODC domain is 90 percent identical with the carboxy-terminal 250 amino acids of the human UMPS protein.[65] Within this region there are only 26 nonidentical amino acids and 7 of these are neutral substitutions (i.e., changes between Ala or Gly and Ile, Leu, or Val).

Homology of OPRT Proteins. Alignment of the *E. coli* monofunctional OPRT with the amino-terminal 214 amino acids of the UMPS protein gives several regions of strong homology. In the region between residues 96 and 155, the two sequences are 43 percent identical, and if amino acids of similar hydration potential are considered equivalent, this region is 73 percent homologous.[66] This region of the OPRT domain includes a stretch of amino acids that is highly conserved in a set of mammalian enzymes that have the phosphoribosyltransferase function in common (see Figure 5 of reference 59).[65,68,69] This sequence has been predicted to be part of a phosphoribosyltransferase catalytic site.[70] Thus, it appears that the UMPS enzyme in mammals is the result of a fusion process that occurred between the separate genes for OPRT and ODC that are present in the lower eukaryotes and prokaryotes.

Expression of Recombinant cDNA Vector in Urd-C Cells. The most convincing proof that a DNA sequence encodes a specific protein is by expression of the sequence and production of the protein. The complete coding region for UMP synthase, including a 450-base pair stretch of nontranslated 3′ region, was inserted into a mammalian shuttle vector and transfected into Urd$^-$ cells.[47,71] Urd$^-$ cells were selected for resistance to 5-fluorouracil (5FU) and are deficient in both OPRT and ODC, requiring uridine in the medium for growth.[72] Isolated colonies of transfected cells were selected for their ability to grow in the absence of uridine. Enzyme assays of the selected cells show both OPRT and ODC activity to be two- to fourfold higher than that found in the V79 cell line of Chinese hamster lung cells.[71] This experiment gave definitive evidence that the cDNA sequence is sufficient to code for both OPRT and ODC activity.

Chromosome Location of UMPS Gene. The chromosomal location of the UMPS gene was initially determined through the use of somatic cell hybrids between human lymphocytes and the mutant Urd$^-$C Chinese hamster cells.[72,73] Hybrid cells were isolated that did not require uridine for growth and were sensitive to 5FU. These cells were analyzed cytogenetically for chromosome 3 and for concordance between the human ODC activity and chromosome-specific markers (ACY-1, β-galactosidase, D3S1, and transferrin receptor). Very high concordance was demonstrated between the presence of the long arm of chromosome 3, transferrin receptor, human ODC activity, and uridine independent growth, providing strong evidence for the location of the UMPS gene on the long arm of chromosome 3.[73] The location of the gene was later narrowed to 3cen-3q21 by analysis of deletion mutants in hamster-human hybrids containing chromosome 3 as the only human chromosome.

In order to sublocalize the UMPS gene on the long arm of chromosome 3, *in situ* hybridization of the human UMPS cDNA probe to human metaphase spreads of lymphocytes was carried out.[74] Analysis of the spreads showed 20 percent of the silver grains to be localized in the region 3q13. By this procedure the UMPS gene is positioned between the transferrin receptor and the D3S1 DNA sequence. No other region of significant hybridization was detected, indicating only one locus for the UMPS gene sequence.

Pyrimidine Metabolism

Transport. OA is not transported into nucleated cells, but there is a high capacity, nonsaturable transport system for OA into erythrocytes, with the rate-limiting step being the conversion of OA to UMP.[75] If nucleated cells (fibroblasts, lymphoblasts) are incubated with erythrocytes, the erythrocytes take up OA and excrete uridine into the medium, where it is utilized by the nucleated cells.[75]

Uridine enters animal cells by means of a carrier-mediated nucleoside transport process[76,77] that is concentrative.[78,79] Uridine transport in murine splenocytes involves cotransport.[79] It has been difficult to measure rates of transport separate from the rate of uridine utilization, but modern techniques[77] indicate that the kinetic parameters for transport are about 100 times that for phosphorylation, while the first-order rate constants are about the same. This means that in rat hepatoma cells at physiological (less than 10 μM) concentrations of uridine, uridine is phosphorylated inside the cell at about 70 percent of its rate of entry into the cell, so neither phosphorylation nor transport is rate-limiting and the cells effectively deplete the medium of substrate. At higher concentrations, phosphorylation becomes rate-limiting and intracellular uridine concentrations approach those in the medium. Also at higher concentrations (10 to 30 μM), the rate of uptake decreases with time, possibly due to some feedback inhibition or depletion of substrate.[77] Uracil, 5FU, and thymine are transported into rat intestine by an active process that requires Na^+.[80]

Blood levels of uridine in mice following oral uridine doses are significantly higher over a longer time if benzylacyclouridine (an inhibitor of uridine phosphorylase) is also given.[81] Dipyridamole (an inhibitor of nucleoside transport) reduces plasma uridine concentrations in humans[82] and increases tissue uridine concentrations in murine spleen.[83] The accumulation of uridine occurred in all tissues if exogenous uridine was also given or if *de novo* pyrimidine synthesis was increased by inhibiting the urea cycle.[83]

Utilization. Levels of pyrimidine nucleotides in cultured and blood cells have been measured by high performance liquid chromatography (HPLC).[84,85] The UTP level is 100 to 300 pmol per 10^6 cells, 10 to 20 percent of the level of ATP. Exogenous uridine is rapidly incorporated into nucleotides in nucleated cells but not in erythrocytes, and the increased uracil nucleotide pool size may be associated with a reduction in *de novo* synthesis.[18,19]

Differential incorporation of labeled OA and uridine into UMP in rat hepatoma cells has indicated that there may be two separate UTP pools, one formed from *de novo* synthesis that is used for RNA incorporation and uridine sugar nucleotide production and one from pyrimidine salvage which is the primary source of cytidine nucleotides. The two pools are interconnected.[86] Compartmentation of UTP pools but not of the CTP pool has also been demonstrated in rat hepatocytes. Expansion of the UTP and CTP pools did not alter the amount of OA incorporation into RNA.[87] Double-label studies of perfused rat liver slices and measurement of OA, uracil, uridine, and UMP have also indicated marked compartmentalization of uridine, uracil, and UMP.[88]

It has been suggested that PP-ribose-P availability may coordinate purine and pyrimidine metabolic activity, because it is an important intermediate in both systems.[16] Pyrimidine nucleotides are increased in cells from patients with Lesch-Nyhan syndrome, and PP-ribose-P is elevated in these cells.[89] Reduction in pyrimidine synthesis in erythrocytes by adenosine may be mediated by PP-ribose-P because adenosine does not inhibit OPRT or ODC, but these experiments were at high adenosine concentrations.[90]

Pharmacologic Inhibition of UMPS

The usual pharmacologic effect of inhibitors of UMPS is to increase the urinary excretion of OA and orotidine. Paradoxically, there is often a concomitant increase in the measured level of OPRT and ODC activity in blood cells. A similar increase is also seen in human fibroblasts grown in the presence of various drugs or enzyme inhibitors, including allopurinol and oxypurinol, 5-azaorotic acid (5AZOA), 6AZUR, and barbituric acid (BA).[91,92]

Allopurinol. Allopurinol and its metabolite oxypurinol cause orotic aciduria and orotidinuria while increasing OPRT and ODC activity in patients. In vitro, these compounds (or their metabolites) inhibit OPRT and/or ODC. Early reports indicated that allopurinol caused substantial increases in levels of urinary OA and orotidine in gouty patients and control subjects.[93,94] Normal subjects receiving 200 to 300 mg allopurinol per day showed an increase in urinary orotidine from <3 mg/day to 24 to 55 mg/day and in OA from <2 mg/day to 6 to 30 mg/day.[94] Allopurinol (800 mg/day) and oxypurinol (800 mg/day) reduced expired $[^{14}C]CO_2$ from $[7\text{-}^{14}C]$-OA and increased urinary metabolite excretion. It was suggested that the inhibitory compound may be oxypurinol-1-ribotide or oxypurinol-7-ribotide.[95]

Allopurinol-induced orotic aciduria can be reduced by dietary pyrimidines, RNA, or RNA hydrolysates, and by dietary purines.[96] Pigs given allopurinol showed increased urinary levels of orotidine and OA, but these declined with time even though the allopurinol dose was kept constant.[97]

Allopurinol also causes increased levels of erythrocyte OPRT and ODC activity, with exposure times varying from a few days to 2 weeks.[93,98–100] The increase of ODC activity with allopurinol was not associated with a reduction of ODC inhibition in vivo in either nucleated cells or erythrocytes. Data are consistent with enzyme activation, stabilization of the enzyme in the extraction procedure,[99,101] or to stabilization of enzymes in the aging erythrocyte.[98] It was suggested that there may be "pseudosubstrate" stabilization of UMPS by oxypurinol ribonucleotide, synthesized by OPRT.

A concentration-dependent increase in OPRT and ODC in fibroblasts and lymphoblasts incubated with oxypurinol occurred within 2 to 3 h, implying enzyme stabilization during extraction from the cells or direct activation of enzyme rather than inhibition of normal enzyme catabolism. Oxipurinol incubated with lymphoblasts caused inhibition of OA incorporation within 90 min, and OPRT and ODC activity increased within this time.[102] This is consistent with oxypurinol ribonucleotide alteration of quaternary structure and increased stability and activity of the enzyme complex.

Rat liver studies suggested allopurinol is converted to an inhibitor which promotes formation of a more stable form of UMPS with a higher molecular weight.[103] In 1975, Grobner and colleagues showed that allopurinol ribonucleotide and oxypurinol-7-ribonucleotide cause alterations in the molecular weight form of UMPS, so that the most stable forms predominate. Thus, the apparent increase in enzyme activity is related to the stabilization of an enzyme complex during lysis and extraction.[104]

Allopurinol ribonucleotide inhibits ODC in dialyzed erythrocyte lysate.[94] A compound that inhibits ODC is produced when erythrocytes from normal, OPRT-deficient, and HPRT-deficient individuals are incubated with oxypurinol. This required PP-ribose-P, and implied the inhibitory compound was oxypurinol-1-ribotide or oxypurinol-7-ribotide.[95] OA excretion also increased in xanthinuric patents, who do not form oxypurinol, implying allopurinol-1-ribotide also inhibits ODC in vivo, although not as effectively as the oxypurinol nucleotides.[105] High levels of oxypurinol-7-ribotide have been found in renal failure, and this has been correlated with high levels of plasma, urine, and erythrocyte orotidine.[106]

Allopurinol reduces PP-ribose-P in fibroblasts and OA utilization in normal and HPRT-deficient fibroblasts. Oxipurinol does not alter PP-ribose-P, but reduces OA incorporation into acid-precipitable material. Neither compound altered uridine incorporation.[107,108] Oxipurinol increased ODC in fibroblasts, including OPRT-deficient cells.[92]

6-Azauridine (6AZUR). 6AZUR is converted to 6-azauridine-5′-monophosphate (6AZUMP) by uridine kinase.[109] In its monophosphate form, 6AZUR is a competitive inhibitor of the ODC activity of UMPS. Inhibition of UMPS by 6AZUR has been demonstrated in tumor slices, cell-free preparations, yeast, and leukocytes.[110,111] The inhibition is reversible and pH-dependent.[111]

Intravenous 6AZUMP given to chronic myelogenous leukemia patients (180 to 240 mg/(kg/day)) produced 8 to 19 mM OA per day and 5 to 9 mM orotidine per day. Three patients had $[6\text{-}^{14}C]$OA infused and its incorporation into pseudouridine determined. *De novo* pyrimidine production was 4 to 16 mM/day. Patients given $[7\text{-}^{14}C]$OA and 6AZUR excreted 50 to 66 percent of label as OA, 3 to 13 percent as orotidine, 1 to 7 percent as other urine compounds, and 14 to 26 percent as expired CO_2. They showed a sevenfold increase in *de novo* pyrimidine production with 6AZUR, but a decrease in UMP production estimated by respiratory expired isotopic CO_2.[1] In other similar studies increased orotic aciduria and enzyme inhibition in leukocytes were observed.[111,112] Clinical response to 6AZUR was correlated with inhibition of UMPS in intact leukocytes, but no effect on UMPS could be shown in cell-free systems. Development of drug resistance was correlated with lack of enzyme inhibition in intact leukocytes. Urinary excretion of OA and orotidine did not correlate with enzyme inhibition or antileukemic effects.[113,114]

Mouse tumor response to 6AZUR did correlate with in vitro inhibition of OA decarboxylation by tissue slices, but after initial suppression of OA metabolism, enzyme activity returned to pretreatment levels despite continued 6AZUR.[115] Response to 6AZUR did not correlate with inhibition of UMPS in other mouse tumors.[116] Mouse salivary glands stimulated with isoproterenol have increased incorporation of OA into RNA and thymidine into DNA, both of which are inhibited by 6AZUR, but uridine incorporation into RNA was not inhibited.[117] 6AZUR reduced OA incorporation into RNA in cat brain.[118]

Barbituric Acid (BA). BA competitively inhibits dihydroorotate dehydrogenase (DHODH) and OPRT (directly or indirectly), and has been shown to increase OPRT and ODC in human fibroblasts. It was suggested that the molecule active in augmenting enzyme activity may be dihydroorotic acid.[119] The ribonucleotide of BA, 6-hydroxyuridine-5′-monophosphate, inhibits uridine monophosphate kinase and is a powerful competitive inhibitor of ODC. BA is a competitive inhibitor itself of ODC if PP-ribose-P is present.[120]

Niedzwicki[121] evaluated 80 pyrimidine base analogs as inhibitors of OPRT and found 4,6-dihydroxypyrimidine to be a potent inhibitor of the enzyme activity. 5-Azauridine, 5-azaorotic acid, and BA inhibited ODC significantly only after preincubation with PP-ribose-P and MgCl, in the presence of cytosol.

5-Fluorouracil (5FU). 5FU can be metabolized to 5FUMP by action of OPRT in the presence of PP-ribose-P.[41,122,123] OPRT will utilize 5FU or orotate as a substrate with similar efficiency.[41] The conversion of 5FUMP to 5FdUMP or 5FUTP is required for cytotoxicity. 5FdUMP acts as an inhibitor of thymidylate synthase, which is required for the production of dTMP *de novo*. 5FUTP can be incorporated into RNA.

Cells in culture can be selected for resistance to the cytotoxic action of 5FU.[31,72,124,125] The 5FU-resistant cells are deficient in OPRT and ODC activity. The level of activity of remaining enzyme in the resistant cells varies from undetectable[72] to up to 50 percent.[125] The level of 5FU resistance should correlate inversely with the amount of OPRT activity in the cells.

Stabilization of UMPS Protein. Human fibroblasts grown in 10^{-5} M 6AZUR had increased specific activities of ODC and OPRT.[91,124] The increase in enzyme activity occurred also when cytidine was present in the cultures. Pinsky and Krooth[91] found that direct addition of 6AZUMP to human fibroblast extracts inhibited the activity of ODC, but inhibition could be overcome by excess OMP. The activity obtained with addition of excess substrate was no higher than in extracts assayed without addition of the drug. Mixtures of extracts from cells grown with or without

6AZUR had an average value for the enzyme, and dialysis of extracts grown in the presence or absence of 6AZUR did not alter the enzyme specific activity. These results were interpreted as indicating the increased ODC activity was due to increased enzyme in the cell.

The same workers also showed that 5AZOA (which inhibits OPRT but not ODC) in the culture medium increased both activities in fibroblast extracts. The concentrations of 5AZOA used did not inhibit cell growth. BA also had no effect on growth but augmented enzyme activity levels. They suggested that dihydroorotic acid may be the active precursor that stimulates OPRT and ODC activities.[119]

Purines. Adenosine toxicity to cultured mammalian cells has been associated with increased purine nucleotide pools and decreased pyrimidine nucleotide pools. The toxic effects are reversible by the addition of uridine to the culture medium and are thought to be mediated by PP-ribose-P concentration changes.[126–128] Altered PP-ribose-P concentration was correlated with inhibition of UMPS by adenosine in fibroblasts and erythrocytes.[90] Other work suggests that the effect of adenosine at low concentrations (less than 10 μM in lymphoid cells) is depletion of PP-ribose-P, UTP and CTP, and a G_1.S transition block, while higher concentrations neither inhibit cell growth nor alter nucleotide levels.[129,130]

Hereditary Orotic Aciduria (MIM 25890)

Clinical Aspects. There are several inherited diseases in which excessive amounts of OA may be excreted in the urine, but the term hereditary orotic aciduria was first applied to a case of UMPS deficiency[131] and is best restricted to that deficiency. Homozygous UMPS deficiency is rare in human beings, and we know of only 15 cases (in sufficient detail) for review, of which 14 have been established by direct measurement of UMPS. These cases are summarized in Table 113-2. Huguley and colleagues reported the first patient in 1959, J.P., a child who died at age 2 years 9 months, before enzyme assays were performed.[132] The authors' prediction of the nature of the metabolic defect was later confirmed by the demonstration of partial deficiencies of OPRT and ODC in the child's parents and other presumed family heterozygotes.[114,131,133] By 1973, six further patients with confirmed enzyme deficiency had been reported, summarized as cases 2 to 7 in Table 113-2.[99] We have excluded from our series two possible cases reported in the literature[16,134,135] because the enzyme deficiencies were not confirmed. We agree with the comments by the author of one of the reports[136] that they appear to represent different disorders. We know of only seven patients with confirmed enzyme deficiency reported since 1973, cases 8 through 12 and 14 in Table 113-2: YS, RS, XX, DM, YY, HB, YF,[137–141] and only one other enzymatically confirmed but unpublished case, patient AM born in 1990.[142] From our review of the information available on each of the 15 cases, we conclude that a majority of homozygotes for UMPS deficiency have a uniform clinical presentation in which the consistent features are megaloblastic anemia and OA crystalluria frequently associated with some degree of physical and intellectual retardation. These features will respond to appropriate pyrimidine replacement therapy, and most cases will be uncomplicated and have a good prognosis in the short term.

A minority of cases have additional features, particularly congenital malformations and immune deficiencies, which may adversely affect this prognosis. These variations occur with sufficient frequency to suggest that they are not coincidental but are the result of a poorly understood heterogeneity in the UMPS gene or its expression.

For the seventh edition of MMBID we also directed inquiries to the authors of the previous reports on 10 living patients listed in the sixth edition. Eight replied and as a result we had recent information on 10 patients in all, including 7 surviving to age 15 to 32 years.[143–146] This information confirmed our impression of a good prognosis into early adult life for the "typical" patient. However, the appearance of progressive neurologic deterioration continuing into the late teenage years of one treated patient is a cause for concern.[147]

There is a notable lack of published follow-up information on those patients who initially did well. For this reason and as a basis for discussion of the clinical manifestations in all 15 cases, we will first summarize the history of DG. This patient, now 38 years old was the first to be treated with uridine and has been the subject of a number of reports of clinical and laboratory studies over the years.[21,65,71,92,124,148–153]

Case Report. DG, male, mother Maori/part white, father white, was born in October 1961.[148] His birth weight was 4.15 kg. He grew normally until about 3 months of age, when he became pale and lethargic and his motor development slowed. At 13 months during an admission to hospital with bronchopneumonia he was found to be severely anemic (hemoglobin 46 g/liter) and leukopenic. His bone marrow showed megaloblastosis, and he had a low serum iron level. Treatment with iron, folic acid, cobalamin, pyridoxine, and thyroxine caused a slight rise in the hemoglobin level, but the marrow remained megaloblastic. At 17 months he was assessed at a children's hospital when his weight (9.5 kg) was below the 3rd percentile. He was pale, had expressionless facies, and an alternating convergent strabismus. His hair was sparse, short, and fine and his nails had not grown during previous months. He showed little interest in his surroundings, could not sit up, but was able to maintain a sitting position. He did not say words. Psychometric assessment indicated abilities in the 7- to 11-month range. The spleen was just palpable. There was no glossitis or specific neurologic findings. His peripheral blood had a hemoglobin of 80 g/liter with normal platelet, neutrophil, and lymphocyte counts. The erythrocytes showed a marked degree of anisocytosis and poikilocytosis with numerous macrocytes up to 16 μm in diameter and other morphological abnormalities consistent with megaloblastosis (Fig. 113-4A). Many macrocytes were hypochromic. The bone marrow was megaloblastic with a predominance of erythroid cells. Serum vitamin B_{12} and folate levels were above normal for age. Urine specimens were clear when fresh but when left to stand for several hours produced an abundant white flocculent precipitate which microscopic analysis revealed to be colorless, fine, needle-shaped crystals (Fig. 113-5). A feature of the deposit was the firm adherence of the particles to the sides of glass containers. This deposit was identified as OA. There was an average of 1.5 g OA excreted daily during the initial period of assessment. Orotidine, carbamylaspartate, and dihydroorotate were also increased in the urine. Studies initiated before treatment showed that the activities of OPRT and ODC were very low in his erythrocytes and cultured fibroblasts, and there was no ODC activity demonstrable in leukocytes. Later studies showed that growth of cultured skin fibroblasts was stimulated by addition of uridine or cytidine to the culture medium.[152]

His initial treatment is summarized in Fig. 113-6. Cytidylic acid, 2.6 mM/day orally for 12 days, caused only a slight rise in hemoglobin and the average daily OA excretion decreased to 58 percent of the pretreatment level. An equivalent dose of uridine, 3.1 mM/day orally in five doses, had similar slight effects, but there was a marked response when uridine was increased to 6.1 mM/day (150 mg/kg/day). There was a prompt reticulocytosis and return of blood hemoglobin levels to normal. The bone marrow became normoblastic, and erythrocytes were normal (Fig. 113-4B). OA excretion decreased to a mean of 0.30 g/day, 26 percent of the pretreatment level, and was not further reduced by temporary doubling of the dose of uridine. Previously elevated levels of aspartate transcarbamylase (ATC) and dihydroorotase (DHO) in red cells returned to normal with therapy.[154] The clinical response was impressive, with a rapid improvement in his color, activity, alertness, and appetite, and immediate weight gain. There was a sudden spurt in the growth of his hair and nails. At 2 years he

Table 113-2 Cases of Hereditary Orotic Aciduria: UMPS Deficiency

Name*	Sex	Age at presen-tation	Presenting features†	MA	CR	OU	GD	DD	MAL	SQ	CM	MInf	ID	Age at treat-ment	Age at last report	Status	Refs
1 JR	M	3 m	Pallor, diarrhea	+	+	−	−	−	+		−	+		18 m	2 y, 9 m	Dead	131–133
2 DG	M	3 m	Pale, retarded development	+	+	−	+	+		+	−	+	−	19 m	38 y	Well	21, 148, 149, 155
3 JP	M	10 m	Weakness, anemia, poor development	+	+	+	−	+		+	?	−	+	20 m	30 y	Well	158
4 TH	F	2 m	Anemia, strabismus	+	+	−	+	−		+	+	−		11 m	26 y	Well	163
5 DB	F	7 y	Fatigue, hematuria, back and flank pain	+	+	+	−	−			?	−		7 y	31 y	Well	150
6 KP	M	1 d	Multiple malformations	+	+	+		+			+	+		4 m	6 m	Dead	164, 208
7 PM	M	6 m	Failure to thrive, anemia	+	+	−	+	+				−		6 m	24 m	Well	164, 208
8 DM	M	6 m	Cough, anemia, failure to thrive	+	+	+	+	+				−		2 y	18 y	Progressive neurological impairment	138, 165
9 YS	M	7y	Diarrhea, hematuria, stomatitis, anemia	+	+	−	+−	+				+	+	7 y	8 y	Dead	137, 157, 169
10 RS	F	3 m	Sib of YS, pallor, transient diarrhea	+		−	−	−				−	+	3 m	12 y	Well	137, 157, 169
11 XX§	F		Anemia, failure to thrive	+		−	+	+		+					9 y	Well	166
12 HB	F	4 d	Congenital heart disease	+	+	−	−	+			+	−	+	23 m	9 y	Well	139, 146, 177
13 YF	F	1 m	Congenital heart disease, failure to thrive, anemia	+	+	−	+				+	−	+	3 m	18 m	Well	140
14 YY§	M	28 y	Anemia	+	+	+	−	−	−	−	−	−	−	Untreated	32 y	Well	141
15 AM	F	5 m	Failure to thrive, anemia	+	+	−	+	+	−	−	−	−	+	20 m	21 m	Well	175

*Number shown indicates the case number.
§XX, YY = patient's name is unknown.
†Abnormalities abbreviations: MA = megaloblastic anemia; MAL = malabsorption; CR = crystalluria; SQ = squint; OU = obstructive nephropathy; CM = cardiac malformation (? = heart murmur was present which may have been hemic); GD = growth deficiency; MInf = major infection; DD = developmental delay; ID = immune dysfunction (refers to the results of laboratory studies); + = a feature documented as present; − = a feature documented as absent.

began to feed himself; he spoke single words at 2 years 2 months; and he walked at 2 years 5 months.

This clinical improvement was maintained but after 8 months of treatment, because of weight gain, his oral uridine dose had fallen to 100 mg/kg/day. At this uridine level there were signs of hematologic relapse, which were reversed by increasing uridine to 150 mg/kg/day (in three doses). This was the recommended dose of uridine during the next three decades except for a short and unsuccessful trial of uracil as alternative therapy (Fig. 113-4C).[21] His progress during these years has been monitored clinically, hematologically, and by assay of urinary OA levels. In the first 18 months of treatment his weight increased from the 3rd to the 90th percentile, after which this growth spurt diminished, and he has maintained average adult height and weight. He had the usual childhood infections, including measles, but no major illnesses. His intelligence at the last formal assessment at age 7 years was in the range of 73 to 81 on the Weschler scale, and his subsequent performance suggests he is functioning at or above this level. He had normal schooling, has been employed as a warehouseman-driver, appears well-adjusted socially, is married, and has two living children and one stillborn infant dying of Rh isoimmunization.

His compliance with treatment has been variable. When taking uridine, although not necessarily at the recommended dose, he has blood hemoglobin levels in the range 115 to 135 g/L (average 120 g/L), and there is minimal anisocytosis of red cells with normal white cell and platelet counts. The mean urinary OA excretion has been 0.38 mM/mM creatinine. Periodically he has stopped taking his uridine and has presented after ill-defined time intervals with recurrences of macrocytosis, hemoglobin levels falling to as low as 68 g/L, and urinary OA excretion as high as 3.2 mM/mM creatinine. He has felt some loss of energy during these episodes, but there have been no urinary or other specific symptoms. His urine has normal cell and protein content, and at

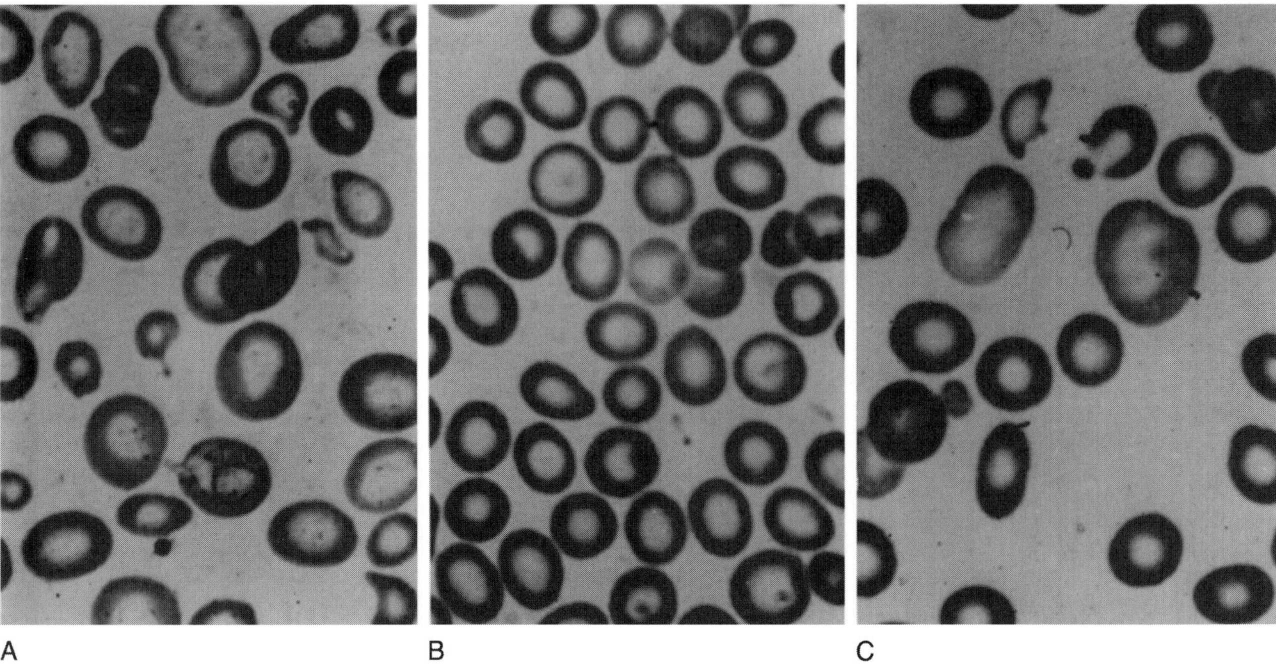

Fig. 113-4 Blood films from a patient (DG) with hereditary orotic aciduria: (A) Before uridine treatment; (B) After 6 months of uridine treatment; (C) During relapse on uracil therapy.

various times his creatinine clearance, urinary concentrating capacity, and intravenous pyelogram have been normal.[155]

A more detailed in vivo study of purine and pyrimidine metabolism and the effect of allopurinol was made when he was 17 years old.[155,156] Uridine therapy and a caffeine-free diet were maintained while the effects of oral allopurinol and diets with high or low nucleoprotein content were investigated. Allopurinol produced up to a 70 percent reduction in urinary OA excretion and more than a 50 percent reduction in the previously elevated urinary uric acid and oxypurine excretion, irrespective of the purine content of the diet. The study confirmed that allopurinol could reduce the excretion of potentially crystal-forming components in the urine, but this treatment was not continued because he had no urinary symptoms and normal renal function. Further studies of the relationship of purines and pyrimidines to immune function were undertaken in 1983 and 1984 following reports[137,157] of abnormal cellular immunity in other cases of hereditary orotic aciduria. These studies of immune function in DG were undertaken during periods of compliance and noncompliance with uridine therapy. All results were normal and consistent with the clinical impression of his immunologic competence and general good health.[149,151,155]

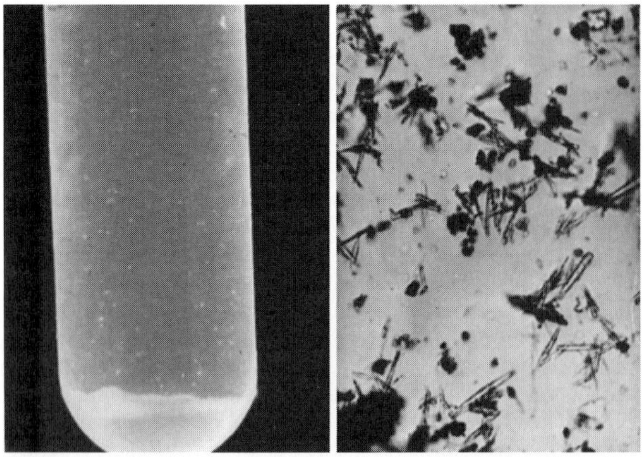

Fig. 113-5 OA crystals in the urinary sediment of a patient (DG) with hereditary orotic aciduria.

Clinical Diagnosis.

Megaloblastic Anemia. The 14 cases of hereditary orotic aciduria identified in childhood have had a variety of clinical presentations but in all cases the eventual detection of an anemia and bone marrow megaloblastosis has predicated the biochemical investigations leading to the confirmed diagnosis. Anemia has first been detected at ages ranging from 1 month to 7 years. Hemoglobin levels in nine patients presenting between 3 months and 7 years of age were in the range 60 to 80 g/liter. Four young children[139,142,148,158] had more severe anemia, including two infants only 1.5 and 2 months old with hemoglobin levels about 50 g/liter. The anemia was of moderate severity and not rapidly progressive in several patients untreated for several months. In some patients, the anemia has improved after treatment with various vitamins, steroids, and hematinics but without reversal of megaloblastosis. Rapid falls in hemoglobin occurred in the terminal phases of illness in JR and YS.[132,137,157] Reticulocyte counts have been in the normal to low range. Most reports have described or illustrated striking abnormalities of erythrocyte morphology including severe anisocytosis, poikilocytosis, and other cytologic abnormalities indicative of marrow megaloblastosis (Fig. 113-4). Anisocytosis and macrocytosis of this degree is very unusual in young children, and will be easily detected by modern blood cell analyzers. Several authors have commented on the degree of associated hypochromia (Fig. 113-4) despite normal serum iron levels or iron therapy. The total leukocyte counts have usually been low at presentation, accompanied by varying degrees of neutropenia and lymphopenia, with counts less than 2.0×10^6 per liter. A few patients have had normal or even higher neutrophil and lymphocyte counts prior to specific therapy, while in others the neutropenia or lymphopenia was intermittent. Platelet counts have been normal in all patients. Bone marrows, when differentials have been reported, have had levels of erythroid precursors 60 to 80 percent of normal and megaloblastic changes which in most patients have been considered atypical but in others were not commented on as differing from those of megaloblastosis of other causes. Myeloid precursors and megakaryocytes have been specified as having megaloblastic features in some patients.

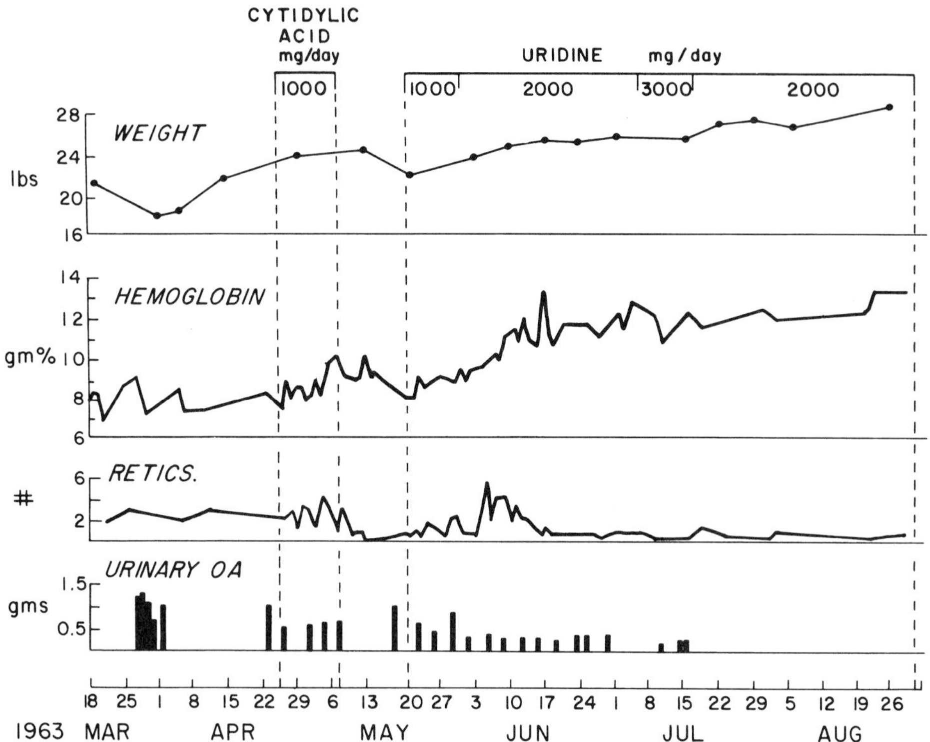

Fig. 113-6 Changes in weight, hemoglobin, reticulocytes, and urinary OA in a 19-month-old patient (DG) with hereditary orotic aciduria during treatment with cytidylic acid and with uridine.

YY, the only patient first identified in adult life was admitted to hospital aged 28 years in a critical condition after a car accident.[141] Severe anemia was attributed to blood loss and possibly an underlying hemoglobinopathy, but persistence of hematologic abnormalities and splenomegaly in the next year led to the identification of megaloblastosis and orotic aciduria. Other hematologic investigations in this patient showed decreased red cell survival with the spleen acting as the major site for removal of erythrocytes, and there was ineffective erythropoiesis of moderate degree and limited erythropoietic expansion. Elevation of HbA2 and HbF in this patient and one other (AM) at presentation raised the possibility of thalassemia, but this was not supported by studies on the parents of YY. The association with hereditary orotic aciduria is unexplained. JR at 2 years of age had 6.1 percent HbF, but normal hemoglobin electrophoresis was reported in three patients (JR, JP, and HB).

The differential diagnosis of the anemia is mainly from other causes of megaloblastosis in infancy and early childhood.[159,160] The more common "nutritional" megaloblastic anemias due to dietary deficiencies or congenital or acquired defects in absorption of folate or vitamin B_{12} will usually be considered first, and in most reported cases of hereditary orotic aciduria were readily excluded by measurement of plasma folate and vitamin B_{12} levels and/or by the failure to obtain a response to therapeutic amounts of folate or cobalamin. The hematologic problem that has emerged in many cases is the further investigation of a "refractory" megaloblastic anemia. We do not intend to review in detail the conditions of childhood in which there may be megaloblastosis unrelated to folate or vitamin B_{12} deficiency. These include the leukemias and other forms of dyshematopoiesis, anemias responsive to pyridoxine or thiamine, drug-induced megaloblastosis, Lesch-Nyhan syndrome, and the inborn errors of folate or vitamin B_{12} metabolism. The latter are discussed in detail in Chapter 155 and may have clinical features similar to those described for hereditary orotic aciduria, including onset in infancy of megaloblastic anemia, retarded motor and intellectual development, and sparse hair. Differentiation from hereditary orotic aciduria will be based on the additional clinical and biochemical features (see Chap. 155) and more specifically the absence of orotic aciduria. Page et al.[161] have reported the case of a 3-year-old girl with megaloblastic anemia, developmental delay, alopecia, and mild immunodeficiency believed to be the result of excessive degradation of pyrimidine nucleotides; and this alternative cause of pyrimidine "starvation" can be excluded by the absence of orotic aciduria. Orotic aciduria has been described in a child with formiminotransferase-cyclodeaminase deficiency.[162] This might cause diagnostic difficulty, but the slight increase in OA excretion (6.4 to 21.4 mM/mol creatinine) was considerably less than that in UMPS deficiency and formiminoglutamic acid (FIGLU) excretion was increased. The child in whom Niemann and colleagues[134] diagnosed hereditary orotic aciduria had a megaloblastic anemia responsive to high doses of folic and folinic acid, and although OA crystals were demonstrable, this was after in vitro concentration of urine samples. FIGLU excretion was increased, and this patient is more likely to have an inborn error of folate metabolism than UMPS deficiency and has been excluded from our list of cases. We also exclude a child with presumed PRPP-synthetase deficiency[135] who had megaloblastic anemia, severe mental retardation, and hyperuricemia and who excreted small amounts of OA in the urine. Both megaloblastosis and orotic aciduria disappeared after ACTH treatment.

Orotic Acid Crystalluria and Obstructive Uropathy. The excretion of large amounts of OA in the urine is a constant feature of UMPS deficiency. OA is present in the urine in amounts that may result in crystalluria both within the urinary tract and, more consistently, in voided urine. Urine may be clear initially but on standing produces deposits similar to those illustrated in Fig. 113-5. Methods for the quantification of urinary OA, including differentiating hereditary orotic aciduria from other causes of orotic aciduria, will be presented in the following section on laboratory diagnosis. Although orotic aciduria from other causes may reach levels comparable with those associated with UMPS deficiency, symptoms or signs resulting from OA crystalluria have been reported only with UMPS deficiency. The clinical manifestations have been diverse and have occurred in 11 of the 15 patients. Crystalluria and the subsequent identification of the crystals as OA provided the lead to the identification of the underlying metabolic error in the first-reported patient, JR,[132] and later in JH.[163] When JR became dehydrated, he suffered from precipitation of crystals in his bladder and episodes of urethral and ureteral obstruction. KP aged 4 months required catheterization to relieve urethral obstruction.[164] DM developed urethral obstruction at 22 months and required meatotomy.[138,165] Patient JP at 19 months old[158] had an upper respiratory tract infection followed by hematuria, crystalluria, oliguria, and azotemia. An intravenous pyelogram showed intrarenal retention of radio-opaque material, which was interpreted as due to blockage of collecting tubules by crystals. Both DB and YS presented at age 7 years[137,150,157] with hematuria presumably caused by crystals injuring the renal tract. A preceding history of back pain in DB is likely to have been due to intermittent partial obstruction of the upper urinary tract and YY[141] is believed to have had renal colic. The mothers of DM and AM noticed a powdery or crystalline deposit in their infants' diapers.[142,165]

Growth Deficiency. A history of weight loss or "failure to thrive" is common but not invariable in hereditary orotic aciduria. DG had a typical history of above-average birth weight and failure to thrive in later infancy, so that by 1 year his weight was below the 3rd percentile for his age. Seven of the affected children whose birth weights are known were delivered at term and averaged 3.4 kg, and three delivered prematurely had average birth weights for their gestations of 30 to 35 weeks. Subsequently, 6 of the 14 affected children (at ages between 3 months and 7 years) had weights at or below the 3rd percentiles for age. In addition, XX[166] failed to thrive in infancy, and the weight of TH dropped from the 50th to the 10th percentiles between 6 and 9 months of age.[163] In contrast, JR was described as well-developed and well-nourished at 9 months of age[132] and JP, DB, and HB had weights above the 25th percentile for age when 10 months, 7 years, and 23 months old, all before treatment.[139,150,158] RS had normal growth in early infancy,[137,157] and YY, presenting at 28 years old, appears to have grown normally.[141] The growth of YF improved after a cardiac defect was repaired at age 2 years.[167] Body heights have not been severely affected.

Intellectual and Motor Impairment. Developmental delay was not observed during the first year of life of JR, the first patient with hereditary orotic aciduria,[132] but has been noted in at least seven subsequent cases before replacement therapy was begun. However, both the frequency and specificity of this developmental delay remain in doubt. Formal assessments have been made in three young children before treatment: DG at 17 months had abilities in the 7- to 11- month range; JP at 1 year old was functioning at a 66 percent level as assessed by Gessell development testing;[158] and PM at 5 months old was functioning at the 3-month-old level.[168] Before treatment XX at five months old and DM at two years old were described as having poor development.[165,166] HB had marked developmental delay at 18 months old, although a previous episode of bacterial meningitis may have contributed.[139] AM is described as being slightly delayed in comparison with a sibling.[142] The central nervous system effects were difficult to assess in KP,[164] who was severely handicapped, with multiple congenital malformations and hypertonia from birth until death in infancy. In contrast, there are six affected children, including JR, in whom developmental delay was either excluded or not mentioned at time of presentation. Those with normal development included two 7-year-olds, DB and YS, one of whom (DB) had an IQ of 133 on the Stanford-Binet intelligence scale.[137,157,169] YY, untreated at 28 years old, had worked as a farmer and had served in the Army, but his intelligence has not been formally assessed.[141]

The assessment of the level of retardation in some infants may have been affected adversely by an associated effect on their muscular or motor functions. Weakness, hypotonia, lack of activity, and sluggish movements have received special comment in some affected infants, as has the prompt reversal of these features with specific therapy. The motor effect may be progressive, as PM had good head control at age 5 weeks but lost the control at age 4 months.[168] An unusually high incidence of strabismus may be another manifestation of abnormal motor activity. Strabismus has been recorded in four children, described in three as alternating or bilateral[148,158,163] and as unilateral in one.[166] DG's strabismus resolved spontaneously as he grew older, and surgical correction was performed in TH.[163] The incidence of strabismus in the general population has been conservatively estimated at 5 percent.[170]

Prenatal Development and Malformations. Normal birth weights for gestation of children with hereditary orotic aciduria suggest that there are no major effects on late fetal growth. There is stronger evidence that there may be an effect during organogenesis causing an increased incidence of malformations, particularly cardiac. Systolic cardiac murmurs reported in some anemic children may have been hemic. Four cases had stronger evidence for a cardiac malformation. HB had a severe abnormality, including pulmonary atresia, hypoplastic right ventricle, and a large atrial septal defect, for which a Blalock-Taussig shunt had been performed.[139] TH had a probable interventricular septal defect.[163] KP had other malformations in addition to a presumed intraventricular septal defect and died without a necropsy.[164] YF had an intraventricular septal defect and had a patent ductus arteriosis closed at 2 years of age.[140,167] This is an unusual incidence when structural heart defects overall have an incidence of 6 to 7 per 1000 births.[171,172]

Minor congenital abnormalities, outward torsion of the left tibia, and coloboma of the eyelid were each noted in a single case. KP was the only patient with multiple congenital defects. In addition to the presumed intraventricular septal defect he had defects of the thoracic and abdominal musculature which caused herniation of the lung into the supraclavicular regions and umbilical and inguinal hernias. There was dorsolumbar kyphoscoliosis and a scaphoid skull and severe hypertonia, and the infant was grossly handicapped from birth. This spectrum of skeletal muscle abnormalities, including a pleural "dome" in the neck, closely resemble those of amyoplasia, a nonfamilial form of muscular abnormality causing multiple congenital contractures.[173]

Malabsorption. There are theoretical reasons for believing that the untreated genetic defect might have an effect on epithelial function in the gastrointestinal tract, but the majority of cases have shown no evidence of this. The two exceptional cases had other factors that may have contributed to the observed malabsorption. Diarrhea with bulky stools suggestive of malabsorption was the presenting symptom in the first reported case of hereditary orotic aciduria.[132] However, a recurrence of diarrhea late in the patient's course was attributed to the high phosphate and salt content of the yeast extract that had induced hematologic remission. Another affected child[137,157] also had periods of diarrhea and chronic stomatitis during the first years of his life, but an underlying immunodeficiency and infection may have contributed to these symptoms. His diarrhea recurred after 3 months of apparently successful treatment with oral and intramuscular uridine. The diarrhea became severe and was associated with intestinal candidiasis, partial intestinal villous atrophy, and malabsorption. Parenteral nutrition was instituted, but the patient died of meningitis.

Immunodeficiency and Susceptibility to Infection. The majority of cases of hereditary orotic aciduria did not show undue susceptibility to infection before or after treatment. Three patients died of infection, but there were other predisposing factors including severe malabsorption and anemia in two cases when uridine therapy could not be maintained, and severe immobilizing physical handicap in the third. Girot and colleagues[157] raised the possibility of immune dysfunction in UMPS deficiency, analogous to that found in purine nucleoside phosphorylase and adenosine deaminase deficiencies,[16] when they reported two siblings who had UMPS deficiency with impaired cell-mediated immunity.[137,157,169] Patient YS before treatment at age seven years had severe lymphopenia and negative tests for delayed skin hypersensitivity to several antigens. He had depressed lymphocyte proliferative responses to mitogens and depressed cell-mediated lymphocytolysis. Plasma-cell generation by pokeweed mitogen (PWM) was absent and did not improve with the addition of uridine to the culture system. He had increased serum immunoglobulins and normal antibody formation. These findings were not altered when the patient received uridine therapy, to which he had a poor clinical response. He developed diarrhea, malabsorption, and intestinal candidiasis, and died from purulent meningitis. RS, his sister, tested before and after uridine therapy commenced at age three months, had normal humoral immunity. At various times she had impaired in vitro mitogenic responses, impaired skin hypersensitivity reactions, and impaired cell-mediated lymphocytolysis. There was no lymphopenia, but several T-cell subsets were markedly reduced when first analyzed three months after her treatment began. She remained well, but percentages of mature T-cell subsets were mildly subnormal at 12 years old and T-cell-mediated lymphocytolysis was still profoundly decreased.[174]

Four other affected individuals (HB, YF, YY, AM) had studies of immune function before treatment began.[139–141,175] HB had bacterial meningitis at 7 months of age, but otherwise the four had not shown unusual susceptibility to infections. HB had depressed levels of serum immunoglobulins, which, with the exception of IgA, returned to normal after treatment with uridine.[139] The possibility that the hypogammaglobulinemia was unrelated to the metabolic defect was debated.[176,177] Immunoglobulins were normal in AM, YY, and YF except for a low serum IgA in AM. All four patients had abnormalities of various parameters of T-cell function, but the findings are difficult to interpret because of their inconsistency and the variable effects of the treatment on each. DG when 21 years old had normal T-cell and T-cell subset levels and normal delayed skin hypersensitivity reactions to antigens both when in remission on uridine treatment and in hematologic relapse when he had stopped taking uridine.[151]

Treatment

Uridine. Pyrimidine replacement with the nucleoside uridine has been used for all patients except JR. The salvage pathway for uridine utilization has been discussed previously. Uridine can be taken as a mildly bitter but otherwise flavorless powder and appears to have no gastrointestinal or other side effects at the usual doses. DG responded to 150 mg uridine per kilogram body weight per day given orally in five divided doses. Eight further children treated with oral doses of between 100 and 200 mg/kg/day have shown improvement in their anemias, disappearance of megaloblastosis, decrease in orotic aciduria, and immediate improvement in strength, activity, alertness, and general well-being. At 2 years old, DG. showed early bone marrow relapse when his uridine dose fell to 100 mg/kg/day, although other patients have responded to lower uridine amounts. Uridine at 50 mg/kg/day was sufficient to produce hematologic and clinical remission in RS,[137,157] and a similar effect of 300 mg/day in XX at 5 months old[166] probably represents another response to a lesser dose. AM also achieved remission on 50 mg/kg/day given as a single dose daily.[142] YF responded to 150 mg/kg/day in infancy but at 6 years old became anemic and the dose was increased to 300 mg/kg/day.[178]

YS showed no response to oral uridine at a dose increasing from 75 to 150 mg/kg/day over a 9-month period.[137,157] He is the only patient known to have been treated with intramuscular uridine. The previous oral dose of 150 mg/kg/day, divided approximately equally between the oral and intramuscular routes, stabilized the hemoglobin level, improved the bone marrow to show only minimal megaloblastosis, and decreased orotic aciduria, but leukopenia persisted.

The rate of relapse after stopping uridine appears to be relatively slow. The return of orotic aciduria to pretreatment levels and full hematologic relapse took 3 weeks when DG's uridine was replaced by uracil. The dependency on uridine appears to be lifelong. DG, JP,[144] TH,[179] and DB[180] at 20 years of age or older still showed hematologic relapse and increased orotic aciduria when uridine was stopped, either intentionally or against advice. However, the dose of uridine required to maintain remission may be less in later life. We doubt DG's compliance with his recommended dose of 150 mg/kg/day (9 g/day). In other patients, doses have not been increased to match growth, and as teenagers or adults they are said to be maintaining good control, TH on a dose of 25 mg/kg/day,[181] and DB on 1.5 g/day.[180] RS has had a progressively increased dose and now takes 30 mg/kg/day.[174]

The decision that DG should take uridine in divided doses five or three times daily was arbitrary, because there was no available information on uridine pharmacokinetics or more importantly on whether the presumed cumulative effect on "pyrimidine starvation," might allow less frequent dosage. Pharmacokinetic studies of oral and iv uridine have been done in conjunction with the use of uridine rescue in 5FU chemotherapy.[182] In six healthy volunteers and three patients with advanced colorectal cancer given oral doses of 0.3 to 12 g/M^2, peak plasma uridine levels of 13 to 87 μM at 2 to 3 h were found. The area under the concentration-time curve increased linearly with doses in the range 48 to 476 mM/h/liter. The total plasma clearance varied between 25 and 76 ml/kg/min, while the volume of distribution was 4.3 to 16.6 ml/kg. The mean residence time was 200 to 300 min. Dose-limiting toxicity was diarrhea at 12 g/M^2. Plasma uracil increased from 4 h at doses of 8 to 12 g/M^2.[182] Other studies confirm the very rapid metabolism of uridine and tissue concentration of uridine.[82,183] Normal blood levels of uridine in adults are approximately 2 to 10 μM. DG has had levels between 30 and 50 μM while in hematologic remission.[149]

The bioavailability of oral uridine in healthy adults was 6 to 9 percent relative to a 1-h infusion.[182,184] In mice doses of 350 and 3500 mg/kg orally produced blood uridine levels 7 percent of those achieved following equal subcutaneous doses.[185] Since oral bioavailability is low, defects in intestinal absorption or increased degradation could be an important limitation on treatment. Information on this point would have been of particular interest in YS,[137,157] who had no response to a long trial of a seemingly adequate oral dose of uridine. He had a history of episodic diarrhea, and late in his illness there was evidence of malabsorption and partial intestinal villous atrophy. Circulating uridine diffuses readily into cells and is quickly metabolized. There are no relevant published studies in hereditary orotic aciduria, but in cancer patients, infused uridine has a terminal half-life of between 18 and 118 min,[82,186] and this may depend on the uridine dose. Peak plasma levels increased with dose in one study.[186] Infused uridine at large doses (up to 12 g/m^2) was excreted 24 percent unchanged and 3 percent as uracil.[186] Weissman has shown that uridine is normally reutilized in humans and that the renal clearance is 0.5 to 2 percent of the creatinine clearance.[187] DG excreted 2 to 7 percent of his daily dose as uridine and uracil in the urine.[156] A normal adult also excreted less than 5 percent of a daily dose at the usual therapeutic level.[188]

There does not appear to be a strong case for divided daily oral doses. On the basis of the results of initial treatment of AM we would suggest that in previously untreated patients, the effective dose of uridine should be sought by gradually increasing a single daily dose beginning with between 25 and 50 mg/kg body weight. Well-controlled trials are needed to determine the frequency of the dose and to determine the dosage and frequency in older patients. Treatment can be monitored by occasional checks on hemoglobin and erythrocyte morphology. Urinary OA levels can also be measured, but in retrospect this was not essential for DG's later management. Sumi et al.[178] have suggested that blood uridine may be a useful index for clinical treatment.

YY, first diagnosed aged 28 years, has not been treated because he is well and normally active despite a significant anemia with hemoglobin levels as low as 6.7 g/dl. We believe all such cases should have a trial of uridine to assess the effect on general well-being expected not only from reversal of the anemia but also from the more immediate effect of uridine on activity, energy, and alertness noted in several cases to precede correction of anemia.

Side effects of uridine therapy have been reported only in the high doses used in uridine rescue. Diarrhea was the dose-limiting toxic effect at 10–12 g/m^2 oral uridine,[184] and mild rises in body temperature occurred with iv uridine.[183]

Uridine in Pregnancy. All children of affected individuals will be heterozygous and it is not known if some or all will have unusual requirement for exogenous pyrimidines in utero or whether this hypothetical need could be met by the homozygous mother, with or without the assistance of uridine therapy. DB, treated with uridine from seven years old and now aged thirty-two years, has had four pregnancies resulting in the births of three normal females and one normal male.[179] During these pregnancies she was on her usual uridine dose of 1.5 g daily in six divided doses, but in the last two pregnancies this was increased to 2.5 g daily at seven months gestation.[179] In contrast, Bensen and colleagues[181] have reported the management of two pregnancies in TH, first treated aged 11 months and now twenty- six years old, and in each pregnancy the dose of uridine was increased progressively, in the first from 1.5 g per day up to 24 g per day at term, and in the second from 4 g per day up to 28 g per day at term. This increase was said to have been an adjustment based on hemoglobin levels. However, the changes in hemoglobin were not very different from the physiological fall expected during pregnancy. Other causes of anemia do not appear to have been excluded and the concurrent measurements of urinary OA excretion did not suggest that these changes were related to inadequate pyrimidine supplementation. Blood levels of pyrimidines including uridine were not measured. There was concern about the possible teratogenic effects of this high uridine dosage when the first infant had a number of congenital abnormalities, but these were later shown to be due to aneuploidy derived from a familial balanced chromosome translocation found in the mother and several family members and not segregating with the carrier state for UMP synthase deficiency. The experience with DB supports our belief that uridine requirements will not increase greatly during pregnancy and although we have no expectation that high doses of uridine will be harmful, we believe that these are best avoided. The dose of uridine giving good control in the nonpregnant state should be continued during pregnancy and blood and urine should be monitored more frequently; and the uridine dose increased only if there is an increase in macrocytosis or OA excretion above the range usual before pregnancy or a significant fall in blood uridine level.

A female heterozygote received uridine supplementation during one of two pregnancies monitored for further homozygous conceptuses and the results suggest that uridine had transferred to the amniotic fluid.[167]

Other Pyrimidines. A yeast extract containing uridylic and cytidylic acids was effective in inducing hematologic and clinical remission in JR.[132] The maximum dose used provided about 6 mM of the nucleotides per day. This dose of about 0.6 mM/kg/day was equal in molar terms to uridine at 150 mg/kg/day. The response could not be maintained because the yeast extract was poorly tolerated and caused diarrhea that seemed directly related to the dose. The diarrhea was assumed to be due to the high phosphate and salt content of the yeast extract. DG showed a reduction in orotic aciduria in response to treatment with cytidylic acid at 900 mg per day orally in six doses continued for 12 days (0.26 mM/kg/day).[148] This is a further indication that pure nucleotides in higher weight (equimolar) doses could be as effective as uridine, but their cost is much greater and their effect may involve degradation to nucleosides before absorption. A prolonged trial of uracil at 2.5 g/day (approximately 2 mM/kg/day) was ineffective in JR.[132] A trial of uracil when DG was 4 years old was similarly unsuccessful. Frank relapse occurred with a daily oral dose of 3 g (1.3 mM/kg/day), followed by prompt remission with the reintroduction of oral uridine at 0.6 mM/kg/day.[21] Assuming that uracil is adequately absorbed, the lack of response is consistent with other information suggesting that the normal utilization of uracil through salvage pathways is less efficient than that of uridine (see "Pyrimidine Metabolism"). If OPRT is important for normal uracil salvage, this would be impaired in hereditary orotic aciduria. There is in vitro evidence that uridine had a much greater stimulating effect on DG's cultured fibroblasts than did uracil.[28,92,124]

Allopurinol. Allopurinol increases blood OPRT and ODC activities in humans (see "Pharmacologic Inhibition of UMPS," above) and has been given to three patients with hereditary orotic aciduria. Allopurinol 2.2 mM/day for 6 days did not increase OPRT or ODC activity in DG's erythrocytes, but urine OA was markedly reduced in parallel with a significant reduction in urate excretion.[155] This reduction was possibly caused by in vivo enzyme stabilization by allopurinol or a metabolite. No orotidine was observed in the urine at any time during this study.[155] Allopurinol in two other cases did not decrease urinary OA but caused an increase in orotidinuria.[99] Uridine alone reduces orotic aciduria to a level where there appears to be no long-term effects on the renal tract or renal function. At present, allopurinol does not have a therapeutic role.

Nonspecific Therapy. Patients with orotic aciduria have received a variety of hematinics and vitamins, but the only consistent response has been to adrenal corticosteroids. Reticulocytosis and improvement in anemia to near-normal hemoglobin levels were obtained in JR with cortisone and prednisone, 10 to 51 mg/day,[132] and in JP with prednisone, 30 mg/day.[158] The bone marrows remained megaloblastic in both cases. When steroids were stopped, hemoglobin levels fell sharply in both, but there was a second response when these were reintroduced. Conversely, 1 mg/kg/day prednisone over 6 weeks had no clinical or hematologic effect in YS.[137,157] Amelioration of anemia by adrenal steroids has been reported in pernicious anemia and in megaloblastic anemia of other causes.[159] The mode of action of steroids in these situations has been described as complex and probably not the same in all patients,[159] and therefore the effect in hereditary orotic aciduria may be nonspecific. Possible modes of action include improved absorption or availability of pyrimidines from dietary sources and increased salvage from increased cell catabolism.

Prognosis. Reversal of megaloblastosis and reduction of orotic aciduria with uridine is not necessarily an indication that the effects of the metabolic defect have been ameliorated in other tissues, nor does monitoring these parameters exclude the possibility of other long-term sequelae. Two of the 13 hereditary orotic aciduria patients treated with uridine in childhood died of infections as described above. The other 11 were in hematologic remission and clinically improved at the time case reports were published or available to us; in most cases this was after a treatment period of 2 years or less. Therefore, we inquired about the current status of all surviving patients and have additional unpublished information in varying detail on seven cases: DB, 31 years;[179] DG, 38 years; JP, 30 years;[144] TH, 26 years;[181] PM, 24 years;[147] DM, 15 years;[165] SR, 12 years;[174] and HB, 7 years.[146] All except PM were well physically and there was no mention of recurrence of anemia, urinary symptoms, infections or other medical complications while uridine treatment was maintained. Despite the frequency of urinary tract symptoms before treatment and continuing but reduced orotic aciduria during treatment[149] there have been no reports of long-term effects on renal function or structure (DG, SR[174]). The question of whether there is long-term intellectual impairment in some cases if treatment is delayed or because uridine does not reach the central nervous system[21] is not resolved. One patient, who was not regarded as retarded before treatment at 11 months of age (TH), at 13 years of age was assessed as having an intelligence quotient of 85 and dyslexia was diagnosed.[181] HB, who was severely retarded before treatment at 2 years old, was found on psychological assessment at 6 years of age to have a borderline low intellect and mild to moderate attention deficit. Of particular concern is PM, who was first treated aged 5 months but did not regain an earlier developmental deficit,[168] and at three years was lagging considerably.[145] Ataxic gait and movements were noted at four years old, and there was progressive neurologic deterioration so that at age 18 years he was unable to walk unaided.[147] He had pronounced dysarthria, dystonic posturing, and slow athetoid movements of arms and face. Tone was increased in all the limbs and the plantar responses are extensor. He had a mild peripheral neuropathy. It is possible that this exceptional course is because he is the only case of the "Type 2" hereditary orotic aciduria but there are other possible causes, including poor compliance with treatment in his early years,[145] and the presence of mental retardation in other family members and his possible consanguineous birth suggest alternative diagnoses.[168]

Other treated patients have shown no late deterioration and even those whose early development had appeared retarded have achieved a normal education and lifestyle. Growth and sexual development have been normal and one male (DG) and two female (TH and DB) patients have had a total of nine children, suggesting that fertility is not affected. DG and his wife had been trying to conceive but this was only successful, perhaps coincidentally, after he was advised to comply fully with his uridine dose. The untreated disease in YY appears to have had no serious consequences during his first 32 years of life. Therefore, the prognosis into early adult life is excellent in the majority of treated cases and even in some cases in which treatment is delayed. This good prognosis may be modified by severe congenital malformations (KP) or by undue susceptibility to infection (JR and YS) and, possibly progressive late neurologic changes if those shown by PM are a consequence of the disease.

Biochemical Features

Urinary Orotic Acid. The simplest method for measurement of urinary OA is that of Rogers and Porter,[189] but this colorimetric method is subject to interference from a variety of compounds.[190] Interfering compounds are unlikely to be a problem when OA is measured for the diagnosis or monitoring of therapy in hereditary orotic aciduria because the concentrations involved are high. The specificity of this method can be increased by the use of a nonbrominated blank sample,[191] and when the urine has a chromatographic cleanup before analysis the method gives an excellent correlation with a HPLC method.[192] Both OA and orotidine are measured unless these compounds are separated chromatographically before analysis. The modified colorimetric assay[192] or other more specific method, for example, chromatographic,[193–195] isotope dilution,[196,197] gc-ms,[198] enzymatic,[199] or capillary zone electrophoresis[200] should be used when a precise measurement is needed for determination of carrier status in hereditary orotic aciduria or the urea cycle disorders.

While fresh or frozen urine is generally used for OA measurements, OA in urine dried on filter paper has been shown to be stable for up to two weeks and this makes transport of samples cheap and easy.[197]

Urinary excretion of OA is less than 10 μM/mM of creatinine[190,193,201,202] in normal individuals. Absolute excretion has been reported as 10.3 ± 6.0 μM/24h in 8 adults[141] and 9.28 ± 1.02 μM/day in 18 adults.[203] The level is higher in newborns than in older children or adults.[190,192,193,201,204,205] The range is 1.3 to 5.3 μM/mM of creatinine in newborns, 1.0 to 3.2 in children 2 weeks to 1 year old, and 0.5 to 3.3 in children from 1 to 10 years old.[190] Van Gennip and colleagues report urine OA 3.9 to 20.3 μM in six children aged 0.3 to 5.9 years.[194] A recent study of 1011 adults (using HPLC) gave a normal range of 0.26 to 3.20 μM per mM creatinine.[206]

OA excretion is about half normal in periods of starvation.[192,207] Slight elevations in some other disorders (including hypertension, cerebral infection, malignancy) have been reported.[206]

In contrast, urine OA levels in hereditary orotic aciduria are several orders of magnitude greater than normal. Levels have been reported in nine untreated cases: JR, age 9 months, 9.6 mM/24 h;[132] DG, age 17 months, 4.4 and 8.6 mM/24 h, and at 23 years, 1.4, 3.2, and 1.9 mM/mM of creatinine;[148,149] JP, age 11 months, 6.0 mM/24 h;[158] PM, 1.8 mM/24 h;[164] YS, age 7 years, 5.4 mM/24 h;[137] RS, age 3 months, 1.0 mM/24 h;[137] YF at 3 months, about 1.9 mM/day;[140] HB, age 18 months, 5.6 mM/mM of creatinine;[139] YY age 28 years, 1 to 7 g orotic acid/24 hours[141] and AM age 2 years, 10 mM.[175]

Orotidine has been very low to undetectable; for example TH excreted 6 to 27 μM/mM creatinine during pregnancy,[181] and AM, 0.017 mM pretreatment;[175] except in PM (weight 5 kg), who excreted 1.8 mM OA per day and 0.2 mM orotidine per day before treatment.[208]

Orotic aciduria has been reported in a number of other metabolic diseases and as a consequence of pharmacologic agents.

Urea Cycle Defects. These are discussed elsewhere in this volume (see Chap. 85). They are the only metabolic diseases in which the magnitude of the orotic aciduria is comparable to that observed in UMPS deficiency. Blocks in the urea cycle after CPS I can cause accumulation of intramitochondrial carbamyl phosphate. This diffuses into the cytosol and is available for entry into the *de novo* pyrimidine synthetic pathway. In ornithine transcarbamylase deficiency, argininosuccinate synthetase deficiency (citrullinemia),[194,209] and argininemia,[209] urine OA levels are increased and can be comparable to those found in hereditary orotic aciduria. The levels can be 3 to 10 mM OA per mM of creatinine in hemizygous affected males and 0.1 to 9 mM per mM of creatinine in heterozygotes.[209] These conditions can be differentiated from hereditary orotic aciduria as they are associated with hyperammonemia and abnormal plasma amino acid levels. Also, levels of uridine and uracil are also raised and this is not found in untreated hereditary orotic aciduria. In patients with argininosuccinate lyase deficiency only slightly elevated urinary OA levels are seen, while uridine and uracil are within the normal range.[194]

Heterozygous carriers for these disorders are thought to have increased *de novo* pyrimidine metabolism and this has been detected by slightly raised urine OA concentrations, especially after high protein meals or amino acid loading, but this is not always the case.[210] Normal individuals also show a slight increase in OA after high protein meals or amino acid loading, but the increase is of smaller magnitude. Amino acid induced orotic aciduria has also been observed in rats.[211] The increase in pyrimidine metabolism has also been detected by the measurement of orotidine following inhibition of ODC with allopurinol.[212] Carpenter[198] and colleagues report benign persistent orotic aciduria increasing with allopurinol loading not due to urea cycle defects.

Orotic aciduria and orotidinuria following allopurinol administration has also been observed in the HHH (hyperornithinemia, hyperammonemia, and homocitrullinuria) syndrome (MIM 238970, see Chap. 83). This condition is caused by a defect in mitochondrial transport of ornithine; and the resulting low mitochondrial ornithine levels increase *de novo* pyrimidine metabolism by the same mechanism as ornithine transcarbamylase deficiency.[213] Some girls with Rett syndrome and some of their mothers have increased levels of urinary OA following an alanine load, which suggests a possible urea cycle defect in this condition.[214]

Nutrition and Liver Damage. Arginine depletion causes increased urinary OA in many species.[215] It has been postulated that this is due to inhibition of urea cycle activity, accumulation of carbamyl phosphate and increased *de novo* pyrimidine synthesis. Liver carbamyl phosphate increased dramatically in mice fed an arginine-deficient diet and the level of carbamyl phosphate correlated with the urinary OA level.[216] Arginine infusion reduced urinary OA in sheep only when a high nitrogen diet was given.[215] However, Carey and colleagues[217] found an arginine-deficient diet did not produce hyperammonemia or orotic aciduria in humans, and concluded that "the adult human's capacity for *de novo* arginine synthesis when fed a dietary deficiency of arginine is sufficient for the maintenance of normal cellular metabolism."

As mentioned above, starvation reduces the level of orotic aciduria in humans.[192,207] A separate study has shown that blood uridine levels are decreased on a 400-kilocalorie carbohydrate diet.[218] Male alcoholics showed elevated urinary OA: creatinine ratios early after drinking episodes, suggesting liver damage as the cause of the orotic aciduria.[207] One patient with hepatocellular carcinoma (in a noncirrhotic liver) had excretions of OA similar to those seen in hereditary orotic aciduria (3.1 to 8.3 mM/day) accompanied by high ammonia levels.[219] Increased levels of OA excretion in other malignancies has been reported.[206,219] Jeffers and coworkers postulated that tumor destruction was the source of the ammonia and excess pyrimidines in their patient.[219] Hyperammonemia was also thought to be the cause of the orotic aciduria observed in rats after liver damage with CCl_4.[220] Mild orotic aciduria and uricosuria was demonstrated in catabolic trauma victims.[203]

Lysinuric Protein Intolerance. Patients with this inherited disorder of diamino acid transport (see Chap. 192) may have increased urine OA concentrations (controls-mean 7.9, range 6.5 to 10.8 μM/mM of creatinine; homozygotes-mean 44, range 0.7 to 639 μM/mM of creatinine on a self-chosen diet). All had orotic aciduria outside the control range following alanine loading. The postulated mechanism for this is the same as that in the urea cycle enzyme defects.[221]

Formiminotransferase/Cyclodeaminase Deficiency. A moderate orotic aciduria (6.4 to 21.4 μM/mM of creatinine) has been described in this condition and attributed to increased pyrimidine synthesis.[162] It is possible that orotic aciduria of this magnitude is present in other disorders of folate metabolism or absorption, and the OA crystalluria may not be apparent until the urine is concentrated.[134]

PP-Ribose-P Synthetase Deficiency. One 11-month-old patient had a urine excretion of 0.2 mM OA per day. This child had persistently low levels of uric acid in body fluids, low erythrocyte PP-ribose-P concentrations, and markedly decreased PP-ribose-P synthetase activity in erythrocytes.[135]

Other Purine Metabolic Disorders. There is a report that children with purine nucleoside phosphorylase deficiency[222] have raised levels of urinary OA, although this has not been confirmed.[223,224] One patient studied on various purine and pyrimidine dietary supplements and allopurinol has urinary OA and orotidine excretions sometimes within, and sometimes just outside, the normal range.[194] Children with adenosine deaminase deficiency[223,225] have normal levels of urinary OA. Some other immunodeficiency conditions may have slightly increased urinary OA.[225]

Pregnancy. Slight to moderate increases in urinary OA and orotidine were found in pregnancy in one study,[226] but not in two others.[201,206]

Drugs. Allopurinol given in regular doses to gouty patients has been found to increase urine OA and OA levels; 200 to 400 mg/day of allopurinol produced 0.09 to 0.42 mM orotidine per day and 0.05 to 0.19 mM OA per day.[94,99] A similar effect was found with oxypurinol.

The monophosphate form of 6AZUR inhibits the ODC activity of UMPS, resulting in accumulation of orotidine and OA. In patients with nonterminal malignant disease, 6AZUR at 70 mg/day resulted in urinary OA of 0.12 mM/day. Doses of 450 mg 6AZUR per day resulted in excretion of 1.12 mM orotidine and 0.42 mM OA per day.[112] Another study reported that 180 to 240 mg/kg/day 6AZUR gave 5 to 9 mM orotidine and 8 to 19 mM OA per day.[1] When normalized for body weight, the amount of OA excreted with 6AZUR-induced orotic aciduria may be greater than that found in hereditary orotic aciduria, but since 6AZUMP inhibits ODC, significant amounts of orotidine are also excreted.[112] Patients receiving both 6AZUR and allopurinol excreted less OA and orotidine than when 6AZUR was given alone.

Blood Orotic Acid. OA levels in blood have not been used for the diagnosis of hereditary orotic aciduria. The concentration of OA in normal plasma is less than 0.5 μM and the HPLC technology for the measurement has been available only in the last three decades. AM pretreatment had 68 μM;[175] DG on treatment has OA levels around 20 to 30 μM,[149] so increased blood OA could then be helpful in diagnosis. Blood OA is increased in the urea cycle defects,[227] but as in urine, uracil and uridine levels are also increased and hyperammonemia is present. The observation of fractional OA clearances greater than 1 in hereditary orotic aciduria and ornithine carbamyltransferase deficiency[227] suggests the presence of an active renal secretory mechanism for OA is involved.

Other Pyrimidine Metabolites. Dihydroorotic acid was undetectable in urine from normal adults, normal children, and patients JP and DM. Carbamylaspartate concentrations were slightly increased in hereditary orotic aciduria.[175]

Urine pseudouridine was 0.13 mM and uracil not detected in patient AM.[138] Urine uracil is normally undetectable (less than 6 μM per mM of creatinine).[228] A wider range in measurement of all these compounds is obtained when the measurement is not corrected for the concentration of urine or the size of the child. In six children aged between 0.3 and 5.9 years, van Gennip and colleagues report urine values of orotidine 9 to 26 μM, uridine < 44 μM, uracil 30 to 90 μM, and pseudouridine < 601 μM.[194]

Plasma pyrimidines can be measured by simple HPLC techniques.[194,227] Care should be taken to ensure peak identity and purity as with all HPLC methods. Serum and plasma uridine is normally in the range 2 to 10 μM,[186,227,229,230] and is not affected by fasting.[229] Plasma uracil is less than 0.5 μM.[227,231] Plasma OA is normally less than 0.5 μM.[227]

A microbiologic assay measuring blood "uridine + uracil" indicated that about 15 μM of these compounds was present,[232] while a recent HPLC method involving extraction and derivatization gave uridine levels about 2 μM and uracil about 8 μM.[233] CSF uridine levels have been measured at 3.3 μM (2 SD, range 0.6 to 6.3 μM) in newborn infants and 1.6 μM (2 SD, range 0.2 to 8.2 μM) in adults.[234] Amniotic fluid uridine is 0.8 to 2.7 μM and OA is 0.19 to 0.37 μM in pregnancies with no identified risk factors.[196,235] The same authors report 0.33 to 0.84 μM uracil levels but do not report either uridine or pseudouridine present. It is possible these compounds may have been hydrolyzed to uracil by the derivatization process used.

Purine metabolites have not been studied in most cases of hereditary orotic aciduria reported to date. Patient AM untreated had blood levels of 78 μM urate, 2 μM hypoxanthine, and 1 μM xanthine.[175] At age 17 years, DG's plasma urate was 160 and 140 μM on a low purine diet, and he excreted 4.30 and 6.03 mM urate per 24 h on the same diet. At age 23 years, on a normal diet, his plasma urate was 130 μM, and urine urate 2.5 mM/24 h. Plasma and urine hypoxanthine and xanthine were not abnormal.[149,155] These results give fractional urate clearances ($C_{urate}/C_{creatine}$) of 14.7 and 18.3 at age 17 years and 14.3 at age 23 years. This high fractional (and absolute) urate clearance could be due to the uricosuric action of OA.[236,237] It has been suggested that this results from the competition between urate and orotate for the same transport mechanism for tubular resorption.[112,237] Purine metabolites are normal in a sheep model of orotic aciduria.[237]

Conversely, JR showed a slight rise in urine urate excretion while OA excretion declined during the initial course of nucleotide treatment.[132] The increased urine urate may have been caused by increased dietary purine taken with the nucleotide preparation.[238] JP had normal urinary urate following a histidine load.[158] Fallon and coworkers note the absence of hyperuricemia or any abnormality of urate clearance members of the R. family.[114]

Enzymes. The two activities of UMPS catalyze the conversion of OA to OMP, and OMP to UMP. The most commonly used assay of OPRT and ODC activity is the release of $^{14}CO_2$ from labeled OA or OMP. The activities can be measured separately or together. OPRT activity is determined when OA is the substrate and OMP is the measured product, or if CO_2 release or UMP is quantitated in the presence of added ODC. ODC activity is determined when OMP is the substrate and CO_2 release or UMP is quantitated. UMPS activity, that is both activities combined, is measured when OA is the substrate and CO_2 release or UMP is quantitated in the absence of added ODC. Since the specific activity of ODC is at least twofold greater than OPRT in the normal UMPS protein,[32] OPRT is the rate-limiting step in the combined reaction. Thus, assays of UMPS activity usually reflect the level of OPRT activity. However, this would not be the case if the endogenous ODC activity were deficient or inhibited.

These assays are usually done on lysed cell preparations at high substrate concentrations. It is also possible to separate and quantitate substrate and/or products by HPLC.[239,240] A direct spectrophotometric assay using thio-substituted substrates has been published.[241] In interpreting measurements of OPRT in tissue extracts it is necessary to consider possible competition for PP-ribose-P by other enzymes, especially hypoxanthine phosphoribosyltransferase.[239] PP-ribose-P levels are not increased in hereditary orotic aciduria erythrocytes measured directly[242] or by adenine utilization.[149]

Erythrocytes. It is difficult to compare results between laboratories, as different measures of erythrocyte or hemolysate amount and different methods of lysate preparation are used. Standard methods for preparation of lysates for enzyme assays have been suggested.[243] Standardization is important for these enzymes because their activity levels are much higher in younger than in older cell populations.

Erythrocyte OPRT is about 130 nM/h/ml of erythrocytes and ODC about 280 nM/h/ml of erythrocytes.[98] Other estimates include: UMPS in 19 normal controls, 2.4 to 14.9 nM/h per 10^9 erythrocytes;[163] ODC 1.18 ± 0.52 nM/h/10^9 erythrocytes;[141] UMPS 1.35 ± 0.43, OPRT 1.7 ± 0.99, and ODC 4.2 ± 2.2 nM/min/ml erythrocytes;[166] OPRT 34 to 109 and ODC 52 to 285 nM/h/ml of red cells;[155] OPRT, 131 ± 35 and ODC 288 ± 77 nM/h/ml of erythrocytes;[98] OPRT 923 and ODC 152, 107 nM/h/mg of hemoglobin;[150] OPRT 0.12 ± 0.06 and ODC 0.13 ± 0.06 nM/h/mg of erythrocyte protein for adults, and OPRT 0.26 ± 0.16 and ODC 0.18 ± 0.15 nM/h/mg of erythrocyte protein for children.[99]

Some patients have had small but measurable OPRT and ODC activities (DG, KP, DB, YF, TH, HB[139,140,148,150,163,164]) in erythrocytes. JP had ODC "markedly reduced" in erythrocytes.[158] YS and RS had undetectable OPRT and low ODC.[137,157] YY had undetectable ODC activity.[141] In 1971 Fox demonstrated coordinate activity between erythrocyte OPRT and ODC activities and showed specific activity decreases with increased erythrocyte age.[98] This was confirmed by a study that showed that the net orotidylate activity was directly related to the maturity of the peripheral erythrocyte population.[244] The relationship of cell age to enzyme activity has also been shown for adenosine phosphoribosyl transferase,[245] G6PD,[244] and UMP kinase.[246] The decrease in enzyme activity with cell age observed in children with reticulocytosis is much greater than in individuals without measurable reticulocytosis.[188] As has been found for other enzymes, the amount of the increase per percent reticulocytes is less in cells from cord blood than from older individuals.[247] Levels of OPRT and ODC are elevated in patients with congenital hypoplastic anemia.[248] ODC is elevated in Diamond-Blackfan anemia to about the same extent as in cord blood or hemolytic anemia.[249] UMPS activity is reduced in vitamin B_{12} and folate deficiency, possibly due to a population of older erythrocytes.

Other Tissues. It is possible to measure OPRT and ODC in saliva, but there is a wide range of normal values, and it was not possible to distinguish levels found in a UMPS heterozygote from normal levels.[133] There is measurable UMPS in amniocentesis-derived cells.[166] The activity in white cells was OPRT 0.79, 0.87, and ODC 4.3, 5.1 nM/h/mg of leukocyte protein.[155] Control liver samples had OPRT, 0.79 and 1.9; ODC, 5.4, 4.1, and 3.6; and UMPS, 0.83, 1.5, and 2.4 nM/h/mg wet liver.[168]

Fibroblasts from hereditary orotic aciduria patients also have had low enzyme activity,[92,124,150,152,166,250] but these activities are variable and depend on the culture growth.[152] The low levels are close to blank values and difficult to interpret.

Other Enzymes in UMPS Deficiency. DHO was not different from normal in fibroblasts from DG and JP,[152] and DHODH was also normal in fibroblasts from the same patients and not altered by growth in BA or 6AZUR.[153]

The Molecular Defect in UMP Synthase Deficiency

Structural Organization of the Human UMP Synthase Gene. As previously discussed ("Erythrocytes" and "Other Tissues" above) cells from most patients with UMPS deficiency have low but detectable enzyme activity. The residual OPRT and ODC activities in fibroblasts from JP and DG are thermolabile and nondialyzable.[152] Fibroblasts from TH have residual ODC more thermolabile and of different electrophoretic mobility than the enzyme from normal cells, but with the same kinetic characteristics, suggesting a structural gene mutation.[250]

The ODC activity in fibroblasts from PM and DG increased severalfold when cells were grown with BA or oxypurinol.[92,124] Cells from DG show increased enzyme activity when grown with dihydroorotic acid, 6AZUR, or 5AZOA.[91,119] This increase in activity is not prevented when cytidine is added to the growth media. DG and JP cells are more sensitive to adenosine than normal cells, but this can be prevented by addition of uridine or cytidine to the growth medium.

Fibroblasts from DG, DB and XX have been characterized for defects in the gene or mRNA for UMPS.[251] Normal fibroblasts were used as the control. Southern blot analysis of DNA digested with five different restriction enzymes revealed no alteration of the UMPS gene in the deficient cells. In each case the restriction pattern was quite simple with only two to five fragments. The minimum total fragment size of approximately 15 kb can be used as an estimate of the size of the UMPS gene.

The amount of UMPS mRNA was estimated by quantification of the amount of UMPS probe hybridizing to cell mRNA. There was no significant decrease in the quantity of UMPS mRNA in the orotic aciduria cells.[251] Northern blot analysis showed the mRNA to be of the same size in the deficient cells as in normal cells. An SI nuclease analysis of the mRNA did not reveal any alteration in the structure, sequence, or processing of the UMP synthase mRNA. From these studies it is confirmed that the orotic aciduria cells do express the UMPS gene at normal levels, that the mRNA transcript is stable, and that the mRNA is processed in a manner that results in the proper size for the mature mRNA.

In fibroblasts derived from patient DG, Perry and Jones demonstrated by immunoblotting techniques that a UMPS protein is synthesized and comigrates with the normal protein in polyacrylamide gel electrophoresis.[252] In the absence of substrate, the deficient cell UMPS exhibits an altered pattern of inactivation at 57°C. This is similar to the results reported by Worthy et al.,[250] which showed alterations in enzyme stability in cells from orotic aciduria patient TH. These results provide evidence that the UMPS deficiency is the result of the production of a structurally altered protein.

The hypothesis is put forth[251] that the defect may result from an altered amino acid sequence that has changed the ability of the subunits to form the 5.6 S altered dimer conformation necessary for optimal ODC activity (see discussion under "Conformation"). Alteration of the amino acids that form the interacting surface(s) of the monomer could result in weakened association and loss of stability of the dimer. If the active form of the enzyme in vivo is the dimer, the inability of the protein to form competent dimers could greatly reduce the catalytic activity. The addition of inhibitors that increase functional activity might stabilize or induce the formation of the 5.6 S altered dimer.

Characterization of UMP synthase Mutations in Patients with Orotic Aciduria. The OPRT and ODC from lower eukaryotes and bacteria exist as independent proteins transcribed from different loci, but human UMP synthase is encoded by a single gene mapped to 3q13.[65,74] The human UMP synthase gene is a single copy gene and spans approximately 15 kb.[253] It is composed of six exons with lengths ranging from 115 to 627 bp and all introns contain the conserved 5′-GT splice donor and 3′-AG splice acceptor sites. When compared with fly and slime mould UMP synthase, the amino acid sequence of human UMP synthase showed a high degree of similarity with more than 30 percent amino acid identity across all three proteins.

The proline at position 92 in the human UMP synthase sequence is conserved in *Drosophlia* UMPS and in *E. coli* OPRT. The isoleucine at position 286 in the human UMPS is conserved in 13 of 16 eukaryotic sequences representing UMPS or ODC from other species.[67] The conservation of the isoleucine at this position indicates that this residue may play a critical role in the function or structure of the protein.

The determination of the actual mutation that is responsible for the deficiency of UMPS requires the direct sequencing of UMPS cDNAs from the orotic aciduria patient. Starting with RNA isolated from virus-transformed lymphoblasts, this strategy[254] has shown the mutant alleles in HB and her parents to be 378C > T, resulting in a P92S missense mutation, and 961T > A, resulting in an I286N missense mutation.[255] These mutations have been shown to result in loss of ODC activity.[256]

Mutations have been identified in other patients. Fore example, in DG the same 378C > T that was present in patient HB and her mother was identified.

The analysis of a family presenting a patient with complete UMP synthase deficiency at the molecular level revealed the presence of three mutations. One allele had two mutations in cis: R96G (286A > G) and G429R (1285G > C); the second allele had a V109G (326T > G) missense mutation.[253] Expression analysis of the cDNAs containing R96G, R96G + G429R and V109G in pyrimidine auxotrophic *E. coli* bacteria demonstrated no detectable OPRT activity in contrast to *E. coli* transfected with the wild-type allele. Conversely, a cDNA with the G429R mutation had normal OPRT activity. Thus, R96G and V109G are most likely the disease-causing mutations in this family.

Orotic Aciduria Type 2. In all cases of orotic aciduria except two, a deficiency in both OPRT and ODC activities has been described. In one patient (YY), only ODC was measured.[141] The other patient (PM) has been referred to as having "Type 2" hereditary orotic aciduria[164] because the first measured values of erythrocyte OPRT activity (after 3 months of uridine therapy) were 0.83 and 0.24 nM/h/mg of protein (one high and one normal value), while ODC was barely detectable. At 2 years of age, while on uridine therapy, OPRT was 0.005 nM/h/mg of red cell protein[208] and was undetectable in fibroblasts.[168] Later assays measured fibroblast ODC at 0.02 nM/h/mg of protein.[92] At 13 years he had detectable OPRT and no ODC in erythrocytes. The finding of normal OPRT was corroborated by high urine orotidine excretion. When OPRT levels decreased, orotidine excretion was also reduced.

Although it has now been shown that a single gene encodes the bifunctional protein UMPS, it may still follow that one activity can be deficient and the other normal. The work of Jones and coworkers has demonstrated that the ODC activity is predominantly associated with the 5.6S altered dimer form, whereas the OPRT activity is found in all of the conformations of the enzyme.[36,37] Thus if dimer formation were blocked or otherwise inhibited, ODC activity would be lost or diminished while OPRT activity might be unaffected. For deficiency in both activities, one could postulate an altered amino acid sequence that would result in a protein that does not form the proper monomer configuration. An alternative would be a mutation that results in a protein that is more susceptible to proteolytic action or that is more heat labile.

Prenatal Diagnosis. There are no reports of prenatal diagnosis of hereditary orotic aciduria. Normal UMPS activity was found in chorionic villi and amniocytes during a further pregnancy in the mother of YS and RS.[22] The pregnancy concluded with the delivery of a child with normal erythrocyte enzyme activities. Amniocentesis-derived cells grown in culture from a further pregnancy of the mother of XX had 26 percent of the UMPS activity of a control,[166] and subsequent investigations suggest the infant was heterozygous. Any consideration of termination of affected pregnancies should recognize that most infants with hereditary orotic aciduria are normal at birth and have a good prognosis following simple treatment. Maternal uridine supplementation might be considered, although, if intended for prevention of malformations, this would have to be initiated before fetal diagnosis is currently possible. It is unlikely that OA levels in amniotic fluid would be diagnostic. Ornithine transcarbamylase deficiency is another condition with postnatal orotic aciduria (see Chap. 85), and OA, orotidine, uridine or uracil were undetectable in amniotic fluid from a pregnancy with an affected male fetus.[257] Two further pregnancies in the mother of YS were monitored by estimation of ODC activity in chorionic villi and cultured amniocytes, and of orotic acid, uracil and uridine in amniotic fluids.[167] Both were confirmed as heterozygotes but because of difficulty in interpreting ODC levels it was suggested that quantitation of amniotic fluid OA is necessary for definitive diagnosis.

Neonatal Diagnosis. None of the cases of hereditary orotic aciduria to date have been diagnosed in the neonatal period. McClard and colleagues report exclusive neonatal diagnosis in an unaffected sib of XX,[166] and prenatal diagnosis of an unaffected child was confirmed by OPRT and ODC measurements after birth in another case.[22] It seems likely that an increase in urinary OA would be detectable soon after birth. Care would need to be exercised in interpretation of OPRT and ODC levels in the presence of the neonatal reticulocytosis, as discussed earlier.

Pathogenesis of Clinical Features of Hereditary Orotic Aciduria

Precursor Toxicity. The high levels of urinary OA imply that a marked increase in the rate of OA synthesis, may cause obstructive uropathy, and probably have a uricosuric effect. Blood levels of OA are only slightly increased, and there is no information on whether or not intracellular levels would be sufficiently elevated to exert pharmacologic effects. OA has been used therapeutically as a pyrimidine source in the treatment of neonatal jaundice, myocardial infarction, pernicious anemia,[258] and degenerative retinal diseases.[259] Oral OA reduces both blood urate and cholesterol levels.[259] OA inhibits *de novo* purine synthesis, probably by depleting intracellular PP-ribose-P,[260] and has been used as a therapeutic agent in gout.[236,258] OA has had pharmacologic use to lower plasma β-lipoprotein and triglyceride.[258] This is in contrast to the production of grossly fatty livers in rats receiving diets supplemented with OA. These animals have an associated increase in uridine nucleotides and reduced adenine nucleotides. The biochemical changes and the fatty liver are prevented by the addition of allopurinol to the diet.[261] Both dietary and endogenous OA in excess produce carcinogenesis in rodent liver.[262] Most of these effects of OA are likely to be related to its further metabolism to OMP and UMP causing nucleotide imbalance or PP-ribose-P depletion.[16] Therefore the enzymatic block in hereditary orotic aciduria should be protective, probably explaining the lack of corresponding effects in the disease.

Product Deficiency. The depletion of pyrimidine nucleotides is assumed to be the cause of the majority of clinical features of the disorder. Again, there are no direct measurements of the severity of this depletion, and it is not known whether all tissues are affected equally. The consistent occurrence of bone marrow megaloblastosis is a strong indication of important consequences at the cellular level. Megaloblastosis is evidence of slowed DNA synthesis per unit time and of the arrest of the process of cell division, particularly in S phase.[263] There are lesser effects on RNA and protein synthesis, giving the characteristic asynchronous "young nucleus-old cytoplasm" appearance at all stages of erythrocyte maturation.[263] Kelley[16] has postulated that certain reported cytologic variations from the usual pattern in megaloblastosis in hereditary orotic aciduria might be because RNA synthesis is more severely affected, but not all observers regard the megaloblastosis as atypical. The defective DNA synthesis in megaloblastic states is usually present in all proliferating cells and is particularly marked in rapidly dividing cells such as those in the alimentary tract and vagina.[159,263] This could account for the malabsorption in some of the treated cases of hereditary orotic aciduria and the intestinal villous atrophy observed in one patient. It also could account for DG's deficient hair and nail growth, although this has been described in only one other case.[164] There are some inconstant features of hereditary orotic aciduria in which the possible contribution of genetic variation in enzyme function cannot be separated from the modifying effects of pyrimidines obtained from dietary and salvage sources or from chance events unrelated to the genetic defect. Growth deficiency responds immediately to therapy, but this may be an indirect effect of improved appetite, motor activity, or general well-being rather than a reversal of pyrimidine "starvation." The difficulty of assessing intellectual impairment as either a short- or long-term effect of the disease has been referred to above. There is no firm theoretical basis for effects of the metabolic error on the developing nervous system. Some other inborn errors of metabolism causing megaloblastosis may be associated with mental retardation,[16] and there may be periods at which the developing brain has critical requirements for pyrimidine synthesis. This appears to be the case during restorative brain growth after under nutrition in neonatal animals.[264]

Girot and colleagues[157,169] drew an analogy between the pathogenesis of the immune deficiencies in their patients with hereditary orotic aciduria and the immune deficiency associated with inherited deficiencies of two enzymes of the purine degradative pathway, adenosine deaminase and purine nucleoside phosphorylase. Selective toxicity to immunocytes of deoxyadenosine, adenosine, deoxyguanosine, and their metabolites is the currently favored explanation for the immune impairment in the latter deficiencies. Adenosine causes OA accumulation and pyrimidine nucleotide depletion in cultured cells, possibly by inhibition of PP-ribose-P synthetase. Therefore, pyrimidine starvation could be the basis for the immune impairments in both adenosine deaminase and UMPS deficiencies and the explanation for the mild immunodeficiency in a child with excessive pyrimidine nucleotide degradation.[161] Dietary nucleotide depletion has been associated with reduced cell-mediated immunity in mice[265] possibly because circulating pyrimidine levels cause low dCTP pools and reduced cell proliferation.[130,266] Yasaki and colleagues[140] found that in vitro uridine supplementation increased protein synthesis in lectin-stimulated lymphocytes and EB virus-transformed B-cell lines from a uridine treated patient while a control remained unchanged. However, mechanisms other than pyrimidine starvation are now preferred for the immune impairment in ADA deficiency. Uridine in vitro did not prevent the blocking effect of adenosine on the mitogenic response of human lymphocytes or prevent adenosine toxicity to a human B-cell line.[267]

No features of the disease have been related to defective synthesis of specific cofactors. Depletion of UDP-sugars and CDP-choline, necessary for galactose utilization and glycogen formation, or depletion of CDP-ethanolamine, necessary for phospholipid synthesis, might be the basis for the skeletal muscle weakness in some cases.

There appears to be an increased incidence of cardiac and other malformations in patients with hereditary orotic aciduria. Teratogenic or other effects of the enzyme deficiency in the homozygous embryo or fetus will depend on the relative contribution of *de novo* synthesis and placental transfer of circulating maternal pyrimidines and either may vary at different stages of pregnancy. There is a "normal" megaloblastic phase of erythropoiesis in the embryo prior to the commencement of hepatic blood formation,[159] which may indicate susceptibility to additional deficiencies during that phase. Evidence from other species suggests that *de novo* pyrimidine synthesis is of major importance to the embryo during organogenesis, when there is maximum teratogenic susceptibility. 6AZUR inhibits ODC and is a potent teratogenic and embryo-lethal agent when given to pregnant animals during the phase of organogenesis.[268] Uridine protects against this effect. In the bovine model of UMPS deficiency, the homozygous state is usually lethal around forty days postconception.[269,270] Embryo-lethality has not been demonstrated in human homozygotes but a slightly less severe effect would be expected to cause an increased incidence of malformations in the survivors. Shanks and Robinson[269] suggest that placental transfer of pyrimidines may be less efficient in bovines than in humans, but there is no supporting data. The enzyme defect may also affect the function of the fetal component of placental tissue. 6AZUR administered to pregnant women induced degenerative changes in placental trophoblast at gestations of 1 to 2 months, but not later in gestation,[271] and this is a further indication that certain tissues have particular pyrimidine requirements that may change during pregnancy. The normal birth weights for gestation found in most cases of hereditary orotic aciduria imply that there was no pyrimidine starvation during late gestation. Studies in sheep have shown that 40 to 60 percent of uridine in fetal blood in pregnancy is maternally derived,[272] and a similar lack of dependence on *de novo* synthesis in late pregnancy could protect the human fetus with UMPS deficiency and allow normal growth.

Genetics and Gene Frequency

Cases of hereditary orotic aciduria have been widely distributed geographically, and include patients of Polynesian, Oriental, white, American Indian, and black origin. Immunologic, molecular, biochemical, and genetic evidence indicates that the structural gene coding for UMPS activity is located on the long arm of chromosome 3 in the region 3q13.[74] This is consistent with the presumption of autosomal recessive inheritance of hereditary orotic aciduria[131,163,168,208] based on the facts that patients with hereditary orotic aciduria have been both male (eight cases) and female (seven cases), that one family had two siblings affected, and that it is possible to assign heterozygote status by biochemical observation.

Hereditary orotic aciduria is a rare disorder whose exact incidence is unknown. Estimates of gene frequency based on screening (by measurement of enzyme levels or urinary orotic acid) have been inconclusive because of the large number of subjects required, the population selected for study and the difficulty of defining heterozygote levels. One case was identified by the biochemical investigation of 2269 hospitalized Chinese children.[273] Most family studies have shown that obligate heterozygotes have blood enzyme levels or urinary OA levels different from those of normal individuals.[16,131,140,150,166,189,272] However, Fox and coworkers showed that the frequency histogram for erythrocyte ODC was non-Gaussian and that the levels of both OPRT and ODC in obligate heterozygotes overlapped the lower end of the normal distribution.[208] This observation has been confirmed by other workers.[16,188] Fox and coworkers suggests that assignation of heterozygote status should require both a low enzyme activity and a raised urine OA level.[208] The combined criterion is necessary since there are many other causes of slightly elevated urine OA.

Cattle heterozygous for UMPS deficiency have intermediate levels of enzyme activity in liver, spleen, kidneys, skeletal muscle, and mammary gland.[274] Deficiency of UMPS (acronym DUMPS) is estimated to be present in 1 to 2 percent of Black and White Holstein cattle in the United States and in a higher percentage of Red and White Holsteins, largely because of the popularity of artificial insemination programs using a few sires later shown to be heterozygotes.[274,275] The homozygous state has not been identified in Holstein cattle and breeding studies; and studies of UMPS levels in 35-day fetuses support the suggestion that this is usually lethal in utero around 40 days gestation.[270,274,275] Reproductive efficiency is impaired and Holstein breeding societies introduced screening programs with the intention of progressive elimination of DUMPS from the bovine gene pool.[275]

PYRIMIDINE-5′-NUCLEOTIDASE DEFICIENCY (MIM 266120)

Enzymology

Pyrimidine-5′-nucleotidase (P5N, enzyme 25, Fig. 113-1), sometimes called UMP hydrolase, catalyzes the dephosphorylation of pyrimidine-5′-ribomonophosphates to the corresponding nucleosides (Fig. 113-7). The enzyme was first identified in the soluble fraction of erythrocytes.[276,277] It has been separated from acid phosphatase and electrophoretically characterized.[278,279] P5N does not dephosphorylate purine nucleotides or the 2′- or cyclic pyrimidine nucleotides. The activity with thymidine monophosphate (TMP) is about half that found with UMP and CMP (K_ms 0.33 mM, UMP; 0.15 mM, CMP; and 1.0 mM, TMP).[277] The pH optimum is 7.5[276,280] and the enzyme is most stable between pH 6 and 7.5.[280] Optimal activity requires the presence of magnesium and cannot be achieved with manganese. The enzyme is heat-sensitive and inhibited by AMP, some purine bases, purine and pyrimidine nucleosides, divalent cations of heavy metals, and agents active against sulfhydryl groups.[277]

Purification. The enzyme has been purified 250,000-fold by DEAE-cellulose chromatography, ammonium sulfate precipitation, gel filtration through Sephacryl S-200, and isoelectric focusing. Electrophoresis of the purified fraction revealed two major and two faint bands.[280] The enzyme has a pI of 5.0. The molecular weight was estimated by gel filtration to be 28 kDa. The purified enzyme has a K_m of 10 μM for CMP. This was lower than that measured in hemolysates (10 μM Vs 40 μM), suggesting the possible presence of an inhibitor in the preparations.[280]

Isozymes. More recent reports indicate that specific isozymes of P5N exist. Erythrocytes from classic P5N-deficient patients that exhibited the expected loss of activity with UMP or CMP as substrate had activity with TMP as substrate.[281,282] Hydrolytic activity of erythrocytes from a P5N-deficient patient toward TMP and dUMP led Swallow and colleagues[281,282] to postulate two separate structural gene loci, and the gene for the enzyme which hydrolyzes deoxynucleotides has been localized to the long arm of chromosome 17.[283] Further evidence for a number of isozymes came from the study of four more families.[284] Somatic cell hybridization studies showed the presence of two isozymes catalyzing UMP hydrolysis, one of which is more active against deoxynucleotides.[285]

One isozyme (MW 52kDa) separated from normal erythrocytes is active for UMP and CMP, but not for TMP. Two other isozymes (MW 52kDa and 48 kDa) were more active for TMP than for UMP or CMP.[286] The isoelectric points were 5.22, 4.90, and 4.68 respectively. None of these isozymes appear to correspond with the high purified enzyme of Torrance and colleagues (pI 5.0 and MW 28kDa).[279]

A 5′-nucleotidase that is specific for OMP has been isolated from mouse liver microsomes.[287] This enzyme has negligible activity for UMP, CMP, dTMP or purine monophosphates. The molecular weight is estimated to be 53 kDa. This activity may be responsible in part for the low levels of intracellular OMP and the accumulation of orotidine in cells treated with 6-AZUR. Studies in rat hepatocytes suggest an immature form (MW 67 kDa), which converts to a mature form (72 kDa). The half-life of the enzyme after the level reached plateau was 22.8 h.[287]

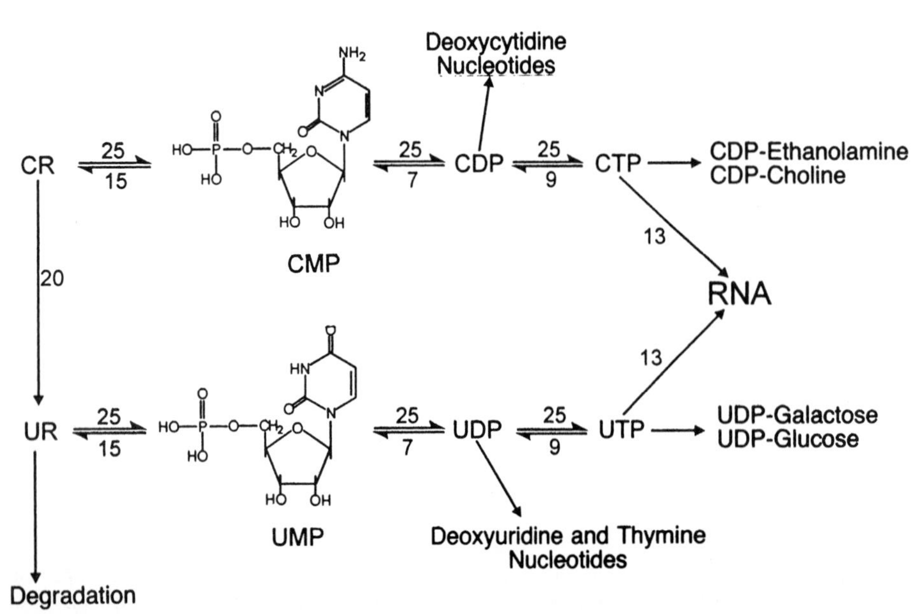

Fig. 113-7 Chemical structure of metabolic intermediates involved in pyrimidine-5′s-nucleotidase deficiency. Enzyme numbers refer to Table 113-1.

Table 113-3 Erythrocyte Nucleotide Levels (μM) in Pyrimidine-5′-Nucleotidase Deficiency in Two Patients and Three Different Control Series

	Patients (2)		Controls (3)		
Nucleotide	Ref 431		Ref 307	Ref 308	Ref 431
AMP	0.01	0.01	0.084		0.01–0.02
ADP	0.16	1.18	0.610	0.260	0.13–0.19
ATP	1.73	1.87	1.063	1.270	1.41–2.04
IMP	< 0.02	< 0.02			< 0.02
GMP	< 0.01	< 0.01			< 0.01
GDP	0.02	0.02		0.17	0.01–0.39
GTP	0.08	0.07		0.060	0.05–0.09
UMP	0.05	0.04		0.108	< 0.01
UDP	0.10	0.08	0.276	0.024	< 0.01
UTP	0.94	0.86	0.220	0.380	< 0.01
CMP	0.09	0.07	0.757	0.025	< 0.01
CDP	0.35	0.31	0.278	0.130	< 0.01
CTP	1.74	1.54	0.831	0.770	< 0.01
UDP-glucose	0.66	0.61	0.237	0.310	< 0.10
UDP-N-Ac-glucosamine	0.61	0.59			< 0.10
CDP-choline	1.51	1.50		0.930	< 0.05
CDP-ethanolamine	0.57	0.56		0.410	< 0.01
NAD	0.09	0.09			0.04–0.07

Work by Hirono and colleagues[288] suggested there may be two totally separate enzymes of similar molecular weight, only one of which is important in the hydrolysis of nucleotides in the developing erythrocyte. They refer to these as P5N-I (hydrolyses nucleotides) and P5N-II (similar to the 5′-nucleotidase in rat liver cytosol). The properties of the enzymes are so different it was felt they are different species, not isozymes.[288]

Two cytoplasmic forms have been purified from erythrocytes.[289] PN-I (MW 34 kDa) preferentially hydrolyses 5′-monophosphates, and PN-II 3′-monophosphates. PN-I is specific for pyrimidines, but PN-II will also hydrolyze IMP and GMP although the affinity is greater for pyrimidines.

Clinical Studies

Presentation. P5N deficiency as a cause of hereditary hemolytic anemia was reported first by Valentine and colleagues in 1974.[290] They described four members of three kindreds who had hemolytic anemia with splenomegaly, and erythrocytes having prominent basophilic stippling. By 1980, 33 cases from 24 unrelated families had been reported.[291] Presentation is with a mild to moderate, usually well-compensated anemia. Splenomegaly is usually present, and sometimes hepatomegaly is noted. Hemoglobin concentrations are around 10 g/dl with reticulocytosis and marrow hyperplasia. There is unconjugated hyperbilirubinemia, increased erythrocyte glutathione, and decreased serum haptoglobins. There may be exacerbations during acute infections or pregnancy. Two siblings reported by Hansen and colleagues[291] had hemolysis, hemoglobinuria, and enlarged kidneys with considerable iron accumulation. The association with mental retardation in a minority of cases is of uncertain significance. The presenting details of 23 patients are summarized by Paglia and coworkers.[292] Two siblings with P5N deficiency had an acute aplastic crisis following B19 parvovirus infection.[293]

Diagnosis. The diagnosis is often suspected because of basophilic stippling of erythrocytes and may be made simply by measurement of the ultraviolet (UV) absorption spectrum of deproteinized erythrocytes. The presence of high levels of cytidine and uridine ribonucleotides causes a pronounced shift in the UV absorption maximum and magnitude. At pH 2.0, control extracts had a maximum absorbance between 255 to 260 nm, while patient extracts had maxima at 266 to 270 nm.[276] The method is the recommended screening test for P5N deficiency.[294] The elevated levels of pyrimidine nucleotides may be confirmed by chromatographic separation of erythrocyte nucleotides.[295,296] Quantification of erythrocyte nucleotides (Table 113-3) shows large increases in cytidine nucleotides and cytidine phosphodiesters (3 to 4 mM). Smaller but substantial increases are seen in uridine nucleotides and nucleotide sugars (2 to 3 mM). Levels of purine nucleotides are not elevated. The elevated levels of pyrimidine nucleotides may also be detected using nuclear magnetic resonance spectroscopy.[297]

Diagnosis may be confirmed by measurement of erythrocyte enzyme activity. Affected individuals have activity from 0 to 30 percent of normal mean. However, these levels are sometimes difficult to interpret, as the enzyme is much more active in young cells[291,298,299] and patients typically have 5 to 25 percent reticulocytes. It is necessary to prepare erythrocytes free of leukocytes and platelets by a standard methodology so as to obtain preparations of equivalent density and hence cell age. The enzyme may be assayed by separation of [^{14}C]CMP from cytidine by binding of the CMP to the barium sulfate precipitate that forms in the deproteinization procedure. The soluble cytidine can then be counted.[243,280] The products of the enzyme assay may also be quantified by chemical, other radiochemical,[300,301] or chromatographic methods.[280,302,303] A comprehensive discussion of methodology has been written by Paglia and colleagues.[291] The inherited enzyme deficiency can be distinguished from the acquired deficiency by the differential decrease in P5N-II.[304] An anion-exchange HPLC method adapted for the measurement of both nucleotide profiles and enzyme activity has been described.[295]

Mononuclear leukocytes from a patient with P5N deficiency have approximately twice control levels of pyrimidine nucleotides and granulocytes 4-6 times control levels.[305] Lymphocytes had about 60 percent of control activity of P5N (inhibitable by AOPCP) while granulocytes had about 10 percent of control activity (inhibitable by β-GP).[305] Hopkinson and colleagues report minor but significant increases in pyrimidine nucleotides in lymphoblastoid cell lines of patients with P5N deficiency.[306]

Treatment. There is no specific treatment at present for P5N deficiency, and there is no improvement with splenectomy. The erythrocyte hemolysis is probably caused by the accumulated pyrimidine nucleotides, and it has been shown that most of these nucleotides come from circulating preformed pyrimidines.[307] Kinetic analysis suggests that most of the pyrimidines are likely to be from orotate rather than from uridine, so a likely prospect for therapy of this condition is an inhibitor of orotate transport across erythrocyte membranes.[296] A trial of allopurinol in one patient increased the levels of erythrocyte pyrimidine nucleotides after 2 to 3 weeks. This is consistent with allopurinol in vivo inhibition of UMPS, increase of circulating orotate, increased orotate salvage, and therefore, increased pyrimidine nucleotides.[307]

Pathophysiology. Chromatographic separation of the two enzyme activities by Hirono and coworkers[292] showed P5N-II activity to be the same in patients as in controls. P5N-I had very different enzymatic characteristics in patients from controls, and different patients had different abnormalities. It was suggested that the basic enzyme defect is caused by a structural gene mutation.[292]

The striking biochemical abnormality is the vastly increased amounts of erythrocyte pyrimidine nucleotides. Chromatographic separation and quantification (Table 113-3) showed that the increase was greater for the cytidine nucleotides,[308,309] and the increase is greatest in the trinucleotides. The cytidine diphosphodiesters, CDP-ethanolamine and CDP-choline, were identified by Fourier transform-nuclear magnetic resonance and mass spectrometry.[309] These are found in high concentration, although no abnormality was reported in erythrocyte membrane phospholipids in one patient.[309] The mechanism by which the increased concentration of pyrimidine nucleotides causes hemolysis remains unknown.

Lachant and coworkers[309] have studied pyrimidine nucleoside monophosphate kinase (PNMK, enzyme 7) activity in P5N deficiency. The enzyme has about double the activity in young cells compared with older erythrocytes, and is increased about fourfold in patients with P5N deficiency. PNMK activity in normal hemolysates is increased by UMP and CDP-ethanolamine. This suggests that in P5N deficiency increase of PNMK activity by UMP causes accumulation of UDP and CDP, which are subsequently phosphorylated by pyrimidine nucleoside diphosphate kinase (enzyme 9) to accumulate as triphosphates.[309] The triphosphates may compete with ATP to inhibit glycolysis[276] or compete with ATP for ATPase.[308]

Erythrocytes have been shown to readily increase uridine nucleotides when incubated with orotate,[310] and this increase goes into a separate cell compartment from the increase after uridine incubation.[310] Erythrocytes of two patients were found to have decreased pentose phosphate shunt activity. UTP and CTP inhibited glucose-6-phosphate dehydrogenase (G6PD) and pentose phosphate shunt activity about 50 percent at 5.5 mM, suggesting this may contribute to the pathogenesis of hemolysis.[311] Further kinetic analysis indicated that the K_is are above the intra-erythrocytic concentrations in P5N deficiency and that it is unlikely this was a contributory factor in the hemolysis. Work by David and colleagues[312] on red cells of different age from P5N patients also showed reduced G6PD and stimulated pentose phosphate shunt activity compared to controls.

Patients with P5N deficiency have a high erythrocyte concentration of glutathione, although the reduced glutathione synthesis rate is normal. It was thought the increase was due to decreased transport of oxidized glutathione out of the cells.[313]

It has been suggested that since pyrimidine nucleotides avidly bind magnesium, the hemolytic anemia may be due to a state of functional magnesium depletion in erythrocytes. The addition of 6 to 10 mM magnesium to intact red cells from a patient with P5N deficiency did not improve the autohemolysis test, the incubated Heinz body assay, or the rate of glucose oxidation by the pentose phosphate shunt. This lack of effect may have been due to the slow rate of uptake by the red cells.[313,314] Further work by Lachant and colleagues showed PP-ribose-P synthetase activity is decreased in P5N deficiency due to reduced subunit aggregation caused by magnesium deficiency.[315]

Intraerythrocytic accumulation of CDP-choline to levels 15 to 25 times normal, but without increases in other pyrimidine nucleotides, has been found in 7 cases[316,317] presenting with a syndrome of low grade hemolysis, splenomegaly, unconjugated hyperbilirubinemia, elevated NAD levels and erythrocyte stippling, which is very similar to that caused by P5N deficiency. Inherited deficiency of CDP-choline phosphotransferase in erythroid precursors has been assumed but not proven. Other patients presenting with hemolytic anemia have been shown to have elevated CDP-ethanolamine and normal NAD. These results suggest there are different enzymes for metabolism of CDP-choline and CDP-ethanolamine.[317]

Studies of a family with both Hb E/β-thalassemia and pyrimidine-5′-nuculeotidase deficiency show a marked decrease in the stability of Hb E in pyrimidine-5′-nucleotidase deficient red cells, possibly because of oxidant damage to the mildly unstable hemoglobin variant.[318]

Genetics

P5N deficiency is inherited as an autosomal recessive trait. Although affected individuals can be identified by assay of P5N activity in erythrocytes, detection of heterozygotes is less reliable. A large family study could not identify all carriers by enzyme kinetic studies, electrophoresis, chromatographic examination of nucleotide extracts, or measurement of enzyme in cells of different ages due to overlap of obligate heterozygote levels with the normal range.[319] P5N activity was the same in males and females.[299] The measurement of pyrimidine nucleotides, especially UDP-N-acetylglucosamine, in combination with enzyme assays may improve the precision of carrier detection.[304]

Although it has been suggested that the disease is more common in Ashkenazim and blacks, it has also been reported in South Africans,[279] Norwegians,[291] Turks,[320] and Spaniards.[319] There are several reports of families with different P5N enzyme mutants. Hirono[288] reports three families with different kinetic-thermostability properties: $P5N_{KUNAMOTO}$, $_{NAGANO}$, and $_{KURUME}$. Japanese families with different mutations are also reported by Fujii[321] ($P5N_{KAGUSHIMA}$) and Rosa[277,278] ($P5N_{ISHIDA}$). A Guadaloupe family was found to have about 14 percent normal activity.

Acquired Pyrimidine-5′-Nucleotidase Deficiency

In 1975, Paglia and colleagues[322] noted the similarity of the hematologic picture in lead poisoning to that in hereditary P5N deficiency. In 1976[323] they found reduced nucleotidase activity and increased pyrimidine nucleotides in erythrocytes in patients with lead poisoning. The severity of the enzyme inhibition was correlated with blood lead levels.[324] Lieberman and Gordon-Smith reported decreased P5N and increased glutathione in a variety of myeloproliferative disorders.[325] No correlation was found between the P5N and glutathione levels.

Acquired P5N deficiency has been reported in thalassemia. The mechanism for this is thought to be oxidation of sulfhydryl groups on the enzyme by aldehydes produced by membrane lipid peroxidation.[326,327] The inhibition of P5N can be produced in vitro by incubating red cells with hydrogen peroxide, when the oxidizing agent is thought to be malonyldialdehyde. The inhibition was only partly reversible by the addition of mercaptoethanol to the incubation medium.[328] The acquired defect can be distinguished from heterozygote levels of P5N by the decreased activity of P5N-II in erythrocytes.[303]

Pyrimidine 5′-Nucleotidase Superactivity (MIM 311850)

Pyrimidine 5′nucleotidase superactivity has been described in four unrelated patients with a syndrome that included developmental delay, seizures, ataxia, recurrent infections, severe language deficit, hyperactivity, short attention span and poor social interaction.[329] No unusual metabolites were found in plasma and urine except for persistent hypouricosuria. The patients were detected by six- to tenfold increased activity of P5N in their

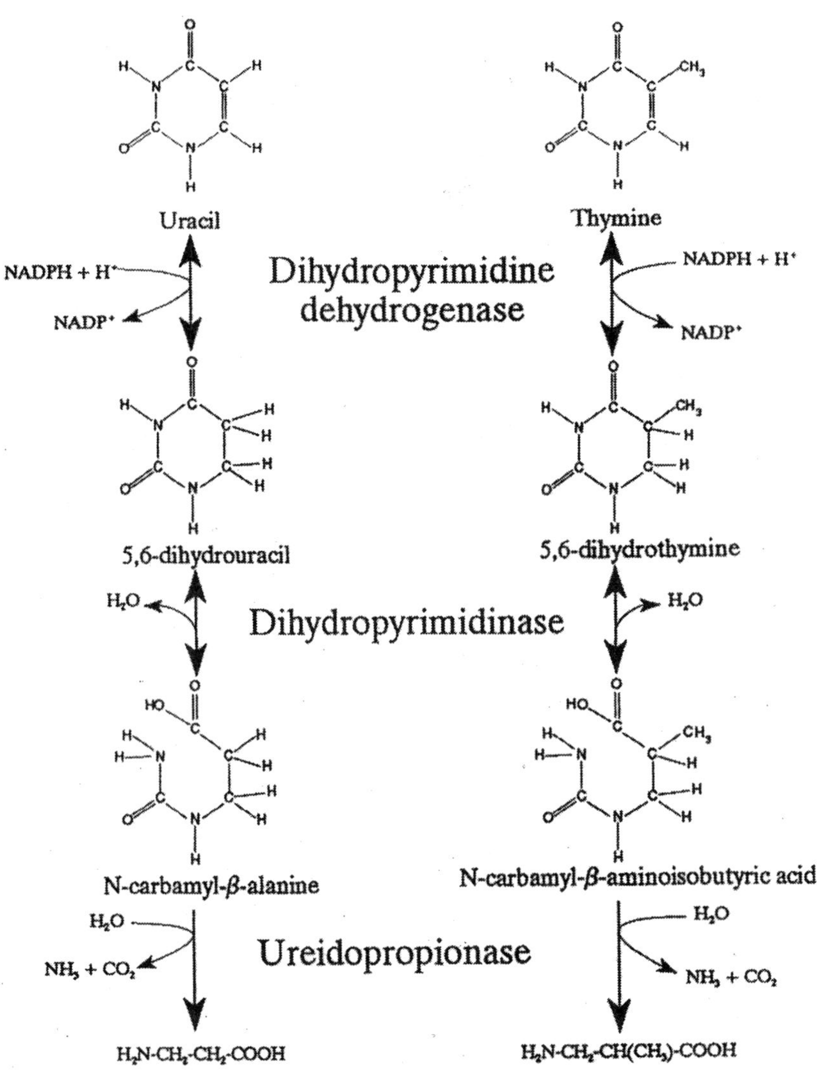

Fig. 113-8 Scheme of pyrimidine degradation pathways showing the four compounds and the enzymes involved in the catalysis of each step. Numbers are as in Fig. 113-1.

fibroblasts. Treatment with uridine resulted in remarkable improvement of the clinical condition.

THYMIDINE PHOSPHORYLASE DEFICIENCY (MIM 550900)

Thymidine phosphorylase (TP) catalyzes the conversion of thymidine into thymine. The enzyme is also called "platelet-derived endothelial cell growth factor (PD-ECGF)" or "endothelial growth factor 1 (ECGF1)," because of its angiogenic properties, or "gliostatin" to denote its inhibitory effects on glial cell proliferation. Examination of 12 patients with mitochondrial neurogastrointestinal encephalopathy (MNGIE) revealed homozygous or compound-heterozygous mutations in the gene specifying TP. This gene is located on chromosome 22q13.32-qter. The activity in leukocytes from six MNGIE patients was less than 5 percent of controls, indicating that loss of function mutations in TP cause the disease.[330]

DIHYDROPYRIMIDINE DEHYDROGENASE DEFICIENCY (MIM 274270)

Dihydropyrimidine dehydrogenase (EC 1.3.1.2; DPD) catalyzes the rate-limiting step in the degradation of the pyrimidine bases uracil and thymine. This NADPH-dependent reaction converts the bases to their dihydro derivatives (enzyme 22, Fig. 113-1). The dihydrouracil and dihydrothymine are then further catabolized to CO_2 and β-alanine or β-aminoisobutyric acid respectively (Fig. 113-8).

Enzymology

The highest activity of DPD is found in monocytes, liver, and lymphocytes, with less activity in granulocytes, thrombocytes, skin fibroblasts, kidney, lung, pancreas, colon, and breast. The DPD enzyme in human tissues is known to be dependent on NADPH as a cosubstrate, but some substantial NADH-dependent DPD activity in human liver and fibroblasts with only a very low activity in lymphocytes has been reported.[331] The significance of this finding is still not clear. Until recently conflicting data existed on the subcellular localization of DPD. However, investigation of the distribution profile of the activity of DPD and of various marker enzymes in crude subcellular fractions obtained by differential centrifugation of a rat liver homogenate clearly indicated that DPD is exclusively located in the cytosol.[332]

Purification. DPD has been purified form several sources including bacteria[333] and liver tissue from rats,[334,335] pig,[336] cattle,[337,338] and human.[339] The purified mammalian enzymes are composed of two similar subunits of MW 107 kDa. The pig enzyme contains FMN, FAD, and two iron-sulfur [4Fe-4S] prosthetic groups[336,340] and exhibits a nonclassical two-site ping-pong mechanism with two separate binding sites for

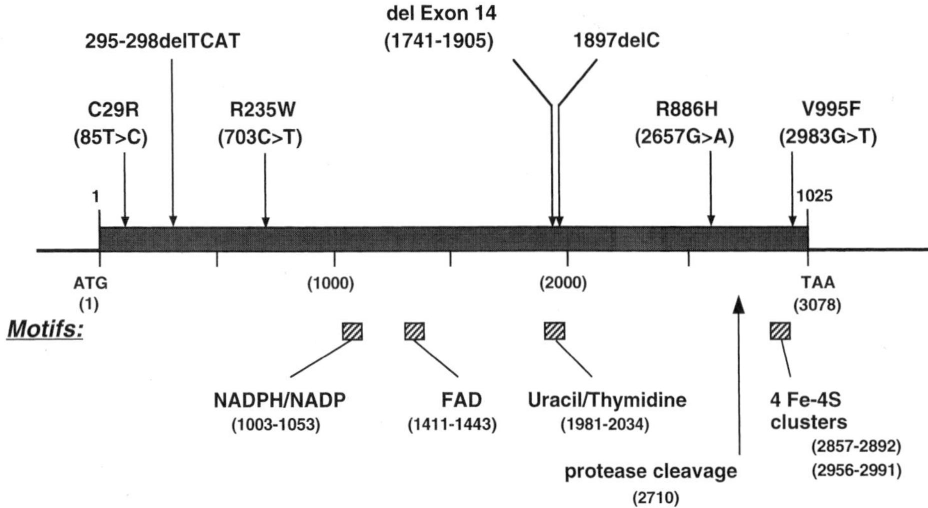

Fig. 113-9 The human DPD cDNA showing localization of segments encoding functional motifs of the enzymes and location of the mutations causing DPD. The DPD open reading frame is indicated by the gray rectangle; the motifs by the hatched rectangles below. The mutations are shown above. Nucleotide numbers are shown in parentheses.

NADPH/NADP and uracil/5,6-dihydrouracil.[341] The NADPH reduces the enzyme at site 1, and electrons are transferred to site 2 to reduce uracil to 5,6-dihydrouracil. DPD activity is decreased in regenerating and differentiating rat liver, rat hepatomas, and colon tumor in mouse.[342,343]

Kinetics. Substrate inhibition was shown for the pig liver enzyme by NADPH that is competitive with uracil and by uracil that is uncompetitive with NADPH. The predictive mechanism is corroborated by exchange between [^{14}C] NADP and NADPH, as well as [^{14}C] thymine and dihydrothymine in the absence of the other substrate-product pair. A model for DPD activity incorporating an acid-base catalytic mechanism has been described.[344]

The optimal pH for the reaction is 7.4, with an apparent K_m of 2.6 μM for thymine and 1.8 μM for uracil in the presence of NADPH. Very similar values have been obtained for ammonium sulphate-precipitated liver extracts.[334] The rates of degradation of 5′-substituted analogues were highest for 5FU and 5-bromouracil, and lowest for 5-nitrouracil. The degradation rate of uracil was slightly faster than for thymine, but significantly slower than for 5FU. Uridine is a noncompetitive inhibitor of pyrimidine base degradation in vitro, with total inhibition of 5-FU degradation at 10 μM. Thymidine is a less potent inhibitor of 5FU degradation.[345]

The Molecular Basis of DPD Deficiency

The Human DPD Gene. The cDNAs coding for human DPD, pig DPD, and bovine DPD have been isolated and sequenced.[346,347] The mammalian DPD sequence is relatively conserved; bovine DPD has 93 percent and 92 percent identity with pig and human DPD, respectively. The human DPD cDNA encodes a protein containing 1025 amino acids with a calculated molecular weight of 111 kDa (Fig. 113-9). Conserved domains corresponding to a possible NADPH-binding site and FAD-binding site are present in the N-terminal and middle region of the enzyme. In the C-terminal region typical motifs for [4Fe-4S] clusters are present between residues 953 and 964 and residues 986 and 997. On the basis of chemical modification studies the putative uracil-binding site of DPD is between Gly661 and Arg678. Thus, the functional domains of DPD can be arranged from the N-terminus in the order of NADPH-FAD-uracil-[4Fe-4S].

The human DPD gene has been mapped to chromosome 1p22 and is present as a single copy.[348,349] The gene consists of 23 exons with exon 15 (69 bp) the smallest one and exon 23 (961 bp) the largest.[53] The human DPD gene is at least 950 kb in length with 3 kb of coding sequence and a minimal average intron size of about 43 kb.[54]

The Molecular Basis of DPD Deficiency. The analysis of 17 families presenting 22 patients with a complete deficiency of DPD identified 7 different mutations including 1 splice-site mutation, 2 deletions, and 4 missense mutations (Table 113-4). The G → A splice-site mutation in intron 14 changes an invariant GT splice donor site into AT and leads to skipping of exon 14. Consequently, a 165 bp segment encoding amino acid residues 581 to 635 of the primary sequence of the DPD protein is lacking in the mature DPD mRNA.[350,351] Both the four base deletion 295-298delTCAT and the 1897delC mutation cause a frameshift leading to a premature stop codon shortly thereafter.[352,353] The 295-298delTCAT deletion is located in a TCAT tandem-repeat sequence and most likely results from polymerase slippage. Expression of the missense mutations C29R, R235W, R886H, and V995F in *E. coli* demonstrated that C29R, R235W, and V995F resulted in mutant DPD proteins without significant residual enzyme activity.[354,355] However, the R886H allele possessed a residual activity of 25 percent and it is therefore unlikely that this mutation is responsible for the observed complete deficiency in a patient who proved to be homozygous for both the C29R and R886H mutations.[354] The mutations identified so far are more or less randomly distributed along the cDNA and there are no apparent hot spots present (Fig. 113-9). All mutations are located outside those regions known to be involved in the binding of the various substrates and prosthetic groups with the exception of the V995F, which is located in the C-terminal region of DPD, thought to be involved in the binding of a [4Fe-4S] cluster.

The majority of the patients (68 percent) were homozygous for one of the identified mutations while the remaining patients were compound heterozygotes. Analysis of family members of the index patients for the presence of mutant alleles showed segregation of the mutant alleles in accordance with the pattern observed for the DPD activity in mononuclear cells and fibroblasts.[350,353,354,356] Analysis of the prevalence of the various mutations among DPD patients showed that the G → A point mutation in the invariant splice donor site leading to the skipping of exon 14 is by far the most common, whereas the other 6 mutations are less frequently observed (Table 113-4).

Clinical Presentation

Intensive investigation of clinical symptoms in the patients with a complete or nearly complete DPD deficiency[357,358] showed a considerable variation among these patients (Table 113-5). Convulsive disorders (seizures and epileptic insults), motor retardation and mental retardation were observed in approximately half of the patients, whereas growth retardation, microcephaly, autism and dysmorphy were less frequently observed. In this

Table 113-4 Mutations in Patients with DPD Deficiency

Name*	Genotype†	Effect‡	Location§	Allele frequency
Splicing				
*DPYD*2A*	IVS14 + 1G > A	del(exon 14)	IVS14	23/44 (52%)
Frameshift				
*DPYD*7*	295-298delTCAT	frameshift	EX4	7/44 (16%)
*DPYD*3*	1897delC	frameshift	EX14	3/44 (7%)
Missense				
*DPYD*9A*	85T > C	C29R	EX2	7/44 (16%)
*DPYD*8*	703C > T	R235W	EX7	1/44 (2%)
	2657G > A	R886H	EX21	2/44 (4%)
*DPYD*10*	2983G > T	V995F	EX23	2/44 (4%)
	Unknown	–	–	1/44 (2%)

*Nomenclature according to McLeod et al. (1998).[432]
†Nomenclature according to Antonarakis (1998).[433]
‡Effect of the mutation on DPD protein or mRNA.
§According to Wei et al. (1998).[348]

respect, it is worthwhile to note that five out of 17 intensively investigated families had a history of epilepsy (Table 113-5). A remarkable finding was the presence of ocular abnormalities in five patients. In one of the patients the ocular symptoms was part of a Kearns-Sayre syndrome with a verified mtDNA deletion, but the finding of four other cases still indicates a possible association with DPD deficiency. Surprisingly, one other patient suffered from DPD deficiency and Bartter's syndrome. The phenotypic variability of DPD deficiency is demonstrated by the fact that two asymptomatic patients have been identified and that seven other patients did not show the previously mentioned neurologic and developmental abnormalities. However, six out of these seven patients presented with other (neurologic) abnormalities such as lethargy, dizziness, monoplegia, acute life threatening event (ALTE) with hypothermia, and minor difficulties in learning speech and language. The latter abnormality has recently been described in two other families with otherwise healthy DPD-deficient siblings.[359,360] The possible pathophysiological mechanisms in patients with DPD deficiency are discussed below ("Pathophysiology").

In all patients the onset of clinical symptoms occurred during childhood with the majority of patients showing clinical abnormalities during the first years of life (Table 113-6). The important role of DPD in the chemotherapy with 5FU has been shown in cancer patients with a complete or near-complete deficiency of this enzyme. These patients suffered from severe (neuro)toxicity including death, following 5FU chemotherapy.[345,361–373] In this way, two cancer patients with a complete deficiency of DPD,[361,362] three patients with a suspected deficiency of DPD[345,363] and 17 patients with a very low activity of DPD have been reported.[364–373] The two patients with a complete DPD deficiency had been in excellent health (with only minor unrelated illnesses) prior to the appearance of a tumor.

Diagnosis. The diagnosis of DPD deficiency in most patients was suspected when urine (the preferred body fluid for diagnosis), examined as part of a screening protocol for inborn errors of metabolism, showed the presence of high concentrations of uracil and thymine. In some cases 5-hydroxymethyluracil is also elevated. As expected the dihydropyrimidines, the N-carbamyl-β-amino acids (β-ureidoisobutyrate and β-ureidopropionate) and β-amino acids are present in low concentrations or these metabolites are even absent.

The five known pyrimidine degradation defects can be detected by gas chromatography-mass spectometry (GC-MS) analysis of urinary trimethylsilylated organic acid extracts,[228] by amino acid analysis of urine before and after acid hydrolysis,[374] and by proton NMR spectroscopy.[375]

Strongly elevated concentrations of the pyrimidine bases and dihydropyrimidines can be detected and identified by gas chromatography (GC) or GC-MS,[376,377] but quantification is not possible because of variable extraction yields. Specific methods like two-dimensional thin layer chromatography (TLC),[378] HPLC with or without prefractionation of urine,[379] and proton nuclear magnetic resonance (NMR) spectroscopy[375] are more sensitive. Quantification requires such sophisticated methods as isotope dilution GC-MS,[380] HPLC with (diode-array), UV detection at various wave-lengths in off-line fractions obtained by isolation, and prefractionation of the bases and nucleosides, or on-line (dual-column methods) prepared fractions,[381] and proton NMR spectroscopy.[375] Isotope dilution GC-MS measurement of uracil and thymine in ethyl acetate extracts of amniotic fluid as their trimethylsilyl ethers with $^{15}N_2$-labeled uracil as internal standard has been reported.[380] In urine from a patient with DPD deficiency the elevated excretion of uracil and thymine could easily be detected by GC, TLC, and NMR as well as HPLC, but 5-hydroxymethyluracil was found only by TLC and HPLC. In the patients with DPD deficiency we found the following ranges by HPLC for the excretion (mM/mol creatinine) of the index compounds: uracil 56 to 683 (controls: 3 to 33, n = 100), thymine 7 to 439 (controls: 0 to 4, n = 100) and 5-hydroxymethyl uracil 0 to 54 (controls: not detectable, n = 100)

Screening for elevated urinary dihydropyrimidines and/or N-carbamyl-β-amino acids can easily be performed by amino acid analysis after conversion of these compounds into their corresponding β-amino acids by acid hydrolysis.[382] Differential analysis of these compounds can be done by the same procedure after isolation of the dihydropyrimidines, N-carbamyl-β-amino acids and β-amino acids in separate fractions by cation- and anion-exchange chromatography.[374] Application of this method on the urine of three DPH-deficient patients revealed dihydrouracil to be 393 to 626 and dihydrothymine 108 to 451 mM/mol creatinine. Alternatively, dihydropyrimidines in urine can also be measured by HPLC/FAB-MS with selected protonated molecular ion monitoring[382] and by proton NMR spectroscopy.[375]

Urine OA and uric acid were normal in 22 patients detected in The Netherlands[357,358] and urine urate was also normal in another patient.[376]

Localization of the enzyme block in the first patient was made by oral loading studies.[383] Most (75 percent) of the dose of uracil and thymine was excreted unchanged, while only 7 percent of corresponding doses of dihydrouracil and 40 percent of dihydrothymine (given as a mixture of R and S forms) were not metabolized.

The diagnosis of DPD deficiency can be confirmed by analysis of DPD activity in liver tissue, fibroblasts, and

Table 113-5 Genotype and Phenotype of Patients with DPD Deficiency at Diagnosis

Patient*	Genotype	Convulsions	Motor retardation	Mental retardation	Growth retardation	Microcephaly	Dysmorphy	Autism	Ocular abnormalities	Others
1 (NL)	ΔEX14/ΔEX14	–	+	++	–	–	–	–	+	1
2 (NL)	ΔEX14/ΔEX14	+	+	+	–	–	–	+	–	2
3 (DK)	ΔEX14/ΔEX14	+	+	+	–	–	–	–	–	3
4 (DK)	ΔEX14/ΔEX14	–	–	–	–	–	–	–	–	4
5 (S)	ΔEX14/ΔEX14	–	+	–	+	–	–	–	+	5
6 (DK)	ΔEX14/ΔEX14	++	++	++	–	–	–	–	–	
7 (NL)	ΔEX14/ΔEX14	–	–	–	–	–	–	–	–	6
8.1 (SF)	ΔEX14/ΔEX14	+	–	–	–	–	–	–	–	7
8.2 (SF)	ΔEX14/ΔEX14	–	–	–	–	–	–	–	–	8
9.1 (NL)	ΔTCAT/ΔTCAT	+	+	–	–	+	–	–	–	
9.2 (NL)	ΔTCAT/ΔTCAT	–	–	–	–	–	–	–	–	
9.3 (NL)	ΔTCAT/ΔTCAT	+	–	+	–	–	–	–	–	9
10 (IT)	C29R/C29R	–	+	++	–	–	+	++	–	10
11 (NL)	V995F/V995F	+	–	+	–	–	–	+	–	11
12.1 (TUR)	ΔC1897/ΔC1897	–	–	–	–	–	–	–	–	12
12.2 (TUR)	ΔC1897/R235W	+	++	++	++	++	+	–	+	13
13 (TUR)	C29R, R886H/ C29R, R886H	–	–	–	+	–	–	–	–	14
14.1 (NL)	C29R/ΔEX14	+	–	–	–	–	–	–	–	15
14.2 (NL)	C29R/ΔEX14	–	–	–	–	–	–	–	–	
15 (NL)	ΔEX14/ΔTCAT	+	++	++	–	+	–	++	+	16
16 (NL)	ΔEX14/C29R	–	–	–	–	–	–	–	–	17
17 (NL)	ΔEX14/?	–	+	+	+	–	+	–	+	18
Total		10/22 (45%)	10/22 (45%)	10/22 (45%)	4/22 (18%)	3/22 (14%)	3/22 (14%)	4/22 (18%)	5/22 (23%)	

*nationality of the patient is given in parenthesis
– = none; + = mild; ++ = severe
1) Ocular abnormalities (bilateral microphthalmia, iris and chorioidea coloboma) and nystagmus.[434]
2) CT scan showed strong contrast between white and gray matter.
3) Delayed development of speech.[435]
4) Lethargy.[435]
5) Bilateral ptosis, progressive external ophthalmoplegia, retinitis pigmentosa and muscle weakness due to Kearns-Sayre syndrome with a verified mtDNA deletion. Hemolytic anemia due to hereditary spherocytosis.
6) Initially suffering from dizziness.
7) Status epilepticus, dizziness, minor difficulties in learning and in mathematics at school.[436]
8) Minor difficulties in learning speech and language.[436]
9) Generalized tonic clonic seizures. EGG showed generalized epileptic activity.[377,391]
10) Slight white matter hyperintensity.[437]
11) Delayed development of speech and hyperactivity.[383,400]
12) Suspected for monoplegia.
13) Mild dysmorphic features (low set and posteriorly rotated ears, high arched palate) were noted. The child was in a state of unconsciousness without any response to verbal, sensory, or physical stimuli. Only massive motor reaction to pain was noted. There was no reaction to light with preserved corneal reflexes. Bilateral optic atrophy was present. Superficial abdominal and anal reflexes were absent. Tetraspasticity and flexion contractures were present. EEG revealed severe dysrhythmia and multifocal sharp/spike waves. Generalized loss of white and gray matter and diffuse cerebral atrophy was observed on cranial MRI. Deceased at the age of 8 years.
14) Upper airway infection, Bartter syndrome (hypokalemia, 2.5 mM), enuresis nocturna.
15) Paroxysmal vertigo with attacks of 30 min up to 2 h, hemiparesthesia, diplopia, hemiparesis, headache.
16) Severe behavioral disorder and delayed development of speech, episodic tempers, chronic hypernatremia, spastic diplegia, partial agenesis of corpus callosum, delayed myelination, hamartoid cerebral lesion, epileptic discharges, megalocorneae, hypopigmentation of the fundus and pallor of optic discs[438].
17) ALTE with hypothermia (29°C) and shock.
18) Pseudostrabismus, abnormally formed, coarse, notched, and fawn-colored teeth.[439]

lymphocytes.[356,377,384–386] The results of the loading studies in the first patient were confirmed by the observation that no substantial activity of DPD could be detected in the patient's leukocytes.[387] Very recently, DPD activity was also demonstrated in human monocytes, granulocytes and platelets, but not in erythrocytes.[388] In the Dutch pediatric patients with DPD deficiency, no activity with NADPH cosubstrate was found in leukocytes and fibroblasts.

A prenatal diagnosis of DPD deficiency by analyzing DPD activity in fetal liver has been reported, but in this case the activity of DPD in a control liver was also rather low. However, the diagnosis was confirmed by measurement of significantly elevated concentrations of thymine and uracil in amniotic fluid.[380]

In the adult patients with severe neurotoxicity due to 5FU, activities of DPD have been reported varying from very low to about 30 percent of normal.[361,362,389] For comparison of the results of patients with controls and the interpretation of the results one has to be aware of the fact that DPD activity shows a circadian rhythm, there being a factor of two difference between top and valley activities in humans.

Enzyme studies are essential for diagnosis because there are other causes of uracil thyminuria such as dihydropyrimidinase deficiency. High concentrations of uracil are also excreted in urea cycle defects, but are accompanied by increased urine uridine and OA (see Chap. 85). High urinary concentrations of uracil can also originate from bacterial degradation of pseudouridine[301,374] resulting in low concentrations of pseudouridine. Patients with malignancies and elevated excretion of pyrimidines usually excrete purines and degradation products such as uric acid, β-aminoisobutyric acid and pseudouridine.[390] One child with medulloblastoma showed high urinary thymine and uracil levels and had fibroblast DPD levels about half those in controls but the pyrimidine over excretion was difficult to explain on the basis of either enzyme deficiency or overproduction by neoplastic tissue.[390] A patient with Burkitt Lymphoma presented with severe uracil thyminuria simulating DPD deficiency after starting of treatment with cytostatic drugs, but the uracil thyminuria normalized within three days.[301,374] The orotic aciduria reported in malignancy is of much less magnitude (normal <7 μM/day, malignancy 4 to 28 μM/day).[219] Six other children with neoplastic

Table 113-6 Ages of Onset and of Diagnosis, Treatment, and Family History of 22 Patients in 17 Families with DPD Deficiency

Patient	Age of onset of symptoms	Age of diagnosis	Epilepsy in family	Consanguinity	Treatment
1	at birth	2 y, 1 m	No	No	
2	3 y	7 y	Yes	No	1
3	1 to 2 y	2 y	No	No	
4	at birth	at birth	NA	No	
5	10 y, 2 m	14 y, 6 m	No	No	
6	0 y, 6 m	6 y, 2m	No	No	2
7	childhood	NA	NA	NA	
8.1	7 y, 5 m	8 y, 1 m	Yes	No	3
8.2	childhood	4 y, 5 m	Yes	No	
9.1	3 y	6 y	Yes	Yes	4
9.2	AS	4 y	Yes	Yes	
9.3	12 y	28 y	Yes	Yes	5
10	1 y	3 y	No	No	
11	1 y, 6 m	3 y, 1 m	No	No	
12.1	NA	30 y	Yes	No	
12.2	0 y, 4 m	6 y, 2 m	Yes	Yes	
13	8 y	8 y	NA	NA	
14.1	17 y, 6 m	18 y, 2 m	Yes	No	
14.2	AS	26 y, 4 m	Yes	No	
15	0 y, 6 m	1 y, 3 m	No	No	6
16	5 weeks	5 weeks	No	No	
17	at birth	1 y, 10 m	NA	No	

AS = Asymptomatic
NA = Data not available for analysis
1) Responded to valproate.
2) No response to treatment with valproate. Good response to carbamazepine and lamotrigine. After interruption of medication symptoms of complex partial epilepsy recurred. After reintroduction of medication the patient is again seizure free.
3) Good response to oxcarbazepine.
4) Phenobarbital and ethosuximide.
5) Phenytoin and phenobarbitone.
6) Responded to pipamperon, clonazepam.
References of the literature in which detailed information is given concerning individual cases are reviewed by Van Kuilenburg et al.[357]

disease produced normal or only slightly elevated uracil and thymine levels.[390]

Treatment.
No treatment specific for the enzyme defect or consequences of the defect has been described, except for withdrawal of fluoridated pyrimidines in case of increased toxicity. In general a good response was noted when patients with convulsions/epileptic attacks were treated with anti-epileptic medication.

Pathophysiology

Braakhekhe and colleagues[391] present several possible mechanisms by which DPD deficiency might affect neurologic function and cause epilepsy. Moreover, all enzyme defects of pyrimidine degradation except BAIBPAT deficiency will lead to altered β-alanine concentrations. In case of DPD, DPH, or UP deficiency β-alanine will be decreased, in case of BAKAT or BAPAT deficiency β-alanine will accumulate. The altered concentrations of the neurotransmitter β-alanine may be of relevance with respect to the cerebral dysfunction often seen in patients with these defects. In DPD- and DPH-deficient patients, exposure of the nervous system to high concentrations of uracil and/or thymine may be a contributing factor.[357]

β-Alanine Homeostasis. β-Alanine is a structural analogue of glycine and γ amino butyric acid (GABA), which are the major inhibitory neurotransmitters in the central nervous system. It has been shown in chick spinal cord neurons and in mouse brain that β-alanine activates both glycine and $GABA_A$ receptors with a similar efficiency as glycine and GABA, respectively.[392–394] In addition it has been demonstrated that β-alanine is a potent blocker of the uptake of GABA in glial cells.[395]

β-Alanine and its acid, GABA, are metabolized by transaminases (BAKAT and GABA transaminase, respectively), which show activity towards both compounds. Altered levels of β-alanine due to pyrimidine degradation defects might therefore have a profound effect on the degree of activation of glycine and $GABA_A$ receptors as well as in GABA transport into glial cells. Moreover, GABA uptake blockers such as β-alanine have shown to possess profound anticonvulsant effects.[396]

The neurotransmitters β-alanine and GABA play also a role in the visual system[397] and recently a new GABA receptor has been detected in the retina which is sensitive to β-alanine and glycine.[398] Therefore, the ocular abnormalities seen in five patients with DPD deficiency and the one patient with putative UP deficiency may be related to the decreased β-alanine production in these patients.[357]

5FU Toxicity. The severe neurotoxicity seen in patients with a (partial) deficiency of DPD under treatment with 5FU may result from the exposure of the nervous system to relatively high concentrations of this drug leading to its increased incorporation into cellular RNA. However, shortage of β-alanine caused by complete DPD deficiency or by competition of 5FU as substrate in case of partial DPD deficiency may also contribute to this condition.

A study of 5FU metabolism in DPD deficiency confirmed that 5FU had a prolonged elimination half-life of 159 minutes versus 13 ± 7 minutes for controls and was largely excreted in the urine (89.7 percent of a 50 mg radiolabeled dose versus 9.8 ± 1.6 percent for controls).[361] Diasio and colleagues[361] concluded that there was a markedly prolonged exposure causing increased toxicity and that CNS toxicity in his patient was due to 5FU and not as has previously been suggested to 5FU catabolites, because of a complete deficiency in this patient. The kinetics of 5FU metabolism were studied by Coustere and colleagues[399] who concluded that their compartmental model fitted the data from a patient[361] deficient in DPD.

Genetics

DPD appears to be inherited in an autosomal recessive fashion. Carrier detection of DPD deficiency by analysis of enzyme activity in lymphocytes or fibroblasts has been reported to be unreliable. However, it is our experience that carrier detection in mononuclear cells may be possible if differential blood cell count and circadian rhythm is taken into consideration. Therefore, we recommend collection of samples from suspected carriers, patients, and noncarriers at the same time of day.

Some obligate heterozygotes may have reduced DPD in fibroblasts, although two of six parents studied had enzyme levels within the normal range.[400] Studies of two families showed low levels of enzyme activity in the mononuclear leukocytes of all three parents studied and in 7 of 11 possible carriers, and no overlap with the control range.[361,362] The mother of one patient had no significant residual enzyme activity, similar to that of her affected child but there was complex consanguinity consistent with her also being homozygous deficient.[231,391]

There appears to be some homogeneity for the intron 14 G>A splice-site mutation in Northern Europe, as homozygosity for this mutation has been observed in 9 individuals from Denmark, Sweden, Finland and The Netherlands. Furthermore, the majority of the DPD patients are of Dutch origin (55 percent), which probably reflects the fact that in The Netherlands screening for inborn errors of pyrimidine degradation is part of an intensive diagnostic program for inborn errors in general. The condition might be much more prevalent in other populations also.

So far, the frequency of these mutations in a normal population is not known. Based on the analysis of the DPD activity in various populations it has been estimated that the frequency of heterozygotes might be as high as 3 percent.[401] Fortunately, the G>A splice-site mutation destroys a unique MaeII restriction site present in an amplified genomic DNA fragment encompassing the skipped exon and its flanking sequences, allowing the rapid screening of this mutation in patients.[351,369] Screening for the presence of the G>A splice-site mutation in a limited number of individuals of various nationalities revealed heterozygosity for this mutation in 1 percent of the Finnish population (180 alleles analyzed) but none in British (60 alleles), Japanese (100 alleles), African-American (210 alleles), or Dutch populations (100 alleles).[348,351,369] Initially, an allele frequency of 5 percent had been found for the G>A splice-site mutation in Taiwanese subjects (72 alles analyzed).[369] However, in subsequent studies, the G>A splice site mutation could not be detected in a larger group of Taiwanese subjects (262 alleles analyzed).[348] In addition, neither the splice-site nor the 1897delC were detected in 60 Caucasian subjects.[402]

Pharmacogenetics

Severe 5FU toxicity is another manifestation to be added to the list of pharmacogenetic conditions.[403] DPD is responsible for the breakdown of this widely used antineoplastic agent. The catabolic route plays a significant role since more than 80 percent of the administered 5FU is catabolized by DPD.[404] In this light, a pharmacogenetic disorder has been described concerning cancer patients with a complete or partial deficiency of DPD suffering from a severe or even life-threatening toxicity after the administration of 5FU. Recently, it has been shown that three such patients were genotypically heterozygous for a mutant allele of the gene encoding DPD.[369,371,372,405,406]

DIHYDROPYRIMIDINURIA: DEFICIENCY OF DIHYDROPYRIMIDINASE

Enzymology

DPH (dihydropyrimidinase, 5,6-dihydropyrimidineamidohydrolase, hydantoinase or dihydropyrimidine hydrase) (MIM 222748) catalyzes the hydrolytic cleavages of dihydropyrimidines, hydantoins, phthalmide, and 1RCF-187. The latter compound needs DPH for its ring opening to become therapeutically active. For some substrates under experimental conditions the reaction is reversible.

Purification

DHP has been found in both mammalian kidney and liver and has been purified to homogeneity from bovine liver,[407] calf liver,[408] pig liver,[409] and rat liver.[410]

The native enzyme is a tetramer with molecular weight of 217 kDa consisting of four subunits of 54 kDa each. DPH is a metalloenzyme containing one zinc atom in each subunit, which can be removed by chelating agents.

Kinetics

There is evidence for stereoselectivity and for stereospecificity for some substrates and N-carbamyl β-alanine is a significant inhibitor.[410]

The optimal pH of the reaction for the several substrates appears to correlate qualitatively with the pKa of the amide proton. The chemical acid-base catalytic mechanisms for pig[409] and rat liver DPH[410] have been studied intensely.

Molecular Genetics

A human liver DPH cDNA contained a 1,560-bp open reading frame encoding a protein of 519 amino acids with a predicted molecular mass of 56.6kDa.[411] The human DPH protein showed 90 percent amino acid identity with that of rat DPH. The human DPH structural gene was found to span >80 kb and contained 10 exons with lengths of 131–420 bp.[412] All introns contained the conserved 5′-GT splice donor and 3′-AG splice acceptor sites. Southern blot analysis of total human genomic DNA restriction fragments showed that the DPH gene is single copy and is located at 8q22.[412]

The mutation analysis of genomic DNA in one symptomatic and five asymptomatic individuals presenting with dihydropyrimidinuria revealed the presence of one frameshift mutation and five missense mutations (Table 113-7).[412] The single base insertion at nucleotide positions 812–814 leads to a frameshift at codon 272 and causes premature termination of translation at codon 287. Expression of the frame shift mutation (InsA) and the five

Table 113-7 Mutations in Patients with DHP Deficiency

Genotype	Effect*	Location†	Allele frequency
812–814 Ins A	Frameshift‡	Exon 5	1/12 (8%)
1001 A > G	Q334R	Exon 6	6/12 (50%)
1303 G > A	G435R	Exon 8	1/12 (8%)
203 G > C	T68R	Exon 1	1/12 (8%)
1468 C > G	R490T	Exon 9	1/12 (8%)
1078 T > C	W360R	Exon 6	2/12 (16%)

*Effect of the mutation on DHP protein or mRNA.
†According to Hamajima et al. (1998).[412]
‡Single-base insertion of A at nucleotide position +812 to +814 leading to a frameshift from codon 272 and to a premature termination of translation at codon 287.

missense mutations (T85R, Q334R, W360R, G435R, R490T) in COS7 cells revealed that all mutant alleles exhibited a severely reduced DPH activity compared to that of wild type. Western blot analysis showed a profound reduction of DPH immuno-stainable protein in the COS7 cells transfected with the DPH mutants InsA, W360R and G435R suggesting that the stability or biosynthesis of these mutant proteins is reduced since the mutant mRNAs were equally well expressed as the wild-type DPH construct. The InsA frameshift mutation is likely to result in a truncated protein that is either unstable or no longer recognized by the antibody. W360R is located near the amino-terminal end of the strongly conserved region in DPH and DPH-related proteins[411] and this region has been shown to be essential for in vitro heterotetramerisation with DPH-related proteins.[413] Therefore, W360R might cause instability of the subunit by preventing tetramerization. The G435 DPH mutant possessed a higher residual activity when compared to other DPH mutants despite a reduced level of protein. Thus, G435 might be essential for the stability but not for catalytic activity of the DPH enzyme. The T68R and Q334R mutations are located in those regions suggested to be involved in the binding of zinc ions, which are obligatory for catalytic activity. In addition, the T68R, Q334R, and R490T mutations are located at completely conserved residues between human and rat DPH as well as in mammalian and avian DPH related proteins.

Clinical Presentation

In contrast to DPD deficiency of which 50 cases have been described, so far only 6 cases have been described with DPH deficiency.[331] Therefore, a general conclusion concerning the clinical picture of DPH deficiency cannot be drawn. So far, symptomatology of DPH-deficient individuals seems to be as variable as in DPD deficiency. Epileptic and convulsive attacks have been reported in three,[359,414,415] and mental retardation, motor retardation, and microcephaly in two of these individuals.[331,359] Dysmorphic features and retarded growth were seen in one case.[415] Also one patient suffered from intractable diarrhea due to congenital atrophy, but had no other symptoms.[416] Two of these patients were of Turkish origin, one of Moroccan and one of Pakistani origin. The first patient[414] had only one attack of seizures and is still developing normally. Two individuals are healthy and were detected by mass-screening in Japan.[417,418]

Diagnosis. Suspected patients can be screened for the presence of the defect by analysis of the relevant metabolites in their body fluids (as described for DPD deficiency above). The diagnosis can only be confirmed by analysis of the enzyme activity in liver, because the enzyme is not expressed in other more accessible tissues. Confirmation is important because the dihydropyrimidines may be converted into the corresponding N-carbamyl-β-amino acids when the urine is contaminated by bacteria due to urinary tract infection.[301,374] The measurement of DPH activity in liver of two patients with dihydropyrimidinuria has been reported.[331]

Treatment. Supplementation of β-alanine has been tried in the patient described by Putman[415] but until now the effect is not clear.

Pathophysiology

As discussed with DPD deficiency, a deficiency of β-alanine may cause the neurologic problems in DPH deficiency.

For similar reasons to those discussed for DPD deficiency, although not reported yet, increased sensitivity for 5FU neurotoxicity can also be expected in patients with DPH deficiency. Moreover, patients treated with Adriamycin in combination with IRCF-187 [1,2-bis (3,5-dioxopiperazinyl-1-yl) propane] need DPH activity for the ring opening of IRCF-187 to provide a chelator and reduce the toxicity of iron bound to the Adriamycin.[419]

Genetics

The first two reported cases were of Turkish and Pakistani origin respectively and consanguinity in both families suggested an autosomal recessive basis for the DPH deficiency. So far the frequency of the mutations in a normal population is not known. Screening for the presence of the Q334R and W360R mutation in 100 Japanese and 200 Caucasian subjects, respectively, did not reveal carriers for these two mutations suggesting that Q334 is not common in the Japanese population and the W360R is not common in the Caucasian population.[412]

N-CARBAMYL-β-AMINOACIDURIA: DEFICIENCY OF UREIDOPROPIONASE (MIM 210100)

Excessive urinary excretion of N-carbamyl-β-alanine and N-carbamyl-β-aminoisobutyric acid has been reported in a 17 month old girl born to consanguineous parents who presented with muscular hypotonia, dystonic movements and severe developmental delay.[420] From the first days of life on, the child was hyperexcitable with dystonic movements of the upper limbs and showed abnormal eye movements without visual responses. At 11 months, optic atrophy was diagnosed, but some visual contacts and smiles were noticed. The patient had reduced tendon reflexes, scoliosis, tremor of the head, frequent sweating, and chest infections. There was progress in motor development. Despite thriving normally, head circumference dropped below P3. MRI at age 5 months showed aplasia of the inferior cerebellum vermis, hypoplasia of the brainstem, a thin corpus callosum, and normal myelination. Analysis of the patient's urine by proton NMR spectroscopy[375] and amino acid analysis of the isolated dihydropyrimidines and N-carbamyl-β-amino acids after acid hydrolysis[301,374] showed moderate dihydropyrimidinuria and strongly increased N-carbamyl-β-alanine (ureidopropionate) and N-carbamyl-β-amino-isobutyric acid (ureidoisobutyric acid), but the corresponding β-amino acids were nearly absent. The enzyme deficiency has been confirmed in liver tissue, being the only tissue in which the enzyme is expressed.[421]

Increased excretion of β-ureidopropionate has also been reported in a patient with severe propionic acidemia, probably due to inhibition of UP by propionate.[422] N-carbamyl-β-amino aciduria simulating UP deficiency has been seen in a patient with DPH deficiency during urinary tract infection.[374]

R(−)β-AMINOISOBUTYRATE-PYRUVATE AND β-ALANINE-α-KETOGLUTARATE AMINOTRANSFERASE DEFICIENCIES

Two enzymes are involved in the fourth step of the pyrimidine degradation pathway: R(-)β-aminoisobutyrate-pyruvate aminotransferase (BAIBPAT) (MIM 210100) and β-alanine-α-ketoglutarate aminotransferase (BAKAT). A deficiency of BAIBPAT in liver has been proposed as the cause of a permanent high excretion of β-aminoisobutyric acid in urine of some healthy individuals.[423,424] These genetic high excretors have less than 10 percent of normal activity in the liver.[424] They are found with a frequency of 1 to 10 percent in Western European populations and up to 80 percent among Mongoloid races in Southeast Asia. Hyper β-aminoisobutyric aciduria is thought to be a benign polymorphism and therefore the measurement of BAIBPAT in patients is not indicated. The β-aminoisobutyric acid found in urine is almost exclusively the R-isomer.

A deficiency of BAKAT is hypothesized in patients with primary hyper-β-alaninemia.[425] The one reported case concerns a boy with hypotonia, hyporeflexia, generalized tonic-clonic seizures, and intermittent lethargy, who eventually died in infancy.[425] The patient also had increased β-alanine concentrations in cerebrospinal fluid and elevated concentrations of β-alanine, β-aminoisobutyric acid, (GABA) and taurine in urine. Recently hyper-β-alaninemia has also been associated with Cohen's syndrome.[426] The patient with this syndrome had a partial deficiency (50 percent of normal) of the enzyme in skin fibroblasts. The symptoms in patients with hyper-β-alaninemia presumably reflect the effect of β-alanine on nervous tissue.

BAKAT is generally supposed to be the same enzyme as GABA transaminase, although Mendelian phenotypes imply that they are different.[427]

Hyper-β-alaninuria combined with hyper-β-aminoisobutyric aciduria can simulate BAKAT deficiency, and isolated hyper-β-aminoisobutyric aciduria can simulate BAIBPAT deficiency. However, both conditions can also occur in cancer patients due to increased tissue degradation.[428] Hyper-β-alaninuria with hyper-β-aminoaciduria can also be caused by γ-vinyl-GABA, a drug that inhibits the relevant transaminase. Excessive urinary excretion of β-alanine and RS-β-aminoisobutyric acid in combination with β-hydroxypropionate, 3-hydroxyisobutyrate and S-2-(hydroxymethyl)butyrate has also been reported in a patient with reduced malonic semialdehyde dehydrogenase activity and deficient methylmalonic semialdehyde dehydrogenase.[429,430]

Clinical Presentation

Diagnosis. The patient with BAKAT deficiency[425] and the patient with proven partial BAKAT deficiency[426] both presented with persistently elevated concentrations of β-alanine in plasma (patients: range 20 to 51 μM; N < 14), CSF (patient 1:45 μM; patient 2: elevated; N < 0.06) and urine (patient 1: 100 × N; patient 2: 28 μM/24 hr; N: trace). GABA was also reported to be elevated in the urines of both patients, and in plasma and CSF of patient 1. In patient 1 also urinary β-aminoisobutyric acid and taurine were elevated. Individuals with BAIBPAT deficiency are only characterized by elevated concentration of β-aminoisobutyric acid in their urine. The patients with BAKAT deficiency or individuals with BAIBPAT deficiency can easily be detected by urine amino acid analysis. No patients with BAPAT deficiency have been reported to date, but in principle they can also be detected by the methods described above.

Treatment. Patients with BAIBPAT deficiency need not be treated. Treatment for hyper-β-alaninemia may be effective: in the first patient, the metabolic but not the clinical phenotype improved by treatment with 10 mg/day of pyridoxine orally,[425] in the second patient both the metabolic as well as clinical phenotype improved dramatically on 100 mg/day of pyridoxine.[426]

REFERENCES

1. Bono V, Weissman S, Frei E: The effect of 6-azauridine administration on de novo pyrimidine production in chronic myelogenous leukemia. *J Clin Invest* **43**:1486, 1964.
2. Smith LJ: Pyrimidine metabolism in man. *N Engl Med J* **238**:764, 1973.
3. Henderson J, Paterson A: *Nucleotide Metabolism. An Introduction.* New York, Academic Press, 1973.
4. Makoff A, Radford A: Genetics and biochemistry of carbamoyl phosphate biosynthesis and its utilisation in the pyrimidine biosynthetic pathway. *Microbiol Rev* **42**:307, 1978.
5. Coleman P, Suttle D, Stark G: Purification from hamster cells of the multifunctional protein that initiates de novo synthesis of pyrimidine nucleotides. *J Biol Chem* **252**:6379, 1977.
6. Davidson J, Patterson D: Alteration in structure of multifunctional protein form Chinese hamster ovary cells defective in pyrimidine biosynthesis. *Proc Natl Acad Sci U S A* **76**:1731, 1979.
7. Davidson J, Niswander L: Partial cDNA sequence to a hamster gene corrects defects in Escherichia coil pyrB mutant. *Proc Natl Acad Sci U S A* **80**:6897, 1983.
8. Shigesada K, Stark G, Maley J, Niswander L, Davidson J: Construction of a cDNA to the hamster CAD gene and its application toward defining the domain for aspartate transcarbamylase. *Mol Cell Biol* **5**:1735, 1985.
9. Mori M, Tatibana M: Purification of homogeneous glutamine-dependent carbamyl phosphate synthetase from ascites hepatoma cells as a complex with aspartate transcarbamylase and dihydroorotase. *J Biochem* **78**:239, 1975.
10. Lee L, Kelly R, Pastra-Landis S, Evans D: Oligomeric structure of the multifunctional protein CAD that initiates pyrimidine biosynthesis in mammalian cells. *Proc Natl Acad Sci U S A* **82**:6802, 1985.
11. Rumsby P, Campbell P, Niswander L, Davidson J: Organization of a multifunctional protein in pyrimidine biosynthesis. *Biochem J* **217**:435, 1984.
12. Grayson D, Evans D: The isolation and characterization of the aspartate transcarbamylase domain of the multifunctional protein CAD. *J Biol Chem* **258**:4123, 1983.
13. Padgett R, Wahl G, Stark G: Structure of the gene for CAD, the multifunctional protein that initiates UMP synthesis in Syrian hamster cells. *Mol Cell Biol* **2**:293, 1982.
14. Wahl G, Padgett R, Stark G: Gene amplification causes overproduction of the first three enzymes of UMP synthesis in *N*-(phosphonoacetyl)-L-aspartate-resistant hamster cells. *J Biol Chem* **264**:8679, 1979.
15. Jones M: Regulation of pyrimidine and arginine biosynthesis in mammals, in Advances, in Weber G (ed): *Enzyme Regulations.* New York, Pergamon Press, 1971, p 19.
16. Kelley W: Hereditary orotic aciduria, in Stanbury JB, Wyngaarden JB, Fredrickson DS, Goldstein JL, Brown MS (eds): *The Metabolic Basis of Inherited Disease.* New York, McGraw-Hill, 1983, p 1202.
17. Dileepan K, Kennedy J: Rapid conversion of newly synthesized orotate to uridine-5-monophosphate by rat liver cytosolic enzymes. *FEBS Lett* **153**:1, 1983.
18. Hoogenraad N, Lee D: Effect of uridine on de novo pyrimidine biosynthesis in rat hepatoma cells in culture. *J Biol Chem* **249**:2763, 1974.
19. Karle J, Cowan K, Chisena C, Cysyk R: Uracil nucleotide synthesis in a human breast cancer cell line (MCF-7) and in two drug-resistant sublines that contain increased levels of enzymes of the de novo pyrimidine pathway. *Mol Pharmacol* **30**:136, 1986.
20. Sugiura Y, Fujioka S, Yoshida S: Biosynthesis of pyrimidine nucleotides in human leukemic cells. *Jpn J Cancer Res* **77**:664, 1986.
21. Becroft D, Phillips L, Simmonds A: Hereditary orotic aciduria: Long term therapy with uridine and a trial of uracil. *J Pediatr* **75**:885, 1969.
22. Perignon J-L, Bories D, Houllier A-M, Thuillier L, Cartier P: Metabolism of pyrimidine bases and nucleosides by pyrimidine-nucleoside phosphorylases in cultured cells. *Biochim Biophys Acta* **928**:130, 1987.
23. Reichard P: The enzymatic synthesis of pyrimidines. *Adv Enzymol* **21**:623, 1959.
24. Shoaf W, Jones M: Uridylic acid synthesis in Ehrlich ascites carcinoma. Properties, subcellular distribution, and nature of enzyme complexes of the six biosynthetic enzymes. *Biochemistry* **12**:4039, 1973.
25. Kavipurapu P, Jones M: Purification, size, and properties of the complex of orotate phosphoribosyltransferase: Orotidylate decarboxylase from mouse Ehrlich ascites carcinoma. *J Biol Chem* **251**:5589, 1976.
26. Kasbekar D, Nagabhushanam A, Greenberg D: Purification and properties of orotic acid-decarboxylating enzymes from calf thymus. *J Biol Chem* **239**:4245, 1964.
27. Brown G, Fox R, O'Sullivan W: Interconversion of different molecular weight forms of human erythrocyte orotidylate decarboxylase. *J Biol Chem* **250**:7352, 1975.
28. Krooth R, Pan Y-L, Pinsky L: Studies of the orotidine 5′-monophosphate decarboxylase activity of crude extracts of human cells. *Biochem Genet* **8**:133, 1973.
29. Mclard R, Black M, Livingstone L, Jones M: Isolation and initial characterization of the single polypeptide that synthesizes uridine 5′-monophosphate from orotate in Ehrlich ascites carcinoma. Purification by tandem affinity chromatography of uridine-5′-monophosphate synthase. *Biochemistry* **19**:4699, 1980.
30. Livingstone L, Jones M: The purification and preliminary characterization of UMP synthase from human placenta. *J Biol Chem* **262**:15726, 1987.
31. Levinson B, Ullman B, Martin DJ: Pyrimidine pathway variants of cultured mouse lymphoma cells with altered levels of both orotate phosphoribosyltransferase and orotidylate decarboxylase. *J Biol Chem* **254**:4396, 1979.
32. Suttle D, Stark G: Coordinate overproduction of orotate phosphoribosyltransferase and orotidine-5′-phosphate decarboxylase in hamster cells resistant to pyrazofurin and 6-azauridine. *J Biol Chem* **254**:4206, 1979.
33. Suttle D: Increased levels of UMP synthase protein and mRNA in pyrazofurin-resistant rat hepatoma cells. *J Biol Chem* **258**:7707, 1983.
34. Suttle D: Unpublished data.

35. Kanalas J, Hutton J, Suttle D: Characterization of pyrazofurin-resistant HeLa cells with amplification of UMP synthase gene. *Somat Cell Mol Genet* **11**:359, 1985.
36. Traut T, Payne R, Jones M-E: Dependence of the aggregation and conformation states of uridine 5′-phosphate synthase on pyrimidine nucleotides. Evidence for a regulatory site. *Biochemistry* **19**:6062, 1980.
37. Traut T, Jones M: Interconversion of different molecular weight forms of the orotate phosphoribosyltransferase. Orotidine-5′-phosphate decarboxylase enzyme complex from mouse Erlich ascites cells. *J Biol Chem* **254**:1143, 1979.
38. Traut T, Payne R: Dependence of the catalytic activities on the aggregation and conformation states of uridine 5′-phosphate synthase. *Biochemistry* **19**:6068, 1980.
39. Schminke-Ott E, Bisswanger H: Multifunctional proteins, in Schmincke-Ott E, (ed): *H Bisswanger*. New York, John Wiley and Sons, 1980, p 1.
40. Stark G: Structure of the multifunctional CAD protein. *TIBS* **7**:134, 1977.
41. Reyes P, Guganig M: Studies on a pyrimidine phosphoribosyltransferase from murine leukemia P1534J. *J Biol Chem* **250**:5097, 1975.
42. Floyd E, Jones M: Isolation and characterisation of the orotidine 5′-monophosphate decarboxylase domain of the multifunctional protein uridine 5′-phosphate synthase. *J Biol Chem* **260**:9443, 1985.
43. Rose M, Grisafi P, Botstein D: Structure and function of the yeast URA3 gene: Expression in *Escherichia coli*. *Gene* **29**:113, 1984.
44. Ohmstede C-A, Lanngdon S, Chae C-B, Jones M: Expression and sequence analysis of a cDNA encoding the orotidine 5′-monophosphate decarboxylase domain from Ehrlich ascites uridylate synthase. *J Biol Chem* **261**:4276, 1986.
45. Langdon S, Jones M: Study of the kinetic and physical properties of the orotidine-5′-monophosphate decarboxylase domain from mouse UMP synthase produced in *Saccharomyces cerevisiae*. *J Biol Chem* **262**:13359, 1987.
46. Lin T, Suttle D: Expression of catalytic domains of human UMP synthase in uridine auxotrophic bacteria. *Somat Cell Mol Genet* **19**(2):193, 1993.
47. Lin T, Suttle D: UMP synthase activity expressed in deficient hamster cells by separate transferase and decarboxylase proteins or by linker-deleted bifunctional protein. *Somat Cell Mol Genet* **21**(3):161, 1995.
48. Victor J, Leo-Mensah A, Sloan D: Divalent metal ion activation of the yeast orotate phosphoribosyltransferase catalyzed reaction. *Biochemistry* **18**:3597, 1979.
49. Syed D, Strauss R, Sloan D: Orotate phosphoribosyltransferase and hypoxanthine/guanine phosphoribosyltransferase from yeast: Nuclear magnetic relaxation studies of enzyme-bound phosphoribosyl 1-pyrophosphate. *Biochemistry* **26**:1051, 1987.
50. Victor J, Greenberg L, Sloan D: Studies of the kinetic mechanism of orotate phosphoribosyltransferase from yeast. *J Biol Chem* **254**:2647, 1979.
51. Bell J, Jones M, Carter C: Crystallization of yeast orotidine 5′-monophosphate decarboxylase complexed with 1-(5′-phospho-B-D-ribofuranosyl) barbituric acid. *Proteins* **9**:143, 1991.
52. Beak P, Siegel B: Mechanism of decarboxylation of 1,3 dimethylorotic acid. *J Am Chem Soc* **98**:3601, 1976.
53. Silverman R, Groziak M: Model chemistry for a covalent mechanism of action of orotidine 5′-phosphate decarboxylase. *J Am Chem Soc* **104**:6434, 1982.
54. Acheson S, Bell J, Jones M, Wolfenden R: Orotidine-5′-monophosphate decarboxylase catalysis: Kinetic isotope effects and the state of hybridization of a bound transition state analogue. *Biochemistry* **29**:3198, 1990.
55. Smiley J, Paneth P, O'Leary M, Bell J, Jones M: Investigation of the enzymatic mechanism of yeast orotidine-5′-monophosphate decarboxylase using 13C kinetic isotope effects. *Biochemistry* **30**:6216, 1991.
56. Levine H, Brody R, Westheimer F: Inhibition of orotidine-5′-phosphate decarboxylase by 1-(5′-phospho-B-D-ribofuranosyl) barbituric acid, 6-azauridine 5′-phosphate and uridine 5′-phosphate. *Biochemistry* **19**:4993, 1980.
57. Jones M: Orotidylate decarboxylase of yeast and man. *Curr Top Cell Regul* **33**:331, 1992.
58. Jones M: Pyrimidine pathways: News concerning the mechanism of orotidine-5′-monophosphate decarboxylase. *Adv Exp Med Biol* **309B**:305, 1991.
59. Traut T: UMP synthase: The importance of quaternary structure in channeling intermediates. *TIBS* **7**:255, 1982.
60. Traut T, Jones M: Kinetic and conformational studies of the orotate phosphoribosyltransferase: Orotidine-5′-phosphate decarboxylase enzyme complex from mouse Ehrlich ascites cells. *J Biol Chem* **252**:8374, 1977.
61. Traut T: Significance of the enzyme complex that synthesizes UMP in Ehrlich ascites cells. *Arch Biochem Biophys* **200**:590, 1980.
62. Mcclard R, Shokat K: Does the bifunctional uridylate synthase channel orotidine 5′-monophosphate? Kinetics of orotate phosphoribosyltransferase and orotidylate decarboxylase activities fit a non-interacting sites model. *Biochemistry* **26**:3378, 1987.
63. Kanalas J, Suttle D: Amplification of the UMP synthase gene and enzyme overproduction in pyrazofurin-resistant rat hepatoma cells. Molecular cloning of a cDNA for UMP synthase. *J Biol Chem* **259**:1848, 1984.
64. Wiginton D, Adrian G, Friedman R, Suttle D, Hutton J: Cloning of cDNA sequences of human adenosine deaminase. *Proc Natl Acad Sci U S A* **80**:7481, 1983.
65. Suttle D, Bugg B, Winkler J, Kanalas J: Molecular cloning and nucleotide sequence for the complete coding region of UMP synthase. *Proc Natl Acad Sci U S A* **84**:1754, 1988.
66. Poulsen P, Jensen K, Valentin-Hansen P, Carlsson P, Lundberg L: Nucleotide sequence of the *Escherichia coli* pyrE gene and of the DNA in front of the protein-coding region. *Eur J Biochem* **135**:223, 1983.
67. Kimsey H, Kaiser D: The orotidine-5′-decarboxylase gene of *Myxococcus xanthus*. Comparison to the OMP decarboxylase gene family. *J Biol Chem* **267**:819, 1992.
68. Dush M, Sikela J, Khan S, Tischfield J, Stambrook P: Nucleotide sequence and organization of the mouse adenine phosphoribosyltransferase gene: Presence of a coding region common to animal and bacterial phosphoribosyltransferases that has a variable intron/exon arrangement. *Proc Nalt Acad Sci U S A* **82**:2731, 1985.
69. Broderick T, Schaff D, Bertino A, Dush M, Tischfield J: Comparative anatomy of the human APRT gene and enzyme: Nucleotide sequence divergence and conservation of a nonrandom CpG dinucleotide arrangement. *Proc Natl Acad Sci U S A* **84**:3349, 1987.
70. Argos P, Hanei M, Wilson J, Kelly W: A possible nucleotide-binding domain in the tertiary fold of phosphoribosyltransferases. *J Biol Chem.* **258**:6450, 1983.
71. Stepanik P, Bugg B, Suttle D: Construction of a UMP synthase (UMPS) expression vector capable of selection, amplification, and deamplification. *FASEB J* 1992.
72. Patterson D: Isolation and characterization of 5-fluorouracil-resistant mutants of Chinese hamster ovary cells deficient in the activities of orotate phosphoribosyltransferase and orotidine 5′-monophosphate decarboxylase. *Somat Cell Genet* **6**:101, 1980.
73. Patterson D, Jones C, Morse H, Rumsby P, Miller Y, Davis R: Structural gene coding for multifunctional protein carrying orotate phosphoribosyltransferase and OMP decarboxylase activity is located on the long arm of human chromosome 3. *Somat Cell Genet* **9**:359, 1983.
74. Qumsiyeh M, Valentine M, Suttle D: Localization of the gene for uridine monophosphate synthase to human chromosome region 3q13 by in situ hybridisation. *Genomics* **5**:160, 1989.
75. Berman P, Harley E: Orotate uptake and metabolism by human erythrocytes. *Adv Exp Biol Med A* **165**:367, 1984.
76. Young J, Jarvis S: Nucleoside transport in animal cells. *Biosci Rep* **3**:309, 1983.
77. Plagemann P, Wohlheuter R: Nucleoside transport in mammalian cells and interaction with intracellular metabolism, in Berne RM, Rall TW, Rubio R, (eds): *Regulatory Function of Adenosine*. The Hague, Martinus Nijhoff, 1983, p 179.
78. Darnowski J, Handschumacher R: Tissue uridine pools: Evidence in vivo of a concentrative mechanism for uridine uptake. *Cancer Res* **46**:3490, 1986.
79. Darnowski J, Holdridge C, Handschumacher R: Concentrative uridine transport by murine splenocytes: Kinetics, substrate specificity, and sodium dependency. *Cancer Res* **47**:2614, 1987.
80. Bronk J, Hastewell J: The transport of pyrimidines into tissue rings cut from rat small intestine. *J Physiol* **382**:475, 1987.
81. Martin D, Stolfi R, Sawyer R: Use of oral uridine as a substitute for parenteral uridine rescue of 5-fluorouracil therapy, with and without the uridine phosphorylase inhibitor 5-benzylacycloruridine. *Cancer Chemother Pharmacol* **24**:9, 1989.

82. Chan T, Markman M, Pfeifle C, Taetle R, Abramson I, Howell S: Uridine pharmacokinetics in cancer patients. *Cancer Chemother Pharmacol* **22**:83, 1988.
83. Darnowski J, Handschumacher R, Wiegand R, Goulette F, Calabresi P: Tissue-specific expansion of uridine pools in mice. Effects of benzylacyclouridine, dipyridamole and exogenous uridine. *Biochem Pharmacol* **41**:2301, 1991.
84. Taylor M, Kothari R, Holland G, Martinez-Valdez H, Zeige G: A comparison of purine and pyrimidine pools in Bloom's syndrome and normal cells. *Cancer Biochem Biophys* **7**:19, 1983.
85. Korte D, Haverkorte W, Van Gennip A, Roos D: Nucleotide profiles of normal human blood cells determined by high performance liquid chromatography. *Anal Biochem* **147**:197, 1985.
86. Losman M, Harley E: Evidence for compartmentation of uridine nucleotide pools in rat hepatoma cells. *Biochim Biophys Acta* **521**:762, 1978.
87. Rasenack J, Pausch J, Gerok W: De novo pyrimidine biosynthesis in isolated rat hepatocytes. *J Biol Chem* **260**:4145, 1985.
88. Tseng J, Gurpide E: Compartmentalisation of uridine and uridine 5′-monophosphate in rat liver slices. *J Biol Chem* **248**:5634, 1973.
89. Nuki G, Astrin K, Brenton D, Cruikshank M, Lever J, Seegmiller J: *Purine and pyrimidine nucleotides in some mutant human lymphoblasts*. Amsterdam, Elsevier, 1977, Purine and Pyrimindine Metabolism, Ciba Foundation Symposium 48 (New Series).
90. Fox I, Burk L, Planet G, Goren M, Kaminska J: Pyrimidine nucleotide biosynthesis. A study of normal and purine-enzyme deficient cells. *J Biol Chem* **253**:6794, 1978.
91. Pinsky L, Krooth R: Studies on the control of pyrimidine biosynthesis in human diploid cell strains, I effect of 6-azauridine on cellular phenotype. *Proc Natl Acad Sci U S A* **57**:925, 1967.
92. Krooth R, Lam G, Chen Kiang S: Oxipurinol and orotic aciduria: effect on the orotidine-5′-monophosphate decarboxylase activity of cultured human fibroblasts. *Cell* **3**:55, 1974.
93. Kelley W, Beardmore T: Allopurinol: Alteration of pyrimidine metabolism in man. *Science* **169**:388, 1970.
94. Beardmore T, Fox I, Kelley W: Effect of allopurinol on pyrimidine metabolism in the Lesch-Nyhan syndrome. *Lancet* **830**:93, 1970.
95. Beardmore T, Kelley W: Mechanism of allopurinol-mediated inhibition of pyrimidine biosynthesis. *J Lab Clin Med* **78**:696, 1971.
96. Grobner W, Zollner N: The influence of dietary purines and pyrimidines on human pyrimidine biosynthesis. *Klin Wochenschr* **61**:1191, 1983.
97. Hatfield P, Simmonds H, Cameron J, Jones A, Cadenhead A: Effects of allopurinol and oxonic acid on pyrimidine metabolism in the pig. *Adv Exp Med Biol B* **41**:637, 1974.
98. Fox R, Wood M, O'Sullivan W: Studies on the coordinate activity and lability of orotidylate phosphoribosyltransferase and decarboxylase in human erythrocytes, and the effect of allopurinol administration. *J Clin Invest* **50**:10050, 1971.
99. Beardmore T, Cashman J, Kelley W: Mechanism of allopurinol-mediated increase in pyrimidine metabolism in man. *J Clin Invest* **51**:1823, 1972.
100. Foster D, Lee C, O'Sullivan W: Allopurinol and enzymes of de novo pyrimidine biosynthesis. *Biochem Med* **7**:61, 1973.
101. Beardmore T, Kelley W: Effects of allopurinol and oxipurinol on pyrimidine biosynthesis in man. *Adv Exp Med Biol* **41**:609, 1974.
102. Becker M, Argubright K, Fox R, Seegmiller J: Oxypurinol-associated inhibition of pyrimidine synthesis in human lymphoblasts. *Mol Pharmacol* **10**:657, 1974.
103. Brown G, Fox R, O'Sullivan W: Alteration of quaternary structural behaviour of an hepatic orotate phosphoribosyltransferase-orotidine-5′-phosphate decarboxylase complex in rats following allopurinol therapy. *Biochem Pharmacol* **21**:2469, 1972.
104. Grobner W, Kelley W: Effect of allopurinol and its metabolic derivatives on the configuration of human orotate phosphoribosyltransferase and orotidine 5′-phosphate decarboxylase. *Biochem Pharmacol* **24**:379, 1975.
105. Reiter S, Zollner N, Braun S, Knedel M: Allopurinol-induced oroticaciduria in a xanthinuric patient not forming allopurinol. *Klin Wochenschr Suppl X* **65**:13, 1987.
106. Davies P, Simmonds H, Mulligan P: Orotidine accumulates in the erythrocytes of patients with renal failure or gout during allopurinol therapy. *Klin Wochenschr Suppl X* **65**:10, 1987.
107. Kelley W, Fox I, Beardmore T, Meade J: Allopurinol and oxipurinol: Alteration of purine and pyrimidine metabolism in cell culture. *Ann N Y Acad Sci* **179**:588, 1971.
108. Kelley W, Beardmore T, Fox I, Meade J: Effect of allopurinol and oxipurinol on pyrimidine synthesis in cultured human fibroblasts. *Biochem Pharmacol* **20**:1471, 1971.
109. Pasternak C, Handschumacher R: The biochemical activity of 6-azauridine: Interference with pyrimidine metabolism in transplantable mouse tumors. *J Biol Chem* **234**:2992, 1959.
110. Handschumacher R, Pasternak C: Inhibition of orotidylic acid decarboxylase, a primary site of carcinostasis by 6-azauracil. *Biochim Biophys Acta* **30**:451, 1958.
111. Handschumacher R: Orotidylic acid decarboxylase: Inhibition studies with azauridine 5′-phosphate. *J Biol Chem* **235**:2917, 1960.
112. Fallon H, Frei E, Block J, Seegmiller J: The uricosuria and orotic aciduria induced by 6-azauridine. *J Clin Invest* **40**:1906, 1961.
113. Fallon H, Frei E, Freireich E: Correlations of biochemical and clinical effects of 6-azauridine in patients with leukemia. *Am J Med* **33**:526, 1962.
114. Fallon H, Lotz M, Smith L: Congenital orotic aciduria: Demonstration of an enzyme defect in leukocytes and comparison with drug-induced orotic aciduria. *Blood* **20**:700, 1962.
115. Conn H, Creasey W, Calabresi P: Effect of 6-azauridine on plasma cell tumours of mice: Correlation of antitumour effect with inhibition of orotic acid metabolism. *Cancer Res* **27**:618, 1967.
116. Bruemmer N, Holland J, Sheehe P: Drug effects on a target metabolic pathway and on mouse tumour growth: Azauridine and decarboxylation of orotic acid-7-C14. *Cancer Res* **22**:113, 1962.
117. Roux J, Hoogenraad N, Kretchmer N: Biosynthesis of pyrimidine nucleotides in mouse salivary glands stimulated with isoproterenol. *J Biol Chem* **248**:1196, 1973.
118. Wells W, Gaines D, Koenig H: Studies of pyrimidine nucleotide metabolism in the central nervous system I metabolic effects and metabolism of 6-azauridine. *J Neurochem* **10**:709, 1963.
119. Pinsky L, Krooth R: Studies on the control of pyrimidine biosynthesis in human diploid cell strains, II. Effects of 5-azaorotic acid, barbituric acid and pyrimidine precursors on cellular phenotype. *Proc Natl Acad Sci U S A* **57**:1267, 1967.
120. Potvin B, Stern H, May S, Lam G, Krooth R: Inhibition by barbituric acid and its derivatives of the enzymes in rat brain which participate in the synthesis of pyrimidines ribotides. *Biochem Pharmacol* **27**:655, 1978.
121. Niedzwicki J, Iltzsch M, El Kouni M, Cha S: Structure-activity relationship of pyrimidine base analogs as ligands of orotate phosphoribosyltransferase. *Biochem Pharm* **33**:2383, 1984.
122. Ardalan B, Glazer R: An update on the biochemistry of 5-fluorouracil. *Cancer Treatment Rev* **8**:157, 1981.
123. Kessel D, Hall T, Peyes P: Metabolism of uracil and 5-fluorouracil in P388 murine leukemia cells. *Mol Pharmacol* **5**:481, 1969.
124. Krooth R: Molecular models for pharmacological tolerance and addiction. *Ann N Y Acad Sci* **179**:548, 1971.
125. Mulkins M, Heidelberger C: Isolation of fluoropyrimidine-resistant murine leukemic cell lines by one-step mutation and selection. *Cancer Res* **42**:956, 1982.
126. Ishii K, Green H: Lethality of cultured mammalian cells by interference with pyrimidine biosynthesis. *J Cell Sci* **13**:429, 1973.
127. Green H, Chan T-S: Pyrimidine starvation induced by adenosine in fibroblasts and lymphoid cells; role of adenosine deaminase. *Science* **182**:836, 1973.
128. Danks M, Scholar E: Regulation of phosphoribosylpyrophosphate synthase by purine and pyrimidine compounds and synthetic analogues in normal and leukemic white blood cells. *Biochem Pharmacol* **31**:1687, 1982.
129. Van Der Kraan P, Van Zandvoort P, De Abreu R, Van Baal J, Bakkeren J: Inhibition of lymphoid cell growth by adenine ribonucleotide accumulation. The role of phosphoribosylpyrophosphate-depletion induced pyrimidine starvation. *Biochim Biophys Acta* **927**:213, 1987.
130. Faller J, Palella T, Dean P, Fox I: Altered cell cycle distributions of cultured human lymphoblasts during cytotoxicity related to adenosine deaminase inhibition. *Metabolism* **33**:369, 1984.
131. Fallon H, Smith LJ, Graham J, Burnett C: A genetic study of hereditary orotic aciduria. *N Engl J Med* **270**:878, 1964.
132. Huguley C, Bain J, Rivers S, Scoggins R: Refractory megaloblastic anaemia associated with excretion of orotic acid. *Blood* **14**:615, 1959.
133. Smith LJ, Sullivan M, Huguley C: Pyrimidine metabolism in man. IV The enzymatic defect of orotic aciduria. *J Clin Invest* **40**:656, 1961.
134. Neimann N, Najean Y, Scialom C, Boulard M, Pierson M, Bernard J: Étude d'un cas d'anemie megaloblastique de l'enfant avec excretion anormale d'acide orotique. *Nouv Rev Fr Hematol* **5**:445, 1963.

135. Wada Y, Nishimura Y, Tanabu M, Yoshimura Y, Iinuma K, Yoshida T, Arakawa T: Hypouricemic, mentally retarded infant with a defect of 5-phosphoribosyl-1-pyrophosphate synthetase of erythrocytes. *Tohoku J Exp Med* **113**:149, 1974.
136. Wada Y: Personal communication, 1986.
137. Girot R, Durandy A, Perignon J-L, Griscelli C: Hereditary orotic aciduria: A defect of pyrimidine metabolism with cellular immunodeficiency. *Birth Def Orig Art Series* **19**:313, 1983.
138. Smith LJ, Gilmour L: Determination of urinary carbamoylaspartate and dihydro-orotate in normal subjects and in patients with hereditary orotic aciduria. *J Lab Clin Med* **86**:1047, 1975.
139. Alvarado C, Livingstone L, Jones M, Ravielle A, McKolanis J, Elsas L: Uridine-responsive hypogammaglobulinemia and congenital heart disease in a patient with hereditary orotic aciduria. *J Pediatr* **113**:867, 1988.
140. Yazaki M, Okajima K, Suchi M, Morishita H, Wada Y: Increase of protein synthesis by uridine supplement in lectin-stimulated peripheral blood lymphocytes and EB virus-transformed B cell line of hereditary orotic aciduria type I. *Tohoku J Exp Med* **153**:189, 1987.
141. Fessas P, Papadakis D, Rombos Y, Tassiopoulos T: Hereditary orotic aciduria (uridine monophosphate synthase deficiency) in an adult: The broadening spectrum of a rare disorder, in Bartsocas C, Loukopoulos D (eds): *Genetics of Hematological Disorders*. New York, Hemisphere, 1992, p 103.
142. Price R, Wilson R: Personal Communication, 1992.
143. Young S: Personal communication, 1992.
144. Bordelon J: Personal communication, 1992.
145. Yu J: Personal communication, 1992.
146. Alvarado C: Personal communication, 1992.
147. McLeod J: Personal communication, 1992.
148. Becroft D, Phillips L: Hereditary orotic aciduria and megaloblastic anaemia: A second case with response to uridine. *BMJ* **1**:547, 1965.
149. Becroft D, Webster D, Simmonds H, Fairbanks L, Wilson J, Phillips L: Hereditary orotic aciduria: Further biochemistry. *Adv Exp Med Biol* **195**:67, 1986.
150. Tubergen D, Krooth R, Heyn R: Hereditary orotic aciduria with normal growth and development. *Am J Dis Child* **118**:864, 1969.
151. Becroft D, Phillips L, Webster D, Wilson J: Absence of immune deficiency in hereditary orotic aciduria. *N Engl J Med* **310**:1333, 1984.
152. Howell R, Klinenberg J, Krooth R: Enzyme studies on diploid cell strains developed from patients with hereditary orotic aciduria. *J Hopkins Med J* **120**:81, 1967.
153. Wuu K-D, Krooth R: Dihydroorotic acid dehydrogenase activity of human diploid cell strains. *Science* **160**:539, 1968.
154. Smith LJ, Huguley CJ, Bain J: Hereditary orotic aciduria, in Stanbury J, Wyngaarden J, Frederickson D, (eds): *The Metabolic Basis of Inherited Disease*, 2d ed. New York, McGraw-Hill, 1966, p 739.
155. Simmonds H, Webster D, Becroft D, Potter C: Purine and pyrimidine metabolism in hereditary orotic aciduria: some unexpected effects of allopurinol. *Eur J Clin Invest* **10**:333, 1980.
156. Webster D, Simmonds H, Potter C, Becroft D: Purine and pyrimidine metabolism in hereditary orotic aciduria during a 15-year followup study. *Adv Exp Med Biol* **122**:203, 1980.
157. Girot R, Hamet M, Perignon J-L, Guesnu M, Fox R, Cartier P, Durnady A, et al: Cellular immune deficiency in two siblings with hereditary orotic aciduria. *N Engl J Med* **308**:700, 1983.
158. Haggard ME, Lockhart LH: Megaloblastic anemia and orotic aciduria. A hereditary disorder of pyrimidine metabolism responsive to uridine. *Am J Dis Child* **113**:733, 1967.
159. Chanarin I: *The Megaloblastic Anemias*, 2d ed. Oxford, Blackwell Scientific, 1979.
160. Cooper B, Rosenblatt D, Whitehead V: Megaloblastic anemia, in Nathan D, Oski F (eds): *Hematology of Infancy and Childhood*, 4th ed. Philadelphia, WB Saunders, 1993, p 354.
161. Page T, Nyhan W, Yu A, Yu J: A syndrome of megaloblastic anemia, immunodeficiency and excessive nucleotide degradation. *Int J Pur Pyr Res* **2(Suppl 1)**:74, 1991.
162. Shin Y, Reiter S, Zelger O, Brunstler I, V. Rucker A: Orotic aciduria, homocystinuria, formiminoglutamic aciduria and megaloblastosis associated with the formiminotransferase/cyclodeaminase deficiency. *Adv Exp Med Biol* **195**:71, 1986.
163. Rogers L, Warford L, Patterson B, Porter F: Hereditary orotic aciduria. I. A new case with family studies. *Pediatrics* **42**:415, 1968.
164. Fox R, O'Sullivan W, Firkin B: Orotic aciduria, differing enzyme patterns. *Am J Med* **47**:332, 1969.
165. Lahey M: Personal communication, 1987.
166. Mcclard R, Black M, Jones M, Young S, Berkowitz G: Neonatal diagnosis of orotic aciduria: An experience with one family. *J Pediatr* **102**:85, 1983.
167. Ohba S, Kidouchi K, Toyama J, Oda T, Tsuboi T, Ichiki T, Sobajima H, et al: Quantitative analysis of pyrimidines for the prenatal diagnosis of hereditary orotic aciduria. *J Inherit Metab Dis* **16**:872, 1993.
168. Soutter J, Yu J, Lovric A, Stapleton T: Hereditary orotic aciduria. *Aust Paediatr J* **6**:47, 1970.
169. Girot R, Durandy A, Perignon J-L, Griscelli C: Absence of immune deficiency in hereditary orotic aciduria. *N Engl J Med* **310**:1334, 1984.
170. Reineke R: Current concepts in opthalmology — Strabismus. *N Engl J Med* **300**:1139, 1979.
171. Insley J: The heritability of congenital heart disease. *BMJ* **294**:662, 1987.
172. Kenna A, Smithells R, Fielding D: Congenital heart disease in Liverpool: 1960–1969. *QJM* **44**:17, 1975.
173. Reid C, Hall J, Anderson C, Bocian M, Carey J, Costa, Curry C, et al: Association of amyoplasia with gastroschisis, bowel atresia, and defect of muscular layer of the trunk. *Am J Med Genet* **24**:701, 1986.
174. Ogier H: Personal communication, 1992.
175. Price R, Wilson R, Simmonds H: Personal communication, 1992.
176. Etzioni A: Hypogammaglobulinemia in orotic aciduria. *J Pediatr* **115**:332, 1989.
177. Alvarado C, McKolanis J: Hypogammaglobulinemia in orotic aciduria. *J Pediatr* **115**:333, 1989.
178. Sumi S, Suchi M, Kidouchi K, Morishita H, Ohba S, Wada Y: Pyrimidine metabolism in hereditary orotic aciduria. *J Inherit Metab Dis* **20**:104, 1997.
179. Heyn R: Personal communication, 1992.
180. Tubergen D: Personal communication, 1992.
181. Bensen J, Nelson L, Pettenati M, Block S, Brusilow S, Livingstone L, Burton B: First report of management and outcome of pregnancies associated with hereditary orotic aciduria. *Am J Med Genet* **41**:426, 1991.
182. Peters J, Van Groeningen C, Nadal J, Leyva A, Laurensse E, Pinedo H: Metabolism, excretion and bioavailability of orally administered uridine in man. *Klin Wochenschr Suppl X* **65**:15, 1987.
183. Van Groeningen C, Peters G, Leyva A, Laurensse E, Pinedo H: Reversal of 5-fluorouracil induced myelosuppression by prolonged administration of high-dose uridine. *J Natl Cancer Inst* **81**:157, 1989.
184. Van Groeningen C, Peters G, Nadal J, Laurensse E, Pinedo H: Clinical and pharmacological study of orally administered uridine. *J Natl Cancer Inst* **83**:437, 1991.
185. Klubes P, Geffen D, Cysyk R: Comparison of the bioavailability of uridine in mice after either oral or parenteral administration. *Cancer Chemother Pharmacol* **17**:236, 1987.
186. Leyva A, Van Groeningen C, Kraal I, Peters J, Lankelma J, Pinedo H: Phase I and pharmacokinetic studies of high-dose uridine intended for rescue from 5-fluorouracil toxicity. *Cancer Res* **44**:5928, 1984.
187. Weissman S, Lewis M, Karon M: The metabolism of isotopically labelled uracil and uridine in man. *Metabolism* **12**:60, 1963.
188. Webster D, Simmonds H, Becroft D: Unpublished observations, 1988.
189. Rogers LE, Porter F: Hereditary orotic aciduria II: A urinary screening test. *Pediatrics* **42**:423, 1968.
190. Harris M, Oberholzer V: Conditions affecting the colorimetry of orotic acid and orotidine in urine. *Clin Chem* **26**:473, 1980.
191. Kamoun P, Coude M, Deprun C, Rabier D: Source of error in the assay of urinary orotic acid. *Clin Chem* **33**:713, 1987.
192. Jeevanandam M, Shoemaker J, Horowitz G, Lowry S, Brennan M: Orotic acid excretion during starving and after refeeding in normal men. *Metabolism* **34**:325, 1985.
193. Glasgow A: A new method for measuring urinary orotic acid. *Am J Clin Path* **77**:452, 1982.
194. Van Gennip A, Van Bree-Blom E, Grift J, De Bree P, Wadman S: Urinary purines and pyrimidines in patients with hyperammonemia of various origins. *Clin Chim Acta* **104**:227, 1980.
195. Kidouchi K, Ohba S, Nakamura C, Katoh T, Kibe T, Wada Y: Automated quantitative analysis for orotidine and uracil/thymine in urine. *Int J Pur Pyr Res* **2(Suppl1)**:58, 1992.
196. Jakobs C, Sweetman L, Nyhan W, Gruenke L, Craig J, Wadman S: Stable isotope dilution analysis of orotic acid and uracil in amniotic fluid. *Clin Chim Acta* **143**:123, 1984.
197. McCann M, Thompson M, Gueron I, Tuchman M: Quantitation of orotic acid in dried filter-paper urine samples by stable isotope dilution. *Clin Chem* **41(5)**:739, 1995.

198. Carpenter K, Potter M, Hammond J, Wilcken B: Benign persistent orotic aciduria and the possibility of misdiagnosis of ornithine carbamoyltransferase deficiency. *J Inherit Metab Dis* **20**:354, 1997.
199. Allen M, Glasgow M: Urinary orotic acid in pregnancy. *Am J Clin Pathol* **77**:452, 1982.
200. Sevcik J, Adam T, Sazel V: A rapid and simple screening method for detection of orotic aciduria by capillary zone electrophoresis. *Clin Chim Acta* **259**:73, 1997.
201. Glasgow A, Larsen J: Urinary orotic acid in pregnancy. *Am J Obstet Gynecol* **149**:464, 1984.
202. Visek W, Long D, Wellik D, Nelson R: Urinary orotic acid (UOA) compared to other urinary metabolites for adult volunteers. *Fed Proc* **39**:1116, 1980.
203. Jeevanandam M, Hsu Y-C, Ramais L, Schiller W: Mild orotic aciduria and uricosuria in severe trauma victims. *Am J Clin Nutr* **53**:1242, 1991.
204. Tax W, Veerkamp J, Schretlen E: The urinary excretion of orotic acid and orotidine, measured by isotope dilution assay. *Clin Chim Acta* **90**:217, 1978.
205. Ohba S, Kidouchi K, Nakamura C, Katoh T, Kobayashi M, Wada Y: Reference values of orotic acid, uracil and pseuduridine in urine. *Int J Pur Pyr Res* **2(Suppl 1)**:73, 1992.
206. Sumi S, Kidouchi K, Imadea M, Asai M, Ito T, Wada Y: Urinary Orotic acid in healthy adults and patients with various diseases. *Clin Chim Acta* **266**:195, 1997.
207. Visek W, Shoemaker J: Orotic acid, arginine and hepatotoxicity. *J Am Coll Nutr* **5**:153, 1986.
208. Fox R, Wood M, Royse-Smith D, O'Sullivan W: Hereditary orotic aciduria: Types I and II. *Am J Med* **55**:791, 1973.
209. Bachmann C, Colombo J: Diagnostic value of orotic acid in heritable disorders of the urea cycle and hyperammonemia due to organic acidurias. *Eur J Paediatr* **134**:109, 1980.
210. Becroft D, Barry D, Webster D, Simmonds H: Failure of protein loading tests to identify heterozygosity for ornithine carbamoyltransferase deficiency. *J Inherit Metab Dis* **7**:157, 1984.
211. Hatchwell L, Milner J: Amino-acid induced orotic aciduria. *J Nutr* **108**:578, 1978.
212. Hauser E, Finkelstein J, Valle D, Brusilow S: Allopurinol-induced orotidinuria. A test for mutations at the ornithine carbamyltransferase locus in women. *N Engl J Med* **322**:1641, 1990.
213. Tuchman M, Knopman D, Shih V: Episodic hyperammonemia in adult siblings with hyperornithinemia, hyperammonemia and homocitrullinuria syndrome. *Arch Neurol* **47**:1134, 1990.
214. Thomas S, Oberholzer V, Wilson J, Hjelm M: The urea cycle in the Rett syndrome. *Brain Dev* **12**:93, 1990.
215. Boedeker D, Martens H: Urinary orotic acid excretion in sheep: Effects of nitrogen, glucose and arginine. *J Nutr* **120**:1001, 1990.
216. Alonso E, Rubio V: Orotic aciduria due to arginine deprivation: Changes in the levels of carbamoylphosphate and other urea cycle intermediates in mouse liver. *J Nutr* **119**:1188, 1989.
217. Carey G, Kime Z, Rogers Q, Morris J, Hargrove D, Buffington C, Brusilow S: An arginine deficient diet in humans does not evoke hyperammonemia or orotic aciduria. *J Nutr* **117**:1734, 1987.
218. Stene R, Spector R: Effect of a 400-kilocalorie carbohydrate diet on human plasma uridine and hypoxanthine concentrations. *Biochem Med Metab Biol* **38**:44, 1987.
219. Jeffers L, Dubow R, Zieve L, Reddy K, Livingston A, Neimark S, Viamonte M, et al: Hepatic encephalopathy and orotic aciduria associated with hepatocellular carcinoma in a noncirrhotic liver. *Hepatology* **8**:78, 1988.
220. Shoemaker J, Visek W: Orotic acid overproduction in experimental cirrhosis of rats. *Exp Mol Pathol* **50**:371, 1989.
221. Rajantie J: Orotic aciduria in lysinuric protein intolerance: dependence on urea cycle intermediates. *Pediatr Res* **15**:115, 1981.
222. Cohen A, Stahl G, Ammann A, Martin DJ: Orotic aciduria in two unrelated patients with inherited deficiencies of purine nucleoside phosphorylase deficiency. *J Clin Invest* **60**:491, 1977.
223. Simmonds H, Potter C, Sahota A, Cameron J, Webster D, Becroft D: Absence of orotic aciduria in adenosine deaminase deficiency and purine nucleoside phosphorylase deficiency. *Clin Exp Immunol* **34**:42, 1978.
224. Edwards N, Gelfand E, Biggar D, Fox I: Partial deficiency of purine nucleoside phosphorylase: studies of purine and pyrimidine metabolism. *J Lab Clin Med* **91**:736, 1978.
225. Mills G, Schmalsteig F, Newkirk K, Goldblum R: Cytosine and orotic acid in urine of immunodeficient children. *Clin Chem* **25**:419, 1979.
226. Wood M, O'Sullivan W: The orotic aciduria of pregnancy. *Am J Obstet Gynecol* **116**:57, 1973.
227. Webster D, Simmonds H, Barry D, Becroft D: Purine and pyrimidine metabolites in ornithine carbamoyltransferase deficiency. *J Inherit Metab Dis* **4**:27, 1981.
228. Wadman S, Beemer F, De Bree P, Duran M, Van Gennip A, Ketting D, Van Sprang F: New defects of pyrimidine metabolism. *Adv Exp Med Biol* **165**:109, 1984.
229. Karle J, Anderson L, Dietrick D, Cysyk R: Determination of serum and plasma uridine levels in mice rats and humans by high-pressure liquid chromatography. *Anal Biochem* **109**:41, 1980.
230. Chan T, Markman M, Cleary S, Howell S: Plasma uridine changes in cancer patients treated with the combination of dipyridamole and *N*-phosphonoacetyl-l-aspartate. *Cancer Res* **46**:3168, 1986.
231. De Abreu R, Bakkeren J, Braakhekke J, Gabreels F, Maas J, Sengers R: Dihyrothymine dehydrogenase deficiency in a family, leading to elevated levels of uracil and thymine. *Adv Exp Med Biol* **195**:77, 1986.
232. Parry T, Blackmore J: Serum "uracil + uridine" levels in pernicious anaemia. *Br J Haematol* **34**:567, 1976.
233. Yoshida S, Hirose S: Use of 4-bromomethyl-7-methoxycoumarin for derivatisation of pyrimidine compounds in serum analysed by high-performance liquid chromatography with fluorometric detection. *J Chromatog* **383**:61, 1986.
234. Harkness R, Lund R: Cerebrospinal fluid concentrations of hypoxanthine, xanthine, uridine and inosine: High concentrations of the ATP metabolite hypoxanthine after hypoxia. *J Clin Pathol* **36**:1, 1983.
235. Harkness R, Geirsson R, Mcfadyen I: Concentrations of hypoxanthine, xanthine, uridine and urate in amniotic fluid at caesarean section and the association of raised levels with prenatal risk factors and foetal distress. *Br J Obstet Gynaecol* **90**:815, 1983.
236. Delbarre F, Auscher C: Traitement de la goutte par l'acide uracil-6-carboxylique et ses derives. *Presse Med* **71**:11765, 1963.
237. Motyl T, Siwecka B, Kukulska W, Orzechowski A: Urinary excretion of purines in a sheep with experimental orotic aciduria. *J Vet Med A* **38**:198, 1991.
238. Zollner N, Grobner W: *Dietary feedback regulation of purine and pyrimidine biosynthesis in man.* Amsterdam, Elsevier, 1977, Purine and Pyrimidine Metabolism, Ciba Foundation Symposium 48.
239. Chung SH, Sloan DL: Enzymatic kinetic analyses that employ high performance liquid chromatography. Competition between orotate- and hypoxanthine/guanine phosphoribosyltransferase for a common substrate. *J Chromatog* **371**:71, 1986.
240. Fairbanks L, Duley J, Shores A, Simmonds H: HPLC assay of uridine monophosphate synthase (UMPS) activity in chorionic villus samples (CVS) and erythrocytes (RBC). *Int J Pur Pyr Res* **2(Suppl 1)**:44, 1992.
241. Shostak K, Christopherson R, Jones M: Direct spectrophotometric assays for orotate phosphoribosyltransferase and orotidylate decarboxylase. *Anal Biochem* **191**:365, 1990.
242. Fox I, Kelley W: Phosphoribosylpyrophosphate in man: Biochemical and clinical significance. *Ann Intern Med* **74**:424, 1971.
243. Beutler E, Blume K, Kaplan J, Lohr G, Ramot B, Valentine W: International committee for standardisation in haematology: Recommended methods for red cell enzyme analysis. *Br J Haematol* **35**:331, 1977.
244. Van Der Weyden M, Cooper M, Firkin B: Altered erythrocyte pyrimidine activity in vitamin B12 or folate deficiency. *Br J Haematol* **42**:85, 1979.
245. Borden M, Nyhan W, Bakay B: Increased activity of adenine phosphoribosyltransferase in erythrocytes of normal newborn infants. *Pediatr Res* **8**:31, 1974.
246. Teng Y-S, Chen S-H, Giblett E: Red cell uridine monophosphate kinase: effects of red cell aging on the activity of the two UMPK gene products. *Am J Hum Genet* **28**:138, 1986.
247. Konrad P, Valentine W, Paglia D: Enzymatic activities and glutathione content of erythrocytes in the newborn: Comparison with red cells of older normal subjects and those with comparitive reticulocytosis. *Acta Haemat* **48**:193, 1972.
248. Zielke H, Ozand P, Luddy R, Zinkham W, Schwartz A, Sevdalian D: Elevation of pyrimidine enzyme activities in the rbc of patients with congenital hypoplastic anemia and their parents. *Br J Haematol* **42**:381, 1979.
249. Glader B, Backer K: Comparative activity of erythrocyte adenosine deaminase and orotidine decarboxylase in Diamond-Blackfan anemia. *Am J Hematol* **23**:135, 1986.
250. Worthy T, Grobner W, Kelley W: Hereditary orotic aciduria: Evidence for a structural genê mutation. *Proc Nat Acad Sci U S A* **71**:3031, 1974.
251. Winkler J, Suttle D: Analysis of UMP synthase gene and mRNA structure in hereditary orotic aciduria fibroblasts. *Am J Hum Genet* **43**:86, 1988.

252. Perry M, Jones M: Orotic aciduria fibroblasts express a labile form of UMP synthase. *J Biol Chem* **264**:15522, 1989.
253. Suchi M, Mizuno H, Kawai Y, Tsuboi T, Sumi S, Okajima K, Hodgson M, et al: Molecular cloning of the human UMP synthase gene and characterisation of point mutations in two hereditary orotic aciduria families. *Am J Hum Genet* **60**:525, 1997.
254. Perry M, Livingston L: Unpublished data.
255. Reed R, Lin T, Suttle D: Unpublished observations.
256. Webster D, Becroft D, Suttle DP : Hereditary orotic aciduria and other disorders of pyrimidine metabolism, in Scriver CR, Beaudet AL, Sly WS, Valle D (eds): *The Molecular and Metabolic Bases of Inherited Disease*, 7th ed, vol II. New York, McGraw-Hill, 1995, p 1799.
257. Rodeck C, Patrick A, Pembrey M, Tzannatos C, Whitfield A: Fetal liver biopsy for prenatal diagnosis of ornithine carbamoyltransferase deficiency. *Lancet* **ii**:297, 1982.
258. O'Sullivan W: Orotic acid. *Aust N Z J Med* **3**:417, 1973.
259. Collipp P: Orotic acid, inosine and nucleotides in the treatment of degenerative retinal diseases: a double blind study. *Curr Ther Res* **41**:135, 1987.
260. Kelley W, Fox I, Wyngaarden J: Regulation of purine biosynthesis in cultured human cells I effects of orotic acid. *Biochim Biophys Acta* **215**:512, 1970.
261. Windmueller H, Van Euler L: Prevention of orotic acid induced fatty liver with allopurinol. *Proc Soc Exp Biol Med* **136**:98, 1971.
262. Vasudevan S, Laconi E, Rao PM, Rajalakshmi S, Sarma D: Perturbations of endogenous levels of orotic acid and carcinogenesis: Effect of an arginine-deficient diet and carbamyl aspartate on hematogenesis in the rat and the mouse. *Carcinogenesis* **15(11)**:2497, 1994.
263. Herbert V: Biology of disease. Megaloblastic anemias. *Lab Invest* **52**:3, 1985.
264. Weischel M, Clark B: Pyrimidine metabolism during restorative brain growth after neonatal undernutrition in the rat. *Pediatr Res* **11**:293, 1977.
265. Van Buren C, Kulkarni A, Schandle V, Rudolph F: The influence of dietary nucleotides on cell-mediated immunity. *Transplantataion* **36**:350, 1983.
266. Bhalla K, Grant S: Effect of deoxycytidine on the in vitro response of human leukemia cells too inhibitors of de novo pyrimidine biosynthesis. *Cancer Chemother Pharmacol* **19**:226, 1987.
267. Gutova M, Elis J, Raskova H: Teratogenic effect of 6-azauridine in rats. *Teratology* **4**:287, 1971.
268. Shanks R, Robinson J: Embryonic mortality attributed to inherited deficiency of uridine monophosphate synthase. *J Dairy Sci* **72**:3035, 1989.
269. Vojta M, Jirasek J: 6-Azauridine-induced changes of the trophoblast of early human pregnancy. *Clin Phamacol Ther* **7**:162, 1966.
270. Shanks R, Popp R, McCoy G, Nelson D, Robinson J: Identification of the homozygous recessive genotype for the deficiency of uridine monophosphate synthase in 35-day bovine embryos. *J Reprod Fertil* **94**:5, 1992.
271. Gurpide E, Tseng J, Escarcena L, Fahning M, Gibson C, Fehr P: Fetomaternal production and transfer of progesterone and uridine in sheep. *Am J Obstet Gynecol* **113**:21, 1972.
272. Lotz M, Fallon H, Smith LJ: Excretion of orotic acid and orotidine in heterozygotes of congenital orotic aciduria. *Nature* **197**:194, 1963.
273. Pang C, Law L, Mak Y, Shek C, Cheung K, Mak T, Lam C, et al: Biochemical investigation of young hospitalized Chinese children: results over a 7-year period. *Am J Med Genet* **72**:417, 1997.
274. Harden K, Robinson J: Deficiency of UMP synthase in dairy cattle, a model for hereditary orotic aciduria. *J Inherit Metab Dis* **10**:201, 1987.
275. Shanks D, Robinson J: Deficiency of uridine monophosphate synthase among Holstein cattle. *Cornell Vet* **80**:119, 1990.
276. Paglia D, Valentine W: Characteristics of a pyrimidine-specific 5′-nucleotidase in human erythrocytes. *J Biol Chem* **250**:7973, 1975.
277. Rosa R, Rochant H, Dreyfus B, Valentin C, Rosa J: Electrophoretic and kinetic studies of human erythrocytes deficient in pyrimidine 5′-nucleotidase. *Hum Genet* **38**:209, 1977.
278. Rosa R, Valentin C, Rosa J: Electrophoretic characterisation of pyrimidine 5′-nucleotidase of human erythrocytes and its distinction from acid phosphatase. *Clin Chim Acta* **79**:115, 1977.
279. Torrance J, West C, Beutler E: A simple rapid radiometric assay for pyrimidine 5′-nucleotidase. *J Lab Clin Med* **90**:563, 1977.
280. Paglia D, Valentine W, Keitt A, Brockway R, Nakatani M: Pyrimidine nucleotidase deficiency with active dephosphorylation of dTMP: Evidence for existence of thymidine nucleotidase in human erythrocytes. *Blood* **62**:1147, 1983.
281. Swallow M, Aziz I, Hopkinson D, Miwa S: Analysis of human erythrocyte 5′-nucleotidases in healthy individuals and a patient deficient in pyrimidine 5′-nucleotidase. *Ann Hum Genet* **47**:19, 1983.
282. Wilson D, Swallow D, Povey S: Assignment of the gene for uridine 5′-monophosphate phosphohydrolase (UMPH2) to the long arm of chromosome 17. *Ann Hum Genet* **50**:223, 1986.
283. Paglia D, Valentine W, Brockway R: Identification of thymidine nucleotidase and deoxyribonucleotidase activities among normal isozymes of 5′-nucleotidase in human erythrocytes. *Proc Natl Acad Sci U S A* **81**:588, 1984.
284. Hopkinson D, Swallow D, Turner V, Aziz I: Evidence for a distinct deoxypyrimidine 5′-nucleotidase in human tissues. *Adv Exp Med Biol* **165**:535, 1984.
285. Oda T, Nagao M, Shirono K, Kagimoto T, Takatsuki K: Isozymes of human erythrocyte pyrimidine 5′-nucleotidase. *J Lab Clin Med* **106**:646, 1985.
286. El Kouni M, Cha S: Isolation and partial characterization of a 5′-nucleotidase specific for orotidine-5′-monophosphate. *Proc Natl Acad Sci U S A* **79**:1037, 1982.
287. Baron M, Luzio J: The synthesis and turnover of 5′-nucleotidase in primary cultured hepatocytes. *Biochim Biophys Acta* **927**:81, 1987.
288. Hirono A, Fujii H, Miyajima H, Kawakatsu T, Hiyoshi Y, Miwa S: Three families with hereditary hemolytic anemia and pyrimidine 5′-nucleotidase deficiency: electrophoretic and kinetic studies. *Clin Chim Acta* **130**:189, 1983.
289. Amici A, Emanuelli M, Magni G, Rafaelli N, Ruggieri S: Pyrimidine nucleotidases from human erythrocyte possess phosphotransferase activities specific for pyrimidine nucleotides. *FEBS Lett* **419**:263, 1997.
290. Valentine W, Fink K, Paglia D, Harris S, Adams W: Hereditary hemolytic anemia with human erythrocyte pyrimidine 5′-nucleotidase deficiency. *J Clin Invest* **54**:866, 1974.
291. Hansen T, Siep M, De Verdier C-H, Ericson A: Erythrocyte pyrimidine 5′-nucleotidase deficiency. Report of 2 new cases, with a review of the literature. *Scand J Hematol* **31**:122, 1983.
292. Paglia D, Fink K, Valentine W: Additional data from two kindreds with genetically-induced deficiencies of erythrocyte pyrimidine nucleotidase. *Acta Haematol* **63**:262, 1980.
293. Rechavi G, Vonsover A, Manor Y, Mileguir F, Shpilberg O, Kende G, Brok-Simoni F, et al: Aplastic crisis due to human B-19 parvovirus infection in red cell pyrimidine-5′-nucleotidase deficiency. *Acta Hematol (Basel)* **82**:46, 1989.
294. International Committee for Standardisation in Hematology: Recommended screening test for pyrimidine-5′-nucleotidase deficiency. *Clin Lab Haematol* **11**:55, 1989.
295. Harley E, Berman P: Diagnostic and therapeutic approaches in pyrimidine 5′-nucleotidase deficiency. *Adv Exp Med Biol* **165**:1003, 1984.
296. Adair C, Elder E, Lappin T, Bridges J, Nelson M: Red cell pyrimidine 5′-nucleotidase deficiency: Determination of nucleotidase activity and nucleotide content using HPLC. *Clin Chim Acta* **171**:75, 1988.
297. Kagimoto T, Shirono K, Higaki T, Oda T, Matsuzaki H, Nagata K, Nakaji T, et al: Detection of pyrimidine 5′-nucleotidase deficiency using 1H or 31P nuclear magnetic resonance. *Experentia* **42**:69, 1986.
298. Torrance J, Whittaker D, Jenkins T: Erythrocyte pyrimidine 5′-nucleotidase. *Br J Haematol* **45**:585, 1980.
299. Buc H, Kaplan J-C: A radioassay for pyrimidine-5′-nucleotidase activity. *Clin Chim Acta* **85**:193, 1978.
300. Ellims P, Bailey L, Van Der Weyden M: An improved method for the determination of human erythrocyte pyrimidine 5′-nucleotidase activity. *Clin Chim Acta* **88**:99, 1978.
301. Torrance J, Karabus C, Shnier M, Meltzer M, Katz J, Jenkins T: Haemolytic anaemia due to erythrocyte pyrimidine 5′-nucleotidase deficiency. Report of the first South African family. *S Afr Med J* **671**:243, 1977.
302. Zerez C, Tanaka K: A continuous spectrophotometric assay for pyrimidine 5′-nucleotidase. *Anal Biochem* **151**:282, 1985.
303. Cook L, Kubitschek C, Stohs S, Angle C: Erythrocyte pyrimidine 5′-nucleotidase and deoxynucleotidase isozymes. Metallosensitivity and kinetics. *Drug Chem Toxicol* **11**:195, 1988.
304. De Korte D, Van Doorn C, Sijstermans J, Van Gennip A, Roos D: Deficiency of pyrimidine 5′-nucleotidase in human leukocytes. *J Inherit Metab Dis* **12**:267, 1989.
305. Hopkinson D, Swallow D, Marinaki A, Harley E: Pyrimidine 5′-nucleotidase activity in normal and deficient human lymphoblastoid cells. *J Inherit Metab Dis* **13**:701, 1990.

306. Harley E, Heaton A, Wicomb W: Pyrimidine metabolism in hereditary erythrocyte pyrimidine 5′-nucleotidase deficiency. *Metabolism* **27**:1743, 1978.
307. Torrance J, Whittaker D: Distribution of erythrocyte nucleotides in pyrimidine 5′-nucleotidase deficiency. *Br J Haematol* **43**:423, 1979.
308. Swanson M, Markin R, Stohs S, Angle C: Identification of cytidine diphosphodiesters in erythrocytes from a patient with pyrimidine nucleotidase deficiency. *Blood* **63**:665, 1984.
309. Lachant N, Zerez C, Tanaka K: Pyrimidine nucleoside monophosphate hyperactivity in hereditary pyrimidine 5′-nucleotidase deficiency. *Br J Haematol* **66**:91, 1987.
310. Harley E, Zetler P, Neal S: Kinetics and compartmentation of erythrocyte pyrimidine metabolism. *Adv Exp Med Biol* **122**:217, 1980.
311. Oda E, Oda S, Tomoda A, Lachant N, Tanaka K: Hemolytic anemia in hereditary pyrimidine 5′-nucleotidase deficiency. II. Effect of pyrimidine nucleotides and their derivatives on glycolytic and pentose phosphate shunt enzyme activity. *Clin Chim Acta* **141**:93, 1984.
312. David O, Ramenghi U, Camaschella C, Vota M, Comino L, Pescarmona G, Nicola P: Inhibition of hexose monophosphate shunt in young erythrocytes by pyrimidine nucleotides in hereditary pyrimidine 5′-nucleotidase deficiency. *Eur J Haematol* **47**:48, 1991.
313. Lachant N, Tanaka K: Red cell metabolism in hereditary pyrimidine 5′-nucleotidase deficiency: Effect of magnesium. *Br J Haematol* **63**:615, 1986.
314. Harley E, Sacks S, Berman P, Cohen L, Simmonds H, Fairbanks L, Black D: Source and fate of circulating pyrimidines. *Adv Exp Med Biol* **195**:109, 1986.
315. Lachant N, Zerez C, Tanaka K: Pyrimidine nucleotides impair phosphoribosylpyrophosphate (PRPP) synthetase subunit aggregation by sequestering magnesium. A mechanism for decreased PRPP synthetase activity in hereditary erythrocyte pyrimidine 5′-nucleotidase deficiency. *Biochim Biophys Acta* **994**:81, 1989.
316. Paglia D, Valentine W, Nakatani M, Rauth B: Selective accumulation of CDP-choline as an isolated erythrocyte defect in chronic hemolysis. *Proc Natl Acad Sci U S A* **80**:3081, 1983.
317. Laurence A, Duley J, Simmonds H, Layton M, Rees D: Characteristic changes in erythrocyte nucleotides in hemolytic anemia with basophilic stippling of differing aetiology. *Cell Mol Biol Lett* **4**:406, 1999.
318. Rees D, Duley J, Simmonds H, Wonke B, Thein S, Clegg J, Weatherall D: Interaction of hemoglobin E and pyrimidine 5′-nucleotidase deficiency. *Blood* **88**:2761, 1996.
319. Vives-Corrons J, Montserrat-Costa E, Rozman C: Hereditary hemolytic anemia with erythrocyte pyrimidine 5′-nucleotidase deficiency in Spain. Clinical, biological and familial studies. *Hum Genet* **34**:285, 1976.
320. Ozsoylu S, Gurgey A: A case of hemolytic anaemia due to erythrocyte pyrimidine 5′-nucleotidase deficiency. *Acta Haematol* **66**:56, 1981.
321. Fujii H, Nakashima K, Miwa S, Nomura K: Electrophoretic and kinetic studies of a mutant red cell pyrimidine 5′-nucleotidase. *Clin Chim Acta* **95**:98, 1979.
322. Paglia D, Valentine W, Dahlgren J: Effects of low-level lead exposure on pyrimidine 5′-nucleotidase and other erythrocyte enzymes. *J Clin Invest* **56**:1164, 1975.
323. Valentine W, Paglia D, Fink K, Madokoro G: Lead poisoning. Association with hemolytic anemia, basophilic stippling, erythrocyte pyrimidine 5′-nucleotidase deficiency and intraerythrocytic accumulation of pyrimidines. *J Clin Invest* **58**:926, 1976.
324. Paglia D, Valentine W, Fink K: Lead poisoning. Further observations on erythrocyte pyrimidine nucleotidase deficiency and intracellular accumulation of pyrimidine nucleotides. *J Clin Invest* **60**:1362, 1977.
325. Lieberman J, Gordon-Smith E: Red cell pyrimidine 5′-nucleotidase and glutathione in myeloproliferative and lymphoproliferative disorders. *Br J Haematol* **44**:425, 1980.
326. David O, Vota M, Piga A, Ramenghi U, Bosia A, Pescarmona G: Pyrimidine 5′-nucleotidase acquired deficiency in β-thalassemia: Involvement of enzyme-SH groups in the inactivation process. *Acta Haematol (Basel)* **82**:69, 1989.
327. David O, Sacchetti L, Vota M, Comino L, Pescarmona G: Pyrimidine 5′-nucleotidase and oxidative damage in red blood cells transfused to B-thalassemic children. *Haematologica* **75**:313, 1990.
328. Vives-Corrons J, Pujades M, Colomer D: Pyrimidine 5′-nucleotidase acquired deficiency in β-thalassemia: Involvement of enzyme-SH groups in the inactivation process. *Acta Haematol (Basel)* **83**:215, 1990.
329. Page T, Yu A, Fontanesi J, Nyhan W: Developmental disorder associated with increased cellular nucleotidase activity. *Proc Natl Acad Sci U S A* **94**:11601, 1997.
330. Nishono I, Spinazolla A, Hirano M: Thymidine phosphorylase gene mutations in MNGIE, a human mitochondrial disorder. *Science* **283**:689, 1999.
331. Van Gennip A, Abeling N, Vreken P, Van Kuilenburg A: Inborn errors of pyrimidine degradation: Clinical, biochemical and molecular aspects. *J Inherit Metab Dis* **20**:203, 1997.
332. Van Kuilenburg A, Van Lenthe H, Wanders R, Van Gennip A: Subcellular localisation of dihydropyrimidine dehydrogenase. *Biol Chem* **378**:1047, 1997.
333. Campbell L: Reductive degradation of pyrimidines. III Purification and properties of dihydrouracil dehydrogenase. *J Biol Chem* **227**:693, 1957.
334. Shiotani T, Weber G: Purification and properties of dihydrothymine dehydrogenase from rat liver. *J Biol Chem* **256**:219, 1981.
335. Fujimoto S, Matsuda K, Kikugama M, Kameko M, Tamak N: Effect of vitamin B2 deficiency on rat liver dihydropyrimidine dehydrogenase activity. *J Nutr Sci Vitaminol (Tokyo)* **37**:89, 1991.
336. Podschun B, Wahler G, Schnackerz K: Purification and characterisation of dihydropyrimidine dehydrogenase from pig liver. *Eur J Biochem* **185**:219, 1989.
337. Porter D, Chestnut W, Taylor L, Merrill B, Spector T: Inactivation of dihydropyrimidine dehydrogenase by 5-iodouracil. *J Biol Chem* **266**:19988, 1991.
338. Sanna Y, Holzed M, Schmike R: Studies of a mutation affecting pyrimidine degradation in inbred mice. *J Biol Chem* **245**:56, 1970.
339. Lu Z, Zhang R, Diasio R: Purification and characterisation of dihydropyrimidine dehydrogenase from human liver. *J Biol Chem* **267**:17102, 1992.
340. Rosenbaum K, Schaffrath B, Hagen W, Jahnke K, Gonzales F, Cook P, Schnackerz K: Purification, characterization and kinetics of porcine recombinant dehydrogenase. *Protein Expr Purif* **10**:185, 1997.
341. Podschun B, Cook P, Schnackerz K: Kinetic Mechanism of dihydropyrimidine dehydrogenase from pig liver. *J Biol Chem* **265**: 12966, 1990.
342. Potter V, Potit H, Ono T, Morris H: The comparative enzymology and cell origin of rat hepatoma. I. Deoxycytidylate deaminase and thymine degradation. *Cancer Res* **20**:1255, 1960.
343. Queener S, Morris H, Weber G: Dihyourical dehydrogenase activity in normal, differentiating, and regenerating liver and in hepatomas. *Cancer Res* **31**:1004, 1971.
344. Podschun B, Jahnke K, Schnackerz K, Cook P: Acid base catalytic mechanism of the dihydropyrimidine dehydrogenase from pH studies. *J Biol Chem* **268**:3407, 1993.
345. Tuchman M, Stoeckeler J, Kiang D, O'Dea R, Ramnaraine M, Mirken B: Familial pyridinaemia and pyrimidinuria associated with severe fluorouracil toxicity. *N Engl J Med* **313**:245, 1985.
346. Yokota H, Fernandez-Salguero P, Furuya H, Lin K, McBride O, Podschun B, Schnackerz K, et al: cDNA cloning and chromosome mapping of human dihydropyrimidine dehydrogenase, an enzyme associated with 5-fluorouracil toxicity and congenital thymine uraciluria. *J Biol Chem* **269**:23192, 1994.
347. Albin N, Johnson M, Diasio R: cDNA cloning of bovine liver dihydropyrimidine dehydrogenase. *DNA Seq* **6**:243, 1996.
348. Wei X, Elizondo G, Sapone A, McLeod H, Raunio H, Fernandez-Salguero P, Gonzalez F: Characterisation of the human dihydropyrimidine dehydrogenase gene. *Genomics* **51**:391, 1998.
349. Takai S, Fernandez-Salguero P, Kimura S, Gonzalez F, Yamada K: Assignment of the human dihydropyrimidine dehydrogenase gene (DPYD) to chromosome region 1p22 by fluorescence in situ hybridisation. *Genomics* **24**:613, 1994.
350. Meinsma R, Fernandez-Salguero P, Van Kuilenburg A, Van Gennip A, Gonzalez F: Human polymorphism in drug metabolism: Mutation in the dihydropyrimidine dehydrogenase gene results in exon skipping and thymine uraciluria. *DNA Cell Biol* **14**:1, 1995.
351. Vreken P, Van Kuilenburg A, Meinsma R, Smit G, Bakker H, De Abreu R, Van Gennip A: A point mutation in an invariant splice donor site leads to exon skipping in two unrelated Dutch patients with dihydropyrimidine dehydrogenase deficiency. *J Inherit Metab Dis* **19**:645, 1996.
352. Vreken P, Van Kuilenburg A, Meinsma R, De Abreu R, Van Gennip A: Identification of a four-base deletion (delTCAT296-299) in the dihydropyrimidine dehydrogenase gene with variable clinical expression. *Hum Genet* **100**:263, 1997.

353. Vreken P, Van Kuilenburg A, Meinsma R, Van Gennip A: Identification of novel point mutations in the dihydropyrimidine dehydrogenase gene. *J Inherit Metab Dis* **20**:335, 1997.
354. Vreken P, van Kuilenburg A, Meinsma R, Van Gennip A: Dihydropyrimidine dehydrogenase (DPD) deficiency: Identification and expression of missense mutations C29R, R886H and R235W. *Hum Genet* **101**:333, 1997.
355. Vreken P, Van Kuilenburg A, Meinsma R, Beemer F, Duran M, Van Gennip A: Dihydropyrimidine dehydrogenase deficiency; a novel mutation and expression of missense mutations in *E. coli*. *J Inherit Metab Dis* **21**:276, 1998.
356. Van Gennip A, Van Lenthe H, Abeling N, Bakker H, Van Kuilenburg A: Combined deficiencies of NADPH- and NADH-dependent dihydropyrimidine dehydrogenases, a new finding in a family with thymine-uraciluria. *J Inherit Metab Dis* **18**:185, 1995.
357. Van Kuilenburg A, Vreken P, Abeling N, Bakker H, Meinsma R, Van Lenthe H et al: Genotype and phenotype in patients with dihydropyrimidine dehydrogenase deficiency. *Hum Genet* **104**:1, 1999.
358. Van Gennip A, Abeling N, Stroomer A, Van Lenthe H, Bakker H: Clinical and biochemical findings in six patients with pyrimidine degradation defects. *J Inherit Metab Dis* **17**:130, 1994.
359. Henderson M, Ward K, Simmonds H, Duley J, Davies P: Dihydropyrimidines deficiency presenting in infancy with severe developmental delay. *J Inherit Metab Dis* **16**:574, 1993.
360. Fernandez-Salguero P, Sapone A, Wei X, Holt J, Jones S, Idle J, Gonzalez F: Lack of correlation between phenotype and genotype for the polymorphically expressed dihydropyrimidine dehydrogenase in a family of Pakistani origin. *Pharmacogenetics* **7**:161, 1997.
361. Diasio R, Beavers T, Carpenter J: Familial deficiency of dihydropyrimidine dehydrogenase. *J Clin Invest* **81**:47, 1988.
362. Harris B, Carpenter J, Diasio R: Severe 5-fluorouracil toxicity secondary to dihydropyrimidine dehydrogenase deficiency: A potentially more common pharmacogenetic syndrome. *Cancer* **68**:499, 1991.
363. Fleming R, Milano G, Gaspard M, Bargnoux P, Thyss A, Plagne R, Renee M, et al: Dihydropyrimidine dehydrogenase activity in cancer patients. *Eur J Cancer* **29A**:740, 1993.
364. Houyau P, Gay C, Chatelut E, Canal P, Roche H, Milano G: Severe fluorouracil toxicity in a patient with dihydropyrimidine dehydrogenase deficiency. *J Natl Cancer Inst* **85**:1602, 1993.
365. Lyss A, Lilenbaum R, Harris B, Diasio R: Severe 5-fluorouracil toxicity in a patient with decreased dihydropyrimidine dehydrogenase activity. *Cancer Invest* **11**:239, 1993.
366. Lu Z, Zhang R, Diasio R: Dihydropyrimidine dehydrogenase activity in human peripheral blood mononuclear cells and liver: Population characteristics, newly identified deficient patients, and clinical implication in 5-fluorouracil chemotherapy. *Cancer Res* **53**:5433, 1993.
367. Stephan F, Etienne M, Wallays C, Milano G, Clergue F: Depressed hepatic dihydropyrimidine dehydrogenase activity and fluorouracil related toxicities. *Am J Med* **99**:685, 1995.
368. Beuzeboc P, Pierga J-Y, Stoppa-Lyonnet D, Etienne M, Milano G: Severe 5-fluorouracil toxicity possibly secondary to dihydropyrimidine dehydrogenase deficiency in a breast cancer patient with osteogenesis imperfecta. *Eur J Cancer* **32A**:370, 1996.
369. Wei X, McLeod H, McMurrough J, Gonzalez F, Fernandez-Salguero P: Molecular basis of the human dihydropyrimidine dehydrogenase deficiency and 5-fluorouracil toxicity. *J Clin Invest* **3**:610, 1996.
370. Van Kuilenburg A, Vreken P, Beex L, De Abreu R, Van Gennip A: Heterozygosity for a point mutation in an invariant splice donor site of dihydropyrimidine dehydrogenase and severe 5-fluorouracil related toxicity. *Eur J Cancer* **33**:2258, 1997.
371. Van Kuilenburg A, Vreken P, Beex L, De Abreu R, Van Gennip A: Severe 5-fluorouracil toxicity caused by reduced dihydropyrimidine dehydrogenase activity due to heterozygosity for a G $\rightarrow$ A point mutation. *J Inherit Metab Dis* **21**:280, 1998.
372. Kouwaki M, Hamajima N, Sumi S, Nonaka M, Sasaki M, Dobashi K, Kidouchi K, et al: Identification of novel mutations in the dihydropyrimidine dehydrogenase gene in a Japanese patient with 5-fluorouracil toxicity. *Clin Cancer Res* **4**:2999, 1998.
373. Shehata N, Pater A, Tang S-H: Prolonged severe 5-fluorouracil associated neurotoxicity in a patient with dihydropyrimidine dehydrogenase deficiency. *Cancer Invest* **17**:201, 1999.
374. Van Gennip A, Busch S, Wlzinga L, Stroomer A, Van Cruchten A, Scholten E, Abeling N: Application of simple chromatographic methods for the diagnosis of defects in pyrimidine degradation. *Clin Chem* **39**:380, 1993.
375. Wevers R, Engelke U, Rottveel J, Heerschap A, De Jong D, Abeling N, Van Gennip A, et al: H-NMR spectroscopy in body fluids of patients with inborn errors of purine and pyrimidine metabolism. *J Inherit Metab Dis* **20**:345, 1997.
376. Wilcken B, Hammond J, Berger R, Wise G, James C: Dihydropyrimidine dehydrogenase deficiency — A further case. *J Inherit Metab Dis* **2(Suppl 8)**:115, 1985.
377. Bakkeren J, De Abreu R, Sengers R, Gabreels F, Maas J, Renier R: Elevated urine, blood and cerebrospinal fluid levels of uracil and thymine in a child with dihydrothymine dehydrogenase deficiency. *Clin Chim Acta* **140**:247, 1984.
378. Van Gennip A, Abeling N, De Korte D: Application of TLC for the detection of aberrant purine and pyrimidine metabolism in man, in Sherma J, Fried B (eds): *Handbook of Thin Layer Chromatography*, vol 55. New York, Marcel Dekker, 1990, p 863.
379. Van Gennip A, Abeling N, Elzinga-Zoetekouw L, Scholten E, Van Cruchen A: Comparative study of thymine and uracil metabolism in healthy persons and in a patient with dihydropyrimidine dehydrogenase deficiency. *Adv Exp Biol Med* **253A**:111, 1989.
380. Jakobs C, Stellaard F, Smit L, Van Vugt J, Duran M, Berger R, Rovers P: The first prenatal diagnosis of dihydropyrimidine dehydrogenase deficiency. *Eur J Pediatr* **150**:291, 1991.
381. Van Gennip A: Screening for inborn errors of purine and pyrimidine metabolism by bi-dimensional TLC and HPLC, in Zwieg G, Sherma J, Krstulovic A (eds): *Handbook of Chromatography*, vol 1, part A. Boca Raton, Florida, CRC Press, 1987.
382. Duran M, Rovers P, De Bree P, Schreuder C, Beukenhorst H, Dorland L, Berger R: Dihydropyrimidinuria: A new error of pyrimidine metabolism. *J Inherit Metab Dis* **14**:367, 1991.
383. Van Gennip A, Van Bree-Blom E, Wadman S, De Bree P, Duran M, Beemer F: Liquid chromatography of urinary pyrimidines for the evaluation of primary and secondary abnormalities of pyrimidine metabolism: Biological/biomedical applications of liquid chromatography, in Hawk G, Champlin P, Hutton R, Mol C (eds): *Chromatographic Science*, 3rd ed, vol 18. New York, Marcel Dekker, 1981.
384. Diasio R, Van Kuilenburg A, Lu Z, Zhang R, Van Lenthe H, Van Gennip A: Determination of dihydropyrimidine dehydrogenase (DPD) in fibroblasts of a DPD deficient pediatric patient and family members using a polyclonal antibody to human DPD. *Adv Exp Med Biol* **370**:7, 1994.
385. Van Kuilenburg A, Van Lenthe H, Van Gennip A: Identification and tissue-specific expression of a NADH-dependent activity of dihydropyrimidine dehydrogenase deficiency in man. *Anticancer Res* **16**:389, 1996.
386. Van Kuilenburg A, Van Lenthe H, Blom M, Mul E, Van Gennip A: Profound variation in dihydropyrimidine dehydrogenase activity in human blood cells; major implications for the detection of partly deficient patients. *Br J Cancer* **79**:620, 1999.
387. Wadman S, Berger R, Duran M, De Bree P, Stoker-De Vries S, Beemer F, Weits-Binnerts J, et al: Dihydropyrimidine dehydrogenase deficiency leading to thymine-uraciluria. An inborn error of pyrimidine metabolism. *J Inherit Metab Dis* **2(Suppl 8)**:113, 1984.
388. Van Kuilenburg A, Blom M, Van Lenthe H, Mul E, Van Gennip A: The activity of dihydropyrimidine dehydrogenase deficiency in human blood cells. *J Inherit Metab Dis* **20**:331, 1997.
389. Lu Z, Zhang R, Diasio R: Dihydropyrimidine dehydrogenase deficiency in human peripheral blood mononuclear cells and liver; population characteristics, newly identified deficient patients, and clinical implication of 5-fluorouracil chemotherapy. *Biochem Pharmacol* **46**:945, 1994.
390. Berglund G, Greter J, Lindstedt S, Steen G, Waldenstrom J, Wass U: Urinary excretion of thymine and uracil in a two-year-old child with a malignant tumor of the brain. *Clin Chem* **25**:1325, 1979.
391. Braakhekke J, Renier W, Gabreels F, De Abreu R, Bakkeren J, Sengers R: Dihydropyrimidine dehydrogenase deficiency, Neurological aspects. *J Neurol Sci* **78**:71, 1987.
392. Choquet D, Korn H: Does β-alanine activate more than one chloride channel associated receptor? *Neurosci Lett* **84**:329, 1988.
393. Horikoshi T, Asanuma A, Yanagisawa K, Anzai K, Goto S: Taurine and β-alanine act on both GABA and glycine receptors in Xenopus oocyte injected with mouse brain messenger RNA. *Mol Brain Res* **4**:97, 1988.
394. Wu F, Gibbs T, Farb D: Dual activation of GABAA and glycine receptors by β-alanine: inverse modulation by progesterone and 5α-pregnan-3α-ol-20-one. *Eur J Pharmacol* **246**:239, 1993.
395. Mabjeesh N, Frese M, Rauen T, Jeserich G, Kanner B: Neuronal and glial γ-aminobutyric acid+ transporters are distinct proteins. *FEBS Lett* **299**:99, 1992.

396. Pfeiffer M, Draguhn A, Meierkord H, Heineman U: Effects of γ-aminobutyric acid (GABA) agonists and GABA uptake inhibitors on pharmacosensitive and pharmacoresistent epileptiform activity in vitro. *Br J Pharmacol* **119**:569, 1996.
397. Sandberg M, Jacobsen I: β-Alanine, a possible neurotransmitter in the visual system? *J Neurochem* **37**:1353, 1981.
398. Calvo D, Miledi R: Activation of GABAp1 receptors by glycine and β-alanine. *Neuroreport* **6**:1118, 1995.
399. Coustere C, Mentre F, Sommadossi J-P, Diasio R, Steimer J-L: A mathematical model of the kinetics of 5-fluorouracil and its metabolites in cancer patients. *Cancer Chemother Pharmacol* **28**:123, 1991.
400. Berger R, Stoker-De Vries S, Wadman S, Duran M, Beemer F, De Bree P, Weits-Binnerts J, et al: Dihydropyrimidine dehydrogenase deficiency leading to thymine-uraciluria. An inborn error of pyrimidine metabolism. *Clin Chim Acta* **141**:227, 1984.
401. Gonzalez F, Fernandez-Salguero P: Diagnostic analysis, clinical importance and molecular basis of dihydropyrimidine dehydrogenase deficiency. *Trends Pharmacol Sci* **16**:325, 1995.
402. Ridge S, Sludden J, Brown O, Robertson L, Wei X, Sapanone A, Fernandez-Salguero P, et al: Dihydropyrimidine dehydrogenase pharmacogenetics in Caucasian subjects. *Br J Clin Pharmacol* **46**:151, 1998.
403. Vessell E: Genetic host factors: Determinants of drug response. *N Engl J Med* **313**:261, 1985.
404. Heggie G, Sommadossi J-P, Cross D, Huster W, Diasio R: Clinical pharmacokinetics of 5-fluorouracil and its metabolism in plasma, urine and bile. *Cancer Res* **47**:2203, 1987.
405. Van Kuilenburg A, Vreken P, Beex L, Meinsma R, Van Lenthe H, De Abreu R, Van Gennip A: Heterozygosity for a point mutation in an invariant splice donor site of dihydropyrimidine dehydrogenase and severe 5-fluorouracil associated toxicity. *Eur J Cancer* **33**:2258, 1997.
406. Van Kuilenburg A, Vreken P, Beex L, Meinsma R, Van Lenther H, De Abreu R, Van Gennip A: Heterozygosity for a point mutation in an invariant splice donor site of dihydropyrimidine dehydrogenase deficiency and severe 5-fluorouracil associated toxicity. *Adv Exp Med Biol* **431**:293, 1998.
407. Lee M, Crowling R, Sander E, Pettigrew D: Bovine liver dihydropyrimidine aminohydrolase: pH dependencies of inactivation by chelators and steady-state kinetic properties. *Arch Biochem Biophys* **248**:368, 1986.
408. Kautz J, Schnackerz K: Purification and properties of 5,6-dihydropyrimidine amindohydrolase from calves' liver. *Eur J Biochem* **181**:431, 1989.
409. Jahnke K, Podschun B, Schnackerz K, Kautz J, Cook P: Acid-base catalytic mechanism of dihydropyrimidines from pH studies. *Biochemistry* **32**:5160, 1993.
410. Yang Y-S, Sengoda R, Jakoby W: Rat liver imidase. *J Biol Chem* **268**:10870, 1993.
411. Hamajima N, Matsuda K, Sakata S, Tamaki N, Sasaki M, Nonaka M: A novel gene family defined by human dihydropyrimidines and three related proteins with differential tissue distribution. *Gene* **180**:157, 1996.
412. Hamajima N, Kouwaki M, Vreken P, Matsuda K, Sumi S, Iameda M, Ohba S, et al: Dihydropyrimidinase deficiency: Structural organisation, chromosomal localization, and mutation analysis of the human dihydropyrimidinase gene. *Am J Hum Genet* **63**:717, 1998.
413. Wang L, Strittmatter S: Brain CRMP forms heterotetramers similar to liver dihydropyrimidinase. *J Neurochem* **69**:2261, 1997.
414. Duran M, Rovers P, De Bree P, Schreuder C, Beukenhorst H, Dorland L, Berger R: Dihydropyrimidinuria. *Lancet* **336**:817, 1990.
415. Putman C, Rotteveel J, Wevers R, Van Gennip A, Bakkeren J, De Abreu R: Dihydropyrimidine dehydrogenase deficiency, a progressive neurological disorder? *Neuropaediatrics* **28(2)**:106, 1997.
416. Assmann B, Hoffmann G, Wagner L, Seyberth H, Berger R: Microvillous atrophy and elevated excretion of pyrimidines. *J Inherit Metab Dis* **19(Suppl 1)**:10, 1996.
417. Ohba S, Kidouchi K, Sumi S, Imaeda M, Takeda N, Yoshizumi H, Tatematsu A, et al: Dihydropyrimidinuria: The first case in Japan. *Adv Exp Med Biol* **370**:383, 1994.
418. Sumi S, Kidouchi K, Hayashi K, Ohba S, Wada Y: Dihydropyrimidinuria without symptoms. *J Inherit Metab Dis* **19**:701, 1996.
419. Hasinoff B, Reinders F, Clark V: The enzymatic hydrolysis-activation of the adriamycin cardioprotective agent (=)-1,2-bis(3,5-duoxopiperazinyl-1-yl)propane. *Drug Metab Dispos* **19(1)**:74, 1991.
420. Assmann B, Gohlich-Ratmann G, Brautigam C, Wagner L, Moolenaar S, Engelke U, Wevers R, et al: Presumptive ureidopropionase deficiency as a new defect in pyrimidine catabolism found with in vitro H-NMR spectroscopy. *J Inherit Metab Dis* **21(Suppl 2)**:1, 1998.
421. Van Gennip A, Van Lenthe H, Assmann B, Gohlich-Ratman G, Hoffmann G, Brautigam C, Vreken P, et al: Confirmation of the enzyme defect in the first case of β-alanine synthase deficiency. *J Inher Metab Dis* (In press).
422. van Gennip A, Van Lenthe H, Abeling N, Scholten E, Van Kuilenburg A: Inhibition of β-ureido-propionase by propionate may contribute to the neurological complications in patients with propionic acidemia. *J Inherit Metab Dis* **20**:379, 1997.
423. Kakimoto Y, Taniguchi K, Sano I: δ-β-Aminoisobutyrate:pyruvate aminotransferase in mammalian liver and excretion of β-aminoisobutyrate by man. *J Biol Chem* **244**:335, 1969.
424. Tanaguchi K, Tsujio T, Kakimoto Y: Deficiency of β-aminoisobutyrate:pyruvate aminotransferase in the liver of genetic high excreters of δ-β-aminoisobutyrate. *Biochim Biophys Acta* **279**:475, 1972.
425. Scriver C, Pueschel S, Davies E: Hyper-β-alaninemia associated with β-amino-aciduria and δ-aminoaciduria, somnolence and seizures. *N Engl J Med* **274**:635, 1966.
426. Higgins J, Kaneski C, Bernadini I, Brady R, Barton N: Pyridoxine responsive hyper β-alaninemia with Cohen's syndrome. *Neurology* **44**:1728, 1994.
427. Scriver C, Gibson K: Disorders of beta and gamma amino acids in free and peptide linked forms, in Scriver C, Beaudet A, Sly S, Valle D (eds): *The Metabolic and Molecular Bases of Inherited Disease*, 7th ed, vol 1. New York, McGraw-Hill, 1995, p 1349.
428. Van Gennip A, Van Bree-Blom E, Abeling N, Van Erven A, Voutre P: β-Aminoisobutyric acid as a marker of thymine catabolism in malignancy. *Clin Chim Acta* **165**:365, 1987.
429. Pollitt R, Green A, Mith R: Excessive excretion of β-alanine and 3-hydroxypropionic, R-and S-3-aminoisobutyric and S-2-(hydroxymethyl)butyric acids probably due to a defect in the metabolism of the corresponding malonic semialdehydes. *J Inherit Metab Dis* **8**:75, 1985.
430. Gray R, Pollitt J, Webley J: Methylmalonic semialdehyde dehydrogenase deficiency: Demonstration of defective valine and β-alanine metabolism and reduced malonic semialdehyde dehydrogenase activity in cultured fibroblasts. *Biochem Med Metab Biol* **38**:121, 1987.
431. Ericson A, De Verdier C-H, Hansen T, Siep M: Erythrocyte nucleotide pattern in two children in a Norwegian family with pyrimidine 5′-nucleotidase deficiency. *Clin Chim Acta* **134**:25, 1983.
432. McLeod H, Collie-Duguid E, Vreken P, Johnson M, Wei X, Sapone A, Diasio R, et al: Nomenclature for human DPYD alleles. *Pharmacogenetics* **8**:455, 1998.
433. Antonarakis S: Recommendations for a nomenclature system for human gene mutations. Nomenclature Working Group. *Hum Mutat* **11(1)**:1, 1998.
434. Bakker H, Gonzalbo M, Van Gennip A: Dihydropyrimidine dehydrogenase deficiency presenting with psychomotor retardation and ocular abnormalities. *J Inherit Metab Dis* **17**:640, 1994.
435. Christensen E, Cezanne I, Kjaergaard S, Horlyk H, Faurholt-Pedersen V, Vreken P, Van Kuilenburg A, et al: Clinical variability in three Danish patients with dihydropyrimidine dehydrogenase deficiency all homozygous for the same mutation. *J Inherit Metab Dis* **21**:272, 1998.
436. Holopainen I, Pulkki K, Heinonen O, Nanto-Salonen K, Haataja L, Greter J, Holme E, et al: Partial epilepsy in a girl with a symptom-free sister, first two Finnish patients with dihydropyrimidine dehydrogenase deficiency. *J Inherit Metab Dis* **20**:719, 1997.
437. Van Kuilenburg A, Vreken P, Riva D, Botteon G, Abeling N, Bakker H, Van Gennip A: Clinical and biochemical abnormalities in a girl with dihydropyrimidine dehydrogenase deficiency due to homozygosity for the C29R mutation. *J Inherit Metab Dis* **22**:191, 1999.
438. Brockstedt M, Jakobs C, Smit L, Van Gennip A, Berger R: A new case of dihydropyrimidine dehydrogenase deficiency. *J Inherit Metab Dis* **13**:121, 1990.
439. Van Gennip A, Zoetekouw A, Abeling N: A new case of thymine-uraciluria. *Klin Wochenschr Suppl X* **65**:14, 1987.

LIPIDS

PART 12

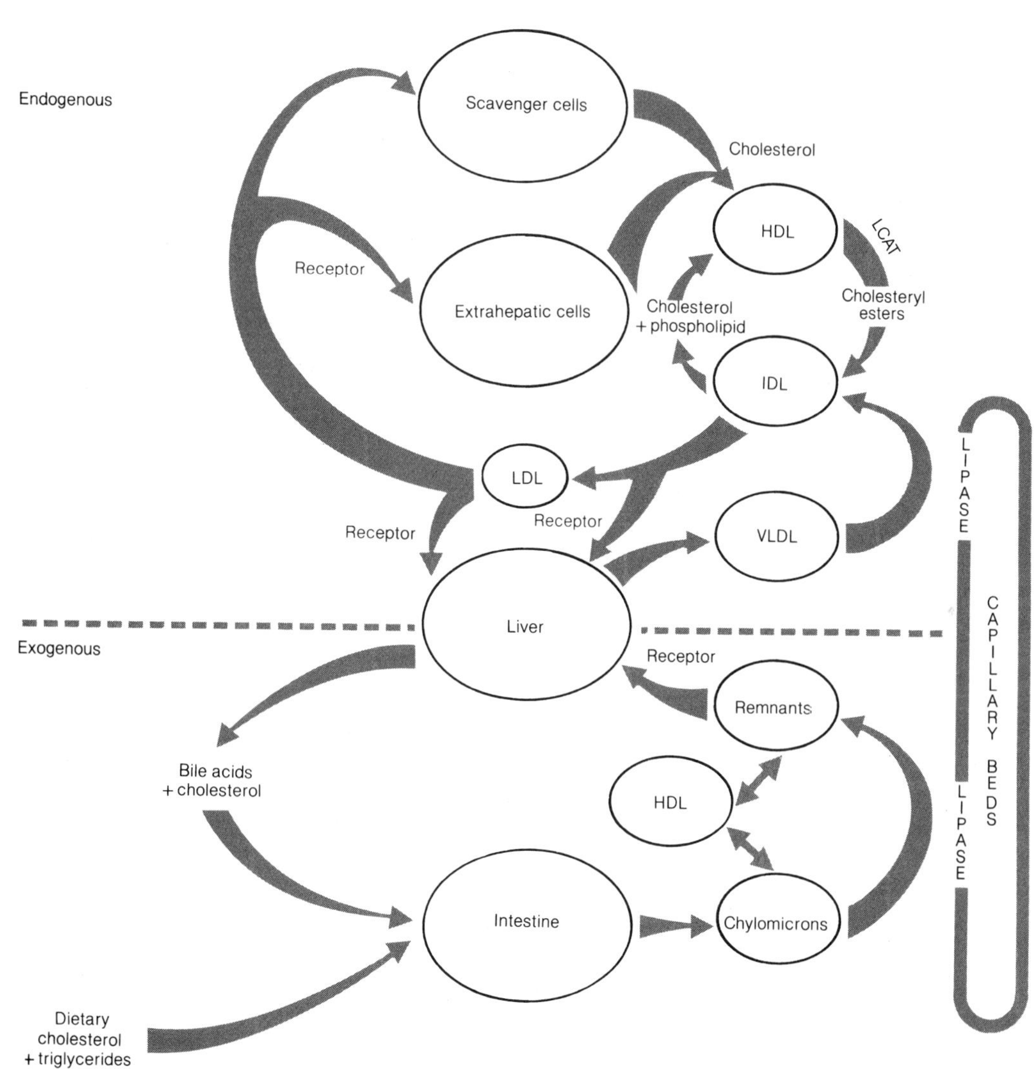

CHAPTER 114

Introduction: Structure and Metabolism of Plasma Lipoproteins

Richard J. Havel ▪ John P. Kane

Although it was appreciated at the turn of the century that the lipids of plasma are solubilized by protein,[1] it was another 28 years before the first lipoproteins, high-density lipoproteins (HDL), were isolated.[2] During the comprehensive efforts to isolate human plasma proteins during World War II, lipoproteins of low density and β electrophoretic mobility were clearly identified and separated from HDL with α mobility.[3] Within the next decade, the major antigenic determinants of α and β lipoproteins were shown to be distinct.[4,5] Studies of their hydrodynamic behavior demonstrated the existence of the larger, less dense, very low density lipoproteins (VLDL) and intermediate density lipoproteins (IDL);[6] it was established that a strongly antigenic protein was common to these lipoproteins and low density lipoproteins (LDL).[7] The presence of glutamic acid as the principal N-terminus in LDL[8,9] and one of several in VLDL[10] gave chemical support to the concept that one protein, distinct from the principal proteins in HDL, is virtually the only apolipoprotein in LDL and is present in significant amounts with other apolipoproteins in VLDL. This common protein constituent of LDL and its lipoprotein precursors was termed "apolipoprotein (apo) B" to distinguish it from the protein moiety of HDL (apo A) and the newly recognized proteins of VLDL (apo C).

Current knowledge of the processes of lipid transport in the blood owes much to discoveries of major gene mutations affecting the apolipoproteins, the key enzymes and transfer proteins that control lipid transport, and the cellular receptors that recognize specific apolipoproteins. Indeed, it is difficult to imagine how this field could have reached its present state in the absence of these discoveries, which resulted from clinical investigations of patients manifesting qualitative or quantitative abnormalities of the plasma lipoproteins.

Despite extraordinary advances during the past few years, the basis of much of the variation in lipoprotein concentrations among humans remains poorly understood. However, the primary structure of almost all the proteins that direct the processes of lipid transport in blood plasma is now known, and the discovery of polymorphisms among these proteins and the availability of transgenic mice expressing these proteins and mice in which genes have been deleted by homologous recombination holds much promise for elucidating this variation.

To facilitate understanding of the disorders described in this section, a brief overview of lipoprotein structure, composition, and metabolism is given here (for more extensive discussions, see references 11 to 14). The general clinical approach to determining the presenting phenotype is also included (see also references 15 and 16).

GENERAL STRUCTURE AND CLASSIFICATION OF PLASMA LIPOPROTEINS

The lipoproteins normally present in blood plasma vary widely in size, but virtually all but the smallest appear to be microemulsions.[17] Lipoprotein particles are thus spherical and contain a central core of nonpolar lipids (primarily triglycerides and cholesteryl esters) and a surface monolayer of polar lipids (primarily phospholipids) and apoproteins. Unesterified cholesterol is also present mainly in the surface monolayer, but with increasing particle size, it is distributed progressively into the core. Small amounts of nonpolar lipids are also distributed into the monolayer in accordance with their phase behavior. Most of the protein components of the monolayer, like the phospholipids, have amphipathic (detergent-like) properties. These properties are conferred by regions containing both polar and nonpolar amino acid residues, which are often distributed on opposite sides of an α helix.[11] The association of the polar lipids and proteins with lipoproteins is thus driven by hydrophobic forces whereby the fatty acyl chains and the nonpolar amino acid side chains are excluded from the aqueous environment. With the exception of the B apoproteins, the apoproteins, together with unesterified cholesterol, have appreciable water solubility and can exchange readily between lipoprotein particles or with other lipid surfaces. Phospholipids and the nonpolar lipids have little potential for exchange, but may be transferred between lipoproteins by specific transfer proteins.

Most of the apolipoproteins possess repeated amphipathic helical regions (apoproteins A-I, A-II, A-IV, C-I, C-II, C-III, and E). These proteins belong to a multigene family in which the coding regions are composed of tandem repeats of 11 codons, indicating that these genes evolved through duplications of a primordial gene.[18] Some of the proteins, however, do not belong to this family and contain few amphipathic helices. The B apoproteins (B-100 and B-48), which are by far the largest of the apolipoproteins, and which are the products of a single gene, evidently derive their lipophilicity in large part from stretches of hydrophobic amino acid residues and amphipathic β structure (see Chap. 115). Apo D (a member of the $\alpha 2\mu$-globulin gene family, which includes retinol binding protein) and the cholesteryl ester transfer protein (CETP) and phospholipid transfer protein (PLTP) (members of a gene family of lipid-binding proteins) also contain many nonpolar amino acid residues.[19–21] The failure of apo B to transfer between lipoprotein particles is presumably related to the large number of nonpolar amino acid side chains that penetrate the

A list of standard abbreviations is located immediately preceding the index in each volume. Additional abbreviations used in this chapter include: CETP = cholesteryl ester transfer protein; IDL = intermediate density lipoprotein; LCAT = lecithin:cholesterol acyltransferase; LP(a) = lipoprotein (a); LRP = LDL-receptor-related protein; PLTP = phospholipid transfer protein; and SR-B1 = scavenger receptor B1.

Table 114-1 Characteristics of Major Plasma Apolipoproteins and Transfer Proteins in Normal Fasting Humans

	Plasma Concentration		Distribution in Lipoproteins %†					
	(mg/dl)	(mol %)*	HDL	LDL	IDL	VLDL	Major Tissue Source	Molecular Weight of Amino Acid Chain
Apolipoproteins								
Apo A-I	130	40	100				Liver and intestine	29,016
Apo A-II	40	20	100				Liver and intestine	17,414
Apo A-IV	18	5					Liver and intestine	44,465
Apo B-48	0.2	–				>70	Intestine	241,000
Apo B-100	80	5		88	6	6	Liver	512,723
Apo C-I	6	8	97		1	2	Liver	6,630
Apo C-II	3	3	60		10	30	Liver	8,900
Apo C-III	12	12	60	10	10	20	Liver	8,800
Apo D	10	5	100				Many sources	19,000
Apo E-II, Apo E-III, Apo E-IV	5	2	50	10	20	20	Liver	34,145
Transfer Proteins								
CETP	0.17	–	>80				Many sources	53,000
PLTP	?	–	>80				Many sources	54,719

*Total plasma concentration
†For each apoprotein or transfer protein

SOURCE: Modified from Gotto et al.[11] Used with permission of the publisher. Data on CETP are from Tall.[44] Data on PLTP are from Albers et al.[21]

surface monolayer. The smaller apo D and CETP have relatively low affinities for lipoproteins and can be dissociated by procedures such as ultracentrifugation. A number of plasma proteins are partially bound to lipoproteins; this binding may have functional consequences.[22] Some properties of the apolipoproteins and transfer proteins and their origin and distribution in plasma lipoproteins are summarized in Table 114-1.

The density of lipoprotein particles is inversely related to their size, reflecting the relative contents of low-density, nonpolar core lipid, and high-density surface protein. Based on density and certain compositional and functional properties, the lipoproteins are usually separated into several classes (Table 114-2). The two largest classes contain mainly triglycerides in their cores. These are the chylomicrons, secreted from absorptive enterocytes, in which the B apoprotein is primarily or exclusively apo B-48, and the VLDL, secreted by hepatocytes, which contain apo B-100. LDL, HDL2, and HDL3, contain mainly cholesteryl esters in their cores. The mature forms of these particles are not secreted directly from cells but rather are produced by metabolic processes within the blood plasma. LDL are mainly produced as end products of the metabolism of VLDL. Components of HDL are secreted with chylomicrons and VLDL, as well as independently as HDL precursors. IDL, which contain appreciable amounts of both triglycerides and cholesteryl esters in their core, are produced during the conversion of VLDL to LDL. Pre $\beta 1$ HDL is a precursor of mature α-HDL. LP(a) lipoprotein is present in highly variable amounts in plasma. It is composed of a particle of LDL complexed via disulfide bonding to a large, polymorphic glycoprotein, apo A (see Chap. 116). The composition of the lipoprotein classes is summarized in Table 114-3.

In certain pathologic states, lamellar lipoproteins, which are lipoproteins with a different structure, are found. These particles lack a nonpolar core and are composed of a bilayer of lipids and proteins, as in cell membranes. They occur in two distinct forms: disks and vesicles. In the disks, amphipathic apoproteins are thought to comprise a peripheral annulus.[23] These particles occur in familial lecithin:cholesterol acyltransferase (LCAT) deficiency and in liver disease in which this enzyme is deficient. Similar particles, found in perfusates of isolated livers and in intestinal and peripheral lymph, are thought to represent a form of nascent HDL. The vesicles are composed of a lipid bilayer with apoproteins adsorbed to the surface. In biliary obstruction, such particles ("lipoprotein X") are formed as a result of reflux of biliary lipids into the blood.[24] Similar particles also occur in familial LCAT deficiency (see Chap. 118).

KEY ENZYMES OF LIPOPROTEIN-LIPID TRANSPORT

Three enzymes have important roles in lipoprotein-lipid transport — lipoprotein lipase, hepatic lipase, and LCAT (Table 114-4). Lipoprotein lipase and hepatic lipase are members of a multigene family that includes pancreatic lipase.[25,26]

Lipoprotein lipase is synthesized in a variety of tissues, but most is present in adipose tissue and striated muscle (see Chap. 117). The enzyme is synthesized in tissue parenchymal cells and is secreted and transported to the endothelial surface of blood

Table 114-2 Physical Properties of Human Plasma Lipoprotein Classes

Class	Density (g/ml)	Electrophoretic Mobility	Diameter (nm)	Molecular Weight
Chylomicrons	~0.93	Remains at origin	75–1200	$50–1000 \times 10^6$
VLDL	0.93–1.006	Preβ-lipoproteins	30–80	$10–80 \times 10^6$
IDL	1.006–1.019	Slow preβ-lipoproteins	25–35	$5–10 \times 10^6$
LDL	1.019–1.063	β-Lipoproteins	18–25	2,300,000
HDL_2	1.063–1.125	α-Lipoproteins	9–12	360,000
HDL_3	1.125–1.210	α-Lipoproteins	5–9	175,000
Preβ-HDL	~1.28	Preβ-lipoproteins	~5	67,000
LP(a)	1.040–1.090	Slow preβ-lipoproteins	25–30	~2,800,000

Table 114-3 Chemical Composition of Normal Human Plasma Lipoproteins

	Surface Components			Core Lipids	
	Cholesterol	Phospholipids	Apolipoprotein	Triglycerides	Cholesteryl Esters
Chylomicrons	2	7	2	86	3
VLDL	7	18	8	55	12
IDL	9	19	19	23	29
LDL	8	22	22	6	42
HDL_2	5	33	40	5	17
HDL_3	4	25	55	3	13
Preβ 1-HDL	5	5	90	0	0

Surface components and core lipids given as percentage of dry mass.

capillaries, where it is bound to heparan sulfate proteoglycans. Lipoprotein lipase is required for the efficient hydrolysis of triglycerides in chylomicrons and most VLDL particles. Its action requires the presence of apo C-II, an activator protein, on the surface of lipoproteins. In adipose tissue, enzyme activity is induced by insulin and is high in anabolic conditions. In muscle, particularly red skeletal muscle and cardiac muscle, the activity remains high or increases under catabolic conditions. These changes in activity contribute to the storage of triglyceride fatty acids in adipose tissue in the postprandial state and to the provision of these fatty acids to contracting muscles in the postabsorptive state.

Hepatic lipase resembles lipoprotein lipase in acting at cell surfaces, bound to heparan sulfate proteoglycans. It is synthesized in hepatocytes and is transported to the cell surface and to cells in the adrenals and gonads as well. Hepatic lipase participates in the lipolysis of VLDL and IDL during the later stages of the formation of LDL,[27] in the hydrolysis of phospholipids and triglycerides in HDL,[28] and in the clearance of partially degraded chylomicrons by the liver.[27,29] Its activity is increased by androgens and reduced by estrogens.

LCAT is responsible for the synthesis of most cholesteryl esters in plasma lipoproteins (see Chap. 118). LCAT is synthesized in hepatocytes and secreted into the blood, where it acts on species of HDL to esterify cholesterol with a fatty acyl residue of phosphatidyl choline (lecithin). In some mammals, including humans, the product cholesteryl esters are rapidly transferred to acceptor lipoproteins by CETP.[14] The major normal acceptor is LDL, but VLDL and HDL also derive their cholesteryl esters by this route. The system comprising LCAT and CETP, acting on species of HDL, is thought to have a key role in the process of reverse cholesterol transport by which cholesterol is transported from extrahepatic cells to hepatocytes.[14]

LIPOPROTEIN RECEPTORS

The terminal catabolism of lipoproteins that contain B apolipoproteins occurs by receptor-mediated endocytosis (see Chap. 120). The mechanism of the terminal catabolism of HDL particles is less well understood. The best-defined lipoprotein receptor is the LDL receptor, a member of an expanding gene family, most of which bind lipoproteins through apo E. The LDL receptor binds apo B-100 as well as apo E, and thus mediates the endocytosis of partially catabolized VLDL, IDL and LDL. Like other receptors that mediate macromolecular endocytosis, the LDL receptor is a transmembrane protein. The lipoprotein particles bound to the receptor via apo B-100 or apo E are endocytosed via coated pits on the plasma membrane. The lipoproteins dissociate from the receptor in the acidic internal environment of endosomes and are eventually catabolized in secondary lysosomes. The receptor separates from the endosome in prelysosomal compartments and recycles to the cell surface for another round of endocytosis. The number of LDL receptors in cells is tightly regulated by the availability of cholesterol. Excess cellular cholesterol inhibits the proteolytic release from the ER of soluble domains of transcription factors called SREBPs which downregulate transcription of the LDL receptor and cholesterol biosynthetic enzymes (see Chap. 120). These events contribute to maintenance of cellular cholesterol concentrations within narrow limits.

The terminal catabolism of partially degraded chylomicrons in hepatocytes is likewise mediated by receptor-dependent endocytosis, chiefly via the LDL receptor, but another member of the LDL receptor-gene family (LRP) can also bind and endocytose apo E-rich remnant particles.[29] LRP is a multifunctional receptor that mediates the catabolism of several proteins, including activated $\alpha 2$ macroglobulin.

Scavenger receptor B1 (SR-B1), a member of the scavenger receptor gene family, mediates selective uptake of cholesteryl esters of HDL particles into cells.[30] SR-B1, which recognizes lipids as well as protein components of HDL, is chiefly expressed in steroid-secreting endocrine cells and hepatocytes. Selective uptake depletes HDL particles of cholesteryl esters. The mechanism of the selective uptake process is poorly understood.

Certain modified lipoproteins, including oxidized LDL, are taken up into cells, such as macrophages, by class A and certain other scavenger receptors.[31,32] These receptors appear to be

Table 114-4 Key Enzymes of Plasma Lipid Transport

Enzyme	Molecular Weight of Amino Acid Chain	Major Tissue Source	Substrates
Lipoprotein lipase	50,394	Adipose tissue (adipocytes)	Triglycerides and phospholipids of chylomicrons and large VLDL
		Striated muscle	
Hepatic lipase	53,222	Liver (hepatocytes)	Triglycerides and phospholipids of small VLDL, IDL, and large HDL
Lecithin: cholesterol acyltransferase	47,090	Liver	Cholesterol and phosphatidylcholine of species of HDL

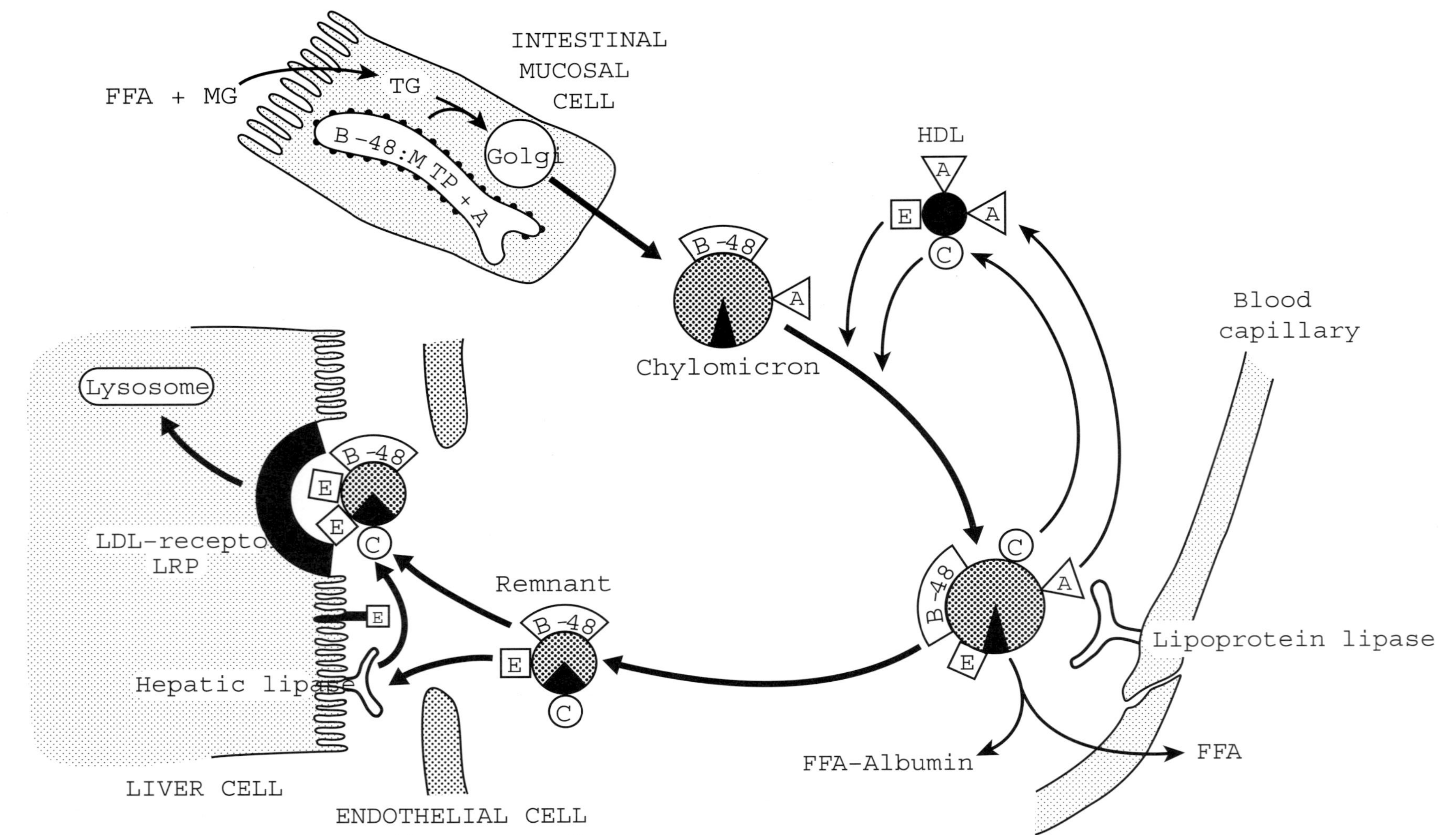

Fig. 114-1 Chylomicron pathway. Dietary triglycerides are hydrolyzed in the intestine by pancreatic lipase to fatty acids (FFA) and monoglycerides (MG), which are reesterified to form triglycerides (TG) in intestinal mucosal cells. Dietary cholesterol is likewise esterfied with long chain fatty acids in the mucosal cells to form cholesteryl esters. The triglycerides and cholesteryl esters are assembled in the ER with other lipids and proteins to form the core of nascent chylomicrons. Apo B-48, acting in concert with microsomal triglyceride transfer protein (MTP), is required for chylomicron particle assembly, which is completed in the Golgi apparatus. After secretion into intestinal lymph, the nascent chylomicrons are delivered into the blood, where the proteins synthesized in the absorptive cells (apo B-48 and the A apoproteins) are augmented by transfer of apo E and C apoproteins from HDL. The first step in chylomicron catabolism occurs in extrahepatic tissues, where most of the component triglycerides (shaded area in particles) are rapidly hydrolyzed by lipoprotein lipase to yield chylomicron remnants (see text). The remnants, which retain their component cholesteryl esters (black area in particles) are released from the enzyme and are then taken up onto the surface of hepatocytes by the LDL receptor and hepatic lipase. Hepatic lipase-bound remnants may be further processed enzymatically and may acquire additional apo E residing on the cell surface. The LDL receptor and the LDL receptor-related protein (LRP) bind remnants via apo E, leading to endocytosis of the particles and catabolism in lysosomes from which cholesterol can enter metabolic pathways in hepatocytes, including excretion into the bile. (*Modified from Havel RJ.*[15] *Used with the permission of the publisher.*)

involved in cholesterol accumulation in atherosclerotic plaques, but there is little evidence that they participate in normal lipoprotein metabolism.

LIPOPROTEIN METABOLISM

Biosynthesis and Catabolism of Lipoproteins Containing Apo B

Apo B, in concert with microsomal triglyceride transfer protein (MTP), is required for the assembly of chylomicrons and VLDL in the ER of enterocytes and hepatocytes, respectively. The nascent lipoproteins are transported to the Golgi apparatus, packaged in secretory vesicles, and delivered into the extracellular space by exocytosis (see Chap. 115). Chylomicrons enter lacteals in the intestinal villi, and VLDL pass through the fenestrae of the hepatic sinusoidal endothelium to enter the blood.

Nascent chylomicrons contain newly absorbed fatty acids as triglycerides. Their protein components include the smaller form of apo B (B-48) and the A apoproteins (A-I, A-II, and A-IV) (Fig. 114-1). After secretion, chylomicrons acquire C apoproteins and apo E by transfer from HDL. Following delivery via the thoracic duct into the blood, chylomicrons bind to lipoprotein lipase on the surface of capillary endothelial cells, where most of the triglycerides are rapidly hydrolyzed together with some of the surface glycerophospholipids. Concomitantly, some phospholipids and the A apoproteins are transferred to HDL. With these changes, the particles gradually lose their affinity for C apoproteins, which are also transferred to HDL; the residual particle, now called a "chylomicron remnant," is released into the blood. The remnant binds to proteins located on the sinusoidal surface of hepatocytes, chiefly the LDL receptor and hepatic lipase. Hepatic lipase further hydrolyzes remnant lipids, and the particles may acquire additional apo E, which is bound, like hepatic lipase, to heparan sulfate proteoglycans on the cell surface. Such modifications are not required for effective binding of remnants to the LDL receptor, but facilitate binding to a second receptor (LRP). After endocytosis via coated pits, components of the particle are hydrolyzed in lysosomes.

During the first step of chylomicron metabolism in extrahepatic tissues, most of the triglyceride fatty acids enter adipocytes for storage or cells of other tissues for oxidation. In addition, some of the released fatty acids become bound to plasma albumin and are transported to a variety of tissues, including the liver. During the second step of chylomicron metabolism, the residual triglycerides, and virtually all dietary cholesterol, are delivered to hepatocytes. The cholesterol released from lysosomes in hepatocytes can enter pathways leading to the formation of bile acids, be secreted into the bile as such, be incorporated into nascent lipoproteins, or be esterified with a long chain fatty acid and stored in lipid droplets within the cell.

VLDL provide a pathway for export from hepatocytes of excess triglycerides (derived from lipogenesis, from plasma free fatty acids, or from chylomicron remnants taken up from the blood), which would otherwise be stored within the cells. As they enter the blood, nascent VLDL contain the larger form of apo B (B-100) and small amounts of E and C apoproteins (Fig. 114-2). Additional amounts of the latter proteins are added after secretion, as in the case of nascent chylomicrons. Thereafter, the initial phase of metabolism resembles that of chylomicrons—hydrolysis by lipoprotein lipase and the formation of VLDL remnants. The rate of hydrolysis of VLDL triglycerides is slower than that of chylomicron triglycerides. This is probably related to the smaller size of the average VLDL particle, which can bind fewer lipoprotein lipase molecules than the larger chylomicron particle. The normal residence time for chylomicron triglycerides in the blood is 5 to 10 min, whereas for VLDL triglycerides it is 15 to 60 min.

VLDL remnants can interact with LDL receptors on hepatocytes via apo E. The presence of several molecules of apo E on larger remnant particles results in high-affinity binding and rapid removal of the remnants from the blood followed by lysosomal catabolism. Smaller VLDL particles yield smaller remnants, with fewer molecules of apo E; these have lower affinity for hepatic LDL receptors and remain longer in the blood. The smaller remnants include particles that are isolated as IDL. Many of these particles are further lipolyzed after binding to hepatic lipase on the hepatocyte surface to form LDL. LDL contain little or no apo E, but can bind to the LDL receptor monovalently via component apo B-100.

Although nascent VLDL contain apo E, the binding domain is not initially exposed for interaction with LDL receptors. During the formation of VLDL remnants, and particularly with the loss of C apoproteins, the binding domain becomes exposed, permitting uptake by LDL receptors. Similarly, the binding domain of apo B is not exposed in nascent VLDL, but eventually becomes exposed during lipolysis, so that as apo E is lost, the particle retains some affinity for the LDL receptor. The relatively low affinity of LDL for the LDL receptor, as compared with that of VLDL remnants, presumably accounts for the long residence time of LDL particles (about 3 days), as compared with that of VLDL remnants (minutes to hours).

The endocytosis of chylomicron remnants into hepatocytes is also mediated by apo E and, as with nascent VLDL, exposure of the binding domain of apo E requires lipolysis, accompanied by loss of C apoproteins. In contrast to VLDL, particles equivalent to LDL are not formed during the lipolysis of chylomicron remnants. In addition, the B-48 protein of chylomicrons lacks the receptor-binding domain present in apo B-100, and consequently is thought not to participate in remnant uptake into the liver (see Chap. 120).

In most mammals, VLDL remnants are taken up mainly into the liver and only a small fraction is converted to LDL. In humans, more remnants, perhaps about half, are eventually converted to LDL. Whereas remnants are taken up almost entirely into the liver, some LDL particles are taken up into extrahepatic tissues, mainly via the LDL receptor. Normally, the liver is also the principal site of removal of LDL from the blood. In general, the higher the activity of LDL receptors on hepatocytes, the greater the efficiency of removal of VLDL remnants and the lower the fraction of remnants converted to LDL (see Chap. 120).

FORMATION OF HDL AND PLASMA CHOLESTEROL TRANSPORT

The A apoproteins (apo A-I, A-II, and A-IV) are the major protein components of plasma HDL. These proteins are secreted primarily as components of nascent chylomicrons and VLDL. Some HDL apoproteins may also be secreted in a lipid-poor form, but plasma HDL, as such, are assembled extracellularly as surface components of triglyceride-rich lipoproteins, including phospholipids and cholesterol, and certain apoproteins become dissociated during lipolysis.[33] These components are organized into certain HDL particles, where cholesterol can be esterified by LCAT to yield lysolecithin and cholesteryl ester. The lysolecithin is transferred to albumin and removed from the blood, whereas the cholesteryl esters are transferred via CETP between HDL particles from these to LDL or triglyceride-rich lipoproteins. The size of HDL particles increases as LCAT-derived cholesteryl esters accumulate; triglyceride-rich lipoproteins and LDL can become enriched in cholesteryl esters transferred from HDL. Triglycerides transfer reciprocally via CETP from apo B-containing lipoproteins to HDL, in which they are gradually hydrolyzed by hepatic lipase. Efficient lipolysis is associated with increased size and cholesteryl ester content of HDL owing to transfer of surface components from triglyceride-rich lipoproteins and increased LCAT activity; accordingly, HDL cholesterol levels rise. The transfer of cholesteryl esters out of HDL by CETP and the hydrolysis of HDL triglycerides and phospholipids by hepatic lipase reduce HDL size. Large HDL particles are often called HDL2 and smaller HDL particles are called HDL3, but this distinction is somewhat

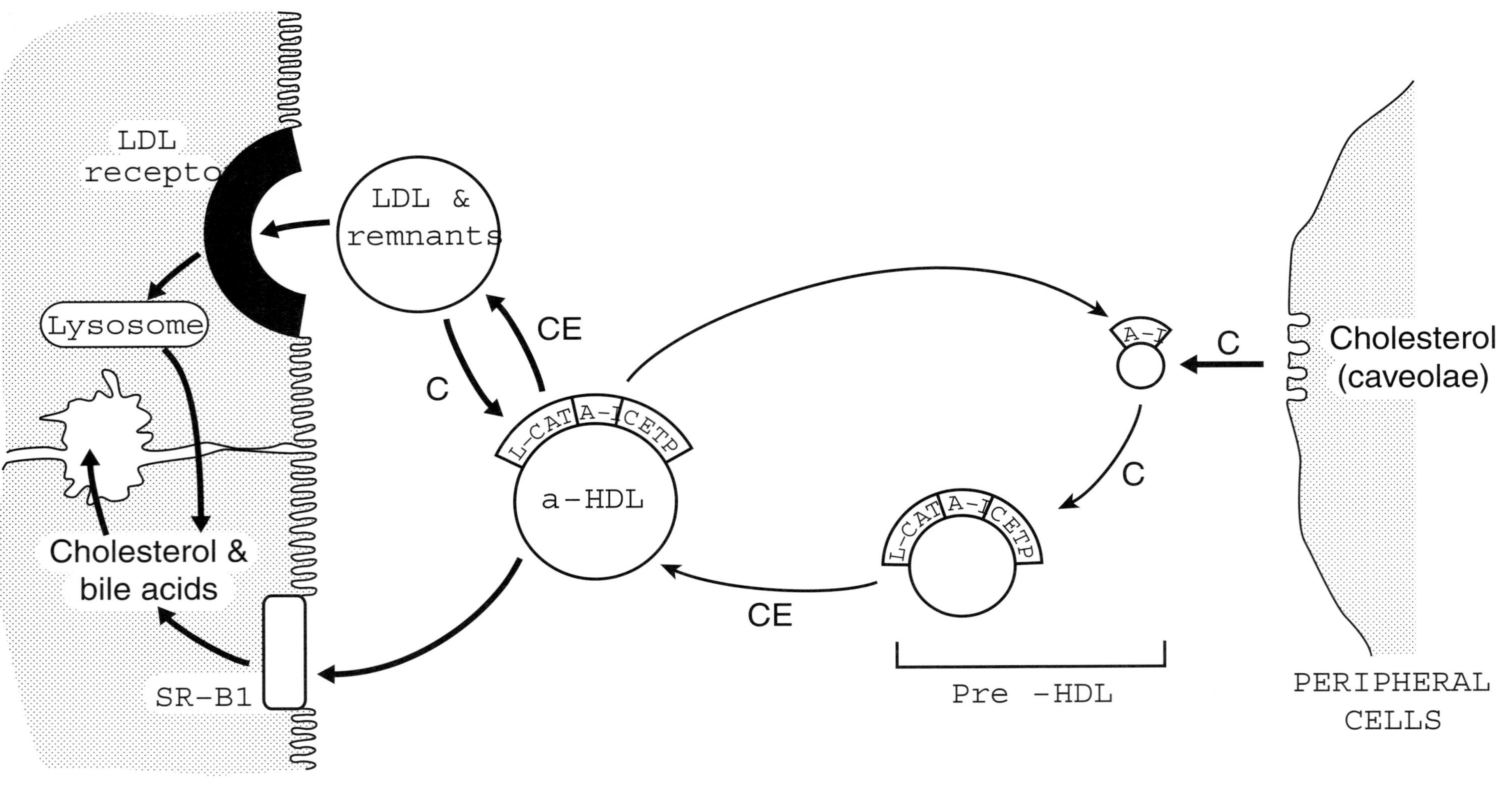

Fig. 114-2 VLDL-LDL pathways. The formation of VLDL in hepatocytes resembles that of chylomicrons in intestinal absorptive cells. VLDL provide a pathway for exit of surplus fatty acids as triglycerides (shaded area in lipoprotein particles) from the liver (see text). VLDL also transport cholesteryl esters from the liver (black areas), but most of these esters are synthesized by LCAT in species of HDL and transferred to the VLDL particles in the blood. The liver synthesizes a larger form of apo B (B-100) than the B-48 protein synthesized in the intestine, and also synthesizes apo E and C apoproteins, which enter the blood with nascent VLDL. As with chylomicrons, most VLDL triglycerides are hydrolyzed in extrahepatic tissues by lipoprotein lipase to yield remnant particles. LDL receptors on hepatocytes recognize apo E on VLDL remnants and mediate the endocytosis of a substantial fraction of these particles. Some, however, are further processed by hepatic lipase, also located on the hepatocyte surface, to yield LDL. LDL can also be taken up into hepatocytes by LDL receptors (which recognize a binding domain on apo B-100) or by LDL receptors on extrahepatic cells. Unlike their remnant precursors, which have a short life span, LDL circulate in the blood for days (see text). (*Modified from Havel RJ.*[15] *Used with the permission of the publisher.*)

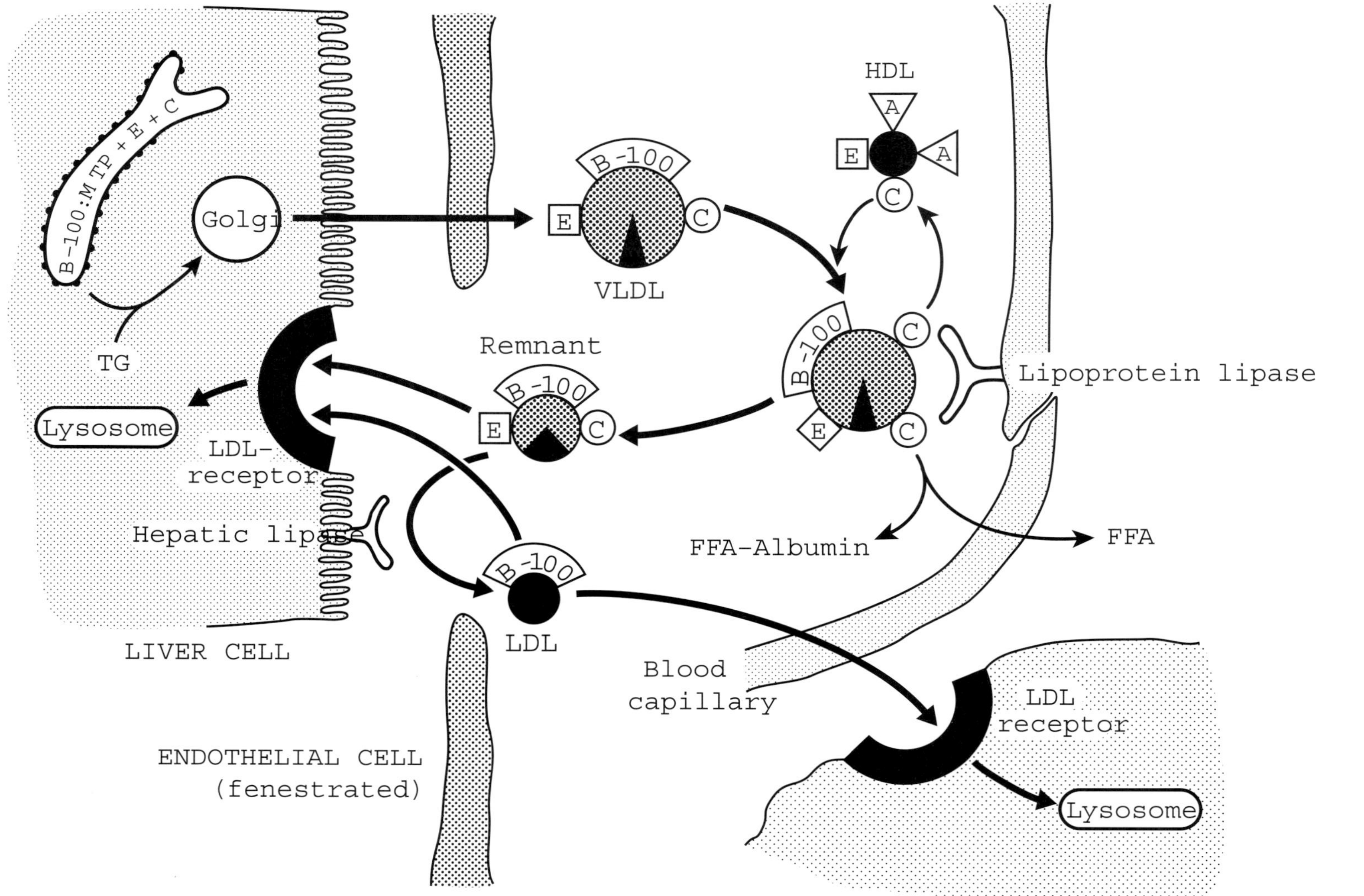

Fig. 114-3 Reverse cholesterol transport. The process of reverse cholesterol transport, whereby cholesterol in extrahepatic cells is delivered to the liver, is initiated by the delivery of cellular cholesterol and phospholipid from cholesterol-rich domains on the cell surface (caveolae) to small preβ-HDL particles that contain apo A-I. The resulting larger preβ-HDL, which may be a lamellar discoidal particle, is a preferred substrate for LCAT, which esterifies the cholesterol with long chain fatty acids derived from phosphatidyl choline (see text). The product cholesteryl esters are rapidly transferred to other lipoproteins including α-HDL and to lipoproteins containing apo B (LDL and remnant particles). The former can deliver the cholesteryl esters selectively to the liver through interaction with SR-B1 on the hepatocyte surface. The latter are taken up with the entire particle by receptor-mediated endocytosis and delivered to lysosomes. Preβ-HDL are regenerated from α-HDL by actions involving hepatic lipase, CETP, and PLTP (see text). The esterification of cholesterol by LCAT creates a gradient that permits cellular cholesterol to be transferred into the blood. Cholesterol on the surface of lipoproteins can also be esterified by LCAT after transfer to species of α-HDL and the cholesteryl esters formed can also be delivered to the liver. Within the liver, the cholesteryl esters are hydrolyzed to yield cholesterol, which can be excreted into the bile as such or after conversion to bile acids.

Table 114-5 Normal Values (mg/dl) for Total Cholesterol

	White Males			White Females (Sex Hormone Nonusers)		
		Percentiles			Percentiles	
Age (years)	Mean	5	95	Mean	5	95
0–4	155	114	203	156	112	200
5–9	160	121	203	163	126	205
10–14	158	119	202	160	124	201
15–19	150	113	197	157	119	200
20–29	174	129	231	167	125	219
30–39	197	142	262	180	135	236
40–49	209	155	272	198	150	259
50–59	213	157	277	224	167	293
60–69	213	159	275	231	171	300
70–79	206	153	265	230	169	292
≥80	207	144	275	222	165	279

arbitrary and many HDL species with differing composition (and, possibly, distinct functions) exist.[34]

The cholesterol substrate for LCAT is also derived in part from the plasma membrane of cells.[14] Recent studies indicate that transfer of cellular cholesterol to the external leaflet of the plasma membrane requires the ATP-binding cassette transporter, ABC1. ABC1, which is induced by cellular cholesterol-loading, may act as a cholesterol "flippase."[35] Mutations of ABC1 have been shown to underlie Tangier disease, in which cholesteryl esters accumulate in lymphoid and other cells and only trace amounts of HDL are present in the blood.[35–39] ABC1 thus mediates an early step of *reverse cholesterol transport*, whereby cholesterol in extrahepatic cells in delivered into the bile (Fig. 114-3). Actual removal of cholesterol from cells is promoted by small pre-β migrating HDL particles, which bind to cholesterol-rich domains of the plasma membrane. In quiescent cells, the domains are often organized into flask-like invaginations (caveolae) by a group of proteins called caveolins.[36] Preβ HDL are a preferred substrate for LCAT, which, by esterifying the cellular cholesterol, traps it within the apopolar core of HDL particles. The cholesteryl esters of α-migrating HDL thus formed can then be delivered to the liver by two major routes. One is via CETP-mediated transfer to lipoproteins containing apo B, as described above, and receptor-mediated uptake and catabolism in hepatocytes. The other is via a process of selective uptake of cholesteryl esters into hepatocytes, mediated by SR-B1 (SR-B1 is also highly expressed in steroid-secreting endocrine cells, providing cholesterol via selective uptake for hormone synthesis).[30] Selective uptake may be facilitated through hydrolysis of HDL-phospholipids by hepatic lipase, the activity of which is inversely related to the plasma concentration of HDL. This action of hepatic lipase, together with CETP-mediated transfer of cholesteryl esters[40] and PLTP-mediated transfer of phospholipids from HDL to other lipoproteins,[41] is also thought to contribute the conversion of α HDL to preβ HDL, thereby maintaining the flow of cholesterol to the liver.[14] In addition, hepatic lipase, by increasing the chemical potential of HDL-cholesterol, may promote net transfer of cholesterol as such from the surface of HDL to the liver. Finally, a small fraction of HDL particles that contain apo E may be taken up by hepatocytes directly via the LDL receptor.[42]

DEFINITION AND CLASSIFICATION OF HYPERLIPIDEMIA

The concentrations of lipids in blood plasma and in the major lipoprotein classes are continuous, widely distributed functions in the population. Hence, any definition of hyperlipidemia is

Table 114-6 Normal Values (mg/dl) for Total Triglycerides

	White Males			White Females (Sex Hormone Nonusers)		
		Percentiles			Percentiles	
Age (years)	Mean	5	95	Mean	5	95
0–4	56	29	99	64	34	112
5–9	56	30	101	60	32	105
10–14	66	32	125	75	36	131
15–19	78	37	148	72	39	124
20–29	108	45	225	74	37	138
30–39	137	52	293	82	40	163
40–49	152	57	324	101	46	203
50–59	147	58	303	120	54	248
60–69	140	58	279	129	58	241
70–79	129	58	263	131	59	237
≥80	132	55	255	135	60	242

Table 114-7 Normal Values (mg/dl) for LDL Cholesterol

	White Males			White Females (Sex Hormone Nonusers)		
		Percentiles			Percentiles	
Age (years)	Mean	5	95	Mean	5	95
5–9	93	67	126	100	67	133
10–15	96	62	130	96	66	134
15–19	97	65	149	100	69	146
20–29	116	73	163	106	68	158
30–39	132	83	190	113	72	168
40–49	141	89	198	128	81	189
50–59	143	83	211	150	96	219
60–69	143	87	208	159	97	227
70–79	136	81	202	157	98	330

necessarily arbitrary. For diagnostic purposes, the concentration of total cholesterol and triglycerides in blood plasma and the concentration of total cholesterol in major lipoprotein classes forms the basis for clinical classification of hyperlipidemia and hyperlipoproteinemia. Hypolipidemia and hypolipoproteinemia are similarly classified. Arbitrarily, values in the upper and lower 5 percent of the distribution are usually taken to define an abnormality, but prevalence of the monogenic disorders considered here increases at more restrictive cutoff points. Age- and sex-specific values for American and Canadian populations based on data from the Lipid Research Clinics Program are shown in Tables 114-5 to 114-8.

In general, VLDL triglyceride concentrations are highly correlated with triglyceride levels in plasma and provide a useful estimate of VLDL concentration, but it must be remembered that the composition of VLDL varies considerably, even in the absence of a lipoprotein disorder. Chylomicrons contribute little to triglycerides in plasma obtained during the postabsorptive state except when the lipoprotein lipase system is deficient or overwhelmed. The presence of chylomicrons is simply evaluated by the presence of a creamy layer on the surface of plasma or serum that has been stored overnight in the cold.

LDL cholesterol normally accounts for about two-thirds of plasma total cholesterol, but the correlation between the two is insufficient for use of plasma levels as an index of LDL concentration. LDL cholesterol is usually estimated from the difference between plasma and HDL cholesterol, with an additional correction for VLDL cholesterol, which is usually estimated to be one-fifth of the plasma triglyceride level. The correlation with directly measured LDL cholesterol is good, except in conditions such as familial dysbetalipoproteinemia in which the composition of VLDL is altered, or in patients with very high triglyceride levels. However, in such individuals, LDL levels are usually depressed. For more accurate estimation of LDL cholesterol, VLDL are first removed by ultracentrifugation of plasma at its native small-molecule density (1.006 g/ml). Thus, after subtraction of HDL cholesterol, the calculated LDL fraction includes IDL ($1.006 < d < 1.019$ g/ml). This is satisfactory in normal situations because "true" LDL ($1.019 < d < 1.063$ g/ml) are present in much higher concentrations than IDL. However, in pathologic states, IDL levels may be substantial, and the usual method becomes inaccurate. In addition, LDL separated by ultracentrifugation include a small but variable amount of the LP(a) lipoprotein, in which the B apoprotein of LDL is complexed with the LP(a) protein (see Chap. 116).

HDL levels are most commonly measured as the cholesterol remaining in plasma after precipitation of VLDL, IDL, and LDL with a polyanion such as heparin or phosphotungstate in the presence of a divalent cation. HDL cholesterol is an imperfect measure of total HDL mass or particle number because of the heterogeneity of HDL size and composition. In addition, with increasing plasma triglyceride levels, HDL become progressively enriched in triglycerides at the expense of cholesteryl esters. The low HDL cholesterol levels in most hypertriglyceridemic patients reflect mainly this phenomenon, as well as predominance of small HDL_3 particles, and, to a lesser extent, a reduction of HDL particle number.[43] The number of HDL particles is better reflected by measurement of the major protein of HDL, apo A-I, in whole plasma.

With the presence of abnormal lipoproteins, as in LCAT deficiency states, measurement of unesterified (free) cholesterol concentrations as well as total cholesterol may be useful. There are

Table 114-8 Normal Values (mg/dl) for HDL Cholesterol

	White Males			White Females (Sex Hormone Nonusers)		
		Percentiles			Percentiles	
Age (years)	Mean	5	95	Mean	5	95
5–9	56	39	73	53	33	72
10–14	54	37	73	52	35	70
15–19	45	29	68	52	33	74
20–29	45	30	64	55	35	77
30–39	44	27	64	56	35	81
40–49	44	29	67	57	35	87
60–69	46	28	70	57	35	85
70–79	47	29	84	55	34	79

Table 114-9 Hyperlipidemic Disorders

Generic Designation and Elevated Lipoprotein Class	Synonym	Primary Disorders	Secondary Disorders*
Exogenous hyperlipemia (chylomicrons)	Type I	Familial lipoprotein lipase deficiency C-II apolipoprotein deficiency Unclassified	Dysglobulinemias Systemic lupus erythematosus
Endogenous hyperlipemia (VLDL)	Type IV	Familial hypertriglyceridemia (mild form) Familial multiple lipoprotein-type hyperlipidemia Sporadic hypertriglyceridemia Tangier disease	§ Dysglobulinemias Systemic lupus erythematosus Diabetic hyperlipemia† Glycogenosis, type I Lipodystrophies Uremia Hypopituitarism Nephrotic syndrome (Diabetes mellitus)‡ (Alcoholism)
Mixed hyperlipemia (VLDL + chylomicrons)	Type V	Familial hypertriglyceridemia (severe form) Familial lipoprotein lipase deficiency C-II apolipoprotein deficiency	(Estrogen use) (Glucocorticoid use) (Stress-induced)
Hypercholesterolemia (LDL)	Type II-a	Familial hypercholesterolemia (LDL receptor defects) Familial multiple lipoprotein-type hyperlipidemia Polygenic hypercholesterolemia (includes exogenous hypercholesterolemia)	Nephrotic syndrome Hypothyroidism Dysglobulinemias Cushing syndrome Acute intermittent porphyria
Combined hyperlipidemia (LDL + VLDL)	Type II-b	Familial multiple lipoprotein-type hyperlipidemia Unclassified	Nephrotic syndrome Hypothyroidism Dysglobulinemias Cushing syndrome (Glucocorticoid use) (Stress-induced)
Remnant hyperlipidemia (β-VLDL)	Type III	Familial dysbetalipoproteinemia Unclassified	Hypothyroidism Systemic lupus erythematosus
Lamellar hyperlipoproteinemia (Vesicular and discoidal lipoproteins)		Familial lecithin: cholesterol acyltransferase deficiency	Cholestasis (with LP-X) Hepatic failure (with lamellar HDL)

* All conditions associated with VLDL or β-VLDL are aggravated by hypertrophic obesity.
† Denotes mixed hyperlipemia caused by severe, prolonged insulin deficiency.
‡ Parentheses indicate conditions that frequently aggravate a primary hyperlipemia but that seldom cause hyperlipemia de novo. These conditions cause some cases of primary hypertriglyceridemia (mild form) to present as mixed hyperlipemia.
§ Bracket indicates secondary disorders that can cause type IV or type V hyperlipidemia.
SOURCE: From RJ Havel.[15] Reprinted with permission.

few clinical indications, however, for estimation of other plasma lipids, such as phospholipids. Lipoprotein electrophoresis can help to document the presence of abnormal lipoproteins, especially when applied to ultracentrifugally separated fractions such as VLDL, but it is seldom needed for diagnosis of the genetic disorders discussed in this section.

The initial measurements of plasma triglycerides, LDL cholesterol, and HDL cholesterol, together with a qualitative estimate of chylomicronemia, are usually sufficient to determine the nature and severity of hyperlipidemia. This is commonly expressed as a lipoprotein "phenotype," which denotes the class or classes of lipoproteins whose concentration is abnormal. With this information, the physician should exclude abnormalities reflecting systemic disorders associated with altered lipoprotein concentrations (Table 114-9). Well-defined monogenic disorders account for only a small fraction of the primary hyperlipoproteinemias, and all of the monogenic hypolipoproteinemias are rare (Table 114-10). In some cases, other clinical information, especially the presence of xanthomas of skin or tendons, narrows the diagnostic possibilities and occasionally permits a specific diagnosis to be made (Table 114-11). For example, xanthomas of the Achilles tendons in a patient with a very high LDL cholesterol level are usually caused by familial hypercholesterolemia, and occasionally by familial defective apo B. However, for most of the disorders considered here, special diagnostic tests are needed to detect abnormal amounts or structure of apolipoproteins or enzymes of lipid transport.

Most apoproteins can be estimated in whole plasma by immunoassay. However, qualitative abnormalities of apolipoproteins and gross changes in their concentration are usually evaluated by electrophoresis of apolipoproteins from ultracentrifugally separated lipoprotein fractions in polyacrylamide gels containing sodium dodecyl sulfate or by isoelectric focusing electrophoresis. The activities of lipoprotein lipase and hepatic lipase are usually estimated in blood plasma obtained after IV injection of heparin, which releases these enzymes from their binding sites on cell surfaces. The activity of lipases and LCAT is usually assayed with artificial emulsions or liposomes containing radioactive substrate. CETP activity is assayed by measuring the transfer of cholesteryl esters between HDL and LDL + VLDL. Immunoassays for these enzymes, CETP and PLTP, and assay of LDL-receptor activity in freshly isolated leukocytes, or in cultured

Table 114-10 Monogenic Disorders of the Plasma Lipoproteins

Apolipoprotein disorders*	
Apo A-1 (121, 122)	A-I deficiency (multiple mutants) A-I/C-III deficiency
Apo B (115)	Familial hypobetalipoproteinemia (apo B truncation mutants) Familial defective apo B
Apo C-II (117)	C-II deficiency (multiple mutants)
Apo E (119)	E deficiency Dysfunctional apo E (multiple mutants)
Enzyme disorders	
Lipoprotein lipase (117)	Lipoprotein lipase deficiency Lipoprotein lipase inhibitor
Hepatic lipase (117)	Hepatic lipase deficiency
Lecithin: cholesterol acyltransferase (118)	LCAT deficiency (multiple mutants) Fish-eye disease
Receptor disorders	
LDL receptor (120)	Familial hypercholesterolemia (multiple mutants)
Transfer/transport protein disorders	
Cholesteryl ester transfer protein (121)	Cholesteryl ester transfer protein deficiency
Microsomal triglyceride transfer protein (115)	Classic abetalipoproteinemia
ABC1 (122)	Tangier disease
Unknown (115)	Chylomicron retention disease

*Numbers refer to relevant chapters in this section.

Table 114-11 Associations of Visible Xanthomas and Lipid Infiltrates with Lipoprotein Disorders

Xanthoma	Genetic Disorder	Secondary Disorder
Eruptive	Familial lipoprotein lipase deficiency C-II apolipoprotein deficiency Familial lipoprotein lipase inhibitor Familial hypertriglyceridemia (severe forms of, aggravated by alcohol, estrogen use, or diabetes)	Diabetic hyperlipemia Cholestasis Lipodystrophies Glycogenosis type I Monoclonal gammopathies
Tuberoeruptive	Familial hypertriglyceridemia (as above) Familial dysbetalipoproteinemia	Cholestasis Monoclonal gammopathies
Tuberous	Familial dysbetalipoproteinemia Familial hypercholesterolemia Phytosterolemia	Monoclonal gammopathies
Tendinous	Familial hypercholesterolemia Familial defective apo B Familial dysbetalipoproteinemia Phytosterolemia Cerebrotendinous xanthomatosis	
Planar		
Palmar-digital creases	Familial dysbetalipoproteinemia	Cholestasis
Intertriginous	Familial hypercholesterolemia (homozygotes)	
Diffuse	A-I apolipoprotein deficiency	Monoclonal gammopathies
Subcutaneous	Familial hypercholesterolemia	Monoclonal gammopathies
Xanthelasma*	Familial hypercholesterolemia Familial defective apo B Familial dysbetalipoproteinemia	Monoclonal gammopathies
Corneal arcus*	Familial hypercholesterolemia	
Tonsillar	Tangier disease	

*May occur in normolipidemic individuals.

fibroblasts, are currently available in only a few research laboratories. The application of these diagnostic tests is described in the chapters that follow.

REFERENCES

1. Nerking J: Fetterweissverbindungen. *Pflugers Arch* **85**:330, 1901.
2. Machebouef MA: Recherches sur les phosphoaminolipids et les sterides du serum et du plasma sanguins. *Bull Soc Chim Biol* **11**:268, 1929.
3. Oncley JL, Scatchard G, Brown A: Physical-chemical characteristics of the certain proteins of normal human plasma. *J Phys Chem* **51**:184, 1947.
4. Levine L, Kauffman DL, Brown RK: The antigenic similarity of human low-density lipoproteins. *J Exp Med* **102**:105, 1955.
5. Aladjem J, Leiberman M, Gofman JW: Immunochemical studies on human plasma lipoproteins. *J Exp Med* **105**:49, 1957.
6. Gofman JW, Lindgren FT, Elliott H: Ultracentrifugal studies of lipoproteins of human serum. *J Biol Chem* **179**:973, 1949.
7. Briner WW, Riddle JW, Cornwell DG: Studies on the immunochemistry of human low-density lipoproteins utilizing an hemaglutination technique. *J Exp Med* **110**:113, 1959.
8. Shore B: C- and N-terminal amino acids of human serum lipoproteins. *Arch Biochem* **71**:1, 1957.
9. Rodbell M: N-terminal amino acid and lipid composition of lipoproteins from chyle and plasma. *Science* **127**:701, 1958.
10. Gustafson A, Alaupovic P, Furman RH: Preliminary notes—Studies of the composition and structure of serum lipoproteins: Physical-chemical characterization of phospholipid-protein residues obtained from very-low-density human serum lipoproteins. *Biochim Biophys Acta* **84**:767, 1964.
11. Gotto AM Jr, Pownall HR, Havel RJ: Introduction to the plasma lipoproteins. *Methods Enzymol* **128**:3, 1986.
12. Havel RJ: Origin, metabolic fate and metabolic function of plasma lipoproteins, in Steinberg D, Olefsky JM (eds): *Contemporary Issues in Endocrinology and Metabolism.* New York, Churchill Livingstone, 1987, vol 3, p 117.
13. Eisenberg S: High-density lipoprotein metabolism. *J Lipid Res* **25**:1017, 1984.
14. Fielding CJ, Fielding PE: Molecular physiology of reverse cholesterol transport. *J Lipid Res* **36**:211, 1995.
15. Havel RJ: Approach to the patient with hyperlipidemia. *Med Clin North Am* **66**:319, 1982.
16. Brown WV, Ginsberg H: Classification and diagnosis of the hyperlipidemias, in Steinberg D, JM Olefsky (eds): *Contemporary Issues in Endocrinology and Metabolism.* New York, Churchill Livingstone, 1987, vol 3, p 143.
17. Edelstein C, Kezdy F, Scanu AM, Shen BW: Apolipoproteins and the structural organization of plasma lipoproteins: Human plasma high-density lipoprotein-3. *J Lipid Res* **20**:143, 1979.
18. Luo C-C, Li W-H, Moore MN, Chan L: Structure and evolution of the apolipoprotein multigene family. *J Mol Biol* **187**:325, 1986.
19. Drayna D, Fielding C, McLean J, Baer B, Castro G, Chen E, Comstock L, Henzel W, Kohr W, Rhee L, Wion K, Lawn R: Cloning and expression of human apolipoprotein D cDNA. *J Biol Chem* **216**:165355, 1986.
20. Drayna D, Jarnagin AS, McLean J, Henzel W, Kohr W, Fielding C, Lawn R: Cloning and sequencing of human cholesteryl ester transfer protein cDNA. *Nature* **327**:632, 1987.
21. Albers JJ, Tu A-Y, Wolfbauer G, Cheung MC, Marcovina SM: Molecular biology of phospholipid transfer protein. *Curr Opin Lipidol* **2**:88, 1996.
22. Kunitake ST, Carilli CT, Lau K, Protter AA, Naya-Vigne J, Kane JP: Identification of proteins associated with apolipoprotein A-I-containing lipoproteins purified by selected affinity immunosorption. *Biochemistry* **33**:1988, 1994.
23. Tall AR, Small DM, Deckelbaum RJ, Shipley G: Structure and thermodynamic properties of high-density lipoprotein recombinants. *J Biol Chem* **252**:4702, 1977.
24. Felker TE, Hamilton RL, Vigne J-L, Havel RJ: Properties of lipoproteins in blood plasma and liver perfusates of rats with cholestasis. *Gastroenterology* **83**:652, 1982.
25. Wion KL, Kirchgessner TG, Lusis AJ, Schotz JC, Lawn RM: Human lipoprotein lipase complementary DNA sequence. *Science* **235**:1638, 1987.
26. Komarony MC, Schotz MC: Cloning of rat hepatic lipase cDNA: Evidence for a lipase gene family. *Proc Natl Acad Sci U S A* **84**:1526, 1987.
27. Qiu S, Bergeron N, Kotite L, Krauss RM, Bensadoun A, Havel RJ: Metabolism of lipoproteins containing apolipoprotein B in hepatic lipase-deficient mice. *J Lipid Res*, **39**:1661, 1998.
28. Jackson RL: Lipoprotein lipase and hepatic lipase, in Boyer PD (ed): *The Enzymes*. New York, Academic, 1983, vol 16, p 141.
29. Havel, RJ: Receptor and non-receptor mediated uptake of chylomicron remnants by the liver. *Atherosclerosis*, **141 suppl:S1**, 1998.
30. Krieger, M: The "best" of cholesterols, and "worst" of cholesterols: A tale of two receptors. *Proc Natl Acad Sci U S A* **95**:4077, 1998.
31. Krieger M, Herz, J: Structure and functions of multiligand lipoprotein receptors: Macrophage scavenger receptors and LDL receptor-related protein (LRP). *Annu Rev Biochem* **63**:601, 1994.
32. Suzuki H, Kurihara Y, Takeya M, Kamada N, Kataoka M, Jishage K, Ueda O, et al: A role for macrophage scavenger receptors in atherosclerosis and susceptibility to infection. *Nature* **386**:292, 1997.
33. Hamilton RL, Moorehouse A, Havel RJ: Isolation and properties of nascent lipoproteins from highly purified rat hepatocytic Golgi fractions. *J Lipid Res* **32**:529, 1991.
34. Kunitake ST, La Sala KJ, Kane JP: Apoprotein A-I-containing lipoproteins with pre-beta electrophoretic mobility. *J Lipid Res* **26**:549, 1985.
35. Lawn RM, Wade DP, Garvin MR, Wang X, Schwartz K, Porter JG, Seilhamer JJ, Vaughan AM, Oram JF. The Tangier disease gene product ABC1 controls the cellular apolipoprotein-mediated lipid removal pathway. *J Clin Invest* **104**:R25, 1999.
36. Fielding CJ, Fielding PE: Intracellular cholesterol transport. *J Lipid Res* **38**:1503, 1997.
37. Brooks-Wilson A, Marcil M, Clee S, Zhang L-H, Roomp K, van Dam M, Yu L, et al.: Mutations in ABC1 in Tangier disease and familial high-density lipoprotein deficiency. *Nat Genet* **22**:336, 1999.
38. Bodzioch M, Orso E, Klucken J, Langmann T, Böttcher A, Diederich W, Drobnik W, et al.: The gene encoding ATP-binding cassette transporter 1 is mutated in Tangier disease. *Nat Gen* **22**:347, 1999.
39. Rust S, Rosier M, Funke H, Real J, Amoura Z, Piette J-C, Deleuze J-F, et al.: Tangier disease is caused by mutations in the gene encoding ATP-binding cassette transporter 1. *Nat Gen* **22**:352, 1999.
40. Kunitake ST, Mendel, CM, Hennessy, LK: Interconversion between apolipoprotein A-I-containing lipoproteins of pre-beta and alpha electrophoretic mobilities. *J Lipid Res* **33**:1807, 1992.
41. Jiang XC, Francone OL, Bruce C, Milne R, Mar J, Walsh A, Breslow JL, Tall AR: Increased Preβ-high density lipoprotein, apolipoprotein AI, and phospholipid in mice expressing the human phospholipid transfer protein and human apolipoprotein AI transgenes. *J Clin Invest* **98**:2373, 1996.
42. Hennessy LK, Kunitake, ST, Jarvis M, Hamilton RL, Endeman G, Protter A, Kane JP: Isolation of subpopulations of high-density lipoproteins: Three particle species containing apo E and two species devoid of apo E that have affinity for heparin. *J Lipid Res* **38**:1859, 1997.
43. Phillips NR, Havel RJ, Kane JP: Serum apolipoprotein A-I levels: relationship to lipoprotein lipid levels and selected demographic variables. *Am J Epidemiol* **116**:302, 1982.
44. Tall AR: Plasma cholesteryl ester transfer protein. *J Lipid Res* **34**:1255, 1993.

CHAPTER 115

Disorders of the Biogenesis and Secretion of Lipoproteins Containing the B Apolipoproteins

John P. Kane ▪ Richard J. Havel

1. VLDL and chylomicrons, which transport triglycerides to peripheral tissues via the bloodstream, are major lipoprotein secretory products of the liver and intestine, respectively. Each class of these lipoproteins contains a protein of very-high molecular weight (a B apolipoprotein) that is essential for the secretion of the lipoprotein particle and that has very high affinity for lipids, remaining with the lipoprotein complex throughout its metabolic processing in plasma or lymph.
2. There are two translation products of a single structural gene for B apolipoproteins. In humans, the exclusive B apoprotein of VLDL and LDL is apo B-100, a single polypeptide chain of 4536 amino acid residues and the full-length translation product of the gene. The predominant species of apo B in chylomicrons is apo B-48, a single chain of 2152 amino acid residues identical to the N-terminal portion of apo B-100. This protein is translated from an edited mRNA transcript containing a single base substitution that produces a stop codon corresponding to residue 2153 of apo B-100. Several disorders are now recognized in which the secretion of apo B-containing lipoproteins or the structure of apo B itself is abnormal.
3. Abetalipoproteinemia (MIM 200100) is an autosomal recessive disorder characterized by the virtual absence of VLDL and LDL from plasma. Fat malabsorption is severe and triglyceride accumulation occurs in enterocytes and, to some extent, in liver. Acanthocytosis of erythrocytes is common. Spinocerebellar ataxia with degeneration of the fasciculus cuneatus and fasciculus gracilis, peripheral neuropathy, degenerative pigmentary retinopathy, and ceroid myopathy all appear to be secondary to defects of transport of tocopherol in blood. It is possible that mechanisms underlying the failure to secrete VLDL and chylomicrons differ among kindreds. However, intracellular accumulation of B protein points to defects in the processing of B apoproteins or impairment of the assembly or secretion of triglyceride-rich lipoproteins. The first molecular defect now recognized is the absence of activity of microsomal triglyceride transfer protein, a factor critical to the lipidation of B proteins. Treatment involves reduction of dietary fat to prevent steatorrhea and supplementation with tocopherol to prevent progression of the neuromuscular and retinal degenerative disease.
4. In the homozygous state, clinical manifestations of familial hypobetalipoproteinemia (HBL) (MIM 107730) are indistinguishable from those of abetalipoproteinemia: acanthocytosis, neuromuscular disability, and malabsorption. Clinically, this disorder is distinguished from recessive abetalipoproteinemia by the appearance of hypolipidemia in heterozygotes. The defects underlying this disorder involve the gene for apo B in most cases. A number of mutations have been described that lead to the secretion of truncated forms of the protein. In some cases, the phenotype does not cosegregate with apo B haplotypes. Defects affecting the rate of synthesis or the rate of removal of apo B are emerging.
5. Fat malabsorption and the absence of chylomicrons in plasma after fat ingestion characterize chylomicron retention disease (MIM 246700). Apo B-100 is found in LDL; however, total LDL levels are about half of normal. Acanthocytosis and neurologic manifestations occur in some patients. The defect appears to be recessive. Large numbers of particles resembling nascent chylomicrons crowd the enterocyte, accompanied by high levels of apo B-48, suggesting a specific defect in the secretion of chylomicrons.
6. Apo B-100 carries a ligand domain for the LDL receptor. Several mutations in apo B-100 affecting the binding affinity of LDL for the receptor have been identified. Levels of LDL in plasma are increased in many but not all individuals who bear one mutant allele. The hyperlipidemia is usually less severe than that observed with LDL receptor defects because LDL precursors can be endocytosed via the ligand in apolipoprotein E.
7. Familial combined hyperlipidemia is probably the most prevalent genetically determined disorder of lipoproteins now recognized. It carries a significantly increased risk of coronary arteriosclerosis. It appears to be an autosomal

A list of standard abbreviations is located immediately preceding the index in each volume. Additional abbreviations used in this chapter include: ABL = abetalipoproteinemia; ABL-HDL$_4$ = abetalipoproteinemia-HDL$_4$; ACAT = acylCoA:cholesterol acyltransferase; CD = circular dichroism; C/EBP = CCAAT/enhancer-binding protein; CETP = cholesteryl ester transfer protein; FCH = familial combined hyperlipidemia; FLDB = familial ligand-defective apo B; HBL = hypobetalipoproteinemia; HNF-1 = hepatic nuclear factor 1; IDL = intermediate-density lipoproteins; LCAT = lecithin:cholesterol acyltransferase; Lp(a) = lipoprotein(a); LPL = lipoprotein lipase; MTP = microsomal triglyceride transfer protein; T-1, T-2, etc. = and thrombin cleavage fragments of apo B; TRL = triglyceride-rich lipoproteins.

dominant trait with high penetrance that leads to increased levels of apo B-100 and elevated levels of VLDL, LDL, or both in plasma. The phenotypic pattern can shift among these types over time. Kinetic studies suggest that increased production of apo B-100 may be a common underlying metabolic characteristic.

INTRODUCTION

All vertebrates appear to have proteins evolutionarily related to human apolipoprotein B. Several sequence regions in these proteins show homologies with vitellogenins.[1] In mammals, B apolipoproteins are chiefly secreted by the liver and intestine for the transport of endogenous and exogenous lipids, respectively. Expression of apo B-100 and secretion of apo B-containing lipoproteins by the heart has also been demonstrated.[2] Gene knockout experiments in mice demonstrated an essential role for secretion of apo B-100-containing lipoproteins by the yolk sac during gestation.[3]

The essential roles of the B apolipoproteins in the secretion of triglyceride-rich lipoproteins from liver and intestine were brought to light by the discovery of autosomal recessive abetalipoproteinemia and familial hypobetalipoproteinemia (HBL). A more recently discovered disorder, chylomicron retention disease, provides evidence that tissue-specific events in the secretion of chylomicrons may involve different gene products than are required for the secretion of VLDL by liver. A general pattern is emerging with respect to the genetic bases of these disorders. The dominant disorders appear in the majority of cases to represent abnormalities at the apo B gene locus, whereas the recessive hypolipidemic states are the result of genetic impairment of elements that function in the machinery of the lipidation and secretory pathways. The apo B-100 molecule contains a receptor-ligand domain that is essential for the receptor-mediated endocytosis of LDL. Mutations affecting ligand function are now known. As additional functional domains are recognized in apo B, it is likely that other disorders of lipoprotein metabolism will be attributable to mutations in B apoproteins. Familial combined hyperlipidemia, a common disorder of lipoproteins and a major cause of arteriosclerotic disease, involves several classes of lipoproteins that contain apo B-100. The full elucidation of its causes, probably multifactorial, will only come with further exploration of the mechanisms that regulate the assembly, secretion, and metabolic processing of these lipoproteins.

The characterization of apo B proceeded very slowly, in contrast to that of the smaller apolipoproteins. Chief among the obstacles to its chemical manipulation was its extreme self-association upon removal of lipids.[4] Soluble, lipid-free preparations were achieved only by chemical modification, followed by extraction of lipids, or by laborious extractions in the presence of chaotropic or amphipathic compounds.[4,5] A further obstacle was the marked susceptibility of the molecule to scission by proteases from serum or microbial proteases acquired casually during purification. Thus, a number of investigators reported the isolation of putative protomeric units varying in estimated size from 8 to more than 250 kDa. However, later studies designed to inhibit self-association and protease attack yielded apparent molecular weights in good agreement with aminoacyl mass calculated from cDNA sequence.[6]

STRUCTURE OF apo B

Apo B in Lipoproteins

Recognition of Multiple Forms of Apo B. In 1980, it was found that there are two primary forms of apo B in human plasma and thoracic duct lymph.[7] One, found in LDL and VLDL, had an apparent molecular mass of 549 kDa, whereas the other, found in chylomicrons from thoracic duct lymph and plasma, had an apparent molecular mass of 264 kDa. The amino acid compositions were distinct, but immunochemical cross-reactivity was prominent. To facilitate comparison of apparent molecular weights of apo B species, a centile system of nomenclature was proposed in which the predominant form of apo B in human LDL is termed "apo B-100" and each other species or fragment of apo B is assigned a centile designation reflecting its apparent M_r relative to apo B-100 (Fig. 115-1). In this system, the smaller species of human apo B was designated "apo B-48."

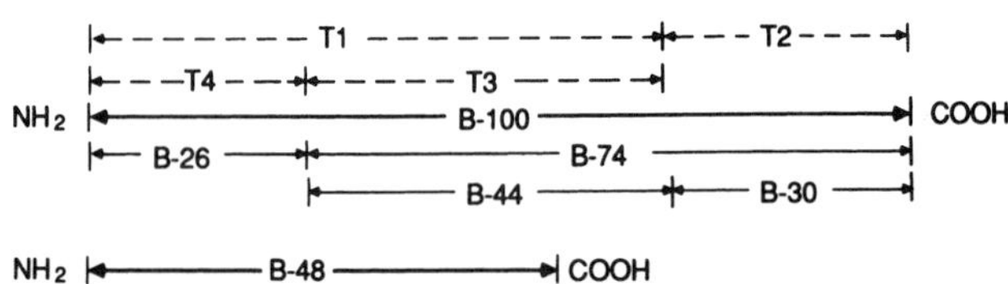

Fig. 115-1 B apolipoproteins and their large proteolytic fragments. The proteins and fragments are aligned according to sequence, with the amino termini of the B-100 and B-48 proteins indicated at left. Thrombin-derived fragments are indicated with broken lines, above the B-100 line; kallikrein-derived fragments with solid lines, below the B-100 line.

The Molar Representation of Apo B Species in Lipoproteins. As described below, the distribution of the primary species of apo B among the lipoproteins of plasma in humans appears to resemble that found in many mammals. That is, apo B-100 appears in hepatogenous triglyceride-rich lipoproteins and in LDL, whereas apo B-48 is the predominant, and nearly exclusive, B apolipoprotein produced by the intestine of adult animals. A number of mammalian species can edit apo B mRNA in liver to produce apo B-48 as well. One other class of particles, the (a) lipoprotein [Lp(a)], also contains apo B-100 as the sole B-apoprotein species, linked to the (a) apoprotein by disulfide bridging (see Chaps. 114 and 116).[8,9] All the lipoproteins that contain B apolipoproteins are organized as microemulsion particles, having a hydrophobic core surrounded by a monolayer of amphipathic lipids. The B apolipoproteins interact with the surface monolayer and in some regions penetrate to contact the hydrophobic core.[10]

A content of 540 × 10^3 daltons of protein per LDL particle has been found, based on amino acyl mass (Kane JP, Hardman DA, unpublished observations), a value that is in relatively close agreement with the mass based on sequence (512,937 daltons) indicating that LDL, and by inference VLDL, contain a single copy of apo B-100. These data are in agreement with other data based on composition.[10,11] This is supported by the observation, in individuals heterozygous for a polymorphism of apo B, that a specific discriminating monoclonal antibody is capable of precipitating only half of the LDL particles, indicating that the product of only one allele is present on each.[12] Strong additional evidence comes from studies of the stoichiometries of the reactions of eight anti-apo B monoclonal antibodies with LDL.[13] The stoichiometries range from 0.5 to 1.2 mol of antibody per particle of LDL, with a mean of 0.75 mol. When the mass ratio of lipid to apo B is known, the number average molecular weight for particles obtained from a narrow density interval can be calculated accurately.[10] If sphericity is assumed, the particle diameter can likewise be calculated. Measurements of intrinsic viscosity of LDL reveal values close to those of the Einsteinian minimum for perfect spheres, strongly supporting that assumption (Kane JP, unpublished data). Thus, the mean particle diameter of LDL with a modal density of 1.030 g/cm^3 is 202 Å.

Determination of the number of copies of apo B-48 per chylomicron particle is a much more formidable task because of the extreme heterogeneity of particle size, the relatively small percentage of total mass attributed to B protein, and the likelihood of contamination with VLDL. Employing a determination of mass of chemical constituents and estimating particle volume by electron microscopy, Battacharya and Redgrave estimated a content of apo B-48 of 4.8 × 10^5 daltons per particle, a figure that would nearly accommodate two copies of the protein.[14] However, the estimate of mean particle volume is particularly difficult due to extensive flattening of the particles on electron microscope grids. To the contrary, data from immunoelectron microscopy strongly support a ratio of one copy of apo B-48 per chylomicron remnant particle.[15] Because of the inability of B proteins to migrate between particles, it may be presumed that the ratio holds for nascent chylomicrons as well.

Disposition of Apo B in Lipoproteins. Virtually all the data available on the conformation of B apoproteins and their relationship to lipids in lipoproteins were obtained by study of LDL and VLDL. Some inference may be drawn for apo B-48 based on its sequence homology with apo B-100, but direct observation is required to determine with confidence its conformation in chylomicrons. B apoprotein is thought to be disposed largely at the interface of the surface monolayer with the aqueous environment, hydrophobic side chains interacting with lipid, and hydrophilic side chains extending into the aqueous phase. This model is supported by the relative completeness of modification of hydrophilic side chains by hydrophilic reagents[16] and by accessibility to trypsin. LDL exhibits three major thermal transitions during unfolding.[17] NMR studies indicate constraint by apo B-100 on the phospholipids of LDL.[18] It appears that apo B-100 is also capable of constraining the motion of core cholesteryl esters, either directly or indirectly, because scission of the protein by trypsin in native LDL causes an increase of disorder as detected by a decrease of induced circular dichroism (CD) of intrinsic carotenoids.[19] Analyses of CD indicate that apo B in LDL contains approximately 41 percent helix, 22 percent β structure, 20 percent β turns, and 17 percent random coil structure,[16,20–22] in close agreement with secondary structure predicted from cDNA sequence.[23] Allowing for the CD contribution of non-B apoproteins, it appears that apo B-100 is more helical in VLDL than in LDL.[24]

Studies of recombination of delipidated apo B-100 with lipids have shed useful light on the nature of its interaction with lipid. Krieger et al.[25] were able to produce an apo B-100-phospholipid complex in which hydrophobic core lipids could be replaced, reforming LDL-like particles. Further evidence of affinity of apo B for surface phospholipids is the association of apo B-100 with lecithin to form complexes in which the protein conformation resembles that of native LDL.[26] Apo B-100 solubilized with deoxycholate forms a complex with dimyristoylphosphatidylcholine liposomes,[26,27] but the complex has less thermal stability than native LDL.

Delipidated apo B-100 also recombines with microemulsions to form LDL-like particles.[27,28] Thermal analysis revealed that apo B influences the transitions of core lipids in the recombinant particles and that greater thermal stability of the protein was achieved in the microemulsion complexes than when it reacted with phospholipid alone.[28] Secondary structure of the protein in these complexes was similar to that in LDL. Recombination of proteolytic fragments of apo B-100 with microemulsions of phospholipid and cholesteryl esters indicates that lipid-binding properties are broadly distributed within the apo B molecule. Virtually all the larger polypeptides (14 to 100 kDa) in arrays of fragments produced by specific endoproteases bind to microemulsion particles, yielding LDL-like particles with similar helicity to native LDL but with less β conformation.[29] This affinity of apo B for lipid is reflected by a high average hydrophobicity (0.916 kcal/residue).[30]

Domain Structure of Apo B-100. Both kallikrein and thrombin cleave apo B-100, producing large fragments that have been useful in sequence determination. They promise to be of much further use in exploring structural domains because of the large molecular weights of the B proteins. LDL as commonly prepared from human blood often contains two fragments of apo B-100, termed "apo B-74" and "apo B-26" in the centile system.[7] This scission is the result of proteolysis mediated by kallikrein.[31,32] The addition of appropriate inhibitors to freshly drawn blood prevents the appearance of the fragments, indicating that proteolysis by kallikrein is probably minimal or absent in vivo. The observation that C1 esterase inhibitor is the natural inhibitor of this reaction[33] suggests that LDL apo B of individuals deficient in that protein may be subject to scission in vivo.

Thrombin also cleaves apo B-100 of LDL and, to a lesser extent, apo B of VLDL into large fragments. The primary fragments T1 and T2 were at first confused with B-74 and B-26, respectively, because they have similar molecular weights. However, the scission sites are on opposite ends of the B-100 chain[34,35] (see Fig. 115-1). T1 is cleaved further into two polypeptides, T3 and T4. T2 and T3 remain joined by a disulfide bridge unless reduced.

Exploration of the domain structure of apo B in LDL using 12 specific endoproteases revealed 3 nearly equal superdomains, separated by interdomain loops of 40 and 100 amino acids, respectively, at residues 1280 to 1320 and 3180 to 3280.[36] Limited digestion with trypsin defines five superdomains.[37] Apo B-100 is also cleaved by cathepsin D.[38] It is likely that this protease initiates endosomal hydrolysis of apo B in lipoproteins after endocytosis.[39] Endoprotease probe studies identified a local sequence, near residue 1076 in apo B-100 of LDL, that undergoes a helix to β structure transition as the triglyceride content of the particles changes.[40] Reactivities of several monoclonal antibodies with epitopes on apo B-100 also reflect the lipid composition of the particles.

Calculations based on the composition of LDL indicate that protein must participate in the surface monolayer. Electron photomicrographs of apo B crosslinked on LDL with glutaraldehyde and extracted free of lipids, reveal a ring-like structure, suggesting an equatorial disposition in the LDL particle.[41] Three-dimensional mapping with monoclonal antibodies by immunoelectron microscopy has yielded an accurate model of apo B-100 disposed in a kinked circumferential fashion around the LDL lipid microemulsion particle.[42] Further studies have demonstrated a redundant loop or "bow" at the C-terminus that crosses over the chain at the approximate region of the sequence believed to be central to the LDL receptor ligand domain.[43] Apo B-100 contains 39 short hydrophobic sequences that could exist in the monolayer.[44] As described below, the circumferential disposition of apo B could account for the monotonic relationship of chain length of apo B to the diameters of lipoprotein particles that contain apo B molecules truncated either by puromycin or as a result of transfection with constructs coding for foreshortened apo B chains.[45–47] However, to accommodate larger contents of lipid, the conformation of the B apoproteins in large triglyceride-rich VLDL and chylomicrons must involve major differences from that of apo B-100 in LDL. The length of the equatorial belt of apo B as described for LDL-like particles is about 700 Å. In contrast, the circumferences of normal VLDL particles average approximately 1200 Å and range as high as 1800 Å in the largest VLDL. The disparity is even greater for chylomicrons in which an apo B species of less than half the chain length of apo B-100 must accommodate particle circumferences of 3000 Å or more. Studies comparing the accessibility of susceptible sequences to endoprotease attack[36] and of epitopes to monoclonal antibodies[48,49] support major conformational differences in apo B-100 between VLDL and LDL. Although only a few sequences capable of forming amphipathic helixes are present, sequences capable of forming β structure are common, including four regions rich in proline.[50,51]

Apo B-100 contains 25 cysteine residues, chiefly located in the N-terminal domain, of which at least 22 are involved in intrachain disulfide bridges.[37,52] Both apo B-100 and apo B-48 are glycoproteins. At least 16 sites in apo B-100 are glycosylated, with concentrations in the N-terminal region and around the putative LDL receptor-ligand domain.[37] Removal of carbohydrate does not appear to change affinity for the receptor, however.[53] The presence of several moles of fatty acids in ester or thioester linkage may facilitate interaction with lipids.[54,55] Phosphorylation of apo B-48 has also been described.[56]

Biochemical Functions of B Apolipoproteins. The binding domain for the B-100:E receptor (LDL receptor) appears to reside in the portion of apo B-100 that is not homologous with apo B-48.[57] Modification of Arg or Lys residues interrupts binding.[58,59] Heparin, a polyanion, displaces LDL from the receptor, adding further support to a model in which ligand sequences with a number of cationic residues interact electrostatically with polyanionic sites on the receptor. Several monoclonal antibodies that block binding react with epitopes in the C-terminal half of B-100,[60–62] particularly those with epitopes near the T2-T3 junction.[63] In agreement with this, the peptide sequence from residues 3345 to 3381 partially restores binding of trypsinized VLDL, indicating that at least one element of the receptor-binding domain is at that site.[23] Furthermore, truncations of apo B shorter than apo B-67 (which contains 3040 amino acid residues) completely lose affinity for the receptor, whereas the longer truncations, apo B-75 and apo B-89, have increased affinity.[64–70] The binding of chylomicron and VLDL remnants to the LDL receptor involves other ligands. Apo E-deficient remnants of chylomicrons and VLDL bind poorly to the receptor,[71] as do remnants of chylomicrons from individuals homozygous for apo E-2, a defective ligand. Thrombin proteolysis of VLDL, which attacks receptor-interactive apo E, eliminates binding.[72] Apo B tends to be cleaved as well, but this, at least in LDL, does not inhibit binding. Addition of intact apo E restores binding of the triglyceride-rich particles. Kallikrein proteolysis of LDL also does not interfere with receptor-binding.[73] Thus, apo B of VLDL is not a ligand for the LDL receptor.[60,72] This suggests that conformational changes attendant to intravascular lipolysis are required to establish this domain.[74]

Although all the sequence elements that participate in receptor binding are probably not yet known, a highly conserved cluster of Arg and Lys residues near the T2-T3 junction is involved (site B). Studies with monoclonal antibodies suggest that sequences between residues 1480 and 1693 and between residues 2152 and 2377 influence binding to the receptor.[75] This requires a complicated folding of apo B to juxtapose those sequences or to influence the conformation of the protein in the region of site B. In keeping with the finding that deletions of the C-terminal portion of apo B-100 may enhance binding to the receptor, a monoclonal antibody directed at that region also appeared to enhance binding.[75] Elegant mutagenesis experiments in mice by Boren et al., contrasting various apolipoprotein B mutants with wild-type human apo B-100, defined the elements participating in binding with greater clarity.[76] Replacement of positively charged amino acids between residues 3359 and 3367 with neutral amino acids largely abolishes binding, suggesting that sequence in site B which has strong homology with the ligand sequence of apo E is essential. Furthermore, replacement of site B sequence by the ligand sequence of apo E retained receptor affinity. Mutation of Arg 3500 to Glu, which mimics a natural ligand-defective mutation, greatly reduces binding to the receptor, and truncations at apo B-77 and apo B-80 enhanced affinity, as noted in natural human mutations. Finally, the combination of the Arg 3500 → Glu substitution with the apo B-80 truncation has enhanced binding, indicating that Arg 3500 is not part of the ligand but normally interacts with the C-terminal "bow" of apo B-100, exposing site B. In the absence of the C-terminus, site B is exposed and free to interact with the receptor, whereas when the C-terminus is present, Glu 3500 fails to interact with the C-terminal bow region, leading to occlusion of site B. It is thus likely that the C-terminal bow is the conformational regulator that modulates ligand activity in VLDL and IDL (intermediate-density lipoprotein) by acting as an operculum over site B. The observation that individuals who lack mutations in site B or at codons 3500 or 3531 may have LDL with very low affinity for the LDL receptor suggests that elements of the receptor may reside elsewhere in apo B-100 or that they may influence conformation in the C-terminal region.

Observations in human apo B transgenic mice add further to knowledge of the ligand behavior of triglyceride-rich lipoproteins. When mice secreting only apo B-48 or only apo B-100 are crossed with mice lacking apo E, the mice carrying the apo B-100 transgene have moderately increased levels of cholesterol and normal levels of apo B-100, whereas those carrying the apo B-48 transgene have very high levels of cholesterol and of apo B-48 in plasma. This suggests that in the absence of the apo E ligand the apo B-100-containing particles can still be removed via the LDL receptor, whereas apo B-48 does not contain a ligand domain.[77]

The heparin-binding property, common to both primary forms of apo B,[78–81] may play an important role in the hydrolysis of circulating triglycerides by lipoprotein lipase and may facilitate the activity of hepatic lipase. Subfractions of heparin with high affinity for LDL also bind thrombin, apo E, and the antithrombin III-thrombin complex with high affinity.[80] Proteolysis of apo B-100 in LDL results in enhanced heparin-binding while reducing interaction with the B-100:E receptor, indicating that some heparin-binding sites are not involved in receptor-ligand interaction.[82] Apo B-100 appears to contain as many as eight heparin-interactive sites[81,83,84] distributed rather evenly through the length of the chain, three of which are present in apo B-48. Three of the putative heparin-binding sites have been shown to interact with arterial glycosaminoglycans.[85] Despite the observation that a number of sites exist in apo B-100 that can be shown to interact with glycosaminoglycans, the sequence including residue 3359–3369 (site B) appears to be critical. Mutagenesis of Arg 3363 to Glu virtually abolishes binding to biglycan and versican.[86] It is possible that the other sites may play physiological roles selectively in VLDL or chylomicrons.

As described below, both apo B-100 and B-48 appear to play essential roles in the organization and secretion of their respective lipoproteins from liver and intestinal epithelium, as evidenced by the absence of corresponding lipoproteins in abetalipoproteinemia and homozygous HBL. Furthermore, certain sequences may function specifically in a pause-transfer mechanism of lipidation in the ER and some portion of apo B, which is deleted from the C-terminal region in disorders associated with truncated B proteins, may be essential to the normal processing of VLDL to LDL.[87,88]

Species variation in apo B may account in part for differences in the rate of atherogenesis between humans and other mammalian species. Expression of human apo B transgene in mice dramatically increases the rate of atherogenesis in mice when the animals are fed a high fat diet. The combination of the human transgene and the diet resulted in a large increase in plasma non-HDL cholesterol.[89] That much, if not all, of the increase in atherosclerosis is attributable to effects on circulating lipoproteins is supported by experiments with transgenic mice selectively expressing apo B-48 alone or apo B-100[90] cross bred with apo E knockouts. The B 48/48; E −/− mice had the highest levels of plasma cholesterol and the most severe atherosclerosis, whereas the apo B 100/100; E −/− mice had lower plasma cholesterol levels and less atherosclerosis, probably reflecting retention of the ligand domain for the LDL receptor in apo B-100.

Polymorphisms of Apo B. A number of common structural variations in apo B were first identified immunologically as five allotypes of the (Ag) antigen system. The underlying genomic bases for four polymorphisms of this system have been identified,[91–97] and population genoclines have been observed for some of the dimorphs. The genetic basis of the fifth polymorphism (X/Y) remains obscure because of the linkage disequilibrium between two dimorphs.[97–99] The two dimorphs result in a pair of single residue substitutions such that Leu 2712/Ser 4311 are associated with the Ag(X) epitope and the allelic Pro 2712/Asn 4311 with the more prevalent Ag(Y) epitope.[97,100] It is of interest that individuals with homozygosity for the less common allele had significantly reduced levels of VLDL cholesterol and of the fraction of VLDL containing apo E and apo B.[100] An insertion-deletion polymorphism of the signal peptide has also been identified.[101,102] A number of associations have been made between these dimorphs (and other RFLP) and the levels of LDL or triglycerides in plasma or risk of coronary disease in various populations. Because the Ag polymorphisms involve changes in amino acid sequence, it is probable that some will have sufficient effect on the conformation of apo B that at least subtle alterations in metabolic behavior will result. Over 30 polymorphisms of the coding sequences of the apo B gene are recognized and 10 in noncoding DNA.[10,103]

Cloning of Apo B

The application of molecular genetic techniques to elucidate the structure of apo B was retarded by the chemical intractability of the B proteins. Because of their strong self-association, the isolation of internal peptides for sequencing was extremely difficult. The first cDNA sequence for B protein was reported by Lusis et al.[104] based on antibody screening of rat hepatic cDNA libraries. They reported an mRNA of approximately 20 kb in both liver and intestine. Others found a message of similar length in human, monkey, and baboon liver,[34,105] in HepG2 cells,[106] and in human and monkey intestine.[34] A message of approximately half that length was also observed in intestine with varying amounts of mRNA of intermediate lengths. Additional cDNA clones were then reported.[34,107–112] One series of overlapping clones yielded the sequence of the C-terminal third of the B-100 protein.[34] Another series[111,112] yielded the sequence of the N-terminal third and a signal peptide sequence (GenBank M14162, J02610).

Structure of the Apo B Gene. Analysis of genomic DNA in the 5′ flanking region revealed two classic promotor elements, a TATA box 29 nucleotides upstream of the transcription initiation site and a CAAT box 31 nucleotides upstream from the TATA box. A further sequence associated with promotors — CCGCCC — is repeated twice in the 80 bases preceding the ATG site.[111,112] The entire cDNA sequence was subsequently reported by several laboratories,[30,50,113–115] establishing apo B-100 as a single polypeptide chain of 4536 amino acids, corresponding to an aminoacyl mass of 513 kDa. The gene for apo B is on chromosome 2 in the 2p23-p24 region.[34,116] It is 43 kb in length with 29 exons, 24 of which are in the 5′ third. Two exons, 26 and 29, are extremely large, containing 7572 and 1906 bases, respectively. Two tandem repetitive elements 5′ and 3′ to the coding region are identified.[117] DNase I protection studies identified the boundaries of the gene[118] and homologies with the mouse gene have been studied.[119] Both enhancer and suppressor sites are identified in the 5′ region of the gene,[120–123] and differences in transcriptional control are observed between HepG2 and CaCo-2 cells. Two positive regulatory elements appear to confer hepatic-specific expression.[124] Two nuclear proteins, LIT 1 and LIT 2, bind to the major positive element of the apo B promotor.[124] An enhancer in the second intron containing four protein-binding sequences interacts with several nuclear proteins, including HNF-1 and a C/EBP-like element.[123,125,126] Tissue-specific transcription of apo B in liver and intestine appears to be related to undermethylation in the 5′ flanking region.

Analysis of a hypervariable region in the 3′ flanking region comprising 15-bp AT-rich tandem repeats greatly facilitated haplotyping of apo B alleles. At least 14 alleles have been identified at this site.[117]

The evolutionary history of the apo B gene may be complex because it contains 8 sequences of 22 codons that code for amphipathic helices with homology to a family of small apolipoproteins (A-I, A-II, A-IV, C-I, C-II, C-III, C-IV, and E). There are also 6 52-amino-acid sequences that are hydrophobic and rich in proline that have high potential for beta structure, and that appear to be unique to apo B. One sequence (residues 3352 to 3371) is highly homologous to the ligand domain in apolipoprotein E for the LDL receptor. Covalent attachment of the (a) protein moiety to apo B-100 in the Lp(a) lipoprotein complex is specific for a single Cys, residue 4326.[127]

The Origin of Apo B-48: Two Proteins From a Single Gene. Studies of the protein sequence of apo B-48 determined by N-terminal sequence analysis,[112] by the study of peptide fragments,[128,129] and by reactivity with monoclonal and sequence-specific polyclonal antibodies,[128] demonstrated that the sequence of apo B-48 corresponds to the N-terminal portion of apo B-100, yet there was only one gene for apo B in the human genome. Thus, some tissue-specific mechanism must be involved in the production of apo B-48. Alternative splicing was ruled out because there was no appropriately placed intron. It then became apparent that the mRNA of intestine differs by a single base, a C-to-U change at nucleotide 6666, changing a Gln codon to a stop.[130–133] If this represented the critical editing process, then the C-terminus of apo B-48 should be coded by methionine, which is the next codon in the 5′ direction. The finding that methionine was, indeed, the C-terminus, confirmed the site and the proposed mechanism.[133] It was also found that the editing process activates polyadenylation signals downstream from the stop, resulting in a message of about 7 kb in the human and rabbit intestine.[130] The rat apparently lacks the cryptic polyadenylation sites, consequently producing a message of 14.5 kb.[130] Alteration of codon 2153 from CAA to CTA blocked the reaction.[134] Editing occurs posttranscriptionally,[131] but largely before polyadenylation,[135] and is tissue-specific.[135,136] Studies of the sequence required to produce the editing signal reveal three components: a mooring sequence 3′ to codon 6666; a spacer sequence on the 3′ side; and a regulator sequence adjacent on the 5′ side.[131,135,137,138] Several protein components appear to be involved in the editing complex.[139] The process of editing in human intestine is nearly complete. However, some mRNA for apo B-100 can be detected.[140] The editing event is the conversion of a C nucleotide at position 6666 to U by a cytidine deaminase (APOBEC-1) in the nucleus.[141] The human enzyme coded by a single locus at chromosome 12 p13.1-p13.2 contains 229 amino acids and is restricted to the intestine.[142,143] The human gene differs in many respects from that of the rat, notably in lacking a far upstream promotor that may function in expression in tissues other than intestine.[144,145] Several species including rats, mice, horses, and dogs can form apo B-48 in the liver.[146] A number of hormonal and dietary factors appear to influence hepatic editing.[147–150] Targeted disruption of the APOBEC-1 gene in the mouse abolishes the production of apo B-48.[145,151] McCormick, Young, and collaborators showed that the sequence elements that regulate the expression of apo B in intestine are far removed from those required for hepatic synthesis.[152] Mating of apo B knockout mice with mice carrying a human apo B transgene restored apo B-100 secretion in the liver. In the embryo, it also restored expression of apo B-100 in the yolk sac, rescuing the animals from the severe developmental anomalies of brain associated with ablation of apo B-100 synthesis in the yolk sac.[153]

BIOSYNTHESIS OF LIPOPROTEINS CONTAINING APOLIPOPROTEIN B

Assembly and Secretion of Lipoprotein Particles

The secretion of lipoproteins containing apo B follows the pathway identified for other proteins in constitutive secretory cells: apo B-100 and apo B-48 are synthesized on attached ribosomes of the ER. The typical signal peptide of 27 amino acids[111] is presumably cleaved cotranslationally. Apo B was identified in rat hepatocytes associated with ribosomes and elsewhere in the rough ER by immunoelectron microscopy.[154] However, particles resembling nascent VLDL associated with the immunoreactive apo B are evident only at the smooth-surfaced terminals of this organelle. Because similar particles lacking apo B immunoreactivity are also seen in cisternae of the smooth ER, it has been proposed that nascent VLDL-sized particles are formed in the SER independent of apo B (possibly by a process of budding inward from the organelle membrane[155]) and that these particles migrate to junctions with the rough ER, where apo B is added.[154] Similar observations have been made for nascent chylomicrons in mucosal cells of human jejunum.[156] In both cells, the nascent particles are transported to the Golgi apparatus, where the protein components may be further processed and where they are eventually terminally glycosylated in the *trans*-cisternae. The particles accumulate in the expanded ends of the *trans*-cisternae, which are thought to bud off as secretory vesicles that migrate to and fuse with the cell membrane (the basolateral membrane in enterocytes and hepatocytes), resulting in exocytosis of the nascent lipoproteins.[157] Recent studies during early suckling in mice genetically deficient in intestinal apo B provide strong support for this two-step model of VLDL assembly. Particles resembling large nascent chylomicrons are abundant in smooth ER of absorptive enterocytes in those mice, but few particles are found in Golgi cisternae and even fewer in extracellular spaces as compared with wild-type mice.[158] Thus, formation of a nascent chylomicron competent for transport to the Golgi apparatus is largely dependent on addition of apo B in the ER.

In pulse-chase experiments, the translation of apo B-100 in chicken hepatocytes[159] and human hepatoma cells[160] was found to require about 10 to 14 min, transport to the Golgi apparatus 5 to 10 min, and secretion from the cell another 10 min. Phospholipids (mainly phosphatidylcholine) are added to apo B to form an initial lipoprotein complex during or shortly after translation, prior to acquisition of newly synthesized triglycerides, and presumably are also added to the nascent VLDL-sized particle as it forms in the smooth ER. Some phospholipids may also be added later, presumably in the Golgi apparatus.[161] When the addition of puromycin prematurely terminates translation of apo B in chicken hepatocytes, newly secreted VLDL contains truncated forms of apo B, which evidently can sustain the secretory mechanism.[159]

Although the biogenesis of nascent lipoproteins containing apo B is complex and several details remain controversial, recent studies from several laboratories illuminate important and clinically relevant aspects of the early steps in this process. Consistent with the earlier immunomicroscopic observations, biochemical studies indicate that the assembly of nascent VLDL particles in hepatocytes proceeds in two discrete steps.[162] In the first step, a nascent triglyceride-rich particle is generated at the luminal aspect of the rough ER that contains only a small fraction of the core lipids found in nascent VLDL isolated from Golgi cisternae. In the second step, the major portion of core lipids is added in a pre-Golgi (ER) compartment. Effective generation of the first-step particle requires microsomal triglyceride transfer protein (MTP). MTP is a heterodimer, composed of protein disulfide isomerase, a ubiquitous protein of 55 kDa and a 97-kDa subunit expressed primarily in cells that secrete lipoproteins containing apo B. In addition to hepatocytes and absorptive enterocytes, these include yolk sac visceral endoderm[3] and cardiac myocytes.[2] Mutations of the 97-kDa subunit are associated with abetalipoproteinemia,[163–165] in which apo B is translated, but virtually no lipoproteins competent for secretion are formed. MTP has considerable homology with Xenopus lipovitellin and some domains are homologous with apo B-100 and cholesteryl ester transfer protein (CETP).[165] The MTP gene is on chromosome 4q22-q24 and includes 18 exons.[166,167] MTP can transfer both triglycerides as well as cholesteryl esters, and to some extent, phospholipids between lipid vesicles, and it is thought to promote the acquisition of nonpolar lipids during or just after completion of translation of apo B.[168] At least in cultured hepatic cells, however, a substantial fraction of apo B is degraded prior to secretion. Two types of degradation have been observed: first, by proteasomes in the cytosol following ubiquitination, and second, by intraluminal ER protease(s).[169] In addition, apo B contains numerous "stop-transfer" sequences, which sequences have been proposed to be associated with transient interruption of translocation during translation.[170] These pauses could facilitate cotranslational addition of phospholipids within the translocon or subsequent MTP-mediated lipid addition at the luminal interface. A number of studies suggest that, perhaps related to the stop-transfer process,[171] continuing translation of apo B leaves portions exposed to the cytosol and thus subject to proteasomal degradation. Other studies, however, fail to confirm appreciable cytosolic exposure of apo B during translation.[169] The second form of degradation is thought to occur posttranslationally, depending on the availability of lipid to produce a secretion-competent particle.[169] The extent to which degradation occurs *in vivo* is unclear, but it provides a potentially important mechanism of control of apo B secretion, inasmuch as apo B messenger RNA appears to be constitutive, at least in the short term (see "Regulation of Synthesis and Secretion of Apo B-Containing Lipoproteins" below).

The mechanism by which MTP facilitates the formation of a lipoprotein particle containing nonpolar lipids in the first step of assembly has been partially elucidated by use of an MTP inhibitor in pulse-chase studies. As described earlier, the N-terminal 15 percent of apo B is globular and organized by disulfide bonds. Constructs of this portion of apo B are translated and secreted in a lipid-poor form[168] independent of MTP. In the absence of this portion of the molecule, however, downstream regions of the protein cannot form a lipoprotein particle. MTP is physically associated with apo B, probably the N-terminal region,[168] and it is tempting to speculate that the protein disulfide isomerase subunit promotes folding of this portion of the protein, whereas the 97-kDa subunit subsequently enables acquisition of neutral lipids that associate with the amphipathic domains of the molecule. Other studies suggest that MTP stabilizes apo B posttranslationally (i.e., within the lumen of the ER) as the lipid-binding domains fold and are able to receive neutral lipids.[168] It is also possible that MTP adds lipids to amphipathic domains as they enter the lumen before translation is complete. In the absence of MTP, apo B may be degraded within the ER lumen or following retrograde translocation to the cytosol.[169] In cultured hepatoma cells (Hep G2), in which the second step of VLDL assembly is deficient,[172] secreted lipoprotein particles presumably reflect predominantly the first step. When truncated forms of apo B are thus secreted from cells incubated with puromycin, or when truncated forms are produced by appropriately transfected cells, the diameter of these particles, isolated at densities of 1.03 to 1.17 g/ml, is a linear function of the length of the apo B chains with which they are associated.[46,47] These findings and other evidence are consistent with a model in which apo B is disposed as an equatorial belt surrounding the nonpolar core.[42] Thus, for apo B-100, the diameter of this particle is about 227 Å, close to that of LDL; for apo B-48, the diameter is close to 125 Å.[47]

The role of MTP in the second step of VLDL (and presumably chylomicron) assembly is less clear, although it is likely that this process also requires one or more chaperones. However, MTP may also mediate a posttranslational step required to "adjust" the structure of the first-step particle so that it can acquire additional lipid in the second step.[162]

Properties of Nascent Lipoprotein Particles

VLDL. Nascent lipoproteins have been isolated from Golgi apparatus-rich fractions of the liver of several species.[157] Some of these fractions were contaminated with multivesicular bodies and other endosomal structures that contain lipoproteins taken up into the liver by receptor-mediated endocytosis,[173] making it difficult to evaluate their properties. Apo B-containing particles isolated from Golgi-rich fractions from rat liver in which endosomal contamination is very limited have been shown to be almost entirely VLDL that resemble those found in blood plasma.[174]

Rat plasma VLDL contains appreciable amounts of apo B-48 as well as apo B-100, and both of these are secreted by the liver in this species.[175] The B-48 protein is also secreted in a particle in the

HDL density range; secretion of this putative first-step particle is not abolished in rats fed orotic acid, which inhibits hepatic secretion of VLDL.[176] By contrast, in other species (monkeys and rabbits) in which apo B-100 is virtually the sole apo B component of plasma VLDL, only this form of apo B is secreted by the liver.[175] Although Golgi VLDL also contains apo E and the several C apoproteins found in plasma VLDL,[174] the content of C apoproteins is considerably lower in Golgi VLDL. All the proteins found in Golgi VLDL appear to be newly synthesized; there is no evidence that plasma apolipoproteins can be reutilized in the intracellular assembly of the nascent particles. Golgi VLDL also differs from plasma VLDL in lipids of the particle surface: Golgi VLDL contains much less unesterified cholesterol and more phospholipids.[174] When Golgi VLDL are incubated with blood plasma from which VLDL have been removed by ultracentrifugation, they acquire C apoproteins from HDL.[174] They also acquire cholesterol and lose phospholipids by transfers with other lipoproteins so that they then closely resemble plasma VLDL in surface composition. In rats, Golgi VLDL contains an appreciable complement of cholesteryl esters, reflecting the high activity of acyl CoA cholesterol acyltransferase (ACAT) in this species.[174,177] In guinea pigs and rabbits, in which only apo B-100 is secreted from the liver and the activity of this enzyme is low, the Golgi apparatus and perfusate VLDL contain much lower amounts of cholesteryl esters.[178,179] In humans, the activity of hepatic ACAT is low.[180] Therefore, nascent human VLDL presumably resembles that of species like guinea pigs and rabbits, which contain few cholesteryl esters. In all species, triglycerides are the major constituent of nascent VLDL, accounting for 50 percent or more of particle mass.

Chylomicrons. It is considerably more difficult to isolate nascent chylomicrons from enterocytes, but it is thought that, like nascent VLDL, the size and core lipid composition of triglyceride-rich lipoproteins secreted from enterocytes are similar to those of lymph chylomicrons. Chylomicrons isolated from prenodal intestinal lymph are changed least from those secreted from the cells, but some modification of surface components clearly occurs in the interstitial space and lacteals, as plasma HDL and other lipoproteins are present at these sites.[181] In the several mammalian species examined, apo B-48 was the sole form of apo B present in chylomicrons.[175] The other major apoproteins of nascent chylomicrons of rats are apo A-I and apo A-IV, which, although synthesized in the liver as well, are present in only trace amounts in nascent VLDL.[177,181,182] This difference between chylomicrons and VLDL is not solely a matter of the large size of chylomicrons during active fat absorption, because the protein composition of small chylomicrons secreted in the absence of dietary fat is not appreciably different.[182] Apo E and the C apoproteins are also present on intestinal lymph chylomicrons of rats, but they are thought to be acquired mainly from HDL after secretion because synthesis of these proteins by enterocytes is very limited.[181] Both rat and human enterocytes, however, have some capacity to synthesize C apoproteins.[183] Acquisition of apoproteins from HDL continues after chylomicrons enter the blood plasma, and some of the apoproteins may concomitantly be transferred to HDL, together with some chylomicron phospholipids.[182] In addition to the apoproteins found in rat lymph chylomicrons, human plasma chylomicrons contain at least two additional apoproteins: complement 4b-binding protein[184] and a large carbohydrate-rich protein, apoprotein (a), which is normally found in disulfide linkage with apo B-100 in dense LDL particles as the Lp(a) lipoprotein (see Chap. 116).

Specificity of Apo B Synthesis in Human Liver and Intestine

Triglyceride-rich lipoproteins (TRL) obtained from healthy postabsorptive subjects contain small amounts of apo B-48 ($\approx$5 percent of total apo B mass).[185] Only apo B-100 was found to accumulate in the culture medium of a human hepatoma cell line (HepG2).[186] Furthermore, newly synthesized apo B in samples of human liver consists exclusively of apo B-100, in fetuses as well as adults.[187] Therefore, the apo B-48 found in plasma TRL evidently reflects the continued secretion of small chylomicrons in the absence of dietary fat. Apo B-48 is the predominant form of apo B in human thoracic duct lymph chylomicrons.[7] Although apo B-100 is present, this could reflect the presence of lipoproteins derived from hepatic lymph. Apo B has been localized in normal human enterocytes, particularly the apical regions, with monoclonal antibodies that react with epitopes exclusive to apo B-100 as well as those that recognize regions common to apo B-100 and apo B-48.[188] By contrast, monoclonal antibodies that recognize both apo B-100 and B-48, but not those that recognize apo B-100 alone, identified apo B in isolated enterocytes from patients with chylomicron retention disease.[189] In one report, the only form of newly synthesized apo B identified in experiments with isolated human jejunal enterocytes from normal adults was apo B-48.[187] However, in another study, about 2 percent of tracer label was found in apo B-100 formed by human intestinal explants (Oksenkühn T, Kane J, unpublished observations), newly synthesized apo B-100 was also found in enterocytes from fetuses up to the sixteenth week of gestation.[187] After liver transplantation, distinct allotypes of apo B-100, but not those of apo B-48, are changed to those of the liver donor.[190] This observation suggests that the amount of apo B-100 synthesized by the intestine must be very small. Estimates based on the content of fed retinyl palmitate in separated apo B-48 and apo B-100 particles during active absorption of dietary fat indicate that fewer than 5 percent of TRL particles of intestinal origin contain apo B-100 (Kovar J, Havel RJ, unpublished data).

Hepatic Production of LDL. Kinetic studies of apo B metabolism in rabbits[191] and other species[192] have been interpreted to indicate that LDL particles are secreted by the liver independently of VLDL. However, in rabbits, other studies challenge this interpretation.[193] Furthermore, virtually all apo B-containing lipoproteins isolated from Golgi fractions or isolated perfusates of rabbit and rat liver are VLDL.[174,179] LDL-sized particles are, however, secreted from perfused livers of cholesterol-fed animals and in certain other pathologic states.[157,178,194] Although some nascent VLDL or IDL may be rapidly converted to LDL, available kinetic data on apo B metabolism have failed to establish independent secretion of LDL from human liver.[195] This issue is important for understanding the pathophysiology of a number of disorders involving apo B. Available evidence strongly suggests that VLDL is the sole or major form in which apo B is secreted from the liver of normal individuals. Additional information is needed for patients with diseases affecting the synthesis or catabolism of apo B.

Regulation of Secretion of Chylomicrons and VLDL

Plasticity of VLDL and Chylomicrons in Lipid Transport. As evidenced by the paucity of chylomicrons and VLDL in classical abetalipoproteinemia,[196] apo B-100 and apo B-48 are required for these lipoproteins to be appropriately assembled and secreted. As described above, nascent VLDL and chylomicrons contain a single copy of apo B. This constancy evidently applies to all VLDL particles, regardless of their size.[197] Increased transport of triglycerides can be accomplished by expansion of the core of chylomicrons or VLDL without a necessary increase in the number of particles synthesized and secreted. Feeding fat to rats for up to 48 h increases the transport of triglycerides in intestinal lymph chylomicrons by a factor of 20, but transport of apo B is increased no more than twofold.[181] This is accomplished by increasing mean particle diameter by approximately 2.5 times. Synthesis of apo B-48 in jejunal and ileal enterocytes is not altered when rats are fed isocaloric diets containing no fat or up to 30 percent by weight of triglycerides.[198] Thus, transport of dietary fat seems to be accomplished mainly by incorporating many more triglyceride molecules into chylomicron particles, which continue to be synthesized and secreted independently of dietary fat absorption. Similarly, in the liver, the size of secreted VLDL increases in response to increased rates of hepatic triglyceride synthesis. This is evident from rates of accumulation of apo B and triglycerides in perfusates of isolated livers from rats fed carbohydrate-rich diets.[199,200] In fetal guinea pigs, livers accumulate fat toward the end of gestation as a result of the uptake of large amounts of free fatty acids transported across the placenta.[201] Secreted VLDL containing apo B-100 then becomes very large, approaching the size of chylomicrons normally secreted after administration of a dietary fat load.[202] Likewise, in transgenic mice that secrete only apo B-100 from the intestine, chylomicrons within enterocytes appear to enlarge normally during fat absorption.[203]

The core of VLDL can also expand to accommodate more cholesteryl esters in animals fed cholesterol-rich diets.[157] This is particularly striking in animals such as the rabbit and guinea pig,[178] in which cholesterol feeding is accompanied by accumulation of large amounts of cholesteryl esters in the liver. Under these conditions, some newly secreted VLDL contain many more cholesteryl ester molecules than can be accommodated in a particle the size of LDL (≈200 Å in diameter). Consequently, removal of VLDL triglycerides by lipolysis yields particles whose diameters and densities remain predominantly in the VLDL or IDL range. Although these particles, like LDL, contain little triglyceride, they may retain substantial amounts of apo E and some C apoproteins.

Regulation of Synthesis and Secretion of Apo B-Containing Lipoproteins. Although the upstream region and the second intron of the apo B gene contain a number of potential regulatory elements,[204,205] apo B mRNA is expressed constitutively in a variety of conditions in which VLDL-triglyceride secretion varie widely.[206,207] Apo B mRNA is increased, however, by certain cytokines in HepG2 cells.[208] In livers from two patients with abetalipoproteinemia, the concentration of apo B-100 mRNA was found to be increased several-fold,[209] suggesting the potential for substantial transcriptional regulation of apo B synthesis. As discussed earlier, synthesis of apo B is evidently not rate-limiting for secretion of apo B-containing lipoproteins from isolated liver cells; rather much newly synthesized apo B is degraded if an adequate supply of triglyceride is not immediately available for particle assembly. Increased flux of fatty acids into the liver may underlie increased secretion of VLDL in insulin-resistant states and familial disorders associated with increased plasma concentrations of apo B-100.[210,211] Some, but not all studies have shown that availability of cholesteryl ester may also regulate secretion of apo B-containing lipoproteins from the liver.[212]

A common human variant in which the length of the signal peptide of apo B is reduced from 27 to 24 amino acids is associated with a lower postprandial increase in the concentrations of large particles containing apo B-48 and apo B-100.[213] This supports data indicating that this variant is associated with a reduced rate of translocation of apo B across the ER in a yeast expression system,[214] suggesting that deletion of a hydrophobic segment of the signal peptide (Leu-Ala-Leu) may affect the secretion of apo B-containing lipoproteins postprandially.

Recent observations in genetically modified mice heterozygous for MTP deficiency suggest that the availability of MTP in the ER lumen may regulate apo B-containing lipoprotein assembly. In these mice, levels of MTP mRNA were 50 percent of normal and the concentration of apo B-100 in plasma was reduced by about 30 percent.[215] Secretion of apo B into the blood was comparably reduced. These results, which suggest that MTP deficiency is codominant in mice, run counter to the general conclusion that human abetalipoproteinemia is a recessive trait. Available data are not adequate to establish the expression of the phenotype in human MTP-deficient heterozygotes. Apo B concentrations in genetically confirmed heterozygotes may be low in some patients,[216] but are within the normal range in others. A recently described MTP inhibitor can reduce plasma triglyceride secretion in fasted or fed rats in a dose-dependent manner by up to 97 percent, lower the concentration of plasma lipoproteins containing apo B comparably in hamsters, and normalize plasma cholesterol and triglyceride concentrations in LDL receptor-deficient rabbits.[217] Taken together, the animal data on MTP deficiency and inhibition suggest that MTP concentration in the ER may be rate-limiting for secretion of lipoproteins containing apo B. In this respect, it is of interest that the mRNA and protein for MTP are increased in intestine and liver of hamsters fed a high fat diet.[218,219] Insulin inhibits synthesis and secretion of apo B from cultured rat hepatocytes,[220,221] and from jejunal explants from human fetuses without altering apo B mRNA levels.[222] A functional negative insulin response element has been described in the MTP gene,[223,224] which could explain the short-term reduction in apo B secretion after insulin administration. In insulin-deficient rats, however, greatly reduced hepatic triglyceride secretion occurs with no appreciable changes in hepatic MTP levels.[225] In contrast to apo B, MTP mRNA levels are reduced by certain cytokines in hamster liver.[226] Strong evidence that MTP is rate-limiting for the synthesis of lipoproteins containing apo B has come from studies with an irreversible photoaffinity inhibitor in liver cells: apo B secretion was reduced in proportion to inhibition of MTP activity.[227]

A recently described common polymorphism of the MTP gene provides further support for the concept that MTP activity regulates VLDL synthesis in humans, and at the same time illustrates the complexity of the associated phenotype. In a Swedish population, 25 percent of individuals are heterozygous or homozygous for T rather than G at position −493 from the transcriptional start site. Constructs containing this variant yield an almost twofold enhancement of transcriptional activity.[228] VLDL apo B-100 concentrations are reduced by 50 percent in TT homozygotes with no change in VLDL triglycerides, and LDL-cholesterol concentrations are reduced by 22 percent. TT homozygotes are thought to secrete larger triglyceride-rich VLDL that are more likely to be cleared from the blood as VLDL remnants, thereby reducing LDL formation. Although the rate of MTP synthesis in human MTP deficiency heterozygotes is unknown, heterozygotes may secrete smaller triglyceride-poor VLDL that are more likely to form LDL, minimizing the tendency to hypocholesterolemia.

The relative importance of the various regulatory mechanisms for apo B synthesis and the secretion of lipoproteins containing apo B in vivo is currently unclear. Although a role for apo B proteolysis in the ER has not been demonstrated in vivo, availability of triglycerides and, possibly, cholesteryl esters for core lipidation of apo B are likely to be significant factors. Physiological regulation of apo B and particularly MTP gene expression clearly have the potential for important consequences. Altered regulation of these genes could be involved in some of the complex genetic disorders of plasma lipoproteins containing apo B.

ABETALIPOPROTEINEMIA

Early Descriptions

The first description of this syndrome appeared in 1950.[229] Bassen and Kornzweig described an 18-year-old female with an atypical pigmented retinopathy and abnormalities of red-cell morphology not previously described. The "star-shaped" erythrocytes that abounded in peripheral blood were noted to form rouleaux very poorly. Ataxia and loss of deep-tendon reflexes were also present. During childhood, the patient was thought to have celiac disease, based on the presence of chronic diarrhea. The appearance of similar erythrocytes and retinopathy in the patient's brother, consanguineous parentage, and the absence of findings in the parents suggested autosomal recessive inheritance of a rare allele. In 1958, Jampel and Falls,[230] studying another case with acanthocytosis, fat malabsorption, retinopathy, and advanced neurologic disability, made the critical observation that the content of cholesterol in the serum was extremely low. They also observed, using free electrophoresis, that the β-globulin fraction of serum proteins, then known to be associated with cholesterol transport, was deficient. This discovery linked the malabsorption of lipid to impaired lipid transport in plasma.

Hypocholesterolemia was soon found in another case,[231] and in 1960, three reports described the absence of β- and pre-β-migrating lipoproteins from plasma,[232–234] though one of these,[234] actually represented the homozygous form of HBL because both parents had markedly low levels of cholesterol in plasma. The fundamental clinical distinction between homozygous abetalipoproteinemia (ABL) and homozygous HBL—that obligate heterozygotes for ABL do not usually have severe hypolipidemia—was made in the following year.[235] Preparative ultracentrifugation confirmed the virtual absence of LDL in patients with homozygous ABL. Normal pancreatic lipase activity and bile acid levels in duodenal contents and of high levels of free fatty acids in stool[232] indicated that the malabsorption involved triglycerides, with a defect at the level of the intestinal epithelium. With these key observations, a syndrome encompassing fat malabsorption, acanthocytosis, retinopathy, and progressive neurologic disease was identified. Though not all patients described subsequently had all these features at the time they were studied, the absence of β-lipoproteins was at once a unifying feature and the first clue to underlying mechanisms. Whereas most cases present in early childhood, the diagnosis may be delayed until adulthood in the absence of diarrhea.

Lipoproteins and Lipid Transport in Abetalipoproteinemia

Structure and Composition of Plasma Lipoproteins. As techniques for isolation and identification of plasma lipoproteins improved, it became apparent that the lipoproteins that were absent from blood in ABL included chylomicrons and all the lipoproteins of the VLDL cascade, that is, all lipoproteins that contain B apolipoproteins.[236–240] Because these lipoproteins carry most of the cholesterol and triglycerides in plasma, the levels of both classes of lipids are markedly reduced. Levels of triglycerides in plasma are frequently only a few milligrams per deciliter and cholesterol levels are usually less than half of normal, often 20 to 45 mg/dl. Plasma triglyceride levels fail to rise after ingestion of fat, although some polyunsaturated fatty acids eventually appear in plasma.[240] The content of exogenous polyunsaturated fatty acids such as linoleate is decreased in plasma and in adipose tissue, reflecting inefficiency in the uptake of dietary fat.[240] There is a striking shift away from the normal distribution of generic species of phospholipids in plasma. The relative content of phosphatidylcholine is decreased and that of sphingomyelin is increased.[236,241]

Examination of the lipoproteins of blood showed the presence of some lipoprotein material in the ultracentrifugal density intervals in which chylomicrons, VLDL, IDL, and LDL are found (Fig. 115-2). Early efforts to detect circulating apo B were unsuccessful;[242–244] however, sensitive detection methods reveal small amounts of apo B of normal molecular weight including a complex with apo(a).[196,245] Much of the circulating apo B appears to consist of truncated molecules that include the N-terminus consistent with the concept that failure to lipidate apo B 100 results in cotranslational proteolysis.[246]

Among the lipoproteins of the $d < 1.006$ g/ml and $1.006 < d < 1.063$ g/ml ultracentrifugal fractions, apo A-I is a major constituent,[243,244] but apo A-II and apo E are also present.[244] As with the other lipoproteins of ABL, the most anionic isoform of apo C-III, apo C-III_2, which carries two residues of sialic acid, is the only isoform present in the LDL interval.[243,244,247] This pattern is also observed when VLDL secretion from liver is inhibited by administration of orotic acid, suggesting that the more highly sialated form of apo C-III may enter plasma via pathways other than by the secretion of VLDL. The lipoproteins of the LDL and VLDL density intervals in ABL have a distinct cuboidal, square-packing appearance with an 80- to 90-Å periodicity[244,248] (see Fig. 115-2). A possible mechanism for the development of particles of this type is suggested by the observation that when bovine HDL acquire dimyristoylphosphatidylcholine they lose a portion of their complement of apo A-I, becoming less dense and assuming cuboidal shape.[249,250] Like the more abundant HDL particles, the lipoproteins of the LDL density interval show a decreased ratio of lecithin to sphingomyelin (nearly 1 in contrast to a normal ratio of 2). The phosphatidyl choline of ABL plasma and erythrocytes is relatively deficient in sn-2-18:2 fatty acids.[250] Nearly half the cholesterol is unesterified, compared with less than one-third in normal LDL.[244]

The HDL density interval contains about half the normal amount of lipoprotein mass. As with the lipoproteins of lower density, the HDL have an abnormally high ratio of free to esterified cholesterol (0.7 compared with 0.3) and a lecithin:sphingomyelin ratio of about 5:4 (compared with a normal ratio of about 8:1).[244] By electron microscopy, they resemble normal HDL except that they tend to larger particle diameters.[248,249] Rate zonal ultracentrifugation shows that most of the particles have the flotation characteristics of HDL_2, with mean diameters of 135 Å. A second population has mean diameters of about 100 Å, and a third, designated ABL- HDL_4 is also spherical, with a mean diameter of 60 Å. Apo A-I is the predominant protein constituent of all three particle types. Levels of pre-β_1 HDL are about half of normal (Malloy MJ, personal communication). Apo A-II comprises about one-eighth of the apoprotein mass of the HDL_2-like fraction and about one-third of that of the ABL-HDL_4. All the isoforms of apo A-II are present, but their distribution differs from the normal pattern.[251] Apo E is almost as abundant in the HDL_2-like particles as apo A-II, and it is present to the extent of 1 to 3 percent of protein mass in the HDL_3-like particles, but only in trace amounts in the ABL-HDL_4 particle.[252]

Because apolipoproteins, especially apo E, may become dissociated from lipoprotein particles during ultracentrifugation, it is important to verify their distribution among lipoprotein particles by nonultracentrifugal techniques. Using gel permeation chromatography, Gibson et al.[253] found that apo E was not associated with the LDL-size particles of ABL, indicating that its appearance in the HDL particles was not a consequence of the disintegration during ultracentrifugation of particles of lower density. Much of the apo E appears to be present in the form of an apo E:apo A-II dimer.[254] The apolipoproteins that appear in plasma in ABL all appear to be structurally normal. Absence of the nonsialated and monosialated forms of apo C-III characterizes the HDL species as well as the lipoproteins of lower density. Apo E also appears to be maximally sialated in ABL.[255] Apo(a) is present in ABL plasma, largely unattached to lipoproteins.[256] Platelet-activating factor acetylhydrolase, normally associated with LDL, is found in association with HDL in ABL.[257]

In contrast to the decreased levels of apo A-I, plasma levels of apo E are normal in abetalipoproteinemia. Production rates and the fractional catabolic rate for apo-A-I are increased whereas the production rate for apo E is normal.[255] The mean residence time for apo E is moderately shorter than in normals. In contrast with the normal metabolism of HDL, the apo A-I in particles that also contain apo A-II is catabolized faster than in particles lacking apo A-II. HDL particles with apo E are also catabolized rapidly, especially those carrying the apo E monomer. Because apo E associates with apo A-I:A-II HDL particles[258] it is probable that the apo A-II-containing particles are catabolized rapidly due to their content of apo E. In the absence of apo B-100, apo E becomes the sole ligand for the LDL receptor. Extraction of apo E-containing particles by up-regulated receptors thus probably accounts in large part for the HDL deficiency in abetalipoproteinemia, providing cholesterol for steroidogenesis and to the liver.

Viewed mechanistically, the circulating lipoproteins in ABL reflect the lack of transport of both exogenous and endogenous triglycerides. The lipid constituents that are normally transferred

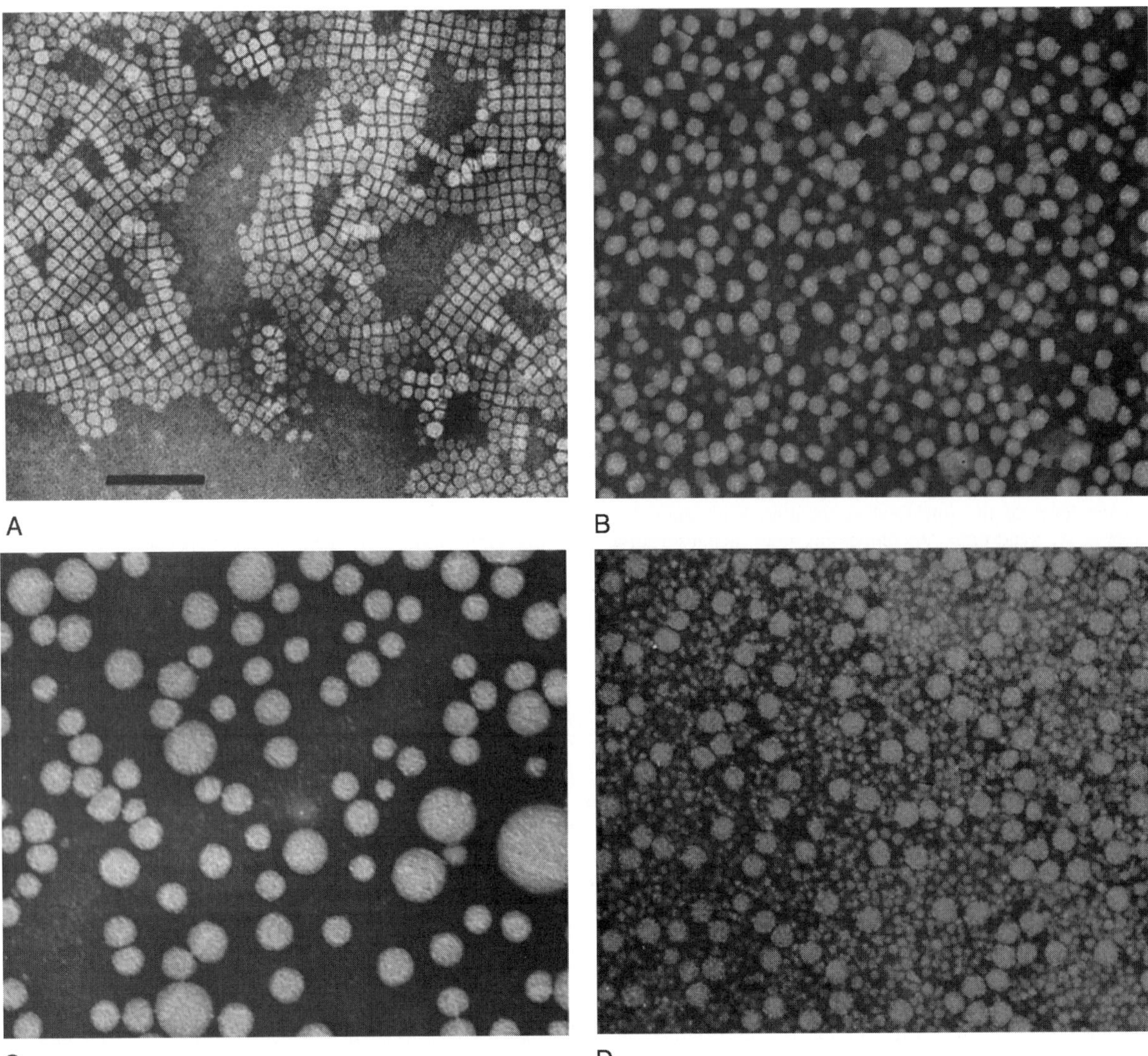

Fig. 115-2 Electron-microscopic appearance of abnormal serum lipoproteins in two forms of hypolipidemia and in Lp(a) hyperlipidemia. (*Original magnification indicated.*) A. "Square packing" lipoproteins from the LDL density interval in recessive abetalipoproteinemia ×195,000. (*Courtesy of Dr. Trudy Forte.*) B. Lipoproteins of the LDL density interval from a patient with normotriglyceridemic adetalipoproteinemia, showing irregular outlines and some cuboidal forms. ×180,000. C. Lipoproteins of the d < 1.006 g/ml fraction of serum in normotriglyceridemic abetalipoproteinemia. ×180,000. (*Courtesy of Dr. Mary Malloy.*) D. Lipoproteins of the HDL density interval from a patient with hyper Lp(a) lipoproteinemia, showing numerous Lp(a) particles among normal-appearing HDL particles. ×180,000 Lipoproteins in all panels are visualized by negative staining with phosphotungstate.

to HDL in the course of intravascular lipolysis are lacking. Also, the transport of dietary cholesterol is impaired. The appearance of most of the normal apolipoproteins other than the two molecular forms of apo B indicates that they can be secreted independently of the apo B-containing lipoproteins, the exception being the apo C-III_0 and the C-III_1 isoforms. Sphingomyelin, which normally is acquired from tissues by HDL and transferred to apo B-containing lipoproteins,[259] accumulates in HDL. Free cholesterol also accumulates in HDL, perhaps as a consequence of the lack of appropriate acceptor particles for the transfer of cholesteryl esters generated by the lecithin:cholesterol acyltransferase reaction. The accumulation of lipid in some of the HDL particles causes a reordering and loss of a portion of the complement of apo A-I, forming particles that enter the low-density interval.

Activities of Lipoprotein Lipase and LCAT

Lipoprotein lipase (LPL) activity has been found to be very low in ABL.[240,260] Illingworth et al. found heparin-releasable activities of LPL and hepatic lipase to be about half normal.[261] It is likely that this reflects reduced induction of the enzymes consequent to fat malabsorption because extremely low dietary intake of fat[262] or malabsorption[263] results in reduction of LPL activity.

Decreased LCAT activity likewise has been observed in ABL.[243,244,264,265] This may be due in part to the relatively poor substrate activity of HDL_2.[266] However, the observation that the addition of normal LDL results in marked stimulation of cholesterol esterification in plasma from patients with ABL[267] suggests that deficiency of acceptor lipoproteins is a major factor. The esters formed are relatively deficient in sn-2-18:2 fatty acids in contrast to cholesteryl esters of normal plasma.[268] Even though the addition of normal LDL or VLDL as acceptor lipoproteins accelerated esterification, it did not change the fatty acid composition of the esters, probably reflecting the abnormal fatty acid composition of phosphatidyl choline in this disorder.[250]

Sterol Metabolism and the Interaction of Plasma Lipoproteins with Receptors

Several studies of sterol balance have been reported in ABL. In two of these studies,[269,270] slightly elevated production rates of about 15 mg/kg/day were observed. In two other subjects,[271] rates somewhat higher were observed, which could be accounted for by the impaired reabsorption of biliary cholesterol alone. In long-term cholesterol turnover studies in two individuals, Goodman et al.[272] showed rates of cholesterol production of 0.82 and 0.89 g/day, well within the normal range. The data fit a three-pool model. The most rapidly exchanging pool was markedly reduced, whereas the total exchangeable cholesterol pool was essentially normal. Studies in freshly isolated lymphocytes from one patient with ABL showed cholesterol synthesis to be normal,[273] but in others, an elevated rate was observed.[274,275] Activity of HMG-CoA reductase was normal in hair roots from one subject.[276] However, a twofold increase in urinary mevalonate excretion in both ABL and homozygous HBL suggests that de novo sterol biosynthesis is increased.[277] Freshly isolated mononuclear cells from one patient were found to bind and degrade LDL at a rate comparable to that of cells from normal individuals.[278]

The delivery of cholesterol to cells in ABL is apparently accomplished with efficiency via apo E-containing HDL particles.[275,279,280] These particles compete effectively with LDL for binding and endocytosis via the B-100:E receptors, down-regulating them. Apo E-containing HDL from subjects with ABL were capable of inducing a three- to fivefold increase in the cholesteryl ester content of cultured fibroblasts,[280,281] indicating their effectiveness in the delivery of cholesterol to peripheral cells. HDL allows plasma in ABL to deliver cholesterol to the periphery with the same efficiency as would occur at a LDL cholesterol level of approximately 100 mg/dl.

Delivery of cholesterol to peripheral cells appears to be nearly normal in the absence of VLDL and LDL. In the adrenal cortex, delivery of cholesterol also appears to be normal in the basal state, but the maximum secretion of cortisol is reduced during corticotropin stimulation.[282,283] Similarly, the production of progesterone during the luteal phase of the menstrual cycle appears to have been abnormally low in one patient with homozygous HBL.[284] Thus, the extraction of cholesterol from plasma via the abnormal lipoproteins appears to be insufficient to support maximum steroidogenesis. In spite of this, at least one patient has carried a pregnancy to term, delivering a normal infant.[285]

Clinical Features

Hematologic Manifestations. The markedly abnormal form of erythrocytes has attracted the attention of investigators since the earliest descriptions of the disorder. Singer et al.[286] created the term acanthrocytosis (from acantha, "thorn" in Greek), which soon became modified to acanthocytosis.

Acanthocytes comprise from 50 to 100 percent of circulating erythrocytes (Fig. 115-3). They are not found in bone marrow, suggesting that the membranous changes leading to malformation are acquired by contact with plasma. Their structure strongly inhibits rouleau formation, leading to extremely low erythrocyte sedimentation rates.[287] The lipid composition of their envelopes reflects the abnormal composition of the plasma lipoproteins.[288–291] The contents of total phospholipids and cholesterol are greater than in normal cells, and the sphingomyelin:lecithin ratio is increased from 0.9 to over 1.4. There is a shift to more saturated fatty acids among the sphingomyelins.[290] The erythrocytes apparently assume the acanthocytic form because of a maldistribution of lipids between the bilayer leaflets.[292] The redundant exterior leaflet drives outward curvature, a phenomenon that is rapidly reversible in the presence of chlorpromazine, which expands the cytoplasmic leaflet.

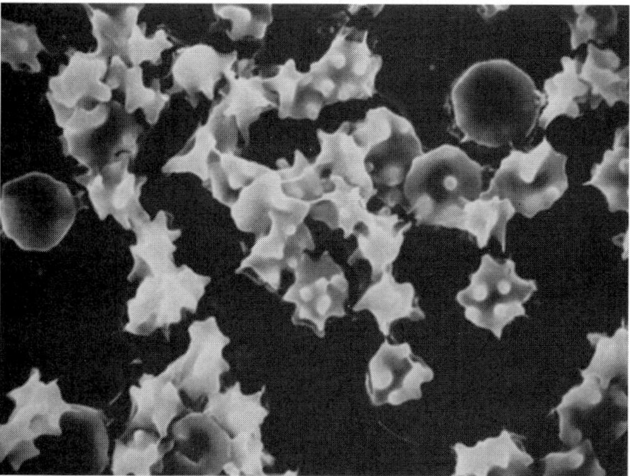

Fig. 115-3 Acanthocytosis of erythrocytes from a patient with homozygous recessive abetalipoproteinemia. (*Scanning electron micrograph courtesy of Dr. Mary Malloy.*)

Red-cell survival is frequently shortened,[231,289,293] and hyperbilirubinemia[231,236,293] has been described. Many patients demonstrate erythroid hyperplasia[231,241,294,295] and reticulocytosis,[237,296] suggesting that erythropoiesis per se is not notably impaired in ABL.

Anemia and Abnormalities of Hemostasis. Severe anemia has been described in a number of children with ABL,[286,293,297,298] many of whom appear to respond to replacement therapy with iron or folic acid.[296,299,300] It is likely that most cases of severe anemia principally reflect deficiencies of iron, folate, and perhaps other nutrients secondary to fat malabsorption, but probably not deficiency of cobalamin.[241,293] Autohemolysis of erythrocytes, which appears to result from accelerated hydroperoxidation of olefinic fatty acids secondary to tocopherol deficiency, may also contribute to the anemia.[278,291,296,301,302]

A number of descriptions of cases in which vitamin K deficiency resulted in significant prothrombin deficiency[291,295–298,303,304] have appeared. In two other cases, significant gastrointestinal bleeding was present in infancy or childhood, associated with severe vitamin K deficiency (Malloy MJ, unpublished observation).[305]

Like erythrocytes, the platelet membranes show compositional changes, notably an increase in free cholesterol.[306] Because the lipoproteins bearing apo B-100 appear to stimulate platelet aggregation and serotonin release in response to collagen and ADP, it is expected that the platelet response in ABL is attenuated. However, HDL from patients with ABL binds to platelets, activating them as LDL normally do.[307] This finding is of interest because normal HDL inhibits platelet reactiveness to those stimuli. It is likely that the apo E-containing HDL are the particles responsible for the stimulatory effect. Plasma levels of the lipoprotein-associated coagulation inhibitor, which functions to regulate the extrinsic coagulation pathway, are greatly reduced in patients with ABL and HBL.[308]

Gastrointestinal Manifestations. Malabsorption of fat is a central pathophysiological feature of ABL. It is usually observed in the neonatal period, with vomiting, diarrhea, and failure to gain weight normally. It is no doubt the reason for the somatic underdevelopment described in the majority of cases. Radiographic examination of the intestine frequently demonstrates clumping of contrast material.[232,293,309] The intestinal symptoms correlate directly with the amount of fat in the diet and tend to diminish with age, reflecting in part a striking aversion of many patients to dietary fat.

Studies of Intestinal Absorption. Despite the inability to secrete chylomicrons, some absorption of long chain fatty acids occurs.[241,291,310] Some fatty acids, especially polyunsaturated ones, are probably transported directly to the liver as free fatty acids. Lysosomal hypertrophy in enterocytes has been described with fat feeding, suggesting that some alternative processes are induced. In adult life, loss of fatty acids in stool may represent as little as 20 percent of the ingested mass. The long-term excretion of fatty acids is apparently enough to induce oxalate urolithiasis,[311] however, which might be prevented by increasing dietary calcium and fluid intake.

In normal individuals, vitamin A is esterified in the enterocyte and its esters are secreted into the intestinal lymphatics in chylomicrons.[312] The absorption of vitamin A is diminished in patients with ABL.[289,291,294] Although the concentration in plasma tends to be low,[237,313,314] administration of supplemental vitamin restores normal levels.

Unlike vitamins A and K, where even modest supplementation serves to achieve normal plasma levels, the transport of tocopherol is severely inhibited in ABL.[314–318] Normally, tocopherol enters plasma via the chylomicrons and, apparently, directly via the portal system.[319,320] The bulk of plasma tocopherol is found in LDL, which deliver the vitamin, at least in part, to peripheral tissues by endocytosis via the B-100:E receptor.[320,321] The abnormal lipoproteins of ABL appear incapable of incorporating normal amounts of tocopherol even in the face of relatively large oral supplements[318] or intramuscular injection. Massive supplementation, however, somehow increases the flux into the body, eventually increasing the tocopherol content of adipose tissue appreciably.[316] Low plasma and tissue levels of tocopherol in homozygous HBL with apo B-49.6,[88] in which chylomicrons are apparently formed normally, suggest that LDL plays a vital role in the transport of tocopherol and that the impairment of transport in ABL is not entirely due to failure to produce chylomicrons. The physiological effects of vitamin E deficiency are best demonstrated by the phenotype of autosomal recessive deficiency of α-tocopherol transfer protein (see Chap. 232).[321,321a] This deficiency causes malabsorption and deficiency of vitamin E with a phenotype that closely resembles that of Friedreich ataxia.

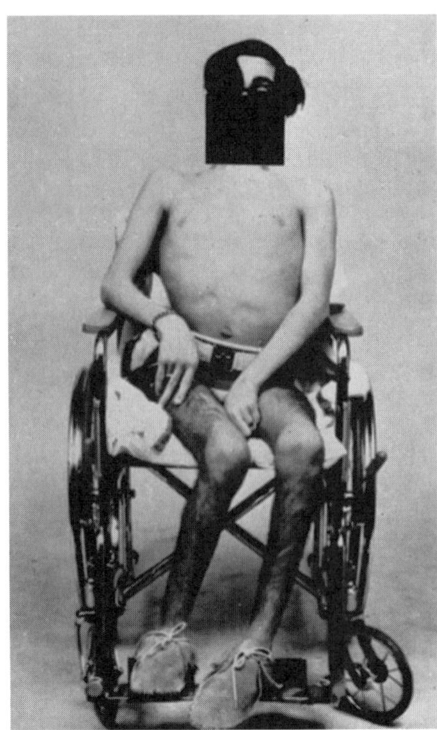

Fig. 115-4 A 17-year-old patient with abetalipoproteinemia with generalized weakness, kyphoscoliosis, and lordosis. (*Courtesy of Drs. Peter Herbert, Gerd Assmann, Antonio M. Gotto, Jr., and Donald Fredrickson.*)

The Intestinal Mucosa. Yellow discoloration of duodenal mucosa has been observed on endoscopy.[322] The findings in biopsy specimens are highly characteristic. Unlike celiac disease, with which ABL is frequently confused, the villi are formed normally. Extensive hyaline vacuolization of the villus cells is evident when stained conventionally.[237,309] The lipid content of the mucosa is several times normal,[296] even when no fat was ingested for days. Electron microscopy reveals numerous fat droplets within the mucosal cells.[323] However, they are not clearly withinathe Golgi apparatus as are the lipoprotein particles seen during normal fat absorption. Early immunofluorescence studies in intestinal biopsies failed to demonstrate apo B.[324,325] However, more sensitive analyses reveal apo B in both liver and intestine.[188,209,326]

Hepatic Manifestations. Despite the inability of the liver to secrete VLDL, abnormalities of liver function are uncommon in ABL. Several patients have had abnormal levels of transaminases in serum[241,327] and three have had cirrhosis.[304,326,327] Two of these patients, however, had been given medium-chain triglycerides. Accumulation of lipid droplets in two different dispositions was observed in hepatocytes. In some patients,[241,310,323–326] the lipid droplets in the cytoplasm are membrane-bound and the rough ER and smooth ER appear dilated and vesiculated. In another case, liver tissue from an adult not treated with medium-chain triglycerides was also found to have numerous lipid droplets in hepatocytes. They were not membrane-bound, nor were they associated with the Golgi apparatus. Peroxisomes have been noted to be pleomorphic, containing electron-dense nucleoids.[328] Because peroxisomes appear to interact with apo E (329) in addition to their roles in the metabolism of long chain fatty acids and cholesterol, morphologic abnormalities of peroxisomes in ABL may reflect abnormalities of intracellular lipid trafficking.

Neuromuscular Manifestations. The neurologic manifestations of ABL place it among the hereditary spinocerebellar degenerative syndromes (Fig. 115-4). In fact, it is only the recognition of disordered lipoprotein metabolism that has permitted a clear separation of ABL from the other disorders of that group. Early cases were frequently considered variants of Friedreich ataxia. In retrospect, many of the reported cases of Freidreich ataxia with pigmented retinopathy must have been ABL. Prior to the advent of intensive tocopherol therapy, the onset of neurologic disease usually began in the first or second decade of life and often progressed to catastrophic disability, although some patients inexplicably escaped serious affliction until much later. The most characteristic degenerative sites in the nervous system are the large sensory neurons of the spinal ganglia and their heavily myelinated axons, which enter the cord lateral to the posterior funiculus. The pathologic appearance is that of an axonopathy[295,297,330] (Fig. 115-5). Extensive demyelination of the fasciculus cuneatus and fasciculus gracilis may occur.[295,297]

The first neurologic signs are diminution in intensity of deep-tendon reflexes, which may appear in the first few years of life,[289,299] probably due primarily to loss of function in spinocerebellar pathways and posterior columns. Vibratory sense and proprioception tend to be lost progressively, and an ataxic gait appears. The Romberg sign is frequently present. Untreated patients are often unable to stand unaided by the third decade. Movements may become highly dysmetric, and dysarthria may become severe. Muscle contractions are common, leading to pes cavus, pes equinovarus, and kyphoscoliosis.

The presence of Babinski responses in some patients has been attributed to pyramidal tract disease;[229,241,295] spastic paralysis, however, has not been seen. Mental retardation or dullness was described in a number of cases. Attribution of this phenomenon to the metabolic defect of ABL is difficult because specific neuropathologic evidence of cerebral cortical disease is lacking. Furthermore, slow neuromuscular development observed in neonates is often associated with steatorrhea and general growth failure and may reflect multiple nutritional deficiencies. Also, because approximately one-third of patients described to date appear to be the products of consanguineous

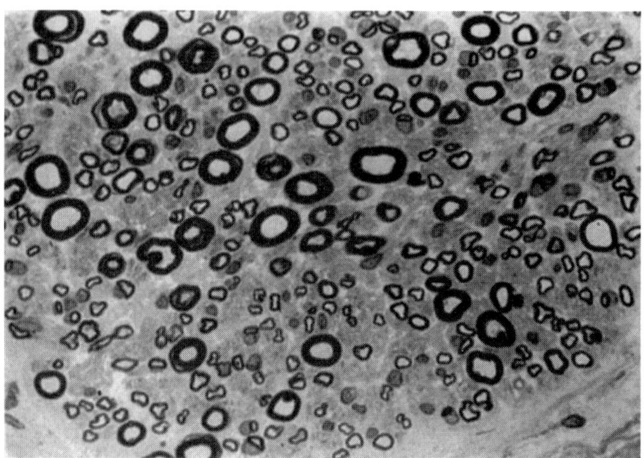

Fig. 115-5 Abetalipoproteinemia. Section of a sural nerve from a 14-year-old patient with homozygous ABL showing a marked decrease in the numbers of large-caliber neurons. (*Courtesy of Sokol, Free Radic Biol Med 6:189, 1989. Reproduced with the permission of Pergamon Press.*)

matings, other rare alleles may be responsible for mental retardation.

Clinical evidence of peripheral neuropathy was described infrequently, but included classic stocking-and-glove distribution of hypesthesia.[232,237,331,332] Patients frequently show diminished response to local anesthetics. Studies of somatosensory conduction revealed abnormalities in 9 of 10 patients with ABL, whereas brainstem evoked potentials were normal in all patients.[333] Marked diminution in amplitude of sensory potentials was found in tibial and sural nerves, with slowing of conduction velocity. Electromyographic studies revealed evidence of denervation of skeletal muscle.[334] In general, the cranial nerves are spared, but oculomotor nerve involvement and denervation of the tongue are observed.[332]

The principal finding in biopsies of sural nerves is loss of large myelinated fibers (see Fig. 115-5). Paranodal demyelination appears to correlate with the severity and duration of disease, whereas unmyelinated fibers appear to be relatively unaffected.[334] In all, there is a striking resemblance between the neurologic lesions of ABL and those encountered in various malabsorption syndromes involving tocopherol deficiency[335–338] and in vitamin E-deficient animals.[339–342] The appearance of a metastatic glioma in an adult patient with ABL raises the interesting possibility that the deficiency of tocopherol may lead to free radical-mediated mutagenesis in the central nervous system.[343]

Muscle weakness is a frequent feature of ABL, but the clinical determination that myopathy is present tends to be obscured by the frequent presence of denervative neuropathy. Myopathy characterized by the presence of ceroid pigment in the muscle fibers was described, however, in a 26-year-old man.[344] The granules in muscle reacted with periodic acid-Schiff (PAS) reagent, and were electron-dense and autofluorescent, resembling closely the ceroid pigment observed in the muscle tissue of tocopherol-deficient animals. Cardiomyopathy leading to death has been described at 10 and 13 years.[295,345] Again, the pathologic appearance of perinuclear deposits of lipochrome pigment suggests tocopherol deficiency.

Ophthalmic Manifestations. The most prominent ophthalmic abnormality in ABL is pigmentary retinal degeneration, which clinically resembles other forms of retinitis pigmentosa not associated with deficiency of lipoproteins. Commonality of mechanism with the neurologic abnormalities in ABL is suggested by the general observation that more severe examples of retinopathy tend to occur in individuals with severe neurologic disability.[229,230,237,332] Major pathologic features are loss of photoreceptors, loss of pigment epithelium, and relative preservation of submacular pigment epithelium. Lipofuscin pigment is present, and macrophage-like cells that invade the retina contain trilaminar structures that probably represent ingested lipofuscins.[346,347] These retinal alterations closely resemble the retinopathy of experimental tocopherol deficiency.[339,348,349] The presence of angioid streaks in some patients indicates the involvement of Bruch's membrane.[350] Deficiency of vitamin A may also contribute to the retinopathy. Clinical descriptions of improvement in dark adaptation and electrophysiological behavior of the retina with vitamin A supplementation suggest this.[314,351–353] Because retinitis pigmentosa is not typical of the pathology observed in experimental[354,355] or in human[356] vitamin A deficiency, it appears that this vitamin probably does not play a central role in the retinal disease in ABL. That progression of retinopathy has been described despite vitamin A supplementation[357] tends to support this view. Thus, it is likely, especially in the light of the abundance of lipofuscin pigment in the retina, that tocopherol deficiency plays a central role, although vitamin A supplements may be of some benefit.

The onset of symptoms is variable. Visual acuity was significantly compromised during the first decade in a few cases,[237,300,358] although many patients are asymptomatic until adulthood. Loss of night vision is frequently a presenting symptom,[229,359] and loss of color vision has also been described.[346] The retinopathy often produces slowly enlarging annular scotomas with macular sparing, such that patients are relatively unaware of the progression of the disease. Complete loss of vision can ultimately occur. Nystagmus often develops.

Ophthalmoplegia has been described in a number of cases.[293,331,346,359,360] A neural basis for this symptom is suggested by the occurrence of primary aberrant regeneration of the oculomotor nerve.[332] Ptosis[237,289] and anisocoria[285,295,322] likewise are most likely the result of neuropathy. Although lenticular opacities are frequently encountered in other forms of retinitis pigmentosa, they are observed infrequently in ABL.

Associated Clinical Abnormalities. A number of diverse clinical abnormalities have been described in isolated cases or in a few instances. Among these are aminoaciduria,[299] hypogammaglobulinemia,[291,313] extra digits and webbing of the fingers,[360] deformities of the digits,[229,231,346,361] and microcephaly.[361] It is likely that these abnormalities either reflect contiguous gene syndromes or some effect of the gestational environment. On the other hand, hypoalbuminemia[359] and low levels of gamma globulins[291,313] may reflect severe calorie and amino acid malabsorption, and acrodermatitis enteropathica[362] is probably due to deficiency of essential fatty acids.

Mechanism and Genetics

All pedigrees described to date are compatible with an autosomal recessive mode of inheritance. There are no examples of an affected parent and child. It is of interest, however, that males outnumber females about 3:2. Few karyotypes have been reported.[300,313] A number of studies provide evidence that the apo B gene is not involved.[345,363,364] Furthermore, the apo B detected in liver and intestine in ABL includes a full-length product. Very small amounts of apo B were detected in a poorly lipidized state, either in association with or without apo(a).[245] N-terminal fragments represent some of the apo B in plasma. Reactivity with monoclonal antibodies to apo B-100 demonstrate that many epitopes are present in liver and intestine, suggesting that at least some full-length apo B is synthesized.[188] In two studies, the quantities of B proteins in liver[326] and intestine[187,326] were less than in normal tissues, but levels of apo B message were greatly increased. In these studies, the intestinal message was appropriately edited. Apo B-48 formed in the intestine in another study was found to be of appropriate length, but was absent from the Golgi apparatus.[345] Thus, ABL is probably due in most cases to defects of one or more proteins involved in processing apo B through the secretory pathway for VLDL and chylomicrons.

Defects in the microsomal triglyceride transfer protein, MTP, as a cause of abetalipoproteinemia, were first suggested by the absence of that protein from intestinal and hepatic microsomes in affected homozygotes.[163] Truncations of the C-terminus resulting from nonsense mutations,[164,216] point substitutions,[216,365] and a splice mutant,[165] all involving the MTP gene (GenBank X59657), were found in association with abetalipoproteinemia. In several cases, the mutant subunit of MTP did not associate normally with the protein disulfide isomerase subunit.[216,365,366] It is possible that defects in other elements involved in the assembly, processing, and secretion of apo B-containing lipoproteins could also underlie some cases of ABL. Defects in the pause-transfer process of lipidation of apo B, in the protein disulfide isomerase moiety of the MTP complex, of proteins involved in movement of nascent VLDL particles and chylomicrons to the cell surface via the Golgi apparatus, or defects affecting the stability of message for apo B or the folding and stability of the B-protein are potentially also responsible in some cases. It is likely that apo-B interacts physically with MTP during the initial lipidation step, because MTP and apo-B can be co-immunoprecipitated.[367] Therefore, it is possible that mutations in an MTP binding domain of the B apoproteins could produce a phenocopy disorder. However, all published studies report defects in the large subunit of MTP in ABL. The induction of a phenotype that approaches that of ABL by potent MTP inhibitors lends mechanistic support to the role of MTP defects.[217]

Treatment

Clinical experience conclusively shows that the gastrointestinal symptoms respond to restriction of triglycerides containing long chain fatty acids to about 15 g per day. Fatty acids derived from medium-chain triglycerides do not require the formation of chylomicrons for absorption but are transported mainly by albumin as free fatty acids via the hepatic portal system. They are an energy substrate for liver but are not necessary nutrients. Reports of hepatic fibrosis associated with their use in patients with ABL[304,327] suggest that they should not be used routinely. However, in extremely malnourished infants, temporary use might be undertaken as long as liver function is followed carefully.

The assessment of the effects of tocopherol supplementation in treatment of ABL requires prolonged observation. However, it is now apparent that such supplementation does inhibit the progression of the neurologic disease and probably leads to some regression of symptoms, even if it is started in adulthood.[314,368–373] The retinopathy[353,374] can also be prevented if therapy is started early, or stabilized if disease is already present when therapy commences. The myopathy, too, appears to be reversed with tocopherol treatment.[372] Further support for the rationale of therapy with tocopherol comes from similar observations on the effect of tocopherol in other malabsorption states that produce clinical effects in the central nervous system similar to those associated with ABL.[375] Until the reliability and safety of parenteral vitamin E preparations are established, treatment requires the use of large oral doses of the vitamin. Concentrated preparations now permit the convenient administration of 1000 to 2000 mg/day to infants and 5000 to 10,000 mg/day to older children and adults. In most cases, institution of tocopherol therapy before the appearance of neurologic symptoms will prevent them. Some reversal of existing neurologic disease can often be achieved as well. In view of the low blood levels of vitamin A and β-carotene in untreated patients, supplementation with water-soluble preparations of vitamin A would appear to be a reasonable adjunct to treatment with vitamin E. Because vitamin D has its own transport mechanism, and because signs and symptoms of deficiency are lacking in ABL, no specific therapy appears necessary in this regard. Supplementation with vitamin K should be undertaken if hypoprothrombinemia is present.

FAMILIAL HYPOBETALIPOPROTEINEMIA

Early Descriptions and Discovery of the Role of Mutations of Apo B

Probably the first example of the syndrome of HBL was a child who was at first thought to have ABL and who was born to parents who both had abnormally low levels of cholesterol in serum.[234] A few years later a sibship in which three brothers had hypocholesterolemia without any of the classic clinical findings of ABL was described.[376] A lack of accumulation of lipid droplets was shown by intestinal biopsy in one of the subjects. In 1969, Mars et al. described a kindred in which nine individuals with hypocholesterolemia were found in three generations.[377] The propositus was a 37-year-old woman with ataxia and resistance to local anesthetics. She showed only minimal increases in plasma triglycerides after the ingestion of fat, and abnormal fat droplet accumulation was seen in jejunal biopsy specimens taken after a 12-h fast. Erythrocytes from the individuals with serum cholesterol levels below 100 mg/dl became acanthocytocytic on incubation. Another kindred was described in the same year in which two generations were affected, again suggesting an autosomal dominant mode of inheritance.[378] Over the next 7 years, individuals with HBL were identified in five additional kindreds.[379–382] Fasting chylomicronemia was noted in one kindred.[379]

In 1974[383] and 1975,[384] it was reported that individuals totally lacking apo B-containing lipoproteins could be found in kindreds containing individuals with HBL. This defined a new autosomal disorder in which low levels of LDL and minimal sequelae are present in the heterozygous state, and in which the homozygous state is clinically indistinguishable from homozygous recessive ABL. This concept was soon supported by additional case reports.[385,386]

The finding of small amounts of apo B in the plasma of an apparent homozygote[387] was the first suggestion that this syndrome might be due to disorders at the apo B locus that could influence the production, stability, or half-life of lipoproteins containing apo B. The subsequent recognition by Young et al.[87] of a truncated apo B protein in plasma in a kindred with HBL led to the recognition of a number of distinct apo B truncations in this disorder. It is now evident that many cases of dominantly transmitted HBL are due to truncations of apo B, although evidence is already at hand to suggest that other mechanisms exist, some of which do not involve the apo B locus. In most instances, simple heterozygosity does not appear to be deleterious, resulting only in a level of plasma LDL about half that of normal. Many of the presumed heterozygotes who also manifest more severe HBL are probably compound heterozygotes, carrying a second mutation.[388–390] Simple heterozygosity will probably prove to be prevalent. Among 19,800 free-living adolescents and adults in California who volunteered for measurement of serum cholesterol levels, 67 (about 1 in 300) were found to have plasma cholesterol levels below 100 mg/dl (Kane JP, Malloy MJ, Pullinger CR, unpublished data). From current experience in screening for HBL, as many as 10 percent of such individuals could carry truncations of apo B. Thus, the incidence could be about 1 in 3000. Other causes of HBL would contribute an additional as yet undefined number of cases.

Genetics

Truncations of Apo B. In 1979, Steinberg et al. reported a complex kindred in which several individuals had serum cholesterol levels compatible with heterozygous familial HBL, and others had a more severe deficiency of LDL suggestive of the presence of two mutant alleles;[391] several had fasting hypertriglyceridemia. Serum cholesterol levels in the proband varied between 33 and 42 mg/dl and triglyceride levels between 61 and 103 mg/dl, despite wide variations in his diet. There was no neurologic disease, and only rare acanthocytes were observed. The apo B content of the lipoproteins of the LDL density interval was only 7.4 mg/dl, and that of the VLDL interval was 0.9 mg/dl. The HDL interval contained apo B as well, unlike normal plasma. The plasma levels of apo A-I and apo A-II were somewhat low at 77 and 17 mg/dl, respectively. Apo C-III was undetectable in any of the lipoproteins. Triglyceride turnover measured by [^{3}H]glycerol kinetics showed delayed and diminished secretion followed by slow decay from plasma. Chylomicron kinetics studied by the technique of constant duodenal infusion indicated a removal defect. Neutral sterol excretion was about twice normal.

Further studies of this kindred[87,392] demonstrated apo B-37, a truncated form of apo B. It was found in chylomicrons as well as in particles that are probably hepatogenous VLDL, along with apparently normal apo B-100. In contrast with apo B-100, apo B-37 was found in the HDL density interval as well, on particles discrete from typical HDL.[393] The N-terminal sequence of apo B-37 was identical to that of B-100.

An additional mutation was found in this kindred that allowed limited production of apo B-100, but was also expressed as apo B-86.[389,392,394] Apo B-48 in the plasma of affected individuals was shown to be the product of the allele that produced B-100. The apo B-86 mutation is a 1-bp deletion that causes a frameshift mutation leading to a premature stop codon following 20 novel amino acids. The probable basis for expression of both apo B-86 and apo B-100 is that the deletion results in a continuous sequence of eight adenines. The production of some normal message is probably then the result of limited fidelity of the polymerase reaction leading to restoration of reading frame.[394]

Another disorder with virtual absence of LDL but with nearly normal levels of triglyceride-rich lipoproteins, termed "normotriglyceridemic abetalipoproteinemia," was described by Malloy et al.[88] Chylomicrons were present in plasma after a high-fat meal. Serum cholesterol levels remained around 25 mg/dl, whereas serum triglycerides rose from 30 mg/dl to 250 mg/dl after fat feeding, and to 76 mg/dl after feeding of a high-carbohydrate, low-fat diet for 5 days. Jejunal biopsy showed no retention of lipid in intestinal epithelium 16 h after a high-fat meal (Fig. 115-6). The patient, an 8-year-old female, was obese. She had esotropia, genu valgum, and a wide-based, ataxic gait. She was retarded, with a mental age of 2 to 3 years. Dark-adapted retinograms showed low normal responses. On a typical American diet, her excretion of fat in the stool averaged 10 g/day. Her serum carotene level was low, but vitamin A levels were normal. When she was first studied, tocopherol was undetectable in plasma, but increased to the normal range with oral supplementation of 400 mg per day. Over several years of observation while she received tocopherol supplementation, her ataxia improved significantly.

Analysis of lipoproteins showed spherical particles resembling VLDL in serum after a 12-h fast. Very small amounts of somewhat cuboidal lipoprotein particles were present in the LDL density interval, along with larger spherical particles of ≈1300 Å diameter, resembling VLDL remnants (see Fig. 115-2). In contrast to ABL and homozygous HBL, spherical particles with diameters and hydrodynamic properties typical of HDL_3 predominated in the HDL-density interval.

Each of the lipoprotein fractions showed an increase in the ratio of sphingomyelin to phosphatidylcholine similar to that in recessive ABL. Apo C-I, C-II, C-III, E, A-I, A-II, and D were present, but apo C-III_0 and apo C-III_1 isoforms were nearly absent. The total apo A-I content of plasma was 96 mg/dl. By high-resolution SDS gel electrophoresis a B protein very close to the molecular weight of apo B-48 was detected on triglyceride-rich lipoproteins and in lipoproteins of the HDL density interval. Only traces were present in the LDL interval. This protein was found to be the product of mutant alleles bearing a point substitution that introduces a premature stop codon.[395] The patient is homozygous for this mutation that yields apo B-49.6. The fact that the mutation spares the portion of the gene responsible for apo B-48 explains the ability of the patient to form chylomicrons normally, thus absorbing and transporting dietary fat in a normal fashion. Reinfusion studies showed a half-time for removal of radiolabeled

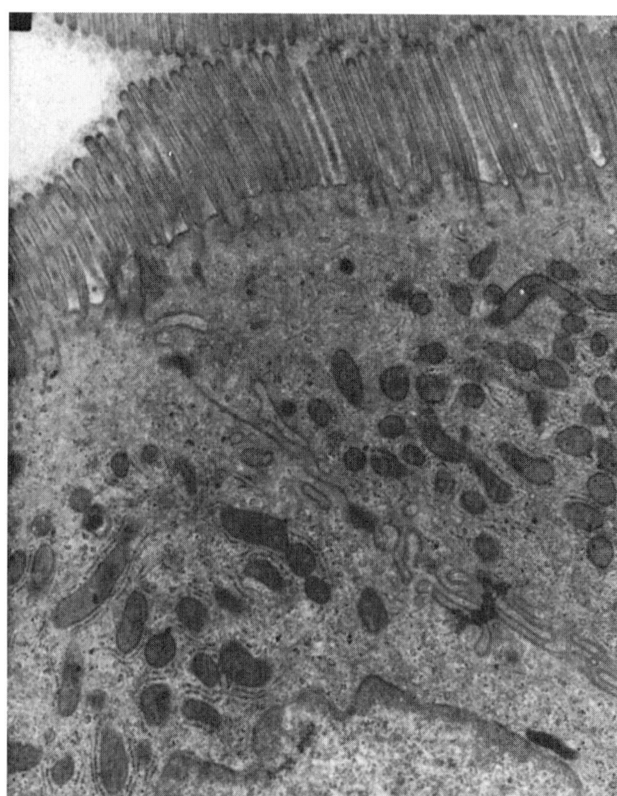

Fig. 115-6 Electron-microscopic appearance of intestinal epithelium in normotriglyceridemic abetalipoproteinemia. Biopsy was taken 16 h following a fat-rich meal. (*Electron microscopy courtesy of Dr. Albert L. Jones.*)

apo B protein in the triglyceride-rich lipoproteins of approximately 50 min, with virtually no detectable label in the LDL interval. Thus, either the truncation has altered the B protein such that LDL cannot be formed from triglyceride-rich precursors or the LDL formed is removed at a very high rate. Additional similar cases have been described.[396–399] A similar phenotypic picture, in which apo B-48 is present in chylomicrons but apo B-100 is absent after infancy was described in which it could be demonstrated unequivocally that the apo B locus is not involved.[400] This raises the possibility that a tissue-specific abnormality in liver can interdict the secretion of VLDL. Another fascinating possibility is that the liver may be secreting apo B-48 as the result of an atavistic mutation involving mRNA editing.

Many truncations of apo B have been identified in the past 5 years.[390] The underlying gene defects and metabolic characteristics of these disorders are presented in Table 115-1. Many result from substitutions or deletions that cause frameshifts leading to premature stop codons. The frameshifts may introduce novel sequences that could exert specific effects on the conformation of apo B. Two apo B-52.8 species have been found to have different C-termini because frameshifts commence at different points. Furthermore, truncations per se may cause conformational changes at the new C-terminus because of removal of protein sequence.[395] Clearly, some deletions other than truncations may be expected to result from gene rearrangements and splice errors. The study of truncations will be, no doubt, important in identifying functional domains of apo B.

Other Mechanisms. There is evidence at hand that genetic disorders other than truncations can cause HBL. Several kindreds have already been identified in which HBL cosegregates with a haplotype of apo B in which truncated apo B species could not be detected.[388,401,402] Decreased content of apo B within hepatocytes

Table 115-1 Apo B Truncating Mutations

Apo B chain length	Mutation	Lipoprotein Species in Which Truncation Found	Ref.
Apo B-2	G to T transversion, intron 5	Absent from plasma	590
Apo B-9	C to T substitution, terminates after codon 411	Absent from plasma	590
Apo B-25	694 bp deletion in exon 21	Absent from plasma	591
Apo B 29	C to T substitution nucleotide 4125	Absent from plasma	64
Apo B 31	Deletion of cDNA nucleotide 4480	HDL and d > 1.21 g/cm^3 fraction	592
Apo B-32	C to T substitution in codon 1450	HDL, LDL	65
Apo B-32.5	T to G substitution at nucleotide 4631	HDL and d > 1.21 g/cm^3 fraction	593
Apo B-37	Deletion of cDNA nucleotides 5391–5394	VLDL, LDL, HDL	389
Apo B-38.7	C to T transversion at nucleotide 5472		594
Apo B 38.95	14-nucleotide deletion at nucleotide 1768	VLDL, LDL	426
Apo B-39	Deletion cDNA nucleotide 5591	VLDL, LDL	64
Apo B-40	Deletion of cDNA nucleotides 5693–5694	VLDL, LDL, HDL	66, 595
Apo B-43.7	C to T transversion, nucleotide 6162	VLDL, IDL, HDL	606
Apo B-44.4	2014 amino acids 11 bp insertion	(VLDL), LDL, HDL	596
Apo B-45.2	T to A transversion at nucleotide 6368		597
Apo B-46	C to T substitution at cDNA nucleotide 6381	VLDL, LDL, HDL	598
Apo B-49.6	C to T substitution at cDNA nucleotide 6963	VLDL, HDL, (LDL)	395
Apo B-52	Short deletion	VLDL, LDL	599
Apo B-52*	5 bp deletion	(VLVL, IDL) LDL	408
Apo B-52.8	deletion of cDNA nucleotide 7295	VLDL, LDL	593
Apo B-52.8	deletion of cDNA nucleotide 7359	VLDL, LDL,	593
Apo B-54.8	C to T substitution at cDNA nucleotide 7665	VLDL, LDL	600
Apo B-55	C to T transition nucleotide 7692	LDL	596, 601
Apo B-61	37 bp deletion at nucleotide 8525	VLDL, LDL	388
Apo B-67	deletion of cDNA nucleotide 9327	LDL, VLDL	602
Apo B-70.5	Insertion of A between nucleotides 9754 and 9760 (dysbetalipoproteinemia also present)	(LDL)	603
Apo B-74.7	deletion of cDNA nucleotide 10366	LDL, VLDL	69
Apo B-82	C to A substitution at nucleotide 11411	VLDL, IDL	Young SG, personal commun.
Apo B-83	C to A transversion at nucleotide 11458	VLDL	604
Apo B-86	deletion of cDNA nucleotide 11840	VLDL, LDL	605
Apo B-87	deletion of cDNA nucleotide 12032	VLDL, LDL	70
Apo B-89	deletion of cNDA nucleotide 12309	VLDL, LDL	66, 595

has been described in homozygous HBL.[403,404] Presumably, mutations involving initiation sites, regulatory sequences, or signal peptide, or mutations resulting in an unstable message can be anticipated in some instances in which truncations are absent. In such cases, an allele product may be completely absent. It is possible that defects of pause-transfer sequences may also be found. However, findings based on haplotypes have clearly demonstrated that some cases of HBL are based on mechanisms that do not directly involve the apo B locus.[402,405] Also, Hobbs et al. described a kindred in which hypercholesterolemia was prevented in some heterozygotes with a genetic defect of the LDL receptor by the concomitant inheritance of HBL that did not cosegregate with the apo B gene.[406] A case in which a very large fraction of VLDL was removed directly from plasma leading to a low production rate for LDL has also been identified.[407] Bile acid biosynthesis was about three times normal, suggesting that up-regulation of the hepatic LDL receptors secondary to increased bile acid synthesis could underlie the abnormal catabolism of VLDL. It is also possible that HBL results from a pathologic increase in the fraction of apo B that is degraded within the hepatocyte. In one patient, activity of microsomal triglyceride transfer protein was normal.[163] Although the majority of mutations leading to truncation of the apo B gene product are point substitutions, short deletions based on a misaligned pairing have been reported.[408]

Effect of Truncations of Apo B on Lipoprotein Metabolism. Certain patterns are beginning to emerge from the study of truncations. Those shorter than apo B-27 have not been described in plasma. This may reflect deletion of sequences required for translocation and assembly of lipoproteins. However, instability of secreted lipoproteins or apo B itself resulting in rapid removal could also account for this observation. Further, as with the findings based on transfections of cells with constructs containing abbreviated apo B genes, the shorter truncations form smaller, denser particles. Progressively larger particles of lower density are formed by longer truncated species with LDL-like particles appearing somewhere in the interval between apo B-31 and apo B-37. Curiously, with the apo B-49.6 mutation, virtually no apo B-containing LDL is present in blood even though the protein is present in significant quantities in VLDL. The truncations from apo B-46 through apo B-67 are found predominantly in VLDL, suggesting that either some element of sequence required to facilitate conversion of VLDL to LDL was deleted, or that the LDL formed is catabolized very rapidly. Lipoproteins bearing apo B with truncations from apo B-74.7 to apo B-89 are found chiefly in the LDL interval. Particles bearing apo B-75, apo B-87, and apo B-89 bind to the LDL receptors of cultured fibroblasts with abnormally high affinity.[64–67] This reflects the existence of sequence in the C-terminal portion of apo B that modulates binding to the receptor. Alternatively, particles with foreshortened apo B may bind apo E, as do chylomicron remnants. Kinetic studies on apo B-75, apo B-87, and apo B-89 demonstrate more rapid clearance than for their apo B-100-containing analogues.[68–70] In the case of LDL, this is consistent with increased affinity for the LDL receptor. In some truncations, decreased production rates seem to be the dominant mechanism responsible for low levels of the affected gene product in plasma. Production of an apo B-67-containing VLDL, for instance, was found to be approximately 6 percent of apo B-containing VLDL in heterozygous patients in addition to an increased fractional catabolic rate for B-67 LDL.[409] Decreased production rates have also been found for VLDL apo B-100 in patients heterozygous for truncations varying from apo B-31 to apo B-89.[410] Low production rates were also noted for IDL and LDL in these cases. In heterozygous subjects from a kindred with HBL in which no truncation could be observed, decreased production of apo B-100 was also noted,[411] whereas in another case, the sole kinetic abnormality was an increased fractional catabolic rate for both VLDL and LDL.[412] In the latter subjects, editing of apo B mRNA and apo B-48 production were normal in intestinal biopsy specimens.[413]

Patterns are emerging from the study of the metabolism of both naturally occurring truncations of apo B and of the products of transfected cell lines that reveal several mechanisms that underlie the lipoprotein deficiencies in familial HBL. Study of the products of rat hepatoma cells transfected with mutant apo B clearly indicate that the lipidation of apo B is progressively limited as the extent of truncation increased.[414,415] Kinetic studies in humans heterozygous for a series of truncations showed progressively decreased production rates as the truncations became more severe.[416] A mouse model heterozygous for a B-70 truncation mimics many of the biochemical abnormalities seen in human hypobetalipoproteinemia.[417] In another mouse model, apo B-83 is removed rapidly from plasma, as in humans.[418]

To detect the organs in which lipoproteins bearing apo B truncations are catabolized, labeled, purified human lipoproteins containing apo B-31, apo B-38.9, and apo B-43.8 were injected into rabbits. All were catabolized significantly faster than human apo B-100 LDL. Whereas the apo B-LDL was catabolized in liver, kidney was the catabolic site for the particles bearing the mutant allele products.[419]

Thus, truncated forms of apo B are poorly lipidized and are secreted at greatly reduced rates. Truncations involving the C-terminus of apo B delete a region that modulates binding of LDL to the LDL receptor, resulting in increased affinity and increased endocytosis, further decreasing the plasma levels of the lipoproteins bearing the mutant apo B species. A poorly understood phenomenon appears also to be involved in some cases, causing decreased secretion of the wild-type allele product, apo B-100. However, it is possible that in these cases a second defect made the recognition of the truncation more likely, creating a preselection bias. In general, patients homozygous for truncations of apo B usually have little or no LDL in plasma. It appears that a single wild-type allele is sufficient to provide for normal absorption of dietary fat and formation of chylomicrons.[420]

Lipoprotein Composition and Metabolism

In the heterozygous state, serum cholesterol levels range from 40 to 180 mg/dl, and average approximately 90 mg/dl. Serum triglycerides range from 15 mg/dl into the normal range. In contrast to patients with ABL, the ratio of free to esterified cholesterol in plasma is normal, as is the distribution of fatty acids in phospholipids and cholesteryl esters.[376–378] The levels of LDL in plasma are probably best compared with those of family members to control for other genetic determinants and diet. As compared with first-degree relatives, heterozygotes appear to have clearly distinguishable LDL levels, usually 50 percent or less of the mean for the unaffected members.[379,381,421] HDL cholesterol levels are widely scattered over the normal range.[377,378,380,381,383,387,407,421] LDL lipid composition is normal.[378,381]

In the homozygous state, the lipoprotein pattern closely resembles that in homozygous recessive ABL. Lipoproteins with β or pre-β mobility are absent on electrophoresis of serum, and chylomicrons do not appear after fat feeding.[234,383,384] However, very small amounts of apo B-100-containing lipoproteins have been isolated that also contain apo E and other small apolipoproteins and that are also enriched in tocopherols.[196] Scant amounts of cuboidal lipoproteins containing apo A-I, like those of recessive ABL, are found in the LDL density interval (Forte TM, personal communication), and the apoprotein composition of HDL also resembles that of recessive ABL.[254]

Cholesterol synthesis was moderately increased in one patient with homozygous HBL.[386] Absorption of cholesterol from the gastrointestinal tract was below normal. The increases in cholesterogenesis could be accounted for by decreased absorption of biliary cholesterol in this case.

In heterozygotes, the (a) protein forms Lp(a) complexes normally with the wild-type apo B-100. Truncations of apo B-89 and shorter do not complex with protein (a) because they lack the appropriate cysteine residue.

Clinical Features

Most patients with simple heterozygosity do not present with clinical signs. The features described here are usually associated with severe HBL as encountered with compound heterozygosity or in the homozygous state.

Hematologic Manifestations. Several instances of acanthocytosis have been described[384,422] in heterozygotes, but usually the fraction of the red cells affected is lower than in recessive ABL. That some subtle changes in erythrocytes may be present is suggested by the finding of extremely low erythrocyte sedimentation rates in other individuals in whom frank acanthocytosis was not seen. Homozygous patients, lacking circulating B apolipoproteins, however, have all had acanthocytosis, as have some patients with severe HBL associated with truncations of apo B.[88] The content of free cholesterol is increased, as is the ratio of sphingomyelin to phosphatidylcholine, and the content of linoleate is low among the esterified fatty acids of plasma. Prothrombin deficiency was observed in homozygotes in two instances,[383,384] with significant hemorrhage in one subject. Levels of the lipoprotein-associated coagulation inhibitor were found to be very low in homozygous HBL.[404]

Gastrointestinal Manifestations. In heterozygotes, there has been only limited clinical evidence of impaired fat absorption.[377,403] Fat malabsorption may be transiently present in infancy.[423] Minor abnormalities of intestinal mucosa were described in one case,[377] but were not found in others,[376,381,407] and the absorption of dietary fat appears to proceed normally.[378,383] However, prolonged chylomicronemia after meals suggests that the rate of chylomicron release may be abnormal in some subjects.[424] Similarly, the appearance of a limited steatosis of liver in one case may indicate impaired release of VLDL.[377]

The histologic findings in homozygous subjects lacking significant amounts of B apolipoproteins in plasma are in general indistinguishable from those in homozygous recessive ABL, with numerous fat droplets in the intestinal epithelium[234,383,385] and liver.[383] Chylomicrons are absent from plasma after a fat meal,[234,383–385] and fat is found in abnormal amounts in the stool.[383,384]

Hepatic steatosis[196,425–427] and hepatic fibrosis[428] have been reported in severely affected individuals. The use of medium-chain triglycerides may be implicated in hepatic fibrosis.

Neuromuscular Manifestations. In contrast to the hematologic and gastrointestinal manifestations, neurologic disease can be found in heterozygotes.[376,378,380,403,405,429] Absent or diminished deep-tendon reflexes are most frequently described, but ataxia and proprioceptive deficits have also been observed. In the few cases reported to date, neurologic disease in homozygotes appears to be less severe than it is in recessive ABL.[383–385]

Ophthalmic Manifestations. Classic retinitis pigmentosa has been reported in several cases of HBL,[403] including in the patient with increased bile acid synthesis.[407] Some structural abnormalities of the retina were described in two others[407,430] who had no impairment of visual acuity. Typical retinitis has also been described in homozygotes.[357,377]

Treatment

Treatment for the disease in homozygotes is the same as for recessive ABL, restriction of dietary fat and intensive supplementation of vitamin E. Administration of moderate doses (400 to 800 mg/day) of tocopherol is recommended for heterozygotes because neurologic deficits can develop. In heterozygotes, restriction of fat in the diet appears judicious if evidence of malabsorption or oxalate urolithiasis is present.

HYPOBETALIPOPROTEINEMIA WITH SELECTIVE DELETION OF APO B-48 (CHYLOMICRON RETENTION DISEASE)

In 1961, Anderson et al. reported an infant in whom fat malabsorption was present and fat droplets abounded in intestinal epithelium[431] (Fig. 115-7). Chylomicrons were absent from plasma after meals, and both LDL and HDL levels were low, as were plasma levels of fat-soluble vitamins and carotenoids. Additional reports have further characterized the disorder.[189,432–437] Bouma et al. studied seven patients.[189,432] All presented with severe diarrhea in childhood and had varying degrees of growth retardation. Serum cholesterol levels ranged from 33 to 116 mg/dl, with all but one below 95 mg/dl. Some patients had hypocalcemia and signs of rickets. The diagnosis was established by the finding of fat-laden enterocytes in small-bowel biopsies. Monoclonal antibodies directed at apo B-48 reacted intensely with the enterocytes of patients, but those selectively reactive with apo B-100 showed no binding. LDL levels in plasma were about half normal, as was the plasma content of apo B and apo A-I. The LDL was rich in triglycerides. The triglyceride content of plasma increased modestly after a high-fat meal, but no chylomicronemia ever appeared. A protein with an apparent molecular weight appropriate for apo B-100 was found in LDL. All isoforms of apo C-III and apo E were found in the VLDL interval. Apo A-I, A-II, and A-IV were present in plasma. An abnormally large percentage of the apo A-I appeared to be in the pro A-I form, and semiquantitative analysis suggested that the relative content of apo E and apo E:apo A-II dimer was increased.

In a study of eight additional subjects, Roy et al. also found increased amounts of immunoreactivity in enterocytes with antibodies against apo B.[438] All patients showed severe growth retardation, steatorrhea, and malnutrition. Three had hypoalbuminemia, and five had undetectably low levels of vitamin E in plasma. One had mild acanthocytosis, and neurologic symptoms were present in three patients who were in the second decade of life. Deep-tendon reflexes were diminished or absent, and vibratory sense was diminished. Among three patients, one was clearly retarded and two were considered to have normal intelligence. Additional patients with neurologic defects have been identified.[432,433] Whereas the mental retardation may be the consequence of pairing of other recessive alleles because of consanguinity, the neurologic findings are compatible with hypovitaminosis E.

Following a fat load, plasma triglyceride levels rose only about 10 mg/dl and levels of LDL apo B and apo A-I in HDL were unchanged.[438] Activities of LPL and hepatic lipase after heparin injection were significantly lower than normal. Total LDL apo B levels in plasma averaged 61 mg/dl, as compared with 76 mg/dl in controls. Total apo A-I levels were more strikingly abnormal, with an average of 50 mg/dl in comparison to an average of 137 mg/dl in the plasma of controls. The LDL was found to be markedly depleted in cholesterol (22 percent of mass as compared with 41 percent in control LDL) and somewhat enriched in triglyceride, phospholipid, and protein. The cholesterol content of HDL was halved (23 percent vs. 43 percent in controls). The percent of total plasma phospholipid represented by sphingomyelins was moderately higher (20 percent vs. 17 percent), and the percentage of phosphatidylcholine was lower (66 percent) than in normal subjects (71 percent).[439] As in other forms of fat malabsorption, essential fatty acid levels were lower among total plasma fatty acids than in normal subjects.

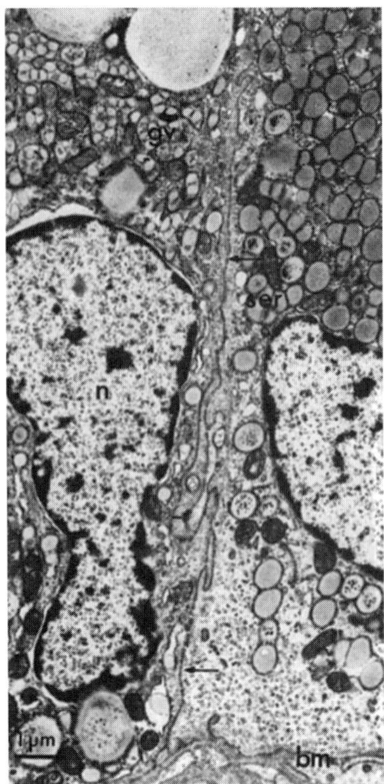

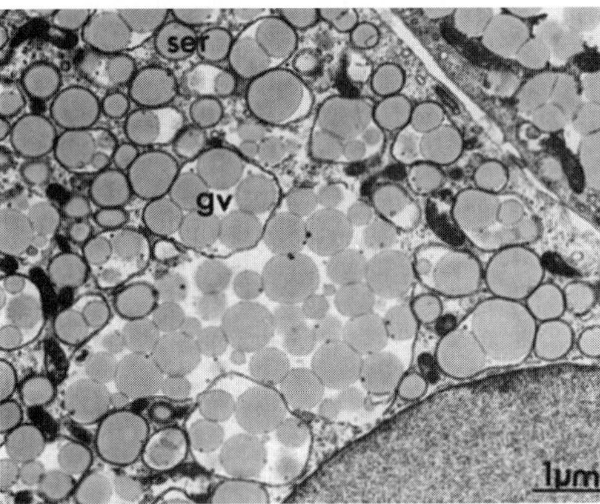

Fig. 115-7 Electron-photomicrographic appearance of intestinal epithelium in chylomicron retention disease. (*Courtesy of Dr. Claude Roy.*) *Top panel*: Accumulation of lipid droplets in the supranuclear region of the cell. n = nucleus; ser = endoplasmic membranes; gv = possible Golgi vesicle; bm = basement membrane. *Bottom panel*: Clustering of lipid droplets within membranous structure in the supranuclear region.

Levy et al.[439] studied in vitro explants obtained by intestinal biopsy in short-term culture. Total protein synthesis appeared normal in the explants, but glycosylation was significantly decreased in comparison with normal control tissue. A monoclonal antibody to apo B-100 reacted with a protein from an extract of explant tissue, labeling a band that comigrated precisely with authentic apo B-48. Secretion of triglyceride into the medium by explants of tissue from patients with the disorder was impaired in comparison with normal tissue, though phospholipid secretion appeared normal.[439] These results strongly suggest that apo B-48 synthesis may be normal in this disorder, but the formation and secretion of chylomicrons are impaired, perhaps as part of a generalized defect in glycosylation. Findings from the EM studies by two groups[432,438] suggest possible heterogeneity of underlying mechanisms. Whereas Roy et al.[438] described a plethora of chylomicron-sized lipid droplets surrounded by membranes of the ER, Lacaille et al.[432] reported droplets apparently in the cytoplasm, with the Golgi apparatus appearing empty. Thus, it is possible that defects at several steps in the lipidation, translocation, and secretion of apo B-48 may emerge. Activity of microsomal triglyceride transfer protein was found to be normal in one case.[163] Studies in kindreds of Arab and Pakistani origin have excluded the apo B locus as the site of the defect.[440,441] Studies in one kindred showed the presence of normally edited message for apo B-48.[441] Thus, in at least one kindred each, errors in mRNA editing or defects in MTP have not been found, suggesting that the formation of apo B-48 proceeds normally, but that the disorder reflects a defect in some additional gene product unique to the secretion of chylomicrons from the intestine. Until more observations are made, it is impossible to rule out mRNA-editing defects or defects in the apo B gene in some kindreds that might produce phenocopy disorders.

The finding of several kindreds with multiple affected sibs establishes the familial nature of this disorder, and the lack of vertical transmission of the phenotype suggests it is a recessive trait. The presence of the disorder in females indicates it is not predominantly X-linked, but the predominance of males (3:1 in the two largest kindreds reported) suggests that complex mechanisms of inheritance could be involved. Treatment should include restriction of dietary fat, especially in infancy. Adequate amounts of essential fatty acids should be supplied. The appearance of neurologic manifestations in several patients indicates that supplementation with vitamin E and perhaps vitamin A should be maintained in all cases as described for ABL.

FAMILIAL LIGAND-DEFECTIVE APO B

Defects in the ligand domain in apo B for the LDL receptor are a relatively common cause of hypercholesterolemia. Because defects in other functional domains of apo B may occur, the term heretofore applied to this disorder, familial defective apo B, should be modified to indicate the specific functional deficit. We suggest that the term familial ligand-defective apo B (FLDB) is more descriptive of the specific pathophysiology. Defects of the ligand domain in apo B-100 for the LDL receptor would be predicted to cause preferential accumulation in blood of LDL particles bearing the defective protein because each LDL particle bears a single copy of apo B-100. Because apo B does not appear to be a significant ligand for the removal of VLDL remnants by the liver (see Chap. 114), ligand defects in apo B are not predicted to alter the fractional conversion of remnants to LDL. In this respect, the hyperlipidemia associated with such defects should produce a less severe hypercholesterolemia than defects in the receptor, and only LDL should accumulate. The combined prevalence of these defects equals that of heterozygous familial hypercholesterolemia in populations of western European origin.[442–445]

The R3500Q and R3500W Mutations

The first observations supporting the existence of functional ligand defects came from studies comparing the removal kinetics of autologous and homologous preparations of human LDL from plasma by Vega and Grundy.[446] Donor LDL were identified that were cleared slowly in receptor-competent recipients. Impaired binding of the LDL to receptors on normal human fibroblasts was subsequently demonstrated.[447] Defective binding of LDL was associated with decreases in endocytosis, degradation, and accumulation of cholesteryl esters. It was possible to separate ligand-defective LDL in patients heterozygous for the polymorphism of apo B detectable with monoclonal antibody MB19.[448] These particles had less than 10 percent of the receptor-binding activity found in LDL carrying the product of the normal allele. There were no detectable differences in particle dimensions or chemical composition of the LDL. Markedly enhanced reactivity of the ligand-defective LDL with monoclonal antibody MB47, known to react with an epitope in the region of apo B sequence involved in binding to the LDL receptor, provided strong evidence for a structural abnormality of apo B.[449] The genomic DNA from affected individuals contained a CGG-to-CAG mutation at the codon for amino acid 3500, which results in an Arg to Gln substitution (R3500Q).[450] A mutation at codon 3500, which results in an Arg to Trp substitution (R3500W), that produces hypercholesterolemia that is a phenocopy of the R3500Q disorder was discovered.[451–453] This mutation appears to be rare among individuals of European origin. The R3500W mutation in the context of a different haplotype appears to be common among Chinese.[453] It was not found among 309 normolipidemic individuals, but it did occur at a frequency of approximately 1:40 among a cohort of 373 hyperlipidemic patients in Taiwan, suggesting that it may be a significant cause of hyperlipidemia among Chinese.[453] Haplotype studies of this mutation are consistent with a founder gene effect.

Data from ^{13}C NMR studies suggest that the R3500Q mutation has effects on the disposition of charged residues in apo B of much greater potential consequence to ligand function than would be expected with the loss of a single unit of cationic charge at a receptor-interactive site.[454] Approximately seven lysine residues in the mutant protein that normally exhibit a pK $\approx$8.9, redistribute to the population of lysines with apparent pK $\approx$10.5, and thus are shifted out of a basic microenvironment. However, no gross changes in secondary structure are evident between the mutant and normal proteins by circular dichroism. The affected allele can be detected by hybridization with allele-specific oligonucleotide probes,[450] by differential introduction of restriction sites,[455–457] by an amplification refractory-mutation system,[444] by single-stranded DNA mobility shift analysis,[458] and by direct measurement of receptor binding of LDL.[459]

The salient biochemical abnormality in patients with the R3500Q mutation has been hypercholesterolemia.[442,447,460] LDL cholesterol levels have varied from about 100 mg/dl to more than 400 mg/dl. Mean LDL cholesterol levels have varied considerably among study populations, but the average of levels reported for 266 individuals in 5 surveys[442,446,458,460–462] was 281 mg/dl, in keeping with the mechanistic prediction that the hypercholesterolemia would be less severe than that associated with major defects of the LDL receptor. Total triglyceride and HDL cholesterol levels are not altered. No clinical stigmata serve to separate patients with this disorder from those with heterozygous familial hypercholesterolemia; those with higher plasma levels of LDL cholesterol may have corneal arcus or tendon xanthomas.[460] Some individuals with higher LDL cholesterol levels may be double heterozygotes with mutations for FH or other forms of hypercholesterolemia. Several polymorphisms of the LDL receptor appear to exert a modest effect on LDL levels in patients with the R3500Q mutations.[460] Individuals with homozygosity for ligand-defective apo B have been identified.[463,464] Combined heterozygosity with familial hypercholesterolemia has also been documented.[465] Among these subjects, LDL cholesterol levels were not higher than those commonly associated with heterozygous FH. A study of stable isotope kinetics in a patient homozygous for the R3500Q mutation revealed, as expected, a prolonged residence time for LDL apo B, as well as a markedly decreased production rate for LDL.[463] The residence time for VLDL particles that contain apo E was reduced by half in comparison with normal subjects. Similarly, stable isotope kinetic studies in heterozygotes bearing the R3500Q allele showed that the fractional catabolic rate for IDL is increased, and the production rate and fractional catabolic rates for LDL are decreased.[466] These observations support the view that LDL receptors are up-regulated by diminished ingress of LDL cholesterol into hepatocytes, and that the increased receptor population abstracts VLDL remnants bearing apo E at an increased rate, reducing conversion of these precursors to LDL. In general, the R3500Q defect is associated with less coronary arteriosclerosis than is heterozygous FH.[103,443,460] This probably reflects quantitative differences in plasma LDL levels, because the severity of coronary arteriosclerosis was indistinguishable when subjects were matched for gender and LDL levels.[467]

Calculations based on the frequency of the R3500Q mutation among hypercholesterolemic individuals suggest a prevalence of 1:500 to 1:600 individuals in populations of European descent.[442,446] The mutation is rare among individuals of non-European origin, and it appears to be rare or absent in Finland. Haplotype analysis in several populations suggests a strong founder gene effect[103,117,461] despite the fact that the mutation occurs at a CpG dinucleotide in which frequent spontaneous mutations might be anticipated. It is estimated that this mutation descended over a period of 6000 to 7000 years from a single European founder.[468]

The R3531C Mutation

A mutation at codon 3531 of apo B was originally found by differential DNA melting of genomic DNA from patients whose LDL was found to have impaired affinity for the LDL receptor in cultured fibroblasts.[458] A C to T transition at nucleotide 10,800 was found to cause an Arg to Cys (R3531C) substitution of cysteine for arginine. In the original study, 2 probands and 8 affected individuals were found on screening 1400 sequential patients with hyperlipidemia. The mean serum cholesterol level for the patients was 263 mg/dl, compared with a level of 150 mg/dl for relatives who lacked the mutation. Subsequently, more than 40 cases were identified, representing 22 kindreds.[103,443,445,469,470] Receptor affinity of the patients' LDL, representing a mixture of apo B allele products was found to be about 49 percent of normal using a double isotope competition assay in which R3500Q-containing LDL had a mean affinity of 37 percent.[445] In other subjects, mixed LDL was found to be about 50 percent as good a competitor as normal LDL.[103] In support of these findings, R3531C-containing LDL was found to produce a very significant reduction in growth rate among cholesterol-dependent U937 cells.[445]

Evidence that the reduced affinity of the R3531C apo B allele product for the LDL receptor has physiological importance comes from the determination of the relative abundance of LDL particles bearing the mutant and wild-type allele products in human plasma. This was accomplished by employing a discriminating monoclonal antibody coupled with detection by laser light scattering.[459] The mutant apo B was predominant among the nine patients studied by this method.[445] Predominance of the mutant LDL was also noted in heterozygous subjects who had normal LDL levels. The decreased affinity of the R3531C gene product for the LDL receptor also appears to affect the level of LDL in blood. Analysis of 44 affected individuals[103,445,469,470] yielded a mean serum cholesterol level of 253 mg/dl ($p < 0.003$) compared to 202 mg/dl among 29 unaffected family members, an average increase of 51 mg/dl. The mean LDL cholesterol level was 171 mg/dl for 40 heterozygotes, an increase of 27 percent over the mean level in affected relatives.

In a large Danish population, the prevalence of the R3531C mutation was found to equal that of the R3500Q mutation, approximately 1 in 1000.[443] The prevalence among patients selected for primary hypercholesterolemia has been reported at 1 in 373.[445] In the Danish population, the R3531C mutation was not associated with higher LDL levels than the nonaffected subjects. However, the entire population had much higher LDL levels than an average American population, a characteristic that might tend to minimize the impact of the mutation. A relatively low incidence of arteriosclerotic heart disease among the R3531C heterozygotes in this study may reflect in part that almost 90 percent were females. Coronary artery disease or other atherosclerotic disease is prevalent among the other cases reported. Though preselection bias may be present in cases detected in lipid clinic populations, it is likely that this mutation contributes to the risk of arteriosclerosis. It clearly impairs the binding of LDL to the LDL receptor and accounts for a significant increment of LDL cholesterol, albeit more mild than that associated with the R3500Q mutation and still smaller than that observed with major defects in the receptor.

In contrast with the R3500Q mutation, which among individuals of European origin appears to have originated as a single founder gene, a limited number of distinct haplotypes for the R3531C mutation are known.[103,445,469,470]

The observation that one haplotype appears to predominate among individuals of Celtic ancestry with the R3531C mutation suggests a founder gene effect in that population.[445] Several additional mutations in the putative receptor ligand domain of apo B are known to lack impact on ligand properties or plasma lipoprotein levels.[445,469] However, it is probable that mutations in other domains of apo B may alter ligand properties, because a number of patients have been identified whose LDL binds poorly to the receptor but in whom no mutations were detectable in the region of the apo B gene between codons 3187 and 3715 (Pullinger C, Kane JP, unpublished observations).

Treatment

Treatment of patients with ligand-defective apo B using HMGCoA reductase inhibitors results in appreciable lowering of LDL levels in most cases.[471–474] In large part, this probably reflects increased endocytoses of apo E containing intermediate density lipoproteins by up-regulated hepatic receptors.[475,476]

FAMILIAL COMBINED HYPERLIPIDEMIA

Clinical Features

Familial combined hyperlipidemia (FCH) was independently identified as a new phenotype in studies of survivors of myocardial infarction and their relatives.[477–480] Patients were found to present with one of three patterns of lipoprotein distribution: elevated plasma levels of VLDL or LDL or a combination of both. Within a kindred, affected individuals often have different lipoprotein patterns, and the pattern may change over time. However, most patients manifest the combined pattern at some time. It is notable that affected individuals who present with isolated elevations of plasma LDL may develop significant hypertriglyceridemia if treated with a bile acid-binding resin. Family pedigrees are usually compatible with autosomal dominant inheritance.[477,478] The disorder is seen in childhood, but expression is limited until approximately the third decade. Penetrance appears to be higher among sibs of phenotypically affected children.[481] The progeny of mating between normal individuals and affected spouses who present with predominant hypertriglyceridemia may have isolated elevations of LDL. Conversely, the mating of a normal spouse with an affected individual who presents with hypercholesterolemia can produce offspring with hypertriglyceridemia.[477] Among hypercholesterolemic subjects, levels of LDL cholesterol tend to be somewhat lower than in heterozygous FH. Among hypertriglyceridemic subjects, plasma triglyceride levels tend to distribute between 200 and 400 mg/dl but may be much higher. Unlike patients with primary endogenous hypertriglyceridemia, patients with FCH seldom have LDL cholesterol levels below 100 mg/dl.[482,483] Most affected family members have total serum apo B levels greater than 85 mg/dl.[484,485] Few patients have xanthomas, even when they have LDL cholesterol levels comparable to those typical of heterozygous FH. Xanthelasma has been found to cosegregate with the trait in one kindred (Kane JP, Malloy MJ, Pullinger CR, unpublished data). A few individuals may also have tuberous xanthomata. Some progeny from mating between individuals with heterozygous FH and FCH have unusually severe hyperlipidemia, often with both tuberous and tendinous xanthomata and premature coronary disease, suggesting that combined heterozygosity for the two disorders can exist, producing a highly atherogenic double-heterozygote genotype. The prevalence of FCH can be estimated roughly from the fraction of patients randomly selected for myocardial infarction who are found to have the phenotype.[478,479] Based on such data, FCH may be present in 1 to 2 percent of the population of North America and Europe, and accounts for about 10–15 percent of myocardial infarctions in those populations. The phenotype shares some features with disorders termed dyslipidemic hypertension[486,487] and the "metabolic syndrome."[488]

Pathophysiology

Plasma Lipoproteins. The plasma concentrations of VLDL, LDL, or both are elevated in FCH. The content of intermediate density lipoproteins is usually increased as well.[489,490] The mass of cholesterol in HDL is reduced.[489–491] In large part, this is probably a reflection of the increased movement of cholesteryl esters from HDL particles to triglyceride-rich lipoproteins with increasing plasma triglyceride levels[492] and is consistent with a shift of HDL to smaller diameters seen on gradient gel electrophoresis.[491] Apolipoprotein A-I levels in plasma tend to be normal or slightly lower than normal.[493,494] The content of pre-β_1 HDL in plasma is increased in FCH and is monotonically related to plasma triglyceride levels (Malloy MJ, O'Connor P, Kane JP, unpublished observations).

Heterogeneity of Lipoprotein Diameters. The LDL particles in FCH tend to be of smaller diameter and higher density than in normal individuals.[489,490,493,495–500] The term *hyperapobetalipoproteinemia* is applied to LDL particles with a high ratio of protein to lipid,[498] and the constellation of elevated plasma triglyceride levels, decreased HDL cholesterol levels and dense LDL of smaller diameter than normal is termed the *atherogenic lipoprotein phenotype*.[501] The LDL particles contain less cholesteryl ester, unesterified cholesterol, and phospholipid than normal LDL. Whether the triglyceride content is increased remains unresolved.[490,493] Ultracentrifugal flotation velocity measurements assign a S*f* of about 6.3 to the predominant LDL particle species in normal individuals, in contrast with a S*f* of about 4.7 for the chief LDL particle species in FCH. Nondenaturing gradient gel electrophoresis clearly shows an increase in mobility consistent with smaller particles. However, the absolute diameters assigned are considerably larger than those that would be appropriate for the chemical compositions of the particles, assuming microemulsion structure, and are also inconsistent with the hydrodynamic data.[489,490,493] This is probably attributable to the lack of appropriate molecular weight standards in the range of LDL diameters.

The distribution of LDL toward smaller particle diameters in FCH is relative.[493] In normal humans, LDL particles appear to be distributed among five or more quantized species rather than in a continuum of diameters.[502–504] The conformation of apo B-100 differs among the species, with distinct diminution of ligand properties for the LDL receptor in the smallest particles (LDL-5).[504] Diameters of LDL particles are larger among normal young women than among men and after menopause approach the smaller diameters seen in men.[505,506] Small dense LDL are a general concomitant of elevated plasma triglyceride levels in normal subjects and those with a number of phenotypes of hyperlipidemia.[491,502,504] This probably reflects two mechanisms. One is the movement of cholesteryl esters to triglyceride-rich lipoproteins, with some reverse transfer of triglycerides, which then can be hydrolyzed by hepatic triglyceride lipase.[507–509] This mechanism may include impairment of the transfer of cholesteryl esters from HDL to LDL and LDL precursors as well.[510] A second mechanism may be operative in which altered precursor lipoproteins, both IDL and small diameter VLDL, lead to the production of small dense LDL.[511] High-density lipoproteins may also play a role in the speciation of IDL.[512] The particle diameters of LDL are dependent on plasma triglyceride levels in patients with FCH, as well as in normal subjects.[489,490] Small dense LDL are reported in individuals whose triglyceride levels are not elevated. This could reflect in part transitory hypertriglyceridemia because of the relatively short half-life of triglyceride-rich lipoproteins, but suggests that another mechanism contributes significantly to the phenomenon.[490,513]

Small-diameter LDL particles have moderately increased susceptibility to copper-catalyzed oxidation, in vitro, a property that could increase the atherogenicity of the particles.[493,514–516] Curiously, in one study the difference in oxidative lag phase between LDL from normals and patients with FCH was most striking in the LDL-3 fraction, which is the predominant species in normal subjects.[493] Treatment of FCH patients with several lipid-lowering regimens increases the buoyant density of their LDL particles.[494] Treatment with bile-acid-binding resins alone has the opposite effect, probably reflecting their propensity to increase triglyceride levels.

Lipoprotein Kinetics

It is well-known that very few of the larger VLDL particles (S*f* 100 to 400) in plasma are converted to LDL-size particles in normal subjects or in hyperlipidemic individuals, despite their conversion to smaller VLDL particles (S*f* 20 to 100) by intravascular lipolysis.[517–520] On the other hand, much more of the apo B-100 in the S*f* 20 to 100 fraction is converted to LDL, suggesting that there is metabolically significant particle heterogeneity among small VLDL. Most studies using either reinfusion of radioiodinated lipoproteins or endogenous labeling with stable isotopes have shown an approximate doubling of the secretion rate for apo B-100 in patients with FCH.[521–525] The observation that VLDL particles in FCH tend to be of small diameter[496] would be compatible with an increased production rate of LDL. A common underlying theme in FCH may be increased lipidation of apo B-100 in the smooth ER of liver, sparing apo B from degradation and resulting in secretion of a larger mass of apo B-100, perhaps in VLDL of smaller than normal particle diameter. Obesity, which is frequently present among patients who present with FCH, is expected to aggravate the hyperlipidemia because it is associated with increased flux of VLDL particles.[526] The report of a kindred whose affected individuals meet the requirements for the FCH phenotype, but whose kinetic defect is impaired clearance of both VLDL and LDL, strongly supports mechanistic heterogeneity among kindreds displaying the FCH phenotype.[527] The binding properties of the LDL receptor for LDL from patients with FCH are normal.[528] However, a defect in the receptor could increase the severity of FCH by impairing the removal of LDL precursors, thereby increasing the production rate of LDL.

Metabolic Correlates of FCH

Insulin resistance occurs in many patients with FCH including individuals who are not obese,[529–536] although obesity, per se, would be expected to further augment insulin resistance. The disorder termed familial dyslipidemic hypertension also includes insulin resistance and may overlap FCH phenotypically.[486,537] Insulin resistance in FCH is associated with impaired suppression of lipolysis by hormone sensitive lipase in adipocytes, producing an increased flux of free fatty acids into the blood, and in turn, increased extraction by liver.[538,539] This increases production of triglyceride fatty acids for lipidation of apo B-100, and thus increases hepatic secretion of VLDL.[540,541] Increased levels of free fatty acids have been found in FCH in association with insulin resistance.[529,539] Elevated levels of free fatty acids can stimulate hepatic gluconeogenesis, thereby augmenting insulin secretion.[541–543] Lack of appropriate stimulation of uptake and esterification by adipocytes of free fatty acids derived from intravascular lipolysis is an additional postulated mechanism that could increase the flux of fatty acids to the liver.[544] Diminished activity of lipoprotein lipase, reflecting insulin resistance,[545] could intensify the hypertriglyceridemia in some patients with FCH.

Genetics of FCH

Specific mutations responsible for FCH are unknown. However, mutations that affect its phenotypic expression are emerging and evidence for complex inheritance has been adduced.[546,547] An elevated plasma level of apo B-100 is one of the best markers for the phenotype, though the apo B gene on chromosome 2 is clearly not directly involved.[534,548,549] Complex segregation analysis implies the existence of a locus with large effects on the levels of apo B-100 in plasma[550,551] and the appearance of small dense LDL.[500,552] Genetic analysis also supports other mendelian loci that are associated with small dense LDL.[553] These loci may interact in complementary fashion.[500,551] By segregation analysis, the effect of elevated triglyceride levels per se on LDL particle size can be shown not to account alone for the phenomenon of small dense LDL.[500,554] These data are compatible with a recessive autosomal locus that interacts with polygenic determinants. Complex segregation analysis supports the existence of at least one major dominant gene locus influencing plasma triglyceride levels.[555] Insulin resistance in FCH is not associated with the codon 54 polymorphism that is associated with insulin resistance in Pima Indians; however, that polymorphism may influence lipid levels in FCH.[535]

Several studies demonstrate linkage disequilibrium between haplotypes at the AI-CII-AIV apolipoprotein cluster and FCH,[556–563] although one study yielded strongly negative results.[564] Among French Canadian patients with FCH, no association could be demonstrated, suggesting either that this gene cluster does not include a primary determinant or that the genetic basis of FCH is heterogeneous in terms of major gene effects.[565] In several studies, haplotypes of the AI-CIII-AIV gene cluster were found to influence lipid values among patients with FCH, but not to account for the phenotype.[559,562] Demonstration of synergistic interaction of haplotypes at this site suggests that influence of this gene cluster is complex.[563]

Despite the fact that CETP activity measured in an *in vitro* system and CETP mass are increased in FCH,[566] net transfer of cholesteryl esters from HDL to LDL does not occur.[510] Increased CETP activity is not unique to FCH, having been reported also in primary hypercholesterolemia.[566] Nonetheless, a possible role of the CETP locus in FCH is suggested by linkage analyses.[500,549]

Although the LPL locus cannot account for FCH alone,[547,567] the possibility that genetic variation in the coding or regulatory regions of the lipoprotein lipase (LPL) gene might act as modifiers was raised by the observation that some heterozygous relatives of patients with the chylomicronemia syndrome due to homozygosity for LPL mutations present with the FCH phenotype.[568–571] In one survey, approximately one-third of patients with the FCH phenotype were found to have levels of LPL activity in the range observed in patients heterozygous for mutations that significantly reduce LPL activity.[569] Several studies show a significantly elevated representation of mutations in the coding region of the LPL gene[572–575] or sequence variations in the promoter region[571] as compared with normal controls. These mutations tend to be associated with increased plasma lipid levels, particularly triglycerides and an increased representation was also described for the LPL (Asp 9 to Asn;D9N) mutation among patients with endogenous lipemia.[573] In several of the studies, cosegregation with the FCH phenotype could not be demonstrated. Thus, LPL mutations do not appear to cause the FCH phenotype, but do augment the hyperlipidemia, and the increased representation of LPL mutations probably reflects an increased likelihood of detection attributable to higher lipid levels. Among Finnish families with the FCH phenotype, no major gene effects could be attributed to the LPL, hepatic lipase, or hormone-sensitive lipase loci.[567] Mutations in the apo A-IV gene could contribute to phenotypic enhancement in a similar fashion.[576]

A spontaneous mouse strain that closely resembles the human FCH phenotype has been identified. It has increased plasma levels of triglycerides and apo B, in which the primary defect appears to be an increased secretion rate for VLDL.[577] This trait (*Hyplip1*) maps to the distal region of mouse chromosome 3. Linkage analyses focused on 10 chromosomal regions containing genes related to lipid metabolism and employing a dominant model yielded a significant association with a region close to the apo A-II gene locus on 1q21-q23 in 31 Finnish kindreds with the FCH phenotype.[578] However, the apo A-II gene was outside the region of maximal linkage. The locus identified is syntenic with the region of mouse chromosome 3 that is linked to the *Hyplip1* phenotype. The emerging view of the genetic basis of FCH in humans is that it is oligogenic but with a complex pattern of inheritance involving a number of modifying genes.[546,551,554,555,579] The small dense LDL trait has been associated in FCH patients and in families with a high prevalence of coronary disease, with the loci for manganese superoxide dismutase, the CI-CIII-AIV locus, cholesterol ester transfer protein, and lecithin cholesterol acyl transferase.[500] An association of small dense LDL with the LDL receptor locus reported in some studies,[579] has not been confirmed in others.[500] An interactive oligogenic rabbit model resembling FCH has also been reported.[580] It is of interest that genome search in Pima Indians[581] and studies of pedigrees in individuals of European background[582] have both shown linkage of type II diabetes with chromosomal region 1q21-q23.

Coronary Heart Disease

The association of the FCH phenotype with increased risk of coronary heart disease was evident even from the first studies.[477–479] Several studies have also related the phenomenon of small dense LDL to coronary disease.[502,583–585] However, it remains unclear to what extent this is simply a reflection of the associated elevation of VLDL and IDL levels, and reduced HDL levels. Clearly, small dense LDL are not a uniform concomitant of coronary disease in the population.[586]

Treatment

Dietary restriction of saturated fats and cholesterol has limited impact on the hyperlipidemia of FCH. Perhaps more important are dietary determinants of increased VLDL secretion rates: alcohol and caloric excess. Weight reduction to ideal body weight and abstinence from alcohol both effect significant reductions in plasma VLDL levels, although they seldom eliminate the hyperlipidemia without the addition of drug treatment. Dietary modification appears to act synergistically with the effect of medications.

The administration of bile acid resins alone often results in significant increases in plasma triglyceride levels; however, the combination of niacin, which probably decreases VLDL production, with resins is an effective regimen.[494] Fibric acid derivatives can reduce triglyceride levels in FCH[509,587] but may increase LDL levels. Treatment with fibrates does not restore normal buoyant density to LDL.[587] It has been reported that HMGCoA reductase inhibitors increase the fractional catabolic rate of LDL without altering the secretion rate of VLDL.[587,588] However, others have shown a decreased production rate for VLDL apo B during treatment with atorvastatin.[589] The most effective drug regimen appears to be a reductase inhibitor with niacin, a combination that is capable of normalizing lipoprotein values in many patients.[494]

REFERENCES

1. Banaszak L, Sharrock W, Timmins P: Structure and function of a lipoprotein: Lipovitellin. *Annu Rev Biophys Biophys Chem* **20**:221, 1991.
2. Boren J, Veniant MM, Young SG: Apo B100-containing lipoproteins are secreted by the heart. *J Clin Invest* **101**:1197, 1998.
3. Farese RV Jr, Cases S, Ruland SL, Kayden HJ, Wong JS, Young SG, Hamilton RL: A novel function for apolipoprotein B: Lipoprotein synthesis in the yolk sac is critical for maternal-fetal lipid transport in mice. *J Lipid Res* **37**:347, 1996.

4. Kane JP: Apolipoprotein B: Structural and metabolic heterogeneity. *Annu Rev Physiol* **45**:637, 1983.
5. Walsh MT, Atkinson D: Solubilization of low-density lipoprotein with sodium deoxycholate and recombination of apoprotein B with dimyristoylphosphatidylcholine. *Biochemistry* **22**:3170, 1983.
6. Hardman DA, Kane JP: Isolation and characterization of apolipoprotein B-48. *Methods Enzymol* **128**:262, 1986.
7. Kane JP, Hardman DA, Paulus HE: Heterogeneity of apolipoprotein B: Isolation of a new species from human chylomicrons. *Proc Natl Acad Sci U S A* **77**:2465, 1980.
8. Gaubatz JW, Heideman C, Gotto AM Jr, Morrisett JD, Dahlen GH: Human plasma lipoprotein [a]. Structural properties. *J Biol Chem* **258**:4582, 1983.
9. Fless GM, ZumMallen ME, Scanu AM: Isolation of apolipoprotein(a) from lipoprotein(a). *J Lipid Res* **26**:1224, 1985.
10. Schumaker VN, Phillips ML, Chatterton JE: Apolipoprotein B and low-density lipoprotein structure: Implications for biosynthesis of triglyceride-rich lipoproteins. *Adv Protein Chem* **45**:205, 1994.
11. Elovson J, Chatterton JE, Bell GT, Schumaker VN, Reuben MA, Puppione DL, Reeve JR Jr, Young NL: Plasma very low density lipoproteins contain a single molecule of apolipoprotein B. *J Lipid Res* **29**:1461, 1988.
12. Robinson MT, Schumaker VN, Butler R, Berg K, Curtiss LK: Ag(c): Recognition by a monoclonal antibody. *Arteriosclerosis* **6**:341, 1986.
13. Wiklund O, Dyer CA, Tsao BP, Curtiss LK: Stoichiometric binding of apolipoprotein B-specific monoclonal antibodies to low density lipoproteins. *J Biol Chem* **260**:10956, 1985.
14. Bhattacharya S, Redgrave TG: The content of apolipoprotein B in chylomicron particles. *J Lipid Res* **22**:820, 1981.
15. Phillips ML, Pullinger C, Kroes I, Kroes J, Hardman DA, Chen G, Curtiss LK, Gutierrez MM, Kane JP, Schumaker VN: A single copy of apolipoprotein B-48 is present on the human chylomicron remnant. *J Lipid Res* **38**:1170, 1997.
16. Scanu A, Hirz R: Human serum low-density lipoprotein protein: Its conformation studied by circular dichroism. *Nature* **218**:200, 1968.
17. Walsh MT, Atkinson D: Calorimetric and spectroscopic investigation of the unfolding of human apolipoprotein B. *J Lipid Res* **31**:1051, 1990.
18. Lund-Katz S, Phillips MC: Packing of cholesterol molecules in human low-density lipoprotein. *Biochemistry* **25**:1562, 1986.
19. Chen GC, Chapman MJ, Kane JP: Secondary structure and thermal behavior of trypsin-treated low-density lipoproteins from human serum, studied by circular dichroism. *Biochim Biophys Acta* **754**:51, 1983.
20. Gotto AM, Levy RI, Fredrickson DS: Observations on the conformation of human beta lipoprotein: evidence for the occurrence of beta structure. *Proc Natl Acad Sci U S A* **60**:1436, 1968.
21. Chen GC, Kane JP: Temperature dependence of the optical activity of human serum low density lipoprotein. The role of lipids. *Biochemistry* **14**:3357, 1975.
22. Chen GC, Kane JP: Circular dichroism of lipoprotein lipids. *Methods Enzymol* **128**: 519, 1986.
23. Yang CY, Chen SH, Gianturco SH, Bradley WA, Sparrow JT, Tanimura M, Li WH, Sparrow DA, DeLoof H, Rosseneu M, et al: Sequence, structure, receptor-binding domains and internal repeats of human apolipoprotein B-100. *Nature* **323**:738, 1986.
24. Chen GC, Kane JP: Secondary structure in very low density and intermediate density lipoproteins of human serum. *J Lipid Res* **20**:481, 1979.
25. Krieger M, Brown MS, Faust JR, Goldstein JL: Replacement of endogenous cholesteryl esters of low-density lipoprotein with exogenous cholesteryl linoleate. Reconstitution of a biologically active lipoprotein particle. *J Biol Chem* **253**:4093, 1978.
26. Watt RM, Reynolds JA: Interaction of apolipoprotein B from human serum low-density lipoprotein with egg yolk phosphatidylcholine. *Biochemistry* **20**:3897, 1981.
27. Ginsburg GS, Small DM, Atkinson D: Microemulsions of phospholipids and cholesterol esters. Protein-free models of low density lipoprotein. *J Biol Chem* **257**:8216, 1982.
28. Ginsburg G., Walsh MT, Small DM, Atkinson D: Reassembled plasma low-density lipoproteins. Phospholipid-cholesterol ester-apoprotein B complexes. *J Biol Chem* **259**:6667, 1984.
29. Chen GC, Hardman DA, Hamilton RL, Mendel CM, Schilling JW, Zhu S, Lau K, Wong JS, Kane JP: Distribution of lipid-binding regions in human apolipoprotein B-100. *Biochemistry* **28**:2477, 1989.
30. Chen SH, Yang CY, Chen PF, Setzer D, Tanimura M, Li WH, Gotto AM Jr, Chan L: The complete cDNA and amino acid sequence of human apolipoprotein B-100. *J Biol Chem* **261**:12918, 1986.
31. Cardin AD, Witt KR, Chao J, Margolius HS, Donaldson VH, Jackson RL: Degradation of apolipoprotein B-100 of human plasma low-density lipoproteins by tissue and plasma kallikreins. *J Biol Chem* **259**:8522, 1984.
32. Cardin AD, Jackson RL, Donaldson VH, Chao J, Margolius HS: Processing of apolipoprotein B-100 of human plasma low density lipoproteins by tissue and plasma kallikreins. *Adv Exp Med Biol* **198(Pt A)**:195, 1986.
33. Gustafson A, Kane JP, Havel RJ: Determinants of kallikrein proteolysis of apolipoprotein B-100 in human blood plasma. *Eur J Clin Invest* **18**:75, 1988.
34. Knott TJ, Rall SC Jr, Innerarity TL, Jacobson SF, Urdea MS, Levy-Wilson B, Powell LM, Pease RJ, Eddy R, Nakai H, et al: Human apolipoprotein B: Structure of carboxyl-terminal domains, sites of gene expression, and chromosomal localization. *Science* **230**:37, 1985.
35. Cardin AD, Price CA, Hirose N, Krivanek MA, Blankenship DT, Chao J, Mao SJ: Structural organization of apolipoprotein B-100 of human plasma low density lipoproteins. Comparison to B-48 of chylomicrons and very low-density lipoproteins. *J Biol Chem* **261**:16744 1986.
36. Chen GC, Zhu S, Hardman DA, Schilling JW, Lau K, Kane JP: Structural domains of human apolipoprotein B-100. Differential accessibility to limited proteolysis of B-100 in low density and very low density lipoproteins. *J Biol Chem* **264**:14369, 1989.
37. Yang CY, Gu ZW, Weng SA, Kim TW, Chen SH, Pownall HJ, Sharp PM, Liu SW, Li WH, Gotto AM Jr, et al: Structure of apolipoprotein B-100 of human low-density lipoproteins. *Arterioscler Thromb Vasc Biol* **9**:96, 1989.
38. Chen GC, Lau K, Hamilton RL, Kane JP: Differences in local conformation in human apolipoprotein B-100 of plasma low density and very low-density lipoproteins as identified by cathepsin D. *J Biol Chem* **266**:12581 1991.
39. Runquist EA, Havel RJ: Acid hydrolases in early and late endosome fractions from rat liver. *J Biol Chem* **266**:22557, 1991.
40. Kunitake ST, Young SG, Chen GC, Pullinger CR, Zhu S, Pease RJ, Scott J, Hass P, Schilling J, Kane JP: Conformation of apolipoprotein B-100 in the low-density lipoproteins of Tangier disease. Identification of localized conformational response to triglyceride content. *J Biol Chem* **265**:20739, 1990.
41. Phillips ML, Schumaker VN: Conformation of apolipoprotein B after lipid extraction of low density lipoproteins attached to an electron microscope grid. *J Lipid Res* **30**:415, 1989.
42. Chatterton JE, Phillips ML, Curtiss LK, Milne RW, Marcel YL, Schumaker VN: Mapping apolipoprotein B on the low density lipoprotein surface by immunoelectron microscopy. *J Biol Chem* **266**:5955, 1991.
43. Chatterton JE, Phillips ML, Curtiss LK, Milne R, Fruchart JC, Schumaker VN: Immunoelectron microscopy of low density lipoproteins yields a ribbon and bow model for the conformation of apolipoprotein B on the lipoprotein surface. *J Lipid Res* **36**:2027, 1995.
44. Olofsson SO, Bjursell G, Boström K, Carlsson P, Elovson J, Protter AA, Reuben MA, Bondjers G: Apolipoprotein B: structure, biosynthesis and role in the lipoprotein assembly process. *Atherosclerosis* **68**:1, 1987.
45. Borén J Graham L, Wettesten M, Scott J, White A, Olofsson SO: The assembly and secretion of ApoB 100-containing lipoproteins in Hep G2 cells. ApoB 100 is cotranslationally integrated into lipoproteins. *J Biol Chem* **267**:9858, 1992.
46. Yao ZM, Blackhart BD, Linton MF, Taylor SM, Young SG, McCarthy BJ: Expression of carboxyl-terminally truncated forms of human apolipoprotein B in rat hepatoma cells. Evidence that the length of apolipoprotein B has a major effect on the buoyant density of the secreted lipoproteins. *J Biol Chem* **266**:3300, 1991.
47. Spring DJ, Chen-Liu LW, Chatterton JE, Elovson J, Schumaker VN: Lipoprotein assembly. Apolipoprotein B size determines lipoprotein core circumference. *J Biol Chem* **267**:14839, 1992.
48. Tsao BP, Curtiss LK, Edgington TS: Immunochemical heterogeneity of human plasma apolipoprotein B. II. Expression of apolipoprotein B epitopes on native lipoproteins. *J Biol Chem* **257**:15222, 1982.
49. Marcel YL, Hogue M, Weech PK, Davignon J, Milne RW: Expression of apolipoprotein B epitopes in lipoproteins. Relationship to conformation and function. *Arterioscler Thromb Vasc Biol* **8**:832, 1988.

50. Knott TJ, Pease RJ, Powell LM, Wallis SC, Rall SC Jr, Innerarity TL, Blackhart B, Taylor WH, Marcel Y, Milne R, et al: Complete protein sequence and identification of structural domains of human apolipoprotein B. *Nature* **323**:734, 1986.
51. Scott J, Pease RJ, Powell LM, Wallis SC, McCarthy BJ, Mahley RW, Levy-Wilson B, Knott TJ: Human apolipoprotein B: Complete cDNA sequence and identification of structural domains of the protein. *Biochem Soc Trans* **15**:195, 1987.
52. Cardin AD, Witt KR, Barnhart CL, Jackson RL: Sulfhydryl chemistry and solubility properties of human plasma apolipoprotein B. *Biochemistry* **21**:4503:1982.
53. Shireman RB, Fisher WR: The absence of a role for the carbohydrate moiety in the binding of apolipoprotein B to the low density lipoprotein receptor. *Biochim Biophys Acta* **572**:537, 1979.
54. Hoeg JM, Meng MS, Ronan R, Demosky SJ Jr, Fairwell T, Brewer HB Jr: Apolipoprotein B synthesized by Hep G2 cells undergoes fatty acid acylation. *J Lipid Res* **29**:1215, 1988.
55. Huang G, Lee DM, Singh S: Identification of the thiol ester linked lipids in apolipoprotein B. *Biochemistry* **27**:1395, 1988.
56. Davis RA, Clinton GM, Borchardt RA, Malone-McNeal M, Tan T, Lattier GR: Intrahepatic assembly of very low density lipoproteins. Phosphorylation of small molecular weight apolipoprotein B. *J Biol Chem* **259**:3383, 1984.
57. Scott J: The molecular and cell biology of apolipoprotein-B. *Mol Biol Med* **6**:65, 1989.
58. Mahley RW, Innerarity TL, Pitas RE, Weisgraber KH, Brown JH, Gross E: Inhibition of lipoprotein binding to cell surface receptors of fibroblasts following selective modification of arginyl residues in arginine-rich and B apoproteins. *J Biol Chem* **252**:7279, 1977.
59. Weisgraber KH, Innerarity TL, Mahley RW: Role of lysine residues of plasma lipoproteins in high affinity binding to cell surface receptors on human fibroblasts. *J Biol Chem* **253**:9053, 1978.
60. Krul ES, Tikkanen MJ, Cole TG, Davie JM, Schonfeld G: Roles of apolipoproteins B and E in the cellular binding of very low-density lipoproteins. *J Clin Invest* **75**:361-, 1985.
61. Hui DY, Innerarity TL, Milne RW, Marcel YL, Mahley RW: Binding of chylomicron remnants and beta-very low density lipoproteins to hepatic and extrahepatic lipoprotein receptors. A process independent of apolipoprotein B48. *J Biol Chem* **259**:15060, 1984.
62. Marcel, YL, Innerarity TL, Spilman C, Mahley RW, Protter AA, Milne RW: Mapping of human apolipoprotein B antigenic determinants. *Arterioscler Thromb Vasc Biol* **7**:166, 1987.
63. Milne R, Théolis R Jr, Maurice R, Pease RJ, Weech PK, Rassart E, Fruchart JC, Scott J, Marcel YL: The use of monoclonal antibodies to localize the low-density lipoprotein receptor-binding domain of apolipoprotein B. *J Biol Chem* **264**:19754, 1989.
64. Collins DR, Knott TJ, Pease RJ, Powell LM, Wallis SC, Robertson S, Pullinger CR, Milne RW, Marcel YL, Humphries SE, et al: Truncated variants of apolipoprotein B cause hypobetalipoproteinaemia. *Nucleic Acids Res* **16**:8361, 1988.
65. McCormick SP, Fellowes AP, Walmsley TA, George PM: Apolipoprotein B-32: A new truncated mutant of human apolipoprotein B capable of forming particles in the low-density lipoprotein range. *Biochim Biophys Acta* **1138**:290, 1992.
66. Talmud P, King-Underwood L, Krul E, Schonfeld G, Humphries S: The molecular basis of truncated forms of apolipoprotein B in a kindred with compound heterozygous hypobetalipoproteinemia. *J Lipid Res* **30**:1773, 1989.
67. Tennyson GE, Gabelli C, Baggio G, Bilato C, Brewer HBJ: Molecular defect in the apolipoprotein B gene in a patient with hypobetalipoproteinemia and three distinct apoB species. *Clin Res* **38**:482A, 1990.
68. Parhofer KG, Daugherty A, Kinoshita M, Schonfeld G: Enhanced clearance from plasma of low-density lipoproteins containing a truncated apolipoprotein, apoB-89. *J Lipid Res* **31**:2001, 1990.
69. Krul ES, Parhofer KG, Barrett PH, Wagner RD, Schonfeld G: ApoB-75, a truncation of apolipoprotein B associated with familial hypobetalipoproteinemia: genetic and kinetic studies. *J Lipid Res* **33**:1037, 1992.
70. Gabelli C, Bilato C, Martini S, Tennyson GE, Zech LA, Corsini A, Albanese M, Brewer HB Jr, Crepaldi G, Baggio G: Homozygous familial hypobetalipoproteinemia. Increased LDL catabolism in hypobetalipoproteinemia due to a truncated apolipoprotein B species, apo B-87 Padova. *Arterioscler Thromb Vasc Biol* **16**:1189, 1996.
71. Schaefer EJ, Gregg RE, Ghiselli G, Forte TM, Ordovas JM, Zech LA, Brewer HB Jr: Familial apolipoprotein E deficiency. *J Clin Invest* **78**:1206, 1986.
72. Bradley WA, Gianturco SH: ApoE is necessary and sufficient for the binding of large triglyceride-rich lipoproteins to the LDL receptor; apo B is unnecessary. *J Lipid Res* **27**:40, 1986.
73. Yamamoto M, Ranganathan S, Kottke BA: Structure and function of human low density lipoproteins. Studies using proteolytic cleavage by plasma kallikrein. *J Biol Chem* **260**:8509, 1985.
74. Bradley WA, Hwang SL, Karlin JB, Lin AH, Prasad SC, Gotto AM Jr, Gianturco SH: Low-density lipoprotein receptor binding determinants switch from apolipoprotein E to apolipoprotein B during conversion of hypertriglyceridemic very-low-density lipoprotein to low-density lipoproteins. *J Biol Chem* **259**:14728, 1984.
75. Fantappiè S, Corsini A, Sidoli A, Uboldi P, Granata A, Zanelli T, Rossi P, Marcovina S, Fumagalli R, Catapano AL: Monoclonal antibodies to human low-density lipoprotein identify distinct areas on apolipoprotein B-100 relevant to the low density lipoprotein-receptor interaction. *J Lipid Res* **33**:1111, 1992.
76. Boren J, Lee I, Zhu W, Arnold K, Taylor S, Innerarity TL: Identification of the low density lipoprotein receptor-binding site in apolipoprotein B100 and the modulation of its binding activity by the carboxyl terminus in familial defective apo-B100. *J Clin Invest* **101**:1084, 1998.
77. Farese R, Véniant MM, Cham CM, Flynn LM, Pierotti V, Loring JF, Traber M, Ruland S, Stokowski RS, Huszar D, Young SG: Phenotypic analysis of mice expressing exclusively apolipoprotein B48 or apolipoprotein B100. *Proc Natl Acad Sci U S A* **93**:6393, 1996.
78. Iverius PH: The interaction between human plasma lipoproteins and connective tissue glycosaminoglycans. *J Biol Chem* **247**:2607, 1972.
79. Mahley RW, Weisgraber KH, Innerarity TL: Interaction of plasma lipoproteins containing apolipoproteins B and E with heparin and cell surface receptors. *Biochim Biophys Acta* **575**:81, 1979.
80. Cardin AD, RL Barnhart, KR Witt, RL Jackson: Reactivity of heparin with the human plasma heparin-binding proteins thrombin, antithrombin III, and apolipoproteins E and B-100. *Thromb Res* **34**:541, 1984.
81. Weisgraber KH, Rall SC Jr: Human apolipoprotein B-100 heparin-binding sites. *J Biol Chem* **262**:11097, 1987.
82. Cardin AD, Ranganathan S, Hirose N, Wallhausser L, Harmony JA, Jackson RL: Effect of trypsin treatment on the heparin- and receptor-binding properties of human plasma low-density lipoproteins. *Biochemistry* **25**:5258, 1986.
83. Hirose N, Blankenship DT, Krivanek MA, Jackson RL, Cardin AD: Isolation and characterization of four heparin-binding cyanogen bromide peptides of human plasma apolipoprotein B. *Biochemistry* **26**:5505, 1987.
84. Olsson U, Camejo G, Hurt-Camejo E, Elfsber K, Wiklund O, Bondjers G: Possible functional interactions of apolipoprotein B-100 segments that associate with cell proteoglycans and the ApoB/E receptor. *Arterioscler Thromb Vasc Biol* **17**:149, 1997.
85. Camejo G, Olofsson SO, Lopez F, Carlsson P, Bondjers G: Identification of Apo B-100 segments mediating the interaction of low density lipoproteins with arterial proteoglycans. *Arterioscler Thromb Vasc Biol* **8**:368, 1988.
86. Borén J, Olin K, Lee I, Chait A, Wight TN, Innerarity TL: Identification of the principal proteoglycan-binding site in LDL. A single-point mutation in apo-B100 severely affects proteoglycan interaction without affecting LDL receptor binding. *J Clin Invest* **101**:2658, 1998.
87. Young SG, Bertics SJ, Curtiss L K, Witztum JL: Characterization of an abnormal species of apolipoprotein B, apolipoprotein B-37, associated with familial hypobetalipoproteinemia. *J Clin Invest* **79**:1831, 1987.
88. Malloy MJ, Kane JP, Hardman DA, Hamilton RL, Dalal KB: Normotriglyceridemic abetalipoproteinemia. Absence of the B-100 apolipoprotein. *J Clin Invest* **67**:1441, 1981.
89. Purcell-Huynh DA, Farese RV Jr, Johnson DF, Flynn LM, Pierotti V, Newland DL, Linton MF, Sanan DA, Young SG: Transgenic mice expressing high levels of human apolipoprotein B develop severe atherosclerotic lesions in response to a high-fat diet. *J Clin Invest* **95**:2246, 1995.
90. Véniant MM, Pierotti V, Newland D, Cham CM, Sanan DA, Walzem RL, Young SG: Susceptibility to atherosclerosis in mice expressing exclusively apolipoprotein B48 or apolipoprotein B100. *J Clin Invest* **100**:180, 1997.
91. Huang LS, Ripps ME, Breslow JL: Molecular basis of five apolipoprotein B gene polymorphisms in noncoding regions. *J Lipid Res* **31**:71, 1990.

92. Ma YH, Schumaker VN, Butler R, Sparkes RS: Two DNA restriction fragment length polymorphisms associated with Ag(t/z) and Ag(g/c) antigenic sites of human apolipoprotein B. *Arterioscler Thromb Vasc Biol* **7**:301, 1987.
93. Wang XB, Schlapfer P, Ma YH, Bütler R, Elovson J, Schumaker VN: Apolipoprotein B: The Ag(a1/d) immunogenetic polymorphism coincides with a T-to-C substitution at nucleotide 1981, creating an Alu I restriction site. *Arterioscler Thromb Vasc Biol* **8**:429, 1988.
94. Young SG, HublST: An ApaLI restriction site polymorphism is associated with the MB19 polymorphism in apolipoprotein B. *J Lipid Res* **30**:443, 1989.
95. Xu CF, Nanjee N, Tikkanen MJ, Huttunen JK, Pietinen P, Bütler R, Angelico F, Del Ben M, Mazzarella B, Antonio R, et al: Apolipoprotein B amino acid 3611 substitution from arginine to glutamine creates the Ag (h/i) epitope: The polymorphism is not associated with differences in serum cholesterol and apolipoprotein B levels. *Hum Genet* **82**:322, 1989.
96. Berg K, Powell LM, Wallis SC, Pease R, Knott TJ, Scott J: Genetic linkage between the antigenic group (Ag) variation and the apolipoprotein B gene: Assignment of the Ag locus. *Proc Natl Acad Sci U S A* **83**:7367, 1986.
97. Dunning AM, Renges HH, Xu CF, Peacock R, Brasseur R, Laxer G, Tikkanen MJ, Bütler R, Saha N, Hamsten A, et al: Two amino acid substitutions in apolipoprotein B are in complete allelic association with the antigen group (x/y) polymorphism: Evidence for little recombination in the 3′ end of the human gene. *Am J Hum Genet* **50**:208, 1992.
98. Huang LS, Gavish D, Breslow JL: Sequence polymorphism in the human apo B gene at position 8344. *Nucleic Acids Res* **18**:5922, 1990.
99. Wu MJ, Bütler E, Bütler R, Schumaker VN: Identification of the base substitution responsible for the Ag(x/y) polymorphism of apolipoprotein B-100. *Arterioscler Thromb Vasc Biol* **11**:379, 1991.
100. Moreel JF, Roizes G, Evans AE, Arveiler D, Cambou JP, Souriau C, Parra HJ, Desmarais E, Fruchart JC, Ducimetière P, et al: The polymorphism Apo B/4311 in patients with myocardial infarction and controls: The ECTIM Study. *Hum Genet* **89**:169, 1992.
101. Visvikis S, Chan L, Siest G, Drouin P, Boerwinkle E: An insertion deletion polymorphism in the signal peptide of the human apolipoprotein B gene. *Hum Genet* **84**:373, 1990.
102. Boerwinkle E, Lee SS, Butler R, Schumaker VN, Chan L: Rapid typing of apolipoprotein B DNA polymorphisms by DNA amplification. Association between Ag epitopes of human apolipoprotein B-100, a signal peptide insertion/deletion polymorphism, and a 3′ flanking DNA variable number of tandem repeats polymorphism of the apolipoprotein B gene. *Atherosclerosis* **81**:225, 1990.
103. Ludwig EH, Hopkins PN, Allen A, Wu LL, Williams RR, Anderson JL, Ward RH, Lalouel JM, Innerarity TL: Association of genetic variations in apolipoprotein B with hypercholesterolemia, coronary artery disease, and receptor binding of low density lipoproteins. *J Lipid Res* **38**:1361, 1997.
104. Lusis AJ, West R, Mehrabian M, Reuben MA, LeBoeuf RC, Kaptein JS, Johnson DF, Schumaker VN, Yuhasz MP, Schotz MC, et al: Cloning and expression of apolipoprotein B, the major protein of low and very low density lipoproteins. *Proc Natl Acad Sci U S A* **82**:4597, 1985.
105. Deeb SS, Motulsky AG, Albers JJ: A partial cDNA clone for human apolipoprotein B. *Proc Natl Acad Sci U S A* **82**:4983, 1985.
106. Carlsson P, Olofsson SO, Bondjers G, Darnfors C, Wiklund O, Bjursell G: Molecular cloning of human apolipoprotein B cDNA. *Nucleic Acids Res* **13**:8813, 1985.
107. Law SW, Lackner KJ, Hospattankar AV, Anchors JM, Sakaguchi AY, Naylor SL, Brewer HB Jr: Human apolipoprotein B-100: Cloning, analysis of liver mRNA, and assignment of the gene to chromosome 2. *Proc Natl Acad Sci U S A* **82**:8340, 1985.
108. Wei CF, Chen SH, Yang CY, Marcel YL, Milne RW, Li WH, Sparrow JT, Gotto AM Jr, Chan L: Molecular cloning and expression of partial cDNAs and deduced amino acid sequence of a carboxyl-terminal fragment of human apolipoprotein B-100. *Proc Natl Acad Sci U S A* **82**:7265, 1985.
109. Huang LS, Bock SC, Feinstein SI, Breslow JL: Human apolipoprotein B cDNA clone isolation and demonstration that liver apolipoprotein B mRNA is 22 kilobases in length. *Proc Natl Acad Sci U S A* **82**:6825, 1985.
110. Deeb SS, Disteche C, Motulsky AG, Lebo RV, Kan YW: Chromosomal localization of the human apolipoprotein B gene and detection of homologous RNA in monkey intestine. *Proc Natl Acad Sci U S A* **83**:419, 1986.
111. Protter AA, Hardman DA, Schilling JW, Miller J, Appleby V, Chen GC, Kirsher SW, McEnroe G, Kane JP: Isolation of a cDNA clone encoding the amino-terminal region of human apolipoprotein B. *Proc Natl Acad Sci U S A* **83**:1467, 1986.
112. Protter AA, Hardman DA, Sato KY, Schilling JW, Yamanaka M, Hort YJ, Hjerrild KA, Chen GC, Kane JP: Analysis of cDNA clones encoding the entire B-26 region of human apolipoprotein B. *Proc Natl Acad Sci U S A* **83**:5678, 1986.
113. Knott TJ, Wallis SC, Powell LM, Pease RJ, Lusis AJ, Blackhart B, McCarthy BJ, Mahley RW, Levy-Wilson B, Scott J: Complete cDNA and derived protein sequence of human apolipoprotein B-100. *Nucleic Acids Res* **14**:7501, 1986.
114. Law SW, Grant SM, Higuchi K, Hospattankar A, Lackner K, Lee N, Brewer HB Jr: Human liver apolipoprotein B-100 cDNA: Complete nucleic acid and derived amino acid sequence. *Proc Natl Acad Sci U S A* **83**:8142, 1986.
115. Cladaras C, Hadzopoulou-Cladaras M, Nolte RT, Atkinson D, Zannis VI: The complete sequence and structural analysis of human apolipoprotein B-100: Relationship between apo B-100 and apo B-48 forms. *EMBO J* **5**:3495, 1986.
116. Mehrabian M, Sparkes RS, Mohandas T, Klisak IJ, Schumaker VN, Heinzmann C, Zollman S, Ma YH, Lusis AJ: Human apolipoprotein B: Chromosomal mapping and DNA polymorphisms of hepatic and intestinal species. *Somat Cell Mol Genet* **12**:245, 1986.
117. Ludwig EH, McCarthy BJ: Haplotype analysis of the human apolipoprotein B mutation associated with familial defective apolipoprotein B100. *Am J Hum Genet* **47**:712, 1990.
118. Levy-Wilson B, C Fortier: The limits of the DNase I-sensitive domain of the human apolipoprotein B gene coincide with the locations of chromosomal anchorage loops and define the 5′ and 3′ boundaries of the gene. *J Biol Chem* **264**:21196, 1989.
119. Ludwig EH, Levy-Wilson B, Knott T, Blackhart BD, McCarthy BJ: Comparative analysis of sequences at the 5′ end of the human and mouse apolipoprotein B genes. *DNA Cell Biol* **10**:329, 1991.
120. Ross RS, Li AC, Hoeg JM, Schumacher UK, Demosky SJ Jr, Brewer HB Jr: Apolipoprotein B upstream suppressor site: Identification of an element which can decrease apolipoprotein B transcription. *Biochem Biophys Res Commun* **176**:1116, 1991.
121. Paulweber B, Sandhofer F, B Levy-Wilson: The mechanism by which the human apolipoprotein B gene reducer operates involves blocking of transcriptional activation by hepatocyte nuclear factor 3. *Mol Cell Biol* **13**:1534, 1993.
122. Zannis VI, Kardassis D, Ogami K, Hadzopoulou-Cladaras M, Cladaras C: Transcriptional regulation of the human apolipoprotein genes. *Adv Exp Med Biol* **285**:1, 1991.
123. Carlsson P, Eriksson P, Bjursell G: Two nuclear proteins bind to the major positive element of the apolipoprotein B gene promoter. *Gene* **94**:295, 1990.
124. Das HK, Leff T, Breslow JL: Cell type-specific expression of the human apo B gene is controlled by two cis-acting regulatory regions. *J Biol Chem* **263**:11452, 1988.
125. Brooks AR, Levy-Wilson B: Hepatocyte nuclear factor 1 and C/EBP are essential for the activity of the human apolipoprotein B gene second-intron enhancer. *Mol Cell Biol* **12**:1134, 1992.
126. Kardassis D, Hadzopoulou-Cladaras M, Ramji DP, Cortese R, Zannis VI, Cladaras C: Characterization of the promoter elements required for hepatic and intestinal transcription of the human apo B gene: Definition of the DNA-binding site of a tissue-specific transcriptional factor. *Mol Cell Biol* **10**:2653, 1990.
127. McCormick SP, Ng JK, Taylor S, Flynn LM, Hammer RE, Young SG: Mutagenesis of the human apolipoprotein B gene in a yeast artificial chromosome reveals the site of attachment for apolipoprotein(a). *Proc Natl Acad Sci U S A* **92**:10147, 1995.
128. Hardman DA, Protter AA, Chen GC, Schilling JW, Sato KY, Lau K, Yamanaka M, Mikita T, Miller J, Crisp T, et al: Structural comparison of human apolipoproteins B-48 and B-100. *Biochemistry* **26**:5478, 1987.
129. Innerarity TL, Young SG, Poksay KS, Mahley RW, Smith RS, Milne RW, Marcel YL, Weisgraber KH: Structural relationship of human apolipoprotein B48 to apolipoprotein B100. *J Clin Invest* **80**:1794, 1987.
130. Powell LM, Wallis SC, Pease RJ, Edwards YH, Knott TJ, Scott J: A novel form of tissue-specific RNA processing produces apolipoprotein-B48 in intestine. *Cell* **50**:831, 1987.
131. Chen SH, Habib G, Yang CY, Gu ZW, Lee BR, Weng SA, Silberman SR, Cai SJ, Deslypere JP, Rosseneu M, et al: Apolipoprotein B-48 is

the product of a messenger RNA with an organ-specific in-frame stop codon. *Science* **238**:363, 1987.

132. Hospattankar AV, Higuchi K, Law SW, Meglin N, Brewer HB Jr: Identification of a novel in-frame translational stop codon in human intestine apo B mRNA. *Biochem Biophys Res Commun* **148**:279, 1987.
133. Hardman DA, Protter AA, Schilling JW, Kane JP: Carboxyl terminal analysis of human B-48 protein confirms the novel mechanism proposed for chain termination. *Biochem Biophys Res Commun* **149**:1214, 1987.
134. Yao ZM, Blackhart BD, Johnson DF, Taylor SM, Haubold KW, McCarthy BJ: Elimination of apolipoprotein B48 formation in rat hepatoma cell lines transfected with mutant human apolipoprotein B cDNA constructs. *J Biol Chem* **267**:1175, 1992.
135. Boström K, Lauer SJ, Poksay KS, Garcia Z, Taylor JM, Innerarity TL: Apolipoprotein B48 RNA editing in chimeric apolipoprotein EB mRNA. *J Biol Chem* **264**:15701, 1989.
136. Davies MS, Wallis SC, Driscoll DM, Wynne JK, Williams GW, Powell LM, Scott J: Sequence requirements for apolipoprotein B RNA editing in transfected rat hepatoma cells. *J Biol Chem* **264**:13395, 1989.
137. Backus JW, Smith HC: Apolipoprotein B mRNA sequences 3′ of the editing site are necessary and sufficient for editing and editosome assembly. *Nucleic Acids Res* **19**:6781. 1991.
138. Shah RR, Knott TJ, Legros JE, Navaratnam N, Greeve JC, Scott J: Sequence requirements for the editing of apolipoprotein B mRNA. *J Biol Chem* **266**:16301, 1991.
139. Innerarity TL, Borén J, Yamanaka S, Olofsson SO: Biosynthesis of apolipoprotein B48-containing lipoproteins. Regulation by novel post-transcriptional mechanisms. *J Biol Chem* **271**:2353, 1996.
140. Tennyson GE, Sabatos CA, Higuchi K, Meglin N, Brewer HB Jr: Expression of apolipoprotein B mRNAs encoding higher- and lower-molecular weight isoproteins in rat liver and intestine [published erratum appears in *Proc Natl Acad Sci U S A* **86(8)**:2657, 1989]. *Proc Natl Acad Sci U S A* **86**:500, 1989.
141. Teng B, Burant CF, Davidson NO: Molecular cloning of an apolipoprotein B messenger RNA editing protein. *Science* **260**:1816, 1993.
142. Nakamuta M, Oka K, Krushkal J, Kobayashi K, Yamamoto M, Li WH, Chan L: Alternative mRNA splicing and differential promoter utilization determine tissue-specific expression of the apolipoprotein B mRNA-editing protein (Apobec1) gene in mice. Structure and evolution of Apobec1 and related nucleoside/nucleotide deaminases. *J Biol Chem* **270**:13042, 1995.
143. Hadjiagapiou C, Giannoni F, Funahashi T, Skarosi SF, Davidson NO: Molecular cloning of a human small intestinal apolipoprotein B mRNA editing protein. *Nucleic Acids Res* **22**:1874, 1994.
144. Fujino T, Navaratnam N, Scott J: Human apolipoprotein B RNA editing deaminase gene (APOBEC1). *Genomics* **47**:266, 1998.
145. Hirano K, Min J, Funahashi T, Davidson NO: Cloning and characterization of the rat apobec-1 gene: A comparative analysis of gene structure and promoter usage in rat and mouse. *J Lipid Res* **38**:1103, 1997.
146. Greeve J, Altkemper I, Dieterich JH, Greten H, Windler E: Apolipoprotein B mRNA editing in 12 different mammalian species: Hepatic expression is reflected in low concentrations of apo B-containing plasma lipoproteins. *J Lipid Res* **34**:1367, 1993.
147. Funahashi T, Giannoni F, DePaoli AM, Skarosi SF, Davidson NO: Tissue-specific, developmental and nutritional regulation of the gene encoding the catalytic subunit of the rat apolipoprotein B mRNA editing enzyme: Functional role in the modulation of apo B mRNA editing. *J Lipid Res* **36**:414, 1995.
148. Leighton JK, Joyner J, Zamarripa J, Deines M, Davis RA: Fasting decreases apolipoprotein B mRNA editing and the secretion of small molecular weight apo B by rat hepatocytes: Evidence that the total amount of apo B secreted is regulated post-transcriptionally. *J Lipid Res* **31**:1663, 1990.
149. Sjöberg A, Oscarsson J, Boström K, Innerarity TL, Edén S, Olofsson SO: Effects of growth hormone on apolipoprotein-B (apo B) messenger ribonucleic acid editing, and apo B 48 and apo B 100 synthesis and secretion in the rat liver. *Endocrinology* **130**:3356, 1992.
150. Baum CL, Teng BB, Davidson NO: Apolipoprotein B messenger RNA editing in the rat liver. Modulation by fasting and refeeding a high carbohydrate diet. *J Biol Chem* **265**:19263, 1990.
151. Nakamuta M, Chang BHJ, Zsigmond E, Kobayashi K, Lei H, Ishida BY, Oka K, Li E, Chan L: Complete phenotypic characterization of apobec-1 knockout mice with a wild-type genetic background and a human apolipoprotein B transgenic background, and restoration of apolipoprotein B mRNA editing by somatic gene transfer of Apobec-1. *J Biol Chem* **271**:25981, 1996.
152. McCormick SP, Ng JK, Véniant M, Borén J, Pierotti V, Flynn LM, Grass DS, Connolly A, Young SG: Transgenic mice that overexpress mouse apolipoprotein B. Evidence that the DNA sequences controlling intestinal expression of the apolipoprotein B gene are distant from the structural gene. *J Biol Chem* **271**:11963, 1996.
153. Young SG, Cham CM, Pitas RE, Burri BJ, Connolly A, Flynn L, Pappu AS, Wong JS, Hamilton RL, Farese RV Jr: A genetic model for absent chylomicron formation: Mice producing apolipoprotein B in the liver, but not in the intestine. *J Clin Invest* **96**:2932, 1995.
154. Alexander CA, Hamilton RL, Havel RJ: Subcellular localization of B apoprotein of plasma lipoproteins in rat liver. *J Cell Biol* **69**:241, 1976.
155. Norum KR, Berg T, Helgerud P, Drevon CA: Transport of cholesterol. *Physiol Rev* **63**:1343, 1983.
156. Christensen NJ, Rubin CE, Cheung MC, Albers JJ: Ultrastructural immunolocalization of apolipoprotein B within human jejunal absorptive cells. *J Lipid Res* **24**:1229, 1983.
157. Hamilton RL: Hepatic Secretion of Plasma Lipoproteins. *Plasma Protein Secretion by the Liver.* New York, Academic Press, 1983.
158. Hamilton RL, Wong JS, Cham CM, Nielsen LB, Young SG: Chylomicron-sized lipid particles are formed in the setting of apolipoprotein B deficiency. *J Lipid Res* **39**:1543, 1998.
159. Janero DR, Siuta-Mangano P, Miller KW, Lane MD: Synthesis, processing, and secretion of hepatic very low-density lipoprotein. *J Cell Biochem* **24**:131, 1984.
160. Olofsson SO, Boström K, Carlsson P, Borén J, Wettesten M, Bjursell G, Wiklund O, Bondjers G: Structure and biosynthesis of apolipoprotein B. *Am Heart J* **113**:446, 1987.
161. Higgins JA, Fieldsend JK: Phosphatidylcholine synthesis for incorporation into membranes or for secretion as plasma lipoproteins by Golgi membranes of rat liver. *J Lipid Res* **28**:268, 1987.
162. Rustaeus S, Lundberg K, Stillemark P, Claesson C, Asp L, Larsson T, Boren J, Olofsson O: Assembly of VLDL—a two step process of apolipoprotein B core lipidation. *J Nutr* **129(2S Suppl)**:463S, 1999.
163. Wetterau JR, Aggerbeck LP, Bouma ME, Eisenberg C, Munck A, Hermier M, Schmitz J, Gay G, Rader DJ, Gregg RE: Absence of microsomal triglyceride transfer protein in individuals with abetalipoproteinemia. *Science* **258**:999, 1992.
164. Sharp D, Blinderman L, Combs KA, Kienzle B, Ricci B, Wager-Smith K, Gil CM, Turck CW, Bouma ME, Rader DJ, et al: Cloning and gene defects in microsomal triglyceride transfer protein associated with abetalipoproteinaemia. *Nature* **365**:65, 1993.
165. Shoulders CC, Brett DJ, Bayliss JD, Narcisi TM, Jarmuz A, Grantham TT, Leoni PR, Bhattacharya S, Pease RJ, Cullen PM, et al: Abetalipoproteinemia is caused by defects of the gene encoding the 97-kDa subunit of a microsomal triglyceride transfer protein. *Hum Mol Genet* **2**:2109, 1993.
166. Sharp D, Ricci B, Kienzle B, Lin MC, Wetterau JR.: Human microsomal triglyceride transfer protein large subunit gene structure. *Biochemistry* **33**:9057, 1994.
167. Shoulders CC, Narcisi TM, Read J, Chester A, Brett DJ, Scott J, Anderson TA, Levitt DG, Banaszak LJ: The abetalipoproteinemia gene is a member of the vitellogenin family and encodes an alpha-helical domain [Letter]. *Nat Struct Biol* **1**:285, 1994.
168. Gordon DA: Recent advances in elucidating the role of the microsomal triglyceride transfer protein in apolipoprotein B lipoprotein assembly. *Curr Opin Lipidol* **8**:131, 1997.
169. Shelness GS, Ingram MF, Huang XF, DeLozier JA: Apolipoprotein B in the rough endoplasmic reticulum: translation, translocation and the initiation of lipoprotein assembly. *J Nutr* **129 (2S Suppl)**:456S, 1999.
170. Chuck SL, Yao Z, Blackhart BD, McCarthy BJ, Lingappa VR: New variation on the translocation of proteins during early biogenesis of apolipoprotein B. *Nature* **346**:382, 1990.
171. Hegde RS, Voigt S, Rapoport TA, Lingappa VR: TRAM regulates the exposure of nascent secretory proteins to the cytosol during translocation into the endoplasmic reticulum. *Cell* **92**:6211998.
172. Thrift RN, Forte TM, Cahoon BE, Shore VG: Characterization of lipoproteins produced by the human liver cell line, Hep G2, under defined conditions. *J Lipid Res* **27**:236, 1986.
173. Hornick CA, Hamilton RL, Spaziani E, Enders GH, Havel RJ: Isolation and characterization of multivesicular bodies from rat hepatocytes: An organelle distinct from secretory vesicles of the Golgi apparatus. *J Cell Biol* **100**:1558, 1985.

174. Hamilton RL, Moorehouse A, Havel RJ: Isolation and properties of nascent lipoproteins from highly purified rat hepatocytic Golgi fractions. *J Lipid Res* **32**:529, 1991.
175. Havel RJ: *Metabolism of Triglyceride-Rich Lipoproteins. Atherosclerosis VI.* Berlin-Heidelberg, Springer-Verlag, 1983.
176. Hamilton RL, Guo LS, Felker TE, Chao YS, Havel RJ: Nascent high density lipoproteins from liver perfusates of orotic acid-fed rats. *J Lipid Res* **27**:967, 1986.
177. Hamilton RL, Williams MC, Fielding CJ, Havel RJ: Discoidal bilayer structure of nascent high density lipoproteins from perfused rat liver. *J Clin Invest* **58**:667, 1976.
178. Guo LS, Hamilton RL, Ostwald R, Havel RJ: Secretion of nascent lipoproteins and apolipoproteins by perfused livers of normal and cholesterol-fed guinea pigs. *J Lipid Res* **23**:543, 1982.
179. Hornick CA, Kita T, Hamilton RL, Kane JP, Havel RJ: Secretion of lipoproteins from the liver of normal and Watanabe heritable hyperlipidemic rabbits. *Proc Natl Acad Sci U S A* **80**:6096, 1983.
180. Erickson SK, AD Cooper: Acyl-coenzyme A:cholesterol acyltransferase in human liver. In vitro detection and some characteristics of the enzyme. *Metabolism* **29**:991, 1980.
181. Imaizumi K, Havel RJ, Fainaru M, Vigne JL: Origin and transport of the A-I and arginine-rich apolipoproteins in mesenteric lymph of rats. *J Lipid Res* **19**:1038, 1978.
182. Imaizumi K, Fainaru M, Havel RJ: Composition of proteins of mesenteric lymph chylomicrons in the rat and alterations produced upon exposure of chylomicrons to blood serum and serum proteins. *J Lipid Res* **19**:712, 1978.
183. Schonfeld G, Grimme N, Alpers D: Detection of apolipoprotein C in human and rat enterocytes. *J Cell Biol* **86**:562, 1980.
184. Matsuguchi T, Okamura S, Aso T,Sata T, Niho Y: Molecular cloning of the cDNA coding for proline-rich protein (PRP): Identity of PRP as C4b-binding protein. *Biochem Biophys Res Commun* **165**:138, 1989.
185. Kotite L, Bergeron N, Havel RJ: Quantification of apolipoproteins B-100, B-48, and E in human triglyceride-rich lipoproteins. *J Lipid Res* **36**:890, 1995.
186. Rash JM, Rothblat GH, Sparks CE: Lipoprotein apolipoprotein synthesis by human hepatoma cells in culture. *Biochim Biophys Acta* **666**:294, 1981.
187. Glickman RM, Rogers M, Glickman JN: Apolipoprotein B synthesis by human liver and intestine in vitro. *Proc Natl Acad Sci U S A* **83**:5296, 1986.
188. Dullaart RP, Speelberg B, Schuurman HJ, Milne RW, Havekes LM, Marcel YL, Geuze HJ, Hulshof MM, Erkelens DW: Epitopes of apolipoprotein B-100 and B-48 in both liver and intestine. Expression and evidence for local synthesis in recessive abetalipoproteinemia. *J Clin Invest* **78**:1397, 1986.
189. Bouma ME, Beucler I, Aggerbeck LP, Infante R, Schmitz J: Hypobetalipoproteinemia with accumulation of an apoprotein B-like protein in intestinal cells. Immunoenzymatic and biochemical characterization of seven cases of Anderson's disease. *J Clin Invest* **78**:398, 1986.
190. Linton MF, Gish R, Hubl ST, Bütler E, Esquivel C, Bry WI, Boyles JK, Wardell MR, Young SG: Phenotypes of apolipoprotein B and apolipoprotein E after liver transplantation. *J Clin Invest* **88**:270, 1991.
191. Ghiselli G: Evidence that two synthetic pathways contribute to the apolipoprotein B pool of the low-density lipoprotein fraction of rabbit plasma. *Biochim Biophys Acta* **711**:311, 1982.
192. Huff MW, Telford DE: Direct synthesis of low-density lipoprotein apoprotein B in the miniature pig. *Metabolism* **34**:36, 1985.
193. Havel RJ, Yamada N, Shames DM: Watanabe heritable hyperlipidemic rabbit. Animal model for familial hypercholesterolemia. *Arterioscler Thromb Vasc Biol* **9**:133, 1989.
194. Johnson FL, Swift LL, Rudel LL: Nascent lipoproteins from recirculating and nonrecirculating liver perfusions and from the hepatic Golgi apparatus of African green monkeys. *J Lipid Res* **28**:549, 1987.
195. Shames DM, Havel RJ: De novo production of low density lipoproteins: Fact or fancy. *J Lipid Res* **32**:1099, 1991.
196. Aguie GA, Rader DJ, Clavey V, Traber MG, Torpier G, Kayden HJ, Fruchart JC, Brewer HB Jr, Castro G: Lipoproteins containing apolipoprotein B isolated from patients with abetalipoproteinemia and homozygous hypobetalipoproteinemia: Identification and characterization. *Atherosclerosis* **118**:183, 1995.
197. Kane JP, Sata T, Hamilton RL, Havel RJ: Apoprotein composition of very low density lipoproteins of human serum. *J Clin Invest* **56**:1622, 1975.
198. Davidson NO, Magun AM, Brasitus TA, Glickman RM: Intestinal apolipoprotein A-I and B-48 metabolism: Effects of sustained alterations in dietary triglyceride and mucosal cholesterol flux. *J Lipid Res* **28**:388, 1987.
199. Schonfeld G, B Pfleger: Utilization of exogenous free fatty acids for the production of very low-density lipoprotein triglyceride by livers of carbohydrate-fed rats. *J Lipid Res* **12**:614, 1971.
200. Davis RA, Engelhorn SC, Pangburn SH, Weinstein DB, Steinberg D: Very low density lipoprotein synthesis and secretion by cultured rat hepatocytes. *J Biol Chem* **254**:2010, 1979.
201. Bohmer T, Havel RJ, Long JA: Physiological fatty liver and hyperlipemia in the fetal guinea pig: Chemical and ultrastructural characterization. *J Lipid Res* **13**:371, 1972.
202. Bohmer T, Havel RJ: Genesis of fatty liver and hyperlipemia in the fetal guinea pig. *J Lipid Res* **16**:454, 1975.
203. Kim E, Young SG: Genetically modified mice for the study of apolipoprotein B. *J Lipid Res* **39**:703, 1998.
204. Blackhart BD, Ludwig EM, Pierotti VR, Caiati L, Onasch MA, Wallis SC, Powell L, Pease R, Knott TJ, Chu ML, et al: Structure of the human apolipoprotein B gene. *J Biol Chem* **261**:15364, 1986.
205. Paulweber B, Brooks AR, Nagy BP, Levy-Wilson B: Identification of a negative regulatory region 5′ of the human apolipoprotein B promoter. *J Biol Chem* **266**:21956, 1991.
206. Davidson NO, Carlos RC, Drewek MJ, Parmer TG: Apolipoprotein gene expression in the rat is regulated in a tissue-specific manner by thyroid hormone. *J Lipid Res* **29**:1511, 1988.
207. Pullinger CR, North JD, Teng BB, Rifici VA, Ronhild de Brito AE, Scott J: The apolipoprotein B gene is constitutively expressed in HepG2 cells: Regulation of secretion by oleic acid, albumin, and insulin, and measurement of the mRNA half-life. *J Lipid Res* **30**:1065, 1989.
208. Yokoyama K, Ishibashi T, Yi-qiang L, Nagayoshi A, Teramoto T, Maruyama Y: Interleukin-1beta and interleukin-6 increase levels of apolipoprotein B mRNA and decrease accumulation of its protein in culture medium of HepG2 cells. *J Lipid Res* **39**:103, 1998.
209. Lackner KJ, Monge JC, Gregg RE, Hoeg JM, Triche TJ,.Law SW, Brewer HB Jr: Analysis of the apolipoprotein B gene and messenger ribonucleic acid in abetalipoproteinemia. *J Clin Invest* **78**:1707, 1986.
210. Arner P: Is familial combined hyperlipidaemia a genetic disorder of adipose tissue? *Curr Opin Lipidol* **8**:89, 1997.
211. Lewis GF: Fatty acid regulation of very low density lipoprotein production. *Curr Opin Lipidol* **8**:89, 1994.
212. Pease RJ, Leiper JM: Regulation of hepatic apolipoprotein-B-containing lipoprotein secretion. *Curr Opin Lipidol* **7**:132, 1996.
213. Peacock RE, Karpe F, Talmud PJ, Hamsten A, Humphries SE: Common variation in the gene for apolipoprotein B modulates postprandial lipoprotein metabolism: A hypothesis generating study. *Atherosclerosis* **116**:135, 1995.
214. Sturley SL, Talmud PJ, Brasseur R, Culbertson MR, Humphries SE, Attie AD: Human apolipoprotein B signal sequence variants confer a secretion-defective phenotype when expressed in yeast. *J Biol Chem* **269**:21670, 1994.
215. Raabe M, Flynn LM, Zlot CH, Wong JS, Véniant MM, Hamilton RL, Young SG: Knockout of the abetalipoproteinemia gene in mice: Reduced lipoprotein secretion in heterozygotes and embryonic lethality in homozygotes. *Proc Natl Acad Sci U S A* **95**:8686, 1998.
216. Narcisi TM, Shoulders CC, Chester SA, Read J, Brett DJ, Harrison GB, Grantham TT, Fox MF, Povey S, de Bruin TW, et al: Mutations of the microsomal triglyceride-transfer-protein gene in abetalipoproteinemia. *Am J Hum Genet* **57**:1298, 1995.
217. Wetterau JR, Gregg RE, Harrity TW, Arbeeny C, et al: An MTP inhibitor that normalizes atherogenic lipoprotein levels in WHHL rabbits. *Science* **282**:751, 1998.
218. Lin MC, Arbeeny C, Bergquist K, Kienzle B, Gordon DA, Wetterau JR: Cloning and regulation of hamster microsomal triglyceride transfer protein. The regulation is independent from that of other hepatic and intestinal proteins which participate in the transport of fatty acids and triglycerides. *J Biol Chem* **269**:29138, 1994.
219. Bennett AJ, Billett MA, Salter AM, White DA: Regulation of hamster hepatic microsomal triglyceride transfer protein mRNA levels by dietary fats. *Biochem Biophys Res Commun* **212**:473, 1995.
220. Patsch W, Franz S, Schonfeld G: Role of insulin in lipoprotein secretion by cultured rat hepatocytes. *J Clin Invest* **71**:1161, 1983.
221. Sparks CE, Sparks JD, Bolognino M, Salhanick A, Strumph PS, J. Amatruda M: Insulin effects on apolipoprotein B lipoprotein synthesis and secretion by primary cultures of rat hepatocytes. *Metabolism* **35**:1128, 1986.

222. Levy E, Sinnett D, Thibault L, Nguyen TD, Delvin E, Ménard D: Insulin modulation of newly synthesized apolipoproteins B-100 and B-48 in human fetal intestine: Gene expression and mRNA editing are not involved. *FEBS Lett* **393**:253, 1996.
223. Hagan DL, Kienzle B, Jamil H, Hariharan N: Transcriptional regulation of human and hamster microsomal triglyceride transfer protein genes. Cell type-specific expression and response to metabolic regulators. *J Biol Chem* **269**:28737, 1994.
224. Lin MC, Gordon D, Wetterau JR: Microsomal triglyceride transfer protein (MTP) regulation in HepG2 cells: Insulin negatively regulates MTP gene expression. *J Lipid Res* **36**:1073, 1995.
225. Brett DJ, Pease RJ, Scott J, Gibbons GF: Microsomal triglyceride transfer protein activity remains unchanged in rat livers under conditions of altered very-low-density lipoprotein secretion. *Biochem J* **310**:11, 1995.
226. Navasa M, Gordon DA, Hariharan N, Jamil H, Shigenaga JK, Moser A, Fiers W, Pollock A, Grunfeld C, Feingold KR: Regulation of microsomal triglyceride transfer protein mRNA expression by endotoxin and cytokines. *J Lipid Res* **39**:1220, 1998.
227. Jamil H, Chu C-H, Dickson JKJ, Chen Y, Yan M, Biller SA, Gregg RE, Wetterau JR, Gordon DA: Evidence that microsomal triglyceride transfer protein is limiting in the production of apolipoprotein B-containing lipoproteins in hepatic cells. *J Lipid Res* **39**:1448, 1998.
228. Karpe F, Lundahl B, Ehrenborg E, Eriksson P, Hamsten A: A common functional polymorphism in the promoter region of the microsomal triglyceride transfer protein gene influences plasma LDL levels. *Arterioscler Thromb Vasc Biol* **18**:756, 1998.
229. Bassen FA, Kornzweig AL: Malformation of the erythrocytes in a case of atypical retinitis pigmentosa. *Blood* **5**:381, 1950.
230. Jampel RS, Falls HF: Atypical retinitis pigmentosa, acanthocytosis, and heredogenerative neuromuscular disease. *Arch Ophthalmol* **59**:818, 1958.
231. Druez G: Un nouveau cas d'acanthocytose; Dysmorphie erythrocytaire congenitale avec retinite, troubles nerveux et stigmates degeneratifs. *Rev Hematol* **14**:3, 1959.
232. Lamy M, Frezal J, Polonovski J, Rey J: L'Absence congenitale de beta lipoproteins. *CR Soc Biol (Paris)* **154**:1974, 1960.
233. Mabry CC, George AMD, Auerbach VH: Studies concerning the defect in a patient with acanthocytosis. *Clin Res* **8**:371, 1960.
234. Salt HB, Wolff OH, Lloyd JK, Fosbrooke AS, Cameron AH, Hubble DV: On having no beta-lipoprotein: A syndrome comprising abetalipoproteinemia, acanthocytosis, and steatorrhea. *Lancet* **2**:325, 1960.
235. Wolff JA, Bauman WA: Studies concerning acanthocytosis: A new genetic syndrome with absent beta lipoprotein. *Am J Dis Child* **102**:478, 1961.
236. Jones JW, Ways P: Abnormalities of high density lipoproteins in abetalipoproteinemia. *J Clin Invest* **46**:1151, 1967.
237. Schwartz JF, Rowland LP, Eder H, Marks PA, Osserman EF, Hirschberg E, Anderson H: Bassen-Kornzweig syndrome: Deficiency of serum beta-lipoprotein. *Arch Neurol* **8**:438, 1963.
238. Levy RI, Fredrickson DS, Laster L: The lipoproteins and lipid transport in abetalipoproteinemia. *J Clin Invest* **45**:531, 1966.
239. Fredrickson DS, Levy RI, Lindgren FT: A comparison of heritable abnormal lipoprotein patterns as defined by two different techniques. *J Clin Invest* **47**:, 1969.
240. Barnard G, Fosbrooke AS, Lloyd JK: Neutral lipids of plasma and adipose tissue in abetalipoproteinaemia. *Clin Chim Acta* **28**:417, 1970.
241. Hooghwinkel GJM, Bruyn GW: Congenital lack of beta-lipoproteins. A study of blood phospholipids in a patient and his family. *J Neurol Sci* **3**:374, 1966.
242. Gotto AM, Levy RI, John K, Fredrickson DS: On the nature of the protein defect in abetalipoproteinemia. *N Engl J Med* **284**:, 1971.
243. Kostner G, Holasek A, Bohlmann HG, Thiede H: Investigation of serum lipoproteins and apoproteins in abetalipoproteinaemia. *Clin Sci Mol Med* **46**:457, 1974.
244. Scanu AM, Aggerbeck LP, Kruski AW, Lim CT, Kayden HJ: A study of the abnormal lipoproteins in abetalipoproteinemia. *J Clin Invest* **53**:440-453. 1974.
245. Menzel HJ, Dieplinger H, Lackner C, Hoppichler F, Lloyd JK, Muller DR, Labeur C, Talmud PJ, Utermann G: Abetalipoproteinemia with an ApoB-100-lipoprotein(a) glycoprotein complex in plasma. Indication for an assembly defect. *J Biol Chem* **265**:981, 1990.
246. Du EZ, Wang SL, Kayden HJ, Sokol R, Curtiss LK, Davis RA: Translocation of apolipoprotein B across the endoplasmic reticulum is blocked in abetalipoproteinemia. *J Lipid Res* **37**:1309, 1996.
247. Gotto AM, Levy RI, John K, Fredrickson DS: On the protein defect in abetalipoproteinemia. *N Engl J Med* **284**:813, 1971.
248. Forte T, Nichols AV: Application of electron microscopy to the study of plasma lipoprotein structure. *Adv Lipid Res* **10**:1, 1972.
249. Forte TM, Luming Ren C, Nordhausen RW, Nichols AV: Formation of phospholipid-rich HDL: A model for square-packing lipoprotein particles found in interstitial fluid and in abetalipoproteinemic plasma. *Biochim Biophys Acta* **834**:386, 1985.
250. Banerji B, Subbaiah PV, Gregg RE, Bagdade JD: Molecular species of phosphatidylcholine in abetalipoproteinemia: Effect of lecithin:cholesterol acyltransferase and lysolecithin acyltransferase. *J Lipid Res* **30**:1907, 1989.
251. Schmitz G, Ilsemann K, Melnik B, Assmann G: Isoproteins of human apolipoprotein A-II: Isolation and characterization. *J Lipid Res* **24**:1021, 1983.
252. Deckelbaum RJ, Eisenberg S, Oschry Y, Cooper M, Blum C: Abnormal high density lipoproteins of abetalipoproteinemia: Relevance to normal HDL metabolism. *J Lipid Res* **23**:1274, 1982.
253. Gibson JC, Rubinstein A, Brown WV, Ginsberg HN, Greten H, Norum R, Kayden H: Apo E-containing lipoproteins in low or high density lipoprotein deficiency. *Arterioscler Thromb Vasc Biol* **5**:371, 1985.
254. Herbert PN, Heiner RJ, Bausserman LL, Henderson LO, Musliner TA: *Abetalipoproteinemia and Hypobetalipoproteinemia: Questions Still Exceed Insights. Atherosclerosis V.* Proceedings of the Fifth International Symposium on Atherosclerosis. New York, Springer-Verlag, 1980.
255. Ikewaki K, Rader DJ, Zech LA, Brewer HB Jr: In vivo metabolism of apolipoproteins A-I and E in patients with abetalipoproteinemia: Implications for the roles of apolipoproteins B and E in HDL metabolism. *J Lipid Res* **35**:1809, 1994.
256. Holmquist L, Hamsten A, Dahlén GH: Free apolipoprotein (a) in abetalipoproteinaemia. *J Intern Med* **225**:285, 1989.
257. Stafforini DM, Carter ME, Zimmerman GA, McIntyre TM, Prescott SM: Lipoproteins alter the catalytic behavior of the platelet-activating factor acetylhydrolase in human plasma. *Proc Natl Acad Sci U S A* **86**:2393, 1989.
258. Hennessy LK, Kunitake ST, Jarvis M, Hamilton RL, Endeman G, Protter A, Kane JP: Isolation of subpopulations of high density lipoproteins: Three particle species containing apo E and two species devoid of apo E that have affinity for heparin. *J Lipid Res* **38**:1859, 1997.
259. Blumenfeld OO, Schwartz E, Adamany AM: Efflux of phospholipids from cultured aortic smooth muscle cells. Selectivity of the process. *J Biol Chem* **254**:7183, 1979.
260. Kuo PT, Bassett DR, Di George AM, Carpenter GG: Lipolytic activity of post-heparin plasma in hyperlipemia and hypolipemia. *Circ Re.* **16**:221, 1965.
261. Illingworth DR, Alam SS, Alam NA: Lipoprotein lipase and hepatic lipase activity after heparin administration in abetalipoproteinemia and hypobetalipoproteinemia. *Metabolism* **32**:869, 1983.
262. Frederickson DS, Ono D, Davis LL: Lipolytic activity of post heparin plasma in hypertriglyceridemia. *J Lipid Res* **4**:24. 1963.
263. Slack J, Nair S, Traisman H: Lipoprotein lipase in cystic fibrosis of the pancreas. *J Lab Clin Med* **59**:302, 1962.
264. Cooper RA, Gulbrandsen CL: The relationship between serum lipoproteins and red cell membranes in abetalipoproteinemia: deficiency of lecithin:cholesterol acyltransferase. *J Lab Clin Med* **78**:323, 1971.
265. Holmquist L, Carlson LA, Lloyd JK: Substrate specificity of plasma lecithin: cholesterol acyltransferase in abetalipoproteinemia. *Acta Med Scand* **224**:135, 1988.
266. Fielding CJ, Fielding PE: Purification and substrate specificity of lecithin-cholesterol acyltransferase from human plasma. *FEBS Lett* **15**:355, 1971.
267. Subbaiah PV: Requirement of low density lipoproteins for the lysolecithin acyl transferase activity in human plasma: Assay of enzyme activity in abetalipoproteinemic patients. *Metabolism* **31**:294, 1982.
268. Subbaiah PV, Banerji B, Gregg RE, Bagdade JD: Molecular species of cholesteryl esters formed in abetalipoproteinemia: Effect of apoprotein B-containing lipoproteins. *J Lipid Res* **31**:927, 1990.
269. Myant NB, Reichl D, Lloyd JK: Sterol balance in a patient with abetalipoproteinaemia. *Atherosclerosis* **29**:509, 1978.
270. Kayden HJ: *Abetalipoproteinemia-Abnormalities of Serum Lipoproteins. Protides of the Biological Fluids* (Proceedings of the 25th Coll, Bruges, 1977). Oxford, Pergamon, 1978.

271. Illingworth DR, Connor WE, Lin DS, Diliberti J: Lipid metabolism in abetalipoproteinemia: A study of cholesterol absorption and sterol balance in two patients. *Gastroenterology* **78**:68, 1980.
272. Goodman DS, Deckelbaum RJ, Palmer RH, Dell RB, Ramakrishnan R, Delpre G, Beigel Y, Cooper M: Cholesterol turnover and metabolism in two patients with abetalipoproteinemia. *J Lipid Res* **24**:1605, 1983.
273. Reichl D, Myant NB, Lloyd JK: Surface binding and catabolism of low-density lipoprotein by circulating lymphocytes from patients with abetalipoproteinaemia, with observations on sterol synthesis in lymphocytes from one patient. *Biochim Biophys Acta* **530**:124, 1978.
274. Ho YK, Faust JR, Bilheimer DW, Brown MS, Goldstein JL: Regulation of cholesterol synthesis by low-density lipoprotein in isolated human lymphocytes. Comparison of cells from normal subjects and patients with homozygous familial hypercholesterolemia and abetalipoproteinemia. *J Exp Med* **145**:1531, 1977.
275. Alam NA, Illingworth DR, Sundberg EE Alam SS: Regulation of cholesterol synthesis by plasma lipoproteins from patients with abetalipoproteinemia. *Atherosclerosis*, **49**:295, 1983.
276. Brannan PG, Goldstein JL, Brown MS: 3-hydroxy-3-methylglutaryl coenzyme A reductase activity in human hair roots. *J Lipid Res* **16**:7, 1975.
277. Illingworth DR, Pappu AS, Gregg RE: Increased urinary mevalonic acid excretion in patients with abetalipoproteinemia and homozygous hypobetalipoproteinemia. *Atherosclerosis* **76**:21, 1989.
278. Lees AM, Lees RS: Low density lipoprotein degradation by mononuclear cells from normal and dyslipoproteinemic subjects. *Proc Natl Acad Sci U S A* **80**:5098, 1983.
279. Illingworth DR, Alam NA, Sundberg EE, Hagemenas FC, Layman DL: Regulation of low density lipoprotein receptors by plasma lipoproteins from patients with abetalipoproteinemia. *Proc Natl Acad Sci U S A* **80**:3475, 1983.
280. Innerarity TL, Bersot TP, Arnold KS, Weisgraber KH, Davis PA, Forte TM, Mahley RW: Receptor binding activity of high-density lipoproteins containing apoprotein E from abetalipoproteinemic and normal neonate plasma. *Metabolism* **33**:186, 1984.
281. Hagemenas FC, Illingworth DR: The influence of plasma lipoproteins from patients with abetalipoproteinemia on cellular cholesterol esterification. *Atherosclerosis* **68**:105, 1987.
282. Illingworth DR, Kenny TA, Orwoll ES: Adrenal function in heterozygous and homozygous hypobetalipoproteinemia. *J Clin Endocrinol Metab* **54**:27, 1982.
283. Illingworth DR, Kenny TA, Connor WE, Orwoll ES: Corticosteroid production in abetalipoproteinemia: Evidence for an impaired response ACTH. *J Lab Clin Med* **100**:115, 1982.
284. Illingworth DR, Corbin DK, Kemp ED, Keenan EJ: Hormone changes during the menstrual cycle in abetalipoproteinemia: Reduced luteal phase progesterone in a patient with homozygous hypobetalipoproteinemia. *Proc Natl Acad Sci U S A* **79**:6685, 1982.
285. Ehlers N, Hansen HJ: Abetalipoproteinaemia. Ocular involvement in a Danish case. *Acta Ophthalmol (Copenh)* **59**:747, 1981.
286. Singer K, Fisher B, Perlstein MA: Acanthrocytosis: A generic erythrocytic malformation. *Blood* **7**:577, 1952.
287. Kayden HJ, Bessis M: Morphology of normal erythrocyte and acanthocyte using Nomarski optics and the scanning electron microscope. *Blood* **35**:427, 1970.
288. Phillips GB: Quantitative chromatographic analysis of plasma and red blood cell lipids in patients with acanthocytosis. *J Lab Clin Med* **59**:357, 1962.
289. Ways P, Reed CF, Hanahan DJ: Red cell and plasma lipids in acanthocytosis. *J Clin Invest* **42**:1248, 1963.
290. Iida H, Takashima Y, Maeda S, Sekiya T, Kawade M, Kawamura M, Okano Y, Nozawa Y: Alterations in erythrocyte membrane lipids in abetalipoproteinemia: Phospholipid and fatty acyl composition. *Biochem Med* **32**:79, 1984.
291. Bach C, Polonovski J, Polonovski C, Leluc R, Jolly G, Moszer M: Congenital absence of beta-lipoproteins. A further case. *Arch Fr Pediatr* **24**:1093, 1967.
292. Lange Y, Steck TL: Mechanism of red blood cell acanthocytosis and echinocytosis in vivo. *J Membr Biol* **77**:153, 1984.
293. Mier M, Schwartz SO, Boshes B: Acanthocytosis, pigmentary degeneration of the retina and ataxic neuropathy: A genetically determined syndrome with associated metabolic disorder. *J Biol Chem* **5**:1586, 1960.
294. Farquhar JW, Ways P: Abetalipoproteinemia. *The Metabolic Basis of Inherited Disease* 2nd ed. New York, McGraw-Hill, 1966.
295. Sobrevilla LA, Goodman ML, Kane CA: Demyelinating central nervous system disease, macular atrophy and acanthocytosis (Bassen-Kornzweig syndrome). *Am J Med* **37**:821, 1964.
296. Ways PO, Parmentier CM, Kayden HJ, Jones JW, Saunders DR, Rubin CE: Studies on the absorptive defect for triglyceride in abetalipoproteinemia. *J Clin Invest* **46**:35, 1967.
297. Dische MR, Porro RS: The cardiac lesions in Bassen-Kornzweig syndrome. Report of a case with autopsy findings. *Am J Med* **49**:568, 1970.
298. Leyland FC, Fosbrooke AS, Lloyd JK, Segall MM, Tamir I, Tomkins R, Wolff OH: Use of medium-chain triglyceride diets in children with malabsorption. *Arch Dis Child* **44**:170, 1969.
299. Becroft DMO, Costello JM, Scott PJ: Abetalipoproteinemia (Bassen-Kornzweig syndrome). *Arch Dis Child* **40**:40, 1965.
300. Forsyth CC, Lloyd JK, Fosbrooke AS: A-beta-lipoproteinemia. *Arch Dis Child* **40**:47, 1965.
301. Simon ER, Ways P: Incubation hemolysis and red cell metabolism in acanthocytosis. *J Clin Invest* **43**:1311, 1964.
302. Kayden HJ, Silber R: The role of vitamin E deficiency in the abnormal autohemolysis of acanthocytosis. *Trans Assoc Am Physicians* **78**:334, 1965.
303. Caballero FM, Buchanan GR: Abetalipoproteinemia presenting as severe vitamin K deficiency. *Pediatrics* **65**:161, 1980.
304. Illingworth DR, Connor WE, Miller RG: Abetalipoproteinemia. Report of two cases and review of therapy. *Arch Neurol* **37**:659, 1980.
305. Willemin B, Coumaros D, Zerbe S, Weill-Bousson M, Annonier P, Hirsch E, Aby MA, Schmutz G, Bockel R: Abetalipoproteinemia. Apropos of two cases. *Gastroenterol Clin Biol* **11**:704, 1987.
306. Shastri KM, Carvalho AC, Lees RS: Platelet function and platelet lipid composition in the dyslipoproteinemias. *J Lipid Res* **21**:467, 1980.
307. Aviram M, Deckelbaum RJ, Brook JG: Platelet function in a case with abetalipoproteinemia. *Atherosclerosis* **57**:313, 1985.
308. Novotny WF, Brown SG, Miletich JP, Rader DJ, Broze GJ Jr: Plasma antigen levels of the lipoprotein-associated coagulation inhibitor in patient samples. *Blood* **78**:387, 1991.
309. Weinstein MA, KD Pearson, Agus SG: Abetalipoproteinemia. *Radiology* **108**:269, 1973.
310. Isselbacher KJ, Scheig R, Plotkin GR, Caufield JB: Congenital betalipoprotein deficiency: An hereditary disorder involving a defect in the absorption and transport of lipids. *Medicine* **43**:347,1964.
311. Grise P, Le Luyer B, Mitrofanoff P: Oxalate lithiasis associated with abetalipoproteinemia. Report of a case. *Chir Pediatr* **24**:411, 1983.
312. Huang HS, Goodman DS: Vitamin A and carotenoids. I. Intestinal absorption and metabolism of 14C-labeled vitamin A alcohol and betacarotene in the rat. *J Biol Chem* **240**:2839, 1965.
313. Bélanger M, Tremblay M, Lapointe JR: Congenital absence of beta-lipoproteins: Unusual and peculiar syndrome. A recent case. *Laval Med* **42**:332, 1971.
314. Bieri JG, Hoeg JM, Schaefer EJ, Zech LA, Brewer HB Jr: Vitamin A and vitamin E replacement in abetalipoproteinemia. *Ann Intern Med* **100**:238, 1984.
315. Wallis K, Gross M, Zaidman JL, Julsary A, Szeinberg A, Kook AI: Tocopherol therapy in acanthocytosis. *Pediatrics* **48**:669, 1971.
316. Kayden HJ, Hatam LJ, Traber MG: The measurement of nanograms of tocopherol from needle aspiration biopsies of adipose tissue: Normal and abetalipoproteinemic subjects. *J Lipid Res* **24**:652, 1983.
317. Muller DR, Harries JT, Lloyd JK: Vitamin E therapy in abetalipoproteinaemia. *Arch Dis Child* **45**:, 1970.
318. Muller DP, Harries JT, Lloyd JK: The relative importance of the factors involved in the absorption of vitamin E in children. *Gut* **15**:966, 1974.
319. MacMahon MT, Neale G, Thompson GR: Lymphatic and portal venous transport of alpha-tocopherol and cholesterol. *Eur J Clin Invest* **1**:288, 1971.
320. Kayden HJ, Traber MG: Absorption, lipoprotein transport, and regulation of plasma concentrations of vitamin E in humans. *J Lipid Res* **34**:343, 1993.
321. Traber MG, Kayden HJ: Vitamin E is delivered to cells via the high affinity receptor for low-density lipoprotein. *Am J Clin Nutr* **40**:747, 1984.
321a. Cavalier L, Ouahchi K, Kayden HJ, Di Donato S, Reutenauer L, Mandel JL, Koenig M: Ataxia with isolated vitamin E deficiency: Heterogeneity of mutations and phenotypic variability in a large number of families. *Am J Hum Genet* **62**:301, 1998.

322. Delpre G, Kadish U, Glantz I, Avidor I: Endoscopic assessment in abetalipoproteinemia (Bassen-Kornzweig-syndrome). *Endoscopy* **10**:59, 1978.
323. Dobbins WO: An ultrastructural study of the intestinal mucosa in congenital betalipoprotein deficiency with particular emphasis upon the intestinal absorptive cell. *Gastroenterology* **50**:195, 1966.
324. Glickman RM, Green PH, Lees RS, Lux SE, Kilgore A: Immunofluorescence studies of apolipoprotein B in intestinal mucosa. Absence in abetalipoproteinemia. *Gastroenterology* **76**:288, 1979.
325. Levy E, Marcel YL, Milne RW, Grey VL, Roy CC: Absence of intestinal synthesis of apolipoprotein B-48 in two cases of abetalipoproteinemia. *Gastroenterology* **93**:1119, 1987.
326. Black DD, Hay RV, Rohwer-Nutter PL, Ellinas H, Stephens JK, Sherman H, Teng B-B, Whitington PF, Davidson NO: Intestinal and hepatic apolipoprotein B gene expression in abetalipoproteinemia. *Gastroenterology* **67**:520, 1991.
327. Partin, JS, Partin JC, Schubert WK, McAdams AJ: Liver ultrastructure in abetalipoproteinemia: Evolution of micronodular cirrhosis. *Gastroenterology* **67**:107, 1974.
328. Collins JC, Scheinberg IH, Giblin DR, Sternlieb I: Hepatic peroxisomal abnormalities in abetalipoproteinemia. *Gastroenterology* **97**:766, 1989.
329. Hamilton RL, Wong JS, Guo LS, Krisans S, Havel RJ: Apolipoprotein E localization in rat hepatocytes by immunogold labeling of cryothin sections. *J Lipid Res* **31**:1589, 1990.
330. Brin MF, Nelson JS, Roberts WC, Marquardt MD, Suswankosai P, Petito CK: Neuropathology of abetalipoproteinemia: A possible complication of the tocopherol (vitamin E) deficiency state. *Neurology* **33**: 142, 1983.
331. Kornzweig AL, Bassen FA: Retinitis pigmentosa, acanthocytosis, and heredogenerative neuromuscular disease. *Arch Ophthalmol* **58**:183, 1957.
332. Cohen DA, Bosley TM, Savino PJ, Sergott RC, Schatz NJ: Primary aberrant regeneration of the oculomotor nerve. Occurrence in a patient with abetalipoproteinemia. *Arch Neurol* **42**:821, 1985.
333. Brin MF, Pedley TA, Lovelace RE, Emerson RG, Gouras P, MacKay C, Kayden HJ, Levy J, Baker H: Electrophysiologic features of abetalipoproteinemia: Functional consequences of vitamin E deficiency. *Neurology* **36**:669, 1986.
334. Wichman A, Buchthal F, Pezeshkpour GH, Gregg RE: Peripheral neuropathy in abetalipoproteinemia [published erratum appears in *Neurology* **36(7)**:1009, 1986]. *Neurology* **35**:1279, 1985.
335. Werlin SL, Harb JM, Swick H, Blank E: Neuromuscular dysfunction and ultrastructural pathology in children with chronic cholestasis and vitamin E deficiency. *Ann Neurol* **13**:291, 1983.
336. Kobayashi Y, Tazawa Y, Nakagawa M, Suzuki H, Konno T, Yamamoto TY: Ultrastructural changes in skeletal muscle of a patient with familial intrahepatic cholestasis associated with vitamin E deficiency. *Tohoku J Exp Med* **142**:337, 1984.
337. Harding AE, Matthews S, Jones S, Ellis CJ, Booth IW, Muller DP: Spinocerebellar degeneration associated with a selective defect of vitamin E absorption. *N Engl J Med* **313**:32, 1985.
338. Stumpf DA, Sokol R, Bettis D: Clinical picture mimicking Friedreich's ataxia associated with vitamin E deficiency and normal fat absorption. *Neurology* **35(Suppl)**:145, 1985.
339. Hays KC: Retinal degeneration in monkeys induced by deficiencies of vitamin E or A. *Invest Ophthalmol* **13**:499, 1974.
340. Robison WG Jr, Kuwabara T, Bieri JG: Deficiencies of vitamins E and A in the rat. Retinal damage and lipofuscin accumulation. *Invest Ophthalmol Vis Sci* **19**:1030, 1980.
341. Nelson JS: *Pathology of vitamin E deficiency. Vitamin E: A Comprehensive Treatise*. New York, Marcel Dekker, 1980.
342. Nelson JS, Fitch CD, Fische VW, Broun GD, Chou AC: Progressive neuropathologic lesions in vitamin E deficient rhesus monkeys. *J Neuropathol Exp Neurol* **40**:166, 1981.
343. Newman RP, Schaefer EJ, Thomas CB, Oldfield EH: Abetalipoproteinemia and metastatic spinal cord glioblastoma. *Arch Neurol* **41**:554, 1984.
344. Kott E, Delpre G, Kadish U, Dziatelovsky M, Sandbank U: Abetalipoproteinemia (Bassen-Kornzweig syndrome). Muscle involvement. *Acta Neuropathol (Berl)* **37**:255, 1977.
345. Bouma ME, Beucler I, Pessah M, Heinzmann C, Lusis AJ, Naim HY, Ducastelle T, Leluyer B, Schmitz J, Infante R, et al: Description of two different patients with abetalipoproteinemia: Synthesis of a normal-sized apolipoprotein B-48 in intestinal organ culture. *J Lipid Res* **31**:1, 1990.
346. Khachadurian AK, Freyha R, Shamma'a MM, Baghdassarian SA: A-beta-lipoproteinaemia and colour-blindness. *Arch Dis Child* **46**:871, 1971.
347. Von Sallmann L, Gelderman AH, Laster L: Ocular histopathologic changes in a case of a-beta-lipoproteinemia (Bassen-Kornzweig syndrome). *Doc Ophthalmol* **26**:451, 1969.
348. Robison WG, Kuwabara T, Bieri JG: The roles of vitamin E and unsaturated fatty acids in the visual process. *Retina* **2**:263, 1982.
349. Robison WG Jr, Kuwabara T, Bieri JG: Vitamin E deficiency and the retina: Photoreceptor and pigment epithelial changes. *Invest Ophthalmol Vis Sci* **18**:683, 1979.
350. Dieckert JP, White M, Christmann L, Lambert HM: Angioid streaks associated with abetalipoproteinemia. *Ann Ophthalmol* **21**:173, 1989.
351. Gouras P, Carr RE, Gunkel RD: Retinitis pigmentosa in abetalipoproteinemia: Effects of vitamin A. *Invest Ophthalmol* **10**:784, 1971.
352. Sperling MA, Hiles DA, Kennerdell JS: Electroretinographic responses following vitamin A therapy in A-beta-lipoproteinemia. *Am J Ophthalmol* **73**:342, 1972.
353. Bishara S, Merin S, Cooper M, Aziz G, Delpre G, Deckelbaum RJ: Combined vitamin A and E therapy prevents retinal electrophysiological deterioration in abetalipoproteinemia. *Br J Ophthalmol* **12**:767, 1971.
354. Dowling JE: Nutritional and inherited blindness in the rat. *Ex. Eye Res* **3**:348, 1964.
355. Scott PP, Greaves JP, Scott MG: Nutritional blindness in the cat. *Exp Eye Res* **3**:357, 1964.
356. Rodger RC: The ocular effects of vitamin A deficiency in man in the tropics. *Exp. Eye Res* **3**:367, 1963.
357. Wolff OH, Lloyd JK, Tonks EL: A-beta-lipoproteinemia with special reference to the visual defect. *Exp Eye Res* **3**:439, 1964.
358. Cogan DG, Rodrigues M, Chu FC, Schaefer EJ: Ocular abnormalities in abetalipoproteinemia. A clinicopathologic correlation. *Ophthalmology* **91**:991, 1984.
359. Sperling MA, Hengstenberg F, Yunis E, Kenny FM, Drash AL: Abetalipoproteinemia: Metabolic, endocrine, and electron-microscopic investigations. *Pediatrics* **48**:91, 1971.
360. Friedman IS, Cohn H, Zymoris M, Goldman AMG: Hypocholesterolemia in idiopathic steatorrhea. *Arch Intern Med* **105**:112, 1960.
361. Bohlmann HG, Thede H, Rosentiel K, Herdemerten S, Pantz D, Tackman W: A-beta-Lipoproteinamie bei drei Geschwistern. *Dtsch Med Wochenschr* **97**:892, 1972.
362. Zaidman JL, Julsary A, Kook AI,Szeinberg A, Wallis K, Azizi E: Abetalipoproteinemia in acrodermatitis enteropathica. *N Engl J Med* **284**:1387, 1971.
363. Talmud PJ, Lloyd JK, Muller DP, Collins DR, Scott J, Humphries S: Genetic evidence from two families that the apolipoprotein B gene is not involved in abetalipoproteinemia. *J Clin Invest* **82**:1803, 1988.
364. Huang LS, Jänne PA, de Graaf J, Cooper M, Deckelbaum RJ, Kayden H, Breslow JL, Decklebaum RJ:. Exclusion of linkage between the human apolipoprotein B gene and abetalipoproteinemia [published erratum appears in *Am J Hum Genet* **47(1)**:172, 1990]. *Am J Hum Genet* **46**:1141, 1990
365. Rehberg EF, Samson-Bouma ME, Kienzle B, Blinderman L, Jamil H, Wetterau JR, Aggerbeck LP, Gordon DA: A novel abetalipoproteinemia genotype. Identification of a missense mutation in the 97-kDa subunit of the microsomal triglyceride transfer protein that prevents complex formation with protein disulfide isomerase. *J Biol Chem* **271**:29945, 1996.
366. Ricci B, Sharp D, O'Rourke E, Kienzle B, Blinderman L, Gordon D, Smith-Monroy C, Robinson G, Gregg RE, Rader DJ, et al: A 30-amino acid truncation of the microsomal triglyceride transfer protein large subunit disrupts its interaction with protein disulfide-isomerase and causes abetalipoproteinemia. *J Biol Chem* **270**:14281, 1995.
367. Wu X, Zhou M, Huang LS, Wetterau J, Ginsberg HN: Demonstration of a physical interaction between microsomal triglyceride transfer protein and apolipoprotein B during the assembly of apo B-containing lipoproteins. *J Biol Chem* **271**:10277, 1996.
368. Kayden HJ, Traber MG: Clinical, nutritional and biochemical consequences of apolipoprotein B deficiency. *Adv Exp Med Biol* **201**:67, 1986.
369. Muller DP, Lloyd JK, Bird AC: Long-term management of abetalipoproteinaemia. Possible role for vitamin E. *Arch Dis Child* **52**:209, 1977.
370. Azizi E, Zaidman JL, Eschar J, Szeinberg A: Abetalipoproteinemia treated with parental and oral vitamins A and E, and with medium chain triglycerides. *Acta Paediatr Scand* **67**:796, 1978.

371. Muller DP, Lloyd JK, Wolff OH: Vitamin E and neurological function. *Lancet* **1**:225, 1983.
372. Hegele RA, Angel A: Arrest of neuropathy and myopathy in abetalipoproteinemia with high-dose vitamin E therapy. *Can Med Assoc J* **132**:41, 1985.
373. Muller DP, Lloyd JK: Effect of large oral doses of vitamin E on the neurological sequelae of patients with abetalipoproteinemia. *Ann N Y Acad Sci* **393**:133, 1982.
374. Runge P, Muller DP, McAllister J, Calver D, Lloyd JK, Taylor D: Oral vitamin E supplements can prevent the retinopathy of abetalipoproteinaemia. *Br J Ophthalmol* **70**:166, 1986.
375. Sung J H, Park SH, Mastri AR, Warwick WJ: Axonal dystrophy in the gracile nucleus in congenital biliary atresia and cystic fibrosis (mucoviscidosis): beneficial effect of vitamin E therapy. *J Neuropathol Exp Neurol* **39**:584, 1980.
376. Van Buchem FSP, Pol G, De Gier J, Botticher CJF, Pries C: Congenital-beta-lipoprotein deficiency. *Am J Med* **40**:794, 1966.
377. Mars H, Lewis LA, Robertson AL Jr, Butkus A, Williams GH Jr: Familial hypo-beta-lipoproteinemia: A genetic disorder of lipid metabolism with nervous system involvement. *Am J Med* **46**:886, 1969.
378. Richet G, Durepaire H, Hartmann L, Ollier MP, Polonovski J, Maitrot B: Asymptomatic familial hypolipoproteinemia involving mainly beta-lipoproteins revealed during the study of an isolated proteinuria. *Presse Med* **77**:2045, 1969.
379. Levy RI, Langer T, Gotto AM, Frederickson DS: Familial hypobetalipoproteinemia, a defect in lipoprotein synthesis. *Clin Res* **18**:539. 1970.
380. Mawatari S, Iwashita H, Kuroiwa Y: Familial hypo-beta-lipoproteinaemia. *J Neurol Sci* **16**:93, 1972.
381. Fosbrooke A, Choksey S, Wharton B: Familial hypo-beta-lipoproteinaemia. *Arch Dis Child* **48**:729, 1973.
382. Brown BJ, Lewis LA, Mercer RD: Familial hypobetalipoproteinemia: Report of a case with psychomotor retardation. *Pediatrics* **54**:111, 1974.
383. Cottrill C, Glueck CJ, Leuba V, Millett F, Puppione D, Brown WV: Familial homozygous hypobetalipoproteinemia. *Metabolism* **23**:779, 1974.
384. Biemer JJ, McCammon RE: The genetic relationship of abetalipoproteinemia and hypobetalipoproteinemia: a report of the occurrence of both diseases within the same family. *J Lab Clin Med* **85**:556, 1975.
385. Feit JP, David M, Macabéo V, Divry P, Bernard JC, Lambert D, Beucler I, Jeune M: Abetalipoproteinemia. Clinical, genetic, endocrine and metabolic study of a recent familial case. *Pediatrics* **32**:753, 1977.
386. Illingworth DR, Connor WE, Buist NR, Jhaveri BM, Lin DS, McMurry MP: Sterol balance in abetalipoproteinemia: Studies in a patient with homozygous familial hypobetalipoproteinemia. *Metabolism* **28**:1152, 1979.
387. Berger GM, Brown G, Henderson HE, Bonnici F: Apolipoprotein B detected in the plasma of a patient with homozygous hypobetalipoproteinaemia: Implications for aetiology. *J Med Genet* **20**:189, 1983.
388. Pullinger CR, Hillas E, Hardman DA, Chen GC, Naya-Vigne JM, Iwasa JA, Hamilton RL, Lalouel JM, Williams RR, Kane JP: Two apolipoprotein B gene defects in a kindred with hypobetalipoproteinemia, one of which results in a truncated variant, apoB-61, in VLDL and LDL. *J Lipid Res* **33**:699, 1992.
389. Young SG, Bertics SJ, Curtiss LK, Dubois BW, Witztum JL: Genetic analysis of a kindred with familial hypobetalipoproteinemia. Evidence for two separate gene defects: One associated with an abnormal apolipoprotein B species, apolipoprotein B-37; and a second associated with low plasma concentrations of apolipoprotein B-100. *J Clin Invest* **79**:1842, 1987.
390. Linton MF, Farese RV Jr, Young SG: Familial hypobetalipoproteinemia. *J Lipid Res* **34**:521, 1993.
391. Steinberg D, Grundy SM, Mok HY, Turner JD, Weinstein DB, Brown WV, Albers JJ: Metabolic studies in an unusual case of asymptomatic familial hypobetalipoproteinemia with hypolphalipoproteinemia and fasting chylomicronemia. *J Clin Invest* **64**:292, 1979.
392. Young SG, Northey ST, McCarthy BJ: Low plasma cholesterol levels caused by a short deletion in the apolipoprotein B gene. *Science* **241**:591, 1988.
393. Young SG, Peralta FP, Dubois BW, Curtiss LK, Boyles JK, Witztum JL: Lipoprotein B37, a naturally occurring lipoprotein containing the amino-terminal portion of apolipoprotein B100, does not bind to the apolipoprotein B, E (low density lipoprotein) receptor. *J Biol Chem* **262**:16604, 1987.
394. Linton MF, Pierotti V, Young SG: Reading-frame restoration with an apolipoprotein B gene frameshift mutation. *Proc Natl Acad Sci U S A* **89**:11431, 1992.
395. Hardman DA, Pullinger CR, Hamilton RL, Kane JP, Malloy MJ: Molecular and metabolic basis for the metabolic disorder normotriglyceridemic abetalipoproteinemia. *J Clin Invest* **88**:1722, 1991.
396. Takashima Y, Kodama T, Iida H, Kawamura M, Aburatani H, Itakura H, Akanuma Y, Takaku F, Kawade M: Normotriglyceridemic abetalipoproteinemia in infancy: An isolated apolipoprotein B-100 deficiency. *Pediatrics* **75**:541, 1985.
397. Herbert PN, Hyams JS, Bernier DN, Berman MM, Saritelli AL, Lynch KM, Nichols AV, Forte TM: Apolipoprotein B-100 deficiency. Intestinal steatosis despite apolipoprotein B-48 synthesis. *J Clin Invest* **76**:403, 1985.
398. Huet G, Dieu MC, Martin A, Grard G, Bard JM, Fossati P, Degand P: Heterozygous hypobetalipoproteinemia with fasting chylomicronemia. *Clin Chem* **37**:296, 1991.
399. Harano Y, Kojima H, Nakano T, Harada M, Kashiwagi A, Nakajima Y, Hidaka TH, Ohtsuki T, Suzuki T, Tamura A, et al: Homozygous hypobetalipoproteinemia with spared chylomicron formation. *Metabolism* **38**:1, 1989.
400. Naganawa S, Kodama T, Aburatani H, Matsumoto A, Itakura H, Takashima Y, Kawamura M, Muto Y: Genetic analysis of a Japanese family with normotriglyceridemic abetalipoproteinemia indicates a lack of linkage to the apolipoprotein B gene. *Biochem Biophys Res Commun* **182**:99, 1992.
401. Leppert M, Breslow JL, Wu L, Hasstedt S, O'Connell P, Lathrop M, Williams RR, White R, Lalouel JM: Inference of a molecular defect of apolipoprotein B in hypobetalipoproteinemia by linkage analysis in a large kindred. *J Clin Invest* **82**:847, 1988.
402. Pulai JI, Neuman RJ, Groenewegen AW, Wu J, Schonfeld G: Genetic heterogeneity in familial hypobetalipoproteinemia: linkage and nonlinkage to the apo B gene in Caucasian families. *Am J Med Genet* **76**:79, 1998.
403. Ross RS, Gregg RE, Law SW, Monge JC, Grant SM, Higuchi K, Triche TJ, Jefferson J, Brewer HB Jr: Homozygous hypobetalipoproteinemia: A disease distinct from abetalipoproproteinemia at the molecular level. *J Clin Invest* **81**:590, 1988.
404. Gay G, Pessah M, Bouma ME, Roche JF, Aymard JP, Beucler I, Aggerbeck LP, Infante R: Familial hypobetalipoproteinemia. Familial study of 4 cases. *Rev Med Interne* **11**:273, 1990.
405. Fazio S, Sidoli A, Vivenzio A, Maietta A, Giampaoli S, Menotti A, Antonini R, Urbinati G, Baralle FE, Ricci G: A form of familial hypobetalipoproteinaemia not due to a mutation in the apolipoprotein B gene. *J Intern Med* **229**:41, 1991.
406. Hobbs HH, Leitersdorf E, Leffert CC, Cryer DR, Brown MS, Goldstein JL: Evidence for a dominant gene that suppresses hypercholesterolemia in a family with defective low density lipoprotein receptors. *J Clin Invest* **84**:656, 1989.
407. Vega GL, von Bergmann K, Grundy SM, Beltz W, Jahn C, East C: Increased catabolism of VLDL-apolipoprotein B and synthesis of bile acids in a case of hypobetalipoproteinemia. *Metabolism* **36**:262, 1987.
408. Groenewegen WA, Krul ES, Schonfeld G: Apolipoprotein B-52 mutation associated with hypobetalipoproteinemia is compatible with a misaligned pairing deletion mechanism. *J Lipid Res* **34**:971, 1993.
409. Welty F., Lichtenstein AH, Barrett PH, Dolnikowski GG, Ordovas JM, Schaefer EJ: Production of apolipoprotein B-67 in apolipoprotein B-67/B-100 heterozygotes: Technical problems associated with leucine contamination in stable isotope studies. *J Lipid Res* **38**:1535, 1997.
410. Aguilar-Salinas CA, Barrett PH, Parhofer KG, Young SG, Tessereau D, Bateman J, Quinn C, Schonfeld G: Apoprotein B-100 production is decreased in subjects heterozygous for truncations of apoprotein B. *Arterioscler Thromb Vasc Biol* **15**:71, 1995.
411. Malmendier CL, Lontie JF, Delcroix C, Sérougne C, Férézou J, Lee DM: Receptor-dependent and -independent catabolism of low-density lipoprotein in a kindred with familial hypobetalipoproteinemia. *Metabolism* **41**:571, 1992.
412. Latour MA, Patterson BW, Pulai J, Chen Z, Schonfeld G: Metabolism of apolipoprotein B-100 in a kindred with familial hypobetalipoproteinemia without a truncated form of apoB. *J Lipid Res* **38**:592, 1997.
413. Pulai JI, Averna M, Srivastava RA, Latour MA, Clouse RE, Ostlund RE, Schonfeld G: Normal intestinal dietary fat and cholesterol absorption, intestinal apolipoprotein B (apo B) mRNA levels, and apo

B-48 synthesis in a hypobetalipoproteinemic kindred without any apo B truncation. *Metabolism* **46**:1095, 1997.

414. Graham DL, Knott TJ, Jones TC, Pease RJ, Pullinger CR, Scott J: Carboxyl-terminal truncation of apolipoprotein B results in gradual loss of the ability to form buoyant lipoproteins in cultured human and rat liver cell lines. *Biochemistry* **30**:5616, 1991.
415. McLeod RS, Zhao Y, Selby SL, Westerlund J, Yao Z: Carboxyl-terminal truncation impairs lipid recruitment by apolipoprotein B100 but does not affect secretion of the truncated apolipoprotein B-containing lipoproteins. *J Biol Chem* **269**:2852, 1994.
416. Parhofer KG, Barrett PH, Aguilar-Salinas CA, Schonfeld G: Positive linear correlation between the length of truncated apolipoprotein B and its secretion rate: In vivo studies in human apo B-89, apo B-75, apo B-54.8, and apo B-31 heterozygotes. *J Lipid Res* **37**:844, 1996.
417. Homanics GE, Smith TJ, Zhang SH, Lee D, Young SG, Maeda N: Targeted modification of the apolipoprotein B gene results in hypobetalipoproteinemia and developmental abnormalities in mice. *Proc Natl Acad Sci U S A* **90**:2389, 1993.
418. Kim E, Cham CM, Véniant MM, Ambroziak P, Young SG: Dual mechanisms for the low plasma levels of truncated apolipoprotein B proteins in familial hypobetalipoproteinemia. Analysis of a new mouse model with a nonsense mutation in the apo B gene. *J Clin Invest* **101**:1468, 1998.
419. Zhu XF, Noto D, Seip R, Shaish A, Schonfeld G: Organ loci of catabolism of short truncations of apo B. *Arterioscler Thromb Vasc Biol* **17**:1032, 1997.
420. Averna M, Seip RL, Mankowitz K, Schonfeld G: Postprandial lipemia in subjects with hypobetalipoproteinemia and a single intestinal allele for apo B-48. *J Lipid Res* **34**:1957, 1993.
421. Tamir I, Levtow O, Lotan D, Legum C, Heldenberg D, Werbin B: Further observations on familial hypobetaliproteinaemia. *Clin Genet* **9**:149, 1976.
422. Scott BB, Miller JP, Losowsky MS: Hypobetalipoproteinaemia—A variant of the Bassen-Kornzweig syndrome. *Gut* **20**:163–168, 1979.
423. Levy E, Roy CC, Thibault L, Bonin A, Brochu P, Seidman EG: Variable expression of familial heterozygous hypobetalipoproteinemia: Transient malabsorption during infancy. *J Lipid Res* **35**:2170, 1994.
424. Sigurdsson G, Nicoll A, Lewis B: Turnover of apolipoprotein-B in two subjects with familial hypobetalipoproteinemia. *Metabolism* **26**:25, 1977.
425. Hagve TA, Myrseth LE, Schrumpf E, Blomhoff JP, Christophersen B, Elgjo K, Gjone E, Prydz H: Liver steatosis in hypobetalipoproteinemia. A case report. *J Hepatol* **13**:104, 1991.
426. Tarugi P, Lonardo A, Ballarini G, Grisendi A, Pulvirenti M, Bagni A, Calandra S: Fatty liver in heterozygous hypobetalipoproteinemia caused by a novel truncated form of apolipoprotein B. *Gastroenterology* **111**:1125 1996.
427. Ogata H, Akagi K, Baba M, Nagamatsu A, Suzuki N, Nomiyama K, Fujishima M: Fatty liver in a case with heterozygous familial hypobetalipoproteinemia [see comments]. *Am J Gastroenterol* **92**:339, 1997.
428. Scoazec JY, Bouma ME, Roche JF, Blache D, Verthier N, Feldmann G, Gay G: Liver fibrosis in a patient with familial homozygous hypobetalipoproteinaemia: Possible role of vitamin supplementation. *Gut* **33**:414, 1992.
429. Frederickson DS, Gotto AM, Levy RI: Familial lipoprotein deficiency, in Stanbury JB, Wyngaarden JB, Fredrickson DS (eds): *The Metabolic Basis of Inherited Disease*, 3rd ed. New York, McGraw-Hill, 1972, p. 493
430. Yee RD, Herbert PN, Bergsma DR, Beimer JJ: Atypical retinitis pigmentosa in familial hypobetalipoproteinemia. *Am J Ophthalmol* **82**:64, 1976.
431. Anderson CM, Townley RRW, Freeman JP: Unusual causes of steatorrhea in infancy and childhood. *Med J Aust* **11**:617, 1961.
432. Lacaille F, Bratos M, Bouma ME, Jos J, Schmitz J, Rey J: Anderson's disease. Clinical and morphologic study of 7 cases. *Arch Fr Pediatr* **46**:491-498, 1989.
433. Silverberg M, Kessler J, Neumann PZ, Wiglesworth FW: An intestinal lipid transport defect. A possible variant of hypobetalipoproteinemia. *Gastroenterology* **54**:1221, 1968.
434. Lamy M, Frezal J, Rey J, Jos J, Nezelot C, Herrault A, Cohen-Solal J: Diarrhee chronique par trouble du transport intracellulaire des lipides. *Arch Fr Pediatr* **24**:1079, 1967.
435. Partin JC, Schubert WK: Jejunal mucosa biopsy studies in two new types of hypobetalipoproteinemia: Light, electron microscopical and biochemical analysis. *Gastroenterology* **58**:1022, 1970.
436. Polonovski C, Navarro J, Fontaine JL, Gouyon FD, Saudubray JM, Cathelineau L: Anderson's disease. *Ann Pediatr (Paris)* **17**:342, 1970.
437. Polanco I, Mellado MJ, Lama R, Larrauri J, Zapata A, Redondo E, Vázquez C: Anderson's disease. Apropos of a new case. *An Esp Pediatr* **24**:185, 1986.
438. Roy CC, Levy E, Green PH, Sniderman A, Letarte J, Buts JP, Orquin J, Brochu P, Weber AM, Morin CL, et al: Malabsorption, hypocholesterolemia, and fat-filled enterocytes with increased intestinal apoprotein B. Chylomicron retention disease. *Gastroenterology* **92**:390, 1987.
439. Levy E, Marcel Y, Deckelbum RJ, Milne R, Lepage G, Seidman E, Bendayan M, Roy CC: Intestinal apo B synthesis, lipids and lipoproteins in chylomicron retention disease. *J Lipid Res* **28**:1263, 1987.
440. Pessah M, Benlian P, Beucler I, Loux N, Schmitz J, Junien C, Infante R: Anderson's disease: Genetic exclusion of the apolipoprotein-B gene in two families. *J Clin Invest* **87**:367, 1991.
441. Patel S, Pessah M, Beucler I, Navarro J, Infante R: Chylomicron retention disease: Exclusion of apolipoprotein B gene defects and detection of mRNA editing in an affected family. *Atherosclerosis* **108**:201, 1994.
442. Tybjaerg-Hansen A, Gallagher J, Vincent J, Houlston R, Talmud P, Dunning AM, Seed M, Hamsten A, Humphries SE, Myant NB: Familial defective apolipoprotein B-100: Detection in the United Kingdom and Scandinavia, and clinical characteristics of ten cases. *Atherosclerosis* **80**:235, 1990.
443. Tybjaerg-Hansen A, Steffensen R, Meinertz H, Schnohr P, Nordestgaard BG. Association of mutations in the apolipoprotein B gene with hypercholesterolemia and the risk of ischemic heart disease. *N Engl J Med* **338**:1577, 1998.
444. Wenham PR, Newton CR, Houlston RS, Price WH. Rapid diagnosis of familial defective apolipoprotein B-100 by amplification refractory mutation system. *Clin Chem* **37**:1983, 1991.
445. Pullinger C, Gaffney D, Gutierrez M, Malloy M, Schumaker V, Packard C, Kane J: The apolioprotein B R3531C mutation: characteristics of 24 subjects from 9 kindreds. *J Lipid Res* **40**:318, 1999.
446. Vega GL, Grundy SM: In vivo evidence for reduced binding of low density lipoproteins to receptors as a cause of primary moderate hypercholesterolemia. *J Clin Invest* **78**:1410, 1986.
447. Innerarity TL, Weisgraber KH, Arnold KS, Mahley RW, Krauss RM, Vega GL, Grundy SM: Familial defective apolipoprotein B-100: Low density lipoproteins with abnormal receptor binding. *Proc Natl Acad Sci U S A* **84**:6919, 1987.
448. Innerarity TL, Balestra ME, Arnold KS, Mahley RW, Vega GL, Grundy SM, Young SG: Isolation of defective receptor-binding low density lipoproteins from subjects with familial defective apolipoprotein B-100. *Arterioscler Thromb Vasc Biol* **8**:551a, 1988.
449. Weisgraber KH, Innerarity TL, Newhouse YM, Young SG, Arnold KS, Krauss RM, Vega GL, Grundy SM, Mahley RW: Familial defective apolipoprotein B-100: Enhanced binding of monoclonal antibody MB47 to abnormal low density lipoproteins. *Proc Natl Acad Sci U S A* **85**:9758, 1988.
450. Soria LF, Ludwig EH, Clarke HR, Vega GL, Grundy SM, McCarthy BJ: Association between a specific apolipoprotein B mutation and familial defective apolipoprotein B-100. *Proc Natl Acad Sci U S A* **86**:587, 1989.
451. Gaffney D, Reid JM, Cameron IM, Vass K, Caslake MJ, Shepherd J, Packard CJ: Independent mutations at codon 3500 of the apolipoprotein B gene are associated with hyperlipidemia. *Arterioscler Thromb Vasc Biol* **15**:1025, 1995.
452. Tai D-Y, Pan J-P, Lee-Chen GJ: Identification and haplotype analysis of apolipoprotein B-100 Arg3500-Trp mutation in hyperlipidemic Chinese. *Clin Chem* **44**:1659, 1998.
453. Choong ML, Koay ES, Khoo KL, Khaw MC, Sethi SK: Denaturing gradient-gel electrophoresis screening of familial defective apolipoprotein B-100 in a mixed Asian cohort: two cases of arginine3500 → tryptophan mutation associated with a unique haplotype. *Clin Chem* **43**:916, 1997.
454. Lund-Katz S, Innerarity TL, Arnold KS, Curtiss LK, Phillips MC: 13C NMR evidence that substitution of glutamine for arginine 3500 in familial defective apolipoprotein B-100 disrupts the conformation of the receptor-binding domain. *J Biol Chem* **266**:2701, 1991.
455. Motti C, Funke H, Rust S, Dergunov A, Assmann G: Using mutagenic polymerase chain reaction primers to detect carriers of familial defective apolipoprotein B-100. *Clin Chem* **37**:1762, 1991.

456. Geisel J, Schleifenbaum T, Weibhaar B, Oette K: Rapid diagnosis of familial defective apolipoprotein B-100. *Eur J Clin Chem Clin Biochem* **29**:395, 1991.
457. Hansen PS, Rüdiger N, Tybjaerg-Hansen A, Faergeman O, Gregersen N: Detection of the apoB-3500 mutation (glutamine for arginine) by gene amplification and cleavage with MspI. *J Lipid Res* **32**:1229, 1991.
458. Pullinger CR, Hennessy LK, Chatterton JE, Liu WQ, Love JA, Mendel CM, Frost PH, Malloy MJ, Schumaker VN, Kane JP: Familial ligand-defective apolipoprotein B — Identification of a new mutation that decreases LDL receptor binding affinity. *J Clin Invest* **95**:1225, 1995.
459. Chatterton JE, Schlapfer P, Butler E, Guitierriz M, Puppoine DL, Pullinger CR, Kane JP, Curtiss LK, Schumaker VN: Identification of apolipoprotein B-100 polymorphisms which affect low density lipoprotein metabolism: Description of a new approach involving monoclonal antibodies and dynamic light scattering. *Biochemistry* **34**:9571, 1995.
460. Hansen PS, Defesche JC, Kastelein JJ, Gerdes LU, Fraza L, Gerdes C, Tato F, Jensen HK, Jensen LG, Klausen IC, Faergeman O, Schuster H: Phenotypic variation in patients heterozygous for familial defective apolipoprotein B (FDB) in three European countries. *Arterioscler Thromb Vasc Biol* **17**:741, 1997.
461. Rauh G, Schuster H, Fischer J, Keller C, Wolfram G, Zöllner N: Familial defective apolipoprotein B-100: haplotype analysis of the arginine(3500) — glutamine mutation. *Atherosclerosis* **88**:219, 1991.
462. Corsini A, McCarthy BJ, Granata A, Soria LF, Fantappiè S, Bernini F, Romano C, Romano L, Fumagalli R, Catapano AL: Familial defective apo B-100, characterization of an Italian family. *Eur J Clin Invest* **21**:389, 1991.
463. Schaefer JR, Scharnagl H, Baumstark MW, Schweer H, Zech LA, Seyberth H, Winkler K, Steinmetz A, März W: Homozygous familial defective apolipoprotein B-100. Enhanced removal of apolipoprotein E-containing VLDLs and decreased production of LDLs. *Arterioscler Thromb Vasc Biol* **17**:348, 1997.
464. März W, Ruzicka C, Pohl T, Usadel KH, Gross W: Familial defective apolipoprotein B-100: mild hypercholesterolaemia without atherosclerosis in a homozygous patient [Letter]. *Lancet* **340**:1362, 1992.
465. Rauh G, Schuster H, Fischer J, Keller C, Wolfram G, Zöllner N: Identification of a heterozygous compound individual with familial hypercholesterolemia and familial defective apolipoprotein B-100. *Klin Wochenschr* **69**:320, 1991.
466. Pietzsch J, Wiedemann B, Julius U, Nitzsche S, Gehrisch S, Bergmann S, Leonhardt W, Jaross W, Hanefeld M: Increased clearance of low density lipoprotein precursors in patients with heterozygous familial defective apolipoprotein B-100: A stable isotope approach. *J Lipid Res* **37**:2074, 1996.
467. Maher VM, Gallagher JJ, Thompson GR, Myant NB: Does the presence of the 3500 mutant apolipoprotein B-100 in low density lipoprotein particles affect their atherogenicity? *Atherosclerosis* **118**:105, 1995.
468. Myant NB, Forbes SA, Day IN, Gallagher J: Estimation of the age of the ancestral arginine3500 → glutamine mutation in human apoB-100. *Genomics* **45**:78, 1997.
469. Rabès JP, Varret M, Saint-Jore B, Erlich E, Jondeau G, Krempf M, Giraudet P, Junien C, Boileau C: Familial ligand-defective apolipoprotein B-100: Simultaneous detection of the ARG3500 → GLN and ARG3531 → CYS mutations in a French population. *Hum Mutat* **10**:160, 1997.
470. Wenham PR, Henderson BG, Penney MD, Ashby JP, Rae PW, Walker SW: Familial ligand-defective apolipoprotein B-100: Detection, biochemical features and haplotype analysis of the R3531C mutation in the UK. *Atherosclerosis* **129**:185, 1997.
471. Mamotte CD, Sturm M, Foo JI, van Bockxmeer FM, Taylor RR: Familial defective apolipoprotein B-100 (FDB): Effect of simvastatin therapy on LDL-receptor binding. *Atherosclerosis* **125**:103, 1996.
472. Raal FJ, Pilcher G, Rubinsztein DC, Lingenhel A, Utermann G: Statin therapy in a kindred with both apolipoprotein B and low density lipoprotein receptor gene defects. *Atherosclerosis* **129**:97, 1997.
473. Maher VM, Gallagher J, Gallagher JJ, Thompson GR, Myant NB: Response to cholesterol-lowering drugs in familial defective apolipoprotein B-100. *Atherosclerosis* **91**:73, 1991.
474. Illingworth DR, Vakar F, Mahley RW, Weisgraber KH: Hypocholesterolaemic effects of lovastatin in familial defective apolipoprotein B-100. *Lancet* **339**:598, 1992.
475. Berglund L, Witztum JL, Galeano NF, Khouw AS, Ginsberg HN, Ramakrishnan R: Three-fold effect of lovastatin treatment on low density lipoprotein metabolism in subjects with hyperlipidemia: Increase in receptor activity, decrease in apo B production, and decrease in particle affinity for the receptor. Results from a novel triple-tracer approach. *J Lipid Res* **39**:913, 1998.
476. Burnett JR, Wilcox LJ, Telford DE, Kleinstiver SJ, Hugh P, Barrett P, Newton RS, Huff MW: Inhibition of HMG-CoA reductase by atorvastatin decreases both VLDL and LDL apolipoprotein B production in miniature pigs. *Arterioscler Thromb Vasc Biol* **17**:2589, 1997.
477. Goldstein JL, Schrott HG, Hazzard WR, Bierman EL, Motulsky AG: Hyperlipidemia in coronary heart disease. II. Genetic analysis of lipid levels in 176 families and delineation of a new inherited disorder, combined hyperlipidemia. *J Clin Invest* **52**:1544, 1973.
478. Hazzard WR, Goldstein JL, Schrott HG, Motulsky AG, Bierman EL: Evaluation of lipoprotein phenotypes of 156 genetically defined survivors of myocardial infarction. *J Clin Invest* **52**:1569, 1973.
479. Nikkila EA, Aro A: Family study of serum lipids and lipoproteins in coronary heart disease. *Arterioscler Thromb Vasc Biol* **1**:82, 1981.
480. Rose HG, Kranz P, Weinstock M, Juliano J, Haft JI: Inheritance of combined hyperlipoproteinemia: evidence for a new lipoprotein phenotype. *Am J Med* **54**:148, 1973.
481. Cortner JA, Coates PM, Gallagher PR: Prevalence and expression of familial combined hyperlipidemia in childhood. *J Pediatr* **116**:514, 1990.
482. Vaverková H, Weinbergová O, Horcicka V, Kubasta M, Vrublovsky P: Familial combined hyperlipidemia. Part I. Lipid values and the lipoprotein pattern. *Acta Univ Palacki Olomuc Fac Med* **113**:193, 1986.
483. Vaverková H, Weinbergová O, Horcicka V, Kubasta M, Vrublovsky P: Familial combined hyperlipidemia. Part II. Clinical picture. *Acta Univ Palacki Olomuc Fac Med* **114**:243, 1986.
484. Austin MA, Horowitz H, Wijsman E, Krauss RM, Brunzell J: Bimodality of plasma apolipoprotein B levels in familial combined hyperlipidemia. *Atherosclerosis* **92**:67, 1992.
485. Chait A, Brunzell JD: Severe hypertriglyceridemia: role of familial and acquired disorders. *Metabolism* **32**:209, 1983.
486. Hunt SC, Wu LL, Hopkins PN, Stults BM, Kuida H, Ramirez ME, Lalouel JM, Williams RR: Apolipoprotein, low density lipoprotein subfraction, and insulin associations with familial combined hyperlipidemia. Study of Utah patients with familial dyslipidemic hypertension. *Arterioscler Thromb Vasc Biol* **9**:335, 1989.
487. Williams RR, Hunt SC, Hopkins PN, Wu LL, Hasstedt SJ, Berry TD, Barlow GK, Stults BM, Schumacher MC, Ludwig EH, et al: Genetic basis of familial dyslipidemia and hypertension: 15-year results from Utah. *Am J Hypertens* **6**:319S, 1993.
488. Reaven GM: Banting lecture 1988. Role of insulin resistance in human disease. *Diabetes* **37**:1595, 1988.
489. Hokanson JE, Austin MA, Zambon A, Brunzell JD: Plasma triglyceride and LDL heterogeneity in familial combined hyperlipidemia. *Arterioscler Thromb Vasc Biol* **13**:427, 1993.
490. Hokanson JE, Krauss RM, Albers JJ, Austin MA, Brunzell JD: LDL physical and chemical properties in familial combined hyperlipidemia. *Arterioscler Thromb Vasc Biol* **15**:452, 1995.
491. Williams PT, Krauss RM, Vranizan KM, Stefanick ML, Wood PD, Lindgren FT: Associations of lipoproteins and apolipoproteins with gradient gel electrophoresis estimates of high density lipoprotein subfractions in men and women. *Arterioscler Thromb Vasc Biol* **12**:332, 1992.
492. Myers LH, Phillips NR, Havel RJ: Mathematical evaluation of methods for estimation of the concentration of the major lipid components of human serum lipoproteins. *J Lab Clin Med* **88**:491, 1976.
493. Dejager S, Bruckert E, Chapman MJ: Dense low density lipoprotein subspecies with diminished oxidative resistance predominate in combined hyperlipidemia. *J Lipid Res* **34**:295, 1993.
494. Brown BG, Zambon A, Poulin D, Rocha A, Maher VM, Davis JW, Albers JJ, Brunzell JD: Use of niacin, statins, and resins in patients with combined hyperlipidemia. *Am J Cardiol* **81**:52B, 1998.
495. Reaven GM, Chen YD, Jeppesen J, Maheux P, Krauss RM: Insulin resistance and hyperinsulinemia in individuals with small, dense low density lipoprotein particles [see comments]. *J Clin Invest* **92**:141, 1993.
496. Brunzell JD, Albers JJ, Chait A, Grundy SM, Groszek E, McDonald GB: Plasma lipoproteins in familial combined hyperlipidemia and monogenic familial hypertriglyceridemia. *J Lipid Res* **24**:147, 1983.
497. Kwiterovich PO: Genetics and molecular biology of familial combined hyperlipidemia. *Curr Opin Lipidol* **4**:133, 1993.

498. Sniderman A, Shapiro S, Marpole D, Skinner B, Teng B, Kwiterovich PO Jr: Association of coronary atherosclerosis with hyperapobetalipoproteinemia [increased protein but normal cholesterol levels in human plasma low density (beta) lipoproteins]. *Proc Natl Acad Sci U S A* **77**:604, 1980.
499. Bredie SJ, Demacker PN, Stalenhoef AF: Metabolic and genetic aspects of familial combined hyperlipidaemia with emphasis on low-density lipoprotein heterogeneity. *Eur J Clin Invest* **27**:802, 1997.
500. Allayee H, Aouizerat BE, Cantor RM, Dallinga-Thie GM, Krauss RM, Lanning CD, Rotter JI, Lusis AJ, de Bruin TWA: Families with familial combined hyperlipidemia and families enriched for coronary artery disease share genetic determinants for the atherogenic lipoprotein phenotype. *Am J Hum Genet* **63**:577, 1998.
501. Austin MA, King MC, Vranizan KM, Newman B, Krauss RM: Inheritance of low-density lipoprotein subclass patterns: Results of complex segregation analysis. *Am J Hum Genet* **43**:838, 1988.
502. Swinkels DW, Demacker PN, Hendriks JC, van 't Laar A: Low density lipoprotein subfractions and relationship to other risk factors for coronary artery disease in healthy individuals [published erratum appears in *Arterioscler Thromb Vasc Biol* **10(3)**:491, 1990]. *Arterioscler Thromb Vasc Biol* **9**:604, 1989.
503. Williams PT, Krauss RM, Nichols AV, Vranizan KM, Wood PD: Identifying the predominant peak diameter of high-density and low-density lipoproteins by electrophoresis. *J Lipid Res* **31**:1131, 1990.
504. Chen G, Liu W, Duchateau P, Allaart J, Hamilton R, Mendel C, Lau K, Hardman D, Frost P, Malloy M, Kane J: Conformational differences in human apolipoprotein B-100 among subspecies of low density lipoproteins. *J Biol Chem* **269**:29121, 1994.
505. Nichols AV: Human serum lipoproteins and their interrelationships. *Adv Biol Med Phys* **11**:109, 1967.
506. Tilly-Kiesi MK, Tikkanen MJ: Differential low density lipoprotein hydrated density distribution in female and male patients with familial hypercholesterolemia. *Clin Chim Acta* **201**:65, 1991.
507. Tall AR: Plasma cholesteryl ester transfer protein. *J Lipid Res* **34**:1255, 1993.
508. Zambon A, Austin MA, Brown BG, Hokanson JE, Brunzell JD: Effect of hepatic lipase on LDL in normal men and those with coronary artery disease. *Arterioscler Thromb Vasc Biol* **13**:147, 1993.
509. Eisenberg S, Gavish D, Oschry Y, Fainaru M, Deckelbaum RJ: Abnormalities in very low, low and high density lipoproteins in hypertriglyceridemia. Reversal toward normal with bezafibrate treatment. *J Clin Invest* **74**:470, 1984.
510. Guérin M, Bruckert E, Dolphin PJ, Chapman MJ: Absence of cholesteryl ester transfer protein-mediated cholesteryl ester mass transfer from high-density lipoprotein to low-density lipoprotein particles is a major feature of combined hyperlipidaemia. *Eur J Clin Invest* **26**:485, 1996.
511. Musliner TA, Giotas C, Krauss RM: Presence of multiple subpopulations of lipoproteins of intermediate density in normal subjects. *Arterioscler Thromb Vasc Biol* **6**:79, 1986.
512. Gambert P, Bouzerand-Gambert C, Athias A, Farnier M, Lallemant C: Human low density lipoprotein subfractions separated by gradient gel electrophoresis: composition, distribution, and alterations induced by cholesteryl ester transfer protein. *J Lipid Res* **31**:1199, 1990.
513. Krauss RM, Burke DJ: Identification of multiple subclasses of plasma low density lipoproteins in normal humans. *J Lipid Res* **23**:97, 1982.
514. de Graaf J, Hak-Lemmers HL, Hectors MP, Demacker PN, Hendriks JC, Stalenhoef AF: Enhanced susceptibility to in vitro oxidation of the dense low density lipoprotein subfraction in healthy subjects. *Arterioscler Thromb Vasc Biol* **11**:298, 1991.
515. Tribble DL, Holl LG, Wood PD, Krauss RM: Variations in oxidative susceptibility among six low density lipoprotein subfractions of differing density and particle size. *Atherosclerosis* **93**:189, 1992.
516. de Rijke YB, Bredie SJ, Demacker PN, Vogelaar JM, Hak-Lemmers HL, and Stalenhoef AF: The redox status of coenzyme Q10 in total LDL as an indicator of in vivo oxidative modification. Studies on subjects with familial combined hyperlipidemia. *Arterioscler Thromb Vasc Biol* **17**:127, 1997.
517. Packard CJ, Munro A, Lorimer AR, Gotto AM, Shepherd J: Metabolism of apolipoprotein B in large triglyceride-rich very low density lipoproteins of normal and hypertriglyceridemic subjects. *J Clin Invest* **74**:2178, 1984.
518. Stalenhoef AF, Malloy MJ, Kane JP, Havel RJ: Metabolism of apolipoproteins B-48 and B-100 of triglyceride-rich lipoproteins in normal and lipoprotein lipase-deficient humans. *Proc Natl Acad Sci U S A* **81**:1839, 1984.
519. Grundy SM, Vega GL: What is meant by overproduction of apo B-containing lipoproteins? *Adv Exp Med Biol* **285**:213, 1991.
520. Marzetta CA, Foster DM, Brunzell JD: Relationships between LDL density and kinetic heterogeneity in subjects with normolipidemia and familial combined hyperlipidemia using density gradient ultracentrifugation. *J Lipid Res* **30**:1307, 1989.
521. Chait A, Albers JJ, Brunzell JD: Very low density lipoprotein overproduction in genetic forms of hypertriglyceridaemia. *Eur J Clin Invest* **10**:17, 1980.
522. Janus ED, Nicoll A, Wootton R, Turner PR, Magill PJ, Lewis B: Quantitative studies of very low density lipoprotein: Conversion to low density lipoprotein in normal controls and primary hyperlipidaemic states and the role of direct secretion of low density lipoprotein in heterozygous familial hypercholesterolaemia. *Eur J Clin Invest* **10**:149, 1980.
523. Kissebah AH, Alfarsi S, Evans DI: Low density lipoprotein metabolism in familial combined hyperlipidemia: Mechanism of the multiple lipoprotein phenotype expression. *Arterioscler Thromb Vasc Biol* **24**:199, 1976.
524. Grundy SM, Chait A, Brunzell JD: Familial combined hyperlipidemia workship. *Arterioscler Thromb Vasc Biol* **7**:203, 1987.
525. Venkatesan S, Cullen P, Pacy P, Halliday D, Scott J: Stable isotopes show a direct relation between VLDL apoB overproduction and serum triglyceride levels and indicate a metabolically and biochemically coherent basis for familial combined hyperlipidemia. *Arterioscler Thromb Vasc Biol* **13**:1110, 1993.
526. Kesäniemi YA, Beltz WF, Grundy SM: Comparisons of metabolism of apolipoprotein B in normal subjects, obese patients, and patients with coronary heart disease. *J Clin Invest* **76**:586, 1985.
527. Aguilar-Salinas CA, Hugh P, Barrett R, Pulai J, Zhu XL, Schonfeld G: A familial combined hyperlipidemic kindred with impaired apolipoprotein B catabolism. Kinetics of apolipoprotein B during placebo and pravastatin therapy. *Arterioscler Thromb Vasc Biol* **17**:72, 1997.
528. Goldstein JL, Dana SE, Brunschede GY, Brown MS: Genetic heterogeneity in familial hypercholesterolemia: Evidence for two different mutations affecting functions of low-density lipoprotein receptor. *Proc Natl Acad Sci U S A* **72**:1092, 1975.
529. Bredie SJ, Tack CJ, Smits P, Stalenhoef AF: Nonobese patients with familial combined hyperlipidemia are insulin resistant compared with their nonaffected relatives. *Arterioscler Thromb Vasc Biol* **17**:1465, 1997.
530. Castro Cabezas M, de Bruin TW, de Valk HW, Shoulders CC, Jansen H, Willem Erkelens D: Impaired fatty acid metabolism in familial combined hyperlipidemia. A mechanism associating hepatic apolipoprotein B overproduction and insulin resistance. *J Clin Invest* **92**:160, 1993.
531. Ascaso JF, Sales J, Merchante A, Real J, Lorente R, Martinez-Valls J, Carmena R: Influence of obesity on plasma lipoproteins, glycaemia and insulinaemia in patients with familial combined hyperlipidaemia. *Int J Obes Relat Metab Disord* **21**:360, 1997.
532. Sijbrands EJ, Westendorp RG, Hoffer MJ, Havekes LM, Frants RR, Meinders AE, Frölich M, Smelt AH: Effect of insulin resistance, apoE2 allele, and smoking on combined hyperlipidemia. *Arterioscler Thromb Vasc Biol* **14**:1576, 1994.
533. Ascaso JF, Lorente R, Merchante A, Real JT, Priego A, Carmena R: Insulin resistance in patients with familial combined hyperlipidemia and coronary artery disease. *Am J Cardiol* **80**:1484, 1997.
534. Austin MA, Wijsman E, Guo SW, Krauss RM, Brunzell JD, Deeb S: Lack of evidence for linkage between low-density lipoprotein subclass phenotypes and the apolipoprotein B locus in familial combined hyperlipidemia. *Genet Epidemiol* **8**:287, 1991.
535. Pihlajamäki J, Rissanen J, Heikkinen S, Karjalainen L, Laakso M: Codon 54 polymorphism of the human intestinal fatty acid binding protein 2 gene is associated with dyslipidemias but not with insulin resistance in patients with familial combined hyperlipidemia. *Arterioscler Thromb Vasc Biol* **17**:1039, 1997.
536. de Graaf J, Stalenhoef AF: Defects of lipoprotein metabolism in familial combined hyperlipidaemia. *Curr Opin Lipidol* **9**:189, 1998.
537. Williams RR, Hunt SC, Hopkins PN, Stults BM, Wu LL, Hasstedt SJ, Barlow GK, Stephenson SH, Lalouel JM, Kuida H: Familial dyslipidemic hypertension. Evidence from 58 Utah families for a syndrome present in approximately 12% of patients with essential hypertension. *JAMA* **259**:3579, 1988.
538. Reynisdottir S, Eriksson M, Angelin B, Arner P: Impaired activation of adipocyte lipolysis in familial combined hyperlipidemia. *J Clin Invest* **95**:2161, 1995.

539. Aitman TJ, Godsland IF, Farren B, Crook D, Wong HJ, Scott J: Defects of insulin action on fatty acid and carbohydrate metabolism in familial combined hyperlipidemia. *Arterioscler Thromb Vasc Biol* **17**:748, 1997.
540. Sniderman AD, Cianflone K: Substrate delivery as a determinant of hepatic apo B secretion. *Arterioscler Thromb Vasc Biol* **13**:629, 1993.
541. Lewis GF, Uffelman KD, Szeto LW, Weller B, Steiner G: Interaction between free fatty acids and insulin in the acute control of very low density lipoprotein production in humans. *J Clin Invest* **95**:158, 1995.
542. Nuutila P, Koivisto VA, Knuuti J, Ruotsalainen U, Teräs M, Haaparanta M, Bergman J, Solin O, Voipio-Pulkki LM, Wegelius U, et al: Glucose-free fatty acid cycle operates in human heart and skeletal muscle in vivo. *J Clin Invest* **89**:1767, 1992.
543. González-Manchón C, Martín-Requero A, Ayuso MS, Parrilla R: Role of endogenous fatty acids in the control of hepatic gluconeogenesis. *Arch Biochem Biophys* **292**:95, 1992.
544. Baldo A, Sniderman AD, St-Luce S, Avramoglu RK, Maslowska M, Hoang B, Monge JC, Bell A, Mulay S, Cianflone K: The adipsin-acylation stimulating protein system and regulation of intracellular triglyceride synthesis. *J Clin Invest* **92**:1543, 1993.
545. Simsolo RB, Ong JM, Saffari B, Kern PA: Effect of improved diabetes control on the expression of lipoprotein lipase in human adipose tissue. *J Lipid Res* **33**:89, 1992.
546. Williams WR, Lalouel JM: Complex segregation analysis of hyperlipidemia in a Seattle sample. *Hum Hered* **32**:24, 1982.
547. Aouizerat BE, Allayee H, Dallinga-Thie GM, Cantor RM, Vora HR, Lusis AJ: Evidence for a multilocus contribution to familial combined hyperlipidemia (FCHL). *Circulation* **96(Suppl)**: 545, 1997.
548. Rauh G, Schuster H, Müller B, Schewe S, Keller C, Wolfram G, Zöllner N: Genetic evidence from 7 families that the apolipoprotein B gene is not involved in familial combined hyperlipidemia. *Atherosclerosis* **83**:81, 1990.
549. Rotter JI, Bu X, Cantor RM, Warden CH, Brown J, Gray RJ, Blanche PJ, Krauss RM, Lusis AJ: Multilocus genetic determinants of LDL particle size in coronary artery disease families. *Am J Hum Genet* **58**:585, 1996.
550. Bredie SJ, van Drongelen J, Kiemeney LA, Demacker PN, Beaty TH, Stalenhoef AF: Segregation analysis of plasma apolipoprotein B levels in familial combined hyperlipidemia. *Arterioscler Thromb Vasc Biol* **17**:834, 1997.
551. Jarvik GP, Brunzell JD, Austin MA, Krauss RM, Motulsky AG, Wijsman E: Genetic predictors of FCHL in four large pedigrees. Influence of ApoB level major locus predicted genotype and LDL subclass phenotype. *Arterioscler Thromb Vasc Biol* **14**:1687, 1994.
552. Juo S-HH, Bredie SJH, Kiemeney LA, Dmacker PNM, Stalenhoef AFH: A common genetic mechanisms determines plasma apolipoprotein B levels and dense LDL subfraction distribution in familial combined hyperlipidemia. *Am J Hum Genet* **63**:586, 1998.
553. Austin MA, Brunzell JD, Fitch WL, Krauss RM: Inheritance of low density lipoprotein subclass patterns in familial combined hyperlipidemia. *Arterioscler Thromb Vasc Biol* **10**:520, 1990.
554. Bredie SJ, Kiemeney LA, de Haan AF, Demacker PN, Stalenhoef AF: Inherited susceptibility determines the distribution of dense low-density lipoprotein subfraction profiles in familial combined hyperlipidemia. *Am J Hum Genet* **58**:812, 1996.
555. Cullen P, Farren B, Scott J, Farrall M: Complex segregation analysis provides evidence for a major gene acting on serum triglyceride levels in 55 British families with familial combined hyperlipidemia. *Arterioscler Thromb Vasc Biol* **14**:1233, 1994.
556. Ribalta J, La Ville AE, Vallvé JC, Humphries S, Turner PR, Masana L. A variation in the apolipoprotein C-III gene is associated with an increased number of circulating VLDL and IDL particles in familial combined hyperlipidemia. *J Lipid Res* **38**:1061, 1997.
557. Tybjaerg-Hansen A, Nordestgaard B, Gerdes L, Faergeman O, Humphries S: Genetic markers in the apo AI-CIII-AIV gene cluster for combined hyperlipidemia, hypertriglyceridemia, and predisposition to atherosclerosis. *Atherosclerosis* **100**:157, 1993.
558. Wojciechowski AP, Farrall M, Cullen P, Wilson TM, Bayliss JD, Farren B, Griffin BA, Caslake MJ, Packard CJ, Shepherd J, et al: Familial combined hyperlipidaemia linked to the apolipoprotein AI-CII-AIV gene cluster on chromosome 11q23-q24. *Nature* **349**: 161, 1991.
559. Dallinga-Thie GM, Bu XD, van Linde-Sibenius Trip M, Rotter JI, Lusis AJ, de Bruin TW: Apolipoprotein A-I/C-III/A-IV gene cluster in familial combined hyperlipidemia: Effects on LDL-cholesterol and apolipoproteins B and C-III. *J Lipid Res* **37**:136, 1996.
560. Hayden MR, Kirk H, Clark C, Frohlich J, Rabkin S, McLeod R, Hewitt J: DNA polymorphisms in and around the Apo-A1-CIII genes and genetic hyperlipidemias. *Am J Hum Genet* **40**:421, 1987.
561. Patsch W, Sharrett AR, Chen IY, Lin-Lee YC, Brown SA, Gotto AM Jr, Boerwinkle E: Associations of allelic differences at the A-I/C-III/A-IV gene cluster with carotid artery intima-media thickness and plasma lipid transport in hypercholesterolemic-hypertriglyceridemic humans. *Arterioscler Thromb Vasc Biol* **14**:874, 1994.
562. Xu CF, Talmud P, Schuster H, Houlston R, Miller G, Humphries S: Association between genetic variation at the APO AI-CIII-AIV gene cluster and familial combined hyperlipidaemia. *Clin Genet* **46**:385, 1994.
563. Dallinga-Thie GM, van Linde-Sibenius Trip M, Rotter JI, Cantor RM, Bu X, Lusis AJ, de Bruin TW: Complex genetic contribution of the Apo AI-CIII-AIV gene cluster to familial combined hyperlipidemia. Identification of different susceptibility haplotypes. *J Clin Invest* **99**:953, 1997.
564. Wijsman EM, Brunzell JD, Jarvik GP, Austin MA, Motulsky AG, Deeb SS: Evidence against linkage of familial combined hyperlipidemia to the apolipoprotein AI-CIII-AIV gene complex. *Arterioscler Thromb Vasc Biol* **18**:215, 1998.
565. Marcil M, Boucher B, Gagné E, Davignon J, Hayden M, Genest J Jr: Lack of association of the apolipoprotein A-I-C-III-A-IV gene XmnI and SstI polymorphisms and of the lipoprotein lipase gene mutations in familial combined hyperlipoproteinemia in French Canadian subjects. *J Lipid Res* **37**:309, 1996.
566. Tatò F, Vega GL, Tall AR, Grundy SM: Relation between cholesterol ester transfer protein activities and lipoprotein cholesterol in patients with hypercholesterolemia and combined hyperlipidemia. *Arterioscler Thromb Vasc Biol* **15**:112, 1995.
567. Pajukanta P, Porkka KV, Antikainen M, Taskinen MR, Perola M, Murtomäki-Repo S, Ehnholm S, Nuotio I, Suurinkeroinen L, Lahdenkari AT, Syvänen AC, Viikari JS, Ehnholm C, Peltonen L: No evidence of linkage between familial combined hyperlipidemia and genes encoding lipolytic enzymes in Finnish families. *Arterioscler Thromb Vasc Biol* **17**:841, 1997.
568. Wilson DE, Emi M, Iverius PH, Hata A, Wu LL, Hillas E, Williams RR, Lalouel JM: Phenotypic expression of heterozygous lipoprotein lipase deficiency in the extended pedigree of a proband homozygous for a missense mutation. *J Clin Invest* **86**:735, 1990.
569. Babirak SP, Brown BG, Brunzell JD: Familial combined hyperlipidemia and abnormal lipoprotein lipase. *Arterioscler Thromb Vasc Biol* **12**:1176, 1992.
570. Nevin DN, Brunzell JD, Deeb SS: The LPL gene in individuals with familial combined hyperlipidemia and decreased LPL activity. *Arterioscler Thromb Vasc Biol* **14**:869, 1994.
571. Yang WS, Nevin DN, Iwasaki L, Peng R, Brown BG, Brunzell JD, Deeb SS: Regulatory mutations in the human lipoprotein lipase gene in patients with familial combined hyperlipidemia and coronary artery disease. *J Lipid Res* **37**:2627, 1996.
572. de Bruin TW, Mailly F, van Barlingen HH, Fisher R, Castro Cabezas M, Talmud P, Dallinga-Thie GM, Humphries SE: Lipoprotein lipase gene mutations D9N and N291S in four pedigrees with familial combined hyperlipidaemia. *Eur J Clin Invest* **26**:631, 1996.
573. Mailly F, Tugrul Y, Reymer PW, Bruin T, Seed M, Groenemeyer BF, Asplund-Carlson A, Vallance D, Winder AF, Miller GJ, et al: A common variant in the gene for lipoprotein lipase (Asp9 → Asn). Functional implications and prevalence in normal and hyperlipidemic subjects. *Arterioscler Thromb Vasc Biol* **15**:468, 1995.
574. Hoffer MJ, Bredie SJ, Boomsma DI, Reymer PW, Kastelein JJ, Knijff Pd, Demacker PN, Stalenhoef AF, Havekes LM, Frants RR: The lipoprotein lipase (Asn291 → Ser) mutation is associated with elevated lipid levels in families with familial combined hyperlipidaemia. *Atherosclerosis* **119**:159, 1996.
575. Reymer PW, Groenemeyer BE, Gagné E, Miao L, Appelman EE, Seidel JC, Kromhout D, Bijvoet SM, van de Oever K, Bruin T, et al: A frequently occurring mutation in the lipoprotein lipase gene (Asn291Ser) contributes to the expression of familial combined hyperlipidemia. *Hum Mol Genet* **4**:1543, 1995.
576. Deeb SS, Nevin DN, Iwasaki L, Brunzell JD: Two novel apolipoprotein A-IV variants in individuals with familial combined hyperlipidemia and diminished levels of lipoprotein lipase activity. *Hum Mutat* **8**:319, 1996.
577. Castellani LW, Weinreb A, Bodnar J, Goto AM, Doolittle M, Mehrabian M, Demant P, Lusis AJ: Mapping a gene for combined hyperlipidaemia in a mutant mouse strain. *Nat Genet* **18**:374, 1998.

578. Pajukanta P, Nuotio I, Terwilliger JD, Porkka KV, Ylitalo K, Pihlajamäki J, Suomalainen AJ, Syvänen AC, Lehtimäki T, Viikari JS, Laakso M, Taskinen MR, Ehnholm C, Peltonen L: Linkage of familial combined hyperlipidaemia to chromosome 1q21-q23. *Nat Genet* **18**:369, 1998.
579. Nishina PM, Johnson JP, Naggert JK, Krauss RM: Linkage of atherogenic lipoprotein phenotype to the low density lipoprotein receptor locus on the short arm of chromosome 19. *Proc Natl Acad Sci U S A* **89**:708, 1992.
580. Beaty TH, Prenger VL, Virgil DG, Lewis B, Kwiterovich PO, Bachorik PS: A genetic model for control of hypertriglyceridemia and apolipoprotein B levels in the Johns Hopkins colony of St. Thomas Hospital rabbits. *Genetics* **132**:1095, 1992.
581. Baier LJ, Wiedrich C, Dobberfuhl A, Traurig M, Thuillez P, Bogardus C, Hanson RL: Sequence analysis of candidate genes in a region of chromosome 1 linked to type 2 diabetes. *Diabetes* **47**:A171, 1998.
582. Elbein SC, Yount PA, Teng K, Hasstedt SJ: Genome-wide search for type 2 diabetes susceptibility genes in Caucasians; evidence for a recessive locus on chromosome 1. *Diabetes* **47**:A15, 1998.
583. Austin MA, Breslow JL, Hennekens CH, Buring JE, Willett WC, Krauss RM: Low-density lipoprotein subclass patterns and risk of myocardial infarction. *JAMA* **260**:1917, 1988.
584. Campos H, Genest JJ Jr, Blijlevens E, McNamara JR, Jenner JL, Ordovas JM, Wilson PW, Schaefer EJ: Low density lipoprotein particle size and coronary artery disease. *Arterioscler Thromb Vasc Biol* **12**:187, 1992.
585. Swinkels DW, Demacker PN, Hendriks JC, Brenninkmeijer BJ, Stuyt PM: The relevance of a protein-enriched low density lipoprotein as a risk for coronary heart disease in relation to other known risk factors. *Atherosclerosis* **77**:59, 1989.
586. Vega GL, Grundy SM: Comparison of apolipoprotein B to cholesterol in low density lipoproteins of patients with coronary heart disease. *J Lipid Res* **25**:580, 1984.
587. Bredie SJ, de Bruin TW, Demacker PN, Kastelein JJ, Stalenhoef AF: Comparison of gemfibrozil versus simvastatin in familial combined hyperlipidemia and effects on apolipoprotein-B-containing lipoproteins, low-density lipoprotein subfraction profile, and low-density lipoprotein oxidizability. *Am J Cardiol* **75**:348, 1995.
588. Schonfeld G, Aguilar-Salina C, Elias N: Role of 3-hydroxy-3-methylglutaryl coenzyme A reductase inhibitors ("statins") in familial combined hyperlipidemia. *Am J Cardiol* **81**:43B, 1998.
589. Forster LF, Steward G, Bedford DK, Stewart JP, Caslake MJ, Packard CJ, et al: Stable isotope turnover studies of apolipoprotein B in combined hyperlipidemia before and after treatment with atorvastatin, a new HMGCoA reductase inhibitor. *Circulation* **94**:583, 1996.
590. Huang LS, Kayden H, Sokol RJ, Breslow JL: ApoB gene nonsense and splicing mutations in a compound heterozygote for familial hypobetalipoproteinemia. *J Lipid Res* **32**:1341, 1991.
591. Huang LS, Ripps ME, Korman SH, Deckelbaum RJ, Breslow JL: Hypobetalipoproteinemia due to an apolipoprotein B gene exon 21 deletion derived by Alu-Alu recombination. *J Biol Chem* **264**:11394, 1989.
592. Young SG, Hubl ST, Smith RS, Snyder SM, Terdiman JF: Familial hypobetalipoproteinemia caused by a mutation in the apolipoprotein B gene that results in a truncated species of apolipoprotein B (B-31). A unique mutation that helps to define the portion of the apolipoprotein B molecule required for the formation of buoyant, triglyceride-rich lipoproteins. *J Clin Invest* **85**:933, 1990.
593. Young SG, Pullinger CR, Zysow BR, Hofmann-Radvani H, Linton MF, Farese RV Jr, Terdiman JF, Snyder SM, Grundy SM, Vega GL, et al: Four new mutations in the apolipoprotein B gene causing hypobetalipoproteinemia, including two different frameshift mutations that yield truncated apolipoprotein B proteins of identical length. *J Lipid Res* **34**:501, 1993.
594. Ohashi K, Ishibashi S, Yamamoto M, Osuga J, Yazaki Y, Yukawa S, Yamada N: A truncated species of apolipoprotein B (B-38.7) in a patient with homozygous hypobetalipoproteinemia associated with diabetes mellitus. *Arterioscler Thromb Vasc Biol* **18**:1330, 1998.
595. Krul ES, Kinoshita M, Talmud P, Humphries SE, Turner S, Goldberg AC, Cook K, Boerwinkle E, Schonfeld G: Two distinct truncated apolipoprotein B species in a kindred with hypobetalipoproteinemia. *Arterioscler Thromb Vasc Biol* **9**:856, 1989.
596. Welty FK, Ordovas J, Schaefer EJ, Wilson PW, Young SG: Identification and molecular analysis of two apoB gene mutations causing low plasma cholesterol levels. *Circulation* **92**:2036, 1995.
597. Young SG, Bihain B, Flynn LM, Sanan DA, Ayrault-Jarrier M, Jacotot B: Asymptomatic homozygous hypobetalipoproteinemia associated with apolipoprotein B45.2. *Hum Mol Genet* **3**:741, 1994.
598. Young SG, Hubl ST, Chappell DA, Smith RS, Claiborne F, Snyder SM, Terdiman JF: Familial hypobetalipoproteinemia associated with a mutant species of apolipoprotein B (B-46). *N Engl J Med* **320**:1604, 1989.
599. Groenewegen WA, Krul ES, Schonfeld G: Deletion ambiguities in a novel apolipoprotein B truncation, apo B-52 [Abstract]. *Circulation* **86**:I-690, 1992.
600. Wagner RD, Krul ES, Tang J, Parhofer KG, Garlock K, Talmud P, Schonfeld G: ApoB-54.8, a truncated apolipoprotein found primarily in VLDL, is associated with a nonsense mutation in the apoB gene and hypobetalipoproteinemia. *J Lipid Res* **32**:1001, 1991.
601. Talmud PJ, Converse C, Krul E, Huq L, McIlwaine GG, Series JJ, Boyd P, Schonfeld G, Dunning A, Humphries S: A novel truncated apolipoprotein B (apo B55) in a patient with familial hypobetalipoproteinemia and atypical retinitis pigmentosa. *Clin Genet* **42**:62, 1992.
602. Welty FK, Hubl ST, Pierotti VR, Young SG: A truncated species of apolipoprotein B (B67) in a kindred with familial hypobetalipoproteinemia. *J Clin Invest* **87**:1748, 1991.
603. Groenewegen WA, Krul ES, Averna MR, Pulai J, Schonfeld G: Dysbetalipoproteinemia in a kindred with hypobetalipoproteinemia due to mutations in the genes for Apo B (Apo B-70.5) and Apo E (Apo E2). *Arterioscler Thromb Vasc Biol* **14**:1695, 1994.
604. Farese RV Jr, Garg A, Pierotti VR, Vega GL, Young SG: A truncated species of apolipoprotein B, B-83, associated with hypobetalipoproteinemia. *J Lipid Res* **33**:569, 1992.
605. Linton MF, Pierotti VR, Hubl ST, Young SG: An apo-B gene mutation causing familial hypobetalipoproteinemia analyzed by examining the apo-B cDNA amplified from the fibroblast RNA of an affected subject. *Clin Res* **38**:286A, 1990.
606. Srivastava N, Noto D, Averna M, Pulai J, Srivastava RA, Cole TG, Latour MA, et al: A new apolipoprotein B truncation (apo B-43.7) in familial hypobetalipoproteinemia: Genetic and metabolic studies. *Metabolism* **45**:1296, 1996.

CHAPTER 116

Lipoprotein(a)

Gerd Utermann

1. Lipoprotein(a), or Lp(a), is a complex particle in human plasma. It combines elements of the lipid transport and the blood-clotting system in its structure. It is assembled from one LDL which carries all the lipid, and one glycoprotein called apolipoprotein(a) or apo(a). Apo(a) has a high degree of homology to plasminogen (PLG) and a high degree of internal repeat structure due to the presence of multiple repeats of plasminogen-like kringle IV modules. In the Lp(a) particle, LDL and apo(a) are linked by a single disulfide bridge between apo B-100 from LDL and one of the repeated kringle IV structures (K IV-9).
2. Plasma apo(a) is secreted exclusively by the liver. Assembly of Lp(a) from LDL and apo(a) occurs in plasma or at the hepatocyte plasma membrane surface. Plasma Lp(a) concentrations are primarily determined by the rate of synthesis rather than by catabolism. The mechanism and sites of Lp(a) catabolism are unknown. The LDL-receptor (LDLR) pathway seems to play only a minor role, if any, but members of the LDLR gene family (including megalin/GP 330) have been implicated in Lp(a)/apo(a) degradation, and some data indicate that the kidney may be involved in Lp(a)/apo(a) catabolism. Apo(a) fragments have been demonstrated in plasma and urine, but their significance is unclear.
3. Lp(a) is a quantitative genetic trait. The distribution of Lp(a) concentrations in most populations is highly positively skewed and very broad varying over one thousand-fold (from less than 0.2 to more than 200 mg/dl) among subjects. There exist striking but unexplained differences in the concentration and distribution of Lp(a) concentrations across populations. African populations have severalfold-higher average Lp(a) levels than do Caucasian and most Asian populations.
4. The human apo(a) gene is closely linked to the gene for plasminogen on chromosome 6q27 from which it evolved during primate evolution by duplication, deletion, gene conversion, and mutation. Most striking is the enormous expansion of the plasminogen-like kringle IV modules in the gene. Ten types of kringle IV repeats (K IV-1 to K IV-10), which vary in sequence, exist in apo(a), one of which (K IV-2) occurs in variable number (K IV-2 VNTR). Apo(a)/Lp(a) evolved twice independently during vertebrate evolution. An apo(a) gene that has evolved from a PLG K III and contains a variable number of K III repeats is present in the hedgehog. Insectivore apo(a) also forms a disulfide-linked complex with LDL.
5. The number of K IV-2 repeats in apo(a) may vary from 2 to >40, resulting in a genetic size polymorphism of the apo(a) DNA, mRNA, and protein. Determination of the numbers, frequencies, sequence variations, and effects of apo(a) alleles on Lp(a) levels has resulted into some insights into the genetic architecture of the Lp(a) trait, which differs between Africans and Caucasians. Sib-pair linkage and family analyses demonstrated that from 70 percent to >90 percent of the within-population variance in Lp(a) levels is explained by variation at the apo(a) gene locus, but that transacting factors may exist in Africans. The apo(a) effect has been dissected into two components, the K IV-2 repeat variation at the apo(a) locus, which is inversely correlated with Lp(a) levels and explains from 30 to 70 percent of the variability in Lp(a) levels depending on the population, and sequence variation in regulatory and coding sequences. Among these are a +93 C/T polymorphism that introduces an alternative ATG start codon, a 5′ pentanucleotide repeat polymorphism (5′-PNRP) and a splice mutation resulting in a null allele. Mutations in the genes for the LDLR and apo B that cause familial hypercholesterolemia (MIM 143890) or defective apo B (MIM 107730), respectively, may also affect Lp(a) levels.
6. Numerous epidemiologic studies have shown that high Lp(a) in plasma is a primary genetic risk factor for coronary heart disease (CHD), stroke, and peripheral vascular disease, but the suggested mechanisms are largely speculative. Most *in vitro* functions attributable to Lp(a) have also been suggested as an explanation for the pathophysiological properties of Lp(a), and may be responsible for the fatal consequences of excessive Lp(a) levels in human subjects. One is the modulation of the balance between clotting and fibrinolysis at the endothelial cell layer of the blood vessel wall, which results in a prothrombic state. The *in vitro* studies also suggest that a forming fibrin thrombus at a damaged vessel wall has the capacity to bind Lp(a), and an apo(a)/Lp(a) binding site in fibrinogen has been defined. High homocysteine concentrations enhance fibrin binding of Lp(a) and might accelerate thrombus formation. Deposition of apo(a)/apo B complexes in atherosclerotic plaques and coronary vein grafts has been demonstrated. Apo(a)/Lp(a) also induce cellular responses of endothelial cells and smooth muscle cells which are proatherogenic and the identification of ligands for apo(a)/Lp(a) (e.g. β_2-glycoprotein I, fibronectin) may result in new insights into the (patho-)physiological functions of Lp(a). Studies in mice that are transgenic for human apo(a), or double transgenics for the human apo(a) and apo B-100 genes, have generated contradictory results.
7. Lp(a) concentrations may be affected by disease (e.g., end-stage renal disease) and some rare genetic conditions (e.g., familial hypercholesterolemia, MIM 143890) but are only moderately influenced by diet, exercise, or other environmental factors. Most lipid-lowering drugs have no effect on Lp(a) concentration, the only exception being nicotinic acid.

A list of standard abbreviations is located immediately preceding the index in each volume. Additional abbreviations used in this chapter include: apo(a) = apolipoprotein(a); CHD = coronary heart disease; FH = familial hypercholesterolemia; IDL = intermediate-density lipoprotein; K = kringle including K I, K II, etc; LBS = lysine-binding site; LDLR = LDL receptor; Lp(a) = lipoprotein(a); LPL = lipoprotein lipase; MDBP = methylated DNA-binding protein; 5′-PNRP = 5′ pentanucleotide repeat polymorphism; PAI-1 = plasminogen activator inhibitor-1; PLG = plasminogen; SDS-AGE = SDS agarose gel electrophoresis; TGF- = transforming growth factor ; tPA = tissue-plasminogen activator; and VLDLR = VLDL receptor.

Therapeutic plasmapheresis or LDL-/Lp(a)-apheresis may be used in the treatment of severe dyslipidemia with high Lp(a).

HISTORY AND OVERVIEW

Lipoprotein(a) or Lp(a) was detected in 1963 by Kåre Berg[1] and considered an autosomal dominant trait.[2] Shortly after it became apparent that Lp(a) is a distinct particle rather than an allelic variant of LDL.[3–7] This particle occurs in extremely different concentrations, which are genetically determined in the plasma of humans and Old World monkeys.[8] Lp(a) was rediscovered several times and designated "sinking-prebeta lipoprotein,"[9] pre-beta-1 lipoprotein,[10] LDL-a-1,[11] or just a "new" or "atypical" lipoprotein.[12,13]

Lp(a) was purified to homogeneity and characterized in some detail already in the early 1970s,[6,11,14–16] but the nature of the protein components of the complex hindered further detailed studies of Lp(a) until the development of molecular biology techniques. Lp(a) contains a lipoprotein moiety that is essentially a low-density lipoprotein (LDL) and a high-molecular-weight glycoprotein designated apolipoprotein(a) or apo(a).[15,17–19] A breakthrough in Lp(a) research was the cloning and sequencing of apo(a) by Lawn and colleagues that revealed a high degree of homology of apo(a) with plasminogen (PLG).[20] This homology triggered studies on the still elusive function of Lp(a) that demonstrated that both Lp(a) and apo(a) interact with the fibrinolytic cascade at several points *in vitro* and *in vivo* in transgenic mice and may modulate blood clotting[21–25] (Fig. 116-1). Lp(a) has been described as an interloper into the fibrinolytic system.[26] Effects on endothelial and smooth muscle cell functions and the identification of apo(a)/Lp(a) ligands have raised speculations on other roles of Lp(a).[27–32] Whether these *in vitro* findings are of physiological significance that may explain some of the pathogenicity of Lp(a) is still unclear. No deficiency state associated with any pathology has yet been described, but it is known that true congenital Lp(a) deficiency caused by molecularly defined null alleles exists in humans. Rather, high levels of Lp(a) have been implicated in the pathogenesis of atherothrombotic disease.[10,33–40]

Kostner and coworkers[33] were the first to demonstrate high Lp(a) concentrations in patients with myocardial infarction using a quantitative assay. Dozens of case-control studies in different ethnic groups using different quantification methods have confirmed and extended these original observations (see reviews in references 41 to 50), but two of the first published prospective studies[51–55] failed to identify high Lp(a) as an independent risk factor for myocardial infarction.[52,55] Most subsequent prospective studies have, however, identified Lp(a) as an independent predictor of coronary heart disease (CHD) and/or myocardial infarction.[39,40,56–64] Association studies have also related apo(a) isoforms and genomic K IV-2 repeat number in apo(a) to the risk for CHD, thus providing direct evidence for the role of the apo(a) gene in CHD.[62,65–68]

Lp(a) is a quantitative genetic trait. Major gene models[69,70] and a pure polygenic model[71] were proposed to explain the inheritance of Lp(a) concentrations. Today, it is certain that Lp(a) concentrations in the population at large are controlled by a single gene with multiple alleles, each coding for a different concentration.[72–76] This gene is the apo(a) gene that was localized to chromosome 6q27.[77–80] Alleles at the apo(a) locus, which differ in the number of K IV-2 intragenic repeats and in sequence, affect Lp(a) concentrations in an additive fashion, but the effect of many alleles is small or negligible. Other genes, environment, and disease may also effect Lp(a) concentrations. Although not relevant for the general population this may be significant for individuals with some rare genetic conditions such as familial hypercholesterolemia (FH) (MIM 143890; Chap. 120) and genetic defects in apo B (MIM 107730; Chap. 115), or more common disorders such as end-stage renal disease.[81]

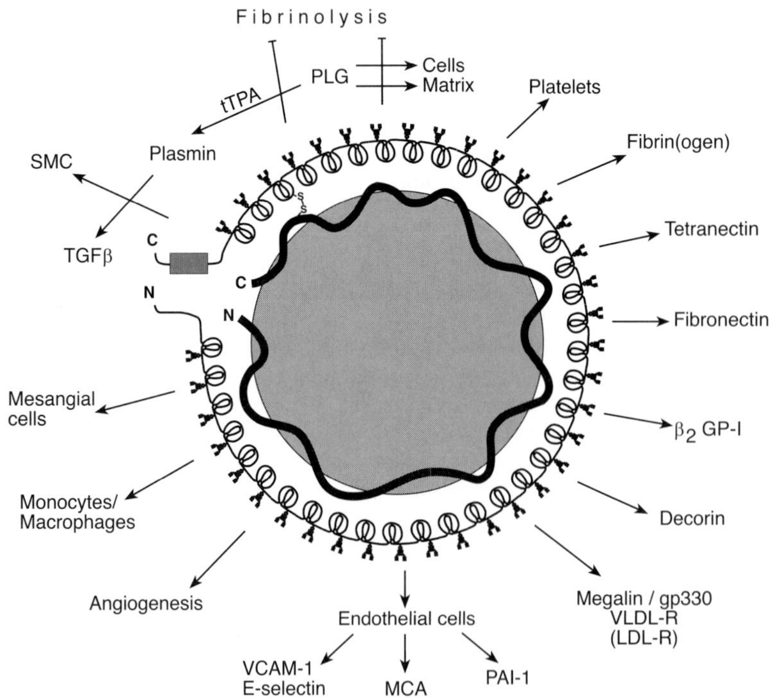

Fig. 116-1 Model of Lp(a) and reported interactions of Lp(a)/apo(a) with components of the fibrinolytic system, cells, receptors and other binding proteins (for explanation see text). The central LDL particle, with its core of neutral lipids and the apo B-100 molecule, is attached to one molecule of apo(a) by a single disulfide bond between one of the K IV repeats (K IV-9) in apo(a) and the C-terminal region of apo B. The exact spatial orientation of the components is unknown and the regularity of carbohydrate chains is a simplification. (*Modified from Utermann.*[8] *Used with permission.*)

STRUCTURE OF LIPOPROTEIN(a)

Lp(a) is a complex that is assembled from two very different components. One component is an LDL particle that contains all the lipid and the 512-kDa hydrophobic apo B-100, which is essentially insoluble in water. The second component is a hydrophilic glycoprotein with a uniquely high degree of conserved internal repeat structure and an enormous size-heterogeneity. Both components, LDL and apo(a), are linked by a single disulfide bond that was localized in one of the repeat structures of apo(a) (kringle IV-9)[20] and in the N-terminal region of apo B-100 (Fig. 116-1).

Isolation of Lipoprotein(a)

The isolation of Lp(a) usually combines stepwise, density gradient, or rate zonal ultracentrifugation[19,82] with chromatographic procedures.[6,11,18,83,84] Lp(a) has a density from 1.04 g/ml to 1.125 g/ml.[85] Fractions from ultracentrifugation are usually contaminated with LDL and HDL components. These are then removed by size-exclusion chromatography,[6,11,18] ion-exchange chromatography,[86,87] passage over lysine-sepharose,[88] hydroxyapatite,[7] or anti-apo(a) affinity columns.[89] These procedures yield a single Lp(a) species from subjects who are homozygous for apo(a) size, but may yield two species with different physicochemical properties in apo(a) heterozygotes. A problem in working with isolated Lp(a) is the ease with which Lp(a) precipitates in the cold or disintegrates once isolated.[15,84,90]

Lp(a) floats as a single or double peak on ultracentrifugation, the density of which depends on the genetic apo(a) type.[85,91] The Lp(a) particle is spherical and approximately 4 million daltons in size with a diameter of approximately 250Å in negative-staining electron microscopy (Table 116-1). Lipids comprise 64 to 74 percent of the particle and 26 to 36 percent of the protein with a relatively large carbohydrate moiety.[18] Lp(a) contains approximately six times more sialic acid than LDL.[15,18] Apo(a) contains *N*- and *O*-linked carbohydrate chains.[82] Under nonreducing conditions, Lp(a) from homozygotes moves as a single band on native gel electrophoresis[92,93] and denaturing SDS-polyacrylamide gel electrophoresis. The mobility in agarose gel electrophoresis of native Lp(a) is between LDL (β-lipoprotein) and VLDL (pre-β-lipoprotein).[14] Upon reduction, Lp(a) disintegrates into an LDL component and apolipoprotein(a).[18,19,82,83,89] Estimated molecular masses for apo(a) range from 280 kDa to greater than 800 kDa.[8,82,94] Studies of circular dichroism demonstrated 8 to 14 percent α helix, 13 to 20 percent β-pleated sheet, and 66 to 71 percent disordered structure in apo(a).[18,82] Some authors have described other protein components as a minor part of Lp(a), including albumin, apo C, apo E, and apo D.[15,16,84,90] It is, however, unclear whether this is due to contamination or reflects transient interactions or the presence of subpopulations of Lp(a).

Table 116-1 Some Characteristics of Lp(a) and Apo(a)

Lp(a)	
IElectrophoretic mobility (agarose)	beta
Buoyant density (g/ml)	1.040–1.131
Isoelectric point (ph)	4.9
Molecular mass (Da)	3.8–4.66 × 10^6
Molecular diameter (Å)	~250
Plasma concentration (mg/dl)*	0.1–120
Protein(g/mol)	~800.000–1.350.000
Free cholesterol (mol/mol)	750
Cholesteryl ester (mol/mol)	2000
Triglycerides (mol/mol)	350
Phospholipids (mol/mol)	1110
Fractional catabolic rate (per day)	0.26–0.306
Plasma $T_{0.5}$ (days)	3.32–3.93
Synthetic rate (mg/kg/day)	4.60 ±3.64 (0.54–11.39)
Apo (a)	
Molecular mass (Da)	300.000–800.000
Amino acids in mature protein$^+$	4529
Carbohydrate (%)	28
Sialic acid (%)	21

*Given as Lp(a) mass in healthy subjects; $^+$ isoform With 37 K IV repeats.[20]

SOURCE: From References 18, 82, 89, 93, 191, 210, 564

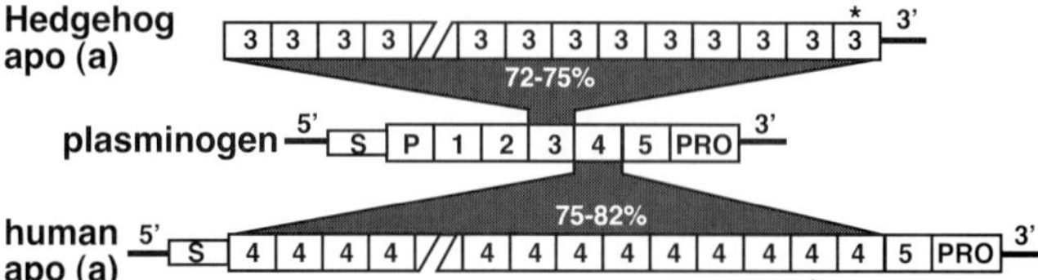

Fig. 116-2 cDNA structures of plasminogen and apo(a) illustrating the convergent evolution of primate and insectivore apo(a). Numbers denote kringle types. Pro = protease domain. The stars indicate the sites of unpaired Cys residues that form the disulfide bridge with apo B in LDL. (*Reproduced from Lawn et al.*[190] *Used with permission.*)

Structure of the LDL Moiety of Lp(a)

The LDL moiety from Lp(a) is obtained by reductive cleavage of Lp(a) with thiols followed by ultracentrifugal separation of the LDL and apo(a).[82,83,89] The lipoprotein contains apo B-100 as the only protein-component, and has been designated Lp(a−).[82] The lipid moiety of Lp(a)-derived LDL is similar to authentic LDL.[82,83] Reportedly, the LDL from Lp(a) is not identical to homologous LDL in that it is larger in size, higher in lipid content, and its density is slightly lower than LDL isolated from the same individual.[19]

Structure of Apolipoprotein(a)

Sequencing of apo(a) at the protein[95,96] and cDNA level[20] revealed a high degree of homology with plasminogen (PLG) (Fig. 116-2). This plasma serine protease of the fibrinolytic system contains a signal sequence followed by five so-called kringle structures (K I to K V) and a protease domain. Kringles are modules whose shape resembles a Danish bretzel (baked good), hence their name.[97] They are sequences of 80 to 90 amino acids arranged in a triple-loop tertiary structure rigidly stabilized by three disulfide bridges. In PLG and apo(a), they are connected by spacer regions, most, but not all, of which are glycosylated in apo(a). Apo(a) is much larger than PLG. This is due to an amplification of one of the plasminogen-like kringles in apo(a) (K IV) which is present in multiple copies with minor sequence variation designated K IV-1 to K IV-10[98] (Fig. 116-3). K IV-1 and K IV-6 have small deletions.[20] The Cys residues in all kringles are conserved. One K IV repeat (K IV-2) does, however, occur in variable numbers, which explains the apo(a) size polymorphism (Fig. 116-3 and see below).

K I to K III homologues are not present and K V is present once in human apo(a), as is the protease domain. The homology at the cDNA level between plasminogen and apo(a) modules is from 75 to 85 percent for the K IV domains, to 94 percent for the protease domain. The signal sequences from both proteins are 100 percent identical.[20] There are, however, also some remarkable structural differences that may have functional significance. One notable difference exists between the protease domains of PLG and apo(a). The activation site Arg-Val in positions 561 to 562 of PLG is exchanged for Ser-Ile [positions 4308 to 4309 in the original apo(a) sequence].[20] This position is the cleavage site essential for maturation of plasminogen to the active protease plasmin. Lack of this site in apo(a) suggests that apo(a) is not involved in plasmin-like protease activity. It has been reported that an alternative site for the proteolytic activation exists in apo(a).[98] The catalytic triad

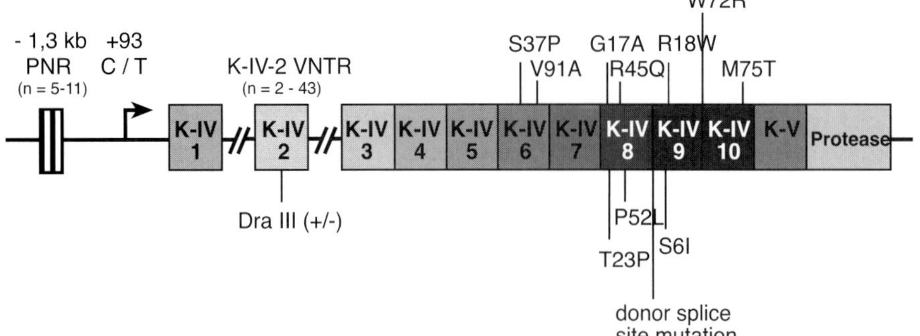

Fig. 116-3 Structure of the apo(a) gene with some polymorphisms. K IV-1 to -10 denote the 10 different types of PLG K IV-related domains and K V, the single K V domain in human apo(a). PNR denotes the pentanucleotide repeat polymorphism in the apo(a) promoter and K IV-2 VNTR denotes the variable number of tandem K IV type 2 repeats. (*Reproduced from Utermann.*[563] *Used with permission.*)

Ser-His-Asp is conserved in the protease domain of human apo(a) but is altered by two substitutions in rhesus apo(a).[99] This suggests that apo(a) has an altered protease activity, if any.

K IV-9 contains an extra, unpaired Cys residue that facilitates disulfide bond formation with a Cys residue in apo B-100. The type of homology of K IV-10 with the lysine-binding K IV from plasminogen suggests that this kringle has lysine binding capacity. Comparative functional studies of Rhesus and human apo(a), which differ at critical positions in the K IV-10 lysine-binding site, and a mutant in human apo(a) support this conclusion.[100,101] Thus the unique kringles K IV-3 to K IV-10 may have distinct functional properties. One is complex formation with LDL.[102–106]

Single apo(a) kringles type IV-1, -2, -9, and -10 have been expressed in bacteria and mammalian cell culture systems and characterized for functional properties (e.g., lysine and fibrin binding).[107–109]

The kringles of apo(a) are joined by linkers that likely influence the structural flexibility of the kringle domains. With the exception of the linkers between the identical K IV-2 repeats, those joining the nonidentical kringles differ in length of the peptide chain from 26- to 36-amino-acid residues. There are also differences in glycosylation status between linkers. Most linkers are predicted to be heavily glycosylated with a predominance of *O*-glycosylation.[110] However linker 4 (which joins K IV-4 and K IV-5) is not predicted to have glycosylation sites, whereas linker 7 also contains one *N*-glycosylation site in addition to being highly *O*-glycosylated. Linker 4 also contains the primary site for elastase cleavage (Ile 3520–Leu 3521 bond). Enzymes of the elastase family have been used to dissect apo(a) and Lp(a) into structural and functional domains.[110,111]

The Lp(a) Particle

Apo(a) can be separated from the LDL moiety of Lp(a) only after reductive cleavage, and apo(a) contains one unpaired Cys residue in its sequence. It has been, therefore, suggested that apo(a) and apo B in LDL are covalently linked by a single disulfide bridge[17–19] and that apo(a) and apo B exist in a molar ratio of 1:1 in Lp(a). This is consistent with most biochemical analysis on the stoichiometry of Lp(a), and also with the finding that apo(a) heterozygotes have two distinct Lp(a) particles in plasma, each containing only one of the respective isoforms.[85,91,112] Physicochemical studies using fluorescent probes that selectively label sulfhydryl groups for quantification of free SH groups in LDL and Lp(a) also indicate that one single disulfide bond exists between apo(a) and apo B-100.[113,114] The most direct evidence for the role of Cys was obtained in experiments in which Hep G2 cells were transfected to express apo(a) corresponding to wild-type apo(a) or to altered apo(a)-containing mutations, which changed the critical Cys residue in K IV-9 (Cys 67; position 4057 in the sequenced apo(a)) to Ser, Gly, or Arg, respectively. Although mutant apo(a) was secreted by the cells, it did not form Lp(a) particles, showing that the Cys residue in K IV-9 is essential for Lp(a) formation.[105,115,116] The Cys residue in apo B, which is critical for formation of the Lp(a) particle, was identified by studies in transgenic mice containing the human apo(a) gene. Such mice do not form an Lp(a) particle due to the inability of mouse apo B to form a stable Lp(a) complex.[117] Lp(a) is only formed if human LDL is injected into such mice,[118] or if the mice are made double transgenics by crossing them with mice transgenic for human apo B-100.[119,120] Injection of VLDL into apo(a)-transgenic mice does not result in a stable covalent VLDL apo(a) complex.[118] By generating mice containing truncated and mutated forms of human apo B and crossing them with the apo(a) transgenic mice, it was shown that the critical Cys residue resides in the C-terminal 10 percent of the apo B sequence.[121,122] Callow et al.[123] and McCormick et al.[124] identified apo B Cys 4326 as the essential residue for Lp(a) complex formation. The data from the transgenic mice work are consistent with cell culture studies and observations in humans with hypobetalipoproteinemia (MIM 107730) due to truncated forms of apo B.[125] The results from the transgenics are, however, in conflict with earlier biochemical and biophysical data that identified apo B Cys 3734 in mediating disulfide linkage with apo(a),[114] and with recent studies of binding of recombinant apo(a) to synthetic apo B peptides.[126] The true site, therefore, is yet to be identified. It is presently unclear how much noncovalent binding contributes to apo(a) binding to LDL after the particle has formed. It has been shown that K IV types 5 to 8 are involved in the noncovalent docking of apo(a) to LDL that precedes the disulfide-bridge formation.[102,103,105,115,127–129] Images from atomic force microscopy suggest that apo(a) is attached to LDL at two sites, with its N- and C-terminal domains. The sequences and mode of interaction of the putative C-terminal binding region have not been further studied. Transfection studies have identified in apo B-100 another apo(a) binding site that is involved in noncovalent binding in N-terminal sequences in apo B between amino acid residues 680 and 781.[130] Besides the apo(a)/apo B interactions, there also seem to exist interkringle interactions that are stabilized by chloride ions and are critical for the mechanisms of Lp(a) particle assembly.[131] Results from small-angle x-ray-scattering studies of Lp(a) suggest that apo(a) is placed above the surface of the LDL moiety and is wrapped around the particle. No evidence for major globular domains projecting into the aqueous phase was obtained.[132] This also strongly suggests that in addition to the covalent disulfide linkage, other noncovalent interactions between apo(a) and LDL are required to maintain apo(a) close to the lipoprotein surface. Lp(a) can, however, undergo a conformational change from this compact form to an open, extended structure on binding the lysine analogue 6-aminohexamoic acid and several other amino acid analogs.[131]

A study using hydrodynamic techniques and electron microscopy also suggested that in addition to the apo(a)-apo B disulfide bond, strong noncovalent forces hold the Lp(a) molecule together.[133] These authors did, however, conclude that the bulk of apo(a) is extended away from the lipoprotein surface. This model is attractive because it allows ready interaction of a floating "N-terminal tail" of apo(a) with ligands.

It has been shown that Lp(a) binds to LDL and VLDL *in vitro*,[134,135] suggesting noncovalent binding of apo(a) to LDL/VLDL. The binding of Lp(a)/apo(a) to other apo B-containing lipoproteins is probably mediated by the K IV domains of apo(a). L-Proline and hydroxyproline, but not L-lysine, inhibit the binding of apo(a) to LDL.[136]

Apo(a) and Apo(a) Fragments in Non-Lp(a) Plasma Fractions

Apo(a) has been demonstrated in triglyceride-rich lipoproteins and as "free" apo(a) in lipoprotein-deficient serum prepared by ultracentrifugation ["bottom" fraction apo(a)].[137–140] In most healthy subjects, the relative concentration of apo(a) in these fractions is comparatively small, ranging from <1 percent to ~16 percent in the triglyceride-rich lipoproteins and from <1 percent to ~17 percent in the lipid-poor bottom.[137,141,142] The nature and origin of apo(a) in triglyceride-rich lipoproteins and the significance of its presence in this fraction has remained controversial. Apo(a) was demonstrated in triglyceride-rich postprandial lipoproteins believed to represent chylomicrons, and an intestinal origin of Lp(a) was postulated.[138] However, >95 percent of Lp(a) in plasma is derived from the liver and not from the intestine or other sources.[143]

The percentage of apo(a) associated with triglyceride-rich lipoprotein (including IDL) is moderately elevated and two- to threefold higher in patients with lipoprotein (LPL) deficiency (MIM 238600; Chap. 117) and type III hyperlipoproteinemia (MIM 107741; Chap. 119) as compared to controls.[141] This increase has been explained to result from the affinity of Lp(a) particles to triglyceride-rich lipoproteins, which has been demonstrated *in vitro*.[134,135,141] Apo(a)/Lp(a) with high-molecular-weight isoforms does preferentially associate with triglyceride-rich lipoproteins.[139,141] This was demonstrated in healthy fasting subjects[141] in the postprandial phase,[138,139] and in subjects with type III hyperlipoproteinemia (MIM 107741).[138,141] The association of Lp(a) with triglyceride-rich lipoproteins may have pathophysiological consequences. Kostner and Grillhofer[144] showed that apo(a)/Lp(a) stimulates the binding of LDL to fibroblasts several-fold by an LDLR-independent mechanism.

The origin, and relation to Lp(a) of apo(a) in the lipid-poor fractions is also unclear. Recent studies demonstrate that most, if not all, free apo(a) in plasma exists as apo(a) fragments.[145] Apo(a) fragments are also excreted into human urine.[145–148] Plasma apo(a) fragments range in size from ~125 kDa to 360 kDa.[145] Smaller fragments (~85 kDa to 215 kDa) are present in the urine from healthy individuals.[145,147] The concentration of apo(a) fragments in plasma and urine correlates with Lp(a) plasma concentration. However, even individuals with no detectable apo(a) in plasma had apo(a) fragments in urine. NH_2-terminal sequence analysis revealed sequences specific for the K IV-1 repeat and clarified that the fragments represent N-terminal sequences and contain the repetitive K IV-2 domain. Immunoblot analysis showed that they do not contain the protease domain and K IV-9.[147] These findings are intriguing for two reasons. First, they have resulted in speculations about a possible role of apo(a) fragments as active peptides because they share a high degree of homology with angiostatin, a proteolytic fragment of PLG K IV. Angiostatin inhibits angiogenesis, vascularization, and cell proliferation.[149] Although no such activity has yet been reported for proteolytic apo(a) fragments, it has been proposed that Lp(a) can induce angiogenesis *in vitro*.[150]

Second, occurrence of apo(a) fragments in urine may support claims that the human kidney is involved in Lp(a)/apo(a) catabolism.[81] It is unclear how the apo(a) fragments in plasma and urine are generated and whether they are cleavage products of unassembled free apo(a) or of apo(a) from Lp(a). Scanu and coworkers extensively studied the susceptibility of Lp(a) to protease digestion and demonstrated that cleavage by enzymes (e.g., elastase) may generate a "mini Lp(a)" containing LDL and the C-terminal kringles and protease domain of apo(a). The cleavage site was identified in the linker region between K IV-4 and K IV-5.[110] Kostner et al.[151] suggested that Lp(a) might be converted by a collagenase-like activity to a "mini-Lp(a)" containing the C-terminus of apo(a), which is rapidly removed by the liver, and a N-terminal apo(a) fragment, which is further degraded by an activity in the kidney followed by excretion of the fragments into the urine.

A special situation exists in patients with autosomal recessive abetalipoproteinemia (MIM 200100; Chap. 115) in which intact apo(a) is almost exclusively present in the lipid-deficient fraction and most apo(a) forms a complex with apo B-100.[152] An apo(a)/apo B complex has also been demonstrated in the lipoprotein-free fraction of supernatants from Hep G2 cells that were transfected to express apo(a).[153] Patients with abetalipoproteinemia (MIM 200100) have a deficiency in the intracellular triglyceride transfer protein[154] and Hep G2 cells are defective in the secretion of triglyceride-rich lipoproteins (VLDL). Apo B is entirely water insoluble and degraded intracellularly if not assembled with lipids. Scanu and coworkers[155] studied the properties of a lipid-free apo(a)/apo B-100 complex and demonstrated that this complex is essentially soluble in water. The occurrence of a lipid-free apo(a) apo B-100 complex in abetalipoproteinemia plasma may, therefore, indicate that apo(a) can assemble with apo B in the ER if apo B is not assembled into VLDL.

Chromosomal Localization, Structure, and Regulatory Elements of the Apo(a) Gene Region

Apo(a) is a member of a superfamily of trypsin-like serine proteases.[45,156] There exist at least seven genes or pseudogenes that are closely related to apo(a), including plasminogen,[20] hepatocyte growth factors I and II on chromosome 7,[157] and apo(a)-related genes or pseudogenes.[158–164] The genes for plasminogen and apo(a) were assigned to the telomeric region of chromosome 6 (6q27) by *in situ* hybridization.[77,165] Linkage analysis has shown that apo(a) is in close proximity to plasminogen.[78–80] These linkage data have been confirmed by the analysis of YAC clones.[158,166–168] The apo(a) and plasminogen genes are about 50 kb apart and oriented in opposite directions.[158] The analysis of YAC and P 1 clones further demonstrated that the leader sequence of apo(a) is separated from the first kringle in apo(a) by a ~14-kb intron.[158,161] The complete genomic structure of the apo(a) gene, which spans >120 kb, will become available with the sequencing of the human genome.

The intron-exon structure of the K IV repeats 1 and 3 to 10 has been reported,[169] and the intron-exon structure of the variable apo(a) K IV-2 repeat domain in apo(a) has been studied by PCR-amplification. The coding region for one K IV-2 is split into two exons of 162 bp (exon 1) and 180 bp (exon 2) by the 4.2-kb intron 1. A 1.4-kb intron 2 is located between the 3′ end of exon 2 and the 5′ end of exon 1.[73,170] The total size of a genomic kringle K IV-2 repeat is ~5.6 kb.[8,73,170] Southern blotting of genomic DNA digested with different restriction enzymes (*Pvu*II, *Eco*RI, *Bam*H1, *Bgl*II) and probing with an apo(a) K IV-specific oligonucleotide results in only one major 5.6-kb fragment. This suggests that not only the exon but also the intron sequences in the K IV-2 repeats have a high degree of internal homology that most likely is a result of gene conversions or unequal crossing over. There exist, however, at least three types of K IV-2 repeats, designated K IV-2A, B, and C[20] (W. Parson, H.G. Kraft, G. Utermann, unpublished), which differ by silent base substitutions in exons, and a polymorphic *Dra*III site that is present in some K IV-2 introns.[171]

The regulatory 5′ region of the gene has been characterized to some extent.[172,173] Binding sites for several transcription factors, including hepatocyte nuclear factor-1α (HNF-1α),[174] and sex hormones have been identified.[175] A retinoid response element has also been identified in the apo(a) promoter.[176] An apo(a) enhancer region that resides in a LINE element has been observed in the intergenic region between apo(a) and PLG.[177,178]

APO(A) IN NON-HUMAN SPECIES AND EVOLUTION OF THE APO(a) GENE

The primate apo(a) gene most likely arose from a plasminogen gene by duplication, deletion, gene conversion, and point mutations.[20]

It has been calculated that these genes diverged some 40 million years ago during primate evolution at a time when Old and New World monkey lineages also diverged.[20] This agreed with the observation at the time that apo(a) is present in humans, nonhuman primates, and Old World monkeys, but not in New World monkeys, prosimians, or lower mammals. Lp(a) has been demonstrated in chimpanzee,[179] gorilla, orangutan,[180] gibbon, rhesus,[99,181] baboon,[182,183] cynomolgus monkey,[181,184] savannah monkey, pig-tailed monkey, Japanese monkey, and crab-eating monkey.[185,186] There exist striking sequence differences in apo(a) from different species, which differences affect critical residues (see "Structure of Apolipoprotein(a)" above). K V is not present in rhesus apo(a).[99] The view that Lp(a) did not evolve before the evolution of Old World monkeys was challenged when Laplaud et al.[187] demonstrated apo(a) and Lp(a) in the hedgehog (*Erinnaceus europeans*), which is an insectivore that diverged from other mammals about 140 million years ago.[156] This species distribution is unusual and resulted in some confusion. Using the published apo(a) sequence data, Ikeo et al.[188] and Pesole et al.[189] recalculated the time of divergence between apo(a) and PLG and arrived at a dating of ~80 million years ago. This dating implied that apo(a) appeared at almost the same time as the mammalian divergence. Thus, the evolutionary origin of apo(a) from PLG seemed clear, but not the time of the occurrence of this gene in evolution. The cloning of hedgehog apo(a) and the elucidation of its cDNA structure by Lawn et al.[156,190] yielded a surprising and important result, and clarified the situation. Apo(a) and Lp(a) were invented twice during mammalian evolution (Fig. 116-2). However, whereas PLG K I to K III was lost and K IV has expanded during primate apo(a) evolution, the insectivore apo(a) is made exclusively from K III-like repeats with 74 to 100 percent homology to plasminogen K III. The hedgehog apo(a) contains neither PLG KI, KII, KIV, or KV homologues, nor a protease domain. As true of its primate counterpart, the hedgehog apo(a) seems variable in the number of kringle repeats, as suggested by its protein-size polymorphism.[187] It does, however, contain a single unpaired Cys in one of the K III repeats, which presumably forms the disulfide bridge with apo B in hedgehog LDL. This detail is of special relevance. Whereas primate PLG K IV does not contain an unpaired Cys, hedgehog K III does. Thus, one expanded K IV repeat in the primate lineage had to acquire an unpaired Cys, whereas in the insectivore, all expanded K III repeats except one had to loose their unpaired Cys to create an apo(a) molecule with the ability to form a single disulfide bond with apo B and, hence, an Lp(a) particle. This is a striking example of recurrent and convergent evolution and supports the idea that strong selective pressure has resulted in the evolution of Lp(a). The nature of this selective pressure is unknown, but if it is understood, it may shed light on the physiological function of Lp(a).[156]

Presence of two different "apo(a)" genes in different mammalian species raises the intriguing possibility that still other forms of apo(a) may be present in species believed not to have apo(a)/Lp(a). Such genes or their products may be undetectable by human DNA probes or by antibodies against the human protein.

METABOLISM OF LP(a)

Synthesis and Assembly of Lp(a)

The major determinant of plasma Lp(a) concentration is the rate of synthesis of apo(a),[191,192] rather than the degradation of Lp(a). Apo(a) mRNA is present in significant amounts only in liver, and in minor amounts in testis, brain, adrenals, lung, and pituitary from humans and monkeys.[20,99] Because the liver is the only one of these organs that also produces apo B, it is the only organ that has the potential to assemble Lp(a). Direct evidence for the role of the liver in apo(a) production comes from studies of patients undergoing therapeutic liver transplantation. Such patients may change their genetic apo(a) type completely following transplantation and acquire the phenotype of the liver donor.[143] Primary baboon hepatocytes produce Lp(a)[193] when cultured in serum-free medium. Although this has established the liver as the major site of apo(a) synthesis, it is less clear where apo(a) is assembled with lipoproteins to form Lp(a). Theoretically, assembly of Lp(a) may occur within liver cells or in the plasma compartment. Because both apo(a)- and apo B-containing lipoproteins exit the cell through the secretory pathway, there seems no *a priori* reason why assembly should not occur in the ER or Golgi where many other macromolecules are formed. The development of a line of mice transgenic for the human apo(a) gene suggests that assembly of Lp(a) may occur in plasma. The mice expressed a single apo(a) isoform containing K IV-9 with the only unpaired Cys residue in apo(a). Less than 5 percent of apo(a) in mouse plasma was associated with lipoproteins, whereas most was present as free apo(a). Mouse LDL apparently lacks structural elements required for association with human apo(a).[117,118,194] Intravenous injections into the mice of human LDL, but not of mouse LDL or human HDL, resulted in the rapid association of apo(a) with the human LDL.[118] The apo(a) LDL complexes formed within 1 min and were resistant to boiling in the presence of SDS and urea but, as in authentic Lp(a), dissociated upon disulfide reduction. Apo(a) LDL-complexes with the same characteristics and stability could also be formed *in vitro* by incubation of transgenic mouse plasma with human LDL. This suggests that the specific interaction between human apo(a) and human LDL may occur in plasma also *in vivo*. A further interesting aspect of the lipoprotein/apo(a) association studies in transgenic mice is that human VLDL when injected into the animals associated with apo(a) at a much slower rate than LDL. Increase of apo(a) binding parallels the loss of apo E from VLDL suggesting that apo(a) associates with a catabolic product of VLDL and not with VLDL itself. This catabolic product most likely is LDL. This observation is consistent with results in humans with type I hyperlipidemia (MIM 238600; Chap. 117) and type III hyperlipidemia (MIM 107741; Chap. 119), which suggest that there is no triglyceride-rich VLDL-like precursor of Lp(a) in human plasma.[141]

Although all these data perfectly agree with the idea that Lp(a) is formed in plasma by association of secreted free apo(a) with circulating LDL, there are, unfortunately, some findings that do not support such a scenario. *In vivo* turnover studies using stable isotopes recently demonstrated that apo B in Lp(a) is derived from a pool that is metabolically different from the pool from which LDL is derived.[195] The synthetic rates of apo(a) and apo B in Lp(a) are identical and different from the synthetic rate of apo B in LDL.[196] In earlier studies, Krempler et al.[197] showed that ^{131}I-labeled apo B in VLDL is not converted into apo B in Lp(a), and concluded that VLDL apo B is not a precursor for Lp(a) apo B. Together these turnover studies suggest that *in vivo* human apo(a) is not associated with preexisting LDL in plasma. Although this suggests an intracellular assembly of Lp(a), most investigators were unable to find evidence for intracellular apo(a)/apo B complexes.[198,199] Instead, there is increasing evidence from cell-culture experiments that Lp(a) is assembled at the hepatocyte cell surface.[200]

Original studies in apo(a)-transfected CHO cells demonstrated that apo(a) is secreted into the cell media and can form a covalent (Cys 4057 mediated) complex with exogenously added LDL.[127] However, CHO cells do not synthesize apo B. Therefore, such experiments could not rule out an intracellular assembly and other cell model systems had to be used. Two types of experiments were performed to investigate the site of assembly in cells that produce both apo(a) and apo B-100. One was the addition of antibodies against apo B or apo(a) to the cell culture media during secretion, which completely blocked Lp(a) formation in the baboon hepatocyte model and apo(a) transfected HepG2 cells.[200,201] These results strongly argue for an extracellular Lp(a) assembly. The second were studies in HepG2 cells stably transfected to express apo(a) in which the secretory pathway was inhibited at restricted temperatures. Neither at 15°C, where secretory proteins are retained in the ER, nor at 20°C, where the exit of proteins from the *trans*-Golgi network is blocked, were there any apo(a)/apo B-100 complexes detectable in the cell lysates although apo(a) accumulated in the respective cellular compartments (in particular at +20°C as mature protein in the *trans*-Golgi network (TGN)).

Further, transient transfection of HepG2 cells with to express apo(a) containing a KDEL tag as an ER retention signal did result in the expected accumulation of apo(a) precursor in the ER, but not in intracellular apo(a)/apo B complex formation.[198] Apo(a)/B-100 complexes were also not detected in lysates from human liver biopsies.[198] In contrast, Bonen et al.[202] reported the occurrence of an intracellular apo(a)/apoB complex in transfected HepG2 cells, and Edelstein et al.[203] observed such complexes in lysates from primary human liver cultures. The formation of apo(a)/apo B-100 complexes was stimulated by oleate which is known to prevent apo B-100 intracellular degradation and increase apo B-100 secretion from cells.[204] Oleate also stimulated the secretion of apo(a) from transfected HepG2 cells, which suggests that apo(a) secretion and Lp(a) production are coupled to triglyceride synthesis.[205] However Bonen et al.[202] used a recombinant apo(a) construct in their experiments that codes for an apo(a) minigene containing only some of the kringles present in human apo(a). Their data may therefore not reflect a physiological situation. Together the cell culture studies therefore provide strong evidence against an intracellular assembly of Lp(a). Hence there is a conflict between the *in vitro* cell culture results that have excluded intracellular assembly of Lp(a) and the *in vivo* turnover data that are incompatible with the assembly of newly secreted apo(a) with circulating LDL. One reason for the conflicting results is that the cell systems used do not secrete LDL under the experimental conditions, but rather secrete VLDL that is converted to LDL only after secretion. Hence, there is no intracellular LDL for assembly.

Another possible solution to the puzzle is the recent observation by White et al.[200] that Lp(a) assembly may take place at the hepatocyte cell surface where apo(a) is transiently attached to the plasma membrane. A scenario in which newly secreted apo(a) and LDL meet at the site of exit from the cell would be compatible with most experimental data but there is no known example for a similar mechanism. Recently, it was demonstrated that a drug (Neomycin) that is known to reduce Lp(a) concentrations *in vivo*[206] inhibits the release of apo(a) from the baboon hepatocyte plasma membrane.[207] These data support the concept of a cell surface assembly of Lp(a) and may also guide the way to more potent Lp(a)-lowering drugs.

The assembly of Lp(a) is a two-step process that starts with the docking of apo(a) to the LDL. This first step is mediated by the unique K IV-5 to K IV-9 domain of apo(a).[102,103,105,127] Sequences in K IV-6 and K IV-8, as well as the spacing between these kringle, are believed to be critical.[104] As a second step, the disulfide between K IV-9 Cys 67 and apo B Cys 4326 is formed.[115,123,124] Complex formation occurs *in vivo* in human apo(a) and apo B-100 transgenic mice[119,120] as well as *in vitro*, and seems not to require enzymatic activity or chaperoning.

The rate of secretion of apo(a)/Lp(a) by liver cells determines the concentration of Lp(a) in plasma,[191] which, in turn, is under almost complete genetic control by the apo(a) locus. This means that the rate of synthesis of apo(a)/Lp(a) in a subject is genetically fixed.

Catabolism of Lp(a)

The site(s) and mechanism(s) of Lp(a) removal from plasma are still unclear. Lp(a) contains apo B-100, which is a ligand for the LDLR.[208] Hence, the LDLR, which is most abundant on liver cells, had been considered as a prime candidate for Lp(a) clearance from plasma. Unfortunately, evidence for the role of the LDLR in Lp(a) removal is controversial. Studies on the binding of Lp(a) to LDL receptors in cell culture indicate that Lp(a) is a poor ligand for the receptor.[83,209–213] Mice transgenic for the human LDL receptor under the control of the metallothionein-promoter do, however, rapidly clear Lp(a) when Rs are up-regulated and Lp(a) binds to LDL-receptors on ligand blots.[211] The situation in the LDLR transgenics may be rather unphysiological compared to the *in vivo* situation in humans. Mice have very-low LDL concentrations and human LDLRs were overexpressed in the animals. Accordingly, injected Lp(a) was cleared within 20 min, whereas the half-life of Lp(a) in human plasma is 3 to 4 days.[191,192,210] In line with the results in the transgenic mice, initial studies of unrelated patients with defects in the LDLR gene (familial hypercholesterolemia, MIM 143890; Chap. 120) have shown two- to threefold elevated Lp(a) concentrations in plasma.[214–216] However, these observations in unrelated FH patients were not or only partially confirmed by initial family studies.[217–219] Only recent investigations using a sib-pair approach and apo(a) genotype information have clarified the situation and shown that Lp(a) levels are, indeed, elevated in FH (MIM 143890)[220] and also in familial defective apo B-100 (FDB) (MIM 107730).[221] These studies have also shown that the variability in Lp(a) levels is increased in patients with FH and FDB.[220,221] The elevation of Lp(a) in FH patients is not evidence for a role for this receptor in Lp(a) removal from plasma. Rather, the higher levels and greater variability of Lp(a) might be a consequence of a more general metabolic disturbance in FH. This conclusion is supported by the lack of any significant effect of HMG CoA reductase inhibitors on Lp(a) levels. These drugs effectively lower LDL concentrations through an up-regulation of LDLR activity, but have no effect on Lp(a). Kostner and coworkers suggested that Lp(a) may associate with LDL and is removed by an LDL-mediated hitch-hike mechanism.[222,223]

Some recent observations implicate the kidney as a site for apo(a)/Lp(a) degradation and removal. Lp(a) levels are significantly elevated in kidney disease[81] and proteolytic apo(a) fragments occur in the urine of healthy individuals.[145–147,224] The size of the largest apo(a) fragments in urine (215 kDa) suggests an active transport mechanism. The quantitative contribution of the kidney to Lp(a) removal calculated from urinary excretion of apo(a) fragments is, however, far too small to account for the total decay in Lp(a). Kronenberg et al.[225] have measured the arteriovenous difference in Lp(a) concentrations between the ascending aorta and renal vein in patients with normal kidney function and found a significant decrease in Lp(a) levels in the venous branch of the renal circulation. This could suggest an active role of the kidney in Lp(a) removal, although the quantitative aspects need to be clarified as well as the site and mechanism of a potential uptake. Renal cells are exposed to the blood flow and hence to circulating Lp(a) in the glomeruli. Immunohistochemistry of renal tissue sections has detected apo(a) immunoreactivity in glomerular areas,[226,227] and uptake of Lp(a) by cultural human mesangial cells has been demonstrated.[228] Glomerular apo(a) deposits were only present in tissues from patients with renal disease, and mesangial uptake was less for Lp(a) than LDL. Therefore, it is unclear whether these observations, which may have pathophysiological implications, are of any physiological relevance.

As alternative routes for Lp(a) clearance several other mechanisms and receptors have been proposed but none operate *in vivo*. Among these are binding to and uptake by macrophages.[229]

Uptake and degradation of native Lp(a) and apo(a) by the macrophage apo(a) receptor requires preloading of macrophages with cholesterol which converts them to foam cells.[230] Receptor activity is down-regulated by γ-interferon.[231] The physiological significance of the regulation by cholesterol and cytokine and the molecular identity of the receptor are unclear. Studies using deletion mutants of apo(a) suggest that binding of apo(a) to the macrophage site is mediated by K IV domains 6 to 7.[232,233] Other members from the LDLR family have also been identified to bind Lp(a)/apo(a) *in vitro*. These multifunctional receptors which bind several ligands include the VLDLR[234] and gp 300/megalin.[235] The VLDLR is expressed predominantly in heart and skeletal muscle and, to a lesser extent, in ovaries, kidneys, endothelial cells, and macrophages in humans.[236–238] *In vitro* the apo(a)-mediated binding, internalization and degradation of Lp(a) by the VLDLR leads to lipid accumulation in macrophages, which indicates this receptor in atherogenesis. Niemeier et al.[235] recently used mouse embryonic yolk sac cells from normal and gp 330 knockout mice to demonstrate Lp(a) binding to gp 330 that was blocked by RAP, an inhibitor of ligand binding to several members of the LDLR family, including gp 330.

For several reasons gp 330/megalin is an attractive candidate for a physiological role in Lp(a)/apo(a) metabolism. This receptor, which is expressed by polarized cells, is the only LDLR family member known to bind LDL and the apo(a) homologue plasmin. However, because gp 330 is exclusively expressed in polarized epithelial cells that are not known to be exposed to Lp(a) *in vivo*, it is unclear whether Lp(a) binding to gp 330 is of physiological significance. An appealing idea is that gp 330 might be involved in renal metabolism of apo(a) fragments. In the kidney, gp 330 is expressed in the apical domain of proximal tubular cells.[239] Although these cells are not exposed to intact Lp(a) *in vivo* their apical site is flooded by primary urine, which contains proteolytic peptides of apo(a).[147] Hence this receptor might be involved in the reuptake of apo(a) fragments from urine.

An interesting observation is that lipoprotein lipase (LPL) seems to have a profound effect on Lp(a) uptake and degradation by cells *in vitro*. The cellular degradation of Lp(a) was found increased by 277 percent $\pm$ 3.8 percent and cell association by 509 percent $\pm$ 8.7 percent in the presence of LPL.[240] The effect of LPL on Lp(a) degradation did not require LPL enzymatic activity and had two components, one LDLR-dependent and the other LDLR independent. The LPL-enhanced LDLR-independent cell association and degradation of Lp(a) was heparinase-sensitive. The enhanced degradation was entirely lysosomal. This suggests that LPL promotes the binding of Lp(a) to cell-surface heparan sulfate proteoglycans. Other lipoproteins (e.g., chylomicron remnants) are taken up by cells through a concerted interaction with proteoglycans, lipase, and LDLR-related protein.[241,242] In analogy, Lp(a) uptake may be mediated by a novel catabolic pathway allowing substantial cellular and interstitial removal of Lp(a), independent of feedback inhibition by cellular sterol content.[240]

The *in vivo* metabolism of radioiodinated Lp(a) has been studied by Krempler et al.[191,197,210] and Rader et al..[192,243,244] The rate of Lp(a) catabolism was slower than for LDL but did not correlate with Lp(a) plasma concentration suggesting that differences in synthesis rather than in catabolism determine genetic differences in Lp(a) levels. Similar results were obtained when the reoccurrence of Lp(a) in plasma after therapeutic LDL-plasmapheresis was studied.[245] Furthermore, Lp(a) species containing apo(a) isoforms with different numbers of K IV-2 repeats were identical in their fractional catabolic rate.[243]

The regulation of Lp(a) concentrations is independent from the regulation of other apo B-containing lipoprotein and Lp(a) levels are not associated or correlated with any other lipoproteins or metabolic markers except triglycerides.[246–248] Several conditions exist where Lp(a) and other apo B-containing lipoprotein are regulated in opposite directions (e.g., in kidney disease, Lp(a) concentrations rise, whereas LDL and apo B concentrations fall). The opposite is true following renal transplantation. Several drugs affect Apo B but not Lp(a) metabolism (see "Therapeutic Approach to High Lp(a)").

PHYSIOLOGY AND PATHOPHYSIOLOGY OF LP(a)

Most *in vitro* functional properties attributed to Lp(a) have also been related to its pathophysiology. These aspects are discussed here.

The extensive homology of apo(a) with plasminogen raises the possibility that Lp(a) may function as a modulator of the blood-clotting process. If so, this might also partly explain the pathogenicity of the Lp(a) particle. The role of Lp(a) in blood coagulation/fibrinolysis has been extensively studied,[21–26,249] but attempts to demonstrate a physiological function in humans have not met with unequivocal results. Observations in apo(a) transgenic mice have demonstrated an *in vivo* effect of apo(a) on fibrinolysis,[250] but the situation in the transgenics may not reflect the physiological situation in humans because the mice (a) express apo(a) but do not form Lp(a) and (b) may express apo(a) in cells (e.g., endothelial cells) that do not express apo(a) in humans. Under *in vitro* conditions both Lp(a) and apo(a) interfere with several steps in the complex biochemical cascades that, in their concerted action, regulate the balance between clotting and fibrinolysis (Fig. 116-1). The reported *in vitro* functions of Lp(a)/apo(a) may shift this balance either way and thereby result in more or less tendency for clotting.

Apo(a) itself has no plasmin-like fibrinolytic activity. It does however inhibit the streptokinase-mediated activation of human plasminogen[21] and the conversion of plasminogen to plasmin. Streptokinase is a nonphysiological plasminogen activator, but these initial studies suggested that Lp(a) may also inhibit physiological activators such as urokinase and tissue-type plasminogen activator (t-PA). Inhibition of t-PA and urokinase-mediated activation of plasminogen by Lp(a) has been demonstrated.[46,251–254] Lp(a) inhibits t-PA in solution in the presence of soluble fibrin and competes with plasminogen and t-PA binding for soluble fibrin. As a result, Lp(a) is expected to inhibit the stimulation of plasminogen activation by t-PA.[251,254–256]

Rouy et al.[257] demonstrated that Lp(a) impairs the generation of plasmin by fibrin-bound t-PA. Their *in vitro* study was performed in a plasma milieu. In similar experiments, it was shown that hedgehog Lp(a) is a modulator of activation of plasminogen at the fibrin surface supporting the data obtained in the human system.[258] This is of particular interest in view of the recent demonstration that hedgehog apo(a) has evolved by independent evolution and, compared to primate apo(a), contains a PLG K III instead of a PLG K IV homologue.[190]

Fibrinolysis is a surface-controlled process resulting in the plasmin-catalyzed proteolysis of fibrin and hence in clot dissolution. The fibrinolytic system connected to the surface of endothelial cells plays a critical role in thromboregulation *in vivo*. Endothelial cells secrete t-PA in culture that binds to different sites at the endothelial cell plasma membrane.[259–261] Glu-PLG, which is the main circulating fibrinolytic zymogen, also binds specifically to PLG receptors that have a very high density at the endothelial cell surface.[262] Lp(a) inhibits Glu-PLG binding to the endothelial cell receptor and consequently plasmin generation and thereby interferes with endothelial cell-surface-connected fibrinolysis.[23,24] Gonzalez-Grondow et al.[22] showed that the PLG-2 isoform of PLG binds with a much higher affinity to the receptor than PLG-1. It is the binding of the PLG-2 isoform that is inhibited by Lp(a).[22]

A particularly attractive hypothesis is that Lp(a) may bind to fibrin by the kringles in apo(a), thus delivering cholesterol to sites of recent injury and wound healing.[263] Indeed, apo(a) has been immunolocalized in wounded tissues.[264] Several studies investigated the interaction of Lp(a) and apo(a) with fibrin and its effect on fibrinolysis and dissolution of fibrin clots. Plasminogen activators enhance the binding of Glu-PLG to a fibrin clot.[265–267] It is the plasmin that is formed by plasminogen activation that induces modification in fibrin, which, in turn, creates plasminogen-binding sites.[267] Thus the serine protease plasmin participates in a positive feedback control mechanism that increases the binding of its zymogen, plasminogen, to fibrin and also to fibrinogen. Harpel and collegues[25] demonstrated that plasmin treatment of immobilized fibrinogen and fibrin also results in the exposure of binding sites for Lp(a). They reported, however, that fibrin-bound Lp(a) promotes plasminogen binding but inhibits fibrin degradation by plasmin.[268] As for PLG, this binding is dependent from a lysine-binding site (LBS) and is inhibited by ε-aminocaproic acid. PLG and Lp(a) compete for this site(s) because Lp(a) inhibits the binding of Glu-PLG to immobilized plasmin-modified fibrinogen. This indicates that Lp(a) binds to the dissolving clot. Originally, it was suggested that Lp(a) does not bind to unmodified fibrin or fibrinogen. Recombinant apo(a) containing 17 K IV repeats, including all the unique K IV sequences, however, binds to native and plasmin degraded fibrin.[269]

The domain in apo(a) that mediates binding to fibrin/fibrinogen is still in dispute. Rouy et al.[269] concluded that the K IV domains of apo(a) are functionally heterogeneous in terms of fibrin binding. Putative lysine-binding sites have been identified in kringles IV-5, -6, -8, and -10 by modeling studies using plasminogen K IV for comparison.[270] K IV-10 contains the LBS that most closely resembles that of plasminogen K IV.

The prototype fibrin binding kringle from PLG contains anionic Asp 55 and Asp 57 interacting with cationic Arg 34 and Arg 71. Furthermore, hydrophobic aromatic residues Trp 62, Phe 64, and especially Trp 72 are believed to play an important role in fibrin binding. All apo(a) K IV modules contain Arg at position 31 and most at position 71. The critical Trp 72 is also conserved in each K IV from apo(a). Only K IV-10 from apo(a) contains the important pair of Asp residues at positions 55 and 57, suggesting that this kringle is responsible for lysine binding. An LBS has been identified in K IV-10 and this site is believed to mediate the interaction with plasmin modified fibrin, although this view is not shared by all.[100] Several studies provide clear evidence that apo(a) K IV-10 is involved in the lysine-binding properties of Lp(a).[101,108,128,271,272] Moreover, a natural Trp72 → Arg mutation in human K IV-10, and the same substitution introduced into recombinant apo(a) by *in vitro* mutagenesis, results in a loss of binding of apo(a) to lysine-sepharose.[128] In contrast, Scanu and Edelstein[273] and Klezovitch[100] concluded from binding studies with human and rhesus apo(a) (which has Trp 72 replaced by Arg in the analogous kringle) that the binding to plasmin-modified fibrin is facilitated by a Lys/Pro-sensitive site in the K IV-6 to 9 domain of apo(a) and that the K IV-10 LBS is not involved in fibrin binding. Recently, deletion analysis identified K IV-8 as a critical domain mediating the binding of apo(a) to the extracellular matrix[274] and it has been suggested that K IV-6 contains the lysine-binding site II identified by Ernst et al.[128,201] The same sites are believed to be involved in the interaction of apo(a) with apo B-100 as a first step in Lp(a) assembly.[102,103,105] Therefore, these sites are largely masked in the Lp(a) particle, contradicting the proposal that the Lys/Pro-sensitive site in K IV-6 is an important fibrin-binding site in intact Lp(a). Chenivesse et al.[272] found that the chimpanzee K IV-10 analogue differs from the human counterpart by an Asp 57 → Asn mutation. The mutation of this amino acid, which is critical to the LBS of K IV-10 in human apo(a), is associated with a poor lysine-specific interaction of chimpanzee Lp(a) with both intact and plasmin-degraded fibrin as compared to human Lp(a), supporting the notion that K IV-10 is the important fibrin-binding kringle in Lp(a).

The postulated fibrin binding that mediates transport of Lp(a) cholesterol to sites of injury and facilitates wound healing may be beneficial, but as a side effect might also trigger deposition of cholesterol in growing atherosclerotic plaques and inhibit fibrinolysis. It has been reported that Lp(a), or more specifically the apo(a) portion of Lp(a) but not LDL, is a substrate for tissue transglutaminase and for factor XIIIa.[275] These enzymes catalyze cross-linking between endo-γ-glutamyl and endo-ε-lysyl residues of proteins. Known substrates for transglutaminases include fibrinogen, fibrin, and fibronectin.[276,277] Because of the intimate interaction of Lp(a) with fibrin and other cell-surface oriented structures, factor XIIIa or tissue transglutaminase may catalyze cross-linking of Lp(a) to these surface structures with the final result of deposition of Lp(a) in a growing atherosclerotic plaque.

Recently, covalent binding of Lp(a) with fibrin and endothelial cells that is mediated by the pseudoprotease domain of apo(a) and K IV-independent has been described.[278] Another mechanism by which Lp(a) might be trapped in atherosclerotic plaque is through its ability to bind to glycosaminoglycans[31,279] or macrophage receptors.[229,230,232,233]

The interaction of Lp(a) and apo(a) with fibrin, fibrinolysis, and dissolution of clots is well documented *in vitro* under appropriate conditions. The only evidence to date that apo(a) interacts with fibrinolysis *in vivo* is from studies in apo(a) transgenic mice in which an antifibrinolytic activity of the transgene was demonstrated.[280] If such an interaction occurs *in vivo* in humans, it is not likely to modulate the process of fibrinolysis according to physiological needs. Lp(a) concentrations are not subject to any kind of fibrinolysis-related or other regulation, but are genetically fixed in an individual. Thus, they are set at a given level that may vary by a factor of a thousand or more among subjects. This would mean that each individual has his or her own genetically fixed balance between clot formation and clot lysis dependent on its Lp(a) concentration which seems unlikely. A comparison of conventional parameters for evaluation of the fibrinolytic system and of D-dimer levels in plasma and in serum after standardized coagulation did not show a difference between individuals with high and low levels of Lp(a).[281] That such a difference is not apparent in blood-clotting assays, suggests that Lp(a) acts locally, if at all, *in vivo*.

The affinity of Lp(a) to unmodified and plasmin-activated fibrin is increased several-fold by low concentrations of homocysteine.[282] Other sulfhydryl compounds, including cysteine, glutathione, and *N*-acetylcysteine, also increase the affinity between Lp(a) and fibrin. At the concentration used in the experiments, homocysteine partially reduces Lp(a). Therefore, it has been suggested that homocysteine changes the properties of intact Lp(a) so as to increase the reactivity of the apolipoprotein(a) moiety of the complex. Typ 72 in the lysine-binding pocket is sensitive to oxidation, which explains the sensitivity of the lysine-binding properties of Lp(a) to oxidative modification, for example, by homocysteine. In this context, it is of interest that the recessive disease homocystinuria (MIM 236200, Chap. 88) is characterized by severe atherosclerotic and thromboembolic phenomena, and that even heterozygotes may be at an increased risk for atherosclerotic vascular disease.

Lp(a) has also been shown to bind to tetranectin ($K_d = 0.013$ μM) a plasma protein which reversibly binds to kringle IV of plasminogen and enhances plasminogen activation by t-PA.[283] Lp(a) binding to tetranectin is of higher affinity than the binding of either Glu- or Lys-PLG (0.5 μM).[284] This capacity of Lp(a) again might result in less plasmin formation and hence less clot lysis. Still another mechanism by which Lp(a) may interfere with the endothelial cell surface associated fibrinolysis is by regulating the expression of plasminogen activator inhibitor-1 (PAI-1) expression. Lp(a) enhances PAI-1 antigen, activity, and steady-state mRNA levels in human cultured endothelial cells. The effect of Lp(a) is cell-specific, and no coordinate rise in PAI-1 mRNA is found for other lipoproteins.[285] This molecular mechanism would support a specific prothrombic situation at the endothelial cell surface.

In summary, the results show that Lp(a) and/or apo(a) can interfere *in vitro* with several key reactions in the regulation of fibrinolysis. These include competition for plasminogen binding to fibrinogen and fibrin, competition for plasminogen activation by t-PA, competition of plasminogen binding to cellular binding sites, competition of plasminogen binding to tetranectin, and enhancement of PAI-1 activity (Fig. 116-1). Because of these multiple interactions, Lp(a) has been described as an interloper into the fibrinolytic system.[26]

Besides the different interactions with the fibrinolytic system, other functions have been ascribed to apo(a)/Lp(a), some of which may also have pathophysiological consequences (Fig. 116-1). Lp(a) has chemoattractant activity for human peripheral monocytes[286] and induces the release of monocyte chemotactic activity (MCA) from endothelial cells.[287] Through its inhibition of plasmin generation from plasminogen, apo(a)/Lp(a) also inhibits the plasmin catalyzed activation of transforming growth factor β (TGFβ).[27,288] Decreased activity of this inhibitor of cell proliferation results in an enhanced proliferation and migration of smooth muscle cells, which has been demonstrated *in vitro*[27] and *in vivo* in apo(a) transgenic mice.[28] Stimulating effects of Lp(a) on proliferation of a variety of other cells, including endothelial cells[289] and mesangial cells,[290] has also been reported. The effect of Lp(a) on umbilical vein endothelial cell migration and proliferation may be mediated at least in part by fibroblast growth factor-2.[289] Such a mechanism could result in angiogenesis during wound healing.

Recently it was shown that Lp(a) also stimulates the expression of adhesion molecules, including intercellular adhesion molecule-1 (ICAM-1), vascular cell adhesion molecule-1 (VCAM-1), and E-selectin, at the surface of endothelial cells.[29,30] Leucocyte recruitment to the vessel wall is believed to be an important step in early atherogenesis and has been postulated as a novel mechanism explaining the atherogenicity of Lp(a). Apo(a)/Lp(a) interacts with several components of the extracellular matrix including fibrin,[25,249,267,268] fibronectin,[291] tetranectin,[283,284] and proteoglycans (e.g., decorin).[31] To find additional apo(a) protein ligands that are not predicted by the homology of apo(a) with plasminogen Köchl et al.[32] have employed the GAL5 Two Hybrid Library Interaction Trap System and identified β_2-glycoprotein I as a novel ligand that interacts with the K IV domain of apo(a). This interaction indicates new potential roles for Lp(a) in fibrinolysis but also autoimmunity.

β_2- Glycoprotein I binds to negatively charged phospholipids which creates novel antigenic epitopes recognized by certain antiphospholipid antibodies. There is a strong association between significantly increased Lp(a) levels and the occurrence of thrombotic events in patients with immune-mediated diseases characterized by antiphospholipid antibodies (i.e., systemic lupus erythematosus (SLE), rheumatoid arthritis, and antiphospholipid syndrome). Hence, the Lp(a) β_2-glycoprotein I interaction may be a link between thrombosis and autoimmune disease.[32]

Other potential functions have been attributed to apo(a)/Lp(a). Recombinant apo(a) binds to the complement component C3.[292] However, neither Lp(a) nor recombinant-apo(a) affect complement activation or degradation of activated C3. The significance of the interaction of apo(a)/Lp(a) with iC3b, which was demonstrated by an altered electrophoretic migration of iC3b in the presence of apo(a), is unclear.

Is Lp(a) an Active Protease?

Two particularly relevant questions are: Is the protease domain of apo(a) active? and does Lp(a) have protease activity? Analysis of the cDNA structure of human and rhesus apo(a) suggests that the protease domain of apo(a) is inactive and that Lp(a) does not have protease activity.[20,99] The kringle domains of PLG are connected to the protease domains by a sequence containing the activation cleavage site Arg 561-Val 562. In human apo(a), the arginine of the activation cleavage site in PLG has been replaced by a serine. This substitution impairs the generation of plasmin-like activity by activators.[20]

The catalytic triad Ser-His-Asp is, however, present in the human apo(a) protease domain. This situation is reversed in the rhesus apo(a) where the activation cleavage site is preserved but there are amino acid substitutions at two of the critical sites of the catalytic triad.[99] In agreement with expectation from the structural analysis, functional studies with purified apo(a) or Lp(a) fail to demonstrate plasmin-like activity.[20,95] Aminolytic activity of purified apo(a) against artificial substrates *N*-α-tosyl-L-arginine-methylester-HCl and *N*-α-benzoyl-L-arginine-4-nitroamilide-HCl was observed in an early report.[293] Salonen et al.[291] reported that Lp(a) and apo(a) bind to the C-terminal heparin-binding domain of immobilized fibronectin. This interaction leads to proteolytic cleavage of fibronectin. The amino acid specificity for Lp(a)/apo(a) was arginine rather than lysine as demonstrated by the use of synthetic peptide substrates, and the cleavage pattern was different from that generated with plasmin or kallikrein. Experiments with inhibitors indicate that the proteolytic activity of apo(a) is that of a serine protease.[291,294] In addition to being able to degrade the adhesive glycoprotein fibronectin, it has been suggested that Lp(a) has autocatalytic activity towards the apo B in the LDL-moiety,[295] thereby producing proteolytically digested LDL. Macrophages are known to avidly take up such particles. This might result in foam-cell formation and atherogenesis.

GENETICS OF LP(a)

Early Studies

Lp(a) was originally demonstrated by the Ouchterlony double diffusion assay,[1] which detects Lp(a) only in sera in which concentrations are high. A study of 175 Norwegian families with 646 children suggested that Lp(a) is inherited as an autosomal dominant trait.[2,3] Only a few clear exceptions from dominant inheritance were reported.[2,296] Harvie and Shultz[5] and Utermann and Wiegandt[297] postulated that Lp(a) is a quantitative rather than a qualitative trait. The development of semiquantitative and quantitative assays for Lp(a) enabled population, family, and twin studies using Lp(a) levels as the trait and applying the methodology of quantitative biometrical genetics. Several authors concluded that Lp(a) levels are determined by a major dominant gene but with polygenic background.[69,298] From a study of Lp(a) levels in 300 mother-father-offspring triplets, it was concluded that the observed quantitative Lp(a) variation is determined by a polygenic model of inheritance.[71] Morton et al.[70] proposed that an additional recessive allele determines low levels of Lp(a). Hasstedt and Williams supported the three-allele hypothesis.[299] The genetic models for Lp(a) delineated in these early studies were dependent on whether Lp(a) was determined as a qualitative or quantitative trait and on the method of statistical analysis. Morton et al.[300] were unable to confirm the major gene effect and Iselius et al.[301] the polygenic effect, although both applied similar likelihood analysis using the mixed model but on qualitative and quantitative Lp(a), respectively. All early studies on Lp(a) agree that the heritability of the trait is high ranging from 0.88 to 0.95 in family studies to 1.0 in twin studies.[302–308]

Population Genetics of the Quantitative Lp(a) Trait

Genetic epidemiologic studies show that the distribution of Lp(a) concentrations is heterogeneous across populations (Fig. 116-4).

The distributions of Lp(a) levels are broad in all populations with more than one thousandfold differences between the extremes within a group (e.g., $<$0.2 mg/dl to $>$200 mg/dl in unselected Caucasian population samples). They are highly nonnormal and positively skewed in all Caucasian and most Asian populations. They are closer to a Gaussian distribution in African populations.[8,309–313] In American Blacks, Lp(a) levels are also very high.[314,315]

As a general rule African populations have the highest Lp(a) plasma levels and Caucasians, some east Asians, Native Americans, and Eskimos the lowest. There is, however, heterogeneity within Asian populations. Whereas very low Lp(a) concentrations were consistently found in different samples of Chinese from Singapore,[65,311] mainland Chinese from Wuhan reportedly have Lp(a) concentrations the same as Caucasians;[310] American Chinese and Chinese from Hong Kong have high Lp(a) as compared to Caucasians.[312,313] The reasons for the large interindividual and interpopulation differences in average Lp(a) levels and their distributions are presently unknown.

Family, twin, and sib-pair linkage studies in Caucasians, Japanese, and Africans together have demonstrated that Lp(a) is an inherited quantitative trait.[69,72–76,299,300,316] The genetic architecture of a quantitative trait is defined by the number and type of

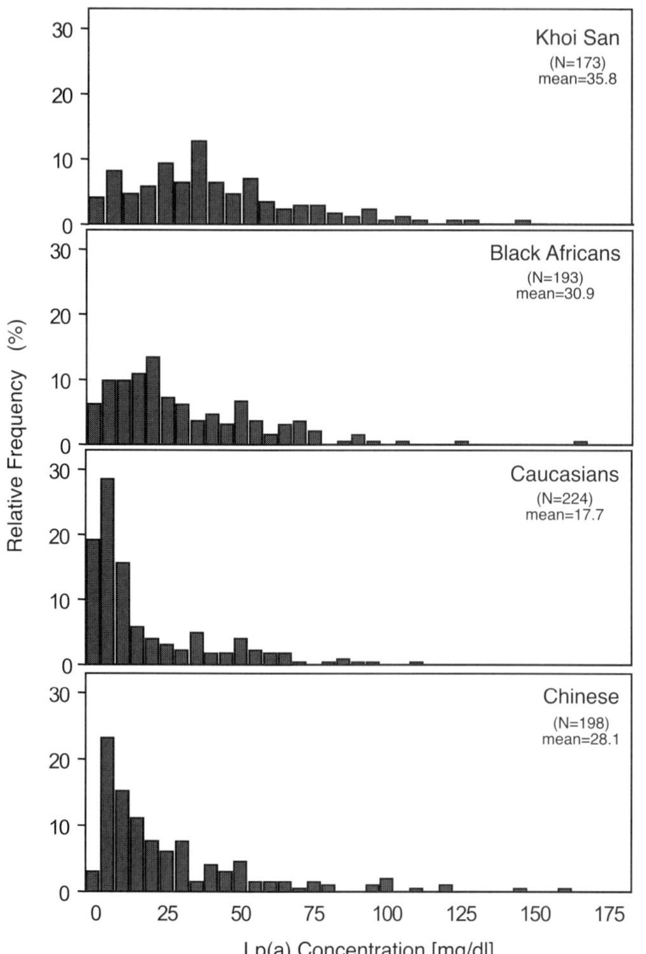

Fig. 116-4 Histogram showing the distributions of plasma Lp(a) concentrations in four populations. (*Reproduced from Kraft et al.*[313] *Used with permission.*)

genes that affect the trait, by allele numbers and frequencies at the respective loci, and by the effects of the alleles on the trait.[317] Further interactions between the genes, as well as interactions of genes with environmental factors, may contribute to a quantitative character. This was proposed for the Lp(a) trait to occur in Africans.[318]

The ongoing analysis of the apo(a) gene and its polymorphisms have enabled clarification of the genetic architecture of Lp(a) to some extent.[8,20,72,73,94,170,311,319] In Caucasian and Asian populations, the apo(a) structural gene is a major determinant of Lp(a) plasma concentrations.[72–76,312,313] In Africans, the apo(a) gene effect is less pronounced, and two groups found evidence for (a) transacting factor(s).[74,76] Furthermore, other genes may be involved in special situations such as rare genetic disorders and some common diseases.[141,214,320–322]

Size Polymorphism of Apolipoprotein(a)

Using separation of reduced total plasma by SDS-PAGE and SDS agarose gel-electrophoresis (SDS-AGE) followed by immunoblotting with apo(a)-detecting antibodies, several apo(a) isoforms, ranging in apparent molecular mass from <300 to >800 kDa, have been identified.

Originally, Utermann and coworkers[94] demonstrated six apo(a) isoforms of different size by SDS-PAGE/immunoblotting. According to their relative mobilities compared with apo B-100 (~520 kDa), apo(a) was categorized into isoforms F (faster than apo B-100), B (similar to apo B-100), S1, S2, S3, and S4 (all slower than apo B-100), a nomenclature that is still used in some laboratories. The number of isoforms has increased with improvement of the techniques.[323,324] Several modified immunoblotting techniques for phenotyping apo(a) have been described.[325–328] By high-resolution SDS agarose gel-electrophoresis (SDS-AGE) isoforms differing by one K IV-2 repeat can be separated and more than 35 isoforms have been identified.[323,324] Family studies showed isoforms were inherited in a simple codominant manner.[73,94,319,329] (Fig. 116-5). Individuals

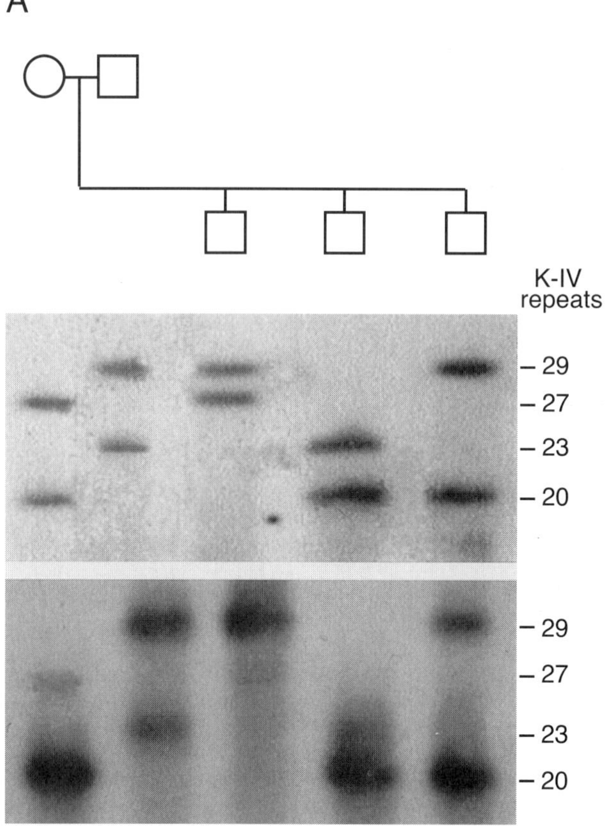

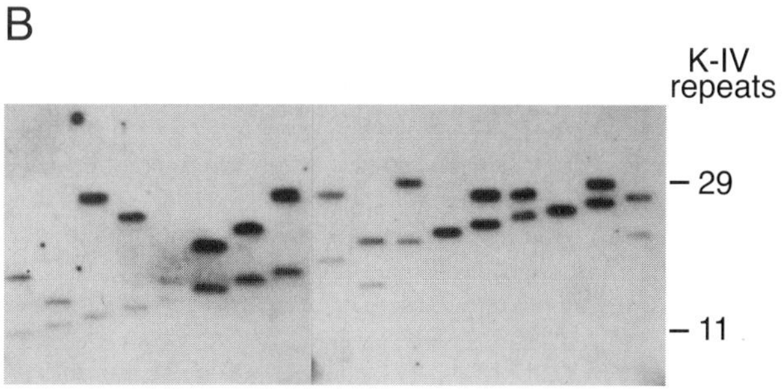

Fig. 116-5 Genetic size polymorphism of apo(a) caused by a variable number of transcribed and translated K IV-2 repeats. *A*, Pedigree illustrating the cosegregation of genomic apo(a) DNA fragments containing the K IV-2 repeat domain (*Kpn*I fragments) and of apo(a) isoforms in plasma and the large differences in expression in plasma of individual alleles. Upper panel: pedigree; Middle panel: demonstration of DNA fragments by pulsed-field gel-electrophoresis (PFGE)/Southern blotting using an apo(a) K IV-2-specific probe; Lower panel: demonstration of apo(a) isoforms by SDS-agarose gel-electrophoresis followed by immunoblotting with the monoclonal anti-apo(a) antibody 1A^2. *B*, Southern blot of genomic DNA separated by PFGE. DNA from 17 selected subjects was digested with *Kpn*I and samples were arranged to create a stepladder demonstrating the increment in the size of the *Kpn*I fragments. The DNA in the tenth lane was initially misclassified. The size difference between two adjacent fragments in the ladder is 5.6 kb. (*Reproduced from Kraft et al.*[73] *Used by permission.*)

have either two, one, or no apo(a) isoform. The intensities of apo(a) isoforms on the immunoblot vary considerably, even within the same subject (Fig. 116-5). As a general rule isoforms of lower molecular mass are more abundant on the blots than those of higher molecular mass. The absence of a detectable apo(a) isoform on the immunoblot was interpreted to result from homozygosity for an "operational" null allele (the term "operational" was chosen[319] because it was apparent that the detectability of isoforms greatly depends on the sensitivity of the immunoblotting procedure and because, until recently, no molecular basis for the apparent nonexpression of an apo(a) allele was known). The introduction of more powerful separation techniques and the increase in the sensitivity of the blotting procedure have increased the number of apo(a) isoforms to more than 35 and decreased the number of subjects with no detectable apo(a) isoforms (and hence the frequency of null alleles) from 40 percent to less than 5 percent.[313,323,324] This has not changed the principal genetic interpretation. The apo(a) size polymorphism is controlled by a large number (>35) of codominant alleles that do vary widely in their expressivity, with some being apparent null alleles. The average heterozygosity at the apo(a) structural locus is 94 percent.

Apparent exceptions from the Mendelian codominant model were observed in two families.[72,330] Lack of Hardy-Weinberg equilibrium in the sample, together with the family data, let Gaubatz et al.[330] conclude that inheritance of apo(a) isoforms is not strictly Mendelian. Reanalysis of their family, including apo(a) genotyping (see next paragraph), revealed that the exceptions were explained by mistyping (G. Utermann, J. Morrisett, H.G. Kraft, unpublished). The other exception was due to a new mutation of one apo(a) allele out of a total of 376 meioses.[72]

Molecular Basis of Apo(a) Polymorphism

The cDNA structure of the apo(a) gene with its high number of identical or near identical plasminogen-like K IV repeats (Figs. 116-2 and 116-3) immediately suggested that the protein-size polymorphism may result from inherited differences in the number of K IV repeats in the apo(a) gene. This hypothesis was strengthened by quantitative Southern blotting experiments.[8,331,332] The molecular basis of apo(a) protein-size variability has also been studied by analysis of apo(a) mRNA in humans[333] and in baboons.[183] Liver RNA from individuals with different apo(a) isoforms was analyzed by northern blot analysis. Transcripts of 8.0 to 12.0 kb corresponded to proteins of 590 to 850 kDa.[183,333] The apparent molecular mass of apo(a) from SDS-PAGE is, however, far from its true molecular weight due to the high carbohydrate content of apo(a) that results in anomalous mobility in SDS-PAGE. Therefore, the number of K IV repeats in apo(a) cannot be deduced from such data. Koschinsky et al.[333] used expression of recombinant apo(a) with a known number of K IV repeats to calculate the number of K IV units in plasma apo(a) isoforms, and found from <17 to >30 tandemly repeated K IV units. This is within the range determined by the analysis of apo(a) DNA.

Ten different types of K IV repeats, which are commonly designated K IV-1 to K IV-10,[98] were identified. A direct approach to demonstrate that the protein-size polymorphism is due to a variable number of K IV repeats in the gene capitalized on restriction enzymes (e.g., *Kpn*I) that cut outside the repeat domain.[73,170,334] Because the resulting fragments are very large, PFGE/genomic blotting was used to separate and identify apo(a) fragments which has limited application of this technique. Digestion with *Sva*I, *Hpa*I, or *Kpn*I results in fragments of ~35 kb to > 200 kb depending on the apo(a) allele; an apo(a) DNA-typing system based on *Kpn*I-digested DNA has been developed.[73,170] The 5′ restriction site for *Kpn*I was localized in the 14-kb intron preceding the first K IV repeat. One 3′ *Kpn*I site is between K V and the protease domain,[170] but a further site was found in an intron separating the unique kringles K IV-4 and K IV-5.[334] Thus, apo(a) *Kpn*I fragments contain K IV-1, all the common K IV-2 A and K IV-2 B repeats, and kringles IV-3 and IV-4. PFGE of *Kpn*I-digested DNA demonstrated the existence of >30 apo(a) DNA-size alleles. Neighboring alleles differed in size by ~5.6 kb (Fig. 116-5*B*). This corresponds to the size of one K IV repeat in genomic DNA.[73,170] A stepladder is created by applying samples ordered by size to the pulsed-field gels (Fig. 116-5*B*). Recently, the number of K IV-2 repeats in apo(a) alleles was determined by fiber-FISH.[335]

Family studies showed the expected codominant inheritance of DNA fragments. The size variation of DNA fragments corresponded to the size heterogeneity of protein isoforms in plasma; both cosegregate in families (Fig. 116-5*A*). A 42-kb allele has been cloned and contains 12 K IV repeats.[334] Based on the *Kpn*I restriction map, the number of K IV-encoding repeats is estimated to range from 11 to >42, which corresponds to 2 to >33 identical K IV-2 repeats. The complete correspondence in size between DNA fragments and protein isoforms demonstrated that the size polymorphism in apo(a) is generated by a variable number of K IV type 2 repeats.[73,334] This was confirmed by direct studies of the K IV types 3 to 10 region of the apo(a) gene.[166] PFGE/genomic blotting enabled the direct correlation of the DNA and protein polymorphisms, and resulted in a typing system at the DNA level. The K IV-2 repeat polymorphism was instrumental in determining the contribution of the apo(a) gene locus to Lp(a)concentration by sib-pair analysis (see "Sib-Pain Linkage Analysis" below). To date, more than 40 alleles have been identified in the pooled samples from several ethnic groups,[312,313] but there are significant differences in the frequency distribution of apo(a) K IV-2 alleles across populations (Fig. 116-6).

Together with apo(a) sequence variation, this makes the apo(a) gene one of the most polymorphic known in humans. Formally, it may be described as a transcribed VNTR locus.[73] The best way to describe apo(a) size alleles is by their K IV-2 repeat number.[336,337]

Relation of Apo(a) Polymorphism to Lp(a) Concentrations

The first report of the apo(a) protein-size polymorphism noted a strong negative correlation of apo(a) size with Lp(a) concentrations.[94] All subsequent studies confirmed this finding. The finding has been extended to various ethnic groups, including several Caucasian populations (Austrians, Hungarians, Welsh, Danes, Icelandic, Germans, Scots, Italians, and Americans); Africans (South African Blacks, Sudanese, Ghanaians, Nigerians, and Khoi-San); American Blacks; Asians from China, Japan, Hong Kong (Chinese), Singapore (Chinese, Indians, Malays); and Inuits from Greenland.[65,66,89,94,310,311,315,330,338,339] The protein-size variation of apo(a) explained a fraction of the total variability in Lp(a) levels ranging from a low of 0.19 (Sudanese) to a high of 0.77 (Malays).

More recently, the variation in the number of K IV repeats in apo(a) as demonstrated by PFGE has been related to Lp(a) concentrations, confirming the conclusion from the apo(a) protein studies[73,170,312,313] and extending them to Russian, Finnish, Thai, and Asian Indian populations (H.G. Kraft, G. Utermann, unpublished). Family studies have demonstrated cosegregation of apo(a) isoforms with Lp(a) concentrations.[73,319,329]

Because of the high number of alleles in the samples (26 in Kraft et al.[73] and 19 in Lackner et al.[170]) and the high degree of heterozygosity, no average Lp(a) values for each DNA allele or DNA phenotype have been calculated. Instead, results have been presented graphically (Fig. 116-7). This has impressively demonstrated the general inverse correlation of apo(a) allele size with Lp(a) plasma concentration. The effect of apo(a) alleles on Lp(a) levels appears to be additive.[85,319,340] Heterozygotes for different apo(a) isoforms have two different Lp(a) particles in plasma, each containing one of the isoforms and each occurring with a concentration that is characteristic for the isoform.[85,91] Therefore, the sum of the K IV-2 repeats in an individual has been taken as a measure to calculate the correlation of apo(a) alleles with Lp(a) levels.

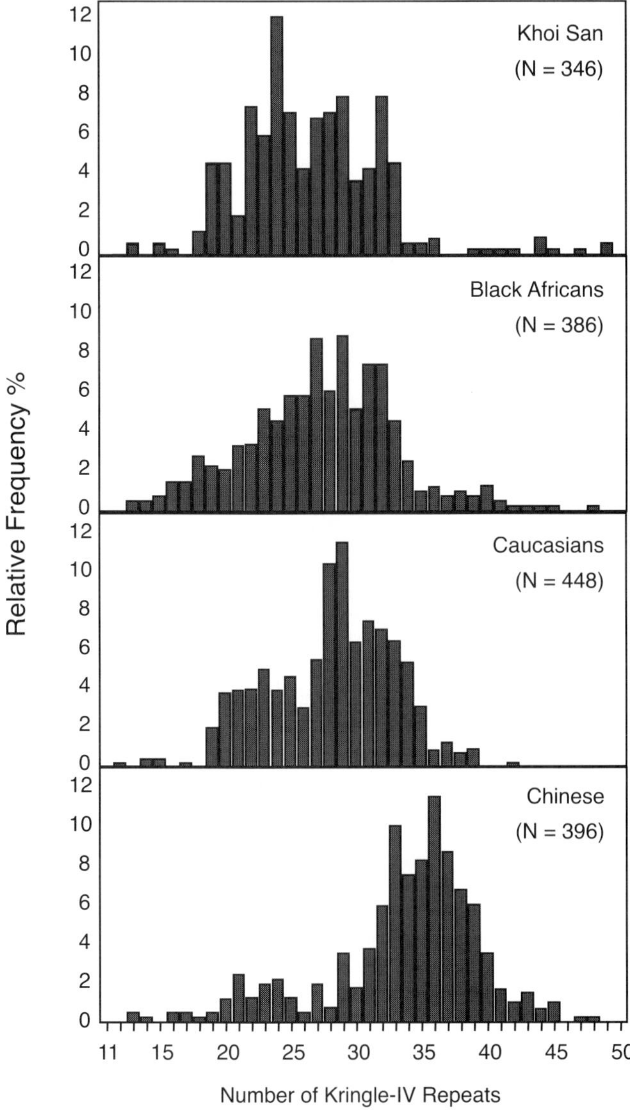

Fig. 116-6 Frequency distributions of K IV-2 repeat alleles in four ethnic groups. The total number of K IV repeats including the unique kringles is given. (*Reproduced from Kraft et al.*[313] *Used by permission.*)

The following scenario has emerged from these investigations. The number of K IV-2 repeats in apo(a) is inversely associated with Lp(a) plasma concentrations (Fig. 116-7). Apo(a) alleles with low K-IV copy numbers tend to be associated with high Lp(a), whereas those with high K IV repeat numbers tend to be associated with low Lp(a). There are notable exceptions, particularly in the group with low copy numbers. Some small apo(a) alleles are associated with low Lp(a). Moreover, family studies demonstrate that apo(a) isoforms of identical size may cosegregate with very different Lp(a) concentrations.[329] The relation between plasma Lp(a) concentration and apo(a) alleles is, therefore, more complex than indicated by the inverse relation with apo(a) K IV-2 repeats.

Isoforms with few K IV repeats are associated with a much larger range in Lp(a) levels than long isoforms. Kraft et al.[313] calculated the average allele-associated Lp(a) concentrations for different ethnic groups. Kraft et al. made two observations: (a) the relation between apo(a) size and Lp(a) concentration is not linear and (b) the relation between apo(a) size and Lp(a) concentration differs across populations. The variability of Lp(a) levels is also not homogeneous across K IV-2 repeat length. Gaw et al. analyzed this relationship in detail.[341] When expressed as the R^2 from the analysis of variance, the apo(a) K IV-VNTR explains from a low of <30 percent to a high of 70 percent of the variation in Lp(a) concentrations.[72,73,312,313] The association is notoriously stronger in Asian and Caucasian populations than in Africans (Blacks, Khoi-San). Analysis of the Spearman rank correlation coefficients between K IV repeat number and Lp(a) levels, which is significantly stronger in Chinese (Rs = −0.672) and Caucasians (Rs = −0.505) than in Blacks (Rs = −0.400) and Khoi-San (Rs = −0.464),[313] has confirmed this. This indicates that other factors — besides the size polymorphism — determine Lp(a) levels to a larger extent in Africans than in Asians and Caucasians. Recently, Gaw et al.[341] claimed that the effect of the K IV-2 VNTR on Lp(a) was overestimated in previous studies and concluded from their statistical analysis that the polymorphism explains only 9 to 10 percent of the variance in Lp(a) concentrations (instead of the ~40 percent in Caucasians estimated by others). There are some objections to their conclusions. One objection is that average Lp(a) levels (mean 41 mg/dl) in their cohort are at least twofold higher than in any other Caucasian population (only Africans have been reported with Lp(a) in this range), which either questions the validity of their assay or suggests bias by sample selection. Due to the unusual distribution of Lp(a) concentrations and their nonlinear and heterogeneous association with K IV repeat numbers,[313] calculation of the R^2 of variance from raw or logarithmically transformed data may be questionable, and numbers should not be taken too seriously.

The association of K IV repeat number/apo(a) isoform with Lp(a) concentrations had suggested that the large variation in the distribution and mean concentration of Lp(a) across populations (in particular the higher Lp(a) in Blacks) is caused by different frequencies of apo(a) size alleles, but it turned out that this prediction was wrong. Three large studies, either on protein isoforms[311] or determining DNA-phenotypes[312,313] have demonstrated that frequency differences of apo(a) size alleles do not explain the differences in Lp(a) concentrations between populations. In fact, what differs between populations are the mean apo(a)-size allele-associated Lp(a) concentrations.[313] Large apo(a) alleles are associated with much higher Lp(a) in Blacks than in Caucasians. In contrast, small apo(a) alleles are associated with several-fold higher Lp(a) in Chinese and Caucasians than in Africans. One reasonable explanation for this is that apo(a) isoforms of identical size differ in sequence and that the frequencies of sequence variants differ between populations. Another is that there exist *trans*-acting factors. There is now evidence for both mechanisms.

Sib-Pair Linkage Analysis

The above studies established that apo(a) is a major gene for Lp(a) in Asian and Caucasian populations. However, the size polymorphism explained neither all of the interindividual variation of Lp(a) levels in a population nor the differences across populations, and the situation in African populations remained unclear. Independent twin studies have claimed that Lp(a) is virtually entirely under genetic control in Caucasians.[316] So, what determines the fraction of the variance in Lp(a) concentration that is not explained by the K IV-2 VNTR?

To estimate the contribution of variation at the apo(a) locus to Lp(a) concentrations, sib-pair linkage studies have been performed.[72–76] Sib-pair linkage methods are more commonly applied to detect linkage between a marker and a qualitative trait locus. They can also be used to estimate the overall contribution of a candidate gene to a quantitative phenotype. The apo(a) K IV-2 VNTR is particularly informative for such a study because the number of alleles is high and most individuals are heterozygous for different combinations of apo(a) alleles, which allows distinction of all four parental alleles in most families. In addition, apo(a) typing of parents allows the determination of whether DNA fragments identical in size are identical by descent as opposed to identical by state. Five sib-pair linkage studies have been reported and all came to very similar conclusions.[72–76]

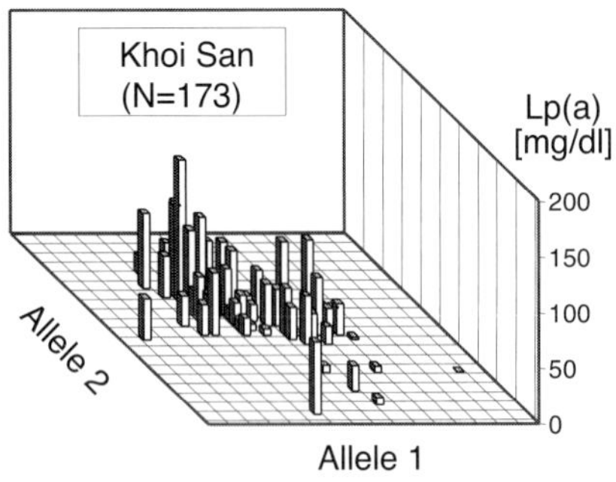

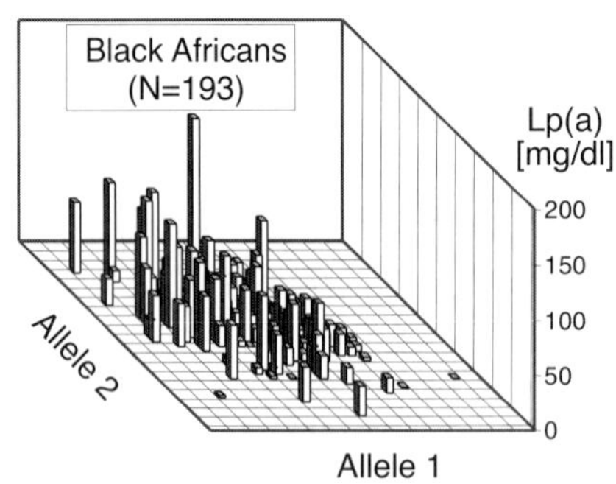

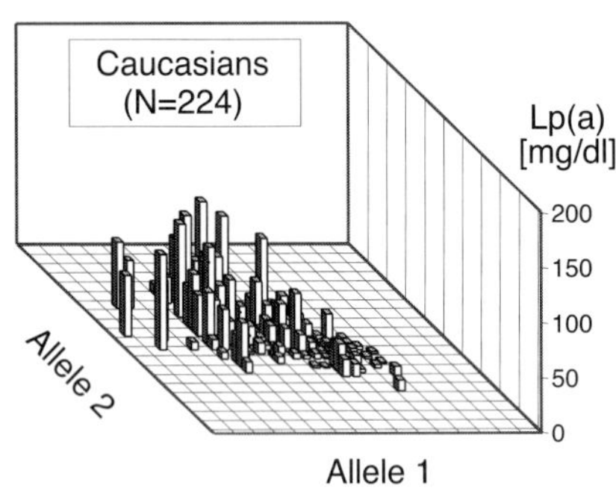

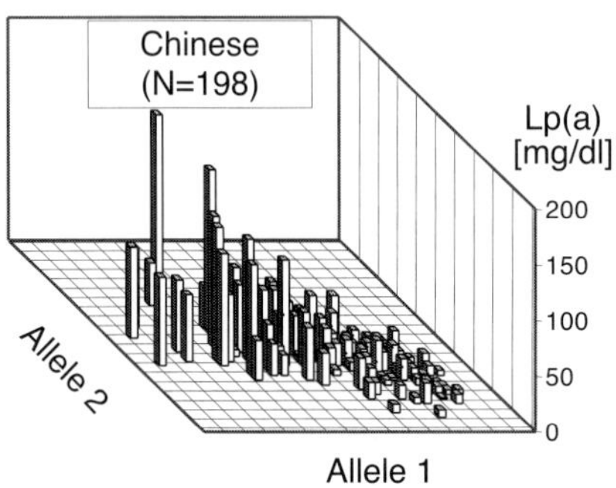

Fig. 116-7 Representation of the relation between apo(a) K IV-2 variation and Lp(a) concentrations in plasma from four ethnic groups. The two *KpnI* fragments in a subject are denoted as allele number 1 and allele number 2 and given at the y- and z-axes. Lp(a) concentrations in a subject is represented by the height of the bar (x-axis). (*Reproduced from Kraft et al.*[313] *Used by permission.*)

The magnitude of the apo(a) gene effect on Lp(a) level variation was estimated from 74 to >90 percent in three independent studies of Caucasian families.[72,73,75,76] These estimates were confirmed by a variance components analysis of two of these family sets.[75,76] Sib-pair linkage studies and variance components analyses in North American Blacks, African Blacks, and Khoi-San demonstrated that both the total genetic component and the effect of the apo(a) gene are smaller in Africans. The studies provided evidence for the existence of *trans*-acting factor(s) in Africans that needs to be identified. Each study, however, suggested that there might be variation at the apo(a) gene locus beyond the K IV-2 VNTR that also effects Lp(a) levels.

Sequence Variation in Apo(a)

The above observations prompted an extensive search for sequence polymorphism in apo(a) with potential effects on Lp(a) levels,[161,171,172,329,342–347] which search is hampered by the repeat structure of the gene. Sequence variation has been detected in noncoding and coding regions of apo(a). These include SSCP-polymorphisms in introns of the apo(a) gene,[329] a pentanucleotide repeat polymorphism (5′PNRP) in the apo(a) promoter,[343,344] point mutations in the 5′prime region of the gene,[172,173,345,346] including a C/T polymorphism at +93,[347] and sequence variants in K IV-6 to K IV-10 exons[348] (M. Ogorelkova and G. Utermann, unpublished) (Fig. 116-3). Particularly interesting for an understanding of the evolutionary dynamics of the K IV-2 VNTR is a *Dra*III restriction-site polymorphism in the K IV type 2 repeat.[171] A restriction site is present in the introns of some of the K IV-2 repeats, but not in others. Depending on the number of K IV repeats, the number of *Dra*III restriction sites, and the distribution of repeats with or without a *Dra*III site, different complex patterns are observed. This together with a polarity in the distribution resembles the structure of minisatellites, suggesting that the mechanism that has driven the evolution of these repeats may be similar for apo(a) and minisatellites.[171] Polymorphisms and rare variants that show a population-specific distribution have been identified in the coding sequence of the K IV-6 to K IV-10 repeats. An apparently rare mutation affecting the lysine binding of apo(a) has been observed in some American Blacks.[349] Among the polymorphism in the coding sequence for apo(a) is a Met/Thr polymorphism in K IV type 10 that is of no physiological significance.[342,350] Several of the sequence variants are in linkage disequilibrium with each other.[342,347,351] There exist strong allelic associations between markers across the K IV-2 VNTR that suggest that this polymorphism is rather stable[351] (H.G. Kraft, G. Utermann, unpublished).

Furthermore, there exist null alleles that result in a failure to express apo(a) isoforms in plasma. In baboons, transcript-negative and transcript-positive null alleles have been distinguished.[352] Only two molecularly defined apo(a) null alleles have been described, one in baboons[353] and one in humans.[353a] Both are due to splice-site mutations and result in truncated isoforms.

Apo(a) Sequence Variation and Lp(a) Plasma Concentration

Both, the 5′ PNRP and the *Dra*III polymorphism are associated with Lp(a) levels.[171,343,344] For the 5′-PNRP this association exists in Caucasians but not in Blacks.[343] Direct analysis of promoter activity in a luciferase reporter gene assay has revealed no differences in promoter activity between constructs containing different 5′PNRP numbers.[172,344] This demonstrates that the 5′-PNRP is in allelic association with unknown sequence variation affecting Lp(a) concentrations.

The situation is also complex for the +93 C/T polymorphism.[347] The T at this position creates an alternative ATG translational start codon which explains that the *in vitro* translational activity of the +93 T allele is 60 percent lower than that of the +93 C allele.[345] Therefore, it is expected that +93 T alleles are associated with lower Lp(a) *in vivo*. This is, indeed, observed in Africans (Blacks, Khoi-San). On average, Lp(a) levels are 50 to 60 percent lower in carriers of the T alleles than in those with +93 T. The +93 C/T polymorphism has a strong effect on Lp(a) in Africans, which explains about 7 percent of the variation in Lp(a) concentration. It came as a surprise that no such effect was observed in two independent Caucasian samples (Austrians, Danes). Upon close analysis of the data, a strong allelic association of the +93 C/T polymorphism with the K IV-2 VNTR was observed that might explain the seemingly contradictory results.[347] The +93 T site was found in association with alleles characterized by a large number of K IV-2 repeats and 9 repeats for the 5′-PNRP (Fig. 116-8) that reportedly are associated with very low Lp(a) (~2 mg/dl) in Caucasians.[343,344]. Hence any Lp(a)-lowering

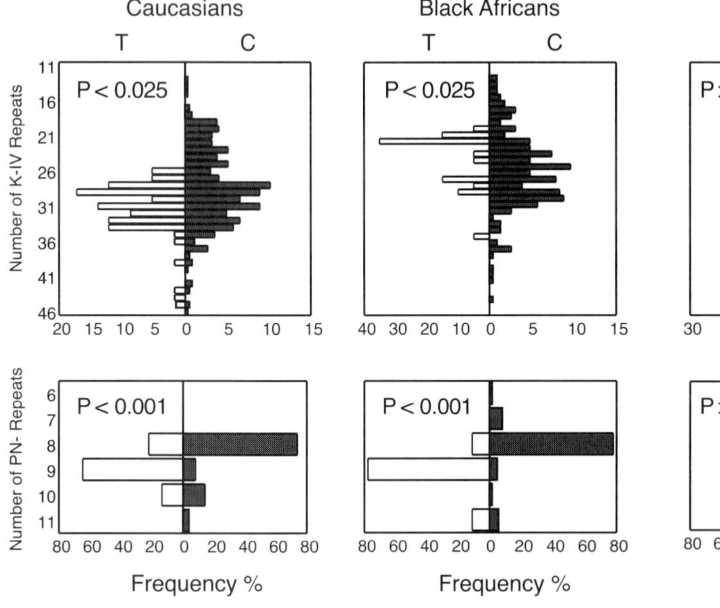

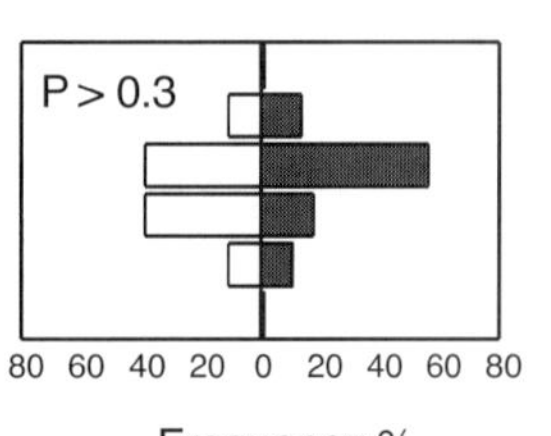

Fig. 116-8 Frequency distributions of +93 T/C alleles on K IV-2 repeat alleles and 5′-pentaneucleotide repeat alleles illustrating allelic associations of the +93 T allele with intermediate/high K IV-2 repeat number in Caucasians and with 9-pentaneucleotide repeats in Black Africans and Caucasians. (*Reproduced from Kraft et al.*[347] *Used with permission.*)

effect of the +93 T, if present, will be difficult to detect for alleles that segregate with low Lp(a) anyhow. Furthermore, they will have no significant impact on Lp(a) concentration in the population at large. Here we face the unusual situation in which an allelic association masks a biologic effect of an allele in one population but not in another population.

There are two conclusions to be drawn from this: (a) The sequence variation in apo(a) effects Lp(a) can only be assessed in population studies when full information for the K IV-2 VNTR is also available and stratification for the large K IV-2 VNTR effect can be performed. This seems justified because the K IV-2 effect is causal. (b) The widely held belief that heterogeneity of a gene effect across populations indicates that the observed effect is not causal but rather results from an allelic association is not necessarily true. Together the analysis of apo(a) intragenic variations in relation to Lp(a) concentrations has provided some insights into the genetic architecture of the trait (Fig. 116-9).

Mechanism of Genetic Regulation of Lp(a) Levels

In vivo turnover studies using purified labeled Lp(a) have demonstrated that differences in Lp(a) concentrations between individuals result from differences in the rate of production of apo(a)/Lp(a) rather than from differences in catabolism.[191,243] Hence a relation must exist between the synthesis/production of Lp(a) and the number of K IV-2 repeats in the apo(a) gene. However, even for healthy individuals with the same apo(a) isoform but different plasma Lp(a) levels, synthesis and not catabolism is responsible for the difference.[192] An answer to the following questions was therefore sought: How does variation at the apo(a) gene locus and in particular the number of K IV-2 repeats in apo(a) influence the production of Lp(a)? Is it at the level of transcription, mRNA stability, translation, intracellular processing, secretion, or assembly? To address these questions animal models and *in vitro* cell culture systems, some in combination with transfections, were used. Together, the results suggest that the regulation occurs at different levels. Studies in cynomolgus monkeys indicate that plasma Lp(a) concentration is related to the abundance of hepatic mRNA implicating regulation at the level of transcription and/or mRNA stability.[184] In line with this, results from luciferase and CAT assays show that human apo(a) promoters that differ in sequence affect transcriptional activity.[173,346] The same site (+93) implicated to affect

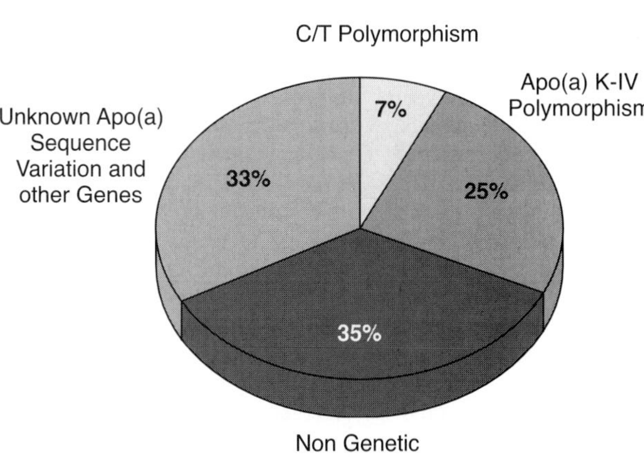

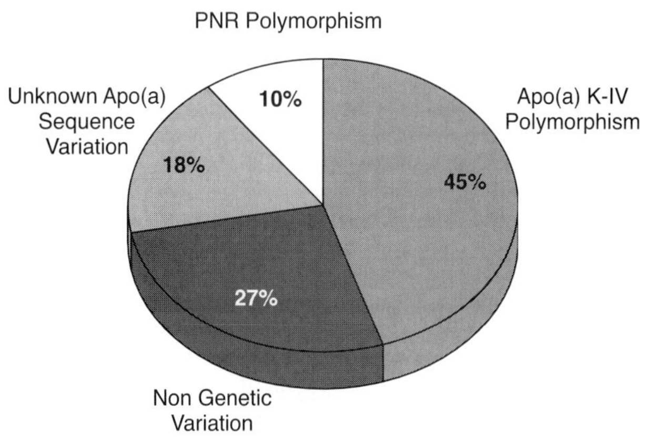

Fig. 116-9 Genetic architecture of Lp(a). Pie diagram illustrating the contribution of genetic and nongenetic variation to plasma Lp(a) levels in Black Africans and caucasian Europeans. Data used are from references 72 to 74, 313, 343, and 347. (*Reproduced from Utermann.*[563] *Used by permission.*)

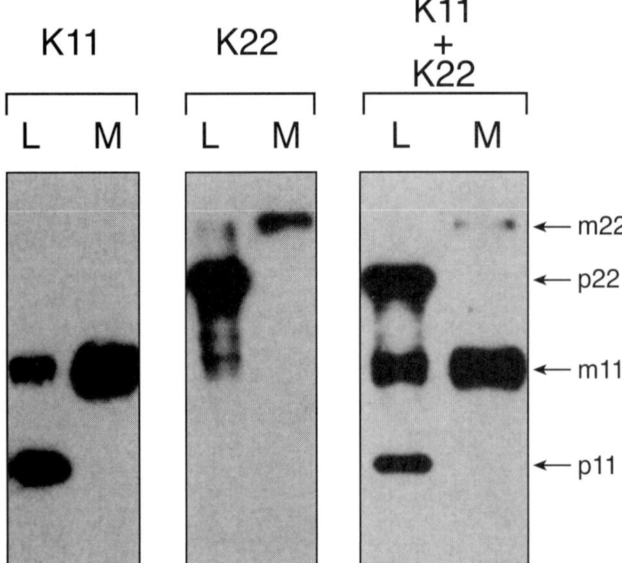

Fig. 116-10 Immunoblots with monoclonal anti-apo(a) antibody 1A[2] from lysates (L) and media (M) from HepG2 cells transiently transfected to express apo(a) containing different numbers (11 and 22) of K IV-repeats. The apo(a) precursor is denoted as p and the mature protein as m. The panel at the right shows the results from a cotransfection of differently sized recombinant apo(a) constructs. Note the difference in expressivity of the apo(a) isoforms in the medium. (*Reproduced from Brunner et al.*[355] *Used by permission.*)

transcriptional activity has, however, also been related to the efficiency of apo(a) in *in vivo* translation.[345]

Two cell culture model systems have been used extensively to study posttranslational aspects of apolipoprotein(a) biosynthesis: baboon primary hepatocytes and the human hepatocarcinoma cell line Hep G2. More recently, hepatocytes from Lp(a) transgenic mice have also been used.[354]

Hep G2 cells synthesize and secrete most apolipoproteins and lipoproteins but do not produce significant amounts of apo(a)/Lp(a). When transfected with constructs expressing apo(a), these cells synthesize and secrete apo(a), most of which is found as Lp(a) in the cell culture media.[153] Studies in HepG2 cells which were either transiently[355] or stably[198] transfected to express apo(a), in primary cell cultures from baboons,[356,357] and in hepatocytes from apo(a) transgenic mice,[354] demonstrate that apo(a) is synthesized as an intracellular precursor with a lower molecular weight than the mature secreted form (Fig. 116-10). Compared to other secreted proteins, the apo(a) precursor has an unusually long retention time in the endoplasmic reticulum, which is associated with aggregate formation and degradation of the proteins,[358] suggesting a complex maturation process. Degradation of apolipoprotein(a) is mediated by the proteasome pathway. Binding of newly synthesized apo(a) to the ER chaperon calnexin and conditions that enhance the apo(a)/calnexin interaction prevent apo(a) degradation. This suggests that calnexin can protect apo(a) from proteolysis.[359] The fully glycosylated mature Golgi-form is rapidly secreted from the hepatocyte. Inhibition of *N*-linked glycosylation results in retention of intracellular apo(a) in hepatoma cells.[360] The time needed for an apo(a) isoform to travel through the secretory pathway and exit from the cell is determined by the number of K IV-2 repeats it carries.[352,355] The more K IV-2 repeats there are in apo(a), the longer is the retention time in the ER, the more intracellular aggregates are formed, and the more apo(a) precursor is degraded before maturation.[198,352,355] It is still not known what precisely causes the isoform-size-dependent retention and degradation in the ER. Folding intermediates occur at the same rate for isoforms of different length.[357] The K IV-2 dependent differential retention of apo(a) isoforms in liver cells does, however, explain at least in part the inverse relation of K IV-2 repeat number with plasma Lp(a) levels and provides a new mechanism for the genetic regulation of the concentrations of a protein.

An interesting observation is the interaction of methylated DNA-binding proteins (MDBP) with the highly repeated sites in the apo(a) gene.[361] MDBP is a ubiquitous mammalian sequence-specific DNA-binding protein that recognizes a highly degenerated 14-bp consensus sequence. Some sites require methylation of cytosine residues for binding. MDBP binds to sites in several viral enhancers, and it is predicted that many methylated MDBP sites matching the consensus sequence exist in mammalian DNA. Three different types of nucleotide sequence that match the MDBP consensus sequence were detected by computer-assisted search of the mammalian DNA database in the highly repeated K IV domain of the apo(a) gene. A consensus sequence for the AP-2 transcription factor, another enhancer-binding protein, was also identified in 29 of the human apo(a) K IV units that contain MDBP sites in the sequenced apo(a) cDNA.[361] The finding of so many intragenic copies of MDBP sites in apo(a) is unique, but the functional significance is presently unclear. It has been suggested, however, that MDBP may help to down-modulate apolipoprotein(a) gene expression by acting from a distance and in concert with other sequence-specific DNA-binding proteins, such as AP-2, on the transcription complex. If so, less MDBP molecules binding over a smaller region of chromatin or more MDBP binding over a longer region might also contribute to the observed inverse relationship between the numbers of K IV repeats in the apo(a) gene and the plasma levels of Lp(a).[361]

Non-apo(a) Mediated Genetic Effects

The quantitative data describing the genetic control of Lp(a) levels were obtained by studying unselected population samples, healthy families, and twins. In these analyses, the large effect of rare alleles, or even frequent disorders that are not represented or underrepresented in the samples, may go undetected. Some rare genes as well as environmental factors and diseases (see "Disease Associations and Exogenous Effects" below) have been shown to affect Lp(a) levels. In abetalipoproteinemia (MIM 200100; Chap. 115), no Lp(a) is present in plasma.[152] Only low levels of apo(a) are detected in lipid-free plasma fractions.[152] Patients with autosomal recessive lipoprotein lipase deficiency (MIM 238600; Chap. 117)[141] and lecithin-cholesterol acyltransferase deficiency (MIM 245900; Chap. 118)[321] have markedly reduced Lp(a) levels in plasma. The mechanisms by which these gene defects affect Lp(a) levels are unknown. Lp(a) has been reported to be absent in patients with Zellweger syndrome (MIM 214100; Chap. 129),[362] but this may be secondary to the severe impairment of liver functions (G. Utermann, unpublished). De Knijff et al.[363] described an effect of the apo E polymorphism on Lp(a) levels that was confirmed by others.[364] Several types of dyslipidemia are associated with elevated or subnormal Lp(a) levels, but the mechanisms are largely unclear.[141,365,366] Lipid and lipoprotein factors are also associated with variation in Lp(a) density and composition.[367]

Lp(a) in Familial Hypercholesterolemia

Elevated levels of Lp(a) have been found in the plasma of unrelated patients with heterozygous familial hypercholesterolemia (MIM 143890; Chap. 120) from England,[214,216,368] South Africa,[369] and Sweden.[215] One study showed that Lp(a) levels are elevated in FH patients independent from apo(a) phenotype.[214] Lp(a) levels were also found elevated in South African patients with homozygous familial hypercholesterolemia, but mean concentrations were not higher than in heterozygous FH.[369] High Lp(a) concentrations were further reported in a group of eight unrelated French homozygous FH patients.[370]

Subsequent family studies of Lp(a) in FH kindreds and in kindreds with familial defective apo B-100 (MIM 107730; Chap.

115) have resulted in a confusing picture. Soutar et al.[217] studied the relationship between apolipoprotein(a) phenotype, lipoprotein(a) concentration in plasma, and LDLR function in a large Pakistani kindred with familial hypercholesterolemia due to the Pro 664→Leu mutation in the LDLR gene. They found no significant difference in Lp(a) concentration between groups of FH and non-FH of the same apo(a) phenotype. However, the subjects were not all identical by descent at the apo(a) gene locus, and Lp(a) values from individuals with identical isoforms but extreme deviations of their Lp(a) values were removed from the analysis, which might have obscured the results. Moreover, they found a higher mean value for the FH group in each apo(a) phenotype class. They also found evidence for an apo(a) gene and LDLR-independent factor that markedly increased Lp(a) concentration and that was also present in unrelated spouses. In contrast, Lp(a) concentrations were found significantly higher in five heterozygous subjects with familial defective apo B-100 (MIM 107730) as compared to their unaffected siblings or close relatives with the same apo(a) phenotype.[371] Nonetheless the authors concluded from biochemical and turnover studies that defective apo B-100 is not associated with elevated Lp(a).[371]

In 14 FH kindreds from Israel who had different LDLR mutations, Lp(a) levels were found elevated in FH cases from all kindreds, although to a different degree.[218] Mean plasma Lp(a) levels were significantly higher in the cases from the combined kindreds than in the controls. Lp(a) was raised only moderately (by 30 to 33 percent) in FH cases from Druze, Christian-Arab, and Ashkenazi Jewish groups, but significantly (by 110 percent) in the -Sephardic Jewish group. The finding was assumed to reflect a diverse effect of ethnicity (or LDLR mutation) on plasma Lp(a) levels in heterozygous FH patients and possibly multiple gene interactions.[218] Segregation analysis of Lp(a) in molecularly defined FH families from Israel identified the apo(a) locus, polygenes, and an untransmitted major environmental factor.[219]

A further family study investigated Lp(a) levels and apo(a) phenotypes in French-Canadian FH kindreds with the 10-kb deletion. Lp(a) levels were found significantly higher in FH affected family members than in unrelated controls, but only moderately and insignificantly increased over the unaffected blood relatives.[372] Lp(a) levels were higher in the unaffected family members as compared to controls from the general population. This seems to be a consistent but unexplained finding. Independent from the population, higher Lp(a) has been observed in non-FH blood relatives over controls from the same area in three independent studies. In these studies, some spouses also had extremely high Lp(a) concentrations and some apo(a) alleles in the kindreds were associated with unusually high Lp(a) levels. Together the data from the different family studies is inconclusive.

The *in vivo* catabolism of Lp(a) in FH patients was studied by three groups.[210,244,373] Krempler et al.[210] found a decreased fractional clearance rate of Lp(a) in one homozygous FH patient, but the decrease was not to the same extent as that of LDL and argued against a major role of the LDLR in the removal of LDL. The same conclusion was reached by Knight et al.[373] and Rader et al.[244] who studied Lp(a) catabolism in four FH heterozygotes. The fractional clearance rate of Lp(a) was the same in FH heterozygous subjects as in non-FH controls despite a large difference in the fractional clearance rate of LDL between the groups.[373] These data were interpreted to mean that Lp(a) metabolism is not affected by LDLR variation.

Recently, two large family-studies, one in FH and one in familial defective apo B-100 kindreds were done in which LDLR genotype/apo B genotypes, apo(a) genotypes and phenotypes, and Lp(a) concentrations were determined.[220,221] Using various approaches including a comparison of sib-pairs that were identical by descent for apo(a) alleles but nonidentical for FH/familial defective apo B status, it was clearly demonstrated that Lp(a) concentrations are elevated in FH as well as in familial defective apo B. These studies, which are the only ones that have rigorously stratified for the effect of the apo(a) locus, also demonstrate that

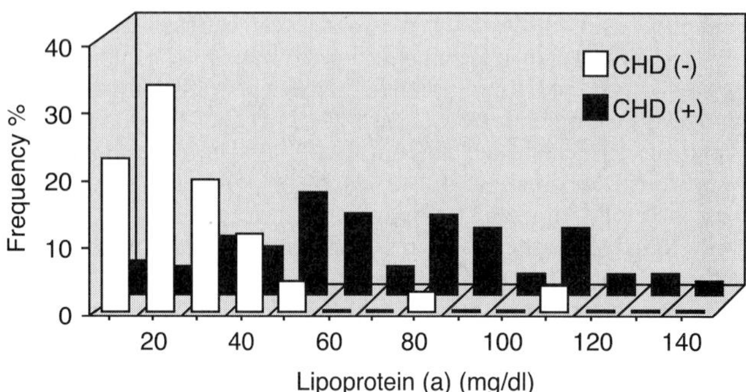

Fig. 116-11 Frequency distribution of serum lipoprotein(a) concentrations among patients with familial hypercholesterolemia who did and did not have CHD. (*Reproduced from Seed et al.[216] Used with permission.*)

the variability of Lp(a) concentration is affected by the two forms of familial hypercholesterolemia. The mechanism and nature of this effect is presently unclear, but if known, may shed light on the *in vivo* regulation of Lp(a) concentrations.

Familial hypercholesterolemia (MIM 143890) carries a marked increase in the risk of CHD, but there is considerable variation between individuals in disease susceptibility. One possible factor that may increase the risk for CHD in FH patients is elevated Lp(a). Two studies document that Lp(a) levels are markedly elevated in FH patients with CHD as compared to those patients without CHD[215,216] (Fig. 116-11). In both studies, discriminant function analysis showed that Lp(a) level was the best discriminator between the two groups as compared with other lipid and lipoprotein levels, age, sex, and smoking habits. In one study, apo(a) phenotypes were also determined, and the frequencies of those apo(a) isoforms that are associated with high Lp(a) levels were found significantly more frequently among the FH patients with CHD.[216] These findings were not confirmed by a recent family study from Canada.[372]

DISEASE ASSOCIATIONS AND EXOGENOUS EFFECTS

Age, gender, exercise, diet, and other environmental factors have long been considered to be without effect on Lp(a) levels, but it is now clear that they may have moderate effects.[246] In cord blood plasma, Lp(a) levels are low. They rise significantly from birth until day 7 postpartum and reach adult levels within 6 months.[374] Lp(a) concentrations do not correlate significantly with age in adult populations.[246,375] Diet affects Lp(a) levels in newborns. A Finnish study of coronary risk in babies included healthy infants and revealed that breast-fed babies on average had 40 percent lower Lp(a) than formula-fed babies. Upon weaning Lp(a) levels increased.[376] Recent, carefully controlled, dietary intervention studies have shown that elaidic acid or other *trans*-fatty acids from vegetables and marine sources significantly elevate Lp(a) levels.[377–379] Notably, these changes were only observed for high intakes of these compounds, which may explain why previous studies failed to detect the effect. The intake of *trans*-fatty acids produced by industrial hydrogenation of edible oils and fats also raises Lp(a) levels.[380] Intake of other dietary compounds lowers Lp(a) levels in comparison to a habitual diet. These include palm oil[381] and n-3 polyunsaturated fatty acids.[382,383] Saturated fatty acids reportedly have differential effects on Lp(a) concentrations.[384]. The effect of exercise on Lp(a) is dose dependent. Endurance and power athletes who exercise on a daily basis have elevated Lp(a),[385] but moderate exercise does not affect Lp(a) plasma levels in adults.[386,387] Heavy alcohol consumption does lower Lp(a),[388] and ethanol withdrawal in alcoholic men results in a rapid increase in Lp(a) levels.[389]

Direct and indirect evidence suggests that both male and female steroid sex hormones influence Lp(a) plasma levels. There are only small differences in Lp(a) levels between genders.[246] Lp(a) is, however, elevated in pregnancy[390] and in postmenopausal women.[247] Estrogen-progesterone replacement therapy in postmenopausal women lowers Lp(a).[196,391–394] The anabolic steroids stanozolol, danazol, and norethisterone, used in postmenopausal osteoporosis decrease Lp(a) levels by approximately 50 to 60 percent[395–397] In males with prostatic carcinoma, Lp(a) levels were found to drastically decrease upon estrogen treatment and to increase after orchidectomy, suggesting that sex hormones exert a regulatory role on Lp(a) levels in men.[398] Testosterone replacement does not change Lp(a) levels in hypogonadal men,[399] but when normal men receive testosterone supplements, Lp(a) concentrations decrease.[400] Thus, there is ample evidence that Lp(a) is under sex hormone control but precise actions and mechanisms are not yet defined. Thyroid hormone also has an effect on plasma Lp(a).[401] Hypothyroidism is associated with decreased Lp(a) and hyperthyroidism is associated with a significant increase Lp(a) concentration.[402–408]

Acute phase reaction,[409,410] and in particular that following a myocardial infarction, were reported to increase Lp(a).[411] The latter has been of particular concern because of the possibility that elevated Lp(a) in myocardial infarction might be secondary to the event.

A study in mice transgenic with an apo(a) YAC demonstrated a decrease rather than an increase in apo(a) following the induction of an acute phase reaction.[175] Because the dramatic response of apo(a)levels to puberty in male mice indicates that transgenic mice may react differently than do humans in their Lp(a) response to sex hormones, the findings in apo(a) YAC-transgenic mice do not rule out the possibility that Lp(a) is increased by acute phase induction in humans.

Renal disease is among the established conditions associated with significantly increased Lp(a) levels (see review in reference 81), which may be termed secondary hyper-Lp(a)-emia. This is of interest in view of the dramatically increased risk for coronary atherosclerosis in patients with end-stage kidney disease, and because it has, together with other evidence, implicated the kidney in Lp(a) catabolism (see Catabolism or Lp(a)). Plasma Lp(a) levels are markedly elevated in patients with proteinuria or nephrotic syndrome.[412–417] In such patients, extreme values of Lp(a) of over 400 mg/dl have been measured. These high Lp(a) levels decrease following remission of the nephrotic syndrome.[413–416] Whether or not there is a threshold for proteinuria at which Lp(a) levels start to increase is unknown. There seems to be no relation of Lp(a) response to apo(a) isoforms.[414] A turnover study using stable isotopes suggests that the increased Lp(a) levels in the patients are caused by increased synthesis[418] A plethora of studies has consistently demonstrated elevated Lp(a) concentrations in patients with end-stage renal disease, whether treated by hemodialysis or continuous ambulatory peritoneal dialysis (see review in reference 81). A large multicenter study that included 534 hemodialysis patients and 168 peritoneal dialysis patients showed significantly higher Lp(a) levels in peritoneal dialysis patients.[419] Interestingly the elevation of Lp(a) in patients with kidney disease is associated with apo(a) phenotype. Lp(a) is clearly and significantly elevated only in patients with phenotypes characterized by high-molecular-weight isoforms.[419–421] Hemodialysis patients with low-molecular-weight isoforms have Lp(a) levels similar to controls matched for apo(a) phenotype. The mechanism underlying this isoform-associated secondary elevation of Lp(a) in endstage renal disease is unclear. Lp(a) levels fall to a normal range following renal transplantation of patients with end-stage renal disease.[422–430]

The situation is less clear in diabetes mellitus. Some initial studies did report elevated Lp(a) in metabolically poorly controlled type II diabetics[431] and type I diabetics, and a decrease of Lp(a) with improved glycemic control in insulin-dependent diabetes mellitus (IDDM) subjects.[432] These and numerous other small case-control studies are likely to be biased and have obscured the field. If only large studies are considered, it becomes clear that Lp(a) is not elevated in patients with non-insulin-dependent diabetes (NIDDM).[433–438] Although the situation is more controversial in IDDM, all case-control and longitudinal studies together suggest that IDDM exerts only a moderate, if any, effect on Lp(a) concentration.[431,432,437,439–444] A study of identical twins did not find differences in Lp(a) levels between IDDM-affected and their unaffected cotwins with an interpair correlation of $r = 0.90$,[445] which is close to the correlation of $r = 0.94$ in identical twins without diabetes.[316] Thus, there is neither an effect on Lp(a) of NIDDM nor of IDDM that is large enough to explain the increased risk of diabetes patients for arteriosclerotic vascular disease. This should not be confused with the finding that, as in nondiabetics, Lp(a) is associated with ischemic heart disease and macroangiopathy.[442] The situation is different in diabetics who develop nephropathy. In such patients, Lp(a) plasma levels may rise, conferring additional risk to this group of diabetics.[414]

Lp(a) levels are low in severe liver disease.[446,447] Increased Lp(a) levels have been reported in cancer patients, but the significance of this observation is unclear.[448] Recently, a positive correlation of the degree of target-organ damage in arterial hypertension and Lp(a) plasma levels was described; multivariate analysis identified Lp(a) concentration as the best discriminator between patients with and without target-organ damage.[449] This finding needs confirmation by an independent study. Primary gout has also been associated with elevated Lp(a).[450]

LP(a) AND ATHEROTHROMBOTIC VASCULAR DISEASE

Epidemiology

Shortly after the discovery of the Lp(a) system by Berg,[1] it was recognized that high concentrations of Lp(a) in plasma are associated with CHD and early myocardial infarction.[10,34,35] Lp(a) was measured as a qualitative marker, either by immunodiffusion, agarose gel-electrophoresis, or polyacrylamide gel-electrophoresis, and atherosclerotic vascular disease was defined by angina pectoris, a previous myocardial infarction, or by the presence of coronary artery occlusion at coronary angiography.[10,302,451–455]

These original reports were confirmed by numerous studies in different ethnic groups, using different endpoints for definition of CHD and different methods to measure Lp(a) in plasma. Some recent studies included apo(a) phenotyping[66,67] and genotyping[456] (Fig. 116-12). The vast majority of these studies are cross-sectional case-control studies, but recent prospective studies, some of which included apo(a) phenotyping, confirm the role of Lp(a) as an independent risk factor for CHD. High Lp(a) is also associated with peripheral vascular disease and stroke (see recent reviews in references 457,458).

Coronary Heart Disease

In the first study considering Lp(a) as a quantitative trait, Kostner et al.[33] observed that Lp(a) levels above 30 mg/dl represent a 1.75-fold risk for myocardial infarction and that levels above 50 mg/dl represent a two- to threefold risk in normolipidemic men aged 40 to 60 years. From their study they concluded that Lp(a) concentrations greater than 30 mg/dl represent an independent risk factor for myocardial infarction. Although some authors have concluded that there is an apparent threshold for coronary risk at Lp(a) concentrations of 30 to 40 mg/dl, this has never been rigorously shown. This does not mean that for practical reasons values above a certain level should not be considered as critical; a concentration of 30 mg/dl does seem most appropriate.

Studies in Caucasian[36,248,459–462] and Asian[65,463] populations demonstrate the independence of Lp(a) from most other known cardiovascular risk factors. In most studies, no associations were observed between other lipoproteins including apo B and Lp(a) and between fibrinolytic parameters and Lp(a).[464] Some reports found a weak correlation between Lp(a) and triglycerides,[246–248] and associations between low HDL cholesterol[247,460] and

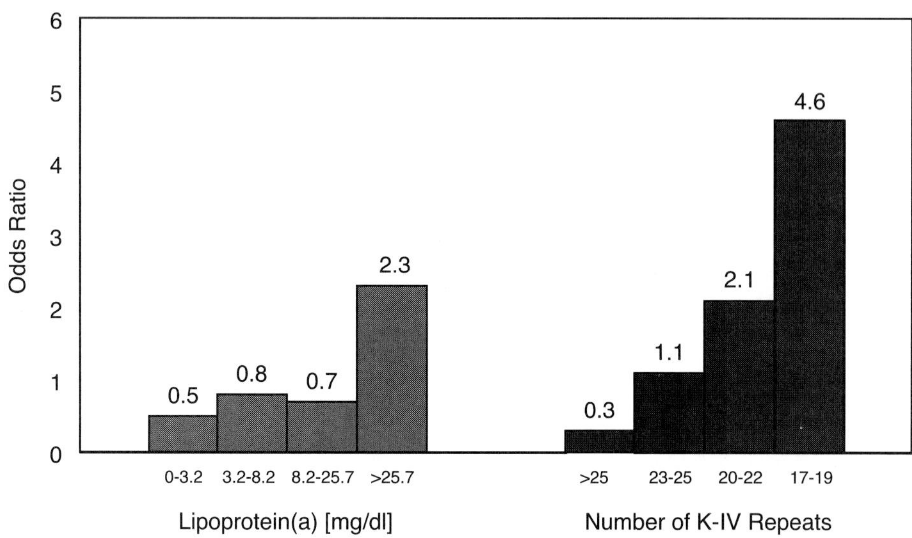

Fig. 116-12 The relative odds ratios for CHD associated with quintiles of Lp(a) concentrations and of apo(a) K IV-repeat number in Austrians. (Data from Kraft et al.[456])

hypoalphalipoproteinemia[247] with Lp(a). Although most studies did not find strong correlations between Lp(a) and other lipoprotein concentrations, it is noteworthy that several reports suggest an association of Lp(a) with dyslipidemic states.[33,214,365,366,368,460] Some of these may be explained by selection bias, but it seems unlikely that all are due to bias.

Compared to controls, higher levels of Lp(a) were measured in myocardial infarction patients from Austria,[33] Germany,[459,465] France,[462] Northern Ireland,[462] and Hawaii (Japanese).[37] An association of levels of Lp(a) with CHD documented by angiography was observed in several studies from different countries (U.S. Caucasians,[36,248] Koreans,[463] Tyroleans, Welsh, Singapore Chinese, and Singapore Indians).[66] By multivariate analysis, levels of Lp(a) were associated significantly and independently with the presence of CHD and tended to correlate with lesion scores in U.S. Caucasians.[36] Lp(a) levels were found associated with CHD in women and men.[36,248] Some studies indicate that Lp(a) may be a risk factor for early myocardial infarction, particularly in young men.[36,37,459] Others concluded that high Lp(a) is associated with rapid angiographic progression of CHD.[466] Considering only Lp(a) and no other risk factors, odds ratios ranging from ~1.5 to ~3.5 were reported for subjects with elevated Lp(a). [FES14]In an angiographic study that considered all of the major risk factors for CHD, multivariate predictors were age, family history, apo B, and Lp(a), in that order.[461] Together these studies suggest that plasma Lp(a) levels in Caucasian patients are a major risk factor with an importance that appears to approach that of the level of LDL or HDL cholesterol. In contrast to these variables, Lp(a) is strictly genetically controlled. Independence of Lp(a) from other risk factors does not mean, however, that Lp(a) and conventional risk factors do not interact. This issue is sometimes confused (e.g. interaction with LDL levels taken as evidence for dependence of Lp(a)). It is, therefore, important to note that the risk conferred by Lp(a) needs to be considered in the context of other independent risk factors.

A dependence on LDL and HDL levels has been demonstrated. Armstrong et al.[465] found an odds ratio of 2.7 for Lp(a) levels above 30 mg/dl versus Lp(a) levels below 5 mg/dl in a study of angiographed CHD-positive and CHD-negative patients from Germany. At concentrations above the median of LDL-cholesterol levels, the odds ratio increased to 6.0. An angiographic study in Wales demonstrated an odds ratio for CHD of ~5.0 in subjects with Lp(a) above the median and LDL-cholesterol in the upper quartile. The odds ratio increased to 38 if HDL-levels were also below the median (A. Rees, R. Morgan, Ch. Sandholzer, G. Utermann, unpublished). One study concluded that high Lp(a) increases the risk of familial CHD only if the ratio of total HDL cholesterol is elevated.[467] One study found that the odds ratio for CHD increased to 25 when the plasma total cholesterol cholesterol/HDL-cholesterol was >5.8 in individuals with Lp(a) over 40 mg/dl and to 122 when two or more nonlipid risk factors were also present.[468] Two studies in unrelated patients with FH (MIM 143890) identified significantly elevated Lp(a) in FH patients with CHD and concluded that Lp(a) levels are the best discriminator between FH patients with and without CHD.[215,216] Hence elevated Lp(a) may be a strong risk factor especially if associated with certain dyslipidemic states.

Some studies found an association between Lp(a) levels in offspring and myocardial infarction in their parents.[38,469] In the European Atherosclerosis Research Study (EARS), no relation of parental myocardial infarction with either Lp(a) level or apo(a) phenotype in offspring was found.[470] Another study observed that Lp(a) concentrations accounted for much of the familial predisposition to cardiac ischemia.[38] An increased prevalence of high Lp(a) has also been observed in families of CHD patients.[248]

In the Bogalusa Heart Study, the distribution Lp(a) level in children (8 to 17 years old) from two racial groups of a biracial community (U.S. Blacks and U.S. Caucasians) were related to parental myocardial infarction.[471] Caucasian children with parental myocardial infarction had increased levels of Lp(a) as compared to Caucasian children without parental myocardial infarction. The prevalence of parental myocardial infarction was higher in those with Lp(a) levels of more than 25 mg/dl than in those with 25 mg/dl or less. In contrast, a relation of Lp(a) to parental myocardial infarction was not seen in Black children. In view of the much higher Lp(a) levels in Blacks as compared to Caucasians, this finding is intriguing. The question of whether Lp(a) is a risk factor in Black populations has been studied only recently, and controversial results were obtained. No association was found in one study,[472] whereas another reported an association of Lp(a) with CHD in Black women but not in Black men.[473]

There are only a few case-control studies that did not find an association of Lp(a) level with atherosclerotic vascular disease in Caucasians,[474] and in some reports an association was found only in one gender (e.g., in Israeli men but not in Israeli women).[66] Such negative results are expected to occur considering the many studies that have been performed.

The strong genetic component in the determination of Lp(a) levels in conjunction with the results from the epidemiologic studies have led to the conclusion that high Lp(a) concentrations are an independent genetic risk factor for CHD. Strong support for this conclusion came from studies in which Lp(a) levels, apo(a) phenotype,[62,65–68,475,476] and apo(a) genotype[456] were analyzed in patients with CHD and controls, including one large multicenter study representing six different populations.[66] Low molecular apo(a) isoforms (designated B, S1, and S2), which are associated

Table 116-2 Prospective Studies Investigating Lp(a) As a Risk Factor for Coronary Heart Disease

Author (ref No.)	Number of patients/controls		Lp(a) (mg/dl) patients/controls		P	Years of follow-up
Rosengren, 1990[54] (Gothenberg Study)	26	109	27.8	17.3	0.01	6
Jauhiainen, 1991[52] (Helsinki Heart Study)	138	130	13.1	11.1	NS	5
Sigurdsson, 1992[53]	104	1228	23.0	17.0	0.014	8.6
Cressman, 1992[56]	26	103	78.9	35.4	<0.001	4
Coleman, 1992[57] (Guernsey Study)	51	3583	40.2	28.8	NS	?
Ridker, 1993[55] (Physicians' Health Study)	296	296	10.3	10.25	NS	5
Cremer, 1994[40] (GRIPS)	107	5124	18.0	9.0	<0.001	5
Bostom, 1994[60] (Framingham Study)	174	2679	8.2%*	4.1%*	<0.05	12
Alfthan, 1994[478] (North Carelia Project)	256	269	9.3	9.9	NS	9
Bostom, 1996[39] (Framingham Study)	129	2062	8.0%*	4.3%*	<0.05	15.4
Assmann, 1996[61] (PROCAM Study)	33	828	9.0	5.0	<0.011	8
Klausen, 1997[67] (MONICA Study)	74	190	12.4	9.4	<0.05†	8
Wild, 1997[62] (Stanford 5-City Project)	90	90	41.8	21.2	<0.01	13 (males)
	44	44	32.5	24.3	NS	13 (females)

*Given as percentage of cases/controls with Lp(a) >30 mg/dl.
†OR = 3.82, 95% CI: 1.47–9.96 for men aged below 60 Yrs

with high Lp(a) plasma concentrations, were more frequent in the CHD patients in all ethnic groups (Tyrolean, Germans, Danes, Welsh, Singapore Chinese, and Singapore Indian). The effects of the apo(a) size polymorphism on Lp(a) levels were similar in CHD patients and control subjects from the different populations.[66] The odds ratios for subjects with low-molecular-mass isoforms (B, S1, S2) to be in the CHD group ranged from 1.39 in Singapore Indians to 2.61 in Tyroleans from Austria, and the Mantel-Haenszel summary odds ratio was 1.78 in the pooled sample from six populations.[66] The data also suggest that odds ratios are similar in different populations. Results from stepwise logistic regression analysis indicated that apo(a) type is a significant predictor of CHD, independent of total cholesterol and HDL-cholesterol, but not independent of Lp(a) levels.[65] This suggests that alleles at the apo(a) locus determine the risk for CHD through their effects on Lp(a) levels.

There are now 18 prospective studies on Lp(a) in CHD with follow-up ranging from 5 to 13 years (see review in reference 477 and bibliographies in references 39, 40, 51–64, 67, and 478) (Table 116-2). Only four studies were unable to identify Lp(a) as a predictor of CHD, and Lp(a) levels were never lower in cases than controls in any study. All other studies yielded significant positive findings. The reasons for the negative findings of four of the prospective studies are unclear. Some had limitations in design that may have biased the outcome (e.g., included only patients with increased non-HDL-cholesterol[52] or excluded all individuals with known cardiovascular disease and/or younger subjects) and may have contributed to an underestimation of genetic risk factors like Lp(a). In some studies, the systematic use of lipid-lowering[52] or antithrombotic[55] drugs may have obscured the relation between Lp(a) and CHD. In all negative and in some other studies, Lp(a) was measured in samples frozen for long times. Dependent on the Lp(a) assay used, this may also have biased results.[479] These differences evoked provocative editorials on the "passing fashion" of "shrinking" lipoprotein "little" (a) that appeared in reputed journals.[480,481] For a time, Lp(a) was discredited as an independent risk factor for CHD, but with an increasing number of well-designed positive studies, Lp(a) regained its bad reputation as a vascular pathogen. The three studies that determined Lp(a) plasma concentrations or "sinking pre-β lipoprotein" (which is equivalent to a Lp(a) concentration above approximately 30 mg/dl) in fresh plasma samples, found Lp(a) as an independent predictor of CHD.[39,60,61] Apo(a) phenotypes were considered in one recent prospective study.[62] A higher frequency of low-molecular-weight isoforms was observed in cases versus controls. This study is the only one to date that used quantitative assay, which measures Lp(a) independent from apo(a) isoform size.[62] The plasma Lp(a) level is also a predictor of vein graft stenosis after coronary artery bypass surgery.[482,483]

Patients with renal disease seem to be particularly prone to high Lp(a) concentrations in plasma, and may develop a "galloping form of atherosclerosis"[484] if preexisting high Lp(a) concentrations and risk factors associated with end-stage renal disease coexist.[56,485–487] Three studies demonstrated that low-molecular-weight apo(a) isoforms are associated with increased risk for CHD in hemodialysis patients,[485–487] and stepwise logistic regression analysis has resulted in the surprising result that apo(a) phenotype is a better predictor of CHD than Lp(a) level in hemodialysis patients.[485] This has been explained as a consequence of the lifelong high Lp(a) in patients with low-molecular-weight isoforms as distinct from the disease-related elevation in high-molecular-weight isoforms.[485] A longitudinal study that included 440 patients over a follow-up period of 5 years confirmed that apo(a) phenotype is one of the best predictors for major coronary events in hemodialysis patients (F. Kronenberg, personal communication).

Cerebrovascular Disease

Besides its role in CHD, Lp(a) seems to have a significant role in the pathogenesis of carotid atherosclerosis and stroke.[488–491]

Case-control studies from Austria,[488] China,[489] Spain,[490] and Yugoslavia[491] all found significantly elevated Lp(a) levels in cases as compared to controls. There is a positive correlation of Lp(a) serum levels with the degree of carotid atherosclerosis.[484,488,491–493] Serum concentrations of Lp(a) have been related to the presence of asymptomatic echographic plaques in the carotid arteries of untreated middle-aged hypercholesterolemic men and in hemodialysis patients.[484,494] Lp(a) was found to be associated with carotid plaques, independent of other risk factors.

In the Bruneck Study, which follows random samples of 885 men and women, subjects with Lp(a) levels above the 85th percentile (32 mg/dl) had a 4.7-fold increased risk for stenotic and a 1.8-fold increased risk for nonstenotic carotid atherosclerosis.[495] An association with stroke was not confirmed in the prospective Physicians Health Study,[496] but the cohort of this study also did not reveal the established association of Lp(a) with CHD. Apo(a) phenotypes were considered in some of the stroke case control studies.[484,492,497] Two studies have related Lp(a) concentrations and apo(a) phenotypes to carotid atherosclerosis, the Atherosclerosis Risk in Community (ARIC) Study[492] and a study in hemodialysis patients.[484] In both studies, arterial wall thickness and numbers of affected sites correlated with Lp(a) concentration, but in only one study[484] was there a correlation with apo(a) phenotype.

Evidence for the Role of Lp(a) in Atherosclerosis from Pathology

Apolipoprotein(a) deposition in the arterial wall, and especially in areas of atherosclerotic plaque formation, was demonstrated by immunohistochemistry.[24,498,499] Colocalization with apo B and extraction of apo(a)/apo B complexes from atherosclerotic plaques suggest that Lp(a) is deposited in the plaque as an intact particle.[499] The amount of Lp(a) in the atherosclerotic plaques correlates with the concentration of Lp(a) in plasma. The ratio of apo(a) over apo B in a plaque is much higher than the ratio of apo(a)/apo B in plasma. This suggests that either there is more deposition of Lp(a) in an atherosclerotic plaque as compared to LDL or that uptake/binding mechanisms for Lp(a) by components of the growing plaque are different for Lp(a) and LDL resulting in a preferential degradation of apo B from LDL. The data can not be interpreted to suggest that Lp(a) is more important in the formation of plaques than is LDL. Lp(a) is also deposited in vein grafts following coronary artery bypass surgery.[483]

Apo(a) Transgenic Animals

Evidence that apo(a) promotes development of atherosclerosis came from an initial study in mice that were transgenic for the human apo(a) gene.[194] The apo(a) transgenics developed plaques when fed a high-cholesterol atherogenic diet. It was amazing that the mice developed plaques, although most apo(a) was present in the free form in their plasma because mouse LDL does not form Lp(a) particles with human apo(a). This might suggest that apo(a) does contribute to the development of atherosclerosis even as a free uncomplexed glycoprotein. Apo(a) immunoreactivity was, however, localized precisely at sites where cholesterol also was deposited. There are several interpretations for this finding that were discussed in the original report[194] and an accompanying comment.[500] A feedback mechanism in which an initial accumulation of apo(a) inhibits local TGF-β activity, leading to further apo(a) accumulation and activation of smooth muscle cells that subsequently accumulate lipid to form lesions if the mice are fed a high-fat diet, has been postulated.[501] Unfortunately, and reminiscent of the situation with prospective studies in humans, later reports on the potential of apo(a) or Lp(a) to precipitate atherosclerosis in transgenic animals were controversial. In line with the original observations, atherosclerotic lesions were shown to be significantly reduced in mice that were double transgenic for apo(a) and human apo A-I.[502] Transgenics for a mutagenized human apo(a) in which the lysine-binding site had been destroyed also failed to develop lesions,[503] and a reduction in lesions was observed in transgenics where wild-type human apo(a) was expressed on the background of a fibrinogen knockout.[504] This suggests that the binding of apo(a)/Lp(a) demonstrated *in vitro* may occur *in vivo* and could be responsible for mediating the binding of apo(a) to the vessel wall. Mancini et al.[505] were unable to confirm the results from the initial investigation. These authors also observed only a modest and insignificant increase in lesions in mice coexpressing human apo(a) and apo B.[120] Such mice assemble Lp(a) in plasma, making them a more appropriate model to study the atherogenic potential of Lp(a) than mice transgenic for apo(a) alone. In contrast, Callow et al.[506] reported a significant increase in the number and size of lesions of Lp(a) transgenic mice (apo(a)/apo B double transgenics). Finally, Sanan et al.,[507] in a study of LDLR knockout mice, demonstrated a significant effect of human apo B-100 on atherosclerotic lesion formation, even with a low-fat diet. However, addition of Lp(a) to the plasma of these animals by coexpression of human apo(a) did not further accelerate atherosclerosis.

Whatever the reasons for the conflicting data in transgenic mice might be, it seems clear that other animal models are needed. Mice do not have the genetic machinery to produce Lp(a) and may also lack appropriate apo(a)/Lp(a)-binding proteins. The lipoprotein metabolism in mice is different from that in humans, and the hormonal regulation of human apo(a) expression in mice is different from the regulation in humans.[175] Together this indicates that mice may not be an optimal model for addressing the question of whether and how Lp(a) is atherogenic. Apo(a) transgenic rabbits have been developed, but their plasma Lp(a) is very low.[508]

Quantification of Plasma Lp(a)

The inherent characteristics of the apo(a)/Lp(a) system make the quantification of Lp(a) a challenging task, and this is reflected in the development of a plethora of assays and methods. Several potential pitfalls and sources of variation need consideration (see reviews in references 509 to 511). Two major problems that do not exist for most other proteins are encountered when measuring Lp(a). Both relate to the size polymorphism of apo(a). First, the mass of Lp(a) particles is not identical due to the wide variation in the sizes of isoforms. Many samples contain two Lp(a) species of different mass. Therefore, standards are not identical. This problem may be overcome by expressing Lp(a) concentrations in moles rather than in mass units as is presently the convention in most laboratories. This is not trivial and requires knowledge of the precise protein molecular mass in the standard.

Second, most available antibodies against apo(a) recognize repeated immunodominant epitopes of the multiple K IV units.[512] Because of the dependence on the isoform size in the sample and because of the different standards, such antibodies will give different values. Lp(a) containing high-molecular-mass isoforms is likely to be overestimated as compared to Lp(a) with a low-molecular-mass isoform. Further problems relate to the occurrence of some apo(a) in free form (as opposed to complexed to LDL) and to the instability of the Lp(a) particle, which is easily proteolytically cleaved and oxidized. A working group of the International Federation of Clinical Chemistry (IFCC) was established to deal with these problems. The group is currently testing several commercial calibrators for use as secondary reference standards.[513]

To overcome problems of particle heterogeneity, assays based on the measurement of Lp(a) cholesterol were developed,[514,515] but they are not widely used. Several immunochemical methods are currently in use to measure Lp(a) in plasma, and for the above mentioned reasons none of these is ideal. No generally accepted reference standard and no universally applicable antibodies are currently available. Radial immunodiffusion,[6,375] electroimmunodiffusion,[33,516] various ELISA methods,[152,517,518] nephelometry,[519] latex immunoassay,[520] radioimmunoassays, and fluorescence immunoassay[521] all have been applied. Polyclonal and monoclonal antibodies against Lp(a) or apo(a) sometimes in combination with anti-apo B are used in the ELISA assays (see reviews in references 510 and 522).

It has been suggested that the apo B in Lp(a), rather than the apo(a), could be measured to overcome the problem of isoform heterogeneity. ELISA methods based on anti-Lp(a) capture antibodies and anti-apo B-detecting antibodies have been developed.[523–525] Although ideal in theory, these assays have some drawbacks. One drawback is that the molar ratio of apo(a):apo B may not be always 1:1 in apo(a)-containing particles. A sizable amount of Lp(a) may be associated with triglyceride-rich lipoproteins,[141] and complexes of Lp(a) with LDL may exist in unfractionated plasma. Moreover, the stability of Lp(a) in the standard and samples must be guaranteed, which, again, is not trivial in view of the properties of the particle. Monoclonal antibodies or polyclonal antipeptide antibodies against epitopes that exist just once in apo(a) (e.g., K V or protease domain) are considered the reagents of choice. One such assay has been published[526] and a another assay was recently developed (M. Hohenegger, G. Utermann, H. Dieplinger, unpublished). Cross-reactivities of monoclonal antibodies with PLG are recognized and no longer pose a problem in assays for plasma Lp(a) quantification.[326] The immunochemical reactivity of Lp(a) is reduced by thiols and cysteine-containing compounds, and the reactivity of apo(a) dissociated from the particle by reductive cleavage is markedly reduced.[527] This may be relevant when measuring Lp(a) in plasma from subjects with high concentrations of cysteine-containing compounds. Long-term storage and lyophilization may also effect Lp(a) immunoreactivity depending on the assay method.[479,528–530] Lp(a) measurement in dried blood spots from newborns has been recommended as a screening procedure.[531,532] Although technically feasible, this recommendation seems premature. Measuring Lp(a) is trickier than for other plasma proteins, but the results of most Lp(a) assays are sufficient for practical medicine. Precision and reproducibility of most ELISA/delayed fluorescence immunoassay (Delfia) are good (precision = ±5 percent)[533] and much of the epidemiologic work has been done using these assays. Therefore, it is certainly possible to use them for prediction of risk.

A particular problem is sample storage. Existing data on the influence of long-term storage and multiple thawing and freezing on the stability of Lp(a) are conflicting[52,479,529,533–537] but together show that each assay has to be evaluated carefully before it can be used to measure Lp(a) in stored plasma samples.

Perhaps more important than how to measure Lp(a) is the question of whose Lp(a) should be measured. Four groups have been suggested for screening for elevated Lp(a) concentrations: (a) all patients with elevated LDL-cholesterol levels and those patients with other forms of dyslipoproteinemia for whom pharmacologic therapy is being considered; (b) young patients with atherosclerotic cardiovascular or cerebrovascular disease; (c) patients from families with a strong history of early cardiovascular or cerebrovascular disease; and (d) patients with renal failure. Although there is currently no satisfactory pharmacologic method to lower Lp(a), knowing the level of this compound may guide the therapeutic schedule.

Apo(a) Genotyping and Phenotyping

Apo(a) genotyping (i.e., determination of genomic apo(a) K IV-2 repeat number) is performed by PFGE/Southern blotting of *Kpn*I- or *Hpa*I-restricted genomic DNA.[73,170,334] The method of choice for apo(a) phenotyping is high-resolution SDS agarose gel-electrophoresis, which permits typing of all expressed apo(a) alleles.[323] These procedures are not for routine use. Commercial kits for apo(a) phenotyping by SDS-PAGE are available. Their resolution and sensitivity are not sufficient to allow separation and identification of all isoforms, but they may well be adequate for some clinical studies (e.g., for risk assessment in patients with kidney disease). Extreme care in the choice of adequate standards must be taken to make the results of such assays comparable.[337]

THERAPEUTIC APPROACHES TO HIGH LP(a)

In general, pharmacologic approaches to lower Lp(a) have met with frustrating results. No drug that has a high potency to lower LDL lowers Lp(a), with the only exception being nicotinic acid. HMG-CoA reductase inhibitors that are most effective in reducing LDL-cholesterol levels have no consistent effect on Lp(a) levels in hypercholesterolemic subjects.[215,538–544] No difference between the various reductase inhibitors was noted in these studies. The same is true for bile acid sequestrants or a combination of HMG-CoA reductase inhibitors and resins.[215,545] Some steroid hormones lower Lp(a) dramatically, but their side effects prevent their use as Lp(a) lowering drugs.[395,397,546]

Recently, the antiestrogen tamoxifen was shown to reduce Lp(a) levels.[547,548] The synthetic steroid tibolone decreases Lp(a) by 26 to 39 percent, but this is accompanied by a decrease in HDL-cholesterol that may counteract the potentially positive action on Lp(a).[549]

Lp(a) levels have been significantly lowered by nicotinic acid in a group ($N = 31$) of hyperlipidemic subjects.[550] There was a strong negative relationship between the percentage reduction of Lp(a) and the serum triglyceride level before treatment in this study ($r = -0.78$). Lp(a) levels increased in subjects with triglycerides above 7.5 mM. Thus, nicotinic acid may not be the drug of choice for all patients with high Lp(a). Treatment of hyperlipidemic patients with α-tocopheryl nicotinate decreased Lp(a) levels in patients with initial high Lp(a) levels.[551]

A combination of nicotinic acid with neomycin may also lower high Lp(a) levels, and neomycin alone reportedly has a moderate Lp(a)-lowering effect.[206] Neomycin interferes with Lp(a) assembly at the hepatocyte cell surface.[200] Because this drug raised total cholesterol and apo B levels, it cannot be recommended for treatment of high Lp(a).

The potential of several substances to lower Lp(a) by interfering with Lp(a) assembly has been tested *in vitro* and *in vivo*. An initial trial with *N*-acetylcysteine seemed promising,[552] but there is evidence now that application of the drug may have altered the immunoreactivity of apo(a)/Lp(a) rather than lowering it.[553,554] This subject is still in dispute.[555] Related substances (e.g., carbocysteine) reportedly do not lower Lp(a).[556] Tranexamic acid, which showed a significant inhibition of Lp(a) assembly *in vitro*, has been tested *in vivo*, resulting in a moderate response average (−18.5 percent) in eight patients.[557] ACTH also has a strong potential to reduce Lp(a) concentrations (up to −65 percent).[558–560]

Because there is no safe drug that effectively and reproducibly reduces Lp(a) levels, and because there are no current data indicating that lowering Lp(a) levels is beneficial, it is not possible at this time to make firm recommendations concerning whether patients with high Lp(a) concentrations should be treated. Lower Lp(a) is strongly recommended, however, as a secondary prevention strategy in patients with established premature CHD and high Lp(a) levels.[561] Therapeutic LDL-apheresis and plasmapheresis have been effectively used to lower LDL and Lp(a) in patients with FH (MIM 143890). This may be the method of choice for patients in whom both lipoproteins are markedly elevated and CHD is present.[562] Lp(a)-apheresis has also been developed to reduce Lp(a) in patients with excessive Lp(a) and CHD but without high LDL. No data are available that justify recommendations to lower Lp(a) in patients with isolated Lp(a) elevations without overt CHD except for those with a strong family history of premature CHD.

REFERENCES

1. Berg K: A new serum type system in man: The Lp-system. *Acta Pathol Microbiol Scand* **59**:369, 1963.
2. Berg K, Mohr J: Genetics of the Lp System. *Acta Genet* **13**:349, 1963.
3. Berg K: Further studies on the Lp-System. *Vox Sang* **11**:419, 1966.

4. Wiegandt H, Lipp K, Wendt G: Identifizierung eines Lipoproteins mit antigenwirksamkeit im Lp-system. *Hoppe-Seyler's Z Physiol Chem* **349**:489, 1968.
5. Harvie NR, Schultz JS: Studies of Lp-lipoprotein as a quantitative trait. *Proc Natl Acad Sci U S A* **66**:99, 1970.
6. Ehnholm C, Garoff H, Simons K, Aro H: Purification and quantification of the human plasma lipoprotein carrying the Lp(a) antigen. *Biochim Biophys Acta* **239**:431, 1971.
7. Utermann G, Wiegand H: Separation and characterization of a lipoprotein with antigenic activity in the Lp(a) system. *Hum Genet* **8**:39, 1969.
8. Utermann G: The mysteries of lipoprotein(a). *Science* **246**:904, 1989.
9. Rider AK, Levy RI, Fredrickson DS: "Sinking" prebeta lipoprotein and the Lp antigen. *Circulation* **42(Suppl 3)**:10, 1970.
10. Dahlen G: The pre-beta1 lipoprotein phenomenon in relation to serum cholesterol and triglyceride levels, the Lp(a) lipoprotein and coronary heart disease. *Acta Med Scand* **570(Suppl)**:1, 1974.
11. Albers JJ, Chen C-H, Aladjem F: Human serum lipoproteins. Evidence for three classes of lipoproteins in Sf 9-2. *Biochemistry* **11**:57, 1972.
12. Sodhi HS: New lipoprotein differing in charge and density from known plasma lipoproteins. *Metabolism* **18(10)**:852, 1969.
13. Wille LE, Phillips GB: Demonstration of an atypical pre-β-lipoprotein in human serum. *Clin Genet* **2**:242, 1971.
14. Simons K, Ehnholm C, Renkonen O, Bloth B: Characterization of the Lp(a) lipoprotein in human plasma. *Acta Path Microbiol Scand* **78**:459, 1970.
15. Ehnholm C, Garoff H, Renkonen O, Simons K: Protein and carbohydrate composition of Lp(a) lipoprotein from human plasma. *Biochemistry* **11**:3229, 1972.
16. Seidel D, Geisen HP, Roelcke D: Identification of the protein moiety of the Lp(a)-lipoprotein in human plasma. *FEBS Lett* **18**:43, 1971.
17. Utermann G, Weber W: Protein composition of Lp(a) lipoprotein from human plasma. *FEBS Lett* **154**:357, 1983.
18. Gaubatz JW, Heideman C, Gotto AMJr, Morrisett JD, Dahlen GH: Human plasma lipoprotein (a): Structural properties. *J Biol Chem* **258**:4582, 1983.
19. Fless GM, Zum Mallen ME, Scanu AM: Isolation of apolipoprotein (a) from lipoprotein (a). *J Lipid Res* **26**:1224, 1985.
20. McLean JW, Tomlinson JE, Kuang W-J, Eaton DL, Chen EY, Fless GM, Scanu AM, et al: cDNA sequence of human apolipoprotein(a) is homologous to plasminogen. *Nature* **300**:132, 1987.
21. Edelberg JM, Gonzales-Gronow M, Pizzo SV: Lipoprotein(a) inhibits streptokinase-mediated activation of human plasminogen. *Biochemistry* **28**:2370, 1989.
22. Gonzales-Gronow M, Edelberg J, Pizzo S: Further characterization of the cellular plasminogen binding site: Evidence that plasminogen 2 and lipoprotein(a) compete for the same site. *Biochemistry* **28**:2374, 1989.
23. Miles LA, Fless GM, Levin EG, Scanu AM, Plow EF: A potential basis for the thrombotic risks associated with lipoprotein(a). *Nature* **339**:301, 1989.
24. Hajjar KA, Gavish D, Breslow JL, Nachman RL: Lipoprotein(a) modulation of endothelial cell surface fibrinolysis and its potential role in atherosclerosis. *Nature* **339**:303, 1989.
25. Harpel P, Gordon B, Parker T: Plasmin catalyzes binding of lipoprotein(a) to immobilized fibrinogen and fibrin. *Proc Natl Acad Sci U S A* **86**:3847, 1989.
26. Miles LA, Plow EF: Lp(a): An interloper into the fibrinolytic system? *Thromb Haemost* **63**:331, 1990.
27. Grainger DJ, Kirschenlohr HL, Metcalfe JC, Weissberg PL, Wade DP, Lawn RM: Proliferation of human smooth muscle cells promoted by lipoprotein(a). *Science* **260**:1655, 1993.
28. Grainger DJ, Kemp PR, Liu AC, Lawn RM, Metcalfe JC: Activation of transforming growth factor-b is inhibited in transgenic apolipoprotein(a) mice. *Nature* **370**:460, 1994.
29. Takami S, Yamashita S, Kihara S, Ishigami M, Takemura K, Kume N, Kita T, et al: Lipoprotein(a) enhances the expression of intercellular adhesion molecule-1 in cultured human umbilical vein endothelial cells. *Circulation* **97**:721, 1998.
30. Allen S, Khan S, Tam Sp, Koschinsky M, Taylor P, Yacoub M: Expression of adhesion molecules by lp(a): A potential novel mechanism for its atherogenicity. *FASEB J* **12**:1765, 1998.
31. Klezovitch O, Edelstein C, Zhu L, Scanu AM: Apolipoprotein(a) binds via its C-terminal domain to the protein core of the proteoglycan decorin. Implications for the retention of lipoprotein(a) in atherosclerotic lesions. *J Biol Chem* **273**:23856, 1998.
32. Köchl S, Fresser F, Lobentanz E, Baier G, Utermann G: Novel interaction of apolipoprotein(a) with b-2 glycoprotein I, mediated by the kringle IV domain. *Blood* **90**:1482, 1997.
33. Kostner GM, Avogaro P, Cazzolato G, Marth E, Bittolo-Bon G, Quinci GB: Lipoprotein Lp(a) and the risk for myocardial infarction. *Atherosclerosis* **38**:51, 1981.
34. Berg K, Dahlen G, Frick MH: Lp (a) lipoprotein and pre-beta lipoprotein in patients with coronary heart disease. *Clin Genet* **6**:230, 1974.
35. Rhoads GG, Morton NE, Gulbrandsen, Kagan A: Shrinking pre-beta lipoprotein and coronary heart disease in Japanese-American men in Hawaii. *Am J Epidemiol* **108**:350, 1978.
36. Dahlen G, Guyton JR, Arrar M, Farmer JA, Kautz JA, Gotto AM Jr: Association of levels of lipoprotein Lp (a), plasma lipids, and other lipoproteins with coronary artery disease documented by angiography. *Circulation* **74**:758, 1986.
37. Rhoads GG, Dahlen G, Berg K, Morton NE, Dannenberg AL: Lp (a) lipoprotein as a risk factor for myocardial infarction. *JAMA* **256**:2540, 1986.
38. Durrington PN, Ishola M, Hunt L, Arrol S, Bhatnagar D: Apolipoproteins (a), AI, and B and parental history in men with early onset ischaemic heart disease. *Lancet* **i**:1070, 1988.
39. Bostom AG, Cupples LA, Jenner JL, Ordovas JM, Seman LJ, Wilson PWF, Schaefer EJ, et al: Elevated plasma lipoprotein(a) and coronary heart disease in men aged 55 years and younger—A prospective study. *JAMA* **276**:544, 1996.
40. Cremer P, Nagel D, Labrot B, Mann H, Muche R, Elster H, Seidel D: Lipoprotein Lp(a) as predictor of myocardial infarction in comparison to fibrinogen, LDL cholesterol and other risk factors: Results from the prospective Göttingen Risk Incidence and Prevalence Study (GRIPS). *Eur J Clin Invest* **24**:444, 1994.
41. Scanu AM, Fless GM: Lipoprotein (a). Heterogeneity and biological relevance. *J Clin Invest* **85**:1709, 1990.
42. Mbewu AD, Durrington PN: Lipoprotein(a): Structure, properties and possible involvement in thrombogenesis and atherogenesis. *Atherosclerosis* **85**:1, 1990.
43. Scanu AM, Lawn RM, Berg K: Lipoprotein(a) and atherosclerosis. *Ann Intern Med* **115**:209, 1991.
44. Scanu AM: Lipoprotein(a): A genetically determined cardiovascular pathogen in search of a function. *J Lab Clin Med* **116**:142, 1990.
45. Lawn RM: Lipoprotein(a) in heart disease. *Sci Am* **266**:54, 1992.
46. Loscalzo J: Lipoprotein(a). A unique risk factor for atherothrombotic disease. *Arteriosclerosis* **10**:672, 1990.
47. Rees A: Lipoprotein (a): A possible link between lipoprotein metabolism and thrombosis. *Br Heart J* **65**:2, 1991.
48. Scott J: Lipoprotein(a). *BMJ* **303**:663, 1991.
49. Scanu AM: Lipoprotein(a): A genetic risk factor for premature coronary heart disease. *JAMA* **267**:3326, 1992.
50. Utermann G: Lipoprotein(a): A genetic risk factor for premature coronary heart disease. *Nutr Metab Cardiovasc Dis* **1**:7, 1991.
51. Dahlen GH: Lipoprotein(a) in relation to atherosclerotic diseases. *Prog Clin Biol Res* **255**:27, 1988.
52. Jauhiainen M, Koskinen P, Ehnholm C, Frick HM, Mänttäri M, Manninen V, Huttunen JK: Lipoprotein(a) and coronary heart disease risk: A nested case-control study of the Helsinki Heart Study participants. *Atherosclerosis* **89**:59, 1991.
53. Sigurdsson G, Baldursdottir A, Sigvaldason H, Agnarsson U, Thorgeirsson G, Sigfusson N: Predictive value of apolipoproteins in a prospective survey of coronary artery disease in men. *Am J Cardiol* **69**(16):1251, 1992.
54. Rosengren A, Wilhelmsen L, Eriksson E, Risberg B, Wedel H: Lipoprotein (a) and coronary heart disease: A prospective case-control study in a general population sample of middle aged men. *BMJ* **301**:1248, 1990.
55. Ridker PM, Hennekens CH, Stampfer MJ: A prospective study of lipoprotein(a) and the risk of myocardial infarction. *JAMA* **270**:2195, 1993.
56. Cressman MD, Heyka RJ, Paganini EP, O'Neil J, Skibinski CI, Hoff HF: Lipoprotein(a) is an independent risk factor for cardiovascular disease in hemodialysis patients. *Circulation* **86**:475, 1992.
57. Coleman MP, Key TJ, Wang DY, Hermon C, Fentiman IS, Allen DS, Jarvis M, et al: A prospective study of obesity, lipids, apolipoproteins and ischaemic heart disease in women. *Atherosclerosis* **92**:177, 1992.
58. Wald NJ, Law M, Watt HC, Wu T, Bailey A, Johnson AM, Craig WY, et al: Apolipoproteins and ischaemic heart disease: Implications for screening. *Lancet* **343**:75, 1994.

59. Schaefer EJ, Lamon-Fava S, Jenner JL, McNamara JR, Ordovas JM, Davis CE, Abolafia JM, et al: Lipoprotein(a) levels and risk of coronary heart disease in men: The lipid research clinics coronary primary prevention trial. *JAMA* **271**:999, 1994.
60. Bostom AG, Gagnon DR, Cupples LA, Wilson PWF, Jenner JL, Ordovas JM, Schaefer EJ, et al: A prospective investigation of elevated lipoprotein (a) detected by electrophoresis and cardiovascular disease in women: The Framingham Heart Study. *Circulation* **90**:1688, 1994.
61. Assmann G, Schulte H, Von Eckardstein A: Hypertriglyceridemia and elevated lipoprotein(a) are risk factors for major coronary events in middle-aged men. *Am J Cardiol* **77**:1179, 1996.
62. Wild SH, Fortmann SP, Marcovina SM: A prospective case-control study of lipoprotein(a) levels and apo(a) size and risk of coronary heart disease in Stanford Five-City Project participants. *Arterioscler Thromb Vasc Biol* **17**:239, 1997.
63. Nguyen TT, Ellefson RD, Hodge DO, Bailey KR, Kottke TE, Abu-Lebdeh HS: Predictive value of electrophoretically detected lipoprotein(a) for coronary heart disease and cerebrovascular disease in a community-based cohort of 9936 men and women. *Circulation* **96**:1390, 1997.
64. Cantin B, Gagnon F, Moorjani S, Despres JP, Lamarche B, Lupien PJ, Dagenais GR: Is lipoprotein(a) an independent risk factor for ischemic heart disease in men? The Quebec Cardiovascular Study. *J Am Coll Cardiol* **31**:519, 1998.
65. Sandholzer C, Boerwinkle E, Saha N, Tong C, Utermann G: Apolipoprotein(a) phenotypes, Lp(a) concentration and plasma lipid levels in relation to coronary heart disease in a chinese population: Evidence for the role of the apo(a) gene in coronary heart disease. *J Clin Invest* **89**:1040, 1992.
66. Sandholzer C, Saha N, Kark JD, Rees A, Jaross W, Dieplinger H, Hoppichler F, et al: Apo(a) isoforms predict risk for coronary heart disease: A study in six populations. *Arterioscler Thromb* **12**:1214, 1992.
67. Klausen IC, Sjol A, Hansen PS, Gerdes LU, Moller L, Lemming L, Schroll M, et al: Apolipoprotein(a) isoforms and coronary heart disease in men: A nested case-control study. *Atherosclerosis* **132**:77, 1997.
68. Parlavecchia M, Pancaldi A, Taramelli R, Valsania P, Galli L, Pozza G, Chierchia S, et al: Evidence that apolipoprotein(a) phenotype is a risk factor for coronary artery disease in men <55 years of age. *Am J Cardiol* **74**:346, 1994.
69. Sing CF, Schultz JS, Shreffler DC: The genetics of the LP antigen II. A family study and proposed models of genetic control. *Ann Hum Genet* **38**:47, 1974.
70. Morton NE, Berg K, Dahlen G, Ferrel RE, Rhoads GG: Genetics of the Lp lipoprotein in Japanese-Americans. *Genet Epidemiol* **2**:113, 1985.
71. Albers JJ, Wahl P, Hazzard WR: Quantitative genetic studies of the human plasma Lp(a) lipoprotein. *Biochem Genet* **11**:475, 1974.
72. Boerwinkle E, Leffert CC, Lin J, Lackner C, Chiesa G, Hobbs HH: Apolipoprotein(a) gene accounts for greater than 90% of the variation in plasma lipoprotein(a) concentrations. *J Clin Invest* **90**:52, 1992.
73. Kraft HG, Köchl S, Menzel HJ, Sandholzer C, Utermann G: The apolipoprotein(a) gene: A transcribed hypervariable locus controlling plasma lipoprotein(a) concentration. *Hum Genet* **90**:220, 1992.
74. Scholz M, Kraft HG, Lingenhel A, Delport R, Vorster EH, Bickeböller H, Utermann G: Genetic Control of lipoprotein(a) concentrations is different in Africans and Caucasians. *Eur J Hum Genet* **7**:169, 1999.
75. DeMeester CA, Bu X, Gray RJ, Lusis AJ, Rotter JI: Genetic variation in lipoprotein(a) levels in families enriched for coronary artery disease is determined almost entirely by the apolipoprotein(a) gene locus. *Am J Hum Genet* **56**:287, 1995.
76. Mooser V, Scheer D, Marcovina SM, Wang J, Guerra R, Cohen J, Hobbs HH: The apo(a) gene is the major determinant of variation in plasma Lp(a) levels in African Americans. *Am J Hum Genet* **61**:402, 1997.
77. Frank SL, Klisak I, Sparkes RS, Mohandas T, Tomlinson JE, McLean JW, Lawn RM, et al: The apolipoprotein (a) gene resides on human chromosome 6q26-27 in close proximity to the homologous gene for plasminogen. *Hum Genet* **79**:352, 1988.
78. Drayna DT, Hegele RA, Hass PE, Wu LL, Emi M, Eaton DL, Lawn RM, et al: Genetic linkage between lipoprotein (a) phenotype and a DNA polymorphism in the plasminogen gene. *Genomics* **3**:230, 1988.
79. Lindahl G, Gersdorf E, Menzel HJ, Duba C, Cleve H, Humphries S, Utermann G: The gene for the Lp (a) specific glycoprotein is closely linked to the gene for plasminogen on chromosome 6. *Hum Genet* **81**:149, 1989.
80. Weitkamp LR, Guttormsen SA, Schultz JS: Linkage between the loci for the Lp (a) lipoprotein (LP) and plasminogen. *Hum Genet* **79**:80, 1988.
81. Kronenberg F, Utermann G, Dieplinger H: Lipoprotein(a) in renal disease. *Am J Kidney Dis* **27**:1, 1996.
82. Fless GM, Zum Mallen ME, Scanu AM: Physicochemical properties of apolipoprotein (a) and lipoprotein (a−) derived from the dissociation of human plasma lipoprotein (a). *J Biol Chem* **261**:8712, 1986.
83. Armstrong VW, Walli AK, Seidel D: Isolation, characterization and uptake in human fibroblasts of apo (a)-free lipoprotein obtained on reduction of lipoprotein (a). *J Lipid Res* **26**:1314, 1985.
84. Jürgens G, Kostner GM: Studies on the structure of the Lp(a) lipoprotein: Isolation and partial characterization of the Lp(a)-specific antigen. *Immunogenetics* **1**:560, 1975.
85. Kraft HG, Sandholzer C, Menzel HJ, Utermann G: Apolipoprotein(a) alleles determine lipoprotein(a) particle density and concentration in plasma. *Arterioscler Thromb* **12(3)**:302, 1992.
86. Roelcke D, Weicker H: Physikochemische, immunologische und biochemische Charakterisierung des Proteinanteils der low-density lipoproteins. *Z Klin Chem Klin Biochem* **7**:467, 1969.
87. Roelcke D, Krah E, Fahimian A: Die Unterteilbarkeit menschlicher Lipoproteine niederer Dichte (LDL) hinsichtlich ihrer Lp(a)-Eigenschaft durch Ionenaustauscher-Säulenchromatographie. *Blut* **18**:160, 1968.
88. Armstrong VW, Harrach B, Robenek H, Helmhold M, Walli AK, Seidel D: Heterogeneity of human lipoprotein Lp(a): Cytochemical and biochemical studies on the interaction of two Lp(a) species with the LDL receptor. *J Lipid Res* **31**:429, 1990.
89. Gaubatz JW, Chari MV, Nava L, Guyton JR, Morrisett JD: Isolation and characterization of the two major apoproteins in human lipoprotein(a). *J Lipid Res* **28**:69, 1987.
90. Utermann G, Lipp K, Wiegandt H: Studies on the Lp(a)-lipoprotein of human serum. IV. The disaggregation of the Lp(a)-lipoprotein. *Humangenetik* **14**:142, 1972.
91. Reblin T, Rader DJ, Beisiegel U, Greten H, Brewer HBJr: Correlation of apolipoprotein(a) isoproteins with Lp(a) density and distribution in fasting plasma. *Atherosclerosis* **94**:223, 1992.
92. Garoff H, Simons K, Ehnholm C, Berg K: Demonstration by disc electrophoresis of the lipoprotein carrying the Lp(a) antigen in human plasma. *Acta Path Microbiol Scand* **78**:253, 1970.
93. Fless GM, Rolik CA, Scanu AM: Heterogeneity of human plasma lipoprotein (a). Isolation and characterization of the lipoprotein subspecies and their apoproteins. *J Biol Chem* **259**:11470, 1984.
94. Utermann G, Menzel HJ, Kraft HG, Duba HC, Kemmler HG, Seitz C: Lp(a) glycoprotein phenotypes. Inheritance and relation to Lp(a)-lipoprotein concentrations in plasma. *J Clin Invest* **80**:458, 1987.
95. Eaton DL, Fless GM, Kohr WJ, McLean JW, Xu Q-T, Miller CG, Lawn RM, et al: Partial amino acid sequence of apolipoprotein (a) shows that it is homologous to plasminogen. *Proc Natl Acad Sci U S A* **84**:3224, 1987.
96. Kratzin H, Armstrong VW, Niehaus M, Hilschman N, Seidel D: Structural relationship of an apolipoprotein (a) phenotype (570 kDa) to plasminogen: Homologous kringle domains are linked by carbohydrate-rich regions. *Biol Chem Hoppe-Seyler* **368**:1533, 1987.
97. Patthy L: Evolution of the proteases of the blood coagulation and fibrinolysis by assembly from modules. *Cell* **41**:657, 1985.
98. Guevara J Jr, Knapp RD, Honda S, Northup SR, Morrisett JD: A structural assessment of the apo(a) protein of human lipoprotein(a). *Proteins* **12**:188, 1992.
99. Tomlinson JE, McLean JW, Lawn RM: Rhesus monkey apolipoprotein(a). Sequence, evolution, and sites of synthesis. *J Biol Chem* **264**:5957, 1989.
100. Klezovitch O, Edelstein C, Scanu AM: Evidence that the fibrinogen binding domain of Apo(a) is outside the lysine binding site of kringle IV-10: A study involving naturally occurring lysine binding defective lipoprotein(a) phenotypes. *J Clin Invest* **98**:185, 1996.
101. Scanu AM, Miles LA, Fless GM, Pfaffinger D, Eisenbart J, Jackson E, Hoover-Plow JL, et al: Rhesus monkey lipoprotein(a) binds to lysine sepharose and U937 monocytoid cells less efficiently than human lipoprotein(a). Evidence for the dominant role of kringle 4_{37}. *J Clin Invest* **91**:283, 1993.
102. Gabel BR, Koschinsky ML: Sequences within apolipoprotein(a) kringle IV types 6–8 bind directly to low-density lipoprotein and

mediate noncovalent association of apolipoprotein(a) with apolipoprotein B-100. *Biochemistry* **37**:7892, 1998.

103. Gabel BR, May LF, Marcovina SM, Koschinsky ML: Lipoprotein(a) assembly. Quantitative assessment of the role of apo(a) kringle IV types 2–10 in particle formation. *Arterioscler Thromb Vasc Biol* **16**:1559, 1996.
104. Frank S, Kostner GM: The role of apo-(a) kringle-IVs in the assembly of lipoprotein-(a). *Protein Eng* **10**:291, 1997.
105. Frank S, Durovic S, Kostner GM: Structural requirements of apo-a for the lipoprotein-a assembly. *Biochem J* **304**:27, 1994.
106. Trieu VN, McConathy WJ: A two-step model for lipoprotein(a) formation. *J Biol Chem* **270**:15471, 1995.
107. Li Z, Gambino R, Fless GM, Copeland RA: Expression and purification of kringle 4-type 2 of human apolipoprotein(a) in *Escherichia coli. Protein Expr Purif* **3**:212, 1992.
108. Sangrar W, Marcovina SM, Koschinsky ML: Expression and characterization of apolipoprotein(a) kringle IV types 1, 2 and 10 in mammalian cells. *Protein Eng* **7**:723, 1994.
109. Chung FZ, Wu LH, Lee HT, Mueller WT, Spahr MA, Eaton SR, Tian Y, et al: Bacterial expression and characterization of human recombinant apolipoprotein(a) kringle IV type 9. *Protein Expr Purif* **13**:222, 1998.
110. Scanu AM, Edelstein C: Learning about the structure and biology of human lipoprotein (a) through dissection by enzymes of the elastase family: Facts and speculations. *J Lipid Res* **38**:2193, 1997.
111. Edelstein C, Italia JA, Klezovitch O, Scanu AM: Functional and metabolic differences between elastase-generated fragments of human lipoprotein(a) and apolipoprotein(a). *J Lipid Res* **37**:1786, 1996.
112. Albers JJ, Kennedy H, Marcovina SM: Evidence that Lp(a) contains one molecule of apo(a) and one molecule of apoB: Evaluation of amino acid analysis data. *J Lipid Res* **37**:192, 1996.
113. Sommer A, Gorges R, Kostner GM, Paltauf F, Hermetter A: Sulfhydryl-selective fluorescence labeling of lipoprotein(a) reveals evidence for one single disulfide linkage between apoproteins(a) and B-100. *Biochemistry* **30**:11245, 1991.
114. Guevara J, Spurlino J, Jan AY, Yang CY, Tulinsky A, Prasad BVV, Gaubatz JW, et al: Proposed mechanism for binding of apo(a) kringle type-9 to apo-B-100 in human lipoprotein(a). *Biophys J* **64(3)**:686, 1993.
115. Brunner Ch, Kraft HG, Utermann G, Müller HJ: Cys4057 of apolipoprotein(a) is essential for lipoprotein(a) assembly. *Proc Natl Acad Sci U S A* **90**:11643, 1993.
116. Koschinsky ML, Côté GP, Gabel B, Van der Hoek YY: Identification of the cysteine residue in apolipoprotein(a) that mediates extracellular coupling with apolipoprotein B-100. *J Biol Chem* **268**:19819, 1993.
117. Trieu VN, McConathy WJ: The binding of animal low-density lipoproteins to human apolipoprotein(a). *Biochem J* **309**:899, 1995.
118. Chiesa G, Hobbs HH, Koschinsky ML, Lawn RM, Maika SD, Hammer RE: Reconstitution of lipoprotein(a) by infusion of human low density lipoprotein into transgenic mice expressing human apolipoprotein(a). *J Biol Chem* **267**:24369, 1992.
119. Callow MJ, Stoltzfus LJ, Lawn RM, Rubin EM: Expression of human apolipoprotein B and assembly of lipoprotein(a) in transgenic mice. *Proc Natl Acad Sci U S A* **91**:2130, 1994.
120. Linton MF, Farese RV Jr, Chiesa G, Grass DS, Chin P, Hammer RE, Hobbs HH, et al: Transgenic mice expressing high plasma concentrations of human apolipoprotein B100 and lipoprotein(a). *J Clin Invest* **92**:3029, 1993.
121. McCormick SPA, Linton MF, Hobbs HH, Taylor S, Curtiss LK, Young SG: Expression of human apolipoprotein B90 in transgenic mice. Demonstration that apolipoprotein B90 lacks the structural requirements to form lipoprotein(a). *J Biol Chem* **269**:24284, 1994.
122. McCormick SP, Ng JK, Cham CM, Taylor S, Marcovina SM, Segrest JP, Hammer RE, et al: Transgenic mice expressing human ApoB95 and ApoB97. Evidence that sequences within the carboxyl-terminal portion of human apoB100 are important for the assembly of lipoprotein. *J Biol Chem* **272**:23616, 1997.
123. Callow MJ, Rubin EM: Site-specific mutagenesis demonstrates that cysteine 4326 of apolipoprotein B is required for covalent linkage with apolipoprotein(a) *in vivo*. *J Biol Chem* **270**:23914, 1995.
124. McCormick SP, Ng JK, Taylor S, Flynn LM, Hammer RE, Young SG: Mutagenesis of the human apolipoprotein B gene in a yeast artificial chromosome reveals the site of attachment for apolipoprotein(a). *Proc Natl Acad Sci U S A* **92**:10147, 1995.
125. Gabel B, Yao Z, McLeod RS, Young SG, Koschinsky ML: Carboxyl-terminal truncation of apolipoprotein B-100 inhibits lipoprotein(a) particle formation. *FEBS Lett* **350**:77, 1994.
126. Koschinsky ML, Marcovina SM, May LF, Gabel BR: Analysis of the mechanism of lipoprotein(a) assembly. *Clin Genet* **52**:338, 1997.
127. Frank S, Krasznai K, Durovic S, Lobentanz E, Dieplinger H, Wagner E, Zatloukal K, et al: High-level expression of various apolipoprotein(a) isoforms by "transfer infection": The role of kringle IV sequences in the extracellular association with low-density lipoprotein. *Biochemistry* **33**:12329, 1994.
128. Ernst A, Helmhold M, Brunner C, Pethö-Schramm A, Armstrong VW, Müller HJ: Identification of two functionally distinct lysine-binding sites in kringle 37 and in kringles 32–36 of human apolipoprotein(a). *J Biol Chem* **270**:6227, 1995.
129. Frank S, Durovic S, Kostner GM: The assembly of lipoprotein Lp(a). *Eur J Clin Invest* **26**:109, 1996.
130. Gabel BR, McLeod RS, Yao Z, Koschinsky ML: Sequences within the amino terminus of ApoB100 mediate its noncovalent association with apo(a). *Arterioscler Thromb Vasc Biol* **18**:1738, 1998.
131. Fless GM, Santiago JY, Furbee JJr, Meredith SC: Specificity of ligand-induced conformational change of lipoprotein(a). *Biochemistry* **36**:11304, 1997.
132. Prassl R, Schuster B, Abuja PM, Zechner M, Kostner GM, Laggner P: A comparison of structure and thermal behavior in human plasma lipoprotein(a) and low-density lipoprotein. Calorimetry and small-angle X-ray scattering. *Biochemistry* **34**:3795, 1995.
133. Phillips ML, Lembertas AV, Schumaker VN, Lawn RM, Shire SJ, Zioncheck TF: Physical properties of recombinant apolipoprotein(a) and its association with LDL to form an Lp(a)-like complex. *Biochemistry* **32**:3722, 1993.
134. Trieu VN, McConathy WJ: Lipoprotein(a) binding to other apolipoprotein B containing lipoproteins. *Biochemistry* **29**:5919, 1990.
135. Ye SQ, Trieu VN, Stiers DL, McConathy WJ: Interactions of low density lipoprotein 2 and other apolipoprotein B-containing lipoproteins with lipoprotein(a). *J Biol Chem* **263**:6337, 1988.
136. Trieu VN, Zioncheck TF, Lawn RM, McConathy WJ: Interaction of apolipoprotein(a) with apolipoprotein B-containing lipoproteins. *J Biol Chem* **266**:5480, 1991.
137. Gries A, Nimpf J, Nimpf M, Wurm H, Kostner GM: Free and Apo-B-associated Lpa-specific protein in human serum. *Clin Chim Acta* **164**:93, 1987.
138. Bersot TP, Innerarity T, Pitas RE, Rall SCJr, Weisgraber KH, Mahley RW: Fat feeding in humans induces lipoproteins of density less than 1.006 that are enriched in Apolipoprotein (a) and that cause lipid accumulation in macrophages. *J Clin Invest* **77**:622, 1986.
139. Pfaffinger D, Schuelke J, Kim C, Fless GM, Scanu AM: Relationship between apo(a) isoforms and Lp(a) density in subjects with different apo(a) phenotype: A study before and after a fatty meal. *J Lipid Res* **32**:679, 1991.
140. Scanu AM, Fless G: The apoB100-apo(a) complex: Relation to triglyceride-rich particles. *Adv Exp Med Biol* **285**:295, 1991.
141. Sandholzer C, Feussner G, Brunzell J, Utermann G: Distribution of apolipoprotein(a) in the plasma from patients with lipoprotein lipase deficiency with type III hyperlipoproteinemia. No evidence for a triglyceride-rich precursor of lipoprotein(a). *J Clin Invest* **90**:1958, 1992.
142. Trenkwalder E, Gruber A, Konig P, Dieplinger H, Kronenberg F: Increased plasma concentrations of LDL-unbound apo(a) in patients with end-stage renal disease. *Kidney Int* **52**:1685, 1997.
143. Kraft HG, Menzel HJ, Hoppichler F, Vogel W, Utermann G: Changes of genetic apolipoprotein phenotypes caused by liver transplantations. Implications for apolipoprotein synthesis. *J Clin Invest* **83**:137, 1989.
144. Kostner GM, Grillhofer HK: Lipoprotein(a) mediates high affinity low density lipoprotein association to receptor negative fibroblasts. *J Biol Chem* **266**:21287, 1991.
145. Mooser V, Marcovina SM, White AL, Hobbs HH: Kringle-containing fragments of apolipoprotein(a) circulate in human plasma and are excreted into the urine. *J Clin Invest* **98**:2414, 1996.
146. Oida K, Takai H, Maeda H, Takahashi S, Shimada A, Suzuki J, Tamai T, et al: Apolipoprotein(a) is present in urine and its excretion is decreased in patients with renal failure. *Clin Chem* **38**:2244, 1992.
147. Mooser V, Seabra MC, Abedin M, Landschulz KT, Marcovina S, Hobbs HH: Apolipoprotein(a) kringle 4-containing fragments in human urine. Relationship to plasma levels of lipoprotein(a). *J Clin Invest* **97**:858, 1996.

148. Kostner KM, Maurer G, Huber K, Stefenelli T, Dieplinger H, Steyrer E, Kostner GM: Urinary excretion of apo(a) fragments. Role in apo(a) catabolism. *Arterioscler Thromb Vasc Biol* **16**:905, 1996.
149. O'Reilly MS, Holmgren L, Shing Y, Chen C, Rosenthal RA, Moses M, Lane WS, et al: Angiostatin: A novel angiogenesis inhibitor that mediates the suppression of metastases by a Lewis lung carcinoma. *Cell* **79**:315, 1994.
150. Ribatti D, Vacca A, Giacchetta F, Cesaretti S, Anichini M, Roncali L, Damacco F: Lipoprotein (a) induces angiogenesis on the chick embryo chorioallantoic membrane. *Eur J Clin Invest* **28**:533, 1998.
151. Kostner GM, Wo X, Frank S, Kostner K, Zimmermann R, Steyrer E: Metabolism of Lp(a): Assembly and excretion. *Clin Genet* **52**:347, 1997.
152. Menzel H-J, Dieplinger H, Lackner C, Hoppichler F, Lloyd JK, Muller DR, Labeur C, et al: Abetalipoproteinemia with an ApoB-100-lipoprotein(a) glycoprotein complex in plasma. Indication for an assembly defect. *J Biol Chem* **265**:981, 1990.
153. Koschinsky ML, Tomlinson JE, Zioncheck TF, Schwartz K, Eaton DL, Lawn RM: Apolipoprotein(a): Expression and characterization of a recombinant form of the protein in mammalian cells. *Biochemistry* **30**:5044, 1991.
154. Wetterau JR, Aggerbeck LP, Bouma M-E, Eisenberg C, Munck A, Hermier M, Schmitz J, et al: Absence of microsomal triglyceride transfer protein in individuals with abetalipoproteinemia. *Science* **258**:999, 1992.
155. Fless GM, Pfaffinger DJ, Eisenbart JD, Scanu AM: Solubility, immunochemical, and lipoprotein binding properties of apoB-100-apo(a), the protein moiety of lipoprotein(a). *J Lipid Res* **31**:909, 1990.
156. Lawn RM, Schwartz K, Patthy L: Convergent evolution of apolipoprotein(a) in primates and hedgehog. *Proc Natl Acad Sci U S A* **94**:11992, 1997.
157. Weidner KM, Arakaki N, Hartmann G, Vandekerckhove J, Weingart S, Rieder H, Fonatsch C, et al: Evidence for the identity of human scatter factor and human hepatocyte growth factor. *Proc Natl Acad Sci U S A* **88**:7001, 1991.
158. Malgaretti N, Acquati F, Magnaghi P, Bruno L, Pontoglio M, Rocchi M, Saccone S, et al: Characterization by yeast artificial chromosome cloning of the linked apolipoprotein(a) and plasminogen genes and identification of the apolipoprotein(a) 5′ flanking region. *Proc Natl Acad Sci U S A* **89**:11584, 1992.
159. Magnaghi P, Citterio E, Malgaretti N, Acquati F, Ottolenghi S, Taramelli R: Molecular characterisation of the human apo(a)-plasminogen gene family clustered on the telomeric region of chromosome 6 (6q26-27). *Hum Mol Genet* **3**:437, 1994.
160. Byrne CD, Schwartz K, Lawn RM: Loss of a splice donor site at a 'skipped exon' in a gene homologous to apolipoprotein(a) leads to an mRNA encoding a protein consisting of a single kringle domain. *Arterioscler Thromb* **15**:65, 1995.
161. Ichinose A: Multiple members of the plasminogen-apolipoprotein(a) gene family associated with thrombosis. *Biochemistry* **31**:3113, 1992.
162. Takabatake N, Souri M, Ichinose A: Multiple novel transcripts for apolipoprotein(a)-related gene II generated by alternative splicing in tissue and cell type-specific manners. *J Biochem (Tokyo)* **124**:540, 1998.
163. Ichinose A: Characterization of the apolipoprotein(a) gene. *Biochem Biophys Res Commun* **209**:365, 1995.
164. Byrne CD, Schwartz K, Meer K, Cheng J-F, Lawn RM: The human apolipoprotein(a)/plasminogen gene cluster contains a novel homologue transcribed in liver. *Arterioscler Thromb* **14**:534, 1994.
165. Murray JC, Buetow KH, Donovan M, Hornung S, Motulsky AG, Disteche C, Dyer K, et al: Linkage disequilibrium of plasminogen polymorphisms and assignment of the gene to human chromosome 6q26-6q27. *Am J Hum Genet* **40**:338, 1987.
166. Haibach C, Kraft HG, Kochl S, Abe A, Utermann G: The number of kringle IV repeats 3-10 is invariable in the human apo(a) gene. *Gene* **208**:253, 1998.
167. Acquati F, Malgaretti N, Hauptschein R, Rao P, Gaidano G, Taramelli R: A 2-Mb YAC contig linking the plasminogen-apolipoprotein(a) gene family to the insulin-like growth factor 2 receptor (IGF2R) gene on the telomeric region of chromosome 6 (6q26-q27). *Genomics* **22**:664, 1994.
168. Kraft HG, Malgaretti N, Köchl S, Acquati F, Utermann G, Taramelli R: Demonstration of physical linkage between the promoter region and the polymorphic kringle IV domain in the apo(a) gene by pulsed field gel electrophoresis. *Genomics* **17**:260, 1993.
169. Mihalich A, Magnaghi P, Sessa L, Trubia M, Acquati F, Taramelli R: Genomic structure and organization of kringles type 3 to 10 of the apolipoprotein(a) gene in 6q26-27. *Gene* **196**:1, 1997.
170. Lackner C, Boerwinkle E, Leffert CC, Rahmig T, Hobbs HH: Molecular basis of apolipoprotein (a) isoform size heterogeneity as revealed by pulsed-field gel electrophoresis. *J Clin Invest* **87**:2153, 1991.
171. Mancini FP, Mooser V, Guerra R, Hobbs HH: Sequence microheterogeneity in apolipoprotein(a) gene repeats and the relationship to plasma Lp(a) levels. *Hum Mol Genet* **4**:1535, 1995.
172. Bopp S, Kochl S, Acquati F, Magnaghi P, Petho Schramm A, Kraft HG, Utermann G, et al: Ten allelic apolipoprotein(a) 5′ flanking fragments exhibit comparable promoter activities in HepG2 cells. *J Lipid Res* **36**:1721, 1995.
173. Wade DP, Clarke JG, Lindahl GE, Liu AC, Zysow BR, Meer K, Schwartz K, et al: 5′ control regions of the apolipoprotein(a) gene and members of the related plasminogen gene family. *Proc Natl Acad Sci U S A* **90**:1369, 1993.
174. Wade DP, Lindahl GE, Lawn RM: Apolipoprotein(a) gene transcription is regulated by liver-enriched *trans*-acting factor hepatocyte nuclear factor 1a. *J Biol Chem* **269**:19757, 1994.
175. Frazer KA, Narla G, Zhang JL, Rubin EM: The apolipoprotein(a) gene is regulated by sex hormones and acute-phase inducers in YAC transgenic mice. *Nat Genet* **9**:424, 1995.
176. Ramharack R, Wyborski RJ, Spahr MA: The apolipoprotein(a) promoter contains a retinoid response element. *Biochem Biophys Res Commun* **245**:194, 1998.
177. Wade DP, Puckey LH, Knight BL, Acquati F, Mihalich A, Taramelli R: Characterization of multiple enhancer regions upstream of the apolipoprotein(a) gene [Erratum J Biol Chem 272(48):30387, 1997]. *J Biol Chem* **272**:30387, 1997.
178. Yang Z, Boffelli D, Boonmark N, Schwartz K, Lawn R: Apolipoprotein(a) gene enhancer resides within a LINE element. *J Biol Chem* **273**:891, 1998.
179. Doucet C, Wickings J, Chapman J, Thillet J: Chimpanzee lipoprotein(A): Relationship between apolipoprotein(A) isoform size and the density profile of lipoprotein(A) in animals with different heterozygous apo(A) phenotypes. *J Med Primatol* **27**:21, 1998.
180. Berg K: The Lp System. *Series Haematologica* **I(1)**:111, 1968.
181. Nachman RL, Gavish D, Azrolan N, Clarkson TB: Lipoprotein(a) in diet-induced atherosclerosis in nonhuman primates. *Arteriosclerosis* **11**:32, 1991.
182. Rainwater DL, Manis GS, Vandeberg L: Hereditary and dietary effects on apolipoprotein(a) isoforms and Lp(a) in baboons. *J Lipid Res* **30**:549, 1989.
183. Hixson JE, Britten ML, Manis GS, Rainwater DL: Apolipoprotein (a) glycoprotein isoforms result from size differences in apo(a) mRNA in baboons. *J Biol Chem* **264**:6013, 1989.
184. Azrolan N, Gavish D, Breslow JL: Plasma lipoprotein(a) concentration is controlled by apolipoprotein(a) (Apo(a)) protein size and the abundance of hepatic Apo(a) mRNA in a cynomolgus monkey model. *J Biol Chem* **266**:13866, 1991.
185. Makino K, Abe A, Maeda S, Noma A, Kawade M, Takenaka O: Lipoprotein(a) in nonhuman primates: Presence and characteristics of Lp(a) immunoreactive material using anti-human Lp(a) serum. *Atherosclerosis* **78**:81, 1989.
186. Makino K, Scanu AM: Lipoprotein(a): Nonhuman primate models. *Lipids* **26**:679, 1991.
187. Laplaud PM, Beaubatie L, Rall SC, Luc G, Saboureau M: Lipoprotein (a) is the major apoB-containing lipoprotein in the plasma of a hibernator, the hedgehog (*Erinaceus europaeus*). *J Lipid Res* **29**:1157, 1988.
188. Ikeo K, Takahashi K, Gojobori T: Evolutionary origin of numerous kringles in human and simian apolipoprotein(a). *FEBS Lett* **287**:146, 1991.
189. Pesole G, Gerardi A, Di Jeso F, Saccone C: The peculiar evolution of apolipoprotein(a) in human and rhesus macaque. *Genetics* **136**:255, 1994.
190. Lawn RM, Boonmark NW, Schwartz K, Lindahl GE, Wade DP, Byrne CD, Fong KJ, et al: The recurring evolution of lipoprotein(a). Insights from cloning of hedgehog apolipoprotein(a). *J Biol Chem* **270**:24004, 1995.
191. Krempler F, Kostner GM, Bolzano K, Sandhofer F: Turnover of lipoprotein(a) in man. *J Clin Invest* **65**:1483, 1980.
192. Rader DJ, Cain W, Zech LA, Usher D, Brewer HBJr: Variation in lipoprotein(a) concentrations among individuals with the same apolipoprotein(a) isoform is determined by the rate of lipoprotein(a) production. *J Clin Invest* **91**:443, 1993.

193. Rainwater DL, Lanford RE: Production of lipoprotein(a) by primary baboon hepatocytes. *Biochim Biophys Acta* **1003**:30, 1989.
194. Lawn RM, Wade DP, Hammer RE, Chiesa G, Verstuyft JG, Rubin EM: Atherogenesis in transgenic mice expressing human apolipoprotein(*a*). *Nature* **360**:670, 1992.
195. Morrisett J, Gaubatz J, Nava M, Guyton J, Hoffmann A, Opekum A, Hachey D: Metabolism of apo(a) and apoB-100 in human lipoprotein(a) [Abstract]. *Sec Int Conf Lipoprotein(a)* 71**,** 1992.
196. Su W, Campos H, Judge H, Walsh BW, Sacks FM: Metabolism of apo(a) and apo B-100 of lipoprotein(a) in women: Effect of postmenopausal estrogen replacement. *J Clin Endocrinol Metab* **83**:3267, 1998.
197. Krempler F, Kostner GM, Bolzano K, Sandhofer F: Lipoprotein(a) is not a metabolic product of other lipoproteins containing apolipoprotein B. *Biochim Biophys Acta* **575**:63, 1979.
198. Lobentanz EM, Krasznai K, Gruber A, Brunner C, Muller HJ, Sattler J, Kraft HG, et al: Intracellular metabolism of human apolipoprotein(a) in stably transfected Hep G2 cells. *Biochemistry* **37**:5417, 1998.
199. White AL, Rainwater DL, Hixson JE, Estlack LE, Lanford RE: Intracellular processing of apo(a) in primary baboon hepatocytes. *Chem Phys Lipids* **67–68**:123, 1994.
200. White AL, Lanford RE: Cell surface assembly of lipoprotein(a) in primary cultures of baboon hepatocytes. *J Biol Chem* **269**:28716, 1994.
201. Ernst A, Brunner C, Pethö-Schramm A, et al: Assembly and lysine binding of recombinant lipoprotein(a), in Woodford FP, Davignon J, Sniderman A(eds): *Atherosclerosis X. Proceedings of the 10th International Symposium on Atherosclerosis, Montreal, October 9–14, 1994*. Amsterdam, Elsevier, 1995, p 879.
202. Bonen DK, Hausman AML, Hadjiagapiou C, Skarosi SF, Davidson NO: Expression of a recombinant apolipoprotein(a) in HepG2 cells. Evidence for intracellular assembly of lipoprotein(a). *J Biol Chem* **272**:5659, 1997.
203. Edelstein C, Davidson NO, Scanu AM: Oleate stimulates the formation of triglyceride-rich particles containing APOB100-APO(a) in long-term primary cultures of human hepatocytes. *Chem Phys Lipids* **67–68**:135, 1994.
204. Dixon JL, Furukawa S, Ginsberg HN: Oleate stimulates secretion of apolipoprotein B-containing lipoproteins from Hep G2 cells by inhibiting early intracellular degradation of apolipoprotein B. *J Biol Chem* **266**:5080, 1991.
205. Nassir F, Bonen DK, Davidson NO: Apolipoprotein(a) synthesis and secretion from hepatoma cells is coupled to triglyceride synthesis and secretion. *J Biol Chem* **273**:17793, 1998.
206. Gurakar A, Hoeg JM, Kostner GM, Papadopoulos NM, Brewer BH Jr: Levels of lipoprotein Lp (a) decline with neomycin and niacin treatment. *Atherosclerosis* **57**:293, 1985.
207. Lanford RE, Estlack L, White AL: Neomycin inhibits secretion of apolipoprotein(a) by increasing retention on the hepatocyte cell surface. *J Lipid Res* **37**:2055, 1996.
208. Brown MS, Goldstein JL: A receptor-mediated pathway for cholesterol homeostasis. *Science* **232**:34, 1986.
209. Havekes L, Vermeer BJ, Brugman T, Emeis J: Binding of Lp (a) to the low density lipoprotein receptor of human fibroblast. *FEBS Lett* **132**:169, 1981.
210. Krempler F, Kostner GM, Roscher A, Haslauer F, Bolzano K: Studies on the role of specific cell surface receptors in the removal of lipoprotein (a) in man. *J Clin Invest* **71**:1431, 1983.
211. Hofmann SL, Eaton DL, Brown MS, McConathy WJ, Goldstein JL, Hammer RE: Overexpression of human low-density lipoprotein receptors leads to accelerated catabolism of Lp(a) lipoprotein in transgenic mice. *J Clin Invest* **85**:1542, 1990.
212. Maartman-Moe K, Berg K: Lp (a) lipoprotein enters cultured fibroblasts independently of the plasma membrane low-density lipoprotein receptor. *Clin Genet* **20**:352, 1981.
213. Floren CH, Albers JJ, Bierman EL: Uptake of Lp(a) lipoprotein by cultured fibroblasts. *Biochem Biophys Res Commun* **102**:636, 1981.
214. Utermann G, Hoppichler F, Dieplinger H, Seed M, Thompson G, Boerwinkle E: Defects in the LDL receptor gene affect Lp (a) lipoprotein levels: Multiplicative interaction of two gene loci associated with premature atherosclerosis. *Proc Natl Acad Sci U S A* **86**:4171, 1989.
215. Wiklund O, Angelin B, Olofsson SO, Eriksson M, Fager G, Berglund L, Bondjers G: Apolipoprotein(a) and ischaemic heart disease in familial hypercholesterolaemia. *Lancet* **335**:1360, 1990.
216. Seed M, Hoppichler F, Reaveley D, McCarthy S, Thompson GR, Boerwinkle E, Utermann G: Relation of serum lipoprotein(a) concentration and apolipoprotein(a) phenotype to coronary heart disease in patients with familial hypercholesterolemia. *N Engl J Med* **322**:1494, 1990.
217. Soutar AK, McCarthy SN, Seed M, Knight BL: Relationship between apolipoprotein(a) phenotype, lipoprotein(a) concentration in plasma, and low density lipoprotein receptor function in a large kindred with familial hypercholesterolemia due to the $Pro_{664} \rightarrow$ Leu mutation in the LDL receptor gene. *J Clin Invest* **88**:483, 1991.
218. Leitersdorf E, Friedlander Y, Bard J-M, Fruchart J-C, Eisenberg S, Stein Y: Diverse effect of ethnicity on plasma lipoprotein(a) levels in heterozygote patients with familial hypercholesterolemia. *J Lipid Res* **32**:1513, 1991.
219. Friedlander Y, Leitersdorf E: Segregation analysis of plasma lipoprotein(a) levels in pedigrees with molecularly defined familial hypercholesterolemia. *Genet Epidemiol* **12**:129, 1995.
220. Lingenhel A, Kraft HG, Kotze M, Peeters AV, Kronenberg F, Kruse R, Utermann G: Concentrations of the atherogenic Lp(a) are elevated in FH. *Eur J Hum Genet* **6**:50, 1998.
221. Van der Hoek YY, Lingenhel A, Kraft HG, Defesche JC, Kastelein JJP, Utermann G: Sib-pair analysis detects elevated Lp(a) levels and large variation of Lp(a) concentration in subjects with familial defective apo B. *J Clin Invest* **99**:2269, 1997.
222. Hofer G, Steyrer E, Kostner GM, Hermetter A: LDL-mediated interaction of Lp(a) with HepG2 cells: A novel fluorescence microscopy approach. *J Lipid Res* **38**:2411, 1997.
223. Kostner GM: Interaction of Lp(a) and of apo(a) with liver cells. *Arterioscler Thromb* **13**:1101, 1993.
224. Kostner KM, Clodi M, Bodlaj G, Watschinger B, Horl W, Derfler K, Huber K: Decreased urinary apolipoprotein (a) excretion in patients with impaired renal function. *Eur J Clin Invest* **28**:447, 1998.
225. Kronenberg F, Trenkwalder E, Lingenhel A, Friedrich G, Lhotta K, Schober M, Moes N, et al: Renovascular arteriovenous differences in Lp(a) plasma concentrations suggest removal of Lp(a) from the renal circulation. *J Lipid Res* **38**:1755, 1997.
226. Sato H, Suzuki S, Ueno M, Shimada H, Karasawa R, Nishi S-I, Arakawa M: Localization of apolipoprotein(a) and B-100 in various renal diseases. *Kidney Int* **43**:430, 1993.
227. Suzuki S, Takahashi H, Sato H, Takashima N, Arakawa M, Gejyo F: Significance of glomerular deposition of apolipoprotein (a) in various glomerulopathies. *Am J Nephrol* **17**:499, 1997.
228. Kramer-Guth A, Greiber S, Pavenstadt H, Quaschning T, Winkler K, Schollmeyer P, Wanner C: Interaction of native and oxidized lipoprotein(a) with human mesangial cells and matrix. *Kidney Int* **49**:1250, 1996.
229. Zioncheck TF, Powell LM, Rice GC, Eaton DL, Lawn RM: Interaction of recombinant apolipoprotein(a) and lipoprotein(a) with macrophages. *J Clin Invest* **87**:767, 1991.
230. Bottalico LA, Keesler GA, Fless GM, Tabas I: Cholesterol loading of macrophages leads to marked enhancement of native lipoprotein(a) and apoprotein(a) internalization and degradation. *J Biol Chem* **268**:8569, 1993.
231. Skiba PJ, Keesler GA, Tabas I: Interferon-gamma down-regulates the lipoprotein(a)/apoprotein(a) receptor activity on macrophage foam cells. Evidence for disruption of ligand-induced receptor recycling by interferon-gamma. *J Biol Chem* **269**:23059, 1994.
232. Keesler GA, Li Y, Skiba PJ, Fless GM, Tabas I: Macrophage foam cell lipoprotein(a)/apoprotein(a) receptor: Cell-surface localization, dependence of induction on new protein synthesis, and ligand specificity. *Arterioscler Thromb* **14**:1337, 1994.
233. Keesler GA, Gabel BR, Devlin CM, Koschinsky ML, Tabas I: The binding activity of the macrophage lipoprotein(a)/apolipoprotein(a) receptor is induced by cholesterol via a post-translational mechanism and recognizes distinct kringle domains on apolipoprotein(a). *J Biol Chem* **271**:32096, 1996.
234. Argraves KM, Kozarsky KF, Fallon JT, Harpel PC, Strickland DK: The atherogenic lipoprotein Lp(a) is internalized and degraded in a process mediated by the VLDL receptor. *J Clin Invest* **100**:2170, 1997.
235. Niemeier A, Willnow T, Dieplinger H, Jacobsen C, Meyer N, Hilpert J, Beisiegel U: Identification of megalin/gp330 as a receptor for lipoprotein(a). *Arterioscler Thromb Vasc Biol* **19**:552, 1999.
236. Webb JC, Patel DD, Jones MD, Knight BL, Soutar AK: Characterization and tissue-specific expression of the human "very low density lipoprotein (VLDL) receptor" mRNA. *Hum Mol Genet* **3**:531, 1994.
237. Nakazato K, Ishibashi T, Shindo J, Shiomi M, Maruyama Y: Expression of very-low-density lipoprotein receptor mRNA in rabbit atherosclerotic lesions. *Am J Pathol* **149**:1831, 1996.

238. Multhaupt HA, Gafvels ME, Kariko K, Jin H, Arenas-Elliot C, Goldman BI, Strauss JF, et al: Expression of very-low-density lipoprotein receptor in the vascular wall. Analysis of human tissues by in situ hybridization and immunohistochemistry. *Am J Pathol* **148**:1985, 1996.
239. Lundgren S, Carling T, Hjalm G, Juhlin C, Rastad J, Pihlgren U, Rask L, et al: Tissue distribution of human gp330/megalin, a putative Ca(2+)-sensing protein. *J Histochem Cytochem* **45**:383, 1997.
240. Williams KJ, Fless GM, Petrie KA, Snyder ML, Brocia RW, Swenson TL: Mechanisms by which lipoprotein lipase alters cellular metabolism of lipoprotein(a), low-density lipoprotein, and nascent lipoproteins. Roles for low-density lipoprotein receptors and heparan sulfate proteoglycans. *J Biol Chem* **267**:13284, 1992.
241. Beisiegel U: New aspects on the role of plasma lipases in lipoprotein catabolism and atherosclerosis. *Atherosclerosis* **124**:1, 1996.
242. Mahley RW, Ji Z-S: Remnant lipoprotein metabolism: Key pathways involving cell-surface heparan sulfate proteoglycans and apolipoprotein E. *J Lipid Res* **40**:1, 1999.
243. Rader DJ, Cain W, Ikewaki K, Talley G, Zech LA, Usher D, Brewer HBJr: The inverse association of plasma lipoprotein(a) concentrations with apolipoprotein(a) isoform size is not due to differences in Lp(a) catabolism but to differences in production rate. *J Clin Invest* **93**:2758, 1994.
244. Rader DJ, Mann WA, Cain W, Kraft H-G, Usher D, Zech LA, Hoeg JM, et al: The low-density lipoprotein receptor is not required for normal catabolism of Lp(a) in humans. *J Clin Invest* **95**:1403, 1995.
245. Armstrong VW, Schleef J, Thiery J, Muche R, Schuff-Werner P, Eisenhauer T, Seidel D: Effect of HELP-LDL-apheresis on serum concentrations of human lipoprotein(a). *Eur J Clin Invest* **19**:235, 1989.
246. Jenner JL, Ordovas JM, Lamon-Fava S, Schaefer MM, Wilson PWF, Castelli WP, Schaefer EJ: Effects of age, sex, and menopausal status on plasma lipoprotein(a) levels: The Framingham Offspring Study. *Circulation* **87**:1135, 1993.
247. Schriewer H, Assmann G, Sandkamp M: The Relationship of Lipoprotein(a) (Lp(a)) to Risk Factors of Coronary Heart Disease: Initial results of the prospective epidemiological study on company employees in Westfalia. *J Clin Chem Clin Biochem* **22**:591, 1984.
248. Genest J Jr, Jenner JL, McNamara JR, Ordovas JM, Silberman SR, Wilson PWF, Schaefer EJ: Prevalence of lipoprotein (a) [Lp(a)] excess in coronary artery disease. *Am J Cardiol* **67**:1039, 1991.
249. Harpel PC, Hermann A, Zhang X, Ostfeld I, Borth W: Lipoprotein(a), plasmin modulation, and atherogenesis. *Thromb Haemost* **74**:382, 1995.
250. Palabrica TM, Liu AC, Aronovitz MJ, Furie B, Lawn RM, Furie BC: Antifibrinolytic activity of apolipoprotein(a) *in vivo*: Human apolipoprotein(a) transgenic mice are resistant to tissue plasminogen activator-mediated thrombolysis. *Nat Med* **1**:256, 1995.
251. Edelberg JM, Gonzalez-Gronow M, Pizzo SV: Lipoprotein(a) inhibition of plasminogen activation by tissue-type plasminogen activator. *Thromb Res* **57**:155, 1990.
252. Edelberg J, Pizzo SV: Why is lipoprotein(a) relevant to thrombosis? *Am J Clin Nutr* **56(Suppl)**:791S, 1992.
253. Edelberg JM, Reilly CF, Pizzo SV: The inhibition of tissue type plasminogen activator by plasminogen activator inhibitor-1. The effects of fibrinogen, heparin, vitronectin, and lipoprotein(a). *J Biol Chem* **266**:7488, 1991.
254. Loscalzo J, Weinfeld M, Fless GM, Scanu AM: Lipoprotein(a), fibrin binding, and plasminogen activation. *Arteriosclerosis* **10**:240, 1990.
255. Simon DI, Fless GM, Scanu AM, Loscalzo J: Tissue-type plasminogen activator binds to and is inhibited by surface-bound lipoprotein(a) and low-density lipoprotein. *Biochemistry* **30**:6671, 1991.
256. Liu J, Harpel PC, Pannell R, Gurewich V: Lipoprotein(a): A kinetic study of its influence on fibrin-dependent plasminogen activation by prourokinase or tissue plasminogen activator. *Biochemistry* **32**:9694, 1993.
257. Rouy D, Grailhe P, Nigon F, Chapman J, Anglés-Cano E: Lipoprotein(a) impairs generation of plasmin by fibrin-bound tissue-type plasminogen activator: *In vitro* studies in a plasma milieu. *Arteriosclerosis* **11**:629, 1991.
258. Rouy D, Laplaud PM, Saboureau M, Anglés-Cano E: Hedgehog lipoprotein(a) is a modulator of activation of plasminogen at the fibrin surface: An *in vitro* study. *Arterioscler Thromb* **12**:146, 1992.
259. Hajjar KA, Hamel NM, Harpel PC, Nachman RL: Binding of tissue plasminogen activator to cultured human endothelial cells. *J Clin Invest* **80**:1712, 1987.
260. Beebe DP: Binding of tissue plasminogen activator to human umbilical vein endothelial cells. *Thromb Res* **46**:241, 1987.
261. Barnathan ES, Kuo A, Van der Keyl H, McCreae KR, Larsen GR, Clines DB: Tissue-type plasminogen activator binding to human endothelial cells. *J Biol Chem* **263**:7792, 1988.
262. Miles LA, Fless GM, Scanu AM, Baynham P, Sebald MT, Skocir P, Curtiss LK, et al: Interaction of Lp(a) with plasminogen binding sites on cells. *Thromb Haemost* **73**:458, 1995.
263. Brown MS, Goldstein JL: Teaching old dogmas new tricks. *Nature* **83**:113, 1987.
264. Yano Y, Shimokawa K, Okada Y, Noma A: Immunolocalization of lipoprotein(a) in wounded tissues. *J Histochem Cytochem* **45**:559, 1997.
265. Tran-Than C, Kruithof EKO, Bachman F: Tissue-type plasminogen activator increases the binding of Glu-plasminogen to clots. *J Clin Invest* **74**:2009, 1984.
266. Suenson E, Lützen O, Thorsen S: Initial plasmin-degradation of fibrin as the basis of a positive feed-back mechanism in fibrinolysis. *Eur J Biochem* **140**:513, 1984.
267. Harpel PC, Chang T-S, Verderber E: Tissue plasminogen activator and urokinase mediate the binding of Glu-plasminogen to plasma fibrin I. *J Biol Chem* **260**:4432, 1985.
268. Liu J, Harpel PC, Gurewich V: Fibrin-bound lipoprotein(a) promotes plasminogen binding but inhibits fibrin degradation by plasmin. *Biochemistry* **33**:2554, 1994.
269. Rouy D, Koschinsky ML, Fleury V, Chapman J, Anglés-Cano E: Apolipoprotein(a) and plasminogen interactions with fibrin: A study with recombinant apolipoprotein(a) and isolated plasminogen fragments. *Biochemistry* **31**:6333, 1992.
270. Guevara J Jr, Jan AY, Knapp R, Tulinsky A, Morrisett JD: Comparison of ligand-binding sites of modeled apo(a) kringle-like sequences in human lipoprotein(a). *Arterioscler Thromb* **13**:758, 1993.
271. LoGrasso PV, Cornell-Kennon S, Boettcher BR: Cloning, expression, and characterization of human apolipoprotein(a) Kringle IV37. *J Biol Chem* **269**:21820, 1994.
272. Chenivesse X, Huby T, Wickins J, Chapman J, Thillet J: Molecular cloning of the cDNA encoding the carboxy-terminal domain of chimpanzee apolipoprotein(a): An Asp57 → Asn mutation in kringle IV-10 is associated with poor fibrin binding. *Biochemistry* **37**:7213, 1998.
273. Scanu AM, Edelstein C: Kringle-dependent structural and functional polymorphism of apolipoprotein(a). *Biochim Biophys Acta* **1256**:1, 1995.
274. Trieu VN, McConathy WJ: Functional characterization of T7 and T8 of human apolipoprotein (a). *Biochem Biophys Res Commun* **251**:356, 1998.
275. Borth W, Chang V, Bishop P, Harpel PC: Lipoprotein (a) is a substrate for Factor XIIIa and tissue transglutaminase. *J Biol Chem* **266**:18149, 1991.
276. Mosher DF: Action of fibrin-stabilizing factor on cold-soluble globulin and alpha-2 macroglobulin in clotting plasma. *J Biol Chem* **251**:1639, 1976.
277. Mosher DF: Cross-linking of fibronectin to collagenous proteins. *Mol Cell Biochem* **58**:63, 1984.
278. Liu JN, Kung W, Harpel PC, Gurewich V: Demonstration of covalent binding of lipoprotein(a) [Lp(a)] to fibrin and endothelial cells. *Biochemistry* **37**:3949, 1998.
279. Dahlen G, Ericson C, Berg K: *In vitro* studies of the interaction of isolated Lp(a) lipoprotein and other serum lipoproteins with glycosaminoglycans. *Clin Genet* **14**:36, 1978.
280. Palabrica TM, Liu AC, Aronovitz MJ, Furie B, Lawn RM, Furie BC: Antifibrinolytic activity of apolipoprotein(a) *in vivo*: Human apolipoprotein(a) transgenic mice are resistant to tissue plasminogen activator-mediated thrombolysis. *Nat Med* **1**:256, 1995.
281. Halvorsen S, Skjonsberg OH, Berg K, Ruyter R, Godal HC: Does Lp(a) lipoprotein inhibit the fibrinolytic system? *Thromb Res* **68**:223, 1992.
282. Harpel PC, Chang VT, Borth W: Homocysteine and other sulfhydryl compounds enhance the binding of lipoprotein(a) to fibrin: A potential biochemical link between thrombosis, atherogenesis, and sulfhydryl compound metabolism. *Proc Natl Acad Sci U S A* **89**:10193, 1992.
283. Clemmensen I, Petersen LC, Kluft C: Purification and characterization of a novel, oligomeric, plasminogen kringle 4 binding protein from human plasma: Tetranectin. *Eur J Biochem* **156**:327, 1986.

284. Kluft C, Jie AFH, Los P, De Wit E, Havekes L: Functional analogy between lipoprotein(a) and plasminogen in the binding to the kringle 4 binding protein, tetranectin. *Biochem Biophys Res Commun* **161**:427, 1989.
285. Etingin OR, Hajjar DP, Hajjar KA, Harpel PC, Nachman RL: Lipoprotein (a) regulates plasminogen activator inhibitor-1 expression in endothelial cells. A potential mechanism in thrombogenesis. *J Biol Chem* **266**:2459, 1991.
286. Syrovets T, Thillet J, Chapman MJ, Simmet T: Lipoprotein(a) is a potent chemoattractant for human peripheral monocytes. *Blood* **90**: 2027, 1997.
287. Poon M, Zhang X, Dunsky KG, Taubman MB, Harpel PC: Apolipoprotein(a) induces monocyte chemotactic activity in human vascular endothelial cells. *Circulation* **96**:2514, 1997.
288. Kojima S, Harpel PC, Rifkin DB: Lipoprotein (a) inhibits the generation of transforming growth factor β: An endogenous inhibitor of smooth muscle cell migration. *J Cell Biol* **113**:1439, 1991.
289. Yano Y, Seishima M, Tokoro Y, Noma A: Stimulatory effects of lipoprotein(a) and low-density lipoprotein on human umbilical vein endothelial cell migration and proliferation are partially mediated by fibroblast growth factor-2. *Biochim Biophys Acta* **1393**:26, 1998.
290. Morishita R, Yamamoto K, Yamada S, Matsushita H, Tomita N, Sakurabayashi I, Kaneda Y, et al: Stimulatory effect of lipoprotein (a) on proliferation of human mesangial cells: Role of lipoprotein (a) in renal disease. *Biochem Biophys Res Commun* **249**:313, 1998.
291. Salonen EM, Jauhiainen M, Zardi L, Vaheri A, Ehnholm C: Lipoprotein(a) binds to fibronectin and has a serine proteinase activity capable of cleaving it. *EMBO J* **8**:4035, 1989.
292. Seifert PS, Roth I, Zioncheck TF: The apolipoprotein(a) moiety of lipoprotein(a) interacts with the complement activation fragment iC3b but does not functionally affect C3 activation or degradation. *Atherosclerosis* **93**:209, 1992.
293. Jürgens G, Marth E, Kostner GM, Holasek A: Investigation of the Lp(a) lipoprotein: Lipoprotein aggregation and enzymatic activity associated with the Lp(a) polypeptide. *Artery* **3**:13, 1977.
294. Jauhiainen M, Metso J, Koskinen P, Ehnholm C: Characterization of the enzyme activity of human plasma lipoprotein (a) using synthetic peptide substrates. *Biochem J* **274**:491, 1991.
295. Ehnholm C, Jauhiainen M, Kovanen PT: Proteolytic activity of lipoprotein(a) [Abstract]. *Sec Intern Conf Lipoprotein(a)* 18, 1992.
296. Wendt GG: International Lp-Workshop. *Hum Genet* **3**:269, 1967.
297. Utermann G, Wiegandt H: Disk-elektrophoretischer Nachweis des Lp(a)—Proteins in Lipoproteinfraktionen. *Humangenetik* **11**:66, 1970.
298. Schultz JS, Shreffler DC, Sing CF: The genetics of the Lp antigen. *Ann Hum Genet* **38**:39, 1974.
299. Hasstedt SJ, Williams RR: Three alleles for the quantitative Lp (a). *Genet Epidemiol* **3**:53, 1986.
300. Morton NE, Gulbrandsen CL, Rhoads GG, Kagan A: The Lp lipoprotein in Japanese. *Clin Genet* **14**:2097, 1978.
301. Iselius L, Dahlen G, de Faire U, Lindman T: Complex segregation analysis of the Lp(a) (pre-β)-lipoprotein trait. *Clin Genet* **20**:147, 1981.
302. de Faire U, Dahlen G, Liljefors I, Lundman T, Theorell T: Pre-beta1-lipoprotein in patients with ischemic heart disease: Genetic determination and relation to early insulin response. *Acta Med Scand* **209**:65, 1981.
303. de Faire U, Dahlen G, Lundman T, et al: Serum pre-β1-lipoprotein fraction in twins discordant and concordant for ischemic heart disease, in Nance WE, Allen G, Parisi P (eds): *Progress in Clinical and Biological Research*. New York, Alan R Liss, 1978, p 193.
304. Hewitt D, Milner J, Breckenridge C, Maguire G: Heritability of "sinking" pre-beta lipoprotein level: A twin study. *Clin Genet* **11**:224, 1977.
305. Hasstedt SJ, Wilson DE, Edwards CQ, Cannon WN, Carmelli D, Williams RR: The genetics of quantitative plasma Lp (a): Analysis of a large pedigree. *Am J Med Genet* **16**:179, 1983.
306. Hewitt D, Milner J, Owen ARG, Breckenridge WC, Maguire GF, Jones GJL, Little JA: The inheritance of sinking-pre-beta lipoprotein and its relation to the Lp(a) antigen. *Clin Genet* **21**:301, 1982.
307. Lamon-Fava S, Jimenez D, Christian JC, Fabsitz RR, Reed T, Carmelli D, Castelli WP, et al: The NHLBI twin study: heritability of apolipoprotein A-I, B, and low-density lipoprotein subclasses and concordance for lipoprotein (a). *Atherosclerosis* **91**:97, 1991.
308. Boomsma DI, Kaptein A, Kempen HJM, Gevers Leuven JA, Princen HMG: Lipoprotein(a): Relation to other risk factors and genetic heritability. Results from a Dutch parent-twin study. *Atherosclerosis* **99**:23, 1993.
309. Parra HJ, Luyéyé I, Bouramoué C, Demarquilly C, Fruchart JC: Black-white differences in serum Lp(a) lipoprotein levels. *Clin Chim Acta* **167**:27, 1987.
310. Helmhold M, Bigge J, Muche R, Mainoo J, Thiery J, Seidel D, Armstrong VW: Contribution of the apo(a) phenotype to plasma Lp(a) concentrations shows considerable ethnic variation. *J Lipid Res* **32**:1919, 1991.
311. Sandholzer C, Hallman DM, Saha N, Sigurdsson G, Lackner C, Császár A, Boerwinkle E, et al: Effects of the apolipoprotein(a) size polymorphism on the lipoprotein(a) concentration in 7 ethnic groups. *Hum Genet* **86**:607, 1991.
312. Gaw A, Boerwinkle E, Cohen JC, Hobbs HH: Comparative analysis of the *apo(a)* gene, apo(a) glycoprotein, and plasma concentrations of Lp(a) in three ethnic groups. Evidence for no common "null" allele at the apo(a) locus. *J Clin Invest* **93**:2526, 1994.
313. Kraft HG, Lingenhel A, Pang RWC, Delport R, Trommsdorff M, Vermaak H, Janus ED, et al: Frequency distributions of apolipoprotein(a) kringle IV repeat alleles and their effects on lipoprotein(a) levels in Caucasian, Asian, and African Populations: The distribution of null alleles is non-random. *Eur J Hum Genet* **4**:74, 1996.
314. Guyton JR, Dahlen GH, Patsch W, Kautz JA, Gotto AMJr: Relationship of plasma lipoprotein Lp(a) levels to race and to apolipoprotein B. *Arteriosclerosis* **5(3)**:265, 1985.
315. Marcovina SM, Albers JJ, Wijsman E, Zhang Z, Chapman NH, Kennedy H: Differences in Lp(a) concentrations and apo(a) polymorphs between black and white Americans. *J Lipid Res* **37**:2569, 1996.
316. Austin MA, Sandholzer C, Selby JV, Newman B, Krauss RM, Utermann G: Lipoprotein(a) in women twins: Heritability and relationship to apolipoprotein(a) phenotypes. *Am J Hum Genet* **51**:829, 1992.
317. Sing CF, Moll PP: Genetics of atherosclerosis. *Annu Rev Genet* **24**:171, 1990.
318. Rotimi CN, Cooper RS, Marcovina SM, McGee D, Owoaje E, Ladipo M: Serum distribution of lipoprotein(a) in African Americans and Nigerians: Potential evidence for a genotype-environmental effect. *Genet Epidemiol* **14**:157, 1997.
319. Utermann G, Duba Ch, Menzel HJ: Genetics of the quantitative Lp(a) lipoprotein trait. II. Inheritance of Lp(a) glycoprotein phenotypes. *Hum Genet* **78**:47, 1988.
320. Menzel HJ, Assmann G, Rall SCJr, Weisgraber KH, Mahley RW: Human Apolipoprotein A-I polymorphism: Identification of the amino acid substitution in three electrophoretic variants of the Muenster-3 type. *J Biol Chem* **259**:3070, 1984.
321. Steyrer E, Durovic S, Frank S, Giessauf W, Burger A, Dieplinger H, Zechner R, et al: The role of lecithin: cholesterol acyltransferase for lipoprotein (a) assembly. Structural integrity of low-density lipoproteins is a prerequisite for Lp(a) formation in human plasma. *J Clin Invest* **94**:2330, 1994.
322. Kronenberg F, Utermann G, Dieplinger H: Lipoprotein(a) in renal disease. *Am J Kidney Dis* **27**:1, 1996.
323. Kamboh MI, Ferrell RE, Kottke BA: Expressed hypervariable polymorphism of apolipoprotein (a). *Am J Hum Genet* **49**:1063, 1991.
324. Marcovina SM, Zhang ZH, Gaur VP, Albers JJ: Identification of 34 apolipoprotein(a) isoforms: Differential expression of apolipoprotein(a) alleles between American Blacks and Whites. *Biochem Biophys Res Commun* **191**:1192, 1993.
325. Huang CM, Kraft HG, Gregg RE: Modified immunoblotting technique for phenotyping lipoprotein(a). *Clin Chem* **37**:576, 1991.
326. Kraft HG, Dieplinger H, Hoye E, Utermann G: Lp (a) phenotyping by immunoblotting with polyclonal and monoclonal antibodies. *Arteriosclerosis* **8**:212, 1988.
327. Farrer M, Game FL, Adams PC, Laker MF, Alberti KGMM: A simple, sensitive technique for classification of apolipoprotein(a) isoforms by sodium dodecyl sulphate-polyacrylamide gel electrophoresis. *Clin Chim Acta* **207**:215, 1992.
328. Abe A, Noma A: Studies on apolipoprotein(a) phenotypes. Part 1. Phenotype frequencies in a healthy Japanese population. *Atherosclerosis* **96**:1, 1992.
329. Cohen JC, Chiesa G, Hobbs HH: Sequence polymorphisms in the apolipoprotein (a) gene. Evidence for dissociation between apolipoprotein(a) size and plasma lipoprotein(a) levels. *J Clin Invest* **91**:1630, 1993.

330. Gaubatz JW, Ghanem KI, Guevara J Jr, Nava ML, Patsch W, Morrisett JD: Polymorphic forms of human apolipoprotein(a): Inheritance and relationship of their molecular weights to plasma levels of lipoprotein(a). *J Lipid Res* **31**:603, 1990.
331. Lindahl G, Gersdorf E, Menzel HJ, Seed M, Humphries S, Utermann G: Variation in the size of human apolipoprotein(a) is due to a hypervariable region in the gene. *Hum Genet* **84**:563, 1990.
332. Gavish D, Azrolan N, Breslow JL: Plasma Lp(a) concentration is inversely correlated with the ratio of kringle IV/kringle V encoding domains in the apo(a) gene. *J Clin Invest* **84**:2021, 1989.
333. Koschinsky ML, Beisiegel U, Henne-Bruns D, Eaton DL, Lawn RM: Apolipoprotein(a) size heterogeneity is related to variable number of repeat sequences in its mRNA. *Biochemistry* **29**:640, 1990.
334. Lackner C, Cohen JC, Hobbs HH: Molecular definition of the extreme size polymorphism in apolipoprotein(a). *Hum Mol Genet* **2**:933, 1993.
335. Erdel M, Hubalek M, Lingenhel A, Kofler K, Duba H-C, Utermann G: Counting the repetitive kringle IV repeats in the gene encoding human apolipoprotein(a) by fibre-FISH. *Nat Genet* **21**:357, 1999.
336. Marcovina SM, Hobbs HH, Albers JJ: Relation between number of apolipoprotein(a) kringle 4 repeats and mobility of isoforms in agarose gel: Basis for a standardized isoform nomenclature. *Clin Chem* **42**:436, 1996.
337. Kraft HG, Lingenhel A, Bader G, Kostner GM, Utermann G: The relative electrophoretic mobility of apo(a) isoforms depends on the gel system: Proposal of a nomenclature for apo(a) phenotypes. *Atherosclerosis* **125**:53, 1996.
338. Klausen IC, Gerdes LU, Schmidt EB, Dyerberg J, Faergeman O: Differences in apolipoprotein(a) polymorphism in West Greenland Eskimos and Caucasian Danes. *Hum Genet* **89**:384, 1992.
339. Marcovina SM, Albers JJ, Jacobs DR Jr, Perkins LL, Lewis CE, Howard BV, Savage P: Lipoprotein(a) concentrations and apolipoprotein(a) phenotypes in Caucasians and African Americans: The CARDIA Study. *Arterioscler Thromb* **13**:1037, 1993.
340. Utermann G: Lipoprotein(a): A genetic risk factor for premature coronary heart disease. *Curr Opin Lipid* **1**:404, 1990.
341. Gaw A, Brown EA, Ford I: Impact of apo(a) length polymorphism and the control of plasma Lp(a) concentrations: Evidence for a threshold effect. *Arterioscler Thromb Vasc Biol* **18**:1870, 1998.
342. Kraft HG, Haibach C, Lingenhel A, Brunner C, Trommsdorff M, Kronenberg F, Müller HJ, et al: Sequence polymorphism in kringle IV 37 in linkage disequilibrium with the apolipoprotein(a) size polymorphism. *Hum Genet* **95**:275, 1995.
343. Trommsdorff M, Köchl S, Lingenhel A, Kronenberg F, Delport R, Vermaak H, Lemming L, et al: A pentanucleotide repeat polymorphism in the 5′ control region of the apolipoprotein(a) gene is associated with lipoprotein(a) plasma concentrations in Caucasians. *J Clin Invest* **96**:150, 1995.
344. Mooser V, Mancini FP, Bopp S, Schramm AP, Guerra R, Boerwinkle E, Müller HJ, et al: Sequence polymorphisms in the apo(a) gene associated with specific levels of Lp(a) in plasma. *Hum Mol Genet* **4**:173, 1995.
345. Zysow BR, Lindahl GE, Wade DP, Knight BL, Lawn RM: C/T polymorphism in the 5′ untranslated region of the apolipoprotein(a) gene introduces an upstream ATG and reduces *in vitro* translation. *Arterioscler Thromb* **15**:58, 1995.
346. Suzuki K, Kuriyama M, Saito T, Ichinose A: Plasma lipoprotein(a) levels and expression of the apolipoprotein(a) gene are dependent on the nucleotide polymorphisms in its 5′-flanking region. *J Clin Invest* **99**:1361, 1997.
347. Kraft HG, Windegger M, Menzel HJ, Utermann G: Significant impact of the +93 C/T polymorphism in the apolipoprotein(a) gene on Lp(a) concentrations in Africans but not in Caucasians: confounding effect of linkage disequilibrium. *Hum Mol Genet* **7**:257, 1998.
348. Prins J, Leus FR, Van der Hoek YY, Kastelein JJ, Bouma BN, van Rijn HJ: The identification and significance of a Thr→Pro polymorphism in kringle IV type 8 of apolipoprotein(a). *Thromb Haemost* **77**:949, 1997.
349. Scanu AM: Identification of mutations in human apolipoprotein(a) kringle 4–37 from the study of the DNA of peripheral blood lymphocytes: Relevance to the role of lipoprotein(a) in atherothrombosis. *Am J Cardiol* **75**:58B, 1995.
350. Van der Hoek YY, Wittekoek ME, Beisiegel U, Kastelein JJP, Koschinsky ML: The apolipoprotein(a) kringle IV repeats which differ from the major repeat kringle are present in variably-sized isoforms. *Hum Mol Genet* **2**:361, 1993.
351. Puckey LH, Lawn RM, Knight BL: Polymorphisms in the apolipoprotein(a) gene and their relationship to allele size and plasma lipoprotein(a) concentration. *Hum Mol Genet* **6**:1099, 1997.
352. White AL, Hixson JE, Rainwater DL, Lanford RE: Molecular basis for "null" lipoprotein(a) phenotypes and the influence of apolipoprotein(a) size on plasma lipoprotein(a) level in the baboon. *J Biol Chem* **269**:9060, 1994.
353. Cox LA, Jett C, Hixson JE: Molecular basis of an apolipoprotein(a) null allele: A splice site mutation is associated with deletion of a single exon. *J Lipid Res* **39**:1319, 1998.
353a. Ogorelkova M, Gruber A, Utermann G: Molecular basis of congenital Lp(a) deficiency: a frequent apo(a) "null" mutation in Caucasians. *Hum Mol Genet* **8**:2087, 1999.
354. White AL: Biogenesis of Lp(a) in transgenic mouse hepatocytes. *Clin Genet* **52**:326, 1997.
355. Brunner C, Lobentanz EM, Petho-Schramm A, Ernst A, Kang C, Dieplinger H, Muller HJ, et al: The number of identical kringle IV repeats in apolipoprotein(a) affects its processing and secretion by HepG2 cells. *J Biol Chem* **271**:32403, 1996.
356. White AL, Rainwater DL, Lanford RE: Intracellular maturation of apolipoprotein(a) and assembly of lipoprotein(a) in primary baboon hepatocytes. *J Lipid Res* **34**:509, 1993.
357. White AL, Guerra B, Lanford RE: Influence of allelic variation on apolipoprotein(a) folding in the endoplasmic reticulum. *J Biol Chem* **272**:5048, 1997.
358. White AL, Guerra B, Lanford RE: Influence of allelic variation on apolipoprotein(a) folding in the endoplasmic reticulum. *J Biol Chem* **272**:5048, 1997.
359. White AL, Guerra B, Wang J, Lanford RE: Presecretory degradation of apolipoprotein(a) is mediated by the proteasome pathway. *J Lipid Res* **40**:275, 1999.
360. Bonen DK, Nassir F, Hausman AM, Davidson NO: Inhibition of N-linked glycosylation results in retention of intracellular apo(a) in hepatoma cells, although nonglycosylated and immature forms of apolipoprotein(a) are competent to associate with apolipoprotein B-100 *in vitro*. *J Lipid Res* **39**:1629, 1998.
361. Ehrlich KC, Ehrlich M: Highly repeated sites in the apolipoprotein(a) gene recognized by methylated DNA-binding protein, a sequence-specific DNA-binding protein. *Mol Cell Biol* **10**:4957, 1990.
362. Van der Hoek YY, Wanders RJ, Van den Ende AE, Kraft HG, Gabel BR, Kastelein JJ, Koschinsky ML: Lipoprotein(a) is not present in the plasma of patients with some peroxisomal disorders. *J Lipid Res* **38**:1612, 1997.
363. Knijff P, Kaptein A, Boomsma D, Princen HMG, Frants RR, Havekes LM: Apolipoprotein E polymorphism affects plasma levels of lipoprotein(a). *Atherosclerosis* **90**:169, 1991.
364. Klausen IC, Gerdes LU, Hansen PS, Lemming L, Gerdes C, Faergeman O: Effects of apo E gene polymorphism on Lp(a) concentrations depend on the size of apo(a): A study of 466 white men. *J Mol Med* **74**:685, 1996.
365. Elisaf MS, Bairaktari ET, Tzallas CS, Siamopoulos KC: Lipoprotein (a) concentrations in patients with various dyslipidaemias. *Ann Med* **29**:305, 1997.
366. Bartens W, Rader DJ, Talley G, Brewer HB Jr: Decreased plasma levels of lipoprotein(a) in patients with hypertriglyceridemia. *Atherosclerosis* **108**:149, 1994.
367. Rainwater DL, Ludwig MJ, Haffner SM, VandeBerg JL: Lipid and lipoprotein factors associated with variation in Lp(a) density. *Arterioscler Thromb* **15**:313, 1995.
368. Mbewu AD, Bhatnagar D, Durrington PN, Hunt L, Ishola M, Arrol S, Mackness M, et al: Serum lipoprotein(a) in patients heterozygous for familial hypercholesterolemia, their relatives, and unrelated control populations. *Arterioscler Thromb* **11**:940, 1991.
369. Hughes JK, Mendelsohn D: Serum lipoprotein (a) levels in 'normal' individuals, those with familial hypercholesterolaemia, and those with coronary artery disease. *S Afr Med J* **78**:567, 1990.
370. Guo HC, Chapman MJ, Bruckert E, Farriaux JP, De Gennes JL: Lipoprotein Lp(a) in homozygous familial hypercholesterolemia: Density profile, particle heterogeneity and apolipoprotein(a) phenotype. *Atherosclerosis* **31**:69, 1991.
371. Perombelon YFN, Gallagher JJ, Myant NB, Soutar AK, Knight BL: Lipoprotein(a) in subjects with familial defective apolipoprotein B_{100}. *Atherosclerosis* **92**:203, 1992.
372. Carmena R, Lussier-Cacan S, Roy M, Minnich A, Lingenhel A, Kronenberg F, Davignon J: Lp(a) levels and atherosclerotic vascular disease in a sample of patients with familial hypercholesterolemia

sharing the same gene defect. *Arterioscler Thromb Vasc Biol* **16**:129, 1996.
373. Knight BL, Perombelon YFN, Soutar AK, Wade DP, Seed M: Catabolism of lipoprotein(a) in familial hypercholesterolaemic subjects. *Atherosclerosis* **87**:227, 1991.
374. Van Biervliet JP, Labeur C, Michiels G, Usher DC, Rosseneu M: Lipoprotein (a) profiles and evolution in newborns. *Atherosclerosis* **86**:173, 1991.
375. Albers JJ, Hazzard WR: Immunochemical quantification of human plasma Lp(a) lipoprotein. *Lipids* **9**:15, 1974.
376. Routi T, Ronnemaa T, Lapinleimu H, Salo P, Viikari J, Leino A, Valimaki I, et al: Effect of weaning on serum lipoprotein(a) concentration: The STRIP baby study. *Pediatr Res* **38**:522, 1995.
377. Katan MB, Zock PL, Mensink RP: Trans fatty acids and their effects on lipoproteins in humans. *Annu Rev Nutr* **15**:473, 1995.
378. Mensink RP, Zock PL, Katan MB, Hornstra G: Effect of dietary *cis* and *trans* fatty acids on serum lipoprotein(a) levels in humans. *J Lipid Res* **33**:1493, 1992.
379. Nestel P, Noakes M, Belling B, McArthur R, Clifton P, Janus E, Abbey M: Plasma lipoprotein lipid and Lp(a) changes with substitution of elaidic acid for oleic acid in the diet. *J Lipid Res* **33**:1029, 1992.
380. Almendingen K, Jordal O, Kierulf P, Sandstad B, Pedersen JI: Effects of partially hydrogenated fish oil, partially hydrogenated soybean oil, and butter on serum lipoproteins and Lp(a) in men. *J Lipid Res* **36**:1370, 1995.
381. Hornstra G, van Houwelingen AC, Kester AD, Sundram K: A palm oil-enriched diet lowers serum lipoprotein(a) in normocholesterolemic volunteers [Letter]. *Atherosclerosis* **90**:91, 1991.
382. Herrmann W, Biermann J, Kostner GM: Comparison of effects of N-3 to N-6 fatty acids on serum level of lipoprotein(a) in patients with coronary artery disease. *Am J Cardiol* **76**:459, 1995.
383. Eritsland J, Arnesen H, Berg K, Seljeflot I, Abdelnoor M: Serum Lp(a) lipoprotein levels in patients with coronary artery disease and the influence of long-term n-3 fatty acid supplementation. *Scand J Clin Lab Invest* **55**:295, 1995.
384. Tholstrup T, Marckmann P, Vessby B, Sandstrom B: Effect of fats high in individual saturated fatty acids on plasma lipoprotein(a) levels in young healthy men. *J Lipid Res* **36**:1447, 1995.
385. Mackinnon LT, Hubinger L, Lepre F: Effects of physical activity and diet on lipoprotein(a). *Med Sci Sports Exerc* **29**:1429, 1997.
386. Lobo RA, Notelovitz M, Bernstein L, Khan FY, Ross RK, Paul WL: Lp(a) lipoprotein: Relationship to cardiovascular disease risk factors, exercise, and estrogen. *Am J Obstet Gynecol* **166**:1182, 1992.
387. Thomas TR, Ziogas G, Harris WS: Influence of fitness status on very-low-density lipoprotein subfractions and lipoprotein(a) in men and women. *Metabolism* **46**:1178, 1997.
388. Marth E, Cazzolato G, Bon B, Avogaro P, Kostner GM: Serum concentrations of Lp(a) and other lipoprotein parameters in heavy alcohol consumers. *Ann Nutr Metab* **26**:56, 1982.
389. Kervinen K, Savolainen MJ, Antero Kesäniemi Y: A rapid increase in lipoprotein (a) levels after ethanol withdrawal in alcoholic men. *Life Sci* **48**:2183, 1991.
390. Kostner GM: Lp(a) lipoproteins and the genetic polymorphisms of lipoprotein B, in Day C (ed): *Low-Density Lipoproteins*,New York, Plenum Press, , 1976, p 229.
391. Soma M, Fumagalli R, Paoletti R, Meschia M, Maini MC, Crosignani P, Ghanem K, et al: Plasma Lp(a) concentration after oestrogen and progestogen in postmenopausal women. *Lancet* **337**:612, 1991.
392. Espeland MA, Marcovina SM, Miller V, Wood PD, Wasilauskas C, Sherwin R, Schrott H, et al: Effect of postmenopausal hormone therapy on lipoprotein(a) concentration. PEPI Investigators. Postmenopausal estrogen/progestin interventions. *Circulation* **97**:979, 1998.
393. Kim CJ, Jang HC, Cho DH, Min YK: Effects of hormone replacement therapy on lipoprotein(a) and lipids in postmenopausal women. *Arterioscler Thromb* **14**:275, 1994.
394. Tuck CH, Holleran S, Berglund L: Hormonal regulation of lipoprotein(a) levels: Effects of estrogen replacement therapy on lipoprotein(a) and acute phase reactants in postmenopausal women. *Arterioscler Thromb Vasc Biol* **17**:1822, 1997.
395. Albers JJ, Taggart HM, Appelbaum-Bowden D, Haffner F, Chesnut CH, Hazzard WR: Reduction of LCAT, apo D and the Lp (a) lipoprotein with the anabolic steroid stanozolol. *Biochim Biophys Acta* **795**:293, 1984.
396. Farish E, Rolton HA, Barnes JF, Hart DM: Lipoprotein (a) concentrations in postmenopausal women taking norethisterone. *BMJ* **303**:694, 1991.
397. Crook D, Sidhu M, Seed M, O'Donnell M, Stevenson JC: Lipoprotein Lp(a) levels are reduced by danazol, an anabolic steroid. *Atherosclerosis* **92**:41, 1992.
398. Henriksson P, Angelin B, Berglund L: Hormonal regulation of serum Lp (a) levels: Opposite effects after estrogen treatment and orchidectomy in males with prostatic carcinoma. *J Clin Invest* **89**:1166, 1992.
399. Ozata M, Yildirimkaya M, Bulur M, Yilmaz K, Bolu E, Corakci A, Gundogan MA: Effects of gonadotropin and testosterone treatments on Lipoprotein(a), high-density lipoprotein particles, and other lipoprotein levels in male hypogonadism. *J Clin Endocrinol Metab* **81**:3372, 1996.
400. Zmunda JM, Thompson PD, Dickenson R, Bausserman LL: Testosterone decreases lipoprotein(a) in men. *Am J Cardiol* **77**:1244, 1996.
401. Klausen IC, Nielsen FE, Hegedüs L, Gerdes LU, Charles P, Faergeman O: Treatment of hypothyroidism reduces low-density lipoproteins but not lipoprotein(a). *Metabolism* **41**:911, 1992.
402. De Bruin TWA, Van Barlingen H, Van Linde-Sibenius Trip M, Van Vuurst de Vries A-RR, Akveld MJ, Erkelens DW: Lipoprotein(a) and apolipoprotein B plasma concentrations in hypothyroid, euthyroid, and hyperthyroid subjects. *J Clin Endocrinol Metab* **76**:121, 1993.
403. Kung AWC, Pang RWC, Lauder I, Lam KSL, Janus ED: Changes in serum lipoprotein(a) and lipids during treatment of hyperthyroidism. *Clin Chem* **41**:226, 1995.
404. Hoppichler F, Sandholzer C, Moncayo R, Utermann G, Kraft HG: Thyroid hormone (fT4) reduces lipoprotein(a) plasma levels. *Atherosclerosis* **115**:65, 1995.
405. Engler H, Riesen WF: Effect of thyroid function on concentrations of lipoprotein(a). *Clin Chem* **39**:2466, 1993.
406. Kurbaan AS, Barbir M, Ilsley GDJ: Normalization of lipoprotein (a) following successful treatment of hypothyroidism. *QJM* **88**:221, 1995.
407. Yamamoto K, Ozaki I, Fukushima N, Setoguchi Y, Kajihara S, Mizuta T, Yanagita T, et al: Serum lipoprotein(a) levels before and after subtotal thyroidectomy in subjects with hyperthyroidism. *Metabolism* **44**:4, 1995.
408. Klausen IC, Hegedüs L, Hansen PS, Nielsen FE, Gerdes LU, Faergeman O: Apolipoprotein(a) phenotypes and lipoprotein(a) concentrations in patients with hyperthyroidism. *J Clin Invest* **73**:41, 1995.
409. Maeda S, Abe A, Seishima M, Makino K, Noma A, Kawade M: Transient changes of serum lipoprotein(a) as an acute phase protein. *Atherosclerosis* **78**:145, 1989.
410. Craig WY, Ledue TB: Lipoprotein(a) and the acute phase response. *Clin Chim Acta* **210**:231, 1992.
411. Slunga L, Johnson O, Dahlén GH, Eriksson S: Lipoprotein(a) and acute-phase proteins in acute myocardial infarction. *Scand J Clin Lab Invest* **52**:95, 1992.
412. Karádi I, Romics L, Palos G, Doman J, Kaszas I, Hesz A, Kostner GM: Lp(a) lipoprotein concentration in serum of patients with heavy proteinuria of different origin. *Clin Chem* **35**:2121, 1989.
413. Faucher C, Doucet C, Baumelou A, Chapman J, Jacobs C, Thillet J: Elevated lipoprotein (a) levels in primary nephrotic syndrome. *Am J Kidney Dis* **22**:808, 1993.
414. Wanner C, Rader D, Bartens W, Krämer J, Brewer HB, Schollmeyer P, Wieland H: Elevated plasma lipoprotein(a) in patients with the nephrotic syndrome. *Ann Intern Med* **119**:263, 1993.
415. Stenvinkel P, Berglund L, Heimbürger O, Pettersson E, Alvestrand A: Lipoprotein(a) in nephrotic syndrome. *Kidney Int* **44**:1116, 1993.
416. Joven J, Simo JM, Vilella E, Camps J, Espinel E, Villabona C: Accumulation of atherogenic remnants and lipoprotein(a) in the nephrotic syndrome: relation to remission of proteinuria. *Clin Chem* **41**:908, 1995.
417. Kanno H, Saito E, Fujioka T, Yasugi T: Lipoprotein(a) levels in the nephrotic syndrome. *Intern Med* **31**:1004, 1992.
418. De Sain-Van Der Velden MG, Reijngoud DJ, Kaysen GA, Gadellaa MM, Voorbij H, Stellaard F, Koomans HA, et al: Evidence for increased synthesis of lipoprotein(a) in the nephrotic syndrome. *J Am Soc Nephrol* **9**:1474, 1998.
419. Kronenberg F, König P, Neyer U, Auinger M, Pribasnig A, Lang U, Reitinger J, et al: Multicenter study of lipoprotein(a) and apolipoprotein(a) phenotypes in patients with end-stage renal disease treated

by hemodialysis or continous ambulatory peritoneal dialysis. *J Am Soc Nephrol* **6**:110, 1995.
420. Dieplinger H, Lackner C, Kronenberg F, Sandholzer Ch, Lhotta K, Hoppichler F, Graf H, et al: Elevated plasma concentrations of lipoprotein(a) in patients with end-stage renal disease are not related to the size polymorphism of apolipoprotein(a). *J Clin Invest* **91**:397, 1993.
421. Zimmermann J, Herrlinger S, Pruy A, Wanner C: Mechanism of high serum lipoprotein(a) in hemodialysis patients [Abstract]. *J Am Soc Nephrol* **8**:260A, 1997.
422. Murphy BG, McNamee PT: Apolipoprotein(a) concentration decreases following renal transplantation. *Nephrol Dial Transplant* **7**:174, 1992.
423. Gault MH, Longerich LL, Purchase L, Harnett J, Breckenridge C: Comparison of Lp(a) concentrations and some potential effects in hemodialysis, CAPD, transplantation, and control groups, and review of the literature. *Nephron* **70**:155, 1995.
424. Black IW, Wilcken DEL: Decreases in apolipoprotein(a) after renal transplantation: Implications for lipoprotein(a) metabolism. *Clin Chem* **38**:353, 1992.
425. Kronenberg F, König P, Lhotta K, Königsrainer A, Sandholzer Ch, Utermann G, Dieplinger H: Cyclosporin and serum lipids in renal transplant recipients. *Lancet* **341**:765, 1993.
426. Segarra A, Chacón P, Martin M, Vilardell M, Vila J, Cotrina M, Fort J, et al: Serum lipoprotein (a) levels in patients with chronic renal failure—Evolution after renal transplantation and relationship with other parameters of lipoprotein metabolism: A prospective study. *Nephron* **69**:9, 1995.
427. Azrolan N, Brown CD, Thomas L, Hayek T, Zhao ZH, Roberts KG, Scheiner C, et al: Cyclosporin A has divergent effects on plasma LDL cholesterol (LDL-C) and lipoprotein(a) (Lp(a)) levels in renal transplant recipients: Evidence for renal involvement in the maintenance of LDL-C and the elevation of Lp(a) concentrations in hemodialysis patients. *Arterioscler Thromb* **14**:1393, 1994.
428. Kronenberg F, König P, Lhotta K, Öfner D, Sandholzer C, Margreiter R, Dosch E, et al: Apolipoprotein(a) phenotype-associated decrease in lipoprotein(a) plasma concentrations after renal transplantation. *Arterioscler Thromb* **14**:1399, 1994.
429. von Ahsen N, Helmhold M, Eisenhauer T, Armstrong VW, Oellerich M: Decrease in lipoprotein(a) after renal transplantation is related to the glucocorticoid dose. *Eur J Clin Invest* **26**:668, 1996.
430. Kandoussi AM, Hugue V, Cachera C, Hazzan M, Dracon M, Tacquet A, Noel C: Apo(a) Phenotypes and Lp(a) Concentrations in Renal Transplant Patients. *Nephron* **80**:183, 1998.
431. Bruckert E, Davidoff P, Grimaldi A, Truffert J, Giral P, Doumith R, Thervet F, et al: Increased serum levels of lipoprotein(a) in diabetes mellitus and their reduction with glycemic control. *JAMA* **263**:35, 1990.
432. Haffner SM, Tuttle KR, Rainwater DL: Decrease of lipoprotein(a) with improved glycemic control in IDDM subjects. *Diabetes Care* **14(4)**:302, 1991.
433. Haffner SM, Morales PA, Stern MP, Gruber MK: Lp(a) concentrations in NIDDM. *Diabetes* **41**:1267, 1992.
434. Velho G, Erlich D, Turpin E, Néel D, Cohen D, Froguel P, Passa P: Lipoprotein(a) in diabetic patients and normoglycemic relatives in familial NIDDM. *Diabetes Care* **16**:742, 1993.
435. Imperatore G, Rivellese A, Galasso R, Celentano E, Iovine C, Ferrara A, Riccardi G, et al: Lipoprotein(a) concentrations in non-insulin-dependent diabetes mellitus and borderline hyperglycemia: A population-based study. *Metabolism* **44**:1293, 1995.
436. Heller FR, Jamart J, Honore P, Derue G, Novik V, Galanti L, Parfonry A, et al: Serum lipoprotein(a) in patients with diabetes mellitus. *Diabetes Care* **16**:819, 1993.
437. Császár A, Dieplinger H, Sandholzer Ch, Karádi I, Juhász E, Drexel H, Halmos T, et al: Plasma lipoprotein(a) concentration and phenotypes in diabetes mellitus. *Diabetologia* **36**:47, 1993.
438. Chang CJ, Kao JT, Wu TJ, Lu FH, Tai TY: Serum lipids and lipoprotein(a) concentrations in Chinese NIDDM patients. Relation to metabolic control. *Diabetes Care* **18**:1191, 1995.
439. Klausen IC, Berg Schmidt E, Lervang HH, Gerdes LU, Ditzel J, Faergeman O: Normal lipoprotein(a) concentrations and apolipoprotein(a) isoforms in patients with insulin-dependent diabetes mellitus. *Eur J Clin Invest* **22**:538, 1992.
440. Couper JJ, Bates DJ, Cocciolone R, Magarey AM, Boulton TJC, Penfold JL, Ryall RG: Association of lipoprotein(a) with puberty in IDDM. *Diabetes Care* **16**:869, 1993.
441. Salzer B, Stavljenic A, Jürgens G, Dumic M, Radica A: Polymorphism of apolipoprotein E, lipoprotein(a), and other lipoproteins in children with type I diabetes. *Clin Chem* **39**:1427, 1993.
442. James RW, Boemi M, Sirolla C, Amadio L, Fumelli P, Pometta D: Lipoprotein (a) and vascular disease in diabetic patients. *Diabetologia* **38**:711, 1995.
443. Purnell JQ, Marcovina SM, Hokanson JE, Kennedy H, Cleary PA, Steffes MW, Brunzell JD: Levels of lipoprotein(a), apolipoprotein B, and lipoprotein cholesterol distribution in IDDM. Results from follow-up in the Diabetes Control and Complications Trial. *Diabetes* **44**:1218, 1995.
444. Perez A, Carreras G, Caixas A, Castellvi A, Caballero A, Bonet R, Ordonez-Llanos J, et al: Plasma lipoprotein(a) levels are not influenced by glycemic control in type 1 diabetes. *Diabetes Care* **21**:1517, 1998.
445. Dubrey SW, Reaveley DR, Seed M, Lane DA, Ireland H, O'Donnell M, O'Connor B, et al: Risk factors for cardiovascular disease in IDDM. A study of identical twins. *Diabetes* **43**:831, 1994.
446. Feely J, Barry M, Keeling PWN, Weir DG, Cooke T: Lipoprotein(a) in cirrhosis. *BMJ* **304**:545, 1992.
447. Gregory WL, Game FL, Farrer M, Idle JR, Laker MF, James OFW: Reduced serum lipoprotein(a) levels in patients with primary biliary cirrhosis. *Atherosclerosis* **105**:43, 1994.
448. Wright LC, Sullivan DR, Muller M, Dyne M, Tattersall HN, Mountford CE: Elevated apolipoprotein(a) levels in cancer patients. *Int J Cancer* **43**:241, 1989.
449. Sechi LA, Kronenberg F, De Carli S, Falleti E, Zingaro L, Catena C, Utermann G, et al: Association of serum lipoprotein(a) levels and apolipoprotein(a) size polymorphism with target-organ damage in arterial hypertension. *JAMA* **277**:1689, 1997.
450. Takahashi S, Yamamoto T, Moriwaki Y, Tsutsumi Z, Higashino K: Increased concentrations of serum Lp(a) lipoprotein in patients with primary gout. *Ann Rheum Dis* **54**:90, 1995.
451. Berg K, Dahlén G, Borresen AL: Lp(a) phenotypes, other lipoprotein parameters, and a family history of coronary heart disease in middle-aged males. *Clin Genet* **16**:347, 1979.
452. Dahlén G, Ericson C, Furberg C, Lundkvist L, Svärsudd K: Angina of effort and an extra pre-beta lipoprotein in fraction. *Acta Med Scand* **II(Suppl 531)**:11, 1972.
453. Dahlen G, Berg.K., Gillnas T, Ericson C: Lp(a) lipoprotein/prebeta1,-lipoprotein in Swedish middle-aged males and in patients with coronary heart disease. *Clin Genet* **7**:334, 1975.
454. Dahlen G, Berg K, Frick MH: Lp(a) lipoprotein/pre-b1-lipoprotein, serum lipids and atherosclerotic disease. *Clin Genet* **9**:558, 1976.
455. Ose L, Kalager T, Grundt IK: Serum beta-lipoprotein subfractions in polyacrylamide gel electrophoresis associated with coronary Heart Disease. *Scand J Clin Lab Invest* **36**:75, 1976.
456. Kraft HG, Lingenhel A, Kochl S, Hoppichler F, Kronenberg F, Abe A, Muhlberger V, et al: Apolipoprotein(a) kringle IV repeat number predicts risk for coronary heart disease. *Arterioscler Thromb Vasc Biol* **16**:713, 1996.
457. Kronenberg F, Steinmetz A, Kostner GM, Dieplinger H: Lipoprotein(a) in health and disease. *Crit Rev Clin Lab Sci* **33**:495, 1996.
458. Stein JH, Rosenson RS: Lipoprotein Lp(a) excess and coronary heart disease. *Arch Intern Med* **157**:1170, 1997.
459. Sandkamp M, Funke H, Schulte H, Köhler E, Assmann G: Lipoprotein(a) is an independent risk factor for myocardial infarction at a young age. *Clin Chem* **36**:20, 1990.
460. Albers JJ, Cabana VG, Warnick R, Hazzard WR: Lp(a) lipoprotein: relationship to sinking pre-b-lipoprotein, hyperlipoproteinemia, and apolipoprotein B. *Metabolism* **24**:1047, 1975.
461. Hearn JA, DeMaio SJJr, Roubin GS, Hammarstrom M, Sgoutas D: Predictive value of lipoprotein (a) and other serum lipoproteins in the angiographic diagnosis of coronary artery disease. *Am J Cardiol* **66**:1176, 1990.
462. Parra HJ, Arveiler D, Evans AE, Cambou JP, Amouyel P, Bingham A, McMaster D, et al: A case-control study of lipoprotein particles in two populations at contrasting risk for coronary heart disease: The ECTIM study. *Arterioscler Thromb* **12**:701, 1992.
463. Kim JQ, Song JH, Lee MM, Park YB, Chung HK, Tchai BS, Kim SI: Evaluation of Lp(a) as a risk factor of coronary artery disease in the Korean population. *Ann Clin Biochem* **29**:226, 1992.
464. Frade LJG, Alvarez JJ, Rayo I, Torrado MC, Lasunción MA, Avello AG, Hernandez A: Fibrinolytic parameters and lipoprotein(a) levels in plasma of patients with coronary artery disease. *Thromb Res* **63**:407, 1991.

465. Armstrong VW, Cremer P, Eberle E, Manke A, Schulze F, Wieland H, Kreuzer H, et al: The association between serum Lp (a) concentrations and angiographically assessed coronary atherosclerosis—dependence on serum LDL-levels. *Atherosclerosis* **62**:249, 1986.
466. Terres W, Tatsis E, Pfalzer B, Beil F, Beisiegel U, Hamm ChW: Rapid angiographic progression of coronary artery disease in patients with elevated lipoprotein(a). *Circulation* **91**:948, 1995.
467. Hopkins PN, Hunt SC, Schreiner PJ, Eckfeldt JH, Borecki IB, Ellison CR, Williams RR, et al: Lipoprotein(a) interactions with lipid and non-lipid risk factors in patients with early onset coronary artery disease: Results from the NHLBI Family Heart Study. *Atherosclerosis* **141**:333, 1998.
468. Hopkins PN, Wu LL, Hunt SC, James BC, Vincent GM, Williams RR: Lipoprotein(a) interactions with lipid and nonlipid risk factors in early familial coronary artery disease. *Arterioscler Thromb Vasc Biol* **17**:2783, 1997.
469. Hoefler G, Harnoncourt F, Paschke E, Mirtl W, Pfeiffer KH, Kostner GM: Lipoprotein(a). A risk factor for myocardial infarction. *Arteriosclerosis* **8**:398, 1988.
470. Klausen IC, Beisiegel U, Menzel HJ, Rosseneu M, Nicaud V, Faergeman O: Apo(a) phenotypes and Lp(a) concentrations in offspring of men with and without myocardial infarction. The EARS Study. European Atherosclerosis Research Study. *Arterioscler Thromb Vasc Biol* **15**:1001, 1995.
471. Srinivasan SR, Dahlen GH, Jarpa RA, Webber LS, Berenson GS: Racial (black-white) differences in serum lipoprotein (a) distribution and its relation to parental myocardial infarction in children: Bogalusa Heart Study. *Circulation* **84**:160, 1991.
472. Moliterno DJ, Jokinen EV, Miserez AR, Lange RA, Willard JE, Boerwinkle E, Hillis LD, et al: No association between plasma lipoprotein(a) concentrations and the presence or absence of coronary atherosclerosis in African-Americans. *Arterioscler Thromb Vasc Biol* **15**:850, 1995.
473. Sorrentino MJ, Vielhauer C, Eisenbart JD, Fless GM, Scanu AM, Feldman T: Plasma lipoprotein(a) protein concentration and coronary artery disease in black patients compared with white patients. *Am J Med* **93**:658, 1992.
474. Schumacher M, Tiran A, Eber B, Toplak H, Wilders-Truschnig M, Klein W: Lipoprotein (a) is not a risk factor for restenosis after percutaneous transluminal coronary angioplasty. *Am J Cardiol* **69**:572, 1992.
475. Linden T, Taddei-Peters W, Wilhelmsen L, Herlitz J, Karlsson T, Ullstrom C, Wiklund O: Serum lipids, lipoprotein(a) and apo(a) isoforms in patients with established coronary artery disease and their relation to disease and prognosis after coronary by-pass surgery. *Atherosclerosis* **137**:175, 1998.
476. Amemiya H, Arinami T, Kikuchi S, Yamakawa-Kobayashi K, Li L, Fujiwara H, Hiroe M, et al: Apolipoprotein(a) size and pentanucleotide repeat polymorphisms are associated with the degree of atherosclerosis in coronary heart disease. *Atherosclerosis* **123**:181, 1996.
477. Dieplinger H, Kronenberg F: Genetics and metabolism of lipoprotein(a) and their clinical implications (Part 2). *Wien Klin Wochenschr* **111**:46, 1999.
478. Alfthan G, Pekkanen J, Jauhiainen M, Pitkäniemi J, Karvonen M, Tuomilehto J, Salonen JT, et al: Relation of serum homocysteine and lipoprotein(a) concentrations to atherosclerotic disease in a prospective Finnish population based study. *Atherosclerosis* **106**:9, 1994.
479. Kronenberg F, Trenkwalder E, Dieplinger H, Utermann G: Lipoprotein(a) in stored plasma samples and the ravages of time. Why epidemiological studies might fail. *Arterioscler Thromb Vasc Biol* **16**:1568, 1996.
480. Barnathan ES: Has lipoprotein "little" (a) shrunk? *JAMA* **270**:2224, 1993.
481. Simons LA: Lipoprotein(a): Important risk factor or passing fashion? *Med J Aust* **158**:512, 1993.
482. Hoff HF, Beck GJ, Skibinsky CI, Jürgens G, O'Neil JA, Kramer J, Lytle B: Serum Lp(a) levels as a predictor of vein graft stenosis after coronary artery bypass surgery in patients. *Circulation* **77**:1238, 1988.
483. Cushing GL, Gaubatz JW, Nava ML, Burdick BJ, Bocan TMA, Guyton JR, Weilbaecher DDB, et al: Quantitation and localization of apolipoproteins (a) and B in coronary artery bypass vein grafts resected at reoperation. *Arteriosclerosis* **9**:593, 1989.
484. Kronenberg F, Kathrein H, König P, Neyer U, Sturm W, Lhotta K, Gröchenig E, et al: Apolipoprotein(a) phenotypes predict the risk for carotid atherosclerosis in patients with end-stage renal disease. *Arterioscler Thromb* **14**:1405, 1994.
485. Koch M, Kutkuhn B, Trenkwalder E, Bach D, Grabensee B, Dieplinger H, Kronenberg F: Apolipoprotein B, fibrinogen, HDL cholesterol, and apolipoprotein(a) phenotypes predict coronary artery disease in hemodialysis patients. *J Am Soc Nephrol* **8**:1889, 1997.
486. Wanner C, Bartens W, Walz G, Nauck M, Schollmeyer P: Protein loss and genetic polymorphism of apolipoprotein(a) modulate serum lipoprotein(a) in CAPD patients. *Neph Dial Transplant* **10**:75, 1995.
487. Webb AT, Reaveley DA, O'Donnell M, O'Connor B, Seed M, Brown EA: Lipids and lipoprotein(a) as risk factors for vascular disease in patients on renal replacement therapy. *Neph Dial Transplant* **10**:354, 1995.
488. Költringer P, Jürgens G: A dominant role of lipoprotein(a) in the investigation and evaluation of parameters indicating the development of cervical atherosclerosis. *Atherosclerosis* **58**:187, 1985.
489. Woo J, Lau E, Lam CWK, Kay R, Teoh R, Wong HY, Prall WY, et al: Hypertension, lipoprotein(a), and apolipoprotein A-I as risk factors for stroke in the Chinese. *Stroke* **22**:203, 1991.
490. Pedro-Botet J, Senti M, Nogués X, Rubiés-Prat J, Roquer J, D'Olhaberriague L, Olivé J: Lipoprotein and apolipoprotein profile in men with ischemic stroke: Role of lipoprotein(a), triglyceride-rich lipoproteins, and apolipoprotein E polymorphism. *Stroke* **23**:1556, 1992.
491. Jovicic A, Ivanisevic V, Ivanovic I: Lipoprotein(a) in patients with carotid atherosclerosis and ischemic cerebrovascular disorders. *Atherosclerosis* **98**:59, 1993.
492. Brown SA, Morrisett JD, Boerwinkle E, Hutchinson R, Patsch W: The relation of lipoprotein(a) concentrations and apolipoprotein(a) phenotypes with asymptomatic atherosclerosis in subjects of the Atherosclerosis Risk in Communities (ARIC) study. *Arterioscler Thromb* **13**:1558, 1993.
493. Wendelhag I, Wiklund O, Wikstrand J: Atherosclerotic changes in the femoral and carotid arteries in familial hypercholesterolemia: Ultrasonographic assessment of intima-media thickness and plaque occurrence. *Arterioscler Thromb* **13**:1404, 1993.
494. Cambillau M, Simon A, Amar J, Giral P, Atger V, Segond P, Levenson J, et al: Serum Lp(a) as a discriminant marker of early atherosclerotic plaque at three extracoronary sites in hypercholesterolemic men. *Arterioscler Thromb* **12**:1346, 1992.
495. Willeit J, Kiechl S, Santer P, Oberhollenzer F, Egger G, Jarosch E, Mair A: Lipoprotein(a) and asymptomatic carotid artery disease. Evidence of a prominent role in the evolution of advanced carotid plaques: The Bruneck Study. *Stroke* **26**:1582, 1995.
496. Ridker PM, Stampfer MJ, Hennekens CH: Plasma concentration of lipoprotein(a) and the risk of future stroke. *JAMA* **273**:1269, 1995.
497. Jurgens G, Taddei-Peters WC, Koltringer P, Petek W, Chen Q, Greilberger J, Macomber PF, et al: Lipoprotein(a) serum concentration and apolipoprotein(a) phenotype correlate with severity and presence of ischemic cerebrovascular disease. *Stroke* **26**:1841, 1995.
498. Walton KW, Hitchens J, Magnani HN, Khan M: A study of methods of identification and estimation of Lp(a) lipoprotein and of its significance in health, hyperlipidaemia and atherosclerosis. *Atherosclerosis* **20**:323, 1974.
499. Rath M, Niendorf A, Reblin T, Dietel M, Krebber HJ, Beisiegel U: Detection and quantification of lipoprotein(a) in the arterial wall of 107 coronary bypass patients. *Arteriosclerosis* **9**:579, 1989.
500. Scott J: Medical genetics: Arterial hardening in mice. *Nature* **360**:631, 1992.
501. Lawn RM, Pearle AD, Kunz LL, Rubin EM, Reckless J, Metcalfe JC, Grainger DJ: Feedback mechanism of focal vascular lesion formation in transgenic apolipoprotein(a) mice. *J Biol Chem* **271**:31367, 1996.
502. Liu AC, Lawn RM, Verstuyft JG, Rubin EM: Human apolipoprotein A-I prevents atherosclerosis associated with apolipoprotein(a) in transgenic mice. *J Lipid Res* **35**:2263, 1994.
503. Boonmark NW, Lou XJ, Yang ZJ, Schwartz K, Zhang JL, Rubin EM, Lawn RM: Modification of apolipoprotein(a) lysine binding site reduces atherosclerosis in transgenic mice. *J Clin Invest* **100**:558, 1997.
504. Lou XJ, Boonmark NW, Horrigan FT, Degen JL, Lawn RM: Fibrinogen deficiency reduces vascular accumulation of apolipoprotein(a) and development of atherosclerosis in apolipoprotein(a) transgenic mice. *Proc Natl Acad Sci U S A* **95**:12591, 1998.
505. Mancini FP, Newland DL, Mooser V, Murata J, Marcovina S, Young SG, Hammer RE, et al: Relative contributions of apolipoprotein(a) and apolipoprotein-B to the development of fatty lesions in the proximal aorta of mice. *Arterioscler Thromb Vasc Biol* **15**:1911, 1995.

506. Callow MJ, Verstuyft J, Tangirala R, Palinski W, Rubin EM: Atherogenesis in transgenic mice with human apolipoprotein B and lipoprotein (a). *J Clin Invest* **96**:1639, 1995.
507. Sanan DA, Newland DL, Tao R, Marcovina S, Wang J, Mooser V, Hammer RE, et al: Low density lipoprotein receptor-negative mice expressing human apolipoprotein B-100 develop complex atherosclerotic lesions on a chow diet: No accentuation by apolipoprotein(a). *Proc Natl Acad Sci U S A* **95**:4544, 1998.
508. Rouy D, Duverger N, Lin SD, Emmanuel F, Houdebine LM, Denefle P, Viglietta C, et al: Apolipoprotein(a) yeast artificial chromosome transgenic rabbits. Lipoprotein(a) assembly with human and rabbit apolipoprotein B. *J Biol Chem* **273**:1247, 1998.
509. Albers JJ, Marcovina SM: Lipoprotein(a) quantification: comparison of methods and strategies for standardization. *Curr Opin Lipidol* **5**:417, 1994.
510. Albers JJ, Marcovina SM, Lodge MS: The unique lipoprotein(a): Properties and immunochemical measurement. *Clin Chem* **36**:2019, 1990.
511. Kostner GM: Standardization of Lp(a) assays. *Clin Chim Acta* **211**:191, 1992.
512. Dieplinger H, Gruber G, Krasznai K, Reschauer S, Seidel C, Burns D, Müller HJ, et al: Kringle 4 of human apolipoprotein(a) shares a linear antigenic site with human catalase. *J Lipid Res* **36**:813, 1995.
513. Tate JR, Rifai N, Berg K, Couderc R, Dati F, Kostner GM, Sakurabayashi I, et al: International Federation of Clinical Chemistry standardization project for the measurement of lipoprotein(a). Phase I. Evaluation of the analytical performance of lipoprotein(a) assay systems and commercial calibrators. *Clin Chem* **44**:1629, 1998.
514. Seman LJ, Jenner JL, McNamara JR, Schaefer EJ: Quantification of lipoprotein(a) in plasma by assaying cholesterol in lectin-bound plasma fraction. *Clin Chem* **40**:400, 1994.
515. Nauck M, Winkler K, Wittmann C, Mayer H, Luley C, März W, Wieland H: Direct determination of lipoprotein(a) cholesterol by ultracentrifugation and agarose gel electrophoresis with enzymatic staining for cholesterol. *Clin Chem* **41**:731, 1995.
516. Kostner GM, Gries A, Pometta M, Molinari E, Pichler P, Aicher H: Immunochemical determination of lipoprotein Lp(a): Comparison of Laurell electrophoresis and ELISA. *Clin Chim Acta* **188**:187, 1990.
517. Yeo KHJ, Walmsley TA, Owen MC, George PM: A competitive ELISA for lipoprotein(a). *Clin Chim Acta* **205**:213, 1992.
518. Wong WLT, Eaton DL, Berloui A, Fendly B, Hass PE: A monoclonal-antibody-based enzyme-linked immunosorbent assay of lipoprotein(a). *Clin Chem* **36(2)**:192, 1990.
519. Cazzolato G, Prakasch G, Green S, Kostner GM: The determination of lipoprotein(a) by rate and endpoint nephelometry. *Clin Chim Acta* **135**:203, 1983.
520. Vu Dac NG, Chekkor A, Parra H, Duthilleul P, Fruchart JC: Latex immunoassay of human serum Lp(a) lipoprotein. *J Lipid Res* **26**:267, 1985.
521. Jürgens G, Hermann A, Aktuna D, Petek W: Dissociation-enhanced lanthanide fluorescence immunoassay of lipoprotein(a) in serum. *Clin Chem* **38**:853, 1992.
522. Labeur C, Rosseneu M: Methods for the measurement of lipoprotein(a) in the clinical laboratory. *Curr Opin Lipid* **3(6)**:372, 1992.
523. Labeur C, Michiels G, Bury J, Usher DC, Rosseneu M: Lipoprotein(a) quantified by an enzyme-linked immunosorbent assay with monoclonal antibodies. *Clin Chem* **35**:1380, 1989.
524. Vu Dac N, Mezdour H, Parra HJ, Luc G, Luyeye I, Fruchart JC: A selective bi-site immunoenzymatic procedure for human Lp(a) lipoprotein quantification using monoclonal antibodies against apo(a) and apo B. *J Lipid Res* **30**:1437, 1989.
525. Fless GM, Snyder ML, Scanu AM: Enzyme-linked immunoassay for Lp(a). *J Lipid Res* **30**:651, 1989.
526. Marcovina SM, Albers JJ, Gabel B, Koschinsky ML, Gaur VP: Effect of the number of apolipoprotein(a) kringle 4 domains on immunochemical measurements of lipoprotein(a). *Clin Chem* **41**:246, 1995.
527. Scanu AM, Pfaffinger D, Fless GM, Makino K, Eisenbart J, Hinman J: Attenuation of immunologic reactivity of lipoprotein(a) by thiols and cysteine-containing compounds: Structural implications. *Arterioscler Thromb* **12**:424, 1992.
528. Craig WY, Ledue TB: The effects of long term storage on serum Lp(a) levels. *Atherosclerosis* **93**:261, 1992.
529. Craig WY, Poulin SE, Forster NR, Neveux LM, Wald NJ, Ledue TB: Effect of sample storage on the assay of lipoprotein(a) by commercially available radial immunodiffusion and enzyme-linked immunosorbent assay kits. *Clin Chem* **38**:550, 1992.
530. Sgoutas DS, Tuten T: Effect of lyophilization on determinations of lipoprotein(a) in serum. *Clin Chem* **38**:1355, 1992.
531. Van Biervliet J-P, Michiels G, Rosseneu M: Quantification of lipoprotein(a) in dried blood spots and screening for above-normal lipoprotein(a) concentrations in newborns. *Clin Chem* **37**:706, 1991.
532. Wang XL, Wilcken DEL, Dudman NPB: Neonatal apo A-I, apo B, and apo(a) levels in dried blood spots in an Australian population. *Pediatr Res* **28**:496, 1990.
533. Kronenberg F, Lobentanz E-M, König P, Utermann G, Dieplinger H: Effect of sample storage on the measurement of lipoprotein(a), apolipoproteins B and A-IV, total and high-density lipoprotein cholesterol and triglycerides. *J Lipid Res* **35**:1318, 1994.
534. Sgoutas DS, Tuten T: Effect of freezing and thawing of serum on the immunoassay of lipoprotein(a). *Clin Chem* **38**:1873, 1992.
535. Usher DC, Swanson C, Rader DJ, Krämer J, Brewer HB: A comparison of Lp(a) levels in fresh and frozen plasma using ELISAs with either anti-apo(a) or anti-apo B reporting antibodies. *Chem Phys Lipids* **67–68**:243, 1994.
536. Desmarais RL, Sarembock IJ, Ayers CR, Vernon SM, Powers ER, Gimple LW: Elevated serum lipoprotein(a) is a risk factor for clinical recurrence after coronary balloon angioplasty. *Circulation* **91**:1403, 1995.
537. Evans RW, Sankey SS, Hauth BA, Sutton Tyrrell K, Kamboh MI, Kuller LH: Effect of sample storage on quantitation of lipoprotein(a) by an enzyme-linked immunosorbent assay. *Lipids* **31**:1197, 1996.
538. Fieseler H-G, Armstrong VW, Wieland E, Thiery J, Schütz E, Walli AK, Seidel D: Serum Lp(a) concentrations are unaffected by treatment with the HMG-CoA reductase inhibitor pravastatin: Results of a 2-year investigation. *Clin Chim Acta* **204**:291, 1991.
539. Slunga L, Johnson O, Dahlén GH: Changes in Lp(a) lipoprotein levels during the treatment of hypercholesterolaemia with simvastatin. *Eur J Clin Pharmacol* **43**:369, 1992.
540. Berg K, Leren TP: Unchanged serum lipoprotein(a) concentrations with lovastatin. *Lancet* **30**:812, 1989.
541. Crook D, Sidhu M, Bruce R: Simvastatin and lipoprotein(a). *Lancet* **339**:313, 1992.
542. Thiery J, Armstrong VW, Schleef J, Creutzfeldt C, Creutzfeldt W, Seidel D: Serum lipoprotein Lp (a) concentration are not influenced by an HMG CoA reductase inhibitor. *Klin Wochenschr* **66**:462, 1988.
543. McDowell IF, Smye M, Trinick T: Simvastatin in severe hypercholesterolaemia: A placebo controlled trial. *Br J Clin Pharmacol* **31**:340, 1991.
544. Leren TP, Hjermann I, Foss OP, Leren P, Berg K: Long-term effect of lovastatin alone and in combination with cholestyramine on lipoprotein (a) level in familial hypercholesterolemic subjects. *Klin Wochenschr* **70**:711, 1992.
545. Vessby B, Kostner G, Lithell H, Thomis J: Diverging effects of cholestyramine on apolipoprotein B and lipoprotein Lp(a). *Atherosclerosis* **44**:61, 1982.
546. Hiraga T, Harada K, Kobayashi T, Murase T: Reduction of serum lipoprotein(a) using estrogen in a man with familial hypercholesterolemia. *JAMA* **267**:2328, 1992.
547. Love RR, Wiebe DA, Feyzi JM, Newcomb PA, Chappell RJ: Effects of tamoxifen on cardiovascular risk factors in postmenopausal women after 5 years of treatment. *J Natl Cancer Inst* **86**:1534, 1994.
548. Shewmon DA, Stock JL, Rosen CJ, Heiniluoma KM, Hogue MM, Morrison A, Doyle EM, et al: Tamoxifen and estrogen lower circulating lipoprotein(a) concentrations in healthy postmenopausal women. *Arterioscler Thromb* **14**:1586, 1994.
549. Farish E, Barnes JF, Rolton HA, Spowart K, Fletcher CD, Hart DM: Effects of tibolone on lipoprotein(a) and HDL subfractions. *Maturitas* **20**:215, 1994.
550. Carlson LA, Hamsten A, Asplund A: Pronounced lowering of serum levels of lipoprotein Lp(a) in hyperlipidemic subjects treated with nicotinic acid. *J Intern Med* **226**:271, 1989.
551. Noma A, Maeda S, Okuno M, Abe A, Muto Y: Reduction of serum lipoprotein(a) levels in hyperlipidaemic patients with alpha-tocopheryl nicotinate. *Atherosclerosis* **84**:213, 1990.
552. Gavish D, Breslow JL: Lipoprotein(a) reduction by *N*-acetylcysteine. *Lancet* **337**:203, 1991.
553. Scanu AM: N-acetylcysteine and immunoreactivity of lipoprotein(a). *Lancet* **337**:1159, 1991.
554. Stalenhoef AFH, Kroon AA, Demacker PNM: *N*-acetylcysteine and lipoprotein. *Lancet* **337**:491, 1991.
555. Breslow JL, Azrolan N, Bostom A: *N*-acetylcysteine and lipoprotein(a). *Lancet* **339**:126, 1992.

556. Mbewu AD, Durrington PN, Bhatnagar D, Miller JP, Mackness MI: Oral carbocysteine does not lower serum lipoprotein(a) levels. *Atherosclerosis* **90**:219, 1991.
557. Frank S, Durovic S, Kostner K, Kostner GM: Inhibitors for the *in vitro* assembly of Lp(a). *Arterioscler Thromb Vasc Biol* **15**:1774, 1995.
558. Arnadottir M, Berg AL, Kronenberg F, Lingenhel A, Hugosson T, Hegbrandt J, Nilsson-Ehle P: Corticotropin-induced reduction of plasma lipoprotein(a) concentrations in healthy individuals and hemodialysis patients: Relation to apo(a) size polymorphism. *Metabolism* **48**:342, 1999.
559. Berg AL, Nilsson-Ehle P: ACTH lowers serum lipids in steroid-treated hyperlipemic patients with kidney disease. *Kidney Int* **50**:538, 1996.
560. Arnadottir M, Berg AL, Dallongeville J, Fruchart JC, Nilsson-Ehle P: Adrenocorticotrophic hormone lowers serum Lp(a) and LDL cholesterol concentrations in hemodialysis patients. *Kidney Int* **52**:1651, 1997.
561. Rader DJ, Brewer HBJr: Lipoprotein(a): Clinical approach to a unique atherogenic lipoprotein. *JAMA* **267**:1109, 1992.
562. Schenck I, Keller C, Hailer S, Wolfram G, Zöllner N: Reduction of Lp(a) by different methods of plasma exchange. *Klin Wochenschr* **66**:1197, 1988.
563. Utermann G: Genetic architecture and evolution of the lipoprotein(a) trait. *Curr Opin Lipid* **10**:133, 1999.
564. Eigner D, Schurz J, Jürgens G, Holasek A: Molecular parameters of Lp(a)-lipoprotein by light scattering. *FEBS Lett* **106**:165, 1979.

CHAPTER 117

Familial Lipoprotein Lipase Deficiency, Apo C-II Deficiency, and Hepatic Lipase Deficiency

John D. Brunzell ▪ Samir S. Deeb

1. Three inherited disorders have been described in which chylomicrons accumulate in plasma: familial lipoprotein lipase deficiency (MIM 238600), familial apolipoprotein C-II deficiency (MIM 207750), and familial inhibitor to lipoprotein lipase (MIM 118830). Chylomicronemia can also occur in individuals with common familial forms of hypertriglyceridemia who also have an acquired cause of hypertriglyceridemia such as untreated diabetes mellitus, estrogen or antihypertensive drug therapy, or alcohol use.

2. Familial lipoprotein lipase deficiency is a rare autosomal recessive disorder characterized by absence of LPL activity and a massive accumulation of chylomicrons in plasma and a corresponding increase of plasma triglyceride concentration. The concentration of VLDL may be fairly normal. The disease is usually detected in childhood based on repeated episodes of abdominal pain, recurrent attacks of pancreatitis, eruptive cutaneous xanthomatosis, and hepatosplenomegaly. The severity of symptoms is proportional to the degree of chylomicronemia, which, in turn, is dependent on dietary fat intake. Over 60 structural defects in the lipoprotein lipase gene have been demonstrated to cause deficiency of the activity of lipoprotein lipase. This lipolytic enzyme is present on vascular endothelial cells of extrahepatic tissues and is essential for hydrolysis of chylomicron and VLDL triglycerides to provide free fatty acids to tissues for energy. The enzyme is released into the blood by heparin and can be assayed in postheparin plasma or directly in biopsies of adipose tissue. Diagnosis is based on low or absent enzyme activity in an assay system that excludes other lipolytic enzymes and contains normal plasma or apoprotein C-II, a necessary cofactor of the enzyme; diagnosis is confirmed by demonstration of a defect in the structure of the lipoprotein lipase gene. The disorder is probably not associated with atherosclerotic vascular disease, but recurrent pancreatitis may threaten the patient's life. Restriction of dietary fat to 20 g/day or less is usually sufficient to reduce plasma triglyceride levels and keep the patient free of symptoms. Available lipid-lowering drugs are not effective. Heterozygotes exhibit a 50 percent decrease of lipoprotein lipase in postheparin plasma but have normal or only slightly abnormal plasma lipid levels.

3. Familial apolipoprotein C-II deficiency is a very rare autosomal recessive disorder in which apo C-II is absent, the clearance of chylomicrons from the blood is greatly impaired, and triglycerides accumulate in plasma. VLDL may also be elevated. The disorder is diagnosed in children or adults based on recurrent attacks of pancreatitis or by detection of milky fasting plasma on screening. Over 10 structural defects in the apolipoprotein C-II gene have been associated with absence of or production of defective apolipoprotein C-II, a cofactor for lipoprotein lipase. Absence of this protein creates a functional enzyme deficiency with accumulation of the substrate lipoproteins in the blood. The diagnosis is based on assay of lipoprotein lipase activity in postheparin plasma and on gel electrophoresis of VLDL apolipoproteins. Transfusion of normal plasma into the patient is followed by a dramatic fall in the plasma triglyceride level. Treatment involves use of a moderate fat-restricted diet throughout life. In the case of severe pancreatitis, transfusion of normal plasma may be helpful. Heterozygotes have a 50 percent reduction in apo C-II levels, but normal lipid levels.

4. Familial hepatic lipase deficiency (MIM 151670) is a rare autosomal recessive disorder characterized by moderate hypertriglyceridemia and premature coronary artery disease. Low-density and high-density lipoproteins are very triglyceride-rich with an accumulation of apo B containing lipoproteins that range from small, very low-density lipoproteins to buoyant LDL. These VLDL have β motility on agarose gel. Twelve individuals in six families have been reported with hepatic lipase deficiency; most have onset of clinical atherosclerosis in their forties and fifties. Treatment consists of diet and the use of lipid-lowering drugs. Heterozygotes and individuals with a fairly common promoter variant have reduced hepatic lipase activity. Men have higher hepatic lipase activity than women, particularly centrally obese men. High hepatic lipase activity is associated with accumulation of small dense LDL and decreases in HDL_2-C, changes that increase risk for early atherosclerosis.

A list of standard abbreviations is located immediately preceding the index in each volume. Additional abbreviations used in this chapter include: C/EBP = CAAT enhancer-binding protein; FCHL = familial combined hyperlipidemia; GP330/LRP-2 = lipoprotein receptor-related protein 2; HL = hepatic lipase; IDL = intermediate-density lipoprotein; *LIPC* = gene symbol for hepatic lipase; LPL = lipoprotein lipase; LRP = lipoprotein receptor-related protein; Oct-1 = octamer-binding transcription factor 1; OxLDL = oxidized LDL; PPARα and γ = peroxisome proliferator-activated receptors α and γ; SMC = smooth muscle cell; SREBP = sterol regulatory-binding protein; VLDLR = VLDL receptor.

HISTORICAL ASPECTS

Milky (lipemic) plasma was noted in 1799[1] and eruptive xanthomas were described as early as 1851.[2] The eruptive xanthomas were called "xanthomata diabeticorum" because of their occurrence in diabetic patients[3] with lipemic plasma. The lipemic serum that occasionally occurred in the untreated diabetic patient cleared with successful therapy of the hyperglycemia.[4] Now it is realized that the untreated diabetic state is accompanied by lipemic plasma, with signs and symptoms of the chylomicronemia syndrome only when an independent familial form of hypertriglyceridemia is also present.[5]

In 1921, patients were noted who had eruptive xanthomata who did not have diabetes,[6] and in 1932, the first patient with a familial form of chylomicronemia was described.[7] He was a young boy with extensive eruptive xanthomas, hepatosplenomegaly, and milky plasma. The lipemia and all symptoms cleared after switching to a fat-free diet. The familial nature of the disorder was suggested because the parents were cousins. These patients were included in a group with what was then entitled "idiopathic familial lipemia,"[8,9] later called "essential hyperlipidemia,"[10] "fat-induced lipemia,"[11] and, finally, "type I hyperlipoproteinemia."[12] In 1960, lipoprotein lipase deficiency[13] was noted as a cause of familial chylomicronemia in children with this syndrome, and in 1978, a patient with deficiency of apo C-II, which is required for activation of LPL, was reported as another cause of familial chylomicronemia.[14] In 1974, it was realized that more than one lipase activity is present in postheparin plasma with the separation of lipoprotein lipase and hepatic lipase activities.[15] The first patient with hepatic lipase deficiency was reported in 1982.[16]

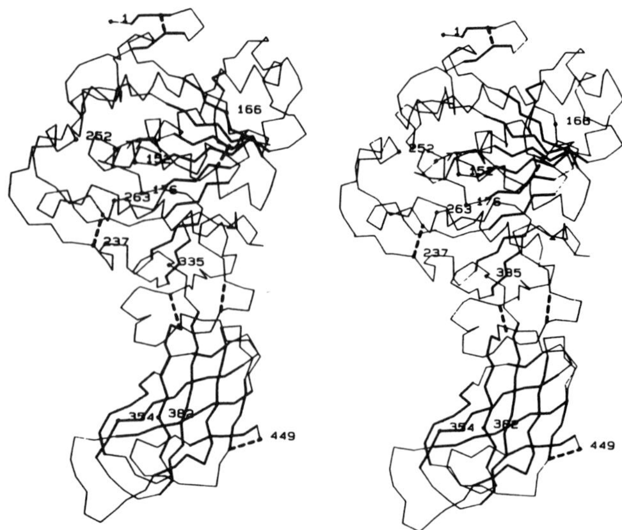

Fig. 117-1 Stereo view of the active site region of human pancreatic lipase. Alpha carbon traces of the segments forming the active site are drawn together with the side chains of the Asp 176-His 263-Ser 152 catalytic triad. The corresponding residues in human LPL are Asp 156, His 241, and Ser 132 for the triad. The segment between the disulfide-linked residues 237 to 261 (indicated by dotted lines) forms the flap over the active site. (*From Winkler et al.*[18] *Used with permission.*)

THE LIPASE FAMILY: EVOLUTION AND STRUCTURE FUNCTION RELATIONSHIPS

The vertebrate family of lipase genes includes lipoprotein lipase (LPL), hepatic lipase (HL), and pancreatic lipase (PL). These lipase genes have similar exon/intron boundaries, and the encoded proteins have significant amino acid sequence similarity, which led to the proposal that they have evolved from a common ancestral gene.[17] Based on these similarities, it is evident that PL diverged earlier than LPL and HL, which share a more recent ancestor. Interestingly, the sequence of LPL is the most highly conserved among mammalian species (2.0 percent difference between human and mouse vs 24 percent for HL and PL). The dipteran yolk proteins 1 to 3 also share limited homology with these lipases but lack enzymatic activity.

Examination of sequence homologies among the lipases revealed the presence of functionally and structurally important aspects. The Ser-Asp-His catalytic triad (Asp 176-His 263-Ser 152 in human PL) of the three vertebrate lipases is conserved in all species and is necessary for catalytic activity. Additional stretches of amino acid residues in these lipases are highly conserved, indicating that they form functionally important domains. The most highly conserved stretch is the nine-amino acid sequence of VHLLGYSLG, which surrounds the catalytic triad serine. Another completely conserved feature is the distribution of the eight cysteine residues in all members of the lipase family. Six of these eight residues are found in the very highly conserved central region of the lipase molecule, indicating that they form disulfide bridges critical for structure and function. The positions of two potential N-linked glycosylation sites are conserved in mammalian LPL and HL. LPL and HL bind to cell surface heparan sulfate proteoglycans. This feature has been ascribed to a conserved C-terminus segment with relatively high content of basic amino acids.

The three-dimensional structure of pancreatic lipase (Fig. 117-1), and the similar structure inferred for LPL and HL, reveals two major domains: a larger N-terminus domain linked by a short region to a C-terminus domain of approximately half its size.[18] HL/LPL chimeric proteins have been used to assign certain functions to the two major structural domains.[19–21] The results of these studies indicate that the globular N-terminus domain, which contains the catalytic triad, specifies the catalytic properties of the lipase, whereas the C-terminus domain specifies substrate specificity and heparin-binding properties.

One important structural domain present in both HL and LPL is the lipase lid or "flap," which is postulated to cover the active site and prevent access to the substrate. A conformational change that repositions the lid occurs before the lipases can bind substrate. There is limited amino acid sequence homology between the lids of HL, LPL, and pancreatic lipase. The lipase lid is essential for the hydrolysis of lipid substrates and plays a role in determining substrate preference. The lid of LPL favors hydrolysis of triglycerides, whereas that of HL favors hydrolysis of phospholipids.[22,23]

LPL, APO C-II, AND CHYLOMICRONEMIA—THE STRUCTURE AND FUNCTION OF LIPOPROTEIN LIPASE

Normal LPL Gene and Protein

Lipoprotein lipase (LPL) (GenBank cDNA M15856, M26380) is a glycoprotein located on the luminal surface of capillary endothelial cells. The active enzyme is a noncovalent homodimer.[24,25] The enzyme has an apparent monomeric molecular mass of 60 kDa on SDS-PAGE and between 41.7 kDa[26] and 48.4 kDa[24] by sedimentation equilibrium ultracentrifugation. The human LPL gene is approximately 30 kb in length and is located on chromosome 8p22.[27] This gene contains 10 exons[28–30] from which two messenger RNAs of about 3350 and 3750 nucleotides[31] are transcribed in human adipose tissue due to alternative sites of polyadenylation. The mRNA has a short 5′ untranslated region and a long (~1.5 kb) 3′ untranslated region. The cDNA for the human enzyme encodes a mature protein of 448 amino acids with a molecular mass of 50.4 kDa.[31] The cDNA for bovine mammary LPL predicts a protein of 450 amino acids and a molecular mass of 50.5 kDa.[32] Because bovine LPL is about 8 percent carbohydrate,[24] the molecular mass of the glycosylated monomeric subunit is approximately 54.5 kDa.

LPL mRNA has been found in human adipose tissue, and also in muscle, adrenal, kidney, intestine, and neonatal liver, but not in adult liver. The mRNA for LPL in humans is highly homologous with that of mice, rats, and cattle.[31,32] It also has 46 percent homology with the mRNA for hepatic triglyceride lipase (HL).

This homology between LPL and HL might represent similar catalytic, heparin-, and lipid-binding sites, while the apo C-II binding site of LPL might represent an area of difference. Studies of the molecular size of LPL and its mRNA in various tissues suggest that a similar or identical enzyme is present in adipose tissue, heart, skeletal muscle, lung, and lactating mammary gland.[33]

The production of LPL is highly regulated by transcriptional, postranscriptional, and postranslational mechanisms. Transcriptional regulation was shown to be responsible for changes in LPL production during differentiation of adipocytes, myocytes, and macrophages. Much of LPL regulation, being nutritional or hormonal, is thought to involve posttranscriptional and posttranslational mechanisms. In addition to mRNA stability, regulation could involve rates of translation as well as modification and secretion of the protein. Translational regulation often involves specific sequences in the untranslated regions (UTRs) of the mRNA. The 3′-UTR of LPL mRNA is approximately 2 kb in length and its sequence is approximately 75 percent homologous to that in bovine and mouse LPL mRNA. An interesting case of posttranscriptional regulation of LPL was recently described in which the nonrandom choice of polyadenylation signals in LPL mRNA was proposed to play a role in tissue-specific expression of the protein.[34] Human muscle contains predominantly the longer mRNA transcript, whereas adipose tissue contains the short and long transcripts. Further, it was shown that the longer transcript was translated more efficiently than the shorter one. The same group[35] recently showed that inhibition of LPL synthesis by epinephrine in 3T3-L1 adipocytes is mediated by a transacting factor (probably a protein) that binds to a specific segment of the 3′ untranslated region of LPL mRNA.

In studies of normal twins, a highly significant intrapair resemblance was noted for adipose tissue LPL activity in monozygotic male twins before and during short-term overfeeding.[36] In a comparison between monozygotic and dizygotic male twins, a high pairwise correlation for postheparin plasma hepatic lipase was found for monozygotic twins, but the intrapair correlation for postheparin plasma LPL in monozygotic twins was low.[37] The high degree of heritability for adipose tissue LPL, but not postheparin LPL, may reflect the multiple tissue sites that contribute to postheparin plasma LPL, several of which may be under opposite physiological regulation.[38,39]

Functional analysis of the human LPL promoter was made by transient transfection of the human monocytic leukemia cell line THP-1 (which can be differentiated into macrophage-like cells) and the murine skeletal muscle cell line C2C12.[40,41] Three motifs that interact with the transcription factors Oct 1, C/EBP, and Sp1, located within 100 bp upstream from the transcription start site, were shown to be critical for basal promoter activity (Fig. 117-2).

A silencer element (from -169 to -152) was implicated in suppression of LPL promoter activity in Hela and CHO cells (42). Two motifs, LP-α (between -702 and -666) and LP-β (between -468 and -430), which bind hepatic nuclear factor 3-like proteins, were suggested to contribute to differentiation-dependent promoter activity during adipogenesis of 3T3-f442A cells.[43] A nuclear factor 1-like binding site (between -517 and -491) was implicated in postnatal extinction of LPL expression in rat liver.[44]

Overexpression of a truncated (active) sterol regulatory element binding protein (SREBP)1a in transgenic mice resulted in a 25× induction of liver LPL mRNA,[45] suggesting a role of SREBP in inducing LPL gene transcription. In conjunction with this finding, the LPL promoter was shown to be synergistically transactivated by SREBP and the ubiquitous transcription factor shown Sp1 in transfection assays.[41] This observation points to a potential role of SREBP in coordinating regulation of cholesterol and triglyceride metabolic pathways. SREBP was also shown to play such a role by activating the LDL receptor, fatty acid synthase,[46] and acetyl coenzyme a carboxylase[47] genes in vitro and in transgenic mice overexpressing SREBP1c.[45]

The hypotriglyceridemic effects of fibrates and thiazolidinediones, which activate peroxisome proliferator-activated receptors α and γ (PPARα and γ), were shown to be at least partially due to activation of LPL gene transcription.[48] A PPAR-responsive *cis*-DNA element in the human LPL promoter (Fig. 117-2) was shown to mediate functional responsiveness to fibrates and thiazolidinediones. Whereas, fibrates exert their activation primarily in the liver via activation of PPARα, thiazolidinediones predominantly activate LPL in adipose tissue through PPARγ.

Functional Domains and Properties of LPL

Many functional domains for LPL have been postulated. The catalytic Ser 132 forms part of the catalytic triad with Asp 156 and

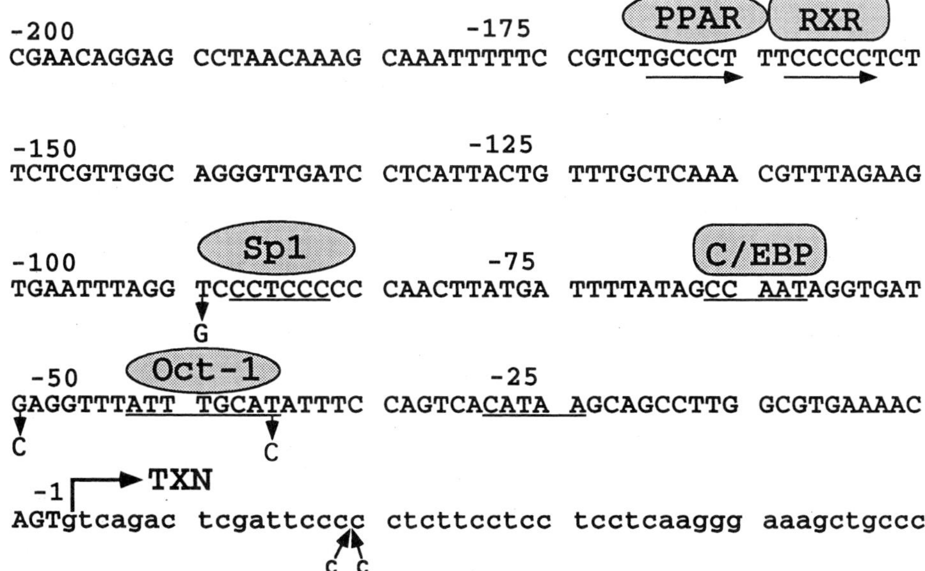

Fig. 117-2 Sequence of the human LPL gene promoter and location of naturally occurring mutations. Underlined are binding sites for the transcription factors shown above the sequences. Arrows indicate mutations. Letters in lowercase belong to exon 1.

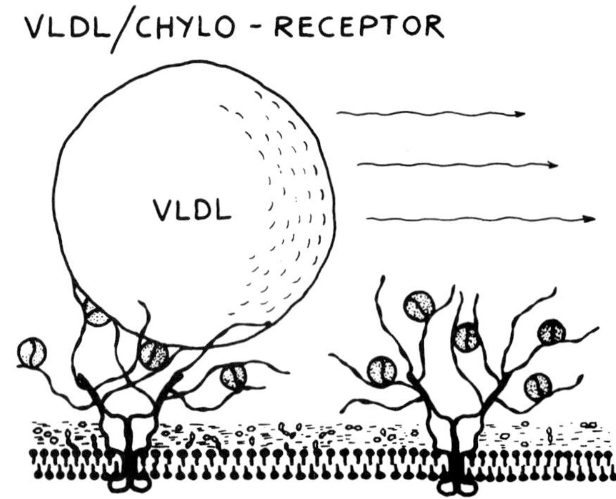

Fig. 117-3 Schematic of the action of LPL at the capillary endothelium. Heparan sulfate proteoglycans are intercalated onto the surface of the endothelial cell. LPL (small spheres) bound to heparan sulfate is extended into the lumen, where chylomicrons and VLDL can be bound. (*Modified from Olivecrona and Bengtsson-Olivecrona.*[96] *Used with permission.*)

His 241 of human LPL.[49–52] Ser 132 is located in one of two proposed lipid-binding domains, which extends from residue 126 to 135.[50,53,54] Alternatively, this domain may form part of the bottom of a hydrophobic channel, covered by a lid or flap, in which the substrate is inserted.[18,55] The other lipid-binding domain is proposed to involve residues 245 to 253.[17,54,56] The flap, with low homology between species, has been described[18] as extending from Cys 216 to Cys 239 (between which a disulfide bond exists) and plays an important role in substrate specificity. The heparin-binding site is an arginine-lysine-rich region in exon 6, particularly involving residues 292 to 304[49,50,57] and possibly residues 279 to 282. A domain that might bind free fatty acids has been suggested to involve residues 257 to 274, which is similar to a domain in intracellular fatty acid binding proteins.[29,56] A number of cysteine disulfide bonds appear to be important in the tertiary structure of LPL.[50,53] Asn 43 is an important site for N-linked glycosylation and enzyme activation.[50,56,58] The apo C-II binding site on LPL is confined to the C-terminal end of the protein.[19] A monoclonal antibody to bovine milk LPL has been developed[59] that binds to residues in the vicinity of amino acid 400 of human LPL[60] and totally inactivates the enzyme, without having an effect on hepatic lipase activity.

LPL binds to heparan sulfate[61–63] on the surface of endothelial cells via the heparin-binding site (Fig. 117-3), which allows the LPL molecule to be extended into the plasma.[64] By administration of intravenous heparin, LPL can be displaced from the endothelial surface into plasma where enzyme activity can be measured. The active enzyme bound to heparan sulfate on the capillary endothelium is predominantly in the dimeric form. The dimeric enzyme is less susceptible to degradation than the monomeric enzyme.[65] Apparently, the active monomeric enzyme is in equilibrium with the dimeric form,[25] with heparin[66] and heparan sulfate helping to maintain the enzyme as a dimer. The monomeric enzyme irreversibly loses activity and ultimately is degraded by the liver.[67,68]

Triglyceride and monoglyceride are preferred substrates for LPL, while lecithin is hydrolyzed at a slower rate. LPL preferentially hydrolyzes the 1- and 3-ester bonds in triglyceride, generating 2-monoglyceride, which is converted to 1-monoglyceride by isomerization for further hydrolysis.

Synthesis, Secretion, and Processing of LPL

LPL is synthesized in adipose tissue, cardiac and skeletal muscle cells, in monocyte-derived macrophages, and in Kupffer cells. LPL is secreted from the adipocyte and transported[69] in an unknown fashion to heparan sulfate on the luminal surface of the capillary endothelium.[67,70] The details of LPL synthesis and secretion (Fig. 117-4) have been demonstrated in studies of isolated and cultured adipocytes[71–73] and cultured heart cells.[74] An inactive proenzyme is synthesized in the ER and is transported to the Golgi apparatus. Glycosylation of LPL, which occurs in the endoplasmic reticulum, is critical for processing and secretion of an active enzyme.[75] Human LPL has two N-glycosylation sites: Asn 43 and Asn 359. Substitution of N43 by A completely abolishes activity[58] and results in accumulation of the inactive protein in the ER.[76] Secretory vesicles and the microtubular system are involved in the secretion of the active enzyme from the cell, a process that is enhanced by heparin in cultured cell systems. The active enzyme may also be degraded by lysosomes intracellularly. An inactive form of the enzyme, presumably one that has not undergone all steps of glycosylation, can also be secreted from the cell. Immunoreactive enzyme can be demonstrated in adipocytes, in connective tissue cells, and in endothelial cells of capillaries and larger vessels.[77]

The synthesis, processing, and secretion of LPL from various cell types seems to be under hormonal control.[71,73] In rats, feeding leads to a marked increase in LPL activity in adipose tissue and to a reciprocal decrease in activity in heart and skeletal muscle. Although addition of insulin to rat adipose tissue in vitro is associated with an increase in LPL activity,[71,73] the role of insulin as a primary regulator of LPL synthesis and secretion in vivo is not clear. In humans, adipose-tissue LPL activity does not vary much when meals of normal composition are consumed,[78] but when high carbohydrate meals are ingested, an increase in adipose LPL activity is seen after 3 to 6 h. A similar increase is seen when

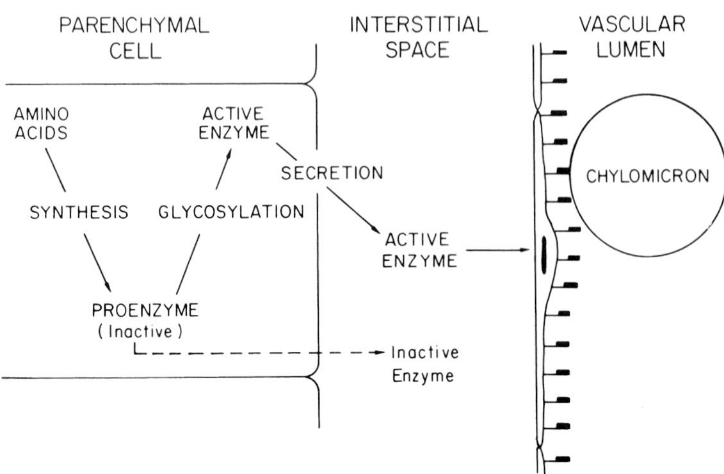

Fig. 117-4 Posttranslational processing and extracellular transit of LPL. LPL is synthesized in parenchymal cells in inactive form. Activation of the enzyme occurs in the Golgi apparatus. The active enzyme is released from the cell and bound to the endothelial cell surface. Inactive enzyme can also be released from the cell. (*From Garfinkel and Schotz.*[73] *Used with permission.*)

insulin and glucose are given intravenously to humans.[79–81] However, it has been difficult to demonstrate a primary regulatory role of insulin for adipose-tissue LPL in humans.[82] At a minimum, insulin may be permissive for the synthesis of LPL in many tissues, as might thyroxine and glucocorticoid hormones.[71] An alternative mechanism of feedback regulation of adipose and muscle LPL might be via the β-adrenergic system, which is activated with feeding. β-Adrenergic stimulation decreases LPL activity in adipose tissue[71,83] and increases LPL in muscle cells in culture.[74] A combination of the neuroadrenergic systems and the hypothalamic-adrenal axis might be important in central regulation of peripheral LPL.

Role of LPL in Lipoprotein Metabolism

LPL bound to the endothelial cell, in conjunction with apo C-II contained in chylomicrons and VLDL, is a major focal point in the processing of lipoproteins. Apo C-II is synthesized in the liver and secreted into plasma. Apo C-II recycles between HDL and the triglyceride-rich lipoproteins, chylomicrons, and VLDL.[84] Apo C-II is present in excess in plasma; it has been estimated that only 10 percent of normal values are needed for maximal LPL activity.[85] The hydrolysis of triglycerides in the core of these lipoproteins provides free fatty acids to be utilized as energy by muscle and other tissues or to be stored in adipose tissue. The enzyme seems to play a gatekeeper role for energy storage,[86] because fat-cell size is proportional to enzyme activity in adipose tissue.[78,87] With reduction of body fat content and fat-cell size by dieting, adipose-tissue LPL activity measured after an overnight fast is increased in males[88] but not in females.[87] However, in formerly obese women, adipose-tissue LPL is increased in the fed state.[89,90] An increase in LPL mRNA has been noted in formerly obese men and women.[91] This paradoxical increase in LPL activity in the reduced-obese state has been suggested to be a feedback mechanism for maintenance of body weight or fat-cell size.[88]

The role of LPL in clearing plasma triglyceride can be demonstrated in both fasted and fed states. The fractional clearance of triglyceride-rich lipoproteins from plasma is correlated with adipose tissue[92–94] and postheparin plasma LPL activity[93] in the fasting state. The decrease in plasma triglyceride levels following high-carbohydrate meals is correlated with a meal-induced increase in adipose-tissue LPL activity,[82,94] when one would expect adipose tissue to predominate. The amount of LPL available to hydrolysis of triglyceride seems to be limited, because triglyceride-rich lipoprotein removal is a kinetically saturable process.[95]

LPL activity increases markedly in the lactating mammary gland, presumably to allow for hydrolysis of plasma lipoprotein triglyceride for the formation of milk,[96,97] and is regulated by prolactin levels.[97] In response to endotoxin, macrophages in vitro secrete into the medium tumor necrosis factor, which, when added in culture, decreases LPL synthesis in adipose tissue.[75,98] The role this system has in regulating adipose tissue mass in animals and humans is not well understood.[99]

The lipoprotein core remnants remaining after hydrolysis of triglycerides in chylomicrons and VLDL are further processed in the liver (see Chap. 119). Chylomicron remnants are completely degraded, while some of the VLDL remnants are processed to form LDL particles. It has been suggested that some LPL may dissociate from the endothelium bound to the remnant lipoprotein.[100,101] This LPL-remnant complex can then be taken up by the putative remnant receptor,[101] perhaps with LPL as the ligand. It has also been suggested that hepatic lipoprotein uptake mediated by LPL modulates subsequent hepatocyte apo B secretion.[102]

A small portion of the core triglyceride from chylomicrons and VLDL can be transferred to the HDL. However, more important contributors to the formation of HDL are the surface remnants of the triglyceride-rich lipoproteins that are produced as a result of hydrolysis of core triglycerides. A relationship between LPL activity and HDL cholesterol concentration has been noted in many clinical situations by Nikkila and his coworkers.[103] The transfer of the lipoprotein surface containing unesterified cholesterol and phospholipid prolongs the residence time of these apo A-I- and A-II-containing particles, accentuating the increase in HDL cholesterol.[92,104] Thus, LPL functions at an important junction in lipoprotein metabolism, regulating the distribution of energy in the form of free fatty acids and the distribution of cholesterol to LDL and HDL.

Small amounts of LPL activity and protein are present in preheparin plasma. These preheparin activity levels are said to be proportional to the amount of LPL activity present in postheparin plasma,[105] although this remains controversial. The LPL in plasma is bound to circulating lipoproteins.[106–108] When in vitro triglyceride hydrolysis of the carrier lipoproteins occurring after the blood draw is blocked with an LPL inhibitor, the dimeric LPL is bound to VLDL both in preheparin and postheparin plasma.[108]

It is proposed that the triglyceride-rich lipoproteins leave the endothelial wall with an LPL dimer attached.[108] The very low levels in preheparin plasma suggest that this particle is rapidly removed, presumably by the liver. The 10^2- to 10^3-fold increase in activity and dimeric LPL in postheparin plasma[105] also bound to lipoproteins[108] reflects those lipoproteins presumably bound to LPL on the endothelium. In postheparin plasma only 1 to 5 percent of VLDL particles have LPL bound to them,[109] indicating a limited amount of endothelial LPL available for triglyceride hydrolysis.[95]

The early steps leading to atherosclerosis are not clearly understood. Williams and Tabas[110] have proposed that atherosclerotic plaques may originate by a mechanism they called "response-to-retention." They hypothesized that subendothelial retention of atherogenic lipoproteins is both necessary and sufficient to initiate lesion formation, while other factors such as dyslipidemia, smoking, increased endothelial permeability to lipoproteins due to injury[111] and blood flow turbulence play contributory roles (reviewed in reference 110). Indeed, many studies have shown that apo B-rich lipoproteins accumulate at "prelesional" atherosclerosis-susceptible sites. In vivo studies with cholesterol-fed rabbits have indicated that prefatty streak accumulation of atherogenic lipoproteins occurs preferentially at sites that are known to be prone to development of plaques, and that this accumulation is due to increased retention rather than increased permeability.[112,113] If this is the case, then lipid accumulation may depend on expression, at atherosclerosis-susceptible sites, of molecules that are responsible for intimal lipoprotein retention (reviewed in reference 110). In the absence of the protective effects of plasma antioxidants, retained lipoproteins may become oxidized and trigger an inflammatory response leading to plaque progression.[111]

A number of studies indicate that accumulation of atherogenic lipoproteins within the vessel wall involves cell surface and extracellular matrix components, primarily proteoglycans (reviewed in reference 114), as well as lipases, primarily LPL[114–118] (reviewed in reference 110), which act as "bridges" anchoring lipoprotein particles to proteoglycans. Increased retention of apo B-rich lipoproteins in the vessel wall appears to be related, in part, to the higher relative content of proteoglycans with longer glycosaminoglycan chains secreted by intimal smooth muscle cells.[119–121] LPL is present at very low concentrations in the normal vessel wall, but is abundant in human atherosclerotic lesions, being synthesized and secreted primarily by macrophages that are recruited in response to lipid retention and, subsequently, by macrophage foam cells of advanced lesions.[122–124]

LPL has been suggested to play a particularly important role in mediating retention of oxidatively modified LDL (OxLDL) on extracellular matrix.[125] Previous studies had shown that LPL increased the binding of LDL to matrix produced by cultured aortic endothelial cells.[126,127] More recently, it was shown that LPL is even more effective at binding OxLDL to endothelial cell matrix,[128] and that oxidized protein, rather than the oxidized lipid of OxLDL, mediates this binding. These in vitro results suggest that LPL-anchored arterial wall proteoglycans might be particularly effective in inducing retention of OxLDL in the artery wall. However, no in vivo studies have been done to test this hypothesis.

Role of LPL in Cellular Uptake of Plasma Lipoproteins

Insights have been obtained recently into the mechanisms by which LPL promotes cellular uptake of lipoprotein particles, thereby leading to foam cell formation from precursor macrophages and SMC. Mechanisms for lipid accumulation in these cells include endocytosis of intact VLDL or triglyceride-depleted VLDL produced by the action of LPL, and direct uptake of free fatty acids. LPL remodels both VLDL[129] and IDL-LDL to forms with increased rates of uptake by macrophages. Reduction in the triglyceride content of LDL particles appears to increase their affinity for the LDL receptor.[130] However, because LDL receptor density on the cell surface is down-regulated by cell cholesterol accumulation, other mechanisms must be invoked to account for the effect of LPL on increased uptake of plasma lipoproteins. One of these involves the observation by several groups that LPL can mediate receptor-independent uptake of the atherogenic apo B-containing lipoproteins, LDL and Lp(a).[102,131,132] LPL also has been shown to promote uptake of protein-free triglyceride emulsion particles by macrophages.[131] Schissel et al. have suggested that the catalytic activity of LPL may alter LDL particles to make them more susceptible to the action of arterial wall sphingomyelinases, which induce lipoprotein aggregation by producing ceramide from LDL-associated sphingomyelin.[133]

Additionally, LPL has been shown to markedly increase the affinity of apo E-containing lipoproteins, such as VLDL, for three cell-surface receptors that recognize apo E, the low-density lipoprotein receptor-related protein (LRP),[101] GP330/LRP-2,[134] and the recently cloned VLDL receptor (VLDLR).[135] The expression of LRP by cells of both normal and atherosclerotic vessels, including SMC and macrophages, was demonstrated recently by two groups.[136,137] Because SMC lack scavenger receptors and because LDL receptors are down-regulated by cell cholesterol accumulation, the LRP and receptor-independent pathways of lipoprotein uptake, both of which are enhanced by LPL, may be particularly important mechanisms for SMC foam cell formation. Further, while apo B-containing lipoproteins have long been known to accumulate in atherosclerotic plaques, VLDL remnants were recently detected in plaques,[138,139] thus making LRP, GP330/LRP-2, and VLDLR relevant pathways by which SMCs and macrophages could accumulate excessive cholesterol.

Finally, recent studies confirm the importance of LPL in VLDL particle uptake by cellular receptors.[128,140] In particular, these studies have identified tryptophan residues at positions 393 and 394 of the LPL molecule as being essential for binding to cellular receptors.[128] Further, site-directed mutagenesis of these tryptophan residues to alanines converted an LPL C-terminal fragment from a promoter to an inhibitor of VLDL binding to cellular receptors,[140] and a recent study has demonstrated that this LPL mutant can be expressed and secreted as a full-length, dimeric protein.[141] These observations raise the possibility that overexpression by macrophages in the artery wall of a mutant LPL protein containing alanines rather than tryptophans at residues 393 and 394 might inhibit both lipoprotein retention on extracellular matrix as well as LRP-, GP330/LRP-2-, and VLDLR-mediated lipoprotein uptake by cells.

LPL deficiency in the homozygous LPL gene knockout mouse is lethal.[142] However, this mouse can be rescued by tissue-specific expression of LPL in muscle[143] or the liver.[144] It has been proposed that the knockout mouse dies of hypoglycemia at birth and is rescued by hepatic free fatty acids in the hepatic transgenic and glucose intermediates in the muscle transgenic mouse.[144] It is of interest that adipose tissue accumulates in all of these animals, in the absence of adipose-tissue LPL, due to adipocyte lipogenesis.[145] Similar accumulations of adipose tissue with triglycerides enriched in nonessential fatty acids made from glucose occurs in humans with LPL deficiency.[146] This explains the normal amount and distribution of adipose tissue reported in these subjects.[147]

THE STRUCTURE AND FUNCTION OF APO C-II

Apo C-II is one of a family of apolipoproteins in which the gene has four exons and three introns.[148,149] The gene for apo C-II is on chromosome 19[150] and is closely linked to the genes for apo E and apo C-I. The similarity of gene structure for apo A-I, apo C-III, and apo A-IV, which are present on chromosome 11, with the apolipoprotein genes on chromosome 19 suggests a common ancestry for all of these apolipoproteins.[151] The human apo C-II gene spans 3.3 kb, divided into four exons,[152] while the mRNA deduced from complementary DNA is 494 nucleotides in length. Messenger RNA for apo C-II is found in the liver and intestine in human and nonhuman primates and is also found in HepG2 cells, a liver-cell line. Preproapo C-II contains 101 amino acids and undergoes intracellular removal of 22 amino acids, leaving the remaining 79-amino acid proapo C-II. The proapo C-II may undergo further posttranslational processing, deglycosylation, and further proteolysis to remove 6 amino acids to become the mature apo C-II of 73 amino acids.[153] Most apo C-II in plasma is 79 residues in length and contains no carbohydrate. Amino acids 56 to 79 may contain the lipoprotein lipase binding and activation domain, while amino acids 44 to 51 appear to contain the site for binding to VLDL and chylomicrons.[154] The apo C-II is present on HDL and is transferred to nascent chylomicrons and VLDL to act as an activator for lipoprotein lipase.[84] Apo C-III may cause abnormalities in LPL-mediated triglyceride hydrolysis through an indirect mechanism. Mice that overexpress apo C-III have defective apo E-mediated hepatic remnant lipoprotein removal, which leads to accumulation of remnant lipoproteins, which are poor LPL substrate.[155,156] Apolipoprotein A-IV has been implicated as a facilitator of transfer of apo C-II from HDL to the triglyceride-rich lipoproteins.[157]

CLINICAL MANIFESTATIONS OF THE CHYLOMICRONEMIA SYNDROME

The chylomicronemia syndrome can occur due to many different causes of marked hypertriglyceridemia. "Chylomicronemia" is defined as the presence in plasma of large lipoprotein particles that originate from dietary fat. Chylomicrons appear in the circulation shortly after the ingestion of meals containing fat. However, these particles are cleared rapidly from plasma and are not normally present after an overnight fast. In individuals with moderate hypertriglyceridemia, a postprandial state of 10 to 12 h is also long enough to clear chylomicrons from plasma. Moderately hypertriglyceridemic individuals without chylomicrons in the fasting state have been arbitrarily divided into subgroups type IIB and type IV hyperlipoproteinemia, depending on the presence or absence of elevated levels of LDL cholesterol.[158] Individuals with dysbetalipoproteinemia or type III hyperlipoproteinemia (Chap. 119) may not have chylomicrons in their plasma in the postabsorptive state; but do have detectable chylomicrons 10 to 12 h after their last meal. Subjects with fasting chylomicronemia have been arbitrarily divided into subgroups (types I and V hyperlipoproteinemia) depending on the level of VLDL;[158] however, this distinction appears to have had little clinical utility or genetic basis. A more helpful clinical measure is the absolute level of plasma triglyceride.

Although fasting chylomicronemia often occurs at plasma triglyceride levels between 1000 and 2000 mg/dl, the symptoms and signs associated with the chylomicronemia syndrome almost always occur at higher triglyceride levels. We define the chylomicronemia syndrome as the presence of one or more of a set of symptoms or signs occurring in a patient with a plasma triglyceride level of 2000 mg/dl or higher (Fig. 117-5).[159] For

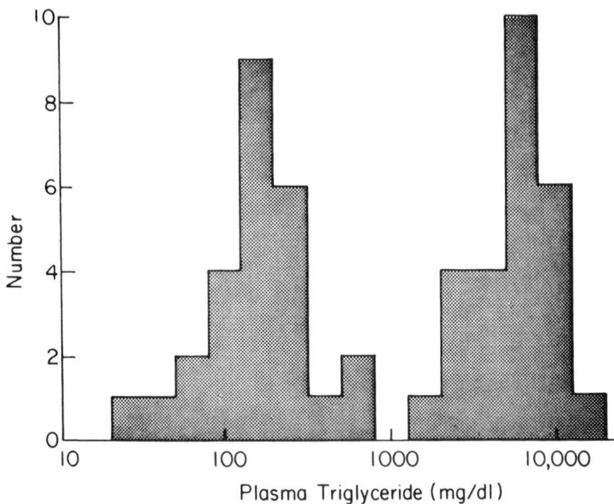

Fig. 117-5 Frequency distribution of plasma triglyceride levels in patients with possible pancreatitis at the University of Washington Hospital. Note bimodal distribution of triglyceride levels—the highest triglyceride level in the lower mode was 759 mg/dl and the lowest in higher mode was 1925 mg/dl. (*From Brunzell and Bierman.*[159] *Used with permission.*)

unexplained reasons, some individuals with massive hypertriglyceridemia, up to triglyceride levels of 29,000 mg/dl, have no symptoms or signs at all. More commonly, eruptive xanthomata, lipemia retinalis, and pancreatitis occur together.

For many years, the clinical sequelae of chylomicronemia have been known to occur in individuals with classic LPL deficiency.[12] The association of abdominal pain and pancreatitis with hypertriglyceridemia in other situations also has long been appreciated; however, it was once thought that the pancreatitis caused the hypertriglyceridemia. The opposite appears to be the case.[160–162] Marked hypertriglyceridemia has been reported in from 12 to 22 percent of patients admitted to a hospital for acute pancreatitis.[161–163] The pancreatitis is usually of acute onset and often is recurrent, occasionally leading to total pancreatic necrosis and death. Mild fat malabsorption can occur, but pancreatic calcification is unusual. The abdominal pain of the chylomicronemia syndrome is usually midepigastric and migrates through to the back, but it can also be present in the right or left upper abdominal quadrants, or even the midanterior chest. The pain can vary from a mild, bothersome ache to one that causes severe incapacitation. It has been difficult to determine whether the pain reported in the chylomicronemia syndrome always reflects classic pancreatitis, because both serum and urinary amylase levels are frequently normal. Indeed, amylase levels have been found to be normal in some patients with hemorrhagic pancreatitis documented at laparotomy.[160,161,164] However, many patients with particularly severe pancreatitis due to the chylomicronemia syndrome have elevated serum or urine amylase levels. Normal amylase levels in the presence of marked hypertriglyceridemia might be due to the interference of the plasma lipids with the assay[165] or to an inhibitor of the amylase assay present in the plasma and urine.[166,167] Recognition and treatment of the abdominal pain as part of the chylomicronemia syndrome in a patient with marked hypertriglyceridemia leads to reduced morbidity and mortality, if plasma triglyceride levels are maintained at levels somewhat lower than 2000 mg/dl.[160] The recognition of the etiology of the marked hypertriglyceridemia and the lack of recurrent pain with maintenance of low triglyceride levels has led to the conclusion that the pain is due to the chylomicronemia and that pancreatitis does not cause significant hypertriglyceridemia. Hepatomegaly is commonly found with chronic chylomicronemia,[12] as well as with many milder forms of hypertriglyceridemia. Splenomegaly is less commonly present, but the spleen can be remarkably hard. The enlarged spleen can return to normal size within 1 week of lowering of triglyceride levels in patients with LPL deficiency who are placed on a very-low-fat diet.

Eruptive xanthomas are deposits of lipid in the skin (Fig. 117-6) that result from the extravascular phagocytosis of chylomicrons by macrophages in the skin.[168] These lesions reflect chronic chylomicronemia. The xanthomas are localized over the buttocks, knees, and extensor surfaces of the arms, and may become generalized. They are small yellow papular cutaneous lesions. As a single lesion they may be several millimeters in diameter; when they coalesce, they may form plaques but retain their individual papular component. These lesions are usually not tender unless they occur at a site susceptible to repeated trauma. The xanthomas initially are composed of chylomicrons leading to triglyceride enrichment of lipid-laden foam cells.[168] With lowering of plasma triglyceride levels, the xanthomas clear over the course of weeks to several months. Recurrent or persistent eruptive xanthomas are indications of inadequate triglyceride-lowering therapy. As they regress, the triglyceride is mobilized, leaving transient, erythematous lesions that are rich in cholesteryl ester.

With triglyceride levels above 4000 mg/dl, "lipemia retinalis" can be detected by examination of the fundus of the eye. The retinal arterioles and venules, and often the fundus itself, develop a pale pink color. This change is due to the light scattering of the large chylomicrons and is reversible. Vision is not affected, and there appear to be no clinical sequelae of lipemia retinalis. Neuropsychiatric findings, including dementia, depression, and memory loss, have also been reported with chylomicronemia.[169]

Both objective and subjective dyspnea have been noted in patients with chylomicronemia,[169] and symptoms resolve with lowering of triglyceride levels. The observed relationship between hyperlipidemia and angina led to the hypothesis that hypertriglyceridemia might impair both oxygen uptake from the lungs and oxygen delivery to tissues.[170] Subsequent studies on oxygenation in hyperlipemia focused on the finding of arterial hypoxemia[171] and an increased affinity of hemoglobin for oxygen associated with normal 2,3-diphosphoglycerate (2,3-DPG) levels.[172] It now appears that these abnormalities were artifactual, related to the interference by lipemic plasma with the blood O_2 electrode[173] and with the measurement of hemoglobin levels.[174] Thus, the explanation for the dyspnea of the chylomicronemia remains unknown.

Other laboratory tests can also be misleading in the presence of marked hypertriglyceridemia. Chylomicrons may interfere directly with measurement of amylase and hemoglobin levels, as noted earlier. Bilirubin levels also are artifactually elevated in chylomicronemic plasma. Chylomicrons also replace water volume, which leads to artifactual decreases in plasma components by dilution.

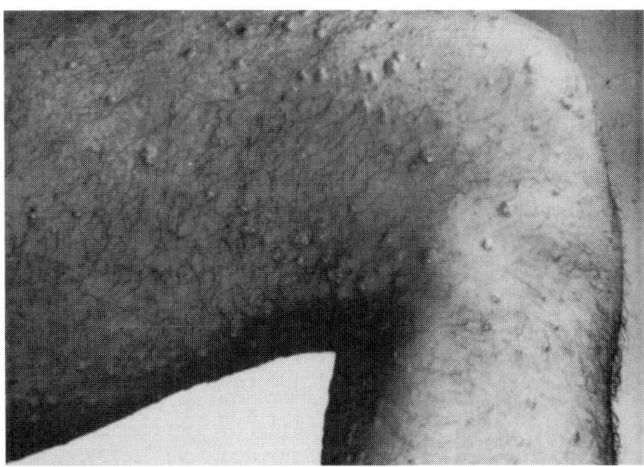

Fig. 117-6 Eruptive xanthomas of the skin in patients with chronic chylomicronemia. (*From Brunzell and Bierman.*[159] *Used with permission.*)

For example, serum sodium levels decreased between 2 and 4 mEq/liter for each 1000 mg/dl of plasma triglyceride.[175,176] Although hemolytic anemia has been reported with marked hypertriglyceridemia, this has not been confirmed when red blood cell life span was determined. Thus, a variety of clinical and biochemical findings have been reported with the chylomicronemia syndrome, although some are artifacts. The spectrum of acute and chronic symptoms and signs may be quite puzzling.

For clinical purposes, two practical approaches for the detection and evaluation of chylomicronemia can be used. First, the presence of chylomicrons in plasma after an overnight fast is usually related to the absolute plasma triglyceride level. Fasting plasma with triglyceride levels below 1000 mg/dl usually does not contain chylomicrons, whereas plasma with triglyceride concentrations above 1500 mg/dl almost always does contain them. Second, because the large fat particles scatter light and cause turbidity ("lactescence" or "lipemia"), visual inspection of serum or plasma can often lead to a fairly accurate estimation of plasma triglyceride levels in the presence of chylomicrons. Plasma with the appearance of 4 percent whole milk has a triglyceride level about equal to that of whole milk, that is, 4000 mg/dl; 2 percent milk, about 2500 mg/dl; 1 percent milk, about 1500 mg/dl; and nonfat skim milk, about 1000 mg/dl.

LIPOPROTEIN LIPASE DEFICIENCY

History

Burger and Grutz first described the clinical syndrome associated with lactescent plasma in childhood in 1932 in a young male offspring of a consanguineous marriage.[7] In 1960, Havel and Gordon[13] demonstrated defective clearance of triglyceride-rich lipoproteins in this disorder related to diminished lipolytic activity in plasma after intravenous heparin. Harlan et al.[177] found decreased LPL activity in adipose tissue to be associated with the decrease in postheparin plasma lipolytic activity in two patients. In 1974, Krauss et al.[15] separated the postheparin plasma activities into LPL and hepatic lipase and noticed very low levels of LPL with normal levels of hepatic lipase in this disease. Many of these patients have been noted to have a catalytically defective enzyme protein.[178] In 1989, the first of many lipoprotein lipase structural gene defects was described.[179]

Clinical Phenotype

Familial LPL deficiency is a rare disease,[180] estimated to occur about once per million population.[181] This rough estimate is based on the number of patients and families described, assuming that early, complete detection of patients with this defect is possible. The disease is usually manifested in childhood. Of 43 cases in one review,[182] 13 were detected in the first year of life, another 22 before the age of 10, and 8 at a later age. The age of detection may be related to the ability of the patient to avoid dietary fat intake.[181] Some adult patients present for the first time during pregnancy[183–186] or following a period of dietary excess. The disease has been described among Caucasians, Blacks, and Asians, and it affects both sexes equally.[182] The disease often presents in infancy with colicky pain, failure to thrive, and the other symptoms and signs of the chylomicronemia syndrome. At all ages, the most common clinical manifestation is episodic abdominal pain. The pain may be epigastric, with radiation to the back, or it may be diffuse, with the appearance of an emergent acute abdomen. This has often led to surgery where either no abnormality or pancreatitis was noted. Young patients learn to prevent the abdominal pain by avoiding foods with high fat contents. It is unusual for diabetes, steatorrhea, or pancreatic calcification to develop in these patients, even after recurrent bouts of acute pancreatitis until middle age. Hepatomegaly is very common in LPL deficiency, and splenomegaly is often present during periods when plasma triglyceride levels are markedly increased. The organomegaly occurs as a result of triglyceride uptake by macrophages, which become foam cells, and may rapidly regress with a decrease in dietary fat intake.

About half of the patients with LPL deficiency were noted to have eruptive xanthomas of the skin. These are the only xanthomas that occur in LPL deficiency. They are not specific for this disorder, but reflect the presence, or recent presence, of chylomicronemia. These xanthomas can appear rapidly with plasma triglyceride levels over 2000 mg/dl and can clear over several weeks after plasma triglyceride levels have been lowered. Patients with complete LPL deficiency do not seem to be predisposed to atherosclerosis although this was questioned recently.[187] In the past, many patients died of pancreatitis at an early age. With the recognition of the disease, the avoidance of unnecessary abdominal surgery, and the maintenance of a low-fat diet, these patients can lead a fairly normal life.

Mutant Gene and Genetics

The frequency of LPL deficiency is about one per million in the general population,[181] but is much higher in some areas of Quebec, Canada due to a founder effect.[188] Consanguinity is fairly common in LPL deficiency,[178,180,181] suggesting that the abnormal alleles for the defective LPL activity are rare. Multiple affected sibs, the lack of parent-to-child transmission, and equal involvement of both sexes are observations consistent with an autosomal recessive pattern of inheritance. There is 100 percent penetrance for the individual with mutations that abolish LPL activity.

The first structural defects in the LPL gene were reported in a young male who had neither LPL activity nor LPL immunoreactive mass in postheparin plasma.[179] He was found to be a compound heterozygote with two major gene arrangements: a 6-kb deletion involving exons 3 to 5 and a 2-kb gene duplication involving exon 6.[179,189] This patient, as might be expected, also had no detectable mRNA for LPL in adipose tissue.[189] Since that time, over 60 additional structural mutations in the LPL gene have been reported.[190,191] At least 28 missense mutations associated with markedly reduced or absent LPL activity have been described (Fig. 117-7). Five single base-pair substitutions

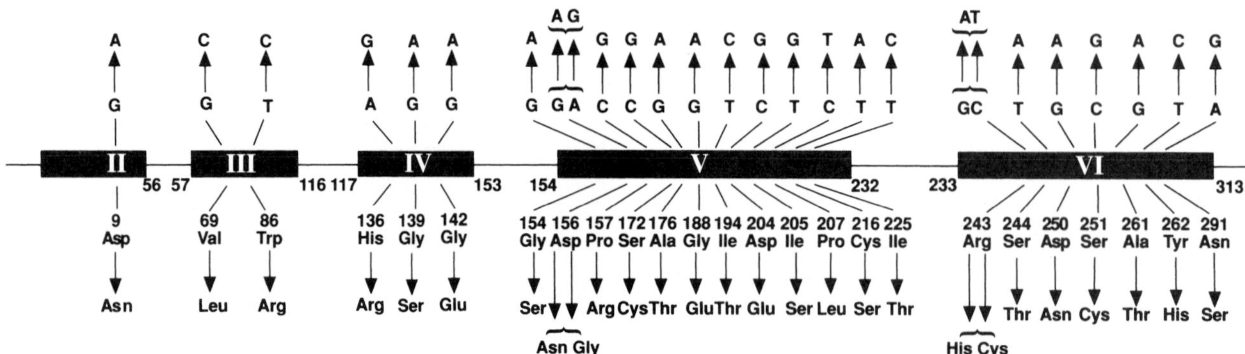

Fig. 117-7 Location of known missense mutations in the human LPL gene. Only 5 of 10 exons are shown. Both the nucleotide substitutions and the amino acid changes are shown.

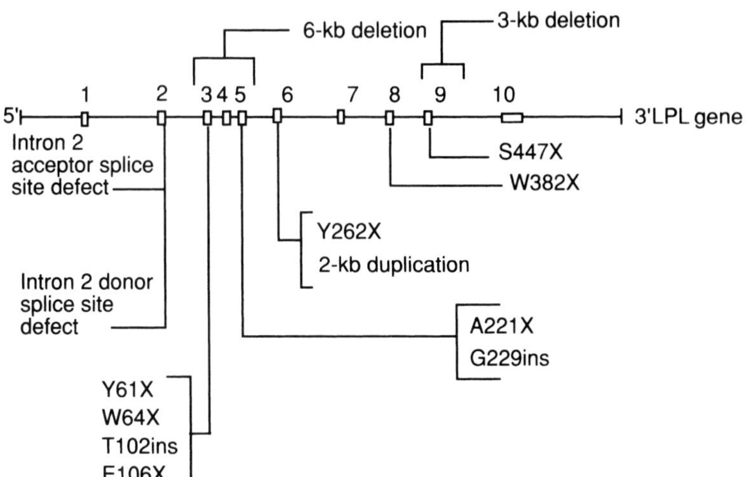

Fig. 117-8 Location of known nonsense, insertion, deletion, and splice-site mutations in the human LPL gene. (Modified from Santamarina-Fojo,[251] by permission of *Current Opinion in Lipidology*.)

causing stop codons have been noted (Fig. 117-8). One involves residue 447 and may be associated with elevated LPL activity (192). In addition to the original patient with two major gene rearrangements, a 3-kb deletion involving exon 9 and four smaller insertion-deletion defects have been noted (Fig. 117-8). Finally, an acceptor splice-site defect and a donor splice-site defect, both involving intron 2, have been reported. To date, very few LPL mutant alleles from patients with classic lipoprotein deficiency remain uncharacterized. This suggests that regulatory abnormalities do not lead commonly to LPL deficiency or that the phenotype associated with potential regulatory abnormalities is milder than that of classic LPL deficiency.

The insertion-deletion mutations, the splice-site defects, and the nonsense mutations presumably lead to absent or truncated LPL protein with defective catalytic activity. Insights into how the mutations with single amino acid substitutions cause deficiency of LPL activity were deduced with the aid of the tertiary structure of pancreatic lipase as a model[18] (see Fig. 117-1). A number of the LPL missense mutations have been examined.[193] Most of the mutations are in the highly conserved central homology region,[53] involving LPL exons 4, 5, and 6. The two mutations at residue 156 involve aspartic acid of the catalytic triad. Many of the mutations change hydrophobic residues to ones that are less so, particularly those involving residues 142, 157, 176, 188, 194, 205, and 225. Some are part of beta-sheet strands (residues 154, 204, 205, and 207) and some involve alpha-helical structures (residues 136, 139, 142, 243, 244, 250, and 251). It would seem likely that milder forms of hypertriglyceridemia will be found to be associated with as-yet-undetected defects in the LPL gene.

Reymer et al.[194] reported an association of the common LPL mutation N291S with reduced levels of HDL cholesterol in male coronary artery disease patients as well as controls, and with reduced HDL and elevated triglyceride levels in male familial combined hyperlipidemia (FCHL) patients. This mutation, which reduces LPL activity by approximately 40 percent,[195] was found at a frequency of 11.8 percent in 169 male FCHL patients and in 4.6 percent among 215 male controls in a Dutch population. It was also reported that familial hypercholesterolemia heterozygotes (FH) who were also heterozygous carriers of the N291S mutation, had significantly higher triglycerides and lower HDL-C levels and a higher ratio of total to HDL-cholesterol, when compared to FH heterozygotes who did not carry this mutation.[196] However, a meta-analysis of studies of the N291S variant did not reveal an association with coronary artery disease.[197]

On the other hand, the relatively common S447X variant was shown to be associated with increased HDL-C levels. In a study of healthy men with lower-, middle-, and upper-decile concentrations of plasma HDL-C, the stop allele was significantly more represented in the high HDL-C group.[198] The mechanism by which this variant may affect HDL-C levels is unknown. Results of in vitro analyses as to the functional consequences of the S447X truncation indicated no effect on activity or stability,[198] moderate decrease in specific activity,[199] and increased activity.[200] The effect of the S447X variant on LPL activity and HDL-C levels was investigated in coronary artery disease patients. Carriers of the S447X allele had higher postheparin plasma LPL activity HDL-C and triglyceride concentrations than noncarriers.[201] Interestingly, the effect on LPL was confined to those patients using β-blockers. This finding is consistent with the in vitro observation that the truncated enzyme has higher activity. The possibility that the S447X mutation may be in linkage disequilibrium with other substitutions at the LPL gene locus that causes the associated lipid and lipoprotein phenotypes has not been formally excluded. This variant appears to be associated with a decrease in coronary disease.[197]

In addition to the structural mutations, regulatory variants of the LPL promoter were identified (Fig. 117-2). The T→C substitution at position −39, which lies within the critical Oct-1 binding site, results in loss of approximately 85 percent of promoter activity.[202] The G→C substitution at position −53 leads to a reduction of approximately 70 to 75 percent of promoter activity. This nucleotide does not seem to lie within any known transcription factor-binding site, but may influence binding of either Oct-1 or C/EBP. The −93G promoter allele (frequency of 0.008 among Caucasians, $N = 183$) was shown to have approximately 40 percent reduction in activity in vitro[40] and a similar reduction in affinity to the transcription factor Spl, which binds to the functionally important and conserved CT box (5′-CCTCCCCCC-3′, nucleotides −91 to −83) in the LPL promoter[41] (Fig. 117-2). This mutation was found to be quite prevalent among unselected population samples of African Americans ($N = 96$) and Africans (Gambians, $N = 39$), with allele frequencies of 0.32 and 0.41, respectively.[202] The T-93G and a relatively common D9N substitution are in almost complete linkage disequilibrium among Caucasians but not Africans.[202,203] These two substitutions were not observed among 130 Chinese.[203] The D9N substitution has very little, if any, effect on catalytic activity of LPL.[204]

Kastelein et al.[205] reported that healthy normolipidemic Caucasians who carry the −93G/9N haplotype had higher plasma total cholesterol, lower mean HDL-C, lower LPL activity, and tended to have higher TG levels. Moreover, this haplotype appears to be associated with an increased risk for coronary artery disease.[197,205] In a study of South African Blacks, who, in general, have lower cholesterol and TG levels than Caucasians, Ehrenberg et al.[203] observed a marginally significant association of the −93G allele with a mild decrease in TG levels. Furthermore, there was no significant association between the 9N allele (independently of the −93G allele) and TG levels in this population. More studies are needed to assess the influence of the T-93G substitution on plasma lipids and coronary artery disease. It would be interesting to investigate whether this mutation exacerbates the effects of other genetic or environmental risk factors for dyslipidemia.

Pathophysiology

Several hundred patients with a familial abnormality in LPL activity have been described. A familial syndrome of chylomicronemia can characterize most of these patients, with clinical onset in childhood. Variations of this syndrome with autosomal dominant inheritance have been reported.[206] The lactescent or lipemic plasma seen in LPL deficiency is due to the accumulation of dietary fat in plasma as triglyceride-rich chylomicrons. The severity of the hypertriglyceridemia is related to the amount of ingested long-chain fatty acids—thus the term fat-induced or exogenous hypertriglyceridemia.[11] Although it is difficult to separate endogenous, triglyceride-rich VLDL from chylomicrons (particularly when the latter are markedly elevated), VLDL are usually not very elevated in children and young adults with LPL deficiency. However, compelling data exist that indicate that VLDL triglyceride is nonetheless catabolized abnormally in LPL deficiency,[207] and, therefore, factors in addition to LPL deficiency must exist for the presence (phenotype V) or absence (phenotype I) of VLDL. Low-density and high-density lipoproteins have altered composition and are decreased in amount in either case.[180] Of note, one subject with LPL deficiency who also was heterozygous for familial hypercholesterolemia had no low-density lipoproteins due to the block in VLDL catabolism.[208]

LPL activity in plasma is low or absent in these patients with LPL deficiency following a bolus of heparin[15,181] and is not responsive to higher doses or prolonged infusions of heparin.[209] In contrast, postheparin plasma HL activity is present in low or normal amounts.[15,181] Adipose-tissue LPL activity is very low[177] or undetectable.[209] LPL activity also was not detected in cultured monocyte-derived macrophages from subjects with the classic form of LPL deficiency.[210,211] Thus, the patient with LPL deficiency presents in childhood with chylomicronemia, has very low to absent levels of LPL activity in all tissues, and has normal HL activity. While LPL immunoreactivity was not detected in the plasma of the patient without detectable gene transcription due to two major gene rearrangements,[179,189] plasma LPL mass appears in many patients following the intravenous administration of heparin[59,178,212] as detected by ELISA. The Ile-to-Thr missense mutation at position 194 (I194T) is associated with high levels of postheparin plasma LPL mass.[213,214] This catalytically defective protein has normal affinity for heparin-Sepharose and appears to be relatively stable.[215] In contrast, the defective protein seen with the A176T[216] and G188E[217] mutations is associated with a mild decrease in heparin affinity. It appears that this change in affinity is secondary to the structural instability of the A176T and G188E mutations.[215] When evaluating the mutated LPL protein, the care taken in processing the protein for study may be critical in understanding why the protein is defective.

Variant Phenotypes. A significant number of patients have been reported with LPL deficiency in which LPL-like immunoreactivity is present in preheparin plasma.[211,212] Whether this is intact LPL protein, LPL peptide fragments, or some other epitope is not known. One LPL-deficient patient has been described in whom no LPL activity was seen in postheparin plasma, while abundant LPL activity was present intracellularly in adipose tissue.[218] This patient may be similar to the patient who was homozygous for a missense mutation involving N43S, the N linked glycosylation site.[197] This patient apparently can synthesize active LPL but cannot secrete and transport the enzyme to the vascular endothelium. The molecular defect in this patient is unknown. In addition to the individuals with the classic forms of LPL deficiency, there are unusual patients with unique variations in the syndrome (reviewed in reference 206). Several patients have been noted who may have an abnormality in the enzyme in one tissue but normal activity in other tissues.[209,219] The molecular basis of these abnormalities is unknown. Very low levels of LPL activity in postheparin plasma were found in a 9-year-old boy several weeks after he recovered from an episode of pancreatitis associated with lactescent plasma.[220] Following institution of moderately severe dietary fat restriction, his LPL activity and plasma triglyceride returned to normal. One patient was noted to have very low levels of postheparin lipolytic activity after moderate doses of intravenous heparin, but normal lipolytic activity after high doses of heparin,[221] which suggests a state of heparin resistance. Several patients were reported to have absence of LPL activity in postheparin plasma, with reappearance of LPL after ingestion of omega-3 fatty acids.[222] One of these patients was found not to have a mutation in the LPL gene and was felt to have a posttranslational defect in LPL.[222]

The Defective LPL Heterozygote State

The obligate heterozygote parents and other family members of LPL-deficient patients have been noted to have normal LPL activity[223,224] or decreased LPL activity[59,225,226] in postheparin plasma. With the development of an ELISA to measure LPL immunoreactivity in plasma, it has been possible to demonstrate that the postheparin plasma activity and mass in heterozygotes is intermediate between those of normal controls and LPL-deficient probands.[59] Mild hyperlipidemia and variable lipid phenotype, predominantly an increase in triglyceride and a decrease in HDL cholesterol, have been observed in the parents and relatives in some families of probands with LPL deficiency,[59,178,223–225,227–231] while the families of other probands are normolipidemic.[178,223,224,226] It appears that abnormalities exist across the lipoprotein density spectrum, with an increase in VLDL and small, dense LDL on some occasions manifested as an increase in triglyceride and an increase in IDL,[228,231,232] and small, dense LDL[231,233] on other occasions manifested as an increase in cholesterol. Thus, this increase in LDL is not typical, buoyant LDL, but a variable combination of IDL and small, dense LDL[228,231,232] measured in the usual total LDL density fraction. Similar mild lipoprotein abnormalities were noted in a large Utah kindred to be due to an interaction at the single defective LPL allele with environmental or other familial factors.[234] In this large pedigree, the LPL heterozygous genotype appeared to segregate independently from a gene for hypertriglyceridemia. Recently, it was demonstrated that LDL size is linked to the LPL gene in families with known defects in the LPL gene.[233]

More severe hypertriglyceridemia can occur when other known genetic defects occur in addition to the heterozygous LPL state. Although the N291S LPL gene variant does not seem to have much effect on lipids or risk for coronary disease in the general population, it may allow for expression of marked hypertriglyceridemia in association with other genetic defects. It may contribute to hyperlipidemia in the presence of an apo E-2 allele,[235] in diabetes,[236] in familial combined hyperlipidemia,[237,238] and in hepatic lipase deficiency (Table 117-1, patient Seattle #1). We also have noted excessive hypertriglyceridemia in a young male with glycogen storage disease type Ib, who had decreased LPL activity and one N291S allele.[239] It is possible that the effect of the N291S is only a reflection of the relatively high frequency of this allele in the population in the reports of the unusual disorders noted above.

Some mutations in the LPL gene may cause mild dyslipidemia in the heterozygous state,[59,234] and contribute to common familial forms of dyslipidemia. In a group of 56 patients with FCHL, 20 had a 50 percent reduction in postheparin plasma LPL activity.[240] None of these 20 patients had LPL mutations that are found in individuals homozygous for total LPL deficiency.[241] Others also have found structural mutations in the LPL gene to be uncommon in FCHL.[242,243] Three promoter-variant alleles (base substitutions at nucleotides -39, -53 and -93) were found in 3 of 20 FCHL patients who had reduced plasma LPL activity[40,202] (Fig. 117-2). These variants significantly reduced promoter activity in transient

Table 117-1 Hepatic Lipase-Deficient Patients

Source		Gender	Genotype	Reference	Atherosclerosis
Ontario	1	M	T383M/S267F	359	MI late 40s
	2	M	T383M/S267F		CABG 53
	3	M	T383M/S267F		CABG 57
Stockholm	1	M		324, 331	None age 63
	2	M			
Seattle	1	M	Intron 1 acceptor splice-site mutation —homoz.	232, 323, 328	MI age 41
Quebec	1	F	T383M/not found	322	None age 32
	2	M	T383M/not found		None age 25
	3	M	T383M/not found		None age 24
Providence	1	M		360	MI age 45
	2	M			Long hx angina CABG age 75
Seattle	2	M	G225R/not found	*	MI age 37
	3	M	Deletion exon 1 and promoter, homoz.	*	MI age 42

*Not previously reported

transfection assays in THP-1 and C2C12 cells. In contrast, only one promoter variant, which had little affect on promoter function, was identified among the 20 FCHL patients who had normal LPL levels.[241] Furthermore, the variants with base substitution at nucleotides -39 and -53 were not found among either 115 patients with coronary artery disease or among 183 control subjects.[40] Taken together, these results strongly suggest that LPL promoter mutations are not rare and may contribute to the etiology of FCHL, at least in the subset of patients who have reduced postheparin plasma LPL activity. LPL regulatory sequence variants might be one of the factors that contribute to the development of FCHL and atherosclerosis.

It has been suggested that apo A-IV plays a role in modulating the activation of lipoprotein lipase (LPL) by apo C-II.[157] Therefore, the role of genetic variation at the apolipoprotein A-IV locus in a subset of FCHL patients with half the level of plasma LPL activity was investigated. Two of 20 such patients were found to be heterozygous carriers of previously undescribed amino acid substitutions: S158L and R244Q substitutions.[244] These substitutions were not detected among 20 other FCHL patients with normal LPL levels and among 97 unselected medical students. The finding of these two alleles among only the 20 patients with FCHL with reduced levels of LPL suggests an association with this phenotype. It is hypothesized that these two alleles may contribute, along with alleles of other genes or environmental factors, to the development of dyslipoproteinemia.

Thus, in FCHL, mutations in the LPL gene contribute to the lipoprotein phenotype. Gene-gene and gene-environment interactions need to be considered in attempting to explain heterogeneity in lipoprotein phenotypes associated with common and complex diseases. Foreknowledge of these interactions that may predispose to dyslipoproteinemia in patients would form the basis for early detection (in the case of first-degree relatives) and for the design of a treatment regimen.

Diagnosis and Treatment

Familial LPL deficiency should be considered in anyone with the chylomicronemia syndrome. The absence of secondary causes of hypertriglyceridemia (diabetes, alcohol, estrogen, glucocorticoid, Zoloft, or isotretinoin therapy, certain antihypertensive agents, and paraproteinemic disorders) increases the possibility of LPL deficiency. A presumptive diagnosis can be made if a marked decrease in plasma triglyceride occurs after a week on a severely restricted low-fat diet. In this instance, apo C-II deficiency also has to be considered.

The clinical diagnosis of LPL deficiency requires the specific assay of LPL activity in postheparin plasma or adipose tissue.[245,246] Because it contains no HL activity as seen in plasma, measurement of adipose tissue enzyme has an advantage over postheparin plasma. Plasma LPL activity obtained 10 to 15 min after the intravenous injection of heparin (60 to 100 units/kg body weight) is stable if immediately refrigerated and quickly frozen. LPL activity has to be differentiated from the HL activity because both are released simultaneously with heparin. These enzymatic activities can be separated in several ways. Specific antibodies to the enzyme can remove HL; the residual activity is LPL. Alternatively, the activity removed as LPL can be estimated: (a) an antibody to LPL can be added; (b) protamine sulfate, which inhibits LPL, can be included; or (c) the assay can be performed with high ionic strength to inhibit LPL activity.

A more laborious, but precise, technique involves the separation of postheparin plasma HL and LPL by heparin-Sepharose chromatography.[246] Once decreased LPL activity is demonstrated, one has to distinguish between absent catalytic activity due to an enzyme defect, and absent apo C-II activating capacity. The diagnosis of LPL deficiency is often confirmed by the demonstration of structural defects in the LPL gene.

Treatment of familial LPL deficiency is predominantly by dietary fat restriction. The aim of therapy is to reduce the chylomicronemia to a level associated with clearance of symptoms and signs of the chylomicronemia syndrome. Success depends on the patient's acceptance of a diet, often extremely low in both animal and vegetable fats. It is critical for the patient and his or her family to realize that unsaturated, as well as saturated, fat must be restricted. Often dietary restriction of fat to 15 percent of calories is adequate for control of symptoms, usually to plasma triglyceride levels consistently below 1000 to 2000 mg/dl. Medium-chain triglycerides can be used for cooking, because they are absorbed into the portal vein without becoming incorporated into chylomicron triglyceride. Additional measures in the prevention of excessive hypertriglyceridemia are avoidance of agents known to increase endogenous triglyceride levels, such as alcohol, estrogens, diuretics, isotretinoin, Zoloft and β-adrenergic blocking agents. During pregnancy, extreme dietary fat restriction with close monitoring of triglyceride levels has resulted in normal term delivery.[129–132] We have restricted dietary intake to less than 2 g per day during the second and third trimester in one patient. The infant was normal and had normal levels of essential fatty acids in plasma. When VLDL levels are increased in a patient with LPL deficiency, such as might occur in adults, fibric acid derivatives may lower triglyceride levels slightly, especially when the patient is on a low-fat, high-carbohydrate diet.[247] One unique patient who had LPL deficiency in the absence of a molecular defect in the LPL gene responded to ingestion of omega-3 fatty acids in fish oil.[222]

Investigations are underway aimed at determining the feasibility of gene-replacement therapy for LPL deficiency. In one study, ectopic liver expression of human LPL was achieved through infusion of a replication-deficient adenovirus vector expressing human LPL into mice heterozygous for targeted inactivation of the LPL gene.[248] Human LPL was detected in both liver and postheparin plasma and caused a significant reduction in plasma VLDL triglycerides, which persisted for approximately 42 days. Furthermore, administration of the recombinant adenovirus-LPL resulted in correction of the impaired tolerance to fat feeding exhibited by the heterozygous LPL-deficient mice. In another study, a recombinant adenovirus vector expressing human LPL under the control of the cytomegalovirus promoter was infused into either apo E $-/-$ or LDL receptor $-/-$ mice.[249] The high level of expression of human LPL in liver postheparin plasma of these mice caused marked reduction in VLDL/chylomicron remnant cholesterol and triglycerides. The results of these studies are encouraging in that liver-targeted LPL cDNA expression may be an effective method of correcting the lipoprotein abnormalities in LPL deficient patients.

APOLIPOPROTEIN C-II DEFICIENCY

History

In 1978, Breckenridge et al.[14] reported a 59-year-old male with gross hypertriglyceridemia and absent postheparin lipolytic activity. He had recurrent abdominal pain since the age of 18, and diabetes mellitus and steatorrhea developed. Despite insulin therapy, he remained markedly hypertriglyceridemic. On a low-fat diet, his triglyceride levels dropped from about 4000 to below 1000 mg/dl. Following a transfusion for anemia he had a marked decrease in triglyceride levels into the normal range, suggesting that a plasma component for which he was deficient was supplied by the transfusion. Breckenridge et al. demonstrated that the patient was deficient in apo C-II, and that the addition of apo C-II to his plasma corrected his postheparin lipolytic activity. Other individuals in his family have been found to have apo C-II deficiency. The relatives heterozygous for the defect have half the normal levels of apo C-II in plasma, establishing the familial nature of this disorder.

Clinical Phenotype

Because apo C-II deficiency results in the functional deficiency of LPL, it is not surprising that the clinical manifestations are similar to those in primary LPL deficiency. However, some interesting differences have been found between apo C-II deficiency and the classic form of LPL deficiency. As compared with the patients with familial LPL deficiency, the homozygous apo C-II-deficient subject generally has been detected at a later age, ranging from 13 to 60 years of age. Even so, the symptoms often can be traced back to earlier childhood or adolescence.

The predominant symptom reported in apo C-II-deficient patients is recurrent abdominal pain, apparently caused by repeated attacks of pancreatitis. The prevalence of pancreatitis in the Toronto kindred was found to be 64 percent among 14 affected patients, which is higher than that reported for the pancreatitis in familial LPL deficiency.[14,250] It is possible that patients with LPL deficiency learn to avoid dietary fat early in life, while those with apo C-II deficiency, even as adults, consume more dietary fat and subsequently suffer more frequent episodes of pancreatitis. The index patient in the Toronto family had repeated attacks of pancreatitis, which resulted in chronic pancreatic insufficiency with steatorrhea and insulin-dependent diabetes. It has been suggested that the apo C-II-deficient patients do not have eruptive xanthomas or hepatosplenomegaly as often as those with LPL deficiency. As in LPL deficiency, there is little evidence for premature atherosclerosis in individuals with apo C-II deficiency.

The delay in onset of symptoms and the higher dietary fat tolerance in apo C-II deficiency might be related to a less severe defect in the clearance of chylomicrons and VLDL, because some residual LPL activity might exist. The homozygous apo C-II-deficient patients may have markedly elevated fasting plasma triglyceride levels ranging from 500 to 10,000 mg/dl. Most of this triglyceride is in the form of chylomicrons, but there is also an increase in VLDL triglyceride. The VLDL cholesterol levels are elevated above the normal range, while the levels of LDL and HDL are very low, similar to that seen in familial LPL deficiency. Immunoassays have revealed low plasma levels of A-I, A-II, and B, and high concentrations of apo C-III and E in these patients. Activation of LPL in the homozygote by the intravenous infusion of plasma rapidly reduces the concentrations of chylomicrons and VLDL. These changes were associated with reciprocal increases in LDL, HDL, and the plasma levels of apo A-I and apo B.

Mutant Gene and Genetics

Apo C-II deficiency is inherited as an autosomal recessive disorder. The gene structure is known (GenBank cDNA J02698; gDNA X05151). The disorder appears to be less common than LPL deficiency. Consanguinity is common among patients, who to date were reported to be homozygotes. Families have been reported from a worldwide distribution.

At least 14 kindreds with apo C-II deficiency have been described.[206] In many, a structural defect in the apo C-II gene was described.[251] Four kindreds have single base substitution mutations leading to stop codons (Fig. 117-9), while one patient has a single base substitution in the initiation methionine codon. One patient has been found to have a donor splice-site mutation in intron 2. All these patients have markedly reduced to absent apo C-II, as determined by immunoblotting or immunoassay.

Four frameshift mutations secondary to a single base deletion or insertion have been described (reviewed in reference 190) (Fig. 117-9). Three presumably lead to stop codons and truncated proteins; one seems to lead to an extension of the defective protein to 96 residues. Two involving Val 18 and Gln 2 have no detectable plasma apo C-II, while normal amounts of defective apo C-II are present in the plasma in the patients with longer apo C-II. The Japanese and Venezuelan kindreds have additional, but different, structural changes in their apo C-II genes.[252]

Individuals heterozygous for a defective apo C-II allele have normal plasma lipid levels.[14,253] Thus, it appears that apo C-II in plasma is not rate limiting for the clearance of chylomicron and VLDL triglyceride. One heterozygote member of the Toronto kindred was reported to be markedly hypertriglyceridemic. This has been suggested to be due to an interaction with apo E-4 in this patient with apo C-II Toronto.[254] An interaction between apo E and apo C-II has also been reported in Nigerians.[255] In rare

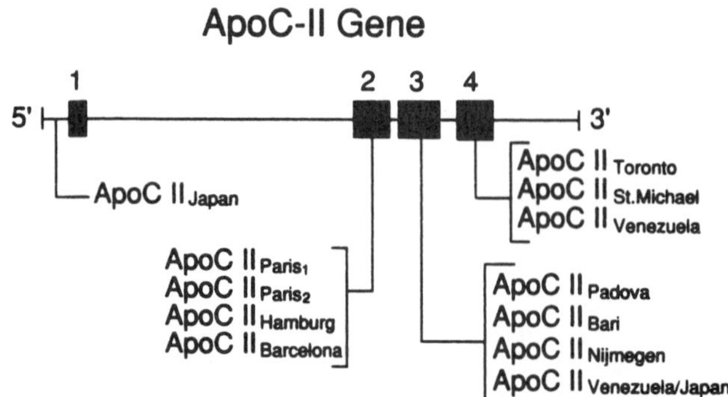

Fig. 117-9 Location of known mutations in the human apo C-II gene. (Modified from Santamarina-Fojo,[251] by permission of *Current Opinion in Lipidology*.)

homozygous apo E-4 subjects, marked hypertriglyceridemia has been reported;[255,256] in two brothers, this was associated with an Arg-for-Cys substitution at codon 228 of the apo E gene.[257]

The decrease in LPL activity in the postheparin plasma of patients with apo C-II deficiency is corrected by the addition of normal apo C-II in vitro, or by the intravenous infusion of apo C-II in all the families in which it has been reported.[14,253,258] Adipose-tissue LPL was mildly increased in the Vancouver patient,[259] but was not increased in the Milan family.[260] For unknown reasons, moderate decreases in HL activity have been reported in at least three of the probands with apo C-II deficiency.

Pathophysiology

When apo C-II is absent or nonfunctional, the function of LPL is severely impaired, with a marked increase in the K_m of LPL for the hydrolysis of triglyceride-rich lipoproteins. It may be that minimal LPL activity is still present, allowing hydrolysis of some of the triglyceride contained in these lipoproteins. As a result of apo C-II deficiency, triglyceride, predominantly in the form of chylomicrons and endogenously synthesized VLDL, accumulate in plasma. There is no difficulty with the accumulation of triglyceride in fat cells, suggesting pathways for energy uptake by fat cells through mechanisms other than the LPL-apo C-II system. There is a decrease in LDL and HDL, due, in part, to a decrease in the input of core and surface components from the triglyceride-rich lipoprotein remnants normally produced during triglyceride hydrolysis.

Diagnosis and Treatment

The deficiency of apo C-II manifests itself as diminished postheparin plasma LPL activity when assayed in the absence of apo C-II. With the addition of normal apo C-II to the assay, the decrease in postheparin plasma lipolytic activity corrects to normal. One can also use a source of LPL such as bovine milk LPL, which is free of apo C-II, to evaluate the plasma of a patient with potential apo C-II deficiency. One can then titrate the amount of apo C-II needed to correct the LPL activity. Deficiency of apo C-II can be verified by electrophoresis of the apolipoproteins contained in VLDL and chylomicrons on two-dimensional gels.[251] The treatment of apo C-II deficiency is the same as that outlined above for LPL deficiency.

CHYLOMICRONEMIA OF RELATED DISORDERS—PHENOCOPIES

History

Fredrickson and Lees[12] first separated patients with fasting chylomicronemia into those who had elevated levels of VLDL (the type V lipoprotein pattern) and those who did not (the type I lipoprotein pattern). Type I hyperlipoproteinemia was subsequently modified to include the absence of postheparin plasma LPL activity.[158] Type V hyperlipoproteinemia is a highly diverse group of primary and secondary disorders with moderate to severe hypertriglyceridemia. Many individuals with monogenic familial hypertriglyceridemia have moderate hypertriglyceridemia with chylomicrons present in plasma after an overnight fast on some occasions (type V) and not on others (type IV).

The families of probands with chylomicronemia often contain hypertriglyceridemic relatives.[261,262] Frequently, the proband has a secondary cause for hypertriglyceridemia such as alcohol intake; isotretinoin, diuretic, β-adrenergic blocker, HIV protease inhibitor, Zoloft, or estrogen treatment; or diabetes,[261] which increases the difficulty in determining the overall metabolic defect in the family. It has been demonstrated that the majority of probands with plasma triglyceride levels above 2000 mg/dl have both a common familial form of hypertriglyceridemia and a common secondary cause,[160] which accounts for the lesser degree of hypertriglyceridemia seen in the affected relatives who do not have the secondary cause for the increase in plasma triglyceride. When probands with a type V pattern with secondary causes of hypertriglyceridemia were excluded,[262] hypertriglyceridemia was found in 61 of 181 first-degree relatives, of whom 29 had fasting chylomicronemia. Because the median plasma triglyceride level was 770 mg/dl in the male probands, it is difficult to assess how many of these families represented monogenic familial hypertriglyceridemia. Neither in this study[262] nor in a study of the relatives of families with familial hypertriglyceridemia[263] was an increase in atherosclerosis seen.

Clinical Phenotype and Pathophysiology

Each of the primary familial disorders with plasma triglyceride levels over 2000 mg/dl and chylomicronemia is rare, but collectively they may account for up to 10 percent of individuals referred to a lipid clinic with the chylomicronemia syndrome. The vast majority of patients with chylomicronemia and plasma triglyceride levels above 2000 mg/dl do not have one of these rare genetic disorders. Rather, they appear to have one of the more common genetic disorders of triglyceride metabolism occurring simultaneously with, and independently of, a common, acquired, secondary form of hypertriglyceridemia.[159] The combination of the primary familial and the secondary acquired abnormality, each alone capable of causing mild to moderate hypertriglyceridemia, seems to lead to massive hypertriglyceridemia and the chylomicronemia syndrome.

Two genetic disorders—familial combined hyperlipidemia and monogenic familial hypertriglyceridemia—are commonly seen in the chylomicronemia syndrome. Remnant removal disease, or dysbetalipoproteinemia, is also occasionally seen. The most prevalent, acquired form of hypertriglyceridemia associated with these genetic disorders is related to the mild-to-moderate defect in LPL documented in untreated or recently treated diabetes mellitus.[5,169] The increase in triglyceride synthesis in familial hypertriglyceridemia and the increase in VLDL apo B synthesis seen in familial combined hyperlipidemia appear to interact with the LPL-related removal defect of the diabetic state to cause chylomicronemia. Such massive elevations in plasma triglyceride levels are rare with other acquired abnormalities of adipose-tissue LPL, such as in hypothyroidism or uremia, occurring concomitantly with one of the common familial forms of hypertriglyceridemia.[264]

Obesity seems to be associated with elevated VLDL triglyceride synthesis and leads to further increased triglyceride levels in familial hypertriglyceridemia, but not to the levels seen in the chylomicronemia syndrome. Other acquired forms of hypertriglyceridemia related to drugs or hormones that appear to be associated with increased VLDL triglyceride synthesis, such as estrogen therapy, the third trimester of pregnancy, glucocorticoid therapy, and alcohol use, may, in themselves, be associated with mild-to-moderate hypertriglyceridemia, but not with chylomicronemia. However, we commonly see plasma triglyceride levels above 2000 mg/dl in individuals with one of these drug- or hormone-related causes of increased VLDL triglyceride production who also have familial hypertriglyceridemia.

Whether massive hypertriglyceridemia can occur as the result of two separate but concurrent acquired causes of hypertriglyceridemia is unknown. Massive hypertriglyceridemia has been reported with multiple myeloma, with systemic lupus erythematosus, and with lymphoma, which reversed with therapy aimed at the acquired disease, and may have been due to the one acquired disease alone.[180] Diuretics and β-adrenergic blocking agents, which mildly increase triglyceride levels in normolipidemic subjects with hypertension, may play a significant role in the chylomicronemia syndrome when these drugs are given to patients with familial forms of hypertriglyceridemia.[265]

Of the 123 patients referred with marked idiopathic hypertriglyceridemia studied in our laboratory,[264] all but 13 had a known acquired cause of hypertriglyceridemia. Five of these 13 were found to have familial LPL deficiency. Five other patients had a genetic form of hypertriglyceridemia in the families of both parents. These patients could quite possibly be homozygous for a common familial form of hypertriglyceridemia or a double heterozygote of two common familial disorders. In the remaining three patients, the cause of the marked hypertriglyceridemia remained unknown. When the LPL gene was screened for structural mutations, heterozygosity for functional mutations was found in about 10 percent of these patients, similar to that reported by others.[266]

There is no doubt that families exist in which marked hypertriglyceridemia exists among multiple relatives[93,261,262,264] who do not have a defect in LPL, but the nature of the disorder(s) remains obscure. Fallat and Glueck[261] and Greenberg et al.[262] studied individuals with marked hypertriglyceridemia, many with plasma triglyceride levels above 2000 mg/dl. They noted a high prevalence of acquired forms of hypertriglyceridemia among these individuals. Because these patients have hypertriglyceridemic relatives, their disorder was characterized as "familial type V." It appears that they were studying the same phenomenon reported here — that is, chylomicronemia syndrome in the index patients caused by an interaction of a common familial disorder with an acquired form of hyperlipidemia. Triglyceride levels in their relatives rarely exceeded 2000 mg/dl, and acquired disorders among relatives were less common, suggesting that many of the index patients with "familial type V" come from families with one of the common genetic hypertriglyceridemias.

Prevalence

It is difficult to measure directly the prevalence of plasma triglyceride levels over 2000 mg/dl. In the Lipid Research Clinics' Prevalence Study, 7 individuals with this degree of hypertriglyceridemia were found among a population of 39,090 randomly chosen adult Caucasians. This is 1.8 such individuals per 10,000 population, or about 20,000 such individuals in the adult Caucasian population in the United States. Although no data are available, it appears that the prevalence and incidence of massive hypertriglyceridemia is more common in diabetes clinics and in hospitals that treat alcoholism. Based on the conservative estimated prevalence of familial hypertriglyceridemia of 1 to 2 percent and of familial combined hyperlipidemia of 2 to 3 percent, one might expect that up to 5 percent of untreated symptomatic diabetic patients could have massive hypertriglyceridemia.

Treatment

All of the clinical manifestations of the chylomicronemia syndrome are reversible with the reduction of plasma triglyceride levels. Thus, therapy is directed toward elimination of the causes of the hypertriglyceridemia. As in individuals with the rare genetic defects in LPL, most of those who appear to have inherited a common familial form of hypertriglyceridemia from each parent (homozygotes or compound heterozygotes) require a low-fat diet. Such individuals usually learn to avoid certain fat-containing foods, such as milk, on their own. To be pain-free, however, they often need to restrict dietary fat intake severely. Patients with hypertriglyceridemia inherited from both parents may respond dramatically to therapy with nicotinic acid alone, or in combination with a fibric acid or HMG-CoA reductase inhibitor.

Treatment of the hypertriglyceridemia in the more common patients, with concomitant familial and acquired disorders, should be directed first toward the acquired disorder. With symptomatic, untreated diabetes, insulin or oral sulfonylurea therapy is almost always required. Younger, thin individuals with insulin-dependent diabetes mellitus, with or without ketosis, may require no therapy other than insulin to keep triglyceride levels lowered. Many with insulin-dependent diabetes will have mild residual elevations in plasma triglyceride or cholesterol levels. Patients with noninsulin-dependent diabetes and marked hypertriglyceridemia are often more difficult to treat than those with insulin-independent diabetes. This difficulty is often associated with obesity and its resultant potential for hypertriglyceridemia and with the use of other drugs that might affect triglyceride metabolism. Some individuals with noninsulin-dependent diabetes respond to insulin therapy alone, while others require a fibric acid, in addition, to significantly lower triglyceride levels. Occasionally, a patient with noninsulin-dependent diabetes will have lower triglyceride levels when taking a fibric acid and an oral sulfonylurea than when given insulin with the fibric acid. Difficult patients with noninsulin-dependent diabetes may require therapy in addition to the oral sulfonylurea and fibric acid. Long-term nicotinic acid therapy should be used with caution in the presence of diabetes because of its hyperglycemic effect. We believe that weight loss is contraindicated in obese patients with noninsulin-dependent diabetes and the chylomicronemia syndrome. Although weight loss and maintenance of the weight loss are extremely effective forms of therapy, the maintenance of reduced weight is unusual; the often-inevitable weight regain leads to extreme hypertriglyceridemia and recurrent pancreatitis.

The marked hypertriglyceridemia that occurs in individuals with a familial form of hypertriglyceridemia treated with estrogens, glucocorticoids, isotretinoin, or alcohol almost always responds to the discontinuation of the drug or alcohol, with no further antihyperlipidemic therapy required. In general, marked hypertriglyceridemia that is unresponsive to a low-fat diet and/or treatment of the acquired disease is a definite indication for the addition of a fibric acid to the therapeutic program.

Most of the minor symptoms of the chylomicronemia syndrome do not require urgent therapy. However, in the presence of moderate-to-severe abdominal pain or pancreatitis, immediate therapy is indicated. Pancreatitis associated with the chylomicronemia syndrome is treated in the same way as are the usual forms of pancreatitis.[160–162] The discontinuation of oral intake stops chylomicron triglyceride formation, and replacement with hypocaloric parenteral nutrition decreases VLDL triglyceride production. The administration of excess calories, as in hyperalimentation, is contraindicated in the acute state, and the intravenous administration of lipid emulsions may lead to persistent or recurrent pancreatitis. On this regimen, subjects with alcohol-induced hypertriglyceridemia respond rapidly; those with estrogen- or glucocorticoid-induced hypertriglyceridemia respond less quickly. The noninsulin-dependent diabetic, however, presents a special situation. Although triglyceride levels will fall with hypocaloric intravenous fat-free fluids in combination with antihyperglycemic drugs and a fibrate, the defect in LPL does not correct rapidly with treatment of the diabetes, and the patient on a low-fat diet may need to be watched closely for 2 to 3 months.

HEPATIC LIPASE, DYSLIPIDEMIA, AND ATHEROSCLEROSIS

Structure and Function of Hepatic Lipase

Normal Hepatic Lipase Gene and Protein. Hepatic lipase (HL) is a glycoprotein that catalyzes the hydrolysis of mono-, di-, and triacylglycerols, phosphatidylcholines, and phosphatidylethanolamines[268] (reviewed in references 269–271). N-linked glycosylation at residue Asn 57 of HL and the corresponding amino acid (Asn 43) in LPL were shown to be required for maximal secretion of an active enzyme.[58,272] The majority of HL is synthesized and secreted by the liver and is bound to heparan sulfate proteoglycans on the surfaces of sinusoidal endothelial cells and external surfaces of microvilli of parenchymal cells in the space of Disse.[273–275]

The human hepatic lipase gene (*LIPC*) (GenBank cDNA D83548; gDNA M29186) spans over 30 kb, is comprised of 9 exons and 8 introns,[276,277] and is located on chromosome 15q21.[54] The gene encodes a protein of 499 amino acids from which a 22-amino acid signal peptide is cleaved to form the mature enzyme of 477 residues and a predicted molecular mass of 53 kDa.[54,278,279] Verhoeven et al.[280] showed that steroidogenic organs express a truncated version of HL (a result of alternate splicing) that is retained intracellularly.

Regulation by Sterols. Data from the Familial Atherosclerosis Treatment Study (FATS)[281] indicate that HMG-CoA reductase inhibitors or nicotinic acid in combination with bile acid sequestrants decrease HL activity.[282] In contrast, bile acid sequestrants alone increased HL levels. The effects of these intensive and long-term treatments suggest a relationship between cholesterol homeostasis and HL activity. However, these effects may have been indirect and may have involved transcriptional or posttranscriptional steps. In two studies with female Zucker rats, dietary enrichment with 2 percent cholesterol caused a 34 percent decrease in HL lipase activity and mRNA level,[283,284] which were even greater when both cholesterol and cholate were supplemented.[283] Again, these effects may or may not involve direct regulation of *LIPC* transcription, yet they also point to a link between cholesterol metabolism and HL production.

Results of experiments with HepG2 cells also point to a link between regulation of the cholesterol biosynthetic pathway and HL production. Busch et al.,[285] working with HepG2 cells cultured in lipoprotein-deficient serum, reported that blocking cholesterol biosynthesis by greater than 85 percent with mevinolin, *induced* HL mRNA levels by twofold and HL secretion by four- to fivefold. Conversely, incubation of untreated or mevinolin-treated HepG2 cells with mevalonic acid raised intracellular cholesterol concentrations, *decreased* HL secretion to levels below control values, and abrogated mevinolin-induction of HL mRNA. Interestingly, exposure of cells simultaneously to mevinolin and 25-hydroxy cholesterol further enhanced HL mRNA levels and HL secretion. These results suggest that a metabolite in the cholesterol biosynthetic pathway suppresses HL production, and that both transcriptional and posttranscriptional mechanisms may be involved.

Nimmo et al.[286] showed that HL secretion is markedly *increased* on culture of HepG2 cells in lipoprotein-deficient serum. This activation was reversed in the presence of increasing concentrations of LDL. Berg et al.[287] also showed that the secretion of HL from HepG2 cells is *inhibited* on addition of LDL to the medium (supplemented with 10 percent fetal calf serum). However, they also observed a decrease in HL secretion in the presence of compactin. Although apparently in partial conflict (perhaps due to the culture conditions: confluency and presence or absence of delipidated serum), these results strongly suggest a complex regulatory link between the cholesterol biosynthetic pathway and HL production. Whether the effects of sterols are at least in part due to direct effects on transcription of the *LIPC* gene remains to be investigated in a more defined system.

Regulation by Sex Steroids. Estrogens were observed to decrease postheparin plasma HL activity in humans,[288–291] whereas androgens had the opposite effect.[289] Androgen administration resulted in reduced HDL_2-cholesterol, which was preceded by an increase in HL activity in men and women.[292,293] The mechanisms by which these sex steroids influence HL activity are unknown.

Function of Hepatic Lipase.

Hepatic Lipase and Remodeling of Remnant and Low-Density Lipoproteins. HL catalyses the hydrolysis of triglyceride and phospholipid of intermediate-density lipoprotein remnants and large-buoyant low-density lipoproteins resulting in more dense lipoprotein particles (Fig. 117-10). As shown below, the absence of HL activity leads to large-buoyant, triglyceride- and phospholipid-enriched LDL particles.[232] In normal males and those with coronary artery disease, HL activity is related to decreasing size and increasing density of LDL particles.[294] Women have larger, more buoyant LDL[295] and lower hepatic lipase activity than men,[296–298] and HL activity seems to account for the gender differences in peak LDL density.[299,300] Although men have more intra-abdominal fat than women, both men[301,302] and women with increased intra-abdominal fat have increased HL activity.[303] Depending on the level of triglyceride and the degree of triglyceride enrichment of VLDL, hepatic lipase and cholesteryl ester transfer protein (CETP) are the major determinants of LDL size and density.[302] The promoter variant of the hepatic lipase gene is associated with decreased HL activity and more buoyant LDL.[304] And finally, intensive lipid-lowering therapy decreases HL activity and increases LDL buoyancy, predicting regression of preexisting atherosclerosis.[305] Each of these differences suggests that hepatic lipase is proatherogenic (see below).

Hepatic Lipase and Remodeling of HDL. In addition to its acylglycerol hydrolase activity, HL acts as a phospholipase. The phospholipase activity may play an important role in the ability of HL, as opposed to LPL, to convert the phospholipid-rich HDL_2 to HDL_3 particles. Therefore, one would expect an inverse relationship between HL activity and plasma HDL_2 cholesterol concentrations.[306–308] As described below, a number of population-based studies recently demonstrated a direct correlation between HL activity, and HDL-C concentrations. Plasma HDL levels are influenced by genetic and environmental (obesity, cigarette smoking, and a sedentary life style) factors. Family[309–311] and twin[295,312] studies suggest that between 40 percent and 60 percent of the interindividual variation in HDL-C is accounted for by genetic factors. The evidence from studies on identical twins raised apart is particularly compelling because they minimize the confounding effects of shared environmental factors.[312,313] There is now good evidence for a role of polymorphisms in the promoter of the HL gene in influencing HL and HDL levels (see below).

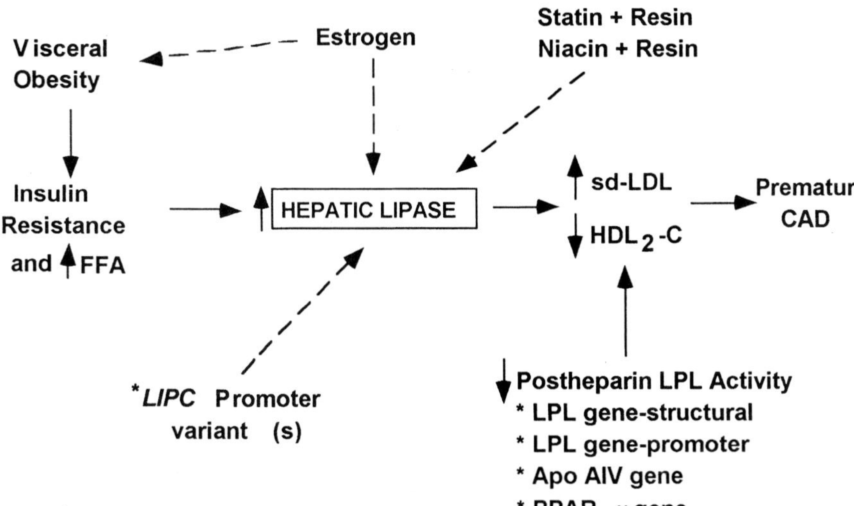

Fig. 117-10 Variation in HL activity can predispose to coronary artery disease by effecting size and density of LDL and HDL. Many clinical situations have positive (→) or negative (- - - >) effects in the transcription of the hepatic lipase gene. (*From Zambon et al.*[304] *Used with permission.*)

Table 117-2 Lipoproteins in Hepatic Lipase Deficiency

		TG	TC	Apo B	VLDL C/TG	LDL C/TG	HDL C/TG	HDL-C 2/TOTAL	IDL MASS	β VLDL	VLDL-C TG	Apo E isoform
Ontario	1	↑	↑	↑	212/494	134/94	81/51	.32	↑	+	.12	3/3
	2	↑	↑	↑	80/261	127/165	62/60	.57	↑	+	.17	3/3
	3	↑↑	↑	↑	25/67	77/119	31/51	NA	NA	+	.28	3/3
Stockholm	1	↑	↑	↑	104/234	70/125	76/103	NA	NA	+	.22	3/4
	2	↑±	↑	↑	23/45	171/124	132/71	NA	NA	+	.10	
Seattle	1	↑↑*		↑	209/788	107/190	42/51	NA	↑	+	.12	3/3
Quebec	1	↑	↑	NA	NA	NA	NA	NA	NA	NA	NA	NA
	2	↑	±	NA	NA	NA	NA	NA	NA	NA	NA	NA
	3	NL	±	NA	NA	NA	NA	NA	NA	NA	NA	NA
Providence	1	↑	↑	↑	NA	NA	NA	.70	NA	NA	NA	NA
	2	↑	↑	↑	NA	NA	NA	.69	NA	NA	NA	NA
Seattle	2	↑↑*	↑	↑	23/43	139/126	50/52	.40	↑		.10	4/3
	3	↑	↑	↑	104/266	188/257	45/52	NA	↑		.18	3/3

*Lipids on fibrate therapy

Studies in animals have also clearly demonstrated an important role of HL in HDL metabolism. For example, inactivation of HL by infusion of rats with antibodies against HL or targeted HL gene inactivation in mice caused an increase in HDL_2-C levels.[314,315] Conversely, overexpression of human HL in transgenic rabbits resulted in a dramatic (85 percent) decrease in the level of both large (HDL_1 and HDL_2) and small, dense (HDL_3) HDL particles.[316] Similarly, overexpression of human HL in transgenic mice was associated with a 30 percent lowering of plasma HDL-C and a decrease in HDL particle size.[285] The ligand-binding and catalytic activities of HL contribute to lowering plasma HDL concentration.

Hepatic Lipase as a Ligand for Lipoprotein Uptake. Recent in vitro data suggest HL participates with cell surface heparan sulfate proteoglycans and the LDL receptor-like protein (LRP) in promoting uptake of apolipoprotein B-containing remnant lipoproteins and HDL. The enhancement of hepatic uptake of apo B-containing lipoproteins was independent of lipolytic activity and did not require apolipoprotein E.[317–319] Several groups have demonstrated direct binding of HL to LRP.[317,319] To test whether these effects occur in vivo, Dichek et al.[320] generated transgenic mice overexpressing catalytically active human HL in the liver. Both apo B-containing remnant lipoproteins and HDL were reduced in these transgenic mice when fed a high fat diet or after crossing them to apo B-overexpressing or apo E-deficient mice. While the apo B-containing lipoproteins were reduced in mice overexpressing catalytically inactive HL, HDL was minimally reduced.

Clinical Manifestations of Hepatic Lipase Deficiency

History. Hepatic lipase activity in postheparin plasma was first separated from lipoprotein lipase activity in 1974.[15] The first patient with hepatic lipase deficiency was reported in 1982.[321] Two additional brothers were found to have hepatic lipase deficiency in this family in Ontario, Canada.[322] Since that time 12 patients in 6 families have been detected (Tables 117-1 and 117-2).

Classical Phenotype. The original Ontario patient presented with hypertriglyceridemia.[321] This patient and Seattle patients #1 and #2 intermittently had severe hypertriglyceridemia with eruptive xanthomata and pancreatitis.[232,321] Although most patients with hepatic lipase deficiency have mild hypertriglyceridemia, one affected brother in the Quebec family had a normal plasma triglyceride level. One feature found in all patients is triglyceride enrichment of total LDL (1.006 to 1.063 g/ml) and HDL (Table 117-2), with the mass of TG being equal to cholesterol both in LDL and in HDL. There seems to be an increase in the number of apo B-containing particles as reflected by an increase in plasma apo B levels. HDL_2 cholesterol is particularly increased with the proportion of HDL_2 of total HDL cholesterol reaching over 50 percent in affected males.

Beta-migrating VLDL on agarose gel was reported in the first patient[321] and has been present in most patients where reported. As in remnant removal disease (type III) (Chap. 119), the presence of β VLDL is associated with increased intermediate density lipoprotein mass. In contrast to remnant removal disease, patients with hepatic lipase deficiency do not have the apo E-2 isoform, or elevated plasma VLDL cholesterol to total triglyceride ratio, but do have elevated apo B levels. The lipoprotein distribution by density gradient ultracentrifugation[232,321,323,324] or gel chromatography,[325] has revealed changes in lipoprotein cholesterol distribution (Fig. 117-11). A fairly sharp peak of apo B-containing lipoprotein in the density 1.006 to 1.063 g/ml range typical of LDL occurs but with a decrease in lipoprotein peak density.[232,321] This increase is associated with triglyceride and phospholipid enrichment of this lipoprotein.[232] In addition, a buoyant shoulder on the LDL-like lipoprotein peak[325] can occur. The mechanism of accumulation of the more buoyant shoulder in the LDL-like

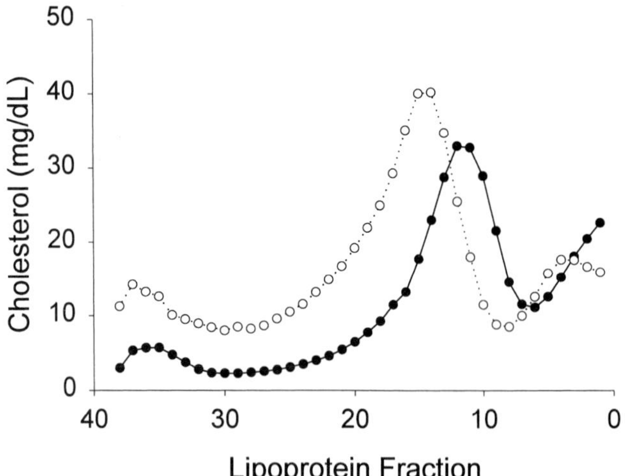

Fig. 117-11 Mean distribution of cholesterol by nonequilibrium density gradient ultracentrifugation in 32 normal males (●—●) and 3 patients (○—○) with HL deficiency in Seattle (Tables 117-1, 117-2). Note increased buoyancy of LDL peak (10 to 20) and HDL (0 to 10) peaks in HL deficiency. Also note accumulation of buoyant remnants (15 to 25) and VLDL in HL deficiency.

Table 117-3 Hepatic Lipase Sequence Variants

Exon	Change*		Frequency	Activity	Reference
1	**Del of prom & exon 1**		Rare	**Defective**	Deeb & Brunzell†
Intr 1	**A-13G accept. splice site**		Rare	**Defective**	Brand et al. (328)
3	G290A	V73M	0.05	NL	Hegele et al. (329)
4	G472T	V133V	0.45	NL	Hegele et al. (329)
5	A598G	G175G	0.35	NL	Mori et al. (361)
5	G630T	**R186H**	Rare	**Defective**	Knudson et al. (362)
5	A651G	N193S	0.46	NL	Hegele et al. (329)
5	C679G	T202T	0.48	NL	Hegele et al. (329)
5	G736C	**G225R**	Rare	**Defective**	Deeb & Brunzell†
6	C873T	**S267F**	Rare	**Defective**	Hegele et al. (322,329)
7	A1075C	**L334F**	Rare	**Defective**	Knudsen et al. (345,362)
7	A1105G	T344T	0.32	NL	Knudsen et al. (345)
8	C1221T	**T383M**	Rare	**Defective**	Hegele et al. (322,329)
9	C1444A	T457T	0.23	NL	Knudsen et al. (345)

* cDNA nucleotide positions and codon numbers of mature protein
† Not previously published

lipoprotein peak is not evident, but might be related to defective HL-mediated uptake of remnant lipoproteins.

Although the patients usually present with dyslipidemia, 8 of 10 patients above age 35 years developed coronary artery disease in their forties or early fifties (Table 117-1). One patient (Seattle #1) also had type II diabetes, but cardiovascular risk factors other than the dyslipidemia do not seem to account for the very early onset of coronary artery disease in hepatic lipase deficiency. Several patients presented with severe hypertriglyceridemia and were found to have $\frac{1}{2}$ normal levels of postheparin plasma LPL activity and mass (Seattle #1 and Seattle #2). The Seattle #1 patient was heterozygote for the LPL missense mutation N9D, which, in the presence of hepatic lipase deficiency, might cause the severe hypertriglyceridemia. Seattle #3 was one of the subjects in the Familial Atherosclerosis Treatment Study.[281]

Mutant Gene and Genetics. The three affected brothers in the original Ontario family are compound heterozygotes for rare missense mutations[322,326,327] (Table 117-1). The two brothers and one sister in the Quebec family, and the patient in the Seattle 2 family, were heterozygous carriers of a rare missense mutation involving one chromosome.[326,327] The second mutation in these patients has not been found.[322] One patient was homozygous for an intron 1 acceptor splice-site mutation (Seattle #1)[328] and one was homozygous for a deletion involving exon 1 and part of the gene promoter (Seattle #3). Evidence that the missense mutations are causative include: (a) the mutation alleles are not found among randomly selected individuals; (b) they are associated with phenotypic changes in lipoproteins; (c) they cosegregate with the phenotype; and (d) they are associated with severely diminished activity when expressed in vitro. In addition to these mutations, polymorphisms of the HL gene that have no apparent impact on activity have been reported (Table 117-3).[329]

Of the 12 patients with hepatic lipase deficiency only 1 is female. This imbalance in gender ratio may reflect the difficulty in identifying affected females compared to normal females who have lower hepatic lipase activity than males.[296,297] The pattern of inheritance for the full phenotype is autosomal recessive. It is possible that the Quebec family and the Seattle #2 family, where only one defective allele was found, might indicate autosomal dominant inheritance. However, the probands in these two families were much more hyperlipidemic than in the relatives who had mild abnormalities and carried one or the other of the missense mutations.[322,330] It is likely that an additional defect of HL will be found in the probands of these two families.

Pathophysiology

The triglyceride enrichment of LDL and HDL in total hepatic lipase deficiency reflects the defect in hydrolysis of triglyceride (and phospholipid) in the lipoproteins. A defect in hepatic lipase-mediated uptake of the remnants of chylomicrons and VLDL by the liver, which seems to be independent of lipolytic activity, also might play a role in the dyslipidemia. The lipolytic defect would increase the buoyancy of all lipoproteins across the usual lipoprotein spectrum based on size and density (Fig. 117-12). Thus, the terminal apo B-containing lipoprotein in the VLDL to LDL cascade, which is in the 1.019 to 1.063 g/ml density fraction, extends into the IDL range (1.006 to 1.019 g/ml).[232,321] The lipid enrichment of VLDL remnants typically seen in IDL extends into the more buoyant fraction usually termed VLDL and is responsible for the β-migrating remnants in the VLDL density fraction. The defect in hepatic lipase recognition and enhancement of remnant uptake by the liver might aggravate the above, delay the clearance of these remnants (in VLDL and IDL) (Fig. 117-11), and further increase "VLDL" levels.[324]

The premature coronary disease that occurs in these individuals might reflect arterial wall uptake and retention of the increased numbers of apo B-containing lipoproteins of abnormal composition and/or HDL might be defective and unable to participate in reverse cholesterol transport because of the compositional abnormalities seen in HDL.

Diagnosis and Treatment. The typical patient with hepatic lipase deficiency might present with moderate hypertriglyceridemia, mild elevations in total cholesterol, elevated apo B, and premature coronary artery disease. If one only measured total plasma triglyceride, total cholesterol, and HDL cholesterol, and estimated the LDL cholesterol, such a patient might be confused with a patient with familial combined hyperlipidemia. One difference might be a mild increase in HDL-cholesterol in HL deficiency and a mild decrease in HDL in FCHL. The patients reported with HL deficiency have been ascertained through more extreme phenotypes. Some were extremely hypertriglyceridemic and hepatic lipase deficiency was discovered while evaluating postheparin plasma LPL activity.[232,321] One was found by noting extreme elevations in HDL cholesterol,[331] while others were formed by noting β VLDL were present as an atypical form of remnant removal disease.

The definitive way to diagnose HL deficiency is to demonstrate absent HL activity in postheparin plasma associated with defects

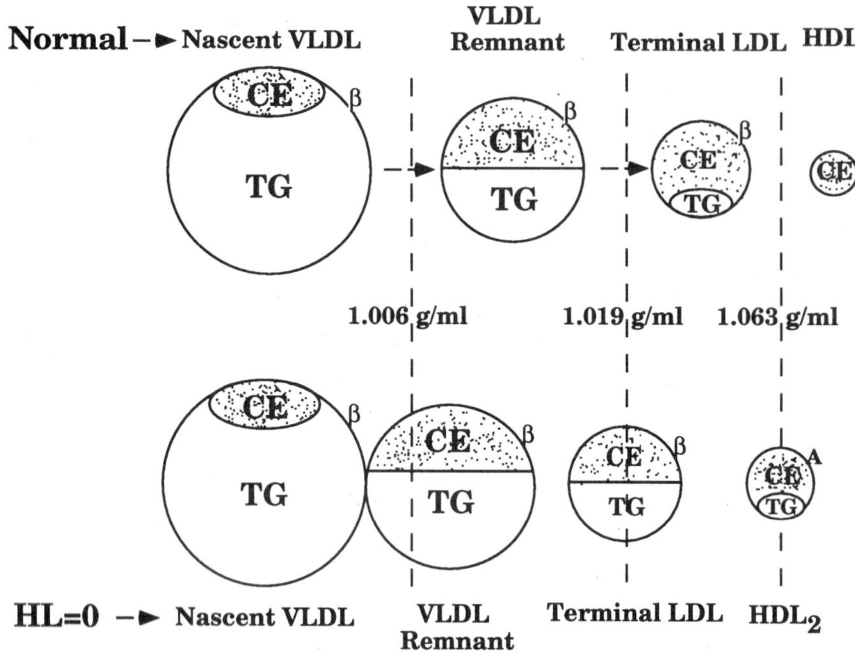

Fig. 117-12 The hydrated density of lipoproteins has been used to separate major lipoprotein subclasses. In normals, 1.006 g/ml separates VLDL and IDL, 1.019 g/ml separates IDL and LDL, and 1.063 g/ml separates LDL and HDL. If hepatic lipase deficiency leads to triglyceride and phospholipid enrichment of lipoproteins that have been generated by the effect of LPL on chylomicrons and VLDL, these physiologic counterparts of VLDL, IDL, LDL, and HDL[358] would be more buoyant than the normal lipoproteins and would violate the traditional lipoprotein boundaries defined by hydrated density.

in both HL alleles. The presence of marked triglyceride enrichment of LDL and HDL can be determined by measurement of triglyceride in the 1.006 g/ml bottom fraction, or in LDL and HDL separated by sequential ultracentrifugation. The presence of β VLDL in agarose electrophoresis with elevated apo B and normal VLDL-cholesterol/total triglyceride ratio, also supports the diagnosis.

The unusual presentation of some of the probands with HL deficiency caused by additional abnormalities suggests that many other HL-deficient patients might be diagnosed as moderate hypertriglyceridemia or familial combined hyperlipidemia. Indeed, to test this hypothesis, postheparin plasma hepatic lipase activity was measured in 80 of the probands of the Familial Atherosclerosis Treatment Study.[281] One new HL-deficient patient was found (Seattle #3),[332] implying the disease may be more common than thought.

No unique treatment of the hyperlipidemia has yet been recommended. If severe hypertriglyceridemia is present, one should consider fibrate or nicotinic acid therapy. Lipids have been shown to improve with HMG-CoA reductase inhibitor therapy.

Hepatic lipase deficiency is a good candidate disease for gene therapy. Studies are ongoing in animal models. Hepatic lipase-deficient mice were infused with a recombinant adenovirus vector expression, the human hepatic lipase cDNA.[267] The transiently expressed human HL, bound to the mouse vascular endothelium, caused a marked decrease (50 to 80 percent) in total cholesterol, triglycerides, phospholipids, cholesteryl ester, and HDL cholesterol. The successful delivery of HL to the vascular endothelium opens the door for correction of human HL deficiency.

THE HETERPZYGOTE STATE AND OTHER CAUSES OF PARTIAL HEPATIC LIPASE DEFICIENCY

Most individuals with heterozygous hepatic lipase deficiency have a 50 percent reduction in postheparin plasma hepatic lipase activity.[322,323] Although many individuals with one defective hepatic lipase allele have normal lipid levels,[322,323] some have triglyceride enrichment of HDL and LDL,[322,333] which are large and buoyant.[333] The clinical significance of this heterozygote state is unknown at present.

Given the involvement of HL in HDL metabolism and the observation that the level of plasma HDL-C is inversely correlated with hepatic lipase activity in humans,[306,308] regulatory or structural variants in the gene encoding hepatic lipase are logical candidates in accounting for interindividual variation in HDL-C. The first suggestive evidence for involvement of the hepatic lipase locus in influencing HDL-C levels was provided by Cohen et al.[298] Using sibling-pair linkage analysis in 73 normotriglyceridemic Caucasian nuclear families, they observed that allelic variation at the hepatic lipase locus and apo A-I/C-III/A-IV loci accounted for 25 percent and 22 percent, respectively, of the total interindividual variation in plasma HDL-C levels. In another study, Mahaney et al.[334] performed linkage analysis using data from 526 Mexican American individuals from 25 randomly ascertained pedigrees in the San Antonio Family Heart Study and found evidence for a major locus effect (with a codominant mixed model) on plasma HDL-C levels. However, linkage was excluded between the observed major locus and markers at the following candidate gene loci: apo A-I/C-II/A-IV, apo B, hepatic lipase ($P = 0.001$), lipoprotein lipase, and the LDL receptor.

Cohen's group,[335] using sibling-pair analysis of data from a much larger sample (1465 individuals from 218 nuclear families) of Caucasian Americans, confirmed their own earlier results that variation at the hepatic lipase locus was associated with HDL-C levels ($P = 0.01$). Variation at the hepatic lipase locus accounted for a significant fraction (approximately 25 percent) of variation in HDL-C levels.

Guerra and colleagues[335] observed four polymorphisms in the 5′ flanking region of hepatic lipase gene: G → A at position −250, C → T at −514, T → C at −710, and A → G at −763. The four polymorphisms are in complete linkage disequilibrium in Caucasians and, therefore, define two haplotypes. The frequency of the less common haplotype was found to be 0.15 among 272 unrelated Caucasian Americans. Their results indicated that heterozygosity for the less common haplotype was associated with moderate elevation in plasma HDL-C (41 ± 11 vs. 37 ± 10 mg/dl) and apo A-I (131 ± 23 vs. 122 ± 21 mg/dl) in *men* but not in women. Men homozygous for the less common haplotype had markedly elevated (63 ± 3 mg/dl) HDL-C.

These results prompted investigation of a possible association of hepatic lipase gene promoter variants with HL, HDL, and LDL size and density in relation to our results from the FATS.[304] First, the less common allele of the gene promoter disease polymorphism was associated with high HDL_2, but not HDL_3, cholesterol levels and with buoyant LDL particles among Caucasian normals and men with coronary artery disease. Second, these associations were mediated by differences in HL activity between individuals with different hepatic lipase promoter genotypes in both groups of subjects. The hepatic lipase genotype accounted for 20 to 32 percent of the variance in HL levels.

In two subsequent studies on male coronary artery disease patients from Holland ($N = 782$)[336] and Finland ($N = 395$),[337] the less common HL promoter, haplotype was also found to be highly associated with lower HL activity. Heterozygotes for the less common allele had a 25 percent reduction in HL and homozygotes had up to 50 percent reduction. Whereas Jansen et al.[336] found the polymorphism to be associated with coronary artery disease and with HDL-C levels, Tahvanainen et al.[337] observed an association with only the triglyceride content of LDL, IDL, and HDL. In both studies, polymorphisms in the coding sequence of hepatic lipase gene could not account for these associations. Therefore, it seems likely that one or more of the four promoter polymorphisms is responsible for variation in HL activity. Alternatively, the observed promoter polymorphisms may be in linkage disequilibrium with other variants within an adjacent gene encoding a protein that regulates hepatic lipase gene expression. In a fourth study of 95 Finnish students (of *both sexes*) whose fathers had documented premature myocardial infarction and 194 matched control subjects, the less common haplotype was again associated with elevated HDL, Apo A-I, and Lp(a)-I values.[338]

The less common haplotype of the hepatic lipase gene promoter was observed to be approximately threefold greater among African Americans and Japanese Americans than among Caucasians.[304] This raised the possibility that the higher frequency of this polymorphism among individuals of African and Japanese descent may explain the relatively high levels of HDL observed in these two ethnic groups,[339–342] that could not be explained by differences in lifestyle.[343] Vega et al.[344] tested this hypothesis in African American *men* and found that HDL-C levels were significantly higher and plasma HL activity was significantly lower in African Americans than in Caucasian American men. The less common haplotype was associated with lower HL activity and higher HDL-C levels but it accounted for only part of the ethnic differences in these phenotypes, indicating that these two ethnic groups differ in other genetic factors that influence these parameters. The difference in HDL-C between African and Caucasian Americans is restricted to men, and appears to be largely due to the difference in magnitude of the decrease which occurs during puberty.[339,340] These results indicate that sex steroids may play an important role in regulating HL levels, and that the two promoter alleles may respond differently to these hormones.

In sum, there seems to be agreement that the hepatic lipase gene promoter polymorphisms are associated with HL activity and with the triglyceride content of IDL, LDL, and HDL. These observations are consistent with findings among heterozygous carriers of nonfunctional HL alleles. For example, heterozygotes for the R186H and L334F mutations were observed to have triglyceride-rich LDL and HDL, but no elevation in HDL-C concentration.[345] However, there is disagreement on the association of the hepatic lipase gene promoter polymorphisms with total HDL-C concentrations. Because HDL-C levels are influenced by a number of genetic and environmental factors, this variability in findings may be due to differences in genetic background or in lifestyle. Because HL is known to be directly involved in remodeling of HDL particles, and that HL levels are more significantly correlated with HDL_2-C concentrations,[304,306] it is more appropriate to examine association and linkage of hepatic lipase gene polymorphisms with HDL_2-C concentrations rather than with total HDL-C.

HEPATIC LIPASE AND ATHEROSCLEROSIS

Hepatic lipase has been proposed to be both proatherogenic and antiatherogenic. Patients with familial HL deficiency and absent HL activity have definite premature coronary artery disease (Table 117-1). Normolipidemic males[346,347] and hypercholesterolemic males[347] with premature coronary artery disease have significantly decreased postheparin plasma HL activity, while males with hypertriglyceridemia or central obesity[347,348] or elevated apo B levels[304,305] have normal or elevated HL activity. The common hepatic lipase gene promoter variants associated with lower HL activity were found to be more common in individuals with coronary artery disease in one study,[336] but not in others.[304,338] The association of low HL activity with coronary disease might be mediated by a defect in HL-enhanced remnant uptake by the liver; however, one then would expect to see an association of low HL activity with coronary disease in the hypertriglyceridemic patients.

The proatherogenic effects of excess HL probably are mediated through the lipolytic processing of intermediate and buoyant low-density lipoproteins, and the conversion of HDL_2 to HDL_3 particles. Many clinical situations imply that elevated HL activity causes adverse lipoprotein changes. Men have higher hepatic lipase activity than women,[296–298] which is associated in men with smaller, denser LDL[349] and less HDL_2.[350] Central obesity is associated with increased hepatic lipase activity,[303] smaller, denser LDL,[350] and decreased HDL_2.[306,307] Studies of individuals after weight loss demonstrate a decrease in HL activity, an increase in size and buoyancy of LDL particles, and an increase in HDL_2 cholesterol.[351] The relationship of central obesity to the clinical findings seems to be mediated by the amount of intra-abdominal fat present.[303,350,351]

Dyslipoproteinemia characterized by reduced HDL and HDL_2 cholesterol levels and elevated levels of small, dense LDL particles are risk factors for coronary artery disease. The high concentration of the large HDL_2 particles has been reported to underlie the protective effect of HDL-C.[352,353] Conversely, high concentrations of very small HDL_3 particles are positively correlated with the severity of coronary artery disease.[354,355] Katzel et al.[301] reported reduced HDL_2-C levels and elevated postheparin HL activity in men with central obesity and asymptomatic coronary artery disease.

Small, dense LDL particles are associated with coronary artery disease and appear to predict angiographic changes in response to intensive lipid-lowering therapy. Intensive lipid-lowering therapy with double-drug therapy in the Familial Atherosclerosis Treatment Study[281] resulted in significant improvement in coronary stenosis. The clinical relevance of these changes in LDL density on coronary stenosis regression has led to a focus on HL as the mechanism which links lipid-lowering therapy to coronary disease via changes in LDL density. The changes in LDL buoyancy and in HL activity both predicted changes in disease severity ($p < 0.001$). In a multivariate analysis, the change in LDL buoyancy was the best predictor of coronary disease regression accounting for 38.3 percent of variance ($p < 0.01$). In subjects with coronary artery disease, HL-mediated changes in LDL density strongly affected coronary artery disease regression, highlighting a new and potentially important pathophysiological mechanism linking lipid-lowering therapy to clinical improvement of cardiovascular disease. These results suggest that a relatively high level of postheparin plasma HL activity is expected to increase the risk for atherosclerosis.

In contrast to humans, HL-deficient mice do not have increased atherosclerosis.[315] However, HL deficiency in mice is protective against atherosclerosis in apo E-deficient[356] and LCAT-over-expressing transgenic mice[357] despite significant increases in plasma cholesterol concentrations. Whether a low level of HL is atherogenic or antiatherogenic may depend on a number of genetic and environmental factors that influence lipoprotein metabolism.

REFERENCES

1. Thannhauser SJ: *Lipidoses: Diseases of the Intracellular Lipid Metabolism* 3rd ed. New York, Grune and Stratton, 1958, p 296.
2. Addison T, Gull W: On a certain affection of the skin, vitiligoidea (a) plana, (b) tuberosa, with remarks. *Guys Hosp Rep* **7**:265, 1851.
3. Jensen J: The story of xanthomatosis in England prior to the First World War. *Clio Med* **2**:289, 1967.
4. Joslin EP: *The Treatment of Diabetes Mellitus*. Philadelphia, Lea and Febiger, 1916.
5. Brunzell JD, Hazzard WR, Motulsky AG, Bierman EL: Evidence for diabetes mellitus and genetic forms of hypertriglyceridemia as independent entities. *Metabolism* **24**:1115, 1975.
6. Siemans HW: Zur kenntnis der xanthoma. *Arch Dermatol Syph* **136**:159, 1921.
7. Burger M, Grutz O: Uber Hepatosplenomegale lipoidose mit xanthomatosen veranderungen in haut und schleimhaut. *Arch Dermatol Syph* **166**:542, 1932.
8. Holt LE Jr, Aylward FX, Timbres HG: Idiopathic familial lipemia. *Bull Johns Hopkins Hosp* **64**:279, 1939.
9. Poulsen HM: Familial lipemia, a new form of lipoidosis showing increase in neutral fats combined with attacks of acute pancreatitis. *Acta Med Scand* **138**:413, 1950.
10. Malmros H, Swahn B, Truedsson E: Essential hyperlipidaemia. *Acta Med Scand* **149**:91, 1954.
11. Ahrens EH Jr, Hirsch J, Oette K, Farquhar JW, Stein Z: Carbohydrate-induced and fat-induced lipemia. *Trans Assoc Am Physicians* **74**:134, 1961.
12. Fredrickson DS, Lees RS: Familial hyperlipoproteinemia, in: Stanbury JB, Wyngaarden JB, Fredrickson DS (eds): *The Metabolic Basis of Inherited Disease* 2nd ed. New York, McGraw-Hill, 1966, p 429.
13. Havel RJ, Gordon RS Jr. Idiopathic hyperlipemia: Metabolic studies in an affected family. *J Clin Invest* **39**:1777, 1960.
14. Breckenridge WC, Little JA, Steiner G, Chow A, Poapst M: Hypertriglyceridemia associated with deficiency of apolipoprotein C-II. *N Engl J Med* **298**:1265, 1978.
15. Krauss RM, Levy RI, Fredrickson DS: Selective measurement of two lipase activities in post-heparin plasma from normal subjects and patients with hyperlipoproteinemia. *J Clin Invest* **54**:1107, 1974.
16. Breckenridge WC, Little JA, Alaupovic P, Wang C-S, Kuksis A, Kakis G, Lindgren F, Gardiner G: Lipoprotein abnormalities associated with a familial deficiency of hepatic lipase. *Atherosclerosis* **45**:161, 1982.
17. Hide WA, Chan L, Li W-H: Structure and evolution of the lipase superfamily. *J Lipid Res* **33**:167, 1992.
18. Winkler FK, D'Arcy A, Huzinkas W: Structure of human pancreatic lipase. *Nature* **343**:771, 1990.
19. Wong H, Davis RC, Nikazy J, Seebart KE, Schotz MC: Domain exchange: Characterization of a chimeric lipase of hepatic lipase and lipoprotein lipase. *Proc Natl Acad Sci U S A* **88**:11290, 1991.
20. Davis RC, Wong H, Nikazy J, Wang K, Han QQ, Schotz MC: Chimeras of hepatic lipase and lipoprotein lipase. Domain localization of enzyme-specific properties. *J Biol Chem* **267**:21499, 1992.
21. Dichek HL, Parrott C, Ronan R, Brunzell JD, Brewer HB, Santamarina-Fojo S: Functional characterization of chimeric lipase genetically engineered from human lipoprotein lipase and human hepatic lipase. *J Lipid Res* **34**:1393, 1993.
22. Dugi KA, Dichek HL, Santamarina-Fojo S: Human hepatic and lipoprotein lipase: The loop covering the catalytic site mediates lipase substrate specificity. *J Biol Chem* **270**:25396, 1995.
23. Kobayashi J, Applebaum-Bowden DM, Dugi KA, Brown DR, Kashyap VS, Parrott C, Duarte C, et al: Analysis of protein structure-function in vivo: Adenovirus-mediated transfer of lipase lid mutants in hepatic lipase-deficient mice. *J Biol Chem* **272**:26296, 1996.
24. Iverius P-H, Ostlund-Lindqvist A-M: Lipoprotein lipase from bovine milk. *J Biol Chem* **251**:7791, 1976.
25. Peterson J, Fujimoto WY, Brunzell JD: Human lipoprotein lipase: Relationship of activity, heparin affinity, and conformation as studied with monoclonal antibodies. *J Lipid Res* **33**:1165, 1992.
26. Olivecrona T, Bengtsson G, Osborne JC Jr.: Molecular properties of lipoprotein lipase: Effects of limited trypsin digestion on molecular weight and secondary structure. *Eur J Biochem* **124**:629, 1982.
27. Sparkes RS, Zollner S, Klisak I, Kirchgessner TG, Komaromy MC, Mohandas T, Schotz MC, Lusis AJ: Human genes involved in lipolysis of plasma lipoproteins: Mapping of loci for lipoprotein lipase to 8p22 and hepatic lipase to 15q21. *Genomics* **1**:138, 1987.
28. Deeb SS, Peng RL: Structure of the human lipoprotein lipase gene [published erratum appears in *Biochemistry* **28**:6786, 1989]. *Biochemistry* **28**:4131, 1989.
29. Enerbäck S, Bjursell G: Genomic organization of the region encoding guinea pig lipoprotein lipase; Evidence for exon fusion and unconventional splicing. *Gene* **84**:391, 1989.
30. Kirchgessner TG, Chuat JC, Heinzman C, Etienne J, Guilhot S, Svenson K, Ameis D et al: Organization of the human lipoprotein gene and evolution of the lipase family. *Proc Natl Acad Sci U S A* **86**:9647, 1989.
31. Wion KL, Kirchgessner TG, Lusis AJ, Schotz MC, Lawn RM: Human lipoprotein lipase complementary DNA sequence. *Science* **235**:1638, 1987.
32. Senda M, Oka K, Brown WV, Qasba PK, Furushi Y: Molecular cloning and sequence of a cDNA coding for bovine lipoprotein lipase. *Proc Natl Acad Sci U S A* **84**:4369, 1987.
33. Semb H, Olivecrona T: Lipoprotein lipase in guinea pig tissues. *Biochim Biophys Acta* **878**:330, 1986.
34. Ranganathan G, Ong JM, Yukht A, Saghizadeh M, Simsolo RB, Pauer A, Kern PA: Tissue-specific expression of human lipoprotein lipase. Effect of the 3′-untranslated region on translation. *J Biol Chem* **270**:7149, 1995.
35. Yukht A, Davis RC, Ong JM, Ranganathan G, Kern PA: Regulation of lipoprotein lipase translation by epinephrine in 3T3-L1 cells. Importance of the 3′ untranslated region. *J Clin Invest* **96**:2438, 1995.
36. Poehlman ET, Desprès J-P, Marcotte M, Tremblay A, Theriault G, Bouchard C: Genotype dependency of adaptation in adipose tissue metabolism after short-term overfeeding. *Am J Physiol* 250:E480, 1986.
37. Kuusi T, Kesaniemi YA, Vuoristo M, Miettinen TA, Koskenvuo M: Inheritance of high-density lipoprotein and lipoprotein lipase and hepatic lipase activity. *Arteriosclerosis* **7**:421, 1987.
38. Borensztajn J: Heart and skeletal muscle lipoprotein lipase, in: Borensztajn J (ed): *Lipoprotein Lipase*, Chicago, Evener Publishers, 1987, p 133.
39. Ben-Zeev O, Lusis AJ, LeBoeuf RC, Nikazy J, Schotz MC: Evidence for independent genetic regulation of heart and adipose lipoprotein lipase activity. *J Biol Chem* **258**:13632, 1983.
40. Yang WS, Nevin DN, Peng R, Brunzell JD, Deeb SS: A mutation in the promoter of the lipoprotein lipase gene in a patient with familial combined hyperlipidemia and low LDL activity. *Proc Natl Acad Sci U S A* **92**:4462, 1995.
41. Yang WS, Deeb SS: Sp1 and Sp3 transactivate the human lipoprotein lipase gene promoter: Synergy with the sterol response element binding protein and reduced transactivation of a naturally occurring promoter variant. *J Lipid Res* **39**:2054, 1998.
42. Tanuma Y, Nakabayashi H, Esumi M, Endo H: A silencer element for the lipoprotein lipase gene promoter and cognate double- and single-stranded DNA-binding proteins. *Mol Cell Biol* **15**:517, 1995.
43. Enerbäck S, Ohlsson BG, Samuelsson L, Bjursell G: Characterization of the human lipoprotein lipase (LPL) promoter: Evidence of two *cis*-regulatory regions, LP-alpha and LP-beta, of importance for the differentiation-linked induction of the LPL gene during adipogenesis. *Mol Cell Biol* **12**:4622, 1992.
44. Schoonjans K, Staels B, Devos P, Szpirer J, Szpirer C, Deeb SS, Verhoeven G, Auwerx J: Developmental extinction of liver lipoprotein lipase mRNA expression might be regulated by an NF-1-like site. *FEBS Lett* **329**:89, 1993.
45. Shimano H, Horton JD, Hammer RE, Shimomura I, Brown MS, Goldstein JL: Overproduction of cholesterol and fatty acids causes massive liver enlargement in transgenic mice expressing truncated SREBP-1a. *J Clin Invest* **98**:1575, 1996.
46. Bennett MK, Lopez JM, Sanchez HB, Osborne TF: Sterol regulation of fatty acid synthase promoter. Coordinate feedback regulation of two major lipid pathways. *J Biol Chem* **270**:25578, 1995.
47. Lopez JM, Bennett MK, Sanchez HB, Rosenfeld JM, Osborne TE: Sterol regulation of acetyl coenzyme A carboxylase: A mechanism for coordinate control of cellular lipid. *Proc Natl Acad Sci U S A* **93**:1049, 1996.

48. Schoonjans K, Peinado-Onsurbe J, Lefebvre AM, Heyman RA, Briggs M, Deeb SS, Staels B, Auwerx J: PPARalpha and PPARgamma activators direct a distinct tissue-specific transcriptional response via a PPRE in the lipoprotein lipase gene. *EMBO J* **15**:5336, 1996.
49. Enerbäck S, Semb H, Bengtsson-Olivecrona G, Carlsson P, Hermansson M-L, Olivecrona T, Bjursell G: Molecular cloning and sequence analysis of cDNA encoding lipoprotein lipase of guinea pig. *Gene* **58**:1, 1987.
50. Yang C-Y, Gu Z-W, Yang H-X, Rohde MF, Gotto AM Jr, Pownall HJ: Structure of bovine milk lipoprotein lipase. *J Biol Chem* **264**:16822, 1989.
51. Faustinella F, Smith LC, Semenkovich CF, Chan L: Structural and functional roles of highly conserved serines in human lipoprotein lipase. *J Biol Chem* **266**:9481, 1991.
52. Emmerich J, Beg OU, Peterson J, Previato L, Brunzell JD, Brewer HB Jr, Santamarina-Fojo S: Human lipoprotein lipase: Analysis of the catalytic triad by site-directed mutagenesis of Ser-132, Asp-156, and His-241. *J Biol Chem* **267**:4161, 1992.
53. Persson B, Bengtsson-Olivecrona G, Enerbäck S, Olivecrona T, Jörnvall H: Structural features of lipoprotein lipase. Lipase family relationships, binding interactions, non-equivalence of lipase cofactors, vitellogenin similarities and functional subdivision of lipoprotein lipase. *Eur J Biochem* **179**:39, 1989.
54. Datta S, Luo C-C, Li W-H, VanTuinen P, Ledbetter DH, Brown MA, Chen S-H et al: Human hepatic lipase: Cloned cDNA sequence, restriction fragment length polymorphisms, chromosomal localization, and evolutionary relationships with lipoprotein lipase and pancreatic lipase. *J Biol Chem* **263**:1107, 1988.
55. Persson B, Jörnvall H, Olivecrona T, Bengtsson-Olivecrona G: Lipoprotein lipases and vitellogenins in relation to the known three-dimensional structure of pancreatic lipase. *FEBS Lett* **288**:33, 1991.
56. Cooper DA, Stein JC, Strieleman PJ, Bensadoun A: Avian adipose lipoprotein lipase: cDNA sequence and reciprocal regulation of mRNA levels in adipose and heart. *Biochim Biophys Acta* **1008**:92, 1989.
57. Bengtsson-Olivecrona G, Olivecrona T, Jörnvall H: Lipoprotein lipase from cow, guinea-pig and man: Structural characterization and identification of protease-sensitive internal regions. *Eur J Biochem* **161**:281, 1986.
58. Semenkovich CF, Luo C-C, Nakanishi MK, Chen S-H, Smith LC, Chan L: In vitro expression and site-specific mutagenesis of the cloned human lipoprotein lipase gene: Potential N-linked glycosylation site asparagine 43 is important for both enzyme activity and secretion. *J Biol Chem* **265**:5429, 1990.
59. Babirak SP, Iverius P-H, Fujimoto WY, Brunzell JD: Detection and characterization of the heterozygote state for lipoprotein lipase deficiency. *Arteriosclerosis* **9**:326, 1989.
60. Liu M-S, Ma Y, Hayden MR, Brunzell JD: Mapping of the epitope on lipoprotein lipase recognized by a monoclonal antibody (5D2) which inhibits lipase activity. *Biochim Biophys Acta* **1128**:113, 1992.
61. Clarke AR, Luscombe M, Holbrook JJ: The effect of chain length of heparin on its interaction with lipoprotein lipase. *Biochim Biophys Acta* **747**:130, 1983.
62. Klinger MM, Margolis RU, Margolis RK: Isolation and characterization of the heparan sulfate proteoglycans of brain. Use of affinity chromatography on lipoprotein lipase-agarose. *J Biol Chem* **260**:4082, 1985.
63. Hoogewerf AJ, Cisar LA, Evans DC, Bensadoun A: Effect of chlorate on the sulfation of lipoprotein lipase and heparan sulfate proteoglycans. Sulfation of heparan sulfate proteoglycans affects lipoprotein lipase degradation. *J Biol Chem* **266**:16564, 1991.
64. Pedersen ME, Cohen M, Schotz MC: Immunocytochemical localization of the functional fraction of lipoprotein lipase in the perfused heart. *J Lipid Res* **24**:512, 1983.
65. Olivecrona T, Bengtsson-Olivecrona G, Osborne JC Jr, Kempner ES: Molecular size of bovine lipoprotein lipase as determined by radiation inactivation. *J Biol Chem* **280**:6888, 1985.
66. Cupp M, Bensadoun A, Melford K: Heparin decreases the degradation rate of lipoprotein lipase in adipocytes. *J Biol Chem* **262**:6383, 1987.
67. Cheng C-F, Oosta GM, Bensadoun A, Rosenberg RD: Binding of lipoprotein lipase to endothelial cells in culture. *J Biol Chem* **256**:12893, 1981.
68. Wallinder LA, Peterson J, Olivecrona T, Bengtsson-Olivecrona G: Hepatic and extrahepatic uptake of intravenously injected lipoprotein lipase. *Biochim Biophys Acta* **795**:513, 1984.
69. Scow RO, Desnuelle P, Verger R: Lipolysis and lipid movement in a membrane model. Action of lipoprotein lipase. *J Biol Chem* **254**:6456, 1979.
70. Saxena U, Klein MG, Goldberg IJ: Identification and characterization of the endothelial cell surface lipoprotein lipase receptor. *J Biol Chem* **266**:17516, 1991.
71. Robinson DS, Parkin SM, Speake BK, Little JA: Hormonal control of rat adipose tissue lipoprotein lipase activity, in: Angel A, Hollenberg CH, Roncari DAK (eds): *The Adipocyte and Obesity: Cellular and Molecular Mechanisms*, New York, Raven Press, 1983, p 127.
72. Ailhaud G, Ez-Zoubir A, Etienne J, Negrel R, Vannier C: Development and maturation of lipoprotein lipase in cultured adipose cells, in: Freysz L, Dreyfus H, Massarelli R, Gatt S (eds): *Enzymes of Lipid Metabolism II*, New York, Plenum Publishing, 1986, p 485.
73. Garfinkel AS, Schotz MC: Lipoprotein lipase, in: Gotto AM Jr. (ed): *Plasma Lipoproteins*, Amsterdam, Elsevier Science, 1987, p 335.
74. Stein O, Stein Y, Friedman G, Chajek-Shaul T: Lipoprotein lipase, synthesis and regulation, in: Schlierf G, Morl H (eds): *Expanding Horizons in Atherosclerosis Research*, Berlin, Springer-Verlag, 1987, p 204.
75. Semb H, Peterson J, Tavernier J, Olivecrona T: Multiple effects of tumor necrosis factor on lipoprotein lipase in vivo. *J Biol Chem* **262**:8390, 1987.
76. Busca R, Pujana MA, Pognone P, Auwerx J, Deeb SS, Reina M, Vilaro S: Absence of N-glycosylation at asparagine 43 in human lipoprotein lipase induces its accumulation in the rough endoplasmic reticulum and alters this cellular compartment. *J Lipid Res* **36**:939, 1995.
77. Jonasson L, Hansson GK, Bondjers G, Bengtsson G, Olivecrona T: Immunohistochemical localization of lipoprotein lipase in human adipose tissue. *Atherosclerosis* **51**:313, 1984.
78. Pykalisto OJ, Smith PH, Brunzell JD: Determinants of human adipose tissue LPL. *J Clin Invest* **56**:1108, 1975.
79. Taskinen M-R, Nikkila EA: Lipoprotein lipase of adipose tissue and skeletal muscle in human obesity: Response to glucose and to semistarvation. *Metabolism* **30**:810, 1981.
80. Sadur CN, Eckel RH: Insulin stimulation of adipose tissue lipoprotein lipase: Use of the euglycemic clamp technique. *J Clin Invest* **69**:1119, 1982.
81. Yki-Jarvinen H, Taskinen M-R, Koivisto VA, Nikkila EA: Response of adipose tissue lipoprotein lipase activity and serum lipoproteins to acute hyperinsulinemia in man. *Diabetologia* **27**:364, 1984.
82. Brunzell JD, Schwartz RS, Eckel RH, Goldberg AP: Insulin and adipose tissue lipoprotein lipase in humans. *Int J Obes Relat Metab Disord* **5**:685, 1981.
83. Speake BK, Parkin SM, Robinson DS: Degradation of lipoprotein lipase in rat adipose tissue. *Biochim Biophys Acta* **840**:419, 1985.
84. Havel RJ, Kane JP, Kashyap ML: Interchange of apolipoproteins between chylomicrons and high-density lipoproteins during alimentary lipemia in man. *J Clin Invest* **52**:32, 1973.
85. Jackson RL, Tajima S, Yamamura T, Yokoyama S, Yamamoto A: Comparison of apolipoprotein C-II deficient triacylglycerol-rich lipoproteins and trioleoylglycerol/phosphatidylcholine-stabilized particles as substrates for lipoprotein lipase. *Biochim Biophys Acta* **875**:211, 1986.
86. Greenwood MRC: The relationship of enzyme activity to feeding behavior in rats: Lipoprotein lipase as the metabolic gatekeeper. *Int J Obes Relat Metab Disord* **9**:67, 1985.
87. Eckel RH: Adipose tissue lipoprotein lipase, in: Borensztajn J (ed): *Lipoprotein Lipase*, Chicago, Evener Publishers, 1987, p 79.
88. Schwartz RS, Brunzell JD: Increase of adipose tissue lipoprotein lipase activity with weight loss. *J Clin Invest* **67**:1425, 1981.
89. Taskinen M-R, Nikkila EA: Basal and postprandial lipoprotein lipase activity in adipose tissue during caloric restriction and refeeding. *Metabolism* **36**:625, 1987.
90. Eckel RH, Jost TJ: Weight reduction increases adipose tissue lipoprotein lipase responsiveness in obese women. *J Clin Invest* **80**:992, 1987.
91. Kern PA, Ong JM, Saffari B, Carty J: The effects of weight loss on the activity and expression of adipose-tissue lipoprotein lipase in very obese humans. *N Engl J Med* **322**:1053, 1990.
92. Magill P, Rao SN, Miller NE, Nicoll AM, Brunzell JD, St. Hilaire RJ, Lewis B: Relationships between the metabolism of high-density and very low-density lipoproteins in man: Studies of apolipoprotein kinetics and adipose tissue lipoprotein lipase activity. *Eur J Clin Invest* **12**:113, 1982.
93. Taskinen M-R: Lipoprotein lipase in hypertriglyceridemiasin: Borensztajn J (ed): *Lipoprotein Lipase*, Chicago, Evener, 1987, p 201.
94. Pagano M-O, Havekes L, Terpstra J, Frolich M, VanGent CM, Jansen H: Diurnal changes in serum triglycerides as related to changes in lipolytic enzymes, apolipoproteins and hormones in normal subjects on a carbohydrate-rich diet. *Eur J Clin Invest* **13**:301, 1983.

95. Brunzell JD, Hazzard WR, Porte D Jr, Bierman EL: Evidence for a common saturable triglyceride removal mechanism for chylomicrons and very-low-density lipoproteins in man. *J Clin Invest* **52**:1578, 1973.
96. Olivecrona T, Bengtsson-Olivecrona G: Lipoprotein lipase from milk—The model enzyme in lipoprotein lipase research, in: Borensztajn J (ed): *Lipoprotein Lipase*, Chicago, Evener, 1987, p 149.
97. Scow RO, Chernick SS: Role of lipoprotein lipase during lactation, in: Borensztajn J (ed): *Lipoprotein Lipase*, Chicago, Evener Publishers, 1987, p 149.
98. Kawakami M, Pekala PH, Lane MD, Cerami A: Lipoprotein lipase suppression in 3T3-L1 cells by an endotoxin-induced mediator from exudate cell. *Proc Natl Acad Sci U S A* **79**:912, 1982.
99. Kern PA: Potential role of TNFa and lipoprotein lipase as candidate genes for obesity. *J Nutr* **127**:1917S, 1997.
100. Felts JM, Itakura H, Crane RT: The mechanism of assimilation of constituents of chylomicrons, very-low-density lipoproteins, and remnants—A new theory. *Biochem Biophys Res Commun* **66**:1467, 1975.
101. Beisiegel U, Weber W, Bengtsson-Olivecrona G: Lipoprotein lipase enhances the binding of chylomicrons to low-density lipoprotein receptor-related protein. *Proc Natl Acad Sci U S A* **88**:8342, 1991.
102. Williams KJ, Petrie KA, Brocia RW, Swenson TL: Lipoprotein lipase modulates net secretory output of apolipoprotein B in vitro. A possible pathophysiologic explanation for familial combined hyperlipidemia. *J Clin Invest* **88**:1300, 1991.
103. Nikkila EA, Taskinen M-R, Kekki M: Relation of plasma high-density lipoprotein cholesterol to lipoprotein-lipase activity in adipose tissue and skeletal muscle of man. *Atherosclerosis* **29**:497, 1978.
104. Brinton EA, Eisenberg S, Breslow JL: Elevated high density lipoprotein cholesterol levels correlate with decreased apo A-I and apo A-II fractional catabolic rate in women. *J Clin Invest* **84**:262, 1989.
105. Glaser DS, Yost TJ, Eckel RH: Preheparin lipoprotein lipolytic activities: Relationship to plasma lipoproteins and postheparin lipolytic activities. *J Lipid Res* **33**:209, 1992.
106. Goldberg IJ, Kandel JJ, Blum CB, Ginsberg HN: Association of plasma lipoproteins with post-heparin lipase activity. *J Clin Invest* **78**:1523, 1986.
107. Vilella E, Joven J, Fernandez M, Vilaro S, Brunzell JD, Olivecrona T, Bengtsson-Olivecrona G: Lipoprotein lipase in human plasma is mainly inactive and associated with cholesterol-rich lipoproteins. *J Lipid Res* **34**:1555, 1993.
108. Zambon A, Schmidt I, Beisiegel U, Brunzell JD: Dimeric lipoprotein lipase is bound to triglyceride-rich plasma lipoproteins. *J Lipid Res* **37**:2394, 1996.
109. Schmidt I, Brunzell JD: 2000.(Submitted)
110. Williams KJ, Tabas I: The response-to-retention hypothesis of early atherogenesis. *Arterioscler Thromb Vasc Biol* **15**:551, 1995.
111. Ross R: The pathogenesis of atherosclerosis: A perspective for the 1990s. *Nature* **362**:801, 1993.
112. Schwenke DC, Carew TE: Initiation of atherosclerotic lesions in cholesterol-fed rabbits. II. Selective retention of LDL vs. selective increases in LDL permeability in susceptible sites of arteries. *Arteriosclerosis* **9**:908, 1989.
113. Schwenke DC, Carew TE: Initiation of atherosclerotic lesions in cholesterol-fed rabbits. I. Focal increases in arterial LDL concentration precede development of fatty streak lesions. *Arteriosclerosis* **9**:895, 1989.
114. Camejo G, Hurt-Camejo E, Olsson U, Bondjers G: Proteoglycans and lipoproteins in atherosclerosis. *Arteriosclerosis* **4**:385, 1993.
115. Rutledge JC, Goldberg IJ: Lipoprotein lipase (LPL) affects low-density lipoprotein (LDL) flux through vascular tissue: Evidence that LPL increases LDL accumulation in vascular tissue. *J Lipid Res* **35**:1152, 1994.
116. Corey JE, Zilversmit DB: Effect of cholesterol feeding on arterial lipolytic activity in the rabbit. *Atherosclerosis* **27**:201, 1977.
117. Williams KJ, Fless GM, Petrie KA, Snyder ML, Brocia RW, Swenson TL: Mechanisms by which lipoprotein lipase alters cellular mechanism of lipoprotein(a), low-density lipoprotein, and nascent lipoproteins. *J Biol Chem* **267**:13284, 1992.
118. Tabas I, Li Y, Brocia RW, Xu SW, Swenson TL, Williams KJ: Lipoprotein lipase and sphingomyelinase synergistically enhance the association of atherogenic lipoproteins with smooth muscle cells and extracellular matrix. A possible mechanism for low-density lipoprotein and lipoprotein(a) retention and macrophage foam cell formation. *J Biol Chem* **268**:20419, 1993.
119. Wight TN, Curwen KD, Litrenta MM, Alonso DR, Minick CR: Effect of endothelium on glycosaminoglycan accumulation in injured rabbit aorta. *Am J Pathol* **113**:156, 1983.
120. Hoff HF, Wagner WD: Plasma low-density lipoprotein accumulation in aortas of hypercholesterolemic swine correlates with modifications in aortic glycosaminoglycan composition. *Atherosclerosis* **258**:9086, 1994.
121. Cardoso LE, Mourao PA: Glycosaminoglycan fractions from human arteries presenting diverse susceptibilities to atherosclerosis have different binding affinities to plasma LDL. *J Biol Chem* **258**:9086, 1994.
122. O'Brien KD, Gordon D, Deeb SS, Ferguson M, Chait A: Lipoprotein lipase is synthesized by macrophage-derived foam cells in human coronary atherosclerotic plaques. *J Clin Invest* **89**:1544, 1992.
123. Ylä-Herttuala S, Lipton BA, Rosenfeld ME, Goldberg IJ, Steinberg D, Witztum JL: Macrophages and smooth muscle cells express lipoprotein lipase in human and rabbit atherosclerotic lesions. *Proc Natl Acad Sci U S A* **88**:10143, 1991.
124. O'Brien KD, Deeb SS, Ferguson M, McDonald TO, Allen MD, Alpers CE, Chait A: Apolipoprotein E localization in human coronary atherosclerotic plaques by in situ hybridization and immunohistochemistry and comparison with lipoprotein lipase. *Am J Pathol* **144**:538, 1994.
125. Auerbach BJ, Bisgaier CL, Wolle J, Saxena U: Oxidation of low-density lipoproteins greatly enhances their association with lipoprotein lipase anchored to endothelial cell matrix. *J Biol Chem* **271**:1329, 1996.
126. Saxena U, Ferguson E, Auerbach BJ, Bisgaier CL: Lipoprotein lipase facilitates very-low-density lipoprotein binding to the subendothelial cell matrix. *Biochem Biophys Res Commun* **194**:769, 1993.
127. Saxena U, Auerbach BJ, Ferguson E, Wolle J, Marcel YL, Weisgraber KH, Hegele RA, Bisgaier CL: Apolipoprotein B and E basic amino acid clusters influence low-density lipoprotein association with lipoprotein lipase anchored to the subendothelial matrix. *Arterioscler Thromb Vasc Biol* **15**:1240, 1995.
128. Williams SE, Inoue I, Tran H, Fry GL, Pladet MW, Iverius P-H, Lalouel J-M et al: The carboxyl-terminal domain of lipoprotein lipase binds to the low-density lipoprotein receptor-related protein/alpha 2-macroglobulin receptor (LRP) and mediates binding of normal very-low-density lipoproteins to LRP. *J Biol Chem* **269**:8653, 1994.
129. Lindqvist P, Ostlund-Lindqvist A-M, Witztum JL, Steinberg D, Little JA: The role of LPL in the metabolism of TG-rich lipoproteins by macrophages. *J Biol Chem* **258**:9086, 1998.
130. Aviram M, Lund-Katz S, Phillips MC, Chait A: The influence of the triglyceride content of low-density lipoprotein on the interaction of apolipoprotein B-100 with cells. *J Biol Chem* **263**:16842, 1988.
131. Rumsey SC, Obunike JC, Arad Y, Deckelbaum RJ, Goldberg IJ: Lipoprotein lipase-mediated uptake and degradation of low-density lipoprotein by fibroblasts and macrophages. *J Clin Invest* **90**:1504, 1992.
132. Mulder M, Lombardi P, Jansen H, van Berkel TJC, Frants RR, Havekes LM: Low-density lipoprotein receptor internalizes low-density and very-low-density lipoproteins that are bound to heparan sulfate proteoglycans via lipoprotein lipase. *J Biol Chem* **268**:9369, 1993.
133. Schissel SL, Tweedie-Hardman J, Rapp JH, Graham G, Williams KJ, Tabas I: Rabbit aorta and human atherosclerotic lesions hydrolyze the sphingomyelin of retained low-density lipoprotein. Proposed role for arterial-wall sphingomyelinase in subendothelial retention and aggregation of atherogenic lipoproteins. *J Clin Invest* **98**:1455, 1996.
134. Kounnas MZ, Chappell DA, Strickland DK, Agraves WS: Glycoprotein 330, a member of the low-density lipoprotein receptor family, binds lipoprotein lipase in vitro. *J Biol Chem* **268**:14176, 1993.
135. Takahashi S, Suzuki J, Kohno M, Oida K, Tamai T, Miyabo S, Yamamoto T, Nakai T: Enhancement of the binding of triglyceride-rich lipoproteins to the very-low-density lipoprotein receptor by apolipoprotein E and lipoprotein lipase. *J Biol Chem* **270**:15747, 1995.
136. Luoma J, Hiltunen T, Sarkioja T, Moestrup SK, Gliemann J, Kodama T, Nikkari T, Ylä-Herttuala S: Expression of alpha 2-macroglobulin receptor/low-density lipoprotein receptor-related protein and scavenger receptor in human atherosclerotic lesions. *J Clin Invest* **93**:2014, 1994.
137. Lupu F, Heim D, Bachmann F, Kruithof EK: Expression of LDL receptor-related protein/alpha 2-macroglobulin receptor in human normal and atherosclerotic arteries. *Arterioscler Thromb* **14**:1438, 1994.
138. Rapp JH, Lespine A, Hamilton RL, Colyvas N, Chaumeton AH, Tweedie-Hardman J, Kotite L et al: Triglyceride-rich lipoproteins isolated by selected-affinity anti-apolipoprotein B *immunosorption* from human atherosclerotic plaque. *Arterioscler Thromb* **14**:1767, 1994.

139. Chung BH, Tallis G, Yalamoori V, Anantharamaiah GM, Segrest JP: Liposome-like particles isolated from human atherosclerotic plaques are structurally and compositionally similar to surface remnants of triglyceride-rich lipoproteins. *Arterioscler Thromb* **14**:622, 1994.
140. Medh JD, Bowen SL, Fry GL, Ruben S, Andracki M, Inoue I, Lalouel J-M et al: Lipoprotein lipase binds to low-density lipoprotein receptors and induces receptor-mediated catabolism of very low-density lipoproteins in vitro. *J Biol Chem* **271**:17073, 1996.
141. Lookene A, Groot NB, Kastelein J, Olivecrona G, Bruin T: Mutation of tryptophan residues in lipoprotein lipase. Effects on stability, immunoreactivity, and catalytic properties. *J Biol Chem* **272**:766, 1997.
142. Weinstock PH, Bisgaier CL, Aalto-Setälä K, Radner H, Ramakrishnan R, Levak-Frank S, Essenburg AE, Zechner R: Severe hypertriglyceridemia, reduced high-density lipoprotein, and neonatal death in lipoprotein lipase knockout mice. *J Clin Invest* **96**:2555, 1995.
143. Levak-Frank S, Weinstock PH, Hayek T, Verdery R, Hofmann W, Ramakrishnan R, Sattler W, et al: Induced mutant mice expressing lipoprotein lipase exclusively in muscle have subnormal triglycerides yet reduced high-density lipoprotein cholesterol levels in plasma. *J Biol Chem* **272**:17182, 1997.
144. Merkel M, Weinstock PH, Chajek-Shaul T, Radner H, Yin B, Breslow JL, Goldberg IJ: Lipoprotein lipase expression exclusively in liver: A mouse model for metabolism in the neonatal period and during cachexia. *J Clin Invest* **102**:893, 1998.
145. Weinstock PH, Levak-Frank S, Hudgins LC, Radner H, Friedman JM, Zechner R, Breslow JL: Lipoprotein lipase controls fatty acid entry into adipose tissue, but fat mass is preserved by endogenous synthesis in mice deficient in adipose tissue lipoprotein lipase. *Genetics* **94**:10261, 1997.
146. Ullrich NFE, Purnell JQ, Brunzell JD: Adipose tissue fatty acid composition in humans with lipoprotein lipase deficiency: Evidence for increased fatty acid synthesis as a source for maintaining adipose tissue stores. 2000 (submitted).
147. Peeva E, Brun LD, Ven Murthy MR, Despres JP, Normand T, Gagne C, Lupien PJ, Julien P: Adipose cell size and distribution in familial lipoprotein lipase deficiency. *Int J Obes Relat Metab Disord* **16**:737, 1992.
148. Jackson CL, Bruns GA, Breslow JL: Isolation and sequence of a human apolipoprotein C-II cDNA clone and its use to isolate and map to human chromosome 19 the gene for apolipoprotein C-II. *Proc Natl Acad Sci U S A* **81**:2945, 1984.
149. Das HK, Jackson CL, Miller DA, Leff T, Breslow JL: The human apolipoprotein C-II gene sequence contains a novel chromosome 19-specific mini-satellite in its third intron. *J Biol Chem* **262**:4787, 1987.
150. Humphries SE, Berg K, Gill L, Cumming AM, Robertson FW, Stalenhoef AFH, Williamson R, Borresen A-L: The gene for apolipoprotein C-II is closely linked to the gene for apolipoprotein E on chromosome 19. *Clin Genet* **26**:389, 1984.
151. Luo C-C, Li W-H, Moore MN, Chan L: Structure and evolution of the apolipoprotein multigene family. *J Mol Biol* **187**:325, 1986.
152. Wei C-F, Tsao Y-K, Robberson DL, Gotto AM Jr, Brown K, Chan L: The structure of the human apolipoprotein C-II gene: Electron microscopic analysis of RNA:DNA hybrids, complete nucleotide sequence, and identification of 5′ homologous sequences among apolipoprotein genes. *J Biol Chem* **260**:15211, 1985.
153. Fojo SS, Taam L, Fairwell T, Ronan R, Bishop C, Meng MS, Hoeg JM, et al: Human preproapolipoprotein C-II: Analysis of major plasma isoforms. *J Biol Chem* **261**:9591, 1986.
154. Wang C-S: Structure and functional properties of apolipoprotein C-II. *Prog Lipid Res* **30**:253, 1991.
155. de Silva HV, Lauer SJ, Wang J, Simonet WS, Weisgraber KH, Mahley RW, Taylor JM: Overexpression of human apolipoprotein C-III in transgenic mice results in an accumulation of apolipoprotein B48 remnants that is corrected by excess apolipoprotein E. *J Biol Chem* **269**:2324, 1994.
156. Aalto-Setälä K, Weinstock PH, Bisgaier CL, Wu L, Smith JD, Breslow JL: Further characterization of the metabolic properties of triglyceride-rich lipoproteins from human and mouse apo C-III transgenic mice. *J Lipid Res* **37**:1802, 1996.
157. Goldberg IJ, Scheraldi CA, Yacoub LY, Saxena U, Bisgaier CL: Lipoprotein apo C-II activation of lipoprotein lipase: Modulation by apolipoprotein A-IV. *J Biol Chem* **265**:4266, 1990.
158. Beaumont JL, Carlson LA, Cooper GR, Fejfar Z, Fredrickson DS, Strasser T: Classification of hyperlipidemias and hyperlipoproteinemias. *Bull World Health Organ* **43**:891, 1970.
159. Brunzell JD, Bierman EL: Chylomicronemia syndrome. Interaction of genetic and acquired hypertriglyceridemia. *Med Clin North Am* **66**:455, 1982.
160. Brunzell JD, Schrott HG: The interaction of familial and secondary causes of hypertriglyceridemia: Role in pancreatitis. *Trans Assoc Am Physicians* **86**:245, 1973.
161. Cameron JL, Capuzzi DM, Zuidema GD, Margolis S: Acute pancreatitis with hyperlipidemia: The incidence of lipid abnormalities in acute pancreatitis. *Ann Surg* **177**:483, 1973.
162. Farmer RG, Winkelman EI, Brown HB, Lewis LA: Hyperlipoproteinemia and pancreatitis. *Am J Med* **54**:161, 1973.
163. Greenberger NJ, Hatch FT, Drummey GD, Isselbacher KJ: Pancreatitis and hyperlipemia: A study of serum lipid alterations in 25 patients with acute pancreatitis. *Medicine* **45**:161, 1966.
164. Howard JM, Ehrlich E, Spitzer JJ, Singh LM: Hyperlipemia in patients with acute pancreatitis. *Ann Surg* **160**:210, 1964.
165. Fallat RW, Vestor JW, Glueck CJ: Suppression of amylase activity by hypertriglyceridemia. *JAMA* **225**:1331, 1973.
166. Lesser PB, Warshaw AL: Diagnosis of pancreatitis masked by hyperlipemia. *Ann Intern Med* **82**:795, 1975.
167. Warshaw AL, Bellini CA, Lesser PB: Inhibition of serum and urine amylase activity in pancreatitis with hyperlipemia. *Ann Surg* **182**:72, 1975.
168. Parker F, Bagdade JD, Odland GF, Bierman EL: Evidence for the chylomicron origin of lipids accumulating in diabetic eruptive xanthomas: A correlative lipid biochemical, histochemical and electron microscopic study. *J Clin Invest* **49**:2172, 1970.
169. Chait A, Robertson HT, Brunzell JD: Chylomicronemia syndrome in diabetes mellitus. *Diabetes Care* **4**:343, 1981.
170. Kuo PT, Whereat AF, Horowitz O: The effect of lipemia upon coronary and peripheral arterial circulation in patients with essential hyperlipemia. *Am J Med* **26**:68, 1959.
171. Talbot GD, Frayser R: Hyperlipidaemia: A cause of decreased oxygen saturation. *Nature* **200**:684, 1963.
172. Ditzel J, Dyerberg J: Hyperlipoproteinemia, diabetes, and oxygen affinity of hemoglobin. *Metabolism* **26**:141, 1977.
173. Robertson HT, Chait A, Hlastala MP, Brunzell JD: Red cell oxygen affinity in severe hypertriglyceridemia. *Proc Soc Exp Biol Med* **159**:437, 1978.
174. Shah PC, Patel AR, Rao KR: Hyperlipemia and spuriously elevated hemoglobin levels. *Ann Intern Med* **82**:382, 1975.
175. Simons LA, Williams PF, Turtle JR: Type V hyperlipoproteinemia revisited: Findings in a Sydney population. *Aust N Z J Med* **5**:210, 1975.
176. Steffes MW, Freier EF: A simple and precise method of determining true sodium, potassium and chloride concentrations in hyperlipemia. *J Lab Clin Med* **88**:683, 1976.
177. Harlan WR Jr, Winesett PS, Wasserman AJ: Tissue lipoprotein lipase in normal individuals and in individuals with exogenous hypertriglyceridemia and the relationship of this enzyme to assimilation of fat. *J Clin Invest* **46**:239, 1967.
178. Brunzell JD, Iverius P-H, Scheibel MS, Fujimoto WY, Hayden MR, McLeod R, Frohlich JJ: Primary lipoprotein lipase deficiency, in: Angel A, Frohlich J (eds): *Lipoprotein Deficiency Syndromes*, New York, Plenum Press, 1986, p 227.
179. Langlois S, Deeb SS, Brunzell JD, Kastelein JJP, Hayden MR: A major insertion accounts for a significant proportion of mutations underlying human lipoprotein lipase deficiency. *Proc Natl Acad Sci U S A* **86**:948, 1989.
180. Nikkila EA: Familial lipoprotein lipase deficiency and related disorders of chylomicron metabolism, in: Stanbury JB, Wyngaarden JB, Fredrickson DS, Goldstein JL. Brown MS (eds): *The Metabolic Basis of Inherited Disease*, 5th ed. New York, McGraw-Hill, 1983, p 622.
181. Fredrickson DS, Goldstein JL, Brown MS: The familial hyperlipoproteinemias, in: Stanbury JB, Wyngaarden JB, Fredrickson DS (eds): *The Metabolic Basis of Inherited Disease*, 4th ed. New York, McGraw-Hill, 1978, p 604.
182. Lees RS, Wilson DE, Schoenfeld G, Fleet S: The familial dyslipoproteinemias, in: Steinberg AG, Bearn AG (eds): *Progress in Medical Genetics*, New York, Grune and Stratton, 1973, p 237.
183. Ma Y, Liu M-S, Ginzinger D, Frohlich J, Brunzell JD, Hayden MR: Gene-environment interaction in the conversion of a mild to severe phenotype in a patient homozygous for a Ser^{172}-Cys mutation in the lipoprotein lipase gene. *J Clin Invest* **91**:1953, 1993.
184. Berger GMB, Spark A, Baillie PM, Huskisson J, Stockwell G, Van der Merwe E: Absence of serum-stimulated lipase activity and altered lipid content in milk from a patient with type I hyperlipoproteinemia. *Pediatric Res* **17**:835, 1983.
185. Watts GF, Morton K, Jackson P, Lewis B: Management of patients with severe hypertriglyceridemia during pregnancy: Report of two cases with familial lipoprotein lipase deficiency. *Br J Obstet Gynaecol* **99**:163, 1992.

186. Steiner G, Myher JJ, Kuksis A: Milk and plasma lipid composition in a lactating patient with type I hyperlipoproteinemia. *Am J Clin Nutr* **41**:121, 1985.
187. Benlian P, DeGennes JL, Foubert L, Zhang H, Gagne SE, Hayden M: Premature atherosclerosis in patients with familial chylomicronemia caused by mutations in the lipoprotein lipase gene. *N Engl J Med* **335**:848, 1996.
188. Bergeron J, Normand T, Bharucha A, Ven Murthy MR, Julien P, Gagné C, Dionne C, et al: Prevalence, geographical distribution and genealogical investigations of mutation 188 of lipoprotein lipase gene in the French Canadian population of Quebec. *Clin Genet* **41**:206, 1992.
189. Devlin RH, Deeb SS, Brunzell JD, Hayden MR: Partial gene duplication involving exon-Alu interchange results in lipoprotein lipase deficiency. *Am J Hum Genet* **46**:112, 1990.
190. Brunzell JD: Lipoprotein lipase deficiency and other causes of the chylomicronemia syndrome, in: Scriver CR, Beaudet AL, Sly WS, Valle D (eds): *The Metabolic and Molecular Bases of Inherited Disease* 7th ed. New York, McGraw-Hill, 1995, p 1913.
191. Brunzell JD, Deeb SS, Ling RO: www.crc.washington.edu/lipase.htm (Lipoprotein lipase and hepatic lipase gene variants), 1998.
192. Hata A, Robertson M, Emi M, Lalouel J-M: Direct detection and automated sequencing of individual alleles after electrophoretic strand separation: Identification of a common nonsense mutation in exon 9 of the human lipoprotein lipase gene. *Nucleic Acids Res* **18**:5407, 1990.
193. Derewenda ZS, Cambillau C: Effects of gene mutations in lipoprotein and hepatic lipases as interpreted by a molecular model of the pancreatic triglyceride lipase. *J Biol Chem* **266**:23112, 1991.
194. Reymer PWA, Groenemeyer BE, Gagne E, Miao L, Appelman EE, Seidel JC, Kromhout D, et al: A frequently occurring mutation in the lipoprotein lipase gene (Asn291Ser) contributes to the expression of familial combined hyperlipidemia. *Hum Mol Genet* **4**:1543, 1995.
195. Busca R, Pienado J, Vilella E, Auwerx J, Deeb SS, Vilaro S, Reina M: The mutant Asn^{291}(rho)Ser human lipoprotein lipase is associated with reduced catalytic activity and does not influence binding to heparin. *FEBS Lett* **367**:257, 1995.
196. Wittekoek ME, Pimstone SN, Reymer PW, Feuth L, Botma GJ, Defesche JC, Prins M, et al: A common mutation in the lipoprotein lipase gene (N291S) alters the lipoprotein phenotype and risk for cardiovascular disease in patients with familial hypercholesterolemia. *Circulation* **97**:729, 1998.
197. Hokanson JE: Lipoprotein lipase gene variants and risk of coronary disease: a quantitative analysis of population-based studies. *Int J Clin Lab Res* **27**:24, 1997.
198. Kuivenhoven JA, Groenemeyer BE, Boer JM, Reymer PW, Berghuis R, Bruin T, Jansen H, et al: Ser447stop mutation in lipoprotein lipase is associated with elevated HDL cholesterol levels in normolipidemic males. *Arterioscler Thromb Vasc Biol* **17**:595, 1997.
199. Previato L, Guardamagna O, Dugi KA, Ronan R, Talley GD, Santamarina-Fojo S, Brewer HB Jr. A novel missense mutation in the C-terminal domain of lipoprotein lipase (Glu410 → Val) leads to enzyme inactivation and familial chylomicronemia. *J Lipid Res* **35**:1552, 1994.
200. Kozaki K, Gotoda T, Kawamura M, Shimano H, Yazaki Y, Ouchi Y, Orimo H, Yamada N: Mutational analysis of human lipoprotein lipase by carboxy-terminal truncation. *J Lipid Res* **34**:1765, 1993.
201. Groenemeyer BE, Hallman MD, Reymer PW, Gagne E, Kuivenhoven JA, Bruin T, Jansen H, et al: Genetic variant showing a positive interaction with beta-blocking agents with a beneficial influence on lipoprotein lipase activity, HDL cholesterol, and triglyceride levels in coronary artery disease patients. The Ser447-stop substitution in the lipoprotein lipase gene. REGRESS Study Group. *Circulation* **95**:2628, 1997.
202. Yang WS, Nevin DN, Iwasaki L, Peng R, Brown BG, Brunzell JD, Deeb SS: Regulatory mutations in the human lipoprotein lipase gene in patients with familial combined hyperlipidemia and coronary artery disease. *J Lipid Res* **37**:2627, 1996.
203. Ehrenborg E, Clee SM, Pimstone SN, Reymer PWA, Benlian P, Hoogendijk CF, Davis HJ, et al: Ethnic variation and in vivo effects of the —93— >g promoter variant in the lipoprotein lipase gene. *Arterioscler Thromb Vasc Biol* **17**:2672, 1997.
204. Mailly F, Tugrul Y, Reymer PWA, Bruin T, Seed M, Groenemeyer BF, Asplund-Carlson A, et al: A common variant in the gene for lipoprotein lipase (Asp9 → Asn): functional implications and prevalence in normal and hyperlipidemic subjects. *Arterioscler Thromb Vasc Biol* **15**:468, 1995.
205. Kastelein JJ, Groenemeyer BE, Hallman DM, Henderson H, Reymer PW, Gagne SE, Jansen H, et al: The Asn9 variant of lipoprotein lipase is associated with the −93G promoter mutation and an increased risk of coronary artery disease. The Regress Study Group. *Clin Genet* **53**:27, 1998.
206. Brunzell JD: Lipoprotein lipase deficiency and other causes of the chylomicronemia syndrome, in: Scriver CR, Beuadel AL, Sly WS, Valle D (eds): *The Metabolic Basis of Inherited Disease*, 6th ed. New York, McGraw-Hill, 1989, p 1165.
207. Chait A, Brunzell JD: Very-low-density lipoprotein kinetics in familial forms of hypertriglyceridemia, in: Berman M, Grundy S, Howard B (eds): *Lipoprotein Kinetics and Modeling*, New York, Academic Press, 1982, p 69.
208. Zambon A, Torres A, Bijvoet S, Gagne C, Moorjani S, Lupien PJ, Hayden MR, Brunzell JD et al: Prevention of raised low density lipoprotein cholesterol in a patient with familial hypercholesterolaemia and lipoprotein lipase deficiency. *Lancet* **341**:1119, 1993.
209. Brunzell JD, Chait A, Nikkila EA, Ehnholm C, Huttunen JK, Steiner G: Heterogeneity of primary lipoprotein lipase deficiency. *Metabolism* **29**:624, 1980.
210. Chait A, Iverius P-H, Brunzell JD: Lipoprotein lipase secretion by human monocyte-derived macrophages. *J Clin Invest* **69**:490, 1982.
211. Skarlatos SI, Dichek HL, Fojo SS, Brewer HB, Kruth HS: Absence of triglyceride accumulation in lipoprotein lipase-deficient human monocyte-macrophages incubated with human very-low-density lipoprotein. *J Clin Endocrinol Metab* **76**:793, 1993.
212. Ikeda Y, Takagi A, Ohkaru Y, Nogi K, Iwanaga T, Kurooka S, Yamamoto A: A sandwich-enzyme immunoassay for the quantification of lipoprotein lipase and hepatic triglyceride lipase in human postheparin plasma using monoclonal antibodies to the corresponding enzymes. *J Lipid Res* **31**:1911, 1990.
213. Henderson HE, Ma Y, Hassan MF, Monsalve MV, Winkler FK, Gubernator K, Marais AD, et al: Amino acid substitution (Ile194 - Thr) in exon 5 of the lipoprotein lipase deficiency in three probands support for a multicenteric origin. *J Clin Invest* **87**:2005, 1991.
214. Dichek HL, Fojo SS, Beg OU, Skarlatos SI, Brunzell JD, Cutler GB, Brewer HB: Identification of two separate allelic mutations in the lipoprotein lipase gene of a patient with the familial hyperchylomicronemic syndrome. *J Biol Chem* **266**:473, 1991.
215. Hata A, Ridinger DN, Sutherland SD, Emi M, Kwong LK, Shuhua J, Lubbers A, et al: Missense mutations in exon 5 of the human lipoprotein lipase gene. Inactivation correlates with loss of dimerization. *J Biol Chem* **267**:20132, 1992.
216. Beg OU, Meng MS, Skarlatos SI, Previato L, Brunzell JD, Brewer HB Jr, Fojo SS: Lipoprotein lipase Bethesda: A single amino acid substitution (Ala176 - Thr) leads to abnormal heparin binding and loss of enzymatic activity. *Proc Natl Acad Sci U S A* **87**:3474, 1990.
217. Emi M, Wilson DE, Iverius P-H, Wu LL, Hata A, Hegele R, Williams RR, Lalouel J-M: Missense mutation (Gly-Glu188) of human lipoprotein lipase imparting functional deficiency. *J Biol Chem* **265**:5910, 1990.
218. Fager G, Semb H, Enerbäck S, Olivecrona T, Jonasson L, Bengtsson-Olivecrona G, Camejo G, et al: Hyperlipoproteinemia type I in a patient with active lipoprotein lipase in adipose tissue and indications of defective transport of the enzyme. *J Lipid Res* **31**:1187, 1990.
219. Burton BK, Nadler HL: Primary type I hyperlipoproteinemia with normal lipoprotein lipase activity. *J Pediatr* **90**:777, 1977.
220. Goldberg IJ, Paterniti JR Jr, Franklin BH, Ginsberg HN, Ginsberg-Fellner F, Brown WV: Transient lipoprotein lipase deficiency with hyperchylomicronemia. *Am J Med Sci* **286**:28, 1983.
221. Horst A, Paluszak J, Zawilska K, Sobisz S: Three variants of postheparin lipoprotein lipase activity in idiopathic hyperlipoproteinemia. *Bull Acad Pol Sci Biol* **21**:199, 1973.
222. Rouis M, Dugi KA, Previato L, Patterson AP, Brunzell JD, Brewer HB, Santamarina-Fojo S: Therapeutic response to medium-chain triglycerides and omega-3 fatty acids in a patient with the familial chylomicronemia syndrome. *Arterioscler Thromb Vasc Biol* **17**:1400, 1997.
223. Gagnë C, Brun D, Moorjani S, Lupien PJ: Familial hyperchylomicronemia: Study of lipolytic activity in a family. *Union Med Can* **106**:333, 1977.
224. Wilson DE, Edward CQ, Chan I-F: Phenotypic heterogeneity in the extended pedigree of a proband with lipoprotein lipase deficiency. *Metabolism* **32**:1107, 1983.
225. Fellin R, Baggio G, Poli A, Augustin J, Baiocchi MR, Baldo G, Sinigaglia M, et al: Familial lipoprotein lipase and apolipoprotein C-II deficiency: Lipoprotein and apoprotein analysis, adipose tissue and hepatic lipoprotein lipase levels in seven patients and their first degree relatives. *Atherosclerosis* **49**:55, 1983.

226. Kondo Y, Kurobane I, Omura K, Sano R, Abe R, Chida N, Tada K: Postheparin plasma lipoprotein lipase activity in heterozygotes of familial lipoprotein lipase deficiency. *Tohoku J Exp Med* **145**:1, 1985.
227. Potter JM, MacDonald WB: Primary type I hyperlipoproteinaemia: A metabolic and family study. *Aust N Z J Med* **9**:688, 1979.
228. Bijvoet S, Gagne SE, Moorjani S, Gagne C, Henderson HE, Fruchart J, Dallongville J, et al: Alterations in plasma lipoproteins and apolipoproteins before the age of 40 in heterozygotes for lipoprotein lipase deficiency. *J Lipid Res* **37**:640, 1996.
229. Sprecher DL, Harris BV, Stein EA, Bellet PS, Keilson LM, Simbartl LA: Higher triglycerides, lower high-density lipoprotein cholesterol, and higher systolic blood pressure in lipoprotein lipase-deficient heterozygotes: A preliminary report. *Circulation* **94**:3239, 1996.
230. Nordestgaard BG, Abildgaard S, Wittrup HH, Steffensen R, Jensen G, Tybjaerg-Hansen A: Heterozygous lipoprotein lipase deficiency: Frequency in the general population, effect on plasma lipid levels, and risk ischemic heart disease. *Circulation* **96**:1737, 1997.
231. Miesenbock G, Holzl B, Foger B, Brandstatter E, Paulweber B, Sandhofer F, Patsch JR: Heterozygous lipoprotein lipase deficiency due to a missense mutation as the cause of impaired triglyceride tolerance with multiple lipoprotein abnormalities. *J Clin Invest* **91**:448, 1993.
232. Auwerx J, Marzetta CA, Hokanson JE, Brunzell JD: Large-buoyant LDL-like particles in hepatic lipase deficiency. *Arteriosclerosis* **9**:319, 1989.
233. Hokanson JE, Brunzell JD, Jarvik GP, Wijsman EM, Austin MA: Linkage of low-density lipoprotein size to the lipoprotein lipase gene in heterozygous lipoprotein lipase deficiency. *Am J Hum Genet* **64**:608, 1999.
234. Wilson DE, Emi M, Iverius P-H, Hata A, Wu LL, Hillas E, Williams RR, Lalouel J-M: Phenotypic expression of heterozygous lipoprotein lipase deficiency in the extended pedigree of a proband homozygous for a missense mutation. *J Clin Invest* **86**:735, 1990.
235. Zhang H, Reymer PWA, Liu M, Forsythe IJ, Groenemeyer BE, Frolich J, Brunzell JD, et al: Patients with apo E3 deficiency (E2/2, E3/2, and E4/2) who manifest with hyperlipidemia have increased frequency of an ASN291SER mutation in the human LPL gene. *Arterioscler Thromb Vasc Biol* **15**:1695, 1995.
236. Knudsen P, Murtomaki S, Antikainen M, Ehnholm S, Lahdenpera S, Enholm C, Taskinen M-R: The Asn-291 → Ser and Ser-477 → stop mutations of the lipoprotein lipase gene and their significance for lipid metabolism in patients with hypertriglyceridaemia. *Eur J Clin Invest* **27**:928, 1997.
237. De Bruin TWA, Mailly F, Van Barlingen HHJJ, Fisher R, Castro M, Cabezas P, Talmud P, et al: Lipoprotein lipase gene mutations D9N and N291S in four pedigrees with familial combined hyperlipidaemia. *Eur J Clin Invest* **26**:631, 1996.
238. Hoffer MJV, Bredie SJH, Boomsma DI, Reymer PWA, Kastelein JJP, de Knijff P, Demacker PNM, et al: The lipoprotein lipase (Asn291 → - Ser) mutation is associated with elevated lipid levels in families with familial combined hyperlipidaemia. *Atherosclerosis* **119**:159, 1996.
239. Greene HL, Swift LL, Knapp HR: Hyperlipidemia and fatty acid composition in patients treated for type IA glycogen storage disease. *J Pediatr* **119**:398, 1991.
240. Babirak S, Brown BG, Brunzell JD: Familial combined hyperlipidemia and abnormal lipoprotein lipase. *Arterioscler Thromb* **12**:1176, 1992.
241. Nevin DN, Brunzell JD, Deeb SS: The lipoprotein lipase gene in individuals with familial combined hyperlipidemia and decreased lipoprotein lipase activity. *Arterioscler Thromb* **14**:869, 1994.
242. Gagne E, Genest J Jr, Zhang H, Clark LA, Hayden MR: Analysis of DNA changes in the LPL gene in patients with familial combined hyperlipidemia. *Arterioscler Thromb* **14**:1250, 1994.
243. Hoffer MJV, Bredie SJH, Boomsma D, Reymer PWA, Kastelein JJP, deKnijff P, Demacker PNM, et al: The lipoprotein lipase (Asn291Ser) mutation is associated with elevated lipid levels in families with familial combined hyperlipidemia. *Atherosclerosis* **119**:159, 1995.
244. Deeb SS, Nevin DN, Iwasaki L, Brunzell JD: Two novel apolipoprotein A-IV variants in individuals with familial combined hyperlipidemia and diminished levels of lipoprotein lipase activity. *Hum Mutat* **8**:319, 1996.
245. Nilsson-Ehle P: Measurements of lipoprotein lipase activity, in: Borensztajn J (ed): *Lipoprotein Lipase*, Chicago, Evener Publishers, 1987, p 59.
246. Iverius P-H, Ostlund-Lindqvist A-M: Preparation, characterization and measurement of lipoprotein lipase. *Methods Enzymol* **129**:691, 1986.
247. Bierman EL, Brunzell JD, Bagdade JD, Lerner RL, Hazzard WR, Porte D Jr: On the mechanism of action of Atromid-S on triglyceride transport in man. *Trans Assoc Am Physicians* **83**:211, 1970.
248. Excoffon KJ, Liu G, Miao L, Wilson JE, McManus BM, Semenkovich CF, Coleman T, et al: Correction of hypertriglyceridemia and impaired fat tolerance in lipoprotein lipase-deficient mice by adenovirus-mediated expression of human lipoprotein lipase. *Arterioscler Thromb Vasc Biol* **17**:2532, 1997.
249. Zsigmond E, Kobayashi K, Tzung KW, Li L, Fuke Y, Chan L: Adenovirus-mediated gene transfer of human lipoprotein lipase ameliorates the hyperlipidemias associated with apolipoprotein E and LDL receptor deficiencies in mice. *Hum Gene Ther* **8**:1921, 1997.
250. Levy RI, Fredrickson DS: Familial hyperlipoproteinemia, in: Stanbury JB, Wyngaarden JB, Fredrickson DS (eds): *The Metabolic Basis of Inherited Disease*, 3rd ed. New York, McGraw-Hill, 1972, p 545.
251. Santamarina-Fojo S: Genetic dyslipoproteinemias: Role of lipoprotein lipase and apolipoprotein C-II. *Curr Opin Lipidol* **3**:186, 1992.
252. Xiong WJ, Li W-H, Posner I, Yamamura T, Yamamoto A, Gotto AM Jr, Chang L: No severe bottleneck during human evolution: Evidence from two apolipoprotein C-II deficiency alleles. *Am J Hum Genet* **48**:383, 1991.
253. Miller NE, Rao SN, Alaupovic P, Noble N, Slack J, Brunzell JD, Lewis B: Familial apolipoprotein C-II deficiency: Plasma lipoproteins and apolipoproteins in heterozygous and homozygous subjects and the effects of plasma infusion. *Eur J Clin Invest* **11**:69, 1981.
254. Hegele RA, Breckenridge WC, Cox DW, Maguire GF, Little JA, Connelly PW: Interaction between variant apolipoproteins C-II and E that affects plasma lipoprotein concentrations. *Arterioscler Thromb* **11**:1303, 1991.
255. Sepehrnia B, Kamboh MI, Adams-Campbell LL, Bunker CH, Nwankwo M, Majumder PP, Ferrell RE: Genetic studies of human apolipoproteins. XI: The effect of the apolipoprotein C-II polymorphism on lipoprotein levels in Nigerian Blacks. *J Lipid Res* **30**:1349, 1989.
256. Ghiselli G, Schaefer J, Zech LA, Gregg RE, Brewer HB Jr: Increased prevalence of apolipoprotein E_4 in type V hyperlipoproteinemia. *J Clin Invest* **70**:474, 1982.
257. Wardell MR, Rall SC Jr, Brennan SO, Nye ER, George PM, Janus ED, Weisgraber KH: Apolipoprotein E2-Dunedin (228 Arg - Cys): An apolipoprotein E2 variant with normal receptor-binding activity. *J Lipid Res* **31**:535, 1990.
258. Baggio G, Manzato E, Gabelli C, Fellin R, Martini S, Enzi GB, Verlato F, et al: Apolipoprotein C-II deficiency syndrome. Clinical features, lipoprotein characterization, lipase activity, and correction of hypertriglyceridemia after apolipoprotein C-II administration in two affected patients. *J Clin Invest* **77**:520, 1986.
259. Brunzell JD, Auwerx JH, Babirak SP, Deeb SS, Fujimoto WY, Hayden MR: Familial lipoprotein lipase deficiency, in: Gotto AM Jr, Manzaro E (eds): *Atherosclerosis VIII*, New York, Excerpta Medica, 1989, p 265.
260. Catapano AL, Mills GL, Roma P, La Rosa M, Capurso A: Plasma lipids, lipoproteins and apoproteins in a case of apo C-II deficiency. *Clin Chim Acta* **130**:317, 1983.
261. Fallat RW, Glueck CJ: Familial and acquired type V hyperlipoproteinemia. *Atherosclerosis* **23**:41, 1976.
262. Greenberg BH, Blackwelder WC, Levy RI: Primary type V hyperlipoproteinemia. A descriptive study in 32 families. *Ann Intern Med* **87**:526, 1977.
263. Brunzell JD, Schrott HG, Motulsky AG, Bierman EL: Myocardial infarction in the familial forms of hypertriglyceridemia. *Metabolism* **25**:313, 1976.
264. Chait A, Brunzell JD: Severe hypertriglyceridemia: Role of familial and acquired disorders. *Metabolism* **32**:209, 1983.
265. Brunzell JD, Chait A: Lipoprotein pathophysiology and treatment, in: Rifkin H, Porte D Jr (eds): *Ellenberg and Rifkin's Diabetes Mellitus*, 4th ed. New York, Elsevier Science, 1990, p 756.
266. Zhang Q, Cavallero E, Hoffmann MM, Cavanna J, Kay A, Charles A, Braschi S, et al: Mutations at the lipoprotein lipase gene locus in subjects with diabetes mellitus, obesity and lipaemia. *Clin Sci* **93**:335, 1997.
267. Applebaum-Bowden D, Kobayashi J, Kashyap VS, Brown DR, Berard A, Meyn S, Parrott C, et al: Hepatic lipase gene therapy in hepatic lipase-deficient mice. Adenovirus-mediated replacement of a lipolytic enzyme to the vascular endothelium. *J Clin Invest* **97**:799, 1996.
268. Jensen GL, Daggy B, Bensadoun A: Triacylglycerol lipase, monoacylglycerol lipase, and phospholipase activities of highly purified rat hepatic lipase. *Biochim Biophys Acta* **710**:464, 1982.
269. Applebaum-Bowden DM: Lipases and lecithin: Cholesterol acyltransferase in the control of lipoprotein metabolism. *Curr Opin Lipidol* **6**:130, 1995.

270. Bensadoun A, Berryman DE: Genetics and molecular biology of hepatic lipase. *Curr Opin Lipidol* **7**:77, 1996.
271. Santamarina-Fojo S, Haudenschild C, Amar M: The role of hepatic lipase in lipoprotein metabolism and atherosclerosis. *Curr Opin Lipidol* **9**:211, 1998.
272. Ben-Zeev O, Stahnke G, Liu G, Davis RC, Doolittle MH: Lipoprotein lipase and hepatic lipase: the role of asparagine-linked glycosylation in the expression of a functional enzyme. *J Lipid Res* **35**:1511, 1994.
273. Doolittle MH, Wong H, Davis RC, Schotz MC: Synthesis of hepatic lipase in liver and extrahepatic tissue. *J Lipid Res* **28**:1326, 1987.
274. Sanan DA, Fan J, Bensadoun A, Taylor JM: Hepatic lipase is abundant on both hepatocyte and endothelial cell surfaces in the liver. *J Lipid Res* **38**:1002, 1997.
275. Breedveld B, Schoonderwoerd K, Verhoeven AJ, Willemsen R, Jansen H: Hepatic lipase is localized at the parenchymal cell microvilli in rat liver. *Biochem J* **321**:425, 1997.
276. Cai S-J, Wong DM, Chen S-H, Chan L: Structure of the human hepatic lipase gene. *Biochemistry* **28**:8966, 1989.
277. Ameis D, Stahnke G, Kobayashi J, Mclean J, Lee G, Busher M, Schotz MC: Isolation and characterization of the human hepatic lipase gene. *J Biol Chem* **265**:6552, 1990.
278. Stahnke G, Sprengel R, Augustin J, Will H: Human hepatic triglyceride lipase: cDNA cloning, amino acid sequence and expression in a cultured cell line. *Differentiation* **35**:45, 1987.
279. Martin GA, Busch SJ, Meredith GD, Cardin AD, Blankenship DT, Mao SJ, Rechtin AE, et al: Isolation and cDNA sequence of human postheparin plasma hepatic triglyceride lipase. *J Biol Chem* **263**:10907, 1988.
280. Verhoeven AJM, Jansen H: Hepatic lipase mRNA is expressed in rat and human steroidogenic organs. *Biochim Biophys Acta* **1211**:121, 1994.
281. Brown G, Albers JJ, Fisher LD, Schaefer SM, Lin J-T, Kaplan C, Zhao X-Q, et al: Regression of coronary artery disease as a result of intensive lipid-lowering therapy in men with high levels of apolipoprotein B. *N Engl J Med* **323**:1289, 1990.
282. Zambon A, Hokanson JE, Brown BG, Brunzell JD: Evidence for a new pathophysiological mechanism for coronary artery disease regression: Hepatic lipase-mediated changes in LDL density. *Circulation* **99**:1959, 1999.
283. Benhizia F, Lagrange D, Malewiak M-I, Griglio S: In vivo regulation of hepatic lipase activity and mRNA levels by diets which modify cholesterol influx to the liver. *Biochim Biophys Acta* **1211**:181, 1994.
284. Sultan F, Benhizia F, Lagrange D, Will H, Griglio S: Effect of dietary cholesterol on the activity and mRNA levels of hepatic lipase in rat. *Life Sci* **56**:31, 1995.
285. Busch SJ, Barnhart RL, Martin GA, Fitzgerald MC, Yates MT, Mao SJT, Thomas CE, Jackson RL: Human hepatic triglyceride lipase expression reduces high density lipoprotein and aortic cholesterol in cholesterol-fed transgenic mice. *J Biol Chem* **269**:16376, 1994.
286. Nimmo L, McColl AJ, Rosankiewicz JZ, Richmond W, Elkeles RS: Regulation of hepatic lipase expression in HepG2 cells. *Biochem Soc Trans* 25:S689, 1997.
287. Berg AL, Floren CH, Nilsson-Ehle P: Hepatic lipase secretion in the human hepatoblastoma cell line HepG2 is not related to cellular cholesterol homeostasis. *Horm Metab Res* **27**:523, 1995.
288. Applebaum DM, Goldberg AP, Pykalisto OJ, Brunzell JD, Hazzard WR: The effect of estrogen on post-heparin lipolytic activity. Selective decline in hepatic triglyceride lipase. *J Clin Invest* **59**:601, 1977.
289. Tikkanen MJ, Nikkila EA: Regulation of hepatic lipase and serum lipoproteins by sex steroids. *Am Heart J* **113**:562, 1987.
290. Brinton EA: Oral estrogen replacement therapy in postmenopausal women selectively raises levels and production rates of lipoprotein A-I and lowers hepatic lipase activity without lowering the fractional catabolic rate. *Arterioscler Thromb Vasc Biol* **16**:431, 1996.
291. Turpin G, Bruckert E, Dairou F: Substitutive hormonal treatment of menopause. Effects on lipoprotein metabolism. *Presse Med* **24**:905, 1995.
292. Kantor MA, Bianchini A, Bernier D, Sady SP, Thompson PD: Androgens reduce HDL_2-cholesterol and increase hepatic triglyceride lipase activity. *Med Sci Sports Exerc* **17**:462, 1985.
293. Applebaum-Bowden DM, Haffner SM, Hazzard WR: The dyslipoproteinemia of anabolic steroid therapy: Increase in hepatic triglyceride lipase precedes the decrease in high-density lipoprotein 2 cholesterol. *Metabolism* **36**:949, 1987.
294. Zambon A, Austin MA, Brown BG, Hokanson JE, Brunzell JD: Effect of hepatic lipase on LDL in normal men and those with coronary heart disease. *Arterioscler Thromb* **13**:147, 1993.
295. Austin MA, King M-C, Bawol RD, Hully SB, Friedman GD: Risk factors for coronary heart disease in adult female twins. Genetic heritability and shared environmental influences. *Am J Epidemiol* **125**:308, 1987.
296. Hokanson JE, Zambon A, Brunzell JD: Hepatic lipase and gender differences in dyslipidemia. *Abstracts of the 38th Annual Conference on Cardiovascular Disease Epidemiology and Prevention* 26, 1998.
297. Applebaum-Bowden DM, Haffner SM, Wahl PW, Hoover JJ, Warnick GR, Albers JJ, Hazzard WR: Postheparin plasma triglyceride lipases: relationships with very-low-density lipoprotein triglyceride and high density $lipoprotein_2$ cholesterol. *Arteriosclerosis* **5**:273, 1985.
298. Cohen JC, Wang Z, Grundy SM, Stoesz MR, Guerra R: Variation at the hepatic lipase and apolipoprotein AI/CIII/AIV loci is a major cause of genetically determined variation in plasma HDL cholesterol levels. *J Clin Invest* **94**:2377, 1994.
299. Capell WH, Zambon A, Austin MA, Brunzell JD, Hokanson JE: Compositional differences of low density lipoprotein particles in normal subjects with LDL subclass A and LDL subclass B. *Arterioscler Thromb Vasc Biol* **16**:1040, 1996.
300. Hokanson JE, Zambon A, Capell WH, Brunzell JD: Small, dense LDL is associated with low lipoprotein lipase and high hepatic lipase activities, and alterations in IDL and VLDL composition. *Atherosclerosis* **134**:25, 1997.
301. Katzel LI, Coon PJ, Busby J, Gottlieb SO, Krauss RM, Goldberg AP: Reduced HDL_2 cholesterol subspecies and elevated postheparin lipase activity in older men with abdominal obesity and asymptomatic myocardial ischemia. *Arterioscler Thromb* **12**:814, 1992.
302. Brunzell JD, Hokanson JE: Dyslipidemia of central obesity and insulin resistance. *Diabetes Care* **22 (Suppl 3)**:C10, 1999.
303. Després J-P, Ferland M, Moorjani S, Nadeau A, Tremblay A, Lupien PJ, Theriault G, Bouchard C: Role of hepatic-triglyceride lipase activity in the association between intra-abdominal fat and plasma HDL cholesterol in obese women. *Arteriosclerosis* **9**:485, 1989.
304. Zambon A, Deeb SS, Hokanson JE, Brown BG, Brunzell JD: Common variants in the promoter of the hepatic lipase gene are associated with lower levels of hepatic lipase activity, buoyant LDL and higher HDL_2 cholesterol. *Arterioscler Thromb Vasc Biol* **18**:1723, 1998
305. Zambon A, Hokanson JE, Brown G, Brunzell JD: Evidence for a new pathophysiological mechanism for coronary artery disease regression: Hepatic lipase mediated changes in LDL density. *Circulation* **99**:1959, 1999
306. Kuusi T, Saarinen P, Nikkila EA: Evidence for the role of hepatic endothelial lipase in the metabolism of plasma high-density lipoprotein-2 in man. *Atherosclerosis* **36**:589, 1980.
307. Cominacini L, Garbin U, Davoli A, Campagnola M, de Santis A, Pasini C, Pastorino AM, Bosello O: High-density lipoprotein cholesterol concentrations and postheparin hepatic and lipoprotein lipases in obesity: relationships with plasma insulin levels. *Ann Nutr Metab* **37**:175, 1993.
308. Blades B, Vega GL, Grundy SM: Activities of lipoprotein lipase and hepatic triglyceride lipase in postheparin plasma of patients with low concentrations of HDL cholesterol. *Arterioscler Thromb* **13**:1227, 1993.
309. Bucher KD, Friedlander Y, Kaplan EB, Namboodiri KK, Kark JD, Eisenberg S, Stein Y, Rifkind BM: Segregation analysis of low levels of high-density lipoprotein cholesterol in the collaborative Lipid Research Clinics Program Family Study. *Genet Epidemiol* **5**:17, 1988.
310. Rao DC, Laskarzewski PM, Morrison JA, Khoury P, Kelly K, Wette R, Russel J, Glueck CJ: The Cinicinnati Lipid Research Clinic family study: Cultural and biological determinants of lipids and lipoprotein concentrations. *Am J Hum Genet* **34**:888, 1982.
311. Rice T, Vogler GP, Perry TS, Laskarzewski PM, Rao DC: Familial aggregation of lipids and lipoproteins in families ascertained through random and nonrandom probands in the Minnesota Lipid Research Clinic Family Study. *Hum Hered* **41**:107, 1991.
312. Heller DA, deFaire U, Pedersen NL, Dahlen G, McClern GE: Genetic and environmental influences on serum lipid levels in twins. *N Engl J Med* **328**:1150, 1993.
313. Heller DA, Pedersen NL, deFaire U, McClern GE: Genetic and environmental correlations among serum lipids and apolipoproteins in elderly twins reared together and apart. *Am J Hum Genet* **55**:1255, 1994.
314. Daggy BP, Bensadoun A: Enrichment of apolipoprotein B48 in the LDL density class following in vivo inhibition of hepatic lipase. *Biochim Biophys Acta* **877**:252, 1986.

315. Homanics GE, de Silva HV, Osada J, Zhang SH, Wong H, Borensztajn J, Maeda N: Mild dyslipidemia in mice following targeted inactivation of the hepatic lipase gene. *J Biol Chem* **270**:2974, 1995.
316. Fan J, Wang J, Bensadoun A, Lauer SJ, Dang Q, Mahley RW, Taylor JM: Overexpression of hepatic lipase in transgenic rabbits leads to a marked reduction of plasma high density lipoproteins and intermediate density lipoproteins. *Proc Natl Acad Sci U S A* **91**:8724, 1994.
317. Krapp A, Ahle S, Kersting S, Hua Y, Kneser K, Nielsen M, Gliemann J, Beisiegel U: Hepatic lipase mediates the uptake of chylomicrons and beta-VLDL into cells via the LDL receptor-related protein (LRP). *J Lipid Res* **37**:926, 1996.
318. Huff MW, Miller DB, Wolfe BM, Connelly PW, Sawyez CG: Uptake of hypertriglyceridmic very-low-density lipoproteins and their remnants by HepG2 cells: The role of lipoprotein lipase, hepatic triglyceride lipase, and cell surface proteoglycans. *J Lipid Res* **38**:1318, 1997.
319. Ji ZS, Dichek HL, Miranda RD, Mahley RW: Heparan sulfate proteoglycans participate in hepatic lipase and apolipoprotein E-mediated binding and uptake of plasma lipoproteins, including high-density lipoproteins. *J Biol Chem* **272**:1285, 1997.
320. Dichek HL, Brecht W, Fan J, Ji ZS, McCormick SP, Akeefe H, Conzo L, et al: Overexpression of hepatic lipase in transgenic mice decreases apolipoprotein B-containing and high-density lipoproteins. Evidence that hepatic lipase acts as a ligand for lipoprotein uptake. *J Biol Chem* **273**:1896, 1998.
321. Kokoglu E, Ulakoglu E: The transport of vitamin E in plasma and its correlation to plasma lipoproteins in non-insulin-dependent diabetes mellitus. *Diabetes Res Clin Pract* **14**:175, 1991.
322. Hegele RA, Little JA, Vezina C, Maquire GF, Tu L, Woleveer TS, Jenkins DJA, Connelly, PW: Hepatic lipase deficiency. Clinical, biochemical, and molecular genetic characteristics. *Arterioscler Thromb* **13**:720, 1993.
323. Auwerx JH, Babirak SP, Hokanson JE, Stahnke G, Will H, Deeb SS, Brunzell JD: Coexistence of abnormalities of hepatic lipase and lipoprotein lipase in a large family. *Am J Hum Genet* **46**:470, 1990.
324. Demant T, Carlson LA, Holmquist L, Karpe F, Nilsson-Ehle P, Packard CJ, Shepherd J: Lipoprotein metabolism in hepatic lipase deficiency: Studies on the turnover of lipoprotein B and on the effect of hepatic lipase on high density lipoprotein. *J Lipid Res* **29**:1603, 1988.
325. Rubinstein A, Gibson JC, Paterniti JR Jr, Kakis G, Little A, Ginsberg H, Brown WV: Effect of heparin-induced lipolysis on the distribution of apolipoprotein E among lipoprotein subclasses. *J Clin Invest* **75**:710, 1985.
326. Hegele RA, Little JA, Connelly PW: Compound heterozygosity for mutant hepatic lipase in familial hepatic lipase deficiency. *Biochem Biophys Res Commun* **179**:78, 1991.
327. Hegele RA, Vezina C, Moorjani S, Lupien PJ, Gagne C, Brun LD, Little JA, Connelly PW: A hepatic lipase gene mutation associated with heritable lipolytic deficiency. *J Clin Endocrinol Metab* **72**:730, 1991.
328. Brand K, Dugi KA, Brunzell JD, Nevin DN, Santamarina-Fojo S: A novel A → G mutation in intron 1 of the hepataic lipase gene leads to alternative splicing resulting in enzyme deficiency. *J Lipid Res* **37**:1213, 1996.
329. Hegele RA, Tu L, Connelly PW: Human hepatic lipase mutations and polymorphisms. *Hum Mutat* **1**:320, 1992.
330. Connelly PW, Maguire GF, Lee M, Little JA: Plasma lipoproteins in familial hepatic lipase deficiency. *Arteriosclerosis* **10**:40, 1990.
331. Carlson LA, Holmquist L, Nilsson-Ehle P: Deficiency of hepatic lipase activity in post-heparin plasma in familial hyper-α-triglyceridemia. *Acta Med Scand* **219**:435, 1986.
332. Nevin DN, Zambon A, Brown BG, Brunzell JD: Hepatic lipase deficiency in a coronary artery disease population. *J Invest Med* **43**:172A, 1995.
333. Auwerx JH, Marzetta CA, Hokanson JE, Brunzell JD: Large buoyant LDL-like particles in hepatic lipase deficiency. *Arteriosclerosis* **9**:319, 1989.
334. Mahaney MC, Blagero J, Rainwater DL, Commuzzie AG, VandeBerg JL, Stern MP, MacCluer JW, Hixon JE: A major locus influencing plasma high-density lipoprotein cholesterol levels in the San Antonio Family Heart Study. Segregation and linkage analyses. *Arterioscler Thromb Vasc Biol* **15**:1730, 1995.
335. Guerra RG, Wang SM, Grundy SM, Cohen JC: A hepatic lipase (LIPC) allele associated with high plasma concentrations of high-density lipoprotein cholesterol. *Proc Natl Acad Sci U S A* **94**:4532, 1997.
336. Jansen H, Verhoeven AJ, Weeks L, Kastelein JJP, Halley DJJ, van den Ouweland A, Jukema JW, et al: Common C-to-T substitution at position -480 of the hepatic lipase promoter associated with a lowered HL activity in coronary artery disease patients. *Arterioscler Thromb Vasc Biol* **17**:2837, 1997.
337. Tahvanianen E, Syvanne M, Frick MH, Murtomaki-Repo S, Antikainen M, Kesaniemi YA, Kauma H, et al: Association of variation in hepatic lipase activity with promoter variation in the hepatic lipase gene. *J Clin Invest* **101**:956, 1998.
338. Murtomaki S, Tahvanianen E, Antikainen M, Tiret L, Nicaud V, Jansen H, Ehnholm C: Hepatic lipase gene polymorphism influence plasma HDL levels: Results from Finnish EARS participants. *Arterioscler Thromb Vasc Biol* **17**:1879, 1997.
339. Tyroler HA, Glueck CJ, Christiansen B, Kwiterovich PO Jr: Plasma high-density lipoprotein cholesterol comparisons in black and white populations. The Lipid Research Clinics Program Prevalence Study. *Circulation* **62**:IV99, 1980.
340. Brown SA, Hutchinson R, Morrisett J, Boerwinkle E, Davis CE, Gotto AM Jr, Patsch W: Plasma lipid, lipoprotein cholesterol, and apoprotein distribution in selected U.S. communities (ARIC) study. *Arterioscler Thromb* **13**:1139, 1993.
341. Burchfiel CM, Abbott RD, Sharp DS, Curb JD, Rodriguez BL, Yano K: Distribution and correlates of lipids and lipoproteins in elderly Japanese-American men. The Honolulu Heart Program. *Arterioscler Thromb Vasc Biol* **16**:1356, 1996.
342. Committee on Serum Lipid Level Survey 1990 in Japan: Current state of and recent trends in serum lipid levels in the general Japanese population. *Arterioscler Thromb* **2**:122, 1996.
343. Sprafka JM, Norsted SW, Folsom AR, Burke GL, Luepker RV: Life-style factors do not explain racial differences in high-density lipoprotein cholesterol: the Minnesota Heart Survey. *Epidemiology* **3**:156, 1992.
344. Vega GL, Clark LT, Tang A, Marcovina S, Grundy SM, Cohen JC: Hepatic lipase activity is lower in African American men than white American men: effect of 5′ flanking polymorphism in the hepatic lipase gene (LIPC). *J Lipid Res* **39**:228, 1998.
345. Knudsen P, Antikainen M, Ehnholm S, Uusi-Oukari M, Tenkanen H, Lahdenpera S, Kahri J, et al: A compound heterozygote for hepatic lipase gene mutations Leu334Phe and Thr383Met: Correlation between hepatic lipase activity and phenotypic expression. *J Lipid Res* **37**:825, 1996.
346. Groot PHE, van Stiphout WAHJ, Krauss XH, Jansen H, van Tol A, van Ramshorst E, Chin-On S, et al: Postprandial lipoprotein metabolism in normolipidemic men with and without coronary artery disease. *Arterioscler Thromb* **11**:653, 1991.
347. Johansson J, Nilsson-Ehle P, Carlson LA, Hamsten A: The association of lipoprotein and hepatic lipase activities with high-density lipoprotein subclass levels in men with myocardial infarction at a young age. *Atherosclerosis* **86**:111, 1991.
348. Salisbury BG, Falcone DJ, Minick CR: Insoluable low-density lipoprotein-proteoglycan complexes enhance cholesteryl ester accumulation in macrophages. *Am J Pathol* **120**:6, 1985.
349. Austin MA, King M-C, Vranizan KM, Krauss RM: Atherogenic lipoprotein phenotype. A proposed genetic marker for coronary heart disease risk. *Circulation* **82**:495, 1990.
350. Fujimoto WY, Abbate SL, Kahn SE, Hokanson JE, Brunzell JD: The visceral adiposity syndrome in Japanese-American men. *Obes Res* **2**:364, 1994.
351. Nevin DN, Schwartz RS, Kahn SE, Brunzell JD: Metabolic associations in insulin resistance syndrome: Effect of weight perturbation. *American Heart Association: 66th Scientific Sessions* 1993.
352. Fievet C, Fruchart J: HDL heterogeneity and coronary heart disease. *Diabetes Metab Rev* **7**:155, 1991.
353. Miller NE: Association of high-density lipoprotein subclasses and apolipoproteins with ischemic heart disease and coronary atherosclerosis. *Am Heart J* **113**:589, 1987.
354. Cheung MC, Brown BG, Wolf AC, Albers JJ: Altered particle size distribution of apolipoprotein A-I-containing lipoproteins in subjects with coronary artery disease. *J Lipid Res* **32**:383, 1991.
355. Johansson J, Carlson LA, Landou C, Hamsten A: High-density lipoproteins and coronary atherosclerosis. A strong inverse relation with the largest particles is confined to normotriglyceridemic patients. *Arterioscler Thromb* **11**:174, 1991.
356. Mezdour H, Jones R, Dengremont C, Castro G, Maeda N: Hepatic lipase deficiency increases plasma cholesterol but reduces susceptibility to atherosclerosis in apolipoprotein E-deficient mice. *J Biol Chem* **272**:13570, 1997.

357. Amar MJ, Vaisman BL, Foger B, Paigen B, Talley GD, Brewer HB Jr, Santamarina-Fojo S: The effect of hepatic lipase deficiency on the plasma lipids, lipoproteins and diet-induced atherosclerosis in LCAT transgenic mice. *Circulation* **96**:1, 1997.

358. Cheung MC, Wolf AC: In vitro transformation of apoA-I-containing lipoprotein subpopulations: Role of lecithin:cholesterol acyltransferase and apo B-containing lipoproteins. *J Lipid Res* **30**:499, 1989.

359. Babineau TJ, Borlase BC, Blackburn GL: Applied total parenteral nutrition in the critically ill, in: Rippe JM, Irwin RS, Alpert JS, Fink MP (eds): *Intensive Care Medicine* 2nd ed. Boston, Little, Brown, 1991, p 1675.

360. Bausserman LL, Saritelli AL, Herbert PN: Effects of short-term stanozolol administration on serum lipoproteins in hepatic lipase deficiency. *Metabolism* **46**:992, 1997.

361. Mori A, Takagi A, Ikeda Y, Ashida Y, Yamamoto A: An AvaII polymorphism in exon 5 of the human hepatic triglyceride lipase gene. *Mol Cell Probes* **10**:309, 1996.

362. Knudsen P, Antikainen M, Uusi-Oukari M, Ehnholm S, Lahdenpera S, Bensadoun A, Funke H, et al: Heterozygous hepatic lipase deficiency, due to two missense mutations R186H and L334F, in the HL gene. *Atherosclerosis* **128**:165, 1996.

CHAPTER 118

Lecithin Cholesterol Acyltransferase Deficiency and Fish Eye Disease

Silvia Santamarina-Fojo ▪ Jeffrey M. Hoeg†
Gerd Assmann ▪ H. Bryan Brewer, Jr.

1. **Lecithin cholesterol acyltransferase (LCAT) is a plasma enzyme that esterifies free cholesterol present in circulating plasma lipoproteins.**
2. **LCAT deficiency leads to the development of two clinically distinct syndromes: familial LCAT deficiency (FLD) and fish eye disease (FED).**
3. **FLD is characterized by corneal opacities, anemia, and proteinuria that may progress to renal failure. Foam cells and membrane-bound vesicles, which appear to be composed of cholesterol and phospholipid, accumulate in many tissues including the cornea, kidneys, liver, spleen, bone marrow, and arteries. Target cells containing abnormally high amounts of unesterified cholesterol and lecithin are present. Plasma contains high levels of unesterified cholesterol and phospholipids and low concentrations of plasma cholesteryl esters and lysophosphatidylcholine. Plasma triglycerides are normal to increased, low density lipoprotein (LDL) levels are reduced, and high-density lipoprotein (HDL) levels are markedly decreased. The morphology of the lipoproteins is abnormal, with the presence in plasma of multilamellar vesicles, rouleaux, LpX-like particles, discs, and small spherical particles. The diagnosis of FLD is confirmed by a virtual absence of plasma LCAT activity in patients presenting with hypoalphalipoproteinemia, anemia, proteinuria, or renal disease.**
4. **FED is characterized by corneal opacities. The plasma triglyceride levels are normal to increased, and HDL levels are markedly decreased. The diagnosis of FED is confirmed by finding a partial deficiency of LCAT activity in the plasma of patients presenting with corneal opacities and marked hypoalphalipoproteinemia.**
5. **The LCAT gene is organized into six exons interrupted by five introns and is located on the long arm of chromosome 16. Approximately 40 different mutations in the LCAT gene leading to either FLD or FED have been described to date.**
6. **Characterization of FLD and FED patients as well as different LCAT-transgenic and knockout animal models has demonstrated an important role for LCAT in modulating the metabolism of both HDLs and LDLs, as well as the development of atherosclerosis.**

LECITHIN CHOLESTEROL ACYLTRANSFERASE

History

The existence of an enzyme that esterifies cholesterol in plasma was first postulated by Sperry et al.[1] Glomset[2] provided evidence that a plasma enzyme mediated the esterification of plasma cholesterol by a mechanism that involved the transfer of fatty acids from phosphatidylcholine (PC) to free cholesterol (FC), generating cholesteryl esters (CEs) and lysophosphatidylcholine. The enzyme was termed *lecithin cholesterol acyltransferase* (LCAT).

Glomset et al.[3] first proposed a role for LCAT in reverse cholesterol transport, a process by which cholesterol from peripheral cells is transferred to the liver for catabolism. Cellular FC is taken up by high-density lipoprotein (HDL) where it is esterified by LCAT.[4] The newly generated CEs are packaged in the core of the lipoprotein, resulting in the maturation of discoidal pre-β-HDL to spherical α-HDL.[5,6] Subsequently, the CE may be exchanged for very low density lipoprotein (VLDL)-triglycerides by the cholesteryl ester transfer protein (CETP)[7,8] for transport to the liver. Alternatively, the CE may be taken up directly by the liver or steroidogenic tissues by receptor-mediated selective uptake of the neutral lipids.[9,10] Thus, by helping to maintain a concentration gradient for the diffusion of FC from peripheral cells to HDL, LCAT appears to be necessary for reverse cholesterol transport, one of several important mechanisms by which this antiatherogenic lipoprotein modulates the development of atherosclerosis.

The identification and characterization of patients with familial LCAT deficiency (FLD) and fish eye disease (FED) presenting with marked hypoalphalipoproteinemia and abnormal cholesterol and phospholipid tissue deposition by Norum and Gjone[11] and Carlson and Philipson[12] have confirmed the important role that LCAT plays in cholesterol and lipoprotein metabolism in humans.

STRUCTURE AND FUNCTION OF THE LCAT PROTEIN

Human LCAT is a 416-amino-acid glycoprotein of approximately 63 kDa, synthesized mainly by the liver.[13] The enzyme circulates in plasma reversibly bound to lipoproteins, especially HDL and LDL.[14–16] LCAT plays a major role in HDL metabolism by catalyzing the esterification of FC generating CEs and lysophosphatidylcholine (Fig. 118-1).[2,3] Human LCAT preferentially transfers an unsaturated sn-2 chain from PC to cholesterol;

†Deceased July 21, 1998.

A list of standard abbreviations is located immediately preceding the index in each volume. Additional abbreviations used in this chapter include: CE, cholesteryl ester; CETP, cholesteryl ester transfer protein; FC, free cholesterol; FED, fish eye disease; FLD, familial LCAT deficiency; LCAT, lecithin cholesterol acyltransferase; PC, phosphatidylcholine.

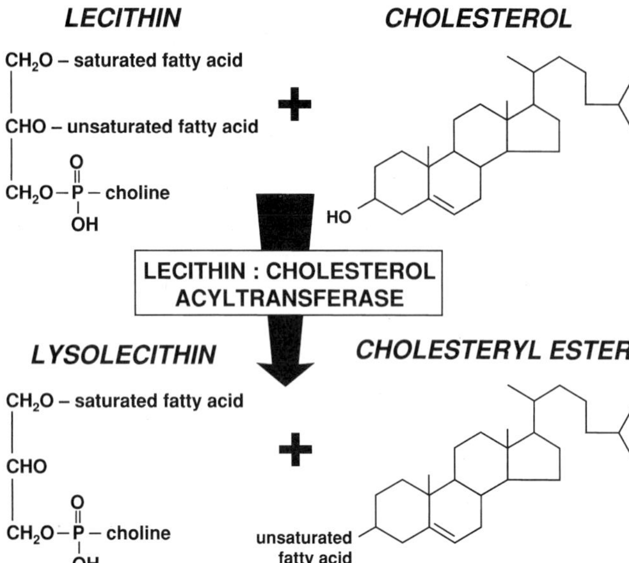

Fig. 118-1 The plasma lecithin cholesterol acyltransferase reaction.

however, the specificity of the enzyme for the phospholipid head group, the sn position or the nature of the acyl group, is not absolute.[17] The preferred lipoprotein substrates of LCAT are HDLs, which contain its major activator, apolipoprotein (apo) A-I,[18] although apo A-II, apo A-IV, apo C-II, and apo C-III also may activate the enzyme.[19]

The primary structure of LCAT is highly conserved among different species,[20–25] suggesting that the full intact protein is required for activity. The secondary and tertiary structures of LCAT have yet to be determined. However, studies involving either chemical or genetic modification of specific amino acid residues as well as molecular modeling have provided some insights into the structural domains required for normal LCAT function. Rosseneu and colleagues[26] have recently proposed a three-dimensional model for LCAT structure based on the known x-ray structures of pancreatic lipase and *Candida antarctica* lipase as well as sequence homologies to known lipases (Fig. 118-2). The model predicts a structure similar to that of the lipases containing an α/β hydrolase fold with the central LCAT domain consisting of seven conserved parallel β strands connected by four α helices and separated by loops. This model accounts for approximately 45 percent of the secondary structure of LCAT and has provided a framework for further analysis of LCAT structure–function.

By combining this molecular modeling approach[26] with site-directed mutagenesis,[26–28] the active site residues of LCAT have been identified. LCAT contains the Gly-X-Ser-X-Gly motif identified as the serine component of the active site triad in different lipases.[29,30] Strong evidence that LCAT serine 181, which lies within this motif, forms part of the active site of LCAT has been provided by chemical modification[27,28] and by the substitution of serine 181.[31] Both approaches abolished LCAT activity. The other two residues that comprise the catalytic triad of LCAT, aspartic acid 345 and histidine 377, have been identified by molecular modeling based on known lipase x-ray structures[26] and confirmed by site-directed mutagenesis.[26,32]

Another important structural domain found in lipases is a flexible helical lid that covers the active site and is displaced following substrate binding.[30] Francone et al.[31] have suggested that serine 216, which lies within a Gly-Gly-Ser motif that forms the interfacial binding site in different lipases,[29,30] may be part of this flap and thus may play a role in orienting the substrate for effective catalysis by LCAT. However, based on homology to the lipase lid, Peelman et al.[26] have proposed that the 25 amino acids spanned by a disulfide bridge between cysteines 50 and 74 represent the LCAT lid domain.[26,33] Deletion of residues 53 to 71,[17,34] as well as substitution of tryptophan 51,[26] produced mutant enzymes that retain activity against monomeric substrates, indicating that the catalytic site is intact. However, these variants are unable to bind reconstituted HDL or react with lipoprotein substrates.[26,34] Thus, similar to the lipase lid,[35,36] LCAT residues 50 to 70 appear to play an important role in mediating LCAT–substrate interaction. In separate studies, Fielding et al.[4] and Peelman et al.[26] have proposed that the putative amphipathic α helix (residues 151 to 174 of LCAT) binds to phospholipids and apo A-I in HDL. LCAT residues threonine 123 and asparagine 228 also may be important for apo A-I activation and binding of the lipid substrate to the active site.[37] Definite localization of the LCAT lid may require the elucidation of the LCAT structure by x-ray crystallography.

The functional domain responsible for conferring substrate specificity in LCAT appears to be located in the middle segment of the protein. Studies involving site-directed mutagenesis and the synthesis of a human/rat chimeric LCAT[38] have shown that residues 130 to 306 are responsible for phospholipid binding and acyl chain selectivity of LCAT. Substitution of a single residue (lysine 149 to alanine) within this region changed the selectivity of the human enzyme for PC 16:0 to 20:4 to that of the rat LCAT, thus synthesizing more 16:0 than 20:4 CEs.[39] The positional specificity of LCAT determines the generation of saturated versus unsaturated CEs, which may in turn influence the overall atherogenic risk.[38–40] In separate studies, substitution of the N-glycosylation residues, asparagine 272 as well as alanine 274, converted LCAT to a phospholipase generating fatty acids instead of CE, indicating an important role for these residues in determining the substrate specificity of the enzyme.[41,42]

These combined studies indicate that LCAT is a structurally complex enzyme consisting of multiple functional domains that are required for LCAT activity (Fig. 118-3). These include a large active site, defined by serine 181, aspartic acid 345, and histidine 377, capable of binding phospholipids and CE simultaneously. A lipid-binding lid region, encompassing residues 50 to 74, covers the active site that may participate in interfacial activation. Finally,

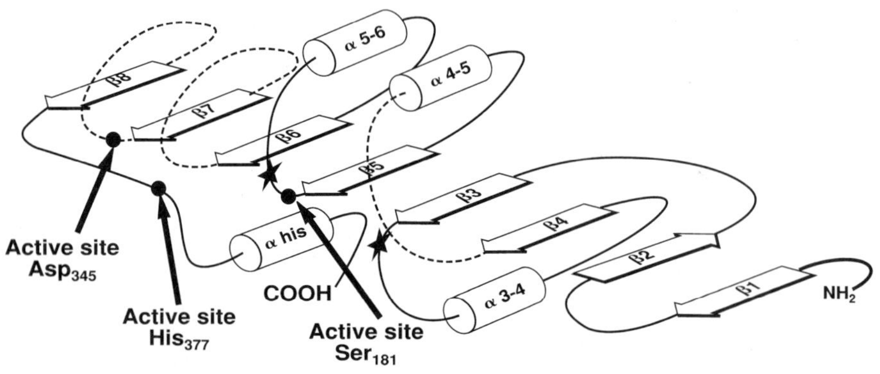

Fig. 118-2 Schematic representation of the predicted three-dimensional structure of LCAT. The α/β hydrolase fold is shown. The dots indicate the predicted location of the catalytic triad residues, and the stars indicate the predicted oxyanion residues phenylalanine 103 and leucine 182. (*Reprinted with permission from Peelman et al.*[26])

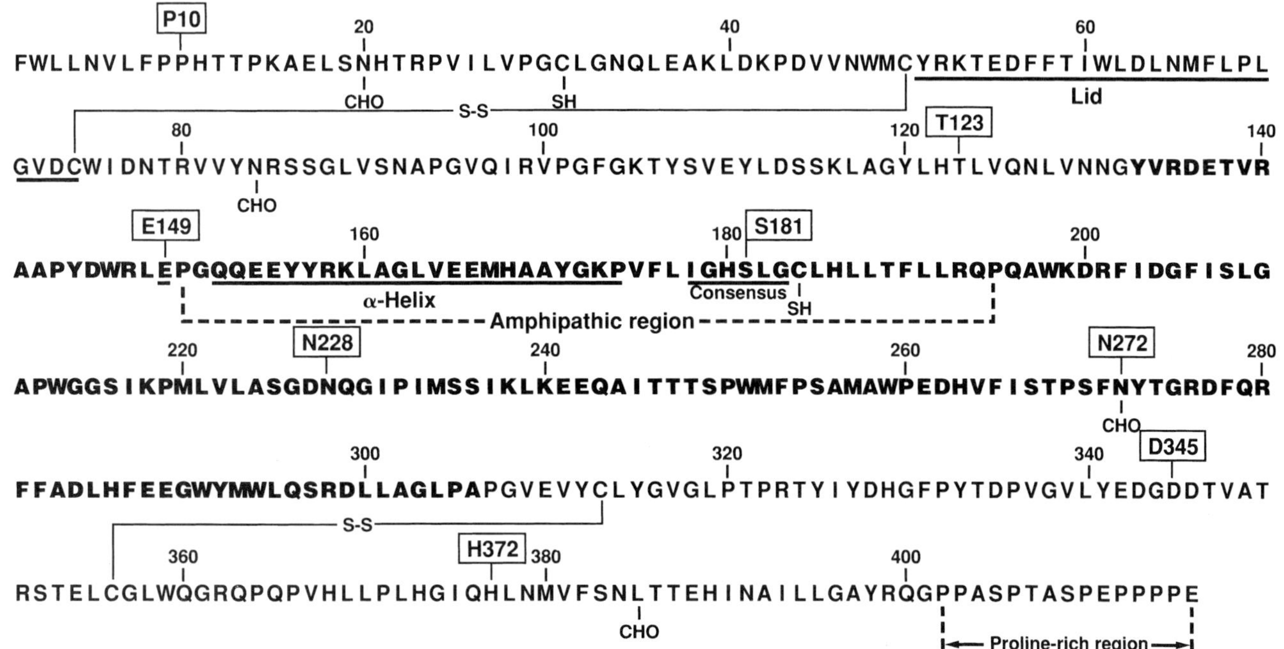

Fig. 118-3 Primary structure of human LCAT. The 416-amino-acid sequence of the mature enzyme is encoded by six exons: exon I, amino acids 1 to 27; exon II, amino acids 28 to 80; exon III, amino acids 81 to 118; exon IV, amino acids 119 to 160; exon V, amino acids 161 to 226; and exon VI, amino acids 227 to 416. The enzyme contains two disulfide bridges and three N-glycosylation sites (indicated by CHO). Residues proposed to be involved in apo A-I activation (P10, T123, and N228), PC selectivity (E149), and phospholipase/transesterase function (N272) as well as the catalytic triad residues (S181, D345, and H372) are boxed. The GXSXG active site serine motif found in lipases is underlined (consensus). Residues that may mediate the PL and acyl chain selectivity (130 to 306) are highlighted in bold. Amino acids that comprise the putative α-helix (151 to 174) that mediates binding to PL and apo A-I are indicated by the dotted line. The C-terminal proline-rich region is also shown.

a lipoprotein-binding domain, including residues 130 to 306, which may play a role in apo A-I binding as well as modulation of LCAT substrate specificity, has been defined.

LCAT activity in plasma can be measured by using either exogenous or endogenous substrates. Common exogenous substrates are radiolabeled HDL, reconstituted HDL, proteoliposomes, and vesicles containing apo A-I.[43] These provide a relative measure of LCAT-mediated cholesterol esterification in HDL. The cholesterol esterification rate, a measure of plasma LCAT activity using endogenous lipoprotein substrates, can be obtained by incubating plasma at 37°C and measuring the decrease in unesterified cholesterol.[44,45] Measurement of LCAT concentration in plasma permits the most accurate quantification of the circulating plasma enzyme.[46] Albers and colleagues[47] and Moriyama et al.[48] have reported the LCAT concentrations in normal men and women 20 to 59 years of age to be 5.49 ± 0.89 and 5.90 ± 1.06 μg/ml, respectively. In contrast, the plasma LCAT concentrations in individuals heterozygous or homozygous for LCAT deficiency are reduced (3.59 ± 0.69 and 0.73 ± 0.70 μg/ml, respectively). LCAT concentrations remain relatively stable with increasing age.[47]

LCAT GENE STRUCTURE, FUNCTION, AND REGULATION

The human LCAT gene is located on the long arm of chromosome 16 in the 16q22.1 region.[13,21,49,50] It is organized into six exons interrupted by five introns that encode the 440 amino acids, including 24 signal peptide residues, that comprise the LCAT protein. In humans and experimental animal models, LCAT is expressed primarily in the liver.[20–25,51] However, LCAT messenger RNA (mRNA) also can be detected at much lower levels in the brain and testes of mice, rabbits, and nonhuman primates.[21–23,52,53] Alternative splicing resulting in the insertion of an Alu cassette between exons 5 and 6 has been reported for both human and nonhuman primate mRNA.[54] Protein synthesis from the alternatively spliced transcripts has not been demonstrated.

Relatively little is known about the regulation of LCAT gene expression. The LCAT gene is under the control of a minimal, 71-bp promoter that includes a TATA box, two Sp1 binding sites, and an LFAI motif.[55] LCAT mRNA levels increase during embryonal development, peak at birth, and then remain constant in adult humans and rats.[21] LCAT expression appears to be fairly resistant to dietary challenges. One study observed a two- to fivefold increase in plasma LCAT activity and hepatic mRNA levels in rabbits fed a high-cholesterol diet.[25] However, most studies in humans, rabbits, and rats[21,56] have failed to demonstrate changes in LCAT expression or activity in response to high-fat and high-cholesterol diets. Plasma LCAT activity is unaffected by weight reduction in obese subjects.[57] Decreased plasma LCAT activity has been reported in patients with diabetes,[58,59] uremia,[60] and hepatobiliary obstruction.[61]

The response of LCAT gene expression and plasma levels to different hormonal and drug treatments is variable. Moderate alcohol ingestion and smoking do not affect plasma LCAT activity in humans.[62–64] Fibrates have been shown to decrease the hepatic mRNA levels by 50 percent[65] and LCAT activity by 20 percent.[66] In contrast, treatment of rats with eicosapentaenoic acid or dexamethasone[67,68] and simvastatin therapy in heterozygous familial hypercholesterolemic patients[69] increased plasma LCAT activity by 21 to 33 percent. In a separate study, probucol, simvastatin, nicotinic acid, ethinylestradiol, L-thyroxine, and hydrocortisone have been reported to have little effect on hepatic LCAT expression in rat livers.[65] As part of the acute-phase response, endotoxin and tumor necrosis factor appear to nonspecifically reduce plasma LCAT activity and hepatic mRNA levels in Syrian hamsters.[70] In vitro studies have demonstrated direct inhibition of LCAT by antihypertensive agents such as propanolol, metaprolol, prazosin, and chlorthalidone,[71] as well as diazepam[72] and cigarette smoke.[73] These combined results suggest

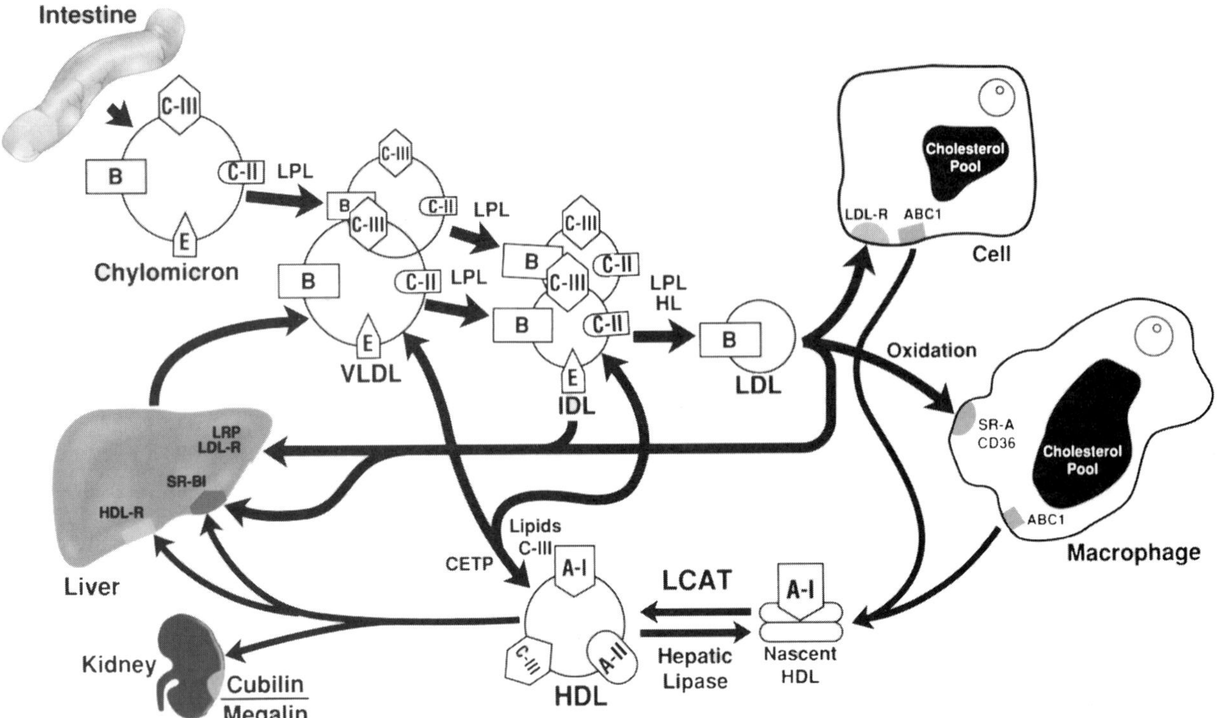

Fig. 118-4 Schematic overview of the role of LCAT in lipoprotein metabolism. Triglyceride-rich apo B–containing lipoproteins are secreted from the intestine and liver. The triglycerides on plasma lipoproteins are hydrolyzed by lipoprotein lipase (LPL) and the particles are remodeled to smaller, very low density lipoproteins (VLDLs) and finally to intermediate-density lipoproteins (IDLs). VLDLs and IDLs may be removed by the liver by the low-density lipoprotein receptor (LDL-R) and low-density lipoprotein–related protein (LRP), or the cholesterol may be selectively removed from the apo B-containing lipoproteins by the scavenger receptor BI (SR-BI). IDLs are converted to low-density lipoproteins (LDLs) by the combined action of LPL and hepatic lipase (HL). LDL is taken up by cells by LDL-R–mediated endocytosis or becomes oxidized and removed from plasma by scavenger receptor A (SRA) or CD36. Nascent HDL facilitates the removal of cellular cholesterol from peripheral cells via the newly described ABC1 transporter.[87] LCAT catalyzes the esterification of cholesterol to cholesterol esters (CEs), which is associated with the maturation of the nascent disk-shaped HDL to spherical particles. Cholesterol ester transfer protein (CETP) exchanges HDL-CE and triglycerides on apo B–containing lipoproteins. HDL-CE may be selectively taken up by SR-BI in the liver, and the major sites of catabolism of HDL are the liver and kidney.

that LCAT gene expression is relatively resistant to dietary challenges and drug treatments.

ROLE OF LCAT IN LIPOPROTEIN METABOLISM

A schematic overview of lipoprotein metabolism and the role of LCAT in cholesterol transport is shown in Fig. 118-4. Lipoprotein metabolism can be conceptually divided into two major pathways, the apo B–containing lipoprotein (apo B-Lp) and HDL pathways.[74] The apo B-Lp pathway consists of a cascade of lipoproteins containing either apo B-48 or apo B-100. The human intestine secretes triglyceride-rich apo B-48, containing chylomicrons whose major function is to transport dietary lipids from the intestine to peripheral tissues and the liver. Shortly after secretion, the triglyceride-rich chylomicrons acquire apo C-II and apo E from HDL. Apo C-II activates lipoprotein lipase, which hydrolyzes the triglycerides on chylomicrons, resulting in the formation of remnants that have a hydrated density of VLDL, and then intermediate-density lipoprotein (IDL). Chylomicron remnants are taken up by the liver primarily by the LDL and low-density lipoprotein–related protein (LRP) receptors, which have a high affinity for apo E.[75,76] The liver secretes triglyceride-rich lipoproteins containing apo B-100. Detailed kinetic and metabolic studies have established that the liver may secrete both large and small triglyceride-rich lipoproteins with a hydrated density of VLDL to IDL.[77,78] After secretion, VLDLs acquire apo E from apo E present on the proteoglycans on the surface of the hepatocyte and in the space of Disse,[79] as well as from HDL.[80] Apo C-II is also transferred from HDL to VLDL. The triglycerides on VLDL, like intestinally derived chylomicrons, undergo hydrolysis by lipoprotein lipase and VLDL and are converted to lipoproteins having the density of IDL. Some particles are further remodeled to LDL. A second lipolytic enzyme, hepatic lipase, which functions as both a phospholipase and triacylglycerol hydrolase, has been proposed to play an important role in the conversion of IDL to LDL. During the conversion to LDL, the majority of the C-II and E apolipoproteins dissociate from VLDL remnants and IDL, reassociating with HDL. The end product of the cascade, LDL, contains virtually only apo B-100. VLDL remnants and IDL containing apo E are removed by the hepatic LDL and LRP receptors.[75,76,81] The apo B-100 containing LDL has two potential metabolic fates. LDL may undergo receptor-mediated endocytosis by the LDL receptor in the liver, adrenal cell, and peripheral cells, including smooth muscle cells and fibroblasts.[81] Alternatively, LDL may become modified or oxidized and may be removed by the scavenger receptor A or CD-36 scavenger receptors on macrophages.[76,82]

The second major pathway in lipoprotein metabolism involves HDL. A central role proposed for HDL in lipoprotein metabolism is the transport of excess cholesterol from cells back to the liver by the process termed *reverse cholesterol transport*. Reverse cholesterol transport is initiated by the removal of FC from cells. Efflux of FC from cells occurs by two mechanisms. The first mechanism involves passive diffusion of FC between cellular membranes and acceptors, which include albumin, LDL, and lipid-rich HDL.[4,83] In the presence of LCAT, the bidirectional movement of cholesterol between plasma membranes and HDL results in net cholesterol efflux.[4,84,85] The second mechanism depends on the specific interaction of cells with extracellular acceptors, which include lipid-free apolipoproteins and lipid-poor HDL subclasses such as nascent or pre-β-HDL.[4,85,86] These particles are formed by several routes, including direct secretion from the liver and intestine, as well as remodeling of HDL and triglyceride-rich lipoproteins.[85,88] This form of cholesterol efflux involves the translocation of intracellular cholesterol to the plasma membrane and is paralleled by phospholipid efflux. [89–91] It requires energy and is mediated by the newly described ATP-binding cassette transporter 1 (ABC1)[87] defective in Tangier disease (see Chap. 122). Interestingly, this form of cholesterol efflux is not increased by the presence of LCAT. [84]

LCAT plays a pivotal role in cholesterol transport by catalyzing the esterification of FC to CE on plasma lipoproteins.[3,92] Together with additional factors, LCAT is important for the maturation of the initially discoidal apolipoprotein–lipid complexes into spherical HDL.[92] LCAT in human plasma is present on HDL as well as apo B-Lps. Esterification of FC on these lipoproteins has been designated α-LCAT activity and β-LCAT activity, respectively.[93] Kinetic studies in humans have shown that approximately 70 percent and 30 percent of plasma CE are synthesized on HDL and apo B-Lps, respectively.[94] The CE formed on lipoproteins is transferred to the hydrophobic core, providing additional surface area for FC. During this process, pre-β-HDL is converted to spherical HDL. HDL also acquires additional lipids, including cholesterol as well as apolipoproteins from the remodeling of plasma triglyceride-rich lipoproteins and HDL. In this regard, HDL in plasma functions as a reservoir for apolipoproteins (e.g., apo C-II and apo E) during lipoprotein metabolism, as outlined above. The CE synthesized in HDL can be transferred to the apo B-Lps by CETP in exchange for triglycerides.[7,8]

Cholesteryl esters are taken up by hepatocytes and other cells from HDL and apo B-Lps by two different receptor-mediated mechanisms. Classically, CE in apo B-Lps are delivered to cells by whole lipoprotein particle uptake by receptor-mediated endocytosis involving either the LDL or LRP receptors.[75,76,81] The receptors involved in the CE uptake and whole particle uptake of HDL have not been reported. Recently, the scavenger receptor BI (SR-BI) has been identified as a separate receptor-mediated mechanism for the delivery of CE to cells.[9,95] In contrast to whole particle uptake, SR-BI functions to selectively remove CE from both HDL and apo B-Lps without lipoprotein particle degradation. In rodents without CETP in which the major plasma lipoproteins are HDL, selective uptake of CE from HDL is a major pathway for CE delivery to the liver.

In summary, in the process of reverse cholesterol transport, the cholesterol in lipoproteins is transported to the liver as FC and CE. Cholesterol kinetic studies in humans conducted by Schwartz and colleagues showed that both HDL and apo B-Lps each transport approximately 50 percent of the total cholesterol to the liver.[94,96,97] In humans, approximately 90 percent of the FC is transported to the liver by HDL, and more than 90 percent of the CE is transported by the apo B-Lps.[94,96,97] A large fraction of the CE in the apo B-Lps transported to the liver is derived from HDL through the action of CETP.

LCAT DEFICIENCY SYNDROMES

Familial LCAT Deficiency

Familial LCAT deficiency was first recognized as a new inborn error of metabolism by Norum and Gjone.[11] They described the clinical features of a 33-year-old woman from western Norway presenting with corneal opacities, anemia, proteinuria, mild hypoalbuminemia, and hyperlipidemia. Although the patient had normal renal function, a renal biopsy revealed accumulation of foam cells in the glomerular tufts. Plasma cholesterol, triglyceride, and phospholipid levels were increased, but CE and lysophosphatidylcholine were decreased and HDL (pre-β and α-lipoproteins) could not be detected on gel electrophoresis. Similar clinical and biochemical abnormalities were subsequently described in the proband's two sisters.[98,99] All three sibs were ultimately shown to lack LCAT activity in plasma, a biochemical hallmark of FLD. The underlying molecular defect that led to LCAT deficiency in this kindred, as well as in three other Norwegian families, was identified as a single T-to-A transversion in codon 252, converting methionine (ATG) to lysine (AAG).[100] Although the clinical features of FLD patients are highly variable, most patients develop corneal opacities, anemia, and some degree of proteinuria or renal dysfunction that can progress to complete renal failure. To date, approximately 30 different LCAT gene defects have been identified in patients presenting with this rare genetic disorder (Table 118-1).

Fish Eye Disease

Carlson and Philipson[12] first described a 61-year-old Swedish woman presenting with massive corneal opacities. The patient had normal plasma cholesterol and CE levels, increased triglycerides, and low HDL. There was no evidence of anemia or proteinuria. Similar features were found in the patient's father and two older sisters, as well as in members of a separate Swedish kindred.[93,101] The plasma LCAT activity was normal, and the syndrome, which was felt to be distinct from FLD, was named fish eye disease.[12] Subsequent biochemical studies demonstrated that although LCAT from patients with FED could esterify cholesterol in plasma, the enzyme was unable to esterify FC in HDL.[93] This suggested that FED resulted from a partial α-LCAT deficiency. The underlying molecular defect leading to FED in the first two Swedish kindreds was subsequently identified as a C-to-T transition in codon 10 of the LCAT gene, converting proline (CCG) to leucine (CTG).[102] Unlike subjects with FLD, FED patients present with corneal opacities and hypoalphalipoproteinemia but no anemia or renal disease. FED appears to be less common than FLD, with only 10 different LCAT gene defects described to date (Table 118-2).

Clinical Features

Ocular Findings. Lipoprotein disorders are frequently associated with alterations in the morphology and lipid composition of the cornea. Corneal opacities are found in several syndromes that lead to HDL deficiency, including Tangier disease,[103] apo A-I deficiency,[104] and apo A-I/C-III deficiency,[105] as well as FLD and FED. Although often detected early in childhood, the onset and severity of the corneal findings in FLD or FED are variable. In a subset of patients, severe visual impairment has required corneal transplantation.[106–108] Grossly, the cornea has a dull, pale, nebulous appearance with more pronounced opacity near the limbus (Fig. 118-5). Slit-lamp examination of the cornea reveals small grayish, granular dots in all layers of the cornea except for the epithelium, giving the cornea a cloudy appearance. Accumulation near the limbal area may lead to the formation of diffuse, grayish, circular bands that resemble, but are distinct from, arcus senilis.[109] Structural analysis of the cornea by electron microscopy has revealed the presence of numerous vacuoles containing electron-dense deposits present in the Bowman layer and the anterior stroma.[110–113] Similar membrane-bound vesicles have been noted in the spleen, liver, aorta, and muscular arteries.[114–116] These membranous deposits probably consist of FC and phospholipids that accumulate in the corneas of FLD and FED patients.[106–108,113] Analysis of the corneal lipids demonstrates a three- to sixfold increase in concentration of the major LCAT substrates, FC and phospholipids, as well as a 50 percent reduction in CE, the product of the LCAT reaction.[104] These findings indicate that LCAT-mediated removal of FC and phospholipids from the cornea is inadequate in FLD and FED and suggest a role for LCAT in modulating the distribution of these lipids between the plasma and peripheral tissues.

Other reported ocular abnormalities include angioid streaks,[117] aneurysmal dilatations in retinal venules near the optic nerve, and papilledema with impaired ocular blood supply leading to functional visual loss.[109,118]

Renal Manifestations. Renal disease is the major cause of morbidity and mortality in FLD patients.[119,120] Proteinuria, often detected in the early twenties, remains mild to moderate until the

Table 118-1 LCAT Gene Defects in FLD

Mutation	Genotype	Location	LCAT* Mass	α-LCAT* Activity	Clinical Symptoms	References
• Asn^{5} → Ile A → T	Homozygote	Exon 1	8%	18%	Corneal opacities, anemia, proteinuria	***
• Leu^{7} 30 bp insertion (bp 889)	Compound heterozygote	Exon 1	—	4%	Corneal opacities, proteinuria, CAD	137
• Pro^{9} C insertion (bp 938)	Homozygote	Exon 1	4%	0–9%	Corneal opacities, anemia, proteinuria	166,171,172
• Gly^{30} → Ser G → A	Homozygote	Exon 2	50%	0%	Corneal opacities, CAD, anemia, proteinuria, renal disease	138,139
• Leu^{32} → Pro T → C	Compound heterozygote	Exon 2	—	< 10%	NA	171
• Gly^{33} → Arg C → A	Compound heterozygote	Exon 2	—	4%	Corneal opacities, proteinuria, CAD	137
• Tyr^{83} → Stop C → A	Homozygote and	Exon 3	0%	7%	Corneal opacities, anemia, proteinuria, renal disease	168
	Compound heterozygote		4%	2%	Corneal opacities, anemia, proteinuria	173
• Ala^{93} → Thr G → A	Homozygote	Exon 3	0%	5%	Corneal opacities, anemia, proteinuria, renal disease	168
• Tyr^{120} → AC → T del (bp 2175)	Compound heterozygote	Exon 4	4%	2%	Corneal opacities, anemia, proteinuria	171
• Arg^{135} → Trp C → T	Compound heterozygote	Exon 4	0%	0%	Corneal opacities, anemia, proteinuria, renal disease	168
• Arg^{140} → His G → A	Homozygote	Exon 4	—	0%	Corneal opacities, anemia, renal disease	174
• Gly^{141}, GGC insertion (bp 2234)	Homozygote	Exon 4	0%	2%	Corneal opacities, anemia, proteinuria, renal disease	175
• Arg^{147} → Trp C → T	Homozygote	Exon 4	60%	0%	Corneal opacities, proteinuria	176
	Compound heterozygote		10%	2%	Corneal opacities, anemia, proteinuria, renal disease	177
• Tyr^{156} → Asn T → A	Compound heterozygote	Exon 5	4%	2%	Corneal opacities, anemia, proteinuria	173
• Arg^{158} → Cys C → T	Homozygote	Exon 5	0%	5%	Corneal opacities, proteinuria, anemia, renal disease	168
• His^{168} C deletion (bp 2399)	Compound heterozygote	Exon 5	1%	0%	Anemia, proteinuria	178
• Tyr^{171} → Stop T → G	Compound heterozygote	Exon 5	10%	2%	Corneal opacities, anemia, proteinuria, renal disease	177
• Gly^{183} → Ser G → A	Compound heterozygote	Exon 5	4%	2%	Corneal opacities, anemia, proteinuria	171
• Leu^{209} → Pro T → C	Homozygote	Exon 5	2%	0–15%	Corneal opacities, anemia, proteinuria, renal disease	179
• Asn^{228} → Lys C → A	Homozygote	Exon 6	35%	0%	Corneal opacities, anemia, proteinuria	175
• Gly^{228} → Arg G → C	Homozygote	Exon 6	—	6%	Anemia	180
• Met^{234} → Ile G → A	Homozygote	Exon 6	8%	50%	NA	166
• Arg^{244} → Gly C → G	Homozygote	Exon 6	27% 26%	12% 13%	Corneal opacities, renal disease	166 171
• Met^{252} → Lys T → A	Homozygote	Exon 6	10–25%	0%	Corneal opacities, anemia, proteinuria	181
• Val^{264} G deletion (bp 873)	Homozygote	Exon 6	10%	0%	Corneal opacities, anemia, proteinuria	182
• Met^{293} → Ile G → A	Homozygote	Exon 6	—	12%	Corneal opacities, anemia	183
			40–46%	8–9%	Corneal opacities, anemia, proteinuria	171, 175
• Thr^{321} → Met C → T	Homozygote	Exon 6	6%	5%	Corneal opacities, anemia, proteinuria	168
	Compound heterozygote		2%	0–10%	Corneal opacities, anemia, proteinuria	171, 178
• Gly^{344} → Ser G → A	Homozygote	Exon 6	0%	0%	Corneal opacities, anemia, proteinuria	182
• Gln^{376}A insertion (bp 4906)	Compound heterozygote	Exon 6	10%	0%	Corneal opacities, anemia, proteinuria, renal disease	168
• Arg^{399} → Cys C → T	Homozygote	Exon 6	—	17%	Corneal opacities, anemia, proteinuria	180
	Compound heterozygote		—	2%	Corneal opacities, anemia, proteinuria	184

*Percentage of controls.
CAD, coronary artery disease.

Table 118-2 LCAT Gene Defects in FED

Mutation	Genotype	Location	LCAT* Mass	α-LCAT* Activity	Clinical Symptoms	References
$Pro^{10} \rightarrow$ Leu C → T	Homozygote	Exon 1	—	15%	Corneal opacities	98
$Pro^{10} \rightarrow$ Gln C → T	Compound heterozygote	Exon 1	64%	8%	Corneal opacities, CAD	135
$Arg^{99} \rightarrow$ Cys C → T	Homozygote	Exon 3	49%	26%	Corneal opacities	104
$Thr^{123} \rightarrow$ Ile C → T	Homozygote	Exon 4	52%	1–3%	Corneal opacities, CAD	140, 141
	Compound heterozygote		—	3–5%	Corneal opacities	185, 186, 189
$Asn^{131} \rightarrow$ Asp A → G	Homozygote	Exon 4	100%	4%	Corneal opacities, CAD	136
$Arg^{135} \rightarrow$ Gln G → A	Compound heterozygote	Exon 4	64%	8%	Corneal opacities, CAD	135
$Tyr^{144} \rightarrow$ Cys A → G	Compound heterozygote	Exon 4	—	5%	Corneal opacities	186
T → C (bp 2327)	Compound heterozygote	Intron 4	—	3%	Corneal opacities	187, 189
Leu^{300}(CTC) del bp 4679	Homozygote	Exon 6	21%	14%	Corneal opacities	188
$Thr^{347} \rightarrow$ Met C → T	Compound heterozygote	Exon 6	—	3%	Corneal opacities	185

*Percentage of controls.
CAD, coronary artery disease.

development of renal failure in the fourth or fifth decade of life. Plasma albumin, serum creatinine, and blood urea nitrogen levels, as well as the clearance of creatinine, inulin, and paraaminohippuric acid, can remain normal for years. Urine may contain hyaline and granular casts, red blood cells, and protein consisting mainly of albumin. Nephrotic syndrome and hypertension develop with the onset of renal failure, which can occur rapidly and without warning.

Histologic examination of renal biopsies in FLD patients reveals lipid deposits in the kidneys with expansion of the mesangial area, foam cell accumulation in the glomeruli and interstitial tissues, as well as thickening of Bowman's capsule and of the glomerular capillary basement membrane (Fig. 118-6*A* and *B*).[116,119–127] Lipid analysis of isolated glomeruli shows marked increases in the amount of FC and phospholipids.[115] Ultrastructurally, deposition of electron-dense membranes in the capillary lumen, the basement membrane, mesangial regions, and pericapsular areas are evident (Fig. 118-6*C*). The capillary walls are abnormal, showing loss of endothelial cells, irregular thickening of the basement membrane, and fused endothelial foot processes.[116,119–121,123–125,127] Membrane-surrounded particles are present both in the subepithelial and subendothelial regions. Immunofluorescence microscopy reveals bright granular staining for C3 in the capillary loops, mesangium, and arteriolar walls, whereas peripheral capillary loops stain weakly with antibodies for C1q and fibrinogen.[120,122,127]

The pathogenesis of renal injury in FLD is not totally understood. It has been suggested that large molecular weight LDL (LM-LDL) particles that are trapped in capillary loops induce endothelial damage and vascular injury.[122,128–130] However, these lipoproteins are not always detected in FLD patients with renal disease.[120] The detection of C3 and of electron-dense deposits indistinguishable from those present in immune complex diseases[120,122,127] has led to the suggestion that a component of the renal damage in FLD may be immune complex and complement mediated.

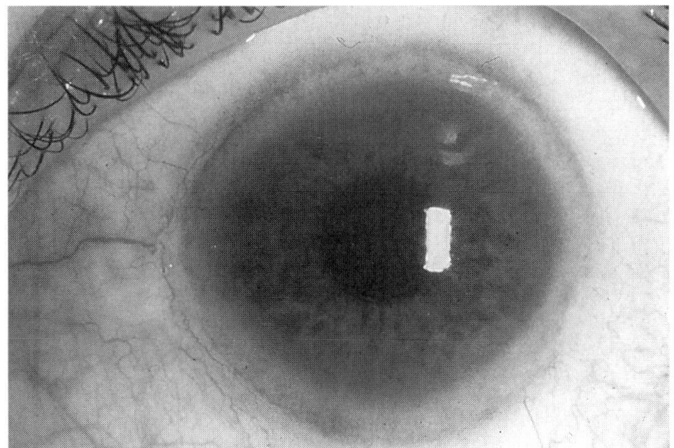

Fig. 118-5 Corneal opacities in a patient with FLD. Note central stromal haze and prominent peripheral opacification, resembling corneal arcus. The corneal infiltrate composed of numerous minute grayish dots is localized to the parenchyma. See Color Plate 4.

Hematologic Findings. Most patients with FLD develop normochromic normocytic anemia with hemoglobin levels of approximately 10 to 11 g/dl.[131] Reticulocytosis and target cells are evident on the peripheral smear. The anemia is secondary to both moderate hemolysis and reduced erythropoiesis. The FLD erythrocyte life span is reduced to one half that of normal individuals (23 to 45 days), partly due to splenic sequestration. Bone marrow biopsy specimens reveal the presence of foam cells, "sea-blue" histiocytes, and increased numbers of nucleated red blood cells.[126,132] Ultrastructural studies indicate that the histiocyte granules are composed of membranes in a lamellar arrangement.[116] FLD erythrocytes and isolated red blood cell membranes have abnormal lipid content, with a twofold increase in unesterified cholesterol and PC but reduced amounts of sphingomyelin and phosphatidylethanolamine.[133–135] There is also a marked decrease in both acetylcholinesterase activity and sodium influx.[136,137] Thus, the mild hemolytic anemia in FLD appears to be secondary to altered red blood cell membrane lipids resulting from altered plasma cholesterol metabolism.

Atherosclerosis. Despite reduced plasma HDL levels, most patients with FLD and FED do not appear to be at increased risk for developing premature cardiovascular disease. Nevertheless, coronary heart disease has been documented angiographically and clinically in a subset of both FLD and FED patients.[138–145] In some cases, other cardiac risk factors, including diabetes and hypertension associated with renal failure, have been identified.

Postmortem examination has revealed atherosclerosis in the aorta and large arteries, including renal and iliac arteries.[115,116,131] Calcification of the aorta before the age of 40 has been described.[131] Ultrastructurally, deposition of electron-dense membranes similar to those present in other tissues can be detected in the different layers of the vessel wall. Lipid analysis of the atheroma from renal arteries revealed increased saturated and monounsaturated fatty acids as well as reduced CE, which amounted to only 35 percent of the total cholesterol.[115]

Other Findings. Despite the accumulation of lipid-laden foam cells and increased content of FC and PC lipids in the liver, spleen, and reticuloendothelial system, adenopathy, hepatosplenomegaly,

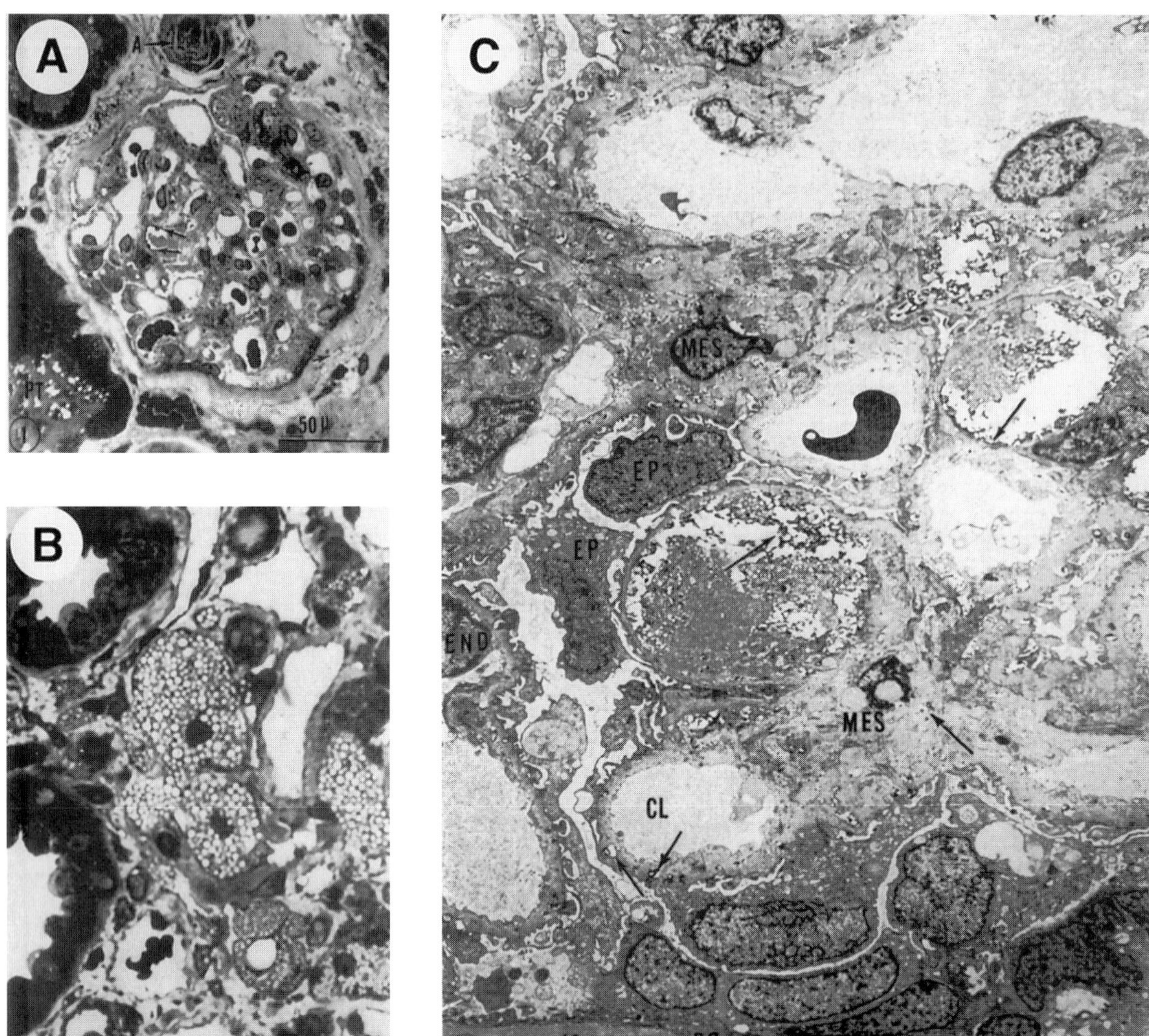

Fig. 118-6 Analysis of a renal biopsy specimen from a patient with FLD. A typical glomerulus with prominent mesangial regions (*A*) and foam cells present in the interstitial tissue (*B*) are shown. The location of foreign material is indicated by the arrow. The presence of electron-dense material within the capillary lumen as well as in other structural parts of the glomerulus are shown by electron microscopy (*C*). Note the increase in the mesangial matrix and irregular thickening of the capillary basement membrane (× 2700). BC, Bowman's capsule; CL, capillary lumen; EP, epithelial cells; MES, mesangial cells. (*Reprinted with permission from Hovig and Gjone.*[116])

and hepatic dysfunction are not commonly seen in FLD.[115,116] Peripheral neuropathy has been described in one patient.[146] However, symptoms suggesting CNS as well as other neurologic abnormalities are absent. Xanthelasmas have been observed, especially in FLD patients with end-stage renal disease.

Treatment. Dietary fat restriction has been shown to decrease the levels of the LM-LDL in patients with FLD.[131,147] Because these abnormal lipoproteins may be associated with the development of renal injury, it seems advisable for FLD patients to restrict their dietary fat intake. However, the value of this approach in either preventing tissue lipid deposition or delaying the development of kidney damage remains unknown.[148] Whole blood and plasma transfusions[137,148,149] resulted in normalization of the plasma lipid and lipoprotein pattern, as well as partial reversal of red blood cell plasma membrane abnormalities, in FLD patients. These changes were transient, and no improvement in anemia or renal function was observed.

Severe visual impairment secondary to corneal opacities has led to successful corneal transplantation[106–108,111,113,150] in FED and FLD patients. Patients with FLD and end-stage renal failure require renal transplantation. Despite evidence of early lipid deposition and histomorphologic changes found in renal grafts,[119,121,151] excellent long-term results and kidney graft function have been reported. However, transplantation does not increase the circulating plasma LCAT levels or reverse the anemia and abnormal lipid profile in these patients.

Future potentially curative therapeutic approaches for the treatment of FLD patients include liver transplantation and gene therapy.

PLASMA LIPIDS AND LIPOPROTEINS IN LCAT DEFICIENCY

Plasma lipids and lipoproteins show multiple abnormalities in patients with LCAT deficiency (Table 118-3). Total plasma cholesterol is increased, and triglycerides are normal to increased in FLD. All patients have elevated plasma FC and PC and decreased CE and lysophosphatidylcholine. The plasma CEs contain decreased proportions of linoleic acid and an increased

Table 118-3 Plasma Lipid Profile, LCAT Activity, and LCAT Concentration in Patients with FLD and FED

	FLD	FED	Controls
TC (mg/dl)	172 (89–185)	215 (185–253)	163 ± 24
TG (mg/dl)	723 (110–723)	149 (60–408)	65 ± 18
HDL-C (mg/dl)	8 (0–12)	8 (0–7)	65 ± 17
Apo A-1 (mg/dl)	39 (36–48)	42 (29–45)	145 ± 24
Apo A-II (mg/dl)	6 (4–8)	12 (10–15)	34 ± 6
CE/TC	6 (6–49)	46 (57–65)	69 ± 2
α-LCAT activity (nmol/ml/h)	1.5 (0)	0.9 (0–14)	99 ± 5
CER (nmol/ml/h)	0 (0–16)	51 (25–74)	59 ± 11
LCAT concentration (μg/ml)	0.2 (0–0.3)	4.0 (0–4)	5.2 ± 0.7
Reference	(173, 168)	(185, 188)	(188)

TC = total cholesterol; TG = triglycerides; CE/TC = cholesteryl ester/total cholesterol; LCAT = lecithin cholesteryl acyltransferase; CER = cholesteryl esterification rate. FLD and FED data for individual patients are shown (range in parentheses). Control data (n = 7) are expressed as mean ± SEM.

percentage of palmitic and oleic acids. VLDLs are increased, LDLs are reduced, and HDLs are decreased to approximately 25 percent of normal.[11,129,152]

The major plasma lipoprotein classes in FLD show several morphologic and biochemical changes when compared with control lipoproteins. The VLDL density fraction from FLD patients contains lipoproteins varying from 275 to 2000 Å in diameter and includes relatively normal spherical VLDL particles as well as large irregular multivesicular trilaminar structures that resemble sheets of bilayer membranes.[152,153]

Low-density lipoproteins are polydisperse and contain three separate lipoprotein particles[153] (Fig. 118-7). Normal 200- to 250-Å spherical lipoproteins are present that resemble normal LDL. These lipoproteins contain apo B-100 and apo E, but are enriched in triglycerides and reduced in CEs. The second particles are 400 to 600 Å in diameter, often in routeaux formation, and similar to LpX lipoproteins present in patients with obstructive liver disease.[153,154] The LpX-like particles contain primarily FC, phospholipids, albumin, and C apolipoproteins.[152,153] The third particles in LDL are large flattened structures approximately 1,000 Å in diameter. These abnormal LDL lipoproteins elute in the void volume when separated by gel filtration in 2 percent agarose columns, and they were designated LM-LDLs by Gjone et al.[128] These abnormal particles decrease with fasting and fat restriction and have thus been proposed to be generated from chylomicron remnant surface components.[155] As discussed above, these abnormal LM-LDL lipoproteins have been proposed to be important in the pathogenesis of the renal disease characteristic of patients with FLD.

The changes in HDL morphology and composition in patients with FLD have been of particular interest[152,153] (Fig. 118-8). Two major types of lipoprotein particles are present in HDLs in FLD. The first type are discoidal particles 40 Å by 150 to 200 Å in dimension, and they have a hydrated density of HDL_2 and often form rouleaux. These disk-shaped lipoprotein particles that are similar to nascent HDL in structure are enriched in FC and phospholipids. Some of these disk-shaped particles contain apo A-I and apo A-II, whereas other particles contain primarily apo E.[153,156,157] Other abnormal lipoproteins which accumulate in FLD are the small 45- to 80-Å spherical particles which contain primarily FC, phospholipids, and two moles of apo A-I per particle.[158]

METABOLISM OF HDL IN LCAT DEFICIENCY

Metabolism of LpA-I and LpA-I:A-II in Normal Subjects and Patients with FLD and FED

High-density lipoproteins are a heterogeneous population of particles that differ in size, hydrated density, apolipoprotein composition, and physicochemical properties. The two major density subfractions, HDL_2 and HDL_3, have been found to differ in their utility as epidemiologic markers: plasma levels of HDL_2 have a stronger inverse correlation with coronary artery disease risk than the levels of HDL_3.[159] The major apolipoproteins in HDL are apo A-I and apo A-II. Using immunabsorption techniques, lipoprotein particles within HDL have been isolated according to their apolipoprotein content. There are two major classes of apo A-I–containing lipoproteins: those that contain both apo A-I and apo A-II (LpA-I:A-II) and those that contain apo A-I but no

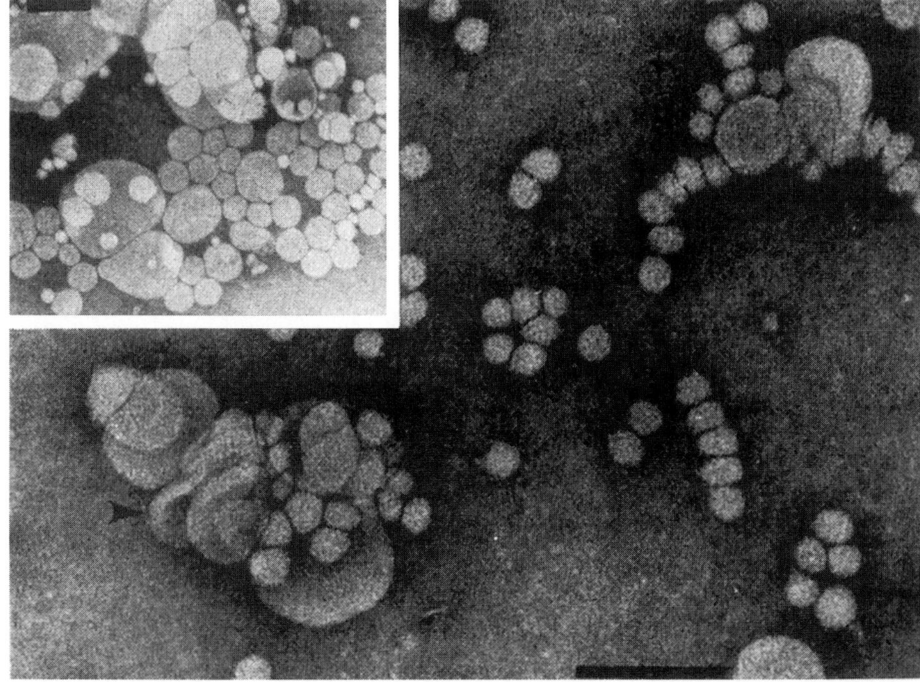

Fig. 118-7 Negatively stained LDL from a patient with FLD. Three types of lipoproteins are present, including very large flattened particles approximately 1000 Å in diameter, intermediate particles of 400 to 600 Å (inset), and small normal LDLs of 200 to 250 Å. (*Reprinted with permission from Forte et al.*[153])

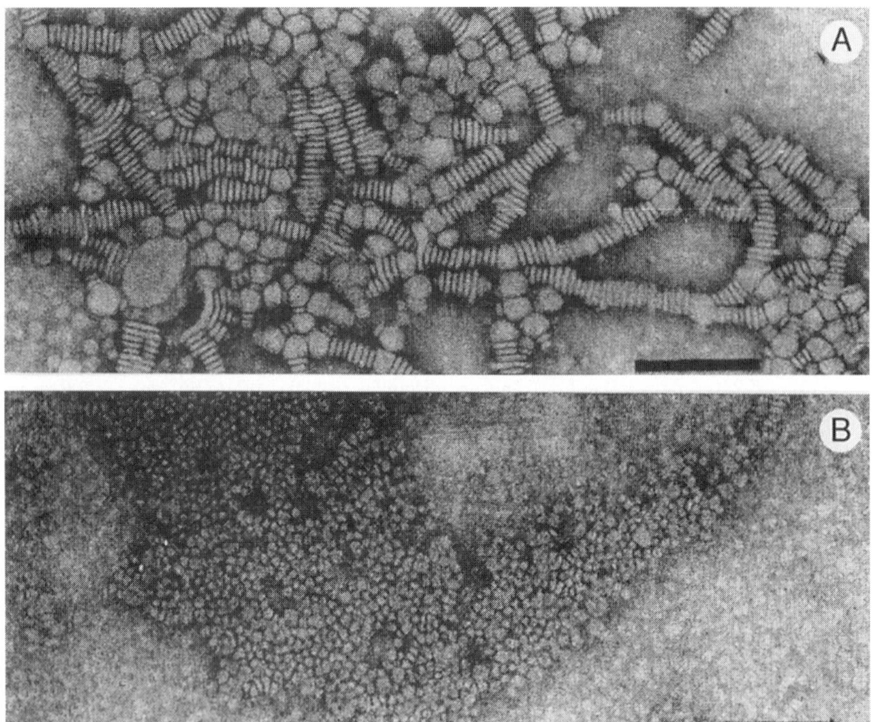

Fig. 118-8 Negatively stained HDL from an FLD patient. Two types of lipoproteins are shown. *A*. Disk-shaped particles in rouleaux. *B*. Small spherical particles approximately 6 Å in diameter. (*Reprinted with permission from Forte et al.*[153])

apo A-II.[160–162] Nascent pre–β-HDL or nascent LpA-I particles have been proposed as the most effective lipoproteins for removing cholesterol from cells[4] and to be the most potentially antiatherogenic lipoprotein particles within HDL.[163] The in vivo kinetics of apo A-I on LpA-I and LpA-I:A-II were investigated in normolipidemic human subjects using radiolabeled apolipoproteins as well as isolated LpA-I and LpA-I:A-I:A-II lipoprotein particles.[164,165] These studies established that LpA-I is catabolized much faster than LpA-I:A-II (Fig. 118-9). In addition, there was a precursor product relationship between LpA-I and LpA-I:A-II. LpA-I was converted to LpA-I:A-II, but there was no significant conversion from LpA-I:A-II to LpA-I (Fig. 118-9 inset). These results emphasize the divergent metabolic pathways for the metabolism of the major LpA-I and LpA-I:A-II lipoprotein particles in HDL.

The hallmark of the plasma lipoproteins in both FLD and FED is decreased plasma HDL-cholesterol levels as well as reduced plasma levels of both apo A-I and apo A-II. The metabolic basis for the hypoalphalipoproteinemia and the absence of premature cardiovascular disease has been investigated by in vivo metabolism studies of apo A-I, apo A-II, LpA-I, and LpA-I:A-II.

Initial in vivo kinetic studies established that the reduced plasma levels of apo A-I and apo A-II in LCAT deficiency were due to increased catabolism.[166,167] As outlined in Table 118-3, the plasma apo A-II levels are decreased to a proportionately greater extent than apo A-I levels.[166] In addition, the plasma levels of LpA-I:A-II were markedly reduced when compared with the LpA-I levels. Initial studies established that the reason for the proportionally greater decrease in apo A-II was due to a much faster catabolism of apo A-II than apo A-I.[166] The synthesis

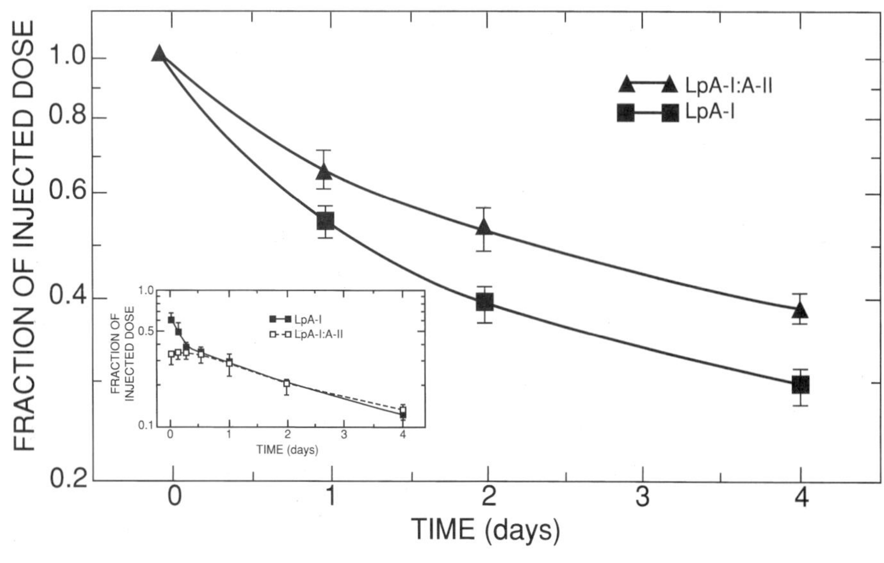

Fig. 118-9 Metabolism of LpA-I and LpA-I:A-II in control subjects. Radiolabeled apo A-I in LpA-I (squares) and LpA-I:A-II (triangles) in three control subjects (mean ± SD). *Inset*. Radiolabeled apo A-I injected on LpA-I followed by resolution on LpA-I (closed squares) and LpA-I:A-II (open squares).

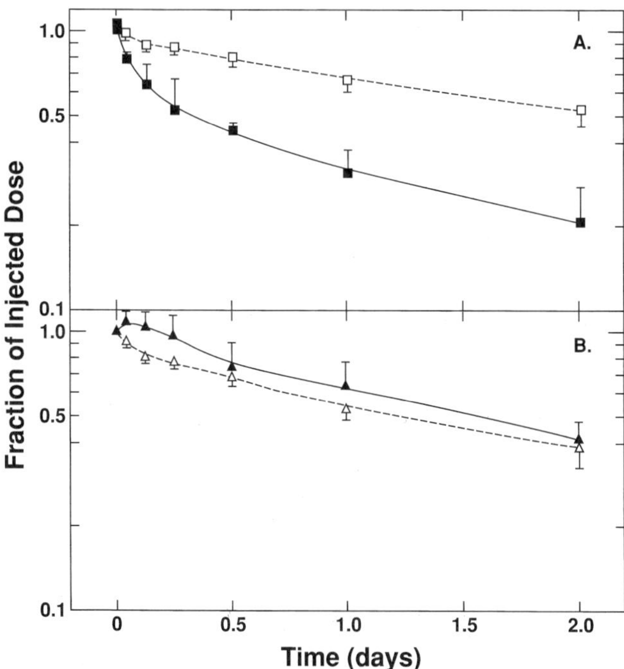

Fig. 118-10 Metabolism of LpA-I and LpA-I:A-II in LCAT-deficient patients and control subjects. Radiolabeled apo A-I in LpA-I:A-II (*A*) and LpA-I (*B*) in four LCAT-deficient patients (solid symbols) and 10 controls (open symbols).

of both apo A-I and apo A-II was similar to that of controls. Of particular interest was the unusual finding that the catabolism of the LpA-I:A-II particles was substantially faster than that of LpA-I in these patients[166] (Fig. 118-10). In normal subjects the reverse is observed, with LpA-I catabolism being faster than that of LpA-I:A-II.[164,165]

In summary, in both FLD and FED the low plasma levels of HDL are due to preferential hypercatabolism of apo A-II and HDL particles containing apo A-II. The metabolism of LpA-I and the plasma levels of pre-β-HDL are relatively normal. In addition, because LpA-I has been proposed to be more protective than LpA-I:A-II against atherosclerosis, this selective effect of increased catabolism on LpA-I:A-II may explain the low incidence of atherosclerosis in LCAT deficiency. Furthermore, in cell culture studies, cholesterol efflux using plasma from patients with FLD is decreased.[168,169] The FC effluxed from cells is readily exchanged to apo B-Lps, suggesting that a major pathway for cholesterol transport in reverse cholesterol transport in FLD and FED may be in the form of FC transport to the liver by the apo B-Lps.

FLD and FED LCAT Gene Defects

Although phenotypically distinct, FLD and FED are autosomally inherited disorders caused by different mutations on the same LCAT gene.[138,170–173] To date, approximately 40 different defects in the LCAT gene have been described (Tables 118-1 and 118-2).[102,108,139–145,170,172,174–193] The functional significance of only some of these mutations has been established by either cosegregation analysis[144,172,187] or in vitro expression.[43,108,139,142,145,170,177,178,182,184,186,188,189,191,192] Although most of the gene defects involve point mutations that lead to single amino acid substitutions, deletions and insertions resulting in frameshift and premature termination have been described (Tables 118-1 and 118-2). Most mutations in the LCAT gene affect the enzyme's activity, suggesting that normal LCAT function requires the structural integrity of the entire molecule.

Analysis of the location of these mutations within the LCAT gene indicates that for both disorders, all regions of the enzyme are involved. Thus, substitutions of LCAT residues 5, 30, 32, 33, 83, 93, 135, 140, 147, 156, 158, 171,183, 209, 228, 230, 234, 244, 252, 293, 321, 344, and 399 (Table 118-1) have been associated with the development of FLD, whereas those in residues 10, 99, 123, 135, 144, and 347 (Table 118-2) lead to FED. Until recently, it was not possible to determine whether the FLD or FED gene defects clustered around different functional domains of LCAT, because the three-dimensional structure of the enzyme had not been elucidated. However, using their proposed model for LCAT structure Rosseneu et al.[26] have been able to show that FLD mutations cluster near the catalytic site or the N-terminal region, where they may interfere with either enzyme activity or enzyme–substrate interaction. In contrast, FED mutations are localized on the hydrophilic surface of the enzyme, where they can affect the binding of small substrates such as HDL and cholesterol. Classically, FED has been associated with a selective deficiency of α-HDL LCAT activity, whereas FLD has been characterized by total (α and β) absence of plasma LCAT activity. However, more recent studies[173,192] indicate that the heterogeneity of phenotypic expression in FLD and FED is dictated primarily by the residual level of LCAT activity, rather than its location within the different lipoproteins.

ANIMAL MODELS

LCAT Knockout Mice

A mouse model for human LCAT deficiency has been generated by targeted disruption of the LCAT gene.[194,195] Like human FLD patients, homozygous LCAT-deficient mice have reduced total cholesterol, HDL-cholesterol, and apo A-I (7 to 25 percent of normal) and increased plasma triglycerides (212 percent of normal),[194,195] whereas heterozygous animals had lower total and HDL-cholesterol values (approximately 60 percent of normal) (Table 118-4). Small, discoidal, pre-β migrating HDL particles that form the classical rouleaux structures observed in patients with FLD are the major lipoproteins present in LCAT-deficient mice.[194,195] On a high-fat, high-cholesterol diet, homozygous animals had lower plasma concentrations of cholesterol, reflecting reduced levels of both HDL and the pro-atherogenic apo B–containing lipoproteins.[194] This latter finding may explain in part the low incidence of atherosclerosis associated with mouse[196] and human LCAT deficiency. No evidence of corneal opacities was detected in this mouse model. However, on a high-fat, high-cholesterol diet, homozygous LCAT-deficient mice developed renal lesions characterized by lipid accumulation in the glomeruli, expansion of the mesangial area, mesangial sclerosis, and endothelial cell inclusions. The availability of homozygous LCAT-deficient mice permits further evaluation of the role that LCAT plays in the development of renal insufficiency and

Table 118-4 Plasma Lipid Profile, LCAT Activity, and LCAT Concentration in LCAT-Deficient Mice

	LCAT Deficient	Controls
TC (mg/dl)	31 ± 12	134 ± 22
TG (mg/dl)	111 ± 16	109 ± 23
HDL-C (mg/dl)	6 ± 6	92 ± 17
Apo A-1 (mg/dl)	14 ± 5	99 ± 19
Apo A-II (mg/dl)	9 ± 7	19 ± 11
CE/TC (mg/dl)	34 ± 11	79 ± 3
α-LCAT (nmol/ml/h)	0.3 ± 0.0	44 ± 3
CER (nmol/ml/h)	0.0 ± 0.0	70 ± 7
Reference	(190)	(190)

TC = total cholesterol; TG = triglycerides; CE/TC = cholesteryl ester/total cholesterol; LCAT = lecithin cholesteryl acyltransferase; CER = cholesteryl esterification rate. Data expressed as mean ± SEM. LCAT deficient (n = 11); controls (n = 9).

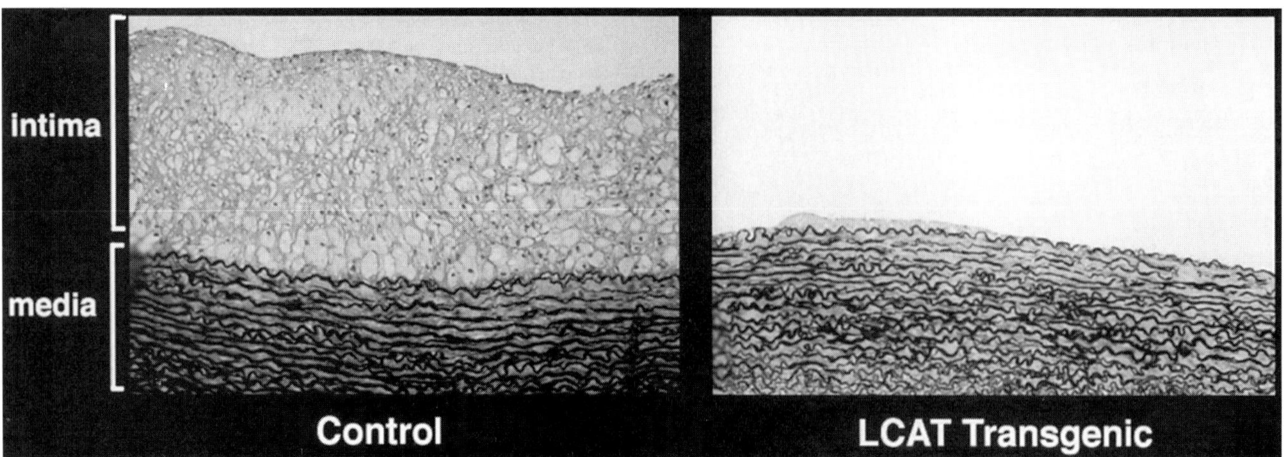

Fig. 118-11 Atherosclerosis in the descending aorta of control and LCAT-transgenic rabbits. The intimal thickness and degree of foam cell accumulation in control animals is markedly reduced in LCAT-transgenic rabbits. (*Reprinted with permission from Hoeg et al.*[53])

atherosclerosis as well as the feasibility of performing gene transfer in human LCAT deficiency states.

LCAT Overexpression and the Risk of Atherosclerosis

Little is known about LCAT's role in modulating plasma levels of different lipoproteins and the development of atherosclerosis in humans. Some, but not all,[47,197] studies have shown a positive correlation between HDL plasma levels and LCAT activity[198–201] and mass in plasma.[202,203] Interestingly, in the Pacific Northwest Bell Telephone Company study, women and nonsmokers, two groups known to have a lower risk of developing cardiovascular disease, had significantly higher plasma LCAT concentrations than men or smokers, respectively.[47] The effect of LCAT expression on plasma levels of the pro-atherogenic lipoproteins (LDLs) has not been well studied; however, LCAT mass has been positively correlated with LDL-cholesterol levels in two human studies.[48,199] Similarly, few studies have addressed the role of LCAT in modulating atherosclerosis in humans. Although LCAT deficiency in most patients has not been associated with premature atherosclerosis, some mutations in the LCAT gene may result in enhanced cardiovascular disease risk.[138–145] LCAT activity has been shown to be significantly reduced (24 to 50 percent of controls) in patients with angiographically documented coronary artery disease[201] and in survivors of myocardial infarction.[45,200,204] In contrast, Wells et al.[205] reported a positive correlation between the levels of plasma LCAT activity and the severity of angiographically proven coronary artery disease.

Recent studies involving the characterization of different animal models that overexpress human LCAT have provided a new understanding of the potential role that LCAT plays in modulating the development of cardiovascular disease risk. LCAT expression in transgenic rabbits increases plasma concentrations of cholesterol, CE, and antiatherogenic HDL-cholesterol and apo A-I (1.5 to 4-fold)[206] by delaying the catabolism of apo A-I HDL.[207,208] A totally unexpected finding was the lowering of the cholesterol present in pro-atherogenic apo B-Lps as well a decrease in plasma apo B by 50 to 66 percent.[206,208] Detailed kinetic studies established that the reduced plasma apo B-Lp levels in LCAT-transgenic rabbits were due to increased catabolism.[208] Furthermore, of particular importance was the marked reduction in diet-induced atherosclerosis in LCAT-transgenic rabbits when compared with control rabbits on a high-cholesterol diet (Fig. 118-11).[53]

Cross-breeding of LCAT-transgenic rabbits with LDL receptor–deficient rabbits has demonstrated that LCAT can, in part, correct the hypoalphalipoproteinemia and increased LDL-cholesterol levels in these animals.[209] However, the presence of functional LDL receptors is required for the LCAT-mediated lowering of apo B-Lps, suggesting that the LDL receptor pathway may play a major role in the LCAT-mediated lowering of LDL. As predicted from the antiatherogenic lipoprotein profile, LCAT significantly reduces the development of diet-induced aortic atherosclerosis in New Zealand White and heterozygous LDL receptor–deficient rabbits.[210]

Like LCAT-transgenic rabbits, mice overexpressing human LCAT have increased plasma concentrations of cholesterol, CEs, HDL-cholesterol, and apo A-I.[52,211,212] Paradoxically, despite elevated HDL, LCAT-transgenic mice have either no protection against atherosclerosis[213] or have enhanced development of aortic lesions.[214] This difference in the atherosclerosis susceptibility between the two LCAT-transgenic animal models is only partially due to the absence of apo B-Lp lowering in LCAT-transgenic mice.[214] In addition, LCAT-transgenic mice accumulate abnormal, dysfunctional HDL, with a reduced ability to mediate reverse cholesterol transport.[214] Expression of CETP[215] as well as the induction of hepatic lipase deficiency[216] normalize the dysfunctional properties of LCAT-HDL and significantly reduce or abolish the diet-induced atherosclerosis observed in LCAT-transgenic mice. Thus, expression of CETP and hepatic lipase can modulate the LCAT-mediated effect on HDL metabolism and atherosclerosis. The LCAT-mediated effect on the plasma lipoproteins has now been confirmed in a third animal model. Adenovirus-mediated transient expression of human LCAT in nonhuman primates increases plasma HDL and apo A-I levels and reduces the concentrations of apo B-Lps and apo B.[217]

In summary, these combined findings emphasize that the plasma concentrations of HDL and apo A-I do not always predict the capacity of HDL to function as an antiatherogenic lipoprotein. LCAT overexpression in rabbits and nonhuman primates leads to elevated HDL, reduced apo B-Lp, and an ideal antiatherogenic lipoprotein profile. With this lipoprotein phenotype, transgenic rabbits had a marked reduction in diet-induced atherosclerosis. Based on these results, LCAT is an ideal candidate gene for gene therapy as well as a target for drug development for the treatment of atherosclerosis in humans.

REFERENCES

1. Sperry WM: Cholesterol esterase in blood. *J Biol Chem* **111**:467–478, 1935.
2. Glomset JA: The mechanism of the plasma cholesterol esterification reaction: Plasma fatty acid transferase. *Biochim Biophys Acta* **65**:128–135, 1962.
3. Glomset JA: The plasma lecithin:cholesterol acyltransferase reaction. *J Lipid Res* **9**:155–167, 1968.

4. Fielding CJ, PE Fielding: Molecular physiology of reverse cholesterol transport. *J Lipid Res* **36**:211–228, 1995.
5. Forte T, Norum KR, JA Glomset, AV Nichols: Plasma lipoproteins in familial lecithin:cholesterol acyltransferase deficiency: structure of low and high density lipoproteins as revealed by electron microscopy. *J Clin Invest* **50**:1141–1148, 1971.
6. Schmitz G, Assmann G, Melnik B: The role of lecithin:cholesterol acyltransferase in high density lipoprotein3/high density lipoprotein2 interconversion. *Clin Chim Acta* **119**:225–236, 1982.
7. Marzetta CA, Meyers TJ, Albers JJ: Lipid transfer protein-mediated distribution of HDL-derived cholesteryl esters among plasma apo B–containing lipoprotein subpopulations. *Arterioscler Thromb* **13**:834–841, 1993.
8. Tall AR: Plasma cholesteryl ester transfer protein. *J Lipid Res* **34**:1255–1274, 1993.
9. Acton S, Rigotti A, Landschulz KT, Xu S, Hobbs HH, Krieger M: Identification of scavenger receptor SR-BI as a high density lipoprotein receptor. *Science* **271**:518–520, 1996.
10. Wang N, Weng W, Breslow JL, Tall AR: Scavenger receptor BI (SR-BI) is up-regulated in adrenal gland in apolipoprotein A-I and hepatic lipase knock-out mice as a response to depletion of cholesterol stores: in vivo evidence that SR-BI is a functional high density lipoprotein receptor under feedback control. *J Biol Chem* **271**:21001–21004, 1996.
11. Norum KR, Gjone E: Familial plasma lecithin:cholesterol acyltransferase deficiency. Biochemical study of a new inborn error of metabolism. *Scand J Clin Lab Invest* **20**:231–243, 1967.
12. Carlson LA, Philipson B: Fish-eye disease: a new familial condition with massive corneal opacities and dyslipoproteinemia. *Lancet* **2**:921–923, 1979.
13. McLean J, Wion K, Drayna D, Fielding C, Lawn R: Human lecithin-cholesterol acyltransferase gene: complete gene sequence and sites of expression. *Nucleic Acids Res* **14**:9397–9406, 1986.
14. Francone OL, Gurakar A, Fielding C: Distribution and functions of lecithin:cholesterol acyltransferase and cholesteryl ester transfer protein in plasma lipoproteins. Evidence for a functional unit containing these activities together with apolipoproteins A-I and D that catalyzes the esterification and transfer of cell-derived cholesterol. *J Biol Chem* **264**:7066–7072, 1989.
15. Cheung MC, Wolf AC, Lum KD, Tollefson JH, Albers JJ: Distribution and localization of lecithin:cholesterol acyltransferase and cholesteryl ester transfer activity in A-I-containing lipoproteins. *J Lipid Res* **27**:1135–1144, 1986.
16. Duverger N, Rader D, Duchateau P, Fruchart JC, Castro G, Brewer HB Jr: Biochemical characterization of the three major subclasses of lipoprotein A-I preparatively isolated from human plasma. *Biochemistry* **32**:12372–12379, 1993.
17. Jonas A: Regulation of lecithin cholesterol acyltransferase activity. *Prog Lipid Res* **37**:209–234, 1998.
18. Fielding CJ, Shore VG, Fielding PE: A protein cofactor of lecithin:cholesterol acyltransferase. *Biochem Biophys Res Commun* **46**:1493–1498, 1972.
19. Jonas A: Lecithin-cholesterol acyltransferase in the metabolism of high-density lipoproteins. *Biochim Biophys Acta* **1084**:205–220, 1991.
20. McLean J, Fielding C, Drayna D, Dieplinger H, Baer B, Kohr W, Henzel W, et al.: Cloning and expression of human lecithin-cholesterol acyltransferase cDNA. *Proc Natl Acad Sci U S A* **83**:2335–2339, 1986.
21. Warden CH, CA Langner, JI Gordon, BA Taylor, JW McLean, AJ Lusis: Tissue-specific expression, developmental regulation, and chromosomal mapping of the lecithin:cholesterol acyltransferase gene. Evidence for expression in brain and testes as well as liver. *J Biol Chem* **264**:21573–21581, 1989.
22. Smith KM, Lawn RM, Wilcox JN: Cellular localization of apolipoprotein D and lecithin:cholesterol acyltransferase mRNA in rhesus monkey tissues by in situ hybridization. *J Lipid Res* **31**:995–1004, 1990.
23. Hixson JE, Driscoll DM, Birnbaum S, Britten ML: Baboon lecithin cholesterol acyltransferase (LCAT): cDNA sequences of two alleles, evolution, and gene expression. *Gene* **128**:295–299, 1993.
24. Meroni G, Malgaretti N, Magnaghi P, Taramelli R: Nucleotide sequence of the cDNA for lecithin-cholesterol acyl transferase (LCAT) from the rat. *Nucleic Acids Res* **18**:5308, 1990.
25. Murata Y, Maeda E, Yoshino G, Kasuga M: Cloning of rabbit LCAT cDNA: increase in LCAT mRNA abundance in the liver of cholesterol-fed rabbits. *J Lipid Res* **37**:1616–1622, 1996.
26. Peelman F, Vinaimont N, Verhee A, Vanloo B, Verschelde JL, Labeur C, Seguret-Mace S, et al.: A proposed architecture for lecithin:cholesterol acyltransferase (LCAT): identification of the catalytic triad and molecular modeling. *Protein Sci* **7**:587–599, 1998.
27. Farooqui JZ, Wohl RC, Kezdy FJ, Scanu AM: Identification of the active-site serine in human lecithin:cholesterol acyltransferase. *Arch Biochem Biophys* **261**:330–335, 1988.
28. Jauhiainen M, Dolphin PJ: Human plasma lecithin-cholesterol acyltransferase. An elucidation of the catalytic mechanism. *J Biol Chem* **261**:7032–7043, 1986.
29. Hide WA, Chan L, Li WH: Structure and evolution of the lipase superfamily. *J Lipid Res* **33**:167–178, 1992.
30. Winkler FK, D'Arcy A, Hunziker W: Structure of human pancreatic lipase. *Nature* **343**:771–774, 1990.
31. Francone OL, Fielding CJ: Structure-function relationships in human lecithin:cholesterol acyltransferase. Site-directed mutagenesis at serine residues 181 and 216. *Biochemistry.* **30**:10074-10077, 1991.
32. Adimoolam S, Lee YP, Jonas A: Mutagenesis of highly conserved histidines in lecithin:cholesterol acyltransferase: identification of an essential histidine (His 377). *Biochem Biophys Res Commun* **243**:337–341, 1998.
33. Brasseur R, Pillot T, Lins L, Vandekerckhove J, Rasseneu M: Peptides in membranes: tipping the balance of membrane stability. *Trends Biochem Sci* **22**:167–171, 1997.
34. Adimoolam S, Jonas A: Identification of a domain of lecithin-cholesterol acyltransferase that is involved in interfacial recognition. *Biochem Biophys Res Commun* **232**:783–787, 1997.
35. Kobayashi J, Applebaum-Bowden D, Dugi KA, Brown D, Kashyap V, Parrott C, Maeda N, et al.: Analysis of protein structure-function in vivo: adenovirus-mediated transfer of lipase mutants in hepatic lipase deficient mice. *J Biol Chem* **271**:26296–26301, 1996.
36. Dugi KA, Dichek HL, Santamarina-Fojo S: Human hepatic and lipoprotein lipase: the loop covering the catalytic site mediates lipase substrate specificity. *J Biol Chem* **270**:25396–25401, 1995.
37. Adimoolam S, Jin L, Grabbe E, Shieh JJ, Jonas A: Structural and functional properties of two mutants of lecithin:cholesterol acyltransferase (T123I and N228K). *J Biol Chem* **273**:32561–32567, 1998.
38. Subbaiah PV, Liu M, Senz J, Wang X, Pritchard PH: Substrate and positional specificities of human and mouse lecithin-cholesterol acyltransferase. Studies with wild type recombinant and chimeric enzymes expressed in vitro. *Biochim Biophys Acta* **1215**:150–156, 1994.
39. Wang J, Gebre AK, Anderson RA, Parks JS: Amino acid residue 149 of lecithin:cholesterol acyltransferase determines phospholipase A_2 and transacylase fatty acyl specificity. *J Biol Chem* **272**:280–286, 1997.
40. Liu M, Bagdade JD, Subbaiah PV: Specificity of lecithin:cholesterol acyltransferase and atherogenic risk: Comparative studies on the plasma composition and in vitro synthesis of cholesteryl esters in 14 vertebrate species. *J Lipid Res* **36**:1813–1824, 1995.
41. Francone OL, Evangelista L, Fielding CJ: Lecithin-cholesterol acyltransferase: effects of mutagenesis at N-linked oligosaccharide attachment sites on acyl acceptor specificity. *Biochim Biophys Acta* **1166**:301–304, 1993.
42. Hill JS, Wang X, McLeod R, Pritchard PH: Lecithin:cholesterol acyltransferase: Role of N-linked glycosylation in enzyme function. *Biochem J* **294**:879–884, 1993.
43. Chen CH, Albers JJ: Characterization of proteoliposomes containing apoprotein A-I: a new substrate for the measurement of lecithin: cholesterol acyltransferase activity. *J Lipid Res* **23**:680–691, 1982.
44. Stokke KT, Norum KR: Determination of lecithin:cholesterol acyltransferase in human blood plasma. *Scand J Clin Lab Invest* **27**:21–27, 1971.
45. Dobiasova M: Lecithin:cholesterol acyltransferase and the regulation of endogenous cholesterol transport. *Adv Lipid Res* **20**:107–194, 1983.
46. Albers JJ, Adolphson JL, Chen C-H: Radioimmunoassay of human plasma lecithin-cholesterol acyltransferase. *J Clin Invest* **67**:141–148, 1981.
47. Albers JJ, Bergelin RO, Adolphson JL, Wahl PW: Population-based reference values for lecithin-cholesterol acyltransferase (LCAT). *Atherosclerosis* **43**:369–379, 1982.
48. Moriyama K, Sasaki J, Takada Y, Matsunaga A, Fukui J, Albers JJ, Arakawa K: A cysteine-containing truncated apo A-I variant associated with HDL deficiency. *Arterioscler Thromb Vasc Biol* **16**:1416–1423, 1996.
49. Azoulay M, Henry I, Tata F, Weil D, Grzeschik KH, Chaves ME, McIntyre N, et al.: The structural gene for lecithin:cholesterol acyl transferase (LCAT) maps to 16q22. *Ann Hum Genet* **51**:129–136, 1987.

50. Frengen E, Brede G, Larsen F, Skretting G, Prydz H: Physical linkage of the gene cluster containing the LCAT gene to the DNA marker D16S124 at human chromosome region 16q22.1. *Cytogenet Cell Genet* **68**:194–196, 1995.
51. Hengstschlager-Ottnad E, Kuchler K, Schneider WJ: Chicken lecithin-cholesterol acyltransferase: molecular characterization reveals unusual structure and expression pattern. *J Biol Chem* **270**:26139–26145, 1995.
52. Vaisman BL, Klein H-G, Rouis M, Berard AM, Kindt MR, Talley GD, Meyn SM, et al.: Overexpression of human lecithin cholesterol acyltransferase leads to hyperalphalipoproteinemia in transgenic mice. *J Biol Chem* **270**:12269–12275, 1995.
53. Hoeg JM, Santamarina-Fojo S, Berard AM, Cornhill JF, Herderick EE, Feldman SJ, Haudenschild CC, et al.: Overexpression of lecithin: cholesterol acyltransferase in transgenic rabbits prevents diet-induced atherosclerosis. *Proc Natl Acad Sci U S A* **93**:11448–11453, 1996.
54. Miller M, Zeller K: Alternative splicing in lecithin:cholesterol acyltransferase mRNA: an evolutionary paradigm in humans and great apes. *Gene* **190**:309–313, 1997.
55. Meroni G, Malgaretti N, Pontoglio M, Ottolenghi S, Taramelli R: Functional analysis of the human lecithin cholesterol acyltransferase gene promoter. *Biochem Biophys Res Commun* **180**:1469–1475, 1991.
56. Meijer GW, Demacker PNM, van Tol A, Groener JEM, Van der Palen JGP, Stalenhoef AFH, Van Zutphen LFM, et al.: Plasma activities of lecithin:cholesterol acyltransferase, lipid transfer proteins and post-heparin lipases in inbred strains of rabbits hypo- or hyper-responsive to dietary cholesterol. *Biochem J* **293**:729–734, 1993.
57. Weisweiler P: Plasma lipoproteins and lipase and lecithin:cholesterol acyltransferase activities in obese subjects before and after weight reduction. *J Clin Endocrinol Metab* **65**:969–973, 1987.
58. Kiziltunc A, Akcay F, Polat F, Kuskay S, Sahin YN: Reduced lecithin:cholesterol acyltransferase (LCAT) and Na^+, K^+, ATPase activity in diabetic patients. *Clin Biochem* **30**:177–182, 1997.
59. Weight MJ, Coetzee HS, Smuts CM, Marais MP, Maritz JS, Hough FS, Benade AJ, et al.: Lecithin:cholesterol acyltransferase activity and high-density lipoprotein subfraction composition in type 1 diabetic patients with improving metabolic control. *Acta Diabetol* **30**:159–165, 1993.
60. Gillett MP, Teixeira V, Dimenstrein R: Decreased plasma lecithin: cholesterol acyltransferase and associated changes in plasma and red cell lipids in uraemia. *Nephrol Dial Transplant* **8**:407–411, 1993.
61. Danielsson B, Ekman R, Johansson BG, Nilsson-Ehle P, Petersson BG: Lipoproteins in plasma from patients with low LCAT activity due to biliary obstruction. *Scand J Clin Lab Invest* **38**:214–217, 1978.
62. Nishiwaki M, Ishikawa T, Ito T, Shige H, Tomiyasu K, Nakajima K, Kondo K, et al.: Effects of alcohol on lipoprotein lipase, hepatic lipase, cholesteryl ester transfer protein, and lecithin:cholesterol acyltransferase in high-density lipoprotein cholesterol elevation. *Atherosclerosis* **111**:99–109, 1994.
63. Riemens SC, van Tol A, Hoogenberg K, van Gent T, Scheek LM, Sluiter WJ, Dullaart RP: Higher high density lipoprotein cholesterol associated with moderate alcohol consumption is not related to altered plasma lecithin:cholesterol acyltransferase and lipid transfer protein activity levels. *Clin Chim Acta* **258**:105–115, 1997.
64. Mero N, van Tol A, Scheek LM, van Gent T, Labeur C, Rosseneu M, Taskinen MR: Decreased postprandial high density lipoprotein cholesterol and apolipoproteins A-I and E in normolipidemic smoking men: relations with lipid transfer proteins and LCAT activities. *J Lipid Res* **39**:1493–1502, 1998.
65. Staels B, van Tol A, Skretting G, Auwerx J: Lecithin:cholesterol acyltransferase gene expression is regulated in a tissue-selective manner by fibrates. *J Lipid Res* **33**:727–735, 1992.
66. Homma Y, Ozawa H, Kobayashi T, Yamaguchi H, Sakane H, Mikami Y, Nakamura H: Effects of bezafibrate therapy on subfractions of plasma low-density lipoprotein and high-density lipoprotein, and on activities of lecithin:cholesterol acyltransferase and cholesteryl ester transfer protein in patients with hyperlipoproteinemia. *Atherosclerosis* **106**:191–201, 1994.
67. Chiang MT, Otomo MI, Ito H, Furukawa Y, Kimura S: Lipoprotein, lecithin:cholesterol acyltransferase and acetyl CoA carboxylase in stroke-prone spontaneously hypertensive rats fed a diet high in eicosapentaenoic acid. *Atherosclerosis* **106**:21–28, 1994.
68. Jansen H, van Tol A, Auwerx J, Skretting G, Staels B: Opposite regulation of hepatic lipase and lecithin:cholesterol acyltransferase by glucocorticoids in rats. *Biochim Biophys Acta* **1128**:181–185, 1992.
69. Desager JP, Horsmans Y, Harvengt C: Lecithin:cholesterol acyltransferase activity in familial hypercholesterolemia treated with simvastatin and simvastatin plus low-dose colestipol. *J Clin Pharmacol* **31**:537–542, 1991.
70. Ly H, Francone OL, Fielding CJ, Shigenaga JK, Moser AH, Grunfeld C, Feingold KR: Endotoxin and TNF lead to reduced plasma LCAT activity and decreased hepatic LCAT mRNA levels in Syrian hamsters. *J Lipid Res* **36**:1254–1263, 1995.
71. Bell FP: Effects of antihypertensive agents propranolol, metoprolol, nadolol, prazosin, and chlorthalidone on ACAT activity in rabbit and rat aortas and on LCAT activity in human plasma in vitro. *J Cardiovasc Pharmacol* **7**:437–442, 1985.
72. Bell FP: Diazepam inhibits cholesterol esterification by arterial ACAT and plasma LCAT, in vitro. *Atherosclerosis* **50**:345–352, 1984.
73. Bielicki JK, Forte TM, McCall MR: Gas-phase cigarette smoke inhibits plasma lecithin-cholesterol acyltransferase activity by modification of the enzyme's free thiols. *Biochim Biophys Acta* **1258**:35–40, 1995.
74. Brewer HB Jr, Santamarina-Fojo S, Hoeg JM: Disorders of lipoprotein metabolism, in DeGroot LJ, Besser M, Jameson JL, Loriaux D, Marshall JC, Odell WD, Potts JT Jr, et al. (eds): *Endocrinology.* Philadelphia: WB Saunders, 1995, pp 2731–2753.
75. Herz J, Hamann U, Rogne S, Myklebos O, Gausepohl H, Stanley KK: Surface location and high affinity for calcium of a 500 kDa liver membrane protein closely related to the LDL receptor suggest a physiological role as a lipoprotein receptor. *EMBO J* **7**:4119–4127, 1988.
76. Krieger M, Herz J: Structures and functions of multiligand lipoprotein receptors: Macrophage scavenger receptor and LDL receptor–related protein (LRP). *Annu Rev Biochem* **63**:601–637, 1994.
77. Packard CJ, Shepherd J: Lipoprotein heterogeneity and apolipoprotein B metabolism. *Arterioscler Thromb Vasc Biol* **17**:3542–3556, 1997.
78. Krauss RM: Atherogenicity of triglyceride-rich lipoproteins. *Am J Cardiol* **81**:13B–17B, 1998.
79. Mahley RW, Ji ZS: Remnant lipoprotein metabolism. Key pathways involving cell-surface heparin sulfate proteoglycans and apolipoprotein. *J Lipid Res* **40**:1–16, 1999.
80. Davignon J, Gregg RE, Sing CF: Apolipoprotein E polymorphism and atherosclerosis. *Arteriosclerosis* **8**:1–21, 1988.
81. Goldstein JL, Brown MS, Anderson RG, Russell DW, Schneider WJ: Receptor-mediated endocytosis: Concepts emerging from the LDL receptor system. *Annu Rev Cell Biol* **1**:1–39, 1985.
82. Steinberg D, Parthasarathy S, Carew TE, Khoo JC, Witztum JL: Beyond cholesterol: Modifications of low-density lipoprotein that increase its atherogenicity. *N Engl J Med* **230**:915–924, 1989.
83. Phillips MC, Gillotte KL, Haynes MP, Johnson WJ, Lund-Katz S, Rothblat GH: Mechanisms of high density lipoprotein-mediated efflux of cholesterol from cell plasma membranes. *Atherosclerosis* **137**(suppl):13–17, 1998.
84. Czarnecka H, Yokoyama S: Regulation of cellular cholesterol efflux by lecithin:cholesterol acyltransferase reaction through nonspecific lipid exchange. *J Biol Chem* **266**:2023–2028, 1996.
85. von Eckardstein A: Cholesterol efflux from macrohpages and other cells. *Curr Opin Lipidol* **7**:308–319, 1996.
86. Castro GR, Fielding CJ: Early incorporation of cell-derived cholesterol into pre-beta-migrating high-density lipoprotein. *Biochemistry* **27**:25–29, 1988.
87. Santamarina-Fojo S, Peterson K, Knapper C, Qiu Y, Freeman L, Cheng JF, Osorio J, et al.: Complete genomic sequence of the human ABCA1 gene: Analysis of the human and mouse ATP-binding cassette A promoter. *Proc Natl Acad Sci U S A* **97**:7987, 2000.
88. Barrans A, Jaspard B, Barbaras R, Chap H, Perret B, Collet X: Pre-HDL: Structure and metabolism. *Biochim Biophys Acta* **1300**:73–83, 1996.
89. Oram JF, Yokoyama S: Apolipoprotein-mediated removal of cellular cholesterol and phospholipids. *J Lipid Res* **37**:2473–2491, 1996.
90. von Eckardstein A, Chirazi A, Schuler-Luttmann S, Walter M, Kastelein JJP, Geisel J, Real T, et al.: Plasma and fibroblasts of Tangier disease patients are disturbed in transferring phospholipids onto apolipoprotein A-I. *J Lipid Res* **39**:987–998, 1998.
91. Remaley AT, Schumacher UK, Stonik JA, Farsi BD, Nazih H, Brewer HB Jr: Decreased reverse cholesterol transport from Tangier disease fibroblasts. Acceptor specificity and effect of brefeldin on lipid efflux. *Arterioscler Thromb Vasc Biol* **17**:1813–1821, 1997.
92. Glomset JA, Janssen ET, Kennedy R, Dobbins J: Role of plasma lecithin:cholesterol acyltransferase in the metabolism of high density lipoproteins. *J Lipid Res* **7**:638–648, 1966.

93. Carlson LA, Holmquist L: Evidence for deficiency of high density lipoprotein lecithin:cholesterol acyltransferase activity (alpha-LCAT) in fish eye disease. *Acta Med Scand* **218**:189–196, 1985.
94. Lacko AG, Pritchard PH: 2nd International Symposium on Reverse Cholesterol Transport: Report on a meeting. *J Lipid Res* **35**:351–356, 1994.
95. Krieger M: The other side of scavenger receptors: Pattern recognition for host defense. *Curr Opin Lipidol* **8**:275–280, 1997.
96. Schwartz CC, Vlahcevic ZR, Berman M, Meadows JG, Nisman RM, Swell L: Central role of high density lipoprotein in plasma free cholesterol metabolism. *J Clin Invest* **70**:105–116, 1982.
97. Schwartz CC, Berman M, Vlahcevic ZR, Swell L: Multicompartmental analysis of cholesterol metabolism in man. Quantitative kinetic evaluation of precursor sources and turnover of high density lipoprotein cholesterol esters. *J Clin Invest* **70**:863–876, 1982.
98. Gjone E, Norum KR: Familial serum cholesterol ester deficiency. Clinical study of a patient with a new syndrome. *Acta Med Scand* **183**:107–112, 1968.
99. Torsvik H, Gjone E, Norum KR: Familial plasma cholesterol ester deficiency. Clinical studies of a family. *Acta Med Scand* **183**:387–391, 1968.
100. Skretting G, Blomhoff JP, Solheim J, Prydz H: The genetic defect of the original Norwegian lecithin:cholesterol acyltransferase deficiency families. *FEBS Lett* **309**:307–310, 1992.
101. Frohlich J, Hoag G, McLeod R, Hayden M, Godin DV, Wadsworth LD, Critchley JD, et al.: Hypoalphalipoproteinemia resembling fish eye disease. *Acta Med Scand* **221**:291–298, 1987.
102. Skretting G, Prydz H: An amino acid exchange in exon I of the human lecithin:cholesterol acyltransferase (LCAT) gene is associated with fish eye disease. *Biochem Biophys Res Commun* **182**:583–587, 1992.
103. Chu FC, Kuwabara T, Cogan DG, Schaefer EJ, Brewer HB Jr: Ocular manifestations of familial high-density lipoprotein deficiency (Tangier disease). *Arch Ophthalmol* **97**:1926–1928, 1979.
104. Funke H, von Eckardstein A, Pritchard PH, Karas M, Albers JJ, Assmann G, Reckwerth A, et al.: A frameshift mutation in the human apolipoprotein A-I gene causes high density lipoprotein deficiency, partial lecithin:cholesterol acyltransferase deficiency, and corneal opacities. *J Clin Invest* **87**:371–376, 1991.
105. Norum RA, Lakier JB, Goldstein S, Angel A, Goldberg RB, Block WD, Noffze DK, et al.: Familial deficiency of apolipoproteins A-I and C-III and precocious coronary-artery disease. *N Engl J Med* **306**:1513–1519, 1982.
106. Gjone E: Recent research on lecithin:cholesterol acyltransferase II. *Scand J Clin Lab Invest Suppl* **38**:1–232, 1978.
107. Winder AF, Garner A, Sheraidah GA, Barry P: Familial lecithin: cholesterol acyltransferase deficiency. Biochemistry of the cornea. *J Lipid Res* **26**:283–287, 1985.
108. Blanco-Vaca F, Qu SJ, Fiol C, Fan HZ, Pao Q, Marzal-Casacuberta A, Albers JJ, et al.: Molecular basis of fish-eye disease in patient from Spain. Characterization of a novel mutation in the LCAT gene and lipid analysis of the cornea. *Arterioscler Thromb Vasc Biol* **17**:1382–1391, 1997.
109. Gjone E, Bergaust B: Corneal opacity in familial plasma cholesterol ester deficiency. *Acta Ophthalmol (Copenh)* **47**:222–227, 1969.
110. Bron AJ, Lloyd JK, Fosbrooke AS, Winder AF, Tripathi RC: Primary LCAT-deficiency disease. *Lancet* **1**:928–929, 1975.
111. Bethell W, McCulloch C, Ghosh M: Lecithin cholesterol acyltransferase deficiency. Light and electron microscopic finding from two corneas. *Can J Ophthalmol* **10**:494–501, 1975.
112. Barchiesi BJ, Eckel RH, Ellis PP: The cornea and disorders of lipid metabolism. *Surv Ophthalmol* **36**:1–22, 1991.
113. Cogan DG, Kruth HS, Datilis MB, Martin N: Corneal opacity in LCAT disease. *Cornea* **11**:595–599, 1992.
114. Hovig T, Gjone E: Familial lecithin:cholesterol acyltransferase deficiency. Ultrastructural studies on lipid deposition and tissue reactions. *Scand J Clin Lab Invest Suppl* **137**:135–146, 1974.
115. Stokke KT, Bjerve KS, Blomhoff JP, Oystese B, Flatmark A, Norum KR, Gjone E: Familial lecithin:cholesterol acyltransferase deficiency. Studies on lipid composition and morphology of tissues. *Scand J Clin Lab Invest Suppl* **137**:93–100, 1974.
116. Hovig T, Gjone E: Familial plasma lecithin:cholesterol acyltransferase (LCAT) deficiency. Ultrastructural aspects of a new syndrome with particular reference to lesions in the kidneys and the spleen. *Acta Pathol Microbiol Scand* **81**:681–697, 1973.
117. Horven I: Ocular manifestations in familial lecithin:cholesterol acyltransferase deficiency. *Scand J Clin Lab Invest Suppl* **173**:89–91, 1974.
118. Horven I, Egge K, Gjone E: Corneal and fundus changes in familial LCAT deficiency. *Acta Ophthalmol* **52**:201–210, 1974.
119. Myhre E, Gjone E, Flatmark A, Hovig T: Renal failure in familial lecithin:cholesterol acyltransferase deficiency. *Nephron* **18**:239–248, 1977.
120. Borysiewicz LK, Soutar AK, Evans DJ, Thompson GR, Rees AJ: Renal failure in familial lecithin:cholesterol acyltransferase deficiency. *Q J Med* **51**:411–426, 1982.
121. Flatmark AL, Hovig T, Myhre E, Gjone E: Renal transplantation in patients with familial lecithin:cholesterol-acyltransferase deficiency. *Transplant Proc* **9**:1665–1671, 1977.
122. Imbasciati E, Paties C, Scarpioni L, Mihatsch MJ: Renal lesions in familial lecithin:cholesterol acyltransferase deficiency. Ultrastructural heterogeneity of glomerular changes. *Am J Nephrol* **6**:66–70, 1986.
123. Chevet D, Ramee MP, Le Pogamp P, Thomas R, Garre M, Alcindar LG: Hereditary lecithin cholesterol acyltransferase deficiency. Report of a new family with two afflicted sisters. *Nephron* **20**:212–219, 1978.
124. Magil A, Chase W, Frohlich J: Unusual renal biopsy findings in a patient with familial lecithin:cholesterol acyltransferase deficiency. *Hum Pathol* **13**:283–285, 1982.
125. Ohta Y, Yamamoto S, Tsuchida H, Murano S, Saitoh Y, Tohjo S, Okada M: Nephropathy of familial lecithin-cholesterol acyltransferase deficiency. *Am J Kidney Dis* **7**:41–46, 1986.
126. Weber P, Owen JS, Desai K, Clemens MR: Hereditary lecithin-cholesterol acyltransferase deficiency: Case report of a German patient. *Am J Clin Pathol* **88**:510–516, 1987.
127. Lager DJ, Rosenberg BF, Shapiro H, Bernstein J: Lecithin cholesterol acyltransferase deficiency: ultrastructural examination of sequential renal biopsies. *Mod Pathol* **4**:331–335, 1991.
128. Gjone E, Blomhoff JP, Skarbovik AJ: Possible association between an abnormal low density lipoprotein and nephropathy in lecithin:cholesterol acyltransferase deficiency. *Clin Chim Acta* **54**:11–18, 1974.
129. Norum KR, Glomset JA, Nichols AV, Forte T: Plasma lipoproteins in familial licithin:cholesterol acyltransferase deficiency: Physical and chemical studies of low and high density lipoproteins. *J Clin Invest* **50**:1131–1140, 1971.
130. Owen JS, Chaves ME, Chitranukroh A: Lecithin:cholesterol acyltransferase in the physiological system. *Biochem Soc Trans* **13**:20–24, 1985.
131. Gjone E: Familial lecithin:choleterol acyltransferase deficiency — A clinical survey. *Scand J Clin Lab Invest Suppl* **137**:73–82, 1974.
132. Jacobsen CD, Gjone E, Hovig T: Sea-blue histiocytes in familial lecithin:cholesterol acyltransferase deficiency. *Scand J Haematol* **9**:106–113, 1972.
133. Gjone E, Torsvik H, Norum KR: Familial plasma cholesterol ester deficiency. A study of the erythrocytes. *Scand J Clin Lab Invest* **21**:327–332, 1968.
134. Godin DV, Gray GR, Frohlich J: Erythrocyte membrane alterations in licithin:cholesterol acyltransferase deficiency. *Scand J Clin Lab Invest Suppl* **150**:162–167, 1978.
135. Yawata Y, Miyashima K, Sugihara T, Murayama N, Hosoda S, Nakashima S, Iida H, et al.: Self-adaptive modification of red-cell membrane lipids in licithin:cholesterol acyltransferase deficiency. Lipid analysis and spin labeling. *Biochem Biophys Acta* **769**:440–448, 1984.
136. Nordoy A, Gjone E: Familial plasma lecithin:cholesterol acyltransferase deficiency. A study of the platelets. *Scand J Clin Lab Invest* **27**:263–268, 1971.
137. Murayama N, Asano Y, Hosoda S, Maesawa M, Saito M, Takaku F, Sugihara T, et al.: Decreased sodium influx and abnormal red cell membrane lipids in a patient with familial plasma lecithin:cholesterol acyltransferase deficiency. *Am J Hematol* **16**:129–137, 1984.
138. Kuivenhoven JA, Pritchard H, Hill J, Frohlich J, Assmann G, Kastelein J: The molecular pathology of lecithin:cholesterol acyltransferase (LCAT) deficiency syndromes. *J Lipid Res* **38**:191–205, 1997.
139. Kuivenhoven JA, Stalenhoef AFH, Hill JS, Demacker PNM, Errami A, Kastelein JJP, Pritchard PH: Two novel molecular defects in the LCAT gene are associated with fish eye disease. *Arterioscler Thromb Vasc Biol* **16**:294–303, 1996.
140. Kuivenhoven JA, van Voorst tot Voorst EJ, Wiebusch H, Marcovina SM, Funke M, Assmann G, Pritchard PH, et al.: A unique genetic and biochemical presentation of fish-eye disease. *J Clin Invest* **96**:2783–2791, 1995.
141. Wiebusch H, Cullen P, Owen JS, Collins D, Sharp PS, Funke H, Assmann G: Deficiency of lecithin:cholesterol acyltransferase due to compound heterozygosity of two novel mutations (Gly33Arg and 30 bp ins) in the LCAT gene. *Hum Mol Gen* **4**:143–145, 1995.

142. Yang X-P, Inazu A, Honjo A, Koizumi I, Kajinami K, Koizumi J, Marcovina SM, et al.: Catalytically inactive lecithin:cholesterol acyltransferase (LCAT) caused by a Gly 30 to Ser mutation in a family with LCAT deficiency. *J Lipid Res* **38**:585–591, 1997.
143. Owen JS, Wiebusch H, Cullen P, Watts GF, Lima VLM, Funke H, Assmann G: Complete deficiency of plasma lecithin:cholesterol acyltransferase (LCAT) activity due to a novel homozygous mutation (Gly-30-Ser) in the LCAT gene. *Hum Mutat* **8**:79–82, 1996.
144. Funke H, von Eckardstein A, Pritchard PH, Albers JJ, Kastelein JJP, Droste C, Assmann G: A molecular defect causing fish eye disease: An amino acid exchange in lecithin-cholesterol acyltransferase (LCAT) leads to the selective loss of α-LCAT activity. *Proc Natl Acad Sci U S A* **88**:4855–4859, 1991.
145. Karmin O, Hill JS, Wang X, Pritchard PH: Recombinant lecithin: cholesterol acyltransferase containing a Thr123→Ile mutation esterifies cholesterol in low density lipoprotein but not in high density lipoprotein. *J Lipid Res* **34**:81–88, 1993.
146. Iwamoto A, Naito C, Teramoto T, Kato H, Kako M, Kariya T, Shimizu T, et al.: Familial lecithin:cholesterol acyltransferase deficiency complicated with unconjugated hyperbilirubinemia and peripheral neuropathy. The first reported cases in the Far East. *Acta Med Scand* **204**:219–227, 1978.
147. Glomset JA, Norum KR, Nichols AV, Gjone E, King W: Evidence of abnormal disposal of chylomicrons in familial licithin:cholesterol acyltransferase deficiency. *Eur Soc Clin Invest* **3**:231, 1973.
148. Murayama N, Asano Y, Kato K, Sakamoto Y, Hosoda S, Yamada N, Kodama T, et al.: Effects of plasma infusion on plasma lipids, apoproteins and plasma enzyme activities in familial lecithin:cholesterol acyltransferase deficiency. *Eur J Clin Invest* **14**:122–129, 1984.
149. Norum KR, Gjone E: The effect of plasma transfusion on the plasma cholesterol esters in patients with familial plasma lecithin:cholesterol acyltransferase deficiency. *Scand J Clin Lab Invest* **22**:339–342, 1968.
150. Winder AF, Bron AJ: Lecithin:cholesterol acyl transferase deficiency presenting as visual impairment, with hypocholesterolaemia and normal renal function. *Scand J Clin Lab Invest* **38**:151–155, 1978.
151. Horina JH, Wirnsberger G, Horn S, Roob JM, Ratschek M, Holzer H, Pogglitsch H, et al.: Long-term follow-up of a patient with lecithin cholesterol acyltransferase deficiency syndrome after kidney transplantation. *Transplantation* **56**:233–236, 1993.
152. Utermann G, Schoenborn W, Langer KH, Dieker P: Lipoproteins in LCAT-deficiency. *Hum Genet* **16**:295–306, 1972.
153. Forte T, Nichols A, Glomset J, Norum K: The ultrastructure of plasma lipoproteins in lecithin:cholesterol acyltransferase deficiency. *Scand J Clin Lab Invest Suppl* **137**:121–132, 1974.
154. Ritland S, Gjone E: Quantitative studies of lipoprotein-X in familial licithin:cholesterol acyltransferase deficiency and during cholesterol esterification. *Clin Chim Acta* **59**:109–119, 1975.
155. Glomset JA, Norum KR, Nichols AV, Forte T, King WC, Albers J, Mitchell CD, et al.: Plasma lipoprotein metabolism in familial lecithin:cholesterol acyltransferase deficiency. *Scand J Clin Lab Invest Suppl* **137**:165–172, 1974.
156. Utermann G, Menzel HJ, Langer KH, Dieker P: Lipoproteins in lecithin-cholesterol-acyltransferase(LCAT)-deficiency. II. Further studies on the abnormal high-density-lipoproteins. *Hum Genet* **27**:185–187, 1975.
157. Mitchell CD, King WC, Applegate KR, Forte T, Glomset JA, Norum KR, Gjone E: Characterization of apolipoprotein E-rich high density lipoproteins in familial licithin:cholesterol acyltransferase deficiency. *J Lipid Res* **21**:625–634, 1980.
158. Chen C, Applegate K, King WC, Glomset JA, Norum KR, Gjone E: A study of the small spherical high density lipoproteins of patients afflicted with familial licithin:cholesterol acyltransferase deficiency. *J Lipid Res* **25**:269–282, 1984.
159. Miller NE: Associations of high-density lipoprotein subclasses and apolipoproteins with ischemic heart disease and coronary atherosclerosis. *Am Heart J* **113**:589–597, 1987.
160. Cheung MC, Albers JJ: Characterization of lipoprotein particles isolated by immunoaffinity chromatography. Particles containing A-I and A-II and particles containing A-I but no A-II. *J Biol Chem* **259**:12201–12209, 1984.
161. Alaupovic P: Apolipoprotein composition as the basis for classifying plasma lipoproteins. Characterization of ApoA- and ApoB-containing lipoprotein families. *Prog Lipid Res* **30**:105–138, 1991.
162. Duverger N, Rader DJ, Duchateau P, Fruchart JC, Castro G, Brewer HB Jr: Biochemical characterization of the three major subclasses of lipoprotein A-I (LpA-I) preparatively isolated from human plasma. *Biochemistry* **32**:12373–12379, 1993.
163. Fruchart JC, Ailhaud G: Apolipoprotein A-containing lipoprotein particles: Physiological role, quantification, and clinical significance. *Clin Chem* **38**:793-797, 1992.
164. Rader DJ, Castro G, Zech LA, Fruchart JC, Brewer HB Jr: In vivo metabolism of apolipoprotein A-I on high density lipoprotein particles LpA-I and LpA-I, A-II. *J Lipid Res* **32**:1849–1859, 1991.
165. Rader DJ, Ikewaki K, Schaefer JR, Brewer HB Jr: Metabolism of HDL particles LpA-I and LpA-I,A-II in normal and hyperalphalipoproteinemic subjects, in: Catapano AL, Bernini F, Corsini A (eds): *High Density Lipoproteins: Physiopathology and Clinical Relevance*. New York: Raven, 1993, pp 43–55.
166. Rader DJ, Ikewaki K, Duverger N, Schmidt H, Pritchard H, Frohlich J, Clerc M, et al.: Markedly accelerated catabolism of apolipoprotein A-II (ApoA-II) and high density lipoproteins containing ApoA-II in classic lecithin:cholesterol acyltransferase deficiency and fish-eye disease. *J Clin Invest* **93**:321–330, 1994.
167. Elkhalil L, Majd Z, Bakir R, Perez-Mendez O, Castro G, Poulain P, Lacroix B, et al.: Fish-eye disease: Structural and in vivo metabolic abnormalities of high-density lipoproteins. *Metabolism* **46**:474–483, 1997.
168. Ohta T, Nakamura R, Ikeda Y, Frohlich J, Takata K, Saito Y, Horiuchi S, et al.: Evidence for impaired cellular cholesterol removal mediated by apo A-I containing lipoproteins in patients with familial lecithin:cholesterol acyltransferase deficiency. *Biochim Biophys Acta* **1213**:295–301, 1994.
169. von Eckardstein A, Huang Y, Wu S, Funke H, Noseda G, Assmann G: Reverse cholesterol transport in plasma of patients with different forms of familial HDL deficiency. *Arterioscler Thromb Vasc Biol* **15**:691–703, 1995.
170. McIntyre N: Familial LCAT deficiency and fish-eye disease. *J Inherit Metab Dis* **11**:45–56, 1988.
171. Assmann G, von Eckardstein A, Funke H: Lecithin-cholesterol acyltransferase deficiency and fish-eye disease. *Curr Opin Lipidol* **2**:110–117, 1991.
172. Funke H, von Eckardstein A, Pritchard PH, Hornby AE, Wiebusch H, Motti C, Hayden MR, et al.: Genetic and phenotypic heterogeneity in familial licithin:cholesterol acyltransferase (LCAT) deficiency. *J Clin Invest* **91**:677–683, 1993.
173. Klein H-G, Duverger N, Albers JJ, Marcovina S, Brewer HB Jr, Santamarina-Fojo S: In vitro expression of structural defects in the lecithin-cholesterol acyltransferase gene. *J Biol Chem* **270**:9443–9447, 1995.
174. Okubo M, Aoyama Y, Shio H, Albers JJ, Murase T: A novel missense mutation (Asn^5—Ile) in lecithin:cholesterol acyltransferase (LCAT) gene in a Japanese patient with LCT deficiency. *Int J Clin Lab Res* **26**:250–254, 1996.
175. McLean JW: Molecular defects in the lecithin:cholesterol acyltransferase gene, in Miller NE, Tall AR (eds): *High Density Lipoproteins and Atherosclerosis III*. New York: Elsevier Science, 1992, pp 59–65.
176. Bujo H, Kusunoki J, Ogasawara M, Yamamoto T, Ohta Y, Shimada T, Saito Y, et al.: Molecular defect in familial lecithin:cholesterol acyltransferase (LCAT) deficiency: A single nucleotide insertion in LCAT gene causes a complete deficient type of the disease. *Biochem Biophys Res Commun* **181**:933–940, 1991.
177. Klein H-G, Lohse P, Duverger N, Albers JJ, Rader DJ, Zech LA, Santamarina-Fojo S, et al.: Two different allelic mutations in the lecithin:cholesterol acyltransferase (LCAT) gene resulting in classic LCAT deficiency: LCAT (tyr83→stop) and LCAT (tyr156→asn). *J Lipid Res* **34**:49–58, 1993.
178. Steyrer E, Haubenwallner S, Horl G, Giessauf W, Kostner GM, Zechner R: A single G to A nucleotide transition in exon IV of the lecithin:cholesterol acyltransferase (LCAT) gene results in a Arg140 to His substitution and causes LCAT-deficiency. *Hum Genet* **96**:105–109, 1995.
179. Gotoda T, Yamada N, Murase T, Sakuma M, Murayama N, Shimano H, Kozaki K, et al.: Differential phenotypic expression by three mutant alleles in familial lecithin:cholesterol acyltransferase deficiency. *Lancet* **338**:778–781, 1991.
180. Taramelli R, Pontoglio M, Candiani G, Ottolenghi S, Dieplinger H, Catapano A, Albers J, et al.: Lecithin cholesterol acyltransferase deficiency: Molecular analysis of a mutated allele. *Hum Genet* **85**:195–199, 1990.
181. Guerin M, Dachet C, Goulinet S, Chevet D, Dolphin PJ, Chapman MJ, Rouis M: Familial lecithin:cholesterol acyltransferase deficiency: molecular analysis of a compound heterozygote: LCAT (Arg^{147}—Trp) and LCAT (Try^{171}—Stop). *Atherosclerosis* **131**:85–95, 1997.

182. Miller M, Zeller K, Kwiterovich PJ Jr, Albers JJ, Feulner G: Lecithin:cholesterol acyltransferase deficiency: identification of two defective alleles in fibroblast cDNA. *J Lipid Res* **36**:931–938, 1995.

183. Dorval I, Jezequel P, Dubourg C, Chauvel B, Le Pogamp P, Le Gall J-Y: Identification of the homozygous missense mutation in the lecithin:cholesterol-acyltransferase (LCAT) gene, causing LCAT familial deficiency in two French patients. *Atherosclerosis* **105**:251–252, 1994.

184. Miettinen HE, Gylling H, Tenhunen J, Virtamo J, Jauhiainen M, Huttunen JK, Kantola I, et al.: Molecular genetic study of Finns with hypoalphalipoproteinemia and hyperalphalipoproteinemia: A novel Gly^{230} Arg mutation ($LCAT_{Fin}$) of licithin:cholesterol acyltransferase (LCAT) accounts for 5 percent of cases with very low serum HDL cholesterol levels. *Arterioscler Thromb Vasc Biol* **18**:591–598, 1998.

185. Skretting G, Blomhoff JP, Solheim J, Prydz H: The genetic defect of the original Norwegian lecithin:cholesterol acyltransferase deficiency families. *Fed Eur Biochem Soc* **309**:307–310, 1992.

186. Moriyama K, Sasaki J, Arakawa F, Takami N, Maeda E, Matsunaga A, Takada Y, et al.: Two novel point mutations in the lecithin:cholesterol acyltransferase (LCAT) gene resulting in LCAT deficiency: LCAT (G^{873} deletion) and LCAT (Gly^{344} — Ser). *J Lipid Res* **36**:2329–2343, 1995.

187. Maeda E, Naka Y, Matozaki T, Sakuma M, Akanuma Y, Yoshino G, Kasuga M: Lecithin-cholesterol acyltransferase (LCAT) deficiency with a missense mutation in exon 6 of the LCAT gene. *Biochem Biophys Res Commun* **178**:460–466, 1991.

188. Miettinen H, Gylling H, Ulmanen I, Miettinen TA, Kontula K: Two different allelic mutations in a Finnish family with lecithin:cholesterol acyltransferase deficiency. *Arterioscler Thromb Vasc Biol* **15**:460–467, 1995.

189. Klein H-G, Lohse P, Pritchard PH, Bojanovski D, Schmidt H, Brewer HB Jr: Two different allelic mutations in the lecithin-cholesterol acyltransferase gene associated with the fish eye syndrome. Lecithin-cholesterol acyltransferase (Thr_{123}→Ile) and lecithin-cholesterol acyltransferase (Thr_{347}→Met). *J Clin Invest* **89**:499–506, 1992.

190. Contacos C, Sullivan DR, Rye K-A, Funke H, Assmann G: A new molecular defect in the lecithin:cholesterol acyltransferase (LCAT) gene associated with fish eye disease. *J Lipid Res* **37**:35–44, 1996.

191. Li M, Kuivenhoven JA, Ayyobi AF, Pritchard PH: T—G or T—A mutation introduced in the branchpoint consensus sequence of intron 4 of lecithin:cholesterol acyltransferase (LCAT) gene: Intron retention causing LCAT deficiency. *Biochim Biophys Acta* **1391**:256–264, 1998.

192. Klein H-G, Santamarina-Fojo S, Duverger N, Clerc M, Dumon M-F, Albers JJ, Marcovina S, et al.: Fish eye syndrome: a molecular defect in the lecithin-cholesterol acyltransferase (LCAT) gene associated with normal alpha-LCAT specific activity. *J Clin Invest* **92**:479–485, 1993.

193. Kuivenhoven JA, Weibusch H, Pritchard PH, Funke H, Benne R, Assmann G, Kastelein JJ: An intronic mutation in a lariat branchpoint sequence is a direct cause of an inherited human disorder (fish-eye disease). *J Clin Invest* **98**:358–364, 1996.

194. Sakai N, Vaisman BL, Koch CA, Hoyt RF Jr, Meyn SM, Talley GD, Paiz JA, et al.: Targeted disruption of the mouse lecithin:cholesterol acyltransferase (LCAT) gene. *J Biol Chem* **272**:7506–7510, 1997.

195. Ng DS, Francone OL, Forte TM, Zhang J, Haghpassand M, Rubin EM: Disruption of the murine lecithin:cholesterol acyltransferase gene causes impairment of adrenal lipid delivery and up-regulation of scavenger receptor class B type I. *J Biol Chem* **272**:15777–15781, 1997.

196. Sakai N, Vaisman BL, Koch C, Hoyt RF Jr, Meyn S, Paiz JA, Brewer HB Jr, et al.: Lecithin:cholesterol acyltransferase (LCAT) knockout mice: a new animal model for human LCAT-deficiency. *Circulation* **94**:I-274, 1996.

197. Albers JJ, Chen CH, Adolphson JL: Lecithin:cholesterol acyltransferase (LCAT) mass: Its relationship to LCAT activity and cholesterol esterification rate. *J Lipid Res* **22**:1206–1213, 1981.

198. Mowri H-O, Patsch JR, Ritsch A, Föger B, Brown S, Patsch W: High density lipoproteins with differing apolipoproteins: Relationships to postprandial lipemia, cholesteryl ester transfer protein, and activities of lipoprotein lipase, hepatic lipase, and lecithin:cholesterol acyltransferase. *J Lipid Res* **35**:291–300, 1994.

199. Tato F, Vega GL, Grundy SM: Determinants of plasma HDL-cholesterol in hypertriglyceridemic patients: Role of cholesterol-ester transfer protein and lecithin cholesteryl acyltransferase. *Arterioscler Thromb Vasc Biol* **17**:56–63, 1997.

200. Solajic-Bozicevic N, Stavljenic A, Sesto M: Lecithin:cholesterol acyltransferase activity in patients with acute myocardial infarction and coronary heart disease. *Artery* **18**:326–340, 1991.

201. Solajic-Bozicevic N, Stavljenic-Rukavina A, Sesto M: Lecithin-cholesterol acyltransferase activity in patients with coronary artery disease examined by coronary angiography. *Clin Invest* **72**:951–956, 1994.

202. Miller NE, Rajput-Williams J, Nanjee MN, Samuel L, Albers JJ: Relationship of high density lipoprotein composition to plasma lecithin:cholesterol acyltransferase concentration in men. *Atherosclerosis* **69**:123–129, 1988.

203. Williams PT, Albers JJ, Krauss RM, Wood PD: Associations of licithin:cholesterol acyltransferase (LCAT) mass concentrations with exercise, weight loss, and plasma lipoprotein subfraction concentrations in men. *Atherosclerosis* **82**:53–58, 1990.

204. Goldstein JL, Hazzard WR, Schrott HG, Bierman EL, Motulsky AG, Levinski MJ, Campbell ED: Hyperlipidemia in coronary heart disease. I. Lipid levels in 500 survivors of myocardial infarction. *J Clin Invest* **52**:1533–1543, 1973.

205. Wells IC, Peitzmeier G, Vincent JK: Lecithin:cholesterol acyltransferase and lysolecithin in coronary atherosclerosis. *Exp Mol Pathol* **45**:303–310, 1986.

206. Hoeg JM, Vaisman BL, Demosky SJ Jr, Meyn SM, Talley GD, Hoyt RF Jr, Feldman S, et al.: Lecithin:cholesterol acyltransferase overexpression generates hyperalphalipoproteinemia and a nonatherogenic lipoprotein pattern in transgenic rabbits. *J Biol Chem* **271**:4396–4402, 1996.

207. Brousseau ME, Santamarina-Fojo S, Zech LA, Berard AM, Vaisman BL, Meyn SM, Powell D, et al.: Hyperalphalipoproteinemia in human lecithin cholesterol acyltransferase transgenic rabbits: In vivo apolipoprotein A-I catabolism is delayed in a gene dose-dependent manner. *J Clin Invest* **97**:1844–1851, 1996.

208. Brousseau ME, Santamarina-Fojo S, Vaisman BL, Applebaum-Bowden D, Berard AM, Talley GD, Brewer HB Jr, et al.: Overexpression of human lecithin:cholesterol acyltransferase in cholesterol-fed rabbits: LDL metabolism and HDL metabolism are affected in a gene dose-dependent manner. *J Lipid Res* **38**:2537–2547, 1997.

209. Brousseau ME, Wang J, Demosky SJ Jr, Vaisman BL, Talley GD, Santamarina-Fojo S, Brewer HB Jr, et al.: Correction of hypoalphalipoproteinemia in LDL receptor-deficient rabbits by lecithin:cholesterol acyltransferase. *J Lipid Res* **39**:1558–1567, 1998.

210. Brousseau ME, Kauffman RD, Herderick EE, Demosky SJ Jr, Evans W, Marcovina S, Santamarina-Fojo S, et al.: LCAT modulates atherogenic plasma lipoproteins and the extent of atherosclerosis only in the presence of normal LDL receptors in transgenic rabbits. *Arterioscler Thromb Vasc Biol* **20**:450, 2000.

211. Francone OL, Gong EL, Ng DS, Fielding CJ, Rubin EM: Expression of human lecithin-cholesterol acyltransferase in transgenic mice: Effect of human apolipoprotein AI and human apolipoprotein AII on plasma lipoprotein cholesterol metabolism. *J Clin Invest* **96**:1440–1448, 1995.

212. Mehlum A, Staels B, Duverger N, Tailleux A, Castro G, Fievet C, Luc G, et al.: Tissue-specific expression of the human gene for lecithin-cholesterol acyltransferase in transgenic mice alters blood lipids, lipoproteins and lipases towards a less atherogenic profile. *Eur J Biochem* **230**:567–575, 1995.

213. Mehlum A, Muri M, Hagve TA, Solberg LA, Prydz H: Mice overexpressing human lecithin:cholesterol acyltransferase are not protected against diet-induced atherosclerosis. *APMIS* **105**:861–868, 1997.

214. Berard AM, Remaley AT, Vaisman BL, Paigen B, Hoyt RF Jr, Meyn SM, Talley GD, et al.: High plasma HDL concentrations associated with enhanced atherosclerosis in transgenic mice overexpressing lecithin cholesteryl acyltransferase. *Nat Med* **3**:744–749, 1997.

215. Foger B, Chase M, Amar MJ, Vaisman BL, Shamburek RD, Paigen B, Fruchart-Najib J et al.: Cholesteryl ester transfer protein corrects dysfunctional high density lipoproteins and reduces aortic atherosclerosis in lecithin cholesterol acyltransferase transgenic mice. *J Biol Chem* **272**:36912, 1999.

216. Amar MJ, Vaisman BL, Foger B, Paigen B, Talley GD, Brewer HB Jr, Santamarina-Fojo S: The effect of hepatic lipase deficiency on the plasma lipids, lipoproteins and diet-induced atherosclerosis in LCAT transgenic mice. *Circulation* **96**:I-109, 1997.

217. Amar MJA, Shamburek RD, Foger B, Hoyt RF Jr, Wood DO, Santamarina-Fojo S, Brewer HB Jr: Adenovirus-mediated expression of LCAT in non-human primates leads to an antiatherogenic lipoprotein profile with increased HDL and decreased LDL. *Circulation* **98**:I-35, 1998.

CHAPTER 119

Type III Hyperlipoproteinemia (Dysbetalipoproteinemia): The Role of Apolipoprotein E in Normal and Abnormal Lipoprotein Metabolism

Robert W. Mahley ▪ Stanley C. Rall, Jr.

1. Patients with type III hyperlipoproteinemia have elevated concentrations of both plasma cholesterol and triglyceride. A biochemical characteristic of the disorder is the occurrence of β-migrating VLDL (β-VLDL), which are cholesterol-enriched remnants of both intestinal chylomicrons and hepatic VLDL. The β-VLDL are enriched in a variant form of apo E, which, in type III hyperlipoproteinemic subjects, is dysfunctional.

2. Clinical features of the disorder are varied. Many type III subjects have cutaneous xanthomas, particularly tuberoeruptive or tuberous xanthomas and xanthomas of the palmar creases (xanthoma striata palmaris); the latter have not been identified in any other disorder. These patients have a high incidence of premature coronary and (especially) peripheral atherosclerosis. In the most common form of the disease, overt hyperlipidemia is only rarely manifested before adulthood. Type III subjects frequently have other disorders that exacerbate the hyperlipoproteinemia.

3. Apolipoprotein E is a polymorphic protein that results from the existence of multiple alleles at a single gene locus and from varying posttranslational sialylation. The genetically determined polymorphism of apo E has a significant impact on normal variations in lipid, lipoprotein, and apolipoprotein levels in the human population. The primary molecular defect in most patients with type III hyperlipoproteinemia is the presence of a mutant form of apo E (apo E-2) that differs from normal apo E (apo E-3) by only a single amino acid substitution (cysteine for arginine at residue 158). The apo E-2 variant binds poorly to low-density lipoprotein receptors and is associated with a recessive mode of inheritance of type III hyperlipoproteinemia. Other rare forms of mutant apo E causing type III hyperlipoproteinemia appear to be associated with dominant inheritance.

4. The normal catabolism of remnant lipoprotein particles, which is directed by apo E, is altered in type III hyperlipoproteinemia. The presence of the defective apo E results in the accumulation of chylomicron and VLDL remnants (β-VLDL) in plasma. These particles in turn have a propensity for uptake by macrophages in peripheral tissues. As a result of massive cholesterol deposition, these macrophages become foam cells, which may be the progenitors of cholesterol-laden cells in the atherosclerotic lesion.

5. In the recessive form of the disorder, the development of overt hyperlipidemia requires the inheritance of two alleles for the mutant apo E [E-2(Arg 158 → Cys)]. The occurrence of the defective alleles is necessary but not usually sufficient to induce the type III hyperlipoproteinemia. Most E-2/2 subjects are either normolipidemic or even hypocholesterolemic. Thus, the development of the recessive form of the overt hyperlipidemia involves other genetic, hormonal, or environmental influences that, in combination with the defective receptor binding of apo E, precipitate the development of the hypertriglyceridemia and hypercholesterolemia. The secondary factors include hypothyroidism, low-estrogen conditions, obesity, diabetes, and age.

6. In the dominant form of the disorder, subjects possessing a single allele for one of the rare variants of apo E have the overt hyperlipidemia, presumably from birth. Secondary genetic, hormonal, or environmental factors usually are not required to precipitate the accumulation of remnant lipoproteins in the plasma, but secondary factors can sometimes modulate the severity of the disorder.

7. Diagnosis of type III hyperlipoproteinemia is indicated by increased plasma cholesterol and triglyceride, the presence of β-VLDL, xanthomas (especially palmar xanthomas), premature vascular disease (especially of the peripheral

A list of standard abbreviations is located immediately preceding the index in each volume. Additional abbreviations used in this chapter include: IDL = intermediate-density lipoprotein(s); LRP = LDL receptor-related protein; and HSPG = heparan sulfate proteoglycan(s).

arteries), and usually the apo E phenotype E-2/2. The diagnostic hallmark of this disorder is the presence of apo E that is defective in binding to lipoprotein receptors.

8. **Type III hyperlipoproteinemia usually responds well to therapy. Dietary control is the preferred treatment, but a drug regimen may also be required to lower lipid levels. Useful drugs for treatment of type III hyperlipoproteinemia include nicotinic acid, fibric acid derivatives, and HMG-CoA reductase inhibitors. In particular, gemfibrozil seems to be the drug of choice in treating this disorder.**

HISTORY AND OVERVIEW

The lipoprotein disorder now known as type III hyperlipoproteinemia was first described by Gofman et al.[1,2] in the 1950s and was originally termed "xanthoma tuberosum," based on the occurrence of xanthomatous lesions of the skin over extensor tendons and planar xanthomas of the volar surfaces of the hands. In affected patients, the distinctively abnormal lipoprotein profile, as determined by analytical ultracentrifugation, was characterized by an increase in the concentration of lipoproteins with flotation rates of S_f = 12 to 20 [small VLDL and intermediate-density lipoproteins (IDL)] and S_f = 0 to 12 (especially LDL).[1,2] Gofman and coworkers also recognized that this disorder was probably familial.

It was later appreciated that xanthoma tuberosum was identical to one of the distinct classes of familial hyperlipoproteinemias (type III hyperlipoproteinemia) established by Fredrickson et al.[3] in 1967. As a result of classifying hyperlipidemic subjects by using a combination of ultracentrifugation and paper electrophoresis, they found one group that had a VLDL fraction ($d < 1.006$ g/ml) with β, rather than the normal pre-β, electrophoretic mobility. These lipoproteins, referred to as β-VLDL,[4] were enriched in cholesterol. These observations were confirmed by others, and the association with accelerated or premature atherosclerosis became well established.[5–8] Through the years, other designations were used for this disorder, most notably *broad-beta disease*,[3] based on the peculiar migration pattern of the abnormal β-VLDL on paper electrophoresis, and *dysbetalipoproteinemia*, used to denote the unusual chemical and physical properties of the VLDL. More recently, the β-VLDL have been shown to represent two different lipoproteins that accumulate in the plasma—chylomicron remnants of intestinal origin and VLDL remnants of hepatic origin.[9,10] In fact, the disorder has also been referred to as *remnant removal disease*.[11]

The abnormal cholesterol-enriched β-VLDL were the diagnostic hallmark of type III hyperlipoproteinemia for some years, until an apolipoprotein abnormality came to light. In 1973, Havel and Kane[12] showed that type III subjects had an absolute increase in the plasma levels of apo E, or *arginine-rich apoprotein*. Apolipoprotein E is one of several protein components that occur normally on VLDL, chylomicrons, and certain subclasses of HDL (for review, see references 8 and 13). Later, in a pioneering series of studies, Utermann and associates[14–18] demonstrated, by isoelectric focusing, that a particular isoform of apo E was invariably absent in type III subjects. These observations suggested that the primary genetic defect in type III hyperlipoproteinemia was homozygosity for a mutant isoform of apo E (referred to as apo E-2 to distinguish it from the normal apo E-3). The genetics and mode of inheritance of apo E, as first described by Utermann et al.[14–18] and later refined by Zannis and Breslow,[19,20] clarified the basis of apo E polymorphism and helped to establish the association of the mutant apo E with type III hyperlipoproteinemia.

Studies by Mahley and coworkers identified the amino acid structural differences among the various apo E isoforms[21–23] and defined, at a molecular level, the role of the mutant apo E in the development of type III hyperlipoproteinemia (for review, see references 8, 13, and 24–26). Apolipoprotein E was discovered to be a major ligand for the LDL receptor[27–29] and the apolipoprotein responsible for mediating the cellular uptake of chylomicron remnants and VLDL remnants (the lipoproteins referred to collectively as β-VLDL that accumulate in the plasma in type III hyperlipoproteinemia).[30–33] These findings focused attention on the role of apo E in regulating the plasma levels of these lipoproteins. These data, in association with the observation that the mutant apo E did not bind normally to the lipoprotein receptors,[30,34,35] also suggested that the primary defect in type III hyperlipoproteinemia was the defective interaction of mutant apo E with the lipoprotein receptors, leading to the accumulation of β-VLDL in the plasma. However, in most subjects with the common mutant form of apo E, the overt expression of hyperlipidemia is modulated by other genetic and environmental factors.

BIOCHEMICAL FEATURES OF THE DISORDER

Blood Lipids, Lipoproteins, and Apolipoproteins

The lipid, lipoprotein, and apolipoprotein values vary widely in subjects with the hallmark biochemical defects of type III hyperlipoproteinemia: β-VLDL and the mutant apo E. The most dramatic demonstration of the abnormalities is found in untreated patients who express the most overt hyperlipidemia (Table 119-1). In severely affected patients, plasma cholesterol levels are usually greater than 300 mg/dl and may approach 1000 mg/dl.[5] Plasma triglyceride concentrations are within the same range and tend to equal or exceed the total cholesterol concentration in any given subject. The diagnosis of type III hyperlipoproteinemia should be considered in hyperlipidemic subjects when the cholesterol and triglyceride levels are both elevated and approximately equal.

As determined by ultracentrifugal analysis and lipoprotein electrophoresis, there is a prominent β band (β-VLDL) in the $d <$ 1.006 g/ml fraction (Fig. 119-1) and a dramatic absolute increase (as compared with normal) in the β-migrating lipoproteins found

Table 119-1 Plasma Lipoprotein Concentrations in Subjects with Untreated Type III Hyperlipoproteinemia*

Subject	Number	Cholesterol (mg/dl)	Triglycerides (mg/dl)	Cholesterol Content (mg/dl)		
				VLDL	LDL+IDL	HDL
Type III hyperlipoproteinemia						
All subjects	47	453 ± 21	699 ± 77	287 ± 25	121 ± 8	38 ± 3
Men, mean age 40	27	440 ± 25	694 ± 104	268 ± 32	131 ± 14	37 ± 3
Women, mean age 49	20	470 ± 36	705 ± 117	307 ± 39	131 ± 9	39 ± 5
Control						
Men, age 30–39	50	210 ± 5	78 ± 6	21 ± 2	143 ± 4	48 ± 2
Women, age 40–49	44	217 ± 5	80 ± 6	14 ± 1	130 ± 4	62 ± 2

*Values cited are mean ± SEM; control values are derived from Fredrickson, Levy, and Lindgren.[4]

SOURCE: Adapted from Morganroth, Levy, and Fredrickson.[5]

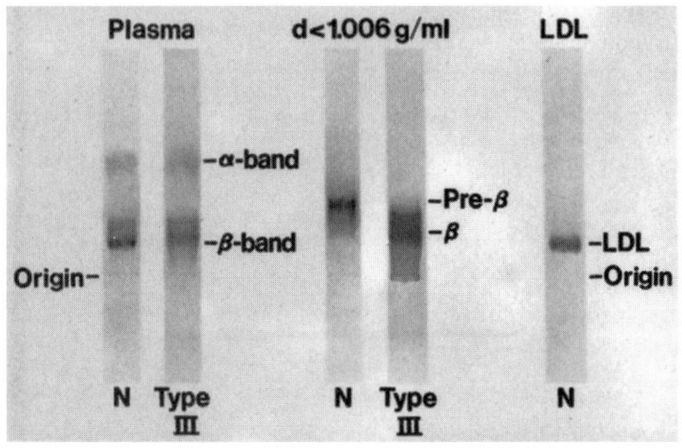

Fig. 119-1 Agarose gel electrophoretic pattern of plasma lipoproteins. Identification of the lanes, from left: total plasma lipoproteins from a normal subject; total plasma lipoproteins from a type III hyperlipoproteinemic subject; VLDL (*d* < 1.006 g/ml) from a normal subject; VLDL (*d* < 1.006 g/ml) from a type III hyperlipoproteinemic subject; LDL (*d* = 1.02 to 1.063 g/ml) from a normal subject. (*Courtesy of Dr. David A. Chappell.*)

in this fraction (as assessed by cholesterol determinations). Pre-β-VLDL are also present in the $d < 1.006$ g/ml fraction and can occur as a single or double electrophoretic band in non–type III subjects.[36] The double pre-β band can sometimes lead to a misinterpretation regarding the presence of β-VLDL. In type III subjects, the $d = 1.006$ to 1.019 g/ml fraction (IDL) is also modestly increased. In contrast, the $d = 1.02$ to 1.063 g/ml fraction (LDL) is almost always significantly reduced.[14] If the ultracentrifugal fractionation is performed so as to include the IDL and LDL ($d = 1.006$ to 1.063 g/ml) within the same fraction, the cholesterol may or may not show a decrease, because of the compensating effects of increased IDL and decreased LDL. The concentration of cholesterol in the $d = 1.063$ to 1.21 g/ml fraction (HDL) is usually also modestly reduced in type III hyperlipoproteinemic subjects. With treatment of the hyperlipidemia, the HDL cholesterol concentration frequently increases, whereas the concentration of the LDL cholesterol may remain low.[5] Table 119-1 lists changes in lipoprotein concentrations seen in type III patients.

Abnormal Lipoproteins

The major abnormal lipoprotein in type III hyperlipoproteinemia is β-VLDL. These particles are remnant lipoproteins that derive from chylomicrons secreted by the intestine and from VLDL secreted by the liver.[9,10] That β-VLDL in humans represent both intestinal and hepatic remnants has been amply demonstrated by the presence of the two forms of apo B. One form, apo B-100, is synthesized in the liver and is secreted as a constituent of VLDL.[37] The other form, apo B-48, synthesized exclusively in the intestine, is secreted as a constituent of chylomicrons.[37,38] Apolipoprotein B-48 represents the N-terminal 48 percent of the 4536-residue apo B-100. In humans, it arises as a result of a unique intestinal mRNA editing mechanism that introduces a stop codon at a position corresponding to amino acid 2153.[39,40] Both forms of apo B can be found in β-VLDL, and the two types of remnants can be separated by biochemical or immunologic techniques.[9,10,41]

Normally, chylomicrons synthesized by the intestine enter the blood and are acted on by lipoprotein lipase, which catalyzes the hydrolysis of the triglyceride, resulting in the formation of chylomicron remnants (cholesterol-rich particles lacking some of their triglyceride). The chylomicron remnants are rapidly and efficiently cleared from the circulation via the liver (for review, see references 8 and 13). Their uptake is mediated by apo E (for review, see references 42 and 43). Likewise, the normal pre-β-VLDL are processed through a lipolytic cascade, resulting in progressively smaller and more cholesterol-rich lipoproteins as the VLDL remnants become IDL and finally LDL.[8] A certain portion of these hepatic VLDL remnants ($\approx$50 percent) is also removed from the circulation via the liver before reaching the final stage in the cascade—the formation of LDL. Hepatic uptake of VLDL remnants, including IDL, is mediated by apo E.

In type III hyperlipoproteinemia, the remnants accumulate in the plasma (for review, see references 13, 24, 44, and 45). The intestinal β-VLDL appear to be derived directly from chylomicrons. The hepatic β-VLDL probably represent a cholesterol-enriched intermediate derived from the hepatic pre-β-VLDL.[46] Both forms of β-VLDL may be normal intermediates of chylomicron and pre-β-VLDL catabolism that, in type III hyperlipoproteinemia, accumulate in the plasma to abnormally high levels secondary to impaired catabolism or impaired lipolysis of these lipoproteins. This is more thoroughly discussed under "Pathogenesis of Type III Hyperlipoproteinemia," below.

The physical and chemical characteristics of β-VLDL found in type III hyperlipoproteinemia are quite distinct from those of normal pre-β-VLDL (Table 119-2). Although hepatic β-VLDL tend to be only slightly smaller in diameter than normal pre-β-VLDL, these lipoproteins are strikingly dissimilar in chemical composition. The β-VLDL are considerably more enriched in cholesterol (mostly as cholesteryl esters) and are relatively depleted of triglycerides.[41,46–48] In addition, the complement of apolipoproteins differs both quantitatively and qualitatively.[12,41,49] Whereas β-VLDL and VLDL have a roughly similar total protein content, β-VLDL have much less of the C apolipoproteins. In contrast, there is a relative and absolute increase in apo E on β-VLDL.[12,41] In addition, the mutant apo E of type III subjects is defective in binding to specific cell-surface receptors (see "Pathogenesis of Type III Hyperlipoproteinemia," below).

The IDL fraction in the plasma of type III subjects is also abnormal in that it is increased and contains some apo B-48, indicating the presence of intestinal remnants. Thus, the IDL in these subjects probably represents the lower end of the spectrum of particle sizes of β-VLDL, as well as normal IDL, although this conclusion can be disputed.[50]

Other lipoproteins in patients with type III hyperlipoproteinemia do not appear to be abnormal in size, shape, or chemical composition.[51] This applies to HDL, LDL ($d = 1.02$

Table 119-2 Chemical Composition of β Very Low Density Lipoproteins from Type III Hyperlipidemic Subjects and Pre-β Very Low Density Lipoproteins from Normal Subjects

Lipoprotein	Mean Particle Diameter (nm)	CE	FC	Composition (% Mass) TG	PL	Protein	Apolipoproteins
Intestinal -VLDL	82	32	7	43	14	4	B(35%) > E > C
Hepatic -VLDL	38	26	7	39	19	9	B(55%) > E > C
Hepatic pre--VLDL	44	12	5	59	16	8	B(45%) > C > E

CE = cholesteryl ester; FC = free cholesterol; TG = triglyceride; PL = phospholipid.

SOURCE: Average of mean values from various sources, including references 5, 9, 10, 41, and 46–48.

to 1.063 g/ml), and probably to pre-β-VLDL, although pre-β-VLDL of type III subjects have not been extensively characterized.

CLINICAL EXPRESSION AND MANIFESTATION OF THE DISORDER

By far the most common variant form of apo E that is associated with type III hyperlipoproteinemia is apo E-2 resulting from a single amino acid substitution of cysteine for the normally occurring arginine at amino acid residue 158 (Arg 158 → Cys). Other rare defective variants of apo E associated with type III hyperlipoproteinemia have been described (for review, see references 13 and 43–45). This section focuses on the effects of the common apo E-2(Arg 158 → Cys) variant on clinical expression of the disorder. Under "Pathogenesis of Type III Hyperlipoproteinemia" below, the impact of this variant on lipoprotein metabolism is contrasted with the effect of the rare variants.

Approximately 1 percent of the North American and Northern European populations is homozygous for the mutant form of apo E (phenotype E-2/2; see "Apolipoprotein E Genetics and the Impact of Allelic Variations on Lipids and Atherosclerosis," below) that is associated with type III hyperlipoproteinemia. All homozygous subjects with this apo E-2(Arg 158 → Cys) phenotype have detectable β-VLDL in their plasma, reflecting the presence of the variant apo E. However, most do not have overt hyperlipoproteinemia; in fact, many are normolipidemic or even hypolipidemic.[14,15,52] It is reasonable to classify these subjects as having *dysbetalipoproteinemia* because they do have β-VLDL in their plasma (although not in sufficient quantities to result in elevated plasma lipid levels) and because they have the genetic predisposition (i.e., the presence of the abnormal apo E variant) for hyperlipidemia. Overt hyperlipoproteinemia, characterized by elevated concentrations of plasma cholesterol and triglyceride, occurs rather rarely, at a frequency of about 1 to 5 per 5000 in the general population.[52] Subjects with overt hyperlipoproteinemia should be classified as having *type III hyperlipoproteinemia* (to distinguish them from those with normal lipid levels but with plasma β-VLDL, i.e., with dysbetalipoproteinemia).

The apparent discrepancy between the relatively high occurrence of the mutant form of apo E-2 and the relatively low expression of overt hyperlipoproteinemia indicates that the disorder is modulated by other genetic and environmental factors that affect the absolute levels of plasma lipids, which range from hypolipidemic to hyperlipidemic. However, it is important to emphasize that an absolute requirement for expression of the disorder is the occurrence of the mutant form of apo E that is defective in binding to the lipoprotein receptors (see "Pathogenesis of Type III Hyperlipoproteinemia," below).

Age of Onset

Type III hyperlipoproteinemia in subjects homozygous for apo E-2(Arg 158 → Cys) rarely manifests itself before adulthood;[5,49,53–58] there are only a few reports of its occurrence in teenagers.[17,53,55,59,60] In light of the more recent discovery of other rare forms of apo E that result in a dominant mode of inheritance of type III hyperlipoproteinemia, it must be suspected that some of the patients presenting with type III hyperlipoproteinemia before adulthood may not have the apo E-2(Arg 158 → Cys) mutation. The disease is much more prevalent in men than in women (Table 119-3), and it tends to occur earlier in men.[5] Women usually do not express the disorder until after menopause. Factors that may result in an earlier onset include obesity and the presence of other clinical disorders, such as diabetes mellitus or hypothyroidism.

Xanthomas

The most striking clinical feature of type III hyperlipoproteinemia is the occurrence of xanthomas (Fig. 119-2), one type of which has not been described in any other disorder and is, therefore, essentially pathognomonic for type III hyperlipoproteinemia (for review, see references 60 and 61). These particular xanthomas, which are termed "xanthoma striata palmaris,"[62] and which also have been called "planar xanthomas" or "palmar xanthomas,"[3] occur as yellowish lipid deposits in the palmar creases. Roughly half of untreated patients have this particular kind of lesion (see Table 119-3). Other types of palmar xanthomas (but never in the palmar creases) have been described in patients with familial hypercholesterolemia.

Table 119-3 Clinical Data on 185 Patients with Type III Hyperlipoproteinemia

No. of patients	185
Male/female	131/54
Age range, years	16 to 95
Mean cholesterol, mg/dl	450
Mean triglyceride, mg/dl	570
Clinical Finding	**Percent of Patients**
Xanthomas	
Striata palmaris	55
Tendon	13
Tuberous and tuberoeruptive	64
Xanthelasma	7
Corneal arcus	11
Coronary heart disease	28
Peripheral vascular disease	21
Cerebrovascular disease	4
Gout	4
Diabetes mellitus (clinical)	4
Hypothyroidism	4

SOURCE: Pooled data from references 5, 53–55, 57, 58.

In addition, subjects with type III hyperlipoproteinemia have other types of xanthomas, especially tuberous and tuberoeruptive xanthomas, but these lesions are not unique to type III hyperlipoproteinemia. The tuberous xanthomas appear most frequently on the elbows, knees, buttocks, and knuckles (see Fig. 119-2). Xanthelasmas and tendinous xanthomas (particularly in the skin over the Achilles tendon) are also sometimes seen, but these occur more frequently in familial hypercholesterolemia. See Table 119-3 for a summary of the results concerning xanthomas in 185 patients. Xanthomas in type III patients usually disappear rather rapidly once treatment is initiated.

Premature Atherosclerosis

Premature or accelerated atherosclerosis occurs in one-third to more than one-half of patients with type III hyperlipoproteinemia[3,53–55,57,58,63,64] but has an unusual distribution. Peripheral vascular disease of the lower extremities is almost as common as coronary artery disease. This is strikingly different from the distribution of vascular disease seen in familial hypercholesterolemia, in which there is less involvement of the lower extremities. Although the mechanism underlying the predisposition for peripheral atherosclerosis in type III hyperlipoproteinemia is unknown, it is noteworthy that certain cholesterol-fed animals that have high levels of β-VLDL also have much more peripheral vascular disease than coronary atherosclerosis.[24,25,65,66]

Morganroth et al.[5] reported that about 43 percent of 47 type III patients had vascular disease, and about one-third had definite coronary artery disease. In a study of 39 patients, Stuyt and Van't Laar[57] described the occurrence of atherosclerotic vascular disease in 22 type III patients (56 percent): 15 had coronary artery disease and 18 had definite peripheral vascular disease. These characteristics have been confirmed in more recent investigations by Feussner and associates.[63,64] In one study of 64 type III patients, 39 percent had atherosclerosis, especially peripheral vascular disease (31 percent),[63] and in another study of 78 type III patients,

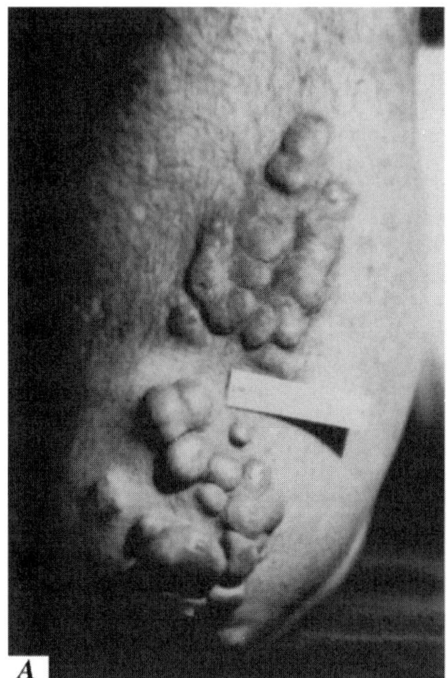

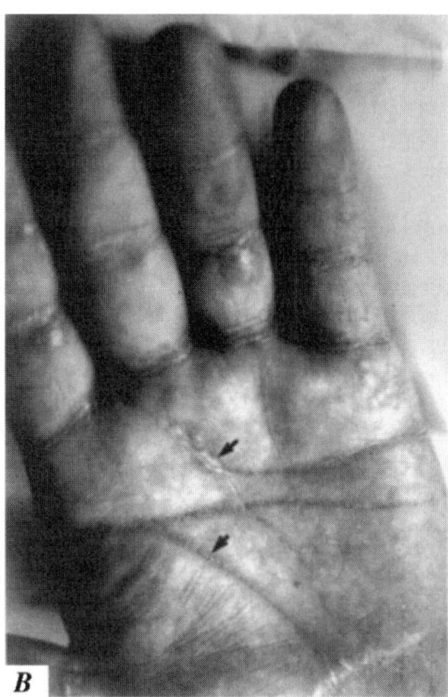

Fig. 119-2 Examples of xanthomas in type III hyperlipoproteinemic subjects. A, Tuberoeruptive xanthomas of the elbows. B, Tuberous xanthomas of the digits and xanthomas of the palmar creases (xanthoma striata palmaris) (arrows). (*Courtesy of Dr. Thomas P. Bersot.*)

41 percent had atherosclerosis and a highly predictive association of carotid artery atherosclerosis with peripheral atherosclerosis of the legs.[64] Vascular disease generally becomes symptomatic earlier in men than in women (mean age, ≈40 versus ≈50 years).[5] Less than 1 percent of all myocardial infarction survivors were found to have type III hyperlipoproteinemia;[67] however, overt hyperlipoproteinemia imposes a high risk of premature vascular disease.

Associated Disorders

Other disorders are also frequently associated with type III hyperlipoproteinemia, which suggests that their presence may exacerbate the hyperlipidemia. Asymptomatic hyperuricemia is present in up to half of the subjects, but only about 4 percent have clinical gout[5] (see Table 119-3). Glucose intolerance is also common in type III subjects, but again, only a small percentage (about 4 percent) have clinical diabetes. Obesity is common in type III hyperlipoproteinemia,[3,63] and this may be associated with the high level of glucose intolerance. Hypothyroidism markedly exacerbates the lipid and lipoprotein abnormalities in type III hyperlipoproteinemia;[5,68] in contrast, hyperthyroidism can essentially eliminate overt hyperlipidemia.

PATHOLOGIC FINDINGS IN TYPE III HYPERLIPOPROTEINEMIA

Autopsy reports on 10 patients with type III hyperlipoproteinemia have appeared in the literature.[69–75] The first report, by Roberts et al.,[69] described findings from a 57-year-old woman with severe coronary artery atherosclerosis. The lumen of all three major coronary arteries was severely narrowed by deposits of lipid-laden foam cells rather than the more typical complicated plaques. The entire aorta and the iliac arteries contained numerous foam-cell lesions, and plaques also narrowed the small arteries of the kidney, adrenal glands, and pancreas. Lipid deposits were also seen in the mural endocardium of the left atrium and in the mitral valve leaflets. Foam cells, presumably macrophages, also characterized the atheroma of a 64-year-old woman with diffuse coronary and peripheral artery atherosclerosis.[72] In the same study, foam cells were seen in the endocardium of the left atrium and ventricle, and in the spleen. Foam cells have also been found in renal glomeruli.[72,76] However, other reports describe the atherosclerosis as being more typical, characterized by extensive fibrotic, complicated lesions.[70,73,74]

At the National Institutes of Health, Cabin et al.[74] and Schwartz[75] reviewed the anatomic data on six patients with type III hyperlipoproteinemia. Four were women, who died between 50 and 74 years of age. All six patients had ischemic heart disease, and four had intermittent claudication. One of the six was the woman described in the original report.[69] All six patients had severe coronary, aortic, and common iliac atherosclerosis. There was a strikingly high incidence of left main coronary artery narrowing; however, the atherosclerosis involved the coronary arteries diffusely. Almost half the patients had coronary artery narrowing of greater than 76 percent. Only one of the six patients (presumably the one from the original report) had foam-cell atherosclerosis. Lesions from the other patients were more fibrous and complicated and resembled atherosclerosis seen in patients with other types of hyperlipidemia.

It is likely that the morphologic appearance of the atherosclerotic lesions changes with time and the extent of disease. Atherosclerotic lesions begin with an abundance of foam cells—that is, lipid-laden macrophages[77]—that evolve into more complicated plaques. However, there is also reason to believe that macrophage foam cells may play a unique role in the development of lipid-laden lesions in type III hyperlipoproteinemia. The β-VLDL from patients with type III hyperlipoproteinemia and from animals fed high levels of fat and cholesterol are uniquely capable of causing cholesterol accumulation in macrophages in cell culture[78,79] (see also "Pathogenesis of Type III Hyperlipoproteinemia," below). Laboratory studies have demonstrated that β-VLDL are the only naturally occurring lipoproteins that cause a 100- to 200-fold increase in the cholesterol content of mouse peritoneal macrophages. Macrophages are major progenitors of atherosclerosis and xanthomatous foam cells. The β-VLDL appear to be the atherogenic lipoproteins in these patients and in animals fed diets high in fat and cholesterol.[24,25,65,66]

APOLIPOPROTEIN E GENETICS AND THE IMPACT OF ALLELIC VARIATIONS ON LIPIDS AND ATHEROSCLEROSIS

The Molecular Basis for Apolipoprotein E Polymorphism

Because the development of type III hyperlipoproteinemia is dependent on the inheritance of an abnormal form of apo E, an understanding of the genetics, structure, and function of apo E is crucial in the consideration of the disease (for review, see references 13, 29, 43–45, and 80). The polymorphic nature of apo E was first appreciated in the studies of Utermann and associates,[14–18] who used isoelectric focusing to demonstrate the polymorphism. These studies clearly established the familial nature of the polymorphism and also demonstrated that one of the isoforms of apo E was invariably deficient or absent in subjects with type III hyperlipoproteinemia. Their studies suggested that this missing isoform was the normal apo E and that type III hyperlipoproteinemia resulted from the inheritance of two abnormal apo E alleles.

Subsequently, Zannis and Breslow,[19,20] using a two-dimensional electrophoretic technique, made two important observations that helped to clarify the polymorphism of apo E. They found that there were actually two types of apo E polymorphism — one genetically determined and one not. The latter polymorphism was shown to be the result of posttranslational sialylation of the apo E polypeptide, giving rise to one or several more acidic isoforms.[19] These minor isoforms could be readily distinguished in the second dimension of the gel analysis by their slightly higher apparent molecular weight, caused by the addition of sialic acids. When the apo E was treated with neuraminidase (an enzyme that cleaves sialic acid residues), these higher-molecular-weight forms disappeared and comigrated with the major, genetically determined apo E isoforms. The appreciation of this complexity of apo E isoform patterns (multiple sialylated and nonsialylated forms) allowed a more thorough understanding of the genetically determined polymorphism.[81]

It was established that the three major isoforms of apo E were all products of the same gene and that apo E genetics could be explained by the existence of three typical alleles at a single gene locus.[20] As a result, six phenotypes are possible, three homozygous and three heterozygous, with the heterozygous phenotypes arising from the inheritance of any two different alleles.[52] The occurrence of these six common phenotypes and their pattern of inheritance has been amply confirmed in a large number of family studies by many investigators (see "Population Studies of Apolipoprotein E Polymorphism," below).

A standard nomenclature for apo E genetics and polymorphism was established in 1982.[81] The three genetically determined isoforms are designated E-4, E-3, and E-2, with E-4 being the most basic (pI $\approx$ 6.1). The corresponding alleles for these three gene products are termed $\varepsilon4$, $\varepsilon3$, and $\varepsilon2$. The six common phenotypes are E-4/4, E-3/3, or E-2/2 (homozygous) and E-4/3, E-3/2, or E-4/2 (heterozygous). The minor sialylated isoforms are designated with a subscript *s* (e.g., E-4_s, E-3_s). It is the apo E phenotype E-2/2 that is associated most commonly with type III hyperlipoproteinemia. Other rare variants of apo E associated with the development of type III hyperlipoproteinemia have been described (discussed below).

The molecular basis for apo E polymorphism was established by Mahley and coworkers.[8,21–25] They determined the primary structure of apo E and found that the isoforms E-4, E-3, and E-2 differed from one another by single amino acid substitutions at two sites in the protein (Fig. 119-3). The existence of these substitutions confirmed that E-4, E-3, and E-2 arose from separate alleles at a single gene locus. These substitutions also explain the single unit charge differences among the three isoforms, because they involve the substitution of the neutral amino acid cysteine for the basic amino acid arginine. The molecular basis has also been determined for the second type of apo E polymorphism — that conferred by posttranslational glycosylation. The glycosylated (sialylated) isoforms in plasma apo E result from the attachment of a carbohydrate chain to a single site at threonine residue 194 in apo E.[82] The asialo isoform, which accounts for about 80 percent of the total apo E in plasma, was found to have no carbohydrate moiety at all. It is unclear whether the major apo E isoform without carbohydrate represents an end product of deglycosylation or whether the major biosynthetic pathway does not result in glycosylation. It is possible that the minor glycosylated isoforms, including those that are multiply sialylated, are products of a subset of cells synthesizing apo E.

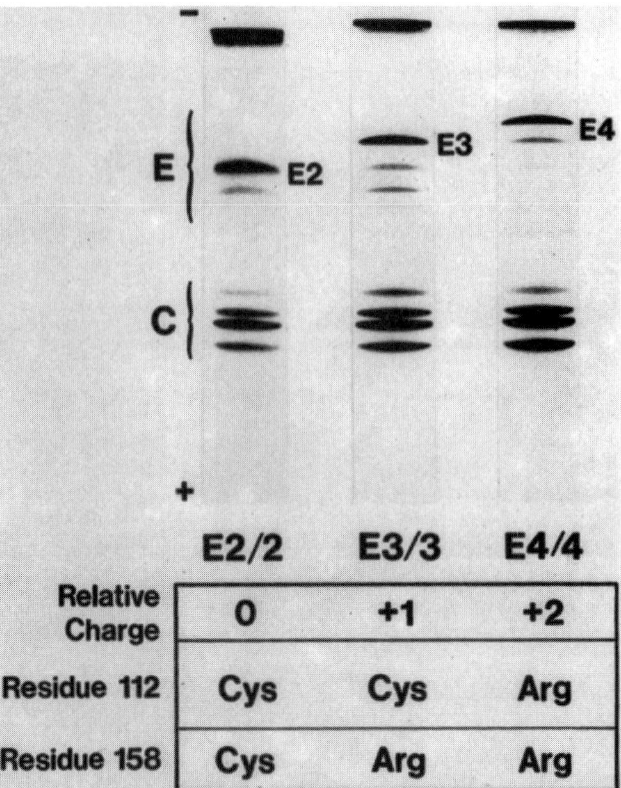

Fig. 119-3 Isoelectric focusing of apo-VLDL demonstrating the three homozygous apo E phenotypes. The amino acid substitutions that account for the charge differences among the isoforms are shown. The minor, more acidic apo E isoforms in each case represent sialylated isoforms. The E-2/2 phenotype is from a type III hyperlipoproteinemic subject. (*From Mahley and Angelin.*[83] *Used by permission of* Advances in Internal Medicine.)

Population Studies of Apolipoprotein E Polymorphism

Studies of apo E phenotype and allelic frequency among various populations worldwide reveal interesting ethnic differences and demonstrate that the apo E genotype has a major effect on plasma lipid levels and possibly on cardiovascular risk. In almost all populations, the apo E-3/3 phenotype is by far the most common (typically $\approx$50 to 70 percent of the population), and the $\varepsilon3$ allele makes up a large majority of the apo E gene pool (typically $\approx$70 to 80 percent). The less frequent $\varepsilon4$ and $\varepsilon2$ alleles nonetheless contribute significantly to the gene pool (typically 10 to 15 percent for $\varepsilon4$ and $\approx$5 to 10 percent for $\varepsilon2$). As a result of the lower frequencies of the $\varepsilon4$ and $\varepsilon2$ alleles, the phenotypes E-4/4, E-4/2, and E-2/2 are relatively rare (Table 119-4).

Initially, the prominence of apo E-3 suggested that it was the parent ("wild-type") form of the protein and that apo E-4 and apo E-2 were variants. However, it now appears that $\varepsilon4$ is most likely the ancestral allele. Almost all animals,[92] including the higher primates, such as the baboon,[93] possess the equivalent of apo E-4 homozygosity (arginine at the residue corresponding to amino acid 112 in the sequence). In addition, aboriginal human groups, such as the Huli of the Papua New Guinea highlands, have $\varepsilon4$ as the most common allelic form.[94] The evolution of the allelic forms of apo E is of considerable interest to population geneticists and suggests that there is a selective advantage to the occurrence of apo E-3, and possibly apo E-2, in humans. Alternatively, genetic drift could be responsible for the disparities in allelic frequency

Table 119-4 Apolipoprotein E Phenotype and Allele Frequencies in Various Populations

	Phenotype and Allele Frequencies (%)															
													Singapore			
	U S A (n=152)	Canada (n=102)	Germany (n=1000)	Germany (n=1031)	Austria (Tyrolean) (n=469)	Scotland (n=400)	Hungary (n=202)	Iceland (n=185)	Turkey (n=8366)	Finland (n=615)	Sudan (n=103)	New Zealand (n=426)	Malay (n=118)	Indian (n=142)	Chinese (n=190)	Japan (n=319)
Phenotype																
E-4/4	3.0	3.9	2.3	2.8	2.1	1.0	1.0	3.2	1.1	6.3	8.7	0.9	3.4	1.4	1.1	1.3
E-4/3	14.0	20.6	20.2	22.9	17.3	24.8	22.8	12.9	35.5	31.9	35.9	25.1	16.1	21.8	11.6	11.3
E-3/3	58.0	61.8	62.7	59.8	64.0	58.3	65.3	74.2	46.8	54.0	39.8	51.4	60.2	68.3	69.5	72.1
E-3/2	22.0	9.8	11.0	12.0	13.2	12.8	7.9	10.6	9.9	6.7	9.7	20.0	16.9	7.0	15.3	13.8
E-2/2	1.3	2.0	0.8	1.0	1.3	0.5	2.0	0.4	0.5	0.3	1.0	1.4	1.5	0.7	1.6	0.6
E-4/2	2.0	2.0	3.0	1.5	2.1	2.8	1.0	0.8	1.5	0.8	4.9	1.2	0.8	0.7	1.1	0.9
Allele																
$\epsilon 4$	11.0	15.2	13.9	15.0	11.7	15.0	12.9	7.9	24.4	22.7	29.1	14.1	11.9	12.7	7.4	7.4
$\epsilon 3$	76.0	77.0	78.3	77.3	78.9	77.0	80.7	86.0	69.5	73.3	61.9	73.9	76.7	82.7	82.8	84.6
$\epsilon 2$	13.0	7.8	7.8	7.7	9.0	8.0	6.4	6.1	6.2	4.1	8.1	12.0	11.4	4.6	9.7	8.0
Reference	84	85	86	87	88	89	88	88	95	90	88	91	88	88	88	88

between the lower species and humans. Apolipoprotein E has diverse roles in metabolism and normal physiology;[13,43,44] however, the selective pressures are probably unrelated to lipoprotein metabolism or heart disease, but are likely to be related to poorly defined roles of apo E involving cell growth and differentiation, nerve development or repair, or modulation of immunologic responses (for review, see reference 13).

As Table 119-4 illustrates, allelic frequency has interesting variations in different racial groups. The apo E gene frequency in most European and North American populations is rather homogeneous (ε3, 76 to 79 percent; ε4, 11 to 15 percent; and ε2, 6 to 9 percent). An obvious exception is the Finnish population, in which ε4 is much more prevalent (23 to 24 percent). On the other hand, Asians (specifically Chinese and Japanese) have a relatively higher frequency of ε3 ($\approx$82 to 85 percent) and, interestingly, the Turks of Central Asian origin have the highest ε3 frequency (86 percent).[95] In contrast, African nationals from the Sudan[88] and Nigeria[96,97] have lower ε3 ($\approx$61 percent) and higher ε4 ($\approx$30 percent). A study comparing the apo E genotype in Black and Caucasian men in the United States revealed that Blacks resembled the Sudanese and Nigerians (ε3, 80.3 percent in Caucasians vs. 65.3 percent in Blacks; ε4, 11.9 percent in Caucasians vs. 23.2 percent in Blacks; ε2, 7.7 percent in Caucasians vs. 11.5 percent in Blacks).[98] One of the interesting population studies compares the apo E phenotypes of two isolated cultural groups in Papua New Guinea — the Huli and the Pawaia.[94] The Huli are characterized by an extremely high frequency of the ε4 allele and low frequency of the ε3 allele (ε3, 35.6 percent; ε4, 49.0 percent; ε2, 15.4 percent). The Pawaia have a very different apo E phenotype pattern, more similar to that of Blacks (ε3, 60.3 percent; ε4, 25.9 percent; ε2, 13.8 percent).

Impact of the Apolipoprotein E Locus on Plasma Lipids and Lipoproteins. Apolipoprotein E polymorphism is one of the common genetic factors responsible for interindividual differences in lipid and lipoprotein levels. While the ε3 allele showed no deviations from the population mean, Sing and Davignon[99] found that the ε4 and ε2 alleles had significant effects on various lipid and lipoprotein parameters (Fig. 119-4).

The ε2 allele is associated with lower levels of plasma cholesterol, LDL cholesterol, and apo B than the ε3 allele. Conversely, the ε4 allele is associated with higher levels of total cholesterol and LDL cholesterol. Utermann et al.[14,18,52] reported that apo E-2 is significantly more frequent in hypertriglyceridemic subjects, whereas apo E-4 is more frequent in hypercholesterolemic subjects. The original observations made by Utermann et al.,[14,18,52] Bouthillier et al.,[100] and Robertson and Cumming[101] have been confirmed in numerous studies (for review, see reference 102). Davignon et al.[102] evaluated the data in seven

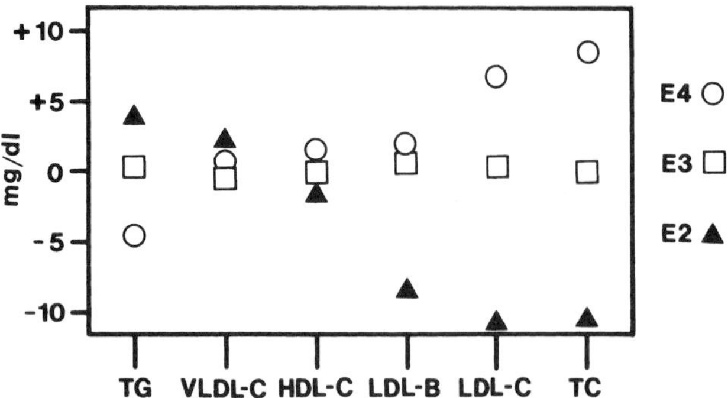

Fig. 119-4 The effects of apo E alleles on various lipoprotein parameters. TG = total plasma triglyceride; VLDL-C = VLDL cholesterol; HDL-C = HDL cholesterol; LDL-B = LDL apo B; LDL-C = LDL cholesterol; TC = total plasma cholesterol. (*Adapted from Sing and Davignon.*[99] *Used by permission of the* American Journal of Human Genetics.)

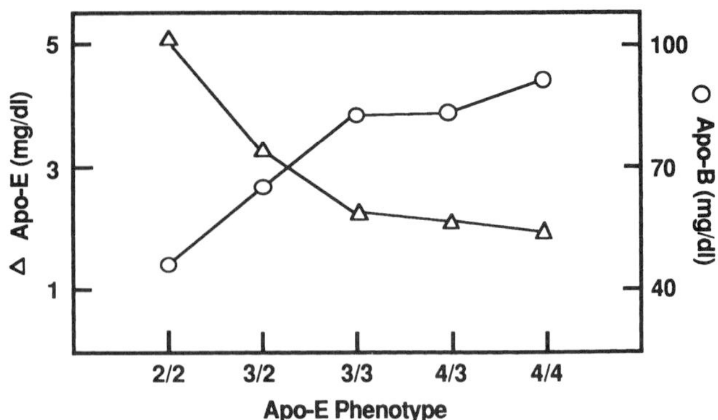

Fig. 119-5 Plasma concentrations of apo E (Δ) and apo B (O) in relation to apo E phenotypes. (*From Utermann.*[52] *Used by permission of Elsevier Science Publishers.*)

different studies that included Caucasian and Asian populations and demonstrated a remarkably consistent pattern: subjects with the E-2/2 phenotype have the lowest plasma cholesterol levels, while those with the E-4/4 phenotype have the highest; the difference in cholesterol levels between E-2/2 and E-4/4 subjects ranges from 25 to 66 mg/dl.

For these same populations, Davignon et al.[102] calculated the average cholesterol effect of each of the common alleles (ε2, ε3, and ε4). The difference in the average effects for ε2 versus ε4 ranged from 13 to 30 mg/dl. Compared to the cholesterol-elevating effect of the ε4 allele, the ε2 allele had a greater impact on lowering plasma cholesterol (by a factor of two- to threefold). This is considered to be an unusually large effect from a single gene on an individual trait. In every study, the ranking of the apo E phenotypes from the lowest to the highest cholesterol levels was E-2/2, E-3/2, E-3/3, E-4/2, E-4/3, and E-4/4. It appears that the apo E allele can explain about 10 percent of the interindividual variation in cholesterol levels in different populations. Using meta-analysis to compare data in 45 populations in 17 countries, Dallongeville and coworkers[103] confirmed and extended these observations. Compared with the ε3 allele, ε2 was associated with lower plasma cholesterol levels, and ε4 was associated with higher cholesterol levels regardless of differences in ethnicity and in metabolic conditions.

Utermann[52] has also shown that one or two doses of ε2 (i.e., E-2/2 or E-3/2 phenotype) correlate with increased plasma apo E levels and decreased apo B levels. Conversely, ε4 (E-4/3 or E-4/4) is associated with lower levels of apo E and higher levels of apo B (Fig. 119-5). The apo B levels primarily reflect the changes in LDL cholesterol. Steinmetz et al.[104] observed similar effects of the apo E alleles on apo E and apo B levels in neonates. Interestingly, recent studies established that the plasma levels of the various apo E isoforms have a major impact on plasma lipids. For example, Salah et al.[105] demonstrated that plasma apo E concentrations account for 20 to 40 percent of the variability of triglyceride levels. Huang et al.[106] showed that high levels of apo E-3 markedly elevated plasma triglyceride in transgenic mice by impairing VLDL lipolysis and stimulating VLDL production.

In a number of studies, ε2 was shown to be significantly associated with hypertriglyceridemia.[107] In their meta-analysis of the effect of the apo E phenotype on triglycerides in various populations, Dallongeville et al.[103] found that subjects with the ε2 allele (E-2/2 or E-3/2) had higher triglyceride levels than those with E-3/3. This is consistent with an association between the ε2 allele and impaired clearance of triglyceride-rich chylomicrons and VLDL remnants and with the observation that the ε2 allele is also associated with defective lipolytic processing of VLDL (discussed in "Effect of Mutant Apolipoprotein E on the Remnant Pathway," below). Gregg and coworkers[108] have shown that apo E-2 is catabolized more slowly in vivo than apo E-3, a difference that has important implications in type III hyperlipoproteinemia (see "Pathogenesis of Type III Hyperlipoproteinemia," below).

The overall impact of apo E alleles on triglyceride levels is a matter of some debate. Although the first studies of Sing and Davignon[99] showed that ε4 was associated with lower triglycerides (Fig. 119-4), this finding has been difficult to confirm. Davignon et al.,[102] in evaluating data from seven studies, found no consistent relationship between apo E and triglyceride levels. Others have reported elevated triglyceride levels in E-4/3[103] but not in E-4/4 subjects.[109] However, patients with type V hyperlipoproteinemia (elevated VLDL and chylomicrons with very high triglycerides) may have an overrepresentation of the ε4 allele.[110]

Metabolic studies have been no less confusing. Gregg et al.[109] demonstrated that apo E-4 perturbs remnant catabolism and is catabolized more rapidly than apo E-3 in vivo. These findings led to speculation that more rapid remnant catabolism downregulates hepatic LDL receptors, thus explaining the association of elevated LDL with the ε4 allele (Fig. 119-4). Weintraub et al.[111] arrived at a similar conclusion from studies showing that apo E-4 carriers cleared dietary fat more rapidly than apo E-3 carriers. However, other studies found no effect of apo E alleles on either postprandial response[112] or triglyceride levels,[113] while yet others found delayed clearance of postprandial triglycerides in association with apo E-4,[114,115] which would suggest at least a transient increase in triglycerides. Clearly, more data are needed to understand the relationship of apo E-4 and triglyceride levels.

Several studies have been unable to demonstrate a consistent effect of the apo E phenotype on HDL cholesterol levels. Likewise, Dallongeville et al.[103] could not demonstrate a clear association between HDL cholesterol and the E-2/2, E-3/2, or E-4/2 phenotypes. However, HDL cholesterol levels were lower in subjects with the E-4/3 phenotype than in those with the E-3/3 phenotype.

Impact of the Apolipoprotein E Locus on Atherosclerosis. The ε4 allele has been suggested as a risk factor for atherosclerosis.[102] This allele is associated with higher cholesterol levels and the E-4/3 phenotype is associated with higher triglyceride levels and lower HDL cholesterol.[103] Studies of patients with coronary artery disease and those who have had myocardial infarctions have yielded conflicting information as to whether apo E-4 increases the risk of cardiovascular disease (for review, see reference 102). Cumming and Robertson[89] and Kuusi et al.[116] demonstrated an association between the ε4 allele and coronary artery disease.

In contrast, it seems clear that the presence of apo E-2 correlates with reduced risk, but only in non-type III subjects, who do not express the overt hyperlipidemia.[102] Most E-2/2 or E-3/2 subjects do not express type III hyperlipoproteinemia and, in fact, display low levels of plasma cholesterol and LDL cholesterol. Subjects with type III hyperlipoproteinemia who have overt hyperlipidemia are at increased risk of both coronary and peripheral artery atherosclerosis (see Table 119-3).

The Pathobiological Determinants of Atherosclerosis in Youth (PDAY) Study correlated atherosclerotic lesions with apo E phenotype in 720 young males (15 to 34 years) who died of external causes.[98] Among both Blacks and Caucasians, subjects with the ε2 allele had the least total involvement and the fewest raised atherosclerotic lesions in the thoracic and abdominal aorta. The ε4 allele tended to be associated with the greatest amount of aortic atherosclerosis. However, coronary artery atherosclerosis could not be well correlated with the ε alleles. The impact of the apo E alleles on aortic atherosclerosis was not explained strictly on the basis of the effect of the alleles on lipid levels. When the cholesterol levels were adjusted, the effect of the apo E genotype on atherosclerosis did not change significantly. Apolipoprotein E is synthesized by macrophages and smooth muscle cells and accumulates in atherosclerotic lesions.[117,118] The different isoforms of apo E may have different roles within the lesion and may actually affect lesion progression or regression by differentially altering cell growth, formation of lipoprotein–artery wall matrix complexes, or cholesterol transport.[13]

Impact of the Apolipoprotein E Locus on Dietary Lipid Absorption and Transport. Several studies demonstrate that the apo E phenotype is not the major determinant of interindividual differences in the response of plasma cholesterol levels to dietary lipids.[112,119] This appears to be especially true when the diets tested were high in fat. However, in studies conducted by Gylling and Miettinen,[120] results using diets with a low fat content, but with either high or low cholesterol, did suggest an effect of the apo E phenotype on LDL cholesterol levels in response to high dietary cholesterol. Subjects with the ε4 allele had increased cholesterol absorption, increased LDL production, and decreased LDL apo B plasma clearance. On the other hand, subjects with the ε2 allele appeared to be less sensitive to high levels of dietary cholesterol and had lower LDL cholesterol levels, increased LDL apo B clearance, and increased bile acid synthesis[120] (see also references 121 and 122).

An additional effect of dietary cholesterol (and dietary saturated fat) on lipoprotein metabolism is to decrease the expression of LDL receptors. This may be affected by apo E phenotype. For example, Weintraub et al.[111] examined the effect of apo E alleles on dietary fat transport by labeling newly synthesized intestinal lipoproteins with vitamin A added to the fat-rich meal and following their metabolism in the plasma. Subjects with the E-3/2 phenotype had a delayed plasma clearance of intestinal lipoproteins and elevated levels of particles thought to be chylomicron remnants. This observation is consistent with a defect in remnant clearance associated with apo E-2; however, in most non-type III hyperlipoproteinemic patients, the plasma cholesterol level is actually low. The postulate is that the reduced clearance of apo E-2–containing lipoproteins is detected in the liver as a deficiency of cholesterol delivery and thus results in an increase in the number of LDL receptors. Upregulation of LDL receptors could account in part for the decrease in LDL cholesterol levels.

APOLIPOPROTEIN E STRUCTURE-FUNCTION CORRELATES

Apolipoprotein E Gene Structure and Mapping

The apo E gene is 3.6 kb in length and contains 4 exons.[123,124] Comparison of the apo E gene structure with those of six other apolipoproteins (apo A-I, apo A-II, apo A-IV, apo C-I, apo C-II, and apo C-III) reveals a strikingly similar location of the introns and suggests a common ancestral origin for this family of genes.[125,126] The apo E gene codes for an mRNA of 1163 nucleotides.[127,128] The primary translation product comprises 317 amino acids, with the N-terminal 18 amino acids serving as a signal peptide. Thus, the mature apo E is secreted as a 299-amino acid protein. The apo E gene is located at the 5′ end of a 44-kb gene cluster[129] on chromosome 19,[123,130] and it is linked closely to apo C-I, an apo C-I pseudogene,[131] and apo C-II.[132] In addition, the LDL receptor[133] has been mapped to chromosome 19, but it is not linked to apo E.

Several different regulatory elements control the expression of the apo E gene in various tissues. Simonet et al.[134,135] mapped the tissue-specific regulatory elements of the 5′ and 3′ regions of the apo E gene, including far-downstream elements that occur in the apo E–C-I intergenic region. There are separate testis- and kidney-positive elements 5′ of the apo E gene and adipose-, skin-, adrenal-, and ovary-positive elements found 3′ of the apo E gene but upstream of the apo C-I gene. A liver control element is located approximately 15 kb 3′ of the apo E gene in the region between the apo C-I gene and the apo C-I′ pseudogene.[135] A second liver control element is located 10 kb further downstream between the apo C-I pseudogene and the apo C-II gene.[136] The liver regulatory elements control the hepatic synthesis of all genes in the apo E gene cluster.

Structure and Function of Apolipoprotein E

Apolipoprotein E, a protein constituent of several plasma lipoproteins, including chylomicrons, chylomicron remnants, VLDL, IDL, and a subclass of HDL (HDL with apo E), participates in the transport of lipids among various tissues and cells.[13] A major physiological role for apo E is to mediate the interaction of apo E-containing lipoproteins with lipoprotein receptors,[13] including the LDL receptor and a putative chylomicron remnant or apo E receptor. The remnant receptor appears now to be the LDL receptor–related protein (LRP) (for review, see references 42, 43, and 137–149).

Apolipoprotein E contains two structural domains that differ in function.[141,142] The N-terminal two-thirds of apo E (residues ≈1 to 165) and the C-terminal one-third (residues ≈200 to 299) are connected by a region (165 to 200) of random structure that serves as a hinge between these two highly structured domains. The C-terminal domain contains a strong amphipathic α-helical region that is thought to represent the major lipid-binding domain. The N-terminal domain contains the region of apo E responsible for its interaction with the LDL receptor and with heparin (heparan sulfate proteoglycans). As discussed below, the LDL receptor- and the heparin-binding sites reside near amino acid residues 130 to 150, a region enriched in basic amino acids (arginine and lysine).

The receptor-binding domain of the apo E molecule has been mapped with six complementary experimental approaches (for review, see references 13, 44, 45, and 80). First, selective chemical modifications of various amino acids established that a limited number of arginine and lysine residues within apo E are critical in mediating its binding to the LDL receptor. Second, identification and sequencing of natural apo E mutants defective in receptor binding (at residues 136, 142, 145, and 146) established that the 136-to-150 region contained several arginine and lysine residues critical for binding. Third, generation of fragments of apo E and testing of their receptor binding localized the binding domain to the middle of the molecule. Fourth, mapping of the epitope of an apo E monoclonal antibody that blocked the interaction of apo E with the LDL receptor demonstrated that the 140-to-150 region was involved. Fifth, analysis of the receptor-binding activity of mutant forms of apo E produced by site-directed mutagenesis revealed that basic residues in the 136-to-150 region, including lysine 143 and arginine 150, were critical. Sixth, the use of x-ray crystallography localized the receptor-binding domain to a basic patch on the surface of the apo E-3 molecule encompassing residues 136 to 150 (Fig. 119-6). Apolipoprotein E appears to bind to the LDL receptor through an ionic interaction between key basic amino acid residues in the 136-to-150 region and acidic amino acid residues of the LDL receptor. The LDL receptor possesses seven repeated segments near its N-terminus that represent the ligand-binding sites and contain the critical acidic amino acids aspartate and glutamate (for review, see references 140 and 143). On the other hand, the LRP contains 31 domains, homologous to the ligand-binding sites of the LDL receptor, that are capable of interacting with apo E (for review, see references 137, 139, and 140). As discussed below, both receptors bind apo E-containing lipoproteins with high affinity and are involved in mediating their uptake.

Analysis of the three-dimensional structures[5] of apo E-3 and its variants apo E-2 and apo E-4 has provided unique insights into the structure of the receptor-binding domain and other functional domains of apo E.[144–146] The N-terminal two-thirds (residues 1 to 191) of apo E-3, containing the receptor-binding domain, occurs as a four-helix bundle. Helix 4 (residues 130 to 164) possesses the critical basic residues responsible for the ionic interaction with the LDL receptor. The crystal structure reveals that basic amino acid residues in the 136-to-150 region are largely solvent exposed and are not involved in either intramolecular or intermolecular salt bridges. These residues form a 20-Å patch of positive potential on the surface of helix 4 and appear to interact directly with the receptor[145] (see Fig. 119-6).

An important observation is that residue 158 of apo E (the site for the common variant that is defective in receptor binding) lies outside the patch of positive potential.[146] Previously, Innerarity et al.[147,148] hypothesized that the substitution of cysteine for arginine at residue 158 disrupts receptor binding secondarily by altering the interaction of this part of the molecule with the critical basic residues in the 136-to-150 region. The crystal structure of apo E-3 versus apo E-2 (the 158 variant) confirms this hypothesis.[146] In apo E-3, the arginine at residue 158 is involved in two salt bridges—one with aspartic acid 154 in helix 4 and the other with glutamic acid 96 in helix 3. However, in apo E-2, where cysteine is substituted for the normally occurring arginine at residue 158, the aspartic acid 154 forms a salt bridge with arginine 150 and swings the side chain of arginine 150 into a new plane. That this new salt bridge is responsible for the apo E-2 receptor-binding defect was elegantly demonstrated by a mutagenesis approach. Dong et al.[149] changed the aspartic acid 154 residue to alanine in apo E-2 to eliminate the possibility of a salt bridge between arginine 150 and residue 154. Receptor-binding activity of the mutated apo E-2 was nearly normal and x-ray analysis showed that arginine 150 no longer formed the abnormal salt bridge but instead adopted a position identical to that in the normally binding apo E-3.

The structural properties of apo E also affect the distribution of its different isoforms among the different plasma lipoproteins.[109,144,150,151] Apolipoproteins E-3 and E-2 preferentially associate with HDL, whereas apo E-4 preferentially associates with VLDL. At residue 112, apo E-4 differs from apo E-3 and apo E-2. Apolipoprotein E-4 has arginine at this position; apo E-3 and apo E-2 have cysteine. Thus, it appears that residue 112 modifies lipoprotein distribution. However, the major lipid-binding domain of apo E lies in the C-terminus of the molecule (residues ≈200 to

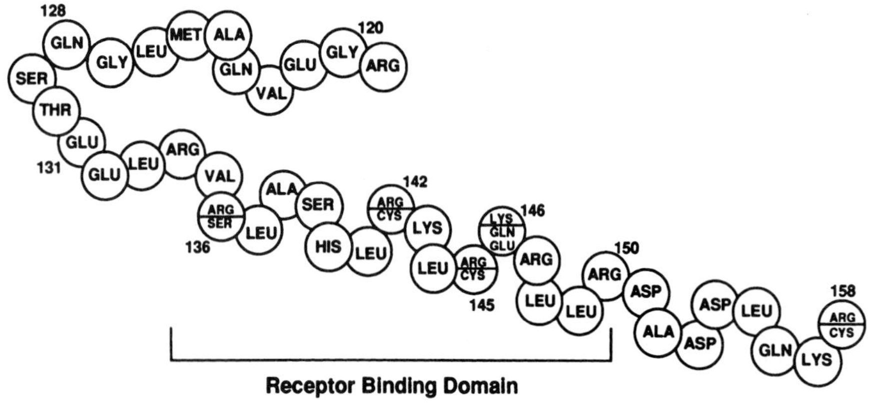

Fig. 119-6 Amino acid sequence of apo E in a region critical for receptor binding. Sites are indicated where neutral amino acids substitute for basic amino acids in receptor binding–defective apo E from type III hyperlipoproteinemic subjects.

280).[23,142,151,152] These observations have led to the hypothesis that the N-terminal and C-terminal domains of apo E interact to determine the specificity of lipid binding.

Analysis of the crystal structure of apo E-4 revealed that the arginine-cysteine interchange at residue 112 causes a profound local change in the structure of the molecule.[144] The occurrence of arginine at residue 112 in apo E-4 results in the formation of a salt bridge between arginine 112 and glutamic acid 109. This ionic interaction causes the side chain of arginine 61 in the adjacent helix to swing into a new plane. By comparison, the cysteine at residue 112 of apo E-3 results in a different orientation for glutamic acid 109 and arginine 61. The repositioning of arginine 61 in apo E-4 leads to an ionic interaction with glutamic acid 255 in the C-terminal domain, and this interaction alone determines the VLDL preference of the apo E-4 isoform.[153,154] In association with the occurrence of specific apo E mutations that affect receptor binding, the distribution of apo E (VLDL vs. HDL preference) impacts the expression of type III hyperlipoproteinemia (see "Pathogenesis of Type III Hyperlipoproteinemia," below).

Sites of Apolipoprotein E Synthesis

Apolipoprotein E is produced in many organs throughout the body (for review, see reference 13). In several different species, significant quantities of apo E mRNA are detected in the liver, brain, spleen, lung, adrenal, ovary, kidney, and muscle.[155–158] Apolipoprotein E mRNA has not been found in the intestinal epithelium, even though the intestine is a major site for lipoprotein biosynthesis. The apo E mRNA is most abundant in the liver, which is the major source for plasma apo E. Hepatic apo E production occurs primarily in the parenchymal cells. The apo E mRNA is most abundant in the brain. Astrocytes are primarily responsible for apo E secretion in the central nervous system.[159] Apolipoprotein E plays a critical role in central nervous system lipid metabolism, and apo E-4 has been shown to be a major susceptibility gene for Alzheimer disease (for review, see references 160–162). In several other organs, macrophages account for the apo E production. Macrophages in culture and *in situ* can produce large quantities of this protein and release it at high concentrations into the medium or interstitial fluid.[163,164] Smooth muscle cells can also produce apo E.[165,166]

Therefore, apo E is present in substantial concentrations in the plasma and interstitial fluid and is available to associate with various lipoproteins. Apolipoprotein E plays a major role in redistributing cholesterol from cells containing excess cholesterol to cells requiring cholesterol for metabolic processes, including membrane biosynthesis for cell proliferation or repair (for review, see reference 13). The apo E–lipid complexes are taken up via the LDL receptors expressed on the cholesterol-deficient cells. This function appears to occur during tissue injury and repair—apo E plays a key role in peripheral nerve regeneration[167–170] and in the maintenance of normal neuronal function.[160–162]

Role of Apolipoprotein E in Normal Remnant Metabolism

Chylomicrons are synthesized by the intestine to transport dietary lipids to peripheral tissues and to the liver (for review, see references 8, 13, 42, 43, 140, and 171). They are triglyceride-rich lipoproteins containing primarily apo B-48, apo A-I, and apo A-IV. They rapidly undergo several modifications, which are associated with triglyceride hydrolysis, and are converted to partially triglyceride-depleted, cholesterol-enriched chylomicron remnants. Triglyceride hydrolysis is mediated primarily by endothelial cell-bound lipoprotein lipase and, to a lesser extent, by hepatic lipase in the liver. The chylomicron remnants are then rapidly cleared from the plasma by the liver (for review, see references 8 and 42). As a consequence of lipolysis, the surface of the particles is reorganized, and some of the apolipoprotein constituents of the newly secreted chylomicrons are lost, particularly apo A-I and apo A-IV. During these changes, apo E and the apo Cs are acquired, resulting in a remnant particle whose protein constituents are now primarily apo B-48, apo E, and the apo Cs. The apo B-48 component of these remnants does not appear to participate in their receptor-mediated catabolism; instead, apo E apparently serves this function.[43]

The liver-derived VLDL undergo lipolytic processing similar to that of chylomicrons, generating smaller particles with a more cholesterol-enriched core (primarily cholesteryl esters) (for review, see references 8 and 171). Eventually this cascade leads to the production of IDL and LDL in a classic precursor-product manner. Unlike chylomicrons, VLDL obtain apo E as they are synthesized in the liver, but during lipolysis their remnants become relatively depleted in all protein components except apo B-100. When further processing converts IDL to LDL, apo E is lost, leaving apo B-100 as the only protein component of LDL. The catabolism of particles along this pathway is complex: a portion of the particles in the lipolytic cascade can be removed from circulation by receptor-mediated processes, whereas others ($\approx$50 percent) proceed completely through this metabolic process to become LDL. Apolipoprotein E serves as the ligand for the removal of these remnants. Farther along the pathway, as more lipolysis occurs and as apo E is lost, apo B-100 becomes the ligand for receptor-mediated catabolism of LDL.[8,13]

Apolipoprotein E is critically important in mediating the catabolism of remnant lipoproteins. This has been established by numerous in vitro and in vivo studies (for review, see references 8, 13, 42, 43, 138, and 140) and highlighted by the role of apo E in type III hyperlipoproteinemia.[45] In patients who lack apo E[172–176] or who have defective apo E (for review, see reference 45), hypertriglyceridemia and hypercholesterolemia characterized by a marked accumulation of both chylomicron remnants and VLDL remnants (collectively called β-VLDL) can develop. Such patients have structurally normal lipoprotein receptors and normal lipases; the critical defect is a structurally abnormal or absent apo E. The necessity of apo E for normal remnant metabolism has been amply confirmed by studies in animals. The knockout of the apo E gene in mice by homologous recombination results in marked remnant accumulation.[177,178] Expression of mutant forms of human apo E in both mice[179–181] and rabbits[182] leads to accumulation of remnants as β-VLDL. Furthermore, in cholesterol-fed rabbits, which have hyperlipidemia associated with increased remnant lipoproteins (β-VLDL), the IV infusion of apo E markedly reduces plasma lipids.[183] In Watanabe heritable hyperlipidemic rabbits, the infusion of apo E rapidly reduces plasma cholesterol levels by 20 to 40 percent, presumably reflecting uptake by the liver.[183,184] It has also been established that the addition of excess apo E to chylomicrons markedly accelerates their clearance from the plasma of normal rabbits, specifically by the liver.[185,186] Over-expression of apo E in mice decreases plasma cholesterol and triglyceride levels and blunts the hyperlipidemia induced in the transgenic mice by diets high in fat and cholesterol.[187] From these studies it has been hypothesized that apo E is not only important for remnant metabolism but can also be rate limiting for remnant clearance, especially during postprandial hyperlipidemia, which is characterized by remnant production.

Several observations have suggested that the enrichment of remnant lipoproteins with apo E is physiologically significant and could signal clearance by a special pathway.[188,189] Cholesterol-induced rabbit β-VLDL, representing both chylomicron remnants and VLDL remnants enriched in apo E, are avidly taken up by cells by a receptor (discussed in "Uptake," below) for which apo E is the ligand.[190,191] The enrichment of the remnant lipoproteins with apo E is necessary for their uptake by this cell-surface receptor. Thus, apo E is important in the remnant clearance process, and the availability of excess apo E may modulate the rate of clearance and the pathway involved in remnant uptake.[42,43,138,192]

Several steps appear to be involved in the plasma clearance and hepatocyte uptake of chylomicron and VLDL remnants.[42,43,192] Chylomicron and VLDL remnants pass through the fenestrae of hepatic sinusoidal endothelial cells into the space of Disse, a

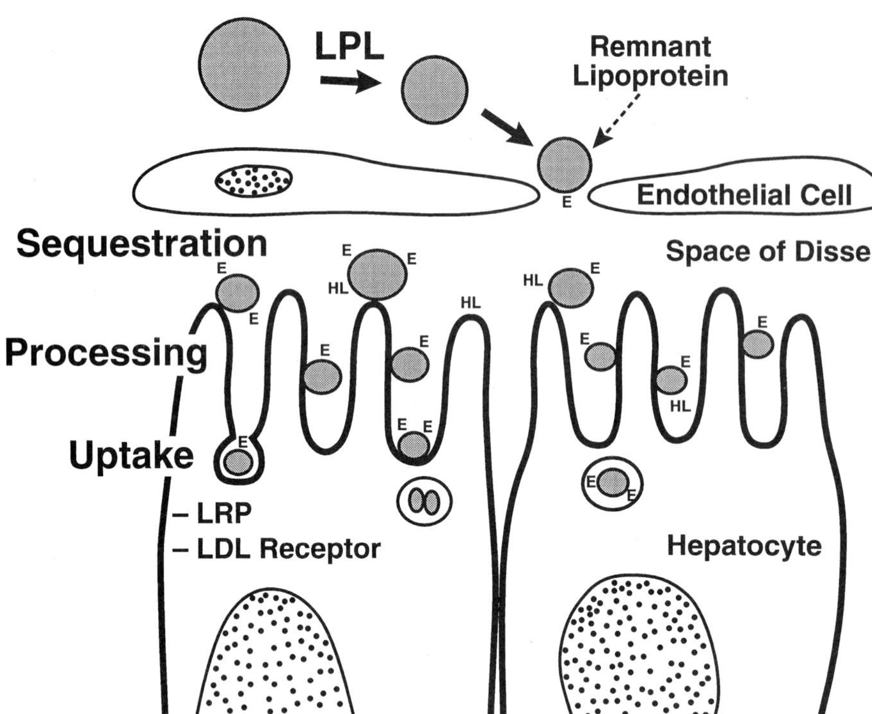

Fig. 119-7 Pathway involved in the clearance of remnant lipoproteins from the plasma. Several steps are involved: *sequestration* of the lipoproteins in the space of Disse accounts for the rapid initial clearance, and HSPG within the space of Disse bind the apo E-enriched remnants; *processing* involves further lipolytic hydrolysis by hepatic lipase (HL) in the liver or lipoprotein lipase (LPL) associated with the remnants when they enter the space of Disse; and *internalization* can be mediated by both the LRP and the LDL receptor.

lymphatic area containing proteoglycans and the microvilli projections of the hepatocytes. Molecules taken up by the liver and secreted from the hepatocytes traverse this space. The control of the molecular traffic into and out of the space of Disse has been the subject of intense investigation in the past 5 years and has led to the demonstration of several steps involved in remnant metabolism. At least three sequential processes — sequestration, processing, and uptake — appear to be required for normal remnant metabolism. These are schematically represented in Fig. 119-7.

Sequestration. An important initial step in the clearance of remnants from the plasma is the sequestration of these particles in the space of Disse.[42,43] The space of Disse possesses abundant heparan sulfate proteoglycans (HSPG), forming a continuous layer on the microvilli of the hepatocytes.[193] Apolipoprotein E is also abundant in this space[193,194] and is known to bind avidly to heparin[195,196] and specifically to heparan sulfate of hepatic origin.[197,198] The enrichment of remnant particles by apo E entrapped by HSPG in the space of Disse appears to be a key step in the catabolic process. Treatment of cells in vitro with heparinase, which removes the sulfated glycosaminoglycans from the HSPG, inhibits up to 90 percent of the binding and uptake of apo E-enriched remnants.[197,198] Intravenous heparinase administration also inhibited plasma clearance of labeled remnants in vivo.[199] In addition, suppression of syndecan (a subset of HSPG) expression in vitro demonstrated the importance of hepatic HSPG in remnant binding.[200] These studies show that HSPG are required for remnant catabolism. One proof of the requirement for apo E in the space of Disse comes from studies in mice. Linton et al.[201] showed that in apo E-null mice, macrophage production of apo E accelerated remnant clearance when LDL receptors were present, but not when they were absent, suggesting that hepatic apo E synthesis, secretion, and sequestration in the space of Disse are required for remnant clearance by non-LDL receptor pathways (i.e., the HSPG/LRP pathway) (Fig. 119-8).

Processing. It is probable that further lipolytic processing of remnants by lipoprotein lipase and/or hepatic lipase occurs in the space of Disse (Fig. 119-7). This is in addition to the presequestration processing that lipoprotein lipase carries out on the capillary endothelial cell surfaces. Hepatic lipase is a heparin-binding protein produced by the liver[202] and is involved in the final processing of remnants at the hepatic surface.[203–206] However, hepatic lipase can also act as a ligand to facilitate the uptake of remnants independently of its catalytic activity[207,208] and interacts with the LRP.[209] Thus, hepatic lipase may participate in remnant metabolism via several mechanisms and may have distinct roles at certain stages of the process.

Similarly, lipoprotein lipase can bind to HSPG[210–212] or the LRP.[213,214] Although some reports also suggest a role for lipoprotein lipase as a ligand,[210,212,213,215] other studies dispute this role,[206] indicating that the quantity of lipoprotein lipase transported on remnants and the relative abundance of lipoprotein lipase in the space of Disse need to be determined before a definitive physiological role for lipoprotein lipase as a ligand can be assigned. Nevertheless, the bulk of the evidence supports a dual role for the lipolytic enzymes in remnant metabolism at various stages of both sequestration and processing in the space of Disse. Furthermore, it is evident that neither the endogenous levels of lipoprotein lipase nor hepatic lipase normalize remnant lipoprotein metabolism in apo E-null mice or type III hyperlipoproteinemic patients with defective apo E.

Uptake. Uptake of the remnants by hepatocytes appears to be receptor mediated (for review, see references 42, 43, 137, 138, and 140) (see Fig. 119-7). It has been shown that chylomicron remnants bind to LDL receptors in vitro. Furthermore, Choi et al.[216] demonstrated that the IV injection of an anti-LDL receptor antiserum significantly delays chylomicron remnant clearance in mice by 25 to 35 percent. Thus, the LDL receptor appears to play an important role in remnant catabolism. However, an alternate pathway also exists that is linked closely to the role of HSPG in remnant catabolism. A unique chylomicron remnant (apo E) receptor is believed to be present in the liver and to play an important role in remnant uptake. The molecule that functions as that receptor has now been identified. Herz et al.[190] cloned a cDNA encoding a 600-kDa protein, the LRP, that has marked structural homology with the LDL receptor. The LRP contains 31 cysteine-rich repeats homologous to the ligand-binding domain of the LDL receptor[190] and functions as a receptor.[217,218] By comparison, the LDL receptor possesses seven of these ligand-binding

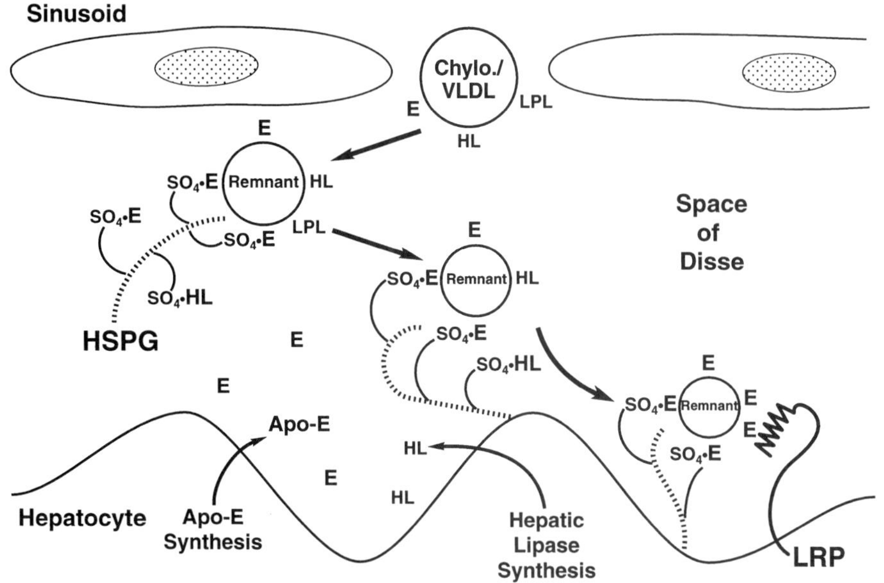

Fig. 119-8 HSPG/LRP pathway. Heparan sulfate proteoglycans are responsible for the initial binding of apo E–enriched remnants. This interaction appears to be required before the involvement of the LRP in the actual internalization of the lipoproteins. The LRP/HSPG may serve as a complex for internalization, or the remnants may be transferred from the HSPG to the LRP before internalization. (*From Mahley.*[8] *Used by permission of W.B. Saunders.*)

domains.[140] Unlike the LDL receptor, for which both apo B-100 and apo E are ligands, apo E is the major apolipoprotein ligand for the LRP. As demonstrated by Kowal et al.,[188] apo E-enriched β-VLDL interact with the LRP on ligand blots and can mediate their uptake, as determined by enhanced cholesteryl ester formation. It is now known that the LRP is the receptor not only for apo E-enriched lipoproteins but also for multiple, diverse ligands, including activated α2-macroglobulin, plasminogen activator inhibitor, lipoprotein lipase/lipoproteins, and lactoferrin.[213,219–225] The multiple cysteine-rich repeats appear to display some specificity for these multiple ligands.

Several lines of evidence have demonstrated that the LRP is involved in the binding and uptake of apo E-enriched remnant lipoproteins. In vitro studies (reviewed in reference 192) implicating the LRP preceded in vivo studies that firmly established the role of the LRP in remnant removal. Injection of α2-macroglobulin reduced the appearance of chylomicron remnants in the liver,[226–228] and the use of an LRP antagonist (the receptor-associated protein, or RAP) further demonstrated the involvement of the LRP in vivo.[229,230] In mice lacking LDL receptors, conditional inactivation of the LRP (LRP inactivation is lethal in embryonic mice, necessitating the use of conditional activation) resulted in the accumulation of remnant lipoproteins in plasma.[231] This finding proved the role of the LRP in vivo and demonstrated that remnant removal is a process shared with the LDL receptor.[232,233]

It now appears that although the LRP is responsible for internalization of apo E-enriched remnants, the initial binding requires the participation of cell-surface HSPG (Fig. 119-8). Studies have established the importance of HSPG in the binding of apo E-enriched remnants and suggest that the LRP alone, in the absence of HSPG, is insufficient to mediate the enhanced binding to the cell surface.[197,198] As illustrated in Fig. 119-8, the HSPG and the LRP may form a complex and be involved jointly in mediating remnant metabolism, the HSPG being responsible for the initial binding and the LRP for internalization. This pathway is referred to as the HSPG/LRP pathway. This theoretical model resembles the proteoglycan receptor binding of basic fibroblast growth factor.[234] Heparinase and heparitinase treatment of the hepatocyte cell lines HepG2 or McA-RH7777 abolish the enhanced binding and uptake of apo E-enriched remnant lipoproteins.[197,198] In addition, CHO mutant cell lines deficient in HSPG do not display the enhanced binding and uptake of apo E-enriched β-VLDL.[197] Most recently, it has come to light that HSPG alone may be sufficient, at least to some extent, to promote the internalization of remnant lipoproteins. In vitro studies suggest HSPG can act as a receptor for lipoprotein internalization without the participation of either the LRP or the LDL receptor,[235,236] although this pathway may be slow in comparison.

The concept that has evolved is a secretion-capture model suggesting that apo E secreted into the space of Disse from hepatocytes becomes associated with the remnant lipoproteins, and thus the apo E-enriched remnants are sequestered in the space of Disse by interacting with HSPG.[42,140] This interaction directs the lipoproteins to the LRP for internalization. Lipoprotein lipase on the surface of the remnants or hepatic lipase associated with HSPG may also direct the remnants to the LRP and mediate their interaction with the receptor. Defective variants of apo E associated with the development of type III hyperlipoproteinemia may have an impact on the catabolism of remnants by interfering with any one of the steps of lipoprotein sequestration, processing, or uptake, as discussed below.

PATHOGENESIS OF TYPE III HYPERLIPOPROTEINEMIA

Effect of Mutant Apolipoprotein E on the Remnant Pathway

Given the importance of apo E in determining the fate of remnants, it is not surprising that a mutant form of apo E, which does not bind normally to hepatic receptors or HSPG, could lead to the accumulation of remnants in the plasma of type III patients. The first evidence that the different apo E isoforms had different abilities to mediate hepatic uptake of lipoproteins came from the studies of Havel and coworkers,[30] who used liver perfusion of estradiol-treated rats as the experimental model. Estradiol increases the expression of hepatic LDL receptors ten- to twentyfold. These investigators found that phospholipid vesicles in which normal apo E had been incorporated were efficiently taken up by the treated rat livers, whereas vesicles containing apo E-2(Arg 158 → Cys) from a patient with type III hyperlipoproteinemia were taken up poorly, suggesting defective receptor recognition of apo E-2.

This phenomenon was subsequently studied directly by comparing how apo E isoforms from various subjects bound to the LDL receptor. Schneider et al.[34] showed that apo E-2 bound poorly in these assays compared with apo E-3. In a similar study, Weisgraber et al.[35] showed that apo E-2 from a type III patient had a binding affinity that was only 1 to 2 percent of that of apo E-3

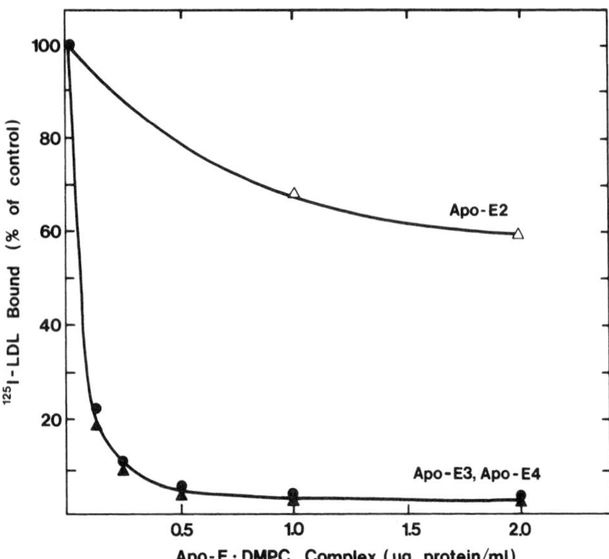

Fig. 119-9 Receptor-binding activity of apo E-2 (△), apo E-3 (▲), and apo E-4 (●) as assessed in an in vitro competition assay. Human ^{125}I-LDL were used as the competitor for the binding of apo E · DMPC (dimyristoyl phosphatidylcholine) complexes to normal human fibroblasts. The apo E-2 is from a type III hyperlipoproteinemic subject. (*From Weisgraber, Innerarity, and Mahley.*[35] *Courtesy of Dr. Karl H. Weisgraber.*)

(Fig. 119-9). In contrast, apo E-4 (the other genetically determined polymorphic form of apo E) had a binding capacity identical to that of apo E-3 (see Fig. 119-9). It was also demonstrated by Gregg et al.[108] that radiolabeled apo E-2 and E-3 were cleared from plasma differently in both normal subjects and type III patients (Fig. 119-10). In both cases, apo E-2 clearance was significantly retarded, suggesting that the clearance impairment was attributable to a defective ligand rather than to defective receptors.

The aforementioned studies directly implicate apo E-2 in the accumulation of the abnormal lipoproteins (β-VLDL) in type III hyperlipoproteinemia. Less readily explained, however, is why type III patients, and E-2/2 homozygotes in general, have significantly lower plasma concentrations of LDL than the population mean. One could argue that the receptor binding-defective apo E-2 might actually reduce the percentage of hepatic VLDL remnants (but not intestinal remnants) that are cleared as VLDL particles, resulting in a higher rate of conversion of these particles to LDL. Thus, one might expect LDL concentrations to increase as a consequence of an enhanced LDL "rate of synthesis." However, the finding that LDL concentrations in E-2/2 subjects are actually decreased very significantly suggests that other mechanisms must be involved. Several hypotheses have been advanced to explain the low LDL levels in E-2/2 subjects. One hypothesis is that the defective apo E-2 causes less remnant uptake (as stated above), which leads to upregulation of hepatic LDL receptors, which, in turn, allows for accelerated clearance (even in the face of increased LDL production) of plasma LDL.[102] One argument against this hypothesis is that the number of hepatic LDL receptors does not seem to be increased in either apo E-2 transgenic rabbits[182] or apo E-null mice.[237] A second possibility is that apo E-2-containing remnants compete less well with LDL (where the ligand is apo B, not apo E) for binding to hepatic LDL receptors, thus accelerating LDL clearance and reducing plasma LDL.[237] Supporting this idea is in vitro evidence demonstrating that while apo E-3 has about 25 times higher affinity than apo B for the LDL receptor,[28] apo E-2 and apo B have approximately the same affinity.[34,35] A third hypothesis is that apo E-2 impairs lipolytic processing of VLDL to LDL. This idea is supported by experimental evidence that lipoprotein lipase-mediated lipolysis is impaired in the presence of apo E-2.[11,238–241] There also is evidence suggesting impairment of hepatic lipase in the presence of apo E-2.[242,243]

Recent studies in transgenic animals have provided strong support for the notion that impairment of lipoprotein lipase-mediated lipolysis by apo E-2 is the major cause of low LDL levels. Huang et al.[244] showed that the low LDL levels in apo E-2 transgenic mice persist in the absence of LDL receptors, suggesting that the LDL-lowering effect of apo E-2 is not dependent on this clearance pathway. Instead, a dramatic lipolytic impairment was found to be due to the effect of apo E-2 on lipoprotein lipase-mediated lipolysis, and displacement of the lipoprotein lipase cofactor apo C-II from the substrate particles by apo E-2 was the major cause of the reduced lipolysis. The displacement of apo C-II and its reduced presence on remnant particles requires high levels of apo E-2, which occur in type III

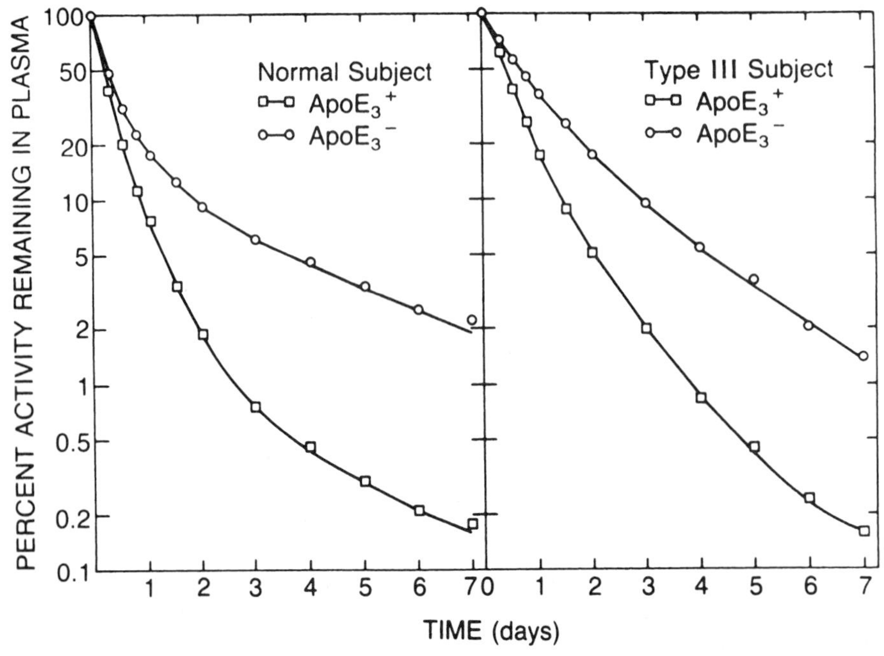

Fig. 119-10 Clearance of simultaneously injected apo E-3 (E_3+) and apo E-2 (E_3-) from the plasma of a normal subject (left) and a type III hyperlipoproteinemic subject (right). (*From Gregg et al.*[108] *Used by permission of* Science.)

Table 119-5 Apolipoprotein E Variants Associated with Type III Hyperlipoproteinemia and Factors Modulating Expression of Hyperlipidemia

Causative Mutation*	Mode of Inheritance	Receptor Binding		Comments	References
		LDLR	LRP/HSPG		
Arg 158 → Cys	Recessive	Very low	Nearly normal	The most common mutation in type III hyperlipoproteinemia; requires secondary factors	35, 245, 246
Arg 136 → Ser	Dominant‡	Moderate	–§	Mutant E:normal E ratio is as high as 4:1 in plasma of heterozygous subjects; one homozygous subject identified; extensive pedigree analyses; influence of age, body mass, gender, but not second apo E allele; increased frequency in Spanish population	13, 247, 248
Arg 136 → Cys	Dominant‡	–	–	Variable expression of hyperlipidemia	249–251
Arg 142 → Leu	Uncertain	–	–	Only two subjects identified	252
Arg 142 → Cys	Dominant	Low	Low	Severe hyperlipidemia; 100% penetrance; very early and severe expression of hyperlipidemia (possibly at birth); VLDL preference for isoform due to second mutation of Cys 112 → Arg; mutuant E:normal E ratio in -VLDL is 3:1	245, 253–255
Arg 145 → Cys	Dominant‡	Moderate	Moderate	Many similarities to apo E-2 homozygosity, including influence of secondary factors; homozygous subjects identified; homozygosity in combination with a second mutation (Glu 13 → Lys) associated with severe hyperlipidemia; increased frequency in Blacks	22, 256–259
Lys 146 → Gln	Dominant	Moderate	–	Extensive pedigree analyses; variable expression of the hyperlipidemia; some influence of secondary factors; very inefficient lipolysis of -VLDL by lipoprotein lipase	260–263
Lys 146 → Glu	Dominant	Very low	Very low	High degree of penetrance	245, 246, 264–266
Lys 146 → Asn, Arg 147 → Trp	Dominant	–	–	Very early expression of hyperlipidemia	267
7-amino-acid duplication of residues 121–127	Dominant	Low	Very low	Extensive pedigree analyses; 100% penetrance; some influence of second apo E allele, body mass, age, but not gender; VLDL preference for isoform due to second mutation of Cys 112 → Arg; mutant E:normal E ratio in plasma is >4:1; commonly referred to as apo E-Leiden	245, 268–270

*Lists changes compared to apo E-3 structure (e.g., Arg 158 → Cys, arginine at residue 158 changed to cysteine at that site).
‡Incomplete dominance or reduced penetrance.
§Dash indicates not yet determined.

hyperlipoproteinemic subjects to a significant extent, and even in normocholesterolemic E-2/2 homozygotes (see Fig. 119-5). This result offers an explanation for why apo E-deficient humans[172] (and apo E-null mice[178,197,198]) have cholesterol-enriched, but not triglyceride-enriched, β-VLDL compared with type III hyperlipoproteinemic humans (and apo E-2–expressing transgenic mice), who have β-VLDL with high triglyceride content.

Mode of Inheritance of Type III Hyperlipoproteinemia

An important insight into type III hyperlipoproteinemia is that the mode of inheritance — dominant vs. recessive — correlates with the specific mutation of apo E (for review, see reference 45). The development of type III hyperlipoproteinemia results from the effects of specific mutations on one or more of the components of remnant metabolism. Factors influencing the mode of inheritance of type III hyperlipoproteinemia include receptor-binding activity, heparin (HSPG) binding, lipoprotein preference, and the impact of apo E-2 on lipolytic processing (see Table 119-5).

Recessive Mode of Inheritance

The most common defective variant associated with type III hyperlipoproteinemia is apo E-2(Arg 158 → Cys) (for review, see references 13, 44, and 45) (Table 119-5). Homozygosity for the defective allele is required for the development of the hyperlipidemia. However, it is estimated that less than 10 percent of E-2 homozygotes have overt type III hyperlipoproteinemia. In fact, most E-2/2 subjects have hypocholesterolemia even though they all have low plasma levels of β-VLDL. The low level of β-VLDL, even in the face of hypocholesterolemia, indicates that defective remnant clearance is associated with the E-2/2 phenotype. Development of type III hyperlipoproteinemia (overt hypertriglyceridemia and hypercholesterolemia) requires the presence of the abnormal apo E-2 plus the occurrence of a secondary genetic, hormonal, or environmental factor to precipitate the hyperlipidemia.[52,83] Homozygosity for apo E-2 appears to induce sensitivity to additional factors that disrupt the normal balance in lipoprotein metabolism. These are factors that may stimulate overproduction of chylomicrons and/or VLDL (obesity, diabetes, excessive calories) or may impair clearance (e.g., decreased LDL receptors as a result of increasing age, hypothyroidism, or low estrogen levels during menopause). Although apo E-2 displays defective binding to LDL receptors in vitro,[13,43,45] Innerarity et al.[147,148] demonstrated that the binding activity of this variant can be modulated from very defective to almost normal under a variety of conditions, which include altered lipid composition of the lipoprotein particles. Thus, this variant may not always display a severe receptor-binding defect in vivo. The variability in response may be explained by the fact that this mutation appears to disrupt receptor binding secondarily by altering the conformation of the 136-to-150 region (see "Structure and Function of Apolipoprotein E," above for a discussion of the three-dimensional structure of apo E-2), and therefore the mutation represents an indirect perturbation (not a direct disruption) of the interaction with LDL receptors.

The impact of apo E-2 on remnant metabolism may also be modulated by the preferential association of apo E-2 with HDL[150] and the ≈1:1 ratio, in heterozygous patients, of mutant apo E-2 to normal apo E-3 in the $d < 1.006$ g/ml fraction. The content of the normal apo E-3 in the remnant particles ($d < 1.006$ g/ml lipoproteins) may be enough, in some circumstances, to allow normal clearance to occur. As discussed below, several other variants of apo E associated with the dominant expression of type III hyperlipoproteinemia have an overabundance of the mutant apo E associated with these triglyceride-rich lipoproteins (VLDL and remnants) (see Table 119-5), and this overabundance could contribute to impaired binding of the $d < 1.006$ g/ml remnants in the dominant hyperlipoproteinemia. Thus, the variability of the hyperlipidemia in patients with apo E-2(Arg 158 → Cys) may be modulated through one or more of the steps involved in remnant metabolism.

Secondary Factors Influencing the Development of Type III Hyperlipoproteinemia in Patients with Apolipoprotein E-2/2. The simultaneous inheritance of two alleles for the abnormal apo E-2(Arg 158 → Cys) is necessary, but not always sufficient, to precipitate the overt hypertriglyceridemia and hypercholesterolemia (see Table 119-5). Utermann[52] hypothesized that other genetic or environmental influences were necessary for the development of type III hyperlipoproteinemia (Fig. 119-11). Among the genetic factors implicated in initiating the hyperlipidemic response are familial combined hyperlipidemia,[271,272] familial hypercholesterolemia,[272–274] familial hypertriglyceridemia,[272] and even lipoprotein lipase mutations.[275] In transgenic mice, expression of apo E-2 at modest levels does not yield the type III hyperlipoproteinemic phenotype, but in the absence of LDL receptors, these animals convert to a typical type III lipoprotein profile.[276] Also, certain genetically determined disturbances in hormonal regulation could influence the development of type III hyperlipoproteinemia. On the other hand, hormonal disturbances need not be strictly genetically driven, but may also arise from environmental influences. The complex relationship of genetic and environmental factors is also exemplified by the frequent association of disorders such as hypothyroidism[277,278] and diabetes (glucose intolerance)[5] with type III hyperlipoproteinemia. Other endogenous and exogenous factors such as age, sex, nutrition, and alcohol consumption can also be aggravating factors. Of the environmental factors, one that seems to be prevalent is obesity. The correspondence between weight and clinical expression of type III hyperlipoproteinemia has been noted.[5,63] Furthermore, the usually prompt response of type III hyperlipoproteinemia to diet control emphasizes the impact of caloric intake (see "Diagnosis and Treatment," below).

One factor that could have a profound modulating effect on hepatic remnant uptake is the absolute level of hepatic lipoprotein receptors. The expression of hepatic LDL receptors is rapidly regulated by diet, drugs, and hormones[8,171,279,280] and is age-dependent, at least in certain animals.[281] It is also possible that the clinical expression of type III hyperlipoproteinemia is influenced by the level of hepatic LDL receptors. First, receptor number decreases with age, and type III hyperlipoproteinemia associated with apo E-2(Arg 158 → Cys) (recessive type III) usually manifests itself during adulthood. Second, that type III hyperlipoproteinemia is more prevalent in men than in women, and that women in whom type III hyperlipoproteinemia develops are primarily postmenopausal, suggest that estrogen balance may be an important factor in expression of the disease. Indeed, estrogen treatment has reversed the hyperlipidemia in several type III subjects.[282,283] Furthermore, estrogens can profoundly increase the level of hepatic LDL receptors in certain animals,[284–286] although this requires pharmacologic doses. A recent study in transgenic rabbits overexpressing apo E-2 supports this notion. Although the major effect of estrogen treatment in these rabbits was on lipolytic processing (see "Effect of Mutant Apolipoprotein E on the Remnant Pathway," above), there was a measurable increase in LDL receptors in estrogen-treated male rabbits compared with

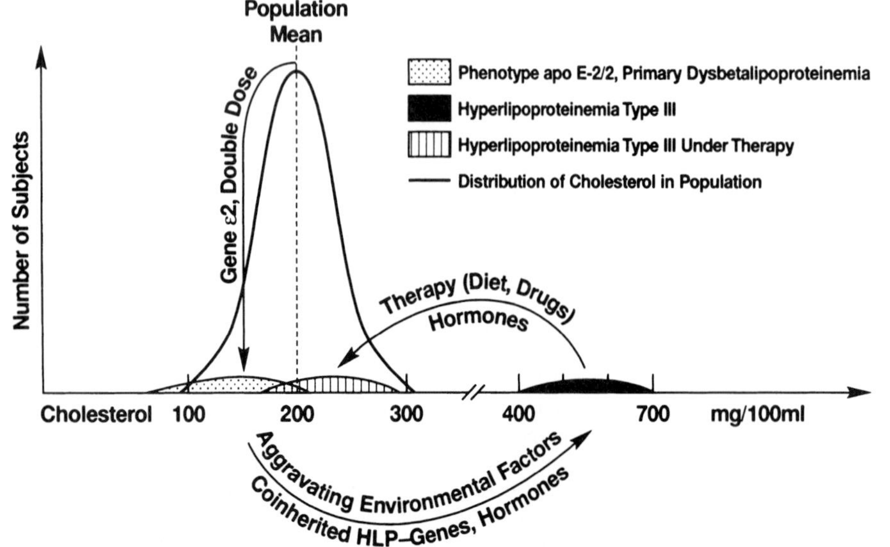

Fig. 119-11 Type III hyperlipoproteinemia as a multifactorial disorder. Factors involved in the pathogenesis and modulation of the expression of type III hyperlipoproteinemia are indicated. HLP = hyperlipoproteinemia. (*From Utermann.*[52] *Used by permission of Elsevier Science Publishers.*)

controls.[182] In humans, the actual changes in hepatic receptor expression needed to reverse or prevent hyperlipidemia may be very slight. Third, the exacerbation of type III hyperlipoproteinemia by hypothyroidism[277] may be related to the decreased receptor-mediated uptake of lipoproteins,[287] which may come about by suppression of hepatic LDL receptor expression. Fourth, the influence of diet on the development of type III hyperlipoproteinemia may also be related to receptor expression. Increased dietary cholesterol and plasma lipoproteins are known to down-regulate LDL receptor expression.[8,171,279,280] Finally, in four families with heterozygous familial hypercholesterolemia (a disease characterized by approximately half-normal levels of LDL receptor activity), the occurrence of a single apo E-2 allele markedly increased the prevalence of type III hyperlipoproteinemia.[273] Thus, the level of LDL receptor expression in the liver may be crucial in regulating intestinal chylomicron and hepatic VLDL remnant accumulation in the circulation. On the other hand, no genetic or environmental factors have been shown to regulate the expression of the LRP,[140] and thus, at present, the level of LRP expression is not thought to be a determinant in the development of type III hyperlipoproteinemia.

Yet another mechanism that may contribute to remnant accumulation is overproduction of lipoproteins. Two factors that may be major contributors to this phenomenon are diet and separate genes for hyperlipidemia. Increased caloric intake would certainly be expected to stimulate intestinal lipoprotein production and probably hepatic VLDL as well, because cholesterol of dietary origin carried in chylomicron remnants is presumed to be a regulator of hepatic cholesterol synthesis.[280,288–290] Although the mechanisms of other genetically determined hyperlipidemias are not well understood, at least some involve hepatic overproduction of VLDL.[291] One of the best examples of the two-gene hypothesis comes from a thorough study of a large family from Seattle,[271] in which the genes for dysbetalipoproteinemia (i.e., the E-2/2 phenotype) and for familial combined hyperlipidemia (probably caused by VLDL overproduction) were shown to segregate independently. The simultaneous occurrence of the gene for familial combined hyperlipidemia and the E-2/2 phenotype resulted in the clinical expression of type III hyperlipoproteinemia, while only other lipoprotein phenotypes (types IIa, IIb, and IV) were associated with other apo E phenotypes. The role of overproduction of apo B-containing lipoproteins in precipitating or exacerbating the hyperlipidemic response is supported by studies in transgenic mice. Expression of moderate levels of apo E-2 did not cause hyperlipidemia, but in combination with human apo B overexpression, which boosted production of apo B-containing lipoproteins, caused a typical type III hyperlipoproteinemic phenotype, including β-VLDL.[181,276]

One additional factor that may trigger the hyperlipidemia in homozygous apo E-2(Arg 158 $\rightarrow$ Cys) patients is increased plasma levels of cholesteryl ester transfer protein. This protein transfers cholesteryl esters from HDL to lower-density lipoproteins, including VLDL and IDL (presumably to remnants). Tall et al.[292] demonstrated a two- to threefold increase in cholesteryl ester transfer protein activity in the plasma of four patients with type III hyperlipoproteinemia (E-2/2 phenotype). In addition, McPherson et al.[293] showed a marked elevation in plasma cholesteryl ester transfer protein levels, as determined by radioimmunoassay, in patients with type III hyperlipoproteinemia. Increased cholesteryl ester transfer protein activity would enrich the lower-density lipoproteins in cholesteryl ester and could exacerbate the formation of β-VLDL in E-2/2 patients already displaying the propensity to accumulate remnants in their plasma. Conversely, the absence of cholesteryl ester transfer protein results in very high levels of large HDL and markedly reduced levels of VLDL and LDL.[294,295]

Dominant Mode of Inheritance

Dominant inheritance of type III hyperlipoproteinemia occurs with several of the rare variants of apo E[296] that, with one exception (apo E-Leiden), involve substitutions of neutral or acidic amino acid residues for basic ones in residues 136 to 150—the region of apo E that interacts directly with the LDL receptor (see Table 119-5 and Fig. 119-6). In these instances, the presence of a single variant allele is sufficient for development of type III hyperlipoproteinemia, and secondary factors are not required. These so-called dominant mutations cause apo E to be defective in binding to lipoprotein receptors.[45] Although the substitution at residue 158 in the recessive variant, apo E-2, results in a rearrangement of salt bridges that indirectly affects receptor binding (see "Structure and Function of Apolipoprotein E," above), substitutions for basic amino acid residues in the 136-to-150 region would not be expected to have such an effect, because all of the basic residues in this region are solvent exposed and not involved in salt bridges[145] (see Fig. 119-6). Thus, it is more likely that the dominant mutations exert their effect on receptor binding by directly affecting the ionic interaction with the receptor. It is also likely that the dominant mutations do not allow for modulation of the receptor-binding activity, as can occur with the recessive apo E-2 variant (see "Recessive Mode of Inheritance," above). One exception to this is apo E-Leiden, which has a tandem duplication of residues 121 to 127.[269,297] This seven-amino acid insertion occurs at the loop connecting helixes 3 and 4 (see "Structure and Function of Apolipoprotein E," above) and probably indirectly affects the binding to lipoprotein receptors by altering the conformation of the receptor-binding region.

It is now apparent that although precipitation of the dominant disorder does not require secondary factors, the severity of the hyperlipidemia can be differentially influenced by many of the secondary factors discussed above (see "Secondary Factors Influencing the Development of Type III Hyperlipoproteinemia in Patients with Apolipoprotein E-2/2"). The influence of these secondary factors ranges from almost none to critically important, which has also led to the evolution of terms such as "incomplete dominance." Pedigree analyses (some of them quite extensive) in kindreds with some of these rare variants highlight the variable influence of secondary factors. For example, both the apo E(142 Arg $\rightarrow$ Cys) and apo E(146 Lys $\rightarrow$ Glu) variants are associated with a very high degree of penetrance and severe hyperlipidemia. The apo E-Leiden variant is associated with a high degree of penetrance and is somewhat influenced by secondary factors, whereas the apo E(136 Arg $\rightarrow$ Ser) variant is associated with "incomplete dominance" (lower penetrance) and is influenced by secondary factors slightly different from those affecting apo E-Leiden. The apo E(136 Arg $\rightarrow$ Cys) and apo E(145 Arg $\rightarrow$ Cys) variants are associated with "incomplete dominance," but the hyperlipidemia can be quite severe, while the apo E(145 Arg $\rightarrow$ Cys) and apo E(146 Lys $\rightarrow$ Gln) variants have lower degrees of penetrance and a highly variable expression of the hyperlipidemia that is profoundly influenced by secondary factors (see Table 119-5).

Therefore, explanations in addition to defective receptor binding must be sought to account for the occurrence and accumulation of remnant lipoproteins in the dominantly expressed hyperlipidemia. Indeed, the magnitude of the receptor-binding defect is opposite of what would be predicted; that is, the recessive variant apo E-2 has the most severely defective binding (see Table 119-5), a hierarchy established by three different in vitro methods.[35,298,299] At least two other properties of apo E have been implicated in the dominant inheritance of type III hyperlipoproteinemia. The first is lipoprotein association preference. Arginine at position 112 of apo E, as occurs in apo E-4, imparts to apo E a preference for binding to triglyceride-rich lipoproteins, whereas cysteine at position 112, as occurs in apo E-3 and apo E-2, imparts a preference for HDL[109,150,151,153,154] (see "Structure and Function of Apolipoprotein E," above). Two of the variants associated with dominant inheritance of type III hyperlipoproteinemia, apo E-Leiden and apo E with cysteine at residue 142, have arginine at position 112; both demonstrate a physical preference for triglyceride-rich lipoproteins (see Table 119-5). Subjects heterozygous for these variants have a markedly increased ratio of defective to normal apo E in their β-VLDL,[254,268] and it has been hypothesized that lipoprotein association preference is largely responsible for this, and that, in turn, the increased ratio of defective apo E exacerbates the accumulation of the β-VLDL.[254,270] In contrast, the recessive apo E-2 variant prefers HDL and does not accumulate preferentially in triglyceride-rich lipoproteins to any significant degree in E-3/2 subjects, who do not accumulate β-VLDL or demonstrate hyperlipidemia.[300]

The second property of apo E that could contribute to dominant inheritance of type III hyperlipoproteinemia is heparin (HSPG) binding. Apolipoprotein E has a high-affinity heparin-binding site that is coincident with its receptor-binding site—residues 136 to 150.[196] A defect in this property could manifest itself at either or both of two sites: the peripheral circulation, where lipolytic processing occurs, and the hepatic surface, where remnant sequestration and uptake occur. In the peripheral circulation, a heparin-binding defect in apo E could lead to impaired lipolytic processing because the lipoprotein would not be held at the vascular wall where HSPG and lipoprotein lipase reside. Because lipolyzed remnants, even those with receptor binding-defective apo E, bind to receptors better than their precursors do,[46] poorly lipolyzed lipoproteins would not be removed from circulation as efficiently. Because the dominant variants, but not apo E-2, have defective heparin binding, this property may be one factor in determining whether an apo E variant will be dominant.

Perhaps a more important consequence of defective heparin binding will be manifested at the hepatic surface. The apo E variants can interact in markedly different ways with the two receptor pathways that are responsible for lipoprotein remnant uptake (Table 119-5). The apo E variants are all defective, to varying degrees, in binding to the LDL receptor, and that is mostly true for binding to the HSPG/LRP pathway.[192,245] The magnitude of the binding defect to the HSPG/LRP correlates approximately with the heparin-binding ability of the apo E protein (i.e., the more defective the heparin binding, the more defective the interaction with the HSPG/LRP pathway). Although the LDL receptor-binding region and the primary heparin-binding region (HSPG/LRP binding) are roughly coincident, the binding activities of the apo E variants to the two receptor systems do not always correlate.[245,246] For example, apo E-2 has the most defective LDL receptor-binding activity, but binds almost normally to the HSPG/LRP. Overall, HSPG/LRP binding activity and LDL receptor-binding activity range from low to moderate. It seems quite likely that these binding differences, summarized in Table 119-5, play a role in determining both the severity of the hyperlipidemia and the mode of inheritance of type III hyperlipoproteinemia. Perhaps most intriguing, apo E variants that associate preferentially with VLDL (see above) and/or interact poorly with HSPG/LRP seem to have the greatest degree of penetrance and cause the most severe hyperlipidemia.

Therefore, it is likely that a combination of properties of apo E is responsible for determining whether type III hyperlipoproteinemia will be inherited as a dominant or recessive trait. It is further likely that the combination of properties important for one variant will not necessarily be the same ones important for other variants. However, whatever properties are involved probably help to exaggerate the accumulation of particles containing relatively more of the defective apo E that ultimately determines whether dominance will occur.

Deposition of β-VLDL in Macrophages

The β-VLDL have an unusual propensity for uptake by macrophages (Fig. 119-12) and for causing a massive accumulation of cholesterol (as cholesteryl esters) in these cells (for review, see references 25, 29, 80, and 301–304). This was first demonstrated in mouse peritoneal macrophages, but it has also been shown to occur in human monocyte-macrophages.[78,79] The foam cells in xanthomas and early atherosclerotic lesions derive, at least in part, from macrophages. The avid uptake of β-VLDL (and especially the intestinal β-VLDL) by macrophages may partly explain the tendency for xanthomas and premature atherosclerosis to develop in type III patients.[9] Thus, the atherogenic nature of β-VLDL probably derives primarily from their uptake by macrophages (for review, see references 24, 25, 66, 303, and 304).

The uptake of β-VLDL by macrophages is a receptor-mediated event, and early studies suggested that there was a specific β-VLDL receptor in these cells.[78,79,305] However, it was demonstrated in mouse macrophages that the LDL receptor is responsible for the uptake of β-VLDL.[306] Furthermore, the LDL receptor is responsible for remnant uptake in human monocyte-macrophages.[307,308] The ligand for the macrophage uptake of β-VLDL is apo E,[309] as demonstrated in animals fed a cholesterol-enriched diet. The β-VLDL induced by the cholesterol feeding have physical and chemical properties similar to those of β-VLDL of human type III patients, except that the animal β-VLDL do not contain a genetically abnormal form of apo E. Human β-VLDL, despite the presence of receptor binding-defective apo E-2, are also taken up by macrophages via apo E-directed binding.[309] At first glance, this would seem paradoxical. However, human β-VLDL from type III patients are generally less efficient than animal β-VLDL in stimulating cholesterol deposition in macrophages, and human β-VLDL uptake by macrophages can be enhanced by the incorporation of normal apo E-3 into these particles. Furthermore, it has been shown that the propensity for β-VLDL uptake by macrophages is greatly enhanced when the particles are oxidized.[310] The oxidized particles induce cholesterol deposition in macrophages in amounts well above those achieved with oxidized LDL, and may be a very important determinant of the atherogenicity of β-VLDL.

Apolipoprotein E almost certainly has a role in the mobilization of cholesterol from peripheral cells, including macrophages.[311,312] Cholesterol accumulation in macrophages stimulates production and secretion of apo E,[163,164] which forms apo E–lipid complexes or is incorporated into HDL particles. These complexes or particles can acquire cholesterol from cholesterol-loaded cells and redistribute it to cells requiring cholesterol. The apo E-enriched HDL (HDL_c) are present in high concentrations in the plasma of cholesterol-fed animals.[29,66,304,313] The HDL_c of cholesterol-fed animals and the HDL with apo E (the comparable particles in humans) are thought to remove cholesterol from peripheral cells (including, but not restricted to, macrophages) and transport it to other cells requiring cholesterol or to the liver, where cholesterol can be excreted from the body in the bile as bile salts or free cholesterol (for review, see references 13, 25, 29, and 304). The uptake of these particles occurs via a receptor-mediated process in which apo E serves as the ligand. This process of redistributing cholesterol is sometimes referred to

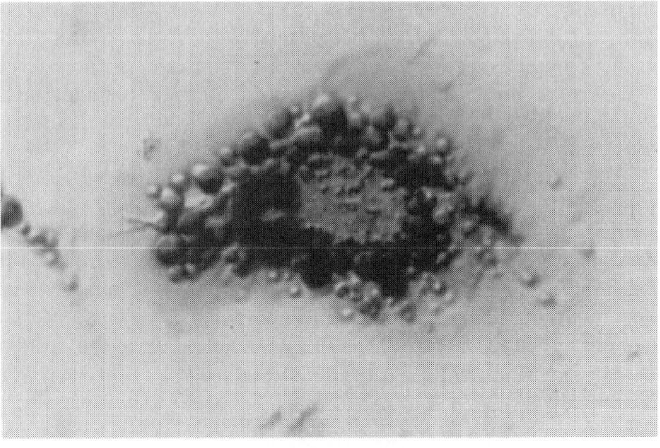

Fig. 119-12 Cultured mouse peritoneal macrophage after incubation with canine β-VLDL. The large droplets are cholesteryl esters. (*Courtesy of Dr. Robert E. Pitas.*)

as a form of reverse cholesterol transport.[314] It is likely that in type III patients with high levels of β-VLDL, the reverse cholesterol transport system is taxed beyond its ability to achieve a normal balance of cholesterol flux.

Atherosclerosis and Apolipoprotein E

Because type III hyperlipoproteinemic subjects are predisposed to the premature development of atherosclerosis (see "Clinical Expression and Manifestation of the Disorder," above), the role of apo E and its mutants in this process is a major consideration. Studies of the atherogenic potential of apo E (and β-VLDL) have been greatly aided by the development of transgenic and gene-targeted animal models. The expression of "normal" apo E, such as human apo E-3 in apo E-null mice[315] or apo E-4[316] or rat apo E[317] in transgenic mice affords protection against diet-induced atherosclerosis. On the other hand, overexpression of human apo E variants in transgenic mice promotes or exacerbates diet-induced atherosclerosis. At high expression levels, both apo E(142 Arg $\rightarrow$ Cys) and apo E-Leiden give rise to a phenotype closely resembling human type III hyperlipoproteinemia, including massive remnant accumulation, hyperlipidemia, and β-VLDL.[179,180,318,319] In addition, both variants cause the transgenic mice to become susceptible to high-fat diet-induced atherosclerosis that is many-fold more extensive and more complicated than in nontransgenic mice.[318,319] These studies establish the atherogenic potential of β-VLDL and are proving useful for the study of both genetic and environmental factors that influence the expression of type III hyperlipoproteinemia. In addition, the overexpression of apo E-2 in transgenic mice[181,276] causes a massive accumulation of β-VLDL in combination with other gene interactions (elimination of endogenous apo E or LDL receptors), producing mice that are also probably more susceptible to atherosclerosis. The potential of apo E-2 expression to promote atherosclerosis has been demonstrated definitively in transgenic rabbits.[182] Expression of high levels of apo E-2 in both male and female rabbits led to spontaneous atherosclerosis that was more pronounced in male rabbits, which also had more severe hyperlipidemia characterized by higher levels of cholesterol- and triglyceride-enriched β-VLDL.

Of great interest for atherosclerosis are the studies on apo E-deficient mice, which are models of human apo E deficiency.[320,321] These mice have massive accumulation of apo B-48-enriched remnants, have very high plasma cholesterol (but not triglyceride) levels similar to those seen in humans with apo E deficiency, and, most significantly, develop both diet-induced and spontaneous atherosclerosis. In addition, these mice develop widespread fibroproliferative lesions that rapidly progress from simple uncomplicated fatty streaks to the most advanced, complex atherosclerotic lesions ever seen in mice.[322] This model has proven to be especially useful because it produces lesions that are very similar to those found in humans.

Other advances in animal models relate to the role of macrophages in the development of atherosclerosis. The impact of macrophage-specific expression of apo E on atherosclerosis has been studied in several ways. Both Linton et al.[323] and Boisvert et al.[324] lethally irradiated apo E-null mice and then repopulated the hematopoietic system with stem cells from normal mice. The plasma apo E levels (produced entirely from circulating or resident macrophages) in these mice were low, but sufficient to reduce the hyperlipidemia and protect against either spontaneous or diet-induced atherosclerosis. Fazio et al.[325] also did the inverse stem cell transplantation experiment, repopulating irradiated wild-type mice with macrophages from apo E-null mice. These mice showed increased susceptibility to atherosclerosis, further demonstrating the crucial role of macrophages in atherosclerosis. Bellosta et al.[326] achieved macrophage-specific expression of human apo E-3 in normal mice using the visna virus long terminal repeat, and then crossed these mice with apo E-null mice to obtain macrophage-specific apo E production. In these mice, apo E in the plasma correlated inversely with plasma cholesterol and afforded significant protection against atherosclerosis. Most importantly, when apo E-null mice and apo E-null mice expressing low levels of human apo E-3 in macrophages were matched for similar degrees of hypercholesterolemia, the mice with macrophage production of human apo E-3 had a marked reduction in foam cell formation in their artery walls. Thus, macrophage apo E-3 synthesis and secretion significantly decrease atherosclerosis in hyperlipidemic mice directly without significantly affecting plasma lipid and lipoprotein levels.[326] Similar results have also been reported by Shimano et al.[317] from studies in mice expressing apo E in the artery wall. All of the animal studies suggest that apo E normally plays a role in protection against lesion development, while dysfunctional or absent apo E has the opposite effect.

DIAGNOSIS AND TREATMENT

Diagnosis

A single simple diagnostic test for type III hyperlipoproteinemia is not available, but there are some diagnostic markers. Nearly equal elevations of plasma total cholesterol and triglyceride concentrations (values above 300 mg/dl) are indicative of possible type III hyperlipoproteinemia.[8] However, the cholesterol and triglyceride levels tend to vary greatly in type III hyperlipoproteinemia. If isolation of VLDL by ultracentrifugation is possible, determination of the ratio of the concentration of VLDL cholesterol to the concentration of plasma triglyceride is very useful. In general, a ratio of $\geq$0.3 reflects the presence of cholesterol-rich β-VLDL and is indicative of type III hyperlipoproteinemia; but this can be misleading in some cases. Demonstration of the broad β band on agarose electrophoresis of whole plasma can also be unreliable. However, when used in combination with ultracentrifugally separated lipoproteins, electrophoretic demonstration of β-migrating particles in the $d <$ 1.006 g/ml fraction is predictive of type III hyperlipoproteinemia (see Fig. 119-1). It should be noted that dysbetalipoproteinemia—the presence of β-VLDL in the plasma—occurs regardless of whether the subject is overtly hyperlipidemic, and therefore can almost always be detected.

The most diagnostic of the clinical features are the xanthomas, but these do not occur in all patients with type III hyperlipoproteinemia.[8] The planar xanthomas in the palmar creases appear to be uniquely associated with type III hyperlipoproteinemia, and their presence is pathognomonic for the disease (see Fig. 119-2). Xanthomas of the tuberous variety, while frequent in type III hyperlipoproteinemia, also occur in other disorders, especially familial hypercholesterolemia (type IIa). The coexistence of premature peripheral vascular disease and hyperlipidemia is also cause for suspecting type III hyperlipoproteinemia.

The most reliable biochemical marker of type III hyperlipoproteinemia is the apo E phenotype.[8] The concurrence of phenotype E-2/2 with any of the other characteristics noted above is virtually diagnostic of type III hyperlipoproteinemia. The vast majority of type III subjects have the E-2/2 phenotype, which can be determined by isoelectric focusing of the $d <$ 1.006 or $d <$ 1.02 g/ml fraction of a small volume of fresh plasma (see Fig. 119-3). Phenotyping can also be performed directly on plasma.[327] In general, one-dimensional isoelectric focusing is sufficient for accurate phenotyping,[87] but in some cases, such as when excess sialylated isoforms are present, the two-dimensional technique may be required for unambiguous assignment.[81] The apo E phenotype persists regardless of other factors or conditions. A more specific genotyping assay that is both convenient and accurate is now available.[328] It relies on the use of DNA probes that distinguish between the presence of arginine or cysteine at residue 112 or 158 to identify the major isoforms—apo E-3, E-2, and E-4.

Because of the familial nature of type III hyperlipoproteinemia, and because affected patients are predisposed to accelerated cardiovascular disease, family members should be screened for hyperlipidemia and should undergo phenotyping. Because the E-2/2 phenotype predisposes individuals to the development of overt hyperlipoproteinemia, family counseling should stress the elimination of factors that exacerbate the expression of type III hyperlipoproteinemia (obesity, regular alcohol consumption, hypothyroidism, glucose intolerance). Particular attention should be given to adolescents and postmenopausal women, because the expression of hyperlipidemia frequently begins in these age groups. In the absence of factors known to influence the expression of type III hyperlipoproteinemia, the E-2/2 phenotype poses little risk for the development of premature vascular disease and probably even affords some protection, owing to the characteristically low levels of plasma LDL in these subjects.

Treatment

Type III hyperlipoproteinemia usually responds well to therapy.[8,329–336] In most cases, dietary therapy alone, or in combination with treatment of a preexisting metabolic condition, normalizes lipid levels. Metabolic conditions that commonly unmask the effect of the E-2/2 phenotype are hypothyroidism, marked weight gain, uncontrolled diabetes mellitus, and regular alcohol consumption. Thyroid hormone replacement, normalization of weight, control of diabetes, and cessation of alcohol consumption usually promptly reduce lipid levels. However, because abnormal apo E-2 is present, small quantities of β-VLDL persist in the plasma even after triglyceride and cholesterol levels are corrected.

Dietary modification should always be the first form of treatment for patients with hyperlipidemia.[329–332,337] The basic approach to diet therapy is to restrict caloric intake in patients who are overweight, and to reduce the intake of saturated fat and cholesterol. The American Heart Association recommends a progressive approach to diet.[338] The goal of the first phase is to reduce total fat in the diet to approximately 30 percent of total calories (from the $\approx$35 to 40 percent in the current U.S. diet) and to decrease saturated fat to 10 percent or less of total calories. It is recommended that cholesterol content of the diet be reduced to 250 to 300 mg/day. Fish oil supplementation in type III patients resulted in a 50 percent reduction in the $d < 1.006$ g/ml cholesterol and triglyceride levels and a reduction in remnant lipoproteins. However, there was no reduction in IDL cholesterol or triglycerides.[339]

Drugs are sometimes required to normalize the triglyceride and cholesterol levels (for review, see references 8 and 340–342); however, drug therapy should be instituted only after an adequate attempt has been made to control lipid levels by diet modification. Useful drugs for type III hyperlipoproteinemia include nicotinic acid (niacin), fibric acid derivatives, and HMG-CoA reductase inhibitors.

Nicotinic acid is effective in treating type III hyperlipoproteinemia.[329–331,335] It usually reduces plasma triglyceride and VLDL cholesterol levels by 40 percent and LDL cholesterol by 20 percent and increases HDL cholesterol by 20 percent. The drug decreases VLDL triglyceride synthesis and increases the VLDL catabolic rate.[343,344] Therapy should be initiated at a dose of 100 mg taken orally two times per day. This can be increased to an average dose of 1.5 g two times per day. Niacin's effect of raising blood glucose levels usually precludes its use in patients with diabetes mellitus. Liver enzymes, uric acid, and glucose levels in the serum should be monitored periodically. Side effects of nicotinic acid—flushing, pruritus, and gastrointestinal distress—can be minimized by taking an aspirin tablet about 30 min before the nicotinic acid and by taking the drug with meals.

Clofibrate has been widely used to treat type III hyperlipoproteinemia because it lowers triglyceride and cholesterol levels and is convenient to administer.[329–332,335,336] Typically, a dose of 1 g twice a day lowers triglyceride and VLDL cholesterol approximately 30 percent and LDL cholesterol slightly. A major effect of clofibrate is a reduction in hepatic cholesterol synthesis and an increase in lipolytic activity.[340–342] Clofibrate was used in a large World Health Organization trial to determine its effect on primary prevention of coronary heart disease.[345] The drug did reduce the rate of coronary disease, but there were more noncoronary deaths. There was also an increase in gastrointestinal diseases and cholelithiasis. Care should be exercised in the long-term use of this drug. In addition, clofibrate potentiates the action of warfarin.

Gemfibrozil is structurally similar to clofibrate[329–331,335] and may be the drug of choice in treating type III hyperlipoproteinemia.[346,347] A dose of 600 mg twice a day usually reduces triglyceride and VLDL cholesterol levels dramatically. The lipid-normalizing effects of gemfibrozil appear to be on the synthesis (production) of remnant particles rather than on clearance.[348] Fenofibrate (300 mg daily) reduces plasma cholesterol and triglycerides, and VLDL cholesterol triglycerides, and increases HDL cholesterol.[349] Micronized fenofibrate is also available (67 mg of the micronized formulation is bioequivalent to 100 mg of the nonmicronized formulation). The β-VLDL usually disappear with fibrate treatment.

The HMG-CoA reductase inhibitors (statins)—lovastatin and simvastatin—are also effective in lowering plasma lipids in type III hyperlipoproteinemia. In addition to inhibiting cholesterol biosynthesis within the liver by serving as a competitive inhibitor of HMG-CoA reductase, these drugs increase LDL receptors in the liver and accelerate lipoprotein clearance from the plasma,[350–354] Lovastatin and simvastatin are also effective in treating patients with type III hyperlipoproteinemia. Vega et al.[355] demonstrated that lovastatin appears to decrease VLDL production by inhibiting the synthesis of apo B-containing lipoproteins and also appears to accelerate the clearance of these lipoproteins. This resulted in a decrease in both VLDL and LDL apo B concentrations in type III hyperlipoproteinemia. Illingworth and O'Malley[356] demonstrated that lovastatin (20 or 40 mg twice/day) effectively lowered plasma cholesterol levels and was more effective than clofibrate alone. Likewise, simvastatin has a prolonged hypolipidemic effect in type III patients: plasma cholesterol levels were reduced 36 to 51 percent and triglycerides 32 to 55 percent, reflecting a decrease in both VLDL and LDL cholesterol levels.[357] Feussner et al.[358] also demonstrated a marked reduction in cholesterol and triglyceride levels with simvastatin and suggested that combination therapy with gemfibrozil may be beneficial when monotherapy does not normalize the lipid levels. Because of the risk of myopathy, this combination of drugs should be used only in refractory cases and with careful monitoring.[359] In general, the dose of a statin used in combination with gemfibrozil should be limited to half of the maximum recommended dose for that particular statin (e.g., 20 mg of simvastatin).

The decline in lipid levels with diet or drug therapy correlates with a decrease in the size of xanthomas or a complete disappearance of these lipid deposits.[60,61] After several months of therapy, blood flow, as determined by plethysmography, was improved in type III patients.[360] In addition, some diminution in intermittent claudication and angina pectoris has been reported.[332] Kuo et al.[361] treated eight type III hyperlipoproteinemic patients with a low-fat diet plus gemfibrozil for 2.5 to 3 years and demonstrated a decrease in the xanthomas, stabilization of coronary lesions by arteriography, and increased exercise tolerance.

REFERENCES

1. McGinley J, Jones H, Gofman J: Lipoproteins and xanthomatous diseases. *J Invest Dermatol* **19**:71, 1952.
2. Gofman JW, deLalla O, Glazier F, Freeman NK, Lindgren FT, Nichols AV, Strisower B, et al.: The serum lipoprotein transport system in health, metabolic disorders, atherosclerosis and coronary heart disease. *Plasma* **2**:413, 1954.
3. Fredrickson DS, Levy RI, Lees RS: Fat transport in lipoproteins—An integrated approach to mechanisms and disorders. *N Engl J Med* **276**:34, 1967.

4. Fredrickson DS, Levy RI, Lindgren FT: A comparison of heritable abnormal lipoprotein patterns as defined by two different techniques. *J Clin Invest* **47**:2446, 1968.
5. Morganroth J, Levy RI, Fredrickson DS: The biochemical, clinical, and genetic features of type III hyperlipoproteinemia. *Ann Intern Med* **82**:158, 1975.
6. Hazzard WR, O'Donnell TF, Lee YL: Broad-β disease (type III hyperlipoproteinemia) in a large kindred. Evidence for a monogenic mechanism. *Ann Intern Med* **82**:141, 1975.
7. Mishkel MA, Nazir DJ, Crowther S: A longitudinal assessment of lipid ratios in the diagnosis of type III hyperlipoproteinaemia. *Clin Chim Acta* **58**:121, 1975.
8. Mahley RW, Weisgraber KH, Farese RV, Jr.: Disorders of lipid metabolism, in Wilson JD, Foster DW, Kronenberg HM, Larsen PR (eds): *Williams Textbook of Endocrinology*. 9th ed. Philadelphia, Saunders, 1998, p 1099.
9. Fainaru M, Mahley RW, Hamilton RL, Innerarity TL: Structural and metabolic heterogeneity of β-very low density lipoproteins from cholesterol-fed dogs and from humans with type III hyperlipoproteinemia. *J Lipid Res* **23**:702, 1982.
10. Kane JP, Chen GC, Hamilton RL, Hardman DA, Malloy MJ, Havel RJ: Remnants of lipoproteins of intestinal and hepatic origin in familial dysbetalipoproteinemia. *Arteriosclerosis* **3**:47, 1983.
11. Chait A, Brunzell JD, Albers JJ, Hazzard WR: Type-III hyperlipoproteinaemia ("remnant removal disease"). Insight into the pathogenetic mechanism. *Lancet* **1**:1176, 1977.
12. Havel RJ, Kane JP: Primary dysbetalipoproteinemia: Predominance of a specific apoprotein species in triglyceride-rich lipoproteins. *Proc Natl Acad Sci U S A* **70**:2015, 1973.
13. Mahley RW: Apolipoprotein E: Cholesterol transport protein with expanding role in cell biology. *Science* **240**:622, 1988.
14. Utermann G, Pruin N, Steinmetz A: Polymorphism of apolipoprotein E. III. Effect of a single polymorphic gene locus on plasma lipid levels in man. *Clin Genet* **15**:63, 1979.
15. Utermann G, Hees M, Steinmetz A: Polymorphism of apolipoprotein E and occurrence of dysbetalipoproteinaemia in man. *Nature* **269**:604, 1977.
16. Utermann G, Jaeschke M, Menzel J: Familial hyperlipoproteinemia type III: Deficiency of a specific apolipoprotein (apo E-III) in the very-low-density lipoproteins. *FEBS Lett* **56**:352, 1975.
17. Utermann G, Vogelberg KH, Steinmetz A, Schoenborn W, Pruin N, Jaeschke M, Hees M, et al.: Polymorphism of apolipoprotein E. II. Genetics of hyperlipoproteinemia type III. *Clin Genet* **15**:37, 1979.
18. Utermann G, Langenbeck U, Beisiegel U, Weber W: Genetics of the apolipoprotein E system in man. *Am J Hum Genet* **32**:339, 1980.
19. Zannis VI, Breslow JL: Human very low density lipoprotein apolipoprotein E isoprotein polymorphism is explained by genetic variation and posttranslational modification. *Biochemistry* **20**:1033, 1981.
20. Zannis VI, Just PW, Breslow JL: Human apolipoprotein E isoprotein subclasses are genetically determined. *Am J Hum Genet* **33**:11, 1981.
21. Weisgraber KH, Rall SC, Jr., Mahley RW: Human E apoprotein heterogeneity. Cysteine-arginine interchanges in the amino acid sequence of the apo-E isoforms. *J Biol Chem* **256**:9077, 1981.
22. Rall SC, Jr., Weisgraber KH, Innerarity TL, Mahley RW: Structural basis for receptor binding heterogeneity of apolipoprotein E from type III hyperlipoproteinemic subjects. *Proc Natl Acad Sci U S A* **79**:4696, 1982.
23. Rall SC, Jr., Weisgraber KH, Mahley RW: Human apolipoprotein E. The complete amino acid sequence. *J Biol Chem* **257**:4171, 1982.
24. Mahley RW, Weisgraber KH, Innerarity TL, Rall SC, Jr.: Genetic defects in lipoprotein metabolism. Elevation of atherogenic lipoproteins caused by impaired catabolism. *JAMA* **265**:78, 1991.
25. Mahley RW: Atherogenic lipoproteins and coronary artery disease: Concepts derived from recent advances in cellular and molecular biology. *Circulation* **72**:943, 1985.
26. Havel RJ: Familial dysbetalipoproteinemia. New aspects of pathogenesis and diagnosis. *Med Clin North Am* **66**:441, 1982.
27. Bersot TP, Mahley RW, Brown MS, Goldstein JL: Interaction of swine lipoproteins with the low-density lipoprotein receptor in human fibroblasts. *J Biol Chem* **251**:2395, 1976.
28. Innerarity TL, Mahley RW: Enhanced binding by cultured human fibroblasts of apo-E-containing lipoproteins as compared with low-density lipoproteins. *Biochemistry* **17**:1440, 1978.
29. Mahley RW, Innerarity TL: Lipoprotein receptors and cholesterol homeostasis. *Biochim Biophys Acta* **737**:197, 1983.
30. Havel RJ, Chao Y-S, Windler EE, Kotite L, Guo LSS: Isoprotein specificity in the hepatic uptake of apolipoprotein E and the pathogenesis of familial dysbetalipoproteinemia. *Proc Natl Acad Sci U S A* **77**:4349, 1980.
31. Sherrill BC, Innerarity TL, Mahley RW: Rapid hepatic clearance of the canine lipoproteins containing only the E apoprotein by a high affinity receptor. Identity with the chylomicron remnant transport process. *J Biol Chem* **255**:1804, 1980.
32. Shelburne F, Hanks J, Meyers W, Quarfordt S: Effect of apoproteins on hepatic uptake of triglyceride emulsions in the rat. *J Clin Invest* **65**:652, 1980.
33. Windler E, Chao Y-S, Havel RJ: Determinants of hepatic uptake of triglyceride-rich lipoproteins and their remnants in the rat. *J Biol Chem* **255**:5475, 1980.
34. Schneider WJ, Kovanen PT, Brown MS, Goldstein JL, Utermann G, Weber W, Havel RJ, et al.: Familial dysbetalipoproteinemia. Abnormal binding of mutant apoprotein E to low-density lipoprotein receptors of human fibroblasts and membranes from liver and adrenal of rats, rabbits, and cows. *J Clin Invest* **68**:1075, 1981.
35. Weisgraber KH, Innerarity TL, Mahley RW: Abnormal lipoprotein receptor-binding activity of the human E apoprotein due to cysteine-arginine interchange at a single site. *J Biol Chem* **257**:2518, 1982.
36. Pagnan A, Havel RJ, Kane JP, Kotite L: Characterization of human very low-density lipoproteins containing two electrophoretic populations: Double pre-beta lipoproteinemia and primary dysbetalipoproteinemia. *J Lipid Res* **18**:613, 1977.
37. Kane JP: Apolipoprotein B: Structural and metabolic heterogeneity. *Annu Rev Physiol* **45**:637, 1983.
38. Kane JP, Hardman DA, Paulus HE: Heterogeneity of apolipoprotein B: Isolation of a new species from human chylomicrons. *Proc Natl Acad Sci U S A* **77**:2465, 1980.
39. Hodges P, Scott J: Apolipoprotein B mRNA editing: A new tier for the control of gene expression. *Trends Biochem Sci* **17**:77, 1992.
40. Innerarity TL, Borén J, Yamanaka S, Olofsson S-O: Biosynthesis of apolipoprotein B48-containing lipoproteins. Regulation by novel post-transcriptional mechanisms. *J Biol Chem* **271**:2353, 1996.
41. Milne RW, Weech PK, Blanchette L, Davignon J, Alaupovic P, Marcel YL: Isolation and characterization of apolipoprotein B-48 and B-100 very low density lipoproteins from type III hyperlipoproteinemic subjects. *J Clin Invest* **73**:816, 1984.
42. Mahley RW, Ji Z-S: Remnant lipoprotein metabolism: Key pathways involving cell-surface heparan sulfate proteoglycans and apolipoprotein E. *J Lipid Res* **40**:1, 1999.
43. Mahley RW, Hussain MM: Chylomicron and chylomicron remnant catabolism. *Curr Opin Lipidol* **2**:170, 1991.
44. Mahley RW, Innerarity TL, Rall SC, Jr., Weisgraber KH, Taylor JM: Apolipoprotein E: Genetic variants provide insights into its structure and function. *Curr Opin Lipidol* **1**:87, 1990.
45. Rall SC, Jr., Mahley RW: The role of apolipoprotein E genetic variants in lipoprotein disorders. *J Intern Med* **231**:653, 1992.
46. Chappell DA: Pre-β-very low density lipoproteins as precursors of β-very low density lipoproteins. A model for the pathogenesis of familial dysbetalipoproteinemia (type III hyperlipoproteinemia). *J Clin Invest* **82**:628, 1988.
47. Sata T, Havel RJ, Jones AL: Characterization of subfractions of triglyceride-rich lipoproteins separated by gel chromatography from blood plasma of normolipemic and hyperlipemic humans. *J Lipid Res* **13**:757, 1972.
48. Hazzard WR, Bierman EL: Broad-β disease versus endogenous hypertriglyceridemia: Levels and lipid composition of chylomicrons and very low density lipoproteins during fat-free feeding and alimentary lipemia. *Metabolism* **24**:817, 1975.
49. Havel RJ, Kotite L, Vigne J-L, Kane JP, Tun P, Phillips N, Chen GC: Radioimmunoassay of human arginine-rich apolipoprotein, apoprotein E. Concentration in blood plasma and lipoproteins as affected by apoprotein E-3 deficiency. *J Clin Invest* **66**:1351, 1980.
50. Patsch JR, Sailer S, Braunsteiner H: Lipoprotein of the density 1.006–1.020 in the plasma of patients with type III hyperlipoproteinaemia in the postabsorptive state. *Eur J Clin Invest* **5**:45, 1975.
51. Quarfordt S, Levy RI, Fredrickson DS: On the lipoprotein abnormality in type III hyperlipoproteinemia. *J Clin Invest* **50**:754, 1971.
52. Utermann G: Genetic polymorphism of apolipoprotein E—Impact on plasma lipoprotein metabolism, in Crepaldi G, Tiengo A, Baggio g (eds): *Diabetes, Obesity and Hyperlipidemias—III*. Amsterdam, Elsevier Science, 1985; p 1.
53. Hazzard WR: Primary type III hyperlipoproteinemia, in Rifkind BM, Levy RI (eds): *Hyperlipidemia. Diagnosis and Therapy*. New York, Grune & Stratton, 1977; p 137.
54. Borrie P: Type III hyperlipoproteinaemia. *Br Med J* **2**:665, 1969.

55. Mishkel MA: Type III hyperlipoproteinaemia with xanthomatosis, in Peeters H (eds): *Protides of the Biological Fluids*. Oxford, Pergamon, 1972; p 283.
56. Vessby B, Hedstrand H, Lundin L-G, Olsson U: Inheritance of type-III hyperlipoproteinemia. Lipoprotein patterns in first-degree relatives. *Metabolism* **26**:225, 1977.
57. Stuyt PMJ, Van't Laar A: Clinical features of type III hyperlipoproteinaemia. *Neth J Med* **26**:104, 1983.
58. Vermeer BJ, Van Gent CM, Goslings B, Polano MK: Xanthomatosis and other clinical findings in patients with elevated levels of very low density lipoproteins. *Br J Dermatol* **100**:657, 1979.
59. Glueck CJ, Fallat RW, Mellies MJ, Steiner PM: Pediatric familial type III hyperlipoproteinemia. *Metabolism* **25**:1269, 1976.
60. Parker F: Xanthomas and hyperlipidemias. *J Am Acad Dermatol* **13**:1, 1985.
61. Haber C, Kwiterovich PO, Jr.: Dyslipoproteinemia and xanthomatosis. *Pediatr Dermatol* **1**:261, 1984.
62. Polano MK: Xanthomatosis and hyperlipoproteinemia. A review. *Dermatologica* **149**:1, 1974.
63. Feussner G, Wagner A, Kohl B, Ziegler R: Clinical features of type III hyperlipoproteinemia: Analysis of 64 patients. *J Clin Invest* **71**:362–366, 1993.
64. Dobmeyer J, Lohrmann J, Feussner G: Prevalence and association of atherosclerosis at three different arterial sites in patients with type III hyperlipoproteinemia. *Atherosclerosis* **119**:89, 1996.
65. Mahley RW: Dietary fat, cholesterol, and accelerated atherosclerosis. *Atheroscler Rev* **5**:1, 1979.
66. Mahley RW: Development of accelerated atherosclerosis. Concepts derived from cell biology and animal model studies. *Arch Pathol Lab Med* **107**:393, 1983.
67. Hazzard WR, Goldstein JL, Schrott HG, Motulsky AG, Bierman EL: Hyperlipidemia in coronary heart disease. III. Evaluation of lipoprotein phenotypes of 156 genetically defined survivors of myocardial infarction. *J Clin Invest* **52**:1569, 1973.
68. Dyerberg J: Type III hyperlipoproteinemia with low plasma thyroxine binding globulin. *Metabolism* **18**:50, 1969.
69. Roberts WC, Levy RI, Fredrickson DS: Hyperlipoproteinemia. A review of the five types with first report of necropsy findings in type 3. *Arch Pathol* **90**:46, 1970.
70. Holimon JL, Wasserman AJ: Autopsy findings in type 3 hyperlipoproteinemia. *Arch Pathol* **92**:415, 1971.
71. Roberts WC, Ferrans VJ, Levy RI, Fredrickson DS: Cardiovascular pathology in hyperlipoproteinemia. Anatomic observations in 42 necropsy patients with normal or abnormal serum lipoprotein patterns. *Am J Cardiol* **31**:557, 1973.
72. Amatruda JM, Margolis S, Hutchins GM: Type III hyperlipoproteinemia with mesangial foam cells in renal glomeruli. *Arch Pathol* **98**:51, 1974.
73. Gown AM, Hazzard WR, Benditt EP: Type III hyperlipoproteinemia and atherosclerosis: A case report and re-evaluation. *Hum Pathol* **13**:506, 1982.
74. Cabin HS, Schwartz DE, Virmani R, Brewer HB, Jr., Roberts WC: Type III hyperlipoproteinemia: Quantification, distribution, and nature of atherosclerotic coronary arterial narrowing in five necropsy patients. *Am Heart J* **102**:830, 1981.
75. Schwartz D (discussant): Type III hyperlipoproteinemia: Diagnosis, molecular defects, pathology, and treatment. Pathology. *Ann Intern Med* **98**:632, 1983.
76. Balson KR, Niall JF, Best JD: Glomerular lipid deposition and proteinuria in a patient with familial dysbetalipoproteinaemia. *J Intern Med* **240**:157, 1996.
77. Ross R: The pathogenesis of atherosclerosis — An update. *N Engl J Med* **314**:488, 1986.
78. Goldstein JL, Ho YK, Brown MS, Innerarity TL, Mahley RW: Cholesteryl ester accumulation in macrophages resulting from receptor-mediated uptake and degradation of hypercholesterolemic canine β-very low density lipoproteins. *J Biol Chem* **255**:1839, 1980.
79. Mahley RW, Innerarity TL, Brown MS, Ho YK, Goldstein JL: Cholesteryl ester synthesis in macrophages: Stimulation by β-very low density lipoproteins from cholesterol-fed animals of several species. *J Lipid Res* **21**:970, 1980.
80. Mahley RW, Innerarity TL, Rall SC, Jr., Weisgraber KH: Plasma lipoproteins: Apolipoprotein structure and function. *J Lipid Res* **25**:1277, 1984.
81. Zannis VI, Breslow JL, Utermann G, Mahley RW, Weisgraber KH, Havel RJ, Goldstein JL, et al.: Proposed nomenclature of apoE isoproteins, apoE genotypes, and phenotypes. *J Lipid Res* **23**:911, 1982.
82. Wernette-Hammond ME, Lauer SJ, Corsini A, Walker D, Taylor JM, Rall SC, Jr: Glycosylation of human apolipoprotein E. The carbohydrate attachment site is threonine 194. *J Biol Chem* **264**:9094, 1989.
83. Mahley RW, Angelin B: Type III hyperlipoproteinemia: Recent insights into the genetic defect of familial dysbetalipoproteinemia. *Adv Intern Med* **29**:385, 1984.
84. Breslow JL: Genetics of the human apolipoproteins, in Scanu AM, Spector AA (eds): *Biochemistry and Biology of Plasma Lipoproteins*. New York, Marcel Dekker, 1986; p 85.
85. Davignon J, Sing CF, Lussier-Cacan S, Bouthillier D: Xanthelasma, latent dyslipoproteinemia and atherosclerosis: Contribution of apo E polymorphism, in de Gennes JL, Polonovski J, Paoletti R (eds): *Latent Dyslipoproteinemias and Atherosclerosis*. New York, Raven, 1984; p 213.
86. Menzel H-J, Kladetzky R-G, Assmann G: Apolipoprotein E polymorphism and coronary artery disease. *Arteriosclerosis* **3**:310, 1983.
87. Utermann G, Steinmetz A, Weber W: Genetic control of human apolipoprotein E polymorphism: Comparison of one- and two-dimensional techniques of isoprotein analysis. *Hum Genet* **60**:344, 1982.
88. Hallman DM, Boerwinkle E, Saha N, Sandholzer C, Menzel HJ, Csázár A, Utermann G: The apolipoprotein E polymorphism: A comparison of allele frequencies and effects in nine populations. *Am J Hum Genet* **49**:338, 1991.
89. Cumming AM, Robertson FW: Polymorphism at the apoprotein-E locus in relation to risk of coronary disease. *Clin Genet* **25**:310, 1984.
90. Ehnholm C, Lukka M, Kuusi T, Nikkilä E, Utermann G: Apolipoprotein E polymorphism in the Finnish population: Gene frequencies and relation to lipoprotein concentrations. *J Lipid Res* **27**:227, 1986.
91. Wardell MR, Suckling PA, Janus ED: Genetic variation in human apolipoprotein E. *J Lipid Res* **23**:1174, 1982.
92. Weisgraber KH: Apolipoprotein E: Structure-function relationships. *Adv Protein Chem* **45**:249, 1994.
93. Hixson JE, Cox LA, Borenstein S: The baboon apolipoprotein E gene: Structure, expression, and linkage with the gene for apolipoprotein C-I. *Genomics* **2**:315, 1988.
94. Kamboh MI, Bhatia KK, Ferrell RE: Genetic studies of human apolipoproteins: XII. Population genetics of apolipoproteins in Papua New Guinea. *Am J Hum Biol* **2**:17, 1990.
95. Mahley RW, Palaoglu KE, Atak Z, Dawson-Pepin J, Langlois A-M, Cheung V, Onat H, et al.: Turkish Heart Study: Lipids, lipoproteins, and apolipoproteins. *J Lipid Res* **36**:839, 1995.
96. Kamboh MI, Sepehrnia B, Ferrell RE: Genetic studies of human apolipoproteins. VI. Common polymorphism of apolipoprotein E in blacks. *Dis Markers* **7**:49, 1989.
97. Sepehrnia B, Kamboh MI, Adams-Campbell LL, Bunker CH, Nwankwo M, Majumder PP, Ferrell RE: Genetic studies of human apolipoproteins. X. The effect of the apolipoprotein E polymorphism on quantitative levels of lipoproteins in Nigerian blacks. *Am J Hum Genet* **45**:586, 1989.
98. Hixson JE, the Pathobiological Determinants of Atherosclerosis in Youth (PDAY) Research Group: Apolipoprotein E polymorphisms affect atherosclerosis in young males. *Arterioscler Thromb* **11**:1237, 1991.
99. Sing CF, Davignon J: Role of the apolipoprotein E polymorphism in determining normal plasma lipid and lipoprotein variation. *Am J Hum Genet* **37**:268, 1985.
100. Bouthillier D, Sing CF, Davignon J: Apolipoprotein E phenotyping with a single gel method: Application to the study of informative matings. *J Lipid Res* **24**:1060, 1983.
101. Robertson FW, Cumming AM: Effects of apoprotein E polymorphism on serum lipoprotein concentration. *Arteriosclerosis* **5**:283, 1985.
102. Davignon J, Gregg RE, Sing CF: Apolipoprotein E polymorphism and atherosclerosis. *Arteriosclerosis* **8**:1, 1988.
103. Dallongeville J, Lussier-Cacan S, Davignon J: Modulation of plasma triglyceride levels by apoE phenotype: A meta-analysis. *J Lipid Res* **33**:447, 1992.
104. Steinmetz A, Thiemann E, Czekelius P, Kaffarnik H: Polymorphism of apolipoprotein E influences levels of serum apolipoproteins E and B in the human neonate. *Eur J Clin Invest* **19**:390, 1989.
105. Salah D, Bohnet K, Gueguen R, Siest G, Visvikis S: Combined effects of lipoprotein lipase and apolipoprotein E polymorphisms on lipid and lipoprotein levels in the Stanislas cohort. *J Lipid Res* **38**:904, 1997.
106. Huang Y, Liu X-Q, Rall SC Jr, Taylor JM, von Eckardstein A, Assmann G, Mahley RW: Overexpression and accumulation of apolipoprotein E as a cause of hypertriglyceridemia. *J Biol Chem* **273**:26388, 1998.

107. Utermann G, Kindermann I, Kaffarnik H, Steinmetz A: Apolipoprotein E phenotypes and hyperlipidemia. *Hum Genet* **65**:232, 1984.
108. Gregg RE, Zech LA, Schaefer EJ, Brewer HB Jr: Type III hyperlipoproteinemia: Defective metabolism of an abnormal apolipoprotein E. *Science* **211**:584, 1981.
109. Gregg RE, Zech LA, Schaefer EJ, Stark D, Wilson D, Brewer HB, Jr.: Abnormal in vivo metabolism of apolipoprotein E4 in humans. *J Clin Invest* **78**:815–821, 1986.
110. Ghiselli G, Schaefer EJ, Zech LA, Gregg RE, Brewer HB, Jr.: Increased prevalence of apolipoprotein E4 in type V hyperlipoproteinemia. *J Clin Invest* **70**:474, 1982.
111. Weintraub MS, Eisenberg S, Breslow JL: Dietary fat clearance in normal subjects is regulated by genetic variation of apolipoprotein E. *J Clin Invest* **80**:1571, 1987.
112. Boerwinkle E, Brown SA, Rohrbach K, Gotto AM Jr, Patsch W: Role of apolipoprotein E and B gene variation in determining response of lipid, lipoprotein, and apolipoprotein levels to increased dietary cholesterol. *Am J Hum Genet* **49**:1145, 1991.
113. Boerwinkle E, Brown S, Sharrett AR, Heiss G, Patsch W: Apolipoprotein E polymorphism influences postprandial retinyl palmitate but not triglyceride concentrations. *Am J Hum Genet* **54**:341, 1994.
114. Brown AJ, Roberts DCK: The effect of fasting triacylglyceride concentration and apolipoprotein E polymorphism on postprandial lipemia. *Arterioscler Thromb* **11**:1737, 1991.
115. Bergeron N, Havel RJ: Prolonged postprandial responses of lipids and apolipoproteins in triglyceride-rich lipoproteins of individuals expressing an apolipoprotein ε4 allele. *J Clin Invest* **97**:65, 1996.
116. Kuusi T, Nieminen MS, Ehnholm C, Yki-Järvinen H, Valle M, Nikkilä EA, Taskinen M-R: Apoprotein E polymorphism and coronary artery disease. Increased prevalence of apolipoprotein E-4 in angiographically verified coronary patients. *Arteriosclerosis* **9**:237, 1989.
117. Vollmer E, Roessner A, Bosse A, Böcker W, Kaesberg B, Robenek H, Sorg C, et al.: Immunohistochemical double labeling of macrophages, smooth muscle cells, and apolipoprotein E in the atherosclerotic plaque. *Pathol Res Pract* **187**:184, 1991.
118. Babaev VR, Dergunov AD, Chenchik AA, Tararak EM, Yanushevskaya EV, Trakht IN, Sorg C, et al.: Localization of apolipoprotein E in normal and atherosclerotic human aorta. *Atherosclerosis* **85**:239, 1990.
119. Glatz JFC, Demacker PNM, Turner PR, Katan MB: Response of serum cholesterol to dietary cholesterol in relation to apolipoprotein E phenotype. *Nutr Metab Cardiovasc Dis* **1**:13, 1991.
120. Gylling H, Miettinen TA: Cholesterol absorption and synthesis related to low-density lipoprotein metabolism during varying cholesterol intake in men with different apoE phenotypes. *J Lipid Res* **33**:1361, 1992.
121. Kesäniemi YA, Ehnholm C, Miettinen TA: Intestinal cholesterol absorption efficiency in man is related to apoprotein E phenotype. *J Clin Invest* **80**:578, 1987.
122. Miettinen TA: Impact of apo E phenotype on the regulation of cholesterol metabolism. *Ann Med* **23**:181, 1991.
123. Das HK, McPherson J, Bruns GAP, Karathanasis SK, Breslow JL: Isolation, characterization, and mapping to chromosome 19 of the human apolipoprotein E gene. *J Biol Chem* **260**:6240, 1985.
124. Paik Y-K, Chang DJ, Reardon CA, Davies GE, Mahley RW, Taylor JM: Nucleotide sequence and structure of the human apolipoprotein E gene. *Proc Natl Acad Sci U S A* **82**:3445, 1985.
125. Luo C-C, Li W-H, Moore MN, Chan L: Structure and evolution of the apolipoprotein multigene family. *J Mol Biol* **187**:325, 1986.
126. Elshourbagy NA, Walker DW, Paik Y-K, Boguski MS, Freeman M, Gordon JI, Taylor JM: Structure and expression of the human apolipoprotein A-IV gene. *J Biol Chem* **262**:7973, 1987.
127. Zannis VI, McPherson J, Goldberger G, Karathanasis SK, Breslow JL: Synthesis, intracellular processing, and signal peptide of human apolipoprotein E. *J Biol Chem* **259**:5495, 1984.
128. McLean JW, Elshourbagy NA, Chang DJ, Mahley RW, Taylor JM: Human apolipoprotein E mRNA. cDNA cloning and nucleotide sequencing of a new variant. *J Biol Chem* **259**:6498, 1984.
129. Allan CM, Walker D, Taylor JM: Evolutionary duplication of a hepatic control region in the human apolipoprotein E gene locus. Identification of a second region that confers high level and liver-specific expression of the human apolipoprotein E gene in transgenic mice. *J Biol Chem* **270**:26278, 1995.
130. Olaisen B, Teisberg P, Gedde-Dahl T, Jr.: The locus for apolipoprotein E (apoE) is linked to the complement component C3 (C3) locus on chromosome 19 in man. *Hum Genet* **62**:233, 1982.
131. Lauer SJ, Walker D, Elshourbagy NA, Reardon CA, Levy-Wilson B, Taylor JM: Two copies of the human apolipoprotein C-I gene are linked closely to the apolipoprotein E gene. *J Biol Chem* **263**:7277, 1988.
132. Jackson CL, Bruns GAP, Breslow JL: Isolation and sequence of a human apolipoprotein CII cDNA clone and its use to isolate and map to human chromosome 19 the gene for apolipoprotein CII. *Proc Natl Acad Sci U S A* **81**:2945, 1984.
133. Francke U, Brown MS, Goldstein JL: Assignment of the human gene for the low-density lipoprotein receptor to chromosome 19: Synteny of a receptor, a ligand, and a genetic disease. *Proc Natl Acad Sci U S A* **81**:2826, 1984.
134. Simonet WS, Bucay N, Pitas RE, Lauer SJ, Taylor JM: Multiple tissue-specific elements control the apolipoprotein E/C-I gene locus in transgenic mice. *J Biol Chem* **266**:8651, 1991.
135. Simonet WS, Bucay N, Lauer SJ, Taylor JM: A far-downstream hepatocyte-specific control region directs expression of the linked human apolipoprotein E and C-I genes in transgenic mice. *J Biol Chem* **268**:8221, 1993.
136. Allan CM, Taylor S, Taylor JM: Two hepatic enhancers, HCR.1 and HCR.2, coordinate the liver expression of the entire human apolipoprotein E/C-I/C-IV/C-II gene cluster. *J Biol Chem* **272**:29113, 1997.
137. Herz J, Willnow TE: Lipoprotein and receptor interactions in vivo. *Curr Opin Lipidol* **6**:97, 1995.
138. Cooper AD: Hepatic uptake of chylomicron remnants. *J Lipid Res* **38**:2173, 1997.
139. Krieger M, Herz J: Structures and functions of multiligand lipoprotein receptors: Macrophage scavenger receptors and LDL receptor-related protein (LRP). *Annu Rev Biochem* **63**:601, 1994.
140. Brown MS, Herz J, Kowal RC, Goldstein JL: The low-density lipoprotein receptor-related protein: Double agent or decoy. *Curr Opin Lipidol* **2**:65, 1991.
141. Wetterau JR, Aggerbeck LP, Rall SC, Jr., Weisgraber KH: Human apolipoprotein E3 in aqueous solution. I. Evidence for two structural domains. *J Biol Chem* **263**:6240, 1988.
142. Aggerbeck LP, Wetterau JR, Weisgraber KH, Wu C-SC, Lindgren FT: Human apolipoprotein E3 in aqueous solution. II. Properties of the amino- and carboxyl-terminal domains. *J Biol Chem* **263**:6249, 1988.
143. Hobbs HH, Brown MS, Goldstein JL: Molecular genetics of the LDL receptor gene in familial hypercholesterolemia. *Hum Mutat* **1**:445, 1992.
144. Wardell MR, Wilson C, Agard DA, Mahley RW, Weisgraber KH: Crystal structures of the common apolipoprotein E variants: Insights into functional mechanisms, in Sirtori CR, Franceschini G, Brewer BH Jr (eds): *Human Apolipoprotein Mutants III. Diagnosis and Treatment.* Berlin, Springer-Verlag, 1993; p 81.
145. Wilson C, Wardell MR, Weisgraber KH, Mahley RW, Agard DA: Three-dimensional structure of the LDL receptor-binding domain of human apolipoprotein E. *Science* **252**:1817, 1991.
146. Wilson C, Mau T, Weisgraber KH, Wardell MR, Mahley RW, Agard DA: Salt bridge relay triggers defective LDL receptor binding by a mutant apolipoprotein. *Structure* **2**:713, 1994.
147. Innerarity TL, Weisgraber KH, Arnold KS, Rall SC, Jr., Mahley RW: Normalization of receptor binding of apolipoprotein E2. Evidence for modulation of the binding site conformation. *J Biol Chem* **259**:7261, 1984.
148. Innerarity TL, Hui DY, Bersot TP, Mahley RW: Type III hyperlipoproteinemia: A focus on lipoprotein receptor-apolipoprotein E2 interactions. *Adv Exp Med Biol* **201**:273, 1986.
149. Dong L-M, Parkin S, Trakhanov SD, Rupp B, Simmons T, Arnold KS, Newhouse YM, et al.: Novel mechanism for defective receptor binding of apolipoprotein E2 in type III hyperlipoproteinemia. *Nat Struct Biol* **3**:718, 1996.
150. Steinmetz A, Jakobs C, Motzny S, Kaffarnik H: Differential distribution of apolipoprotein E isoforms in human plasma lipoproteins. *Arteriosclerosis* **9**:405, 1989.
151. Weisgraber KH: Apolipoprotein E distribution among human plasma lipoproteins: Role of the cysteine-arginine interchange at residue 112. *J Lipid Res* **31**:1503, 1990.
152. Gianturco SH, Gotto AM Jr, Hwang S-LC, Karlin JB, Lin AHY, Prasad SC, Bradley WA: Apolipoprotein E mediates uptake of *Sf* 100–400 hypertriglyceridemic very low density lipoproteins by the low density lipoprotein receptor pathway in normal human fibroblasts. *J Biol Chem* **258**:4526, 1983.
153. Dong L-M, Wilson C, Wardell MR, Simmons T, Mahley RW, Weisgraber KH, Agard DA: Human apolipoprotein E. Role of arginine 61 in mediating the lipoprotein preferences of the E3 and E4 isoforms. *J Biol Chem* **269**:22358, 1994.

154. Dong L-M, Weisgraber KH: Human apolipoprotein E4 domain interaction. Arginine 61 and glutamic acid 255 interact to direct the preference for very low density lipoproteins. *J Biol Chem* **271**:19053, 1996.
155. Blue M-L, Williams DL, Zucker S, Khan SA, Blum CB: Apolipoprotein E synthesis in human kidney, adrenal gland, and liver. *Proc Natl Acad Sci U S A* **80**:283, 1983.
156. Elshourbagy NA, Liao WS, Mahley RW, Taylor JM: Apolipoprotein E mRNA is abundant in the brain and adrenals, as well as in the liver, and is present in other peripheral tissues of rats and marmosets. *Proc Natl Acad Sci U S A* **82**:203, 1985.
157. Lin C-T, Xu Y, Wu J-Y, Chan L: Immunoreactive apolipoprotein E is a widely distributed cellular protein. Immunohistochemical localization of apolipoprotein E in baboon tissues. *J Clin Invest* **78**:947, 1986.
158. Reyland ME, Gwynne JT, Forgez P, Prack MM, Williams DL: Expression of the human apolipoprotein E gene suppresses steroidogenesis in mouse Y1 adrenal cells. *Proc Natl Acad Sci U S A* **88**:2375, 1991.
159. Pitas RE, Boyles JK, Lee SH, Foss D, Mahley RW: Astrocytes synthesize apolipoprotein E and metabolize apolipoprotein E-containing lipoproteins. *Biochim Biophys Acta* **917**:148, 1987.
160. Weisgraber KH, Mahley RW: Human apolipoprotein E: The Alzheimer's disease connection. *FASEB J* **10**:1485, 1996.
161. Mahley RW: Apolipoprotein E: Structure and function in lipid metabolism and neurobiology, in Rosenberg RN, Prusiner SB, DiMauro S, Barchi RL (eds): *The Molecular and Genetic Basis of Neurological Disease*. 2nd ed. Boston, Butterworth-Heinemann, 1997; p 1037.
162. Mahley RW, Nathan BP, Bellosta S, Pitas RE: Apolipoprotein E: Impact of cytoskeletal stability in neurons and the relationship to Alzheimer's disease. *Curr Opin Lipidol* **6**:86, 1995.
163. Basu SK, Brown MS, Ho YK, Havel RJ, Goldstein JL: Mouse macrophages synthesize and secrete a protein resembling apolipoprotein E. *Proc Natl Acad Sci U S A* **78**:7545, 1981.
164. Basu SK, Ho YK, Brown MS, Bilheimer DW, Anderson RGW, Goldstein JL: Biochemical and genetic studies of the apoprotein E secreted by mouse macrophages and human monocytes. *J Biol Chem* **257**:9788, 1982.
165. Driscoll DM, Getz GS: Extrahepatic synthesis of apolipoprotein E. *J Lipid Res* **25**:1368, 1984.
166. Majack RA, Castle CK, Goodman LV, Weisgraber KH, Mahley RW, Shooter EM, Gebicke-Haerter PJ: Expression of apolipoprotein E by cultured vascular smooth muscle cells is controlled by growth state. *J Cell Biol* **107**:1207, 1988.
167. Ignatius MJ, Gebicke-Härter PJ, Skene JHP, Schilling JW, Weisgraber KH, Mahley RW, Shooter EM: Expression of apolipoprotein E during nerve degeneration and regeneration. *Proc Natl Acad Sci U S A* **83**:1125, 1986.
168. Snipes GJ, McGuire CB, Norden JJ, Freeman JA: Nerve injury stimulates the secretion of apolipoprotein E by nonneuronal cells. *Proc Natl Acad Sci U S A* **83**:1130, 1986.
169. Boyles JK, Zoellner CD, Anderson LJ, Kosik LM, Pitas RE, Weisgraber KH, Hui DY, et al.: A role for apolipoprotein E, apolipoprotein A-I, and low density lipoprotein receptors in cholesterol transport during regeneration and remyelination of the rat sciatic nerve. *J Clin Invest* **83**:1015, 1989.
170. Handelmann GE, Boyles JK, Weisgraber KH, Mahley RW, Pitas RE: Effects of apolipoprotein E, β-very low density lipoproteins, and cholesterol on the extension of neurites by rabbit dorsal root ganglion neurons in vitro. *J Lipid Res* **33**:1677, 1992.
171. Brown MS, Goldstein JL: Lipoprotein receptors in the liver. Control signals for plasma cholesterol traffic. *J Clin Invest* **72**:743, 1983.
172. Schaefer EJ, Gregg RE, Ghiselli G, Forte TM, Ordovas JM, Zech LA, Brewer HB Jr: Familial apolipoprotein E deficiency. *J Clin Invest* **78**:1206, 1986.
173. Cladaras C, Hadzopoulou-Cladaras M, Felber BK, Pavlakis G, Zannis VI: The molecular basis of a familial apoE deficiency. An acceptor splice site mutation in the third intron of the deficient apoE gene. *J Biol Chem* **262**:2310, 1987.
174. Lohse P, Brewer HB, III, Meng MS, Skarlatos SI, LaRosa JC, Brewer HB Jr: Familial apolipoprotein E deficiency and type III hyperlipoproteinemia due to a premature stop codon in the apolipoprotein E gene. *J Lipid Res* **33**:1583, 1992.
175. Mabuchi H, Itoh H, Takeda M, Kajinami K, Wakasugi T, Koizumi J, Takeda R, et al.: A young type III hyperlipoproteinemic patient associated with apolipoprotein E deficiency. *Metabolism* **38**:115, 1989.
176. Kurosaka D, Teramoto T, Matsushima T, Yokoyama T, Yamada A, Aikawa T, Miyamoto Y, et al.: Apolipoprotein E deficiency with a depressed mRNA of normal size. *Atherosclerosis* **88**:15, 1991.
177. Zhang SH, Reddick RL, Piedrahita JA, Maeda N: Spontaneous hypercholesterolemia and arterial lesions in mice lacking apolipoprotein E. *Science* **258**:468, 1992.
178. Plump AS, Smith JD, Hayek T, Aalto-Setälä K, Walsh A, Verstuyft JG, Rubin EM, et al.: Severe hypercholesterolemia and atherosclerosis in apolipoprotein E-deficient mice created by homologous recombination in ES cells. *Cell* **71**:343, 1992.
179. Fazio S, Lee Y-L, Ji Z-S, Rall SC, Jr: Type III hyperlipoproteinemic phenotype in transgenic mice expressing dysfunctional apolipoprotein E. *J Clin Invest* **92**:1497, 1993.
180. van den Maagdenberg AMJM, Hofker MH, Krimpenfort PJA, de Bruijn I, van Vlijmen B, van der Boom H, Havekes LM, et al.: Transgenic mice carrying the apolipoprotein E3-Leiden gene exhibit hyperlipoproteinemia. *J Biol Chem* **268**:10540, 1993.
181. Huang Y, Schwendner SW, Rall SC Jr, Mahley RW: Hypolipidemic and hyperlipidemic phenotypes in transgenic mice expressing human apolipoprotein E2. *J Biol Chem* **271**:29146, 1996.
182. Huang Y, Schwendner SW, Rall SC Jr, Sanan DA, Mahley RW: Apolipoprotein E2 transgenic rabbits: Modulation of the type III hyperlipoproteinemic phenotype by estrogen and occurrence of spontaneous atherosclerosis. *J Biol Chem* **272**:22685, 1997.
183. Mahley RW, Weisgraber KH, Hussain MM, Greenman B, Fisher M, Vogel T, Gorecki M: Intravenous infusion of apolipoprotein E accelerates clearance of plasma lipoproteins in rabbits. *J Clin Invest* **83**:2125, 1989.
184. Yamada N, Shimano H, Mokuno H, Ishibashi S, Gotohda T, Kawakami M, Watanabe Y, et al.: Increased clearance of plasma cholesterol after injection of apolipoprotein E into Watanabe heritable hyperlipidemic rabbits. *Proc Natl Acad Sci U S A* **86**:665, 1989.
185. Hussain MM, Mahley RW, Boyles JK, Fainaru M, Brecht WJ, Lindquist PA: Chylomicron-chylomicron remnant clearance by liver and bone marrow in rabbits. Factors that modify tissue-specific uptake. *J Biol Chem* **264**:9571, 1989.
186. Hussain MM, Mahley RW, Boyles JK, Lindquist PA, Brecht WJ, Innerarity TL: Chylomicron metabolism. Chylomicron uptake by bone marrow in different animal species. *J Biol Chem* **264**:17931, 1989.
187. Shimano H, Yamada N, Katsuki M, Shimada M, Gotoda T, Harada K, Murase T, et al.: Overexpression of apolipoprotein E in transgenic mice: Marked reduction in plasma lipoproteins except high density lipoprotein and resistance against diet-induced hypercholesterolemia. *Proc Natl Acad Sci U S A* 89:1750, 1992.
188. Kowal RC, Herz J, Goldstein JL, Esser V, Brown MS: Low density lipoprotein receptor-related protein mediates uptake of cholesteryl esters derived from apoprotein E-enriched lipoproteins. *Proc Natl Acad Sci U S A* 86:5810, 1989.
189. Kowal RC, Herz J, Weisgraber KH, Mahley RW, Brown MS, Goldstein JL: Opposing effects of apolipoproteins E and C on lipoprotein binding to low-density lipoprotein receptor-related protein. *J Biol Chem* 265:10771, 1990.
190. Herz J, Hamann U, Rogne S, Myklebost O, Gausepohl H, Stanley KK: Surface location and high affinity for calcium of a 500-kd liver membrane protein closely related to the LDL-receptor suggest a physiological role as lipoprotein receptor. *EMBO J* **7**:4119, 1988.
191. Beisiegel U, Weber W, Ihrke G, Herz J, Stanley KK: The LDL-receptor-related protein, LRP, is an apolipoprotein E-binding protein. *Nature* **341**:162, 1989.
192. Mahley RW: Heparan sulfate proteoglycan/low density lipoprotein receptor-related protein pathway involved in type III hyperlipoproteinemia and Alzheimer's disease. *Isr J Med Sci* **32**:414, 1996.
193. Stow JL, Kjéllen L, Unger E, Höök M, Farquhar MG: Heparan sulfate proteoglycans are concentrated on the sinusoidal plasmalemmal domain and in intracellular organelles of hepatocytes. *J Cell Biol* **100**:975, 1985.
194. Hamilton RL, Wong JS, Guo LSS, Krisans S, Havel RJ: Apolipoprotein E localization in rat hepatocytes by immunogold labeling of cryothin sections. *J Lipid Res* **31**:1589, 1990.
195. Mahley RW, Weisgraber KH, Innerarity TL: Interaction of plasma lipoproteins containing apolipoproteins B and E with heparin and cell surface receptors. *Biochim Biophys Acta* **575**:81, 1979.
196. Weisgraber KH, Rall SC Jr, Mahley RW, Milne RW, Marcel YL, Sparrow JT: Human apolipoprotein E. Determination of the heparin binding sites of apolipoprotein E3. *J Biol Chem* **261**:2068, 1986.

197. Ji Z-S, Brecht WJ, Miranda RD, Hussain MM, Innerarity TL, Mahley RW: Role of heparan sulfate proteoglycans in the binding and uptake of apolipoprotein E-enriched remnant lipoproteins by cultured cells. *J Biol Chem* **268**:10160, 1993.
198. Ji Z-S, Fazio S, Lee Y-L, Mahley RW: Secretion-capture role for apolipoprotein E in remnant lipoprotein metabolism involving cell surface heparan sulfate proteoglycans. *J Biol Chem* **269**:2764, 1994.
199. Ji Z-S, Sanan DA, Mahley RW: Intravenous heparinase inhibits remnant lipoprotein clearance from the plasma and uptake by the liver: In vivo role of heparan sulfate proteoglycans. *J Lipid Res* **36**:583, 1995.
200. Zeng B-J, Mortimer B-C, Martins IJ, Seydel U, Redgrave TG: Chylomicron remnant uptake is regulated by the expression and function of heparan sulfate proteoglycan in hepatocytes. *J Lipid Res* **39**:845, 1998.
201. Linton MF, Hasty AH, Babaev VR, Fazio S: Hepatic apo E expression is required for remnant lipoprotein clearance in the absence of the low density lipoprotein receptor. *J Clin Invest* **101**:1726, 1998.
202. Doolittle MH, Wong H, Davis RC, Schotz MC: Synthesis of hepatic lipase in liver and extrahepatic tissues. *J Lipid Res* **28**:1326, 1987.
203. Ji Z-S, Lauer SJ, Fazio S, Bensadoun A, Taylor JM, Mahley RW: Enhanced binding and uptake of remnant lipoproteins by hepatic lipase-secreting hepatoma cells in culture. *J Biol Chem* **269**:13429, 1994.
204. Shafi S, Brady SE, Bensadoun A, Havel RJ: Role of hepatic lipase in the uptake and processing of chylomicron remnants in rat liver. *J Lipid Res* **35**:709, 1994.
205. Krapp A, Ahle S, Kersting S, Hua Y, Kneser K, Nielsen M, Gliemann J, et al.: Hepatic lipase mediates the uptake of chylomicrons and β-VLDL into cells via the LDL receptor-related protein (LRP). *J Lipid Res* **37**:926, 1996.
206. Huff MW, Miller DB, Wolfe BM, Connelly PW, Sawyez CG: Uptake of hypertriglyceridemic very low density lipoproteins and their remnants by HepG2 cells: The role of lipoprotein lipase, hepatic triglyceride lipase, and cell surface proteoglycans. *J Lipid Res* **38**:1318, 1997.
207. Dichek HL, Brecht W, Fan J, Ji Z-S, McCormick SPA, Akeefe H, Conzo L, et al.: Overexpression of hepatic lipase in transgenic mice decreases apolipoprotein B-containing and high density lipoproteins. Evidence that hepatic lipase acts as a ligand for lipoprotein uptake. *J Biol Chem* **273**:1896, 1998.
208. Diard P, Malewiak M-I, Lagrange D, Griglio S: Hepatic lipase may act as a ligand in the uptake of artificial chylomicron remnant-like particles by isolated rat hepatocytes. *Biochem J* **299**:889, 1994.
209. Kounnas MZ, Chappell DA, Wong H, Argraves WS, Strickland DK: The cellular internalization and degradation of hepatic lipase is mediated by low density lipoprotein receptor-related protein and requires cell surface proteoglycans. *J Biol Chem* **270**:9307, 1995.
210. Eisenberg S, Sehayek E, Olivecrona T, Vlodavsky I: Lipoprotein lipase enhances binding of lipoproteins to heparan sulfate on cell surfaces and extracellular matrix. *J Clin Invest* **90**:2013, 1992.
211. Mulder M, Lombardi P, Jansen H, van Berkel TJC, Frants RR, Havekes LM: Low density lipoprotein receptor internalizes low density and very low density lipoproteins that are bound to heparan sulfate proteoglycans via lipoprotein lipase. *J Biol Chem* **268**:9369, 1993.
212. Williams KJ, Fless GM, Petrie KA, Snyder ML, Brocia RW, Swenson TL: Mechanisms by which lipoprotein lipase alters cellular metabolism of lipoprotein(a), low-density lipoprotein, and nascent lipoproteins. Roles for low-density lipoprotein receptors and heparan sulfate proteoglycans. *J Biol Chem* **267**:13284, 1992.
213. Beisiegel U, Weber W, Bengtsson-Olivecrona G: Lipoprotein lipase enhances the binding of chylomicrons to low-density lipoprotein receptor-related protein. *Proc Natl Acad Sci U S A* **88**:8342, 1991.
214. Chappell DA, Fry GL, Waknitz MA, Muhonen LE, Pladet MW, Iverius P-H, Strickland DK: Lipoprotein lipase induces catabolism of normal triglyceride-rich lipoproteins via the low-density lipoprotein receptor-related protein/α2-macroglobulin receptor in vitro. A process facilitated by cell-surface proteoglycans. *J Biol Chem* **268**:14168, 1993.
215. Chajek-Shaul T, Friedman G, Stein O, Olivecrona T, Stein Y: Binding of lipoprotein lipase to the cell surface is essential for the transmembrane transport of chylomicron cholesteryl ester. *Biochim Biophys Acta* **712**:200, 1982.
216. Choi SY, Fong LG, Kirven MJ, Cooper AD: Use of an anti-low-density lipoprotein receptor antibody to quantify the role of the LDL receptor in the removal of chylomicron remnants in the mouse in vivo. *J Clin Invest* **88**:1173, 1991.
217. Lund H, Takahashi K, Hamilton RL, Havel RJ: Lipoprotein binding and endosomal itinerary of the low-density lipoprotein receptor-related protein in rat liver. *Proc Natl Acad Sci U S A* **86**:9318, 1989.
218. Herz J, Kowal RC, Ho YK, Brown MS, Goldstein JL: Low-density lipoprotein receptor-related protein mediates endocytosis of monoclonal antibodies in cultured cells and rabbit liver. *J Biol Chem* **265**:21355, 1990.
219. Kristensen T, Moestrup SK, Gliemann J, Bendtsen L, Sand O, Sottrup-Jensen L: Evidence that the newly cloned low-density-lipoprotein receptor related protein (LRP) is the α2-macroglobulin receptor. *FEBS Lett* **276**:151, 1990.
220. Strickland DK, Ashcom JD, Williams S, Burgess WH, Migliorini M, Argraves WS: Sequence identity between the α-macroglobulin receptor and low-density lipoprotein receptor-related protein suggests that this molecule is a multifunctional receptor. *J Biol Chem* **265**:17401, 1990.
221. Nykjaer A, Petersen CM, Møller B, Jensen PH, Moestrup SK, Holtet TL, Etzerodt M, et al.: Purified α2-macroglobulin receptor/LDL receptor-related protein binds urokinase · plasminogen activator inhibitor type-1 complex. Evidence that the α2-macroglobulin receptor mediates cellular degradation of urokinase receptor-bound complexes. *J Biol Chem* **267**:14543, 1992.
222. Huettinger M, Retzek H, Hermann M, Goldenberg H: Lactoferrin specifically inhibits endocytosis of chylomicron remnants but not α-macroglobulin. *J Biol Chem* **267**:18551, 1992.
223. Herz J, Clouthier DE, Hammer RE: LDL receptor-related protein internalizes and degrades uPA–PAI-1 complexes and is essential for embryo implantation. *Cell* **71**:411, 1992.
224. van Dijk MCM, Ziere GJ, van Berkel TJC: Characterization of the chylomicron-remnant-recognition sites on parenchymal and Kupffer cells of rat liver. Selective inhibition of parenchymal cell recognition by lactoferrin. *Eur J Biochem* **205**:775, 1992.
225. Willnow TE, Goldstein JL, Orth K, Brown MS, Herz J: Low-density lipoprotein receptor-related protein and gp330 bind similar ligands, including plasminogen activator-inhibitor complexes and lactoferrin, an inhibitor of chylomicron remnant clearance. *J Biol Chem* **267**:26172, 1992.
226. Hussain MM, Maxfield FR, Más-Oliva J, Tabas I, Ji Z-S, Innerarity TL, Mahley RW: Clearance of chylomicron remnants by the low density lipoprotein receptor-related protein/α2-macroglobulin receptor. *J Biol Chem* **266**:13936, 1991.
227. Choi SY, Cooper AD: A comparison of the roles of the low density lipoprotein (LDL) receptor and the LDL receptor-related protein/α2-macroglobulin receptor in chylomicron remnant removal in the mouse *in vivo*. *J Biol Chem* **268**:15804, 1993.
228. Mortimer B-C, Beveridge DJ, Martins IJ, Redgrave TC: Intracellular localization and metabolism of chylomicron remnants in the livers of low density lipoprotein receptor-deficient mice and apoE-deficient mice. Evidence for slow metabolism via an alternative apoE-dependent pathway. *J Biol Chem* **270**:28767, 1995.
229. Willnow TE, Sheng Z, Ishibashi S, Herz J: Inhibition of hepatic chylomicron remnant uptake by gene transfer of a receptor antagonist. *Science* **264**:1471, 1994.
230. Willnow TE, Rohlmann A, Horton J, Otani H, Braun JR, Hammer RE, Herz J: RAP, a specialized chaperone, prevents ligand-induced ER retention and degradation of LDL receptor-related endocytic receptors. *EMBO J* **15**:2632, 1996.
231. Rohlmann A, Gotthardt M, Hammer RE, Herz J: Inducible inactivation of hepatic LRP gene by Cre-mediated recombination confirms role of LRP in clearance of chylomicron remnants. *J Clin Invest* **101**:689, 1998.
232. de Faria E, Fong LG, Komaromy M, Cooper AD: Relative roles of the LDL receptor, the LDL receptor-like protein, and hepatic lipase in chylomicron remnant removal by the liver. *J Lipid Res* **37**:197, 1996.
233. Jong MC, Dahlmans VEH, van Gorp PJJ, van Dijk KW, Breuer ML, Hofker MH: In the absence of the low-density lipoprotein receptor, human apolipoprotein C1 overexpression in transgenic mice inhibits the hepatic uptake of very low density lipoproteins via a receptor-associated protein-sensitive pathway. *J Clin Invest* **98**:2259, 1996.
234. Klagsbrun M, Baird A: A dual receptor system is required for basic fibroblast growth factor activity. *Cell* **67**:229, 1991.
235. Ji Z-S, Pitas RE, Mahley RW: Differential cellular accumulation/retention of apolipoprotein E mediated by cell surface heparan sulfate proteoglycans. Apolipoproteins E3 and E2 greater than E4. *J Biol Chem* **273**:13452, 1998.
236. Fuki IV, Kuhn KM, Lomazov IR, Rothman VL, Tuszynski GP, Iozzo RV, Swenson TL, et al.: The syndecan family of proteoglycans. Novel

receptors mediating internalization of atherogenic lipoproteins in vitro. *J Clin Invest* **100**:1611, 1997.

237. Woollett LA, Osono Y, Herz J, Dietschy JM: Apolipoprotein E competitively inhibits receptor-dependent low density lipoprotein uptake by the liver but has no effect on cholesterol absorption or synthesis in the mouse. *Proc Natl Acad Sci U S A* **92**:12500, 1995.
238. Chait A, Hazzard WR, Albers JJ, Kushwaha RP, Brunzell JD: Impaired very low density lipoprotein and triglyceride removal in broad beta disease: Comparison with endogenous hypertriglyceridemia. *Metabolism* **27**:1055, 1978.
239. Chung BH, Segrest JP: Resistance of a very low density lipoprotein subpopulation from familial dysbetalipoproteinemia to in vitro lipolytic conversion to the low density lipoprotein density fraction. *J Lipid Res* **24**:1148, 1983.
240. Ehnholm C, Mahley RW, Chappell DA, Weisgraber KH, Ludwig E, Witztum JL: Role of apolipoprotein E in the lipolytic conversion of β-very low density lipoproteins to low density lipoproteins in type III hyperlipoproteinemia. *Proc Natl Acad Sci U S A* **81**:5566, 1984.
241. Demant T, Bedford D, Packard CJ, Shepherd J: Influence of apolipoprotein E polymorphism on apolipoprotein B-100 metabolism in normolipemic subjects. *J Clin Invest* **88**:1490, 1991.
242. Thuren T, Weisgraber KH, Sisson P, Waite M: Role of apolipoprotein E in hepatic lipase catalyzed hydrolysis of phospholipid in high-density lipoproteins. *Biochemistry* **31**:2332, 1992.
243. Thuren T, Wilcox RW, Sisson P, Waite M: Hepatic lipase hydrolysis of lipid monolayers. Regulation by apolipoproteins. *J Biol Chem* **266**:4853, 1991.
244. Huang Y, Liu XQ, Rall SC, Jr., Mahley RW: Apolipoprotein E2 reduces the low density lipoprotein level in transgenic mice by impairing lipoprotein lipase-mediated lipolysis of triglyceride-rich lipoproteins. *J Biol Chem* **273**:17483, 1998.
245. Ji Z-S, Fazio S, Mahley RW: Variable heparan sulfate proteoglycan binding of apolipoprotein E variants may modulate the expression of type III hyperlipoproteinemia. *J Biol Chem* **269**:13421, 1994.
246. Mann WA, Meyer N, Weber W, Greten H, Beisiegel U: Apolipoprotein E isoforms and rare mutations: Parallel reduction in binding to cells and to heparin reflects severity of associated type III hyperlipoproteinemia. *J Lipid Res* **36**:517, 1995.
247. Wardell MR, Brennan SO, Janus ED, Fraser R, Carrell RW: Apolipoprotein E2-Christchurch (136 Arg→Ser). New variant of human apolipoprotein E in a patient with type III hyperlipoproteinemia. *J Clin Invest* **80**:483, 1987.
248. Pocovi M, Cenarro A, Civeira F, Myers RH, Casao E, Esteban M, Ordovas JM: Incomplete dominance of type III hyperlipoproteinemia is associated with the rare apolipoprotein E2 (Arg_{136}→Ser) variant in multigenerational pedigree studies. *Atherosclerosis* **122**:33, 1996.
249. Feussner G, Albanese M, Valencia A, Schuster H: Apolipoprotein $E2_{Heidelberg}$ (Arg_{136}→Cys), a new variant of apolipoprotein E associated with incomplete dominance of type III hyperlipoproteinemia. *Atherosclerosis* **109**:261, 1994. (Abstract)
250. Walden CC, Huff MW, Leiter LA, Connelly PW, Hegele RA: Detection of a new apolipoprotein-E mutation in type III hyperlipidemia using deoxyribonucleic acid restriction isotyping. *J Clin Endocrinol Metab* **78**:699, 1994.
251. Feussner G, Albanese M, Mann WA, Valencia A, Schuster H: Apolipoprotein E2 (Arg_{136}→Cys), a variant of apolipoprotein E associated with late-onset dominance of type III hyperlipoproteinaemia. *Eur J Clin Invest* **26**:13, 1996.
252. Richard P, de Zulueta MP, Beucler I, De Gennes J-L, Cassaigne A, Iron A: Identification of a new apolipoprotein E variant (E_2 Arg_{142}→Leu) in type III hyperlipidemia. *Atherosclerosis* **112**:19, 1995.
253. Havel RJ, Kotite L, Kane JP, Tun P, Bersot T: Atypical familial dysbetalipoproteinemia associated with apolipoprotein phenotype E3/3. *J Clin Invest* **72**:379, 1983.
254. Horie Y, Fazio S, Westerlund JR, Weisgraber KH, Rall SC Jr: The functional characteristics of a human apolipoprotein E variant (cysteine at residue 142) may explain its association with dominant expression of type III hyperlipoproteinemia. *J Biol Chem* **267**:1962, 1992.
255. Rall SC, Jr, Newhouse YM, Clarke HRG, Weisgraber KH, McCarthy BJ, Mahley RW, Bersot TP: Type III hyperlipoproteinemia associated with apolipoprotein E phenotype E3/3. Structure and genetics of an apolipoprotein E3 variant. *J Clin Invest* **83**:1095, 1989.
256. Emi M, Wu LL, Robertson MA, Myers RL, Hegele RA, Williams RR, White R, et al.: Genotyping and sequence analysis of apolipoprotein E isoforms. *Genomics* **3**:373, 1988.
257. Lohse P, Mann WA, Stein EA, Brewer HB, Jr: Apolipoprotein E-$4_{Philadelphia}$ (Glu^{13}→Lys, Arg^{145}→Cys). Homozygosity for two rare point mutations in the apolipoprotein E gene combined with severe type III hyperlipoproteinemia. *J Biol Chem* **266**:10479, 1991.
258. Lohse P, Rader DJ, Brewer HB Jr: Heterozygosity for apolipoprotein E-$4_{Philadelphia}$ (Glu^{13}→Lys, Arg^{145}→ Cys) is associated with incomplete dominance of type III hyperlipoproteinemia. *J Biol Chem* **267**:13642, 1992.
259. de Villiers WJS, van der Westhuyzen DR, Coetzee GA, Henderson HE, Marais AD: The apolipoprotein E2 (Arg145Cys) mutation causes autosomal dominant type III hyperlipoproteinemia with incomplete penetrance. *Arterioscler Thromb Vasc Biol* **17**:865, 1997.
260. Rall SC Jr, Weisgraber KH, Innerarity TL, Bersot TP, Mahley RW, Blum CB: Identification of a new structural variant of human apolipoprotein E, E2(Lys_{146}→Gln), in a type III hyperlipoproteinemic subject with the E3/2 phenotype. *J Clin Invest* **72**:1288, 1983.
261. Smit M, de Knijff P, van der Kooij-Meijs E, Groenendijk C, van den Maagdenberg AMJM, Gevers Leuven JA, Stalenhoef AFH, et al.: Genetic heterogeneity in familial dysbetalipoproteinemia. The E2(lys_{146}→gln) variant results in a dominant mode of inheritance. *J Lipid Res* **31**:45, 1990.
262. de Knijff P, van den Maagdenberg AMJM, Boomsma DI, Stalenhoef AFH, Smelt AHM, Kastelein JJP, Marais AD, et al.: Variable expression of familial dysbetalipoproteinemia in apolipoprotein E*2(Lys_{146}→Gln) allele carriers. *J Clin Invest* **94**:1252, 1994.
263. Mulder M, van der Boom H, de Knijff P, Braam C, van den Maagdenberg A, Gevers Leuven JA, Havekes LM: Triglyceride-rich lipoproteins of subjects heterozygous for apolipoprotein E2(Lys_{146}→Gln) are inefficiently converted to cholesterol-rich lipoproteins. *Atherosclerosis* **108**:183, 1994.
264. Mann WA, Gregg RE, Sprecher DL, Brewer HB Jr: Apolipoprotein E-$1_{Harrisburg}$: A new variant of apolipoprotein E dominantly associated with type III hyperlipoproteinemia. *Biochim Biophys Acta* **1005**:239, 1989.
265. Moriyama K, Sasaki J, Matsunaga A, Arakawa F, Takada Y, Araki K, Kaneko S, et al.: Apolipoprotein E1 Lys-146 →Glu with type III hyperlipoproteinemia. *Biochim Biophys Acta* **1128**:58, 1992.
266. Mann WA, Lohse P, Gregg RE, Ronan R, Hoeg JM, Zech LA, Brewer HB Jr: Dominant expression of type III hyperlipoproteinemia. Pathophysiological insights derived from the structural and kinetic characteristics of apoE-1(Lys^{146}→Glu). *J Clin Invest* **96**:1100, 1995.
267. Hoffer MJV, Niththyananthan S, Naoumova RP, Kibirige MS, Frants RR, Havekes LM, Thompson GR: Apolipoprotein E1-Hammersmith (Lys146→Asn;Arg147→Trp), due to a dinucleotide substitution, is associated with early manifestation of dominant type III hyperlipoproteinaemia. *Atherosclerosis* **124**:183, 1996.
268. de Knijff P, van den Maagdenberg AMJM, Stalenhoef AFH, Leuven JAG, Demacker PNM, Kuyt LP, Frants RR, et al.: Familial dysbetalipoproteinemia associated with apolipoprotein E3-Leiden in an extended multigeneration pedigree. *J Clin Invest* **88**:643, 1991.
269. Wardell MR, Weisgraber KH, Havekes LM, Rall SC Jr: Apolipoprotein E3-Leiden contains a seven-amino acid insertion that is a tandem repeat of residues 121–127. *J Biol Chem* **264**:21205, 1989.
270. Fazio S, Horie Y, Weisgraber KH, Havekes LM, Rall SC, Jr: Preferential association of apolipoprotein E Leiden with very low density lipoproteins of human plasma. *J Lipid Res* **34**:447, 1993.
271. Hazzard WR, Warnick GR, Utermann G, Albers JJ: Genetic transmission of isoapolipoprotein E phenotypes in a large kindred: Relationship to dysbetalipoproteinemia and hyperlipidemia. *Metabolism* **30**:79, 1981.
272. Feussner G, Piesch S, Dobmeyer J, Fischer C: Genetics of type III hyperlipoproteinemia. *Genet Epidemiol* **14**:283, 1997.
273. Hopkins PN, Wu LL, Schumacher MC, Emi M, Hegele RM, Hunt SC, Lalouel J-M, et al: Type III dyslipoproteinemia in patients heterozygous for familial hypercholesterolemia and apolipoprotein E2. Evidence for a gene-gene interaction. *Arterioscler Thromb* **11**:1137, 1991.
274. Sakuma N, Iwata S, Ikeuchi R, Ichikawa T, Hibino T, Kamiya Y, Ohte N, et al.: Coexisting type III hyperlipoproteinemia and familial hypercholesterolemia: A case report. *Metabolism* **44**:460, 1995.
275. Zhang H, Reymer PWA, Liu M-S, Forsythe IJ, Groenemeyer BE, Frohlich J, Brunzell JD, et al.: Patients with apoE3 deficiency (E2/2, E3/2, and E4/2) who manifest with hyperlipidemia have increased frequency of an Asn 291→Ser mutation in the human LPL gene. *Arterioscler Thromb Vasc Biol* **15**:1695, 1995.

276. Huang Y, Rall SC Jr, Mahley RW: Genetic factors precipitating type III hyperlipoproteinemia in hypolipidemic transgenic mice expressing human apolipoprotein E2. *Arterioscler Thromb Vasc Biol* **17**:2817, 1997.
277. Hazzard WR, Bierman EL: Aggravation of broad-β disease (type 3 hyperlipoproteinemia) by hypothyroidism. *Arch Intern Med* **130**:822, 1972.
278. Feussner G, Ziegler R: Expression of type III hyperlipoproteinaemia in a subject with secondary hypothyroidism bearing the apolipoprotein E2/2 phenotype. *J Intern Med* **230**:183, 1991.
279. Angelin B, Raviola CA, Innerarity TL, Mahley RW: Regulation of hepatic lipoprotein receptors in the dog. Rapid regulation of apolipoprotein B,E receptors, but not of apolipoprotein E receptors, by intestinal lipoproteins and bile acids. *J Clin Invest* **71**:816, 1983.
280. Myant NB: *Cholesterol Metabolism, LDL, and the LDL Receptor*. San Diego, Academic Press, 1990.
281. Mahley RW, Hui DY, Innerarity TL, Weisgraber KH: Two independent lipoprotein receptors on hepatic membranes of dog, swine, and man. Apo-B,E and apo-E receptors. *J Clin Invest* **68**:1197, 1981.
282. Falko JM, Schonfeld G, Witztum JL, Kolar J, Weidman SW: Effects of estrogen therapy on apolipoprotein E in type III hyperlipoproteinemia. *Metabolism* **28**:1171, 1979.
283. Kushwaha RS, Hazzard WR, Gagne C, Chait A, Albers JJ: Type III hyperlipoproteinemia: Paradoxical hypolipidemic response to estrogen. *Ann Intern Med* **87**:517, 1977.
284. Chao Y-S, Windler EE, Chen GC, Havel RJ: Hepatic catabolism of rat and human lipoproteins in rats treated with 17α-ethinyl estradiol. *J Biol Chem* **254**:11360, 1979.
285. Kovanen PT, Brown MS, Goldstein JL: Increased binding of low-density lipoprotein to liver membranes from rats treated with 17α-ethinyl estradiol. *J Biol Chem* **254**:11367, 1979.
286. Windler EET, Kovanen PT, Chao Y-S, Brown MS, Havel RJ, Goldstein JL: The estradiol-stimulated lipoprotein receptor of rat liver. A binding site that mediates the uptake of rat lipoproteins containing apoproteins B and E. *J Biol Chem* **255**:10464, 1980.
287. Thompson GR, Soutar AK, Spengel FA, Jadhav A, Gavigan SJP, Myant NB: Defects of receptor-mediated low density lipoprotein catabolism in homozygous familial hypercholesterolemia and hypothyroidism *in vivo*. *Proc Natl Acad Sci U S A* **78**:2591, 1981.
288. Grundy SM: Cholesterol metabolism in man. *West J Med* **128**:13, 1978.
289. Angelin B, Einarsson K: Regulation of HMG-CoA reductase in human liver, in Preiss B (ed): *Regulation of HMG-CoA Reductase*. Orlando, FL, Academic Press, 1985, p 281.
290. Myant NB: *The Biology of Cholesterol and Related Steroids*. London, William Heinemann Medical Books, 1981.
291. Chait A, Albers JJ, Brunzell JD: Very low density lipoprotein overproduction in genetic forms of hypertriglyceridaemia. *Eur J Clin Invest* **10**:17, 1980.
292. Tall A, Granot E, Brocia R, Tabas I, Hesler C, Williams K, Denke M: Accelerated transfer of cholesteryl esters in dyslipidemic plasma. Role of cholesteryl ester transfer protein. *J Clin Invest* **79**:1217, 1987.
293. McPherson R, Mann CJ, Tall AR, Hogue M, Martin L, Milne RW, Marcel YL: Plasma concentrations of cholesteryl ester transfer protein in hyperlipoproteinemia. Relation to cholesteryl ester transfer protein activity and other lipoprotein variables. *Arterioscler Thromb* **11**:797, 1991.
294. Yamashita S, Hui DY, Sprecher DL, Matsuzawa Y, Sakai N, Tarui S, Kaplan D, et al.: Total deficiency of plasma cholesteryl ester transfer protein in subjects homozygous and heterozygous for the intron 14 splicing defect. *Biochem Biophys Res Commun* **170**:1346, 1990.
295. Brown ML, Inazu A, Hesler CB, Agellon LB, Mann C, Whitlock ME, Marcel YL, et al.: Molecular basis of lipid transfer protein deficiency in a family with increased high-density lipoproteins. *Nature* **342**:448, 1989.
296. de Knijff P, van den Maagdenberg AMJM, Frants RR, Havekes LM: Genetic heterogeneity of apolipoprotein E and its influence on plasma lipid and lipoprotein levels. *Hum Mutat* **4**:178, 1994.
297. van den Maagdenberg AMJM, de Knijff P, Stalenhoef AFH, Gevers Leuven JA, Havekes LM, Frants RR: Apolipoprotein E*3-Leiden allele results from a partial gene duplication in exon 4. *Biochem Biophys Res Commun* **165**:851, 1989.
298. Chappell DA: High receptor-binding affinity of lipoproteins in atypical dysbetalipoproteinemia (type III hyperlipoproteinemia). *J Clin Invest* **84**:1906, 1989.
299. Hui DY, Innerarity TL, Mahley RW: Defective hepatic lipoprotein receptor binding of β-very low density lipoproteins from type III hyperlipoproteinemic patients. Importance of apolipoprotein E. *J Biol Chem* **259**:860, 1984.
300. Utermann G: Apolipoprotein E (role in lipoprotein metabolism and pathophysiology of hyperlipoproteinemia type III). *La Ricerca Clin Lab* **12**:23, 1982.
301. Brown MS, Goldstein JL: Lipoprotein metabolism in the macrophage: Implications for cholesterol deposition in atherosclerosis. *Annu Rev Biochem* **52**:223, 1983.
302. Brown MS, Goldstein JL: How LDL receptors influence cholesterol and atherosclerosis. *Sci Am* **251**:58, 1984.
303. Mahley RW, Innerarity TL, Rall SC Jr, Weisgraber KH: Lipoproteins of special significance in atherosclerosis. Insights provided by studies of type III hyperlipoproteinemia. *Ann N Y Acad Sci* **454**:209, 1985.
304. Mahley RW: Atherogenic hyperlipoproteinemia. The cellular and molecular biology of plasma lipoproteins altered by dietary fat and cholesterol. *Med Clin North Am* **66**:375, 1982.
305. Van Lenten BJ, Fogelman AM, Hokom MM, Benson L, Haberland ME, Edwards PA: Regulation of the uptake and degradation of β-very low density lipoprotein in human monocyte macrophages. *J Biol Chem* **258**:5151, 1983.
306. Koo C, Wernette-Hammond ME, Innerarity TL: Uptake of canine β-very low density lipoproteins by mouse peritoneal macrophages is mediated by a low-density lipoprotein receptor. *J Biol Chem* **261**:11194, 1986.
307. Ellsworth JL, Kraemer FB, Cooper AD: Transport of β-very low density lipoproteins and chylomicron remnants by macrophages is mediated by the low-density lipoprotein receptor pathway. *J Biol Chem* **262**:2316, 1987.
308. Koo C, Wernette-Hammond ME, Garcia Z, Malloy MJ, Uauy R, East C, Bilheimer DW, et al.: Uptake of cholesterol-rich remnant lipoproteins by human monocyte-derived macrophages is mediated by low-density lipoprotein receptors. *J Clin Invest* **81**:1332, 1988.
309. Innerarity TL, Arnold KS, Weisgraber KH, Mahley RW: Apolipoprotein E is the determinant that mediates the receptor uptake of β-very low density lipoproteins by mouse macrophages. *Arteriosclerosis* **6**:114, 1986.
310. Whitman SC, Miller DB, Wolfe BM, Hegele RA, Huff MW: Uptake of type III hypertriglyceridemic VLDL by macrophages is enhanced by oxidation, especially after remnant formation. *Arterioscler Thromb Vasc Biol* **17**:1707, 1997.
311. Gordon V, Innerarity TL, Mahley RW: Formation of cholesterol- and apoprotein E-enriched high density lipoproteins in vitro. *J Biol Chem* **258**:6202, 1983.
312. Koo C, Innerarity TL, Mahley RW: Obligatory role of cholesterol and apolipoprotein E in the formation of large cholesterol-enriched and receptor-active high density lipoproteins. *J Biol Chem* **260**:11934, 1985.
313. Mahley RW, Weisgraber KH, Innerarity T: Canine lipoproteins and atherosclerosis. II. Characterization of the plasma lipoproteins associated with atherogenic and nonatherogenic hyperlipidemia. *Circ Res* **35**:722, 1974.
314. Glomset JA: The plasma lecithin:cholesterol acyltransferase reaction. *J Lipid Res* **9**:155, 1968.
315. Kashyap VS, Santamarina-Fojo S, Brown DR, Parrott CL, Applebaum-Bowden D, Meyn S, Talley G, et al.: Apolipoprotein E deficiency in mice: Gene replacement and prevention of atherosclerosis using adenovirus vectors. *J Clin Invest* **96**:1612, 1995.
316. Mortimer B-C, Redgrave TG, Spangler EA, Verstuyft JG, Rubin EM: Effect of human apoE4 on the clearance of chylomicron-like lipid emulsions and atherogenesis in transgenic mice. *Arterioscler Thromb* **14**:1542, 1994.
317. Shimano H, Ohsuga J, Shimada M, Namba Y, Gotoda T, Harada K, Katsuki M, et al.: Inhibition of diet-induced atheroma formation in transgenic mice expressing apolipoprotein E in the arterial wall. *J Clin Invest* **95**:469, 1995.
318. Fazio S, Sanan DA, Lee Y-L, Ji Z-S, Mahley RW, Rall SC Jr: Susceptibility to diet-induced atherosclerosis in transgenic mice expressing a dysfunctional human apolipoprotein E(Arg 112,Cys142). *Arterioscler Thromb Vasc Biol* **14**:1873, 1994.
319. van Vlijmen BJM, van den Maagdenberg AMJM, Gijbels MJJ, van der Boom H, HogenEsch H, Frants RR, Hofker MH, et al.: Diet-induced hyperlipoproteinemia and atherosclerosis in apolipoprotein E3-Leiden transgenic mice. *J Clin Invest* **93**:1403, 1994.
320. Nakashima Y, Plump AS, Raines EW, Breslow JL, Ross R: ApoE-deficient mice develop lesions of all phases of atherosclerosis throughout the arterial tree. *Arterioscler Thromb* **14**:133, 1994.

321. Reddick RL, Zhang SH, Maeda N: Atherosclerosis in mice lacking apo E. Evaluation of lesional development and progression. *Arterioscler Thromb* **14**:141, 1994.
322. Breslow JL, Plump A, Dammerman M: New mouse models of lipoprotein disorders and atherosclerosis, in Fuster V, Ross R, Topol EJ (eds): *Atherosclerosis and Coronary Artery Disease.* Vol. 1, Philadelphia, Lippincott-Raven, 1996, p 363.
323. Linton MF, Atkinson JB, Fazio S: Prevention of atherosclerosis in apolipoprotein E-deficient mice by bone marrow transplantation. *Science* **267**:1034, 1995.
324. Boisvert WA, Spangenberg J, Curtiss LK: Treatment of severe hypercholesterolemia in apolipoprotein E-deficient mice by bone marrow transplantation. *J Clin Invest* **96**:1118, 1995.
325. Fazio S, Babaev VR, Murray AB, Hasty AH, Carter KJ, Gleaves LA, Atkinson JB, et al.: Increased atherosclerosis in mice reconstituted with apolipoprotein E null macrophages. *Proc Natl Acad Sci U S A* **94**:4647, 1997.
326. Bellosta S, Mahley RW, Sanan DA, Murata J, Newland DL, Taylor JM, Pitas RE: Macrophage-specific expression of human apolipoprotein E reduces atherosclerosis in hypercholesterolemic apolipoprotein E-null mice. *J Clin Invest* **96**:2170, 1995.
327. Menzel H-J, Utermann G: Apolipoprotein E phenotyping from serum by Western blotting. *Electrophoresis* **7**:492, 1986.
328. Hixson JE, Vernier DT: Restriction isotyping of human apolipoprotein E by gene amplification and cleavage with *Hha*I. *J Lipid Res* **31**:545, 1990.
329. Gotto AM Jr, Jones PH, Scott LW: The diagnosis and management of hyperlipidemia. *Dis Mon* **32**:245, 1986.
330. Schaefer EJ, Levy RI: Pathogenesis and management of lipoprotein disorders. *N Engl J Med* **312**:1300, 1985.
331. Schaefer EJ (discussant): Type III hyperlipoproteinemia: Diagnosis, molecular defects, pathology, and treatment. Dietary and drug treatment. *Ann Intern Med* **98**:633, 1983.
332. Falko JM, Witztum JL, Schonfeld G, Weidman SW, Kolar JB: Type III hyperlipoproteinemia. Rise in high-density lipoprotein levels in response to therapy. *Am J Med* **66**:303, 1979.
333. Grundy SM: Hypertriglyceridemia: Mechanisms, clinical significance, and treatment. *Med Clin North Am* **66**:519, 1982.
334. Levy RI, Fredrickson DS, Shulman R, Bilheimer DW, Breslow JL, Stone NJ, Lux SE, et al.: Dietary and drug treatment of primary hyperlipoproteinemia. *Ann Intern Med* **77**:267, 1972.
335. Hoogwerf BJ, Bantle JP, Kuba K, Frantz ID Jr, Hunninghake DB: Treatment of type III hyperlipoproteinemia with four different treatment regimens. *Atherosclerosis* **51**:251, 1984.
336. Hoogwerf BJ, Peters JR, Frantz ID Jr, Hunninghake DB: Effect of clofibrate and colestipol singly and in combination on plasma lipids and lipoproteins in type III hyperlipoproteinemia. *Metabolism* **34**:978, 1985.
337. Connor WE, Connor SL: The dietary treatment of hyperlipidemia. Rationale, technique and efficacy. *Med Clin North Am* **66**:485, 1982.
338. American Heart Association: Counseling the Patient with Hyperlipidemia (No. 70-061-A). Dallas, American Heart Association, 1984.
339. Dallongeville J, Boulet L, Davignon J, Lussier-Cacan S: Fish oil supplementation reduces β-very low density lipoprotein in type III dysbetalipoproteinemia. *Arterioscler Thromb* **11**:864, 1991.
340. Choice of cholesterol-lowering drugs. *Med Lett Drugs Ther* **35**:19, 1993.
341. Prihoda JS, Illingworth DR: Drug therapy of hyperlipidemia. *Curr Probl Cardiol* **17**:545, 1992.
342. Illingworth DR: Management of hyperlipidemia: Goals for the prevention of atherosclerosis. *Clin Invest Med* **13**:211, 1990.
343. Grundy SM, Mok HYI, Zech L, Berman M: Influence of nicotinic acid on metabolism of cholesterol and triglycerides in man. *J Lipid Res* **22**:24, 1981.
344. Drood JM, Zimetbaum PJ, Frishman WH: Nicotinic acid for the treatment of hyperlipoproteinemia. *J Clin Pharmacol* **31**:641, 1991.
345. Committee of Principal Investigators: W.H.O. cooperative trial on primary prevention of ischaemic heart disease using clofibrate to lower serum cholesterol: Mortality follow-up. *Lancet* **2**:379, 1980.
346. Stone NJ: Lipid management: Current diet and drug treatment options. *Am J Med* 101(Suppl. 4A):40S, 1996.
347. Larsen ML, Illingworth DR, O'Malley JP: Comparative effects of gemfibrozil and clofibrate in type III hyperlipoproteinemia. *Atherosclerosis* **106**:235, 1994.
348. Mulder M, Smelt AHM, Zhao SP, Frants RR, Havekes LM: Treatment of E2E2 homozygous familial dysbetalipoproteinemic subjects with gemfibrozil does not enhance the binding of their $d < 1.019$ lipoprotein fraction to the low-density lipoprotein receptor. *Metabolism* **42**:327, 1993.
349. Lussier-Cacan S, Bard J-M, Boulet L, Nestruck AC, Grothé A-M, Fruchart J-C, Davignon J: Lipoprotein composition changes induced by fenofibrate in dysbetalipoproteinemia type III. *Atherosclerosis* **78**:167, 1989.
350. Kovanen PT, Bilheimer DW, Goldstein JL, Jaramillo JJ, Brown MS: Regulatory role for hepatic low-density lipoprotein receptors in vivo in the dog. *Proc Natl Acad Sci U S A* **78**:1194, 1981.
351. Bilheimer DW, Grundy SM, Brown MS, Goldstein JL: Mevinolin and colestipol stimulate receptor-mediated clearance of low-density lipoprotein from plasma in familial hypercholesterolemia heterozygotes. *Proc Natl Acad Sci U S A* **80**:4124, 1983.
352. Endo A, Kuroda M, Tsujita Y: ML-236A, ML-236B, and ML-236C, new inhibitors of cholesterogenesis produced by *Penicillium citrinum*. *J Antibiot* **29**:1346, 1976.
353. Illingworth DR, Sexton GJ: Hypocholesterolemic effects of mevinolin in patients with heterozygous familial hypercholesterolemia. *J Clin Invest* **74**:1972, 1984.
354. Gylling H, Relas H, Miettinen TA: Postprandial vitamin A and squalene clearances and cholesterol synthesis off and on lovastatin treatment in type III hyperlipoproteinemia. *Atherosclerosis* **115**:17, 1995.
355. Vega GL, East C, Grundy SM: Lovastatin therapy in familial dysbetalipoproteinemia: Effects on kinetics of apolipoprotein B. *Atherosclerosis* **70**:131, 1988.
356. Illingworth DR, O'Malley JP: The hypolipidemic effects of lovastatin and clofibrate alone and in combination in patients with type III hyperlipoproteinemia. *Metabolism* **39**:403, 1990.
357. Stuyt PMJ, Mol MJTM, Stalenhoef AFH: Long-term effects of simvastatin in familial dysbetalipoproteinaemia. *J Intern Med* **230**:151, 1991.
358. Feussner G, Eichinger M, Ziegler R: The influence of simvastatin alone or in combination with gemfibrozil on plasma lipids and lipoproteins in patients with type III hyperlipoproteinemia. *Clin Investig* **70**:1027, 1992.
359. Wiklund O, Angelin B, Bergman M, Berglund L, Bondjers G, Carlsson A, Lindén T, et al.: Pravastatin and gemfibrozil alone and in combination for the treatment of hypercholesterolemia. *Am J Med* **94**:13, 1993.
360. Zelis R, Mason DT, Braunwald E, Levy RI: Effects of hyperlipoproteinemias and their treatment on the peripheral circulation. *J Clin Invest* **49**:1007, 1970.
361. Kuo PT, Wilson AC, Kostis JB, Moreyra AB, Dodge HT: Treatment of type III hyperlipoproteinemia with gemfibrozil to retard progression of coronary artery disease. *Am Heart J* 116:85, 1988.

CHAPTER 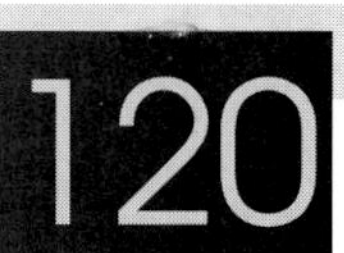

Familial Hypercholesterolemia

Joseph L. Goldstein ▪ Helen H. Hobbs ▪ Michael S. Brown

1. Familial hypercholesterolemia (FH) is characterized clinically by (a) an elevated concentration of LDL, the major cholesterol-transport lipoprotein in human plasma; (b) deposition of LDL-derived cholesterol in tendons and skin (xanthomas) and in arteries (atheromas); and (c) inheritance as an autosomal dominant trait with a gene dosage effect—that is, homozygotes are more severely affected than are heterozygotes.

2. Heterozygotes number about 1 in 500 persons, placing FH among the most common inborn errors of metabolism. Heterozygotes have twofold elevations in plasma cholesterol (350 to 550 mg/dl) from birth. Tendon xanthomas and coronary atherosclerosis develop after ages 20 and 30, respectively.

3. Homozygotes number 1 in 1 million persons. They have severe hypercholesterolemia (650 to 1000 mg/dl). Cutaneous xanthomas appear within the first 4 years of life. Coronary heart disease begins in childhood and frequently causes death from myocardial infarction before age 20.

4. The primary defect in FH is a mutation in the gene specifying the receptor for plasma LDL. Located on the surfaces of cells in the liver and other organs, the LDL receptor binds LDL and facilitates its uptake by receptor-mediated endocytosis and its delivery to lysosomes, where the LDL is degraded and its cholesterol is released for metabolic use. When LDL receptors are deficient, the rate of removal of LDL from plasma declines, and the level of LDL rises in inverse proportion to the receptor number. The excess plasma LDL is deposited in scavenger cells and other cell types, which produces xanthomas and atheromas.

5. The LDL receptor gene is on the short arm of chromosome 19. It comprises 18 exons that span 45 kb. The gene encodes a single-chain glycoprotein that contains 839 amino acids in its mature form. Five classes of mutations at the LDL receptor locus have been identified based on phenotypic behavior of the mutant proteins. Each class has been subdivided into multiple alleles through molecular characterization. More than 420 different mutant alleles distort receptor function in meaningful ways. Class 1 alleles fail to produce an immunoprecipitable protein (null alleles). Class 2 alleles, the most common, encode proteins blocked in intracellular transport between the ER and the Golgi complex (transport-defective alleles). Class 3 alleles encode proteins that are transported to the cell surface, but fail to bind LDL normally (binding-defective alleles). Class 4 alleles, the rarest, encode proteins that reach the cell surface and bind LDL normally, but fail to cluster in coated pits and hence do not internalize bound LDL (internalization-defective alleles). Class 5 alleles encode receptors that bind and internalize LDL in coated pits, but cannot discharge the LDL in the endosome and thus fail to recycle to the cell surface (recycling-defective alleles).

6. FH heterozygotes have one normal allele and one mutant allele at the LDL receptor locus; hence, their cells are able to bind and take up LDL at approximately half the normal rate. Phenotypic homozygotes possess two mutant alleles at the LDL receptor locus; hence, their cells show a total or near-total inability to bind or take up LDL. Some phenotypic homozygotes inherit two identical alleles, whereas others inherit two different mutant alleles and are thus compound heterozygotes. Prenatal diagnosis of receptor-negative homozygotes can be performed by quantitative assays of LDL receptor activity in cultured amniotic fluid cells as well as by direct DNA analysis of the molecular defect. The large number of LDL receptor gene mutations precludes the use of DNA analysis for diagnosis of heterozygotes except in selected populations of the world in which the incidence of a particular mutant allele is high, as in French Canada, Finland, Iceland, Christian Lebanon, and South Africa.

7. Treatment for heterozygotes and homozygotes is directed at lowering the plasma level of LDL. In heterozygotes, the most effective therapy is the administration of a class of drugs called statins, which are inhibitors of 3-hydroxy-3-methylglutaryl CoA reductase. By reducing hepatic cholesterol synthesis, these drugs enhance LDL receptor activity in the liver, which, in turn, increases LDL catabolism and decreases LDL-cholesterol production. Homozygotes with two nonfunctional genes are relatively resistant to drugs that work by stimulating LDL receptors. Their plasma LDLlevels can be effectively lowered by physical or surgical means. Effective treatment in heterozygotes and homozygotes can lead to a reduced rate of progression, and, in some cases, an actual regression of coronary atherosclerosis.

Familial hypercholesterolemia (FH) results from a mutation that affects the structure and function of a cell-surface receptor that normally removes LDL from plasma. The disorder is characterized clinically by a lifelong elevation in the concentration of LDL-bound cholesterol in blood, leading to premature coronary heart disease; pathologically by cholesterol deposits that form xanthomas, arcus corneae, and coronary atherosclerotic plaques; and genetically by autosomal dominant inheritance. FH was the first genetic disorder recognized to cause myocardial infarction.[1,2] To

A list of standard abbreviations is located immediately preceding the index in each volume. Additional abbreviations used in this chapter include: ACAT = acyl-coenzyme A: cholesterol acyltransferase; FDB = familial defective apo B-100; FH = familial hypercholesterolemia; HMG-CoA = 3-hydroxy-3-methylglutaryl coenzyme A; IDL = intermediate-density lipoproteins; LRP = LDL receptor-related protein; Lp(a) = lipoprotein(a); SREBP = sterol regulatory element binding protein; SCAP = SREBP cleavage-activating protein; SRE-1 = sterol regulatory element = 1; WHHL rabbit = Watanabe-heritable hyperlipidemic rabbit.

this day, it remains the most cogent illustration of the causal relation between high blood-cholesterol levels and coronary atherosclerosis.

But beyond its traditional place among diseases of lipid metabolism, FH has acquired importance as a prototype for a class of diseases caused by defects in cell-surface receptor molecules.[3] Discovered more recently than enzymes, receptors are more difficult to study experimentally because they are membrane glycoproteins that reside in a hydrophobic environment and resist standard purification. Important advances in understanding cell-surface receptors are now emerging from analysis of naturally occurring mutations that disrupt their function in human diseases. The LDL receptor is the most extensively studied receptor genetically in that more than 420 mutant alleles have been characterized in different FH patients. Many of these mutations disrupt receptor function in discrete ways that reveal much about the relation between receptor structure and function.

Patients with FH manifest two distinct syndromes, depending on whether the mutant LDL receptor gene is present in the heterozygous or homozygous form. Heterozygotes occur in the population at a frequency of about 1 in 500, placing FH among the most common monogenic diseases in humans. As expected, homozygotes, who inherit two mutant genes at the LDL receptor locus, are much less numerous, occurring with a prevalence of 1 in 1 million. Homozygotes exhibit a syndrome that is more severe than the disease seen in heterozygotes. Homozygotes can inherit two identical mutant genes (true homozygotes) or two different mutant genes (compound heterozygotes). In this chapter, FH homozygotes refers to individuals who have two mutant genes at the LDL receptor locus, whether they are identical or not.

FH is only one of several disorders included in the designation "familial type 2 hyperlipoproteinemia." The simple finding of an elevated LDL cholesterol level, even in an individual with a family history of hypercholesterolemia, does not ensure that this individual has FH. Confirmation of the diagnosis requires either the demonstration of a decrease in LDL receptor activity, the documentation of a mutation in the LDL receptor gene, or the presence of ancillary clinical findings such as tendon xanthomas, autosomal dominant transmission, and expression in childhood.

HISTORICAL ASPECTS

The association of xanthomas in tendons and atheromas in arteries was repeatedly described before 1900.[4] In the 1930s, Müller[1,2] and Thannhauser[5,6] recognized the familial clustering of patients exhibiting xanthomas, premature coronary artery disease, and hypercholesterolemia. Their suggestions of a genetic basis for hypercholesterolemia were substantiated in the 1940s and 1950s by the family studies of Wilkinson et al.,[7] Adlersberg et al.,[8,9] and others.[10–15] Understanding of the genetics was greatly advanced by the extensive observations of Khachadurian, whose studies in Lebanon in the early 1960s delineated the differences between heterozygotes and homozygotes,[16] thereby providing the first unequivocal evidence for the single-gene inheritance of this disorder.

Using analytical ultracentrifugation, in the mid-1950s, Gofman and coworkers showed that the hypercholesterolemia in FH was due to a selective increase in the plasma concentration of one lipoprotein, which is now designated LDL.[17,18] In the 1960s, Fredrickson, Levy, and Lees advanced the concept that FH is a disorder involving the metabolism of both the apoprotein and cholesterol components of LDL.[19] Using cultured fibroblasts from homozygotes to define the basic biochemical defect, Brown and Goldstein, in the 1970s, discovered the cell-surface LDL receptor and demonstrated that FH is caused by mutations in the gene specifying this receptor.[3,20] Subsequent developments led to the purification of the LDL receptor protein in 1982, the cloning of its cDNA in 1983, and the isolation and characterization of its gene in 1985. These advances laid the groundwork for the molecular analysis of the mutations underlying FH. The two most recent developments relate to (a) the crystallization of the ligand binding module of the receptor,[21] and (b) the discovery of the molecular basis for the feedback regulation of LDL receptors, involving the sterol-regulated proteolytic cleavage of membrane-bound transcription factors called sterol regulatory element binding proteins (SREBPs).[22]

CLINICAL FEATURES

Data on the natural history of heterozygous FH have been derived from measurements of the frequency of clinical findings in affected relatives of different ages from large families (Fig. 120-1).[12,13,23,24] The earliest manifestation is hypercholesterolemia, which is present at birth in most affected subjects[25] and remains the only clinical finding throughout the first decade.[26] Arcus corneae and tendon xanthomas appear at the end of the second decade, and by the third decade each is present in about half of all heterozygotes. By the time of death, 80 percent of heterozygotes have xanthomas.[24] Clinical symptoms of coronary heart disease appear in the fourth decade.

The clinical picture in homozygotes is remarkably uniform and distinctly different from that in heterozygotes.[16,27–29] Marked hypercholesterolemia, present at birth, persists throughout life. Unique yellow-orange cutaneous xanthomas, frequently present at birth, develop in almost all homozygotes by age 4.[27–29] Tendon xanthomas, arcus corneae, and generalized atherosclerosis inevitably develop in homozygotes during childhood. Death from myocardial infarction typically occurs before age 30.[27–29] In addition to atherosclerosis of the coronary vessels, xanthomatous infiltration of the aortic valve develops in homozygotes, which produces a picture that is hemodynamically indistinguishable from rheumatic or calcific aortic stenosis.[16,30,31]

Blood Lipids and Lipoproteins

The mean plasma-cholesterol level in large groups of FH heterozygotes is remarkably constant, averaging about 350 mg/dl in various adult populations.[24,27,28,32] Despite this uniformity in mean values, the cholesterol levels in individual patients, even within the same family, may vary as much as twofold. In homozygotes, the plasma cholesterol concentration is uniformly higher than in heterozygotes, ranging from 600 to 1200 mg/dl.[27–29]

Cholesterol esters, which normally make up 70 to 75 percent of the total plasma cholesterol, form a similar proportion in both

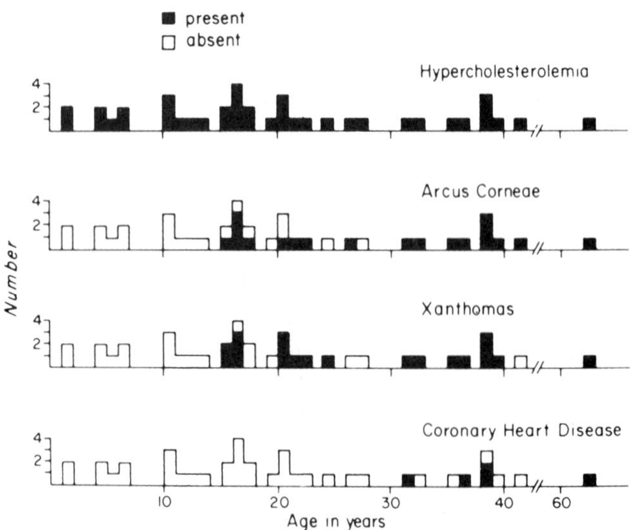

Fig. 120-1 Prevalence of clinical manifestations at different ages in the affected heterozygotes from a single large family with FH. ***(Data redrawn from Schrott et al.[24] by permission of*** **Annals of Internal Medicine.)**

Table 120-1 **Plasma Lipids and Lipoproteins in Familial Hypercholesterolemia**

Genotype	Age, Years	Number of Patients	Plasma Cholesterol, mg/dl				Plasma Triglyceride, mg/dl
			Total	VLDL	LDL	HDL	
Normal	1–19	128	175±28	13±8	110±25	53±13	60±25
Heterozygotes	1–19	105	299±63	15±11	241±60	43±12	82±51
Homozygotes	1–19	10	678±170	19±8	625±160	34±10	101±51
Normal	≥20	76	194±34	16±10	123±31	53±16	83±31
Heterozygotes	≥20	88	368±78	27±17	298±78	44±13	148±75

NOTE: Mean±1 SD.
SOURCE: From Kwiterovich et al.,[26] by permission of the *Journal of Clinical Investigation.*

heterozygotes and homozygotes. Total plasma phospholipids are elevated slightly in heterozygotes and more strikingly in homozygotes.[33] The mean plasma triglyceride concentration is not significantly different from that of the general population (Table 120-1).[24,26,28] In homozygotes, the level of plasma triglycerides may be slightly elevated, but many patients have values in the normal range.[27–29] Occasionally, a heterozygote or a homozygote with documented FH has a plasma triglyceride level of more than 250 mg/dl, which may relate to the function of the LDL receptor in removing remnants of triglyceride-carrying VLDL and intermediate-density lipoproteins (IDL) from the circulation (discussed below).

The excess cholesterol in the plasma of heterozygotes and homozygotes is found entirely in the lipoprotein fraction of density 1.006 to 1.063 g/ml, which includes IDL and LDL.[17,18,28] The mean LDL cholesterol concentration in heterozygotes at all ages is two to three times the mean of normal subjects of similar age. The mean LDL cholesterol concentration in homozygotes is about two to three times that of heterozygotes and about six times that of normal subjects (see Table 120-1). LDL particles are increased in number in the plasma of patients with FH. Most of the particles have normal lipid and protein content, amino acid composition, density, and immunochemical reactivity.[34–36] Some LDL particles show a small decrease in triglyceride content,[33,37] a small difference in hydrated density,[38] and a slight increase in the ratio of cholesterol to phospholipid.[36] It is likely that these slight changes represent minor secondary alterations that result from prolonged circulation of the lipoprotein due to the LDL receptor defect.[36] The minor structural changes do not affect the metabolism of the LDL particles. Thus, when LDL from an FH homozygote was injected into the circulation of a normal subject, the LDL was metabolized normally.[39] Moreover, LDL from homozygotes binds to LDL receptors[40] and suppresses 3-hydroxy-3-methylglutaryl coenzyme A (HMG-CoA) reductase activity[41] in normal fibroblasts in the same manner as LDL from normal subjects.

The HDL cholesterol levels in FH patients are slightly lower, on average, than in normal subjects.[26,42,43] This decrease is seen in heterozygotes, as well as in homozygotes, at all ages (see Table 120-1). The mechanism of this reduction in HDL is not known.

Xanthomas

LDL-derived cholesterol deposits in several tissues of FH patients, especially in skin and tendons (xanthomas) and in arterial plaques (atheromas). The rate of deposition is proportional to the severity and duration of the elevation in LDL, but local trauma and unknown factors, including possible genetic factors, also play a role.[16,28,44] Vergopoulos et al.[44] described a consanguineous Syrian FH family in which some affected heterozygotes and homozygotes have massive xanthomas, whereas others (with the same receptor mutation) have much smaller skin lesions, raising the possibility of a major xanthomatosis-susceptibility gene distinct from the LDL receptor gene.

The types of xanthomas seen in FH are illustrated in Figs. 120-2*A* to *K* and 120-3*A* to *H*. Homozygotes and heterozygotes both may have tendon xanthomas (especially in the Achilles tendons and in the extensor tendons of the hand) (Fig. 120-2*F* to *H*), subcutaneous tuberous xanthomas (especially over the elbows), and subperiosteal xanthomas (commonly below the knee and over the olecranon process) (Fig. 120-2*D*,*E*). Palpebral xanthomas (xanthelasmas) occur commonly in heterozygotes (Fig. 120-2*A*, *B*), but are rare in homozygotes. Xanthelasmas are not specific for FH and can occur in subjects with normal lipid levels.[17,18] The frequency of xanthomas in heterozygotes as a function of age is shown in Table 120-2. These data illustrate the long lag period in heterozygotes before xanthomas appear.

Elevated orange-yellow planar cutaneous xanthomas lying superficially over the extremities, buttocks, and hands (especially in the interdigital web between the first and second fingers) (Fig. 120-3*B,C,E,F*) are unique to FH homozygotes.[27–29] Xanthomas of the tongue and the buccal mucosa occur occasionally in homozygotes.

Patients with cerebrotendinous xanthomatosis, an extremely rare autosomal recessive disorder, may have tendon xanthomas that are indistinguishable from those in FH. Other clinical features, such as cataracts, mental deterioration, and normal plasma-LDL-cholesterol levels, are sufficient to distinguish these patients from FH heterozygotes (Chap. 123). Tendon xanthomas also occur in some patients with phytosterolemia (Chap. 123), familial defective apo B-100 (Chap. 115), an autosomal recessive form of hypercholesterolemia (discussed below), and in a small proportion of individuals with type 3 hyperlipoproteinemia (Chap. 119).

Arcus Corneae

Arcus corneae (Fig. 120-2*B*) appears in about 10 percent of heterozygotes before 30 years of age and is present in about 50 percent of heterozygotes over age 30.[28] It usually occurs before age 10 in homozygotes (Fig. 120-3*A*). Like xanthelasmas, arcus corneae can also be observed in subjects with normal lipid levels.[17,18] Arcus corneae is particularly frequent in healthy black subjects.[45]

Premature Atherosclerosis

In homozygotes, cardiac atherosclerosis involving the supravalvular aorta and the coronary arteries is rapidly progressive, leading to angina pectoris, myocardial infarction, or sudden death before age 30.[27–29,46,47] One homozygote experienced an acute myocardial infarction at 18 months of age,[28] and another died suddenly at age 3 with coronary atherosclerosis at autopsy.[48] Severe atherosclerosis also occurs in the thoracic and abdominal aorta and in the major pulmonary arteries,[16,46,47] but the cerebral vessels are relatively spared.[49] Few homozygotes with a total loss of receptor function survive past age 30.[29,47]

The frequency of deaths attributable to coronary heart disease among homozygotes varies inversely with the number of functional LDL receptors as measured in cultured fibroblasts (Fig. 120-4). Homozygotes can be divided into three broad groups according to the amount of functional LDL receptor activity detected in their cultured fibroblasts. Coronary deaths occurred most frequently and at an earlier age in homozygotes in whom

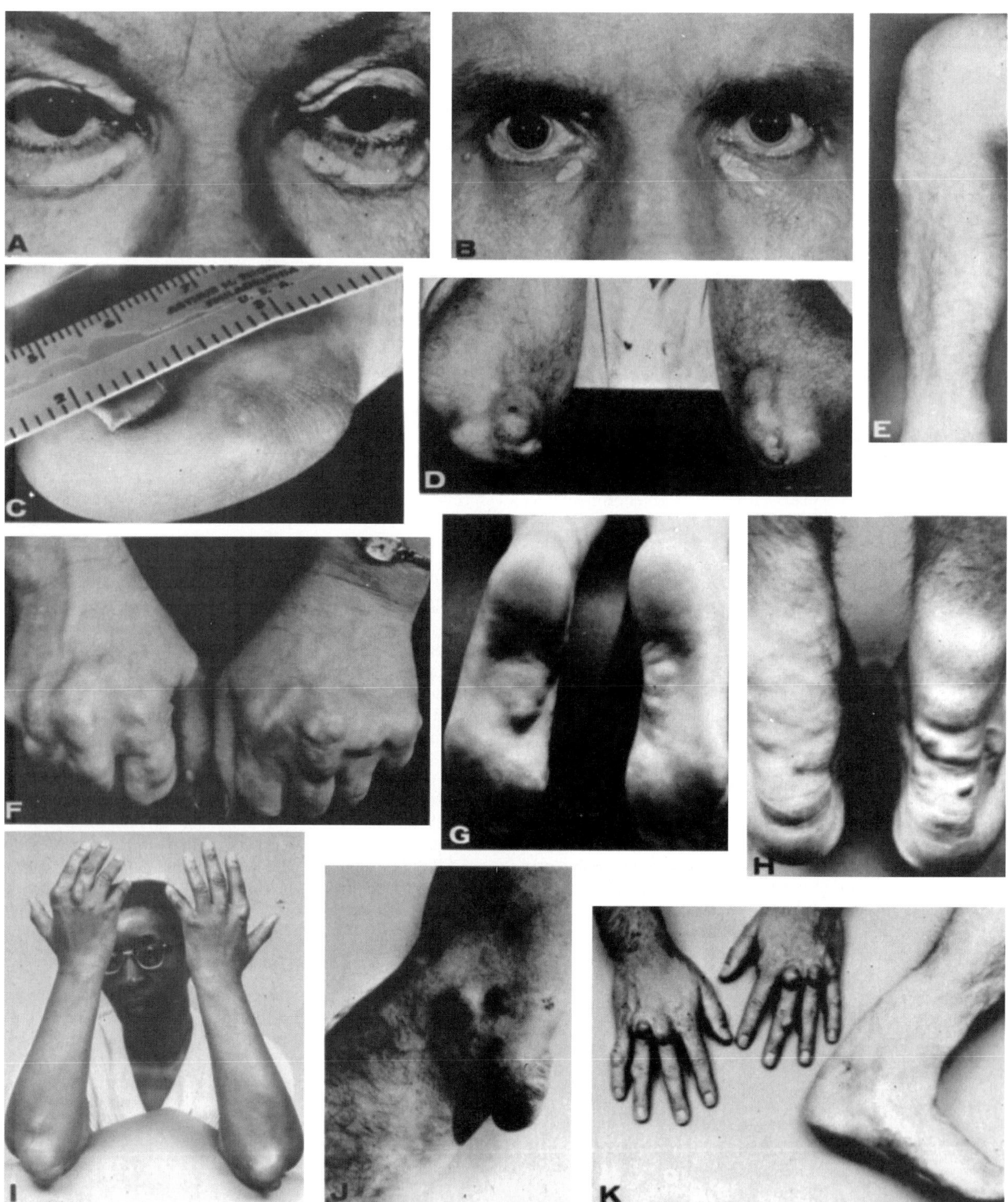

Fig. 120-2 Forms of xanthomas and other lipid deposits frequently seen in FH heterozygotes. *A.* Xanthelasmas. *B.* Arcus corneae and xanthelasmas. *E.* Subperiosteal xanthoma over tibial tuberosity. Others in *C, D,* and *F* through *K* are either tendon xanthomas or a combination of tendon and tuberous xanthomas.

receptor activity was less than 2 percent of normal. In a group of 54 such homozygotes, 17 percent died before age 15 and 19 percent died after age 15. Fewer deaths were seen in the group of 52 homozygotes with 2 to 10 percent of receptor activity in which 7 and 15 percent died before and after age 15, respectively. The most striking finding was in the group of 43 homozygotes with more than 10 percent receptor activity in which no deaths occurred before age 15, and only 2 deaths occurred after age 15 (5 percent of group).

The level of plasma LDL also appears to be higher in the subjects whose cells produce no detectable LDL receptors. Sprecher et al.[50] related the levels of LDL receptor activity in fibroblasts to the pretreatment levels of plasma LDL cholesterol in 13 FH homozygotes. Receptor activity ranged from 2 to 29 percent of normal with LDL cholesterol ranging from 304 to 874 mg/dl. The two parameters were inversely correlated with an r value of -0.89.[50] These data suggest that the earlier onset of symptomatic coronary disease and coronary deaths in FH homozygotes with

Table 120-2 Frequency of Xanthomas as a Function of Age in Heterozygotes with Familial Hypercholesterolemia

Age, Years	Number of Heterozygotes	Percentage with Xanthomas
1–9	38	2.6
10–19	32	12.5
20–29	13	69.2
30–39	30	90.0
40–59	29	70.3

SOURCE: From Kwiterovich et al.,[26] by permission of the *Journal of Clinical Investigation.*

negligible LDL receptor activity is likely due to their higher plasma LDL cholesterol levels.

Both the duration and severity of hypercholesterolemia correlate with the development of atherosclerosis. Hoeg and colleagues[51] determined the total cholesterol-year score (mg-year/dl) by taking the sum of the annual plasma cholesterol levels in 17 FH homozygotes (ages 1 to 17). The cholesterol-year scores, which ranged from 2170 to 32,260 mg-year/dl, correlated with the amount of total body calcific atherosclerosis ($r = 0.77$), as estimated by electron beam tomography. A direct relationship was also seen between the cholesterol-year score and the size of the Achilles tendons, as quantified by computed tomography ($r = 0.81$). Cholesterol-year score was a better predictor of these two variables than age.

In some FH homozygotes, xanthomas form on the endocardial surfaces of the mitral valve.[31,46,47] These may produce findings of mitral regurgitation and mitral stenosis.[46,52] Inasmuch as FH homozygotes may have painful joints,[53] an elevated sedimentation rate,[54] and cardiac murmurs, a misdiagnosis of acute rheumatic fever may be made.[53]

The pattern of cardiac disease in the heterozygote is much more variable than in the homozygote. In Denmark, the prevalence of coronary heart disease among heterozygotes with FH (32 percent) was 25 times greater than among unaffected relatives (1.3 percent).[55] Table 120-3 shows the percentage of heterozygotes who exhibit symptoms of coronary artery disease or death from myocardial infarction at different ages. These values were compiled from 5 large studies involving more than 1000 heterozygotes.[55–59] Women with FH suffer clinical coronary artery disease later than affected men. Thus, in England, Slack found that the mean age of onset of coronary artery disease was 43 years for men and 53 years for women.[56] Among heterozygous men, the risk of a myocardial infarction was 5 percent by age 30, 51 percent by age 50, and 85 percent by age 60. For women the risks at comparable ages were 0, 12, and 58 percent. In Norway, the mean age at death for male and female heterozygotes was 55 and 64 years, respectively.[57]

In the United States, Stone et al.[58] found that the cumulative probability of coronary heart disease in male heterozygotes was 16 percent at age 40 and 52 percent at age 60. In female heterozygotes, the cumulative risk was 32.8 percent by age 60 as compared with only 9.1 percent in unaffected females. Earlier death from coronary artery disease in male heterozygotes (54 years) as compared with female heterozygotes (68 years) was reported in Japan.[60] Interestingly, this sex difference, which is also a characteristic feature of the usual form of normolipidemic atherosclerotic heart disease, does not seem to be operative in homozygotes (see also Fig. 120-4).[46]

Sudhir et al.[61] carried out quantitative coronary angiography in 141 FH heterozygotes (mean age, 43 years) who had no previous history or concurrent symptoms of coronary heart disease. In addition to the expected finding of generalized coronary stenosis (average number of lesions was 5.8 with a mean diameter stenosis of 34 percent), an increased prevalence of coronary ectasia was found. An ectatic segment was defined as one with a luminal diameter > 1.5 times that of the adjacent normal segment. Fifteen percent of the FH heterozygotes had localized or diffuse ectasia of one or more of the coronary arteries. This prevalence of ectasia was sixfold higher than that observed in the coronary arteries of age and sex-matched non-FH patients whose angiograms showed a more severe degree of coronary sclerosis (average number of lesions was 6.2 with a mean diameter stenosis of 57 percent).

A study from Vancouver, Canada involving 208 female and 156 male FH heterozygotes assessed the influence of environmental and genetic factors on the clinical expression of coronary disease.[62] In men, a higher risk was seen in those heterozygotes who smoked (1.8 times increase) and those with HDL cholesterol levels in the lower quartile (2.4 times increase). In women, a higher risk was associated with hypertension (2.9 times increase). This study and a study from Quebec[63] revealed a significant increase in coronary disease in female (but not male) heterozygotes with elevated plasma triglyceride levels. In the study from Quebec, the odds ratio for coronary disease was 3.9 in female heterozygotes with elevated plasma VLDL cholesterol levels. In a study from the Netherlands, FH heterozygotes who were also heterozygous for a polymorphism in lipoprotein lipase (N291S) had lower plasma HDL cholesterol and higher triglyceride levels, which may increase their risk of coronary artery disease.[64]

Analysis of the plasma apo E polymorphism showed no statistically significant difference in the frequency of the *E-2, E-3,* and *E-4* alleles between FH heterozygotes and the control population, regarding either plasma LDL cholesterol levels or coronary disease.[62,63]

One potential factor affecting the incidence of myocardial infarctions in FH heterozygotes may be the plasma level of lipoprotein(a) [Lp(a)], which consists of an LDL particle that bears an additional protein, apo(a), attached by a disulfide bond to the apo B-100 component. Plasma Lp(a) levels vary over a thousandfold range among individuals, and individuals with high Lp(a) levels have an increased risk of myocardial infarction. A review of Lp(a) is given in Chap. 116.

It remains controversial as to whether FH is associated with elevated plasma levels of Lp(a). Although LDL receptors have the capacity to bind and take up Lp(a) in transgenic mice that overexpress receptors in the liver,[65] endogenous LDL receptors appear to play a minor role in the clearance of Lp(a) from the circulation of humans. Rader et al.[66] found the rate of removal of Lp(a) from the plasma of FH homozygotes to be identical to that of controls. Furthermore, administration of HMG-CoA reductase inhibitors, which increase LDL receptor activity, does not lower plasma levels of Lp(a).[67] Rhesus monkeys heterozygous for a mutation in the LDL receptor gene that reduces LDL receptor activity by 50 percent and elevates plasma LDL levels, do not manifest higher Lp(a) levels.[68] Studies comparing plasma Lp(a) levels in FH heterozygotes who were ascertained in lipid clinics versus age- and sex-matched controls, consistently find higher plasma levels of Lp(a) in the FH cohort.[69,70] If high plasma levels of Lp(a) predispose to coronary artery disease, then these studies are potentially flawed by selection bias. Plasma Lp(a) levels in unrelated individuals with the same LDL receptor mutation are higher[71] or the same as[72] a group of non-FH relatives. Moreover, comparisons of Lp(a) levels between FH heterozygotes and unaffected individuals within the same family revealed no significant differences in most,[73–76] but not all, studies.[77]

In the one positive study done by Lingenhel et al.,[77] plasma levels of Lp(a) were compared in FH heterozygotes and non-FH sibs who inherited the same apo(a) alleles from their parents. Inasmuch as the apo(a) gene itself is the major determinant of plasma Lp(a) levels,[78] the independent effect of an LDL receptor mutation can best be evaluated by comparing individuals who inherit identical Lp(a) alleles. No significant difference in plasma Lp(a) levels was seen in 16 Afrikaner sib pairs with apo(a) alleles identical by descent. In contrast, in 10 French Canadian sib pairs, the FH heterozygotes had significantly higher plasma levels of Lp(a) than their unaffected sibs. In view of these inconsistent

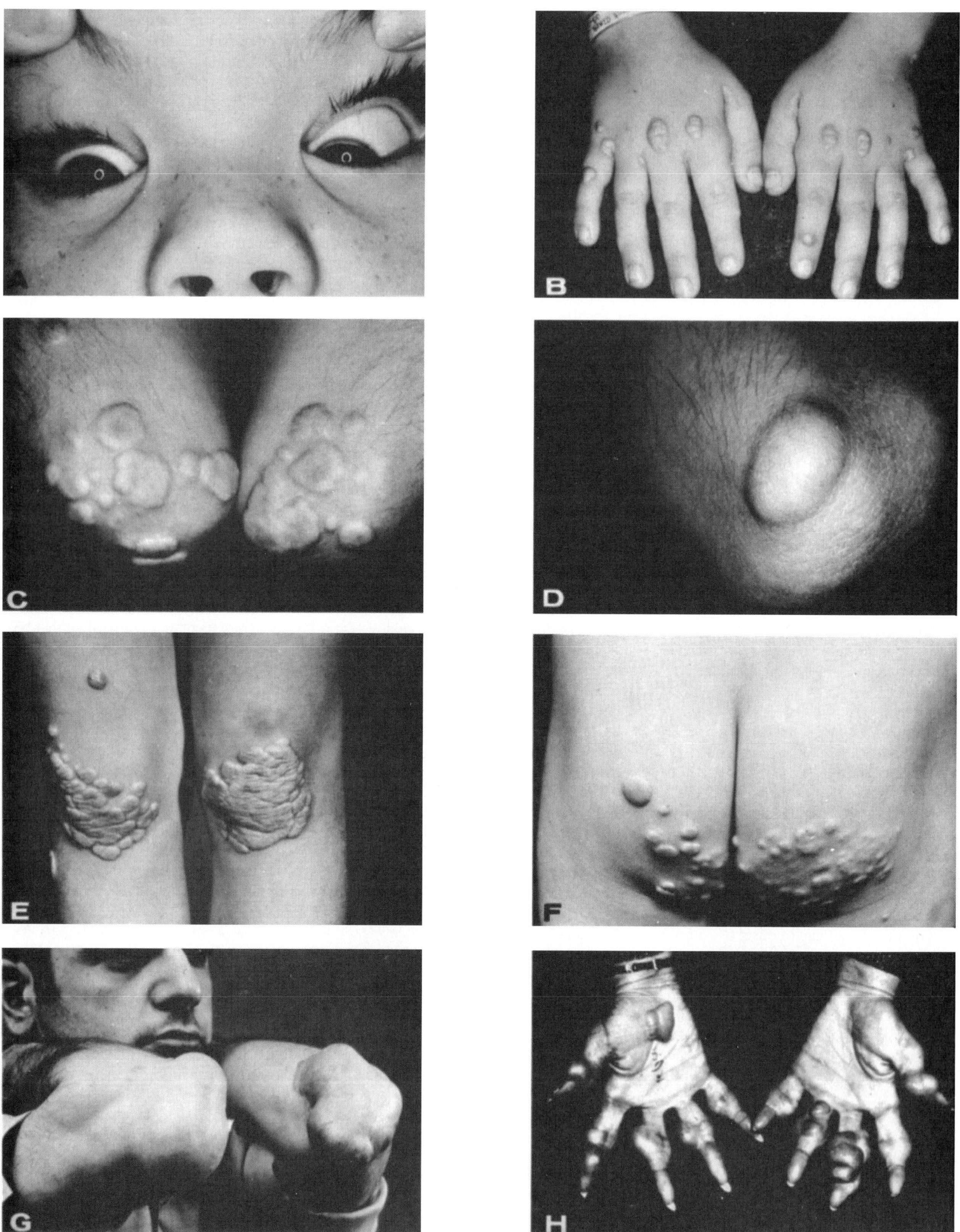

Fig. 120-3 Forms of xanthomas and other lipid deposits frequently seen in FH homozygotes. *A.* Arcus corneae. *B, C, E,* and *F.* Cutaneous planar xanthomas, which usually have a bright orange hue. *C* and *D.* Tuberous xanthomas on the elbows. *H.* Tendon and tuberous xanthomas. (*Panel H reproduced through the courtesy of Dr. A. Khachadurian.*)

results in a well-designed genetic study, it seems unlikely that LDL receptor mutations exert a major influence on the concentration of plasma Lp(a) in FH heterozygotes.

Multiple studies of individuals in the general population have found a synergistic effect of high plasma levels of LDL and Lp(a) on the development of coronary artery disease.[79,80] Thus, high Lp(a) levels might be expected to increase the risk of heart disease in subjects with FH. In two studies, the mean plasma level of Lp(a) was threefold higher in FH heterozygotes with coronary heart disease than in those without the disease,[81,82] but this has not been

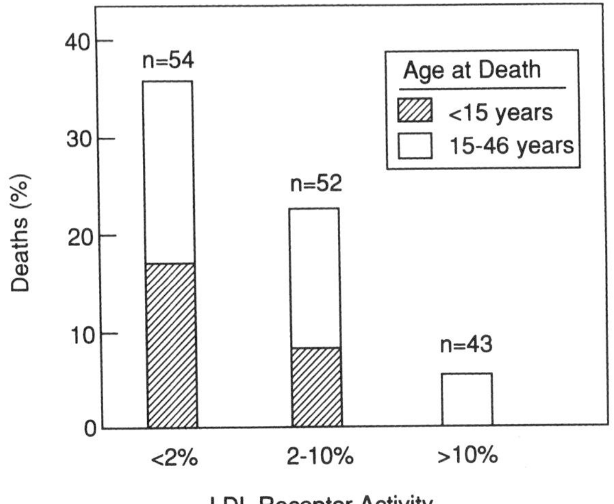

Fig. 120-4 Frequency of deaths at different ages in 149 FH homozygotes with LDL receptor activity of less than 2 percent of normal (n = 54), 2 to 10 percent of normal (n = 52), and >10 percent of normal (n = 43). Receptor activity was measured in cultured fibroblasts in Dallas. The causes of death in the deceased homozygotes were all related to coronary heart disease (i.e., sudden death, myocardial infarction, or acute aortic insufficiency) except for one individual with less than 2 percent receptor activity who died of malignant melanoma at age 32. Clinical information was obtained in 1992 from referring physicians who answered questionnaires.

a universal finding.[63,70,72,83] In one of these studies, the plasma levels of Lp(a) in FH heterozygotes with coronary disease were compared to age- and sex-matched FH heterozygotes without symptomatic disease, and no increase was found.[83] These conflicting results will only be settled by a large prospective study comparing the incidence of myocardial infarction in FH heterozygotes with high and low plasma Lp(a) levels.

An increased frequency of hypertension and of premature cerebrovascular disease is not observed in heterozygotes.[28] Peripheral vascular disease probably does occur at a slightly increased frequency in FH,[28] although it is considerably less prevalent than coronary heart disease. Symptomatic atherosclerosis of peripheral vessels is much more common in patients with familial type 3 hyperlipoproteinemia than in heterozygotes with FH (Chap. 119).

Polyarthritis and Tendinitis

Heterozygotes can have recurrent attacks of polyarthritis and tenosynovitis, especially in the ankles, knees, wrists, and proximal interphalangeal joints.[53,84] In one study, 40 percent of adult heterozygotes had at least one episode of articular pain.[84] Achilles pain or tendinitis occurred in 29 percent, oligoarticular arthritis in 7 percent, and polyarticular or rheumatic fever-like arthritis in 4 percent.[84] Although the joints may be painful and inflamed, fever, leukocytosis, and elevated sedimentation may not always be present in heterozygotes. The typical attack begins quickly, with joint symptoms becoming maximal within 24 h of onset. The signs and symptoms usually persist for 3 to 12 days, after which a complete resolution occurs. Anti-inflammatory drugs do not seem to influence the course of these attacks.[85] In heterozygotes, the joint attacks do not progress to articular damage or deformity.

Homozygotes can have acute joint attacks as well as joint deformities. One homozygote had flexor contractures of the fingers due to tendon and joint xanthomas and required hand surgery for correction.[86] The sedimentation rate and fibrinogen level in homozygotes may be elevated two- to fourfold, even in the absence of joint symptoms.[54] These elevations are presumably related to the high plasma LDL levels.

Table 120-3 Estimated Risk, in Percents, of Heterozygotes Having Symptoms of Coronary Heart Disease and Dying of Myocardial Infarction at Different Ages

	Male Heterozygotes		Female Heterozygotes	
Age	Coronary Symptoms	Coronary Death	Coronary Symptoms	Coronary Death
40 years	20	—	3	0
50 years	45	25	20	2
60 years	75	50	45	15
70 years	—	80	75	30

NOTE: These estimates were compiled from the data of Slack,[56] Jensen et al.,[55] Heiberg,[57] Stone et al.,[58] and Beaumont et al.[59]

GENETIC ASPECTS

Mode of Inheritance

FH is transmitted as a simple autosomal dominant trait.[87] The distribution of plasma cholesterol values in one large family, the Aleutian family reported by Schrott et al.,[24] is shown in Fig. 120-5, and the pedigree is shown in Fig. 120-6.

The first proof that severely affected young individuals are homozygotes rather than severely affected heterozygotes came from the studies of Khachadurian in Lebanon.[16,29] He studied 49 young individuals with juvenile xanthomatosis and rapidly developing atherosclerosis. Their mean cholesterol level (740 mg/dl) was approximately twice that of their heterozygous parents, which, in turn, was twofold greater than that of normal Lebanese control subjects (Fig. 120-7). The frequency of consanguinity among the parents of the apparent homozygotes (58 percent) was much higher than the frequency of consanguinity in the general Lebanese population (10 percent).

In addition to the 49 Lebanese homozygotes, more than 300 other homozygotes from at least 200 families throughout the world have been identified[43,46,47,88,89] (and see below). In virtually all cases, these children were offspring of two clinically identifiable heterozygotes.

Clinical Expression of the FH Gene

When either the plasma total cholesterol or LDL cholesterol level is used as a genetic marker, the FH gene is highly penetrant at all ages.[12,13,23,24] Thus, more than 95 percent of persons carrying the mutant gene have a plasma cholesterol value greater than the 95th percentile value of the population. The LDL cholesterol level appears to be a slightly better marker for the mutant gene than is the total plasma cholesterol level.[26] As discussed below, neither of these elevations is specific for FH.

Inasmuch as symptoms of heterozygous FH do not usually appear until after the childbearing years, the gene does not reduce reproductive fitness.[87] Although homozygotes rarely reproduce, one 36-year-old Japanese woman who is homozygous for a null allele (*FH Niigata*) has successfully delivered four children.[90] The longest-lived biochemically documented homozygote reported to date is a 57-year-old Japanese man who fathered one son.[91] His skin fibroblasts showed normal receptor binding of LDL, but no internalization of the lipoprotein. Angina pectoris was first noted at age 52. The second longest-lived homozygote is also Japanese, a 50-year-old male whose fibroblasts synthesized no immunoprecipitable LDL receptors.[92] Despite his longevity, angina pectoris developed at age 20, and he suffered myocardial infarctions at ages 38, 42, and 48.

Population Prevalence

The prevalence of heterozygotes with FH among patients with coronary heart disease was determined by family analysis of hyperlipidemic survivors of myocardial infarction. The data, collected by three groups of investigators, yielded remarkably

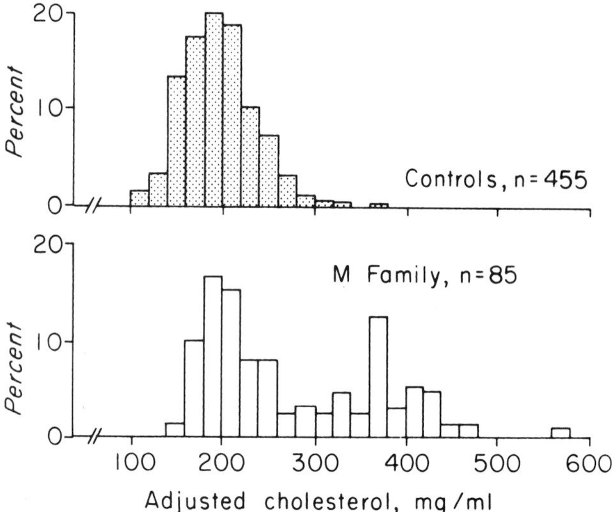

Fig. 120-5 Comparison of the distribution of age- and sex-adjusted total plasma cholesterol levels in control subjects (upper histogram) and in members of a single large family with FH. (*From Schrott et al.*[24] *by permission of* Annals of Internal Medicine.)

similar estimates. Three percent of 193 survivors in London,[93] 4 percent of 366 survivors in Seattle,[94] and 6 percent of 101 survivors in Helsinki[95] appeared to have the heterozygous form of FH.

Among the general population, Goldstein et al.[94] estimated a minimal heterozygote frequency among Caucasians of 1 in 500 with a range of 1 in 200 to 1 in 1000. This figure is in reasonably close agreement with the estimate of Carter, Slack, and Myant, who used the prevalence of homozygotes in London (about 10 in 10 million persons) to derive a heterozygote frequency of about 1 in 200 persons.[96] A revised estimate by Slack, which was based on the Hardy-Weinberg equation and on the identification of seven living homozygotes in England and Wales, suggests a heterozygote frequency of 1 in 500.[97] Similar population frequencies for heterozygotes have been reported from Norway,[98] Denmark,[99] and Japan.[88,100]

A remarkably high prevalence of FH has been noted in three areas of the world. In Lebanon, the estimated prevalence of homozygotes and heterozygotes is 1 in 10,000 and 1 in 171, respectively.[97] In the Quebec province of Canada, the frequency of heterozygotes is 1 in 270 among French Canadians.[101] In South Africa, two populations have a high frequency of FH: the Afrikaners with a heterozygote frequency of 1 in 100,[102] and the Ashkenazi Jews with a frequency of 1 in 67,[103] which is the highest of any population in the world. The molecular basis for the LDL mutations in these populations is discussed below.

Families with FH have been reported from most countries throughout the world. If the disorder is as frequent in other countries as it appears to be in America, Europe, and Japan, it is one of the two most common human diseases caused by a single-gene mutation, the other being hemochromatosis (see Chap. 127).

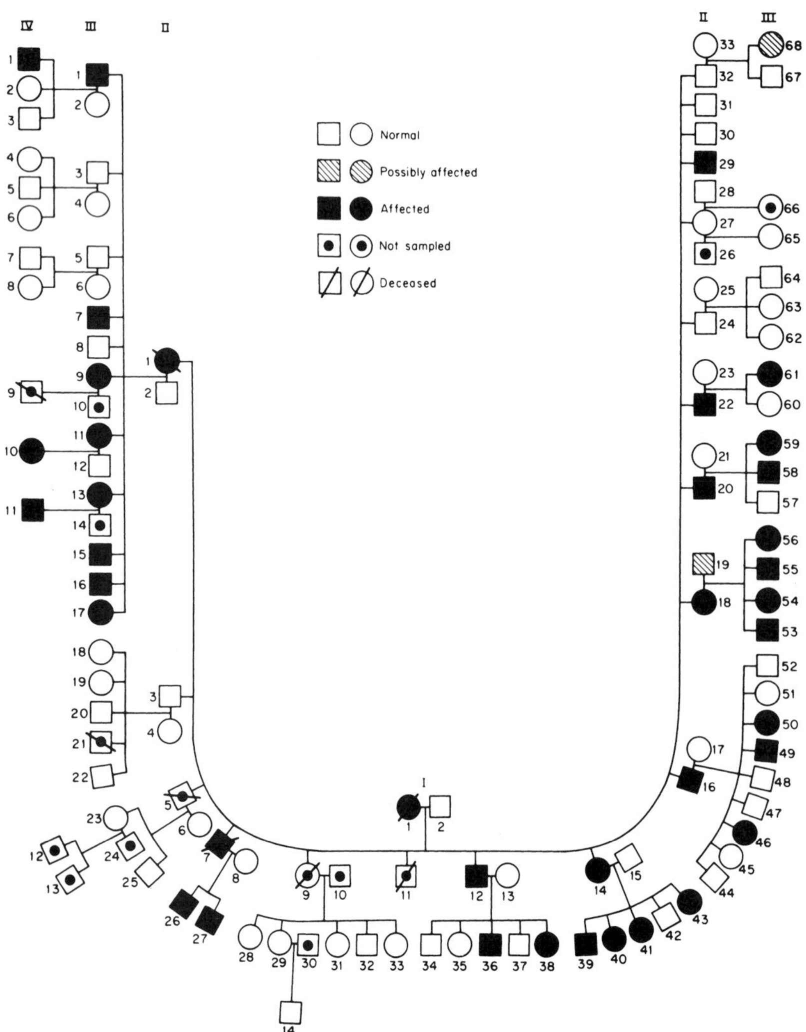

Fig. 120-6 Pedigree of a family with FH. All affected persons are heterozygotes. I-1, II-1, and II-7 each had hypercholesterolemia and tendon xanthomas and died as a result of coronary heart disease. (*From Schrott et al.*[24] *by permission of* Annals of Internal Medicine.)

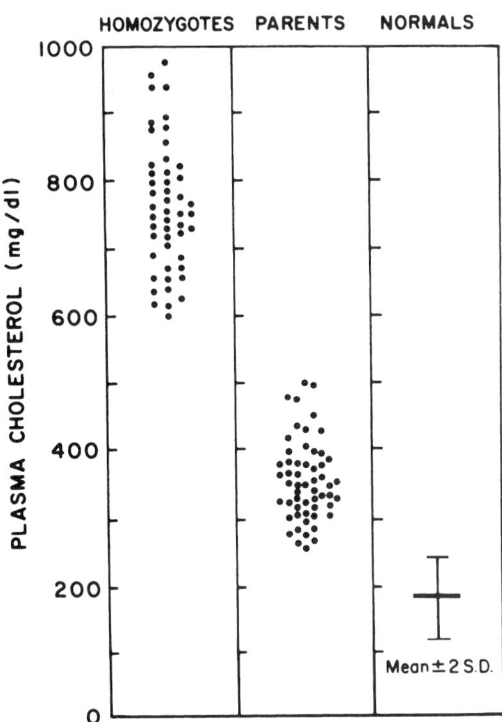

Fig. 120-7 Distribution of total plasma cholesterol levels in 49 FH homozygotes, their parents (obligate heterozygotes), and normal controls. (*Data redrawn from Khachadurian.*[27,29])

PATHOLOGIC ASPECTS

Buja et al.[89] performed extensive pathologic studies of an aborted 20-week-old fetus and three children with homozygous FH and reviewed the pathologic findings in 21 other homozygotes. These data are summarized in Table 33-5 in Chap. 33 of the fifth edition of *The Metabolic Basis of Inherited Disease*.[104] Investigators at the National Institutes of Health have reported additional pathologic findings in four FH homozygotes.[47] Only limited pathologic data are available for heterozygotes.[105]

Initial Pathologic Manifestations: Autopsy Findings in a Homozygous Fetus

Cultured amniotic fluid cells from a woman bearing a fetus at risk for homozygous FH were shown to lack LDL receptors.[106] An autopsy was performed after therapeutic abortion at 20 weeks of gestation.[89] Cord-blood cholesterol in the homozygous fetus was 279 mg/dl, as compared with an average of 31 mg/dl in control fetuses of similar gestational age.[106] The esterified cholesterol content of the thymus was four times that of one control fetus (0.51 mg sterol per g of tissue versus 0.12 mg sterol per g), and the esterified cholesterol content of most other tissues was 1.5 times higher than normal. One small focus of intimal lipid accumulation was found in the aorta and coronary arteries (Fig. 120-8*A*). Multifocal lipid deposition of a mild degree was observed in stromal macrophages in the thymus, spleen (Fig. 120-8*B,C*), skin, and other organs and in stromal and parenchymal cells of the kidneys. The lipid deposits were oil-red O-positive, and showed marked birefringence, indicating a high cholesteryl ester content. By electron microscopy the lipid deposits in the cytoplasm of stromal cells were round, moderately electron dense, and non-membrane-bound. Similar lipid deposits in stromal cells were not observed in three control fetuses.

Atherosclerosis of Aorta and Coronary Arteries

Homozygous children exhibit severe atherosclerosis of the aorta and coronary arteries, ischemic myocardial damage, sclerosis, and lipid deposition in aortic and mitral valves.[46,89] Lipid deposition in stromal macrophages of lymph nodes, spleen, and other organs has been reported in a few homozygotes.[89] However, the degree to which lipid is deposited in extravascular sites other than in xanthomas is not well-defined because most reports have emphasized examination of the cardiovascular system. In young FH homozygotes, the atherosclerotic process appears to involve major arteries selectively and to spare veins despite severe hypercholesterolemia (Fig. 120-9). Atherosclerosis of the aorta

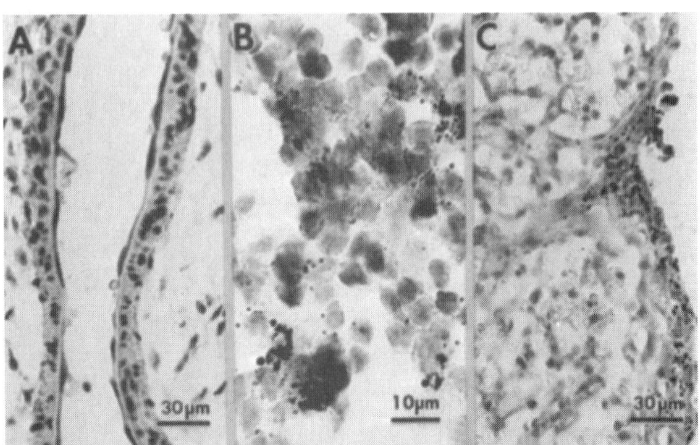

Fig. 120-8 Histologic findings in a 20-week-old fetus with homozygous FH. *A*. Coronary artery is normal. *B*. Thymocytes contain oil-red O-positive (dark) lipid droplets. *C*. Oil-red O-positive lipid deposits are also present in the splenic capsule. (Courtesy of Dr. L. Maximilian Buja.)

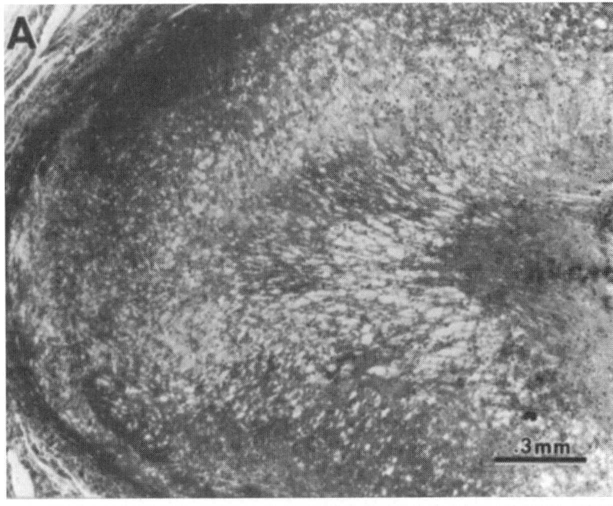

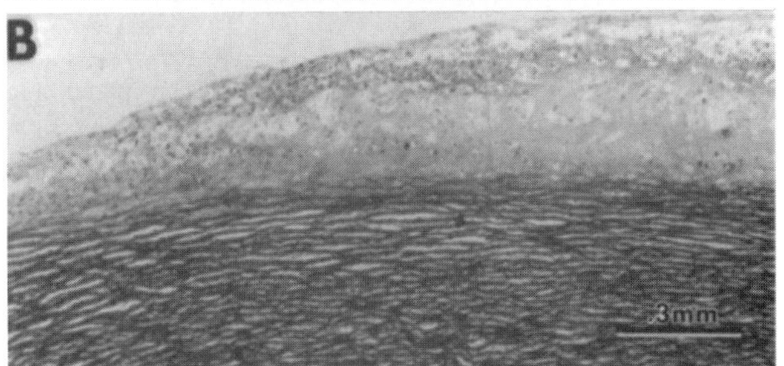

Fig. 120-9 Coronary artery (*A*) and aorta (*B*) from a 4-year-old boy with homozygous FH reported by T. Watanabe, K. Tanake, and N. Yanai (*Acta Pathol Jpn* 18:319, 1968). These photomicrographs were made by Dr. L. Maximilian Buja from histologic sections submitted by Dr. Kenzo Tanaka of Kyushu University, Fukuoka, Japan. *A*. The lumen of the coronary artery is markedly narrowed by an atherosclerotic plaque containing numerous foam cells. The lipid has been removed in the preparation of the paraffin sections. *B*. The aortic intima is thickened by an atherosclerotic plaque. (*Courtesy of Dr. L. Maximilian Buja.*)

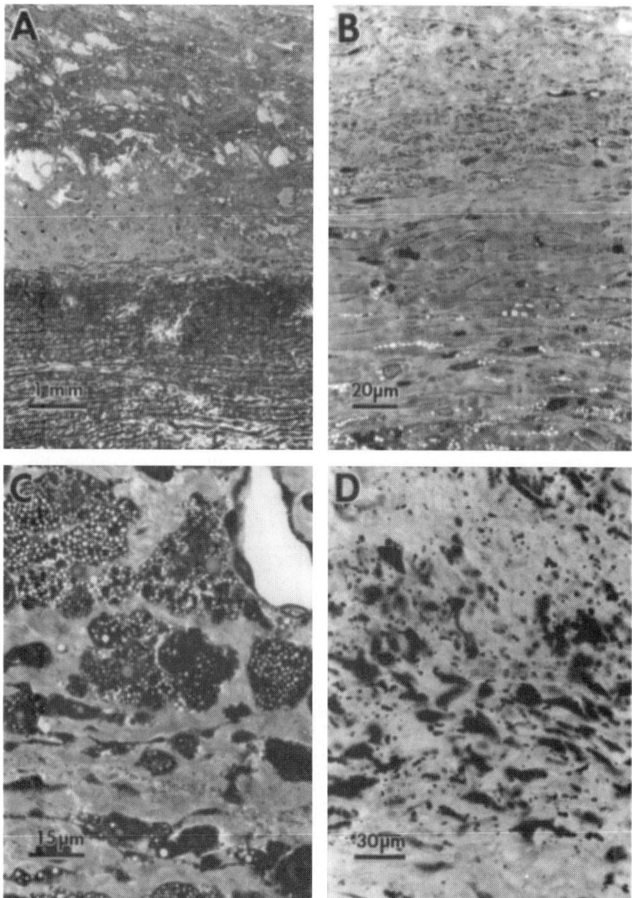

Fig. 120-10 Ascending aorta with atherosclerotic plaque from a 9-year-old girl with homozygous FH. Light micrographs of thin sections from epoxy-embedded tissue (*A* to *C*) and of a frozen section stained with oil red-*O* (*D*). *A*. The plaque core adjacent to the media contains abundant extracellular lipid deposits (clear spaces due to lipid extraction during tissue processing). *B*. Some elongated cells of the fibrous capsule of the plaque contain lipid deposits. *C*. Ovoid foam cells adjacent to the plaque core contain numerous lipid vacuoles. *D*. Frozen section stained with oil red-*O* confirms the presence of neutral lipid in the foam cells. (*Courtesy of Dr. L. Maximilian Buja.*)

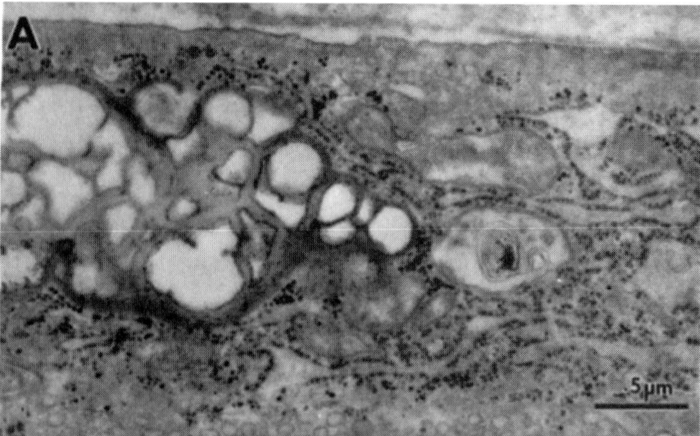

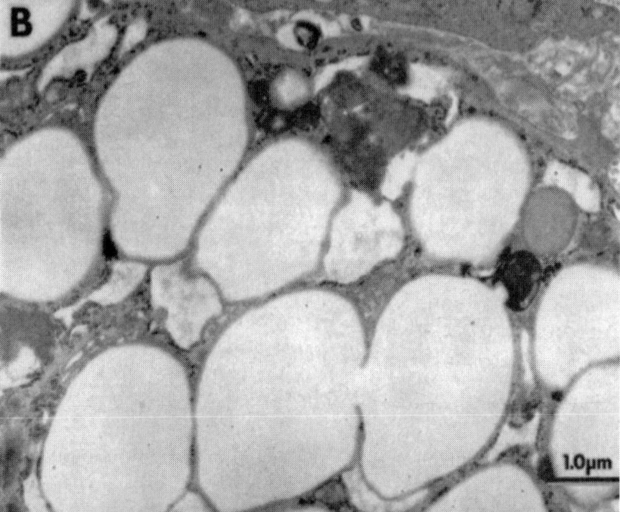

Fig. 120-11 Atherosclerotic plaque from a 9-year-old girl with homozygous FH. *A*. Elongated cell of the plaque capsule exhibits a basement membrane, pinocytotic vesicles, cytoplasmic filaments, rough-surfaced ER, and a large lipid inclusion. *B*. Ovoid foam cell contains numerous non-membrane-bound lipid deposits. (*Courtesy of Dr. L. Maximilian Buja.*)

is typically generalized, but it frequently shows a distinctive, unusually severe predilection for the thoracic aorta, particularly the ascending portion with extension into the coronary ostia.[89] Severe atherosclerosis also occurs in the abdominal aorta and in the major pulmonary arteries.[46]

Figures 120-10 and 120-11 illustrate the features of aortic atherosclerosis in a 9-year-old homozygote. The pathologic findings suggest that plaque cells may originate from multiple sources, including smooth-muscle cells, endothelial cells, intimal histiocytes, and circulating monocytes. A significant proportion of cells in human and experimental atherosclerotic plaques have functional characteristics of macrophages.[107] Inasmuch as lipid-laden foam cells have not been identified in the blood of homozygotes or patients with other conditions predisposing to severe atherosclerosis, it seems likely that macrophages acquire their lipids after the cells have entered the atherosclerotic lesions.

Hoeg et al.[108] reported the use of ultrafast computed tomography (CT) to quantify calcific coronary and aortic lesions in a group of 11 FH homozygotes (3 to 37 years old; mean age of 21 years). Significant calcific atherosclerosis was detected in 7 of 11 homozygotes and in all 9 homozygotes older than 12 years of age. The volume of calcification in the aortic root and coronary ostia showed a strong correlation with the severity and duration of the hypercholesterolemia as well as with symptomatic angina.

Aortic and Mitral Valve Involvement

Atheromatous involvement of the aortic valve leads to significant aortic stenosis more frequently than aortic regurgitation in FH homozygotes.[46] Significant aortic stenosis was reported in 12 (55 percent) of 21 homozygotes and mitral insufficiency in 2 (9.5 percent).[89] FH homozygotes may also have supravalvular left ventricular outflow tract obstruction, owing to bulky atherosclerotic plaques in the ascending aorta.[89] Several homozygotes have undergone successful surgical correction of a severely deformed and atherosclerotic aortic valve,[30,52] and one 7-year-old homozygote had successful replacement of both the aortic and mitral valves.[89]

Cutaneous and Tendon Xanthomas

Cutaneous xanthomas in FH homozygotes are composed of large numbers of histiocytic foam cells in a fibrovascular stroma (Fig. 120-12). It is noteworthy that endothelial cells of small blood vessels in the lesions are devoid of lipid deposits, suggesting selective lipid accumulation in tissue histiocytes of the xanthomas.[89,109]

Cellular lipid accumulation in homozygotes occurs predominantly in the form of cytoplasmic neutral lipid droplets that lack discrete trilaminar membranes. These findings suggest that the cytoplasm is the major site of intracellular lipid storage in this disease. The production of foam cells in homozygotes has been postulated to result from excessive endocytosis of modified or oxidized LDL by an LDL receptor-independent pathway in

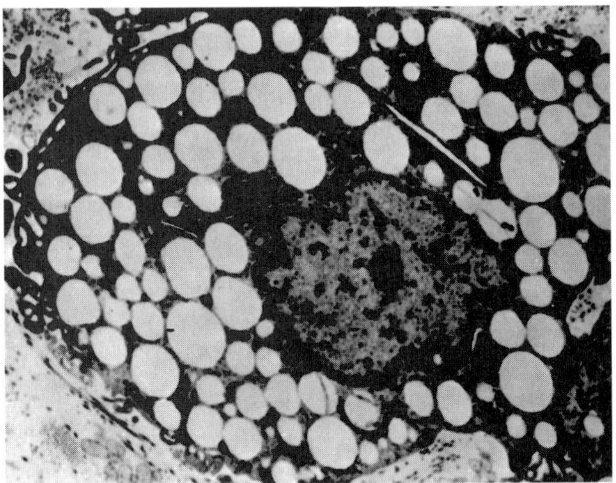

Fig. 120-12 Electron micrograph showing a typical foam cell (scavenger cell) filled with numerous lipid droplets. This mature histiocytic foam cell was observed in a tuberous xanthoma excised from a 17-year-old girl with homozygous FH. (*From Bulkley et al.*[109] *Used by permission of* Archives of Pathology.)

response to chronic hypercholesterolemia, with subsequent lysosomal processing of the LDL and cytoplasmic reesterification of cholesterol.[110,111] The role of macrophage scavenger receptors in mediating the uptake of modified or oxidized LDL is discussed below.

The pattern of intracellular lipid deposition in FH patients is distinctly different from that seen in Wolman disease and cholesteryl ester storage disease. In these two disorders, which are caused by a deficiency in lysosomal cholesteryl ester hydrolase, cholesterol deposits are found within lysosomes of stromal histiocytes as well as parenchymal cells (see Chap. 142).

PATHOGENESIS AT THE CELLULAR LEVEL

LDL Receptor Pathway in Cultured Cells

The genetic defect in FH was unraveled through studies of cholesterol metabolism in human fibroblasts in tissue culture.[3,112] Mammalian cells in tissue culture cannot survive unless they acquire cholesterol, either from a usable exogenous source or as a result of de novo synthesis.[112] The cholesterol is required as a structural component of the plasma membrane of the cell, where it modulates the fluidity of the phospholipid bilayer. Any cholesterol that accumulates within the cell above the amount that can be inserted into the plasma membrane is esterified with a long-chain fatty acid and stored within the cytoplasm as cholesteryl ester droplets.[112]

Sequential Biochemical Steps and Their Ultrastructural Counterparts

When mammalian cells are grown in the presence of animal or human serum, they produce little cholesterol and preferentially utilize the cholesterol of the LDL that is present in the serum of the culture medium.[112] The key to the uptake process is a cell-surface receptor that binds LDL by interacting with its apo B-100 component (Fig. 120-13).[113] Human fibroblasts produce a maximum of about 20,000 to 50,000 LDL receptors per cell,[114] the number varying according to cellular cholesterol requirements[115] (discussed below).

The human LDL receptor is a cell-surface glycoprotein of 839 amino acids that contains approximately 2 asparagine-linked (*N*-linked) oligosaccharide chains of the complex type and approximately 18 serine/threonine-linked (*O*-linked) oligosaccharide chains.[116,117] Two-thirds of the *O*-linked sugars are clustered in the region of the molecule that abuts the plasma membrane.[118] The LDL receptor binds two protein ligands: apo B-100, the 514-kDa glycoprotein that is the sole protein of LDL,[114] and apo E, a 34-kDa protein that is found in multiple copies in VLDL, IDL, chylomicron remnants, and a subclass of HDL.[119,120] Apo E is especially abundant on particles called "β-migrating VLDL" (β-VLDL), which are remnants of chylomicrons and VLDL that accumulate in the plasma of cholesterol-fed rabbits and dogs.[120] Lipoproteins that contain multiple copies of apo E bind to LDL receptors with up to twentyfold higher affinity than LDL, which contains only one copy of apo B-100.[120] The abilities of LDL and apo E-containing lipoproteins to bind to the LDL receptor are abolished when the lysine residues of the lipoproteins are modified by reaction with acetic anhydride[121] or diketone,[122] or when the arginine residues are blocked by reaction with cyclohexanedione.[123] These observations have provided a powerful tool by which to quantify receptor-mediated removal of LDL from human plasma in vivo (discussed below).

Figure 120-14 illustrates the circuitous itinerary that the LDL receptor follows from its site of synthesis to its sites of internalization in coated pits and recycling in endosomes. The receptor is synthesized in the rough ER as a precursor[124] that contains high mannose *N*-linked carbohydrate chains and the core sugar (*N*-acetylgalactosamine) of the *O*-linked chains.[117] The *O*-linked core sugars are added before the mannose residues of the *N*-linked chains are trimmed; that is, while the receptor is still in the endoglycosidase H-sensitive stage. Thus, the *O*-linked sugars must be added either in the ER or in a transitional zone between the ER and the Golgi complex. The receptor precursor migrates on SDS

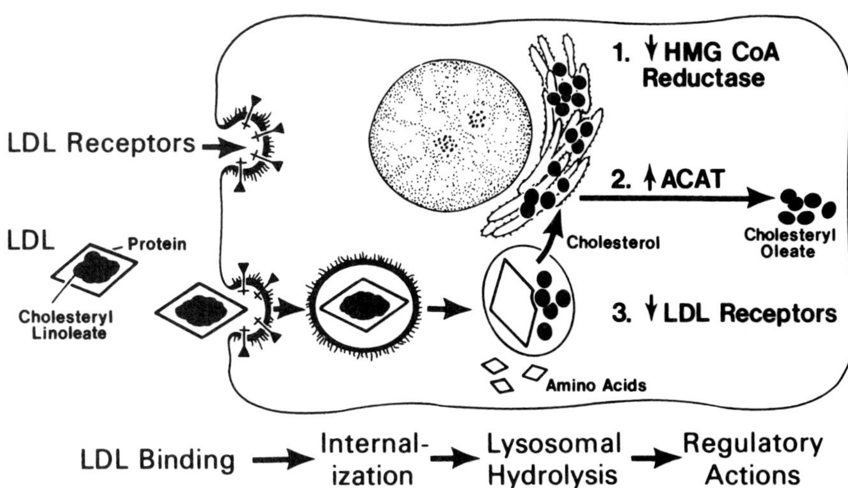

Fig. 120-13 Sequential steps in the LDL receptor pathway in cultured mammalian cells. (*From M. S. Brown and J. L. Goldstein,* Proc Natl Acad Sci U S A *76:3330, 1979. Used by permission.*)

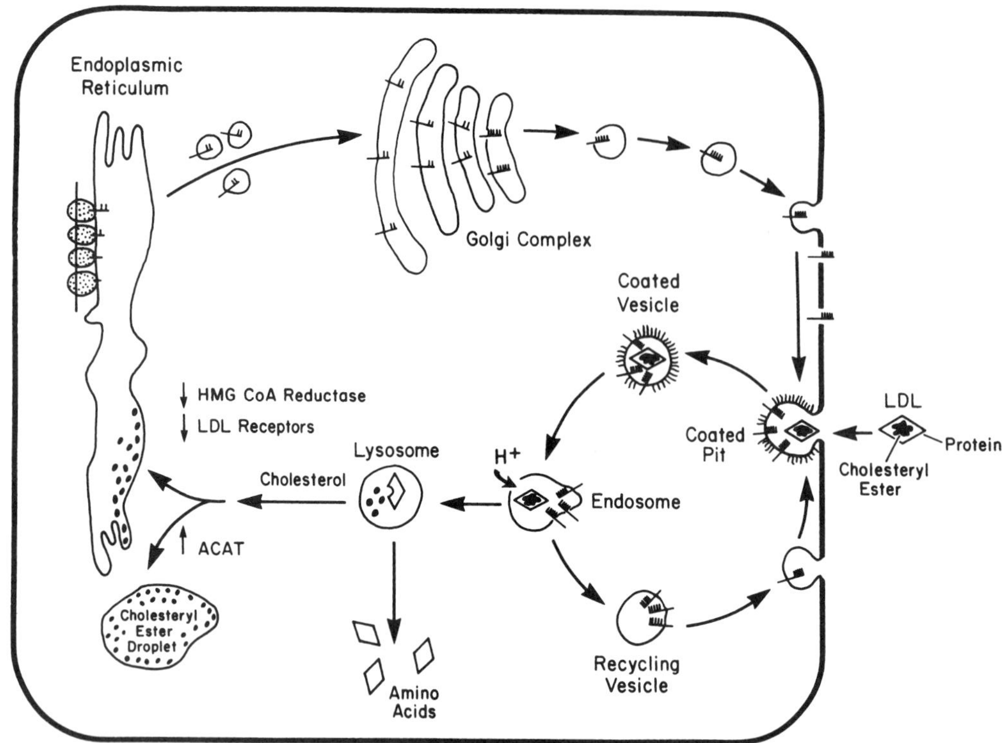

Fig. 120-14 Itinerary of the LDL receptor in mammalian cells. The receptor begins life in the ER from which it travels to the Golgi complex, cell surface, coated pit, endosome, and back to the surface. Vertical arrows indicate the direction of regulatory effects. (*From M. S. Brown and J. L. Goldstein,* Curr Top Cell Reg *27:3, 1985. Used by permission.*)

polyacrylamide gel electrophoresis as a single band corresponding to an apparent molecular weight of 120 kDa.[124]

Within 30 min after its synthesis, the LDL receptor decreases in mobility on SDS gels. The apparent molecular weight increases from 120 to 160 kDa.[124] This change is coincident with the conversion of the high-mannose N-linked oligosaccharide chains to the complex endoglycosidase H-resistant form.[117] At the same time, the addition of one galactose and one or two sialic acid residues elongates each *O*-linked chain.[117] The amount of carbohydrate is not sufficient to account for an increase in molecular mass of 40 kDa. Rather, the decrease in electrophoretic mobility is primarily caused by a change in conformation of the protein that results from the elongation of the clustered *O*-linked sugars.[117,118]

About 45 min after synthesis, LDL receptors appear on the cell surface, where they gather in coated pits, which are specialized regions of the plasma membrane that are lined on the cytoplasmic surface by a protein called "clathrin."[3,125] Within 3 to 5 min of their formation, the coated pits invaginate to form coated endocytic vesicles. Very quickly, the clathrin coat dissociates. Multiple endocytic vesicles then fuse to create larger sacs of irregular contour called "endosomes."[126] The pH of the endosomes falls below 6.5, owing to the operation of ATP-driven proton pumps in the membrane.[125] At this acid pH, the LDL dissociates from the receptor. The latter returns to the surface, apparently by clustering with other receptors in a segment of the endosomal membrane that pinches off to form a recycling vesicle.[127,128] Once it reaches the surface, the receptor binds another lipoprotein particle and initiates another cycle of endocytosis.[127] Each LDL receptor makes one round trip every 10 min in continuous fashion, whether or not it is occupied with LDL.[128] The LDL that dissociates from the receptor is delivered to a lysosome when the membranes of the endosome and lysosome fuse.

Within the lysosomes, acid hydrolytic enzymes degrade the LDL. The apoprotein of LDL is hydrolyzed by proteases to amino acids,[20] and the cholesteryl esters are hydrolyzed by a lysosomal acid lipase.[129] The resulting unesterified cholesterol crosses the lysosomal membrane and enters the cellular compartment, where it is used for membrane synthesis and as a regulator of intracellular cholesterol homeostasis[130] (see below). NPC1, the membrane protein that transports the LDL-derived cholesterol across the lysosomal membrane, is discussed in Chap. 145.

The localization of LDL receptors in coated pits on the surface of human fibroblasts was demonstrated originally by thin-section electron microscopy with the use of LDL coupled to the iron-containing, electron-dense protein ferritin[131,132] and subsequently by ^{125}I-labeled LDL autoradiography.[133] Figure 120-15 shows the visual sequence of events by which LDL-ferritin is bound, internalized, and delivered to lysosomes in human fibroblasts. The techniques of freeze-etching and rotary shadowing allow the visualization of native LDL bound to the LDL receptor on the surface of human fibroblasts. In the freeze-etch micrograph shown in Fig. 120-16, numerous particles of LDL are seen entering the cell through coated pits.

Regulatory Actions of LDL-Derived Cholesterol

The cholesterol derived from the lysosomal hydrolysis of LDL's cholesteryl esters mediates a sophisticated system of feedback control that stabilizes the intracellular cholesterol concentration.[112] First, this cholesterol suppresses the activity of HMG-CoA reductase, the rate-controlling enzyme in cholesterol biosynthesis, thereby turning off cholesterol synthesis in the cell.[134] Second, the cholesterol activates a cholesterol-esterifying enzyme called "acyl-coenzyme A: cholesterol acyltransferase" (ACAT) so that excess cholesterol can be stored as cholesteryl esters.[135] Third, the cholesterol turns off the synthesis of the LDL receptor, preventing further entry of LDL, thereby protecting cells against an overaccumulation of cholesterol[115] (see Fig. 120-13).

The overall effect of this regulatory system is to coordinate the intracellular and extracellular sources of cholesterol so as to maintain a constant level of cholesterol within the cell in the face

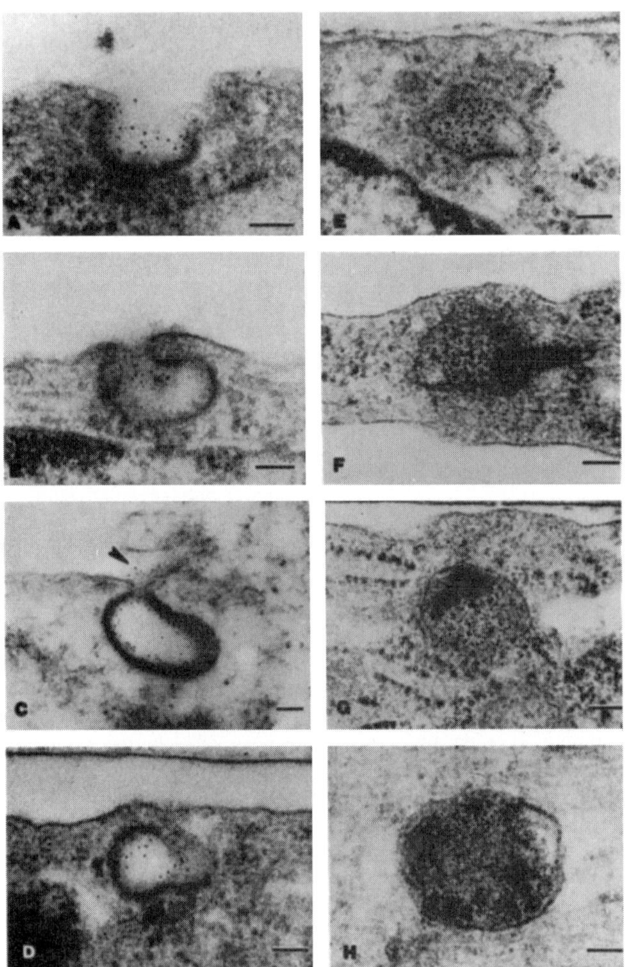

Fig. 120-15 Electron micrographs showing representative stages in the receptor-mediated endocytosis of LDL-ferritin and its subsequent delivery to lysosomes. Normal human fibroblasts were incubated with 47.5 μg protein/ml of LDL-ferritin for 2 h at 4°C, washed extensively, and then warmed to 37°C for various times. Scale bar = 1000 Å. *A.* Typical coated pit (time at 37°C, 1 min), ×67,900. *B.* Coated pit being transformed into an endocytic vesicle with LDL-ferritin included (time at 37°C, 1 min), ×56,700. *C.* Formation of a coated vesicle. As the plasma membrane begins to fuse to form the vesicle, some of the LDL-ferritin is excluded from the interior and is left on the surface of the cell (arrow) (time at 37°C, 1 min), ×38,150. *D.* Fully formed coated vesicle that appears to be losing its cytoplasmic coat on the right side (time at 37°C, 2 min), ×52,500. *E.* Endocytic vesicle that has completely lost its cytoplasmic coat. Note the irregular shape of this vesicle (time at 37°C, 2 min), ×52,500. *F.* Irregularly shaped endocytic vesicle that contains more LDL-ferritin than a typical coated vesicle and also has a region of increased electron density within the lumen (time at 37°C, 6 min), ×52,500. *G.* Endocytic vesicle similar to F, with more electron-dense material in the lumen (time at 37°C, 6 min), ×48,300. *H.* Secondary lysosome that contains LDL-ferritin (time at 37°C, 8 min), ×52,500. (*From Anderson et al.*[132] *Used by permission of* Cell.)

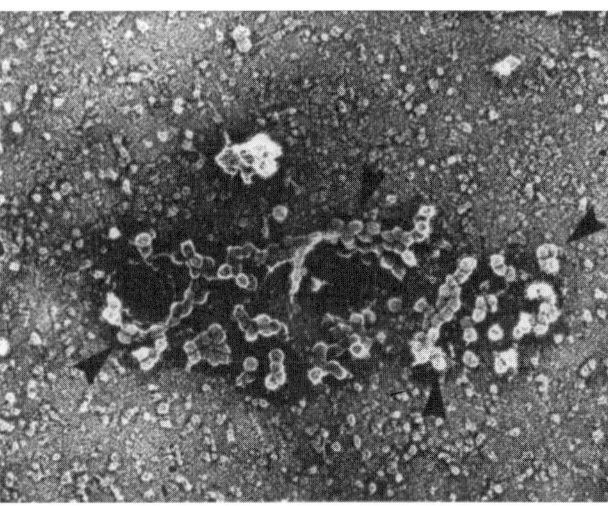

Fig. 120-16 Visualization of LDL bound to receptors on the surface of human fibroblasts. Normal human fibroblasts were incubated with 15 μg protein/ml of native LDL at 4°C for 2 h, after which the cells were washed extensively, warmed to 37°C for 3 min, and then fixed with glutaraldehyde. The cells were then processed by the rapid-freezing, replica technique of Heuser (*J Cell Biol* 84:560, 1980). This picture shows the appearance of native LDL bound to LDL receptors that are clustered around coated pits. The arrows point to typical LDL particles. (×112,000.) (*Courtesy of Dr. Richard G. W. Anderson.*)

of fluctuations in the supply of lipoproteins. Human fibroblasts and other mammalian cells grow in the absence of lipoproteins because they can synthesize cholesterol from acetyl-CoA. When LDL is available, cells preferentially use the receptor to take up LDL and keep their own cholesterol synthesis suppressed.[112,115]

Figure 120-17 summarizes the pattern of regulation of the LDL pathway in cultured human fibroblasts. When the cells are grown in the presence of normal plasma containing LDL, they establish a steady state in which HMG-CoA reductase activity (and hence cholesterol synthesis) is low and the cells derive the small amounts of cholesterol that they need by means of a small number of LDL receptors. Under these conditions, the activity of ACAT is held at an intermediate level so that the rate of synthesis of cholesteryl esters equals their rate of hydrolysis (see Fig. 120-17, "steady state with LDL present"). The delicate balance inherent in this regulated steady state is disclosed when LDL is removed from the culture medium (see Fig. 120-17, "no LDL present"). Under these conditions, the number of LDL receptors and the activity of HMG-CoA reductase greatly increase, while cholesterol-esterifying activity declines. Because LDL is absent from the culture medium, the LDL receptors are not able to supply the cell with cholesterol; hence the cholesterol required for membrane formation is derived both from accelerated *de novo* synthesis and from a net hydrolysis of cholesteryl esters stored within the cell. When LDL is added back to the culture medium (see Fig. 120-17, "initial response to LDL"), the lipoprotein is bound at the receptor site, internalized, and degraded to yield free cholesterol. The liberated sterol, in turn, suppresses *de novo* cholesterol synthesis and stimulates the esterifying system so that excess cholesterol can be reesterified and stored as cholesteryl esters. When sufficient cellular cholesterol has accumulated, the number of LDL receptors becomes suppressed and the cells return to their original steady state (see Fig. 120-17, "steady state with LDL present"), thus completing a metabolic cycle. This "steady state with LDL present" duplicates the condition of most cells in the body.[3,136]

LDL Receptor Gene: Relation of Exons to Protein Domains

The human LDL receptor mRNA is 5.3 kb in length and encodes a protein of 860 amino acids.[137] About half of the mRNA constitutes a long 3′ untranslated region that contains two and a half copies of the *Alu* family of middle repetitive DNAs.[137] The human LDL receptor gene, located on the distal short arm of chromosome 19 (p13.1–p13.3),[138] spans 45 kb and is divided into 18 exons and 17 introns.[139] Many of the exons share an evolutionary history with exons of other genes, suggesting that the gene was assembled by exon shuffling (discussed below). Figure 120-18 shows how the exons of the gene correlate with the functional domains of the mature protein.

Exon 1 encodes a short 5′ untranslated region and 21 hydrophobic amino acids that comprise the signal sequence. This sequence is cleaved from the protein during translocation into

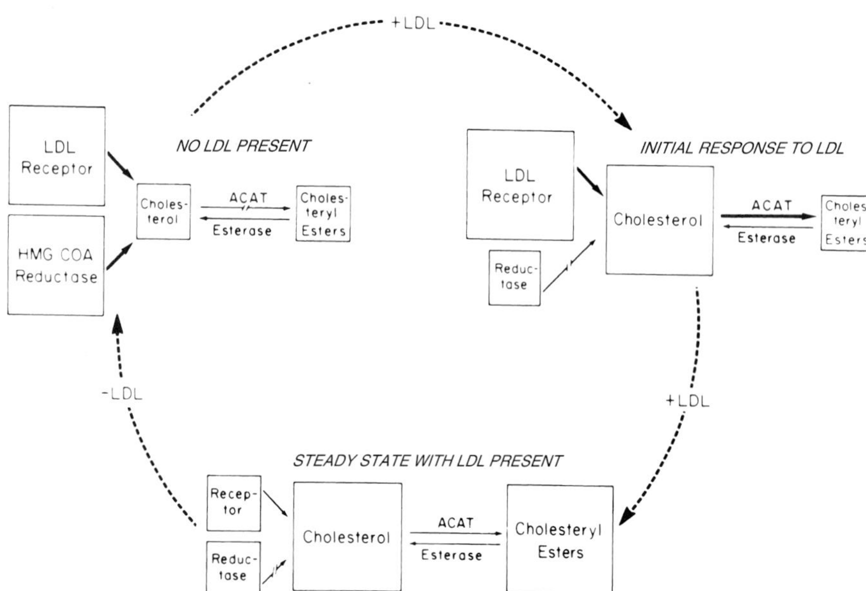

Fig. 120-17 Cyclic changes in cholesterol metabolism that occur in cultured human fibroblasts when LDL is removed from the culture medium (−LDL) and is subsequently returned to the medium (+LDL). The relative level of each constituent is indicated by the size of the square. (*From M. S. Brown and J. L. Goldstein,* Science *191:150, 1976. Used by permission.*)

the ER, leaving a mature protein of 839 amino acids. Exons 2 to 6 encode the ligand binding domain, which is 292 amino acids in length and comprised of 7 tandem repeats of ~40 amino acids each. These repeats show a strong resemblance to sequences in several proteins of the complement cascade[140] and over 100 other proteins in the protein sequence database. Each repeat contains six cysteine residues that form three intrarepeat disulfide bonds. At the C-terminal end of each repeat is a cluster of negatively charged amino acids, Asp-*X*-Ser-Asp-Glu (D*x*SDE). The receptor's two ligands, apo B-100 and apo E, have completely different

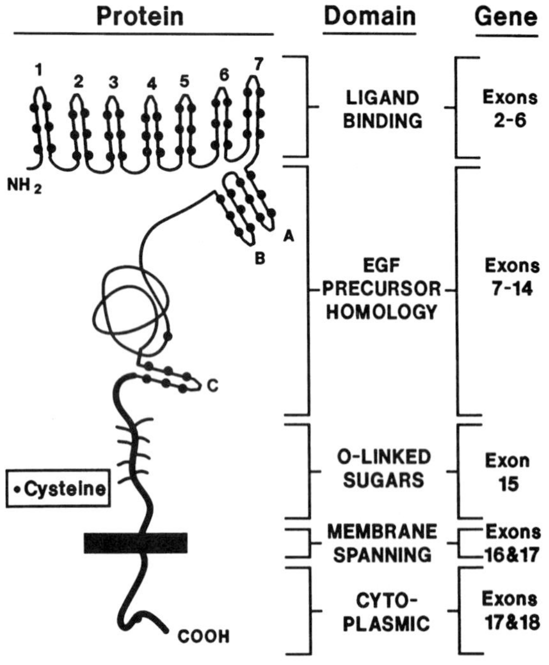

Fig. 120-18 Domain structure of the human LDL receptor protein and its relation to the exon organization of the gene. The domains of the 839-amino acid mature protein are shown at the left and the corresponding exons encoding the protein domains at the right. Exon 1 (not shown) encodes the 21-amino acid signal sequence, which is cleaved from the mature protein during synthesis in the ER. (*From Hobbs et al.*[140] *Used by permission of* Annual Review of Genetics.)

sequences, but both possess short segments rich in basic amino acids[141] that contain the LDL receptor binding site.[142,143] Although it seems likely that these positively charged segments of apo B-100 and apo E would bind the negatively charged D*x*SDE clusters of the LDL receptor through ionic interactions, x-ray crystallography of one of the ligand binding repeats has raised questions about this scenario (discussed below).

Each of the seven cysteine-rich ligand binding repeats (see Fig. 120-18) is encoded by a single exon except repeats 3, 4, and 5, which are all encoded by exon 4.[139] The splice junctions for exons 2 to 7 are in a frame such that if any exons are deleted, the translational reading frame is preserved and the resultant protein is translated normally. Deletional analysis by in vitro mutagenesis revealed that each repeat makes an independent contribution to ligand binding.[144] Deletion of repeat 1 has no effect on binding of either LDL or β-VLDL.[144,145] Deletion of any other single repeat impairs LDL binding by up to 95 percent, but does not impair the binding of β-VLDL. The sole exception is repeat 5, whose deletion reduces β-VLDL binding by 50 percent.[144] The more stringent binding requirements of the receptor for LDL versus β-VLDL create a situation in which an FH individual with an exon deletion in the receptor may have a selective inability to remove LDL but not β-VLDL (or IDL) from the circulation (discussed below).

X-ray crystallography of repeat 5 has been successfully achieved to a resolution of 1.7 Å.[21] The structure of this module is organized around a calcium ion (Fig. 120-19). The Ca^{2+} interacts directly with six residues in the C-terminal half of the repeat, including two of the acidic residues in the highly conserved D*x*SDE sequence. Based on this structure, these acidic residues would not be accessible to form ionic interactions with the short basic segments of apo B-100 and apo E that constitute the putative ligand binding region. It remains possible that apo B-100 and apo E bind to interfaces between the repeats, or that the structure of a single repeat does not accurately reflect its native structure in the context of all seven repeats. Definitive answers require knowledge of the structure of the entire ligand-receptor complex. In any event, the current crystal structure of repeat 5 has revealed a crucial role for Ca^{2+} in the proper folding of the ligand-binding repeats.[21,146]

Exons 7 to 14 of the LDL receptor gene encode a 400-amino acid sequence that is 33 percent identical to a portion of the human epidermal growth factor (EGF) precursor.[139,147] This region includes three growth factor repeats, which are 40-amino acid cysteine-rich sequences that differ from the cysteine-rich sequences in the ligand binding domain by virtue of the spacing of the cysteines and their lack of D*x*SDE sequences[139] (see Fig.

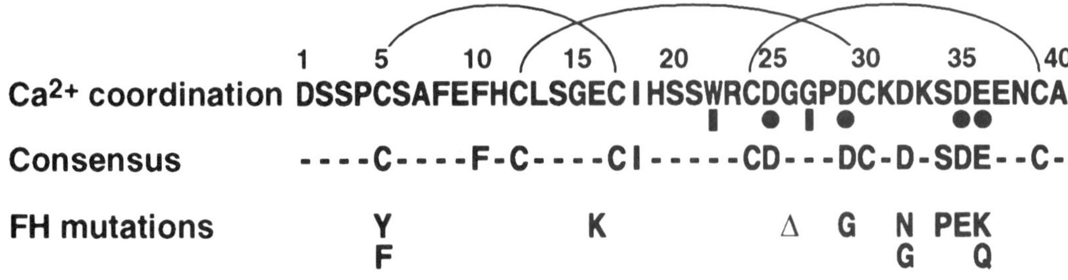

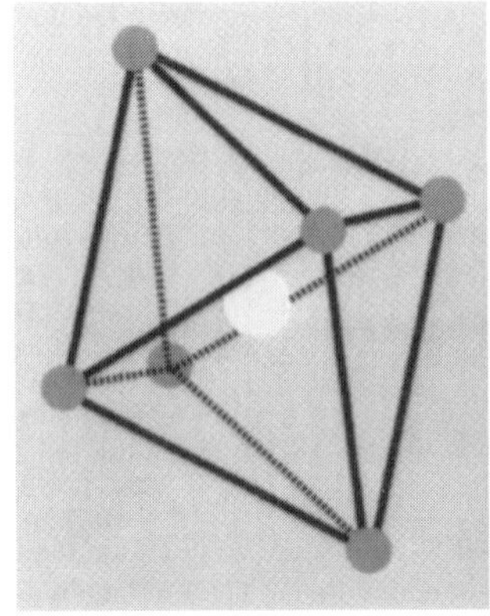
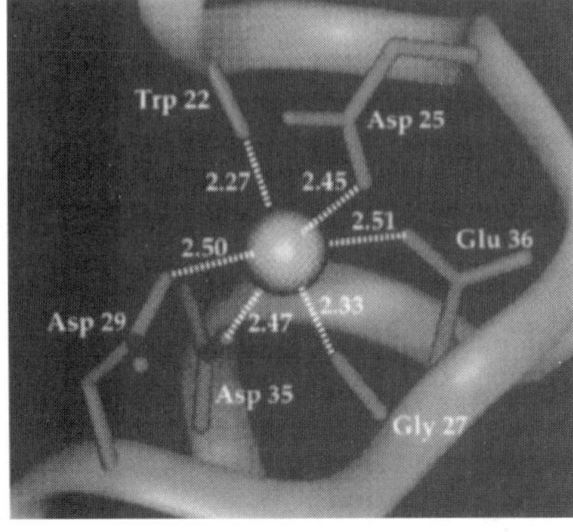

Fig. 120-19 Amino acid sequence (*top*) and X-ray crystallographic structure (*bottom*) of ligand-binding repeat 5 of the LDL receptor. (*Top*) The repeat 5 module of the LDL receptor's ligand-binding domain contains 40 amino acids, 6 of which are cysteine residues. The disulfide bond connectivity between the six cysteines is denoted by the loops. Black circles below the sequence denote the four acidic residues that participate in Ca^{2+} coordination. Vertical bars denote the two residues with backbone carbonyl oxygens that contribute to the Ca^{2+} coordination. Shown below the consensus sequence are the location and identities of point mutations that cause FH by disrupting the structure of repeat 5. The triangle denotes a deletion of a residue. (*Bottom*) The crystal structure of the repeat 5 module reveals an octahedral cage that surrounds a single Ca^{2+} ion that is coordinated by four conserved acidic residues (Asp25, Asp29, Asp35, Glu36) plus two nearby carbonyl oxygens (contributed by Trp22 and Gly27). (*Data from Fass et al.*[21] *Used by permission of* Nature.)

120-18). The first two growth factor repeats, designated A and B, are contiguous and separated from the third growth factor repeat, C, by a 280-amino acid sequence that contains 6 copies of a conserved 40-amino acid sequence that contains motif Tyr-Trp-Thr-Asp (YWTD) (discussed below). The EGF precursor homology domain is required for the acid-dependent dissociation of lipoproteins from the receptor in the endosome during receptor recycling.[148] It also serves to position the ligand-binding domain so that it can bind LDL on the cell surface.[148]

The YWTD-containing region in the LDL receptor is present in multiple members of the LDL receptor gene family (discussed below), the EGF precursor, and many other unrelated proteins. Springer[149] noted that in all these proteins the 40-amino acid YWTD module is tandemly arranged as a group of six repeats. He predicted that the ensemble of repeats folds into a compact circular structure known as a six-bladed β-propeller domain, which brings neighboring modules into close proximity to one another. Point mutations that occur in the YWTD repeats of the LDL receptor would be expected to disrupt the β-propeller architecture, thereby crippling LDL receptor function (discussed below).

Exon 15 encodes 58 amino acids that are enriched in serine and threonine residues, many of which serve as attachment sites for *O*-linked carbohydrate chains.[118] The function of the *O*-linked sugars is not known. This region of the protein can be deleted without adverse effects on receptor function in cultured fibroblasts.[118] However, deletion of this exon in two families with heterozygous FH has been shown to segregate with the hypercholesterolemia,[150,151] suggesting that this domain may play a specific role in receptor function in the liver. In addition to the clustered *O*-linked sugars, the LDL receptor contains a few scattered *O*-linked sugar chains. Their precise location in the molecule is as yet unknown, but they may play a role in stabilizing the receptor.

Exon 16 and the 5′ end of exon 17 encode 22 hydrophobic amino acids that comprise the membrane-spanning domain that anchors the protein to the cell membrane. The remainder of exon 17 and the 5′ end of exon 18 encode the 50 amino acids that make up the cytoplasmic domain. This domain contains two discrete signals, one for localizing the receptor in coated pits[152] and the other for targeting the receptor to the sinusoidal surface of polarized hepatocytes.[153] The remainder of exon 18 specifies the 2.6-kb 3′-untranslated region of the mRNA.

The amino acid sequence of the LDL receptor from eight species (human, cow, rabbit, hamster, rat, swine, the toad *Xenopus laevis* and the banded cat shark *Chiloscyllium plagiosum*) has been determined by cDNA cloning and DNA sequence analysis.[137,154–158] Overall, the protein is highly conserved from humans to shark, suggesting that the receptor was assembled in its modern domain configuration more than 450 million years ago. The most conserved region is the cytoplasmic domain, which is more than 90 percent identical among all mammalian species and 79 percent identical between the human and shark. Next in order of conservation among all species is the EGF precursor domain (70 to 86 percent identity), followed by the ligand binding domain (64 to 78 percent identity), and the transmembrane domain (35 to 62 percent identity).[156,158] Two regions show minimal sequence conservation among the eight species; these are the signal sequence and the *O*-linked sugar domain. Even though the order of amino acids in the latter differs widely among species, this sequence is invariably enriched in threonines and serines.

LDL Receptor Promoter and the SREBP Pathway

In cultured cells, and importantly in liver, the transcription of the LDL receptor gene is regulated by a feedback mechanism that functions to stabilize the lipid composition of cell membranes. This regulatory system is of physiologic importance because it is responsible, at least in part, for the suppression of LDL receptors that is produced by high fat diets, and for the increase in LDL receptors that is achieved by cholesterol-depleting agents such as

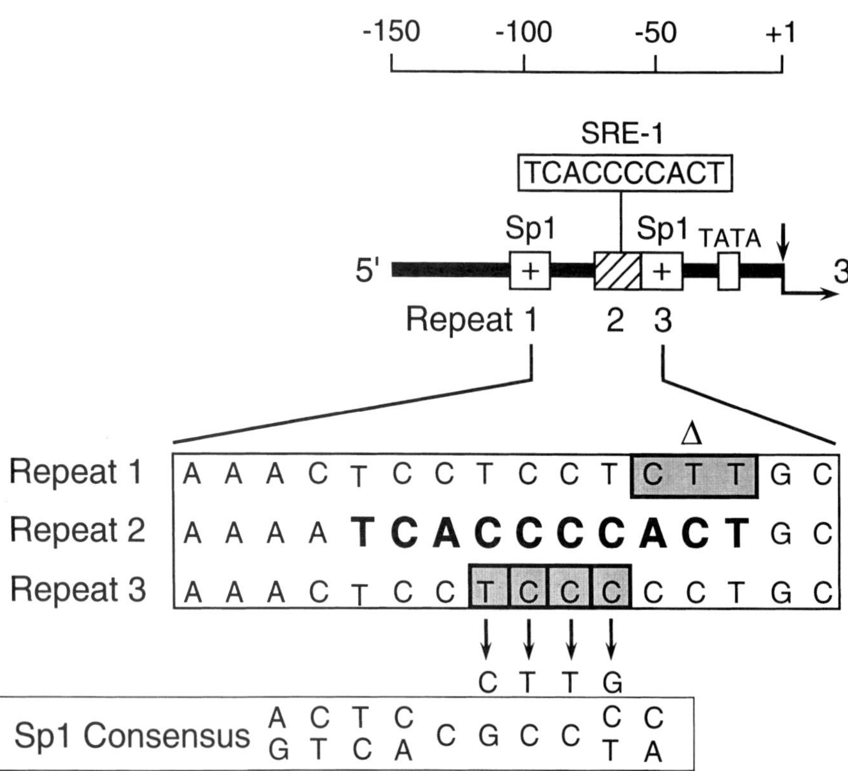

Fig. 120-20 Nucleotide sequence of sterol regulatory element (SRE-1) in the 5′ promoter region of the LDL receptor gene. The core 10 nucleotides comprising the SRE-1 element in repeat 2 that binds SREBP-1a, -1c, or -2 is denoted by bold type. Repeats 1 and 3 are binding sites for transcription factor Sp1. The consensus sequence for Sp1 is shown below the repeat 3 sequence. The shaded boxed nucleotides denote the location of four mutations in individuals with FH (one 3-bp deletion and three point mutations).

HMG CoA reductase inhibitors and bile acid binding resins (discussed below).

The 5′ flanking region of the LDL receptor gene contains most if not all of the *cis*-acting DNA sequences responsible for the sterol-regulated expression of the gene in animal cells.[159,160] Within 200 bp of the initiator methionine codon are three imperfect direct repeats of 16 bp each, two A/T-rich sequences (TATA boxes), and a cluster of mRNA initiation sites, all of which function in transcription (Fig. 120-20). This architecture has been maintained in the promoters of human, rat, hamster, mouse, rabbit, and frog LDL receptor genes.[155,161]

Standard methods of promoter analysis, including hybrid gene construction, transfection into cultured cells, DNase I footprinting, and linker-scanner mutagenesis, were used to dissect the roles of the 5′ flanking sequences in the expression and regulation of the LDL receptor gene.[160] Two of the 16-bp direct repeat sequences (repeats 1 and 3 in Fig. 120-20) interact with transcription factor Sp1 to promote transcription.[160] These sequences in themselves are not sufficient for high-level expression. They require the contribution of the other direct repeat (repeat 2), which contains a conditional-positive sterol regulatory element, termed SRE-1, that is 10 bp in length.[162] SRE-1 is the binding site for a family of transcription factors called sterol regulatory element binding proteins (SREBPs), which are discussed in more detail below. In the absence of sterols, the active form of SREBP synergizes with the two Sp1s to promote transcription of the LDL receptor gene.[160,162] In the presence of sterols, the active form of SREBP is not generated, and transcription of the LDL receptor gene is terminated even though the Sp1s are still bound to the DNA of repeats 1 and 3. Through this regulatory mechanism, cells reduce the amount of receptor mRNA and develop a corresponding decrease in cell-surface LDL receptors when they are cultured in the presence of sterols.[160]

The SREBPs are unique among transcription factors because they are membrane-bound molecules whose activity is controlled by sterol-regulated proteolysis.[22] Each of the three SREBPs (discussed below) is a single-chain polypeptide of ~1100 amino acids that is divided into three domains. The N-terminal domain of ~480 amino acids acts as a transcriptional activator of the basic-helix-loop-helix-leucine zipper (bHLH-Zip) class. The bHLH-Zip sequence allows the receptors to form homo- or heterodimers and to bind to specific sequences in DNA. The N-terminal domain also contains a sequence of acidic amino acids, partially encoded by the first exon, that binds to accessory transcriptional activators, thereby increasing gene transcription.

The N-terminal domain of the SREBPs is followed by a membrane attachment domain that consists of two membrane-spanning sequences separated by a short hydrophilic loop of 31 amino acids (Fig. 120-21, top panel). This is followed by a C-terminal regulatory domain of ~580 amino acids. The SREBPs are bound to membranes of the ER and nuclear envelope in a hairpin fashion with the N-terminal transcription domain and the C-terminal regulatory domain projecting into the cytosol and the 31-amino acid hydrophilic loop projecting into the lumen.

To activate transcription, the N-terminal domain must be released from the membrane so that it can enter the nucleus.[163] This is accomplished by a two-step proteolytic process.[22] In the first step the SREBP is cleaved by a protease, called Site-1 protease (S1P), which cuts between the leucine and serine of the sequence RSVLS, which is in the middle of the luminal loop.[164] Cleavage by S1P requires the action of a regulatory protein designated SREBP-cleavage activating protein (SCAP).[165] SCAP is a polytopic membrane protein with two domains: an N-terminal membrane attachment domain consisting of 8 membrane-spanning helices and a C-terminal domain that contains 5 copies of a 40-amino acid sequence called the WD40 repeat[166] (Fig. 120-21, top panel). WD40 sequences are found in many proteins where they form propeller structures that engage in interactions with other proteins. The WD domain of SCAP projects into the cytosol where it forms a stable complex with the C-terminal regulatory domains of the SREBPs. This complex is essential to maintain the SREBPs in a stable configuration and to allow cleavage by S1P.[167]

At the time of this writing, the cDNA encoding S1P had recently been cloned, and the properties of this protease were just beginning to be studied. The DNA sequence indicates that S1P is a membrane-bound serine protease of the subtilisin superfamily. The

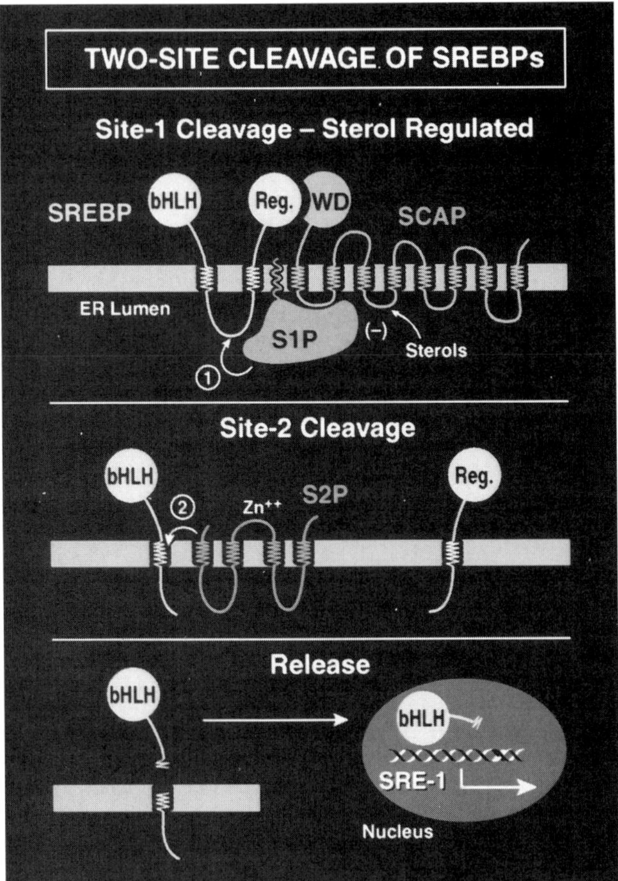

Fig. 120-21 Pathway for the two-site proteolytic cleavage of membrane-bound SREBPs. bHLH, N-terminal basic-helix-loop-helix-leucine zipper transcription factor domain of SREBP; Reg., C-terminal regulatory domain of SREBP; S1P, Site-1 protease; S2P, Site-2 protease; SCAP, SREBP cleavage-activating protein; WD, C-terminal WD-repeat domain of SCAP that interacts with C-terminal regulatory domain of SREBP.

bulk of the protein projects into the lumen of the ER, where it has access to the luminal loop of SREBP. S1P has a single membrane-spanning segment and a short C-terminal cytoplasmic tail.[168]

The activity of S1P is regulated by sterols.[22] In sterol-depleted cells S1P is active. When sterols overaccumulate, the activity of S1P is abolished. The polytopic membrane attachment domain of SCAP mediates this regulation. Five of the eight membrane-spanning helices of SCAP conform to a consensus called the sterol-sensing domain.[165,166] Point mutations at either of two positions within this domain abolish the sterol-sensing function of SCAP and prevent sterol suppression of S1P activity.[165,168] Similar sterol-sensing motifs have been found in three other proteins that are thought to interact with sterols: (a) HMG CoA reductase, whose sterol-sensing domain mediates accelerated degradation of the protein in response to sterols; (b) Niemann-Pick type C protein, whose sterol-sensing domain is required for the transport of LDL-derived cholesterol from the lysosome to the ER[169] (see Chap. 145); and (c) the Patched protein, which serves as a receptor for Sonic Hedgehog, a cell-signaling protein that has a covalently attached cholesterol molecule at its C-terminus.[170,171]

Cleavage by S1P separates the SREBP into halves, each of which remains membrane bound (Fig. 120-21, middle panel). The N-terminal transcription domain is then released by Site-2 protease (S2P), which cleaves within the first transmembrane domain. Current evidence indicates that S2P is an unusual member of a large family of zinc metalloproteases.[172] The sequence of a cloned S2P cDNA indicates that S2P is a highly hydrophobic protein that contains the consensus sequence HE*XX*H, which is characteristic of zinc metalloproteases. Consistent with this hypothesis, substitution of any one of the invariant residues of this consensus blocks the ability of S2P to restore Site-2 cleavage of SREBPs in a mutant line of CHO cells that lacks S2P activity.[172]

S2P cuts SREBPs at a leucine-cysteine bond that is three residues downstream of the sequence DRSR, which are the four amino acids just before the first transmembrane domain.[173] Evidence indicates that this bond is located just within the first membrane-spanning segment. Following this cleavage, the N-terminal domain dissociates from the membrane and enters the nucleus with three hydrophobic amino acids at its C-terminus (Fig. 120-21, bottom panel).

Within the nucleus of cells, the SREBPs trigger a complex program that leads to increased uptake and synthesis of cholesterol and fatty acids through increased transcription of the LDL receptor gene and increases in the transcription of genes encoding multiple enzymes in the cholesterol and fatty acid biosynthetic pathways.[22,174–178a] In the cholesterol biosynthetic pathway, known targets for SREBPs include the genes encoding HMG CoA synthase, HMG CoA reductase, farnesyl diphosphate synthase, squalene synthase, and lanosterol demethylase. In the fatty acid biosynthetic pathway, documented targets include acetyl-CoA carboxylase, fatty acid synthase, and stearoyl CoA desaturase isozymes 1 and 2. In addition, SREBPs lead to activation of the genes encoding ATP citrate lyase, glucose-6-phosphate dehydrogenase, and malic enzyme, which provide acetate units and NADPH as substrates for lipid synthesis,[179] and also to activation of glycerol-3-phosphate acyltransferase, which esterifies excess fatty acids for storage as triglycerides.[180]

Three SREBPs are currently recognized in animal cells.[22] Two of these, SREBP-1a and -1c, are produced from a single gene through alternate promoters that specify alternate first exons.[181] SREBP-1a has a longer first exon than SREBP-1c, and it thus contains a longer acidic transcription-activating sequence. As a result, SREBP-1a is much more proficient than SREBP-1c in activating transcription.[182,183] SREBP-2 is produced by its own gene.[184] It has a long acidic sequence analogous to that of SREBP-1a.

In general, SREBP-1a and -2 activate the same families of genes, but they do so with differing relative efficiencies.[182,183,185] In liver, as well as in tissue culture cells, SREBP-1a favors the fatty acid biosynthetic pathway over the cholesterol biosynthetic pathway, whereas SREBP-2 is somewhat more specific for cholesterol. SREBP-1c has much less transcription-stimulating activity both in cultured cells and in liver. It is somewhat surprising, therefore, that the SREBP-1c transcript is much more abundant than the SREBP-1a transcript in liver and in other organs of adult mice, hamsters, and humans.[185a] All of these organs also produce SREBP-2.

The SREBPs act by binding to two sets of elements in the promoters of the target genes. One set of elements is the SRE-1, which is an asymmetric sequence of 10 bp, the prototype of which is TCACCCCACT (Fig. 120-20). The same SRE-1 sequence is found in the promoters of the LDL receptor and HMG CoA synthase.[186] SREBPs can also bind to "E-boxes," which are palindromic sequences of the form CANNTG.[187,188] The ability to bind to E-boxes is shared with all other members of the bHLH family. The recognition of an asymmetric SRE-1 is unique to SREBPs and results from the insertion of a tyrosine in place of an arginine that is conserved in the basic region of all other bHLH proteins.[187,189]

The ability of SREBPs to interact with SRE-1 elements and E-boxes led to their independent cloning by two laboratories. In Dallas, the SREBPs were purified biochemically based on their binding to the SRE-1 sequence in the LDL receptor promoter,[190] and this permitted cDNA cloning of the three isoforms.[191,192] In Boston, the SREBP-1c isoform was identified in an expression cloning strategy designed to find proteins that bind to E-boxes. The latter protein was named adipocyte determination and differentiation factor (ADD-1).[193]

The mechanism underlying the specificity of SREBPs for certain genes is still poorly understood. SREBPs are able to activate promoters of genes, such as HMG CoA reductase, that contain neither classic SRE-1 elements nor E-boxes.[194] How this occurs and how certain E-boxes are selected over others remains to be elucidated. Selectivity may be mediated in part by the interaction of SREBPs with other transcription factors that recognize nearby sequences. Thus, SREBPs are known to interact with Sp1 in the LDL receptor promoter[186] (Fig. 120-20) and with another ubiquitous transcription factor, NF-Y, in the promoter for farnesyl diphosphate synthase.[176] Undoubtedly, other interactions help specify activities with other promoters.

From the standpoint of FH, the important actions of SREBPs relate to their stimulation of LDL receptor production. In hamsters and mice treated with a combination of an HMG CoA reductase inhibitor and a bile acid binding resin, the amount of SREBP-2 markedly increased in liver nuclei, which was associated with an increase in LDL receptor mRNA.[195,196] It is likely, but not yet proven, that HMG CoA reductase inhibitors lower plasma LDL cholesterol levels in humans, in large part by activating the proteolytic cleavage of hepatic SREBP-2 (discussed below).

LDL Receptor Gene Polymorphisms

Prior to the cloning of the gene, the only genetic marker for the LDL receptor was a protein polymorphism in the third component of complement (C3) loosely linked to FH with a recombination fraction of 0.25.[87] After the receptor cDNA was cloned, multiple RFLPs were identified and are listed online at *www.ucl.ac.uk/fh/polymorph.html*. The polymorphisms span the entire LDL receptor locus and can be used to construct haplotypes to follow the segregation of the gene in families with hypercholesterolemia to establish the diagnosis of FH.[197] Efforts to use the RFLPs to identify common LDL receptor alleles that affect the plasma cholesterol level in the general population are not revealing.

One polymorphism and two mutations in the LDL receptor that produce amino acid substitutions appear to have no clinical consequence. An A to G polymorphism in exon 8 that abolishes a *Stu*I restriction site results in a substitution of threonine for alanine at residue 370.[197,197a] This polymorphism has a frequency of ~6 percent in the North American population and is not associated with a significant difference in plasma cholesterol levels.[197] A rare sequence variant (T705I) that was originally classified as a mutation in a compound FH heterozygote (*FH-Paris-9*)[198] was later identified in homozygous form in a normolipidemic individual.[199] Another silent amino acid substitution (*P84S*) was identified in a Finnish individual with moderate hypercholesterolemia whose plasma LDL cholesterol level was not significantly different from that of his unaffected relatives.[200]

LDL RECEPTOR MUTATIONS CAUSING FH

One Locus with Multiple Alleles

As of August 1, 1998, 421 LDL receptor mutations had been identified in subjects with FH. Of these 421 mutations, 68 are large insertions, deletions, or rearrangements that are detectable by genomic blotting (*www.ucl.ac.uk/fh/*). In most populations, large structural rearrangements comprise 2 to 10 percent of the LDL receptor mutations.[201–203] The remaining 353 mutant alleles include bp substitutions, small deletions, and small insertions; these are compiled online at two Web sites: *www.ucl.ac.uk*[204,205] and *www.umd.necker.fr*.[206,207] The locations of each of the 313 point mutations and small deletions/insertions relative to the exon/intron structure of the LDL receptor gene are shown in Fig. 120-22.

Classification of Mutations

LDL receptor mutations can be divided into five classes based on their phenotypic effects on the protein (Fig. 120-23). Class 1 mutations fail to produce immunoprecipitable protein (null alleles). Class 2 mutations encode proteins that are blocked, either completely (Class 2A) or partially (Class 2B), in transport between the ER and the Golgi apparatus (transport-defective alleles). Class 3 mutations encode proteins that are synthesized and transported to the cell surface, but fail to bind LDL normally (binding-defective alleles). Class 4 mutations encode proteins that move to the cell surface and bind LDL normally, but are unable to cluster in clathrin-coated pits and thus do not internalize LDL (internalization-defective alleles). Class 5 mutations encode receptors that bind and internalize ligand in coated pits, but fail to discharge the ligand in the endosome and fail to recycle to the cell surface (recycling-defective alleles). These classifications are somewhat arbitrary since many LDL receptor alleles fall into more than a single class. For example, some transport-defective alleles are also recycling- and/or binding-defective.

For most LDL receptor mutations, no biosynthetic or functional studies of the receptor protein have been performed. The seventh edition of this textbook (see pages 1997 to 2001)[208] contain tables listing the 127 LDL receptor mutations that have been characterized in sufficient detail (i.e., analysis of cellular

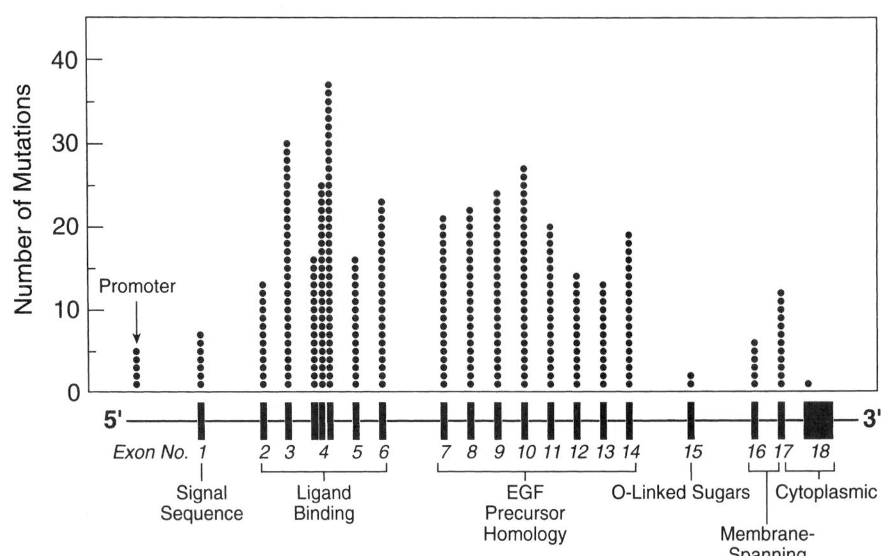

Fig. 120-22 Location of 353 point mutations and small deletions/insertions (< 25 bp) in the LDL receptor gene in individuals with FH (compiled on August 1, 1998). Exons are shown as vertical boxes and introns as the lines connecting them. The map is drawn approximately to scale.

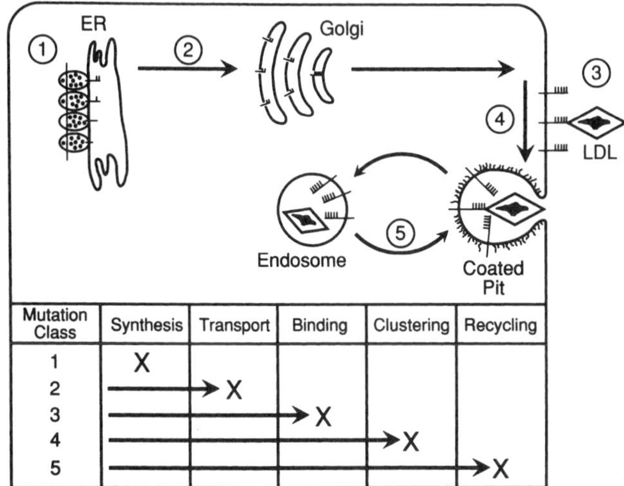

Fig. 120-23 Classification of LDL receptor mutations based on abnormal function of the mutant protein. These mutations disrupt the receptor's synthesis in the ER, transport to the Golgi complex, binding of apoprotein ligands, clustering in coated pits, and recycling in endosomes. Each class is heterogenous at the DNA level. (*From Hobbs et al.*[140] *Used by permission of* Annual Review of Genetics.)

LDL uptake, receptor biosynthesis, receptor transport, and gene structure) to allow classification according to the above scheme. These mutant alleles include 109 mutations identified in cultured fibroblasts obtained from skin biopsy specimens of 157 unrelated FH homozygotes and 13 FH heterozygotes that were collected over a 20-year period (1972 to 1992) in our laboratory. These cell strains are designated the Dallas collection.[198,208] In each cell line, LDL receptor biosynthetic and functional activity studies were performed, the promoter and coding regions of the receptor gene were screened for sequence variations, and the size and quantity of the receptor mRNAs were determined. Thus, the functional effects of the molecular defects in the LDL receptor gene can be deduced for many alleles in the Dallas collection, but not for most of the other LDL receptor mutations in the current online database.

Class 1 Mutations: Null Alleles. Class 1 fibroblasts exhibit less than 2 percent of the normal amount of high affinity binding, uptake, and degradation of ^{125}I-LDL, which is the lowest amount that can be reliably detected. In these cells, LDL does not suppress HMG-CoA reductase activity or cholesterol synthesis, nor does it activate cholesteryl ester formation.[3] Figure 120-24 shows the striking biochemical differences in these LDL-mediated processes in fibroblasts derived from a normal subject and a homozygote with two null alleles. Ultrastructural studies using ferritin-labeled LDL have confirmed the absence of LDL receptors in these receptor-negative cells.[131]

Twenty-seven of 157 FH homozygote fibroblast strains in the Dallas collection (17 percent) produce no immunoprecipitatable LDL receptor protein, and thus have two null alleles of the Class 1 type[209] (and unpublished data). In the Dallas collection, a significantly higher percentage of the Class I FH homozygotes are true homozygotes as compared with the overall sample — 85 versus 41 percent — which is consistent with the relative rarity of the null alleles in the general population.

Multiple molecular defects in the LDL receptor gene produce null alleles. These include deletions that remove the LDL receptor promoter and thus produce no mRNA (example: *FH French Canadian-1*[210]) as well as nonsense, frameshift, and splicing mutations.

Class 2 Mutations: Transport-Defective Alleles. The rate of transport of the LDL receptor from the ER to the Golgi can be measured in pulse-chase experiments in which fibroblasts are incubated with [^{35}S]methionine, and the receptor is isolated by immunoprecipitation and SDS polyacrylamide gel electrophoresis.[124] The normal receptor is synthesized in the ER as a partially glycosylated precursor that migrates with an apparent molecular mass of 120 kDa. When the receptor reaches the Golgi, the *N*- and *O*-linked sugars are processed so that the receptor migrates with an apparent mass of 160 kDa.[124,211] In normal fibroblasts, this transport and processing occur within 60 min after synthesis. In Class 2 fibroblasts, transport to the Golgi is markedly delayed or

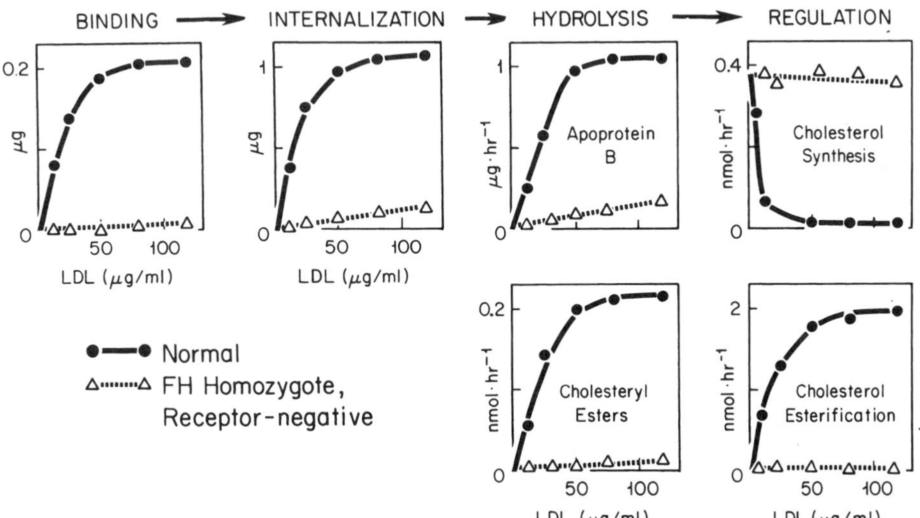

Fig. 120-24 Actions attributable to the LDL receptor in fibroblasts from a normal subject (●) and from a homozygote with the receptor-negative form of FH (△) incubated with varying concentrations of ^{125}I-LDL or unlabeled LDL at 37°C for 5 h. Assays were performed in growing cells in monolayers.[391] All data are normalized to 1 mg of total cell protein. The units for each assay are as follows: *Binding*, μg of ^{125}I-LDL bound to cell surface; *internalization*, μg of ^{125}I-LDL contained within the cell; *hydrolysis of Apo B-100*, μg of ^{125}I-LDL degraded to ^{125}I-monoiodotyrosine per hour; *hydrolysis of cholesteryl esters*, nM of [^{3}H]cholesterol formed per hour from the hydrolysis of LDL labeled with [^{3}H]cholesteryl linoleate; *cholesterol synthesis*, nM of [^{14}C]acetate incorporated into [^{14}C]cholesterol per hour by intact cells; *cholesterol esterification*, nM of [^{14}C]oleate incorporated into cholesteryl [^{14}C]oleate per hour by intact cells. (*From M. S. Brown and J. L. Goldstein,* Proc Natl Acad Sci U S A *76:3330, 1979. Used by permission.*)

abolished, and the apparent molecular mass of the receptor remains at 120 kDa.[124,142,211] Eventually, the receptor is degraded without ever having reached the cell surface.[212] Two subsets of Class 2 mutations are recognized.[140] The more common Class 2B alleles are "leaky" in that a variable portion of the newly synthesized receptor is transported at a reduced rate to the Golgi and then to the cell surface. Class 2A alleles produce a protein that fails to be transported out of the ER so there is no detectable 160-kDa mature form of the receptor.

Class 2A and 2B alleles contain missense mutations or short in-frame deletions that partially or completely disrupt folding of the receptor. The failure of surface transport suggests that cells have a fail-safe mechanism that detects misfolded proteins and prevents their movement from the ER to the Golgi.[154] A similar conclusion has been reached from the study of other cellular and viral proteins that follow the same transport pathway.[213]

A total of 85 (54 percent) of the 157 FH homozygotes in the Dallas collection have at least one Class 2 allele, making it the most common phenotype in the sample. Most Class 2 defects cluster in the exons that encode the ligand-binding domain, and most of the remainder are in the EGF precursor homology domain (see Fig. 120-22). The mutations are not evenly distributed among the ligand-binding repeats. Repeat 5 (the last repeat encoded by exon 4) contains more mutations than any other repeat. This suggests that repeat 5 occupies a crucial structural position so that any alteration in its sequence interferes with folding. The preferential involvement of this repeat may also reflect selection bias. In vitro mutagenesis studies showed that repeat 5 is the only repeat in which missense mutations reduce the binding of lipoproteins containing apo E as well as apo B-100.[144] Thus, Class 2B receptors with missense mutations in repeat 5 that reach the cell surface should interfere with plasma clearance of IDL as well as LDL and produce a more severe phenotype than do mutations in other repeats (discussed below).

In the Dallas collection, of the 32 Class 2 mutations within the ligand-binding domain, 29 involve amino acid residues that are highly conserved between multiple animal species.[156] A more recent analysis of point mutations at the LDL receptor locus revealed that 74 percent of the mutations in the ligand-binding domain involved highly conserved amino acid residues that tended to be located in the 3′ half of the repeat.[207]

Insight into the mechanism by which sequence variations in the ligand-binding domain lead to a Class 2 phenotype has emerged from the crystal structure of repeat 5.[21] Amino acid substitutions of any of the six residues that coordinate the binding of Ca^{2+} in the repeat interfere with the folding of the protein (Fig. 120-19). Short in-frame deletions or insertions of part of a repeat, such as occurs in *FH Lithuania* (*G197del*),[140,214] change the spacing between highly conserved cysteine residues, thus interfering with disulfide bond formation. This is in contrast to the deletion of an entire cysteine-rich repeat, such as the *FH Paris-1* (*del exon 5*)[215] where repeat 6 is deleted, which does not impair its transport to the cell surface.

Most of the remaining Class 2 alleles bear mutations in the EGF precursor homology domain, and many of these map to one of the three growth factor repeats (A, B, and C). All missense mutations in the C repeat in the Dallas collection produce a Class 2 phenotype. The *FH Lebanese* (*C660X*) allele is a nonsense mutation in the third of six cysteine residues in repeat C.[216] The mutant gene produces a reduced amount of receptor protein with an apparent molecular mass of 100 kDa that lacks the *O*-linked sugar, membrane spanning, and cytoplasmic domains. The truncated protein is apparently misfolded, and it fails to reach the Golgi.[212,216] In vitro mutagenesis studies showed that the observed lack of transport of the mutant receptor out of the ER cannot be attributed simply to mispairing of the first two cysteine residues; when the first two cysteine residues were mutated to serines, the receptor protein was still sequestered in the ER.[212] The remainder of Class 2 mutations in the EGF precursor domain are located in the region between the B and C growth factor repeats, which contains the six YWTD repeats that form the compact β-propeller structure.

Approximately 20 percent of the Class 2 mutations in the Dallas collection produce a complete block in transport of the receptor protein out of the ER (Class 2A), and most of these mutations are located within the EGF precursor homology domain. This region of the human receptor protein is 84 percent identical to the same region in the Xenopus receptor[156] and is the second most highly conserved sequence of all domains in the receptor protein. Considered together, these findings suggest that this domain has a compact structure that is easily disrupted if only a single amino acid is changed.

In addition to FH, several other inborn errors of metabolism are caused by mutations that produce transport-defective proteins.[140,217] These mutations involve genes for membrane proteins, such as leukocyte adhesion protein, sucrase-isomaltase, the insulin receptor, the cystic fibrosis transmembrane conductance regulator (CFTR), and rhodopsin. They also involve secretory proteins, including α_1-antitrypsin, fibrillin, pro-α1(I) collagen, and pro-α2(I) collagen. Together with the observations on the LDL receptor, these findings suggest that a transport-defective phenotype may frequently underlie mutations involving cell-surface or secreted proteins. This high frequency is attributable to the ability of the cell to detect small regions of misfolding within a protein and thereby to interdict its movement to the cell surface.[154,213]

Class 3 Mutations: Binding Defective Alleles. Many of the mutant alleles at the LDL receptor locus produce proteins that exhibit more than one type of functional defect. For example, in many Class 2B alleles, the receptor that reaches the cell surface is also defective in ligand binding. The failure of transport precludes study of the ligand-binding capacity, and thus the overall frequency of Class 3 alleles is difficult to estimate. Some mutant alleles produce receptors with defective ligand binding but normal intracellular transport, and thus are designated Class 3. Most of these alleles contain in-frame rearrangements in the cysteine-rich repeats of the ligand-binding domain or in the adjacent growth factor repeats of the EGF precursor domain.

Deletions of individual ligand binding repeats have different effects on the ability of the receptor to bind LDL and β-VLDL. For example, in *FH Paris-1* (*del exon 5*) repeat 6 is deleted in its entirety, and the mutant LDL receptor binds β-VLDL with normal affinity but fails to bind LDL.[215]

In vitro mutagenesis studies have shown that replacement of a single conserved amino acid in a ligand-binding repeat produces the same functional abnormality as does deletion of the entire repeat.[144] Thus, when the isoleucine adjacent to the third cysteine residue in each of the seven repeats was individually changed to an aspartic acid, the resultant receptors had the same binding characteristics as did receptors lacking each of those repeats.[144] *FH Puerto Rico* (*S156L*)[218] and *FH French Canadian-3* (*E207K*),[219] two slowly processed Class 2B alleles, have replacements in the highly conserved D*x*SDE sequence in repeats 4 and 5, respectively. The *FH Puerto Rico* (*S156L*) receptor fails to bind LDL, but binds β-VLDL with near-normal affinity.[218] Substitution of a lysine for glutamic acid in the D*x*SDE sequence of repeat 5 as in the *FH French Canadian-3* mutation results in reduced amounts of both β-VLDL and LDL binding.[219] These results match the results obtained when repeats 4 and 5, respectively, were deleted in vitro[144] and are consistent with the suggestion that certain missense mutations have deleterious effects on only a single repeat.

Normal binding of LDL, but not β-VLDL, requires at least one cysteine-rich repeat in the EGF precursor homology domain.[148,220] If the A repeat or the A plus B repeats are deleted (as in *FH Leuven-1* and *FH Cape Town-2*) (*del exons 7 and 8*), β-VLDL binding is maintained, but LDL binding is markedly reduced.[220,221] Deletion of repeat B alone has no effect on binding of either ligand.[220] If the entire EGF precursor domain is deleted, as in *FH Osaka-2* (*del exons 7–14*),[222] the receptor is unable to bind LDL but continues to bind β-VLDL.[148] If such a truncated receptor is denatured in SDS, subjected to electrophoresis under nonreducing conditions, and transferred to nitrocellulose, it recovers its ability to bind LDL.[148] These observations suggest that the EGF precursor homology domain plays a role in allowing the ligand binding domain to gain access to LDL on the cell surface in addition to its role in receptor recycling (discussed below).

Insertions within the ligand-binding domain of the LDL receptor can also produce a Class 3 phenotype. The best-characterized insertion, *FH St. Louis (dup exons 2–8)*, encodes a receptor protein that is 50 kDa larger than normal (apparent molecular mass of 210 versus 160 kDa on SDS gels).[223] The elongated protein results from a 14-kb duplication of exons 2 to 8 (discussed below) and contains 18 contiguous cysteine-rich repeats instead of the usual 9. Seven of these duplicated repeats are derived from the ligand-binding domain, and two come from the EGF precursor homology region. Remarkably, the elongated receptor is transported normally to the cell surface where it binds reduced amounts of LDL[223] and β-VLDL (unpublished data). Thereupon, it undergoes efficient internalization and recycling.[223] Thus, the only effect of the extensive duplication is a reduction in ligand binding.

Class 4 Mutations: Internalization-Defective Alleles. Studies with the electron microscope show that the Class 4 receptors are distributed diffusely over the surface of the cell and are not concentrated in coated pits.[142,224] They, therefore, cannot carry bound LDL into the cell. These rare mutations are of considerable historical interest because they provided the earliest evidence that cell-surface receptors must cluster in clathrin-coated pits in order to carry ligands into cells.[3,224] Six internalization-defective alleles were characterized through cloning and confirmed by functional studies. All have mutations that alter the 50-amino acid cytoplasmic domain.[152,225–228] The mutations were subclassified into two groups, based on whether the mutation involves the cytoplasmic domain alone (Class 4A) or the cytoplasmic domain together with the adjacent membrane-spanning region (Class 4B).[140]

Two internalization-defective mutations, *FH Bahrain (W792X)* and *FH Paris-3 (N796fs)*,[225] have premature stop codons that leave the membrane-spanning region intact, but leave the receptor with only the first 2 or 6 of the normal 50 amino acids in the cytoplasmic tail, respectively. Another Class 4 mutation, the *J.D.* allele (*FH Bari* allele; *Y807C)*, has a single base pair change that substitutes a cysteine for a tyrosine at amino acid residue 807 in the cytoplasmic domain.[152] The latter observation stimulated a series of in vitro mutagenesis experiments, which revealed that position 807 must be occupied by an aromatic amino acid (tyrosine, phenylalanine, or tryptophan) for internalization to occur normally.[229]

Tyr807 is part of a tetrameric sequence NPVY (Asn-Pro-Val-Tyr) that is conserved in LDL receptors from six species.[230] A variant of this sequence, NPxY (where x can be any amino acid), is present in one or more copies in the cytoplasmic tails of other members of the LDL receptor gene family, including LRP,[231] megalin/gp330 protein (Heymann nephritis antigen),[232] the VLDL receptor,[233] and the chicken vitellogenin receptor[234] (discussed below). Extensive in vitro mutagenesis experiments confirmed the importance of the NPxY sequence as a signal for directing the LDL receptor to coated pits.[230] An NPxY sequence is also present in the cytoplasmic domains of at least 13 other cell-surface receptors, including several with tyrosine kinase activity (EGF, c-erb-B/*neu*, insulin, insulin-like growth factor 1), the β-subunits of the integrin receptors, and the amyloid precursor protein.[230]

Sequences other than NPxY are responsible for localization of other receptors in coated pits. In the transferrin receptor and the mannose 6-phosphate receptor, the signal for coated-pit clustering involves sequences of four to six amino acids that contain at least one aromatic residue, usually a tyrosine, but lack the other elements of the NPxY signal.[235] Computer modeling[236] and MRI studies[237] suggest that the common feature in all of these sequences is the ability to form a tight turn that orients the aromatic residue in a fixed configuration. Presumably, the coated-pit assembly proteins recognize the aromatic residue within this tight turn, and they thereby move the receptor to a coated pit.[238]

The second subclass of internalization-defective alleles (Class 4B) produces truncated receptors that lack the membrane-spanning domain as well as the cytoplasmic tail. Most of these molecules are secreted from the cell, but approximately 10 percent remain adherent to the cell membrane where they bind LDL but do not internalize it, thus giving rise to the internalization-defective phenotype. Three deletion mutations—*FH Rochester*,[226] *FH Osaka-1*,[227] and *FH Helsinki*[228]—have this phenotype. All of the deletions extend from intron 15 to the noncoding region of exon 18, but each has a different end point. In each case, the truncated intron 15 is not removed by splicing. Translation of the mRNA continues into intron 15, and this produces an abnormal C-terminal sequence that contains 55 novel amino acids.[227] This sequence includes a cluster of 14 hydrophobic amino acids that may constitute a pseudotransmembrane domain that anchors some of the receptors to the cell membrane.[227] Inasmuch as this novel sequence lacks the NPxY signal, it is unable to direct the receptor to coated pits, hence the lack of internalization.

Class 5 Mutations: Recycling-Defective Alleles. In addition to its role in facilitating the binding of LDL, the EGF precursor homology domain mediates the acid-dependent dissociation of receptor and ligand in the endosome, an event that is essential for receptor recycling.[148] This function was discovered when the EGF precursor homology domain was deleted by in vitro mutagenesis of an expressible LDL receptor cDNA. The truncated LDL receptor bound and internalized β-VLDL, but it failed to release the ligand in the acidic environment of the endosome. The receptor was then degraded, apparently because it was unable to return to the surface in an unoccupied state.[148] A naturally occurring mutation, *FH Osaka-2 (del exons 7–14)*, with the same deletion and phenotype was described by Miyake et al.[222] (discussed above).

Deletion of the A and B growth factor repeats produces a receptor with the same ligand-binding properties as *FH Osaka-2* (that is, ability to bind β-VLDL but not LDL).[220] van der Westhuyzen et al.[221] demonstrated that such a mutant receptor, *FH Cape Town-2 (del exons 7 and 8)* is more rapidly degraded even in the absence of ligand binding, which suggests that the A and B repeats play a role in receptor recycling.

A total of 22 percent of the fibroblast strains in the Dallas collection have a Class 5 phenotype. The relative number of mutant alleles with this phenotype has been underestimated in prior analyses, because Class 5 mutations can produce a phenotype that superficially resembles Class 3 mutations in terms of deficient LDL binding. The Dallas collection contains 11 Class 5 alleles that are caused by missense mutations, all of which occur in the EGF precursor homology domain. Springer[149] noted a disproportionately high number of mutations that are clustered in the region of the β-propeller domain that is predicted to lie in close physical proximity with EGF repeats B and C.

Promoter Mutations. To date, only five naturally occurring mutations (four single-bp changes and one 3-bp deletion) have been mapped to the transcriptional regulatory elements of the LDL receptor gene (Fig. 120-20).[198,239–241] *FH Pedi-2* has a 3-bp deletion, CTT(-92), involving the final C of the consensus sequence of repeat 1, which is adjacent to an Sp1 binding site. The mutation was found in a compound heterozygote whose other LDL receptor allele has a frameshift mutation in exon 2 (*FH Pedi-1; E37fs)*.[198] Functional assays performed on cultured fibroblasts from this homozygote revealed that the amount of LDL binding, uptake, and degradation was ~10 percent of normal (unpublished data). The other four mutant alleles, *FH Columbia-2 [C(-42)G]*,

C(-43)T, FH Albuquerque [C(-44)T], and *C(-45)T*, each contain single-bp substitutions in repeat 3.[198,240,241] These mutations (demarcated by shaded boxes in Fig. 120-20) are located in the most conserved sequence of the Sp1 recognition site (CCGCCC). Changes at these sites are expected to reduce markedly the binding of Sp1, as was documented for one of these mutations that was found in two heterozygotes, one from Finland and the other from Denmark.[239,240] In the Finnish study, a fragment from the LDL receptor promoter containing the C(-43)T nucleotide substitution was transfected into cultured cells. Transcription of a reporter gene was reduced by 95 percent when compared with the wild-type promoter.[240] In the Danish study, the amount of endogenous mRNA generated from the C(-43)T mutant allele was less than 5 percent of that produced from the wild-type allele.[239]

The relative paucity of mutations within the promoter region of the gene is probably attributed to the small number of base pairs that are crucial for promoter function (<50).

General Characteristics of LDL Receptor Gene Mutations

Distribution of Point Mutations. Analysis of the distribution of 353 point mutations and small deletions/insertions in the LDL receptor gene reveals a higher-than-expected frequency of mutations in exon 4 (Fig. 120-22). One-fifth of all the mutations (78 of 353) are located in exon 4, which is larger than all the other exons and encodes ligand-binding repeats 3, 4, and 5. Within exon 4, the region that encodes the fifth ligand-binding repeat is particularly enriched in mutations. As mentioned previously, the overrepresentation of mutations within this region may be due to selection bias because these mutations tend to be associated with more severe disease.[242] Mutations in exon 15 (clustered O-linked sugar domain) are underrepresented in the sample (Fig. 120-22). This region is the least-conserved domain of the receptor and, not surprisingly, contains only one nonsense and one splicing mutation. Deletion of this domain has no effect on LDL receptor function in fibroblasts[118] and is associated with only mild hypercholesterolemia in humans *(FH Espoo; del exon 15)*.[243]

The actual nucleotide sequence of a given repeat may also predispose to mutations. Three different duplications ranging in size from 8 to 21 bp involve the same 8 bp near the C-terminus of ligand-binding repeat 5.[244] All three insertions are flanked by the sequence GAC, which may promote slipped strand mispairing.[245] Day et al.[204] found other hot spots for mutations at sites with short tandemly repeated sequences in exons 6, 11, and 12 of the LDL receptor gene.

Mutations Involving *Alu* Repeats. Many deletions and insertions in the LDL receptor gene arise because of recombination between *Alu*-type elements, the predominant middle repetitive DNA sequences in mammals. The human genome contains about 910,000 *Alu* repeats[246] that are distributed throughout all chromosomes. Most are located in intergenic regions and introns,[247] but some are present in mature mRNAs, as in the 3′ untranslated region of the LDL receptor. Each *Alu* sequence of approximately 300 bp is composed of two tandem repeats designated the left and right arms. *Alu* repeats can be transcribed by RNA polymerase III, which recognizes sequence blocks in each arm that act as a bipartite promoter, resembling those of the 5S ribosomal RNA genes and tRNA genes.[247] The large number of *Alu* repeats in the human genome and the possible instability stemming from their transcription have led to the idea that these sequences might serve as sites for genome rearrangements.[248] This hypothesis has received its strongest support from the almost invariant finding of *Alu* sequences at the junctions of large rearrangements in mutant LDL receptor genes.[215,222,223,226,227,249,250]

Of the 11 deletions that have been sequenced and characterized from genomic DNA, 10 possess an *Alu* repeat at one or both mutation end points. The locations of 10 of these mutations are shown in Fig. 62-22 on p. 2001 of the seventh edition of this book.[208] The other mutation, a 10-kb deletion *(FH Konazawa)* that removes exons 2 and 3[251] is not shown. Two of the *Alu*-mediated deletions, *FH Rochester (del exons 16–18)*[226] and *FH Osaka-2 (del exons 7–14)*[227] resulted from recombination between two *Alu* sequences oriented in opposite directions. In one of these (*FH Rochester*) inverted repeats in the region surrounding the deletion joint may have formed an intrastrand double-stem loop structure that facilitated the recombination.[226] More commonly, the recombination occurs between two *Alu* repeats in the same orientation, as in *FH Paris-1 (del exon 5)*,[215] *FH London-1 (del exons 13 and 14)*,[249] and *FH Aarhus-3 (del exon 5)*.[250] It is presumed that homology between the *Alu* sequences led to a mispairing of chromosome 19 chromatids during meiosis, followed by an unequal crossover that deletes the intervening sequence. The same type of *Alu*-mediated recombination can result in the reciprocal event, namely a duplication of exons as found in *FH St. Louis (dup exons 2–8)*[223] (discussed above and below). Single *Alu* sequences can also instigate gene rearrangements as has been found at the recombination site in at least nine human genes,[140] including one in the LDL receptor gene *FH Potenza (del exons 13–15)*.[252]

An important question is whether the preponderance of *Alu*-mediated recombinations in the LDL receptor gene is caused by an unusually large number of *Alu* sequences in this gene. To date, approximately 25 percent of the 45-kb human LDL receptor gene has been sequenced, and 28 *Alu* repeats have been identified, indicating an average distribution of one *Alu* sequence per 1.6 kb of gene,[140] which is twofold more frequent than the average region of the genome. In the human genome, one *Alu* repeat occurs on average every 3 kb (3 $\times$ 109 bp/900,000 *Alu* repeats). This twofold increase may be significant. It parallels the findings with globin genes. More *Alu*-mediated recombination events have been described in the α-globin locus, where the distribution of *Alu* repeats is 1 per 2 kb,[253] than in the β-globin locus, where the frequency is 1 per 10 kb.[254] Thus, it seems likely that the number of rearrangements in a region of DNA may rise in geometric fashion with the number of *Alu* sequences, each of which may act as a hot spot for recombination.[255]

Recurrent Mutations. Numerous LDL receptor mutations have been identified in two unrelated individuals with different ethnic backgrounds. Receptor haplotype analysis[197a] can be used to determine if the two individuals inherited the same mutant allele from a common ancestor. Unless there has been recombination within the LDL receptor locus, a mutation will remain associated with the haplotype of the allele on which the mutation originally arose. For example, the *FH Afrikaner-1* mutation was also found in an individual from Maine. In *FH Afrikaner-1 (D206E)* and *FH Maine (D206E)*, haplotype analysis with 10 RFLP sites showed an identical restriction pattern except for the 5′-most site.[140] It is likely that these two mutant alleles descended from the same chromosome, and subsequently a recombinational event occurred, accounting for the single RFLP difference between the two alleles.

If identical mutations arose independently, they should be found on chromosomes with different haplotypes. For example, *FH Gujerat (P664L)* was identified in an Indian from Zambia as well as in an Englishman. The haplotypes of the two alleles differed at five of eight RFLP sites examined.[256] Multiple recurrent mutations at the LDL receptor have been described, some of which were reviewed in the seventh edition of this textbook (see pages 1997–2000).[208]

Cytosine (C) to thymidine (T) transitions at a cytosine-guanine (CpG) dinucleotide are a frequent cause of mutations in the human genome.[257] In most genetic disorders ~32 percent of the disease-causing mutations involve CpG dimers,[245] but at the LDL receptor locus only 20 percent of the point mutations are C-to-T substitutions.[207]

Spontaneous *De Novo* Mutations. The marked allelic genetic heterogeneity at the LDL receptor locus suggests a high mutation rate in this gene. Thus, it is surprising that only three FH heterozygotes have been identified with an LDL receptor mutation that is not found in either of their biological parents (proved by paternity testing).[258–260]

Two Mutations in Same LDL Receptor Allele. Jensen et al.[261] described an LDL receptor allele that carried both a missense mutation in exon 11 *(N543H)* and a 9-bp deletion in exon 17 *(del 778–780)*. The relative role of each mutation was determined by recreating each mutation separately in a recombinant LDL receptor expression construct. Both recombinant mutant proteins had only slightly reduced LDL receptor function when expressed in transfected cultured cells. In contrast, when both mutations were placed in the same expression construct, LDL receptor function was reduced by 75 percent. Eleven examples of double mutations in the same receptor allele have been reported and are listed at *www.umd.necker.fr*.[207] Double mutations have also been identified in numerous other disease-causing genes.[262] For most genetic disorders, molecular screening is terminated as soon as one disease-causing mutation in an allele is identified. It is possible that some of the discrepancies observed between genotype and phenotype in genetic diseases, including FH, result from undetected double mutations.

Population Genetics

In most populations of the world, the frequency of heterozygous FH is ~0.2 percent (discussed above). In certain populations, the frequency is much higher, owing to founder effects (Table 120-4). The highest frequency is found in three different populations of South Africa — the Ashkenazi Jews (1 in 67),[103] the South African Indians (estimated at 1 in 100),[263] and the Afrikaners, in whom the prevalence of FH (1 in 100) is fivefold higher than in the European population from which it originated.[43]

The high frequency of FH in the Ashkenazi Jews of South Africa is likely attributable to their origin from a genetically isolated population of ~40,000 Lithuanian Jews who emigrated to South Africa between 1880 and 1910. In support of this hypothesis, a mutation identified in a patient from New Jersey, *FH Lithuania (del G197)*[140] was present in 8 of 10 South African Ashkenazi Jews tested.[214] This same mutation comprises 35 percent of mutant LDL receptor genes in the Ashkenazi Jews of Israel, 64 percent of whom are of Lithuanian origin.[214]

The Indians of South Africa are suspected of having a high frequency of FH because the same LDL receptor mutation *(P664L)* was identified in four unrelated Indians residing in South Africa.[263,264] This mutation was previously identified in a Zambian subject.[265] The Zambian subject and the four South African Indians are all Muslims originating from the province of Gujerat in India. Many Indians from this region emigrated to different parts of the world, so it is likely that this mutation will be identified in Indians with FH in other locales.

In the Afrikaners, three alleles, *FH Afrikaner-1 (D206E), FH Afrikaner-2 (V408M),* and *FH Afrikaner-3 (D154N),* comprise over 90 percent of the mutant LDL receptor genes responsible for FH.[266,266a] The most common allele, *FH Afrikaner-1*, is found in 60 to 70 percent of the FH patients. *FH Afrikaner-2* and *FH Afrikaner-3* alleles are present in 20 to 30 percent and 5 to 10 percent, respectively. The high frequency of these three alleles can also be attributed to founder effects. The Afrikaners are descended from about 2000 original settlers — mostly from Holland, Germany, and France — who emigrated to the Cape of South Africa in the seventeenth and eighteenth centuries. The ancestry of an individual with the *Afrikaner-2* mutation was traced to a small town in the Netherlands (Ankijk), which was the site of departure of some of the original emigrants to South Africa.[267] The other common mutant allele, *FH-Afrikaner-1*, appears to have its origin in England rather than the Netherlands.[267a] In the nineteenth century, the Afrikaners moved into the interior of the country, the Transvaal, where they remained largely isolated from the surrounding populations. The fertility rate was high, and the

Table 120-4 **Inbred Populations with Mutant LDL Receptor Alleles that Account for >15% of the Mutant Alleles in that Population**

Inbred Population	Mutation	Percent of FH Heterozygotes with Mutation
Christian Lebanon	*FH Lebanese (C660X)*	100
South African:		
Ashkenazi Jews	*FH Lithuania (G197del)*	80
Asian Indians	*FH Gujerat (P664L)*	>15*
Afrikaners	*FH Afrikaner-1 (D206E)*	60–70
	FH Afrikaner-2 (V408M)	20–30
French Canada	*FH French Canadian-1 (del 5′ flanking region-intron 1)*	60
	FH French Canadian-4 (W66G)	18
Iceland	*FH Iceland (IVS4+2T>C)*	60
Finland	*FH Helsinki (del exons 15–18)*	34
	FH North Karelia (P288fs)	34
Israel:		
Sephardic Jews	*FH Sephardic (D147H)*	>15*
Druze	*FH Druze (Y167X)*	>15*
Ashkenazi Jews	*FH Lithuania (G197del)*	35
Norway	*FH Elverum (IVS3+1G>A)*	28
Greece	*FH Genoa (D528G)*	23
	FH Afrikaner-2 (V408M)	15
Spain	*E10X*	20
Belgium (Southern)	*C122X*	16
Denmark	*FH French Canadian-4 (W66X)*	15
	FH Cincinnati-5 (W23X)	15

*Too few individuals were tested to determine an accurate frequency.

population grew dramatically to its present size of approximately 3 million. In addition to FH, Afrikaners have a high frequency of several other genetic disorders, owing to founder effects.[267]

Another African country with a high incidence of FH is Tunisia. The incidence of FH in this North African country is ~1 in 165, and approximately 60 percent of the FH homozygotes are offspring of consanguineous marriages.[267a]

The frequency of FH heterozygotes in the French Canadian population is estimated to be 1 in 270 based on the number of FH homozygotes identified in Quebec Province in 1981.[101] An even higher frequency (1 in 154) was found in the northeastern region of the province. The French Canadians have a high frequency of several other genetic disorders,[269] all of which are attributed to founder effects. The 5.3 million modern French Canadians are descended from about 8000 French settlers who emigrated to Quebec Province from western France between 1608 and 1763, founding an agrarian population that has remained physically and socially isolated.[269]

French Canadian-1, a large deletion in the 5′ end of the LDL receptor gene that produces a Class 1 phenotype,[210] was found in 59 percent of 130 French Canadian FH heterozygotes from Montreal.[210,219] The same mutation was identified in only one of 42 FH heterozygotes who lived in the western part of France and in none of 30 Parisian FH heterozygotes.[270] This finding supports the idea that the high frequency of this mutation in French Canadians is due to a founder effect. Screening for the *French Canadian-1* mutation plus five other less common mutations (*French Canadian-2* to *-6*) will detect ~80 percent of the mutant LDL receptor alleles in the French Canadian population.[219,271] Two of these mutations, *FH French Canadian-3 (E207K)* and *FH French Canadian-4 (W66G)*, were identified in FH homozygotes from France who are patients of Professor J. L. deGennes and Dr. F. Dairou of the Hopitaux de Paris.

A total of four mutations are known to be common causes of FH in the Middle East—*FH Lebanese (C660X), FH Lithuania (del G197), FH Sephardic (D174H)*, and *FH Druze (Y167X)*. The *FH Sephardic* and *FH Druze* mutations have been identified in unrelated families in Israel.[272,273] The Druze are a relatively small Islamic sect that has remained remarkably isolated for ~1000 years,[272] but the exact frequency of FH within the group has not been determined.

The Christian Lebanese population played an important role in delineation of the genetics of FH, owing to Khachadurian's pioneering clinical studies (discussed above). The Dallas collection contains eight FH homozygotes with a Christian Lebanese ancestry. All were found to be homozygous for the *FH Lebanese (C660X)* allele[216] (and unpublished observations), which has not yet been identified in any other population. The exact frequency of the mutation in Lebanon has not been determined, but the high frequency of homozygosity suggests that it is common.[97]

In general, European and North American populations have a plethora of LDL receptor mutations, each of low frequency and typically limited to a single family. Exceptions include the Finnish population in which either of two mutant alleles, *FH Helsinki (del exons 16–18)* or *FH North Karelia (frameshift 287)*, is present in two-thirds of individuals with heterozygous FH.[274,275] The prevalence of each of these mutations varies in different geographic regions, *FH Helsinki* predominating in the Northern region and *FH North Karelia* in the Eastern region of Finland. Screening for these two mutations, plus two less frequent mutations, detects over 75 percent of the mutant alleles in Finland.[276] Three mutations accounted for 43 percent of the defective LDL receptor alleles in 476 Norwegian FH heterozygotes.[277] The population of Iceland is largely of Norwegian origin, but a splicing mutation found in 60 percent of Icelandic FH heterozygotes[278] has not been identified in Norway. In Denmark, 42 percent of individuals with FH have one of three LDL receptor mutations: *W23X* (15 percent), *W66G* (15 percent), and *W556S* (12 percent).[279,279a]

Clusters of unrelated FH patients sharing the same mutant allele have been identified in other regions of Europe. In Greece, 60 percent of 150 FH heterozygotes had one of six different mutations.[280,281] Two mutations *(E10X* or *del G518)* were present in 30 percent of FH heterozygotes in the Aragon region of Spain.[282] In southern Belgium, a nonsense mutation of exon 4 was found in 16 percent of individuals suspected of having FH.[283] In two regions of England, Manchester[284] and the southern part of the country,[285] two different mutations each had a frequency of ~10 percent. In Japan, 30 percent of the FH heterozygotes had one of five different mutations, none of which had a frequency >15 percent.[286]

Correlation of Receptor Mutations and Clinical Expression

Clinical Variability Among FH Homozygotes. In individuals with homozygous FH, the concentration of plasma LDL and the severity of coronary atherosclerosis vary, even among individuals who are homozygous for the same mutations, indicating that other genes play important roles. This variability is exemplified by two individuals, both of whom were homozygous for the *French Canadian-1* allele, which abolishes production of receptor mRNA and protein.[210] In one of the homozygotes, FH 49, symptoms of coronary atherosclerosis did not develop until age 17. Despite treatment with multiple lipid-lowering medications and ileal bypass, her cholesterol level remained between 600 and 1200 mg/dl. Nevertheless, she lived until age 33. Although she had longstanding angina pectoris, she did not die of a myocardial infarction, but of malignant melanoma.[210] Another individual, FH 549, also homozygous for the *French Canadian-1* allele, died suddenly at age 3 and at autopsy had severe three-vessel coronary atherosclerotic disease.[48,210]

Some of the clinical variability results from the nature of the particular LDL receptor mutation. FH homozygotes with one or two mutant receptor alleles whose products retain some LDL receptor function have a lower level of plasma cholesterol and have less aggressive coronary atherosclerosis than individuals with two totally nonfunctional receptor alleles (see Fig. 120-4). Moojani[287] compared 10 French Canadians homozygous for a large deletion *(del 5′ flanking region-intron 1; French Canadian-1)* with an equal number of homozygotes with a missense mutation in exon 3 (*W66F; French Canadian-4*). Total plasma cholesterol levels in the FH homozygotes with the deletion were significantly higher than the levels in those with the missense mutation, with no overlap between the two groups (1068 versus 644 mg/dl). Homozygosity for the deletion was associated with earlier age of onset of coronary artery disease (12.7 versus 23.6 years).

In general, the severity of clinical manifestations of homozygous FH tends to correlate with the activity level of the LDL receptor, as assessed in cultured fibroblasts. An exception to this general trend is seen with the *French Canadian-4* mutation. This missense mutation *(W66F)* is the most perplexing of all the mutations in the LDL receptor gene. The *W66F* mutant allele produces a receptor of normal size that is processed at the usual rate, but its functional activity in fibroblasts from patients homozygous for the mutation varies from 25 to 100 percent of controls.[198,288] Yet, despite this variability in fibroblast assays, FH homozygotes with this mutation all share the clinical manifestations of classic homozygous FH. The lack of correlation between the activity of a mutant LDL receptor allele in fibroblasts and the clinical expression of the disease suggests a liver-specific derangement in the function of this particular mutant protein.

Clinical Variability Among FH Heterozygotes. The nature of the molecular defect in the LDL receptor appears to have less effect on the plasma level of LDL cholesterol in FH heterozygotes than in homozygotes. For example, the plasma levels of total cholesterol in subjects heterozygous for the *French Canadian-1* and *-4* alleles (324 versus 288 mg/dl) were much more similar than levels in the corresponding homozygotes (1068 versus

644 mg/dl).[287] In the deletion group (*French Canadian*-1 allele), the plasma cholesterol level of heterozygotes was ~33 percent of that of the homozygotes, whereas in the missense group (*French Canadian-4* allele) the level in the heterozygotes was ~50 percent of that of the homozygotes. The proportionally higher cholesterol level in FH heterozygotes with the missense mutation suggests that the mutant protein may act in a dominant-negative fashion to interfere with the synthesis or function of the wild-type receptor.

Individuals heterozygous for a mutant LDL receptor allele with no receptor activity tend to have higher plasma levels of LDL cholesterol than those having alleles that retain some residual activity. This is illustrated in the Afrikaner population where FH heterozygotes with the *Afrikaner-2* mutation *(V408M)*, which produces no receptor activity, have significantly higher plasma levels of LDL than those with the *Afrikaner-1* mutation *(D206E)*, which has ~20 percent of normal receptor activity (plasma LDL levels of 360 mg/dl versus 308 mg/dl).[289]

The clinical manifestations of heterozygous FH are also modified by environmental factors, especially diet. In Tunisia, many individuals heterozygous for an LDL receptor mutation had plasma levels of LDL cholesterol lower than the 95th percentile when compared to North American controls.[268] Cardiovascular complications are distinctly uncommon, and no tendon xanthomas were found in 27 Tunisian FH heterozygotes (ages 32 to 80), all of whom were parents of FH homozygotes. It is likely that the low-fat Mediterranean diet consumed in this region of the world is responsible for the lower plasma levels of LDL.

The clinical expression of FH in China is markedly attenuated as compared to that of FH in Western countries.[290] Xanthomas are absent, and symptomatic coronary artery disease is rare in Chinese FH heterozygotes. To determine if genetic differences between Chinese and Caucasians were responsible for the milder disease in the Chinese, Pimstone et al.[291] compared the mean levels of plasma LDL cholesterol in 18 FH heterozygotes from mainland China and 16 from Canada. The Chinese heterozygotes had significantly lower mean LDL levels (174 versus 298 mg/dl). The lower plasma levels of LDL in FH subjects living in China reflects the much lower plasma levels of cholesterol in the general population of this country, owing to their low-fat diet.[292]

Variability Caused by Differential Ligand Receptor Interactions. Among individuals with different LDL receptor mutations, one source of clinical variability stems from the relative effect of different mutations on the ability of the receptor to bind lipoproteins containing apo B-100 or apo E. Several mutations in the ligand binding and EGF precursor homology domains of the receptor abolish binding of LDL, without impairing binding of apo E-containing lipoproteins, such as β-VLDL (discussed above).

Normal LDL metabolism begins with the triglyceride-rich particle, VLDL, which is secreted by the liver. In capillaries, the triglycerides of VLDL are removed by lipoprotein lipase, forming a denser, more cholesterol-rich, apo E-containing particle termed "IDL." Approximately 50 percent of this IDL is cleared by hepatic LDL receptors, which recognize apo E with high affinity.[293] Even when receptors are normal, some IDL remains in the plasma, where it is converted into LDL.[293]

In FH homozygotes with a mutation that blocks binding of both IDL and LDL, the synthesis of LDL is increased because the precursor IDL cannot be cleared efficiently by the liver.[293] The degradation of LDL is decreased, owing to the defective receptors. As a result of this combined overproduction and undercatabolism, LDL rises to high levels.[3,293] In contrast, if the mutant LDL receptor retains the ability to bind IDL, but not LDL, the production of LDL may be normal. The major abnormality is a delayed removal of LDL from plasma, and the overall effect is a more moderate elevation in plasma LDL.

Experimentally, it is difficult to obtain sufficient plasma IDL to perform binding studies with human cells. As a substitute for IDL, we use β-VLDL,[144,220] which is a mixture of lipoproteins of d < 1.006 g/ml obtained from the plasma of cholesterol-fed rabbits.[120,141] β-VLDL contains particles that are equivalent to IDL, as well as chylomicron remnants, which also bind to LDL receptors by virtue of the apo E content.

Clinical studies of a few FH individuals who have LDL receptors that retain the ability to bind β-VLDL suggest that these mutations are indeed associated with relatively mild disease. The proband of the O. family[294] is homozygous for the *FH Denver-2 (D283N)* allele, which substitutes asparagine for the first aspartic acid residue of the D*x*SDE sequence in repeat 7 of the ligand binding domain.[140] The mutation produces a Class 2B receptor that reaches the cell surface slowly and binds β-VLDL, but not LDL[294] (and unpublished observations). LDL turnover studies performed in the proband and her obligate heterozygous parents demonstrated a reduced fractional catabolic rate of the injected radiolabeled LDL, but no increase in LDL production.[295] This is in marked contrast to the results with other FH homozygotes and heterozygotes in whom LDL production is increased. Both heterozygous parents of *FH Denver-2* have only a modest elevation in plasma cholesterol[296] and lack symptomatic coronary atherosclerosis, as do the other heterozygotes in the family.

Variability Caused by an LDL-Lowering Gene. Studies of one FH family, the P. family, have provided evidence that some of the variability in clinical expression of FH may be attributable to a dominant LDL-lowering allele that suppresses the effect of receptor mutations.[218] The mutant LDL receptor allele in the P. family has a missense mutation that substitutes leucine for serine in the D*x*SDE sequence of the fourth ligand-binding repeat.[218] The mutant receptor binds β-VLDL, but not LDL. This allele, *FH-Puerto Rico (S156L)*, is present in homozygous form in 1 individual and in heterozygous form in 18 relatives. LDL turnover studies performed in the homozygote as well as in four heterozygotes from the P. family disclosed a phenotype similar to that seen in the O. family (discussed above). The fractional catabolic rate for LDL was decreased without an increase in the production rate.[297]

One-third of the FH heterozygotes in the P. family, including the proband's mother, have concentrations of plasma LDL below the 90th percentile of the population despite their LDL receptor mutation. The remaining 12 heterozygotes have shown LDL levels above the 95th percentile. Genetic analysis suggests the presence of a gene segregating in an autosomal dominant fashion whose effect is to lower the plasma LDL level. This putative suppressor gene is not linked to the LDL receptor locus itself or to the genes for apo B-100, apo E, apo C-I, apo C-II, apo C-III, hepatic lipase, lipoprotein lipase, LRP, VLDL receptor, 7α-hydroxylase, HMG-CoA reductase, SREBP-1, SREBP-2, SCAP, and the ileal bile acid transporter, as determined by linkage analysis[218] (and unpublished observations). Evidence for an LDL-lowering allele has also been found in a French Canadian family with FH due to a deletion of exons 2 and 3 of the LDL receptor gene.[298] Two of the eight carriers of this mutation in this family have a normal LDL cholesterol level.

Production of Half-Normal Number of LDL Receptors in Heterozygotes

In normal fibroblasts, the synthesis of the LDL receptor is regulated by feedback transcriptional suppression.[112,115,160] The number of receptors declines about tenfold when cellular cholesterol stores are increased by incubation of cells with a usable exogenous source of cholesterol, such as LDL or cholesterol dissolved in ethanol.[115] The number of receptors increases again when the exogenous cholesterol is removed and cellular cholesterol levels fall. In the steady state, the number of receptors is adjusted to allow just enough LDL uptake to provide sufficient cholesterol for cell growth and to balance cholesterol losses.[112,115]

Under conditions that induce a maximal rate of receptor synthesis (i.e., vigorous growth in the absence of an exogenous source of cholesterol), FH heterozygote cells in tissue culture produce about half as many functional receptors as do normal cells.[299] More important, when grown in the presence of increasing amounts of exogenous cholesterol, the heterozygote and normal cells suppress their LDL receptor activities in parallel. Over a ten- to twentyfold range of LDL receptor activities, at any given concentration of intracellular cholesterol the heterozygote cells express about half as many receptors as do normal cells.[299] This relationship is evident even in the range of LDL receptor levels in which the heterozygote cells clearly have the capacity to produce as many active LDL receptors as do the normal cells—that is, when the appropriate number of receptors is less than half the maximal number.[299] The lack of compensation by the normal receptor allele is due to the heterozygote cells, at all levels of exogenous cholesterol, expressing a slightly higher activity of HMG-CoA reductase, which compensates for their cellular cholesterol deficit by synthesis rather than receptor-mediated uptake.

These findings indicate that in the heterozygous cells the regulatory mechanism dictates that the normal allele produces only the amount of gene product that it would normally produce at a given level of cellular cholesterol. The failure of the regulatory mechanism to stimulate the normal allele at the LDL receptor locus to produce twice its normal amount of gene product leaves the heterozygote cells with a persistent 50 percent deficiency in LDL receptors under all conditions of cell growth. Pharmacologic interventions can perturb this cellular regulatory mechanism in vivo (discussed below).

LDL Receptor Mutations in Animals

WHHL Rabbit. A rabbit model for FH, the Watanabe-heritable hyperlipidemic (WHHL) rabbit, was discovered in the late 1970s by Yosio Watanabe, a veterinarian at Kobe University in Japan (Fig. 120-25).[300] Homozygous WHHL rabbits are markedly hypercholesterolemic from the time of birth, and severe atherosclerosis develops by 2 to 3 years of age.[293] The mutation is a 12-bp in-frame deletion that removes 4 amino acids from the fourth ligand-binding repeat of the LDL receptor.[154] The mutant protein has a Class 2B/3 phenotype and reaches the cell surface at a markedly reduced rate.[294] The few receptors that reach the surface retain the ability to bind β-VLDL, but not LDL. WHHL rabbits are extremely useful in dissecting the role of the LDL receptor in vivo (discussed below)[293] and in testing strategies for treatment of FH using gene therapy.[301]

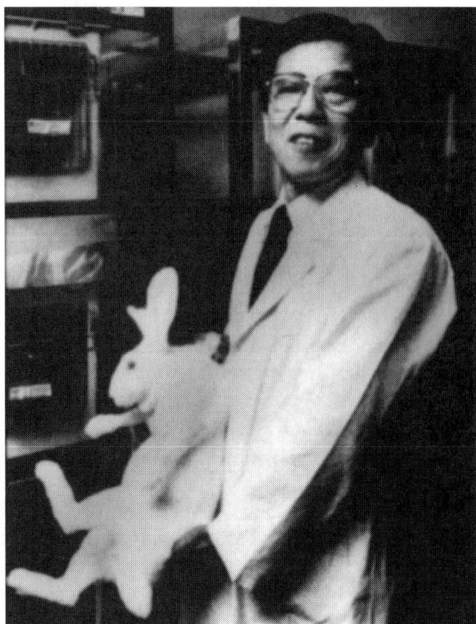

Fig. 120-25 Photograph of Dr. Yoshio Watanabe, Kobe University, Japan, together with one of his WHHL rabbits. (*Courtesy of Dr. Toru Kita.*)

Rhesus Monkey. A second animal model for FH was described by Scanu et al.[302] in a pedigree of rhesus monkeys with hypercholesterolemia inherited in an autosomal dominant pattern. Fibroblasts from the hypercholesterolemic monkeys showed a half-normal level of LDL receptor activity, protein, and mRNA. The responsible mutation, a point mutation that produces a stop codon at amino acid 284, was identified by selectively amplifying and sequencing each exon of the monkey LDL receptor gene with oligonucleotide primers homologous to the human sequences.[303]

Mice. The technique of homologous recombination in cultured embryonic stem cells was used to produce a line of mice that lack functional LDL receptor genes (*LDLR*$^{-/-}$ mice).[304] Homozygous male and female *LDLR*$^{-/-}$ mice are viable and fertile. Total plasma cholesterol levels are twofold higher than those of wild-type littermates, owing to a seven- to ninefold increase in IDL and LDL without a significant change in HDL. Plasma triglyceride levels are normal. The half-lives for intravenously administered ^{125}I-VLDL and ^{125}I-LDL are prolonged by 30 times and 2.5 times, respectively, but the clearance of ^{125}I-HDL is normal in the *LDLR*$^{-/-}$ mice. Unlike wild-type mice, *LDLR*$^{-/-}$ mice responded to moderate amounts of dietary cholesterol (0.2% cholesterol/10% coconut oil) with a major increase in the cholesterol content of IDL and LDL particles.

When the *LDLR*$^{-/-}$ mice were fed a high-cholesterol diet (1.25 percent cholesterol/7.5 percent cocoa butter/7.5 percent casein/0.5 percent cholic acid), the total plasma cholesterol rose from 246 to > 1500 mg/dl, whereas wild-type littermate mice fed the same diet had cholesterol levels < 160 mg/dl.[305] After 7 months on this diet, the *LDLR*$^{-/-}$ mice developed massive xanthomatous infiltration of the skin and subcutaneous tissue (Fig. 120-26*A-D*). The aorta and coronary ostia exhibited gross atheromata, and the aortic and coronary ostia were thickened by cholesterol-laden macrophages (Fig. 120-26*E,F*).

On a regular chow diet, the *LDLR*$^{-/-}$ mice have LDL cholesterol levels that are much lower than those in FH homozygotes,[305] primarily because mouse liver, in contrast to human liver, produces apo B-48 in addition to apo B-100 (Chap. 115). Lipoproteins containing apo B-48 can be removed from plasma by alternate receptors, especially LRP (discussed below). To circumvent this problem, and to create a more exact model of the human disease, *LDLR*$^{-/-}$ mice have been crossed with mice expressing a human apo B-100 transgene[306] and also with mice that produce only mouse apo B-100 (and no apo B-48) in their livers.[307] These two lines of mice manifest plasma levels of LDL cholesterol that are as high as in FH homozygotes and develop extensive complex atherosclerotic lesions, even when the mice consume a regular low-fat chow diet.

The *LDLR*$^{-/-}$ mice offer a new model for the study of environmental and genetic factors that modify the process of atherosclerosis and xanthomatosis. They also provide a useful model to explore somatic-cell gene therapy targeted at the liver. For example, intravenous injection of a recombinant replication-defective adenovirus encoding the human LDL receptor driven by the cytomegalovirus promoter reduced the elevated plasma IDL/LDL level to normal, restored expression of LDL receptor protein in the liver, and increased the clearance of ^{125}I-VLDL.[304]

Swine. A strain of spontaneously hypercholesterolemic pigs was found to have a missense mutation (R94C) in the third ligand repeat of the LDL receptor gene.[157,157a] Biosynthetic studies of the mutant receptor have not been performed, but this allele is likely to have a Class 2 phenotype because insertion of an additional cysteine residue into the repeat is predicted to interfere with its folding. The inheritance pattern of the hypercholesterolemia

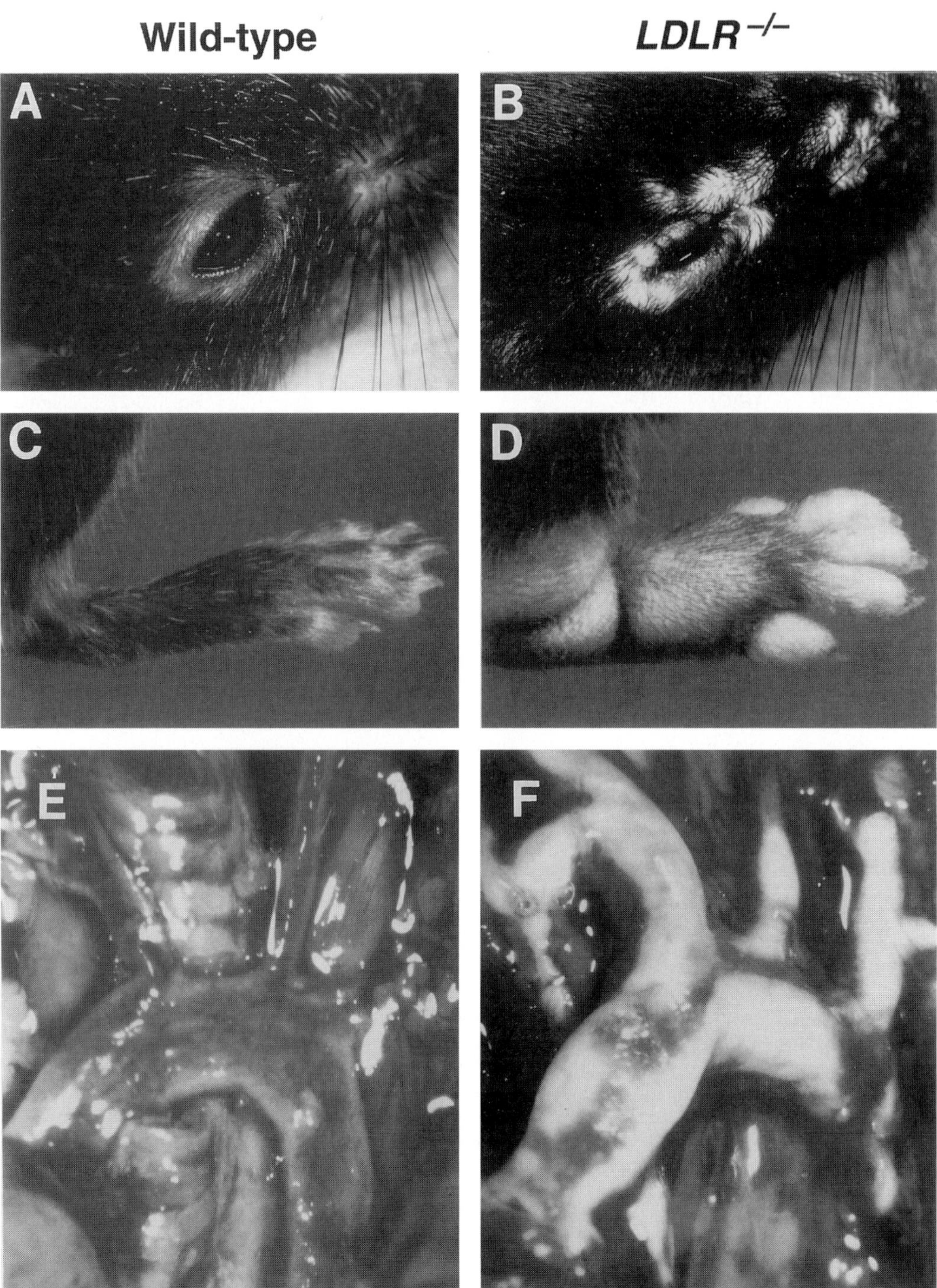

Fig. 120-26 Xanthomas and aortic arch atherosclerosis in LDL receptor knockout mice (*left panels*) as compared with xanthoma-free and atherosclerosis-free wild-type mice (*right panels*). Mice of both genotypes were fed a 1.25 percent cholesterol diet for 8 to 9 months. The *LDLR*$^{-/-}$ mice show xanthomatous involvement of ears and eyelids (xanthelasmas) (*B*), tendon xanthomas of the hind paw (*D*), and extensive aortic plaque formation visible through the thin aortic wall (*F*). The total cholesterol level was 173 to 264 mg/dl in the wild-type mice and 1893 to 2360 mg/dl in the *LDLR*$^{-/-}$ mice. (*Data from Ishibashi et al.*[305] *Used by permission of* Journal of Clinical Investigation.)

associated with this mutation appears to be autosomal recessive; pigs heterozygous for the mutation are normolipidemic.

LDL Receptor Gene Family

The LDL receptor gene is a mosaic of exons shared with several other genes.[139,140,147] These shared sequences fall into three types. The first type is the 40-amino acid cysteine-rich repeat of the LDL-binding domain, which is found in complement factors (C7, C8α, C8β, C9). The second type of shared sequence is the growth factor repeats of the EGF homology region, which are found in plasma proteases of the blood-clotting system (factor IX, factor X, protein C, thrombospondin), cell-surface receptors (TGF-α precursor, ELAM-1, GMP-140, thrombomodulin), adhesive glycoproteins (tenascin, cartilage proteoglycan core protein), and developmental proteins (*Notch, lin-12, delta*).[140] The third type of shared sequence, the six 40-amino acid YWTD repeats that form a β-propeller structure,[149] is interdigitated between clusters of the growth factor repeats. These six YWTD repeats are found in

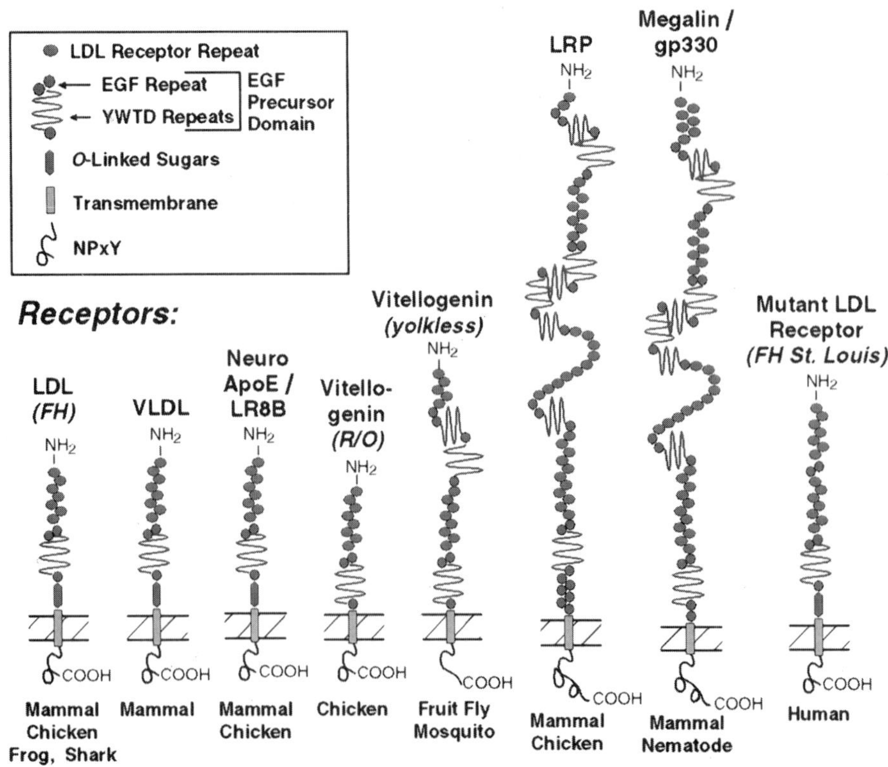

Fig. 120-27 Similarities in shared exons and transmembrane orientation in seven members of the LDL receptor gene family. The mutant human LDL receptor (shown at extreme right) refers to *FH St. Louis (dup exons 2–8)*. The evolutionary significance of this duplication mutation is described in the text. Naturally occurring mutations that disrupt receptor function are denoted in parentheses: *FH*, familial hypercholesterolemia in mammals; *R/O*, restrictor ovulator in chickens; and *yolkless* in *Drosophila melanogaster.*

similar locations in the LDL receptor and the EGF precursor.[139,140,147] In general, all three types of shared sequences are encoded by discrete exons. These findings support Gilbert's exon-shuffling hypothesis[308] in which exons encoding functional protein domains are reused during evolution.

As discussed above, many genes of diverse function possess one or two of the shared types of sequences that are found in the LDL receptor. Only one family of genes shares sequences of all three types. This family is designated the LDL receptor gene family (Fig. 120-27), and all seven known members are cell-surface proteins that bind ligands and transport them into cells by receptor-mediated endocytosis in coated pits. In addition to these three sets of shared exon-encoded sequences, all of these proteins, except the insect receptor, have at least one copy of the NP*x*Y internalization sequence in the cytoplasmic domain (see Fig. 120-27).

Five members of the LDL receptor gene family—the LDL receptor, LRP, the VLDL receptor, the neuro apo E/LR8B receptor, and the chicken vitellogenin receptor—are known to bind and internalize plasma lipoproteins. LRP differs structurally from the LDL receptor primarily because of size. It contains 31 complement-type ligand-binding repeats organized in 4 clusters and 22 growth factor repeats that are separated by 8 YWTD-containing β-propellers. LRP differs functionally from the LDL receptor in that it only binds lipoproteins that are enriched in vitro with excess apo E.[309] LRP is able to bind and internalize at least 20 known ligands, ranging from lipoprotein particles (chylomicron remnants) and protease inhibitors (α-2-macroglobulin) to plasminogen activators.[310] Each ligand probably binds to a unique combination of ligand-binding repeats in LRP.

The VLDL receptor differs functionally from the LDL receptor in that it binds apo E-containing lipoproteins (without the need for enrichment with exogenous apo E), but not LDL.[233] This receptor and the LDL receptor show strikingly different tissue distributions in vivo. The LDL-receptor mRNA is expressed primarily in adrenal cortex and liver with virtually no expression in heart, skeletal muscle, and adipose tissue.[3,154] The VLDL-receptor mRNA is expressed at highest levels in the heart with moderately high expression in skeletal muscle, adipose tissue, and brain, but only in trace amounts in the liver.[233] Although this pattern of expression supports the hypothesis that the VLDL receptor may be involved in uptake of triglycerides from VLDL,[233] a knockout of its gene in mice revealed no abnormality in plasma-lipoprotein levels on normal, high-carbohydrate, or high-fat diets.[310a] The sole abnormality detected was a modest decrease in body weight and adipose tissue mass.

The chicken vitellogenin receptor, expressed exclusively in the developing oocyte, binds and internalizes two yolk proteins: VLDL and vitellogenin. It does not bind LDL.[237] The chicken vitellogenin receptor transports 1.5 g of protein into the chicken oocyte each day, as the single cell grows to the size of a grade AA jumbo egg over seven days. A mutation in this receptor causes the female-sterile "restricted ovulator" phenotype, in which chicken oocytes do not grow to normal size.[311] A mutation in the *Drosophila* homologue of the vitellogenin receptor also produces a female-sterile phenotype, *yolkless*.[312]

Megalin/gp330 is a large protein that resembles LRP.[232] It resides in coated pits on the tubular (apical) surface of epithelial cells in the renal glomerulus and proximal tubule. It is a target for an autoantibody that circulates in rats with Heymann-type autoimmune nephritis.[313] The function of megalin/gp330 is unknown, but it binds most, if not all, of the ligands that are recognized by LRP, including apo E-enriched lipoproteins.[310,314]

The genomic rearrangements that underlie exon shuffling in the LDL receptor gene family may be continuing at the present time owing to the recombinational activity of the *Alu* elements (discussed above). Figure 120-27 shows the structure of a mutant LDL receptor that is produced by the *FH St. Louis (dup exons 2–8)* allele and compares it with the other members of the LDL receptor gene family. As discussed above, this mutant gene has undergone an *Alu*-mediated duplication of 14 kb, which reiterates exons 2 to 8.[223] Although the resulting protein has two complete ligand-binding domains, it binds LDL and β-VLDL poorly. In contrast to the earlier duplications that gave rise to the seven repeats in the ligand-binding domain of the wild-type LDL receptor, this new rearrangement is deleterious, and so is expected to disappear through natural selection. It is possible to envision another duplication that might improve or expand the function of

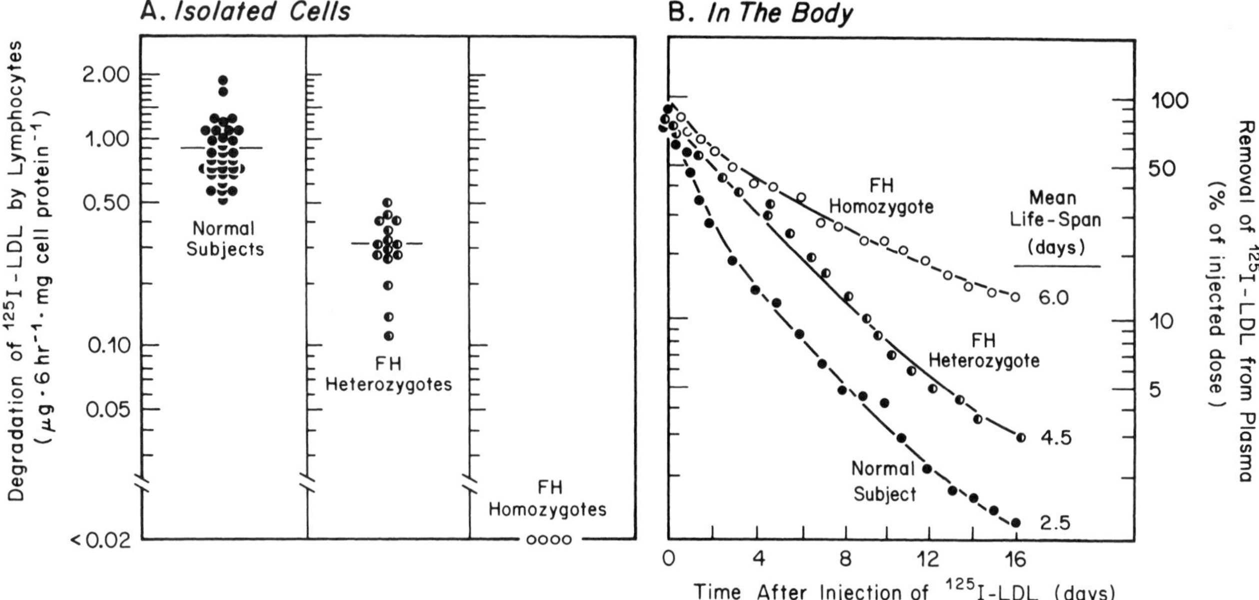

Fig. 120-28 Measurement of the number of LDL receptors in blood lymphocytes (*A*) and in living subjects (*B*). *A*. Lymphocytes were isolated from venous blood of 32 normal patients, 15 FH heterozygotes, and 4 FH homozygotes, as indicated. After incubation for 67 h at 37°C in medium containing 10 percent lipoprotein-deficient serum, LDL receptor activity was assessed by measurement of the high-affinity degradation of ^{125}I-LDL at 37°C. *B*. In the whole-body assay, a tracer amount of ^{125}I-LDL was injected intravenously, and the radioactivity remaining in the circulation over the next 16 days was measured in samples of venous blood. The higher the number of LDL receptors on body cells (*A*), the faster the removal of ^{125}I-LDL from the blood (*B*). (*Data in A replotted from Bilheimer et al.*[318] *Data in B replotted from Bilheimer et al.*[320])

the LDL receptor, especially given that different combinations of cysteine-rich repeats mediate binding of different apoprotein ligands to the LDL receptor.[144]

PATHOGENESIS AT THE WHOLE-BODY LEVEL

The initial demonstration of the LDL receptor pathway in cultured human fibroblasts was followed by its demonstration in virtually all animal cells that grow in culture.[4,112] In each of these cell types, LDL cholesterol is used for membrane synthesis and for the regulation of cholesterol homeostasis. In cultured mouse and bovine adrenal cells, LDL serves an additional function: its cholesterol is a precursor for steroid hormone formation.[315,316]

LDL Receptor Expression in Vivo

The first cells demonstrated to have LDL receptor activity in vivo were circulating blood lymphocytes. When incubated for 67 h in vitro in the absence of exogenous cholesterol so as to derepress receptor synthesis, lymphocytes expressed abundant LDL receptors as determined by measurements of the high-affinity uptake and degradation of ^{125}I-LDL (Fig. 120-28*A*).[317,318] Lymphocytes from receptor-negative FH homozygotes did not express detectable LDL receptor activity and lymphocytes from FH heterozygotes had an intermediate level consistent with the presence of only a single functional gene. LDL receptors were also detectable on lymphocytes immediately after their isolation from the bloodstream, although the level of activity was lower than it was after derepression for 67 h.[318]

Another early clue to the function of LDL receptors in vivo came from studies of the rate of disappearance of intravenously injected ^{125}I-LDL from plasma (Fig. 120-28*B*). Such LDL is removed from the circulation more slowly in FH heterozygotes than it is in normal persons.[319,320] In FH homozygotes, the removal defect is even more profound.[320–322] The sluggishness of LDL catabolism in vivo correlates with the relative deficiency of LDL receptors as determined in isolated lymphocytes (see Fig. 120-28).

More detailed demonstrations of LDL receptor function in vivo have been obtained in experimental animals. An assay to measure the binding of ^{125}I-LDL to membranes from homogenates of animal tissues showed that most organs of the cow had detectable high-affinity ^{125}I-LDL binding; the adrenal gland and ovarian corpus luteum had the highest activity on a per-gram basis.[323] When the organ's weight was considered, the liver was found to produce by far the largest number of LDL receptors. Similar results were obtained in studies of human fetal tissues.[324] In perfused rat livers, ^{125}I-LDL is taken up by a high-affinity receptor-mediated process that is markedly accelerated when LDL receptors are increased by administration of an estrogen, such as 17α-ethinyl estradiol.[325] When radiolabeled LDL is injected into the circulation of experimental animals, approximately 70 percent of the total-body uptake of radiolabeled LDL takes place in the liver by LDL receptor-dependent pathways.[326–330]

A useful method to measure the relative amounts of LDL cleared by LDL receptor-dependent and LDL receptor-independent pathways takes advantage of the observation that chemical modification of lysine or arginine residues on LDL abolishes receptor binding.[121,122] In this method, native LDL is labeled with one isotope, such as ^{125}I, and lysine- or arginine-modified LDL is labeled with another isotope, such as ^{131}I. The mixture is injected intravenously, and the relative rate of the clearance of the native LDL versus the modified LDL gives a measure of the relative contribution of LDL receptors to overall LDL clearance (Table 120-5).[331–333] In healthy young humans, lysine-modified (glycosylated) LDL is removed from the circulation only one-fifth as rapidly as native LDL, indicating that four-fifths of the clearance of LDL is mediated by the receptor pathway (Fig. 120-29).[333,334]

The relative contribution of LDL receptors to LDL clearance can also be estimated by comparing the rate of catabolism of intravenously injected ^{125}I-LDL in normal individuals and in FH homozygotes.[110] The fractional catabolic rate of LDL (i.e., the fraction of the total plasma pool of LDL removed per unit time) is about threefold higher in normal subjects than in FH homozygotes

Table 120-5 Receptor-Mediated Clearance of Plasma LDL in Vivo

Species	Modified LDL Used to Measure Receptor-Independent Degradation	LDL Degraded by Receptors, %
Rat	Methyl-LDL	50–75
Guinea pig	Methyl-LDL	78
	Glucosylated LDL	78
Hamster	Methyl-LDL	72
Rabbit	Methyl-LDL	67
	Glucosylated LDL	62–75
Rhesus monkey	Methyl-LDL	50
Human	Glucosylated LDL	80

NOTE: Modification of the lysine residues on LDL by either methylation or glucosylation abolishes its ability to bind to LDL receptors. Such modified LDL is cleared from the circulation of humans and animals much more slowly than is native LDL, thus providing an in vivo method for quantifying the fraction of LDL clearance attributable to LDL receptors. The original studies from which the data in the table are derived are cited in the reference listed below.

SOURCE: From Brown and Goldstein.[113] Used by permission of the *Journal of Clinical Investigation.*

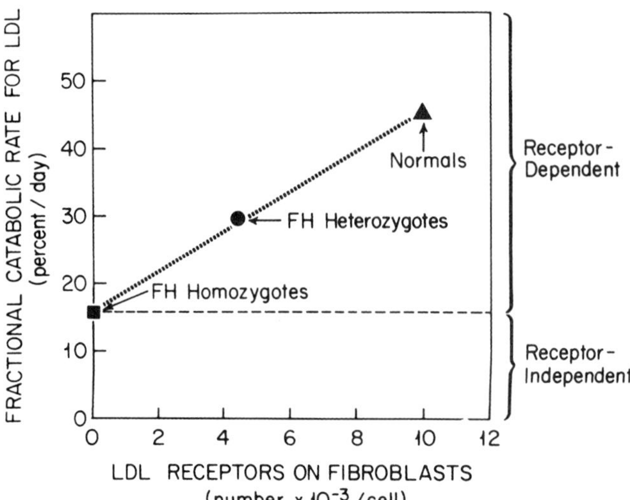

Fig. 120-30 Relation between the fractional catabolic rate (FCR) for plasma LDL and the number of LDL receptors on fibroblasts in patients with FH. The values for the FCR were derived from studies of the turnover of ^{125}I-apo-LDL in the plasma of 6 normal subjects, 6 FH heterozygotes, and 11 FH homozygotes. These turnover studies were performed by Bilheimer et al.[320] and by Myant and co-workers.[321,349] The number of LDL receptors per cell was calculated from experiments in which maximal ^{125}I-LDL binding was measured at 4°C in actively growing fibroblasts that were deprived of LDL for 48 h.

(Fig. 120-30). This method therefore suggests that approximately two-thirds of LDL clearance is normally mediated through the LDL receptor.[110]

In addition to its ability to bind LDL and IDL, which carry endogenous cholesterol, the LDL receptor binds chylomicron remnants, which transport dietary cholesterol from the intestine to the liver (Chap. 115). Although appreciable amounts of chylomicron remnants can be cleared from the circulation by hepatic LDL receptors,[335] a second chylomicron remnant receptor must exist. FH homozygotes,[336] FH heterozygotes,[337] and WHHL rabbits[338] clear chylomicron remnants from the bloodstream at normal rates despite their deficiencies of LDL receptors. The most likely candidate for the second chylomicron remnant receptor is LRP, a multifunctional receptor that binds several ligands, including apo E-enriched chylomicron remnants, and internalizes them into the liver[309,339] (discussed above).

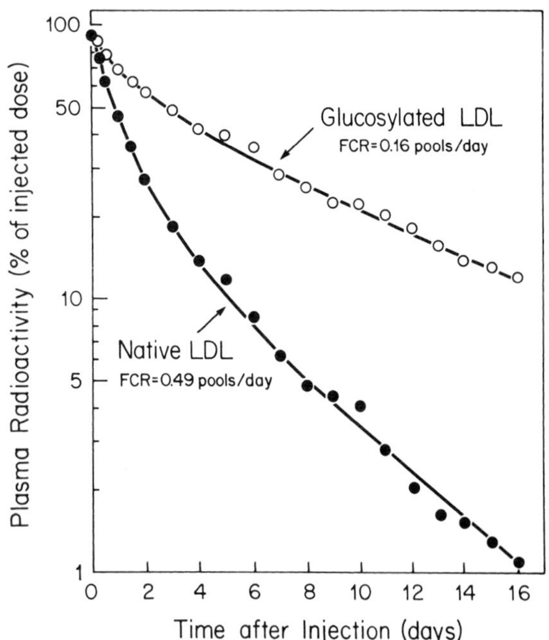

Fig. 120-29 Plasma die-away curves after the IV injection of native ^{125}I-LDL (●) and glucosylated ^{125}I-LDL (○) in a normal subject. FCR = fractional catabolic rate for LDL. *(From D. W. Bilheimer, S. M. Grundy, M. S. Brown, J. L. Goldstein.* Trans Assoc Am Phys *96:1, 1983. Used by permission.)*

Dual Mechanism for Elevated Plasma LDL in FH

An important function of LDL receptors in vivo was first appreciated in studies performed in WHHL rabbits (discussed above; see Fig. 120-25). WHHL rabbits have a mutation in the LDL receptor gene that is similar to the Class 2B/3 mutations in human FH.[154,294,340] In the homozygous form, this mutation gives rise to extremely high LDL cholesterol levels,[341] and atherosclerosis develops early in life.[293,300,342–344]

As discussed in an earlier section, the *WHHL* allele produces a mutant receptor that is transport-deficient and has an altered ligand specificity as studied in cultured cells. In vivo the liver expresses a markedly reduced but detectable number of mutant receptors that can bind apo E-containing lipoproteins. It may also bind reduced, but detectable, amounts of LDL. This mutant receptor gene is subject to regulation, and under certain conditions, it can be increased in amount sufficiently to lower the plasma cholesterol level. Pregnancy in WHHL homozygotes increases the amount of ^{125}I-LDL binding in liver membranes from almost undetectable levels to 20 percent of the values seen in nonpregnant rabbits.[345] This increase in hepatic LDL receptor number was associated with a fall in the plasma LDL-cholesterol level from a mean of 410 to 90 mg/dl.[345] In another study, combined treatment with a bile acid binding resin and an HMG-CoA reductase inhibitor increased LDL receptor mRNA in the WHHL liver 3.4 times, increased receptor activity from 2.5 to 25 percent of that in normal untreated rabbits, and lowered plasma LDL cholesterol by 56 percent.[346] Ethinyl estradiol treatment[347] and partial ileal bypass[348] also raised LDL receptor mRNA and lowered plasma cholesterol levels in WHHL rabbits. Thus, the LDL receptor in WHHL rabbits retains sufficient function to lower plasma cholesterol when its expression is enhanced.

WHHL rabbits have proved invaluable in explaining a previously puzzling feature of homozygous FH. Kinetic studies of ^{125}I-LDL metabolism by Soutar et al.[349] and by Bilheimer et al.[320] indicated that FH subjects have a dual defect. In addition

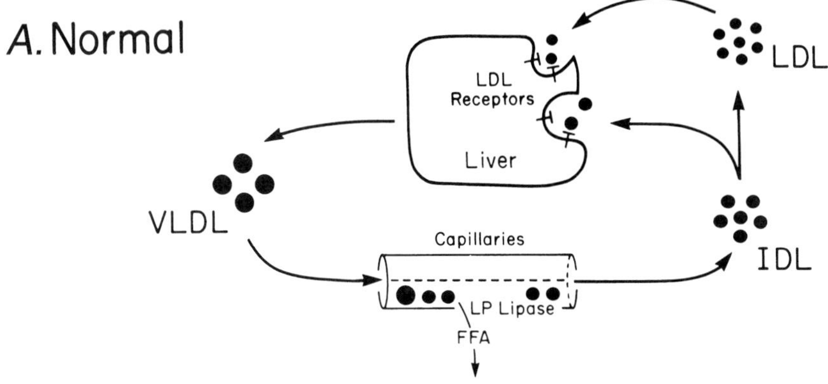

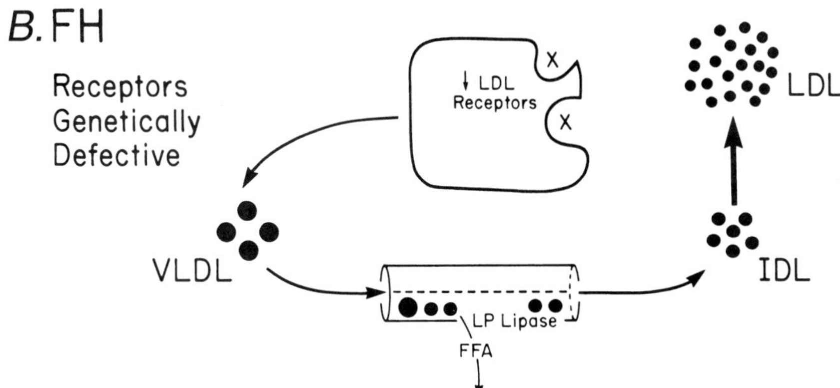

Fig. 120-31 Schematic of the mechanism by which LDL receptors in the liver control both the production and catabolism of plasma LDL in normal human subjects (*A*) and in individuals with FH (*B*). (*From M. S. Brown and J. L. Goldstein.*[3] *Used by permission of* Science.)

to degrading LDL more slowly, FH homozygotes and heterozygotes also appeared to overproduce LDL. How does a genetic defect in the LDL receptor lead simultaneously to overproduction and reduced degradation of LDL? The answer lies in the complex biosynthetic pathway for LDL.

Early studies by Gitlin et al.[350] and later studies by Bilheimer et al.[351] suggested that LDL is not secreted directly from the liver, but that it is, instead, produced in the circulation from a bloodborne precursor, VLDL (Fig. 120-31). VLDL is a large, triglyceride-rich lipoprotein that is secreted by the liver; it transports triglyceride to adipose tissue and muscle. The triglycerides in VLDL are removed in capillaries by the enzyme lipoprotein lipase, and the VLDL is transformed into a smaller particle called IDL (Chaps. 115 and 119). IDL particles have lost most of their triglyceride, but they retain cholesteryl esters. The IDL particles contain multiple copies of apo E in addition to a single copy of apo B-100. As discussed earlier, the multiple copies of apo E allow IDL to bind to the LDL receptor with very high affinity. The liver rapidly takes up some of the IDL particles; others remain in the circulation, where they undergo further triglyceride hydrolysis and are converted to LDL. When IDL is converted to LDL, the apo E leaves the particle and only apo B-100 remains. Thereafter, the affinity for the LDL receptor is much reduced.

The apparent overproduction of LDL in WHHL rabbits is due in large part to the failure of IDL to be removed from the plasma[293,352,353] (see Fig. 120-31*B*). Thus, when ^{125}I-VLDL was administered to WHHL rabbits, the liver did not take up the resultant IDL, as it was in normal rabbits.[352,353] Rather, it remained in the circulation and was converted in increased amounts to LDL. These findings suggest that IDL is normally cleared from plasma by binding to LDL receptors in the liver. Although experiments of similar detail cannot be carried out in humans, the observations of Soutar et al.[349] are consistent with the notion that enhanced conversion of IDL to LDL also occurs in FH homozygotes, thus accounting for much of the apparent overproduction of LDL.

Figure 120-31*A* illustrates the dual role of the LDL receptor in LDL metabolism as determined from the studies of WHHL rabbits. First, the receptor limits LDL production by enhancing the removal of the precursor, IDL, from the circulation. Second, it enhances LDL degradation by mediating cellular uptake of LDL. A deficiency of LDL receptors in FH causes LDL to accumulate as a result both of overproduction and of delayed removal (Fig. 120-31*B*). By this quirk of dual functionality, LDL receptors become crucially important modulators of plasma LDL levels in humans and animals.

Certain tracer studies that compare the metabolism of labeled VLDL, IDL, and LDL suggest that FH homozygotes and WHHL rabbits may secrete enhanced amounts of LDL directly into the circulation.[348,349,354] However, other kinetic studies[353] and direct liver perfusion studies[355] in WHHL rabbits failed to show direct secretion of an LDL particle with apo B-100 as the sole apoprotein. It seems likely, but has not been proved, that the apparent direct overproduction of LDL observed in some studies may be attributable to the existence of a population of VLDL that is rapidly catabolized and is, therefore, underrepresented in the VLDL that is radiolabeled. In LDL receptor deficiency, these VLDL particles may fail to be cleared and may be rapidly converted to LDL, thus explaining the apparent direct production of LDL.

Receptor-Independent Removal of LDL

As discussed above and as illustrated in Fig. 120-30, the fraction of plasma LDL cleared each day by the receptor-independent pathway in FH homozygotes and heterozygotes is inversely related to the number of functional LDL receptors. In homozygotes with no receptors, receptor-independent pathways degrade all the plasma LDL. In heterozygotes with 50 percent of the normal receptor number, about half of plasma LDL is degraded by receptor-independent pathways, whereas in normal subjects only one-third is degraded by this route (see Fig. 120-30). Kinetic studies of ^{125}I-LDL turnover in vivo have demonstrated that the receptor-independent removal pathway is considerably less efficient than the receptor-dependent pathway.[320,354] For example, in FH homozygotes in whom all LDL removal is by receptor-independent pathways, each LDL particle circulates with a life span of 6 days as compared with a life span of 2.5 days in normal subjects.

Despite the potential importance of the receptor-independent pathway in FH patients, virtually nothing is known about the responsible cellular and biochemical mechanisms. Studies in WHHL rabbits suggest that the receptor-independent removal of LDL is divided about equally between the liver and the extrahepatic tissues.[328,356]

Some of the receptor-independent clearance of LDL occurs in macrophages and histiocytes of the reticuloendothelial system, which are referred to collectively as "scavenger cells."[111,357,358] FH homozygotes accumulate considerable amounts of cholesterol in foam cells of the artery wall, splenic macrophages, hepatic Kupffer cells, and bone marrow histiocytes, thus indicating that macrophages have the ability to take up and degrade considerable amounts of LDL in vivo in the absence of LDL receptors.[111,357]

A remaining unsolved problem in the pathogenesis of FH relates to the cellular and biochemical mechanisms by which the elevated plasma LDL cholesterol level leads to accelerated and premature atherosclerosis. In this regard, accumulating evidence suggests that oxidation of the lipids and proteins in LDL may play a role by modifying the LDL particle in such a way that it can now be recognized by a variety of scavenger cell receptors that do not bind and take up native LDL.[111] Steinberg has reviewed the oxidized LDL hypothesis and its pathobiological significance in atherosclerosis.[359]

Cholesterol Synthetic Rates in Heterozygotes and Homozygotes

In cultured fibroblasts from FH individuals, the deficiency of LDL receptors creates a situation in which the rate of cholesterol synthesis is higher in cells from heterozygotes and homozygotes than in cells from normal subjects when all are exposed to the same level of LDL in the incubation medium.[41,134] It has been pointed out, however, that these in vitro findings do not imply that the total-body cholesterol synthetic rate would be elevated in these patients[322] because in vivo the FH individuals do not have normal levels of LDL cholesterol. Heterozygotes, for example, maintain a two- to threefold elevation of plasma LDL levels. In tissue culture, such an increase is sufficient to reduce cholesterol synthesis to almost the same levels that are seen in cells from normal subjects.[299] This type of compensation also seems to take place in vivo. Total-body sterol synthetic rates have been measured in heterozygotes using the sterol balance technique. These studies have shown normal rates of total-body cholesterol synthesis.[320,322,360,361]

It is not clear whether this type of LDL-related compensation can occur in homozygotes. In actively growing fibroblasts from receptor-negative homozygotes, cholesterol synthesis cannot be fully suppressed, even when very high levels of LDL are present in the culture medium.[40,134] However, when fibroblasts become confluent and cease to grow, the rate of cholesterol synthesis falls in homozygote cells as well as in normal cells.[134] Thus, in vivo cholesterol synthesis might be higher than normal in rapidly growing cells, and perhaps in cells that use LDL for the production of steroid hormones. Whether this increase is sufficient to produce a detectable increase in overall total-body cholesterol synthesis is not known.

Studies of cholesterol synthetic rates in homozygotes with the use of sterol balance[320,323,360–364] or isotopic turnover[365] techniques have shown an interesting dichotomy of results. Younger subjects in general appear to have total-body rates of cholesterol synthesis that are two- to threefold above normal, as reflected by an enhanced excretion of cholesterol from the body as compared with normal subjects of the same age. However, in homozygotes who have been studied after the age of 10, the cholesterol synthetic rates are generally at the upper limits of normal. The one exception is a 24-year-old homozygote whose total cholesterol synthetic rate was 34.2 mg/kg/day as compared with a mean normal value of 9.6 mg/kg/day.[362] Bile acid synthetic rates are generally normal in homozygotes. Although the number of subjects studied by these techniques is small, the results suggest that young FH homozygotes may have a total-body overproduction of cholesterol, whereas older homozygotes may not show such overproduction. The tissues in which such overproduction occurs are not known.

Regulation of the LDL Receptor in Dietary Hypercholesterolemia

The vast majority of individuals with elevated LDL cholesterol levels are not FH heterozygotes; hypercholesterolemia develops even though they possess two normal LDL receptor genes. Strong circumstantial evidence suggests that much of this so-called polygenic hypercholesterolemia is attributable to feedback suppression of LDL receptor gene expression. Sterol-mediated feedback suppression of LDL receptors was originally demonstrated in tissue culture cells, and it has now been demonstrated in livers of animals from multiple species, including the toad *Xenopus laevis*.[113,161] As described above, this suppression is mediated transcriptionally by the SREBP family of transcription factors that binds to the 10-bp DNA sequence, the sterol regulatory element, in the promoter of the LDL receptor gene (Figs. 120-20 and 120-21).

A high dietary intake of exogenous saturated fats and cholesterol raises the concentration of LDL, even though this particle has its origin in the liver and not in the intestine.[366–368] In experimental animals, such as hamsters and rabbits, dietary cholesterol raises the plasma LDL level indirectly, primarily through suppression of LDL receptors.[367,368] Dietschy and coworkers[367,369] developed a sophisticated LDL infusion technique to measure LDL receptor activity in cholesterol-fed hamsters. They showed that the feeding of pure cholesterol suppresses hepatic LDL receptors and that this effect is potentiated by a saturated fatty acid (palmitate) and ameliorated by a monounsaturated fatty acid (oleate) or a polyunsaturated fatty acid (linoleate). Stearate, although an 18-carbon saturated fatty acid, had a modest suppressive effect, rather than a potentiating effect like palmitate, presumably because it is readily desaturated in vivo to form oleate. These findings on suppression of hepatic LDL receptors in hamsters are remarkably parallel to observations of the effects of dietary fatty acids on plasma LDL in humans.[370] They provide strong support for the notion that dietary cholesterol and saturated fats raise plasma LDL levels primarily, if not exclusively, by down-regulating hepatic LDL receptors.

Nearly everyone in industrialized societies eats a relatively high-fat diet, yet some individuals suppress their LDL receptors more than others. One source of variability stems from differences in hormonal, nutritional, and pharmacologic factors that influence the expression of hepatic LDL receptors (Table 120-6). Another source of variability may lie in polymorphisms in the genes responsible for the absorption of dietary cholesterol, the metabolism of cholesterol to bile acids, or the transport of cholesterol in plasma. Another source of genetic variation may lie in the genes encoding the regulatory proteins of the SREBP pathway that are responsible for the sterol-mediated feedback regulation of the LDL receptor gene and the genes of cholesterol and unsaturated fatty acid synthesis[22] (discussed above). In some individuals, these regulatory proteins may bind sterols with higher affinity than others, or they may bind to the DNA element more or less tightly. Now that these regulatory proteins have been identified, it will be of great interest to clone their encoding genes and to study their genetic variation in individuals who respond differently to high-fat diets.

Table 120-6 Factors that Influence Expression of LDL Receptors in Liver

Factors increasing LDL receptors
- Hormonal
  - Thyroxine
  - Growth hormone
- Nutritional
  - Cholesterol deprivation
  - Starvation (rats and dogs, but not rabbits)
- Pharmacologic
  - 17α-Ethinyl estradiol
  - Bile acid binding resins (cholestyramine and colestipol)
  - Inhibitors of HMG-CoA reductase (lovastatin, simvastatin, pravastatin, atorvastatin, fluvastatin, cerivastatin)

Factors decreasing LDL receptors
- Genetic
  - Familial hypercholesterolemia
  - Age
- Nutritional
  - Cholesterol feeding (enhanced by saturated but not polyunsaturated fatty acids)
  - Nonfat diet of casein and wheat starch
  - Starvation (rabbits, but not rats and dogs)

Data from refs. 368, 369, 405–407, 419–423, 504–506

DIAGNOSIS

Clinical Diagnosis: Differentiation from Other Disorders that Produce Type 2 Hyperlipoproteinemia

Homozygotes. The clinical diagnosis of FH in the homozygote usually causes no difficulty. Not only is the clinical picture of cutaneous xanthomas and juvenile atherosclerosis distinct, but the finding of a plasma cholesterol level exceeding 650 mg/dl in a nonjaundiced child is virtually pathognomonic. In selected patients, it is sometimes difficult to differentiate a severely affected heterozygote from a homozygote who has two LDL receptor mutations that partially impair but do not abolish receptor function. Individuals doubly heterozygous for an LDL receptor mutation (heterozygous FH) plus an apo B-100 mutation (FDB) can have plasma LDL cholesterol levels as high as that seen in FH homozygotes (discussed below).[371,372]

One disorder that may occasionally be confused clinically with homozygous FH is pseudohomozygous type 2 hypercholesterolemia. This rare disorder was first described in 1974,[373] and 10 affected individuals from 8 unrelated families have been identified.[4,373–375] The clinical picture is that of a child with these abnormalities: (a) severe hypercholesterolemia (total plasma cholesterol level 350 to 700 mg/dl) due to a selective elevation in LDL; (b) a normal triglyceride level; (c) cutaneous planar xanthomas of the type seen in homozygous FH; (d) normal or slightly elevated plasma cholesterol levels in both parents; and (e) a striking response to dietary restriction of cholesterol, with plasma cholesterol levels falling as much as 40 percent, accompanied by regression of the xanthomas.

Pseudohomozygous type 2 hypercholesterolemia can be distinguished clinically from homozygous FH by the absence of heterozygous FH in the parents and other first-degree relatives, and by the remarkable sensitivity to dietary manipulation. The combination of a low-cholesterol diet (< 200 mg/day) and oral cholestyramine (12 g/day) can lower plasma LDL cholesterol levels well into the normal range,[373–375] a completely different result from that obtained with homozygous FH.

Studies of the cultured fibroblasts of one of the two originally described patients with pseudohomozygous type 2 (case 2, B. H.)[4] and several other patients showed no abnormality in any of the steps in the LDL receptor pathway.[374,375] This finding suggests that the elevation in LDL cholesterol levels is not caused by an abnormality in the receptor-mediated catabolism of LDL. In addition, LDL isolated from the plasma of affected patients was taken up, degraded, and metabolized normally by normal human fibroblasts (unpublished observations). Studies of total-body cholesterol and bile acid production and of ^{125}I-labeled LDL turnover in plasma performed while the patients are ingesting low- and high-cholesterol diets should be informative in identifying the reason for the elevated LDL.

The clinical features of pseudohomozygous type 2 hypercholesterolemia are virtually identical to those seen in the autosomal recessive syndrome of phytosterolemia (Chap. 123). We previously suggested that many, if not all, of the children diagnosed as having pseudohomozygous type 2 may actually have phytosterolemia.[4] Low et al.[374] reported two children with the classic clinical syndrome of pseudohomozygous type 2 who had elevated plasma phytosterol levels, which is in keeping with the above suggestion. Plant sterols should be measured in all patients considered to have pseudohomozygous type 2 (Chap. 123). The gene responsible for this disorder has been mapped to chromosome 2p21.[376]

A second autosomal recessive inherited syndrome that clinically resembles homozygous FH but which is distinct from phytosterolemia has been reported.[377,378] Plasma levels of plant sterols were normal in two sibs of an inbred Sardinian family[377] and in a single 38-year-old male whose parents came from the same Turkish village.[378] Genetic polymorphism studies in the Sardinian and Turkish families revealed that the hypercholesterolemia was not linked to the LDL receptor or the apo B-100 gene. Turnover studies of plasma ^{125}I-LDL in the Turkish subject[378] and two additional Sardinian subjects[378a] showed a metabolic picture virtually identical to that seen in homozygous FH—namely, a markedly reduced catabolic rate (30 percent of normal) and a slightly increased LDL production rate (see below). Harada-Shiba et al.[379] described a Japanese sib pair with a phenotypically identical disorder that also had a markedly reduced plasma LDL clearance rate that was not due to the inheritance of mutant LDL receptor alleles. The gene defect responsible for the disorder in these three families is not known.

Heterozygotes. Diagnosis of heterozygous FH begins with the documentation of an elevated plasma level of LDL. In most cases, the finding of hypercholesterolemia without hypertriglyceridemia is sufficient to establish that the LDL cholesterol level is elevated. If the total cholesterol level is at the upper limits of normal (i.e., at or near the 90th percentile cutoff), the HDL cholesterol should be measured to confirm that the elevated plasma cholesterol is in the LDL fraction.[26]

Having documented an elevated LDL level, the physician must then determine whether the cause of the elevation is the heterozygous form of FH. Fewer than 1 in 20 individuals with an elevation in total plasma cholesterol or LDL cholesterol (i.e., a type 2a or type 2b lipoprotein pattern) has FH.[94] Most individuals with a type 2 lipoprotein pattern have polygenic hypercholesterolemia, which derives from a combination of environmental and multiple poorly understood genetic factors.[94] A family history of hypercholesterolemia, tendon xanthomas, and/or premature coronary heart disease makes the diagnosis of heterozygous FH more likely, but necessitates ruling out two other monogenic diseases: familial combined hyperlipidemia[94,95,380,381] and FDB[382,383] (Chap. 115).

Familial combined hyperlipidemia can be confused with FH because both types of patients sometimes have a primary type 2 lipoprotein pattern and no tendon xanthomas. Several clinical clues help make this distinction: (a) Heterozygotes with FH tend to have, on average, higher plasma LDL cholesterol levels. The finding of a plasma LDL cholesterol above 220 mg/dl in children, or above 290 mg/dl in adults, together with a normal triglyceride level in a first-degree relative of a subject with FH is 98 percent specific and 87 percent sensitive for the diagnosis of FH.[384]

(b) Heterozygotes with FH do not usually have relatives with lipoprotein abnormalities of multiple types (i.e., types 2a, 2b, 4, and 5), which is characteristic of familial combined hyperlipidemia. (c) Hypercholesterolemic individuals with familial combined hyperlipidemia never have tendon xanthomas unless they have type 3 hyperlipoproteinemia (Chap. 119). (d) The hypercholesterolemia is not as pronounced in children with familial combined hyperlipidemia as in those with FH.

Differentiating heterozygous FH from FDB is more difficult. FDB is caused by a missense mutation at amino acid position 3500 in apo B-100[383] (Chap. 115). The mutation interferes with the ability of apo B to bind to the LDL receptor and thus results in hypercholesterolemia.[382,383] Most FDB heterozygotes have lower plasma LDL cholesterol levels than FH heterozygotes, but this is not always the case.[385–388] Some patients who were originally classified as having FH were subsequently found to have FDB by direct molecular detection of the base-pair substitution in the apo B-100 gene. Patients with FDB can have a positive family history of hypercholesterolemia, clinically significant coronary atherosclerosis, and tendon xanthomas.[385–387] Thus, the differentiation of FH and FDB cannot be made by clinical criteria alone. The easiest way to differentiate the two disorders is to rule out FDB by direct detection of the mutation in the apo B-100 gene (Chap. 115).

Individuals heterozygous for both FDB and FH have a plasma LDL level intermediate between that of FH heterozygotes and FH homozygotes.[372] Some of these double-heterozygotes have a clinical course that resembles FH homozygotes. One such individual was a 10-year-old boy who suffered a cardiac arrest secondary to coronary atherosclerosis.[371] He had an LDL cholesterol of ~600 mg/dl and tendon xanthomas, but no planar xanthomas. These double-heterozygotes respond well to lipid-lowering therapy, although they may require higher doses of medication than do their relatives with either heterozygous FH or FDB alone.

One patient with autoimmune hyperlipidemia was described with an FH-like syndrome characterized by plasma cholesterol levels of 600 to 900 mg/dl, tendon xanthomas, and premature coronary disease, but with no family history of FH. This 31-year-old Italian male had a monoclonal gammopathy producing an IgA that reacted with the LDL receptor.[389] The autoantibody inhibited binding, uptake, and degradation of ^{125}I-LDL in cultured fibroblasts from a normal subject.

A variety of nongenetic disturbances can cause the plasma LDL cholesterol level to be elevated. For example, a type 2a lipoprotein pattern may be observed in patients with hypothyroidism, nephrotic syndrome, hepatoma, acute intermittent porphyria, anorexia nervosa, and Werner syndrome.[390] Patients with primary biliary cirrhosis and other forms of obstructive jaundice may also manifest a type 2a lipoprotein pattern, but their plasma contains elevated amounts of an unusual lipoprotein called "lipoprotein X."[390]

Laboratory Diagnosis: LDL Receptor Analysis

Four functional tests are available for quantifying LDL receptor function in monolayers of fibroblasts cultured from the skin of patients: (a) measurement of the cell-surface binding and intracellular uptake of ^{125}I-labeled LDL; (b) measurement of the rate of proteolytic degradation of ^{125}I-labeled LDL; (c) measurement of LDL-mediated suppression of the synthesis of [^{14}C]cholesterol from [^{14}C]acetate in intact cells or of HMG-CoA reductase activity as assayed in cell-free extracts; and (d) measurement of LDL-mediated stimulation of the incorporation of [^{14}C]oleate into cellular cholesteryl [^{14}C]oleate.[391] Among these assays, the two most discriminatory are the proteolytic degradation and the measurement of cholesteryl [^{14}C]oleate formation. When both assays are used concomitantly in a family known to have FH, affected and unaffected individuals can be distinguished with an accuracy of about 90 percent. When applied to larger populations, the discriminatory power of these quantitative assays declines because of overlap between the lower limit of receptor activity in normal individuals and in FH heterozygotes with incomplete receptor defects. The number of LDL receptors can also be quantified by immunoblotting techniques[392] or immunoprecipitation of ^{35}S-labeled receptors after growth of cells in [^{35}S]methionine.[124,393] These two assays have the additional virtue of detecting qualitative defects in the LDL receptor.

The LDL receptor defect in FH can also be demonstrated in circulating blood lymphocytes, thus obviating the necessity for long-term culture[318] (see Fig. 120-28*A*). One lymphocyte assay, developed by Cuthbert et al.,[394] is based on the observation that proliferating cells must obtain cholesterol from one of two sources, either by receptor-mediated uptake of LDL or by endogenous sterol synthesis.[3] When freshly isolated lymphocytes are cultured in lipoprotein-deficient medium and endogenous cholesterol synthesis is inhibited with an HMG-CoA reductase inhibitor such as lovastatin, mitogen-stimulated proliferation of lymphocytes becomes dependent on the receptor-mediated uptake of LDL cholesterol.[394] Lymphocytes from FH heterozygotes show the same maximal proliferative response as normal cells, but they require an LDL cholesterol concentration that is two- to threefold higher than that required by normal cells.[394] This assay has not yet been demonstrated to have sufficient discriminatory power to allow use for the general population.

In populations of the world in which particular LDL receptor mutations are frequent, such as the Afrikaners, French Canadians, Finns, Icelanders, and Christian Lebanese (discussed above; see Table 120-4), LDL receptor mutations can be detected directly using DNA extracted from white blood cells and PCR-based techniques. In most populations, however, the plethora of different LDL receptor mutations precludes direct DNA-based diagnosis unless a particular mutation is strongly suspected. Within a single family, genomic markers such as RFLP can be used to follow the segregation of the mutant allele.[197] Development of automated biochip methods to detect sequence variation in DNA may soon make it feasible to screen the LDL receptor gene for all possible mutations.

At this time, it is unclear whether a definitive diagnosis of FH offers the individual hypercholesterolemic patient any prognostic or therapeutic information that is not achieved by accurate measurement of his or her plasma LDL-cholesterol level. Perhaps the most compelling reason to encourage identification of an LDL receptor mutation in a hypercholesterolemic individual is that this knowledge should heighten family awareness of the potential risk for premature coronary heart disease and stimulate all relatives to have their LDL cholesterol levels measured.

Prenatal Diagnosis of Homozygous FH

The first prenatal diagnosis of homozygous FH was made in 1978 using functional assays for quantitative assessment of LDL receptor activity in cultured amniotic fluid cells.[106] Prenatal diagnosis was later made in another case by measurement of the cholesterol concentration in a fetal blood sample obtained at the 24th week of gestation.[395] The total cholesterol level in this sample was 543 mg/dl as compared with the mean value of 66 mg/dl in 48 control fetuses. The diagnosis of homozygous FH was confirmed in skin fibroblasts obtained at the time of therapeutic abortion.[395]

Genomic DNA can be used to make the prenatal diagnosis of FH if the sites of the LDL receptor mutations in the parental alleles are known, or if the haplotype of the chromosome with the mutation is known. The feasibility of such an approach has been documented by the direct detection of heterozygosity for the Lebanese mutation using tissue obtained from a chorionic villus biopsy at the 8th week of gestation.[396] It is likely that these molecular techniques will replace functional assays in making the prenatal diagnosis of homozygous FH.

Neonatal Diagnosis of Heterozygous FH

Neonatal cord-blood screening is not a reliable means for identification of heterozygotes in the general population because, just as with adults, the vast majority of newborns with elevations of LDL cholesterol do not have FH.[397,398] Even in babies born to a parent who is known to have FH, it is not always possible to diagnose heterozygotes at birth. In cord blood samples obtained on 25 neonates born to Finnish FH heterozygotes with molecularly defined LDL receptor mutations, plasma LDL-cholesterol levels were higher in the 14 FH heterozygotes as compared to 11 nonaffected neonates (71 versus 31 mg/dl). However, the individual levels between the two groups showed significant overlap, thus precluding an accurate diagnosis.[399]

TREATMENT

FH Heterozygotes — Adults

An ideal cholesterol-lowering agent in FH would increase the production of LDL receptors in the liver. In FH heterozygotes, this goal can be attained by exploiting the feedback regulatory system that controls transcription of the single normal LDL receptor gene. When the demand for cholesterol is elevated, normal and FH heterozygote cells produce an increased number of LDL receptors as a result of enhanced transcription.[160] This increase is even more pronounced when intracellular cholesterol synthesis is inhibited, thus forcing cells to rely entirely on LDL cholesterol.[400]

The first class of drugs to exploit this regulatory system was the bile acid binding resins, cholestyramine and colestipol. These agents have been used extensively for almost four decades to lower LDL cholesterol by 10 to 20 percent in heterozygous FH and other hypercholesterolemic states.[401–404] Cholestyramine and colestipol are nonabsorbable, anion-exchange resins that bind bile acids in the intestinal lumen, preventing their absorption from the ileum.[403] The increased fecal excretion of bile acids elicits an increased conversion of cholesterol to bile acids in the liver. The liver responds to the cholesterol deficiency by increasing the production of LDL receptors, as revealed by LDL turnover studies. In one such study, treatment of FH heterozygotes with cholestyramine led to an enhanced fractional catabolic rate for ^{125}I-labeled LDL, but not ^{131}I-labeled cyclohexanedione-treated LDL, which cannot bind to the LDL receptor.[405] Similar studies were reported in rabbits.[406] Rudling et al.[407] performed liver biopsies on humans treated with cholestyramine prior to elective surgery. The drug increased the number of LDL receptors twofold, as determined by direct measurement of the binding of ^{125}I-LDL to liver membranes. Similarly, in dogs treated with colestipol, the number of LDL receptors in liver membranes increased, and the fractional catabolic rate for intravenously administered ^{125}I-labeled LDL increased proportionately.[408] Thus, in dogs, rabbits, and humans, bile acid sequestrants lower plasma LDL levels by enhancing the efficiency of receptor-mediated removal of LDL from plasma (Fig. 120-32, left). Animal experiments suggest that this is achieved through increased proteolytic cleavage of SREBP-2 (discussed above).

In humans, bile acid sequestrants generally lower LDL cholesterol levels by only 10 to 20 percent, largely because the liver compensates for the cholesterol deficiency by increasing the rate of cholesterol synthesis (Fig. 120-32, middle).[360,409] By replacing the drained intracellular cholesterol pool, the increase in hepatic cholesterol synthesis blunts the rise in hepatic LDL receptors. The liver also increases the production of VLDL, which can lead to hypertriglyceridemia in some patients.[410] FH heterozygotes who are hypertriglyceridemic should not be treated with bile acid resins.

The above considerations led to the prediction that an inhibitor of cholesterol synthesis should act synergistically with a bile acid sequestrant to lower plasma LDL levels[3] (Fig. 120-32, right). This hypothesis was borne out by studies with a novel class of cholesterol synthesis inhibitors. The prototype, compactin (ML-236B; mevastatin), is a fungal metabolite that was isolated from *Penicillium citrinum* in 1976 by Endo and associates at the Sankyo Drug Company in Japan.[411,412] Compactin, a bicyclic diene with a β-hydroxy-δ-lactone side chain, is a potent competitive inhibitor of HMG-CoA reductase, the rate-controlling enzyme in cholesterol synthesis.[411,413] The K_i for compactin is ~1 nM, which is 10,000 times lower than the K_m for the natural substrate HMG-CoA (about 10 μM). A structurally related compound, lovastatin (also called mevinolin or monacolin K), was isolated from cultures of Aspergillus and Monascus species independently by workers at the Merck Sharp & Dohme Research Laboratories[413] and by Endo.[412] Lovastatin and two chemically modified versions of the natural compounds (pravastatin and simvastatin), as well as three synthetic statins (fluvastatin, cerivastatin, and atorvastatin), are available for human therapy. This class of drugs is referred to as "statins." The pharmacology of the statins is reviewed in Witztum[414] and in *The Medical Letter*.[415,416]

When given to experimental animals and to humans, the reductase inhibitors initially block cholesterol synthesis in the liver, and this elicits two compensatory responses: (a) hepatocytes synthesize increased amounts of HMG-CoA reductase[417,418]; and (b) they synthesize increased numbers of LDL receptors, owing to transcriptional induction.[408,418–423] When a new steady state is attained, the increase in HMG-CoA reductase is almost sufficient to overcome the block by the reductase inhibitor. As a result, total-body cholesterol pool size and production rates do not change appreciably.[424,425] Nevertheless, the plasma LDL level falls as a result of the increase in LDL receptors. In the new steady state, the fall in plasma LDL levels is balanced by the increase in LDL receptors, so the absolute amount of cholesterol entering the liver through the receptor pathway is the same as it was earlier. The difference, however, is that this entry is now occurring at a lower plasma LDL level. Thus, the major net effect of the reductase

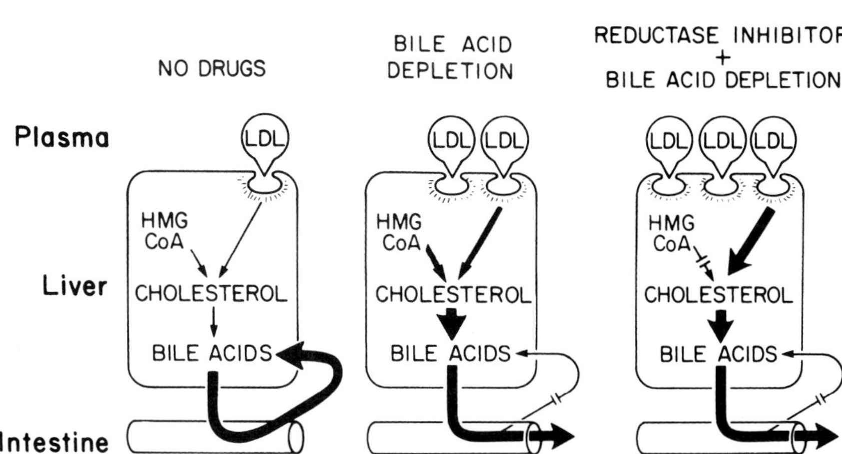

Fig. 120-32 Rationale for the use of a bile acid binding resin and an inhibitor of HMG-CoA reductase in the treatment of FH heterozygotes. A detailed discussion of this figure is presented in the text. (*From M. S. Brown and J. L. Goldstein.*[3] *Used by permission of* Science.)

inhibitors is to lower the concentration of plasma LDL without markedly altering the levels of cholesterol in liver or in other normal tissues. The lowering of the LDL level is predicted to lower the amount of cholesterol in areas of abnormal deposition, such as tendon xanthomas or atheromas, which depend on a high LDL level for their formation.

A major effect of the reductase inhibitors is to enhance LDL receptor-mediated clearance of triglyceride-rich apo B-containing lipoproteins that are the precursors of LDL, thus reducing the rate of LDL production. The strongest evidence for the primary role of LDL receptors in the action of the reductase inhibitors comes from the relative ineffectiveness of these agents in patients with the receptor-negative form of homozygous FH.[426] Even when treated with high doses of lovastatin (2 mg/kg/day for 3 months), these subjects did not exhibit the expected reduction in the concentration of LDL or in its rate of production or catabolism. The most readily detectable effect is a lowering of VLDL cholesterol level. Even though lovastatin may cause a remodeling of VLDL in these patients, it does not lower the rate of LDL production substantially because there are no receptors to bind the resultant IDL. There is one report of a documented LDL-receptor negative FH homozygote who has shown a convincing response to statin therapy. Feber et al.[427] described a 31-year-old FH homozygote with nonsense mutations in both LDL receptor alleles and no immunodetectable receptor protein, who had a 30 percent reduction in total plasma cholesterol (from 800 to 650 mg/dl) after treatment with simvastatin (40 mg/day) for 2 months.

At present, it is controversial as to whether the reductase inhibitors decrease the rates of synthesis or secretion of apo B-100.[419,421,428,429] Marais et al.[430] examined the effect of high-dose atorvastatin therapy (80 mg/day) on the LDL production rate in seven FH homozygotes receiving apheresis or plasma exchange every 2 weeks. Administration of atorvastatin resulted in a significantly slower rate of recovery of the LDL cholesterol level in the 2-week interval between treatments. The slower increase in the LDL level after apheresis was attributed to a decrease in the LDL production rate. However, no direct measurements of the effect of atorvastatin on LDL catabolism were performed, and the molecular characterization of the LDL receptor mutations suggested that each of the homozygotes expressed at least one partially functional receptor allele. A conclusive demonstration that HMG-CoA reductase inhibitors affect lipoprotein synthesis independently of lipoprotein catabolism will require studies to be performed in FH homozygotes who have no LDL receptor mRNA as well as no immunodetectable LDL receptors.

High-dose treatment of FH heterozygotes with reductase inhibitors is associated with a 50 to 60 percent decrease in plasma levels of LDL cholesterol. When given together with cholestyramine, reductase inhibitors block the compensatory increase in cholesterol synthesis, and the increase in LDL receptors is even more profound[431] (see Fig. 120-32, right). The specific type of molecular defect in the LDL receptor gene of heterozygotes appears to play a modest role in the response to therapy with these agents.[432]

To date, six statins have been approved for routine use, as described above. The agents differ in their relative potency, but are similar in their low incidence of side effects. In general, all of the drugs are well tolerated and almost universally effective in lowering plasma LDL cholesterol levels. The major toxicities of these agents include a dose-related asymptomatic elevation in serum hepatic transaminase levels occurring in up to 2 percent of patients on the highest doses, and skeletal muscle disease with myalgias and elevations in serum creatine kinase that may progress to rhabdomyolysis in 0.2 percent of individuals on the highest doses.[433] Both the liver toxicity and rhabdomyolysis are reversible on cessation of the drug. The incidence of rhabdomyolysis is significantly increased when the reductase inhibitor is given in combination with cyclosporine, nicotinic acid, gemfibrozil, or erythromycin.[434–436] With combined therapy the rhabdomyolysis can sometimes be severe enough to produce acute renal failure.

Treatment with reductase inhibitors is associated with a dose-dependent fall in plasma triglycerides and a slight increase in HDL cholesterol levels. In individuals with plasma triglyceride levels over 250 mg/dl, the percentage reduction in triglyceride level is proportional to the reduction in LDL cholesterol, irrespective of the agent employed.[437] The triglyceride-lowering effect of the statins most likely results from the associated increase in the clearance of VLDL and IDL rather than from any effect on VLDL synthesis. Consistent with this scenario is the finding that the reductase inhibitors have a reduced potency in lowering LDL levels in hypertriglyceridemic subjects, presumably because the LDL particles must compete with a large number of circulating apo E-rich and triglyceride-rich particles for receptor-mediated uptake by the liver.

Heterozygotes with FH generally show an impressive response to the combination of a bile acid sequestrant and nicotinic acid.[438,439] Although its mechanism of action has not been definitively established, nicotinic acid probably acts by reducing hepatic secretion of VLDL, which, in turn, reduces LDL production.[403] Treatment with nicotinic acid can be associated with several side effects that include flushing, hepatitis, glucose intolerance, and gout.[403] Triple-drug therapy with nicotinic acid can be extremely effective. When 22 severely affected FH heterozygotes were treated with nicotinic acid in combination with a bile acid sequestrant (colestipol) plus a reductase inhibitor (lovastatin), mean plasma cholesterol levels were lowered from 420 to 184 mg/dl and mean LDL cholesterol levels were lowered from 329 to 107.[439]

Postmenopausal women with heterozygous FH should be treated with estrogen replacement unless there are medical contraindications. In one study of a heterogeneous population of hyperlipidemic women, estrogen administration led to a 14 percent decrease in LDL cholesterol and 15 percent increase in HDL cholesterol.[440]

A surgically created partial ileal bypass prevents bile salt reabsorption and produces essentially the same or somewhat better therapeutic effect in FH heterozygotes as does cholestyramine.[441–443] The major drawbacks are the side effects, which include frequent bowel movements (average of three per day), overt diarrhea (6 percent), kidney stones (4 percent), gallstones (fourfold increase), and symptomatic bowel obstruction (14 percent).[441]

Dietary discretion is generally recommended for every person with hypercholesterolemia, including those with FH. In general, the total cholesterol intake should be limited to 150 mg/day for adults and children (roughly equivalent to the cholesterol content of half of an egg yolk). Total fat intake should be limited, and the intake of saturated fats, especially palmitic acid in dairy products, should be severely restricted.[444] The detrimental effects of saturated fats are attributable to their ability to potentiate the suppression of hepatic LDL receptor activity elicited by a high-cholesterol diet.[367,369,445] FH heterozygotes who rigorously adhere to a low-fat, high-carbohydrate diet usually show a 10 to 20 percent fall in plasma LDL cholesterol concentration, but this is rarely sufficient to produce desirable LDL cholesterol levels. An important consideration in the treatment of FH is the need to identify and treat affected family members of the index case. All first-degree relatives (parents, sibs, children) and available second-degree relatives of FH patients should have plasma cholesterol determinations followed by dietary or drug therapy when indicated.

FH Heterozygotes — Children and Adolescents

Children or adolescents with heterozygous FH should be placed on a low-saturated-fat (<7 percent of total calories), low-cholesterol (<200 mg/day) diet. A dietitian should be involved in the planning to ensure sufficient content of necessary vitamins, minerals, and calories. Drug therapy should be initiated if the LDL cholesterol remains elevated. The goal for treatment should be the achievement of a plasma LDL-cholesterol level of less than

110 mg/dl. Bile acid resins are the first-line drugs of choice because they are not absorbed and are safe and effective in children. Resins in low doses can be initiated as early as age 5. Occasionally, folate or fat-soluble vitamin deficiency develops in association with resin therapy, necessitating the provision of supplemental vitamins to children who do not consume adequate amounts of fruits and vegetables. The major problem associated with bile-acid therapy in children is compliance. In a Norwegian study, 36 children (ages 6 to 11) were placed on cholestyramine. Only 22 of the original subjects continued to take the resin for the 1-year duration of the study.[446] The development of generic forms of resins in multiple different flavors has improved the palatability of this class of drugs. Combined resin therapy with nicotinic acid is associated with an ~40 percent fall in LDL cholesterol levels.[447]

A recent report from Finland showed that daily use of margarine supplemented with an esterified plant sterol, sitostanol ester, was associated with a 15 percent fall in the plasma LDL cholesterol level.[448] If prolonged use of this margarine preparation is shown to be safe in children, this agent will provide another therapeutic option.

Experience with HMG-CoA reductase inhibitors for treatment of children and adolescents is limited, but short-term treatment appears to be safe.[449,450] The longest study involved boys with heterozygous FH (ages 10 to 17) who were treated for 1 year on 10 to 40 mg/day of lovastatin.[451] No significant difference in growth, sexual maturation, or plasma levels of steroids or fat soluble vitamins (except vitamin E, which was reduced secondary to the fall in plasma LDL level) were found between the drug-treated and the placebo groups of 67 and 65 FH heterozygotes, respectively. The drug was well tolerated and associated with up to a 27 percent decrease in plasma LDL cholesterol. Until further data are available, these agents should be used with caution for prolonged treatment of children and adolescents.

The recommendations of the National Cholesterol Education Program are to initiate drug therapy at age 10 if either of these circumstances pertain: the LDL cholesterol level is > 160 mg/dl and there is a positive family history of premature cardiovascular disease, or the LDL cholesterol is > 190 mg/dl and there is no family history.[452] Thus, almost all children with heterozygous FH will qualify for drug therapy. Practitioners often delay the initiation of therapy with an HMG-CoA reductase inhibitor until approximately age 16 in females, owing to their lower risk of developing premature coronary artery disease.

FH Homozygotes

FH homozygotes are generally resistant to the treatments that are effective in heterozygotes. As discussed above, these treatments act by stimulating the normal LDL receptor gene, which is absent or markedly reduced in FH homozygotes. Receptor-negative homozygotes show little response to dietary changes, bile acid binding resins, ileal bypass, or HMG-CoA reductase inhibitors.[404,426,453–456] This resistance was demonstrated clearly in three studies. In one of these, four FH homozygotes failed to respond to doses of compactin that were five to eight times higher than doses that achieved a 33 percent reduction in cholesterol levels in heterozygotes.[454] In a second study, three receptor-negative FH homozygotes had no decrease in LDL cholesterol concentrations or increase in fractional catabolic rate for ^{125}I-LDL after treatment for 3 months with high doses of lovastatin (2 mg/kg/day).[426] In the third study, a bile fistula was created in an FH homozygote so that all biliary cholesterol and bile acids were drained to the exterior for 1 year. Although huge amounts of cholesterol were removed from the body by this route, the plasma LDL cholesterol level did not fall significantly,[456] presumably because LDL receptors could not be induced.

FH homozygotes with genes that produce partially functional LDL receptors may respond to therapy, and they should be treated vigorously with a combination of bile acid binding agent, an HMG-CoA reductase inhibitor, and nicotinic acid in addition to stringent dietary measures. When one FH homozygote with 25 percent of functional receptor activity was treated with triple therapy, the plasma cholesterol level was reduced from 958 to 389 mg/dl, and the LDL cholesterol level was reduced from 809 to 338 mg/dl.[439] Caution must be exercised because of the potential toxicity to muscle and liver that may result from this combination (discussed above).

In two recent studies, 91 FH homozygotes were treated with very high daily doses of statins, either 160 mg of simvastatin ($n = 12$) or up to 80 mg of atorvastatin ($n = 79$).[457,458] Treatment was associated with a mean fall in plasma LDL cholesterol of ~30 percent in both studies. Virtually all of these FH homozygotes had some residual LDL receptor activity. A careful correlation between receptor number and statin responsiveness was not done.

Portacaval Anastomosis. In 1973, Starzl et al.[459] observed that IV hyperalimentation reduced the plasma cholesterol level of one homozygote. Similar results were subsequently obtained in other homozygotes.[362,460] The mechanism for this effect is unknown. Stimulated by this finding, Starzl et al.[459,461,462] created an end-to-side portacaval anastomosis in a homozygous patient, after which the plasma cholesterol level declined from 772 to 240 mg/dl.

At least 45 homozygotes, from 2.5 to 35 years of age, have undergone portacaval shunt surgery, and in most of them, the plasma cholesterol level was reduced 25 to 50 percent.[463] Detailed metabolic studies in one of these homozygotes showed that the portacaval anastomosis reduced these parameters: total-body cholesterol synthesis by 62 percent; synthetic rate for plasma LDL by 48 percent; and bile acid synthesis by 65 percent. The plasma LDL cholesterol level in this patient fell 39 percent despite a 17 percent reduction in the fractional catabolic rate for the lipoprotein.[323] In another homozygote, the procedure lowered total-body cholesterol and bile acid synthesis, and also elicited a net efflux of accumulated tissue cholesterol, as measured by isotopic techniques.[464] Approximately 60 percent of patients experience regression of their xanthomas after this procedure.[463] Portacaval shunting has also been associated with regression of aortic stenotic lesions as well as stabilization or regression of coronary atherosclerotic lesions.[461–463] It is still not clear if the shunting procedure prolongs life because there is no control group with which to compare the shunted patients. Portacaval shunt surgery, though well tolerated, is not associated with enough of a reduction in LDL cholesterol level to be used as a sole therapy in FH homozygotes.

Removal of LDL by Plasma Exchange or LDL Apheresis. The most successful overall therapeutic approach for homozygotes, as well as for severely affected heterozygotes, is the direct removal of LDL from plasma by use of a continuous-flow blood cell-separator. In 1967, DeGennes reported the effectiveness of plasmapheresis in reducing plasma cholesterol levels in FH homozygotes.[465] In one version of this procedure, pioneered by Thompson et al.,[466] plasma is exchanged with normal plasma or albumin. More than 50 FH patients in several medical centers have been treated in this fashion.[466,467] If the procedure is repeated every 1 to 2 weeks and combined with oral nicotinic acid, the mean level of plasma cholesterol can be reduced by about 50 percent on a long-term basis.[468] The procedure is generally well tolerated, but repetition for many years is emotionally difficult.

Long-term plasma exchange produces regression of tendon xanthomas and some amelioration of atherosclerosis in FH homozygotes.[467,469–471] Thompson et al.[472] reported a decreased risk of premature death in 5 homozygotes who were treated every 2 weeks for an average of 8.4 years. These patients survived an average of 5.5 years longer than did their 5 respective homozygous sibs, each of whom presumably had an identical genetic defect, but who died without benefit of plasma exchange.

LDL apheresis has replaced plasma-exchange therapy in most centers. In this method, plasma is passed in a continuous fashion extracorporeally over columns that remove apo B-100-containing lipoproteins (VLDL, IDL, and LDL), but do not absorb HDL or other plasma proteins. These columns employ either heparin agarose,[473] anti-LDL antibody-agarose,[474] or dextran sulfate bound to a cellulose matrix.[475,476] LDL apheresis has been successfully performed on FH homozygotes during childhood[477] and pregnancy.[478] Two homozygous children (ages 7 and 10) underwent apheresis for 2 to 3 h every week, and the mean plasma level of LDL was reduced 71 percent.[477] A reduction of similar magnitude was seen in the plasma levels of vitamins A and E, but the children were maintained on multivitamins, and no clinical or laboratory evidence of a deficiency in either fat-soluble vitamin was detected.

The indications for apheresis have been expanded to include FH heterozygotes in whom adequate lowering of plasma LDL levels cannot be accomplished with diet and lipid-lowering medications. The Food and Drug Administration has approved apheresis therapy for use in these patients: (a) FH heterozygotes with established coronary artery disease and an LDL cholesterol greater than 200 mg/dl; and (b) FH heterozygotes without evidence of ischemic heart disease but with a plasma LDL cholesterol greater than 300 mg/dl on maximum doses of lipid-lowering drugs. Most FH heterozygotes can achieve a reduction in the mean LDL cholesterol level to less than 130 mg/dl by taking lipid-lowering medications and undergoing apheresis every 2 weeks.[479]

Apheresis treatment is often associated with shrinkage of xanthomas. Angiographic regression of coronary atherosclerosis has been reported in about 50 percent of FH patients after long-term LDL apheresis[480,481] (discussed below).

Apheresis has the theoretical added advantage of decreasing another major atherogenic lipoprotein, Lp(a). Two groups studied lipid-lowering therapy coupled with apheresis as compared with lipid-lowering therapy alone.[482,483] Perhaps because of the short duration ($\sim$2 years), neither study demonstrated any significant increase in coronary artery regression in the combined therapy group despite a 20 percent reduction in plasma levels of Lp(a).

As of August 1, 1998, 59 FH homozygotes and heterozygotes were being treated with long-term apheresis at 21 medical centers (Evan Stein, personal communication).

Liver Transplantation. The rationale for liver transplantation is based on experimental data in animals showing that more than 70 percent of the body's LDL receptors are in the liver (discussed above). The first FH homozygote to receive a liver transplant was a 6-year-old girl with a total cholesterol level above 1000 mg/dl who had repeated myocardial infarctions. After she failed to respond to two coronary bypass procedures plus a mitral valve replacement, she underwent heart-liver transplantation by a team of surgeons led by Thomas E. Starzl at the University of Pittsburgh.[484,485] Postoperatively, her total plasma cholesterol level fell from 1100 mg/dl to the range of 200 to 300 mg/dl. Lipoprotein turnover studies performed 6 months after surgery showed an increased fractional catabolic rate for LDL from 0.12 to 0.31 pool/day, confirming that the new LDL receptors furnished by the transplanted liver were responsible for the dramatic drop in plasma cholesterol level.[485] After 13 months, she was started on lovastatin, and her cholesterol fell further, to the range of 150 to 200 mg/dl.[463,485,486] Thus, liver transplantation not only lowered the plasma cholesterol level, but it also restored responsiveness to lovastatin, which requires a normal LDL receptor gene in order to act. Her cutaneous xanthomas resolved after 2 years, and she remained asymptomatic for 6 years with no clinical signs of coronary heart disease. Despite treatment with cyclosporine, she had a liver rejection 6 years after the original heart-liver transplantation, and this necessitated a new liver transplant. She died 6 months later as a result of cardiac rejection. At autopsy, there was no significant atherosclerosis in the arteries of her 6-year-old transplanted heart.

At least six FH homozygotes have been treated with liver transplantation.[463,485–489a] In the five patients who survived the transplant surgery, the plasma LDL fell dramatically. The longest survivor, a boy from Madrid who was 12 at the time of his combined liver-heart transplantation, was alive 9 years later in 1995.[489a] This approach must not be taken lightly. The surgical procedure is hazardous in a patient with advanced atherosclerosis, and the lifelong need for immunosuppression carries a substantial risk.

Gene Therapy. The success of liver transplantation in lowering the plasma level of LDL has stimulated efforts to use gene therapy approaches to express recombinant LDL receptors in the liver. Five FH homozygotes with coronary artery disease have been treated using an *ex vivo* approach.[490,491] In this method, a partial hepatectomy is performed, and a catheter is introduced into the portal vein. The liver cells are transfected *ex vivo* with a retrovirus expressing the LDL receptor. The cells are then reintroduced into the liver via the portal vein three days after the initial surgery.

The first FH homozygote treated by this approach was a 28-year-old French Canadian.[490] Her plasma LDL cholesterol level fell 16 percent within 1 month after the procedure. She was then placed on lovastatin and had an additional 19 percent reduction in the LDL cholesterol level. This subject was homozygous for a missense mutation in exon 3 (*French Canadian-4*; *W66G*), which is associated with LDL receptor activities in fibroblasts that range between 25 and 100 percent of normal (this unique mutation is discussed above). The performance of the surgical procedure in this patient and the subsequent administration of lovastatin is likely to have increased the functional activity of this unusual mutant receptor, making any interpretation of the effectiveness of gene therapy inconclusive.[492]

Four additional FH homozygotes were subsequently treated using the same protocol.[491] Two of the four patients had no significant reduction in their plasma LDL cholesterol levels. One of the four patients, who had an LDL receptor activity in fibroblasts of less than 2 percent of normal, had a 19 percent reduction in the LDL cholesterol level (from 737 to 595 mg/dl) associated with an increase in the fractional catabolic rate of LDL (from 0.182 to 0.280 per day). The molecular defects in this patient's LDL receptor alleles were not defined, and information regarding the presence or absence of immunodetectable LDL receptor protein was not provided.

Based on the results of these preliminary studies, gene therapy cannot currently be advised as a therapeutic option for the treatment of FH homozygotes. The morbidity associated with this procedure is high, including acute myocardial infarction, mesenteric thrombosis, and the need for blood transfusions.[493] The development of more effective methods to deliver and achieve high expression of recombinant LDL receptors will be needed before gene therapy can be justified for use in FH homozygotes.

Regression of Atherosclerosis

Within the past 10 years, 6 teams of investigators have used coronary angiography to demonstrate a reduced rate of progression, and in some cases, an actual regression of atherosclerotic lesions in hypercholesterolemic individuals treated with a variety of cholesterol-lowering regimens.[441,481,494–497] In one of the two studies that focused specifically on FH patients, Kane et al.[494] used various combinations of a bile acid binding resin, nicotinic acid, and lovastatin to lower plasma LDL cholesterol levels in 72 FH heterozygotes by an average of 38 percent while raising HDL cholesterol by 28 percent. At the 2-year follow-up examination in both the control and treated subjects, some of the atherosclerotic plaques had increased in size, whereas others had diminished. To surmount this variability, the investigators determined the average size of all measured plaques in any one individual. The drug-treated patients showed a small but statistically significant net regression in mean plaque size, whereas the control group showed a net progression. The lesions in FH heterozygote women responded as well as those in heterozygote men. The results in individual patients were correlated best with the posttreatment LDL level, and not with the level of HDL. The number of patients and the duration of the study were insufficient to determine an effect on clinical outcome.

In the other study that focused on FH patients, Tatami et al.[481] used LDL apheresis combined with one or more cholesterol-lowering drugs to lower LDL levels in 7 FH homozygotes and 25 heterozygotes. Angiographic evidence of regression was observed in almost 50 percent of the patients—that is, in 4 homozygotes treated for a mean of 6.9 years and in 10 FH heterozygotes treated for a mean of 3 years.

The results of other angiographic studies were similar to those given above, but the treated patients were not evaluated specifically for the diagnosis of FH.[441,495–497] In the most extensive of these studies, Buchwald et al.[441] carried out a 10-year follow-up of 838 moderately hypercholesterolemic patients who had experienced at least one myocardial infarction and were assigned randomly to a control group (some of whom received lipid-lowering drugs) or to partial ileal bypass, which depletes bile acids. In the surgical patients, a 38 percent reduction in LDL cholesterol was associated with a 25 percent reduction in coronary mortality (32 versus 44 deaths), which was not statistically significant. The treatment did produce a statistically significant 36 percent reduction in mortality among those individuals who had relatively normal cardiac function at entry as indicated by a systolic ejection fraction greater than 50 percent. The angiographic follow-up showed a highly significant reduction in the rate of progression of the atherosclerotic lesions ($p < 0.001$). There was also a marked reduction in the number of patients who underwent coronary bypass surgery (137 control versus 52 surgery patients).

In the last five years, four large prospective studies conclusively demonstrated that lowering plasma LDL cholesterol levels is associated with a reduction in coronary events and mortality.[498–501] A striking uniformity in results was seen in these four studies, two of which were primary prevention studies,[500,501] with the other two being secondary prevention studies involving individuals with established coronary artery disease.[498,499] Statins were used as the lipid-lowering agent in the four studies. The four studies involved 21,803 patients who were followed for ~5 years. On average, plasma LDL cholesterol levels were reduced by ~30 percent, and the incidence of myocardial infarctions declined by ~30 percent. In the 4S study from Scandinavia, which was a secondary prevention trial involving patients with a mean total cholesterol of 270 mg/dl, deaths from heart attacks fell 42 percent, and deaths from all causes were reduced 30 percent. The other secondary prevention trial, the CARE study carried out in the U.S. and Canada, showed a clear benefit even in individuals with total plasma cholesterol levels in the "normal" range (~210 mg/dl).

The most recent primary prevention study, reported in 1998 and called the AFCAPS Study, followed 5608 men and 997 women living in Texas who had a mean plasma total cholesterol of 221 mg/dl (corresponding to the 51st percentile in the population), LDL-cholesterol of 150 mg/dl (60th percentile), and HDL cholesterol of 36 mg/dl (5th percentile).[501] These normolipidemic individuals with low plasma HDL cholesterol levels were all treated with lovastatin (20 or 40 mg/day) for ~5 years. A 25 percent reduction in plasma LDL-cholesterol was associated with a 37 percent decrease in myocardial infarctions, sudden death, or unstable angina. The subjects with an initial plasma LDL cholesterol in the lowest quartile benefited as much from lovastatin therapy as those in the highest quartile.

The results of the AFCAPS study have necessitated a reassessment of the definition of a "normal" level of plasma cholesterol. Ingestion of a high-fat diet by an increasing proportion of the world's population has shifted the distribution of plasma cholesterol to the right. The average cholesterol level in a middle-aged individual living in the United States or Europe (~210 mg/dl) is above the 90th percentile value for the human species worldwide.

Considered together with earlier studies, such as the Lipid Research Clinics Coronary Primary Prevention Trial that treated hypercholesterolemic subjects with the less potent resins,[502] these more recent studies with statin therapy strongly suggest that cholesterol-lowering therapy will slow the progression of, and perhaps even reverse, the coronary atherosclerotic process in FH heterozygotes.[503]

REFERENCES

1. Müller C: Xanthomata, hypercholesterolemia, angina pectoris. *Acta Med Scand* **89**:75, 1938.
2. Müller C: Angina pectoris in hereditary xanthomatosis. *Arch Intern Med* **305**:318, 1939.
3. Brown MS, Goldstein JL: A receptor-mediated pathway for cholesterol homeostasis. *Science* **232**:34, 1986.
4. Goldstein JL, Brown MS: Familial hypercholesterolemia, in Scriver CR, Beaudet AL, Sly WS, Valle D (eds): *The Metabolic Basis of Inherited Disease, 6th ed.* New York, McGraw-Hill, 1989, vol 1, p 1215.
5. Thannhauser SJ, Magendantz H: The different clinical groups of xanthomatous diseases: A clinical physiological study of 22 cases. *Ann Intern Med* **11**:1662, 1938.
6. Thannhauser SJ: *Lipidoses*. New York, Oxford, 1950.
7. Wilkinson CE Jr, Hand EA, Fliegelman MT: Essential familial hypercholesterolemia. *Ann Intern Med* **29**:671, 1948.
8. Adlersberg D, Parets AD, Boas EP: Genetics of atherosclerosis. Studies of families with xanthoma and unselected patients with coronary artery disease under the age of fifty years. *JAMA* **141**:246, 1949.
9. Adlersberg D: Inborn errors of lipid metabolism. *Arch Pathol* **60**:481, 1955.
10. Bloom D, Kaufman SR, Stevens RA: Hereditary xanthomatosis: Familial incidence of xanthoma tuberosum associated with hypercholesterolemia and cardiovascular involvement, with report of several cases of sudden death. *Arch Dermatol Syphilol* **45**:1, 1942.
11. Alvord RM: Coronary heart disease and xanthoma tuberosum associated with hereditary hyperlipidemia. *Arch Intern Med* **84**:1002, 1949.
12. Piper J, Orrild L: Essential familial hypercholesterolemia and xanthomatosis. *Am J Med* **21**:34, 1956.
13. Epstein FH, Block WD, Hand EA, Francis T Jr: Familial hypercholesterolemia, xanthomatosis and coronary heart disease. *Am J Med* **26**:39, 1959.
14. Hirschhorn K, Wilkinson CF: The mode of inheritance in essential familial hypercholesterolemia. *Am J Med* **26**:60, 1959.
15. Guravich JL: Familial hypercholesteremic xanthomatosis: A preliminary report. I. Clinical, electrocardiographic and laboratory considerations. *Am J Med* **24**:8, 1959.
16. Khachadurian AK: The inheritance of essential familial hypercholesterolemia. *Am J Med* **37**:402, 1964.
17. Gofman JW, Delalla O, Glazier F, Freeman NK, Lindgren FT, Nichols AV, Strisower B, Tamplin AR: The serum lipoprotein transport system in health, metabolic disorders, atherosclerosis and coronary heart disease. *Plasma* **2**:413, 1954.
18. Gofman JW, Rubin L, McGinley JP, Jones HB: Hyperlipoproteinemia. *Am J Med* **17**:514, 1954.
19. Fredrickson DS, Levy RI, Lees RS: Fat transport in lipoproteins—An integrated approach to mechanisms and disorders. *N Engl J Med* **276**:32, 1967.
20. Goldstein JL, Brown MS: Binding and degradation of low density lipoproteins by cultured human fibroblasts: Comparison of cells from a normal subject and from a patient with homozygous familial hypercholesterolemia. *J Biol Chem* **249**:5153, 1974.
21. Fass D, Blacklow S, Kim PS, Berger JM: Molecular basis of familial hypercholesterolaemia from structure of LDL receptor module. *Nature* **388**:691, 1997.
22. Brown MS, Goldstein JL: The SREBP pathway: Regulation of cholesterol metabolism by proteolysis of a membrane-bound transcription factor. *Cell* **89**:331, 1997.
23. Harlan WR Jr, Graham JB, Estes EH: Familial hypercholesterolemia: A genetic and metabolic study. *Medicine (Baltimore)* **45**:77, 1966.
24. Schrott HG, Goldstein JL, Hazzard WR, McGoodwin MM, Motulsky AG: Familial hypercholesterolemia in a large kindred. Evidence for a monogenic mechanism. *Ann Intern Med* **76**:711, 1972.
25. Kwiterovich PO Jr, Levi RI, Fredrickson DS: Neonatal diagnosis of familial type-II hyperlipoproteinaemia. *Lancet* **1**:118, 1973.
26. Kwiterovich PO Jr, Fredrickson DS, Levy RI: Familial hypercholesterolemia (one form of familial type II hyperlipoproteinemia). A

study of its biochemical, genetic, and clinical presentation in childhood. *J Clin Invest* **53**:1237, 1974.
27. Khachadurian AK: A general review of clinical and laboratory features of familial hypercholesterolemia (type II hyperbetalipoproteinemia). *Protides Biol Fluids* **19**:315, 1971.
28. Fredrickson DS, Levy RI: Familial hyperlipoproteinemia, in Stanbury JB, Wyngaarden JB, Fredrickson DS (eds): *The Metabolic Basis of Inherited Disease, 3rd ed.* New York, McGraw-Hill, 1972, p 545.
29. Khachadurian AK, Uthman SM: Experiences with homozygous cases of familial hypercholesterolemia. A report of 52 patients. *Nutr Metab* **15**:132, 1973.
30. Haitas B, Baker SG, Meyer TE, Joffe BI, Seftel HC: Natural history and cardiac manifestations of homozygous familial hypercholesterolaemia. *Q J Med* **76**:731, 1990.
31. Beppu S, Minura Y, Sakakibara H, Nagata S, Park Y-D, Nambu S, Yamamoto A: Supravalvular aortic stenosis and coronary ostial stenosis in familial hypercholesterolemia: Two-dimensional echocardiographic assessment. *Circulation* **67**:878, 1983.
32. Nevin NC, Slack J: Hyperlipidaemic xanthomatosis. II: Mode of inheritance in 55 families with essential hyperlipidaemia and xanthomatosis. *J Med Genet* **5**:9, 1968.
33. Slack J, Mills GL: Anomalous low density lipoproteins in familial hyperbetalipoproteinaemia. *Clin Chim Acta* **29**:15, 1970.
34. Gotto AM Jr, Brown WV, Levy RI, Birnbaumer ME, Fredrickson DS: Evidence for the identity of the major apoprotein in low density and very low density lipoproteins in normal subjects and patients with familial hyperlipoproteinemia. *J Clin Invest* **51**:1486, 1972.
35. Fisher WR, Hammond MG, Warmke GL: Measurements of the molecular weight variability of plasma low density lipoproteins among normals and subjects with hyper-β-lipoproteinemia. Demonstration of macromolecular heterogeneity. *Biochemistry* **11**:519, 1972.
36. Jadhav AV, Thompson GR: Reversible abnormalities of low density lipoprotein composition in familial hypercholesterolaemia. *Eur J Clin Invest* **9**:63, 1979.
37. Bagnall TF, Lloyd JK: Composition of low-density lipoprotein in children with hyperlipoproteinaemia. *Clin Chim Acta* **59**:271, 1975.
38. Grant EH, Sheppard RJ, Mills GL, Slack J: A dielectric investigation of the water of hydration of low-density lipoproteins in familial hyperbetalipoproteinaemia. *Lancet* **1**:1159, 1972.
39. Reichl D, Simons LA, Myant NB: The metabolism of low-density lipoprotein in a patient with familial hyperbetalipoproteinaemia. *Clin Sci Mol Med* **47**:635, 1974.
40. Patsch W, Witztum JL, Ostlund R, Schonfeld G: Structure, immunology, and cell reactivity of low density lipoprotein from umbilical vein of a newborn type II homozygote. *J Clin Invest* **66**:123, 1980.
41. Goldstein JL, Brown MS: Familial hypercholesterolemia: Identification of a defect in the regulation of 3-hydroxy-3-methylglutaryl coenzyme A reductase activity associated with overproduction of cholesterol. *Proc Natl Acad Sci U S A* **70**:2804, 1973.
42. Streja D, Steiner G, Kwiterovich PO Jr: Plasma high-density lipoproteins and ischemic heart disease: Studies in a large kindred with familial hypercholesterolemia. *Ann Intern Med* **89**:871, 1978.
43. Seftel HC, Baker SG, Sandler MP, Forman MB, Joffe BI, Mendelsohn D, Jenkins T, Mieny CJ: A host of hypercholesterolaemic homozygotes in South Africa. *Br Med J* **281**:633, 1980.
44. Vergopoulos A, Bajari T, Jouma M, Knoblauch H, Aydin A, Bahring S, Mueller-Myhsok B, Dresel A, Joubran R, Luft FC, Schuster H: A xanthomatosis-susceptibility gene may exist in a Syrian family with familial hypercholesterolemia. *Eur J Hum Genet* **5**:315, 1997.
45. Macaraeg PVJ Jr, Lasagna L, Snyder B: Arcus not so senilis. *Ann Intern Med* **68**:345, 1968.
46. Goldstein JL: The cardiac manifestations of the homozygous and heterozygous forms of familial type II hyperbetalipoproteinemia. *Birth Defects* **8**:202, 1972.
47. Sprecher DL, Schaefer EJ, Kent KM, Gregg RE, Zech LA, Hoeg JM, McManus B, Roberts WC, Brewer HB Jr: Cardiovascular features of homozygous familial hypercholesterolemia: Analysis of 16 patients. *Am J Cardiol* **54**:20, 1984.
48. Rose V, Wilson G, Steiner G: Familial hypercholesterolemia: Report of coronary death at age 3 in a homozygous child and prenatal diagnosis in a heterozygous sibling. *J Pediatr* **100**:757, 1982.
49. Postiglione A, Nappi A, Brunetti A, Soricelli A, Rubba P, Gnasso A, Cammisa M, Frusciante V, Cortese C, Salvatore M, Weber G, Mancini M: Relative protection from cerebral atherosclerosis of young patients with homozygous familial hypercholesterolemia. *Atherosclerosis* **90**:23, 1991.
50. Sprecher DL, Hoeg JM, Schaefer EJ, Zech LA, Gregg RE, Lakatos E, Brewer HB Jr: The association of LDL receptor activity, LDL cholesterol level, and clinical course in homozygous familial hypercholesterolemia. *Metabolism* **34**:294, 1985.
51. Schmidt HHJ, Hill S, Makariou EV, Feuerstein IM, Dugi KA, Hoeg JM: Relation of cholesterol-year score to severity of calcific atherosclerosis and tissue deposition in homozygous familial hypercholesterolemia. *Am J Cardiol* **77**:575, 1996.
52. Hendry WG, Seed M: Homozygous familial hypercholesterolaemia with supravalvar aortic stenosis treated by surgery. *J R Soc Med* **78**:334, 1985.
53. Khachadurian AK: Migratory polyarthritis in familial hypercholesterolemia (type II hyperlipoproteinemia). *Arthritis Rheum* **11**:385, 1968.
54. Khachadurian AK: Persistent elevation of the erythrocyte sedimentation rate (ESR) in familial hypercholesterolemia. *J Med Liban* **20**:31, 1967.
55. Jensen J, Blankenhorn DH, Kornerup V: Coronary disease in familial hypercholesterolemia. *Circulation* **36**:77, 1967.
56. Slack J: Risks of ischaemic heart disease in familial hyperlipoproteinaemic states. *Lancet* **2**:1380, 1969.
57. Heiberg A: The risk of atherosclerotic vascular disease in subjects with xanthomatosis. *Acta Med Scand* **198**:249, 1975.
58. Stone NJ, Levy RI, Fredrickson DS, Verter J: Coronary artery disease in 116 kindreds with familial type II hyperlipoproteinemia. *Circulation* **49**:476, 1974.
59. Beaumont V, Jacotot B, Beaumont J-L: Ischaemic disease in men and women with familial hypercholesterolaemia and xanthomatosis. A comparative study of genetic and environmental factors in 274 heterozygous cases. *Atherosclerosis* **24**:441, 1976.
60. Mabuchi H, Miyamoto S, Ueda K, Oota M, Takegoshi T, Wakasugi T, Takeda R: Causes of death in patients with familial hypercholesterolemia. *Atherosclerosis* **61**:1, 1986.
61. Sudhir K, Ports TA, Amidon TM, Goldberger JJ, Bhushan V, Kane JP, Yock P, Malloy MJ: Increased prevalence of coronary ectasia in heterozygous familial hypercholesterolemia. *Circulation* **91**:1375, 1995.
62. Hill JS, Hayden MR, Frohlich J, Pritchard PH: Genetic and environmental factors affecting the incidence of coronary artery disease in heterozygous familial hypercholesterolemia. *Arteriosclerosis* **11**:290, 1991.
63. Ferrieres J, Lambert J, Lussier-Cacan S, Davignon J: Coronary artery disease in heterozygous familial hypercholesterolemia patients with the same LDL receptor gene mutation. *Circulation* **92**:290, 1995.
64. Wittekoek ME, Pimstone SN, Reymer PWA, Feuth L, Botma G-J, Defesche JC, Prins M, Hayden MR, Kastelein JJP: A common mutation in the lipoprotein lipase gene (N291S) alters the lipoprotein phenotype and risk for cardiovascular disease in patients with familial hypercholesterolemia. *Circulation* **97**:729, 1998.
65. Hofmann SL, Eaton DL, Brown MS, McConathy WJ, Goldstein JL, Hammer RE: Overexpression of human low density lipoprotein receptors leads to accelerated catabolism of Lp(a) lipoprotein in transgenic mice. *J Clin Invest* **85**:1542, 1990.
66. Rader DJ, Mann WA, Cain W, Kraft H-G, Usher D, Zech LA, Hoeg JM, Davignon J, Lupien P, Grossman M, Wilson JM, Brewer HB Jr: The low density lipoprotein receptor is not required for normal catabolism of Lp(a) in humans. *J Clin Invest* **95**:1403, 1995.
67. Thiery J, Armstrong VW, Schleef J, Creutzfeldt C, Creutzfeldt W, Seidel D: Serum lipoprotein Lp(a) concentrations are not influenced by an HMG CoA reductase inhibitor. *Klin Wochenschr* **66**:462, 1988.
68. Neven L, Khalil A, Pfaffinger D, Fless GM, Jackson E, Scanu AM: Rhesus monkey model of familial hypercholesterolemia: relation between plasma Lp(a) levels, apo(a) isoforms, and LDL-receptor function. *J Lipid Res* **31**:633, 1990.
69. Utermann G, Hoppichler F, Dieplinger H, Seed M, Thompson G, Boerwinkle E: Defects in the low density lipoprotein receptor gene affect lipoprotein (a) levels: Multiplicative interaction of two gene loci associated with premature atherosclerosis. *Proc Natl Acad Sci U S A* **86**:4171, 1989.
70. Bowden J-F, Pritchard PH, Hill JS, Frohlich JJ: Lp(a) concentration and apo(a) isoform size: relation to the presence of coronary artery disease in familial hypercholesterolemia. *Arterioscler Thromb* **14**:1561, 1994.
71. Leitersdorf E, Friedlander Y, Bard J-M, Fruchart J-C, Eisenberg S, Stein Y: Diverse effect of ethnicity on plasma lipoprotein(a) levels in

heterozygote patients with familial hypercholesterolemia. *J Lipid Res* **32**:1513, 1991.

72. Carmena R, Lussier-Cacan S, Roy M, Minnich A, Lingenhel A, Kronenberg F, Davignon J: Lp(a) levels and atherosclerotic vascular disease in a sample of patients with familial hypercholesterolemia sharing the same gene defect. *Arterioscler Thromb Vasc Biol* **16**:129, 1996.
73. Soutar AK, McCarthy SN, Seed M, Knight BL: Relationship between apoprotein(a) phenotype, lipoprotein(a) concentration in plasma and low density lipoprotein receptor function in a large kindred with familial hypercholesterolemia due to the Pro_{664}-Leu mutation in the LDL-receptor gene. *J Clin Invest* **88**:483, 1991.
74. Defesche JC, van de Ree MA, Kastelein JJP, van Diermen DE, Janssens NWE, van Doormaal JJ, Hayden MR: Detection of the Pro_{664}-Leu mutation in the low-density lipoprotein receptor and its relation to lipoprotein(a) levels in patients with familial hypercholesterolemia of Dutch ancestry from The Netherlands and Canada. *Clin Genet* **42**:273, 1992.
75. Perombelon YFN, Soutar AK, Knight BL: Variation in lipoprotein(a) concentration associated with different apolipoprotein(a) alleles. *J Clin Invest* **93**:1481, 1994.
76. Ghiselli G, Gaddi A, Barozzi G, Ciarrocchi A, Descovich G: Plasma lipoprotein(a) concentration in familial hypercholesterolemic patients without coronary artery disease. *Metabolism* **41**:833, 1992.
77. Lingenhel A, Kraft HG, Kotze M, Peeters AV, Kronenberg F, Kruse R, Utermann G: Concentrations of the atherogenic Lp(a) are elevated in FH. *Eur J Hum Genet* **6**:50, 1998.
78. Boerwinkle E, Leffert CC, Lin J, Lackner C, Chiesa G, Hobbs HH: Apolipoprotein(a) gene accounts for greater than 90% of the variation in plasma lipoprotein(a) concentrations. *J Clin Invest* **90**:52, 1992.
79. Armstrong VW, Cremer P, Eberle E, Manke A, Schulze F, Wieland H, Kreuzer H, Seidel D: The association between serum Lp(a) concentrations and angiographically assessed coronary atherosclerosis: Dependence on serum LDL levels. *Atherosclerosis* **62**:249, 1986.
80. Cremer P, Nagel D, Mann H, Labrot B, Müller-Berninger R, Elster H, Seidel D: Ten-year follow-up results from the Goettingen Risk, Incidence and Prevalence Study, (GRIPS). 1. Risk factors for myocardial infarction in a cohort of 5790 men. *Atherosclerosis* **129**:221, 1997.
81. Seed M, Hoppichler F, Reaveley D, McCarthy S, Thompson GR, Boerwinkle E, Utermann G: Relation of serum lipoprotein(a) concentration and apolipoprotein(a) phenotype to coronary heart disease in patients with familial hypercholesterolemia. *N Engl J Med* **322**:1494, 1990.
82. Wiklund O, Angelin B, Olofsson S-O, Eriksson M, Fager G, Berglund L, Bondjers G: Apolipoprotein(a) and ischaemic heart disease in familial hypercholesterolaemia. *Lancet* **335**:1360, 1990.
83. Mbewu AD, Bhatnagar D, Durrington PN, Hunt L, Ishola M, Arrol S, Mackness M, Lockley P, Miller JP: Serum lipoprotein(a) in patients heterozygous for familial hypercholesterolemia, their relatives, and unrelated control populations. *Arterioscler Thromb* **11**:940, 1991.
84. Mathon G, Gagne C, Brun D, Lupien P-J, Moorjani S: Articular manifestations of familial hypercholesterolaemia. *Ann Rheum Dis* **44**:599, 1985.
85. Rooney PJ, Third J, Madkour MM, Spencer D, Dick WC: Transient polyarthritis associated with familial hyperbetalipoproteinaemia. *Q J Med* **47**:249, 1978.
86. Gunther SF, Gunther AG, Hoeg JM, Kruth HS: Multiple flexor tendon xanthomas and contractures in the hands of a child with familial hypercholesterolemia. *J Hand Surg [Am]* **11**:588, 1986.
87. Goldstein JL, Brown MS: The LDL receptor locus and the genetics of familial hypercholesterolemia. *Annu Rev Genet* **13**:259, 1979.
88. Mabuchi H, Tatami R, Haba T, Ueda K, Ueda R, Kametani T, Itoh S, Koizumi J, Oota M, Miyamoto S, Takeda R, Takeshita H: Homozygous familial hypercholesterolemia in Japan. *Am J Med* **65**:290, 1978.
89. Buja LM, Kovanen PT, Bilheimer DW: Cellular pathology of homozygous familial hypercholesterolemia. *Am J Pathol* **97**:327, 1979.
90. Mabuchi H: Personal communication, 1992.
91. Komuro I, Kato H, Nakagawa T, Takahashi K, Mimori A, Takeuchi F, Nishida Y, Miyamoto T: Case report: The longest-lived patient with homozygous familial hypercholesterolemia secondary to a defect in internalization of the LDL receptor. *Am J Med Sci* **294**:341, 1987.
92. Ishii K, Matsumura T, Hori K, Kita T: A 50-year-old patient with homozygous familial hypercholesterolemia. *J Clin Biochem Nutr* **7**:161, 1989.
93. Patterson D, Slack J: Lipid abnormalities in male and female survivors of myocardial infarction and their first-degree relatives. *Lancet* **1**:393, 1972.
94. Goldstein JL, Schrott HG, Hazzard WR, Bierman EL, Motulsky AG: Hyperlipidemia in coronary heart disease. II. Genetic analysis of lipid levels in 176 families and delineation of a new inherited disorder, combined hyperlipidemia. *J Clin Invest* **52**:1544, 1973.
95. Nikkila EA, Aro A: Family study of serum lipids and lipoproteins in coronary heart disease. *Lancet* **1**:954, 1973.
96. Carter CO, Slack J, Myant NB: Genetics of hyperlipoproteinaemias. *Lancet* **1**:400, 1971.
97. Slack J: Inheritance of familial hypercholesterolemia. *Atheroscler Rev* **5**:35, 1979.
98. Heiberg A, Berg K: The inheritance of hyperlipoproteinaemia with xanthomatosis. A study of 132 kindreds. *Clin Genet* **9**:203, 1976.
99. Andersen GE, Lous P, Friis-Hansen B: Screening for hyperlipoproteinemia in 10,000 Danish newborns. Follow-up studies in 522 children with elevated cord serum VLDL-LDL-cholesterol. *Acta Paediatr Scand* **68**:541, 1979.
100. Mabuchi H, Tatami R, Ueda K, Ueda R, Haba T, Kametani T, Watanabe A, Wakasugi T, Ito S, Koizumi J, Ohta M, Miyamoto S, Takeda R: Serum lipid and lipoprotein levels in Japanese patients with familial hypercholesterolemia. *Atherosclerosis* **32**:435, 1979.
101. Moorjani S, Roy M, Gagne C, Davignon J, Brun D, Toussaint M, Lambert M, Campeau L, Blaichman S, Lupien P: Homozygous familial hypercholesterolemia among French Canadians in Quebec Province. *Arteriosclerosis* **9**:211, 1989.
102. Jenkins T, Nicholls E, Gordon E, Mendelsohn D, Seftel HC, Andrew MJA: Familial hypercholesterolaemia — A common genetic disorder in the Afrikaans population. *S Afr Med J* **57**:943, 1980.
103. Seftel HC, Baker SG, Jenkins T, Mendelsohn D: Prevalence of familial hypercholesterolemia in Johannesburg Jews. *Am J Med Genet* **34**:545, 1989.
104. Goldstein JL, Brown MS: Familial hypercholesterolemia, in Stanbury JB, Wyngaarden JB, Fredrickson DS, Goldstein JL, Brown MS (eds): *The Metabolic Basis of Inherited Disease, 5th ed.* New York, McGraw-Hill, 1983, p 672.
105. Roberts WC, Ferrans VJ, Levy RI, Fredrickson DS: Cardiovascular pathology in hyperlipoproteinemia. Anatomic observations in 42 necropsy patients with normal or abnormal serum lipoprotein patterns. *Am J Cardiol* **31**:557, 1973.
106. Brown MS, Kovanen PT, Goldstein JL, Eeckels R, Vandenberghe K, Berghe HVD, Fryns JP, Cassiman JJ: Prenatal diagnosis of homozygous familial hypercholesterolaemia: Expression of a genetic receptor disease in utero. *Lancet* **1**:526, 1978.
107. Ross R: The pathogenesis of atherosclerosis: A perspective for the 1990s. *Nature* **362**:801, 1993.
108. Hoeg JM, Feuerstein IM, Tucker EE: Detection and quantitation of calcific atherosclerosis by ultrafast computed tomography in children and young adults with homozygous familial hypercholesterolemia. *Arterioscler Thromb* **14**:1066, 1994.
109. Bulkley BH, Buja LM, Ferrans VJ, Bulkley GB, Roberts WC: Tuberous xanthoma in homozygous type II hyperlipoproteinemia: A histologic, histochemical, and electron microscopical study. *Arch Pathol* **99**:293, 1975.
110. Goldstein JL, Brown MS: Atherosclerosis: The low-density lipoprotein receptor hypothesis. *Metabolism* **26**:1257, 1977.
111. Brown MS, Goldstein JL: Lipoprotein metabolism in the macrophage: Implications for cholesterol deposition in atherosclerosis. *Annu Rev Biochem* **52**:223, 1983.
112. Goldstein JL, Brown MS: The low-density lipoprotein pathway and its relation to atherosclerosis. *Annu Rev Biochem* **46**:897, 1977.
113. Brown MS, Goldstein JL: Lipoprotein receptors in the liver: Control signals for plasma cholesterol traffic. *J Clin Invest* **72**:743, 1983.
114. Goldstein JL, Basu SK, Brunschede GY, Brown MS: Release of low density lipoprotein from its cell surface receptor by sulfated glycosaminoglycans. *Cell* **7**:85, 1976.
115. Brown MS, Goldstein JL: Regulation of the activity of the low density lipoprotein receptor in human fibroblasts. *Cell* **6**:307, 1975.
116. Schneider WJ, Beisiegel U, Goldstein JL, Brown MS: Purification of the low density lipoprotein receptor, an acidic glycoprotein of 164,000 molecular weight. *J Biol Chem* **257**:2664, 1982.
117. Cummings RD, Kornfeld S, Schneider WJ, Hobgood KK, Tolleshaug H, Brown MS, Goldstein JL: Biosynthesis of the *N*- and *O*-linked oligosaccharides of the low density lipoprotein receptor. *J Biol Chem* **258**:15261, 1983.

118. Davis CG, Elhammer A, Russell DW, Schneider WJ, Kornfeld S, Brown MS, Goldstein JL: Deletion of clustered *O*-linked carbohydrates does not impair function of low density lipoprotein receptor in transfected fibroblasts. *J Biol Chem* **261**:2828, 1986.
119. Bersot TP, Mahley RW, Brown MS, Goldstein JL: Interaction of swine lipoproteins with the low density lipoprotein receptor in human fibroblasts. *J Biol Chem* **251**:2395, 1976.
120. Mahley RW: Apolipoprotein E: Cholesterol transport protein with expanding role in cell biology. *Science* **240**:622, 1988.
121. Basu SK, Goldstein JL, Anderson RGW, Brown MS: Degradation of cationized low density lipoprotein and regulation of cholesterol metabolism in homozygous familial hypercholesterolemia fibroblasts. *Proc Natl Acad Sci U S A* **73**:3178, 1976.
122. Weisgraber KH, Innerarity TL, Mahley RW: Role of the lysine residues of plasma lipoproteins in high affinity binding to cell surface receptors on human fibroblasts. *J Biol Chem* **253**:9053, 1978.
123. Mahley RW, Innerarity TL, Pitas RE, Weisgraber KH, Brown JH, Gross E: Inhibition of lipoprotein binding to cell surface receptors of fibroblasts following selective modification of arginyl residues in arginine-rich and B apoproteins. *J Biol Chem* **252**:7279, 1977.
124. Tolleshaug H, Goldstein JL, Schneider WJ, Brown MS: Posttranslational processing of the LDL receptor and its genetic disruption in familial hypercholesterolemia. *Cell* **30**:715, 1982.
125. Goldstein JL, Anderson RGW, Brown MS: Coated pits, coated vesicles, and receptor-mediated endocytosis. *Nature* **279**:679, 1979.
126. Helenius A, Mellman I, Wall D, Hubbard A: Endosomes. *TIBS* **8**:245, 1983.
127. Brown MS, Anderson RGW, Goldstein JL: Recycling receptors: The round-trip itinerary of migrant membrane proteins. *Cell* **32**:663, 1983.
128. Basu SK, Goldstein JL, Anderson RGW, Brown MS: Monensin interrupts the recycling of low density lipoprotein receptors in human fibroblasts. *Cell* **24**:493, 1981.
129. Goldstein JL, Dana SE, Faust JR, Beaudet AL, Brown MS: Role of lysosomal acid lipase in the metabolism of plasma low density lipoprotein: Observations in cultured fibroblasts from a patient with cholesteryl ester storage disease. *J Biol Chem* **250**:8487, 1975.
130. Brown MS, Faust JR, Goldstein JL: Role of the low density lipoprotein receptor in regulating the content of free and esterified cholesterol in human fibroblasts. *J Clin Invest* **55**:783, 1975.
131. Anderson RGW, Goldstein JL, Brown MS: Localization of low density lipoprotein receptors on plasma membrane of normal human fibroblasts and their absence in cells from a familial hypercholesterolemia homozygote. *Proc Natl Acad Sci U S A* **73**:2434, 1976.
132. Anderson RGW, Brown MS, Goldstein JL: Role of the coated endocytic vesicle in the uptake of receptor-bound low density lipoprotein in human fibroblasts. *Cell* **10**:351, 1977.
133. Carpentier J-L, Gorden P, Goldstein JL, Anderson RGW, Brown MS, Orci L: Binding and internalization of ^{125}I-LDL in normal and mutant human fibroblasts: A quantitative autoradiographic study. *Exp Cell Res* **121**:135, 1979.
134. Brown MS, Dana SE, Goldstein JL: Regulation of 3-hydroxy-3-methylglutaryl coenzyme A reductase activity in cultured human fibroblasts: Comparison of cells from a normal subject and from a patient with homozygous familial hypercholesterolemia. *J Biol Chem* **249**:789, 1974.
135. Goldstein JL, Dana SE, Brown MS: Esterification of low density lipoprotein cholesterol in human fibroblasts and its absence in homozygous familial hypercholesterolemia. *Proc Natl Acad Sci U S A* **71**:4288, 1974.
136. Dietschy JM, Wilson JD: Regulation of cholesterol metabolism. *N Engl J Med* **282**:1128, 1970.
137. Yamamoto T, Davis CG, Brown MS, Schneider WJ, Casey ML, Goldstein JL, Russell DW: The human LDL receptor: A cysteine-rich protein with multiple *Alu* sequences in its mRNA. *Cell* **39**:27, 1984.
138. Lindgren V, Luskey KL, Russell DW, Francke U: Human genes involved in cholesterol metabolism: Chromosomal mapping of the loci for the low density lipoprotein receptor and 3-hydroxy-3-methylglutaryl-coenzyme A reductase with cDNA probes. *Proc Natl Acad Sci U S A* **82**:8567, 1985.
139. Südhof TC, Goldstein JL, Brown MS, Russell DW: The LDL receptor gene: A mosaic of exons shared with different proteins. *Science* **228**:815, 1985.
140. Hobbs HH, Russell DW, Brown MS, Goldstein JL: The LDL receptor locus and familial hypercholesterolemia: Mutational analysis of a membrane protein. *Annu Rev Genet* **24**:133, 1990.
141. Mahley RW, Innerarity TL, Weisgraber KH, Rall SC Jr, Hui DY, Lalazar A, Boyles JK, Taylor JM, Levy-Wilson B: Cellular and molecular biology of lipoprotein metabolism: Characterization of lipoprotein receptor-ligand interactions. *Cold Spring Harb Symp Quant Biol* **51**:821, 1986.
142. Goldstein JL, Brown MS, Anderson RGW, Russell DW, Schneider WJ: Receptor-mediated endocytosis: Concepts emerging from the LDL receptor system. *Annu Rev Cell Biol* **1**:1, 1985.
143. Brown MS, Herz J, Goldstein JL: Calcium cages, acid baths, and recycling receptors. *Nature* **388**:629, 1997.
144. Russell DW, Brown MS, Goldstein JL: Different combinations of cysteine-rich repeats mediate binding of low density lipoprotein receptor to two different proteins. *J Biol Chem* **264**:21682, 1989.
145. van Driel IR, Goldstein JL, Südhof TC, Brown MS: First cysteine-rich repeat in ligand-binding domain of low density lipoprotein receptor binds Ca^{2+} and monoclonal antibodies, but not lipoproteins. *J Biol Chem* **262**:17443, 1987.
146. Blacklow SC, Kim PS: Protein folding and calcium binding defects arising from familial hypercholesterolemia mutations of the LDL receptor. *Nature Struct Biol* **3**:758, 1996.
147. Südhof TC, Russell DW, Goldstein JL, Brown MS, Sanchez-Pescador R, Bell GI: Cassette of eight exons shared by genes for LDL receptor and EGF precursor. *Science* **228**:893, 1985.
148. Davis CG, Goldstein JL, Südhof TC, Anderson RGW, Russell DW, Brown MS: Acid-dependent ligand dissociation and recycling of LDL receptor mediated by growth factor homology region. *Nature* **326**:760, 1987.
149. Springer TA: An extracellular β-propeller module predicted in lipoprotein and scavenger receptors, tyrosine kinases, epidermal growth factor precursor, and extracellular matrix components. *J Mol Biol* **283**:837, 1998.
150. Kajinami K, Mabuchi H, Itoh H, Michishita I, Takeda M, Wakasugi T, Koizumi J, Takeda R: New variant of low density lipoprotein receptor gene *FH-Tonami*. *Arteriosclerosis* **8**:187, 1988.
151. Koivisto PVI, Koivisto U-M, Miettinen TA, Kontula K: Diagnosis of heterozygous familial hypercholesterolemia. DNA analysis complements clinical examination and analysis of serum lipid levels. *Arterioscler Thromb* **12**:584, 1992.
152. Davis CG, Lehrman MA, Russell DW, Anderson RGW, Brown MS, Goldstein JL: The J.D. mutation in familial hypercholesterolemia: Amino acid substitution in cytoplasmic domain impedes internalization of LDL receptors. *Cell* **45**:15, 1986.
153. Yokode M, Pathak RK, Hammer RE, Brown MS, Goldstein JL, Anderson RGW: Cytoplasmic sequence required for basolateral targeting of LDL receptor in livers of transgenic mice. *J Cell Biol* **117**:39, 1992.
154. Yamamoto T, Bishop RW, Brown MS, Goldstein JL, Russell DW: Deletion in cysteine-rich region of LDL receptor impedes transport to cell surface in WHHL rabbit. *Science* **232**:1230, 1986.
155. Bishop RW: Structure of the hamster low density lipoprotein receptor gene. *J Lipid Res* **33**:549, 1992.
156. Mehta KD, Chen W-J, Goldstein JL, Brown MS: The low density lipoprotein receptor in Xenopus laevis: I. Five domains that resemble the human receptor. *J Biol Chem* **266**:10406, 1991.
157. Hasler-Rapacz J, Ellegren H, Fridolfsson A-K, Kirkpatrick B, Kirk S, Andersson L, Rapacz J: Identification of a mutation in the low density lipoprotein receptor gene associated with recessive familial hypercholesterolemia in swine. *Am J Med Genet* **76**:379, 1998.
157a. Grunwald KAA, Schueler K, Uelmen PJ, Lipton BA, Kaiser M, Buhman K, Attie AD: Identification of a novel Arg → Cys mutation in the LDL receptor that contributes to spontaneous hypercholesterolemia in pigs. *J Lipid Res* **40**:475, 1999.
158. Mehta KD, Chang R, Norman J: *Chiloscyllium plagiosum* low-density lipoprotein receptor: Evolutionary conservation of five different functional domains. *J Mol Evol* **42**:264, 1996.
159. Südhof TC, Russell DW, Brown MS, Goldstein JL: 42-bp element from LDL receptor gene confers end-product repression by sterols when inserted into viral TK promoter. *Cell* **48**:1061, 1987.
160. Goldstein JL, Brown MS: Regulation of the mevalonate pathway. *Nature* **343**:425, 1990.
161. Mehta KD, Brown MS, Bilheimer DW, Goldstein JL: The low density lipoprotein receptor in *Xenopus laevis*: II. Feedback repression mediated by conserved sterol regulatory element. *J Biol Chem* **266**:10415, 1991.
162. Smith JR, Osborne TF, Goldstein JL, Brown MS: Identification of nucleotides responsible for enhancer activity of sterol regulatory element in low density lipoprotein receptor gene. *J Biol Chem* **265**:2306, 1990.

163. Wang X, Sato R, Brown MS, Hua X, Goldstein JL: SREBP-1, a membrane-bound transcription factor released by sterol-regulated proteolysis. *Cell* **77**:53, 1994.
164. Duncan EA, Brown MS, Goldstein JL, Sakai J: Cleavage site for sterol-regulated protease localized to a Leu-Ser bond in lumenal loop of sterol regulatory element binding protein-2. *J Biol Chem* **272**:12778, 1997.
165. Hua X, Nohturfft A, Goldstein JL, Brown MS: Sterol resistance in CHO cells traced to point mutation in SREBP cleavage activating protein (SCAP). *Cell* **87**:415, 1996.
166. Nohturfft A, Brown MS, Goldstein JL: Topology of SREBP cleavage-activating protein, a polytopic membrane protein with a sterol-sensing domain. *J Biol Chem* **273**:17243, 1998.
167. Sakai J, Nohturfft A, Goldstein JL, Brown MS: Cleavage of sterol regulatory element binding proteins (SREBPs) at site-1 requires interaction with SREBP cleavage-activating protein. Evidence from in vivo competition studies. *J Biol Chem* **273**:5785, 1998.
168. Sakai J, Rawson RB, Espenshade PJ, Cheng D, Seegmiller AC, Goldstein JL, Brown MS: Molecular identification of the sterol-regulated luminal protease that cleaves SREBPs and controls lipid composition of animal cells. *Mol Cell* **2**:505, 1998.
168a. Nohturfft A, Hua X, Brown MS, Goldstein JL: Recurrent G-to-A substitution in a single codon of SREBP cleavage-activating protein causes sterol resistance in three mutant CHO cell lines. *Proc Natl Acad Sci U S A* **93**:13709, 1996.
169. Loftus SK, Morris JA, Carstea ED, Gu JZ, Cummings C, Brown A, Ellison J, Ohno K, Rosenfeld MA, Tagle DA, Pentchev PG, Pavan WJ: Murine model of Niemann-Pick C disease: Mutation in a cholesterol homeostasis gene. *Science* **277**:232, 1997.
170. Tabin CJ, McMahon AP: Recent advances in Hedgehog signaling. *Trends Cell Biol* **7**:442, 1997.
171. Porter JA, Young KE, Beachy PA: Cholesterol modification of hedgehog signaling proteins in animal development. *Science* **274**:255, 1996.
172. Rawson RB, Zelenski NG, Nijhawan D, Ye J, Sakai J, Hasan MT, Chang T-Y, Brown MS, Goldstein JL: Complementation cloning of *S2P*, a gene encoding a putative metalloprotease required for intramembrane cleavage of SREBPs. *Mol Cell* **1**:47, 1997.
173. Duncan EA, Dave UP, Sakai J, Goldstein JL, Brown MS: Second-site cleavage in sterol regulatory element-binding protein occurs at transmembrane junction as determined by cysteine panning. *J Biol Chem* **273**:17801, 1998.
174. Kim JB, Spiegelman BM: ADD1/SREBP1 promotes adipocyte differentiation and gene expression linked to fatty acid metabolism. *Genes Dev* **10**:1096, 1996.
175. Lopez JM, Bennett MK, Sanchez HB, Rosenfeld JM, Osborne TF: Sterol regulation of acetyl CoA carboxylase: A mechanism for coordinate control of cellular lipid. *Proc Natl Acad Sci U S A* **93**:1049, 1996.
176. Ericsson J, Jackson SM, Edwards PA: Synergistic binding of sterol regulatory element-binding protein and NF-Y to the farnesyl diphosphate synthase promoter is critical for sterol-regulated expression of the gene. *J Biol Chem* **271**:24359, 1996.
177. Guan G, Dai P, Shechter I: Differential transcriptional regulation of the human squalene synthase gene by sterol regulatory element-binding proteins (SREBP) 1a and 2 and involvement of 5′ DNA sequence elements in the regulation. *J Biol Chem* **273**:12526, 1998.
178. Shimano H, Horton JD, Hammer RE, Shimomura I, Brown MS, Goldstein JL: Overproduction of cholesterol and fatty acids causes massive liver enlargement in transgenic mice expressing truncated SREBP-1a. *J Clin Invest* **98**:1575, 1996.
178a. Tabor DE, Kim JB, Spiegelman BM, Edwards PA: Transcriptional activation of the stearoyl-CoA desaturase 2 gene by sterol regulatory element-binding protein/adipocyte determination and differentiation factor 1. *J Biol Chem* **273**:22052, 1998.
179. Shimomura I, Shimano H, Korn BS, Bashmakov Y, Horton JD: Nuclear sterol regulatory element binding proteins activate genes responsible for entire program of unsaturated fatty acid biosynthesis in transgenic mouse liver. *J Biol Chem* **273**:35299, 1998.
180. Ericsson J, Jackson SM, Kim JB, Spiegelman BM, Edwards PA: Identification of glycerol-3-phosphate acyltransferase as an adipocyte determination and differentiation factor 1 and sterol regulatory element-binding protein-responsive gene. *J Biol Chem* **272**:7298, 1997.
181. Hua X, Wu J, Goldstein JL, Brown MS, Hobbs HH: Structure of human gene encoding sterol regulatory element binding protein-1 (*SREBF1*) and localization of *SREBF1* and *SREBF2* to chromosomes 17p11.2 and 22q13. *Genomics* **25**:667, 1995.
182. Pai J-T, Guryev O, Brown MS, Goldstein JL: Differential stimulation of cholesterol and unsaturated fatty acid biosynthesis in cells expressing individual nuclear sterol regulatory element binding proteins. *J Biol Chem* **273**:26138, 1998.
183. Shimano H, Horton JD, Shimomura I, Hammer RE, Brown MS, Goldstein JL: Isoform 1c of sterol regulatory element binding protein is less active than isoform 1a in livers of transgenic mice and in cultured cells. *J Clin Invest* **99**:846, 1997.
184. Miserez AR, Cao G, Probst L, Hobbs HH: Structure of the human gene encoding sterol regulatory element binding protein 2 (SREBF2). *Genomics* **40**:31, 1997.
185. Horton JD, Shimomura I, Brown MS, Hammer RE, Goldstein JL, Shimano H: Activation of cholesterol synthesis in preference to fatty acid synthesis in liver and adipose tissue of transgenic mice overproducing SREBP-2. *J Clin Invest* **101**:2331, 1998.
185a. Shimomura I, Shimano H, Horton JD, Goldstein JL, Brown MS: Differential expression of exons 1a and 1c in mRNAs for sterol regulatory element binding protein-1 in human and mouse organs and cultured cells. *J Clin Invest* **99**:838, 1997.
186. Briggs MR, Yokoyama C, Wang X, Brown MS, Goldstein JL: Nuclear protein that binds sterol regulatory element of low density lipoprotein receptor promoter I. Identification of the protein and delineation of its target nucleotide sequence. *J Biol Chem* **268**:14490, 1993.
187. Kim JB, Spotts GD, Halvorsen Y-D, Shih H-M, Ellenberger T, Towle HC, Spiegelman BM: Dual DNA binding specificity of ADD1/SREBP1 controlled by a single amino acid in the basic helix-loop-helix domain. *Mol Cell Biol* **15**:2582, 1995.
188. Magana MM, Lin SS, Dooley KA, Osborne TF: Sterol regulation of acetyl coenzyme A carboxylase promoter requires two interdependent binding sites for sterol regulatory element binding proteins. *J Lipid Res* **38**:1630, 1997.
189. Parraga A, Bellsolell L, Ferre-D'Amare AR, Burley SK: Co-crystal structure of sterol regulatory element binding protein 1a at 2.3 Å resolution. *Structure* **6**:661, 1998.
190. Wang X, Briggs MR, Hua X, Yokoyama C, Goldstein JL, Brown MS: Nuclear protein that binds sterol regulatory element of LDL receptor promoter: II. Purification and characterization. *J Biol Chem* **268**:14497, 1993.
191. Yokoyama C, Wang X, Briggs MR, Admon A, Wu J, Hua X, Goldstein JL, Brown MS: SREBP-1, a basic helix-loop-helix leucine zipper protein that controls transcription of the LDL receptor gene. *Cell* **75**:187, 1993.
192. Hua X, Yokoyama C, Wu J, Briggs MR, Brown MS, Goldstein JL, Wang X: SREBP-2, a second basic-helix-loop-helix-leucine zipper protein that stimulates transcription by binding to a sterol regulatory element. *Proc Natl Acad Sci U S A* **90**:11603, 1993.
193. Tontonoz P, Kim JB, Graves RA, Spiegelman BM: ADD1: a novel helix-loop-helix transcription factor associated with adipocyte determination and differentiation. *Mol Cell Biol* **13**:4753, 1993.
194. Osborne TF: Single nucleotide resolution of sterol regulatory region in promoter for 3-hydroxy-3-methylglutaryl coenzyme A reductase. *J Biol Chem* **266**:13947, 1991.
195. Sheng Z, Otani H, Brown MS, Goldstein JL: Independent regulation of sterol regulatory element binding proteins 1 and 2 in hamster liver. *Proc Natl Acad Sci U S A* **92**:935, 1995.
196. Shimomura I, Bashmakov Y, Shimano H, Horton JD, Goldstein JL, Brown MS: Cholesterol feeding reduces nuclear forms of sterol regulatory element binding proteins in hamster liver. *Proc Natl Acad Sci U S A* **94**:12354, 1997.
197. Kotze MJ, Retief AE, Brink PA, Welch HFH: A DNA polymorphism in the human low-density lipoprotein receptor gene. *S Afr Med J* **70**:77, 1986.
197a. Leitersdorf E, Chakravarti A, Hobbs HH: Polymorphic DNA haplotypes at the LDL receptor locus. *Am J Hum Genet* **44**:409, 1989.
198. Hobbs H, Brown MS, Goldstein JL: Molecular genetics of the LDL receptor gene in familial hypercholesterolemia. *Hum Mut* **1**:445, 1992.
199. Lombardi P, Sijbrands EJG, Kamerling S, Leuven JAG, Havekes LM: The T7051 mutation of the low density lipoprotein receptor gene (FH Paris-9) does not cause familial hypercholesterolemia. *Hum Genet* **99**:106, 1997.
200. Vuorio AF, Turtola H, Kontula K: A novel point mutation (Pro84 → Ser) of the low density lipoprotein receptor gene in a family with moderate hypercholesterolemia. *Clin Genet* **51**:191, 1997.

201. Horsthemke B, Dunning A, Humphries S: Identification of deletions in the human low density lipoprotein receptor gene. *J Med Genet* **24**:144, 1987.
202. Langlois S, Kastelein JJP, Hayden MR: Characterization of six partial deletions in the low-density-lipoprotein (LDL) receptor gene causing familial hypercholesterolemia (FH). *Am J Hum Genet* **43**:60, 1988.
203. Kajinami K, Mabuchi H, Inazu A, Fujita H, Koizumi J, Takeda R, Matsue T, Kibata M: Novel gene mutations at the low density lipoprotein receptor locus: FH-Kanazawa and FH-Okayama. *J Intern Med* **227**:247, 1990.
204. Day INM, Whittall RA, O'Dell SD, Haddad L, Bolla MK, Gudnason V, Humphries SE: Spectrum of LDL receptor gene mutations in heterozygous familial hypercholesterolemia. *Hum Mutat* **10**:116, 1997.
205. Wilson DJ, Gahan M, Haddad L, Heath K, Whittall RA, Williams RR, Humphries SE, Day INM: A World Wide Web site for low-density lipoprotein receptor gene mutations in familial hypercholesterolemia: Sequence-based, tabular, and direct submission data handling. *Am J Cardiol* **81**:1509, 1998.
206. Varret M, Rabes J-P, Collod-Beroud G, Junien C, Boileau C, Beroud C: Software and database for the analysis of mutations in the human LDL receptor gene. *Nucleic Acids Res* **25**:172, 1997.
207. Varret M, Rabes J-P, Thiart R, Kotze MJ, Baron H, Cenarro A, Descamps O, Ebhardt M, Hondelijn J-C, Kostner GM, Miyake Y, Pocovi M, Schmidt H, Schuster H, Stuhrmann M, Yamamura T, Junien C, Beroud C, Boileau C: LDLR database (second edition): New additions to the database and the software, and results of the first molecular analysis. *Nucleic Acids Res* **26**:248, 1998.
208. Goldstein JL, Hobbs HH, Brown MS: Familial hypercholesterolemia, in Scriver CR, Beaudet AL, Sly WS, Valle D (eds): *The Metabolic and Molecular Bases of Inherited Disease, 7th ed.* New York, McGraw-Hill, 1995, vol 2, p 1981.
209. Hobbs HH, Leitersdorf E, Goldstein JL, Brown MS, Russell DW: Multiple crm-mutations in familial hypercholesterolemia: Evidence for 13 alleles, including four deletions. *J Clin Invest* **81**:909, 1988.
210. Hobbs HH, Brown MS, Russell DW, Davignon J, Goldstein JL: Deletion in the gene for the LDL receptor in majority of French Canadians with familial hypercholesterolemia. *N Engl J Med* **317**:734, 1987.
211. Pathak RK, Merkle RK, Cummings RD, Goldstein JL, Brown MS, Anderson RGW: Immunocytochemical localization of mutant low density lipoprotein receptors that fail to reach the Golgi complex. *J Cell Biol* **106**:1831, 1988.
212. Esser V, Russell DW: Transport-deficient mutations in the low density lipoprotein receptor: Alterations in the cysteine-rich and cysteine-poor regions of the protein block intracellular transport. *J Biol Chem* **263**:13276, 1988.
213. Gething M-J, Sambrook J: Protein folding in the cell. *Nature* **355**:33, 1992.
214. Meiner V, Landsberger D, Berkman N, Reshef A, Segal P, Seftel HC, van der Westhuyzen DR, Jeenah MS, Coetzee GA, Leitersdorf E: A common Lithuanian mutation causing familial hypercholesterolemia in Ashkenazi Jews. *Am J Hum Genet* **49**:443, 1991.
215. Hobbs HH, Brown MS, Goldstein JL, Russell DW: Deletion of exon encoding cysteine-rich repeat of LDL receptor alters its binding specificity in a subject with familial hypercholesterolemia. *J Biol Chem* **261**:13114, 1986.
216. Lehrman MA, Schneider WJ, Brown MS, Davis CG, Elhammer A, Russell DW, Goldstein JL: The Lebanese allele at the LDL receptor locus: Nonsense mutation produces truncated receptor that is retained in endoplasmic reticulum. *J Biol Chem* **262**:401, 1987.
217. Amara JF, Cheng SH, Smith AE: Intracellular protein trafficking defects in human disease. *Trends Cell Biol* **2**:145, 1992.
218. Hobbs HH, Leitersdorf E, Leffert C, Cryer DR, Brown MS, Goldstein JL: Evidence for a dominant gene that suppresses hypercholesterolemia in a family with defective low density lipoprotein receptors. *J Clin Invest* **84**:656, 1989.
219. Leitersdorf E, Tobin EJ, Davignon J, Hobbs HH: Common low-density lipoprotein receptor mutations in the French Canadian population. *J Clin Invest* **85**:1014, 1990.
220. Esser V, Limbird LE, Brown MS, Goldstein JL, Russell DW: Mutational analysis of the ligand-binding domain of the low density lipoprotein receptor. *J Biol Chem* **263**:13282, 1988.
221. van der Westhuyzen DR, Stein ML, Henderson HE, Marais AD, Fourie AM, Coetzee GA: Deletion of two growth-factor repeats from the low-density-lipoprotein receptor accelerates its degradation. *Biochem J* **278**:677, 1991.
222. Miyake Y, Tajima S, Funahashi T, Yamamoto A: Analysis of a recycling-impaired mutant of low density lipoprotein receptor in familial hypercholesterolemia. *J Biol Chem* **264**:16584, 1989.
223. Lehrman MA, Goldstein JL, Russell DW, Brown MS: Duplication of seven exons in LDL receptor gene caused by Alu-Alu recombination in a subject with familial hypercholesterolemia. *Cell* **48**:827, 1987.
224. Goldstein JL, Anderson RGW, Brown MS: Coated pits, coated vesicles, and receptor-mediated endocytosis. *Nature* **279**:679, 1979.
225. Lehrman MA, Goldstein JL, Brown MS, Russell DW, Schneider WJ: Internalization-defective LDL receptors produced by genes with nonsense and frameshift mutations that truncate the cytoplasmic domain. *Cell* **41**:735, 1985.
226. Lehrman MA, Schneider WJ, Südhof TC, Brown MS, Goldstein JL, Russell DW: Mutation in LDL receptor: Alu-Alu recombination deletes exons encoding transmembrane and cytoplasmic domains. *Science* **227**:140, 1985.
227. Lehrman MA, Russell DW, Goldstein JL, Brown MS: Alu-Alu recombination deletes splice acceptor sites and produces secreted LDL receptor in a subject with familial hypercholesterolemia. *J Biol Chem* **262**:3354, 1987.
228. Aalto-Setala K, Helve E, Kovanen PT, Kontula K: Finnish type of low density lipoprotein receptor gene mutation (FH-Helsinki) deletes exons encoding and carboxy-terminal part of the receptor and creates an internalization-defective phenotype. *J Clin Invest* **84**:499, 1989.
229. Davis CG, van Driel IR, Russell DW, Brown MS, Goldstein JL: The LDL receptor: Identification of amino acids in cytoplasmic domain required for rapid endocytosis. *J Biol Chem* **262**:4075, 1987.
230. Chen W-J, Goldstein JL, Brown MS: NPXY, a sequence often found in cytoplasmic tails, is required for coated pit-mediated internalization of the low density lipoprotein receptor. *J Biol Chem* **265**:3116, 1990.
231. Herz J, Hamann U, Rogne S, Myklebost O, Gausepohl H, Stanley KK: Surface location and high affinity for calcium of a 500-kd liver membrane protein closely related to the LDL-receptor suggest a physiological role as lipoprotein receptor. *EMBO J* **7**:4119, 1988.
232. Raychowdhury R, Niles JL, McCluskey RT, Smith JA: Autoimmune target in Heymann nephritis is a glycoprotein with homology to the LDL receptor. *Science* **244**:1163, 1989.
233. Takahashi S, Kawarabayasi Y, Nakai T, Sakai J, Yamamoto T: The rabbit very low density lipoprotein receptor: A low density lipoprotein receptor-like protein with distinct ligand specificity. *Proc Natl Acad Sci U S A* **89**:9252, 1992.
234. Barber DL, Sanders EJ, Aebersold R, Schneider WJ: The receptor for yolk lipoprotein deposition in the chicken oocyte. *J Biol Chem* **266**:18761, 1991.
235. Vaux D: The structure of an endocytosis signal. *Trends Cell Biol* **2**:189, 1992.
236. Collawn JF, Kuhn LA, Sue-Liu LF, Tainer JA, Trowbridge IS: Transplanted LDL and mannose-6-phosphate receptor internalization signals promote high-efficiency endocytosis of the transferrin receptor. *EMBO J* **10**:3247, 1991.
237. Bansal A, Gierasch LM: The NPXY internalization signal of the LDL receptor adopts a reverse-turn conformation. *Cell* **67**:1195, 1991.
238. Pearse BMF, Robinson MS: Clathrin, adaptors, and sorting. *Annu Rev Cell Biol* **6**:151, 1991.
239. Jensen LG, Jensen HK, Nissen H, Kristiansen K, Faergeman O, Bolund L, Gregersen N: An LDL receptor promoter mutation in a heterozygous FH patient with dramatically skewed ratio between the two allelic mRNA variants. *Hum Mutat* **7**:82, 1996.
240. Koivisto U-M, Palvimo JJ, Janne OA, Kontula K: A single-base substitution in the proximal Sp1 site of the human low density lipoprotein receptor promoter as a cause of heterozygous familial hypercholesterolemia. *Proc Natl Acad Sci U S A* **91**:10526, 1994.
241. Sun X-M, Neuwirth C, Wade DP, Knight BL, Soutar AK: A mutation (T-45C) in the promoter region of the low-density-lipoprotein (LDL)-receptor gene is associated with a mild clinical phenotype in a patient with heterozygous familial hypercholesterolaemia (FH). *Hum Mol Genet* **4**:2125, 1995.
242. Gudnason V, Day INM, Humphries SE: Effect on plasma lipid levels of different classes of mutations in the low-density lipoprotein receptor gene in patients with familial hypercholesterolemia. *Arterioscler Thromb* **14**:1717, 1994.
243. Koivisto PVI, Koivisto U-M, Kovanen PT, Gylling H, Miettinen TA, Kontula K: Deletion of exon 15 of the LDL receptor gene is associated with a mild form of familial hypercholesterolemia FH-Espoo. *Arterioscler Thromb* **13**:1680, 1993.

244. Kotze MJ, Thiart R, Loubser O, de Villiers JNP, Santos M, Vargas MA, Peeters AV: Mutation analysis reveals an insertional hotspot in exon 4 of the LDL receptor gene. *Hum Genet* **98**:476, 1996.
245. Cooper DN, Krawczak M: Mechanisms of insertional mutagenesis in human genes causing genetic disease. *Hum Genet* **87**:409, 1991.
246. Hwu HR, Roberts JW, Davidson EH, Britten RJ: Insertion and/or deletion of many repeated DNA sequences in human and higher ape evolution. *Proc Natl Acad Sci U S A* **83**:3875, 1986.
247. Jelinek WR, Schmid CW: Repetitive sequences in eukaryotic DNA and their expression. *Annu Rev Biochem* **51**:813, 1982.
248. Britten RJ, Baron WF, Stout DB, Davidson EH: Sources and evolution of human Alu repeated sequences. *Proc Natl Acad Sci U S A* **85**:4770, 1988.
249. Horsthemke B, Beisiegel U, Dunning A, Havinga JR, Williamson R, Humphries S: Unequal crossing-over between two Alu-repetitive DNA sequences in the low-density-lipoprotein-receptor gene. A possible mechanism for the defect in a patient with familial hypercholesterolaemia. *Eur J Biochem* **164**:77, 1987.
250. Rudiger NS, Hansen PS, Jorgensen M, Faergeman O, Bolund L, Gregersen N: Repetitive sequences involved in the recombination leading to deletion of exon 5 of the low-density-lipoprotein receptor gene in a patient with familial hypercholesterolemia. *Eur J Biochem* **198**:107, 1991.
251. Kigawa K, Kihara K, Miyake Y, Tajima S, Funahashi T, Yamamura T, Yamamoto A: Low-density lipoprotein receptor mutation that deletes exons 2 and 3 by Alu-Alu recombination. *J Biochem* **113**:372, 1993.
252. Lehrman MA, Russell DW, Goldstein JL, Brown MS: Exon-Alu recombination deletes 5 kilobases from low density lipoprotein receptor gene, producing null phenotype in familial hypercholesterolemia. *Proc Natl Acad Sci U S A* **83**:3679, 1986.
253. Orkin SH, Kazazian HH Jr: The mutation and polymorphism of the human β-globin gene and its surrounding DNA. *Annu Rev Genet* **18**:131, 1984.
254. Henthorn PS, Smithies O, Mager DL: Molecular analysis of deletions in the human β-globin gene cluster: Deletion junctions and locations of breakpoints. *Genomics* **6**:226, 1990.
255. Stoppa-Lyonnet D, Carter PE, Meo T, Tosi M: Clusters of intragenic Alu repeats predispose the human C1 inhibitor locus to deleterious rearrangements. *Proc Natl Acad Sci U S A* **87**:1511, 1990.
256. King-Underwood L, Gudnason V, Humphries S, Seed M, Patel D, Knight B, Soutar A: Identification of the 664 proline to leucine mutation in the low density lipoprotein receptor in four unrelated patients with familial hypercholesterolemia in the UK. *Clin Genet* **40**:17, 1991.
257. Cooper DN, Youssoufian H: The CpG dinucleotide and human genetic disease. *Hum Genet* **78**:151, 1988.
258. Cassanelli S, Bertolini S, Rolleri M, De Stefano F, Casarino L, Elicio N, Naselli A, Calandra S: A "de novo" point mutation of the low-density lipoprotein receptor gene in an Italian subject with primary hypercholesterolemia. *Clin Genet* **53**:391, 1998.
259. Kotze MJ, Theart L, Peeters A, Langenhoven E: A de novo duplication in the low density lipoprotein receptor gene. *Human Mutation* **6**:181, 1995.
260. Koivisto U-M, Gylling H, Miettinen TA, Kontula K: Familial moderate hypercholesterolemia caused by Asp235 → Glu mutation of the LDL receptor gene and co-occurrence of a de novo deletion of the LDL receptor gene in the same family. *Arterioscler Thromb Vasc Biol* **17**:1392, 1997.
261. Jensen HK, Jensen TG, Faergeman O, Jensen LG, Andresen BS, Corydon MJ, Andreasen PA, Hansen PS, Heath F, Bolund L, Gregersen N: Two mutations in the same low-density lipoprotein receptor allele act in synergy to reduce receptor function in heterozygous familial hypercholesterolemia. *Hum Mutat* **9**:437, 1997.
262. Savov A, Angelicheva D, Balassopoulou A, Jordanova A, Noussia-Arvanitakis S, Kalaydjieva L: Double mutant alleles: Are they rare? *Hum Mol Genet* **4**:1169, 1995.
263. Rubinsztein DC, van der Westhuyzen DR, Coetzee GA: Monogenic primary hypercholesterolaemia in South Africa. *S Afr Med J* **84**:339, 1994.
264. Rubinsztein DC, Coetzee GA, Marais AD, Leitersdorf E, Seftel HC, van der Westhuyzen DR: Identification and properties of the proline$_{664}$-leucine mutant LDL receptor in South Africans of Indian origin. *J Lipid Res* **33**:1647, 1992.
265. Soutar AK, Knight BL, Patel DD: Identification of a point mutation in growth factor repeat C of the low density lipoprotein-receptor gene in a patient with homozygous familial hypercholesterolemia that affects ligand binding and intracellular movement of receptors. *Proc Natl Acad Sci U S A*. **86**:4166, 1989.
266. Leitersdorf E, van der Westhuyzen DR, Coetzee GA, Hobbs HH: Two common low density lipoprotein receptor gene mutations cause familial hypercholesterolemia in Afrikaners. *J Clin Invest* **84**:954, 1989.
266a. Kotze MJ, Langenhoven E, Warnich L, Du Plessis L, Retief AE: The molecular basis and diagnosis of familial hypercholesterolaemia in South African Afrikaners. *Ann Hum Genet* **55**:115, 1991.
267. Defesche JC, van Diermen DE, Hayden MR, Kastelein JPP: Origin and migration of an Afrikaner founder mutation $FH_{Afrikaner-2}$ (V408M) causing familial hypercholesterolemia. *Gene Geogr* **10**:1, 1996.
267a. Botha MC, Beighton P: Inherited disorders in the Afrikaner population of southern Africa. Part 1. Historical and demographic background, cardiovascular, neurological, metabolic and intestinal conditions. *S Afr Med J* **64**:609, 1983.
268. Slimane MN, Pousse H, Maatoug F, Hammami M, Ben Farhat MH: Phenotypic expression of familial hypercholesterolaemia in central and southern Tunisia. *Atherosclerosis* **104**:153, 1993.
269. Laberge C: Prospectus for genetic studies in the French Canadians, with preliminary data on blood groups and consanguinity. *Bull Johns Hopkins Hosp* **118**:52, 1966.
270. Fumeron F, Grandchamp B, Fricker J, Krempf M, Wolf L-M, Khayat M-C, Bioffard O, Apfelbaum M: Presence of the French Canadian deletion in a French patient with familial hypercholesterolemia. *N Engl J Med* **326**:69, 1991.
271. Simard J, Moorjani S, Vohl M-C, Couture P, Torres AL, Gagne C, Despres J-P, Labrie F, Lupien PJ: Detection of a novel mutation (stop 468) in exon 10 of the low-density lipoprotein receptor gene causing familial hypercholesterolemia among French Canadians. *Hum Mol Genet* **3**:1689, 1994.
272. Landsberger D, Meiner V, Reshef A, Levy Y, Van Der Westhuyzen DR, Coetzee GA, Leitersdorf E: A nonsense mutation in the LDL receptor gene leads to familial hypercholesterolemia in the Druze Sect. *Am J Hum Genet* **50**:427, 1992.
273. Leitersdorf E, Reshef A, Meiner V, Dann EJ, Beigel Y, van Roggen FG, van der Westhuyzen DR, Coetzee GA: A missense mutation in the low density lipoprotein receptor gene causes familial hypercholesterolemia in Sephardic Jews. *Hum Genet* **91**:141, 1993.
274. Koivisto U-M, Turtola H, Aalto-Setala K, Top B, Frants RR, Kovanen PT, Syvanen A-C, Kontula K: The familial hypercholesterolemia (FH)-north Karelia mutation of the low density lipoprotein receptor gene deletes seven nucleotides of exon 6 and is a common cause of FH in Finland. *J Clin Invest* **90**:219, 1992.
275. Aalto-Setala K, Koivisto U-M, Miettinen TA, Gylling H, Kesaniemi YA, Pyorala K, Ebeling T, Mononen I, Turtola H, Viikari J, Kontula K: Prevalence and geographical distribution of major LDL receptor gene rearrangements in Finland. *J Intern Med* **231**:227, 1992.
276. Koivisto U-M, Viikari JS, Kontula K: Molecular characterization of minor gene rearrangements in Finnish patients with heterozygous familial hypercholesterolemia: identification of two common missense mutations (Gly823 → Asp and Leu380 → His) and eight rare mutations of the LDL receptor gene. *Am J Hum Genet* **57**:789, 1995.
277. Leren TP, Tonstad S, Gundersen KE, Bakken KS, Rodningen OK, Sundvold H, Ose L, Berg K: Molecular genetics of familial hypercholesterolaemia in Norway. *J Intern Med* **241**:185, 1997.
278. Gudnason V, Sigurdsson G, Nissen H, Humphries SE: Common founder mutation in the LDL receptor gene causing familial hypercholesterolaemia in the Icelandic population. *Hum Mutat* **10**:36, 1997.
279. Jensen HK, Jensen LG, Hansen PS, Faergeman O, Gregersen N: The Trp^{23} → Stop and Trp^{66} → Gly mutations in the LDL receptor gene: common causes of familial hypercholesterolemia in Denmark. *Atherosclerosis* **120**:57, 1996.
279a. Jensen HK, Holst H, Jensen LG, Jorgensen MM, Andreasen PH, Jensen TG, Andresen BS, Heath F, Hansen PS, Neve S, Kristiansen K, Faergeman O, Kolvraa S, Bolund L, Gregersen N: A common W556S mutation in the LDL receptor gene of Danish patients with familial hypercholesterolemia encodes a transport-defective protein. *Atherosclerosis* **131**:67, 1997.
280. Mavroidis N, Traeger-Synodinos J, Kanavakis E, Drogari E, Matsaniotis N, Humphries SE, Day INM, Kattamis C: A high incidence of mutations in exon 6 of the low-density lipoprotein receptor gene in Greek familial hypercholesterolemia patients, including a novel mutation. *Hum Mutat* **9**:274, 1997.

281. Traeger-Synodinos J, Mavroidis N, Kanavakis E, Drogari E, Humphries SE, Day INM, Kattamis C, Matsaniotis N: Analysis of low density lipoprotein receptor gene mutations and microsatellite haplotypes in Greek FH heterozygous children: Six independent ancestors account for 60% of probands. *Hum Genet* **102**:343, 1998.
282. Cenarro A, Jensen HK, Civeira F, Casao E, Ferrando J, Gonzalez-Bonillo J, Pocovi M, Gregersen N: Two novel mutations in the LDL receptor gene: common causes of familial hypercholesterolemia in a Spanish population. *Clin Genet* **49**:180, 1996.
283. Descamps O, Hondekijn J-C, Van Acker P, Deslypere J-P, Heller FR: High prevalence of a novel mutation in the exon 4 of the low-density lipoprotein receptor gene causing familial hypercholesterolemia in Belgium. *Clin Genet* **51**:303, 1997.
284. Webb JC, Sun X-M, Patel DD, McCarthy SN, Knight BL, Soutar AK: Characterization of two new point mutations in the low density lipoprotein receptor genes of an English patient with homozygous familial hypercholesterolemia. *J Lipid Res* **33**:689, 1992.
285. Day INM, Haddad L, O'Dell SD, Day LB, Whittall RA, Humphries SE: Identification of a common low density lipoprotein receptor mutation (R329X) in the south of England: complete linkage disequilibrium with an allele of microsatellite D19S394. *J Med Genet* **34**:111, 1997.
286. Maruyama T, Miyake Y, Tajima S, Harada-Shiba M, Yamamura T, Tsushima M, Kishino B-I, Horiguchi Y, Funahashi T, Matsuzawa Y, Yamamoto A: Common mutations in the low-density-lipoprotein-receptor gene causing familial hypercholesterolemia in the Japanese population. *Arterioscler Thromb Vasc Biol* **15**:1713, 1995.
287. Moorjani S, Roy M, Torres A, Betard C, Gagne C, Lambert M, Brun D, Davignon J, Lupien P: Mutations of low-density-lipoprotein-receptor gene, variation in plasma cholesterol, and expression of coronary heart disease in homozygous familial hypercholesterolaemia. *Lancet* **341**:1303, 1993.
288. Levy E, Minnich A, Lussier-Cacan S, Thibault L, Giroux L-M, Davignon J, Lambert M: Association of an exon 3 mutation (Trp66 → Gly) of the LDL receptor with variable expression of familial hypercholesterolemia in a French-Canadian family. *Biochem Molec Med* **60**:59, 1997.
289. Kotze MJ, De Villiers WJS, Steyn K, Kriek JA, Marais AD, Langenhoven E, Herbert JS, van Roggen JFG, van der Westhuyzen DR, Coetzee GA: Phenotypic variation among familial hypercholesterolemics heterozygous for either one of two Afrikaner founder LDL receptor mutations. *Arterioscler Thromb* **13**:1460, 1993.
290. Sun X-M, Patel DD, Webb JC, Knight BL, Fan L-M, Cai H-J, Soutar AK: Familial hypercholesterolemia in China. *Arterioscler Thromb* **14**:85, 1994.
291. Pimstone SN, Sun X-M, du Souich C, Frohlich JJ, Hayden MR, Soutar AK: Phenotypic variation in heterozygous familial hypercholesterolemia. A comparison of Chinese patients with the same or similar mutations in the LDL receptor gene in China or Canada. *Arterioscler Thromb Vasc Biol* **18**:309, 1998.
292. Kesteloot H, Huang DX, Yang XS, Claes J, Rosseneu M, Geboers J, Joossens JV: Serum lipids in the People's Republic of China: Comparison of Western and Eastern populations. *Arteriosclerosis* **5**:427, 1985.
293. Goldstein JL, Kita T, Brown MS: Defective lipoprotein receptors and atherosclerosis: Lessons from an animal counterpart of familial hypercholesterolemia. *N Engl J Med* **309**:288, 1983.
294. Schneider WJ, Brown MS, Goldstein JL: Kinetic defects in the processing of the LDL receptor in fibroblasts from WHHL rabbits and a family with familial hypercholesterolemia. *Mol Biol Med* **1**:353, 1983.
295. Bilheimer DW, East C, Grundy SM, Nora JJ: II. Clinical studies in a kindred with a kinetic LDL receptor mutation causing familial hypercholesterolemia. *Am J Med Genet* **22**:593, 1985.
296. Nora JJ, Lortscher RM, Spangler RD, Bilheimer DW: I. Familial hypercholesterolemia with "normal" cholesterol in obligate heterozygotes. *Am J Med Genet* **22**:585, 1985.
297. Vega GL, Hobbs HH, Grundy SM: Low density lipoprotein kinetics in a family having defective low density lipoprotein receptors in which hypercholesterolemia is suppressed. *Arterioscler Thromb* **11**:578, 1991.
298. Sass C, Giroux L-M, Ma Y, Roy M, Lavigne J, Lussier-Cacan S, Davignon J, Minnich A: Evidence for a cholesterol-lowering gene in a French-Canadian kindred with familial hypercholesterolemia. *Hum Genet* **96**:21, 1995.
299. Goldstein JL, Sobhani MK, Faust JR, Brown MS: Heterozygous familial hypercholesterolemia: Failure of normal allele to compensate for mutant allele at a regulated genetic locus. *Cell* **9**:195, 1976.
300. Watanabe Y: Serial inbreeding of rabbits with hereditary hyperlipidemia (WHHL-rabbit). Incidence and development of atherosclerosis and xanthoma. *Atherosclerosis* **36**:261, 1980.
301. Chowdhury JR, Grossman M, Gupta S, Chowdhury NR, Baker JR Jr, Wilson JM: Long-term improvement of hypercholesterolemia after ex vivo gene therapy in LDLR-deficient rabbits. *Science* **254**:1802, 1991.
302. Scanu AM, Khalil A, Neven L, Tidore M, Dawson G, Pfaffinger D, Jackson E, Carey KD, McGill HC, Fless GM: Genetically determined hypercholesterolemia in a rhesus monkey family due to a deficiency of the LDL receptor. *J Lipid Res* **29**:1671, 1988.
303. Hummel M, Li Z, Pfaffinger D, Neven L, Scanu AM: Familial hypercholesterolemia in a rhesus monkey pedigree: Molecular basis of low density lipoprotein receptor deficiency. *Proc Natl Acad Sci U S A* **87**:3122, 1990.
304. Ishibashi S, Brown MS, Goldstein JL, Gerard RD, Hammer RE, Herz J: Hypercholesterolemia in LDL receptor knockout mice and its reversal by adenovirus-mediated gene delivery. *J Clin Invest* **92**:883, 1993.
305. Ishibashi S, Goldstein JL, Brown MS, Herz J, Burns DK: Massive xanthomatosis and atherosclerosis in cholesterol-fed LDL receptor-negative mice. *J Clin Invest* **93**:1885, 1994.
306. Sanan DA, Newland DL, Tao R, Marcovina S, Wang J, Mooser V, Hammer RE, Hobbs HH: Low density lipoprotein receptor-negative mice expressing human apolipoprotein B-100 develop complex atherosclerotic lesions on a chow diet: No accentuation by apolipoprotein(a). *Proc Natl Acad Sci U S A* **95**:4544, 1998.
307. Powell-Braxton L, Véniant M, Latvala RD, Hirano K-I, Won WB, Ross J, Dybdal N, Zlot CH, Young SG, Davidson NO: A mouse model of human familial hypercholesterolemia: Markedly elevated low density lipoprotein cholesterol levels and severe atherosclerosis on a low-fat, chow diet. *Nat Med* **4**:934, 1998.
308. Gilbert W: Genes-in-pieces revisited. *Science* **228**:823, 1985.
309. Brown MS, Herz J, Kowal RC, Goldstein JL: The low-density lipoprotein receptor-related protein: Double agent or decoy? *Curr Opin Lipidol* **2**:65, 1991.
310. Krieger M, Herz J: Structures and functions of multiligand lipoprotein receptors: macrophage scavenger receptors and LDL receptor-related protein (LRP). *Annu Rev Biochem* **63**:601, 1994.
310a. Frykman PK, Brown MS, Yamamoto T, Goldstein JL, Herz J: Normal plasma lipoproteins and fertility in gene-targeted mice homozygous for a disruption in the gene encoding very low density lipoprotein receptor. *Proc Natl Acad Sci U S A* **92**:8453, 1995.
311. Schneider WJ: Vitellogenin receptors: Oocyte-specific members of the low-density lipoprotein receptor supergene family. *Int Rev Cytol* **166**:103, 1996.
312. Schonbaum CP, Lee S, Mahowald AP: The Drosophila yolkless gene encodes a vitellogenin receptor belonging to the LDL receptor superfamily. *Proc Natl Acad Sci U S A* **92**:1485, 1995.
313. Kerjaschki D, Farquhar MG: Immunocytochemical localization of the Heymann nephritis antigen (GP330) in glomerular epithelial cells of normal Lewis rats. *J Exp Med* **157**:667, 1983.
314. Willnow TF, Goldstein JL, Orth K, Brown MS, Herz J: Low density lipoprotein receptor-related protein (LRP) and gp330 bind similar ligands, including plasminogen activator/inhibitor complexes and lactoferrin, an inhibitor of chylomicron remnant clearance. *J Biol Chem* **267**:26172, 1992.
315. Faust JR, Goldstein JL, Brown MS: Receptor-mediated uptake of low density lipoprotein and utilization of its cholesterol for steroid synthesis in cultured mouse adrenal cells. *J Biol Chem* **252**:4861, 1977.
316. Kovanen PT, Faust JR, Brown MS, Goldstein JL: Low density lipoprotein receptors in bovine adrenal cortex. I. Receptor-mediated uptake of low density lipoprotein and utilization of its cholesterol for steroid synthesis in cultured adrenocortical cells. *Endocrinology* **104**:599, 1979.
317. Ho YK, Brown MS, Bilheimer DW, Goldstein JL: Regulation of low density lipoprotein receptor activity in freshly isolated human lymphocytes. *J Clin Invest* **58**:1465, 1976.
318. Bilheimer DW, Ho YK, Brown MS, Anderson RGW, Goldstein JL: Genetics of the low density lipoprotein receptor: Diminished receptor activity in lymphocytes from heterozygotes with familial hypercholesterolemia. *J Clin Invest* **61**:678, 1978.
319. Langer T, Strober W, Levy RI: The metabolism of low density lipoprotein in familial type II hyperlipoproteinemia. *J Clin Invest* **51**:1528, 1972.
320. Bilheimer DW, Stone NJ, Grundy SM: Metabolic studies in familial hypercholesterolemia: Evidence for a gene-dosage effect in vivo. *J Clin Invest* **64**:524, 1979.

321. Simons LA, Reichl D, Myant NB, Mancini M: The metabolism of the apoprotein of plasma low density lipoprotein in familial hyperbeta-lipoproteinaemia in the homozygous form. *Atherosclerosis* **21**:283, 1975.
322. Bilheimer DW, Goldstein JL, Grundy SM, Brown MS: Reduction in cholesterol and low density lipoprotein synthesis after portacaval shunt surgery in a patient with homozygous familial hypercholesterolemia. *J Clin Invest* **56**:1420, 1975.
323. Kovanen PT, Basu SK, Goldstein JL, Brown MS: Low density lipoprotein receptors in bovine adrenal cortex. II. Low density lipoprotein binding to membranes prepared from fresh tissue. *Endocrinology* **104**:610, 1979.
324. Brown MS, Kovanen PT, Goldstein JL: Receptor-mediated uptake of lipoprotein-cholesterol and its utilization for steroid synthesis in the adrenal cortex. *Recent Prog Horm Res* **35**:215, 1979.
325. Windler EET, Kovanen PT, Chao Y-S, Brown MS, Havel RJ, Goldstein JL: The estradiol-stimulated lipoprotein receptor of rat liver: A binding site that mediates the uptake of rat lipoproteins containing apoproteins B and E. *J Biol Chem* **255**:10464, 1980.
326. Brown MS, Kovanen PT, Goldstein JL: Evolution of the LDL receptor concept — From cultured cells to intact animals. *Ann N Y Acad Sci* **348**:48, 1980.
327. Pittman RC, Carew TE, Attie AD, Witztum JL, Watanabe Y, Steinberg D: Receptor-dependent and receptor-independent degradation of low density lipoprotein in normal rabbits and in receptor-deficient mutant rabbits. *J Biol Chem* **257**:7994, 1982.
328. Spady DK, Bilheimer DW, Dietschy JM: Rates of receptor dependent and independent low density lipoprotein uptake in the hamster. *Proc Natl Acad Sci U S A* **80**:3499, 1983.
329. Meddings JB, Dietschy JM: Regulation of plasma low density lipoprotein levels: New strategies for drug design. *Prog Clin Biochem Med* **5**:1, 1988.
330. Steinberg D: Lipoproteins and atherosclerosis: A look back and a look ahead. *Arteriosclerosis* **3**:283, 1983.
331. Shepherd J, Bicker S, Lorimer AR, Packard CJ: Receptor-mediated low density lipoprotein catabolism in man. *J Lipid Res* **12**:596, 1979.
332. Mahley RW, Weisgraber KH, Melchior GW, Innerarity TL, Holcombe KS: Inhibition of receptor-mediated clearance of lysine- and arginine-modified lipoproteins from the plasma of rats and monkeys. *Proc Natl Acad Sci U S A* **77**:225, 1980.
333. Steinbrecher UP, Witztum JL, Kesaniemi YA, Elam RL: Comparison of glycosylated low density lipoprotein with methylated or cyclohexanedione-treated low density lipoprotein in the measurement of receptor-independent low density lipoprotein catabolism. *J Clin Invest* **71**:960, 1983.
334. Bilheimer DW, Grundy SM, Brown MS, Goldstein JL: Mevinolin stimulates receptor-mediated clearance of low density lipoprotein from plasma in familial hypercholesterolemia heterozygotes. *Proc Natl Acad Sci U S A* **80**:4124, 1983.
335. Nagata Y, Chen J, Cooper AD: Role of low density lipoprotein receptor-dependent and -independent sites in binding and uptake of chylomicron remnants in rat liver. *J Biol Chem* **263**:15151, 1988.
336. Rubinsztein DC, Cohen JC, Berger GM, van der Westhuyzen DR, Coetzee GA, Gevers W: Chylomicron remnant clearance from the plasma is normal in familial hypercholesterolemic homozygotes with defined receptor defects. *J Clin Invest* **86**:1306, 1990.
337. Eriksson M, Angelin B, Henriksson P, Ericsson S, Vitols S, Berglund L: Metabolism of lipoprotein remnants in humans: Studies during intestinal infusion of fat and cholesterol in subjects with varying expression of the low density lipoprotein receptor. *Arterioscler Thromb* **11**:827, 1991.
338. Kita T, Goldstein JL, Brown MS, Watanabe Y, Hornick CA, Havel RJ: Hepatic uptake of chylomicron remnants in WHHL rabbits: A mechanism genetically distinct from the low density lipoprotein receptor. *Proc Natl Acad Sci U S A* **79**:3623, 1982.
339. Rohlmann A, Gotthardt M, Hammer RE, Herz J: Inducible inactivation of hepatic LRP gene by cre-mediated recombination confirms role of LRP in clearance of chylomicron remnants. *J Clin Invest* **101**:689, 1998.
340. Kita T, Brown MS, Watanabe Y, Goldstein JL: Deficiency of LDL receptors in liver and adrenal gland of the WHHL rabbit, an animal model of familial hypercholesterolemia. *Proc Natl Acad Sci U S A* **78**:2268, 1981.
341. Havel RJ, Kita T, Kotite L, Kane JP, Hamilton RL, Goldstein JL, Brown MS: Concentration and composition of lipoproteins in blood plasma of WHHL rabbits. *Arteriosclerosis* **3**:467, 1982.
342. Buja LM, Kita T, Goldstein JL, Watanabe Y, Brown MS: Cellular pathology of progressive atherosclerosis in the WHHL rabbit, an animal model of familial hypercholesterolemia. *Arteriosclerosis* **3**:87, 1983.
343. Atkinson JB, Swift LL, Virmani R: Animal model of human disease: Watanabe heritable hyperlipidemic rabbits. *Am J Pathol* **140**:749, 1992.
344. Rosenfeld ME, Ross R: Macrophage and smooth muscle cell proliferation in atherosclerotic lesions of WHHL and comparably hypercholesterolemic fat-fed rabbits. *Arteriosclerosis* **10**:680, 1990.
345. Shiomi M, Ito T, Watanabe Y: Increase in hepatic low-density lipoprotein receptor activity during pregnancy in Watanabe heritable hyperlipidemic rabbits; an animal model for familial hypercholesterolemia. *Biochim Biophys Acta* **917**:92, 1987.
346. Kuroda M, Matsumoto A, Itakura H, Watanabe Y, Ito T, Shiomi M, Fukushige J, Nara F, Fukami M, Tsujita Y: Effects of pravastatin sodium alone and in combination with cholestyramine on hepatic, intestinal and adrenal low density lipoprotein receptors in homozygous Watanabe heritable hyperlipidemic rabbits. *Jpn J Pharmacol* **59**:65, 1992.
347. Demacker PNM, Staels B, Stalenhoef AFH, Auwerx J: Increased removal of β-very low density lipoproteins after ethinyl estradiol is associated with increased mRNA levels for hepatic lipase, lipoprotein lipase, and the low density lipoprotein receptor in Watanabe heritable hyperlipidemic rabbits. *Arterioscler Thromb* **11**:1652, 1991.
348. Mol MJTM, Stalenhoef AFH, Demacker PNM, van't Laar A: Alterations in the metabolism of very-low- and low-density lipoproteins after partial ileal-bypass surgery in the Watanabe heritable hyperlipidaemic rabbit. *Biochem J* **278**:651, 1991.
349. Soutar AK, Myant NB, Thompson GR: Simultaneous measurement of apolipoprotein B turnover in very-low- and low-density lipoproteins in familial hypercholesterolaemia. *Atherosclerosis* **28**:247, 1977.
350. Gitlin D, Cornwell DG, Nakasato D, Oncley JL, Hughes WL Jr, Janeway CA: Studies on the metabolism of plasma proteins in the nephrotic syndrome. II. The lipoproteins. *J Clin Invest* **37**:172, 1958.
351. Bilheimer DW, Eisenberg S, Levy RI: The metabolism of very low density lipoprotein proteins. I. Preliminary in vitro and in vivo observations. *Biochim Biophys Acta* **260**:212, 1972.
352. Kita T, Brown MS, Bilheimer DW, Goldstein JL: Delayed clearance of very low density and intermediate density lipoproteins with enhanced conversion to low density lipoprotein in WHHL rabbits. *Proc Natl Acad Sci U S A* **79**:5693, 1982.
353. Yamada N, Shames DM, Havel RJ: Effect of LDL receptor deficiency on the metabolism of apolipoprotein B-100 in blood plasma: Kinetic studies in normal and Watanabe heritable hyperlipidemic rabbits. *J Clin Invest* **80**:507, 1987.
354. Shepherd J, Packard CJ: Lipoprotein metabolism in familial hypercholesterolemia. *Arteriosclerosis (Suppl)* **9**:I39, 1989.
355. Hornick CA, Kita T, Hamilton RL, Kane JP, Havel RJ: Secretion of lipoproteins from the liver of normal and Watanabe heritable hyperlipidemic rabbits. *Proc Natl Acad Sci U S A* **80**:6096, 1983.
356. Spady DK, Huettinger M, Bilheimer DW, Dietschy JM: Role of receptor-independent low density lipoprotein transport in the maintenance of tissue cholesterol balance in the normal and WHHL rabbit. *J Lipid Res* **28**:32, 1987.
357. Goldstein JL, Brown MS: Familial hypercholesterolemia: Pathogenesis of a receptor disease. *Johns Hopkins Med J* **143**:8, 1978.
358. Goldstein JL, Ho YK, Basu SK, Brown MS: Binding site of macrophages that mediates uptake and degradation of acetylated low density lipoprotein, producing massive cholesterol deposition. *Proc Natl Acad Sci U S A* **76**:333, 1979.
359. Steinberg D: Low density lipoprotein oxidation and its pathobiological significance. *J Biol Chem* **272**:20963, 1997.
360. Grundy SM, Ahrens EH Jr, Salen G: Interruption of the enterohepatic circulation of bile acids in man: Comparative effects of cholestyramine and ileal exclusion on cholesterol metabolism. *J Lab Clin Med* **78**:94, 1971.
361. Miettinen TA: Cholesterol and bile acid synthesis in two families with homozygous and heterozygous hypercholesterolemia. *Arteriosclerosis* **4**:383, 1984.
362. Stacpoole PW, Grundy SM, Swift LL, Greene HL, Slonim AE, Burr IM: Elevated cholesterol and bile acid synthesis in an adult patient with homozygous familial hypercholesterolemia: Reduction by a high glucose diet. *J Clin Invest* **68**:1166, 1981.
363. Lewis B, Myant NB: Studies in the metabolism of cholesterol in subjects with normal plasma cholesterol levels and in patients with essential hypercholesterolaemia. *Clin Sci* **32**:201, 1967.

364. Schwarz KB, Witztum J, Schonfeld G, Grundy SM, Connor WE: Elevated cholesterol and bile acid synthesis in a young patient with homozygous familial hypercholesterolemia. *J Clin Invest* **64**:756, 1979.

365. Samuel P, Perl W, Holtzman CH, Rochman ND, Lieberman S: Long-term kinetics of serum and xanthoma cholesterol radioactivity in patients with hypercholesterolemia. *J Clin Invest* **51**:266, 1972.

366. McNamara DJ: Effects of fat-modified diets on cholesterol and lipoprotein metabolism. *Annu Rev Nutr* **7**:273, 1987.

367. Dietschy JM, Woollett LA, Spady DK: Dietary fatty acids and the regulation of plasma low-density lipoprotein cholesterol levels. *Atheroscler Rev* **23**:7, 1991.

368. Kovanen PT, Brown MS, Basu SK, Bilheimer DW, Goldstein JL: Saturation and suppression of hepatic lipoprotein receptors: A mechanism for the hypercholesterolemia of cholesterol-fed rabbits. *Proc Natl Acad Sci U S A* **78**:1396, 1981.

369. Daumerie CM, Woollett LA, Dietschy JM: Fatty acids regulate hepatic low density lipoprotein receptor activity through redistribution of intracellular cholesterol pools. *Proc Natl Acad Sci U S A* **89**:10797, 1992.

370. Grundy SM, Denke MA: Dietary influences on serum lipids and lipoproteins. *J Lipid Res* **31**:1149, 1990.

371. Benlian P, Luc de Gennes J, Dairou F, Hermelin B, Ginon I, Villain E, Lagarde JP, Federspiel MC, Bertrand V, Bernard C, Bereziat G: Phenotypic expression in double heterozygotes for familial hypercholesterolemia and familial defective apolipoprotein B-100. *Hum Mutat* **7**:340, 1996.

372. Rubinsztein DC, Raal FJ, Seftel HC, Pilcher G, Coetzee GA, van der Westhuyzen DR: Characterization of six patients who are double heterozygotes for familial hypercholesterolemia and familial defective Apo B-100. *Arterioscler Thromb* **13**:1076, 1993.

373. Morganroth J, Levy RI, McMahon AE, Gotto AM Jr: Pseudohomozygous type II hyperlipoproteinemia. *J Pediatr* **85**:639, 1974.

374. Low LCK, Lin HJ, Lau KS, Kung AWC, Yeung CY: Phytosterolemia and pseudohomozygous type II hypercholesterolemia in two Chinese patients. *J Pediatr* **118**:746, 1991.

375. Fujita M, Okamoto S, Shirai K, Saito Y, Yoshida S: Pseudohomozygous type II hyperlipoproteinemia. *Dermatologica* **182**:94, 1991.

376. Patel SB, Salen G, Hidaka H, Kwiterovich PO Jr, Stalenhoef AFH, Miettinen TA, Grundy SM, Lee M-H, Rubenstein JS, Polymeropoulos MH, Brownstein MJ: Mapping a gene involved in regulating dietary cholesterol absorption; the sitosterolemia locus is found at chromosme 2p21. *J Clin Invest* **102**:1041, 1998.

377. Zuliani G, Vigna GB, Corsini A, Maioli M, Romagnoni F, Fellin R: Severe hypercholesterolaemia: unusual inheritance in an Italian pedigree. *Eur J Clin Invest* **25**:322, 1995.

378. Schmidt HHJ, Stuhrmann M, Shamburek R, Schewe CK, Ebhardt M, Zech LA, Buttner C, Wendt M, Beisiegel U, Brewer HB Jr, Manns MP: Delayed low density lipoprotein (LDL) catabolism despite a functional intact LDL-apolipoprotein B particle and LDL-receptor in a subject with clinical homozygous familial hypercholesterolemia. *J Clin Endocrinol Metab* **83**:2167, 1998.

378a. Zuliani G, Arca M, Signore A, Bader G, Fazio S, Chianelli M, Bellosta S, Campagna F, Montali A, Maioli M, Pacifico A, Ricci G, Fellin R: Characterization of a new form of inherited hypercholesterolemia: The familial recessive hypercholesterolemia. *Arterioscler Thromb Vasc Biol* **19**:802, 1999.

379. Harada-Shiba M, Tajima S, Yokoyama S, Miyake Y, Kojima S, Tsushima M, Kawakami M, Yamamoto A: Siblings with normal LDL receptor activity and severe hypercholesterolemia. *Arterioscler Thromb* **12**:1071, 1992.

380. Brunzell JD, Albers JJ, Chait A, Grundy SM, Groszek E, McDonald GB: Plasma lipoproteins in familial combined hyperlipidemia and monogenic familial hypertriglyceridemia. *J Lipid Res* **24**:147, 1983.

381. Austin MA, Horowitz H, Wijsman E, Krauss RM, Brunzell J: Bimodality of plasma apolipoprotein B levels in familial combined hyperlipidemia. *Atherosclerosis* **92**:67, 1992.

382. Innerarity TL, Weisgraber KH, Arnold KS, Mahley RW, Krauss RM, Vega GL, Grundy SM: Familial defective apolipoprotein B-100: Low density lipoproteins with abnormal receptor binding. *Proc Natl Acad Sci U S A* **84**:6919, 1987.

383. Innerarity TL, Mahley RW, Weisgraber KH, Bersot TP, Krauss RM, Vega GL, Grundy SM, Friedl W, Davignon J, McCarthy BJ: Familial defective apolipoprotein B-100: A mutation of apolipoprotein B that causes hypercholesterolemia. *J Lipid Res* **31**:1337, 1990.

384. Williams RR, Hunt SC, Schumacher MC, Hegele RA, Leppert MF, Ludwig EH, Hopkins PN: Diagnosing heterozygous familial hypercholesterolemia using new practical criteria validated by molecular genetics. *Am J Cardiol* **72**:171, 1993.

385. Tybjaerg-Hansen A, Gallagher J, Vincent J, Houlston R, Talmud P, Dunning AM, Seed M, Hamsten A, Humphries SE, Myant NB: Familial defective apolipoprotein B-100: Detection in the United Kingdom and Scandinavia, and clinical characteristics of ten cases. *Atherosclerosis* **80**:235, 1990.

386. Schuster H, Rauh G, Kormann B, Hepp T, Humphries S, Keller C, Wolfram G, Zollner N: Familial defective apolipoprotein B-100: Comparison with familial hypercholesterolemia in 18 cases detected in Munich. *Arteriosclerosis* **10**:577, 1990.

387. Myant NB, Gallagher JJ, Knight BL, McCarthy SN, Frostegard J, Nilsson J, Hamsten A, Talmud P, Humphries SE: Clinical signs of familial hypercholesterolemia in patients with familial defective apolipoprotein B-100 and normal low density lipoprotein receptor function. *Arterioscler Thromb* **11**:691, 1991.

388. Miserez AR, Keller U: Differences in the phenotypic characteristics of subjects with familial defective apolipoprotein B-100 and familial hypercholesterolemia. *Arterioscler Thromb Vasc Biol* **15**:1719, 1995.

389. Corsini A, Roma P, Sommariva D, Fumagalli R, Catapano AL: Autoantibodies to the low density lipoprotein receptor in a subject affected by severe hypercholesterolemia. *J Clin Invest* **78**:940, 1986.

390. Havel RJ, Goldstein JL, Brown MS: Lipoproteins and lipid transport, in Bondy PK, Rosenberg LE (eds): *Metabolic Control and Disease*. Philadelphia, Saunders, 1980, p 393.

391. Goldstein JL, Basu SK, Brown MS: Receptor-mediated endocytosis of LDL in cultured cells. *Methods Enzymol* **98**:241, 1983.

392. Daniel TO, Schneider WJ, Goldstein JL, Brown MS: Visualization of lipoprotein receptors by ligand blotting. *J Biol Chem* **258**:4606, 1983.

393. Tolleshaug H, Hobgood KK, Brown MS, Goldstein JL: The LDL receptor locus in familial hypercholesterolemia: Multiple mutations disrupting the transport and processing of a membrane receptor. *Cell* **32**:941, 1983.

394. Cuthbert JA, East CA, Bilheimer DW, Lipsky PE: Detection of familial hypercholesterolemia by assaying functional low-density-lipoprotein receptors on lymphocytes. *N Engl J Med* **314**:879, 1986.

395. deGennes JL, Daffos F, Dairou F, Forestier F, Capella-Pavlosky M, Truffert J, Gaschard JC, Darbois Y: Direct fetal blood examination for prenatal diagnosis of homozygous familial hypercholesterolemia. *Arteriosclerosis* **5**:440, 1985.

396. Reshef A, Meiner V, Dann EJ, Granat M, Leitersdorf E: Prenatal diagnosis of familial hypercholesterolemia caused by the "Lebanese" mutation at the low density lipoprotein receptor locus. *Hum Genet* **89**:237, 1992.

397. Goldstein JL, Albers JJ, Schrott HG, Hazzard WR, Bierman EL, Motulsky AG: Plasma lipid levels and coronary heart disease in adult relatives of newborns with normal and elevated cord blood lipids. *Am J Human Genet* **26**:727, 1974.

398. Darmady JM, Fosbrooke AS, Lloyd JK: Prospective study of serum cholesterol levels during first year of life. *Br Med J* **2**:685, 1972.

399. Vuorio AF, Turtola H, Kontula K: Neonatal diagnosis of familial hypercholesterolemia in newborns born to a parent with a molecularly defined heterozygous familial hypercholesterolemia. *Arterioscler Thromb Vasc Biol* **17**:3332, 1997.

400. Goldstein JL, Helgeson JAS, Brown MS: Inhibition of cholesterol synthesis with compactin renders growth of cultured cells dependent on the low density lipoprotein receptor. *J Biol Chem* **254**:5403, 1979.

401. Hashim SA, Van Itallie TB: Cholestyramine resin therapy for hypercholesterolemia: Clinical and metabolic studies. *JAMA* **192**:289, 1965.

402. Grundy SM: Treatment of hypercholesterolemia by interference with bile acid metabolism. *Arch Intern Med* **130**:638, 1972.

403. Brown MS, Goldstein JL: Drugs used in treatment of hyperlipoproteinemias, in Gilman AG, Rall TW, Nies AS, Taylor P (eds): *Goodman and Gilman's The Pharmacological Basis of Therapeutics, 8th ed.* New York, McGraw-Hill, 1990, p 874.

404. Levy RI, Fredrickson DS, Stone NJ, Bilheimer DW, Brown WV, Glueck CJ, Gotto AM Jr, Herbert PN, Kwiterovich PO, Langer T, LaRosa J, Lux SE, Rider AK, Shulman RS, Sloan HR: Cholestyramine in type II hyperlipoproteinemia. *Ann Intern Med* **79**:51, 1973.

405. Shepherd J, Packard CJ, Bicker S, Lawrie TDV, Morgan HG: Cholestyramine promotes receptor-mediated low-density-lipoprotein catabolism. *N Engl J Med* **302**:1219, 1980.

406. Slater HR, Packard CJ, Bicker S, Shepherd J: Effects of cholestyramine on receptor-mediated plasma clearance and tissue uptake of human low density lipoproteins in the rabbit. *J Biol Chem* **255**:10210, 1980.

407. Rudling MJ, Reihner E, Einarsson K, Ewerth S, Angelin B: Low density lipoprotein receptor-binding activity in human tissues: Quantitative importance of hepatic receptors and evidence for regulation of their expression *in vivo*. *Proc Natl Acad Sci U S A* **87**:3469, 1990.
408. Kovanen PT, Bilheimer DW, Goldstein JL, Jaramillo JJ, Brown MS: Regulatory role for hepatic low density lipoprotein receptors *in vivo* in the dog. *Proc Natl Acad Sci U S A* **78**:1194, 1981.
409. Moutafis CD, Simons LA, Myant NB, Adams PW, Wynn V: The effect of cholestyramine on the faecal excretion of bile acids and neutral steroids in familial hypercholesterolaemia. *Atherosclerosis* **26**:329, 1977.
410. Beil U, Crouse JR, Einarsson K, Grundy SM: Effects of interruption of the enterohepatic circulation of bile acids on the transport of very low density-lipoprotein triglycerides. *Metabolism* **31**:438, 1982.
411. Endo A, Kuroda M, Tanzawa K: Competitive inhibition of 3-hydroxy-3-methylglutaryl coenzyme A reductase by ML-236A and ML-236B fungal metabolites, having hypocholesterolemic activity. *FEBS Lett* **72**:323, 1976.
412. Endo A: The discovery and development of HMG-CoA reductase inhibitors. *J Lipid Res* **33**:1569, 1992.
413. Alberts AW, MacDonald JS, Till AE, Tobert JA: Lovastatin. *Cardiovasc Drug Rev* **7**:89, 1989.
414. Witztum JL: Drugs used in the treatment of hyperlipoproteinemias, in Hardman, JG, Limbird, LE, Molinoff, PB, Ruddon, RW (eds): *Goodman and Gilman's The Pharmacological Basis of Therapeutics*. New York, McGraw-Hill, 1995, p 1981.
415. Atorvastatin — A new lipid-lowering drug. *The Medical Letter* **39**:29, 1997.
416. Cerivastatin for hypercholesterolemia. *The Medical Letter* **40**:13, 1998.
417. Brown MS, Faust JR, Goldstein JL, Kaneko I, Endo A: Induction of 3-hydroxy-3-methylglutaryl coenzyme A reductase activity in human fibroblasts incubated with compactin (ML-236B), a competitive inhibitor of the reductase. *J Biol Chem* **253**:1121, 1978.
418. Bergstrom JD, Bostedor RG, Rew DJ, Geissler WM, Wright SD, Chao Y-S: Hepatic responses to inhibition of 3-hydroxy-3-methylglutaryl-CoA reductase: A comparison of atorvastatin and simvastatin. *Biochim Biophys Acta* **1389**:213, 1998.
419. Bilheimer DW, Grundy SM, Brown MS, Goldstein JL: Mevinolin stimulates receptor-mediated clearance of low density lipoprotein from plasma in familial hypercholesterolemia heterozygotes. *Proc Natl Acad Sci U S A* **80**:4124, 1983.
420. Ma PTS, Gil G, Südhof TC, Bilheimer DW, Goldstein JL, Brown MS: Mevinolin, an inhibitor of cholesterol synthesis, induces mRNA for low density lipoprotein receptor in livers of hamsters and rabbits. *Proc Natl Acad Sci U S A* **83**:8370, 1986.
421. Malmendier CL, Lontie J-F, Delcroix C, Magot T: Effect of simvastatin on receptor-dependent low density lipoprotein catabolism in normocholesterolemic human volunteers. *Atherosclerosis* **80**:101, 1989.
422. Matsunaga A, Sasaki J, Takada Y, Hidaka K, Arakawa K: Effect of simvastatin on receptor mediated metabolism of low density lipoprotein in guinea pigs. *Atherosclerosis* **90**:31, 1991.
423. Reihnér E, Rudling M, Ståhlberg D, Berglund L, Ewerth S, Björkhem I, Einarsson K, Angelin B: Influence of pravastatin, a specific inhibitor of HMG-CoA reductase, on hepatic metabolism of cholesterol. *N Engl J Med* **323**:224, 1990.
424. Grundy SM, Bilheimer DW: Inhibition of 3-hydroxy-3-methylglutaryl-CoA reductase by mevinolin in familial hypercholesterolemia heterozygotes: Effects on cholesterol balance. *Proc Natl Acad Sci U S A* **81**:2538, 1984.
425. Goldberg IJ, Holleran S, Ramakrishnan R, Adams M, Palmer RH, Dell RB, Goodman DS: Lack of effect of lovastatin therapy on the parameters of whole-body cholesterol metabolism. *J Clin Invest* **86**:801, 1990.
426. Uauy R, Vega GL, Grundy SM, Bilheimer DW: Lovastatin therapy in receptor-negative homozygous familial hypercholesterolemia: Lack of effect on low-density lipoprotein concentrations or turnover. *J Pediatr* **113**:387, 1988.
427. Feher MD, Webb JC, Patel DD, Lant AF, Mayne PD, Knight BL, Soutar AK: Cholesterol-lowering drug therapy in a patient with receptor-negative homozygous familial hypercholesterolaemia. *Atherosclerosis* **103**:171, 1993.
428. Grundy SM, Vega GL: Influence of mevinolin on metabolism of low density lipoproteins in primary moderate hypercholesterolemia. *J Lipid Res* **26**:1464, 1985.
429. Grundy SM: Multifactorial etiology of hypercholesterolemia: Implications for prevention of coronary heart disease. *Arterioscler Thromb* **11**:1619, 1991.
430. Marais AD, Naoumova RP, Firth JC, Penny C, Neuwirth CKY, Thompson GR: Decreased production of low density lipoprotein by atorvastatin after apheresis in homozygous familial hypercholesterolemia. *J Lipid Res* **38**:2071, 1997.
431. Mabuchi H, Sakai T, Sakai Y, Yoshimura A, Watanabe A, Wakasugi T, Koizumi J, Takeda R: Reduction of serum cholesterol in heterozygous patients with familial hypercholesterolemia: Additive effects of compactin and cholestyramine. *N Engl J Med* **308**:609, 1983.
432. Couture P, Brun LD, Szots F, Lelievre M, Gaudet D, Despres J-P, Simard J, Lupien PJ, Gagne C: Association of specific LDL receptor gene mutations with differential plasma lipoprotein response to simvastatin in young French Canadians with heterozygous familial hypercholesterolemia. *Arterioscler Thromb Vasc Biol* **18**:1007, 1998.
433. Bradford RH, Shear CL, Chremos AN, Dujovne C, Downton M, Franklin FA, Gould AL, Hesney M, Higgins J, Hurley DP, Langendorfer A, Nash DT, Pool JL, Schnaper H: Expanded clinical evaluation of lovastatin (EXCEL) study results: I. Efficacy in modifying plasma lipoproteins and adverse event profile in 8245 patients with moderate hypercholesterolemia. *Arch Intern Med* **151**:43, 1991.
434. East C, Alivizatos PA, Grundy SM, Jones PH, Farmer JA: Rhabdomyolysis in patients receiving lovastatin after cardiac transplantation. *N Engl J Med* **318**:47, 1988.
435. Reaven P, Witztum JL: Lovastatin, nicotinic acid, and rhabdomyolysis. *Ann Intern Med* **109**:597, 1988.
436. Manoukian AA, Bhagavan NV, Hayashi T, Nestor TA, Rios C, Scottolini AG: Rhabdomyolysis secondary to lovastatin therapy. *Clin Chem* **36**:2145, 1990.
437. Stein EA, Lane M, Laskarzewski P: Comparison of statins in hypertriglyceridemia. *Am J Cardiol* **81**:66B, 1998.
438. Kane JP, Malloy MJ, Tun P, Phillips NR, Freedman DD, Williams ML, Rowe JS, Havel RJ: Normalization of low-density-lipoprotein levels in heterozygous familial hypercholesterolemia with a combined drug regimen. *N Engl J Med* **304**:251, 1981.
439. Malloy MJ, Kane JP, Kunitake ST, Tun P: Complementarity of colestipol, niacin, and lovastatin in treatment of severe familial hypercholesterolemia. *Ann Intern Med* **107**:616, 1987.
440. Walsh BW, Schiff I, Rosner B, Greenberg L, Ravnikar V, Sacks FM: Effects of postmenopausal estrogen replacement on the concentrations and metabolism of plasma lipoproteins. *N Engl J Med* **325**:1196, 1991.
441. Buchwald H, Varco RL, Matts JP, Long JM, Fitch LL, Campbell GS, Pearce MB, et al., and the POSCH Group: Effect of partial ileal bypass surgery on mortality and morbidity from coronary heart disease in patients with hypercholesterolemia: Report of the program on the surgical control of the hyperlipidemias (POSCH). *N Engl J Med* **323**:946, 1990.
442. Koivisto P, Miettinen TA: Long-term effects of ileal bypass on lipoproteins in patients with familial hypercholesterolemia. *Circulation* **70**:290, 1984.
443. Schouten JA, Beynen AC: Partial ileal bypass surgery in the treatment of heterozygous familial hypercholesterolemia: A review. *Artery* **13**:240, 1986.
444. Connor WE, Connor SL: Dietary treatment of familial hypercholesterolemia. *Atherosclerosis (Suppl)* **9**:I91, 1989.
445. Spady DK, Dietschy JM: Interaction of dietary cholesterol and triglycerides in the regulation of hepatic low density lipoprotein transport in the hamster. *J Clin Invest* **81**:300, 1988.
446. Tonstad S, Knudtzon J, Sivertsen M, Refsum H, Ose L: Efficacy and safety of cholestyramine therapy in peripubertal and prepubertal children with familial hypercholesterolemia. *J Pediatr* **129**:42, 1996.
447. Stein EA: Treatment of familial hypercholesterolemia with drugs in children. *Arteriosclerosis (Suppl)* **9**:I145, 1989.
448. Gylling H, Siimes MA, Miettinen TA: Sitostanol ester margarine in dietary treatment of children with familial hypercholesterolemia. *J Lipid Res* **36**:1807, 1995.
449. Lambert M, Lupien P-J, Gagne C, Levy E, Blaichman S, Langlois S, Hayden M, Rose V, Clarke JTR, Wolfe BMJ, Clarson C, Parsons H, Stephure DK, Potvin D, Lambert J: Treatment of familial hypercholesterolemia in children and adolescents: Effect of lovastatin. *Pediatrics* **97**:619, 1996.
450. Knipscheer HC, Boelen CCA, Kastelein JJP, van Diermen DE, Groenemeijer BE, Van den Ende A, Buller HR, Bakker HD:

Short-term efficacy and safety of pravastatin in 72 children with familial hypercholesterolemia. *Pediat Res* **39**:867, 1996.

451. Stein EA, Illingworth DR, Kwiterovich PO, Jr., Liacouras CA, Siimes MA, Jacobson MS, Brewster TG, Hopkins P, Davidson M, Graham K, Arensman F, Knopp RH, DuJovne C, Williams CL, Isaacsohn JL, Jacobsen CA, Laskarzewski PM, Ames S, Gormley GJ: Efficacy and safety of lovastatin in adolescent males with heterozygous familial hypercholesterolemia: A randomized controlled trial. *JAMA* **281**:137, 1998.
452. National Cholesterol Education Program. Report of the expert panel on blood cholesterol levels in children and adolescents. *Pediatrics* **89**:525, 1992.
453. Khachadurian AK: Cholestyramine therapy in patients homozygous for familial hypercholesterolemia (familial hypercholesterolemic xanthomatosis). *J Atheroscler Res* **8**:177, 1968.
454. Yamamoto A, Yamamura T, Yokoyama S, Sudo H, Matsuzawa Y: Combined drug therapy—cholestyramine and compactin—for familial hypercholesterolemia. *Int J Clin Pharmacol Ther Toxicol* **22**:493, 1984.
455. Thompson GR, Gotto AM Jr: Ileal bypass in the treatment of hyperlipoproteinaemia. *Lancet* **2**:35, 1973.
456. Deckelbaum RJ, Lees RS, Small DM, Hedberg SE, Grundy SM: Failure of complete bile diversion and oral bile acid therapy in the treatment of homozygous familial hypercholesterolemia. *N Engl J Med* **296**:465, 1977.
457. Raal FJ, Pilcher GJ, Illingworth DR, Pappu AS, Stein EA, Laskarzewski P, Mitchel YB, Melino MR: Expanded-dose simvastatin is effective in homozygous familial hypercholesterolaemia. *Artherosclerosis* **135**:249, 1997.
458. Heinonen TM, Marais AD, Raal FJ, Stalenhoef A, Thompson GR, Rader D, Gaudet D, Gagne C, Davignon J, Keilson L, McBride S, Black DM, Stein E, Hudgins L, Capuzzi D, Salisbury S, McQueen M: Utility of atorvastatin in homozygous familial hypercholesterolemia. Manuscript in preparation.
459. Starzl TE, Chase HP, Putnam CW, Porter KA: Portacaval shunt in hyperlipoproteinaemia. *Lancet* **2**:940, 1973.
460. Torsvik H, Feldman HA, Fischer JE, Lees RS: Effects of intravenous hyperalimentation on plasma-lipoproteins in severe familial hypercholesterolaemia. *Lancet* **1**:601, 1975.
461. Starzl TE, Chase HP, Putnam CW, Nora JJ: Follow-up of patient with portacaval shunt for the treatment of hyperlipidaemia. *Lancet* **2**:714, 1974.
462. Starzl TE, Putnam CW, Koep LJ: Portacaval shunt and hyperlipidemia. *Arch Surg* **113**:71, 1978.
463. Bilheimer DW: Portacaval shunt and liver transplantation in treatment of familial hypercholesterolemia. *Arteriosclerosis (Suppl)* **9**:I158, 1989.
464. McNamara DJ, Ahrens EH Jr, Kolb R, Brown CD, Parker TS, Davidson NO, Samuel P, McVie RM: Treatment of familial hypercholesterolemia by portacaval anastomosis: Effect on cholesterol metabolism and pool sizes. *Proc Natl Acad Sci U S A* **80**:564, 1983.
465. deGennes JL, Touraine R, Maunand B, Truffert J, Laudat P: Formes homozygotes cutanéo-tendineuses de xanthomatose hypercholestérolémique dans une observation familiale exemplaire—essai de plasmaphérèse à titre du traitement héroique. *Société Médicale du Hôpital de Paris* **118**:1377, 1967.
466. Thompson GR, Lowenthal R, Myant NB: Plasma exchange in the management of homozygous familial hypercholesterolaemia. *Lancet* **1**:1208, 1975.
467. Thompson GR, Barbir M, Okabayashi K, Trayner I, Larkin S: Plasmapheresis in familial hypercholesterolemia. *Arteriosclerosis (Suppl)* **9**:I152, 1989.
468. Postiglione A, Thompson GR: Experience with plasma-exchange in homozygous familial hypercholesterolaemia. *Prog Clin Biol Res* **188**:213, 1985.
469. Keller C, Schmitz H, Theisen K, Zollner N: Regression of valvular aortic stenosis due to homozygous familial hypercholesterolemia following plasmapheresis. *Klin Wochenschr* **64**:338, 1986.
470. Stein EA, Adolph R, Rice V, Glueck CJ, Spitz HB: Nonprogression of coronary artery atherosclerosis in homozygous familial hypercholesterolemia after 31 months of repetitive plasma exchange. *Clin Cardiol* **9**:115, 1986.
471. Myant NB: Regression of coronary atherosclerosis in man. *Adv Exp Med Biol* **168**:139, 1984.
472. Thompson GR, Miller JP, Breslow JL: Improved survival of patients with homozygous familial hypercholesterolaemia treated with plasma exchange. *Br Med J* **291**:1671, 1985.
473. Lupien P-J, Moorjani S, Gagne C, Brun L-D, Lou M, Dagenais G: Long term treatment of two familial hypercholesterolemic heterozygote patients with batch affinity chromatography (BAC). *Artery* **10**:286, 1982.
474. Stoffel W, Demant T: Selective removal of apolipoprotein B-containing serum lipoproteins from blood plasma. *Proc Natl Acad Sci U S A* **78**:611, 1981.
475. Yokoyama S, Hayashi R, Satani M, Yamamoto A: Selective removal of low density lipoprotein by plasmapheresis in familial hypercholesterolemia. *Arteriosclerosis* **5**:613, 1985.
476. Homma Y, Mikami Y, Tamachi H, Nakaya N, Nakamura H, Araki G, Goto Y: Comparison of selectivity of LDL removal by double filtration and dextran-sulfate cellulose column plasmapheresis. *Atherosclerosis* **60**:23, 1986.
477. Zwiener RJ, Uauy R, Petruska ML, Huet BA: Low-density lipoprotein apheresis as long-term treatment for children with homozygous familial hypercholesterolemia. *J Pediatr* **126**:728, 1995.
478. Teruel JL, Lasuncion MA, Navarro JF, Carrero P, Ortuno J: Pregnancy in a patient with homozygous familial hypercholesterolemia undergoing low-density lipoprotein apheresis by dextran sulfate adsorption. *Metabolism* **44**:929, 1995.
479. Gordon BR, Kelsey SF, Dau PC, Gotto AM, Graham K, Illingworth DR, Isaacsohn J, Jones PH, Leitman SF, Saal SD, Stein EA, Stern TN, Troendle A, Zwiener RJ: Long-term effects of low-density lipoprotein apheresis using an automated dextran sulfate cellulose adsorption system. *Am J Cardiol* **81**:407, 1998.
480. Koga N, Iwata Y: Pathological and angiographic regression of coronary atherosclerosis by LDL-apheresis in a patient with familial hypercholesterolemia. *Atherosclerosis* **90**:9, 1991.
481. Tatami R, Inoue N, Itoh H, Kishino B, Koga N, Nakashima Y, Nishide T, Okamura K, Saito Y, Teramoto T, Yasugi T, Yamamoto A, Goto Y: Regression of coronary atherosclerosis by combined LDL-apheresis and lipid-lowering drug therapy in patients with familial hypercholesterolemia: A multicenter study. *Atherosclerosis* **95**:1, 1992.
482. Thompson GR, Maher VMG, Matthews S, Kitano Y, Neuwirth C, Shortt MB, Davies G, Rees A, Mir A, Prescott RJ, de Feyter P, Henderson A: Familial hypercholesterolaemia regression study: A randomised trial of low-density-lipoprotein apheresis. *Lancet* **345**:811, 1995.
483. Kroon AA, Aengevaeren WRM, van der Werf T, Uijen GJH, Reiber JHC, Bruschke AVG, Stalenhoef AFH: LDL-apheresis atherosclerosis regression study (LAARS). Effect of aggressive versus conventional lipid-lowering treatment on coronary atherosclerosis. *Circulation* **93**:1826, 1996.
484. Starzl TE, Bilheimer DW, Bahnson HT, Shaw BW Jr, Hardesty RL, Griffith BP, Iwatsuki S, Zitelli BJ, Gartner JC Jr, Malatack JJ, Urbach AH: Heart-liver transplantation in a patient with familial hypercholesterolaemia. *Lancet* **1**:1382, 1984.
485. Bilheimer DW, Goldstein JL, Grundy SC, Starzl TE, Brown MS: Liver transplantation provides low density lipoprotein receptors and lowers plasma cholesterol in a child with homozygous familial hypercholesterolemia. *N Engl J Med* **311**:1658, 1984.
486. East C, Grundy SM, Bilheimer DW: Normal cholesterol levels with lovastatin (mevinolin) therapy in a child with homozygous familial hypercholesterolemia following liver transplantation. *JAMA* **256**:2843, 1986.
487. Hoeg JM, Starzl TE, Brewer HJ Jr: Liver transplantation for treatment of cardiovascular disease: Comparison with medication and plasma exchange in homozygous familial hypercholesterolemia. *Am J Cardiol* **59**:705, 1987.
488. Valdivielso P, Escolar JL, Cuervas-Mons V, Pulpon LA, Chaparro MAS, Gonzalez-Santos P: Lipids and lipoprotein changes after heart and liver transplantation in a patient with homozygous familial hypercholesterolemia. *Ann Intern Med* **108**:204, 1988.
489. Barbir M, Khaghani A, Kehely A, Tan K-C, Mitchell A, Thompson GR, Yacoub M: Normalisation of lipoproteins including Lp(a) after liver-heart transplantation in homozygous familial hypercholesterolaemia. *Q J Med* **85**:807, 1992.

489a. Téllez de Peralta G, Burgos Lázaro, R: Trasplantes multiorgánicos. *Rev Esp Cardiol* **48**:46, 1995.

490. Grossman M, Raper SE, Kozarsky K, Stein EA, Engelhardt JF, Muller D, Lupien PJ, Wilson JM: Successful *ex vivo* gene therapy directed to liver in a patient with familial hypercholesterolaemia. *Nat Genet* **6**:335, 1994.
491. Grossman M, Rader DJ, Muller DWM, Kolansky DM, Kozarsky K, Clark BJ III, Stein EA, Lupien PJ, Brewer HB, Jr, Raper SE, Wilson

JM: A pilot study of *ex vivo* gene therapy for homozygous familial hypercholesterolaemia. *Nat Med* **1**:1148, 1995.

492. Brown MS, Goldstein JL, Havel RJ, Steinberg D: Gene therapy for cholesterol. *Nat Genet* **7**:349, 1994.
493. Raper SE, Grossman M, Rader DJ, Thoene JG, Clark BJ, Kolansky DM, Muller DWM, Wilson JM: Safety and feasibility of liver-directed *ex vivo* gene therapy for homozygous familial hypercholesterolemia. *Ann Surg* **223**:116, 1996.
494. Kane JP, Malloy MJ, Ports TA, Phillips NR, Diehl JC, Havel RJ: Regression of coronary atherosclerosis during treatment of familial hypercholesterolemia with combined drug regimens. *JAMA* **264**:3007, 1990.
495. Blankenhorn DH, Nessim SA, Johnson RL, Sanmarco ME, Azen SP, Cashin-Hemphill L: Beneficial effects of combined colestipol-niacin therapy on coronary atherosclerosis and coronary venous bypass grafts. *JAMA* **257**:3233, 1987.
496. Brown G, Albers JJ, Fisher LD, Schaefer SM, Lin J-T, Kaplan C, Zhao X-Q, Bisson BD, Fitzpatrick VF, Dodge HT: Regression of coronary artery disease as a result of intensive lipid-lowering therapy in men with high levels of apolipoprotein B. *N Engl J Med* **323**:1289, 1990.
497. Watts GF, Lewis B, Brunt JNH, Lewis ES, Coltart DJ, Smith LDR, Mann JI, Swan AV: Effects on coronary artery disease of lipid-lowering diet, or diet plus cholestyramine, in the St Thomas' Atherosclerosis Regression Study (STARS). *Lancet* **339**:563, 1992.
498. Scandinavian Simvastatin Survival Study Group: Randomised trial of cholesterol lowering in 4444 patients with coronary heart disease: The Scandinavian Simvastatin Survival Study (4S). *Lancet* **344**:1383, 1994.
499. Sacks FM, Pfeffer MA, Moye LA, Rouleau JL, Rutherford JD, Cole TG, Brown L, Warnica JW, Arnold JMO, Wun C-C, Davis BR, Braunwald E: The effect of pravastatin on coronary events after myocardial infarction in patients with average cholesterol levels. *N Engl J Med* **335**:1001, 1996.
500. Shepherd J, Cobbe SM, Ford I, Isles CG, Lorimer AR, MacFarlane PW, McKillop JH, Packard CJ: Prevention of coronary heart disease with pravastatin in men with hypercholesterolemia. *N Engl J Med* **333**:1301, 1995.
501. Downs JR, Clearfield M, Weis S, Whitney E, Shapiro DR, Beere PA, Langendorfer A, Stein EA, Kruyer W, Gotto AM Jr: Primary prevention of acute coronary events with lovastatin in men and women with average cholesterol levels: Results of AFCAPS/TexCAPS. *JAMA* **279**:1615, 1998.
502. Lipid Research Clinics Program: The lipid research clinics coronary primary prevention trial results. II. The relationship of reduction in incidence of coronary heart disease to cholesterol lowering. *JAMA* **251**:365, 1984.
503. Brown MS, Goldstein JL: Heart attacks: Gone with the century? *Science* **272**:629, 1996.
504. Brown MS, Kovanen PT, Goldstein JL: Regulation of plasma cholesterol by lipoprotein receptors. *Science* **212**:628,1981.
505. Ericsson S, Eriksson M, Vitols S, Einarsson K, Berglund L, Angelin B: Influence of age on the metabolism of plasma low density lipoproteins in healthy males. *J Clin Invest* **87**:591, 1991.
506. Rudling M, Norstedt G, Olivecrona H, Gustafsson J-A, Angelin B: Induction of hepatic LDL receptors: Importance of growth hormone. *Proc Natl Acad Sci U S A* **89**:6983, 1992.

CHAPTER 121

Genetic Disorders Affecting Plasma High-Density Lipoproteins

Alan R. Tall ▪ Jan L. Breslow ▪ Edward M. Rubin

1. Plasma high-density lipoproteins (HDL) consist of about 50 percent protein and 50 percent lipids. The principal apolipoproteins of HDL, apo A-I and apo A-II, are synthesized in the liver (apo A-I and apo A-II) or small intestine (apo A-I), secreted as components of triglyceride (TG)-rich lipoproteins (TRL), and then transferred into HDL during lipolysis, along with phospholipid and cholesterol. Alternatively, they may be secreted as free apoproteins, then acquire lipids by interaction with the cellular ATP binding cassette transporter, ABC1. The plasma cholesterol-esterifying enzyme lecithin: cholesterol acyltransferase (LCAT) circulates bound to HDL and uses free cholesterol and phospholipids as substrates in the generation of cholesteryl esters (CE). HDL also contains a phospholipid transfer protein (PLTP) and a cholesteryl ester transfer protein (CETP), which mediate the transfer of phospholipid and cholesterol into HDL and the removal of cholesteryl esters from HDL, respectively. CETP mediates a hetero-exchange of HDL CE for TG of TRL, and the HDL TG is subsequently hydrolyzed by hepatic lipase (HL). The coordinate activities of PLTP, CETP, LCAT, and HL promote the formation and turnover of HDL CE, which is a central event in the transport of cholesterol from peripheral tissues to the liver, that is, reverse cholesterol transport. The return of plasma HDL CE to the liver may involve transfer to TRL by CETP, selective uptake of free and esterified cholesterol (i.e., cellular uptake of HDL lipid without protein degradation), or uptake of holo-HDL particles. An authentic HDL receptor, scavenger receptor BI (SR-BI), is highly expressed in the liver and steroidogenic tissues, where it mediates the selective uptake of HDL lipids.
2. Plasma HDL levels show an inverse relationship to atherosclerotic cardiovascular disease. Underlying this relationship is the ability of HDL to promote the efflux of cholesterol from foam cells in the arterial wall and to mediate reverse cholesterol transport. Transgenic mouse studies strongly support an antiatherogenic role of HDL, and are consistent with increased reverse cholesterol transport as the underlying mechanism. Antiatherogenic properties of HDL may also be related to its ability to inhibit the retention, aggregation, and oxidation of LDL in the arterial wall. Humans with low HDL often have increased levels of TRL; in some cases, low HDL is likely a marker for a metabolic predisposition to accumulate atherogenic remnants of TRL. Subjects with low HDL typically have increased catabolism of apo A-I, a process that may be driven by increased core lipid exchange between HDL and TRL. In other cases low HDL may be a marker of an inflammatory state involving the vessel wall.
3. Transgenic mouse models have proven invaluable in elucidating the metabolism of HDL and its relationships to atherosclerosis. Human apo A-I transgenic mice show increased HDL cholesterol and have human-like subspecies of HDL in plasma. Importantly, apo A-I transgenic mice are resistant to the development of early atherosclerotic lesions in response to an atherogenic diet. Moreover, the apo A-I transgene inhibits the development of both early and late complex atherosclerotic lesions in apo E knockout (KO) mice. These experiments provide compelling evidence for a direct antiatherogenic function of HDL. Similar results have been reported when another HDL apolipoprotein, apo A-IV, is overexpressed in mice. However, human apo A-II transgenic mice do not have increased HDL cholesterol levels, and are not protected from atherosclerosis. Gene knockout of apo A-I results in decreased HDL cholesterol levels but does not increase atherosclerosis susceptibility in response to diet or the apo E KO background; apo A-I KO mice show a modest increase in atherosclerosis susceptibility in the presence of an atherogenic stimulus provided by the apo B transgene. These results suggest that multiple genes (apo A-I, apo A-IV) with redundant functions mediate antiatherogenic properties of HDL in response to specific atherogenic stimuli.
4. Genetic manipulation of the HDL processing factors (enzymes, lipid transfer proteins, and receptors) has also provided insight into their role in HDL metabolism. Mice or rabbits transgenic for LCAT show increased HDL cholesterol levels, and LCAT transgenic rabbits are protected from atherosclerosis. CETP transgenic mice have decreased HDL cholesterol and apo A-I levels, increased clearance of HDL CE in the liver, and variable atherosclerosis depending on the metabolic context. Crossbreeding of CETP transgenic mice with hypertriglyceridemic apo C-III transgenic mice results in a synergistic lowering of HDL cholesterol and decrease in HDL size and illustrates how hypertriglyceridemia causes decreased HDL cholesterol levels in the presence of CETP. Gene KO of PLTP results in decreased HDL cholesterol and apo A-I levels, reflecting diminished transfer of phospholipids from TRL into HDL. Mice and rabbits transgenic for HL show reduced HDL cholesterol and apo A-I levels; conversely, HL KO mice have increased levels of HDL. HL KO/apo E KO mice have decreased atherosclerosis compared to apo E KO mice, perhaps due to higher HDL levels. Recent transgenic studies have shown a major role for SR-BI in HDL

metabolism, in the selective uptake of HDL lipids in the liver and steroidogenic tissues, and a protective effect of SR-BI on atherosclerosis.

5. **Reduced HDL cholesterol levels (hypoalphalipoproteinemia) are often familial, may be accompanied by increased triglyceride levels, and are associated with increased CHD risk. In most instances, the genetic basis is unknown. Occasionally, hypoalphalipoproteinemia results from mutations in the apo A-I/apo C-III/apo A-IV gene complex, or from the rare recessive disorders, LCAT deficiency or Tangier disease (see Chaps. 118 and 122). Tangier disease is caused by homozygous mutations in ABC1 and heterozygous mutations may cause familial hypoalphalipoproteinemia. In some families, a gene inversion of apo A-I/apo C-III/apo A-IV has resulted in deletion of the whole cluster and leads to profoundly decreased HDL levels and premature atherosclerosis. Approximately 13 different functionally significant isolated mutations of the apo A-I gene have been described. These result in markedly decreased HDL cholesterol and apo A-I levels and are often associated with corneal opacities and a predisposition to premature coronary heart disease. However, the latter is not uniform and subjects are frequently healthy. A missense mutation of apo A-I (apo A-I Milano) is associated with reduced HDL and LDL cholesterol and has been anecdotally associated with a reduced predisposition to CHD. As in transgenic mouse studies, it appears that the levels of atherogenic lipoproteins may be important contributing factors to the impact of hypoalphalipoproteinemia on CHD in humans; that is, low HDL only appears to be a risk factor in the context of an accompanying atherogenic stimulus. Apo A-II deficiency is extremely rare and does not appear to be associated with altered HDL cholesterol or CHD susceptibility.**
6. **Increased HDL levels (hyperalphalipoproteinemia) commonly have a genetic basis. In the Japanese, heterozygous mutations in the CETP gene are present in 5 to 7 percent of the general population and represent a common cause of increased HDL levels. Homozygous deficiency of CETP results in massive elevations of HDL cholesterol and apo A-I and the accumulation of large CE- and apo E-rich HDL species. Heterozygous deficiency of CETP results in milder (10 to 30 percent) increases in HDL cholesterol. An evaluation of the relationship of CETP mutations to coronary heart disease in Japanese-American men of the Honolulu Heart Program cohort indicates an overall increase in risk of coronary heart disease in subjects with the mutations, consistent with the idea that the protective role of HDL may be related to reverse cholesterol transport. However, the relationship of CETP mutations to CHD appears complex, as subjects with CETP mutations and HDL cholesterol >60 mg/dl enjoy a low prevalence of CHD. Rare null or missense mutations in the HL gene are also a cause of increased HDL levels. Subjects with these mutations have increased HDL cholesterol, apo A-I, and triglyceride levels. They accumulate large, buoyant LDL species, representing VLDL remnants. Although some subjects with HL deficiency accumulate beta-VLDL and have premature CHD, this may reflect concomitant genetic defects in these families.**
7. **Twin and family studies suggest that about 50 percent of the variance of HDL cholesterol levels in the general population is attributable to genetic factors. In the Japanese, about 10 percent of the variance in HDL cholesterol levels is attributable to CETP gene mutations (see above). Recently, sib-pair linkage analysis has demonstrated that common variations at the HL and apo A-I/apo C-III/apo A-IV gene loci are responsible for the major portion of the genetic component of the variance in HDL cholesterol in healthy, normolipidemic Caucasians. These genetic variants are not associated with coding sequence changes and may represent common promoter mutations. A haplotype of the HL gene that is associated with increased HDL cholesterol levels has been defined. Moreover, this haplotype of HL is common in African-Americans and in part explains their higher HDL cholesterol levels.**

HDL GENERAL CONSIDERATIONS

Although a low level of HDL-C is a major risk factor for coronary heart disease (CHD) in westernized societies, the genetic control of HDL-C levels is only partly understood. This chapter critically reviews this subject. However, it is first necessary to review the structure and composition of HDL, the evidence that a reduced level of HDL is a risk factor for CHD, and aspects of HDL metabolism. Major emphasis is placed on transgenic mouse models because they have provided crucial information on the role of different genes in HDL metabolism. Several comprehensive reviews with extensive bibliographies on the subject of HDL have been published.[1–4]

STRUCTURE AND COMPOSITION OF HDL

HDLs are macromolecular complexes of proteins and lipids that range in diameter from 70 to 100 Å and in mass from 200,000 to 400,000 daltons. They sediment in the density region 1.063 to 1.21 g/ml. Analytical ultracentrifugation reveals lighter and heavier particles in this region, called HDL2 and HDL3, respectively. The former are defined as those in the density region 1.063 to 1.12 g/ml, whereas the latter are those in the density region 1.12 to 1.21 g/ml. HDLs contain, on the average, 50 percent lipid and 50 percent protein. The lipid is 32 percent cholesterol ester, 5 percent free cholesterol, 55 percent phospholipid, and 8 percent triglyceride. The protein consists principally of apo A-I (70 percent) and apo A-II (20 percent). HDL2 is relatively lipid-rich and protein-poor compared with HDL3. HDL heterogeneity in apolipoprotein composition also exists with apo A-I-only, apo A-I plus apo A-II, and apo E-rich particles. The apo A-I-only particles contain four apo A-Is per particle and float predominantly in the HDL2 region. The apo A-I plus apo A-II particles contain two of each of these apolipoproteins and are enriched in the HDL3 region. The apo E-rich HDL particles contain apo E as a major apolipoprotein. These particles have a density distribution that is lighter than HDL2. Although they may be quite important metabolically, apo E-rich HDLs are not included in the clinical assays quantitating HDL-C levels.

HDL AS A RISK FACTOR FOR CORONARY HEART DISEASE

The distribution of HDL-C levels in the population was determined by the Lipid Research Clinic Prevalence Study (Table 121-1). For men ages 45 to 49 years, the average HDL-C level is 45 mg/dl, with the bottom decile below 33 mg/dl and the top decile above 60 mg/dl. In women, the average is 56 mg/dl, with the bottom decile below 39 mg/dl and the top decile above 78 mg/dl. From a clinical perspective, the principal interest in HDL stems from the association of low HDL-C levels with an increased risk of coronary heart disease.[5] This association was first noted 40 years ago.[6] However, perhaps because HDL-C is normally a minor constituent (20 to 25 percent) of total plasma cholesterol, the importance of HDL-C levels in predicting coronary heart disease susceptibility was largely ignored until attention was focused on this subject in 1975.[7] Since then dozens of studies have verified the inverse correlation between HDL-C

Table 121-1 Plasma High-Density Lipoprotein Cholesterol Concentration*

	Normal values, mg/dl													
	Males, percentile							Females, percentile						
Age, yr	5	10	25	50	75	90	95	5	10	25	50	75	90	95
5–9	38	42	49	54	63	70	74	36	38	47	52	61	67	73
10–14	37	40	46	55	61	71	74	37	40	45	52	58	64	70
15–19	30	34	39	46	52	59	63	35	38	43	51	61	68	73
20–24	30	32	38	45	51	57	63	†	37	43	50	60	68	†
25–29	31	32	37	44	50	58	63	37	40	47	55	64	73	81
30–34	28	32	38	45	52	59	63	38	40	46	55	64	71	75
35–39	29	31	36	43	49	58	62	34	38	44	52	63	74	82
40–44	27	31	36	43	51	60	67	33	39	48	55	64	78	87
45–49	30	33	38	45	52	60	64	33	39	46	56	66	78	86
50–54	28	31	36	44	51	58	63	37	40	49	59	70	77	89
55–59	28	31	38	46	55	64	71	36	39	47	58	68	82	86
60–64	30	34	41	49	61	69	74	36	43	49	60	73	85	91
65–69	30	33	39	49	62	74	78	34	38	46	60	71	79	89
70†	31	33	40	48	56	70	75	33	37	48	60	69	82	91

*Values are based on Lipid Research Clinics population studies in the U.S. and Canada. The data include 3524 white males and 2545 white females (not using sex hormones) as derived from NIH Publication 80-1527, 1980. All subjects were sampled in the fasting state.
†No data because there were fewer than 100 cases in the cell.

levels and coronary heart disease incidence in westernized societies.[5] For example, in a prospective study, the Framingham Study reported a highly significant inverse relationship between coronary heart disease incidence and HDL-C levels based on a 12-year follow-up.[8] The relationship held after multivariate adjustment for total cholesterol, systolic blood pressure, cigarette smoking, and body-mass index. It was also found that HDL-C levels showed a strong inverse relationship with coronary heart disease risk at low (<200 mg/dl), medium, and high (>260 mg/dl) total cholesterol levels.

It must be pointed out that the decreased level of HDL-C associated with coronary heart disease is usually accompanied by other abnormalities in the plasma lipoprotein pattern.[9] In fact, isolated low HDL-C levels are relatively uncommon. In the majority of cases, the low HDL-C levels are associated with elevated levels of triglycerides, VLDL-C, and IDL-C, and the presence of dense LDL.[10] Low HDL-C levels have also been found to be associated with increased levels of postprandial lipoproteins.[11] In one case control study, the low HDL-C–high triglycerides, VLDL-C- and IDL-C-dense LDL pattern was present in 50 percent of patients with first myocardial infarction and 26 percent of sex- and age-matched neighborhood controls.[10] In this study, it was not possible to statistically separate the coronary heart disease risk of each of these lipoprotein abnormalities, and it is possible that the heart disease risk of low HDL-C levels might be due in part to increased levels of other lipoproteins, which are themselves atherogenic. Finally, in epidemiologic studies HDL-C levels are not correlated with total LDL-C levels that are independently related to coronary heart disease risk.[12] Consequently, the ratio of the levels of LDL-C (or non HDL-C) to HDL-C is a better predictor of risk than is either measurement alone.

HDL PHYSIOLOGY

Synthesis and Secretion of the Components of HDL

The major apolipoproteins of human HDL, apo A-I and apo A-II, are synthesized in the liver. Apo A-I is also synthesized in the small intestine along with apo A-IV, a lesser component of human HDL. These apolipoproteins enter the circulation as components of the triglyceride-rich lipoproteins, that is, chylomicrons arising from the small intestine or VLDL from the liver. In addition, nascent forms of HDL, consisting of phospholipids, free cholesterol, and apo A-I, have been identified in liver perfusates or in intestinal (mesenteric) lymph, suggesting either intracellular assembly and secretion of nascent HDL or its formation at the cell surface. The ATP binding cassette transporter, ABC1, interacts specifically with free apoproteins, such as apo A-I, adding phospholipids and cholesterol and generating a nascent HDL particle. Nascent HDL may consist of phospholipid bilayer discs, stabilized by a peripheral ring of apolipoproteins. In the circulation they are acted on by lecithin:cholesterol acyltransferase, generating hydrophobic cholesteryl esters that split the bilayer and give rise to the mature spherical HDL that predominates in plasma.

Intravascular Metabolism of HDL

An important source of HDL and its components is the intravascular transfer of lipids and apolipoproteins from triglyceride-rich lipoproteins (TRL) into HDL. During the lipolysis of TRL in peripheral tissues (heart, muscle, adipose), surface components of TRL (phospholipids, cholesterol, soluble apolipoproteins) are transferred into HDL (Fig. 121-1). These components may give rise to new HDL species or may be incorporated into preexisting HDL particles. The transfer of phospholipids and free cholesterol from TRL into HDL is facilitated by a plasma phospholipid transfer protein (PLTP).[13–15] Phospholipids and free cholesterol transferred into HDL provide substrates for the LCAT reaction, generating cholesteryl esters and lysolecithin. A portion of the cholesteryl esters formed in HDL is exchanged with triglycerides of TRL, in a process mediated by the plasma cholesteryl ester transfer protein (CETP). HDL triglyceride is then hydrolyzed by hepatic lipase (HL),[16–18] an enzyme found predominantly on the microvilli of hepatocytes.[19,20] Peripheral cells such as macrophages may also donate free cholesterol, phospholipid, and apo E to existing HDL (Fig. 121-2) or may secrete phospholipids and cholesterol via ABC1 onto free apo A-I. Although this is probably not a major source of plasma HDL, it represents an important part of HDL metabolism, as it constitutes a mechanism for the removal of cholesterol from macrophage foam cells in the arterial wall. In the absence of ABC1-mediated transport, cholesterol accumulates in macrophages, forming foam cells, as in Tangier disease.

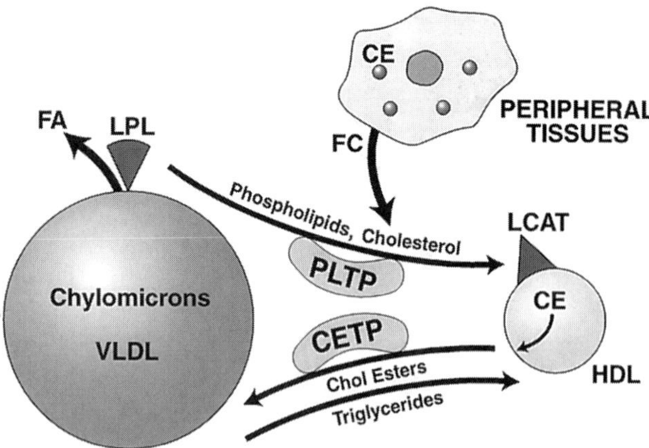

Fig. 121-1 Transfer of lipids from triglyceride-rich lipoproteins into HDL. During lipolysis of the triglyceride-rich lipoproteins (chylomicrons, VLDL), there is transfer of phospholipids and free cholesterol into HDL. A plasma phospholipid transfer protein (PLTP) facilitates this transfer. The enzyme lecithin:cholesterol acyltransferase (LCAT) uses phospholipids and free cholesterol as substrate and forms cholesteryl esters. The resulting depletion of HDL free cholesterol enhances the influx of cellular free cholesterol into HDL. HDL cholesteryl esters (CE) may be transferred from HDL into the triglyceride-rich lipoproteins by cholesteryl ester transfer protein (CETP), by exchanging with triglycerides. The transfer of lipids and apolipoproteins from TRL to HDL represents an important source of HDL components. The formation and transfer of HDL CE is an essential part of reverse cholesterol transport (see text).

The HDL Cycle and Cellular Cholesterol Efflux

The turnover of cholesteryl esters within HDL gives rise to an HDL cycle[21] (Fig. 121-3). The removal of cholesteryl esters from HDL by CETP-mediated CE-TG interchange, followed by the hydrolysis of the TG by HL, converts HDL from a larger, cholesteryl ester-rich form with alpha-migration in agarose gels into a smaller, cholesteryl ester-depleted form with pre-beta mobility.[22,23] In cell culture, pre-beta HDL has increased ability to initiate the efflux of cellular cholesterol, compared to the bulk of alpha-HDL. This may be because pre-beta HDL includes free apo A-I which interacts specifically with ABC1, generating nascent HDL. The action of LCAT on nascent HDL increases their cholesteryl ester content and regenerates alpha-HDL. The plasma phospholipid transfer protein also plays a role in facilitating the conversion of alpha- into pre-beta HDL.

Reverse Cholesterol Transport

Reverse cholesterol transport is initiated by the removal of cholesterol from peripheral cells, involving either ABC1-mediated lipid efflux to apo A-I, or passive diffusion to HDL. LCAT then increases the CE content of HDL. There are three routes by which cholesteryl esters formed within HDL may be returned to the liver (Fig. 121-3). First, HDL cholesteryl esters may be transferred to triglyceride-rich lipoproteins, which are further metabolized to remnant lipoproteins and are then removed from the circulation by proteoglycans and hepatic receptors (LDL receptors and the LDL receptor-related protein, LRP). The activity of this pathway is illustrated by human genetic deficiency of CETP, which causes marked increases in HDL cholesteryl ester levels (see below). Second, HDL cholesteryl esters may be taken up by the liver in a process of selective lipid uptake; that is, cellular uptake of HDL cholesteryl esters without concomitant uptake and degradation of HDL protein.[21,22] Recently, it was shown that selective uptake of HDL cholesteryl esters is mediated by a member of the scavenger receptor gene family, scavenger receptor BI (SR-BI).[24] SR-BI is highly expressed in steroidogenic tissues and the liver, the tissues that are most active in the selective uptake of HDL lipids. Recent evidence indicates that SR-BI is the major mediator of selective uptake of HDL lipids in the liver and adrenal.[25,26] Cholesteryl esters that enter the cell by selective uptake undergo hydrolysis by an extralysosomal cholesteryl ester hydrolase,[27] and provide free sterol for use in corticosteroid or sex hormone synthesis, or for excretion into bile. Mice do not have CETP activity in plasma, and thus may be especially dependent on the SR-BI pathway for the metabolism of HDL lipids. In mammals with CETP such as rabbits, both CETP and selective uptake pathways make a significant contribution to the catabolism of HDL cholesteryl esters.[28] The human homolog of SR-BI, CLA-1, is abundantly expressed in steroidogenic tissues and liver, particularly during embryonic development, suggesting a role for the selective uptake pathway in humans.[29] The third route of return of HDL cholesteryl esters to the liver is in association with the major HDL apolipoproteins (apo A-I and apo A-II), that is, particulate HDL uptake. In humans, the turnover time of HDL cholesteryl esters is rapid (3 to 12 times per day) compared to apo A-I and apo A-II ($t/2 \approx 5$ days), but HDL particles are eventually taken up by tissues.[1,30,31] The catabolism of apo A-I and apo A-II plays an important role in regulating HDL levels in humans[1,31–34] and there is evidence in humans and other species that the hepatic catabolism of apo A-I and apo A-II is a regulated process (see below).

In addition to the reverse transport of HDL cholesteryl esters from plasma to the liver, there is also a pathway for the preferential uptake of HDL free cholesterol in the liver, with its subsequent excretion in bile.[31,34] SR-BI can facilitate the bidirectional exchange of free cholesterol between HDL and cells, and may be partly responsible for the rapid uptake of HDL free cholesterol in the liver.[35] Mice with hepatic overexpression of SR-BI have an increased content of biliary cholesterol, indicating an overall role of SR-BI in stimulating reverse cholesterol transport.[36]

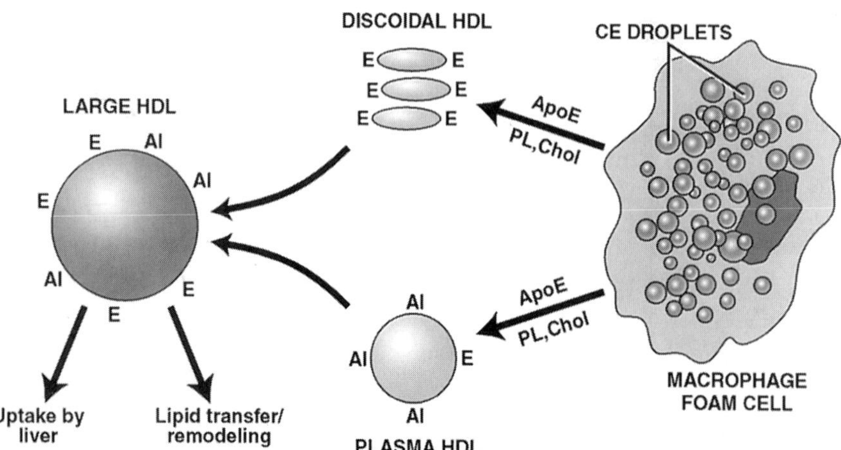

Fig. 121-2 Role of HDL and apo E in the efflux of cholesterol from macrophage foam cells. Macrophage foam cells synthesize increased amounts of apo E, which may be secreted as nascent HDL particles, or incorporated into preexisting HDL. The HDL is acted on by LCAT, giving rise to larger CE and apo E-rich HDL species that are either taken up in the liver or remodeled into smaller particles. Apo E in macrophages plays a crucial role in reverse cholesterol transport and the prevention of atherosclerosis. Also, the interaction of apo A-I with the macrophage ABC1 transporter is important in reversing foam cell formation.

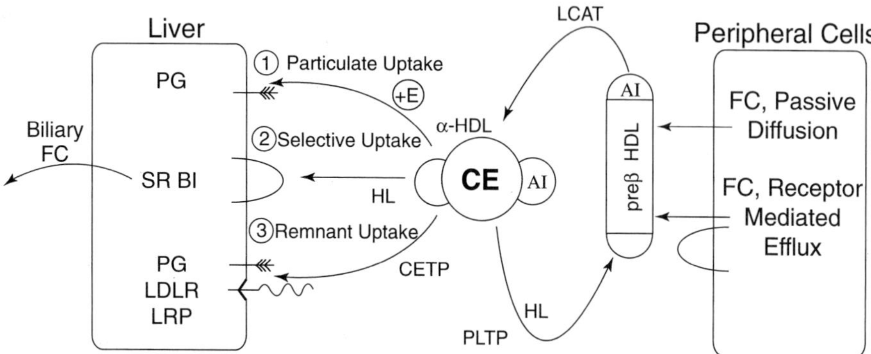

Fig. 121-3 The role of HDL in reverse cholesterol transport. Free cholesterol undergoes efflux from peripheral cells into HDL. Subspecies of HDL, such as pre-beta particles, may be particularly adept at mediating free cholesterol efflux, which may occur by passive diffusion, or may be mediated by interaction with ABC1. LCAT action on pre-beta HDL may generate larger CE-rich HDL. HDL CE returns to the liver (1) as part of an HDL particle uptake mechanism, probably involving proteoglycans, apo E, and unknown receptors; (2) via a process of selective uptake of CE and free cholesterol, mediated by hepatic SR-BI; or (3) by CETP-mediated transfer to TRL, with subsequent uptake of TRL remnants in the liver, involving proteoglycans, LDL receptors, or the LDL receptor-related protein (LRP).

HDL Particle Catabolism

The major sites of catabolism of apo A-I are the liver and kidney. In the kidney, this may involve a size-dependent filtration process leading to degradation of HDL proteins.[37] In the presence of hypertriglyceridemia, the combined activities of CETP and hepatic lipase lead to a decreased size of HDL and increased degradation of HDL protein in the kidney. The molecular mechanisms of HDL particle uptake in the liver are poorly understood. Large, cholesteryl ester-rich HDL can acquire apo E and then be removed from the circulation by apo E-dependent mechanisms in the liver. In liver cell culture experiments, apo E and hepatic lipase enhance the cellular uptake of HDL protein by both a heparan sulfate proteoglycan-dependent LDL receptor-related protein (LRP) pathway and a heparan sulfate proteoglycan-dependent LRP-independent pathway.[38] The latter pathway predominates and could involve the direct uptake of HDL by hepatic syndecan proteoglycans, as has been demonstrated for LDL.[39] Experiments with primary hepatocyte cultures demonstrate the uptake and degradation of HDL apo A-I by a lysosomally mediated, non-LDL-receptor process.[40] In hepatocytes there is substantial recycling of HDL, associated with selective removal of HDL CE. Antibody experiments indicate that SR-BI is the primary receptor mediating uptake and degradation or recycling of HDL.[41]

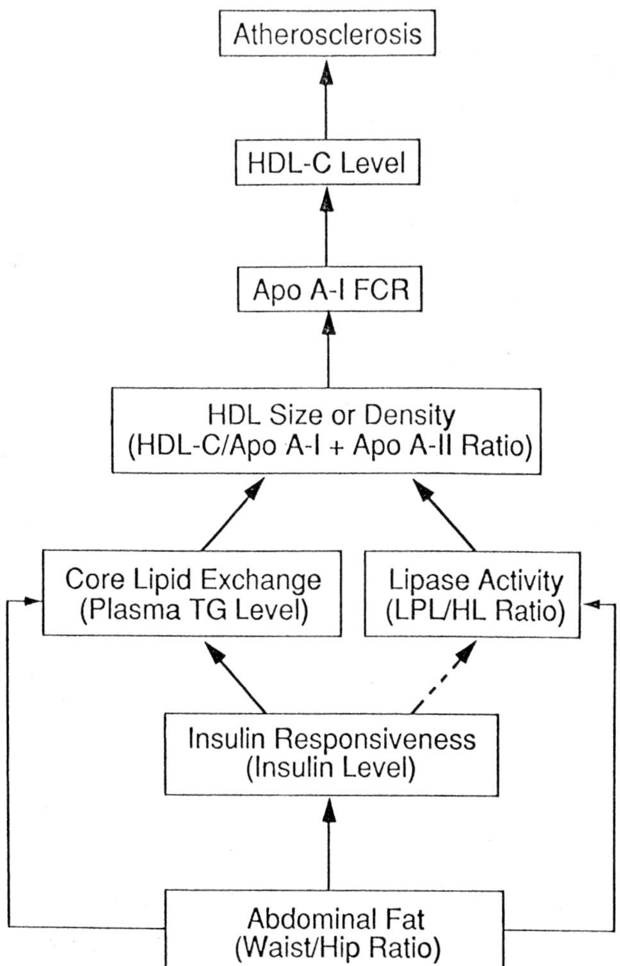

Fig. 121-4 Hypothetical scheme of the factors influencing the levels of HDL and thereby atherosclerosis.

Regulation of HDL Levels

In humans, plasma levels of HDL cholesterol and apo A-I are inversely related to the fractional catabolic rate of apo A-I, indicating an important role for apo A-I catabolism in regulating HDL levels. In contrast to apo A-I, plasma apo A-II levels are poorly correlated with HDL cholesterol levels and variation in plasma apo A-II levels is correlated with apo A-II production rates.[41] The composition and content of the HDL core lipids play important roles in determining the rate of catabolism of the HDL protein. In humans, reduced HDL cholesterol levels are often associated with hypertriglyceridemia. Hypertriglyceridemia stimulates lipid exchange and accelerated catabolism of HDL protein. Thus, disorders that increase levels of TRL — such as insulin resistance, diabetes, and obesity — may indirectly affect HDL levels (Fig. 121-4). Recent studies in obese mice with mutations in leptin (ob/ob mice), the hypothalamic receptor for leptin (db/db mice), or in downstream hypothalamic components in the leptin-signaling pathway (melanocortin receptor 4 knockout mice) suggest that the leptin-signaling pathway plays a role in regulating HDL homeostasis, affecting both synthesis and catabolism of apo A-I.[42] In ob/ob mice, HDL levels are markedly increased due to a predominant catabolic defect that reflects down-regulation of the hepatic HDL receptor.

MECHANISMS RESPONSIBLE FOR THE ANTIATHEROGENIC PROPERTIES OF HDL

Atherogenesis is a complex process that may be viewed as a chronic inflammatory response to the deposition of lipoprotein cholesterol in the arterial wall. Central to this process is the

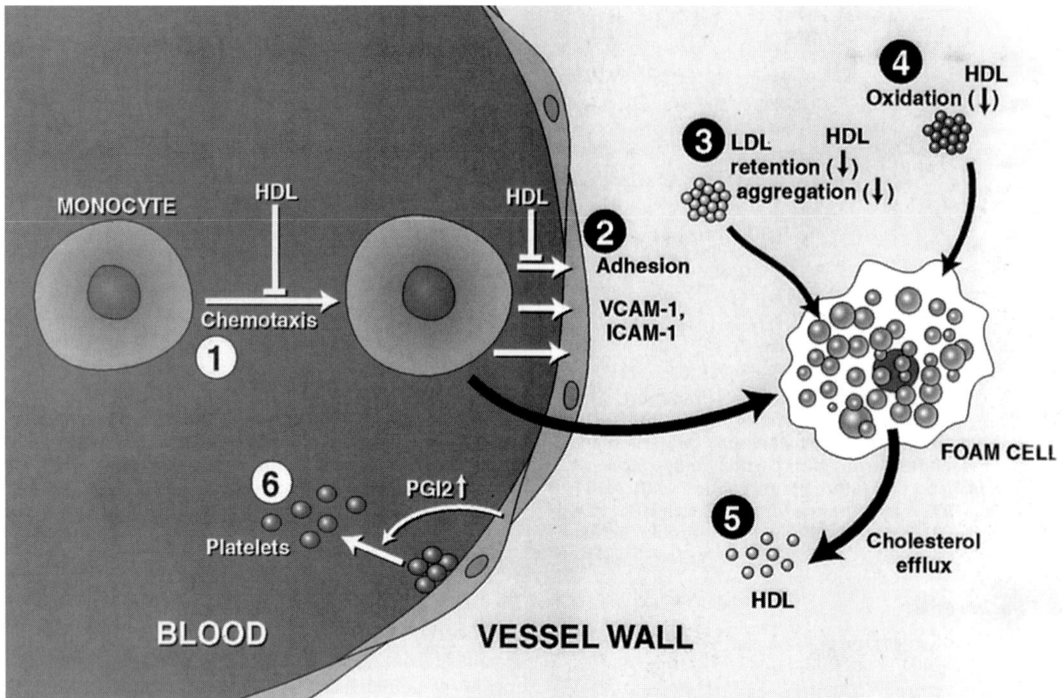

Fig. 121-5 Multiple potential antiatherogenic functions of HDL in the vessel wall. HDL may exert antiatherogenic effects at multiple steps. These include (1) inhibition of monocyte chemotaxis; (2) inhibition of monocyte adhesion to endothelial cells; (3) decreased retention or aggregation of LDL in the arterial wall; (4) decreased oxidation of LDL; (5) increased cholesterol efflux from macrophages; and (6) increased endothelial synthesis of prostacyclin (PGI2). Although each of these properties of HDL has been shown in vitro, there is little information on in vivo relevance. However, evidence in cell culture and transgenic mouse model supports a role of HDL in cholesterol efflux and reverse cholesterol transport.

accumulation of cholesterol and cholesteryl esters in macrophage foam cells in the intima of large- and medium-sized arteries. Foam cells are derived from blood monocytes that become trapped in the subendothelial space at susceptible points in the artery. HDL has been shown to retard at least six different steps in the process of atherogenesis in vitro (Fig. 121-5). These include (1) the chemotaxis of monocytes into the subendothelial space, a process promoted by release of chemokines (notably MCP-1); (2) the adhesion of monocytes to the arterial endothelium, mediated by VCAM-1 and ICAM-1; (3) the modification of LDL in the arterial wall by retention and aggregation; and (4) oxidation. Thus, HDL may inhibit both the accumulation of monocyte-macrophages in the arterial wall and modifications of LDL that lead to foam cell formation. (5) HDL has the ability to prevent or reverse foam cell formation by promoting cholesterol efflux, and can mediate the transport of this cholesterol through the bloodstream to the liver; that is, reverse cholesterol transport. (6) Finally, HDL has the ability to promote the formation and stabilization of the anti-platelet eicosanoid, prostaglandin I_2 (prostacyclin or PGI2), secreted by endothelial cells. This may inhibit the formation of platelet aggregates over atheromatous lesions, potentially inhibiting both the progression of lesions and the formation of an occlusive thrombus over a complex atheroma. A more detailed discussion of several of the potential antiatherogenic properties of HDL follows.

Antioxidant, Anti-inflammatory, and Antiaggregatory Effects of HDL

Several of the antiatherogenic properties of HDL may be related to its antioxidant properties.[43–45] In a coculture system of endothelial cells on smooth muscle cells, the migration of monocytes into the subendothelial space is promoted by minimally oxidized LDL; this process is inhibited by HDL (Step 1).[44] There are several mechanisms underlying the antioxidant properties of HDL. HDL may sequester oxidized lipids away from LDL,[45] transport lipid hydroperoxides to the liver,[46] and bind pro-oxidant transition metals.[47] Moreover, apo A-I has the ability to reduce hydroperoxides of cholesteryl esters and phosphatidylcholine; this likely involves the oxidation of two methionine residues to methionine sulfoxide.[48,49] This activity may supplement the activity of the selenium-dependent plasma glutathione peroxidase activity, and could be particularly important in pathophysiological states where the latter activity is reduced.

The enzyme paraoxonase circulates bound to HDL, and promotes the breakdown of the oxidized phospholipids that accumulate in minimally oxidized LDL.[50] In several mouse models, there are correlations between paraoxonase activity in HDL and the development of atherosclerosis.[51] For example, C57BL/6J mice are susceptible to diet-induced aortic fatty streak lesions, whereas C3H/HeJ mice are resistant to such lesions. When the two strains received a low-fat diet that fails to promote atherosclerosis, their HDL protected against LDL oxidation in vitro. In contrast, HDL isolated from susceptible B6 mice fed a high-fat, high-cholesterol diet was unable to inhibit LDL oxidation, whereas HDL from resistant C3H mice retained this property. Moreover, paraoxonase mRNA levels cosegregated with the extent of atherosclerosis in recombinant inbred strains of mice derived from B6 and C3H. These studies support the notion that paraoxonase plays a role in atherogenesis.

In humans, the relationship of paraoxonase to the protective effect of HDL is complex. Common genetic variation in the coding sequence of paraoxonase leads to altered activity toward the artificial substrate paraoxon. An allelic association between paraoxonase variants and coronary heart disease was found in six of nine cross-sectional studies.[51] PON1B (codon 912), the allele most commonly associated with increased risk of CHD, elevates paraoxonase activity in plasma. This seems inconsistent with the notion that paraoxonase has antiatherogenic properties as a result of its ability to degrade oxidized phospholipids. However, the natural substrates of this enzyme and the relationship of this activity to the enzyme's ability to degrade oxidized phospholipids are poorly understood. Further research is needed to clarify the potential role of paraoxonase activity in the protective properties of HDL.

HDL can inhibit the up-regulation of endothelial cell expression of ICAM-1 and VCAM-1 that is induced by exposure to TNF-alpha.[52] Because these cell-adhesion molecules are expressed over fatty streak lesions, these properties of HDL could potentially inhibit the adhesion of monocytes to the endothelium overlying atherosclerotic lesions (Step 2). Following the entry of LDL into the arterial wall, the LDL is retained on proteoglycans and may undergo oxidation or aggregation. Large HDL-containing apo E has been shown to inhibit the binding of HDL to proteoglycans.[53] The aggregation of LDL in the arterial wall is promoted by the activity of a sphingomyelinase that is secreted by endothelial cells and macrophages.[54] HDL or its apolipoproteins can inhibit the aggregation of LDL produced by vortexing, phospholipase C or sphingomyelinase treatments.[54,55] Sphingomyelinase is secreted by endothelial cells and foam cells and is active in human atherosclerotic lesions. Thus, the ability of HDL to inhibit the aggregation of LDL by local sphingomyelinase activity in lesions may be important (Step 3). HDL stimulates the synthesis of PGI2 by endothelial cells and the synthesis of prostaglandin E-2 by smooth muscle cells.[56–58] PGI2 inhibits platelet aggregation and adherence to the endothelium. The mechanisms of these effects of HDL are complex and may involve delivery of HDL arachidonate moieties to the cell, which subsequently are incorporated into prostaglandins (a substrate effect), and an increase in cyclooxygenase-2 mRNA and protein.[59]

HDL and Reverse Cholesterol Transport

Glomset first proposed that HDL acts in conjunction with LCAT to mediate the reverse transport of cholesterol from peripheral tissues to the liver.[60] There is now substantial evidence for the existence of such a pathway. The initial step of reverse cholesterol transport involves the efflux of cholesterol from peripheral cells onto HDL. Under cell culture conditions, HDL can reverse the accumulation of cholesterol and cholesteryl esters in macrophage foam cells.[61] The ability of human serum to promote efflux of cellular cholesterol is well correlated with its content of HDL,[62] and removal of HDL components from serum reduces its ability to promote cellular cholesterol efflux. The efflux of cellular cholesterol may involve simple diffusion or it may be mediated by HDL receptors. The HDL receptor SR-BI can facilitate the efflux of cellular cholesterol in the presence of HDL. Although expression of SR-BI by macrophages is low, SR-BI mRNA has been detected in atherosclerotic lesions.[35] Tangier disease is characterized by low HDL and the accumulation of cholesterol in macrophages in the spleen and reticuloendothelial system. Cells from Tangier disease subjects display a defect in the efflux of cholesterol and phospholipids to apo A-I or HDL.[63] This disorder indicates the existence of a key cellular molecule involved in efflux of cholesterol and phospholipid from macrophages to apo A-I. Recently, this was identified as the ATP-binding cassette transporter ABC1.[63a–63c]

The efflux of cholesterol from macrophages is promoted by apo E. Apo E is secreted in increased amounts from cholesterol-loaded macrophages, and apo E may be secreted in association with phospholipids and cholesterol, giving rise to nascent HDL particles (Fig. 121-2).[64,65] Moreover, macrophages transfected with apo E show increased efflux of cholesterol to HDL-3, especially following treatment with cAMP analogs.[66] The latter may increase cellular cholesterol esterase activity or up-regulate a cell surface binding site for HDL. Subclasses of serum HDL containing apo E, like pre-beta HDL, appear to have special ability to promote cholesterol efflux from cells.[67] Studies in transgenic mice clearly indicate the ability of macrophage-produced apo E to protect against the development of atherosclerosis.[68] Macrophage-specific expression of apo E in the arterial wall results in decreased atherosclerosis in apo E knockout mice, even when compared to animals with equivalent levels of plasma cholesterol.[69,70] Studies of cholesterol efflux from macrophages of humans homozygous for the various apo E isoforms suggest that net cholesterol efflux is greater from apo E2/E2 and apo E3/E3 macrophages than from apo E4/E4 macrophages, a finding that correlates with an increased prevalence of coronary heart disease in subjects with an apo E4 allele.[71,72]

Thus, there are likely to be multiple antiatherogenic effects of HDL in the arterial wall. Unfortunately, most of the experiments addressing the protective mechanisms of HDL have been carried out in vitro, and the importance of these different properties of HDL in vivo is largely unknown. Although the direct protective properties of HDL on atherosclerosis are clear from transgenic mouse experiments (see below), there is a paucity of information on the mechanisms involved. Moreover, in humans, low HDL levels are often present in association with elevated levels of blood triglycerides. In these circumstances, low HDL may be a marker for a metabolic predisposition to accumulate increased levels of atherogenic remnants of chylomicrons or VLDL. In addition, recent evidence indicates a strong association between inflammatory markers, such as C-reactive protein or IL6, with atherosclerosis. In some instances, low HDL may also be a marker of an inflammatory state involving the vessel wall.

INSIGHTS INTO METABOLISM AND ATHEROGENESIS FROM STUDIES IN TRANSGENIC ANIMALS

To address the function of HDL, many of the major genes postulated to participate in determining the structure and metabolism of this lipoprotein have been manipulated in animals. The levels of expression of these genes have been altered in vivo using gene transfers to somatic tissues and germline manipulations. Transgenic and/or gene-targeted mouse lines have been established with altered levels of expression of apo A-I, apo A-II, PLTP, CETP, HL, and SR-BI. In addition, transgenic rabbits have been created expressing human apo A-I and HL, and transgenic rats expressing human apo A-I. Analysis of the various animals has helped decipher the role of specific genes in complex physiological processes involving HDL in ways not feasible in humans.

Transgenic Animals with Altered Plasma Levels of Apo A-I

Transgenic mice,[73,74] rabbits,[75] and rats[76] expressing human apo A-I have been produced. In all cases, the expression of the human apo A-I transgene with associated increases in total apo A-I were accompanied by increases in plasma HDL-C levels. In addition to germ line manipulations, there have been short-term somatic gene transfer studies in which apo A-I constructs have been delivered in vivo via adenoviral vectors.[77,78] The results of these short-term studies agreed with those of the germ line transgenesis studies, specifically, increased apo A-I expression is accompanied by increases in HDL-C plasma concentrations. These findings are compatible with studies in humans, which show that HDL-C cholesterol levels correlate with apo A-I levels and support pharmacologic interventions that increase apo A-I production as a means to increase HDL-C levels.

The opposite of creating animals with increased plasma apo A-I levels due to high expression of apo A-I transgenes was achieved by inactivation of the murine apo A-I gene via gene targeting in embryonic stem cells.[79,80] Animals both heterozygous and homozygous for the inactivated apo A-I gene show a reduction in total plasma cholesterol and HDL-C concentrations by approximately 50 percent and 80 percent, respectively. The large reduction of HDL-C in the apo A-I-deficient mice resembles the significant reduction of plasma HDL-C in human subjects with mutations inactivating their apo A-I gene. This observation further supports the importance of apo A-I expression as a major determinant of HDL-C plasma levels.

In addition to the increases in HDL concentrations in mice expressing the human apo A-I transgene, changes were detected in its size, composition, and metabolism of HDL.[74,81] While control mouse plasma contains a monodisperse population of HDL particles with a diameter of approximately 10 nm, similar to human HDL_{2b}, expression of the human apo A-I transgene caused polydispersity of HDL, generating three populations with particle sizes of 11.4 nm, 10.2 nm, and 8.7 nm, similar to human HDL_1, HDL_2, and HDL_3. Interestingly, this trend toward a more human-like HDL profile is associated with a nearly complete loss of murine apo A-I from the plasma and its replacement by human apo A-I. These studies in human apo A-I transgenic mice suggest that the primary structure of apo A-I contributes to determining HDL particle size and possibly HDL subspeciation in humans (human and murine apo A-I differ by approximately 30 percent at the amino acid level).

Mice transgenic for human apo A-I have been exploited to analyze the physiological response to pharmacologic agents and diet. The advantage of using transgenic animals containing human transgenes to study the effects of drugs in a manner relevant to humans is illustrated in studies of human apo A-I transgenic mice following fenofibrate administration.[82] As with humans, treatment of the human apo A-I transgenic animals with fenofibrate results in increased human apo A-I as well as HDL plasma levels. In contrast, mouse apo A-I concentrations were decreased after fenofibrate treatment. These differences in human and mouse apo A-I levels following the fenofibrate treatment was directly reflected in their respective mRNA levels (97 percent increase in human apo A-I, 51 percent decrease in murine apo A-I mRNA levels). The increase in human apo A-I mRNA is due to increased transcription of the human transgene, whereas the opposite occurs from the endogenous mouse apo A-I gene. The different responses of the human and murine apo A-I genes to fenofibrate treatment illustrate a limitation in cross-species analysis of drug effects on the one hand, and the power and relevance of studying in transgenic animals the response of human transgenes to pharmacologic agents on the other hand.

The apo A-I transgenic mice have also been used to study the effect of dietary fat on HDL-C and apo A-I levels.[83] A high-fat western-type diet that increases HDL-C and apo A-I levels in humans has a similar effect on the apo A-I in transgenic mice. Turnover studies revealed that the increase in HDL levels in the apo A-I transgenics was not due to increased apo A-I transcription, but instead resulted from mechanisms operating at the posttranscriptional level, including increased transport rate and decreased fractional catabolic rate (FCR) of HDL-C and apo A-I.

Multiple studies in mice, as well as one study in rabbits, have examined the effect of the expression of apo A-I transgenes on atherogenesis. Mice expressing human apo A-I transgenes have been shown to exhibit relative resistance to atherogenesis in a variety of proatherogenic settings. This includes resistance to (a) the fatty streak lesions that occur in C57BL/6 mice when subjected to an atherogenic diet (1.25 percent cholesterol, 15 percent fat, and 0.5 percent cholic acid),[84,85] (b) the diet-independent atherogenesis that occurs in mice homozygous for the apo E knockout allele,[86,87] and (c) the heightened diet-induced atherogenesis associated with expression of the human apo(a) transgene.[88] Because rabbits have served as a well-characterized model for human atherosclerosis, human apo A-I transgenic rabbits were created to examine the impact that high plasma levels of human apo A-I had on atherogenesis in this organism.[75] While plasma cholesterol levels of atherogenic apo B-containing lipoproteins were similar in transgenic and control rabbits fed a cholesterol-rich diet, plasma levels of HDL-C in the transgenic group were about twice that of the control group. Following a 14-week exposure to the diet, the amount of aortic surface area covered by lesions, as well as the amount of lipid accumulation in the aorta, were significantly less (twofold) in the transgenic rabbits than in the control groups.[89] The consistency of results in several mouse studies and one rabbit study demonstrating the antiatherogenic properties of human apo A-I adds additional support to an already large body of information suggesting that increasing the expression of this apolipoprotein is likely to reduce heart disease risk.

Based on the decreased atherogenesis observed in animals with increased expression of apo A-I, a logical prediction is that decreased apo A-I caused by the inactivation of the murine apo A-I gene will result in increased atherogenesis. This proved not to be the case when diet-induced atherogenesis was compared in apo A-I knockout and control animals.[90] Both groups developed small fatty streak aortic lesions, which did not significantly differ in size. Because HDL is the major cholesterol carrier in the mouse, animals with and without apo A-I both had equivalently low levels of non-HDL-C. To more closely mimic the human situation, two groups of investigators followed up this initial apo A-I knockout mouse atherogenesis study with assessments of atherogenesis in mice homozygous for the apo A-I knockout allele, but also containing a human apo B transgene.[91,92] The presence of the human apo B transgene is associated with marked elevations of LDL-C. When diet-induced atherogenesis was compared in mice homozygous for the apo A-I knockout allele and also carrying the human apo B transgene versus mice containing the human apo B transgene alone, the KO mice carrying the human apo B transgene were noted to have significantly larger aortic fatty streak lesions. These results are consistent with the several human studies, which suggests that low levels of HDL-C, although frequently associated with increased atherogenesis susceptibility, is not an obligatory precipitator of heightened susceptibility.

Transgenic Mice with Altered Plasma Levels of Apo A-II

The influence of apo A-II on lipoprotein metabolism has been explored in mice with human and mouse apo A-II transgenes. Unlike findings in mice expressing human apo A-I transgenes, high concentrations of human apo A-II did not noticeably affect HDL-C concentrations.[93] While nontransgenic mice have a unimodal HDL size distribution of HDL particles (9.6 nm), transgenic mice overproducing human apo A-II display a bimodal size distribution of HDL particles with a major size population (9.6 nm) and a population of smaller particles (8.0 nm). Thus, unlike human apo A-I, human apo A-II does not affect the size of the predominant mouse HDL particle (9.6 nm). Analysis of the apoprotein composition of the smaller 8.0-nm particle revealed this particle as composed exclusively of human apo A-II. This human apo A-II only 8.0-nm particle is similar to that which has been previously described in a patient with a structural mutation in the human apo A-I gene (apo A-I Seattle)[94] and in Tangier disease.[95] Individuals with both Tangier disease and the apo A-I Seattle mutation experience a profound decrease in plasma apo A-I.

Lines of mice containing both human apo A-I and human apo A-II transgenes have also been created and the association of these different human HDL-associated apolipoproteins with HDL in the mouse plasma was explored.[85,93] In the plasma of humans, as well as in mice expressing both human apo A-I and human apo A-II transgenes, the majority of the human apo A-II is associated with the HDL particle also containing human apo A-I. The combined human apo A-I/human apo A-II transgenic mice display a unique HDL particle size distribution profile when compared with mice expressing either the human apo A-I or human apo A-II transgenes independently. The combined transgenics have HDL-C consisting of a minor population, $\approx$8.1 nm, and two major populations of $\approx$8.9 nm and $\approx$9.5 nm. This size distribution is similar to that of the immunopurified HDL containing both human apo A-I and human apo A-II present in human plasma. The HDL apolipoprotein composition and size in the combined transgenics suggest that in the absence of human apo A-I, human apo A-II will form significant amounts of human apo A-II only particles, but in the presence of apo A-I it preferentially associates with human apo A-I, resulting in the formation of predominantly human apo A-I/apo A-II HDL particles.

Mice expressing murine apo A-II transgenes have also been created and demonstrate several features that distinguish them from mice transgenic for human apo A-II.[96] Increases in plasma levels of murine apo A-II, unlike those of human apo A-II, are associated with an increase in plasma HDL cholesterol levels. In contrast to mice transgenic for human apo A-II, the murine apo A-II transgenic animals had larger HDL particles, a twofold increase in HDL-C levels, and a two- to threefold increase in plasma triglycerides. The differences in the effects of the human and murine apo A-II on HDL size and levels may be related to differences in primary sequence between human and murine apo A-II (human and murine apo A-II differ by 40 percent at the amino acid level). Related to these sequence differences, murine apo A-II exists in the plasma of mice as a monomer, whereas human apo A-II exists in the plasma of humans and transgenic mice as a disulfide-linked dimer of two identical polypeptide chains. To examine the issue of whether the monomeric versus dimeric differences between human and murine apo A-II alone are responsible for their contrasting effects on HDL, a human apo A-II genomic clone was engineered by site-specific mutagenesis to eliminate the cysteine required for the formation of apo A-II dimer.[97] Several lines of transgenic mice were created with this transgene that had differing plasma levels of the variant human apo A-II protein product. Despite increasing plasma levels of the human apo A-II variant, no increases in HDL cholesterol concentration were observed. Thus, the different effect on HDL of these two apo A-II orthologs is likely the result of other sequence differences between the human and mouse proteins, and not just due to dimeric versus monomeric structural difference.

In other studies, mice deficient in apo A-II were created by gene targeting in embryonic stem cells.[98] Homozygous knockout animals had a 60 percent and 52 percent reduction in HDL cholesterol levels in fasted and fed states, respectively, and HDL particle size was reduced. Metabolic turnover studies revealed that the HDL decrease was due both to decreased HDL cholesterol ester and apo A-I transport rates, and to increased HDL cholesterol ester and apo A-I fractional catabolic rates. Species-specific differences between the effect of HDL on human and murine apo A-II is further exemplified by the difference in HDL levels in mice versus those in humans deficient in apo A-II. Two sisters with apo A-II deficiency were reported to have normal HDL cholesterol concentrations.[99] Thus, there appears to be a direct relationship between plasma levels of mouse apo A-II and HDL in mice, while altering the level of human apo A-II either in mice or in humans seems to have little effect on HDL cholesterol concentration.

Several studies have examined the effect of expression of human and mouse apo A-II transgenes on murine atherosclerosis susceptibility. Expressing human apo A-II transgenes to produce significant plasma levels of human apo A-II does not lower an animal's atherogenic susceptibility.[85] In one study, it increased susceptibility to diet-induced atherogenesis.[100] Expression of murine apo A-II transgenes increased the animal's atherogenic susceptibility[96] significantly more than expression of human apo A-II transgenes. Although laboratory mice do not normally develop aortic fatty streak lesions when maintained on standard mouse chow, male transgenic mice expressing a murine apo A-II transgene, with increased HDL levels compared to controls, developed a significant number of proximal aortic fatty streak lesions when fed a mouse chow diet.

HDL containing primarily apo A-I and HDL containing apo A-I plus apo A-II HDL are the major apolipoprotein-specific HDL populations present in the plasma of humans. To determine whether these two HDL-C populations have different effects on atherogenesis in mice, mice expressing human apo A-I alone and mice expressing both human apo A-I/human apo A-II transgenes were studied.[85] The HDL particles in plasma from the apo A-I and the combined apo A-I/apo A-II transgenic mice no longer resemble those of a nontransgenic mouse. Instead, with regard to apolipoprotein composition and size, they share features with the apo A-I-only and the apo A-I/apo A-II HDL particles, respectively, present in human plasma. Following a 4-month exposure to the atherogenic diet, despite similar total cholesterol and HDL-C concentrations, the area of atherogenic lesions in the combined apo A-I/apo A-II transgenic animals was fifteenfold greater than that observed in the human apo A-I transgenic mice. In vitro studies have also examined properties of the different apolipoprotein-specific HDL particles isolated from the plasma of the various lines of transgenic mice.[101] These studies suggest that apo A-I-only HDL is more effective than HDL containing both apo A-I and apo A-II in mediating cholesterol efflux from cells in vitro, a postulated component of how HDL acts to inhibit atherogenesis in vivo. The results of these studies are consistent with several human observational studies, suggesting that apo A-I-only HDL particles may be more antiatherogenic than HDL particles containing both human apo A-I and human apo A-II. However, not all studies of human lipoprotein (Lp)A-I and LpA-I/A-II are in agreement on this point.

Apo A-IV Transgenic Mice

Recent studies explored the effect of increased expression of apo A-IV, a minor HDL-associated apolipoprotein, on atherogenesis in transgenic mice.[102,103] In the one study in which a human apo A-IV transgene was expressed in mice, marked increases of apo A-IV (three- and sixfold normal plasma levels) were not associated with major increases in HDL-C levels.[103] What differed between the transgenic and nontransgenic control mice was the substantial reduction in the size of aortic fatty streak lesions present in the apo A-IV transgenics. Both the diet-induced atherogenesis in C57BL/6 mice, as well as diet-independent atherogenesis in apo E knockout mice, were lessened in animals expressing apo A-IV transgenes. A similar antiatherogenic effect of high plasma levels of human apo A-IV was noted in a second study examining an apo A-IV transgenic line. When fed the atherogenic diet, this line exhibited significant increases in plasma triglycerides, total cholesterol, and HDL cholesterol.[102] These results indicate that overexpression of human apo A-IV also protects against atherosclerosis.

Mice Transgenic for SR-BI

An important advance in the understanding of HDL metabolism was the identification of SR-BI, the first HDL receptor to be well defined at a molecular level and shown to participate in selective cholesterol uptake. Many of the insights concerning the properties of this receptor on HDL metabolism come from studies of mice whose SR-BI expression has been altered by somatic cell gene transfer or germ line genetic manipulations. Adenovirus-mediated overexpression of SR-BI in mice on both sinusoidal and canalicular surfaces of hepatocytes resulted in a virtual disappearance of plasma HDL and an increase in biliary cholesterol.[36] Transgenic mice with liver-specific overexpression of SR-BI show a marked decrease in HDL cholesterol, apo A-I, and apo A-II, a marked increase in selective uptake in the liver, and an increase in biliary cholesterol.[104] Thus, SR-BI overexpression reduces HDL plasma cholesterol, while increasing reverse cholesterol transport to the liver. Moreover, SR-BI transgenic mice have decreased VLDL and LDL cholesterol and apo B levels, and are resistant to increases in plasma apo B levels produced by an atherogenic diet. These results indicate that SR-BI may also play a role in modulation of apo B and LDL cholesterol levels.

The transgenic studies are consistent with results in SR-BI-deficient mice produced by targeted disruption of this gene in ES cells.[25,26] There was a marked increase in plasma HDL levels in animals homozygous or heterozygous for the targeted alleles. Consistent with SR-BI's suggested role in selective cholesterol uptake by the adrenal gland, mice with decreased expression of SR-BI demonstrated a decrease in adrenal gland cholesterol accumulation. Moreover, the marked decrease in selective uptake of HDL cholesteryl esters in the liver in mice with decreased expression of SR-BI shows that this is the principal molecule mediating selective uptake of HDL cholesteryl esters in vivo.

Additional evidence of the role of HDL and SR-BI in murine adrenal physiology has accrued from studies of SR-BI expression and adrenal cholesteryl accumulation in mice with altered expression of genes that participate in HDL structure and metabolism. Mice deficient in apo A-I, apo A-II, and apo E were assessed for adrenal SR-BI expression and/or adrenal cholesteryl ester accumulation. The apo E- and apo A-II-deficient mice,[105,106] the latter with a profound decrease in HDL levels, did not differ from control animals in adrenal cholesteryl ester accumulation or SR-BI expression. In contrast, apo A-I deficiency resulted in a profound decrease in the accumulation of adrenal cholesteryl ester and an increase in adrenal SR-BI expression. The lack of apo A-I had other important effects on adrenal gland physiology, including diminished basal corticosteroid production, a blunted steroidogenic response to stress, and increased expression of compensatory pathways to provide cholesterol substrate for steroid production. While multiple regulated pathways provide cholesterol to steroidogenic cells, the analysis of the apo A-I knockout mice suggests that the selective uptake pathway for HDL is a primary determinant of cholesteryl ester accumulation in steroidogenic cells, as well as adrenal gland physiology. Related studies involve the analysis of SR-BI expression and adrenal cholesterol accumulation in mice with altered levels of expression of several nonapolipoprotein genes participating in the metabolism of lipoproteins. These include gene-targeted mice deficient in the LDL receptor, LCAT,[107] and hepatic lipase,[106] as well as mice expressing a human CETP transgene.[106] While the LDL receptor-deficient and the CETP transgenic mice did not differ from the control animals, both the HL- and LCAT-deficient animals had a marked decrease in adrenal cholesteryl ester accumulation and increased expression of adrenal SR-BI. Hepatic lipase has been previously shown to increase selective uptake of cholesterol from HDL in vitro, while LCAT deficiency affects HDL size and profoundly decreases total HDL concentration. These findings in the apo A-I-, hepatic lipase-, and LCAT-deficient animals add to the increasing body of evidence that suggests that SR-BI is indeed a functional HDL receptor under feedback control and that hepatic lipase, LCAT, and apo A-I all facilitate SR-BI-mediated uptake of HDL lipids. The feedback control of SR-BI expression in the adrenal may be largely mediated by alterations in adrenal cholesterol stones and consequent altered corticosteroid and ACTH synthesis; ACTH affects transcription of the SR-BI gene via the transcription factor steroidogenic factor 1 (SF-1). There may also be a direct effect of adrenal cholesterol stores on SR-BI expression.

CETP Transgenic Mice

Mice normally lack CETP activity, and the introduction of a human CETP transgene into mice results in reduced HDL cholesterol and apo A-I levels.[108] The human CETP transgene causes more marked reductions in HDL cholesterol and apo A-I in mice also expressing the human apo A-I transgene. A similar species-specific interaction has also been seen between human apo A-I and human LCAT and PLTP transgenes. In the presence of hypertriglyceridemia produced by a human apo C-III transgene, CETP transgenic mice display profound reductions in HDL cholesterol, apo A-I levels, and HDL size.[109] Studies in CETP transgenic mice show either an increase or decrease in early atherosclerotic lesions, depending on the presence of other transgenes in the model.[110–112] In apo E and LDL receptor knockout backgrounds, where atherosclerosis is complex and extensive, the CETP transgene increases the extent of atherosclerotic lesions, suggesting that CETP expression may increase atherosclerosis in settings where there is impaired clearance of remnants or LDL.[113]

Hepatic Lipase

Reminiscent of the human disorder (see below), HL knockout mice have a mild dyslipidemia characterized by accumulation of IDL and large HDL species.[18] Female mice with combined knockouts of hepatic lipase and apo E have higher plasma cholesterol levels but an approximately twofold reduction in extent of atherosclerosis; the double KO mice also have higher HDL cholesterol levels than apo E KO mice,[114] and their HDL supports increased cellular cholesterol efflux compared to apo E KO mice. Circulating pre-beta HDL is present in all mutants, indicating that there is a non-CETP, non-HL pathway for pre-beta HDL formation.

Transgenic Mouse Models as a Test of the Reverse Cholesterol Transport Hypothesis

Mice with altered expression of genes regulating HDL metabolism have been used to test the reverse cholesterol transport hypothesis. Apo A-I transgenic mice, which are protected from atherosclerosis, show increased transport of HDL CE in plasma (equivalent to increased synthesis of CE), and appear to show increased transport of HDL CE to the liver. Conversely, apo A-I KO mice show decreased transport of plasma HDL CE to the liver. These mice have increased atherosclerosis in the context of increased LDL levels produced by overexpression of apo B (i.e., apo B transgenic/apo A-I KO mice have increased atherosclerosis compared to apo B transgenic mice). However, apo A-I KO/apo E KO mice do not show a decrease in atherosclerosis compared to apo E KO mice. Serum from apo AI transgenic rats and from apo A-IV transgenic mice shows increased ability to promote cholesterol efflux from macrophage foam cells. Apo A-I KO mice show decreased efflux of cholesterol from an experimental cholesterol deposit in muscle, suggesting that antiatherogenic properties of apo A-I could be related to reverse cholesterol transport.

LCAT overexpression in mice and rabbits results in increased HDL CE formation and increased levels of HDL CE and apo A-I. In rabbits, LCAT overexpression is markedly antiatherogenic, while in mice LCAT overexpression increases the extent of atherosclerosis and results in a decreased fractional clearance of HDL CE in the liver. The latter defect is reversed in mice expressing both LCAT and CETP transgenes, in association with a decrease in atherosclerosis. In summary, multiple lines of evidence are consistent with the hypothesis that antiatherogenic effects of HDL are related to its ability to mediate reverse cholesterol transport. This process is facilitated by specific HDL apoproteins, such as apo A-I and apo A-IV, acting in conjunction with LCAT and CETP.

GENETIC DISTURBANCES CAUSING DECREASED HDL LEVELS (HYPOALPHALIPOPROTEINEMIA)

Apo A-I and Apo A-II Genetic Variations That Alter HDL Levels

The apo A-I gene codes for the major structural protein of HDL. This gene is located on chromosome 11q23 in a cluster with two other apolipoprotein genes, apo C-III and apo A-IV.[115] The gene order is apo A-I, apo C-III, and apo A-IV, with the apo C-III gene in the opposite orientation to the other two genes as shown in Fig. 121-6. The apo A-I gene contains 4 exons and encodes a primary transcript of 267 amino acids that includes an 18-amino-acid prepeptide, a 6-amino-acid propeptide of unusual sequence that is cleaved extracellularly, and a 243-amino-acid mature protein.[116] The protein sequence consists mainly of 22-amino-acid-long amphipathic alpha helical imperfect repeats separated by helix-breaking proline residues.[117] The nonpolar face of the amphipathic alpha helix is thought to bind lipid, whereas the polar face interacts with the aqueous environment.[118] Similar amphipathic alpha helical repeats have been found in other apolipoproteins and constitute a common feature of this class of lipid-binding proteins.[119] The apo A-I gene is transcribed mainly in liver and intestine.[120] The *cis*-acting DNA element required for liver expression is 5′ to the gene within the proximal 256 bp of the promoter, and the element required for intestinal expression is 3′ to

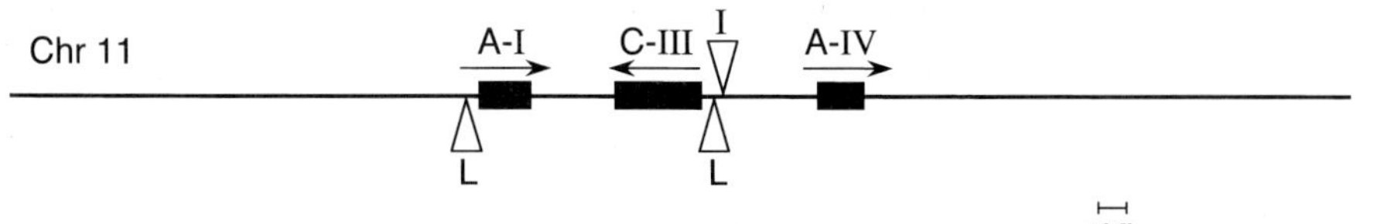

Fig. 121-6 Apolipoprotein gene cluster on chromosome 11q23. The arrows indicate the direction of transcription. L = liver transcription element; I = intestinal transcription element.

the gene in the intergenic region between the apo C-III and apo A-IV genes.[121] In addition to serving as the main structural protein of HDL, apo A-I serves as a major activator of LCAT.

Apo A-I gene mutations have been described that influence HDL-C levels and, in some cases, coronary heart disease susceptibility. These are summarized in Table 121-2. Several categories of mutations have occurred, including gene disruptions, nonsense mutations, frameshifts, and missense mutations.

There are two documented occurrences of major disruptions of the apo A-I/apo C-III/apo A-IV gene locus. Norum described two sisters with apo A-I deficiency and very low HDL-C levels.[122] Both patients had planar xanthomas, which began in childhood, and one had a tendon xanthoma. In contrast to patients with Tangier disease, the tonsils were normal in color and were atrophic. Both patients had mild diffuse corneal clouding. Symptoms of congestive heart failure developed in one patient at age 31 and in the other during childbirth at age 25. Coronary angiography demonstrated extensive obstruction in all three major vessels. HDL-C levels were between 0 and 7 mg/dl, LDL-C levels were 75th percentile, and triglyceride levels were between the 5th and the 25th percentiles. Immunoassay showed undetectable apo A-I and apo C-III. The levels of apo B were normal and the other apolipoproteins were present, but at reduced levels. The small amount of HDL present was spherical and contained apo A-II and

Table 121-2 Characteristics of Apo A-I-Deficient Patients

Mutation	Cholesterol (mg/dl)	HDL-C (mg/dl)	Apo A-I	Xanthoma	Corneal Clouding	CHD	Comments	Reference
Apo A-I, C-III inversion	130	0	0	+	+	+	Two sisters; onset CHD ages 31 and 25	122
Apo A-I, C-III, A-IV deletion	111	1	0	−	+	+	Female; died of CHD age 45	124,125
Codon 84 stop	154	3	0	+	−	+	Female; onset CHD age 52	126
Codon 5, C insertion: Frameshift, stop codon 33	222	2	0	+	+	−	Female; no CHD age 11	130
Codon 202, G deletion	243	0	3	−	+	−	Male; no CHD age 42	131
45-bp deletion (codons 146-160)	209	4	15	−	−	−	Male; no CHD age 34	94
Codon 2, C:T, Q → stop	248	3	0	+	+	+	4 homozygotes, including 2 sisters with CHD ages 34 and 39	127
Codon 107, 3-bp deletion K → 0	215	30	107	−	−	+	10 heterozygotes in a family with premature CHD	143,144
Codon 32, C:T, Q → stop	184	26	83	−	−	−	Female heterozygote, 31. No family history CHD	128
Codon 8, G:A, Trp → stop	202	6	<3	−	+	−	Male 39, no CHD	129
Partial Apo A-1 gene duplication → frameshift mutation, premature stop after aa 207		6	1	+	+	−	Female 50, predicted protein with 2 cysteines	132
Codon 159, T:G, leu → arg	226	12	32	−	−	−	Family with 7 heterozygotes; dominant mutation	138
Codon 156, T:A, val → glu	202	5	5	−	+	+	Male, 67	139

apo E/apo A-II dimers. The other lipoproteins besides HDL were of normal size and density. DNA analysis revealed the probands to be homozygotes for an intrastrand DNA inversion of 5.5 kb of DNA, which resulted in an apo A-I gene that was interrupted in the fourth exon at residue 80 by apo C-III intron 1 sequence, and an apo C-III gene that was interrupted in the midst of intron 1 by apo A-I exon 4 sequence.[123] This inversion prevents both genes from coding for complete polypeptides, effectively inactivating them, and explains the occurrence of both apo A-I and apo C-III deficiency in this kindred.

A second family was described by Schaefer (Table 121-2).[124] The female proband had corneal clouding but no xanthomas. At age 45 she developed congestive heart failure and coronary angiography revealed obstructions in the three major coronary vessels. The patient then underwent coronary artery bypass surgery, but expired 1 week after the procedure. Autopsy showed atherosclerotic lesions in the descending aorta and carotid, pulmonary, and coronary arteries. Diffuse extracellular lipid deposition was observed in the corneal stroma. The HDL-C level was 1 mg/dl and LDL-C and triglyceride levels were 25th percentile. Immunoassay revealed absence of apo A-I, apo C-III, and apo A-IV, with normal levels of apo B, but low levels of the other apolipoproteins. Upon genetic analysis, this patient was homozygous for a deletion that included the entire apo A-I apo/C-III/apo A-IV gene locus.[125]

A disruption of the apo A-I gene has been described in a 39-year-old male patient from Seattle that does not affect the neighboring apolipoprotein genes.[94] This man had HDL-C and apo A-I levels less than 15 percent of normal, but aside from premature bilateral arcus senilis, there were no other signs or symptoms of coronary heart disease. Cholesterol, LDL-C, and HDL-C were 209, 154, and 4 mg/dl, respectively, and triglycerides were 411 mg/dl. Apo A-I levels were 15 mg/dl (12 percent of normal), apo A-II levels were 12 mg/dl (36 percent of normal), apo B was elevated, and LCAT activity was reduced. The proband's HDL was triglyceride-rich and cholesterol ester-poor. DNA analysis revealed the patient as heterozygous for an apo A-I mutation, which was an in-frame deletion of 45 base pairs encoding apo A-I amino acids 146 to 160. As the reduction of HDL-C and apo A-I is greater than 50 percent, this mutation appears to exert a dominant effect. Because each HDL contains more than one apo A-I molecule, it is possible that the mutant apo A-I exerts a *trans*-dominant effect; for example, by stimulating catabolism of the whole HDL particle.

Several patients have been reported with isolated apo A-I deficiency due to nonsense mutations in the apo A-I gene. The first was a 60-year-old Japanese woman who had planar xanthomas beginning at age 18 and angina pectoris starting at age 52.[126] Coronary angiography at age 55 revealed severe atherosclerotic disease. Cholesterol, LDL-C, and HDL-C were 154, 147, and 3 mg/dl, respectively, and triglycerides were 84 mg/dl. Immunoassay revealed no apo A-I, reduced apo A-II, and normal apo C-III. Apo A-IV was not measured. DNA analysis revealed the patient was homozygous for a C to T transition within the codon (CAG) for amino acid 84 (Gln) that produced a nonsense codon (TAG).

A Canadian kindred with apo A-I deficiency due to a nonsense mutation has also been reported.[127] The 34-year-old female proband, a product of a consanguineous marriage, had bilateral cataracts and tendon xanthomas. Cholesterol, LDL-C, and HDL-C were 220, 190, and 3 mg/dl, respectively, and triglycerides were 96 mg/dl. Immunoassay revealed undetectable apo A-I, reduced apo A-II, normal apo C-III, and elevated apo B levels. HDL contained apo A-II-only particles with a diameter of 7.9 nm. DNA analysis revealed the proband to be homozygous for a nonsense mutation in codon −2 with respect to the mature protein coding sequence (signal peptide). Genotyping first-degree relatives revealed four other homozygotes and four heterozygotes. Heterozygotes had half-normal HDL-C and apo A-I levels. The proband did not have symptoms of coronary heart disease. However, her father died of a myocardial infarction at age 64; one homozygous sister, who smoked and had hypercholesterolemia and planar and tendinous xanthomas, had a myocardial infarction at age 34 followed by two-vessel bypass surgery; and one heterozygous sister with hypertension, obesity, and hyperlipidemia had angina and documented reversible myocardial ischemia at age 39.

Another report was of a 31-year-old Italian woman who developed bilateral xanthelasmas at age 22 during pregnancy, but who had no symptoms of CHD.[128] Cholesterol, LDL-C, and HDL-C were 130, 118, and 3 mg/dl, respectively, and triglycerides were 40 mg/dl. Apo A-I was undetectable by immunoassay, and apo A-II and apo B levels were reduced by two-thirds and one-third, respectively. DNA analysis revealed that the patient was homozygous for a nonsense mutation in codon 32 of the mature protein coding sequence. Six heterozygotes were identified in the same family. They, too, had no sign of cardiovascular disease, but had half-normal HDL-C levels and one-third reduced apo A-I levels.

The final report of this type of mutation was of a 39-year-old Japanese man.[129] He had corneal opacification, but no symptomatic coronary heart disease and only minimal changes on coronary angiography. Cholesterol, LDL-C, and HDL-C levels were 202, 175, and 6 mg/dl, respectively, and triglycerides were 104 mg/dl. Apo A-I levels were below 3 mg/dl and apo A-II levels were reduced, but apo B levels were normal. DNA analysis revealed that the patient was homozygous for a nonsense mutation in codon 8 of the mature protein coding sequence.

There have been three reports of frameshift mutations in the apo A-I gene. In the first, an 11-year-old Turkish girl with apo A-I deficiency was described.[130] She had planar xanthomas starting at age 7 and corneal clouding. There was no evidence of CHD. Total cholesterol, LDL-C, and HDL-C were 222, 198, and 2 mg/dl, respectively, and triglycerides were 107 mg/dl. Immunoassay revealed no apo A-I, very low apo A-II levels, elevated levels of apo B, and normal levels of apo A-IV, apo C-III, and apo E. Analysis of the apo A-I gene showed the patient to be homozygous for a cytosine insertion into the codon for amino acid 5 of the mature apo A-I protein. This results in a frameshift altering the amino acid 5 to 33 coding sequence whereupon a premature termination codon is encountered.

The second case of an apo A-I gene frameshift mutation was reported from Germany and actually resembled fish eye disease.[131] The proband was a 42-year-old male with massive corneal opacifications, complete absence of HDL, and half-normal LCAT activity. CHD was not evident. Total cholesterol and LDL-C were 243 and 203 mg/dl, respectively, and triglycerides were 196 mg/dl. Immunoassay showed only 2 percent of normal apo A-I levels, with apo A-I in the LDL and lipoprotein-free fractions. The isoelectric point of apo A-I was changed by preincubation with dithiothreitol, and apo A-I/apo A-II heterodimers were demonstrated, both suggesting an abnormal cysteine containing apo A-I. Upon DNA sequence analysis, the patient was found homozygous for a G deletion in codon 202 of the apo A-I gene. This changes the reading frame, resulting in abnormal amino acids 203 to 229, and a codon 230 stop. Apo A-I is normally devoid of cysteines, but the new C-terminal amino acid sequence contains three cysteines, which explains the unusual patterns observed. The patient's LCAT gene was sequenced and found to be normal, and it is uncertain why he had reduced LCAT activity and the massive corneal opacities more characteristic of fish eye disease.

The third report was of a 50-year-old Japanese female with an HDL of 5 mg/dl and apo A-I of less than 1 mg/dl.[132] She had corneal clouding and extensive tendon xanthomas, the first one appearing at age 9. A stress EKG was normal and there were no symptoms of CHD. DNA analysis revealed she was homozygous for a 23-nucleotide duplication in the apo A-I gene. This resulted in a shift of the normal reading frame and alteration of the apo A-I amino acid sequence beyond residue 162 with premature termination after amino acid 207. The abnormal C-terminal end of the patient's apo A-I had a predicted protein sequence containing two cysteines. The patient's plasma showed evidence of apo A-I heterodimers, perhaps due to intermolecular disulfide bonds, and decreased LCAT activity and mass and decreased CETP activity.

Apo A-I missense mutations causing structural variation in the protein have also been found. Most of these cause no change in HDL-C levels and are not described here. The first missense mutation described that was functionally significant occurred in an extensive Italian kindred from the village of Limone sul Garda.[133–136] Individuals in this kindred have low levels of HDL-C cosegregating with an electrophoretic variant of apo A-I, which has been called apo A-I Milano. Clinically, despite the low HDL-C levels, individuals with apo A-I Milano do not have increased coronary heart disease. In fact, the opposite is suspected, with longevity noted in affected family members. Plasma lipid, lipoprotein, and apolipoprotein levels were compared between individuals with the apo A-I Milano variant and age- and sex-matched unaffected subjects of the same kindred. The variant was associated with a 67 percent decrease in HDL-C levels and a 40 percent decrease in apo A-I and apo A-II levels. Individuals with the variant had a 75 percent increase in triglycerides and VLDL-C levels. Levels of LDL-C, apo B, apo C-II, apo C-III, and apo E were the same as in unaffected family members. VLDL composition was normal, but both LDL and HDL had reduced cholesterol esters and increased triglycerides. HDL consisted exclusively of HDL3, with no HDL2 observed. The smaller HDL3 particles contained apo A-I Milano monomers and the larger HDL3 particles contained apo A-I Milano/apo A-II complexes and apo A-I Milano dimers. In affected subjects, LCAT activity was reduced 25 percent, and there was a significant increase in the ratio of plasma free cholesterol to cholesterol ester. Metabolic turnover studies indicate that the apo A-I Milano protein has an increased FCR, compatible with reduced apo A-I levels in affected subjects. The defect in apo A-I Milano is a missense mutation causing a 173 Arg to Cys change in the primary amino acid sequence. This changes the physical properties of one of the amphipathic alpha helical regions of apo A-I involved in lipid binding, and allows apo A-I Milano to disulfide bond with other proteins altering their metabolism.

Another structural apo A-I variant consistently associated with low HDL-C levels is characterized by a 165 Pro to Arg change.[137] This variant was initially detected by population screening and 17 carriers have been identified. The variant is associated with a mild decrease in HDL-C and apo A-I levels, but there is no known association with coronary heart disease susceptibility.

Recently, three apo A-I gene missense mutations were described that are associated with moderate to severe decreases in plasma HDL-C and apo A-I levels. A 65-year-old Finnish woman with HDL-C and apo A-I of 8 and 22 mg/dl, respectively, was reported who was found heterozygous for a mutation in codon 159 changing leucine to arginine.[138] Six similarly affected family members were also identified. That heterozygotes in this family had a greater than 50 percent lowering of HDL-C and apo A-I, suggesting a dominant effect. Metabolic studies indicated increased in vivo catabolism of apo A-I, suggesting that the mutant apo A-I might increase the catabolism of the whole HDL particle, which also contains normal apo A-I. None of the family with the mutation had corneal clouding, xanthomas, or symptoms of CHD. A 67-year-old Japanese male was discovered with HDL-C and apo A-I of 8 and 11 mg/dl, respectively, who was homozygous for a mutation in codon 156 changing valine to glutamic acid.[139] The proband had corneal clouding and symptomatic coronary heart disease, but no xanthomas. A brother also homozygous for the mutation had similar HDL-C and apo A-I levels and corneal clouding but no symptomatic coronary heart disease. The heterozygous son of the proband had normal HDL-C levels and only a 40 percent decrease in apo A-I. Finally, a family from Italy was reported that segregated an apo A-I null allele of unspecified type and another apo A-I allele characterized by a missense mutation that altered codon 141 from leucine to arginine, the latter resulting in half-normal HDL-C and apo A-I levels.[140] In this kindred, there were three male genetic compounds for both of these defects who were between 45 and 52 years of age, and all had CHD.

Finally, there is some controversy surrounding the significance of a structural variant of apo A-I characterized by a deletion of Lys 107. This variant was initially found in 35 Germans by population screening (population frequency approximately 1 in 5000) and was not associated with altered HDL-C levels.[141,142] Reanalysis of the German data revealed 30 percent lower HDL-C and 48 percent higher triglycerides in men, but not in women, who were carriers of this mutation.[143] More recently, a Finnish family containing 10 carriers of this mutation (6 males and 4 females) was described. Compared to noncarrier family members, they had 36 percent lower HDL-C and 18 percent lower apo A-I levels, and normal triglycerides.[144] No sex differences were noted. There was considerable premature CHD in this family, but it is not clear that it was coinherited with the apo A-I variant.

Apo A-II is the second most abundant HDL structural protein. Its gene is located on the long arm of chromosome 1 in the region designated q21-q23.[145] The gene is 1330 bp in length, contains 4 exons, and encodes a 100-amino-acid-long primary transcript that includes an 18-amino-acid prepeptide, a 5-amino-acid propeptide, and a 77-amino-acid mature protein. Human apo A-II contains a single cysteine at residue 6 and exists in plasma largely in a homodimeric form due to disulfide bond formation. Apo A-II is synthesized primarily in the liver,[146] and may act as a physiological inhibitor of hepatic lipase.[147]

Takata has reported the only cases of apo A-II deficiency in two sisters ages 62 and 59.[99] These sisters were clinically normal and had no evidence of vascular disease by coronary angiography. Biochemical measurements indicated immunologically undetectable levels of apo A-II. In spite of the absence of apo A-II, HDL-C levels in the sisters were in the normal range (47 and 43 mg/dl). The sisters had a 33 percent reduction in apo A-I levels, but normal levels of total cholesterol, triglycerides, and apo B. DNA sequence analysis of their apo A-II gene revealed that the sisters were homozygous for a G to A mutation in the first base of the intron 3 splice-donor site. This would preclude normal intron splicing from the primary transcript and was undoubtedly the cause of the apo A-II deficiency.

Tangier Disease

Tangier disease is a rare recessive disorder characterized by profoundly decreased HDL cholesterol, apo A-I, and apo A-II levels, moderate hypertriglyceridemia, and reduced levels of LDL cholesterol and apo B. The apo A-I gene is normal in Tangier disease. Apo A-I production is unaffected, but there is hypercatabolism of apo A-I. A characteristic feature is the accumulation of cholesteryl ester-laden macrophage foam cells in the tonsils and spleen, suggesting a defect in cellular cholesterol efflux to HDL. In cell culture experiments, fibroblasts from Tangier patients show decreased efflux of cholesterol and phospholipids in response to apo A-I or HDL in the media.[63] Recently, Tangier disease has been shown to be caused by mutations in the ATP binding cassette transporter, ABC1. Tangier disease is described in detail in Chap. 122.

Lecithin:Cholesterol Acyltransferase (LCAT) Deficiency

Classical LCAT deficiency and the related disorder fish eye disease are caused by mutations in the LCAT gene that result, respectively, in complete or partial deficiency of LCAT in plasma. Affected subjects have corneal opacities, markedly reduced HDL levels, reduced or normal LDL levels, and hypertriglyceridemia. The composition and morphology of the plasma lipoproteins is markedly abnormal, reflecting the absence of cholesteryl esters. When the underlying mutation results in a severe defect of LCAT activity, these subjects may develop hemolytic anemia and renal failure. LCAT deficiency is described in detail in Chap. 118.

Lipoprotein Lipase Deficiency

Lipoprotein lipase is responsible for the lipolysis of the triglyceride-rich lipoproteins, chylomicrons, and VLDL. Homozygous deficiency is associated with marked hypertriglyceridemia and the development of pancreatitis in childhood. These subjects typically have substantial reductions in HDL and LDL cholesterol levels. Heterozygous deficiency produces a milder hypertriglyceridemia that is associated with moderate reductions in HDL and LDL cholesterol levels.[148] Familial LPL deficiency is described in Chap. 117.

GENETIC DISTURBANCES CAUSING INCREASED HDL LEVELS (HYPERALPHALIPOPROTEINEMIA)

Increased Production of Apo A-I

A family with marked hyperalphalipoproteinemia associated with overproduction of apo A-I has been described.[149] The apo A-I gene, however, appears normal and the nature of the underlying defect is unknown.

Cholesteryl Ester Transfer Protein Deficiency

Mutations in the cholesteryl ester transfer protein (CETP) gene result in increased HDL levels. The first CETP gene mutation that was characterized was an intron 14 splicing defect (Fig. 121-7) discovered in a Japanese family.[150–152] This is a null mutation with semidominant effects on plasma CETP and HDL levels. It is common in Japan and represents a paradigm for other mutations of the CETP gene that have subsequently been characterized in Japanese and other populations (Fig. 121-7).[153–156] Homozygotes with the intron 14 defect have no detectable plasma CETP, massive elevations of HDL cholesterol levels (2 to 6 times normal levels), moderate increases in apo A-I (1.8 times normal), and normal apo A-II levels. HDL is markedly enriched in cholesteryl esters and depleted of triglycerides. There is a marked increase in the larger HDL species, HDL-2 and HDL-1, which are enriched in apo E[157] and free cholesterol.[158] Characterization of the lipoproteins by immunoaffinity analysis reveals an increase in cholesteryl ester and apo A-I levels in both LpA-I and LpA-I/A-II. Thus, the ratio of apo A-I/apo A-II is increased in LpA-I/A-II. Other apolipoproteins of HDL (apo Cs and apo A-IV) are also increased. These changes reflect the primary role of CETP in regulating the clearance of HDL CE in humans; increases in HDL size and apoprotein content are secondary to delayed clearance of HDL CE from plasma.

Homozygotes with the intron 14 splicing defect have decreased mean plasma apo B levels (about 60 percent of normal), and cholesteryl ester levels in VLDL, IDL, and LDL are diminished by about one-third.[151,159] However, these changes are inconsistent, and homozygotes often have values for these parameters that overlap the normal range. Moreover, the decrease in LDL cholesterol and apo B levels is only observed in the absence of plasma CETP.[160] In this setting, LDL subspeciation is also markedly altered: whereas normal LDL consists of a population of particles within a relatively narrow size range, LDL from CETP-deficient subjects is polydisperse, and contains four or five distinct subspecies ranging in size from 23 to 29 nm.[151] Mean fasting plasma triglyceride levels are increased in homozygotes.[151] A subject with a homozygous null mutation of CETP with a profound increase in plasma triglyceride levels in the postprandial state has been described.[155]

Heterozygotes with the intron 14 splicing defect have mean reductions of 35 percent in plasma CETP levels. Initially, heterozygotes with CETP mutations were characterized as having marked increases in HDL levels.[161] However, in population samples, the impact of heterozygosity on HDL levels appears much milder.[161] In a population of elderly Japanese-American men, the mean HDL cholesterol level of heterozygotes was 67 mg/dl, compared to 50 mg/dl in unaffected subjects, and there was substantial overlap between the groups.[161] In affected families, apo A-I levels and HDL-2/HDL-3 ratios are also increased in heterozygotes, but apo B and LDL cholesterol levels are not altered.[151]

Metabolic turnover studies carried out in a small number of subjects homozygous for the intron 14 mutation showed normal production but delayed fractional clearance of apo A-I and apo A-II.[162] There was also a substantial increase in clearance of apo B from LDL, and moderately decreased production rates of apo B in VLDL and IDL.[163] These findings suggest up-regulation of hepatic LDL receptors, and are consistent with data in CETP transgenic mice suggesting that CETP expression, by enhancing the transfer of HDL cholesteryl esters into the liver, decreases LDL-receptor activity.[164]

A second CETP gene mutation (D442:G) is very common in the Japanese, Chinese, and Korean populations.[160,165,166] Expression studies indicate that this missense variant is secreted by cells in decreased amounts and has reduced specific activity.[165] However, the defective allele still produces some active plasma CETP, and thus the effects of the mutation on plasma lipoproteins are less severe than the intron 14 splicing defect. In the Japanese-American men in the Honolulu Heart Program, mean increases were about 10 percent for HDL cholesterol.[161] Heterozygotes also had significant decreases in mean plasma triglyceride and blood glucose levels. Homozygotes with the D442:G mutation also have moderately increased HDL levels. Compound intron 14/D442:G subjects have markedly increased HDL levels that are not quite as high as homozygous intron 14-deficient individuals.[160]

Although genetic CETP deficiency was initially characterized as a mutation associated with low apparent morbidity from atherosclerosis and possible longevity,[151] this was subsequently called into question.[168] Several subjects with combined CETP and hepatic lipase deficiency and very high HDL who have coronary artery disease and corneal arcus have been described.[168] Moreover, in a population-based sample of 3469 Japanese-American men (in which 5.1 percent had the D442G mutation and 0.5 percent the intron 14 splicing defect), the overall prevalence of definite CHD was 21 percent in men with mutations and 16 percent in men without mutations.[60] Using logistic regression methods to calculate the risk of CHD, the relative risk was found to be 1.43 for men with mutations ($p < .05$), 1.55 ($p = .02$) after adjustment for other risk factors, and 1.68 ($p = .008$) following adjustment for risk factors and HDL levels. Increased CHD risk

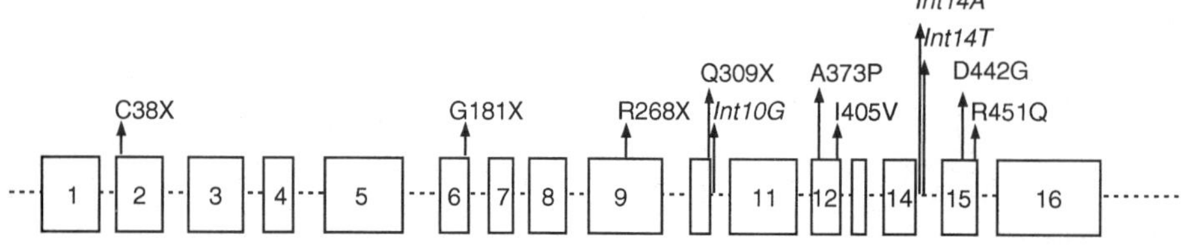

Fig. 121-7 Summary of different CETP gene mutations in human populations. The 16-exon CETP gene is shown schematically, and the location of various missense, nonsense, or splicing mutations is indicated.

was primarily observed for men with HDL cholesterol of 41 to 60 mg/dl; for HDL chol >60 mg/dl, men with and without mutations had a similar low CHD prevalence. The low prevalence of CHD in subjects with CETP deficiency and high HDL cholesterol levels has been replicated in another population based survey.[169] Also, a *Taq*I polymorphism of the CETP gene that is associated with decreased CETP and increased HDL levels[170] is associated with no change in CHD prevalence in the normal range of HDL values; however, subjects with the low CETP variant showed decreased CHD within deciles of increasing HDL levels, associated with increasing alcohol intake.[171] This suggests a gene-environment interaction that modifies the effect of CETP deficiency on CHD. The increase in CHD in CETP-deficient heterozygotes with HDL levels in the normal range probably reflects a defect in reverse cholesterol transport, and provides a crucial piece of evidence in humans that the antiatherogenic function of HDL is related to its role in reverse cholesterol transport. Mechanistic studies indicate a moderate decrease in plasma cholesterol ester formation in heterozygous CETP deficiency,[172] as well as a decreased ability of HDL-2 from CETP homozygotes to mediate cellular cholesterol efflux.[173] Both of these findings suggest a qualitative defect in the ability to promote cellular cholesterol efflux. These deleterious effects are compensated for by increased HDL particle number at higher HDL levels (e.g., in homozygotes), resulting in a net antiatherogenic effect. In summary, the relationship of genetic CETP deficiency to CHD is complex. There is increased CHD at intermediate HDL levels. However, at higher HDL levels CETP-deficient subjects enjoy a low prevalence of CHD similar to other subjects with high HDL.

Hepatic Lipase (HL) Deficiency

The first subjects described with HL deficiency were characterized as having hypertriglyceridemia, hypercholesterolemia, increased HDL levels, and a predisposition to premature CHD.[174–176] In these Toronto families, two different missense mutations are present, S267F (0 percent of wild-type activity in cell transfection experiments) and T383M (38 percent of wild-type activity).[177] Individuals with severe HL deficiency in these families have been characterized as having beta-migrating VLDL (but only when plasma TG levels were greater than 1 mM/liter) and normal or increased LDL and HDL cholesterol.[178] The phenotype of HL deficiency is somewhat obscured by the likely existence of additional genes causing hyperlipidemia in these families.[174] Studies of the beta-VLDL show that it contains predominantly apo B-100 and apo E, and, in cell culture, has a marked ability to stimulate macrophage foam cell formation.[178,179] A Finnish family with 18 members was found to have two missense mutations of HL, R186H (zero activity in cell expression studies) and L334F (30 percent activity).[180] However, both these mutations are on the same chromosome, so the affected family members are heterozygotes for HL insufficiency. These subjects have moderate elevations of total plasma triglycerides, IDL and LDL triglycerides, and large TG-rich, cholesterol-poor LDL. Other HL-deficient subjects who are compound heterozygotes, L334F/T383M, were found to have a subtle phenotype with a slight increase in buoyant LDL and an increase in the larger HDL subclasses, HDL-2a and HDL-2b.[181] A detailed study of LDL subclasses in 3 subjects with HL deficiency versus 18 normal controls showed that deficient subjects had buoyant large LDL, with decreased density and increased diameter, compared to normal LDL.[182] These large "LDL" particles contained apo B-100 and were TG-enriched. A detailed metabolic study of a Swedish subject with complete HL deficiency (and also a 50 percent decrease in lipoprotein lipase activity) showed beta-VLDL, markedly increased IDL, decreased classical LDL, and increased HDL-2.[183] Metabolic turnover studies revealed a 50 percent decrease in the conversion of small VLDL into IDL and a severe block in the conversion of IDL into LDL; the conversion of large VLDL into small VLDL and the pathways of direct catabolism of small VLDL, IDL, and LDL were not affected by the enzyme defect. A subject with hypertriglyceridemia and premature cardiovascular disease was found homozygous for an A to G change in intron 1 of the HL gene, resulting in a splicing defect and premature termination of the coding sequence.[184] Two affected brothers with HL deficiency, CHD, and increased triglycerides, cholesterol, HDL cholesterol, and apo A-I were described.[185] They were found to have a partial lowering of HDL-2 cholesterol, and apo A-I in response to treatment with a synthetic androgen (stanozolol), but no change in HDL-3 levels, indicating that not all of the HDL-lowering effects of androgen treatment are mediated via increased HL activity.

In summary, the major features of HL deficiency appear to be increased IDL levels (equivalent to large buoyant LDL), decreased levels of classical LDL, and accumulation of large, triglyceride-enriched HDL species. These findings are consistent with animal and in vitro studies[54] showing that HL plays a role in the conversion of small VLDL into IDL and of IDL into LDL, and in the remodeling of large, triglyceride-rich HDL-2 into smaller particles.[17,186,187] In some HL-deficient individuals with additional poorly defined metabolic defects, there may be increased accumulation of beta-VLDL and a predisposition to CHD. The relationship of HL insufficiency to atherosclerosis and CHD is complex and additional studies are required to clarify these relationships.

GENETIC DETERMINANTS OF PLASMA HDL LEVELS IN THE GENERAL POPULATION

Although environmental and hormonal influences account for a significant fraction of the variance of HDL cholesterol levels in the population, there is evidence from family studies that genetic factors are also important. For example, twin studies have indicated a high degree of heritability of HDL cholesterol levels. These studies showed a much higher correlation between HDL cholesterol levels of monozygotic than dizygotic twin pairs. In three different studies, the correlation of HDL cholesterol levels in monozygotic twins ranged from 0.68 to 0.74, whereas in dizygotic twins, the correlation was only 0.34 to 0.46.[188–190] Other studies of familial aggregation of HDL cholesterol values, using path analysis, have estimated the heritability of HDL cholesterol values at 0.55, divided between genetic (0.36) and cultural (0.19) components.[188] Together these studies suggest a large genetic component in the determination of HDL cholesterol levels.

Recently, there have been major advances in elucidating the common genetic determinants of HDL cholesterol in the general population. Progress has been on two fronts. First, variants of several genes known to affect HDL processing have turned out to be sufficiently common to have an impact on HDL cholesterol levels in certain populations; examples include CETP deficiency and variants of LPL and LCAT genes. Second, robust sib-pair linkage analysis, using informative microsatellite markers for candidate genes, revealed that common genetic variation in the HL and apo A-I/apo C-III/apo A-IV gene loci account for a substantial portion of the genetic component of the variability in HDL cholesterol levels in healthy normotriglyceridemic Caucasians.[191] Strikingly, while the correlation between sibs who had inherited the identical alleles for these loci from their parents was high, sibs who had zero HL or apo A-I/apo C-III/apo A-IV allele identity-by-descent showed no significant correlation of their HDL cholesterol levels. Although this does not exclude a role for other genes, it suggests that they will have relatively minor effects in similar normolipidemic populations. It is likely that other common genetic determinants of HDL cholesterol levels may be present in other ethnic groups, or in groups of subjects selected for CHD or dyslipidemia (particularly elevated triglycerides or extremes of HDL levels).

A population-based study of families in which the proband was selected based on hypoalphalipoproteinemia indicated that this condition might be present with or without concomitant hypertriglyceridemia, but more commonly without.[192] Other family members of probands most often have hypoalphalipoproteinemia alone, and less often have accompanying hypertriglyceridemia. This contrasts with studies of subjects with CHD in whom low HDL is common and is usually accompanied by hypertriglyceridemia.[193] Although substantial progress has been made in identifying common genetic causes of HDL variation in the general normolipidemic population, the genetic determinants of the common forms of hypoalphalipoproteinemia are unknown.

Cholesteryl Ester Transfer Protein (CETP). Two mutations of the CETP gene are sufficiently common to influence HDL cholesterol levels in the general Japanese population. In a general population sample of Japanese, 2 percent of subjects were heterozygous for the CETP gene intron 14 splicing defect, and 5 percent were heterozygous for the D442:G missense mutation.[160] Together these mutations accounted for about 10 percent of the total variance of HDL cholesterol levels in this population, and they contributed to upward skewing of the distribution of HDL cholesterol values. The high frequency of these two mutations was confirmed in Japanese-American men of the population-based Honolulu Heart Program cohort.[161] While the D442G mutation appears to be widespread in Japan, Korea, and China,[167] the intron 14 splicing defect has a more restricted distribution. In some regions of northern Japan (Omagari), the intron 14 defect, a founder mutation,[151] has been found at extraordinarily high frequency (20 percent of the general population).[194]

It is likely that common genetic variation at or near the CETP locus influences HDL cholesterol levels in the general Caucasian population. A *Taq*I polymorphism in the CETP gene has been consistently associated with variation in HDL cholesterol levels; the presence of the *Taq*IB allele has been associated with 10 to 30 percent lower plasma CETP levels and 5 to 15 percent higher levels of HDL cholesterol.[171,195,196] However, this polymorphism is located at the two hundred forty-fourth nucleotide of the first intron of the CETP gene and it seems unlikely that the mutation has direct effects on CETP and HDL levels. Similarly, msp-1 and 405V:I polymorphisms involving the CETP gene have been associated with lower CETP and higher HDL levels,[196–198] but again, the location and nature of these polymorphisms suggest that they are not directly responsible. These different polymorphisms are in partial linkage disequilibrium with each other and may be linked to unknown functionally significant CETP promoter mutations. A small sib-pair linkage study using a polymorphic microsatellite marker near the CETP locus detected linkage to HDL cholesterol levels,[199] while a larger study with many more informative sib pairs found no linkage.[191] Apart from sample size, other differences in the studies were related to ascertainment of probands, who were selected for coronary artery disease in the first study but not the second. Despite the lack of linkage to HDL cholesterol levels,[191] sib-pair studies reveal a significant linkage of the CETP locus to plasma CETP levels.[200] The failure to detect linkage of the CETP locus to HDL levels in the general population of normal Caucasians suggests that the effect on HDL levels is small. However, the impact of CETP genetic variation on HDL levels may be magnified by concomitant dyslipidemia. Consistent with this idea, the impact of the V405:I variant on HDL levels is brought out by the existence of concomitant hypertriglyceridemia, and is only significant in men with plasma triglycerides > 160 mg/dl.[201] Correlational studies indicate inverse relationships between plasma CETP and HDL cholesterol levels that are only detectable or are more pronounced in subjects with hypertriglyceridemia.[202,203]

Hepatic Lipase. There is strong evidence that common genetic variation at the HL locus plays a major role in determining plasma HDL cholesterol levels in several ethnic groups.[191] Cohen et al.[191,204] carried out sib-pair linkage analysis in 73 normotriglyceridemic Caucasian families, and found that allelic variation in the HL gene explained 22 percent of the interindividual variation in HDL cholesterol between sib pairs. These findings were confirmed in a subsequent larger study of 1465 subjects.[205] Sequencing of the HL gene and promoter revealed a normal coding sequence and the presence of four polymorphisms in the promoter that were in complete linkage disequilibrium. Association studies showed that heterozygosity for the rare allele (designated as −514T) was associated with modestly increased concentrations of HDL cholesterol (41 vs. 37 mg/dl) in men but not in women.[205] Homozygosity was associated with more marked increases in HDL cholesterol (63 mg/dl) and apo A-I (153 mg/dl). The same allele of the HL gene has also been associated with lower hepatic lipase activity (−15 percent, heterozygotes; −20 percent homozygotes) and higher HDL cholesterol levels in a Dutch population,[206] and similar results have been obtained in Finns[207] (in these studies the mutation is designated as −480T). HL activity was found to rise with increasing plasma insulin levels in noncarriers of the rare promoter variant, but not in carriers, suggesting that a promoter variant associated with this haplotype may endow insensitivity of the HL promoter to increases in plasma insulin levels. However, in another study hepatic lipase activity was found to increase in parallel with body mass index, but the actions of body mass index and the −514 polymorphism on hepatic lipase activity were found to be additive and independent.[208] In one study, the allele frequency of the −480 T variant was significantly greater in coronary artery disease patients than in controls, even though it was associated with higher HDL cholesterol levels.[206] These results are reminiscent of the increase in CHD in subjects with heterozygous CETP deficiency in the Honolulu Heart Program cohort[161] and could suggest that mutations that interfere with reverse cholesterol transport and increase HDL levels by a small amount may actually increase the risk of CHD.

Genetic variation in HL may partly account for differences in HDL cholesterol in different ethnic groups. African-Americans have 10 to 15 mg/dl higher HDL cholesterol than Caucasian Americans.[209] The effect is more pronounced in males than females, and appears at puberty, suggesting an androgen effect because androgens increase HL activity and decrease HDL levels. The −514T HL allele, associated with lower HL activity, is three times more common in African-Americans than in Caucasians, suggesting that genetic variation in HL may partly account for the different levels of HDL.[210] In Turks, plasma HDL cholesterol levels are 10 to 15 percent lower than in other Europeans; this effect appears to be genetically mediated, and is associated with higher HL activity.[211]

ApoA-I/apo C-III/apo A-IV Locus. In addition to a major effect of the hepatic lipase gene locus, a sib-pair analysis of 73 normotriglyceridemic, Caucasian, nuclear families found that allelic variation at the apo A-I/apo C-III/apo A-IV locus accounted for 25 percent of the total interindividual variation in plasma HDL cholesterol levels.[191] The mechanism underlying this major contribution to genetic variation in HDL cholesterol levels is obscure. Functionally significant coding mutations of the apo A-I gene (Table 121-2) are far too rare to account for the relationship. A common polymorphism in the apo A-I gene promoter involving a G/A polymorphism at a position 76 bp upstream of the transcription start site affects promoter activity and G/A heterozygotes have 11 percent lower apo A-I production rates than G homozygotes. However, this promoter variant is not associated with changes in plasma HDL cholesterol and apo A-I levels.[212] Common genetic variation at the apo C-III locus has also been described, and could potentially influence HDL cholesterol levels via an effect on plasma triglycerides.[213,214] Paradoxically, variation in HDL cholesterol levels in the general population is correlated with interindividual differences in FCR of apo A-I rather than in production rates.[32] Genetic variation of apo A-IV is not associated with alterations in HDL cholesterol in humans. In summary, there is a major effect of the locus on HDL cholesterol levels that is most likely related to differences in apo A-I production rates. Paradoxically, variation in HDL cholesterol levels in the general population is correlated with interindividual differences in FCRs of apo A-I rather than in production rates.[32] However, the failure to detect this effect in cross-sectional metabolic studies is probably due to selection of subjects with extremes of HDL levels; in such settings, factors other than apo A-I production rate appear to be more important in explaining variability in HDL levels.

Lipoprotein Lipase Gene. A common variant in the lipoprotein lipase (LPL) gene (S447X) is present in about 20 percent of healthy Europeans and is associated with significantly higher postheparin LPL activity, lower plasma triglycerides, lower postprandial hypertriglyceridemia, lower VLDL cholesterol, lower apo C-III, slightly higher HDL cholesterol levels (heterozygotes have a mean increase in HDL cholesterol of 3 to 4 percent), and reduced CHD risk.[215–218] Conversely, less common LPL variants involving N291:S and D9:N may be associated with higher triglyceride and lower HDL cholesterol levels. A common *Hin*dIII polymorphism in intron 8 of the LPL gene is also associated with altered plasma triglycerides, HDL levels, and CHD risk, possibly because of linkage disequilibrium with a functionally significant LPL gene variant.[219] Compared to the wild-type allele, the S447Ter mutation is associated with significantly smaller within-pair differences in HDL cholesterol in male monozygotic twin pairs, indicating attenuated variability in response to environmental stimuli; thus, LPL exerts a restrictive variability gene effect on HDL cholesterol levels.[220]

Lecithin:Cholesterol Acyltransferase Gene. Although LCAT deficiency is generally considered to be a rare recessive cause of low HDL cholesterol, a survey of Finnish smokers with hypoalphalipoproteinemia revealed that carriers of a missense mutation of the LCAT gene (G230:R) represented 5 percent of the cases with very low serum HDL cholesterol levels.[221]

REFERENCES

1. Eisenberg S: High density lipoprotein metabolism. *J Lipid Res* **25**:1017, 1984.
2. Tall AR, Breslow JL: *Atherosclerosis and Coronary Artery Disease. Plasma High-Density Lipoproteins and Atherogenesis*. Philadelphia, Lippincott-Raven, 1996, pp 1, 105.
3. Tall AR: Plasma high density lipoproteins—Metabolism and relationship to atherogenesis. *J Clin Invest* **86**:379–384, 1990.
4. Zannis VI, Kardassis D, Zanni EE: Genetic mutations affecting human lipoproteins, their receptors, and their enzymes. *Adv Hum Genet* **21**:145, 1993.
5. Miller NE: Associations of high-density lipoprotein subclasses and apolipoproteins with ischemic heart disease and coronary atherosclerosis. *Am Heart J* **113**:589, 1987.
6. Gofman JWO, De Lalla H, Glazier NK, Freeman PT, Lindgren AV, Nichols P, Strisower H, et al.: The serum lipoprotein transport system in health, metabolic disorders, atherosclerosis and coronary artery disease. *Plasma* **2**:413, 1954.
7. Miller GJ, Miller NE: Plasma-high-density-lipoprotein concentration and development of ischaemic heart-disease. *Lancet* **1**:16, 1975.
8. Castelli W, Garrison RJ, Wilson PW, Abbott RD, Kalousdian S, Kannel WB: Incidence of coronary heart disease and lipoprotein cholesterol levels. The Framingham Study. *JAMA* **256**:2835, 1986.
9. Genest JJJ, Martin-Munley SS, McNamara JR, Ordovas JM, Jenner J, Myers RH, Silberman SR, Wilson PW, Salem DN, Schaefer EJ: Familial lipoprotein disorders in patients with premature coronary artery disease. *Circulation* **85**:2025, 1992.
10. Austin MA, Breslow JL, Hennekens CH, Buring JE, Willett WC, Krauss RM: Low-density lipoprotein subclass patterns and risk of myocardial infarction. *JAMA* **260**:1917,1988.
11. Patsch JR, Karlin JB, Scott LW, Smith LC, Gotto AMJ Jr: Inverse relationship between blood levels of high density lipoprotein subfraction 2 and magnitude of postprandial lipemia. *Proc Natl Acad Sci U S A* **80**:1449, 1983.
12. Castelli WP, Abbott RD, McNamara PM: Summary estimates of cholesterol used to predict coronary heart disease. *Circulation* **67**:730,1983.
13. Tall AR, Abreu E, Shuman JS: Separation of a plasma phospholipid transfer protein from cholesterol ester/phospholipid exchange protein. *J Biol Chem* **258**:2174, 1983.
14. Day JR, Albers JJ, Lofton-Day CE, Gilbert TE, Ching AFT, Grant FJ, O'Hara PJ, Marcovina SM, Adolphson JL: Complete cDNA encoding human phospholipid transfer protein from human endothelial cells. *J Biol Chem* **269**:9388, 1994.
15. Jiang X, Francone OL, Bruce C, Milne R, Mar J, Walsh A, Breslow JL, et al.: Increased prebeta-high density lipoprotein, apolipoprotein AI, and phospholipid in mice expressing the human phospholipid transfer protein and human apolipoprotein AI transgenes. *J Clin Invest* **98**:2373, 1996.
16. Newnham HH, Barter PJ: Synergistic effects of lipid transfers and hepatic lipase in the formation of very small high-density lipoproteins during incubation of human plasma. *Biochim Biophys Acta* **1044**:57, 1989.
17. Fan J, Wang J, Bensadoun A, Lauer SJ, Diang Q, Mahley RW, Taylor JM: Overexpression of hepatic lipase in transgenic rabbits leads to a marked reduction of plasma high density lipoproteins and intermediate density lipoproteins. *Proc Natl Acad Sci U S A* **91**:8724,1994.
18. Homanics GE, de Silva HV, Osada J, Zhang SH, Wong H, Borensztajn J, Maeda N: Mild dyslipidemia in mice following targeted inactivation of the hepatic lipase gene. *J Biol Chem* **270**:2974, 1995.
19. Breedveld B, Schoonderwoerd K, Verhoeven AJ, Willemsen R, Jansen H: Hepatic lipase is localized at the parenchymal cell microvilli in rat liver. *Biochem J* **321(Pt 2)**:425, 1997.
20. Sanan DA, Fan J, Bensadoun A, Taylor JM: Hepatic lipase is abundant on both hepatocyte and endothelial cell surfaces in the liver. *J Lipid Res* **38**:1002, 1997.
21. Kunitake ST, Mendel CM, Hennessy LK: Interconversion between apolipoprotein A-I containing lipoproteins of pre-beta and alpha electrophoretic mobilities. *J Lipid Res* **33**:1807, 1992.
22. Castro GR, Fielding CJ: Early incorporation of cell-derived cholesterol into pre-β-migrating high-density lipoprotein. *Biochemistry* **27**:25, 1988.
23. Fielding CJ, Fielding PE: Molecular physiology of reverse cholesterol transport. *J Lipid Res* **36**:211, 1995.
24. Acton SL, Scherer PE, Lodish HF, Krieger M: Expression cloning of SR-BI, a CD36-related class B scavenger receptor. *J Biol Chem* **269**:21003, 1994.
25. Varban ML, Rinninger F, Wang N, Fairchild-Huntress V, Dunmore JH, Fang Q, Gosselin ML, et al.: Targeted mutation reveals a central role for SR-BI in hepatic selective uptake of high density lipoprotein cholesterol. *Proc Natl Acad Sci U S A* **95**:4619, 1998.
26. Rigotti A, Trigatti BL, Penman M, Rayburn H, Herz J, Krieger M: A targeted mutation in the murine gene encoding the high density lipoprotein (HDL) receptor scavenger receptor class B type I, reveals its key role in HDL metabolism. *Proc Natl Acad Sci U S A* **94**:12610, 1997.
27. Sparrow CP, Pittman RC: Cholesterol esters selectively taken up from high-density lipoproteins are hydrolyzed extralysosomally. *Biochim Biophys Acta* **1043**:203, 1990.
28. Goldberg DI, Beltz WF, Pittman RC: Evaluation of pathways for the cellular uptake of high density lipoprotein cholesterol esters in rabbits. *J Clin Invest* **87**:331, 1991.
29. Cao G, Garcia CK, Wyne KL, Schultz RA, Parker KL, Hobbs HH: Structure and localization of the human gene encoding SR-BI/CLA-1. Evidence for transcriptional control by steroidogenic factor 1. *J Biol Chem* **272**:33068, 1997.
30. Schwartz CC, Berman M, Vlahcevic ZR, Swell L: Multicompartmental analysis of cholesterol metabolism in man. Quantitative kinetic evaluation of precursor sources and turnover of high density lipoprotein cholesterol esters. *J Clin Invest* **70**:863, 1982.
31. Schwartz CC, Halloran LG, Vlahcevic ZR, Gregory DH, Swell L: Preferential utilization of free cholesterol from high-density lipoproteins for biliary cholesterol secretion in man. *Science* **200**:62, 1978.
32. Brinton EA, Eisenberg S, Breslow JL: Human HDL cholesterol levels are determined by apoA-I fractional catabolic rate, which correlates inversely with estimates of HDL particle size. *Arterioscler Thromb* **14**:707, 1994.
33. Brinton EA, Eisenberg S, Breslow JL: Human HDL cholesterol levels are determined by apoA-I fractional catabolic rate, which correlates inversely with estimates of HDL particle size. Effects of gender, hepatic and lipoprotein lipases, triglyceride and insulin levels, and body fat distribution. *Arterioscler Thromb* **14**:707, 1994.
34. Schwartz CC, Zech LA, Vandenbroek JM, Cooper PS: Reverse cholesterol transport measured in vivo in man: The central roles of

HDL, in Miller NE (ed.): *High Density Lipoproteins and Atherosclerosis II* (Excerpta Medica Intl. Congress no. 826). Amsterdam, Elsevier, 1989, pp. 321–330.
35. Ji Y, Jian B, Wang N, Sun Y, Moya ML, Phillips MC, Rothblat GH, et al.: Scavenger receptor BI promotes high density lipoprotein-mediated cellular cholesterol efflux. *J Biol Chem* **272**:20982, 1997.
36. Kozarsky KF, Donahee MH, Rigotti A, Iqbal SN, Edelman ER, Krieger M: Overexpression of the HDL receptor SR-BI alters plasma HDL and bile cholesterol levels. *Nature* **387**:414, 1997.
37. Horowitz BS, Goldberg IJ, Merab J, Vanni TM, Ramakrishnan R, Ginsberg HN: Increased plasma and renal clearance of an exchangeable pool of apolipoprotein A-I in subjects with low levels of high density lipoprotein cholesterol. *J Clin Invest* **91**:1743, 1993.
38. Ji ZS, Dichek HL, Miranda RD, Mahley RW: Heparan sulfate proteoglycans participate in hepatic lipase and apolipoprotein E-mediated binding and uptake of plasma lipoproteins, including high density lipoproteins. *J Biol Chem* **272**:31285, 1997.
39. Fuki IV, Kuhn KM, Lomazov IR, Rothman VL, Tuszynski GP, Iozzo RV, Swenson TL, et al.: The syndecan family of proteoglycans. Novel receptors mediating internalization of atherogenic lipoproteins in vitro. *J Clin Invest* **100**:1611, 1997.
40. Jackle S, Rinninger F, Lorenzen T, Greten H, Windler E: Dissection of compartments in rat hepatocytes involved in the intracellular trafficking of high-density lipoprotein particles or their selectively internalized cholesteryl esters. *Hepatology* **17**:455, 1993.
41. Ikewaki K, Zech LA, Brewer HBJ, Rader DJ: ApoA-II kinetics in humans using endogenous labeling with stable isotopes: Slower turnover of apoA-II compared with the exogenous radiotracer method. *J Lipid Res* **37**:399, 1996.
42. Silver D, Jiang X-C, Tall AR: Stimulation of HDL metabolism by leptin signaling in *obese* and lean mice. *J Clin Invest* **105**:151, 2000.
43. Hessler JR, Robertson AL Jr, Chisholm GM III: LDL induced cytotoxicity and its inhibition by HDL in human vascular smooth muscle and endothelial cell in culture. *Arteriosclerosis* **32**:213, 1979.
44. Fielding PE, Kawano M, Catapano A, Zoppo A, Marcovina S, Fielding CJ: Unique epitope of apolipoprotein A-I expressed in pre-β-1 high density lipoprotein and its role in the catalyzed efflux of cellular cholesterol. *Biochemistry* **33**:6981, 1994.
45. Parthasarathy S, Barnett J, Fong LG: High-density lipoprotein inhibits the oxidative modification of low-density lipoprotein. *Biochim Biophys Acta* **1044**:275, 1990.
46. Bowry W, Stanley KK, Stocker R: High density lipoprotein is the major carrier of lipid hydroperoxides in human blood plasma from fasting donors. *Proc Natl Acad Sci U S A* **89**:10316, 1992.
47. Kunitake ST, Jarvis MR, Hamilton RL, Kane JP: Binding of transition metals by apolipoprotein A-I containing plasma lipoproteins: Inhibition of oxidation of low density lipoproteins. *Proc Natl Acad Sci U S A* **89**:6993, 1992.
48. Garner B, Waldeck AR, Witting PK, Rye KA, Stocker R: Oxidation of high density lipoproteins. II. Evidence for direct reduction of lipid hydroperoxides by methionine residues of apolipoproteins AI and AII. *J Biol Chem* **273**:6088, 1998.
49. Garner B, Witting PK, Waldeck AR, Christison JK, Raftery M, Stocker R: Oxidation of high density lipoproteins. I. Formation of methionine sulfoxide in apolipoproteins AI and AII is an early event that accompanies lipid peroxidation and can be enhanced by alpha-tocopherol. *J Biol Chem* **273**:6080, 1998.
50. Mackness MI, Arrol S, Abott C, Durrington PN: Protection of low-density lipoprotein against oxidative modification by high-density lipoprotein associated paraoxonase. *Arteriosclerosis* **104**:129, 1993.
51. Heinecke JW, Lusis AJ: Paraoxonase-gene polymorphisms associated with coronary heart disease: support for the oxidative damage hypothesis [Editorial; Comment]? *Am J Hum Genet* **62**:20, 1998.
52. Cockerill GW, Rye KA, Gamble JR, Vadas MA, Barter PJ: High-density lipoproteins inhibit cytokine-induced expression of endothelial cell adhesion molecules. *Arterioscler Thromb Vasc Biol* **15**:1987, 1995.
53. Saxena U, Ferguson E, Bisgaier CL: Apolipoprotein E modulates low density lipoprotein retention by lipoprotein lipase anchored to the subendothelial matrix. *J Biol Chem* **268**:14812, 1993.
54. Williams KJ, Tabas I: The response-to-retention hypothesis of early atherogenesis. *Arterioscler Thromb Vasc Biol* **15**:551, 1995.
55. Khoo JC, Miller E, McLoughlin P, Steinberg D: Prevention of low density lipoprotein aggregation by high density lipoprotein or apolipoprotein A-I. *J Lipid Res* **31**:645, 1990.
56. Fleisher LN, Tall AR, Witte LD, Miller RW, Cannon PJ: Stimulation of arterial endothelial cell prostacyclin synthesis by high density lipoproteins. *J Biol Chem* **257**:6653, 1982.
57. Pomerantz K, Tall AR, Feinmark SJ, Cannon P: Stimulation of vascular smooth muscle prostacyclin and prostaglandin E2 synthesis by plasma high and low density lipoproteins. *Circulation Res* **54**:554, 1984.
58. Pomerantz K, Fleisher L, Tall AR, Cannon PJ: Enrichment of endothelial cell arachidonate by lipid transfer from high density lipoproteins: Relationship to prostaglandin I2 synthesis. *J Lipid Res* **26**:1269, 1985.
59. Vinals M, Martinez-Gonzalez J, Badimon JJ, Badimon L: HDL-induced prostacyclin release in smooth muscle cells is dependent on cyclooxygenase-2 (Cox-2). *Arterioscler Thromb Vasc Biol* **17**:3481, 1997.
60. Glomset JA: The plasma lecithin: cholesterol ester acyltransferase reaction. *J Lipid Res* **9**:155, 1968.
61. Ho YK, Brown MS, Goldstein JL: Hydrolysis and excretion of cytoplasmic cholesteryl esters by macrophages: Stimulation by high density lipoprotein and other agents. *J Lipid Res* **21**: 391, 1980.
62. de la Llera Moya M, Atger V, Paul JT, Fournier N, Moatti N, Giral P, Friday KE, et al.: A cell culture system for screening human serum for ability to promote cellular cholesterol efflux. Relations between serum components and efflux, esterification, and transfer. *Arterioscler Thromb* **14**:1056, 1994.
63. Francis GA, Knopp RH, Oram JF: Defective removal of cellular cholesterol and phospholipids by apolipoprotein A-I in Tangier disease. *J Clin Invest* **96**:78, 1995.
64. Mazzone T, Reardon C: Expression of heterologous human apolipoprotein E by J774 macrophages enhances cholesterol efflux to HDL3. *J Lipid Res* **35**:1345, 1994.
65. Kruth HS, Skarlatos SI, Gaynor PM, Gamble W: Production of cholesterol-enriched nascent high density lipoproteins by human monocyte-derived macrophages is a mechanism that contributes to macrophage cholesterol efflux. *J Biol Chem* **269**:24511, 1994.
66. Smith JD, Miyata M, Ginsberg M, Grigaux C, Shmookler E, Plump AS: Cyclic AMP induces apolipoprotein E binding activity and promotes cholesterol efflux from a macrophage cell line to apolipoprotein acceptors. *J Biol Chem* **271**:30647, 1996.
67. Huang Y, von Eckardstein A, Wu S, Maeda N, Assmann G: A plasma lipoprotein containing only apolipoprotein E and with gamma mobility on electrophoresis releases cholesterol from cells. *Proc Natl Acad Sci U S A* **91**:1834, 1994.
68. Shimano H, Ohsuga J, Shimada M, Namba Y, Gotoda T, Harada K, Katsuki M, Yazaki Y, Yamada N: Inhibition of diet-induced atheroma formation in transgenic mice expressing apolipoprotein E in the arterial wall. *J Clin Invest* **95**:469, 1995.
69. Linton MF, Atkinson JB, Fazio S: Prevention of atherosclerosis in apolipoprotein E-deficient mice by bone marrow transplantation. *Science* **267**:1034, 1995.
70. Bellosta S, Mahley RW, Sanan DA, Murata J, Newland DL, Taylor JM, Pitas RE: Macrophage-specific expression of human apolipoprotein E reduces atherosclerosis in hypercholesterolemic apolipoprotein E-null mice. *J Clin Invest* **96**:2170, 1995.
71. Cullen P, Cignarella A, Brennhausen B, Mohr S, Assmann G, von Eckardstein A: Phenotype-dependent differences in apolipoprotein E metabolism and in cholesterol homeostasis in human monocyte-derived macrophages. *J Clin Invest* **101**:1670, 1998.
72. Huang Y, von Eckardstein A, Wu S, Assmann G: Effects of the apolipoprotein E polymorphism on uptake and transfer of cell-derived cholesterol in plasma. *J Clin Invest* **96**:2693, 1995.
73. Walsh A, Ito Y, Breslow JL: High levels of human apolipoprotein A-I in transgenic mice result in increased plasma levels of small high density lipoprotein (HDL) particles comparable to human HDL3. *J Biol Chem* **264**:6488, 1989.
74. Rubin EM, Ishida BY, Clift SM, KraussRM: Expression of human apolipoprotein A-I in transgenic mice results in reduced plasma levels of murine apolipoprotein A-I and the appearance of two new high density lipoprotein size subclasses. *Proc Natl Acad Sci U S A* **88**:434, 1991.
75. Duverger N, Viglietta C, Berthou L, Emmanuel F, Tailleux A, Parmentier-Nihoul L, Laine B, et al.: Transgenic rabbits expressing human apolipoprotein A-I in the liver. *Arterioscler Thromb Vasc Biol* **16**:1424, 1996.
76. Swanson ME, Hughes TE, Denny IS, France DS, Paterniti JRJ, Tapparelli C, Gfeller P, Burki K: High level expression of human apolipoprotein A-I in transgenic rats raises total serum high density lipoprotein cholesterol and lowers rat apolipoprotein A-I. *Transgenic Res* **1**:142, 1992.

77. Tangirala RK, Tsukamoto K, Chun SH, Usher D, Pure E, Rader DJ: Regression of atherosclerosis induced by liver-directed gene transfer of apoliporotein A-I in mice. *Circulation* **100**:1816, 1999.
78. Kopfler WP, Willard M, Betz T, Willard JE, Gerard RD, Meidell RS: Adenovirus-mediated transfer of a gene encoding human apolipoprotein A-I into normal mice increases circulating high-density lipoprotein cholesterol. *Circulation* **90**:1319, 1994.
79. Williamson R, Lee D, Hagaman J, Maeda N: Marked reduction of high density lipoprotein cholesterol in mice genetically modified to lack apolipoprotein A-I. *Proc Natl Acad Sci U S A* **89**:7134, 1992.
80. Plump AS, Azrolan N, Odaka H, Wu L, Jiang X, Tall A, Eisenberg S, Breslow JL: ApoA-I knockout mice: Characterization of HDL metabolism in homozygotes and identification of a post-RNA mechanism of apo A-I up-regulation in heterozygotes. *J Lipid Res* **38**:1033, 1997.
81. Chajek-Shaul T, Hayek T, Walsh A, Breslow J: Expression of the human apolipoprotein A-I gene in transgenic mice alters high density lipoprotein (HDL) particle size distribution and diminishes selective uptake of HDL cholesteryl esters. *Proc Natl Acad Sci U S A* **88**:6731, 1991.
82. Berthou L, Duverger N, Emmanuel F, Langouet S, Auwerx J, Guillouzo A, Fruchart JC, et al.: Opposite regulation of human versus mouse apolipoprotein A-I by fibrates in human apolipoprotein A-I transgenic mice. *J Clin Invest* **97**:2408, 1996.
83. Hayek T, Azrolan N, Verdery RB, Walsh A, Chajek-Shaul T, Agellon LB, Tall AR, Breslow JL: Hypertriglyceridemia and cholesteryl ester transfer protein interact to dramatically alter high density lipoprotein levels, particle sizes, and metabolism. Studies in transgenic mice. *J Clin Invest* **92**:1143, 1993.
84. Rubin EM, Krauss RM, Spangler EA, Verstuyft JG, Clift SM: Inhibition of early atherogenesis in transgenic mice by human apolipoprotein AI. *Nature* **353**:265, 1991.
85. Schultz JR, Versuyft JG, Gong EL, Nichols AV, Rubin EM: Protein composition determines the anti-atherogenic properties of HDL in transgenic mice. *Nature* **364**:73, 1993.
86. Paszty C, Maeda N, Verstuyft J, Rubin EM: Apolipoprotein AI transgene corrects apolipoprotein e deficiency-induced atherosclerosis in mice. *J Clin Invest* **94**:899, 1994.
87. Plump AS, Scott CJ, Breslow JL: Human apolipoprotein A-I gene expression increases high density lipoprotein and suppresses atherosclerosis in the apolipoprotein E-deficient mouse. *Proc Natl Acad Sci U S A* **91**:9607, 1994.
88. Liu AC, Lawn RM, Verstuyft JG, Rubin EM: Human apolipoprotein A-I prevents atherosclerosis associated with apolipoprotein[a] in transgenic mice. *J Lipid Res* **35**:2263, 1994.
89. Duverger N, Kruth H, Emmanuel F, Caillaud JM, Viglietta C, Castro G, Tailleux A, et al.: Inhibition of atherosclerosis development in cholesterol-fed human apolipoprotein A-I-transgenic rabbits. *Circulation* **94**:713, 1996.
90. Li H, Reddick RL, Maeda N: Lack of apo A-I is not associated with increased susceptibility to atherosclerosis in mice. *Arterioscler Thromb* **13**:1814, 1993.
91. Hughes SD, Verstuyft J, Rubin EM: HDL deficiency in genetically engineered mice requires elevated LDL to accelerate atherogenesis. *Arterioscler Thromb Vasc Biol* **17**:1725, 1997.
92. Voyiaziakis E, Goldberg IJ, Plump AS, Rubin EM, Breslow JL, Huang LS: ApoA-I deficiency causes both hypertriglyceridemia and increased atherosclerosis in human apo B transgenic mice. *J Lipid Res* **39**:313, 1998.
93. Schultz JR, Gong EL, McCall MR, Nichols AV, Clift SM, Rubin EM: Expression of human apolipoprotein A-II and its effect on high density lipoproteins in transgenic mice. *J Biol Chem* **267**:21630, 1992.
94. Deeb SS, Cheung MC, Peng RL, Wolf AC, Stern R, Albers JJ, Knopp RH: A mutation in the human apolipoprotein A-I gene. Dominant effect on the level and characteristics of plasma high density lipoproteins. *J Biol Chem* **266**:13654, 1991.
95. Assmann G, Herbert PN, Fredrickson DS, Forte T: Isolation and characterization of an abnormal high density lipoprotein in Tangier disease. *J Clin Invest* **60**:242, 1977.
96. Warden CH, Hedrick CC, Qiao JH, Castellani LW, Lusis AJ: Atherosclerosis in transgenic mice overexpressing apolipoprotein A-II [Erratum published in *Science* 262(5131):164, 1993]. *Science* **261**:469, 1993.
97. Gong EL, Stoltfus LJ, Brion CM, Murugesh D, Rubin EM: Contrasting in vivo effects of murine and human apolipoprotein A-II. Role of monomer versus dimer. *J Biol Chem* **271**:5984, 1996.
98. Weng W, Breslow JL: Dramatically decreased high density lipoprotein cholesterol, increased remnant clearance, and insulin hypersensitivity in apolipoprotein A-II knockout mice suggest a complex role for apolipoprotein A-II in atherosclerosis susceptibility. *Proc Natl Acad Sci U S A* **93**:14788, 1996.
99. Deeb SS, Takata K, Peng RL, Kajiyama G, Albers JJ: A splice-junction mutation responsible for familial apolipoprotein A-II deficiency. *Am J Hum Genet* **46**:822, 1990.
100. Escola-Gil JC, Marzal-Casacuberta A, Julve-Gil J, Ishida BY, Ordonez-Llanos J, Chan L, Gonzalez-Sastre F, Blanco-Vaca F: Human apolipoprotein A-II is a pro-atherogenic molecule when it is expressed in transgenic mice at a level similar to that in humans: Evidence of a potentially relevant species-specific interaction with diet. *J Lipid Res* **39**:457, 1998.
101. Castro G, Nihoul LP, Dengremont C, de Geitere C, Delfly B, Tailleux A, Fievet C, Duverger N, Denefle P, Fruchart JC, Rubin EM: Cholesterol efflux, lecithin-cholesterol acyltransferase activity, and pre-beta particle formation by serum from human apolipoprotein A-I and apolipoprotein A-I/apolipoprotein A-II transgenic mice consistent with the latter being less effective for reverse cholesterol transport. *Biochemistry* **36**:2243, 1997.
102. Cohen RD, Castellani LW, Qiao JH, Van Lenten BJ, Lusis AJ, Reue K: Reduced aortic lesions and elevated high density lipoprotein levels in transgenic mice overexpressing mouse apolipoprotein A-IV. *J Clin Invest* **99**:1906, 1997.
103. Duverger N, Tremp G, Caillaud JM, Emmanuel F, Castro G, Fruchart JC, Steinmetz A, Denefle P: Protection against atherogenesis in mice mediated by human apolipoprotein A-IV. *Science* **273**:966, 1996.
104. Wang NT, Arai Y, Rinninger JiF, Tall AR: Liver-specific overexpression of scavenger receptor BI decreases levels of VLDL apo B, LDL apo B and HDL in transgenic mice. *J Biol Chem* **273**:32920, 1998.
105. Plump AS, Erickson SK, Weng W, Partin JS, Breslow JL, Williams DL: Apo A-I is required for cholesteryl ester accumulation in steroidogenic cells and for normal adrenal steroid production. *J Clin Invest* **97**:2660, 1996.
106. Wang N, Weng W, Breslow JL, Tall AR: Scavenger receptor BI (SR-BI) is up-regulated in adrenal gland in apolipoprotein A-I and hepatic lipase knock-out mice as a response to depletion of cholesterol stores. *J Biol Chem* **271**:21001, 1996.
107. Ng DS, Francone OL, Forte TM, Zhang J, Haghpassand M, Rubin EM: Disruption of the murine lecithin:cholesterol acyltransferase gene causes impairment of adrenal lipid delivery and up-regulation of scavenger receptor class B type I. *J Biol Chem* **272**:15777, 1997.
108. Agellon LB, Walsh A, Hayek T, Moulin P, Jiang X, Shelanski SA, Breslow JL, Tall AR: Reduced high density lipoprotein cholesterol in human cholesteryl ester transfer protein transgenic mice. *J Biol Chem* **266**:10796, 1991.
109. Hayek T, Azrolan N, Verdery RB, Walsh A, Chajek-Shaul T, Agellon LB, Tall AR, Breslow JL: Hypertriglyceridemia and cholesteryl ester transfer protein interact to dramatically alter high density lipoprotein levels, particles sizes, and metabolism. *J Clin Invest* **92**:1143, 1993.
110. Hayek T, Masucci-Magoulas L, Jiang X, Walsh A, Rubin E, Breslow JL, Tall AR: Decreased early atherosclerotic lesions in hypertriglyceridemic mice expressing cholesteryl ester transfer protein transgene. *J Clin Invest* **96**:2071, 1996.
111. Marotti KR, Castle CK, Boyle TP, Lin AH, Murray RW, Melchior GW: Severe atherosclerosis in transgenic mice expressing simian cholesteryl ester transfer protein. *Nature* **364**:73, 1993.
112. Foger B, Vaisman BL, Paigen B, Hoyt RF Jr, Brewer HB Jr, Santamarina-Fojo S: CETP modulates the development of aortic atherosclerosis in LCAT transgenic mice. *Circulation* **96**:1, 1997.
113. Plump AS, Masucci-Magoulas L, Bisgaier C, Breslow JL, Tall AR: Increased atherosclerosis in apo E and LDL receptor gene knock-out mice as a result of human cholesteryl ester transfer protein transgene expression. *Arterioscler Thromb Vasc Biol* **19**:1105,1998.
114. Mezdour H, Jones R, Dengremont C, Castro G, Maeda N: Hepatic lipase deficiency increases plasma cholesterol but reduces susceptibility to atherosclerosis in apolipoprotein E-deficient mice. *J Biol Chem* **272**:13570, 1997.
115. Karathanasis SK: Apolipoprotein multigene family: tandem organization of human apolipoprotein AI, CIII, and AIV genes. *Proc Natl Acad Sci U S A* **82**:6374, 1985.
116. Zannis VI, Karathanasis SK, Keutmann HT, Goldberger G, Breslow JL: Intracellular and extracellular processing of human apolipoprotein A-I: Secreted apolipoprotein A-I isoprotein 2 is a propeptide. *Proc Natl Acad Sci U S A* **80**:2574, 1983.

117. Barker WC, Dayhoff MO: Evolution of homologous physiological mechanisms based on protein sequence data. *Comp Biochem Physiol B Biochem Mol Biol* **62**:1, 1979.
118. Segrest JP, Jackson RL, Morrisett JD, Gotto AMJ: A molecular theory of lipid-protein interactions in the plasma lipoproteins. *FEBS Lett* **38**:247, 1974.
119. Li WH, Tanimura M, Luo CC, Datta S, Chan L: The apolipoprotein multigene family: Biosynthesis, structure, structure-function relationships, and evolution. *J Lipid Res* **29**:245, 1988.
120. Zannis VI, Cole FS, Jackson CL, Kurnit DM, Karathanasis SK: Distribution of apolipoprotein A-I, C-II, C-III, and E mRNA in fetal human tissues. Time-dependent induction of apolipoprotein E mRNA by cultures of human monocyte-macrophages. *Biochemistry* **24**:4450, 1985.
121. Bisaha JG, Simon TC, Gordon JI, Breslow JL: Characterization of an enhancer element in the human apolipoprotein C-III gene that regulates human apolipoprotein A-I gene expression in the intestinal epithelium. *J Biol Chem* **270**:19979, 1995.
122. Norum RA, Lakier JB, Goldstein S, Angel A, Goldberg RB, Block WD, Noffze DK, et al.: Familial deficiency of apolipoproteins A-I and C-III and precocious coronary-artery disease. *N Engl J Med* **306**:1513, 1982.
123. Karathanasis SK, Ferris E, Haddad IA: DNA inversion within the apolipoproteins AI/CIII/AIV-encoding gene cluster of certain patients with premature atherosclerosis. *Proc Natl Acad Sci U S A* **84**:7198, 1987.
124. Schaefer EJ, Heaton WH, Wetzel MG, Brewer HBJ: Plasma apolipoprotein A-1 absence associated with a marked reduction of high density lipoproteins and premature coronary artery disease. *Arteriosclerosis* **2**:16, 1982
125. Ordovas JM, Cassidy DK, Civeira F, Bisgaier CL, Schaefer EJ: Familial apolipoprotein A-I, C-III, and A-IV deficiency and premature atherosclerosis due to deletion of a gene complex on chromosome 11. *J Biol Chem* **264**:16339, 1989.
126. Matsunaga T, Hiasa Y, Yanagi H, Maeda T, Hattori N, Yamakawa K, Yamanouchi Y, et al.: Apolipoprotein A-I deficiency due to a codon 84 nonsense mutation of the apolipoprotein A-I gene. *Proc Natl Acad Sci U S A* **88**:2793, 1991.
127. Ng DS, Leiter LA, Vezina C, Connelly PW, Hegele RA: Apolipoprotein A-I Q[-2]X causing isolated apolipoprotein A-I deficiency in a family with analphalipoproteinemia. *J Clin Invest* **93**:223, 1994.
128. Romling R, von Eckardstein A, Funke H, Motti C, Fragiacomo GC, Noseda G, Assmann G: A nonsense mutation in the apolipoprotein A-I gene is associated with high-density lipoprotein deficiency and periorbital xanthelasmas. *Arterioscler Thromb* **14**:1915, 1994.
129. Takata K, Saku K, Ohta T, Takata M, Bai H, Jimi S, Liu R, et al.: A new case of apo A-I deficiency showing codon 8 nonsense mutation of the apo A-I gene without evidence of coronary heart disease. *Arterioscler Thromb Vasc Biol* **15**:1866, 1995.
130. Lackner KJ, Dieplinger H, Nowicka G, Schmitz G: High density lipoprotein deficiency with xanthomas. A defect in reverse cholesterol transport caused by a point mutation in the apolipoprotein A-I gene. *J Clin Invest* **92**:2262, 1993.
131. Funke H, von Eckardstein A, Pritchard PH, Karas M, Albers JJ, Assmann G: A frameshift mutation in the human apolipoprotein A-I gene causes high density lipoprotein deficiency, partial lecithin: Cholesterol-acyltransferase deficiency, and corneal opacities. *J Clin Invest* **87**:371, 1991.
132. Moriyama K, Sasaki J, Takada Y, Matsunaga A, Fukui J, Albers JJ, Arakawa K: A cysteine-containing truncated apo A-I variant associated with HDL deficiency. *Arterioscler Thromb Vasc Biol* **16**:1416, 1996.
133. Franceschini G, Sirtori CR, Capurso A, Weisgraber KH, Mahley RW: A-IMilano apoprotein. Decreased high-density lipoprotein cholesterol levels with significant lipoprotein modifications and without clinical atherosclerosis in an Italian family. *J Clin Invest* **66**:892, 1980.
134. Gualandri V, Orsini GB, Cerrone A, Franceschini G, Sirtori CR: Familial associations of lipids and lipoproteins in a highly consanguineous population: The Limone sul Garda study. *Metabolism* **34**:212, 1985.
135. Roma P, Gregg RE, Meng MS, Ronan R, Zech LA, Franceschini G, Sirtori CR, Brewer HBJ: In vivo metabolism of a mutant form of apolipoprotein A-I, apo A-IMilano, associated with familial hypoalphalipoproteinemia. *J Clin Invest* **91**:1445, 1993.
136. Weisgraber KH, Rall SCJ, Bersot TP, Mahley RW, Franceschini G, Sirtori CR: Apolipoprotein A-IMilano. Detection of normal A-I in affected subjects and evidence for a cysteine for arginine substitution in the variant A-I. *J Biol Chem* **258**:2508, 1983.
137. von Eckardstein A, Funke H, Henke A, Altland K, Benninghoven A, Assmann G: Apolipoprotein A-I variants. Naturally occurring substitutions of proline residues affect plasma concentration of apolipoprotein A-I. *J Clin Invest* **84**:1722, 1989.
138. Miettinen HE, Gylling H, Miettinen TA, Viikari J, Paulin L, Kontula K: Apolipoprotein A-IFin. Dominantly inherited hypoalphalipoproteinemia due to a single base substitution in the apolipoprotein A-I gene. *Arterioscler Thromb Vasc Biol* **17**:83, 1997.
139. Huang W, Sasaki J, Matsunaga A, Nanimatsu H, Moriyama K, Han H, Kugi M, et al.: A novel homozygous missense mutation in the apo A-I gene with apo A-I deficiency. *Arterioscler Thromb Vasc Biol* **18**:389, 1998.
140. Miccoli R, Bertolotto A, Navalesi R, Odoguardi L, Boni A, Wessling J, Funke H, et al.: Compound heterozygosity for a structural apolipoprotein A-I variant, apo A-I(L141R)Pisa, and an apolipoprotein A-I null allele in patients with absence of HDL cholesterol, corneal opacifications, and coronary heart disease. *Circulation* **94**:1622, 1996.
141. Rall SCJ, Weisgraber KH, Mahley RW, Ogawa Y, Fielding CJ, Utermann G, Haas J, Steinmetz A, Menzel HJ, Assmann G: Abnormal lecithin:cholesterol acyltransferase activation by a human apolipoprotein A-I variant in which a single lysine residue is deleted. *J Biol Chem* **259**:10063, 1984.
142. von Eckardstein A, Funke H, Walter M, Altland K, Benninghoven A, Assmann G: Structural analysis of human apolipoprotein A-I variants. Amino acid substitutions are nonrandomly distributed throughout the apolipoprotein A-I primary structure. *J Biol Chem* **265**:8610, 1990.
143. Nofer JR, von Eckardstein A, Wiebusch H, Weng W, Funke H, Schulte H, Kohler E, Assmann G: Screening for naturally occurring apolipoprotein A-I variants: Apo A-I(delta K107) is associated with low HDL-cholesterol levels in men but not in women. *Hum Genet* **96**:177, 1995.
144. Tilly-Kiesi M, Zhang Q, Ehnholm S, Kahri J, Lahdenpera S, Ehnholm C, Taskinen MR: Apo A-IHelsinki (Lys107 → 0) associated with reduced HDL cholesterol and LpA-I:A-II deficiency. *Arterioscler Thromb Vasc Biol* **15**:1294, 1995.
145. Moore MN, Kao FT, Tsao YK, Chan L: Human apolipoprotein A-II: Nucleotide sequence of a cloned cDNA, and localization of its structural gene on human chromosome 1. *Biochem Biophys Res Commun* **123**:1, 1984.
146. Hussain MM, Zannis VI: Intracellular modification of human apolipoprotein AII (apo AII) and sites of apo AII mRNA synthesis: Comparison of apo AII with apo CII and apo CIII isoproteins. *Biochemistry* **29**:209, 1990.
147. Zhong S, Goldberg IJ, Bruce C, Rubin E, Breslow J, Tall A: Human apo A-II inhibits the hydrolysis of HDL triglyceride and the decrease of HDL size induced by hypertriglyceridemia and cholesteryl ester transfer protein in transgenic mice. *J Clin Invest* **94**:2457, 1994.
148. Bijvoet S, Gagne SE, Moorjani S, Gagne C, Henderson HE, Fruchart JC, Dallongeville J, Alaupovic P, Prins M, Kastelein JJ, Hayden MR: Alterations in plasma lipoproteins and apolipoproteins before the age of 40 in heterozygotes for lipoprotein lipase deficiency. *J Lipid Res* **37**:640, 1996.
149. Rader DJ, Schaefer J, Lohse P, Ikewaki K, Thomas F, Harris WA, Zech LA, Dujovne CA, Brewer HBJ: Increased production of apolipoprotein A-I associated with elevated plasma levels of high-density lipoproteins, apolipoprotein A-I, and lipoprotein A-I in a patient with familial hyperalphalipoproteinemia. *Metabolism* **42**:1429, 1993.
150. Brown ML, Inazu A, Hesler CB, Agellon LB, Mann C, Whitlock ME, Marcel YL, et al.: Molecular basis of lipid transfer protein deficiency in a family with increased transfer protein deficiency in a family with increased high density lipoproteins. *Nature* **342**:448, 1989.
151. Inazu A, Brown ML, Hesler CB, Agellon LB, Koizumi J, Takata K, Maruhama Y, Mabuchi H, Tall AR: Increased high density lipoprotein caused by a common cholesteryl ester transfer protein gene mutation. *N Engl J Med* **323**:1234, 1990.
152. Gotoda T, Kinoshita M, Ishibashi S, Inaba T, Harada K, Shimada M, Osuga J, et al.: Skipping of exon 14 and possible instability of both the mRNA and the resultant truncated protein underlie a common cholesteryl ester transfer protein deficiency in Japan. *Arterioscler Thromb Vasc Biol* **17**:1376, 1997.
153. Teh EM, Dolphin PJ, Breckenridge WC, Tan MH: Human plasma CETP deficiency: Identification of a novel mutation in exon 9 of the CETP gene in a Caucasian subject from North America. *J Lipid Res* **39**:442, 1998.
154. Arai T, Yamashita S, Sakai N, Hirano K, Okada S, Ishigami M, Maruyama T, et al.: A novel nonsense mutation (G181X) in the human

cholesteryl ester transfer protein gene in Japanese hyperalphalipoproteinemic subjects. *J Lipid Res* **37**:2145, 1996.

155. Ritsch A, Drexel H, Amann FW, Pfeifhofer C, Patsch JR: Deficiency of cholesteryl ester transfer protein. Description of the molecular defect and the dissociation of cholesteryl ester and triglyceride transport in plasma. *Arterioscler Thromb Vasc Biol* **17**:3433, 1997.
156. Sakai N, Santamarina-Fojo S, Yamashita S, Matsuzawa Y, Brewer HBJ: Exon 10 skipping caused by intron 10 splice donor site mutation in cholesteryl ester transfer protein gene results in abnormal downstream splice site selection. *J Lipid Res* **37**:2065, 1996.
157. Yamashita S, Sprecher DL, Sakai N, Matsuzawa Y, Tarui S, Hui DY: Accumulation of apolipoprotein E-rich density lipoproteins in hyperalphalipoproteinemic human subjects with plasma cholesteryl ester transfer protein deficiency. *J Clin Invest* **86**:688, 1990.
158. Chiba H, Akita H, Tsuchihashi K, Hui SP, Takahashi Y, Fuda H, Suzuki H, et al.: Quantitative and compositional changes in high density lipoprotein subclasses in patients with various genotypes of cholesteryl ester transfer protein deficiency. *J Lipid Res* **38**:1204, 1997.
159. Koizumi J,. Inazu A, Kunimas Y, Ichiro K, Uno Y, Kajinami K, Miyamoto S, et al.: Serum lipoprotein lipid concentration and composition in homozygous and heterozygous patients with cholesteryl ester transfer protein deficiency. *Atherosclerosis* **90**:189, 1991.
160. Inazu A, Jiang X-C, Haraki T, Kamon N, Koizumi J, Mabuchi H, Takeda R, et al.: Genetic cholesteryl ester transfer protein deficiency caused by two prevalent mutations as a major determinant of increased levels of high density lipoprotein cholesterol. *J Clin Invest* **94**:1872, 1994.
161. Zhong S, Sharp DS, Grove JS, Bruce C, Katsuhiko Y, Curb JD, Tall AR: Increased coronary heart disease in Japanese-American men with mutations in the cholesteryl ester transfer protein gene despite increased HDL levels. *J Clin Invest* **97**:2917, 1996.
162. Ikewaki K, Rader DJ, Sakamoto T, Nishiwaki M, Wakimoto N, Schaefer JR, Ishikawa T, et al.: Delayed catabolism of high density lipoprotein apolipoproteins A-I and A-II in human cholesteryl ester transfer protein deficiency. *J Clin Invest* **92**:1650, 1993.
163. Ikewaki K, Nishiwaki M, Sakamoto T, Ishikawa T, Fairwell T, Zech LA, Nagano M, et al.: Increased catabolic rate of low density lipoproteins in humans with cholesteryl ester transfer protein deficiency. *J Clin Invest* **96**:1573, 1995.
164. Jiang X-C, Masucci-Magoulas L, Mar J, Lin M, Walsh A, Breslow JL, Tall AR: Down-regulation of LDL receptor mRNA in human cholesteryl ester transfer protein transgenic mice: Mechanism to explain accumulation of lipoprotein B particles. *J Biol Chem* **268**:27406, 1993.
165. Takahashi K, Jiang X-C, Sakai N, Yamashita S, Hirano K, Bujo H, Yamazaki H, et al.: A missense mutation in the cholesteryl ester transfer protein gene with possible dominant effects on plasma high density lipoprotein. *J Clin Invest* **92**:2060, 1993.
166. Akita H, Chiba H, Hui SP, Takahashi Y, Matsuno K, Kobayashi K: Cholesteryl ester transfer protein deficiency: Identification in the Chinese [Letter]. *Am J Med Genet* **59**:399, 1995.
167. Manninen V, Elo MO, Frick MH: Lipid alterations and decline in the incidence of coronary heart disease in the Helsinki Heart Study. *JAMA* **260**:641, 1988.
168. Hirano K, Yamashita S, Sakai N, Arai T, Yoshida Y, Nozaki S, Kameda-Takemura K, Matsuzawa Y: Molecular defect and atherogenicity in cholesteryl ester transfer protein deficiency. *Ann N Y Acad Sci* 599, 1995.
169. Moriyama YT, Okamura A, Inazu M, Doi H, Iso Y, Mouri Y, Ishikawa H, et al.: A low prevalence of coronary heart disease among subjects with increased high-density lipoprotein cholesterol levels, including those with plasma cholesteryl ester transfer protein deficiency. *Prev Med* **27**:659, 1998.
170. Kondo I, Berg K, Drayna D, Lawn R: DNA polymorphism at the locus for human cholesteryl ester transfer protein (CETP) is associated with high density lipoprotein cholesterol and apolipoprotein levels. *Clin Genet* **35**:49, 1989.
171. Fumeron F, Betoulle D, Luc G, Behague I, Ricard S, Poirier O, Jemaa R, et al.: Alcohol intake modulates the effect of a polymorphism of the cholesteryl ester transfer protein gene on plasma high density lipoprotein and the risk of myocardial infarction. *J Clin Invest* **96**:1664, 1995.
172. Ohta T, Nakamura R, Takata K, Saito Y, Yamashita S, Horiuchi S, Matsuda I: Structural and functional differences of subspecies of apo A-I-containing lipoprotein in patients with plasma cholesteryl ester transfer protein deficiency. *J Lipid Res* **36**:696, 1995.
173. Ishigami M, Yamashita S, Sakai N, Arai T, Hirano K, Hiraoka H, Kameda-Takemura K, Matsuzawa Y: Large and cholesteryl ester-rich high-density lipoproteins in cholesteryl ester transfer protein (CETP) deficiency cannot protect macrophages from cholesterol accumulation induced by acetylated low-density lipoproteins. *J Biochem (Tokyo)* **116**:257, 1994.
174. Connelly PW, Maguire GF, Lee M, Little JA: Plasma lipoproteins in familial hepatic lipase deficiency. *Arteriosclerosis* **10**:40, 1990.
175. Hegele RA, Little JA, Vezina C, Maguire GF, Tu L, Wolever TS, Jenkins DJ, Connelly PW: Hepatic lipase deficiency. Clinical, biochemical, and molecular genetic characteristics. *Arterioscler Thromb* **13**:720, 1993.
176. Hegele RA, Tu L, Connelly PW: Human hepatic lipase mutations and polymorphisms. *Hum Mutat* **1**:320, 1992.
177. Durstenfeld A, Ben-Zeev O, Reue K, Stahnke G, Doolittle MH: Molecular characterization of human hepatic lipase deficiency. In vitro expression of two naturally occurring mutations. *Arterioscler Thromb* **14**:381, 1994.
178. Huff MW, Sawyez CG, Connelly PW, Maguire GF, Little JA, Hegele RA: Beta-VLDL in hepatic lipase deficiency induces apo E-mediated cholesterol ester accumulation in macrophages. *Arterioscler Thromb* **13**:1282, 1993.
179. Connelly PW, Ranganathan S, Maguire GF, Lee M, Myher JJ, Kottke BA, Kuksis A, Little JA: The beta very low density lipoprotein present in hepatic lipase deficiency competitively inhibits low density lipoprotein binding to fibroblasts and stimulates fibroblast acyl-CoA:cholesterol acyltransferase. *J Biol Chem* **263**:14184, 1988.
180. Knudsen P, Antikainen M, Uusi-Oukari M, Ehnholm S, Lahdenpera S, Bensadoun A, Funke H, et al.: Heterozygous hepatic lipase deficiency, due to two missense mutations R186H and L334F, in the HL gene. *Atherosclerosis* **128**:165, 1997.
181. Knudsen P, Antikainen M, Ehnholm S, Uusi-Oukari M, Tenkanen H, Lahdenpera S, et al.: A compound heterozygote for hepatic lipase gene mutations Leu334 → Phe and Thr383 → Met: Correlation between hepatic lipase activity and phenotypic expression. *J Lipid Res* **37**:825, 1996.
182. Auwerx JH, Marzetta CA, Hokanson JE, Brunzell JD: Large buoyant LDL-like particles in hepatic lipase deficiency. *Arteriosclerosis* **9**:319, 1989.
183. Demant T, Carlson LA, Holmquist L, Karpe F, Nilsson-Ehle P, Packard CJ, Shepherd J: Lipoprotein metabolism in hepatic lipase deficiency: studies on the turnover of apolipoprotein B and on the effect of hepatic lipase on high density lipoprotein. *J Lipid Res* **29**:1603, 1988.
184. Brand K, Dugi KA, Brunzell JD, Nevin DN, Santamarina-Fojo S: A novel A → G mutation in intron I of the hepatic lipase gene leads to alternative splicing resulting in enzyme deficiency. *J Lipid Res* **37**:1213, 1996.
185. Bausserman LL, Saritelli AL, Herbert PN: Effects of short-term stanozolol administration on serum lipoproteins in hepatic lipase deficiency. *Metabolism* **46**:992, 1997.
186. Shirai K, Barnhart RL, Jackson RL: Hydrolysis of human plasma high density lipoprotein$_2$ phospholipids and triglycerides by hepatic lipase. *Biochem Biophys Res Commun* **100**:591, 1981.
187. Goldberg IJ, Le N-A, Paternity JR, Ginsberg HN, Lindgren FT, Brown WV: Lipoprotein metabolism during acute inhibition of hepatic triglyceride lipase in the cynomolgus monkey. *J Clin Invest* **70**:1184, 1982.
188. McGue M, Rao DC, Iselius L, Russell JM: Resolution of genetic and cultural inheritance in twin families by path analysis: Application to HDL-cholesterol. *Am J Hum Genet* **37**:998, 1985.
189. Feinleib M, Garrison RJ, Fabsitz R, Christian JC, Hrubec Z, Borhani NO, Kannel WB, et al.: The NHLBI twin study of cardiovascular disease risk factors: methodology and summary of results. *Am J Epidemiol* **106**:284, 1977.
190. Austin MA, King MC, Bawol RD, Hulley SB, Friedman GD: Risk factors for coronary heart disease in adult female twins. Genetic heritability and shared environmental influences. *Am J Epidemiol* **125**:308, 1987.
191. Cohen JC, Wang Z, Grundy SM, Stoez MR, Guerra R: Genetically determined variation in plasm HDL cholesterol levels. *J Clin Invest* **94**:2377, 1994.
192. Sprecher DL, Hein MJ, Laskarzewski PM: Conjoint high triglycerides and variation at the hepatic lipase and apolipoprotein AI/CIII/AIV loci is a major cause of low HDL cholesterol across generations. Analysis of proband hypertriglyceridemia and lipid/lipoprotein disorders in first-degree family members. *Circulation* **90**:1177, 1994.

193. Genest JJ Jr, Martin-Munley SS, McNamara JR, Ordovas JM, Jenner J, Myers RH, Siberman SR, et al.: Familial lipoprotein disorders in patients with premature coronary artery disease. *Circulation* 85:2025, 1992.
194. Hirano K, Yamashita S, Nakajima N, Arai T, Maruyama T, Yoshida Y, Ishigami M, Sakai N, K-T Kaoru, Matsuzawa Y: Genetic cholesteryl ester transfer protein deficiency is extremely frequent in the Omagari area of Japan. *Arterioscler Thromb Vasc Biol* **17**:1053, 1997.
195. Freeman DJ, Packard CJ, Shepherd J, Gaffney D: Polymorphisms in the gene coding for cholesteryl ester transfer protein are related to plasma high-density lipoprotein cholesterol and transfer protein activity. *Clin Sci (Colch)* **79**:575, 1990.
196. Kuivenhoven JA, de Knijff P, Boer JM, Smalheer HA, Botma GJ, Seidell JC, Kastelein JJ, Pritchard PH: Heterogeneity at the CETP gene locus. Influence on plasma CETP concentrations and HDL cholesterol levels. *Arterioscler Thromb Vasc Biol* **17**:560, 1997.
197. Ruiz-Noreiga M, Silva-Cardenas I, Delgado-Coello B, Zentella-Dehesa A, Mas-Oliva J: Membrane-bound CETP mediates the transfer of free cholesterol between lipoproteins and membranes. *Biochem Biophys Res Commun* **202**:1322, 1994.
198. Funke H, Wiebusch H, Fuer L, Muntoni S, Schulte H, Assman G: Identification of mutations in the cholesterol ester transfer protein in Europeans with elevated high density lipoprotein cholesterol. *Circulation* **90**:1, 1994.
199. Bu X, Warden CH, Xia YR, DeMeester C, Puppione DL, Teruya S, Lokensgard B, Daneshmand S, Brown J, Gray RJ: Linkage analysis of the genetic determinants of high density lipoprotein concentrations and composition: Evidence for involvement of the apolipoprotein A-II and cholesteryl ester transfer protein loci. *Hum Genet* **93**:639, 1994.
200. McPherson R, Grundy SM, Guerra R, Cohen JC: Allelic variation in the gene encoding the cholesteryl ester transfer protein is associated with variation in the plasma concentrations of cholesteryl ester transfer protein. *J Lipid Res* **37**:1743, 1996.
201. Bruce C, Sharp DS, Tall AR: Relationship of HDL and coronary heart disease to a common amino acid polymorphism in the cholesteryl ester transfer protein in men with and without hypertriglyceridemia. *J Lipid Res* **39**:1071, 1998.
202. Tato F, Vega GL, Grundy SM: Determinants of plasma HDL-cholesterol in hypertriglyceridemic patients. Role of cholesterol-ester transfer protein and lecithin cholesteryl acyl transferase. *Arterioscler Thromb Vasc Biol* **17**:56, 1997.
203. Foger B, Ritsch A, Doblinger A, Wessels H, Patsch JR: Relationship of plasma cholesteryl ester transfer protein to HDL cholesterol. Studies in normotriglyceridemia and moderate hypertriglyceridemia. *Arterioscler Thromb Vasc Biol* **16**:1430, 1996.
204. Tahvanainen E, Syvanne M, Frick MH, Murtomaki-Repo S, Antikainen M, Kesaniemi YA, Kauma H, et al.: Association of variation in hepatic lipase activity with promoter variation in the hepatic lipase gene. The LOCAT Study Invsestigators. *J Clin Invest* **101**:956, 1998.
205. Guerra R, Wang J, Grundy SM, Cohen JC: A hepatic lipase (LIPC) allele associated with high plasma concentrations of high density lipoprotein cholesterol. *Proc Natl Acad Sci U S A* **94**:4532, 1997.
206. Jansen H, Verhoeven AJ, Weeks L, Kastelein JJ, Halley DJ, van den Ouweland A, Jukema JW, Seidell JC, Birkenhager JC: Common C-to-T substitution at position −480 of the hepatic lipase promoter associated with a lowered lipase activity in coronary artery disease patients. *Arterioscler Thromb Vasc Biol* **17**:2837, 1997.
207. Murtomaki S, Tahvanainen E, Antikainen M, Tiret L, Nicaud V, Jansen H, Ehnholm C: Hepatic lipase gene polymorphisms influence plasma HDL levels. Results from Finnish EARS participants. European Atherosclerosis Research Study. *Arterioscler Thromb Vasc Biol* **17**:1879, 1997.
208. Nie L, Wang J, Clark LT, Tang A, Vega GL, Grundy SM, Cohen JC: Body mass index and hepatic lipase gene (LIPC) polymorphism jointly influence postheparin plasma hepatic lipase activity. *J Lipid Res* **39**:1127, 1998.
209. Gordon DJ, Rifkind BM: High density lipoprotein—The clinical implications of recent studies. *N Engl J Med* **321**:1311, 1989.
210. Vega GL, Clark LT, Tang A, Marcovina S, Grundy SM, Cohen JC: Hepatic lipase activity is lower in African American men than in white American men: Effects of 5′ flanking polymorphism in the hepatic lipase gene (LIPC). *J Lipid Res* **39**:228, 1998.
211. Mahley RW, Palaoglu KE, Atak Z, Dawson-Pepin J, Langlois AM, Cheung V, Onat H, Fulks P, Mahley LL, Vakar F: Turkish heart study: Lipids, lipoproteins, and apolipoproteins. *J Lipid Res* **36**:839, 1995.
212. Smith JD, Brinton EA, Breslow JL: Polymorphism in the human apolipoprotein A-I gene promoter region. Association of the minor allele with decreased production rate in vivo and promoter activity in vitro. *J Clin Invest* **89**:1796, 1992.
213. Dammerman N, Sandkuijl LA, Halaas J, Chung W, Breslow JL: An apolipoprotein CIII haplotype protective against hypertriglyceridemia is specified by promoter and 3′ untranslated region polymorphisms. *Proc Natl Acad Sci U S A* **90**:4562, 1993.
214. Dammerman M, Breslow JL: Genetic basis of lipoprotein disorders. *Circulation* **91**:505, 1995.
215. Groenemeijer BE, Hallman MD, Reymer PW, Gagne E, Kuivenhoven JA, Bruin T, Jansen H, et al.: Genetic variant showing a positive interaction with beta-blocking agents with a beneficial influence on lipoprotein lipase activity, HDL cholesterol, and triglyceride levels in coronary artery disease patients. The Ser447-stop substitution in the lipoprotein lipase gene. REGRESS Study Group. *Circulation* **95**:2628, 1997.
216. Humphries SE, Nicaud V, Margalef J, Tiret L, Talmud PJ: Lipoprotein lipase gene variation is associated with a paternal history of premature coronary artery disease and fasting and postprandial plasma triglycerides: the European Atherosclerosis Research Study (EARS). *Arterioscler Thromb Vasc Biol* **18**:526, 1998.
217. Jemaa R, Fumeron F, Poirier O, Lecerf L, Evans A, Arveiler D, Luc G, et al.: Lipoprotein lipase gene polymorphisms: Associations with myocardial infarction and lipoprotein levels, the ECTIM study. Étude cas temoin sur l'infarctus du myocarde. *J Lipid Res* **36**:2141, 1995.
218. Kuivenhoven JA, Groenemeyer BE, Boer JM, Reymer PW, Berghuis R, Bruin T, Jansen H, et al.: Ser447 stop mutation in lipoprotein lipase is associated with elevated HDL cholesterol levels in normolipidemic males. *Arterioscler Thromb Vasc Biol* **17**:595, 1997.
219. Mattu RK, Needham EW, Morgan R, Rees A, Hackshaw AK, Stocks J, Elwood PC, Galton DJ: DNA variants at the LPL gene locus associate with angiographically defined severity of atherosclerosis and serum lipoprotein levels in a Welsh population. *Arterioscler Thromb* **14**:1090, 1994.
220. Thorn JA, Needham EW, Mattu RK, Stocks J, Galton DJ: The Ser447-Ter mutation of the lipoprotein lipase gene relates to variability of serum lipid and lipoprotein levels in monozygotic twins. *J Lipid Res* **39**:437, 1998.
221. Miettinen HE, Gylling H, Tenhunen J, Virtamo J, Jauhiainen M, Huttunen JK, Kantola I, et al.: Molecular genetic study of Finns with hypoalphalipoproteinemia and hyperalphalipoproteinemia: A novel Gly230 Arg mutation (LCAT[Fin]) of lecithin:cholesterol acyltransferase (LCAT) accounts for 5% of cases with very low serum HDL cholesterol levels. *Arterioscler Thromb Vasc Biol* **18**:591, 1998.

CHAPTER 122

Familial Analphalipoproteinemia: Tangier Disease

Gerd Assmann ■ Arnold von Eckardstein ■ H. Bryan Brewer, Jr.

1. **Tangier disease is characterized by the virtual absence of high-density lipoproteins (HDL) in plasma and by the accumulation of cholesteryl esters in many tissues throughout the body. These include tonsils, liver, spleen, lymph nodes, thymus, intestinal mucosa, peripheral nerves, and the cornea. Tangier patients have a moderately increased risk for coronary heart disease.**
2. **The major clinical signs are hyperplastic orange tonsils, hepatosplenomegaly, and relapsing neuropathy. Pathognomonic is the finding of HDL deficiency, low plasma cholesterol concentration accompanied by normal or elevated triglyceride levels in patients with hyperplastic orange-yellow tonsils, and adenoidal tissue.**
3. **Plasma apolipoprotein (apo) A-I concentration is extremely low (<3 percent that of controls) due to the lack of mature, lipid-rich HDL, that is, α-HDL, which have electrophoretic alpha-mobility and represent the majority of HDL in normolipidemic plasma. Apparently normal amounts of apo A-I reside in a lipid-poor particle with electrophoretic pre-beta-mobility, that is, pre-β_1-HDL, which in normal plasma represents approximately 5 percent of apo A-I and is a precursor of mature HDL.**
4. **Tangier fibroblasts are characterized by defective lipid efflux and by disturbed signal transduction processes. Compared to normal fibroblasts, Tangier fibroblasts are completely defective in releasing phospholipids and cholesterol in the extracellular presence of lipid-free apolipoproteins and exhibit reduced capacity to release cholesterol in the presence of HDL. Agonist-mediated breakdown of phospholipids by phospholipases is disturbed in Tangier fibroblasts. Artificial increase of cellular levels of diacylglycerol or phosphatidic acid partially corrects the cholesterol efflux defect of Tangier fibroblasts.**
5. **Obligate heterozygotes have no clinical manifestations and are characterized biochemically by half-normal serum concentrations of HDL-cholesterol, apo A-I, and apo A-II, and by half-normal lipid efflux from fibroblasts.**
6. **Tangier disease is caused by mutations in the gene of the ATP-binding cassette transporter 1 (ABC1), which is located on the long arm of chromosome 9 (9q31).**
7. **Although the pathomechanism is not known, the findings in Tangier disease demonstrate that ABC1 plays a pivotal role in the secretion of cellular lipids and in the formation of mature HDL. Defective lipid efflux appears to facilitate foam cell formation. Defective HDL maturation seems to underlie the enhanced catabolism of apo A-I and apo A-II resulting in HDL deficiency.**
8. **There is no specific treatment for Tangier disease.**

A list of standard abbreviations is located immediately preceding the index in each volume. Additional abbreviations used in this chapter include: ABC = ATP-binding cassette transporter; ATP = adenosine triphosphate; ACAT = acyl-coenzyme A:cholesterol-acyltransferase; apo = apolipoprotein; cAMP = cyclic AMP; CETP = cholesteryl ester transfer protein; CFTR = cystic fibrosis transmembrane conductance regulator; DAG = diacylglycerol; ER = endoplasmic reticulum; HDL = high-density lipoprotein; HL = hepatic lipase; IL-1 = interleukin-1; LCAT = lecithin:cholesterol-acyltransferase; LDL = low-density lipoprotein; LpA-I = apoA-I-containing lipoprotein; LPL = lipoprotein lipase; MDR = multidrug-resistant protein; NCEH = neutral cholesteryl ester hydrolase; NPC = Niemann Pick disease type C; PA = phosphatidic acid; PC = phosphatidylcholine; PI = phosphatidylinositol; PKC = protein kinase C; PLC = phospholipase C; PLD = phospholipase D; PLTP = phospholipid transfer protein; SR-BI = scavenger receptor BI; TGN = trans-Golgi network; VLDL = very-low-density lipoprotein.

DEFINITION AND HISTORY

Tangier disease is a rare inborn error of metabolism which is characterized by severe deficiency or absence of normal high-density lipoproteins (HDL) in plasma and by the accumulation of cholesteryl esters in many tissues including tonsils, peripheral nerves, intestinal mucosa, spleen, liver, bone marrow, lymph nodes, thymus, skin, and cornea. The finding of virtual HDL deficiency, a low plasma cholesterol concentration accompanied by normal or elevated triglyceride levels in individuals with hyperplastic orange-yellow tonsils and adenoidal tissue is pathognomonic for the condition. The plasma concentration of apolipoprotein (apo) A-I is extremely low (<3 percent that of controls).[1–6] Heterozygotes present with no clinical symptoms but with half-normal levels of HDL cholesterol and apo A-I.[1–6]

Tangier disease is named after the island in the Chesapeake Bay (Virginia, U.S.A.) which was home to the first two probands who were described by D.S. Fredrickson in 1961.[7] Tangier disease has since been diagnosed in about 70 patients from 60 families in the United States, England, New Zealand, Australia, Switzerland, Germany, Poland, Pakistan, Japan, Denmark, Italy, Canada, France, Spain, The Netherlands, and Egypt.[8–61] Nearly all children with Tangier disease were identified on the basis of large, yellow-orange tonsils. One-third of the adult patients came to medical attention because of symptoms of neuropathy. Diagnosis in the remaining cases was related to the clinical features of hepatomegaly, splenomegaly, premature myocardial infarction or stroke, thrombocytopenia, anemia, gastrointestinal problems, corneal opacities, hypocholesterolemia, low HDL cholesterol, or to screening families of affected subjects.

HDL AND REVERSE CHOLESTEROL TRANSPORT

HDL Subclasses

High-density lipoproteins (HDLs) encompass a heterogenous class of lipoproteins that have in common a high density (>1.063 g/ml) and a small size (Stokes' diameter: 5 to 17 nm). The majority of the HDL particles contain apo A-I. Differences in the quantitative and qualitative content of lipids, apolipoproteins, and lipid transfer proteins result in the presence of various HDL subclasses that are characterized by differences in shape, density, size, charge, and antigenicity.[62]

HDL can be separated by ultracentrifugation into HDL_2 (d = 1.063 to 1.125 g/ml) and HDL_3 (1.125 to 1.21 g/ml).[63] Nondenaturing polyacrylamide gradient gel electrophoresis (PAGGE) further discriminates by size HDL_2 into HDL_{2b} and HDL_{2a}, as well as HDL_3 into HDL_{3a}, HDL_{3b}, and HDL_{3c}.[64] Immunoaffinity chromatography fractionates HDL by apolipoprotein composition. The serial use of anti-apo A-I- and apo A-II-immunoaffinity-chromatography separates HDL into two subclasses, namely one particle that contains apo A-I and apo A-II (i.e., LpA-I/A-II), and a second particle containing apo A-I but no apo A-II (i.e., LpA-I).[62,65,66]

Following agarose gel electrophoresis of plasma and anti-apo A-I-immunoblotting, the majority of apo A-I is present in a fraction which migrates with α-electrophoretic mobility and is designated α-LpA-I. This fraction eventually contains all of the cholesterol that is quantified in the routine laboratory as HDL-cholesterol. It consists of various particles that differ by size and density, as well as by the stoichiometric content of various apolipoproteins. Approximately 5 to 15 percent of apo A-I in human plasma is associated with particles that have electrophoretic pre-β-mobility and that can be further distinguished by subsequent PAGGE and anti-apo A-I-immunoblotting into pre-β_1-LpA-I, pre-β_2-LpA-I, and pre-β_3-LpA-I (Fig. 122-1*A, C,* and *E*).[62,67–72] Pre-β_1-LpA-I are the smallest particles, are discoidal in shape, and contain apo A-I either as a lipid-free apolipoprotein or in association with a few molecules of sphingomyelin and phosphatidylcholine. Studies in which plasma was initially incubated with ^{3}H-cholesterol-labeled fibroblasts followed by separation by two-dimensional PAGGE identified pre-β_1-LpA-I as the predominant initial acceptor of cell-derived cholesterol. From this particle, cholesterol appears to be transferred first to pre-β_2-LpA-I and then to pre-β_3-LpA-I. The presence of lecithin:cholesterol-acyltransferase (LCAT) and cholesteryl ester transfer protein (CETP) enables this particle to esterify cell-derived cholesterol and transfer the cholesteryl esters to α-HDL.[62,68,70–73] The major fraction of cell-derived cholesterol, however, appears to be transferred to α-LpA-I without prior esterification in preβ_3-LpA-I.[70] The combination of agarose gel electrophoresis, PAGGE, and immunoblotting has facilitated the detection of other lipid-poor HDL subclasses that occur at relatively low plasma concentrations. These particles contain only apo E (γ-LpE) or apo A-IV (LpA-IV-1 and LpA-IV-2) as their only apolipoproteins, and serve, like pre-β_1-LpA-I, as initial acceptors of cell-derived cholesterol into the plasma compartment.[62,74–77] It is also important to note that relative to the concentration of lipid-rich α-HDL the concentration of these lipid-poor particles is increased in extravasal compartments, including the lymph where reverse cholesterol transport is initiated in vivo.[72,78–80]

HDL Metabolism

Lipid-rich α-HDLs arise from lipid-poor particles or from lipid-free apolipoproteins.[62,71,72,81,82] These lipid-poor HDL-precursors are produced as nascent HDL by hepatocytes[83–88] and the intestinal mucosa,[89–91] dissociate from chylomicrons and VLDL during lipolysis,[92–94] or are generated by the remodeling of HDL by CETP,[95–99] phospholipid transfer protein (PLTP),[100,101] and hepatic lipase (HL)[102] (Fig. 122-2). Nascent HDL of intestinal origin contain apo A-I and apo A-IV, and nascent HDL of hepatic origin contain apo A-I, apo A-II, and/or apo E. It is not yet known whether nascent HDL are assembled intracellularly in the endoplasmic reticulum or extracellularly by association of lipid-free apolipoproteins with phospholipids and cholesterol released from the plasma membrane. In agreement with the latter model, lipid-free apolipoproteins A-I, A-IV, and E promote efflux of phospholipids and cholesterol from cultured hepatocytes, macrophages, and fibroblasts, resulting in the formation of lipid-containing HDL-like particles.[58,71,72,82,103–108]

These lipid-poor HDL precursors are converted into mature, lipid-rich, and spherical α-LpA-I by the combined effects exerted

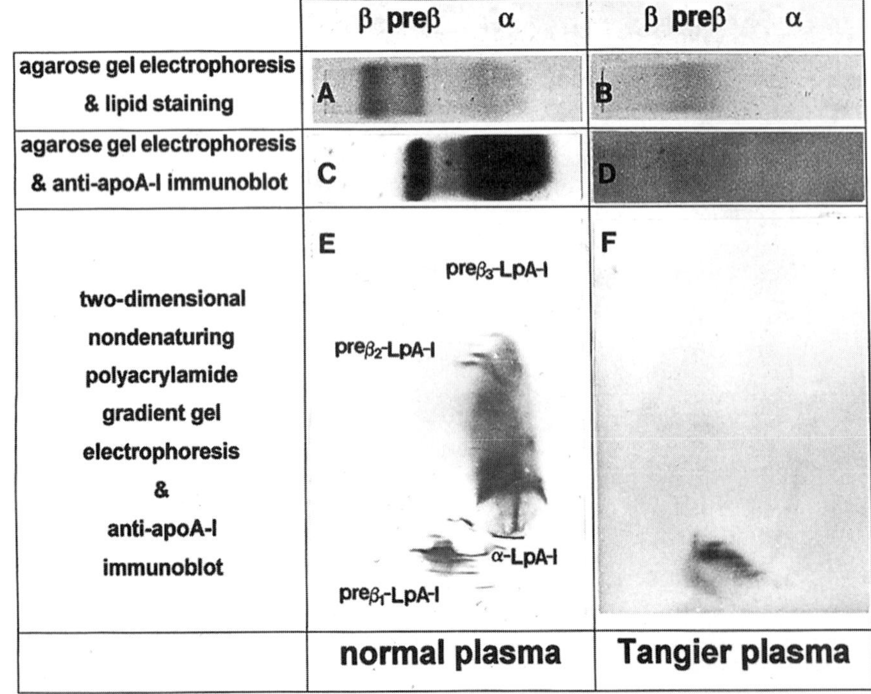

Fig. 122-1 Agarose gel electrophoresis (*A,B,C,D*) and two-dimensional nondenaturing polyacrylamide gradient gel electrophoresis (*E,F*) of plasma from a normolipidemic control (*A,C,E*) and a patient with Tangier disease (*B,D,F*). Lipoproteins were stained either with fat red (*A,B*) or anti-apo A-I antibodies (*C,D,E,F*). In normal plasma, the majority of apo A-I is found in a particle with electrophoretic α-mobility, and a minority in particles with electrophoretic pre-β-mobility (*C,E*). In Tangier plasma, apo A-I is only found in pre-β_1-LpA-I (*F*). For details of the method see references 60 and 67 to 70.

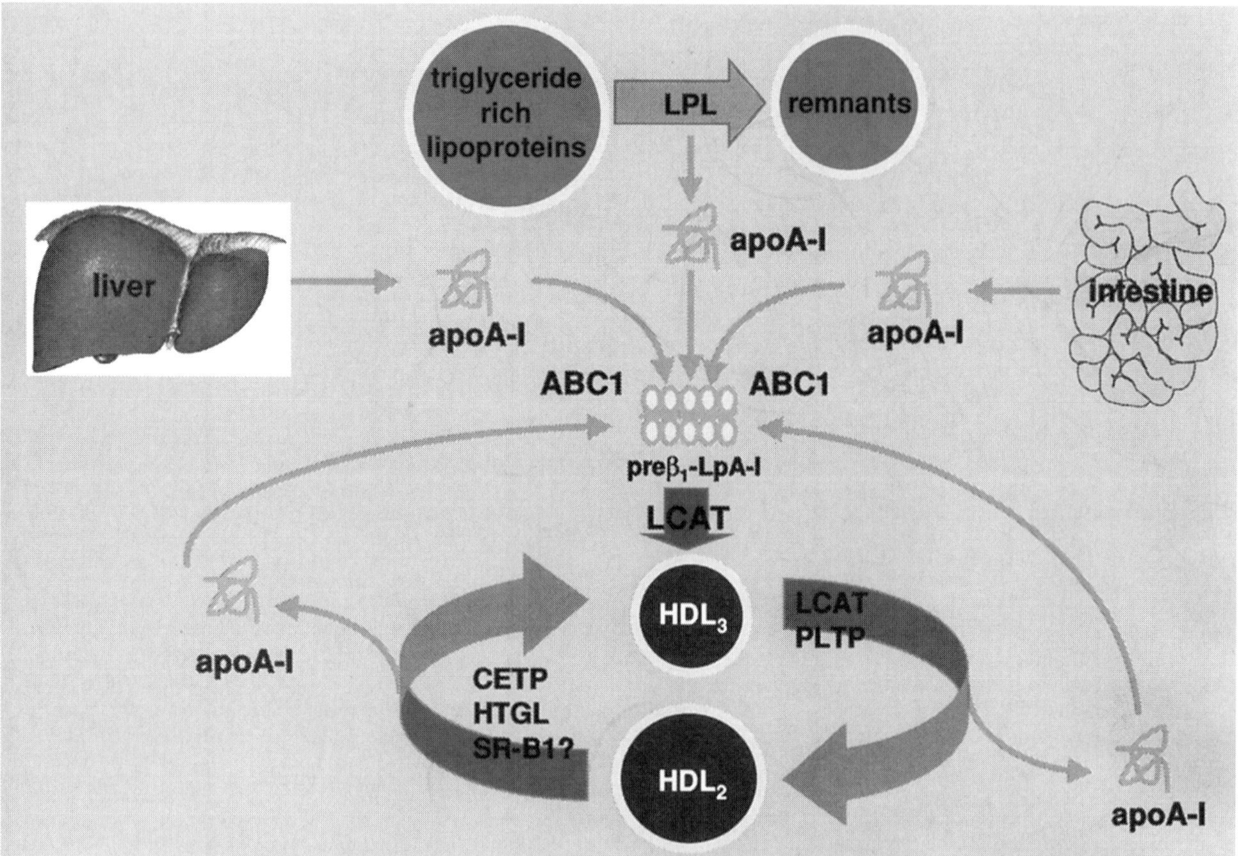

Fig. 122-2 Pathways involved in the generation and conversion of HDL. Mature HDL_3 and HDL_2 are generated from lipid-free apo A-I and lipid-poor pre-β_1-HDL as precursors. These precursors are produced as nascent HDL by the liver or intestine or are released from lipolyzed VLDL and chylomicrons or by interconversion of HDL_3 and HDL_2. ABC1 may be involved in the initial lipidation of apo A-I into pre-β_1-LpA-I (*F*). For details see text. ABC1 = ATP-binding cassette transporter 1; CETP = cholesteryl ester transfer protein; HL = hepatic lipase; LCAT = lecithin:cholesterol-acyltransferase; LPL = lipoprotein lipase; PLTP = phospholipid transfer protein; SR-BI = scavenger receptor BI.

by the acquisition of phospholipids and unesterified cholesterol, the LCAT-mediated esterification of cholesterol, and the association of additional apolipoproteins.[107,109–114] In this process, plasma membranes of peripheral cells serve as donors of lipids, and apo B containing plasma lipoproteins, as well as their remnants, are a source of apolipoproteins and lipids.[60,61,107,115] The initial products are small HDL_3. The particles mature into HDL_2 following esterification of cholesterol through LCAT[81,116,117] and PLTP-mediated fusion of α-HDL_3 particles[118–120] (Fig. 122-2).

Cholesteryl esters of α-HDL are removed from the circulation by two major direct pathways and one indirect pathway: (a) Hepatocytes and steroid hormone-producing cells express scavenger receptor BI (SR-BI), which binds HDL and mediates the selective uptake of cholesteryl esters without internalizing HDL proteins.[121–123] (b) A subpopulation of HDL containing apo E are internalized by hepatic apo E receptors.[124–127] (c) CETP exchanges cholesteryl esters of HDL_2 with triglycerides of VLDL, IDL, and LDL, and the HDL-derived cholesteryl esters are removed from the circulation via the LDL-receptor pathway.[128,129] As products of this process, smaller HDL_3, as well as lipid-free apo A-I or pre-β_1-LpA-I, are formed.[95–99] HDL_3 and pre-β_1-LpA-I are also generated by the hydrolysis of triglycerides and phospholipids of HDL_2 by hepatic lipase (HL), which appears to serve as a coreceptor for HDL binding sites on hepatocytes.[102,130]

The interconversion of HDL_3 into HDL_2 by PLTP, as well as the removal of lipids from HDL_2 by SR-BI, CETP, and HL, regenerates pre-β_1-LpA-I or lipid-free apo A-I.[95–102] These small lipoprotein particles can easily leave the plasma for the extravascular space.[71,72,82] There it can serve as an acceptor of cellular lipids and thus, again, start the generation of HDL. However, in the kidney, these small particles are filtered and removed from the plasma.[131] Cubilin, the receptor for intrinsic factor, mediates the reuptake of apo A-I from the lumen of the proximal tubule.[132]

Regulation of the Cellular Cholesterol Homeostasis

The compartmentalization of cholesterol within the cell is regulated.[133–135] The plasma membrane of mammalian cells accounts for 60 to 90 percent of cellular unesterified cholesterol, 95 percent of which is localized in the cytofacial leaflet of the bilayer membrane.[133,135–137] The lateral distribution of cholesterol within the plasma membrane is organized in microdomains. Coated pits, that is, clathrin-stabilized plasma membrane invaginations that contain lipoprotein receptors, have less cholesterol and sphingolipids than the rest of the plasma membrane. In contrast, caveolae, detergent-resistant plasma membrane invaginations, which are characterized by the presence of caveolins but the absence of clathrin, are enriched in both cholesterol and sphingolipids. Relatively small amounts of unesterified cholesterol are found in intracellular organelles except in those that communicate with the plasma membrane (endosomes, lysosomes and *trans*-Golgi network [TGN]).[133,135,138] The TGN is an acceptor of newly synthesized cholesterol from the endoplasmic reticulum (ER) and exogenous cholesterol from endocytic vesicles, lysosomes, and caveolae,[133–139] and subsequently distributes cholesterol and phospholipids either in the form of detergent-resistant and caveolin-containing vesicles (rafts or

Table 122-1 Intracellular Transport Pathways of Cholesterol

	Cell type	Metabolism	Inhibitors	Mechanism	Involvement of Golgi apparatus/TGN
ER → plasma membrane	Ubiquitous	Membrane integrity, RCT	Nocodazole, progesterone (brefeldin A)*	Rafts, caveolins? ABC1? (vesicles)*	Yes
Lysosome → plasma membrane	Ubiquitous	Membrane integrity, RCT	NPC mutation, progesterone, imipramine, bafilomycin	NPC1, caveolins?	Possibly
Lysosome → ER	Ubiquitous, especially in macrophages and hepatocytes	ACAT bile acid synthesis	NPC mutation, progesterone	NPC1, caveolins? rafts?	Probably
plasma membrane → ER	Ubiquitous	Membrane integrity, ACAT	Progesterone, imipramine	ABC1?	Yes

*In cholesterol-enriched fibroblasts, brefeldin inhibited transfer of cholesterol from the ER to the plasma membrane. For details, see references 133–135, 138, 140–143, 146, 149, 153, and 165–167. Transfers of cholesterol between ER and peroxisomes, ER and mitochondria, and peroxisomes and plasma membranes are also taking place but are not described here.

cytolipoproteins),[133,135,140,141] or as secretory detergent-soluble vesicles[133,134,141–143] (Table 122-1).

High levels of unesterified cholesterol are cytotoxic.[144] Therefore, the concentration of cholesterol in the cell is precisely regulated by *de novo* synthesis, influx, efflux, esterification, and, in some specialized cells, by synthesis and secretion of lipoproteins, steroid hormones, bile acids, or vitamin D.

Endogenous cholesterol is synthesized through several intermediates from acetyl-CoA as the precursor. The rate-limiting step of cholesterol synthesis is the reduction of β-hydroxy, β-methylglutaryl CoA (HMG CoA) to mevalonate[145] (see Chap. 120). Transfer of newly synthesized cholesterol from the ER to the plasma membrane is rapid (half-time: 10 min) and ATP-dependent. The inhibition by amphiphilic drugs such as progesterone, as well as inhibitors of microtubule formation including nocodazole, suggests the involvement of a raft pathway.[133,135,146] Consistent with this concept is the finding of biosynthetic cholesterol in caveolae.[133,135,147,148] However, in lipid-enriched cells this transfer was also inhibited by brefeldin A or monensin, which indicates that at least under certain conditions secretory vesicles are involved in the transport of cholesterol from the Golgi apparatus to the plasma membrane.[143,149]

As a component of plasma lipoproteins, exogenous cholesterol can be internalized by specific lipoprotein receptors and directed to mature lysosomes via a series of clathrin-coated endocytic vesicles for subsequent degradation.[150,151] Within the lysosomes, cholesteryl esters are hydrolyzed by acid lipase followed by incorporation of unesterified cholesterol into lysosomal membranes (see Chap. 142). The majority of lysosomal cholesterol, however, is transferred to the plasma membrane and then to the ER for reesterification by acylCoA:cholesterol-acyltransferase (ACAT)[133,152,153] (see Chap. 120), or in specialized cells, to other locations for the synthesis of bile acids, lipoproteins, or steroid hormones. Up to 30 percent of lysosomal cholesterol may even be directly transferred to the ER.[133] The release of cholesterol from lysosomes and its subsequent translocation to other cellular cholesterol pools depends on regulated transfer mechanisms[133,134] because export of lysosomal cholesterol is impaired in Niemann-Pick disease type C (NPC) (see Chap. 145),[154,155] in a mutant hamster ovary cell line,[156] and in the presence of amphiphilic drugs.[157] Unesterified cholesterol in NPC cells or fibroblasts treated with amphiphiles accumulates in lysosomes, late endosomes, and the TGN, indicating that the latter organelle is involved in the transport of lysosomal cholesterol to the plasma membrane, probably by vesicle formation.[133–136,158,159]

In addition to receptor-mediated pathways, cells selectively take up unesterified and esterified cholesterol from lipoproteins independent of their protein constituents. The HDL receptor SR-BI mediates the selective uptake of esterified cholesterol into hepatic and steroidogenic cells.[121–123] Cholesterol-binding proteins located within the caveolae, so-called caveolins, appear to be involved in the selective uptake of unesterified cholesterol from plasma lipoproteins into many cell types.[70,135,160] Unesterified cholesterol is then directed from the plasma membrane to the TGN via endocytic vesicles.[135,139,161]

Both endogenous and exogenous cholesterol initiate a negative feedback mechanism. An increase in the concentration of intracellular cholesterol down-regulates the expression of the genes for HMG CoA reductase and the LDL receptor, preventing the overloading of cholesterol in many cells that cannot take up exogenous cholesterol independently of the LDL-receptor pathway[145,150] (see Chap. 120). By contrast, the uptake of modified LDL, triglyceride-rich lipoproteins, and their remnants by class A scavenger receptors (SR-A), LDL-receptor-related protein (LRP), and the VLDL-receptor, as well as the phagocytic uptake of cholesterol into macrophages, is not regulated by the intracellular cholesterol concentration.[151,162] Increasing levels of unesterified cholesterol in the plasma membrane stimulate esterification of cholesterol by ACAT in the ER.[151,153] Although most of the esterified cholesterol is *de novo* synthesized, some is of lysosomal origin and transferred to the ER either directly or indirectly via the plasma membrane. The transfer of cholesterol from the plasma membrane to the ER depends on an intact cytoskeleton and is blocked by progesterone.[133,134,164–167] Cholesteryl esters formed by ACAT appear as cytosolic lipid droplets, which give lipid-laden macrophages their foamy appearance.[153] Cytosolic cholesteryl esters can be hydrolyzed by neutral cholesteryl ester hydrolase (NCEH), which is activated by a cAMP-dependent protein kinase A.[168,169] Cholesterol released by NCEH is transferred to the cell membrane where it can be transported to the ER for reesterification by ACAT.[133,134,153] This cycle of cholesterol and cholesteryl esters between ACAT and NCEH is interrupted by the presence of extracellular cholesterol acceptors, such as HDL, which cause cholesterol efflux.[170,171]

Cholesterol Efflux

Cholesterol efflux from cells is a central step in the regulation of the cellular cholesterol homeostasis and the result of unspecific and passive as well as specific and active processes (Fig. 122-3).[71,82,137,172,173]

Protein-free phospholipid vesicles, synthetic cyclodextrins, and trypsinized HDL mediate a slow and unsaturable cholesterol efflux from all cell types investigated thus far.[137,173–181] This form of cholesterol efflux is not prevented by partial proteolysis of plasma

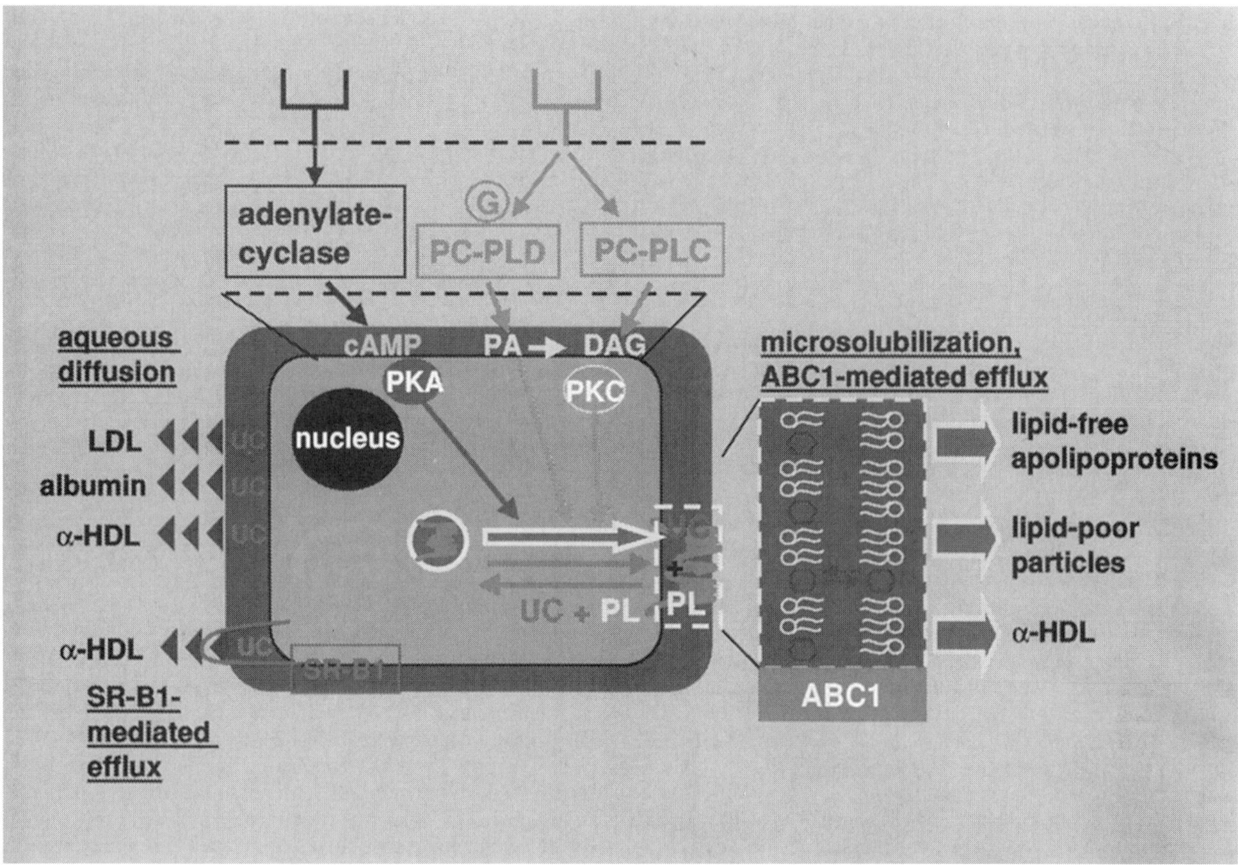

Fig. 122-3 Regulation of cholesterol efflux from cells. Cholesterol efflux by aqueous diffusion onto lipid-rich lipoproteins, albumin, phospholipid vesicles, or cyclodextrins is slow and not inhibited by brefeldin A or proteolysis of cells. Expression of SR-BI can facilitate this process. Efflux by lipid-free apolipoproteins or lipid-poor particles is fast and sensitive to proteolysis or treatment of cells with brefeldin A. It is defective in Tangier cells and therefore depends on ABC1. The intracellular mobilization of cholesterol for specific efflux appears to involve a signal transduction process.

membranes or by preincubation of cells with inhibitors of intracellular vesicular transport such as brefeldin A.[58,182,183] It does not involve specific interactions with cell-surface receptors or the specific activation of cellular transport processes, but simply reflects aqueous diffusion of cholesterol out of the plasma membrane onto acceptor molecules.[137,173] Although the loss in cholesterol from the plasma membrane can be replenished, this form of cholesterol efflux has little effect in depleting cells of intracellularly stored cholesteryl esters.[170,173,183–185]

By contrast, lipid-free apolipoproteins A-I, A-II, A-IV, Cs, and E, as well as amphipathic synthetic peptides without sequence homology to these apolipoproteins, cause an efflux of both phospholipids and cholesterol, which is fast, saturable, unidirectional, independent of LCAT, and efficient in reducing the content of cytosolic cholesteryl esters.[58,71,82,103,104,106,172,183–185] Phospholipid efflux appears to precede cholesterol efflux.[106] As a result, apolipoprotein-mediated lipid efflux lipidates apolipoproteins, producing HDL-like lipoproteins with electrophoretic pre-β- and pre-α-mobilities.[103–105,107] Because two-dimensional PAGGE does not readily separate lipid-free apo A-I and lipid-poor pre-β-LpA-I, it is not possible to say whether pre-β-LpA-I functions like lipid-free apolipoproteins, that is, induces cholesterol efflux, or if this particle is itself the primary product of apo A-I-induced lipid efflux.[68,70,82] Similarly LpA-IV-1 and γ-LpE appear to be immediate precursors or products of the lipid efflux induced by apo A-IV and apo E, respectively.[74,75,77,82]

Apolipoprotein-mediated lipid efflux involves nonspecific desorption of plasma membrane lipids, that is, microsolubilization, and specific interactions with plasma membrane proteins.[174] It is cell-specific and only takes place in growth-arrested and cholesterol-enriched cells.[82,104] Lipid-free apolipoproteins remove phospholipids and cholesterol from normal human skin fibroblasts, macrophages, and smooth-muscle-cell-derived foam cells,[58,71,82,103,104,106,172,183–186] but not from erythrocytes, native smooth muscle cells of various species, and fibroblasts of Tangier disease patients.[58,186–189] Moreover, lipid-free apolipoprotein mediated cholesterol efflux is completely suppressed by low temperature, by partial proteolysis of cell membranes, and by treatment of cells with monensin or brefeldin A which interfere with the regular function of the Golgi apparatus and with intracellular vesicular transport.[58,142,148,183] It has been suggested that lipid-free apolipoproteins and pre-β_1-LpA-I specifically release cholesterol which is located in caveolae.[134,146] Activation of protein kinase C (PKC) enhances and inhibition of PKC suppresses apolipoprotein-mediated cholesterol efflux.[186,190–192] Cyclic AMP (cAMP) was also found to increase apolipoprotein-induced cholesterol efflux from two mouse macrophage cell lines.[193–195] In RAW264 cells this was associated with internalization and resecretion of apo A-I.[193] For these reasons and because apo A-I binds to cell membrane proteins and induces the generation of the PKC-activator diacylglycerol, it has been hypothesized that apo A-I binds to a signal-transducing cell-surface receptor, and that this binding facilitates the translocation of cholesterol from intracellular compartments to the plasma membrane.[82,172,196–199] The nature of this receptor is unknown. Because both cholesterol efflux from cells and the ATP binding cassette transporter 1 (ABC1) are defective in Tangier disease, it is likely that ABC1 plays an important role in apolipoprotein-mediated efflux.[200–205] In support of this, apo A-I-mediated cholesterol efflux was severely decreased by inhibition of ABC1 with either antisense oligonucleotides or pharmacologic compounds (4,4-diisothiocyanostilbene-2,2-disulfonic acid or sulfobromophthalein) and increased by overexpression of ABC1.[203]

Native and reconstituted lipid-rich HDL induce both specific and nonspecific forms of cholesterol efflux. Partial proteolysis of either HDL or cells does not fully prevent HDL-mediated cholesterol efflux, which is slow, unsaturable, and bidirectional, and thus appears to occur by aqueous diffusion.[71,82,136,172,173,181] Esterification of the released cholesterol by LCAT prevents the rediffusion of cholesterol from HDL back to the plasma membrane, and thus enhances net cholesterol efflux.[206] Expression of SR-BI increases HDL-mediated cholesterol efflux.[207] Binding of HDL to SR-BI appears to reorganize the lipid organization in the plasma membrane and to facilitate the bidirectional flux between HDL and plasma membrane.[208] The net movement of cholesterol appears to depend on the relative activities of extracellular lipid transfer enzymes (LCAT, PLTP, CETP) and intracellular enzymes which metabolize cholesterol (e.g., ACAT).[173]

HDL-mediated cholesterol efflux also shares some properties of lipid-free apolipoprotein-mediated cholesterol efflux. In the presence of HDL, intracellularly stored cholesteryl esters are reduced.[170,171,194,195] After incubation of lipid-enriched cells with brefeldin A or the PKC inhibitor sphingosine, HDL-mediated cholesterol efflux is reduced by about 50 percent.[58,142,148,191] Both native and reconstituted HDL elicit various signal transduction pathways that may activate intracellular lipid transfer processes.[186,190–192,209–217] HDL induces the hydrolysis of phosphatidylcholine (PC) and phosphatidylinositol (PI) by phospholipases C and D, and thereby the generation of diacylglycerol (DAG), phosphatidic acid (PA), and inositolphosphates (IP). DAG activates PKC, which was shown to stimulate the translocation of newly synthesized cholesterol to the plasma membrane as well as cholesterol efflux.[190,192,209,212,214] In macrophages, HDL increases the concentration of cAMP, resulting in activation of protein kinase A, which may activate the hydrolysis of cytosolic cholesteryl esters by NCEH.[169,218–221] It is not known whether these specific effects of HDL on cellular cholesterol metabolism are induced by the intact particle or by apolipoproteins that have dissociated during the incubation with cells.

Another controversial mechanism of HDL-mediated cholesterol efflux is retroendocytosis. After uptake into clathrin-coated endosomes, it is postulated that HDL are directed into a nonlysosomal route and enriched with lipids for final resecretion.[193,222,223]

CLINICAL FINDINGS AND MORPHOLOGICAL CORRELATES

In addition to the classic findings of abnormal tonsils and peripheral neuropathy, the clinical expression of Tangier disease is variable. Table 122-2 summarizes the frequency of clinical symptoms in 68 Tangier patients.[7–61] The symptoms of Tangier disease patients result from cholesteryl ester deposition in many organs, which are frequently part of the reticuloendothelial system (RES). Cells other than histiocytes accumulating cholesteryl esters in Tangier disease include fibroblasts of the cornea, melanocytes, Schwann cells, neurons, and nonvascular smooth muscle cells (Table 122-3).

Histiocytic Manifestations

Morphologically, Tangier histiocytes appear as foam cells that contain sudanophilic lipid droplets and occasionally as crystalline material.[1–7,14,18] Most of the droplets within the cytoplasm are not bound by membranes and consist of deposits of cholesteryl esters (mostly cholesteryl oleate) outside of lysosomes (Fig. 122-4). This is in contrast to lipid storage diseases that result from deficiencies of lysosomal enzymes, such as Wolman disease and Niemann-Pick disease, where cholesteryl esters accumulate within lysosomes (see Chaps. 142 to 146).

Table 122-2 Frequencies of Clinical Symptoms and Findings in Tangier Disease

	Number of cases		
Symptoms	Present	Absent	Not examined/ not reported
Yellowish tonsils or pharyngeal plaques	44	6	18
Peripheral neuropathy	36	20	12
Splenomegaly	33	17	18
Abnormal rectal mucosa	28	4	36
Hepatomegaly	19	24	25
Corneal opacities	15	28	25
Coronary heart disease	15	33	20
Thrombocytopenia	14	1	44
Anemia and/or stomatocytes	9	6	53
Lymphadenopathy	6	26	36
Unexplained diarrhea	5	1	62

The data were obtained from the case reports of 68 patients with Tangier disease whose ages range between 2 and 72 years. For details see references 7 to 61.

Tonsils. The unique appearance of the tonsils makes it possible to diagnose Tangier disease by the examination of the oropharynx. The tonsils are large and lobulated and have a distinctive orange or yellowish-gray color that contrasts with the normal red mucosa. Microscopic examination of tonsil tissue reveals the presence of large foam cells located predominantly in the fibrous septa, but also in small numbers within the follicles.[18] When the tonsils have been removed, small plaques or tags of mucosa having the same appearance will usually reveal the diagnosis. Several patients have had a history of recurrent "tonsillitis" or symptoms of obstruction, which have led to tonsillectomy.[1–6]

Spleen. Splenomegaly is accompanied by mild thrombocytopenia and reticulocytosis in many patients. Splenectomy was deemed necessary in some patients because of progressive anemia and thrombocytopenia. Upon splenectomy or autopsy of deceased Tangier patients, the spleen was speckled yellow. The cells of the excised spleen were filled with intracytoplasmic lipid droplets and scattered clusters of cholesterol crystals.[8]

Lymph Nodes and Thymus. In most Tangier patients, lymphadenopathy is not clinically apparent, but both normal-sized and enlarged lymph nodes exhibit bright-yellow streaks and morphologic characteristics similar to those present in the tonsils, and the cholesteryl ester content is increased by a factor of 100 compared to control lymph nodes.[5–7,12–14] In the thymus, large pale macrophages with extensive lipid deposits almost completely replace the lobulated cortex.[5–7,224]

Table 122-3 Cholesteryl Ester Storage in Tangier Disease

Cell type	Affected organs
Histiocytes	Tonsils, mucosa of the small and large intestine, bone marrow, renal pelvis and ureters, gallbladder and bile ducts, lymph nodes, thymus
Schwann cells	Nerves of skin and colon submucosa
Neurons	Spinal ganglion, sacral spinal cord
Nevus cells	Pigmented nevi
Smooth muscle cells	Muscularis mucosae, peritoneal soft tissue (inguinal herniae)
Fibroblasts	Subepidermis, gingiva, cornea, colonic mucosa

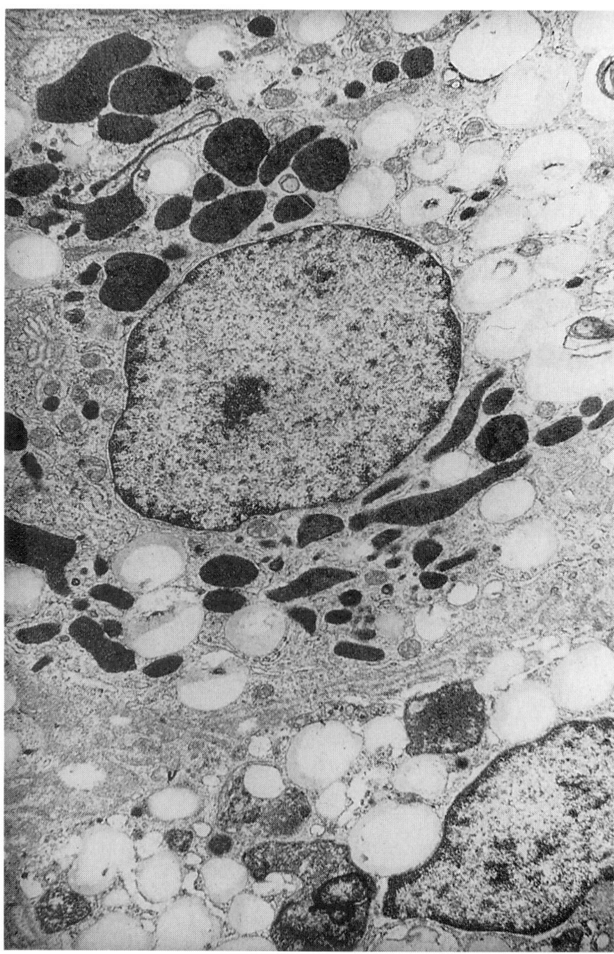

Fig. 122-4 Electron micrograph of a histiocytic foam cell. Note the presence of multiple membrane-free cytosolic lipid-droplets.

Liver and Bile Tract. Enlargement of the liver has been noted in approximately one-third of the patients, but it may be a transient finding.[7,11,12,17,18,21,22,24,29,30,36,39,42,43,49,51,59] Hepatic parenchymal cells are usually not infiltrated with lipids. Liver function tests are usually normal[8,12] and histologic examination of the liver reveals only occasional clusters of intralobular foam cells identified as histiocytes. Moderate numbers of foam cells have also been identified in the gallbladder mucosa.[12] In one homozygous Tangier patient, reduced cholesterol concentration in bile was reported, but the pattern of glyco- and tauro-conjugated bile acids was normal.[31]

Intestinal Mucosa. Bowel habits and food tolerance are usually normal in Tangier disease, although complaints of frequent stools, intermittent diarrhea, and abdominal pain have been reported.[22,30,48] The gross appearance of the rectal mucosa is abnormal in every case examined and may be the most reliable physical finding when palatine and pharyngeal tonsils have been previously completely removed (Fig. 122-5). Proctoscopy of Tangier disease patients revealed a pale mucosa studded with 1- to 2-mm discrete orange-brown spots.[1–6,8–10,12,13,21,22,27,38,45,47,48,52,59] Coloscopy of Tangier disease patients showed that the entire colonic mucosa has a cobblestone-like appearance due to an irregular yellow-orange discoloration and the presence of numerous dark, brown or violet dots 1 to 3 mm in diameter.[51,52] Biopsy of the rectal mucosa or colonic polyps will reveal foamy histiocytes throughout the mucosa and submucosa. The gastric mucosa is covered with yellowish dots.[51] The ileum and colon also have numerous mucosal elevations, but the jejunum is grossly normal.[7] The jejunal mucosal villi are free of foam cells, the latter being found only below the muscularis mucosae.[18] Radiologic examination of the gastrointestinal tract does not reveal any diagnostic features, although mild uniform thickening of the mucosal folds has been observed throughout the jejunum. The pattern is not unlike that found in amyloidosis, giardiasis, and intestinal lymphangiectasia.[9]

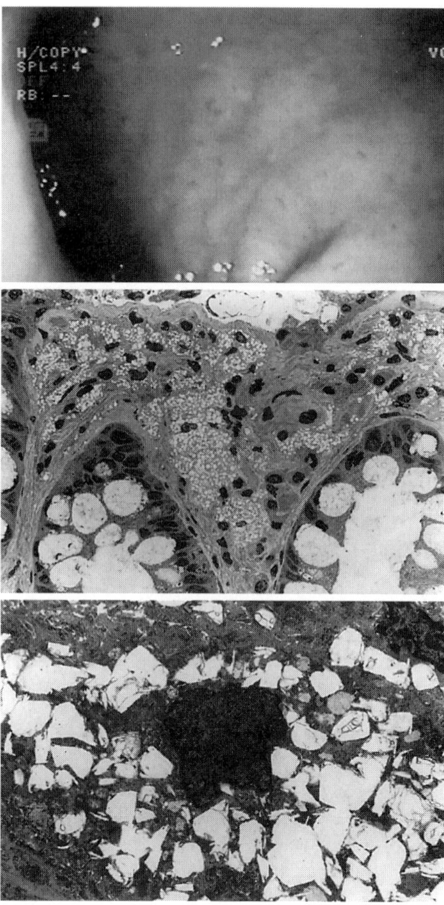

Fig. 122-5 Rectal mucosa in a patient with Tangier disease. The endoscopic view of the rectal mucosa (*top*) shows characteristic orange-brown colored focal depositions. Upon light microscopy (×63 magnification) the lamina propria is found to contain many foamy macrophages with regular vacuoles (middle). The foamy histiocytes of the rectal mucosa are filled with slightly angular or irregular lipid deposits (*bottom*: ultrathin section at ×10,000 magnification) (*Pictures are used by courtesy and permission of Drs. J.J.P. Kastelein and H.O.F. Molhuizen, Amsterdam, The Netherlands.*)

Bone Marrow. Needle biopsies of the bone marrow from the iliac spine as well as aspiration biopsies from the sternal bone marrow from 9 of 13 patients examined[7,8,10,12,18] contained numerous foam cells full of lipid droplets in the cytoplasm. These foam cells appeared smaller than those observed in other lipid storage diseases.

Other Histiocytic Lipid Depositions. Focal collections of foamy histiocytes have been reported in otherwise normal skin,[7,11,12,18,35] ureters, renal pelvises, tunica albuginea of testicles, mitral and tricuspid valves,[18] aorta, coronary arteries, and the pulmonary artery.[47,48]

Neuropathy

Peripheral neuropathy is the most frequent symptom that leads to the identification of adult patients with Tangier disease. Clinical symptoms include weakness, paresthesias, dysesthesias, increased sweating, diplopia, reduced strength, ptosis, ocular muscle palsies, diminished or absent deep-tendon reflexes, muscle atrophy, and loss of pain and temperature sensation. The clinical sequelae of

Table 122-4 Differentiation of Neuropathy in Tangier Disease

Type	Multiple mononeuropathy	Syringomyelia-like syndrome
Number of case reports	17	10
References	7–9, 12, 18–20, 28, 31, 36, 37, 42, 44, 49, 50, 52, 54	10, 13, 21, 23, 30, 34, 35, 38, 46, 57
	Morphologic presentation	
	Demyelination, remyelination	Axonal degeneration
Early fiber loss	Unmyelinated fibers	Small myelinated and unmyelinated fibers
Lipid inclusions	Remak cells	All cells
	Clinical presentation	
Age of onset (years)	8–25	20–50
Motor symptoms	Weakness of muscles of the limbs or face, isolated or asymmetric deficits	Weakness and atrophy of muscles of the face and upper limb
Sensory symptoms	Sensory losses of the limbs or face, asymmetric, distal, not dissociated, all modalities	Facio-brachial sensory losses, asymmetric, central initially dissociated (impaired thermo- and nociception), later all modalities
Other symptoms		Hyperhydrosis, pain
Course	Mostly transient, sometimes subclinical, sometimes permanent	Progressive
Prognosis	Benign	Debilitating
	Electrophysiology	
Denervation	+	+++
Sensory potential amplitude	Normal	Unrecordable
Latency	Prolonged	Normal

these symptoms may be subtle or overt, transient or permanent. At least two prototypes and some atypical forms of neuropathy in Tangier disease have been reported, which interestingly have never been found coexisting within one patient (Table 122-4).[1–6,30,34]

Multifocal Remitting Demyelinating Neuropathy. The multifocal remitting demyelinating neuropathy is often asymptomatic and careful examination may be necessary to demonstrate the abnormalities. In the cases examined, nerve conduction velocities were normal and only distal latency was occasionally prolonged. If clinically manifest, the symptoms were either mononeuropathic or asymmetrically polyneuropathic and sometimes included isolated cranial nerve deficits.[7–9,12,18–20,28,31,36,37,42,44,49,50,52,54] The symptoms were frequently transient or relapsing. The course of this type of Tangier neuropathy is benign.[1–6,26] Morphologically, the mononeuropathic or asymmetric form was characterized by de- and remyelination of peripheral nerves without evidence of axonal degeneration. Lipid vacuoles were almost confined to Schwann cells.[30]

Syringomyelia-like Type. The syringomyelia-like type is slowly progressing but presents with early loss of pain and thermal sensation, atrophy, and paresis especially in the face and the distal parts of the upper limbs. Sensory loss may, however, progress downward to the trunk and to the lower limbs, and thus lead to global anesthesia.[10,13,21,23,30,34,35,38,46,57] Electrophysiological examination reveals prolonged distal motor latencies and slow conduction velocities.[10,23,34,35] In most cases, the syringomyelia-like syndrome in Tangier disease had an early onset and was progressive and debilitating. Morphologically, the syringomyelia-like Tangier neuropathy is characterized by axonal degeneration of small myelinated and unmyelinated fibers, and small dorsal-root ganglion cells.[16,23,30,38,46] This may explain the preferential loss of thermo- and nociception. The involvement of dorsal root ganglions may also explain the spontaneous pain in the upper limbs, which has been reported for some Tangier patients with syringomyelia-like neuropathy.[13,35,57] A spinal ganglion and the sacral spinal cord of a Tangier patient investigated at autopsy showed a motor neuron loss. Numerous neurons, but not glial cells, contained membrane-bound lipid inclusions presumably representing secondary lysosomes or residual bodies. The authors suggested that the syringomyelia-like neuropathy in Tangier disease may represent a lysosomal storage disorder preferentially affecting small dorsal root ganglion cells.[34] Lipid storage was not found in neurons or macrophages of the central nervous system of another patient who was examined postmortem.[14]

Three Tangier patients older than 45 years presented with atypical symmetric sensomotor polyneuropathy of the distal lower limbs which had a rapid progression and led to premature retirement from work. Nerve conduction velocities have been normal. Biopsies of the sural nerve have shown the abundance of abnormal nonmembrane-bound vacuoles in Schwann cells mostly in unmyelinated fibers, and some endoneurial fibroblasts, macrophages, and perineurial cells. Demyelination and remyelination coexisted with axonal degeneration.[26,225] Lipid accumulation was also found in cells of the vasa nervorum, so that the authors speculated that this may contribute to the pathogenesis of neuropathy in Tangier disease.[50]

Abnormal lipid deposition in Schwann cells is proposed to be responsible for the peripheral neuropathy. The origin of lipid deposition in Schwann cells and the resulting neuropathy in Tangier disease is as yet unsolved. Recent studies demonstrate that subsequent to injury, apolipoproteins A-I, A-IV, D, and E accumulate in remyelinating peripheral nerves.[226–228] Apo D and apo E were synthesized in the remyelinating nerve by neurons and by neurolemmal and fibroblastic cells, whereas apo A-I and apo A-IV apparently entered the nerve from the plasma.[227] In addition, apo E has been reported to regulate neural growth.[229–231] Because neuropathy does not occur in apo A-I deficiencies, LCAT deficiency, and fish eye disease, the neuropathy in Tangier disease is unlikely to be due to deficiencies of HDL and apo A-I (see Chaps. 118 and 121). Because lipid metabolism is disturbed in Tangier macrophages and fibroblasts, and because both cell types are involved in the myelination of peripheral nerves, it is most likely that the neuropathy is a primary consequence of the disturbed lipid metabolism in endoneurial and perineurial cells of peripheral nerves.[232]

Arteriosclerosis

In view of the important role of low HDL cholesterol as a risk factor for myocardial infarction,[233] a dramatically increased prevalence of premature atherosclerotic vessel diseases is expected in homozygotes for Tangier disease. In seven Tangier disease patients, coronary heart disease became manifest before age 50.[11,27,36,43,49,54,60] Moreover, in a review of 54 Tangier patients, Serfaty-Lacrosniere et al. reported atherosclerotic vessel disease in 20 percent of the Tangier disease subjects as compared to 5 percent in a population of 3130 controls.[54] In the age range of 35 to 65 years, 44 percent of 25 male Tangier patients, but only 6.5 percent of 1533 controls, had cardiovascular disease. These data suggest that Tangier disease increases the risk for atherosclerosis. Most of these patients, however, had additional risk factors including diabetes mellitus, hypertension, smoking, and obesity. It thus appears that, as in patients with apo A-I deficiency or LCAT-deficiency, the absence of HDL facilitates the manifestation of cardiovascular disease in the presence of additional cardiovascular risk factors[234,235] (see Chaps. 118 and 121). Because Tangier patients frequently have low LDL cholesterol, one important risk factor is missing in Tangier patients *per se*. In contrast to these associations of Tangier disease with premature atherosclerosis, there are also case reports of Tangier patients older than 60 years who did not present with clinical symptoms of coronary heart disease.[13,36,54] In one 60-year-old Tangier patient without any additional risk factors, coronary angiography and intravasal ultrasonography did not identify any atherosclerotic lesion; instead, they were indicative of a retarded coronary sclerosis.[236] In conclusion, Tangier disease appears to cause a moderate increase in cardiovascular risk, which becomes relevant especially in the presence of additional risk factors. Alternatively, it has been suggested that the genetic defect determines the cardiovascular risk of Tangier patients.[201]

Ocular Abnormalities

Ocular abnormalities in Tangier disease include corneal opacifications, ectropion, retinal pigment mottling in the macula and/or periphery, and diplopia on lateral gaze.[36,56,65] The most frequent ocular manifestations in Tangier disease are corneal infiltrations, either diffuse or dot-like, which do not impair vision.[8,9,12,22,23,29,30,36,44,56,57,59] No corneal opacities have been reported for patients younger than 20 years. In most cases, corneal infiltrations of Tangier patients were evident only on slit-lamp examination. In some patients older than 40 years, corneal opacifications were visible on physical examination. However, even in these exceptional cases, corneal opacities were much less intense than in patients with fish eye disease, familial LCAT deficiency, and some forms of apo A-I deficiency (see Chaps. 118 and 121). Transmission electron microscopy of the cornea from a deceased Tangier patient revealed membranous myelin-like lamellar bodies in the stroma. Biochemical analysis demonstrated the enrichment with phospholipids and cholesteryl esters. This is in contrast to the cornea of patients with LCAT deficiency or fish eye disease, which is enriched with unesterified cholesterol.[56,237,238]

Circulating Blood Cells

The most frequent anomaly of peripheral blood in Tangier disease is thrombocytopenia with platelet counts ranging between 30,000 and 120,000 cells per microliter.[12,14,17,22,29,36,37,39,42,48,54,56,59,60] In one patient with Tangier disease the bleeding time was prolonged but was corrected by 1-deamino-8-D-arginine vasopressin, which also indicated a qualitative platelet dysfunction.[239]

Hemolysis and hemolytic anemia have been observed in four Tangier patients. In three Tangier patients, stomatocytes have been found.[19,43,44] This erythrocyte anomaly is characterized by deep membrane invaginations. It has also been found in some patients with apo A-I deficiency,[234] and thus may be secondary to HDL deficiency. The altered erythrocyte morphology may be explained by the decrease of cholesterol and increase of phosphatidylcholine in the membranes of Tangier erythrocytes, because red blood cells underwent stomatocytic transformation when they were depleted of cholesterol in vitro.[43] The reduced cholesterol/phosphatidylcholine ratio in Tangier erythrocytes has also been held responsible for their functional changes: The osmotic resistance was decreased, the dimyristoylphosphatidylcholine-induced vesiculation was delayed, and the anion transport capacity, which is mediated by the anion exchange protein band 3, was impaired. Sodium and potassium fluxes were normal in Tangier erythrocytes. Based on the decreased cholesterol/phosphatidylcholine ratio, stomatocytes in Tangier disease are a counterpart of the echinoacanthocytes present in abetalipoproteinemia (see Chap. 115).[43]

Another peripheral blood anomaly in Tangier disease is a reduced number of circulating monocytes.

PLASMA LIPOPROTEIN METABOLISM IN TANGIER DISEASE

Lipids

Tangier homozygotes have a low plasma concentration of total cholesterol (Table 122-5). The percentage of esterified cholesterol is normal. The plasma triglyceride levels vary considerably in Tangier disease, depending on the diet. Especially in adult Tangier patients, triglycerides are frequently elevated to 300 to 400 mg/dl (Table 122-5). Plasma phospholipid concentrations in Tangier disease are decreased to 30 to 50 percent of normal values. The serum concentration of glycosphingolipids is slightly reduced, and the sphingomyelin to phosphatidylcholine ratio is decreased.[1–6]

Lipoproteins

Lipoprotein electrophoresis of Tangier plasma is characterized by the absence of α-migrating lipoproteins, as well as the loss of a distinct pre-β band and the presence of a diffuse β-pre-β band, which is frequently the only lipoprotein band to be visualized by lipid staining (Fig. 122-1*B*). Quantification of lipids in fractions obtained by sequential or density-gradient ultracentrifugation, as well as gel filtration, confirms the virtual absence of HDL.[1–6,22,240–242]

Chylomicrons. Fasting chylomicronemia is often observed in homozygotes for Tangier disease and may be the result of reduced

Table 122-5 Mean Values, Medians, and Ranges of Serum Concentrations of Lipids, HDL Cholesterol, and Apolipoproteins in Tangier Disease Patients

	mean	median	minimum	maximum
	(mg/dl)			
Total cholesterol (N = 62)	78	73	18	177
Triglycerides (N = 59)	210	175	40	580
HDL cholesterol (N = 57)	2.5	1.5	0	9
Apolipoprotein A-I (N = 21)	4	2.5	0.5	9
Apolipoprotein A-II (N = 12)	3.5	2.5	1.5	8
Apolipoprotein B (N = 9)	86	98	24	140

The data were obtained from the case reports of 62 patients. For details see references 7 to 61. To convert into μM, divide cholesterol and HDL cholesterol by 38.6 and triglycerides by 86.9.

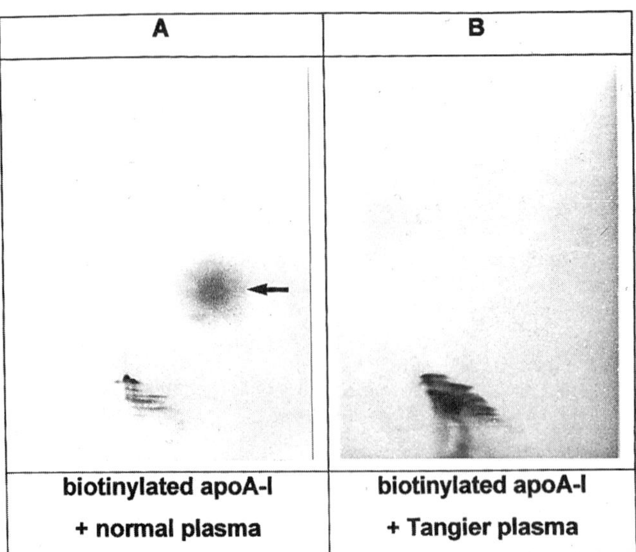

Fig. 122-6 Conversion of exogenous biotinylated apo A-I by plasmas from a normolipidemic proband (*A*) and a patient with Tangier disease (*B*). Note the generation of a larger particle resembling α-LpA-I by normal plasma (*A: arrow*) but not by Tangier plasma. For details of the method see reference 60.

lipoprotein lipase (LPL) activity in these patients and/or impaired substrate properties of Tangier chylomicrons. Bizarre chylomicron remnants were observed in a Tangier patient following splenectomy. The gross lipid and lipoprotein compositions of the chylomicrons are normal.[1–6,224]

Very-Low-Density Lipoproteins (VLDL). Tangier VLDL differ from normal VLDL by their reduced mobility when analyzed by lipoprotein electrophoresis, a relatively high concentration of apo A-II and C apolipoproteins,[243] and a decreased reactivity towards LPL.[244] Immunoaffinity chromatography of Tangier VLDL separated a lipoprotein with apo A-II (LpA-II:B) from another without apo A-II.[245] According to the apo B content, LpA-II:B accounted for 90 percent of VLDL. LpA-II:B was a poor substrate for LPL, whereas the apo A-II-free VLDL of Tangier patients reacted normally with LPL.[245] These findings may partly explain the hypertriglyceridemia seen in these patients.

Low-Density Lipoproteins (LDL). Tangier LDL contain 27 percent triglycerides by mass compared to 7 percent in normal LDL. A monoclonal anti-apo B antibody reacted with an epitope on the surface of Tangier LDL, which otherwise is present only in normal VLDL and lacking in normal LDL. Both the enrichment in triglycerides and the presence of an apo B epitope normally observed in triglyceride-rich lipoproteins may result from the missing cholesteryl ester/triglycerides exchange between LDL and HDL. Another difference compared to normal LDL is the presence of small amounts of apo A-II in Tangier LDL.[45,246]

High-Density Lipoproteins (HDL). The plasma concentration of HDL-C in Tangier homozygotes is reduced to virtually zero due to the absence of mature α-HDL (Figs. 122-1*C* and *F*).[1–8,60,247] Residual amounts of HDL-like particles in Tangier plasma were analyzed by electron microscopy, immunoaffinity chromatography, gel filtration, and electrophoresis.[22,49,60,240–242,247–249] In general, these particles are small, lipid-poor, and contain particles with apo A-I, apo A-II, apo A-IV, or apo E as single apolipoproteins, which have been termed pre-β-LpA-I, LpA-II, LpA-IV, and γ-LpE, respectively.[49,60,240–242,247–249] These particles were shown to release cholesterol from cells and may explain the significant 50 to 70 percent residual cholesterol efflux capacity of Tangier plasma despite virtual HDL deficiency.[49,247] In contrast to plasmas of patients with apo A-I-deficiency, LCAT-deficiency, or fish eye disease, plasma of Tangier patients cannot convert pre-β-LpA-I or exogenous lipid-free apo A-I into an α-migrating particle (Fig. 122-6).[60,249] Thus, the exclusive presence of apo A-I in pre-β-HDL together with the failure of Tangier plasma to convert exogenous apo A-I into α-HDL are specific biochemical hallmarks which distinguish Tangier disease from other familial HDL deficiency syndromes.[60]

Apolipoproteins

Apo A-I. In Tangier homozygotes the plasma concentration of apo A-I is reduced to approximately 1 to 3 percent of normal (Table 122-5).[1–3,22,246] Human apo A-I is synthesized in enterocytes and hepatocytes as a 267-amino-acid-long preproapolipoprotein (preproapo A-I) containing an 18-amino-acid prepeptide and a 6-amino-acid propeptide.[250–252] Isoelectric focusing of apo A-I in Tangier homozygotes reveals a relatively increased concentration of proapo A-I relative to mature apo A-I (Fig. 122-7).[253,254]

Apo A-II. In Tangier disease, the plasma concentration of apo A-II is severely reduced to 5 to 10 percent as compared to normal.[22,49,242,255] Characteristic features of Tangier disease are the presence of apo A-II in apo B-containing lipoproteins and the finding of apo A-II-containing lipoproteins that do not contain apo A-I.[246]

Other Apolipoproteins. In several Tangier patients, the plasma concentrations of apo C-I, C-II, C-III, D, and E were reduced.[255]

Enzymes and Transfer Proteins

Lipoprotein Lipase and Hepatic Lipase. Both reduced postheparin plasma activity of LPL and lower reactivity of Tangier VLDL as a substrate of LPL due to its abnormal apolipoprotein composition contribute to hypertriglyceridemia in Tangier patients.[45,244,245] Postheparin activity of HL was either elevated or normal in Tangier patients.[244]

Lecithin:Cholesterol Acyltransferase. In the plasma of Tangier patients, the ratio of cholesterol to cholesteryl esters as well as the rate of esterification of cholesterol either in VLDL and LDL or in endogenous lipoproteins (i.e., β-LCAT activity or endogenous

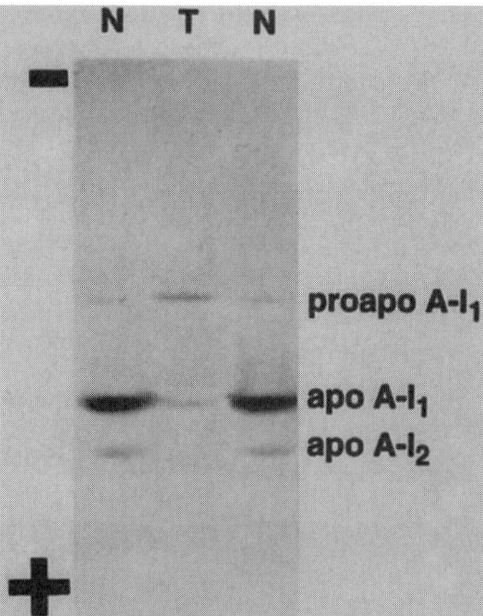

Fig. 122-7 Isoelectric focusing and immunoblotting of apo A-I isoproteins in plasma of a normal (N) and a Tangier plasma (T). Note the low concentration of proapo A-I relative to mature apo A-I in normal plasma (N) and the increased concentration of Tangier-proapo A-I relative to mature Tangier apo A-I (T).

cholesterol esterification rate; see Chap. 118) are approximately normal.[15,19,245,258–265] By contrast, the α-LCAT activity of Tangier plasma, that is, the rate of esterification of cholesterol in either exogenous HDL or artificial apo A-I-containing proteoliposomes (see Chap. 118), and LCAT enzyme mass concentration are reduced by 60 to 70 percent.[261,264,265] The parallel reduction of α-LCAT activity and LCAT mass is also observed in apo A-I deficiency[265–268] and reflects the absence of HDL or specific HDL subclasses, which apparently are necessary for the maintenance of normal LCAT plasma concentrations.[268,269] Cholesterol esterification in Tangier plasma takes place in apo A-I-free lipoproteins, which in both normal and Tangier plasma carry equal absolute amounts of LCAT.[95] In Tangier plasma, LCAT contained by apo A-I-free lipoproteins accounted for 95 percent of LCAT mass and 100 percent of LCAT activity compared to 26 ± 7 percent and 22 ± 11 percent, respectively, in normal plasma. Cholesterol esterified by LCAT in normal plasma has been reported to originate from LDL in normal plasma, but from both LDL and VLDL in Tangier plasma.[247,261,270]

Cholesterol Ester Transfer Protein. By contrast to the reduced CETP activity of plasmas from patients with familial LCAT deficiency and fish eye disease (see Chap. 118), Tangier plasma was reported to exhibit increased CETP activity.[271] This may reflect a secondary and adaptive mechanism rather than the cause of HDL deficiency in Tangier disease.

Phospholipid Transfer Proteins. The activity of PLTP in Tangier plasma, which has been quantified as the transfer of radiolabeled phospholipids from vesicles onto HDL, does not differ significantly from normal plasma.[60,115] By contrast, the transfer of glycerophospholipids from donor vesicles onto immobilized apo A-I or reconstituted HDL was significantly reduced by 50 percent in Tangier plasma compared to normal or apo A-I-deficient plasma.[115] In this assay, homogenates or cell culture media of Tangier fibroblasts also exhibited a reduced activity to transfer phospholipids onto apo A-I. Because maturation of HDL involves transfer of lipids onto apo A-I, it has been hypothesized that defective transfer of phospholipids from donor lipoproteins such as VLDL, or from cell membranes onto lipid-free apo A-I, prevents the conversion of lipid-poor HDL precursors into lipid-rich mature HDL, and thereby causes HDL deficiency.[115]

Metabolism of HDL, Apo A-I, and Apo A-II in Tangier Disease

Several kinetic studies using radiolabeled HDL, apo A-I, proapo A-I, and apo A-II have been performed to unravel whether HDL deficiency in Tangier patients is caused by decreased synthesis or enhanced catabolism of these apolipoproteins. Initial kinetic studies using radiolabeled normal HDL in Tangier patients revealed a markedly increased catabolism of apo A-I, apo A-II, and HDL in Tangier patients.[246] Also, in Tangier heterozygotes, radiolabeled HDL were more rapidly catabolized than in normal controls.[246] The increased catabolism persisted even after increasing the pool size of HDL by infusion of normal HDL into Tangier patients.[272,273] A more detailed crossover study compared the kinetics of mature apo A-I and apo A-II from Tangier and normal subjects in both normal subjects and Tangier patients, and observed that both normal and Tangier A-I and A-II apolipoproteins were more rapidly catabolized in the Tangier patients than in normal controls.[274,275] These studies established that the metabolic basis of Tangier disease is a rapid catabolism of apo A-I and HDL, rather than a defect in the biosynthesis of HDL apolipoproteins.

CELLULAR LIPID METABOLISM IN TANGIER DISEASE

The accumulation of cholesteryl esters in many reticuloendothelial tissues of Tangier patients probably results from a disorder of trafficking of lipids between cellular membranes.[276] In agreement with this, lysosomes of cultivated and acetyl-LDL loaded macrophages of some Tangier patients were characterized by the occurrence of two kinds of abnormal lysosomes, which are filled either with flocculent and fibrillar material (type I vacuoles) or with spiral or lamellar structures (type II vacuoles) (Fig. 122-8), and by the presence of a Golgi apparatus that is dilated and hyperplastic compared to control cells (Fig. 122-9).[277] These morphologic abnormalities have also been observed in cultivated skin fibroblasts of Tangier patients,[277] which are also characterized by anomalies in lipid efflux and signal transduction.

Cholesterol Efflux from Fibroblasts

Cholesterol and phospholipid efflux from Tangier fibroblasts were shown to be defective depending on the nature of the acceptor and on the labeling technique used.[58,82,189,203,212] Compared to control cells, growth-arrested and lipid-enriched Tangier fibroblasts regularly released cholesterol in the presence of cyclodextrins and phospholipid vesicles.[58] Lipid-free apolipoproteins A-I, A-II, A-IV, Cs, or E, or artificial amphipathic polypeptides, were reported to be completely defective in mediating efflux of cholesterol, phosphatidylcholine, or sphingomyelin from Tangier fibroblasts.[58,189] The cholesterol efflux defect was observed, irrespective of whether cholesterol was radiolabeled by incubating the cells with ^{14}C-mevalonate (i.e., during synthesis), by incubation with ^{3}H-cholesteryl ester containing LDL (i.e., via the endosomal-lysosomal pathway), or by equilibration with ^{3}H-cholesterol.[58,189] Moreover, analogues of cAMP stimulated apolipoprotein-mediated cholesterol efflux from normal fibroblasts, but not from Tangier cells.[203,278] In the presence of native or reconstituted HDL, cholesterol efflux from Tangier fibroblasts was reduced by approximately 50 percent, in some experiments, independent of the labeling technique,[58,189] in others at least if biosynthetic cholesterol was radiolabeled by incubation of cells with ^{14}C-mevalonate.[212,279] Although the specific results are not totally consistent, the combined data indicate that in Tangier cells the specific lipid efflux induced by lipid-free apolipoproteins and HDL is defective, whereas the nonspecific cholesterol desorption from the plasma membrane by HDL and apolipoprotein-free acceptor

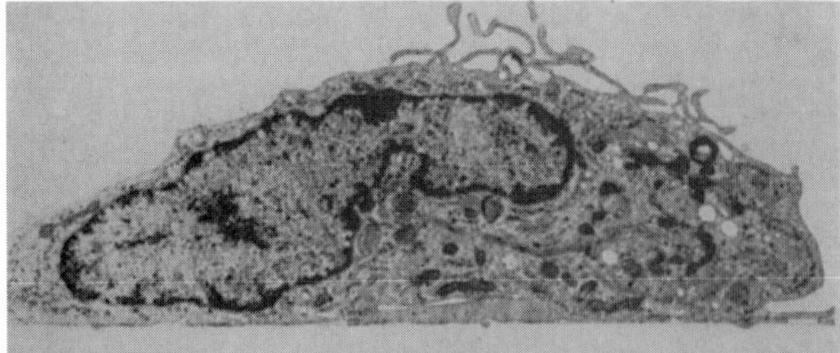

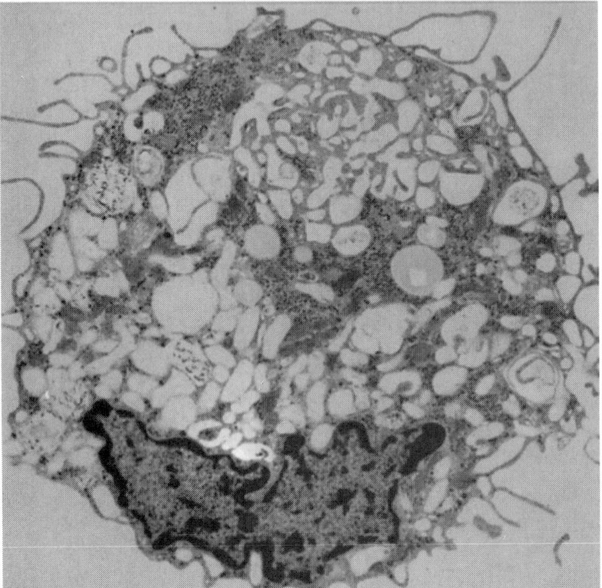

Fig. 122-8 Transmission electron photomicrographs of mononuclear phagocytes from a Tangier patient without (*top*) and with exposure to acetyl LDL. Note the appearance of two types of vacuoles in lipid-laded Tangier mononuclear phagocytes. Type I vacuoles appear to be filled with flocculent and fibrillar structures in a electron-lucent matrix, whereas type II vacuoles contain more electron-dense material. Transmission electron microscopy was performed after 24 h cultivation of mononuclear phagocytes from a normal donor in the presence of 70 μg/ml acetyl LDL at 37°C. (*Micrograph used by courtesy and permission of Dr. H. Robenek, Münster, Germany.*)

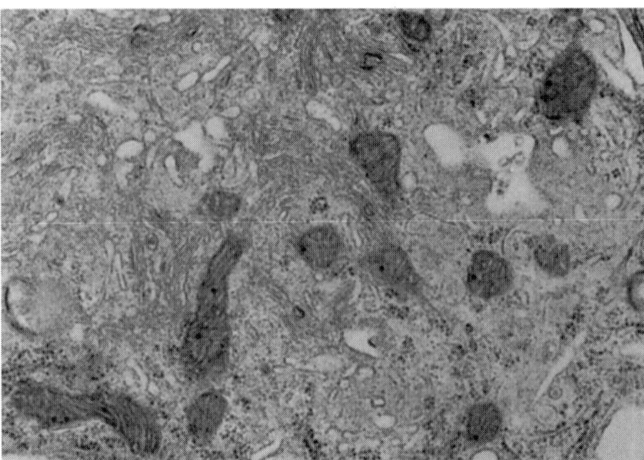

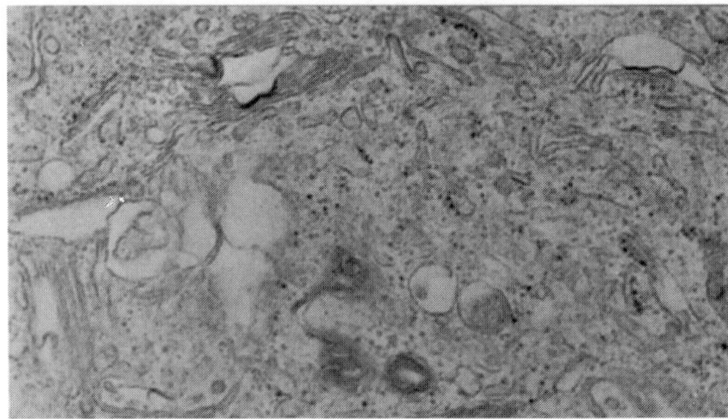

Fig. 122-9 Transmission electron photomicrograph of control (*top*) and Tangier mononuclear phagocytes (*bottom*) under normal culture conditions. In control cells (*top*), the cisternae of Golgi apparatuses are small. In macrophages of Tangier patients (*bottom*), the Golgi apparatuses are dilated and hyperplastic. Similar anomalies of the Golgi apparatus are seen in cultured skin fibroblasts of Tangier disease patients.[277] (*Micrographs used by permission of Dr. H. Robenek, Münster, Germany.*)

molecules is intact.[82] Interestingly, brefeldin A, an inhibitor of the secretory vesicular lipid transport, completely inhibits apolipoprotein-mediated lipid efflux and partially inhibits HDL induced cholesterol efflux from normal fibroblasts, but does not further impair HDL-induced cholesterol efflux from Tangier fibroblasts.[58,143,149,183] Thus, the cholesterol efflux defect in Tangier disease appears to affect the transport between the Golgi apparatus and the plasma membrane. Such a defect would also explain the finding of a hyperplastic Golgi apparatus in lipid-loaded Tangier cells (Fig. 122-9).[277] As the result of this defect, cholesteryl estersin Tangier fibroblasts are resistant to apolipoprotein-induced hydrolysis and, to a lesser extent, to HDL-induced hydrolysis.[58,189]

Signal Transduction in Tangier Fibroblasts

Further evidence for defective translocation of cholesterol from an intracellular pool to the plasma membrane is provided by experiments on HDL-induced signal transduction in normal and Tangier cells.[211–213] Both HDL-induced generation of diacylglycerol (DAG) and inositol phosphates from phosphatidylinositol (PI) phosphates by a PI-specific phospholipase C (PI-PLC) and HDL-induced generation of phosphatidic acid (PA) from phosphatidylcholine (PC) by a phospholipase D (PLD) were reduced in Tangier fibroblasts.[211,213] HDL-induced generation of DAG from PC by PC-PLC, by contrast, was enhanced.[213] Similar effects were seen when Tangier cells were incubated with endothelin instead of HDL as the agonist, suggesting a more general disturbance in Tangier disease.[213] A Tangier-like cholesterol efflux defect was induced by incubation with pertussis toxin, which ADP-ribosylates and inactivates G_i and G_o proteins, thereby disrupting the action of phospholipases.[211] Pharmacologic inhibition of DAG and PA formation markedly reduced HDL-mediated cholesterol efflux from normal cells but had a less pronounced effect on Tangier cells. Conversely, both coincubation of Tangier fibroblasts with a DAG analogue as well as the pharmacologic increase of PA by inhibition of its hydrolysis attenuated the cholesterol efflux defect in Tangier fibroblasts.[212,213] From these data it was concluded that a G-protein-dependent process upstream from protein kinase C (PKC), which is involved in the translocation of cholesterol from intracellular compartments to the plasma membrane, is not properly activated in Tangier cells.[213] Defective binding of apo A-I to Tangier cells was ruled out as the basis of the disturbances in signal transduction and cholesterol efflux by one laboratory,[58] but not by another.[189]

FINDINGS IN HETEROZYGOTES

Heterozygotes for Tangier disease have no symptoms; in particular, tonsil anomalies and neuropathy are not found. Although foam cells were present in the bone marrow of three of six obligate heterozygotes, and lipid-laden histiocytes were identified in rectal biopsies of several heterozygous patients, it is doubtful that these changes effectively identify heterozygotes.[280] Several obligate heterozygotes older than 45 years were reported to have symptoms of coronary heart disease.[54,240,281]

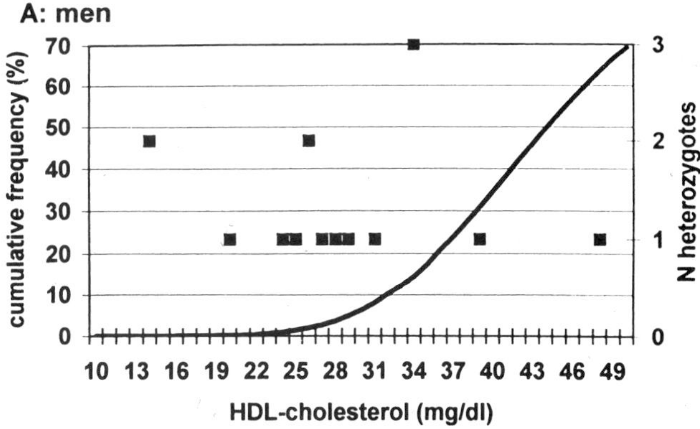

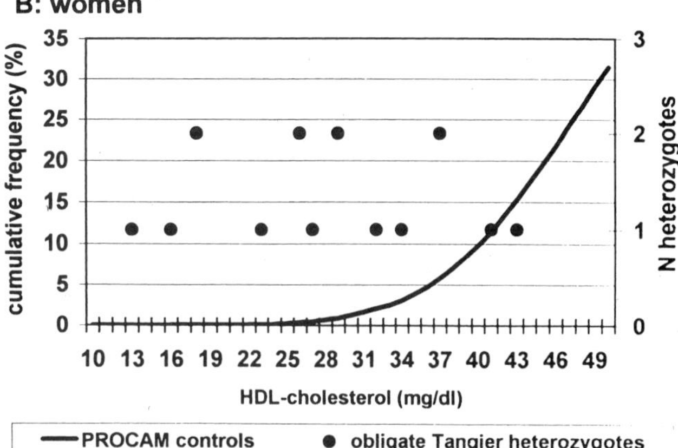

Fig. 122-10 Comparison of HDL cholesterol levels in obligate heterozygotes for Tangier disease (right Y-axis gives the number of probands)[12,14,17,21,22,24,29,47,49] with the cumulative frequency distribution of HDL cholesterol in the German population (N = 22,644 men and 10,954 women from the Prospective Cardiovascular Münster [PROCAM] Study cohort [left Y-axis]).

Heterozygotes are biochemically characterized by half-normal serum concentrations of HDL-cholesterol, apo A-I, and apo A-II,[12,14,17,21,22,24,29,47,49,246,255,280,282,283] which are frequently below the fifth percentiles of sex-matched controls. However, because HDL metabolism is regulated by many genetic, hormonal, and environmental factors, several obligate heterozygotes had higher HDL cholesterol levels (Fig. 122-10). The structure and composition of HDL in Tangier heterozygotes was not different from control HDL.

Cultivated skin fibroblasts of obligate heterozygotes have a half-normal capacity to release radiolabeled cholesterol and phospholipid in the presence of lipid free apo A-I.[284,285]

GENETICS

The clinical phenotype of Tangier disease is inherited as an autosomal recessive trait, and the biochemical phenotype is inherited as an autosomal codominant trait.[6,283] The limited number of recently identified cases, despite the enormous popularity of HDL cholesterol measurements, attests to the rarity of this disease.

The ABC1 Gene Harbors the Defect Underlying Tangier Disease

Using a genome-wide graphical linkage exclusion strategy and by excluding individuals with an ambiguous biochemical phenotype, that is, with HDL levels between the 10th and 25th percentiles, the Tangier locus (HDLDT1; HDL-deficiency Tangier type 1) was mapped to 9q31 on the long arm of chromosome 9.[286] Refinement of this linkage and differential display analysis of mRNA expression in macrophages loaded with cholesterol by incubation with modified LDL and depleted of cholesterol by incubation with HDL led to the identification of the ATP-binding cassette transporter 1 (ABC1) as the defective gene in Tangier disease.[200–203] Defects found in 13 families are listed in Table 122-6.

It is hypothesized that the specific defect determines the clinical phenotype, for example, the presence or absence of coronary heart disease.[201] However, mutations that interfere with the synthesis of full-length ABC1 have been identified in patients with and without coronary heart disease or neuropathy (Table 122-6).[200,202]

Heterozygosity for ABC1 defects, like heterozygosity for LCAT defects or for apo A-I defects, contributes to familial hypoalphalipoproteinemia[201,202,284] (Table 122-6).

ABC1 and the ABC Family

The ABC1 transporter belongs to a large gene family that encompasses more than 30 members. Complete ABC transporters are characterized by the presence of two highly conserved cytoplasmic ATP-binding cassettes, consisting each of a Walker A and a Walker B motif and a nucleotide binding fold (NBF), which provided the name of the gene family, and two transmembrane domains (Fig. 122-11).[287] They are involved in the transmembrane transport of a broad variety of substances, such as ions, amino acids, carbohydrates, phospholipids, steroids, bile acids, vitamins, hormones, peptides, and proteins.[288,289] Defects in ABC transporter genes have been identified in a wide spectrum of inherited diseases, including cystic fibrosis (see Chap. 201);[290] hyperinsulinemic hypoglycemia (see Chap. 68);[291] X-linked adrenoleukodystrophy (see Chap. 131);[292] Zellweger syndrome (see Chap. 129);[293] Stargardt macular dystrophy, autosomal recessive retinitis pigmentosa, and cone rod dystrophy;[294,295] progressive familial intrahepatic cholestasis;[296,297] and Dubin-Johnson hyperbilirubinemia (see Chap. 125).[298]

The human ABC1 gene on chromosome 9q31 encompasses 49 exons within more than 70 kb of genomic sequence.[299] The cDNA encodes for 2201 amino acids.[300] The ATP-binding cassettes are formed by amino acid residues 866 to 1047 and 1879 to 2060, respectively.[300] Each of the two transmembrane domains consists of six transmembrane-spanning segments. The two domains are linked by a hydrophobic segment.[300] By analogy to the multidrug resistance protein 1 whose low-resolution structure is known,[301] it has been suggested that the transmembrane segments form the wall of an aqueous chamber within the plasma membrane. This chamber is opened to the extracellular space and to the lipid phase of the plasma membrane, but not to the cytosol. Substrates of ABC1 may be transported through this channel.[205]

ABC1 was originally characterized in mouse macrophages as the mediator of engulfment and clearance of apoptotic cells especially during embryonal development, anion efflux, and the secretion of interleukin-1β (IL-1β).[302–304] ABC1 is expressed in many organs. The highest expression was found in fetal tissues, placenta, liver, lung, and adrenals.[300] In cell culture, ABC1 was expressed in confluent but not in growing fibroblasts, indicating that ABC1-mediated cholesterol efflux is needed in cell quiescence and other conditions of low cholesterol need.[203] In macrophages, ABC1 expression was up-regulated by cholesterol loading through exposition to acetylated LDL and down-regulated by cholesterol depletion through exposition to HDL.[300] In fibroblasts, ABC1 expression was increased by incubation with cholesterol and 8-Br-cAMP and down-regulated by incubation with apo A-I.[203] As the name suggests, post-translational activation occurs by binding and hydrolysis of ATP at the binding cassettes. The linker segment of ABC1 has several serine and threonine residues that can be phosphorylated and thereby modulate ABC1 activity posttranslationally.[300] ABC1-mediated secretion of anions, lipids, and IL-1β is activated

Table 122-6 Defects in ABC1

Origin	References	Zygosity	Defects	Clinical presentation*
Defects found in patients with Tangier disease				
Canada	37,200,203	homo	Gln537Arg	N, S, T
Germany	60,115,201,202	homo	G1764del, frameshift start aa 548, end aa 574	C
The Netherlands	60,115,200,286	hetero	Cys1417 Arg, G-C mutation in splice donor site of exon 24	C
Pakistan	35,201	homo	deletion of exons 39 to 48 (truncation at aa 1774)	N
Germany	22,69,201,232,236	homo	Asn875Ser	H, S
Germany	201	hetero	Ala877Val, Val339Arg and Ile823Met	?
Germany	201	hetero	Ala877Val, W530Ser	?
Chile	202	homo	110-bp Alu sequence replaces 14 bp in exon 12	C
Spain	60,115,202	homo	Asn875Ser	H, O, S, T
USA	7,18,202,299	homo	2-bp deletion in exon 22, truncation at residue 1085	H, N, T
Switzerland	12,202	hetero	1-bp insertion in exon 22, truncation at residue 1085, 567Stop	H, N, O, T
USA	203	hetero	14-bp insertion following nt 5697, frameshift, stop at residue; 138-bp insertion following nt 5062, in-frame stop at residue	N, T
USA	49,189,203	hetero	Arg527Trp, deletion of several exons?	C, H, N, O, T
Defects found in families with hypoaphalipoproteinemia				
Canada	284	hetero	Arg2048STOP	
Canada	284	hetero	in-frame deletion of aa residues 1833 and 1834	
Canada	284	hetero	Pro849STOP	
The Netherlands	284	hetero	Met1031Thr	

*C = premature coronary heart disease; H = hepatomegaly; N = neuropathy; O = corneal opacities; S = splenomegaly; T = abnormal tonsils.

by analogues of cAMP and is inhibited by sulfonylurea derivatives.[203,302–304]

PATHOPHYSIOLOGY OF TANGIER DISEASE

HDL deficiency and cholesterol accumulation in macrophages of Tangier disease patients clearly indicate that ABC1 plays a key role in the formation of HDL and in the regulation of cholesterol homeostasis in macrophages. However, the mechanism is not known. Current hypotheses are built on analogies with other members of the ABC gene family, namely the multidrug resistance proteins (MDRs) 1 and 3 that mediate the export of lipids out of hepatocytes into the bile,[305] and the cystic fibrosis transmembrane conductance regulator (CFTR) that, in addition to its function as a chloride channel, is involved in the regulation of intracellular trafficking of vesicles between intracellular organelles and the plasma membrane.[306,307]

By analogy to MDRs, it has been suggested that ABC1 forms a channel within the plasma membrane through which phospholipids (sphingomyelin, phosphatidylserine, phosphatidylinositol) and cholesterol are transferred ("flopped") from the inner leaflet to the outer leaflet of the plasma bilayer membrane.[205,308] There they may be picked up by lipid-free apolipoproteins or lipid-poor particles that may even bind to ABC1. In exchange, phospholipids, being more abundant in the outer leaflet (phosphatidylcholine), may be transferred ("flipped") from the outer leaflet to the inner leaflet.[308]

Both HDL and apo A-I were previously found to be internalized by macrophages into an endosomal compartment from which they are resecreted together with lipids.[193,222] Tangier macrophages appear to have a defect in resecretion and erroneously target internalized HDL to lysosomes for degradation.[276] For this reason and because of the presence of hyperplastic Golgi structures within lipid-laden Tangier macrophages (Fig. 122-9),[277] ABC1 may not only translocate lipids between the two leaflets of the plasma membrane, but may also serve as a protein component of vesicles or rafts that target lipids and proteins between lipid-rich intracellular organelles (lysosomes, TGN) and the plasma membrane. In fact, several ABC transporters, such as CFTR, Rim, or MDRs, are important for the trafficking of proteins and lipids between intracellular organelles and the plasma membrane.[306,307,309] ABC1 has been implicated as a targeting protein that mediates the intracellular trafficking and exocytosis of IL-1β by endolysosome-related vesicles.[310]

Both the "floppase/flippase" model and the trafficking model explain defective lipid efflux.[58,189,203,212,279] In these models, the disturbances in signal transduction of Tangier cells[211–213] are secondary to inadequate supply of either substrate (i.e., phospholipids) or proteins (e.g., phospholipases, small G-proteins) to distinct sites of the plasma membrane. Likewise, the failure of Tangier plasma to convert lipid-free apo A-I into mature HDL[60,107,115] is secondary to the lack of lipids and/or proteins that are exported with the help of ABC1 and mediate the maturation of HDL in the plasma compartment.

Whatever the mechanism, defective lipid efflux from ABC1-deficient Tangier cells presumably interferes with the formation of

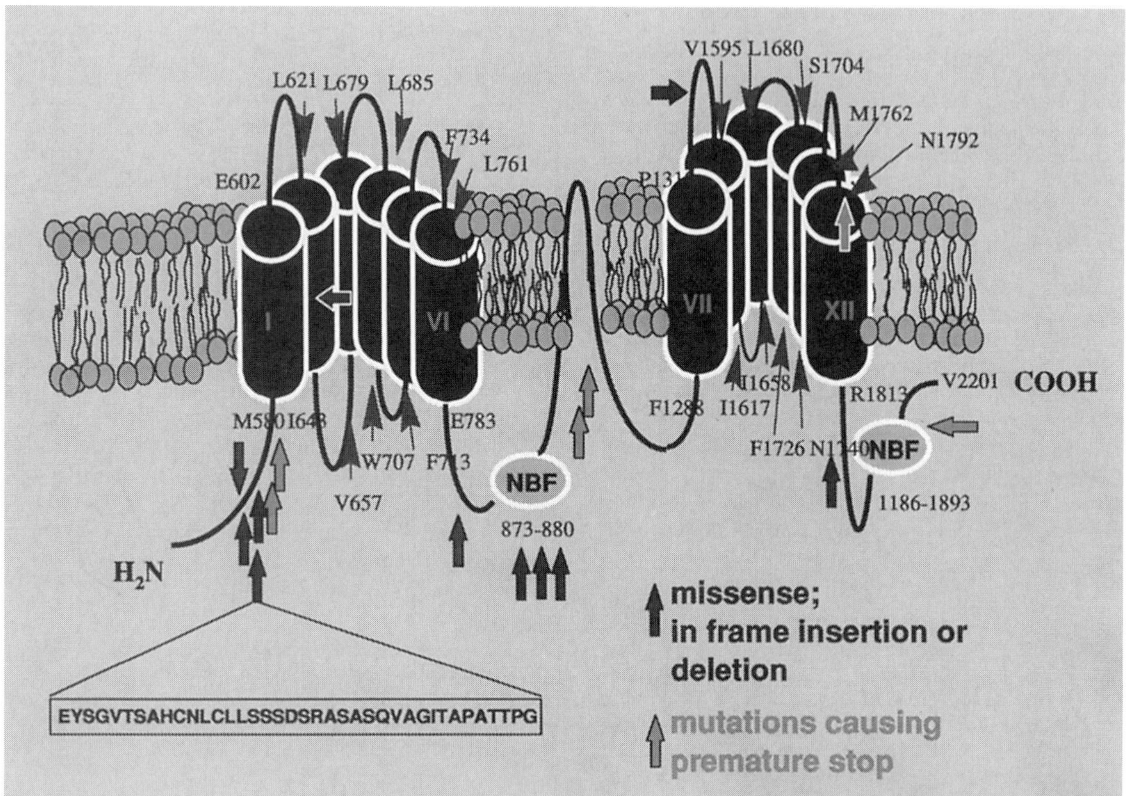

Fig. 122-11 Proposed model for the structure of ABC1 within the plasma membrane (modified from reference 202). The two symmetric halves consisting of six membrane-spanning domains (enumerated with roman numerals) are shown. The two putative nucleotide-binding folds (NBF) are also shown. Bold arrows indicate the localization of defects underlying Tangier disease. Other arrows with numbers refer to amino acid residues which are bordering important structural domains.

lipid-rich HDL.[82,204,205] ABC1 is expressed in both hepatocytes and peripheral cells.[300] ABC1 may hence mediate not only the lipidation of lipid-poor particles that are generated in the circulation by hydrolysis of triglyceride-rich particles or interconversion of HDL (Fig. 122-2),[81] but also the lipidation of nascent HDL in the liver. Without this initial lipidation the HDL particles do not become a substrate for LCAT and cannot mature into α-HDL but instead undergo rapid catabolism (Fig. 122-12).

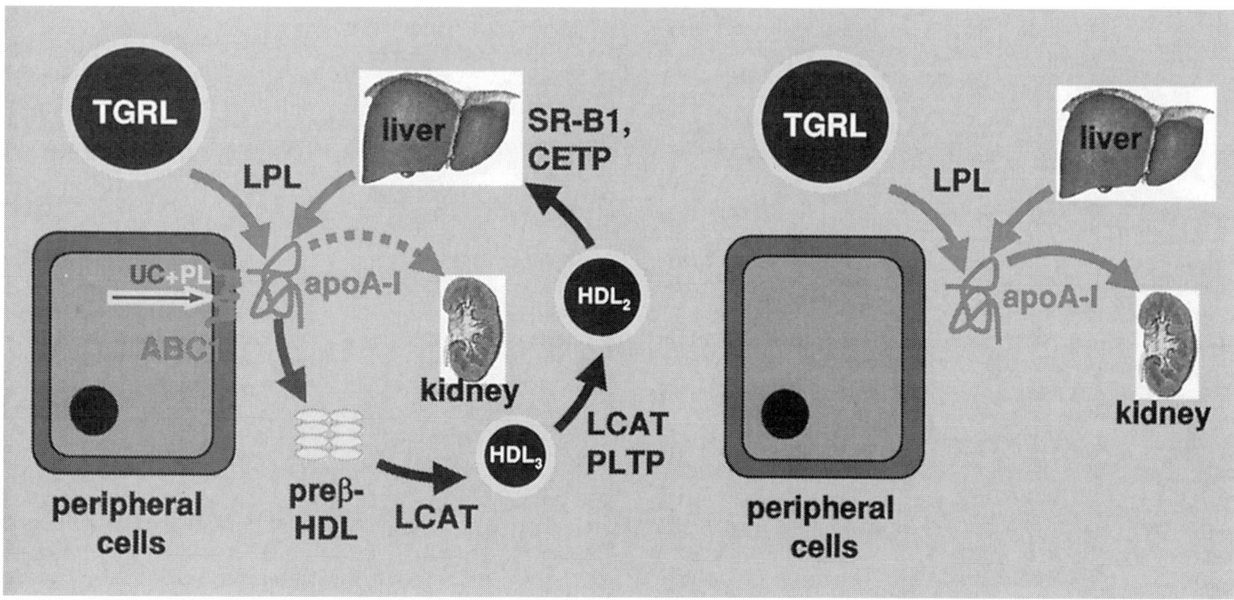

Fig. 122-12 Drawing of HDL metabolism in normolipidemic individuals (*A*) and patients with Tangier disease (*B*). In normal subjects, cellular lipid efflux by ABC1 helps to lipidate apo A-I. The resulting pre-β_1-LpA-I particles mature to HDL with the help of LCAT and PLTP. CETP and SR-BI mediate the removal of HDL lipids. These conversion processes generate new HDL precursors (not shown, but see Fig. 122-2). In Tangier disease, defective ABC1 prevents the lipidation of apo A-I and subsequent maturation of HDL. The consequence is that apo A-I undergoes enhanced catabolism by the kidney.

DIAGNOSIS AND DIFFERENTIAL DIAGNOSIS

In any patient with unexplained hepatic or splenic enlargement, corneal deposits, or neuropathy, a close examination of the oropharynx and rectal mucosa and quantification of serum concentrations of cholesterol, triglycerides, and HDL cholesterol are indicated. HDL cholesterol concentrations below 5 mg/dl, as routinely determined using precipitation techniques or homogenous assays, total cholesterol levels below 150 mg/dl, and moderately elevated triglyceride levels are characteristic of Tangier disease (Table 122-5).[1–6] Serum concentrations of apo A-I and apo A-II are typically below 5 mg/dl (Table 122-5).[1–3,22,246] Analysis of apo A-I isoproteins by isoelectric focusing reveals the increase in proapo A-I that is indicative of HDL deficiency syndromes characterized by increased catabolism (Fig. 122-8).[253,254] On lipoprotein electrophoresis, lipoproteins with α-mobility are not present in even trace amounts. On immunoblotting, residual amounts of apo A-I are found in pre-β-HDL, but virtually none in α-HDL (Fig. 122-1).[60,247,249] Family studies are important to demonstrate that HDL deficiency is of genetic origin because the Tangier phenotype is mimicked in some secondary forms of HDL deficiency (see below).

Other diseases that should be considered in the differential diagnosis of Tangier disease include:

1. Absent or severely reduced serum concentrations of HDL-cholesterol and apo A-I characterize several familial dyslipidemias including apo A-I deficiency, familial LCAT deficiency, and fish eye disease[311–313] (for details see Chaps. 118 and 121). Even if the clinical phenotype is not unequivocal, the genetic and biochemical characteristics of apo A-I deficiencies, fish eye disease, familial LCAT deficiency, and Tangier disease are very different. Thus, these syndromes are easily discriminated in homozygotes (Table 122-7). The clinical and biochemical presentation in heterozygotes for defects in the genes of apo A-I and LCAT is indistinguishable from heterozygosity for Tangier disease.
2. There are several reports of patients with severe HDL deficiency with autosomal codominant inheritance who presented with premature coronary heart disease but not with the

Table 122-7 Comparison of Clinical, Genetic, and Biochemical Characteristics in Tangier Disease, Apo A-I Deficiencies, LCAT Deficiency, and Fish Eye Disease

	Tangier disease	Apo A-I deficiency	Familial LCAT deficiency	Fish eye disease
Affected gene	ABC1	APOLP1	LCAT	LCAT
Tonsil anomalies	yes	no	no	no
Hepato- or splenomegaly	yes	no	no	no
Neuropathy	yes	no	no	no
Corneal opacities	+	+/+++*	+++	+++
Xanthomas	no	no/yes*	no	no
Nephropathy	no	no	yes	no
Serum cholesterol	low	normal	normal	normal
% Cholesterol esters	normal	normal	low	low normal
Serum triglycerides	increased	low - increased	increased	increased
LDL-C	low	normal	normal	normal
HDL-C (%)	none	none	10	10
Apo A-I (%)	2–5	0–2*	15–30	15–30
Apo A-I-containing particles	pre-β_1-HDL	none or pre-β_1-HDL and small α-HDL*	pre-β_1-HDL and small α-HDL	pre-β_1-HDL and small α-HDL
Conversion of apo A-I into α-HDL	no	yes	yes	yes
β-LCAT activity(%)	100	50–80	0	50–100
α-LCAT activity (%)	50	50	0–10	0
LCAT mass (%)	50	50	0–50	10–50
Specific LCAT activity	normal	normal	decreased	decreased
Cholesterol efflux by lipid-free apo A-I	absent	normal	normal	normal
Cholesterol efflux by HDL	reduced	normal	normal	normal

*Apo A-I deficiency because of null alleles causes absence of apo A-I and is usually associated with xanthomatosis but little corneal opacities. Homozygotes for structural apo A-I variants have very low levels of apo A-I and small apo A-I-containing particles in their plasma and clinically present with corneal opacities but not with xanthomatosis. For details, see Chaps. 118 and 121.

typical clinical symptoms seen in apo A-I-deficiency, LCAT-deficiency, fish eye disease, or Tangier disease.[285,314–318] In some cases, defects in the genes of apo A-I and LCAT have been ruled out. In one patient, hypercatabolism of apo A-I could be demonstrated.[316] Cultured fibroblasts of other patients had half-normal cholesterol efflux capacity in the presence of lipid-free apo A-I, instead of the complete efflux defect seen in Tangier disease.[285,318] Genotyping of ABC1 will have to demonstrate whether these forms of HDL deficiency are unusual clinical presentations of Tangier disease.

3. Patients with other storage diseases associated with foam cells and hepatosplenomegaly including Niemann-Pick disease, Wolman disease, and Gaucher disease[319] exhibit HDL-cholesterol levels that are higher than those seen in Tangier disease, and present with distinct clinical symptoms. Moreover, tonsillar abnormalities seen in Tangier patients are absent (for details see Chaps. 142, 144, 145, and 146).
4. The low plasma cholesterol concentrations in Tangier disease are similar to those observed in patients with abetalipoproteinemia, but the presence of normal to elevated triglyceride levels and the absence of HDL in Tangier disease readily differentiate these two conditions (for details see Chap. 115).
5. In obstructive liver disease, the plasma concentrations of HDL and the A apolipoproteins may be reduced to the same extent as in Tangier disease. In contrast to Tangier disease, obstructive jaundice is characterized by hypercholesterolemia.[320]
6. Hepatic parenchymal diseases (e.g., during the course of transient virus infections), hepatic infiltration by tumors, and right heart failure may produce plasma lipoprotein patterns indistinguishable from that observed in Tangier disease.[321]
7. Severe malnutrition and functional loss of the intestine due to inflammatory enteropathies or surgical interventions may cause HDL deficiency due to impaired synthesis of chylomicrons and HDL precursors.[321]
8. Dysglobulinemia may be associated with the development of antibodies against apolipoproteins, enzymes, or receptors involved in HDL metabolism and thereby lead to acquired HDL deficiency.[322]
9. Some patients with severely consumptive and inflammatory disorders (e.g., severe infections, burns, hemophagocytic lymphohistiocytosis, and Hodgkin disease) may present with clinical and biochemical features that are indistinguishable from Tangier disease.[323–328]

TREATMENT

There is no specific treatment for Tangier disease. Drugs known to increase HDL levels in normal individuals, such as estrogens, fibrates, nicotinic acid, statins, or phenytoin, are ineffective in Tangier disease patients.[329]

To minimize the risk of atherosclerotic vessel disease, which may be increased in Tangier disease, cardiovascular risk factors such as smoking, hypertension, diabetes mellitus, obesity, hypertriglyceridemia, and homocysteinemia should be identified and treated.[330] In general, Tangier disease patients have very low levels of LDL cholesterol, so hypercholesterolemia is rarely a cardiovascular risk factor in Tangier disease. By contrast, hypertriglyceridemia, which has emerged as an independent risk factor for myocardial infarction,[331–333] is a frequent finding in Tangier disease patients. In addition to dietary intervention with reduction of intake of total fat and especially saturated fatty acids, fibrates have been found effective in lowering triglycerides in Tangier disease.[54] Lowering of triglyceride-rich lipoproteins and their remnants by dietary and/or drug intervention may also be beneficial to avoid their uptake into cells of the reticuloendothelial system and, hence, hepato- and splenomegaly.

No treatment has been found effective to prevent the progression of neurologic symptoms in Tangier disease, including trials of omega-3-fatty acids, antioxidants, and vitamin E.[329]

ACKNOWLEDGMENTS

The authors thank Drs. Paul Cullen, Thomas Engel, Stefan Rust, and Michael Walter (University of Münster) for their helpful comments in the preparation of this manuscript, and Drs. Horst Robenek (University of Münster), and John J.P. Kastelein and Henry O.F. Molhuizen (University of Amsterdam) for providing photographs.

REFERENCES

1. Assmann G, von Eckardstein A, Brewer HB Jr: Familial high density lipoprotein deficiency. Tangier Disease, in Scriver CR, Beaudet AL, Sly WS, Valle D (eds): *The Metabolic and Molecular Bases of Inherited Disease*, 7th ed, Chap. 65. New York, McGraw-Hill, 1995, p 2053.
2. Assmann G, Schmitz G, Brewer HB Jr: Familial high density lipoprotein deficiency. Tangier Disease, in Scriver CR, Beaudet AL, Sly WS, Valle D (eds): *The Metabolic and Molecular Bases of Inherited Disease*, 6th ed, Chap. 50. New York, McGraw-Hill, 1989, p 1267.
3. Herbert PN, Assmann G, Fredrickson DS: Familial lipoprotein deficiency: Abetalipoproteinemia, hypobetalipoproteinemia, and Tangier disease, in Stanbury JB, Fredrickson DS, Goldstein JL, Brown MS (eds): *The Metabolic and Molecular Bases of Inherited Disease*, 5th ed, Chap. 29. New York, McGraw-Hill, 1983, p 589.
4. Herbert PN, Assmann G, Fredrickson DS: Familial lipoprotein deficiency (abetalipoproteinemia and Tangier disease), in Stanbury JB, Fredrickson DS (eds): *The Metabolic and Molecular Bases of Inherited Disease*, 4th ed, Chap. 28. New York, McGraw-Hill, 1978, p 554.
5. Fredrickson DS, Gotto AM, Levy RI: Familial lipoprotein deficiency, in Stanbury JB, Wyngaarden JB, Fredrickson DS (eds): *The Metabolic and Molecular Bases of Inherited Disease*, 3d ed. New York, McGraw-Hill, 1972, p 493.
6. Fredrickson DS: Familial high density lipoprotein deficiency: Tangier disease, in Stanbury JB, Wyngaarden JB, Fredrickson DS (eds): *The Metabolic and Molecular Bases of Inherited Disease*, 2d ed. New York, McGraw-Hill, 1966, p 486.
7. Fredrickson DS, Altrocchi PH, Avioli LV, Goodman DS, Goodman HC: Tangier disease — Combined clinical staff conference at the National Institutes of Health. *Ann Intern Med* **55**:1016, 1961.
8. Hoffman HN, Fredrickson DS: Tangier disease (familial high-density lipoprotein deficiency): Clinical and genetic features in two adults. *Am J Med* **39**:582, 1965.
9. Engel WK, Dorman JD, Levy RI, Fredrickson DS: Neuropathy in Tangier disease: α-Lipoprotein deficiency manifesting as familial recurrent neuropathy and intestinal lipid storage. *Arch Neurol* **17**:1, 1967.
10. Kocen RS, Lloyd JK, Lascelles PT, Fosbrooke AS, Williams D: Familial α-lipoprotein deficiency (Tangier disease) with neurological abnormalities. *Lancet* **1**:1341, 1967.
11. Waldorf DS, Levy RI, Fredrickson DS: Cutaneous cholesterol ester deposition in Tangier disease. *Arch Dermatol* **95**:161, 1967.
12. Kummer H, Laissur J, Spiess H, Pflugshaupt R, Bucher U: Familiäre Analphalipoproteinämie (Tangier-Krankheit). *Schweiz Med Wochenschr* **98**:406, 1968.
13. Haas LF, Bergin JD: Alpha lipoprotein deficiency with neurological features. *Aust Ann Med* **19**:76, 1970.
14. Bale PM, Clifton-Bligh P, Benjamin BN, White HM: Pathology of Tangier disease. *J Clin Pathol* **24**:609, 1971.
15. Clifton-Bligh P, Nestel PJ, Whyte HM: Tangier disease: Report of a case and studies of lipid metabolism. *N Engl J Med* **286**:567, 1972.
16. Kocen RS, King RHM, Thomas PK, Haas LF: Nerve biopsy findings in two cases of Tangier disease. *Acta Neuropathol* **26**:317, 1973.
17. Greten H, Hannemann T, Gusek W, Vivell O: Lipoproteins and lipolytic plasma enzymes in a case of Tangier disease. *N Engl J Med* **291**:548, 1974.
18. Ferrans VJ, Fredrickson DS: The pathology of Tangier disease: A light and electron microscopic study. *Am J Pathol* **78**:101, 1975.
19. Utermann G, Menzel HJ, Schoenborn W: Plasma lipoprotein abnormalities in a case of primary high-density lipoprotein (HDL) deficiency. *Clin Genet* **8**:258, 1975.
20. Assmann G: Tangier Krankheit, in Schettler G, Greten H, Schlierf G, Seidel D (eds): *Handbuch der Inneren Medizin. Fettstoffwechsel*, vol. 7. Heidelberg, Springer, 1976, p 461.

21. Brooke JG, Lees RS, Yules JH, Cusack B: Tangier disease (α-lipoprotein deficiency). *JAMA* **238**:332, 1977.
22. Assmann G, Smootz E, Adler K, Capruso A, Oette K: The lipoprotein abnormality in Tangier disease. Quantitation of A apoproteins. *J Clin Invest* **59**:565, 1977.
23. Dyck PM, Ellefson RD, Yao JK, Herbert PN: Adult-onset Tangier disease. I. Morphometric and pathologic studies suggesting delayed degradation of neutral lipids after fiber degeneration. *J Neuropathol Exp Neurol* **37**:119, 1978.
24. Chu FC, Kuwabara T, Cogan DG, Schaefer EJ, Brewer HB JR: Ocular manifestations of familial high-density lipoprotein deficiency (Tangier disease). *Arch Ophthalmol* **97**:1926, 1979.
25. Assmann G: Tangier disease and the possible role of high-density lipoproteins in atherosclerosis. *Atheroscl Rev* **6**:1, 1979.
26. Hager H, Zimmermann P: Licht-und elektronenmikroskopische sowie cytometrische Untersuchungen an peripheren Nerven bei Morbus Tangier. *Acta Neurophathol (Berl)* **45**:53, 1979.
27. Suarez BK, Schonfeld G, Sparkes RS: Tangier disease: Heterozygote detection and linkage analysis. *Hum Genet* **60**:150, 1982.
28. Frith RW, Hannan SF, Simcock JP, Scott PJ: Tangier disease with normal serum cholesterol. *Aust N Z J Med* **12**:515, 1982.
29. Ohtaki S, Nakagawa H, Kida N, Nakamura H, Tsuda K, Yokoyama S, Yamamura T, Tajima S, Yamamoto A: A Japanese family with high-density lipoprotein deficiency. *Atherosclerosis* **49**:79, 1983.
30. Pollock M, Nukada H, Frith RW, Simcock, Allpress S: Peripheral neuropathy in Tangier disease. *Brain* **106**:911, 1983.
31. Vergani C, Plancher AC, Zuin M, Cattaneo M, Tramaloni C, Maccari S, Roma P, Catapano AL: Bile lipid composition and haemostatic variables in a case of high density lipoprotein deficiency (Tangier disease). *Eur J Clin Invest* **14**:49, 1983.
32. Dechelotte P, Labbé A, Kantelip B: La maladie de Tangier. *Arch Anat Cytol Pathol* **32**:376, 1984.
33. Tarao K, Iwamura K, Fujii K, Miyake H: Japanese adult siblings with Tangier disease and statistical analysis of reported cases. *Tokai J Exp Clin Med* **9**:379, 1984.
34. Pietrini V, Rizzuto N, Vergani C, Zen F, Milone FF: Neuropathy in Tangier disease: A clinicopathologic study and a review of the literature. *Acta Neurol Scand* **72**:495, 1985.
35. Gibbels E, Schaefer HE, Runne U, Schröder JM, Haupt WF, Assmann G: Severe polyneuropathy in Tangier disease mimicking syringomyelia or leprosy. Clinical, biochemical, electrophysiological, and morphological evaluation, including electron microscopy of nerve, muscle, and skin biopsies. *J Neurol* **232**:283, 1985.
36. Pressly TA, Scott WJ, Ide CH, Winkler A, Reams GP: Ocular complications of Tangier disease. *Am J Med* **83**:991, 1987.
37. Frohlich J, Fong B, Julien P, Despres JP, Angel A, Hayden M, Mcleod R, Chow C, Davison RH, Pritchard H: Interaction of high density lipoprotein with adipocytes in a new patient with Tangier disease. *Clin Invest Med* **10**:377, 1987.
38. Schmalbruch H, Stender H, Boysen G: Abnormalities in spinal neurons and dorsal root ganglion cells in Tangier disease presenting with a syringomyelia-like syndrome. *J Neuropathol Exp Neurol* **46**:533, 1987.
39. Bracco G, Dotti G, Levis F, David E, Saracco G, Rizetto M, Verme G: Familial high density lipoprotein deficiency (Tangier disease): The third Italian case. *J Inherit Metab Dis* **11(Suppl 2)**:155, 1988.
40. Dumon MF, Clerc M, Clerc M: Apolipoprotein A-I: Deficiency in Tangier disease. *Adv Exp Med Biol* **243**:67, 1988.
41. Takizaw A, Okano K, Komoda T, Sakagishi Y, Okano K, Doi Y, Tanaka A, Oguro T: Serum lipoprotein analysis of a patient with Tangier disease. *Jpn J Clin Pathol* **37**:285, 1989.
42. Luna AL, Vaca FB, Gerique JAG, Gallofren A, Peral PM, Romero FF: Tangier disease study of the first case in Spain. *Med Clin (Barc)* **93**:301, 1989.
43. Reinhart WH, Gössi U, Bütikofer P, Ott P, Sigrist H, Schatzmann H-J, Lutz HU, Straub W: Haemolytic anaemia, in analphalipoproteinaemia (Tangier disease): Morphological, biochemical, and biophysical properties of the red blood cell. *Br J Haematol* **72**:272, 1989.
44. Lo WD, Sloan HR, Fahey BP, Donat JF, Strobl W, Patsch JR, Gotto AM, Patsch W: Tangier disease in a black patient: An unusual clinical presentation. *Am J Med* **89**:105, 1990.
45. Kunitake ST, Young S, Chen GC, Pullinger CR, Zhu S, Pease RJ, Scott J, Schilling J, Kane JP: Conformation of apolipoprotein B-100 in the low density lipoproteins of Tangier disease. *J Biol Chem* **265**:20739, 1990.
46. Antoine JC, Tommasi M, Boucheron S, Convers P, Laurent B, Michel D: Pathology of roots, spinal cord and brainstem in syringomyelia-like syndrome of Tangier disease. *J Neurol Sci* **106**:179, 1991.
47. Haust D: Aortic features in Tangier disease and pathogenetic considerations. Part I. Fatty dots and streaks. *Eur J Epidemiol* **8 (Suppl)1**:36, 1992.
48. Mautner SL, Sanchez JA, Rader DJ, Mautner GC, Ferrans VJ, Fredrickson DS, Brewer HB, Jr, Roberts WC: The heart in Tangier disease. Severe coronary atherosclerosis with near absence of high-density lipoprotein cholesterol A. *J Clin Pathol* **98**:191, 1992.
49. Cheung MC, Mendez AJ, Wolf AC, Knopp RH: Characterization of apolipoprotein A-I- and A-II-containing lipoproteins in a new case of high density lipoprotein deficiency resembling Tangier disease and their effects on intracellular cholesterol efflux. *J Clin Invest* **91**:522, 1993.
50. Fazio R, Nemni R, Quattrini A, Rotulo G, Iannaccone S, Mamoli D, Lodi M, Canal N: Acute presentation of Tangier polyneuropathy: A clinical and morphological study. *Acta Neuropathol (Berl)* **86**:90, 1993.
51. Frosini G, Marini M, Galgani P, Carnicelli N, Farnetani L, Pettorali M: Tangier disease, an unusual diagnosis for the endoscopist. *Endoscopy* **26**: 373, 1994.
52. Barnard GF, Jafri IH, Banner BF, Bonkovsky HL: Colonic mucosal appearance of Tangier disease in a new patient. *Gastrointest Endosc* **40**:628, 1994.
53. Burnett JR, Law AJJ, Yeong ML, Crooke, MJ, Sharma AK: Severe aortic stenosis and atherosclerosis in a young man with Tangier disease. *Am J Cardiol* **73**:923, 1994.
54. Serfaty-Lacrosniere C, Civeira F, Lanzberg A, Isaia P, Berg J, Janus ED, Smith MP Jr, Pritchard PH, Frohlich J, Lees RS, Barnard GF, Ordovas JM, Schaefer EJ: Homozygous Tangier disease and cardiovascular disease. *Atherosclerosis* **107**:85, 1994.
55. Lachaux A, Sassolas A, Bouvier R, La Gall C, Loras I, Regnier F, Plauchu H, Froelich P, Hermier M: Early manifestations of Tangier disease. *Arch Pediatr* **2**: 447, 1995.
56. Winder AF, Alexander R, Garner A, Johnston D, Vallance D, Mc Creanor G, Frohlich J: The pathology of the cornea in Tangier disease. *J Clin Pathol* **49**: 407, 1996.
57. Anonymous: Case reports of the Massachusetts General Hospital. Weekly clinicopathological exercises. Case 16-1996. A 36-year-old woman with bilateral facial and hand weakness and impaired truncal sensation. *N Engl J Med* **334**:1389, 1996.
58. Remaley AT, Schumacher K, Stonik JA, Farsi BD, Nazih H, Brewer HB Jr: Decreased reverse cholesterol transport from Tangier disease fibroblasts. Acceptor specificity and effect of brefeldin on lipid efflux. *Arterioscler Thromb Vasc Biol* **17**:1813, 1997.
59. Real JT, Ascaso JF, Sanchis J, Aranda A, von Eckardstein A, Carmena R: Clinical and biochemical characteristics of a new case of Tangier disease in Spain. *Med Clin (Barc)* **110**:344, 1998.
60. von Eckardstein A, Huang Y, Kastelein JJP, Geisel J, Réal J, Miccoli R, Noseda G, Kuivenhoven JA, Assmann G: Lipid-free apolipoprotein (apo) A-I is converted into alpha-migrating high-density lipoproteins by lipoprotein depleted plasma of normolipidemic donors and apo A-I-deficient patients but not of Tangier Disease patients. *Atherosclerosis* **138**:25, 1998.
61. Huth K, Kracht J, Schoenborn W, Fuhrmann W: [Tangier disease (Hyp-α-lipoproteinemia)]. *Dtsch Med Wochenschr* **95**:2357, 1970.
62. von Eckardstein A, Huang Y, and Assmann G: Physiological role and clinical relevance of high-density lipoprotein subclasses. *Curr Opin Lipidol* **5**:404, 1994.
63. Cheung BH, Segrest JP, Ray M, Brunzell JD, Hokanson JE, Krauss RM, Beaudrie K, Cone JT: Single vertical spin density gradient ultracentrifugation. *Methods Enzymol* **128**:181, 1986.
64. Nichols AV, Krauss RM, Musliner TA: Nondenaturing polyacrylamide gradient gel electrophoresis. *Methods Enzymol* **128**:417, 1986.
65. Fruchart JC, Ailhaud G: Apolipoprotein A-containing particles: Physiological role, quantification and clinical significance. *Clin Chem* **38**:793, 1992.
66. Fruchart JC, Ailhaud G, Bard JM: Heterogeneity of high-density lipoprotein particles. *Circulation* **87(Suppl III)**:22, 1993.
67. Kunitake ST, La Sala KI, Kane JP: Apolipoprotein A-I containing lipoproteins with prebeta electrophoretic mobility. *J Lipid Res* **26**:549, 1985.
68. Castro GR, Fielding CJ: Early incorporation of cell-derived cholesterol into pre-β-migrating high density lipoprotein. *Biochemistry* **27**:25, 1988.
69. Asztalos BF, Sloop CH, Wong L, Roheim PS: Two-dimensional electrophoresis of plasma lipoproteins: Recognition of new apoA-I containing subpopulations. *Biochim Biophys Acta* **1169**:291, 1993.

70. Huang Y, von Eckardstein A, Assmann G: Cell-derived cholesterol cycles between different HDLs and LDL for its effective esterification in plasma. *Arterioscler Thromb* **13**:445, 1993.
71. Fielding C, Fielding PE: Molecular physiology of reverse cholesterol transport. *J Lipid Res* **36**:211, 1995.
72. Barrans A, Jaspard B, Barbaras R, Chap H, Perret B, Collet X: Pre-β HDL: Structure and metabolism. *Biochim Biophys Acta* **1300**:73, 1996.
73. Francone OL, Gurakar A, Fielding CJ: Distribution and functions of lecithin:cholesterol acyltransferase and cholesterol ester transfer protein in plasma lipoproteins. *J Biol Chem* **264**:7066, 1989.
74. Huang Y, von Eckardstein A, Wu S, Maeda N, Assmann G: A solely apolipoprotein E containing plasma lipoprotein with electrophoretic gamma-mobility takes up cellular cholesterol. *Proc Natl Acad Sci U S A* **91**:1834, 1994.
75. Huang Y, von Eckardstein A, Wu S, Assmann G: Effects of the apolipoprotein E-polymorphism on uptake and transfer of cell-derived cholesterol in plasma. *J Clin Invest* **96**:2693, 1995.
76. Krimbou JL, Tremblay M, Jacques H, Davignon J, Cohn JS: In vitro factors affecting the concentration of gamma-LpE (γ-LpE) in human plasma. *J Lipid Res* **39**:861, 1998.
77. von Eckardstein A, Huang Y, Wu S, SaadatSarmadi A, Schwarz S, Steinmetz A, Assmann G: Lipoproteins containing apolipoprotein A-IV but not apolipoprotein A-I take up and esterify cell-derived cholesterol in plasma. *Arterioscler Thromb Vasc Biol* **15**:1755, 1995.
78. Asztalos BF, Sloop CH, Wong L, Roheim PS: Comparison of apo A-I-containing subpopulations of dog plasma and prenodal peripheral lymph: Evidence for alteration in subpopulations in the interstitial space. *Biochim Biophys Acta* **1169**:301, 1993.
79. Lefevre M, Sloop CH, Roheim PS: Characterization of dog prenodal peripheral lymph lipoproteins. Evidence for the peripheral formation of lipoprotein unassociated apo A-I with slow pre-b electrophoretic mobility. *J Lipid Res* **29**:1139, 1988.
80. Jaspard B, Collet X, Barbaras R, Manent J, Vieu C, Pontonnier G, Chap. H, Perret B: Biochemical characterization of preβ1-high-density lipoprotein from human ovarian follicular fluid: evidence for the presence of a lipid core. *Biochemistry* **35**:1352, 1996.
81. Rye KA, Clay MA, Barter PJ: Remodelling of high-density lipoproteins by plasma factors. *Atherosclerosis* **145**:227, 1999.
82. Oram JF, Yokoyama S: Apolipoprotein-mediated removal of cellular cholesterol and phopsholipids. *J Lipid Res* **37**:2473, 1997.
83. Hamilton RL, Williams MC, Fielding CJ, Havel RJ: Discoidal bilayer structure of nascent high density lipoproteins from perfused rat liver. *J Clin Invest* **58**:667, 1976.
84. Forte TM, Nichols AV, Selmek-Halsey J, Caylor L, Shore VG: Lipid-poor apolipoprotein A-I in HepG2 cells: Formation of lipid-rich particles by incubation with dimyristoylphosphatidylcholine. *Biochim Biophys Acta* **920**:185, 1987.
85. Thrift RN, Forte TM, Cahoon BE, Shore VG: Characterization of lipoproteins produced by the human liver cell line HepG2 under defined conditions. *J Lipid Res* **27**:236, 1986.
86. McCall MR, Forte TM, Shore VG: Heterogeneity of nascent high-density lipoproteins secreted by the hepatoma-derived cell line HepG2. *J Lipid Res* **29**:1127, 1988.
87. Castle CK, Pape ME, Marotti KR, Melchior GW: Secretion of pre-beta-migrating apo A-I by cynomolgus monkey hepatocytes in culture. *J Lipid Res* **32**:439, 1991.
88. McCall MR, Nichols AV, Blanche PJ, Shore VG, Forte TM: Lecithin:cholesterol acyltransferase-induced transformation of HepG2 lipoproteins. *J Lipid Res* **30**:1579, 1989.
89. Green PHR, Tall AR, Glickman RM: Rat intestine secretes discoid high density lipoprotein. *J Clin Invest* **61**:528, 1978.
90. Forester GP, Tall AR, Bisgaier CL, Glickman RM: Rat intestine secretes spherical high density lipoproteins. *J Biol Chem* **258**:5938, 1983.
91. Danielsen EM, Hansen GH, Poulsen MD: Apical secretion of apolipoproteins from enterocytes. *J Cell Biol* **120**:1347, 1993.
92. Musliner TA, Long DL, Forte TM, Nichols AV, Gong EL, Blanche, Krauss RM: Dissociation of high density lipoprotein precursors from apolipoprotein B-containing lipoproteins in the presence of unesterified fatty acids and a source of apolipoprotein A-I. *J Lipid Res* **32**:917, 1991.
93. Tam SP, Breckenridge WC: Apolipoprotein and lipid distribution between vesicles and HDL-like vesicles formed during lipolysis of human very-low-density lipoproteins by perfused rat heart. *J Lipid Res* **24**:1343, 1983.
94. Schaefer EJ, Wetzel MG, Bengtsson G, Scow RO, Brewer HB, Olivecona T: Transfer of human lymph chylomicron constituents to other lipoprotein density fractions during in vitro lipolysis. *J Lipid Res* **23**:1259, 1982.
95. Clay MA, Newnham HH, Forte TM, Barter PJ: Cholesteryl ester transfer protein and hepatic lipase activity promote shedding of apoA-I from HDL and subsequent formation of discoidal HDL. *Biochim Biophys Acta* **1124**:52, 1992.
96. Liang H-Q, Rye K-A, Barter PJ: Dissociation of lipid-free apolipoprotein A-I from high density lipoproteins. *J Lipid Res* **35**:1187, 1994.
97. Liang H-Q, Rye K-A, Barter PJ: Cycling of apolipoprotein A-I between lipid-associated and lipid-free pools. *Biochim Biophys Acta* **1257**:31, 1995.
98. Francone OL, Royer L, Haghpassand M: Increased preβ-HDL levels, cholesterol efflux, and LCAT mediated esterification in mice expressing the human cholesteryl ester transfer protein (CETP) and human apolipoprotein A-I (apoA-I) transgenes. *J Lipid Res* **37**:1268, 1996.
99. Hennessy LK, Kunitake ST, Kane JP: Apolipoprotein A-I-containing lipoproteins, with or without apolipoprotein A-II, as progenitors of preβ high-density lipoprotein particles. *Biochemistry* **32**:5759, 1993.
100. von Eckardstein A, Jauhiainen M, Huang Y, Metso J, Langer C, Pussinen P, Wu S, Ehnholm C, Assmann G: Phospholipid transfer protein mediated conversion of high density lipoproteins (HDL) generates preβ_1-HDL. *Biochim Biophys Acta* **1301**:255, 1996.
101. Jiang X-J, Francone OL, Bruce C, Milne R, Mar J, Walsh A, Breslow JL, Tall AR: Increased preβ high-density lipoprotein, apolipoprotein AI, and phospholipid in mice expressing the human phospholipid transfer protein and human apolipoprotein AI transgenes. *J Clin Invest* **98**:2373, 1996.
102. Barrans A, Collet X, Barbaras R, Jaspard B, Manent J, Vieu C, Chap H, Perret B: Hepatic lipase induces the formation of preβ1 high-density lipoprotein (HDL) from triacylglycerol-rich HDL2. *J Biol Chem* **269**:11572, 1994.
103. Hara H, Yokoyama S: Interaction of free apolipoproteins with macrophages: Formation of high density lipoprotein-like lipoproteins and reduction of cellular cholesterol. *J Biol Chem* **266**:3080, 1991.
104. Bielicki JK, Johnson WJ, Weinberg RB, Glick JM, Rothblat GM: Efflux of lipid from fibroblasts to apolipoproteins: Dependence on elevated levels of cellular unesterified cholesterol. *J Lipid Res* **33**:1699, 1992.
105. Forte TM, Goth-Goldstein R, Nordhausen RW, McCall MR: Apolipoprotein A-I-cell membrane interaction: Extracellular assembly of heterogeneous nascent HDL particles. *J Lipid Res* **34**:317, 1993.
106. Yancey PG, Bielicki JK, Johnson WJ, Lund-Katz S, Palgunachari MN, Anantharamaiah GM, Segrest JP, Phillips MC, Rothblat GH: Efflux of cellular cholesterol and phospholipid to lipid-free apolipoproteins and class A amphipathic peptides. *Biochemistry* **34**:7955, 1995.
107. Huang Y, von Eckardstein A, Wu S, Assmann G: Generation of preβ_1-high density lipoprotein (HDL) and conversion into α-HDL: Evidence for disturbed preβ_1-HDL conversion in Tangier disease. *Arterioscler Thromb Vasc Biol* **15**:1746, 1995.
108. Asztalos B, Zhang W, Roheim PS, Wong L: Role of free apolipoprotein A-I in cholesterol efflux. Formation of pre-β-migrating high density lipoprotein particles. *Arterioscler Thromb Vasc Biol* **17**:1630, 1997.
109. Kunitake ST, Mendel CM, Hennessy LK: Interconversion between apolipoproteins of pre-beta and alpha electrophoretic mobilities. *J Lipid Res* **33**:1807, 1992.
110. Ishida BY, Albee D, Paigen B: Interconversion of preβ migrating lipoproteins containing apoA-I and HDL. *J Lipid Res* **31**:227, 1990.
111. Neary R, Bhatnagar D, Durrington P, Ishola M, Arrol S, Mackness M: An investigation of the role of lecithin:cholesterol acyltransferase and triglyceride-rich lipoproteins in the metabolism of high density lipoproteins. *Atherosclerosis* **89**:35, 1991.
112. Miida T, Kawano M, Fielding CJ, Fielding PE: Regulation of the concentration of preβ high density lipoprotein in normal plasma by cell membranes and lecithin:cholesterol acyltransferase. *Biochemistry* **31**:11112, 1992.
113. Liang H-Q, Rye K-A, Barter PJ: Remodelling of reconstituted high density lipoproteins by lecithin:cholesterol acyltransferase. *J Lipid Res* **37**:1962, 1996.
114. Clay MA, Barter PJ: Formation of new HDL particles from lipid-free apolipoprotein A-I. *J Lipid Res* **37**:1722, 1996.
115. von Eckardstein A, Chirazi A, Walter M, Kastelein JJP, Kuivenhoven JA, Geisel J, Réal J, Miccoli R, Noseda G, Höbbel G, Assmann G: Plasmas and fibroblasts of tangier disease patients are disturbed in transferring phospholipids onto apolipoprotein A-I. *J Lipid Res* **39**:987, 1998.
116. Cheung MC, Wolf AC: In vitro transformation of apo A-I-containing lipoprotein subpopulations: Role of lecithin:cholesterol acyltransferase. *J Lipid Res* **30**:499, 1989.

117. Dieplinger H, Zechner R, Kostner GM: The in vitro formation of HDL2 during the action of LCAT: the role of triglyceride-rich lipoproteins. *J Lipid Res* **26**:273, 1985.
118. Jauhiainen M, Metso J, Pahlman R, Blomqvist S, van Tol A, Ehnholm C: Human plasma phospholipid transfer protein causes high-density lipoprotein conversion. *J Biol Chem* **268**:4032, 1993.
119. Tu AY, Nishida HI, Nishida T: High-density lipoprotein conversion mediated by human phospholipid transfer protein. *J Biol Chem* **268**:23098, 1993.
120. Lusa S, Jauhiainen M, Metso J, Somerharju P, Ehnholm C: The mechanism of human plasma phospholipid transfer protein-induced enlargement of high-density lipoprotein particles: Evidence for particle fusion. *Biochem J* **313**:275, 1996.
121. Acton S, Rigotti A, Landschulz KT, Xu S, Hobbs HH, Krieger M: Identification of scavenger receptor SR-BI as a high density lipoprotein receptor. *Science* **271**:518, 1996.
122. Kozarsky KF, Donahee MH, Rigotti A, Iqbal SN, Edelman ER, Krieger M: Overexpression of the HDL receptor SR-BI alters plasma HDL and bile cholesterol levels. *Nature* **387**:414, 1997.
123. Rigotti A, Trigatti BL, Penman M, Rayburn H, Herz J, Krieger, M: A targeted mutation in the murine gene encoding the high density lipoprotein (HDL) receptor scavenger receptor class B type I reveals its key role in HDL metabolism. *Proc Natl Acad Sci U S A* **94**:12610, 1997.
124. Mahley RW: Apolipoprotein E: Cholesterol transport protein with expanding role in cell biology. *Science* **240**:622, 1988.
125. Koo C, Innerarity TL, Mahley RW: Obligatory role of cholesterol and apolipoprotein E in the formation of large cholesterol enriched and receptor-active high-density lipoproteins. *J Biol Chem* **260**:11934, 1985.
126. Gordon V, Innerarity TL, Mahley RW: Formation of cholesterol- and apoprotein E-enriched high-density lipoproteins in vitro. *J Biol Chem* **258**:6202, 1983.
127. Funke H, Boyles J, Weisgraber KH, Ludwig EH, Hui DY, Mahley RW: Uptake of apolipoprotein E containing high-density lipoproteins by hepatic parenchymal cells. *Arteriosclerosis* **4**:452, 1984.
128. Tall AR: Plasma lipid transfer enzymes. *Ann Rev Biochem* **64**:235, 1995.
129. Tall AR: Plasma cholesteryl ester transfer protein. *J Lipid Res* **34**:1255, 1993.
130. Garcia A, Barbaras R, Collet X, Bogyo A, Chap H, Perret-B: High-density lipoprotein 3 receptor-dependent endocytosis pathway in a human hepatoma cell line (HepG2). *Biochemistry* **35**:13064, 1996.
131. Horowitz BS, Goldberg IJ, Merab J, Vanni TM, Ramakrishnan R, Ginsberg HN: Increased plasma and renal clearance of an exchangeable pool of apolipoprotein A-I in subjects with low levels of high density lipoprotein cholesterol. *J Clin Invest* **91**:1743, 1993.
132. Kozyraki R, Fyfe J, Kristiansen M, Gerdes C, Jacobsen C, Cui SY, Christensen EI, Aminoff M, de la Chapelle A, Krahe R, Verroust PJ, Moestrup SK: The intrinsic factor-vitamin B-12 receptor, cubilin, is a high-affinity apolipoprotein A-I receptor facilitating endocytosis of high-density lipoprotein. *Nat Med* **5**:656, 1999.
133. Liscum L, Munn NJ: Intracellular cholesterol transport. *Biochim Biophys Acta* **1438**:19, 1999.
134. Lange Y, Steck TL: The role of intracellular cholesterol transport in cholesterol homeostasis. *Trends Cell Biol* **6**:205, 1996.
135. Fielding CJ, Fielding PE: Intracellular cholesterol transport. *J Lipid Res* **38**:1503, 1997.
136. Schroeder F, Jefferson JR, Kier AB, Knittel J, Scallen TJ, Wood, WG, Hapala I: Membrane cholesterol dynamics — cholesterol domains and kinetic pools. *Proc Soc Exp Biol Med* **196**:235, 1991.
137. Rothblat GH, Mahlberg FH, Johnson WJ, Phillips MC: Apolipoproteins, membrane cholesterol domains, and the regulation of cholesterol efflux. *J Lipid Res* **33**:1091, 1992.
138. Bretscher MS, Munro S: Cholesterol and the Golgi apparatus. *Science* **261**:1280, 1993.
139. Fielding PE, Fielding CJ: Intracellular transport of low-density lipoprotein-derived free cholesterol begins at clathrin-coated pits and terminates at cell surface caveolae. *Biochemistry* **35**:14932, 1996.
140. Reinhart MP: Intracellular sterol trafficking. *Experientia* **46**:599, 1990.
141. Simons K, Ikonen E: Functional rafts in cell membranes. *Nature* **387**:569, 1997.
142. Rothman JE, Wieland FT: Protein sorting by transport vesicles. *Science* **272**:227, 1996.
143. Mendez AJ: Monensin and brefeldin A inhibit high-density lipoprotein mediated cholesterol efflux from cholesterol-enriched cells. Implications for intracellular cholesterol trafficking. *J Biol Chem* **270**:5891, 1995.
144. Warner GJ, Stoudt G, Bamberger M, Johnson WJ, Rothblat GH: Cell toxicity induced by inhibition of acyl coenzyme A:cholesterol acyltransferase and accumulation of unesterified cholesterol. *J Biol Chem* **270**:5772, 1995.
145. Brown MS, Goldstein JL: A proteolytic pathway that controls the cholesterol content of membranes, cells, and blood. *Proc Natl Acad Sci U S A* **96**:11041, 1999.
146. Lange Y, Steck TL: Cholesterol homeostasis. Modulation by amphiphiles. *J Biol Chem* **269**:29371, 1994.
147. Fielding PE, Fielding CJ: Plasma membrane caveolae mediate the efflux of cellular free cholesterol. *Biochemistry* **34**:14288, 1995.
148. Smart EJ, Ying Y-S, Donzell WC, Anderson RGW: A role for caveolin in transport of cholesterol from endoplasmic reticulum to plasma membrane. *J Biol Chem* **271**:29427, 1996.
149. Mendez AJ, Uint L: Apolipoprotein mediated cellular cholesterol and phospholipid efflux depends on a functional Golgi apparatus. *J Lipid Res* **37**:2510, 1996.
150. Brown MS, Goldstein, JL: A receptor mediated pathway for cholesterol homeostasis. *Science* **232**:34, 1986.
151. Krieger M, Herz J: Structures and functions of multiligand lipoprotein receptors: macrophage scavenger receptors and LDL receptor-related protein (LRP). *Ann Rev Biochem* **63**:601, 1994.
152. Tabas I: The stimulation of the cholesterol esterification pathway by atherogenic lipoproteins. *Curr Opin Lipidol* **6**:260, 1995.
153. Chang TY, Chang CY, Cheng D: Acyl coenzyme A: Cholesterol acyltransferase. *Ann Rev Biochem* **66**:237, 1997.
154. Liscum L, Ruggiero RM, Faust JR: The intracellular transport of low-density lipoprotein derived cholesterol is defective in Niemann Pick type C fibroblasts. *J Cell Biol* **108**:1625, 1989.
155. Sokol J, Blanchette-Mackie EJ, Kruth HS, Dwyer NK, Amende LM, Butler JD, Robinson E, Brady RO, Comly ME, Vanier MT, Pentchev PG: Type C Niemann-Pick disease: Lysosomal accumulation and defective intracellular mobilization of low-density lipoproteins. *J Biol Chem* **263**:3411, 1988.
156. Cadigan KM, Spillane DM, Chang TY: Isolation and characterization of Chines Hamster ovary cell mutants defective in intracellular low-density lipoprotein cholesterol trafficking. *J Cell Biol* **110**:295, 1990.
157. Liscum L: Pharmacological inhibition of the intracellular transport of low-density lipoprotein-derived cholesterol in Chinese hamster ovary cells. *Biochim Biophys Acta* **1045**:40, 1990.
158. Kobayashi T, Gu F, Gruenberg J: Lipids, lipid domains and lipid-protein interactions in endocytic membrane traffic. *Semin Cell Dev Biol* **9**:517, 1998.
159. Coxev RA, Pentchev PG, Campbell G, Blanchette-Mackie EJ: Differential accumulation of cholesterol in Golgi compartments of normal and Niemann-Pick type C fibroblasts incubated with LDL a cytochemical freeze-fracture study. *J Lipid Res* **34**:1165, 1993.
160. Fielding CJ, Fielding PE: Role of an N-ethylmaleimide-sensitive factor in the selective cellular uptake of low density lipoprotein free cholesterol. *Biochemistry* **34**:14237, 1995.
161. Smart EJ, Ying Y-S, Conrad PA, Anderson RGW: Caveolin moves from caveolae to the Golgi apparatus in response to cholesterol oxidation. *J Cell Biol* **127**:1185, 1994.
162. Brown MS, Goldstein JL: Lipoprotein metabolism in the macrophage: Implications for cholesterol deposition in atherosclerosis. *Annu Rev Biochem* **52**:223, 1983.
163. Tabas I, Zha X, Beatini N, Myers JN, Maxfield FR: The actin cytoskeleton is important for the stimulation of cholesterol esterification in macrophages. *J Biol Chem* **269**:22547, 1994.
164. Mazzone T, Krishna M, Lange Y: Progesterone blocks intracellular translocation of free cholesterol derived from cholesteryl ester in macrophages. *J Lipid Res* **36**:544, 1995.
165. Metherall JE, Waugh K, Li H: Progesterone inhibits cholesterol biosynthesis in cultured cells. Accumulation of cholesterol precursors. *J Biol Chem* **271**:2627, 1996.
166. Metherall JE, Li H, Waugh K: Role of multidrug resistance P-glycoproteins in cholesterol synthesis. *J Biol Chem* **271**:2634, 1996.
167. Lange Y: Cholesterol movement from plasma membrane to rough endoplasmic reticulum. *J Biol Chem* **269**:3411, 1994.
168. Brown MS, Ho YK, Goldstein JL: The cholesteryl ester cycle in macrophage foam cells. Continual hydrolysis and re-esterification of cytoplasmic cholesteryl esters. *J Biol Chem* **255**:9344, 1980.
169. Bernard D, Rodriguez A, Rothblat GH, Glick JM: cAMP stimulates cholesteryl ester clearance to high-density lipoproteins in J774 macrophages. *J Biol Chem* **266**:710–716, 1991.

170. Ho YK, Brown MS, Goldstein JL: Hydrolysis and excretion of cytoplasmic cholesteryl esters by macrophages: Stimulation by high-density lipoprotein and other agents. *J Lipid Res* **21**:391, 1980.
171. Bernard DW, Rodriguez A, Rothblat GH, GLick JM: Influence of high-density lipoproteins on esterified cholesterol stores in macrophages and hepatoma cells. *Arteriosclerosis* **10**:135, 1990.
172. von Eckardstein A: Cholesterol efflux from macrophages and other cells. *Curr Opin Lipidol* **7**:308, 1996.
173. Rothblat GH, de la Llera-Moya M, Atger V, Kellner-Weibel G, Williams DL, Phillipis MC: Cell cholesterol efflux: Integration of old and new observations provides new insight. *J Lipid Res* **40**:781, 1999.
174. Davidson WS, Gillotte KL, Lund-Katz S, Johnson WJ, Rothblat GH, Phillips MC: Effects of acceptor particle size on the efflux of cellular free cholesterol. *J Biol Chem* **270**:5882, 1995.
175. Davidson WS, Rodriguez WV, Lund-Katz S, Johnson WJ, Rothblat GH, Phillips MC: Effects of acceptor particle size on the efflux of cellular free cholesterol. *J Biol Chem* **270**:17106, 1995.
176. Johnson WJ, Fischer RT, Phillips MC, Rothblat GH: Efflux of newly synthesized cholesterol and biosynthetic sterol intermediates from cells. Dependence on acceptor type and enrichment of cells with cholesterol. *J Biol Chem* **270**:25037, 1995.
177. Kilsdonk EPC, Yancey PG, Stoudt GW, Bangerter FW, Johnson WJ, Phillips MC, Rothblat GH: Cellular cholesterol efflux mediated by cyclodextrins. *J Biol Chem* **270**:17250, 1995.
178. Bartholow LC, Geyer RP: Sterol efflux from mammalian cells induced by human serum albumin phospholipid complexes: Dependence on phospholipid acyl-chain length, degree of saturation, and net charge. *J Biol Chem* **257**:3126, 1982.
179. Fielding CJ, Moser A: Evidence for the separation of albumin- and apo A-I-dependent mechanisms of cholesterol efflux from cultured fibroblasts into human plasma. *J Biol Chem* **257**:10955, 1982.
180. Zhao Y, Marcel YL: Serum albumin is a significant intermediate in cholesterol transfer between cells and lipoproteins. *Biochemistry* **35**:7174, 1996.
181. De Lamatre J, Wolfbauer G, Phillips MC, Rothblat GH: Role of apolipoproteins on cellular cholesterol efflux. *Biochim Biophys Acta* **875**:419, 1986.
182. Kawano M, Miida T, Fielding CJ, Fielding PE: Quantitation of preβ-HDL-dependent and nonspecific components of the total efflux of cellular cholesterol and phospholipid. *Biochemistry* **32**:5025, 1993.
183. Mendez AJ: Cholesterol efflux mediated by apolipoproteins is an active cellular process distinct from efflux mediated by passive diffusion. *J Lipid Res* **38**:1807, 1997.
184. Mendez AJ, Anantharamaiah GM, Segrest JP, Oram JF: Synthetic amphipathic helical peptides that mimic apolipoprotein A-I in clearing cellular cholesterol. *J Clin Invest* **94**:1698, 1994.
185. Hara H, Yokoyama S: Role of apolipoproteins in cholesterol efflux from macrophages to lipid microemulsion: proposal of a putative model for the pre-beta high-density lipoprotein pathway. *Biochemistry* **31**:2040, 1992.
186. Li Q, Yokoyama S: Independent regulation of cholesterol incorporation into free apolipoprotein-mediated cellular lipid efflux in rat vascular smooth muscle cells. *J Biol Chem* **269**:26216, 1995.
187. Czarnecka H, Yokoyama S: Regulation of cellular cholesterol efflux by lecithin:cholesterol acyltransferase reaction through nonspecific lipid exchange. J Biol Chem **266**:2023, 1996.
188. Li Q, Komaba A, Yokoyama S: Cholesterol is poorly available for apolipoprotein-mediated cellular lipid efflux from smooth muscle cells. *Biochemistry* **32**:4597, 1993.
189. Francis GA, Knopp RH, Oram JF: Defective removal of cellular cholesterol and phospholipids by apolipoprotein A-I in Tangier disease. *J Clin Invest* **96**:78, 1995.
190. Theret N, Delbart C, Aquie G, Fruchart JC, Vassaux G, Ailhaud G: Cholesterol efflux from adipose cells is coupled to diacylglycerol production and protein kinase C activation. *Biochem Biophys Res Commun* **137**:1361, 1990.
191. Mendez AJ, Oram JF, Bierman EL: Protein kinase C as a mediator of high-density lipoprotein dependent efflux of intracellular cholesterol. *J Biol Chem* **266**:10104, 1991.
192. Dusserre E, Pulcini T, Bourdillon MC, Berthezene F: High density lipoprotein 3 stimulates phosphatidylcholine breakdown and sterol translocation by a phospholipase C/protein kinase C process. *Biochem Med Metab Biol* **52**:45, 1994.
193. Takahashi Y, Smith JL: Cholesterol efflux to apolipoprotein A-I involves endocytosis and resecretion in a calcium-dependent pathway. *Proc Natl Acad Sci U S A* **96**:11358, 1999.
194. Sakr SW, Williams DL, Stoudt GW, Phillipis MC, Rothblat GH: Induction of cholesterol efflux to lipid-free apolipoprotein A-I by cAMP. *Biochim Biophys Acta* **1438**:85, 1999.
195. Smith JD, Miyata M, Ginsberg M, Grigaux C, Shmookler E, Plump AS: Cyclic AMP induces apolipoprotein E binding activity and promotes cholesterol efflux from a macrophage cell line to apolipoprotein acceptors. *J Biol Chem* **271**:30647, 1996.
196. Schmitz G, Niemann R, Brennhausen B, Krause R, Assmann G: Regulation of high-density lipoprotein receptors in cultured macrophages: Role of acyl-CoA: cholesterol acyltransferase. *EMBO J* **4**:2773, 1985.
197. Aviram M, Biermann EL, Oram J: High-density lipoprotein stimulated sterol translocation between intracellular and plasma membrane pools in human monocyte derived macrophages. *J Lipid Res* **30**:65, 1989.
198. Slotte JP, Oram JF, Bierman EL: Binding of high density lipoproteins to cell receptors promotes translocation of cholesterol from intracellular membranes to the cell surface. *J Biol Chem* **262**:12904, 1987.
199. Oram JF, Mendez AJ, Slotte JP, Johnson TF: High-density lipoproteins mediate removal of sterol from intracellular pools but not from plasma membranes of cholesterol loaded fibroblasts. *Arteriosclerosis Thromb* **11**:403, 1991.
200. Brooks-Wilson A, Marcil M, Clee SM, Zhang LH, Roomp K, van Dam M, Yu L, Brewer C, Collins JA, Molhuizen HOF, Loubser O, Ouelette BFF, Fichter K, Ashbourne-Excoffon KJD, Sensen CW, Scherer S, Mott S, Denis M, Martindale D, Frohlich J, Morgan K, Koop B, Pimstone S, Kastelein JJP, Genest J, Hayden MR: Mutations in ABC1 in Tangier disease and familial high-density lipoprotein deficiency. *Nat Genet* **22**:336, 1999.
201. Bodzioch, M, Orso, E, Klucken, J, Langmann, T, Böttcher, A, Diedrich, W, Drobnik, W, Barlage, S, Büchler, C, Porsch-Özcürümez M, Kaminski W, Hahmann HW, Oette K, Rothe G, Aslanidis C, Lackner KJ, Schmitz G: The gene encoding ATP binding cassette transporter 1 is mutated in Tangier disease. *Nat Genet* **22**:347, 1999.
202. Rust S, Rosier M, Funke H, Real J, Amoura Z, Piette JC, Deleuze JF, Brewer HB, Duverger N, Denefle P, Assmann G: Tangier disease is caused by mutations in the gene encoding ATP-binding cassette transporter 1. *Nat Genet* **22**:352, 1999.
203. Lawn RM, Wade DP, Garvin MR, Wanfg X, Schwarttz K, Porter JG, Seiilhamer JJ, Vaughan AM, Oram JF: The Tangier disease gene product controls the cellular apolipoprotein-mediated lipid removal pathway. *J Clin Invest* **104**:R25, 1999.
204. Young SG, Fielding CJ: The ABCs of cholesterol efflux. *Nat Genet* **22**:316, 1999.
205. Scott J: Good cholesterol news. *Nature* **400**:816, 1999.
206. Czarnecka H, Yokoyama S: Lecithin:cholesterol acyltransferase reaction on cellular lipid released by free apolipoprotein-mediated efflux. *Biochemistry* **34**:4385, 1995.
207. Ji Y, Jian B, Wang N, Sun Y, Moya ML, Phillips MC, Rothblat GH, Swaney JB, Tall AR: Scavenger receptor BI promotes high density lipoprotein-mediated cellular cholesterol efflux. *J Biol Chem* **272**:20982, 1997.
208. De La Llera-Moya M, Rothblat GH, Connelly MA, Kellner-Weibel G, Sakr SW, Phillipis MC, Williams DL: Scavenger receptor B1 mediates free cholesterol flux independent of HDL tethering to the cell surface. *J Lipid Res* **40**:575, 1999.
209. Walter M, Reinecke H, Nofer J-R, Seedorf U, Assmann G: HDL_3 stimulates multiple signaling pathways in human skin fibroblasts. *Arterioscler Thromb Vasc Biol* **15**:1975, 1995.
210. Nofer JR, Walter M, Kehrel B, Seedorf U, Assmann G: HDL_3 activates phospholipase D in normal but not in glycoprotein IIb/IIIa-deficient platelets. *Biochem Biophys Res Commun* **207**:148, 1995.
211. Walter M, Reinecke H, Gerdes U, Nofer JR, Höbbel G, Seedorf U, Assmann G: Defective regulation of phosphatidylcholine-specific phospholipases C and D in a kindred with Tangier disease. Evidence for the involvement of phosphatidylcholine breakdown in HDL-mediated cholesterol efflux mechanisms. *J Clin Invest* **98**:2315, 1996.
212. Rogler GB, Trümbach B, Klima B, Lackner KJ, Schmitz G: HDL-mediated efflux of intracellular cholesterol is impaired in fibroblasts from Tangier disease patients. *Arterioscler Thromb Vasc Biol* **15**:683, 1995.
213. Drobnik W, Möllers C, Resink T, Schmitz G: Activation of phosphatidylinositol-specific phospholipase C in response to HDL3 and LDL is markedly reduced in cultured fibroblasts from Tangier patients. *Arterioscler Thromb Vasc Biol* **15**:1369, 1995.
214. Pörn MI, Ackerman KEO, Slotte JP: High density lipoprotein induces a rapid and transient release of $Ca2^{+}$ in cultured fibroblasts. *Biochem J* **279**:29, 1991.

215. Mollers C, Drobnik W, Resink T, Schmitz G: High density lipoprotein and low-density lipoprotein-mediated signal transduction in cultured human skin fibroblasts. *Cell Signal* **7**:695, 1995.
216. Voyno-Yaenetskaya TA, Dobbs LG, Erickson SK, Hamilton RL: Low-density lipoprotein and high-density lipoprotein-mediated signal transduction and exocytosis in alveolar type II cells. *Proc Natl Acad Sci U S A* **90**:4256, 1993.
217. Wu YQ, Handwerger S: High-density lipoproteins stimulate molecular weight 80K protein phosphorylation in human trophoblast cells: Evidence for a protein kinase C-dependent pathway in human placental lactogen release. *Endocrinology* **131**:2935, 1992.
218. Morishita H, Yui Y, Hattori R, Aoyama T, Kawai C: Increased hydrolysis of cholesteryl ester with prostacyclin is potentiated by high-density lipoprotein through the prostacyclin stabilization. *J Clin Invest* **86**:1885, 1990.
219. Hajjar DP: Regulation of neutral cholesteryl esterase in arterial smooth muscle cells: Stimulation by antagonists of adenylate cyclase and cyclic AMP-dependent protein kinase. *Arch Biochem Biophys* **247**:49, 1986.
220. Khoo JC, Mahoney EM, Steinberg DS: Neutral cholesterol esterase activity in macrophages and its enhancement by cyclic AMP-dependent protein kinase. *J Biol Chem* **256**:12659, 1981.
221. Hajjar Dp, Weksler Bb, Falcone DJ, Hefton JM, Tack-Goldmann K, Minick CR: Prostacyclin modulates cholesteryl ester hydrolytic activity by its effect on cyclic adenosine monophosphate in rabbit aortic smooth muscle cells. *J Clin Invest* **70**:479, 1982.
222. Schmitz G, Robenek, H, Lohmann, U, Assmann G: Interaction of high density lipoproteins with cholesteryl ester-laden macrophages: Biochemical and morphological characterization of cell surface receptor binding, endocytosis and resecretion of high density lipoproteins by macrophages. *EMBO J* **4**:613, 1985.
223. Oram, JF, Johnson, CJ, Brown, TA: Interaction of high density lipoprotein with its receptor on cultured fibroblasts and macrophages. Evidence for reversible binding at the cell surface without internalization. *J Biol Chem* **262**: 2405, 1987.
224. Herbert PN, Forte T, Heinen RJ, Fredrickson DS: Tangier disease. One explanation for lipid storage. *N Engl J Med* **299**:519, 1978.
225. Marbini A, Gemignani, F, Ferranini G, Maccari S, Bragaglia MM, Plancher C, Vergani MC: Tangier disease. A case with sensorimotoric distal polyneuropathy and lipid accumulation in striated muscle and vasa nervorum. *Acta Neuropathol* **67**:121, 1985.
226. Boyles JK, Zoellner CD, Anderson LJ, Kosik LM, Pitas P, Weisgraber KH, Hui DY, Mahley RW, Gebicke-Härter PJ, Ignatius MJ, Shooter EM: A role for apolipoproteins E, apolipoprotein A-I, and low density lipoprotein receptors in cholesterol transport during regeneration and remyelinization of the rat sciatic nerve. *J Clin Invest* **83**:1015, 1989.
227. Boyles JK, Notterpek, LM, Anderson, LJ: Accumulation of apolipoproteins in the regenerating remyelinating mammalian peripheral nerve. Identification of apolipoprotein D, apolipoprotein A-IV, apolipoprotein E, and apolipoprotein A-I. *J Biol Chem* **265**:17805, 1990.
228. Kivatinitz SC, Pelsman MA, Alonso AC, Bagatolli L, Quiroga S: High-density lipoprotein aggregated by oxidation induces degeneration of neuronal cells. *J Neurochem* **69**:2102, 1997.
229. de-Chaves EI, Rusinol AE, Vance DE, Campenot RB, Vance JE: Role of lipoproteins in the delivery of lipids to axons during axonal regeneration. *J Biol Chem* **272**:30766, 1997.
230. DeMattos RB, Curtiss LK, Williams DL: A minimally lipidated form of cell-derived apolipoprotein E exhibits isoform-specific stimulation of neurite outgrowth in the absence of exogenous lipids or lipoproteins. *J Biol Chem* **273**:4206, 1998.
231. Nathan BP, Bellosta S, Sanan DA, Weisgraber KH, Mahley RW, Pitas RE: Differential effects of apolipoproteins E3 and E4 on neuronal growth in vitro. *Science* **264**:850, 1994.
232. Schmitz G, Fischer H, Beuck M, Hoecker K-P, Robenek H: Dysregulation of lipid metabolism in Tangier monocyte derived macrophages. *Arteriosclerosis* **10**:1010, 1990.
233. Gordon D, Rifkind BM: Current concepts: High density lipoproteins—The clinical implications of recent studies. *N Engl J Med* **321**:1311, 1989.
234. Miccoli R, Bertolotto A, Navalesi R, Odoguardi L, Boni A, Wessling J, Funke H, Wiebusch H, von Eckardstein A, Assmann G: Hemizygosity for a structural apolipoprotein A-I-variant—apoA-I(L141R)$_{Pisa}$—causes high-density lipoprotein deficiency, corneal opacifications, and coronary heart disease. *Circulation* **94**:1622, 1996.
235. Kuivenhoven JA, Stalenhoef AF, Hill JS, Demacker PN, Errami A, Kastelein JJ, Pritchard PH: Two novel molecular defects in the LCAT gene are associated with fish eye disease. *Arterioscler Thromb Vasc Biol* **16**:294, 1996.
236. Walter M, Kerber S, Fechtrup C, Seedorf U, Breithardt G, Assmann G: Characterization of atherosclerosis in a patient with familial high-density lipoprotein deficiency. *Atherosclerosis* **110**:203, 1994.
237. Barchiesi BJ, Eckel RH, Ellis PP: The cornea and disorders of lipid metabolism. *Surv Ophthalmol* **36**:1, 1991.
238. Blanco-Vaca F, Qu SJ, Fiol C, Fan HZ, Pao Q, Marzal-Casacuberta A, Albers JJ, Hurtado I, Gracia V, Pinto X, Marti T, Pownall HJ: Molecular basis of fish-eye disease in a patient from Spain. Characterization of a novel mutation in the LCAT gene and lipid analysis of the cornea. *Arterioscler Thromb Vasc Biol* **17**:1382, 1997.
239. Di Michele DM, Hathaway WE: Use of DDAVP in inherited and acquired platelet dysfunction. *Am J Hematol* **33**:39, 1990.
240. Schaefer EJ: Clinical, biochemical, and genetic features in familial disorders of high-density lipoprotein deficiency. *Arteriosclerosis* **4**:303, 1984.
241. Lux SE, Levy RI, Gotto AM, Fredrickson DS: Studies on the protein defect in Tangier disease: Isolation and characterization of an abnormal high-density lipoprotein. *J Clin Invest* **51**:2505, 1972.
242. Assmann G, Herbert PN, Fredrickson DS, Forte T: Isolation and characterization of an abnormal high-density lipoprotein in Tangier disease. *J Clin Invest* **60**:242, 1977.
243. Heinen RS, Herbert P, Fredrickson DS, Forte T, Lindgren FT: Properties of the plasma very-low- and low-density lipoproteins in Tangier disease. *J Clin Invest* **61**:120, 1978.
244. Wang C-S, Alaupovic P, Gregg RE, Brewer HB Jr: Studies on the mechanism of hypertriglyceridemia in Tangier disease. Determination of plasma lipolytic activities, k_1 values and apolipoprotein composition of the major lipoprotein density classes. *Biochim Biophys Acta* **920**:9, 1987.
245. Alaupovic P, Knight-Gibson C, Wang C-S, Downs D, Koren E, Brewer HB Jr, Gregg RE: Isolation and characterisation of an apo A-II containing lipoprotein (Lp-A-II:B) complex) from plasma very low density lipoproteins of patients with Tangier disease and type V hyperlipoproteinemia. *J Lipid Res* **32**:9, 1991.
246. Schaefer EJ, Blum CB, Levy RI, Jenkins LL, Alaupovic P, Foster DM, Brewer BH JR: Metabolism of high density apolipoproteins in Tangier disease. *N Engl J Med* **299**:905, 1978.
247. von Eckardstein A, Huang Y, Wu S, Funke H, Noseda G, Assmann G: Reverse cholesterol transport in plasmas of patients with different forms of familial high-density lipoprotein deficiency. *Arterioscler Thromb Vasc Biol* **15**:691, 1995.
248. Duverger N, Theret N, De Geitere, Brewer HB Jr, Fruchart JC, Castro G: Tangier disease isolation and characterization of LpA-I, LpA-II, LpA-I:A-II and LpA-IV particles from plasma. *Biochim Biophys Acta* **1182**:30, 1993.
249. von Eckardstein A, Huang Y, Wu S, Funke H, Noseda G, Assmann G: Reverse cholesterol transport in plasmas of patients with different forms of familial high density lipoprotein deficiency. *Arterioscler Thromb Vasc Biol* **15**:691, 1995.
250. Law SW, Gray G, Brewer HB JR: cDNA cloning of human apo A-I: Amino acid sequence of preproapo A-I. *Biochem Biophys Res Commun* **112**:257, 1983.
251. Karathanasis SK, Zannis VI, Breslow JL: Isolation and characterization of the human apolipoprotein A-I gene. *Proc Natl Acad Sci U S A* **80**:6147, 1983.
252. Shoulders CC, Kornblihtt AR, Munro BS, Baralle FE: Gene structure of human apolipoprotein A-I. *Nucleic Acids Res* **11**:2877, 1983.
253. Zannis VI, Lees AM, Lees RS, Breslow JL: Abnormal apolipoprotein A-I isoprotein composition in patients with Tangier disease. *J Biol Chem* **257**:4978, 1982.
254. Brewer HB Jr, Fairwell T, Meng MS, Kay L, Ronan R: Human proapo A-I: Isolation of proapoA-I and amino acid sequence of the peptide. *Biochem Biophys Res Commun* **113**:934, 1983.
255. Alaupovic P, Schaefer EJ, Mcconathy WJ, Fesmire JD, Brewer HB Jr: Plasma apolipoprotein concentrations in familial apolipoprotein A-I and A-II deficiency (Tangier disease). *Metabolism* **30**:805, 1981.
256. Assmann G, Schmitz G, Heckers H: Lecithin-cholesterol acyltransferase in Tangier disease. *Scand J Clin Lab Invest* **38(Suppl)**:98, 1978.
257. Assmann G: Structure-function relationship of lipoproteins, in Tangier disease, in Greten H (ed): *Lipoprotein Metabolism*. Berlin, Springer-Verlag, 1976, p 106.
258. Yao JK, Dyck PJ: In vitro cholesterol esterification in human serum. *Clin Chem* **23**:447, 1977.
259. Scherer R, Ruhenstroth-Bauer G: Untersuchung der lecithin-cholesterin acyltransferase-aktivität im serum von drei patienten mit Tangier-Krankheit (hyp-alpha-liproteinämie). *Klin Wochenschr* **51**:1059, 1973.

260. Pritchard PH, Frohlich J: Apoprotein A-I and lecithin: Cholesterol acyltransferase in a patient with Tangier disease. *Adv Exp Med Biol* **201**:105, 1987.
261. Pritchard PH, Mcleod RM, Frohlich J, Park MC, Kudchodkar BJ, Lacko AG: Lecithin: Cholesterol acyltransferase metabolism in familial HDL deficiency (Tangier disease). *Biochim Biophys Acta* **958**:227, 1988.
262. Carlson LA: Fish eye disease: A new familial condition with massive corneal opacities and dyslipoproteinaemia. *Eur J Clin Invest* **12**:41, 1982.
263. Carlson LA, Holmquist L: Evidence for deficiency of high-density lipoprotein lecithin: Cholesterol acyltransferase activity (α-LCAT) in fish eye disease. *Acta Med Scand* **218**:189, 1985.
264. Carlson LA, Holmquist L: Evidence for the presence in human plasma of lecithin: Cholesterol acyltransferase activity (β-LCAT) specifically esterifying free cholesterol of combined pre-β and β-lipoproteins. Studies on fish eye disease patients and control subjects. *Acta Med Scand* **218**:197, 1985.
265. Carlson LA, Holmquist L, Assmann G: Different substrate specificities of plasma lecithin: Cholesterol acyl transferase in fish eye disease and Tangier disease. *Acta Med Scand* **222**:345, 1987.
266. Forte TM, Nichols AV, Krauss RM, Norum RA: Familial apolipoprotein A-I and C-III deficiency. Subclass distribution, composition and morphology of lipoproteins in a disorder associated with premature atherosclerosis. *J Clin Invest* **74**:1601, 1984.
267. Funke H, von Eckardstein A, Pritchard PH, Karas M, Albers JJ, Assmann G: A frameshift mutation in the apo A-I gene causes corneal opacities, HDL deficiency and partial LCAT deficiency a syndrome that is distinct from fish eye disease. *J Clin Invest* **87**:375, 1991.
268. Assmann G, von Eckardstein A, Funke H: Lecithin:cholesterol acyltransferase deficiency and fish eye disease. *Curr Opin Lipidol* **2**:110, 1991.
269. Jonas A: Regulation of lecithin cholesterol acyltransferase activity. *Prog Lipid Res* **37**:209, 1998.
270. Cheung MC, Wang D, Lum KD, Albers JJ: Cholesterol esterification by lecithin:cholesterol acyltransferase in A-I free plasma. *Biochim Biophys Acta* **962**:258, 1988.
271. Sparks DL, Frohlich J, Pritchard PH: Cholesteryl ester transfer activity in plasma of patients with familial high density lipoprotein deficiency. *Clin Chem* **34**:1812, 1988.
272. Assmann G, Smootz E: High-density lipoprotein infusion and partial plasma exchange in Tangier disease. *Eur J Clin Invest* **8**:131, 1978.
273. Schaefer EJ, Anderson DW, Zech LA, Lindgren FT, Bronzert TB, Rubalcaba EA, Brewer HB JR: Metabolism of high density lipoprotein subfractions and constituents in Tangier disease following the infusion of high-density lipoproteins. *J Lipid Res* **22**:217, 1981.
274. Schaefer EJ, Kay LL, Zech LA, Lindgren FT, Brewer HB JR: Tangier disease: High-density lipoprotein deficiency due to defective metabolism of an abnormal apolipoprotein apo A-I (apo A-I). *J Clin Invest* **70**:934, 1982.
275. Bojanovski D, Gregg RE, Zech LA, Meng MS, Bishop C, Ronan R, Brewer HB JR: In vivo metabolism of proapolipoprotein A-I in Tangier disease. *J Clin Invest* **80**:1742, 1987.
276. Schmitz G, Assmann G, Robenek H, Brennhausen B: Tangier disease: A disorder of intracellular membrane traffic. *Proc Natl Acad Sci U S A* **82**:6305, 1985.
277. Robenek H, Schmitz G: Abnormal processing of Golgi elements and lysosomes in Tangier disease. *Arteriosclerosis Thromb* **11**:1007, 1991.
278. Oram JF, Mendez AJ, Lymp J, Kavanagh TJ, Halbert CL: Reduction in apolipoprotein-mediated removal of cellular lipids by immortalization of human fibroblasts and its reversion by cAMP: Lack of effect with Tangier disease cells. *J Lipid Res* **40**:1769, 1999.
279. Walter M, Gerdes U, Seedorf U, Assmann G: The high-density lipoprotein- and apolipoprotein A-I-induced mobilization of cellular cholesterol is impaired in fibroblasts from Tangier disease subjects. *Biochem Biophys Res Commun* **205**:850, 1994.
280. Assmann G, Simantke O, Schaefer HE, Smootz E: Characterization of high density lipoproteins in patients heterozygous for Tangier disease. *J Clin Invest* **60**:1025, 1977.
281. Schaefer EJ, Zech LA, Schwartz DE, Brewer HB JR: Coronary heart disease prevalence and other clinical features in familial high-density lipoprotein deficiency (Tangier disease). *Ann Intern Med* **93**:261, 1980.
282. Henderson LO, Herbert PN, Fredrickson DS, Heinen RJ, Easterling JC: Abnormal concentration and anomalous distribution of apolipoprotein A-I in Tangier disease. *Metabolism* **27**:165, 1978.
283. Fredrickson DS: The inheritance of high-density lipoprotein deficiency (Tangier disease). *J Clin Invest* **43**:228, 1964.
284. Marcil M, Brooks-Wislon A, Clee SM, Roomp K, Zhang LH, Yu L, Collins JA, van Dam M, Molhuizen HOF, Loubster O, Ouellette BFF, Sensen CW, Fichter K, Mott S, Denis M, Boucher B, Pimstone S, Genest J, Kastelein JJP, Hayden MR: Mutations in the ABC1 gene in familial HDL deficiency with defective cholesterol efflux. *Lancet* **354**:1341, 1996.
285. Eberhardt E, Mendez AJ, Freeman WM: Decreased cholesterol efflux from fibroblasts of a patient without Tangier disease, but with markedly reduced high density lipoprotein cholesterol levels. *J Clin Endocrinol Metab* **83**:836, 1998.
286. Rust S, Walter M, Funke H, von Eckardstein A, Cullen P, Kroes HY, Hordijk R, Geisel J, Kastelein JJP, Molhuizen HOF, Schreiner M, Mischke A, Hahmann HW, Assmann G: Assignment of Tangier disease (familial deficiency of high density lipoprotein) to chromosome 9 by a graphical linkage exclusion strategy. *Nat Genet* **20**:96, 1998.
287. Dean M, Allikmets R: Evolution of ATP binding cassette transporter genes. *Curr Opin Genet Dev* **5**:79, 1995.
288. Higgins CF: ABC transporters: From microorganisms to man. *Ann Rev Cell Biol* **8**:67, 1992.
289. Higgins CF: The ABC of channel regulation. *Cell* **82**:693, 1995.
290. Riordan JR, Rommens JM, Kerem B, Alon N, Rozmahel R, Grzelczak Z, Zielenski J, Lok S, Plavsic N, Chou JL: Identification of the cystic fibrosis gene—Cloning and characterisation of complementary cDNA. *Science* **245**:1066, 1989.
291. Thomas PM, Cote GJ, Wohllk N, Haddad B, Mathew PM, Rabl W, Aguilar Bryan L, Gagel RF, Bryan J: Mutations in the sulfonylurea receptor gene in familial persistent hyperinsulinemic hypoglycemia of infancy. *Science* **268**:426, 1995.
292. Mosser J, Douar AM, Sarde CO, Kioschis P, Feil R, Moser H, Poustka AM, Mandel JL, Aubourg P: Putative X-liked adrenoleukodystrophy gene shares unexpected homology to ABC transporters. *Nature* **361**:726, 1993.
293. Gartner J, Moser H, Valle D: Mutations in the 70K peroxisomal membrane protein gene in Zellweger syndrome. *Nat Genet* **1**:16, 1992.
294. Allikmets R: A photoreceptor-cell specific ATP-binding transporter gene (ABCR) is mutated in Stargardt macular dystrophy. *Nat Genet* **17**:122, 1997.
295. Cremers FP, van de Pol DJ, van Driel M, den Hollander AI, van Haren FJ, Knoers NV, Tijmes N, Bergen AA, Rohrschneider K, Blankenagel A, Pinckers AJ, Deutman AF, Hoyng CB: Autosomal recessive retinitis pigmentosa and cone rod dystrophy caused by splice site mutations in the Stargardt's disease gene ABCR. *Hum Mol Genet* **7**:355, 1998.
296. de Vree JM, Jacquemin E, Sturm E, Cresteil D, Bosma PJ, Aten J, Deleuze JF, Desrochers M, Burdelski M, Bernard O, Oude Elferink RP, Hadchouel M: Mutations in the MDR3 gene cause progressive familial intrahepatic cholestasis. *Proc Natl Acad Sci U S A* **95**:282, 1998.
297. Strautnieks SS, Bull LN, Knisely AS, Kocoshis SA, Dahl N, Arnell H, Sokal E, Dahan K, Shilds S, Ling V, Tanner MS, Kagalwalla AF, Nemeth A, Pawlowska J, Baker A, Mieli-Vergani G, Freimer NB, Gardiner RM, Thompson RJ: A gene encoding a liver-specific ABC transporter is mutated in progressive familial intrahepatic cholestasis. *Nat Genet* **20**:233, 1998.
298. Wada M, Toh S, Taniguchi K, Nakamura T, Uchiumi T, Kohno K, Yoshida I, et al.: Mutations in the canilicular multispecific organic anion transporter (cMOAT) gene, a novel ABC transporter, in patients with hyperbilirubinemia II Dubin-Johnson syndrome. *Hum Mol Genet* **7**:203, 1998.
299. Remaley AT, Rust S, Rosier M, Knapper C, Naudin L, Broccardo C, Peterson KM, Koch C, Arnould I, Prades C, Duverger N, Funke H, Assmann G, Dinger M, Dean M, Chimini G, SantamarinA-Fojo S, Fredrickson DS, Denefle P, Brewer HB: Human ATP binding cassette transporter 1 (ABC1): Genomic organisation and identification of the genetic defect in the original Tangier disease kindred. *Proc Natl Acad Sci U S A* **96**:12685, 1999.
300. Langmann T, Klucken J, Reil M, Liebisch G, Luciani M-F, Chimini G, Kaminski WE, Schmitz G: Molecular Cloning of the human ATP binding cassette transporter 1 (hABC1): Evidence for sterol-dependent regulation in macrophages. *Biochem Biophys Res Commun* **257**:29, 1999.
301. Rosenberg MF, Callaghan R, Ford RC, Higgins CF: Structure of the multidrug resistance P-glycoprotein to 2.5 nm resolution determined by electron microscopy and image analysis. *J Biol Chem* **272**:10685, 1997.
302. Luciani M-F, Chimini G: The ATP binding cassette transporter ABC1 is required for the engulfment of corpses generated by apoptotic cell death. *EMBO J* **15**:226, 1996.

303. Becq F, Hamon Y, Bajetto A, Gola M, Verrier B, Chimini G: ABC1, an ATP-binding cassette transporter required for phagocytosis of apoptotic cells, generates a regulated anion flux after expression in *Xenopus laevis* oocytes. *J Biol Chem* **272**:2695, 1997.
304. Hamon Y, Luciani M-F, Becq F, Verrier B, Rubartelli A, Chimini G: Interleukin 1b secretion is impaired by inhibitors of the ATP binding cassette transporter ABC1. *Blood* **90**:211, 1997.
305. Van Helvoort A, Smith AJ, Sprong H, Fritzsche I, Schinkel AH, Borst P, van Meer G: MDR1 P-glycoprotein is a lipid translocase of broad specificity, while MDR3 p-glycoprotein specifically translocates phosphatidylcholine. *Cell* **87**:507, 1996.
306. Schwiebert Em, Benos DJ, Egan ME, Stutts MJ, Guggino WB: CFTR is a conductance regulator as well as a chloride channel. *Physiol Rev* 79:S145, 1999.
307. Bradbury NA: Intracellular CFTR: Localization and function. *Physiol Rev* **79**:S175, 1999.
308. Bevers EM, Comfurius P, Dekkers DWC, Zwaal RFA: Lipid translocation across the plasma membrane of mammalian cells. *Biochim Biophys Acta* **1439**:317, 1999.
309. Weng J, Mata NL, Azarian SM, Tzekov RT, Birch DG, Travis GH: Insights into the function of Rim protein in photoreceptors and etiology of Stargardt's disease from the phenotype in abcr knockout mice. *Cell* **98**:13, 1999.
310. Adrei C, Dazzi C, Lotti L, Torrisi MR, Chimini G, Rubartelli A: The secretory route of the leaderless protein interleukin 1β involves exocytosis of endolysosome-related vesicles. *Mol Biol Cell* **10**:1463, 1999.
311. Funke H: Familial HDL deficiency syndromes. Atherosclerosis XI. *Excerpta Medica* **1155**:713, 1998.
312. Kuivenhoven JA, Pritchard PH, Frohlich JJ, Assmann G, Kastelein JJP: The molecular pathology of LCAT deficiency syndromes. *J Lipid Res* **38**:191, 1997.
313. Assmann G, von Eckardstein A, Funke H: High-density lipoproteins, reverse transport of cholesterol, and coronary heart disease: insights from mutations. *Circulation* **87(Suppl III)**:III-28, 1993.
314. Lindeskog GR, Gustafson A: Serum lipoprotein deficiency in diffuse normolipemic plane xanthoma. *Arch Dermatol* **106**:529, 1972.
315. Gustavson A, McConathy WJ, Alaupovic P, Curry MD, Persson B: Identification of apoprotein families in a variant of human plasma apolipoprotein A deficiency. *Scand J Clin Lab Invest* **39**:377, 1979.
316. Emmerich J, Verges B, Tauveron I, Rader D, Santamarina-Fojo S, Schaefer J, Ayrault-Jarrier M, Thieblot P, Brewer HB Jr: Familial HDL deficiency due to marked hypercatabolism of normal apoA-I. *Arterioscler Thromb* **13**:1299, 1993.
317. Marcil M, Boucher B, Krimbou L, Solymoss BC, Davignon J, Frohlich J, Genest J Jr: Severe familial HDL deficiency in French Canadian kindreds. Clinical, biochemical, and molecular characterization. *Arterioscler Thromb Vasc Biol* **15**:1015, 1995.
318. Marcil M, Yu L, Krimbou L, Boucher B, Oram JF, Cohn JS, Genest J Jr: Cellular cholesterol transport and efflux in fibroblasts are abnormal in subjects with familial HDL deficiency. *Arterioscler Thromb Vasc Biol* **15**:1015, 1999.
319. Pocovi M, Cenarro A, Civeira F, Torralba MA, Perez-Calvo JI, Mozas P, Giraldo P, Giralt M, Myers RH, Cupples LA, Ordovas JM: β-glucocerebrosidase gene locus as a link for Gaucher's disease and familial hypo-α-lipoproteinemia. *Lancet* **351**:1919, 1998.
320. McIntyre N, Owen JS: Plasma lipids and lipoproteins in liver disease, in Cohen RD, Lewis B, Alberti KGMM, Denamn AM: *The Metabolic and Molecular Basis of Acquired Disease*. London, Baillière Tindall, 1991, p 1176.
321. Lewis B: Hyperlipidemia, in Cohen RD, Lewis B, Alberti KGMM, Denamn AM: *The Metabolic and Molecular Basis of Acquired Disease*. London, Baillière Tindall, 1991, p 860.
322. Noseda G, Riesen W, Schlumpf E, Morell A: Hypo-α-lipoproteinaemia associated with auto-antibodies against α-lipoproteins. *Eur J Clin Invest* **2**:342, 1972.
323. De Buyzere M, Delanghe J, Labeur C, Noens L, Benoit Y, Baert J, Rosseneu M: Acquired hypoalphalipoproteinemia. *Clin Chem* **38**:776, 1992.
324. Janka GE: Familial hemophagocytic lymphohistiocytosis. *Eur J Pediatr* **140**:221, 1983.
325. Henter JI, Carlson LA, Söder O, Nilson-Ehle P, Elinder G: Lipoprotein alterations and plasma lipoprotein lipase reduction in familial hemophagocytic lymphohistiocytosis. *Acta Paediatr Scand* **80**:675, 1991.
326. Gallin JI, Kaye DO, O'Leary W: Serum lipids in infection. *N Engl J Med* **281**:1081, 1970.
327. Akerlund B, Carlson LA, Jarstrand C: Dyslipoproteinemia in patients with severe bacterial infections. *Scand J Infect Dis* **18**:539, 1986.
328. Walter M, Seedorf U, Assmann G: Acquired HDL deficiency with Tangier-like phenotype induced by a soluble factor. *Circulation (Suppl)* **96**: I-723, 1997.
329. Franceschini G, Werba JP, D'Acquarica AL, Gianfranceschi G, Michelagnoli S, Sirtori CR: Microsomal enzyme inducers raise plasma high density lipoprotein cholesterol levels in healthy control subjects but not in patients with primary hypoalphalipoproteinemia. *Clin Pharmacol Ther* **57**:434, 1995.
330. International Task Force for Prevention of Coronary Heart Disease: Coronary heart disease: Reducing the risk. The scientific background to primary and secondary prevention of coronary heart disease. A worldwide view. *Nutr Metab Cardiovasc Dis* **8**:205, 1998.
331. Jeppesen J, Hein HO, Suadicani P, Gyntelberg F: Triglyceride concentration and ischemic heart disease. An eight-year follow-up in the Copenhagen male study. *Circulation* **97**:1029, 1998.
332. Austin MA: Plasma triglyceride and coronary artery disease. *Arterioscler Thromb* **11**:2, 1991.
333. Assmann G, Schulte H, von Eckardstein A: Hypertriglyceridemia and elevated levels of lipoprotein(a) are risk factors for major coronary events in middle-aged men. *Am J Cardiol* **77**:1179, 1996.

CHAPTER 123

Inborn Errors in Bile Acid Biosynthesis and Storage of Sterols Other than Cholesterol

Ingemar Björkhem ■ Kirsten Muri Boberg ■ Eran Leitersdorf

1. 3β-Hydroxysteroid-Δ^5-oxidoreductase/isomerase deficiency is a very rare cholestatic disease characterized by jaundice, hepatomegaly, pale stools, and dark urine. No normal bile acids are present in plasma. Sulfated 3β,7α-dihydroxy- and 3β,7α,12α-trihydroxy-5-cholenoic acids are excreted in urine and bile. Untreated the disease may lead to early development of liver cirrhosis. Treatment with chenodeoxycholic acid inhibits the rate-limiting enzyme in bile acid biosynthesis, the cholesterol 7α-hydroxylase, and diminishes the production of toxic metabolites from cholesterol.

2. 3-Oxo-Δ^4-steroid 5β-reductase deficiency is also a very rare cholestatic disease with symptoms similar to those above. Bile, serum, and urine contain 7α-hydroxylated bile acids with a 3-oxo-Δ^4-structure. These patients also respond favorably to bile acid therapy.

3. 27-Hydroxylase deficiency (cerebrotendinous xanthomatosis (CTX)) is a rare familial sterol storage disease with accumulation of cholestanol and cholesterol in most tissues, and in particular in xanthomas, bile, and brain. Clinically, this disorder is characterized by dementia, spinal cord paresis, cerebellar ataxia, tuberous and tendon xanthomas, early atherosclerosis, and cataracts.

More than 20 different mutations have been defined in the sterol 27-hydroxylase gene of CTX patients. The defect leads to a block in bile acid biosynthesis, with accumulation of substrates for the mitochondrial 27-hydroxylase such as 5β-cholestane-3α,7α,12α-triol and 7α-hydroxy-4-cholestene-3-one. The former metabolite is metabolized into 5β-cholestane-3α,7α,12α,25-tetrol, 5β-cholestane-3α,7α,12α,23-tetrol, and 5β-cholestane-3α,7α,12α,24,25-pentol.

These bile alcohols are excreted in gram amounts in bile and feces. At least part of the excess cholestanol in patients with CTX is formed from the accumulated 7α-hydroxy-4-cholesten-3-one. The reason for the accumulation of cholesterol in tissues is not known with certainty. In general, the levels of cholesterol in serum are normal, whereas the levels of cholestanol are markedly increased. Patients with CTX should be treated with chenodeoxycholic acid which reduces the 7α-hydroxylation of cholesterol, thereby reducing the formation of cholestanol and the excretion of bile alcohols in feces and urine.

4. In addition to the above defects in bile acid synthesis, one fatal case with a defined mutation in the gene coding for the oxysterol 7α-hydroxylase has been reported. A patient with a unique inborn error in bile acid conjugation involving a deficiency in amidation has also been described.

5. Phytosterolemia (sitosterolemia) is a rare inherited sterol storage disease characterized by tendon and tuberous xanthomas and by a strong predisposition to premature coronary atherosclerosis. Some patients may develop hemolytic syndromes. Increased amounts of phytosterols (plant sterols), such as sitosterol and campesterol and their 5α-stanols, are found in blood, plasma, erythrocytes, and different tissues, in particular in the xanthomas and arteries of affected patients. Increased serum cholesterol and cholestanol have also been found in many patients.

The basic biochemical defect in this autosomal recessive disease has not been defined. Increased intestinal absorption of phytosterols and shellfish sterols has been observed in some cases. Evidence has also been presented for decreased biliary and fecal excretion of cholesterol, phytosterols, and shellfish sterols.

Patients with phytosterolemia should be treated with diets low in plant and shellfish sterols. In addition, they should be given cholestyramine, which causes increased excretion and lowered plasma levels of phytosterols.

NORMAL BIOSYNTHESIS AND METABOLISM OF BILE ACIDS

The hepatic conversion of cholesterol into bile acids involves almost all the conceivable mechanisms for conversion of a lipophilic compound into an excretable water-soluble product (for general reviews, see references 1–3). The more than 15 different enzymes participating in the conversion belong to the groups of hydroxylases, oxidoreductases, reductases, ligases, oxidases, thiolases, and transferases. The enzymes modifying the steroid nucleus are able to convert the unpolar 3β-hydroxy-Δ^5-steroid in cholesterol into a considerably more polar 5β-cholestane-3α,7α-dihydroxy- or 5β-cholestane-3α,7α,12α-trihydroxy steroid. The enzymes involved in these nuclear conversions are mainly located to the endoplasmic reticulum and the cytosol. The enzymes involved in the steroid side-chain degradation are able to convert the highly unpolar C_{27}-steroid side-chain into a chain-shortened carboxylic acid conjugated to an amino acid. These enzymes are mainly located in the mitochondria and in the peroxisomes.

Neutral Pathway to Cholic and Chenodeoxycholic Acid

According to current concepts, the major pathway for conversion of cholesterol into bile acids in mammals starts with the nuclear transformations and most or all of these changes precede those of the steroid side-chain ("neutral pathway"). The sequence of reactions in this pathway from cholesterol to the two primary bile acids cholic acid and chenodeoxycholic acid is shown in Fig. 123-1. During the last few years an alternative

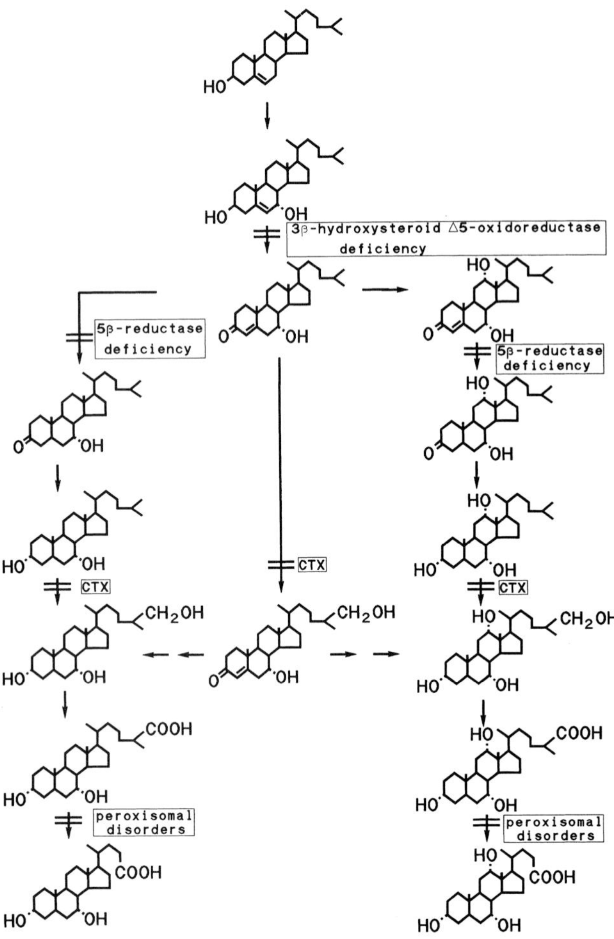

Fig. 123-1 Neutral pathway for the normal synthesis of cholic acid and chenodeoxycholic acid in humans. The known metabolic defects are indicated. CTX = cerebrotendinous xanthomatosis.

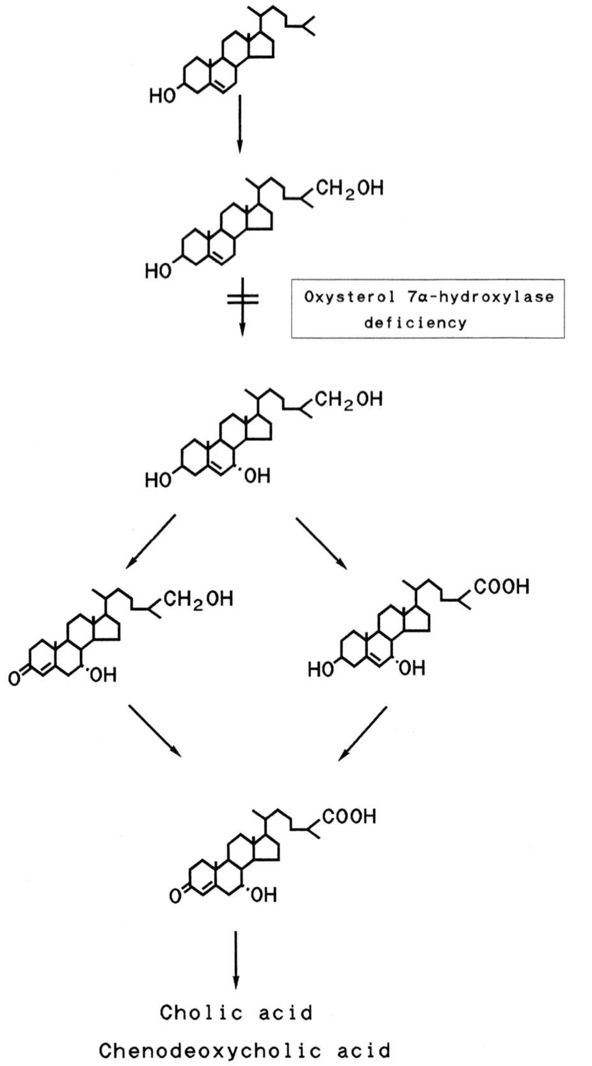

Oxysterol 7α-hydroxylase deficiency

Cholic acid

Chenodeoxycholic acid

Fig. 123-2 Acid pathway for the normal synthesis of cholic acid and chenodeoxycholic acid. The known metabolic defect in this pathway is indicated.

pathway starting with oxidation of the side-chain has been demonstrated to be important in mammals (Fig. 123-2). Under basal conditions this latter pathway (also called "acidic pathway") seems to be responsible for formation of 30 to 50 percent of the synthesis in adults. In early life, the acidic pathway seems to be more important than the neutral pathway, however.

Up to now, five of the different enzymes involved in the major pathway have been reported to be missing or to have reduced activity due to an inborn defect.

The first and rate-limiting reaction in the sequence, conversion of cholesterol into 7α-hydroxy-cholesterol, is catalyzed by the *cholesterol 7α-hydroxylase*. The cDNA encoding this cytochrome P-450 enzyme in human liver has been characterized.[4]

This enzyme regulates the overall conversion of cholesterol into bile acids in the major pathway. The most important mechanism for regulation of the enzyme seems to be a negative feedback by bile acids reabsorbed from the intestine, returning to the liver via the portal vein. As a consequence, interruption of the enterohepatic circulation (bile duct fistulation, treatment with resins such as cholestyramine) leads to a marked increase in the activity. It has been shown in rats that this up-regulation occurs at the transcriptional level.[3,5] The enzymatic activity is of great importance for cholesterol homeostasis and is influenced by a number of dietary and hormonal factors.[1–3] There is a close coupling between this enzyme and the rate-limiting enzyme in cholsterol biosynthesis, the HMG CoA reductase (for a review, see reference 5). Thus, under most experimental conditions, the activity of these two enzymes changes in parallel. This means that changes in cholesterol synthesis are paralleled by the corresponding changes in cholesterol degradation and vice versa. As a consequence, the cholesterol level is kept constant. No inborn defect in the cholesterol 7α-hydroxylase has been reported.

The next step in the sequence, oxidation of 7α-hydroxycholesterol into 7α-hydroxy-4-cholesten-3-one, is catalyzed by a microsomal NAD-dependent *3β-hydroxysteroid-Δ⁵-oxidoreductase/isomerase*. It should be noted that the enzyme catalyzes two reactions, both an oxidation of the 3β-hydroxy group and an isomerization of the double bond.[1] This enzyme is present both in liver and fibroblasts. The enzyme has been purified to homogeneity from pig liver and characterized.[6] The possibility has been discussed that this enzyme may be regulated to some extent by the flux of bile acids in the enterohepatic circulation,[7] but no evidence has been presented yet for this. An inborn error of this enzyme has been described, but this defect has not yet been defined at a molecular level (see below).

The third step in the sequence to cholic acid, conversion of 7α-hydroxy-4-cholestene-3-one into 7α,12α-dihydroxy-4-cholestene-3-one, is catalyzed by a microsomal cytochrome P-450-containing *sterol-12α-hydroxylase*. This enzyme was recently purified to homogeneity and cloned from rabbit liver.[8] The enzyme seems to be up-regulated to some extent in human liver in connection with interruption of the enterohepatic circulation[9] and at least in rats and rabbits the enzyme is also up-regulated by starvation.[10]

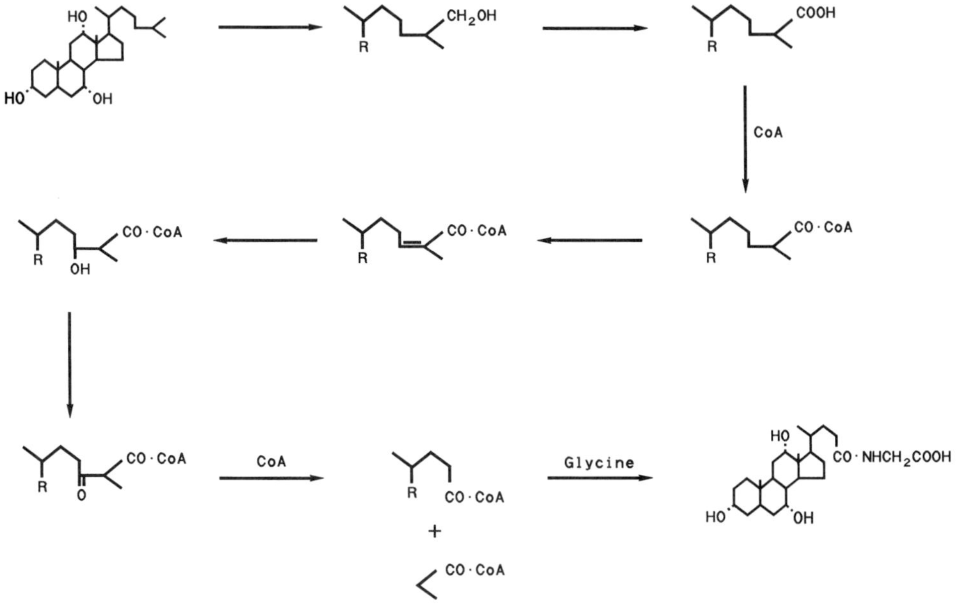

Fig. 123-3 Normal mechanism for degradation of the steroid side-chain in the biosynthesis of bile acid from cholesterol (27-hydroxylase pathway).

There is no firm evidence for the occurrence of a defect in this specific enzyme. If it exists, such a defect may not be associated with clinical symptoms, and may therefore go undetected.

The next step in the sequence, conversion of 7α,12α-dihydroxy-4-cholestene-3-one into 7α,12α-hydroxy-5β-cholestane-3-one, is catalyzed by a *soluble 3-oxosteroid* Δ^4*-steroid 5β-reductase*. A cDNA coding for this enzyme in human liver was recently characterized.[11] The enzyme does not seem to be of regulatory importance. A few cases with an apparent inborn defect in this enzyme have been reported (see below). The mutations have not yet been defined at a molecular level, however.

The next step in the sequence, conversion of 7α,12α-dihydroxy-5β-cholestane-3-one into 5β-cholestane-3α,7α,12α-triol, is catalyzed by a *3α-hydroxysteroid dehydrogenase*. This enzyme has been purified to homogeneity from rat liver and characterized.[12] There are no reports on inborn defects in this enzyme.

The next step in the sequence, conversion of 5β-cholestane-3α,7α,12α-triol into 5β-cholestane-3α,7α,12α,27-tetrol, is catalyzed by a mitochondrial *sterol 27-hydroxylase* (the enzyme was previously called 26-hydroxylase). This cytochrome P-450-containing hydroxylase has been extensively characterized in several species, including man (for a review, see reference 13). There is an inborn defect of this hydroxylase called cerebrotendinous xanthomatosis (CTX) which is described below.

The subsequent enzymatic reactions involve oxidation of the 27-hydroxyl group to yield 3α,7α,12α-trihydroxy-5β-cholestanoic acid (trihydroxycoprostanoic acid or THCA). These conversions may be catalyzed by the above mitochondrial 27-hydroxylase,[14] or by soluble or mitochondrial alcohol dehydrogenase (for a review see reference 13).

THCA is activated with CoA by a *microsomal CoA ligase*[15] (Fig. 123-3). The CoA activated THCA is then β-oxidized in the peroxisomes to yield the CoA ester of cholic acid in reactions similar to those involved in β-oxidation of fatty acids. The detailed mechanism for the side-chain degradation is shown in Fig. 123-3. The first step in this sequence of reactions is rate limiting and catalyzing by a specific peroxisomal *THCA CoA acyl oxidase*. The gene coding for this enzyme was recently cloned and it was shown that it is different from the peroxisomal acyl CoA oxidases involved in β-oxidation of fatty acids.[16,17] Peroxisomes are also able to catalyze oxidation of 3α,7α-dihydroxy-5β-cholestanoic acid (dihydroxycoprostanoic acid or DHCA) into the CoA ester of chenodeoxycholic acid. It is not known, however, if the enzymes involved are different from those involved in the biosynthesis of cholic acid.[17] The end product of the peroxisomal reactions is thus the CoA esters of cholic acid or chenodeoxycholic acid (Fig. 123-1) or the corresponding glycine or taurine conjugate (Fig. 123-3). The conjugation reactions may also take place in the peroxisomes or in the endoplasmic reticulum.[13,18] A number of peroxisomal disorders are known in which THCA CoA acyl oxidase, and probably also some of the other peroxisomal enzymes, are lacking (see below). One case with a deficient amidation has also been reported (see below).

The end products of the above major pathway are amino acid conjugates of the primary bile acids cholic acid and chenodeoxycholic acid. After secretion in bile these bile acids may, however, be deconjugated and also dehydroxylated at C-7 by intestinal microorganisms.[1] Deoxycholic acid is the 7α-dehydroxylated product of cholic acid and lithocholic acid is the corresponding dehydroxylated product of chenodeoxycholic acid.

Lithocholic acid and also to some extent chenodeoxycholic acid may be hydroxylated in the liver.[1]

Acidic Pathways

Because the mitochondrial 27-hydroxylase has broad substrate specificity, pathways exist where the 27-hydroxyl group is introduced at a stage where only part of the nuclear changes have occurred.

At present there is experimental support for the presence of three specific such pathways in human liver (for a review, see reference 13). The most important of these pathways starts with a mitochondrial 27-hydroxylation followed by a microsomal 7α-hydroxylation by a specific *oxysterol 7α-hydroxylase*[19–21] (Fig. 123-2). The gene coding for the latter enzyme in humans was recently cloned.[21] As mentioned above, evidence has been presented to support the contention that this pathway may be responsible for up to 50 percent of the biosynthesis of bile acids in adults under normal conditions. Regardless of the quantitative importance, a block of this pathway at the specific level of the oxysterol 7α-hydroxylase leads to severe consequences.[21] It is evident that the acid pathway is regulated separately from the major pathway. Thus, the pathway, starting with a 27-hydroxylation of cholesterol, is not increased by, for example, interruption of the enterohepatic circulation of bile acids.

There is a pathway in which 7α-hydroxy-4-cholestene-3-one formed in the major pathway is 27-hydroxylated to yield

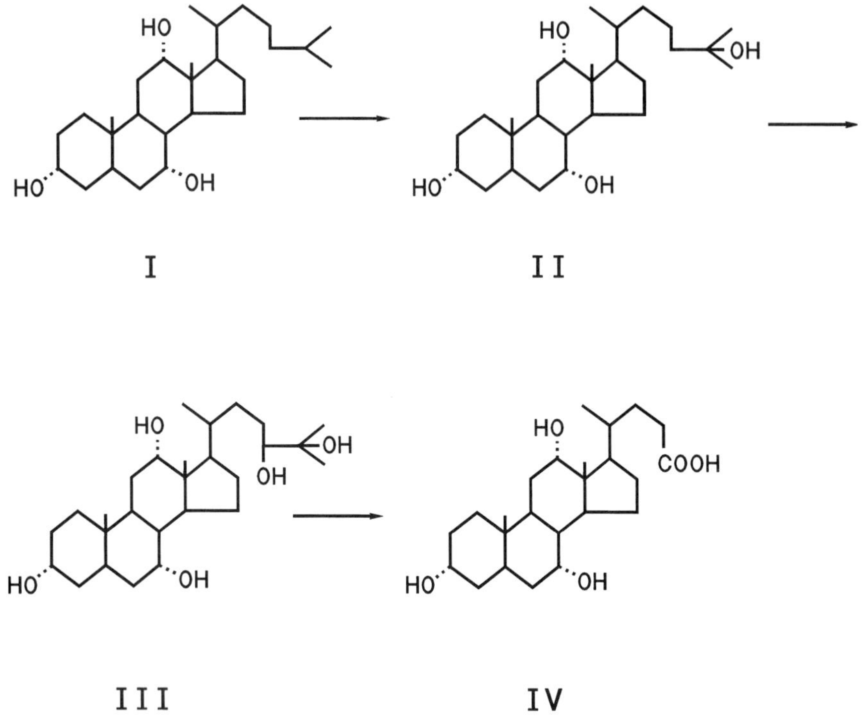

I

II

III

IV

Fig. 123-4 Formation of cholic acid from 5β-cholestane-3α,7α,12α-triol by the pathway described by Salen et al.[170]

7α,27-dihydroxy-4-cholesten-3-one.[13] In this pathway, the 5β-reductase and the 3α-hydroxysteroid dehydrogenase are acting on 27-oxygenated or C_{24}-carboxylic acid intermediates.

There is a pathway in which 7α,12α-dihydroxy-4-cholesten-3-one is 27-hydroxylated to yield 7α,12α,27-trihydroxy-4-cholesten-3-one.[13] Also in this pathway the 5β-reductase and the 3α-hydroxysteroid dehydrogenase are active on 27-oxygenated or C_{24}-carboxylic acid intermediates.

Alternative Pathways

In addition to the above major pathways, there is an alternative microsomal pathway for cleavage of the steroid side-chain in 5β-cholestane-3α,7α,12α-triol which does not involve any mitochondrial or peroxisomal enzymes.

This pathway starts with a microsomal 25-hydroxylation of 5β-cholestane-3α,7α,12α-triol followed by an additional 24-hydroxylation to yield 5β-cholestane-3α,7α,12α,24β,25-pentol (Fig. 123-4). The latter compound is converted into cholic acid by soluble enzymes. This conversion must be assumed to involve acetone. The importance of the "25-hydroxylase pathway" has been a matter of controversy (for reviews, see the seventh edition of this book and reference 1). It has now been established, however, in both rat and man, that the 25-hydroxylase pathway is responsible for less than 5 percent of the cholic acid formed under normal conditions.[22,23] This pathway seems to be important under conditions when the normal 27-hydroxylase pathway is blocked (see below). It is noteworthy that the 25-hydroxylase pathway is only active on 12α-hydroxylated compounds; thus, chenodeoxycholic acid is never formed in this pathway.

NORMAL BIOSYNTHESIS AND METABOLISM OF CHOLESTANOL

Because cholestanol is accumulated in one of the inborn errors of metabolism in bile acid biosynthesis (CTX) and in sitosterolemia, it is important to know the mechanism behind the normal biosynthesis of cholestanol.

Small amounts of cholestanol accompany cholesterol in most mammalian tissues. Cholesterol is also the precursor of cholestanol in experimental animals, in healthy subjects, and in subjects with CTX. It is generally believed that the major pathway in the normal biosynthesis of cholestanol involves a rate-limiting oxidation of cholesterol into 4-cholestene-3-one by a microsomal NAD-dependent 3β-hydroxy-Δ^5-dehydrogenase (Fig. 123-5). 4-Cholesten-3-one is then converted into cholestanol by a microsomal 5α-reductase and a 3β-hydroxysteroid oxidoreductase. This reaction sequence from cholesterol to cholestanol does not share any intermediates with the pathways for biosynthesis of cholesterol and bile acids.

The possibility has been discussed, however, that the microsomal NAD-dependent 3β-hydroxy-Δ^5-dehydrogenase involved in cholestanol synthesis is the same as that involved in bile acid biosynthesis.[7]

As detailed in the sixth edition this book,[24] we have described an alternative, normally minor pathway for formation of cholestanol involving intermediates in bile acid biosynthesis as precursors. This pathway starts with dehydration of 7α-hydroxy-4-cholesten-3-one by a specific enzyme in the liver,[25] to yield cholesta-4,6-dien-3-one. The latter steroid is rapidly converted into 4-cholesten-3-one, 5α-cholestan-3-one and 5α-cholestane-3β-ol by microsomal enzymes (Fig. 123-5). The mechanism and stereochemistry in connection with these conversions have been elucidated.[26] The quantitative significance of this pathway for biosynthesis of cholestanol has been studied with use of 7α-^{3}H-labeled cholesterol.[24] If such cholesterol is converted into cholestanol by the above pathway involving 7α-hydroxylated bile acid intermediates, the ^{3}H label can be expected to be lost. Using this technique we could show that under normal conditions the pathway from cholesterol to cholestanol involving 7α-hydroxylated intermediates is responsible for at most 20 percent of the cholestanol formed in rat, rabbit, and man. In a patient with CTX, however, this pathway is much more important.[27]

Like cholesterol, cholestanol is transported mainly in the LDL fraction[28] and part of the cholestanol in plasma is esterified. LCAT (plasma lecithin:cholesterol acyltransferase) is the enzyme responsible for esterification of cholestanol. Cholestanol is degraded to 5α-bile acids (allocholic acid and allochenodeoxycholic acid) by the same or similar enzymes as those involved in the biosynthesis of normal 5β-bile acids.[1]

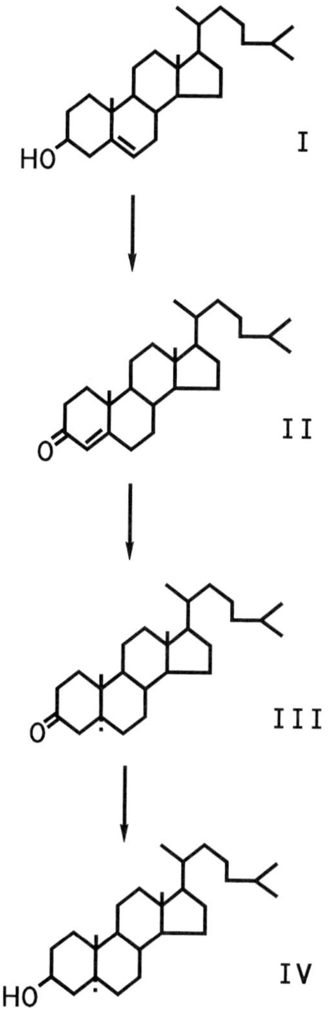

Fig. 123-5 Major pathway for the normal synthesis of cholestanol from cholesterol.

CHEMISTRY, ABSORPTION, AND METABOLISM OF PHYTOSTEROLS (PLANT STEROLS)

Chemistry of Plant Sterols

Plant sterols are constituents of the lipids of plants. A variety of plant sterols have been described, but the most common are sitosterol, campesterol, and stigmasterol.[29,30] These sterols are structurally similar to cholesterol, possessing a steroid nucleus with a Δ^5-double-bond and a 3β-hydroxyl group. The structure of the side-chain is different from that of cholesterol (Fig. 123-6). Sitosterol is a C_{29}-sterol (containing 29 carbon atoms, as compared with the 27 carbon atoms of cholesterol), with an ethyl substituent at C-24. Campesterol is a C_{28}-sterol, containing a methyl group at the C-24 position. Stigmasterol has the same structure as sitosterol, except for a double-bond at C-22. The plant sterols react similarly to cholesterol in colorimetric assays. They are also measured by methods based on cholesterol oxidase. They can be separated by different high-performance liquid chromatography methods or by gas chromatography.

Plant oils, nuts, seeds, and fat-rich vegetables and fruits are important dietary sources of plant sterols.[31] The intake varies with the diet. In the United States, the daily intake of plant sterols is estimated to be about 180 mg,[32] while the average plant sterol content in Japanese diets is approximately 400 mg/day.[33] Plant sterols constitute about 20 percent of the total sterols consumed.[34] Sitosterol is the most abundant plant sterol in the diet, contributing about 65 percent, whereas campesterol constitutes about 32 percent and stigmasterol the remaining 3 percent.[35]

There is no evidence that plant sterols can be synthesized in mammalian tissues.[36,37]

Absorption of Plant Sterol

The intestinal absorption of plant sterols is normally limited. About 5 percent or less of ingested sitosterol is absorbed in man[36,38] and other mammals (e.g., the rat).[39,40] In contrast, the cholesterol absorption amounts to about 40 percent. Campesterol is more easily absorbed than sitosterol.[41–43] The absorption rates of sitosterol, stigmasterol, and campesterol were 4.2, 4.8, and 9.6 percent, respectively, in a study of ten healthy human subjects.[43] Intestinal bacteria metabolize unabsorbed plant sterols in principally the same way as cholesterol,[44,45] but to a moderately lower extent.[41] Metabolites corresponding to coprostanol, coprostanone, and cholestanol are thus formed from plant sterols in the intestine.[44]

Because of the restricted absorption, sitosterol has been used as an internal standard in cholesterol balance studies.[46,47] Sitostanol (the 5α-saturated derivative of sitosterol) is even less absorbable than sitosterol in rats[48] and is practically nonabsorbable in humans.[48] Sitostanol is, therefore, an even better marker of cholesterol absorption.[48] The serum level of sitosterol may also be an indicator of cholesterol absorption and synthesis.[49]

Several hypotheses have been proposed to explain the mechanism of intestinal sterol discrimination, but the poor absorbability of sitosterol is still not fully understood. In perfusion studies of the jejunum of healthy volunteers, the absorption of sitosterol was limited by its solubility in micellar solutions.[50] On the other hand, in vitro studies have indicated that cholesterol and sitosterol have approximately the same micellar solubility.[51,52] Some studies support discrimination between cholesterol and sitosterol at the brush border membrane.[53–55] Still another possibility is a slower rate of transfer of sitosterol than cholesterol from the cell surface to the intracellular site of use.[56] Furthermore, the esterification rate of sitosterol in the intestinal mucosa is very low as compared with that of cholesterol,[55,57,58] and sitosterol appears largely unesterified in the lymph of experimental animals.[55,59]

The limited absorption of sitosterol might thus be caused by a combination of several discriminatory steps.

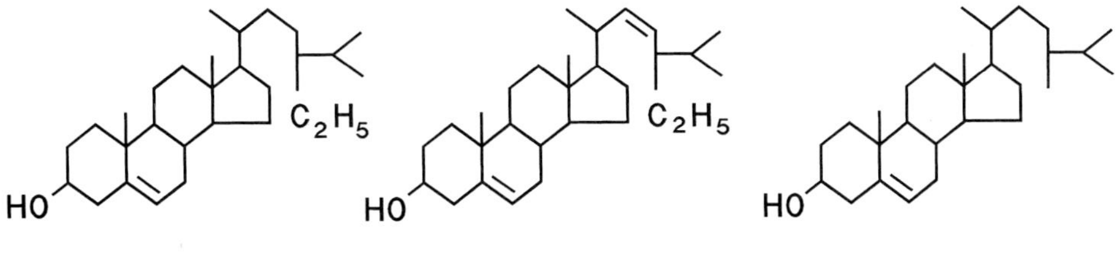

Fig. 123-6 Structures of the major plant sterols.

Interference of Sitosterol with Cholesterol Absorption

Plant sterols interfere with the absorption of cholesterol[40,60] and have been used as agents in the treatment of hypercholesterolemia.[61–71] Sitosterol in daily doses of 3 to 20 g may reduce plasma cholesterol concentration by 5 to 20 percent.[64–70] The exact mechanism by which sitosterol inhibits cholesterol absorption has not been clarified. In experiments with rats, sitosterol restricted the micellar solubility of cholesterol.[54] Other possible mechanisms include formation of a nonabsorbable complex with cholesterol in the intestinal lumen,[63] inhibition of cholesterol uptake at the absorptive site, and interference with cholesterol esterification or chylomicron formation in the intestinal mucosal cell. In experiments with a human intestinal cell line, sitosterol interfered with the uptake of micellar cholesterol causing a decreased influx of plasma membrane cholesterol to the endoplasmic reticulum and, subsequently, a reduced secretion of cholesteryl esters.[71] Cholesterol synthesis and HMG-CoA reductase activity were decreased in cells incubated with sitosterol. Sitosterol did not influence the ACAT activity under these experimental conditions.[71]

Sitostanol may be even more effective than sitosterol in reducing the cholesterol level in both experimental animals[72,73] and man.[61,74,75] In a study of nine children with severe familial hypercholesterolemia, a daily 6-g dose of sitosterol for 3 months reduced LDL cholesterol levels by 20 percent.[61] During subsequent treatment with sitostanol 1.5 g/day for 3 months, the LDL cholesterol levels decreased further by 33 percent. In a randomized double-blind study of 153 patients with mild hypercholesterolemia, addition of sitostanol ester to margarine to the diet reduced the mean total serum cholesterol concentration by 10.2 percent after 1 year.[62] Despite the reports of a favorable effect of plant sterols in hypercholesterolemia, the role of plant sterols in this condition remains to be established.[64]

Organ Distribution of Plant Sterols

Small levels of sitosterol can be detected in normal human plasma. The total plasma plant sterols in healthy adults range from 7 to 24 μM (0.3 to 1.0 mg/dl), thus accounting for less than 1 percent of the total plasma sterols.[35]

After absorption, only about 12 to 25 percent of sitosterol in the thoracic lymph is esterified, compared with 70 to 90 percent esterification of cholesterol.[55,59] Sitosterol in plasma is esterified to almost the same extent as cholesterol (60 to 75 percent).[33] LCAT is the most important enzyme for formation of circulating plant sterol esters.[76]

The organ distribution and excretion of plant sterols have been studied in experimental animals after oral[77] or parenteral[78–80] administration. Sitosterol,[77,79,80] campesterol,[77] and 24-ethyl-4-cholesten-3-one[80] were enriched in rat liver as compared with cholesterol. The lysosomal and microsomal fractions contained slightly more plant sterols than the other subcellular fractions,[77,80] but the subcellular distribution was quite similar to that of cholesterol. The adrenal glands, ovaries, and testes contained the greatest amounts of plant sterols among the organs examined.[79,80] Relative to the plasma concentration, the accumulation of plant sterols in the endocrine organs was even larger than that of cholesterol. Plant sterols are incorporated into lipoproteins in the liver[81] and accumulate in organs rich in lipoprotein receptors (e.g., the adrenal glands). In the rat, more than 80 percent of the plant sterols in plasma is carried in the HDL-fraction, in similarity with cholesterol. In humans, 75 to 85 percent of the total plasma plant sterols is found in LDL.[82,83] Most of the remainder is present in HDL, while VLDL only contains traces.

Metabolism of Plant Sterols

Studies in Animals. Several authors have reported that sitosterol is converted into acidic products in rat bile,[78–80] but the identities of these compounds have been difficult to establish. The conversion of sitosterol into bile acids in rats is less efficient than that of cholesterol.[78–80,84] In the metabolism of cholesterol to bile acids, the side-chain degradation involves formation of a Δ^{24}-unsaturated steroid (3α,7α,12α-trihydroxy-24-en-5β-cholestanoic acid), as described above. The presence of an ethyl group at C-24 in sitosterol should prevent, or at least obstruct, a side-chain oxidation according to this mechanism. The possibility has been considered that sitosterol is first dealkylated to cholesterol and then converted into bile acids. Dealkylation of sitosterol, yielding desmosterol, has been reported in tobacco hornworms,[85] Florida land crabs,[86] and insects.[87] It has not been possible to demonstrate such a pathway in either rats[79] or man.[88] Compounds identified as C_{29}-bile acids with intact side-chains were isolated from the feces of monkeys fed sitosterol.[89] Attempts to demonstrate conversion of sitosterol into natural bile acids in animals have failed.[78,79,90]

Previously unknown di- and trihydroxylated C_{21}-bile acids have been identified in our laboratory as the major degradation products of sitosterol in bile-fistulated female Wistar rats after injection of 4-^{14}C-labeled sitosterol and sitosterol labeled with ^{3}H in specific positions.[90] The major trihydroxylated C_{21}-bile acids were identified as 5β-pregnan-3α,11β,15β-triol-21-oic acid and 5β-pregnan-3α,11β,15α-triol-21-oic acid.[91,92] Experiments with isolated perfused rat liver gave direct evidence that the overall conversion of sitosterol into C_{21}-bile acids takes place in this organ.[90] Injected 7α,7β-$^{3}H_2$-campesterol gave a product pattern identical to that of 4-^{14}C-labeled sitosterol. The proximal cleavage of the side-chain of sitosterol might involve an initial hydroxylation at C-21,[90] and further β-oxidation of this compound in the mitochondrial or peroxisomal fraction would yield a C_{21}-bile acid, but intermediates in this hypothetical pathway have not yet been isolated.

Human Studies. In an early investigation, Salen et al. reported that intravenously injected 22,23-^{3}H-sitosterol was converted into cholic- and chenodeoxycholic acid at approximately the same rate as cholesterol in humans.[36] This result could not be reproduced, however, in a later study in our laboratory. Thus, no labeled C_{24}-bile acids could be detected in the bile of healthy individuals after intravenous injection of 4-^{14}C-sitosterol.[88] The major part (>90 percent) of the radioactivity was present as unmetabolized sitosterol. Minor amounts of the excreted compounds had chromatographic properties that could possibly represent hydroxylated products of sitosterol. No conversion of sitosterol into highly polar C_{21}-bile acids could be detected in the human studies, as opposed to the findings in rats.[90] It may also be mentioned that no significant conversion of sitosterol into 7α-hydroxysitosterol could be detected in human liver microsomes, even after stimulation of the enzyme by cholestyramine.[88] These results are in accordance with experiments in rat liver microsomes in which the rate of 7α-hydroxylation of sitosterol is very low, amounting to less than 2 percent of that of cholesterol.[93–96] Bypassing the rate-limiting enzymatic step by injection of ^{3}H-7α-hydroxysitosterol resulted in a significant conversion of the precursor into acidic products in human bile.[88] The major part of these acid products were, however, not identical to the normal C_{24}-bile acids.

7α-Hydroxysitosterol was metabolized in the same manner as cholesterol in rat liver experiments.[97] Among the isolated products were small amounts of 24-ethyl-7α,12α-dihydroxy-4-cholesten-3-one, 24-ethyl-7α,12α-dihydroxy-5β-cholestan-3-one, and 24-ethyl-5β-cholestane-3α,7α,12α-triol. The only significant conversion of plant sterols that occurred in rat liver in vitro was mitochondrial ω-hydroxylation of the side-chain with formation of the 27- and 29-hydroxylated derivatives.[98] Initial ω-hydroxylation of the steroid side-chain might represent a minor pathway in the metabolism of sitosterol.[90]

In isotope-kinetic studies in normal individuals, the fractional turnover rate of sitosterol was more rapid than that of cholesterol.[36,99] This may be explained by the restricted intestinal absorption of sitosterol, combined with a rapid excretion into the bile. Under normal circumstances, the liver has the ability to preferentially excrete plant sterols into the bile.[36,83] A rapid turnover rate may explain why plant sterols do not normally accumulate in the organism. Plant sterols may also to some extent be excreted into to skin surface lipids.[100]

Sitosterol may also serve as a precursor of steroid hormones. Administration of ^{3}H-sitosterol led to excretion of labeled cortisol in the urine of guinea pigs.[101] The rate of this conversion is, however, lower than with cholesterol as precursor.[102] Sitosterol can be converted into pregnenolone and progesterone in mitochondrial preparations from rat adrenals, testes, ovaries, and placenta.[102,104] Also, human endocrine tissues form these C_{21}-steroids from sitosterol.[102]

5α-Sitostanol is a quantitatively important metabolite of sitosterol which is formed in the liver.[84] The most important pathway seems to involve a primary conversion of sitosterol to 24-ethyl-4-cholesten-3-one, in accordance with the normal pathway of formation of cholestanol from cholesterol.

REDUCED BILE ACID SYNTHESIS DUE TO DEFECT IN CHOLESTEROL SYNTHESIS

Recently, an inborn error in cholesterol synthesis was described. It was shown that the basal biochemical defect causing the Smith-Lemli-Opitz syndrome is a deficient 7-dehydrocholesterol-7-reductase. The reduced formation of cholesterol in this disease may cause a lack of substrate for bile acid synthesis and thus a reduced formation of bile acids. This disease is discussed in detail in Chap. 249.

3β-HYDROXYSTEROID-Δ⁵-OXIDOREDUCTASE/ ISOMERASE DEFICIENCY

General

Clayton et al. first described this very rare disease in 1986.[105] The Saudi Arabian patient was the fifth child of parents who were first cousins, and he was the third child in the family to be affected by progressive liver disease. Jaundice, pale stools, and dark urine were noted on the third day of life. At the time of the investigation conjugated bilirubin, aminotransferases, and alkaline phosphatase were elevated, and fat-soluble vitamins were low. Surprisingly, cholate and chenodeoxycholate were not found in plasma. Using modifications of previously used methods for analysis of bile acids it was shown that the major bile acids excreted in urine were sulfate esters of $3\beta,7\alpha$-dihydroxy-5-cholenoic acid and $3\beta,7\alpha,12\alpha$-trihydroxy-5-cholenoic acid.

On the basis of the above findings, it was suggested that the child had a specific defect in the 3β-hydroxysteroid-Δ^5-oxidoreductase/isomerase activity. The possibility could not be completely excluded, however, that the apparent loss of enzyme activity was secondary to some other factor. It was not possible to take a liver biopsy in order to measure directly the enzyme activity. We have previously shown that fibroblasts express 3β-hydroxysteroid-Δ^5-oxidoreductase/isomerase activity.[106] It could be shown that cultured fibroblasts from the patient were practically devoid of this activity (see Table 123-1).[107] Cultured fibroblasts from the patient's parents had an activity about half that of normal. Thus, it can be concluded that the patient must have an inherited defect in the enzyme and that the disorder is not secondary to some other disease.

This defect is different from another previously described 3β-hydroxysteroid-Δ^5-oxidoreductase/isomerase defect in the metabolism of C_{19}- and C_{21}-steroids.[108] The enzyme involved in oxidation of C_{19}- and C_{21}-3β-hydroxy-Δ^5-steroids is different from that involved in bile acid biosynthesis.[109]

As of February, 1998, at least 20 additional similar cases have been observed (K.D.R. Setchell, unpublished observations). It has been diagnosed in a 10-year-old boy with chronic cholestasis, indicating that late-onset chronic liver disease may be accounted for by this inborn error.

Table 123-1 **3β-Hydroxysteroid-Δ^5-Oxidoreductase/Isomerase Activity in Cultured Human Fibroblasts***

	nM/mg protein/h
Control values	6.22–21.57
Mother	6.8
Father	2.50
Patient U	<0.10

*Fibroblasts were cultured from 18 different healthy subjects. Enzyme activity was assayed with 1 mg protein, incubated with 0.1 mM 7α-hydroxycholesterol, 1.5 mM NAD in 0.1 M phosphate buffer (pH 7.5) for 20 min.

SOURCE: Buchmann et al.[107]

Basic Defect

In view of the broad substrate specificity of the enzymes involved in steroid side-chain cleavage, a specific defect in the 3β-hydroxysteroid-Δ^5-oxidoreductase/isomerase could be expected to yield the C_{24}-bile acids with 3β-hydroxysteroid-Δ^5-structure found in urine of the patients. Futhermore, the bile contains a variety of sulfated bile alcohols and C_{27}-bile acids all having the 3β-hydroxy-Δ^5-structure.[110] High concentrations of 5-cholestene-$3\beta,7\alpha$-diol were also found in serum of the first patient.[107] Fig. 123-7 shows the mechanism behind the formation of the 3β-hydroxy-Δ^5-bile acids excreted in urine.

If the end products in the pathway are less effective as suppressors of the cholesterol 7α-hydroxylase than cholic acid and chenodeoxycholic acid, one would expect an up-regulation of the rate-limiting enzyme in bile acid biosynthesis. There is as yet no information on this, but it is probable that the cholestatic condition induced by the defect may uncouple the normal mechanism for regulation of bile acid biosynthesis. It has been speculated that the di- and trihydroxycholenoic acids and their sulfates are unable to produce a bile-acid-dependent bile flow, which results in failure to secrete conjugated bilirubin and other constituents in the bile.[110] That $3\beta,7\alpha$-dihydroxy-5-cholenoic acid does not cause cholestasis in the normal hamster[111] does not exclude this possibility. If this hypothesis is correct, oral administration of bile salts could be expected to improve the condition.[110] In addition to effects on fat absorption, exogenous bile acids could inhibit the cholesterol 7α-hydroxylase and reduce the production of toxic metabolites from cholesterol. This has proven correct (see below). Untreated, the disease led to cirrhosis by the age of 2 to 3 years in the family of the first described patient.

Clinical Phenotype and Pathological Findings

The patients hitherto described have had clinical and laboratory signs of cholestatic liver disease (see above), hepatic dysfunction, and vitamin D malabsorption. Increased levels of conjugated bilirubin, aspartate aminotransferase, alkaline phosphatase, and low levels of vitamin E in plasma are common findings. Giant cells are found in liver biopsy in most patients. In one patient, there was a progression to micronodular cirrhosis despite treatment (P.T. Clayton, personal communication). In addition, there was growth failure associated with clinical rickets, with widening of wrists and a rachitic rosary in addition to bowed legs.[110,112] There is, however, no specific clinical finding that makes it possible to differentiate this specific disorder from other cholestatic disorders, and to get a diagnosis, some specific investigations must be made.

Diagnosis

3β-hydroxysteroid-Δ^5-oxidoreductase/isomerase deficiency may be suspected in cholestatic infants in whom little or no bile acids are found in serum. The most convenient diagnostic method is negative-ion Fast Atomic Bombardment-Mass Spectrometry (FAB-MS) of a urinary bile acid fraction obtained by adsorption to octadecyl-bonded silica followed by extraction with ethanol.[110,113]

cholesterol → HO ... OH ⫲→ O ... OH → → cholic acid

COOH HO OH   HO COOH HO OH

3-monosulfate
monosulfate-glycine conjugate

Fig. 123-7 Metabolic consequences of the 3β-hydroxysteroid-Δ^5-oxidoreductase deficiency.

A very characteristic mass spectrometric pattern is obtained corresponding to the sulfate esters of 3β,7α-dihydroxy-5-cholestenoic acid and 3β,7α,12α-trihydroxy-5-cholestenoic acid (Fig. 123-8). A more time-consuming method is to make a group separation of the urinary bile acids on Lipidex-DEAP.[105] The sulfate fraction is then solvolyzed.[110] Many standard methods used for solvolysis give an almost complete degradation of the compounds. The two 3β-hydroxy-Δ^5-bile acids can then be identified by GC-MS as methyl ester trimethylsialyl derivatives.

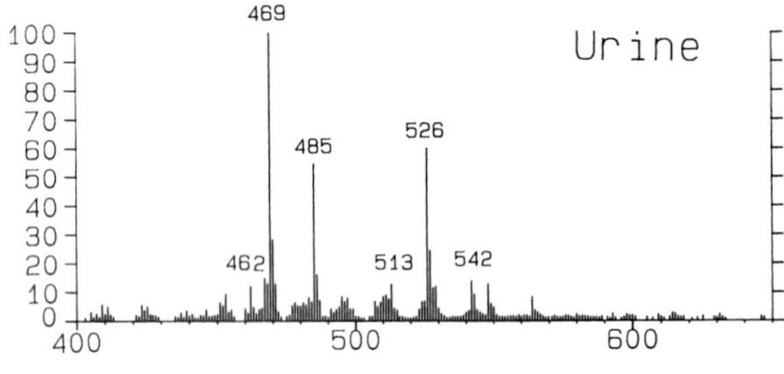

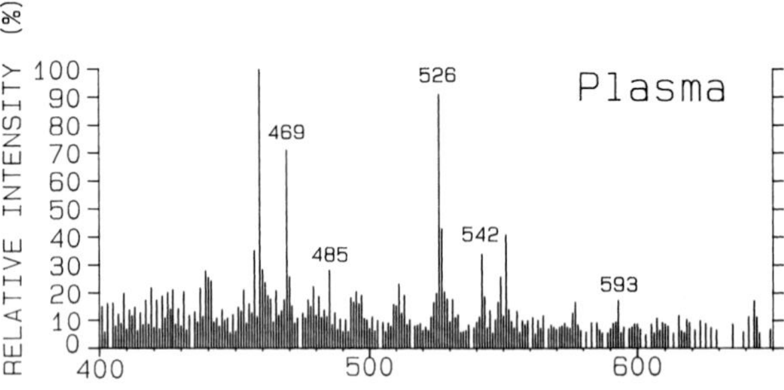

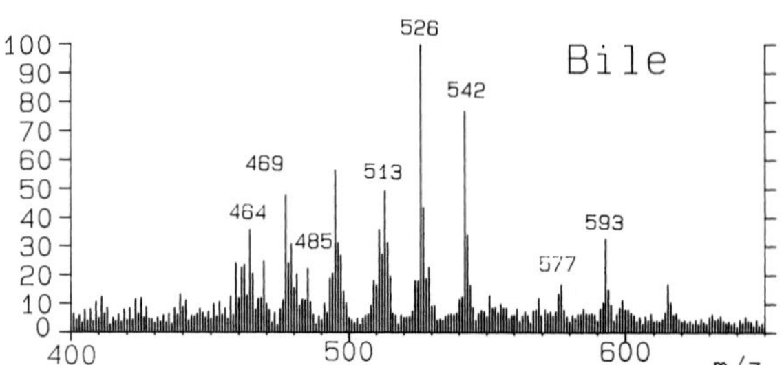

Fig. 123-8 The high-mass regions of negative ion FAB mass spectra of urine, plasma, and bile collected from a patient with 3β-hydroxysteroid-Δ^5-oxidoreductase/isomerase deficiency. (*From Ichimiya et al.*[110] *Used by permission.*)

Because the large amounts of 3β-hydroxy-Δ^5-bile acids present in urine of the affected patients give a positive Lifschütz reaction,[110] a very simple colorimetric test can be used to get a preliminary diagnosis. A positive result of such a test must, however, always be followed by a more specific investigation.

Another diagnostic method is to use cultivated skin fibroblasts and incubate a homogenate of such cells with labeled 7α-hydroxycholesterol and NAD+ under standardized conditions.[107] It is advisable to have parallel control incubation with fibroblasts from a healthy subject. If the patient suffers from a 3β-hydroxysteroid-Δ^5-oxidoreductase/isomerase defect, there should be little or no conversion into 7α-hydroxy-4-cholesten-3-one.[107] In Table 123-1, the results are shown from the first case investigated by this method.

In spite of the cholestatic condition, patients with this deficiency have normal levels of γ-glutamyl-transpeptidase.[114] This is also a feature of patients with familial progressive intrahepatic cholestasis or Byler disease.

Because bile acid synthesis is well developed in early gestation, prenatal diagnosis of this enzyme defect is, in principle, possible from the analysis of the bile acid composition of amniotic fluid.[114]

Treatment

Administration of 250 mg/day of chenodeoxycholic acid to a 10-year-old boy with this disease resulted in a decrease in the concentration of bile acids with the 3β-hydroxy-Δ^5-structure in all biological fluids, concomitant with a rapid normalization of the serum bilirubin and transaminase levels (Fig. 123-9).[114]

Comparable clinical and biochemical responses to chenodeoxycholic acid were also observed in the original Saudi Arabian infant diagnosed with 3β-hydroxysteroid dehydrogenase/isomerase deficiency.[112,113] Since then, several more cases have been treated with primary bile acids.[114]

Early diagnosis of this defect is important because these patients respond to primary bile acid therapy. The experience to date indicates that, providing cirrhosis is not advanced, a normalization of liver enzymes, resolution of jaundice, and an improvement in liver histology are attained with primary bile acid therapy, thereby circumventing the need for liver transplantation.[114]

3-OXO-Δ^4-STEROID 5β-REDUCTASE DEFICIENCY

General

In 1988, Setchell et al. described two monochorionic male twins with cholestatic liver disease, presenting with jaundice, pale

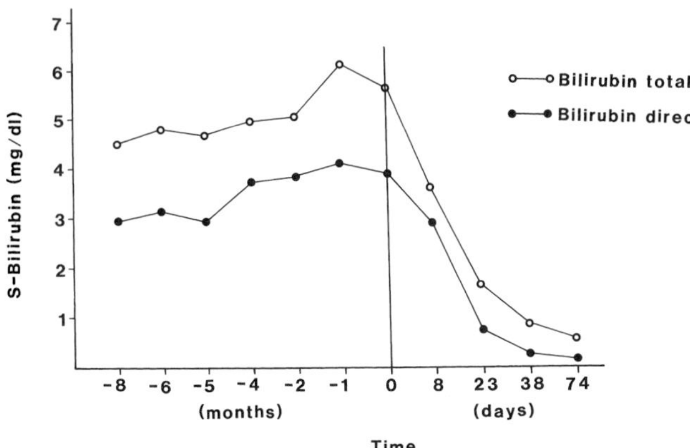

Fig. 123-9 Effect of chenodeoxycholic acid feeding on the bilirubin levels of a 10-year-old boy with 3β-hydroxy-Δ5-oxidoreductase/isomerase deficiency. (*From Setchell et al.*[114] *Used by permission.*)

stools, and dark urine on the first day of life.[115] The parents were not consanguineous. The twins were born at term after an uncomplicated pregnancy. They had marked conjugated hyperbilirubinemia and coagulopathy, while serum aminotransferases initially were normal or only slightly increased. A previous male sib with an identical clinical history had died of liver failure at the age of 4 months.

The patients excreted taurine conjugated 7α-hydroxy-3-oxo-4-cholenoic acid and 7α,12α-dihydroxy-3-oxo-4-cholenoic acid as the major bile acids in the urine. Fasting serum bile acid concentrations were elevated, with 3-oxo-Δ^4-bile acids accounting for about 17 percent of the total. Chenodeoxycholic acid was the predominating bile acid in serum, but significant amounts (about 30 percent) of allochenodeoxycholic and allocholic acid were also present. These findings could be explained by reduced activity of the enzyme 3-oxo-Δ^4-steroid 5β-reductase catalyzing the conversion of 7α-hydroxy-4-cholesten-3-one and 7α,12α-dihydroxy-4-cholesten-3-one to the corresponding 3-oxo-5β (H) structures, and it was suggested that the infants suffered from an inborn error of this enzyme.[115] Excretion of large amounts of 3-oxo-Δ^4-bile acids has also been detected in the urine of children with severe liver disease of causes other than primary defects in bile acid metabolism, as, for example, fumarylacetoacetase deficiency (tyrosinemia), α_1-antitrypsin deficiency, and hepatitis B.[116] Thus, it must be considered that reduced activity of 3-oxo-Δ^4-steroid 5β-reductase may be a secondary phenomenon in severe liver damage in children.[117]

Fibroblasts do not express 3-oxo-Δ^4-steroid 5β-reductase activity, and more direct evidence of a primary defect of this enzyme has not yet been obtained. In a preliminary joint study together with Setchell and Okuda, we performed immunoblotting of the 5β-reductase in normal liver cells and liver cells from two patients with 5β-reductase deficiency.[118] A monoclonal antibody directed against the cytosolic rat liver 3-oxo-Δ^4-steroid 5β-reductase was used. The antibody recognized the human 5β-reductase in livers from control subjects and from subjects with liver disease, but did not recognize the enzyme in the liver from two patients biochemically diagnosed with this error. Whether the 5β-reductase is not expressed at all in the liver cells of the patients or whether a deficient enzyme is synthesized cannot be evaluated from these results.

Basic Defect

Deficiency of 3-oxo-Δ^4-steroid 5β-reductase results in failure to convert the bile acid intermediates 7α-hydroxy-4-cholesten-3-one and 7α,12α-dihydroxy-4-cholesten-3-one to the corresponding 3-oxo-5β (H) saturated derivatives in the pathway to chenodeoxycholic acid and cholic acid (Fig. 123-10). Normally, the modifications of the C_{27}-steroid nucleus are completed prior to oxidation of the side-chain and formation of a C_{24}-bile acid. The finding of significant amounts of 7α-hydroxy-3-oxo-4-cholenoic acid and 7α,12α-dihydroxy-3-oxo-4-cholenoic acid in serum and urine of the patients indicates that the side-chain of the accumulated 3-oxo-Δ^4-bile acid precursors may be oxidized in a pathway which is active despite incomplete transformation of the nucleus.

The occurrence of elevated amounts of *allo*-bile acids is most likely explained by metabolism of the accumulated 3-oxo-Δ^4-intermediates by a microsomal 3-oxo-Δ^4-steroid 5α-reductase[119] (Fig. 123-10). Normally this pathway is of minor quantitative importance. If the 3-oxo-Δ^4-steroid 5β-reductase activity is reduced, significant amounts of 3-oxo-Δ^4-precursors may be diverted into the pathway to *allo*-bile acids.

Primary bile acids have important choleretic properties whereas 3-oxo-Δ^4-bile acids are poorly secreted into the bile.[115] The lack of normal production of bile acids could thus possibly explain the cholestasis. It may also be speculated that accumulated 3-oxo-Δ^4-bile acids and *allo*-bile acids have hepatotoxic effects, contributing to reduced secretion of conjugated bilirubin and other components into the bile.

The total serum concentration of bile acids was elevated in the above two infants, and chenodeoxycholic acid was the major bile acid identified. The existence of several 3-oxo-Δ^4-steroid 5β-reductases could explain the preferential formation of chenodeoxycholic acid. This hypothesis has not been confirmed, however, and other explanations must also be considered.[115]

Clinical Phenotype and Pathologic Findings

The two patients reported by Setchell et al. had manifestations of cholestatic liver disease at birth.[115] They had pale stools, dark urine, and progressive jaundice. Initial tests revealed elevated levels of conjugated bilirubin. Serum aminotransferase levels were normal or only slightly elevated, and serum alkaline phosphatase

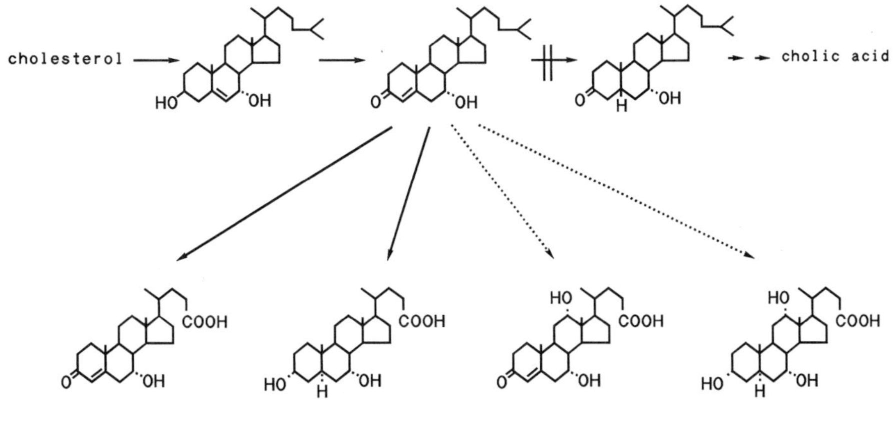

cholesterol → → cholic acid

Fig. 123-10 Metabolic consequences of the 3-oxo-Δ^4-steroid 5β-reductase deficiency.

was within the normal range. They had a coagulopathy with prothrombin time 13 to 15 s. The liver size was small, and liver biopsies showed giant-cell hepatitis. On electron microscopy, bile canaliculi were small with few or absent microvilli.

Urine. Analysis of urine samples from the twins by FAB-MS revealed the presence of two prominent ions at *m/z* 494 and *m/z* 510, consistent with taurine conjugates of unsaturated monooxo-monohydroxy- and monooxo-dihydroxy-cholenoic acids.[115] GC-MS analysis of the urine identified these as 3-oxo-7α-hydroxy-4-cholenoic acid and 3-oxo-7α,12α-dihydroxy-4-cholenoic acid. The urinary bile acid excretion was elevated, with the above compounds amounting to 75 to 92 percent of the total.

Serum. Serum bile acid concentration was elevated in both infants (37 to 52 μM). Chenodeoxycholic acid was the predominating bile acid in serum, but significant amounts of allochenodeoxycholic and allocholic acid (about 30 percent) and 3-oxo-Δ^4-bile acids (12 to 17 percent) were also identified.[115,120]

Bile. The biliary bile acid concentration measured in one of the patients was extremely low (<2 μM). Chenodeoxycholic acid, allochenodeoxycholic, and allocholic acid were the major bile acids present. In contrast to the urine, no 3-oxo-Δ^4-bile acids could be detected in the bile.[115]

Diagnosis

The possibility of 3-oxo-Δ^4-steroid 5β-reductase deficiency may be considered in infants with impaired liver function and cholestasis. Screening of the urine with the FAB-MS technique reveals a spectrum dominated by ions, which is characteristic of taurine or glycine conjugates of 3-oxo-7α-hydroxy-4-cholenoic acid and 3-oxo-7α,12α-dihydroxy-4-cholenoic acid. GC-MS analysis of the urine samples after extraction, solvolysis, hydrolysis, and derivatization confirms the presence of these compounds.[115]

Definitive evidence that the reduced activity of 3-oxo-Δ^4-steroid 5β-reductase represents an inborn error of metabolism with a primary defect in this enzyme, however, is still lacking. Reduced activity of the 3-oxo-Δ^4-steroid 5β-reductase thus might be secondary to another defect. The enzyme is labile and under severe cholestasis it may become the rate-limiting enzyme for bile acid synthesis, particularly if the cholesterol 7α-hydroxylase is up-regulated.[114] A high proportion of 3-oxo-Δ^4-bile acids has been observed in patients with chronic, profuse diarrhea.[114] Several patients diagnosed with neonatal hemochromatosis were also found to exhibit biochemical profiles consistent with a deficiency of the 3-oxo-Δ^4-reductase.[114] The recent sequencing of a human cDNA encoding the human 3-oxo-Δ^4-steroid 5β-reductase[11] will probably soon permit a definitive identification of the defect by molecular genetic techniques. At least 14 cases with deficiency of 3-oxo-Δ^4-steroid 5β-reductase have been diagnosed.[2,121]

Treatment

If the end products in the alternative pathways suppress the rate-limiting enzyme cholesterol 7α-hydroxylase less efficiently than the normal products of cholic acid and chenodeoxycholic acid, an up-regulation of this enzymatic step would be expected. In analogy to the considerations in the case of 3β-hydroxysteroid Δ^5-oxidoreductase deficiency (see above) and 27-hydroxylase deficiency (see below), treatment with exogenous bile acids would inhibit cholesterol 7α-hydroxylase activity, thereby preventing the accumulation of potentially toxic bile acid intermediates. In addition, oral administration of bile acids may have a choleretic effect and it improves intestinal fat absorption.

The above two infants were initially treated with a combination of chenodeoxycholic acid and cholic acid (100 mg of each/day).[114] The treatment resulted in suppression of the endogenous production of 3-oxo-Δ^4-bile acids. A combination of ursodeoxycholic acid with cholic acid seemed to be even more effective, resulting in reduction of serum bilirubin levels with eventual normalization after 6 months.[114,122] However, in one patient excreting 3-oxo-Δ^4-bile acids, treatment with chenodeoxycholic acid resulted in deterioration of liver function.[114,122]

27-HYDROXYLASE DEFICIENCY (CEREBROTENDINOUS XANTHOMATOSIS)

General

Van Bogaert, Scherer, and Epstein first reported this rare disease in 1937.[123] The patient they described suffered from dementia, ataxia, cataracts, and xanthomas in the tendons and nervous system. The same group later reported that a relative of this patient had the same symptoms.[124,125] Patients with this "van Bogaert disease" were subsequently also described by Epstein and Lorenz[126] and Epstein and Kreitner.[127] In 1968, Menkes, Schimshock, and Swanson reported that the central nervous system of two patients with CTX contained increased levels of cholestanol.[128] It was later shown that blood, xanthomas, and bile from these patients also contained elevated levels of cholestanol.[129–139]

The levels of cholesterol were found to be elevated in tissues, but not in blood. In 1971, Salen reported that the composition of bile from CTX was abnormal, with very low concentrations of chenodeoxycholic acid.[131]

In 1974, Setoguchi et al. made the key discovery that these patients have a defect in bile acid biosynthesis with incomplete oxidation of the C_{27}-steroid side-chain, leading to excretion of great amounts of C_{27}-bile alcohols in bile, feces, and urine.[140] In 1980, Oftebro et al. reported that a liver biopsy from a patient with CTX had an almost complete lack of the mitochondrial 27-hydroxylase involved in the normal biosynthesis of bile acids.[141] The same group of authors also reported that the hepatic levels of different substrates for the mitochondrial 27-hydroxylase were increased in patients with CTX.[142] Furthermore, it was shown that the relative rate of conversion of a number of intermediates in bile acid biosynthesis was consistent with a metabolic block at the level of the 27-hydroxylase.[143] The same group of authors also demonstrated that skin fibroblasts cultured from CTX patients have a deficient 27-hydroxylase activity[106] and that there is a metabolic link between the 27-hydroxylase deficiency and the accumulation of cholestanol.[27]

In 1991, Cali and Russell cloned the human sterol 27-hydroxylase cDNA, mapped the human gene to chromosome 2, and described the first two missense mutations in the gene causing CTX.[144,145] Following the cloning of the human gene and determination of its intron-exon boundaries,[146] numerous mutations were identified in different populations[146–160] (Fig. 123-11, Table 123-2).

Basic Defect and Metabolic Consequences

The major clinical manifestations of CTX are due to the generalized accumulation of cholestanol and cholesterol in almost every tissue, including the central nervous system. This accumulation may be due to increased synthesis and/or increased influx of the two sterols from the circulation. Another alternative is a reduced rate of efflux from the tissues and/or reduced degradation. Salen and collaborators have shown convincingly that both cholesterol and cholestanol synthesis are increased in the livers of patients with CTX.[28] This group of authors also reported that, when grown in a cholesterol-free medium, fibroblasts from CTX patients synthesize cholesterol but not cholestanol.[161] In addition, the fibroblasts did respond normally to LDL with a suppression of the rate-limiting enzyme in cholesterol synthesis, the HMG CoA reductase. In view of this, it seems most probable that either cholestanol or a precursor of cholestanol is transported to the different tissues after synthesis elsewhere.

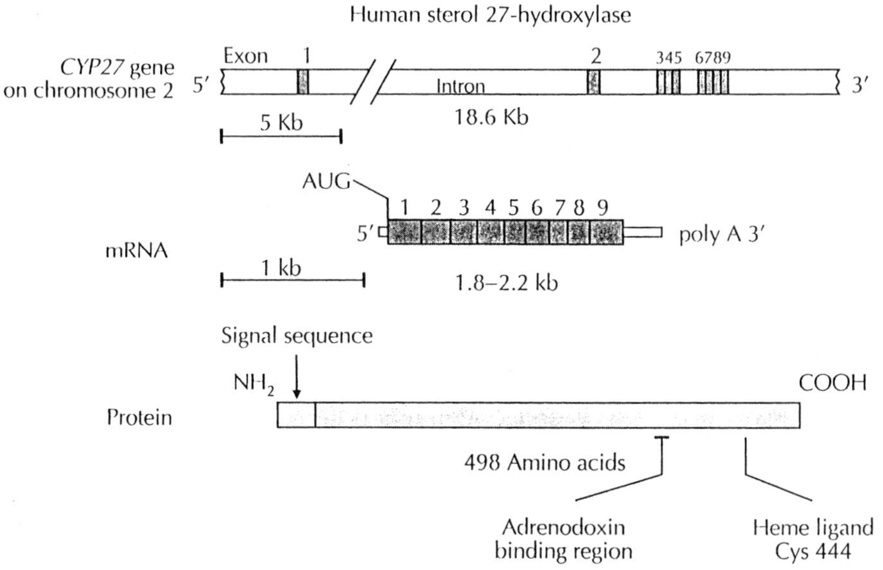

Fig. 123-11 The CYP27 gene, the messenger RNA, and the sterol 27-hydroxylase enzyme. The gene contains 9 exons and spans 18.6 kb of DNA. The size of the mRNA is 1.8 to 2.2 kb, and the mature enzyme (8498 amino acids) contains putative binding sites for adrenodoxin and heme. ***(From Leitersdorf et al.[146] Used by permission.)***

The mechanism behind the increased synthesis of cholesterol and cholestanol is discussed below. There is now a general agreement that the primary defect in patients with CTX is localized to bile acid biosynthesis and that the increased biosynthesis and accumulation of neutral sterols are secondary to this defect.

There has been past controversy with respect to the location of the defect in the side-chain cleavage in connection with bile acid biosynthesis. It is now well established that the basic metabolic defect is located at the mitochondrial 27-hydroxylase. Our demonstration that cultured skin fibroblasts from CTX patients lack 27-hydroxylase activity, and that fibroblasts from apparently healthy parents of such patients have about 50 percent reduced 27-hydroxylase activity, gave strong evidence for the location of the basic metabolic defect. In 1991, the human 27-hydroxylase cDNA was cloned and the gene mapped to chromosome 2.[145] Cali et al. isolated mRNA from fibroblasts from two CTX patients and synthesized the corresponding cDNA by reverse transcription.[144] The latter was sequenced and two point mutations were detected. Transfection of mutant cDNAs containing these two mutations into cultured COS cells resulted in greatly diminished sterol 27-hydroxylase activity and provided the proof for the causative

Table 123-2 Published CYP27 Mutations

Type	References	Origin
Missense		
R94Q	153	England
R104W	149	Japan
A183P	157	Italy
T306M	148	Israel (Algeria, Jewish)
R362C*,†	144, 156	The Netherlands, USA (Black)
R362H†	155	Japan
P368R	154	Japan
R372G*	159	Japan
R441G*,‡	159	Japan
R441W‡	150	Japan
R446C*,‡	144	USA (Canada)
Nonsense		
G126Stop	156	The Netherlands
R237Stop	158	Pakistan
K251Stop	147	South Africa (Afrikans)
Frameshift		
InsC6	152	France
delC376	151	Israel (Druze)
delG546	156	The Netherlands
delT840	146	Moroccan
Splice Junction		
G to A Intron 4 donor site	160	The Netherlands
G to A Intron 4 acceptor site	146	Israel (Morocco, Jewish)
G to A Intron 7 donor site	157	Italy

*Mutations verified by COS cells transfection
†Mutations mapped to the adrenodoxin binding region
‡Mutations mapped to the heme ligand-binding site

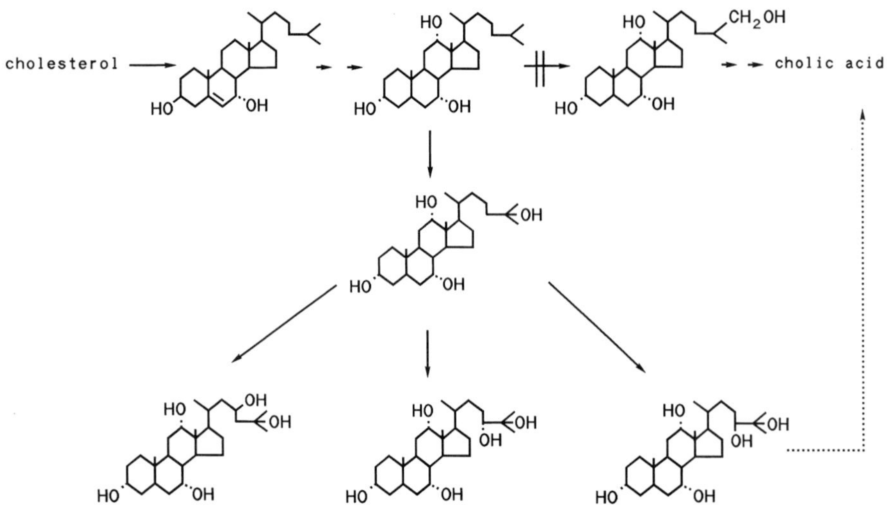

Fig. 123-12 Metabolic consequences of the accumulation of 5β-cholestane-$3\alpha,7\alpha,12\alpha$-triol in patients with CTX.

nature of these mutations. In 1993, we characterized the human gene structure and identified two common mutations in Moroccan Jews.[146] Subsequently, an additional 17 novel mutations in the Cyp27 gene[147–160] were found. Known Cyp27 mutations include now 11 missense and 10 null mutations (3 nonsense, 4 minor insertions/deletions, and 3 splice-junction mutations). Several missense mutations map to the adrenodoxin binding site or to the heme ligand binding region. These critical regions are considered essential for the proper function of this enzyme, as for other members of the P-450 family[144] (Table 123-2). Cyp27 mutations were identified in CTX patients from four continents (except Australia). Interestingly, only one mutation, R362C, was found in two different populations. It is yet to be shown whether this mutation occurred twice or the two patients share a common ancestor.

The lack of the mitochondrial 27-hydroxylase activity leads to extensive accumulation of a number of substrates for the enzyme such as 7α-hydroxy-4-cholesten-3-one and 5β-cholestane-$3\alpha,7\alpha,12\alpha$-triol.[142] Because there is a reduced formation of normal bile acids, in particular, chenodeoxycholic acid, the rate-limiting enzyme in bile acid biosynthesis, the cholesterol 7α-hydroxylase is markedly up-regulated. As a consequence the accumulation of 7α-hydroxylated bile acid, intermediates will be even greater and these intermediates will be metabolized in pathways not normally used.

The accumulated 5β-cholestane-$3\alpha,7\alpha,12\alpha$-triol cannot be metabolized by the usual pathway to bile acids, which means that the 25-hydroxylase pathway may be utilized (Fig. 123-4). Because the enzymes involved in this pathway appear to have limited capacity, some of the intermediates in this pathway accumulate and are excreted in bile and feces (Fig. 123-12). Thus patients with CTX excrete high amounts of 5β-cholestane-$3\alpha,7\alpha,12\alpha,25$-tetrol.[140] Several other metabolites of 5β-cholestane-$3\alpha,7\alpha,12\alpha$-triol, such as 5β-cholestane-$3\alpha,7\alpha,12\alpha,24\alpha,25$-pentol and 5β-cholestane-$3\alpha,7\alpha,12\alpha,23,25$-pentol, are excreted.[140] Hoshita et al. made an extensive characterization of a number of bile alcohols and their metabolites in urine and feces from patients with CTX.[162,163] It is evident that the high accumulation of 5β-cholestane-$3\alpha,7\alpha,12\alpha$-triol leads to exposure of this substrate to the normally less active microsomal 23-, 24-, and 25-hydroxylases. In total, gram amounts of all the above alcohols may be excreted daily in urine and feces.[164]

Because 7α-hydroxy-4-cholesten-3-one cannot be metabolized by the usual pathway to bile acids, more unusual pathways may be utilized for this steroid also (Fig. 123-13). As mentioned above, we have shown that one product of 7α-hydroxy-4-cholesten-3-one is cholestanol. As a consequence of the accumulation of 7α-hydroxy-4-cholesten-3-one, this pathway may be utilized to a higher extent.

Salen et al. reported that the activity of the microsomal 12α-hydroxylase is increased about threefold in liver biopsies from CTX patients.[165] In the liver biopsy we studied, 12α-hydroxylase activity was high and was also present in the mitochondrial fraction.[166] The increased 12α-hydroxylase activity may be a consequence of the reduced feedback regulation by bile acids in CTX. We have recently shown that, for example, cholestyramine treatment leads to a significant stimulation of the microsomal 12α-hydroxylase activity in humans.[9] The increased 12α-hydroxylase activity in CTX may contribute to the very high proportion of cholic acid formed in relation to cholic acid.

Evidence has accumulated that the mitochondrial 27-hydroxylase is able to catalyze 25-hydroxylation of vitamin D (for a review, see reference 13). In the patient we studied, a liver biopsy contained a low but significant vitamin D 25-hydroxylase activity, but no measurable 27-hydroxylase activity,[141] and it is possible that there is more than one 25-hydroxylase active toward vitamin D in human liver mitochondria. The importance of the mitochondrial 27-hydroxylase for circulating levels of 25-hydroxyvitamin D is, however, not known and has been a matter of controversy. Reduced serum levels of 25-hydroxyvitamin D have been shown in some,[167] but not in all,[168] CTX patients. Low levels of vitamin D metabolites may thus be the explanation for the osteoporosis found in some patients with CTX.[167] In a mouse with a disrupted Cyp27 gene, however, there is no defect in vitamin D metabolism.[169]

Salen et al. have also reported an increased 3β-hydroxysteroid-Δ^5-dehydrogenase activity[7] and reduced 24S-hydroxylase activity[170] in liver biopsies from patients with CTX. The former finding may be one of the causes for the accumulation of cholestanol in this disease (see below).

Mechanisms Behind the Increased Synthesis of Cholestanol

Increased biosynthesis of cholestanol may not be completely unique for patients with CTX. Increased levels of cholestanol have also been reported in some hepatic disorders, particularly in primary biliary cirrhosis.[171]

There are three hypotheses for the mechanism behind the increased synthesis of cholestanol in patients with CTX:

1. The activity of the rate-limiting enzyme in the normal biosynthesis of cholestanol, the microsomal 3β-hydroxysteroid-Δ^5-oxidoreductase active on cholesterol, may be increased in patients with CTX.

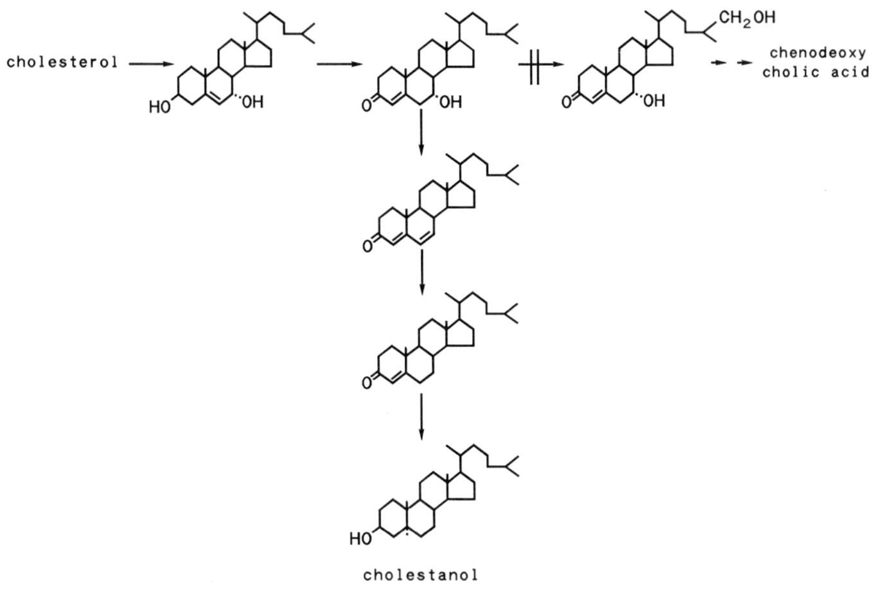

cholesterol → ... chenodeoxy cholic acid

cholestanol

Fig. 123-13 Metabolic consequences of the accumulation of 7α-hydroxy-4-cholesten-3-one in patients with CTX.

2. The increased biosynthesis of cholestanol may be secondary to the increased biosynthesis of cholesterol.
3. The increased biosynthesis of cholestanol may be due to increased utilization of bile acid intermediates as precursors for cholestanol. As a consequence of the metabolic block, considerable amounts of such intermediates accumulate in CTX.

The first hypothesis was put forward by Salen et al.,[7] who showed that the apparent formation of 4-cholesten-3-one from cholesterol by hepatic microsomes from one subject with CTX was about threefold higher than that obtained with control microsomes. In view of the great difficulties of assaying this low activity (see reference 172), the result may, however, be difficult to evaluate. In contrast to Salen et al., we did not find any significant difference between the activity of the 3β-hydroxysteroid-Δ^5-oxidoreductase in liver biopsies from control subjects and from patients with CTX.[173] In our experiments, 7α-hydroxycholesterol was used as substrate because we were unable to accurately measure the very low conversion obtained with cholesterol as substrate.

The second hypothesis is difficult to fit with most known facts concerning cholesterol and cholestanol metabolism. If an increased rate of cholesterol synthesis is the cause of the increased rate of cholestanol synthesis, other conditions with increased cholesterol biosynthesis would also be expected to stimulate synthesis of cholestanol.

According to the third hypothesis, the bile acid intermediates accumulating in patients with CTX due to the lack of the 27-hydroxylase may be shunted into the cholestanol pathway (Fig. 123-13). In accordance with this hypothesis, we were able to show that cholestanol isolated from serum, bile, and feces from a CTX patient treated with a mixture of 4-^{14}C-cholesterol and 7α-^{3}H-cholesterol had lost about 75 percent of the ^{3}H label.[27] This indicates that about 75 percent of the cholestanol had been formed by a pathway involving 7α-hydroxylation and 7α-dehydroxylation. In addition, it was shown that there was a significant conversion of intravenously administered 7β-^{3}H-labeled 7α-hydroxy-cholesterol into cholestanol in a patient with CTX.[27,174] 7α-Hydroxy-4-cholesten-3-one would be expected to be an intermediate in the conversion of 7α-hydroxycholesterol into cholestanol.

When labeled 7α-hydroxy-4-cholesten-3-one was administered to a CTX patient, however, little or no conversion could be demonstrated into cholestanol.[143] This may be due to compartmentation and dilution of the administered labeled steroid. Thus, plasma contains relatively high concentrations of this steroid,[175] and the administered 7α-hydroxy-4-cholesten-3-one may not equilibrate with the small intrahepatic pool of this compound utilized for cholestanol biosynthesis.[175] It should be noted that only a very small shunting (2 to 4 percent) of the 7α-hydroxycholesterol formed into the cholestanol pathway is required to explain the increased synthesis of cholestanol in patients with CTX.

At present, the third hypothesis has the best experimental support, and it is evident that at least part of the cholestanol is synthesized by this pathway in patients with CTX. This hypothesis can also explain the effects of different treatments on the synthesis of cholestanol. Treatment with chenodeoxycholic acid is the therapy of choice (see below) and reduces plasma levels of cholestanol dramatically in patients with CTX. Due to feedback inhibition, treatment with chenodeoxycholic acid inhibits the cholesterol 7α-hydroxylase, which leads to reduction in the amounts of 7α-hydroxylated precursors to cholestanol. We have shown that the elevated levels of 7α-hydroxy-4-cholesten-3-one and cholesta-4,6-dien-3-one in patients with CTX decrease dramatically after treatment with chenodeoxycholic acid.[175] It has been reported that treatment of patients with CTX with cholestyramine leads to increased levels of cholestanol. This effect can also be explained by the third hypothesis. Thus, treatment with cholestyramine leads to increased 7α-hydroxylation of cholesterol, and, therefore, to increased levels of 7α-hydroxylated precursors for biosynthesis of cholestanol.

It has been reported that treatment of CTX patients with an inhibitor of cholesterol synthesis causes a considerable reduction in the levels of cholestanol in plasma.[176] Such treatment has also been used in combination with bile acids.[177,178] This effect is consistent with the second of the three above hypotheses. On the other hand, a marked reduction of cholesterol synthesis in the liver can be expected to reduce the formation of bile acid intermediates such as 7α-hydroxy-4-cholesten-3-one, which is a precursor for cholestanol. Such an effect can be expected to be more pronounced if the cholesterol 7α-hydrolase is up-regulated.

Mechanisms Behind the Increased Synthesis and Accumulation of Cholesterol

The increased biosynthesis of cholesterol in patients with CTX is likely to be secondary to the markedly up-regulated cholesterol 7α-hydroxylase, similar to the effect of cholestyramine on cholesterol homeostasis. Because 27-hydroxycholesterol is a potent suppressor of cholesterol synthesis in various cell systems, the possibility has been discussed that the lack of 27-hydroxy-cholesterol in CTX is one reason for the accelerated synthesis of cholesterol.[179] It has also been suggested that the increased synthesis may be secondary to the accumulation of cholestanol.[180] In this connection, it is of interest that mice deficient in sterol 27-hydroxylase have a marked up-regulation of the cholesterol 7α-hydroxylase (ninefold), but only a twofold up-regulation of the rate-limiting enzyme in cholesterol synthesis HMG CoA reductase.[169] These mice do not have an overproduction of cholestanol as a consequence of the enzymatic defect.

It was recently suggested that one reason for the accumulation of cholesterol and the development of premature atherosclerosis in patients with CTX is related to a transport function of the sterol 27-hydroxylase.[181] Cultured human alveolar macrophages were shown to have a high capacity to eliminate intracellular cholesterol by oxidation into 27-hydroxycholesterol and 3β-hydroxy-5-cholestenoic acid.[181,182] The latter two products are more polar than cholesterol and are easily transported out of the cells. The relative importance of this mechanism is difficult to evaluate in the present state of knowledge. In this connection, it is of interest that sterol 27-hydroxylase deficient mice on a normal diet do not develop xanthomas. The development of xanthomas in patients with CTX may be due to several factors, resulting in an imbalance between cholesterol synthesis, cholesterol uptake, and cholesterol efflux from the cells.

Mechanisms for the Accumulation of Cholesterol and Cholestanol in the Brain

It is clear that explanations can be offered for the increased biosynthesis of cholesterol and cholestanol in the liver in patients with CTX. Due to the blood-brain barrier, it is not evident, however, that increased levels of cholesterol and cholestanol, or their precursors, in the circulation, lead to an accumulation in the brain. In view of this, it is interesting that Salen et al. reported drastically increased levels of apolipoprotein B (about one hundredfold) with smaller increase in concentrations of other lipoproteins (1.5 to 3 times) and of albumin (three- to fourfold) in the cerebrospinal fluid of patients with CTX.[183]

The concentration of cholestanol was about 20 times higher in CTX than in controls. Treatment of the CTX patients with chenodeoxycholic acid decreased the levels of cholestanol in cerebrospinal fluid about threefold. Thus, the permeability of the blood-brain barrier seems to be affected in CTX by an unknown mechanism.

Buchmann and Clausen showed that rabbits fed diets enriched with cholestanol (3.5 g/week) for 8 weeks had cholestanol levels in the brain about twofold higher than in controls.[184] After an additional regression period with cholestyramine for 8 weeks, the increased content of cholestanol in the brain was unchanged. Buyn et al. showed that feeding mice with 1 percent cholestanol for 32 weeks resulted in significant incorporation of this sterol in cerebellum.[185] The level of cholestanol in the cerebellum increased almost linearly with feeding time and no decline was observed. It is thus clear that cholestanol to some extent can pass the blood-brain barrier in experimental animals. The possibility must also be considered that a precursor to cholestanol might pass the blood-brain barrier and be converted into cholestanol in the brain. We have shown that the microsomal fraction of a homogenate of rat brain is able to catalyze formation of cholestanol from cholesta-4,6-dien-3-one.[186]

Clinical Phenotype

A few hundred patients with this disease had been reported in 1998 including 52 who were molecularly characterized.[144,146–160] Most of the patients reside in Japan, the United States, the Netherlands, and Israel. Sporadic cases were reported in additional countries (Table 123-2).

A multitude of clinical signs develop gradually during life in CTX patients. These include Achilles tendon xanthomas, tuberous xanthomas, neurologic dysfunction, low intelligence, and cataracts. In addition, some patients have respiratory insufficiency and cardiovascular disease. A few cases were reported to have endocrinological disturbances. A recent investigation in two large Druze families residing in one village allowed for detailed investigation into the age-related manifestations of the disease. In these families, a single-base deletion mutation (delC376) caused CTX in 10 patients.[151] Although age stratification demonstrated gradual development of almost all major clinical signs of the disease during life, some exceptions do exist. Some patients do not develop xanthomas or epilepsy even at an advanced age.[151] Other investigators have also reported that the development of symptoms in patients with CTX may be variable. Some of the patients may be mentally retarded already in childhood, whereas some patients have normal intelligence even in the sixth decade of life.[187] Tendon xanthomas are most often developed in the third or fourth decade, but may occur as early as age 15.[188,189] The Achilles tendon is the most common site but xanthomas may also occur on the tibial tuberosities, the extensor tendons of the fingers, and in the triceps (Fig. 123-14). The xanthomas are histologically similar to those developed in familial hypercholesterolemia (Chap. 120), and chemical analysis for cholestanol content is necessary to separate the two types.

In a recent study in molecularly confirmed CTX cases, we showed that early neurologic manifestations may include mild cognitive impairment and peripheral neuropathy.[168] Spasticity, often associated with ataxia, most often develops during the second and third decades of life and becomes more severe with increasing age. During the fourth or fifth decade, the patient may become incapacitated.[123,127,187] In the final stage of CTX, spasticity, tremor, and ataxia increase in parallel with the enlargement of the xanthomas. Epilepsy may occur and the patients may develop bladder and bowel incontinence. In addition they can lose pain and vibratory sensation and may develop difficulty swallowing. Death usually occurs between the fourth and sixth decades due to myocardial infarction or progressive neurological deterioration including pseudobulbar paralysis.[187] In the fifth edition of this book,[187] three patients between age 44 and 46 were reported to have tendon xanthomas and spastic gaits but were otherwise functioning normally. We studied one patient who, at age 59, had large xanthomas but no neurologic symptoms apart from a mild distal peripheral neuropathy.[175] This patient, however, had symptoms of angina pectoris from age 53 (two-vessel coronary artery disease).

Osteoporosis is reported to be common in CTX and may predispose to early bone fractures.[167]

Psychiatric disorders may also appear in CTX, and may precede the onset of neurologic disturbances.[190] Some patients may have delusions, hallucinations, or catatonia similar to features seen in schizophrenia.[190]

Pathologic Findings

Nervous System. van Bogaert et al. have given a detailed description of the central nervous system in CTX.[123–125,129] The most prominent changes occur in the cerebellum where yellow xanthomas sometimes can replace most of the white matter. The adjacent folia may be atrophic and there is demyelination of specific parts of the white matter.[123,191] In these areas of demyelination, there can be cystic spaces and needle-shaped clefts. The cysts and clefts contain large mononuclear cells with foamy, vacuolated cytoplasm. Multinucleated giant cells may also surround the clefts and cysts.[123,192] In general, there is a loss of Purkinje cells and granule cells in the demyelinated zones. In addition, there may be degeneration of the olivocerebellar fibers.[123,192]

In spite of the dementia and mental retardation in many patients, the cerebral cortex seems to be almost free from morphologic and histologic changes. The forebrain, however, may contain xanthomas in the cerebral peduncles and globus pallidus.[123,124] Mononuclear cells with foamy cytoplasm are also found in caudate nucleus, basal ganglia, and thalamus and in the

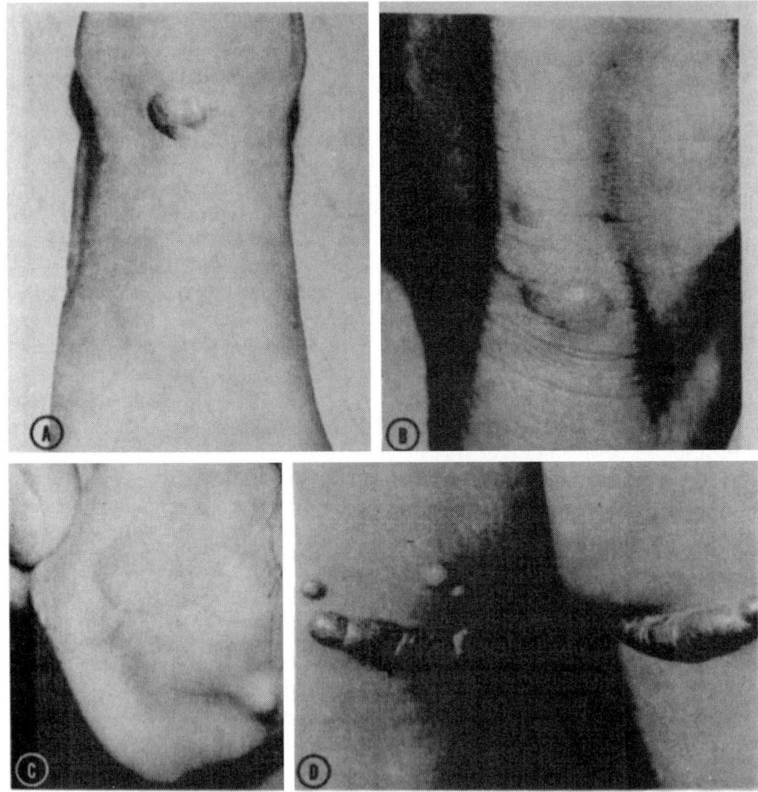

Fig. 123-14 Xanthomas in the area of the anterior ankle (*A*), Achilles tendon (*B*), posterior aspect of ear (*C*), and buttocks area (*D*). (From McArthur et al.[285] Used by permission.)

white matter adjacent to the lateral ventricles.[123,124] Demyelination has been reported in the cerebral peduncles, in the fibers of ansa lenticularis,[123,129,192] and in parts of the globus pallidus and corona radiata.[129] The optic pathway is often atrophic.[123]

Lesions have also been reported in the midbrain and the brain stem,[123,124] as well as in the spinal cord.[123,191] In one study of nerve biopsies from patients with CTX, demyelination and remyelination were reported, as well as production of onion bulbs.[127]

In the report by Menkes,[128] up to 25 percent of the total free sterol fraction from affected parts of the cerebellum was composed of cholestanol. In morphologically and histologically normal parts of the gray and white matter of the cerebrum, the corresponding cholestanol content was 20 percent. The total esterified sterol fraction from affected parts of cerebellum contained 49 percent cholestanol ester. Other groups have reported similar findings in brain as well as in peripheral nerves.[129,132] Increased content of cholesteryl esters has been found both in normal and abnormal brain tissue from patients with CTX.[131,192]

Computerized tomographic (CT) scanning and magnetic resonance imaging (MRI) of the brain may demonstrate brain atrophy, as well as focal or diffuse cerebral, cerebellar, and basal ganglia lesions (reviewed in reference 193). The findings are usually milder than expected according to the neurologic manifestations of the disease.[193] Positron emission tomography (PET) was used in one case and demonstrated functional abnormality in presynaptic dopaminergic neurons.[194]

Tendons. Light microscopy of the tendon xanthomas shows birefringent crystalline clefts surrounded by multinucleated giant cells with foamy cytoplasm.[123,126,187]

Philippart and van Bogaert were the first to demonstrate accumulation of cholestanol in tendon xanthoma.[129] Salen et al. reported that cholestanol accounted for 11 percent of the total sterols in an Achilles tendon xanthoma and 7.3 percent of the sterols in a tuberous xanthoma.[187] The tendon xanthoma from one of our patients contained 17 percent cholestanol in the sterol fraction.[141] Bhattacharyya and Connor[132] reported similar findings. It has been reported that one CTX patient with hyperapobetalipoproteinemia had a marked accumulation of apolipoprotein B in a xanthoma.[195] Such accumulation is not seen in xanthomas from patients with familial hypercholesterolemia.

Cardiovascular System. Premature atherosclerosis is a characteristic feature in CTX and at least 18 cases with angina pectoris or myocardial infarction have been reported.[196] In the fifth edition this book, four patients were reported to have died after myocardial infarction.[187] The aorta and the atheromatous plaque obtained at autopsy of one patient contained cholestanol corresponding to 2 percent and 2.8 percent, respectively, of the total sterols. One case with aneurysmal coronary artery disease has been reported.[196]

Lens. Cataract is common in CTX and may appear as early as age 5 to 6 years.[123,129] Small irregular corticonuclear opacities, anterior polar cataracts, and dense posterior subcapsular cataracts are found in various ages. Some patients may show clinical signs of optic neuropathy (reviewed in reference 130). By electron microscopy, electron-lucent areas were found in the anterior cortex and vacuoles in the epithelial cells of the lens in one of our patients.[197] The cataractous lens contains elevated levels of cholestanol.[198]

Liver. It has been reported[199] that hepatocytes from two patients with CTX contained a light golden pigment, which at high magnification appeared in two forms: either as diffuse, amorphous electron-dense material enveloped by the smooth endoplasmic reticulum or as free-floating bodies in the cytosol. The cytosol also contained free rhomboid-shaped crystals.

Lung and Skeleton. Granulomatous lesions containing multinucleated giant cells and large foam cells have been seen in the lung, in the femur, and in the bodies of the lumbar vertebrae.[123,124,191]

Plasma. In most cases, plasma cholesterol levels are normal (115 to 220 mg/dl). Elevated levels (up to 400 mg/dl) have been reported in a few patients. With few exceptions, plasma triglyceride levels are normal. Plasma cholestanol levels are, however, always elevated in untreated CTX patients.

The values range from 1.3 to 15 mg/dl and are generally between 3 and 15 times higher than mean values in normal plasma (0.1 to 0.6 mg/dl).[187] One case has been reported with a very moderate increase in the ratio between cholestanol and cholesterol.[200] According to a study by Seyama et al.,[201] the ratio between cholestanol and cholesterol gives a better discrimination than the concentration of cholestanol alone. The serum levels of some accumulated bile acid intermediates, such as 7α-hydroxy-4-cholesten-3-one, and a potential cholestanol precursor, cholesta-4,6-dien-3-one, are also increased in untreated patients with CTX.[175] As a consequence of the high activity of the rate-limiting enzyme in bile acid biosynthesis, cholesterol 7α-hydroxylase (see below), the level of 7α-hydroxy-cholesterol in serum is also increased.[202] As a consequence of the high activity of the rate-limiting enzyme in cholesterol biosynthesis, HMG CoA reductase, the level of some cholesterol precursors such as lathosterol are also elevated in plasma.[202] As could be expected from the decreased pool of bile acids, the levels of bile acids in serum are low.[204] It has been shown that patients with CTX have increased levels in plasma of bile alcohol glucuronides.[205]

Shore et al.[206] have reported decreased mean levels of HDL cholesterol in 8 CTX subjects (14.5 ± 3.2 mg/dl versus normally 48.0 ± 9.0 mg/dl). The ratio between apoprotein to total cholesterol in the HDL of these patients was also two to three times greater than normal. The above abnormalities have not been confirmed by other groups,[146,148,151] however, and cannot easily be explained by the basic metabolic defect (see below). Two Norwegian patients had normal levels of HDL cholesterol. One had a slightly increased level of VLDL, but the other lipoprotein fractions, as isolated by ultracentrifugation, did not deviate from the normal pattern. A normal pattern of lipoproteins has been documented in at least one additional patient.[175]

Cerebrospinal Fluid. Salen et al. reported that mean cholesterol and cholestanol levels in cerebrospinal fluid from CTX patients are about 1.5 and 20 times, respectively, higher than normal.[183] Drastic changes were observed with respect to the protein pattern. The concentration of apolipoprotein B was increased about one hundredfold, and the level of albumin about three- to fourfold as compared to normal.[183]

Bile. In patients with CTX, considerable amounts of cholestanol are excreted in bile, and cholestanol constitutes from 4 to 11 percent of total biliary neutral sterols.[131] In normal bile, the corresponding figure is less than 1 percent. Bile from patients with CTX also contains excessive amounts of some cholesterol precursors such as lanosterol and 7-cholesten-3β-ol.[131]

The composition of bile acids in bile is also abnormal in CTX. Cholic acid constitutes the majority (about 80 percent) and the content of chenodeoxycholic acid is very low (only a few percent of the total bile acids).[131] There is almost no deoxycholic acid. Normally, there are about equal amounts of cholic acid and chenodeoxycholic acid in bile. The low content of chenodeoxycholic acid is a direct consequence of the metabolic block. The low content of deoxycholic acid may be due to an inhibitory effect of bile alcohols on the microbial 7α-dehydroxylation of cholic acid.[207] It has been reported that about 2 percent of the total bile acids in CTX consists of allocholic acid.[131,132] Allocholic is a 5α-bile acid derived from cholestanol and is present in trace amounts only in normal bile.[1]

The most unique finding in bile from subjects with CTX is the high concentrations of different 25-hydroxylated C_{27}-bile alcohols containing four or five hydroxyl groups.[140,208–210] 5β-Cholestane-3α,7α,12α,23-tetrol, 5β-cholestane-3α,7α,12α,25-tetrol, and 5β-cholestane-3α,7α,12α,24R,25-pentol are the dominant bile alcohols (Fig. 123-12). These steroids are excreted in the bile mainly as conjugates of glucuronic acid.[205,211] In feces, however, they are found in deconjugated form.

Urine. Patients with CTX excrete considerable amounts of glucuronidated bile alcohols in urine.[212–214] In contrast to bile, where the predominant bile alcohol is 5β-cholestane-3α,7α,12β,25-tetrol, 5β-cholestane-pentols dominate in urine. The pentols have hydroxyl groups at C-22, C-23, or C-25, in addition to the hydroxyl groups at C-3, C-7, and C-12. Most probably there is also some urinary excretion of C_{27}-hexols and heptols (Sjövall et al., unpublished observation). Batta et al.[214] reported 5β-cholestane-3α,7α,12α,23,25-pentol to be the dominating urinary bile alcohol (56 percent). 5β-Cholestane-3α,7α,12α,24S,25-pentol was not detected in bile, but was isolated from the urine of all patients studied. In addition to these unusual alcohols, abnormal bile acids, such as 23-hydroxycholic acid and 23-norcholic acid, can also be found in urine of patients with CTX.[200,214] Koopman et al. reported that CTX patients treated with chenodeoxycholic acid excrete significant amounts of 23-hydroxychenodeoxycholic acid.[215] Treatment with ursodeoxycholic acid leads to excretion of 23-hydroxyursodeoxycholic acid and 23-norursodeoxy-cholic acid.[216] These findings seem to reflect increased 23-hydroxylase activity.

Diagnosis

CTX should be suspected in all patients with tendon xanthomas and normal or only elevated serum cholesterol. The diagnosis must also be considered in all cases of unexplained juvenile cataracts. These characteristic features may precede the neurologic disturbances by decades. Due to the slow progression of the disease, the diagnosis is seldom obtained before the second decade of life, except in cases where CTX is suspected for genetic reasons. The diagnosis may be made by quantitation of cholestanol in serum by gas chromatography. Preferably, also bile and xanthoma should be analyzed. It may be difficult to separate cholestanol from cholesterol by a simple gas-chromatographic step, and a prepurification step may be necessary. Because the trimethylsilylether of cholestanol contains a specific ion at m/z 306 in its mass spectrum, which is not present in the mass spectrum of the corresponding derivative of cholesterol, selected ion monitoring is a suitable method for quantitation of cholestanol in serum.[137] High-performance liquid chromatography of the benzoyl derivative of cholestanol[201] and reverse-phase thin-layer chromatography[216] are also suitable methods for quantitation. In specialized laboratories, the diagnosis may be obtained by quantitation of, for example, 5β-cholestane-3α,7α,12α,23,25-pentol in the urine. Koopman et al. suggested a very simple urinary screening test for CTX suitable for larger populations. In this method, a simple commercial kit for assay of 7α-hydroxylated bile acids is used for detection of elevated levels of 7α-hydroxylated bile alcohols in urine.[217] In all positive cases, the diagnosis must be confirmed by more specific means. FAB-MS is an excellent method to use for diagnosis confirmation.[218] A definitive identification of the lack of the 27-hydroxylase can be done with fibroblast cultures[106] or by determination of 27-hydroxycholesterol in plasma.[179]

In principle, it should also be possible to identify heterozygotes by assay of the level of 27-hydroxylase activity in cultured fibroblasts.[106] This method is very impractical because control fibroblasts from several individuals must be used. Koopman et al.[219] suggested a simpler method. They showed that when carriers and noncarriers for the disease were subjected to cholestyramine treatment, by which endogenous bile acid synthesis was stimulated, the urinary excretion of 5β-cholestane-3α,7α,12α,23,25-pentol in the carrier increased considerably, but remained essentially the same in noncarriers. This test may be of value for the genetic counseling of carriers for CTX and for detection of newborn infants with CTX in families where the Cyp27 gene mutation has not yet been identified.

Common Cyp27 gene mutations have been identified in several world populations. The increased prevalence of these mutations in some countries may be related to the founder gene effect[146,148,151] or other, as yet undefined, mechanisms. In these populations, DNA diagnosis may provide a rapid and inexpensive tool for clinical diagnosis and genetic counseling. It is expected that a large number of cases will be identified in the near future due to increased awareness of the disease and because of DNA-based screening of suspected families.

The importance of an early diagnosis of CTX cannot be overemphasized. If the disease is detected in early childhood, treatment with chenodeoxycholic acid and HMG CoA reductase inhibitors may prevent the occurrence of irreversible CNS-damage and at least some of the other major manifestations of the disease.

Treatment

Salen was the first to treat a CTX patient with chenodeoxycholic acid.[220] He showed that the expansion of the deficient bile acid pool resulted in a marked drop in plasma cholestanol. It was also demonstrated that cholesterol and cholestanol production rates were suppressed. In addition, HMG CoA reductase, the rate-controlling enzyme in cholesterol synthesis, was inhibited fourfold during the therapy and bile alcohols almost disappeared from the bile. It has been reported that a number of patients on therapy with chenodeoxycholic acid showed reversal of their neurologic disability, with clearing of the dementia, better orientation, a rise in IQ, and improved strength and independence.[221] Cholic acid and deoxycholic acid can be used to depress cholestanol formation in patients with CTX.[222]

Treatment with HMG CoA reductase inhibitors may further decrease plasma cholestanol levels in CTX.[176–178] The combined treatment with chenodeoxycholic acid may decrease the formation of bile acid precursors that could be converted to cholestanol.

Disruption of Cyp27 in the Mouse

Recently, in an attempt to create a mouse model for CTX, we disrupted the mouse Cyp27.[169] These mice had normal circulating levels of cholesterol and triglycerides. Serum levels of vitamin A, vitamin E, and 1,25-dihydroxy vitamin D were normal, and serum levels of 25-hydroxyvitamin D were above normal. Excretion of bile acids in feces was decreased to less than 20 percent of normal, and formation of bile acids from intraperitoneally injected tritium-labeled 7α-hydroxycholesterol was less than 15 percent of normal. There was a compensatory up-regulation of the cholesterol 7α-hydroxylase as judged from a ninefold increase in its mRNA level and a tenfold increase in the levels of 7α-hydroxycholesterol in the circulation and in the liver. In humans, the pathway involving 25-hydroxylated bile alcohols as intermediates can partly compensate for the loss of the sterol 27-hydroxylase. Only traces of 25-hydroxylated bile alcohols were found in bile and feces of the Cyp27 -/- mice, however. CTX patients are known to have an accumulation of cholestanol. This was not found in the mice with a disrupted Cyp27. The mice did not develop any neurologic abnormality, atherosclerosis, or xanthomatosis even if placed on a high-cholesterol high-fat diet for up to 7 months.

PEROXISOMAL DISORDERS

In some peroxisomal disorders (Zellweger syndrome, adrenoleukodystrophy, juvenile Refsum disease) peroxisomal trihydroxycoprostanic acid acyl CoA oxidase is missing or defective, resulting in accumulation of trihydroxycoprostanic acid and its metabolites (Fig. 123-1). Several other important peroxisomal enzymes are also missing, and only part of the symptoms is due to the defect in bile acid biosynthesis. It has been reported that Zellweger patients may respond favorably to bile acid therapy.[223] The peroxisomal disorders are described in Chap. 129. For more information concerning peroxisomal disorders that emphasizes their consequences for bile acid biosynthesis, the reader is referred to some recent articles.[224,225]

AMIDATION DEFECT

Setchell et al. recently reported, in preliminary form, a case with a unique inborn error in bile acid conjugation, involving a deficiency of amidation.[226] This defect was identified in a 14-year-old boy of Laotian descent who, in the first 3 months of life, presented with hyperbilirubinemia, elevated serum transaminases, a normal GGT, and a form of α-thalassemia resulting in severe hemolysis. A liver biopsy at 5 months of age demonstrated significant periportal fibrosis, marked proliferation of small bile ducts, cholestasis, and bile plugs. At 1 year of age, the patient was admitted with anemia, hypocalcemia, and elevated alkaline phosphatase. Bone X-rays demonstrated moderate rickets. The patient responded to ergocalciferol and calcium supplements. He required transfusions many times throughout life. Later clinical investigations revealed abnormally low serum concentrations of 25-hydroxyvitamin D, 1,25-dihydroxy vitamin D, carotene, and vitamin K. Liver function tests were normal. A liver biopsy showed severe hemosiderosis within hepatocytes and Kupffer cells, minimal periportal fibrosis, and focal mild inflammation. The cholestasis and ductular proliferation have resolved.

Analysis of the urinary bile acids by FAB-MS revealed an increased urinary bile acid excretion, but a lack of the ions corresponding to glyco- and tauro-conjugated cholanic acids. Fractionation of the urinary bile acids according to the conjugation state by lipophilic anion exchange chromatography confirmed the majority of the bile acids to be unconjugated. Similar findings were obtained in analyses of serum and biliary bile acids. Small amounts of sulfate and glucuronide conjugates were present.

GC-MS analysis showed that unconjugated cholic acid dominated the unconjugated bile acid fraction.

It remains uncertain whether the specific point of the defect involves the bile acid CoA ligase or the amino acid N-acyltransferase. The elevated serum bile acid concentrations suggest that it is at the level of bile acid CoA ligase and no evidence could be obtained for the presence of choloyl CoA in any of the samples from the patient analyzed by HPLC or GC-MS.

DEFECT IN OXYSTEROL 7α-HYDROXYLASE

Very recently, Setchell et al. reported on one unique case with severe neonatal liver disease due to mutation of the oxysterol 7α-hydroxylase gene.[21]

The patient was a Hispanic male infant whose parents were first cousins. His postnatal course was remarkable for transient tachypnea of the newborn requiring oxygen therapy and the development of jaundice at 6 days of age, which resolved by phototherapy. At 10 weeks of age, bright red blood was passed via rectum and a spontaneous episode of epistaxis occurred. On physical examination at 10 weeks of age at a children's hospital, the patient was alert and icteric. There were no dysmorphic features and neurologic examination was normal. Initial laboratory studies revealed markedly elevated transaminases and alkaline phosphatase. Serum α-tocopherol and retinol concentrations were reduced. Hepatobiliary scintigraphy showed delayed hepatic clearance and no biliary excretion. Percutaneous liver biopsy performed after correction of coagulopathy suggested biliary tract obstruction. The patient was treated with medium chain triglyceride-containing formula, fat-soluble vitamin supplementation, and ursodeoxycholic acid.

Following the recognition of a defect in primary bile acid synthesis, the patient was treated with oral cholic acid at 15 mg/kg body weight/day. There was, however, no response after 49 days of cholic acid therapy with continued deterioration of hepatic synthetic function. Because of progressive hepatosplenomegaly, hypoalbuminemia, and coagulopathy, the patient underwent orthotopic liver transplantation from a cadaver donor at 4.5 months of age. Acute allograft rejection occurred on day 9 posttransplantation. On day 19, the patient developed rapidly progressive cerebral edema and died 24 hours later. Autopsy revealed disseminated lymphoproliferative disease (Epstein-Barr virus related) in all body tissues, including brain and liver, and mild allograft rejection.

FAB-MS revealed elevated urinary bile acid excretion. Most of the bile acids were sulfate and monoglucuronidate of monounsaturated monohydroxycholenic acids, and no primary bile acids were detected. The major products of hepatic synthesis were found to be 3β-hydroxy-5-cholestenoic acids and 3β-hydroxy-5-cholenoic acid, which accounted for 96 percent of total bile acids in serum. Levels of 27-hydroxycholesterol were more than 4500 times normal. The biochemical findings were thus consistent with a deficiency in 7α-hydroxylation, leading to the accumulation of hepatotoxic unsaturated monohydroxy-bile acids. Hepatic microsomal oxysterol 7α-hydroxylase was undetectable. Gene analysis revealed a cytosine to thymidine transition mutation in exon 5 that converts an arginine codon at position 388 to a stop codon. The truncated protein was inactive when expressed in 293 cells.

This is the first example of an inborn error of an enzyme specific for the acidic pathway for bile acid formation and illustrates the importance of this pathway in early life.

PHYTOSTEROLEMIA (SITOSTEROLEMIA)

General

Sitosterolemia is a rare familial disorder of sterol metabolism, which was first described by Bhattacharyya and Connor in 1973.[227] They reported two sisters who developed extensive tendon and subcutaneous xanthomas during childhood, despite normal levels of plasma cholesterol. The condition was characterized by high plasma levels of the plant sterols sitosterol, campesterol, and stigmasterol, and accumulation of plant sterols in the tissues (tendon xanthomas, adipose tissue, skin surface lipids). Plant sterols constituted about 16 and 11 percent of their respective total plasma sterols. The intestinal absorption of sitosterol was greatly increased in the two patients. Increased absorption of plant sterols, possibly combined with impaired excretion, was suggested as a cause of the disease.

In June 1998, we knew of 45 patients with this disease[228] for which we use the term *phytosterolemia.* Bhattacharyya and Connor suggested *sitosterolemia and xanthomatosis* as an alternative. The above terms, used alternatively here, should, however, be made more precise when the biochemical defect is defined.

Basic Defect

The primary metabolic defect in sitosterolemia has not yet been identified, but several possible mechanisms behind the plant sterol accumulation have been considered.

Increased Plant Sterol Absorption. In the patients originally described by Bhattacharyya and Connor, the intestinal absorption of sitosterol was greatly increased.[227] Normally, about 5 percent or less of ingested sitosterol is absorbed, while these patients absorbed 24 percent and 28 percent, respectively. Increased absorption of sitosterol, ranging from 15 to 63 percent, has been confirmed in several patients.[83,99,229,230] Using a highly accurate method based on deuterium-labeled sterols and combined gas-liquid chromatography-mass spectrometry, we found that the sitosterol absorption averaged 16 percent in three patients with sitosterolemia as opposed to 5 percent in healthy volunteers.[43] Campesterol absorption was also significantly elevated to 24 percent in the patients, versus 16 percent in the controls. Absorption of cholesterol was higher in the patients (53 percent) than in the volunteers (43 percent), but it was still within the normal range.[43] Cholesterol absorption in the high normal range has also been described in other cases of sitosterolemia.[82,83,99,230,231] Thus, the enhanced sitosterol absorption does not seem to inhibit the cholesterol absorption. One patient absorbed increased amounts of shellfish sterols,[232] indicating a more general abnormality in sterol absorption. The mechanism behind the accelerated sterol absorption is not known, but possible explanations include altered solubilization of plant sterols in intestinal micelles, increased uptake by mucosal cell membranes, decreased sterol specificity of mucosal cell acyl CoA:cholesterol acyltransferase (ACAT), or changes in intracellular transport processes.

Gregg et al. proposed that sitosterolemia results from a general loss of discrimination between various sterols for esterification.[232] Sitosterol is normally a poor substrate for the intestinal ACAT,[58] as well as for ACAT in the liver.[233] According to Gregg et al.'s hypothesis increased mucosal esterification of sitosterol could lead to increased absorption, while increased esterification in the liver could prevent secretion of this sterol into the bile. There is no evidence, however, of alteration in any specific ACAT activity in this disease, and sitosterol does not stimulate the ACAT reaction in macrophages or in cultured intestinal cells.[71,234]

Decreased Biliary Plant Sterol Excretion. Kinetic studies show that the half-life of sitosterol is prolonged[99,230,235,236] and that the sitosterol elimination constant is considerably decreased[231] in patients with sitosterolemia as compared to controls. The total exchangeable sitosterol pool is expanded from 120 to 290 mg in healthy subjects to levels of 3500 to 6200 mg in patients.[99,235,236] This greatly increased sitosterol pool cannot be accounted for by enhanced absorption alone and is considered to be the result of a combined hyperabsorption and impaired biliary excretion.[82,83,99,230,235,237] Decreased biliary sterol excretion has been reported in several patients with sitosterolemia.[83,232,235] The patient investigated by Gregg et al. had a relative inability to concentrate both plant sterols and shellfish sterols in the bile.[232] Miettinen found that the biliary excretion of sitosterol in one patient was less than 20 percent of normal.[83] There was also a low rate of biliary cholesterol excretion, which would decrease the intestinal dilution of plant sterols. The micellar solubilization of plant sterols might then increase, facilitating the absorption. The mechanism of the reduced biliary sterol elimination in sitosterolemia is currently unknown.

Reduced Cholesterol Synthesis. Nguyen et al. proposed that the primary metabolic defect in sitosterolemia is inadequate cholesterol biosynthesis, due to reduced formation of HMG-CoA reductase,[238,239] and that the absorption defect is secondary to this. The cholesterol turnover rate in two patients was reduced by about 60 percent[99] in accordance with a previous finding.[236] Considering the tendency to enhanced rather than reduced cholesterol absorption in sitosterolemia, a diminished cholesterol synthesis was postulated to explain the reduced turnover rate.[237] It was calculated that the cholesterol synthesis in the patients was reduced to about 30 to 50 percent of the controls.[99] In mononuclear leukocytes from patients with sitosterolemia, the HMG-CoA reductase activity was reduced to about 30 percent of the control levels, and was found to be associated with about 65 percent less enzyme protein than in control preparations.[239] Furthermore, HMG-CoA reductase activity was reduced to 12 percent of control levels in liver-cell microsomes[238,240] and to less than half of control levels in ileal mucosal cells from patients with sitosterolemia.[241] The HMG-CoA reductase mRNA was decreased to barely detectable levels in the sitosterolemic livers.[238,240] LDL receptors were up-regulated in the sitosterolemic liver cells.[238] In contrast, cultured fibroblasts from four Amish subjects with sitosterolemia had normal LDL receptor function.[242] On the basis of the above observations,[99,238–241] an enhanced intestinal plant sterol absorption in conjunction with augmented LDL receptor function and reduced plant sterol excretion were suggested to represent compensatory mechanisms to supply the cells with sterols due to a reduced cholesterol synthesis.[238]

Reduced cholesterol synthesis has also been found in other patients with sitosterolemia.[43,83,235] In the study by Lütjohann et al.,[43] cholesterol synthesis was about five times lower in the patients than in controls. The plasma sitosterol concentration seems to be inversely correlated with cholesterol synthesis.[49,243,244] These observations are in accordance with the hypothesis that reduced cholesterol synthesis is the primary defect in sitosterolemia, but the findings may as well represent a secondary phenomenon. If reduced activity of HMG-CoA reductase is the primary defect, treatment with inhibitors of this enzyme should provide a model for sitosterolemia and result in elevated plasma sitosterol levels. In normal human subjects treated with HMG-CoA inhibitors, however, plasma sitosterol levels appear to be reduced, rather than increased.[245] In the patients with sitosterolemia investigated by Nguyen et al.,[238] a greater reduction of the cholesterol concentration in whole liver and liver microsomes (24 and 14 percent, respectively) would be expected if insufficient cholesterol synthesis is the primary abnormality. Nevertheless, the reduced HMG-CoA reductase activity in sitosterolemia does not seem to be merely due to feedback inhibition by elevated tissue sitosterol levels.[240,241] HMG-CoA reductase activity was reduced in liver and ileal mucosal cell preparations from patients with sitosterolemia,[238,240,241] but not in liver microsomes[96,240] or ileal mucosal tissues[241] from rats infused with or fed sitosterol to obtain tissue concentrations comparable to those of the patients.

Reduced conversion of mevalonic acid to cholesterol has also been observed in the sitosterolemic livers.[238] The possibility that more than one enzyme in the synthetic pathway to cholesterol may be deficient was, therefore, suggested.[238] The studies were recently extended to include several enzymes in the cholesterol biosynthetic pathway.[246] Acetoacetyl-CoA thiolase, HMG-CoA synthase, HMG-CoA reductase, and squalene synthase activities were all significantly decreased (by 39 percent, 54 percent, 76 percent, and 57 percent, respectively), and cholesterol Δ^7-reductase activity tended to be lower in liver tissue from four patients with sitosterolemia compared with control subjects.[246] The levels of the cholesterol precursors desmosterol and lathosterol were markedly lower in three patients with sitosterolemia than in controls.[43] Down-regulation of several enzymes in the cholesterol synthesis makes a single inherited gene defect less likely in this pathway.[246]

The relationship between the increased intestinal absorption of plant sterols, the reduced hepatic excretion of these compounds, and a diminished cholesterol synthesis remains unexplained.

Other Potential Metabolic Defects. Increased quantities of bile alcohols in feces and urine have been described in one specific patient with sitosterolemia.[247] The major bile alcohol was 26 (or 27)-nor-5β-cholestane-3α,7α,12α, 24,25-pentol, and the 5β-cholestane-tetrols and -pentols as described in CTX were also present. Because of this finding the possibility has been discussed that bile acid formation might be impaired in sitosterolemia.[247] The activity of C_{27}-steroid 27-hydroxylase was, however, found to be normal in cultured skin fibroblasts from a sitosterolemic patient,[248] ruling out an enzyme deficiency of the same nature as in CTX. Patients with cholestasis or other types of liver disease may also excrete the above bile alcohols.[249] In any case, bile alcohols are not present in all sitosterolemia patients.[250]

Metabolic Consequences of Elevated Plasma Plant Sterol Levels

The xanthomas in sitosterolemia resemble those of familial hypercholesterolemia, both with respect to localization and histologic features[251] (Fig. 123-14). The pathogenesis of the lipid depositions is unknown. They develop despite normal or moderately elevated plasma cholesterol concentrations. One possibility is that the presence of structurally altered sterols affects the stability of the lipoproteins and make them more vulnerable to tissue uptake and degradation.[82,252] Monocytes and leukocytes from patients with sitosterolemia degraded LDL more actively than cells from controls in experiments performed by Nguyen et al.[253] The possibility was discussed that the presence of increased amounts of plant sterols and 5α-stanols in LDL, or the presence of these sterols in the cell membrane, might alter the affinity of sitosterolemic LDL for the LDL receptor.[253] Sitosterolemic cells might fail to down-regulate the LDL receptor synthesis despite a high cellular sterol content.

A striking feature of sitosterolemia is the increased incidence of coronary heart disease at an early age. The mechanism behind the atherosclerosis is unexplained, but a high content of plant sterols in the circulating lipoproteins might promote accumulation of such sterols in the arterial wall. In experimental animals, C_{29}-sterols are retained in the liver to a higher extent than C_{27}-sterols, and they seem to accumulate also in other lipoprotein receptor-rich organs.[80,84] Some studies have indicated that sitosterol might interfere with cell viability. High concentrations of sitosterol caused cytotoxic effects in experiments with cultured human umbilical vein endothelial cells.[254] Sitosterol also increased synthesis and secretion of plasminogen activator from cultured bovine carotid artery endothelial cells.[255]

Episodes of hemolysis have been reported in several patients with sitosterolemia.[83,84,256] The erythrocytes contain increased amounts of sitosterol, corresponding to the elevated plasma level.[82] The presence of sitosterol might render the erythrocyte membrane more rigid and increase the fragility. Enrichment of rat liver microsomes with sitosterol and campesterol resulted in rigidization of the membrane,[257] and this effect might possibly occur in erythrocytes as well.

Patients with sitosterolemia also have increased levels of 5α-stanols.[32,84,258,259] 5α-Sitostanol and 5α-campestanol are most likely synthesized endogenously[32,84,259] (see above). In addition to the 5α-derivatives of the plant sterols, the cholestanol concentration is also increased. The mechanism of the hypercholestanolemia is most probably different from that in CTX. In the latter disease, hyperproduction of cholestanol is at least partly caused by the drainage of a small fraction of early bile acid intermediates into a pathway involving cholesta-4,6-dien-3-one as an intermediate.[24] The analogous route for synthesis of 5α-phytostanols is probably almost inactive.[84] That there are different mechanisms for the hypercholestanolemia in sitosterolemia and CTX is further supported by the effect of cholestyramine, which causes a decrease of plasma cholestanol in sitosterolemia[32,258] and an increase in CTX. It is believed that the majority of cholestanol is produced endogenously from cholesterol[32,260] and that cholestanol is retained along with sitosterol and cholesterol.[260] Studies in three sitosterolemic females seemed to suggest that cholestanol is derived from 4-cholesten-3-one rather than from 7α-hydroxycholesterol.[260] The significance of the increased levels of 5α-stanols in the pathogenesis of the lipid depositions is unknown.

Even though hypercholesterolemia is not a constant finding in sitosterolemia, several patients have cholesterol levels above the values of control individuals.[237] As discussed above, the cholesterol absorption tends to be increased and the biliary output tends to be reduced. Another possible mechanism is that high levels of sitosterol interfere with the cholesterol metabolism, either at the level of its biosynthesis or at some step in the degradation to bile acid. The increased cholesterol synthesis observed both in rats[261–263] and humans[264] after increased intake of plant sterol, could be caused by reduced feedback inhibition of hepatic HMG-CoA reductase in the presence of sitosterol. Increased hepatic microsomal sitosterol concentrations in rats tended to increase HMG-CoA reductase activity in one report,[96] but did not significantly affect either the enzyme activity or the HMG-CoA reductase mRNA levels in other similar experiments.[240] In cultured cells of a human intestinal cell line (CaCo-2-cells), sitosterol inhibited cholesterol synthesis by decreasing HMG-CoA reductase mRNA levels.[71] Thus, the results of such studies are not completely concordant. Sitosterol may also interfere with the metabolism of cholesterol at sites other than in the liver, but the results of such studies have been conflicting. Intraperitoneal[265] and subcutaneous[266] injection of sitosterol in rats and subcutaneous administration to chicken[267] resulted in lower plasma cholesterol levels, while feeding rabbits with sterols caused a 60 percent increase.[267] After intravenous infusions of sitosterol in rats, the cholesterol concentration increased to about twice the normal level.[96] The activity of the cholesterol 7α-hydroxylase in the livers of these animals was significantly depressed by about 30 percent. Sitosterol also depressed the 7α-hydroxylase activity towards cholesterol in human liver microsomes.[88] These results are in accordance with those of Shefer et al., who found that sitosterol competitively inhibited cholesterol 7α-hydroxylase in both rat and human liver microsomes.[95,262] In patients with sitosterolemia, the cholesterol 7α-hydroxylase activity was reduced to about 70 percent of the controls.[95,240] The observations that the cholesterol 7α-hydroxylase activity increased to normal levels in a reconstituted sitosterol-free system[240,260] and that cholesterol 7α-hydroxylase mRNA levels were equal in livers from patients with sitosterolemia and controls[260] support the contention of competitive inhibition by high microsomal sitosterol concentrations.

Cholestanol is an even more potent inhibitor of cholesterol 7α-hydroxylase.[95] Presence of elevated levels of both sitosterol and cholestanol in sitosterolemia might therefore inhibit transformation of cholesterol to bile acids and contribute to the hypercholesterolemia frequently observed. A reduced cholesterol 7α-hydroxylase activity in patients with sitosterolemia would be expected to lead to reduced bile acid biosynthesis. Miettinen[83] found, however, that the bile acid synthesis was quantitatively normal or even higher in a sitosterolemic subject compared to controls.

Recently, a reduced hepatic mitochondrial sterol 27-hydroxylase activity was described in three patients with sitosterolemia, and experimental studies gave support to a competitive inhibitory mechanism.[268] It was suggested that elevated sitosterol levels in the patients reduce the conversion of cholesterol to bile acids by inhibition of both the cholesterol 7α-hydroxylase and the sterol 27-hydroxylase.[268] Addition of serum from patients with sitosterolemia to cultured human macrophages did not, however, inhibit the sterol 27-hydroxylase activity in these cells.[269]

Genetics

The parents of the two sisters originally reported by Bhattacharyya and Connor were clinically unaffected and had normal levels of plasma plant sterols. It was suggested that sitosterolemia is inherited in an autosomal recessive pattern.[82] Kwiterovich et al. investigated both the original family and the family of a 13-year-old Amish boy who died from coronary heart disease and who had five siblings with characteristics of sitosterolemia.[270] The authors suggested that individuals exhibiting xanthomas, elevated plasma levels of plant sterols, and hyperapobetalipoproteinemia were homozygotes for a mutant allele and that an increased LDL B protein level identified the heterozygotes in these families. From a detailed genetic investigation, including determination of plasma plant sterols in 240 relatives of the above Amish patient, Beaty et al. concluded that the phenotype of sitosterolemia is controlled by a rare autosomal recessive gene.[271] The plasma sitosterol levels in the parents and six children of the five sitosterolemia probands were within the normal range. In contrast to these studies, investigations in a Japanese family with sitosterolemia demonstrated moderately increased plasma levels of plant sterols as well as cholestanol in heterozygotes.[272] The children and mother of a Chinese man with sitosterolemia (and coexisting CTX) also had small but significant elevations in their plant sterol levels.[256] In a family consisting of two obligate heterozygote parents and their homozygous daughter, Salen et al. found that the sitosterol and cholestanol concentrations in the mother were significantly higher than in the controls (0.95 mg/dl versus 0.22 mg/dl for sitosterol and 0.65 mg/dl versus 0.20 mg/dl for cholestanol), whereas these values were within reference limits in the father.[230] The different observations in the sitosterolemia heterozygotes might be due to a genetic heterogeneity.[272] The absorption of sitosterol in the heterozygotes was about three times that in a control subject, but still lower than in the homozygous patient.[230] Absorption of plant sterols in sitosterolemia heterozygotes was not different from controls in another report.[231] In the study by Salen et al., cholesterol absorption was similar in the heterozygotes and the homozygotes and tended to be in the high-normal range, whereas cholesterol synthesis was reduced to 27 percent of the control values in the homozygous patient and was normal in the parents.[230]

Potential gene defects in sitosterolemia have been investigated,[273] but still remain to be identified. Defects in the genes for HMG-CoA reductase, HMG-CoA synthase, and LDL receptor were excluded as a cause of the disease by segregation analyses in three sitosterolemic families.[273] Furthermore, no mutations could be localized in the genes for ACAT, microsomal triglyceride transfer protein (MTP), or sterol regulatory element binding proteins (SREBP-1 and -2).[273]

Clinical Phenotype

The major clinical manifestations of sitosterolemia include development of tendon and tuberous xanthomas at an early age, a predisposition for early development of atherosclerosis, and episodes of hemolysis and painful arthritis. In one of the two sisters reported by Bhattacharyya and Connor, tendon xanthomas, localized to the extensor tendons of both hands, were first noted at age 8.[82] Subsequently, xanthomas developed in the patellar, plantar, and Achilles tendons. As a university student, she presented with pains in the heels and knees. Her sister also had extensive tendon xanthomas, dating back to childhood. In addition, she had tuberous xanthomas of the elbows. Most of the sitosterolemic patients described have developed subcutaneous and tendon xanthomas during the first years of life, in one case as early as age 1.5 years.[229] The xanthomas are typically localized to the Achilles tendon and the extensor tendons of the hands.[82,274] Subcutaneous xanthomas have been noted in different regions, such as the buttocks and the abdomen (Fig. 123-14).[275,276] One patient had generalized eruptive xanthomatosis at the age of 5 years.[277] Xanthelasmas and arcus corneae are observed less frequently.

Early development of atherosclerosis has been present in several cases of sitosterolemia. In particular, the coronary vessels and the aorta are affected, but the vessel wall lipid depositions may also be more generalized.[83] Some patients with sitosterolemia have died as a consequence of coronary atherosclerosis at ages 13, 18, and 32.[270,278,279] Coronary bypass surgery was performed in a 29-year-old male patient, due to extensive coronary atherosclerosis causing angina pectoris,[83] and a 33-year-old male underwent combined coronary bypass and aortic root replacement surgery.[280] Male patients with sitosterolemia especially seem to be predisposed to early development of vascular complications, but angina pectoris developed in a 12-year-old girl,[281] and a 16-year-old girl had coronary bypass surgery.[282]

Some patients with sitosterolemia have exhibited episodic hemolysis or chronic hemolytic anemia.[83,84,256] Splenomegaly and platelet abnormalities were also present in these cases. Recurrent arthritis of the knee and ankle joints has been described.[229] One patient with sitosterolemia who had neurologic symptoms has been reported.[283] Paraplegia developed in this 48-year-old woman as a result of spinal cord compression by multiple intradural, extramedullary xanthomas.

Table 123-3 summarizes the main clinical symptoms in the 16 first-described cases of sitosterolemia.[132]

Pathologic Anatomy

An 18-year-old male with sitosterolemia who died suddenly has been described in detail.[278] Postmortem examination revealed extensive coronary atherosclerosis with about 60 percent occlusion of the proximal left main and proximal right coronary arteries. Diffuse atherosclerotic lesions were also present in other coronary vessels as well as in the thoracic and abdominal aorta and the iliac vessels. Histologic evidence of acute infarction was not found, but

Table 123-3 Clinical Findings in 16 Patients with Phytosterolemia

	No. of patients		
	Documented	Absent	Not mentioned
Tendon xanthomas			
Achilles	16	–	–
Other	16	–	–
Xanthelasma	2	6	8
Arcus corneae	2	6	8
Atherosclerosis			
Coronary	2	7	7
Large vessel	3	8	5
Hemolysis	3	7	6
Hypersplenism	3	7	6
Platelet abnormalities	4	3	9
Arthralgia-arthritis	3	3	10
Hypercholesterolemia	9	7	–

SOURCE: From Salen et al.[187]

many areas of myocardial fibrosis suggested previous infarctions, and death was attributed to cardiac arrhythmia and myocardial infarction. In other patients, extensive coronary atherosclerosis has been documented by angiography.[83,256] Surgical exploration in the patient with neurologic symptoms revealed multiple intradural, extramedullary yellowish, oval tumors that could be completely removed.[283] The histologic appearance of liver biopsies from two patients was largely normal.[238]

Pathophysiology

Blood. All the reported patients with sitosterolemia characteristically have had increased concentrations of sitosterol and campesterol in plasma. The plant sterols constitute from 7 to 27 percent of the total sterols in the patients.[35,43] Stigmasterol may also be detected, and in some cases, avenasterol has been present.[83,231] A new plant sterol, tentatively identified as episterol or fecosterol, was detected in a 14-year-old girl with sitosterolemia.[231] The concentration of sitosterol in normal plasma is in the range of 0.005 to 0.024 mM (0.2 to 1.0 mg/dl).[35,43] In a group of 14 patients, the mean sitosterol level was 0.85 mM (35 mg/dl) with a range from 0.34 to 1.57 mM (14 to 65 mg/dl).[35] The sitosterol level is thus about one hundredfold higher in the patients than in controls.[43] In normal subjects, the campesterol concentration may be as high as that of sitosterol,[43] whereas campesterol levels amount to approximately half that of sitosterol in the patients.[35,43] The mean plasma campesterol concentration in the 14 patients was 0.40 mM, with a range of 0.20 to 0.72 mM.[35]

In most patients, the 5α-saturated derivatives of the plant sterols are also present.[84] The concentrations of sitostanol and campestanol in the above group of patients were 0.1 and 0.07 mM (4.1 and 2.9 mg/dl), respectively. The mean cholestanol concentration was 0.10 mM (4.2 mg/dl), more than tenfold higher than in the controls. While sitostanol and campestanol represented 18 and 13 percent of their respective unsaturated derivatives, cholestanol amounted to only 1.6 percent of the plasma cholesterol level.

The plant sterols and their 5α-saturated stanols are mainly (75 to 85 percent) carried in the LDL fraction.[35,82,83] HDL contains most of the remainder. The plasma plant sterols, particularly the 5α-saturated derivatives, are esterified to a lower extent than cholesterol in patients with sitosterolemia. About 60 percent of plasma sitosterol and campesterol was esterified in the two original patients. According to the fatty acid pattern, the plasma plant sterol esters in sitosterolemia originate both from synthesis in plasma via LCAT and from synthesis in the tissues via ACAT.[284]

Some patients with sitosterolemia have plasma cholesterol levels within the normal limits,[272] while about 50 percent have moderately elevated values.[35,83] In the patients investigated by Salen et al., the mean plasma cholesterol concentration was 6.7 mM (258 mg/dl) (range: 3.5 to 12.5 mM), as compared with 4.9 mM (187 mg/dl) in controls.[35] In one patient, plasma cholesterol was as high as 19.4 mM (750 mg/dl).[285] Hyperapobetalipoproteinemia has been described in several cases.[270] Two Chinese patients were reported to have a combination of elevated plasma plant sterols and pseudohomozygous type II hypercholesterolemia.[286] In a patient with sitosterolemia who was fed a diet rich in shellfish, high plasma levels of shellfish sterols resulted (13.1 mg/dl versus 1.9 mg/dl in normal subjects).[232]

Tissues. The plant sterols and 5α-stanols are deposited in virtually all tissues, in approximately the same proportions as found in plasma.[232,281]

In the xanthomas, the plant sterols account for 15 to 20 percent of the total sterols, while cholesterol is the predominating sterol.[82,278] This is also the case in the atheromatous depositions. In one lethal case, the aorta was extensively atherosclerotic and contained more than twice the quantity of sterols of a control aorta, with increased amounts of cholesterol, plant sterols, and 5α-stanols.[278] Sterol quantitation in a biopsy of aortic tissue from a 33-year-old male patient gave similar results.[280] In the brain of the patient who died, only trace amounts of unsaturated plant sterols and cholestanol were present.[278] Thus, cholestanol is not deposited in the brain as in CTX. The intradural tumors in the patient reported by Hatanaka et al. contained increased levels of sitosterol, campesterol, and cholestanol.[283] The plant sterols deposited in the tissues are less esterified than cholesterol.[278]

Bile. The bile has been examined in some patients with sitosterolemia, and only C_{24}-bile acids (cholic, chenodeoxycholic, and deoxycholic acid) have been identified.[83,235,256] In one case, a relative deficiency of chenodeoxycholic acid (as in CTX) was reported.[83] Cholic acid constituted about 60 percent of the total bile acids in this patient, while deoxycholic acid was the major bile acid in another case.[256] In the patient described by Miettinen, bile acid synthesis was quantitatively normal or even higher than in the controls. The total excretion of sterols in the bile was less than 50 percent of the controls. Plant sterols comprised about 30 percent of the biliary sterols. Low excretion of sitosterol into the bile, resulting in low sitosterol to cholesterol ratios, has been reported in several patients with sitosterolemia.[232,235,236] The ability of the liver to preferentially excrete plant sterols into the bile is apparently impaired.[36] As described above, this might be a pathophysiological factor in sitosterolemia.

In one patient fed shellfish sterols, a relative deficiency to concentrate these compounds in the bile was also detected.[232] The biliary phospholipid output in sitosterolemia is normal.[83]

Feces. In the patient studied by Miettinen, the bile acid excretion was normal, while the fecal neutral sterols were exceptionally low.[83] Fecal excretion of 26-nor-5β-cholestane-3α,7α,12α, 24,25-pentol, 5β-cholestane-3α,7α,12α,24-tetrol, 5β-cholestane-3α,7α,12α,25-tetrol, and 5β-cholestane-3α,7α,12α,25,26-pentol has been described in one patient.[247] The total amount of bile alcohols was 1 mg/g of feces. Significant amounts of bile alcohols were not, however, present in another patient.[250]

Urine. In the patient described by Dayal et al., small amounts (about 2 mg/L) of the 26-nor pentol and the 25,26-pentol were also excreted in the urine.[247]

Diagnosis

Phytosterolemia should be suspected in patients who develop xanthomas in early childhood, despite normal or only moderately elevated plasma cholesterol concentration. Some of the reported cases have been misinterpreted for a time as heterozygotes for familial hypercholesterolemia. Low et al. identified two patients with pseudohomozygous type II hypercholesterolemia who also had elevated plant sterol levels, so these conditions may be associated.[286] The diagnosis can be established by gas chromatographic examination of the plasma sterols.[35,287–289] Normally, the plasma sitosterol concentration is less than 0.024 mM (1 mg/dl),[35] but it may increase to 0.216 mM (9 mg/dl) in normal infants fed commercial formulas rich in vegetable oil.[290] In sitosterolemia, levels of 0.34 to 1.57 mM (10 to 65 mg/dl) have been reported. Increased levels of campesterol, stigmasterol, and the 5α-saturated derivatives of plant sterols and cholestanol are also regularly present.[32,82,270]

Treatment

Patients with sitosterolemia should consume a diet low in cholesterol and with the lowest possible amount of plant sterols. When such a regimen is instituted, the plasma plant sterol levels usually decrease rapidly,[132,235,284] but full normalization is difficult to achieve.[83,84] Some patients may, however, respond poorly to a low-sterol diet.[235,291,292]

To compose a diet low in plant sterols, all sources of vegetable fats should be eliminated, and all plant foods with high contents of fat should be avoided. Thus, the diet should not contain vegetable oils, shortening, or margarine. Likewise, nuts, seeds, chocolate, olives, and avocados should be avoided. Only cereal products without the germ should be used. The diet may contain fruits, vegetables, and refined cereal products. Food derived from animal sources with cholesterol as the dominating sterol is allowed (e.g., meat, butter, lard, cheese, eggs, and milk powder). Shellfish should also be avoided.[232] Compositions of suitable diets and sample menus were given in the third edition of this book.[132]

Cholestyramine is an effective treatment in addition to the diet because this combination causes a significant reduction of plasma plant sterols, cholesterol, and cholestanol.[35,83,291,293,294] This bile acid binding resin interrupts the enterohepatic circulation of bile acids and promotes bile acid excretion in the feces. Bile acid synthesis is stimulated, and the output of fecal plant sterols increases.[83] In one report, treatment with cholestyramine (up to 12g/day for 1 month) reduced the levels of cholesterol and plant sterols by 45 percent and the 5α-saturated stanols by 55 percent.[35] The xanthomas may regress and the attacks of arthritis may become less frequent.[231,256,293,295] Interruption of cholestyramine treatment causes the sterol levels to increase to the previous levels.[231] Colestipol is a bile acid resin with the same effects as cholestyramine.[296]

Increased intestinal bile acid loss can also be induced by ileal bypass surgery. In subjects with sitosterolemia following ileal bypass surgery, a considerable reduction of total plasma sterols was obtained.[253,296] The plasma plant sterol and 5α-saturated stanol concentrations declined by 55 percent in two patients.[296] Plasma apolipoprotein B levels declined to the same extent. The reduction of sterol concentrations was associated with clinical improvement, including disappearance of aortic systolic murmur.[296] The observations that cholesterol synthesis and microsomal HMG-CoA reductase activity were not stimulated in mononuclear leukocytes isolated from sitosterolemia patients after ileal bypass[296] or cholestyramine treatment[291] have been interpreted to support the hypothesis of an inherent defect in cholesterol synthesis in sitosterolemia.[237,291,296] Lovastatin treatment has no effect on plasma sterol concentrations in sitosterolemia.[237,291,296]

Sitostanol inhibits cholesterol absorption, but is not absorbed itself.[46] In two patients with sitosterolemia fed sitostanol for 4 weeks, Lütjohann et al. noted a marked reduction of serum levels of sitosterol and campesterol, in addition to the expected reduction of cholesterol levels.[43] Sitostanol thus might prove to be a new therapeutic approach in sitosterolemia.[43]

The response to treatment emphasizes the importance of early diagnosis and treatment of phytosterolemia.

ACKNOWLEDGMENTS

We are most grateful to the following colleagues for unpublished material referred to in this review and, in some cases, for critical reading of the manuscript: Dr. K. von Bergmann, Dr. P. Clayton, Dr. D. Lütjohann, Dr. G. Salen, Dr. K. Setchell, and Dr. J. Sjövall. The work referred to as carried out in the authors' laboratories has been supported by grants from the Swedish Medical Research Council, the Norwegian Council on Cardiovascular Disease, the United States-Israel Binational Science Foundation (BSF), and the Sarah and Moshe Mayer Foundation for Research.

REFERENCES

1. Björkhem I: Mechanism of bile acid biosynthesis in mammalian liver (review), in Danielsson H, Sjövall J (eds): *Comprehensive Biochemistry*, Vol 12. Amsterdam, Elsevier, 1985, p 231.
2. Russell DW, Setchell KDR: Bile acid biosynthesis. *Biochemistry* **31**:4737, 1992.
3. Princen HMG, Post SM, Twisk J: Regulation of bile acid biosynthesis. *Curr Pharmaceut Design* **3**:59, 1997.
4. Noshiro M, Okuda K: Molecular cloning and sequence analysis of a cDNA encoding human cholesterol 7α-hydroxylase. *FEBS Lett* **1**:137, 1990.
5. Björkhem I, Lund E, Rudling M: Coordinate regulation of HMG CoA reductase and cholesterol 7α-hydroxylase, in: *Subcellular Biochemistry*. Vol. 28. New York, Plenum, 1997, p 23.
6. Furster C, Zhang J, Toll A: Purification of a 3β-hydroxy-Δ^5-C_{27}-steroid dehydrogenase from pig liver microsomes active in major and alternative pathways of bile acid biosynthesis. *J Biol Chem* **271**:20907, 1996.
7. Salen G, Shefer S, Tint GS: Transformation of 4-cholesten-3-one and 7α-hydroxy-4-cholesten-3-one into cholestanol and bile acids in CTX. *Gastroenterology* **87**:276, 1984.
8. Eggertsen G, Olin M, Andersson U, Ishida H, Kubota S, Hellman U, Okuda K, Björkhem I: Molecular cloning and expression of rabbit sterol 12α-hydroxylase *J Biol Chem* **271**:32269, 1996.
9. Einarsson K, Åkerlund J-E, Reihnér E, Björkhem I: 12α-Hydroxylase activity in human liver and its relation to cholesterol 7α-hydroxylase activity. *J Lipid Res* **33**:1591, 1992.
10. Johansson G: Effect of cholestyramine and diet on hydroxylations in the biosynthesis and metabolism of bile acids. *Eur J Biochem* **17**:292, 1970.
11. Kondo K, Kai M, Setoguchi Y, Eggertsen G, Sjöblom P, Setoguchi T, Okuda K, Björkhem I: Cloning and expression of cDNA of human Δ^4-4-3-oxysteroid-5β-reductase and substrate specificity of the expressed enzyme. *Eur J Biochem* **219**:357, 1994.
12. Penning TM, Abrams WR, Pawlowski JE: 3α-Hydroxysteroid dehydrogenase. *J Biol Chem* **266**:8826, 1991.
13. Björkhem I: Mechanism of degradation of the steroid side-chain in the formation of bile acids. Review. *J Lipid Res* **33**:455, 1992.
14. Holmberg-Betzholtz I, Lund E, Björkhem I, Wikvall K: Sterol 27-hydroxylase in bile acid biosynthesis. *J Biol Chem* **268**:11079, 1993.
15. Prydz K, Kase BF, Björkhem I, Pedersen J-I: Subcellular localization of 3α,7α-dihydroxy and 3α,7α,12α-trihydroxy-5β-cholestanoyl-CoA-ligase (s) in rat liver. *J Lipid Res* **29**:997, 1988.

16. Baumgart E, Vanhooren JCT, Fransén M, Marynen P, Puype M, Vandekerckhove J, Leunissen JAM, Fahimi HD, Mannaerts GP, van Veldhoven PP: Molecular characterization of the human peroxisomal branched chain acyl-CoA oxidase: cDNA cloning, chromosomal assignment, tissue distribution, and evidence for the absence of the protein in Zellweger syndrome. *Proc Natl Acad Sci U S A* **93**:13748, 1996.
17. Pedersen JI, Eggertsen G, Hellman U, Andersson A, Björkhem I: Molecular cloning and expression of cDNA encoding THCA CoA oxidase from rabbit liver. *J Biol Chem* **272**:18481, 1997.
18. Kase BF, Prydz K, Björkhem I: Peroxisomal bile acid CoA: amino acid N-acyltransferase in rat liver. *J Biol Chem* **264**:9220, 1989.
19. Björkhem I, Nyberg B, Einarsson K: 7α-Hydroxylation of 27-hydroxycholesterol in human liver microsomes. *Biochim Biophys Acta* **1128**:73, 1992.
20. Shoda J, Toll A, Axelson M, Pieper F, Wikvall K, Sjövall J: Formation of 7α- and 7β-hydroxylated bile acid precursors from 26-hydroxycholesterol in human liver microsomes and mitochondria. *Hepatology* **17**:395, 1993.
21. Setchell KDR, Schwartz M, O'Connell NC, Lund EG, Davis DL, Thompson HR, Thyson W, Sokol RJ, Russell DW: Identification of a new inborn error in bile acid biosynthesis. Mutation of the oxysterol 7α-hydroxylase gene causing severe neonatal disease. *J Clin Invest* **102**:1690, 1998.
22. Duane E, Björkhem I, Hamilton JN, Mueller SM: Quantitative importance of the 25-hydroxylase pathway for bile acid biosynthesis in the rat. *Hepatology* **8**:613, 1988.
23. Duane WE, Pooler PA, Hamilton JN: Bile acid synthesis in man. In vivo activity of the 25-hydroxylase pathway. *J Clin Invest* **82**:82, 1988.
24. Björkhem I, Skrede S: Cerebrotendinous xanthomatosis and phytosterolemia, in Scriver CR, Beaudet AL, Sly WS, Valle D (eds). *The Metabolic Basis of Inherited Disease*, 6th ed. New York, McGraw-Hill, 1989, p 1283.
25. Skrede S, Buchmann MS, Björkhem I: Hepatic 7α-dehydroxylation of bile acid intermediates and its significance for the pathogenesis of cerebrotendinous xanthomatosis. *J Lipid Res* **29**:157, 1988.
26. Björkhem I, Buchmann MS, Byström S: Mechanism and stereochemistry in the sequential enzymatic saturation of two double bonds in cholesta-4,6-dien3-one. *J Biol Chem* **267**:19872, 1992.
27. Skrede S, Björkhem I, Buchmann MS, Hopen G, Fausa S: A novel pathway for biosynthesis of cholestanol with 7α-hydroxysteroids as intermediates, and its importance for the accumulation of cholestanol in CTX. *J Clin Invest* **75**:448, 1985.
28. Salen G, Grundy SM: The metabolism of cholestanol, cholesterol and bile acids in CTX. *J Clin Invest* **52**:2822, 1973.
29. Fedeli E, Lanzani A, Capella P, Jacini G: Triterpene alcohols and sterols of vegetable oils. *J Am Oil Chem Soc* **43**:254, 1966.
30. Pollak OJ, Kritchevsky D: Sitosterol, in Clarkson TB, Kritchevsky D, Pollak OJ (eds): *Monographs on Atherosclerosis*. Vol. 10. Basel, Karger, 1981, p 4.
31. Weihrauch JL, Gardner JM: Sterol content of foods of plant origin. *J Am Diet Assoc* **73**:39, 1978.
32. Connor WE: Dietary sterols: Their relationship to atherosclerosis. *J Am Diet Assoc* **52**:202, 1968.
33. Hirai K, Shimazu C, Takezoe R, Ozeki Y: Cholesterol, phytosterol and polyunsaturated fatty acid levels in 1982 and 1957 Japanese diets. *J Nutr Sci Vitaminol* **32**:363, 1986.
34. Subbiah MTR: Significance of dietary plant sterols in man and experimental animals. *Mayo Clin Proc* **46**:549, 1971.
35. Salen G, Kwiterovich PO Jr, Shefer S, Tint GS, Horak I, Shore V, Dayal B, Horak E: Increased plasma cholesterol and 5α-saturated plant sterol derivatives in subjects with sitosterolemia and xanthomatosis. *J Lipid Res* **26**:203, 1985.
36. Salen G, Ahrens EH Jr, Grundy SM: Metabolism of β-sitosterol in man. *J Clin Invest* **49**:952, 1970.
37. Nicholas HJ: The biogenesis of terpenes in plants, in Bernfeld P (ed): *Biogenesis of Natural Compounds*, 2nd ed. New York, Pergamon, 1967, p 829.
38. Gould RG, Jones RJ, LeRoy GV, Wissler RW, Taylor CB: Absorbability of β-sitosterol in humans. *Metabolism* **18**:652, 1969.
39. Sylvén C, Borgström B: Absorption and lymphatic transport of cholesterol and sitosterol in the rat. *J Lipid Res* **10**:179, 1969.
40. Vahouny GV, Connor WE, Subramaniam S, Lin DS, Gallo LL: Comparative lymphatic absorption of sitosterol, stigmasterol, and fucosterol and differential inhibition of cholesterol absorption. *Am J Clin Nutr* **37**:805, 1983.
41. Subbiah MTR, Kottke BA, Carlo IA, Naylor MC: Human intestinal specificity toward dietary sterols studied by balance methods. *Nutr Metabol* **18**:23, 1975.
42. Tilvis RS, Miettinen TA: Serum plant sterols and their relation to cholesterol absorption. *Am J Clin Nutr* **43**:92, 1986.
43. Lütjohann D, Björkhem I, Beil UF, Berman K: Sterol absorption and sterol balance in phytosterolemia evaluated by deuterium-labeled sterols: Effect of sitostanol treatment. *J Lipid Res* **36**:1763, 1995.
43a. Heinemann T, Axtmann G, von Bergmann K: Comparison of intestinal absorption of cholesterol with different plant sterols in man. *Eur J Clin Invest* **23**:827, 1993.
44. Eneroth P, Hellström K, Ryhage R: Identification and quantification of neutral fecal steroids by gas-liquid chromatography and mass spectrometry: Studies of human excretion during two dietary regimens. *J Lipid Res* **5**:245, 1964.
45. McNamara DJ, Proia A, Miettinen TA: Thin-layer and gas-liquid chromatographic identification of neutral steroids in human and rat feces. *J Lipid Res* **22**:474, 1981.
46. Grundy SM, Ahrens EH Jr, Salen G: Dietary β-sitosterol as an internal standard to correct for cholesterol losses in sterol balance studies. *J Lipid Res* **9**:374, 1968.
47. Newton DF, Mansbach CM: β-Sitosterol as a nonabsorbable marker of dietary lipid absorption in man. *Clin Chim Acta* **89**:331, 1978.
48. Hassan AS, Rampone AJ: Intestinal absorption and lymphatic transport of cholesterol and β-sitostanol in the rat. *J Lipid Res* **20**:646, 1979.
48a. Czubakayko F, Beumers B, Lammsfuss S, Lütjohann D, von Bergmann K: A simplified micro-method for quantification of fecal excretion of neutral and acidic sterols for outpatient studies in humans. *J Lipid Res* **32**:1861, 1991.
48b. Lütjohann D, Meese CO, Crouse III JR, von Bergmann K: Evaluation of deuterated cholesterol and deuterated sitostanol for measurement of cholesterol absorption in humans. *J Lipid Res* **34**:1039, 1993.
49. Miettinen TA, Tilvis RS, Kesüniemi YA: Serum plant sterols and cholesterol precursors reflect cholesterol absorption and synthesis in volunteers of a randomly selected male population. *Am J Epidemiol* **131**:20, 1990.
50. Slota T, Kozlov NA, Ammon HV: Comparison of cholesterol and β-sitosterol: Effects on jejunal fluid secretion induced by oleate, and absorption from mixed micellar solutions. *Gut* **24**:653, 1983.
51. Borgström B: Partition of lipids between emulsified oil and micellar phases of glyceride-bile salt dispersions. *J Lipid Res* **8**:598, 1967.
52. Chijiiwa K: Distribution and partitioning of cholesterol and β-sitosterol in micellar bile salt solutions. *Am J Physiol* **253**:G268, 1987.
53. Child P, Kuksis A: Uptake of 7-dehydro derivatives of cholesterol, campesterol, and β-sitosterol by rat erythrocytes, jejunal villus cells, and brush border membranes. *J Lipid Res* **24**:552, 1983.
54. Ikeda I, Sugano M: Some aspects of mechanism of inhibition of cholesterol absorption by β-sitosterol. *Biochim Biophys Acta* **732**:651, 1983.
55. Ikeda I, Tanaka K, Sugano M, Vahouny GV, Gallo LL: Discrimination between cholesterol and sitosterol for absorption in rats. *J Lipid Res* **29**:1583, 1988.
55a. Compassi S, Werder M, Weber FE, Boffelli D, Hauser H, Schulthess G: Comparison of cholesterol and sitosterol uptake in different brush border membrane models. *Biochemistry* **36**:6643, 1997.
56. Ikeda I, Sugano M, Scallen TJ, Vahouny GV, Gallo LL: Transfer of cholesterol and sitosterol from rat intestinal brush border membranes to phospholipid liposomes: Effects of SCP_2. *Agric Biol Chem* **54**:2649, 1990.
57. Field FJ, Mathur SN: β-Sitosterol: esterification by intestinal acylcoenzyme A: cholesterol acyltransferase (ACAT) and its effect on cholesterol esterification. *J Lipid Res* **24**:409, 1983.
58. Norum KR, Berg T, Helgerud P, Drevon CA: Transport of cholesterol. *Physiol Rev* **63**:1343, 1983.
59. Dunham LW, Fortner RE, Moore RD, Culp HW, Rice CN: Comparative lymphatic absorption of β-sitosterol and cholesterol by the rat. *Arch Biochem Biophys* **82**:50, 1959.
60. Peterson DW: Effect of soybean sterols in the diet on plasma and liver cholesterol in chicks. *Proc Soc Exp Biol Med* **78**:143, 1951.
61. Becker M, Staab D, von Bergmann K: Treatment of severe hypercholesterolemia in childhood with sitosterol and sitostanol. *J Pediatr* **122**:292, 1993.
62. Miettinen TA, Puska P, Gylling H, Vanhanen H, Vartiainen E: Reduction of serum cholesterol with sitostanol-ester margarine in a mildly hypercholesterolemic population. *N Engl J Med* **333**:1308, 1995.

63. Mattson FH, Grundy SM, Crouse JR: Optimizing the effect of plant sterols on cholesterol absorption in man. *Am J Clin Nutr* **35**:697, 1982.
64. Denke MA: Lack of efficacy of low-dose sitostanol therapy as an adjunct to a cholesterol-lowering diet in men with moderate hypercholesterolemia. *Am J Clin Nutr* **61**:392, 1995.
65. Grundy SM, Ahrens EH Jr, Davignon J: The interaction of cholesterol absorption and cholesterol synthesis in man. *J Lipid Res* **10**:304, 1969.
66. Kudchodkar BJ, Horlick L, Sodhi HS: Effects of plant sterols on cholesterol metabolism in man. *Atherosclerosis* **23**:239, 1976.
67. Grundy SM, Mok HYI: Effects of low dose phytosterols on cholesterol absorption in man, in Greten H (ed): *Lipoprotein Metabolism*. Berlin, Springer-Verlag, 1976, p 112.
68. Lees AM, Mok HYI, Lees RS, McCluskey MA, Grundy SM: Plant sterols as cholesterol-lowering agents: Clinical trials in patients with hypercholesterolemia and studies of sterol balance. *Atherosclerosis* **28**:325, 1977.
69. Drexel H, Breier C, Lisch H-J, Sailer S: Lowering plasma cholesterol with beta-sitosterol and diet. *Lancet* **1**:1157, 1981.
70. Pollak OJ: Effect of plant sterols on serum lipids and atherosclerosis. *Pharmacol Ther* **31**:177, 1985.
71. Field FJ, Born E, Mathur SN: Effect of micellar β-sitosterol on cholesterol metabolism in CaCo-2 cells. *J Lipid Res* **38**:348, 1997.
72. Sugano M, Morioka H, Ikeda I: A comparison of hypocholesterolemic activity of β-sitosterol and β-sitostanol in rats. *J Nutr* **107**:2011, 1977.
73. Ikeda I, Kawasaki A, Samezima K, Sugano M: Antihypercholesterolemic activity of β-sitostanol in rabbits. *J Nutr Sci Vitaminol* **27**:243, 1981.
74. Heinemann T, Pietruck B, Kullak-Ublick G, von Bergmann K: Comparison of sitosterol and sitostanol on inhibition of intestinal cholesterol absorption. *Agents Actions Suppl* **26**:117, 1988.
75. Heinemann T, Kullak-Ublick G-A, Pietruck B, von Bergmann K: Mechanisms of action of plant sterols on inhibition of cholesterol absorption. Comparison of sitosterol and sitostanol. *Eur J Clin Pharmacol* **40**(Suppl 1):S59, 1991.
76. Nordby G, Norum KR: Substrate specificity of lecithin: Cholesterol acyltransferase. Esterification of desmosterol, β-sitosterol, and cholecalciferol in human plasma. *Scand J Clin Lab Invest* **35**:677, 1975.
77. Sugano M, Morioka H, Kida Y, Ikeda I: The distribution of dietary plant sterols in serum lipoproteins and liver subcellular fractions of rats. *Lipids* **13**:427, 1978.
78. Swell L, Treadwell CR: Metabolic fate of injected C^{14}-phytosterols. *Proc Soc Exp Biol Med* **108**:810, 1961.
79. Subbiah MTR, Kuksis A: Differences in metabolism of cholesterol and sitosterol following intravenous injection in rats. *Biochim Biophys Acta* **306**:95, 1973.
80. Boberg KM, Skrede B, Skrede S: Metabolism of 24-ethyl-4-cholesten-3-one and 24-ethyl-5-cholesten-3β-ol (sitosterol) after intraperitoneal injection in the rat. *Scan J Clin Lab Invest* **46**(Suppl 184):47, 1986.
81. Boberg KM, Skrede S: Content of sitosterol, cholestanol, and cholesterol in very low density lipoproteins of rat liver perfusate. *Scand J Gastroenterol* **23**:442, 1988.
82. Bhattacharyya AK, Connor WE: β-Sitosterolemia and xanthomatosis. A newly described lipid storage disease in two sisters. *J Clin Invest* **53**:1033, 1974.
83. Miettinen TA: Phytosterolaemia, xanthomatosis and premature atherosclerotic arterial disease: A case with high plant sterol absorption, impaired sterol elimination and low cholesterol synthesis. *Eur J Clin Invest* **10**:27, 1980.
84. Skrede B, Björkhem I, Bergesen O, Kayden HJ, Skrede S: The presence of 5α-sitostanol in the serum of a patient with phytosterolemia, and its biosynthesis from plant steroids in rats with bile fistula. *Biochim Biophys Acta* **836**:368, 1985.
85. Svoboda JA, Thompson MJ, Robbins WE: Desmosterol, an intermediate in dealkylation of β-sitosterol in the tobacco hornworm. *Life Sci* **6**:395, 1967.
86. Douglass TS, Connor WE, Lin DS: The biosynthesis, absorption, and origin of cholesterol and plant sterols in the Florida land crab. *J Lipid Res* **22**:961, 1981.
87. Fujimoto Y, Morisaki M, Ikekawa N: Enzymatic dealkylation of phytosterols in insects. *Methods Enzymol* **111**:346, 1985.
88. Boberg KM, Einarsson K, Björkhem I: Apparent lack of conversion ofsitosterol into C_{24}-bile acids in humans. *J Lipid Res* **31**:1083, 1990.
89. Kritchevsky D, Davidson LM, Mosbach EH, Cohen BI: Identification of acidic steroids in feces of monkeys fed β-sitosterol. *Lipids* **16**:77, 1981.
90. Boberg KM, Lund E, Ölund J, Björkhem I: Formation of C_{21}-bile acids from plant sterols in the rat. *J Biol Chem* **265**:7967, 1990.
91. Lund E, Boberg KM, Byström S, Ölund J, Carlström K, Björkhem I: Formation of novel C_{21}-bile acids from cholesterol in the rat. *J Biol Chem* **266**:4929, 1991.
92. Björkhem I, Muri-Boberg K, Lund E, Byström S, Carlström K, Ölund J: Formation of novel C_{21}-bile acids from plant sterols and cholesterol in rat liver, in Paumgartner G, Stiehl A, Gerok W (eds): *Bile Acids as Therapeutic Agents. From Basic Science to Clinical Practice*. Falk Symposium 58, Freiburg. Dordrecht, Kluwer, 1991, p 77.
93. Aringer L, Eneroth P: Studies on the formation of C_7-oxygenated cholesterol and β-sitosterol metabolites in cell-free preparations of rat liver. *J Lipid Res* **14**:563, 1973.
94. Boyd GS, Brown MJG, Hattersley NG, Suckling KE: Studies on the specificity of the rat liver microsomal cholesterol 7α-hydroxylase. *Biochim Biophys Acta* **337**:132, 1974.
95. Shefer S, Salen G, Nguyen L, Batta AK, Packin V, Tint GS, Hauser S: Competitive inhibition of bile acid synthesis by endogenous cholestanol and sitosterol in sitosterolemia with xanthomatosis. Effect on cholesterol 7α-hydroxylase. *J Clin Invest* **82**:1833, 1988.
96. Boberg KM, Åkerlund J-E, Björkhem I: Effect of sitosterol on the rate-limiting enzymes in cholesterol synthesis and degradation. *Lipids* **24**:9, 1989.
97. Aringer L: Conversion of 7α-hydroxycholesterol and 7α-hydroxy-β-sitosterol to 3α,7α-dihydroxy- and 3α,7α,12α-trihydroxy-5β-steroids in vitro. *J Lipid Res* **16**:426, 1975.
98. Aringer L, Eneroth P, Nordström L: Side-chain hydroxylation of cholesterol, campesterol, and β-sitosterol in rat liver mitochondria. *J Lipid Res* **17**:263, 1976.
99. Salen G, Shore V, Tint GS, Forte T, Shefer S, Horak I, Horak E, Dayal B, Nguyen L, Batta AK, Lindgren FT, Kwiterovich PO Jr: Increased sitosterol absorption, decreased removal, and expanded body pools compensate for reduced cholesterol synthesis in sitosterolemia with xanthomatosis. *J Lipid Res* **30**:1319, 1989.
100. Bhattacharyya AK, Connor WE, Lin DS: The origin of plant sterols in the skin surface lipids in humans: from diet to plasma to skin. *J Invest Dermatol* **80**:294, 1983.
101. Werbin H, Chaikoff IL, Jones EE: The metabolism of H^3-β-sitosterol in the guinea pig: its conversion to urinary cortisol. *J Biol Chem* **235**:1629, 1960.
102. Aringer L, Eneroth P, Nordström L: Side-chain cleavage of 4-cholesten-3-one, 5-cholesten-3α-ol, β-sitosterol, and related steroids in endocrine tissues from rat and man. *J Steroid Biochem* **11**:1271, 1979.
103. Subbiah MT, Kuksis A: Oxidation of 4-^{14}C-β-sitosterol by mitochondria of rat liver and testes. *Fed Proc* **28**:515, 1969.
104. Subbiah MTR, Kuksis A: Conversion of β-sitosterol to steroid hormones in rat testes in vitro. *Experientia* **31**:763, 1975.
105. Clayton PT, Leonard JV, Lawson AM, Setchell KDR, Andersson S, Egestad B, Sjövall J: Familial giant cell hepatitis associated with synthesis of 3β,7α-dihydroxy- and 3β,7α,12α-trihydroxy-5-cholenoic acid. *J Clin Invest* **79**:1031, 1987.
106. Skrede S, Björkhem I, Kvittingen EA, Buchmann MS, East C, Grundy S: Demonstration of 26-hydroxylation of C-27-steroids in human skin fibroblasts and a deficiency of this activity in CTX. *J Clin Invest* **78**:729, 1986.
107. Buchmann MS, Kvittingen EA, Nazer H, Gunasekaran T, Clayton PT, Sjövall J, Björkhem I: Lack of 3β-hydroxy-Δ^5-C_{27}-steroid dehydrogenase/isomerase in fibroblasts from a child with urinary excretion of 3β-hydroxy-Δ^5-bile acids: A new inborn error of metabolism. *J Clin Invest* **86**:2034, 1990.
108. Laatikainen T, Perheentupa J, Vihko R, Makino I, Sjövall J: Bile acids and hormonal steroids in bile of a boy with 3β-hydroxysteroid deficiency. *J Steroid Biochem* **3**:715, 1972.
109. Björkhem I, Einarsson K, Gustafsson J-Å: 3β-Hydroxy-Δ^5-C_{19}- and C_{21}-Δ^5-steroid oxidoreductase activity in rat liver. *Steroids* **19**:471, 1972.
110. Ichimiya H, Egestad B, Nazer H, Baginski ES, Clayton P, Sjövall P: Bile acids and bile alcohols in a child with hepatic 3β-hydroxy-Δ^5-C_{27}-steroid dehydrogenase deficiency: effects of chenodeoxycholic acid treatment. *J Lipid Res* **32**:829, 1991.
111. Kulkarni B, Javitt NB: Chenodeoxycholic acid synthesis in the hamster: A metabolic pathway via 3β,7α-dihydroxy-5-cholen-24-oic acid. *Steroids* **40**:581, 1982.
112. Ichimiya H, Nazer H, Gunasekaran T, Clayton P, Sjövall J: Treatment of chronic liver disease caused by 3β-hydroxy-Δ^5-C_{27}-steroid dehydrogenase deficiency with chenodeoxycholic acid. *Arch Dis Child* **65**:1121, 1990.

113. Horslen SP, Lawson AM, Malone M, Clayton PT: 3β-Hydroxysteroid dehydrogenase deficiency. Effect of chenodeoxycholic acid on liver histology. *J Inherit Metab Dis* **15**:38, 1992.
114. Setchell KDR, Balistreri WF, Piccoli DA, Clerici C: Oral bile acid therapy in the treatment of inborn errors in bile acid synthesis associated with liver disease, in Paumgartner G, Stiehl A, Gerok W (eds): *Bile Acids as Therapeutic Agents. From Basic Science to Clinical Practice.* Falk Symposium 58, Freiburg. Dordrecht, Kluwer, 1991, p. 367.
115. Setchell KDR, Suchy FJ, Welsh MB, Zimmer-Nechemias L, Heubi J, Balistreri WF: Δ^4-3-Oxosteroid 5β-reductase deficiency described in identical twins with neonatal hepatitis. *J Clin Invest* **82**:2148, 1988.
116. Clayton PT, Patel E, Lawson AM, Carruthers RA, Tanner MS, Strandvik B, Egestad B, Sjövall J: 3-Oxo-Δ^4 bile acids in liver disease. *Lancet* **I**:1283, 1988.
117. Clayton PT: Inborn errors of bile acid metabolism. *J Inherit Metab Dis* **14**:478, 1991.
118. Setchell KDR, Björkhem I, Okuda K. Unpublished observation.
119. Björkhem I, Einarsson K: Formation and metabolism of 7α-hydroxy-5α-cholestan-3-one and 7α,12α-dihydroxy-5α-cholestan-3-one in rat liver. *Eur J Biochem* **13**:174, 1970.
120. Setchell KDR, Suchy FJ, Welsh MB, Zimmer-Nechemias L, Heubi JE, Hofmann AF, Balistreri WF: A new inborn error in bile acid synthesis-Δ^4-3-oxosteroid 5β-reductase deficiency described in identical twins with neonatal hepatitis, in Paumgartner G, Stiehl A, Gerok W (eds): *Trends in Bile Acid Research.* Falk Symposium 52, Freiburg. Dordrecht, Kluwer, 1988, p 197.
121. Setchell KDR: Disorders of bile acid synthesis and metabolism, in *Pediatric Gastrointestinal Disease: Pathophysiology, Diagnosis, Management.*, Philadelphia, BC Decker, 1996, p 1205.
122. Balistreri WF: Fetal and neonatal bile acid synthesis and metabolism: clinical implications. *J Inherit Metab Dis* **14**:459, 1991.
123. Van Bogaert L, Scherer HJ, Epstein E: *Une forme cerebrale de la cholestérinose géneralisée.* Paris, Mason et Cie, 1937.
124. Van Bogaert L, Scherer HJ, Froelich A, Epstein E: Une deuxième observation de cholestérinose tendineuse symétrique avec symptomes cérébraux. *Ann Med* **42**:69, 1973.
125. Van Bogaert L: Les Aspects neurologiques des cholestérinoses généralisées. *Prog Med (Paris)* **22**:785, 1938.
126. Epstein E, Lorenz K: Beitrag zur Pathologie und Pathochemie der cholesterinigen Lipidose vom Typus van Bogaert-Scherer. *Klin Wochenschr* **16**:1320, 1937.
127. Epstein E, Kreitner H: Beitrag zu einer vergleichenden Pathologie und Pathochemie der allgemeinen Cholesterin-lipoidosen. *Virchows Arch (Zellpathol)* **306**:53, 1940.
128. Menkes J, Schimshock JR, Swanson PD: Cerebrotendinous xanthomatosis: The storage of cholestanol within the nervous system. *Arch Neurol* **19**:47, 1968.
129. Philippart M, Van Bogaert L: Cholestanolosis (cerebrotendinous xanthomatosis): A follow-up study on the original family. *Arch Neurol* **21**:603, 1969.
130. Cruysberg JR, Wevers RA, van Engelen BG, Pinckers A, van Spreeken A, Tolboom-JJ: Ocular and systemic manifestations of cerebrotendinous xanthomatosis. *Am J Ophthalmol* **120**:597, 1995.
131. Salen G: Cholestanol deposition in cerebrotendinous xanthomatosis: A possible mechanism. *Ann Intern Med* **75**:843, 1971.
132. Bhattacharyya AK, Connor WE: Familial diseases with storage of sterols other than cholesterol: Cerebrotendinous xanthomatosis, and β-sitosterolemia and xanthomatosis, in Stanbury JB, Wyngaarden JB, Fredrickson DS (eds): *The Metabolic Basis of Inherited Diseases*, 3rd ed. New York, McGraw-Hill, 1978, p 656.
133. Farpour H, Mahloudji M: Familial cerebrotendinous xanthomatosis. *Arch Neurol* **32**:223, 1975.
134. Bergner V, Korczyn AP, Mayersdore A: Cerebrotendinous xanthomatosis. *Harefuah* **92**:537, 1977.
135. De Jong JGY, Van Gent CM, Dellman JW: Cerebrotendinous cholestanolosis in relation to other cerebral xanthomatosis. *Clin Neurol Neurosurg* **79**:253, 1977.
136. Brasseur G, Marx P, Langlois J, Houdent G: Cerebrotendinous xanthomatosis. *Bull Soc Ophtalmol Fr* **78**:913, 1978.
137. Seyama Y, Ichikawa K, Yamakawa T: Quantitative determination of cholestanol in plasma with mass fragmentography. Biochemical diagnosis of cerebrotendinous xanthomatosis. *J Biochem* **80**:223, 1976.
138. Ohnishi A, Yamashita Y, Goto I, Kuroiwa Y, Murakami S, Ikeda M: De- and remyelination and onion bulb in cerebrotendinous xanthomatosis. *Acta Neuropathol* **45**:43, 1979.
139. Kuritzy A, Berginer VM, Korczyn AD: Peripheral neuropathy in cerebrotendinous xanthomatosis. *Neurology* **29**:880, 1979.
140. Setoguchi T, Salen G, Tint GS, Mosbach EH: A biochemical abnormality in cerebrotendinous xanthomatosis: Impairment of bile acid biosynthesis associated with incomplete degradation of the cholesterol side chain. *J Clin Invest* **531**:1395, 1974.
141. Oftebro H, Björkhem I, Skrede S, Schreiner A, Pedersen J: Cerebrotendinous xanthomatosis: A defect in mitochondrial 26-hydroxylase required for normal biosynthesis of cholic acid. *J Clin Invest* **65**:1418, 1980.
142. Björkhem I, Oftebro H, Skrede S, Pedersen JI: Assay of intermediates in bile acid biosynthesis using isotope dilution-mass spectrometry: Hepatic levels in the normal state and in cerebrotendinous xanthomatosis. *J Lipid Res* **22**:191, 1981.
143. Björkhem I, Fausa O, Hopen G, Oftebro H, Pedersen JI, Skrede S: Role of the 26-hydroxylase in the biosynthesis of bile acids in the normal state and in CTX. An in vivo study. *J Clin Invest* **71**:142, 1983.
144. Cali JJ, Hsieh C-L, Francke U, Russell DW: Mutations in the bile acid biosynthetic enzyme sterol 27-hydroxylase underlie cerebrotendinous xanthomatosis. *J Biol Chem* **266**:7779, 1991.
145. Cali JJ, Russell DW: Characterization of human sterol 27-hydroxylase: A mitochondrial cytochrome P-450 that catalyzes multiple oxidations in bile acid biosynthesis. *J Biol Chem* **266**:7774, 1991.
146. Leitersdorf E, Reshef A, Meiner V, Levitzki R, Schwartz SP, Dann EJ, Berkman N, Cali JJ, Klapholz L, Berginer VM: Frameshift and splice-junction mutations in the sterol 27-hydroxylase gene cause cerebrotendinous xanthomatosis in Jews of Moroccan origin. *J Clin Invest* **91**:2488, 1993.
147. Meiner V, Marais DA, Reshef A, Bjorkhem I, Leitersdorf E. Premature termination codon at the sterol 27-hydroxylase gene causes cerebrotendinous xanthomatosis in an Afrikaner family. *Hum Mol Genet* **3**:193, 1994.
148. Reshef A, Meiner V, Berginer VM, Leitersdorf E: Molecular genetics of cerebrotendinous xanthomatosis in Jews of North African origin. *J Lipid Res* **35**:478, 1994.
149. Nakashima N, Sakai Y, Sakai H, Yanase T, Haji M, Umeda F, Koga S, Hoshita T, Nawata H: A point mutation in the bile acid biosynthetic enzyme sterol 27-hydroxylase in a family with cerebrotendinous xanthomatosis. *J Lipid Res* **35**:663, 1994.
150. Kim KS, Kubota S, Kuriyama M, Fujiyama J, Bjorkhem I, Eggertsen G, Seyama Y: Identification of new mutations in sterol 27-hydroxylase gene in Japanese patients with cerebrotendinous xanthomatosis (CTX). *J Lipid Res* **35**:1031, 1994.
151. Leitersdorf E, Safadi R, Meiner V, Reshef A, Bjorkhem I, Friedlander Y, Morkos S, Berginer VM. Cerebrotendinous xanthomatosis in the Israeli Druze: Molecular genetics and phenotypic characteristics. *Am J Hum Genet* **55**:907, 1994.
152. Segev H, Reshef A, Clavey V, Delbart C, Routier G, Leitersdorf E: Premature termination codon at the sterol 27-hydroxylase gene causes cerebrotendinous xanthomatosis in a French family. *Hum Genet* **95**:238, 1995.
153. Watts GF, Mitchell WD, Bending JJ, Reshef A, Leitersdorf E: Cerebrotendinous xanthomatosis: A family study of sterol 27-hydroxylase mutations and pharmacotherapy. *QJM* **89**:55, 1996.
154. Okuyama E, Tomita S, Takeuchi H, Ichikawa Y: A novel mutation in the cytochrome P450 (27) (CYP27) gene caused cerebrotendinous xanthomatosis in a Japanese family. *J Lipid Res* **37**:631, 1996.
155. Chen W, Kubota S, Nishimura Y, Nozaki S, Yamashita S, Nakagawa T, Kameda-Takemura K, Menju M, Matsuzawa Y, Bjorkhem I, Eggertsen G, Seyama Y. Genetic analysis of a Japanese cerebrotendinous xanthomatosis family: Identification of a novel mutation in the adrenodoxin binding region of the CYP 27 gene. *Biochim Biophys Acta* **1317**:119, 1996.
156. Verrips A, Steenbergen-Spanjers GC, Luyten JA, van den Heuvel LP, Keyser A, Gabreels FJ, Wevers RA: Two new mutations in the sterol 27-hydroxylase gene in two families lead to cerebrotendinous xanthomatosis. *Hum Genet* **98**:735, 1996.
157. Garuti R, Lelli N, Barozzini M, Tiozzo R, Dotti MT, Federico A, Ottomano AM, Croce A, Bertolini S, Calandra S: Cerebrotendinous xanthomatosis caused by two new mutations of the sterol-27-hydroxylase gene that disrupt mRNA splicing. *J Lipid Res* **37**:1459, 1996.
158. Ahmed MS, Afsar S, Hentati A, Ahmad A, Pasha J, Juneja T, Hung WY, Ahmad A, Choudhri A, Saya S, Siddique T: A novel mutation in the sterol 27-hydroxylase gene of a Pakistani family with autosomal recessive cerebrotendinous xanthomatosis. *Neurology* **48**:258, 1997.
159. Chen W, Kubota S, Kim KS, Cheng J, Kuriyama M, Eggertsen G, Bjorkhem I, Seyama Y: Novel homozygous and compound hetero-

zygous mutations of sterol 27-hydroxylase gene (CYP27) cause cerebrotendinous xanthomatosis in three Japanese patients from two unrelated families. *J Lipid Res* **38**:870, 1997.

160. Verrips A, Steenbergen-Spanjers GC, Luyten JA, Wevers RA, Wokke JH, Gabreels FJ, Wolthers BG, van den Heuvel LP: Exon skipping in the sterol 27-hydroxylase gene leads to cerebrotendinous xanthomatosis. *Hum Genet* **100**:284, 1997.
161. Tint GS, Salen G: Synthesis of cholesterol and its precursors but not cholestanol in cultured fibroblasts from patients with cerebrotendinous xanthomatosis. *J Lipid Res* **23**:597, 1982.
162. Yasuhara M, Kuramoto T, Hoshita T: Identification of 5β-cholestane-3α,7α,12α,26-tetrol, 5β-cholestane-3α,7α,12α,24α-tetrol and 5β-cholestane-3α,7α,12β-tetrol in CTX. *Steroids* **31**:333, 1978.
163. Kuramoto T, Furukawa Y, Nishina T, Sugimoto T, Mahara R, Tohma M, Kihara K, Hoshita T: Identification of short side-chain bile acids in urine of patients with CTX. *J Lipid Res* **31**:1895, 1990.
164. Sjövall J, Setchell KDR, Lawson A, Karlaganis G, Skrede S. Unpublished observation.
165. Salen G, Shefer S, Tint GS, Nicolav G, Dayal B, Batta AK: Biosynthesis of bile acids in CTX. Relationship of bile acid pool sizes and synthesis rates to hydroxylations at C-12, C-25 and C-26. *J Clin Invest* **76**:744, 1985.
166. Oftebro H, Björkhem I, Stormer FC, Pedersen JI: CTX: Detective liver mitochondrial hydroxylation of chenodeoxycholic acid precursors. *J Lipid Res* **22**:632, 1981.
166a. Salen G, Shefer S, Beginer VM: Familial disease with storage of sterols other than cholesterol: Cerebrotendinous xanthomatosis and sitosterolemia with xanthomatosis, in Stanbury JB, Wyngaarden JB, Fredrickson DS, Brown MS, Goldstein JL (eds): *Metabolic Basis of Inherited Disease*, 5th ed. New York, McGraw-Hill, 1983, p 713.
167. Berginer VM, Salen G, Shefer S: Cerebrotendinous xanthomatosis. *Neurol Clin* **7**:55, 1989.
168. Meiner V, Meiner Z, Reshef A, Bjorkhem I, Leitersdorf E, Cerebrotendinous xanthomatosis: Molecular diagnosis enables presymptomatic detection of a treatable disease. *Neurology* **44**:288, 1994.
169. Rosen H, Reshef A, Maeda N, Lippoldt A, Shpizen S, Triger L, Eggertsen G, Björkhem I, Leitersdorf E: Markedly reduced bile acid synthesis but maintained levels of cholesterol and vitamin D metabolites in mice with disrupted sterol 27-hydroxylase gene. *J Biol Chem* **273**:14805, 1998.
170. Salen G, Shefer S, Cheng FW, Dayal B, Batta AK, Tint GS: Cholic acid biosynthesis. The enzymatic defect in cerebrotendinous xanthomatosis. *J Clin Invest* **63**:38, 1979.
171. Koopman BJ, Molen JC, Wolthers BG, Jager AEJ, Watterus RJ, Gips CH: Capillary gas chromatographic determination of cholestanol/cholesterol ratio in biological fluids. *Clin Chim Acta* **137**:305, 1984.
172. Björkhem I, Karlmar KE: Biosynthesis of cholestanol: Conversion of cholesterol into 4-cholesten-3-one by rat liver microsomes. *Biochim Biophys Acta* **337**:129, 1947.
173. Skrede S, Björkhem I, Buchmann MS, Fausa O: Studies on the mechanism of the increased biosynthesis of cholestanol in CTX: The activity of Δ^5-3β-hydroxysteroid dehydrogenase. *Scand J Gastroenterol* **20**:1262, 1985.
174. Buchmann MS, Björkhem I, Lund AM, Skrede S: On the mechanism of biosynthesis of cholestanol from 7α-hydroxycholesterol. *Scand J Clin Lab Invest* **46**(Suppl 184):41, 1986.
175. Björkhem I, Skrede S, Buchmann MS, East C, Grundy S: Accumulation of 7α-hydroxy-4-cholesten-3-one and cholesta-4,6-dien-3-one in patients with CTX. Effect of treatment with chenodeoxycholic acid. *Hepatology* **7**:266, 1987.
176. Lewis B, Mitchell WD, Marenah CB, Cortese C: Cerebrotendinous xanthomatosis: Biochemical response to inhibition of cholesterol synthesis. *Br Med J* **287**:21, 1983.
177. Nakamura T, Matsuzawa Y, Takemura K, Kubo M, Miki H, Tarui S: Combined treatment with chenodeoxycholic acid and pravastatin improves plasma cholestanol levels associated with marked regression of tendon xanthomas in cerebrotendinous xanthomatosis. *Metabolism* **40**:741, 1991.
178. Salen G, Batta AK, Tint GS, Shefer S: Comparative effects of lovastatin and chenodeoxycholic acid on plasma cholestanol levels and abnormal bile acid metabolism in cerebrotendinous xanthomatosis. *Metabolism* **43**:1018, 1994.
179. Javitt NB: 26-Hydroxycholesterol: Synthesis, metabolism and biologic activities. *J Lipid Res* **31**:1527, 1990.
180. Shefer S, Hauser S, Salen G, Zaki FG, Bullock J, Salgado E, Shevitz J: Comparative effects of cholestanol and cholesterol on hepatic sterol and bile acid metabolism in the rat. *J Clin Invest* **74**:1773, 1984.
181. Björkhem I, Andersson O, Diczfalusy U, Sevastik B, Xiu RJ, Duan C, Lund E: Atherosclerosis and sterol 27-hydroxylase: Evidence for a role of this enzyme in elimination of cholesterol from human macrophages. *Proc Natl Acad Sci U S A* **91**:8592, 1994.
182. Babiker A, Andersson O, Lund E, Xiu RJ, Deeb S, Reshef A, Leitersdorf E, Diczfalusy U, Björkhem I: Elimination of cholesterol in macrophages and endothelial cells by the sterol 27-hydroxylase mechanism. *J Biol Chem* **272**:26253, 1997.
183. Salen G, Tint S, Shefer S: Increased cerebrospinal fluid cholestanol and apolipoprotein B concentrations in CTX: Effect of chenodeoxycholic acid. *Abstract IX* International Bile Acid Meeting, Basel, 1986, p 59.
184. Buchmann MS, Clausen OP: Effects of cholestanol feeding and cholestyramine treatment on the tissue sterols in the rabbit. *Lipids* **21**:738, 1986.
185. Byun DS, Kasama T, Shimizu T, Yorifuji H, Seyama Y: Effect of cholestanol feeding on sterol concentrations in the serum, liver and cerebellum of mice. *J Biochem* **103**:375, 1988.
186. Buchmann MS, Björkhem I, Skrede S: Conversion of the cholestanol precursor cholesta-4,6-dien-3-one in different tissues of the rat. *Biochim Biophys Acta* **922**:111, 1987.
187. Salen G, Shefer S, Berginer VM: Familial diseases with storage of sterols other than cholesterol: Cerebrotendinous xanthomatosis and sitosterolemia with xanthomatosis, in Stanbury JB, Wyngaarden JB, Fredrickson DS, Brown MS, Goldstein JL (eds): *The Metabolic Basis of Inherited Disease*, 5th ed. New York, McGraw-Hill, 1983, p 713.
188. Giampalmo A: Uber einen Fall von cholesterinlipidose vom Typus van Bogaert-Scherer. *Verh Dtsch Ges Pathol* **34**:227, 1950.
189. Vinditti D: Una rara Lipidosi di interesse ortopedico: Forma cerebrotendinea della cholesterinosi generalizzata. *Chir Organi Mov* **34**:429, 1950.
190. Berginer VM, Foster NLF, Sadowsky M, Townsend JA, Siegel GJ, Salen G: Psychiatric disorders in patients with CTX. *Am J Psychiatry* **145**:354, 1988.
191. Schimschock JR, Alvord EC Jr, Swanson PD: Cerebrotendinous xanthomatosis: Clinical and pathological studies. *Arch Neurol* **18**:688, 1968.
192. Giampalmo A: Les lipoidoses cholesteriniques due système nerveaux. *Acta Neurol Belg* **54**:786, 1954.
193. Hokezu Y, Kuriyama M, Kubota R, Nakagawa M, Fujiyama J, Osame M. Cerebrotendinous xanthomatosis: cranial CT and MRI studies in eight patients. *Neuroradiology* **34**:308, 1992.
194. Kuwabara K, Hitoshi S, Nukina N, Ishii K, Momose T, Kubota S, Seyama Y, Kanazawa I: PET analysis of a case of cerebrotendinous xanthomatosis presenting hemiparkinsonism. *J Neurol Sci* **138**:145, 1996.
195. Lussier-Cacan S, Cantin M, Roy CC, Snidermann AD, Nestruck AC, Davidnon I: Tendon xanthomas associated with cholestanolosis and hyperbetalipoproteinemia. *Clin Invest Med* **9**:94, 1986.
196. Kuriyama M, Fujiyama J, Yoshidome H, Takenaga S, Matsumuro K, Kasama T, Fukuda K, et al.: CTX: Clinical and biochemical evaluation of eight patients and review literature. *J Neurol Sci* **102**:225, 1991.
196a. Potkin BN, Hoeg JM, Connor WE, Salen G, Quyyumi AA, Brush JE Jr, Roberts WC, Brewer HB Jr: Aneurysmal coronary artery disease in CTX. *Am J Cardiol* **61**:1150, 1988.
197. Seland JH, Slagsvold JE: The ultrastructure of lens and iris in cerebrotendinous xanthomatosis. *Acta Ophtalmol* **55**:201, 1977.
198. McKenna P, Morgan SJ, Bosanquet RC, Laker MF: A case of CTX: the sterol, content of a cataracteous lens. *Br J Opthalmol* **74**:629, 1990.
199. Salen G, Zaki FG, Sabesin S, Boehme D, Shefer S, Mosbach EH: Intrahepatic pigment and crystal forms in patients with cerebrotendinous xanthomatosis (CTX). *Gastroenterology* **74**:82, 1978.
200. Koopman BJ, Wolthers BG, Molen JC, Nagel GT, Waterreus RJ, Oosterhuis HJGH: Capillary gas chromatographic determinations of urinary bile acids and bile alcohols in CTX patients proving the ineffectiveness of ursodeoxycholic acid treatment. *Clin Chim Acta* **142**:103, 1984.
201. Kasama T, Byun DS, Seyama Y: Quantitative analysis of sterols by HPLC. Application to the biochemical analysis of CTX. *J Chromatogr* **400**:241-6, 1987.
202. Koopman BJ, Molen JC, Wolthers BG: Determination of some hydroxycholesterols in human serum samples. *J Chromatogr* 416, 1987.
203. Wolthers BG, Walrecht HT, Molen JC, Nagel GT, Doormal JJ, Wijnandts PN: Use of determination of 7-lathosterol and other

cholesterol precursors in serum in the study and treatment of disturbances of sterols metabolism, particular CTX. *J Lipid Res* **32**:603, 1991.

204. Beppu T, Seyama Y, Kasama T, Serizawa S, Yamakawa T: Serum bile acid profiles in CTX. *Clin Chim Acta* **118**:167, 1982.
205. Batta AK, Salen G, Shefer S, Tint GS, Batta M: Increased plasma bile alcohol glucuronides in patients with CTX: Effect of chenodeoxycholic acid. *J Lipid Res* **28**:1006, 1987.
206. Shore V, Salen G, Cheng FW, Forte T, Shefer S, Tint GS, Lindgren F: Abnormal high-density lipoproteins in cerebrotendinous xanthomatosis. *J Clin Invest* **68**:1295, 1981.
207. Lindqvist A, Midtvedt T, Skrede S, Sjövall J: Effect of bile alcohols on the microbial 7α-dehydroxylation of chenodeoxycholic acid. *Microb Ecol Health Dis* **3**:25, 1990.
208. Shefer S, Dayal B, Tint GS, Salen G, Mosbach EH: Identification of pentahydroxy bile alcohols in cerebrotendinous xanthomatosis: Characterization of 5β-cholestane-3α,7α,12α,24,25-pentol and 5β-cholestane 3α,7α,12α,23,25-pentol. *J Lipid Res* **16**:280, 1975.
209. Dayal B, Salen G, Tint GS, Toome V, Mosbach EH: Absolute configuration of pentahydroxy bile alcohols excreted by patients with cerebrotendinous xanthomatosis: A circular dichroism study. *J Lipid Res* **19**:187, 1978.
210. Hoshita T, Yasuhara M, Kihira K, Kuramoto T: Identification of (23S)-5β-cholestane-3α,7α,12α,23,25-pentol excreted by patients with cerebrotendinous xanthomatosis. *Steroids* **27**:657,1976.
211. Hoshita T, Yasuhara M, Une M, Kibe A, Itoga E, Kito S, Kuramoto T: Occurrence of bile alcohol glucuronides in bile of patients with cerebrotendinous xanthomatosis. *J Lipid Res* **21**:1015, 1980.
212. Karlaganis G, KarlaganisV, Sjövall J: Bile alcohol glucuronides in urine: secondary intermediates in the formation of bile acids from cholesterol? Proceedings of the 33rd Falk Symposium held during the VIIth International Bile Acid Meeting, Basel. Boston, MTP Press, 1982, p 119.
213. Wolthers BG, Volmer M, van der Molen J, Koopman BJ, Jager AEJ, Watterreus RJ: Diagnosis of cerebrotendinous xanthomatosis (CTX) and effect of chenodeoxycholic acid therapy by analysis of urine using capillary gas chromatography. *Clin Chim Acta* **131**:53, 1983.
214. Batta AK, Shefer S, Batta M, Salen G: Effect of chenodeoxycholic acid on biliary and urinary bile acids and bile alcohols in CTX: Monitoring by high performance liquid chromatography. *J Lipid Res* **26**:690, 1985.
215. Koopman BJ, Wolthers BG, Molen JC, Nagel GT, Rutgers H, Strijtveen B, Kaptein B: Increased (23R)-hydroxylase activity in patients suffering from cerebrotendinous xanthomatosis, resulting in (23R)-hydroxylation of bile acid. *Biochim Biophys Acta* **883**:585, 1986.
216. Kasama T, Seyama Y: Biochemical diagnosis of CTX using reversed phase thin layer chromatography. *J Biochem* **99**:771, 1986.
217. Koopman BJ, Molen JC, Wolthers BG, Waterreus RJ: Screening for CTX by using an enzymatic assay for 7α-hydroxylated steroids in urine. *Clin Chem* **33**:142, 1987.
218. Egestad B, Petterson P, Skrede S: Fast atomic bombardment in the diagnosis of CTX. *Scand J Clin Lab Invest* **45**:443, 1985.
219. Koopman BJ, Waterreus RJ, Brekel HWC, Wolthers BG: Detection of carriers of CTX. *Clin Chim Acta* **158**:179, 1986.
220. Salen G, Meriwether TW, Nicolav G: Chenodeoxycholic acid inhibits increased cholesterol and cholestanol synthesis in patients with CTX. *J Clin Invest* **75**:448, 1985.
221. Berginer VM, Salen G, Shefer S: Long-term treatment of CTX with chenodeoxycholic acid. *N Engl J Med* **26**:1649, 1984.
222. Wolthers LFGM, Molen JC, Walrecht H, Hesselmans LFGM: Reduction of urinary bile alcohol excretion and serum cholestanol in CTX after oral administration of deoxycholic acid. *Clin Chem* **193**:113, 1990.
223. Setchell KDR, Bragetti P, Zimmer-Nechemias, Daugherty C, Pelli MA, Vaccaro R, Gentili G, Distrutti E, Dozzini G, Morelli A, Clerici C: Oral bile acid treatment and the patient with Zellweger syndrome. *Hepatology* **15**:198, 1992.
224. Björkhem I, Kase BF, Pedersen JI: Role of peroxisomes in the synthesis of bile acids. *Scand J Clin Invest* **43**:163, 1985.
225. Setchell KDR, Street JM: Inborn errors of bile acid synthesis. *Semin Liver Dis* **7**:85, 1987.
226. Setchell KDR, Heubi JE, O'Connell NC, Hofmann AF, Lavine JE: Identification of a unique inborn error in bile acid conjugation involving a deficiency in amidation, in Paumgartner G, Stiehl A, Gerok W. (eds): *Bile Acids in Hepatobiliary Disease*. London, Kluwer Academic, 1997, p 43.
227. Battacharyya AK, Connor WE: β-Sitosterolemia and xanthomatosis: A newly described lipid storage disease in two sisters. *J Clin Invest* **52**:9a, 1973.
228. Bergman K. Personal communication.
229. Shulman RS, Bhattacharyya AK, Connor WE, Fredrickson DS: β-Sitosterolemia and xanthomatosis. *N Engl J Med* **294**:482, 1976.
230. Salen G, Tint GS, Shefer S, Shore V, Nguyen L: Increased sitosterol absorption is offset by rapid elimination to prevent accumulation in heterozygotes with sitosterolemia. *Arterioscler Thromb* **12**:563, 1992.
231. Lütjohann D, Björkhem I, Ose L: Phytosterolaemia in a Norwegian family: Diagnosis and characterization of the first Scandinavian case. *Scand J Clin Lab Invest* **56**:229, 1996.
232. Gregg RE, Connor WE, Lin DS, Brewer HB Jr: Abnormal metabolism of shellfish sterols in a patient with sitosterolemia and xanthomatosis. *J Clin Invest* **77**:1864, 1986.
233. Tavani DM, Nes WR, Billheimer JT: The sterol substrate specificity of acyl CoA:cholesterol acyltransferase from rat liver. *J Lipid Res* **23**:774, 1982.
234. Tabas I, Feinmark SJ, Beatini N: The reactivity of desmosterol and other shellfish- and xanthomatosis-associated sterols in the macrophage sterol esterification reaction. *J Clin Invest* **84**:1713, 1989.
235. Bhattacharyya AK, Connor WE, Lin DS, McMurry MM, Shulman RS: Sluggish sitosterol turnover and hepatic failure to excrete sitosterol into bile cause expansion of body pool of sitosterol in patients with sitosterolemia and xanthomatosis. *Arterioscler Thromb* **11**:1287, 1991.
236. Lin H-J, Wang C, Salen G, Lam K-C, Chan T-K: Sitosterol and cholesterol metabolism in a patient with coexisting phytosterolemia and cholestanolemia. *Metabolism* **32**:126, 1983.
237. Salen G, Shefer S, Nguyen L, Ness GC, Tint GS, Shore V: Sitosterolemia. *J Lipid Res* **33**:945, 1992.
238. Nguyen LB, Shefer S, Salen G, Ness GC, Tint GS, Zaki FG, Rani I: A molecular defect in hepatic cholesterol biosynthesis in sitosterolemia with xanthomatosis. *J Clin Invest* **86**:923, 1990.
239. Nguyen LB, Salen G, Shefer S, Tint GS, Shore GS, Shore V, Ness GC: Decreased cholesterol biosynthesis in sitosterolemia with xanthomatosis: diminished mononuclear leukocyte 3-hydroxy-3-methylglutaryl coenzyme A reductase activity and enzyme protein associated with increased low-density lipoprotein receptor function. *Metabolism* **39**:436, 1990.
240. Shefer S, Salen G, Bullock J, Nguyen LB, Ness GC, Vhao Z, Belamarich PF, Chowdhary I, Lerner S, Batta AK, Tint GS: The effect of increased hepatic sitosterol on the regulation of 3-hydroxy-3-methylglutaryl-coenzyme A reductase in the rat and sitosterolemic homozygotes. *Hepatology* **20**:213, 1994.
241. Nguyen LB, Salen G, Shefer S, Bullock J, Chen T, Tint GS, Chowdhary IR, Lerner S: Deficient ileal 3-hydroxy-3-methylglutaryl coenzyme A reductase activity in sitosterolemia: Sitosterol is not a feedback inhibitor of intestinal cholesterol biosynthesis. *Metabolism* **43**:855, 1994.
242. Khachadurian AK, Clancy KF: Familial phytosterolemia (β-sitosterolemia): Report of five cases and studies in cultured skin fibroblasts. *Clin Res* **26**:329A, 1978.
243. Gylling H, Miettinen TA: Serum noncholesterol sterols related to cholesterol metabolism in familial hypercholesterolemia. *Clin Chim Acta* **178**:41, 1988.
244. Kempen HJM, de Knijff P, Boomsma DI, van der Voort HA, Gevers Leuven JA, Havekes L: Plasma levels of lathosterol and phytosterols in relation to age, sex, anthropometric parameters, plasma lipids, and apolipoprotein E phenotype, in 160 Dutch families. *Metabolism* **40**:604, 1991.
245. Björkhem I: Unpublished results.
246. Honda A, Salen G, Nguyen LB, Tint GS, Batta AK, Shefer S: Down-regulation of cholesterol biosynthesis in sitosterolemia: diminished activities of acetoacetyl-CoA thiolase, 3-hydroxy-3-methylglutaryl-CoA synthase, reductase, squalene synthase, and 7-dehydrocholesterol Δ^7-reductase in liver and mononuclear leukocytes. *J Lipid Res* **39**:44, 1998.
247. Dayal B, Tint GS, Toome V, Batta AK, Shefer S, Salen G: Synthesis and structure of 26 (or 27)-nor-5β-cholestane-3α,7α,12α,24S,25-pentol isolated from the urine and feces of a patient with sitosterolemia and xanthomatosis. *J Lipid Res* **26**:298, 1985.
248. Boberg KM, Björkhem I, Skrede S: Normal activity of C_{27}-steroid 26-hydroxylase in cultured sitosterolaemia fibroblasts. *Scand J Clin Lab Invest* **47**:701, 1987.
249. Karlaganis G, Nemeth A, Hammarskjöld B, Strandvik B, Sjövall J: Urinary excretion of bile alcohols in normal children and patients with

α_1-antitrypsin deficiency during development of liver disease. *Eur J Clin Invest* **12**:399, 1982.
250. Setchell KDR, Ives JA, Lawson AM, Kayden JH: Fecal bile acid and sterol excretion in a case of phytosterolemia. Falk Symposium 42, VIIIth International Bile Acid Meeting, Berne, p 84.
251. Bhattacharyya AK: The pathogenesis of xanthomata: The role of sterols. *Artery* **2**:2, 1976.
252. Parker F: Normocholesterolemic xanthomatosis. *Arch Dermatol* **122**:1253, 1986.
253. Nguyen LB, Shefer S, Salen G, Horak I, Tint GS, McNamara DJ: The effect of abnormal plasma and cellular sterol content and composition on low density lipoprotein uptake and degradation by monocytes and lymphocytes in sitosterolemia with xanthomatosis. *Metabolism* **37**:346, 1988.
254. Boberg KM, Pettersen KS, Prydz H: Toxicity of sitosterol to human umbilical vein endothelial cells in vitro. *Scand J Clin Lab Invest* **51**:509, 1991.
255. Hagiwara H, Shimonaka M, Morisaki M, Ikekawa N, Inada Y: Sitosterol-stimulative production of plasminogen activator in cultured endothelial cells from bovine carotid artery. *Thromb Res* **33**:363, 1984.
256. Wang C, Lin HJ, Chan T-K, Salen G, Chan W-C, Tse T-F: A unique patient with coexisting cerebrotendinous xanthomatosis and β-sitosterolemia. *Am J Med* **71**:313, 1981.
257. Leikin AI, Brenner RR: Fatty acid desaturase activities are modulated by phytosterol incorporation in microsomes. *Biochim Biophys Acta* **1005**:187, 1989.
258. Whitington GL, Ragland JB, Sabesin SM, Kuiken LB: Neutral sterolemia and xanthomas. *Circulation* 60:(II)33, 1979.
259. Dayal B, Tint GS, Batta AK, Speck J, Khachadurian AK, Shefer S, Salen G: Identification of 5α-stanols in patients with sitosterolemia and xanthomatosis: Stereochemistry of the protonolysis of steroidal organoboranes. *Steroids* **40**:233, 1982.
260. Salen G, Batta AK, Tint GS, Shefer S, Ness GC: Inverse relationship between plasma cholestanol concentrations and bile acid biosynthesis in sitosterolemia. *J Lipid Res* **35**:1878, 1994.
261. Fishler-Mates Z, Budowski P, Pinsky A: Effect of soy sterols on cholesterol synthesis in the rat. *Lipids* **8**:40, 1973.
262. Shefer S, Hauser S, Lapar V, Mosbach EH: Regulatory effects of sterols and bile acids on hepatic 3-hydroxy-3-methylgutaryl CoA reductase and cholesterol 7α-hydroxylase in the rat. *J Lipid Res* **14**:573, 1973.
263. Raicht RF, Cohen BI, Shefer S, Mosbach EH: Sterol balance studies in the rat. Effects of dietary cholesterol and β-sitosterol on sterol balance and rate-limiting enzymes of sterol metabolism. *Biochim Biophys Acta* **388**:374, 1975.
264. Grundy SM, Ahrens EH Jr, Davignon J: The interaction of cholesterol absorption and cholesterol synthesis in man. *J Lipid Res* **10**:304, 1969.
265. Geron T, Shorland FB, Duckling GG: The effect of β-sitosterol on the metabolism of cholesterol and lipids in rats on a diet low in fat. *Biochem J* **92**:385, 1964.
266. Malini T, Vanithakumari G: Rat toxicity studies with β-sitosterol. *J Ethnopharmacol* **28**:221, 1990.
267. Konlande JE, Fisher H: Evidence for a nonabsorptive antihyperch-olesterolemic action of phytosterols in the chicken. *J Nutr* **98**:435, 1969.
267a. Bhattacharyya AK, Lopez LA: Absorbability of plant sterols and their distribution in rabbit tissues. *Biochim Biophys Acta* **574**:146, 1979.
268. Nguyen LB, Shefer S, Salen G, Tint SG, Batta AK: Competitive inhibition of hepatic sterol 27-hydroxylase by sitosterol: Decreased activity in sitosterolemia. *Proc Assoc Am Physicians* **110**:32, 1998.
269. Babiker A, Björkhem I: Unpublished observation.
270. Kwiterovich PO Jr, Bachorik PS, Smith HH, McKusick VA, Connor WE, Teng B, Sniderman AD: Hyperapobetalipoproteinemia in two families with xanthomas and phytosterolaemia. *Lancet* **1**:466, 1981.
271. Beaty TH, Kwiterovich PO Jr, Khoury MJ, White S, Bachorik PS, Smith HH, Teng B, Sniderman A: Genetic analysis of plasma sitosterol, apoprotein B, and lipoproteins in a large Amish pedigree with sitosterolemia. *Am J Hum Genet* **38**:492, 1986.
272. Hidaka H, Nakamura T, Aoki T, Kojima H, Nakajima Y, Kosugi K, Hatanaka I, Harada M, Kobayashi M, Tamura A, Fujii T, Shigeta Y: Increased plasma plant sterol levels in heterozygotes with sitoster-olemia and xanthomatosis. *J Lipid Res* **31**:881, 1990.
273. Patel SB, Honda A, Salen G: Sitosterolemia: Exclusion of genes involved in reduced cholesterol biosynthesis. *J Lipid Res* **39**:1, 1998.
274. Berger GMB, Deppe WM, Marais AD, Biggs M: Phytosterolemia in three unrelated South African families. *Postgrad Med J* **70**:631, 1994.
275. Matsuo I, Yoshino K, Ozawa A, Ohkido M: Phytosterolemia and type IIa hyperlipoproteinemia with tuberous xanthomas. *J Am Acad Dermatol* **4**:47, 1981.
276. Nye ER, Sutherland WHF, Mortimer JG, Stringer HCW: Sitoster-olaemia and heterozygous familial hypercholesterolaemia in a three-year-old girl: A case report. *N Z Med J* **101**:418, 1988.
277. Hidaka H, Sugiura H, Nakamura T, Kojima H, Fujita M, Sugie N, Okabe H: β-Sitosterolemia with generalized eruptive xanthomatosis. *Endocrine J* **44**:59, 1997.
278. Salen G, Horak I, Rothkopf M, Cohen JL, Speck J, Tint GS, Shore V, Dayal B, Chen T, Shefer S: Lethal atherosclerosis associated with abnormal plasma and tissue sterol composition in sitosterolemia with xanthomatosis. *J Lipid Res* **26**:1126, 1985.
279. Grahlke BK: Xanthome der Achillessehnen als Leitsymptom der Siosterinümie. *Dtsch Med Wochenschr* **116**:335, 1991.
280. Watts GF, Mitchell WD: Clinical and metabolic findings in a patient with phytosterolemia. *Ann Vlin Biochem* **29**:231, 1992.
281. Kottke BA, Cornicelli JA; Didisheim P, Kazmier FJ, Barham SS, Weidman WH: Phyto-sterolemia, xanthomatosis, and acquired aortic valve stenosis (Abstract). *Arteriosclerosis* **1**:58, 1981.
282. Kolovou G, Voudris V, Drogari E, Palatianos G, Cokkinos DV: Coronary bypass grafts in a young girl with sitosterolemia. *Eur Heart J* **17**:965, 1996.
283. Hatanaka I, Yasuda H, Hidaka H, Harada N, Kobayashi M, Okabe H, Matsumoto K, Hukuda, S, Shigeta Y: Spinal cord compression with paraplegia in xanthomatosis due to normocholesterolemic sitoster-olemia. *Ann Neurol* **28**:390, 1990.
284. Kuksis A, Myher JJ, Marai L, Little JA, McArthur RG, Roncari DAK: Fatty acid composition of individual plasma steryl esters in phytosterolemia and xanthomatosis. *Lipids* **21**:371, 1986.
285. McArthur RG, Roncardi DAK, Little JA, Kuksis A, Myher JJ, Marai L: Phytosterolemia and hypercholesterolemia in childhood. *J Pediatr* **108**:254, 1986.
286. Low LCK, Lin HJ, Lau KS, Kung AWC, Yeung CY: Phytosterolemia and pseudohomozygous type II hypercholesterolemia in two Chinese patients. *J Pediatr* **118**:746, 1991.
287. Govind Rao MK, Perkins EG: Identification of β-sitosterol, campesterol, and stigmasterol in human serum. *Lipids* **10**:566, 1975.
288. Kuksis A, Myher JJ, Marai L: Usefulness of gas chromatographic profiles of plasma total lipids in diagnosis of phytosterolemia. *J Chromatogr* **381**:1, 1986.
289. Tvrzická E, Mares P, Písaríková A, Novakovic J, Hrabák P: Simplified gas chromatographic method for the simultaneous determination of phytosterols and cholesterol. *J Chromatogr* **563**:188, 1991.
290. Mellies M, Glueck CJ, Sweeney C, Fallat RW, Tsang RC, Ishikawa TT: Plasma and dietary phytosterols in children. *Pediatrics* **57**:60, 1976.
291. Nguyen LB, Cobb M, Shefer S, Salen G, Ness GC, Tint GS: Regulation of cholesterol biosynthesis in sitosterolemia: Effect of lovastatin, cholestyramine, and dietary sterol restriction. *J Lipid Res* **32**:1941, 1991.
292. Cobb MM, Salen G, Tint GS: Comparative effect of dietary sitosterol on plasma sterols and cholesterol and bile acid synthesis in a sitosterolemic homozygote and heterozygote subject. *J Am Coll Nutr* **16**:605, 1997.
293. Parsons HG, Jamal R, Baylis B, Dias VC, Roncari D: A marked and sustained reduction in LDL sterols by diet and cholestyramine in β-sitosterolemia. *Clin Invest Med* **18**:389, 1995.
294. Cobb MM, Salen G, Tint GS, Greenspan J, Nguyen LB: Sitoster-olemia: Opposing effects of cholestyramine and lovastatin on plasma sterol levels in a homozygous girl and her heterozygous father. *Metabolism* **45**:673, 1996.
295. Belamarich PF, Deckelbaum RJ, Starc TJ, Dobrin BE, Tint GS, Salen G: Response to diet and cholestyramine in a patient with sitosterolemia. *Pediatrics* **86**:977, 1990.
296. Nguyen L, Salen G, Shefer S, Shore V, Tint GS, Ness G: Unexpected failure of bile acid malabsorption to stimulate cholesterol synthesis in sitosterolemia with xanthomatosis. Comparison with lovastatin. *Arteriosclerosis* **10**:289, 1990.

PART 13

PORPHYRINS

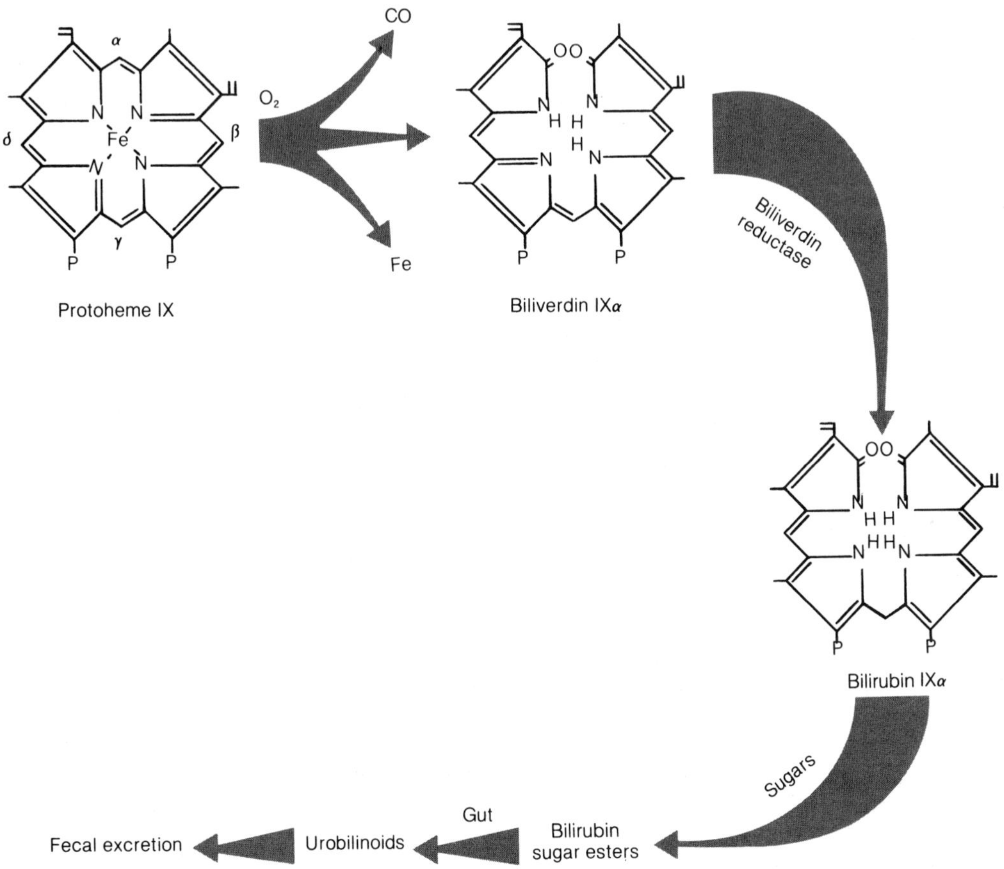

Protoheme IX

O_2

CO

Fe

Biliverdin IXα

Biliverdin reductase

Bilirubin IXα

Sugars

Bilirubin sugar esters

Gut

Urobilinoids

Fecal excretion

Heme metabolism

CHAPTER 124

Disorders of Heme Biosynthesis: X-Linked Sideroblastic Anemia and the Porphyrias

Karl E. Anderson ▪ Shigeru Sassa
David F. Bishop ▪ Robert J. Desnick

1. **X-linked sideroblastic anemia (XLSA) and the porphyrias are inherited metabolic disorders resulting from the decreased activities of specific enzymes in the heme biosynthetic pathway. Porphyrias are classified as "hepatic" or "erythroid," reflecting the predominant accumulation site of metabolic intermediates, and as "acute" or "cutaneous" depending on the major clinical features (Table 124-1). In addition to the underlying enzymatic defect, the clinical severity of the hepatic porphyrias is greatly influenced by environmental and endogenous factors, including drugs, hormones and diet, while disease severity in the erythropoietic disorders depends primarily on the specific mutation(s).**
2. **XLSA is an X-linked recessive disorder due to deficient activity of erythroid-specific 5-aminolevulinic acid synthase (ALAS2), the first enzyme in the pathway. Reduced heme synthesis stimulates erythropoiesis, which is ineffective, increasing erythron iron turnover and causing nonferritin iron accumulation in the mitochondria that surround proerythroblast nuclei, giving rise to the characteristic ring sideroblasts. Clinical onset is variable, usually occurring in the second or third decade of life, although later-onset forms can result from milder mutations. The defective enzyme and associated anemia is typically pyridoxine-responsive, but responsiveness can be impaired by significant iron accumulation.**
3. **5-Aminolevulinic acid dehydratase porphyria (ADP), an autosomal recessive hepatic disorder, results from the deficient activity of 5-aminolevulinic acid dehydratase (ALAD), the second enzyme in the pathway. In the few reported cases, clinical manifestations were primarily neurologic, without cutaneous photosensitivity.**
4. **Acute intermittent porphyria (AIP), the most common acute hepatic porphyria, is an autosomal dominant disorder resulting from the half-normal activity of porphobilinogen deaminase (PBGD, also known as hydroxymethylbilane synthase). Although most carriers (>80 percent) do not develop symptoms, other carriers have neurologic manifestations that are usually intermittent, but no cutaneous photosensitivity. Symptoms usually develop after puberty, are more frequent in women than in men, and are often exacerbated by certain sex steroids, drugs, and diet that induce the housekeeping form of 5-aminolevulinic acid synthase (ALAS1) in the liver, causing increased synthesis of heme pathway intermediates. Neurologic manifestations, which are poorly understood, may result from excess intermediates or from heme deficiency in the nervous system. Glucose and heme administration decreases ALAS1 activity and provides effective therapy.**
5. **Congenital erythropoietic porphyria (CEP), an autosomal recessive disorder, results from the markedly deficient activity of uroporphyrinogen III synthase (UROS, also known as uroporphyrinogen III cosynthase). Clinical**

A list of standard abbreviations is located immediately preceding the index in each volume. Additional abbreviations used in this chapter include: *ABC7* = ATP-binding cassette transporter gene 7; ADP = 5-aminolevulinic acid dehydratase-deficient porphyria; AIA = 2-allyl-2-isopropylacetamide; AIP = acute intermittent porphyria; ALAD = 5-aminolevulinic acid dehydratase (also known as δ-aminolevulinic acid dehydratase); *ALAD* = 5-aminolevulinic acid dehydratase gene; ALA = 5-aminolevulinic acid (also known as δ-aminolevulinic acid); ALAS = 5-aminolevulinic acid synthase (also known as δ-aminolevulinic acid synthase); ALAS1 = housekeeping 5-aminolevulinic acid synthase; *ALAS1* = housekeeping 5-aminolevulinic acid synthase gene; ALAS2 = erythroid-specific 5-aminolevulinic acid synthase; *ALAS2* = erythroid-specific 5-aminolevulinic acid synthase gene; CEP = congenital erythropoietic porphyria; CPO = coproporphyrinogen oxidase; *CPO* = coproporphyrinogen oxidase gene; DDC = 3,5-diethoxycarbonyl-1,4-dihydrocollidine; DFO = deferoxamine (desferrioxamine); DMSO = dimethylsulfoxide; ECR = erythroid control region; EPP = erythropoietic protoporphyria; GABA = γ-aminobutyric acid; GnRH = gonadotropin-releasing hormone; GATA-1 = erythroid-specific transcription factor-1; HCP = hereditary coproporphyria; HEP = hepatoerythropoietic porphyria; *HFE* = hereditary hemochromatosis gene; HH = hereditary hemochromatosis; HRM = heme regulatory motif; INH = isonicotinic acid hydrazide; IRE = iron-response element; IRP1 = IRE binding protein 1; IRP2 = IRE binding protein 2; kDa = kilodalton; MEL = murine erythroleukemia; NF = nuclear factor; PBG = porphobilinogen; PBGD = porphobilinogen deaminase (also known as hydroxymethylbilane synthase); *PBGD* = porphobilinogen deaminase gene; PPO = protoporphyrinogen oxidase; *PPO* = protoporphyrinogen oxidase gene; PCT = porphyria cutanea tarda; PLP = pyridoxal 5′-phosphate; SIADH = syndrome of inappropriate antidiuretic hormone secretion; RARS = refractory anemia with ring sideroblasts; RDW = red cell distribution width; TCDD = 2,3,7,8-tetrachlorodibenzo-p-dioxin; TdT = terminal deoxynucleotidyl transferase; UROD = uroporphyrinogen decarboxylase; *UROD* = uroporphyrinogen decarboxylase gene; UROS = uroporphyrinogen III synthase (also known as uroporphyrinogen III cosynthase); *UROS* = uroporphyrinogen III synthase gene; VP = variegate porphyria; XLSA = X-linked sideroblastic anemia.

Table 124-1 Classification of the Human Porphyrias Associated with Deficiencies of Specific Enzymes of the Heme Biosynthetic Pathway

Porphyria	Deficient enzyme	Classification	Inheritance[†]	Principal symptomatology	Biochemical Findings*		
					Erythrocytes	Urine	Stool
5-Aminolevulinate dehydratase-deficient porphyria (ADP)	5-Aminolevulinate dehydratase (ALAD)	Hepatic[‡]	AR	Neurovisceral	Zn-protoporphyrin	ALA, coproporphyrin	
Acute intermittent porphyria(AIP)	Porphobilinogen deaminase (PBGD)	Hepatic	AD	Neurovisceral		ALA, PBG, uroprphyrin	
Congenital erythropoietic porphyria (CEP)	Uroporphyrinogen III synthase (UROS)	Erythropoietic	AR	Cutaneous photosensitivity	Uroporphyrin I; coproporphyrin I	Uroporphyrin I; Coproporphyrin I	Coproporphyrin I[§]
Porphyria cutanea tarda (PCT)	Uroporphyrinogen decarboxylase (UROD)	Hepatic	AD[¶]	Cutaneous photosensitivity		Uroporphyrin, Heptacarboxyl-porphyrin	Isocoproporphyrin
Hepatoerythropoietic porphyria (HEP)	Uroporphyrinogen decarboxylase (UROD)	Hepatic[‡]	AR	Cutaneous photosensitivity	Zn-protoporphrin	Uroporphyrin, Heptacarboxyl-porphyrin	Isocoproporphyrin
Hereditary coproporphyria (HCP)	Coproporphyrinogen oxidase (CPO)	Hepatic	AD	Neurovisceral & occasional cutaneous photosensitivity		ALA, PBG, coproporphyrin	
Variegate porphyria (VP)	Protoporphyrinogen oxidase (PPO)	Hepatic	AD	Neurovisceral & cutaneous photosensitivity		ALA, PBG, coproporphyrin	Coproporphyrin; protoporphyrin
Erythropoietic protoporphyria (EPP)	Ferrochelatase	Erythropoietic	AD	Cutaneous photosensitivity	Free protoporphyrin		Protoporphyrin

*Only major increases are listed.
†AR = Autosomal recessive; AD = Autosomal dominant.
‡These porphyrias also have erythropoietic features including increased erythrocyte porphyrins.
§Type Isomers; ALA = 5′-aminolevulinic acid; PBG = porphobilinogen.
¶Inherited deficiency of UROD is partially responsible for familial (type II) PCT.

severity can range from nonimmune hydrops *in utero* to transfusion-dependent anemia with severe photosensitivity in early childhood and to relatively mild cutaneous photosensitivity in adults. Skin lesions may become infected leading to scarring and deformities. Chronic transfusions for anemia will reduce erythropoiesis and porphyrin accumulation, whereas bone marrow transplantation can be curative.

6. **Porphyria cutanea tarda (PCT), the most common porphyria, results from the decreased activity of uroporphyrinogen decarboxylase (UROD). The clinically indistinguishable subtypes include type 1 (sporadic, most common), type 2 (familial, autosomal dominant), and type 3 (familial, very rare). Only type 2 results from inherited systemic UROD deficiency. In the other types, UROD activity is inhibited or inactivated only in the liver. Factors that can precipitate all subtypes include excess hepatic iron, ethanol use, hepatitis C, HIV infection, estrogen administration, and induction of cytochrome P450 enzymes, as occurs in smokers. Hemochromatosis (*HFE*) gene mutations also may predispose to PCT. All subtypes respond to repeated phlebotomy or low-dose chloroquine or hydroxychloroquine. Hepatoerythropoietic porphyria (HEP) is an autosomal recessive disease resulting from the marked systemic deficiency of UROD, and clinically resembles CEP with hemolysis, anemia, increased erythrocyte porphyrins, and cutaneous photosensitivity, usually from birth.**
7. **Hereditary coproporphyria (HCP) is an autosomal dominant hepatic porphyria resulting from the half-normal activity of coproporphyrinogen oxidase (CPO). The clinical features, precipitating factors, and treatment are essentially identical to those of AIP. Occasional skin photosensitivity occurs.**
8. **Variegate porphyria (VP) is an autosomal dominant hepatic porphyria due to the half-normal activity of protoporphyrinogen oxidase (PPO). The clinical features, precipitating factors, and treatment are similar to those of AIP. Photosensitivity is more common than in HCP. The skin lesions are readily confused with PCT and do not respond to phlebotomy or chloroquine. A founder mutation is responsible for its high prevalence in South Africa.**
9. **Erythropoietic protoporphyria (EPP) is an autosomal dominant disorder due to the decreased activity of ferrochelatase. EPP is characterized by high levels of protoporphyrin in erythrocytes, bone marrow, and plasma, and mild to moderate cutaneous photosensitivity. Skin redness and swelling commonly occur after sunlight exposure, in contrast to the chronic, blistering lesions that characterize other cutaneous porphyrias. *β*-Carotene, and especially avoidance of sunlight, are important for prevention of cutaneous symptoms. Hepatic failure, sometimes associated with severe blistering and motor neuropathy, is an uncommon complication and may require liver transplantation.**
10. **Genotype/phenotype correlations have been established for certain porphyrias, each having a variety of severe to mild mutations. Rare homozygous autosomal dominant porphyrias have been described. "Dual porphyria" results from simultaneous occurrence of two porphyrias.**
11. **Treatment and genetic counseling depend on accurate diagnosis. Initial diagnostic screening for symptomatic acute porphyrias should include urinary porphyrin precursors (5-aminolevulinic acid and porphobilinogen) and plasma total porphyrins for cutaneous porphyrias. Enzyme assays and DNA analyses are useful for diagnostic confirmation, detection of asymptomatic individuals, and genetic counseling.**

THE HEME BIOSYNTHETIC PATHWAY

Heme is a key constituent of the cellular hemoproteins that carry out such important functions as the transport and storage of oxygen (e.g., hemoglobin, myoglobin), electron transport (e.g., respiratory cytochromes), and oxidation-reduction reactions (e.g., the cytochrome P450 enzymes). The bone marrow and liver are the major sites for heme synthesis, where heme is utilized primarily for synthesis of hemoglobin and cytochrome P450 enzymes, respectively. Because heme is also required for other important cellular hemoproteins, such as catalase, peroxidase, tryptophan pyrrolase, prostaglandin endoperoxide synthase, indoleamine 2,3-dioxygenase, and guanylate cyclase, heme is synthesized in most, if not all, cells.

Enzymes and Intermediates of the Heme Biosynthetic Pathway

The heme biosynthetic pathway consists of eight enzymes that sequentially convert glycine and succinyl CoA to heme (Fig. 124-1). The first and last three enzymes are found in mitochondria and the others in the cytosol. All of these enzymes are encoded by nuclear genes, and their full-length human cDNA and genomic sequences have been isolated and characterized, and their respective chromosomal locations established (Table 124-2). Both erythroid-specific and non-erythroid or "housekeeping" transcripts have been identified for each of the first four enzymes in the pathway. Erythroid-specific and housekeeping transcripts for ALAS are encoded by separate genes on different chromosomes, whereas erythroid and housekeeping transcripts for ALAD, PBGD, and UROS are each transcribed from the same gene.

5-Aminolevulinic acid synthase (ALAS), the first enzyme in the pathway, catalyzes the condensation of glycine and succinyl coenzyme A to form 5-aminolevulinic acid (ALA), which is exclusively committed to the synthesis of heme (Fig. 124-1). ALAS is encoded by two nuclear genes, a housekeeping gene (*ALAS1*) expressed in all cells, and an erythroid-specific gene (*ALAS2*) expressed only in fetal liver and adult bone marrow. They are located in mitochondria where succinyl coenzyme A (CoA) is produced by the tricarboxylic acid cycle. ALAD then catalyzes the condensation of two molecules of ALA to form the monopyrrole porphobilinogen (PBG). The third enzyme, PBGD, catalyzes the stepwise condensation of four molecules of PBG to form hydroxymethylbilane (HMB), a linear tetrapyrrole. UROS, the fourth enzyme, is responsible for an intramolecular rearrangement and ring closure of HMB to form uroporphyrinogen III, a cyclic tetrapyrrole with eight carboxyl side chains. UROD and then CPO catalyze the stepwise decarboxylation of uroporphyrinogen III to form protoporphyrinogen IX, which has two carboxyl side chains, and is then oxidized to protoporphyrin IX by the seventh enzyme, PPO. The final enzymatic step in heme synthesis is the insertion of iron by the enzyme ferrochelatase. Each of the enzymes and their respective deficiency diseases are described in subsequent sections.

Porphyrinogens and Porphyrins

The nomenclature for porphyrins proposed by Hans Fischer[1] is used in this chapter and in the literature. Nomenclature revisions have been recommended by the International Union of Pure and Applied Chemistry (IUPAC) and the International Union of Biochemistry (IUB).[2] Fig. 124-2 shows the structure and nomenclature of the porphyrin macrocycle, and Table 124-3 compares the Fischer and the IUPAC-IUB nomenclatures. All of the cyclic tetrapyrrole intermediates of the heme biosynthetic pathway, with the exception of protoporphyrin IX, the last intermediate, are porphyrinogens, which are reduced forms that are rapidly oxidized to porphyrins when exposed to air with loss of six protons (Fig. 124-3). The porphyrin isomers differ by the

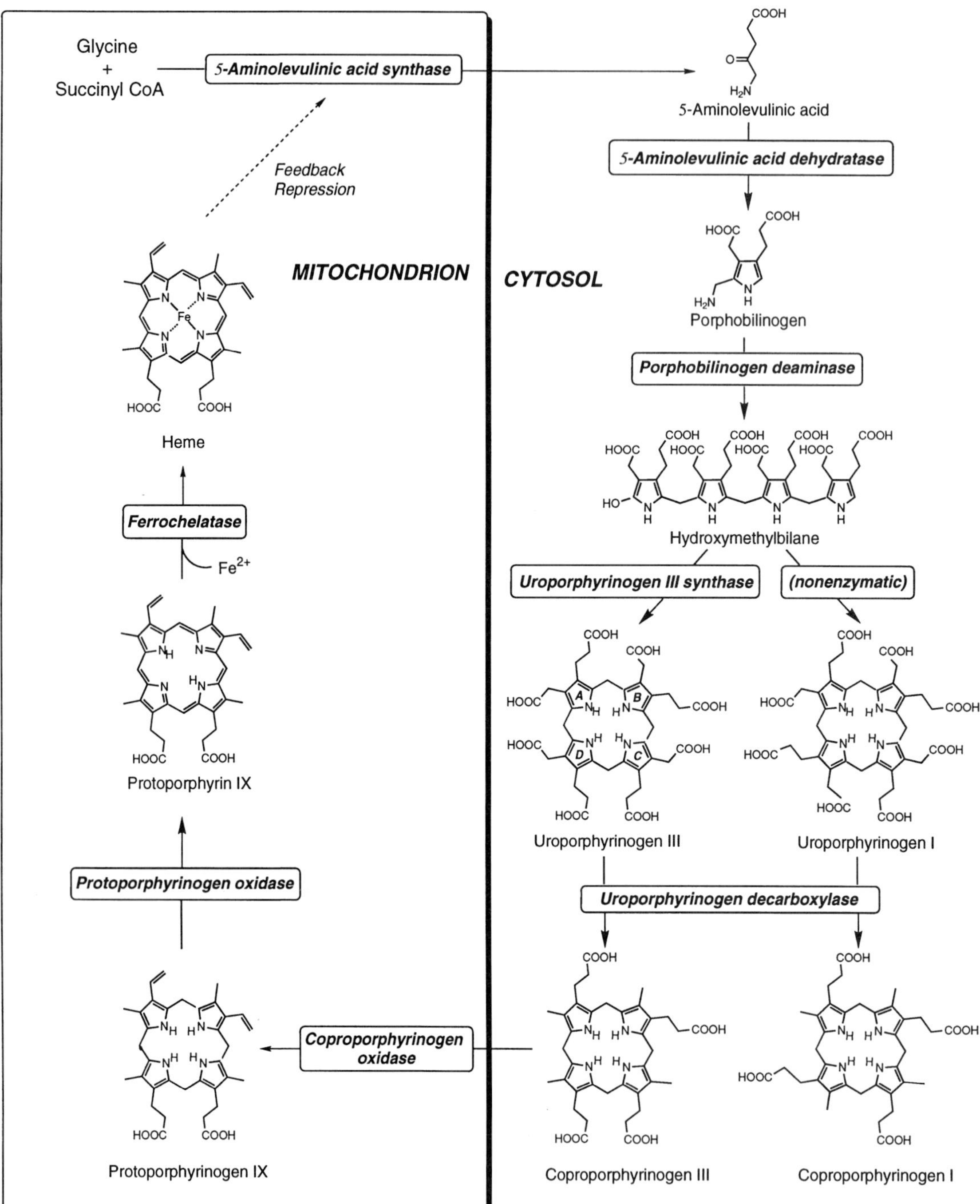

Fig. 124-1 The heme biosynthetic pathway. The pathway consists of eight enzymes, four localized in mitochondria and four in the cytosol. Only the type III isomers of uroporphyrinogen and coproporphyrinogen are metabolized to heme. Heme is exported from mitochondria for incorporation into cellular hemoproteins and, particularly in liver, exerts feedback regulation on 5-aminolevulinic acid synthase.

arrangement of the side chain substituents. The structures of uroporphyrins I, II, III, and IV are shown in Fig. 124-4, and the substituents of additional biologically important porphyrins and their isomers are listed in Table 124-3.

Porphyrins emit intense red fluorescence when exposed to light at around 400 nm. When dissolved in acid they display two strong emission bands, one at 600 to 610 nm and the other at 640 to 660 nm. Thus, spectrofluorometric methods provide very sensitive detection and quantitation of porphyrins. Heme (Fe-protoporphyrin IX) and porphyrins chelated to other paramagnetic metals (e.g., Mn, Co) do not fluoresce, whereas porphyrin chelates of diamagnetic metals (e.g., Zn, Sn, Mg) are fluorescent. Porphyrins or metalloporphyrins that lack fluorescence can be measured by their characteristic absorbance properties. All porphyrins display an absorption spectrum consisting of a major band near 400 nm, called the Soret band, and four smaller absorption bands between 500 nm and 630 nm, with decreasing intensity toward the red wavelengths.[3]

Water solubility of porphyrins is favored by the presence of carboxylic acid side chains. Uroporphyrin (an octacarboxyl porphyrin) is the most water-soluble of the porphyrins derived from the heme biosynthetic pathway, and protoporphyrin (a dicarboxyl porphyrin) the least soluble. Routes of excretion are determined in part by the degree of porphyrin solubility in water. Uroporphyrin is excreted predominantly in urine and coproporphyrin (a tetracarboxyl porphyrin) mostly in urine but partly in

Table 124-2 Human Heme Biosynthesis Enzymes and Genes

				Genome	
Enzyme	**Gene symbol**	**Chromosomal location**	**cDNA (bp) protein (aa)**	**Size (kb)**	**Organization***
5-Aminolevulinate synthase:					
Housekeeping	*ALAS1*	3p21.1	2199 bp/640 aa	17 kb	11 exons
Erythroid-specific	*ALAS2*	Xp11.21	1937 bp/587 aa	22 kb	11 exons
5-Aminolevulinate dehydratase:	*ALAD*	9q34			13 exons
Housekeeping			1149 bp/330 aa	15.9 kb	Exons 1A + 2–12
Erythroid-specific			1154 bp/330 aa		Exons 1B + 2–12
Porphobilinogen deaminase:	*PBGD*	11q23.3		11 kb	15 exons
Housekeeping			1086 bp/361 aa		Exons 1 + 3–15
Erythroid-specific			1035 bp/344 aa		Exons 2–15
Uroporphyrinogen III synthase:	*UROS*	10q25.2 → q26.3		34 kb	10 exons
Housekeeping			1296 bp/265 aa		Exons 1 + 2B–10
Erythroid-specific			1216 bp/265 aa		Exons 2A + 2B–10
Uroporphyrinogen decarboxylase	*UROD*	1p34	1104 bp/367 aa	3 kb	10 exons
Corproporphyrinogen oxidase	*CPO*	3q12	1062 bp/354 aa	14 kb	7 exons
Protoporphyrinogen oxidase	*PPO*	1q23	1431 bp/477 aa	5.5 kb	13 exons
Ferrochelatase	*FECH*	18q21.3	1269 bp/423 aa	45 kb	11 exons

*Number of exons and those encoding housekeeping and erythroid-specific forms.

bile, whereas protoporphyrin is so hydrophobic that it is excreted only in bile.

Regulation of Heme Biosynthesis

Tissues that make heme in the largest amounts are the bone marrow and liver. ALA is the first intermediate in the heme biosynthetic pathway exclusively committed to heme synthesis, and the rate of ALA synthesis is an important controlling step for heme formation, especially in the liver. Heme biosynthesis in the liver and erythroid cells is regulated in part by separate housekeeping and erythroid-specific genes that encode ALAS isozymes ALAS1 and ALAS2, respectively. The bulk of heme produced in bone marrow is used for hemoglobin formation. Of the ALA and heme produced in rat liver, as much as 65 percent is utilized for the formation of the microsomal cytochrome P450 enzymes, about 15 percent for the synthesis of catalase, which is localized in peroxisomes, 6 percent for the formation of mitochondrial cytochromes, and 8 percent for the formation of cytochrome b_5.[4] Bilirubin, which is derived exclusively from heme breakdown, is normally produced in humans at a rate of approximately 5 to 8 μmol bilirubin/kg body weight/day.[5] Liver cells make about 15 percent of the heme that is synthesized in the body.[6] Thus, under normal conditions, approximately 54 mg of ALA per day is required for hepatic heme synthesis. For comparison, heme formation in bone marrow for hemoglobin synthesis requires approximately 304 mg of ALA per day. However, during an acute attack of the hepatic porphyrias, such as AIP, ALAS1 is markedly induced, and the liver may form as much ALA as does the normal bone marrow.

ALAS1 Controls Hepatic Heme Biosynthesis. In the liver, ALAS1 has many features of a rate-limiting enzyme in the production of heme under a variety of conditions.[7,8] ALAS1 activity in normal liver is the lowest (30 to 100 nmol ALA/h/g liver in mice)[9] among all enzymes in the heme biosynthetic pathway. The activity of PBGD, the third enzyme in the pathway, is close to that of ALAS1 (35 to 60 nmol PBG/h/g liver in mice, which is equivalent to 70 to 120 nmol ALA/h/g).[9] Under conditions of ALAS1 induction and increased ALA production, such as in an acute attack of AIP, HCP, or VP, PBGD can become a rate-limiting metabolic step. This and the half-normal level of PBGD would account for the especially marked increases in ALA

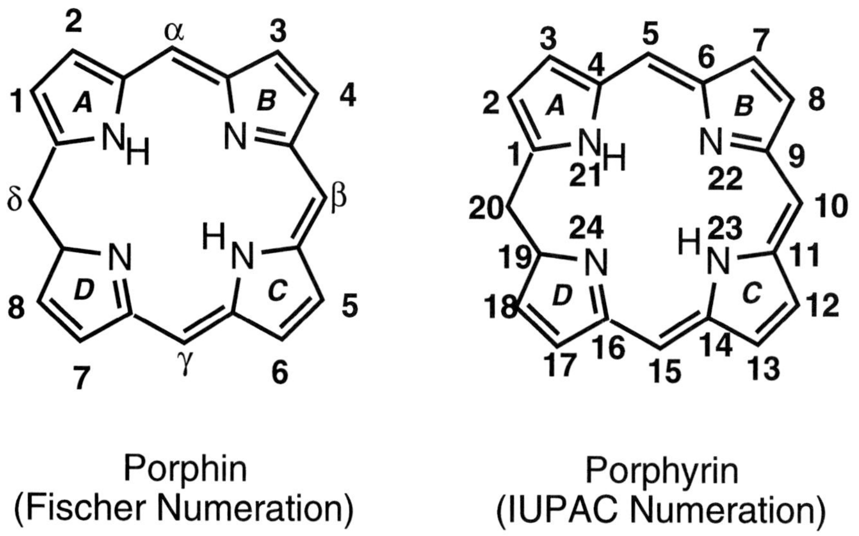

Porphin (Fischer Numeration)

Porphyrin (IUPAC Numeration)

Fig. 124-2 Structure and nomenclatures of the porphyrin macrocycle. The *porphin* (Fischer) and more recently proposed *porphyrin* (IUPAC-"1-24") nomenclatures portray the basic structure of naturally occurring ring tetrapyrroles, and differ in the numeration of the carbon and nitrogen atoms (shown in bold).

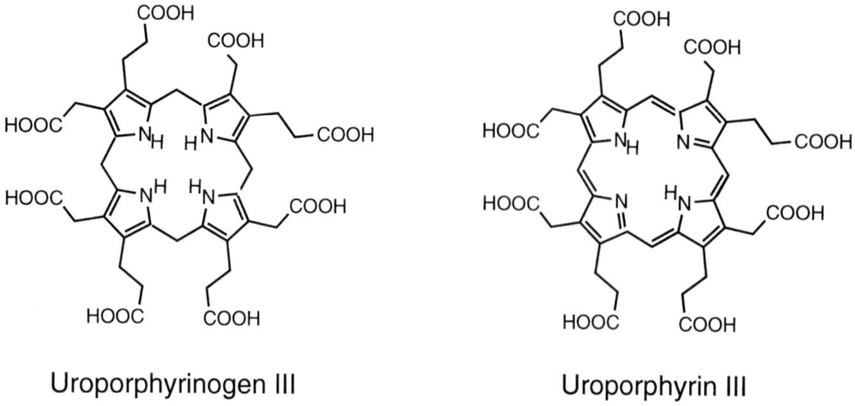

Uroporphyrinogen III

Uroporphyrin III

Fig. 124-3 Chemical structures of a typical porphyrinogen (uroporphyrinogen III) and the corresponding porphyrin (uroporphyrin III). The porphyrinogen is the reduced form of the porphyrin and is oxidized to the porphyrin with loss of six protons.

and PBG that are produced and excreted in AIP. Ferrochelatase also has a somewhat low hepatic activity (0.4 nmol/min of heme/mg mitochondria protein in rat liver, or ~1200 nmol of heme/h/g liver).[10] However, because this activity is much higher than that of ALAS1 and PBGD, it rarely is rate limiting in the liver. Activities of other enzymes in the pathway greatly exceed the activities of ALAS1, PBGD, and ferrochelatase.[11]

Second, the rate of ALAS1 turnover is very rapid, a property appropriate for an enzyme catalyzing a rate-limiting reaction. The half-life of ALAS1 in rat liver is approximately 70 min,[12] and 3 h in mouse liver and in cultured chick embryo liver cells.[13,14] The half-life of mitochondrial ALAS1 is among the shortest of all mitochondrial proteins, which generally turn over with a half-life of approximately 5 days.

Third, basal or uninduced hepatic ALAS1 provides sufficient ALA and heme to maintain normal levels of liver hemoproteins, but when the synthesis of the cytochrome P450 enzymes is induced and more heme synthesis is required, ALAS1 is induced, which strongly suggests a rate-limiting role. Hepatic ALAS1 induction also results in the accumulation of porphyrin precursors or porphyrins. Experimental porphyrias, for example, are accompanied by hepatic ALAS1 induction and increased excretion of porphyrins, and sometimes by ALA and PBG. During attacks of AIP and other acute porphyrias, hepatic ALAS1 activity is elevated at least several-fold and is accompanied by overproduction and excretion of ALA, PBG, and porphyrins. Thus, under many conditions, the excess accumulation of heme biosynthetic intermediates is accompanied by the induction of ALAS1. Finally, the effects of experimental ALA loading suggest that the formation of ALA is a rate-limiting step. For example, administration of ALA to rats and mice results in increased heme formation in liver, as evidenced by induction of heme oxygenase,[15]

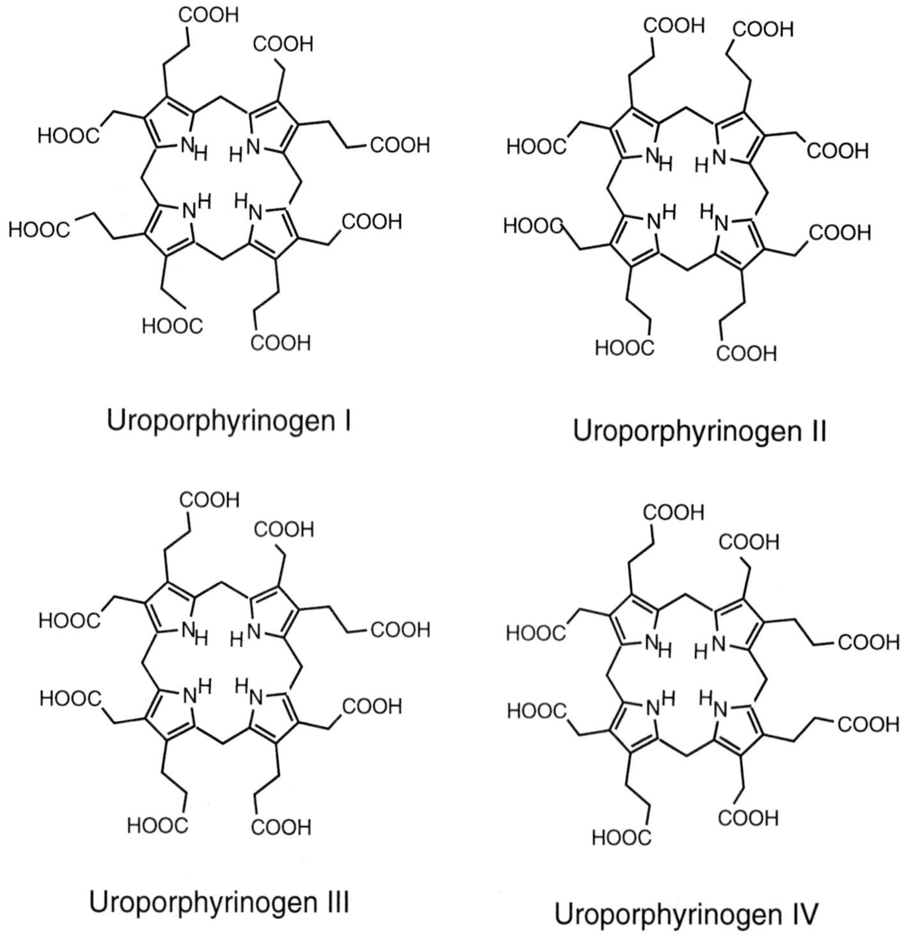

Uroporphyrinogen I

Uroporphyrinogen II

Uroporphyrinogen III

Uroporphyrinogen IV

Fig. 124-4 The four isomers of uroporphyrinogen. Only isomers I and III are synthesized enzymatically in biologic systems, and only isomer III can ultimately proceed to form heme.

Table 124-3 Structures and Trivial Names of Porphyrins

Name	Substituent							
IUPAC numeration:	**2**	**3**	**7**	**8**	**12**	**13**	**17**	**18**
Fischer numeration:	**1**	**2**	**3**	**4**	**5**	**6**	**7**	**8**
Etioporphyrin I	M	E	M	E	M	E	M	E
Etioporphyrin II	M	E	E	M	M	E	E	M
Etioporphyrin III	M	E	M	E	M	E	E	M
Etioporphyrin IV	M	E	E	M	E	M	M	E
Uroporphyrin I	A	P	A	P	A	P	A	P
Uroporphyrin III	A	P	A	P	A	P	P	A
Heptacarboxyl porphyrin III	M	P	A	P	A	P	P	A
Hexacarboxyl porphyrin III	M	P	M	P	A	P	P	A
Pentacarboxyl porphyrin III	M	P	M	P	A	P	P	M
Dehydroisocoproporphyrin III	M	V	M	P	A	P	P	M
Coproporphyrin I	M	P	M	P	M	P	M	P
Coproporphyrin III	M	P	M	P	M	P	P	M
Protoporphyrin IX	M	V	M	V	M	P	P	M
Mesoporphyrin IX	M	E	M	E	M	P	P	M
Hematoporphyrin IX	M	HE	M	HE	M	P	P	M
Deuteroporphyrin IX	M	H	M	H	M	P	P	M

M = $-CH_3$; E = $-C_2H_5$; A = $-CH_2COOH$; P = $-CH_2CH_2COOH$; V = $-CH{=}CH_2$; HE = $-CHOHCH_3$

increased bilirubin production,[16] and, ultimately, in the repression of ALAS1 activity.[17,18] Together, these observations suggest that ALA is readily converted to heme and bilirubin in liver, and that the remaining enzymes in the heme biosynthetic and catabolic pathways are in excess compared to the rate-limiting activity of hepatic ALAS1.

Effect of Heme on Hepatic Heme Biosynthesis. Heme exerts multiple regulatory effects on hepatic heme biosynthesis (Fig. 124-5). Heme inhibits ALAS1 synthesis at both transcriptional and translational steps as well as its transfer from cytosol into mitochondria, but does not significantly inhibit its catalytic activity in vivo. Intracellular heme concentration can be altered by intravenous heme administration or by heme treatment of cells in vitro. Direct inhibition of ALAS1 activity by hemin ($K_i = 2 \times 10^{-5}$ M)[19] does not appear to be a physiologically significant process because ALAS1 synthesis in liver is suppressed at substantially lower heme concentrations. Complete repression of ALAS1 in cultured chick embryo liver cells maintained in a serum-free medium, for example, takes place at a hemin concentration of 10^{-7} M.[20,21] The K_i, that is, the concentration of hemin which reduces the rate of ALAS1 synthesis by half, was $1 - 2 \times 10^{-8}$ M[22,23] under these conditions (Fig. 124-5). It was also shown that heme generated in mitochondria was not sufficient to inhibit ALAS1 activity[24].

Several heme-binding proteins in the cytosol of liver and intestinal cells facilitate heme uptake. Heme-binding proteins in the cytosol may also facilitate efflux of newly synthesized heme from mitochondria. Heme efflux is also inversely related to mitochondrial energy levels.[25] In liver cell cultures treated with hemin, ALAS1 decays with a half-life of approximately 3 h; a similar half-life was determined by the use of inhibitors of protein synthesis.[14] Findings in cultured avian embryonic liver cells suggest that hemin may repress the synthesis of the mRNA for ALAS1,[26] shorten the life span of the messenger RNA for ALAS1, or interfere specifically with the synthesis of ALAS1 at the posttranscriptional level (Fig. 124-5).[14,27] A conserved motif, termed the heme regulatory motif (HRM), is present in the presequence of both the ALAS1 and ALAS2 precursors, and has been shown to be involved in hemin inhibition of transport of these enzymes into mouse mitochondria in vitro.[28,29] The effect of hemin on the HRM-mediated inhibition of enzyme transfer appears stronger for ALAS1 than for ALAS2.[29]

The regulatory role of heme with respect to its own biosynthesis and catabolism can be best explained by assuming the existence of one or more "free" heme pools, as outlined in the hypothetical scheme shown in Fig. 124-5. Free heme can be considered as heme that is either synthesized very recently and not yet bound as the prosthetic group of specific hemoproteins, or possibly heme that has just been released from hemoproteins. Free heme pools probably exist in mitochondria, cytosol, and the endoplasmic reticulum. All free heme pools are presumed to be very small and probably turn over very rapidly. For example, almost all the heme in hepatic microsomes can be accounted for by heme contained in cytochrome P450 enzymes and cytochrome b_5. Although the existence of free heme pools remains hypothetical, there is good evidence to suggest that rapidly synthesized free heme pools exist as functional entities in liver cells.[30,31]

Free heme pools may affect heme biosynthesis and catabolism in a number of ways. First, free heme in mitochondria may regulate the rate of synthesis of cytochrome oxidase. Second, cytosolic free heme may repress the rate of synthesis of ALAS1 (Fig. 124-5). Because this heme fraction plays a critically important role in heme biosynthesis, it can be considered as a "regulatory" heme pool. Third, microsomal free heme may regulate the activity of heme oxygenase in addition to serving as substrate for the enzyme.

Tryptophan pyrrolase, the rate-limiting enzyme for tryptophan metabolism, is a hemoprotein that may serve as a sensitive marker for cytosolic free heme because it exists as both a heme-free apoenzyme and a heme-containing holoenzyme. The amounts of the free and heme-containing enzyme forms can be determined by comparing the enzyme activity with and without adding hemin. Inhibition of heme synthesis or increased destruction or utilization of heme is believed to decrease cytosolic free heme, and will decrease the saturation of tryptophan pyrrolase. Added heme increases the saturation of tryptophan pyrrolase in a dose-dependent manner. Moreover, the relative distribution of ALAS1 in the liver cytosol and mitochondria changes significantly, and this effect correlates well with the degree of heme saturation of tryptophan pyrrolase.[20,32]

Compounds that destroy free heme or inhibit heme synthesis are generally strong inducers of ALAS1 in hepatocytes. The most marked induction of ALAS1 occurs when animals are treated with a combination of compounds that affect heme biosynthesis by separate mechanisms, such as 3,5-diethoxycarbonyl-1,4-dihydrocollidine (DDC) and phenobarbital,[33,34] or DDC and allylisopropylacetamide (AIA).[35] Induction of ALAS1 by AIA or phenobarbital, which is representative of the many drugs that exacerbate acute hepatic porphyrias, can also be potentiated by simultaneous treatment with chemicals that only partially inhibit ferrochelatase activity, such as deferoxamine (desferrioxamine, DFO),[36] CaMg EDTA,[37] or a small dose of DDC.[38,39]

Partial inhibition of heme synthesis by chelators or a small dose of DDC is analogous to the latent stages of the acute hepatic porphyrias, and treatment with an additional agent has an exacerbating effect that is biochemically similar to that observed in an acute crisis of these conditions. In latent gene carriers of AIP, half-normal PBGD activity is sufficient to maintain normal hepatic heme synthesis. However, when the liver increases heme and cytochrome P450 synthesis in response to certain drugs, such as barbiturates, the primary enzyme deficiency can become rate limiting for heme formation, resulting in a decrease in the regulatory free heme concentration. ALAS1 synthesis is then freed from heme repression and an overproduction of ALAS1 ensues.

The activity of heme oxygenase, the rate-limiting enzyme for heme degradation to bile pigment, can also influence the level of regulatory free heme in hepatocytes. Thus, mechanisms for both heme synthesis and degradation can regulate heme formation.

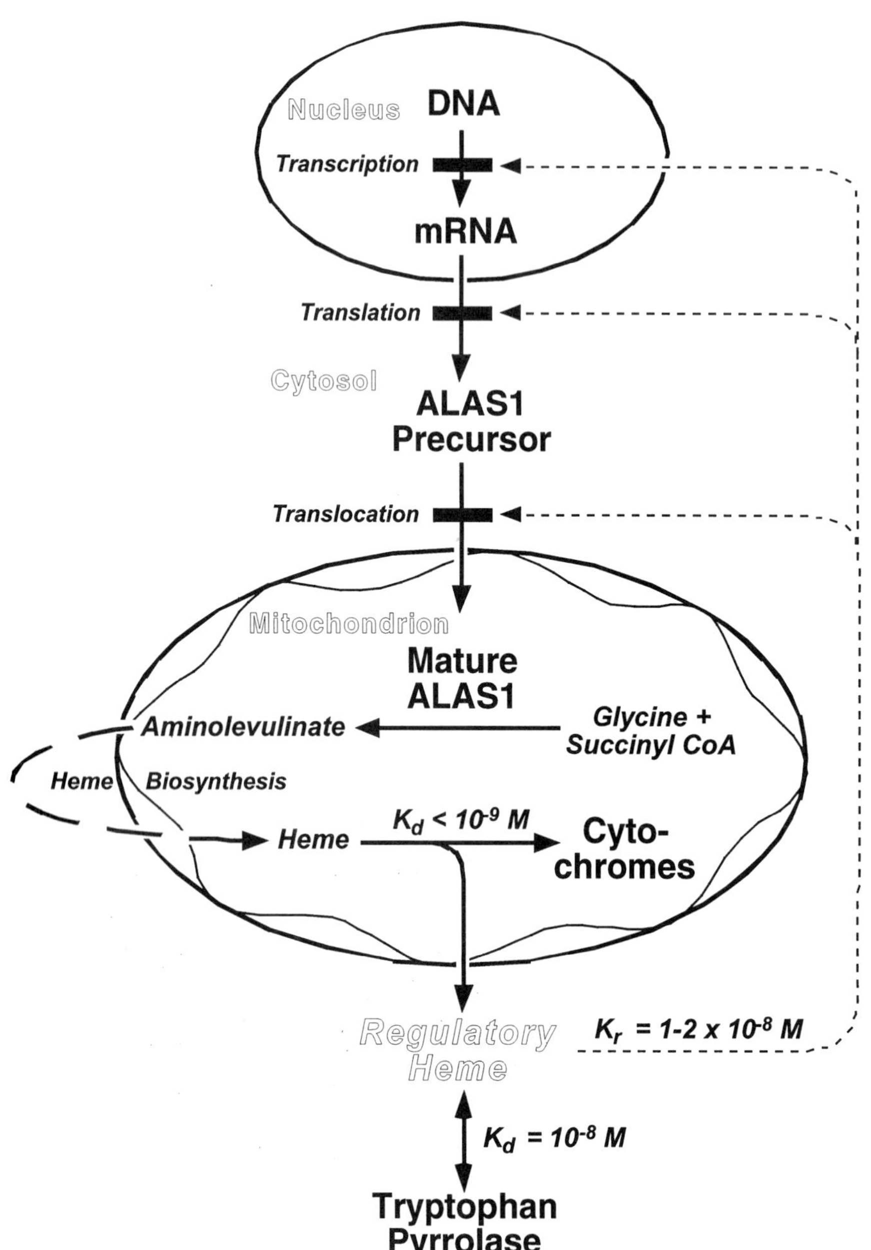

Fig. 124-5 Regulation of heme biosynthesis in liver by heme. Regulatory or "free" heme (not incorporated into hemoproteins) presumably is present in small pools in various subcellular locations and the amount of free heme is responsible for regulating the synthesis and mitochondrial translocation of ALAS1, the initial and rate-limiting enzyme in liver. ALAS1 = housekeeping form of 5-aminolevulinic acid synthase.

For example, divalent metals,[40–44] endotoxin,[17] organic chemicals,[45,46] and nutritional deprivation can stimulate the *de novo* synthesis of heme oxygenase leading to depletion of the regulatory free heme pool. Starvation leads to increased heme oxygenase activity,[47] which by depleting heme may contribute to developing a crisis in acute hepatic porphyrias.[48,49] Conversely, attacks of these disorders can be prevented by a high carbohydrate diet.[50]

Heme Synthesis in Erythroid Cells. Regulatory influences on the heme biosynthetic pathway in the erythron act during cell differentiation. Thus, in contrast to the liver, the erythron responds to stimuli for heme synthesis in part by increasing its cell numbers to meet changing requirements for hemoglobin. In the erythron, certain of the heme pathway enzymes are subject to erythroid-specific regulatory mechanisms. For example, as noted above, ALAS is regulated in a tissue-specific manner. ALAS1 is important in the liver, whereas ALAS2 is critical for heme formation in erythroid cells,[51–53] and there are differences in regulation of the synthesis of these ALAS isozymes in the erythron and the liver.[54–57] First, ALAS2 is not inducible by the drugs that induce ALAS1,[58] and is not repressed by hemin treatment. Therefore, in erythroid cells, heme biosynthesis is not regulated by feedback repression of ALAS2 synthesis by heme. The lack of heme feedback on ALAS2 is evident from studies in murine erythroleukemia (MEL) cells, human erythroleukemia (K562), and normal bone marrow colonies in vitro. For example, when MEL cells are treated with dimethylsulfoxide (DMSO), or a variety of other compounds, cells increase their heme content and ALAS2 levels.[51,59] Unlike the liver, the stimulation of heme synthesis in erythroid cells is accompanied not only by increases in ALAS, but also by induction of other heme biosynthetic enzymes.[56,60] Heme also exerts a strong positive role in hemoglobin formation. Although hemin treatment has been reported to suppress ALAS2 synthesis in human reticulocytes,[61] hemin treatment of MEL cells not only increases synthesis of hemoglobin,[62,63] but also increases levels of ALAS2, ALAD, PBGD, and ^{59}Fe incorporation into heme.[60,64] Increases in ALAS2 activity in response to hemin in MEL cells are in striking contrast to effects in the liver, where hemin treatment suppresses the synthesis of ALAS1. Hemin-mediated induction of the heme pathway enzymes, including ALAS2, has also been reported in human K562 erythroleukemia cells.[65] Hemin, but not ALA, stimulates hemoglobin formation in normal mouse bone marrow cultures.[66] In addition, hemin-mediated induction of ALAS2 in MEL cells occurs both at transcriptional[51] and translational levels.[67,68]

Ferrochelatase, the final enzyme of heme biosynthesis, may also play a significant role in controlling the rate of heme formation in erythroid cells. First, hemin, but not its precursors, such as ALA, PBG, and protoporphyrin, can increase hemoglobin content in undifferentiated MEL cells.[62–64] Second, a mutant MEL cell line that can induce (with DMSO) ALAS1, ALAD, and PBGD, but fails to make hemoglobin, can be corrected by the addition of DMSO plus hemin.[54,55] Third, ferrochelatase deficiency in human protoporphyria results in the accumulation of protoporphyrin almost exclusively in erythroid tissue, even though ferrochelatase is deficient in all other tissues in these patients. This clinical finding suggests that ferrochelatase activity can become rate limiting in erythroid cells, but not in other tissues, when the enzyme is partially deficient. Although protoporphyrin accumulates in the liver in some patients with EPP and in a murine model of the disease, the protoporphyrin presumably originated in the bone marrow.[69]

Heme Synthesis in Nonerythroid Cells. Regulation of heme biosynthesis in other tissues and cell types remains largely unknown, but may be significantly different from that in the liver and erythroid cells. For example, potent inducers of ALAS1 in liver do not increase ALAS activity in the Harderian gland of mice;[70] in the heart,[71] adrenal glands,[72] testes,[73] brain,[74] or spleen[58] of the rat; or in cultured human amniotic cells.[75] On the other hand, certain hormones increase ALAS activity in specific nonhepatic target tissues. For example, adrenocorticotropic hormone increases ALAS activity in the adrenal gland,[72] human chronic gonadotrophin increases the enzyme activity in the testes,[73] and erythropoietin increases ALAS activity in the spleen.[58] A recent study showed that ALAS1 mRNA in the rat Harderian gland is not inducible by AIA, a potent inducer of ALAS1 in the liver.[76]

The effect of hemin on ALAS activity in these nonhepatic tissues also differs from that in liver. Hemin does not suppress ALAS in mouse Harderian gland,[70] or in rat heart,[71] adrenal gland,[72] or testes.[73] ALAS1 mRNA in the rat Harderian gland is refractory to hemin treatment, even though hemin induced heme oxygenase mRNA in the gland.[76] The constitutive expression of the *ALAS1* gene suggests a novel transcriptional control mechanism for this gene in the Harderian gland.

ALAS in fetal liver, which largely consists of erythroid cells, is also refractory to inhibition by hemin.[77] Moreover, changes in ALAS activity in fetal guinea pig liver are correlated with changes in erythropoietic activity.[78] Thus, regulation of ALAS in fetal liver reflects mostly that of erythroid cells.

Nonhepatic cells, such as skin fibroblasts or lymphocytes in culture obtained from patients with acute hepatic porphyrias, fully express the deficiency of the relevant heme pathway enzyme, and the degree of enzymatic deficiency in these cells is similar to that found in the liver. Cultured skin fibroblasts[79,80] or mitogen-stimulated lymphocytes[81] from patients with AIP do not show elevated ALAS activity in spite of the half-normal activity of PBGD. These findings suggest that heme deficiency in these nonhepatic cells in culture is less marked than in the liver of patients with active AIP, or that ALAS in cells from nonhepatic tissues is not controlled by the cellular free heme concentration.

Watson[82] postulated that a heme deficiency involving cytochrome P450 might develop in central nervous system tissues in acute porphyrias, leading to a decrease in the activity of cytochrome P450-associated mixed-function oxidases. Although it is not known whether such a deficiency of cytochrome P450 enzymes occurs, there is evidence that cells in the central nervous system contain these enzymes,[83] can form porphyrins from ALA,[15] and might be capable of forming heme from appropriate precursors. For example, cultured dorsal root ganglion cells from chick embryo[84] and mouse[85] can form protoporphyrin from ALA. Thus, the heme pathway enzymes, at least from ALAD to ferrochelatase, are present in these cells. Ferrochelatase activity appears to be predominant in Schwann cells rather than in neuronal cells,[84] and is subject to inhibition by potent inhibitors of heme biosynthesis such as lead.[85,86] Hemin treatment of dorsal root ganglion cells can limit the extent of the demyelination produced by lead.[87] It is possible, therefore, that neuronal cells may depend to some extent on the supply of heme or heme precursors that may be provided by surrounding nonneuronal elements, such as Schwann cells or other supporting cells. It also may be possible that a heme deficiency in central nervous system tissues can be corrected by exogenous hemin.

X-LINKED SIDEROBLASTIC ANEMIA (XLSA)

XLSA is an X-linked recessive disorder of heme biosynthesis resulting from the deficient activity of the erythroid-specific form of 5-aminolevulinate synthase (ALAS, also known as δ-aminolevulinate synthase; EC 2.3.1.37) in the mitochondria of erythroid cells in fetal liver and adult bone marrow. The resultant reduction in heme synthesis stimulates erythropoiesis, which is ineffective, increasing erythron iron turnover. Iron accumulates in the erythroid marrow because there is insufficient protoporphyrin IX for its incorporation into heme by the enzyme ferrochelatase. The excess iron in the marrow is deposited as nonferritin iron in the mitochondria that surround the nuclei of proerythroblasts, giving rise to the descriptive term ring sideroblasts—the pathologic hallmark of the disease. Increased iron absorption, stimulated by ineffective erythropoiesis, leads to progressive iron accumulation in many tissues with fatal consequences if untreated. The disorder, first recognized by Cooley in 1945,[88] typically presents in the second or third decade of life, but onset may occur in infancy or as late as the ninth decade of life.[89] XLSA is typically pyridoxine-responsive, but can be pyridoxine refractory, especially in patients with significant iron accumulation.

XLSA has also been known as congenital sideroblastic anemia, hereditary anemia, hereditary hypochromic anemia, hereditary iron-loading anemia, hereditary sideroblastic anemia, pyridoxine-responsive anemia, sideroachrestic anemia, and X-linked hypochromic anemia. It is distinct from Xq13-linked sideroblastic anemia with ataxia,[90] which is caused by mutations in the human *ABC7* iron-transporter gene.[91]

XLSA is a rare genetic disorder. Since the discovery of the gene defect,[92] about 25 different mutations have been identified. Because several of these mutations have occurred more than once, the total number of unrelated XLSA families identified to date is only approximately 35.[93,94]

Clinical Manifestations

The clinical manifestations of XLSA result from anemia due to reduced heme synthesis and cellular toxicity involving various organs due to the elevated iron levels. When anemia is severe, presenting features may include pallor, shortness of breath, fatigue, and weakness.[89,92,94–99] When the underlying *ALAS2* defect is less severe, the anemia may be adequately compensated and clinical pathology delayed until the progressive iron accumulation causes toxicity later in life. Affected females typically present a decade later than males, being partially protected from iron overload by blood loss due to menstruation. Clinically affected patients may present with hepatomegaly and/or splenomegaly,[92,95,96,99,100] cirrhosis, hepatocellular carcinoma, nausea/abdominal pain,[92,99] weight loss,[97] diabetes,[100] skin pigmentation,[100] growth delay,[95] arthropathy, body hair loss, decreased libido in males, and missed menses in females. Cardiac myopathy ranges in severity from systolic murmur[92,98] and tachycardia[92] to end-stage cardiac failure.[99,100] Iron toxicity to hormone production may result in growth delay[95] and, more

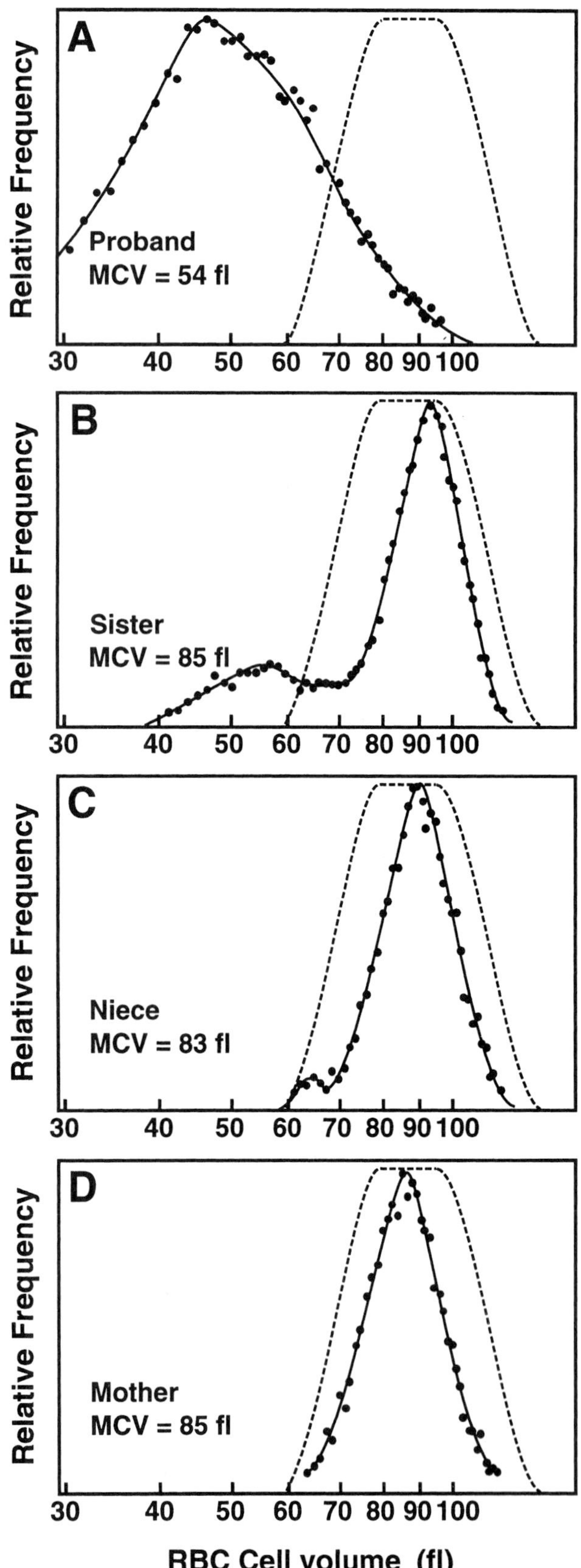

Fig. 124-6 Erythrocyte size distribution histogram for: (A) an affected male with XLSA and his heterozygous (B) sister, (C) niece, and (D) mother. The dashed line indicates the distribution of erythrocyte cell size for the normal population. (*Reproduced from Cotter et al.*[94] *Used by permission.*)

frequently, in diabetes.[100] Associated symptoms such as palpitations, fatigue, and weakness may relate to cardiac involvement and overlap with the symptoms of anemia.

The Metabolic Defect in XLSA

Biochemical Abnormalities. The major biochemical abnormalities in XLSA are decreased blood hemoglobin concentration and increased serum and tissue iron concentrations. In the XLSA patients with proven *ALAS2* mutations, the hemoglobin concentrations at presentation ranged from about 3.5 to 10 g/dl, MCV averaged 63 fl, and MCH averaged 20.3 pg. Serum ferritin ranged from 400 to 14,500 μg/dl and transferrin saturation ranged from 51 percent to 100 percent. ALAS2 enzymatic activity in erythroblasts is decreased in XLSA, but requires a bone marrow biopsy and may be normal or increased under some circumstances.[96,98]

Ringed sideroblasts are present in the marrow at levels generally greater than 15 percent. Peripheral erythrocytes are typically microcytic and hypochromic with frequent poikilocytes, including teardrop-, cigar-, and/or pencil-shaped cells, ovalocytes, and target cells. Erythrocyte-size dimorphism is frequent in males and can include both microcytes and macrocytes, but is usually strongly skewed towards microcytic cells. In female carriers, the dimorphic-size distribution can be skewed to mostly microcytes or to nearly all normalocytes due to random X inactivation. While the erythrocyte anisocytosis typically results in an abnormal red cell distribution width (RDW), the sometimes small populations of microcytic cells in heterozygotes can be missed by MCV and RDW values (see Fig. 124-6).

The Enzymatic Defect in XLSA. The enzymatic defect in XLSA is the deficient activity of ALAS2, the erythroid-specific form of ALAS. ALAS is a mitochondrial enzyme that requires pyridoxal 5′-phosphate (PLP) as cofactor and catalyzes the condensation of succinyl-CoA and glycine to form the aminoketone, ALA, and CO_2 (Fig. 124-7). PLP forms a covalent Schiff's base linkage with the active site lysine (Lys 313) in the murine erythroid enzyme[101] or Lys 391 in human ALAS2 (numbered as per SWISSPROT accession number P22557). Although the cofactor remains bound to the murine enzyme if Lys 313 is mutated, the enzyme is inactive, demonstrating participation of this amino acid in catalysis.[102] Fig. 124-7 shows a theoretic reaction mechanism based on kinetic studies of transaminases and bacterial ALAS.[103] *Trans*-aldimation between the substrate glycine and the lysyl-pyridoxal enzyme results in an external aldimine. The *pro R* proton on the α-carbon atom of the pyridoxal-activated glycine is removed, and the resulting stabilized carbanion undergoes a stereospecific nucleophilic condensation with the carbonyl of the CoA-activated succinate. An α-amino β-ketoadipic acid/enzyme adduct is formed prior to the release of CO_2 and ALA.[103]

Erythroid-Specific and Housekeeping Isozymes. The existence of erythroid and nonerythroid isozymes of ALAS with different physical and kinetic properties was first recognized in guinea pigs in 1981.[78] Subsequently, erythroid isozymes of chicken and rat ALAS were shown to be immunologically nonidentical with their respective hepatic isozymes.[104,105] Erythroid-specific and hepatic forms of ALAS were also reported in trout.[106] The definitive establishment of tissue-specific ALAS isozymes occurred with the isolation of unique cDNAs for the erythroid-specific and housekeeping chicken *ALAS* genes[107] and the erythroid-specific gene for human ALAS2[108–110] (see "Molecular Genetics" below). The erythroid isozyme has also been termed ALASE and the housekeeping isozyme ALASH or ALASN.

Biosynthesis and Mitochondrial Import. The nuclear-encoded human ALAS2 precursor protein is synthesized on cytoplasmic ribosomes and is targeted to the mitochondria by signals in the polypeptide. After proteolytic processing, human bone marrow ALAS2 is associated with the matrix face of the inner

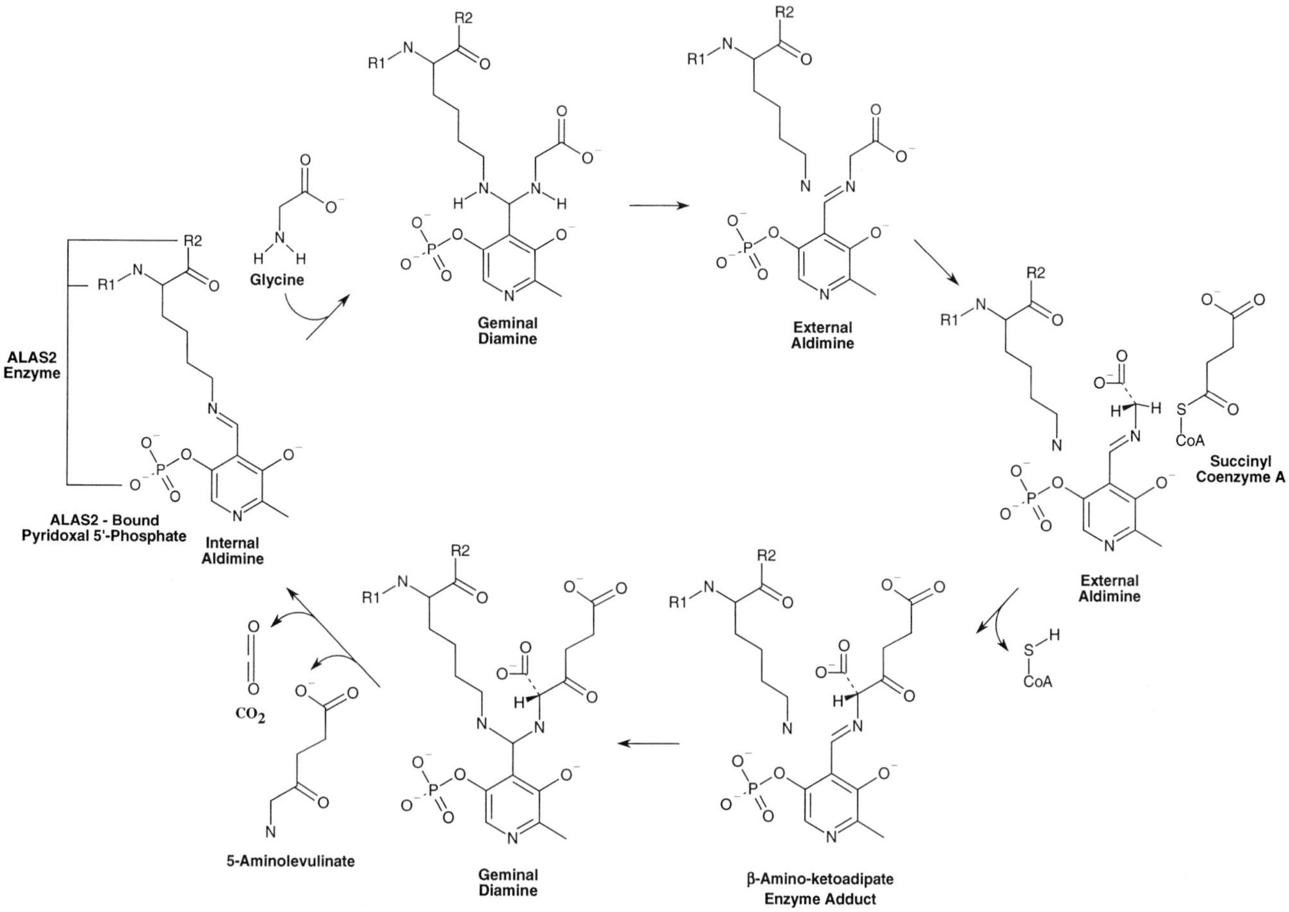

Fig. 124-7 Theoretical reaction mechanism for the enzymatic biosynthesis of 5-aminolevulinic acid.

mitochondrial membrane.[111] The amino-terminal leader sequence of ALAS2 contains multiple positive charges and is cleaved following mitochondrial import, similar to other mitochondrially targeted leader peptides. Interestingly, deletion of the first 75 residues of the yeast ALAS1 isozyme blocked matrix localization but not mitochondrial targeting and import,[112] demonstrating the involvement of internal residues for targeting.

Purification and microsequencing of ALAS1 from rat liver mitochondria identified Gln 57 as the amino-terminal residue of the mature mitochondrial enzyme.[113] In contrast, the leader peptide cleavage site for mouse erythroid ALAS2 was localized between Gln 77 and Asp 78 based on homology to the human ornithine transcarbamylase leader peptide.[114] Similarly, the predicted cleavage site in human ALAS2 was between Gln 78 and Asp 79,[95] yielding a mature subunit size of 56.4 kDa. Immunoblot analysis of ALAS2 from rat reticulocyte lysates and human bone marrow cells estimated the mature form to be 56 kDa,[115,116] while another study found the mature human form to be 49 kDa.[61] The amino-terminus of the mature mitochondrial human ALAS2 isozyme remains to be determined by microsequencing.

The amino-terminal leader peptide of mammalian ALAS2 also contains sequence motifs that may interact with heme to block mitochondrial import of the enzyme. Studies by Kikuchi and coworkers demonstrated that micromolar hemin concentrations blocked mitochondrial uptake of rat ALAS1 with a concomitant increase of the ALAS1 precursor in the hepatic cytosol.[117] Using isolated mouse hepatocyte mitochondria, Lathrop and Timko demonstrated that conserved sequences in the ALAS1 and ALAS2 leader peptides, termed the HRMs, were required for hemin-dependent inhibition of import into isolated liver mitochondria for both mouse ALAS1 and ALAS2.[28] The HRM consensus sequence, $CP(\Phi)X_{12-30}CP$ (Φ = hydrophobic residue) is present in all known eukaryotic ALAS leader sequences. This motif also is required for heme-activated DNA binding by the yeast transcription factor HAP1[118] and for heme-dependent functions of yeast cytochrome c_1 lyase.[119] Although it was suggested that heme may down-regulate ALAS2 mitochondrial import to allow fine-tuning of heme synthesis in the lag period prior to heme-stimulated globin synthesis,[28] it has not been demonstrated that heme binding to the ALAS2 HRM blocks import into mitochondria in erythroid cells. ALAS isolated from the cytosol before mitochondrial internalization and proteolytic processing is enzymatically active in vitro, but is not thought to synthesize ALA in vivo in this compartment, because its substrate, succinyl CoA, is synthesized and found only in the mitochondria. Thus, preventing ALAS import would be an effective means of down-regulating heme biosynthesis.

Purification and Properties of ALAS2. Before the cloning of the *ALAS2* cDNA, only partial purification of the enzyme was achieved from rabbit reticulocytes,[19] fetal rat liver,[77] and guinea pig bone marrow.[78] More recently, murine ALAS2, lacking the amino-terminal 78 residue leader sequence, was expressed in *E. coli* and purified to homogeneity.[120] In contrast, constructs of human ALAS2 lacking the 78-residue amino-terminal sequence formed mostly inclusion bodies when expressed in *E. coli*.[121] To date, expression and purification of soluble, highly active human ALAS2 has only been possible as a fusion protein with the highly soluble *E. coli* maltose-binding protein.[89]

Purified recombinant murine ALAS2 is a homodimer[122] with a subunit molecular weight of 56.2 kDa.[120] Studies with symmetric active-site mutants demonstrate that the active site includes Lys 313 and requires amino acid residues from the opposing subunit for catalytic activity, thereby predicting that the monomer would

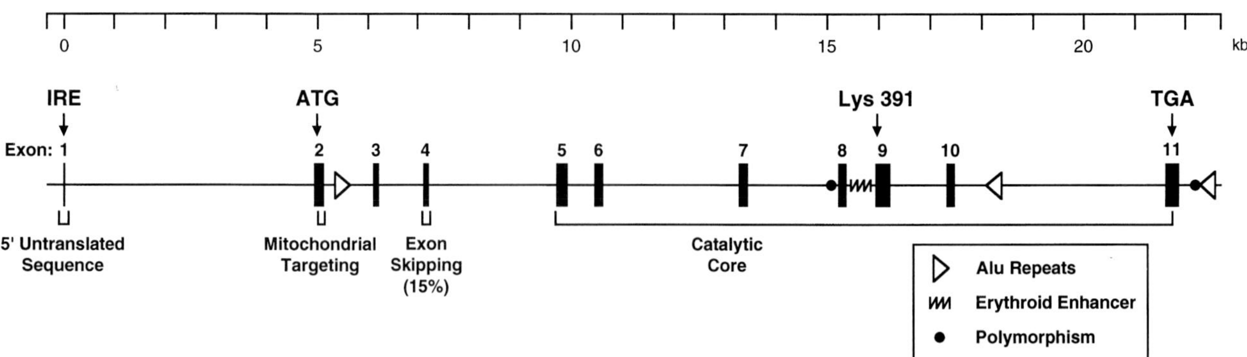

Fig. 124-8 Structure of the human *ALAS2* gene. IRE = iron responsive element; ATG = start codon; Lys[391] = pyridoxal binding site; TGA = stop codon.

be inactive.[123] The enzyme was yellow in color with an absorption maximum at 420 nm, which is characteristic of proteins with covalently bound PLP. Removal of the cofactor by dialysis resulted in complete loss of enzymatic activity, which was restored by addition of 20 μM PLP. The cofactor is covalently bound via a Schiff's base linkage to Lys 313 in the mouse ALAS2 enzyme.[101] The calculated maximal specific activity of the most highly purified preparation of recombinant murine ALAS2 was 42,300 nmol ALA/h/mg.[124] The K_m for glycine was 11.7 mM, and that for succinyl-CoA was 2.03 μM. The specific activity of the purified recombinant human ALAS2 fusion protein was 38,000 nmol ALA/h/mg,[89] indicating that the presence of the maltose-binding protein did not inhibit enzymatic activity, especially because the calculated specific activity based on the ALAS2 peptide protein alone is 66,600 nM ALA/h/mg.

The stability of ALAS2 depends on the presence of PLP.[89] A serine protease that specifically inactivates the apo-forms of various PLP-requiring enzymes, including human ALAS2, has been identified in human bone marrow cells.[111] Because the half-life of rat mitochondrial ALAS2 activity is only 34 min,[125] it is likely that mutations resulting in small changes in PLP affinity and/or protease susceptibility can have dramatic effects on the amount of mitochondrial ALAS2 activity.

Although the effect of iron on pure human ALAS2 is not known, partially purified ALAS2 from rabbit reticulocytes was inhibited about 35 percent by 100 μM ferrous or ferric iron.[19] The normal available iron concentration in human erythroblasts is around 3 μM,[126] but is much higher in sideroblastic marrow proerythroblasts where it is microscopically visible as nonferritin iron deposits in mitochondria.[127]

Hemin inhibited the partially purified rabbit reticulocyte ALAS2 by 37 percent at 10 μM,[19] but activated rat ALAS2 by 111 percent.[128] Because the free heme concentration in rabbit erythroblasts is estimated to be 0.7 μM,[129] it is unlikely that heme inhibits ALAS2 activity in marrow erythroblasts.

Recently, it was shown that ATP-specific succinyl CoA synthetase binds to ALAS2, but not to ALAS1, in mitochondria in vivo.[130] Because ineffective binding was observed for the XLSA mutation D190V, some clinical heterogeneity may relate to the role that succinyl CoA synthetase plays in ALAS2 stabilization and/or activity.

Molecular Genetics and Pathology of XLSA

cDNA and Genomic Sequences. Erythroid-specific chicken and human *ALAS2* cDNAs were isolated and sequenced in 1989,[107,109,131] and shown to be distinct from their respective housekeeping *ALAS1* cDNAs. At that time, it was also recognized that the previously cloned murine "hepatic" ALAS sequence[114,132] was actually the cDNA for the erythroid-specific *ALAS2* gene.[133] The human *ALAS2* gene was assigned to the X chromosome[109,131] and then its locus was refined to Xp11.21,[134] confirming that it was a separate gene from the housekeeping *ALAS1* gene, which mapped to the human chromosomal region 3p21.1.[108,135,136] The full-length human *ALAS2* cDNA has a 52-nt 5′-untranslated region, a coding region of 587 nt encoding a precursor polypeptide of 587 residues with a predicted molecular weight of 64,689, a 3′-untranslated region of 127 nt,[68,109] and is the defective gene in XLSA.[92]

The human *ALAS2* gene is 22 kb in length, contains 11 exons (Fig. 124-8), and undergoes alternative splicing with deletion of exon 4 in about half of the transcripts resulting in an in-frame deletion of 37 amino acids.[137] In mice, alternative splicing of the first 45 nt of exon 3 results in an in-frame deletion of 15 amino acids in about 15 percent of the transcripts,[132] suggesting dispensability of this region in mammalian ALAS2 polypeptides. The intron/exon structure of the *ALAS2* gene is conserved between chicken, mouse, and man, with identical boundaries and exon lengths. as well as high-sequence homology for exons 6 through 10.[68,132,138] Because there is much less sequence homology in exons 1 to 4, because exons 3 and 4 seem dispensable, and because prokaryotic *ALAS2* homologues lack the exon 1 to 4 region, it is presumed that the exon 5 through 11 coding region constitutes the catalytically competent core of the enzyme.[107,139]

Primer extension studies identified the location of the transcription start site 52 nt upstream from the ATG start codon.[137] The entire 22-kb human *ALAS2* genomic sequence with 18 kb of 5′- and 72 kb of 3′-flanking sequence is available (GenBank Z83821). A subsequent 35-kb *ALAS2* genomic sequence (GenBank AF068624) differed from the 112-kb clone by only 217 nt in nonexonic regions.[140]

The human *ALAS2* gene has two well-characterized intragenic polymorphic sites useful for linkage studies in families with unidentified mutations: a 25 percent informative single-nucleotide polymorphism at nucleotide 40351 (GenBank Z83821)[141] and a 78 percent informative CA repeat in intron 7.[142]

Transcriptional Regulation. The *ALAS2* promoter/enhancer region contains numerous erythroid-specific elements and deletion analysis demonstrated that maximal erythroid-specific expression was supported by the first 300 nt upstream of the transcription start site.[143] A canonical CCAAT promoter element was at −93 nt and a TATA-like promoter element was at −23 nt, which bound both erythroid-specific transcription factor I (GATA-1) and the TATA binding proteins in vitro.[143] Functional erythroid-specific GATA-1 enhancer elements have been identified at −97 and −121 nt and a functionally important CACCC element at −51 nt bound the erythroid EKLF enhancer as well as the BKLF and Sp1 factors.[143] Although the erythroid-specific element, nuclear factor NF-E2, was found at −39, functionality was not demonstrated.[143] DNase I hypersensitive sites, indicative of regions of importance for transcriptional regulation, were identified in the proximal promoter and introns 1, 3, and 8 of the murine *ALAS2* gene.[132] The homologous regions in the human *ALAS2* gene are important in transcriptional regulation.[140] Human intron 1 stimulated *ALAS2* promoter activity threefold in erythroid cells, while intron 3 was somewhat inhibitory. Intron 8 enhanced promoter activity twelvefold in human K562 cells, but only 0.9-fold in COS-1 cells.[140] Human intron 8 had a core 239-nt enhancer region that was orientation-dependent and contained two functionally important CACCC elements and one functional GATA-1 site, as well as additional uncharacterized sequences that were conserved in mouse and dog.

The promoter-proximal and intron 8 erythroid control regions (ECRs) of human *ALAS2* are analogous in their sequence motifs and functions to the globin locus control regions, except that they appear to act locally on a single gene during erythroid differentiation. Promoter proximal ECRs also are present in other heme biosynthetic genes including *ALAD*,[144] *PBGD*,[145] and ferrochelatase.[146] A synthetic ECR containing the GATA1 and CACCC or NF-E2 elements confers strong erythroid-specific expression to a minimal TATA-containing promoter.[147]

Although end-product inhibition of transcription of the housekeeping *ALAS1* gene has been documented,[148] heme does not repress *ALAS2* transcription in erythroid cells.[133,149,150]

Translational Control. The 5′ untranslated region of the erythroid-specific ALAS2 mRNA contains an iron-responsive element (IRE) that coordinates ALAS2 synthesis with iron availability.[133,151] A 28-nt region (spanning most of *ALAS2* intron 1) forms a stem-loop structure that acts as a binding site for the IRE-binding protein 1 (IRP1).[152] Because the binding of IRP1 to the *ALAS2* IRE is tenfold greater than that of the IRE-binding protein 2 (IRP2) isoprotein,[152] and because the level of IRP1 protein appears to be greater than that of IRP2 in bone marrow,[153] it is likely that translational control of human *ALAS2* is mediated by IRP1. This protein/mRNA complex blocks translation in iron-deficient erythroid cells,[94,151] whereas in iron-replete cells, the iron/IRP1 complex is released from the *ALAS2* IRE, allowing translation to proceed.

Molecular Pathology of XLSA. The availability of the *ALAS2* cDNA and genomic sequences has permitted the analysis of the mutations causing XLSA. To date, over 25 different mutations have been identified[93,100] (Fig. 124-9). Except for one nonsense mutation, all have been missense mutations in the ALAS2 catalytic core encoded by exons 5 through 11, with the majority occurring in exons 5 and 9. Of note, exon 9 encodes lysine 391, the putative covalent binding site for the PLP cofactor in the human enzyme.

Of the published mutations, most were pyridoxine-responsive in vivo (F165L,[95] R170L,[100] A172T,[89] Y199H,[94] R204Q,[154] G291S,[97] K299Q,[89] T388S,[96] R411C,[94,155] M426V,[116] R448Q,[94] R452C,[94] R452H,[99] I476N,[92] H524D,[156] and S568G[157]). Of the pyridoxine-responsive mutations expressed in *E. coli*, all exhibited pyridoxine-responsiveness in vitro. One had reduced affinity for PLP,[92] two had markedly reduced apoenzyme stability,[89] and seven had decreased enzymatic activity.[92,95–97,116,154,157] Similarly, apo-ALAS2 isolated from two patients with pyridoxine-responsive sideroblastic anemia was much more susceptible to inactivation by an erythroid cell protease than was apo-ALAS2 from normal individuals.[158] *ALAS2* mutations occurred in severely anemic infants (F165L, I476N, M426V, H524D), children (R411C), adolescents (Y199, R448Q, I476N), middle-aged individuals (R170L, T388S, R452C, R452H), and in late-onset cases (A172T, K299Q), with the most pyridoxine-responsive mutations generally found in the late-onset patients. Only one patient, an 18-year-old male with a D190V lesion, was pyridoxine-refractory.[116] Of note, this mutant protein was PLP-responsive in vitro, but a presumed defect in ALAS2 mitochondrial transport prevented pyridoxine supplementation from enhancing the residual ALAS2 enzymatic activity in vivo.[116] Alternatively, the residual activity could have been inhibited due to the severe iron overload in this patient.

Excess mitochondrial iron in the marrow of XLSA patients may further exacerbate the disorder by inhibiting ALAS2 activity as noted above or indirectly by inhibition of energy metabolism in mitochondria. For example, bone marrow ALAS2 activity was only 13 percent of normal in a patient with pyridoxine-responsive XLSA during relapse when serum iron was high, while during remission (16 months after pyridoxine therapy when serum iron levels were low) enzymatic activity was 3.7 times normal.[98,116] These results suggested that the decreased ALAS2 activity in marrow during relapse could be due to excess iron. Likewise, recent studies have shown that high iron levels were inversely correlated with pyridoxine-responsiveness in XLSA patients in vivo.[94] An XLSA hemizygote with a Y199H mutation was responsive to pyridoxine supplementation (Hb concentration rising from 9.5 to 12 g/dl) earlier in life when his serum ferritin was low

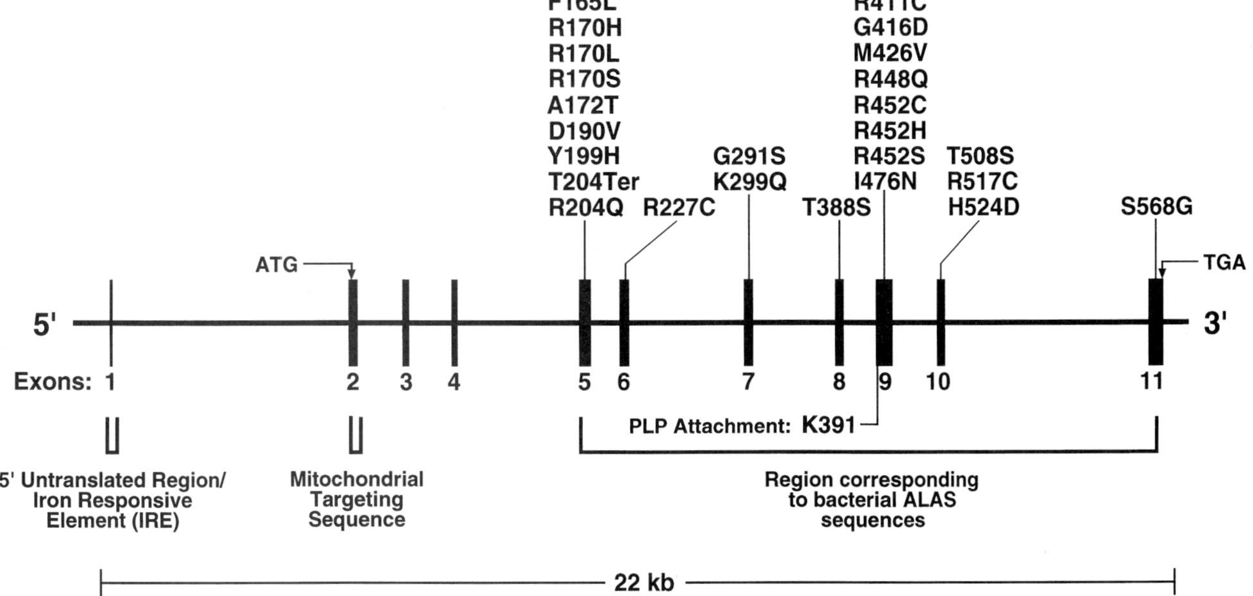

Fig. 124-9 Diagram of the *ALAS2* gene and locations of mutations causing XLSA.

in response to chelation therapy with DFO. Although pyridoxine therapy was continued, as soon as chelation therapy was terminated, iron levels rose and the Hb concentration decreased to 9 g/dl. Only following aggressive removal of iron by phlebotomy did the hemoglobin return to its earlier levels above 11 g/dl.[94]

Chemicals that react with PLP and/or other B6 vitamers have been associated with sideroblastic anemia. Isonicotinic acid hydrazide (INH, isoniazid), commonly used to treat tuberculosis, reacts with PLP to form a hydrazone that inhibits pyridoxal phosphokinase, an enzyme required for intracellular conversion of pyridoxal to PLP.[159] Sideroblastic anemia and reduced bone marrow ALAS2 activity have resulted from INH treatment in humans[160] and in experimental animals,[161] but INH alone rarely causes sideroblastic anemia unless treatment includes a second drug such as para-aminosalicylic acid, cycloserine, or pyrazinamide, all reactants with B6 vitamers.[162]

Recently, the first animal model for erythroid ALAS2 deficiency was established in the zebrafish.[163] The *sauternes (sau)* mutants of zebrafish displayed an embryonic developmental defect that resulted in a hypochromic, microcytic anemia. By positional cloning, *sau* was identified as the erythroid-specific homologue of human *ALAS2*. The two mutant alleles sau^{tb233} and sau^{ty121} were found to have V249D and L305Q mutations, respectively. The sau^{ty121} mutation was less severe than the sau^{tb233} mutation, and sau^{ty121} homozygotes survived to adulthood. In the embryo, the sau^{ty121} zebrafish had a tenfold reduction in heme concentration and reduced, but longer, persistence of β_{e2} hemoglobin expression. In contrast, in the adult, heme was only reduced by 30 percent and globin expression was normal. Phenotypic rescue of the β_{e2} hemoglobin defect was demonstrated by transient expression of the wild-type *alas2* gene in the sau^{ty121} embryo. Interestingly, the adult sau^{ty121} fish did not have the characteristic ring sideroblasts seen in XLSA, suggesting differences in iron metabolism or that the defect in adult zebrafish was too mild to cause mitochondrial iron storage.

Recently, an ALAS2 knockout mouse was generated which was an embryonic lethal.[164] The male hemizygous null mutants could not support primitive hematopoiesis and were not viable beyond embryonic stage E11.5. The heterozygous female mice exhibited ringed sideroblasts in the marrow.[164] These results indicated that the housekeeping gene cannot rescue the ALAS2 deficiency in erythroid cells.

Diagnosis

Clinical Diagnosis. The combined findings of microcytic and hypochromic anemia, elevated iron, pyridoxine-responsiveness, and X-linked inheritance in the absence of ataxia[90] suggest the diagnosis of XLSA. To help establish the mode of inheritance, erythrocytes from putative heterozygous females should be evaluated by histogram or scattergram for the erythrocyte dimorphism due to random X-inactivation. The value and limitations of a careful analysis of erythrocyte size distribution are illustrated in Fig. 124-6. The proband's erythrocyte size distribution is clearly microcytic, but his sister and niece have MCVs in the normal range and were only shown to be heterozygotes by the presence of discrete microcytic populations in the histogram. In contrast, the proband's mother, an obligate heterozygote who had the *ALAS2* mutation in this family, had no detectable microcytic cells and all other blood indices were normal. The latter finding is compatible with most of her cells expressing the normal allele, while the mutation allele was on the inactivated X chromosome. This family highlights the usefulness of histograms or scattergrams in clinical diagnosis, but also demonstrates that gene-based diagnosis is required in heterozygotes to provide a definitive diagnosis.

Due to the ineffective erythropoiesis, the marrow will show erythroid hyperplasia with a decreased myeloid/erythroid ratio, and ferrokinetic studies will show increased erythroid iron turnover. XLSA patients generally have serum ferritin levels >200 μg/dl and transferrin saturation >30 percent. Pediatric cases, mildly affected individuals, and heterozygotes may not have elevated serum ferritin or transferrin saturation, but microscopic examination of the marrow will usually detect ring sideroblasts (typically >15 percent, which are pathognomonic for a defect in heme synthesis) and/or increased reticuloendothelial iron.[165]

Iron-deficiency anemia, which also presents with microcytic, hypochromic erythrocytes, is distinguished from XLSA by the lack of excess storage iron. Bone marrow examination is diagnostic for iron-deficiency anemia with the absence of hemosiderin and ring sideroblasts.

Other conditions that can result in elevated serum ferritin include liver dysfunction, inflammation, and malignancies. The thalassemias also present with microcytic, hypochromic anemia with elevated iron storage and, except for α-thalassemia, can be ruled out by hemoglobin electrophoresis. For α-thalassemia, hemoglobin Bart (β-chain tetramers) may be present, especially in newborns. The presence of >10 percent ring sideroblasts in the marrow is rare for the thalassemias.

Pyridoxine responsiveness should always be evaluated, as most patients are pyridoxine-responsive, if only to a modest extent, and even a small increase in iron utilization and heme production is beneficial. In families with known *ALAS2* mutations, the average increase in hemoglobin concentration was 5.6 g/dl (range: 1.5 to 9) following 2 to 6 weeks of pyridoxine supplementation at doses from 50 to 400 mg/d.[89,94–100,134] There is increasing evidence that iron overload suppresses pyridoxine responsiveness.[94,166] Hemoglobin levels were highly responsive to pyridoxine supplementation when the proband was young, but after iron stores were elevated, pyridoxine had a significantly muted effect. Only after repeated phlebotomy to reduce iron concentrations into the normal range, did the hemoglobin concentration rise in these XLSA patients. Thus, a patient should not be categorized as refractory until pyridoxine responsiveness has been evaluated when iron stores are in the normal range following phlebotomy or iron chelation therapy.

Primary acquired sideroblastic anemia, also classified as a myelodysplastic syndrome (refractory anemia with ring sideroblasts, RARS), is a frequent disorder in the elderly, which presents with hypochromic, refractory anemia with ring sideroblasts. Erythroblasts are typically macrocytic, with MCV values >100 pL. Marrow evaluation frequently demonstrates abnormal lymphocytes and/or granulocytes. Nonetheless, XLSA probands have been misdiagnosed as having RARS when they present at an advanced age.[89] Individuals with pure erythroid dysplasia and any hint of a microcytic cell population, X-linked inheritance, or pyridoxine responsiveness should be evaluated for mutations in the *ALAS2* gene. Note that the X-linked inheritance can be missed due to random X inactivation in heterozygotes and because XLSA mutations can occur *de novo*.[94]

Molecular Diagnosis. The definitive diagnosis of XLSA requires detection of an *ALAS2* mutation and demonstration of its X-linked inheritance in affected relatives or demonstration of altered function of the recombinant mutant enzyme. While point mutations in the coding region can be detected by sequencing reverse-transcribed and amplified reticulocyte ALAS2 mRNA,[93,94] mutations in the promoter, splice sites, and deletions in heterozygotes can be missed. Therefore, the preferred approach is amplification of genomic DNA and direct sequencing of each of the 11 exons, flanking regions, and the intron/exon boundaries. Primer sets for these analyses have been published[94,116] and the complete genomic sequence is available online (GenBank Z83821 and AF068624).

Treatment

Treatment of XLSA currently consists of pyridoxine and folic acid therapy to optimize heme biosynthesis and phlebotomy and/or chelation therapy to reverse iron overload. Splenectomy is seldom recommended for hypersplenism, because of attendant risks such as thrombosis and infection.[95,99]

Pyridoxine Supplementation. Because ALAS2 requires PLP as a cofactor, oral supplementation with pyridoxine should be instituted in all newly diagnosed patients. Pyridoxine responsiveness has been demonstrated in 14 of the 15 mutation-proven XLSA families reported to date. Even for normal individuals, in vitro studies of marrow erythroblasts showed a 25 percent increase in ALAS2 activity following addition of 200 μM PLP.[160,167] A typical pyridoxine treatment regimen is 100 to 300 mg/d initially and then 100 mg/d as maintenance therapy. Caution is warranted as dosages of over 500 mg/d can lead to a peripheral sensory neuropathy[168] with possible irreversible damage, especially at dosages above 1 g/d.[169] Titration of pyridoxine supplementation can define the lower limits for maximal responsiveness in specific cases, the lowest to date being approximately 4 mg/d.[96] Pyridoxine supplementation needs may be increased due to chemical inhibition of PLP synthesis by theophylline[170] or destruction by antituberculosis drugs, as discussed above (see "Molecular Pathology of XLSA").

Iron Removal. The primary cause of morbidity and mortality in XLSA is tissue damage from iron toxicity. Iron storage is insidious, increasing to toxic levels over decades, and should be monitored in mild cases and in heterozygotes. Phlebotomy is the preferred means of iron removal because of its efficiency (0.25 g iron/unit blood removed), low cost, absence of side effects, and stimulation of heme synthesis. In spite of anemia, phlebotomy usually results in increased hemoglobin levels, especially if introduced gradually with pyridoxine therapy.[166,171] Chelation therapy by continuous subcutaneous infusion of DFO[172] is also efficient (0.02 g iron/day removed by urinary and fecal excretion), but is expensive, is associated with ocular and auditory neuropathies, and can result in infections. Aggressive chelation can be life saving when elevated iron stores cause cardiac complications. Ascorbic acid enhances iron mobilization from the reticuloendothelial system and should be avoided unless there is concurrent chelation therapy as it may markedly increase redistribution of iron to the parenchymal cells of liver and heart with increased tissue damage. In contrast, when iron stores are reduced, phlebotomy should replace chelation, as DFO is toxic to certain tissues when in excess of stored iron. Considering that iron depletion by DFO may preferentially target hepatocellular as opposed to reticuloendothelial iron,[173] phlebotomy may be more effective in lowering erythroblast iron than chelation therapy because it increases erythrocyte turnover. Whether iron is depleted by phlebotomy or a combination of chelation and subsequent phlebotomy, removal should continue until the patient reaches an iron-deficiency state as indicated by transferrin saturation levels of less than 15 percent, serum ferritin levels below 20 μg/dl, and/or lowered hemoglobin values that do not recover within 2 weeks after iron removal. De-ironing can take from 6 months to 3 years, depending on the extent of storage and aggressiveness of therapy. Thereafter, iron stores must be regularly monitored and maintained in the normal range to prevent tissue damage.[165] Typically, phlebotomy four times a year will maintain transferrin saturation below 40 percent and serum ferritin below 100 μg/dl.

Due to the high frequency of hereditary hemochromatosis (HH) in individuals of northern European descent caused by the C282Y mutation in the *HFE* gene, there may be an additional risk of iron loading from coinheritance of XLSA and HH. C282Y heterozygotes have higher transferrin saturation than normal individuals.[174–176] Both PCT[177] and XLSA patients[94] have been reported to have an increased frequency of the C282Y allele. One XLSA patient with severe iron overload was also homozygous for HH (C282Y/C282Y).[94] Increased iron loading is also seen in HH patients with the C282Y/H63D or H63D/H63D genotypes.[178,179] XLSA probands and family members should be screened for mutant *HFE* alleles because XLSA heterozygotes who coinherit HH mutant alleles may be at risk for additional iron loading and should be closely followed. Early and lifetime intervention to avoid iron deposition secondary to XLSA and HH can eliminate or minimize pathology associated with iron toxicity and can decrease anemia, and therefore should be encouraged in all XLSA hemizygotes and iron-loading heterozygotes.

Genetic Counseling. Genetic counseling should be provided to all families with XLSA. All relatives should be offered testing and plans should be instituted for lifetime treatment and monitoring of their iron status.

5-AMINOLEVULINIC ACID DEHYDRATASE-DEFICIENT PORPHYRIA (ADP)

ADP is an autosomal recessive disorder due to the markedly deficient activity of 5-aminolevulinic acid dehydratase (ALAD, PBG synthase, E.C.4.2.1.24), the second enzyme in the heme biosynthetic pathway. Clinical manifestations have been primarily neuropathic, while the severity and the age of onset have been highly variable in the few reported cases. It is becoming customary to abbreviate this disorder as ADP (for 5-*a*minolevulinic acid dehydratase *d*eficient *p*orphyria). It is also termed ALAD porphyria and Doss porphyria after the investigator who described the first two cases in 1979.[180,181] The term plumboporphyria emphasizes the clinical similarity of this condition to lead poisoning, but incorrectly implies that it is due to excess lead.

Only about seven cases of ADP, two of which are in one family, have been reported to date, which indicates that this porphyria is very rare. To date, only four cases have been confirmed by immunochemical characterization of the deficient enzyme and/or determination of the underlying *ALAD* mutations.[180–184] The ADP patients were unrelated, except for two brothers from Chile, and were of European, Hispanic, or Japanese descent. Because multiple causes of ALAD deficiency have been described, all cases considered to have ADP should be confirmed by molecular studies. Of the reported cases, the two sibs in Chile[185] and an elderly woman in Japan[186] have not been confirmed by mutation analysis.

ADP undoubtedly occurs elsewhere and is underrecognized. The prevalence of heterozygous ALAD deficiency in Germany, where the first two homozygous cases were recognized, has been estimated to be less than 1 percent.[187] The frequency of ALAD deficiency (less than 50 percent normal enzyme activity) among 880 individuals in Sweden was found to be approximately 2 percent.[182]

Clinical Manifestations

Marked clinical heterogeneity has been observed in the few reported patients with ADP. The first two patients were unrelated male adolescents in Germany with acute symptoms resembling those of AIP (see below), including abdominal pain and neuropathy.[180] After initial acute attacks, both remained well during 20 years of follow-up.[188] The third patient was a Swedish infant who had more severe disease, including failure to thrive.[182] The fourth patient was essentially normal until age 63, when he developed an acute motor polyneuropathy not accompanied by abdominal pain. He concurrently developed a myeloproliferative disorder.[189] The fifth and sixth patients were Chilean siblings (26 and 28 years of age) who presented with symptoms typical of an acute porphyria and ALAD activity less than 4 percent of normal.[185] ADP may be associated with hyponatremia and the syndrome of inappropriate ADH secretion (SIADH), as in a 69-year-old Japanese woman.[186] Heterozygotes identified in family studies have been clinically asymptomatic with normal urinary ALA levels;[180,182,185,190] however, they may have enhanced susceptibility to lead poisoning.[187] In addition, heterozygotes may be at increased risk if exposed to the toxic effects of certain chemicals, for example, iron, trichloroethylene, and styrene, that are known to adversely influence ALAD activity.[191] Indeed,

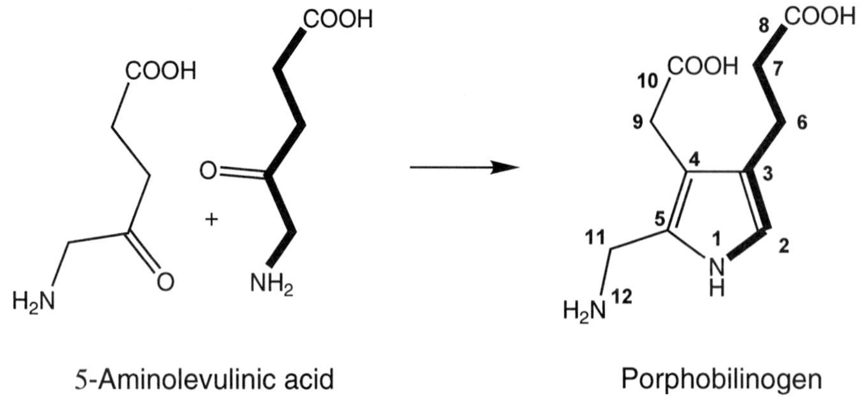

Fig. 124-10 Reaction catalyzed by 5-aminolevulinic acid dehydratase (ALAD), in which 2 molecules of 5-aminolevulinic acid (ALA) form the monopyrrole porphobilinogen (PBG). The ALA molecule that contributes atoms 1, 2, 3, 6, 7, and 8 in PBG, including the propionic acid side, is indicated in bold, and initially binds to the enzyme.

individuals heterozygous for ALAD deficiency and with blood lead levels in the high-normal range have had evidence of subclinical lead poisoning as manifested by increased erythrocyte protoporphyrin.[187] Therefore, heterozygotes for ALAD deficiency may be susceptible to the toxic effects of environmental chemicals that interact with this enzyme.

The Metabolic Defect in ADP

Accumulated Porphyrin Precursor and Porphyrins. The markedly deficient ALAD activity in affected ADP homozygotes results in the accumulation and urinary excretion of large amounts of ALA. Markedly increased coproporphyrin III is also detected in urine, while accumulated protoporphyrin (complexed with zinc) is detected in erythrocytes. Coproporphyrin isomer excretion is substantial in normal subjects after ALA loading and strikingly similar to that seen in patients with ADP and lead poisoning, who accumulate excess amounts of endogenous ALA.[192,193] The increased erythrocyte protoporphyrin may, as in all other homozygous porphyrias, be explained by accumulation of earlier pathway intermediates in bone marrow erythroid cells during hemoglobin synthesis, followed by their transformation to protoporphyrin after hemoglobin synthesis is complete.[194]

The Enzymatic Defect in ADP. The enzymatic defect in ADP is the markedly deficient activity of ALAD, the second enzyme in the heme biosynthetic pathway. ALAD catalyzes the formation of PBG from two molecules of ALA (Fig. 124-10). All patients had <5 percent of normal erythrocyte ALAD activity and several had <1 percent ALAD activity.[184] Heterozygous relatives had about half-normal levels of enzymatic activity. The substrate ALA is an amino acid that is the obligate precursor for porphyrinogens, porphyrins, heme, and other tetrapyrroles.

Purification and Properties of ALAD. In mammalian cells, ALAD is abundant, having eighty- to one hundredfold greater activity in the liver than the activity of ALAS1, the rate-limiting enzyme in heme synthesis.[3] ALAD has been purified and characterized from mammalian erythrocytes and consists of eight identical subunits of ~36 kDa.[195] The enzyme requires an intact sulfhydryl group and one zinc atom per subunit for full activity and is inactivated by the reversible replacement of the zinc atoms by lead. Using [5-^{14}C]-ALA as substrate, it was shown that, of the two molecules of ALA, it is the one contributing the propionic acid side (atoms 1, 2, 3, 6, 7, and 8 in PBG) that is initially bound to the enzyme (Fig. 124-10).[196]

Crystal Structure. The tertiary structure of yeast ALAD has been solved to 2.3-Å resolution, revealing that each subunit adopts a TIM barrel fold with a 39-residue *N*-terminal arm (Fig. 124-11). Pairs of monomers then wrap their arms around each other to form compact dimers, and these associate to form an octamer with 4-2-2 symmetry.[197] All eight active sites are on the surface of the octamer and contain two lysine residues (210 and 263), one of which, Lys263, forms a Schiff's base linkage with the substrate. The two lysine side chains are close to two zinc binding sites, one of which is formed by three cysteine residues (133, 135, and 143), while the other involves Cys234 and His142.

ALAD has also been reported to be identical to the 240-kDa-proteasome inhibitor (CF-2).[198] The dual role of ALAD as CF-2 in both the ATP/ubiquitin-dependent pathway and the heme biosynthetic pathway may be an example of "gene sharing"[199] and may explain the unexpected abundance of this enzyme in the cell, as compared to other heme biosynthetic pathway enzymes.

The Molecular Genetics and Pathology of *ALAD*

cDNA and Genomic Sequence of *ALAD*. The cDNA for *ALAD* was cloned from a human liver library and predicted a protein of 330 amino acid residues.[200,201] An identical zinc-binding domain was conserved in man, rat, and mouse *ALAD* cDNAs.[201] The single *ALAD* gene was localized by *in situ* hybridization to the chromosome 9q34.[202] The human *ALAD* genomic structure was 16 kb in length with 2 promoter regions and 2 alternative noncoding exons, 1A and 1B, that generate housekeeping and erythroid-specific transcripts that include 12 coding exons.[203] The housekeeping transcript, which contains exon 1A fused to coding exons 2 to 12, was isolated from a human adult liver cDNA library, while an erythroid-specific transcript, which contains exon 1B fused to coding exons 2 to 12, was isolated from a human K562 erythroleukemia cDNA library. Both transcripts encode the same amino acid sequence because translation began in exon 2. The promoter region upstream of housekeeping exon 1A is GC-rich, contains three potential Sp1 elements, a CCAAT box, three potential GATA-1 binding sites, and an AP1 site. The promoter region upstream of erythroid-specific exon 1B has several CACCC boxes and two potential GATA-1 binding sites. The mouse *ALAD* gene has similar features.[144] The novel expression of housekeeping and erythroid-specific transcripts apparently evolved to ensure sufficient heme biosynthesis for the high-level tissue-specific production of hemoglobin.[203]

Molecular Pathology. To date, *ALAD* point mutations have been reported in four unrelated patients with ADP (Fig. 124-12). In the two original German ADP cases,[180] patient H had *ALAD* missense mutation V153M and a two-base deletion, 818delTC, that resulted in a frameshift and premature truncation after residue 294.[204] Patient B had *ALAD* missense mutations R240W and A274T.[205,206] When the V153M and 818delTC mutations were expressed in Chinese hamster ovary cells, the missense mutation produced a mutant enzyme with significant, but unstable, activity, while the deletion allele did not produce enzyme protein.[204] Expression of the R240W and A274T alleles in Chinese hamster ovary cells demonstrated that the A274T enzyme had little catalytic activity, while the R240W allele encoded an enzyme protein with partial, but unstable, activity.[206]

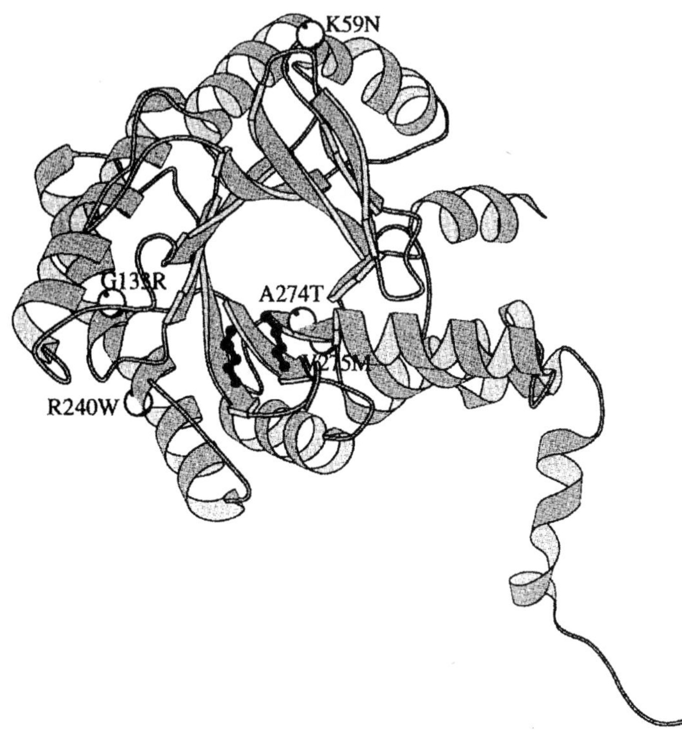

Fig. 124-11 The tertiary structure of yeast ALAD and corresponding sites of mutations found in human ALAD.[197] The small dark side chains indicate the active site lysines 210 (left) and 263 (right). The G133R mutation likely disrupts the enzyme's zinc binding loop which is to the immediate right of this residue in the diagram. The R240W mutation (in α6) removes a buried salt bridge, which occurs in a region of the subunit making quaternary contacts. The A274T and V275M mutations occur in β9 and probably destabilize the buried core of the barrel while the common K59N polymorphism may remove an intramolecular salt bridge. (*Reproduced from Erskine et al.*[197] *Used by permission.*)

Molecular analysis of the *ALAD* gene in a severely affected Swedish child with ADP also revealed two missense mutations, G133R and V275M (Fig. 124-12).[207] Both missense mutations, which occurred at CpG dinucleotides, were confirmed in genomic DNA samples from family members by competitive PCR for the paternal mutation, and by the detection of a *Pst*I restriction site created by the maternal mutation.[207]

Molecular analysis of a 63-year-old Belgian patient[183] identified the lesion in one allele, G133R, a mutation previously identified in the Swedish child.[184] Another point mutation, F12L, was identified in an asymptomatic Swedish girl who had 12 percent of normal erythrocyte ALAD activity.[208]

***ALAD* Polymorphism.** In addition to these mutations that cause ALAD deficiency, a common *ALAD* polymorphism, K59N,[209] has been detected in ~20 percent of the Caucasian population.[210] This polymorphism, termed the *ALAD2* allele, retains normal ALAD activity, and may bind zinc more effectively. When lead enters the bloodstream it is taken up by the erythrocytes, with usually less than 1 percent of the lead remaining in the plasma. Liquid chromatography with inductively coupled plasma mass spectrometry revealed the principal lead-binding protein with a mass of approximately 240 kDa, and adsorption to specific antibodies showed that the protein was ALAD.[211]

Several epidemiologic studies have demonstrated an association of the *ALAD2* allele and high lead levels.[212–215] It is not known, however, whether this difference is reflected in increased or decreased lead toxicity. Although lead in blood and serum was increased 5 to 10 percent in similarly exposed individuals with the *ALAD2* allele, bone lead was not increased.[214] The *ALAD2* allele

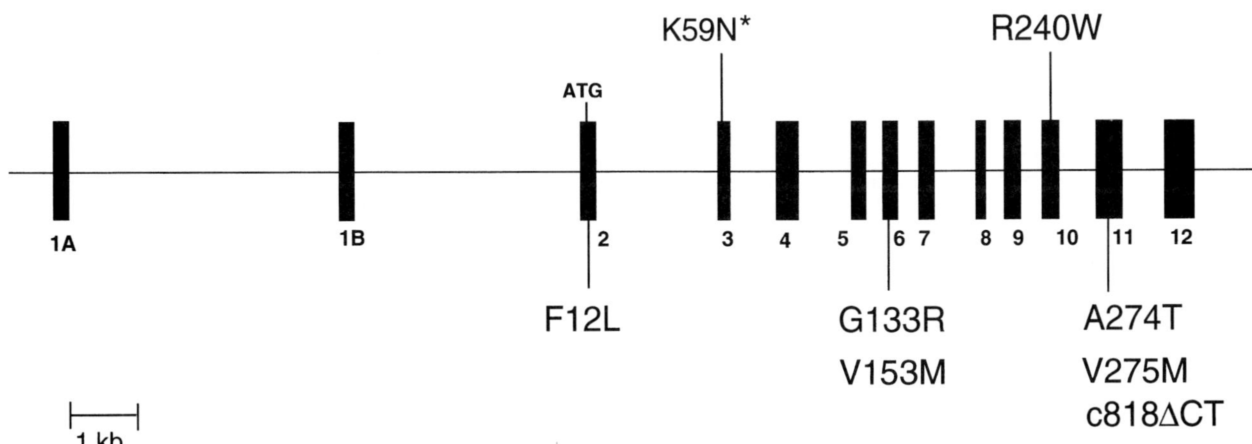

Fig. 124-12 The human *ALAD* gene and locations of mutations causing ADP. (*Courtesy of Dr. K. H. Astrin.*)

may affect disposition of this toxic metal and its delivery to target organs such as brain.

Pathophysiology

It is believed, although not directly demonstrated, that acute attacks of ADP occur in association with the overexpression of ALAS1 in liver due to a loss of heme-mediated repression,[7] leading to accumulation of ALA in liver (see section on AIP). Therefore, ADP, like the other acute porphyrias, is often classified as one of the hepatic porphyrias. However, as in other autosomal recessive porphyrias, erythrocyte porphyrins are substantially increased, which is a feature of an erythropoietic porphyria.

As in other acute porphyrias, the pathogenesis of the neurologic symptoms is poorly understood (see section on AIP). The fact that both ADP and AIP show similar clinical and biochemical abnormalities (see "Acute Intermittent Porphyria") suggests that ALA, rather than PBG, may be a neurotoxic agent. This point is further supported by the finding that patients with hereditary tyrosinemia frequently develop symptoms resembling acute porphyria[216,217] in association with marked inhibition of ALAD by succinylacetone.[218,219]

Diagnosis

ADP should be suspected when symptoms such as abdominal pain and peripheral neuropathy suggest an acute porphyria. ADP is differentiated from other acute porphyrias by normal urinary PBG in the presence of increased ALA, and by markedly decreased ALAD activity, as most conveniently measured in erythrocytes. Increased urinary coproporphyrin and erythrocyte protoporphyrin levels are characteristic but not specific. Unlike other acute porphyrias, the inheritance is autosomal recessive, rather than dominant. Therefore, both parents should have approximately half-normal erythrocyte ALAD activities. ALAD is assayed by incubating tissue homogenates with ALA in the presence of a sulfhydryl reducing reagent such as reduced glutathione or dithiothreitol and then colorimetrically determining the amount of PBG produced using a modified Ehrlich's reagent.[220]

ALAD activity can be deficient in conditions other than ADP. Lead, styrene, and succinylacetone (the latter accumulates in hereditary tyrosinemia and is structurally similar to ALA) inhibit ALAD, causing increased urinary excretion of ALA and clinical manifestations that resemble those of the acute porphyrias.[216,218,221–223] Lead inhibits ALAD activity by displacing zinc atoms from the enzyme. Therefore, the enzymatic activity is diminished in patients with lead poisoning, resulting in excess ALA in blood and urine.[224] Lead poisoning is excluded by finding a normal blood lead level and showing that the deficient enzyme activity is not restored in vitro by addition of zinc and/or sulfhydryl reducing reagents such as dithiothreitol. Lead-poisoned patients often develop neurologic manifestations that resemble those of ADP and other acute porphyrias.[225] The most potent known inhibitor of the enzyme is succinylacetone,[218,219] a structural analogue of ALA found in urine and blood of patients with hereditary tyrosinemia.[222] Idiopathic-acquired ALAD deficiency has been reported.[226] ADP was reported in a lead worker in whom a peripheral neuropathy was initially thought to be due to lead poisoning.[227] Therefore, because ADP is very rare and may be difficult to differentiate from other causes of ALAD deficiency, it is important to confirm the diagnosis unequivocally by biochemical and molecular studies.

Treatment

There is little experience with treatment of this porphyria. Glucose and heme therapy are not uniformly effective[182,189] but were apparently beneficial in both of the original cases reported by Doss.[188] Heme therapy is used to treat other acute porphyrias, is effective in treating porphyria-like symptoms associated with hereditary tyrosinemia,[217,228] and can significantly reduce urinary output of ALA and coproporphyrin in lead poisoning.[229] Avoidance of drugs that are harmful in other acute porphyrias is prudent; however, it is not known if this is helpful.[189] An ADP patient who underwent liver transplantation experienced minimal clinical improvement and little, if any, decrease in ALA and porphyrins.[230]

ACUTE INTERMITTENT PORPHYRIA (AIP)

AIP is an autosomal dominant acute hepatic porphyria that results from the half-normal activity of porphobilinogen deaminase (PBGD, also called HMB synthase; EC 4.3.1.8). Urinary excretion of ALA and PBG is markedly increased, particularly when the disease is clinically expressed. The marked increase in PBG occurs only in AIP, HCP, and VP. The increased urinary excretion of ALA, PBG, and porphyrins in these acute porphyrias reflects their overproduction in the liver.

Clinically, AIP is characterized by visceral, autonomic, peripheral, and central nervous system involvement, which leads to a wide variety of manifestations that are usually intermittent and sometimes life threatening. However, the neurovisceral symptoms and signs are nonspecific and highly variable, and are readily confused with other medical conditions. This and other hepatic porphyrias have been referred to as pharmacogenetic or ecogenetic conditions to emphasize the importance of certain factors, including drugs, hormones, and nutritional alterations, most of which have the capacity to influence the rate of heme biosynthesis in the liver and to precipitate clinical expression of the underlying genetic trait.[231] The great majority of those who inherit PBGD deficiency remain clinically latent, without symptoms or increased urinary excretion of heme pathway intermediates. It is remarkable that Stokvis, the Dutch physician who originally described acute porphyria in 1889, noted exacerbation of the disease by the sedative Sulfonal, and also showed that porphyrinuria could be induced in rabbits with this drug.[232,233] Synonyms for AIP include intermittent acute porphyria, pyrroloporphyria, and Swedish porphyria. The term pyrroloporphyria reflects the predominant accumulation of the monopyrrole PBG. It has been called Swedish porphyria because it is prevalent there and some important early descriptions concerned Swedish patients.

AIP is the most common of the acute porphyrias. Although it occurs in all races, it may be somewhat more common in northern European countries such as Sweden, Britain, and Ireland. The prevalence of AIP in the United States and most other countries is commonly estimated to be about 5 in 100,000.[234,235] The prevalence of manifest AIP in adults in Sweden was calculated to be 7.7 in 100,000.[236] In Finland, the combined prevalence of AIP and VP was calculated to be 3.4 in 100,000.[237] Prevalence is very high in northern Sweden (approximately 60 to 100 in 100,000), where almost all cases are related[238] and have the same *PBGD* mutation.[239] Another mutation has been linked to a founder effect in Nova Scotia.[240]

A high prevalence (210 in 100,000) of AIP was reported in a chronic psychiatric population in the United States based on erythrocyte PBGD screening.[241] Screening of the general population by erythrocyte PBGD activity or DNA analysis revealed an AIP prevalence of ~200 heterozygotes in 100,000 in Finland,[242] and 1 in approximately 1675 (60 in 100,000) in France,[243] suggesting that the prevalence of latent and undetected gene carriers in the population may be considerably higher than previously thought.

Suggestions that historical individuals, such as a patient described by Hippocrates,[244] King George III, Mary Queen of Scots,[245] and Vincent van Gogh,[246] and mythical creatures such as vampires[247] might have had acute porphyria are highly speculative because the diagnosis of acute porphyria requires specific[248] laboratory confirmation. Recent studies of DNA from exhumed tissues of two descendants of George III are of interest but have not established a diagnosis of AIP or VP in any members of the British royal family.[249] Recent proposals that patients with poorly understood conditions, such as multiple chemical sensitivity

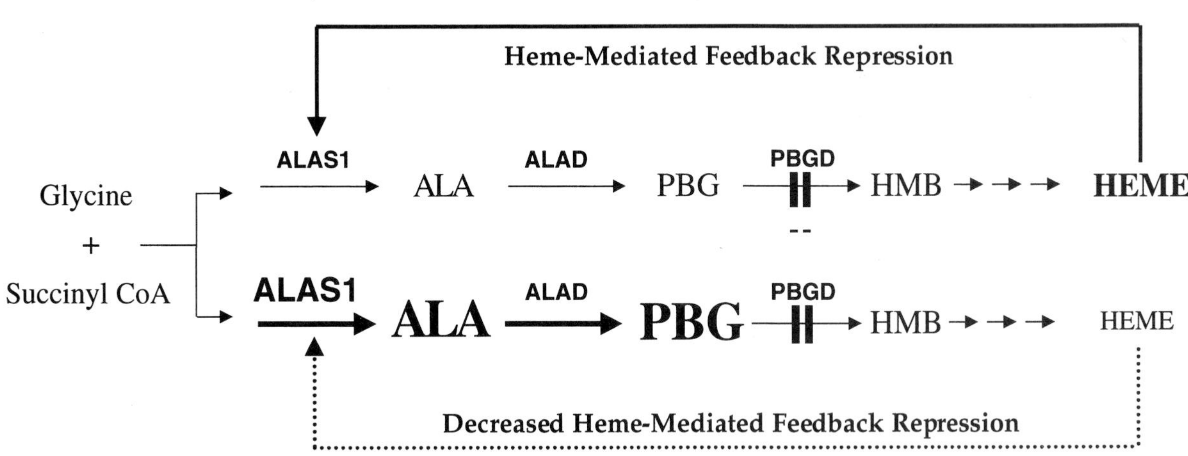

Fig. 124-13 Enzymatic block in AIP and loss of heme-mediated repression of hepatic ALAS1 when the disease is made clinically manifest by precipitating factors such as drugs, steroids, and dietary alterations. In the presence of PBGD deficiency, factors that stimulate heme synthesis result in decreased availability of heme for the regulatory heme pool in hepatocytes. ALA 5-aminolevulinic acid; ALAD = 5-aminolevulinic acid dehydratase; ALAS1 = ALA synthase, housekeeping form; HMB = hydroxymethylbilane; PBG = porphobilinogen; PBGD = porphobilinogen deaminase.

syndrome, actually have acute porphyria also are poorly founded.[250–252]

Clinical Manifestations

The major clinical manifestations of AIP, including abdominal pain and other neurovisceral and circulatory disturbances, are due to effects on the nervous system. Adverse effects on the liver and kidney sometimes occur as well. Symptoms of AIP are associated with marked overproduction and excretion of porphyrin precursors and porphyrins, and increased activity of hepatic ALAS1. In asymptomatic AIP heterozygotes, porphyrin precursor excretion is usually normal, and, presumably, hepatic ALAS1 activity is not increased. Apparently, AIP becomes clinically manifest when there is an increased demand for hepatic heme synthesis due to exposure to a drug or other precipitating factor. Under these conditions, PBGD deficiency becomes limiting for heme synthesis. Because heme synthesis does not increase sufficiently to meet the increased demand, heme-mediated repression of ALAS1 is impaired (Fig. 124-13).

Clinical symptoms in AIP heterozygotes are more common in women than men, and are very rare in children. As already noted, symptoms of AIP before puberty are very rare. A child who died of porphyria at age 8 had severe neurologic and developmental abnormalities, and was later shown to have homozygous AIP.[253] Symptoms may appear any time after puberty, but often not until the third or fourth decade of life. In some women, attacks first appear after menopause. Because the disease so often remains latent, there may be no family history of porphyria.

Acute Attacks. Neurologic and visceral symptoms are usually intermittent and occur in acute attacks that develop over a few hours or days. Because the symptoms and signs are often nonspecific, a high index of suspicion is required to suggest the proper diagnosis. The disease can be disabling, but is only occasionally fatal. The neurovisceral manifestations of the other acute porphyrias are identical to those of AIP.

Abdominal pain has been reported in 85 to 95 percent of cases and is the most common and often the initial symptom of an acute attack.[254–256] Tachycardia is the most common physical sign, occurring in up to 80 percent of acute attacks.[256] Catecholamine secretion can be markedly increased during acute attacks.[257] Abdominal pain is usually severe, steady, and poorly localized, but may be cramping. It is usually accompanied by other gastrointestinal symptoms such as nausea, vomiting, and constipation, and signs of ileus, including abdominal distention and decreased bowel sounds. However, increased bowel sounds and diarrhea may occur. Dysuria and bladder dysfunction may occur, and urinary retention may require catheterization. The urine is often dark red in color. Because the neurovisceral manifestations are neurologic rather than inflammatory, tenderness, fever, and leukocytosis are absent or mild. Tachycardia, hypertension, restlessness, coarse or fine tremors, and excess sweating may be due to sympathetic overactivity or autonomic neuropathy. Postural hypotension and abnormal cardiovascular reflexes may also result from autonomic neuropathy.[258,259] A variety of mental symptoms, pain in limbs, head, neck, or chest, muscle weakness, and sensory loss can occur. Extremity pain is often described as muscle pain, and may be a manifestation of early peripheral neuropathy. Recurrent attacks tend to be similar in a given patient.

Neuropathy and Central Nervous System Involvement. Significant neuropathy does not occur in all patients with acute attacks of porphyria, even when abdominal symptoms are severe. However, sometimes a significant peripheral neuropathy develops in this and other acute porphyrias when there is little or no abdominal pain.[260] Peripheral neuropathy in the acute porphyrias is primarily motor and appears to result from axonal degeneration rather than demyelinization.[261–263] Weakness most commonly begins in the proximal muscles and more often in the arms than in the legs. Detection of proximal muscle weakness often requires a careful neurologic examination. Motor weakness is often symmetric, but may be asymmetric or strikingly focal. Tendon reflexes may be minimally affected or hyperactive in early stages, but are usually decreased or absent when neuropathy is advanced. Impairment of motor conduction velocities, which would primarily reflect impaired conduction in the fastest fibers, may not be prominent. However, an analysis of slow motor fibers by antidromal blocking indicated that conduction in these fibers can be impaired even in latent AIP.[264,265] Cranial nerves, most commonly the tenth and seventh, can be affected. Rarely, involvement of the optic nerves or occipital lobes may produce blindness. Cortical blindness, which may be a presenting manifestation and resolve with therapy, may result from vasospasm.[266,267] There may be sensory involvement with areas of paresthesia, dysesthesia, and loss of sensation. Progression to respiratory and bulbar paralysis and death seldom occurs unless porphyria is not recognized, harmful drugs not discontinued, and appropriate treatment not instituted.

The course of the neurologic manifestations of acute porphyria is highly variable. Advanced motor neuropathy, respiratory and bulbar paralysis, and death due to porphyria were more common in the past than now. Sudden death may occur, presumably due to cardiac arrhythmia.[259,261,268] Acute attacks of porphyria may resolve quite rapidly, with abdominal pain disappearing within a few hours and paresis within a few days. Even advanced motor neuropathy is potentially reversible. After a severe attack, motor function may continue to improve for several years but may leave some residual weakness.[255] Recurrent attacks of porphyria may slow neurologic recovery if the attacks are associated with recurrent nerve damage.

Central nervous system involvement is common and highly variable. Anxiety, insomnia, depression, disorientation, hallucinations, and paranoia can be especially severe during acute attacks, and suggest a primary mental disorder or hysteria. Chronic depression and other continuing mental symptoms may occur. Suicide is reported to be common.[269] It is often difficult to determine if chronic mental symptoms are due to porphyria or other causes. As already noted, the prevalence of AIP may be higher in psychiatric patients than in the general population,[241] although this has not been found in some studies.[270] Some investigators,[271] but not others,[272–274] have suggested that schizophrenia is associated with genetic variation at or near the *PBGD* gene.

Seizures are a particularly difficult problem in patients with acute porphyria. They may be a neurologic manifestation of porphyria itself or may be secondary to hyponatremia or a cause unrelated to porphyria (e.g., coexistent idiopathic epilepsy). A recent survey of 268 AIP patients in Sweden found that 3.7 percent reported epileptic seizures, either tonic-clonic seizures or partial seizures becoming secondarily generalized.[275] Associated hyponatremia was more likely when seizures occurred with an acute attack. As discussed below, almost all antiseizure drugs can exacerbate acute porphyria. Therefore, before committing to prolonged antiseizure treatment, it is important to determine whether seizures are simply a manifestation of an acute attack or are due to another cause and are likely to recur without continued drug treatment.

Electrolyte Abnormalities. The disease may be complicated by electrolyte abnormalities. Hyponatremia is common during acute attacks, and may help to suggest the diagnosis. This is sometimes due to SIADH. Damage to the supraoptic nuclei of the hypothalamus has been noted at autopsy.[276] However, hyponatremia during an acute porphyric attack is not always attributable to inappropriate ADH secretion. Unexplained reductions in total blood and red blood cell volumes occur in some patients.[277] When this is accompanied by hyponatremia and evidence of increased ADH secretion, the latter can be considered an appropriate physiologic response, and morphologic changes in the hypothalamus may reflect a hyperfunctional state rather than a degenerative process.[268] It has been suggested that salt depletion from gastrointestinal loss and poor intake, and excess renal sodium loss are more frequent causes of hyponatremia than inappropriate ADH secretion.[268,278,279] A possible nephrotoxic effect of ALA may explain renal tubular sodium loss and impaired renal function in some patients with acute porphyria.[278,280] Hypomagnesemia and hypercalcemia — the latter as a result of prolonged immobilization — may complicate acute porphyria.[281,282]

Prognosis. The outlook for patients with acute attacks of porphyria was previously regarded as poor, with a mortality rate as high as 80 percent. Morbidity and mortality of the acute porphyrias has improved markedly in the past 20 to 30 years. In a 1992 case series, for example, 74 percent of patients with AIP or VP reported that they lead normal lives.[283] During several years of follow-up, less than one-third of patients had recurrences of attacks and only 6 percent of gene carriers who had never had attacks developed symptoms. In patients who presented with acute symptoms, recurrent attacks were most likely within the subsequent 1 to 3 years.[283] This improved outlook may be due to earlier detection, a decline in use of barbiturates in medical practice, and better management of acute attacks.

Other Manifestations. Other organ systems can be affected. Mild, unexplained and usually chronic abnormalities in liver function tests (especially serum alanine aminotransferase) are common in AIP and other acute porphyrias.[284] More advanced liver disease and hepatocellular carcinoma sometimes complicate the disease.[285–290] When hepatocellular carcinoma develops in AIP, other factors known to predispose to this cancer are seldom present, and the uninvolved liver may be normal histologically.[290,291] AIP may also predispose to chronic hypertension and impaired renal function.[283]

Other metabolic abnormalities have been associated with AIP. Hypercholesterolemia and elevated low-density lipoprotein cholesterol appear to be less common in this disorder than previously thought.[292] Serum thyroxin levels may be increased due to increased thyroxin-binding globulin. Occasionally, true hyperthyroidism and porphyria occur together.[293] Sex hormone-binding globulin, thyroxine-binding globulin, and cortisol-binding globulin may be increased during attacks of AIP; sex hormone-binding globulin is most commonly increased and is likely to fall with treatment and resolution of an attack.[294]

Other endocrine and metabolic abnormalities reported in AIP include paradoxical glucose-stimulated growth hormone release,[295] defective ACTH release,[296] galactorrhea,[281] glucose intolerance,[297] and hyperinsulinemia.[298] Coexistent diabetes mellitus does not appear to exacerbate acute porphyrias, and may even be beneficial.[299] The contribution of endocrine factors to activating the disease is discussed below.

The Metabolic Defect in AIP

Accumulated Porphyrin Precursors and Porphyrins. Urinary ALA and PBG are always markedly increased in symptomatic patients with AIP and even in some asymptomatic individuals with the inherited enzyme deficiency. PBG and porphyrin concentrations are increased in liver, which suggests the liver is the predominant source of these excess compounds. Urinary PBG excretion is generally in the range of 50 to 200 mg/day during an attack. ALA excretion, when also expressed as mg/day, is about half that of PBG.[300] These porphyrin precursors remain increased between attacks in patients who are prone to repeated exacerbations, and increase further at the time of an attack. They may decrease to normal if the disease becomes inactive for a prolonged period. Urinary porphyrins are also markedly increased, which may seem surprising since the deficient enzyme precedes the synthesis of porphyrins in the pathway. Circulating concentrations of ALA and PBG in plasma (or serum) are substantially increased. As expected for a type of porphyria that does not cause photosensitivity, plasma porphyrins are normal or only slightly increased. ALA and PBG decrease rapidly after heme infusions.

ALA and PBG are colorless and therefore their presence does not explain the red or brown urine that is common in AIP. Reddish urine in AIP is due to increased porphyrins. When urinary PBG is increased the predominant porphyrin in urine is uroporphyrin. Coproporphyrin may also be substantially increased. Uroporphyrin can form nonenzymatically from PBG. This may not be the only explanation for increased porphyrins in AIP, because the excess porphyrins in this condition are predominantly type III, which suggests that they are formed enzymatically.[301–303] This might occur if excess ALA produced in liver enters cells in other tissues and is there converted to porphyrins via the heme biosynthetic pathway.[15] It is well known that ALA loading in normal animals and humans increases tissue porphyrin content and urinary coproporphyrin, and it is possible that PBGD deficiency does not preclude excess endogenous ALA from being metabolized to porphyrins in some tissues. Liver abnormalities are common in AIP, which, if sufficient to impair hepatic excretion of coproporphyrin, would explain, at least in part, increased urinary excretion of this porphyrin.

Brownish discoloration of the urine in AIP may be due to porphobilin, a degradation product of porphobilinogen, or dipyrrylmethenes. A combination of these compounds and red-colored porphyrins may account for the commonly described "port wine" color of the urine in acute porphyrias. Acid pH, heat, and exposure to light promote the nonenzymatic formation of these compounds.

Fecal porphyrins are usually normal or minimally increased in AIP, which distinguishes this disorder from HCP and VP. Erythrocyte zinc protoporphyrin concentrations are often mildly or moderately increased in patients with clinically expressed AIP. Iron deficiency and other causes, such as lead poisoning, should be excluded before this finding is attributed to AIP.

The Enzymatic Defect in AIP. The half-normal activity of PBGD is the enzymatic defect in AIP.[304–306] However, about 5 percent of the patients have normal PBGD activity in their erythrocytes.[307] These AIP heterozygotes have the "erythroid variant" due to mutations in or near exon 1 which result in the deficiency of the housekeeping isozyme in all tissues, but not the erythroid isozyme (see below "Molecular Pathology"). The range of erythrocyte PBGD activity in patients without the "erythroid variant" overlaps somewhat the range for normal individuals, as discussed later (see "Decreased PBGD Activity"). To our knowledge, the levels of hepatic PBGD activity have not been compared in patients with active and latent AIP. In the absence of evidence to the contrary, it is presumed that hepatic PBGD is half-normal in AIP in both latent and clinically expressed disease, and the degree of induction of hepatic ALAS1 by the factors such as drugs and steroids determines the degree of clinical expression. However, the possibility that in some circumstances ALAS1 induction is enhanced by a further reduction of PBGD activity is not excluded. Genetic influences that are presently not identified may also influence the clinical expression of inherited PBGD deficiency.[235]

Uroporphyrinogen III is a key intermediate in the biosynthesis of all naturally occurring tetrapyrroles, and is formed from PBG through the sequential action of two enzymes. Four molecules of PBG can also undergo a nonenzymatic condensation to yield four possible uroporphyrinogen isomers[308,309] (Fig. 124-4), while enzyme-catalyzed reactions yield only the type I and III isomers of uroporphyrinogen. The first enzyme, PBGD (or uroporphyrinogen I synthase in the older literature), catalyzes the polymerization of four molecules of PBG in a linear head-to-tail fashion, yielding a linear tetrapyrrole intermediate, HMB[310] (Fig. 124-14). In the absence of the next enzyme in the heme biosynthetic pathway, UROS, the linear tetrapyrrole HMB undergoes spontaneous ring closure to form the uroporphyrinogen I isomer.[310] Thus, the deaminase furnishes a straight chain tetrapyrrole, but is not an enzyme for ring closure.[311] UROS then rapidly converts HMB to uroporphyrinogen III, a reaction that involves an intramolecular rearrangement affecting only ring D and the atoms that become C-15 and C-20 of uroporphyrinogen III. There is also evidence suggesting an association or complex of PBGD and UROS, which

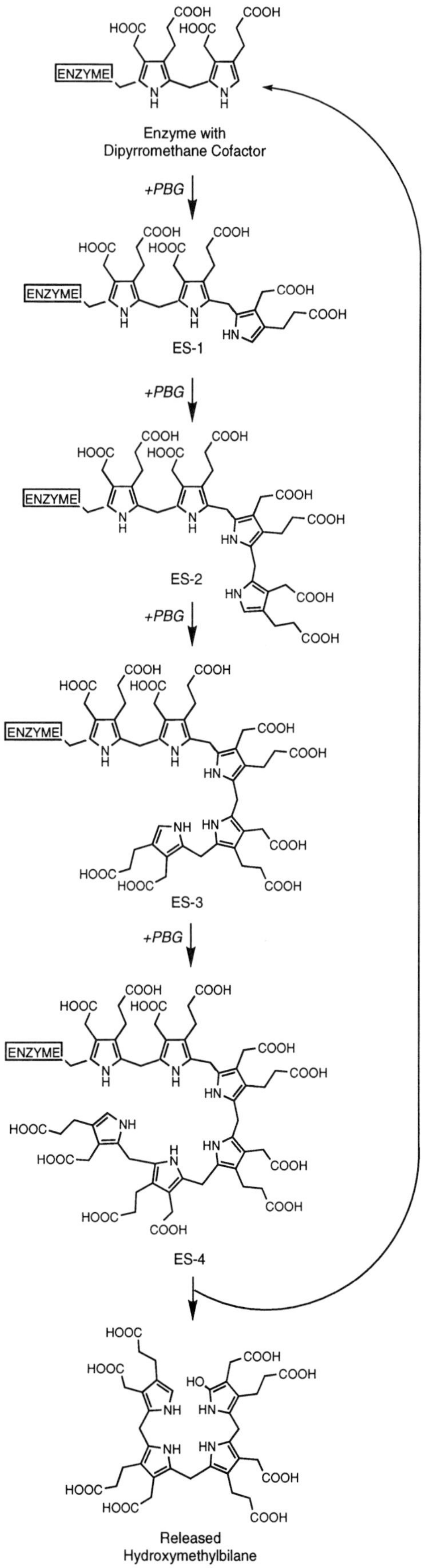

Enzyme with Dipyrromethane Cofactor

+PBG

ES-1

+PBG

ES-2

+PBG

ES-3

+PBG

ES-4

Released Hydroxymethylbilane

Fig. 124-14 Enzymatic formation of hydroxymethylbilane from PBG. The structure of the dipyrromethane cofactor, which is complexed with the enzyme PBGD, and its role in the tetrapolymerization of PBG are shown. Hydroxymethylbilane forms uroporphyrinogen III by the action of uroporphyrinogen III synthase, or after its release from PBGD undergoes nonenzymatic spontaneous closure of the tetrapyrrole ring to become uroporphyrinogen I.

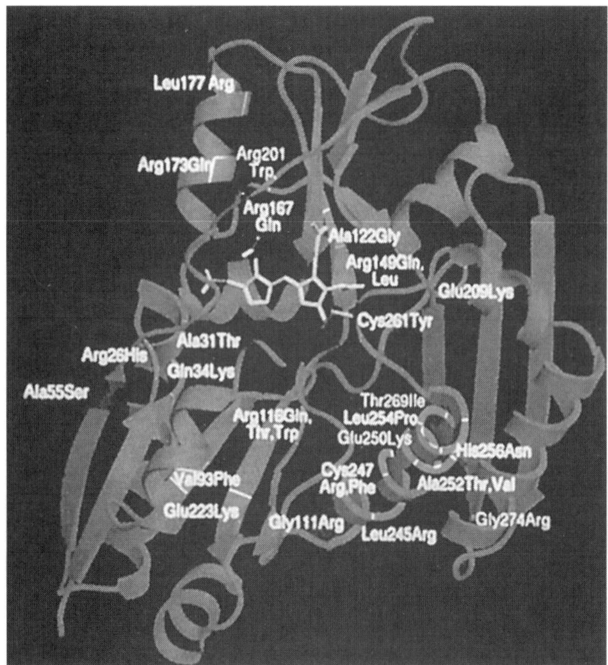

Fig. 124-15 Crystal structure of *E. coli* PBGD showing the polypeptide chain folded into three domains with the dipyrromethane cofactor located in the active site cavity. Suggested locations of the human PBGD mutations causing AIP are shown, as predicted by comparing the aligned amino acid sequences of *E. coli* and human PBGD. The effects of specific mutations on enzyme structure and function can be predicted as described.[325] *(Reproduced from Brownlie et al.[325] Used by permission.)*

would account for the rapid enzymatic formation of uroporphyrinogen III.[312,313]

Purification and Properties of PBGD. Human PBGD purified from erythrocytes has a specific activity of ~2300 units/mg protein.[314] PBGD functions as a monomer and the enzyme from human and other sources has molecular weights ranging from 36 to 40 kDa.[314–316] PBGD is stable when bound covalently to its substrate.[317] Lead inhibits the activity of erythrocyte PBGD in vitro,[318] although the concentrations required are much higher than those found to inhibit ALAD activity in lead poisoning; erythrocyte PBGD activity is not inhibited in patients with plumbism. PBGD from rat liver also is inhibited in vitro by a wide range of di- and trivalent metal ions.[319]

PBGD purified from human erythrocytes forms stable covalent enzyme-substrate complexes with PBG.[314] Using purified PBGD from *E. coli* or *Euglena gracilis*, it was shown that the enzyme contains, at its catalytic site, a dipyrromethane cofactor.[320–322] The cofactor is derived from PBG, but is not subject to catalytic turnover.[323] The function of the dipyrromethane cofactor is to anchor the substrate molecules at the catalytic site, and to direct the condensation of PBG to form the tetrapyrrole.

Crystal Structure. The crystal structure of *E. coli* PBGD revealed that the polypeptide chain of 313 amino acids is folded into 3 domains, each comprising β-strands and α-helices and a discrete hydrophobic core.[324,325] The dipyrromethane cofactor is attached to a loop on domain III and positioned at the mouth of a deep cavity formed between the structurally related domains I and II.[325] Because the *E. coli* and human PBGD amino acid sequences have 35 percent homology and more than 70 percent similarity, it is possible to infer structure/function relationships for certain human *PBGD* mutations (Fig. 124-15).[326]

The Molecular Genetics and Pathology of *PBGD*

cDNA and Genomic Sequences. The cDNA encoding PBGD was first isolated from a rat erythroid library[327] and then used to isolate human *PBGD* cDNAs from erythroid and nonerythroid sources.[328,329] Based on the cDNA sequence, human erythroid PBGD was predicted to consist of 344 amino acid residues. Sequencing of the nonerythroid cDNA predicted the existence of 17 additional amino acid residues at its *N*-terminus, while the remainder was identical to the erythroid cDNA[329] (Fig. 124-16). *PBGD* cDNAs have been cloned from variety of organisms from *E. coli* to humans. There is a high degree of evolutionary conservation in certain regions of the amino acid sequence that may define functional domains.

The gene encoding PBGD initially was localized to chromosome 11 using human/mouse somatic cell hybrids.[330] Subsequently, the regional assignment of the human *PBGD* gene was made to chromosome 11q23 → 11qter using somatic cell hybrids and immunologic, electrophoretic, and cytogenetic techniques.[331,332] The 10-kb human *PBGD* genomic sequence contains 15 exons.[333] The erythroid-specific and housekeeping mRNAs are produced by alternative splicing under the control of two promoters. The upstream promoter is active in all tissues, while the other promoter, located 3 kb downstream, is active only in erythroid cells. The erythroid promoter displays some structural characteristics of other erythroid-specific promoters, including a CACCC motif, two GATA-1 sites, and one NF-E2 binding site.[334] This finding suggests that common *trans*-acting factors may coregulate the transcription of these genes during erythroid development.[335–337]

Molecular Pathology. Over 150 mutations in the *PBGD* gene have been identified (for reviews, see references 235 and 338) (Fig. 124-17) including missense, nonsense, and splicing

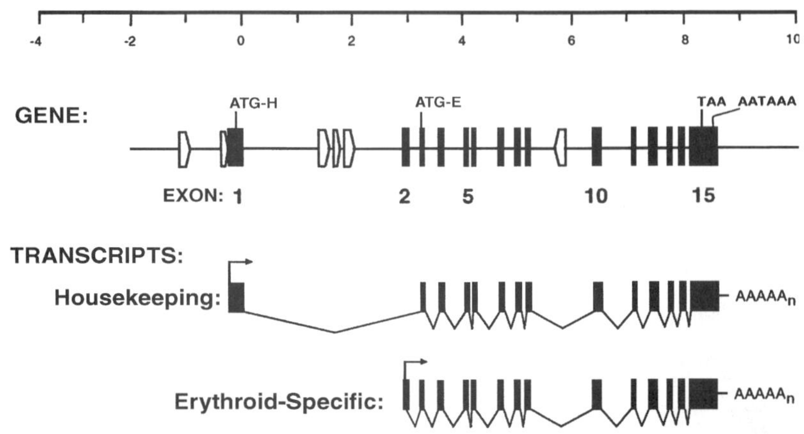

Fig. 124-16 Organization of the *PBGD* gene and alternate splicing of the housekeeping and erythroid-specific transcripts. The 15 exons are represented as solid rectangles, and the positions and orientations of the *Alu* repeat elements are indicated by the pentagonal boxes. The promoter region for the housekeeping transcript is 5′ to exon 1, and the promoter for the erythroid-specific transcript is immediately 5′ to exon 2. Translation initiation methionines for the housekeeping and erythroid-specific enzymes are indicated (ATG-H and ATG-E, respectively).

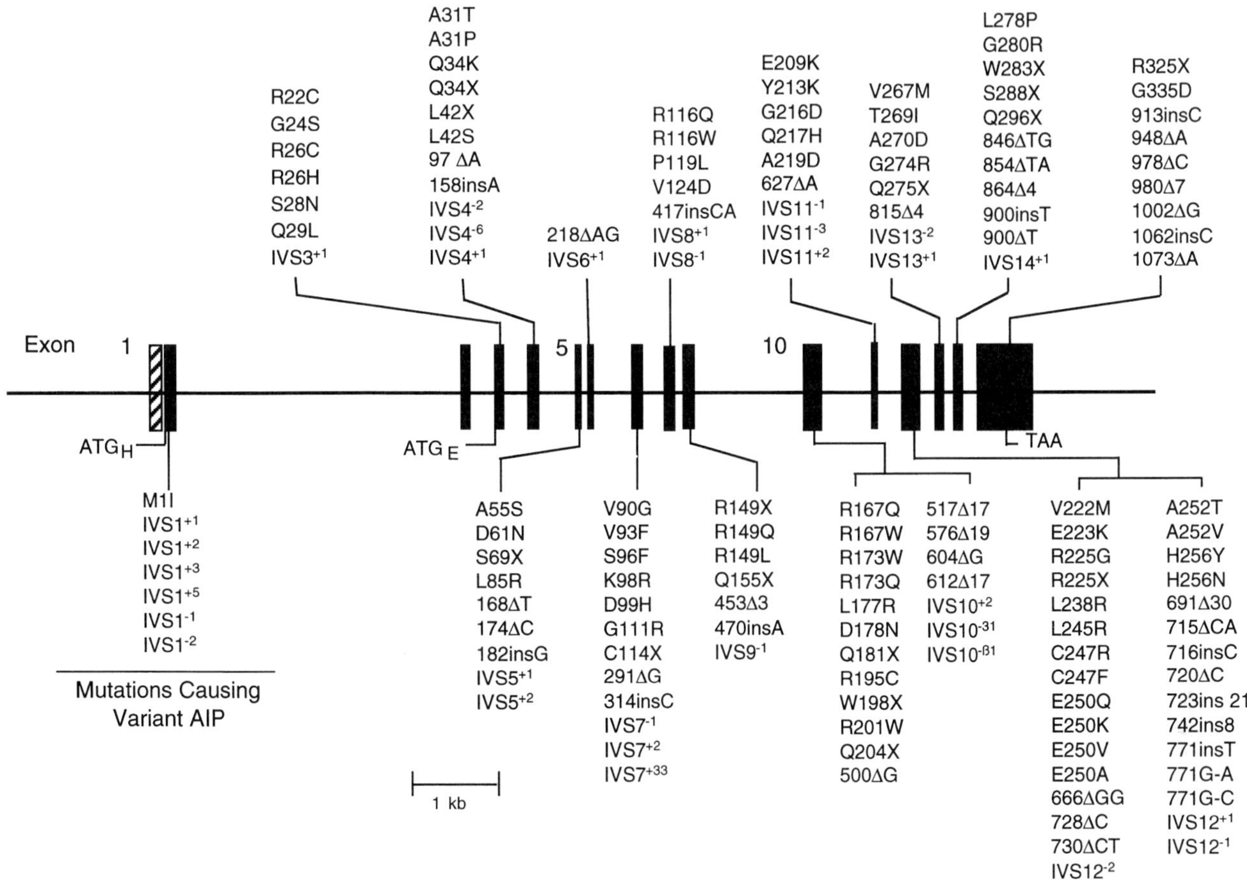

Fig. 124-17 The human *PBGD* gene, with locations of some of the many mutations causing AIP. (*Courtesy of Dr. K. H. Astrin.*)

mutations, as well as insertions and deletions. Most of these mutations are private, having been reported in only one or a few families. However, common mutations have been identified in Swedish (R116W), Dutch (W198X), Argentinean (G116R), and Nova Scotian (R173W) patients.[239,240,339] Based on immunologic studies of the mutant enzyme proteins in erythrocytes, three subtypes of *PBGD* mutations have been identified.[338,340] In type 1 CRIM-negative mutations, the PBGD activity and enzyme protein are decreased by ~50 percent in all tissues. This is the largest category of mutations (~85 percent) that render the enzyme protein unstable. They include missense and nonsense mutations, small deletions, and insertions, and splicing defects that cause frameshifts and early polypeptide truncation.[336,338] Type II mutations also are CRIM-negative and include five mutations that alter the 5′ splice-donor site of intron 1, and a missense mutation in the exon 1 initiation of translation codon.[341–345] These mutations result in the absence of the housekeeping isozyme, but normal levels of the erythroid-specific isozyme. Therefore, the level of erythrocyte PBGD activity in these patients is normal, while the activity in other tissues and cells is half-normal. Less than 5 percent of AIP patients are known to have these mutations that cause the "erythroid variant" form of AIP. Type III mutations are CRIM-positive and include mutations that decrease PBGD activity, but do not alter the mutant enzyme's stability. Examples of type III mutations include the intron 12 point mutation IVS12^{-1} that results in abnormal splicing and skipping of exon 12, producing an abnormal but stable polypeptide lacking the 40 residues encoded by exon 12,[342] and two exon 10 missense mutations, R167Q and R173Q, that produce catalytically impaired, but stable enzyme proteins.[346] The R173Q mutant protein binds PBG and stable enzyme-substrate intermediates accumulate. It has been suggested that these enzyme-substrate intermediates stabilize the mutant enzyme, thereby explaining the CRIM-positive status of this mutation.[326]

As shown in Fig. 124-15, modeling of the AIP lesions to the corresponding residues in the crystal structure of *E. coli*, PBGD provides insight into the structure-function relationships of the human enzyme (see above "Crystal Structure").[324–326] For example, mutations R167Q and R173Q involve highly conserved arginines with R167Q impairing substrate binding.[325] Many other exon 10 mutations occur at conserved amino acids in the active site, while many exon 12 mutations alter the α-helix connecting domains 1 and 3.[306,326,336] Thus, with over 150 reported mutations, there is marked molecular heterogeneity underlying AIP.[235,336] *De novo* mutations occur in approximately 3 percent of cases.[347]

Pathophysiology

Virtually all the symptoms and signs of the acute porphyrias are thought to result from neurologic dysfunction. However, the mechanism of neural damage in these disorders is poorly understood.[348,349] Various hypotheses that are not mutually exclusive have been proposed. It is possible that the formation of heme and important hemoproteins is compromised in nervous tissue due to the inherited enzyme deficiency.[82] However, direct evidence for this hypothesis is lacking.[265] Vasospasm perhaps resulting from decreased production of nitrous oxide by the hemoprotein enzyme nitrous oxide synthase has been suggested to cause cerebral manifestations of the disease.[266,267]

A leading hypothesis is that ALA or PBG, originating in nonneural tissues, is neurotoxic. This possibility is suggested by the increased production of these porphyrin precursors during acute attacks of AIP, HCP, and VP, and by the finding of increased ALA in ADP, lead poisoning, and hereditary tyrosinemia.[265] These levels are virtually never normal during acute attacks of porphyria. Although porphyrin precursor levels are sometimes increased in clinically asymptomatic stages of acute porphyria, they increase further when there are symptoms due to porphyria. If porphyrin precursors do contribute to neural damage in the acute hepatic porphyrias, it is likely that they originate from the liver, where ALAS1 is inducible by factors such as drugs and hormones that are known to exacerbate acute porphyria. ALAS does not appear to be inducible in brain.[74] Most tissues take up ALA more readily than PBG, although PBG appears to cross the blood-brain barrier more readily.[350] Because peripheral nerves are not protected by a blood-brain barrier, they are exposed to levels of ALA comparable to those in blood.[265] ALA can enter cells readily and then be converted to porphyrins, which, in turn, may have toxic potential. ALA loading can increase protoporphyrin in the nervous system, albeit to a lesser degree than in other tissues.[15] A potential role for porphyrins as neurotoxic agents is suggested by the development of neuropathy in some patients with EPP and liver failure, as discussed later (see "EPP, Clinical Manifestations"). ALA is also structurally similar to γ-aminobutyric acid (GABA) and can interact with GABA receptors.[351,352] However, it is unclear how this receptor interaction would lead to neuronal damage. ALA can also undergo metal-catalyzed oxidation, promote lipid peroxidation, and induce iron release from ferritin in liver. It is conceivable that iron released from ferritin can mediate oxidative damage and contribute to cell damage, at least in the liver.[353]

Another hypothesis is that a functional heme deficiency in liver might predispose to unsaturation of hepatic tryptophan pyrrolase and lead to altered tryptophan delivery to nervous tissues.[354] Modestly increased urinary excretion of some tryptophan metabolites during acute attacks of porphyria, which decreased to normal with heme administration, is consistent with this idea.[355] Low nocturnal plasma melatonin levels in patients with recurrent attacks of this disease may suggest disordered pineal function and circadian rhythm.[355] Increased serotonergic activity, perhaps resulting from increased delivery of tryptophan, might contribute to autonomic dysfunction in acute porphyrias.[265] Heme deficiency in the nervous system might also impair the functions of other hemoproteins, such as nitric oxide synthase, and impair formation of cyclic GMP. Central nervous system manifestations of AIP might also result from vasospasm, as suggested by the observation by MRI of reversible cerebral abnormalities.[356] A further suggestion is that the increased activity of ALAS1 may result in depletion of PLP, the cofactor required by this enzyme. Neuropathic manifestations of PLP deficiency and AIP are similar in some respects, and there is evidence suggesting low PLP status in some AIP patients.[357,358]

A mouse model in which PBGD deficiency was induced by gene targeting will be useful to further define the mechanisms of neurologic damage in acute porphyrias.[265,359] These animals display impaired motor function, ataxia, increased levels of ALA in plasma and brain, and decreased heme saturation of liver tryptophan pyrrolase. A recent report indicates that motor neuropathy can develop in these mice with normal or only slightly increased ALA in plasma and urine, which may support a primary role for heme deficiency in porphyric neuropathy.[360]

Precipitating Factors. An inherited deficiency of PBGD is not in itself sufficient to cause clinical expression of AIP. The great majority, perhaps 90 percent, of individuals who inherit a *PBGD* mutation never develop porphyric symptoms. Most precipitating factors have the capacity to induce hepatic cytochrome P450 enzymes and ALAS1, and by increasing the demand for heme synthesis cause the partial deficiency of PBGD to become rate limiting for heme synthesis in the liver. There are certain factors that are well known for precipitating acute attacks, and these often act in an additive fashion. However, the immediate precipitating factor cannot always be identified. It is possible that individual susceptibility to clinical expression is determined by other and presently unknown genetic factors.[235]

Endocrine Factors. There is considerable evidence that endocrine factors and steroid hormones, in particular, are among the most important precipitating factors in AIP. (a) The disease is rarely symptomatic before puberty. Likewise, increased excretion of porphyrin precursors is almost never observed in children with PBGD deficiency. (b) Symptoms are more common in women with this enzyme deficiency than in men, suggesting that adult levels of female hormones are particularly important. (c) Some women develop premenstrual attacks. These are probably due to endogenous progesterone, and can be prevented by the administration of gonadotropin-releasing hormone (GnRH) analogues.[361–365] (d) Acute porphyrias are sometimes exacerbated by exogenous steroids, including oral contraceptive preparations. (e) Pregnancy can exacerbate attacks, albeit in a minority of women with AIP, as discussed below. (f) Attacks seem to be less common in women after menopause, although they can occur. (g) More subtle abnormalities in steroid hormone metabolism, such as a deficiency of hepatic steroid 5α-reductase activity in some patients with AIP, can predispose to the excess production of steroid hormone metabolites that are inducers of ALAS1 in the liver.[366,367]

Pregnancy is usually well tolerated, and is usually not contraindicated in this or other acute porphyrias if harmful drugs are avoided and nutritional status is optimized. For example, Kauppinen and coworkers[283] reviewed the clinical features of 76 women with AIP or VP who had 176 deliveries. Porphyric symptoms did not occur in 92 percent of these pregnancies. Some previous reports of worsening symptoms during pregnancy may have been due to the use of barbiturates and perhaps to reduced caloric intake. Metoclopramide, a contraindicated drug, has been associated with exacerbation of the disease when used to treat hyperemesis gravidarum.[368,369] The generally favorable course during pregnancy is surprising given the considerably increased circulating progesterone levels. Progesterone and its metabolites are potent inducers of the heme biosynthetic pathway in liver.[21,370] As previously described, certain metabolic effects of pregnancy may protect against the development of acute attacks, including potentially favorable changes in progesterone metabolism.[371] However, for reasons that are not clear, some women with these disorders do have attacks more frequently during pregnancy. Urinary excretion of porphyrin precursors and coproporphyrin is increased in normal pregnant women, especially in the month before delivery, but the levels do not approach those seen in the acute porphyrias.[3]

Drugs. Drugs are among the most important factors that precipitate attacks of acute porphyria. Many patients do well after the diagnosis of porphyria is established if they avoid harmful drugs. Barbiturates and sulfonamide antibiotics have been the drugs most commonly implicated in causing attacks of porphyria. Barbiturates are now seldom used as sedatives in medical practice, and this undoubtedly has greatly improved the prognosis of patients with acute porphyrias. While barbiturate-induced attacks are much less common than in the past, sulfonamides and other drugs remain important as precipitating agents.

It is widely agreed that many commonly used drugs are either safe or unsafe in the acute porphyrias, and these are listed in Table 124-4. Knowledge about the safety of many other drugs and chemicals is incomplete, making it impossible to classify them all as definitely safe or unsafe. Clinical observations, although usually sporadic, incompletely reported, and necessarily uncontrolled, and experimental studies in animals and liver cell cultures may provide useful guidance. Some drugs about which opinions vary also are indicated in Table 124-4. More extensive lists of drugs have been prepared.[233,371] An extensive list is also available through the American Porphyria Foundation's Web site (www.enterprise.net/apf). Whenever possible, it is advisable to use drugs established as safe for treating concurrent diseases in patients with porphyria.

Table 124-4 Categories of Safe and Unsafe Drugs in the Acute Porphyrias*

Unsafe	Potentially Unsafe	Probably Safe	Safe
ACE inhibitors (especially enalapril)[380,383]	Alfadolone acetate[985,986]	Adrenaline[383]	Acetaminophen (paracetamol)[383,968]
Antipyrine (phenazone)[383,967,968]	Alfaxolone[985,986]	Azathioprine[988,993]	Acetazolamide[383,386]
Aminopyrine (amidopyrine)[383,967,968]	Alkylating agents [cyclophosphamide, ifosfamide, busulphan, altretamine (hexamethylmelamine); dacarbazine, chlorambucil, and melphalan may be safer)][388,967,981,987,988]	Chloramphenicol[968,969]	Allopurinol[383,386]
Aminoglutethimide[383,969]	Altretamine (hexamethylmelamine, see alkylating agents)	Cisapride[383]	Amiloride[383,386]
Barbiturates[248,254,256,383,968]	Amitriptyline (see tricyclic antidepressants)	Colchicine[233,383]	Aspirin[383,968]
N-Butylscopolammonium bromide[383]	Benzodiazepines[383,989,990]	Cytarabine[987]	Atropine[383,968]
Calcium channel blockers (especially nifedipine)[380–382,384]	Busulphan (see alkylating agents)	Chloroquine[233,383]	Bethanidine[383,384]
Carbamazepine[383,467]	Captopril (see ACE inhibitors)	Digoxin[383]	Bromides[466,974]
Carisoprodol[383]	Cephalosporins[383]	Daunorubicin[987]	Bumetanide[386]
Chlorpropamide[383,967,970–972]	Chlorambucil (see alkylating agents)	Doxazosin[384]	Chloral hydrate[39,255,383]
Danazol[475,476]	Chlordiazepoxide[968,969,991]	Estrogens (natural/ endogenous)[370,469,1006,1007]	Cimetidine[459]
Dapsone[383,973]	Clonidine[15,992]	Ibuprofen[383]	Corticosteroids[279,383]
Diclofenac[383]	Cyclophosphamide (see alkylating agents)	Indomethacin[383]	Coumarins[383]
Enalapril (see ACE inhibitors)	Cyclosporin[383,993]	Labetalol[383]	Fluoxetine[383,386,387]
Diphenylhydantion[256,466,467,974]	Diazepam[968,969,991]	Lithium[383]	Gabapentin[468]
Ethosuximide (see succinimides)	Diltiazem (see calcium channel blockers)	Losartan[380]	Gentamycin[383]
Ergot preparations[383,971]	Colistin[383]	Methenamine[279]	Guanethidine[39,279,384]
Ethchlorvynol[967]	Dacarbazine (see alkylating agents)	Methylphenidate[383,969]	Insulin[383,967]
Ethinamate[970]	Diphenhydramine[383,969]	Naproxen[383]	Narcotic analgesics[39,383]
Felbamate[468]	EDTA (see iron chelators)	Neostigmine[279,383]	Ofloxacin[383]
Glutethimide[279,969,971]	Etomidate[383,986,994]	Nitrous oxide[279,383]	Penicillin and derivatives[279,383,967]
Griseofulvin[49,975]	Estrogens (synthetic)[474,995]	Penicillamine[383]	Phenothiazines[39,383]
Ketoconazole[383]	Erythromycin[383]	Procaine[383]	Propranolol[279,1008]
Lamotrigine[468,976]	5-Fluorouracil[988]	Propanidid[279,383]	Streptomycin[279,383]
Mephenytoin[383,969,977]	Gold compounds (see heavy metals)	Propofol[383]	Succinylcholine[383,967]
Metoclopramide[368,369,978]	Fluroxene[996,997]	Propoxyphene[279,383]	Tetracycline[279]
Meprobamate[39,383,969]	Heavy metals[383,967,971,998]	Rauwolfia alkaloids[279]	
Methyprylon[39,383,969]	Hydralazine[39,383]	6-Thioguanine[987]	
Nefazadone[387]	Hyoscine[383]	Thiouracils[383]	
Nifedipine (see calcium channel blockers)	Ifosfamide (see alkylating agents)	Thyroxine[383]	
Novobiocin[383]	Imipramine (see tricyclic antidepressants)	Tubocurarine[383]	
Phenylbutazone[34,383,967,968]	Iron chelators (DFO, EDTA)	Vigabatrin[468]	
Primidone[383]	Ketamine[383,390]	Vitamin B[279]	
Pargyline[39,383,969]	Lisinopril (see ACE inhibitors)	Vitamin C[279]	
Progesterone & progestins[370,979]			
Rifampin[383,980,981]			
Succinimides[383,969]			
Sulfasalazine[982]			
Sulfonamide antibiotics[256,383]			
Sulfonmethane (Sulfonal) & sulfonethylmethane(Trional)[983]			
Sulfonylureas[383,970]			

(Continued on next page)

Table 124-4 (Continued)

Unsafe	Potentially Unsafe	Probably Safe	Safe
Trimethadione[383,969,977]	Mefenamic acid[383]		
Valproic acid[466,984]	Melphalan (see alkylating agents)		
Tranylcypromine[969]	Mifepristone (RU-486)[999,1000]		
	Methyldopa[383,971]		
	Metyrapone[969]		
	Nalidixic acid[383]		
	Nikethamide[383,967,969,970]		
	Nitrazepam[383,991]		
	Nitrofurantoin[279,383]		
	Nortriptyline (see tricyclic antidepressants)		
	Pentazocine[380,383,971,986,1001]		
	Phenoxybenzamine[39]		
	Procarbazine[988]		
	Pyrazinamide[967,1002]		
	Spironolactone[39,383]		
	Theophylline[383,967]		
	Tiagabine[468]		
	Tramadol[380]		
	Tricyclic antidepressants[383,386,967,968,1003]		
	Troglitazone[1004,1005]		

*Drugs (generic names) are listed in four categories, depending upon the weight of evidence as to their safety. There is considerable evidence for classification of drugs in the Safe and Unsafe categories, but much less evidence, or conflicting evidence, for drugs in the other two categories. This list is not comprehensive and does not reflect all information and opinions about drug safety in acute porphyrias. Some references cited may reflect conflicting opinions rather than supporting the classifications shown here.

Knowing the effects of a drug on hepatic heme metabolism in humans or laboratory animals is often useful in predicting whether a drug is safe or not. Most drugs that exacerbate porphyria have the capacity to induce hepatic ALAS1, which is closely associated with induction of cytochrome P450 enzymes, a process that increases the demand for heme synthesis in the liver.[370] If one of the enzymes in the heme biosynthetic pathway is deficient, ALAS1 induction can occur with lower dosages of inducing drugs.[39,370] In the liver, the response to an increased demand for heme includes induction of ALAS1 and increased synthesis of all heme biosynthetic pathway intermediates, which in turn can lead to the accumulation of pathway intermediates when one of the enzymes in the pathway is partially deficient. Therefore, it is reasonable to consider that any drug that induces hepatic cytochrome P450 enzymes is potentially harmful in acute porphyrias. Drugs that interact with P450 enzymes as substrates or inhibitors rather than as inducers are not necessarily harmful in porphyria.

The mechanism for the harmful effects of sulfonamide antibiotics in acute porphyria has been little studied. These drugs are harmful even though they apparently do not induce ALAS1 and cytochrome P450 enzymes. Although there is evidence that they inhibit PBGD,[372] a recent study questions whether these drugs or others act in this manner.[373] Ethanol intake has been associated with attacks, which is consistent with ethanol and other alcohols found in beverages being inducers of ALAS1 and at least some cytochrome P450 enzymes.[374–376]

Some drugs also can increase heme synthesis by promoting the destruction of cytochrome P450 enzymes, at least in experimental systems.[377] Mechanism-based destruction of cytochrome P450 by some drugs and chemicals can also lead to formation of *N*-alkylated protoporphyrins, some of which are potent inhibitors of ferrochelatase (e.g., *N*-methyl protoporphyrin). Inhibition of ferrochelatase and cytochrome P450 destruction can further limit heme synthesis. Griseofulvin, for example, is known to be harmful in AIP, perhaps at least in part due to the formation of *N*-methyl protoporphyrin. Some synthetic steroids, when given in high doses to laboratory animals, also can cause mechanism-based destruction of cytochrome P450 enzymes.[378]

If a drug is safe or unsafe, it cannot be concluded that other drugs in the same class will have the same properties. Some calcium-channel antagonists have been reported to induce ALAS1 and cytochrome P450 enzymes in rats[379,380] and/or in chick embryo liver cells,[380–382] and have been implicated in some attacks of porphyria.[383] Among these agents, amlodipine was safely administered in one patient[384] but not in another patient.[385] ACE inhibitors also differ in their capacity to induce porphyrin accumulation in cultured liver cells, with enalapril being the most potent.[380] Thiazide diuretics have been generally regarded as safe, but hydrochlorothiazide,[383] and even all thiazides,[386] have been listed as unsafe. Recent evidence indicates that the antidepressant nefazodone is a potent inducer of porphyrins in cultured liver cells.[387] Antineoplastic drugs have been administered safely to patients with acute porphyrias and advanced cancer.[388] There is disagreement regarding safety of several antibiotics, such as chloramphenicol, cephalosporins, erythromycin, and vancomycin.[386]

Anesthetic agents have been studied in animal models, and the clinical experience with these drugs in patients with acute porphyrias has been reviewed.[389,390] Halothane has been recommended as an inhalation agent and propofol or midazolam appear suitable as intravenous induction agents for use in acute porphyria.[390] It is especially important to avoid induction of anesthesia with a barbiturate, the risk for which is great in patients in whom the diagnosis of acute porphyria has not been recognized prior to surgery. By contrast, even major surgery can be carried out safely in patients known to have acute porphyria when appropriate anesthetic drugs are used.[391]

Even when a harmful drug induces an attack of porphyria, other predisposing factors, such as endogenous hormones, nutritional factors, and smoking, have additive effects in a given patient. Multiple inducing factors are usually involved in acute attacks, as suggested by the following clinical observations. (a) Harmful drugs and other precipitating factors are less likely to cause attacks in patients with no recent symptoms of acute porphyria than in those with recent and frequent symptoms.[283] In a large retrospective study of the risk from anesthetic use in patients with acute porphyrias in Finland, barbiturates or other inducing drugs were quite frequently detrimental in patients who already had porphyric symptoms but seldom exacerbated latent disease.[389] (b) Some PBGD-deficient heterozygotes who require long-term anticonvulsants for epilepsy do not develop attacks of porphyria. (c) Drugs are only rarely reported to cause acute symptoms in children with PBGD deficiency. Although such clinical experience suggests that individuals with latent AIP are less likely to develop attacks than patients with recently active disease, exposure to harmful drugs should be avoided in all PBGD-deficient individuals, including children.

Nutritional Factors. Diet and nutritional status are underrecognized as contributors to acute attacks of porphyria, in part because obtaining accurate dietary histories is difficult. In metabolic ward studies, reduced caloric and carbohydrate intakes increased urinary ALA and PBG and precipitated symptoms.[48,49] Reduced energy intake, usually instituted in an effort to lose weight, commonly contributes to attacks of acute porphyria. Therefore, even brief periods of starvation during weight reduction, during postoperative periods, or with intercurrent illnesses should be avoided.[49]

Glucose and other forms of carbohydrate are effective in treating acute attacks of porphyria. In animals, starvation enhances, whereas glucose or protein can repress, the inducing effect of chemicals on ALAS1 and on PBG excretion.[50,392] Increased dietary carbohydrate can reduce cytochrome P450 enzymes in normal animals and humans.[393,394] Therefore, it is possible that the demand on hepatic heme synthesis is decreased during carbohydrate feeding. If so, the carbohydrate effect on ALAS1, and therefore the beneficial carbohydrate effect in acute porphyria, may be secondary, at least in part, to an effect on the synthesis of cytochrome P450 enzymes. Starvation in animals also induces heme oxygenase,[47] which can lead to depletion of the regulatory hepatic heme pools and contribute to ALAS1 induction.

Adequate intake of all nutrients is at least as beneficial in patients with porphyria as it is in normal individuals. Worldwide, the most common nutrient deficiency is iron deficiency, due to multiple causes. In developed countries, borderline iron deficiency, manifested by low serum ferritin concentrations but without anemia, is common in women due to menstrual blood loss and self-selection of foods low in iron (especially red meats). This is accompanied by increased erythrocyte protoporphyrin, which indicates early impairment of bone marrow heme synthesis. Although it is not known if hepatic heme synthesis is impaired in women with AIP who develop borderline iron deficiency, it is reasonable to assure adequate iron status in this disease.

Smoking. Smokers are exposed to chemicals such as polycyclic aromatic hydrocarbons that induce hepatic cytochrome P450 enzymes and heme synthesis.[395] It is well known that drug metabolism by cytochrome P450 enzymes is increased in smokers, reflecting increased amounts of these liver hemoproteins. An association between cigarette smoking and repeated attacks of porphyria was found in a survey of 144 AIP patients in Britain.[396] Therefore, smoking cessation may have particular health benefits in patients with acute porphyrias.

Infections, Surgery, and Stress. Attacks of porphyria may develop during intercurrent infections and other illnesses and after major surgery. The mechanisms involved in situations of increased metabolic stress are not known, but impaired nutrition and the increased production of steroid hormones that induce ALAS1 may play a role.[397] Patients report that psychologic stress can contribute to the exacerbation of porphyria, but underlying mechanisms are not established.

Diagnosis

Acute porphyria must be considered as a possible diagnosis in the presence of clinical features consistent with these disorders. However, the symptoms and signs of an acute attack of porphyria are highly nonspecific. Laboratory studies can reliably establish the diagnosis or exclude it. Screening for acute porphyrias in patients with suggestive symptoms should not be expected to have a high yield, because other diseases that produce similar symptoms are more common. It is sometimes difficult to recognize other diseases such as appendicitis, pancreatitis, and gallstones, in patients with AIP because these conditions have symptoms that resemble those of porphyria. To avoid overdiagnosis of porphyria, it is important to use tests with high sensitivity and specificity. If the patient being screened has a relative with AIP and the laboratory findings in that relative are known, only AIP needs to be considered. In the absence of such information, the other acute porphyrias also need to be excluded.

Increased Porphyrin Precursors. A marked increase in urinary PBG is found only in AIP, HCP, and VP and is, therefore, diagnostic for the presence of one of these conditions. In these porphyrias this finding is accompanied by increases in ALA and porphyrins (usually mostly uroporphyrin and coproporphyrin in AIP), although the increase in ALA is usually less than PBG, when expressed as mg/day or mg/liter. In ADP, urinary ALA and coproporphyrin, but not PBG, are increased. Normal quantitative measurements for urinary ALA, PBG, and total porphyrins can reliably exclude all acute porphyrias as a cause for concurrent symptoms. In screening for these conditions, it is useful to measure total porphyrins as well as ALA and PBG because porphyrins may remain increased longer after an acute attack. However, it should be noted that increases in urinary porphyrins are much less specific than increases in ALA and PBG. Urinary porphyrins are increased in many medical conditions, especially when liver or bone marrow function is affected. A diagnosis of porphyria is commonly made incorrectly based on overinterpretation of minimal abnormalities in porphyrin precursor or porphyrin levels. This can lead to delay in recognizing the actual cause of abdominal pain or other symptoms.

PBG is colorless but is readily detected and measured as the chromogen generated with Ehrlich's reagent (para-dimethylaminobenzaldehyde). Other substances in urine, and especially urobilinogen, also react with Ehrlich's reagent. The chromogen formed with urobilinogen is similar to that formed with PBG. The Watson-Schwartz test[398,399] is a qualitative method for detecting excess PBG that separates the chromogen formed with PBG from that formed with urobilinogen and other substances by a two-step solvent extraction. Another qualitative method, the Hoesch test,[400,401] takes advantage of the fact that the chromogen formed with PBG in strongly acidic Ehrlich's reagent is much more highly colored than that formed with urobilinogen. Disadvantages of these qualitative methods are relative lack of sensitivity and an appreciable incidence of false positive results, usually due to lack of experience in interpreting small changes in color.

A quantitative anion exchange column method proposed by Mauzerall and Granick[402] is the preferred method for documenting increases in urinary PBG. The method is readily modified for serum. Modifications with somewhat greater sensitivity have been described.[403,404] A column method should be used as the primary method, or should be used to verify positive results from a qualitative test, using the same sample. False positive results with the column method are rare, but have been reported following treatment with phenothiazines.[405] As described by Mauzerall and Granick, ALA can be quantitated simultaneously by sequential elution into a second column.[402]

A qualitative method that is based on the method of Mauzerall and Granick was developed in Australia and recently became available in other countries, including the United States. This is the preferred rapid, qualitative screening method for urinary PBG, because it is sensitive and specific.[406] The kit for this screening test (available in the U.S. from Trace America, Arlington, TX) includes color standards for interpretation of the results. This test seems very reliable in emergent situations. Quantitative measurements of PBG, plus ALA and total porphyrins, should be carried out on the same sample at a later time.

Urinary PBG generally remains increased between repeated attacks of AIP, although it increases even more before and during an attack. Such variations with time are difficult to document unless accurate, serial 24-h urine collections are obtained. Even then, precise correlations of PBG levels with symptoms may be difficult to discern. ALA and PBG fall markedly after heme therapy in AIP patients. However, this biochemical response is not always accompanied by clinical improvement, as discussed later (see "Treatment"). Urinary porphyrins are expected to be increased in AIP in association with increases in PBG. Increases in urinary uroporphyrin and coproporphyrin are usually most prominent. Normal or only slightly increased total fecal porphyrins in a patient with high urinary PBG helps to confirm a diagnosis of AIP. HCP and VP are associated with marked increases in fecal porphyrins. Fractionation and measurements of individual porphyrins in feces and urine are seldom helpful for the diagnosis of AIP.

Decreased PBGD Activity. PBGD activity is measured as the amount of uroporphyrinogen formed from PBG, as determined spectrophotometrically[315,407] or fluorometrically[305,408] after oxidation to uroporphyrin. Erythrocyte PBGD activity is approximately half-normal in most (70 to 80 percent) patients with AIP.[409] A low value does not distinguish between latent and clinically manifest AIP. Therefore, symptoms should not be attributed to AIP unless urinary PBG is increased. Enzyme activity may be partially lost, giving a falsely low result, if storage or transport of the sample is compromised before the enzyme measurement. Assays for this enzyme in some large referral laboratories may not be reliable, and it may be advisable for a specialty laboratory to confirm the finding of a low enzyme activity.

For several reasons, a normal erythrocyte PBGD activity does not completely exclude AIP. (a) As already noted, some mutations of the *PBGD* gene cause the enzyme to be deficient only in nonerythroid tissues. In AIP patients with these mutations, erythrocyte PBGD activity is normal. (b) In normal individuals the range for this enzyme activity in erythrocytes is wide and overlaps with the range for patients with AIP. (c) The enzymatic activity in erythrocytes is highly age-dependent.[410] The enzyme is physiologically increased in erythrocytes from infants and children.[411] In addition, an increase in reticulocytes or younger erythroblasts in the circulation can increase the erythrocyte activity. For this reason, erythrocyte PBGD activity can be normal during an attack of AIP and decrease to subnormal levels during remission especially in patients with concurrent conditions such as anemia or hepatic disease.[412,413] Therefore, measurement of erythrocyte PBGD has little role in screening for AIP in patients with acute symptoms. Moreover, when acute porphyria is suspected it is important to exclude the other acute porphyrias in which PBGD activity is normal.

Mutation Analysis. Detecting the specific *PBGD* mutation in each family makes the definitive diagnosis of AIP. If the specific mutation is known in an AIP family, then other heterozygotes can be readily identified by DNA analysis. Restriction fragment length polymorphism (RFLP) studies in informative families may also be useful.[414–418] DNA analysis is more reliable than measuring erythrocyte PBGD activity, and has revealed that 5 to 15 percent of individuals can be misclassified using only the enzymatic assay.[235,306,419] In newly diagnosed families, initial examination of exons 10 and 12 of the *PBGD* gene may prove efficient because about 40 percent of known mutations have been found in these regions.[235] DNA methods are not used to exclude AIP in patients with suggestive acute symptoms.

The prenatal diagnosis of AIP has been accomplished by measuring the enzyme activity in cultured amniotic fluid cells.[420] However, knowledge of the specific mutation in the family would facilitate prenatal DNA diagnosis.

Treatment

Repression of Hepatic ALAS1. Intravenous heme administration and provision of large amounts of carbohydrate are considered specific therapies for acute attacks of porphyria. General and supportive measures are also important. Hospitalization for the acute attack facilitates prompt institution of heme therapy, treatment of pain and nausea, monitoring of nutritional status, provision of adequate amounts of carbohydrate, investigation of the precipitating causes of an attack, and observation for neurologic complications and electrolyte imbalances.

Heme therapy and carbohydrate loading are considered specific therapies because they repress hepatic ALAS1 and reduce urinary ALA and PBG. They therefore address some of the underlying biochemical manifestations rather than the symptoms of acute porphyrias. Glucose polymer solutions are useful for oral carbohydrate loading. Intravenous glucose (at least 300 g daily) has been recommended for patients hospitalized with attacks of porphyria.[279] However, intravenous administration of large volumes of 10 percent glucose may favor the development of hyponatremia. Especially if a severe attack precludes oral or enteral feeding for more than a few days, provision of a more complete nutritional regimen, including intravenous vitamins, lipids, and amino acids should be considered. Safety and efficacy of specific parenteral and enteral nutrition regimens in porphyria have not been studied. Amounts of fat and protein administered parenterally should probably not greatly exceed basic requirements, because increasing dietary fat may increase porphyrin precursor excretion in AIP,[48] and high-protein diets can induce hepatic cytochrome P450 enzymes in animals and humans.[393]

Heme therapy is much more effective than glucose in reducing levels of ALA and PBG.[350,421,422] When infused intravenously, heme binds to plasma hemopexin and albumin and is then taken up primarily in hepatocytes. Within these cells, which are considered the major overproduction sites of porphyrin precursors in acute porphyrias, heme enters the regulatory heme pool where it represses hepatic ALAS1 synthesis. Thus, heme-mediated repression of ALAS1, which is impaired in clinically manifest AIP (Fig. 124-13), can be enhanced by heme therapy. Porphyrin precursor levels in plasma and urine fall promptly after heme therapy. Few controlled studies of efficacy have been done, due to ethical constraints, as well as difficulties in studying a rare disease that causes intermittent and spontaneously remitting symptoms. However, heme therapy (either heme arginate or hematin) is now approved in many countries for treating acute porphyrias. Controlled trials that were attempted with hematin[423] and heme arginate[424] demonstrated biochemical responses and favorable trends in clinical assessments. However, these studies may have failed to better establish clinical efficacy because they lacked statistical power, had incompletely characterized patients and treatment responses, and delayed the start of heme therapy for 2 days or longer.[425–427]

In the past, it was often recommended that heme therapy be started only after there was no response to intravenous glucose administered for several days. Indeed, mild attacks may respond to glucose alone. Nevertheless, it is now recognized that heme therapy should be initiated as soon as possible after the onset of an acute porphyric attack, and that efficacy is compromised if treatment is delayed.[428,429] The clinical response depends on the degree of neuronal damage that occurred prior to initiation of heme therapy. This is supported by observations that advanced neurologic damage and subacute or chronic symptoms are generally unresponsive to heme therapy.[422,430] Heme administered by mouth, subcutaneously, or intramuscularly is not effective for treating porphyria,[422] as it is quickly broken down by small bowel mucosal heme oxygenase and does not reach the liver intact.

Heme therapy should be instituted only after the diagnosis of acute porphyria has been confirmed at least by a marked increase in urinary PBG. The prompt and dramatic fall in porphyrin precursors in plasma and urine after heme administration makes diagnosis much more difficult. If heme therapy is delayed, porphyrin precursors may be reduced, but response in terms of neuropathic manifestations may be poor. Therefore, a biochemical response to heme therapy does not always predict a clinical response.[350,422]

Heme is insoluble at neutral pH but can be prepared as hematin (heme hydroxide), heme albumin, or heme arginate for intravenous infusion. A lyophilized hematin preparation (Panhematin, Abbott) is approved in the U.S. for the treatment and prevention of porphyric attacks. Given its short shelf-life of 3 months, it is generally shipped overnight by the manufacturer when needed. Hematin solutions are unstable and should be infused promptly.[431,432] Even then, the degradation products that form rapidly when hematin is solubilized cause a transient anticoagulant effect and phlebitis at the infusion site.[432,433] Phlebitis leading to loss of venous access is common in patients who receive repeated courses of hematin. Phlebitis is less common if hematin is infused into a large peripheral vein or a central line. However, some patients have developed vena caval thrombosis after repeated hematin dosing through a central line. Infrequently reported side effects of hematin include fever, aching, malaise, hemolysis, and circulatory collapse.[434] Acute renal tubular damage associated with excretion of hematin in urine can occur with excessive doses.[435] Instability of hematin may also reduce its efficacy.[436]

Heme albumin and heme arginate are much more stable than hematin and are seldom associated with phlebitis and coagulopathy. Lyophilized hematin can be stabilized as heme albumin by solubilizing it in 30 percent human albumin rather than in sterile water before infusion.[437] Although not extensively studied, this approach is becoming the preferred method for heme therapy in countries where heme arginate is not available, because the risk of phlebitis appears to be substantially reduced. Increased safety generally outweighs the additional cost and intravascular volume-expanding effects of albumin. Similar safety advantages were observed with a lyophilized heme albumin preparation, which was studied in Germany, but is no longer under development.[438]

Heme arginate (Normosang, Leiras) was initially developed in Finland and is available in a number of European countries and in South Africa.[428,439,440] It is an investigational drug in the U.S. The drug is an incompletely characterized preparation of heme and arginine, and is provided as a concentrated solution with a long shelf-life (2 years vs. 3 months for lyophilized hematin). The concentrated solution must be diluted with saline before infusion. After infusion, the heme and arginine moieties dissociate and the heme becomes bound to circulating hemopexin and albumin. Therefore, heme arginate is similar to hematin and heme albumin with regard to in vivo distribution, and its efficacy appears to be comparable. Phlebitis occurs much less often than with hematin, and coagulation is not impaired. In more than 1250 infusions of heme arginate, less than 1 percent were complicated by phlebitis.[436] The better safety profile and longer shelf-life of heme arginate should enhance the availability of heme therapy for prompt treatment of acute porphyric attacks and facilitate the development of preventive regimens.[441]

The standard treatment regimen for heme arginate is a single dose of 3 mg/kg daily for 4 days.[429] This dose is also appropriate for hematin, although a regimen of 4 mg/kg twice daily has been recommended in the past. Lower-dose regimens (e.g., 1 to 1.5 mg/kg once daily) may be effective[430] but have not been extensively studied. The pharmacokinetics of heme administered intravenously and the duration of response of porphyrin precursors[350,422] suggests that once-daily treatment should be effective.

Because repeated heme administration can induce heme oxygenase, leading to reduced efficacy, an inhibitor of heme oxygenase may be particularly useful in combination with heme for preventive regimens. An investigational approach is to combine heme therapy with a heme oxygenase inhibitor (e.g., tin protoporphyrin or tin mesoporphyrin) to prolong the efficacy of the administered heme. Tin protoporphyrin prevents ALAS1 induction and reduces porphyrin precursor concentrations in AIA-induced porphyria in the rodent.[442] Early experience with tin protoporphyrin in AIP suggests that it may reduce porphyrin precursor excretion to some extent,[443] and when combined with heme may be more effective for treating acute attacks than heme alone.[444] Studies with tin mesoporphyrin are currently in progress. Zinc mesoporphyrin is another potential agent, but has not yet been studied in humans.[445]

Drug metabolism by hepatic cytochrome P450 enzymes is reduced in some patients with acute porphyrias.[446] Rapid normalization of drug oxidation rates after heme therapy suggests that heme is deficient in the liver in acute porphyrias and that there may be an excess of cytochrome P450 apoproteins.[447,448] However, heme infusions can also increase drug oxidation rates in normal subjects, suggesting that heme may increase drug metabolism by other mechanisms, such as stabilizing or enhancing synthesis of cytochrome P450 apoenzymes.[437,448]

Symptomatic Treatment. Adequate treatment of symptoms usually includes narcotic analgesics for abdominal and extremity pain and a phenothiazine such as chlorpromazine for nausea, vomiting, anxiety, and restlessness. Because pain due to porphyria is generally severe, full therapeutic doses of a narcotic analgesic such as meperidine or morphine should be administered on a schedule that reflects the duration of drug action. Addiction potential is small except with prolonged attacks. Phenothiazine is usually administered in small doses as needed for short periods. Large doses of phenothiazines, as commonly used for treating acute psychiatric conditions, are seldom required in acute porphyrias and may produce unpleasant side effects. Chloral hydrate is commonly recommended for insomnia. Diazepam and other commonly used benzodiazepines in low doses are probably safe if a minor tranquilizer is required.

Chlorpromazine is approved in the U.S. for treatment of AIP, and the suggested dosage is 25 to 50 mg by mouth (or 25 mg i.m.) t.i.d. or q.i.d. for several weeks, with maintenance therapy required for some patients.[449] In our experience, considerably smaller dosages are effective for acute attacks, and maintenance therapy is rarely indicated. This and other phenothiazines are not known to reduce the overproduction of porphyrin precursors or to otherwise address the underlying pathophysiology in this disease. As with other symptomatic therapies, dosages administered should be individualized and maintenance treatment should be considered only if required to control continuing psychiatric symptoms.

Many other therapies have been advocated for treating acute porphyric attacks. β-Adrenergic blocking agents may control tachycardia and hypertension in acute attacks of porphyria and were considered by some to hasten recovery.[450,451] Propranolol reduces experimentally induced porphyria in animals and cultured hepatocytes. However, because both *D*- and *L*-propranolol have this effect, nonspecific membrane effects rather than β-adrenergic blockade are probably involved.[452] Propranolol may even be hazardous in patients with hypovolemia and incipient cardiac failure, because increased catecholamine secretion may in this situation be an important compensatory mechanism.[453]

Administration of 3,5,3′-triiodothyronine can partially correct the 5α-reductase defect in patients with AIP. This approach can lead to symptoms of hyperthyroidism, and clinical benefit has not been reported.[454] Studies with thyroid analogues that act primarily on the liver might be warranted. Administration of glucocorticoids to suppress adrenal androgen production is probably not beneficial.[397]

Increased levels of plasma and urinary zinc have been reported during exacerbations of porphyria, possibly due to increased levels of porphyrins that can complex zinc.[455] However, neither EDTA treatment to chelate zinc, nor the administration of zinc in AIP has been convincingly beneficial.[455–457] EDTA and other chelators, such as DFO, can compromise hepatic heme synthesis by binding iron, and have been found to worsen experimental hepatic porphyrias.[36,37,370] Vitamin B_6 status has been of concern because PLP is a coenzyme for ALAS1.[358] However, in the absence of a nutritional deficiency, there is no convincing evidence that administration of vitamin B_6 or other micronutrients is beneficial in acute porphyria. Sorbents have been shown to bind porphyrin precursors in vitro but have been studied little in vivo.[458] Other therapies, such as cimetidine,[459] adenosine monophosphate,[460] vitamin E,[461] folic acid,[462] hemodialysis,[463] and hemoperfusion[464] are not generally regarded as effective. Treatment with antioxidants has been studied but not demonstrated to be clinically effective.[465]

Identifying and removing inciting factors, which are expected to differ in individual patients, including harmful drugs and nutritional deficiencies is important in the management of the acute attack. Cyclic attacks in women occur during the luteal phase of the menstrual cycle and usually resolve with the onset of menses.

Seizures in patients with acute porphyria are difficult to manage, because almost all antiseizure drugs have at least some potential for exacerbating acute porphyria. In patients with idiopathic epilepsy combined with porphyria, it is sometimes necessary to continue antiseizure medications. Clonazepam may be less harmful than phenytoin or barbiturates.[466,467] Bromides are safe but are seldom preferred as treatment for seizures. Studies of newer anticonvulsants in chick embryo liver cells suggest that felbamate, lamotrigine, and tiagabine are inducers of heme synthesis and are likely to be harmful in acute porphyrias, whereas gabapentin and vigabatrin are not.[468]

Prevention of Acute Attacks. Avoiding harmful drugs and other exacerbating factors is often effective in preventing further attacks of acute porphyria. However, in patients who experience repeated attacks, it is important to recognize that multiple harmful factors contribute to exacerbations of porphyria. Therefore, a broad and individualized approach to prevention is important.

Avoiding harmful drugs is often not simple, because it is not known whether many commonly used drugs can be administered safely in this condition. Lists of safe and harmful and drugs are available but are not infallible. Wearing a medical alert bracelet may be advisable for patients prone to repeated attacks, but wording such as "avoid all drugs" should be discouraged because it might impair treatment of other conditions in emergency situations.

Dietary indiscretions are difficult to detect without a careful diet history. Consultation with a dietitian may be useful even if the patient and physician have concluded that there is no obvious dietary problem. If body weight is near normal, patients should be advised to follow a well-balanced diet with sufficient calories to maintain weight. The diet can be somewhat high in carbohydrate (60 to 70 percent of total calories). If such a diet is followed, there is little evidence that additional dietary carbohydrate helps further in preventing attacks. Iron deficiency, if present, should be corrected because at least theoretically it might impair hepatic heme synthesis.

Patients who are overweight and wish to lose weight should do so gradually and after their porphyria has been asymptomatic for several months. A diet that provides about 10 percent fewer calories than what is required to maintain weight appears to be unlikely to exacerbate porphyria. This degree of restriction, which leads to gradual weight loss and encourages long-term development of good dietary habits, is preferred to crash diets even in obese individuals without porphyria, but requires considerable commitment.

Cyclic attacks of AIP as well as HCP and VP are attributed to cyclic production of progesterone, and can be prevented by administration of a GnRH analogue.[361–363,365,469,470] This is a preventive approach, and there is no immediate benefit if ovulation has already occurred or if a premenstrual attack is already in progress. Continued experience suggests that prevention is dramatically effective only in the subset of women with clear-cut cyclic attacks and not in patients with attacks partially associated with the menstrual cycle. Although a low-dose GnRH analogue regimen, which allows some endogenous estrogen production, is associated with fewer side effects than standard high-dose regimens, marketed GnRH analogues are not readily administered in low doses. Therefore, a standard dosage regimen of a GnRH analogue can be combined with an "add-back" of low dose estradiol (transdermal or oral) to control adverse effects of low estrogens.[365,469] Treatment with a GnRH analogue is seldom needed for longer than 1 to 3 years because cyclic attacks do not occur throughout the reproductive period in women with porphyria. Because this and other treatment options are available, oophorectomy is not an acceptable option for preventing cyclic attacks.[364]

Exogenous estrogens, progestins, and androgens, given alone or in combination, have prevented acute cyclical attacks in some women.[279,283,471–473] However, progestins and androgens or their metabolites may induce ALAS1 and sometimes worsen the disease. Synthetic steroids (including estrogens) with an ethynyl substituent can cause a mechanism-based destruction of cytochrome P450 enzymes and should probably be avoided in patients with acute porphyria.[474] Danazol is especially contraindicated.[475,476] In contrast, GnRH analogues are peptides that appear not to have detrimental effects on heme metabolism. There is little evidence that administered estradiol, a natural endogenous estrogen, induces acute attacks of porphyria. Because the risk of exacerbating acute porphyria is greater with an oral contraceptive combination than with a GnRH analogue, it may be preferable to use a GnRH analogue initially. Add-back estradiol or changing to an oral contraceptive can be considered after attacks have been prevented for about 3 months. Continuing a GnRH analogue alone for longer than 6 months is inadvisable due to the risk of irreversible bone loss.

Cyclic attacks also can be prevented by heme therapy given at weekly intervals,[477] or at intervals of several days during the luteal phase of the cycle.[371] Early experience with heme arginate suggests that once- or twice-weekly administration of single doses of heme arginate can prevent repeated attacks of porphyria in some patients.[441] A beneficial effect of heme can be observed in some patients in whom the repeated attacks are noncyclic. Therefore, some women with repeated attacks who do not respond to a GnRH analogue may respond to a preventive heme regimen.

CONGENITAL ERYTHROPOIETIC PORPHYRIA (CEP)

CEP is an autosomal recessive inborn error of heme biosynthesis resulting from the markedly deficient activity of the cytosolic enzyme, uroporphyrinogen III synthase [UROS; EC 4.2.1.75,

HMB hydrolase (cyclizing)].[478,479] The enzymatic defect causes the accumulation of the nonphysiological and pathogenic porphyrin isomers, uroporphyrin I and coproporphyrin I, leading to the clinical manifestations. CEP also has been termed Günther disease, erythropoietic porphyria, congenital porphyria, congenital hematoporphyria, and erythropoietic uroporphyria. CEP is rare and panethnic. As of 1997, about 130 cases had been reported.[480] CEP occurs in animals such as cattle and the fox squirrel.

Clinical Manifestations

The age at onset and clinical severity of CEP are highly variable, ranging from nonimmune hydrops fetalis due to severe hemolytic anemia *in utero* to milder, later-onset forms, that have only cutaneous lesions in adult life. In most cases, photosensitivity develops soon after birth. A number of factors lead to the phenotypic variability in CEP including (a) the amount of residual UROS activity,[481] (b) the degree of hemolysis and consequent stimulation of erythropoiesis, and (c) exposure to ultraviolet light. The major debilitating clinical features in patients with CEP are anemia and cutaneous photosensitivity. Overall life expectancy may be markedly diminished in more severely affected patients due to hematologic complications and the increased risk of infection.

Hematologic Features. Mild to severe hemolysis is a feature of CEP and is accompanied by anisocytosis, poikilocytosis, polychromasia, basophilic stippling, reticulocytosis, increased nucleated red cells, absence of haptoglobin, increased unconjugated bilirubin, increased fecal urobilinogen, and increased plasma iron turnover. Hemolysis presumably results from the accumulated uroporphyrin I in erythrocytes. Secondary splenomegaly develops in response to the increased uptake of abnormal erythrocytes from the circulation, which may contribute to the anemia and may also result in leukopenia and thrombocytopenia. The latter is sometimes associated with significant bleeding and splenectomy may be beneficial in such cases.[482,483] Anemia due to hemolysis can be severe if the bone marrow does not compensate, and some severely affected patients are transfusion dependent.

Dermatologic Involvement. In most cases of CEP, cutaneous photosensitivity usually begins in early infancy and is manifested by increased friability and blistering of the epidermis on the hands and face and other sun-exposed areas. Bullae and vesicles contain serous fluid and are prone to rupture and infection. The skin may be thickened, with areas of hypo- and hyperpigmentation. Hypertrichosis of the face and extremities is often prominent.[484] Sunlight, other sources of ultraviolet light, and minor skin trauma increase the severity of the cutaneous manifestations. Recurrent vesicles and secondary infection can lead to cutaneous scarring and deformities, as well as to loss of digits and facial features such as the eyelids, nose, and ears (Fig. 124-18). Later or adult-onset patients have milder clinical symptoms and often exhibit only the skin manifestations of the disease.[479,485–487]

Other Features. Corneal scarring can lead to blindness. Porphyrins deposited in the teeth produce a reddish brown color in natural light, termed erythrodontia. The teeth may fluoresce on exposure to long wavelength ultraviolet light. Porphyrin deposition in bone also occurs, and bone loss due to demineralization[488] or expansion of the hyperplastic bone marrow[3,489] has been described.

The Metabolic Defect in CEP

Accumulated Porphyrins. Urinary porphyrin excretion is markedly increased (up to 50 to 100 mg daily) and consists mostly of uroporphyrin and coproporphyrin, with lesser increases in hepta-, hexa-, and pentacarboxyl porphyrins.[480] Although the predominant increase is in the type I isomers, type III isomers also are increased. Urinary ALA and PBG excretion is not increased. Fecal porphyrins are markedly increased with a predominance of coproporphyrin I. Fecal isocoproporphyrins are not increased.[490]

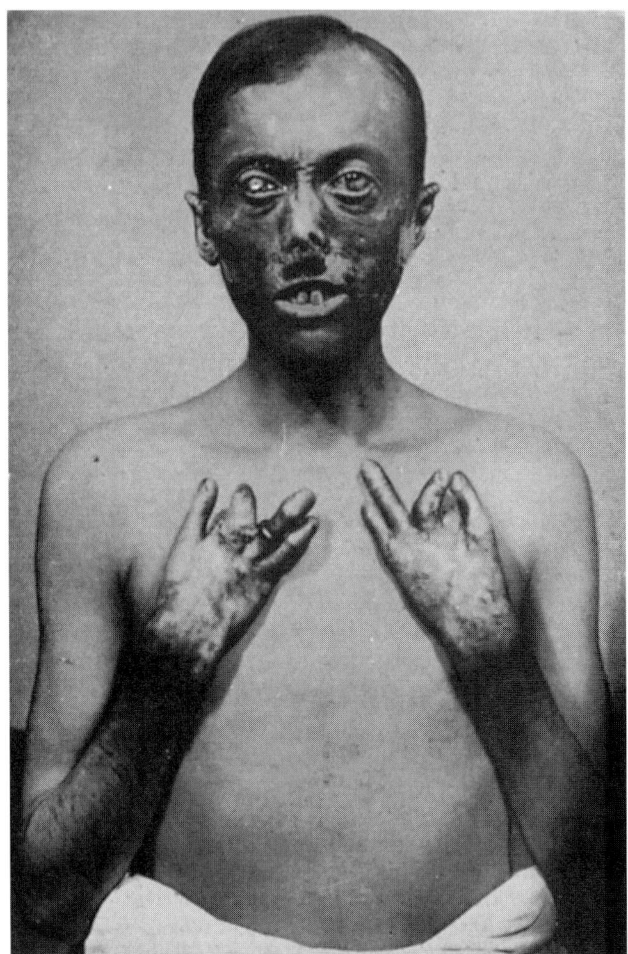

Fig. 124-18 Destructive cutaneous and ocular manifestations of CEP. This is the famous patient, Petry, who survived to age 34 and provided specimens to Hans Fischer for early studies of porphyrin chemistry. (*Reproduced from Günther.[965] Used by permission.*)

Circulating erythrocytes in most reported cases of CEP have contained large amounts of uroporphyrin I, and lesser, but still excessive, amounts of coproporphyrin I. Red cell protoporphyrin may also be increased, and in some reported cases was the predominant porphyrin in erythrocytes, as in the bovine form of this disease. However, other porphyrias, such as HEP, need to be considered if protoporphyrin is the predominant erythrocyte porphyrin. The bone marrow contains much larger amounts of porphyrins than other tissues in this disease, and these consist mostly of uroporphyrin and coproporphyrin. These porphyrins are also found in spleen and to a lesser extent in liver.[491–497] Excess plasma porphyrins, which probably originate from the bone marrow and circulating red cells, are mostly uroporphyrin and coproporphyrin. Erythrocyte PBGD is increased in this disease and is attributable to increased erythropoiesis,[498] as in other disorders associated with hemolysis.[410] Studies of nine Indian CEP patients indicated a close relationship between the degree of porphyrin excess and the severity of disease expression.[499]

The Enzymatic Defect in CEP. The enzymatic defect in CEP is the markedly deficient, but not totally absent, activity of UROS, the fourth enzyme in the heme biosynthetic pathway.[478] Most CEP patients have less than 10 percent of normal erythrocyte UROS activity, while heterozygous carriers have ~50 percent of normal activity.[478,500] UROS is a cytosolic enzyme that catalyzes the conversion of the linear tetrapyrrole, HMB, by inversion of the pyrrole D ring and cyclization to uroporphyrinogen III, which is the physiologic cyclic isomer that is metabolized in subsequent enzymatic steps to heme (Fig. 124-1).[501–503] In the past, this enzyme was termed uroporphyrinogen III cosynthase. In human erythroid cells, there is an excess of UROS activity compared to PBGD, thus favoring the synthesis of uroporphyrinogen III over uroporphyrinogen I.[504] UROS and PBGD may exist in a cytosolic complex.[312,313,505]

Purification and Properties of UROS. Human UROS has been purified to homogeneity from erythrocytes and is a monomeric protein with an apparent molecular weight of 29.5 kDa.[505] The purified enzyme has a specific activity of over 300,000 nmol/hr/mg, an isoelectric point of 5.5, and is remarkably thermolabile ($t_{1/2}$ at 60°C ~1 min). The enzyme's pH optimum is 7.4 and the K_m for HMB is 5 to 20 μM. The enzyme is activated by Na^+, K^+, Mg^{2+}, and Ca^{2+} and is inhibited by Cd^{2+}, Cu^{2+}, Hg^{2+}, and Zn^{2+}. UROS has also been purified from other species including spinach, *Euglena gracilis, E. coli*, and rat liver.[506]

The Molecular Genetics and Pathology of *UROS*

cDNA and Genomic Sequences. The full-length cDNA encoding human UROS has been isolated, sequenced, and expressed in *Escherichia coli*.[507] The cDNA is 1296 bp with 5′ and 3′ untranslated regions of 196 bp and 302 bp, respectively, and an open reading frame of 798 bp that encodes a polypeptide of 265 amino acids. Using the cDNA as a probe, a single *UROS* gene was assigned to the narrow chromosomal region 10q25.3 → q26.3.[508] Analysis of the *UROS* genomic sequence revealed 10 exons and the sequence of each exon-intron junction has been determined.[509] Comparison of the human and mouse cDNAs and the predicted amino acid sequences revealed 80.5 percent nucleotide and 77.8 percent amino acid identity.[510,511] The murine gene was localized to a narrow region on mouse chromosome 7 within 1.5 cM of *Oat*, which is syntenic with the localization of the human gene on chromosome 10q.[511]

The genomic structure of the human *UROS* gene recently was determined.[512] The gene is ~34 kb in length and contains 10 exons, ranging from 75 to 423 bp in length, while the introns were ~0.2 to 8.9 kb. All the intron-exon boundaries conform to the GT-AG rule. Of particular interest, the *UROS* gene has alternative promoters that generate housekeeping and erythroid transcripts. The housekeeping transcript contains the 5′ untranslated exon 1 fused to coding exons 2B through 10 and is present in all tissues and cells, while the erythroid transcript contains the alternative 5′ untranslated exon 2A fused to coding exons 2B through 10 and is present in fetal and adult erythropoietic tissues. The housekeeping proximal promoter region upstream of exon 1 lacked TATA and SP1 sites for initiation of transcriptional activity of the housekeeping transcript, consistent with its observed low level of expression in most cells. The erythroid-specific proximal promoter upstream of exon 2A contained erythroid transcription factor binding sites including GATA1 and NF-E2. Luciferase reporter assays performed in erythroid K562 and HeLa cells, demonstrated that the housekeeping promoter was active in both cell lines, while the erythroid-specific promoter was active in erythroid cells. Thus, *UROS* is similar to *ALAD* and *PBGD* in having alternative housekeeping and erythroid promoters.

Molecular Pathology. The availability of the full-length cDNA and genomic sequence has facilitated the identification of the molecular lesions causing CEP. To date, a variety of mutations that cause CEP have been identified in the *UROS* gene (Fig. 124-19, for reviews see references 513 to 515; for recent mutations see references 516 to 519). These include missense and nonsense mutations, large and small deletions and insertions, splicing defects, and intronic branch point mutations. Of the 18 single base changes, 4 (A66V, A104V, T228M, and G225S,) occurred at CpG dinucleotides, known hotspots for mutation.[520,521] All but one (V82F) of the known CEP missense mutations occurred in amino acid residues that are conserved in both the mouse and human UROS polypeptide sequences.[510,513] Among the mutations, V82F was of particular interest because it was a single base substitution (G to T) in the last nucleotide of exon 4, at the 5′ donor splice site for intron 4, which also caused a splicing defect. A branch point mutation 23 bp upstream from the intron/exon boundary of intron 8 has also been reported.[514]

Most patients were heteroallelic for the *UROS* mutations. The most common mutation, C73R, was found in about 33 percent of the studied alleles. Haplotype analysis of four CEP families using microsatellite markers closely flanking the *UROS* gene showed that the high frequency of C73R is due to its being at a mutational hotspot and not due to a founder effect.[522] The next most common mutations were L4F and T228M (7 percent and 6 percent, respectively). Except for the above mutations, the other mutations have been detected in only one or a few CEP families and therefore were "private." Most of the mutations were panethnic in origin, having been identified in diverse racial and demographic groups. Notably, about 12 percent of the mutant alleles were

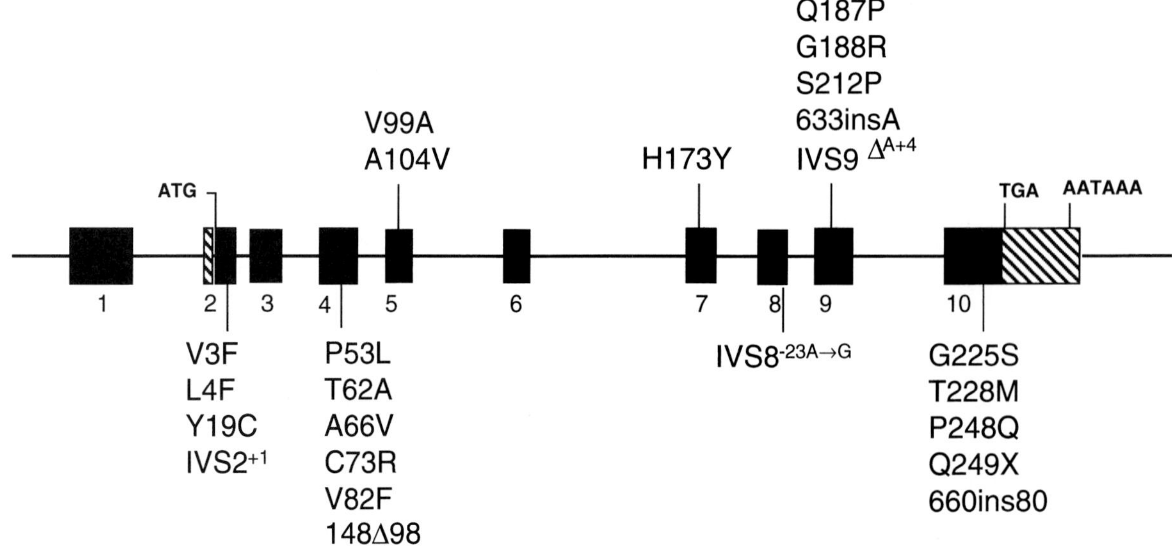

Fig. 124-19 The human *UROS* gene and locations of mutations causing CEP. (*Courtesy of Dr. K. H. Astrin.*)

undetected by sequencing the entire coding region and the intron-exon boundaries, thus suggesting that other sites for the mutations exist.

Genotype/Phenotype Correlations. The expression of the human *UROS* mutations has permitted the estimation of their relative residual activities for genotype/phenotype comparisons. When *UROS* constructs containing missense mutations were expressed in *E. coli*, their mean activities ranged from essentially nondetectable to levels that were about 35 percent of the mean activity expressed in *E. coli* by the normal cDNA. The A66V and V82F alleles had activities greater than 10 percent of the mean normal expressed level. However, both were less stable than the expressed normal enzyme, having half-lives at 37°C of 13.3, 30.5, and 49.5 min, respectively.[514,523,524]

For genotype/phenotype correlations, a series of CEP patients were classified as very mild to severely affected based on age, degree of hemolytic anemia, organomegaly, osteopenia, and cutaneous involvement. Homoallelism for the most common allele, C73R, was correlated with the most severe phenotype, nonimmune hydrops fetalis and/or transfusion dependency from birth. Consistent with the severe phenotype of C73R/C73R homozygotes, expression of the C73R allele in *E. coli* resulted in the detection of less than 1 percent of the activity expressed by the normal allele. Of note, gene targeting of the mouse *UROS* gene resulted in a fetal lethal.[525] The fact that the C73R/C73R homozygotes are viable and do not die early in fetal life indicates that the mutant enzyme retains a very small amount of residual activity that is sufficient to produce enough heme for the biosynthesis of hemoglobin and hemoproteins. Alternatively, if the C73R mutation produced only nonfunctional enzyme, then the fact that affected fetuses survive suggests the possibility of another gene that is responsible for UROS activity during development. Patients heteroallelic for C73R and a mutation that expressed little residual activity, such as P53L, also manifested a severe or moderately severe phenotype. Patients heteroallelic for mutations that expressed residual activity such as V82F (35 percent of normal activity), A104V (7.7 percent of normal activity), and A66V (14.5 percent of normal activity), had milder forms of CEP, even if the other allele was C73R or another mutation that did not express detectable activity. For example, a teenage boy whose genotype was C73R/A66V only had mild cutaneous involvement.[481]

Pathophysiology

The pathogenesis of CEP is readily explained by markedly deficient UROS activity. This enzyme deficiency leads to the accumulation of the substrate HMB, which is converted nonenzymatically to uroporphyrinogen I. Although uroporphyrinogen I can undergo decarboxylation by uroporphyrinogen decarboxylase to form hepta-, hexa-, and pentacarboxyl porphyrinogen I and finally coproporphyrinogen I, further metabolism cannot proceed because the next enzyme in the pathway, coproporphyrinogen oxidase, is stereospecific for the III isomer. Therefore, the isomer I porphyrins are nonphysiological in that they cannot be metabolized to heme, and are pathogenic compounds when they accumulate in large amounts in CEP and are autoxidized to the corresponding porphyrins. The large amounts of isomer I porphyrinogens that accumulate in bone marrow erythroid precursors (especially normoblasts and reticulocytes) and erythrocytes in this disease undergo autoxidation to the corresponding porphyrins, which damage erythrocytes, cause cutaneous photosensitivity, are deposited in tissues and bones, and are excreted in large amounts in urine and feces. Photosensitivity occurs because these porphyrins are photocatalytic compounds. Exposure of the skin to sunlight and other sources of long-wave ultraviolet light results in blistering and vesicle formation, and in increased friability of the skin.[526] Hemolysis is usually present, but may not be accompanied by anemia if erythroid hyperplasia is sufficient to compensate for the increased rate of erythrocyte destruction. The degree of compensation may vary over time. Plasma iron turnover is increased in CEP.[3,496]

Diagnosis

CEP should be suspected when severe photosensitivity presents in infancy or childhood, and porphyrins are markedly increased in both erythrocytes and urine. Pink to dark reddish urine or staining of the diaper noted shortly after birth may be the first clue to the diagnosis. In some cases, the disease is less severe and presents in adult life with hemolytic anemia or skin lesions suggestive of PCT. High levels of urinary uroporphyrin I and coproporphyrin I are consistent with the diagnosis of CEP. Sensitive assays have been developed to measure UROS activity in erythrocytes and cultured cells using both direct and coupled enzyme reactions.[500,527] Determination of the nature of the underlying mutation provides a definitive diagnosis and genotype/phenotype correlations.

CEP can cause nonimmune hydrops or hemolytic anemia *in utero*. The diagnosis can be established by measuring total porphyrins in amniotic fluid or cord blood plasma. Diagnosis of CEP *in utero* can avoid the harmful photosensitizing effects of photodynamic therapy for neonatal hyperbilirubinemia.[490]

CEP is distinguishable from HEP, a porphyria with clinical symptoms similar to CEP but due to the homozygous deficiency of UROD, by the absence of high levels of isocoproporphyrin in feces and urine. HEP is also distinguished by a predominance of protoporphyrin (complexed with zinc) in erythrocytes. Homozygous forms of other porphyrias such as VP and HCP also may be characterized by photosensitivity in childhood and increased erythrocyte zinc protoporphyrin. EPP is readily distinguished by a predominance of free protoporphyrin in erythrocytes and stool and normal urinary porphyrins.

If heterozygous parents have had a child with this disease, the disease can be detected *in utero* in future pregnancies by finding a red-brown discoloration and increased porphyrins (especially uroporphyrin I) in amniotic fluid,[528] by measuring UROS activity in chorionic villi or cultured amniotic fluid cells,[529] or by direct detection of *UROS* gene mutations in chorionic villi or cultured amniotic cells.[530]

Treatment

Skin Protection. Protection of the skin from sunlight and minor trauma is essential in CEP. Sunscreen lotions and β-carotene are sometimes beneficial.[531] Bacterial infections that complicate cutaneous blisters require timely treatment in an effort to prevent scarring and mutilation. Severe infections such as cellulitis and bacteremia may require intravenous antibiotics.

Marrow Suppression. Frequent blood transfusions are sometimes essential. Repeated transfusions can suppress erythropoiesis, and thereby decrease porphyrin production and can greatly reduce porphyrin levels and photosensitivity.[488] Such therapy is likely to be successful if the hematocrit remains above 32 percent and DFO is administered to reduce the resulting iron overload.[532] Treatment with hydroxyurea to reduce the bone marrow porphyrin synthesis may be considered.[533] Splenectomy may substantially reduce transfusion requirements in some patients.[488] Oral charcoal may increase fecal loss of porphyrins[534] and may be useful for patients who are not transfusion-dependent and who have milder disease. It seems less successful in more severe cases.[535,536] Heme therapy, which is effective for treatment of the acute hepatic porphyrias, may be somewhat effective in CEP,[537] but has not been extensively studied, and seems unlikely to provide long-term benefit. Chloroquine has not been beneficial.[538–542]

Bone Marrow Transplantation. Allogenic bone marrow transplantation has proved curative for patients with CEP. To date, four patients have been transplanted, and when successful this has resulted in marked reduction in porphyrin levels and photosensitivity.[518,543–545] The first patient died of intercurrent cytomegalovirus infection emphasizing the morbidity and mortality associated with this approach, even with HLA identical donors. A stem cell transplant was performed in one CEP patient.[546]

Experimental Gene Therapy. The success of bone marrow transplantation in alleviating the severe manifestations of this disease provides the rationale for hematopoietic stem cell gene therapy. Because stable transduction of the patient's own stem cells with vectors containing the *UROS* cDNA would abrogate the need for HLA-identical donors and minimize the risk of rejection, efforts are underway to develop retroviral-mediated transduction of hematopoietic stem cells for treatment of patients with CEP. The *UROS* cDNA has been subcloned into the various retroviral vectors that have been used to transduce a variety of cell types.[547–550] Transduction of CEP fibroblasts and lymphoblasts resulted in significant levels of enzyme expression ranging from 2 to 100 times greater than the endogenous activity in CEP fibroblasts and up to 3 times greater than that in normal lymphoblasts.[547–549] In addition, transduction of hematopoietic progenitor cells and early erythroid cells has also been achieved.[549–551] These studies indicated that in vitro gene transfer and persistent overexpression can indeed be effected in hematopoietic cells. However, the in vivo efficacy of individual retroviral vector constructs may not be predictable from these in vitro experiments, and animal studies are needed. Such in vivo experiments could determine if transduction of hematopoietic stem cells could be efficient enough to minimize the proportion of nontransduced progenitors that produce toxic quantities of porphyrins in their descendants.

PORPHYRIA CUTANEA TARDA (PCT) AND HEPATOERYTHROPOIETIC PORPHYRIA (HEP)

PCT results from decreased uroporphyrinogen decarboxylase (UROD, EC 4.1.1.37) activity in the liver, and is characterized by blistering skin lesions on sun-exposed areas. It has also been known as symptomatic porphyria, porphyria cutanea tarda symptomatica, and idiosyncratic porphyria. The disease has been classified into three subtypes: type I (sporadic), type II (familial, autosomal dominant), and type III (familial, rare). In addition, occasional cases result from environmental exposure to polyhalogenated chemicals. Type II disease is an autosomal dominant disorder due to underlying mutations in the *UROD* gene, which act as a predisposing factor. *UROD* mutations have not been found in patients with types I or III disease. Type III disease is a rare familial form and appears to result from an unknown inherited defect that secondarily affects hepatic UROD activity. All three types have similar clinical features and management. Porphyrins accumulate in large amounts in the liver, and are increased in the plasma and urine (predominantly uroporphyrin and heptacarboxyl porphyrin). Multiple factors can contribute to inactivation or inhibition of hepatic UROD in this disease, probably by an iron-dependent oxidative mechanism, including alcohol, hepatitis C infection, estrogen, HIV, smoking, and factors that increase hepatic iron content, such as mutations of the *HFE* gene.

PCT is the most common porphyria and occurs worldwide. Of the subtypes, type I or "sporadic" PCT is the most common and accounts for about 80 percent of PCT patients. The disease prevalences in the United States and Czechoslovakia have been estimated at about 1 in 25,000 and 1 in 5000, respectively. The incidence in the United Kingdom was estimated at 2 to 5 per million.[552] The prevalence may be higher in regions where alcohol abuse and hepatitis C are more frequent. PCT is prevalent in the Bantus of South Africa in association with iron overload.[553] PCT is generally more common in males, possibly due to greater alcohol intake. When it occurs in women, it is often due in part to estrogen-containing oral contraceptives or postmenopausal estrogen use.

HEP is the homozygous dominant form of type II PCT and results from the markedly deficient activity of UROD.[554,555] The clinical manifestations are very similar to CEP. However, the excess porphyrins are apparently produced in both the liver and bone marrow, hence its designation as "hepatoerythropoietic." HEP is panethnic but it is extremely rare and only 20 cases were reported as of 1994.[556]

Clinical Manifestations in PCT

The clinical features of all three PCT subtypes include cutaneous manifestations and hepatic abnormalities in the absence of neurologic involvement. Symptoms usually develop in adult life. Multiple risk factors are usually readily recognizable in individual patients, supporting the notion that PCT requires exogenous precipitating factors.[552]

Cutaneous Involvement. Chronic blistering lesions develop on sun-exposed areas of skin, mostly commonly the dorsal aspects of the hands, and also on the face, forearms, legs, and, in women, on the dorsa of the feet. The fluid-filled vesicles rupture easily and the denuded areas become crusted and heal slowly (Fig. 124-20). Sun-exposed skin becomes friable, and minor trauma may cause bullae to form or denudation of the skin. Secondary infection can occur. Cutaneous thickening, scarring, and calcification, when striking, are features that have been termed pseudoscleroderma because

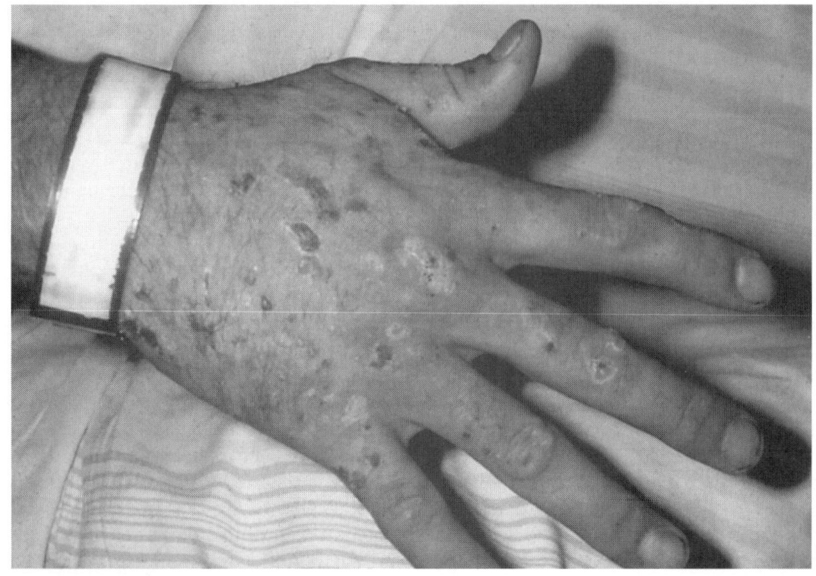

Fig. 124-20 Chronic, crusted lesions resulting from blistering due to photosensitivity on the dorsum of the hand of a patient with porphyria cutanea tarda (PCT). These occur less commonly on other sun-exposed areas, such as the face, neck, ears, forearms, and feet.

they can mimic systemic sclerosis.[557] Previous areas of blisters may appear atrophic, brownish, or violaceous. Small white plaques, termed milia, also are common and may precede or follow vesicle formation. Facial hypertrichosis and hyperpigmentation also are common, and occasionally present in the absence of vesicles.[558] The lesions occur more commonly in the summer than winter. Immediate light-induced urticaria is rare.[559] Onycholysis of the fingernails is sometimes seen.[560] Photodamage to the eyes and particularly to the conjunctivae and sclerae has been described.[561–563]

The skin lesions in VP and HCP are identical to those of PCT. Those in CEP and HEP are also similar but usually more severe. Skin histopathology includes subepidermal blistering, deposition of PAS-positive material around blood vessels and fine fibrillar material at the dermoepithelial junction with IgG, other immunoglobulins, and complement.[564,565] Membrane-limited vacuoles appear in the superficial dermis, and the site of split formation is the lamina lucida.[566,567] Collagen fibrils in scleroderma-like lesions in PCT have been shown to be of decreased diameter as in morphea.[568]

Although the liver is the major source of excess porphyrins in PCT, it was suggested that excess porphyrin synthesis in skin might contribute to the pathology.[569] The phototoxic reaction appears to involve the generation of reactive oxygen species, which may be followed by activation of the complement system and lysosomal damage.[570–574] Activation of complement does not account fully for the phototoxic manifestations of PCT.[575]

Hepatic Involvement. PCT is almost always associated with abnormal liver function tests, especially transaminases and γ-glutamyltranspeptidase, even in cases not associated with hepatitis C. Although many patients have moderately excessive alcohol intake and/or hepatitis C infection, few have advanced liver disease at the time of initial presentation. The degree of excess porphyrins in the liver is much more marked in PCT than in most other porphyrias, with the notable exception of some cases of EPP complicated by massive hepatic protoporphyrin deposition. Fresh liver tissue, unfixed sections, or even fixed sections if processed properly manifest red fluorescence on exposure to long-wave ultraviolet light.[576] Contact of sections with water can cause porphyrins to redistribute artifactually to nuclei.[577] Needlelike inclusions that are fluorescent and birefringent are evident microscopically, and by electron microscopy are located in lysosomes; there are also paracrystalline inclusions in mitochondria. Other histologic findings are much more nonspecific and include necrosis, inflammation, increased iron, and increased fat. Cirrhosis has been reported in up to one-third of cases, but has been much less common in most series. Distorted lobular architecture and cirrhosis are more common in older patients with more long-standing disease and at autopsy.[578,579] Hemosiderosis is usually mild or moderate but can be severe, especially with concurrent HH. The risk of developing hepatocellular carcinoma is clearly increased in this disease; the reported incidence has ranged from 4 to 47 percent and was highest in an autopsy series.[578,579] These tumors seldom contain large amounts of porphyrins. Nonspecific liver abnormalities are seen in patients without heavy alcohol intake and hepatitis C, indicating that PCT itself is associated with liver damage. Serum antibodies directed against hepatocytes have been reported in PCT, but their significance is unknown.[580] A mild or moderate erythrocytosis is found in some patients and is not well understood; smoking and consequent chronic lung disease may contribute.

Precipitating Factors. The risk factors that commonly contribute to the development of PCT include: (a) an increased amount of hepatic iron; (b) excess ethanol consumption; (c) hepatitis C virus infection; (d) HIV infection; (e) estrogen use; (f) smoking; and (g) low vitamin C and carotenoid status. In addition, genetic factors that can contribute include heterozygosity or homozygosity for *HFE* mutations. Exposures to certain chlorinated polycyclic aromatic hydrocarbons are responsible for occasional outbreaks of PCT.

Iron Involvement. Early studies of iron absorption and kinetics have been consistent with normal or increased iron stores and absorption.[581–586] Liver biopsy specimens commonly show increased iron staining.[582,584,587] Serum ferritin levels are usually normal, although generally in the upper part of the normal range, or moderately increased. The degree of increase may correlate with the degree of transaminase elevation.[588] Phlebotomy to decrease hepatic iron is effective in treating PCT, and iron supplementation can lead to relapse.[589,590] Recently, mutations of the *HFE* gene that are associated with HH, an autosomal recessive disorder, have been found to be more common in PCT than in controls.[177,591] These studies suggest that either the homozygous or heterozygous presence of the *HFE* C282Y and H63D mutations may predispose to the development of PCT.[177,592–596] Prevalence of the C282Y mutation is increased in both sporadic (type I) and familial (type II) PCT.[177,592,595] In southern Europe, where the C282Y is less prevalent, the H63D mutation is more commonly associated with PCT.[597] These associations will be more clearly understood when the function of the *HFE* gene is established and the effects of the C282Y and H63D mutations on iron absorption are defined.

Hepatitis C and HIV Infections. An association between PCT and hepatitis C may explain at least in part the chronic liver damage in PCT and the development of hepatocellular carcinoma in some patients (see above "Hepatic Involvement"). In some locations, 80 percent or more of patients with PCT are chronically infected with the hepatitis C virus, particularly in southern Europe and in some locations in the United States.[596,598–600] The prevalence is lower in other areas including some northern European countries.[601,602] There also is an association of PCT with HIV infection.[603,604] While some PCT patients are infected with both HIV and hepatitis C virus,[605,606] others are infected only with HIV.[596] Therefore, HIV appears to be an independent risk factor for PCT, although not as commonly associated as hepatitis C.

Ethanol, Estrogens, Smoking, and Antioxidants. Excess ethanol intake of varying degree has long been associated with PCT.[587] That only a small proportion of alcoholics develops PCT is an indication that factors in addition to alcohol are required. How alcohol exacerbates PCT is unclear. Alcohol may increase iron uptake in PCT patients and in normal subjects,[607,608] and the increased iron may accelerate the development of PCT. Alcohol also may cause oxidative damage in hepatocytes, but whether this can be associated with damage to UROD or oxidization of uroporphyrinogen to uroporphyrin in the presence of iron remains to be established.

Estrogens contained in oral contraceptives or as postmenopausal estrogen replacement are commonly associated with PCT in women.[587] Men treated with estrogens for prostate cancer also have developed the disease. In one series, many of the patients with estrogen-associated PCT had type II disease, as indicated by reduced erythrocyte UROD activity.[609] PCT can develop during pregnancy, although it is not established that the risk is increased. Endogenous estrogens in cirrhotic patients and in Klinefelter syndrome may occasionally contribute to this condition.[610] Estrogens may have an additive effect in animals treated with hexachlorobenzene,[596,611,612] but have never been shown to cause porphyria when administered alone.

Smoking as well as excess alcohol use is very common in patients with PCT, although the relationship to smoking has not been carefully studied. Alcohol and chemicals in cigarette smoke may contribute to oxidative damage in liver via induction of the cytochrome P450 enzymes.[613] Antioxidant status may also play an important role. Vitamin C[614] and carotenoid status[615] are decreased in some PCT patients. A potential role for vitamin

C is supported by animal studies showing that vitamin C treatment can ameliorate chemical induction of uroporphyria in rodents.[616]

Hexachlorobenzene-Induced Porphyria. A large outbreak of cutaneous porphyria occurred in eastern Turkey from ingestion of wheat that was treated with hexachlorobenzene as a fungicide. Approximately 6 months elapsed between ingestion of the contaminated grain and the development of porphyric symptoms. Bullae, scarring, hyperpigmentation, and hypertrichosis of sun-exposed areas of skin were common and resembled PCT. Hexachlorobenzene was shown later in animals to induce a deficiency of hepatic UROD and porphyrin accumulation and excess excretion similar to that in human PCT.[617,618] In the Turkish outbreak, the disease was more common in children than adults, and slightly more common in men than women. Arthritis was common in children. Other symptoms, such as irritability, abdominal colic, anorexia, and weakness, may have been due to neurologic effects of the fungicide itself. Some breast-fed infants died after developing convulsions and cutaneous annular erythema possibly due to hexachlorobenzene in breast milk. Follow-up observations 20 or more years after the initial exposure showed some sequelae such as cutaneous scarring and deformities, but no active skin lesions and normal or nearly normal urinary porphyrins.[619]

PCT has been reported after exposure to other chemicals including di- and trichlorophenols and 2,3,7,8-tetrachlorodibenzo-*p*-dioxin (TCDD, dioxin).[620,621] In most such cases, porphyria developed during exposure to the harmful chemical and improved when the exposure was stopped. However, there have been some apparent instances of delayed onset many years after chemical exposure.[622] The porphyrinogenic effects of these chemicals probably involve metabolic activation by cytochrome P450 enzymes.

Because PCT is not a rare disorder, it is not surprising that it sometimes occurs with other conditions such as diabetes mellitus.[623] It occurs more frequently in patients with systemic lupus erythematosus and other immunologic disorders than would have been expected by chance[624] and can lead to therapeutic challenges.[625]

Clinical Manifestations of HEP

HEP resembles CEP clinically[194] and usually presents in infancy or childhood with red urine, blistering skin lesions, hypertrichosis, and scarring. Sclerodermoid skin changes may be prominent.[626] Erythrocyte porphyrins are increased, and hemolytic anemia is often present, and associated with splenomegaly. HEP is genetically heterogeneous, and unusually mild cases have been described.[627,628] In one case, HEP became manifest at age 2 years in a child with hepatitis A and improved dramatically with resolution of the hepatitis.[629] This indicates that concurrent conditions may contribute to the severity of HEP.

The Metabolic Defect in PCT and HEP

Accumulated Porphyrins in PCT. Porphyrins are markedly increased in liver, plasma, urine, and feces in all patients with PCT. The pattern of porphyrins is complex because UROD deficiency results in the accumulation of porphyrinogens with different numbers of carboxyl groups (including octa-, hepta-, hexa-, and penta-carboxyl porphyrinogens) of both the I and III isomer types, as well as isocoproporphyrinogen. These porphyrinogens undergo nonenzymatic oxidation to the corresponding porphyrins (uro-, hepta-, hexa-, and penta-carboxyl porphyrins, and isocoproporphyrins). Large amounts of uroporphyrin and heptacarboxyl porphyrin are retained in the liver. Urinary porphyrins consist mostly of uroporphyrin and heptacarboxyl porphyrin, with lesser amounts of coproporphyrin and penta- and hexa-carboxyl porphyrin.[630] Although urinary porphyrins are increased to a greater extent than fecal porphyrins (relative to normal values), the total amount of porphyrins excreted in feces exceeds that in urine, and the total excretion of type III isomers exceeds that of type I isomers. This includes isocoproporphyrins, which are mostly derived from the type III series.[630] The excess urinary uroporphyrin in PCT is predominantly isomer I; hepta- and hexacarboxyl porphyrins are mostly isomer III; and pentacarboxyl porphyrin and coproporphyrin are approximately equal mixtures of isomers I and III. Increases in plasma and urinary porphyrins are strongly correlated, and the distribution pattern of plasma porphyrins is similar to that in urine.[631,632] Porphyrins are also increased in skin. The observation that concentrations are highest in areas of skin that have not been exposed to light suggests that light destroys porphyrins in the skin.[633]

Accumulation of isocoproporphyrins is specific for UROD deficiency. This occurs via a normally minor pathway whereby pentacarboxyl porphyrinogen III, the last intermediate in the formation of coproporphyrinogen III, is decarboxylated by CPO, the next enzyme in the pathway, to form dehydroisocoproporphyrinogen. Dehydroisocoproporphyrinogen is metabolized to harderoporphyrinogen (a tricarboxyl porphyrinogen) by UROD, and thereby reenters the heme biosynthetic pathway. If UROD is deficient in the liver, dehydroisocoproporphyrinogen accumulates and undergoes oxidation to dehydroisocoproporphyrin. After biliary excretion, bacterial enzymes in the gut probably act on the vinyl group (at the 2 position) to give isocoproporphyrin and de-ethylisocoproporphyrin, which are the major porphyrins of this series in PCT patients and in rats treated with hexachlorobenzene. Fecal meso- and deuteroporphyrins are normally derived from protoporphyrin by the action of bacterial enzymes in the same manner.[630,634,635]

Elder[630] has calculated that the total porphyrin excretion in urine and feces is approximately 6 μmol/day in PCT, and if porphyrins accumulate at a similar rate it would take months to reach the levels found in patients' livers (0.22 to 2.0 μmol/g wet weight). In the presymptomatic phases of PCT, a smaller proportion of uroporphyrin and heptacarboxyl porphyrin may be excreted,[636] suggesting that these porphyrins are preferentially retained in the liver. The immediate red fluorescence observed in sections of liver from patients with PCT suggests that porphyrins accumulate mostly as the oxidized porphyrins rather than porphyrinogens. Elder has also estimated the total amounts of series I and III porphyrins excreted in PCT to be 4 to 5 μmol/day and 8 to 9 μmol/day, respectively. Comparison of these estimates to the normal overall rate of uroporphyrinogen III production (assumed to be essentially the same as the rate of hepatic heme and bilirubin production, or 90 to 100 μM/day)[637] suggests that excess porphyrin excretion in this disease is only a small fraction of the total amount of uroporphyrinogen III formed in the liver.[630] Therefore, only a very small increase in synthesis of heme pathway intermediates is required to account for the excess porphyrins excreted in this condition.[552] One would also expect that there is little or no increase in hepatic ALAS1, and that heme is probably synthesized at a normal rate in this disease. In this regard, studies with [^{14}C]ALA suggest that heme synthesis is normal in patients with PCT,[638] and the hepatic cytochrome P450 enzymes are normal or even increased, rather than decreased as might be expected if hepatic heme synthesis were substantially impaired.[639,640]

As already noted, the excess uroporphyrin in PCT is predominantly type I. This may be explained by inhibition of UROS by ferrous iron[641] or by porphyrins and porphyrinogens[642] that accumulate in the liver in PCT, which would increase the formation of uroporphyrinogen I. Although isocoproporphyrins are often the major porphyrins in feces in PCT, coproporphyrin, heptacarboxyl porphyrin, and uroporphyrin may also be increased.[635,636,643] In Turkish patients with hexachlorobenzene porphyria, the fecal porphyrins were predominantly coproporphyrins,[644] which presumably included excess isocoproporphyrins. Smaller amounts of isocoproporphyrins may be found in urine and plasma.

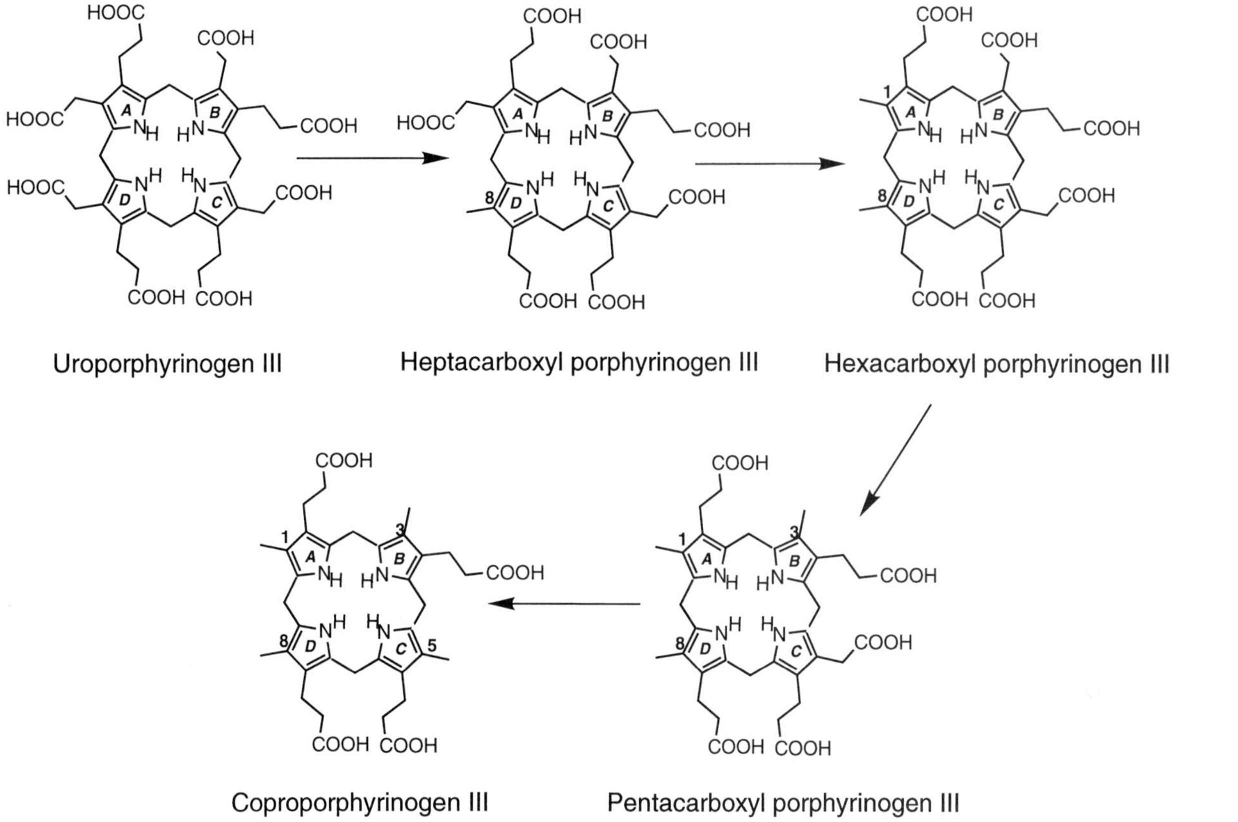

Uroporphyrinogen III   Heptacarboxyl porphyrinogen III   Hexacarboxyl porphyrinogen III

Coproporphyrinogen III   Pentacarboxyl porphyrinogen III

Fig. 124-21 Formation of coproporphyrinogen III from uroporphyrinogen III. Decarboxylation of the four acetic acid groups in uroporphyrinogen III proceeds clockwise around the macrocycle, starting from ring D (position 8), to yield the four methyl groups (at positions 8, 1, 3, and 5) in coproporphyrinogen III.[966]

Accumulated Porphyrins in HEP. The biochemical findings in HEP resemble those in PCT, and include predominant accumulation and excretion of uroporphyrin, heptacarboxyl porphyrin, and isocoproporphyrins. In addition, the erythrocyte protoporphyrin concentration is increased, the excess protoporphyrin in erythrocytes being complexed with zinc.

The Enzymatic Defect in PCT and HEP. The enzymatic defect in PCT and HEP is the deficient activity of UROD. In type II PCT and in HEP, the enzymatic activities are systemically deficient with about 50 percent and 3 to 27 percent of normal activity, respectively, as measured in erythrocytes.[645] In types I and III PCT, only hepatic UROD activity is decreased. Type III PCT resembles type I biochemically, but there is clustering of cases in families.

UROD is a cytosolic enzyme that catalyzes the sequential removal of the carboxyl groups of the four acetic acid side chains in uroporphyrinogen to yield coproporphyrinogen[646] (Fig. 124-21). The enzyme decarboxylates all four uroporphyrinogen isomers, the type III isomer being decarboxylated most rapidly, followed by type IV, II, and I isomers.[646,647] With uroporphyrinogen III as substrate, the order of decarboxylation of the acetate groups on each pyrrolic ring proceeds in a clockwise fashion starting from ring D (Fig. 124-21). The affinity of the enzyme for the substrate decreases with the sequential removal of each carboxyl group from the substrate.

Of note, UROD is active only on porphyrinogen substrates, and not on the corresponding porphyrins.[648] Enzymatic activity is inhibited by metals, such as Cu, Hg, and Pt, and is sensitive to sulfhydryl modification. Evidence for a direct effect of iron on enzyme activity in vitro remains controversial. However, it is well known that iron removal by venesection is beneficial in the treatment of PCT.[649] Experimental porphyria induced with TCDD in mice does not occur if the animals are initially made iron deficient by phlebotomy.[650] Rats with genetic[651] or acquired[652,653] siderosis also are more susceptible to hexachlorobenzene-induced porphyria than nonsiderotic rats.

Purification and Properties of UROD. UROD has been purified to homogeneity from human erythrocytes[654,655] and from yeast, bacterial, and other mammalian species (for review see reference 656). Although these studies suggested that UROD was monomeric, the recent purification of human recombinant UROD expressed in bacteria indicated that UROD was active as a dimer.[657] In contrast to most decarboxylase reactions, no coenzyme or metal requirements have been identified. Of interest, iron does not appear to directly affect UROD activity. Purified UROD is not inhibited by Fe^{+2} or Fe^{+3} under conditions that are likely to be present in vivo.[654] As discussed below (see "Pathophysiology") the effect of iron on hepatic UROD probably results from the formation of reactive oxygen species and cytochrome P450 enzyme induction leading to an oxidation product that is derived from ALA or possibly uroporphyrinogen and that irreversibly inhibits UROD.[552]

Crystal Structure. Recombinant human UROD purified to homogeneity has been crystallized.[658] Light-scattering analysis indicated that the purified protein was a dimer with a dissociation constant of 0.1 μM.[657] The crystal structure was determined at 1.60-Å resolution.[658] As shown in Fig. 124-22, the 40.8-kDa polypeptide forms a single domain with a distorted $(\beta/\alpha)_8$-barrel fold and a distinctive deep cleft for the enzyme's active site formed by loops at the C-terminal ends of the barrel strands. The dimeric form of UROD has two active site clefts adjacent to each other, suggesting that such an arrangement is required for enzyme function. Certain conserved residues, including arginines 37 and

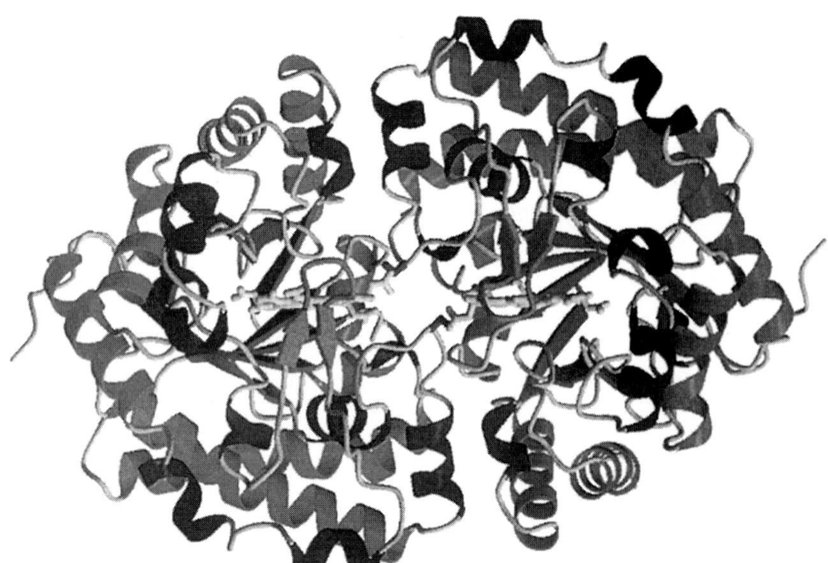

Fig. 124-22 The crystal structure of human UROD, shown as the dimer. The active site clefts of the monomers are adjacent, creating an extended cleft. This large cleft can accommodate one or two substrate molecules, and might enable intermediates to shuttle between monomers during the four-step decarboxylation of uroporphyrinogen. (*Reproduced from Whitby et al.*[658] *Used by permission.*)

41 and histidine 339, presumably are involved in substrate binding and cluster at a cleft that appears large enough for insertion of a porphyrinogen into the active site.

The Molecular Genetics and Pathology of *UROD*

cDNA and Genomic Sequences. The cDNA encoding rat *UROD* was first isolated from an erythroid cDNA library[659] and the cloned rat DNA was used to isolate the human cDNA.[660] The full-length human cDNA contained a coding region of 1104 bp and 5′ and 3′ untranslated regions of 18 and 72 bp, respectively, encoding a polypeptide of 367 amino acids. The human *UROD* gene was mapped to chromosome 1p34.[661,662]

A single ~3-kb human genomic sequence containing 10 exons has been isolated and all intron-exon boundaries are consistent with the boundary consensus sequences.[663] In contrast to the unique expression mechanisms for erythroid regulation of the first four enzymes of the heme biosynthetic pathway, the *UROD* gene has only a single promoter. Analysis of the *UROD* promoter region revealed a TATA-like sequence at −21 and one GC box at −60. The gene contains two initiation-of-transcription sites; however, both sites are apparently used with the same frequencies in all tissues, including erythroid cells, and the gene is transcribed as a single mRNA.[660] Promoter/enhancer elements responsible for increased transcription of the *UROD* gene during erythroid differentiation have not been investigated. Alternative splicing of the UROD mRNA has been described in both normal individuals and PCT patients; however, the significance of these transcripts, which lack between one and seven exons, is not clear.[664]

Molecular Pathology of PCT. A variety of *UROD* mutations causing type II autosomal dominant PCT have been identified including missense, nonsense, and splice site mutations, several small and large deletions, and a small insertion (Fig. 124-23).[554,555,665–669] With the exception of the G281E, IVS6^{+1}, and g10insA mutations, each of which has been identified in several families, the other *UROD* mutations were private, each having been found in only one family.[554,666,668] X-ray crystallography studies suggest that most of the *UROD* mutations identified in type II PCT patients appear to perform important structural roles in regions not involving the active site cleft or dimer interface. Two mutants, however, E167K and H220P, are located near the active site cleft and may disrupt the active site geometry and/or dimerization.[658]

UROD mutations have not been found in type I PCT.[552,670] Type III PCT has been identified in only a few families and is biochemically similar to type I, with low UROD activity in liver, but normal activity in erythrocytes, and is clinically indistinguishable from type I and II disease.[552] Mutations in the *UROD* gene have not been identified in any type III patients, to our knowledge. At present, it is unclear whether the type III cases represent a distinct subtype due to a familial predisposing gene encoding a protein that inactivates hepatic UROD activity.

Molecular Pathology of HEP. A variety of mutations have been identified in HEP patients indicating the molecular heterogeneity underlying this disease.[554,555,671,672] Of note, with a few exceptions, the *UROD* mutations causing HEP were unique and not found in type II PCT (Fig. 124-23).[336,552,554] Although the UROD activity in HEP is markedly deficient, some of the HEP mutations encode residual UROD activity. This is consistent with an essential need for heme synthesis and the finding that the homozygous knockout mouse for UROD is a fetal lethal.[673]

Pathophysiology of PCT

Most patients with PCT have the sporadic (type I) form, in which UROD deficiency is confined to the liver and there is no family history of the disease. Mutations of the *UROD* locus have not been found in type I disease, which appears to be due to a liver-specific enzyme defect.[552,670] Even in type II PCT, hepatic UROD activity is considerably less than the half-normal when there is active disease. As already noted, there is no evidence for tissue-specific isoforms of UROD. The mechanism for UROD inactivation in liver in this disease is not well understood, although an iron-dependent oxidative process is postulated and is supported by studies of experimental uroporphyria in rodents, other animals, and liver cell cultures. These provide useful models for human PCT. In addition to iron, certain cytochrome P450 enzymes, ALA, and ascorbic acid deficiency have been shown to influence uroporphyria in animals and liver cells in culture. Iron-mediated formation of reactive oxygen species apparently leads to generation of an UROD-inhibitory substance derived from uroporphyrinogen or another intermediate of the heme biosynthetic pathway.[552]

As already noted, uroporphyria in rodents is enhanced by iron overload and prevented by iron deficiency, and the effect of iron is probably not mediated by direct inhibition of UROD, but rather by generation of reactive oxygen species.[552,674] Studies in rodents suggest that an iron-dependent process oxidizes uroporphyrinogen to uroporphyrin and nonporphyrin products capable of inhibiting UROD.[674,675] These inhibitors have not been characterized.[552] Marked decreases in UROD activity seem necessary for the development of uroporphyria in rodents.[676] Likewise, a much

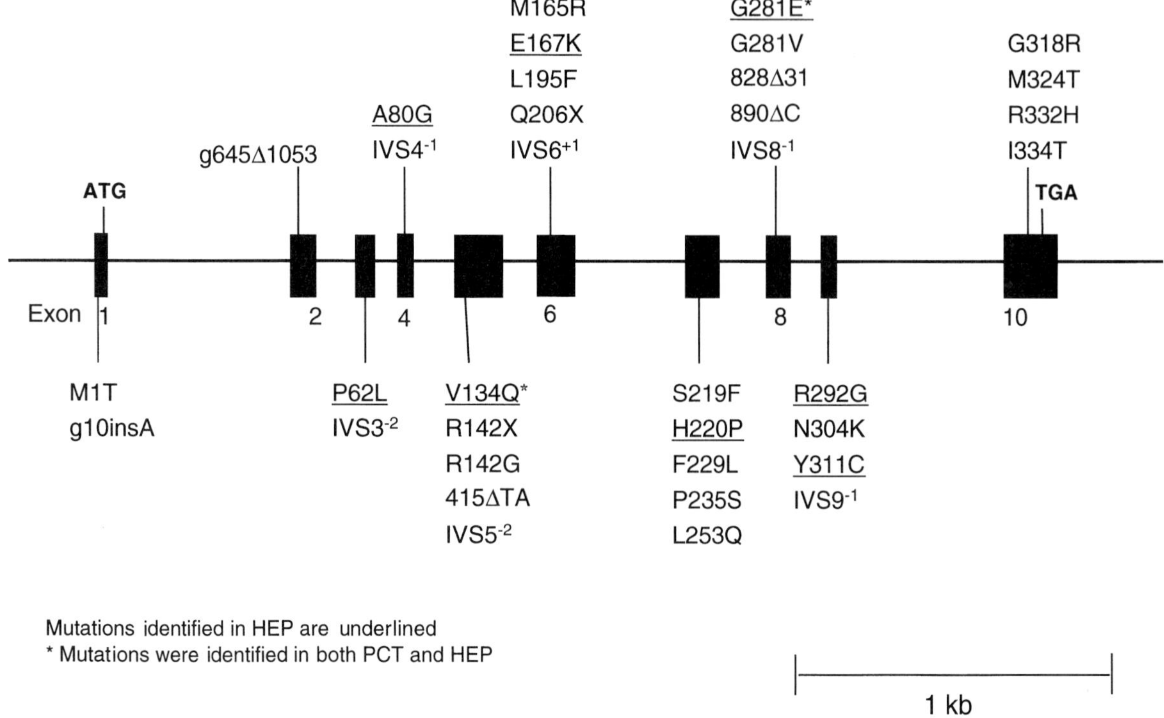

Fig. 124-23 The human *UROD* gene and locations of mutations causing familial (type 2) PCT and HEP. (*Courtesy of Dr. K. H. Astrin.*)

greater than 50 percent deficiency of hepatic UROD is necessary for development of human PCT.[552] Hexachlorobenzene-induced porphyria in rodents is accentuated by estrogens and attenuated by vitamin C.[677,678] Several susceptibility loci for this chemically induced porphyria have been identified in mice by chromosomal linkage analysis, but the nature of these genes is not yet known.[679]

Studies in rodents and hepatocyte cultures also suggest an important role for cytochrome P450 enzymes. Chlorinated cyclic hydrocarbons and polycyclic aromatic hydrocarbons that cause or enhance experimental uroporphyria are inducers of the CYP1A subfamily of these enzymes.[680] CYP1A2 in rodents catalyzed the oxidation of uroporphyrinogen to uroporphyrin, a process that is enhanced by iron and may involve formation of hydroxyl radicals by the flavoprotein enzyme NADPH-cytochrome P450 reductase and increased formation of inhibitors of UROD.[681–683] CYP1A2 knockout mice, in contrast to controls, did not develop uroporphyria when treated with ALA and iron.[684] In humans, in contrast to mice, cytochrome P450 enzymes other than CYP1A2 may be more active in uroporphyrinogen oxidation.[685] Potential influences of other cytochrome P450 enzymes, such as the CYP2E subfamily induced by alcohol, have been less studied.

Antioxidant status may be an important influence on the development of PCT, as indicated by studies of uroporphyria in laboratory animals and of PCT patients. Vitamin C prevents the CYP1A2-mediated oxidation of uroporphyrinogen to uroporphyrin and the accumulation of uroporphyrin in hepatocyte cultures.[616] In an ascorbic acid-requiring strain of rats, when exogenous ALA was provided and CYP1A2 was chemically induced, massive accumulation of uroporphyrin occurred when the animals were ascorbate-deficient. Ascorbate in amounts needed to achieve normal hepatic concentrations prevented uroporphyrin accumulation in these animals.[686] Plasma ascorbate levels were substantially reduced in 84 percent of PCT patients in a recent report.[614] Although ascorbate repletion of PCT patients was not found to influence porphyrin excretion,[687] an immediate response might not be expected given the large amounts of porphyrins stored in the liver in this disease. It remains to be determined whether maintaining normal ascorbate status can prevent the disease. Low levels of serum carotenoids also have been reported in PCT, further suggesting that oxidant stress in hepatocytes may be important in this disease.[615]

Administration of ALA to rodents treated with iron and cyclic hydrocarbons greatly accelerates the development of uroporphyria.[552,688,689] In the SWR strain of mice, long-term administration of ALA alone leads to decreased UROD and uroporphyria.[689] Such observations indicate that ALA or a compound derived from it is required for UROD inactivation.[552,688] A proposed mechanism involves generation of a nonporphyrin oxidation product that irreversibly inhibits UROD. Generation of this product may occur during the oxidation of uroporphyrinogen to uroporphyrin in hepatocytes, which is mediated by CYP1A2 and enhanced by iron.[552]

How important factors such as alcohol, estrogens, and HCV contribute to development of PCT is not well understood. Alcohol and estrogens can generate reactive oxygen species in some experimental systems,[690,691] but have been little studied in experimental uroporphyria or PCT. HCV in humans and chlorinated aromatic hydrocarbons may release storage iron in hepatocytes in a form that enhances formation of reactive oxygen species.[552,692] HCV infection and liver damage do not alone reduce hepatic UROD,[693] which is consistent with the multifactorial nature of PCT.[552,596]

Diagnosis of PCT and HEP

Diagnosis of PCT. PCT is strongly suggested by the characteristic skin lesions in sun-exposed areas, and particularly on the dorsal aspect of the hands (Fig. 124-20). However, the same blistering skin manifestations occur in all other cutaneous porphyrias, with the exception of EPP, and in "pseudoporphyria." Skin histopathology in PCT is similar or identical to that in other cutaneous porphyrias and in pseudoporphyria. Therefore, a skin biopsy does not provide specific diagnostic confirmation. As in other porphyrias, laboratory testing is essential for screening and for confirmation of the diagnosis. The most useful initial diagnostic test is a total plasma porphyrin determination. This is a sensitive and specific means of screening for cutaneous porphyrias, whereas urinary and fecal porphyrins are commonly increased in other medical conditions. A normal plasma porphyrin level is useful for excluding the diagnosis PCT. A high plasma porphyrin level with a fluorescence emission maximum at neutral pH near 619 nm excludes VP and is highly suggestive of PCT. However, several other porphyrias, such as CEP and HCP, can also be associated with a similar fluorescence emission spectrum.[694,695] In pseudoporphyria, skin findings are suggestive of PCT but plasma porphyrins are normal, which is an indication that a nonporphyrin photosensitizer is causing the skin lesions. Some medical conditions, such as end-stage renal disease,[696] HIV infection, and chronic hepatitis C,[697] may be associated with slight increases in plasma porphyrins, but these increases are small compared to those in PCT.

If the plasma total porphyrin level is abnormal, further testing is indicated to establish the type of porphyria. The diagnosis of PCT can be established by chromatographic separation and quantitation of urinary and fecal porphyrins, and demonstrating a predominance of uroporphyrin and heptacarboxyl porphyrin in urine, and excess isocoproporphyrins in feces. Despite an increase in fecal isocoproporphyrins, total fecal porphyrins are often normal or only slightly increased. Fecal isocoproporphyrins are often expressed as the isocoproporphyrin-to-coproporphyrin ratio, based on relative peak heights observed by HPLC or TLC.[698] Urinary ALA may be increased, but only slightly, and PBG is normal.

Most patients with familial (type II) PCT have no family history of the disease, and this form is distinguished by finding low UROD activity in erythrocytes. Erythrocyte UROD is normal in types I and III, and in PCT due to toxic exposures. Therefore, these are difficult to distinguish from each other unless adequate family studies can be carried out or there is clearly an outbreak of toxic porphyria in many unrelated individuals. Although classification of individual patients into types I, II, and III is not essential for clinical management, if the patient has type II PCT, other family members can be screened and counseled. Mild cases of HEP may resemble PCT, but can usually be differentiated by finding markedly deficient erythrocyte UROD activity, and by markedly increased erythrocyte zinc protoporphyrin. In patients with type II PCT or HEP, molecular analysis of the specific *UROD* mutations permits definitive diagnosis and genetic counseling, and provides UROD structure/function information.

Other diagnostic testing is important in PCT, because factors that contribute to the disease may themselves require attention. It is important to screen for various precipitating factors including hepatitis C, HIV, and *HFE* mutations.[177] Liver imaging studies are advisable to exclude complicating hepatocellular carcinoma and to serve as a baseline for follow-up.

Diagnosis of HEP. HEP should be suspected in patients with severe photosensitivity and especially considered in the differential diagnosis of CEP. It can be distinguished from CEP by finding elevated levels of fecal or urinary isocoproporphyrin and erythrocyte zinc protoporphyrin. Marked increases in erythrocyte porphyrins occur in both HEP and CEP, but in CEP there is a predominance of uroporphyrin I or coproporphyrin I, rather than zinc protoporphyrin. In contrast to HEP, EPP is characterized by increased free erythrocyte protoporphyrin and normal urinary porphyrins. Skin manifestations in EPP are generally milder, and blistering is unusual.

Assay. Various assays have been developed to determine the rate of conversion of uroporphyrinogen to coproporphyrinogen.[699] Many methods use uroporphyrinogen I or III as the substrate, which may be prepared either by reducing the appropriate porphyrin with sodium amalgam or by enzymatic synthesis from PBG. Chemical reduction is useful to produce substrates other than uroporphyrinogen I and III. Reaction products and the substrate are separated by HPLC, and quantified by fluorometry after oxidation to corresponding porphyrins. Because a single enzyme catalyzes all four decarboxylation reactions from uroporphyrinogen to coproporphyrinogen, pentacarboxyl porphyrinogen can be used as substrate and provides an assay from which it is easier to interpret the data because it represents a single step forming only a single product, coproporphyrinogen.[654]

Treatment of PCT

Phlebotomy and low-dose chloroquine (or hydroxychloroquine) are specific forms of treatment in PCT that are virtually always effective in all PCT subtypes. VP, HCP, and even mild cases of CEP and HEP, can produce similar cutaneous lesions, but are apparently unresponsive to these therapies. Therefore, it is advisable to establish a diagnosis of PCT and exclude other porphyrias before specific treatment is initiated.

Phlebotomy Therapy. Phlebotomy therapy can be initiated after excluding VP by a screening plasma porphyrin determination (including analysis of the fluorescence spectrum at neutral pH; see above "Diagnosis of PCT") while urine and fecal studies are still pending. Patients should cease exposure to alcohol, estrogens, iron supplements, or other exogenous agents that are judged to have contributed to the disease. Estrogen replacement can be resumed in postmenopausal women after successful treatment of PCT. Drugs such as barbiturates, phenytoin, and sulfonamides, which are harmful to patients with acute porphyrias, are seldom reported to precipitate PCT, but they may contribute and should be avoided as a precaution. Although some patients improve dramatically after the cessation of alcohol,[700] the results are generally unpredictable or slow.[701] Therefore, it is generally advisable to begin phlebotomy or low-dose chloroquine as well. These treatments, which are effective in both children and adults with PCT, lead to complete remission of the skin lesions, although some residual microscopic abnormalities may persist.[702–704]

Ippen introduced phlebotomy for treatment of PCT in 1961, and it is still standard therapy. This approach can induce remissions in almost all patients.[700] The original aim was to normalize the mild or moderately increased hemoglobin that is common in this disease, to stimulate erythropoiesis, and perhaps channel excess heme pathway intermediates to hemoglobin synthesis in the bone marrow.[649] It is now appreciated that the major biochemical pathology in PCT is confined to the liver, and the intermediates that accumulate there are primarily oxidized porphyrins that are not available as reduced porphyrinogens to enter the heme biosynthetic pathway. Thus, the current rationale for phlebotomy is the reduction of total body iron stores and liver iron content in order to interrupt the iron-mediated oxidative inhibition of hepatic UROD and the oxidation of hepatic porphyrinogens to porphyrins. To gradually reduce excess hepatic iron, about 450 ml of blood can be removed at intervals of 1 to 2 weeks. In one series, an average of 5.4 phlebotomies was required to induce a remission.[587] The most valuable guides to the efficacy of phlebotomy therapy are plasma (or serum) levels of ferritin and porphyrins.[705,706] Phlebotomies can be stopped when the serum ferritin reaches the lower limit of normal, and the plasma porphyrin level will then fall to normal, usually within several weeks (Fig. 124-24). Skin lesions are usually improved although not fully resolved at this point; they will continue to gradually improve. Hemoglobin or hematocrit levels should be followed to prevent development of significant anemia during the course of the phlebotomies. The tolerated level of hemoglobin depends upon the initial level and the age and clinical condition of the patient. In most patients, the blood hemoglobin should not fall below 10 to 11 g/dl, and probably should be maintained at a higher level in elderly patients. Pretreatment plasma porphyrin levels are generally 10 to 25 μg/dl. New skin lesions are unlikely after the plasma porphyrin falls below 1 μg/dl, which is near the upper limit of normal. Atrophy, hyperpigmentation, and hypertrichosis improve over periods of weeks or months after normal plasma porphyrin levels are achieved. Even scarring and pseudoscleroderma can disappear,[700] but showed little or no improvement in one series.[557] Liver function abnormalities can also improve.[707] Siderosis, needle-like inclusions, and red fluorescence in liver can

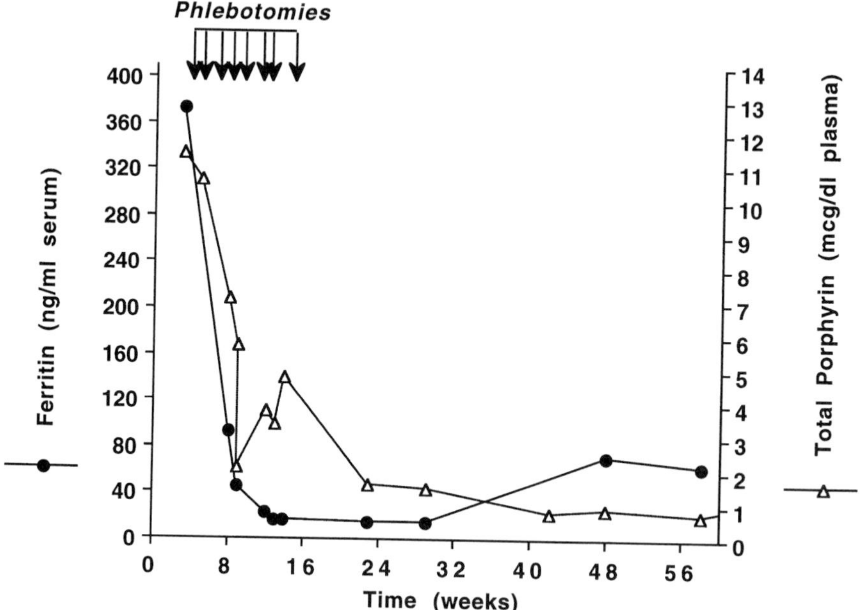

Fig. 124-24 Treatment of PCT by phlebotomy. Each arrow indicates removal of 450 ml of whole blood. Treatment is stopped when serum ferritin is near the lower limit of normal. Plasma porphyrins become normal and appearance of new skin lesions ceases within several months. (Reproduced from Anderson.[1009] Used by permission.)

be expected to improve or disappear, although other histologic abnormalities may not.[578,708] After a remission is obtained, continued phlebotomies are usually not needed even if ferritin levels later return to normal. However, it is advisable to follow porphyrin levels and reinstitute phlebotomies if porphyrin levels begin to rise. In some cases, relapses of PCT do occur and will respond to another course of phlebotomies.

Some patients with coexisting HH have marked increases in ferritin levels prior to phlebotomy, and require many more phlebotomies than most patients with PCT. Therefore, it is important to measure serum ferritin, iron, and transferrin saturation, and to test for the C282Y and H63D mutations in the *HFE* gene prior to the phlebotomies.

Infusions of DFO, an iron chelator, may be an alternative approach when phlebotomy is contraindicated, but is a less efficient means for iron reduction.[709,710] PCT improved when the coexisting hepatitis C infection was treated with interferon.[711,712] However, because interferon treatment of hepatitis C is not highly effective, it is preferable to treat PCT initially by phlebotomy or low-dose chloroquine and assess the need for treatment of hepatitis C later.[713]

Chloroquine Therapy. Low-dose chloroquine (or hydroxychloroquine) is highly effective and a suitable alternative treatment when phlebotomy is contraindicated or difficult, and when there is not marked iron overload, as assessed by serum ferritin or liver biopsy. This is the preferred therapy at some centers, especially for patients without marked iron overload.[714] The larger dosages of chloroquine that are used for other diseases may, in PCT, induce fever, malaise, and nausea, accompanied by marked increases in urinary uroporphyrin and heptacarboxyl porphyrin, plasma porphyrins, serum transaminases, other liver function tests, and ferritin levels. In addition, cutaneous manifestations of PCT can be acutely increased. These are manifestations of acute hepatic damage and the release of large amounts of stored porphyrins from the liver. Indeed, chloroquine administration can unmask previously unrecognized PCT.[715,716] These adverse effects of chloroquine, which are unique to PCT, are transient and followed by complete remission of the disease.[717] Chloroquine-induced remission was observed even with continued estrogen treatment for prostate cancer.[718] A low-dose regimen of either chloroquine (e.g., 125 mg by mouth twice weekly) or hydroxychloroquine (e.g., 100 mg by mouth twice weekly) is much preferred, because porphyrins are mobilized from liver more gradually with little or no increase in plasma porphyrins or hepatocellular damage; treatment is continued until plasma or urinary porphyrins are normalized.[719–721] Some patients may require later treatment with larger doses, and there is at least some risk of retinopathy.[722]

The mechanism of the effects of these antimalarial drugs in PCT is not established. Chloroquine concentrates in liver, particularly in lysosomes and mitochondria, and may form complexes with many different types of porphyrins that are then more readily mobilized from the liver.[723,724] However, recent studies do not support the notion that chloroquine can mobilize a variety of porphyrins from liver and other tissues.[725] Other mechanisms, such as mobilization of hepatic iron, have been suggested.[719,726] Although it is reported that chloroquine does not reduce hepatic siderosis, at least acutely,[718] iron excretion may increase in some patients.[719,722] Low-dose chloroquine may decrease hemosiderin deposition in liver, but otherwise has little effect on liver histology.[727] The lack of efficacy of chloroquine in other porphyrias, such as VP and CEP,[541] indicates that its mechanism of action in PCT is highly specific.

Therapy of PCT with End-Stage Renal Disease. Treatment of PCT associated with end-stage renal disease can be especially difficult. Porphyrin retention may be accentuated because urinary porphyrin excretion is not available, and the excess plasma porphyrins that accumulate in PCT are poorly dialyzable by standard hemodialysis or peritoneal dialysis techniques.[728] As a result, the plasma porphyrin levels can exceed 200 μg/dl. Management was difficult in the past because phlebotomy was contraindicated by anemia in most cases. Chloroquine also is not effective, presumably because kidney failure precludes excretion of excess porphyrins mobilized from liver, and porphyrins in blood plasma are not readily dialyzable. Because the anemia of end-stage renal disease results primarily from erythropoietin deficiency, recombinant erythropoietin with or without phlebotomy has become the treatment of choice for these patients. Erythropoietin administration can correct anemia, mobilize iron, and support phlebotomy in this condition.[729–731] Serial serum ferritin and plasma porphyrin levels are the most useful guides to treatment efficacy, as in patients with PCT and normal renal function.[729] The serum ferritin, which is the best predictor of iron storage in patients on maintenance dialysis,[732] should be reduced to near the lower limit of normal. Plasma porphyrins fall in parallel, and after remission is achieved, the ferritin may increase to a higher level without exacerbating the disease.[729] High-flux hemodialysis removes porphyrins from plasma better than standard hemodialysis and may be of some benefit until a remission is achieved with erythropoietin and phlebotomy.[733] Earlier approaches, such as DFO[734] and plasma exchange,[735] were somewhat effective in a few patients. Response also may occur after renal transplantation,[736] probably due in part to resumption of endogenous erythropoietin production.

Pseudoporphyria. Patients with this condition, which is also known as pseudo-PCT, have photocutaneous lesions that closely resemble PCT, but no significant increases in plasma porphyrins. It can occur in patients with or without end-stage renal disease, and is presumably due to photosensitizers other than porphyrins. Sometimes drugs, such as nonsteroidal anti-inflammatory drugs, are implicated.[737–739] This condition does not respond to the specific therapies that are effective in PCT.

Treatment of HEP

Therapies for HEP, and especially avoiding sunlight, are generally the same as those for CEP, but different from therapies for PCT. Oral charcoal was helpful in a severe case associated with dyserythropoiesis.[740] Phlebotomy is usually not beneficial.[626] Recent studies indicate that gene therapy may be applicable in HEP in the future. Using retrovirus-mediated gene transfer, metabolic correction of porphyria was demonstrated in transduced lymphoblastoid cells from patients with HEP. The genetically corrected cells had normal porphyrin levels, lacked fluorescence when illuminated with UV light, and had a competitive advantage for cellular expansion in vitro and in vivo in immunodeficient mice.[741] These findings suggested that gene therapy may be possible for HEP using transduced hematopoietic stem cells.

HEREDITARY COPROPORPHYRIA (HCP)

HCP is an autosomal dominant hepatic porphyria that results from the half-normal activity of coproporphyrinogen oxidase (CPO, EC 1.3.3.3).[742] Symptoms are identical to those of AIP, except that patients occasionally have cutaneous lesions. Berger and Goldberg named the disease in 1955.[743]

HCP has been reported mostly in Britain, Europe, and North America. Although the prevalence has not been carefully estimated, it is panethnic, and less common than AIP. A severe form of homozygous-dominant HCP has been described, as well as patients with harderoporphyria, a biochemically distinguishable variant of homozygous-dominant HCP that is characterized by the accumulation of coproporphyrin and harderoporphyrin, an intermediate tricarboxyl porphyrin.[744]

Clinical Manifestations

HCP usually presents with symptoms identical to AIP. Photosensitivity similar to that in PCT sometimes occurs. In one series, the most common clinical manifestations were abdominal pain (80 percent), vomiting (34 percent), skin lesions (29 percent), neuropathic involvement (23 percent), psychiatric symptoms (23 percent), and constipation (20 percent).[745] The disease is latent before puberty, and symptoms are more common in adult women than men. Although generally milder than AIP, severe motor neuropathy and death from respiratory paralysis can occur.[260]

Precipitating Factors. This porphyria is exacerbated by many of the same factors that precipitate acute attacks in AIP, including barbiturates and other drugs, and endogenous or exogenous steroid hormones, including oral contraceptive steroids.[745,746] Symptoms can occur in association with the menstrual cycle. Studies of urinary steroid hormone metabolites suggest increased production of 17-oxosteroids and reduced metabolism of androgens by the 5α-reductive pathway in some HCP patients.[747] Concomitant liver diseases, such as hepatitis, may increase porphyrin retention and photosensitivity.[742] HCP, like other acute porphyrias, may be exacerbated by fasting. Of interest, fasting has been shown to decrease hepatic CPO activity in pigs.[748] The risk of hepatocellular carcinoma may be increased in this acute hepatic porphyria, as in AIP and VP.[290]

Several well-documented cases of homozygous-dominant HCP, with cutaneous lesions beginning in early childhood, have been reported.[744,745,749]

The Metabolic Defect in HCP

Accumulated Porphyrin Precursors and Porphyrins. The most prominent biochemical feature of HCP is a marked increase in urinary and fecal coproporphyrin, predominantly isomer type III.[303] Urinary ALA, PBG, and uroporphyrin are increased during acute attacks. With resolution of symptoms, ALA and PBG revert to normal more readily than in AIP. Fecal coproporphyrin may be partially in the form of copper coproporphyrin.[750] In harderoporphyria, fecal excretion of harderoporphyrin (tricarboxyl porphyrin), as well as coproporphyrin, is increased.[744]

The Enzymatic Defect in HCP. The enzymatic defect in HCP is the half-normal activity of CPO, a mitochondrial enzyme that catalyzes the conversion of coproporphyrinogen III to the divinyl compound, protoporphyrinogen IX, by the stereospecific removal of the carboxyl group and the two hydrogens from the propionic groups of pyrrole rings A and B to form vinyl groups at these positions (Fig. 124-25).[751–753] This reaction proceeds through an intermediate tripropionate monovinyl porphyrinogen termed harderoporphyrinogen. The corresponding porphyrin was originally isolated from the Harderian gland of rodents,[754] and was also found in the stool of patients with a variant of HCP named harderoporphyria.[744] The accumulation of harderoporphyrinogen in harderoporphyria presumably is due to the propionate side chain in the 2-position being decarboxylated first and at a faster rate than the side chain in the 4-position, with the mutant enzyme prematurely releasing harderoporphyrinogen.

This mitochondrial enzyme is not membrane bound,[755–757] and was shown to be present in the intermembrane space.[758–760] This localization of CPO implies that either protoporphyrinogen or protoporphyrin must cross the inner membrane because heme is formed within the inner membrane.

Purification and Properties of CPO. CPO has been purified from *S. cerevisiae*, bovine liver, and mouse liver.[760–762] Purified bovine liver CPO has a molecular weight of about 74 kDa and appears to function as a monomer.[760] Human CPO has been expressed in *E. coli* and appears to be a nearly globular homodimer composed of ~39 kDa subunits.[763,764] Oxygen is an absolute requirement for the enzymatic function and other oxidants cannot replace oxygen. Reducing agents such as NADPH are not required for enzyme activity. Prosthetic groups, such as flavin and heme, are not present in the purified enzyme. Thiol groups are not involved in the catalytic site of the enzyme. This oxidase is unusual in that it contains no metals, and therefore its activity is unaffected by treatment with metal chelators.[760,763,764]

Mammalian and yeast CPO differ in their intracellular localization, subunit composition, and metal content. In yeast, CPO is localized in the cytosol, and the purified enzyme has a M_r ~35,000[761] or 37,673, as deduced from the sequence of the isolated yeast *CPO* gene.[765] In contrast to the bovine liver enzyme, the yeast enzyme contains two iron atoms per molecule of native protein. The yeast enzyme uses molecular oxygen as electron acceptor, and thiol-directed reagents partially inhibit the enzyme, indicating the importance of an SH group for activity.[761]

The Molecular Genetics and Pathology of *CPO*

cDNA and Genomic Sequences. The full-length cDNA encoding human CPO was isolated from human placenta and fibroblast libraries.[766,767] The cDNA had an open reading frame of 1062 bp, encoding a polypeptide of 354 amino acids. However, RT-PCR

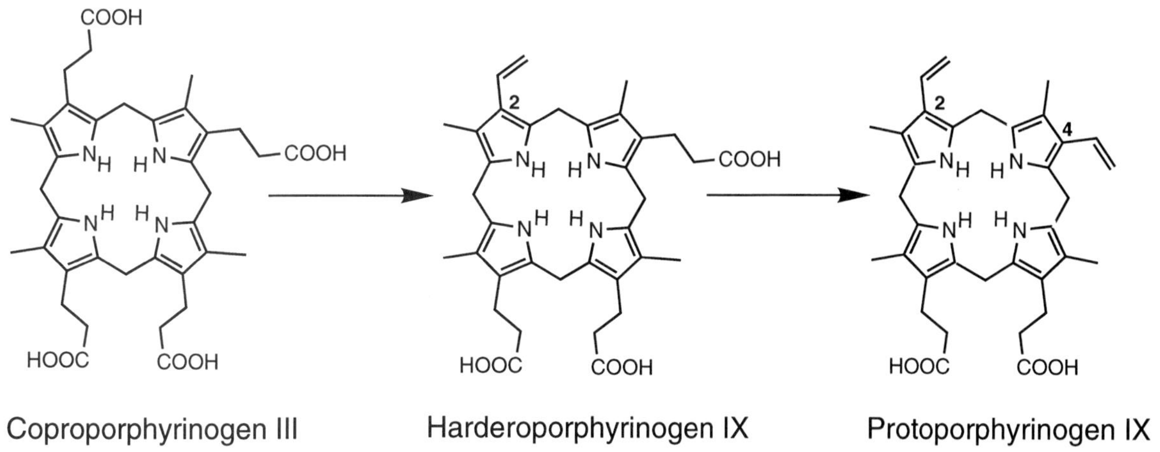

Coproporphyrinogen III   Harderoporphyrinogen IX   Protoporphyrinogen IX

Fig. 124-25 Formation of protoporphyrinogen IX from coproporphyrinogen III as catalyzed by coproporphyrinogen oxidase (CPO). The propionic acid groups of ring A and B (positions 2 and 4) are decarboxylated in the order shown to vinyl groups, yielding first harderoporphyrinogen IX (a tricarboxyl porphyrinogen) and then protoporphyrinogen IX.

studies performed after elucidation of the genomic structure indicated that the first in-frame AUG was 300 bp upstream from the previously described initiation codon;[768] the additional amino acids appear to be the putative mitochondrial leader sequence. Comparison of the human and murine predicted amino acid sequences was consistent with a mature human enzyme of 354 residues (M_r = 36,842), with a putative *N*-terminal signal peptide of 110 residues.[768] The human *CPO* gene was localized to chromosome 3q12,[769] spans approximately 14 kb, and consists of 7 exons.[768] The 6 introns vary in size from 269 bp to 5 kb, and all have AG-GT consensus sequences at their intron/exon boundaries. The *CPO* promoter region is GC-rich, and contains multiple potential Sp1 elements, CACCC boxes and GATA-1 binding sites.[768]

Although there is not a unique erythroid-specific promoter, *CPO* transcripts increase during erythroid cell differentiation.[770,771] Functional analysis of the mouse *CPO* promoter demonstrated the synergistic action of an Sp-1 like element, a GATA-1 site, and a novel regulatory element, CPRE (*CPO* Promoter Regulatory Element), were prerequisite for the promoter activity in erythroid cells.[772] In contrast, in nonerythroid cells, the GATA-1 site was not required, while the CPRE was necessary. These findings indicate that a single promoter contains elements for both the housekeeping and erythroid-specific expression of the *CPO* gene.[772] However, two polyadenylation signals 126 bp apart have been identified in the *CPO* gene and these may also play a role in tissue-specific expression of CPO mRNA.[773]

Molecular Pathology. Molecular analysis of several families with HCP, including the homozygous dominant form and the harderoporphyria variant, has revealed a variety of mutations in the *CPO* gene (Fig. 124-26). These include missense, nonsense, and splice-site defects, as well as insertions and deletions.[336,773] Except for one mutation (K404E) found in two unrelated families with harderoporphyria, the *CPO* mutations found to date are private, each occurring in only one affected family.[336,773] Mutations G197W, Q306X, Q385X, and W427X occur in highly conserved amino acids.[774] A consanguineous patient with homozygous HCP who had a large accumulation of coproporphyrin in his feces and very low CPO activity was homozygous for R331W.[775] Expression of this mutation in *E. coli* showed that the enzyme had decreased activity and heat stability. In two

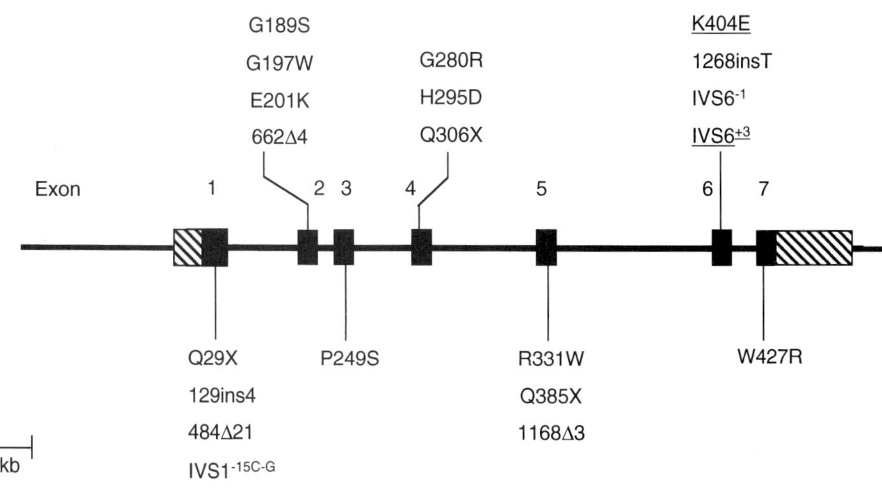

Underlined Mutations Found in Patients with Harderoporphyria

Fig. 124-26 The human *CPO* gene and locations of mutations causing HCP. (*Courtesy of Dr. K. H. Astrin.*)

unrelated families with harderoporphyria, *CPO* mutation analysis revealed homozygosity for K404E in one family, while the second family was heteroallelic for K404E and an exon 6 splice-site mutation (IVS6^{+3}).[776,777] The K404E lesion is located immediately after the most phylogenetically conserved region in the CPO enzyme, which may be involved in substrate binding. Therefore, this mutation may impair substrate binding, leading to the accumulation of the substrate intermediate, harderoporphyrinogen.[773]

Diagnosis

A diagnosis of HCP is readily confirmed by porphyrin analysis when the disease is clinically manifest. The most prominent findings are increased urinary and fecal coproporphyrin III. Fecal porphyrins in HCP are mostly coproporphyrin, whereas in VP coproporphyrin and protoporphyrin are often similarly increased. Excretion of coproporphyrin III in the urine and feces may be increased in some asymptomatic (or latent) heterozygotes. The ratio of fecal coproporphyrin III to coproporphyrin I is more likely to be increased in latent heterozygotes (especially adults) than total fecal coproporphyrin.[778] In homozygous HCP, porphyrin excretion patterns resemble those observed in heterozygotes with manifest disease, but may be more severe. Harderoporphyria is characterized by a marked increase in fecal excretion of harderoporphyrin (tricarboxyl porphyrin), as well as coproporphyrin, low CPO activity, and clinical symptoms of jaundice, severe chronic hemolytic anemia of early onset associated with hepatosplenomegaly, and skin photosensitivity.[744,777]

As noted above, reliable assays for CPO are not widely available. Because the enzyme is localized in mitochondria, cells such as lymphocytes are most commonly used for enzyme assay.[778,779] The diagnosis of HCP is often made incorrectly in patients who have other conditions. To avoid misdiagnosis it must be kept in mind that urinary coproporphyrin can be increased in many conditions other than porphyria, and that minimal increases may not be clinically significant. Increases in urinary or fecal coproporphyrin during drug therapy do not necessarily indicate the presence of a "coproporphyria-like syndrome."[780]

CPO activity has been assayed by the spectrophotometric determination of the product, protoporphyrinogen, after its oxidation to protoporphyrin.[756,757] However, these assays are not sensitive enough to accurately measure CPO activity in small amounts of tissue such as human lymphocytes or cultured fibroblasts. Degradation of protoporphyrinogen or protoporphyrin during extraction presents another problem in the reproducibility of the assay. Elder and Evans[781] have described a more sensitive radiochemical method for the determination of CPO activity. The method measures the rate of production of $^{14}CO_2$ from the radiolabeled substrate, [^{14}C] coproporphyrinogen III. In this method, [^{14}C] coproporphyrinogen III was labeled in the carboxyl carbon atoms of the 2- and 4-propionate groups. Grandchamp and Nordmann[782] circumvented the problem of the tedious and difficult chemical synthesis of the substrate by enzymatically synthesizing [^{14}C] coproporphyrin III from [4-^{14}C] ALA. Both methods appear to be very sensitive as a high specific activity of the substrate can be obtained, and the use of cobalt protoporphyrin as an internal standard permits the reliable measurement of the protoporphyrin IX formed.[783]

A fluorometric assay for CPO has been described[784] in which the enzymatic activity is measured in the presence of a large excess of protoporphyrinogen oxidase provided by yeast mitochondrial membranes isolated from commercial baker's yeast. A sensitive and accurate reverse phase HPLC assay for CPO activity has also been reported.[785]

Treatment

Acute attacks are treated in the same manner as in AIP. It is important to identify and avoid precipitating factors. Heme therapy is useful, as in other acute porphyrias.[786] Cholestyramine may be of some value for photosensitivity occurring with liver dysfunction.[787] Phlebotomy and chloroquine are not effective. Preventive measures are the same as in AIP, including avoidance of harmful drugs and dietary indiscretions, and the use of GnRH analogues in women with cyclic attacks.[470]

VARIEGATE PORPHYRIA (VP)

First described in 1937, VP is an autosomal dominant hepatic porphyria that results from the deficient activity of protoporphyrinogen oxidase (PPO, EC 1.3.3.4).[233,788] The disease was termed variegate because it can present with neurologic manifestations, cutaneous photosensitivity, or both. VP also has been known as porphyria variegata, protocoproporphyria, and South African genetic porphyria. Some cases of VP were described as having "porphyria cutanea tarda hereditaria" before VP and PCT were clearly distinguished. The term "mixed porphyria" referred to either HCP or VP. Several cases of homozygous-dominant VP have also been described.[789,790]

In most countries, this porphyria is less commonly recognized than AIP. VP is especially common in South Africa, where it was first reported in 1945.[233] The high prevalence among South African whites (approximately 3 in 1000) can be traced to a common founding couple who emigrated from Holland and were married in 1688.[248] As many as 20,000 South Africans may carry this trait due to the "founder" mutation (see below).[788,791] In Finland, the prevalence is also high, about 1.3 per 100,000.[792] VP has been termed the "Royal Malady" based on the suggestion that some British royalty may have had this condition.[245] However, as noted earlier (see AIP), this speculation is based on a retrospective analysis of symptoms, which are characteristically nonspecific in this and other acute porphyrias.[248]

Clinical Manifestations

The acute attacks of VP are identical to those in other acute porphyrias.[283] Symptoms may include abdominal pain, tachycardia, vomiting, constipation, hypertension, neuropathy, back pain, confusion, bulbar paralysis, psychiatric symptoms, fever, urinary frequency, and dysuria.[280] Hyponatremia with evidence of sodium depletion or inappropriate ADH secretion can occur during acute attacks.[280] In South Africa, attacks of VP are generally milder and recur much less frequently than in AIP.[788] In the past, VP most commonly presented with neurovisceral symptoms. However, at least in South Africa and Europe, perhaps due to early diagnosis and counseling of asymptomatic patients, acute attacks have become considerably less common, and skin manifestations are more frequently the initial presentation.[788,793] For example, in the recent series of 108 English and French VP patients noted above, 59 percent presented only with skin lesions, 20 percent only with an acute neurovisceral attack, and 21 percent had both symptoms.[793] Improved clinical outcomes have been noted in Finland, presumably due to earlier and improved treatment of acute attacks.

Cutaneous photosensitivity is more common in VP than in HCP. Skin manifestations often occur apart from the neurovisceral symptoms, and are usually of longer duration. They are very similar to those seen in PCT and HCP, and include increased fragility, vesicles, bullae, erosions, milia, hyperpigmentation, and hypertrichosis of sun-exposed areas.[788,794] Histologic changes include PAS-positive thickening and IgG deposition in the vessel walls and reduplication of the basal lamina.[795] Photosensitivity may be less common in more northern countries where sunlight is less intense.[792,796]

Precipitating Factors. Symptoms rarely occur before puberty. However, the disease may present late in life.[797] The same drugs, steroid hormones, and nutritional factors that are detrimental in AIP can provoke exacerbations of VP.[280,798] Restriction of calories can be detrimental, particularly near the time of menses.[798,799] Women taking oral contraceptives are prone to develop cutaneous manifestations of VP.

Chronic liver abnormalities, which are generally mild, may be seen in VP.[800,801] Some patients with VP have developed hepatocellular carcinoma,[290,802,803] which suggests that the risk of this tumor may be increased, as in AIP and PCT.

Homozygous-Dominant VP. Homozygous-dominant VP patients inherited a *PPO* mutation from each parent, have markedly reduced PPO activity, and have severe VP clinical manifestations with onset in childhood.[789] In addition to photosensitivity, they have neurologic symptoms, convulsions, and developmental disturbances. Growth retardation in infancy or childhood has been noted in some patients.[789,804–808] However, for reasons that are unclear, these patients do not have acute attacks.[789]

The Metabolic Defect in VP

Accumulated Porphyrin Precursors and Porphyrins. When VP is clinically active, fecal protoporphyrin and coproporphyrin and urinary coproporphyrin are markedly increased. Pentacarboxyl porphyrin and "pseudo-pentacarboxyl porphyrin" (a modified dicarboxyl porphyrin presumably derived from protoporphyrin) are also increased in feces.[788] Urinary and fecal coproporphyrin is mostly type III.[303] Urinary ALA, PBG, and uroporphyrin are increased during acute attacks, but may be normal or only slightly increased during remission. Plasma porphyrins are commonly increased, particularly when photosensitivity is present. The increased plasma porphyrins in VP consist in part of a dicarboxyl porphyrin tightly bound to plasma proteins.[694,695,809,810] Biliary porphyrins also are increased.[811] It has been suggested that the risk of gallstones may be increased in VP, and that the stones contain protoporphyrin.[812]

The *X porphyrin fraction* (defined as ether-acetic acid-insoluble porphyrins extracted from feces by urea-Triton) is increased in this disease more than in other porphyrias. In VP, this fraction contains a heterogeneous group of porphyrin-peptide conjugates termed *X porphyrins*. X-porphyrins have also been detected in bile in VP.[813,814] In PCT, the fecal X porphyrin fraction consists mostly of uroporphyrin and heptacarboxyl porphyrin.[815,816] Fecal levels of meso- and deuteroporphyrins derived in the gut from protoporphyrin are also increased in VP. These porphyrins are seldom examined for clinical diagnostic purposes.

As in all homozygous porphyrias so far described, homozygous VP patients have markedly increased erythrocyte zinc protoporphyrin levels.[804–806] A less marked increase has been observed in heterozygous cases.[792]

The Enzymatic Defect in VP. This porphyria results from the half-normal activity of PPO as demonstrated in cultured skin fibroblasts, peripheral leukocytes and lymphocytes, cultured lymphocytes, and liver.[817–821] PPO is the penultimate step in the heme biosynthetic pathway and catalyzes the oxidation of protoporphyrinogen IX to protoporphyrin IX by the removal of six hydrogen atoms (Fig. 124-1). This mitochondrial enzyme acts specifically on protoporphyrinogen, and does not catalyze the oxidation of coproporphyrinogen I, coproporphyrinogen III, or uroporphyrinogen I. Sulfhydryl-reducing agents, such as glutathione at low concentrations, stimulate the enzyme activity.[822] PPO from most sources use molecular oxygen as the electron acceptor, but under anaerobic conditions in *E. coli*, fumarate[823] and nitrate[824] can serve as alternative electron acceptors. Because the enzymatic conversion of protoporphyrinogen to protoporphyrin is not inhibited by cyanide, 2,4-dinitrophenol, or azide, disulfide bonds are not essential for activity.[825] Hemin at concentrations of 50 μM inhibits the enzyme activity by approximately 50 percent and the inhibition is apparently noncompetitive and irreversible.[825]

Human skin fibroblasts display PPO activity (2 to 3 nmol/h of protoporphyrin formed per mg protein)[822,826] and rat liver mitochondria have enzyme activity in the range of 10 to 12 nmol protoporphyrin/h per mg protein.[826] PPO activity is decreased in fibroblasts from patients with VP, but not from patients with EPP.[826] Several commercial and experimental herbicides such as *p*-nitrodiphenylesters, oxadiazoles, and cyclic imides inhibit PPO activity, and cells treated with these PPO inhibitors accumulate protoporphyrin in the cytosol, presumably by the accumulation of protoporphyrinogen, its export from mitochondria and autoxidation to protoporphyrin.[827] In plants treated with these herbicides, light-dependent damage occurs and is correlated with the level of accumulated protoporphyrin.[827]

Purification and Properties of PPO. PPO has been purified from rat liver mitochondria and shown to have a molecular weight of 35 kDa, a K_m of 11 μM, a V_{max} of 8.7 nmol/min per mg protein, and an absolute requirement for oxygen. The same enzyme purified from yeast, however, has a molecular weight of approximately 180 kDa and a K_m of 4.8 μM.[825]

The Molecular Genetics and Pathology of *PPO*

cDNA and Genomic Sequences. The human cDNA for PPO was isolated by complementation in vivo of a *hemG* mutant of *E. coli*,[828] and subsequently genomic DNA fragments containing the entire coding sequence for human PPO were isolated and characterized.[828–830] The 5.5-kb gene has 1 noncoding and 12 coding exons, and the exon/intron boundaries all conform to consensus acceptor (GTN) and donor (NAG) sequences.[829,830] The human *PPO* coding sequence is 1431 bp, and encodes a 477-amino-acid polypeptide, a protein with a M_r ~50.8 kDa. Comparison of the predicted human, mouse, and bacterial PPO amino acid sequences reveals a high degree of homology near the *N*-terminus of the polypeptide. This area corresponds to a typical flavin adenine dinucleotide (FAD)-binding motif. Consistent with this finding, human PPO has been shown to contain noncovalently bound FAD.[831] The gene for human PPO has been mapped to chromosomal region 1q22-q23[830,832] by fluorescence *in situ* hybridization.

Northern blot analyses from a variety of tissues indicate that there is a single PPO transcript of 1.8 kb in all tissues.[828,831,833] Although the PPO enzyme was localized to the cytosolic side of the inner mitochondrial membrane,[834,835] the gene does not encode mitochondrial targeting and import sequences or membrane spanning regions.[788,829]

Molecular Pathology. A variety of *PPO* mutations have been reported in families with VP from different ethnic and demographic groups.[336,788,793] These include missense, nonsense, and splice-site mutations, as well as small deletions and insertions as shown in Fig. 124-27 (e.g., references 336 and 793). Of note, a missense *PPO* mutation, R59W, is prevalent in South Africa (~20,000 individuals) where it has originated from a common founder, as most VP cases can be traced to a Dutch immigrant couple who married in Cape Town in 1688.[248,791] A recent study of 108 unrelated English and French VP families identified 60 novel and 6 previously reported mutations. Forty-seven mutations were each detected in single, unrelated families, and 14 in 2 or 3 families. Mutations L15F, E198X, L295P, 1082insC, and Q435X were common, each occurring in four to seven unrelated VP families. These common mutations accounted for 26 percent of the mutations among the 108 families studied.[793] Haplotype analysis of the families with the L15F and Q435X mutations indicated that both were recurrent because neither mutation resulted from a common founder. No genotype/phenotype correlations were identified.

Rare homozygous dominant VP patients have been identified; these patients had *PPO* mutations that were not found in heterozygous VP, suggesting that they were hypomorphs encoding enzyme proteins with residual activity.[790,791,836] For example, one allele in each homozygous dominant patient exhibited 9 to 25 percent of normal PPO activity.[790] These findings suggest that VP mutations with high residual activity may be present in

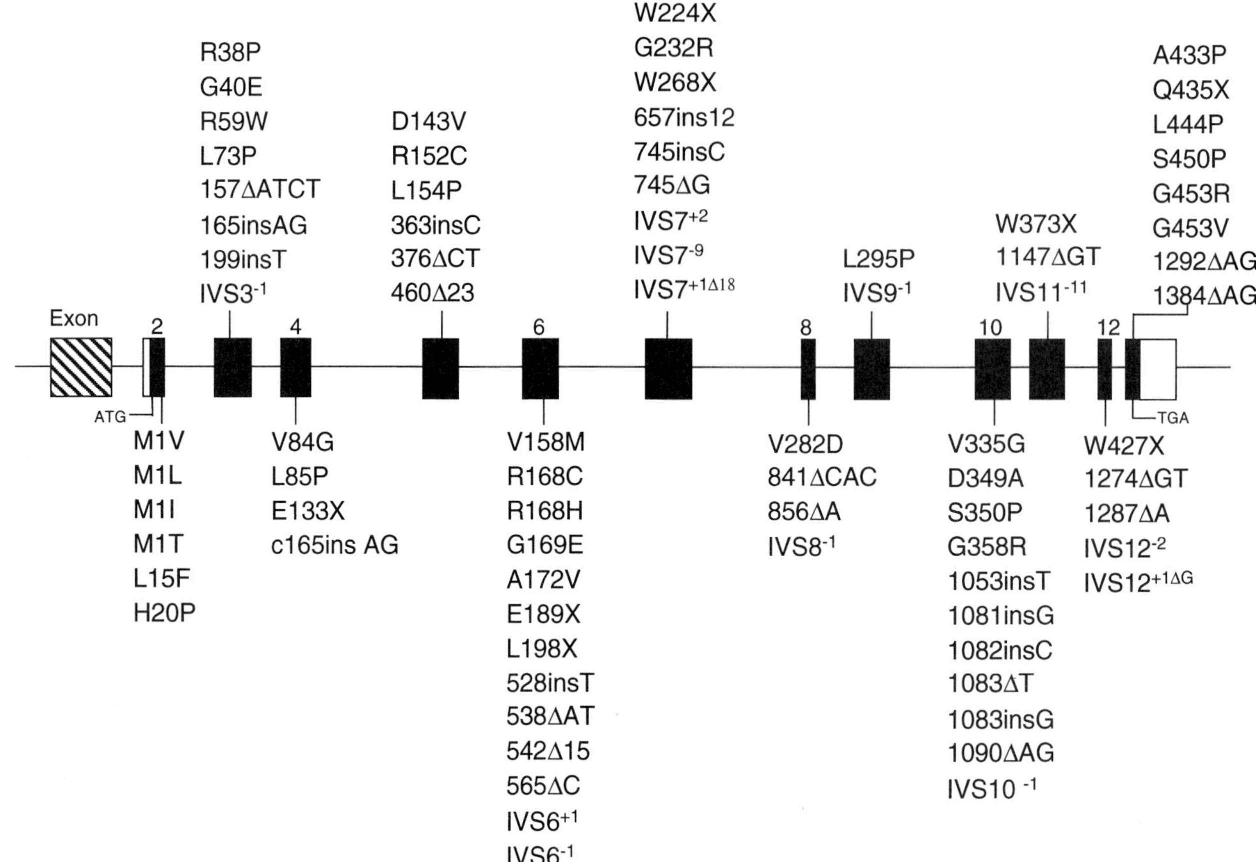

Fig. 124-27 The human *PPO* gene showing locations of mutations causing VP. (*Courtesy of Dr. K. H. Astrin.*)

heterozygous individuals but seldom, if ever, cause clinical symptoms.

Pathophysiology

Most individuals (~75 percent) who inherit PPO deficiency remain asymptomatic throughout life and clinical symptoms may not develop until the third decade of life.[788] How the disease becomes manifest in some individuals is not fully understood. However, additional influences, such as certain drugs and steroids, alcohol, and nutritional alterations, many of which increase hepatic ALAS1, are important, as in other acute porphyrias. This rate-limiting enzyme is increased in the liver in VP.[837–839] Therefore, ALA and PBG are increased during acute attacks due to the induction of ALAS1 and the normal, but rate-limiting activity of hepatic PBGD.[742] In addition, PBGD is inhibited by protoporphyrinogen (but not protoporphyrin),[840] presumably accounting for the low activity levels of PBGD in VP (approximately 25 percent reduction), thereby further contributing to the accumulation of porphyrin precursors.[820] Although many of the same environmental factors induce both AIP and VP attacks, the latter are rarer and occur equally in both males and females, whereas attacks of AIP are seen more frequently in women.[788] Also, attacks recur less frequently in VP than AIP.

Much of the protoporphyrinogen IX that accumulates in VP undergoes autoxidation to protoporphyrin IX before excretion in bile and feces. PPO in the inner mitochondrial membrane and CPO in the intermembrane space are closely associated, which may relate to the excess excretion of both protoporphyrin and coproporphyrin in this disease.[834] In addition, increased coproporphyrinogen may be more readily lost from the liver cell than other intermediates when heme synthesis is stimulated. Because liver porphyrin content is not substantially increased, excess porphyrins must be efficiently removed from the liver or may be generated in part in tissues other than the liver in this disease.[841] The relationship between accumulation of protoporphyrinogen and formation of porphyrin-peptide conjugates, which are an interesting biochemical feature of this disease, is poorly understood.

Diagnosis

VP should be included whenever AIP and other acute porphyrias are considered as a cause of neurovisceral symptoms. During an acute attack of VP, urinary ALA and PBG should be increased, although sometimes less markedly than in AIP. VP can be distinguished from AIP by the finding of increased plasma porphyrins and marked increases in urinary and fecal coproporphyrin. Erythrocyte PBGD is deficient in most cases of AIP, but remains in the normal range in VP. VP is differentiated from HCP by fecal and plasma porphyrin analyses. In patients with cutaneous symptoms, it is important to differentiate VP and PCT, because PCT is considerably more common than VP, but treatments that are effective for PCT are not effective in VP. Plasma porphyrin analysis provides a simple and reliable means of rapidly distinguishing VP from other cutaneous porphyrias. The increased plasma porphyrins in VP include a dicarboxyl porphyrin tightly bound to plasma proteins. As a result, the fluorescence emission spectrum of plasma porphyrins at neutral pH in VP is characteristic and can distinguish this disease from other types of porphyria. The emission maximum occurs at or near 626 nm in VP, 619 nm in PCT and CEP, and when plasma porphyrins are increased in HCP and AIP, and 634 nm in EPP.[694,695,809,810] Also diagnostically useful is an increase in fecal "pseudo-pentacarboxyl porphyrin," a dicarboxyl porphyrin derived from protoporphyrin.[788]

Direct fluorometric measurement of plasma porphyrins may be the best alternate method for detecting asymptomatic VP and is clearly more effective than examination of fecal porphyrins.[842] Fecal porphyrin analysis is very useful for the diagnosis of VP, but timed fecal collections are usually not feasible or meaningful, and results can be confounded by dietary and other substances. For example, a fecal porphyrin excretion pattern suggestive of VP can follow excessive ingestion of porphyrin-containing yeast tablets.[843] Biliary porphyrins are increased in VP and their analysis may be useful in detecting asymptomatic individuals.[811] Obtaining samples for biliary porphyrin analysis is more difficult than plasma porphyrin analysis, and their usefulness has not been compared. In a direct comparison, plasma porphyrin determinations were less sensitive than PPO assays for identifying asymptomatic carriers of VP.[844]

PPO can be measured in cells that contain mitochondria, such as lymphocytes. However, assays for PPO activity are difficult to perform and not widely available for detecting latent cases. Spectrophotometric and fluorometric assays for protoporphyrinogen oxidation have been described for use in rat liver mitochondria and other tissues.[845] The fluorometric assay is more sensitive, while the spectrophotometric assay may be more useful for a wider variety of tissues as enzyme sources. In both assays, three properties of protoporphyrin are important for assay validity. First, protoporphyrin, unlike uroporphyrin, tends to aggregate at neutral pH in aqueous solutions. Therefore, addition of tissue or a neutral detergent is required to circumvent this problem. Second, protoporphyrinogen oxidation occurs at a significant rate in air, and is minimized by the addition of a reducing agent such as glutathione. Third, a chelating agent must be present to prevent the spontaneous formation of certain metalloporphyrin complexes, such as zinc protoporphyrin, or heme.[845]

Treatment

Treatment measures that are effective in AIP, such as glucose and heme therapy, also are effective for acute attacks of VP. Heme arginate has been found to be beneficial in treating acute attacks.[846] Identifying and avoiding exacerbating factors is very important. Heme therapy does not improve cutaneous symptoms.[847] Other therapies such as propranolol, D-penicillamine, hemodialysis, alkalization of urine, and β-carotene are of little or no benefit. Repeated venesections and chloroquine are highly effective in PCT, but not in VP.[788,848] Protection from sunlight is extremely important and may include use of protective clothing, gloves, a broad-brimmed hat, and opaque sunscreen preparations. Increasing the amount of skin pigment by exposure to short wavelength ultraviolet light, which does not excite porphyrins, may provide some protection.[794] Improved treatment, earlier diagnosis, and detection of latent cases have greatly improved the outlook for patients with this disease.[788] Because the prognosis is usually good once the diagnosis is established, a diagnosis of VP or any other acute porphyria should not lead to difficulty obtaining insurance.

ERYTHROPOIETIC PROTOPORPHYRIA (EPP)

EPP is an autosomal dominant disorder resulting from the partially deficient activity of the last enzyme in the heme biosynthetic pathway, ferrochelatase (heme synthase, heme synthetase, or protoheme-ferrolyase, EC4.99.1.1). EPP is also known as protoporphyria, whereas the term erythrohepatic protoporphyria is no longer used. Protoporphyrin accumulates primarily in erythroid cells in the bone marrow, and appears in excess amounts in plasma, circulating erythrocytes, bile, and feces. In affected cases, cutaneous photosensitivity characteristically begins in childhood. Skin manifestations are usually nonblistering, in contrast to the other cutaneous porphyrias. Severe liver damage occurs occasionally.

Although this is the most common erythropoietic porphyria, it was not clearly described until 1961,[849] probably because the cutaneous features are usually mild and there is no excess urinary porphyrin excretion. The prevalence of this disease has not been reliably estimated; however, it is considered the third most common porphyria. As of 1976, more than 300 cases had been reported,[850] mostly in Caucasians, but also in other races, including Blacks.[851]

Clinical Manifestations

Cutaneous Involvement. The major clinical feature of EPP is cutaneous photosensitivity, which begins in childhood, affects sun-exposed areas, and is generally worse in spring and summer. Common symptoms include itching, painful erythema, and swelling that can develop within minutes of sun exposure.[850] Diffuse edema of the skin in sun-exposed areas may resemble angioneurotic edema. On occasion, burning and itching can occur without obvious skin damage. Petechiae and purpuric lesions may occur. Skin lichenification, leathery pseudovesicles, and nail changes can be pronounced (Fig. 124-28).[852–854] Labial grooving is sometimes noted.

The cutaneous manifestations of EPP differ from those of CEP, HEP, and other cutaneous porphyrias. Pigment changes and severe scarring are unusual. Vesicles and bullae are uncommon; in one

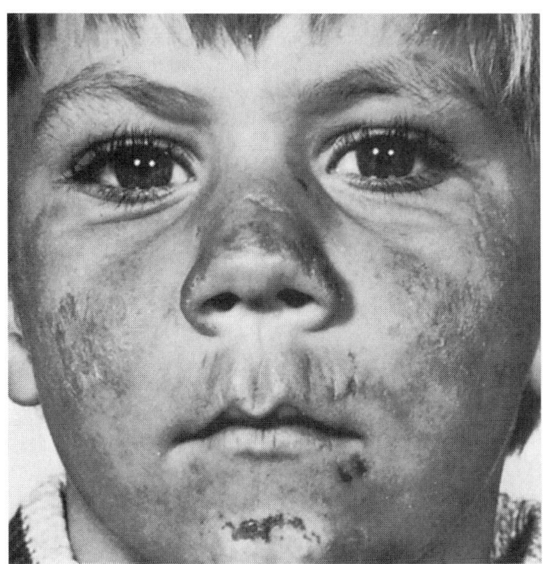

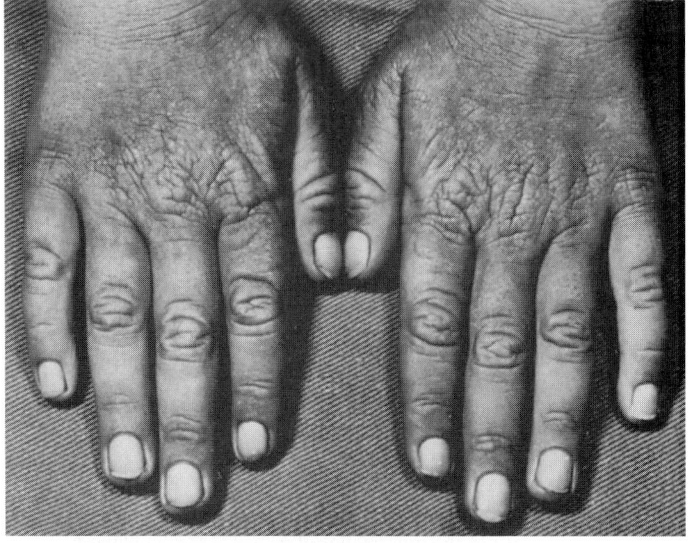

Fig. 124-28 Cutaneous manifestations of EPP in a 6-year-old boy, including ulcerations and scarring on the face, labial grooving, coarse, thickened skin on the hands, and loss of lunulae of the fingernails. (*Reproduced from Schmidt et al.*[852] *Used by permission.*)

series, they occurred in only 10 percent of cases.[850] Deformities of facial features and digits do not occur. Increased fragility and hirsutism are also not characteristic of this disease. The teeth are not fluorescent and there are no neurovisceral symptoms, except in some patients with severe hepatic complications who may develop motor neuropathy.[855]

EPP displays a stable course for many years in most patients with little change in photosensitivity or in levels of porphyrins in erythrocytes, plasma, and feces.[856] There are no known precipitating factors, such as those associated with the hepatic porphyrias. Pregnancy has been associated with somewhat lower levels of erythrocyte protoporphyrin and increased sunlight tolerance, which is unexplained.[857,858]

Hematologic Involvement. Mild anemia with hypochromia and microcytosis or mild anemia with reticulocytosis is sometimes noted in EPP.[343,850,859,860] However, in most uncomplicated cases, hemolysis is absent or very mild. There also is little evidence for impaired erythropoiesis or abnormal iron metabolism in this condition.[582,850,859,861] Moreover, depletion of iron stores may be relatively common even in the absence of iron deficiency anemia in EPP.[582] On the other hand, iron accumulation in erythroblasts and ring sideroblasts has been noted in some EPP patients.[862]

Hepatic Involvement. Hepatobiliary complications are a particular feature of this porphyria, but occur only in a minority of patients. The risk of biliary stones seems to be increased, and the stones contain protoporphyrin.[863] The majority of patients with EPP have normal liver function, and the liver protoporphyrin content is usually normal.[864] The chronic liver disease that sometimes develops in EPP is associated with marked protoporphyrin accumulation in liver, which can begin insidiously and progress rapidly to death from liver failure.[865] EPP sometimes presents with advanced liver disease.[866] Hepatic complications can produce upper abdominal pain that may suggest biliary obstruction; unnecessary laparotomy to exclude this possibility can be detrimental.[865]

The life-threatening hepatic complications of EPP are characteristically preceded by increasing levels of erythrocyte and plasma protoporphyrin levels, abnormal liver function tests, marked deposition of protoporphyrin in liver cells and bile canaliculi, and increased photosensitivity. Artificial lights, such as operating room lights, may cause photosensitivity with extensive burns of the skin and peritoneum and cause photodamage of circulating erythrocytes.[867] End-stage protoporphyric liver disease may even be accompanied by a severe motor neuropathy that resembles that seen in the acute porphyrias.[855] Concurrent viral hepatitis, alcohol abuse, iron deficiency, fasting, or oral contraceptive steroids, which may impair liver function or the metabolism of protoporphyrin to heme, have appeared to contribute to hepatic disease in some EPP patients.[868,869]

The Metabolic Defect in EPP

Accumulated Porphyrins. Protoporphyrin is increased in the bone marrow, erythrocytes, plasma, bile, and feces in EPP patients. This is the only heme pathway intermediate that accumulates significantly in this disease. Erythrocyte protoporphyrin in EPP is free and not complexed with zinc. The erythrocyte protoporphyrin concentration can be increased in homozygous porphyrias (see "Diagnosis"), but the increased protoporphyrin in these porphyrias is in the form of zinc protoporphyrin. Because other heme pathway intermediates do not accumulate, and protoporphyrin is excreted only in bile and feces, urinary porphyrin and porphyrin precursor concentrations are normal in uncomplicated EPP.

The Enzymatic Defect in EPP. The enzymatic defect in EPP is the deficient activity of the mitochondrial enzyme, ferrochelatase. This enzyme catalyzes the final step of heme biosynthesis, which is the insertion of iron into protoporphyrin IX (Fig. 124-1). Ferrochelatase activity is deficient in bone marrow, reticulocytes, liver, cultured fibroblasts, and leukocytes from patients with EPP.[859,870–872] Although hepatic ferrochelatase activity in biopsies from two EPP patients was approximately 17 percent of normal, immunoreactive enzyme protein (as assessed by an ELISA assay) was detected at normal levels, indicating that the mutant enzymes in these patients were catalytically defective, but stable.[872] Many symptomatic patients have ferrochelatase activity as low as 15 to 25 percent of normal, which is less than the 50 percent of normal ferrochelatase activity expected if EPP was inherited strictly as an autosomal dominant trait. For example, in a study of 29 French and Swiss EPP patients, ferrochelatase activity ranged from 15 to 50 percent of normal.[873] Recent molecular studies have provided insight into the lower than expected ferrochelatase activity (see "Molecular Pathology" below).

Ferrochelatase is localized to the inner membrane of mitochondria. The enzyme activity is also found in plant chloroplasts and chromatophores of photosynthetic bacteria. Unlike the three preceding enzymes in the heme biosynthetic pathway, which use porphyrinogens as substrates, ferrochelatase uses protoporphyrin IX, the oxidized form of protoporphyrinogen IX. In addition to protoporphyrin IX, other dicarboxyl porphyrins, such as deutero- and mesoporphyrin IX, serve as good substrates for this enzyme in vitro.[10,874,875] Only the reduced form of iron (Fe^{2+}), and not Fe^{3+}, is incorporated into protoporphyrin IX by the enzyme.[876] Co^{2+} and Zn^{2+} are more efficient substrates than Fe^{2+} for the enzyme.[874] Therefore, various rates of ferrochelatase activity can be obtained in vitro, depending upon which metal and porphyrin substrates are used.[874]

Purification and Properties of Ferrochelatase. Ferrochelatase has been purified from rat and bovine liver.[877–880] The rat liver enzyme is enriched in lysine (11 percent) and hydrophobic amino acid residues (48 percent), is markedly stimulated by the addition of fatty acids, and is inhibited by metals such as Co, Zn, Pb, Cu, or Mn.[877] Bovine ferrochelatase from liver mitochondria has been purified to homogeneity.[878,879] The molecular weight of the homogeneous protein was estimated to be ~42.5 kDa by SDS-polyacrylamide gel electrophoresis, but ~200 kDa by gel filtration.[878,879] Other physical-chemical properties of the bovine enzyme were similar to those of the rat enzyme. An antibody specific for purified bovine ferrochelatase inhibited the incorporation of iron, zinc, and cobalt into protoporphyrin, confirming that the synthetic activities for these metalloporphyrins can be ascribed to a single enzyme protein.[878] Human liver mitochondrial membranes contain a large amount of endogenous metals, especially zinc, which may influence ferrochelatase activity.[880] Thus, endogenous zinc content in biologic samples must be taken into account when measuring ferrochelatase activity.

An iron-sulfur cluster, [2Fe-2S], has been identified in purified ferrochelatase from mouse liver, and in recombinant mouse and human ferrochelatase.[881–883] Both the human and the mouse enzymes contain a putative Fe-S binding site at the C-terminus, a 30-residue region that contains 4 cysteine residues arranged in a sequence ($C\text{-}X_7\text{-}C\text{-}X_2\text{-}C\text{-}X_4\text{-}C$), which is a fingerprint for a [2Fe-2S] binding motif.[884] The Fe-S cluster is thought to be essential for the mammalian enzyme activity,[881] but the putative binding site for the Fe-S cluster is not present in the bacterial and yeast enzymes' predicted *N*-terminal amino acid sequences.[882] Thus, the exact role of the Fe-S cluster in the enzyme reaction remains unclear.

N-methylprotoporphyrin,[885] a potent inhibitor of ferrochelatase activity, has been found in the livers of mice that have been treated with DDC. Synthetic *N*-methylprotoporphyrin also strongly inhibits ferrochelatase activity both in crude and purified enzyme preparations.[879] It has been shown that *N*-alkylated dicarboxyl porphyrins compete reversibly with the protoporphyrin substrate for ferrochelatase, and that structural and steric factors affect the inhibitory activity by modifying the affinity of the *N*-alkyl porphyrin inhibitor for the active site of the enzyme.[886]

Biogenesis. Like most other mitochondrial proteins, ferrochelatase is synthesized in the cytosol as a larger precursor form, and then imported into the mitochondria.[880,887] When the mouse mRNA is expressed in a cell-free system, a 43-kDa precursor polypeptide is synthesized, which in cells is imported into the mitochondria and subsequently processed into the mature form of the enzyme.[888] It has been suggested that ferrochelatase is associated with complex I of the mitochondrial electron transport chain, and that ferrous ion may be produced upon NADH oxidation.[889]

Crystal Structure. Recently, the crystal structure of *Bacillus subtilis* ferrochelatase was determined at 1.9 Å resolution.[890] The polypeptide was folded into two similar domains each with a four-stranded parallel β-sheet flanked by α-helices. Structural elements from both domains formed a cleft containing several amino acid residues, including His 183, which were invariant in ferrochelatases from different organisms. This histidine residue was thought to be involved in ferrous iron binding. Based on these findings, it has been suggested that the porphyrin binds in the cleft, which also contains the metal binding site of the enzyme.[890] More recently, recombinant human ferrochelatase has been purified from bacteria and crystallized to better than 2 Å diffraction with an intact [2Fe-2S] cluster.[891] Gel filtration and dynamic light scattering measurements showed that the enzyme exists in solution as a homodimer.[891]

The Molecular Genetics and Pathology of Ferrochelatase

cDNA and Genomic Sequences. The cDNA encoding human ferrochelatase was isolated from a placental cDNA library.[892] The cDNA had an open reading frame of 1269 bp, which encoded a polypeptide of 423 amino acids, including a leader sequence of 54 residues (MW 47.9 kDa) and a mature enzyme of 369 amino acids. Northern blot analysis showed two mRNAs of ~1.6 and ~2.5 kb for ferrochelatase, due to the use of two alternative polyadenylation signals in the ferrochelatase mRNA.

The single, functional human ferrochelatase gene spans ~45 kb and contains 11 exons.[893] The functional gene was mapped to chromosomal region 18q21.3,[893,894] while a ferrochelatase pseudogene mapped to chromosome 3.[895] Analysis of the promoter region of the functional gene revealed a single promoter sequence with potential Sp1, NF-E2, and GATA-1 binding sites, but no typical TATA or CAAT sequences. The functional gene's transcription initiation site was assigned to an adenine, 89 bp upstream from the translation-initiating ATG. Comparison of the amino acid sequences predicted by the mouse and yeast ferrochelatase cDNAs[896–898] with the predicted human sequence revealed an 88 percent and 46 percent identity, respectively. Analysis of the mouse ferrochelatase gene promoter identified Sp1 sites located at −37 to −32 bp that were essential for housekeeping expression and a region containing a CACCC box and a neighboring GC box that was involved in inducible erythroid expression in MEL cells.[899]

Molecular Pathology. Molecular analysis of the ferrochelatase mutations causing EPP has revealed a variety of lesions including missense, nonsense, and splicing mutations, as well as small and large deletions and an insertion (Fig. 124-29).[336] Among these lesions, splicing mutations that resulted in exon skipping were the most predominant.[336] However, systematic screening of ferrochelatase genomic DNA by denaturing gradient gel electrophoresis and direct sequencing from 29 unrelated Swiss and French patients with EPP found only 4 splice-site mutations.[873] Among the 14 Swiss families, 4 common lesions (Q59X, 213insT, 580delTACAG, and 899delTG) accounted for 86 percent of the mutations

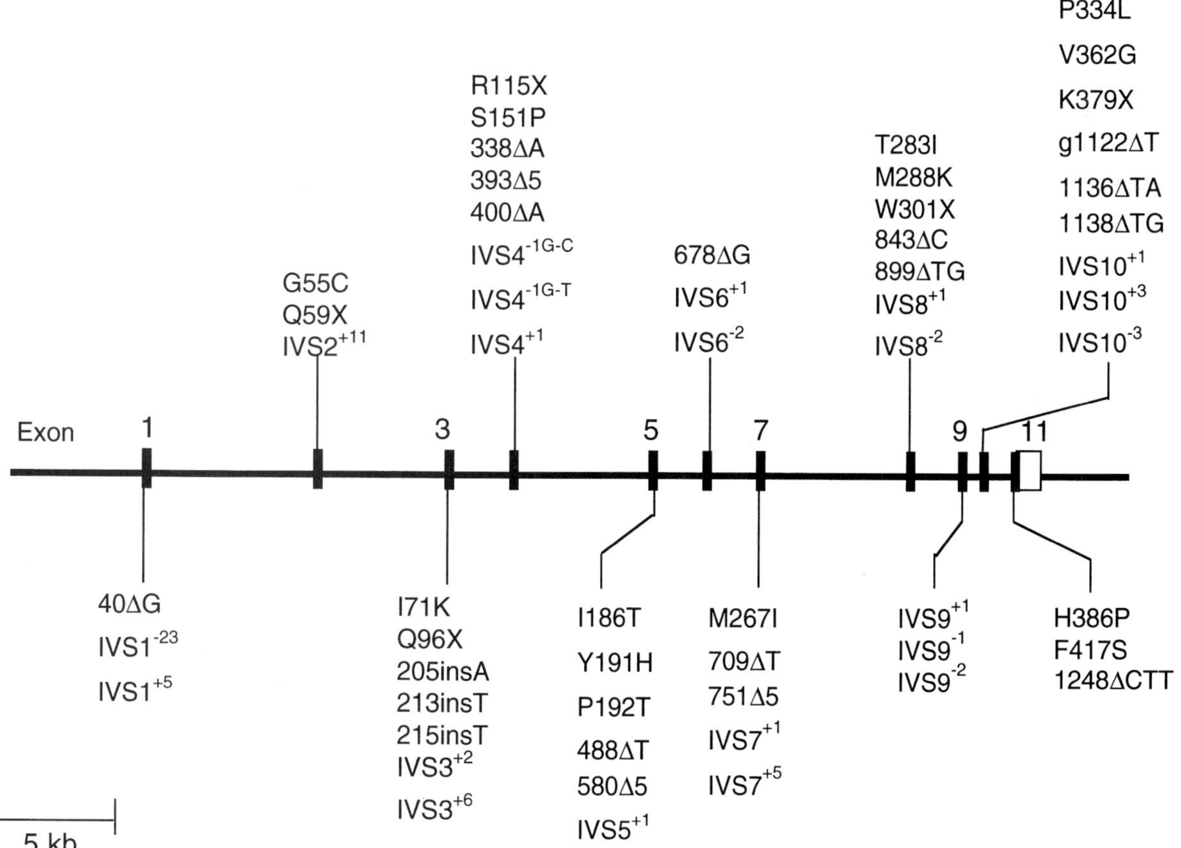

Fig. 124-29 **The human ferrochelatase gene showing locations of mutations causing EPP. (*Courtesy of Dr. K. H. Astrin.*)**

identified. Haplotype analysis was not performed to determine whether these mutations arose in common founders, as might be expected. One possible explanation for the high frequency of exon skipping in other studies is that many mutations were detected in RT-PCR products in which deletions are easily recognizable.[900]

The finding that EPP patients have only 10 to 25 percent of normal ferrochelatase activity has presented a dilemma because the disorder is an autosomal dominant disease. Initial explanations revolved around the concept that the enzyme was a dimer, as recently proven by radiation inactivation studies[901] and more recently by crystallography of the purified human enzyme.[891] If one subunit of a dimer is stable and defective, it may render the dimer nonfunctional. In this case, only dimers composed of two normal subunits would be functional and thereby account for the finding of about 25 percent of normal activity in EPP. However, arguing against this concept is the fact that most identified mutations predict little or no mRNA (due to frameshift, splicing, or nonsense mutations). In addition, mutations that lead to unstable subunits would not interact with the normal enzyme polypeptide, so that only normal subunits would dimerize, resulting in 50 percent of normal activity.

The recent characterization of mutations causing EPP has revealed only one ferrochelatase lesion in most affected families. However, there are notable exceptions.[900,902] Thus, two possible explanations for low ferrochelatase activity in EPP patients have been advanced. In 1996, Gouya et al. identified an EPP family with a normal coding sequence ferrochelatase allele that was expressed at a lower than normal level.[903] Recent studies showed five additional EPP families with a normal low-expressed allele as well as a mutant allele.[904] The low expression normal allele, which had a particular 5′ haplotype (−251A/G, IVS1-23C/T, IVS2μsa-t:An, 798G/C, and 1520C/T), was present in about 10 percent of the Caucasian population. The sequence variation that makes up the haplotype was not believed to be the cause of the lowered expression of the allele. Thus, inheritance of a ferrochelatase mutation in *cis* and the low-expression allele in *trans* could provide an explanation for the low ferrochelatase activity and clinical expression of the disease. This 5′ intragenic haplotype may be predictive of clinical expression among family members who also inherit a ferrochelatase mutation.

The finding that heterozygous knockout mice with ferrochelatase deficiency have about 35 percent residual activity in their tissues, rather than 50 percent, suggests that this model partly mimics the human disease.[873,905] However, the mechanism responsible for the decreased activity is unknown.

Recombinant human ferrochelatase mutant cDNAs that had been engineered to have individual exon deletions of exons 3 through 11 were shown to produce truncated polypeptides lacking significant enzyme activity when expressed in *E. coli*. All these mutants, with the exception of F417S, did not contain the [2Fe-2S] cluster.[906]

Limited information with respect to genotype/phenotype correlations suggests little correlation between the different mutations and the erythrocyte protoporphyrin levels, or between the level of ferrochelatase activity and disease severity. For example, the same mutation found among four unrelated Swiss patients (Q59X) was associated with symptoms ranging from mild photosensitivity to terminal liver failure.[873] However, all EPP patients with liver failure (i.e., the most severe phenotype) had either splice site, insertion, deletion, or nonsense mutations.[873,907] Clearly, genetic modifiers contribute to the variable expression of EPP and environmental factors may influence the development over time of liver failure.

Haplotype analysis using microsatellite markers flanking the ferrochelatase gene was performed in American families with forbears from several European countries who share recurrent mutations ($IVS1^{+5}$ and $IVS7^{+5}$). These studies revealed that these mutations largely represent hotspot mutations for EPP. However, some unrelated families with the same ferrochelatase lesions were found to share the same haplotypes, indicating that there are wide dispersions of ancestral mutant alleles among European populations.[908]

Animal Models. Bovine EPP is an autosomal recessive disease that results from a point mutation that causes a minor to moderate change in enzyme structure.[909,910] A viable autosomal recessive form of EPP has also been identified in the mouse and is due to a specific ferrochelatase mutation (M98K).[905,911] Expression of the murine M98K ferrochelatase cDNA protein in *E. coli* resulted in an enzyme protein with markedly deficient activity. The M98K mutation had a very significant effect in the BALB/c strain with rapid development of liver failure,[905] while it resulted only in a mild disease in the C57BL/6 strain (JC Deybach, unpublished data quoted from reference 873).

Pathophysiology

Bone marrow reticulocytes are thought to be the primary source of the excess protoporphyrin that accumulates in EPP and is excreted in bile and feces. Bone marrow fluorescence is almost entirely in reticulocytes rather than nucleated erythroid cells in this disease, because during erythroid differentiation protoporphyrin accumulation begins just before the loss of cell nuclei.[859,912,913] At times, the liver may be an important source of excess protoporphyrin,[859,861,912–915] but measuring its contribution relative to that of the erythron has not been possible.[914]

Most of the excess protoporphyrin in circulating erythrocytes is found in a small percentage of cells, and the rate of protoporphyrin leakage from these cells is proportional to their protoporphyrin content.[916] Erythrocyte protoporphyrin in EPP is free and not complexed with zinc, unlike that in other porphyrias and conditions associated with increased erythrocyte protoporphyrin content. The content of free protoporphyrin in these cells declines much more rapidly with red cell age than it does in conditions in which erythrocyte zinc protoporphyrin is increased.[912,913] In lead poisoning and iron deficiency, the excess erythrocyte zinc protoporphyrin is bound to hemoglobin and persists in the red cell as long as it circulates, whereas the free protoporphyrin in EPP binds less readily to hemoglobin and diffuses more rapidly into the plasma. Moreover, ultraviolet light may cause free protoporphyrin to photodamage its hemoglobin-binding site and thus be released from the red cell even without disruption of the red cell membrane. In this manner, free protoporphyrin may then diffuse into the plasma, where it is bound to albumin.[917,918] This light-mediated mechanism for the release of free protoporphyrin from hemoglobin in EPP may be important because binding of excess free protoporphyrin to hemoglobin is usually greater than binding to plasma proteins. The capacity of the liver to take up and excrete protoporphyrin into bile may also influence the flux of protoporphyrin from erythroid cells to the plasma in this disease.[851] Hepatocellular uptake of protoporphyrin from plasma is favored by fatty acid binding protein (Z protein) in hepatocytes, which binds protoporphyrin with high affinity and favors hepatocellular uptake of protoporphyrin from plasma.[919]

The skin of patients with EPP is maximally sensitive to light near 400 nm, which corresponds to the so-called Soret band (the narrow peak absorption maximum that is characteristic for protoporphyrin and other porphyrins).[849] When porphyrins absorb light they enter an excited energy state. This energy is released as fluorescence and by formation of singlet oxygen and other oxygen radicals that can produce tissue damage. This may involve lipid peroxidation, oxidation of amino acids, and cross-linking of proteins in cell membranes.[920–922] Photoactivation of the complement system and release of histamine, kinins, and chemotactic factors may mediate skin damage.[923] Histologic changes occur predominantly in the upper dermis and include deposition of amorphous material containing immunoglobulin, complement components, glycoproteins, acid glycosaminoglycans, and lipids around blood vessels.[565,924–927] The histologic changes of the skin in EPP are not specific and may resemble those in PCT. Damage to capillary endothelial cells in the upper dermis has been demonstrated immediately after light exposure in this disease.[928]

As already noted, patients with EPP seem predisposed to develop gallstones that are fluorescent and contain large quantities of protoporphyrin. This and other hepatobiliary complications relate to uptake and excretion of protoporphyrin by the liver. This dicarboxyl porphyrin is not soluble in aqueous solution and is therefore not excreted in urine.

Long-term observations of patients with protoporphyria generally show little change in protoporphyrin levels in erythrocytes, plasma, and feces. On the other hand, severe hepatic complications, when they do occur, often follow increasing accumulation of protoporphyrin in erythrocytes, plasma, and liver. Iron deficiency and factors that impair liver function sometimes contribute.[868,869] Enterohepatic circulation of protoporphyrin may favor its return and retention in the liver, especially when liver function is impaired. Liver damage probably results at least in part from protoporphyrin accumulation itself, as this porphyrin is insoluble, tends to form crystalline structures in liver cells, can impair mitochondrial functions in liver cells, and can decrease hepatic bile formation and flow.[865,929,930] In one patient, hepatic complications and hemolysis were both considerably improved by splenectomy,[931] which suggested that the bone marrow had been the major source of excess protoporphyrin.

Diagnosis

While an increased erythrocyte protoporphyrin concentration is the hallmark of this disease, it is not a specific finding. Erythrocyte protoporphyrin concentrations are increased in many other conditions such as lead poisoning, iron deficiency, anemia of chronic disease,[932] hemolytic disorders[410] and in all homozygous forms of porphyria, and may be somewhat increased in AIP and other acute porphyrias. The increased protoporphyrin in all these conditions, other than EPP, is complexed with zinc. However, many assays for erythrocyte protoporphyrin or "free erythrocyte protoporphyrin" measure both zinc and free protoporphyrin, and assays that specifically measure true "free" erythrocyte protoporphyrin are not widely available. Free protoporphyrin in EPP can be differentiated from zinc protoporphyrin in other disorders by ethanol extraction or HPLC, which is important in confirming a diagnosis of EPP.[779]

Plasma porphyrins are seldom substantially increased in conditions other than porphyrias with cutaneous manifestations. Therefore, a normal plasma porphyrin in a patient with an increased erythrocyte protoporphyrin should exclude EPP as well as other cutaneous porphyrias. However, there is a greater chance of a falsely negative plasma porphyrin result in EPP than in other cutaneous porphyrias, because protoporphyrin in plasma of patients with EPP is particularly subject to photodegradation during the processing of the sample unless great care is taken to avoid exposure of the sample to sunlight or fluorescent lighting.[933] As already noted, urinary porphyrin and porphyrin precursor concentrations are normal in EPP. Protoporphyrin concentrations are increased in bile and feces in EPP, which help to confirm the diagnosis.

Hepatic complications of EPP are difficult to predict by laboratory tests, but may be preceded by increased photosensitivity and by increasing erythrocyte and plasma protoporphyrin levels, abnormal liver function tests, and marked deposition of protoporphyrin in liver cells and bile canaliculi. When hepatic function becomes impaired in EPP, this can contribute to further retention of protoporphyrin in the liver. An increasing ratio of erythrocyte to fecal protoporphyrin and an increasing ratio of biliary protoporphyrin to biliary bile acids also may suggest impending hepatic complications.[865,934,935]

Molecular Diagnosis. The definitive diagnosis of EPP can be made by determining the specific mutation, after results of erythrocyte and plasma porphyrin measurements are compatible with the diagnosis of EPP. Identification of the specific mutation in each family permits the facile diagnosis of other relatives who carry the same mutation. Several neutral polymorphisms in the ferrochelatase gene have been identified that may be useful for screening families in which the specific disease-causing mutation has not been identified. Examples of exonic polymorphisms, with their frequencies shown in parentheses, include 287A/G (9/91), 798G/C (70/30), and 921A/G (72/28).[873] A useful microsatellite polymorphism has also been identified in intron 2 of the ferrochelatase gene, a dinucleotide repeat $(AT)_7(GT)_5$ $(AT)_3(G\text{-}T)_{12}(AT)_3$.[895] The observed heterozygosity was 0.68 in 126 chromosomes.

Assay. Assays for ferrochelatase are not widely available and have not been extensively evaluated for diagnostic purposes. Ferrochelatase activity has been measured by three different methods.[936] (a) ^{59}Fe is used as a metal substrate, and radioactivity is determined in the purified heme fraction after the reaction. This method is the most sensitive,[936] but is tedious and great care must be taken to ascertain the purity and the complete recovery of the radioactive heme product. (b) Formation of heme is determined by the pyridine hemochromogen assay.[38,876] This method gives good results, but has a low sensitivity. Greater sensitivity has been reported using mesoporphyrin, rather than protoporphyrin as substrate.[937] The enzyme activity determined with one type of porphyrin or metal substrate may differ from that determined with another substrate.[938] (c) Disappearance of the porphyrin substrate during the incubation is determined as a measure of ferrochelatase activity. Although this is a simple assay, loss of porphyrin substrate may also occur by reactions other than ferrochelatase, such as photocatalyzed destruction. Moreover, sufficient substrate concentration must be maintained to assure a linear rate of reaction (>90 percent of the substrate should remain at the end of incubation). This makes the porphyrin disappearance assay insensitive.

Treatment

Oral administration of β-carotene was first reported to be useful for treating EPP in 1970.[531,939] Tolerance to sunlight improves in most patients treated with β-carotene, sometimes considerably. Clinical improvement and greater tolerance of graded exposures to long-wave ultraviolet light has been substantiated in large series of patients.[940,941] Improvement is usually maximal 1 to 3 months after initiation of treatment. β-Carotene doses of 120 to 180 mg daily in adults are usually required to maintain serum carotene levels in the recommended range of 600 to 800 mg/dl, but doses up to 300 mg daily may be needed. Better tolerance and longer exposure to sunlight can result in suntanning, which may provide further protection.[531] When pure preparations of β-carotene (e.g., Lumitene, Tishcon) have been used, no side effects other than a mild, dose-related skin discoloration due to carotenemia have been noted.[940] The mechanism of action of β-carotene is not fully established but may involve quenching of singlet oxygen or free radicals. The drug appears less effective in other forms of porphyria associated with photosensitivity, such as CEP and PCT.[531] The potential value of oral cysteine, which like β-carotene may quench excited oxygen species, is under investigation.[942]

Topical dihydroxyacetone and lawsone (naphthoquinone) can darken the skin, thereby partially blocking exposure of the dermis to light and being of some benefit in EPP.[850,943] Subjective improvement has been noted after narrow-band UV-B phototherapy.[944] Cholestyramine, which may interrupt the enterohepatic circulation of protoporphyrin and promote its fecal excretion, has been reported to reduce liver protoporphyrin and improve cutaneous symptoms in some protoporphyria patients.[865,945] Oral bile acid supplementation was beneficial in some animal models of EPP,[946] and may be of some value in the early stages of protoporphyric liver disease.[947] Splenectomy may be beneficial when EPP is complicated by secondary hypersplenism. Caloric restriction and drugs or hormone preparations that impair hepatic excretory function should be avoided, and iron deficiency should be corrected if present.[948,949]

Treatment of hepatic complications must be individualized and the results are unpredictable. Resolution of hepatic complications may occur spontaneously, especially if another reversible cause of liver dysfunction, such as viral hepatitis or alcohol, is contributing.[868,869] Cholestyramine and other porphyrin absorbents such as activated charcoal and perhaps ursodeoxycholic acid should be considered in this situation.[947,950] Other therapeutic options include erythrocyte transfusions, exchange transfusion, and intravenous heme to suppress erythroid and hepatic protoporphyrin production.[951,952] Although liver transplantation can be beneficial,[934] the new liver is susceptible to protoporphyrin-induced damage.[953,954] Unexplained increases in photosensitivity and the development of a motor neuropathy have been observed in some EPP patients with liver failure after they were transfused with blood[955] or received liver transplants.[855,956] This neuropathy is very similar to that which occurs in the acute porphyrias, and is potentially reversible.[957]

A patient who underwent bone marrow transplantation for acute myelocytic leukemia experienced remission of EPP with marked decreases in porphyrin levels.[958] This patient had two different ferrochelatase mutations. After transplant, the disease in the recipient followed the course of the donor, who was a sib with one ferrochelatase mutation and subclinical EPP. This case indicates that bone marrow genotype and not other tissues (e.g., liver) is the primary determinant of EPP severity. Thus, if a sib donor is considered for bone marrow transplantation in an EPP patient, both the donor and recipient should be screened for ferrochelatase mutations by molecular methods.[958]

DUAL PORPHYRIA

Patients with two different porphyrias are classified as having "dual porphyria." For example, kindreds with individuals having both VP and familial PCT have been described.[794,959] Patients with deficiencies of both PBGD and UROD may develop symptoms of AIP, PCT, or both.[960] An infant with severe porphyria was found to have inherited CPO deficiency from one parent and UROS deficiency from both parents.[961] Coexistence of UROS and UROD deficiencies has also been described in a patient with features of an erythropoietic porphyria.[962] A family with deficiencies of both PBGD and CPO has also been described.[963]

PORPHYRIA DUE TO TUMORS

Porphyria is a very rare complication of neoplasms, especially hepatocellular tumors, and the porphyria can be regarded as a paraneoplastic condition if the excess porphyrins are shown to originate in the tumor. The porphyrin excretion patterns in such cases have not been uniform, suggesting that the tumors did not all have the same metabolic defect.[964] Heme biosynthetic pathway enzymes have not been studied in these cases. Hepatocellular carcinoma is a recognized complication of PCT and the acute hepatic porphyrias (AIP, HCP, and VP, see earlier discussions). In these instances, the tumors usually do not contain large amounts of porphyrins.

ACKNOWLEDGMENTS

This work was supported in part by grants to KEA from the FDA (FD-R-001459), the American Porphyria Foundation, and an NIH grant for the University of Texas Medical Center, Galveston, General Clinical Research Center (5 M01 RR00073); by a grant to DFB from NIH (5 R01 DK40895); by grants to SS from NIH (5 R01 DK37890), the American Porphyria Foundation, and the Chugai Fund for Molecular Hematology; and by grants to RJD from the NIH, including a research grant (5 R01 DK26824), a grant (5 M01 RR00071) for the Mount Sinai General Clinical Research Center, and a grant (5 P30 HD28822) for the Mount Sinai Child Health Research Center. We also thank Dr. Kenneth H. Astrin for critical review and assistance in preparation of this manuscript and the indicated figures.

REFERENCES

1. Fischer H, Orth H: *Die Chemie des Pyrrols (reprint).* (Leibzig, Akademische Verlag Gueleschaft m.b.h, 1934.) New York, Johnson, p 1, 1968.
2. IUPAC-IUB Joint Commission on Biochemical Nomenclature (JCBN): Nomenclature of tetrapyrroles: Recommendations 1978. *Eur J Biochem* **108**:1, 1980.
3. Kappas A, Sassa S, Galbraith RA, Nordmann Y: The porphyrias, in Scriver CR, Beaudet AL, Sly WS, Valle D (eds.): *The Metabolic Basis of Inherited Disease*. New York, McGraw-Hill, 1995, p 1305.
4. Sassa S, Kappas A: Genetic, metabolic, and biochemical aspects of the porphyrias, in Harris H, Hirschhorn K (eds.): *Advances in Human Genetics*. New York, Plenum, 1981, p 121.
5. Berk PD, Rodkey FL, Blaschke TF, Collison HA, Waggoner JG: Comparison of plasma bilirubin turnover and carbon monoxide production in man. *J Lab Clin Med* **83**:29, 1974.
6. Granick S, Sassa S: δ-Aminolevulinic acid synthetase and the control of heme and chlorophyll synthesis, in Vogel HJ (ed.): *Metabolic Regulation*. New York, Academic Press, 1971, p 77.
7. Granick S: The induction in vitro of the synthesis of δ-aminolevulinic acid synthetase in chemical porphyria: A response to certain drugs, sex hormones, and foreign chemicals. *J Biol Chem* **241**:359, 1966.
8. Granick S, Urata G: Increase in activity of δ-aminolevulinic acid synthetase in liver mitochondria induced by feeding of 3,5-dicarbethoxy-1,4-dihydrocollidine. *J Biol Chem* **238**:821, 1963.
9. Hutton JJ, Gross SR: Chemical induction of hepatic porphyria in inbred strains of mice. *Arch Biochem Biophys* **141**:284, 1970.
10. Jones MS, Jones OTG: The structural organization of haem synthesis in rat liver mitochondria. *Biochem J* **113**:507, 1969.
11. Bishop DF, Desnick RJ: Assays of the heme biosynthetic enzymes. Preface. *Enzyme* **28**:91, 1982.
12. Tschudy DP, Marver HS, Collins A: A model for calculating messenger RNA half-life: Short-lived messenger RNA in the induction of mammalian δ-aminolevulinic acid synthetase. *Biochem Biophys Res Commun* **21**:480, 1965.
13. Gayathri AK, Rao MR, Padmanaban G: Studies on the induction of δ-aminolevulinic acid synthetase in mouse liver. *Arch Biochem Biophys* **155**:299, 1973.
14. Sassa S, Granick S: Induction of δ-aminolevulinic acid synthetase in chick embryo liver cells in culture. *Proc Natl Acad Sci U S A* **67**:517, 1970.
15. Anderson KE, Drummond GS, Freddara U, Sardana MK, Sassa S: Porphyrogenic effects and induction of heme oxygenase in vivo by δ-aminolevulinic acid. *Biochim Biophys Acta* **676**:289, 1981.
16. Song CS, Moses HL, Rosenthal AS, Gelb NA, Kappas A: The influence of postnatal development on drug-induced hepatic porphyria and the synthesis of cytochrome P-450: A biochemical and morphological study. *J Exp Med* **134**:1349, 1971.
17. Bissell DM, Hammaker LE: Cytochrome P-450 heme and the regulation of hepatic heme oxygenase activity. *Arch Biochem Biophys* **176**:91, 1976.
18. Bissell DM, Hammaker LE: Cytochrome p-450 heme and the regulation of delta-aminolevulinic acid synthetase in the liver. *Arch Biochem Biophys* **176**:103, 1976.
19. Aoki Y, Wada O, Urata G, Takaku F, Nakao K: Purification and some properties of δ-aminolevulinate (ALA) synthetase in rabbit reticulocytes. *Biochem Biophys Res Comm* **42**:568, 1971.
20. Granick S, Sinclair P, Sassa S, Grieninger G: Effects by heme, insulin, and serum albumin on heme and protein synthesis in chick embryo liver cells cultured in a chemically defined medium, and a spectrofluorometric assay for porphyrin composition. *J Biol Chem* **250**:9215, 1975.
21. Sassa S, Bradlow HL, Kappas A: Steroid induction of δ-aminolevulinic acid synthase and porphyrins in liver. Structure-activity studies on the permissive effects of hormones on the induction process. *J Biol Chem* **254**:10011, 1979.
22. Sinclair PR, Granick S: The transport of hemin and protoporphyrin across the plasma membrane of chick embryo liver cells in culture. *Ann Clin Res* **8 (Suppl 17)**:250, 1976.

23. Srivastava G, Brooker JD, May BK, Elliott WH: Haem control in experimental porphyria: The effect of haemin on the induction of δ-aminolevulinate synthase in isolated chick-embryo liver cells. *Biochem J* **188**:781, 1980.
24. Wolfson SJ, Bartczak A, Bloomer JR: Effect of endogenous heme generation of δ-aminolevulinic acid synthase activity in rat liver mitochondria. *J Biol Chem* **254**:3543, 1979.
25. Romslo I, Husby P: Iron, porphyrin and heme transport in mitochondria. *Int J Biochem* **12**:709, 1980.
26. Whiting MJ: Synthesis of δ-aminolaevulinate synthase by isolated liver polyribosomes. *Biochem J* **158**:391, 1976.
27. Tyrrell DL, Marks GS: Drug-induced porphyrin biosynthesis. V. Effect of protohemin on the transcriptional and post-transcriptional phases of δ-aminolevulinic acid synthetase induction. *Biochem Pharmacol* **21**:2077, 1972.
28. Lathrop JT, Timko MP: Regulation by heme of mitochondrial protein transport through a conserved amino acid motif. *Science* **259**:522, 1993.
29. Munakata H, Furuyama K, Hayashi N: Regulation by the heme regulatory motif of mitochondrial import of the non-specific and erythroid-specific 5-aminolevulinate synthase [Abstract]. *J Biochem (Tokyo)* **68**:792, 1996.
30. Yannoni CZ, Robinson SH: Early labeled haem in erythroid and hepatic cells. *Nature* **258**:330, 1975.
31. Grandchamp B, Bissell DM, Licko V, Schmid R: Formation and disposition of newly synthesized heme in adult rat hepatocytes in primary culture. *J Biol Chem* **256**:11677, 1981.
32. Badawy AA: Tryptophan pyrrolase, the regulatory free haem and hepatic porphyrias. Early depletion of haem by clinical and experimental exacerbators of porphyria. *Biochem J* **172**:487, 1978.
33. De Matteis F, Abbritti G, Gibbs AH: Decreased liver activity of porphyrin-metal chelatase in hepatic porphyria caused by 3,5-diethoxycarbonyl-1,4-dihydrocollidine. Studies in rats and mice. *Biochem J* **134**:717, 1973.
34. De Matteis F, Gibbs A: Stimulation of liver 5-aminolaevulinate synthetase by drugs and its relevance to drug-induced accumulation of cytochrome P-450. Studies with phenylbutazone and 3,5-diethoxycarbonyl- 1,4-dihydrocollidine. *Biochem J* **126**:1149, 1972.
35. Whiting MJ, Granick S: δ-Aminolevulinic acid synthase from chick embryo liver mitochondria I. Purification and some properties. *J Biol Chem* **251**:1340, 1976.
36. Sinclair PR, Granick S: Heme control on the synthesis of delta-aminolevulinic acid synthetase in cultured chick embryo liver cells. *Ann N Y Acad Sci* **244**:509, 1975.
37. Sassa S, Kappas A: Induction of δ-aminolevulinate synthase and porphyrins in cultured liver cells maintained in chemically defined medium. Permissive effects of hormones on induction process. *J Biol Chem* **252**:2428, 1977.
38. Rifkind AB: Maintenance of microsomal hemoprotein concentrations following inhibition of ferrochelatase activity by 3,5-diethoxycarbonyl-1,4-dihydrocollidine in chick embryo liver. *J Biol Chem* **254**:4636, 1979.
39. Anderson KE: Effects of antihypertensive drugs on hepatic heme biosynthesis, and evaluation of ferrochelatase inhibitors to simplify testing of drugs for heme pathway induction. *Biochim Biophys Acta* **543**:313, 1978.
40. Maines MD, Kappas A: Cobalt induction of hepatic heme oxygenase; with evidence that cytochrome P-450 is not essential for this enzyme activity. *Proc Natl Acad Sci U S A* **71**:4293, 1974.
41. Maines MD, Kappas A: Cobalt stimulation of heme degradation in the liver. Dissociation of microsomal oxidation of heme from cytochrome P-450. *J Biol Chem* **250**:4171, 1975.
42. Maines MD, Kappas A: Studies on the mechanism of induction of haem oxygenase by cobalt and other metal ions. *Biochem J* **154**:125, 1976.
43. Maines MD, Kappas A: Metals as regulators of heme metabolism. *Science* **198**:1215, 1977.
44. Drummond GS, Kappas A: Metal ion interactions in the control of haem oxygenase induction in liver and kidney. *Biochem J* **192**:637, 1980.
45. Levin W, Sernatinger E, Jacobson M, Kuntzman R: Destruction of cytochrome P 450 by secobarbital and other barbiturates containing allyl groups. *Science* **176**:1341, 1972.
46. Rosenberg DW, Drummond GS, Cornish HC, Kappas A: Prolonged induction of hepatic haem oxygenase and decreases in cytochrome P-450 content by organotin compounds. *Biochem J* **190**:465, 1980.
47. Thaler MM, Dawber NH: Stimulation of bilirubin formation in liver of newborn rats by fasting and glucagon. *Gastroenterology* **72**:312, 1977.
48. Welland FH, Hellman ES, Gaddis EM, Collins A, Hunter GWJ, Tschudy DP: Factors affecting the excretion of porphyrin precursors by patients with acute intermittent porphyria. 1. The effects of diet. *Metabolism* **13**:232, 1964.
49. Felsher BF, Redeker AG: Acute intermittent porphyria: Effect of diet and griseofulvin. *Medicine* **46**:213, 1967.
50. Tschudy DP, Welland FH, Collins A, Hunter GWJ: The effect of carbohydrate feeding on the induction of δ-aminolevulinic acid synthetase. *Metabolism* **13**:396, 1964.
51. Fujita H, Yamamoto M, Yamagami T, Hayashi N, Sassa S: Erythroleukemia differentiation. Distinctive responses of the erythroid-specific and the nonspecific δ-aminolevulinate synthase mRNA. *J Biol Chem* **266**:17494, 1991.
52. Meguro K, Igarashi K, Yamamoto M, Fujita H, Sassa S: The role of the erythroid-specific delta-aminolevulinate synthase gene expression in erythroid heme synthesis. *Blood* **86**:940, 1995.
53. Harigae H, Suwabe N, Weinstock PH, Nagai M, Fujita H, Yamamoto M, Sassa S: Deficient heme and globin synthesis in embryonic stem cells lacking the erythroid-specific delta-aminolevulinate synthase gene. *Blood* **91**:798, 1998.
54. Sassa S, Granick JL, Eisen H, Ostertag W: Regulation of heme synthesis in mouse Friend virus-transformed cells in culture, in Murphy MJ Jr (ed.): *In Vitro Aspects of Erythropoiesis*. New York, Springer-Verlag, 1978, p 135.
55. Eisen H, Keppel-Ballinet F, Georgopoulos CP, Sassa S, Granick JL, Pragnell I, Ostertag W: Biochemical and genetic analysis of erythroid differentiation in Friend virus-transformed murine erythroleukemia cells, in Clarkson B, Marks PA, Till J (eds.): *Cold Spring Harbor Conference on Differentiation of Normal and Neoplasmic Hematopoietic Cells*. Cold Spring Harbor, Cold Spring Harbor Laboratory, 1978, p 277.
56. Rutherford T, Thompson GG, Moore MR: Heme biosynthesis in Friend erythroleukemia cells: Control by ferrochelatase. *Proc Natl Acad Sci U S A* **76**:833, 1979.
57. Sassa S, Nagai T: The role of heme in gene expression. *Int J Hematol* **63**:167, 1996.
58. Wada O, Sassa S, Takaku F, Yano Y, Urata G, Nakao K: Different responses of the hepatic and erythropoietic δ-aminolevulinic acid synthetase of mice. *Biochim Biophys Acta* **148**:585, 1967.
59. Sassa S: Sequential induction of heme pathway enzymes during erythroid differentiation of mouse Friend leukemia virus-infected cells. *J Exp Med* **143**:305, 1976.
60. Sassa S: Control of heme biosynthesis in erythroid cells, in Rossi GB (ed.): *In vitro and In Vivo Erythropoiesis*. Amsterdam, Elsevier/North-Holland, 1980, p 219.
61. Smith SJ, Cox TM: Translational control of erythroid delta-aminolevulinate synthase in immature human erythroid cells by heme. *Cell Mol Biol (Noisy-le-grand)* **43**:103, 1997.
62. Ross J, Sautner D: Induction of globin mRNA accumulation by hemin in cultured erythroleukemic cells. *Cell* **8**:513, 1976.
63. Dabney BJ, Beaudet AL: Increase in globin chains and globin mRNA in erythroleukemia cells in response to hemin. *Arch Biochem Biophys* **179**:106, 1977.
64. Granick JL, Sassa S: Hemin control of heme biosynthesis in mouse Friend virus-transformed erythroleukemia cells in culture. *J Biol Chem* **253**:5402, 1978.
65. Hoffman R, Ibrahim N, Murnane MJ, Diamond A, Forget BG, Levere RD: Hemin control of heme biosynthesis and catabolism in a human leukemia cell line. *Blood* **56**:567, 1980.
66. Porter PN, Meints RH, Mesner K: Enhancement of erythroid colony growth in culture by hemin. *Exp Hematol* **7**:11, 1979.
67. Melefors O, Goossen B, Johansson HE, Stripecke R, Gray NK, Hentze MW: Translational control of 5-aminolevulinate synthase messenger RNA by iron-responsive elements in erythroid cells. *J Biol Chem* **268**:5974, 1993.
68. Cox TC, Bawden MJ, Martin A, May BK: Human erythroid 5-aminolevulinate synthase: Promoter analysis and identification of an iron-responsive element in the mRNA. *EMBO J* **10**:1891, 1991.
69. Nakao K, Wada O, Takaku F, Sassa S, Yano Y, Urata G: The origin of the increased protoporphyrin in erythrocytes of mice with experimentally induced porphyria. *J Lab Clin Med* **70**:923, 1967.
70. Margolis FL: Regulation of porphyrin biosynthesis in the harderian gland of inbred mouse strains. *Arch Biochem Biophys* **145**:373, 1971.

71. Briggs DW, Condie LW, Sedman RM, Tephly TR: δ-Aminolevulinic acid synthetase in the heart. *J Biol Chem* **251**:4996, 1976.
72. Condie LW, Baron J, Tephly TR: Studies on adrenal δ-aminolevulinic acid synthetase. *Arch Biochem Biophys* **172**:123, 1976.
73. Tofilon PJ, Piper WN: Measurement and regulation of rat testicular δ-aminolevulinic acid synthetase activity. *Arch Biochem Biophys* **201**:104, 1980.
74. Paterniti JR, Simone JJ, Beattie DS: Detection and regulation of δ-aminolevulinic acid synthetase in the rat brain. *Arch Biochem Biophys* **189**:86, 1978.
75. Sassa S, Levere RD, Solish G, Kappas A: Studies on the porphyrin-heme biosynthetic pathway in cultured human amniotic cells. *J Clin Invest* **53**:70a, 1974.
76. Nagai M, Nagai T, Yamamoto M, Goto K, Bishop TR, Hayashi N, Kondo H, Seyama Y, Kano K, Fujita H, Sassa S: Novel regulation of delta-aminolevulinate synthase in the rat harderian gland. *Biochem Pharmacol* **53**:643, 1997.
77. Woods JS, Murthy VV: δ-Aminolevulic acid synthetase from fetal rat liver: Studies on the partially purified enzyme. *Mol Pharmacol* **11**:70, 1974.
78. Bishop DF, Kitchen H, Wood WA: Evidence for erythroid and nonerythroid forms of δ-aminolevulinate synthetase. *Arch Biochem Biophys* **206**:380, 1981.
79. Meyer UA: Intermittent acute porphyria. Clinical and biochemical studies of disordered heme biosynthesis. *Enzyme* **16**:334, 1973.
80. Bonkowsky HL, Tschudy DP, Weinbach EC, Ebert PS, Doherty JM: Porphyrin synthesis and mitochondrial respiration in acute intermittent porphyria: studies using cultured human fibroblasts. *J Lab Clin Med* 93, 1975.
81. Sassa S, Zalar GL, Kappas A: Studies in porphyria VII. Induction of uroporphyrinogen-I synthase and expression of the gene defect of acute intermittent porphyria in mitogen-stimulated human lymphocytes. *J Clin Invest* **61**:499, 1978.
82. Watson CJ: Hematin and porphyria. *N Engl J Med* **293**:605, 1975.
83. Cohn JA, Alvares AP, Kappas A: On the occurrence of cytochrome P-450 and aryl hydrocarbon hydroxylase activity in rat brain. *J Exp Med* **145**:1607, 1977.
84. Whetsell WO Jr, Sassa S, Bickers D, Kappas A: Studies on porphyrin-heme biosynthesis in organotypic cultures of chick dorsal root ganglion I. Observations on neuronal and non-neuronal elements. *J Neuronal Exp Neurology* **37**:497, 1978.
85. Whetsell WOJ, Sassa S, Kappas A: Studies on effects of chronic lead exposure upon porphyrin biosynthesis and myelin in cultures of mouse dorsal root ganglia (DRG). *J Neuropathol Exp Neurol* **38**:348, 1979.
86. Sassa S, Whetsell WO Jr, Kappas A: Studies on porphyrin-heme biosynthesis in organotypic cultures of chick dorsal root ganglia II. The effect of lead. *Environ Res* **19**:415, 1979.
87. Whetsell WO Jr, Kappas A: Protective effect of exogenous heme against lead toxicity in organotypic cultures of mouse dorsal root ganglia (DRG): Electron microscopic observations. *J Neuropathol Exp Neurol* **40**:334, 1981.
88. Cooley TB: A severe type of hereditary anemia with elliptocytosis. Interesting sequence of splenectomy. *Am J Med Sci* **209**:561, 1945.
89. Cotter PD, May A, Fitzsimons EJ, Houston T, Woodcock B, Al-Sabah AI, Wong L, Bishop DF: Late onset X-linked sideroblastic anemia: Missense mutations in the erythroid δ-aminolevulinate synthase (ALAS2) gene in two pyridoxine-responsive patients initially diagnosed with acquired refractory sideroblastic anemia and ringed sideroblasts (RARS). *J Clin Invest* **96**:2090, 1995.
90. Raskind WH, Wijsman E, Pagon RA, Cox TC, Bawden MJ, May BK, Bird TD: X-linked sideroblastic anemia and ataxia: Linkage to phosphoglycerate kinase at Xq13. *Am J Hum Genet* **48**:335, 1991.
91. Allikmets R, Raskind WH, Hutchinson A, Schueck ND, Dean M, Koeller DM: Mutation of a putative mitochondrial iron transporter gene (ABC7) in X-linked sideroblastic anemia and ataxia (XLSA/A). *Hum Mol Genet* **8**:743, 1999.
92. Cotter PD, Baumann M, Bishop DF: Enzymatic defect in X-linked sideroblastic anemia: Molecular evidence for erythroid δ-aminolevulinate synthase deficiency. *Proc Natl Acad Sci U S A* **89**:4028, 1992.
93. May A, Bishop D: The molecular biology and pyridoxine responsiveness of X-linked sideroblastic anaemia. *Haematologica* **83**:56, 1998.
94. Cotter PD, May A, Li L, Al-Sabah AI, Fitzsimons EJ, Cazzola M, Bishop DF: Four new mutations in the erythroid-specific 5-aminolevulinate synthase (ALAS2) gene causing X-linked sideroblastic anemia: Increased pyridoxine responsiveness after removal of iron overload by phlebotomy and coinheritance of hereditary hemochromatosis. *Blood* **93**:1757, 1999.
95. Cotter PD, Rucknagel DL, Bishop DF: X-linked sideroblastic anemia: Identification of the mutation in the erythroid-specific δ-aminolevulinate synthase gene (ALAS2) in the original family described by Cooley. *Blood* **84**:3915, 1994.
96. Cox TC, Bottomley SS, Wiley JS, Bawden MJ, Matthews CS, May BK: X-linked pyridoxine-responsive sideroblastic anemia due to a Thr^{388}-to-Ser substitution in erythroid 5-aminolevulinic synthase. *N Engl J Med* **330**:675, 1994.
97. Prades E, Chambon C, Dailey TA, Dailey HA, Briere J, Grandchamp B: A new mutation of the ALAS2 gene in a large family with X-linked sideroblastic anemia. *Hum Genet* **95**:424, 1995.
98. Murakami R, Takumi T, Gouji J, Nakamura H, Kondou M: Sideroblastic anemia showing unique response to pyridoxine. *Am J Pediatr Hematol Oncol* **13**:345, 1991.
99. Edgar AJ, Losowsky MS, Noble JS, Wickramasinghe SN: Identification of an arginine452 to histidine substitution in the erythroid 5-aminolaevulinate synthetase gene in a large pedigree with X-linked hereditary sideroblastic anaemia. *Eur J Haematol* **58**:1, 1997.
100. Edgar AJ, Vidyatilake HM, Wickramasinghe SN: X-linked sideroblastic anaemia due to a mutation in the erythroid 5-aminolaevulinate synthase gene leading to an arginine170 to leucine substitution. *Eur J Haematol* **61**:55, 1998.
101. Ferreira GC, Neame PJ, Dailey HA: Heme biosynthesis in mammalian systems: Evidence of a Schiff base linkage between the pyridoxal 5′-phosphate cofactor and a lysine residue in 5-aminolevulinate synthase. *Protein Sci* **2**:1959, 1993.
102. Ferreira GC, Vajapey U, Hafez O, Hunter GA, Barber MJ: Aminolevulinate synthase: Lysine 313 is not essential for binding the pyridoxal phosphate cofactor but is essential for catalysis. *Protein Sci* **4**:1001, 1995.
103. Abboud MM, Jordan PM, Akhtar M: Biosynthesis of 5-aminolevulinic acid: Involvement of a retention-inversion mechanism. *J Chem Soc Chem Commun* **13**:643, 1974.
104. Watanabe N, Hayashi N, Kikuchi G: δ-Aminolevulinate synthase isozymes in the liver and erythroid cells of chicken. *Biochem Biophys Res Comm* **113**:377, 1983.
105. Yamamoto M, Fujita H, Watanabe N, Hayashi N, Kikuchi G: An immunochemical study of delta-aminolevulinate synthase and delta-aminolevulinate dehydratase in liver and erythroid cells of rat. *Arch Biochem Biophys* **245**:76, 1986.
106. Fernandez J, Gonzalez O, Martin M, Ruiz AM: Erythroid 5-aminolevulinate synthetase from trout (*Salmo gairdneri* R.). *Comp Biochem Physiol [B]* **85**:675, 1986.
107. Riddle RD, Yamamoto M, Engel JD: Expression of δ-aminolevulinate synthase in avian cells: Separate genes encode erythroid-specific and nonspecific isozymes. *Proc Natl Acad Sci U S A* **86**:792, 1989.
108. Astrin KH, Desnick RJ, Bishop DF: Assignment of human δ-aminolevulinate synthase (ALAS) to chromosome 3. *Cytogenet Cell Genet* **46**:573, 1987.
109. Bishop DF: Two different genes encode δ-aminolevulinate synthase in humans: Nucleotide sequences of cDNAs for the housekeeping and erythroid genes. *Nucleic Acids Res* **18**:7187, 1990.
110. Bishop DF, Henderson AS, Astrin KH: Human delta-aminolevulinate synthase: Assignment of the housekeeping gene to 3p21 and the erythroid-specific gene to the X chromosome. *Genomics* **7**:207, 1990.
111. Aoki Y: Crystallization and characterization of a new protease in mitochondria of bone marrow cells. *J Biol Chem* **253**:2026, 1978.
112. Volland C, Urban GD: The presequence of yeast 5-aminolevulinate synthase is not required for targeting to mitochondria. *J Biol Chem* **263**:8294, 1988.
113. Srivastava G, Borthwick IA, Maguire DJ, Elferink CJ, Bawden MJ, Mercer JF, May BK: Regulation of 5-aminolevulinate synthase mRNA in different rat tissues. *J Biol Chem* **263**:5202, 1988.
114. Schoenhaut DS, Curtis PJ: Nucleotide sequence of mouse 5-aminolevulinic acid synthase cDNA and expression of its gene in hepatic and erythroid tissues. *Gene* **48**:55, 1986.
115. Munakata H, Yamagami T, Nagai T, Yamamoto M, Hayashi N: Purification and structure of rat erythroid-specific δ-aminolevulinate synthase. *J Biochem Tokyo* **114**:103, 1993.
116. Furuyama K, Fujita H, Nagai T, Yomogida K, Munakata H, Kondo M, Kimura A, Kuramoto A, Hayashi N, Yamamoto M: Pyridoxine refractory X-linked sideroblastic anemia caused by a point mutation in the erythroid 5-aminolevulinate synthase gene. *Blood* **90**:822, 1997.

117. Yamauchi K, Hayashi N, Kikuchi G: Translocation of δ-aminolevulinate synthase from the cytosol to the mitochondria and its regulation by hemin in the rat liver. *J Biol Chem* **255**:1746, 1980.
118. Zhang L, Guarente L: Heme binds to a short sequence that serves a regulatory function in diverse proteins. *EMBO J* **14**:313, 1995.
119. Steiner H, Kispal G, Zollner A, Haid A, Neupert W, Lill R: Heme binding to a conserved Cys-Pro-Val motif is crucial for the catalytic function of mitochondrial heme lyases. *J Biol Chem* **271**:32605, 1996.
120. Ferreira GC, Dailey HA: Expression of mammalian 5-Aminolevulinate synthase in Escherichia Coli: overproduction, purification, and characterization. *J Biol Chem* **268**:584, 1993.
121. Cotter PD, Bishop DF: unpublished.
122. Dailey HA, Dailey TA: Expression and purification of mammalian 5-aminolevulinate synthase. *Methods Enzymol* **281**:336, 1997.
123. Tan D, Ferreira G: Active site of 5-aminolevulinate synthase resides at the subunit interface. Evidence from in vivo heterodimer formation. *Biochemistry* **35**:8934, 1996.
124. Tan D, Harrison T, Hunter GA, Ferreira GC: Role of arginine 439 in substrate binding of 5-aminolevulinate synthase. *Biochemistry* **37**:1478, 1998.
125. Woods JS: Studies on the role of heme in the regulation of δ-aminolevulinic acid synthetase during fetal hepatic development. *Mol Pharmacol* **10**:389, 1973.
126. Ponka P: Tissue-specific regulation of iron metabolism and heme synthesis: Distinct control mechanisms in erythroid cells [see comments]. *Blood* **89**:1, 1997.
127. Trump BF, Berezesky IK, Jiji RM, Mergner WJ, Bulger RE: Energy dispersive x-ray microanalysis of mitochondrial deposits in sideroblastic anemia. *Lab Invest* **39**:375, 1978.
128. Woods JS, Murthy VV: Delta-aminolevulinic acid synthetase from fetal rat liver: studies on the partially purified enzyme. *Mol Pharmacol* **11**:70, 1975.
129. Neuwirt J, Ponka P, Borova J: Evidence for the presence of free and protein-bound nonhemoglobin heme in rabbit reticulocytes. *Biochim Biophys Acta* **264**:235, 1972.
130. Furuyama K, Sassa S: Interaction between succinyl CoA synthetase and the heme biosynthetic enzyme ALAS-E is disrupted in sideroblastic anemia. *J Clin Invest* **105**:757, 2000.
131. Astrin KH, Bishop DF: Assignment of human erythroid δ-aminolevulinate synthase (ALAS2) to the X chromosome. *Cytogenet Cell Genet* **51**:953, 1989.
132. Schoenhaut DS, Curtis PJ: Structure of a mouse erythroid 5-aminolevulinate synthase gene and mapping of erythroid-specific DNAse I hypersensitive sites. *Nucleic Acids Res* **17**:7013, 1989.
133. Dierks P: Molecular biology of eukaryotic 5-aminolevulinate synthase, in Dailey HA (eds.): *Biosynthesis of Heme and Chlorophylls*. New York, McGraw-Hill, 1990, p 201.
134. Cotter PD, Willard HF, Gorski JL, Bishop DF: Assignment of human erythroid δ-aminolevulinate synthase (ALAS2) to a distal subregion of band xp11.21 by PCR analysis of somatic cell hybrids containing X; autosome translocations. *Genomics* **13**:211, 1992.
135. Sutherland GR, Baker E, Callen DF, Hyland VJ, May BK, Bawden MJ, Healy HM, Borthwick IA: 5-Aminolevulinate synthase is at 3p21 and thus not the primary defect in X-linked sideroblastic anemia. *Am J Hum Genet* **43**:331, 1988.
136. Cotter PD, Drabkin HA, Varkony T, Smith DI, Bishop DF: Assignment of the human housekeeping δ-aminolevulinate synthase gene (ALAS1) to chromosome band 3p21.1 by PCR analysis of somatic cell hybrids. *Cytogenet Cell Genet* **69**:207, 1995.
137. Conboy JG, Cox TC, Bottomley SS, Bawden MJ, May BK: Human erythroid 5-aminolevulinate synthase: Gene structure and species-specific differences in alternative RNA splicing. *J Biol Chem* **267**:18753, 1992.
138. Lim KC, Ishihara H, Riddle RD, Yang Z, Andrews N, Yamamoto M, Engel JD: Structure and regulation of the chicken erythroid delta-aminolevulinate synthase gene. *Nucleic Acids Res* **22**:1226, 1994.
139. Elliott WH, May BK, Bawden MJ, Hansen AJ: Regulation of genes associated with drug metabolism. *Biochem Soc Symp* **55**:13, 1989.
140. Surinya KH, Cox TC, May BK: Identification and characterization of a conserved erythroid-specific enhancer located in intron 8 of the human 5-aminolevulinate synthase 2 gene. *J Biol Chem* **273**:16798, 1998.
141. Jardine PE, Cotter PD, Johnson SA, Fitzsimons EJ, Tyfield L, Lunt PW, Bishop DF: Pyridoxine-refractory congenital sideroblastic anaemia with evidence for autosomal inheritance: Exclusion of linkage to ALAS2 at Xp11.21 by polymorphism analysis. *J Med Genet* **31**:213, 1994.
142. Cox TC, Kozman HM, Raskind WH, May BK, Mulley JC: Identification of a highly polymorphic marker within intron 7 of the ALAS2 gene and suggestion of at least two loci for X-linked sideroblastic anemia. *Hum Mol Genet* **1**:639, 1992.
143. Surinya KH, Cox TC, May B: Transcriptional regulation of the human erythroid 5-aminolevulinase synthase gene. *J Biol Chem* **272**:26585, 1997.
144. Bishop TR, Miller MW, Beall J, Zon LI, Dierks P: Genetic regulation of delta-aminolevulinate dehydratase during erythropoiesis. *Nucleic Acids Res* **24**:2511, 1996.
145. Porcher C, Picat C, Daegelen D, Beaumont C, Grandchamp B: Functional analysis of DNase-I hypersensitive sites at the mouse porphobilinogen deaminase gene locus. Different requirements for position-independent expression from its two promoters. *J Biol Chem* **270**:17368, 1995.
146. Magness ST, Tugores A, Diala ES, Brenner DA: Analysis of the human ferrochelatase promoter in transgenic mice. *Blood* **92**:320, 1998.
147. Walters M, Martin DI: Functional erythroid promoters created by interaction of the transcription factor GATA-1 with CACCC and AP-1/NFE-2 elements. *Proc Natl Acad Sci U S A* **89**:10444, 1992.
148. May BK, Dogra SC, Sadlon TJ, Bhasker CR, Cox TC, Bottomley SS: Molecular regulation of heme biosynthesis in higher vertebrates. *Prog Nucleic Acids Res* **51**:1, 1995.
149. Fujita H, Yamamoto M, Yamagami T, Hayashi N, Bishop TR, Deverneuil H, Yoshinaga T, Shibahara S, Morimoto R, Sassa S: Sequential activation of genes for heme pathway enzymes during erythroid differentiation of mouse Friend virus-transformed erythroleukemia cells. *Biochim Biophys Acta* **1090**:311, 1991.
150. Gardner LC, Smith SJ, Cox TM: Biosynthesis of δ-aminolevulinic acid and the regulation of heme formation by immature erythroid cells in man. *J Biol Chem* **266**:22010, 1991.
151. Bhasker RC, Burgiel G, Neupert B, Emery-Goodman A, Kühn LC, May BK: The putative iron-responsive element in the human erythroid 5-aminolevulinate synthase mRNA mediates translational control. *J Biol Chem* **268**:12699, 1993.
152. Ke Y, Wu J, Leibold EA, Walden WE, Theil EC: Loops and bulge/loops in iron-responsive element isoforms influence iron regulatory protein binding. Fine-tuning of mRNA regulation? *J Biol Chem* **273**:23637, 1998.
153. Guo B, Brown FM, Phillips JD, Yu Y, Leibold EA: Characterization and expression of iron regulatory protein 2 (IRP2). Presence of multiple IRP2 transcripts regulated by intracellular iron levels. *J Biol Chem* **270**:16529, 1995.
154. Harigae H, Furuyama K, Kimura A, Neriishi K, Tahara N, Kondo M, Hayashi N, Yamamoto M, Sassa S, Sasaki T: A novel mutation of the erythroid-specific delta-aminolaevulinate synthase gene in a patient with X-linked sideroblastic anaemia. *Br J Haematol* **106**:175, 1999.
155. Furuyama K, Uno R, Urabe A, Hayashi N, Fujita H, Kondo M, Sassa S, Yamamoto M: R411C mutation of the ALAS2 gene encodes a pyridoxine-responsive enzyme with low activity. *Br J Haematol* **103**:839, 1998.
156. Edgar AJ, Wickramasinghe SN: Hereditary sideroblastic anaemia due to a mutation in exon 10 of the erythroid 5-aminolaevulinae synthase gene. *Br J Haematol* **100**:389, 1998.
157. Harigae H, Furuyama K, Kimura A, Neriishi K, Tahara N, Kondo M, Hayashi N, Yamamoto M, Sassa S, Sasaki T: A novel mutation of the erythroid-specific delta-aminolaevulinate synthase gene in a patient with X-linked sideroblastic anaemia. *Br J Haematol* **106**:175, 1999.
158. Aoki Y, Muranaka S, Nakabayashi K, Ueda Y: δ-Aminolevulinic acid synthetase in erythroblasts of patients with pyridoxine responsive anemia. *J Clin Invest* **64**:1196, 1979.
159. Leklem JE: Vitamin B-6 metabolism and function in humans, in Leklem JE, Reynolds RD (eds.): *Current Topics in Nutrition and Disease* **19**:3, 1988.
160. Konopka L, Hoffbrand AV: Heme synthesis in sideroblastic anaemia. *Br J Haematol* **42**:73, 1979.
161. Tanaka M, Bottomley SS: Bone marrow delta-aminolevulinic acid synthetase activity in experimental sideroblastic anemia. *J Lab Clin Med* **84**:92, 1974.
162. Sharp RA, Lowe JG, Johnston RN: Anti-tuberculous drugs and sideroblastic anaemia. *Br J Clin Pract* **44**:706, 1990.
163. Brownlie A, Donovan A, Pratt SJ, Paw BH, Oates AC, Brugnara C, Witkowska HE, Sassa S, Zon LI: Positional cloning of the zebrafish sauternes gene: A model for congenital sideroblastic anaemia. *Nat Genet* **20**:244, 1998.

164. Nakajima O, Takahashi S, Harigae H, Furuyama K, Hayashi N, Sassa S, Yamamoto M: Heme deficiency in erythroid lineage causes differentiation arrest and cytoplasmic iron overload. *EMBO J* **18**:6282, 1999.
165. Bottomley SS: Sideroblastic anemias, in Lee GR, Foerster J, Lukens J, Paraskevas F, Greer JP, Rodgers GM (eds.): *Wintrobe's Clinical Hematology*. Baltimore, MD, Williams & Wilkins, 1998, p 1022.
166. Hines JD: Effect of pyridoxine plus chronic phlebotomy on the function and morphology of bone marrow and liver in pyridoxine-responsive sideroblastic anemia. *Semin Hematol* **13**:133, 1976.
167. Buchanan GR, Bottomley SS, Nitschke R: Bone marrow delta-aminolaevulinate synthase deficiency in a female with congenital sideroblastic anemia. *Blood* **55**:109, 1980.
168. Bendich A, Cohen M: Vitamin B6 safety issues. *Ann N Y Acad Sci* **585**:321, 1990.
169. Albin RL, Albers JW, Greenberg HS, Townsend JB, Lynn RB, Burke JM Jr, Alessi AG: Acute sensory neuropathy-neuronopathy from pyridoxine overdose. *Neurology* **37**:1729, 1987.
170. Ubbink JB, Delport R, Bissbort S, Vermaak WJH, Becker PJ: Relationship between vitamin B-6 status and elevated pyridoxal kinase levels induced by theophylline therapy in humans. *J Nutr* **120**:1352, 1990.
171. Bottomley SS: Secondary iron overload disorders. *Semin Hematol* **35**:77, 1998.
172. Olivieri NF, Brittenham GM: Iron-chelating therapy and the treatment of thalassemia. *Blood* **89**:739, 1997.
173. Kim BK, Huebers H, Pippard MJ, Finch CA: Storage iron exchange in the rat as affected by deferoxamine. *J Lab Clin Med* **105**:440, 1985.
174. Bulaj ZJ, Griffen LM, Jorde LB, Edwards CQ, Kushner JP: Clinical and biochemical abnormalities in people heterozygous for hemochromatosis. *N Engl J Med* **335**:1799, 1996.
175. Adams PC: Prevalence of abnormal iron studies in heterozygotes for hereditary hemochromatosis: An analysis of 255 heterozygotes. *Am J Hematol* **45**:146, 1994.
176. Garry PJ, Montoya GD, Baumgartner RN, Liang HC, Williams TM, Brodie SG: Impact of HLA-H mutations on iron stores in healthy elderly men and women. *Blood Cells Molec Dis* **23**:277, 1997.
177. Roberts AG, Whatley SD, Morgan RR, Worwood M, Elder GH: Increased frequency of haemochromatosis Cys282Tyr mutation in sporadic porphyria cutanea tarda. *Lancet* **349**:321, 1997.
178. Merryweather-Clarke AT, Pointon JJ, Shearman JD, Robson KJ: Global prevalence of putative haemochromatosis mutations. *J Med Genet* **34**:275, 1997.
179. Sham RL, Ou C-Y, Cappuccio J, Braggins C, Dunnigan K, Phatak PD: Correlation between genotype and phenotype in hereditary hemochromatosis: Analysis of 61 cases. *Blood Cells Mol Dis* **23**:314, 1997.
180. Doss M, von Tiepermann R, Schneider J, Schmid H: New type of hepatic porphyria with porphobilinogen synthase defect and intermittent acute clinical manifestation. *Klin Wochenschr* **57**:1123, 1979.
181. Doss M, Von Tiepermann R, Schneider J: Acute hepatic porphyria syndrome with porphobilinogen synthase defect. *Int J Biochem* **12**:823, 1980.
182. Thunell S: Aminolaevulinate dehydratase porphyria in infancy: A clinical and biochemical study. *J Clin Chem Clin Biochem* **25**:5, 1987.
183. Hassoun A, Verstraeten L, Mercelis R, Martin J-J: Biochemical diagnosis of an hereditary aminolaevulinic dehydratase deficiency in a 63-year-old man. *J Clin Chem Clin Biochem* **27**:781, 1989.
184. Sassa S: ALAD porphyria. *Semin Liver Dis* **18**:95, 1998.
185. Wolff C, Piderit F, Armas-Merino R: Deficiency of porphobilinogen synthase associated with acute crisis. Diagnosis of the first two cases in Chile by laboratory methods. *Eur J Clin Chem Clin Biochem* **29**:313, 1991.
186. Muraoka A, Suehiro I, Fujii M, Murakami K: delta-Aminolevulinic acid dehydratase deficiency porphyria (ADP) with syndrome of inappropriate secretion of antidiuretic hormone (SIADH) in a 69-year-old woman. *Kobe J Med Sci* **41**:23, 1995.
187. Doss M, Laubenthal F, Stoeppler M: Lead poisoning in inherited δ-aminolevulinic acid dehydratase deficiency. *Int Arch Occup Environ Health* **54**:55, 1984.
188. Gross U, Sassa S, Jacob K, Deybach JC, Nordmann Y, Frank M, Doss MO: 5-Aminolevulinic acid dehydratase deficiency porphyria: A twenty-year clinical and biochemical follow-up. *Clin Chem* **44**:1892, 1998.
189. Mercelis R, Hassoun A, Verstraeten L, Debock R, Martin J-J: Porphyric neuropathy and hereditary δ-aminolevulinic acid dehydratase deficiency in an adult. *J Neurol Sci* **95**:39, 1990.
190. Bird TD, Hamernyik P, Nutter JY, Labbe RF: Inherited deficiency of delta-aminolevulinic acid dehydratase. *Am J Hum Genet* **31**:662, 1979.
191. Sassa S, Fujita H, Kappas A: Genetic and chemical influences on heme biosynthesis, in Kotyk A, Skoda J, Paces V, Kostka V (eds.): *Highlights of Modern Biochemistry*. Utrecht, VSP International Science Publishers, 1989, p 329.
192. Shimizu Y, Ida S, Naruto H, Urata G: Excretion of porphyrins in urine and bile after the administration of delta-aminolevulinic acid. *J Lab Clin Med* **92**:795, 1978.
193. Jacob K, Egeler E, Gross U, Doss MO: Investigations on the formation of urinary coproporphyrin isomers I-IV in 5-aminolevulinic acid dehydratase deficiency porphyria, acute lead intoxication and after oral 5-aminolevulinic acid loading. *Clin Biochem* **32**:119, 1999.
194. Elder GH, Smith SG, Herrero C, Lecha M, Mascaro JM, Muniesa AM, Czarnecki DB, Brenan J, Poulos V, de Salamanca RE: Hepatoerythropoietic porphyria: A new uroporphyrinogen decarboxylase defect or homozygous porphyria cutanea tarda? *Lancet* **1**:916, 1981.
195. Anderson PM, Desnick RJ: Purification and properties of δ-aminolevulinate dehydrase from human erythrocytes. *J Biol Chem* **254**:6924, 1979.
196. Jordan PM, Seehra JS: Mechanism of action of δ-aminolevulinic acid dehydratase. Stepwise order of addition of the two molecules of delta-aminolevulinic acid in the enzyme synthesis of porphobilinogen. *J Chem Soc Chem Commun* 240, 1980.
197. Erskine PT, Senior N, Awan S, Lambert R, Lewis G, Tickle IJ, Sarwar M, Spencer P, Thomas P, Warren MJ, Shoolingin-Jordan PM, Wood SP, Cooper JB: X-ray structure of 5-aminolaevulinate dehydratase, a hybrid aldolase. *Nat Struct Biol* **4**:1025, 1997.
198. Guo GG, Gu M, Etlinger JD: 240-kDa proteasome inhibitor (CF-2) is identical to delta-aminolevulinic acid dehydratase. *J Biol Chem* **269**:12399, 1994.
199. Piatigorsky J: The twelfth Frederick H. Verhoeff Lecture: Gene sharing in the visual system. *Trans Am Ophthalmol Soc* **91**:283, 1993.
200. Wetmur JG, Bishop DF, Ostasiewicz L, Desnick RJ: Molecular cloning of a cDNA for human δ-aminolevulinate dehydratase. *Gene* **43**:123, 1986.
201. Wetmur JG, Bishop DF, Cantelmo C, Desnick RJ: Human delta-aminolevulinate dehydratase: Nucleotide sequence of a full-length cDNA clone. *Proc Natl Acad Sci U S A* **83**:7703, 1986.
202. Potluri VR, Astrin KH, Wetmur JG, Bishop DF, Desnick RJ: Human δ-aminolevulinate dehydratase: Chromosomal localization to 9q34 by in situ hybridization. *Hum Genet* **76**:236, 1987.
203. Kaya AH, Plewinska M, Wong DM, Desnick RJ, Wetmur JG: Human δ-aminolevulinate dehydratase (ALAD) gene: Structure and alternative splicing of the erythroid and housekeeping mRNAs. *Genomics* **19**:242, 1994.
204. Akagi R, Shimizu R, Furuyama K, Doss MO, Sassa S: Novel molecular defects of the δ-aminolevulinate dehydratase gene in a patient with inherited acute hepatic porphyria. *Hepatology* **31**:704, 2000.
205. Ishida N, Fujita H, Noguchi T, Doss M, Kappas A, Sassa S: Message amplification phenotyping of an inherited δ-aminolevulinate dehydratase deficiency in a family with acute hepatic porphyria. *Biochem Biophys Res Commun* **172**:237, 1990.
206. Ishida N, Fujita H, Fukuda Y, Noguchi T, Doss M, Kappas A, Sassa S: Cloning and expression of the defective genes from a patient with δ-aminolevulinate dehydratase porphyria. *J Clin Invest* **89**:1431, 1992.
207. Plewinska M, Thunell S, Holmberg L, Wetmur JG, Desnick RJ: δ-Aminolevulinate dehydratase deficient porphyria: Identification of the molecular lesions in a severely affected homozygote. *Am J Hum Genet* **49**:167, 1991.
208. Akagi R, Yasui Y, Harper P, Sassa S: A novel mutation of delta-aminolaevulinate dehydratase in a healthy child with 12% erythrocyte enzyme activity. *Br J Haematol* **106**:931, 1999.
209. Battistuzzi G, Petrucci R, Silvagni L, Urbani FR, Caiola S: delta-Aminolevulinate dehydrase: A new genetic polymorphism in man. *Ann Hum Genet* **45**:223, 1981.
210. Wetmur JG: Influence of the common human δ-aminolevulinate dehydratase polymorphism on lead body burden. *Environ Health Perspect* **102**:215, 1994.
211. Bergdahl IA, Grubb A, Schutz A, Desnick RJ, Wetmur JG, Sassa S, Skerfving S: Lead binding to delta-aminolevulinic acid dehydratase (ALAD) in human erythrocytes. *Pharmacol Toxicol* **81**:153, 1997.

212. Astrin KH, Bishop DF, Wetmur JG, Kaul B, Davidow B, Desnick RJ: delta-Aminolevulinic acid dehydratase isozymes and lead toxicity. *Ann N Y Acad Sci* **514**:23, 1987.
213. Wetmur JG, Lehnert G, Desnick RJ: The δ-aminolevulinate dehydratase polymorphism: Higher blood lead levels in lead workers and environmentally exposed children with the 1-2 and 2-2 isozymes. *Environ Res* **56**:109, 1991.
214. Fleming DE, Chettle DR, Wetmur JG, Desnick RJ, Robin JP, Boulay D, Richard NS, Gordon CL, Webber CE: Effect of the delta-aminolevulinate dehydratase polymorphism on the accumulation of lead in bone and blood in lead smelter workers. *Environ Res* **77**:49, 1998.
215. Alexander BH, Checkoway H, Costa-Mallen P, Faustman EM, Woods JS, Kelsey KT, van Netten C, Costa LG: Interaction of blood lead and delta-aminolevulinic acid dehydratase genotype on markers of heme synthesis and sperm production in lead smelter workers. *Environ Health Perspect* **106**:213, 1998.
216. Mitchell G, Larochelle J, Lambert M, Michaud J, Grenier A, Ogier H, Gauthier M, Lacroix J, Vanasse M, Larbrisseau A, Paradis K, Weber A, Lefevre Y, Melancon S, Dallaire L: Neurologic crises in hereditary tyrosinemia. *N Engl J Med* **322**:432, 1990.
217. Rank JM, Pascual-Leone A, Payne W, Glock M, Freese D, Sharp H, Bloomer JR: Hematin therapy for the neurological crisis of tyrosinemia. *J Pediatr* **118**:136, 1991.
218. Sassa S, Kappas A: Hereditary tyrosinemia and the heme biosynthetic pathway. *J Clin Invest* **71**:625, 1983.
219. Tschudy DP, Hess RA, Frykholm BC: Inhibition of δ-aminolevulinic acid dehydrase by 4,6-dioxoheptanoic acid. *J Biol Chem* **256**:9915, 1981.
220. Sassa S: Delta-aminolevulinic acid dehydratase assay. *Enzyme* **28**:133, 1982.
221. Anderson KE, Fischbein A, Kestenbaum D, Sassa S, Alvares A, Kappas A: Plumbism from airborne lead in a firing range. An unusual exposure to a toxic heavy metal. *Am J Med* **63**:306, 1977.
222. Lindblad B, Lindstedt S, Steen G: On the enzymic defects in hereditary tyrosinemia. *Proc Natl Acad Sci U S A* **74**:4641, 1977.
223. Fujita H, Koizumi A, Furusawa T, Ikeda M: Decreased erythrocyte δ-aminolevulinate dehydratase activity after styrene exposure. *Biochem Pharmacol* **36**:711, 1987.
224. Granick JL, Sassa S, Granick S, Levere RD, Kappas A: Studies in lead poisoning. II. Correlations between the ratio of activated and inactivated δ-aminolevulinic acid dehydratase of whole blood and the blood lead level. *Biochem Med* **8**:149, 1973.
225. Granick JL, Sassa S, Kappas A: Some biochemical and clinical aspects of lead intoxication, in Bodansky O, Latner AL (eds.): *Advances in Clinical Chemistry*. New York, Academic Press, 1978, p 287.
226. Akagi R, Prchal JT, Eberhart CE, Sassa S: An acquired acute hepatic porphyria: A novel type of δ-aminolevulinate dehydratase inhibition. *Clin Chim Acta* **212**:79, 1992.
227. Dyer J, Garrick DP, Inglis A, Pye IF: Plumboporphyria (ALAD deficiency) in a lead worker—A scenario for potential diagnostic confusion. *Br J Ind Med* **50**:1119, 1993.
228. Salo MK, Simell O: Invited lecture: Hemiarginate therapy for porphyria crisis of tyrosinemia [Abstract]. Presented at the Annual Meeting of the European Society for Pediatric Research (Conference Proceedings), Zürich, 1991.
229. Lamon JM, Frykholm BC, Tschudy DP: Hematin administration to an adult with lead intoxication. *Blood* **53**:1007, 1979.
230. Thunell S, Henrichson A, Floderus Y, Groth CG, Eriksson BG, Barkholt L, Nemeth A, Strandvik B, Eleborg L, Holmberg L, Lundgren J: Liver transplantation in a boy with acute porphyria due to aminolaevulinate dehydratase deficiency. *Eur J Clin Chem Clin Biochem* **30**:599, 1992.
231. Desnick RJ, Anderson KE: The porphyrias, in Hoffman R, Benz EJJ, Shattil SJ, Furie B, Cohen H (eds.): *Hematology: Basic Principles and Practice*. New York, Churchill Livingston, 1991, p 350.
232. Wilson JP: Stokvis and acute porphyria. *Mol Aspects Med* **11**:6, 1990.
233. Moore MR, McColl KEL, Rimington C, Goldberg A: *Disorders of Porphyrin Metabolism*. New York, Plenum, 1987.
234. Bonkowsky HL: The porphyrias, in Zakim D, Boyer T (eds.): *Hepatology*. Philadelphia, WB Saunders, 1982, p 351.
235. Grandchamp B: Acute intermittent porphyria. *Semin Liver Dis* **18**:17, 1998.
236. Wetterberg L: *A Neuropsychiatric and Genetical Investigation of Acute Intermittent Porphyria*. Svenska Bokfölaget, Scandinavian University Books, Norstedts, 1967.
237. Mustajoki P, Koskelo P: Hereditary hepatic porphyrias in Finland. *Acta Med Scand* **200**:171, 1976.
238. Goldberg A, Rimington C: *Diseases of Porphyrin Metabolism*. Springfield, IL, Charles C Thomas, 1962.
239. Lee J-S, Anvret M: Identification of the most common mutation within the porphobilinogen deaminase gene in Swedish patients with acute intermittent porphyria. *Proc Natl Acad Sci U S A* **88**:10912, 1991.
240. Greene-Davis ST, Neumann PE, Mann OE, Moss MA, Schreiber WE, Welch JP, Langley GR, Sangalang VE, Dempsey GI, Nassar BA: Detection of a R173W mutation in the porphobilinogen deaminase gene in the Nova Scotian "foreign Protestant" population with acute intermittent porphyria: A founder effect. *Clin Biochem* **30**:607, 1997.
241. Tishler P, Woodward B, O'Connor J, Holbrook DA, Seidman LJ, Hallet M, Knighton DJ: High prevalence of intermittent acute porphyria in a psychiatric patient population. *Am J Psychiatry* **142**:1430, 1985.
242. Mustajoki P, Kauppinen R, Lannfelt L, Lilius L, Koistinen J: Frequency of low erythrocyte porphobilinogen deaminase activity in Finland. *J Intern Med* **231**:389, 1992.
243. Nordmann Y, Puy H, Da Silva V, Simonin S, Robreau AM, Bonaiti C, Phung LN, Deybach JC: Acute intermittent porphyria: prevalence of mutations in the porphobilinogen deaminase gene in blood donors in France. *J Intern Med* **242**:213, 1997.
244. Rimington C: Was Hippocrates the first to describe a case of acute porphyria? *Int J Biochem* **25**:1351, 1993.
245. Macalpine I, Hunter R, Rimington C, Brooke J, Goldberg A: *Porphyria—A Royal Malady*. London, British Medical Association, 1968.
246. Loftus LS, Arnold WN: Vincent van Gogh's illness: Acute intermittent porphyria. *BMJ* **303**:1589, 1991.
247. Winkler M, Anderson KE: Vampires, porphyria and the media: The medicalization of a myth. *Perspect Biol Med* **33**:598, 1990.
248. Dean G: The Porphyrias: *A Study of Inheritance and Environment*, 2nd ed. London, Pitman Medical, 1971.
249. Röhl JCG, Warren M, Hunt D: *Purple Secret—Genes, "Madness" and the Royal Houses of Europe*. Bantam Press, London, Transworld Publishers, 1998.
250. Daniell WE, Stockbridge HL, Labbe RF, Woods JS, Anderson KE, Bissell DM, Bloomer JR, Ellefson RD, Moore MR, Pierach CA, Schreiber WE, Tefferi A, Franklin GM: Environmental chemical exposures and disturbances of heme synthesis. *Environ Health Perspect* **105(Suppl 1)**:37, 1997.
251. Hahn M, Bonkovsky HL: Multiple chemical sensitivity syndrome and porphyria. A note of caution and concern. *Arch Intern Med* **157**:281, 1997.
252. McDonagh AF, Bissell DM: Porphyria and porphyrinology—The past fifteen years. *Semin Liver Dis* **18**:3, 1998.
253. Beukeveld GJJ, Wolthers BG, Nordmann Y, Deybach JC, Grandchamp B, Wadman SK: A retrospective study of a patient with homozygous form of acute intermittent porphyria. *J Inherit Metab Dis* **13**:673, 1990.
254. Waldenström J: The porphyrias as inborn errors of metabolism. *Am J Med* **22**:758, 1957.
255. Goldberg A: Acute intermittent porphyria. A study of 50 cases. *QJM* **28**:183, 1959.
256. Stein JA, Tschudy DP: Acute intermittent porphyria: A clinical and biochemical study of 46 patients. *Medicine* **49**:1, 1970.
257. Beal MF, Atuk NO, Westfall TC, Turner SM: Catecholamine uptake, accumulation, and release in acute porphyria. *J Clin Invest* **60**:1141, 1977.
258. Yeung Laiwah AA, MacPhee GJ, Boyle P, Moore MR, Goldberg A: Autonomic neuropathy in acute intermittent porphyria. *J Neurol Neurosurg Psychiatry* **48**:790, 1985.
259. Blom H, Andersson C, Olofsson BO, Bjerle P, Wiklund U, Lithner F: Assessment of autonomic nerve function in acute intermittent porphyria: A study based on spectral analysis of heart rate variability. *J Intern Med* **240**:73, 1996.
260. Barohn RJ, Sanchez JE, Anderson KE: Acute peripheral neuropathy due to hereditary coproporphyria. *Muscle Nerve* **17**:793, 1994.
261. Ridley A: Porphyric neuropathy, in Dyck PJ, Thomas PK, Lambert EH, Bunge R (eds.): *Peripheral Neuropathy*. Philadelphia, WB Saunders, 1984, p 1704.
262. Cavanagh JB, Mellick RS: On the nature of the peripheral nerve lesions associated with acute intermittent porphyria. *J Neurol Neurosurg Psychiatry* **28**:320, 1965.

263. Sweeney VP, Pathak MA, Asbury AK: Acute intermittent porphyria: increased ALA-synthetase activity during an acute attack. *Brain* **93**:369, 1970.
264. Mustajoki P, Seppalainen AM: Neuropathy in latent hereditary hepatic porphyria. *BMJ* **2**:310, 1975.
265. Meyer UA, Schuurmans MM, Lindberg RLP: Acute porphyrias: Pathogenesis of neurological manifestations. *Semin Liver Dis* **18**:43, 1998.
266. Kupferschmidt H, Bont A, Schnorf H, Landis T, Walter E, Peter J, Krahenbuhl S, Meier PJ: Transient cortical blindness and bioccipital brain lesions in two patients with acute intermittent porphyria. *Ann Intern Med* **123**:598, 1995.
267. Sze G: Cortical brain lesions in acute intermittent porphyria. *Ann Intern Med* **125**:422, 1996.
268. Stein JA, Curl FD, Valsamis M, Tschudy DP: Abnormal iron and water metabolism in acute intermittent porphyria with new morphologic findings. *Am J Med* **53**:784, 1972.
269. Jeans JB, Savik K, Gross CR, Weimer MK, Bossenmaier IC, Pierach CA, Bloomer JR: Mortality in patients with acute intermittent porphyria requiring hospitalization: A United States case series. *Am J Med Genet* **11**:269, 1996.
270. Patience DA, Blackwood DH, McColl KE, Moore MR: Acute intermittent porphyria and mental illness—A family study. *Acta Psychiatr Scand* **89**:262, 1994.
271. Sanders AR, Rinconlimas DE, Chakraborty R, Grandchamp B, Hamilton JD, Fann WE, Patel PI: Association between genetic variation at the porphobilinogen deaminase gene and schizophrenia. *Schizophr Res* **8**:211, 1993.
272. Nimgaonkar VL, Ganguli R, Washington SS, Chakravarti A: Schizophrenia and porphobilinogen deaminase gene polymorphisms: An association study. *Schizophr Res* **8**:51, 1992.
273. Owen MJ, Mant R, Parfitt E, Williams J, Asherson P, O'Mahoney G, Vanos J, Llewellyn D, Collier D, Gill M, McGuffin P: No association between RFLPs at the porphobilinogen deaminase gene and schizophrenia. *Hum Genet* **90**:131, 1992.
274. Wang ZW, Black D, Andreasen NC, Crowe RR: A linkage study of chromosome 11q in schizophrenia. *Arch Gen Psychiatry* **50**:212, 1993.
275. Bylesjo I, Forsgren L, Lithner F, Boman K: Epidemiology and clinical characteristics of seizures in patients with acute intermittent porphyria. *Epilepsia* **37**:230, 1996.
276. Perlroth MG, Tschudy DP, Marver HS, Berard CW, Zeigel RF, Rechcigl M, Collins A: Acute intermittent porphyria: New morphologic and biochemical findings. *Am J Med* **41**:149, 1966.
277. Bloomer JR, Berk PD, Bonkowsky HL, Stein JD, Berlin NI, Tschudy DP: Blood volume and bilirubin production in acute intermittent porphyria. *N Engl J Med* **284**:17, 1971.
278. Eales L, Dowdle EB, Sweeney GD: The electrolyte disorder of the acute porphyric attack and the possible role of delta-aminolaevulic acid. *S Afr J Lab Clin Med* **17**:89, 1971.
279. Tschudy DP, Lamon JM: Porphyrin metabolism and the porphyrias, in Bondy PK, Rosenberg LE (eds.): *Duncan's Diseases of Metabolism*. Philadelphia, WB Saunders, 1980, p 939.
280. Eales L: Porphyria as seen in Cape Town. A survey of 250 patients and some recent studies. *S Afr J Lab Clin Med* **9**:151, 1963.
281. Tschudy DP, Valsamis M, Magnussen CR: Acute intermittent porphyria: Clinical and selected research aspects. *Ann Intern Med* **83**:851, 1975.
282. Barois A, Gajdos P, Lienhart A, Goulon M: Hypercalcémie au cours de la porphyrie aigüe intermittente: A propos de 3 observations. *Semin Hosp Paris* **53**:1115, 1977.
283. Kauppinen R, Mustajoki P: Prognosis of acute porphyria: Occurrence of acute attacks, precipitating factors, and associated diseases. *Medicine* **71**:1, 1992.
284. Ostrowski J, Kostrzewska E, Michalak T, Zawirska B, Medrzejewski W, Gregor A: Abnormalities in liver function and morphology and impaired aminopyrine metabolism in hereditary hepatic porphyrias. *Gastroenterology* **85**:1131, 1983.
285. Lithner F, Wetterberg L: Hepatocellular carcinoma in patients with acute intermittent porphyria. *Acta Med Scand* **215**:271, 1984.
286. Hardell L, Bengtsson NO, Jonsson U, Eriksson S, Larsson LG: Aetiological aspects on primary liver cancer with special regard to alcohol, organic solvents and acute intermittent porphyria—An epidemiological investigation. *Br J Cancer* **50**:389, 1984.
287. Bengtsson NO, Hardell L: Porphyrias, porphyrins and hepatocellular cancer. *Br J Cancer* **54**:115, 1986.
288. Gubler JG, Bargetzi MJ, Meyer UA: Primary liver carcinoma in two sisters with acute intermittent porphyria. *Am J Med* **89**:540, 1990.
289. Kauppinen R, Mustajoki P: Acute hepatic porphyria and hepatocellular carcinoma. *Brit J Cancer* **57**:117, 1987.
290. Andant C, Puy H, Faivre J, Deybach JC: Acute hepatic porphyrias and primary liver cancer [Letter]. *N Engl J Med* **338**:1853, 1998.
291. Bjersing L, Andersson C, Lithner F: Hepatocellular carcinoma in patients from northern Sweden with acute intermittent porphyria: morphology and mutations. *Cancer Epidemiol Biomarkers Prev* **5**:393, 1996.
292. Mustajoki P, Nikkila EA: Serum lipoproteins in asymptomatic acute porphyria: No evidence for hyperbetalipoproteinemia. *Metabolism* **33**:266, 1984.
293. Hollander CS, Scott RL, Tschudy DP, Perlroth M, Waxman A, Sterling K: Increased protein bound iodine and thyroxine binding globulin in acute intermittent porphyria. *N Eng J Med* **277**:995, 1967.
294. Herrick AL, McColl KE, Wallace AM, Moore MR, Goldberg A: Elevation of hormone-binding globulins in acute intermittent porphyria. *Clin Chim Acta* **187**:141, 1990.
295. Perlroth MG, Tschudy DP, Waxman A, Odell WD: Abnormalities of growth hormone regulation in acute intermittent porphyria. *Metabolism* **16**:87, 1967.
296. Waxman AD, Berk PD, Schalch D, Tschudy DP: Isolated adrenocorticotrophic hormone deficiency in acute intermittent porphyria. *Ann Intern Med* **70**:317, 1969.
297. Waxman A, Schalach DS, Odell WD, Tschudy DP: Abnormalities of carbohydrate metabolism in acute intermittent porphyria. *J Clin Invest* **46**:1129, 1967.
298. Sixel-Dietrich F, Verspohl F, Doss M: Hyperinsulinemia in acute intermittent porphyria. *Horm Metab Res* **17**:375, 1985.
299. Andersson C, Bylesjo I, Lithner F: Effects of diabetes mellitus on patients with acute intermittent porphyria. *J Intern Med* **245**:193, 1999.
300. Granick S, Van Den Schreieck HG: Porphobilinogen and δ-aminolevulinic acid in acute porphyria. *Proc Soc Exp Biol Med* **88**:270, 1955.
301. Doss M, Schermuly E: Urinary porphyrin excretion pattern and isomer distribution of I and III in human porphyrin disorders, in Doss M (ed.): *Porphyrins and Human Disease*. Basel, S Karger, 1976, p 189.
302. Doss M, Schermuly E, Look D, Henning H, Hocevar V, Dohmen K, Anlauf M: Studies on the metabolism of δ-aminolevulinic acid and porphobilinogen in liver biopsies from patients with acute intermittent porphyria, in Doss M (ed.): *Porphyrins and Human Disease*. Basel, S Karger, 1976, p 205.
303. Kuhnel A, Gross U, Jacob K, Doss MO: Studies on coproporphyrin isomers in urine and feces in the porphyrias. *Clin Chim Acta* **282**:45, 1999.
304. Meyer UA, Strand LJ, Doss M, Rees AC, Marver HS: Intermittent acute porphyria—Demonstration of a genetic defect in porphobilinogen metabolism. *N Engl J Med* **286**:1277, 1972.
305. Strand LJ, Meyer UA, Felsher BF, Redeker AG, Marver HS: Decreased red cell uroporphyrinogen I synthetase activity in intermittent acute porphyria. *J Clin Invest* **51**:2530, 1972.
306. Puy H, Deybach JC, Lamoril J, Robreau AM, Da Silva V, Gouya L, Grandchamp B, Nordmann Y: Molecular epidemiology and diagnosis of PBG deaminase gene defects in acute intermittent porphyria. *Am J Hum Genet* **60**:1373, 1997.
307. Mustajoki P: Normal erythrocyte uroporphyrinogen I synthase in a kindred with acute intermittent porphyria. *Ann Int Med* **95**:162, 1981.
308. Cookson GH, Rimington C: Porphobilinogen. *Biochem J* **57**:476, 1954.
309. Mauzerall D: The thermostability of porphyrinogens. *J Am Chem Soc* **82**:2601, 1960.
310. Battersby AR, Fookes CJR, Matcham GWJ, McDonald E: Order of assembly of the four pyrrole rings during biosynthesis of the natural porphyrins. *J Chem Soc Chem Commun* 539, 1979.
311. Battersby AR, Fookes CJR, Matcham GWJ, McDonald E: Biosynthesis of the pigments of life: Formation of the macrocycle. *Nature* **285**:17, 1980.
312. Frydman RB, Feinstein G: Studies on porphobilinogen deaminase and uroporphyrinogen III cosynthase from human erythrocytes. *Biochim Biophys Acta* **350**:358, 1974.
313. Higuchi M, Bogorad L: The purification and properties of uroporphyrinogen I synthase and uroporphyrinogen III cosynthase. Interactions between the enzymes. *Ann N Y Acad Sci* **244**:401, 1975.

314. Anderson PM, Desnick RJ: Purification and properties of uroporphyrinogen I synthase from human erythrocytes. *J Biol Chem* **255**:1993, 1980.
315. Jordan PM, Shemin D: Purification and properties of uroporphyrinogen I synthase from Rhodopseudomonas spheroides. *J Biol Chem* **248**:1019, 1973.
316. Miyagi K, Kaneshima M, Kawakami J, Nakada F, Petryka ZJ, Watson CJ: Uroporphyrinogen I synthase from human erythrocytes: Separation, purification, and properties of isoenzymes. *Proc Natl Acad Sci* **76**:6172, 1979.
317. Beaumont C, Grandchamp B, Bogard M, De Verneuil H, Nordmann Y: Porphobilinogen deaminase in unstable in the absence of its substrate. *Biochim Biophys Acta* **882**:384, 1986.
318. Piper WN, Tephly TR: Differential inhibition of erythrocyte and hepatic uroporphyrinogen I synthase activity by lead. *Life Sci* **14**:873, 1974.
319. Farmer DJ, Hollebone BR: Comparative inhibition of hepatic hydroxymethylbilane synthase by both hard and soft metal cations. *Can J Biochem Cell Biol* **62**:49, 1984.
320. Miller AD, Packman LC, Hart GJ, Alefounder PR, Abell C, Battersby AR: Evidence that pyridoxal phosphate modification of lysine residues (Lys-55 and Lys-59) causes inactivation of hydroxymethylbilane synthase (porphobilinogen deaminase). *Biochem J* **262**:119, 1989.
321. Jordan PM, Warren MJ, Williams HJ, Stolowich NJ, Roessner CA, Grant SK, Scott AI: Identification of a cysteine residue as the binding site for the dipyrromethane cofactor at the active site of *Escherichia coli* porphobilinogen deaminase. *FEBS Lett* **235**:189, 1988.
322. Lander M, Pitt AR, Alefounder PR, Bardy D, Abell C, Battersby AR: Studies on the mechanism of hydroxymethylbilane synthase concerning the role of arginine residues in substrate binding. *Biochem J* **275**:447, 1991.
323. Warren MJ, Jordan PM: Investigation into the nature of substrate binding to the dipyrromethane cofactor of *Escherichia coli* porphobilinogen deaminase. *Biochemistry* **27**:9020, 1988.
324. Louie GV, Brownlie PD, Lambert R, Cooper JB, Blundell TL, Wood SP, Warren MJ, Woodcock SC, Jordan PM: Structure of porphobilinogen deaminase reveals a flexible multidomain polymerase with a single catalytic site. *Nature* **359**:33, 1992.
325. Brownlie PD, Lambert R, Louie GV, Jordan PM, Blundell TL, Warren MJ, Cooper JB, Wood SP: The three-dimensional structures of mutants of porphobilinogen deaminase: Toward an understanding of the structural basis of acute intermittent porphyria. *Protein Sci* **3**:1644, 1994.
326. Wood S, Lambert R, Jordan M: Molecular basis of acute intermittent porphyria. *Mol Med Today* **5**:232, 1995.
327. Grandchamp B, Romeo P-H, Dubart A, Raich N, Rosa J, Goossens M: Molecular cloning of a cDNA sequence complementary to porphobilinogen deaminase mRNA from rat. *Proc Natl Acad Sci U S A* **81**:5036, 1984.
328. Raich N, Romeo PH, Dubart A, Beaupain D, Cohen-Solal M, Goossens M: Molecular cloning and complete primary sequence of human erythrocyte porphobilinogen deaminase. *Nucleic Acids Res* **14**:5955, 1986.
329. Grandchamp B, De Verneuil H, Beaumont C, Chretien S, Walter O, Nordmann Y: Tissue specific expression of porphobilinogen deaminase. Two isoenzymes from a single gene. *Eur J Biochem* **162**:105, 1987.
330. Meisler M, Wanner L, Eddy RE, Shows TB: The UPS locus encoding uroporphyrinogen I synthase is located on human chromosome 11. *Biochem Biophys Res Commun* **95**:170, 1980.
331. Wang AL, Arredondo-Vega FX, Giampietro PF, Smith M, Anderson WF, Desnick RJ: Regional gene assignment of human porphobilinogen deaminase and esterase A4 to chromosome 11q23 leads to 11qter. *Proc Natl Acad Sci U S A* **78**:5734, 1981.
332. De Verneuil H, Phung N, Nordmann Y, Allard D, Leprince F, Jerome H, Aurias A, Rethore MO: Assignment of human uroporphyrinogen I synthase locus to region 11qter by gene dosage effect. *Hum Genet* **60**:212, 1982.
333. Chretien S, Dubart A, Beaupain D, Raich N, Grandchamp B, Rosa J, Goossens M, Romeo PH: Alternative transcription and splicing of the human porphobilinogen deaminase gene result either in tissue specific or in housekeeping expression. *Proc Natl Acad Sci U S A* **85**:6, 1988.
334. Mignotte V, Eleout JF, Raich N, Romeo PH: *Cis-* and *trans-*acting elements involved in the regulation of the erythroid promoter of the human porphobilinogen deaminase gene. *Proc Natl Acad Sci U S A* **86**:6548, 1989.
335. Grandchamp B, Nordmann Y: Enzymes of the heme biosynthesis pathway: Recent advances in molecular genetics. *Semin Hematol* **25**:303, 1988.
336. Human Gene Mutation Database: www.uwcm.ac.uk/uwcm/mg/hgmd0.html
337. De Siervi A, Rossetti MV, Parera VE, Astrin KH, Aizencang GI, Glass IA, Battle AM, Desnick RJ: Identification and characterization of hydroxymethylbilane synthase mutations causing acute intermittent porphyria: Evidence for an ancestral founder of the common G111R mutation. *Am J Med Genet* **86**:366, 1999.
338. Astrin KH, Desnick RJ: Molecular basis of acute intermittent porphyria: Mutations and polymorphisms in the human hydroxymethylbilane synthase gene. *Hum Mutat* **4**:243, 1994.
339. Gu XF, De Rooij F, Lee JS, Velde KT, Deybach JC, Nordmann Y, Grandchamp B: High prevalence of a point mutation in the porphobilinogen deaminase gene in Dutch patients with acute intermittent porphyria. *Hum Genet* **91**:128, 1993.
340. Desnick RJ, Ostasiewicz LT, Tishler PA, Mustajoki P: Acute intermittent porphyria: Characterization of a novel mutation in the structural gene for porphobilinogen deaminase. *J Clin Invest* **76**:865, 1985.
341. Grandchamp B, Picat C, Mignotte V, Wilson JHP, Tevelde K, Sandkuyl L, Romeo PH, Goossens M, Nordmann Y: Tissue-specific splicing mutation in acute intermittent porphyria. *Proc Natl Acad Sci U S A* **86**:661, 1989.
342. Grandchamp B, Picat C, De Rooij FWM, Beaumont C, Deybach J-C, Nordmann Y: Molecular analysis of acute intermittent porphyria in a Finnish family with normal erythrocyte porphobilinogen deaminase. *Eur J Clin Invest* **19**:415, 1989.
343. Mathews-Roth MM: Anemia in erythropoietic protoporphyria. *JAMA* **230**:824, 1974.
344. Puy H, Gross U, Deybach JC, Robreau AM, Frank M, Nordmann Y, Doss M: Exon 1 donor splice site mutations in the porphobilinogen deaminase gene in the non-erythroid variant form of acute intermittent porphyria. *Hum Genet* **103**:570, 1998.
345. Mustajoki S, Pihlaja H, Ahola H, Petersen NE, Mustajoki P, Kauppinen R: Three splicing defects, an insertion, and two missense mutations responsible for acute intermittent porphyria. *Hum Genet* **102**:541, 1998.
346. Delfau MH, Picat C, De Rooij FWM, Hamer K, Bogard M, Wilson JHP, Deybach J-C, Nordmann Y, Grandchamp B: Two different point G to point A mutations in exon 10 of the porphobilinogen deaminase gene are responsible for acute intermittent porphyria. *J Clin Invest* **86**:1511, 1990.
347. Whatley SD, Roberts AG, Elder GH: *De novo* mutation and sporadic presentation of acute intermittent porphyria. *Lancet* **346**:1007, 1995.
348. Bonkowsky HL, Schady W: Neurological manifestations of acute porphyria. *Semin Liver Dis* **2**:108, 1982.
349. Yeung Laiwah AC, Moore MR, Goldberg A: Pathogenesis of acute porphyria. *QJM* **241**:377, 1987.
350. Bonkowsky HL, Tschudy DP, Collins A, Doherty J, Bossenmaier I, Cardinal R, Watson CJ: Repression of the overproduction of porphyrin precursors in acute intermittent porphyria by intravenous infusions of hematin. *Proc Natl Acad Sci U S A* **8**:2725, 1971.
351. Müller WE, Snyder SH: δ-Aminolevulinic acid: influences on synaptic GABA receptor binding may explain CNS symptoms of porphyria. *Ann Neurol* **2**:340, 1977.
352. Brennan MJW, Cantrill RC: δ-Aminolaevulinic acid is a potent agonist for GABA autoreceptors. *Nature* **280**:514, 1979.
353. Oteiza PI, Kleinman CG, Demasi M, Bechara EJ: 5-Aminolevulinic acid induces iron release from ferritin. *Arch Biochem Biophys* **316**:607, 1995.
354. Litman DA, Correia MA: Elevated brain tryptophan and enhanced 5-hydroxytryptamine turnover in acute hepatic heme deficiency: Clinical implications. *J Pharmacol Exp Ther* **232**:337, 1985.
355. Puy H, Deybach JC, Baudry P, Callebert J, Touitou Y, Nordmann Y: Decreased nocturnal plasma melatonin levels in patients with recurrent acute intermittent porphyria attacks. *Life Sci* **53**:621, 1993.
356. King PH, Bragdon AC: MRI reveals multiple reversible cerebral lesions in an attack of acute intermittent porphyria. *Neurology* **41**:1300, 1991.
357. Cavanagh JB, Ridley AR: The nature of the neuropathy complicating acute intermittent porphyria. *Lancet* **2**:1023, 1967.
358. Hamfelt A, Wetterberg L: Pyridoxal phosphate in acute intermittent porphyria. *Ann N Y Acad Sci* **166**:361, 1969.
359. Lindberg RL, Porcher C, Grandchamp B, Ledermann B, Burki K, Brandner S, Aguzzi A, Meyer UA: Porphobilinogen deaminase

deficiency in mice causes a neuropathy resembling that of human hepatic porphyria. *Nat Genet* **12**:195, 1996.
360. Lindberg RL, Martini R, Baumgartner M, Erne B, Borg J, Zielasek J, Ricker K, Steck A, Toyka KV, Meyer UA: Motor neuropathy in porphobilinogen deaminase-deficient mice imitates the peripheral neuropathy of human acute porphyria. *J Clin Invest* **103**:1127, 1999.
361. Anderson KE, Spitz IM, Sassa S, Bardin CW, Kappas A: Prevention of cyclical attacks of acute intermittent porphyria with a long-acting agonist of luteinizing hormone-releasing hormone. *N Engl J Med* **311**:643, 1984.
362. Anderson KE: LHRH analogues for hormonal manipulation in acute intermittent porphyria. *Semin Hematol* **26**:10, 1989.
363. Anderson KE, Spitz IM, Bardin CW, Kappas A: A GnRH analogue prevents cyclical attacks of porphyria. *Arch Int Med* **150**:1469, 1990.
364. Anderson KE, Goeger DE: Cyclic attacks of porphyria prevented with a gonadotropin-releasing hormone analogue [Abstract]. *Clin Res* **39**:858A, 1991.
365. De Block CE, Leeuw IH, Gaal LF: Premenstrual attacks of acute intermittent porphyria: hormonal and metabolic aspects—A case report. *Eur J Endocrinol* **141**:50, 1999.
366. Kappas A, Bradlow HL, Gillette PN, Gallagher TF: Studies in porphyria. I. A defect in the reductive transformation of natural steroid hormones in the hereditary liver disease, acute intermittent porphyria. *J Exp Med* **136**:1043, 1972.
367. Anderson KE, Bradlow HL, Sassa S, Kappas A: Studies in porphyria. VIII. Relationship of the 5α-reductive metabolism of steroid hormones to clinical expression of the genetic defect in acute intermittent porphyria. *Am J Med* **66**:644, 1979.
368. Milo R, Neuman M, Klein C, Caspi E, Arlazoroff A: Acute intermittent porphyria in pregnancy. *Obstet Gynecol* **73**:450, 1989.
369. Shenhav S, Gemer O, Sassoon E, Segal S: Acute intermittent porphyria precipitated by hyperemesis and metoclopramide treatment in pregnancy. *Acta Obstet Gynecol Scand* **76**:484, 1997.
370. Anderson KE, Freddara U, Kappas A: Induction of hepatic cytochrome P-450 by natural steroids: relationships to the induction of δ-aminolevulinate synthase and porphyrin accumulation in the avian embryo. *Arch Biochem Biophys* **217**:597, 1982.
371. Kappas A, Sassa S, Anderson KE: The porphyrias, in Stanbury JB, Wyngaarden JB, Fredrickson DS, Goldstein JL, Brown MS (eds.): *The Metabolic Basis of Inherited Disease*. New York, McGraw-Hill, 1983, p 1301.
372. Peters PG, Sharma ML, Hardwicke DM, Piper WN: Sulfonamide inhibition of rat hepatic uroporphyrinogen I synthetase activity and the biosynthesis of heme. *Arch Biochem Biophys* **201**:88, 1980.
373. Tishler PV: The effect of therapeutic drugs and other pharmacologic agents on activity of porphobilinogen deaminase, the enzyme that is deficient in intermittent acute porphyria. *Life Sci* **65**:207, 1999.
374. Sinclair JF, McCaffrey J, Sinclair PR, Bement WJ, Lambrecht LK, Wood SG, Smith EL, Schenkman JB, Guzelian PS, Park SS, Gelboin HV: Ethanol increases cytochromes P450IIE, IIB1/2, and IIIA in cultured rat hepatocytes. *Arch Biochem Biophys* **284**:360, 1991.
375. Thunell S, Floderus Y, Henrichson A, Moore MR, Meissner P, Sinclair J: Alcoholic beverages in acute porphyria. *J Stud Alcohol* **53**:272, 1992.
376. Louis CA, Sinclair JF, Wood SG, Lambrecht LK, Sinclair PR, Smith EL: Synergistic induction of cytochrome-P450 by ethanol and isopentanol in cultures of chick embryo and rat hepatocytes. *Toxicol Appl Pharmacol* **118**:169, 1993.
377. Marks GS: Exposure to toxic agents: the heme biosynthetic pathway and hemoproteins as indicators. *CRC Critical Rev Toxicol* **15**:151, 1985.
378. White INH: Metabolic activation of acetylenic substituents to derivatives in the rat causing the loss of hepatic cytochrome P-450 and haem. *Biochem J* **174**:853, 1978.
379. Koleva M, Stoytchev T: On the enzyme-inducing action of calcium antagonists. *Arch Toxicol* **67**:294, 1993.
380. Lambrecht RW, Gildemeister OS, Williams A, Pepe JA, Tortorelli KD, Bonkovsky HL: Effects of selected antihypertensives and analgesics on hepatic porphyrin accumulation: implications for clinical porphyria. *Biochem Pharmacol* **58**:887, 1999.
381. Schoenfeld N, Aelion J, Beigel Y, Epstein O, Atsmon A: The porphyrogenic effects of calcium channel blocking drugs. *Clin Sci* **69**:581, 1985.
382. Marks GS, Goldman DR, McCluskey SA, Sutherland EP, Lyon ME: The effects of dihydropyridine calcium antagonists on heme biosynthesis in chick embryo liver cell culture. *Can J Physiol Pharmacol* **64**:438, 1986.
383. Moore MR, Hift RJ: Drugs in the acute porphyrias—Toxicogenetic diseases. *Cell Mol Biol (Noisy-le-grand)* **43**:89, 1997.
384. Gorchein A: Drug treatment of hypertension in acute intermittent porphyria: Doxazosin and amlodipine [Letter]. *Br J Clin Pharmacol* **43**:339, 1997.
385. Kepple A, Cernek PK: Amlodipine-induced acute intermittent porphyria exacerbation [Letter]. *Ann Pharmacother* **31**:253, 1997.
386. Gorchein A: Drug treatment in acute porphyria. *Br J Clin Pharmacol* **44**:427, 1997.
387. Lambrecht RW, Gildemeister OS, Pepe JA, Tortorelli KD, Williams A, Bonkovsky HL: Effects of antidepressants and benzodiazepine-type anxiolytic agents on hepatic porphyrin accumulation in primary cultures of chick embryo liver cells. *J Pharmacol Exp Ther* **291**:1150, 1999.
388. Samuels B, Bezwoda WR, Derman DP, Goss G: Chemotherapy in porphyria. *S Afr Med J* **65**:924, 1984.
389. Mustajoki P, Heinonen J: General anesthesia in "inducible" porphyrias. *Anesthesiology* **53**:15, 1980.
390. Harrison GG, Meissner PN, Hift RJ: Anaesthesia for the porphyric patient. *Anaesthesia* **48**:417, 1993.
391. Dover SB, Plenderleith L, Moore MR, McColl KE: Safety of general anaesthesia and surgery in acute hepatic porphyria. *Gut* **35**:1112, 1994.
392. Tschudy DP: The influence of hormonal and nutritional factors on the regulation of liver heme biosynthesis, in De Matteis F, Aldridge WN (eds.): *Heme and Hemoproteins—Handbook of Experimental Pharmacology*. Berlin, Springer-Verlag, 1978, p 255.
393. Anderson KE, Kappas A: Dietary regulation of cytochrome P450. *Annu Rev Nutr* **11**:141, 1991.
394. Anderson KE, Conney AH, Kappas A: Nutrition and oxidative drug metabolism in man: Relative influence of dietary lipids, carbohydrate and protein. *Clin Pharmacol Ther* **26**:493, 1979.
395. Pantuck EJ, Hsiao KC, Maggio A, Nakamura K, Kuntzman R, Conney AH: Effect of cigarette smoking on phenacetin metabolism. *Clin Pharmacol Ther* **15**:9, 1974.
396. Lip GYH, McColl KEL, Goldberg A, Moore MR: Smoking and recurrent attacks of acute intermittent porphyria. *BMJ* **302**:507, 1991.
397. Paxton JW, Moore MR, Beattie AD, Goldberg A: 17-Oxosteroid conjugates in plasma and urine of patients with acute intermittent porphyria. *Clin Sci Mol Med* **46**:207, 1974.
398. Watson CJ, Schwartz S: A simple test for urinary porphobilinogen. *Proc Soc Exp Biol Med* **47**:393, 1941.
399. Watson CJ, Taddeini L, Bossenmaier I: Present status of the Ehrlich aldehyde reaction for urinary porphobilinogen. *JAMA* **190**:501, 1964.
400. Lamon J, With TK, Redeker AG: The Hoesch test: Bedside screening for urinary porphobilinogen in patients with suspected porphyria. *Clin Chem* **11**:1438, 1974.
401. Lamon JM, Frykholm BC, Tschudy DP: Screening tests in acute porphyria. *Arch Neurol* **34**:709, 1977.
402. Mauzerall D, Granick S: The occurrence and determination of δ-aminolevulinic acid and porphobilinogen in urine. *J Biol Chem* **219**:435, 1956.
403. Galbraith RA, Sassa S, Kappas A: A comparison of the utility of Dowex resin and polybenzimidazole Aurorez resin in the determination of urinary porphobilinogen concentrations. *Clin Chim Acta* **164**:235, 1987.
404. Schreiber WE, Jamani A, Pudek MR: Screening tests for porphobilinogen are insensitive: The problem and its solution. *Am J Clin Path* **92**:644, 1989.
405. Reio L, Wetterberg L: False porphobilinogen reactions in the urine of mental patients. *JAMA* **207**:148, 1969.
406. Deacon AC, Peters TJ: Identification of acute porphyria: Evaluation of a commercial screening test for urinary porphobilinogen. *Ann Clin Biochem* **35**:726, 1998.
407. Grandchamp B, Phung N, Grelier M, Nordmann Y: The spectrophotometric determination of uroporphyrinogen I synthetase activity. *Clin Chim Acta* **70**:113, 1976.
408. Sassa S, Granick S, Bickers DR, Bradlow HL, Kappas A: A microassay for uroporphyrinogen I synthase, one of three abnormal enzyme activities in acute intermittent porphyria, and its application to the study of the genetics of this disease. *Proc Natl Acad Sci U S A* **71**:732, 1974.
409. Kauppinen R: Prognosis of acute porphyrias and molecular genetics of acute intermittent porphyria in Finland [Thesis], in 1992.
410. Anderson KE, Sassa S, Peterson CM, Kappas A: Increased erythrocyte uroporphyrinogen-I-synthetase, δ-aminolevulinic acid

dehydratase and protoporphyrin in hemolytic anemias. *Am J Med* **63**:359, 1977.

411. Nordmann Y, Grandchamp B, Grelier M, Phung NG, De Verneuil H: Detection of intermittent acute porphyria trait in children. *Lancet* **2**:201, 1976.
412. Blum M, Koehl C, Abecassis J: Variations in erythrocyte uroporphyrinogen I synthetase activity in nonporphyrias. *Clinica Chimica Acta* **87**:119, 1978.
413. Kostrzewska E, Gregor A: Increased activity of porphobilinogen deaminase in erythrocytes during attacks of acute intermittent porphyria. *Ann Clin Res* **18**:195, 1986.
414. Llewellyn DH, Kalsheker NA, Harrison PR, Goossens M: DNA polymorphism of human porphobilinogen deaminase gene in acute intermittent porphyria. *Lancet* **2**:706, 1987.
415. Lee JS, Anvret M, Lindsten J, Lannefelt L, Gellerfors P, Wetterberg L, Floderus Y, Thunell S: DNA polymorphisms within the porphobilinogen deaminase gene in two Swedish families with acute intermittent porphyria. *Hum Genet* **79**:379, 1988.
416. Schreiber WE, Jamani A, Ritchie B: Detection of a T/C polymorphism in the porphobilinogen deaminase gene by polymerase chain reaction amplification of specific alleles. *Clin Chem* **38**:2153, 1992.
417. Sagen E, Laegreid A, Anvret M, Lundin G, Lannfelt L, Lilius L, Floderus Y, Romslo I: Genetic carrier detection in Norwegian families with acute intermittent porphyria. *Scand J Clin Lab Invest* **53**:687, 1993.
418. Daimon M, Morita Y, Yamatani K, Igarashi M, Fukase N, Ohnuma H, Sugiyama K, Ogawa A, Manaka H, Tominaga M, Sasaki H: Two new polymorphisms in introns 2 and 3 of the human porphobilinogen deaminase gene. *Hum Genet* **92**:115, 1993.
419. Kauppinen R, Mustajoki S, Pihlaja H, Peltonen L, Mustajoki P: Acute intermittent porphyria in Finland: 19 mutations in the porphobilinogen deaminase gene. *Hum Mol Genet* **4**:215, 1995.
420. Sassa S, Solish G, Levere RD, Kappas A: Expression of the gene defect of acute intermittent porphyria in cultured human skin fibroblasts and amniotic cells: Prenatal diagnosis of the porphyric trait. *J Exp Med* **142**:722, 1975.
421. Watson CJ, Pierach CA, Bossenmaier I, Cardinal R: Use of hematin in the acute attack of the "inducible" hepatic porphyrias. *Adv Intern Med* **23**:265, 1978.
422. Lamon JM, Frykholm BC, Hess RA, Tschudy DP: Hematin therapy for acute porphyria. *Medicine* **58**:252, 1979.
423. McColl KEL, Moore MR, Thompson GG, Goldberg A: Treatment with haematin in acute hepatic porphyria. *QJM* **198**:161, 1981.
424. Herrick AL, McColl KEL, Moore MR, Cook A, Goldberg A: Controlled trial of haem arginate in acute hepatic porphyria. *Lancet* **1**:1295, 1989.
425. Pierach CA: Haem and porphyria [Letter]. *Lancet* **2**:213, 1989.
426. Herrick AL, McColl KEL, Moore MR, Goldberg A: Haem and porphyria [Reply]. *Lancet* **2**:213, 1989.
427. Anderson KE: The porphyrias, in Zakim D, Boyer T (eds.): *Hepatology*. Philadelphia, WB Saunders, 1996, p 417.
428. Mustajoki P, Tenhunen R, Tokola O, Gothani G: Haem arginate in the treatment of acute hepatic porphyrias. *BMJ* **293**:538, 1986.
429. Mustajoki P, Nordmann Y: Early administration of heme arginate for acute porphyric attacks. *Arch Int Med* **153**:2004, 1993.
430. Bissell DM: Treatment of acute hepatic porphyria with hematin. *J Hepatol* **6**:1, 1988.
431. Goetsch CA, Bissell DM: Instability of hematin used in the treatment of acute hepatic porphyria. *N Engl J Med* **315**:235, 1986.
432. Jones RL: Hematin-derived anticoagulant. Generation in vitro and in vivo. *J Exp Med* **163**:724, 1986.
433. Green D, Reynolds N, Klein J, Kohl H, Ts'ao CH: The inactivation of hemostatic factors by hematin. *J Lab Clin Med* **102**:361, 1983.
434. Khanderia U: Circulatory collapse associated with hemin therapy for acute intermittent porphyria. *Clin Pharmacy* **5**:690, 1986.
435. Jeelani Dhar G, Bossenmaier I, Cardinal R, Petryka ZJ, Watson CJ: Transitory renal failure following rapid administration of a relatively large amount of hematin in a patient with acute intermittent porphyria in clinical remission. *Acta Med Scand* **203**:437, 1978.
436. Tenhunen R, Mustajoki P: Acute porphyria: Treatment with heme. *Semin Liver Dis* **18**:53, 1998.
437. Bonkovsky HL, Healey BS, Lourie AN, Gerron GG: Intravenous heme-albumin in acute intermittent porphyria: Evidence for repletion of hepatic hemoproteins and regulatory heme pools. *Am J Gastroenterol* **86**:1050, 1991.
438. Fuchs T, Ippen H: Behandlung der akut intermittierenden porphyrie mit einem neuen, an albumin gebundenen lyophilisierten hämatin. *Dtsch Med Wochenschr* **112**:1302, 1987.
439. Tenhunen R, Tokola O, Lindén IB: Haem arginate: A new stable haem compound. *J Pharm Pharmacol* **39**:780, 1987.
440. Sievers G, Hakli H, Luhtala J, Tenhunen R: Optical and EPR spectroscopy studies on haem arginate, a new compound used for treatment of porphyria. *Chem Biol Interact* **63**:105, 1987.
441. Anderson KE, Egger NG, Goeger DE: Heme arginate for prevention of acute porphyric attacks [Abstract]. *Acta Haematol* **98(Suppl 1)**:120, 1997.
442. Galbraith RA, Drummond GS, Kappas A: Sn-protoporphyrin suppresses chemically induced experimental hepatic porphyria: Potential clinical implications. *Clin Invest* **76**:2436, 1985.
443. Galbraith RA, Kappas A: Pharmacokinetics of tin-mesoporphyrin in man and the effects of tin-chelated porphyrins on hyperexcretion of heme pathway precursors in patients with acute inducible porphyria. *Hepatology* **9**:882, 1989.
444. Dover SB, Graham A, Fitzsimons E, Moore MR, McColl KEL: Tin protoporphyrin prolongs the biochemical remission produced by heme arginate in acute hepatic porphyria. *Gastroenterology* **105**:500, 1993.
445. Russo SM, Pepe JA, Cable EE, Lambrecht RW, Bonkovsky HL: Repression of ALA synthase by heme and zinc-mesoporphyrin in a chick embryo liver cell culture model of acute porphyria. *Eur J Clin Invest* **24**:406, 1994.
446. Anderson KE, Alvares AP, Sassa S, Kappas A: Studies in porphyria. V. Drug oxidation rates in hereditary hepatic porphyria. *Clin Pharmacol Ther* **19**:47, 1976.
447. Herrick A, McColl KEL, McLellan A, Moore MR, Brodie MJ, Goldberg A: Effect of haem arginate therapy on porphyrin metabolism and mixed function oxygenase activity in acute hepatic porphyria. *Lancet* **2**:1178, 1987.
448. Mustajoki P, Himberg JJ, Tokola O, Tenhunen R: Rapid normalization of antipyrine oxidation by heme in variegate porphyria. *Clin Pharmacol Ther* **51**:320, 1992.
449. *Physicians' Desk Reference*. Montvale, NJ, Medical Economics, p. 3050, 2000.
450. Atsmon A, Blum I, Fischl J: Treatment of an acute attack of porphyria variegata with propranolol. *S Afr Med J* **46**:46:311, 1972.
451. Beattie AD, Moore MR, Goldberg A, Ward RL: Acute intermittent porphyria: response of tachycardia and hypertension to propranolol. *BMJ* **3**:257, 1973.
452. Schoenfeld N, Epstein O, Atsmon A: The effect of beta-adrenergic blocking agents on experimental porphyria induced by 3,5-diethoxycarbonyl-1,4-dihydrocollidine (DDC) in vivo and in vitro. *Biochim Biophys Acta* **444**:286, 1976.
453. Bonkowsky HL, Tschudy DP: Hazard of propranolol in treatment of acute porphyria. *BMJ* **4**:47, 1974.
454. Kappas A, Bradlow HL: Enhancement of 5α-steroid hormone metabolism in patients with acute intermittent porphyria following treatment with triiodothyronine, in Doss M (ed.): *Porphyrins and Human Disease*. Basel, S Karger, 1976, p 274.
455. Olsson RA, Ticktin HE: Zinc metabolism in acute intermittent porphyria. *J Lab Clin Med* **60**:48, 1962.
456. Peters HA, Cripps DJ, Reese HH: Porphyria: Types of etiology and treatment. *Int Rev Neurobiol* **16**:301, 1974.
457. Roman W, Oon R, West RF, Reid DP: Zinc sulphate in acute porphyria. *Lancet* **2**:716, 1967.
458. Winston SH, Tishler PV: Sorbent therapy of the porphyrias. V. Adsorption of the porphyrin precursors delta-aminolevulinic acid and porphobilinogen by sorbents in vitro. *Methods Find Exp Clin Pharmacol* **8**:233, 1986.
459. Siepmann M, Stolzel U, Sieg I, Leo-Rossberg I, Riecken EO, Doss MO: [Cimetidine in treatment of acute intermittent porphyria]. *Z Gastroenterol* **31**:246, 1993.
460. Gadjos A, Gadjos-Török M: Studies on the porphyrias in France. *S Afr J Lab Clin Med* **9**:295, 1963.
461. Watson CJ, Bossenmaier I, Cardinal R: Lack of significant effect of vitamin E on porphyrin metabolism: Report of four patients with various forms of porphyria. *Arch Intern Med* **131**:698, 1973.
462. Wider de Xifra EA, Del Battle AM, Stella AM, Malamud S: Acute intermittent porphyria: Another approach to therapy. *Int J Biochem* **12**:819, 1980.
463. Rees HA, Goldberg A, Cochrane AL, Williams MJ, Donald KW: Renal haemodialysis in porphyria. *Lancet* **1**:919, 1967.

464. Martasek P, Kordac V, Kotal P, Vacek J, Jirsa M, Horak J, Tomasek R: Recovery from a severe attack of acute intermittent porphyria during coated-resin hemoperfusion. *Intl J Artif Organs* **9**:117, 1986.
465. Thunell S, Andersson D, Harper P, Henrichson A, Floderus Y, Lindh U: Effects of administration of antioxidants in acute intermittent porphyria. *Eur J Clin Chem Clin Biochem* **35**:427, 1997.
466. Bonkowsky HL, Sinclair PR, Emery S, Sinclair JF: Seizure management in acute hepatic porphyria: risks of valproate and clonazepam. *Neurology* **30**:588, 1980.
467. Larson AW, Wasserstrom WR, Felsher BF, Shih JC: Posttraumatic epilepsy and acute intermittent porphyria: Effects of phenytoin, carbamazepine, and clonazepam. *Neurology* **28**:824, 1978.
468. Hahn M, Gildemeister OS, Krauss GL, Pepe JA, Lambrecht RW, Donohue S, Bonkovsky HL: Effects of new anticonvulsant medications on porphyrin synthesis in cultured liver cells: Potential implications for patients with acute porphyria. *Neurology* **49**:97, 1997.
469. Anderson KE, Goeger DE, Nagamani M: Invited lecture: A GnRH analogue for prevention of cyclic attacks of porphyria: Progress and prospects, in Blake D, McManus J, Ratnaike S, Hill J, Poulos V, Rossi E, (eds): Presented at the Porphyrins, Porphyrias and Photodynamic Therapy (Conference Proceedings), Melbourne, Australia, Proceedings: Abstract 52, 1993.
470. Yamamori I, Asai M, Tanaka F, Muramoto A, Hasegawa H: Prevention of premenstrual exacerbation of hereditary coproporphyria by gonadotropin-releasing hormone analogue [see comments]. *Intern Med* **38**:365, 1999.
471. Perlroth MG, Marver HS, Tschudy DP: Oral contraceptive agents and the management of acute intermittent porphyria. *JAMA* **194**:1037, 1965.
472. Schley G, Anlauf M, Bock KD: Orale kontrazeptiva zur prophylaxe akuter schübe der intermittierenden porphyrie. *Dtsch Med Wschr* **101**:1901, 1976.
473. Gross U, Honcamp M, Daume E, Frank M, Dusterberg B, Doss MO: Hormonal oral contraceptives, urinary porphyrin excretion and porphyrias. *Horm Metab Res* **27**:379, 1995.
474. White INH, Muller-Eberhard U: Decreased liver cytochrome P-450 in rats caused by norethindrone or ethynyloestradiol. *Biochem J* **166**:57, 1977.
475. Lamon JM, Frykholm BC, Herrera W, Tschudy DP: Danazol administration to females with menses-associated exacerbations of acute intermittent porphyria. *J Clin Endocrinol Metab* **48**:123, 1979.
476. Hughes MJ, Rifkind AB: Danazol, a new steroidal inducer of δ-aminolevulinic acid synthetase. *J Clin Endocrinol Metab* **52**:549, 1981.
477. Lamon JM, Frykholm BC, Bennett M, Tschudy DP: Prevention of acute porphyric attacks by intravenous haematin. *Lancet* **2**:492, 1978.
478. Romeo G, Levin EY: Uroporphyrinogen III cosynthetase in human congenital erythropoietic porphyria. *Proc Natl Acad Sci U S A* **63**:856, 1969.
479. Deybach JC, De Verneuil H, Phung N, Nordmann Y, Puissant A, Boffety B: Congenital erythropoietic porphyria (Günther's disease): Enzymatic studies on two cases of late onset. *J Lab Clin Med* **97**:551, 1981.
480. Fritsch C, Bolsen K, Ruzicka T, Goerz G: Congenital erythropoietic porphyria. *J Am Acad Dermatol* **36**:594, 1997.
481. Warner CA, Poh-Fitzpatrick MB, Zaider EF, Tsai SF, Desnick RJ: Congenital erythropoietic porphyria: A mild variant with low uroporphyrin I levels due to a missense mutation (A66V) encoding residual uroporphyrinogen III synthase activity. *Arch Dermatol* **128**:1243, 1992.
482. Pain RW, Welch FW, Woodroffe AJ, Handley DA, Lockwood WH: Erythropoietic uroporphyria of Gunther first presenting at 58 years with positive family studies. *BMJ* **3**:621, 1975.
483. Weston MJ, Nicholson DC, Lim CK, Clark KG, Macdonald A, Henderson MA, Williams R: Congenital erythropoietic uroporphyria (Gunther's disease) presenting in a middle aged man. *Int J Biochem* **9**:921, 1978.
484. Poh-Fitzpatrick MB: The erythropoietic porphyrias. *Dermatol Clin* **4**:291, 1986.
485. Kramer S, Viljoen E, Meyer AM, Metz J: The anemia of erythropoietic porphyria with the first description of the disease in an elderly patient. *Br J Haematol* **11**:666, 1965.
486. Rank JM, Straka JG, Weimer MK, Bossenmaier I, Taddeini BL, Bloomer JR: Hematin therapy in late onset congenital erythropoietic porphyria. *Br J Haematol* **75**:617, 1990.
487. Murphy A, Gibson G, Elder GH, Otridge BA, Murphy GM: Adult-onset congenital erythropoietic porphyria (Gunther's disease) presenting with thrombocytopenia. *J R Soc Med* **88**:357P, 1995.
488. Piomelli S, Poh-Fitzpatrick MB, Seaman C, Skolnick LM, Berdon WE: Complete suppression of the symptoms of congenital erythropoietic porphyria by long-term treatment with high-level transfusions. *N Engl J Med* **314**:1029, 1986.
489. Laorr A, Greenspan A: Severe osteopenia in congenital erythropoietic porphyria. *Can Assoc Radiol J* **45**:307, 1994.
490. Verstraeten L, Van Regemorter N, Pardou A, De Verneuil H, Da Silva V, Rodesch F, Vermeylen D, Donner C, Noel JC, Nordmann Y, Hassoun A: Biochemical diagnosis of a fatal case of Gunther's disease in a newborn with hydrops-fetalis. *Eur J Clin Chem Clin Biochem* **31**:121, 1993.
491. Schmid R, Schwartz S, Watson CJ: Porphyrin content of bone marrow and liver in the various forms of porphyria. *Arch Intern Med* **93**:167, 1954.
492. Rosenthal IM, Lipton EL, Asrow G: Effect of splenectomy on porphyria erythropoietica. *Pediatrics* **15**:663, 1955.
493. Aldrich RA, Hawkinson V, Geinstein M, Watson CJ: Photosensitive or congenital porphyria with hemolytic anemia I. Clinical and fundamental studies before and after splenectomy. *J Hematol* **6**:685, 1951.
494. Watson CJ, Perman V, Spurrell FA, Hoyt HH, Schwartz S: Some studies of the comparative biology of human and bovine erythropoietic porphyria. *Arch Int Med* **103**:436, 1959.
495. Heilmeyer VL, Clotten R, Kerp L, Merker H, Parra CA, Wetzel HP: Porphyria erythropoetica congenita Günther: Bericht über zwei familien mit erfassung der merkmalsträger. *Dtsch Med Wschr* **88**:2449, 1963.
496. Schmid R, Schwartz S, Sundberg RD: Erythropoietic (congenital) porphyria: A rare abnormality of the normoblasts. *Blood* **10**:416, 1955.
497. Schwartz S, O'Connor N, Stephenson BD, Anderson AS, Johnson LW, Johnson J: Turnover of erythrocyte protoporphyrin, with special reference to bovine porphyria and iron deficiency anemia. *Ann Clin Res* **8**:203, 1976.
498. Romeo G, Glenn BL, Levin EY: Uroporphyrinogen III cosynthetase in asymptomatic carriers of congenital erythropoietic porphyria. *Biochem Genet* **4**:719, 1970.
499. Freesemann AG, Bhutani LK, Jacob K, Doss MO: Interdependence between degree of porphyrin excess and disease severity in congenital erythropoietic porphyria (Gunther's disease). *Arch Dermatol Res* **289**:272, 1997.
500. Tsai SF, Bishop DF, Desnick RJ: Coupled-enzyme and direct assays for uroporphyrinogen III synthase activity in human erythrocytes and cultured lymphoblasts. *Anal Biochem* **166**:120, 1987.
501. Bogorad L: The enzymatic synthesis of porphyrins from porphobilinogen II. Uroporphyrin III. *J Biol Chem* **233**:1958.
502. Battersby AR, Fookes CJR, Gustafson-Potter KE, McDonald E, Matcham GWJ: Biosynthesis of porphyrins and related macrocycles. Part 18. Proof by spectroscopy and synthesis that unrearranged hydroxymethylbilane is the product from deaminase and substrate for cosynthase in the biosynthesis of uroporphyrinogen III. *J Chem Soc Perkin Trans* **1**:2427, 1982.
503. Battersby AR, Fookes CJR, Gustafson-Potter KE, McDonald E, Matcham GWJ: Biosynthesis of porphyrins and related macrocycles. Part 17. Chemical and enzymatic transformation of isomeric aminomethylbilanes into uroporphyrinogens: Proof that unrearranged bilanes are the preferred enzymatic substrate and detection of a transient intermediate. *J Chem Soc Perkin Trans* **1**:2413, 1982.
504. Stevens E, Frydman RB, Brydman B: Separation of porphobilinogen deaminase and uroporphyrinogen III cosynthase from human erythrocytes. *Biochim Biophys Acta* **158**:496, 1968.
505. Tsai SF, Bishop DF, Desnick RJ: Purification and properties of uroporphyrinogen III synthase from human erythrocytes. *J Biol Chem* **262**:1268, 1987.
506. Shoolingin-Jordan PM: Porphobilinogen deaminase and uroporphyrinogen III synthase: Structure, molecular biology, and mechanism. *J Bioenerg Biomembr* **27**:181, 1995.
507. Tsai SF, Bishop DF, Desnick RJ: Human uroporphyrinogen III synthase: Molecular cloning, nucleotide sequence and expression of a full-length cDNA. *Proc Natl Acad Sci U S A* **85**:7049, 1988.
508. Astrin KH, Warner CA, Yoo HW, Goodfellow PJ, Tsai SF, Desnick RJ: Regional assignment of the human uroporphyrinogen III synthase (UROS) gene to chromosome 10q25.2 $\rightarrow$ q26.3. *Hum Genet* **87**:18, 1991.

509. Warner CA, Yoo H-W, Tsai S-F, Roberts AG, Desnick RJ: Congenital erythropoietic porphyria: Characterization of the genomic structure and identification of mutations in the uroporphyrinogen III synthase gene. *Am J Hum Genet* **47**:83, 1990.
510. Bensidhoum M, Ged CM, Poirier C, Guenet JL, de Verneuil H: The cDNA sequence of mouse uroporphyrinogen III synthase and assignment to mouse chromosome 7. *Mamm Genome* **5**:728, 1994.
511. Xu W, Kozak CA, Desnick RJ: Uroporphyrinogen-III synthase: Molecular cloning, nucleotide sequence, expression of a mouse full-length cDNA, and its localization on mouse chromosome 7. *Genomics* **26**:556, 1995.
512. Aizencang GI, Solis C, Bishop DF, Warner C, Desnick RJ: Human uroporphyrinogen synthase: Alternative promoters generate housekeeping and erythroid transcripts, in review.
513. Xu W, Astrin KH, Desnick RJ: Molecular basis of congenital erythropoietic porphyria: Mutations in the human uroporphyrinogen III synthase gene. *Hum Mutat* **7**:187, 1996.
514. Fontanellas A, Bensidhoum M, Enriquez de Salamanca R, Moruno Tirado A, de Verneuil H, Ged C: A systematic analysis of the mutations of the uroporphyrinogen III synthase gene in congenital erythropoietic porphyria. *Eur J Hum Genet* **4**:274, 1996.
515. Desnick RJ, Glass IA, Xu W, Solis C, Astrin KH: Molecular genetics of congenital erythropoietic porphyria. *Semin Liver Dis* **18**:77, 1998.
516. Moruno Tirado A, Herrera Saval A, Martinez Montero E, Hernandez Hazanas F, Ceballos Aragon J, Ged C, de Verneuil H: Congenital erythropoietic porphyria, description of a new mutation in two brothers [Letter]. *Eur J Pediatr* **156**:817, 1997.
517. Takamura N, Hombrados I, Tanigawa K, Namba H, Nagayama Y, de Verneuil H, Yamashita S: Novel point mutation in the uroporphyrinogen III synthase gene causes congenital erythropoietic porphyria of a Japanese family. *Am J Med Genet* **70**:299, 1997.
518. Tezcan I, Xu W, Gurgey A, Tuncer M, Cetin M, Oner C, Yetgin S, Ersoy F, Aizencang G, Astrin KH, Desnick RJ: Congenital erythropoietic porphyria successfully treated by allogeneic bone marrow transplantation. *Blood* **92**:4053, 1998.
519. Freesemann AG, Gross U, Bensidhoum M, de Verneuil H, Doss MO: Immunological, enzymatic and biochemical studies of uroporphyrinogen III-synthase deficiency in 20 patients with congenital erythropoietic porphyria. *Eur J Biochem* **257**:149, 1998.
520. Barker DF, Shafer M, White R: Restriction sites containing CpG show a higher frequency of polymorphism in human DNA. *Cell* **36**:131, 1984.
521. Cooper DN, Krawczak M: The mutational spectrum of single base-pair substitutions causing human genetic disease: Patterns and predictions. *Hum Genet* **85**:55, 1990.
522. Frank J, Wang X, Lam HM, Aita VM, Jugert FK, Goerz G, Merk HF, Poh-Fitzpatrick MB, Christiano AM: C73R is a hotspot mutation in the uroporphyrinogen III synthase gene in congenital erythropoietic porphyria. *Ann Hum Genet* **62**:225, 1998.
523. Warner CA, Yoo HW, Roberts AG, Desnick RJ: Congenital erythropoietic porphyria: identification and expression of exonic mutations in the uroporphyrinogen III synthase gene. *J Clin Invest* **89**:693, 1992.
524. Xu W, Warner CA, Desnick RJ: Congenital erythropoietic porphyria: identification and expression of 10 mutations in the uroporphyrinogen III synthase gene. *J Clin Invest* **95**:905, 1995.
525. Bensidhoum M, Audine M, Fontanellas A, Gory P, Raymond S, Costet P, Daniel J, de Verneuil H, Ged C: The disruption of mouse uroporphyrinogen III synthase (uros) gene is fully lethal. *Acta Haematol* **98(Suppl 1)**:100, 1997.
526. Bickers DR, Pathak MA: The porphyrias, in Fitzpatrick TB, Eisen AZ, Wolff K, Freedberg IM, Austen KF (eds.): *Dermatology in General Medicine*. New York, McGraw-Hill, 1987, p 1679.
527. Shoolingin-Jordan PM, Leadbeater: Coupled assay for uroporphyrinogen III synthase. *Method Enzymol* **281**:327, 1997.
528. Kaiser IH: Brown amniotic fluid in congenital erythropoietic porphyria. *Obstet Gynecol* **56**:383, 1980.
529. Deybach JC, Grandchamp B, Grelier M, Nordmann Y, Boué J, Boué A, de Berranger P: Prenatal exclusion of congenital erythropoietic porphyria (Günther's disease) in a fetus at risk. *Hum Genet* **53**:217, 1980.
530. Ged C, Moreau-Gaudry F, Taine L, Hombrados I, Calvas P, Colombies P, De Verneuil H: Prenatal diagnosis in congenital erythropoietic porphyria by metabolic measurement and DNA mutation analysis. *Prenat Diagn* **16**:83, 1996.
531. Mathews-Roth MM: Carotenoids in erythropoietic protoporphyria and other photosensitivity diseases. *Ann NY Acad Sci* **691**:127, 1993.
532. Poh-Fitzpatrick MB, Piomelli S, Seaman C, Skolnick LM: Congenital erythropoietic porphyria: complete suppression of symptoms by long-term high-level transfusion with deferoxamine infusion iron rescue, in Orfanos CE, Stadler R, Gollnick H (eds.): *Dermatology in Five Continents*. Berlin, Springer-Verlag, 1988, p 876.
533. Guarini L, Piomelli S, Poh-Fitzpatrick MB: Hydroxyurea in congenital erythropoietic porphyria [Letter]. *N Engl J Med* **330**:1091, 1994.
534. Tishler PV, Winston SH: Rapid improvement in the chemical pathology of congenital erythropoietic porphyria with treatment with superactivated charcoal. *Meth Find Exp Clin Pharmacol* **12**:645, 1990.
535. Minder EI, Schneider-Yin X, Möll F: Lack of effect of oral charcoal in congenital erythropoietic porphyria [Letter]. *N Engl J Med* **330**:1092, 1994.
536. Gorchein A, Guo R, Lim CK, Raimundo A, Pullon HW, Bellingham AJ: Porphyrins in urine, plasma, erythrocytes, bile and faeces in a case of congenital erythropoietic porphyria (Gunther's disease) treated with blood transfusion and iron chelation: lack of benefit from oral charcoal. *Biomed Chromatogr* **12**:350, 1998.
537. Watson CJ, Bossenmaier I, Cardinal R, Petryka ZJ: Repression by hematin of porphyrin biosynthesis in erythrocyte precursors in congenital erythropoietic porphyria. *Proc Natl Acad Sci U S A* **71**:278, 1974.
538. Varadi S: Haematological aspects in a case of erythropoietic porphyria. *Br J Haematol* **4**:270, 1958.
539. Kaufman BM, Vickers HR, Rayne J, Ryan TJ: Congenital erythropoietic porphyria: Report of a case. *Br J Dermatol* **79**:21, 1967.
540. Moore MR, Thompson GG, Goldberg A: The biosynthesis of haem in congenital (erythropoietic) porphyria. *Int J Biochem* **9**:933, 1978.
541. Pimstone NR, Mukerji SK, Saicheur T, Lee J, Invited lecture: Utility of chloroquine therapy in two patients with congenital erythropoietic porphyria (CEP), in Blake D, McManus J, Ratnaike S, Hill J, Poulos V, Rossi E (eds.): Presented at the Porphyrins, Porphyrias and Photodynamic Therapy (Conference Proceedings), Melbourne, Australia, Proceedings. Abstract 62, 1993.
542. Lagarde C, Hamel-Teillac D, De Prost Y, Blanche S, Thomas C, Fischer A, Nordmann Y, Ged C, De Verneuil H: [Allogeneic bone marrow transplantation in congenital erythropoietic porphyria. Gunther's disease]. *Ann Dermatol Venereol* **125**:114, 1998.
543. Kauffman L, Evans D, Stevens R, Weinkove C: Bone-marrow transplantation for congenital erythropoietic porphyria. *Lancet* **337**:1510, 1991.
544. Thomas C, Ged C, Nordmann Y, de Verneuil H, Pellier I, Fischer A, Blanche S: Correction of congenital erythropoietic porphyria by bone marrow transplantation. *J Pediatr* **129**:453, 1996.
545. Zix-Kieffer I, Langer B, Eyer D, Acar G, Racadot E, Schlaeder G, Oberlin F, Lutz P: Successful cord blood stem cell transplantation for congenital erythropoietic porphyria (Gunther's disease). *Bone Marrow Transplant* **18**:217, 1996.
546. Fritsch C, Lang K, Bolsen K, Lehmann P, Ruzicka T: Congenital erythropoietic porphyria. *Skin Pharmacol Appl Skin Physiol* **11**:347, 1998.
547. Moreau-Gaudry F, Mazurier F, Bensidhoum M, Ged C, de Verneuil H: Metabolic correction of congenital erythropoietic porphyria by retrovirus-mediated gene transfer into Epstein-Barr virus-transformed B- cell lines. *Blood* **85**:1449, 1995.
548. Moreau-Gaudry F, Ged C, Barbot C, Mazurier F, Boiron JM, Bensidhoum M, Reiffers J, de Verneuil H: Correction of the enzyme defect in cultured congenital erythropoietic porphyria disease cells by retrovirus-mediated gene transfer. *Hum Gene Ther* **6**:13, 1995.
549. Kauppinen R, Glass IA, Aizencang G, Astrin KH, Atweh GF, Desnick RJ: Congenital erythropoietic porphyria: Prolonged high-level expression and correction of the heme biosynthetic defect by retroviral-mediated gene transfer into porphyric and erythroid cells. *Mol Genet Metab* **65**:10, 1998.
550. Moreau-Gaudry F, Barbot C, Mazurier F, Mahon FX, Reiffers J, Ged C, de Verneuil H: Correction of the enzyme deficit of bone marrow cells in congenital erythropoietic porphyria by retroviral gene transfer. *Hematol Cell Ther* **38**:217, 1996.
551. Mazurier F, Moreau-Gaudry F, Salesse S, Barbot C, Ged C, Reiffers J, de Verneuil H: Gene transfer of the uroporphyrinogen III synthase cDNA into haematopoietic progenitor cells in view of a future gene therapy in congenital erythropoietic porphyria. *J Inherit Metab Dis* **20**:247, 1997.
552. Elder GH: Porphyria cutanea tarda. *Semin Liver Dis* **18**:67, 1998.

553. Barnes HD: Porphyria in the Bantu races on the Witwaterrand. *S Afr Med J* **29**:781, 1955.
554. Roberts AG, Elder GH, De Salamanca RE, Herrero C, Lecha M, Mascaro JM: A mutation (G281E) of the human uroporphyrinogen decarboxylase gene causes both hepatoerythropoietic porphyria and overt familial porphyria cutanea tarda: biochemical and genetic studies on Spanish patients. *J Invest Dermatol* **104**:500, 1995.
555. Moran-Jimenez MJ, Ged C, Romana M, Enriquez De Salamanca R, Taieb A, Topi G, D'Alessandro L, de Verneuil H: Uroporphyrinogen decarboxylase: complete human gene sequence and molecular study of three families with hepatoerythropoietic porphyria. *Am J Hum Genet* **58**:712, 1996.
556. Meguro K, Fujita H, Ishida N, Akagi R, Kurihara T, Galbraith RA, Kappas A, Zabriskie JB, Toback AC, Harber LC, Sassa S: Molecular defects of uroporphyrinogen decarboxylase in a patient with mild hepatoerythropoietic porphyria. *J Invest Dermatol* **102**:681, 1994.
557. Grossman ME, Poh-Fitzpatrick MB: Porphyria cutanea tarda: Diagnosis and management. *Med Clin North Am* **64**:807, 1980.
558. Boffa MJ, Reed P, Weinkove C, Ead RD: Hypertrichosis as the presenting feature of porphyria cutanea tarda. *Clin Exp Dermatol* **20**:62, 1995.
559. Ichihashi M, Hasei K, Horikawa T: A case of porphyria cutanea tarda with experimental light urticaria. *Br J Dermatol* **113**:745, 1985.
560. Byrne JP, Boss JM, Dawber RP: Contraceptive pill-induced porphyria cutanea tarda presenting with onycholysis of the finger nails. *Postgrad Med J* **52**:535, 1976.
561. Proia AD, Anderson KE: The porphyrias, in Gold DH, Weingeist TA (eds.): *The Eye in Systemic Disease*. Philadelphia, JB Lippincott, 1990, p 398.
562. Hammer H, Korom I: Photodamage of the conjunctiva in patients with porphyria cutanea tarda. *Br J Ophthalmol* **76**:592, 1992.
563. Salmon JF, Strauss PC, Todd G, Murray AD: Acute scleritis in porphyria cutanea tarda. *Am J Ophthalmol* **109**:400, 1990.
564. Cormane RH, Szabo E, Hoo TT: Histopathology of the skin in acquired and hereditary porphyria cutanea tarda. *Br J Dermatol* **85**:531, 1971.
565. Epstein JH, Tuffanelli DL, Epstein WL: Cutaneous changes in the porphyrias: A microscopic study. *Arch Dermatol* **107**:689, 1973.
566. Caputo R, Berti E, Gasparini G, Monti M: The morphologic events of blister formation in porphyria cutanea tarda. *Int J Dermatol* **22**:467, 1983.
567. Klein GF, Hintner H, Schuler G, Fritsch P: Junctional blisters in acquired bullous disorders of the dermal-epidermal junction zone: Role of the lamina lucida as the mechanical locus minoris resistentiae. *Br J Dermatol* **109**:1983.
568. Parra CA, de Parra NP: Diameter of the collagen fibrils in the sclerodermatous skin of porphyria cutanea tarda. *Br J Dermatol* **100**:573, 1979.
569. Bickers DR, Keogh L, Rifkind AB, Harber LC, Kappas A: Studies in porphyria. VI. Biosynthesis of porphyrins in mammalian skin and in the skin of porphyric patients. *J Invest Dermatol* **68**:5, 1977.
570. Lim HW, Poh-Fitzpatrick MB, Gigli I: Activation of the complement system in patients with porphyrias after irradiation in vivo. *J Clin Invest* **74**:1961, 1984.
571. Meurer M, Schulte C, Weiler A, Goerz G: Photodynamic action of uroporphyria on the complement system in porphyria cutanea tarda. *Arch Dermatol Res* **277**:293, 1985.
572. Torinuki W, Miura T, Tagami H: Activation of complement by 405-nm light in serum from porphyria cutanea tarda. *Arch Dermatol Res* **277**:174, 1985.
573. Pigatto PD, Polenghi MM, Altomare GF, Giacchetti A, Cirillo R, Finzi AF: Complement cleavage products in the phototoxic reaction of porphyria cutanea tarda. *Br J Dermatol* **114**:567, 1986.
574. Sandberg S, Romslo I, Hovding G, Bjorndal T: Porphyrin-induced photodamage as related to the subcellular localization of the porphyrins. *Acta Derm Venereol Suppl* **100**:75, 1982.
575. Nomura N, Lim HW, Levin JL, Sassa S: Effect of soluble complement receptor type 1 on porphyrin-induced phototoxicity in guinea pigs. *J Photochem Photobiol B* **42**:28, 1998.
576. James KR, Cortes JM, Paradinas FJ: Demonstration of intracytoplasmic needle-like inclusions in hepatocytes of patients with porphyria cutanea tarda. *J Clin Pathol* **33**:899, 1980.
577. Enerbäck L, Lundvall O: Properties and distribution of liver fluorescence in porphyria cutanea tarda (PCT). *Virchows Arch Abt A Path Anat* **350**:293, 1970.
578. Cortés JM, Oliva H, Paradinas FJ, Hernandez-Guío C: The pathology of the liver in porphyria cutanea tarda. *Histopathology* **4**:471, 1980.
579. Kordac V: Frequency of occurrence of hepatocellular carcinoma in patients with porphyria cutanea tarda in long-term followup. *Neoplasma* **19**:135, 1972.
580. Baravalle E, Prieto J: Serum antibodies against porphyric hepatocytes in patients with porphyria cutanea tarda and liver disease. *Gastroenterology* **84**:1483, 1983.
581. Saunders SJ: Iron metabolism in symptomatic porphyria. *S Afr J Lab Clin Med* **9**:277, 1963.
582. Turnbull A, Baker H, Vernon-Roberts B, Magnus IA: Iron metabolism in porphyria cutanea tarda and in erythropoietic protoporphyria. *QJM* **42**:341, 1973.
583. Kramer S: Iron metabolism in the porphyrias. *S Afr J Lab Clin Med* **9**:283, 1963.
584. Lundvall O, Weinfeld A, Lundin P: Iron storage in porphyria cutanea tarda. *Acta Med Scand* **188**:37, 1970.
585. Reizenstein P, Hoglund S, Landegren J, Carlmark B, Forsberg K: Iron metabolism in porphyria cutanea tarda. *Acta Med Scand* **198**:95, 1975.
586. French TJ, Weir H, Dowdle E: Ferrokinetics in symptomatic porphyria. *S Afr J Lab Clin Med* **17**:62, 1971.
587. Grossman ME, Bickers DR, Poh-Fitzpatrick MB, DeLeo VA, Harber LC: Porphyria cutanea tarda. Clinical features and laboratory findings in 40 patients. *Am J Med* **67**:277, 1979.
588. D'Alessandro Gandolfo L, Griso D, Macri A, Biolcati G, Barlattani A, Topi GC: Iron and porphyria cutanea tarda. *Cell Mol Biol (Noisy-le-grand)* **43**:75, 1997.
589. Lundvall O: The effect of replenishment of iron stores after phlebotomy therapy in porphyria cutanea tarda. *Acta Med Scand* **189**:51, 1971.
590. Felsher BF, Jones ML, Redeker AG: Iron and hepatic uroporphyrin synthesis. Relation in porphyria cutanea tarda. *JAMA* **226**:663, 1973.
591. Fargion S, Fracanzani AL, Romano R, Cappellini MD, Fare M, Mattioli M, Piperno A, Ronchi G, Fiorelli G: Genetic hemochromatosis in Italian patients with porphyria cutanea tarda: possible explanation for iron overload. *J Hepatol* **24**:564, 1996.
592. Jackson H, Whatley SD, Morgan RR, Roberts AG, Worwood M, Elder GH: The haemochromatosis C282Y mutation in sporadic and familial porphyria cutanea tarda [Abstract]. *Acta Haematol* **98(Suppl 1)**:114, 1997.
593. Bonkovsky HL, Poh-Fitzpatrick M, Pimstone N, Obando J, Di Bisceglie A, Tattrie C, Tortorelli K, LeClair P, Mercurio MG, Lambrecht RW: Porphyria cutanea tarda, hepatitis C, and HFE gene mutations in North America. *Hepatology* **27**:1661, 1998.
594. Sampietro M, Piperno A, Lupica L, Arosio C, Vergani A, Corbetta N, Malosio I, Mattioli M, Fracanzani AL, Cappellini MD, Fiorelli G, Fargion S: High prevalence of the His63Asp HFE mutation in Italian patients with porphyria cutanea tarda. *Hepatology* **27**:181, 1998.
595. Stuart KA, Busfield F, Jazwinska EC, Gibson P, Butterworth LA, Cooksley WG, Powell LW, Crawford DH: The C282Y mutation in the haemochromatosis gene (HFE) and hepatitis C virus infection are independent cofactors for porphyria cutanea tarda in Australian patients. *J Hepatol* **28**:404, 1998.
596. Egger NG, Goeger DE, Miskovsky EP, Weinman SA, Payne DA, Anderson KE: Multiple risk factors including HFE mutations in porphyria cutanea tarda. *Gastroenterology* **116**:A1206, 1999.
597. Enriquez de Salamanca R, Morales P, Castro MJ, Rojo R, Gonzalez M, Arnaiz-Villena A: The most frequent HFE allele linked to porphyria cutanea tarda in Mediterraneans is His63Asp [Letter]. *Hepatology* **30**:819, 1999.
598. Fargion S, Piperno A, Cappellini MD, Sampietro M, Fracanzani AL, Romano R, Caldarelli R, Marcelli R, Vecchi L, Fiorelli G: Hepatitis-C virus and porphyria cutanea tarda — Evidence of a strong association. *Hepatology* **16**:1322, 1992.
599. Herrero C, Vicente A, Bruguera M, Ercilla MG, Barrera JM, Vidal J, Teres J, Mascaro JM, Rodes J: Is hepatitis C virus infection a trigger of porphyria cutanea tarda? *Lancet* **341**:788, 1993.
600. Chuang TY, Brashear R, Lewis C: Porphyria cutanea tarda and hepatitis C virus: A case-control study and meta-analysis of the literature. *J Am Acad Dermatol* **41**:31, 1999.
601. Stolzel U, Kostler E, Koszka C, Stoffler-Meilicke M, Schuppan D, Somasundaram R, Doss MO, Habermehl KO, Riecken EO: Low prevalence of hepatitis C virus infection in porphyria cutanea tarda in Germany. *Hepatology* **21**:1500, 1995.
602. Lamoril J, Andant C, Bogard C, Puy H, Gouya L, Pawlotsky JM, Da Silva V, Soule JC, Deybach JC, Nordmann Y: Epidemiology of hepatitis C and G in sporadic and familial porphyria cutanea tarda. *Hepatology* **27**:848, 1998.

603. Wissel PS, Sordillo P, Anderson KE, Sassa S, Savillo RL, Kappas A: Porphyria cutanea tarda associated with the acquired immune deficiency syndrome. *Am J Hematology* **25**:107, 1987.
604. Cohen PR: Porphyria cutanea tarda in human immunodeficiency virus-seropositive men: Case report and literature review. *J Acq Immun Defic Syndrome* **4**:1112, 1991.
605. Gafa S, Zannini A, Gabrielli C: Porphyria cutanea tarda and HIV infection — Effect of zidovudine treatment on a patient. *Infection* **20**:373, 1992.
606. Drobacheff C, Derancourt C, Van Landuyt H, Devred D, de Wazieres B, Cribier B, Rey D, Lang JM, Grosieux C, Kalis B, Laurent R: Porphyria cutanea tarda associated with human immunodeficiency virus infection. *Eur J Dermatol* **8**:492, 1998.
607. Felsher BF, Kushner JP: Hepatic siderosis and porphyria cutanea tarda: Relation of iron excess to the metabolic defect. *Semin Hematol* **14**:243, 1977.
608. Charlton RU, Jacobs P, Seftel H, Bothwell TH: Effect of alcohol on iron absorption. *BMJ* **2**:1427, 1964.
609. Sixel-Dietrich F, Doss M: Hereditary uroporphyrinogen-decarboxylase deficiency predisposing porphyria cutanea tarda (chronic hepatic porphyria) in females after oral contraceptive medication. *Arch Dermatol Res* **278**:13, 1985.
610. Saeed-uz-Zafar M, Gronewald WR, Bluhm GB: Co-existent Klinefelter's syndrome, acquired cutaneous hepatic porphyria and systemic lupus erythematosus. *Henry Ford Hosp Med J* **18**:227, 1970.
611. Rizzardini M, Smith AG: Sex differences in the metabolism of hexachlorobenzene by rats and the development of porphyria in females. *Biochem Pharmacol* **31**:3543, 1982.
612. Smith AG, Francis JE, Green JA, Greig JB, Wolf CR, Manson MM: Sex-linked hepatic uroporphyria and the induction of cytochromes P450IA in rats caused by hexachlorobenzene and polyhalogenated biphenyls. *Biochem Pharmacol* **40**:2059, 1990.
613. Morimoto M, Hagbjork AL, Nanji AA, Ingelman-Sundberg M, Lindros KO, Fu PC, Albano E, French SW: Role of cytochrome P4502E1 in alcoholic liver disease pathogenesis. *Alcohol* **10**:459, 1993.
614. Sinclair PR, Gorman G, Shedlofsky SI, Honsinger C, Sinclair JF, Karagas MR, Anderson KE: Ascorbic acid deficiency in porphyria cutanea tarda. *J Lab Clin Med* **130**:197, 1997.
615. Rocchi E, Stella AM, Cassanelli M, Borghi A, Nardella N, Seium Y, Caselgrande G: Liposoluble vitamins and naturally occurring carotenoids in porphyria cutanea tarda. *Eur J Clin Invest* **25**:510, 1995.
616. Sinclair PR, Gorman N, Walton HS, Bement WJ, Jacobs JM, Sinclair JF: Ascorbic acid inhibition of cytochrome P450-catalyzed uroporphyrin accumulation. *Arch Biochem Biophys* **304**:464, 1993.
617. Taljaard JJF, Shanley BC, Deppe WM, Joubert SM: Porphyrin metabolism in experimental hepatic siderosis in the rat. II. Combined effect of iron overload and hexachlorobenzene. *Br J Haematol* **23**:513, 1972.
618. Taljaard JJF, Shanley BC, Deppe WM, Joubert SM: Porphyrin metabolism in experimental hepatic siderosis in the rat. III. Effect of iron overload and hexachlorobenzene on the liver haem biosynthesis. *Br J Haematol* **23**:587, 1972.
619. Cripps DJ, Peters HA, Gocmen A, Dogramici I: Porphyria turcica due to hexachlorobenzene: a 20 to 30 year follow-up study on 204 patients. *Br J Dermatol* **3**:413, 1984.
620. Lynch RE, Lee GR, Kushner JP: Porphyria cutanea tarda associated with disinfectant misuse. *Arch Intern Med* **135**:549, 1975.
621. Doss M, Sauer H, Von Tiepermann R, Colombi AM: Development of chronic hepatic porphyria (porphyria cutanea tarda) with inherited uroporphyrinogen decarboxylase deficiency under exposure to dioxin. *Int J Biochem* **16**:369, 1984.
622. McConnell R, Anderson K, Russell W, Anderson KE, Clapp R, Silbergeld EK, Landrigan PJ: Angiosarcoma, porphyria cutanea tarda, and probable chloracne in a worker exposed to waste oil contaminated with 2,3,7,8-tetrachlorodibenzo-*p*-dioxin. *Br J Ind Med* **50**:699, 1993.
623. Franks AG, Pulini M, Bickers DR, Rayfield EJ, Harber LC: Carbohydrate metabolism in porphyria cutanea tarda. *Am J Med Sci* **277**:163, 1979.
624. Cram DL, Epstein JH, Tuffanelli DL: Lupus erythematosus and porphyria. *Arch Dermatol* **108**:779, 1973.
625. Gibson GE, McEvoy MT: Coexistence of lupus erythematosus and porphyria cutanea tarda in fifteen patients. *J Am Acad Dermatol* **38**:569, 1998.
626. Koszo F, Elder GH, Roberts A, Simon N: Uroporphyrinogen decarboxylase deficiency in hepatoerythropoietic porphyria: further evidence for genetic heterogeneity. *Br J Dermatol* **122**:365, 1990.
627. Fujita H, Sassa S, Toback AC, Kappas A: Immunochemical study of uroporphyrinogen decarboxylase in a patient with mild hepatoerythropoietic porphyria. *J Clin Invest* **79**:1533, 1987.
628. De Verneuil H, Beaumont C, Deybach J-C, Nordmann Y, Sfar Z, Kastally R: Enzymatic and immunological studies of uroporphyrinogen decarboxylase in familial porphyria cutanea tarda and hepatoerythropoietic porphyria. *Am J Hum Genet* **36**:613, 1984.
629. Hift RJ, Meissner PN, Todd G: Hepatoerythropoietic porphyria precipitated by viral hepatitis. *Gut* **34**:1632, 1993.
630. Elder GH: Porphyrin metabolism in porphyria cutanea tarda. *Semin Hematol* **14**:227, 1977.
631. Moore MR, Thompson GG, Allen BR, Hunter JA, Parker S: Plasma porphrin concentrations in porphyria cutanea tarda. *Clin Sci Mol Med* **45**:711, 1973.
632. Moran MJ, Fontanellas A, Santos JL, Enriquez de Salamanca R: Correlation between levels of free and protein-bound plasma porphyrin and urinary porphyrins in porphyria cutanea tarda. *Int J Biochem Cell Biol* **27**:585, 1995.
633. Malina L, Miller V, Magnus LA: Skin porphyrin assay in porphyria. *Clinica Chimica Acta* **83**:55, 1978.
634. Elder GH: Identification of a group of tetracarboxylate porphyrins, containing one acetate and three β-substituents, in faeces from patients with symptomatic cutaneous hepatic porphyria and from rats with porphyria due to hexachlorobenzene. *Biochem J* **126**:877, 1972.
635. Elder GH: The metabolism of porphyrins of the isocoproporphyrin series. *Enzyme* **17**:61, 1974.
636. Doss VM, Look D, Henning H, Lüders CJ, Dölle W, Strohmeyer G: Chronische hepatische porphyrien. *J Clin Chem Clin Biochem* **9**:471, 1971.
637. Berk PD, Blaschke TF, Scharschmidt BF, Waggoner JG, Berlin NI: A new approach to quantitation of the various sources of bilirubin in man. *J Lab Clin Med* **87**:767, 1976.
638. Dowdle E, Mustard P, Spong N, Eales L: The metabolism of [5-^{14}C]δ-aminolevulinic acid in normal and porphyric human subjects. *Clin Sci* **34**:233, 1968.
639. Blekkenhorst GH, Pimstone NR, Webber BL, Eales L: Hepatic haem metabolism in porphyria cutanea tarda (PCT): Enzymatic studies and their relation to liver ultrastructure. *Ann Clin Res* **8**:108, 1976.
640. Blekkenhorst GH, Eales L, Pimstone NR: The nature of hepatic cytochrome P-450 induced in hexachlorobenzene-fed rats. *Clin Sci Mol Med* **55**:461, 1978.
641. Kushner JP, Lee GR, Nacht S: The role of iron in the pathogenesis of porphyria cutanea tarda: an in vitro model. *J Clin Invest* **51**:3044, 1972.
642. Levin EY: Enzymatic properties of uroporphyrinogen III cosynthetase. *Biochemistry* **10**:4669, 1971.
643. Smith SG: Porphyrins found in urine of patients with symptomatic porphyria. *Biochem Soc Trans* **5**:1472, 1977.
644. Watson CJ: The problem of porphyria: some facts and questions. *N Engl J Med* **263**:1205, 1960.
645. Elder GH, Worwood M: Mutations in the hemochromatosis gene, porphyria cutanea tarda, and iron overload. *Hepatology* **27**:289, 1998.
646. Mauzerall D, Granick S: Porphyrin synthesis in erythrocytes: III. Uroporphyrinogen and its decarboxylase. *J Biol Chem* **232**:1141, 1958.
647. Smith AG, Francis JE: Decarboxylation of porphyrinogens by rat liver uroporphyrinogen decarboxylase. *Biochem J* **183**:455, 1979.
648. Neve RA, Labbe RF, Aldrich RA: Reduced uroporphyrin III in the biosynthesis of heme. *J Am Chem Soc* **78**:691, 1956.
649. Ippen H: Treatment of porphyria cutanea tarda by phlebotomy. *Semin Hematol* **14**:253, 1977.
650. Sweeney GD, Jones KG, Cole FM, Basford D, Kretynski F: Iron deficiency prevents liver toxicity of 2,3,7,8-tetrachlorodibenzo-*p*-dioxin. *Science* **204**:332, 1979.
651. Smith AG, Francis JE: Genetic variation of iron-induced uroporphyria in mice. *Biochem J* **291**:29, 1993.
652. Blekkenhorst GH, Day RS, Eales L: The effect of bleeding and iron administration on the development of hexachlorobenzene-induced rat porphyria. *Int J Biochem* **12**:1013, 1980.
653. Louw M, Neethling AC, Percy VA, Carstens M, Shanley BC: Effects of hexachlorobenzene feeding and iron overload on enzymes of haem biosynthesis and cytochrome P450 in rat liver. *Clin Sci Mol Med* **53**:111, 1977.

654. De Verneuil H, Sassa S, Kappas A: Purification and properties of uroporphyrinogen decarboxylase from human erythrocytes. *J Biol Chem* **258**:2454, 1983.
655. Elder GH, Tovey JA, Sheppard DM: Purification of uroporphyrinogen decarboxylase from human erythrocytes. Immunochemical evidence for a single protein with decarboxylase activity in human erythrocytes and liver. *Biochem J* **215**:45, 1983.
656. Elder GH, Roberts AG: Uroporphyrinogen decarboxylase. *J Bioenerg Biomembr* **27**:207, 1995.
657. Phillips JD, Whitby FG, Kushner JP, Hill CP: Characterization and crystallization of human uroporphyrinogen decarboxylase. *Protein Sci* **6**:1343, 1997.
658. Whitby FG, Phillips JD, Kushner JP, Hill CP: Crystal structure of human uroporphyrinogen decarboxylase. *EMBO J* **17**:2463, 1998.
659. Romeo PH, Dubart A, Grandchamp B, de Verneuil H, Rosa J, Nordmann Y, Goossens M: Isolation and identification of a cDNA clone coding for rat uroporphyrinogen decarboxylase. *Proc Natl Acad Sci U S A* **81**:3346, 1984.
660. Roméo PH, Raich N, Dubart A, Beaupain D, Pryor M, Kushner J, Solal MC, Goossens M: Molecular cloning and nucleotide sequence of a complete human uroporphyrinogen decarboxylase cDNA. *J Biol Chem* **261**:9825, 1986.
661. De Verneuil H, Grandchamp B, Foubert C, Weil D, N'Guyen VC, Gross MS, Sassa S, Nordmann Y: Assignment of the gene for uroporphyrinogen decarboxylase to human chromosome 1 by somatic cell hybridization and specific enzyme immunoassay. *Hum Genet* **66**:202, 1984.
662. Dubart A, Mattei MG, Raich N, Beaupain D, Romeo PH, Mattei JF, Goossens M: Assignment of human uroporphyrinogen decarboxylase (URO-D) to the p34 band of chromosome 1. *Hum Genet* **73**:277, 1986.
663. Roméo PH, Raich N, Dubart A, Beaupain D, Mattei MG, Goosens M: Molecular cloning and tissue-specific expression analysis of human porphobilinogen deaminase and uroporphyrinogen decarboxylase, in Nordmann Y (eds.): *Porphyrins and Porphyrias*. London, John Libbey, 1986, p 25.
664. McManus JF, Begley CG, Ratnaike S: Complex pattern of alternative splicing in the normal uroporphyrinogen decarboxylase gene: Implications for diagnosis of familial porphyria cutanea tarda. *Clin Chem* **40**:1884, 1994.
665. Garey JR, Hansen JL, Harrison LM, Kennedy JB, Kushner JP: A point mutation in the coding region of uroporphyrinogen decarboxylase associated with familial porphyria cutanea tarda. *Blood* **73**:892, 1989.
666. Garey JR, Harrison LM, Franklin KF, Metcalf KM, Radisky ES, Kushner JP: Uroporphyrinogen decarboxylase: A splice-site mutation causes the deletion of exon-6 in multiple families with porphyria cutanea tarda. *J Clin Invest* **86**:1416, 1990.
667. McManus JF, Begley CG, Sassa S, Ratnaike S: Five new mutations in the uroporphyrinogen decarboxylase gene identified in families with cutaneous porphyria. *Blood* **88**:3589, 1996.
668. Mendez M, Sorkin L, Rossetti MV, Astrin KH, del C. Batlle AM, Parera VE, Aizencang G, Desnick RJ: Familial porphyria cutanea tarda: Characterization of seven novel uroporphyrinogen decarboxylase mutations and frequency of common hemochromatosis alleles. *Am J Hum Genet* **63**:1363, 1998.
669. Christiansen L, Ged C, Hombrados I, Brons-Poulsen J, Fontanellas A, de Verneuil H, Horder M, Petersen NE: Screening for mutations in the uroporphyrinogen decarboxylase gene using denaturing gradient gel electrophoresis. Identification and characterization of six novel mutations associated with familial PCT. *Hum Mutat* **14**:222, 1999.
670. Garey JR, Franklin KF, Brown DA, Harrison LM, Metcalf KM, Kushner JP: Analysis of uroporphyrinogen decarboxylase complementary DNAs in sporadic porphyria cutanea tarda. *Gastroenterology* **105**:165, 1993.
671. De Verneuil H, Grandchamp B, Beaumont C, Picat C, Nordmann Y: Uroporphyrinogen decarboxylase structural mutant ($Gly^{281} \rightarrow Glu$) in a case of porphyria. *Science* **234**:732, 1986.
672. De Verneuil H, Grandchamp B, Romeo PH, Raich N, Beaumont C, Goossens M, Nicholas H, Nordmann Y: Molecular analysis of uroporphyrinogen decarboxylase deficiency in a family with two cases of hepatoerythropoietic porphyria. *J Clin Invest* **77**:431, 1986.
673. Kushner JP: personal communication.
674. De Matteis F: Drug induced abnormalities of liver heme biosynthesis, in Meeks RG, Harrison SD, Bull RJ (eds.): *Hepatotoxicology*. Boston, CRC Press, 1991, p 437.
675. Francis JE, Smith AG: Oxidation of uroporphyrinogens by hydroxyl radicals. Evidence for nonporphyrin products as potential inhibitors of uroporphyrinogen decarboxylase. *FEBS Lett* **233**:311, 1988.
676. Franklin MR, Phillips JD, Kushner JP: Cytochrome P450 induction, uroporphyrinogen decarboxylase depression, porphyrin accumulation and excretion, and gender influence in a 3-week rat model of porphyria cutanea tarda. *Toxicol Appl Pharmacol* **147**:289, 1997.
677. Legault N, Sabik H, Cooper SF, Charbonneau M: Effect of estradiol on the induction of porphyria by hexachlorobenzene in the rat. *Biochem Pharmacol* **54**:19, 1997.
678. Anderson KE, Vadhanavikit S, Goeger DE: Estrogen and antioxidants in hexachlorobenzene-induced hepatic porphyria in rats [Abstract]. *Hepatology* **22**:378A, 1995.
679. Akhtar RA, Smith AG: Chromosomal linkage analysis of porphyria in mice induced by hexachlorobenzene-iron synergism: A model of sporadic porphyria cutanea tarda. *Pharmacogenetics* **8**:485, 1998.
680. Francis JE, Smith AG: Polycyclic aromatic hydrocarbons cause hepatic porphyria in iron-loaded C57BL/10 mice: Comparison of uroporphyrinogen decarboxylase inhibition with induction of alkoxyphenoxazone dealkylations. *Biochem Biophys Res Comm* **146**:13, 1987.
681. De Matteis F: Role of iron in the hydrogen peroxide-dependent oxidation of hexahydroporphyrins (porphyrinogens): A possible mechanism for the exacerbation by iron of hepatic uroporphyria. *Molec Pharmacol* **33**:463, 1988.
682. Jacobs JM, Sinclair PR, Lambrecht RW, Sinclair JF: Effects of iron-EDTA on uroporphyrinogen oxidation by liver microsomes. *FEBS Lett* **250**:349, 1989.
683. Lambrecht RW, Sinclair PR, Gorman N, Sinclair JF: Uroporphyrinogen oxidation catalyzed by reconstituted cytochrome P450IA2. *Arch Biochem Biophys* **294**:504, 1992.
684. Sinclair PR, Gorman N, Dalton T, Walton HS, Bement WJ, Sinclair JF, Smith AG, Nebert DW: Uroporphyria produced in mice by iron and 5-aminolaevulinic acid does not occur in Cyp1a2(−/−) null mutant mice. *Biochem J* **330**:149, 1998.
685. Sinclair PR, Gorman N, Tsyrlov IB, Fuhr U, Walton HS, Sinclair JF: Uroporphyrinogen oxidation catalyzed by human cytochromes P450. *Drug Metab Dispos* **26**:1019, 1998.
686. Sinclair PR, Gorman N, Sinclair JF, Walton HS, Bement WJ, Lambrecht RW: Ascorbic acid inhibits chemically induced uroporphyria in ascorbate-requiring rats. *Hepatology* **22**:565, 1995.
687. Percy VA, Naidoo D, Joubert SM, Pegoraro RJ: Ascorbate status of patients with porphyria cutanea tarda symptomatica and its effect on porphyrin metabolism. *S Afr J Med Sci* **40**:185, 1975.
688. Sweeney GD: Porphyria cutanea tarda, or the uroporphyrinogen decarboxylase deficiency diseases. *Clin Biochem* **19**:3, 1986.
689. Constantin D, Francis JE, Akhtar RA, Clothier B, Smith AG: Uroporphyria induced by 5-aminolaevulinic acid alone in Ahrd SWR mice. *Biochem Pharmacol* **52**:1407, 1996.
690. Cederbaum AI: Oxygen radical generation by microsomes: Role of iron and implications for alcohol metabolism and toxicity. *Free Radic Biol Med* **7**:559, 1989.
691. Liehr JG: Vitamin C reduces the incidence and severity of renal tumors induced by estradiol or diethylstilbestrol. *Am J Clin Nutr* **54**:S1256, 1991.
692. Van Gelder W, Siersema PD, Voogd A, De Jeu-Jaspars NCM, Van Eijk HG, Koster JF, De Rooy FWM, Wilson JHP: The effect of desferrioxamine on iron metabolism and lipid peroxidation in hepatocytes of C57BL/10 mice in experimental uroporphyria. *Biochem Pharmacol* **46**:221, 1993.
693. Moran MJ, Fontanellas A, Brudieux E, Hombrados I, de Ledinghen V, Couzigou P, de Verneuil H, De Salamanca RE: Hepatic uroporphyrinogen decarboxylase activity in porphyria cutanea tarda patients: the influence of virus C infection. *Hepatology* **27**:584, 1998.
694. Poh-Fitzpatrick MB, Lamola AA: Direct spectrophotometry of diluted erythrocytes and plasma: A rapid diagnostic method in primary and secondary porphyrinemias. *J Lab Clin Med* **87**:362, 1976.
695. Poh-Fitzpatrick MB: A plasma porphyrin fluorescence marker for variegate porphyria. *Arch Dermatol* **116**:543, 1980.
696. Poh-Fitzpatrick MB, Sosin AE, Bemis J: Porphyrin levels in plasma and erythrocytes of chronic hemodialysis patients. *J Am Acad Dermatol* **7**:100, 1982.
697. Nomura N, Zolla-Pazner S, Simberkoff M, Kim M, Sassa S, Lim HW: Abnormal serum porphyrin levels in patients with the acquired immunodeficiency syndrome with or without hepatitis C virus infection. *Arch Dermatol* **132**:906, 1996.

698. Elder GH: Differentiation of porphyria cutanea tarda symptomatica from other types of porphyria by measurement of isocoproporphyrin in faeces. *J Clin Pathol* **28**:601, 1975.
699. Bogorad L: Porphyrin synthesis III. Uroporphyrinogen decarboxylase, in Colowick SP, Kaplan NO (eds.): *Methods in Enzymology*. Vol. 5. New York, Academic Press, 1962, p 885.
700. Ramsay CA, Magnus IA, Turnbull A, Barker H: The treatment or porphyria cutanea tarda by venesection. *QJM* **43**:1, 1974.
701. Topi GC, Amantea A, Griso D: Recovery from porphyria cutanea tarda with no specific therapy other than avoidance of hepatic toxins. *Br J Dermatol* **3**:75, 1984.
702. Timonen K, Niemi KM, Mustajoki P: Skin morphology in porphyria cutanea tarda does not improve despite clinical remission. *Clin Exp Dermatol* **16**:355, 1991.
703. Poh-Fitzpatrick MB: Childhood onset familial porphyria cutanea tarda: Effects of therapeutic phlebotomy. *J Am Academy Dermatol* **27**:896, 1992.
704. Bruce AJ, Ahmed I: Childhood-onset porphyria cutanea tarda: Successful therapy with low-dose hydroxychloroquine (Plaquenil). *J Am Acad Dermatol* **38**:810, 1998.
705. Rocchi E, Gibertini P, Cassanelli M, Pietrangelo A, Borghi A, Ventura E: Serum ferritin in the assessment of liver iron overload and iron removal therapy in porphyria cutanea tarda. *J Lab Clin Med* **107**:36, 1986.
706. Ratnaike S, Blake D, Campbell D, Cowen P, Varigos G: Plasma ferritin levels as a guide to the treatment of porphyria cutanea tarda by venesection. *Australas J Dermatol* **29**:3, 1988.
707. Adjarov D, Ivanov E: Clinical value of serum γ-glutamyl transferase estimation in porphyria cutanea tarda. *Br J Dermatol* **102**:541, 1980.
708. Chlumsky J, Malina L, Chlumská A: The effect of venesection therapy on liver tissue in porphyria cutanea tarda. *Acta Hepato-Gastroenterol* **20**:124, 1973.
709. Rocchi E, Cassanelli M, Ventura E: High weekly intravenous doses of desferrioxamine in porphyria cutanea tarda. *Br J Dermatol* **117**:393, 1987.
710. Rocchi E, Gibertini P, Cassanelli M, Pietrangelo A, Borghi A, Pantaleoni M, Jensen J, Ventura E: Iron removal therapy in porphyria cutanea tarda: phlebotomy versus slow subcutaneous desferrioxamine infusion. *Br J Dermatol* **114**:621, 1986.
711. Siegel LB, Eber BB: Porphyria cutanea tarda remission. *Ann Int Med* **121**:308, 1994.
712. Sheikh MY, Wright RA, Burruss JB: Dramatic resolution of skin lesions associated with porphyria cutanea tarda after interferon-alpha therapy in a case of chronic hepatitis C. *Dig Dis Sci* **43**:529, 1998.
713. Willson RA, Kirby P, Hart J: Association of chronic hepatitis C and porphyria cutanea tarda [Abstract]. *Hepatol* **16**:225A, 1992.
714. Valls V, Ena J, Enriquez-De-Salamanca R: Low-dose oral chloroquine in patients with porphyria cutanea tarda and low-moderate iron overload. *J Dermatol Sci* **7**:169, 1994.
715. Thornsvard MAJCT, Guider BA, Kimball DB: An unusual reaction to chloroquine-primaquine. *JAMA* **235**:1719, 1976.
716. Liu AC: Hepatotoxic reaction to chloroquine phosphate in a patient with previously unrecognized porphyria cutanea tarda. *West J Med* **162**:548, 1995.
717. Sweeney GD, Jones KG: Porphyria cutanea tarda: Clinical and laboratory features. *Can Med Assoc J* **120**:803, 1979.
718. Felsher BF, Redeker AG: Effect of chloroquine on hepatic uroporphyrin metabolism in patients with porphyria cutanea tarda. *Medicine* **45**:575, 1966.
719. Taljaard JJF, Shanley BC, Stewart-Wynne EG, Deppe WM, Joubert SM: Studies on low dose chloroquine therapy and the action of chloroquine in symptomatic porphyria. *Br J Derm* **87**:261, 1972.
720. Kordac V, Semradova M: Treatment of porphyria cutanea tarda with chloroquine. *Br J Derm* **90**:95, 1974.
721. Ashton RE, Hawk JLM, Magnus IA: Low-dose oral chloroquine in the treatment of porphyria cutanea tarda. *Br J Dermatol* **3**:609, 1984.
722. Malkinson FD, Levitt L: Hydroxychloroquine treatment of porphyria cutanea tarda. *Arch Dermat* **116**:1147, 1980.
723. Cohen SN, Phifer KO, Yielding KL: Complex formation between chloroquine and ferrihaemic acid in vitro, and its effect on the antimalarial action of chloroquine. *Nature* **202**:805, 1964.
724. Scholnick PL, Epstein J, Marver HS: The molecular basis of the action of chloroquine in porphyria cutanea tarda. *J Invest Dermatol* **61**:226, 1973.
725. Egger NG, Goeger DE, Anderson KE: Effects of chloroquine in hematoporphyrin-treated animals. *Chem Biol Interact* **102**:69, 1996.
726. Vizethum W, Dahlmann D, Bolsen K, Goerz G: Influence of chloroquine (Resochin) on hexachlorobenzene (HCB) induced porphyria of the rat. *Arch Dermat Res* **264**:125, 1979.
727. Chlumska A, Chlumsky J, Malina L: Liver changes in porphyria cutanea tarda patients treated with chloroquine. *Br J Dermatol* **102**:261, 1980.
728. Hebert AA, Farmer KL, Poh-Fitzpatrick MB: Peritoneal dialysis does not reduce serum porphyrin levels in porphyria cutanea tarda. *Nephron* **60**:240, 1992.
729. Anderson KE, Goeger DE, Carson RW, Lee S-MK, Stead RB: Erythropoietin for the treatment of porphyria cutanea tarda in a patient on long-term hemodialysis. *N Engl J Med* **322**:315, 1990.
730. Yaqoob M, Smyth J, Ahmad R, McClelland P, Fahal I, Kumar KAS, Yu R, Verbov J: Haemodialysis-related porphyria cutanea tarda and treatment by recombinant human erythropoietin. *Nephron* **60**:428, 1992.
731. Peces R, Enriquez de Salamanca R, Fontanellas A, Sanchez A, de la Torre M, Caparros G, Ferreras I, Nieto J: Successful treatment of haemodialysis-related porphyria cutanea tarda with erythropoietin. *Nephrol Dial Transplant* **9**:433, 1994.
732. Bell JD, Kincaid WR, Morgan RG, Bunce H III, Alperin JB, Sarles HE, Remmers AR Jr: Serum ferritin assay and bone-marrow iron stores in patients on maintenance hemodialysis. *Kidney Int* **17**:237, 1980.
733. Carson RW, Dunnigan EJ, DuBose TDJ, Goeger DE, Anderson KE: Removal of plasma porphyrins with high-flux hemodialysis in porphyria cutanea tarda associated with end-stage renal disease. *J Am Soc Nephrol* **2**:1445, 1992.
734. Stockenhuber F, Kurz R, Grimm G, Moser G, Balcke P: Successful treatment of hemodialysis related porphyria cutanea tarda with deferoxamine. *Nephron* **55**:321, 1990.
735. Disler P, Day R, Burman N, Blekkenhorst G, Eales L: Treatment of hemodialysis-related porphyria cutanea tarda with plasma exchange. *Am J Med* **72**:989, 1982.
736. Stevens BR, Fleischer AB, Piering F, Crosby DL: Porphyria cutanea tarda in the setting of renal failure: response to renal transplantation. *Arch Dermatol* **129**:337, 1993.
737. Harber LC, Bickers DR: Porphyria and pseudoporphyria. *J Invest Dermatol* **82**:1984.
738. Harvey E, Bell CH, Paller AS, Lavoo EJ, Hanna W, Balfe JW, Krafchik BR: Pseudoporphyria cutanea tarda: Two case reports on children receiving peritoneal dialysis and erythropoietin therapy. *J Pediatr* **121**:749, 1992.
739. Poh-Fitzpatrick M: Porphyria, pseudoporphyria, pseudopseudoporphyria. . .? *Arch Dermatol* **122**:403, 1986.
740. Pimstone NR, Gandhi SN, Mukerji SK: Therapeutic efficacy of oral charcoal in congenital erythropoietic porphyria. *N Engl J Med* **316**:390, 1987.
741. Fontanellas A, Mazurier F, Moreau-Gaudry F, Belloc F, Ged C, de Verneuil H: Correction of uroporphyrinogen decarboxylase deficiency (hepatoerythropoietic porphyria) in Epstein-Barr virus-transformed B-cell lines by retrovirus-mediated gene transfer: Fluorescence-based selection of transduced cells. *Blood* **94**:465, 1999.
742. Elder GH, Evans JO, Thomas N, Cox R, Brodie MJ, Moore MJ, Goldberg A, Nicholson DC: The primary enzyme defect in hereditary coproporphyria. *Lancet* **2**:1217, 1976.
743. Berger H, Goldberg A: Hereditary coproporphyria. *BMJ* **2**:85, 1955.
744. Nordmann Y, Grandchamp B, De Verneuil H, Phung L, Cartigny B, Fontaine G: Harderoporphyria: A variant hereditary coproporphyria. *J Clin Invest* **72**:1139, 1983.
745. Brodie MJ, Thompson GG, Moore MR, Beattie AD, Goldberg A: Hereditary coproporphyria. Demonstration of the abnormalities in haem biosynthesis in peripheral blood. *QJM* **46**:229, 1977.
746. Andrews J, Erdjument H, Nicholson DC: Hereditary coproporphyria: Incidence in a large English family. *J Med Genet* **21**:341, 1984.
747. Paxton JW, Moore MR, Beattie AD, Goldberg A: Urinary excretion of 17-oxosteroids in hereditary coproporphyria. *Clin Sci Molec Med* **49**:441, 1975.
748. Smith SG, El-Far MA: The effect of fasting and malnutrition on the liver porphyrins. *Int J Biochem* **12**:979, 1980.
749. Grandchamp B, Phung N, Nordmann Y: Homozygous case of hereditary coproporphyria. *Lancet* **2**:1348, 1977.
750. Carlson RE, Dolphin D, Bernstein M: Copper coproporphyrin: Excretion in familial coproporphyria. *Clin Chem* **24**:2009, 1978.
751. Granick S, Mauzerall D: Enzymes of porphyrin synthesis in red blood cells. *Ann N Y Acad Sci* **75**:115, 1958.

752. Zaman Z, Akhtar M: Mechanism and stereochemistry of vinyl-group formation in haem biosynthesis. *Eur J Biochem* **61**:215, 1976.
753. Battersby AR, Baldas J, Collins J, Grayson DH, James KJ, McDonald E: Mechanism of biosynthesis of the vinyl groups of protoporphyrin IX. *J Chem Soc Chem Commun* 1265, 1972.
754. Jackson AH, Jones DM, Philip G, Lash TD, Battle AMdC, Smith SG: Synthetic and biosynthetic studies of porphyrins. IV. Further studies of the conversion of coproporphyrinogen III to protoporphyrin IX: Mass spectrometric investigation of the incubation of specifically deuteriated coproporphyrinogen III with chicken red cell haemolysates. *Int J Biochem* **12**:681, 1980.
755. Sano S, Granick S: Mitochondrial coproporphyrinogen oxidase and protoporphyrin formation. *J Biol Chem* **236**:1173, 1961.
756. Del Batlle AM, Benson A, Rimington C: Purification and properties of coproporphyrinogenase. *Biochem J* **97**:731, 1965.
757. Poulson R, Polglase WJ: Aerobic and anaerobic coproporphyrinogenase activities in extracts from Saccharomyces cerevisiae. *J Biol Chem* **249**:6367, 1974.
758. Elder GH, Evans JO: Evidence that the coproporphyrinogen oxidase activity of rat liver is situated in the intermembrane space of mitochondria. *Biochem J* **172**:345, 1978.
759. Grandchamp B, Phung N, Nordmann Y: The mitochondrial localization of coproporphyrinogen III oxidase. *Biochem J* **176**:97, 1978.
760. Yoshinaga T, Sano S: Coproporphyrinogen oxidase. I. Purification, properties and activation by phospholipids. *J Biol Chem* **255**:4722, 1980.
761. Camadro JM, Chambon H, Jolles J, Labbe P: Purification and properties of coproporphyrinogen oxidase from the yeast Saccharomyces cerevisiae. *Eur J Biochem* **256**:579, 1986.
762. Bogard M, Camadro JM, Nordmann Y, Labbe P: Purification and properties of mouse liver coproporphyrinogen oxidase. *Eur J Biochem* **181**:417, 1989.
763. Medlock AE, Dailey HA: Human coproporphyrinogen oxidase is not a metalloprotein. *J Biol Chem* **271**:32507, 1996.
764. Martasek P, Camadro JM, Raman CS, Lecomte MC, Le Caer JP, Demeler B, Grandchamp B, Labbe P: Human coproporphyrinogen oxidase. Biochemical characterization of recombinant normal and R231W mutated enzymes expressed in E. coli as soluble, catalytically active homodimers. *Cell Mol Biol (Noisy-le-grand)* **43**:47, 1997.
765. Zagorec M, Buhler JM, Treich I, Keng T, Guarente L, Labbe Bois R: Isolation, sequence, and regulation by oxygen of the yeast HEM13 gene coding for coproporphyrinogen oxidase. *J Biol Chem* **263**:9718, 1988.
766. Taketani S, Kohno H, Furukawa T, Yoshinaga T, Tokunaga R: Molecular cloning, sequencing and expression of cDNA encoding human coproporphyrinogen oxidase. *Biochim Biophys Acta Bioenerg* **1183**:547, 1994.
767. Martasek P, Camadro JM, Delfaularue MH, Dumas JB, Montagne JJ, Deverneuil H, Labbe P, Grandchamp B: Molecular cloning, sequencing, and functional expression of a cDNA encoding human coproporphyrinogen oxidase. *Proc Natl Acad Sci U S A* **91**:3024, 1994.
768. Delfau-Larue MH, Martasek P, Grandchamp B: Coproporphyrinogen oxidase: Gene organization and description of a mutation leading to exon 6 skipping. *Hum Mol Genet* **3**:1325, 1994.
769. Cacheux V, Martasek P, Fougerousse F, Delfau MH, Druart L, Tachdjian G, Grandchamp B: Localization of the human coproporphyrinogen oxidase gene to chromosome band 3q12. *Hum Genet* **94**:557, 1994.
770. Conder LH, Woodard SI, Dailey HA: Multiple mechanisms for the regulation of haem synthesis during erythroid cell differentiation. Possible role for coproporphyrinogen oxidase. *Biochem J* **275**:321, 1991.
771. Taketani S, Yoshinaga T, Furukawa T, Kohno H, Tokunaga R, Nishimura K, Inokuchi H: Induction of terminal enzymes for heme biosynthesis during differentiation of mouse erythroleukemia cells. *Eur J Biochem* **230**:760, 1995.
772. Takahashi S, Taketani S, Akasaka J, Kobayashi A, Hayashi H, Yamamoto M, Nagai T: Differential regulation of mouse coproporphyrinogen oxidase gene expression in erythroid and non-erythroid cells. *Blood* **92**:3436, 1998.
773. Martasek P: Hereditary coproporphyria. *Semin Liver Dis* **18**:25, 1998.
774. Rosipal R, Lamoril J, Puy H, Da Silva V, Gouya L, De Rooij FW, Te Velde K, Nordmann Y, Martasek P, Deybach JC: Systematic analysis of coproporphyrinogen oxidase gene defects in hereditary coproporphyria and mutation update. *Hum Mutat* **13**:44, 1999.
775. Martasek P, Nordmann Y, Grandchamp B: Homozygous hereditary coproporphyria caused by an arginine to tryptophane substitution in coproporphyrinogen oxidase and common intragenic polymorphisms. *Hum Mol Genet* **3**:477, 1994.
776. Lamoril J, Martasek P, Deybach JC, Da SV, Grandchamp B, Nordmann Y: A molecular defect in coproporphyrinogen oxidase gene causing harderoporphyria, a variant form of hereditary coproporphyria. *Hum Mol Genet* **4**:275, 1995.
777. Lamoril J, Puy H, Gouya L, Rosipal R, Da Silva V, Grandchamp B, Foint T, Bader-Meunier B, Dommergues JP, Deybach JC, Nordmann Y: Neonatal hemolytic anemia due to inherited harderoporphyria: Clinical characteristics and molecular basis. *Blood* **91**:1453, 1998.
778. Blake D, McManus J, Cronin V, Ratnaike S: Fecal coproporphyrin isomers in hereditary coproporphyria. *Clin Chem* **38**:96, 1992.
779. Elder GH, Smith SG, Jane Smyth S: Laboratory investigation of the porphyrias. *Ann Clin Biochem* **27**:395, 1990.
780. Moder KG: A coproporphyria-like syndrome induced by glipizide. *Mayo Clin Proc* **66**:312, 1991.
781. Elder GH, Evans JO: A radiochemical method for the measurement of coproporphyrinogen oxidase and the utilization of substrates other than coproporphyrinogen III by the enzyme from rat liver. *Biochem J* **169**:205, 1978.
782. Grandchamp B, Nordmann Y: Decreased lymphocyte coproporphyrinogen III oxidase activity in hereditary coproporphyria. *Biochem Biophys Res Commun* **74**:1089, 1977.
783. Grandchamp B, Nordmann Y: Coproporphyrinogen III oxidase assay. *Enzyme* **28**:196, 1982.
784. Labbe P, Camadro JM, Chambon H: Fluorometric assays for coproporphyrinogen oxidase and protoporphyrinogen oxidase. *Anal Biochem* **149**:248, 1985.
785. Li F, Lim CK, Peters TJ: A high-performance-liquid-chromatographic method for the assay of coproporphyrinogen oxidase activity in rat liver. *Biochem J* **239**:481, 1986.
786. Manning DJ, Gray TA: Haem arginate in acute hereditary coproporphyria. *Arch Dis Child* **66**:730, 1991.
787. Hunter JAA, Khan SA, Hope E, Beattie AD, Beveridge GW, Smith AWM, Goldberg A: Hereditary coproporphyria. Photosensitivity, jaundice and neuropsychiatric manifestations associated with pregnancy. *Br J Dermatol* **84**:301, 1971.
788. Kirsch RE, Meissner PN, Hift RJ: Variegate porphyria. *Semin Liver Dis* **18**:33, 1998.
789. Hift RJ, Meissner PN, Todd G, Kirby P, Bilsland D, Collins P, Ferguson J, Moore MR: Homozygous variegate porphyria: an evolving clinical syndrome [published erratum appears in *Postgrad Med J* 70(829):855, 1994]. *Postgrad Med J* **69**:781, 1993.
790. Roberts AG, Puy H, Dailey TA, Morgan RR, Whatley SD, Dailey HA, Martasek P, Nordmann Y, Deybach JC, Elder GH: Molecular characterization of homozygous variegate porphyria. *Hum Mol Genet* **7**:1921, 1998.
791. Meissner PN, Dailey TA, Hift RJ, Ziman M, Corrigall AV, Roberts AG, Meissner DM, Kirsch RE, Dailey HA: A R59W mutation in human protoporphyrinogen oxidase results in decreased enzyme activity and is prevalent in South Africans with variegate porphyria. *Nat Genet* **13**:95, 1996.
792. Mustajoki P: Variegate porphyria. Twelve years' experience in Finland. *QJM* **44**:191, 1980.
793. Whatley SD, Puy H, Morgan RR, Robreau AM, Roberts AG, Nordmann Y, Elder GH, Deybach JC: Variegate porphyria in Western Europe: Identification of PPOX gene mutations in 104 families, extent of allelic heterogeneity, and absence of correlation between phenotype and type of mutation. *Am J Hum Genet* **65**:984, 1999.
794. Day RS: Variegate porphyria. *Semin Dermatol* **5**:138, 1986.
795. Timonen K, Niemi KM, Mustajoki P, Tenhunen R: Skin changes in variegate porphyria. Clinical, histopathological, and ultrastructural study. *Arch Dermatol Res* **282**:108, 1990.
796. Muhlbauer JE, Pathak MA, Tishler PV, Fitzpatrick TB: Variegate porphyria in New England. *JAMA* **247**:3095, 1982.
797. Grabczynska SA, McGregor JM, Hawk JL: Late onset variegate porphyria. *Clin Exp Dermatol* **21**:353, 1996.
798. Perlroth MG, Tschudy DP, Ratner A, Spaur W, Redeker A: The effect of diet in variegate (South African genetic) porphyria. *Metabolism* **17**:571, 1968.
799. Quiroz-Kendall E, Wilson FA, King LE Jr: Acute variegate porphyria following a Scarsdale gourmet diet. *J Am Acad Dermatol* **8**:46, 1983.
800. McGrath H, Taaffe JA, Gilsenan D, Cunnane K: An Irish family with variegate porphyria. *Clin Exp Dermatol* **9**:583, 1984.
801. Mascaro JM, Bruguera M, Herrero C, Lecha M, Muniesa AM: Microscopic abnormalities in the liver of two patients with porphyria variegata. *J Cutan Pathol* **12**:395, 1985.

802. Germanaud J, Luthier F, Causse X, Kerdraon R, Grossetti D, Gargot D, Nordmann Y: A case of association between hepatocellular carcinoma and porphyria variegata. *Scand J Gastroenterol* **29**:671, 1994.
803. Tidman MJ, Higgins EM, Elder GH, MacDonald DM: Variegate porphyria associated with hepatocellular carcinoma. *Br J Dermatol* **121**:503, 1989.
804. Kordac V, Martásek P, Zeman J, Rubín A: Increased erythrocyte protoporphyrin in homozygous variegate porphyria. *Photodermatology* **2**:257, 1985.
805. Murphy GM, Hawk JLM, Magnus IA, Barrett DF, Elder GH, Smith SG: Homozygous variegate porphyria: Two similar cases in unrelated families. *J R Soc Med* **79**:361, 1986.
806. Mustajoki P, Tenhunen R, Niemi KM, Nordmann Y, Kääriäinen H, Norio R: Homozygous variegate porphyria. *Clin Genet* **32**:300, 1987.
807. Coakley J, Hawkins R, Crinis N, McManus J, Blake D, Nordmann Y, Sloan L, Connelly J: An unusual case of variegate porphyria with possible homozygous inheritance. *Aust N Z J Med* **20**:587, 1990.
808. Norris PG, Elder GH, Hawk JL: Homozygous variegate porphyria: A case report. *Br J Dermatol* **122**:253, 1990.
809. Longas MO, Poh-Fitzpatrick MB: A tightly bound protein-porphyrin complex isolated from the plasma of a patient with variegate porphyria. *Clin Chim Acta* **118**:219, 1982.
810. Martasek P, Kordac V, Jirsa M: Variegate porphyria and porphyria cutanea tarda [Letter]. *Arch Dermatol* **119**:537, 1983.
811. Logan GM, Weimer MK, Ellefson M, Pierach CA, Bloomer JR: Bile porphyrin analysis in the evaluation of variegate porphyria. *N Engl J Med* **324**:1408, 1991.
812. Herrick AL, Moore MR, Thompson GG, Ford GP, McColl KE: Cholelithiasis in patients with variegate porphyria. *J Hepatol* **12**:50, 1991.
813. Smith SC, Belcher RV, Mahler R, Yudkin J: Bile and faecal porphyrins in the quiescent phase of variegate porphyria. *Biochem J* **110**:15P, 1968.
814. Smith SG, Belcher RV, Mahler R, Yudkin J: Preliminary studies on bile porphyrins in the quiescent phase of variegate porphyria. *Clin Chim Acta* **23**:241, 1969.
815. Rimington C, Lockwood WH, Belcher RV: The excretion of porphyrin-peptide conjugates in porphyria variegata. *Clin Sci* **35**:211, 1968.
816. Elder GH, Magnus IA, Handa F, Doyle M: Faecal "X porphyrin" in the hepatic porphyrias. *Enzyme* **17**:29, 1974.
817. Brenner DA, Bloomer JR: The enzymatic defect in variegate porphyria: Studies with human cultured skin fibroblasts. *N Engl J Med* **302**:765, 1980.
818. Deybach JC, De Verneuil H, Nordmann Y: The inherited enzymatic defect in porphyria variegata. *Hum Genet* **58**:425, 1981.
819. Viljoen DJ, Cummins R, Alexopoulos J, Kramer S: Protoporphyrinogen oxidase and ferrochelatase in porphyria variegata. *Eur J Clin Invest* **13**:283, 1983.
820. Meissner PN, Day RS, Moore MR, Disler PB, Harley E: Protoporphyrinogen oxidase and porphobilinogen deaminase in variegate porphyria. *Eur J Clin Invest* **16**:257, 1986.
821. Li F, Lim CK, Simpson KJ, Peters TJ: Coproporphyrinogen oxidase, protoporphyrinogen oxidase and ferrochelatase activities in human liver biopsies with special reference to alcoholic liver disease. *J Hepatol* **8**:86, 1989.
822. Poulson R: The enzymic conversion of protoporphyrinogen IX to protoporphyrin IX in mammalian mitochondria. *J Biol Chem* **251**:3730, 1976.
823. Jacobs NJ, Jacobs JM: Fumarate as alternate electron acceptor for the late steps of anaerobic heme synthesis in Escherichia coli. *Biochem Biophys Res Commun* **65**:435, 1975.
824. Jacobs NJ, Jacobs JM: Nitrate, fumarate, and oxygen as electron acceptors for a late step in microbial heme synthesis. *Biochim Biophys Acta* **449**:1, 1976.
825. Poulson R, Polglase WJ: The enzymic conversion of protoporphyrinogen IX to protoporphyrin IX. Protoporphyrinogen oxidase activity in mitochondrial extracts of Saccharomyces cerevisiae. *J Biol Chem* **250**:1269, 1975.
826. Brenner DA, Bloomer JR: A fluorometric assay for measurement of protoporphyrinogen oxidase activity in mammalian tissue. *Clin Chim Acta* **100**:259, 1980.
827. Duke SO, Lydon J, Becerril JS, Sherman TD, Lehnen LP Jr, Matsumoto H: Protoporphyrinogen oxidase-inhibiting herbicides. *Weed Sci* **39**:465, 1991.
828. Nishimura K, Taketani S, Inokuchi H: Cloning of a human cDNA for protoporphyrinogen oxidase by complementation in vivo of a hemG mutant of *Escherichia coli*. *J Biol Chem* **270**:8076, 1995.
829. Puy H, Robreau AM, Rosipal R, Nordmann Y, Deybach JC: Protoporphyrinogen oxidase: Complete genomic sequence and polymorphisms in the human gene. *Biochem Biophys Res Commun* **226**:226, 1996.
830. Taketani S, Inazawa J, Abe T, Furukawa T, Kohno H, Tokunaga R, Nishimura K, Inokuchi H: The human protoporphyrinogen oxidase gene (PPOX): Organization and location to chromosome 1. *Genomics* **29**:698, 1995.
831. Dailey TA, Dailey HA, Meissner P, Prasad AR: Cloning, sequence, and expression of mouse protoporphyrinogen oxidase. *Arch Biochem Biophys* **324**:379, 1995.
832. Roberts AG, Whatley SD, Daniels J, Holmans P, Fenton I, Owen MJ, Thompson P, Long C, Elder GH: Partial characterization and assignment of the gene for protoporphyrinogen oxidase and variegate porphyria to human chromosome 1q23. *Hum Mol Genet* **4**:2387, 1995.
833. Dailey TA, Dailey HA: Human protoporphyrinogen oxidase: Expression, purification, and characterization of the cloned enzyme. *Protein Sci* **5**:98, 1996.
834. Deybach JC, Da Silva V, Grandchamp B, Nordmann Y: The mitochondrial location of protoporphyrinogen oxidase. *Eur J Biochem* **149**:431, 1985.
835. Ferreira GC, Andrew TL, Karr SW, Dailey HA: Organization of the terminal two enzymes of the heme biosynthetic pathway. Orientation of protoporphyrinogen oxidase and evidence for a membrane complex. *J Biol Chem* **263**:3835, 1988.
836. Frank J, McGrath J, Lam H, Graham RM, Hawk JL, Christiano AM: Homozygous variegate porphyria: identification of mutations on both alleles of the protoporphyrinogen oxidase gene in a severely affected proband. *J Invest Dermatol* **110**:452, 1998.
837. Strand LJ, Felsher BF, Redeker AG, Marver HS: Heme biosynthesis in intermittent acute porphyria: Decreased hepatic conversion of porphobilinogen to porphyrins and increased delta-aminolevulinic acid synthetase activity. *Proc Natl Acad Sci U S A* **67**:1315, 1970.
838. Masuya T: Pathophysiological observations on porphyrias. *Acta Hematol Jpn* **32**:465, 1969.
839. Dowdle EB, Mustard P, Eales L: δ-Aminolevulinic acid synthetase activity in normal and porphyric human livers. *S Afr Med J* **41**:1093, 1967.
840. Meissner P, Adams P, Kirsch R: Allosteric inhibition of human lymphoblast and purified porphobilinogen deaminase by protoporphyrinogen and coproporphyrinogen. A possible mechanism for the acute attack of variegate porphyria. *J Clin Invest* **91**:1436, 1993.
841. Day RS, Blekkenhorst GH, Eales L: Hepatic porphyrins in variegate porphyria [Letter]. *N Engl J Med* **303**:1368, 1980.
842. Long C, Smyth SJ, Woolf J, Murphy GM, Finlay AY, Newcombe RG, Elder GH: Detection of latent variegate porphyria by fluorescence emission spectroscopy of plasma. *Br J Dermatol* **129**:9, 1993.
843. Lim CK, Rideout JM, Peters TJ: Pseudoporphyria associated with consumption of brewers' yeast. *BMJ* **288**:1640, 1984.
844. Da Silva V, Simonin S, Deybach JC, Puy H, Nordmann Y: Variegate porphyria: Diagnostic value of fluorometric scanning of plasma porphyrins. *Clin Chim Acta* **238**:163, 1995.
845. Jacobs NJ, Jacobs JM: Assay for enzymatic protoporphyrinogen oxidation, a late step in heme synthesis. *Enzyme* **28**:206, 1982.
846. Hift RJ, Meissner PN, Corrigall AV, Ziman MR, Petersen LA, Meissner DM, Davidson BP, Sutherland J, Dailey HA, Kirsch RE: Variegate porphyria in South Africa, 1688-1996—New developments in an old disease. *S Afr Med J* **87**:722, 1997.
847. Timonen K, Mustajoki P, Tenhunen R, Lauharanta J: Effects of haem arginate on variegate porphyria. *Br J Dermatol* **123**:381, 1990.
848. Cramers M, Jepsen LV: Porphyria variegata: Failure of chloroquin treatment. *Acta Derm Venereol* **60**:89, 1980.
849. Magnus IA, Jarrett A, Prankert TAJ, Rimington C: Erythropoietic protoporphyria: A new porphyria syndrome with solar urticaria due to protoporphyrinaemia. *Lancet* **2**:448, 1961.
850. De Leo VA, Poh-Fitzpatrick M, Mathews-Roth M, Harber LC: Erythropoietic protoporphyria. 10 years experience. *Am J Med* **60**:8, 1976.
851. Poh-Fitzpatrick MB: Erythropoietic porphyrias: Current mechanistic, diagnostic, and therapeutic considerations. *Semin Hematol* **14**:211, 1977.
852. Schmidt H, Snitker G, Thomsen K, Lintrup J: Erythropoietic protoporphyria. A clinical study based on 29 cases in 14 families. *Arch Dermatol* **110**:58, 1974.
853. Bopp C, Bakos L, da Grace Busko M: Erythropoietic protoporphyria. *Int J Biochem* **12**:909, 1980.

854. Eales L: Liver involvement in erythropoietic protoporphyria (EPP). *Int J Biochem* **12**:915, 1980.
855. Rank JF, Carithers R, Bloomer J: Evidence for neurological dysfunction in end-stage protoporphyric liver disease. *Hepatol* **18**:1404, 1993.
856. Poh-Fitzpatrick MB: Human protoporphyria: long-term variance in protoporphyrin balance in RBC and fecal distribution compartments in 24 patients. *J Invest Dermatol* **94**:567, 1990.
857. Poh-Fitzpatrick MB: Human protoporphyria: reduced cutaneous photosensitivity and lower erythrocyte porphyrin levels during pregnancy. *J Am Acad Dermatol* **36**:40, 1997.
858. Bewley AP, Keefe M, White JE: Erythropoietic protoporphyria improving during pregnancy. *Br J Dermatol* **139**:145, 1998.
859. Bottomley SS, Tanaka M, Everett MA: Diminished erythroid ferrochelatase activity in protoporphyria. *J Lab Clin Med* **86**:126, 1975.
860. Suurmond D: Some aspects of erythropoietic protoporphyria in the Netherlands. *Dermatologica* **138**:303, 1969.
861. Gray CH, Kulczycka A, Nicholson DC, Magnus IA, Rimington C: Isotope studies on a case of erythropoietic protoporphyria. *Clin Sci* **26**:7, 1964.
862. Rademakers LHPM, Koningsberger JC, Sorber CWJ, Delafaille HB, Vanhattum J, Marx JJM: Accumulation of iron in erythroblasts of patients with erythropoietic protoporphyria. *Eur J Clin Invest* **23**:130, 1993.
863. Doss MO, Frank M: Hepatobiliary implications and complications in protoporphyria, a 20-year study. *Clin Biochem* **22**:223, 1989.
864. Wilson JHP, Bosdijik AE, Vandenberg JWO, Delafaille HB, Vanhattum J: Liver protoporphyrin in relation to liver disease in erythropoeitic protorphyria. *Gastroenterology* **104**:A1019, 1993.
865. Bloomer JR: The liver in protoporphyria. *Hepatol* **8**:402, 1988.
866. Singer JA, Plaut AG, Kaplan MM: Hepatic failure and death from erythropoietic protoporphyria. *Gastroenterology* **74**:588, 1978.
867. Key NS, Rank JM, Freese D, Bloomer JR, Hammerschmidt DE: Hemolytic anemia in protoporphyria: Possible precipitating role of liver failure and photic stress. *Am J Hemat* **39**:202, 1992.
868. Bonkovsky HL, Schned AR: Fatal liver failure in protoporphyria: Synergism between ethanol excess and the genetic defect. *Gastroenterology* **90**:191, 1986.
869. Poh-Fitzpatrick MB, Whitlock RT, Lefkowitch JH: Changes in protoporphyrin distribution dynamics during liver failure and recovery in a patient with protoporphyria and Epstein-Barr viral hepatitis. *Am J Med* **80**:943, 1986.
870. Bonkowsky HL, Bloomer JR, Ebert PS, Mahoney MJ: Heme synthetase deficiency in human protoporphyria. Demonstration of the defect in liver and cultured skin fibroblasts. *J Clin Invest* **56**:1139, 1975.
871. Norris PG, Nunn AV, Hawk JL, Cox TM: Genetic heterogeneity in erythropoietic protoporphyria: a study of the enzymatic defect in nine affected families. *J Invest Dermatol* **95**:260, 1990.
872. Straka JG, Hill HD, Krikava JM, Kools AM, Bloomer JR: Immunochemical studies of ferrochelatase protein: characterization of the normal and mutant protein in bovine and human protoporphyria. *Am J Hum Genet* **48**:72, 1991.
873. Rufenacht UB, Gouya L, Schneider-Yin X, Puy H, Schafer BW, Aquaron R, Nordmann Y, Minder EI, Deybach JC: Systematic analysis of molecular defects in the ferrochelatase gene from patients with erythropoietic protoporphyria. *Am J Hum Genet* **62**:1341, 1998.
874. Johnson A, Jones OTG: Enzymatic formation of hemes and other metalloporphyrins. *Biochim Biophys Acta* **93**:171, 1964.
875. Porra RJ, Jones OTG: Studies on ferrochelatase: 2. An investigation of the role of ferrochelatase in the biosynthesis of various haem prosthetic groups. *Biochem J* **87**:186, 1963.
876. Porra RJ, Jones OTG: Studies on ferrochelatase: I. Assay and properties of ferrochelatase from a pig liver mitochondrial extract. *Biochem J* **87**:181, 1963.
877. Taketani S, Tokunaga R: Rat liver ferrochelatase: Purification, properties, and stimulation by fatty acids. *J Biol Chem* **256**:12748, 1981.
878. Taketani S, Tokunaga R: Purification and substrate specificity of bovine liver ferrochelatase. *Eur J Biochem* **127**:443, 1982.
879. Dailey HA, Fleming JE: Bovine ferrochelatase: Kinetic analysis of inhibition by *N*-methylprotoporphyrin, manganese, and heme. *J Biol Chem* **258**:11453, 1983.
880. Camadro JM, Ibraham NG, Levere RD: Kinetic studies of human liver ferrochelatase. *J Biol Chem* **259**:5678, 1984.
881. Dailey HA, Finnegan MG, Johnson MK: Human ferrochelatase is an iron sulfur protein. *Biochemistry* **33**:403, 1994.
882. Ferreira GC, Franco R, Lloyd SG, Pereira AS, Moura I, Moura JJ, Huynh BH: Mammalian ferrochelatase, a new addition to the metalloenzyme family. *J Biol Chem* **269**:7062, 1994.
883. Ferreira GC: Mammalian ferrochelatase: Overexpression in *Escherichia coli* as a soluble protein, purification and characterization. *J Biol Chem* **269**:4396, 1994.
884. Ta DT, Vickery LE: Cloning, sequencing, and overexpression of a [2Fe-2S] ferredoxin gene from *Escherichia coli*. *J Biol Chem* **267**:11120, 1992.
885. Ortiz de Montellano PR, Beilan HS, Kunze KL: *N*-Methylprotoporphyrin IX: chemical synthesis and identification as the green pigment produced by 3,5-diethoxycarbonyl-1,4-dihydrocollidine treatment. *Proc Natl Acad Sci U S A* **78**:1490, 1981.
886. De Matteis F, Gibbs AH, Harvey C: Studies on the inhibition of ferrochelatase by *N*-alkylated dicarboxylic porphyrins. Steric factors involved and evidence that the inhibition is reversible. *Biochem J* **226**:537, 1985.
887. Camadro JM, Labbe P: Purification and properties of ferrochelatase from the yeast *Saccharomyces cerevisiae*. Evidence for a precursor form of the protein. *J Biol Chem* **263**:11675, 1988.
888. Karr SR, Dailey HA: The synthesis of murine ferrochelatase in vitro and in vivo. *Biochem J* **254**:799, 1988.
889. Taketani S, Tanaka-Yoshioka A, Masaki R, Tashiro Y, Tokunaga R: Association of ferrochelatase with complex I in bovine heart mitochondria. *Biochim Biophys Acta* **883**:277, 1986.
890. Al-Karadaghi S, Hansson M, Nikonov S, Jonsson B, Hederstedt L: Crystal structure of ferrochelatase: the terminal enzyme in heme biosynthesis. *Structure* **5**:1501, 1997.
891. Burden AE, Wu C, Dailey TA, Busch JL, Dhawan IK, Rose JP, Wang B, Dailey HA: Human ferrochelatase: crystallization, characterization of the [2Fe-2S] cluster and determination that the enzyme is a homodimer. *Biochim Biophys Acta* **1435**:191, 1999.
892. Nakahashi Y, Taketani S, Okuda M, Inoue K, Tokunaga R: Molecular cloning and sequence analysis of cDNA encoding human ferrochelatase. *Biochem Biophys Res Commun* **173**:748, 1990.
893. Taketani S, Inazawa J, Nakahashi Y, Abe T, Tokunaga R: Structure of the human ferrochelatase gene: Exon/intron gene organization and location of the gene to chromosome 18. *Eur J Biochem* **205**:217, 1992.
894. Whitcombe DM, Carter NP, Albertson DG, Smith SJ, Rhodes DA, Cox TM: Assignment of the human ferrochelatase gene (FECH) and a locus for protoporphyria to chromosome 18q22. *Genomics* **11**:1152, 1991.
895. Whitcombe DM, Albertson DG, Cox TM: Molecular analysis of functional and nonfunctional genes for human ferrochelatase: isolation and characterization of a FECH pseudogene and its sublocalization on chromosome 3. *Genomics* **20**:482, 1994.
896. Taketani S, Nakahashi Y, Osumi T, Tokunaga R: Molecular cloning, sequencing, and expression of mouse ferrochelatase. *J Biol Chem* **265**:19377, 1990.
897. Brenner DA, Frasier F: Cloning of murine ferrochelatase. *Proc Natl Acad Sci U S A* **88**:849, 1991.
898. Labbe-Bois R: The ferrochelatase from *Saccharomyces cerevisiae*: Sequence, disruption, and expression of its structural gene Hem15. *J Biol Chem* **265**:7278, 1990.
899. Taketani S, Mohri T, Hioki K, Tokunaga R, Kohno H: Structure and transcriptional regulation of the mouse ferrochelatase gene. *Gene* **227**:117, 1999.
900. Cox TM, Alexander GJ, Sarkany RP: Protoporphyria. *Semin Liver Dis* **18**:85, 1998.
901. Straka JG, Bloomer JR, Kempner ES: The functional size of ferrochelatase determined in situ by radiation inactivation. *J Biol Chem* **266**:24637, 1991.
902. Lamoril J, Boulechfar S, De Verneuil H, Grandchamp B, Nordmann Y, Deybach J-C: Human erythropoietic protoporphyria: Two point mutations in the ferrochelatase gene. *Biochem Biophys Res Commun* **181**:594, 1991.
903. Gouya L, Deybach JC, Lamoril J, Da Silva V, Beaumont C, Grandchamp B, Nordmann Y: Modulation of the phenotype in dominant erythropoietic protoporphyria by a low expression of the normal ferrochelatase allele. *Am J Hum Genet* **58**:292, 1996.
904. Gouya L, Puy H, Lamoril J, Da Silva V, Grandchamp B, Nordmann Y, Deybach JC: Inheritance in erythropoietic protoporphyria: A common wild-type ferrochelatase allelic variant with low expression accounts for clinical manifestation. *Blood* **93**:2105, 1999.
905. Tutois S, Montagutelli X, Dasilva V, Jouault H, Rouyer-Fessard P, Leroy-Viard K, Guénet J-L, Nordmann Y, Beuzard Y, Deybach J-C:

Erythropoietic protoporphyria in the house mouse: A recessive inherited ferrochelatase deficiency with anemia, photosensitivity, and liver disease. *J Clin Invest* **88**:1730, 1991.

906. Sellers VM, Dailey TA, Dailey HA: Examination of ferrochelatase mutations that cause erythropoietic protoporphyria. *Blood* **91**:3980, 1998.
907. Bloomer J, Bruzzone C, Zhu L, Scarlett Y, Magness S, Brenner D: Molecular defects in ferrochelatase in patients with protoporphyria requiring liver transplantation. *J Clin Invest* **102**:107, 1998.
908. Wang X, Yang L, Kurtz L, Lichtin A, DeLeo VA, Bloomer J, Poh-Fitzpatrick MB: Haplotype analysis of families with erythropoietic protoporphyria and novel mutations of the ferrochelatase gene. *J Invest Dermatol* **113**:87, 1999.
909. Bloomer JR, Hill HD, Morton KO, Anderson-Burnham LA, Straka JG: The enzyme defect in bovine protoporphyria: Studies with purified ferrochelatase. *J Biol Chem* **262**:667, 1987.
910. Jenkins MM, LeBoeuf RD, Ruth GR, Bloomer JR: A novel stop codon mutation (X417L) of the ferrochelatase gene in bovine protoporphyria, a natural animal model of the human disease. *Biochim Biophys Acta* **1408**:18, 1998.
911. Boulechfar S, Lamoril J, Montagutelli X, Guenet JL, Deybach JC, Nordmann Y, Dailey H, Grandchamp B, De Verneuil H: Ferrochelatase structural mutant ($Fech^{m1Pas}$) in the house mouse. *Genomics* **16**:645, 1993.
912. Clark KGA, Nicholson DC: Erythrocyte protoporphyrin and iron uptake in erythropoietic protoporphyria. *Clin Sci* **41**:363, 1971.
913. Piomelli S, Lamola AA, Poh-Fitzpatrick MB, Seamon C, Harber LC: Erythropoietic protoporphyria and Pb intoxication: The molecular basis for difference in cutaneous photosensitivity. I. Different rates of disappearance of protoporphyrin from the erythrocytes, both in vivo and in vitro. *J Clin Invest* **56**:1519, 1975.
914. Nicholson DC, Cowger ML, Kalivas J, Thompson RPH, Gray CH: Isotopic studies of the erythropoietic and hepatic components of congenital porphyria and "erythropoietic" protoporphyria. *Clin Sci* **44**:135, 1973.
915. Scholnick P, Marver HS, Schmid R: Erythropoietic protoporphyria: Evidence for multiple sites of excess protoporphyrin formation. *J Clin Invest* **50**:203, 1971.
916. Sassaroli M, Dacosta R, Vaananen H, Eisinger J, Poh-Fitzpatrick MB: Distribution of erythrocyte free porphyrin content in erythropoietic protoporphyria. *J Lab Clin Med* **120**:614, 1992.
917. Sandberg S, Brun A: Light-induced protoporphyrin release from erythrocytes in erythropoietic protoporphyria. *J Clin Invest* **70**:693, 1982.
918. Sandberg S, Talstad I, Hovding G, Bjelland N: Light-induced release of protoporphyrin, but not of zinc protoporphyrin, from erythrocytes in a patient with greatly elevated erythrocyte protoporphyrin. *Blood* **62**:846, 1983.
919. Knobler E, Poh-Fitzpatrick MB, Kravetz D, Vincent WR, Muller-Eberhard U, Vincent SH: Interaction of hemopexin, albumin and liver fatty acid-binding protein with protoporphyrin. *Hepatology* **10**:995, 1989.
920. Sandberg S, Romslo I: Porphyrin-induced photodamage at the cellular and the subcellular level as related to the solubility of the porphyrin. *Clin Chim Acta* **109**:193, 1981.
921. Goldstein BD, Harber LC: Erythropoietic protoporphyria: Lipid peroxidation and red cell membrane damage associated with photohemolysis. *J Clin Invest* **51**:892, 1972.
922. De Goeij AFPM, Van Steveninch J: Photodynamic aspects of protoporphyrin on cholesterol and unsaturated fatty acids in erythrocyte membranes in protoporphyria and in normal red blood cells. *Clin Chim Acta* **68**:115, 1976.
923. Lim HW: Pathophysiology of cutaneous lesions in porphyrias. *Sem Hematol* **26**:114, 1989.
924. Gigli I, Schothorst AA, Soter NA, Pathak MA: Erythropoietic protoporphyria: Photoactivation of the complement system. *J Clin Invest* **66**:517, 1980.
925. Peterka ES, Fusaro RM, Goltz RW: Erythropoietic protoporphyria II. Histological and histochemical studies of cutaneous lesions. *Arch Dermat* **92**:357, 1965.
926. Sasai Y: Erythropoietic protoporphyria: Histochemical study of hyaline material. *Acta Dermatovener* **53**:179, 1973.
927. Ryan EA, Madill GT: Electron microscopy of the skin in erythropoietic protoporphyria. *Br J Dermatol* **80**:561, 1968.
928. Schnait FG, Wolff K, Konrad K: Erythropoietic protoporphyria—Submicroscopic events during the acute photosensitivity flare. *Br J Dermatol* **92**:545, 1975.
929. Avner DL, Lee RG, Berenson MM: Protoporphyrin-induced cholestasis in the isolated in situ perfused rat liver. *J Clin Invest* **67**:385, 1981.
930. Berenson MM, Kimura R, Samowitz W, Bjorkman D: Protoporphyrin overload in unrestrained rats: Biochemical and histopathologic characterization of a new model of protoporphyric hepatopathy. *Int J Exp Pathol* **73**:665, 1992.
931. Porter FS, Lowe BA: Congenital erythropoietic protoporphyria. I. Case reports, clinical studies and porphyrin analyses in two brothers. *Blood* **22**:521, 1963.
932. Hastka J, Lasserre JJ, Schwarzbeck A, Strauch M, Hehlmann R: Zinc protoporphyrin in anemia of chronic disorders. *Blood* **81**:1200, 1993.
933. Poh-Fitzpatrick MB, DeLeo VA: Rates of plasma porphyrin disappearance in fluorescent vs. red incandescent light exposure. *J Invest Dermatol* **69**:510, 1977.
934. Morton KO, Schneider F, Weimer MK, Straka JG, Bloomer JR: Hepatic and bile porphyrins in patients with protoporphyria and liver failure. *Gastroenterology* **94**:1488, 1988.
935. Poh-Fitzpatrick MB: Protoporphyrin metabolic balance in human protoporphyria. *Gastroenterology* **88**:1239, 1985.
936. Bloomer JR, Morton KO: A radiochemical assay for heme synthase activity. *Enzyme* **28**:220, 1982.
937. Porra RJ: A rapid spectrophotometric assay for ferrochelatase (E.C.4.99.1.1) in preparations containing high concentrations of haemoglobin, in Doss M (ed.): *Porphyrins in Human Diseases*. Basel, S. Karger, 1976, p 123.
938. Tephly TR: Inhibition of liver hemoprotein synthesis, in De Matteis F, Aldridge WN (eds.): *Heme and Hemoproteins—Handbook of Experimental Pharmacology*. Berlin, Springer-Verlag, 1978, p 81.
939. Mathews-Roth MM, Pathak MA, Fitzpatrick TB, Harber LC, Kass EH: Beta-carotene as a photoprotective agent in erythropoietic protoporphyria. *N Engl J Med* **282**:1231, 1970.
940. Mathews-Roth MM, Pathak MA, Fitzpatrick TB, Harper LH, Kass EH: Beta carotene therapy for erythropoietic protoporphyria and other photosensitivity diseases. *Arch Dermatol* **113**:1229, 1977.
941. Thomsen K, Schmidt H, Fischer A: Beta-carotene in erythropoietic protoporphyria: 5 years' experience. *Dermatologica* **159**:82, 1979.
942. Roberts JE, Mathews-Roth M: Cysteine ameliorates photosensitivity in erythropoietic protoporphyria. *Arch Dermatol* **129**:1350, 1993.
943. Fusaro RM, Runge WJ: Erythropoietic protoporphyria. IV. Protection from sunlight. *BMJ* **1**:730, 1970.
944. Warren LJ, George S: Erythropoietic protoporphyria treated with narrow-band (TL-01) UVB phototherapy. *Australas J Dermatol* **39**:179, 1998.
945. Kniffen JC: Protoporphyrin removal in intrahepatic porphyrastasis. *Gastroenterology* **58**:1027, 1970.
946. Van Hattum J, Baart de la Faille H, Van den Berg JWO, Edixhoven-Bosdijk A, Wilson JHP: Chenodeoxycholic acid therapy in erythrohepatic protoporphyria. *J Hepatol* **3**:407, 1986.
947. Gross U, Frank M, Doss MO: Hepatic complications of erythropoietic protoporphyria. *Photodermatol Photoimmunol Photomed* **14**:52, 1998.
948. Gordeuk VR, Brittenham GM, Hawkins CW, Mukhtar H, Bickers DR: Iron therapy for hepatic dysfunction in erythropoietic protoporphyria. *Ann Int Med* **105**:27, 1986.
949. Mercurio MG, Prince G, Weber FL, Jacobs G, Zaim MT, Bickers DR: Terminal hepatic failure in erythropoietic protoporphyria. *J Am Acad Dermatol* **29**:829, 1993.
950. Gorchein A, Foster GR: Liver failure in protoporphyria: long-term treatment with oral charcoal [Letter]. *Hepatology* **29**:995, 1999.
951. Van Wijk HJ, Van Hattum J, Delafaille HB, Vandenberg JWO, Edixhoven-Bosdijk A, Wilson JHP: Blood exchange and transfusion therapy for acute cholestasis in protoporphyria. *Dig Dis Sci* **33**:1621, 1988.
952. Reichheld JH, Katz E, Banner BF, Szymanski IO, Saltzman JR, Bonkovsky HL: The value of intravenous heme-albumin and plasmapheresis in reducing postoperative complications of orthotopic liver transplantation for erythropoietic protoporphyria. *Transplantation* **67**:922, 1999.
953. Bloomer JR, Weimer MK, Bossenmaier IC, Snover DC, Payne WD, Ascher NL: Liver transplantation in a patient with protoporphyria. *Gastroenterology* **97**:188, 1989.
954. Meerman L, Haagsma EB, Gouw AS, Slooff MJ, Jansen PL: Long-term follow-up after liver transplantation for erythropoietic protoporphyria. *Eur J Gastroenterol Hepatol* **11**:431, 1999.
955. Todd DJ, Callender ME, Mayne EE, Walsh M, Burrows D: Erythropoietic protoporphyria, transfusion therapy and liver disease. *Br J Dermatol* **127**:534, 1992.

956. Nordmann Y: Erythropoietic protoporphyria and hepatic complications. *J Hepatol* **16**:4, 1992.
957. Muley SA, Midani HA, Rank JM, Carithers R, Parry GJ: Neuropathy in erythropoietic protoporphyrias. *Neurology* **51**:262, 1998.
958. Lichtin A, Anderson K, Bloomer J, Bolwell B, Poh-Fitzpatrick M, Wang X: Correction of erythropoietic protoporphyria (EPP) phenotype by allogenic bone marrow transplant. *American Society of Hematology Annual Meeting*, December 7, 1998.
959. Day RS, Eales L, Meissner D: Coexistent variegate porphyria and porphyria cutanea tarda. *N Engl J Med* **30**:36, 1982.
960. Doss M: Dual porphyria in double heterozygotes with porphobilinogen deaminase and uroporphyrinogen decarboxylase deficiencies. *Clin Genet* **35**:146, 1989.
961. Nordmann Y, Amram D, Deybach JC, Phung LN, Lesbros D: Coexistent hereditary coproporphyria and congenital erythropoietic porphyria (Günther disease). *J Inherit Metab Dis* **13**:687, 1990.
962. Freesemann AG, Hofweber K, Doss MO: Coexistence of deficiencies of uroporphyrinogen III synthase and decarboxylase in a patient with congenital erythropoietic porphyria and in his family. *Eur J Clin Chem Clin Biochem* **35**:35, 1997.
963. Gregor A, Kostrzewska E, Tarczynska-Nosal S, Stachurska H: Coexistence of hereditary coproporphyria with acute intermittent porphyria. *Ann Med* **26**:125, 1994.
964. Poh-Fitzpatrick MB: Is porphyria cutanea tarda a paraneoplastic disorder? *Clin Dermatol* **11**:119, 1993.
965. Günther H: in Schittenhelm A (eds.): *Handbuch der Krankheiten der Blutes und der Blutbildenden Organe*. Berlin, Springer-Verlag, Vol 2, 1925.
966. Jackson AH, Sancovich HA, Ferramola AM, Evans N, Games DE, Matlin SA: Macrocycle intermediates in the biosynthesis of porphyrins. *Philos Trans R Soc Lond [Biol]* **273**:191, 1975.
967. Rifkind AB: Drug-induced exacerbations of porphyria. *Primary Care* **3**:665, 1976.
968. Eales L: Porphyria and the dangerous life-threatening drugs. *S Afr Med J* **56**:914, 1979.
969. Rifkind AB, Gillette PN, Song CS, Kappas A: Drug stimulation of δ-aminolevulinic acid synthetase and cytochrome P-450 in vivo in chick embryo liver. *J Pharmacol Exp Ther* **185**:214, 1973.
970. De Matteis F: Drugs and porphyria. *S Afr Med J* **17**:126, 1971.
971. Wetterberg L: Internationell enkät om farliga och ofarliga läkemedel vid akut intermittent porfyri. *Läkartidningen* **73**:4090, 1976.
972. Canepa ET, Llambias EBC, Grinstein M: Studies on induction of δ-aminolevulinic acid synthase, ferrochelatase, cytochrome P-450 and cyclic AMP by phenformin: Chlorpropamide, allylisopropylacetamide and lead in hepatocytes from normal and experimental diabetic rats. *Biochem Pharmacol* **40**:365, 1990.
973. Mustajoki P, Vuoristo M, Reunala T: Celiac disease or dermatitis herpetiformis in three patients with porphyria. *Dig Dis Sci* **26**:618, 1981.
974. Magnussen CR, Doherty JM, Hess RA, Tschudy DP: Grand mal seizures and acute intermittent porphyria. The problem of differential diagnosis and treatment. *Neurology* **25**:121, 1975.
975. De Matteis F, Marks GS: Cytochrome P450 and its interactions with the heme biosynthetic pathway. *Can J Physiol Pharmacol* **74**:1, 1996.
976. Gregersen H, Nielsen JS, Peterslund NA: [Acute porphyria and multiple organ failure during treatment with lamotrigine]. *Ugeskr Laeger* **158**:4091, 1996.
977. Reynolds NC, Miska RM: Safety of anticonvulsants in hepatic porphyrias. *Neurology* **31**:480, 1981.
978. Doss M, Becker U, Peter HJ, Kaffarnik H: Drug safety in porphyria: Risks of valproate and metoclopramide. *Lancet* **2**:91, 1981.
979. Rifkind AB, Gillette PN, Song CS, Kappas A: Induction of hepatic δ-aminolevulinic acid synthetase by oral contraceptive steroids. *J Clin Endocrinol Metab* **30**:330, 1970.
980. Brodie MJ: Drug safety in porphyria. *Lancet* **1**:86, 1980.
981. Chang TK, Yu L, Maurel P, Waxman DJ: Enhanced cyclophosphamide and ifosfamide activation in primary human hepatocyte cultures: response to cytochrome P-450 inducers and autoinduction by oxazaphosphorines. *Cancer Res* **57**:1946, 1997.
982. Sieg I, Beckh K, Kersten U, Doss MO: Manifestation of acute intermittent porphyria in patients with chronic inflammatory bowel disease. *Z Gastroenterol* **29**:602, 1991.
983. With TK: Toxic porphyria after treatment with sulphonal and trional. *S Afr Med J* 133, 1971.
984. Garcia-Merino JA, Lopez-Lozano JJ: Risks of valproate in porphyria. *Lancet* **2**:856, 1980.
985. Fischer PWF, Ferizovic A, Neilson IR, Marks GS: Porphyrin-inducing activity of alfaxolone and alfadolone acetate in chick embryo liver cells. *Anesthesiology* **50**:350, 1979.
986. Parikh RK, Moore MR: Effect of certain anaesthetic agents on the activity of rat hepatic δ-aminolaevulinate synthase. *Br J Anaesth* **50**:1099, 1978.
987. Wehmeier A, Fischer JT, Goerz G, Schneider W: Polychemotherapy of acute myelogenous leukemia in a patient with acute intermittent porphyria. *Klin Wochenschr* **65**:338, 1987.
988. Cochon AC, Aldonatti C, San Martin de Viale LC, Wainstok de Calmanovici R: Evaluation of the porphyrinogenic risk of antineoplastics. *J Appl Toxicol* **17**:171, 1997.
989. Suzuki A, Aso K, Ariyoshi C, Ishimaru M: Acute intermittent porphyria and epilepsy: safety of clonazepam. *Epilepsia* **33**:108, 1992.
990. Bonkowsky HL, Shedlofsky SI, Sinclair PR: Seizure management and hepatic porphyrias. *Neurology* **32**:1410, 1982.
991. Zimmer S, Taub H, Marks G: A comparison of the porphyrin-inducing activity of barbiturates and benzodiazepines in chick embryo liver cells. *Can J Physiol Pharmacol* **58**:991, 1980.
992. Goerz G, Bolsen K, Bohrer H, Fritsch C, Kalka K, Rominger KL: Effects of clonidine in a primed rat model of acute hepatic porphyria. *Arzneimittelforschung* **47**:731, 1997.
993. Nunez DJ, Williams PF, Herrick AL, Evans DB, McColl KEL: Renal transplantation for chronic renal failure in acute porphyria. *Nephrol Dial Transplant* **2**:271, 1987.
994. Harrison GG, Moore MR, Meissner PN: Porphyrinogenicity of etomidate and ketamine as continuous infusions. Screening in the DDC-primed rat model. *Br J Anaesth* **57**:420, 1985.
995. Welland FH, Hellman ES, Collins A, Hunter GWJ, Tschudy DP: Factors affecting the excretion of porphyrin precursors by patients with acute intermittent porphyria II. The effect of ethinyl estradiol. *Metabolism* **13**:251, 1964.
996. Ziman MR, Bradshaw JJ, Ivanetich KM: The effect of fluroxene [(2,2,2-trifluoroethoxy)ethane] on haem biosynthesis and degradation. *Biochem J* **190**:571, 1980.
997. Ortiz de Montellano PR, Kunze KL, Beilan HS, Wheeler C: Destruction of cytochrome P-450 by vinyl fluoride, fluroxene, and acetylene. Evidence for a radical intermediate in olefin oxidation. *Biochemistry* **21**:1331, 1982.
998. Eiseman JL, Alvares AP: Alterations induced in heme pathway enzymes and monooxygenases by gold. *Mol Pharmacol* **14**:1176, 1978.
999. Cable EE, Pepe JA, Donohue SE, Lambrecht RW, Bonkovsky HL: Effects of mifepristone (RU-486) on heme metabolism and cytochromes P-450 in cultured chick embryo liver cells, possible implications for acute porphyria. *Eur J Biochem* **225**:651, 1994.
1000. He K, Woolf TF, Hollenberg PF: Mechanism-based inactivation of cytochrome P-450-3A4 by mifepristone (RU486). *J Pharmacol Exp Ther* **288**:791, 1999.
1001. Parikh RJ, Moore MR: A comparison of the porphyrinogenicity of di-isopropylphenol (propofol) and phenobarbitone. *Biochem Soc Transactions* **14**:726, 1986.
1002. Treece GL, Magnussen CR, Patterson JR, Tschudy DP: Exacerbation of porphyria during treatment of pulmonary tuberculosis. *Am Rev Respir Dis* **113**:233, 1976.
1003. Goldberg A, Rimington C, Lochhead AC: Hereditary coproporphyria. *Lancet* **1**:632, 1967.
1004. LeCluyse EL, Sahi J, Sinz M, Woolf T, Hawke R, Hamilton G, Lesko LJ, Huang S-M: Troglitazone induces CYP3A4 in cultured human hepatocytes. *Clin Pharmacol Ther* **65**:157, 1999.
1005. Sparano N, Seaton TL: Troglitazone in type II diabetes mellitus. *Pharmacotherapy* **18**:539, 1998.
1006. Sundstrom SA, Sinclair JF, Smith EL, Sinclair PR: Effect of 17α-ethynylestradiol on the induction of cytochrome P-450 by 3-methylcholanthrene in cultured chick embryo hepatocytes. *Biochem Pharmacol* **37**:1003, 1988.
1007. Wetterberg L, Olsson MB, Alm-Agvald I: [Estrogen treatment caused acute attacks of porphyria]. *Lakartidningen* **92**:2197, 1995.
1008. Schoenfeld N, Mamet R, Mevasser R, Atsmon A: Experimental latent and acute porphyria in the non-fasted rat—Preventive effect of propranolol. *Scand J Clin Lab Invest* **51**:667, 1991.
1009. Anderson KE: The porphyrias. In: Goldman L, Benneth CJ (eds.) *Cecil Textbook of Medicine*. Philadelphia, Saunders, 2000, p.1123.

CHAPTER 125

Hereditary Jaundice and Disorders of Bilirubin Metabolism

Jayanta Roy Chowdhury ▪ Allan W. Wolkoff
Namita Roy Chowdhury ▪ Irwin M. Arias

1. Bilirubin is an orange pigment derived from the degradation of the heme moiety of hemoproteins, particularly the hemoglobin of mature circulating erythrocytes.

2. Bilirubin is a potentially toxic waste product that is normally rendered harmless by binding to serum albumin, conjugation in the liver, and efficient excretion into bile by the liver. Bilirubin is an antioxidant, and a protective role of bilirubin against oxidant damage has been suggested. On the other hand, patients with profound unconjugated hyperbilirubinemia are at risk for bilirubin encephalopathy (kernicterus). Accumulation of bilirubin in plasma and tissues results in jaundice, which has attracted the attention of patients and clinicians since antiquity.

3. Following formation in the reticuloendothelial system, bilirubin is released into the circulation, where it avidly binds to serum albumin and is rapidly cleared by the liver. Extraction of bilirubin from the circulation is a specific hepatic function involving facilitated diffusion. Within the hepatocyte, bilirubin binds to cytosolic proteins, primarily to glutathione-S-transferases. The water-insoluble bilirubin molecule is transformed into polar bilirubin monoglucuronide and diglucuronide by the action of bilirubin-UDP-glucuronosyltransferase (bilirubin-UGT) and is excreted into the bile canaliculus against a concentration gradient by energy-consuming mechanisms.

4. Inherited disorders of bilirubin metabolism result in hyperbilirubinemia. These include disorders resulting in predominantly unconjugated hyperbilirubinemia (Crigler-Najjar syndrome types I and II, and Gilbert syndrome) and those resulting in predominantly conjugated hyperbilirubinemia (Dubin-Johnson syndrome, Rotor syndrome, and benign recurrent intrahepatic cholestasis).

5. Bilirubin-UGT (UGT1A1) and several additional isoforms of the UGT1A subfamily that mediate the glucuronidation of other aglycone substrates are expressed from the locus *UGT1A*, located on chromosome 2q37. Genetic lesions in any of the five exons that encode UGT1A1 may lead to complete absence (Crigler-Najjar syndrome type I; MIM 218800) or incomplete deficiency (Crigler-Najjar syndrome type II) of bilirubin glucuronidation. In contrast, Gilbert syndrome (MIM 143500) is associated with an abnormality of the TATAA box within the promoter region upstream to exon 1 of *UGT1A1* that results in reduced expression of structurally normal UGT1A1. Dubin-Johnson syndrome (MIM 237500) is caused by a genetic abnormality of bile canalicular multispecific organic anion transporter, which is involved in the excretion of many non–bile salt organic anions by an adenosine triphosphate (ATP)-requiring active process. Dubin-Johnson syndrome is associated with a characteristic accumulation of pigments in the liver and an abnormality of porphyrin metabolism in which over 80 percent of urinary coproporphyrin is coproporphyrin I, as compared with less than 35 percent in normal individuals. Rotor syndrome (MIM 327450) is primarily a disorder of hepatic storage and differs from Dubin-Johnson syndrome by the lack of hepatic pigmentation, urinary coproporphyrin excretion pattern, and hepatic sulfobromophthalein (BSP) metabolism. Dubin-Johnson syndrome is caused by genetic lesions of the gene *MRP2* (also termed *cMOAT*). Other genetic abnormalities can cause hyperbilirubinemia, secondary to structural abnormalities of the biliary system or derangement of specific excretory functions of the bile canaliculus. These include progressive familial intrahepatic cholestasis, type I (MIM 211600) and benign recurrent intrahepatic cholestasis (MIM 243300), both of which are associated with mutations of the *FIC1* gene on chromosome 18q21. Progressive familial intrahepatic cholestasis type II (MIM 601847) is characterized by abnormality of bile salt excretion and is associated with mutations of the gene *SPGP*, which is located on chromosome 2q24. A third type of progressive familial intrahepatic cholestasis (MIM 602347) involves mutations of the *MDR3* gene, the products of which are needed for phospholipid excretion in bile. Several heritable developmental disorders of the biliary system have been described. Of these, Alagille syndrome (MIM 118450) has been found to be caused by lesions of *JAG1*, a gene located on chromosome 20p12.

6. Crigler-Najjar syndrome types I and II have an autosomal-recessive pattern of inheritance. Patients with Gilbert syndrome are homozygous for the specific promoter

A list of standard abbreviations is located immediately preceding the index in each volume. Additional abbreviations used in this chapter include: BRIC, benign recurrent intrahepatic cholestasis; BSP, bromosulphthalein; cMOAT, canalicular multiorganic anion transporter; DBSP, dibromosulphthalein; EHBR, Eisai hyperbilirubinemic rat; FIC1/*FIC1*, protein/gene for familial intrahepatic cholestasis-1; ICG, indocyanine green; MDR, multidrug resistance protein; MOAT, multiorganic anion transporter; MRP, multidrug resistance-like protein, *MRP2* encodes cMOAT; oatp, organic anion-transporting polypeptide; PFIC, progressive familial intrahepatic cholestasis; SPGP, sister-p-glycoprotein, member of MDR family; TCDD, 2,3,7,8-tetrachloro-dibenzo-p-dioxin; TR$^-$, transport-deficient mutant rat strain; UGT, UDP-glucuronosyltransferase; UGT1A1/*UGT1A1*, protein/gene for UDP-glucuronosyltransferase 1, family member 1A equivalent to bilirubin-UGT; UGT1A6/*UGT1A6*, protein/gene for UDP-glucuronosyltransferase 1, family member A6.

abnormality, but all subjects homozygous for this genotype do not exhibit the clinical picture of Gilbert syndrome. Studies of urinary coproporphyrin excretion reveal autosomal-recessive patterns of inheritance for Dubin-Johnson and Rotor syndromes.

7. **Several animal models of inherited disorders of bilirubin metabolism are important in understanding the pathophysiology of their human counterparts. These models include the Gunn rat (Crigler-Najjar syndrome type I); the Bolivian population of squirrel monkeys (Gilbert syndrome); and mutant albino rats with organic anion excretion defect (TR −\−), golden lion tamarin monkeys, and mutant Corriedale sheep (Dubin-Johnson syndrome).**

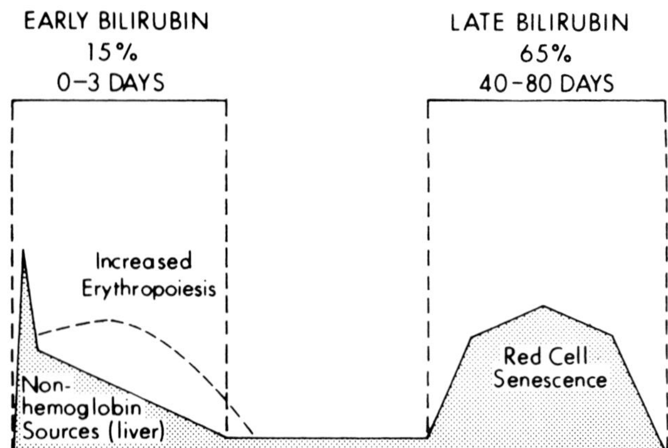

Fig. 125-1 Labeling of plasma bilirubin in UDP-glucuronosyltransferase–deficient rats (Gunn strain) after the injection of [^{14}C]glycine. The early (0 to 3 days) peak has an initial "sharp" and a slower component. [Reprinted with permission from Robinson SH: In Stohlman F Jr (ed): *Hemopoietic Cellular Proliferation.* New York: Grune & Stratton, 1970, p 180.]

Bilirubin is an orange pigment derived from the degradation of heme proteins, particularly the hemoglobin of mature circulating erythrocytes and hepatic hemoproteins. Bilirubin is a potentially toxic waste product that is generally harmless because of binding to serum albumin. However, patients with profound unconjugated hyperbilirubinemia are at risk for bilirubin encephalopathy (kernicterus).

Studies of bilirubin chemistry, synthesis, transport, metabolism, distribution, and excretion have attracted the attention of generations of chemists, biologists, and clinical investigators. Because bilirubin is an organic anion of limited aqueous solubility, it has proved to be a model for the study of the transport, metabolism, and excretion of other biologically important organic anions. Defects in bilirubin formation or disposal are usually manifested by hyperbilirubinemia and jaundice. A number of inherited disorders affecting these pathways have been described in both humans and animals. Study of these disorders has provided important information regarding normal and abnormal metabolic pathways.

Crigler-Najjar syndrome type I, a potentially lethal disorder, requires liver transplantation as a definitive treatment, and transplantation of isolated hepatocytes also has been used. Development of strategies for noninvasive therapy for this condition remains a therapeutic challenge and continues to stimulate research.

BILIRUBIN

Formation of Bilirubin

Bilirubin is exclusively derived from heme. In humans, 250 to 400 mg of bilirubin is formed daily by the breakdown of hemoglobin, other hemoproteins, and free heme.[1] Approximately 80 percent is derived from the hemoglobin of senescent erythrocytes.[2] After injection of radiolabeled porphyrin precursors (glycine or δ-aminolevulinic acid) in humans or rats, radioactivity is incorporated into bile pigments in two peaks[3] (Fig. 125-1). The first peak (early-labeled peak of bilirubin, ELB) appears within 3 days and contains an initial component and a slow later phase. The initial component comprises two thirds of the ELB in humans and is largely derived from hepatic hemoproteins such as cytochromes, catalase, peroxidase, and tryptophan pyrrolase.[4] The labeled bilirubin that appears in bile within 15 min after administration of the precursor may be derived from a rapidly turning over pool of free heme in the cytosol of hepatocytes that is degraded without incorporation into hemoproteins.[5] Myoglobin has a relatively long half-life and is an unlikely source. Induction of hepatic cytochrome P450 enhances the ELB.[6] The slower phase of the ELB is derived from both erythroid and nonerythroid sources and is enhanced in conditions associated with ineffective erythropoiesis, such as congenital dyserythropoietic anemias, megaloblastic anemias, iron-deficiency anemia, and lead poisoning.[4] The ELB is also increased in erythropoietic porphyria[3] but not in porphyria cutanea tarda[7] or acute intermittent porphyria.[8] The erythroid phase is increased in accelerated erythropoiesis, probably because of intramedullary destruction of normoblasts, destruction of reticulocytes in the peripheral circulation, and injury to reticulocytes during maturation.[9] δ-Aminolevulinic acid is preferentially incorporated into hepatic hemoproteins.[10] A late-labeled peak appears at approximately 50 days in rats and by 110 days in humans and is derived from the hemoglobin of senescent erythrocytes.

In the liver, heme derived from exogenously administered hemoglobin is quantitatively converted to bilirubin.[11] A portion of heme associated with hepatic hemoproteins may not be converted to bilirubin.[12] This suggests that exogenous heme and hepatocellular heme may be processed differently by the liver.

Mechanism of Opening of the Heme Ring. Ferroprotoporphyrin IX is the heme prosthetic group (Fig. 125-2) in vertebrate hemoproteins. The porphyrin ring is selectively cleaved at the α-methene bridge. The first step is catalyzed by microsomal heme oxygenase and requires an electrophilic attack at Fe(II) by a reducing agent, such as NADPH and oxygen. This reaction results in formation of α-oxyheme (Fig. 125-2).[13] Heme oxygenase

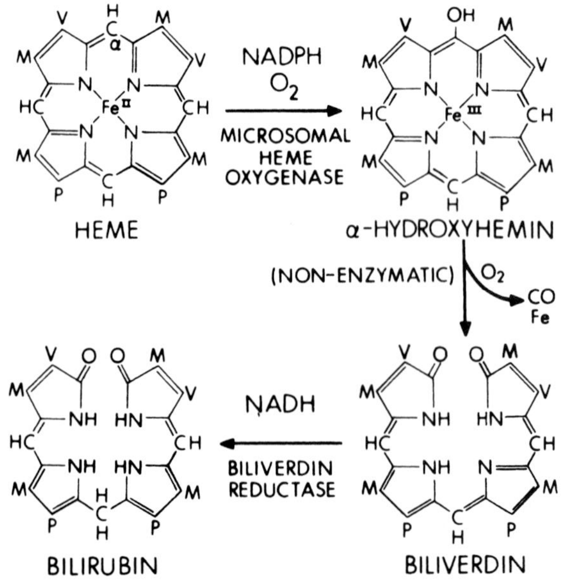

Fig. 125-2 Mechanism of heme ring opening and subsequent reduction of biliverdin to bilirubin.

activity is highest in the spleen, which is involved in sequestration of senescent erythrocytes, and is enhanced in hemolytic states. Within the liver, hepatocytes and Kupffer cells have heme oxygenase activity. In Kupffer cells, the enzyme activity is comparable with that in the spleen.[14] Heme stimulates the synthesis of heme oxygenase,[15] which enhances heme degradation,[16] suggesting that heme oxygenase is rate limiting in heme oxidation and bilirubin formation.[16] However, evidence also has been presented supporting a contrasting view that heme oxygenase is present in excess as compared with its substrate.[17] Heme oxygenase has been purified from microsomal fractions of pig[18] and bovine[19] spleen and rat liver.[20] The binding of purified heme oxygenase to heme requires heme iron and the propionic acid substituents in the C6 and C7 positions. Protoporphyrins that contain other metals, such as tin, bind with even greater affinity[19] but are not degraded by heme oxygenase. Thus, noniron hemes may serve as dead-end inhibitors of heme oxygenase.[19]

The second step in opening the heme ring involves oxidation by molecular oxygen and probably occurs nonenzymatically.[21] Carbons at the angular positions of the porphyrin ring neighboring the α-methene bridge are oxidized, and CO is eliminated. During this step, two oxygen atoms, derived from two different oxygen molecules, are added.[22] These oxygen atoms appear as the lactam oxygens of biliverdin and bilirubin. Release of iron occurs after addition of electrons, suggesting that conversion of ferric to ferrous iron is required.[23] The resulting green pigment is biliverdin.

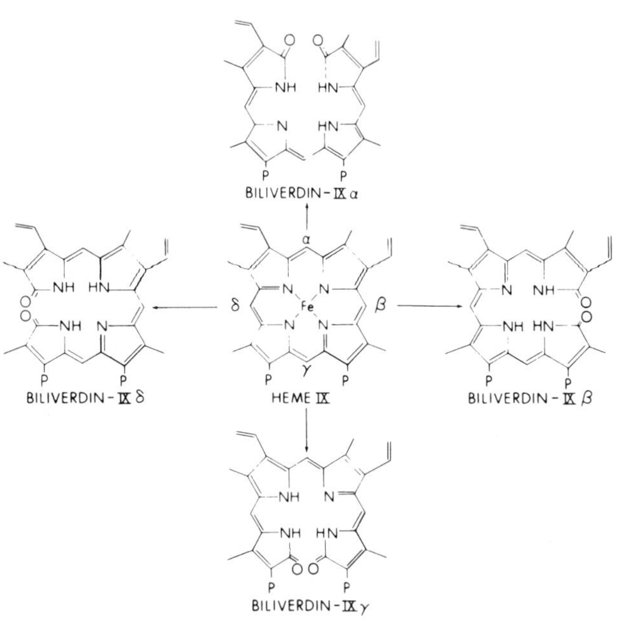

Conversion of Biliverdin to Bilirubin. Biliverdin is readily excreted by the liver and is the major bile pigment in many amphibian, avian, and fish species. However, in most mammals, biliverdin is converted to bilirubin, which requires several energy-consuming metabolic steps for biliary excretion. The physiologic benefits of conversion of biliverdin to bilirubin are not clear. Bilirubin is less polar than is biliverdin and crosses the placental membranes more readily than does biliverdin.[24] However, some placentate animals, such as nutria and rabbits, excrete biliverdin as the main bile pigment,[25] whereas many nonplacentate vertebrates, such as some species of fish, excrete predominantly bilirubin in bile.[26] Bilirubin is an antioxidant and is thought to play an important antioxidant defense for the body.[27–29] The antioxidant activity of bilirubin may be particularly important during the neonatal period, when concentrations of other antioxidants are low in body fluids.

Conversion of biliverdin to bilirubin is catalyzed by a cytosolic enzyme, biliverdin reductase, which requires NADH or NADPH for activity.[30,31] Guinea pig liver biliverdin reductase is a 70-kDa protein.[32] Three interconverting molecular forms of biliverdin reductase have been described in rat liver.[33]

Because of the specificity of heme oxygenase for the α-carbon bridge, the most abundant bile pigment is bilirubin IXα, and only minute amounts of non-α isomers (Fig. 125-3) have been detected in human and animal bile.[34]

Quantification of Bilirubin Production. Bilirubin production reflects turnover of biologically important hemoproteins. At a steady-state condition of blood hemoglobin levels, the rate of bilirubin production approximates the rate of heme synthesis. For these reasons, the quantification of bilirubin production is important in clinical and physiologic investigations.[35] Normally, bilirubin is almost quantitatively excreted in bile; therefore, bilirubin production can be quantified in biliary excretion in animals, but this is not practical in humans. Bilirubin is converted to urobilinogen by bacteria in the gastrointestinal tract, and fecal urobilinogen excretion approximates daily bilirubin production,[36] although conversion to urobilinogen may not be quantitative.

In humans, bilirubin production is conveniently quantified from the turnover of radioisotopically labeled bilirubin. Radiolabeled bilirubin bound to albumin is injected intravenously, blood samples are collected at frequent intervals, and plasma bilirubin concentration and radioactivity are measured.[37] Plasma bilirubin clearance (the fraction of plasma from which bilirubin is irreversibly extracted) is proportional to the reciprocal of the area under the radiobilirubin disappearance curve.[38] Bilirubin removal is quantified as the product of plasma bilirubin concentration and clearance. When plasma bilirubin concentrations remain constant, removal of bilirubin equals the amount of newly synthesized bilirubin entering the plasma pool. This method does not take into account a small portion of bilirubin that is produced in the liver and excreted directly into bile without appearing in the circulation and, therefore, slightly underestimates bilirubin production.

Bilirubin formation also can be quantified from carbon monoxide production. The subject is placed in a closed rebreathing system to prevent CO excretion. CO production is calculated from the CO concentration in the breathing chamber or from an increment in blood carboxyhemoglobin saturation.[39] This method assumes that body CO stores rapidly equilibrate, blood carboxyhemoglobin reflects total body CO, and metabolism of CO is insignificant compared with its rate of production. However, under certain circumstances, such as anoxia, assumption of a steady equilibrium of body stores of CO with blood carboxyhemoglobin may not be correct.[40] CO production exceeds plasma bilirubin turnover by 12 to 18 percent. This discrepancy is partly due to a small portion of bilirubin produced in the liver and excreted into bile without appearing in serum. A portion of CO in expired air may be produced from nonheme sources, such as halogenated methane[41] and polyphenolic compounds, including catecholamines.[42] A small fraction of the CO may be formed by intestinal bacteria.[43]

Fig. 125-3 Nonenzymatic cleavage of heme *in vitro* results in the formation of four isomeric forms of biliverdin owing to the nonequivalence of the four methene bridge positions (α, β, γ, and δ). P, CH_2CH_2COOH.

Pharmacologic Inhibition of Bilirubin Production. Administration of nonmetabolized dead-end inhibitors of heme oxygenase, such as tin-protoporphyrin or tin-mesoporphyrin, results in marked inhibition of the enzyme activity in various organs.[19] A single dose of tin-mesoporphyrin administered in neonates, shortly after birth, resulted in an average of 76 percent reduction of serum bilirubin levels and abolished the need for phototherapy.[44,45]

Chemistry of Bilirubin

The systemic name given to bilirubin IXα is 1,8-dioxo-1,3,6,7-tetramethyl-2,8-divinylbiladiene-a,c-dipropionic acid.[4,5] The gross

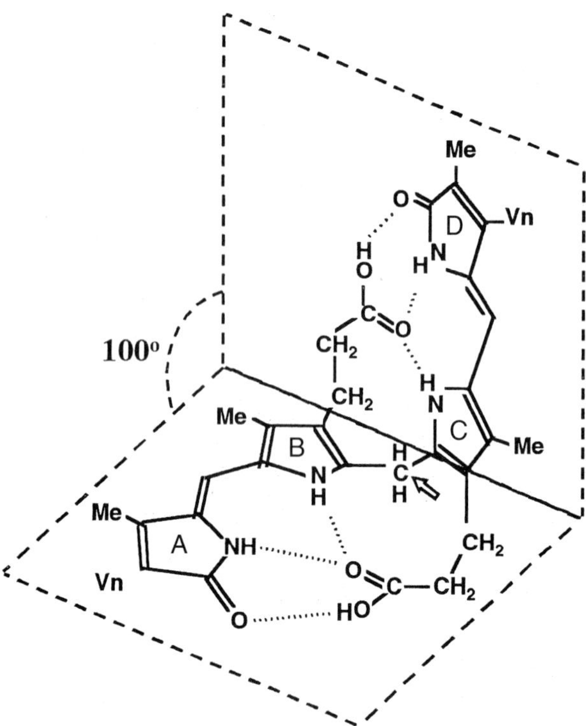

Fig. 125-4 X-ray crystallographic structure of bilirubin showing a ridge-tile configuration caused by internal hydrogen bonding of the propionic acid carboxyls to the amino groups and the lactam oxygen of the pyrrolenone rings of the opposite half of the molecule. The bonds between pyrrolenone rings A, B, C, and D are in the Z (*trans*) configuration.

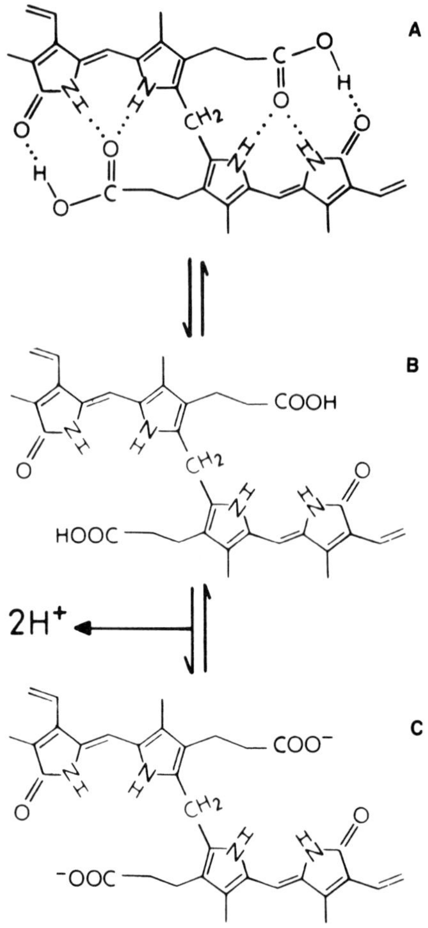

chemical structure (Fig. 125-3) assigned to bilirubin by Fischer and Plieninger[46] has been confirmed by x-ray diffraction analysis (Fig. 125-4).[47] The bonds between pyrrolenone rings A and B (C4 to C5) and C and D (C15 to C16) are in the Z or *trans*-configuration. The oxygen attached to the outer pyrrolenone ring is in a lactam rather than lactim configuration. Titration of bilirubin in aqueous solutions suggests a pK value of 7.0 to 8.0.[48] Because bilirubin tends to form insoluble aggregates below pH 8.0, determination of pK by titration of aqueous solutions of bilirubin may be misleading.[49] Studies using ^{13}C NMR spectra and potentiometric and spectrophotometric titrations in aqueous solutions indicate that bilirubin has four acidic groups. The pK value of the two carboxyl groups is 4.4 and that of the two lactam groups is 13.0.[49]

Physical Conformation and Solubility of Bilirubin IXα. Crystallized bilirubin IXα-*ZZ* with two protonated carboxyl groups is virtually insoluble in water. At acidic, neutral, or mildly alkaline pH, bilirubin can be extracted from aqueous solutions into water-immiscible solvents such as chloroform, ethyl acetate, or methylethyl ketone. After intravenous injection, bilirubin stains phospholipid membranes of brain and those covering adipose tissues. However, bilirubin is not truly lipophilic. Determination of solubility in progressively nonpolar solvents indicates that bilirubin is readily soluble in polar solvents, provided the intramolecular hydrogen bonds can be interrupted.[50] Bilirubin and polar ligands, such as sulfonamides, share a binding site within a polar domain of albumin.[49,51] Thus, despite its insolubility in water at physiologic pH, bilirubin should be considered a relatively polar substance, and its mechanism of toxicity may differ from that of truly lipid-soluble toxins, such as DDT.[51] Although both bilirubin and biliverdin have two propionic acid side chains, bilirubin IXα is less polar than is biliverdin IXα at physiologic pH (Fig. 125-2). An explanation for this was

Fig. 125-5 Ionic species of bilirubin. *A*. Internally hydrogen bonded form. *B*. Bilirubin acid with hydrogen bonds disrupted. *C*. Bilirubin dianion.

suggested initially by Fog and Jellum[52] and Kuenzle et al.,[53] who proposed that bilirubin IXα may be internally stabilized by hydrogen bonding between the carboxyl and the two external pyrrolenone rings (Fig. 125-5). X-ray diffraction studies of crystalline bilirubin confirm hydrogen bonding between each propionic acid side chain and the pyrrolic and lactam sites in the opposite half of the molecule.[47] The molecule takes the form of a ridge tile in which the two dipyrrolic halves of the molecule lie in two different planes with an interplanar angle of 98 to 100 degrees (Fig. 125-4). The integrity of the hydrogen bonded structure requires the interpyrrolic bridges at the 5 and 15 position of bilirubin to be in *trans*- or Z configuration. In nonpolar solvents, the structure of unconjugated bilirubin oscillates between that shown in Fig. 125-5 and its mirror image.[54] A similar conformation has been proposed for bilirubin dianions in aqueous solutions.[55] The hydrogen bonded structure of bilirubin may explain many of its physicochemical properties. The two carboxylic groups, all four NH groups, and the two lactam oxygens are engaged by hydrogen bonding, making the molecule insoluble in water. Addition of methanol, ethanol, or 6 M urea disrupts the hydrogen bonds, thereby making bilirubin water soluble and more labile.[56] The central methene bridge becomes accessible to diazo reagents after disruption of hydrogen bonds, making bilirubin readily reactive to these reagents.

Ultraviolet/Visible Absorption Spectra. The position of the main absorption band (λ_{max}) of bilirubin depends on the bile pigment and the solvent. Unconjugated bilirubin IXα has a λ_{max} of 450 to 474 nm in most organic solvents (Fig. 125-2) and an extinction coefficient (E_{max}) of 48.0 to 63.4/mM. In alkaline aqueous solutions, there is a 10- to 30-nm shift of the λ_{max} toward shorter wavelengths (hypsochromic shift) and a weaker absorption band at 280 to 300 nm.

Helical Conformation of Bilirubin and Biliverdin. Circular dichroism spectroscopy shows that bilirubin preferentially adopts a plus-helicity when bound to human serum albumin, whereas biliverdin prefers a minus helicity.[57]

Fluorescence. Pure bilirubin does not fluoresce. When it is dissolved in detergent, albumin solution, or alkaline methanol, an intense fluorescence is observed at 510 to 530 nm.[58] Determination of fluorescence of bilirubin can be used for rapid quantification of blood bilirubin concentrations and the unsaturated bilirubin binding capacity of albumin.

Geometric Isomerization and Cyclization. As mentioned earlier (Fig. 125-3), the 5 and 15 bridges of bilirubin are in a *trans-* or Z configuration. Exposure of circulating bilirubin to light changes the configuration of one or both of the interpyrrolic bridges at the 5 and 15 positions to an E or *cis*-configuration. The resulting ZE, EZ, or EE isomers lack one or more internal hydrogen bonds, are more polar than is bilirubin IXα-ZZ, and can be excreted in bile without conjugation.[59] The vinyl substituent in the endovinyl half of bilirubin IXα-EZ is subsequently cyclized with the methyl substituent on the internal pyrrole ring, forming the structural isomer E-cyclobilirubin.[60] Although cyclization of bilirubin occurs at a slower rate than formation of configurational isomers, because of the relative stability of cyclobilirubin, this form may be quantitatively more important in phototherapy of neonatal jaundice.[60]

Photooxidation and Degradation. Whether in aqueous solution or bound to proteins or lipids, bilirubin undergoes gradual bleaching in light and oxygen.[61] Bleaching results in formation of colorless fragments, chiefly maleimides and propentdyopent adducts, owing to a self-sensitized reaction involving singlet oxygen. A small amount of biliverdin is also formed by mechanisms that are not established.[61]

Dipyrrolic Scrambling. When bilirubin IXα is irradiated in deoxygenated aqueous solution, free radical disproportionation results in formation of bilirubin IIIα and bilirubin XIIIα (Fig. 125-6), which are nonphysiologic symmetrical isomers of bilirubin.[61] The reaction is faster in the presence of oxygen and is catalyzed by acid[61] and inhibited by ascorbic acid.

Toxicity of Bilirubin

A toxic effect of bilirubin on the brain of neonates has been known for at least five centuries.[62] Yellow discoloration of basal ganglia in babies with intense jaundice was described in 1847, and the term *kernicterus* was coined to describe these changes in 1903.[63,64]

Biochemical Mechanisms of Bilirubin Toxicity. Bilirubin inhibits DNA synthesis in a mouse neuroblastoma cell line.[65] Bilirubin also may uncouple oxidative phosphorylation and inhibit adenosine triphosphatase (ATPase) activity of brain mitochondria.[66] Studies *in vitro* reveal that bilirubin inhibits hydrolytic enzymes,[67] dehydrogenases,[68] and enzymes involved in electron transport.[69] In mutant rats (Gunn strain) with congenital nonhemolytic hyperbilirubinemia, bilirubin inhibited RNA synthesis, protein synthesis, and carbohydrate metabolism in brain and inhibited protein synthesis in liver.[70,71] Bilirubin also decreased respiration of isolated brain mitochondria, uncoupled oxidative phosphorylation, inhibited ATPase activity, and induced swelling in the brain.[72–74] Bilirubin has been shown to inhibit protein kinase-mediated phosphorylation of neural proteins.[75,76] In a cell-free system, bilirubin irreversibly inhibited Ca^{2+}-activated, phospholipid-dependent protein kinase (protein kinase C) activity and cyclic adenosine monophosphate (cAMP)-dependent protein kinase activity.[77] All toxic effects of bilirubin are reduced or

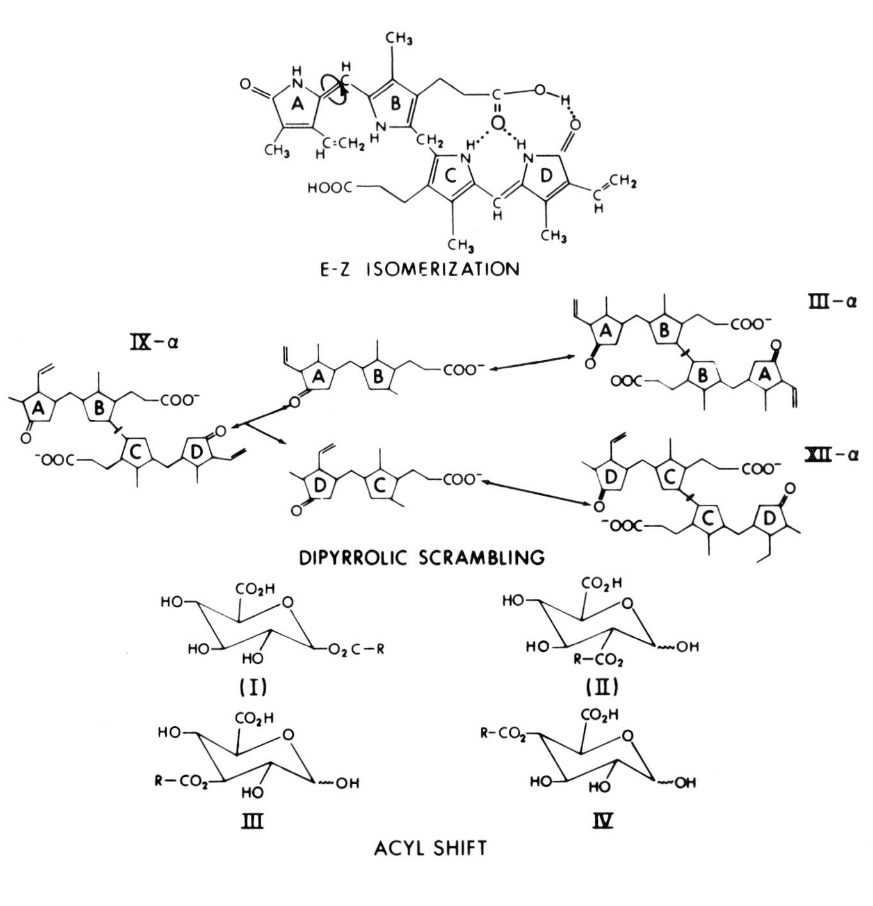

Fig. 125-6 Isomerization of unconjugated and conjugated bilirubin. *Upper panel.* Geometric isomerization: The bond between pyrrolenone rings A and B or C and D can change into an E (*cis*) configuration, as shown here on the left half of the bilirubin molecule, resulting in the EZ, ZE, or EE isomers. E configuration of the bond between the pyrrolenone rings interferes with hydrogen bonding and renders the molecule relatively polar. *Middle panel.* Nonenzymatic dipyrrolic scrambling involves formation of dipyrrolic free radicals and their random reassembly into asymmetric (bilirubin IXα) and symmetric (bilirubin IIIα and XIIIα) tetrapyrroles. *Lower panel.* Acyl shifting of bilirubin glucuronides occurs on nonenzymatic incubation, resulting in conversion of the normal 1-O-acylglucuronide to 2-, 3-, or 4-O-acyl forms. R, propionyl side chain of bilirubin.

reversed by albumin *in vivo* and *in vitro*. Increased plasma concentrations of bilirubin increase the risk of bilirubin encephalopathy in newborn babies. A serum concentration of 20 mg/dl is often quoted as the highest limit of safety, although kernicterus can occur at lower serum bilirubin concentrations.[78] Individual differences in the susceptibility to bilirubin encephalopathy is underscored by the finding that Gunn rats bred against different normal background strains have similar serum bilirubin levels but markedly different incidences of kernicterus and mortality.[79] Serum albumin concentrations, pH, and substances that compete for albumin binding are important in the pathogenesis of bilirubin encephalopathy.[80]

Clinical Features of Bilirubin Encephalopathy. Kernicterus occurs in infants with severe unconjugated hyperbilirubinemia and in young adults with high serum unconjugated bilirubin levels due to severe inherited deficiency of bilirubin-UGT activity. Kernicterus usually presents between the third and sixth days of life, with poor feeding and feeble suck reflex, high-pitched cry, hypertonia or hypotonia, reflex opisthotonus in response to a startling stimulus, convulsion, incomplete Moro reflex, and instability of thermal regulation (hypothermia or hyperthermia).[78] This may progress to lethargy, atonia, and death. Long-term sequelae include delay in motor development, chorioathetosis, asymmetric spasticity, sensorineural hearing loss, paralysis of upward gaze, dental dysplasia, cognitive dysfunction, and mental retardation. The cochlear nucleus is particularly sensitive to bilirubin-induced damage. The affected areas in the cochlear nucleus and superior olive are innervated by large axosomatic end bulbs or caliceal endings. Cells receiving synaptic input from end bulbs or calices appear to be early targets of bilirubin toxicity in the auditory system.[81] Brainstem auditory evoked responses correlate well with plasma free bilirubin levels in humans[82] and with morphologic changes in the cochlear nucleus in Gunn rat pups.[83] There is prolongation of interval between the auditory stimulus and appearance of wave I (latency), indicating delayed auditory nerve conduction. The intervals between wave I and wave III (reflecting the superior olive) and wave I and wave V (reflecting inferior colliculus) are also prolonged (interpeak latency). This test may be made more sensitive by recording binaural difference waves obtained by subtracting the sum of two monaural brainstem auditory evoked potentials from a binaural brainstem auditory evoked potential.[84] Moderately high serum unconjugated bilirubin levels may result in a higher incidence of impaired neurologic or intellectual performance in later life.[85,86] In some children with Crigler-Najjar syndrome type I there may be late clinical presentation of bilirubin encephalopathy with cerebellar symptoms as the presenting feature.[87]

Magnetic resonance imaging of the brain provides a sensitive means of evaluating kernicterus.[86–90] Abnormally high intensity signals are observed over the globus pallidus, particularly over the posteromedial border. In many cases, increased intensity is also seen over the thalamus, internal capsule, and hippocampi. These magnetic resonance imaging abnormalities are also found in several other types of metabolic encephalopathy and must be interpreted in the context of the clinical presentation. Bilirubin staining of the hippocampus, basal ganglia, and nuclei of the cerebellum and brainstem is observed in infants who die from acute kernicterus.[91] In infants who die within 72 h after the onset of kernicterus, there may be no cellular damage of the brain seen by light microscopy. Early histologic changes occur after this period and include cytoplasmic degeneration, loss of Nissl substance, and fine vacuolation and swelling of nuclear chromatin.[92] Evidence of cell death may be present. In children who die in the chronic stage of the disorder, bilirubin staining is not found in the brain,[91] but focal necrosis of neurons and glia are found. Gliosis of the affected areas occurs in later cases.[92]

Role of the Blood–Brain Barrier. Tight junctions between capillary endothelial cells and foot processes of astroglial cells restrict the exchange of water-soluble substances and proteins between blood and brain.[93] In addition, specific transport processes for ions, water, and nutrients from plasma to brain may provide a functional blood–brain barrier. Conventionally, the immaturity of the blood–brain barrier in neonates has been thought to contribute to kernicterus. However, a more rapid passage of labeled markers[94] or lipophilic substances[95] into the immature brain has been difficult to confirm, and there is little evidence to support the concept of immaturity of the blood–brain barrier in the neonate. Moreover, opening of the blood–brain barrier is expected to permit both bilirubin and albumin to enter the brain. Because albumin binding neutralizes the toxic effects of bilirubin, this should not result in increased bilirubin toxicity. Current evidence indicates that the non–albumin-bound (free) fraction of bilirubin enters the brain, and such entry is independent of the intactness of the blood–brain barrier. A special proclivity of the neonatal brain cells to bind bilirubin may facilitate its retention in the brain of newborns with severe unconjugated hyperbilirubinemia. Hyperosmolarity-associated shrinkage of capillary endothelial cells results in temporary and reversible opening of the tight junctions. When the blood–brain barrier is opened in newborn rats by infusion of hypertonic urea[96] or arabinose,[93] intravenously administered albumin–bilirubin complex rapidly enters the brain. Following reversal of opening of the blood–brain barrier, bilirubin is rapidly cleared from the brain in parallel with clearance from the serum, suggesting that bilirubin is cleared by diffusion or transport back into the general circulation.[97] However, damaged and edematous brain may bind bilirubin,[98] may be unable to clear it rapidly, and may be more vulnerable to bilirubin toxicity for that reason.

Binding of Bilirubin to Albumin

In the circulation, bilirubin is tightly but reversibly bound to albumin. Albumin binding plays a critical role in the disposition of bilirubin by the body. It keeps bilirubin in solution and transports the pigment from its sites of production, primarily the spleen and the bone marrow, to its site of excretion, the liver. The tight binding of unconjugated bilirubin to albumin prevents its excretion by the kidney, except during albuminuria. Conjugated bilirubin is bound much less tightly to albumin, and the relatively larger unbound fraction undergoes glomerular filtration and is excreted in the urine. During disease states that are associated with prolonged increase in plasma-conjugated bilirubin levels, a fraction of the pigment becomes irreversibly bound to albumin.[99] This fraction, termed *δ-bilirubin*, is not excreted in the bile or urine and disappears slowly, reflecting the long half-life of albumin.

Albumin-binding protects against all known toxic effects of bilirubin, and a small unbound fraction of bilirubin is thought to be responsible for its toxicity. Coadministration of equimolar amounts of albumin protects against otherwise lethal effects of unconjugated bilirubin following intravenous injection in puppies.[100]

In normal plasma, bilirubin is bound to a primary binding site on albumin, almost exclusively as the dianion. Normal molar concentration of albumin (500–700 μM) exceeds that of bilirubin (upper limit 17 μM). However, during neonatal jaundice, in patients with Crigler-Najjar syndrome, and occasionally in acquired liver diseases, the molar ratio of unconjugated bilirubin to albumin can exceed 1. The molar excess of bilirubin can be accentuated by reduction of serum albumin levels due to inflammatory states, chronic malnutrition, or liver diseases. In these circumstances, bilirubin also can bind weakly to a second, third, and a fourth site. However, such binding is much weaker, so the unbound fraction of bilirubin increases sharply. Use of sulfonamides in newborn babies enhances bilirubin encephalopathy,[101] as a result of dissociation of bilirubin by sulfonamide from its binding to albumin.[102] Infusion of albumin increases the plasma bilirubin concentration because of transfer of bilirubin from tissues to plasma.[103] Because of the clinical importance of estimation of the unbound fraction of unconjugated bilirubin, the binding of bilirubin to albumin has been evaluated by separating bound from free bilirubin by ultrafiltration, ultracentrifugation, gel chromatography, affinity chromatography on albumin agarose polymers, dialysis, and electrophoresis. Unbound bilirubin is rapidly destroyed by treatment with H_2O_2 and horseradish peroxidase, as compared with bound bilirubin. Binding of bilirubin to albumin induces bilirubin fluorescence, circular dichroism, quenching of protein fluorescence, and a shift in the absorbance spectra. In most studies, the primary binding constant at physiologic pH and temperature is slightly below 10^8 M^{-1}. The binding constant for the secondary site is believed to be lower by one order of magnitude.[49,104] Enzymatic hydrolysis and analysis of albumin covalently bound to bilirubin indicate that bilirubin binds to lysine 240 in human albumin and to lysine 238 in bovine serum albumin.[105] Binding of other ligands to albumin plays a major role in determining bilirubin binding capacity. The other ligand may bind at the same site as does bilirubin, resulting in competitive displacement, or it may bind noncompetitively at a different site. Noncompetitive binding may not affect bilirubin binding or may produce conformational changes that enhance (cooperative binding) or decrease (anticooperative) bilirubin binding. Sulfonamides, antiinflammatory drugs, and contrast media used for cholangiography displace bilirubin competitively from albumin and increase the risk of kernicterus in jaundiced newborn babies.[106] Some benzodiazepine drugs and long-chain fatty acids in low concentration bind to human albumin without affecting bilirubin binding.[107,108] Albumin binding of medium-chain fatty acids, such as laureate and myristate, increase the binding constant for bilirubin.[109] Short-chain fatty acids bind to albumin anticooperatively with bilirubin.[110] When large amounts of fatty acid bind to albumin, major conformational changes occur that generally decrease the binding of other ligands, including bilirubin. Acidosis increases the risk of brain damage in neonatal jaundice[111,112] but does not influence bilirubin binding to the primary site of albumin. The increased risk of kernicterus may result from enhanced transport of bilirubin from plasma to selected areas of the central nervous system.[49] Because of the influence of many metabolites and drugs on albumin binding of bilirubin and on its transfer from plasma to the central nervous system, measurement of plasma bilirubin concentration does not accurately estimate the risk of brain damage from unconjugated bilirubin. It is generally believed, although it has not been verified, that unbound bilirubin is transferred from plasma to the central nervous system.[102] Efforts have been made to quantify unbound bilirubin in serum by gel chromatography,[113] peroxidase treatment,[114] electrophoresis on cellulose acetate,[115] and fluorimetry of serum with or without detergent treatment.[116]

Free bilirubin concentration is determined from the equilibrium equation

$$[F] = [B]([RA]K)$$

where [F] is the free bilirubin concentration, [B] is albumin-bound bilirubin concentration, [RA] is the concentration of reserve bilirubin binding sites on albumin, and K is the association constant for bilirubin. Equilibrium between free and bound bilirubin is assumed, and binding of bilirubin to tissues and secondary binding sites on albumin are ignored. The numerical values for binding constants, as determined from experiments with pure albumin and bilirubin, are assumed to be valid in serum. These assumptions may not be valid with icteric serum, so it is not possible to calculate reliably the concentration of unbound bilirubin. The alternative approach is to determine the amount of unoccupied bilirubin binding sites on albumin. Titration of serum with bilirubin or a dye that binds to albumin has been used to estimate unoccupied bilirubin binding sites.

Binding to secondary binding sites begins before primary sites are saturated, and some dyes bind at sites other than the bilirubin site. Binding of bilirubin to erythrocytes depends on the albumin:bilirubin ratio in serum and indirectly reflects reserve bilirubin binding sites on albumin.[117] Competitive binding by a ^{14}C-labeled ligand (monoacetyl-4,4′-diaminodiphenyl sulfone)[118] or a spin-labeled ligand [1-N-(2,2,6,6, tetramethyl-1-oxyl-4-piperidinyl)5-N-(1-aspartate)-2,4,-dinitrobenzene][119] has been used to determine reserve binding capacity. A fluorimetric method has been described for determination of bound albumin and reserve bilirubin binding capacity.[116] Despite inaccuracies, several empirical tests for determination of reserve bilirubin binding capacity of serum albumin correlate clinically with brain damage[120] and may be useful in assessing the risk of bilirubin toxicity.

Uptake of Bilirubin by the Liver

Although tightly bound to albumin, bilirubin is rapidly removed from the circulation by the liver (Fig. 125-7). Kinetic studies of bilirubin uptake in isolated perfused livers of dogs[121] and rats[122] and in intact rats *in vivo*[123] reveal that the process is saturable. Following an intravenous loading dose of bilirubin, the plasma disappearance of a subsequent tracer dose of [^3H]-bilirubin is enhanced,[123] suggesting a carrier-mediated facilitated diffusion. Countertransport of bilirubin (i.e., efflux of radiolabeled ligand from liver after subsequent infusion with unlabeled ligand) has been claimed,[123] but the data also could be interpreted to represent efflux of ligand from intracellular binding sites. Mutual competition for hepatic uptake *in vivo* has been described with respect to bilirubin and other organic anions, such as indocyanine green

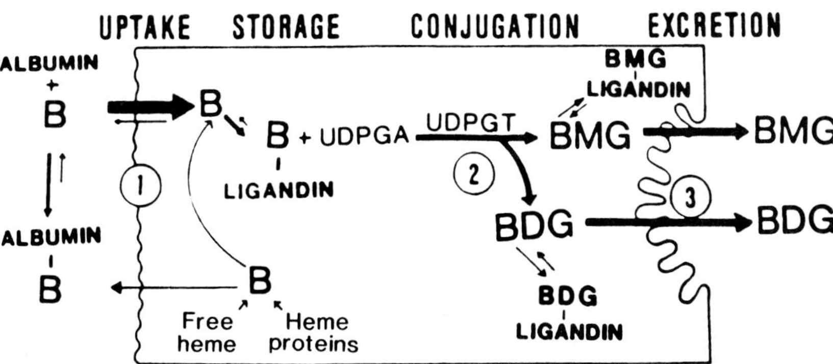

Fig. 125-7 Summary of hepatic metabolism of bilirubin (B). Bilirubin is strongly bound to albumin in the circulation. This complex dissociates, and bilirubin enters hepatocytes by a specific uptake mechanism (1). A fraction of the bilirubin is also derived from catabolism of hepatocellular heme proteins. Within the hepatocyte, bilirubin binds to a group of cytosolic proteins, termed ligandins; this inhibits the efflux of bilirubin from the cell. UDP-glucuronosyltransferase (UDPGT) (2), an ER enzyme, catalyzes the transfer of glucuronic acid from UDP-glucuronate (UDPGA) to bilirubin, forming bilirubin monoglucuronide (BMG) and diglucuronide (BDG). Both conjugates may bind to ligandins in the cytosol. Normally, conjugation is obligatory for biliary excretion (3) of bilirubin; only small amounts of unconjugated bilirubin are found in bile. Canalicular excretion is thought to be an energy-dependent process that is normally rate limiting and may be shared by other organic anions, except bile salts.

(ICG),[123,124] sulfobromophthalein (BSP),[123,124] and conjugated bilirubin.[124] Bile acids do not compete with these compounds for hepatic uptake.[123,125]

Bilirubin dissociates from albumin before entering the hepatocyte, and albumin does not accompany the pigment into the hepatocyte. Five minutes after intravenous injection of a mixture of [^{3}H]-bilirubin and ^{131}I-labeled albumin into rats, approximately 60 percent of injected bilirubin is internalized by the liver, whereas only 10 percent of the injected albumin is present in the liver, probably in the vascular space.[122] In isolated perfused rat and dog livers, simultaneous injection of [^{125}I]-albumin and [^{3}H]-bilirubin discloses rapid bilirubin uptake, with no removal of albumin from the perfusate.[121,126] It is not clear whether free or albumin-bound bilirubin interacts with the hepatocyte. Early studies suggested that the unbound fraction of bilirubin is taken up by the hepatocyte.[127] This view was challenged by investigators who found that uptake of albumin-bound ligands by the perfused rat liver correlated poorly with the expected concentration of unbound ligand.[128,129] For example, increasing the albumin concentration tenfold from 0.5 g/dl to 5 g/dl reduced the concentration of free taurocholate by a factor of five, but reduced uptake by only 50 percent.[129] Similar results were found for uptake of fatty acids, bilirubin, and BSP.[128,130] In addition, uptake of a 1:1 complex of one of these ligands with albumin was saturable and competitively inhibited by albumin.[128] Based on these observations, it was suggested that albumin mediated hepatic uptake of these ligands,[129] and the presence of a receptor for albumin on the liver cell surface was postulated.[128] However, an alternative hypothesis to explain albumin receptor-like kinetics suggests that the unbound ligand interacts with the liver cell plasma membrane, but the rate of dissociation of the ligand from albumin may limit uptake.[131,132] This new model of dissociation-limited uptake of bilirubin is compatible with the existence of an albumin receptor and adequately describes BSP uptake in perfused elasmobranch liver.[133]

To evaluate the role of albumin binding on solute distribution within the zones of the hepatic acinus, Gumucio et al. studied BSP transport in isolated rat liver perfused with 0.01 to 1.0 mM BSP with or without albumin.[134] When steady-state conditions of BSP excretion were established, the liver was frozen and relative BSP concentrations in various zones of the liver acinus were estimated. Without albumin, there was 95 percent extraction of BSP in a single pass; a decreasing concentration gradient from zone 1 (periportal) to zone 3 (pericentral) was observed. Inclusion of 4.5 percent or 1 percent albumin in the perfusate resulted in single-pass extraction of only 8 to 22 percent of BSP, and the zonal gradient of BSP content was abolished. The results demonstrate that albumin binding produces more homogeneous distribution of organic anions within the liver acinus. When the liver was perfused retrogradely (through the hepatic vein) in the absence of albumin, BSP was taken up predominantly by hepatocytes of zone 3 and a decreasing gradient from zone 3 to zone 1 was produced. BSP-glutathione conjugates appeared in bile during antegrade and retrograde perfusion, indicating that hepatocytes of both zones have the ability to conjugate and excrete BSP.

To elucidate the mechanism and driving forces responsible for hepatic organic anion uptake, a number of studies have been performed on isolated rat hepatocytes[135–138] or liver sinusoidal vesicles.[139] These experiments, conducted in the absence of albumin, suggested temperature-dependent, sodium-independent uptake. Studies of [^{35}S]-BSP uptake in short-term cultured rat hepatocytes, performed in the presence of a molar excess of bovine albumin, revealed linear uptake of BSP over at least 15 min with little formation of its glutathione (GSH) conjugate over this time.[140] The initial uptake of [^{35}S]-BSP was depressed by isosmotic substitution of NaCl by sucrose. A specific cation requirement for BSP uptake is unlikely because uptake was unaffected by substitution for NaCl by KCl or LiCl. However, substitution of Cl^- by HCO_3^- or gluconate$^-$ markedly inhibited BSP uptake. Similar observations were made for the uptake of [^{3}H]-bilirubin glucuronides.[141] Studies in rat liver perfused with $NaCl^-$ or Na gluconate-substituted mediums revealed similar inhibition of bilirubin influx.[140] The mechanism by which hepatocyte organic anion transport is stimulated by inorganic anions does not appear to be related to transport of the inorganic anion in or out of the cell.[142] Studies using ^{36}Cl revealed that in short-term cultured rat hepatocytes, BSP uptake requires external Cl^- and is not stimulated by unidirectional Cl^- gradients.[142] Thus, there was no evidence for linkage of chloride transport with organic anion transport. Studies of binding of [^{35}S]-BSP to hepatocytes at 4°C revealed an approximately tenfold higher affinity in the presence of Cl^- as compared with its absence.[142] Whether this is the complete explanation for Cl^--dependent kinetics of BSP transport remains to be determined. In the transfer of organic anions from the space of Disse to the hepatocyte, the liver cell plasma membrane is the first barrier to entry into the cell and presumably is the site of interaction with organic anions that results in carrier-mediated uptake kinetics. Although kinetic evidence has been presented that bilirubin has rapid transit across lipid bilayers,[132,143] the cellular specificity and driving forces of this event suggest a hepatocyte transporter for this ligand.

Several studies of organic anion interaction with liver plasma membrane preparations have been performed in an attempt to describe the nature of the putative carrier. A number of early studies demonstrated saturable binding of BSP to liver plasma membrane.[143–145] Several putative plasma membrane organic binding proteins were isolated. One isolated by Berk, Stremmel, and colleagues was termed a "BSP/bilirubin binding protein."[143,146] These investigators reported that polyclonal antibodies to this protein inhibited uptake of BSP and bilirubin by isolated rat hepatocytes.[147] However, interpretation of these studies is difficult because a relatively large amount of antibody was needed for even a partial inhibition of BSP uptake. A second protein termed *bilitranslocase* was isolated by Tiribelli, Sottocasa, and colleagues.[148] Bilitranslocase is a 170-kDa protein composed of 37-kDa and 35-kDa subunits and has been reported to reconstitute BSP transport in liposomes[148] and in erythrocyte membrane vesicles.[149] In studies by Wolkoff and Chung, a photoaffinity probe was devised in which [^{35}S]-BSP was covalently bound to liver cell plasma membrane after exposure to ultraviolet light.[144] Subsequent sodium dodecyl sulfate polyacrylamide gel electrophoresis and fluorography revealed radioactivity predominantly associated with a single 55-kDa protein.[150] This organic anion-binding protein was purified and characterized immunologically.[144] It appears to differ from the BSP/bilirubin binding protein and bilitranslocase. Using an antibody against this organic acid- binding protein to screen a rat liver λgt11 expression library, a 1550-bp complementary DNA (cDNA) was cloned.[151] On further characterization, it was found that this cDNA encoded the β subunit of mitochondrial F_1-ATPase.

Based on the characteristics of [^{35}S]-BSP extraction from albumin by hepatocytes,[140] an assay was devised that enabled detection of transport in *Xenopus laevis* oocytes that had been injected with rat liver poly(A)+ RNA.[152] These oocytes were able to extract BSP from albumin in a chloride-dependent fashion. Subsequently, a single complementary RNA (cRNA) was isolated that when injected into oocytes resulted in marked enrichment of BSP transport activity. The corresponding cDNA encodes a rat liver protein that has been named organic anion-transporting polypeptide (oatp). The oatp cDNA contains an open reading frame of 2010 nucleotides and suggests that oatp is a hydrophobic protein. The best computer-generated model of oatp predicts that the protein has 12 transmembrane domains and three potential N-glycosylation sites. Northern blot analysis revealed that oatp is expressed in the liver and kidney. Recent data indicate that it is also present in the choroid plexus, a tissue that also expresses several otherwise liver-specific proteins. At low stringency, oatp cDNA also hybridizes with messenger RNA (mRNA) extracted from other organs, including lung, skeletal muscle, and proximal colon. Studies using HeLa cells stably transfected with oatp indicate that oatp-mediated taurocholate transport is Na^+ independent, saturable, and associated with HCO_3^- exchange.[153] However, the role of oatp or one of the related proteins in bilirubin transport has not been directly established, and is being investigated. Oatp appears to be the first member of a family of sodium-independent plasma membrane transport proteins. Other members include transporters for prostaglandins,[154] digoxin, and folic acid.

Intrahepatocellular Storage of Bilirubin

Fifteen minutes following intravenous injection of [^{3}H]-bilirubin into rats, over 90 percent disappeared from plasma and 25 to 30 percent of the injected dose remained in liver.[155] Radioactivity does not appear in bile until 3 to 4 min after injection and subsequently appears at a rate of approximately 3 percent of the injected dose per minute.[156] Thus, from the time bilirubin is cleared from plasma and subsequently excreted into bile, it is stored within hepatocytes. At all times after intravenous injection, a large proportion of [^{3}H]-bilirubin is associated with the cytosolic fraction of liver homogenates.[155,156] Because the water solubility of unconjugated bilirubin is very low at physiologic pH, it is kept in solution by binding to cytosolic proteins. Gel filtration of cytosol containing [^{3}H]-bilirubin or [^{35}S]-BSP reveals that radioactivity is associated with two protein peaks that were originally termed Y and Z (Fig. 125-8).[157] Tracer quantities of anions bind almost exclusively to the Y protein; with larger amounts, binding to the Z protein becomes apparent.[157] This suggests that, under physiologic conditions, Y protein is the principal cytoplasmic protein to which organic anions bind. Purified Y protein was shown to bind many compounds, including drugs, hormones, and organic anions.[157,158] Similar proteins with the ability to bind a cortisol metabolite[159] and an azo-dye carcinogen[160] were identified by various laboratories. These proteins were found to be immunologically cross-reactive and were termed *ligandin*. Ligandin accounts for 5 percent of liver cytosol proteins.[161] Subsequently, ligandin was found to be a family of proteins, identical to the α class of glutathione-S-transferases in the rat liver.[162,163] There are corresponding proteins in human hepatocytes as well. These proteins bind bilirubin and a wide variety of organic anions as nonsubstrate ligands.[163] The high affinity of these proteins for organic anions suggests that they may play a role in transport by the liver. The role of ligandin in transport of bilirubin was studied in isolated perfused liver from rats in which ligandin levels were increased following thyroidectomy or treatment with phenobarbital.[164] There was no correlation between hepatic ligandin concentration and the influx rate of bilirubin.

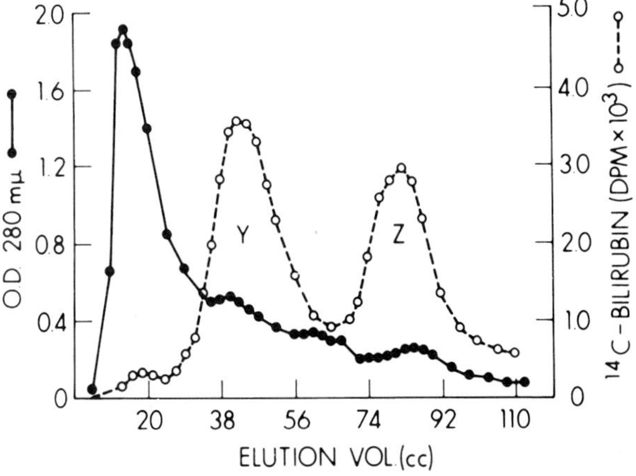

Fig. 125-8 Binding of bilirubin to cytosolic proteins. Sephadex-G75 gel chromatography of 110,000 × g rat liver supernatant to which [^{14}C]bilirubin has been added reveals association of radioactivity with two protein peaks, Y and Z. Y protein was determined to be quantitatively more important in organic anion binding and was named ligandin. Subsequently, ligandin was found to consist of several proteins belonging to the glutathione-S-transferase family.

However, the efflux rate of bilirubin from liver back to plasma varied inversely with hepatic ligandin concentration. Thus, intracellular protein binding of bilirubin appears to play no role in its extraction from serum albumin and subsequent influx into the hepatocyte. However, binding to ligandin increases the net uptake of bilirubin by reducing efflux from the hepatocyte. With respect to organic anion transport, ligandin may function within the hepatocyte much as albumin does in the circulation, binding bilirubin and preventing efflux from the hepatocyte back into the circulation and nonspecific diffusion of bilirubin into compartments of the hepatocyte in which it may do harm. This hypothesis is supported by the finding that bilirubin inhibits mitochondrial respiration *in vitro*, an effect that is prevented by ligandin.[165]

Conjugation of Bilirubin

Bilirubin Conjugates. Efficient excretion of bilirubin across the bile canaliculus requires its conversion to polar conjugates by esterification of the propionic acid carboxyl groups. Esterification of one or both propionic acid side chains forms monoconjugates or diconjugates, respectively. Glucuronic acid is by far the major conjugating group in normal mammalian bile pigments,[166] although smaller amounts of glucosyl and xylosyl conjugates are also found.[167] Bilirubin glucuronides are present as monoconjugates and diconjugates (Fig. 125-9).[168] Bilirubin IXα is asymmetrical; therefore, bilirubin IXα monoglucuronide exists as two isomers, depending on where the glucuronosyl group is attached.[168–171] Bilirubin diglucuronide is the major pigment in normal human bile.[169–171]

Enzyme-Catalyzed Glucuronidation of Bilirubin. Conjugation of bilirubin with glucuronic acid is catalyzed by a specific form of uridine diphosphoglucuronate glucuronosyltransferase, abbreviated as UDP-glucuronosyltransferase or UGT. Protein isolation[172–177] and molecular cloning studies[178–184] revealed that UGTs are a family of enzymes[185] present in the endoplasmic reticulum and nuclear envelope of hepatocytes and many other cells.[186] All UGT isoforms accept uridine diphosphoglucuronic acid as the donor substrate and use a broad range of aglycone acceptor substrates; they catalyze the transfer of the glucuronic acid moiety from uridinediphosphoglucuronic acid (UDP-glucuronic acid), forming ether, ester, thiol, and N-glucuronides.[187] Aglycone substrates of UGTs are diverse, including steroid hormones, thyroid hormones, bile salts, neurotransmitters, bilirubin, and various exogenous substrates, such as drugs, environmental toxins, and laboratory xenobiotics. UGTs are integral membrane proteins that require specific membrane lipids for their function.[188,189] Delipidation results in loss of enzyme activity, which is restored upon addition of appropriate phospholipids.[188,189] UGT activity in microsomal vesicles is partially latent. Membrane perturbation by detergent treatment, sonication, or brief incubation with phospholipase A removes the latency, and full activity of the enzyme is expressed.[188–191] UGT activity in native microsomes is also enhanced by low concentrations of UDP-N-acetylglucosamine, which may be a physiologic activator of the transferase. Two mechanisms have been proposed to explain this activation. In the compartmental model, microsomal lipid membranes are thought to pose a partial barrier between UDP-glucuronic acid and the catalytic site of UGT, which is thought to be located within the endoplasmic reticular lumen. The amino acid sequences of UGTs have been interpreted to indicate a single transmembrane domain of the protein. Transport of UDP-glucuronic acid into the endoplasmic reticulum cisternae by specific mechanisms has been proposed.[192] This model also postulates the presence of a transporter in the microsomal membranes, which facilitates access of UDP-glucuronic acid to the catalytic site of the transferase. UDP-N-acetylglucosamine is envisioned as an activator of the permease. Membrane perturbation is thought to enhance enzyme activity *in vitro* by increasing the permeability of the lipid membranes to UDP-glucuronic acid.[193] The alternative hypothesis, termed the *allosteric model*,

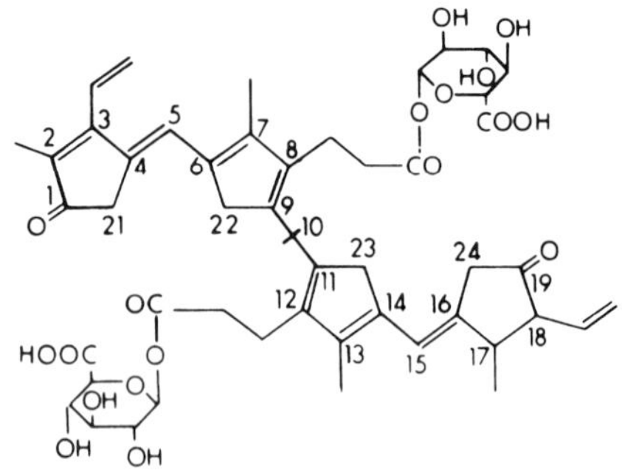

1. BILIRUBIN DIGLUCURONIDE

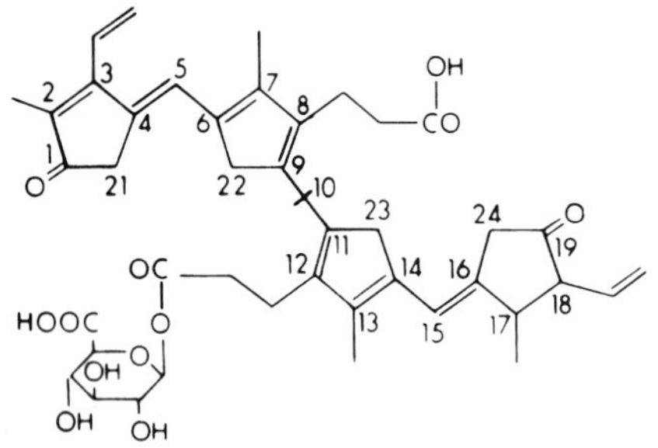

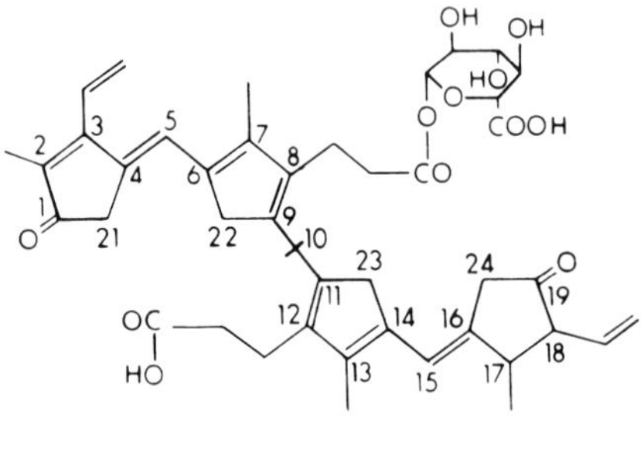

Fig. 125-9 Bilirubin glucuronides. Both propionic acid side chains are glucuronidated in bilirubin diglucuronide. Bilirubin mono-glucuronide can exist as two molecular species, depending on whether the C_{12} or C_8 propionic acid is conjugated.

postulates that the enzyme activity is constrained by the membrane. Activating agents release the enzyme from constraint and thereby enhance enzyme activity.[194]

Structure and Expression of UGT Isoforms. UGT isoforms are expressed from multiple loci. The C-terminal domain of UGT isoforms have a high degree of homology and is responsible for binding of the common donor substrate, UDP-glucuronic acid,[195] whereas the N-terminal domains are more heterogeneous and account for the aglycone substrate specificity of individual isoforms.[196] Based on the degree of homology of the mRNA sequences, UGT genes have been classified among multiple families, and each family into several subfamilies.[185] Only one UGT isoform is physiologically relevant in bilirubin glucuronidation.[196] The locus that expresses bilirubin-UGT is termed *UGT1A* (Fig. 125-10).[197] This locus expresses several UGT isoforms and

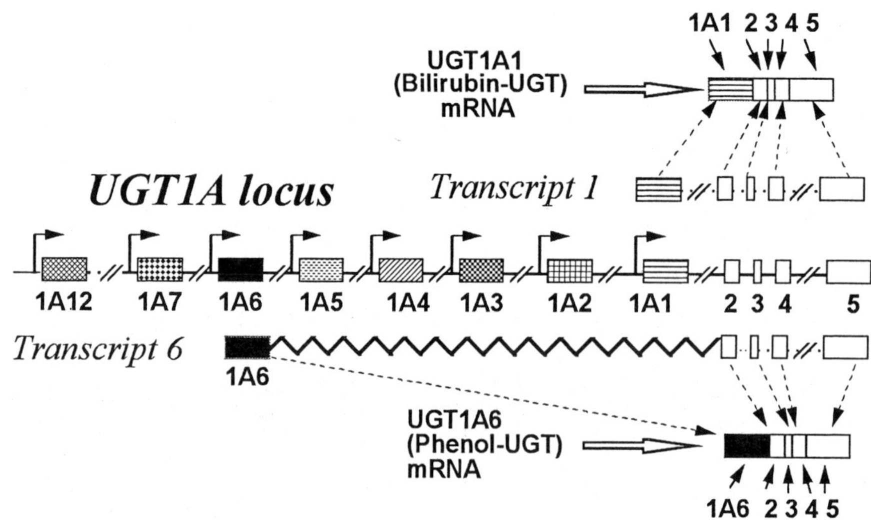

Fig. 125-10 Schematic representation of the human *UGT1A* locus, located at 2q37. This locus contains multiple genes that express bilirubin-UGT and several other UGT isoforms. Exons 2, 3, 4, and 5, located at the 3′ end of *UGT1A*, encode the identical C-terminal domains of all UGT isoforms expressed from this locus. Upstream to these common region exons are a series of unique exons (exons 1A1 through 1A12), each of which encodes the variable N-terminal domain of a different UGT isoform expressed from this locus. Each unique region exon is preceded by a separate promoter region (shown by arrows), permitting independent regulation of gene expression. Transcription can start from any of the promoters, producing transcripts of varying lengths. The unique exon located at the 5′ end of the transcript is spliced to the 3′ end of exon 2, and other unique region exons present in the transcript are spliced out. Thus, based on differential promoter usage, several mRNAs, each encoding a different member of the UGT1A subfamily, are generated. Genes belonging to this locus are named according the unique exon used in the expressed mRNA. Thus, when the transcription starts 5′ to exon 1A1 (transcript 1 in the figure), the mRNA encoding bilirubin-UGT is generated. This gene, which consists of exon 1A1 plus the common region exons 2 to 5, is termed *UGT1A1*, and the expressed enzyme is termed UGT1A1. If, on the other hand, the transcription starts 5′ to exon 1A6 (Transcript 6 in the figure), an mRNA consisting of exon 1A6 plus exons 2 to 5 is generated. This mRNA encodes a UGT isoform that accepts simple phenolic substrates, but not bilirubin. According to the current system of terminology, this gene is named *UGT1A6*, and the expressed isoform is termed UGT1A6.

contains four consecutive exons (exons 2–5) at the 3′ end that are used in all mRNAs expressed from this locus. Upstream from these four common region exons are a series of unique exons, each preceded by a separate promoter. Depending on which promoter is used, transcripts of various sizes are generated. The unique exon, present at the 5′ end of the transcript, is spliced to exon 2, and the intervening sequence is spliced out. Thus, all isoforms expressed from the *UGT1A* locus have identical C-terminal domains (encoded by exons 2–5) but variable N-terminal domains (encoded by a single unique exon). Within the *UGT1A* locus, genes encoding individual isoforms are named according to the unique exon used in the expressed mRNA. Thus, the gene for the bilirubin-UGT mRNA, which consists of the first unique region exon of the *UGT1A* locus (plus exons 2–5), is termed *UGT1A1* according to current terminology, and the enzyme is termed UGT1A1. Another isoform that catalyzes phenolic substrates is encoded by the unique region exon 6 (plus exons 2–5); therefore, this gene is termed *UGT1A6*, and the expressed isoform is termed UGT1A6.

Differential Expression of UGT Isoforms. The presence of a separate promoter upstream from each unique region exon (Fig. 125-10) permits differential regulation of individual UGT isoforms during ontogenic development[198] and enzyme induction.[199,200] Enzyme activity toward 4-nitrophenol and other simple phenolic substrates (catalyzed by UGT1A6) develops in late fetal life, whereas UGT activity toward bilirubin (UGT1A1) develops after birth.[198] Treatment of rats with 3-methylcholanthrene induces UGT1A6.[199,200] In contrast, UGT activity toward bilirubin is specifically induced by clofibrate.[199] Treatment of rats with triiodothyronine results in a threefold increase in transferase activity toward 4-nitrophenol, whereas activity toward bilirubin is decreased by 80 percent.[198]

Quantification of Bilirubin and Its Conjugates

Bile pigments are quantified in body fluids as native or derivatized tetrapyrroles, or after conversion to azoderivatives. Total bilirubin also can be quantified indirectly by quantification of the intensity of yellow discoloration of the skin.

Methods Involving Conversion of Bilirubin to azo Derivatives. Conversion to azodipyrroles by reaction with diazo reagents is used commonly for determination of serum bilirubin levels for clinical purposes. Reaction of bilirubin with diazo reagents begins with electrophilic attack by a diazonium ion at the 9 and 11 positions of bilirubin[201] and converts 1 mole of the tetrapyrrole to 2 moles of diazotized azodipyrrole and 1 mole of formaldehyde (Fig. 125-11). The azoderivatives are more stable than is bilirubin, and its conjugates and can be quantified colorimetrically. Unconjugated bilirubin is converted to two unconjugated dipyrroles. Bilirubin diconjugates form two conjugated azodipyrroles, and bilirubin monoconjugates form one conjugated and one unconjugated azodipyrrole. In 1916, van den Bergh and Muller[202] showed that, on the basis of diazo reaction, serum bile pigments can be classified into a direct and an indirect reacting species. The direct reaction occurs within minutes, and the indirect reaction occurs rapidly only in the presence of accelerator substances such as methanol or caffeine. Subsequently, the direct and indirect reacting components were identified as conjugated and unconjugated bilirubin, respectively.[203] The basis of the direct and indirect van den Bergh reactions can be understood from the crystal structure of bilirubin. Because of internal hydrogen bonding, the central methene bridge of bilirubin is not readily accessible to diazo reagents. Addition of accelerators results in disruption of the hydrogen bonds, and completes the reaction. Bilirubin glucuronides lack some or all of the hydrogen bonds and, therefore, react immediately with diazo reagents, without requiring the addition of accelerators. For confirmation, the conjugated and unconjugated azodipyrroles can be extracted and analyzed by thin-layer chromatography[204] or high-pressure liquid chromatography (HPLC)[205] (Fig. 125-12).

Because 10 to 15 percent of unconjugated bilirubin may give direct diazo reaction, the direct-reacting fraction slightly overestimates the levels of conjugated bilirubin. In addition, the irreversibly albumin-bound fraction of serum bilirubin, which is formed in the serum of patients with prolonged conjugated hyperbilirubinemia, exhibits direct diazo reaction.[99] Because irreversibly protein-bound bilirubin is cleared slowly, it persists in serum for a relatively long period after correction of biliary obstruction. Finding of direct-reacting bilirubin during this period may give a false impression of continued biliary obstruction. In patients with renal failure, indican accumulates in serum and may interfere with the diazo reaction of bilirubin.[206] Finally, the diazo method cannot be applied to separately quantify bilirubin

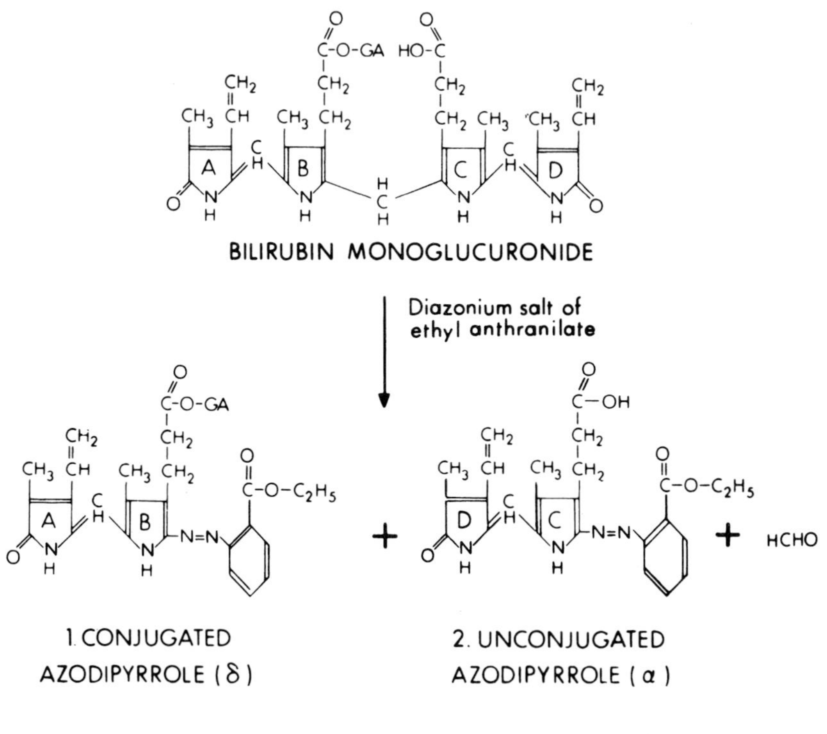

Fig. 125-11 Reaction of bilirubin tetrapyrrole with the diazonium salt of ethylanthranilate results in the formation of equimolar amounts of two azodipyrroles. The central methenyl bridge carbon is converted to formaldehyde. GA, glucuronic acid.

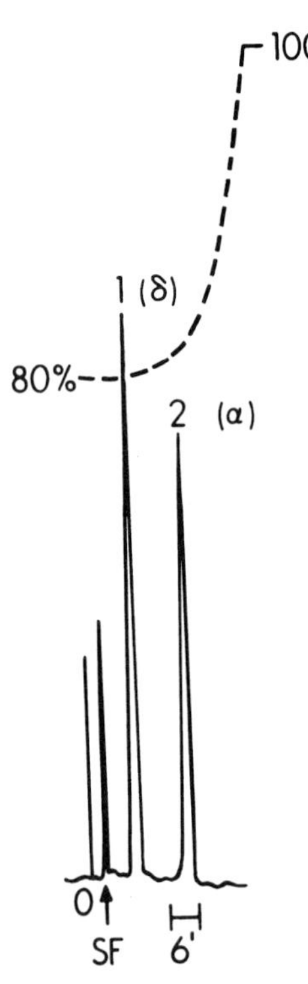

Fig. 125-12 Separation of ethylanthranilate azodipyrroles by HPLC. Wistar rat bile was diazotized with ethylanthranilate diazo reagent, azodipyrroles were extracted,[208] organic solvents were eliminated in reduced pressure, and the pigments were dissolved in methanol and separated by reverse-phase HPLC (μ-Bondapak C-18 column, Waters Associates) using a concave gradient (dashed line) of methanol (80 to 100 percent) in sodium acetate (0.1 M, pH 4.0) containing 5 mM 1-heptane sulfonic acid for 30 min, at 1 ml/min. SF, solvent front. Peak 1 (optical density, 530 nm) represents glucuronidated azodipyrrole, which was designated δ by Heirwegh and his associates,[208] and peak 2 represents the unconjugated azodipyrrole, designated α (see Fig. 125-11).

monoconjugates and diconjugates when they are present in a complex mixture. The latter requires analysis of intact bilirubin tetrapyrroles.

Separation and Quantification of Intact Bilirubin Tetrapyrroles. Chromatographic separation of unmodified bile pigments was attempted by Cole *et al.* as early as in 1954.[207] Subsequently, Heirwegh and associates developed highly resolving thin-layer chromatographic systems for separation of bilirubin and its conjugates.[208] Higher resolution and quantitative recovery of bile pigments is possible by using HPLC. Methyl esters formed by alkaline methanolysis of bilirubin monoconjugates and diconjugates have been separated and quantified by HPLC.[209] Because the conjugating sugars are replaced by methyl groups, the pigments cannot be separated on the basis of their conjugating moieties. Therefore, methods for separation and quantitation of underivatized bilirubin tetrapyrroles by HPLC have been developed[169–171,210] (Fig. 125-13). Reverse-phase HPLC of incompletely deproteinated serum has been used to quantify simultaneously irreversibly protein-bound and other bilirubin fractions.[99] These studies indicate that the irreversibly protein-bound serum bilirubin fraction is present in conditions associated with conjugated hyperbilirubinemia. After successful surgical correction of biliary obstruction, the reversibly protein-bound fraction of serum bilirubin is rapidly excreted in bile; this results in an increase in the proportion of the irreversibly protein-bound fraction of serum bilirubin. If biliary obstruction persists, both reversibly protein-bound and irreversibly protein-bound fractions are retained, and no increase in the proportion of the latter is observed.

Slide Tests. Two slide tests have been introduced for determination of conjugated, unconjugated, and irreversibly protein-bound bilirubin. One slide (Ektachem TIBL) is used for measurement of total bilirubin by a diazo technique.[211] The other slide has a special coating that allows only the free and reversibly protein-bound bilirubins to come in contact with the diazo reagent; conjugated and unconjugated bilirubin are separately quantified by reflectometric measurements at two wavelengths.[212] The difference between total bilirubin and the sum of conjugated and unconjugated bilirubin gives the value for irreversibly protein-bound bilirubin. These results have been verified by HPLC and indicate that the results obtained by the Ektachem slide tests are consistent and reliable.

Transcutaneous Bilirubinometry. The current emphasis on early discharge of neonates makes it imperative to assess the risk of severe neonatal hyperbilirubinemia by evaluating the rate of increase of serum bilirubin levels during the first 24 to 48 hours of life. This requires repeated measurement of serum bilirubin levels, which is painful and expensive. Measurement of the yellow color of the skin by analysis of reflected light provides a noninvasive and relatively inexpensive method for estimating serum bilirubin levels without drawing samples.[213,214] The analyzers use on-board computers programmed to measure the yellow color without interference by underlying skin pigmentation or degree of erythema. In 900 term and premature infants of various races, bilirubin levels estimated by transcutaneous bilirubinometry correlated well with serum billirubin concentrations measured by a standard diazo method.[215]

Fluorimetric Analysis. Fluorescence characteristics of bilirubin have been used in the development of a method for determination of total bilirubin, albumin-bound bilirubin, and reserve bilirubin-binding capacity from as little as 0.1 ml of whole blood. Bilirubin bound to the high-affinity site of albumin has a fluorescence peak at 520 nm when excited at 430 nm. Unbound bilirubin and bilirubin bound to other proteins have negligible fluorescence. Addition of a saturating amount of bilirubin to blood results in maximum fluorescence, allowing determination of total bilirubin-binding capacity. Addition of a detergent, dodecylmethylamine oxide, to whole blood results in hemolysis and quantitative incorporation of bilirubin into the detergent micelles. Fluorescence of detergent-bound bilirubin is used for quantitation of total bilirubin. These parameters can be readily determined using a digital hematofluorometer. Because fluorescence also depends on hemoglobin concentration, hemoglobin values are independently determined by the hematofluorometer and taken into account in calculation of displayed values for total bilirubin and albumin-bound bilirubin and reserve bilirubin binding capacity.[216]

Biliary Secretion of Bilirubin

In mammals, conjugation is essential for the secretion of bilirubin acoss the bile canaliculus. Gunn rats and patients with Crigler-Najjar syndrome type 1 lack bilirubin UGT activity and manifest lifelong unconjugated hyperbilirubinemia. Their bile contains only a small amount of bilirubin. Normally, the conjugating capacity and biliary excretory capacity of bilirubin are closely matched. Thus, drugs and chemicals that reduce the maximal secretory capacity for bilirubin cause the retention of conjugated bilirubin. On the other hand, when bilirubin-UGT activity is partially deficient, conjugation becomes rate limiting in bilirubin secretion.[217] In rats there is approximately a 15-fold functional reserve in the ability to secrete conjugated bilirubin into bile.

Prior to 1991, the major driving force for the transport of bilirubin conjugates from the hepatocyte into the bile was thought to be the electrochemical gradient of −35 mV.[218] Relative intracellular negativity is generated by the sodium pump, which tranports three molecules of sodium out of the cell while transporting two molecules of potassium into the cell. The sodium pump is functional mainly in the basolateral domain of the

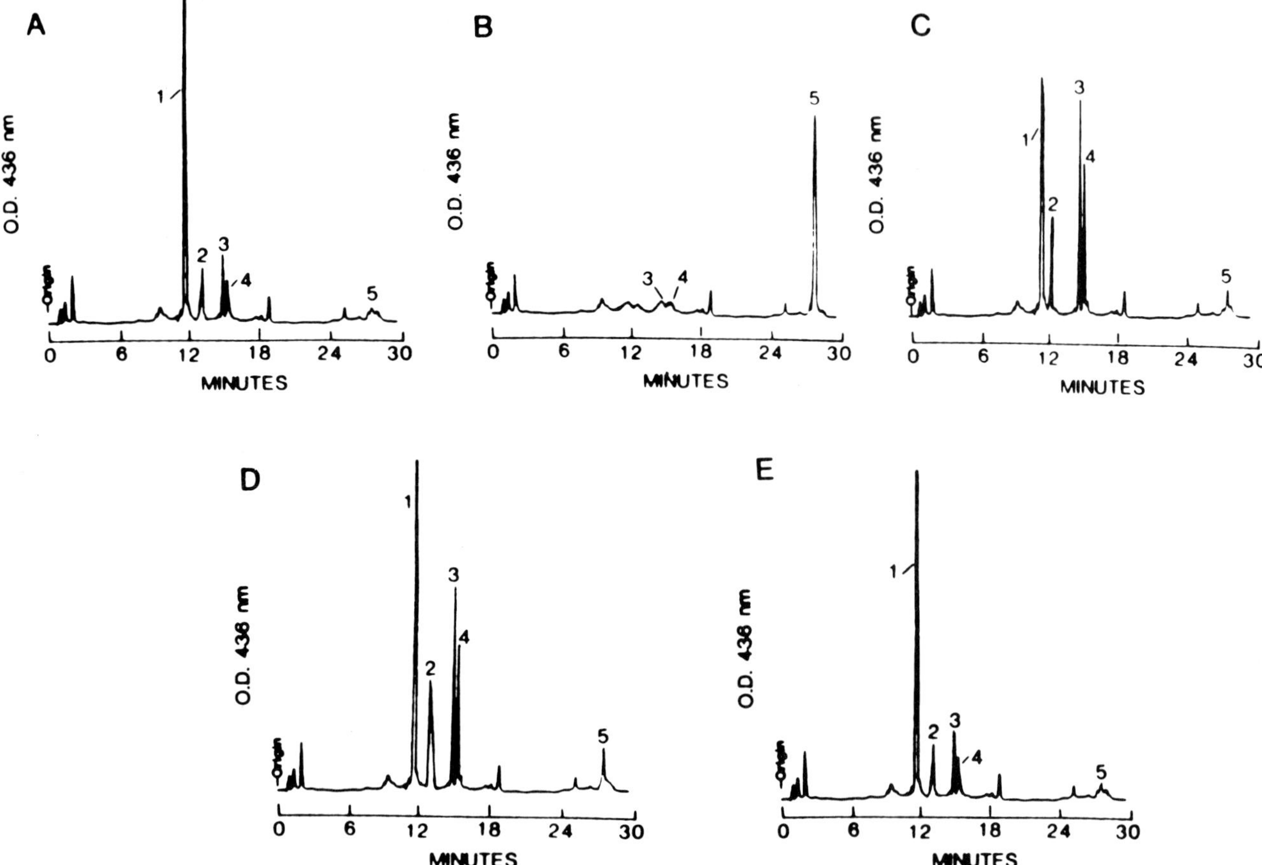

Fig. 125-13 HPLC of intact underivatized bilirubin tetrapyrroles in human bile from a normal individual (*A*) and from patients with Crigler-Najjar syndrome type I (*B*), Crigler-Najjar syndrome type II (Arias syndrome) (*C*), Gilbert syndrome (*D*), and Dubin-Johnson syndrome (*E*). Bile pigments were separated by reverse-phase chromatography. Absorbance at 436 nm (ordinate) and retention time (abscissa) are shown. Peaks are as follows: 1, bilirubin diglucuronide; 2, bilirubin glucoside-glucuronide mixed conjugate; 3 and 4, C-8 and C-12 isomers of bilirubin monoglucuronide; 5, unconjugated bilirubin.

hepatocyte plasma membrane, and is present but inactive in the canalicular domain. The observed potential difference is too small to account for the large bilirubin glucuronide concentration gradients between the hepatocyte and bile, which may be as high as 150-fold. The energy for this uphill transport is provided by an ATP-dependent system in the canalicular membranes that is specific for non–bile acid organic anions, including bilirubin and other glucuronides and glutathione conjugates.[218–223] In contrast to the bidirectional transport at the sinusoidal aspect of the hepatocyte, canalicular transport of organic anions is unidirectional from the cytoplasmic aspect of the hepatocyte into the bile. In addition to the energy-consuming process, the canalicular transport may be assisted by the membrane potential, but the contribution of membrane potential in organic anion transport has not been quantified. The membrane potential–driven canalicular transport of non–bile acid organic anions is distinct from that driven by ATP hydrolysis.[223] Mutant animals that lack ATP-dependent canalicular transport of non–bile acid organic anions retain normal activity with respect to potential-driven canalicular transport of non–bile acid organic anions, including bilirubin glucuronides.[224,225] The benign phenotype of the defect in human and animal mutants may reflect persistence of the potential-driven transport system in the bile canaliculus.

The ATP-dependent canalicular non–bile acid organic anion transporter (also called MOAT, multiorganic anion transporter) is functionally distinct from other canalicular ATP-dependent transporters for organic cations,[226–228] bile acids,[229,230] and phospholipids.[231] Attempts to purify the ATP-dependent transporter for bilirubin glucuronide were unsuccessful. Its identification by cloning followed the serendipitous observation that a drug-resistant cancer cell line expressed an ATP-dependent multidrug resistance–like protein (MRP) that transports various organic cations.[232] The MRP family of ATP-dependent membrane transporters differs from the previously described multidrug resistance (MDR) family of ATP-dependent membrane proteins in amino acid sequence, molecular weight, hydropathy plots, and substrates. Both have multiple transmembrane domains and two nucleotide binding sites that are separated by distinct linker domains. Whereas MRP1 is present in the plasma membrane of many cell types, a family member, MRP2 (initially termed multispecific organic anion transporter, MOAT), is restricted to the bile canalicular membrane, where it is responsible for ATP-dependent transport of a wide variety of non-bile acid organic anions, which are primarily glucuronides and glutathione conjugates.[233]

Patients with the Dubin-Johnson syndrome,[234,235] mutant Corriedale sheep,[224] transport-deficient mutant rat strain (TR^-) and Eisai hyperbilirubinemic rat (EHBR) rats[225] and mutant golden lion tamarin monkeys[236] manifest conjugated hyperbilirubinemia that is transmitted as an autosomal-recessive trait. These mutants share defective capacity to transport bilirubin glucuronide, other organic anionic metabolites (including leukotriene C4 and metanephrine glucuronide), and other organic anions, such as BSP, ICG, iopanoic acid, and phylloerythrin, from hepatocytes into the bile. Affected patients and mutant animals have a normal transport maximum for infused bile acids.[235,237] These observations demonstrated that there are at least two mechanisms for organic anion secretion by the liver, one for bile acids and another for other organic anions. In canalicular membrane vesicles, these processes were functionally distinct and required ATP hydrolysis.[230] The major, and possibly only, canalicular bile acid transporter has been demonstrated to be sister-p-glycoprotein (SPGP), a member of the MDR family of transmembrane transporters.[238]

The predominant member (approximately 90 percent) of MDR family gene products in the canalicular membrane is MDR3 (the human homologue of murine mdr2). MDR3 couples ATP hydrolysis to the selective transfer of phosphatidylcholine from the inner to the outer leaflet of the bile canalicular membrane.[239] Phospholipids are required to form mixed micelles with bile acids, which protects small bile ducts from the detergent action of bile acids.

Maximal bilirubin secretory capacity (T_{max}) depends on bile flow. Flow is increased by infusion of bile acids[240] or by phenobarbital treatment, which enhances bile flow rate by a non–bile acid dependent mechanism.[241] The T_{max} of bilirubin is enhanced in both cases. Several other bile acid–independent choleretics increase bile flow but not the T_{max} for organic anions.[242] The maximal ATP-dependent biliary secretion of bile acids and non–bile acid organic anions greatly exceeds the apparent capacity and amount of SPGP and MRP2 present in the canalicular membrane under basal conditions.[243] Bile acids increase the transfer of MRP2, SPGP, and MDR3 from the Golgi to the apical domain, thereby more than doubling the amount of each transporter in the canalicular membrane.[244] Recruitment of canalicular ATP-dependent transporters involves microtubular-dependent vesicular trafficking, which requires association with and activity of phosphoinositide 3-kinase and its lipid products.

A small amount of unconjugated bilirubin (up to 3% of total bile pigments) is found in normal bile. This may be explained by hydrolysis of bilirubin glucuronide by biliary β-glucuronidase, canalicular ATP-dependent transport of bilirubin, or self-aggregation and incorporation of bilirubin in mixed micelles.

Although bilirubin glucuronides, bile acids, and phospholipids are transported across the canalicular membrane by different ATP-dependent transporters, heritable defects in bile acid or phospholipid transport produce bile secretory failure (i.e., cholestasis), which is manifested by conjugated hyperbilirubinemia. Molecular defects in heritable cholestatic disorders remained unknown until the mechanisms responsible for biliary secretion of bilirubin glucuronide, bile acids, and phospholipids were identified. The discovery of bile canalicular ATP-dependent transporters for bile acids (SPGP), non–bile acid organic anions (MRP2), and phospholipids (MDR3) enabled the molecular characterization of several heritable hyperbilirubinemias, cholestatic or not.

Fate of Bilirubin in the Gastrointestinal Tract

Bilirubin reaches the intestinal tract mainly conjugated and is not substantially absorbed.[245] In some circumstances, there may be enhanced excretion of unconjugated bilirubin into the intestine. Absorption of unconjugated bilirubin from the intestine may contribute to neonatal hyperbilirubinemia.[246] Milk inhibits intestinal absorption of unconjugated bilirubin. However, human milk inhibits this reabsorption less than does infant milk formula.[247] These observations suggest that intestinal absorption of bilirubin may contribute to jaundice associated with breast-feeding. Absorption of bilirubin from the gallbladder occurs in animals.[248] Bilirubin is degraded by intestinal bacteria into a series of urobilinogen and related products.[249] The specific products may relate to strains of bacteria present in the intestine.[250] Urobilinogens are present in the deconjugated state. It is not known whether deconjugation precedes or follows bilirubin degradation, but bacterial β-glucuronidase plays a role in the deconjugation.[246,251] Most of the urobilinogen reabsorbed from the intestine is reexcreted in the bile. A small fraction is excreted by the kidney. Enhanced tubular absorption and instability of the pigment in acid urine makes urobilinogen excretion in urine an unreliable indicator of the status of bilirubin metabolism. Absence of urobilinogen in stool and urine indicates complete obstruction of the bile duct. In liver disease and states of increased bilirubin production, urinary urobilinogen excretion is increased. Urobilinogen is colorless. Oxidation leads to formation of urobilin, which contributes to the color of normal urine and stool.

Alternative Pathways of Bilirubin Elimination

After injection of labeled unconjugated bilirubin, only 3 percent of radioactivity is normally excreted by the kidney in humans. Even in the presence of marked hyperbilirubinemia, bile remains the main route of bilirubin excretion. In patients with Crigler-Najjar syndrome and in Gunn rats, a small amount of unconjugated bilirubin is secreted in bile. Additional unconjugated bilirubin may reach the intestinal lumen by passage across the intestinal wall or by desquamation of intestinal epithelial cells.[252] Ambient light or phototherapy forms geometric isomers of bilirubin (EE, EZ, or ZE forms), which are excreted in unconjugated forms and converted to bilirubin IXα-ZZ in the bile.[253] Considerable amounts of bilirubin are degraded to polar diazo-negative compounds, which are excreted in both bile and urine.[252]

The presence of hydroxylated products of bilirubin in Gunn rat bile suggests a role of enzyme-catalyzed oxidation in the disposition of bilirubin.[254] Induction of a specific isoform of microsomal P450s by administration of 2,3,7,8-tetrachlorodibenzo-p-dioxin (TCDD) in Gunn rats results in a sevenfold increase in the fractional turnover of bilirubin and reduction of the bilirubin pool.[255] A mitochondrial bilirubin oxidase found in rat liver,[256] intestine,[257] and kidney consumes 1 to 1.5 moles of oxygen per mole of bilirubin and forms propentdyopents. The enzyme does not require NADP, NAD, or ATP and is inhibited by potassium cyanide (KCN), thiol reagents, NADH, and albumin.[256] Enzyme-mediated oxidation of bilirubin also has been reported to occur in mitochondrial fractions of brain, lung, heart, and skeletal muscle.

Disposition of Bilirubin by the Kidney. In intrahepatic or extrahepatic cholestasis, the plasma-conjugated bilirubin concentration increases. After injection of radiolabeled bilirubin in animals with experimentally ligated bile ducts[258] and in children with biliary atresia,[259] 50 to 90 percent of injected radioactivity is excreted in urine. In total biliary obstruction, urinary excretion becomes the major pathway of bilirubin excretion.[260] Renal excretion of conjugated bilirubin depends on glomerular filtration of a small non–protein-bound fraction of conjugated bilirubin.[260,261] There is evidence for tubular reabsorption but none for tubular secretion of bilirubin.[261]

Antioxidative Property of Bilirubin

Until recently, bilirubin has been considered a waste product with no known physiologic utility. However, both unconjugated[262] and conjugated[263] bilirubin have been shown to be inhibitors of lipid peroxidation. This property of bilirubin depends on its ability to donate hydrogen ions.[264] Bilirubin bound to hepatic cytosolic proteins has a greater free-radical scavenging effect than does the bilirubin–albumin complex. It has been postulated that bilirubin is converted to its peroxidative product, biliverdin, thereby sparing hepatic endoplasmic reticulum membranes of lipid peroxidation.[265] Regeneration of bilirubin by the action of cytosolic biliverdin reductase may enhance the protective effect of bilirubin. Albumin binding increases the cytoprotective activity of bilirubin,[265] suggesting a possible beneficial role of bilirubin on tissues other than the liver.

DISORDERS OF BILIRUBIN METABOLISM RESULTING IN UNCONJUGATED HYPERBILIRUBINEMIA

General Considerations

The hepatic transport of bilirubin involves four distinct but probably interrelated stages: (1) uptake from the circulation; (2) intracellular binding or storage; (3) conjugation, largely with glucuronic acid; and (4) biliary excretion. Abnormalities in any of these processes may result in hyperbilirubinemia. Complex clinical disorders, such as hepatitis or cirrhosis, may affect multiple processes. In several inherited disorders, the transfer of bilirubin from blood to bile is disrupted at a specific step. Study of these disorders has permitted better understanding of bilirubin metabolism in health and disease. Each disorder is characterized by varied degrees of hyperbilirubinemia of the unconjugated or conjugated type.

Neonatal Jaundice

By adult standards, every newborn baby has hyperbilirubinemia, and about half of all neonates become clinically jaundiced during the first 5 days of life. Serum bilirubin is predominantly unconjugated. Exaggeration of this physiologic jaundice can result in marked hyperbilirubinemia, with an attendant risk of kernicterus (see earlier section on Toxicity of Bilirubin). In 4000 consecutive infants, 16 percent had maximal serum bilirubin concentrations of 10 mg/dl or above, and in 5 percent, bilirubin concentrations exceeded 15 mg/dl.[266] In the normal, full-term human neonate, the serum bilirubin concentration increases rapidly from 1 to 2 to 5 to 6 mg/dl in approximately 72 h and subsequently decreases until normal levels are attained in 7 to 10 days.[267] Physiologic jaundice of the newborn appears to result from a combination of increased bilirubin production and delayed maturation in the capability of the liver to dispose of bilirubin. Severe neonatal unconjugated hyperbilirubinemia results from exaggeration in one or more of the regularly occurring developmental restrictions that are characteristic of the newborn period or from superimposition of additional mechanisms. Although the incidence of cerebral toxicity from neonatal jaundice had decreased markedly after the introduction of immunoglobulin therapy for maternal–fetal Rh blood group incompatibility, the incidence of neonatal kernicterus may be on the increase again. This may be partly related to early discharge after delivery, which is being practiced in a majority of hospitals in the United States and elsewhere. This issue and the current concepts of neonatal jaundice have been reviewed elsewhere.[78] The physiologic basis of neonatal hyperbilirubinemia and mechanisms of its exaggeration to potentially harmful states are discussed briefly below.

Increased bilirubin production in the newborn period is evidenced by increased endogenous carbon monoxide production,[268] increased early-labeled peak from erythroid and nonerythroid sources, and decreased erythrocyte half-life.[269] Meconium contains unconjugated bilirubin derived primarily from hydrolysis of conjugated bilirubin by intestinal β-glucuronidase.[270] As compared with adults, newborns lack intestinal bacteria that degrade bilirubin to urobilinogen and have a greater surface-to-volume ratio of the bowel. As a result, intestinal absorption of unconjugated bilirubin in neonates may be increased.[270] Hemolytic diseases of the fetus increase bilirubin production and may lead to severe neonatal unconjugated hyperbilirubinemia. Rh incompatibility between mother and fetus was formerly a common cause of severe neonatal unconjugated hyperbilirubinemia and kernicterus (erythroblastosis fetalis). This disease can be prevented by treatment of the mother with anti-Rh immunoglobulins.[271] Major blood group (ABO) incompatibility remains a common cause of exaggerated neonatal hyperbilirubinemia that often requires treatment.[272]

Hepatic Bilirubin Uptake During the Neonatal Period. Cumulative hepatic bilirubin uptake capacity is reduced during the first 25 h of life in the rhesus monkey. Relative hepatic uptake deficiency extends beyond the second day of life and correlates with maturation of hepatic ligandin,[273] which influences the net hepatic uptake of bilirubin (see earlier section on Uptake of Bilirubin by the Liver). Delayed closure of the ductus venosus may permit portal blood, which is enriched in unconjugated bilirubin from the intestine, to bypass the liver. Reduced caloric intake, which reduces hepatic bilirubin clearance in adults (see later section on Gilbert Syndrome), may have a similar effect in neonates.

Postnatal Development of Bilirubin-Glucuronidating Activity. In many mammals, including humans, UGT activity toward bilirubin is deficient in fetal liver and rapidly develops to adult levels during the first few days of life.[274] Deficiency of UGT activity may be prolonged and exaggerated in some inherited disorders due to inhibitory factor(s) in maternal milk or serum (see later section on Transient Familial Neonatal Hyperbilirubinemia).

Recently, a variant TATAA element within the promoter region of UGT1A1 has been found to be associated with Gilbert syndrome.[275] This variant promoter reduces the expression of bilirubin-UGT (UGT1A1). The Gilbert genotype has been found to accentuate neonatal hyperbilirubinemia[276] and prolong the duration of neonatal jaundice.[277]

Inhibition of Bilirubin Glucuronidation by Maternal Milk. Plasma bilirubin concentrations tend to be higher in breast-fed infants as compared with formula-fed babies[278] and occasionally rise to maximum concentrations of 15 to 24 mg/dl within 10 to 19 days of life. This transient nonhemolytic, unconjugated hyperbilirubinemia is promptly ameliorated by discontinuation of breast-feeding; otherwise, the hyperbilirubinemia may take up to a month to disappear. Kernicterus is rare, but isolated cases have been reported.[279] Neonatal unconjugated hyperbilirubinemia related to breast-feeding is associated with an inhibitor of UGT activity in maternal milk but not maternal serum.[280] A progestational steroid, $3\alpha,20\beta$-pregnanediol, was isolated from the milk of mothers of infants who had the syndrome. The steroid inhibited bilirubin glucuronidation by rat and rabbit liver,[280] but activity with human liver was not inhibited.[281] Experimental feeding of the steroid to healthy infants yielded contradictory results.[282,283] The free fatty acid concentration in maternal milk correlates positively with its inhibitory effect on human hepatic bilirubin-UGT activity, and free fatty acids inhibit UGT activity *in vitro* in proportion to the number of double bonds in unsaturated fatty acids and in inverse proportion to the chain lengths of saturated fatty acids (C10 to C18).[284] Odievre and associates have postulated that a lipolytic enzyme, which is present in some maternal milk samples, may be responsible for the increased concentration of free fatty acids in the milk.[284] The inhibitory effect of maternal milk on UGT increases on storage and is destroyed by heating at 56°C.

Inhibition of Bilirubin Glucuronidation by Factors Derived from Maternal Plasma. Transient familial neonatal hyperbilirubinemia (Lucey-Driscoll syndrome) was described by Lucey and associates in 1961.[285,286] This syndrome is characterized by jaundice occurring within the first 4 days of life. In 24 infants,[286] peak serum bilirubin concentrations of 8.9 to 65 mg/dl were reached within 7 days. An unidentified inhibitor of UGT was found in the serum of mothers of these infants. One infant died at 36 h. This condition is clinically distinguished from maternal milk jaundice by earlier onset of severe hyperbilirubinemia, a more prolonged course, and occasional kernicterus.

Immaturity of Canalicular Excretion. During the late newborn period, hepatic bilirubin uptake, conjugation, and canalicular excretion attain adult levels, even though the bilirubin load remains increased. In this period of life, canalicular excretion may be rate limiting in the hepatic disposition of bilirubin. Consequently, when the bilirubin load is further increased, conjugated bilirubin accumulates in serum.[287]

Management of Neonatal Unconjugated Hyperbilirubinemia. In the great majority of cases, neonatal hyperbilirubinemia is innocuous, and indeed may provide an important antioxidant defense for the newborn. However, it is critical to be vigilantly prepared for the occasional case in which neonatal jaundice can

Table 125-1 Principal Differential Characteristics of Inherited Unconjugated Hyperbilirubinemia

	Crigler-Najjar Syndrome Type I	Crigler-Najjar Syndrome Type II	Gilbert Syndrome
Histology of liver	Normal	Normal	Normal
Serum bilirubin concentration	20–50 mg/dl	<20 mg/dl	Usually <3 mg/dl
Routine liver function test results	Normal	Normal	Normal
45-min plasma BSP retention	Normal	Normal	Usually normal; may be elevated in some patients
Bile	Usually pale; contains small amounts of unconjugated bilirubin	Increased proportion of bilirubin monoglucuronide	Increased proportion of bilirubin monoglucuronide
Hepatic bilirubin UDP-glucuronosyltransferase activity	Absent	Markedly reduced	Reduced
Effect of phenobarbital on serum bilirubin	None	Reduction	Reduction
Mode of inheritance	Autosomal recessive	Autosomal recessive	Autosomal recessive
Prevalence	Rare	Rare	Common (~9% of caucasians are homozygous for a variant TATAA box; 4–5% have hyperbilirubinemia)
Prognosis	Kernicterus, unless vigorously treated	Usually benign, kernicterus occurs rarely	Benign
Animal model	Homozygous Gunn rat	—	Bolivian squirrel monkey

reach levels that may cause cerebral toxicity.[78] Although a plasma bilirubin concentration of 20 mg/dl is usually considered dangerous, cerebral toxicity can occur at lower concentrations of bilirubin (see earlier section on Toxicity of Bilirubin). The goal of treatment is to decrease serum bilirubin concentrations to an acceptable level until the capacity of the liver to dispose of bilirubin matures. Phototherapy is the most common treatment modality used. In severe cases, exchange transfusion is used to reduce serum bilirubin levels rapidly (see later section on Treatment of Crigler-Najjar Syndrome Type I). Although phototherapy is useful and safe, concern persists about its potential side effects. Ingestion of agar to bind unconjugated bilirubin in the intestine also decreases serum bilirubin concentrations,[270] but the efficacy of this treatment is not certain.[269] Inhibition of heme oxygenase activity by the administration of tin-mesoporphyrin at birth has been shown to prevent the development of significant levels of neonatal jaundice, thereby abolishing the need for phototherapy or exchange transfusion.[44,45] However, the routine use of this compound in all newborns is not generally recommended.

Hyperbilirubinemia Due to Bilirubin Overproduction

Hyperbilirubinemia in the presence of normal liver function often occurs in disorders associated with increased bilirubin production. The serum bilirubin is unconjugated and rarely exceeds 3 to 4 mg/dl. Higher levels usually indicate hepatobiliary dysfunction in addition to bilirubin overproduction.[4] The most common cause of increased bilirubin production is hemolysis such as occurs in sickle cell anemia, hereditary spherocytosis, and toxic or idiosyncratic drug reactions in susceptible individuals. These disorders are associated with premature destruction of erythrocytes; red cell morphology and life span are often abnormal. In the absence of any hepatobiliary disorder, a small amount of conjugated bilirubin, mainly bilirubin monoglucuronide, may accumulate in the serum, in addition to unconjugated bilirubin. In these cases, the proportion of conjugated bilirubin does not usually exceed the normal limits (approximately 4 percent of total bilirubin). The conjugated bilirubin probably appears in the serum by diffusion out of the hepatocyte. In contrast to previous interpretation,[288] this phenomenon does not necessarily indicate that the rate of bilirubin production has exceeded the excretory transport maximum for biliary excretion of conjugated bilirubin. Ineffective erythropoiesis occurs in thalassemia and other hematologic disorders and is often associated with hyperbilirubinemia.[289] Congenital dyserythropoietic anemias are a group of rare hereditary anemias characterized by ineffective erythropoiesis, intramedullary normoblastic hyperplasia, secondary hemochromatosis, and unconjugated hyperbilirubinemia.[290–293]

Crigler-Najjar Syndrome Type I

Clinical Findings. Crigler-Najjar syndrome type I is a rare disorder in which hepatic bilirubin-UGT activity is absent or barely detectable (Table 125-1). The syndrome was described by Crigler and Najjar in 1952 in six infants in three families.[294] All infants manifested severe nonhemolytic icterus within the first few days of life. Jaundice was characterized by increased plasma concentration of indirect-reacting bilirubin and was lifelong. Five of the six infants died of kernicterus by the age of 15 months. Although icteric, the single surviving infant was free of neurologic disease until 15 years of age, when kernicterus suddenly developed, and he died 6 months later.[295] A female cousin also had Crigler-Najjar syndrome; she developed neurologic symptoms at 18 years of age and died at the age of 24.[296] This family had increased consanguinity and several other recessively inherited traits, such as Morquio syndrome, homocystinuria, metachromatic leukodystrophy, and bird-headed dwarfism.[297] However, association with these disorders was not observed in the subsequently reported cases of Crigler-Najjar syndrome type I. The syndrome occurs in all races, is transmitted as an autosomal-recessive trait (Fig. 125-14),[295–298] and is associated with known consanguinity in some, but not all, cases. Until the introduction of phototherapy, almost all patients died with kernicterus during the first 18 months of life.[299] Several individuals have survived only to succumb to kernicterus later in life.[291,294,296,297] With the advent of phototherapy and intermittent plasmapheresis, survival until puberty, without significant brain damage, is not unusual. However, the risk of bilirubin encephalopathy persists, and kernicterus is common around the time of adolescence, when phototherapy becomes less effective. Orthotopic liver transplantation or auxiliary transplantation of a single liver lobe has resulted in long-term survival in several cases.[300] As discussed below, isolated hepatocyte transplantation has been used in a single case with partial amelioration of hyperbilirubinemia.

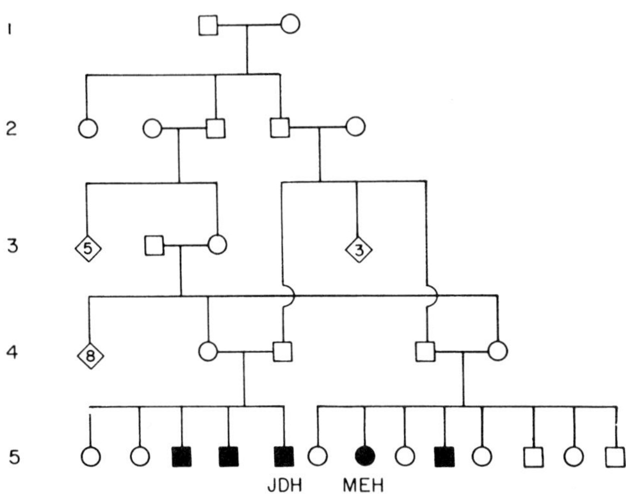

Fig. 125-14 Inheritance of Crigler-Najjar syndrome type I. This family, originally described by Crigler and Najjar in 1962, is unique in that two cousins, J.D.H. and M.E.H., escaped kernicterus in infancy only to die at ages 16 and 24, respectively. (*Reprinted with permission from Blaschke et al.*[363])

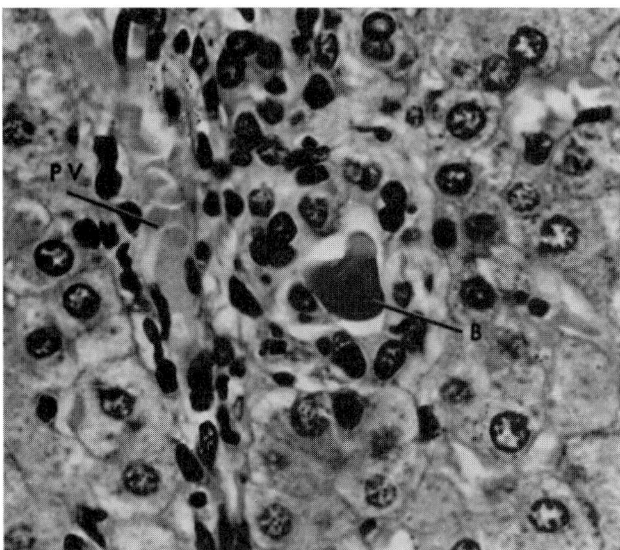

Fig. 125-15 High-power view (hematoxylin and eosin; magnification ×650) of a liver biopsy obtained from a patient with Crigler-Najjar syndrome type I during pregnancy. A portal area is shown with portal vein (PV) and a bile ductule (B) containing amorphous material, which appeared to be bilirubin. (*Reprinted with permission from Wolkoff et al.*[299])

Laboratory Tests. Laboratory test results in Crigler-Najjar syndrome type 1 are normal except for the serum bilirubin level, which is usually 20 to 25 mg/dl, but may be as high as 50 mg/dl.[294–297,299] Virtually all the serum bilirubin is unconjugated, and no serum conjugated bilirubin has been found. There is no bilirubinuria, but the urine may be yellow due to a chloroform-soluble pigment of unknown structure.[300] The level of icterus in a given patient varies—it is lower in summer and on exposure to sun and higher during intercurrent illness.[301] Stool color is normal, but fecal urobilinogen excretion is reduced.[294–301] Bilirubin production, hematocrit, bone marrow morphology, and red cell survival are normal.[250,302] Results of routine liver function tests are normal, including studies of plasma disappearance of BSP and ICG.[294,303] Because the canalicular excretion mechanism is normal in these patients, radiologic visualization of the biliary tree by cholecystographic agents is normal. Jaundice and occasional neurologic impairment are the only abnormal physical findings. Liver biopsy reveals normal histology. In several patients, pigment plugs were observed in bile canaliculi and bile ducts (Fig. 125-15).[294,301,303] Pigment stones have been found in several cases. The pigment plugs and stones probably result from biliary excretion of unconjugated bilirubin as an effect of long-term phototherapy. Electron microscopy of the liver reveals no specific pathologic change.[304]

Molecular Defect in Crigler-Najjar Syndrome Type 1. Of the numerous isoforms of UGT, UGT1A1 (bilirubin-UGT1) is the only isoform that contributes significantly to bilirubin metabolism in humans (GenBank AJ005162).[196] Genetic lesions of exons constituting the *UGT1A1* gene that cause Crigler-Najjar syndrome type 1 were first described in 1992.[196,305–307] Subsequently, several laboratories have reported the genetic lesions in over 60 patients with Crigler-Najjar syndrome type 1 by polymerase chain reaction–based DNA sequence analysis. These genetic lesions and their relationship to Crigler-Najjar syndrome have been reviewed.[308] The genetic lesions can be deletions, insertions, missense mutations, or premature stop codons, and can be located in any of the five exons comprising the UGT1A1 mRNA (Fig. 125-16).[308] In one case the mutation is located in the hydrophobic signal peptide that is cleaved off from the enzyme during synthesis.[309] In two other cases, the mutation was located within the intronic regions of the gene at a splice donor and a splice acceptor region, respectively.[310] These mutations result in the utilization of a cryptic splice site within an exon, which leads to the splicing out of a part of the exon. In most families, with or without known consanguinity, both alleles carry identical mutations, although different genetic lesions on the two alleles are not rare.[308] A 13-nucleotide deletion in exon 2 of *UGT1A1* has been observed in three unrelated families of different ethnic origins. Crigler-Najjar syndrome type 1 is relatively common among the Amish and Mennonite communities of Lancaster County, Pennsylvania.[311] All Crigler-Najjar syndrome type 1 patients within these related communities carry identical mutations in exon 1, indicating a founder effect. Similarly, four apparently unrelated families, originating from Punjab, India, have been fround to carry an identical mutation (unpublished observation, J. Roy Chowdhury and N. Roy Chowdhury). In cases where the genetic lesion is located in exon 1, only bilirubin-UGT (UGT1A1) activity is expected to be abnormal, whereas when the mutation affects one of the common region exons (exons 2 to 5), all UGT isoforms expressed from the *UGT1A* locus are expected to be abnormal.

Diagnosis. The combination of very high levels of serum unconjugated bilirubin and the absence of any other abnormality of routine liver function tests is diagnostic of Crigler-Najjar syndrome type 1. Hemolysis alone does not increase serum bilirubin levels beyond 6 to 8 mg/dl. Differential diagnosis includes Crigler-Najjar syndrome type 2, with or without coexisting hemolysis. Although serum bilirubin levels are relatively lower in Crigler-Najjar syndrome type 2, ranges of bilirubin concentration in the two disorders overlap. In most cases, serum bilirubin concentrations are reduced by more than 25 percent after phenobarbital administration (60 to 120 mg for 14 days) in Crigler-Najjar syndrome type 2, but not in type 1.[301] The two types of Crigler-Najjar syndrome can be differentiated conveniently by chromatographic analysis of bile collected from the duodenum through a perorally placed duodenal catheter or an upper gastrointestinal endoscope. In bile from patients with Crigler-Najjar syndrome type 1, bilirubin glucuronides are absent or are present in traces only (in concentrations less than that of unconjugated bilirubin). In contrast, in Crigler-Najjar syndrome type 2 significant amounts of conjugated bilirubin are excreted in bile, although the proportion of bilirubin diglucuronide is reduced

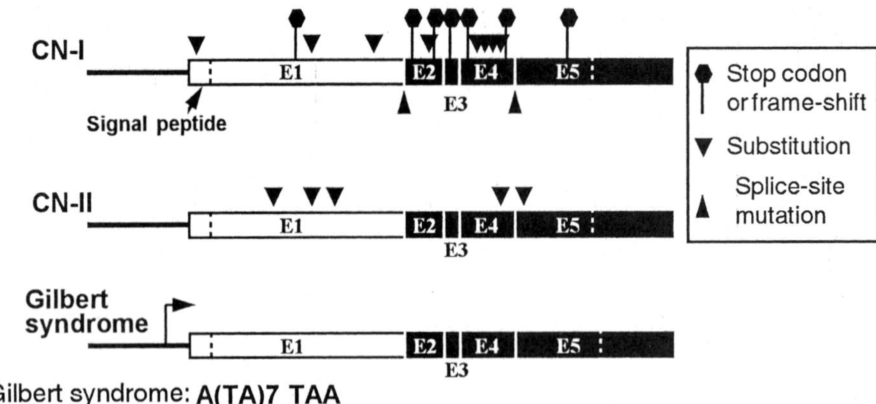

Fig. 125-16 Genetic lesions causing Crigler-Najjar syndrome type I, Crigler-Najjar syndrome type II, and Gilbert syndrome. Crigler-Najjar syndrome type I is produced by mutations, deletions, or insertions within the five exons that constitute the UGT1A1 mRNA. These genetic lesions may cause premature stop codons or substitution of a single amino acid. In two cases, there were mutations in the splice donor sequences on intron 1 and splice acceptor region of intron 4, respectively, resulting in the utilization of cryptic splice sites within exons, with consequent deletion of a segment of an exon from the mRNA. Crigler-Najjar syndrome type II is also caused by genetic lesions within the coding region of *UGT1A1*. In these cases, however, the mutations result in single amino acid substitutions that reduce the catalytic activity of the enzyme, but does not abolish it. In contrast to the two types of Crigler-Najjar syndrome, Gilbert syndrome is associated with a variant TATAA box, which contains two extra nucleotides, TA. This results in reduced expression of structurally normal UGT1A1.

(see below in Crigler-Najjar syndrome type 2). Liver biopsy is not necessary for diagnosis, unless a coexisting liver disease is suspected. If a biopsy is performed, UGT activity toward bilirubin can be determined, and is expected to be undetectable. The diagnosis can be made also on the basis of genetic analysis of DNA extracted from blood, buccal scrapings, or any tissue. The five exons of the *UGT1A1* gene, and the flanking intronic sequences are amplified by polymerase chain reaction and the nucleotide sequences are determined.[305] If the genetic lesion matches one of the previously identified lesions associated with Crigler-Najjar syndrome type 1, the diagnosis is established. If a new mutation is found that predicts the truncation of a major portion of the enzyme or causes a frame-shift, the diagnosis is also established. When a novel mutation predicts the substitution of a single amino acid residue, the mutation can be generated in an expression plasmid by site-directed mutagenesis and the effect of the mutation can be determined after transfection of the plasmid into African Green monkey kidney cell lines (COS cells).[196] Genetic analysis can be utilized to detect heterozygous carriers of one Crigler-Najjar syndrome type 1 allele. Genetic analysis of chorionic villus samples has been used successfully for prenatal identification of the Crigler-Najjar syndrome type 1 genotype in four fetuses in three families (J. Roy Chowdhury and N. Roy Chowdhury, unpublished observation).

Animal Model for Crigler-Najjar Syndrome Type 1: The Gunn Rat. The description by Gunn in 1938 of mutant Wistar rats with nonhemolytic unconjugated hyperbilirubinemia[312] and the wisdom of the late Professor William E. Castle, Emeritus Professor of Genetics at Berkeley, who maintained the mutants for over 15 years, have resulted in major advances in understanding bilirubin metabolism, transport, and encephalopathy.[313,314] Jaundice in these animals is inherited as an autosomal recessive trait.[312] Heterozygotes are anicteric. Depending on the background strain against which a Gunn rat colony is maintained, homozygous Gunn rats have bilirubin levels that range from 3 to 20 mg/dl. Serum bilirubin is all unconjugated,[313] there is no bilirubinuria, and bile is light yellow in color due to the excretion of small amounts of unconjugated bilirubin.[313] Liver histology is normal.[315]

Neurologic Lesions. Homozygous Gunn rats are prototypes of Crigler-Najjar syndrome type I and frequently develop kernicterus.[299,315–317] The Gunn rat is the only experimental model in which endogenously produced bilirubin results in neuropathologic lesions and neurologic deficits. Cytoplasmic neuronal changes develop in these rats on the third day of life, and by 2 weeks, degeneration of Purkinje cells and other neurons occurs. The degenerative changes begin by enlargement of mitochondria and formation of membranous cytoplasmic bodies. By 8 days of age, many mitochondria contain glycogen.[316,317] When a clinically healthy Gunn rat is killed and rapidly perfused with saline or formalin, the brain does not show yellow staining. Administration of sulfadimethoxine, a drug that competes with bilirubin for binding to albumin, to 14-day-old animals results in neurologic deterioration and yellow staining in the brain.[318]

Urinary Concentration Defect. Gunn rats cannot concentrate urine and do not tolerate water deprivation.[319] The renal medullary bilirubin concentration is high and interferes with sodium and water transport.[319] Occasionally, renal papillary necrosis occurs.[320] Treatment of rats with agents or methods designed to lower serum bilirubin, such as cholestyramine, agar, or phototherapy, may ameliorate the renal lesion.[319] Similar concentrating problems have not been described in patients with Crigler-Najjar syndrome type I, although bilirubin is deposited in the kidney.[321]

Abnormalities of UGT Activity and Their Relationship to Genetic Lesions. The rat *UGT1A* locus closely resembles its human counterpart in exon organization.[322] The genetic lesion in Gunn rats consists of the deletion of a single guanosine residue in the common region exon, exon 4, which creates a frameshift and deletes a large segment of the C-terminal domain of all UGT isoforms that are expressed from this locus.[322–324] Consequently, not only bilirubin glucuronidation is absent in this strain, other UGT isoforms expressed from the *UGT1A* locus are also truncated and nonfunctional.[325] As in patients with Crigler-Najjar syndrome type 1, Gunn rats lack bilirubin conjugates in bile.[252,313,315] Gunn rat livers lack UGT activity toward digitoxigenin monodigitoxoside.[326] The transferase activity toward 4-nitrophenol is present at a lower level,[327] suggesting that this activity is partly provided by UGT isoforms expressed from other loci. Several functionally normal forms of UGT have been isolated from the Gunn rat liver,[328] indicating that UGT isoforms expressed from genes that do not belong to the *UGT1A* locus are normal. UGT activities for aniline,[329] steroid substrates,[330] and thyroid hormone[331] are normal in Gunn rat liver. Biliary excretion of substances that do not require glucuronidation, such as BSP,[313] phenol red,[332] and exogenously administered conjugated bilirubin,[125] are normal in Gunn rats.

Treatment of Crigler-Najjar Syndrome Type 1. Unconjugated hyperbilirubinemia in Crigler-Najjar syndrome type 1 is usually associated with bilirubin encephalopathy (kernicterus). Conventional treatment is designed to reduce serum bilirubin levels. Unlike in patients with Crigler-Najjar syndrome type II and Gilbert syndrome, the serum bilirubin levels are not significantly reduced by the administration of UGT enzyme inducing agents, such as phenobarbital.[301,302]

Phototherapy has received widespread acceptance. It is the major treatment for icteric newborns whose serum bilirubin concentrations place them at risk for kernicterus.[253,299,333] Experience with phototherapy in older children and adults is limited to patients with Crigler-Najjar syndrome type 1 and occasional cases of Crigler-Najjar syndrome type 2. An array of 140-W fluorescent lamps with devices for shielding the eyes has been used effectively. However, about the time of puberty, phototherapy becomes relatively less effective because of thickening of the skin, increased skin pigmentation, and decreased surface area in relation to body mass.[299] Phototherapy converts a fraction of bilirubin IXα-ZZ into geometric and structural isomers, that are excreted in bile (see earlier section on Chemistry of Bilirubin). A portion of the unconjugated bilirubin excreted in bile may be reabsorbed in the small intestine. Oral administration of agar, cholestyramine, or calcium salts[333] enhances the effect of phototherapy, probably by inhibiting the reabsorption of unconjugated bilirubin.

Plasmapheresis is the most efficient method for rapidly reducing serum bilirubin concentration during crisis (Fig. 125-17).[296,299,303] This procedure takes advantage of the fact that bilirubin is tightly bound to serum albumin and removal of albumin results in the removal of equimolar amounts of bilirubin.

Liver Transplantation. Orthotopic or auxiliary liver transplantation rapidly normalizes serum bilirubin levels. Currently, liver transplantation is considered the only definitive treatment for Crigler-Najjar syndrome type 1.[334] Although these procedures are not without risk in these individuals, some investigtors have suggested prophylactic liver transplantation in patients with Crigler-Najjar syndrome type 1 to avoid the risk of kernicterus, which once established, may not be fully reversible.[334]

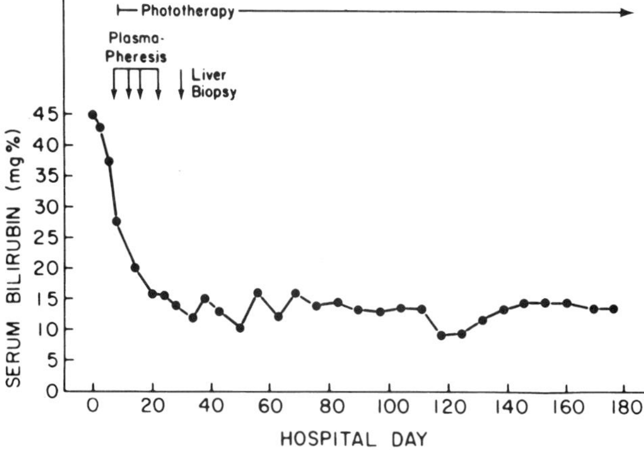

Fig. 125-17 Summary of the hospital course of a 19-year-old patient with Crigler-Najjar syndrome type I who was admitted with acute bilirubin encephalopathy. Before hospitalization, the patient's serum bilirubin ranged between 35 and 45 mg/dl. After an initial course of plasmapheresis and maintenance phototherapy, serum bilirubin was maintained between 10 and 15 mg/dl. (*Reprinted with permission from Wolkoff et al.*[299])

Hepatocyte Transplantation. Because the liver is structurally normal in Crigler-Najjar syndrome type 1 and in Gunn rats, alternatives to the irreversible, expensive, and risky procedure of liver transplantation are being sought. Transplantation of congeneic normal isolated hepatocytes into Gunn rats by infusion into the portal vein,[335] intrasplenic injection,[336,337] or intraperitoneal injection after attachment to microcarrier beads[338] has been used successfully to provide partial correction of bilirubin-UGT deficiency in Gunn rats. It has been shown that after intrasplenic injection, a great majority of the hepatocytes rapidly translocate to the liver, where, in the absence of immune rejection, they exhibit long-term persistence.[336] The liver is the preferred site for long-term survival and function of isolated hepatocytes. Following transplantation by intraportal infusion or intrasplenic injection, hepatocytes migrate out of the sinusoidal space and integrate into the liver chords within days. The transplanted cells survive and function for prolonged periods and respond to normal proliferative stimuli.[337]

Based on the extensive experience in Gunn rats, an 11-year-old girl with Crigler-Najjar syndrome was transplanted with 7.5 billion isolated allogeneic primary human hepatocytes by infusion through a percutaneously placed portal venous catheter.[339,340] Tacrolimus was used for prevention of allograft rejection. The procedure did not cause portal hypertension, and resulted in excretion of bilirubin glucuronides in bile and led to approximately 50 percent reduction of serum bilirubin concentration over the course of several months. The hypobilirubinemic effect persists to date 16 months after the transplantation. Although the experience is limited to one case only, transplantation of isolated hepatocytes appears to be a safe and relatively inexpensive alternative to liver transplantation in patients with Crigler-Najjar syndrome type 1.

Degradation of Bilirubin by Bilirubin Oxidase. Bilirubin oxidase from *Myrothecium verrucaria* catalyzes the oxidation of bilirubin with oxygen to a colorless derivative. Perfusion of filters packed with bilirubin oxidase immobilized on agarose with rat or human blood containing bilirubin resulted in the degradation of 90 percent of the pigment in a single pass.[341] When blood from a Gunn rat was passed through the column and returned to the venous circulation, the serum bilirubin level was reduced to 50 percent in 30 min. However, the use of such columns may be associated with removal of formed elements of blood. As an alternative, systemic administration of bilirubin oxidase has been considered. To circumvent the short half-life of bilirubin oxidase in circulation (2.5 min), the enzyme has been covalently linked to polyethyleneglycol.[342] The linked enzyme has a plasma half-life of 190 min in rats. A single intravenous injection of polyethyleneglycol-conjugated bilirubin oxidase in Gunn rats resulted in substantial reduction of serum bilirubin level for 3 h.

Induction of P450c. As mentioned above, the induction of P450c with TCDD results in a decrease of serum bilirubin levels in Gunn rats, presumably due to oxidation of bilirubin in the liver. This observation has stimulated the search for more innocuous drugs for induction of this enzyme. Several naturally occurring indoles extracted from cruciferous vegetables, such as cabbage, cauliflower, and brussels sprouts induce P4501A1 and P4501A2 in rat liver and intestine.[343] Administration of indole-3-carbinol, an inducer of P4501A2, results in a short-term reduction of serum bilirubin levels in children with Crigler-Najjar syndrome type 1.[343]

Gene Therapy. Because the metabolic defect in Gunn rats and in patients with Crigler-Najjar syndrome type I is caused by molecular lesions of a single gene, introduction of a normal bilirubin-UGT would be an elegant potential therapeutic method.

Although there has been no clinical trial of gene therapy for this disease as yet, significant progress has been made by experiments on Gunn rats. Introduction of a normal bilirubin-UGT gene can be performed by *ex vivo* methods, introduction of the gene into the liver by *in situ* perfusion, or systemic administration of vectors that are capable of carrying the gene to the liver. These approaches are briefly mentioned below.

In *ex vivo* gene therapy, liver cells harvested from a mutant subject by partial hepatectomy are established in primary culture and transduced with a therapeutic gene using a method that permits stable gene expression.[344] These cells are then transplanted into the same mutant subject. This method has been used in low-density lipoprotein (LDL) receptor-deficient rabbits (Watanabe heritable hyperlipidemic strain), with long-term reduction of plasma LDL cholesterol concentration. Because the cells are autologous, immunosuppression is not needed. However, the number of hepatocytes that can be harvested and transduced is limited, and because surgical resection is required, this procedure cannot be readily repeated. Therefore, for the treatment of Gunn rats, hepatocytes have been conditionally immortalized before transduction with the bilirubin-UGT gene and transplantation.[345] In addition to improving gene transduction, this strategy could potentially assure a long-term supply of phenotypically corrected autologous hepatocytes. Additional research is required to assure that the transplanted cells should not become transformed into malignant cells.

Methods are also being developed to directly introduce a normal bilirubin-UGT gene into the liver of mutant Gunn rats, using viral or nonviral vectors. Recombinant murine leukemia viruses have been used to transfer the gene into the liver by perfusing the liver with the recombinant vector after transiently occluding inflow and outflow vessels.[346] Because gene transfer by the murine leukemia viruses requires cell division, these vectors are not very efficient in transferring genes to the intact liver.

Adenoviral vectors have the advantage of spontaneously localizing to the liver after systemic administration and the ability to transfer genes into nondividing cells with high efficiency. However, these viruses are episomal and would require repeated administration for long-term gene therapy. Unfortunately, the vectors evoke both cellular and humoral immunity in the host, precluding repeated injection. Several approaches are being developed to tolerize the host to antigens contained in the vector. These include administration in neonatal animals,[347] intrathymic inoculation,[348] or oral tolerization to adenoviral antigens.[349,350] Specific tolerization to the vector proteins permits long-term gene therapy in Gunn rats using adenoviral vectors. Whether these methods would be effective in nonhuman primates and humans remains to be examined. Newer viral vectors, such as recombinant SV40 and recombinant lentiviruses that can transfer genes into nondividing cells are being developed for trial in Gunn rats.

Receptor-mediated gene delivery to the liver using carrier proteins that deliver systemically administered DNA into the liver also have been used in the treatment of Gunn rats.[351] Transgenes introduced in this manner are expressed transiently. The expression can be prolonged to several months by inducing cell proliferation by partial hepatectomy[352] or by pharmacologic disruption of microtubules.[353]

Site-directed gene conversion is a recently described strategy. RNA-DNA chimeric molecules have been used in an effort to repair genetic mutations.[354] These chimeric molecules are designed to align with specific sequences within the genome and to create a single mismatch. This triggers the host mismatch repair system to correct the mutation. One study has reported that it may be possible to insert the missing guanosine residue into the Gunn rat bilirubin-UGT (*UGT1A1*) gene by this method.[355]

Crigler-Najjar Syndrome Type II (Arias Syndrome)

Clinical Findings. Crigler-Najjar syndrome type II, otherwise known as Arias syndrome, is phenotypically similar to Crigler-Najjar syndrome type I, except that the serum bilirubin concentration is usually below 20 mg/dl, the prognosis is much less severe, serum bilirubin levels are usually reduced after administration of bilirubin-UGT inducing agents, such as phenobarbital, and the bile contains significant amounts of bilirubin glucuronides (Table 125-1). This disorder was first described by Arias in 1962 in a study of chronic unconjugated hyperbilirubinemia in eight patients between 14 and 52 years of age.[356] Although half the patients were icteric before the age of 1 year, one patient was 30 years old before jaundice was noted. In these patients, serum bilirubin concentration ranged from 8 to 18 mg/dl. Each had reduced hepatic glucuronosyltransferase activities using bilirubin, o-aminophenol, or 4-methylumbelliferone as glucuronide acceptor. Survival of ^{51}Cr-labeled red cells was normal.[301] All patients were clinically normal, apart from icterus, except for a 43-year-old woman with a neurologic syndrome resembling kernicterus. The patient died at the age of 44. Autopsy revealed a histologically normal liver. The brain was small and lacked bilirubin staining but demonstrated the typical histology of kernicterus.

Several other cases of neurologic abnormality in Crigler-Najjar syndrome type II have been described subsequently. Three brothers had Crigler-Najjar syndrome type II for over 50 years.[357] Two were neurologically normal. The third had a slight bilateral intention tremor and nonspecific abnormalities on electroencephalogram. These nonspecific neurologic changes had not been noted previously. Another patient was a 15-year-old boy who was icteric from the second day of life.[358] Total serum bilirubin was 24 mg/dl at 10 months and averaged approximately 15 mg/dl thereafter. Development was normal, although psychological testing revealed a perceptual deficit and slightly subnormal intelligence. At age 13, following surgery for acute appendicitis, the serum bilirubin increased to 40 mg/dl, and diplopia, generalized seizures, confusion, and an abnormal electroencephalogram developed. He was treated for hyperbilirubinemia and, after recovering from surgery, resumed a bilirubin level of 15 mg/dl. His neurologic status returned to baseline and he has remained well.

Laboratory Tests. As in Crigler-Najjar syndrome type I, results of laboratory examination are normal except for elevated serum bilirubin, which is usually less than 20 mg/dl but may be as high as 40 mg/dl during fasting[357] or intercurrent illness.[358] Serum bilirubin is unconjugated, and there is no bilirubinuria. The bile is pigmented, although less than 50 percent of estimated daily bilirubin production is excreted into bile.[301,358] Although over 90 percent of conjugated bilirubin in normal bile is bilirubin diglucuronide, the major pigment in this syndrome is bilirubin monoglucuronide.[358,359] The liver has markedly reduced bilirubin-UGT activity.[358]

Effect of Phenobarbital. The reduced levels of hepatic bilirubin-UGT activity in Crigler-Najjar syndrome type II suggested that an inducer of microsomal enzymes could ameliorate the hyperbilirubinemia.[356] Subsequent studies revealed that serum bilirubin concentrations are reduced significantly (greater than 25 percent) following treatment with phenobarbital (Fig. 125-18).[301] Similar results were obtained with other liver microsomal enzyme inducers.[360–364] The response to phenobarbital treatment differentiates Crigler-Najjar syndrome type 1, in which there is no response, from Crigler-Najjar syndrome type II (Fig. 125-19).[301] Although phenobarbital has been used commonly for inducing hepatic bilirubin-UGT activity, clofibrate is equally effective and is associated with fewer side effects.[364] In some patients, the differentiation from Crigler-Najjar syndrome type 1 may be difficult on the basis of serum bilirubin levels and phenobarbital response.[363] In these cases, the differentiation can be made on the basis of chromatographic analysis of pigments excreted in bile.

Inheritance. Crigler-Najjar syndrome type II runs in families.[301,356] There is no sex predilection. Although the pattern

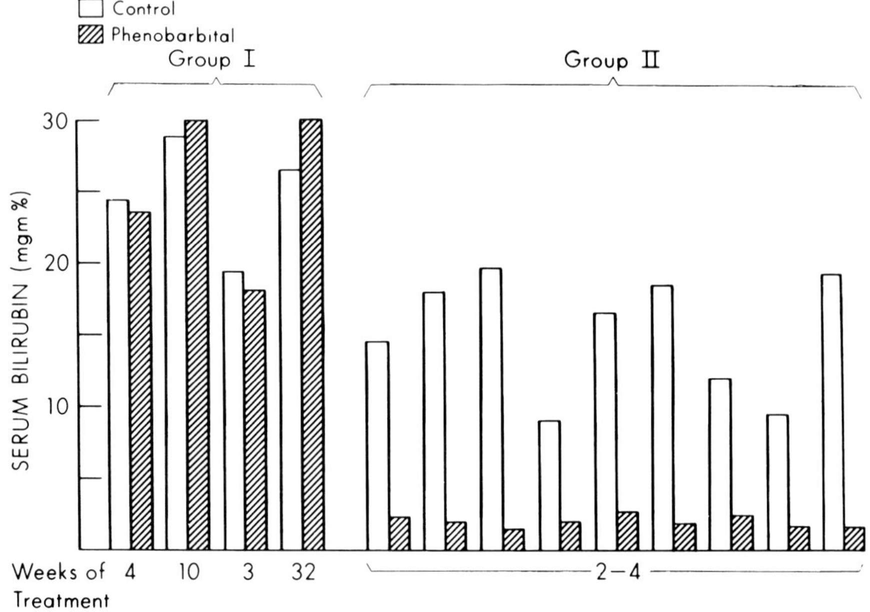

Fig. 125-18 Effect of phenobarbital administration on serum bilirubin concentration, menthol tolerance test, and fecal urobilinogen excretion in a patient with Crigler-Najjar syndrome type II. (*Reprinted with permission from Arias et al.*[299])

of inheritance was not certain for many years, genetic analysis clearly establishes an autosomal-recessive pattern of inheritance. In some heterozygous carriers, the coexistence with a variant promoter associated with Gilbert syndrome may lead to intermediate levels of jaundice (see later section on Gilbert Syndrome), which caused confusion about the mode of inheritance in the past.

Molecular Mechanism. As in Crigler-Najjar syndrome type I, Crigler-Najjar syndrome type II is caused by mutations of one of the five exons that encode bilirubin-UGT (UGT1A1) (Fig. 125-16).[308,365] However, in Crigler-Najjar syndrome type II, the genetic lesion for at least one allele always consists of point mutations that result in substitution of a single amino acid. Such substitutions result in marked reduction, but not a total loss of bilirubin-UGT activity.[365] Phenobarbital works presumably by induction of the residual bilirubin-UGT activity.

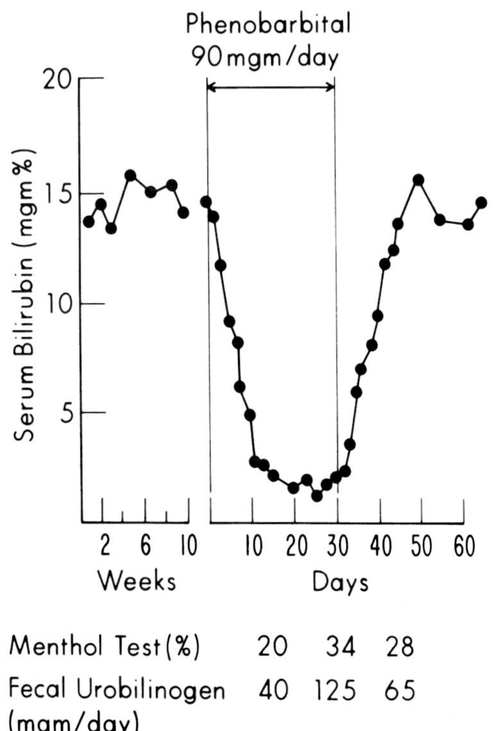

Fig. 125-19 Differentiation of types I and II Crigler-Najjar syndrome on the basis of response to phenobarbital. All patients had chronic unconjugated hyperbilirubinemia and were treated for at least several weeks with phenobarbital. (*Reprinted with permission from Arias et al.*[301])

Gilbert Syndrome

Clinical Findings. The syndrome, described by Gilbert in 1901, also has been called constitutional hepatic dysfunction and familial nonhemolytic jaundice.[366] It is characterized by mild, chronic, unconjugated hyperbilirubinemia (Table 125-1). Familial occurrence is common,[367] although many patients present as isolated cases.

Typically, Gilbert syndrome is diagnosed in young adults, who present with mild, predominantly unconjugated hyperbilirubinemia. Serum bilirubin levels are usually less than 3 mg/dl and fluctuate with time. Bilirubin concentrations can increase during intercurrent illness, but can be normal at other times. Aside from icterus, physical examination is normal. Some patients complain of vague constitutional symptoms, including fatigue and abdominal discomfort[368]; these symptoms are probably unrelated to bilirubin metabolism and may be manifestations of anxiety. Newly presenting patients are rarely symptomatic. Results of routine laboratory tests are normal except for elevated serum bilirubin concentrations. There is no elevation of serum alkaline phosphatase or aminotransferase activities. Oral cholecystography allows visualization of the gallbladder. Although percutaneous liver biopsy is not routinely indicated in patients with Gilbert syndrome, liver histology is normal, except for a nonspecific accumulation of lipofuscin pigment in the centrilobular zones. Electron microscopic studies have not revealed consistent ultrastructural alterations. Hepatic bilirubin-UGT activity is reduced to approximately 30 percent of normal (Fig. 125-20).[369,370]

Organic Anion Transport. Several studies of the disappearance of plasma bilirubin after intravenous injection into patients with Gilbert syndrome have demonstrated reduced clearance (Fig. 125-21). Multicompartmental analysis suggests that reduced plasma clearance results from reduction in hepatic bilirubin uptake as well as bilirubin conjugation.[371] Goresky and associates determined the initial plasma disappearance of radiolabeled bilirubin and then determined an initial space of distribution by

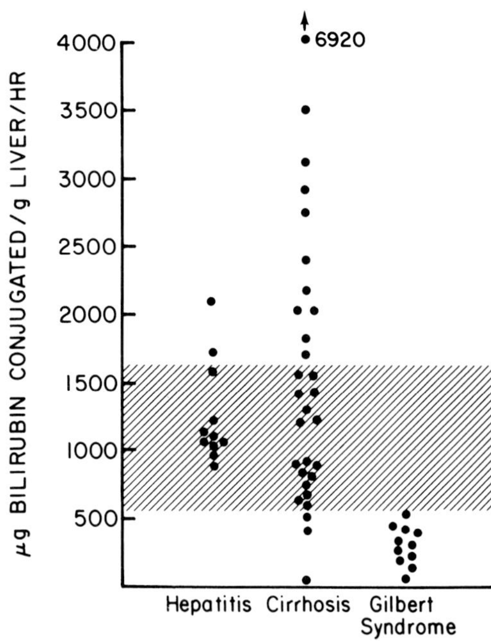

Fig. 125-20 Hepatic bilirubin-UGT activity in patients with hepatitis, cirrhosis, and Gilbert syndrome. The hatched area indicates the normal range. (*Reprinted with permission from Black and Billing.*[369])

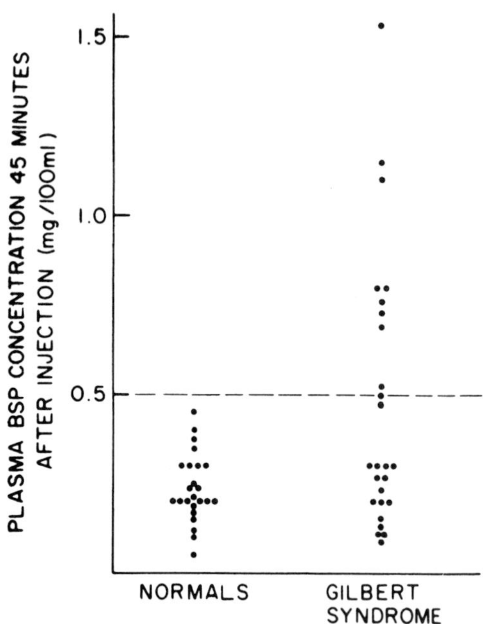

Fig. 125-22 Plasma concentration of BSP 45 min after intravenous administration of 5 mg/kg to normal individuals and patients with Gilbert syndrome. In one subset of patients, BSP retention was elevated. (*Reprinted with permission from Berk et al.*[373])

dividing the injected dose by the plasma volume as determined after radiolabeled albumin injection.[372] The initial plasma disappearance of bilirubin was as rapid in patients with Gilbert syndrome as in normal subjects, suggesting that bilirubin uptake is normal in Gilbert syndrome. Although plasma disappearance of organic anions other than bilirubin is usually normal in Gilbert syndrome (Fig. 125-22), two subsets were described in which BSP[373] and ICG[374] plasma disappearance is abnormal (Fig. 125-23). Because the excretion of neither of these compounds depends on bilirubin-UGT activity, these organic anion clearance abnormalities may not be related to the reduced bilirubin-UGT activity, which is a constant feature of Gilbert syndrome.

The serum bilirubin levels fluctuate in patients with Gilbert syndrome. Factors such as intercurrent illness, physical exertion, and stress have been implicated, and a relationship to the menstrual cycle has been reported in two women.[375] A 48-h fast exaggerates the unconjugated hyperbilirubinemia of Gilbert syndrome.[376] Serum bilirubin levels in normal individuals[377] and in individuals with other hepatobiliary disorders also increase with fasting.[378] Thus, the fasting test appears to be of limited use in the differential diagnosis of Gilbert syndrome. The mechanism of fasting-induced hyperbilirubinemia is unclear. Studies in normal rats revealed no change in hepatic bilirubin-UGT activity during fasting,[378] although there was reduced activity of UDP-glucose dehydrogenase resulting in reduced hepatic content of UDP-glucuronic acid.[379] Fasting also must affect hepatic disposition of bilirubin at a step other than conjugation, because fasting exacerbates hyperbilirubinemia in homozygous Gunn rats.[380] It

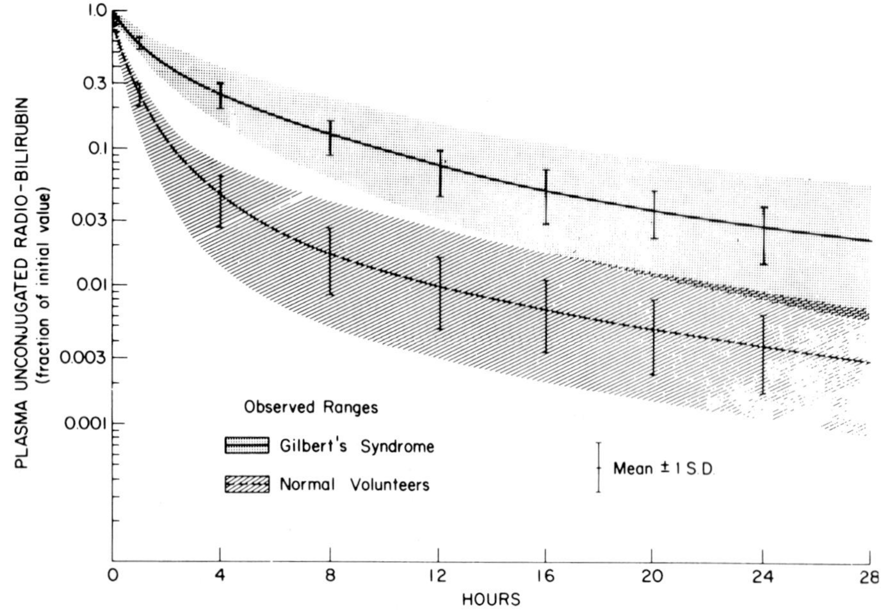

Fig. 125-21 Plasma disappearance of a trace dose of [^{3}H]bilirubin after intravenous administration to patients with Gilbert syndrome and to normal volunteers. There is no overlap between the two groups for the first 16 h after injection. (*Reprinted with permission from Berk et al.*[371])

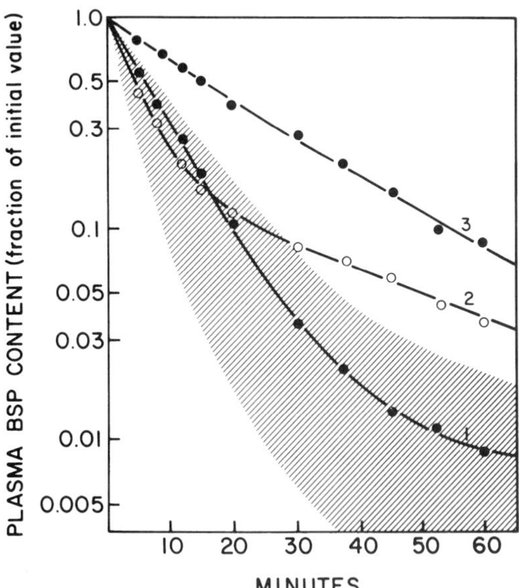

Fig. 125-23 Plasma BSP disappearance curves in three patients with Gilbert syndrome. The shaded area indicates the normal range. Curve 1 is indistinguishable from normal. Curves 2 and 3 are representative of the two subtypes of abnormal BSP disappearance seen in some patients with otherwise typical Gilbert syndrome. (*Reprinted with permission from Berk et al.*[373])

may be a result of several factors, and a role for increased serum nonesterified fatty acid concentration has been suggested.[381]

Intravenous administration of nicotinic acid also has been proposed as a provocative test for the diagnosis of Gilbert syndrome.[382] Its diagnostic value is controversial, and it does not clearly separate patients with Gilbert syndrome from normal subjects or those with hepatobiliary disease. Unconjugated hyperbilirubinemia following nicotinic acid administration does not occur after splenectomy,[382] suggesting that nicotinic acid–induced unconjugated hyperbilirubinemia may result from increased erythrocyte fragility and enhanced splenic heme oxygenase activity, leading to augmentation of splenic bilirubin formation.[383]

Conventionally, The diagnosis of Gilbert syndrome has been applied to individuals with mild unconjugated hyperbilirubinemia without evidence of hemolysis or structural liver disease. However, the coexistence of clinical or subclinical hemolysis may exacerbate the hyperbilirubinemia, thereby bringing the patient to the attention of the physician. The relative content of bilirubin monoglucuronide and diglucuronide in bile is of use in the diagnosis of Gilbert syndrome. Similar to findings in patients with Crigler-Najjar syndrome type II and heterozygous Gunn rats, the proportion of bilirubin monoglucuronide is increased in the bile from patients with Gilbert syndrome. Normally approximately 90 percent of bilirubin excreted in bile is in the form of bilirubin diglucuronide, 7 percent is bilirubin monoglucuronide, and 4 percent is unconjugated bilirubin.[359]

The other significant pigment is a bilirubin monoglucoside-monoglucuronide diester. In Gilbert syndrome the percentage of bilirubin monoglucuronide increases to 14 to 34 percent.[359]

Molecular Mechanism of Gilbert Syndrome. A variant TATAA element within the promoter region upstream to exon 1 of the gene encoding bilirubin UGT (*UGT1A1*) has been found to be associated with Gilbert syndrome.[384] Sequence of the TATAA element in normal subjects is $A[TA]_6TAA$, whereas patients with Gilbert syndrome are homozygous for a longer TATAA element, $A[TA]_7TAA$ (Fig. 125-16). Although this variant promoter was found in all Gilbert syndrome patients studied in the United States and Europe, all subjects who are homozygous for the variant TATAA box do not exhibit hyperbilirubinemia. Expression of the Gilbert genotype appears to require a relatively high level of bilirubin production, in addition to the reduced expression of bilirubin-UGT. For example, most patients diagnosed to have Gilbert syndrome are men, probably because the daily production of bilirubin is greater in men than in women. The incidence of the Gilbert genotype is common in the United States and Europe, approximately 9 percent of the general population being homozygous for the variant promoter, and approximately half the population carrying at least one copy of the variant promoter.

Because of the frequency of the Gilbert type promoter, some heterozygous carriers of a Crigler-Najjar syndrome type I or II mutation are likely to carry the variant TATAA box. If the Gilbert type TATAA element is present on the structurally normal allele of a heterozygous carrier of a Crigler-Najjar syndrome type I or II mutation, the expression of the only normal allele will be reduced to approximately 30 percent of normal, resulting in an intermediate level of jaundice.[385] This explains the frequent finding of intermediate levels of hyperbilirubinemia in the family members of patients with Crigler-Najjar syndrome types I and II.

Inheritance. Subjects who are heterozygous for the Gilbert genotype have higher average serum bilirubin concentrations than subjects who are homozygous for the normal TATAA box. However, all patients in the United States and Europe who were clinically diagnosed to have Gilbert syndrome were homozygous for the variant promoter. On the basis of this, Gilbert syndrome may be considered to have an autosomal-recessive mode of transmission.

Animal Model of Gilbert Syndrome: The Bolivian Squirrel Monkey. The Bolivian population of squirrel monkeys (*Saimiri siureus*) have a higher postcibal serum unconjugated bilirubin concentration and a greater degree of fasting hyperbilirubinemia than does a closely related Brazilian population.[386] Compared with the Brazilian population, Bolivian monkeys have slower plasma clearance of intravenously administered bilirubin, a lower level of hepatic bilirubin-UGT activity, and an increased bilirubin monoglucuronide to diglucuronide ratio in bile.[386] The two populations of squirrel monkeys have a comparable erythrocyte life span and hepatic glutathione-S-transferase activity.[386] In these respects, the Bolivian squirrel monkeys are a model of human Gilbert syndrome. Fasting hyperbilirubinemia is rapidly reversed by oral or intravenous administration of carbohydrates, but not by lipid administration.[387]

DISORDERS OF BILIRUBIN METABOLISM RESULTING IN PREDOMINANTLY CONJUGATED HYPERBILIRUBINEMIA

Dubin-Johnson Syndrome

Clinical Findings. In 1954, Dubin and Johnson[236] and Sprinz and Nelson[388] described patients with chronic nonhemolytic jaundice. The liver was grossly black, but the histology was normal except for an unidentified pigment in hepatocytes. Subsequently, this disorder has been described in both sexes in virtually all nationalities and races.[381–391] Dubin-Johnson syndrome is rare, except in Jews of Middle Eastern origin. Most reports consist of individual cases or small groups. The largest series of 101 cases[391] was reported from Israel on the basis of hospital records from 1955 to 1969. Of these 101 cases, 74 came from families that immigrated from Iran, Iraq, and Afghanistan; nine were of Moroccan origin, and seven were European-Ashkenazim. Among Jews of Persian origin, the incidence is 1:1300.[391] In this population, Dubin-Johnson syndrome is associated with clotting factor VII deficiency.[392]

The syndrome is clinically characterized by mild, predominantly conjugated hyperbilirubinemia (Table 125-2). Except for

Table 125-2 Principal Differential Characteristics of Inherited Chronic Conjugated Hyperbilirubinemias

	Dubin-Johnson Syndrome	Rotor Syndrome
Appearance of liver	Grossly black	Normal
Histology of liver	Dark pigment; predominantly in centrilobular areas; otherwise normal	Normal; no increase in pigmentation
Serum bilirubin	Usually 1.5–5 mg/dl, occasionally as high as 20 mg/dl; predominantly direct reacting	Usually elevated, occasionally as high as 20 mg/dl; predominantly direct reacting
Routine liver function tests	Normal except for bilirubin	Normal except for bilirubin
45-min plasma BSP retention	Normal or elevated; secondary rise at 90 min	Elevated; no secondary increase at 90 min
BSP infusion studies	T_{max} virtually zero; S normal	T_{max} and S both reduced
Oral cholecystogram	Usually does not visualize the gallbladder	Usually visualizes the gallbladder
Urinary coproporphyrin	Normal total; >80% as coproporphyrin I	Elevated total; elevated proportion of coproporphyrin I but <80%
Mode of inheritance	Autosomal recessive	Autosomal recessive
Prevalence	Uncommon (1:1300 in Persian Jews)	Rare
Prognosis	Benign	Benign
Animal model	Mutant TR$^-$ or EHBR rats Mutant Corriedale sheep Mutant golden lion tamarind monkeys	None

jaundice, physical examination is normal. Occasionally a patient may have hepatosplenomegaly. Mild constitutional complaints such as vague abdominal pains and weakness occur, but for the most part patients are asymptomatic.[389–391] Pruritus is absent in Dubin-Johnson syndrome, and serum bile acid levels are normal.[390,393] The degree of icterus is increased by intercurrent illness, oral contraceptives, and pregnancy (Fig. 125-24).[390] Dubin-Johnson syndrome is rarely detected before puberty, although cases have been reported in neonates.[394,395] Often the disorder is not noted until a woman becomes pregnant or receives oral contraceptives with conversion of mild chemical hyperbilirubinemia into overt jaundice.[390]

Laboratory Tests. Routine laboratory examination[389,391] reveals normal complete blood count, serum albumin, cholesterol, transaminases, alkaline phosphatase, and prothrombin time. Serum bilirubin is usually between 2 and 5 mg/dl but can be as high as 20 to 25 mg/dl. Bilirubinuria is frequent, and 50 percent or more of total serum bilirubin is conjugated. The serum bilirubin level fluctuates, and frequently individual determinations may be normal. Both unconjugated and conjugated bilirubin accumulate in serum, and more than half of the bilirubin gives a direct van den Bergh reaction. Prolonged retention of bilirubin glucuronides in plasma results in the formation of irreversible adducts of bilirubin with plasma proteins, particularly albumin. The bilirubin-albumin adduct, termed δ-bilirubin, is found in the serum of patients with Dubin-Johnson syndrome, and various hepatobiliary disorders that are associated with prolonged conjugated hyperbilirubinemia. δ-Bilirubin is not excreted in bile and urine and gives a direct van den Bergh reaction.

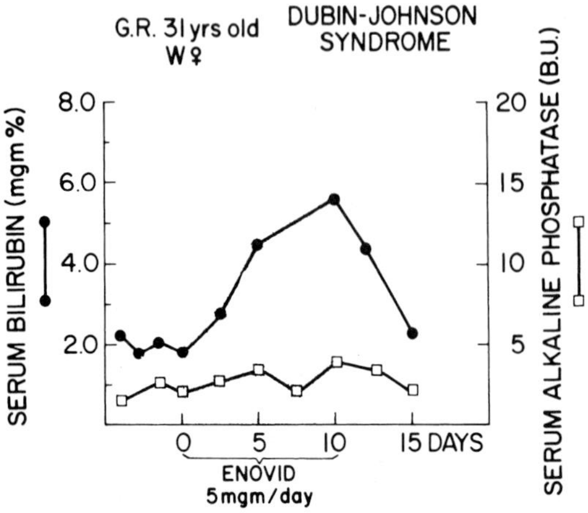

Fig. 125-24 Exacerbation of conjugated hyperbilirubinemia by oral contraceptive administration in a patient with Dubin-Johnson syndrome. Similar findings may be seen in pregnancy.

Excretion of Dyes Used for Imaging of the Biliary System. Oral cholecystography, even using a double dose of contrast material, usually does not allow visualization of the gallbladder, although visualization may occur 4 to 6 h after intravenous injection of iodipamide.[396]

Hepatic Pigmentation. On direct inspection, the liver is black. Light microscopy reveals normal histology except for accumulation of a dense pigment, which on electron microscopy appears to be contained within lysosomes.[397,398] Histochemical staining characteristics and physicochemical properties of extracted pigment resemble those of melanin.[399,400] In the mutant Corriedale sheep, an animal model of Dubin-Johnson syndrome, the hepatic pigment resembles melanin histochemically. Studies performed in mutant Corriedale sheep infused with [^{3}H]-epinephrine revealed reduced biliary excretion of radioactivity and demonstrated incorporation of the isotope into the hepatic pigment,[401] which is consistent with the pigment being a melanin-like derivative. However, electron spin resonance spectroscopy suggests that the Dubin-Johnson pigment differs from authentic melanin, and could be composed of polymers of epinephrine metabolites.[402] The TR$^-$ rat, another animal model for the Dubin-Johnson syndrome, has an identical phenotype except for the absence of pigmentation in the liver.[225] Biliary excretion of [^{3}H]-epinephrine is also disturbed in this rat.[403] When these animals were fed a diet enriched in aromatic amino acids (phenylalanine, tyrosine, and tryptophan), lysosomal pigmentation developed, which was absent in normal rats. Impaired excretion of anionic metabolites of tyrosine, phenylalanine, and tryptophan in the TR$^-$ liver may result in their retention, oxidation, polymerization, and subsequent lysosomal accumulation.[403] One study of computerized tomography of the liver revealed that attenuation values were significantly higher

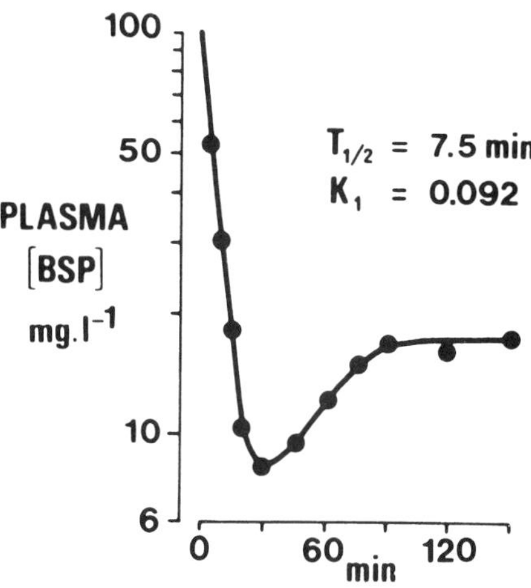

Fig. 125-25 Typical BSP plasma disappearance curve in a patient with Dubin-Johnson syndrome. A secondary increase occurs 45 min after the intravenous injection of the dye. (*Reprinted with permission from Erlinger et al.*[408])

in patients with Dubin-Johnson syndrome as compared with normal controls, although there was considerable overlap between the two groups.[404] The possible relationship of the liver cell pigment to this finding is not known. The degree of hepatic pigmentation may be variable in individuals with the Dubin-Johnson syndrome. Some variability in pigmentation may be due to occurrence of coincidental disease such as acute viral hepatitis, in which the pigment is cleared from the liver only to reaccumulate slowly after recovery.[405]

Organic Anion Transport Defect. In Dubin-Johnson syndrome, initial plasma disappearance of bilirubin,[406,407] BSP,[391,407,408] dibromosulphthalein (DBSP),[408] ICG[407,408] and ^{125}I-labeled rose bengal[408] following intravenous administration are usually normal. Of diagnostic significance is that in approximately 90 percent of patients, the plasma BSP concentration is higher 90 min after intravenous administration than at 45 min (Fig. 125-25).[390,391,395] This is due to reflux of conjugated BSP from the liver cell into the circulation.[409] This secondary increase is not seen following intravenous administration of other organic anions such as DBSP, ^{125}I-labeled rose bengal, and ICG, which are not conjugated prior to excretion by the hepatocytes.[407,408] A similar secondary increase has been described following intravenous administration of unconjugated bilirubin.[402,407] Although the secondary rise of plasma BSP is characteristic of Dubin-Johnson syndrome, it is not diagnostic and occurs in other hepatobiliary disorders.[410]

Studies of BSP transport during constant intravenous infusion reveal that the T_{max} is reduced to only 10 percent of normal, and the relative hepatic storage capacity is normal.[390,391] This finding was also demonstrated directly in a patient with Dubin-Johnson syndrome who had a biliary fistula.[237] In this patient, dehydrocholate choleresis did not augment biliary BSP excretion. Similar studies of BSP transport have been performed in phenotypically normal parents and children (i.e., carriers) of Dubin-Johnson syndrome patients, and it was found to be normal.[390]

Inheritance and Urinary Coproporphyrin Excretion. The familial nature of Dubin-Johnson syndrome was noted in its initial descriptions, but its mode of inheritance was unclear.[389] Subsequently, it was observed that the ratio of coproporphyrin I to coproporphyrin III excreted in the urine of patients with Dubin-Johnson syndrome is greater than that found in other hepatobiliary disorders.[411] Of the two isomeric forms of coproporphyrin, isomer III is the precursor of heme, whereas isomer I is a metabolic by-product without known function.[412] Coproporphyrin isomers I and III are normally found in urine, where approximately 75 percent of total urinary coproporphyrin is coproporphyrin III. In Dubin-Johnson syndrome, total urinary coproporphyrin excretion is normal, but over 80 percent is coproporphyrin I.[411,413] Urinary coproporphyrin excretion has been determined in phenotypically normal relatives of patients with Dubin-Johnson syndrome (Fig. 125-26).[413–415] In obligate heterozygotes (i.e., unaffected parents and children of patients with Dubin-Johnson syndrome), total urinary coproporphyrin excretion was reduced by 40 percent as compared with normal control subjects.[413–415] This was due to a 50 percent reduction in coproporphyrin III excretion. The proportion of coproporphyrin I in urine was intermediate between results in controls and in patients with Dubin-Johnson syndrome. Analysis of data from studies revealed that with respect to urinary coproporphyrin excretion, Dubin-Johnson syndrome is inherited as an autosomal-recessive characteristic (Fig. 125-26 and Table 125-2).[414] A similar mode of inheritance was determined in a

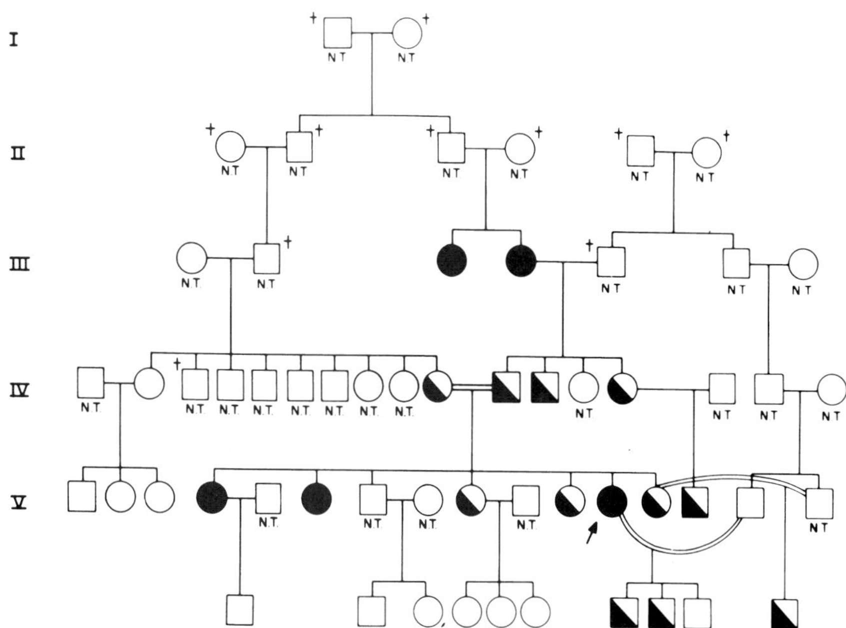

Fig. 125-26 Pedigree of a family in which consanguinity resulted in three children with Dubin-Johnson syndrome (generation V). Solid symbols indicate individuals with Dubin-Johnson syndrome. Partially filled symbols indicate phenotypically normal individuals with urinary coproporphyrin excretion in the heterozygous range. Open symbols represent phenotypically normal individuals with normal urinary coproporphyrin excretion. NT, individuals who were not tested. In this family, the defect was detected in four generations. (*Reprinted with permission from Wolkoff AW, Cohen LE, Arias IM: New Engl J Med 288:113, 1973.*)

study of BSP and bilirubin metabolism in 173 sibs of 44 patients with Dubin-Johnson syndrome.[416] No other hepatobiliary disorder or porphyria has been described in which total urinary coproporphyrin excretion is normal, with over 80 percent of the total as coproporphyrin I. In the presence of a consistent history and physical examination, urinary coproporphyrin excretion appears to be diagnostic of this disorder.

The overlap of results in carriers with those in controls[413–415] makes determination of urinary coproporphyrin excretion less useful in deciding whether an individual carries the gene for the syndrome. However, this disorder is benign, and genetic counseling is rarely required. Urinary coproporphyrin excretion proved useful in diagnosing Dubin-Johnson syndrome in two neonates.[394,395] Although neonates normally have elevated urinary content of coproporphryin I as compared with adults, levels are not as high as seen in Dubin-Johnson syndrome.[417]

The pathogenesis of the abnormal urinary coproporphyrin excretion in this syndrome is unknown, as is its relationship to conjugated hyperbilirubinemia. In addition to being present in urine, coproporphyrins are also found in bile, where isomer I constitutes approximately 65 percent of the total.[412] Normally, total daily biliary coproporphyrin excretion is approximately three times that of total daily urinary excretion. In most hepatobiliary disorders, including cholestasis, coproporphyrin levels are increased in urine.[418] In these disorders, total urinary coproporphyrin excretion is elevated and the proportion of isomer I in urine is usually less than 65 percent. Dubin-Johnson syndrome is unique in that total urinary coproporphyrin is normal, but the proportion of isomer I is over 80 percent. It seems unlikely that the abnormal pattern of coproporphyrin isomers seen in Dubin-Johnson syndrome results simply from reduced biliary excretion, and an alteration in hepatic porphyrin biosynthesis has been postulated (Fig. 125-27).[414,417] Reduced coproporphyrin III formation could result from decreased activity of hepatic uroporphyrin III cosynthetase.[414] Enzyme activity as determined in blood cells and liver from four patients did not differ from normal.[419] Following an intravenous load of δ-aminolevulinic acid, coproporphyrin III content of urine and bile changed very little in patients with Dubin-Johnson syndrome, as compared with results in normal control subjects.[420] Further study of porphyrin biosynthesis is required to elucidate the mechanism of abnormal coproporphyrin excretion and the relationship of the porphyrin abnormality to the conjugated hyperbilirubinemia that characterizes the syndrome.

The differential diagnosis of Dubin-Johnson syndrome includes Rotor syndrome, another benign inherited disorder characterized by the accumulation of both conjugated and unconjugated bilirubin in plasma (see later section on Rotor Syndrome).

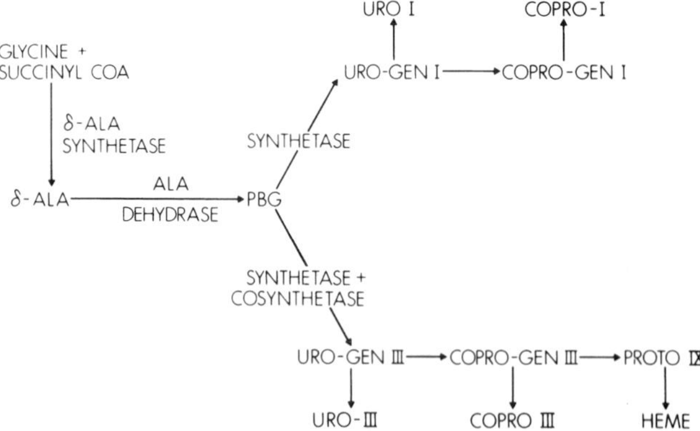

Fig. 125-27 Pathway of porphyrin biosynthesis. δ-Aminolevulinic acid (δ-ALA) condenses to form porphobilinogen (PBG). In the presence of uroporphyrinogen synthetase, PBG forms the isomer I porphyrins, which are excretory products without known function. On addition of uroporphyrinogen cosynthetase, PBG forms the isomer III porphyrins, which are precursors of heme. (*Reprinted with permission from Wolkoff AW, Cohen LE, Arias IM: New Engl J Med 288:113, 1973.*)

Molecular Mechanism of Dubin-Johnson Syndrome. As discussed before, the bile canalicular transport of bilirubin glucuronides occurs against a concentration gradient via an energy-consuming mechanism that is shared with many other organic anions, except bile acids. The functional characteristics of canalicular non–bile acid organic anion transporter, termed the canalicular multispecific organic anion transporter or cMOAT, have been defined largely by studies in mutant animal models with a transport defect for organic anions.[421] cMOAT is also termed MRP2 (GenBank NM_000392).

Animal Models. The first animal model to be described was the mutant Corriedale sheep. The metabolic defect in this strain closely resembles that found in Dubin-Johnson syndrome. Biliary excretion of a large number of organic anions, including conjugated bilirubin, glutathione-conjugated BSP, iopanoic acid, and ICG is decreased, whereas taurocholate transport is normal.[235,422] Although the biliary excretion of the glutathione conjugates of BSP is markedly reduced, the secretion of unconjugated BSP is unimpaired.[240] Serum bilirubin levels are mildly elevated, and 60 percent of the pigments in the serum is glucuronidated. As in Dubin-Johnson syndrome, the liver is pigmented, and the histology is otherwise normal.[422] Total urinary coproporhyrin excretion is normal with increased excretion of coproporphyrin isomer I and decreased isomer III excretion.

The most important animal model for Dubin-Johnson syndrome is the TR^- rat, also known as GY (Groningen yellow) rat.[421] These rats have been used extensively for elucidation of the mechanism of canalicular excretion of conjugated bilirubin and other organic anions. As in Dubin-Johnson syndrome, the biliary excretion of conjugated bilirubin and many other organic anions is impaired, and isomer I of coproporphyrin constitutes the major fraction of porphyrins excreted in the urine.[421] Although the liver of TR^- rats maintained on standard laboratory chow does not contain black pigments, lysosomal pigment accumulation occurs upon feeding a diet enriched in aromatic amino acids.[403] Breeding studies indicated autosomal-recessive inheritance for this disorder and suggested that a single gene is responsible for the defect. For organic anions, such as glutathione-conjugated leukotriene C_4, the canalicular secretion defect is nearly complete, whereas for bilirubin glucuronides, there is a residual transport activity (about 10 percent of normal).[422,423] In contrast, secretion of the synthetic compound bilirubin ditaurate is nearly normal.[422] These observations suggest the presence of additional transport mechanisms for organic anions that may not be affected in TR^- rats.

Energy requirements for cMOAT were investigated using dinitrophenylglutathione, the transport of which is nearly absent in TR^- rats.[421] Dinitrophenylglutathione transport by isolated hepatocytes[421,424] and rat liver plasma membrane vesicles requires ATP.[224,425,426] Similarly, the transport of bilirubin glucuronide,[223] BSP,[220] cysteinyl leukotrienes[221] and p-nitrophenylglucuronide[427] in liver canalicular membrane vesicles is also stimulated by the addition of ATP.

Substrate Specificity of cMOAT. The susbstrate specificity of cMOAT was studied by comparison of the biliary excretion of various compounds in normal and TR^- rats. From these studies a picture emerged of a transporter that recognizes a wide variety of compounds.[421] The common denominator of these substrates is that they are anionic amphipaths. The majority of substrates has more than one negative charge in the molecule. Among the recognized substrates are glucuronide conjugates, like that of bilirubin and triiodothyronine, but also of xenobiotics like naphtol. Glutathione conjugates (including its own conjugate, GSSG) are high-affinity subtrates. The endogenous glutathione conjugate leukotriene C_4 is actually the substrate with the highest affinity known (K_m 0.25 μM) for cMOAT. Sulfate conjugates are also transported but have much lower affinity. There are also a number of anionic substrates that are not metabolized or conjugated in the hepatocyte and that are excreted via cMOAT. Examples of this class are dibromosulphophtalein and the cephalosporin ceftriaxone.[421]

Studies in patients with Dubin-Johnson syndrome and in related animal models (Corriedale sheep and TR$^-$ rats) have shown that bile acids are secreted by a mechanism that is distinct from that of other organic anions. Although both types of compounds undergo primary active (ATP-dependent) transport across the canalicular membrane,[230] their transport processes are clearly mediated by different gene products. The mutant animals as well as patients with Dubin-Johnson syndrome excrete bile salts normally, whereas the biliary excretion of a wide variety of other organic anions is severely impaired. Taurocholate does not compete with the transport of bilirubin glucuronides or BSP in canalicular membrane preparations, further indicating that these compounds use separate transport systems.[219,220] An exception to this is the bile salts that are conjugated at the 3-OH position. In contrast to normal bile salts, these 3-OH conjugated bile acids have a double-negative charge and behave as non–bile acid organic anions.[225,428] There is an ATP-driven and a membrane potential-dependent component of bilirubin glucuronide transport by canalicular plasma membrane vesicles.[223] The ATP-dependent mechanism is absent in membrane vesicles from the livers of TR$^-$ rats, but the membrane potential-dependent mechanism provides the residual transport.

A mutant strain of golden lion tamarins (*Leontopitheous rosalia rosalia*) with Dubin-Johnson–like syndrome has been described.[236]

Molecular Genetics of cMOAT. cMOAT is a member of the family of ATP-binding cassette (ABC) transporters, which are, typically, single polypeptides with two similar halves, each containing at least four and usually six transmembrane helices and an ABC that mediates ATP hydrolysis.[429] The cDNA for cMOAT has been cloned.[430] cMOAT is a 1541–amino acid (200-kDa) integral membrane protein, localized in the apical membrane of the hepatocyte. The protein is highly expressed in the liver and to a much lesser extent in kidney, duodenum, and ileum. Among the other mammalian members of the ABC transporter family, the P-glycoproteins are best characterized. The P-glycoprotein encoded by the human *MDR1* gene mediates ATP-driven extrusion of hydrophobic compounds from cells.[431] Overexpression of this protein in tumor cells makes them multidrug resistant.[432] Another P-glycoprotein, encoded by the *MDR2* gene, is concentrated in the canalicular domain of hepatocyte plasma membranes and is required for the translocation of phospholipids across the canalicular membrane into the bile.[239] The multidrug resistance–related protein, MRP1, is distantly related to the P-glycoproteins and also confers resistance against cytotoxic drugs.[232] MRP1 mediates the canalicular transport of organic anions, such as dinitrophenylglutathione and leukotriene C_4, the transport of which is impaired in TR$^-$ rats.[233,236] However, the expression of MRP1 in the liver is extremely low, and this protein is localized in the basolateral domain of epithelial cell plasma membranes,[433] suggesting that it is not involved in the canalicular transport of organic anions. Direct evidence for the role of the cMOAT in hepatocanalicular organic anion transport came from the discovery of a mutation in this gene in the TR$^-$ rat.[430] The deletion of a single nucleotide leads to a frameshift and a premature stop codon, generating a truncated protein. This mutation also markedly reduces the mRNA level. cMOAT was immunologically undetectable in the plasma membrane preparations of TR$^-$ rats.

More recently, the human cMOAT cDNA has been isolated (GenBank U49248) on the basis of homology with the rat cMOAT,[434] and the gene has been located on chromosome 10q23-q24.[435] Human cMOAT is a 1545–amino acid protein with 78 percent amino acid homology to the rat protein. The first mutation that was described in a Dubin-Johnson syndrome patient was a stop codon, predicted to express a truncated protein.[434] In this patient and a subsequently reported case,[436] immunohistochemical staining of a liver section was negative. Two additional patients with single-base deletions and one with a missense mutation of the cMOAT gene have been reported.[437] Because of its homology with *MRP1*, the *cMOAT* gene is also referred to as *MRP2*.

Inheritance. The male-to-female ratio in clinically diagnosed cases of Dubin-Johnson syndrome is 1.5:1,[389] perhaps because of a greater daily bilirubin production in postpubertal males than in females. With respect to urinary coproporphyrin excretion pattern, Dubin-Johnson syndrome is inherited as an autosomal-recessive characteristic.[412,414] In the TR$^-$ rat, which has a mutation in the same gene, the disease is clearly inherited in an autosomal-recessive manner. This pattern is also confirmed in several patients with Dubin-Johnson syndrome, in whom the genetic lesions have been identified.[435,436]

Clotting Factor VII Deficiency. In a report from Israel, 60 percent of the patients with Dubin-Johnson syndrome were found to have reduced prothrombin activity due to lower levels of clotting Factor VII.[437] Although Factor VII deficiency was most common among the Jews originating from Iran, Iraq, and the neighboring areas, this abnormality was also found in some patients belonging to other Jewish communities. However, in some families the two disorders were found to segregate independently, indicating that the combined disorder may be coincidental and does not represent a true association. The gene for Factor VII is located on chromosome 13,[438] whereas the *cMOAT* gene (*MRP2*) is on chromosome 10,[435] excluding a primary linkage between the two defects.

Rotor Syndrome

Clinical Findings. In 1948, Rotor, Manahan, and Florentin described several individuals from two families in whom there was chronic predominantly conjugated hyperbilirubinemia without any evidence of hemolysis.[439] Serum alkaline phosphatase and cholesterol values were normal. Plasma disappearance of BSP was greatly delayed. Liver histology was normal. Although previously Rotor and Dubin-Johnson syndromes were thought to be variants of a single pathophysiologic disorder,[440] now these disorders are known to be different entities (Table 125-2).[441] Rotor syndrome is benign. The liver is normal on histologic examination and does not have excess pigmentation.[440] Although it has been described in several nationalities and races, Rotor syndrome is rare.

Organic Anion Excretion. Oral cholecystographic agents usually do not visualize the gallbladder in the Dubin-Johnson syndrome, whereas roentgenologic visualization usually is possible in Rotor syndrome.[440] Unlike the findings in Dubin-Johnson syndrome, patients with Rotor syndrome exhibit marked retention of BSP at 45 min after injection, but biphasic plasma BSP peaks are not found (Fig. 125-25) and conjugated BSP does not appear in plasma (Fig. 125-28).[442] There is also marked plasma retention of intravenously administered unconjugated bilirubin and ICG.[443]

With the use of a constant infusion technique, the transport maximum (T_{max}) for BSP and the relative hepatic storage capacity have been determined in patients with Rotor and Dubin-Johnson syndromes (Fig. 125-29).[442,443] In Dubin-Johnson syndrome, the T_{max} is virtually zero, whereas the hepatic storage capacity is normal. In Rotor syndrome, the hepatic storage capacity was reduced by 75 to 90 percent and T_{max} was reduced by 50 percent.[442,443] Determination of T_{max} and relative hepatic storage capacity (S) in phenotypically normal obligate heterozygotes revealed results intermediate between those in patients with Rotor syndrome and controls.[442] The modest reduction in T_{max} accompanied by a larger reduction in hepatic storage is similar to observations in hepatic storage disease, a familial disorder

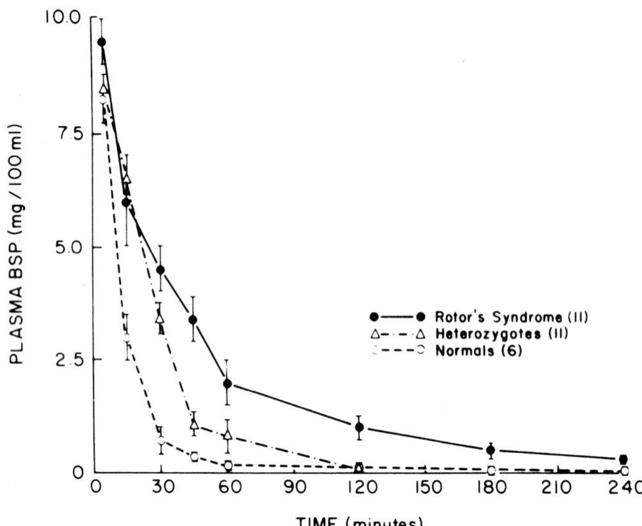

Fig. 125-28 Plasma disappearance of BSP after intravenous injection of a 50 mg/kg dose into 11 patients with Rotor syndrome, 11 phenotypically normal first-degree relatives defined as heterozygotes for the syndrome on the basis of urinary coproporphyrin administration, and six normal controls. There was no secondary increase of plasma BSP, and conjugated BSP was not found in plasma. (*Reprinted with permission from Wolpert et al.*[442])

manifested by predominantly conjugated hyperbilirubinemia and normal liver histology.[444] Because there is little to differentiate Rotor syndrome from hepatic storage disease, they may represent a single pathophysiologic entity.

Urinary Coproporphyrin Excretion. Unlike results for Dubin-Johnson syndrome, total urinary coproporphyrin excretion is increased by 250 to 500 percent as compared with control subjects, and the proportion of coproporphyrin I in urine is approximately 65 percent of total.[441,445] In one report, however, two brothers with clinical Rotor syndrome had over 80 percent of urinary coproporphyrins as isomer I.[446] These results are similar to those seen in many other hepatobiliary disorders.[447] Phenotypically normal obligate heterozygotes have a coproporphyrin excretory pattern that is intermediate between that of control subjects and patients with Rotor syndrome. With respect to urinary coproporphyrin excretion, Rotor syndrome is inherited as an autosomal-recessive characteristic and is distinct from Dubin-Johnson syndrome (Table 125-2, Figs. 125-30, 125-31).[445] The urinary coproporphyrin abnormality in Rotor syndrome, unlike that in

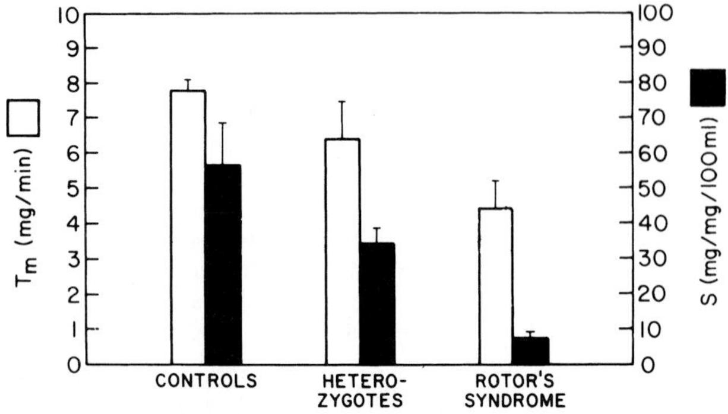

Fig. 125-29 Hepatic relative storage capacity (S) and transport maximum (T_{max}) for BSP in six patients with Rotor syndrome, five phenotypically normal heterozygotes, and six normal controls. (*Reprinted with permission from Wolpert et al.*[442])

Dubin-Johnson syndrome, is most likely caused by a reduced biliary excretion of coproporphyrins, with consequent increase in renal excretion. The nature of the organic anion transport defect in Rotor syndrome is unknown.

Progressive Familial Intrahepatic Cholestasis

Progressive familial intrahepatic cholestasis (PFIC) is a heterogeneous group of autosomal-recessive inherited diseases in infants and children. All are characterized by cholestasis associated with elevated plasma levels of bile acids, defective bile acid secretion in bile, growth failure, and progressive liver damage initially manifested by conjugated hyperbilirubinemia. On the basis of molecular genetic studies, PFIC has been divided into three categories. The availability of DNA expressed sequence tags (ESTs) generated by the Human Genome Project enabled identification of large and frequently inbred families with individual disorders. The findings of the molecular genetic studies overlapped temporally with the discovery of specific ATP-dependent transporters in the bile canaliculus.

Progressive familial intrahepatic cholestasis type I (Byler disease) was described in an old order Amish pedigree of seven generations descended from Jacob Byler.[448] The disease is manifested by variable conjugated hyperbilirubinemia, growth retardation, and progressive, fatal cholestasis. In some patients, intestinal lipid malabsorption is present and not completely ameliorated by liver transplantation. Plasma bile acids are elevated, particularly lithocholate. No unique cholestatic bile acids or metabolites have been demonstrated in blood or urine.

The defective gene was mapped to chromosome 18q21 by screening of the genome for chromosomal sequences shared by patients from the original Byler kindred. Probability calculations indicate that such sharing is unlikely to occur by chance. A mutated gene, designated *FIC1*, that codes for a P-type ATPase was identified (GenBank AF038007).[449] Northern hybridization reveals expression of the normal gene in intestine, liver, and other tissues. Its cellular and subcellular sites have not yet been identified. How defective FIC1 results in cholestasis and abnormal bile acid transport is not known. Normal P-ATPases couple hydrolyis of ATP to the translocation of acidic phospholipids (i.e., phosphatidylserine, phosphatidylethanolamine) from the outer to the inner layer of the plasma membrane of many different cells. Alterations in hepatic or intestinal membrane lipids may affect the function of ATP-dependent tranporters for bile acids, conjugated bilirubin, and other ligands.

Benign Recurrent Intrahepatic Cholestasis (BRIC). This rare disease was described in 1959[450] and is characterized by recurrent episodes of cholestasis followed by complete return to normalcy clinically, biochemically, and by liver histology.[451–453] The disorder may begin in infancy or middle age but predominantly is manifested in adolescence or early adulthood.[452,454] Episodes last from several weeks to months, during which time patients manifest malaise, anorexia, pruritus, weight loss, malabsorption, conjugated hyperbilirubinemia, and biochemical evidence of cholestasis without severe hepatocellular injury.[453–455] Intervals between attacks may last from a few weeks to several years. In a given patient, recurrent attacks resemble each other in symptoms, signs, and duration. Liver histology reveals noninflammatory intrahepatic cholestasis without fibrosis regardless of the number and severity of attacks. During remission, liver histology returns to normal whether examined by light or electron microscopy.[456]

The pathogenesis of this rare disorder is unknown. Recessive inheritance has been demonstrated by family studies in isolated populations in which the disorder is frequently observed. There is no specific treatment to prevent the occurrence of cholestatic episodes or to shorten their duration. Liver transplantation has not been performed because of the episodic and nonprogressive course of the disease.

Unexpectedly, mutated *FIC1* was identified in BRIC by searching for chromosomal sequences shared by only three

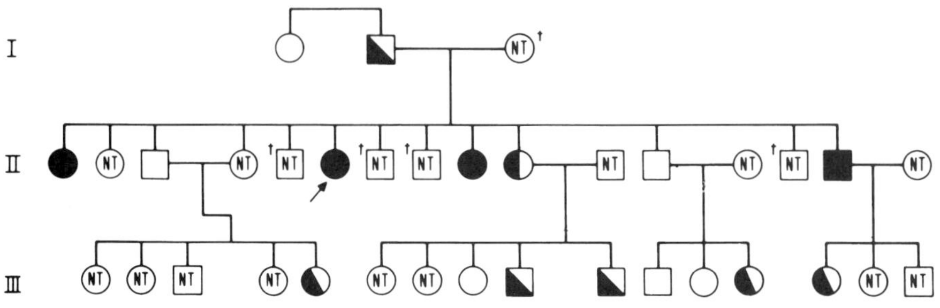

Fig. 125-30 Pedigree of a Philippine family originally described by Rotor in 1948. Solid symbols indicate individuals with Rotor syndrome. Partial symbols indicate phenotypically normal individuals with urinary coproporphyrin excretion in the heterozygote range. Open symbols represent phenotypically normal individuals with normal urinary coproporphyrin excretion. NT, individuals who were not tested. (*Reprinted with permission from Wolkoff et al.*[441])

distantly related patients.[449] Although BRIC and PFIC I have many clinical features in common, the former is progressive whereas the latter is intermittent. How the different phenotypes result from the same genetic defect is unknown.

Progressive Familial Intrahepatic Cholestasis Type II. A second form of PFIC resembles Byler disease clinically but occurs in non-Byler families, mainly in the Middle East and Europe. Homozygosity mapping and genome search in unrelated pedigrees associated the disorder with chromosome 2q24, from which the gene for SPGP (sister of P-glycoprotein) was cloned (GenBank AF091582).[457] Remarkably, at almost the same time, SPGP was shown to be a canalicular ATP-dependent bile acid transporter.[238] Over 20 different point mutations in *SPGP* have been described in patients with PFIC of this type. Liver transplantation ameliorates all manifestations of the disease in concordance with the finding that SPGP is expressed only in the liver.

Progressive Familial Intrahepatic Cholestasis Type III. A third PFIC group involves mutations in the loci encoding class III multidrug resistance (MDR) P-glycoproteins (*mdr2* in mice and

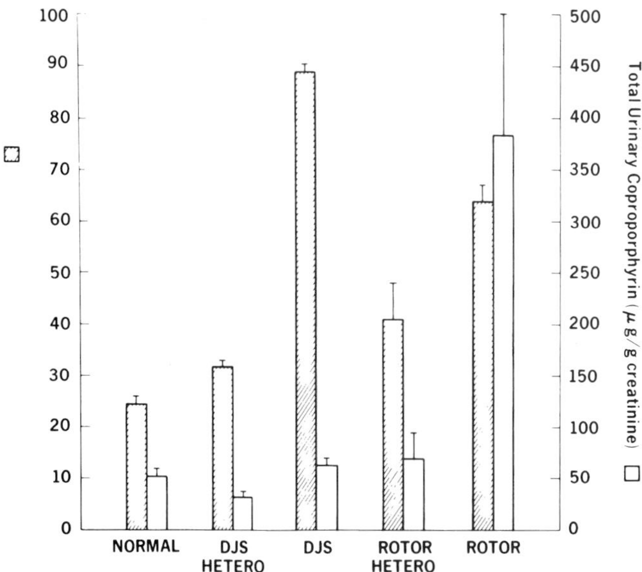

Fig. 125-31 Urinary coproporphyrin excretion in Dubin-Johnson and Rotor syndromes. The shaded bars represent the percentage of total urinary coproporphyrin excreted as coproporphyrin I. The open bars represent total urinary coproporphyrin excretion. Vertical bars represent 1 SEM. Total urinary coproporphyrin excretion is normal in Dubin-Johnson syndrome (DJS), with a markedly elevated proportion of coproporphyrin I (greater than 80 percent). Both variables are elevated in Rotor syndrome, and, with respect to urinary coproporphyrin excretion, the two disorders are distinct. Results in obligate heterozygotes for each of these disorders (DJS hetero, Rotor hetero) lie intermediate between results in normal individuals and in individuals manifesting the respective disorder.

MDR3 in humans), which mediate ATP-dependent translocation of phosphatidylcholine from the inner to the outer leaflet of the bile canalicular plasma membrane.[231] Removal of *mdr2* by homologous recombination in mice results in absence of phosphatidylcholine from bile, progressive destruction of small bile ducts, cholestasis characterized by conjugated hyperbilirubinemia, and eventual biliary cirrhosis. In *mdr2* −/− mice, bile acids are secreted normally by SPGP but are not incorporated into mixed micelles and progressively damage small bile ducts.[430]

Two different point mutations in *MDR3* resulting in a nonfunctioning protein were described in two children with PFIC associated with elevated serum levels of γ-glutamyl transpeptidase activity.[458] Virtual absence of *MDR3* mRNA occurs in Navajo Indian children with PFIC and dysmyelinating peripheral and central neuropathy.[459] The relationship between *MDR3* and neuropathy is unknown. Elevated serum γ-glutamyl transpeptidase activity is proposed to result from small bile duct damage and distinguishes this PFIC group from PFIC I and BRIC.

Alagille Syndrome

Many heritable developmental disorders have been described; however, the Alagille syndrome is the first to be described at the molecular level. The Alagille syndrome is transmitted as an autosomal-recessive inherited characteristic that includes paucity or absence of small bile ducts resulting in progressive intrahepatic cholestasis, and abnormalities of the eye, heart, and vertebrae. Identification of rare patients with cytogenic deletions permitted mapping of the gene to chromosome 20p12, from which *JAG1* was identified.[460] *JAG1* encodes an unidentified ligand that binds to the notch receptor, which is crucial for cell fate development in *Drosophila* and mammals. Analysis of patients with Alagille syndrome who do not have chromosomal deletions (see Chap. 65) revealed several point mutations in *JAG1* (GenBank U73936), each of which abolishes expression of the altered allele.[460]

ACKNOWLEDGMENT

The authors thank Dr. Ajit Kadakol for assistance in preparation of this review. This work was supported in part by National Institutes of Health Grants DK-46057, DK-39137, DK-41296, DK-23026, DK-35652, and DK-34926.

REFERENCES

1. Berk PD, Howe RB, Bloomer JR, Berlin NI: Studies on bilirubin kinetics in normal adults. *J Clin Invest* **48**:2176, 1979.
2. London IM, West R, Shemin D, Rittenberg D: On the origin of bile pigment in normal man. *J Biol Chem* **184**:351, 1950.
3. Schwartz S, Johnson JA, Stephenson BD, Anderson AS, Edmondson PR, Fusaro RM: Erythropoietic defects in protoporphyria: A study of factors involved in labelling of porphyrins and bile pigments from ALA-^{3}H and glycine-^{14}C. *J Lab Clin Med* **78**:411, 1971.
4. Berk PD, Jones EA, Howe RB, Berlin NI: Disorders of bilirubin metabolism, in Bondy PK, Rosenberg LE (eds): *Metabolic Control and Disease*, 8th ed. Philadelphia: WB Saunders, 1980, p 1009.
5. Grandchamp B, Bissel DM, Licko V, Schmidt R: Formation and disposition of newly synthesized heme in adult rat hepatocytes in primary cultures. *J Biol Chem* **256**:11677, 1981.

6. Levitt M, Schacter BA, Zipursky A, Israels LG: The nonerythropoietic component of early bilirubin. *J Clin Invest* **47**:1281, 1968.
7. Gray CH, Scott JJ: The effect of haemorrhage on the incorporation of [^{14}C]glycine into stercobilin. *Biochem J* **71**:38, 1959.
8. Beattie AD, Goldberg A: Acute intermittent porphyria: Natural history and prognosis, in Doss M (ed): *Porphyrins and Human Disease*. Basel, Switzerland: Karger, 1976, p 245.
9. Come SE, Shohet SB, Robinson SH: Surface remodeling vs. whole-cell hemolysis of reticulocytes produced with erythroid stimulation or iron deficiency anemia. *Blood* **44**:817, 1974.
10. Robinson SH: Origins of the early-labeled peak, in Berk PD, Berlin NI (eds): *Bile Pigments: Chemistry and Physiology*. Washington, DC: Department of Health, Education, and Welfare, National Institutes of Health, 1977, p 175.
11. Landaw SA: Quantitative recovery of ^{14}C-labeled carbon monoxide (^{14}CO) from viable heme-labeled red blood cells in the rat. *Blood* **40**:257, 1972.
12. Bissel DM, Guzelian PS: Degradation of endogenous hepatic heme by pathways not yielding carbon monoxide: Studies in normal rat liver and primary hepatocyte culture. *J Clin Invest* **65**:1135, 1980.
13. Tenhunen R, Marver HS, Schmid R: Microsomal heme oxygenase: Characterization of the enzyme. *J Biol Chem* **244**:6388, 1969.
14. Bissel DM, Hammaker L, Schmidt R: Liver sinusoidal cells. Identification of a subpopulation for erythrocyte catabolism. *J Cell Biol* **54**:107, 1972.
15. Sassa S, Kappas A, Bernstein SE, Alvares AP: Heme biosynthesis and drug metabolism in mice with hereditary hemolytic anemia. *J Biol Chem* **254**:729, 1979.
16. Ishizawa S, Yoshida T, Kikuchi G: Induction of heme oxygenase in rat liver. *J Biol Chem* **258**:4220, 1983.
17. Posselt AM, Cowan BE, Kwong LK, Vreman HJ, Stevenson DK: Effect of tin protoporphyrin on the excretion rate of carbon monoxide in newborn rats after hematoma formation. *J Pediatr Gastroenterol Nutr* **4**:650, 1985.
18. Yoshida T, Kikuchi G: Heme oxygenase purified to apparent homogeneity from pig spleen microsomes. *J Biochem (Tokyo)* **81**:265, 1977.
19. Yosinga T, Sassa S, Kappas A: The occurrence of molecular interactions among NADPH-cytochrome C reductase, heme oxygenase and biliverdin reductanse in heme degradation. *J Biol Chem* **257**:7778, 1982.
20. Maines MD, Ibrahim NG, Kappas A: Solubilization and partial purification of heme oxygenase from rat liver. *J Biol Chem* **252**:5900, 1977.
21. Jackson AH, Kenner W: Recent developments in porphyrin chemistry, in Goodwin TW (ed): *Porphyrins and Related Compounds*. London: Academic, 1968, p 5.
22. Brown SB, King RFGJ: The mechanism of heme catabolism: Bilirubin formation in living rats by [^{18}O]oxygen labeling. *Biochem J* **170**:297, 1978.
23. Yoshida T, Kikuchi G: Features of the reaction of heme degradation catalyzed by the reconstituted microsomal heme oxygenase system. *J Biol Chem* **253**:4230, 1978.
24. Cornelius CE: Comparative bile pigment metabolism in vertebrates, in Ostrow JD (ed): *Bile Pigments and Jaundice*. New York: Marcel Dekker, 1986, p 601.
25. McDonagh AF, Palma LA, Schmidt R: Reduction of biliverdin and placental transfer of bilirubin and biliverdin in the pregnant guinea pig. *Biochem J* **194**:273, 1981.
26. Roy Chowdhury J, Roy Chowdhury N, Arias IM: Bilirubin conjugates in the spiny dogfish, *Squalus acanthias*, the small skate, *Raja erinacea* and the winter flounder *Pseudopleuronectes americanas*. *Comp Biochem Physiol [B]* **66**:523, 1980.
27. Stocker R, Yamamoto Y, McDonagh AF, et al.: Bilirubin is an antioxidant of possible physiological significance. *Science* **235**:1043, 1987.
28. Halliwell B, Gutteridge JM, et al.: The antioxidants of human extracellular fluids. *Arch Biochem Biophys* **280**:1, 1990.
29. Dannery PA, McDonagh AF, Spitz DR, et al.: Hyperbilirubinemia results in reduced oxidative injury in neonatal Gunn rats exposed to hyperoxia. *Free Radic Biol Med* **19**:395, 1995
30. Colleran E, O'Carra P: Enzymology and comparative physiology of biliverdin reduction, in Berk PD, Berlin NI (eds): *Bile Pigments: Chemistry and Physiology*. Washington, DC: Department of Health, Education, and Welfare, National Institutes of Health, 1977, p 69.
31. Tenhunen R, Ross ME, Marver HS, Schmid R: Reduced nicotinamide-adenine dinucleotide phosphate dependent biliverdin reductase: Partial purification and characterization. *Biochemistry* **9**:298, 1970.
32. Colleran E, O'Carra P: Enzymology and comparative physiology of biliverdin reduction, in Berk PD, Berlin NI (eds): *Bile Pigments: Chemistry and Physiology*. Washington, DC: Department of Health, Education, and Welfare, National Institutes of Health, 1977, p 69.
33. Frydman RBM, Tomaro ML, Awruch J, Frydman B: Interconversion of the molecular forms of biliverdin reductase from rat liver. *Biochem Biophys Acta* **759**:257, 1983.
34. Heirwegh KPM, Blanckaert N, Compernolle F, Fevery J, Zaman Z: Detection and properties of the non-α isomers of bilirubin-IX. *Biochem Soc Trans* **5**:316, 1977.
35. Bensinger TA, Maisels MJ, Mahmood L, McCurdy PR, Conrad MD: Effect of intravenous urea in invert sugar on heme catabolism in sickle cell anemia. *New Engl J Med* **285**:995, 1971.
36. Howe RB, Berlin NI, Berk PD: Estimation of bilirubin production in man, in Berk PD, Berlin NI (eds): *Bile Pigments: Chemistry and Physiology*. Washington, DC: Department of Health, Education, and Welfare, National Institutes of Health, 1977, p 105.
37. Jones EA, Shrager R, Bloomer JR, Berk PD, Howe RB, Berlin NI: Quantitative studies of the delivery of hepatic synthesized bilirubin to plasma utilizing δ-aminolevulinic acid-4-^{14}C and bilirubin-^{3}H in man. *J Clin Invest* **51**:2450, 1972.
38. Jones EA, Bloomer JR, Berk PD, Carson ER, Owens D, Berlin NI: Quantitation of hepatic bilirubin synthesis in man, in Berk PD, Berlin NI (eds): *Bile Pigments: Chemistry and Physiology*. Washington, DC: Department of Health, Education, and Welfare, National Institutes of Health, 1977, p 189.
39. Berk PD, Rodkey FL, Blaschke TF, Collison HA, Waggoner JG: Comparison of plasma bilirubin turnover and carbon monoxide production in man. *J Lab Clin Med* **83**:29, 1974.
40. Coburn RF, Gondrie P, Abboud F, Ploegmakers E: Myocardial myoglobin oxygen tension. *Am J Physiol* **224**:870, 1973.
41. Stewart RD, Fisher TN, Hosko MJ, Peterson JE, Baretta ED, Dodd HC: Carboxyhemoglobin elevation after exposure to dichloromethane. *Science* **176**:295, 1972.
42. Engel RR: Alternative sources of carbon monoxide, in Berk PD, Berlin NI (eds): *Chemistry and Physiology*. Washington, DC: Department of Health, Education, and Welfare, National Institutes of Health, 1977, p 148.
43. Westlake DWS, Roxburgh JM, Talbot G: Microbial production of carbon monoxide from flavinoids. *Nature* **189**:510, 1961.
44. Valaes T, Petmezaki S, Henschke C, et al.: Control of jaundice in preterm newborns by an inhibitor of bilirubin production: Studies with tin-mesoporphyrin. *Pediatrics* **93**:1, 1994.
45. Kappas A, Drummond GS: Direct comparison of tin-mesoporphyrin, an inhibitor of bilirubin production, and phototherapy in controlling hyperbilirubinemia in term and near-term newborns. *Pediatrics* **95**:468, 1995.
46. Fischer H, Plieninger H: Synthese des biliverdins (uteroverdins) und bilirubins der biliverdine XIII, und III, sowie der Vinulneoxanthosaure. *Hoppe Seyler Z Physiol Chem* **274**:231, 1942.
47. Bonnet RJ, Davis E, Hursthouse MB: Structure of bilirubin. *Nature* **262**:326, 1976.
48. Krasner J, Yaffe SJ: The automatic titration of bilirubin. *Biochem Med* **7**:128, 1973.
49. Broderson R: Binding of bilirubin to albumin. *Crit Rev Clin Lab Sci* **11**:305, 1980.
50. Brodersen R: Aqueous solubility, albumin binding and tissue distribution of bilirubin, in Ostrow JD (ed): *Bile Pigments and Jaundice*. New York; Marcel Dekker, 1986, p 157.
51. Brordersen R: Free bilirubin in the blood plasma of the newborn. Effects of albumin, fatty acids, pH, displacing drugs and phototherapy. Appendix A: Provisional survey of the bilirubin displacing effect of 150 drugs, in Stern L (ed): *Intensive Care of the Newborn*. Vol. 2. New York: Masson, 1978, p 331.
52. Fog J, Jellum E: Structure of bilirubin. *Nature* **198**:88, 1963.
53. Kuenzle CC, Weibel MH, Pelloni RR: A proposed novel structure for the metal chelates of bilirubin. *Biochem J* **130**:1147, 1973.
54. Maritto P, Monti D: Free energy barrier of conformational inversion in bilirubin. *J Chem Soc Chem Commun* **4**:122, 1976.
55. Knell AJ, Johnson B, Hutchinson DW: Intramolecular hydrogen bonds in bilirubin. *Digestion* **6**:288, 1972.
56. Kuenzle CC, Weibel MH, Pelloni RR: The reaction of bilirubin with diazomethane. *Biochem J* **133**:357, 1973.

57. Trull FR, Ibars O, Lightner DA: Conformational inversion of bilirubin formed by reduction of the biliverdin-human serum albumin complex: Evidence from circular dichroism. *Arch Biochem Biophys* **298**:710, 1992.
58. Krasner J, Yaffe SJ: Fluorescent properties of the bilirubin-albumin complex. *Birth Defects* **12**:168, 1976.
59. McDonagh AF, Palma LA, Lightner DA: Phototherapy for neonatal jaundice. Stereospecific and regiospecific photoisomerization of bilirubin bound to human serum albumin and NMR characterization of intromolecularly cyclized photoproducts. *J Am Chem Soc* **104**:6867, 1982.
60. Itho S, Onishi S: Kinetic study of the photochemical changes of (ZZ)-bilirubin IX bound to human serum albumin. Demonstration of (EZ)-bilirubin IX as an intermediate in photochemical changes from (ZZ)-bilirubin IX to (EZ)-cyclobilirubin IX. *Biochem J* **226**:251, 1985.
61. McDonagh AF: Thermal and photochemical reactions of bilirubin IX. *Ann NY Acad Sci* **244**:553, 1975.
62. Schenker S, Hoyumpa AM, McCandless DW: Bilirubin toxicity to the brain (kernicterus) and other tissues, in Ostrow JD (ed): *Bile Pigments and Jaundice*. New York: Marcel Dekker, 1986, p 395.
63. Hervieux J: De l'ictere des nouveau-nes. Paris. These Med. 1847.
64. Schmorl G: Zur Kenntnis des ikterus neonatatorum, inbesondere der dabei auftreten den gehirnveranderungen. *Verh Dtsch Ges Pathol* **6**:109, 1903.
65. Schiff D, Chan G, Poznasky MJ: Bilirubin toxicity in neural cell lines N115 and NBR10A. *Pediatr Res* **19**:908, 1985.
66. Mustafa MG, Cowger ML, Kind TE: Effects of bilirubin on mitochondrial reactions. *J Biol Chem* **244**:6403, 1969.
67. Strumia E: Effect of bilirubin on some hydrolases. *Bull Soc Ital Biol Sper* **35**:2160, 1959.
68. Flitman R, Worth NK: Inhibition of hepatic alcohol dehydrogenase by bilirubin. *J Biol Chem* **251**:669, 1966.
69. Cowger ML, Igo RP, Labbe RF: The mechanism of bilirubin toxicity studied with purified respiratory enzyme and tissue culture systems. *Biochemistry* **4**:2763, 1965.
70. Katoh R, Kashiwamata S, Niwa F: Studies on cellular toxicity of bilirubin. Effect on the carbohydrate metabolism in the young rat brain. *Brain Res* **83**:81, 1975.
71. Greenfield S, Nandi Majumdar AP: Bilirubin encephalopathy. Effect on protein synthesis in the brain of the Gunn rat. *J Neurol Sci* **22**:83, 1974.
72. Nandi Majumdar AP: Bilirubin encephalopathy. Effect on RNA polymerase activity and chromatin template activity in the brain of the Gunn rat. *Neurobiology* **4**:425, 1974.
73. Diamond I, Schmid R: Oxidative phosphorylation in experimental bilirubin encephalopathy. *Science* **155**:1288, 1967.
74. Zetterstrom R, Ernster L: Bilirubin, an uncoupler of oxidative phosphorylation in isolated mitochondria. *Nature* **178**:1335, 1956.
75. Constantopoulos A, Matsaniotis N: Bilirubin inhibition of protein kinase: Its prevention by cyclic AMP. *Cytobios* **17**:17, 1976.
76. Morphis I, Constantopoulos A, Matsaniotis N, Papaphilis A: Bilirubin-induced modulation of cerebral protein phosphorylation in neonate rabbits *in vivo*. *Science* **218**:156, 1982.
77. Sano K, Nakamura H, Tamotsu M: Mode of inhibitory action of bilirubin on protein kinase C. *Pediatr Res* **19**:587, 1985.
78. Gourley GR: Bilirubin metabolism and kernicterus. *Adv Pediatr* **44**:173, 1997.
79. Stobie PE, Hansen CT, Hailey JR, Levine RL: A difference in mortality between two strains of jaundiced rats. *Pediatrics* **87**:88, 1991.
80. Odell GB: Influence of binding on the toxicity of bilirubin. *Ann NY Acad Sci* **226**:225, 1973.
81. Conlee JW, Shapiro SM: Morphological changes in the cochlear nucleus and nucleus of the trapezoid body in Gunn rat pups. *Hear Res* **57**:23, 1991.
82. Funato M, Tamai H, Shimada S, et al.: Viginitiphobia, unbound bilirubin and auditory brainstem responses. *Pediatrics* **93**:50, 1994.
83. Shapiro SW, Conlee JW: Brainstem auditory evoked potentials correlate with morphological changes in Gunn rat pups. *Hear Res* **57**:16, 1991.
84. Shapiro SM: Binaural effects in brainstem auditory evoked potentials of jaundiced Gunn rats. *Hear Res* **53**:41, 1991.
85. Naeye RL: Aminiotic fluid infections, neonatal hyperbilirubinemia and psychomotor impairment. *Pediatrics* **62**:497, 1978.
86. Van De Bor M, Ens-Dokkum M, Schreuder AM, Veen S, Brand R, Verloove-Vanhorick SP: Hyperbilirubinemia in low birth weight infants and outcome at 5 years of age. *Pediatrics* **89**:359, 1992.
87. Labrune PH, Myara A, Francoual J, Trivin F, Odievre M: Cerebellar symptoms as the presenting manifestations of bilirubin encephalopathy in children with Crigler-Najjar type I disease. *Pedicatrics* **89**:768, 1992.
88. Penn AA, Enzmann DR, Hahn JS, et al.: Kernicterus in a full-term infant. *Pediatrics* **93**:1003, 1994.
89. Matrich-Kriss V, Kollins SS, Ball WS Jr: MR findings in kernicterus. *AJNR* **16**:817, 1995.
90. Yokochi K: Magnetic resonance imaging in children with kernicterus. *Acta Pediatr* **84**:937, 1995.
91. Zuelzer WW, Mudgett RT: Kernicterus. Etiologic study based on an analysis of 55 cases. *Pediatrics* **6**:452, 1950.
92. Vaughan VC, Allen FC, Diamond LK: Erythroblastosis fetalis. IV. Further observations on kernicterus. *Pediatrics* **6**:706, 1950.
93. Rappaport SI: *Blood–Brain Barrier in Physiology and Medicine*. New York: Raven, 1976.
94. Purpura DP, Carmichael MW: Characteristics of blood-brain barrier to gamma-aminobutyric acid in neonatal cat. *Science* **131**:410, 1960.
95. Cornford EM, Braun LD, Oldendorp WH, Hill MA: Comparison of lipid-mediated blood–brain barrier penetrability in neonates and adults. *Am J Physiol* **243**:C161, 1982.
96. Laas R, Helmke K: Regional cerebral blood flow following unilateral blood–brain barrier alteration induced by hyperosmolar perfusion in the albino rat, in Cervos-Navarro J, Fritsch E (eds): *Cerebral Circulation and Metabolism*. New York: Raven, 1981, p 317.
97. Levine RL, Fredericks WR, Rappaport SI: Clearance of bilirubin from rat brain after reversible osmotic opening of the blood–brain barrier. *Pediatr Res* **19**:1040, 1985.
98. Lee K-S, Gartner LM: Management of unconjugated hyperbilirubinemia in the newborn. *Semin Liver Dis* **3**:52, 1983.
99. Lauff JJ, Kasper ME, Ambros RT: Quantitative liquid chromatographic estimation of bilirubin species in pathological serum. *Clin Chem* **29**:800, 1983.
100. Bowen WR, Porter E, Waters WF: The protective action of albumin in bilirubin toxicity in newborn puppies. *Am J Dis Child* **98**:568, 1959.
101. Silvermann WA, Andersen DH, Blanc WA, Crozier DN: A difference in mortality rate and incidence of kernicterus among premature infants allotted to two prophylactic antibacterial regimens. *Pediatrics* **18**:614, 1956.
102. Odell GB: The dissociation of bilirubin from albumin and its clinical implications. *J Pediatr* **55**:268, 1959.
103. Bloomer JR, Berk PD, Vergalla J, Berlin NI: Influence of albumin on the extravascular distribution of unconjugated bilirubin. *Clin Sci Mol Med* **45**:517, 1973.
104. Jacobsen J: Binding of bilirubin to human serum albumin. Determination of the dissociation constants. *FEBS Lett* **5**:112, 1969.
105. Jacobsen C: Lysine residue 240 of human serum albumin is involved in high-affinity binding of bilirubin. *Biochem J* **171**:453, 1978.
106. Harris RC, Lucey JF, MacLean Jr: Kernicterus in premature infants associated with low concentrations of bilirubin in plasma. *Pediatrics* **21**:875, 1958.
107. Brodersen R, Sjodin T, Sjoholm I: Independent binding of benzodiazepines and bilirubin to human serum albumin. *J Biol Chem* **252**:5067, 1977.
108. Woolley PW, Hunter M: Binding and circular dichroism data on bilirubin-albumin in the presence of oleate and salicylate. *Arch Biochem Biophys* **140**:197, 1970.
109. Brodersen R: Binding of bilirubin and other ligands of human serum albumin, in Peters T, Sjoholm I (eds): *Albumin, Structure, Biosynthesis, Function. FEBS 11th Meeting, Copenhagen, 1977*. Oxford, England: Pergamon, 1978, p 61.
110. Rudman D, Bixler TJ, Del Rio AE: Effect of free fatty acid on binding of drugs by bovine serum albumin, by human serum albumin and by rabbit serum. *J Pharmacol Exp Ther* **176**:261, 1971.
111. Stern L, Denton RL: Kernicterus in small premature infants. *Pediatrics* **35**:483, 1965.
112. Diamond I, Schmid R: Experimental bilirubin encephalopathy. The mode of entry of bilirubin-^{14}C into the central nervous system. *J Clin Invest* **45**:678, 1966.
113. Kapitulnik J, Valaes T, Kaufmann NA, Blondheim SH: Clinical evaluation of Sephadex gel filtration in estimation of bilirubin binding in serum in neonatal jaundice. *Arch Dis Child* **49**:886, 1974.
114. Brodersen R, Cashore W, Wennberg RP, Ahlfors CE, Rasmussen LF, Shusterman D: Kinetics of bilirubin oxidation with peroxidase, as applied to studies of bilirubin-albumin binding. *Scand J Clin Lab Invest* **39**:143, 1979.

115. Athanassiadis S, Chopra DR, Fisher M, McKenna J: An electrophoretic method for detection of unbound bilirubin and reserve bilirubin binding capacity in serum of newborns. *J Lab Clin Med* **83**:968, 1974.
116. Lamolla AA, Eisinger J, Blumberg WE, Palet SC, Flores J: Fluorometric study of the partition of bilirubin among blood components: Basis for rapid microassays of bilirubin and bilirubin binding capacity in whole blood. *Anal Biochem* **15**:25, 1979.
117. Bratlid D: Reserve albumin binding capacity salicylate saturation index, and red cell binding of bilirubin in neonatal jaundice. *Arch Dis Child* **48**:393, 1973.
118. Brodersen R: Determination of the vacant amount of high affinity bilirubin binding site on serum albumin. *Acta Pharmacol Toxicol* **42**:153, 1978.
119. Hsia JC, Kwan NH, Er SS, Wood DJ, Chance GW: Development of a spin assay for reserve bilirubin loading capacity of human serum. *Proc Natl Acad Sci U S A* **75**:1542, 1978.
120. Porter EG, Waters WJ: A rapid micromethod for measuring the reserve albumin binding capacity in serum for newborn infants with hyperbilirubinemia. *J Lab Clin Med* **67**:660, 1966.
121. Goresky CA: The hepatic uptake process: Its implications for bilirubin transport, in Goresky CA, Fisher MM (eds): *Jaundice*. New York: Plenum, 1975, p 159.
122. Bloomer JR, Zaccaria J: Effect of graded bilirubin loads on bilirubin transport by perfused rat liver. *Am J Physiol* **203**:736, 1976.
123. Scharschmidt F, Waggoner JG, Berk PD: Hepatic organic anion uptake in the rat. *J Clin Invest* **56**:1280, 1975.
124. Hunton DB, Bollman JL, Hoffman HN II: The plasma removal of indocyanine green and sulfobromophthalein: Effect of dosage and blocking agents. *J Clin Invest* **40**:1648, 1961.
125. Shupeck M, Wolkoff AW, Scharschmidt BF, Waggoner JG, Berk PD: Studies of the kinetics of purified conjugated bilirubin-^{3}H in the rat. *Am J Gastroenterol* **70**:259, 1978.
126. Goresky CA: The hepatic uptake and excretion of sulfobromophthalein and bilirubin. *Can Med Assoc J* **92**:851, 1965.
127. Barnhart JL, Clarenburg R: Factors determining clearance of bilirubin in perfused rat liver. *Am J Physiol* **225**:497, 1973.
128. Weisiger RA, Gollan JL, Ockner RK: Receptor for albumin on the liver cell surface may mediate uptake of fatty acids and other albumin-bound substances. *Science* **211**:1048, 1981.
129. Forker EL, Luxon BA: Albumin helps mediate removal of taurocholate by rat liver. *J Clin Invest* **67**:1517, 1981.
130. Fleischer AB, Shurmantine WO, Luxon BA, Forker EL: Palmitate uptake by hepatocyte monolayers. Effect of albumin binding. *J Clin Invest* **77**:964, 1986.
131. Weisiger RA: Dissociation from albumin: A potential rate-limiting step in the clearance of substances by the liver. *Proc Natl Acad Sci U S A* **82**:1563, 1985.
132. Zucker SD, Goessling W, Gollan JL: Kinetics of bilirubin transfer between serum albumin and membrane vesicles. Insight into the mechanism of organic anion delivery to the hepatocyte plasma membrane. *J Biol Chem* **270**:1074, 1995.
133. Weisiger RA, Zacks CM, Smith ND, et al.: Effect of albumin binding on extraction of sulfobromophthalein by perfused elasmobranch liver: Evidence for dissociation-limited uptake. *Hepatology* **4**:492, 1984.
134. Gumucio DL, Gumucio JJ, Wilson JAP: Albumin influences sulfobromophthalein transport by hepatocytes of each acinar zone. *Am J Physiol* **246**:G86, 1984.
135. Schwenk M, Burr R, Schwarz L, Pfaff E: Uptake of bromosulfophthalein by isolated liver cells. *Eur J Biochem* **64**:189, 1976.
136. Van Bezooijen CF, Grell T, Knook DL: Bromosulfophthalein uptake by isolated liver parenchymal cells. *Biochem Biophys Res Commun* **69**:354, 1976.
137. Aperche T, Preaux AM, Berthelot P: Two systems are involved in the sulfobromophthalein uptake by rat liver cells: One is shared with bile salts. *Biochem Pharmacol* **30**:1333, 1982.
138. Schwarz LR, Gotz R, Klassen CD: Uptake of sulphobromophthalein-glutathione conjugates by isolated hepatocytes. *Am J Physiol* **239**:C118, 1980.
139. Potter BJ, Blades BF, Shepard MD, Thung SM, Berk PD: The kinetics of sulfobromophthalein uptake by rat liver sinusoidal vesicles. *Biochim Biophys Acta* **898**:159, 1987.
140. Wolkoff AW, Samuelson SC, Johansen KL, Nakata R, Withers D, Sosiak S: Influence of Cl^- on organic anion transport in short-term cultured rat hepatocytes and isolated perfused rat liver. *J Clin Invest* **79**:1259, 1987.
141. Adachi Y, Roy Chowdhury J, Roy Chowdhury N, Theilman L, Kinne R, Arias IM: Hepatic uptake of bilirubin diglucuronide: Analysis by using sinusoidal plasma membrane vesicles. *J Biochem* **107**:749, 1990.
142. Min AD, Johansen KL, Campbell CG, Wolkoff AW: Role of chloride and intracellular pH on the activity of the rat hepatocyte organic anion transporter. *J Clin Invest* **87**:1496, 1991.
143. Reichen J, Berk PD: Isolation of an organic anion binding protein from rat liver plasma membrane fractions by affinity chromatography. *Biochem Biophys Res Commun* **91**:484, 1979.
144. Wolkoff AW, Chung CT: Identification, purification and partial characterization of an organic anion binding protein from rat liver cell plasma membrane. *J Clin Invest* **65**:1152, 1980.
145. Tiribelli C, Lunazzi G, Luciani GL, Panfili E, Gazzin B, Liut G, Sandri G, Sottocasa G: Isolation of a sulfobromophthalein-binding protein from hepatocyte plasma membrane. *Biochim Biophys Acta* **532**:105, 1978.
146. Stremmel W, Garber MA, Glazerov V, Thung SN, Kochwa S, Berk PD: Physiochemical and immunohistological studies of a sulphobromophtalein and bilirubin-binding protein from rat liver plasma membrane. *J Clin Invest* **71**:1797, 1983.
147. Stremmel W, Berk PD: Hepatocellular uptake of sulfobromophthalein and bilirubin is selectively inhibited by an antibody to the liver plasma membrane sulfobromophthalein/bilirubin binding protein. *J Clin Invest* **78**:822, 1986.
148. Sottocasa GL, Baldini G, Sandri G, Lunazzi G, Tiribelli C: Reconstitution *in vitro* of sulfobromophthalein transport by bilitranslocase. *Biochim Biophys Acta* **685**:123, 1982.
149. Miccio M, Lunazzio GC, Gazzin B, Sottocasa GL: Reconstitution of sulfobromophthalein transport in erythrocyte membranes induced by bilitranslocase. *Biochim Biophys Acta* **1023**:140, 1990.
150. Wolkoff AW, Sosiak A, Greenblatt H, Van Renswoude J, Stockert RJ: Immunological studies of an organic anion-binding protein isolated from rat liver cell plasma membrane. *J Clin Invest* **76**:454, 1985.
151. Goeser T, Nakata R, Braly FL, Sosiak A, Campbell CG, Dermietzel R, Novikoff PM, Stockert RJ, Burk RD, Wolkoff AW: The rat hepatocyte plasma membrane organic anion binding protein is immunologically related to the mitochondrial F_1-adenosine triphosphatase β-subunit. *J Clin Invest* **86**:220, 1990.
152. Jacquemin E, Hagenbuch B, Stieger B, Wolkoff AW, Meier PJ: Expression of the hepatocellular chloride-dependent sulfobromophthalein uptake system in *Xenopus laevis* oocytes. *J Clin Invest* **88**:2146, 1991.
153. Satlin LM, Amin V, Wolkoff AW: Organic anion transporting polypeptide mediates organic anion/HCO_3^- exchange. *J Biol Chem* **272**:26340, 1997.
154. Kanai N, Lu R, Striano JA, Bao Y, Wolkoff AW, Schuster VL: Identification and characterization of a prostaglandin transporter. *Science* **268**:866, 1995.
155. Bernstein LH, Ben-Ezzar JB, Gartner L, Arias IM: Hepatic intracellular distribution of tritium-labeled unconjugated and conjugated bilirubin in normal and Gunn rats. *J Clin Invest* **45**:1194, 1966.
156. Wolkoff AW, Ketley JN, Waggoner JG, Berk PD, Jakoby W: Hepatic accumulation and intracellular binding of conjugated bilirubin. *J Clin Invest* **61**:142, 1978.
157. Levi AJ, Gatmaitan Z, Arias IM: Two hepatic cytoplasmic protein fractions, Y and Z, and their possible role in the hepatic uptake of bilirubin, sulfobromophthalein, and other anions. *J Clin Invest* **48**:2156, 1969.
158. Kamisaka K, Listowsky I, Gatmaitan Z, Arias IM: Interactions of bilirubin and other ligands with ligandin. *Biochemistry* **14**:2175, 1975.
159. Morey KS, Litwack G: Isolation and properties of cortisol metabolite binding proteins of rat liver cytosol. *Biochemistry* **8**:4813, 1969.
160. Ketterer B, Ross-Mansell P, Whitehead JK: The isolation of carcinogen-binding protein from livers of rats given 4-dimethylaminoazobenzene. *Biochem J* **103**:316, 1967.
161. Fleischner G, Robbins J, Arias IM: Immunological studies of Y protein: A major cytoplasmic organic anion binding protein in rat liver. *J Clin Invest* **51**:677, 1972.
162. Hays JD, Pulford DJ: The glutathione S-transferase supergene family: Regulation of GST and the contribution of the isoenzymes to cancer chemoprotection and drug resistance. *Crit Rev Biochem Mol Biol* **30**:445, 1995.

163. Rowe JD, Nieves E and Listowsky I: Subunit diversity and tissue distribution of human glutathione S-transferases: Interpretations based on electrospray ionization-MS and peptide sequence-specific antisera. *Biochem J* **325**:481, 1997.
164. Wolkoff AW, Goresky CA, Sellin J, Gatmaitan Z, Arias IM: Role of ligandin in transfer of bilirubin from plasma into liver. *Am J Physiol* **236**:E638, 1979.
165. Kamisaka K, Gatmaitan Z, Moore CL, Arias IM: Ligandin reverses bilirubin inhibition of liver mitochondrial respiration in vitro. *Pediatr Res* **9**:903, 1975.
166. Gordon ER, Goresky CA, Chan TH, Perlin AS: The isolation and characterization of bilirubin diglucuronide, the major bilirubin conjugate in dog and human bile. *Biochem J* **155**:477, 1976.
167. Heirwegh KPM, Van Hees GP, Leroy P, Van Roy FP, Jansen FH: Heterogeneity of bile pigment conjugates as revealed by chromatography of their ethyl anthranilate azopigments. *Biochem J* **120**:877, 1979.
168. Jansen FH, Billing BH: The identification of mono-conjugates of bilirubin in bile as amide derivatives. *Biochemistry* **1**:917, 1971.
169. Onishi S, Itho S, Kawade N, Isobe K, Sugiyama S: An accurate and sensitive analysis by high pressure liquid chromatography of conjugated and unconjugated bilirubin IXα and in various biological fluids. *Biochem J* **185**:281, 1980.
170. Spivak W, Carey MC: Reverse-phase h.p.l.c. separation, quantification and preparation of bilirubin and its conjugates from native bile. *Biochem J* **225**:787, 1985.
171. Roy Chowdhury J, Roy Chowdhury N: Quantitation of bilirubin and its conjugates by high pressure liquid chromatography. *Falk Hepatol* **11**:1649, 1982.
172. Gorski JP, Kasper CB: Purification and properties of microsomal UDP glucuronyl transferase from rat liver. *J Biol Chem* **252**:1336, 1977.
173. Burchell B: Purification of UDP glucuronyl transferase from untreated rat liver. *FEBS Lett* **78**:101, 1977.
174. Bock KW, Josling D, Lilenblum WM, Pfeil H: Purification of rat liver glucuronyl transferase-separation of two enzyme forms inducible by 3-methyl-cholanthrene or phenobarbital. *Eur J Biochem* **98**:19, 1977.
175. Burchell B: Identification and purification of mutiple forms of UDP-glucuronosyltransferase. *Rev Biochem Toxicol* **3**:1, 1981.
176. Falany CN, Roy Chowdhury J, Roy Chowdhury N, Tephly TW: Steroid 3- and 17-OH-UDP-glucuronosyltransferase activities in rat and rabbit liver microsomes. *Drug Metab Dispos* **11**:426, 1983.
177. Roy Chowdhury J, Roy Chowdhury N, Falany CN, Tephly TW, Arias IM: Isolation and characterization of multiple forms of rat liver UDP-glucuronoate glucuronosyltransferase. *Biochem J* **233**:827, 1986.
178. Harding D, Fournel-Gigleux S, Jackson MR, Burchell B: Cloning and substrate-specificity of a human phenol-UDP-glucuronosyltransferase expressed in COS-7 cells. *Proc Natl Acad Sci U S A* **85**:8381, 1988.
179. Ritter JK, Crawford JM, Owens IS: Cloning of two human liver bilirubin-UDP-glucuronosyltransferase cDNAs with expression in COS-1 cells. *J Biol Chem* **266**:1043, 1991.
180. Wooster R, Sutherland L, Ebner T, Clarke D, Da Cruz E, Silva O, Burchell B: Cloning and stable expression of a new member of a human liver phenol/bilirubin UDP-glucuronosyltransferase cDNA family. *Biochem J* **278**:465, 1991.
181. Iyanagi T, Haniu M, Sogawa K, Fujii-Kuriyama Y, Watanabe S, Shively JE, Anan KF: Cloning and characterization of cDNA encoding 3-methylcholanthrene inducible rat messenger RNA for UDP-glucronosyltransferase. *J Biol Chem* **261**:15607, 1986.
182. Jackson MR, Burchell B: The full length coding sequence of rat liver androsterone UDP-glucuronosyltransferase cDNA and comparison with other members of this gene family. *Nucleic Acids Res* **14**:779, 1986.
183. Jackson MR, McCarthy LR, Corser RB, Barr GC, Burchell B: Cloning of cDNAs coding for rat hepatic microsomal UDP-glucuronosyltransferases. *Gene* **34**:147, 1985.
184. Mackenzie PI: Rat liver UDP-glucuronosyltransferase cDNA sequence and expression of a form glucuronidating 3-hydroxy androgens. *J Biol Chem* **261**:14112, 1986.
185. Mackenzie PI, Owens IS, Burchell B, Bock KW, Bairoch A, Belanger A, Fournel-Gigleux S, Green M, Jum DW, Iyanagi T, Lancet D, Louisot P, Magdalou J, Roy Chowdhury J, Ritter, JK, Schachter H, Tephly TR, Tipton KF, Nebert DW: The UDP glycosyltransferase gene superfamily: Recommended nomenclature update based on evolutionary divergence. *Pharmacogenetics* **7**:255, 1997.
186. Roy Chowdhury J, Novikoff PM, Roy Chowdhury N, Novikoff AB: Distribution of uridinediphosphoglucuronate glucuronosyl transferase in rat tissues. *Proc Natl Acad Sci U S A* **82**:2990, 1985.
187. Dutton GJ, Burchell B: Newer aspects of glucuronidation. *Prog Drug Metab* **2**:1, 1977.
188. Jansen PLM, Arias IM: Delipidation and reactivation of UDP glucuronosyl transferase from rat liver. *Biochim Biophys Acta* **391**:28, 1975.
189. Zakim D, Eibl H: The influence of charge and the distribution of charge in the polar region of phospholipids on the activity of UDP-glucuronosyltransferase. *J Biol Chem* **267**:13166, 1992.
190. Henderson P: The activation *in vitro* of rat hepatic UDP glucuronyl transferase by ultrasound. *Life Sci* **9**:511, 1970.
191. Vassey DA, Zakim D: Regulations of microsomal enzymes by phospholipids. *J Biol Chem* **246**:4649, 1971.
192. Hauser SC, Ziurys JC, Gollan JL: A membrane transporter mediates access of uridine-5-diphosphoglucuronic acid from the cytosol into the endoplasmic reticulum of rat hepatocytes. Implications for glucuronidation reactions. *Biochim Biophys Acta* **967**:149, 1988.
193. Heirwegh KPM, Campbell M, Meuwissen JATP: Compartmentation of membrane bound enzymes. Some basic concepts and consequences for kinetic studies, in Aitio A (ed): *Conjugation Reactions in Drug Biotransformation*. Amsterdam: Elsevier, 1978, p 191.
194. Hallinan T: Comparison of compartmented and of conformational phospholipid-constraint models of the intramembranous arrangement of UDP-glucuronyltransferase, in Aitio A (ed): *Conjugation Reactions in Drug Biotransformation*. Amsterdam: Elsevier, 1978, p 257.
195. Drake RR, Igari Y, Lester R, Elbein AD, Radominska A: Application of 5-azido-UDP-glucose and 5-azido-UDP-glucuronic acid photo-affinity probes for the determination of the active site orientation of microsomal UDP-glucosyltransferases and UDP-glucuronosyltransferases. *J Biol Chem* **267**:11360, 1992.
196. Bosma PJ, Seppen J, Goldhoorn B, Bakker C, Oude Elferink RPJ, Roy Chowdhury J, Roy Chowdhury N, Jansen PLM: Bilirubin UDP-glucuronosyltransferase 1 is the only relevant bilirubin glucuronidating isoform in man. *J Biol Chem* **269**:17960, 1994.
197. Ritter JK, Chen F, Sheen YY, Tran HM, Kimura S, Yeatman MT, Owens IS: A novel complex locus, *UGT1*, encodes human bilirubin, phenol and other UDP-glucuronosyltransferase isozymes with identical carboxy termini. *J Biol Chem* **267**:3257, 1992.
198. Wishart GF: Functional heterogeneity of UDP-glucuronosyl transferase as indicated by its differential development and inducibility by glucocorticoids. *Biochem J* **174**:485, 1978.
199. Lillienblum W, Walli AK, Bock KW: Differential induction of rat liver microsomal UDP-glucuronosyltransferase activities by various inducing agents. *Biochem Pharmacol* **31**:907, 1982.
200. Roy Chowdhury J, Roy Chowdhury N, Moscioni AD, Tukey R, Tephley TR, Arias IM: Differential regulation by triiodothyronine of substrate-specific uridinediphosphoglucuronate glucuronyl transferases in rat liver. *Biochim Biophys Acta* **761**:58, 1983.
201. Hutchinson DW, Johnson B, Knell AJ: The reaction between bilirubin and aromatic diazo compounds. *Biochem J* **127**:907, 1972.
202. van den Bergh AAH, Muller P: Ueber eine direkte und eine indirekte Diazoreaktion auf Bilirubin. *Biochem Z* **77**:90, 1916.
203. Talafant E: Properties and composition of bile pigment giving direct diazo reaction. *Nature* **178**:312, 1956.
204. Heirwegh KPM, Fevery JB, Meuwissen JATP, De Groote J, Compernolle F, Desmet V, Van Roy FP: Recent advances in the separation and analysis of diazo-positive bile pigments. *Methods Biochem Anal* **22**:205, 1974.
205. Trotman BW, Roy Chowdhury J, Wirt GD, Bernstein SE: Azodipyrole analysis of unconjugated and conjugated bilirubin using diazotized ethylanthranilate in dimethylsulfoxide. *Anal Biochem* **121**:175,1982.
206. Poon R, Hinberg IH: Indican interference with six commercial procedures for measuring total bilirubin. *Clin Chem* **31**:92, 1985.
207. Cole PG, Lathe GH, Billing BH: Separation of the bile pigments of serum, bile and urine. *Biochem J* **57**:514, 1954.
208. Heirwegh KPM, Fevery J, Michiels R, Van Hees GP, Compernolle F: Separation of thin layer chromatography and structure elucidation of bilirubin conjugates isolated from dog bile. *Biochem J* **145**:185, 1975.
209. Blanckaert N, Kabra PM, Farina FA, Stafford BE, Marton LJ, Schmidt R: Measurement of bilirubin and its mono- and diconjugates in human serum by alkaline methanolysis and high performance liquid chromatography. *J Lab Clin Med* **96**:198, 1980.

210. Roy Chowdhury J, Roy Chowdhury N, Wu G, Shouval R, Arias IM: Bilirubin monoglucuronide and diglucuronide formation by human liver *in vitro* assay by high pressure liquid chromatography. *Hepatology* **1**:622, 1981.
211. Dappen GM, Sundberg MW, Wu TW, Babb BE, Schaeffer JR: A diazo-based dry film for determination of total bilirubin in serum. *Clin Chem* **29**:37, 1983.
212. Kubasik NP, Mayer TK, Baskar AG, Sine HE, D'Souza JP: The measurement of fractionated bilirubin by Ektachem film slides. Method validation and comparison of conjugated bilirubin measurements with direct bilirubin in obstructive and hepatocellular jaundice. *Am J Clin Pathol* **84**:518, 1985.
213. Schumacher RE, Thornbery JM, Gutcher GR: Transcutaneous bilirubinometry: A comparison of old and new methods. *Pediatrics* **76**:10, 1985.
214. Maisels MJ, Kring E: Transcutaneous bilirubinometry decreases the need for serum billirubin measurement and saves money. *Pediatrics* **99**:599, 1997.
215. Tayba R, Gribetz D, Gribetz I, Holtzman IR: Non-invasive estimation of serum bilirubin. *Pediatrics* **102**:28, 1998.
216. Brown AK, Eisinger J, Blumberg WE, Flores J, Boyle G, Lamola AA: A rapid fluorometric method for determining bilirubin levels and binding in the blood of neonates: Comparison with other methods. *Pediatrics* **65**:767, 1980.
217. Robinson SH, Yannoni C, Nagasawa S: Bilirubin excretion in rats with normal and impaired bilirubin conjugation. Effect of phenobarbital. *J Clin Invest* **50**:2606, 1971.
218. Inoue M, Kinne R, Tran T, Biempica L, Arias IM: Rat liver canalicular membrane vesicles: Isolation and topological characterization. *J Biol Chem* **258**:5183, 1983.
219. Kitamura T, Jansen PLM, Hardenbrook C, Kamimoto Y, Gatmaitan Z, Arias IM: Defective ATP-dependent bile canalicular transport of organic anions in mutant (TR^-) rats with conjugated hyperbilirubinemia. *Proc Natl Acad Sci U S A* **87**:3557,1990.
220. Nishida T, Hardenbrook C, Gatmaitan Z, Arias IM: ATP-dependent multi-specific organic anion transport system in normal and TR^- rat liver canalicular membrane. *Am J Physiol* **262**:4, 1992.
221. Ishikaowa T, Muller M, Klunemann C, Schaub T, Keppler D: ATP-dependent primary active transport of cysteinyl leukotrienes transport system for glutathione S-conjugates. *J Biol Chem* **265**:19279, 1990.
222. Kobayashi K, Sogame Y, Hara H, Hayashi K: Mechanism of glutathione S-conjugate transport in canalicular and basolateral rat liver plasma membranes. *J Biol Chem* **265**:7737, 1990.
223. Nishida T, Gatmaitan Z, Roy Chowdhury J, Arias IM: Two distinct mechanisms for bilirubin glucuronide transport by rat bile canalicular membrane vesicles. *J Clin Invest* **90**:2130, 1992.
224. Cornelius CE: Organic anion transport in mutant sheep with congenital hyperbilirubinemia. *Arch Environ Health* **19**:852, 1969.
225. Jansen PLM, Peters WHM, Lamers WH: Hereditary chronic conjugated hyperbilirubinemia in mutant rats caused by defective hepatic anion transport. *Hepatology* **5**:573 579, 1985.
226. Kamimoto Y, Gatmaitan Z, Hsu J, Arias IM: The function of GP 170, the multidrug resistance gene product in rat liver canalicular membrane vesicles. *J Biol Chem* **264**:11693, 1989.
227. Arias IM: Multidrug resistance genes, P-glycoprotein and the liver. *Hepatology* **12**:159, 1990.
228. Bushman E, Arceci RJ, Croop JM, Che M, Arias IM, Housman DE, Gross P: Mouse mdr2 encodes P-glyprotein expressed in the bile canalicular membrane as determined by isoform-specific antibodies. *J Biol Chem* **267**:18093, 1992.
229. Meier PJ, Ruetz ST, Hugentobler G, Fricker G, Kurtz G: Identification and isolation of the putative canalicular bile acid carrier from rat liver. *Hepatology* **5**:958, 1985.
230. Nishida T, Gatmaitan Z, Che M, Arias IM: Rat liver canalicular membrane vesicles contain an ATP-dependent bile acid transport system. *Proc Natl Acad Sci U S A* **88**:6590, 1991.
231. Nies AT, Gatmaitan Z, Arias IM: ATP-dependent phosphatidylcholine translocation in rat liver canalicular plasma membrane vesicles. *J Lipid Res* **37**:1125, 1996.
232. Cole SPC, Bhardwaj G, Gerlach JH, Mackie JE, Grant CE, Almquist KC, Stewart AJ, Kurz EU, Duncan AMV, Deeley RG: Overexpression of a transporter gene in a multidrug-resistant human lung cancer cell line. *Science* **258**:1650, 1992.
233. Jedlitschky G, Leier I, Buchholz U, Center M, Keppler D: ATP-dependent transport of glutathione S-conjugates by the multidrug resistance-associated protein. *Cancer Res* **54**:4833, 1994.
234. Dubin IN, Johnson FB: Chronic idiopathic jaundice with unidentified pigment in liver cells: A new clinicopathologic entity with a report of 12 cases. *Medicine (Baltimore)* **33**:155, 1954.
235. Alpert S, Mosher M, Shanske A, Arias IM: Multiplicity of hepatic excretory mechanism for organic anions. *J Gen Physiol* **53**:238, 1969.
236. Schulman FY, Montali RJ, Bush M, Citino SD, Tell LA, Ballou JD, Hutson TL, St-Pierre M, Dufour JF, Gatmaitan Z, Arias IM, Johnson FP: Dubin-Johnson-like syndrome in golden lion tamarins (*Leontopithecus rosalia rosalia*). *Vet Pathol* **30**:491, 1993.
237. Gutstein S, Alpert S, Arias IM: Studies of hepatic excretory function. IV. Biliary excretion of sulfobromophthalein in a patient with Dubin-Johnson syndrome and a biliary fistula. *Isr J Med Sci* **4**:46, 1968.
238. Gerloff T, Steiger B, Hagenbuch B, Madon J, Landmann L, Roth J, Hofmann AF, Meier PJ: The sister of P-glycoprotein represents the canalicular bile salt export pump of mammalian liver. *J Biol Chem* **273**:10046, 1998.
239. Smit JJM, Schinkel AH, Elferink RPJO, Groen AK, Wagenaar E, Vandeemter L, Mol CAAM, Ottenhoff R, Vanderlugt NMT, Vanroon MA, Vandervalk MA, Offerhaus GJA, Berns AJM, Borst P: Homozygous disruption of the murine mdr2 P glycoprotein gene leads to a complete absence of phospholipid from bile and to liver disease. *Cell* **75**:451 462, 1993.
240. Upson DW, Gronwall RR, Cornelius CE: Maximal hepatic excretion of bilirubin in sheep. *Proc Soc Exp Biol Med* **134**:9, 1970.
241. Klaassen CD, Plaa GL: Studies on the mechanism of phenobarbital-enhanced sulfobromophthalein disappearance. *J Pharmacol Exp Ther* **161**:361, 1968.
242. Barnhart J, Ritt S, Ware A, Coombes B: A comparison of the effects of taurocholate and theophylline on BSP excretion in dogs, in Paumgartner G, Preisig R (eds): *The Liver: Quantitative Aspects of Structure and Function*. Basel, Switzerland: Karger, 1973, p 315.
243. Gatmaitan ZC, Arias IM: ATP-dependent transport systems in the canalicular membrane of the hepatocyte. *Physiol Rev* **75**:261,1995.
244. Gatmaitan ZC, Nies AT, Arias IM: Regulation and translocation of ATP-dependent apical membrane proteins in rat liver. *Am J Physiol* **272**:G1041, 1997.
245. Lester R, Schmid R: Intestinal absorption of bile pigments. II. Bilirubin absorption in man. *N Engl J Med* **269**:178, 1963.
246. Brodersen R, Herman LS: Intestinal reabsorption of unconjugated bilirubin: A possible contributing factor in neonatal jaundice. *Lancet* **1**:1242, 1963.
247. Alonso EM, Whitington PF, Whitington SH, Rivard WA, Given G: Enterohepatic circulation of nonconjugated bilirubin in rats fed with human milk. *J Pediatr* **118**:425, 1991.
248. Ostrow JD: Absorption of bile pigments by the gall bladder. *J Clin Invest* **46**:2035, 1967.
249. Watson CJ: The urobilinoids: Milestones in their history and some recent developments, in Berk PD, Berlin NI (eds): *Bile Pigments: Chemistry and Physiology*. Washington, DC: Department of Health, Education, and Welfare, National Institutes of Health, 1977, p 469.
250. Moscowitz A, Weiner M, Lightner DA, Petryka ZJ, Davis H, Watson CJ: The *in vitro* conversion of bile pigments to the urobilinoids by a rat clostridia species as compared with the human fecal flora. III. Natural d-urobilin, synthetic I-urobilin, and synthetic I-urobilinogen. *Biochem Med* **4**:149, 1970.
251. Elder G, Gray CH, Nicholson DG: Bile pigment fate in gastro-intestinal tract, in Schmidt R, Jaffe ER, Miescher PA (eds): *Physiology and Disorders of Hemoglobin Degradation. Seminars in Hematology*. New York: Grune & Stratton, 1972, p 71.
252. Schmid R, Hammaker L: Metabolism and disposition of C_{14}-bilirubin in congenital nonhemolytic jaundice. *J Clin Invest* **42**:1720, 1963.
253. Lund HT, Jacobsen J: Influence of phototherapy on the biliary bilirubin excretion patterns in newborn infants with hyperbilirubinemia. *J Pediatr* **85**:262, 1974.
254. Berry CS, Zarembo JE, Ostrow JD: Evidence for conversion of bilirubin to dihydroxyl derivatives in the Gunn rat. *Biochem Biophys Res Commun* **49**:1366, 1972.
255. Kapitulnik J, Ostrow JD: Stimulation of bilirubin catabolism in jaundiced Gunn rats as an inducer of microsomal mixed function mono oxygenases. *Proc Natl Acad Sci U S A* **75**:682, 1978.
256. Cardenas-Vazquez R, Yokosuka O, Billing BH: Enzymic oxidation of unconjugated bilirubin by rat liver. *Biochem J* **236**:625, 1986.
257. Yokosuka O, Billing BH: Catabolism of bilirubin by intestinal mucosa. *Clin Sci* **58**:13, 1980.
258. Cameron JL, Pulaski EJ, Abel T, Iber FL: Metabolism and excretion of bilirubin ^{14}C in experimental obstructive jaundice. *Ann Surg* **163**:330, 1966.

259. Cameron JL, Filler RM, Iber FL, Abel T, Randolph JG: Metabolism and excretion of ^{14}C labeled bilirubin in children with biliary atresia. *N Engl J Med* **274**:231, 1966.
260. Fulop M, Sandson J, Brazeau P: Dialyzabilty, protein binding, and renal excretion of plasma conjugated bilirubin. *J Clin Invest* **44**:666, 1965.
261. Gollan JL, Dallinger KJC, Billing BH: Excretion of conjugated bilirubin in the isolated perfused rat kidney. *Clin Sci Mol Med* **54**:381, 1978.
262. Stocker R, Yamamoto Y, McDonagh AF, Glazer AN, Ames BN: Bilirubin is an antioxidant of possible physiological importance. *Science* **235**:1043, 1987.
263. Stocker R, Peterhans E: Antioxidant properties of conjugated bilirubin and biliverdin; biologically relevant scavenging of hypochlorous acid. *Free Radic Res Commun* **6**:57, 1989.
264. Malik R, Wrehota EM, Brass CA, Gollan JL: Membrane antioxidant activity of bile pigments is dependent on the ability to donate hydrogen ions. *Hepatology* **12**:933, 1990.
265. Wu TW, Carey D, Wu J, Sugiyama H: The cytoprotective effects of bilirubin and biliverdin on rat hepatocytes and human erythrocytes and the impact of albumin. *Biochem Cell Biol* **69**:828, 1991.
266. Hardy JB, Peeples MO: Serum bilirubin levels in newborn infants. Distributions and associations with neurological abnormalities during the first year of life. *Johns Hopkins Med J* **128**:265, 1971.
267. Gartner LM, Lee K, Vaisman S, Lane D, Zarafu I: Development of bilirubin transport and metabolism in the newborn Rhesus monkey. *J Pediatr* **90**:513, 1977.
268. Maisels MJ, Pathak A, Nelson NM, Nathan DG, Smith CA: Endogenous production of carbon monoxide in normal and erythroblastic newborn infants. *J Clin Invest* **50**:1, 1971.
269. Vest M, Strebel L, Hauensiein D: The extent of "shunt" bilirubin and erythrocyte survival in the newborn infant measured by the administration of (^{15}N) glycine. *Biochem J* **95**:11c, 1965.
270. Poland RL, Odell GB: Physiologic jaundice: The enterohepatic circulation of bilirubin. *New Engl J Med* **284**:1, 1971.
271. Clarke CA, Donohoe WTA, Finn R, Lehane D, McConnell RB, Sheppard PM, Towers SH, Woodrow JC, Bowley CC, Tovey LAD, Bias WB, Krevans JR: Combined study: Prevention of Rh hemolytic disease: Final results of the high risk clinical trial. A combined study from centers in England and Baltimore. *BMJ* **2**:607, 1971.
272. Haberman S, Kraft EJ, Leucke PE, Peach RO: ABO isoimmunization: The use of the specific Coombs and best elution tests in the detection of hemolytic disease. *J Pediatr* **56**:471, 1960.
273. Levi AJ, Gatmaitan Z, Arias IM: Deficiency of hepatic organic anion-binding protein, impaired organic anion uptake by liver and "physiologic" jaundice in newborn monkeys. *N Engl J Med* **283**:1136, 1970.
274. Brown AK, Zuelzer WW: Studies on the neonatal development of the glucuronide conjugating system. *J Clin Invest* **37**:332, 1958.
275. Bosma PJ, Roy Chowdhury J, Bakker C, Gantla S, DeBoer A, Oostra BA, Lindhout D, Tytgat GNJ, Jansen PLM, Oude Elferink RPJ and Roy Chowdhury N: The genetic basis of the reduced expression of bilirubin UDP-glucuronosyltransferase 1 in Gilbert's syndrome. *N Engl J Med* **333**:1171, 1995.
276. Bancroft JD, Kreamer B, Gourley GR: Gilbert syndrome accelerates development of neonatal jaundice. *J Pediatr* **132**:656, 1998.
277. Roy Chowdhury N, Deocharan B, Bejjanki HR, Gantla S, Roy Chowdhury J, Koliopoulos C, Petmezaki S, Valaes T: The presence of a Gilbert-type promoter abnormality increases the level of neonatal hyperbilirubinemia. *Hepatology* **26**:370a, 1997.
278. Arthur LJH, Bevan BR, Holton JB: Neonatal hyperbilirubinemia and breast feeding. *Dev Med Child Neurol* **8**:279, 1966.
279. Maisels MJ, Newman TB: Kernicterus in otherwise healthy breast-fed term newborns. *Pediatrics* **96**:730, 1995.
280. Arias IM, Gartner LM, Seifter S, Furman M: Prolonged neonatal unconjugated hyperbilirubinemia associated with breast feeding and a steroid, pregnane-3(alpha), 20(beta)-diol, in maternal milk that inhibits glucuronide formation *in vitro*. *J Clin Invest* **43**:2037, 1964.
281. Holton JB, Lathe GH: Inhibitors of bilirubin conjugation in newborn infant serum and male urine. *Clin Sci* **25**:499, 1963.
282. Arias IM, Gartner LM: Production of unconjugated hyperbilirubinemia in full-term newborn infants following administration of pregnane-3(alpha), 20(beta)-diol. *Nature* **203**:1292, 1964.
283. Ramos A, Silberberg M, Stern I: Pregnanediols and neonatal hyperbilirubinemia. *Am J Dis Child* **111**:353, 1966.
284. Foliot A, Ploussard JP, Housett E, Christoforov B, Luzean R, Odievre M: Breast milk jaundice: *In vitro* inhibition of rat liver bilirubin-uridine diphosphate glucuronyl transferase activity and Z protein-bromosulfophthalein binding by human breast milk. *Pediatr Res* **10**:594, 1976.
285. Lucey JF, Driscol JJ: Physiological jaundice re-examined, in Sass-Kortsak A (ed): *Kernicterus*. Toronto: University of Toronto Press, 1961, p 29.
286. Arias IM, Wolfson S, Lucey JF, McKay RJ Jr: Transient familial neonatal hyperbilirubinemia. *J Clin Invest* **44**:1442, 1965.
287. Hsia DY-T, Patterson P, Allen FH, Diamond LK, Gellis SS: Prolonged obstructive jaundice in infancy: General survey of 156 cases. *Pediatrics* **10**:243, 1952.
288. Snyder AL, Satterlee W, Robinson SH, Schmid R: Conjugated plasma bilirubin in jaundice caused by pigment overload. *Nature* **213**:93, 1967.
289. Robinson S, Vanier T, Desforges JF, Schmid R: Jaundice in thalassemia minor: A consequence of "ineffective erythropoiesis." *New Engl J Med* **267**:512, 1962.
290. Israels LG, Zipursky A: Primary shunt hyperbilirubinemia due to an alternate path of bilirubin production. *Am J Med* **27**:693, 1959.
291. Berendsohn S, Lowman J, Sundberg D, Watson CJ: Idiiopathic dyserythropoietic jaundice. *Blood* **24**:1, 1964.
292. Verwilghen R, Verhaegen H, Waumanns P, Beert J: Ineffective erythropoiesis with morphologically abnormal erythroblasts and unconjugated hyperbilirubinemia. *Br J Haematol* **17**:27, 1969.
293. Verwilghen R, Lewis S, Dacie J, Crookston J, Crookston M: Hempas: Congenital dyserythropoietic anaemia (type II). *Q J Med* **42**:257, 1973.
294. Crigler JF, Najjar VA: Congenital familial non-hemolytic jaundice with kernicterus. *Pediatrics* **10**:169, 1952.
295. Childs B, Sidbury JB, Migeon CJ: Glucuronic acid conjugation by patients with familial non-hemolytic jaundice and their relatives. *Pediatrics* **23**:903, 1959.
296. Berk PD, Martin JF, Blaschke TF, Scharschmidt BF, Plotz PH: Unconjugated hyperbilirubinemia: Physiological evaluation and experimental approaches to therapy. *Ann Intern Med* **82**:552, 1975.
297. Sleisenger MG, Kahn I, Barniville H, Rubin W, Benezzer J, Arias IM: Nonhemolytic unconjugated hyperbilirubinemia with hepatic glucuronyl transferase deficiency: A genetic study in four generations. *Trans Assoc Am Physicians* **80**:259, 1967.
298. Szabo L, Ebrey P: Studies on the inheritance of Crigler-Najjar syndrome by the menthol test. *Acta Paediatr Hung* **4**:153, 1963.
299. Wolkoff AW, Chowdhury JR, Gartner LA, Rose AL, Biempica L, Giblin DR, Fink D, Arias IM: Crigler-Najjar syndrome (Type I) in an adult male. *Gastroenterology* **76**:840, 1979.
300. Kapitulnik J, Kaufmann NA, Goitein K, Cividalli G, Blondheim SH: A pigment found in the Crigler-Najjar syndrome and its similarity to an ultra-filterable photo-derivative of bilirubin. *Clin Chim Acta* **57**:231, 1974.
301. Arias IM, Gartner LM, Cohen M, Benezzer J, Levi AJ: Chronic nonhemolytic unconjugated hyperbilirubinemia with glucuronyl transferase deficiency: Clinical, biochemical, pharmacologic, and genetic evidence for heterogeneity. *Am J Med* **47**:395, 1969.
302. Billing GH, Gray CH, Kulcycka A, Manfield P, Nicholson DC: The metabolism of ^{14}C-bilirubin in congenital nonhaemolytic hyperbilirubinaemia. *Clin Sci* **27**:163, 1964.
303. Blaschke TF, Berk PD, Scharschmidt BF, Guyther JR, Vergalla J, Waggoner JG: Crigler-Najjar syndrome: An unusual course with development of neurologic damage at age eighteen. *Pediatr Res* **8**:573, 1974.
304. Novikoff AB, Essner E: The liver cell. *Am J Med* **19**:102, 1960.
305. Bosma PJ, Roy Chowdhury N, Goldhoorn BG, Hofker MH, Oude Elferink RPJ, Jansen PLM, Roy Chowdhury J: Sequence of exons and the flanking regions of human bilirubin-UDP-glucuronosyltransferase gene complex and identification of a genetic mutation in a patient with Crigler-Najjar syndrome, type I. *Hepatology* **15**:941, 1992.
306. Bosma PJ, Roy Chowdhury J, Huang TJ, Lahiri P, Oude Elferink RPJ, Van ES HHG, Lederstein M, Whitington PF, Jansen PLM, Roy Chowdhury N: Mechanism of inherited deficiencies of multiple UDP-glucuronosyltransferase isoforms in two patients with Crigler-Najjar syndrome, type I. *FASEB J* **6**:2859, 1992.
307. Ritter JK, Yeatman MT, Ferriera P, Owens IS: Identification of a genetic alteration in the code for bilirubin UDP-glucuronosyltransferase in the *UGT1* gene complex of a Crigler-Najjar syndrome, type I. *J Clin Invest* **90**:150, 1992.
308. Kadakol A, Ghosh SS, Sappal BS, Sharma G, Roy Chowdhury J, Roy Chowdhury N: Genetic lesions of bilirubin uridinediphosphoglucuronate glucuronosyltransferase causing Crigler-Najjar Gilbert's syndromes: Correlation of genotype to phenotype. *Hum Mutat* (In Press).

309. Seppen J, Steenken R, Lindhout D, Bosma PJ, Oude Elferink RP: A mutation which disrupts the hydrophobic core of the signal peptide of bilirubin UDP-glucuronosyltransferase, an endoplasmic reticulum membrane protein, causes Crigler-Najjar type II. *FEBS Lett* **390**:294, 1996
310. Gantla S, Bakker CTM, Deocharan B, Thummala NR, Zweiner J, Sinaasappel M, Roy Chowdhury J, Bosma PJ, Roy Chowdhury N: Splice site mutations: A novel genetic mechanism of Crigler-Najjar syndrome type 1. *Am J Hum Genet* **62**:585, 1998.
311. Deocharan B, Gantla S, Morton DH, Rizack L, Roy Chowdhury J, Roy Chowdhury N: Interaction of a Crigler-Najjar syndrome type I mutation and a Gilbert type promoter defect results in two grades of hyperbilirubinemia in members of an Amish and a Mennonite kindred of Lancaster County, Pennsylvania. *Gastroenterology* **112**:1255A, 1997.
312. Gunn CH: Hereditary acholuric jaundice in a new mutant strain of rats. *J Hered* **29**:137, 1938.
313. Roy Chowdhury J, Van Es HHG, Roy Chowdhury N: Gunn rat. An animal model of deficiency of bilirubin conjugation, in Tavoloni N, Berk PD (eds): *Hepatic Transport and Bile Secretion. Physiology and Pathophysiology.* New York: Raven, 1992, p 713.
314. Roy Chowdhury N, Kondapalli R, and Roy Chowdhury J: The Gunn rat: An animal model for inherited deficiency of bilirubin glucuronidation, in Cornelius CE (ed): *Animal Models in Liver Research.* New York: Academic, 1993, p 150.
315. Schmid R, Axelrod J, Hammaker L, Swarn RL: Congenital jaundice in rats due to a defective glucuronide formation. *J Clin Invest* **37**:1123, 1958.
316. Schutta HS, Johnson L: Bilirubin encephalopathy in the Gunn rat: A fine structure study of the cerebellar cortex. *J Neuropathol Exp Neurol* **26**:377, 1967.
317. Rose AL, Johnson A: Bilirubin encephalopathy: Neuropathological and histochemical studies in the Gunn rat model. *Neurology* **22**:420, 1972.
318. Schutta HS, Johnson L: Clinical signs and morphologic abnormalities in Gunn rats treated with sulfadiethoxine. *J Pediatr* **75**:1070, 1969.
319. Call NB, Tisher CC: The urinary concentrating defect in the Gunn strain of rat. Role of bilirubin. *J Clin Invest* **55**:319, 1975.
320. Axelsen RA: Spontaneous renal papillary necrosis in the Gunn rat. *Pathology* **5**:43, 1973.
321. Gardner WA, Konigsmark B: Familial nonhemolytic jaundice: Bilirubinosis and encephalopathy. *Pediatrics* **43**:365, 1969.
322. Iyanagi T: Molecular basis of multiple UDP-glucuronosyltransferase isoenzyme deficiencies in the hyperbilirubinemic rat (Gunn rat). *J Biol Chem* **266**:24048, 1991.
323. Roy Chowdhury J., Huang TJ, Kasari K, Lederstein M, Arias IM, Roy Chowdhury N: Molecular basis for the lack of bilirubin-specific and 3-methylcholanthrene-inducible UDP-glucuronosyltransferase activities in Gunn rats: The two isoforms are encoded by distinct mRNA species that share an identical single base deletion. *J Biol Chem* **266**:18294, 1991.
324. Sato H, Aono S, Kashiwamata S, Koiwai O: Genetic defect of bilirubin UDP-glucuronosyltransferase in the hyperbilirubinemic Gunn rat. *Biochem Biophys Res Commun* **177**:1161, 1991.
325. Elawady M, Roy Chowdhury J, Kesari K, Van Es HHG, Lederstein M, Arias IM, Roy Chowdhury N: Mechanism of the lack of induction of UDP-glucuronosyltransferase activity by 3-methylcholanthrene in Gunn rats. *J Biol Chem* **265**:10752, 1990.
326. Watkins JB, Klassen CD: Induction of UDP-glucuronosyltransferase activities in Gunn, heterozygous and Wistar rat livers by pregnenolone-16 alpha-carbonitrile. *Drug Metab Dispos* **10**:590, 1982.
327. Stevenson IH, Greenwood DT, McEwen J: Hepatic UDP-glucuronosyltransferase in Wistar and Gunn rats—*in vitro* activation by diethylnitrosamine. *Biochem Biophys Res Commun* **32**:866, 1968.
328. Roy Chowdhury N, Gross F, Moscioni AD, Kram M, Arias IM, Roy Chowdhury J: Isolation and purification of multiple normal and functionally defective forms of UDP-glucuronosyltransferase from livers of inbred Gunn rats. *J Clin Invest* **79**:327, 1987.
329. Arias IM: Ethereal and N-linked glucuronide formation by normal and Gunn rats *in vitro* and *in vivo*. *Biochem Biophys Res Commun* **6**:81, 1961.
330. Drucker WD: Glucuronic acid conjugation of tetrahydrocortisone p-nitrophenol in the homozygous Gunn rats. *Proc Soc Exp Biol Med* **129**:308, 1968.
331. Flock EV, Bollman JL, Owen CA, Zollman PE: Conjugation of thyroid hormones and analogues by the Gunn rat. *Endocrinology* **77**:303, 1965.
332. Howan ER, Guarino AM: Biliary excretion of phenol red by Wistar and Gunn rats. *Proc Soc Exp Biol Med* **146**:46, 1974.
333. Van der Veer CN, Schoemaker B, Bakker C, van der Meer R, Jansen PLM, Oude Elferink RP: Influence of dietary calcium phosphate on the disposition of bilirubin in rats with unconjugated hyperbilirubinemia. *Hepatology* **24**:620, 1996.
334. van der Veere CN, Sinaasappel M, McDonagh AF, Rosenthal P, Labrune P, Odievre M, Fevery J, Otte JB, McClean P, Burk G, Masakowski V, Sperl W, Mowat AP, Vergani GM, Heller K, Wilson JP, Shepherd R, Jansen PL: Current therapy for Crigler-Najjar syndrome type 1: Report of a world registry. *Hepatology* **24**:311, 1996.
335. Vroemen JPAM, Blankaert N, Buurman WA, Heirwegh KPM, Koostra G: Treatment of enzyme deficiency by hepatocyte transplantation in rats. *J Surg Res* **39**:267, 1985.
336. Gupta S, Aragona E, Vemuru RP, Bhargava KK, Burk RD, Roy Chowdhury J: Permanent engraftment and functions of hepatocytes delivered to the liver: Implications for gene therapy and liver repopulation. *Hepatology* **14**:144, 1991.
337. Ilan Y, Roy Chowdhury N, Prakash R, Jona V, Attavar P, Guha C, Tada K, Roy Chowdhury J: Massive repopulation of rat liver by transplantation of hepatocytes into specific lobes of the liver and ligation of portal vein branches to other lobes. *Transplantation* **64**:8, 1997.
338. Demetriou AA, Levenson SM, Whiting J, Feldman D, Moscioni AD, Kram M, Roy Chowdhury N, Roy Chowdhury J: Replacement of hepatic functions in rats by transplantation of microcarrier-attached hepatocytes. *Science* **233**:1190, 1986.
339. Fox IJ, Roy Chowdhury J, Kaufman SS, Goertzen TC, Roy Chowdhury N, Warkentin PI, Dorko BS, Sauter BV, Strom SC: Treatment of Crigler-Najjar syndrome type I with hepatocyte transplantation. *New Engl J Med* **338**:1422, 1998.
340. Roy Chowdhury J, Strom S, Fox IJ: Human hepatocyte transplantation: Gene therapy and more? *Pediatrics* **102**:647, 1998.
341. Lavin A, Sung C, Klibanov AM, Langer R: Enzymatic removal of bilirubin from blood: A potential treatment for neonatal jaundice. *Science* **230**:543, 1985.
342. Sugi K, Inoue M, Morino Y: Degradation of plasma bilirubin by a bilirubin oxidase derivative which has a relatively long half-life in the circulation. *Biochim Biophys Acta* **991**:405, 1989.
343. Kapitulnik J: The role of cytochrome P-450 in the alternate pathways of bilirubin metabolism in congenitally jaundiced Gunn rats and infants with the Crigler-Najjar syndrome, type I. International Bilirubin Workshop, Trieste, 1992, p 53.
344. Roy Chowdhury J, Grossman M, Gupta S, Roy Chowdhury N, Baker JR, Wilson JM: Long term improvement of hypercholesterolemia after *ex vivo* gene therapy in LDL-receptor deficient rabbits. *Science* **254**:1802, 1991.
345. Tada K, Roy-Chowdhury N, Prasad V, Kim B-H, Manchikalapudi P, Fox IJ, van Duijvendijk P, Bosma PJ, Roy-Chowdhury J: Long-term amelioration of bilirubin glucuronidation defect in Gunn rats by transplanting genetically modified immortalized autologous hepatocytes. *Cell Transplant* **7**:607, 1998.
346. Tada K, Roy Chowdhury N, Neufeld D, Bosma PJ, Heard M, Prasad VR, Roy Chowdhury J: Long-term reduction of serum bilirubin levels in Gunn rats by retroviral gene transfer *in vivo*. *Liver Transplant Surg* **4**:78, 1998
347. Takahashi M, Ilan Y, Roy Chowdhury N, Guida J, Horwitz MS, Roy Chowdhury J: Long-term correction of bilirubin UDP-glucuronosyltransferase deficiency in Gunn rats by administration of a recombinant adenovirus during the neonatal period. *J Biol Chem* **271**:26536, 1996.
348. Ilan Y, Attavar P, Takahashi M, Davidson A, Horwitz M, Guida J, Roy Chowdhury N, Roy Chowdhury J: Induction of central tolerance by intrathymic inoculation of adenoviral antigens into the host thymus permits long-term gene therapy in Gunn rats. *J Clin Invest* **98**:2640, 1996.
349. Ilan Y, Prakash R, Davidson A, Jona V, Droguett G, Horwitz MS, Roy Chowdhury N, Roy Chowdhury J: Oral tolerization to adenoviral antigens permits long-term gene expression using recombinant adenoviral vectors. *J Clin Invest* **99**:1098, 1997.
350. Ilan Y, Sauter B, Roy Chowdhury N, Reddy B, Thummala NR, Groguett G, Davidson A, Ott M, Horwitz MS, Roy Chowdhury J: Oral tolerization to adenoviral proteins permits repeated adenovirus-mediated gene therapy in rats with preexisting immunity to adenovirus. *Hepatology* **27**:1368, 1998.

351. Wilson JM, Wu GY, Wu CH, Grossman M, Roy Chowdhury N, Roy Chowdhury J: Hepatocyte-directed gene transfer *in vivo* leads to transient improvement of hypercholesterolemia in LDL-receptor-deficient rabbits. *J Biol Chem* **267**:963, 1992.
352. Roy Chowdhury N, Wu CH, Wu GY, Yerneni PC, Bommineni VR, Roy Chowdhury J: Fate of DNA targeted to the liver by asialoglycoprotein receptor-mediated endocytosis *in vivo*: Prolonged persistence in cytoplasmic vesicles after partial hepatectomy. *J Biol Chem* **268**:11265, 1993.
353. Bommineni VR, Roy Chowdhury N, Wu GY, Wu CH, Franki N, Hays RM, Roy Chowdhury J: Depolymerization of hepatocellular microtubules after partial hepatectomy. *J Biol Chem* **269**:25200, 1994.
354. Kren BT, Bandyopadhyay P, Steer CJ: *In vivo* site-directed mutagenesis of the factor IX gene by chimeric RNA/DNA oligonucleotides. *Nat Med* **4**:274, 1998.
355. Kren BT, Parashar B, Bandyopadhyay P, Chowdhury NR, Chowdhury JR, Steer CJ: Correction of the UDP-glucuronosyltransferase gene defect in the Gunn rat model of Crigler-Najjar syndrome type I with a chimeric oligonucleotide. *Proc Natl Acid Sci USA* **96**:10349, 1999.
356. Arias IM: Chronic unconjugated hyperbilirubinemia without overt signs of hemolysis in adolescents and adults. *J Clin Invest* **41**:2233, 1962.
357. Gollan JL, Huang SM, Billing B, Sherlock S: Prolonged survival in three brothers with severe type II Crigler-Najjar syndrome. Ultrastructural and metabolic studies. *Gastroenterology* **68**:1543, 1975.
358. Gordon ER, Shaffer EA, Sass-Kortsak A: Bilirubin secretion and conjugation in the Crigler-Najjar syndrome type II. *Gastroenterology* **70**:761, 1976.
359. Fevery J, Blanckaert N, Heirwegh KPM, Preaux A-M, Berthelot P: Unconjugated bilirubin and an increased proportion of bilirubin monoconjugates in the bile of patients with Gilbert's syndrome and Crigler-Najjar syndrome. *J Clin Invest* **60**:970, 1977.
360. Thompson RPH, Pilcher CWT, Robinson J, Strathers GM, McLean AEM, Williams R: Treatment of unconjugated jaundice with dicophane. *Lancet* **2**:4, 1969.
361. Hunter J, Thompson RPH, Rake MO, Williams R: Controlled trial of phetharbital, a non-hypnotic barbiturate, in unconjugated hyperbilirubinaemia. *BMJ* **2**:497, 1971.
362. Orme MLE: Increased glucuronidation of bilirubin in men and rat by administration of antipyrine (phenazone). *Clin Sci Mol Med* **46**:511, 1974.
363. Blaschke TF, Berk PD, Rodkey FL, Scharschmidt BF, Collison HA, Waggoner JG: Effects of glutethimide and phenobarbital on hepatic bilirubin clearance, plasma bilirubin turnover, and carbon monoxide production in man. *Biochem Pharmacol* **23**:2795, 1974.
364. Gabilan JC, Benattar C, Lindenbaum A: Clofibrate treatment of neonatal jaundice. *Pediatrics* **86**:647, 1990.
365. Seppen J, Bosma P, Roy Chowdhury J, Roy Chowdhury N, Jansen PLM, Oude Elferink R: Discrimination between Crigler-Najjar syndrome type I and II by expression of mutant bilirubin-UDP-glucuronosyltransferase. *J Clin Invest* **94**:2385, 1994.
366. Gilbert A, Lereboullet P: La cholamae simple familiale. *Semin Med* **21**:241, 1901.
367. Thompson RPH: Genetic transmission of Gilbert's syndrome, in Okolicsanyi L (ed): *Familial Hyperbilirubinemia*. New York, Wiley, 1981, p 91.
368. Powell LW, Hemingway E, Billing BH, Sherlock S: Idiopathic unconjugated hyperbilirubinemia (Gilbert's syndrome): A study of 42 families. *New Engl J Med* **277**:1108, 1967.
369. Black M, Billing BH: Hepatic bilirubin UDP glucuronyltransferase activity in liver disease and Gilbert's syndrome. *New Engl J Med* **280**:1266, 1969.
370. Auclair C, Hakim J, Boivin P, Troube H, Boucherrot J: Bilirubin and paranitrophenol glucuronyl transferase activity of the liver in patients with Gilbert's syndrome. *Enzyme* **21**:97, 1976.
371. Berk PD, Bloomer JR, Howe RB, Berlin NI: Constitutional hepatic dysfunction (Gilbert's syndrome): A new definition based on kinetic studies with unconjugated radiobilirubin. *Am J Med* **49**:296, 1970.
372. Goresky CA, Gordon ER, Shaffer EA, Parie P, Carassavas D, Aronoff A: Definition of a conjugation dysfunction in Gilbert's syndrome: Studies of the handling of bilirubin loads and of the pattern of bilirubin conjugates secreted in bile. *Clin Sci Mol Med* **1**:63, 1978.
373. Berk PD, Blaschke TF, Waggoner JG: Defective BSP clearance in patients with constitutional hepatic dysfunction (Gilbert's syndrome). *Gastroenterology* **63**:472, 1972.
374. Cartel GVM, Chisesi T, Cazzavillian M, Barbui T, Battista R, Dini E: Bromsulphthalein-Ausscheidung und Hyperbilirubinamia beim Gilbert Syndrome. *Dtsch Z Verdau Stoffwechselkr* **35**:169, 1975.
375. Cobelli C, Ruggeri A, Toffolo G, Okolicsanyi L, Venuti M, Orlando R: BSP vs bilirubin kinetics in Gilbert's syndrome, in Okolicsanyi L (ed): *Familial Hyperbilirubinemia*. New York: Wiley, 1981, p 121.
376. Felsher BF, Rickard D, Redeker AG: The reciprocal relation between caloric intake and the degree of hyperbilirubinemia in Gilbert's syndrome. *New Engl J Med* **283**:170, 1970.
377. Bloomer JR, Barrett PV, Rodkey FL, Berlin NI: Studies on the mechanisms of fasting hyperbilirubinemia. *Gastroenterology* **61**:479, 1971.
378. Barrett PVD: Hyperbilirubinemia of fasting. *JAMA* **217**:1349, 1971.
379. Felsher BF, Carpio NM, Van Couvering K: Effect of fasting and phenobarbital on hepatic UDP-glucuronic acid formation in the rat. *J Lab Clin Med* **93**:414, 1979.
380. Gollan JL, Hatt KJ, Billing BH: The influence of diet on unconjugated hyperbilirubinemia in the Gunn rat. *Clin Sci Mol Med* **49**:229, 1975.
381. Cowan RE, Thompson RPH, Kaye JP, Clark GM: The association between fasting hyperbilirubinaemia and serum non-esterified fatty acids in man. *Clin Sci Mol Med* **53**:155, 1977.
382. Fromke VL, Miller D: Constitutional hepatic dysfunction (CHD: Gilbert's disease): A review with special reference to a characteristic increase and prolongation of the hyperbilirubinemic response to nicotinic acid. *Medicine (Baltimore)* **51**:451, 1972.
383. Ohkubo H, Musha H, Okuda K: Studies on nicotinic acid interaction with bilirubin metabolism. *Dig Dis Sci* **24**:700, 1979.
384. Bosma PJ, Roy Chowdhury J, Bakker C, Gantla S, DeBoer A, Oostra BA, Lindhout D, Tytgat GNJ, Jansen PLM, Oude Elferink RPJ, Roy Chowdhury N: The genetic basis of the reduced expression of bilirubin UDP-glucuronosyltransferase 1 in Gilbert's syndrome. *N Engl J Med* **333**:1171, 1995.
385. Chalasani N, Roy Chowdhury N, Roy Chowdhury J, Boyer TD: Kernicterus in an adult who is heterozygous for Crigler-Najjar syndrome and homozygous for Gilbert-type genetic defect. *Gastroenterology* **112**:2099, 1997.
386. Portman OW, Roy Chowdhury J, Roy Chowdhury N, Alexander M, Cornelius CE, Arias IM: A non-human primate model for Gilbert's syndrome. *Hepatology* **4**:175, 1984.
387. Portman OW, Alexander M, Roy Chowdhury J, Roy Chowdhury N, Cornelius CE, Arias IM: Effects of nutrition on hyperbilirubinemia in Bolivian squirrel monkeys. *Hepatology* **4**:454, 1984.
388. Sprinz H, Nelson RS: Persistent nonhemolytic hyperbilirubinemia associated with lipochrome-like pigment in liver cells: Report of four cases. *Ann Intern Med* **41**:952, 1954.
389. Dubin IN: Chronic idiopathic jaundice: A review of fifty cases. *Am J Med* **23**:268, 1958.
390. Cohen L, Lewis C, Arias IM: Pregnancy, oral contraceptives, and chronic familial jaundice with predominantly conjugated hyperbilirubinemia (Dubin-Johnson syndrome). *Gastroenterology* **62**:1182, 1972.
391. Shani M, Seligsohn U, Gilon E, Sheba C, Adam A: Dubin-Johnson syndrome in Israel. I. Clinical, laboratory, and genetic aspects of 101 cases. *West J Med* **39**:549, 1970.
392. Levanon M, Rimon S, Shani M, Ramot B, Goldberg E: Active and inactive factor-VII in Dubin-Johnson syndrome with factor-VII deficiency, hereditary factor-VII deficiency and on coumadin administration. *Br J Haematol* **23**:669, 1972.
393. Javitt NB, Konso T, Kuchiba K: Bile acid excretion in Dubin-Johnson syndrome. *Gastroenterology* **75**:931, 1978.
394. Kondo T, Yagi R, Kuchiba K: Dubin-Johnson syndrome in a neonate. *New Engl J Med* **292**:1028, 1975.
395. Nakata F, Oyanagi K, Fujiwara M, Sogawa H, Minain R, Horino K, Nakao T, Kondo T: Dubin-Johnson syndrome in a neonate. *Eur J Pediatr* **132**:299, 1979.
396. Dittrich H, Seifert E: Uber das verhalten des pigmentes sowie der biligrafin ausscheidung bei einem patienten mit Dubin-Johnson syndrom. *Acta Hepatosplenol* **9**:45, 1962.
397. Morita M, Kihava T: Intravenous cholecystography and metabolism of meglumine iodipamide (biligrafin) in Dubin-Johnson syndrome. *Radiology* **99**:57, 1971.
398. Essner E, Novikoff AB: Human hepatocellular pigments and lysosomes. *J Ultrastruct Res* **3**:3764, 1960.
399. Ehrlick JC, Novikoff AB, Platt R, Essner E: Hepatocellular lipofuscin and the pigment of chronic idiopathic jaundice. *Bull NY Acad Med* **36**:488, 1960.

400. Wegmann R, Rangier M, Eteve J, Charbonnier A, Caroli J: Melanose hepatosplenique avec ictere chronique a bilirubine directe: Maladie de Dubin-Johnson? Etude clinique et biologique de la maladie. Etudie histochimique, chimique et spectrographique du pigment anormal. *Semin Hop Paris* **26**:1761, 1960.
401. Arias IM, Bernstein L, Roffler R, Ben Ezzer J: Black liver diseases in Corriedale sheep: Metabolism of tritiated epinephrine and incorporation of isotope into the hepatic pigment *in vivo*. *J Clin Invest* **44**:1026, 1065.
402. Swartz HM, Sarna T, Varma RR: On the nature and excretion of the hepatic pigment in the Dubin-Johnson syndrome. *Gastroenterology* **76**:958, 1979.
403. Kitamura T, Alroy J, Gatmaitan Z, Inoue M, Mikami T, Kansen PLM, Arias IM: Defective biliary excretion of epinephrine metabolites in mutant TR$^-$ rats: Relation to the pathogenesis of rat liver in Dubin-Johnson syndrome and Corriedale sheep with an analogous excretory defect. *Hepatology* **15**:1154, 1992.
404. Rubinstein ZJ, Seligson U, Modan M, Shani M: Hepatic computerized tomography in the Dubin-Johnson syndrome: Increased liver density as a diagnostic acid. *Comput Radiol* **9**:315, 1985.
405. Ware A, Eigenbrodt E, Naftalis J, Combes B: Dubin-Johnson syndrome and viral hepatitis. *Gastroenterology* **67**:560, 1974.
406. Billing BH, Williams R, Richards TG: Defects in hepatic transport of bilirubin in congenital hyperbilirubinaemia. An analysis of plasma bilirubin disappearance curves. *Clin Sci* **27**:245, 1964.
407. Schoenfield LJ, McGill DB, Hunton DB, Foulk MT, Butt HR: Studies of chronic idiopathic jaundice (Dubin-Johnson syndrome). I. Demonstration of hepatic excretory defect. *Gastroenterology* **44**:101, 1963.
408. Erlinger S, Dhumeaux D, Desjeux JF, Benhamou JP: Hepatic handling of unconjugated dyes in the Dubin-Johnson syndrome. *Gastroenterology* **64**:106, 1973.
409. Mandema E, De Fraiture WH, Neiweg HO, Arends A: Familial chronic idiopathic jaundice (Dubin-Sprinz disease), with a note on bromsulphalein metabolism in this disease. *Am J Med* **28**:42, 1960.
410. Rodes J, Zubizarreta A, Bruguera M: Metabolism of the bromsulphalein in Dubin-Johnson syndrome. Diagnostic value of the paradoxical in plasma levels of BSP. *Dig Dis* **17**:545, 1972.
411. Koskelo P, Toivonen I, Adlercreutz H: Urinary coproporphyrin isomer distribution in Dubin-Johnson syndrome. *Clin Chem* **13**:1006, 1967.
412. Kaplowitz N, Javitt N, Kappas A: Coproporphyrin I and III excretion in bile and urine. *J Clin Invest* **51**:2895, 1972.
413. Kondo T, Kuchiba K, Shimizu Y: Coproporphyrin isomers in Dubin-Johnson syndrome. *Gastroenterology* **70**:1117, 1976.
414. Wolkoff AW, Cohen LE, Arias IM: Inheritance of the Dubin-Johnson syndrome. *N Engl J Med* **288**:113, 1973.
415. Ben-Ezzer J, Blonder J, Shani M, Seligsohn U, Post CA, Adam A, Szeinberg A: Dubin-Johnson syndrome. Abnormal excretion of the isomers of urinary coproporphyrin by clinically unaffected family members. *Isr J Med Sci* **9**:1431, 1973.
416. Edwards RH: Inheritance of the Dubin-Johnson-Sprinz syndrome. *Gastroenterology* **68**:734, 1975.
417. Wolkoff AW, Arias IM: Coproporphyrin excretion in amniotic fluid and urine from premature infants: A possible maturation defect. *Pediatr Res* **8**:591, 1974.
418. Aziz MA, Schwartz S, Watson CJ: Studies of coproporphyrin. VIII. Reinvestigation of the isomer distribution in jaundice and liver diseases. *J Lab Clin Med* **63**:596, 1964.
419. Shimizu Y, Kondo T, Kuchiba K, Urata G: Uroporphyrin III cosynthetase in liver and blood in the Dubin-Johnson syndrome. *J Lab Clin Med* **89**:517, 1977.
420. Kondo T, Kuchiba K, Shimizu Y: Metabolic fate of exogenous delta-aminolevulinic acid in Dubin-Johnson syndrome. *J Lab Clin Med* **94**:421, 1979.
421. Oude Elferink RPJ, Meijer DKF, Kuipers F, Jansen PLM, Groen AK, Groothuis GMM: Hepatobiliary secretion of organic compounds; molecular mechanisms of membrane transport. *Biochim Biophys Acta* **1241**:215, 1995.
422. Jansen, PLM, van Klinken JW, van Gelder M, Ottenhoff R, Oude Elferink RPJ: Preserved organic anion transport in mutant TR rats with a hepatobiliary secretion defect. *Am J Physiol* **265**:G445 G452, 1993.
423. Huber M, Guhlmann A, Jansen PLM, Keppler D: Hereditary defect of hepatobiliary cysteinyl leukotriene elimination in mutant rats with defective hepatic anion excretion. *Hepatology* **7**:224, 1987.
424. Oude Elferink RPJ, Ottenhoff R, Liefting WGM, Schoemaker B, Groen AK, Jansen PLM: ATP dependent efflux of GSSG and GS conjugate from isolated rat hepatocytes. *Am J Physiol* **258**:G699, 1990.
425. Kobayashi K, Sogame Y, Hayashi K, Nicotera P, Orrenius S: ATP stimulates the uptake of S dinitrophenylglutathione by rat liver plasma membrane vesicles. *FEBS Lett* **240**:55, 1988.
426. Akerboom TPM, Narayanaswami V, Kunst M, Sies H: ATP dependent S (2,4 dinitrophenyl)glutathione transport in canalicular plasma membrane vesicles from rat liver. *J Biol Chem* **266**:13147, 1991.
427. Kobayashi K, Komatsu S, Nishi T, Hara H, Hayashi K: ATP dependent transport for glucuronides in canalicular plasma membrane vesicles. *Biochem Biophys Res Commun* **176**:622, 1991.
428. Oude Elferink, RPJ, de Haan J, Lambert KJ, Hagey LR, Hofmann AF, Jansen PLM: Selective hepatobiliary transport of nordeoxycholate side chain conjugates in mutant rats with a canalicular transport defect. *Hepatology* **9**:861, 1989.
429. Higgins CF: ABC transporters: From microorganisms to man. *Annu Rev Cell Biol* **867**:1650, 1992.
430. Paulusma CC, Bosma PJ, Zaman GJR, Bakker CTM, Otter M, Scheffer GL, Scheper RJ, Borst P, Oude Elferink RPJ: Congenital jaundice in rats with a mutation in a multidrug resistance-associated protein gene. *Science* **271**:1126, 1996.
431. Ling V: P-glycoprotein: its role in drug resistance. *Am J Med* **99(suppl)**:31, 1995.
432. Muller M, Meijer C, Zaman GJR, Borst P, Scheper RJ, Mulder NH, de Vires EGE, Jansen PLM: Overexpression of the multidrug resistance-associated protein results in increased ATP-dependent glutathione S-conjugate transport. *Proc Natl Acad Sci U S A* **91**:13033, 1994.
433. Evers R, Zaman GJR, van Deemter L, Jansen H, Calafat J, Oomen LCJM, Oude Elferink RPJ, Borst P, Schinkel AH: Basolateral localization and export activity of the human multidrug resistance-associated protein in polarized pig kidney cells. *J Clin Invest* **97**:1, 1996.
434. Paulusma CC, Kool M, Bosma PJ, Scheffer GL, ter Borg F, Scheper RJ, Borst P, Baas F, Oude Elferink RPJ: A mutation in the human *cMOAT* gene causes the Dubin Johnson gene. *Hepatology* **25**:1539, 1997.
435. Allikmets R, Gerrard B, Hutchinson A, Dean M: Characterization of the human ABC superfamily: Isolation and mapping of 21 new genes using the Expressed Sequence Tags database. *Hum Mol Gen* **5**:1649, 1996.
436. Kartenbeck J, Leuschner U, Mayer R, Keppler D: Absence of the canalicular isoform of the MRP-gene encoded conjugate export pump from the hepatocytes in Dubin Johnson syndrome. *Hepatology* **23**:1061, 1996.
436a. Gourley GR: Bilirubin metaboolism and kernicterus. *Adv Pediatr* **44**:173, 1997.
437. Seligsohn U, Shani M, Ramot B, Adam A, Sheba C: Dubin-Johnson Syndrome in Israel. II. Association with factor-VII deficiency. *Q J Med* **39**:569, 1970.
438. De Grouchy J, Dautzenberg M-D, Turleau C, Beguin S, Chavin-Colin F: Regional mapping of clotting factors VII and X to 13q34. Expression of factor VII through chromosome 8. *Hum Genet* **66**:230, 1984.
439. Rotor AB, Manahan L, Florentin A: Familial nonhemolytic jaundice with direct van den Bergh reaction. *Acta Med Phil* **5**:37, 1948.
440. Pereira-Lima JE, Utz E, Rosenberg I: Hereditary nonhemolytic conjugated hyperbilirubinemia without abnormal liver cell pigmentation. A family study. *Am J Med* **40**:628, 1966.
441. Wolkoff AW, Wolpert E, Pascasio FN, Arias IM: Rotor's syndrome: A distinct inheritable pathophysiologic entity. *Am J Med* **60**:173, 1976.
442. Wolpert E, Pascasio FM, Wolkoff AW, Arias IM: Abnormal sulfobromophthalein metabolism in Rotor's syndrome and obligate heterozygotes. *New Engl J Med* **296**:1099, 1977.
443. Kawasaki H, Kinwa N, Irisa T, Hirayama C: Dye clearance studies in Rotor's syndrome. *Am J Gastroenterol* **71**:380, 1979.
444. Dhumeaux D, Berthelot P: Chronic hyperbilirubinemia associated with hepatic uptake and storage impairment: A new syndrome resembling that of the mutant Southdown sheep. *Gastroenterology* **69**:988, 1975.
445. Shimizu Y, Naruto H, Ida S, Kohakura M: Urinary coproporphyrin isomers in Rotor's syndrome. A study in eight families. *Hepatology* **1**:173, 1981.
446. Rapacini GL, Topi GC, Anti M, D'Allasandro GL, Griso D, Amantea A, Devitis I, Fedeli G: Porphyrins in Rotor syndrome: A study on an Italian family. *Hepatogastroenterology* **33**:11, 1986.

447. Localio SA, Schwartz MS, Gannon CF: The urinary/fecal coproporphyrin ratio in liver disease. *J Clin Invest* **20**:7, 1941.
448. Clayton RJ, Iber FL, Ruebner BH, et al.: Byler disease: Fatal familial intrahepatic cholestasis in an Amish kindred. *Am J Dis Child* **117**:112, 1969.
449. Bull LN, van Eijk MJ, Pawlikowaska L, DeYoung JA, Juijn JA, Liao M, Klomp LW, Lomri N, Berger R, Scharshmidt BF, Knisely AS, Houwen RH, Freimer NB: A gene encoding a P-type ATPase mutated in two forms of hereditary cholestasis. *Nat Genet* **18**:219, 1998.
450. Summerskill WHJ, Walshe JM: Benign recurrent intrahepatic obstructive jaundice. *Lancet* **2**:686, 1959.
451. Williams R, Cartter MA, Sherlock S, Sgheuer PJ, Hill KR: Idiopathic recurrent cholestasis: A study of the functional and pathological lesions in four cases. *Q J Med* **33**:387, 1964.
452. De Pagter AGF, Van Berge Henegouwen GP, Bokkel-Huinnuk JA, Brandt K-H: Familial benign recurrent intrahepatic cholestasis. *Gastroenterology* **71**:202, 1976.
453. Summerskill WHJ: The syndrome of benign recurrent cholestasis. *Am J Med* **38**:298, 1965.
454. Tygstrup N, Jensen B: Intermittent intrahepatic cholestasis of unknown etiology in five young males from the Faroe Islands. *Acta Med Scand* **185**:523, 1969.
455. Summerfield JA, Scott J, Berman M, Ghent C, Bloomer JR, Berk PD, Sherlock S: Benign recurrent intrahepatic cholestasis: Studies of bilirubin kinetics, bile acids, and cholangiography. *Gut* **21**:154, 1980.
456. Biempica L, Gutstein S, Arias IM: Morphological and biochemical studies of benign recurrent cholestasis. *Gastroenterology* **52**:521, 1967.
457. Strautnieks SS, Kagalwalla AF, Tanner MS, Knisley AS, Bull L, Freimer N, Kocoshis SA, Gardiner RM, Thompson RJ: Identification of a locus for progressive familial intrahepatic cholestasis PFIC2 on chromosome 2q24. *Am J Hum Genet* **61**:630, 1997.
458. De Vree J, Jacquemin E, Strum E, et al.: Mutations in the MDR3 gene cause progressive familial intrahepatic cholestasis. *Proc Acad Natl Sci U S A* **25**:282, 1998.
459. Zhang N, Arias IM: Deficient MDR3 expression in liver from patients with Navajo neuropathy: A human homologue of mdr2 −/− mice. *Hepatology* **26**:69A, 1997.
460. Oda T, Elkaholoun AG, Meltzer PS, Chandrashekharappa SC: Identification and cloning of the human homolog (*Jag1*) of the rat *jagged 1* gene from the Alagille syndrome critical region at 20p12. *Genomics* **43**:376, 1997.

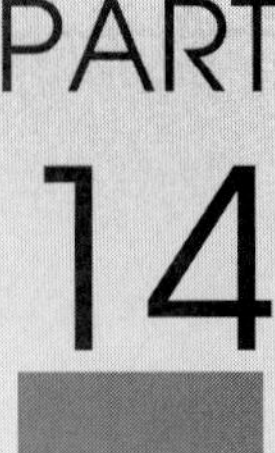

METALS

Erythroid marrow

Absorption and excretion

24

Iron 7 mg/day

17

Transferrin

Extravascular/intravascular

3

22

RE

15

Circulating red cells

5

5

2

2

Parenchymal tissues

Muscles skin, etc. | Liver

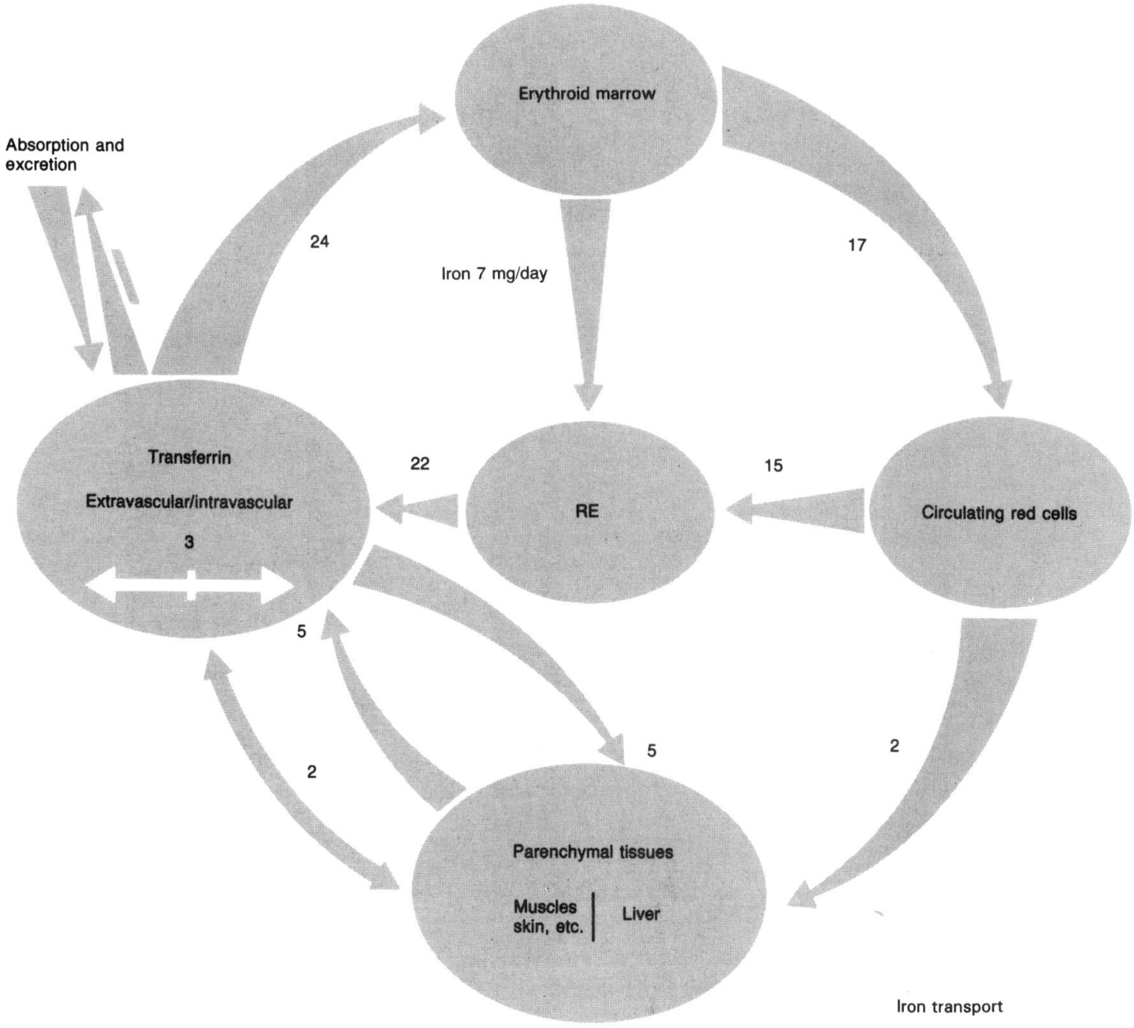

Iron transport

CHAPTER 126

Disorders of Copper Transport

Valeria Cizewski Culotta ▪ Jonathan David Gitlin

1. **Wilson disease and Menkes disease are inherited disorders of copper transport. Each disease results from the absence or dysfunction of homologous copper-transporting adenosine triphosphatases (ATPases) present in the *trans*-Golgi network of cells. The Wilson disease ATPase transports copper into the hepatocyte secretory pathway for incorporation into ceruloplasmin and excretion into the bile. Thus, individuals with this autosomal-recessive disease present with signs and symptoms arising from impaired biliary copper excretion. The Menkes disease ATPase transports copper across the placenta, gastrointestinal tract, and blood–brain barrier, and the clinical features of this X-linked disease arise from copper deficiency. Despite striking differences in the clinical presentation of these two diseases, the respective ATPases function in precisely the same fashion within the cell. The unique clinical features of each disease are the result of the tissue-specific expression of these ATPases.**
2. **Copper is an essential transition element that plays a fundamental role in the biochemistry of all aerobic organisms. Proteins exploit the unique redox nature of this metal to undertake a series of facile electron transfer reactions using copper as a cofactor in a select number of critical enzymatic pathways. The function of these enzymes is essential for cellular respiration, iron homeostasis, pigment formation, neurotransmitter production, peptide biogenesis, connective tissue biosynthesis, and antioxidant defense. The signs and symptoms of copper deficiency are the result of impaired function of these cuproenzymes.**
3. **Copper homeostasis is maintained entirely by gastrointestinal absorption and biliary excretion. Absorbed copper is efficiently removed from the portal circulation by the liver, which is the central organ of copper homeostasis, regulating both storage and excretion. Biliary copper is not absorbed from the gastrointestinal tract, so there is no enterohepatic circulation of this metal. Greater than 95 percent of plasma copper is contained in the multicopper oxidase ceruloplasmin, which is synthesized and secreted by the liver. Despite the abundance of this cuproprotein in the plasma, ceruloplasmin has no essential role in copper transport or metabolism.**
4. **The reactivity of copper in biological systems also accounts for the potential toxicity of this metal when cellular copper homeostasis is disturbed. For this reason, specific pathways have evolved for the trafficking and compartmentalization of copper within cells. The delivery of copper along these pathways is mediated by unique proteins termed copper chaperones. Elucidation of the structure and function of these chaperones has revealed a remarkable evolutionary conservation of the mechanisms of cellular copper metabolism. The inherited disorders of copper transport dramatically underscore both the essential need for copper and the toxicity of this metal, and elucidation of the genetic basis of these diseases permits an understanding of the molecular mechanisms of copper homeostasis.**
5. **In Wilson disease, impaired biliary copper excretion leads to accumulation of this metal in the liver. When the capacity for hepatic storage is exceeded, cell death ensues, with copper release into the plasma resulting in hemolysis and deposition of copper in extrahepatic tissues. Affected individuals usually present in the first or second decade of life with chronic hepatitis and cirrhosis or acute liver failure. Copper accumulation in the cornea results in Kayser-Fleischer rings. Neuropsychiatric symptoms are more common in adults and include dystonia, tremor, personality changes, and cognitive impairment as a result of copper accumulation in the basal ganglia and other brain regions.**
6. **The diagnosis of Wilson disease is confirmed by decreased serum ceruloplasmin, increased urinary copper, and elevated hepatic copper concentration. A large number of different mutations occur in the Wilson disease gene, but allelic heterogeneity does not account for the marked clinical variability among patients. In specific families, haplotype analysis and examination for common mutations can prove diagnostically useful. Copper chelation with penicillamine is effective in most cases, and trientene and zinc are useful alternatives where toxicity is an issue. Hepatic transplantation ameliorates the disease but is reserved for patients with irreversible liver damage.**
7. **In Menkes disease, failure to transport copper to the affected fetus results in copper deficiency *in utero*, and this is compounded after birth by impairment of copper absorption and ineffective copper transport into the central nervous system. The clinical features of Menkes disease result from the loss of function of specific cuproenzymes. These features include abnormal hair and pigmentation, laxity of the skin, metaphyseal dysplasia, cerebellar degeneration, and failure to thrive. Allelic heterogeneity results in milder forms of the disease, including the occipital horn syndrome in which neurologic symptoms are minimal or absent.**
8. **The diagnosis of Menkes disease is confirmed by decreased serum copper and ceruloplasmin, but interpretation of these values is difficult in the first months of life. In such cases, analysis of copper accumulation in the placenta or cultured skin fibroblasts may be helpful in confirming the**

A list of standard abbreviations is located immediately preceding the index in each volume. Nonstandard abbreviations used in this chapter include: CCS, copper chaperone for SOD1; SOD1, intracellular copper zinc superoxide dismutase; SOD3, extracellular copper zinc superoxide dismutase.

diagnosis. Most mutations detected in the Menkes disease gene are unique to an affected family, and about 20 percent of these are rearrangements or partial gene deletions that can be identified by Southern blot analysis. Severe Menkes disease is fatal, and no definitive therapeutic options are currently available. Early treatment with copper histidine may be of value in less severe cases where some residual expression of the Menkes gene occurs.

9. **Aceruloplasminemia is an autosomal-recessive disease characterized by absent serum ceruloplasmin and progressive neurodegeneration of the basal ganglia in association with specific inherited mutations in the ceruloplasmin gene. Affected individuals present with insulin-dependent diabetes and neurologic symptoms, including dysarthria, dystonia, and dementia as a direct result of iron accumulation in affected tissues. Although the basal ganglia symptoms and a lack of serum ceruloplasmin may lead to diagnostic confusion with Wilson disease, magnetic resonance imaging reveals the presence of iron in the basal ganglia. Recognition of this disease reveals an essential role for ceruloplasmin in iron homeostasis and neuronal survival in the central nervous system.**

> ***When I see such things, I'm no longer sure***
> ***that what's important***
> ***is more important than what's not.***
> **Wisława Szymborska, 1993**

Throughout the history of evolution, living organisms have exploited the reactivity of transition metals in biological systems. Copper proved particularly useful in this regard because the orbital structure of this metal permits facile electron transfer reactions. In addition, the relative abundance of copper in the earth's crust provided a powerful driving force for natural selection, resulting in an extraordinary diversity of life forms that use this metal for the binding or activation of dioxygen. For example, in arthropods and mollusks, copper contained in hemocyanin provides the oxygen transport system necessary to sustain life in the myriad environmental niches occupied by these animals. Similarly, plants require copper to respond to environmental cues essential for such processes as stem growth and fruit ripening, and in a remarkable example of evolutionary conservation these metabolic events are dependent on the copper transport function of the plant orthologue of the human Wilson and Menkes disease genes. The past several years have witnessed spectacular advances in our understanding of the molecular and cellular biology of copper metabolism, owing in large part to the elucidation of the genetic basis of the inherited diseases of copper transport. Understanding the basic defect in these rare disorders now provides the opportunity for new approaches to the diagnosis and treatment of affected patients and for the first time permits basic biological insight into the mechanisms of copper metabolism so remarkably conserved among all living species.

COPPER HOMEOSTASIS

Metabolism

Absorption. A healthy adult human maintains a total body copper content of approximately 100 mg. This is accomplished entirely through gastrointestinal uptake and biliary excretion with little or no contribution by other organ systems under normal circumstances. The average daily diet contains about 5 mg of copper; each day about 40 percent of this is absorbed and an equivalent amount is returned to the gastrointestinal tract by biliary secretion[1,2] (Fig. 126-1). Copper can be absorbed through the dermis and the mucosal membranes following prolonged exposure to this metal, as occurs with the use of copper bracelets or certain intrauterine devices, but this is almost always a negligible amount in terms of the total body copper content. Likewise, copper can be excreted via the sweat glands and filtered from the plasma by the kidney for urinary excretion, but these routes are quantitatively unimportant except in the rare circumstance of marked total body copper excess.[3]

Although the precise location within the human gastrointestinal tract where copper is absorbed has not been determined, kinetic studies indicate that a large percentage of an administered dose of copper is absorbed within the stomach and duodenum. Dietary contents may influence copper bioavailability, but in general the efficiency of copper absorption varies little among individuals. Stable isotope studies reveal a specific uptake mechanism that is regulated such that fractional absorption increases as the total body copper content decreases.[4] The regulation of copper absorption in response to total body copper content mitigates against copper deficiency but is not sufficient to maintain copper balance at very low copper intake.

The molecular mechanisms of copper uptake into mammalian cells are unknown. However, studies in the yeast *Saccharomyces cerevisiae* have identified three genes involved in copper uptake, *CTR1*, *CTR2*, and *CTR3*. *CTR1* and *CTR3* are essential for high-affinity copper uptake, and complementation of a *ctr1*Δ strain identified a human gene h*CTR1* encoding a protein homologous to both *CTR1* and an *Arabidopsis thaliana* copper transporter, COPT1.[5–8] In addition to h*CTR1*, a related gene, h*CTR2*, also has been identified in the human genome and, based on sequence homology, is thought to play a role in low-affinity copper uptake.[8]

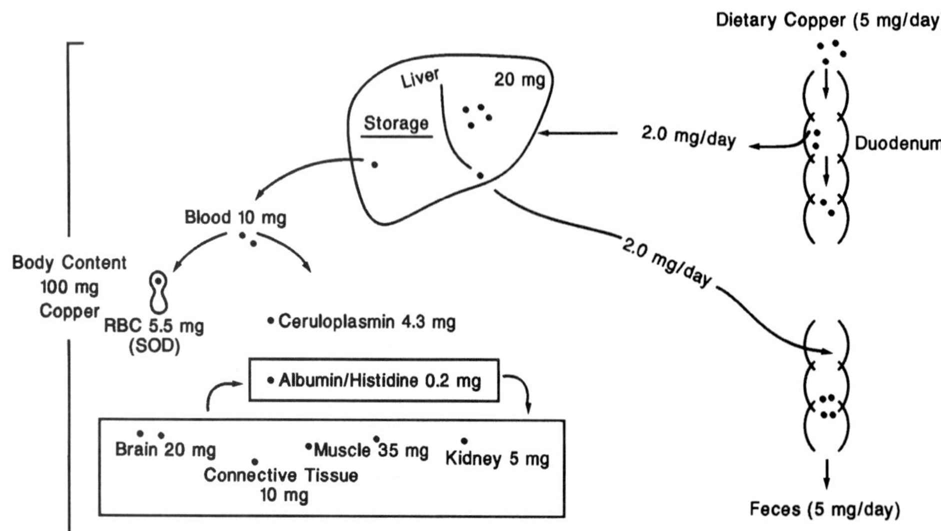

Fig. 126-1 Physiology of copper metabolism in the adult illustrating the pathways of absorption and excretion as well as distribution throughout the body. (*Modified with permission from Harris and Gitlin.*[90])

Transcripts encoding h*CTR1* and h*CTR2* are expressed in multiple tissues, including the intestine, but it remains unclear what role, if any, these proteins play in gastrointestinal copper absorption.

Patients with Menkes disease have a marked impairment in gastrointestinal copper uptake, indicating that the Menkes protein is essential in this process.[9] Based on the known cell biology of the copper-transporting adenosine triphosphatases (ATPases), it is likely that in the gastrointestinal tract this protein functions to transport copper into the enterocyte secretory pathway for subsequent export of copper across the basolateral membrane into the portal venous circulation. Studies in transgenic mice indicate that under normal circumstances metallothionein plays no essential role in gastrointestinal copper uptake.[10,11] Nevertheless, induction of enterocyte metallothionein can inhibit gastrointestinal copper absorption, presumably by sequestration of cytoplasmic copper with impairment of copper trafficking to the secretory pathway. The increased copper bound by metallothionein is subsequently lost during villous shedding of enteric cells.[12]

Distribution. Radioisotope studies reveal that copper absorbed from the gastrointestinal tract appears in the portal venous circulation bound to albumin and amino acids. Newly absorbed copper is rapidly cleared by the liver, and within 24 hours about 10 percent of the administered dose reappears in the circulation incorporated into ceruloplasmin. Kinetic studies suggest that the liver may regulate the distribution of copper to other tissues, but the mechanisms by which this occurs have not been elucidated. Although a significant amount of an administered dose of copper appears in the plasma as ceruloplasmin, this merely reflects the relative abundance of this cuproenzyme because both metabolic studies and data from patients with aceruloplasminemia indicate that this protein plays no role in copper transport to tissues.[13] Similarly, albumin is not essential for copper transport because an absence of this protein in analbuminemia does not result in abnormalities of copper metabolism.[14] Although the precise mechanism of plasma copper transport remains unknown, copper is bound in the plasma complexed with histidine and other small amino acid molecules, and these complexes may be essential for the transport and distribution of this metal to peripheral tissues.[15]

Ceruloplasmin is an abundant α_2-glycoprotein that contains greater than 95 percent of the copper found in plasma. This protein is synthesized in hepatocytes and secreted into the serum as a single polypeptide with six atoms of copper incorporated during biosynthesis. Ceruloplasmin has a serum half-life of 5.5 days, and studies using radioactive copper indicate little or no exchange of ceruloplasmin-bound copper.[16] Although copper has no effect on the rate of synthesis or secretion of ceruloplasmin, failure to incorporate this metal during synthesis results in the secretion of an apoprotein devoid of this metal.[17,18] In the normal adult, approximately 10 percent of circulating ceruloplasmin is found as the apoprotein that is synthesized and secreted from the liver without copper and is rapidly catabolized with a half-life of approximately 5 hours. Because copper availability serves only to determine the ratio of apo- and holoceruloplasmin secreted from the hepatocyte, the steady-state serum ceruloplasmin concentration reflects the sum of these two moieties, determined by intracellular copper availability and the observed differences in half-life. Thus, despite the fact that 90 percent of circulating ceruloplasmin is the holoprotein, given the marked differences in the half-lives of these two forms, under normal circumstances the rate of synthesis and secretion of apo- and holoceruloplasmin is equivalent. As might be anticipated from such a model, an increase in the hepatic copper pool in normal individuals results in a sustained increase in holoceruloplasmin synthesis, and hence the serum ceruloplasmin concentration. Similarly, a decrease in copper availability in the hepatocyte, as occurs in nutritional copper deficiency or Wilson disease, results in a marked decrease in the serum ceruloplasmin concentration secondary to rapid turnover of the secreted apoprotein.

Excretion. The liver is the central organ of copper homeostasis, having an enormous capacity for both storage and excretion of this metal. Biliary excretion is the predominant mechanism determining copper balance and the amount of copper appearing in bile is directly proportional to the size of the hepatic copper pool.[19] Although the molecular nature of the copper appearing in bile remains unknown, radioisotope studies in patients undergoing cholecystectomy suggest that this metal is excreted as a macromolecular complex.[20] Biliary copper is unable to be reabsorbed from the gastrointestinal tract, so enterohepatic recirculation of this metal is negligible. Ceruloplasmin plays no role in copper excretion into bile because patients with aceruloplasminemia have no defect in biliary copper excretion. The absence of ceruloplasmin in the bile of patients with Wilson disease is merely a reflection of the marked decrease in the concentration of this protein in the plasma.

Hepatocytes are the primary site of copper accumulation within the liver. These polarized epithelial cells are able to discern the copper status and regulate copper excretion into the bile, depending on the intracellular concentration of this metal. The molecular mechanisms by which the hepatocyte determines copper homeostasis have been clarified with the elucidation of the genetic defect in Wilson disease. The copper-transporting ATPase encoded at the Wilson disease locus is localized to the *trans*-Golgi network of the hepatocyte.[21,22] As the copper concentration of the hepatocyte increases, this protein moves from the *trans*-Golgi network to a cytoplasmic vesicular compartment near the canalicular pole of the cell[22] (Fig. 126-2). Following the sequestration of copper into this compartment by the Wilson protein, the concomitant decrease in cytosolic copper concentration triggers the return of this ATPase to the *trans*-Golgi network, whereas the copper is discharged at the canalicular membrane. This novel posttranslational mechanism thus ensures that excess cytosolic copper will be excreted rapidly into the bile.

Development. The physiology of copper metabolism during development is relevant to the diagnosis and treatment of the inherited disorders of copper transport. The presence of neurologic symptoms in newborn infants with Menkes disease indicates that copper delivery to the fetus is critical for central nervous system development and that the Menkes protein plays an essential role in copper transport *in utero*. Although the route of copper delivery to the human fetus is not known, the Menkes gene is abundantly expressed in the placenta, suggesting that this ATPase transports copper into the fetal plasma.[23,24] Alternatively, copper may be transported through the membranes into the amniotic fluid and absorbed via the gastrointestinal tract following fetal deglutition. Studies in rodents suggest that there is a critical window during fetal development for copper delivery to the central nervous system;[25,26] thus, elucidation of the mechanisms of copper delivery to the fetus is essential to the development of novel therapeutic approaches in patients with Menkes disease.

Ceruloplasmin can be detected in the human fetus as early as the fifth week of gestation and turnover studies at birth indicate that the ceruloplasmin present in newborn serum is derived entirely from endogenous synthesis with no maternal contribution.[27] Functional studies have demonstrated a marked decrease in biliary excretory capacity in the human fetus and newborn infant.[19] Consistent with these observations, copper accumulates in the fetal and newborn liver, and the concentration of this metal does not begin to decrease until several months after birth. Experimental studies suggest that accompanying this immaturity in biliary function there is a developmental difference in copper handling by the hepatocyte at the level of the secretory pathway.[28] As a result of this difference, the newborn liver synthesizes and secretes almost entirely apoceruloplasmin, and the serum concentration of this protein remains very low for the first 3 to 6 months of life. These developmental changes in copper metabolism mitigate against the use of serum ceruloplasmin concentration as a newborn screening test for Wilson disease or aceruloplasminemia

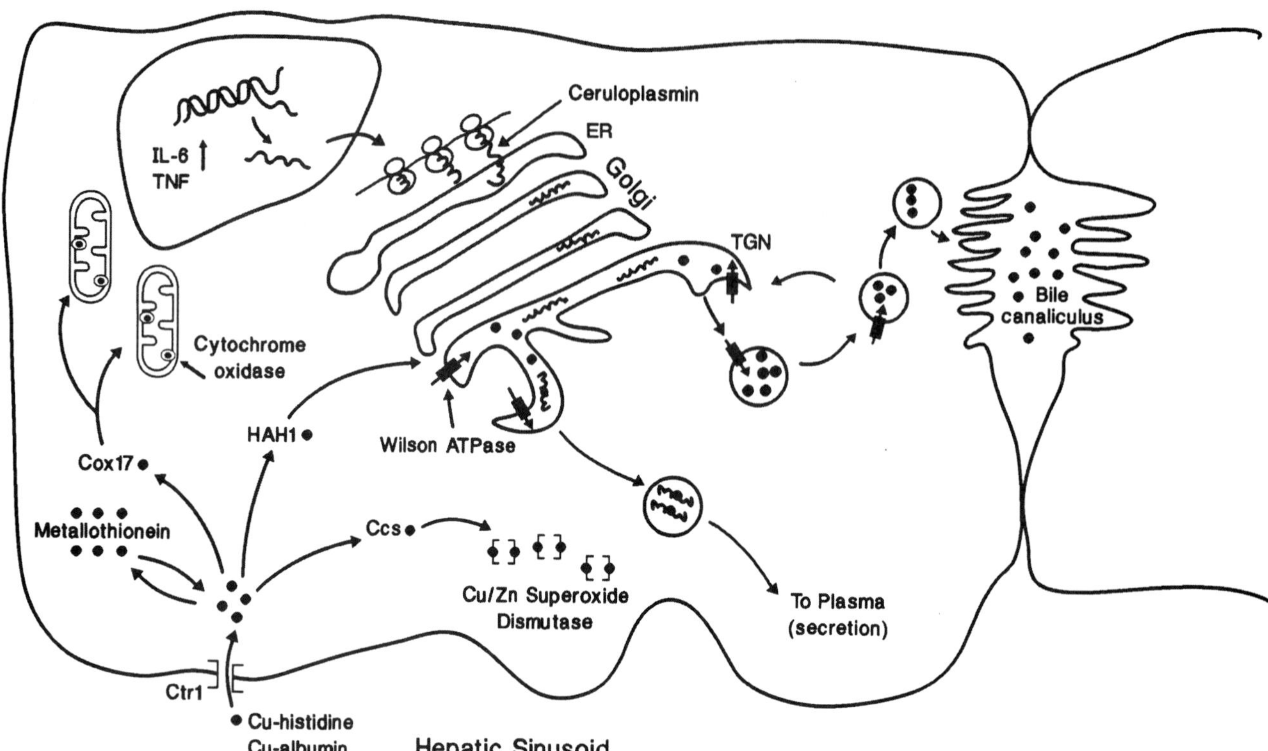

Fig. 126-2 Pathways of intracellular copper metabolism in the hepatocyte, including trafficking to storage proteins and chaperones and the copper-mediated trafficking of the Wilson ATPase from the *trans*-Golgi network to an intracellular vesicular compartment prior to biliary excretion. (*Modified with permission from Harris and Gitlin.*[90])

and complicate the diagnosis of Menkes disease in the neonatal period. The slow increase in serum ceruloplasmin concentration in the first year of life parallels the onset of biliary copper excretion and represents a steady increase in the capacity of the liver for holoceruloplasmin synthesis.

Excess. Copper toxicosis may result from intentional or accidental ingestion and under such circumstances free copper levels are greatly increased in the plasma.[29] Accidental poisoning in young children is associated with circulatory collapse following gastrointestinal damage and bleeding. Because the liver has a marked capacity to excrete copper, chronic copper toxicosis is rare. However, in individuals with liver disease a moderate increase in copper intake may result in copper accumulation when biliary excretion is impaired. Because any process that interrupts biliary flow will result in hepatic copper accumulation, the precise role of copper in subsequent hepatic injury is unclear. However, copper can result in free-radical–mediated damage, and it seems reasonable that such a process may occur once the mechanisms for hepatocyte copper sequestration have been surpassed. Evidence of lipid peroxidation and mitochondrial injury in experimental and clinical hepatic copper overload supports this hypothesis and suggests a potential therapeutic role for α-tocopherol and other antioxidants in situations of hepatic copper overload.[30,31]

Deficiency. The classical signs of copper deficiency, first carefully recorded in a series of malnourished infants in Peru, include hypocupremia, decreased serum ceruloplasmin concentration, neutropenia, anemia, metaphyseal dysplasia, osteoporosis, and fracture of the long bones.[32] Since those original studies, copper deficiency has been reported in various clinical situations where replacement of this metal was inadequate, including premature infants receiving total parenteral nutrition and patients undergoing peritoneal dialysis. Copper deficiency also has been observed in persons treated with large doses of zinc for sickle cell disease or as part of a megavitamin regimen. The signs and symptoms of copper deficiency are similar to those observed in patients with Menkes disease and for the most part can be explained by impaired activity of the well-characterized copper enzymes.[33,34] However, myeloid arrest resulting in neutropenia, consistently observed in copper deficiency, is not found in Menkes disease and cannot be explained by a loss of activity of any currently known cuproenzyme. Furthermore, the neurologic symptoms observed in patients with Menkes disease are not found in nutritional copper deficiency, supporting the concept that these features of Menkes disease are the result of copper deficiency *in utero*. Taken together, these observations suggest that further studies are needed to elucidate the role of copper in myelopoiesis and fetal brain development.

Copper Proteins

Enzymes. Elucidation of the function of the copper-dependent enzymes has come through examination of inherited deficiencies in humans and transgenic animals (Table 126-1). Ceruloplasmin is a ferroxidase that plays an essential role in iron homeostasis. Copper serves as an important metal in two enzymes with roles in antioxidant defense, intracellular copper zinc superoxide dismutase (SOD1),[35,36] and extracellular copper zinc superoxide dismutase (SOD3).[37–39] In mice, a deletion in the gene encoding SOD1 leads to sensitivity to paraquat and defects in neuronal regeneration,[40,41] whereas deletion of the gene encoding SOD3 leads to enhanced sensitivity to oxygen toxicity.[42] No deficiency of these enzymes has been described in humans. Cytochrome c oxidase is a multimeric enzyme that plays an essential role in mitochondrial electron transport.[43] The subunits containing copper-binding sites are encoded in the mitochondria. Defects in cytochrome c oxidase function are found in a number of inherited encephalomyopathies.[44] Dopamine β-hydroxylase converts dopamine to norepinephrine and in mice is essential for *in utero* survival and normal maternal behavior.[45,46] Consistent with the role of norepinephrine in regulation of metabolic rate, dopamine β-hydroxylase deficiency in humans is associated with hypotension, hypoglycemia, and hypothermia.[47,48] Peptidylglycine α-amidating monoxygenase is required for the C-terminal amidation of peptide hormones and neurotransmitters.[49,50] This biochemical

Table 126-1 Human Copper Proteins

Name	Chromosomal Location	Function	Deficiency
Enzymes			
Ceruloplasmin	3q23-25	Ferroxidase	Diabetes, retinal and basal ganglia degeneration secondary to iron accumulation
Copper/zinc superoxide dismutase	21q22.1	Disproportionation of superoxide anions	Paraquat sensitivity and neuronal degeneration
Extracellular copper/zinc superoxide dismutase	4pter-q21	Disproportionation of superoxide anions	Sensitivity to oxygen with pulmonary injury
Cytochrome c oxidase	mtDNA	Electron transport in respiratory chain	Mitochondrial myopathies
MTC01 (CuB)	5904-7444		Encephalomyelopathy
MTC02 (CuA)	7586-8294		
Dopamine β-hydroxylase	9q34	Converts dopamine to norepinephrine	Hypotension, hypoglycemia, hypothermia, *in utero* demise, and impaired maternal behavior
Peptidylglycine α-amidating monoxygenase	5q14-21	Peptide amidation	Lethality in larval stage
Tyrosinase	11q14-21	Converts tyrosine to melanin	Absence of pigment in hair, skin, eyes, nystagmus, photophobia
Lysyl oxidase	5q23.3-31.2	Oxidative deamination of lysines in collagen and elastin	Laxity of skin and joints, wormian bones, hydroureter
Storage/transport proteins			
Metallothionein I (A,B,E,F,G);IIA	16q13	Copper storage via thiolate-metal bonds	Sensitivity to heavy metals
ATOX1 (HAH1)	5q32-33	Copper transport to secretory pathway ATPases	Defective cuproprotein biosynthesis in secretory pathway
CCS	11q13.1	Copper transport to copper/zinc superoxide dismutase (SOD1)	Aerobic sensitivity growth impairment
COX7		Copper transport to cytochrome oxidase	Impairment in oxidative phosphorylation
CTR1	9q31-32	High affinity copper uptake	Growth failure on limited copper
Menkes ATPase (ATP7A)	Xq13.3	Copper export	Menkes disease
Wilson ATPase (ATP7B)	13q14.3-q21.1	Copper export	Wilson disease

modification is necessary for full bioactivity of these peptides, and this enzyme has been shown to be essential for embryonic development in *Drosophila*.[51] Tyrosinase is required for the conversion of tyrosine to melanin. Deficiency of this enzyme results in oculocutaneous albinism with absence of pigment in hair, skin, and eyes, as well as nystagmus and photophobia.[52,53] Lysyl oxidase catalyzes the oxidative deamination of lysine in collagen and elastin and is therefore essential for the cross-linking of these proteins.[54–56] Deficiency of this enzyme results in laxity of the skin and joints, abnormal bone formation, and weakness of the connective tissue in arteries and parenchymal organs.[57] Most recently, a second multicopper oxidase with homology to ceruloplasmin has been identified at the murine sex-linked anemia locus. This membrane-bound enzyme termed hephaestin facilitates iron uptake in the gastrointestinal tract, potentially explaining the anemia associated with copper deficiency.[58] In addition to these well-characterized cuproenzymes, there is evidence that the intracellular enzyme S-adenosylhomocysteine hydrolase binds copper[59,60] and that coagulation factor VIII incorporates copper during biosynthesis.[61,62] However, the precise function of the copper moiety in these proteins remains unclear. Recent studies have identified a number of sequences in the human genome encoding the consensus motif necessary for formation of the copper amine oxidase cofactor topaquinone.[63] The specific function of these putative serum- and tissue-specific amino oxidases is at present unknown.[64–66] A number of genomic sequences also have been identified with homology to tyrosinase[67] and lysyl oxidase,[68–70] but the relationship of these to any functional cuproenzyme activity remains to be determined.

Storage and Transport Proteins. Metallothioneins are small intracellular proteins that are rich in cysteine residues and can coordinate the binding of multiple copper atoms.[12] A cluster of 16 genes encoding these metallothioneins is located on chromosome 16 and functionally divided into two groups, each of which includes several pseudogenes. Studies in transgenic mice reveal that these proteins have no essential role in development or metal metabolism.[10,11] However, experiments in which metallothionein-deficient mice were mated with mottled Menkes-deficient mice demonstrate a critical role for these proteins in metal sequestration when copper homeostasis is perturbed.[71] Presumably, metallothioneins could play a similar role in hepatocytes, mitigating the effects of copper accumulation in Wilson disease.

A series of genetic studies in *S. cerevisiae* have revealed that the delivery of copper to specific pathways within the cell is mediated by a group of intracellular proteins termed copper- or

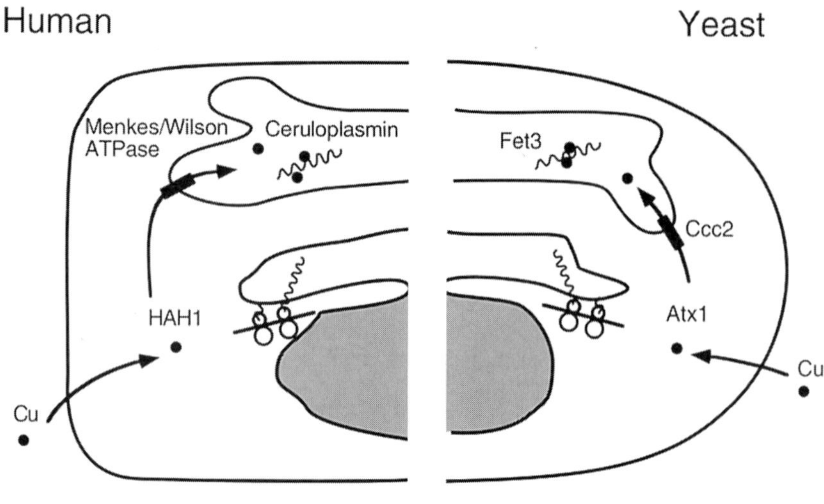

HAH1	Copper Chaperone	ATX1
Menkes/Wilson	Copper Transporter	CCC2
Ceruloplasmin	Essential Ferroxidase	FET3

Fig. 126-3 Evolutionary conservation of the pathways and proteins involved in copper transport into the secretory pathway of yeast and human cells.

metallochaperones.[72] ATX1 encodes a small cytosolic copper-binding protein in *Saccharomyces*, originally identified as a multicopy suppressor of *sod1Δ* mutants.[73] This protein delivers copper to the yeast Menkes/Wilson homologue CCC2 for subsequent transport into the secretory pathway and incorporation into the multicopper oxidase FET3 required for high-affinity iron uptake.[74] The identification of a homologous gene in humans termed *HAH1* has defined a role for this chaperone in mammalian cells and revealed a remarkable evolutionary conservation in the pathways of intracellular copper metabolism[75,76] (Fig. 126-3). Biochemical studies indicate that copper delivery by ATX1 is accomplished via direct protein–protein interaction with CCC2.[77]

Studies in *S. cerevisiae* also have revealed the presence of a small intracellular protein termed COX17, which is essential for the delivery of copper to cytochrome c oxidase in the mitochondria.[78] Absence of this protein leads to impairment in oxidative phosphorylation, and in vitro studies reveal that multiple copper moieties may be bound by COX17.[79] Genetic studies indicate that at least two additional proteins are essential in this copper delivery pathway.[80] A human orthologue of COX17 has been identified, and although no genetic abnormalities of hCOX17 have yet been reported in humans,[81] defects in this pathway might be predicted to be found in the population of patients with mitochondrial myopathies and deficient cytochrome c oxidase activity but lacking mutations in the genes encoding cytochrome c oxidase.

A third copper chaperone, LYS7, has been identified in *S. cerevisiae* and was shown to be essential for the delivery of copper to SOD1.[82] The absence of LYS7 in yeast leads to aerobic sensitivity and marked growth impairment due to the loss of SOD1 activity. A homologous protein in humans termed CCS (copper chaperone for SOD1) can functionally replace LYS7, suggesting that this protein has a similar function in mammalian cells.[82,83] Biochemical studies reveal a marked homology between CCS and its target enzyme SOD1, and in vitro and in vivo studies indicate that copper delivery by CCS to this enzyme is mediated by direct protein–protein interaction dependent on these regions of homology.[84] Gain-of-function mutations in SOD1 have been shown to be responsible for a subset of cases of familial amyotrophic lateral sclerosis.[85,86] Although the mechanism underlying the toxicity of these mutant SOD1 molecules has not been defined, evidence to date supports the role of the bound copper ion. Therefore, manipulation of CCS may represent a novel approach for interrupting copper delivery to this enzyme in such affected patients. Genetic abnormalities in CCS may underlie cases of familial amyotrophic lateral sclerosis where mutations in SOD1 are not present.

Amino acid sequence analysis of the copper chaperones HAH1 and CCS reveals the presence of a single copy of the amino acid sequence MXCXXC in the N-terminal region of each protein. This motif is also present in the N-terminus of the Wilson and Menkes copper transporters, where it has been shown to bind copper in vitro and in vivo.[87,88] Solution structure of this domain in the Menkes protein as well as structure–function studies on the homologous MXCXXC motif in ATX1 and HAH1 reveal a novel linear bicoordinate copper-binding environment capable of rapidly transferring copper.[76,77,89] These findings are consistent with the proposed copper-capturing function of this motif in the copper-transporting ATPases and with observations in yeast, which indicate that the homologous MXCXXC motifs on the yeast copper transporter CCC2 are the site of interaction with ATX1 and copper transfer between these two proteins.[77]

Taken together with the characterization of the Wilson and Menkes genes, the identification of these copper chaperone proteins has permitted the development of a working model of intracellular copper metabolism[90] (Fig. 126-2). Copper in the extracellular space, presumably bound to histidine, is transported across the plasma membrane by h*CTR1*. Once within the cell, copper is distributed between a storage compartment using metallothionein and the various copper chaperones functioning to deliver copper to specific targets. The Wilson and Menkes ATPases reside in the *trans*-Golgi network and transport copper into the secretory pathway for subsequent incorporation into the cuproenzymes tyrosinase, dopamine β-hydroxylase, peptidylglycine α-amidating monoxygenase, lysyl oxidase, SOD3, and ceruloplasmin, as well as for excretion from the cell. Although many details remain unclear, including the factors that determine the distribution of intracellular copper following uptake, the elucidation of this model of cellular copper metabolism provides a molecular blueprint for understanding the pathogenesis of the inherited disorders of copper transport.

WILSON DISEASE

Genetics

Wilson Disease Gene. Wilson disease is an autosomal-recessive disorder resulting in hepatic cirrhosis and neuronal degeneration.

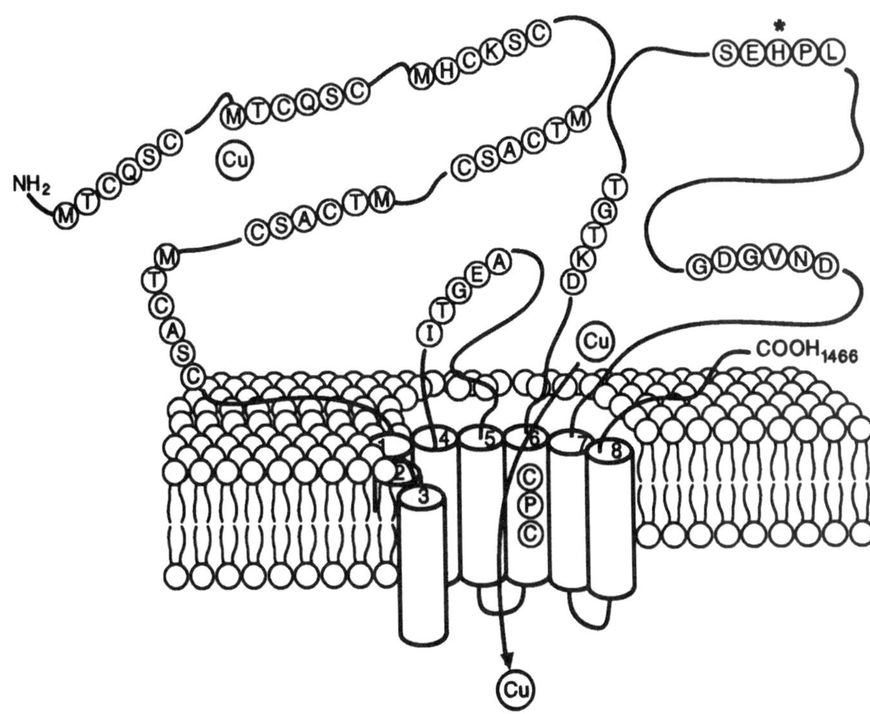

Fig. 126-4 Structural model of the Wilson ATPase in the *trans*-Golgi membrane with conserved functional motifs also present in the homologous Menkes ATPase. Asterisk indicates the conserved histidine, which is the site of the most common mutation in Wilson disease. (*Modified with permission from Payne and Gitlin.*[169])

Although sporadic reports of a similar clinical syndrome appeared in the literature as early as 1850, this disease was recognized as a distinct clinical entity in 1912 by Samuel Alexander Kinnear Wilson, who reported several cases of a new familial disorder resulting in progressive degeneration of the lenticular nuclei invariably associated with hepatic cirrhosis at autopsy.[91] Wilson disease is observed in all ethnic groups and occurs worldwide, with an estimated frequency of 1 in 30,000 individuals and a carrier rate of 1 in 90.[92,93] This frequency is increased in populations from regions of the world where consanguinity was once a more common practice. In 1985, analysis of one such kindred established linkage of the Wilson disease gene to the esterase D locus on chromosome 13.[94]

In 1993, the Wilson disease gene was cloned and shown to encode a novel member of the family of cation-transporting P-type ATPases.[95–97] Sequence comparison and hydropathy analysis of the derived amino acid sequence of the Wilson protein reveals a polytopic membrane protein predicted to transport copper across the lipid bilayer in an ATP-dependent manner (Fig. 126-4). Homologous copper-transporting P-type ATPases have now been identified in a wide variety of prokaryotic and eukaryotic species.[98,99] The Wilson protein contains a number of amino acid motifs characteristic of such ATPases including MXCXXC copper-binding sequences in the N-terminus, a transmembrane CPC thought to be essential for metal transfer across the membrane, an ITGEA phosphatase domain, a conserved DKTGT sequence that is the site of the aspartyl-phosphate intermediate essential for energy transduction, and a GDGVND sequence forming the ATP-binding domain (Fig. 126-4). In addition to these well-defined functional motifs, a highly conserved sequence, SEHPL, is found proximal to the ATP-binding domain. The histidine residue in this sequence, conserved among all known copper-transporting P-type ATPases,[100] is the site of the most common disease mutation (*H1069Q*) in patients with Wilson disease.[101] Although polymerase chain amplification studies suggest the possibility of tissue-specific splicing of the Wilson disease gene, the only isoform of the Wilson protein identified thus far is a truncated species of unknown function generated by alternate promoter usage in the rat pineal gland.[102,102a]

Mutations. The Wilson disease gene is encoded by 21 exons spanning more than 60 kb on chromosome 13q14.3. Analysis of patient mutations reveals an enormous molecular heterogeneity consisting of a very small number of frequent mutations that are population specific, as well as a much greater number of rare individual alleles. To date almost 100 different mutations have been characterized in Wilson disease patients from varying ethnic origins.[103–113] Of these, more than half are missense mutations occurring in transmembrane domains or the ATP-binding region. The remainder of the characterized mutations consist of small deletions or insertions (25 percent), splice site abnormalities (10 percent), and nonsense mutations (10 percent). The inability to identify a specific mutation in about 20 percent of examined alleles suggests the presence of mutations in upstream regions controlling transcription of the Wilson disease gene.[101] Of the common mutations, *H1069Q* accounts for about 40 percent of the alleles in populations of Northern European origin.[101] Similarly, *A778L*, a common missense mutation in transmembrane domain 4, has been identified in up to 30 percent of the alleles in Asian populations.[110,114]

At first pass it is reasonable to assume that the degree of allelic heterogeneity at the Wilson locus might account, at least in part, for the enormous clinical variability observed in patients with Wilson disease. However, as expected from the large number of different mutations, the majority of affected individuals are compound heterozygotes, making it difficult to study any correlation between genotype and clinical phenotype. Nevertheless, such studies have been conducted in individuals homozygous for the *H1069Q* mutation, and the results revealed no correlation between this mutation and the age of onset, clinical manifestations, biochemical markers of disease, or disease activity in affected patients.[111] These findings are consistent with the observation of marked clinical variation among affected sibs, and even identical twins, and supports the notion that additional genetic and environmental factors may significantly influence the outcome of a given disease mutation at the Wilson locus.[115] Although it remains possible that specific mutations such as those leading to variations in splicing may result in a less severe clinical phenotype owing to the presence of residual functional protein, no data are currently available on the abundance of the Wilson protein in tissues from such patients.

Pathogenesis. The Wilson disease gene encodes a 7.5-kb transcript that is abundantly expressed in the human liver.[95–97]

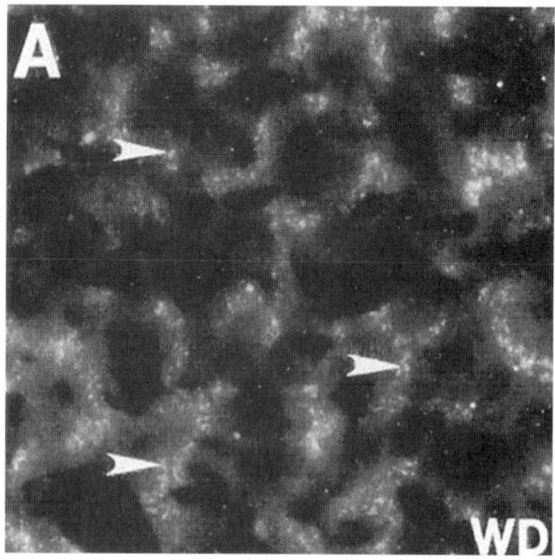

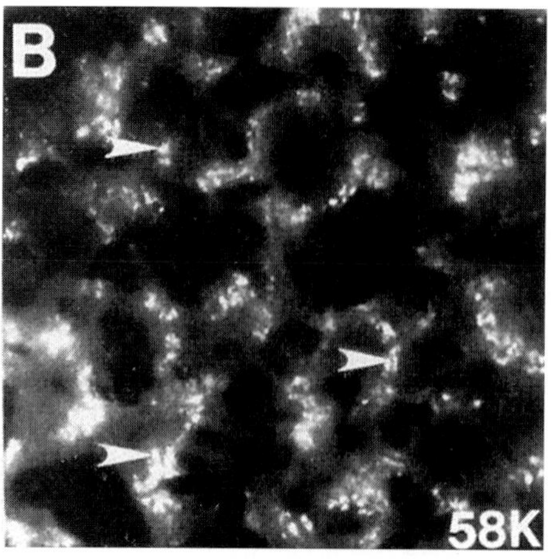

Fig. 126-5 Immunofluorescent colocalization of the Wilson protein (*A*) and the *trans*-Golgi 58-kDa marker (*B*) in the human liver. Arrowheads focus on regions of colocalization within hepatocytes.

Polyclonal antisera generated against the N-terminus of the Wilson ATPase detect a 165-kDa protein that is synthesized in hepatocytes as a single-chain polypeptide localized to the *trans*-Golgi network[22] (Fig. 126-5). Mutations resulting in the absence or dysfunction of the Wilson protein interrupt the transport of copper into the secretory pathway, interfering with holoceruloplasmin synthesis and biliary copper excretion. In support of this model, expression of wild-type but not mutant Wilson proteins in the *ccc2Δ* strain of *S. cerevisiae* restores copper incorporation into the multicopper oxidase FET3,[116] providing direct evidence of copper transport by the Wilson protein.[22]

Although the yeast system is useful to directly evaluate the effect of specific mutations on the copper transport function of the Wilson protein, observations on the cell biology of this ATPase suggest a greater complexity to the pathogenesis of the disease. In normal individuals, an increase in the intracellular copper concentration of the hepatocytes results in translocation of the Wilson protein to a cytoplasmic vesicular compartment. As copper is transported into this compartment by the Wilson ATPase, cytoplasmic copper content decreases, resulting in the redistribution of the protein to the *trans*-Golgi network. This process is rapid and independent of new protein synthesis, providing a mechanism for immediate response of the Wilson protein to changes in the steady-state intracellular copper concentration[22,28] (Fig. 126-6). Analogous to what has been observed in cystic fibrosis,[117] patient mutations might be predicted to affect Wilson protein function not only at the level of transporter activity, but also through alteration of amino acids necessary for proper localization of the transport

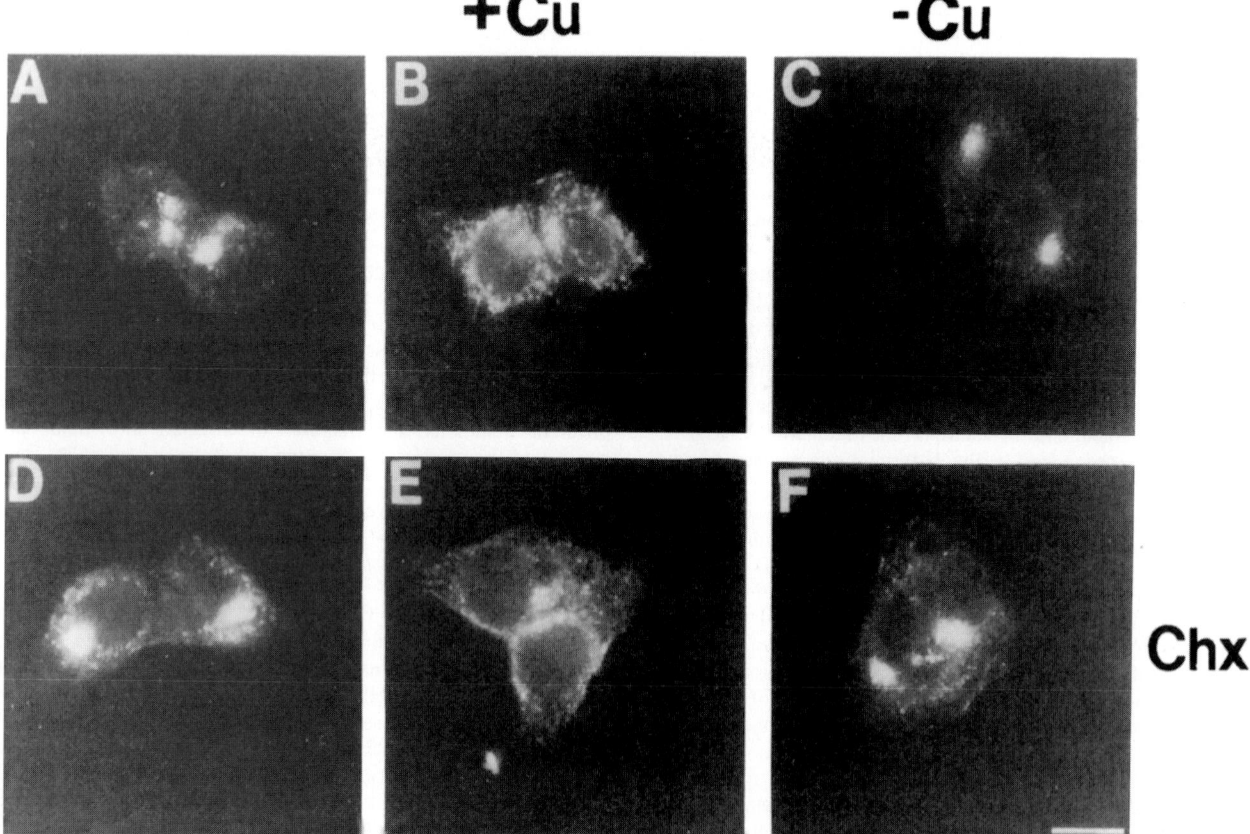

Fig. 126-6 Immunofluorescent detection of the copper-mediated recycling of the Wilson protein in HepG2 cells incubated in calf serum alone (*A and D*), or in the presence of excess copper (*B and E*) or the copper chelator bathocupronine disulfonate (*C and F*). In some experiments (*D–F*), cells were preincubated with cycloheximide prior to incubation. (*Reprinted with permission from Hung et al.*[22])

protein to a specific compartment. In the case of the Wilson protein, mutations also may affect responsiveness to intracellular copper concentrations. In support of this paradigm, expression of the wild-type Wilson protein and the *H1069Q* mutant in a Menkes copper transporter–deficient mottled fibroblast cell line revealed that the *H1069Q* mutation causes a temperature-sensitive defect in protein folding, resulting in mislocalization and rapid degradation of the mutant protein in the endoplasmic reticulum.[118,118a] Additional genetic and environmental factors affecting one or more of these steps are likely candidates to explain the clinical heterogeneity of Wilson disease. Although heterozygotes do not develop signs and symptoms of Wilson disease, the paradigm presented above also raises the possibility that the presence of certain specific single mutant alleles may increase the susceptibility of the liver to damage in other more common liver disorders such as alcoholic cirrhosis.[119]

Animal Models. A spontaneously arising mutant strain, the Long Evans Cinnamon (LEC) rat, develops hepatitis in association with elevated hepatic copper content, decreased serum ceruloplasmin concentration, and impaired biliary copper excretion.[120,121] LEC rats lack expression of the rat orthologue of the Wilson disease gene due to an extensive intragenic deletion, and these rodents are therefore considered to be a bona fide animal model of Wilson disease.[122,123] Most LEC rats present with acute hepatitis accompanied by jaundice, hemolytic anemia, and fulminant liver failure, with survivors progressing to chronic hepatitis and cirrhosis.[124] The hepatic copper toxicosis in LEC rats is responsive to penicillamine chelation therapy,[125] and holoceruloplasmin biosynthesis can be restored by adenovirally mediated expression of the human Wilson disease gene in vivo,[126] making it likely that this rodent model will be useful in further understanding the pathogenesis and treatment of Wilson disease. In contrast to humans, hepatocellular carcinoma is a common event in the LEC rat and appears to be related to a concomitant disturbance in hepatic iron homeostasis.[127]

The "toxic milk mouse" was originally identified by the observation that newborn mice from affected mothers are copper deficient when suckled on their mother's milk.[128] Although neonatal copper deficiency is not observed in the children of women with Wilson disease, adult toxic milk mice do develop progressive liver disease in association with elevated hepatic copper content and decreased serum ceruloplasmin concentration. An *M1356V* missense mutation in a highly conserved methionine in the eighth transmembrane domain of the murine orthologue of the Wilson disease gene in these mice suggests that this strain is also a model of Wilson disease although no functional data on this mutation is currently available.[129] Presumably the unique phenotypic differences in this murine model reflect species-specific environmental and genetic factors that considerably modify disease presentation in comparison with that observed in LEC rats and humans.

Diagnosis

Clinical Features. Although the signs and symptoms of Wilson disease can be protean, the overwhelming majority of patients present with hepatic or neuropsychiatric disease.[92,115] The diverse clinical manifestations of Wilson disease require alertness to the possibility of this diagnosis in any patient with unusual symptoms and tests indicating abnormal hepatic function.[93] Liver dysfunction is the most common initial manifestation of Wilson disease in children.[130] Patients presenting with hepatic disease usually do so at an average age of 10 to 13 years, which is at least 10 years earlier than those initially presenting with neurologic symptoms. Nevertheless, there is considerable overlap, and individual patients have presented with hepatic disease as late as the sixth decade of life. The manifestations of liver disease range from asymptomatic individuals with mild elevation of serum transaminases to chronic active hepatitis and cirrhosis.[131] In some cases the presentation may be fulminant hepatic failure, suggesting that a viral illness or other external factor has triggered the abrupt onset of hepatic degeneration in the copper-loaded liver. Such a fulminant presentation is more common in women and frequently is accompanied by hemolytic anemia due to excess copper abruptly released into the bloodstream.[132] Hepatocellular carcinoma is a rare consequence of cirrhosis in Wilson disease. Regardless of the presenting symptoms, most patients will have evidence of cirrhosis on liver biopsy as a result of many years of hepatocyte copper accumulation prior to clinical symptoms. Initially such biopsy samples may reveal micronodular cirrhosis with variable copper deposition throughout the lobules, but as symptoms worsen, the histology progresses to that of chronic hepatitis with nodular regeneration.[133] The eventual hepatocyte dysfunction from copper overload results in cell death, with release of copper into the bloodstream.[134]

Although neuropsychiatric symptoms are also common at presentation, occurring in upward of 60 percent of all patients, such individuals are generally older than those presenting with liver disease and are most often diagnosed in the third or fourth decade of life. Neurologic manifestations include Parkinsonian symptoms with marked diminution in facial expressions and movement, pseudosclerotic patients with tremors resembling those of multiple sclerosis, and dystonic individuals with hypertonicity and choreoathetosis.[135] These clinical symptoms reflect the changes in the basal ganglia observed at autopsy, which include cavitary degeneration, gliosis, and neuronal loss. The presence of copper in these brain regions as well as specific structural changes can be detected by neuroimaging techniques, which at times may be useful in diagnosis.[136] The mechanisms resulting in the specific involvement of the basal ganglia as well as relative sparing of the motor and sensory cortex in patients with Wilson disease, despite a diffuse increase in copper throughout the central nervous system, are unknown.

Isolated or combined psychiatric illness also may occur in patients with Wilson disease and can include abnormal behavior, personality changes, depression, and marked impairment in cognition with evidence of schizophrenia.[137,138] These neuropsychiatric symptoms are also the result of copper accumulation, although little or no information is available as to the mechanisms leading to specific brain dysfunction in such cases. Because patients initially presenting with psychiatric symptoms will eventually progress to the development of neurologic degeneration and hepatic failure, awareness of Wilson disease as a potential cause of such symptoms is essential to early diagnosis and treatment.

As with hepatic and neuropsychiatric manifestations, signs and symptoms in patients with Wilson disease may arise in any organ in which excess copper is deposited.[115] Such copper often may be detected in the limbus of the cornea by slit-lamp examination (Kayser-Fleischer rings). This finding, frequently present in patients with neuropsychiatric disease, is not pathognomonic and occurs in individuals with increased serum copper resulting from other disorders such as cholestatic liver disease. Similarly, excess copper may occasionally be detected as azure lunulae in the fingernails. Less common clinical manifestations related to copper toxicosis include Fanconi syndrome with aminoaciduria, nephrolithiasis, cardiac dysrhythmias, arthritis and arthralgias, rhabdomyolysis, hemolytic anemia, hypoparathyroidism, and amenorrhea. These symptoms are reversed by systemic chelation therapy, confirming the etiology as copper accumulation rather than any associated hepatic disease.[92,115]

Laboratory Findings. The diagnosis of Wilson disease is based on clinical signs and symptoms in correlation with tests that can detect abnormalities of copper metabolism. Careful diagnostic evaluation should be performed in any individual with isolated elevated serum transaminases, chronic active hepatitis of undetermined etiology, Kayser-Fleischer rings, unexplained psychiatric symptoms including sudden behavioral changes in childhood, or basal ganglia abnormalities on neuroimaging. In patients with

Wilson disease, an inability to efficiently transfer copper into the secretory pathway of hepatocytes results in serum ceruloplasmin concentrations that are generally decreased well below normal values (20 mg/dl) owing to secretion and rapid degradation of the apoprotein. Because ceruloplasmin is an acute-phase reactant, the synthesis of this protein will increase during infection or inflammation, so the serum ceruloplasmin concentration may be in the normal range in some 5 percent of patients.[139] However, in such cases analysis of the ceruloplasmin oxidase activity will reveal that this is circulating apoprotein devoid of copper.[140] Urinary copper concentrations may be elevated (often >100 μg Cu/24 h) and are a cost-effective way of screening individuals. In all cases where it is possible, a liver biopsy should be performed for accurate quantitative measurement of hepatic copper concentration. The normal copper concentration in liver is often increased in affected patients (>250 μg/g dry wt) but it should be remembered that hepatic copper concentration also can be elevated in any condition in which biliary copper excretion is impaired. The measurement of hepatic copper concentration generally permits a definitive diagnosis to be made because even presymptomatic individuals will have elevated levels at the time of diagnosis. Occasionally, when the serum ceruloplasmin concentration is in the normal range and liver biopsy is contraindicated, an oral radioactive copper loading test may be helpful to demonstrate the lack of holoceruloplasmin biosynthesis.[93,140]

Based on physical examination, slit-lamp examination, and laboratory data, the diagnosis of Wilson disease can be made with accuracy in the majority of patients. Nevertheless, the wide range of age of onset and variable symptomatology can make a diagnosis difficult. Although direct molecular diagnosis is problematic due to the degree of molecular heterogeneity at the Wilson locus, analysis for common mutations in patients of specific ethnic origins may be useful.[141] Such analysis is complicated by the fact that most patients will be compound heterozygotes carrying two different mutations of the gene. The identification of unusual haplotypes in affected family members with Wilson disease also may lend support to the diagnosis of this disorder in circumstances where family studies can be used.[101] In such cases these may be followed up by direct identification of the mutation in affected individuals.

Screening. Given the low heterozygote frequency and the lack of a useful biochemical marker in the newborn period, screening for Wilson disease is confined to sibs and first-degree relatives of affected patients.[119] Careful history and physical examination along with ophthalmologic studies and measurement of serum ceruloplasmin, liver transaminases, and urinary copper excretion should be performed. Such an evaluation may suggest the diagnosis of Wilson disease in asymptomatic individuals and may support the need for liver biopsy. In individuals heterozygous for Wilson disease, the results of this evaluation will be entirely normal, with the exception of the serum ceruloplasmin concentration, which may be decreased in 20 percent of heterozygotes. In those cases where the proband mutation has been identified, direct molecular screening can offer a rapid approach to diagnosis. Reproductive genetic counseling should be offered to all identified carriers.

Differential Diagnosis. Indian childhood cirrhosis is a disorder of progressive liver failure in young children associated with marked hepatic copper overload (>800 μg/g dry wt) and hepatocellular necrosis.[142,143] Serum ceruloplasmin concentrations in affected children are always elevated, suggesting impairment in biliary copper excretion at a step beyond the entry of copper into the hepatocyte secretory pathway. This disorder is confined to India and appears to result from increased dietary copper consumption in genetically susceptible individuals; a history of consanguinity and repetitive use of brass and copper cooking vessels is usually present.[143] Consistent with this concept, studies of excess dietary copper intake in otherwise normal individuals reveal no evidence of hepatic copper accumulation or liver disease.[144] Similar disorders termed idiopathic copper toxicosis, endemic Tyrolean cirrhosis, and non-Indian childhood cirrhosis also have been reported and here also epidemiologic studies suggest a combination of genetic and environmental factors in disease pathogenesis.[145,146] Hepatic copper concentrations also may be elevated in cholestatic liver disease, but in these conditions serum ceruloplasmin is elevated, indicating a defect late in the copper excretory pathway.

Treatment

Chelation. The goal of treatment in Wilson disease is to restore normal copper homeostasis through systemic chelation therapy directed at removing or detoxifying accumulated copper. D-penicillamine is the treatment of choice for systemic chelation therapy.[115] The precise mechanism by which penicillamine results in detoxification and elimination of copper remains unclear. Long-term treatment promotes urinary copper excretion and is effective for prophylaxis in presymptomatic patients. Long-term evaluation with neuroimaging often reveals a decrease in copper-related abnormalities, which correlates with clinical improvement.[147,148] Therapy is initiated with a small test dose that if tolerated is then given orally in four divided doses. Penicillamine is taken an hour before eating to prevent chelation with food, and a gradual response in symptoms should occur within the first several months of therapy. If improvement does not ensue, the dose may be increased twofold. Although most patients will become asymptomatic within 4 months after starting penicillamine, occasionally neurologic symptoms may worsen, presumably as a result of increased deposition of mobilized hepatic copper within brain tissue. Once improvement has occurred and decreased total body copper content has been demonstrated, patients should be placed on maintenance therapy at half the initial dose. Assuring compliance with therapy is essential because rapid deterioration can occur following the abrupt discontinuation of penicillamine related to the sudden release of copper from sites where this metal was sequestered in a nontoxic form.[93]

Urinalysis and complete blood counts should be followed at regular intervals in all patients taking penicillamine because hypersensitivity reactions, including fever, lymphadenopathy, and blood dyscrasias, may occur in up to 20 percent of patients. Although these side effects are dose related and can be controlled with corticosteroids, autoimmune symptoms are an indication to discontinue therapy immediately. In such cases, triethylenetetramine dihydrochloride (trientine) is a reasonable alternative therapy.[149,150] Trientine may be taken orally at a dose of 1 to 2 g divided before meals, and although it is a somewhat less effective copper chelating agent, significant improvement has been reported in a number of patients. Neither chelating agent has been reported to have teratogenic effects in humans, and both drugs have been used successfully in pregnant women with Wilson disease.[151]

Adjunct Therapies. The treatment of patients with Wilson disease also should include prevention by dietary restriction of foods rich in copper, such as nuts, liver, chocolate, and shellfish. Absorption of copper also can be limited by the oral administration of zinc salts. The presumed effect of such treatment is the induction of metallothionein within the enterocyte, with subsequent intracellular chelation of copper impairing absorption.[131] Ammonium tetrathiomolybdate also may be used as an adjunct in preventing copper toxicity. Thiomolybdate forms complexes with copper in the diet, resulting in nontoxic complexes of copper within the plasma and tissues. However, the toxicity of molybdate, including bone marrow suppression, has thus far limited the usefulness of this approach in most patients.[92]

Transplantation. Orthotopic liver transplantation is the treatment of choice in individuals with progressive hepatic insufficiency who do not respond to systemic chelation therapy.[93] In addition, this approach is the only reasonable option in patients presenting with fulminant hepatitis. In both cases, patients fare well, with 1-year survival rates exceeding 80 percent in most studies. Hepatic transplantation will result in complete normalization of copper homeostasis within 6 months and usually results in sustained improvement in symptoms.[152] Although many of the neurologic deficits as well as psychiatric symptoms in patients with Wilson disease may resolve following liver transplantation, refractory neurologic disease alone is not currently considered an appropriate criterion for hepatic transplantation.[93]

MENKES DISEASE

Genetics

Menkes Disease Gene. Menkes disease is an X-linked disorder resulting in severe growth failure and profound neurodegeneration in early childhood. The disease was first described in 1962 by John Menkes, who reported on an affected kindred with failure to thrive, peculiar hair, and cerebellar degeneration.[153] In his original study, Menkes noted that this disorder segregated as an X-linked recessive trait, an observation that has since been confirmed in multiple affected kindreds. A decade later, David Danks discovered a defect in copper absorption in affected children, explaining the pleiotropic features of the disease.[154] The occurrence of Menkes disease is rare, with an estimated incidence of 1 in every 250,000 live births.[9] At least a third of such cases represent new mutations occurring in patients with no previous family history. Physical mapping of the Menkes disease gene was accomplished by analysis of a balanced translocation in an affected female that localized the break point to Xq13.2-13.3.[155,156] In 1993, the Menkes disease gene was identified by positional cloning and shown to encode a predicted protein sequence with marked similarity to a cation-transporting P-type ATPase essential for copper homeostasis in *Enterococcus hirae*.[157–159] These important studies, which were the first to identify any mammalian copper transporter and led to cloning of the homologous Wilson disease gene, provide a compelling example of Archibald Garrod's tenet of the lessons of rare maladies.

Mutations. The Menkes disease gene is encoded by 23 exons spanning approximately 140 kb on the X chromosome.[160,161] The spectrum of mutations at the Menkes locus is complex and ranges from easily detectable cytogenetic abnormalities to single-base-pair substitutions.[162] As has been observed for other X-linked disorders, most of these mutations are unique to each affected family. The majority of genetic defects identified thus far in patients with Menkes disease involve very small insertions and deletions (35 percent), nonsense mutations (20 percent), splicing abnormalities (15 percent), and missense mutations (8 percent).[163–165] Approximately 20 percent of mutations in patients with Menkes disease are large deletions or rearrangements that can be readily identified by Southern blot analysis. Detectable cytogenic chromosomal abnormalities account for about 1 to 2 percent of mutations in Menkes disease and consist predominantly of balanced translocations occurring in affected females. Patients with similar but much milder clinical symptoms, including those with the occipital horn syndrome, also have been found to have nucleotide substitutions in the Menkes gene, indicating that allelic heterogeneity at this locus accounts for the observed clinical variability.[164]

Pathogenesis. The Menkes disease gene encodes an 8.0-kb transcript that is expressed in all tissues except the liver.[157–159] The derived amino acid sequence of the Menkes protein is 55 percent identical to the Wilson protein, contains the same functional motifs as this ATPase, and is predicted to form an identical polytopic membrane structure (Fig. 126-4). The Menkes protein is synthesized as a single-chain 178-kDa polypeptide that

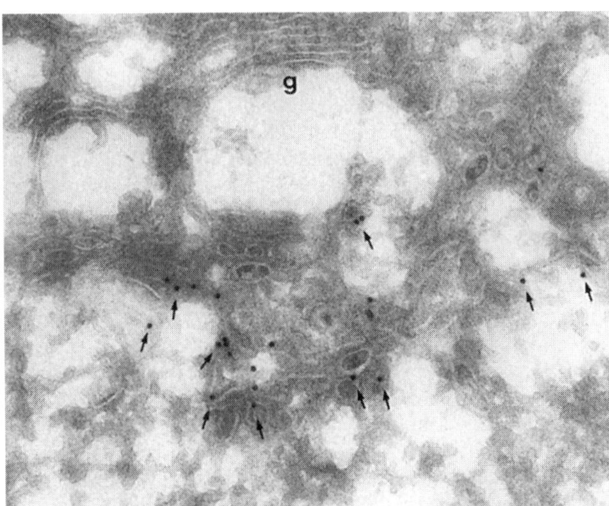

Fig. 126-7 Immunogold electron micrograph of transfected Chinese hamster ovary cells illustrating Menkes protein in the *trans*-Golgi and within vesicular structures. (*Modified with permission from LaFontaine et al.*[171])

is modified by N-linked glycosylation and localized to the *trans*-Golgi network.[166–168] In cells expressing the Menkes protein an increase in the intracellular copper concentration results in redistribution of this protein from the *trans*-Golgi network to a cytoplasmic vesicular compartment clearly visible by immunogold electron microscopy[168] (Fig. 126-7). Expression of the Menkes protein in *ccc2*Δ yeast restores copper incorporation into FET3 in the secretory pathway,[169] and overexpression of the Menkes protein in mammalian cell lines increases the resistance of these cells to extracellular copper.[170,171] These observations and direct evidence of copper transport to vesicles[171a] support the concept that the Menkes and Wilson proteins mediate cellular copper homeostasis by common biochemical mechanisms, transporting copper into the secretory pathway of the cell for subsequent cuproenzyme biosynthesis and copper excretion. In patients with Menkes disease, defective copper transfer into the secretory pathway of cells in the placenta, gastrointestinal tract, and blood–brain barrier results in copper accumulation within these tissues and generalized copper deficiency due to an inability to export copper from these sites into the blood and central nervous system.

Consistent with the severe phenotype observed in patients with Menkes disease, the majority of mutations at this locus would be predicted to completely interrupt transporter function. Nevertheless, milder forms of this disorder do occur, and mutation analysis in such cases has revealed splicing abnormalities and promoter region mutations, suggesting that the presence of residual Menkes protein accounts for the less severe phenotype.[164,172,173] In one well-studied example, a mutation at the splice donor site of exon 10 results in an in-frame deletion of the third and fourth transmembrane domains of the Menkes protein.[174] Interestingly, this alternatively spliced transcript is expressed at low abundance in normal individuals, and immunofluorescence studies in the patient's fibroblasts as well as in normal cells expressing this mutant protein reveal that this transmembrane region is essential for localization of the Menkes protein to the *trans*-Golgi network.[174,175] This finding suggests that variations in the subcellular distribution as well as changes in the abundance of the Menkes protein may result in differences in copper transport that are reflected in the severity of the patient phenotype.

In addition to the analysis of patient mutations, data relevant to the pathogenesis of Menkes disease have come from expression studies using site-directed mutagenesis. Mutation of a conserved histidine to glutamine (*H1086Q*) in the Menkes protein, homologous to the site of the common *H1069Q* mutation in Wilson disease, abrogates the copper transport function of this protein.

The finding that the most commonly occurring mutation in Wilson disease similarly compromises function of the Menkes protein provides further evidence for a commonality of transporter function.[169] Although the mechanisms by which the Menkes and Wilson proteins respond to intracellular copper concentrations remain unclear, expression studies of site-directed mutants of the Menkes protein in mammalian cells suggest that specific residues in the C-terminal cytoplasmic region are critical to this process.[176] Studies demonstrating that the relatively low level of expression of the human Wilson protein can rescue the murine Menkes mottled phenotype support the concept that residual Menkes protein expression in milder disease suffices to prevent the neurologic defects in affected patients.[118] These studies also provide compelling evidence that the molecular pathogenesis of these two diseases is the result of perturbation of identical pathways of cellular copper metabolism.

Animal Models. Variations in the coat color of female mice carrying the X-linked mottled (Mo) locus served as the basis for Mary Lyon's hypothesis of random inactivation of the X chromosome. A number of different alleles occur at the mottled locus, and male hemizygotes have a wide range of phenotypic characteristics, including pale hair, abnormal whiskers, tremor and inactivity, skeletal dysplasia, aortic aneurysms, and perinatal lethality.[24,177] As might be anticipated from these features, mottled mice have a disturbance of copper homeostasis,[178] and molecular analysis of the mottled locus has revealed mutations in the murine orthologue of the Menkes disease gene.[164,179,180] The blotchy mouse (Mo^{blo}) is a mildly affected mutant with abnormalities of connective tissue, and mutation analysis of this allele reveals a splicing defect resulting in partial skipping of exon 11, similar to what has been observed in a patient with occipital horn syndrome.[164,179] More severely affected alleles include brindled (Mo^{br}), viable brindled (Mo^{vbr}) and macular (Mo^{ml}), which show severe copper deficiency at birth with progressive neurologic disease and death by 2 weeks of age. Mutation analysis in these mice has revealed a two-amino-acid in-frame deletion in the cytoplasmic loop between the fourth and fifth transmembrane domains (Mo^{br}), a missense mutation, *K1036T*, in a conserved lysine in the *DKTGT* phosphorylation domain (Mo^{vbr}), and a missense mutation, *S1381P*, in the eighth transmembrane domain of the murine Menkes protein.[181–185]

These molecular studies in mottled mice are relevant to our understanding of the pathogenesis and treatment of Menkes disease. Curiously, administration of copper to the brindled mouse prior to the first week of life permits long-term survival of this animal, suggesting that residual activity of the mutant Menkes protein may be sufficient for the delivery of copper to the newborn mouse brain.[24] Because the administration of copper to the brindled mouse after the first week of life is no longer a successful treatment, these observations also imply the presence of a therapeutic window for copper delivery to the newborn brain. Taken together, these studies suggest that therapeutic approaches aimed at increasing the abundance of functional transporter *in utero* as well as the development of novel approaches to deliver copper directly to the affected fetus warrant further investigation.

Diagnosis

Clinical Features. The distinct clinical features of Menkes disease are present by 3 months of age and are often brought to attention in affected infants by the loss of developmental milestones and failure to thrive.[9,162,186–188] The typical-appearing infant has a cherubic face with pudgy cheeks, sagging jowls, and scant eyebrows (Fig. 126-8*A*). The hair is sparse, resembling steel wool, and on microscopy reveals twisting of the hair shaft (pili torti) as well as fractures and longitudinal splitting (Fig. 126-8*B*). The absence of tyrosinase activity leaves the hair lacking in pigment and appearing white or gray. Loss of lysyl oxidase activity results in connective tissue abnormalities, including wormian skull bones as well as radiographic evidence of osteoporosis and metaphyseal dysplasia, including anterior flaring and fracture of the ribs. As a result of connective tissue weakening, diverticula of the bladder, uterus, and other organs may be present. Vascular complications including aortic aneurysms are commonly present, and neuroimaging techniques reveal tortuosity of the intracranial blood vessels.[189] Histologic examination of these blood vessels reveals thinning of the connective tissue with disruption of the elastic lamina (Fig. 126-8*C*).

Eventually cerebral degeneration ensues, at least in part due to the loss of activity of cytochrome c oxidase, peptidyl α-amidating monoxygenase, and dopamine β-hydroxylase in the central nervous system. Magnetic resonance imaging reveals abnormal myelination and cerebral and cerebellar atrophy, in some cases as early as 5 weeks of age.[190,191] Autopsy of the brain demonstrates subdural hematomas with diffuse atrophy, focal degeneration of gray matter, and prominent neuronal loss in the cerebellum. Purkinje cells are frequently affected, showing abnormal arborization of dendrites and focal swelling of the axons (Fig. 126-8*D*). Not all of these neurologic problems can be explained by the loss of activity of the known copper enzymes, implying that additional cuproenzymes essential for brain development remain to be identified. Diagnosis may be difficult in the neonatal period until the more typical signs and symptoms appear. Premature delivery is common, and affected newborn infants frequently have hypothermia, hypoglycemia, hyperbilirubinemia, umbilical hernias, hypotonia, and seizures.[9,186] Central nervous system abnormalities become more prominent with time and include truncal hypotonia, abnormal head control, and hyperactive reflexes.

Although survival beyond childhood is rare, some children with profound neurologic deficits have survived for many years. In addition, several milder clinical variants have been described, including children who present somewhat later in infancy in whom ataxia and mild intellectual delay are the only neurologic features.[186,192] In the occipital horn syndrome, also known as X-linked cutis laxa or type IX Ehrlers-Danlos syndrome, affected patients have exostoses secondary to calcifications at the insertion sites of muscles attaching to the occiput as well as marked connective tissue abnormalities but little or no neurologic disease. The somewhat atypical presentation of these milder phenotypes suggests that any male infant with connective tissue abnormalities and mental retardation should be evaluated for the possibility of Menkes disease. Reports have appeared in the literature of individuals with clinical features similar to Menkes disease yet displaying differences in biochemical markers of copper absorption and metabolism. At this time it remains unclear if these represent variants of Menkes disease or distinct disorders that have yet to be completely characterized.[193–195]

Laboratory Findings. The marked copper deficiency in affected patients is reflected in very low serum ceruloplasmin and copper concentrations. However, these values are normally quite low in the neonatal period and are diagnostically useful in suspected cases only after the first several months of life. Copper deficiency results in a reduction in the activity of a number of copper-dependent enzymes as well as copper accumulation in tissues where copper export is impaired. The defect in copper export in Menkes disease can be detected by examining copper accumulation in cultured fibroblasts using radioactive copper.[196,197] This technique shows clear differences between affected and unaffected male infants, but does not distinguish between mildly and severely affected patients. Analysis of placental copper concentration, which is increased in affected patients, is often useful if the diagnosis is suspected in the newborn period. Deficiency of dopamine β-hydroxylase activity results in increased plasma and cerebrospinal fluid catecholamines reflective of impaired norepinephrine biosynthesis. Measurement of these metabolites also may be useful in confirming the diagnosis.[198,199] Prenatal diagnosis is possible by examining copper accumulation in cultured amniotic fluid cells, although the results of such studies are variable. First

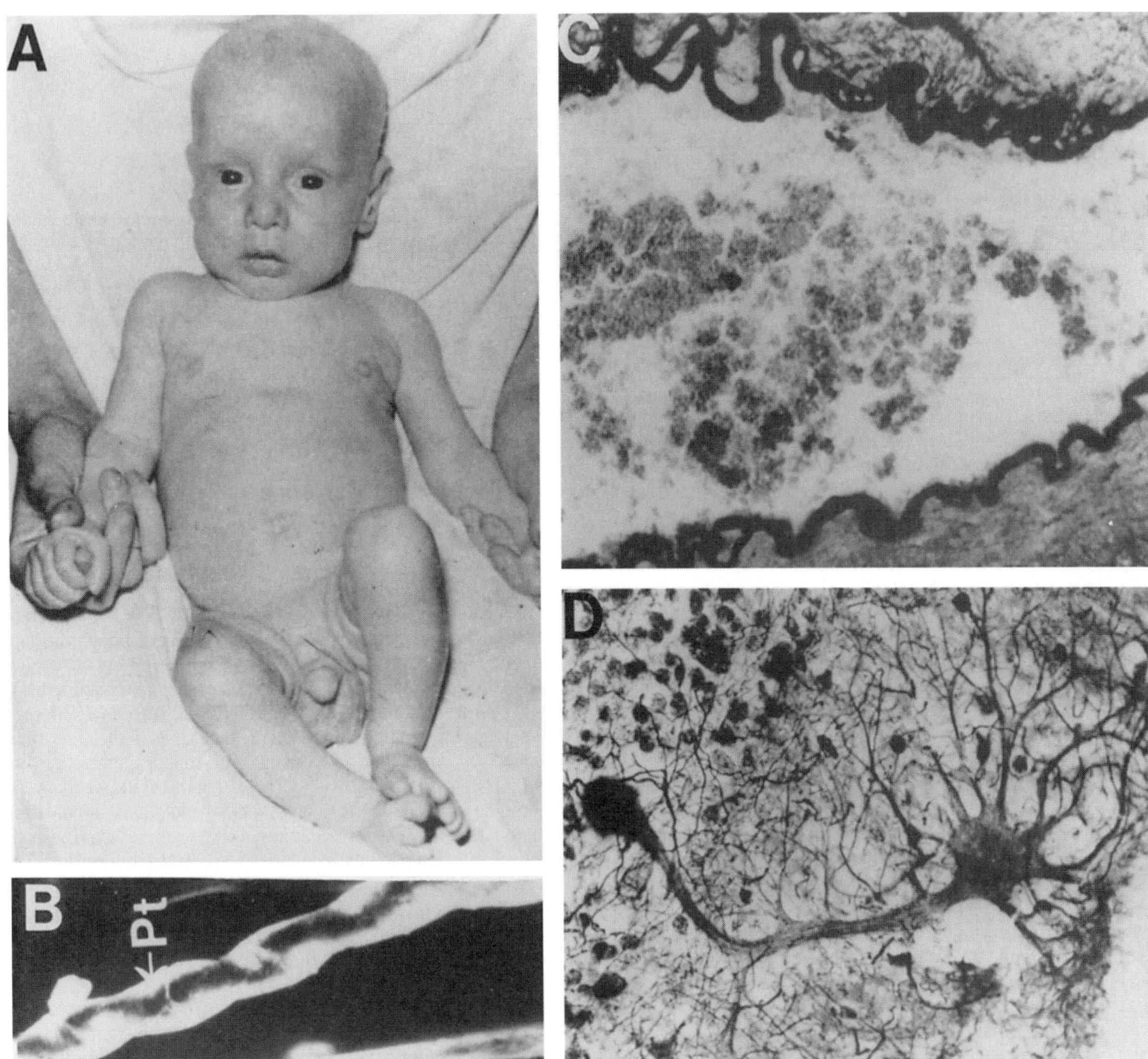

Fig. 126-8 ***A.*** **Clinical features observed in a newborn infant with Menkes disease.** ***B.*** **Pili torti demonstrated by microscopic imaging of hair shaft from an affected patient.** ***C.*** **Microscopic analysis of a cross-section of a large artery from a patient with Menkes disease, illustrating frayed and split elastic lamina.** ***D.*** **Microscopic analysis of Purkinje cells from the cerebellum of a child with Menkes disease, revealing classic axonal swelling. (*Reprinted with permission from Menkes et al.*[188])**

trimester diagnosis also may be made by determining the copper content of chorionic villi.[200]

Molecular diagnosis of Menkes disease is complicated by the heterogeneity at this locus. The development of sensitive methods to rapidly screen for a multiplicity of different mutations will facilitate this diagnostic approach in any given patient. When the mutation in a given family is known, this analysis may be superior to biochemical information, especially in cases of prenatal diagnosis.[201,202] Although carrier detection can be done by measuring copper accumulation in fibroblasts, random X inactivation makes negative results difficult to interpret.[203] Carrier diagnosis is best done with mutation analysis and is readily accomplished when the specific mutation is known. In families where the mutation has not been identified, polymorphic markers and intragenic repeats have been used to facilitate carrier diagnosis.

Treatment

Copper Replacement. There are no effective therapies for the treatment of Menkes disease. Parenteral administration of copper has been attempted using multiple different forms of copper, including copper histidine, copper chloride, and copper sulfate. In such cases this will correct the hepatic copper deficiency and normalize the serum copper and ceruloplasmin concentrations, but clinical studies reveal little or no effect of such treatment on the progressive neurologic deterioration in affected infants.[186] Theoretically, in infants with milder disease where allelic splicing variants may result in some residual Menkes protein, bypassing the gastrointestinal tract with copper injections should result in some movement of copper into the central nervous system prior to a marked abnormality in copper enzymes. In support of this concept, the cumulative experience from therapeutic trials of copper in Menkes disease suggests that infants with severe disease inevitably deteriorate despite any treatment, but patients with milder phenotypes may survive. These data also suggest that patients treated at an earlier age may show better outcomes with regard to neurodevelopmental milestones.[204–206] These patients may experience improvement in general symptoms such as irritability and wakefulness, which presumably reflects at least partial correction of the defect in norepinephrine biosynthesis. Further studies in this area will need to address the relationship of specific mutations to outcome following early copper treatment as well as the additional

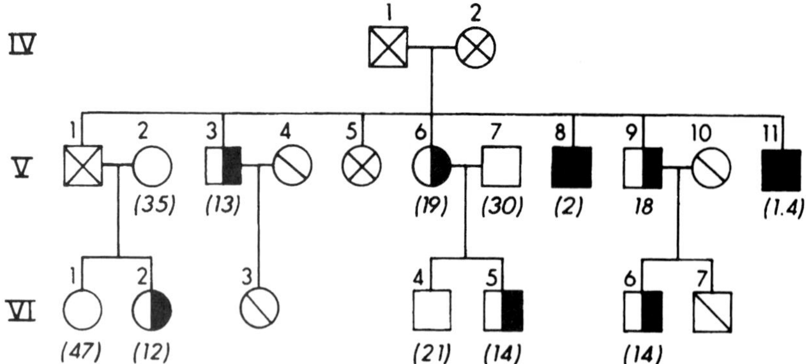

Fig. 126-9 Pedigree and serum ceruloplasmin concentrations in an affected family with aceruloplasminemia. Proband and brother are designated by the filled squares, serum ceruloplasmin concentrations in parentheses (mg/dl). (*Modified with permission from Harris et al.*[221])

environmental and genetic factors that may influence the outcome of such treatment. Although early treatment with copper histidine is not uniformly successful in Menkes disease and is generally considered to be experimental, such treatment should still be offered to affected infants identified at an early age.[186]

Because it is apparent that the metabolic changes that eventually result in the severe neurologic manifestations of Menkes disease are already established *in utero*, any effective therapy must be directed at efforts to get circulating copper into the central nervous system at a time when the affected fetus shows minimal abnormalities. Although no studies have currently addressed approaches to replace copper-transporting activity in affected patients, evidence that the Wilson and the Menkes proteins operate through common biochemical mechanisms may be relevant in this regard. Recent data have revealed that the Wilson protein is abundantly expressed in the liver and other tissues during fetal development.[28] The mechanisms regulating this developmental increase are currently unknown, but experiments demonstrating that the Wilson protein can functionally substitute for the Menkes protein[118] suggest that understanding such mechanisms might permit a novel approach to the treatment of Menkes disease by induction of the Wilson protein in affected cells of Menkes patients during a critical period of development.

ACERULOPLASMINEMIA

Genetics

Ceruloplasmin Gene. Ceruloplasmin is a member of the multicopper oxidase protein family. These enzymes have been highly conserved in evolution and are characterized by the presence of three types of spectroscopically distinct copper ions.[16] In ceruloplasmin, three of these copper ions form a trinuclear copper cluster, which is essential for oxygen binding and activation during the catalytic cycle of the enzyme.[207] Recent determination of the crystal structure of ceruloplasmin has provided support for early biophysical studies of this protein and critically delineates the amino acids in the amino- and C-terminus essential in the formation of the ligands of this trinuclear copper cluster.[208] Although ceruloplasmin can oxidize a number of different substrates in vitro, the recent genetic characterization of patients with aceruloplasminemia has revealed an essential role for this protein as a plasma ferroxidase.

The complete amino acid sequence of ceruloplasmin was determined by Putnam using the methods of protein chemistry.[209] These studies demonstrated the single-chain structure of the protein and revealed a triplicate internal homology in the amino acid sequence. Subsequent isolation of cDNA clones confirmed this sequence and localized the ceruloplasmin gene to chromosome 3q23-25.[210–212] The human ceruloplasmin gene has been isolated and shown to contain 19 exons spanning approximately 50 kb on chromosome 3.[213] A processed pseudogene for ceruloplasmin was detected on chromosome 8 by *in situ* hybridization.[214] Although not expressed, the presence of this pseudogene has methodologic implications that must be considered in the analysis of gene mutations in affected patients.

Mutations. Pedigree analysis in patients with aceruloplasminemia has revealed that this disease is inherited as an autosomal-recessive trait[215,216] (Fig. 126-9). Consanguinity has been observed in most cases studied, and the analysis of serum ceruloplasmin concentrations in family members of affected patients has revealed half-normal serum ceruloplasmin concentrations in obligate heterozygotes (Fig. 126-9). Thus far six different mutations have been identified in the ceruloplasmin gene, each of which is predicted to result in disruption of the open reading frame of the ceruloplasmin gene[217–223] (Table 126-2). In every case these mutations would eliminate the amino acids in the C-terminus essential for formation of the trinuclear copper cluster. Because ceruloplasmin synthesized without this region would be incapable of binding copper, the presence of these mutations is consistent with the lack of detectable ceruloplasmin oxidase activity in the serum of affected patients. The incidence of aceruloplasminemia is unknown, but the disease has been recognized in diverse populations worldwide. Recent screening studies in adults from several prefectures in Japan suggest a frequency of 1 in every 100,000 individuals in this ethnic group.

Pathogenesis. Early experimental studies by Frieden and colleagues[224,225] demonstrated that ceruloplasmin mobilizes iron from reticuloendothelial stores and oxidizes ferrous iron in the plasma for subsequent incorporation into transferrin. These findings were consistent with observations in copper-deficient pigs, revealing that these animals had impaired tissue iron release that could be restored by the administration of ceruloplasmin.[226,227] Recently, support for the role of ceruloplasmin as a ferroxidase has come from genetic experiments in *S. cerevisiae* which showed that high-affinity iron uptake is dependent on the presence of homologous multicopper oxidase FET3.[116,228] As noted above, the Wilson/Menkes homologue CCC2 transports copper with the yeast secretory pathway for incorporation into newly synthesized FET3 (Fig. 126-3), revealing a remarkable evolutionary conservation of the structure and function of these proteins involved in copper and iron homeostasis.[229,230]

Table 126-2 Ceruloplasmin Gene Mutations in Aceruloplasminemia

Mutation	Exon	Predicted Result
Insertion A nt607	3	Frameshift
Insertion TACAC nt1285	7	Frameshift
Splice site 1209-2 A to G	7	Frameshift, truncation
Deletion G nt2389	13	Frameshift
Nonsense Trp858ter	15	Truncation
Splice site 3019-1 G to A	18	Frameshift, truncation

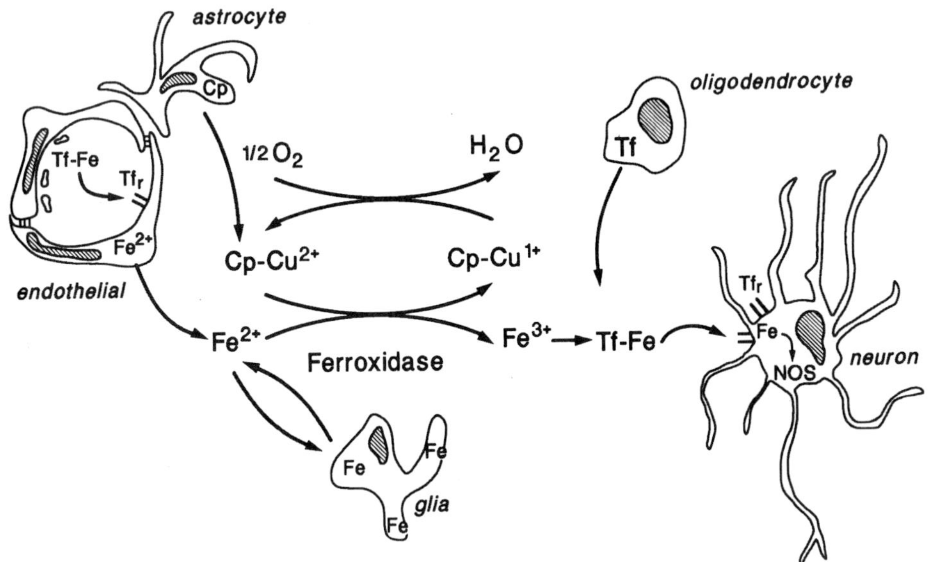

Fig. 126-10 Model of ceruloplasmin functions as a ferroxidase within the central nervous system following synthesis and secretion from astrocytes. (*Modified with permission from Harris et al.*[13])

The disruption of iron homeostasis in patients with aceruloplasminemia can be understood by considering the role of ceruloplasmin as a ferroxidase.[13] The absence of serum ceruloplasmin leads to the slow but constant accumulation of iron within the reticuloendothelial system. In addition, the absence of this ferroxidase activity will result in the accumulation of ferrous iron in the plasma, which is rapidly removed from the circulation by the liver and other tissues, analogous to what is observed in other inherited and acquired iron overload syndromes.[231] Under most circumstances, approximately 5 percent of the normal serum ceruloplasmin concentration is sufficient to sustain plasma iron turnover rates, explaining why abnormalities of iron homeostasis have not been observed in patients with Wilson disease.[227] Although patients with aceruloplasminemia have a low serum copper owing to the absence of serum ceruloplasmin, copper metabolism in such patients is entirely normal, indicating that there is no essential role for ceruloplasmin in copper homeostasis.[215]

Ceruloplasmin does not cross the blood–brain barrier, implying a direct role for this protein in central nervous system iron metabolism. In this regard, recent studies have revealed astrocyte-specific ceruloplasmin gene expression throughout the cerebral microvasculature, surrounding specific neurons in the substantia nigra and other basal ganglia tissues and in the retina.[232,233] Biosynthetic studies confirm this cell-specific expression and reveal that ceruloplasmin is synthesized and secreted by astrocytes with kinetics identical to those previously observed in hepatocytes.[231] The observation that ceruloplasmin is synthesized and secreted within the central nervous system is consistent with the concept that the absence of this protein is directly responsible for the iron accumulation and neuronal degeneration observed in this disease. A mechanistic explanation is envisioned where astrocyte-secreted ceruloplasmin functions both to oxidize ferrous iron after transport of this metal through the cerebral microvasculature as well as to release iron from storage sites within the brain tissue[13,234] (Fig. 126-10). In affected patients, accumulation of iron in glial cells may lead to cell-specific injury with subsequent loss of trophic factors essential for neuronal survival. It is also possible that the accumulation of ferrous iron may result directly in oxidant-mediated central nervous system injury. This latter concept would be consistent with observations in affected patients indicating an increase in plasma lipid peroxidation and interruption of peroxisomal beta oxidation of fatty acids.[235,236] Elucidation of the precise mechanisms of neuronal degeneration in aceruloplasminemia must await the development of a suitable animal model for direct examination of this process.

Diagnosis

Clinical Features. Affected patients generally present in the fourth decade of life due to neurologic symptoms, which include dysarthria, dystonia, and dementia.[215,216] However, at the time of diagnosis, such individuals will frequently have already been diagnosed with insulin-dependent diabetes several years previously. Ophthalmologic examination at presentation reveals photoreceptor loss in the peripheral region of the retina, but visual symptoms are unusual at presentation. Slow progression of neurologic degeneration with worsening of basal ganglia symptoms is described in most patients, although the natural history of this progression is variable among affected individuals. Despite significant iron overload in most tissues, no abnormalities in systemic organs other than the pancreas have been described, and there is usually no evidence of cirrhosis or cardiac abnormalities. Magnetic resonance imaging of the central nervous system reveals marked accumulation of iron within the basal ganglia consistent with the clinical symptoms[237] (Fig. 126-11). Ceruloplasmin is essential for the release of iron from the reticuloendothelial storage sites, and the low serum iron in patients with aceruloplasminemia reflects this impairment of iron release. The mild anemia observed in patients suggests that alternative mechanisms of iron oxidation are available to provide sufficient transferrin-bound iron for erythropoiesis.

Laboratory Findings. At the time of presentation, individuals with aceruloplasminemia manifest a mild normocytic, normochromic anemia with a serum iron concentration approximately one half that of normal.[215,216,237] Serum ferritin concentrations are markedly elevated in the range of 1000 to 1500 ng/ml, similar to what is observed in patients with familial hemochromatosis. Results of liver function tests such as serum transaminases are normal and no other abnormalities in hematologic, renal, or hepatic systems are noted biochemically. Affected patients have normal liver histology on biopsy with no evidence of hepatic copper accumulation, but a marked increase in hepatocellular iron. In most patients at presentation, results of oral glucose tolerance tests are abnormal and hemoglobin A1C levels are elevated, but there are no detectable anti-insulin antibodies and the results of other endocrine tests are normal. The association of basal ganglia symptoms with an absence of serum ceruloplasmin may lead to confusion with the diagnosis of Wilson disease. In such cases, features that may help to confirm the diagnosis of aceruloplasminemia include half-normal serum ceruloplasmin concentrations in parents or sibs, and low serum iron, elevated serum ferritin, and magnetic resonance imaging evidence of iron within the basal ganglia in affected individuals[237] (Fig. 126-11).

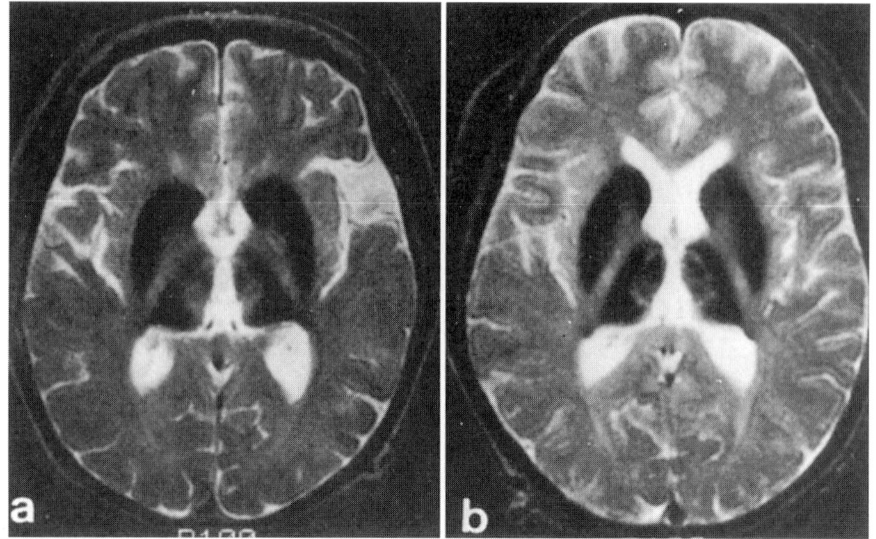

Fig. 126-11 T_2-weighted magnetic resonance imaging in two individuals with aceruloplasminemia revealing increased iron content in the basal ganglia. (*Reprinted with permission from Morita et al.*[237])

Pathologic studies of affected patients[237] reveal accumulation of iron within both the hepatocytes and the reticuloendothelial system of the liver (Fig. 126-12*A*). In addition, as would be suspected from the clinical symptoms of diabetes, analysis of the pancreas reveals abundant iron within the islets of Langerhans and cell-specific dropout of the insulin-producing beta cells (Fig. 126-12*B*). Macroscopic examination of brain tissue reveals cavitary degeneration and discoloration in the basal ganglia. Microscopic analysis of affected basal ganglia tissue reveals abundant neuronal cell loss with no evidence of gliosis or inflammation (Fig. 126-12*C*). Iron staining of basal ganglia reveals a tenfold accumulation of iron within both neurons and glia compared with age-matched controls (Fig. 126-12*D*). Similar findings have been observed in the eye with accumulation of iron in the peripheral regions associated with photoreceptor loss. Although the clinical features of aceruloplasminemia are distinct, the diagnosis has thus far been confirmed by the analysis of ceruloplasmin gene mutations in all reported patients.

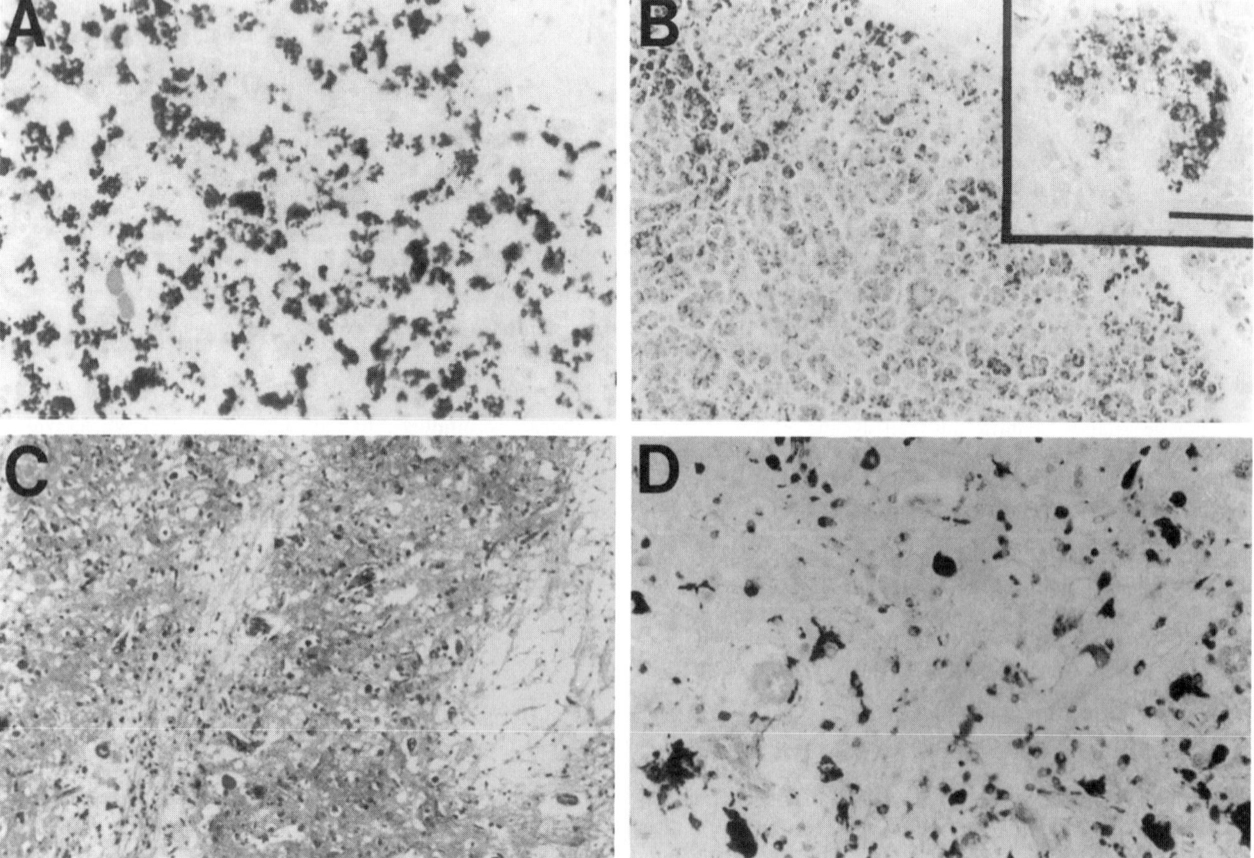

Fig. 126-12 *A.* Prussian blue stain of a liver section from a patient with aceruloplasminemia revealing iron accumulation within hepatocytes. *B.* Prussian blue stain of pancreatic tissue from patient with aceruloplasminemia, revealing iron in the pancreas. Inset shows iron accumulation within an islet of Langerhans. *C.* Section of caudate from a patient with aceruloplasminemia neuronal degeneration. *D.* Prussian blue stain of the prefrontal gyrus in the same patient, illustrating iron accumulation within neurons and glia. (*Modified with permission from Morita et al.*[237])

Treatment

Chelation. Although aceruloplasminemia is a fatal neurologic disease, clinical and laboratory investigations suggest that iron accumulation precedes the onset of neurologic symptoms by several years. These observations have suggested potential therapeutic interventions, particularly in asymptomatic sibs identified through family studies. Preliminary studies using the iron chelator desferroxamine suggest that a reduction in iron body stores as well as amelioration of neurologic symptoms may be possible in severely affected patients.[238] If these observations are supported by further clinical trials, such an approach may be useful as a preventive therapy in asymptomatic individuals. Because the complete absence of serum ceruloplasmin is diagnostic of this disorder, the development of an effective therapy would make it reasonable to consider population screening as a potential preventive approach to this disorder.

The presence of mutations in the ceruloplasmin gene in patients with central nervous system iron accumulation and neuronal degeneration reveals an essential role for ceruloplasmin in human biology. These findings in affected patients suggest the presence of an iron cycle within the central nervous system analogous to that previously characterized within the systemic circulation.[234] Presumably the presence of such a cycle would minimize the effects of systemic iron deficiency on central nervous system function. These findings also have parallels to data on copper homeostasis within the central nervous system and suggest that during development a critical window may exist for both copper and iron repletion within the central nervous system. If confirmed by additional studies this hypothesis has important implications for the cognitive defects observed in children with sustained iron deficiency in the perinatal period. The discovery of aceruloplasminemia taken together with recent data identifying the role of Nramp2 in iron uptake from the gastrointestinal tract[238,239] and frataxin in mitochondrial iron transport[240] provide a starting point for understanding the molecular mechanisms of iron metabolism of direct relevance to a variety of nutritional and genetic disorders of childhood.

EPILOGUE

Elucidation of the molecular genetic basis of the inherited disorders of copper transport completes a circle begun nearly a century ago with the publication of Kinnear Wilson's clinicopathologic description of a novel familial neurologic disease. Knowledge of the structure and function of the copper-transporting ATPases has allowed for a model of cellular copper homeostasis that permits an understanding of disease pathogenesis and provides novel avenues for diagnosis and treatment. As with all important scientific investigation, the insight gained by these advances now leads inevitably to new questions. Recent findings in *S. cerevisiae* that showed an essential role for a chloride ion channel in the copper transport function of CCC2 within the secretory pathway provide a compelling example of potential coming attractions.[241] As for human disease, studies that suggest a distinct role for copper in the pathogenesis of neurodegenerative diseases, including amyotrophic lateral sclerosis,[85,86] Alzheimer disease,[242,243] and the prion-mediated encephalopathies,[244,245] serve as important guides for future investigators in this field. From the advances made in the past few years, it is reasonable to assume that future editions of this text will continue to surprise and delight the reader with novel insights into our understanding of the metabolic and molecular basis of the inherited disorders of copper transport.

ACKNOWLEDGMENT

We are most grateful to our many colleagues who generously provided important data, valuable insights, and useful criticism. Work reported in this chapter from the authors' laboratories was supported in part by National Institutes of Health Grants ES08996 (V.C.C.), GM50016 (V.C.C.), HL41536 (J.D.G.), and DK44464 (J.D.G.). Jonathan D. Gitlin is the recipient of a Burroughs Wellcome Scholar Award in Experimental Therapeutics.

REFERENCES

1. Linder MC, Hazegh-Azam M: Copper biochemistry and molecular biology. *Am J Clin Nutr* **63(suppl)**:797–811, 1996.
2. Turnlund JR: Human whole-body copper metabolism. *Am J Clin Nutr* **67(suppl)**:960–964, 1998.
3. Milne DB: Copper intake and assessment of copper status. *Am J Clin Nutr* **67(suppl)**:1041–1045, 1998.
4. Turnlund JR, Keyes WR, Peiffer GL, Scott KC: Copper absorption, excretion, and retention by young men consuming low dietary copper determined by using the stable isotope 65Cu. *Am J Clin Nutr* **67**:1219–1225, 1998.
5. Dancis A, Yuan DS, Halle D, Askwith C, Eide D, Moehle C, Kaplan J, et al.: Molecular characterization of a copper transport protein in *S. cerevisiae*: An unexpected role for copper in iron transport. *Cell* **76**:393–402, 1994.
6. Kampfenkel K, Kushnir S, Babiychuk E, Inze D, Van Montagu M: Molecular characterization of a putative *Arabidopsis thaliana* copper transporter and its yeast homologue. *J Biol Chem* **270**:28479–28486, 1995.
7. Knight SA, Labbe S, Kwon LF, Kosman DJ, Thiele DJ: A widespread transposable element masks expression of a yeast copper transport gene. *Genes Dev* **10**:1917–1929, 1996.
8. Zhou B, Gitschier J: hCTR1: A human gene for copper uptake identified by complementation in yeast. *Proc Natl Acad Sci U S A* **94**:7481–7486, 1997.
9. Kaler SG: Menkes disease. *Adv Pediatr* **41**:263–304, 1994.
10. Michalska AE, Choo KH: Targeting and germ-line transmission of a null mutation at the metallothionein I and II loci in mouse. *Proc Natl Acad Sci U S A* **90**:8088–8092, 1993.
11. Masters BA, Kelly EJ, Quaife CJ, Brinster RL, Palmiter RD: Targeted disruption of metallothionein I and II genes increases sensitivity to cadmium. *Proc Natl Acad Sci U S A* **91**:584–588, 1994.
12. Palmiter RD: The elusive function of metallothioneins. *Proc Natl Acad Sci U S A* **95**:8428–8430, 1998.
13. Harris ZL, Klomp LW, Gitlin JD: Aceruloplasminemia: An inherited neurodegenerative disease with impaired iron homeostasis. *Am J Clin Nutr* **67(suppl)**:972–977, 1998.
14. Vargas EJ, Shoho AR, Linder MC: Copper transport in the Nagase analbuminemic rat. *Am J Physiol* **267**:G259–G269, 1994.
15. DiDonato M, Sarkar B: Copper transport and its alterations in Menkes and Wilson diseases. *Biochim Biophys Acta* **1360**:3–16, 1997.
16. Harris ZL, Morita H, Gitlin JD: The biology of human ceruloplasmin, in Messerschmidt (ed): *The Multicopper Oxidases*. Singapore: World Scientific Publishing, 1997, pp 285–305.
17. Sato M, Gitlin JD: Mechanisms of copper incorporation during the biosynthesis of human ceruloplasmin. *J Biol Chem* **266**:5128–5134, 1991.
18. Gitlin JD, Schroeder JJ, Lee-Ambrose LM, Cousins RJ: Mechanisms of ceruloplasmin biosynthesis in normal and copper-deficient rats. *Biochem J* **282**:835–839, 1992.
19. Arrese M, Ananthananarayanan M, Suchy FJ: Hepatobiliary transport: Molecular mechanisms of development and cholestasis. *Pediatr Res* **44**:141–147, 1998.
20. Gollan JL, Deller DJ: Studies on the nature and excretion of biliary copper in man. *Clin Sci* **44**:9–15, 1973.
21. Yang X-L, Miura N, Kawarada Y, Terada K, Petrukhin K, Conrad GT, Sugiyama T: Two forms of Wilson disease protein produced by alternative splicing are localized in distinct cellular compartments. *Biochem J* **326**:897–902, 1997.
22. Hung IH, Suzuki M, Yamaguchi Y, Yuan DS, Klausner RD, Gitlin JD: Biochemical characterization of the Wilson disease protein and functional expression in the yeast *Saccharomyces cerevisiae*. *J Biol Chem* **272**:21461–21466, 1997.
23. Paynter JA, Grimes A, Lockhart P, Mercer JF: Expression of the Menkes gene homologue in mouse tissues lack of effect of copper on the mRNA levels. *FEBS Lett* **351**:186–190, 1994.
24. Mercer JFB: Menkes syndrome and animal models. *Am J Clin Nutr* **67(suppl)**:1022–1028, 1998.
25. Prohaska JR, Bailey WR: Persistent regional changes in brain copper, cuproenzymes and catecholamines following perinatal copper deficiency in mice. *J Nutr* **123**:1226–1234, 1993.

26. Prohaska JR, Bailey WR: Alterations of rat brain peptidylglycine alpha-amidating monooxygenase and other cuproenzyme activities following perinatal copper deficiency. *Proc Soc Exp Biol Med* **210**:107–116, 1995.
27. Gitlin D, Biasucci A: Development of gamma G, gamma A, gamma M, beta IC-beta IA, C 1 esterase inhibitor, ceruloplasmin, transferrin, hemopexin, haptoglobin, fibrinogen, plasminogen, alpha 1-antitrypsin, orosomucoid, beta-lipoprotein, alpha 2-macroglobulin, and prealbumin in the human conceptus. *J Clin Invest* **48**:1433–1446, 1969.
28. Schaefer M, Hopkins RG, Failla ML, Gitlin JD: Hepatocyte-specific localization and copper-dependent trafficking of the Wilson's disease protein in the liver. *Am J Physiol* **276**:G639–G646, 1999.
29. Bremner I: Manifestations of copper excess. *Am J Clin Nutr* **67(suppl)**:1069–1073, 1998.
30. Sokol RJ: Antioxidant defenses in metal-induced liver damage. *Semin Liver Dis* **16**:39–46, 1996.
31. Sokol RJ, McKim JM Jr, Devereaux MW: Alpha-tocopherol ameliorates oxidant injury in isolated copper-overloaded rat hepatocytes. *Pediatr Res* **39**:259–263, 1996.
32. Cordano A: Clinical manifestations of nutritional copper deficiency in infants and children. *Am J Clin Nutr* **67(suppl)**:1012–1016, 1998.
33. Uauy R, Olivares M, Gonzalez M: Essentiality of copper in humans. *Am J Clin Nutri* **67(suppl)**:952–959, 1998.
34. Danks DM: Copper deficiency in humans. *Annu Rev Nutr* **8**:235–257, 1988.
35. Fridovich I: Superoxide radical and superoxide dismutases. *Ann Rev Biochem* **64**:97–112, 1995.
36. Fridovich I: Superoxide anion radical (O_2), superoxide dismutases, and related matters. *J Biol Chem* **272**:18515–18517, 1997.
37. Hjalmarsson K, Marklund SL, Engstrom A, Edlund T: Isolation and sequence of complementary DNA encoding human extracellular superoxide dismutase. *Proc Natl Acad Sci U S A* **84**:6340–6344, 1987.
38. Hendrickson DJ, Fisher JH, Jones C, Ho YS: Regional localization of human extracellular superoxide dismutase gene to 4pter-q21. *Genomics* **8**:736–738, 1990.
39. Folz RJ, Crapo JD: Extracellular superoxide dismutase (SOD3): Tissue-specific expression, genomic characterization, and computer-assisted sequence analysis of the human EC SOD gene. *Genomics* **22**:162–171, 1994.
40. Reaume AG, Elliott JL, Hoffman EK, Kowall NW, Ferrante RJ, Siwek DF, Wilcox HM, et al.: Motor neurons in Cu/Zn superoxide dismutase-deficient mice develop normally but exhibit enhanced cell death after axonal injury. *Nat Genet* **13**:43–47, 1996.
41. Ho YS, Gargano M, Cao J, Bronson RT, Heimler I, Hutz RJ: Reduced fertility in female mice lacking copper-zinc superoxide dismutase. *J Biol Chem* **273**:7765–7769, 1998.
42. Carlsson LM, Jonsson J, Edlund T, Marklund SL: Mice lacking extracellular superoxide dismutase are more sensitive to hyperoxia. *Proc Natl Acad Sci U S A* **92**:6264–6268, 1995.
43. Ostermeier C, Iwata S, Michel H: Cytochrome c oxidase. *Curr Opin Struct Biol* **6**:460–466, 1996.
44. Taanman JW: Human cytochrome c oxidase: structure, function, and deficiency. *J Bioenerg Biomembr* **29**:151–163, 1997.
45. Thomas SA, Matsumoto AM, Palmiter RD: Noradrenaline is essential for mouse fetal development. *Nature* **374**:643–646, 1995.
46. Thomas SA, Palmiter RD: Impaired maternal behavior in mice lacking norepinephrine and epinephrine. *Cell* **91**:583–592, 1997.
47. Biaggioni ID, Goldstein S, Atkinson T, Robertson D: Dopamine-beta-hydroxylase deficiency in humans. *Neurology* **40**:370–373, 1990.
48. Craig SP, Buckle VJ, Lamouroux A, Mallet J, Craig IW: Localization of the human dopamine beta hydroxylase (DBH) gene to chromosome 9q34. *Cytogenet Cell Genet* **48**:48–50, 1988.
49. Ouafik LH, Mattei MG, Giraud P, Oliver C, Eipper BA, Mains RE: Localization of the gene encoding peptidylglycine alpha-amidating monooxygenase (PAM) to human chromosome 5q14-5q21. *Genomics* **18**:319–321, 1993.
50. Prigge ST, Kolhekar AS, Eipper BA, Mains RE, Amzel LM: Amidation of bioactive peptides: The structure of peptidylglycine alpha-hydroxylating monooxygenase. *Science* **278**:1300–1305, 1997.
51. Kohhekar AS, Roberts MS, Jiang N, Johnson RC, Mains RE, Eipper BA, Taghert PH: Neuropeptide amidation in *Drosophila*: Separate genes encode the two enzymes catalyzing amidation. *J Neurosci* **17**:1363–1376, 1997.
52. Oetting WS, King RA: Molecular basis of oculocutaneous albinism. *J Invest Dermatol* **103(suppl)**:131–136, 1994.
53. Boissy RE, Nordlund JJ: Molecular basis of congenital hypopigmentary disorders in humans: A review. *Pigment Cell Res* **10**:12–24, 1997.
54. Hamalainen ER, Jones TA, Sheer D, Taskinen K, Pihlajaniemi T, Kivirikko KI: Molecular cloning of human lysyl oxidase and assignment of the gene to chromosome 5q23.3-31.2. *Genomics* **11**:508–516, 1991.
55. Mariani TJ, Trackman PC, Kagan HM, Eddy RL, Shows TB, Boyd CD, Deak SB: The complete derived amino acid sequence of human lysyl oxidase and assignment of the gene to chromosome 5 (extensive sequence homology with the murine *ras* recision gene). *Matrix* **12**:242–248, 1992.
56. Smith-Mungo LI, Kagan HM: Lysyl oxidase: Properties, regulation and multiple functions in biology. *Matrix Biol* **16**:387–398, 1998.
57. Khakoo A, Thomas R, Tropmeter R, Duffy P, Price R, Pope FM: Congenital cutis laxa and lysyl oxidase deficiency. *Clin Genet* **51**:109–114, 1997.
58. Vulpe CD, Kuo Y-M, Murphy TL, Cowley L, Askwith C, Libina N, Gitschier J, et al.: Hephaestin, a ceruloplasmin homologue implicated in intestinal iron transport, is defective in the *sla* mouse. *Nat Genet* **21**:195, 1999.
59. Bethin KE, Cimato TR, Ettinger MJ: Copper binding to mouse liver S-adenosylhomocysteine hydrolase and the effects of copper on its levels. *J Biol Chem* **270**:20703–20711, 1995.
60. Bethin KE, Petrovic N, Ettinger MJ: Identification of a major hepatic copper binding protein as S-adenosylhomocysteine hydrolase. *J Biol Chem* **270**:20698–20702, 1995.
61. Tagliavacca L, Moon N, Dunham WR, Kaufman RJ: Identification and functional requirement of Cu(I) and its ligands within coagulation factor VIII. *J Biol Chem* **272**:27428–27434, 1997.
62. Kaufman RJ, Pipe SW, Tagliavacca L, Swaroop M, Moussalli M: Biosynthesis, assembly and secretion of coagulation factor VIII. *Blood Coagul Fibrinolysis* **8(suppl)**:3–14, 1997.
63. Klinman JP: New quinocofactors in eukaryotes. *J Biol Chem* **271**:27189–27192, 1996.
64. Novotny WF, Chassande O, Baker M, Lazdunski M, Barbry P: Diamine oxidase is the amiloride-binding protein and is inhibited by amiloride analogues. *J Biol Chem* **269**:9921–9925, 1994.
65. Imamura Y, Kubota R, Wang Y, Asakawa S, Kudoh J, Mashima Y, Oguchi Y, et al.: Human retina-specific amine oxidase (RAO): cDNA cloning, tissue expression, and chromosomal mapping. *Genomics* **40**:277–283, 1997.
66. Schwelberger HG, Bodner E: Purification and characterization of diamine oxidase from porcine kidney and intestine. *Biochim Biophys Acta* **1340**:152–164, 1997.
67. DelMarmol V, Beerman F: Tyrosinase and related proteins in mammalian pigmentation. *FEBS Lett* **381**:165–168, 1996.
68. Kenyon K, Modi WS, Contente S, Friedman RM: A novel human cDNA with a predicted protein similar to lysyl oxidase maps to chromosome 15q24-q25. *J Biol Chem* **268**:18435–18437, 1993.
69. Kim Y, Boyd CD, Csiszar K: A new gene with sequence and structural similarity to the gene encoding human lysyl oxidase. *J Biol Chem* **270**:7176–7182, 1995.
70. Saito H, Papaconstantinou J, Sato H, Goldstein S: Regulation of a novel gene encoding a lysyl oxidase-related protein in cellular adhesion and senescence. *J Biol Chem* **272**:8157–8160, 1997.
71. Kelly EJ, Palmiter RJ: A murine model of Menkes disease reveals a physiological function of metallothionein. *Nat Genet* **13**:219–222, 1996.
72. Valentine JS, Gralla EB: Delivering copper inside yeast and human cells. *Science* **278**:817–818, 1997.
73. Lin SJ, Culotta VC: The ATX1 gene of *Saccharomyces cerevisiae* encodes a small metal homeostasis factor that protects cells against reactive oxygen toxicity. *Proc Natl Acad Sci U S A* **92**:3784–3788, 1995.
74. Lin S-J, Pufahl RA, Dancis A, O'Halloran TV, Culotta VC: A role for the *Saccharomyces cerevisiae ATX1* gene in copper trafficking and iron transport. *J Biol Chem* **272**:9215–9220, 1997.
75. Klomp LWJ, Lin S-J, Yuan DS, Klausner RD, Culotta VC, Gitlin JD: Identification and functional expression of HAH1, a novel human gene involved in copper homeostasis. *J Biol Chem* **272**:9221–9226, 1997.
76. Hung IH, Casareno RL, Labesse G, Mathews FS, Gitlin JD: HAH1 is a copper-binding protein with distinct amino acid residues mediating copper homeostasis and antioxidant defense. *J Biol Chem* **273**:1749–1754, 1998.

77. Pufahl RA, Singer CP, Peariso KL, Lin S-J, Schmidt P, Culotta VC, Penner-Hahn JE, et al.: Metal ion chaperone function of the soluble Cu(I) receptor, Atx1. *Science* **278**:853–856, 1997.
78. Glerum DM, Shtanko A, Tzagoloff A: Characterization of COX17, a yeast gene involved in copper metabolism and assembly of cytochrome oxidase. *J Biol Chem* **271**:14504–14509, 1996.
79. Srinivasan C, Posewitz MC, George GN, Winge DR: Characterization of the copper chaperone Cox17 of *Saccharomyces cerevisiae*. *Biochemistry* **37**:7572–7577, 1998.
80. Glerum DM, Shtanko A, Tzagoloff A: SCO1 and SCO2 act as high copy suppressors of a mitochondrial copper recruitment defect in *Saccharomyces cerevisiae*. *J Biol Chem* **271**:20531–20535, 1996.
81. Amaravadi R, Glerum DM, Tzagoloff A: Isolation of a cDNA encoding the human homologue of COX17, a yeast gene essential for mitochondrial copper recruitment. *Hum Genet* **99**:329–333, 1997.
82. Culotta VC, Klomp LWJ, Strain J, Casareno RLB, Krems B, Gitlin JD: The copper chaperone for superoxide dismutase. *J Biol Chem* **272**:23469–23472, 1997.
83. Corson LB, Strain JJ, Culotta VC, Cleveland DW: Chaperone-facilitated copper binding is a property common to several classes of familial amyotrophic lateral sclerosis-linked superoxide dismutase mutants. *Proc Natl Acad Sci U S A* **95**:6361–6366, 1998.
84. Casareno RLB, Waggoner D, Gitlin JD: The copper chaperone CCS directly interacts with copper/zinc superoxide dismutase. *J Biol Chem* **273**:23625–23628, 1998.
85. Siddique T, Deng HX: Genetics of amyotrophic lateral sclerosis. *Hum Mol Genet* **5**:1465–1470, 1996.
86. Bruijn LI, Cleveland DW: Mechanisms of selective motor neuron death in ALS: Insights from transgenic mouse models of motor neuron disease. *Neuropathol Appl Neurobiol* **22**:373–387, 1996.
87. Lutsenko S, Petrukhin K, Cooper MJ, Gilliam CT, Kaplan JH: N-terminal domains of human copper-transporting adenosine triphosphatases (the Wilson's and Menkes disease proteins) bind copper selectively in vivo and in vitro with stoichiometry of one copper per metal-binding repeat. *J Biol Chem* **272**:18939–18944, 1997.
88. DiDonato M, Narindrasorasak S, Forbes JR, Cox DW, Sarkar B: Expression, purification, and metal binding properties of the N-terminal domain from the Wilson disease putative copper-transporting ATPase (ATP7B). *J Biol Chem* **272**:33279–33282, 1997.
89. Gitschier J, Moffat B, Reilly D, Wood WI, Fairbrother WJ: Solution structure of the fourth metal-binding domain from the Menkes copper-transporting ATPase. *Nat Struct Biol* **5**:47–54, 1998.
90. Harris ZL, Gitlin JD: Genetic and molecular basis for copper toxicity. *Am J Clin Nutr* **63(suppl)**:836–841, 1996.
91. Wilson SAK: Progressive lenticular degeneration: A familial nervous disease associated with cirrhosis of the liver. *Brain* **34**:295–507, 1912.
92. Cuthbert JA: Wilson's disease: A new gene and an animal model for an old disease. *J Invest Med* **43**:323–326, 1995.
93. Schilsky ML: Wilson disease: genetic basis of copper toxicity and natural history. *Semin Liver Dis* **16**:83–95, 1996.
94. Frydman M, Bonne-Tamir B, Farrer LA, Conneally PM, Magazanik A, Ashbel S, Goldwitch Z: Assignment of the gene for Wilson disease to chromosome 13: Linkage to the esterase D locus. *Proc Natl Acad Sci U S A* **82**:1819–1821, 1985.
95. Yamaguchi Y, Heiny ME, Gitlin JD: Isolation and characterization of a human liver cDNA as a candidate gene for Wilson disease. *Biochem Biophys Res Commun* **197**:271–277, 1993.
96. Bull PC, Thomas GR, Rommens JM, Forbes JR, Cox DW: The Wilson disease gene is a putative copper transporting P-type ATPase similar to the Menkes gene. *Nat Genet* **5**:327–337, 1993.
97. Tanzi RE, Petrukhin K, Chernov I, Pellequer JL, Wasco W, Ross B, Romano DM, et al.: The Wilson disease gene is a copper transporting ATPase with homology to the Menkes disease gene. *Nat Genet* **5**:344–350, 1993.
98. Lutsenko S, Kaplan JH: Organization of P-type ATPases: significance of structural diversity. *Biochemistry* **34**:15607–15613, 1995.
99. Solioz M, Vulpe C: CPx-type ATPases: A class of P-type ATPases that pump heavy metals. *Trends Biochem* **21**:237–241, 1996.
100. Petrukhin K, Lutsenko S, Chernov L, Ross BM, Kaplan JH, Gilliam TC: Characterization of the Wilson disease gene encoding a P-type copper transporting ATPase: Genomic organization, alternative splicing, and structure/function predicting. *Hum Mol Genet* **3**:1647–1656, 1994.
101. Cox DW: Molecular advances in Wilson disease. *Prog Liver Dis* **14**:245–264, 1996.
102. Li X, Chen S, Wang Q, Zack DJ, Snyder SH, Borjigin J: A pineal regulatory element (PIRE) mediates transactivation by the pineal/retina-specific transcription factor CRX. *Proc Natl Acad Sci U S A* **95**:1876–1881, 1998.
102a. Borjigin J, Payne AS, Deng J, Li X, Wang MM, Ovodenko B, Gitlin JD, et al.: A novel pineal night-specific ATPase encloded by the Wilson disease gene. *J Neurosci* **19**:1018–1026, 1999.
103. Thomas GR, Forbes JR, Roberts EA, Walshe JM, Cox DW: The Wilson disease gene: Spectrum of mutations and their consequences. *Nat Genet* **9**:210–217, 1995.
104. Thomas GR, Jensson O, Gudmundsson G, Thorsteinsson L, Cox DW: Wilson disease in Iceland: A clinical and genetic study. *Am J Hum Genet* **56**:1140–1146, 1995.
105. Thomas GR, Roberts EA, Walshe JM, Cox DW: Haplotypes and mutations in Wilson disease. *Am J Hum Genet* **56**:1315–1319, 1995.
106. Figus A, Angius A, Loudianos G, Bertini C, Dessi V, Loi A, Deiana M, et al.: Molecular pathology and haplotype analysis of Wilson disease in Mediterranean populations. *Am J Hum Genet* **57**:1318–1324, 1995.
107. Waldenstrom E, Lagerkvist A, Dahlman T, Westermark K, Landegren U: Efficient detection of mutations in Wilson disease by manifold sequencing. *Genomics* **37**:303–309, 1996.
108. Loudianos G, Dessi V, Angius A, Lovicu M, Loi A, Deiana M, Akar N, et al.: Wilson disease mutations associated with uncommon haplotypes in Mediterranean patients. *Hum Genet* **98**:640–642, 1996.
109. Nanji MS, Nguyen VT, Kawasoe JH, Inui K, Endo F, Nakajima T, Anezaki T, et al.: Haplotype and mutation analysis in Japanese patients with Wilson disease. *Am J Hum Genet* **60**:1423–1429, 1997.
110. Kim EK, Yoo OJ, Song KY, Yoo HW, Choi SY, Cho SW, Hahn SH: Identification of three novel mutations and a high frequency of the Arg778Leu mutation in Korean patients with Wilson disease. *Hum Mutat* **11**:275–278, 1998.
111. Shah AB, Chernov I, Zhang HT, Ross BM, Das K, Lutsenko S, Parano E, et al.: Identification and analysis of mutations in the Wilson disease gene (ATP7B): Population frequencies, genotype-phenotype correlation, and functional analyses. *Am J Hum Genet* **61**:317–328, 1997.
112. Kalinsky H, Funes A, Zeldin A, Pel-Or Y, Korostishevsky M, Gershoni-Baruch R, Farrer LA, et al.: Novel ATP7B mutations causing Wilson disease in several Israeli ethnic groups. *Hum Mutat* **11**:145–151, 1998.
113. Loudianos G, Dessi V, Lovicu M, Angius A, Nurchi A, Sturniolo GC, Marcellini M, et al.: Further delineation of the molecular pathology of Wilson disease in the Mediterranean population. *Hum Mutat* **12**:89–94, 1998.
114. Chuang L-M, Wu H-P, Jang M-H, Wang T-R, Sue W-C, Lin BJ, Cox DW, et al.: High frequency of two mutations in codon 778 in exon 8 of the ATP7B gene in Taiwanese families with Wilson disease. *J Med Genet* **33**:521–523, 1996.
115. Cuthbert JA: Wilson disease: Update on a systemic disorder with protean manifestations. *Gastroenterol Clin North Am* **27**:655–682, 1998.
116. Askwith C, Eide D, VanHo A, Bernard PS, Li L, Davis-Kaplan S, Sipe DM, Kaplan J: The FET3 gene of *S. cerevisiae* encodes a multicopper oxidase required for ferrous iron uptake. *Cell* **76**:403–410, 1994.
117. Welsh MJ, Smith AE: Molecular mechanisms of CFTR chloride channel dysfunction in cystic fibrosis. *Cell* **73**:1251–1254, 1993.
118. Payne AS, Kelly EJ, Gitlin JD: Functional expression of the Wilson disease protein reveals mislocalization and impaired copper-dependent trafficking of the common H1069Q mutation. *Proc Natl Acad Sci U S A* **95**:10854–10859, 1998.
118a. La Fontaine SL, Firth SD, Camakaris J, Englezou A, Theophilos MB, Petris MJ, Howie M, et al.: Correction of the copper transport defect of Menkes patient fibroblasts by expression of the Menkes and Wilson ATPases. *J Biol Chem* **273**:31375–31380, 1998.
119. Pyeritz RE: Genetic heterogeneity in Wilson disease: Lessons from rare alleles. *Ann Intern Med* **127**:70–72, 1997.
120. Li Y, Togashi Y, Sato S, Emoto T, Kang JH, Takeichi N, Kobayashi H, et al.: Spontaneous hepatic copper accumulation in Long-Evans Cinnamon rats with hereditary hepatitis. A model of Wilson's disease. *J Clin Invest* **87**:1858–1861, 1991.
121. Okayasu T, Tochimaru H, Hyuga T, Takahashi T, Takekoshi Y, Li Y, Togashi Y, et al.: Inherited copper toxicity in Long-Evans cinnamon rats exhibiting spontaneous hepatitis: a model of Wilson's disease. *Pediatr Res* **31**:253–257, 1992.

122. Yamaguchi Y, Heiny ME, Shimizu N, Aoki T, Gitlin JD: Expression of the Wilson disease gene is deficient in the Long-Evans Cinnamon rat. *Biochem J* **301**:1–4, 1994.
123. Wu J, Forbes JR, Chen HS, Cox DW: The LEC rat has a deletion in the copper transporting ATPase gene homologous to the Wilson disease gene. *Nat Genet* **7**:541–545, 1994.
124. Kodama H, Murata Y, Mochizuki D, Abe T: Copper and ceruloplasmin metabolism in the LEC rat, an animal model for Wilson disease. *J Inherit Metab Dis* **21**:203–206, 1998.
125. Jong-Hon K, Togashi Y, Kasai H, Hosokawa M, Takeichi N: Prevention of spontaneous hepatocellular carincoma in Long-Evans Cinnamon rats with hereditary hepatitis by the administration of D-penicillamine. *Hepatology* **18**:614–620, 1993.
126. Terada K, Nakako T, Yang X-L, Iida M, Aiba N, Minamiya T, Nakai M, et al.: Restoration of holoceruloplasmin synthesis in LEC rat after infusion of recombinant adenovirus bearing WND cDNA. *J Biol Chem* **273**:1815–1820, 1998.
127. Kato J, Kobune M, Kohgo Y, Sugawara N, Hisai H, Nakamura T, Sakamaki S, et al.: Hepatic iron deprivation prevents spontaneous development of fulminant hepatitis and liver cancer in Long-Evans Cinnamon rats. *J Clin Invest* **98**:923–929, 1996.
128. Rauch H: Toxic milk, a new mutation affecting copper metabolism in the mouse. *J Hered* **74**:141–144, 1983.
129. Theophilos MB, Cox DW, Mercer JF: The toxic milk mouse is a murine model of Wilson disease. *Hum Mol Genet* **5**:1619–1624, 1996.
130. Walshe JM: Wilson's disease presenting with features of hepatic dysfunction: A clinical analysis of eighty-seven patients. *Q J Med* **70**:253–263, 1989.
131. Brewer GJ, Yuzbasiyan-Gurkan V: Wilson disease. *Medicine* **71**:139–164, 1992.
132. Schilsky ML, Scheinberg IH, Sternlieb I: Liver transplantation for Wilson's disease: Indications and outcome. *Hepatology* **19**:583–587, 1994.
133. Davies SE, Williams R, Portmann B: Hepatic morphology and histochemistry of Wilson's disease presenting as fulminant hepatic failure: A study of 11 cases. *Histopathology* **15**:385–394, 1989.
134. Strand S, Hofmann WJ, Grambihler A, Hug H, Volkmann M, Otto G, Wesch H, et al.: Hepatic failure and liver cell damage in acute Wilson's disease involve CD95 (APO-1/Fas) mediated apoptosis. *Nat Med* **4**:588–593, 1998.
135. Oder W, Grimm G, Kollegger H, Ferenci P, Schneider B, Deecke L: Neurological and neuropsychiatric spectrum of Wilson's disease: A prospective study of 45 cases. *J Neurol* **238**:281–287, 1991.
136. van Wassenaer-van Hall HN: Neuroimaging in Wilson disease. *Metab Brain Dis* **12**:1–19, 1996.
137. Dening TR, Berrios GE: Wilson's disease: Psychiatric symptoms in 195 cases. *Arch Gen Psychiatry* **46**:1126–1134, 1989.
138. Akil M, Schwartz JA, Dutchak D, Yuzbasiyan-Gurkan V, Brewer GJ: The psychiatric presentations of Wilson's disease. *J Neuropsychiatry Clin Neurosci* **3**:377–382, 1991.
139. Steindl P, Ferenci P, Dienes HP, Grimm G, Pabinger I, Madl C, Maier-Dobersberger T, et al.: Wilson's disease in patients presenting with liver disease: A diagnostic challenge. *Gastroenterology* **113**:212, 1997.
140. Schilsky ML, Sternlieb I: Overcoming obstacles to the diagnosis of Wilson's disease. *Gastroenterology* **113**:350–353, 1997.
141. Maier-Dobersberger T, Ferenci P, Polli C, Balac P, Dienes HP, Kaserer K, Datz C, et al.: Detection of the His1069Gln mutation in Wilson disease by rapid polymerase chain reaction. *Ann Intern Med* **127**:21–26, 1997.
142. Pandit A, Bhave S: Present interpretation of the role of copper in Indian childhood cirrhosis. *Am J Clin Nutr* **63(suppl)**:830–835, 1996.
143. Tanner MS: Role of copper in Indian childhood cirrhosis. *Am J Clin Nutr* **67(suppl)**:1074–1081, 1998.
144. Scheinberg IH, Sternlieb I: Wilson disease and idiopathic copper toxicosis. *Am J Clin Nutr* **63(suppl)**:842–845, 1996.
145. Müller T, Feichtinger H, Berger H, Müller W: Endemic Tyrolean infantile cirrhosis: An ecogenetic disorder. *Lancet* **347**:877–880, 1996.
146. Muller T, Muller W, Feichtinger H: Idiopathic copper toxicosis. *Am J Clin Nutr* **67(suppl)**:1082–1086, 1998.
147. Schlaug G, Hefter H, Engelbrecht V, Kuwert T, Arnold S, Stocklin G, Seitz RJ: Neurological impairment and recovery in Wilson's disease: evidence from PET and MRI. *J Neurol Sci* **136**:129–139, 1996.
148. Takahashi W, Yoshii F, Shinohara Y: Reversible magnetic resonance imaging lesions in Wilson's disease: Clinical–anatomical correlation. *J Neuroimaging* **6**:246–248, 1996.
149. Scheinberg IH, Jaffe ME, Sternlieb I: The use of trientine in preventing the effects of interrupting penicillamine therapy in Wilson's disease. *N Engl J Med* **317**:209–213, 1987.
150. Walshe JM: Treatment of Wilson's disease with trientine (triethylene tetramine) dihydrochloride. *Lancet* **1**:643–647, 1982.
151. Walshe JM: The management of pregnancy in Wilson's disease treated with trientine. *Q J Med* **58**:81–87, 1986.
152. Schumacher G, Platz KP, Mueller AR, Neuhaus R, Steinmuller T, Bechstein WO, Becker M, et al.: Liver transplantation: treatment of choice for hepatic and neurological manifestation of Wilson's disease. *Clin Transplant* **11**:217–224, 1997.
153. Menkes JH, Alter M, Steigleder GK, Weakley DR, Sung JH: A sex-linked recessive disorder with retardation of growth, peculiar hair, and focal cerebral and cerebellar degeneration. *Pediatrics* **29**:764–769, 1962.
154. Danks DM, Cartwright E, Stevens BJ, Townley RR: Menkes' kinky hair disease: Further definition of the defect in copper transport. *Science* **179**:1140–1142, 1973.
155. Verga V, Hall BK, Wang S, Johnson S, Higgins JV, Clover TW: Localization of the translocation breakpoint in a female with Menkes syndrome to Xq13.2-q13.3 proximal to PGK-1. *Am J Hum Genet* **48**:1133–1138, 1991.
156. Tümer Z, Tommerup N, Tønnesen T, Kreuder J, Craig IW, Horn N: Mapping of the Menkes locus to Xq13.3 distal to the X-inactivation center by an intrachromosomal insertion of the segment Xq13.3-q21.2. *Hum Genet* **88**:668–672, 1992.
157. Vulpe C, Levinson B, Whitney S, Packman S, Gitschier J: Isolation of a candidate gene for Menkes disease and evidence that it encodes a copper-transporting ATPase. *Nat Genet* **3**:7–13, 1993.
158. Chelly J, Tümer Z, Tønnesen T, Petterson A, Ishikawa-Brush Y, Tommerup N, Horn N, et al.: Isolation of a candidate gene for Menkes disease that encodes a potential heavy metal binding protein. *Nat Genet* **3**:14–19, 1993.
159. Mercer JF, Livingston J, Hall B, Paynter JA, Begy C, Chandrasekhar-appa S, Lockhart P, et al.: Isolation of a partial candidate gene for Menkes disease by positional cloning. *Nat Genet* **3**:20–25, 1993.
160. Tümer Z, Vural B, Tønnesen T, Chelly J, Monaco AP, Horn N: Characterization of the exon structure of the Menkes disease gene using vectorette PCR. *Genomics* **26**:437–442, 1995.
161. Dierick HA, Ambrosini L, Spencer J, Glover TW, Mercer JF: Molecular structure of the Menkes disease gene (ATP7A). *Genomics* **28**:462–469, 1995.
162. Zeynep T, Horn N: Menkes disease: recent advances and new aspects. *J Med Genet* **34**:265–274, 1997.
163. Das S, Levinson B, Whitney S, Vulpe C, Packman S: Diverse mutations in patients with Menkes disease often lead to exon skipping. *Am J Hum Genet* **55**:883–889, 1994.
164. Das S, Levinson B, Vulpe C, Whitney S, Gitschier J, Packman S: Similar splicing mutations of the Menkes/Mottled copper-transporting ATPase gene in occipital horn syndrome and the blotchy mouse. *Am J Hum Genet* **56**:570–576, 1995.
165. Tümer Z, Lund C, Tolshave J, Vural B, Tønnesen T, Horn N: Identification of point mutations in 41 unrelated patients affected with Menkes disease. *Am J Hum Genet* **60**:63–71, 1997.
166. Yamaguchi Y, Heiny ME, Suzuki M, Gitlin JD: Biochemical characterization and intracellular localization of the Menkes disease protein. *Proc Natl Acad Sci U S A* **93**:14030–14035, 1996.
167. Dierick HA, Adam AN, Escara-Wilke JF, Glover TW: Immunocytochemical localization of the Menkes copper transport protein (ATP7A) to the *trans*-Golgi network. *Hum Mol Genet* **6**:409–416, 1997.
168. Petris MJ, Mercer JFB, Culvenor JG, Lockhart P, Gleeson PA, Camakaris J: Ligand-regulated transport of the Menkes copper P-type ATPase efflux pump from the Golgi apparatus to the plasma membrane: A novel mechanism of regulated trafficking. *EMBO J* **15**:6084–6095, 1996.
169. Payne AS, Gitlin JD: Functional expression of the Menkes disease protein reveals common biochemical mechanisms among the copper-transporting P-type ATPases. *J Biol Chem* **273**:3765–3770, 1998.
170. Camakaris J, Petris MJ, Bailey L, Shen P, Lockhart P, Glover TW, Barcroft CL, et al.: Gene amplification of the Menkes (MNK; ATP7A) P-type ATPase gene of CHO cells is associated with copper resistance and enhanced copper efflux. *Hum Mol Genet* **4**:2117–2123, 1995.
171. LaFontaine S, Firth SD, Lockhart PJ, Brooks H, Parton RG, Camakaris J, Mercer JFB: Functional analysis and intracellular localization of the human Menkes protein (MNK) stably expressed from cDNA construct in Chinese hamster ovary cells (CHO-K1). *Hum Mol Genet* **7**:1293–1300, 1998.

171a. Voskoboinik I, Brooks H, Smith S, Shen P, Camakaris J: ATP-dependent copper transport by the Menkes protein in membrane vesicles isolated from cultured Chinese hamster ovary cells. *FEBS Lett* **435**:178–182, 1998.
172. Kaler SG, Gallo LK, Proud VK, Percy AK, Mark Y, Segal NA, Goldstein DS, et al.: Occipital horn syndrome and a mild Menkes phenotype associated with splice site mutations at the MNK locus. *Nat Genet* **8**:195–202, 1994.
173. Levinson B, Conant R, Schnur R, Das S, Packman S, Gitschier J: A repeated element in the regulatory region of the MNK gene and its deletion in a patient with occipital horn syndrome. *Hum Mol Genet* **5**:1737–1742, 1996.
174. Qi M, Byers PH: Constitutive skipping of alternatively spliced exon 10 in the ATP7A gene abolishes Golgi localization of the Menkes protein and produces the occipital horn syndrome. *Hum Mol Genet* **7**:465–469, 1998.
175. Francis MJ, Jones EE, Levy ER, Ponnambalam S, Chelly J, Monaco AP: A Golgi localization signal identified in the Menkes recombinant protein. *Hum Mol Genet* **7**:1245–1252, 1998.
176. Petris MJ, Camakaris J, Greenough M, LaFontaine S, Mercer JFB: A C-terminal di-leucine is required for localization of the Menkes protein in the trans-Golgi network. *Hum Mol Genet* **7**:2063–2071, 1998.
177. Tümer Z, Horn N: Menkes disease: Underlying genetic defect and new diagnostic possibilities. *J Inherit Metab Dis* **21**:604–612, 1998.
178. Hunt DM: Primary defect in copper transport underlies mottled mutants in the mouse. *Nature* **249**:852–854, 1974.
179. Mercer JFB, Grimes A, Ambrosini L, Lockhart P, Paynter JA, Dierick H, Glover TW: Mutations in the murine homologue of the Menkes gene in dappled and blotchy mice. *Nat Genet* **6**:374–378, 1994.
180. Levinson B, Vulpe C, Elder B, Martin C, Verly F, Packman S, Gitschier J: The mottled gene is the mouse homologue of the Menkes disease gene. *Nat Genet* **6**:369–373, 1994.
181. Grimes A, Hearn CJ, Lockhart P, Newgreen DF, Mercer JF: Molecular basis of the brindled mouse mutant (Mo(br)): A murine model of Menkes disease. *Hum Mol Genet* **6**:1037–1042, 1997.
182. Mori M, Nishimura M: A serine-to-proline mutation in the copper-transporting P-type ATPase gene of the macular mouse. *Mamm Genome* **8**:407–410, 1997.
183. Murata Y, Kodama H, Abe T, Ishida N, Nishimura M, Levinson B, Gitschier J, et al.: Mutation analysis and expression of the mottled gene in the macular mouse model of Menkes disease. *Pediatr Res* **42**:436–442, 1997.
184. Cecchi C, Biasotto M, Tosi M, Avner P: The mottled mouse as a model for human Menkes disease: Identification of mutations in the Atp7a gene. *Hum Mol Genet* **6**:829, 1997.
185. Reed V, Boyd Y: Mutation analysis provides additional proof that mottled is the mouse homologue of Menkes' disease. *Hum Mol Genet* **6**:417–423, 1997.
186. Kaler SG: Diagnosis and therapy of Menkes syndrome, a genetic form of copper deficiency. *Am J Clin Nutr* **67(suppl)**:1029–1034, 1998.
187. Menkes JH: Disorders of copper metabolism. In Rosenberg RN, Prusiner SB, DiMauro S, Barchi RL (eds): *Molecular and Genetic Basis of Neurological Disease.* Boston: Butterworth-Heinemann, 1997, p. 1273–1290.
188. Menkes JH: Kinky hair disease, in Gomez MR (ed): *Neurocutaneous Disease: A Practical Approach.* Boston: Butterworth-Heinemann, 1987.
189. Kim OH, Suh JH: Intracranial and extracranial MR angiography in Menkes disease. *Pediatr Radiol* **27**:782–784, 1997.
190. Geller TJ, Pan Y, Martin DS: Early neuroradiologic evidence of degeneration in Menkes' disease. *Pediatr Neurol* **17**:255–258, 1997.
191. Leventer RJ, Kornberg AJ, Phelan EM, Kean MJ: Early magnetic resonance imaging findings in Menkes' disease. *J Child Neurol* **12**:222–224, 1997.
192. Proud VK, Mussell HG, Kaler SG, Young DW, Percy AK: Distinctive Menkes disease variant with occipital horns: Delineation of natural history and clinical phenotype. *Am J Med Genet* **65**:44–51, 1996.
193. Willemse J, Van Den Hamer CJ, Prins HW, Jonker PL: Menkes' kinky hair disease. I. Comparison of classical and unusual clinical and biochemical features in two patients. *Brain Dev* **4**:105–114, 1982.
194. Haas RH, Robinson A, Evans K, Lascelles PT, Dubowitz V: An X-linked disease of the nervous system with disordered copper metabolism and features differing from Menkes' disease. *Neurology* **31**:852–859, 1981.
195. Mehes K, Petrovicz E: Familial benign copper deficiency. *Arch Dis Child* **57**:716–718, 1982.
196. Tønnesen T, Horn N: Prenatal and postnatal diagnosis of Menkes disease, an inherited disorder of copper metabolism. *J Inherit Metab Dis* **1**:207–214, 1989.
197. Herd SM, Camakaris J, Christofferson R, Wookey P, Danks DM: Uptake and efflux of copper-64 in Menkes' disease and normal continuous lymphoid cell lines. *Biochem J* **247**:341–347, 1987.
198. Kaler SG, Goldstein DS, Holmes C, Salerno JA, Gahl WA: Plasma and cerebrospinal fluid neurochemical pattern in Menkes disease. *Ann Neurol* **33**:171–175, 1993.
199. Kaler SG, Gahl WA, Berry SA, Holmes CS, Goldstein DS: Predictive value of plasma catecholamine levels in neonatal detection of Menkes disease. *J Inherit Metab Dis* **16**:907–908, 1993.
200. Tønnesen T, Horn N, Sondergaard F, Jensen OA, Gerdes AM, Girard S, Damsgaard E: Experience with first trimester prenatal diagnosis of Menkes disease. *Prenatal Diagn* **7**:497–509, 1987.
201. Das S, Whitney S, Taylor J, Chen E, Levinson B, Vulpe C, Gitschier J, et al.: Prenatal diagnosis of Menkes disease by mutation analysis. *J Inherit Metab Dis* **18**:364–365, 1995.
202. Tümer Z, Tønnesen T, Böhamann J, Marg W, Horn N: First trimester prenatal diagnosis of Menkes disease by DNA analysis. *J Med Genet* **31**:615–617, 1994.
203. Tümer Z, Tønnesen T, Horn N: Detection of genetic defects in Menkes disease by direct mutation analysis and its implication in carrier diagnosis. *J Inherit Metab Dis* **17**:267–270, 1994.
204. Kaler SG, Buist NR, Holmes CS, Goldstein DS, Miller RC, Gahl WA: Early copper therapy in classic Menkes disease patients with a novel splicing mutation. *Ann Neurol* **38**:921–928, 1995.
205. Tümer Z, Horn N, Tønnesen T, Christodoulou J, Clarke JT, Sarkar B: Early copper-histidine treatment for Menkes disease. *Nat Genet* **12**:11–13, 1996.
206. Christodoulou J, Danks DM, Sarkar B, Baerlocher KE, Casey R, Horn N, Tümer Z, et al.: Early treatment of Menkes disease with parenteral copper-histidine: Long-term follow-up of four treated patients. *Am J Med Genet* **76**:154–164, 1998.
207. Calabrese L, Carbonaro M, Giovanni M: Presence of coupled trinuclear copper cluster in mammalian ceruloplasmin is essential for efficient electron transfer to oxygen. *J Biol Chem* **264**:6183–6187, 1993.
208. Zaitseva I, Zaitsev V, Card G, Moshkov D, Bax B, Ralph A, Lindley PF: The x-ray structure of human ceruloplasmin at 3.1 Å resolution. Nature of the copper centers. *J Biol Inorgan Chem* **1**:15–23, 1996.
209. Takahashi N, Ortel TL, Putnam FW: Single-chain structure of human ceruloplasmin: The complete amino acid sequence of the whole molecule. *Proc Natl Acad Sci U S A* **81**:390–394, 1984.
210. Koschinsky ML, Funk WD, VanOost BA, MacGillivray RT: Complete cDNA sequence of human preceruloplasmin. *Proc Natl Acad Sci U S A* **83**:5086–5090, 1986.
211. Yang F, Naylor SL, Lum JB, Cutshaw S, McCombs JL, Naberhaus KH, McGill JR, et al.: Characterization, mapping, and expression of the human ceruloplasmin gene. *Proc Natl Acad Sci U S A* **83**:3257–3261, 1986.
212. Mercer JF, Grimes A: Isolation of a human ceruloplasmin cDNA that includes the N-terminal leader sequence. *FEBS Lett* **203**:185–190, 1986.
213. Daimon M, Yamatani K, Igarashi M, Fukase N, Kawanami T, Kato T, Tominaga M, et al.: Fine structure of the human ceruloplasmin gene. *Biochem Biophys Res Commun* **208**:1028–1035, 1995.
214. Koschinsky ML, Chow BK, Schwartz J, Hamerton JL, MacGillivray RT: Isolation and characterization of a processed gene for human ceruloplasmin. *Biochemistry* **26**:7760–7767, 1987.
215. Miyajima H, Nishimura Y, Mizoguchi K, Sakanoto M, Shimizu T, Honda N: Familial apoceruloplasmin deficiency associated with blepharospasm and retinal degeneration. *Neurology* **37**:761–767, 1987.
216. Logan JI, Harveyson KB, Wisdom GB, Hughes AE, Archbold GP: Hereditary caeruloplasmin deficiency, dementia and diabetes mellitus. *Q J Med* **87**:663–670, 1994.
217. Harris ZL, Takahashi Y, Miyajima H, Serizawa M, MacGillivray RTA, Gitlin JD: Aceruloplasminemia: Molecular characterization of this disorder of iron metabolism. *Proc Natl Acad Sci U S A* **92**:2539–2543, 1995.
218. Yoshida K, Furihata K, Takeda S, Nakamura A, Yamamoto K, Hiyamuta S, Ikeda S, et al.: A mutation in the ceruloplasmin gene is associated with systemic hemosiderosis humans. *Nat Genet* **9**:267–272, 1995.
219. Takahashi Y, Miyajima H, Shirabe S, Nagataki S, Suenaga A, Gitlin JD: Characterization of a nonsense mutation in the ceruloplasmin gene resulting in diabetes and neurodegenerative disease. *Hum Mol Genet* **5**:81–84, 1996.

220. Daimon M, Kato T, Kawanami T, Tominaga M, Igarashi M, Yamatani K, Sasaki H: A nonsense mutation of the ceruloplasmin deficiency with diabetes mellitus. *Biochem Biophys Res Commun* **217**:89–95, 1995.
221. Harris ZL, Migas MD, Hughes AE, Logan JI, Gitlin JD: Familial dementia due to a frameshift mutation in the caeruloplasmin gene. *Q J Med* **89**:355–359, 1995.
222. Okamoto N, Wada S, Oga T, Kawabata Y, Baba Y, Habu D, Takeda Z, et al.: Hereditary ceruloplasmin deficiency with hemosiderosis. *Hum Genet* **97**:755–758, 1996.
223. Yazaki M, Yoshida K, Nakamura A, Furihata K, Yonekawa M, Okabe T, Yamashita N, et al.: A novel splicing mutation in the ceruloplasmin gene responsible for hereditary ceruloplasmin deficiency with hemosiderosis. *J Neurol Sci* **156**:30–34, 1998.
224. Osaki S, Johnson DA: The possible significance of the ferrous oxidase activity of ceruloplasmin in normal human serum. *J Biol Chem* **241**:2746–2751, 1966.
225. Osaki S, Johnson DA: The mobilization of iron from the perfused mammalian liver by a serum copper enzyme, ferroxidase I. *J Biol Chem* **246**:3018–3023, 1971.
226. Lee GR, Nacht S, Lukens JN, Cartwright GE: Iron metabolism in copper-deficient swine. *J Clin Invest* **47**:2058–2069, 1968.
227. Roeser HP, Lee GR, Nacht S, Cartwright OE: The role of ceruloplasmin in iron metabolism. *J Clin Invest* **49**:2408–2417, 1970.
228. Stearman R, Yuan DS,Yamaguchi-Iwa Y, Klausner RD, Dancis A: A permease-oxidase complex involved in high-affinity iron uptake in yeast. *Science* **271**:1552–1557, 1996.
229. Yuan DS, Stearman R, Dancis A, Dunn T, Beeler T, Klausner RD: The Menkes/Wilson disease gene homologue in yeast provides copper to a ceruloplasmin-like oxidase required for iron uptake. *Proc Natl Acad Sci U S A* **92**:2632–2636, 1995.
230. Yuan DS, Dancis A, Klausner RD: Restriction of copper export in *Saccharomyces cerevisiae* to a late Golgi or post-Golgi compartment in the secretory pathway. *J Biol Chem* **272**:25787–25793, 1997.
231. Craven CM, Alexander J, Eldridge M, Kushner JP, Bernstein S, Kaplan J: Tissue distribution and clearance kinetics of non-transferrin–bound iron in the hypotransferrinemic mouse: A rodent model for hemochromatosis. *Proc Natl Acad Sci U S A* **84**:3457–3461, 1987.
232. Klomp LWJ, Farhangrazi ZS, Dugan LL, Gitlin JD: Ceruloplasmin gene expression in the murine central nervous system. *J Clin Invest* **98**:207–215, 1996.
233. Klomp LWJ, Gitlin JD: Expression of the ceruloplasmin gene in the human retina and brain: Implications for a pathogenic model in aceruloplasminemia. *Hum Mol Genet* **5**:1989–1996, 1996.
234. Gitlin JD: Aceruloplasminemia. *Pediatr Res* **44**:271–276, 1998.
235. Miyajima H, Adachi J, Tatsuno Y, Takahashi Y, Fujimoto M, Kaneko E, Gitlin JD, et al.: Increased very long-chain fatty acids in erythrocyte membranes of patients with aceruloplasminemia HAH1 is a copper-binding protein with distinct amino acid residues mediating copper homeostasis and antioxidant defense. *Neurology* **50**:130–136, 1998.
236. Miyajima H, Takahashi Y, Serizawa M, Kaneko E, Gitlin JD: Increased plasma lipid peroxidation in patients with aceruloplasminemia. *Free Radic Biol Med* **20**:757–760, 1996.
237. Morita H, Ikeda S, Yamamoto K, Morita S, Yoshida K, Nomoto S, Kato M, et al.: Hereditary ceruloplasmin deficiency with hemosiderosis: A clinicopathological study of a Japanese family. *Ann Neurol* **37**:646–656, 1995.
238. Miyajima H, Takahashi Y, Kamata T, Shimizu H, Sakai N, Gitlin JD: Use of desferrioxamine in the treatment of aceruloplasminemia. *Ann Neurol* **41**:404–407, 1997.
239. Fleming MD, Trenor CC III, Su MA, Foernzler D, Beier DR, Dietrich WF, Andrews NC: Microcytic anaemia mice have a mutation in *Nramp2*, a candidate iron transporter gene. *Nat Genet* **16**:383–386, 1997.
240. Gunshin H, Mackenzie B, Berger UV, Gunshin Y, Romero MF, Boron WF, Nussberger S, et al.: Cloning and characterization of a mammalian proton-coupled metal-ion transporter. *Nature* **388**:482–488, 1997.
241. Babcock M, deSilva D, Oaks R, Davis-Kaplan S, Jiralerspong S, Montermini L, Pandolfo M: Regulation of mitochondrial iron accumulation by Yfh1p a putative homolog of frataxin. *Science* **276**:1709–1712, 1997.
242. Gaxiola RA, Yuan DS, Klausner RD, Fink GR: The yeast CLC chloride channel functions in cation homeostasis. *Proc Natl Acad Sci U S A* **95**:4046–4050, 1998.
243. Multhaup G, Schlicksupp A, Hesse L, Beher D, Ruppert T, Masters CL, Beyreuther K: The amyloid precursor protein of Alzheimer's disease in the reduction of copper(II) to copper(I). *Science* **271**:1406–1409, 1996.
244. Atwood CS, Moir RD, Huang X, Scarpa RC, Bacarra NME, Romano DM, Hartshorn M, et al.: Dramatic aggregation of Alzheimer A^{β} by Cu(II) is induced by conditions representing physiological acidosis. *J Biol Chem* **273**:12817–12826, 1998.
245. Brown DR, Qin K, Herms JW, Madlung A, Manson J, Strome R, Fraser PE, et al.: The cellular prion protein binds copper in vivo. *Nature* **390**:684–687, 1997.
246. Stockel J, Safar J, Wallace AC, Cohen FE, Prusiner SB: Prion protein selectively binds copper(II) ions. *Biochemistry* **37**:7185–7193, 1998.

CHAPTER 127

Hereditary Hemochromatosis

Ernest Beutler ▪ Thomas H. Bothwell
Robert W. Charlton ▪ Arno G. Motulsky

1. **Hereditary hemochromatosis is an iron storage disease that results in the impairment of organ structure and function. The iron is stored predominantly as hemosiderin. The liver, heart, pancreas, endocrine organs, skin, and joints are principally affected. Cirrhosis, cardiomyopathy, diabetes mellitus, hypogonadism, skin pigmentation, and arthritis may occur with full clinical expression.**
2. **The iron enters the body via the gastrointestinal tract, because of a failure of the mechanism controlling the absorption of dietary iron. Hereditary hemochromatosis is most commonly the consequence of mutations in a gene that has been designated *HFE*, located approximately 4 megabases telomeric to the HLA-A locus on the short arm of chromosome 6; the gene defect causes the absorption of more iron than is required. Some patients with hereditary hemochromatosis have some other defect, as yet unknown, not linked to the HLA loci. A clinical and pathologic state of iron loading, similar to that of hereditary hemochromatosis, also occurs as a result of the iron burden caused by red cell transfusion and increased gastrointestinal iron absorption in patients with refractory anemias and thalassemia. African iron overload also resembles hereditary hemochromatosis in some respects; it is due to drinking indigenous beers containing large amounts of iron, possibly combined with a non-HLA-linked genetic abnormality.**
3. **The nature of the metabolic defect caused by mutations of *HFE* has not been elucidated. The normal protein appears to bind to the transferrin receptor and to change its affinity for transferrin, but the physiological significance of this interaction is not yet fully understood. Three mutations are known. One of these, 845G → A (C282Y;845A), prevents the formation of a disulfide bond essential for the binding to β_2-microglobulin. This prevents transport of the HFE protein to the cell surface. The 187C → G (H63D) mutation appears to affect the binding of HFE to the transferrin receptor. A third, less common mutation, 193A → T (S65C), is less well studied and of unknown importance, at present. A condition closely resembling human hereditary hemochromatosis can be produced by targeted disruption of a homologous gene in mice.**
4. **The frequency of heterozygotes for the 845A (C282Y) mutations in central, northern, and western Europe ranges between 8 percent to 18 percent, indicating that 1 in 100 to 1 in 625 persons are homozygotes. The clinical manifestation rate (penetrance) and natural history of hemochromatosis among homozygotes for the 845A (C282Y) mutation are not yet known. The 845A (C282Y) mutation is absent from Asian and African populations, and is less frequent among southern Europeans and Ashkenazi Jews. The 187C → G (H63D) mutation is more common (about 24 percent heterozygotes among Europeans) and has a more widespread population distribution than the 845A (C282Y) mutation. The 845A (C282Y) mutation distribution suggests Celtic origin and it may have reached a high frequency because of survival and fertility advantages of 845G (C282Y) heterozygotes vis-a-vis iron deficiency.**
5. **About 75 to 85 percent of clinically recognized hemochromatosis patients of central, northern, and western European origin are homozygotes for the 845A (C282Y) mutation. The penetrance of the compound heterozygous state for the 845A/187G (282Y/463D) mutation is only about 1 percent of that of the homozygotes. An occasional 187G (H63D) homozygote with hemochromatosis has been reported. Some patients with hereditary hemochromatosis have some other defect not linked to the HLA loci and as yet of unknown origin.**
6. **Once clinical manifestations have appeared, hemochromatosis can be fatal unless the iron is removed. If untreated, death may occur as a result of cirrhosis, hepatoma, cardiac failure, arrhythmias, overwhelming infection, or diabetes. Removal of the iron is most conveniently achieved in hereditary hemochromatosis by weekly venesections of 400 to 500 ml of blood. These must be continued until a state of mild iron deficiency is achieved. Thereafter, a venesection every 3 to 4 months or less frequently is sufficient to prevent reaccumulation of iron. In refractory anemias the iron can be eliminated only by administering deferoxamine, which is infused over 10 to 12 h out of every 24, usually subcutaneously.**
7. **Removal of the iron in hereditary hemochromatosis prolongs survival, cures the cardiomyopathy and the skin pigmentation, and arrests the liver damage. Diabetes may improve, but hypogonadism and arthropathy do not, and hepatoma may complicate cirrhosis even years later.**
8. **Because hereditary hemochromatosis is a potentially lethal disease, every effort should be made to achieve early diagnosis. In particular, physicians who specialize in hepatology, cardiology, diabetes, endocrinology, and rheumatology should cultivate a high index of clinical suspicion. It is even more important to diagnose affected homozygotes before the development of significant iron overload. If venesections can be instituted before organ damage has occurred, the consequences of organ damage can be avoided. In this context, appropriate case detection and genetic counseling, especially in sibs, is mandatory.**

Iron is among the most abundant metals in the earth's crust, and all life forms utilize iron in metabolic processes, usually as an electron carrier. Living organisms have therefore developed strategies for extracting iron from their environment. If extraction is insufficient, iron deficiency, a common disorder both in plants and animals, is the result. Yet, an excess of iron must also be avoided, because the reactive nature of iron confers toxic properties. The accumulation of excess iron, when it occurs in humans, is termed hemochromatosis. This term was originally used to describe a disorder with specific pathologic and clinical features, but has gained broader usage more recently to embrace those persons who have the biochemical and genetic evidence of iron overloading, but may lack the clinical manifestations. Most commonly hemochromatosis is the result of a hereditary defect in iron absorption and the disorder that results is termed hereditary hemochromatosis. This reasonably well-defined disorder is the main focus of this chapter. However, hemochromatosis can arise in other ways and may give rise to similar metabolic, pathologic, and clinical consequences. Iron absorption inappropriate to body needs occurs in various anemias, such as thalassemia major. An additional factor in such subjects is the repeated blood transfusions they require. Finally, hemochromatosis occurs in many sub-Saharan Africans who absorb more iron than they require from alcoholic beverages brewed in iron drums.

Table 127-1 Iron-Containing Compounds in Humans

	mg in a 75-kg male* (approximate)	mg/kg (approximate)
Functional compounds		
Hemoglobin	2300	31
Myoglobin	320	4
Heme enzymes	80	1
Nonheme enzymes	100	1
	2800	37
Storage complexes		
Ferritin	700	9
Hemosiderin	300	4
	1000	13
Total	3800	50

*1 mg = 17.9 μmol.

HISTORY

Hemochromatosis was first described by Trousseau in 1865.[1] The massive accumulation of iron that occurred in this disease was recognized as the hallmark of *bronzed diabetes*, the picturesque name by which the disorder was known, but it was thought by some that the toxic metal might be copper,[2] which was also known to accumulate. In 1935 Sheldon helped to focus attention on this disease in a classic monograph.[3] He suggested that the disease might be hereditary and addressed the prevalence of hemochromatosis, proposing that while it was not as rare as had been thought, it was a relatively uncommon disorder. He wrote:

> **Thus McKereth (1932) and Rich (1933) stated that less than 100 cases had been recorded, whereas actually the literature contains references to 345 cases. Even the more correct statement of Nadler and Haugrud, who referred to 200 cases, is still considerably short of the actual number. It may be stated here that many of the case-records are scattered in local journals which are difficult of access, which is the main reason for the general opinion that but few cases have been met with. A difficulty which works the other way is the habit in some places, especially in France, of making use of the same case for a series of papers, often by different authors.**

Sheldon's view that hemochromatosis might have a genetic basis was strongly contested by MacDonald[4,5] who considered the disorder to be caused by increased iron intake, particularly in wine. However, Sheldon's formulation was proven correct when Simon et al.[6] showed the disease to be tightly linked to the HLA locus. These investigators[7] demonstrated both linkage within families and linkage disequilibrium in populations, and realized that it was not the HLA-A or HLA-B gene products themselves that were involved in the pathogenesis of the disease, but that the gene that did cause hemochromatosis was nearby. These findings were soon confirmed.[8] The term *idiopathic hemochromatosis* was gradually supplanted by the more descriptive name, *hereditary hemochromatosis*.

The ingenious development of serial phlebotomy as treatment for the disease by Davis and Arrowsmith in 1952[9] made it clear that iron accumulation was the most important pathogenetic factor. Nowadays it is often forgotten that other metals accumulate as well[10] and may play a subsidiary role.

THE METABOLISM OF IRON

The Distribution of Iron

The body of a healthy adult male contains between 3 and 4 g of iron.[11] The major portion is in the iron porphyrin complexes, hemoglobin, myoglobin, and a variety of heme-containing enzymes (Table 127-1). Erythrocytes contain approximately 1 mg of elemental iron per ml. Also, many nonheme enzymes either contain iron or require it as a cofactor. The remaining iron in the body is present in the relatively inactive storage forms, ferritin and hemosiderin. The size of this reserve of iron normally varies between 0 and 1000 mg.

In normal subjects most of the body's iron reserve is present in roughly equal proportions in the liver, bone marrow, and skeletal muscles.[11] Storage iron in the bone marrow and spleen is confined to macrophages, and this may also be true for skeletal muscles.[12] The iron stored in hepatocytes is derived from the plasma transferrin[13] and to a lesser extent from hemoglobin-haptoglobin and heme-hemopexin complexes,[14] while macrophages derive their iron predominantly from the hemoglobin of broken-down red cells.

Proteins of Iron Transport and Storage

Ferritin

Structure. The diffuse, soluble, mobile fraction of storage iron is ferritin, and the insoluble, aggregated deposits are known as hemosiderin.[15] Most of the storage iron in the body is normally in the form of ferritin, but with increasing degrees of iron overload the proportion in hemosiderin rises progressively. Ferritin serves dual functions of detoxifying and of storing iron.[16] Ferritin consists of a protein shell surrounding an iron core, while hemosiderin results from the breakdown of ferritin in secondary lysosomes.[17,18] Hemosiderin therefore appears to represent the end point of the intracellular storage iron pathway. The apoprotein shell of ferritin is comprised of 24 subunits of 44 kDa, arranged in four/three/two symmetry. They are cylindrical in shape, with specific interactions between them dependent on amino acid sequences that have been highly conserved throughout evolution from amphibia to mammals[15,19–21] (Fig. 127-1). The apoprotein shell encloses a core of polynuclear hydrated ferric oxide phosphate, structurally similar to ferrihydrate, which may contain up to 4500 atoms of iron.[22] The inner cavity of the ferritin molecule communicates with the exterior via eight hydrophilic channels which occur around the threefold axes (see Fig. 127-1). These channels possess metal-binding sites and may therefore be important in the transport of iron in and out of the molecule.[23] There are a further six apolar intersubunit channels around the fourfold axes, but their function is not clear.[24] It has been suggested that the accumulation of iron in apoferritin involves a process in which Fe^{++} binds at sites located in the hydrophilic channels or on the inner surface of the protein, where it is rapidly oxidized (see Fig. 127-1).[25]

Although ferritins are very similar in all species,[26] preparations of ferritin from various tissues exhibit considerable heterogeneity.

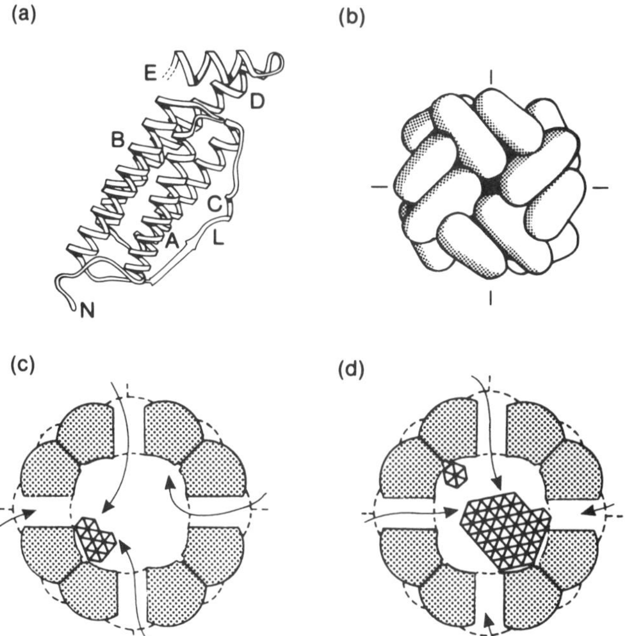

Fig. 127-1 *A*, Schematic drawing of a ferritin subunit showing the five helices A to E and the long interhelix L. *B*, Schematic representation of the ferritin molecule in which 24 subunits surround the iron core. It is viewed down a molecular fourfold axis illustrating four/three/two symmetry. *C*, A model for ferritin iron uptake and release in which Fe^{++} enters the shell through channels and is laid down at sites favoring oxidation (arrows), where an $Fe^{+++}OOH$ iron-core nucleus forms on the bound Fe^{+++}. *D*, The microcrystal builds up by oxidation of further Fe^{++} at its surface. When iron is lost from the microcrystal surface, the last added iron is released first. (*From Harrison et al.*[20] *and Ford et al.*[21] *Used by permission.*)

These differences are due to the presence of differing proportions of two subunits, one heavy (H) with 178 amino acids and the other light (L) with 174.[27] The H subunit predominates in the more acidic ferritins present in the heart, red blood cells, lymphocytes, and monocytes, while the L subunit predominates in the more basic ferritins present in the liver and spleen. The gene for the H subunit is on chromosome 11 (11q13) and that for the L subunit on chromosome 19 (19q13-ter).[28] Numerous H and L pseudogenes have been found. H gene sequences exist on at least eleven different chromosomes (1, 2, 3, 4, 6, 11, 13, 14, 17, 20, and X) and L gene sequences on at least 3 chromosomes (19, 21, and X).[29–36] The finding that H-rich isoferritins have the highest rate of iron uptake[37] is compatible with their presence in tissues such as nucleated red cells and cardiac muscle, which have a high iron requirement for heme synthesis. On the other hand, the storage of excess iron seems to require ferritin rich in L subunits, as iron loading of tissues is associated with an increase in the synthesis of the more basic ferritins.[38]

Regulation of Ferritin Synthesis. Because sufficient iron in an available but nonreactive form is essential for cell proliferation, the regulation of ferritin synthesis is of central importance in cellular metabolism. The principal regulator of ferritin synthesis is the amount of chelatable intracellular iron. Although accelerated synthesis is achieved primarily by an increase in the translation of preformed mRNA coding for H and L subunits,[39,40] there is also increased transcription of the ferritin H and L subunit genes in some cell types.[41] Translation depends on a highly conserved 28-base stem loop structure near the 5′ untranslated region, the iron-responsive element (IRE) (Fig. 127-2)[42,43] When levels of chelatable intracellular iron are low, translation of ferritin mRNA is prevented by a protein that binds specifically to the IRE. Originally designated IRE-binding protein (IRE-BP), iron regulatory factor (IRF), and ferritin repressor protein (FRP), it is now known that there are at least two protein factors, which have been designated IRP-1 and IRP-2.[44] IRP-1 is the cytoplasmic analogue of mitochondrial aconitase.[43,45–47] As the intracellular chelatable iron levels increase, the aconitase binds an iron-sulfur cluster [4Fe-4S], becomes enzymatically active as an aconitase, and dissociates from the ferritin mRNA. The rapid synthesis of ferritin subunits follows. When the iron content is low, loss of the [4Fe-4S] cluster allows the molecule to bind to the 5′-untranslated region of the ferritin mRNA. IRP-2 is 61 percent identical to IRP-1, does not have aconitase activity, but undergoes proteolysis in the presence of iron.[43] Although both IRP-1 and IRP-2 bind the IRE, there are other mRNA motifs that are bound by one or the other protein.[48] However, the natural unique targets of the two IRPs have not been identified. Nitric oxide has an effect opposite to that of iron. It causes the binding of IRP to their RNA targets, repressing the synthesis of ferritin.[49,50]

Other mRNAs, including that for the transferrin receptor, contain IREs very similar to those found in the 5′ untranslated region of ferritin mRNA, and able to bind with the same cytosolic IRPs as does the ferritin IRE (see Fig. 127-2, see "Binding and Release of Iron by Transferrin" below). When the IREs are at the 3′ end of the message, as is the case with the transferrin receptor, binding increases the stability of the mRNA and so protects it from degradation.[43] Thus, a similar process controls opposite mechanisms for the regulation of transferrin receptor and ferritin

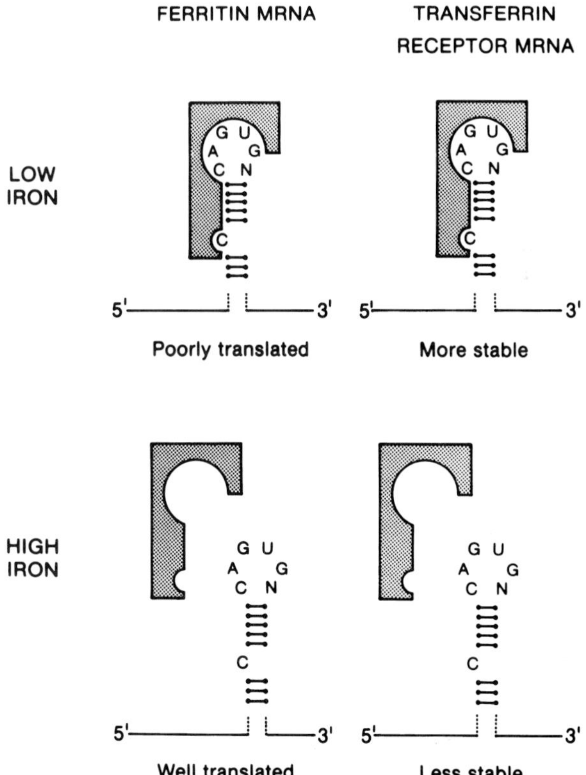

Fig. 127-2 Diagrammatic representation of the coordinated control of central pathways in iron metabolism. The stem-loop structure, with the highly conserved sequence CAGUG at the tip of the loop and a free C at the base of five paired nucleotides, is the iron-responsive element (IRE) which is present in the 5′ untranslated region of ferritin mRNA and as five copies in the 3′ untranslated region of transferrin receptor mRNA. When iron is scarce, an RNA-binding protein, IRP-1 or IRP-2 (shaded figure), binds to the IRE. The binding inhibits translation of ferritin mRNA and prevents degradation of transferrin receptor mRNA. When iron is abundant the opposite occurs. (*Adapted from Hentze et al.*[42] *Used by permission.*)

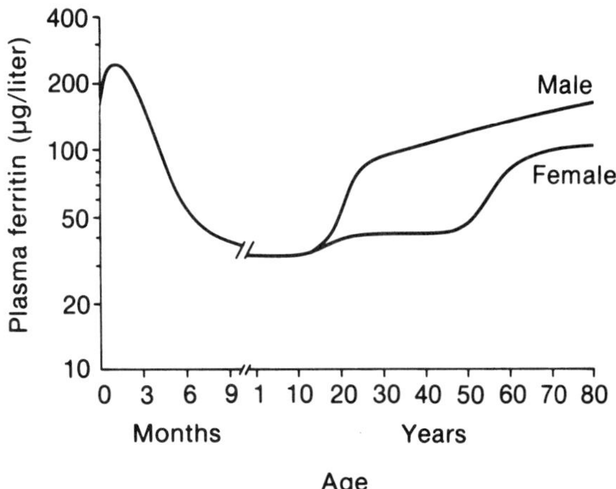

Fig. 127-3 Mean plasma ferritin concentration in American males and females at different ages. (*From Dallman et al.*[62] *Used by permission.*)

synthesis. IREs have been identified in the mRNA of mitochondrial aconitase,[51] Nramp2,[52] and erythroid amino-levulinic acid synthetase.[53]

Plasma Ferritin as a Measure of Storage Iron. Minute amounts of ferritin normally circulate in the plasma.[54] This ferritin has a low iron content and it is rich in L subunits.[27] While its origin is speculative, there is some evidence that plasma ferritin arises from macrophages[55] and hepatic parenchymal cells.[56]

In iron deficiency, the plasma ferritin concentration is always below 12 μg/liter[57] while in iron overload it is greatly elevated. Values are usually in the range of 1000 to 10,000 μg/liter in hemochromatosis.[58] In normal subjects, there is a reasonably close correlation between the plasma ferritin concentration and the size of the body iron stores, with each μg of ferritin per liter being equivalent to about 8 mg of storage iron.[59] The geometric mean value for normal adult males has been found to be approximately 100 μg/liter, and for premenopausal females about one third to one half of this.[60,61] The quite marked variations in the mean values at different ages in the two sexes reflect the changes in iron nutritional status with age (Fig. 127-3). In males consuming Western-type diets there is a steady rise in the plasma ferritin concentration throughout adult life, while a similar trend occurs in females after the menopause. These changes presumably reflect, at least in part, a slightly positive iron balance with a slow accumulation in iron stores.

With increasing degrees of overload, the relationship between the plasma ferritin concentration and the size of the body iron stores becomes less precise.[58] A simple relationship between the plasma ferritin concentration and the size of the iron stores should therefore not be assumed with ferritin values above 4000 μg/liter, or in patients who have received more than 100 units of transfused blood.

There are several situations in which the plasma ferritin concentration may be inappropriately high for the size of the body iron stores. High values have been noted with viral and drug-induced liver disease,[63] infection,[63] other types of inflammatory reaction, such as those produced by endotoxin,[64] rheumatoid arthritis,[65] Gaucher disease,[66,67] and some neoplasms.[68] The hereditary hyperferritinemia-cataract syndrome, due to mutations in the 5′ iron-responsive element of the ferritin light chain, is described under "Hemochromatosis without mutations of *HFE*."

Transferrin and the Transferrin Receptor.

Structure. Proteins specialized for the transport of iron (transferrins) have evolved in parallel with dependence on heme for oxygen transport, and they appear to be essential for the efficient distribution of iron.[11] They include serotransferrin, ovotransferrin, and lactotransferrin.[19] Serotransferrin (transferrin), the iron-binding protein that circulates in the plasma, binds iron from donor cells and delivers it via the plasma to specific receptors on recipient cells. The number of transferrin receptors varies according to the cells' need for iron. Only with such a system can the iron requirements of the erythroid marrow and the placenta be met, because they are as much as a hundredfold greater than those of other tissues. Transferrin is present in lymph fluid, cerebrospinal fluid, and edema fluid as well as plasma; as much as 50 to 60 percent of the total amount is extravascular. Transferrins are all single-polypeptide chains (molecular mass ≈80 kDa) that bind two atoms of Fe^{+++} tightly but reversibly.[19] There are 680 to 700 amino acid residues, 35 to 40 percent of them identical in homologous halves of the molecule with a metal-binding site on the N-terminus and a similar but not identical one on the C-terminus. A number of human genetic variants have been identified but show no differences in molecular weight or content of carbohydrate or iron. The human transferrin gene has been localized to chromosome 3q21-q25.[69]

The half-life of transferrin in the plasma is about 8 days. In normal subjects it is present in amounts capable of binding about 60 mMol of iron. The plasma transferrin concentration rises in iron deficiency states and falls in iron overload; there is thus an inverse relationship with the plasma ferritin concentration.[63] Iron deficiency stimulates the liver transferrin gene, while increased storage iron levels have a negative feedback effect on transferrin synthesis.[70,71] The plasma transferrin concentration is low in the nephrotic syndrome, protein-losing enteropathies, protein malnutrition, hemolysis, and inflammation of various causes, including infections, rheumatoid arthritis, myocardial infarction, and malignant neoplasms. An increased transferrin concentration is found also in pregnancy, even when there is no iron deficiency, and in women taking estrogen-containing contraceptives.[11] The increase is due to a direct effect of estrogen on the transcription of transferrin mRNA.[70]

The iron-binding capacity of transferrin is normally only about one-third saturated, so that the plasma iron concentration is approximately 10 to 30 μM.[61] There is a considerable circadian variation, with a morning peak and an evening trough, due principally to variation in the donation of iron to transferrin by the cells of the macrophage system.[72,73]

The transferrin receptor is a glycoprotein dimer with a single disulfide link, each component capable of binding a diferric transferrin molecule at the pH of the plasma (see Fig. 127-5).[71] Its gene[74] has been mapped to chromosome 3q21-q25.[75] The genes for transferrin and its receptor are thus located close to each other on the same chromosome.

Binding and Release of Iron by Transferrin. Transferrin binds iron at either or both of its binding sites, so that diferric and two monoferric transferrin species coexist with apotransferrin in the plasma, the proportions varying according to the percentage saturation with iron. Tissue uptake of iron is considerably greater from diferric molecules,[77] and is therefore a function of the transferrin saturation as well as of the number of tissue receptors for transferrin. Transferrin releases its iron after binding to specific cell receptors present on essentially all proliferating, differentiating, and hemoglobin-synthesizing cells.[73] The number of surface receptors per erythroid cell is the major factor determining iron uptake during differentiation. There is a peak of 800,000 per cell in intermediate normoblasts, and the number drops to virtually zero in mature erythrocytes. Cell-surface receptors represent only a proportion of the total, and there is a continuous shuttling of receptors between the surface and the interior of the cell.[73]

Regulation of Transferrin Receptor Synthesis. The synthesis of transferrin receptors is closely coordinated with that of ferritin. The 3′ untranslated region of transferrin receptor mRNA contains 5 IREs and these serve to regulate translation as a function of the available iron.[71] Any rise in the chelatable iron concentration leads

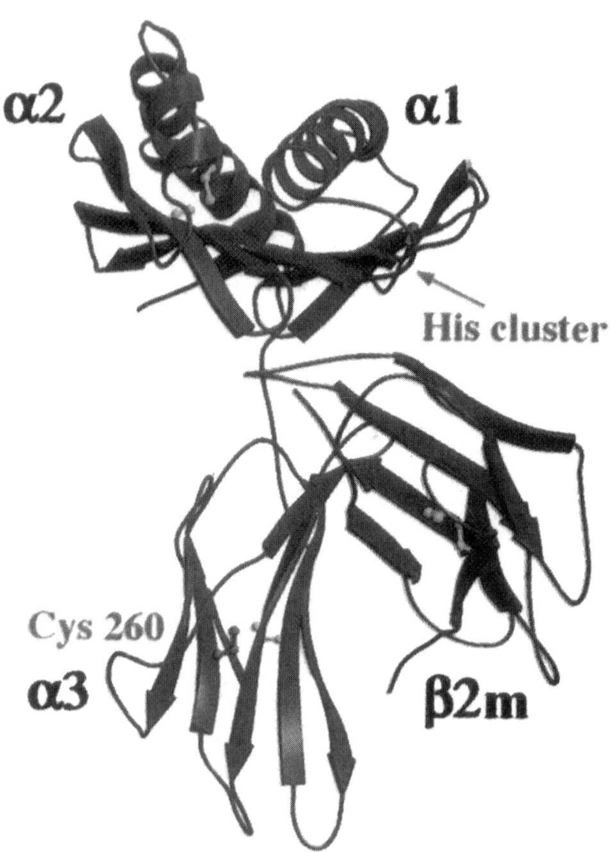

Fig. 127-4 The structure of the HFE molecule complexed with β_2-microglobulin (β_2m). The His cluster is the portion of the molecule in which the 187G(H63D) mutation is found. Cys 260 is another designation for the 845A(C282Y) mutation. The latter mutation prevents the binding of β_2-microglobulin to HFE and thus prevents its transport to the cell surface. (*From Lebrón et al.*[76] *Used with permission.*)

to a decrease in the binding of cytoplasmic aconitase IRP-1 to the IREs of both ferritin and transferrin mRNA (see "Regulation of Ferritin Synthesis"). As a result, the extra chelatable iron within the cell can be sequestered in newly synthesized apoferritin, and fewer iron-loaded transferrin molecules can be bound by reduced numbers of transferrin receptors, so that the rate of delivery of iron from the plasma is reduced.[78]

HFE. *HFE* was discovered by positional cloning of the gene that causes the most common type of hereditary hemochromatosis.[79] The deduced structure of the HFE protein is shown in Fig. 127-4. The *HFE* gene is located about 4 megabases telomeric to the HLA locus. It codes for an HLA-like glycoprotein that contains a β_2-microglobulin-binding site.[79] The primary translated product is comprised of 343 amino acids and it is processed to a mature protein of 321 amino acids.[80] Like other HLA class 1 proteins, HFE has a disulfide bridge in the β_2-microglobulin-binding site. The cysteine-282 that is mutated to tyrosine in the principal mutation that causes hereditary hemochromatosis is one of the two cysteines that forms this bridge, and accordingly it was predicted that the mutant HFE would not bind to β_2-microglobulin. A possible role of β_2-microglobulin in iron metabolism had been suggested earlier by the iron accumulation that occurs in the β_2-microglobulin knockout mouse[81] and before the *HFE* gene was identified it had been proposed that it might be an HLA gene.[82] The crystal structure of HFE has been solved, and it has been concluded that the analogue of the peptide binding groove is nonfunctional in the molecule.[76]

HFE mRNA is found in a broad range of tissues,[79] but relatively little is known about the distribution of the protein in the body. Immunochemical staining for the HFE protein is seen in some epithelial cells in every segment of the alimentary canal. However, its cellular and subcellular expression in the small intestine is mainly intracellular and perinuclear, limited to cells in deep crypts. This is quite distinct from the stomach and colon, where staining is polarized and restricted to the basolateral surfaces, and from the epithelial cells of the esophagus and submucosal leukocytes, which show nonpolarized staining around the entire plasma membrane.[83] Surface localization has also been observed in tissue culture cells, but these have been transfected with *HFE* cDNA, and it is not certain whether it represents the physiological localization of the protein in such cells. HFE has been found to associate with the transferrin receptor[80,84] and to lower its affinity for ligand binding. The effect is strongly pH dependent.[76]

Nramp2. The Nramp (natural resistance-associated m phi) gene was isolated as a candidate for the host resistance locus Bcg/Ity/Lsh, which controls natural resistance of mice to several types of infections.[483] It was soon recognized that this was only one of a small family of proteins, the second of which was designated Nramp2.[87] The iron transport properties of Nramp2 were inferred in 1997 from two entirely independent findings. Fractionation of rat intestine mRNAs that facilitated metal transport when injected into frog oocytes revealed one species which has an unusually broad substrate range that included Fe^{++}, Zn^{++}, Mn^{++}, Co^{++}, Cd^{++}, Cu^{++}, Ni^{++}, and Pb^{++}. The clone was designated *DCT*1 and found to mediate proton-coupled active transport that depends on the cell membrane potential. The sequence of *DCT*1 was that of Nramp2. The other line of evidence that implicated Nramp2 in metal transport was derived from the positional cloning of the locus that causes the mk (microcytic) mouse mutation[88] and subsequently the Belgrade rat mutation.[52] Astonishingly, these two independent mutations both produce a glycine-to-arginine missense mutation in the identical codon in the mouse and rat. Homozygous mk/mk mice have a microcytic, hypochromic anemia due to severe defects in intestinal iron absorption and erythroid iron utilization. Belgrade rats have microcytic, hypochromic anemia associated with abnormal gastrointestinal iron absorption and reticulocyte iron uptake, the latter of which appears to be a failure of iron transport out of endosomes within the transferrin cycle. Thus, although the phenotypes of these two mutations are somewhat different, both are clearly due to a defect in iron transport.

The Nramp2 gene is comprised of 17 exons and spans more than 36 kb. It contains an additional 5′ exon and intron (exon and intron 1) and an additional 3′ exon (exon 17) and intron (intron 16) as compared to the homologous Nramp1. The additional exons and introns account for much of the difference in length between Nramp2 ($>$36 kb) and Nramp 1 (12 kb).[89] The mRNA exists in two major forms. One contains a classical iron-responsive element in the 3′ untranslated region that confers iron-dependent mRNA stabilization. The other has the carboxyl terminal 18 amino acids substituted with 25 novel amino acids and has a new 3′ untranslated region lacking a classical iron-responsive element. Five single nucleotide mutations or polymorphisms were identified within the Nramp2 gene. A 1303 A $\rightarrow$ C resulting in a conservative leucine $\rightarrow$ isoleucine substitution has been found in one patient with non-HFE hemochromatosis, but the significance of this change is unknown.[89] A polymorphism, 1254T/C, also occurs in the coding region of Nramp2 but does not cause an amino acid change. The other three polymorphisms are within introns (IVS2+11A/G, IVS4+44C/A, and IVS6+538G±). In addition, a polymorphic microsatellite was identified in intron 3. At least three different haplotypes are represented.

Mobilferrin. Mobilferrin (named after Mobile, Alabama, where it was described at the University of Alabama) was discovered as a 56-kDa intestinal iron-binding protein. Partial sequence analysis showed it to be identical to calreticulin.[90] Calreticulin/mobilferrin is known to be a chaperone protein that plays a role in the translocation of HLA molecules to the cell surface.[91,92] Mobilferrin isolated from the intestine was found to bind iron with a dissociation constant of 3×10^{-18} M.[93] The binding of iron by mobilferrin is pH dependent, the metal readily dissociating under acidic conditions.

Internal Iron Exchange

Plasma iron follows three main pathways. By far the largest fraction goes to the erythron, virtually all to be incorporated into hemoglobin. The second plasma iron pathway is to parenchymal cells, particularly those of the liver. The quantity is normally small, but if the erythroid marrow uptake is inhibited, virtually all the plasma iron can be deposited in the liver parenchyma.[13] The third pathway is to extravascular fluids.

Most of the iron entering the plasma is contributed by macrophages. This iron is derived mainly from hemoglobin catabolism, but there is also a contribution from storage compounds. A much smaller fraction originates from stores in other tissues. About 3 percent of the plasma iron turnover is normally iron absorbed from the diet by the mucosal cells of the upper small intestine. Unless the body iron stores are exhausted, the supply of iron to the plasma iron pool is capable of adjustment within wide limits to match changing demands. The regulation of macrophage iron release proceeds rapidly so that there are only transient changes in the plasma iron concentration.

The requirement for transferrin iron is determined by the major recipient, the erythroid marrow. In chronic hemolytic states, the quantity of iron passing through the plasma can increase sixfold to eightfold, while it diminishes to one-third of normal when erythropoiesis is inhibited, for example on descending from high altitudes.[13] Erythropoietic demand is reflected by the numbers of transferrin receptors. Independent of requirement, parenchymal uptake of transferrin iron increases with the number of diferric transferrin molecules in the plasma, and hence with the transferrin saturation.[94] The affinity of the binding of diferric transferrin by the transferrin receptor is one to two orders of magnitude greater than that of the monoferric transferrins.[71] The resulting complexes are concentrated in coated pits that bud off to form vesicles (Fig. 127-5). Each endocytic vesicle is transported by saltatory motion along microtubular and microfilamentary tracts to the site of iron delivery. There the pH is lowered by energy-dependent protonation, which releases the iron without disturbing the binding of the apotransferrin to the receptor, so that the apotransferrin is protected from acid hydrolysis.[71] Binding to the transferrin receptor increases the tendency of transferrin to release its iron at a low pH.[86] After the return of the vesicle to the surface of the cell, the rise in pH releases the apotransferrin into the plasma and frees the receptor for binding with another iron-loaded transferrin molecule.

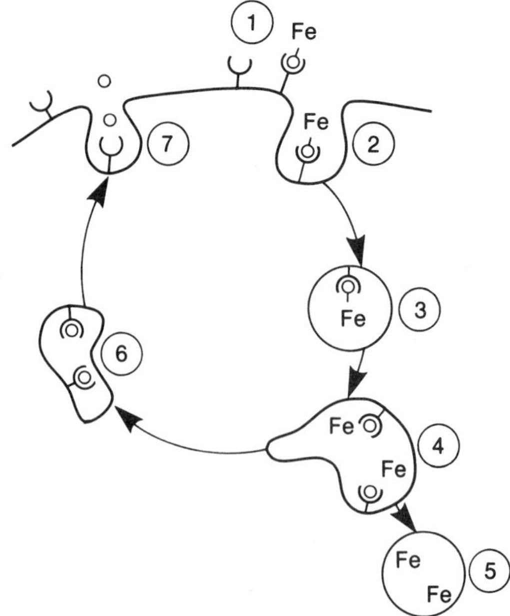

Fig. 127-5 Receptor-mediated endocytic pathway for transferrin. Specific binding of diferric transferrin to the transferrin receptor (step 1) results in the formation of an endocytic vesicle (steps 2 and 3). The vesicle becomes protonated, which results in the uncoupling of the receptor and its ligand (step 4). In this acidic environment, iron is detached from transferrin (step 5). The apotransferrin so released has a high affinity for the transferrin receptor at the acidic pH within the endocytic vesicle and thus escapes digestion (step 6). The vesicle is then exteriorized (steps 6 and 7). On exposure to the physiological pH the apotransferrin loses its affinity for the transferrin receptor and is released into the plasma.

External Iron Exchange

For adequate iron nutrition a positive iron balance is necessary during childhood and adolescence. In this way the growing demand of the body for functional iron is satisfied and storage depots are gradually built up. Thereafter, the amounts absorbed from the diet must at least match the average daily losses from the body. Additional amounts must be absorbed to meet the requirements of pregnancy and to replace any abnormal losses through blood donation or hemorrhage.

Iron Excretion. Iron is lost from the body physiologically by desquamation of surface cells from the skin, gastrointestinal tract, and urinary tract and by the minimal gastrointestinal blood loss that occurs even in healthy individuals. There are also very low concentrations of extracellular iron in the sweat, bile, and urine. In women, the losses incurred through menstruation and pregnancy must be added. Total daily iron losses in adult males amount to between 0.9 and 1 mg (1 mg = 17.9 mmol).[11] The mean normal menstrual losses when expressed in terms of daily iron balance are approximately 0.5 mg, but there is considerable variation, and it has been estimated that in 5 percent of normal women the figure is greater than 1.4 mg.[94]

Iron Absorption. The amount of iron absorbed from the diet at any one time depends on three factors: the quantity of iron, the composition of the diet, and the behavior of the mucosa of the upper small bowel. Although much effort has been expended in attempting to understand the mechanism by which iron is translocated from the intestinal lumen to transferrin in the plasma, the picture that has emerged is still quite incomplete.[1,11] Iron is presented to the intestine as inorganic Fe^{++} or Fe^{+++} salts and as heme. It is very likely that these two forms traverse different pathways, at least until the point at which iron has been released from the heme.[95]

The most active sites of iron absorption are the duodenum and upper jejunum.[96] There are two components to the absorptive mechanism: mucosal uptake and intracellular transport. Some regulation occurs at both phases. Mucosal uptake is the rate-limiting step, the fractional rate being less than 1 percent of subsequent intracellular transport.[97] Within the cell there are two major pathways. Iron is either transported within minutes into the portal circulation or is stored in the cell as ferritin.[98] The relative amounts following these alternate pathways depend on body demands for iron. When demand is high, a large proportion of the iron entering the mucosal cell is transported rapidly into the body. As iron stores expand, an increasing proportion of the iron taken up by the cell is deposited in mucosal ferritin and is subsequently lost to the body at the end of the cell's 2- to 3-day life span.[99,100] Regulation of iron absorption may therefore occur at the point where iron entering from the lumen is directed along one or the other of the two alternative pathways.[98]

Dietary Iron Content and Bioavailability. Typical Western diets usually contain about 6 mg iron per 1000 kcal, with surprisingly little variation from meal to meal.[101] In certain circumstances the iron content is appreciably increased by extrinsic iron, either in the form of dirt or from the surface of containers or cooking vessels. The former is usually of very low bioavailability,[101] but iron derived from pans or containers can add significantly to the absorbable iron intake, especially when the pH of the food being prepared in them is low. This is strikingly illustrated by the traditional alcoholic beverages brewed in iron containers by southern African blacks, whose daily iron intake may be increased from about 15 mg to as much as 100 mg as a result.[11,102]

Variations in the bioavailability of food iron are of greater importance for iron nutrition than is the amount of iron in the diet.[1,103] Heme iron is easily absorbed, whatever the dietary composition, whereas absorption of nonheme iron, usually of low bioavailability, is markedly influenced by other ingredients in the diet. A number of inhibitors of nonheme iron absorption have been recognized. These include phytates present in bran, the tannates in Indian tea, the polyphenols in vegetables, calcium salts, the phosphoprotein in egg yolk, and a factor in soy protein.[101]

The absorptive behavior of the intestinal mucosa changes according to the body iron content, but the amount of dietary iron that can be absorbed is limited because of its restricted bioavailability. Absorption thus rises to only 3 to 4 mg daily when iron deficiency anemia is present and falls to less than 0.5 mg daily with iron overload. These figures underline how small daily external iron exchange is in relation to the total body iron content.

Inorganic Iron Absorption. Ferric iron is very insoluble at alkaline pH levels as are found in the intestine. However, ferric iron complexes with substances in the stomach that allow it to remain soluble when entering the alkaline environment of the intestinal tract.[104–106] The binding substance was designated *gastroferrin* and was believed to play a regulatory role in iron absorption. Initial claims that gastroferrin normally inhibits iron absorption, and that this protein is absent in homozygotes for the HLA-linked iron-loading gene,[105] were not confirmed in subsequent studies.[107] More recent investigations have established that the principal iron-binding substance in the gastrointestinal tract is mucin.[108] Ferrous iron is more soluble at alkaline pH levels and it is not clear whether binding to mucin plays a role in its absorption. Purification of the microvillus membrane-associated proteins indicated that iron is associated with a dimer of polypeptides, one approximately 90 kDa and the other 150 kDa. These reacted with monoclonal antibodies to known integrins.[109] The iron-binding protein mobilferrin binds to the cytosolic carboxy-terminal end of the a chain of an integrin, and pulse-chase experiments suggest that a complex consisting of iron, mobilferrin, integrin(s), a flavin-monooxygenase, and β_2-microglobulin,[110] which has been designated *paraferritin* (based on similarity in chromatographic migration to ferritin), is formed. It is not clear how the iron in the paraferritin complex reaches the transferrin at the abluminal membrane.

The mucin-integrin-mobilferrin pathway delineated by Conrad and his colleagues[93] does not include or take into account the more recently described proteins HFE and Nramp2. At present one can only speculate regarding their roles in iron absorption. HFE, as noted above, is expressed in intestinal cells and its deficiency leads to increased iron absorption. Thus, one may conclude that HFE has an inhibitory effect on iron absorption, but it is not clear whether this effect is exerted directly in the intestine or whether the protein may act at a distance, signaling, in some way, to modulate the absorption of iron. Nramp2 is an iron transport protein. It is found in intestinal cells, and while there is no direct evidence that it participates in the transport of iron across the mucosa, the fact that the mk/mk mouse, which has an abnormality in Nramp2 manifests defective intestinal iron absorption suggests that it does play such a role. The brush border of the intestinal mucosa has been shown to have the capacity to reduce ferric iron to ferrous iron and the rate of reduction is greater in intestinal biopsies obtained from patients with hemochromatosis.[111] It has been suggested that it is only the ferrous form that is absorbed into the cell.[112] The relationship of these pathways to a 160-kDa trimeric protein isolated from microvillous membrane vesicles isolated from human intestine[113] is unknown. Clearly our understanding of the intestinal absorption of inorganic iron is still quite incomplete.

Heme Iron Absorption. A large proportion of iron absorbed from the diet is in the form of heme, especially in Western populations.[114] The chemical properties of heme are quite different from those of the inorganic iron salts that are found in the body. Heme is extremely hydrophobic and most soluble in alkali. Iron salts are more soluble in acid. Desferrioxamine markedly diminishes absorption of inorganic iron but not of hemoglobin iron.[115] It is evident that different mechanisms must have evolved for the absorption of heme iron than those utilized for the absorption of inorganic iron. The percentage absorption of inorganic iron decreases markedly as the dose is increased, but the absorption of heme iron is largely independent of dose.[95,116,117] Both heme and inorganic iron absorption are increased in iron deficiency[95,118] and in hereditary hemochromatosis.[119,120]

Much has been learned about the availability and regulation of the absorption of heme iron, but little is known about the pathway heme traverses in the intestine. Like inorganic iron, particularly in the Fe^{+++} state, pure heme is very poorly soluble, existing largely in miscellar form. The solubility of inorganic iron in the intestine is accomplished by binding to mucin. Heme appears to complex with peptides or amino acids in the intestine; absorption is greatly facilitated by the addition of globin when heme is fed.[95,121] It is likely that a heme receptor exists in the intestine but its characterization is incomplete.[122,123] The subsequent fate of absorbed heme is not understood in detail, but the presumption that the iron is removed from the porphyrin ring by the action of heme oxygenase is supported by the fact that the administration of tin mesoporphyrin, an inhibitor of heme oxygenase, results in diminished uptake of ^{59}Fe from radiolabeled heme. Heme itself has been detected in microendocytic caveolae at the bases of microvilli and in the apical cytoplasm of dogs after hemoglobin was given intraluminally.[124] Studies in patients with portacaval shunts suggested that absorbed iron leaves the intestinal cell as inorganic iron,[125] and it is therefore likely that the distal parts of the pathway of heme and inorganic iron absorption are the same. The fate of the iron after its release from heme is unknown.

Regulation of Iron Absorption. The amount of iron absorbed at any one time is markedly influenced by the body's iron content.[59] In early animal experiments, a direct relationship was also noted between iron absorption and the rate of erythropoiesis,[126] but in humans the situation is more complicated. Absorption is normal or only modestly enhanced in chronic hemolytic states such as hereditary spherocytosis, but is increased in parallel with the rate of erythropoiesis in conditions such as thalassemia major, which are characterized by markedly increased but ineffective erythropoietic activity.[127] As a result, iron overload occurs infrequently in hereditary hemolytic anemias, while it is inevitable in conditions such as thalassemia major, in which maturation of the red cell is disordered.[128] Why this should be so remains an enigma, although it has been suggested that it may relate to different patterns of red cell breakdown.[127]

GENETICS OF HEREDITARY HEMOCHROMATOSIS

Mode of Inheritance

Hereditary hemochromatosis is an inherited disease, and abnormalities in iron metabolism can consistently be demonstrated among some relatives of affected patients.[129] This is not the case in families of patients with alcoholic cirrhosis who exhibit increased liver iron.[130] For many years the finding of detectable abnormalities in iron indices among offspring or parents of patients suggested autosomal dominant inheritance of the disease. More detailed studies of many families, however, established that overt clinical hemochromatosis is less common than minor abnormalities in iron metabolism among children and parents. Genetic analysis of such data led to the hypothesis that hereditary hemochromatosis was an autosomal recessive condition, while the occasional minor abnormalities in iron metabolism apparent in other family members were manifestations of the heterozygous state.[131,132] However, the problems of delayed clinical expression and the low manifestation rate of overt disease in females made interpretation difficult, and no consensus regarding the mode of inheritance existed.

HLA Studies Clarify Autosomal Recessive Transmission. A fortuitous observation that HLA-A3 was frequently found among patients with hemochromatosis[133] was confirmed in many series of patients of European origin clarified the mode of inheritance.[129] While HLA-A3 occurs in no more than 30 percent of persons of European origin, it was present in 73 percent of 384 hemochromatotic patients in a collective series, a finding that was confirmed in many other studies.[129] In contrast, the frequencies of HLA-A3 at the MHC locus in patients with alcoholic cirrhosis and increased liver iron did not differ from those in controls.[135]

Family investigations indicated that the gene for hereditary hemochromatosis was closely linked to the HLA-A locus on the short arm of chromosome 6 (Chr. 6p21).[135,136] Sibs with overt hemochromatosis in a given family usually share both their HLA haplotypes, that is, they have identical HLA alleles on *both* maternal and paternal chromosomes. Thus, a chromosomal segment comprising a gene for hereditary hemochromatosis and a linked group of HLA genes is contributed by both the father and mother of each affected offspring (Fig. 127-6).[137] These data established homozygosity for the disease allele and autosomal recessive inheritance for the disease. Because heterozygotes only share a single haplotype with affected homozygotes, heterozygote status can be established by appropriate family studies that include an overtly affected patient with HLA-linked hemochromatosis.

Identification of the Hemochromatosis Gene

The localization of the hemochromatosis gene to a site closely linked to the MHC locus on 6p21 led many laboratories to search for the abnormal gene. The association with HLA-A3 in several European populations suggested a possible common mutational origin of hemochromatosis. An identical mutational event in a common ancestor (founder effect) became very likely by finding common haplotypes that consisted of several closely linked DNA markers in the MHC region in a large number of unrelated patients.[138–144] With this rationale, linkage disequilibrium mapping was attempted by several research teams. In this method, the presence or absence of closely linked DNA markers around the disease gene was quantitatively assessed to localize the mutational site.[145,146] In hemochromatosis, such an analysis was found to be difficult because of the lack of correspondence between the genetic map (as defined by recombinational events) and actual physical map distances in the hemochromatosis gene region. Markers within 1 centimorgan distance (i.e., 1 percent recombination) were more than 6 megabases apart, a finding explained by a low frequency of recombination in this chromosomal region. Thus, markers that were relatively far apart showed a similar degree of linkage disequilibrium to the hemochromatosis region, making identification of the gene difficult.

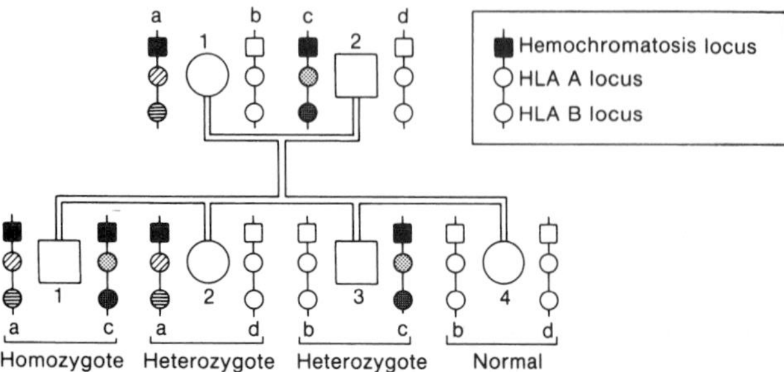

Fig. 127-6 The *HFE* locus and linked HLA and HLA B loci in a male patient with homozygous hereditary hemochromatosis and his family members. The relation between the *HFE* gene and the HLA loci is represented diagrammatically. (The *HFE* locus is located 4kb telomeric to the HLA A locus.) (*From Beaumont et al.*[137] *Used by permission.*)

The isolation of the hemochromatosis gene was ultimately accomplished by a research team at a biotechnology company using disequilibrium mapping, coupled with studies for maximum allelic association of genetic markers and an analysis of historic recombinational events in affected patients.[79] A candidate region of 250 kb was then completely sequenced. A missense mutation (G → A) in an HLA-A2-like gene (first named *HLA-H*, later changed to *HFE*) resulted in a cysteine to tyrosine substitution at amino acid 282 (C282Y) and was detected in the homozygous state in 83 percent of 178 unrelated Caucasian hemochromatosis patients. Six percent of controls were heterozygotes for this mutation, a value consistent with the gene frequency of hemochromatosis in the population. An additional mutation at this gene 187 C → G (H63D) was discovered in the homozygous state in only one of 178 patients with hemochromatosis, but occurred in 17 percent of controls in the heterozygous state. Compound heterozygosity for both the 845A (C282Y) and 187G (H63D) was seen in 4 percent of hemochromatosis patients. The rarity of 187G (H63D) homozygotes among hemochromatosis patients suggests milder or no clinical manifestations among most homozygous individuals for this mutation. Another *HFE* mutation at nucleotide 193 with a gene frequency of 0.015 has been reported, but its involvement in iron loading seems to be minor.[147,148] The absence of further mutations at the *HFE* gene suggests that the remainder of Caucasian hemochromatosis patients owe their disease to yet unidentified mutations that do not reside at the HFE locus, or to other nongenetic factors.

Do Genetic Modifiers Account for Sib Resemblance in Clinical Severity? Familial resemblance in the extent of liver iron storage, particularly among affected male sibs, has been reported.[149] Because affected sibs carry the identical mutation for hemochromatosis, it is likely that (in the absence of environmental factors such as frequent blood donations) such sibs may share identical modifier genes of yet unknown nature to account for such similarities. However, significant clinical differences with the younger sib having more iron storage than an older sib has also been reported.[150] The identification of genetic and other as yet unknown modifiers is awaited with interest.

Frequency of *HFE* Gene Mutations. The findings of a high frequency of homozygosity for the 845A (C282Y) mutation at the *HFE* locus in patients with hemochromatosis were rapidly confirmed in many studies among patients of central, northern, and western European origin. The frequency of homozygosity ranged from 92 percent to 83 percent among Caucasians (see Table 127-2 for references). No more than 2 percent of homozygotes of the 187G (H63D) mutation were found in various studies of affected patients. The detection of compound heterozygotes for both mutations among 2 to 4 percent of hemochromatosis patients is of particular interest. The manifestation rate (penetrance) for clinically recognized hemochromatosis can be calculated to be around 1.5 percent or less for such compound heterozygotes 845A/187G.[79,151] Most studies of hemochromatosis patients also detected occasional heterozygotes (0 to 4.3 percent) for the major 845A (C282Y) mutation. This finding may be unrelated to pathogenesis and may merely reflect the expected high population

Table 127-2 Mutant *HFE* Genotypes in Patients with Hemochromatosis*

			Genotype of Affected Individuals (%)				
Author & reference	Number of patients	Homozygotes 845A (C282Y)	Compound heterozygotes 845A (C282Y)/187G (H63D)	Homozygotes 187G (H63D)	Heterozygotes for 845A (C282Y)	Heterozygotes for 187G (H63D)
Feder (U.S.) 1996[79]	178	83.2%	4.5%	0.6%	0.6%	5.1%
Beutler (U.S.) 1996[151]	147	82.3%	5.4%	1.4%	1.4%	2.7%
Jouanolle (France) 1996[154]	65	90.8%	4.6%	1.5%	0%	3.1%
Robson (U.K.) 1997[155]	115	91.3%	2.6%	0.9%	0.9%	0%
Adams (Canada) 1997[156]	74	91.9%	0%	0%	2.7%	0%
Borot (France) 1997[157]	94	72.3%	4.3%	2.1%	4.3%	8.5%
Carella (Italy) 1997[157]	75	64.0%	6.6%	1.3%	2.7%	4.0%

*Diagnosed by liver biopsy and/or appropriate phlebotomy data.

frequency of heterozygosity for 845A (C282Y) hemochromatosis. Alternately, heterozygosity for this gene may increase the chance of more severe iron loading in those with non-*HFE* mutations. The presence of an additional unrecognized *HFE* allele that causes compound heterozygosity is another possibility,[152] but extensive sequencing so far has failed to detect additional mutations at the *HFE* locus.[79,151,153,248]

The availability of simple molecular tests for *HFE* mutations allowed extensive testing of many populations. The allele frequency for the 845A (C282Y) mutation in central and northern Europe can be roughly classified as a high frequency class, with most values ranging between 0.05 and 0.07, and a lower frequency group, represented by Italians (0.01), Greeks (0.013), and Ashkenazi Jews (0.013) (see Table 127-3 for references).

Many different populations have been studied for the presence of the two *HFE* mutations.[172,174] The major 845A (C282Y) mutation has not been found in populations from Africa, Asia, Southeast Asia (Java, Papua New Guinea), or Micronesia. The few 845A (C282Y) alleles found in Australian aborigines, Melanesians, and Polynesians were accompanied by HLA haplotypes common in Europeans and therefore presumably arose by admixture. *HFE*-linked hemochromatosis is therefore absent or unusual in most non-European populations. Familial hemochromatosis among non-Europeans is likely to be caused by as yet undetected genes.

Hemochromatosis has occasionally been reported among African-Americans.[175] Because the gene pool of African-Americans is about 25 percent of Caucasian origin, the expected frequency of *HFE*-linked homozygous hemochromatosis in the African-American population would be about 1 in 6000 [(845A (C282Y) allele frequency in U.S. Caucasians $\times$ 0.25)^2] or significantly less frequent than among persons of European origin. However, the likely genetic origin of a non-*HFE* related iron-loading disorder among Africans (see "African Iron Loading" below) may be responsible for many cases. The identification of the putative gene for the African iron loading disease and its interactions with *HFE* mutations is awaited with interest.

The frequency of the 187G (H63D) mutation is consistently higher than that of the 845A (C282Y) mutation (Table 127-3). Allelic frequencies range between 13 to 16 percent in European populations. The 187G (H63D) and the 845A (C282Y) mutations are never carried next to each other on the same chromosome and are always in linkage disequilibrium. Because the 187G (H63D) variant is also seen in lower frequencies in many populations who do not carry the 845A (C282Y) allele, and because the 187G allele is in linkage equilibrium with HLA-A, a more ancient origin of the 187G (H63D) mutation has been suggested.[176]

Several polymorphic sites exist in the introns of the *HFE* gene, which together with the 845A and 187G mutations give rise to 10 distinct potential haplotypes. All but one of these haplotypes were detected in "normal" Europeans with distinctly different distributions among "normal" Asians and (as expected) in chromosomes from hemochromatosis patients.[176]

Matings between homozygous individuals and heterozygotes will not be infrequent. With a heterozygote frequency of 10 percent in the population (Table 127-4), 10 percent of all matings by homozygotes would be with a heterozygote. Because 50 percent of the children of homozygote X heterozygote matings are homozygotes, the explanation for observed "vertical" pedigree pattern mimicking autosomal dominant inheritance (i.e., pseudo dominance) is apparent.

Origin of the *HFE* Mutations

The reason for the high frequency of the mutant *HFE* gene is unknown. It is possible that in the past heterozygotes had a selective advantage if they absorbed more dietary iron and were therefore relatively protected against iron deficiency and its deleterious effects.[177,178] The accumulation of larger body iron reserves would improve survival and fertility among heterozygous women particularly. The resultant selective advantage would have led to a gradual increase in the frequency of the gene. Selection against subjects homozygous for hereditary hemochromatosis is minimal, because the condition usually causes overt disease only after the reproductive period is over, at a time when such patients have transmitted the mutant gene to their offspring. However, the commonly reported loss of libido and impotence among affected males may have reduced transmission of the hemochromatosis gene.

The high frequency of the unique 845A (C282Y) mutation associated with a similar haplotypic background in many patients with hemochromatosis suggests a common origin derived from a common ancestor in whom the mutation first occurred. Various data show relatively high frequencies of 845A (C282Y) genes in patients whose ancestors originated from northwest Europe. A Celtic origin, with spread of the gene by migration, has been postulated to account for these findings.[164] In contrast, in most other genetic diseases, especially less common ones, many different specific allelic mutations with unique haplotypes are detected in different patients.

Table 127-3 Allele* Frequencies of *HFE* Mutations in Various Populations of European Origin

845A (C282Y)	187G (H163D)	Population	Number of chromosomes* studied	Reference
Group 1 "High" Frequency				
0.0610	0.136	Caucasian U.S. (New Mexico)	574	Garry et al. 1997[158]
0.075	0.158	Caucasian U.S. (California)	386	Beutler et al. 1996[151]
0.07	0.144	Caucasian U.S. (Alabama)	286	Barton et al. 1997[159]
0.066	0.150	Caucasian U.S. (Maine)	2004	Bradley et al. 1998[160]
0.0425	n.d.	U.K.	400	Willis et al. 1997[161]
—	0.164	U.K.	116	Willis et al. 1997[161]
0.059	0.158	U.K.	202	Robson et al. 1997[155]
0.029	0.147	French	278	Jouanelle et al. 1996[154]
0.042	0.158	French	190	Borot 1997[157]
0.09	n.d.‡	French (Bretons)	188	Mercier et al. 1998[162]
0.0944	0.169	French	508	Jezequel et al. 1998[163]
0.021	n.d.	French (Catalans)	332	Mercier et al. 1997[164]
0.032	0.165	CEPH collection	308	Feder et al. 1996[79]
0.026	0.111	German	306	Gottschalk et al. 1998[165]
0.0625	n.d.	Norway	288	Bell 1997[166]
0.0517	0.166	Swedish	174	Cardoso et al. 1998[167]
0.038	0.136	Europe (all)	2900	Merriweather-Clarke et al. 1997[168]
0.064	n.d.	Australian	4750	Cullen et al. 1998[169]
0.052	n.d.	Finns	346	Beckman et al. 1997[170]
Group 2 "Low" Frequency				
0.01	0.1	Italians	100	Carella et al. 1997[153]
0.013	0.097	Ashkenazi Jews	762	Beutler et al. 1997[171]
0.0163	n.d.	French Basques	184	Mercier et al. 1998[162]
0.013	0.135	Greeks	392	Merriweather-Clarke et al. 1997[168]
0.016	n.d.	Mordvinians	170	Beckman et al. 1997[170]

*Note that frequencies refer to allele and *not* heterozygote frequencies. See Table 127-4 (Explanations) for calculating heterozygote frequencies from allele frequencies.
†Number of individuals studied = 1/2 (number of chromosomes).
‡n.d. - not done.

Frequency of Hemochromatosis by Nongenetic Criteria. In contrast to the expected high frequencies of homozygous 845A (C282Y) hemochromatosis among European populations (Table 127-3), fully developed clinical cases have been considered to be relatively uncommon. By 1935, 350 well-documented cases had been reported,[3] and during the next 20 years another 800 were documented.[179] Since 1955 many further reports have appeared.[1] Phenotypic expression of the gene obviously depends not only on the gene frequency in the population, but also on the amount of iron which can be absorbed from the average diet.

In a study in which the storage iron concentrations in almost 4000 liver specimens from 18 countries were measured, only 3 were found to be more than 5 times normal, and none of these was anywhere near the range of 20 to 50 times normal usually found in

Table 127-4 Expected Frequencies and Significance of Various Genetic Classes for *HFE* Genes in the General U.S. Population (Caucasian)

	Frequency	Remarks
Homozygotes for 845A(C282Y)	0.0043 (4.3/1000)	Hemochromatosis with unknown clinical penetrance.
Homozygotes for 187G(H63D)	0.022 (2.2%)	Rarely affected with clinical hemochromatosis.
Compound heterozygotes 845A(C282Y)/187G(H63D)	0.02 (2%)	Rarely affected with clinical hemochromatosis (penetrance about 1%).
Heterozygotes for 845A(C282Y) allele	0.103 (10.3%)	Occasional heterozygotes (1.5–4%) found among patients with clinical hemochromatosis. Pathogenic significance unknown.
Heterozygotes for 187G(H63D) allele	0.235 (23.5%)	Occasional heterozygotes (0–8.5%) found among patients with clinical hemochromatosis. Pathogenic significance unknown.
Homozygotes for normal allele	0.615 (61.5%)	"Normal" wild-type—not carrying *HFE* mutations.

Explanations:
Frequency for 845A (C282Y) allele 0.066; frequency for 187G (H63D) allele 0.15.[160]
Calculations by the Hardy-Weinberg law. (Note that the 845A allele and the 187G allele are always in linkage disequilibrium, i.e., are never on the same chromosome.)
Population frequencies: $p^2 + q^2 + r^2 + 2pq + 2pr + 2qr = 1$
Allele frequencies: $p + q + r = 1$ where p = normal allele frequency; q = frequency of 845A(C282Y) allele; r = frequency of 187G(H63D) allele. Homozygote frequency for normal allele = p^2.
Homozygote frequency for 845A (C282Y) allele = q^2.
Homozygote frequency for 187G (H63D) allele = r^2.
Heterozygote frequencies for 845A (C282Y) and 187G (H63D) alleles are 2pq and 2pr respectively.
Frequency of compound heterozygote 845A (C282Y)/187G (H63D) is 2qr.

hemochromatosis.[180] In addition, none of more than 3000 apparently normal individuals in the Seattle, Washington area had a plasma ferritin concentration approaching that found in hereditary hemochromatosis.[181] In one comprehensive review, the prevalence of clinically or pathologically identifiable hereditary hemochromatosis was estimated to be 1 in 20,000 hospital admissions and 1 in 7000 deaths.[179] The prevalence in Olmstead County, Minnesota, was calculated to be 4 per 100,000,[1] but in Glasgow, Scotland, it was as high as 1 in 556 male autopsies or about 1 in 2500 male deaths.[182] In Malmo, Sweden, eight cases of hereditary hemochromatosis were detected in a carefully studied autopsy series of 8834 men, for a frequency of 0.1 percent.[183] Several studies based solely on indices of iron metabolism (percent serum iron saturation, serum ferritin) suggested a relatively high frequency of the homozygous state and are more in keeping with the mutation studies. The resultant "disease" frequencies were: Canada, 0.27 percent;[184] Sweden (two different studies), 0.5 percent[185] and 0.24 percent;[186] United Kingdom, 0.3 percent;[187] South Africa (white Afrikaners), 0.95 percent;[188,189] and Iceland, 0.37 percent.[190] These and other studies are discussed further under "Population Screening."

The various data suggest that the hemochromatosis gene is one of the most common disease-producing genes, at least in populations of European origin. However, the frequency by which definitely identified 845A (C282Y) homozygotes will show clinical disease with morbidity and mortality is yet unknown (see Addendum).

ANIMAL MODELS

Three types of animal models for hereditary hemochromatosis exist. The first of these is produced by feeding or injecting large amounts of iron into experimental animals, the second consists of naturally occurring mutant animals with iron storage disease, and the third of genetically engineered mice.

Feeding or Injection of Iron. As long ago as 1918 Peyton Rous attempted to produce hemochromatosis.[191] This and subsequent early efforts to produce the pathologic equivalent of hemochromatosis were unsuccessful.[1] Intramuscular injection of iron dextran produced arthritis in rabbits, but no fibrosis of the liver or other organs was found.[192] More recently, however, investigators have had some success in producing stigmata of hereditary hemochromatosis in experimental animals. Rats and rabbits parenterally treated with a large daily dose of ferric nitrilotriacetate (FeNTA) manifested diabetic symptoms such as hyperglycemia, glycosuria, ketonemia, and ketonuria after approximately 60 days of treatment.[193] Subsequently it was found that prolonged feeding of carbonyl iron produced iron distribution more like that seen in hemochromatosis. FeNTA administration produced excessive iron deposition throughout the hepatic lobule in both hepatocytes and Kupffer cells, whereas dietary carbonyl iron supplementation produced greater hepatic iron overload in a periportal distribution with iron deposition predominantly in hepatocytes.[194,195] After about a year appreciable fibrosis is evident in this model.[196] Chronic alcohol feeding failed to potentiate hepatic fibrosis in iron-overloaded rats, although there was more hepatocyte necrosis, and the serum alanine aminotransferase activity was significantly higher in the iron-alcohol group than in the other groups.[197]

Naturally Occurring Mutant Animals with Hemochromatosis. Massive iron overload and cirrhosis of the liver have been documented in a racing pony[198] and in three horses.[199] Iron loading was observed in macrophages in the pancreas, liver parenchymal cells, and cardiac and intestinal smooth muscle cells. Islets of Langerhans, biliary epithelial cells, and spleen were iron-free. The pancreas was fibrotic with massive macrophage infiltration and loss of secretory epithelium. The liver showed evidence of chronic inflammatory infiltration with increased collagen fibers in the parenchymal region. Unlike in human hemochromatosis, the plasma iron saturation was not greatly increased. Hemochromatosis has also been diagnosed in cattle.[200] Birds have been found to suffer from hemochromatosis. The disorder seems particularly common in mynah birds,[201,202] but has also been documented in a flamingo[203] and a toucan,[204] which were treated by chelation therapy.[205]

Certain types of anemic mutant mouse strains have iron overload. Hypotransferrinemic (hpx/hpx) mice manifest iron loading of the liver preceding that in the pancreas and heart. One-year-old hpx/hpx mice show iron staining in the exocrine pancreas, liver parenchymal cells, and cardiac and intestinal smooth muscle cells. Iron-loaded macrophages are present but the islets of Langerhans, biliary epithelial cells, and spleen are iron-free. There is chronic inflammatory infiltration of the liver with increased collagen fibers in the parenchymal region but no cirrhosis.[206] Mice with homozygous β-thalassemia also show some iron loading, but not to the extent, particularly in the liver, observed in hpx/hpx mice.[207]

Genetically Engineered Mice. Mice with targeted disruption of the β_2-microglobulin gene show accumulation of iron. There is progressive hepatic iron overload, considered to be indistinguishable from that observed in human hemochromatosis.[81] This finding led to the original suggestion that a mutation of an HLA-like gene might be responsible for hemochromatosis.[82] Mucosal uptake of Fe^{+++}, but not of Fe^{++}, by the mutant mice was significantly higher than in control mice. Mucosal transfer in the mutant mice was greater, independent of the iron form tested. No significant differences were found in iron absorption between control and mutant mice when anemia was induced either by repetitive bleeding or by hemolysis through phenylhydrazine treatment. However, iron absorption in mice made anemic by dietary deprivation of iron was significantly greater in the mutant mice, and the mutant mice had an impaired capacity to downmodulate iron absorption when they were iron loaded.[208] With the demonstration that mutations of *HFE* were the cause of hereditary hemochromatosis and the demonstration that a closely homologous gene existed in mice,[209,210] targeted disruption of the gene was achieved. By the time the animals were 10 weeks of age, the fasting transferrin saturation was significantly elevated compared with normal littermates (96 ± 5 percent versus 77 ± 3 percent), and the hepatic iron concentration was eightfold higher than that of wild-type littermates. Stainable hepatic iron in the *HFE* mutant mice was predominantly in hepatocytes in a periportal distribution. Iron concentrations in spleen, heart, and kidney were not significantly different.[211]

PATHOGENESIS AND NATURE OF THE METABOLIC ABNORMALITY

Patients with hereditary hemochromatosis generally have accumulated iron to an extent that the body iron content is between 15 and 40 g, 5 to 10 times the normal quantity. Because all the additional iron is in storage compounds, the iron stores are increased twenty- to fifty-fold.[3,11,179] Because the bioavailable iron content of the diet usually restricts the positive iron balance to a few milligrams per day, the accumulation of 20 to 40 g of surplus iron requires many years. Therefore, most hereditary hemochromatosis subjects are 40 to 60 years of age at the time of diagnosis, although a number of younger patients have been described, including some young adults and even children.[212,213] (See "Juvenile Hemochromatosis" below.) While earlier data suggested that hemochromatosis was encountered approximately 10 times more frequently in males than in females because of a lower iron intake and increased iron losses,[3,179] a much higher proportion of women (27 percent) was reported in one recent study.[214] In one study a later onset was found in women,[215] but in another there was no such difference between male and female patients.[214] On diagnosis, the absorption of iron is usually within the normal range[1,11] but in relation to the grossly enlarged iron stores it is actually inappropriately high.[120,216,217] During venesection therapy, absorption rises to high levels, and it may remain above normal for years after phlebotomies have been discontinued.[218] These observations suggest that iron absorption in homozygotes is subject to the usual influences, but the "absorbostat" is set at an inappropriately high level.

In spite of the identification of the mutation responsible for most cases of hereditary hemochromatosis, the basic abnormality remains obscure, not only in the patients who have not inherited mutations of *HFE*, but also in those in whom the causative mutation is known. Theoretically, hereditary hemochromatosis could be due to a defect or defects at a number of sites. These include the intestinal lumen, the mucosal cells of the upper small intestine, the plasma transport system, the liver, and the macrophage system.

One might have hoped that a part of this distinction would become obvious from the result of liver transplantation into patients with hemochromatosis. Unfortunately the evidence that has been obtained is ambiguous.[219] On the one hand, the inadvertent transplantation of a liver from a patient with hemochromatosis was associated with persistent iron overload in the transplanted liver,[220] but patients with hemochromatosis who underwent liver transplantation also showed iron accumulation in the normal liver.[221]

Some insight into the possible site or sites of the metabolic defect may be gained from the distribution of the excess iron. In various syndromes of secondary iron overload large amounts of iron are present in the macrophages, particularly of the spleen, bone marrow, and liver, with variable involvement of the parenchymal cells of the liver and other organs.[11] In hereditary hemochromatosis the parenchymal cells contain virtually all of the hemosiderin deposits and the macrophage system contains very little. This unique distribution must presumably be a consequence of the metabolic abnormality.[222] It has been suggested that the intestinal and macrophage cells have a common defect leading to reduced iron storage and to the delivery of increased amounts of iron to the plasma.[11] This would raise the transferrin saturation and lead to the deposition of iron in hepatocytes and other parenchymal tissues.[223] A defect in storing iron which is common to the two cell types would account not only for the paucity of iron present in these cells, the increased iron absorption, and the high saturation of circulating transferrin, but also for the fact that the transferrin saturation is found to be raised before the individual has accumulated excess iron. There is some evidence to support this hypothesis. A kinetic study showed enhanced release of macrophage iron to the plasma,[224] and mononuclear cells from homozygotes were found to release increased amounts of ferritin.[225] However, in another series of studies, ferritin synthesis[226] and iron uptake[227] by cultured monocytes from venesected homozygotes were found to be normal. The transport of iron into cells from patients with and without hemochromatosis has been compared.[226–230] The transferrin receptor was also studied.[228,231–238,484] No consistent abnormalities have been found. The export of low molecular weight iron from iron-loaded monocytes of patients with hereditary hemochromatosis was greater than that from iron-loaded monocytes from control patients.[239,240]

The findings in the mucosal cells of the upper small intestine of homozygotes match to some extent those in macrophages and monocytes. Such cells have been shown to contain less ferritin and lower levels of H and L ferritin subunits than would be appropriate in relation to the serum ferritin levels (Fig. 127-7).[241] A larger proportion than normal of the iron taken up by mucosal cells is transferred into the body,[242–244] and kinetic studies have confirmed that the increased iron absorption in homozygotes is mediated primarily by an increase in the rate constant for the transfer of mucosal iron to the plasma.[217]

Alterations in the immune system have been described in hemochromatosis.[245] Some patients with hemochromatosis have abnormally low numbers of CD8+ T cells in their peripheral blood[246] and most patients have lessened activity of an Src receptor related protein kinase that reflects CD8 cell function.[246] Mice with targeted disruption of β_2-microglobulin develop a disorder resembling human hemochromatosis and also are

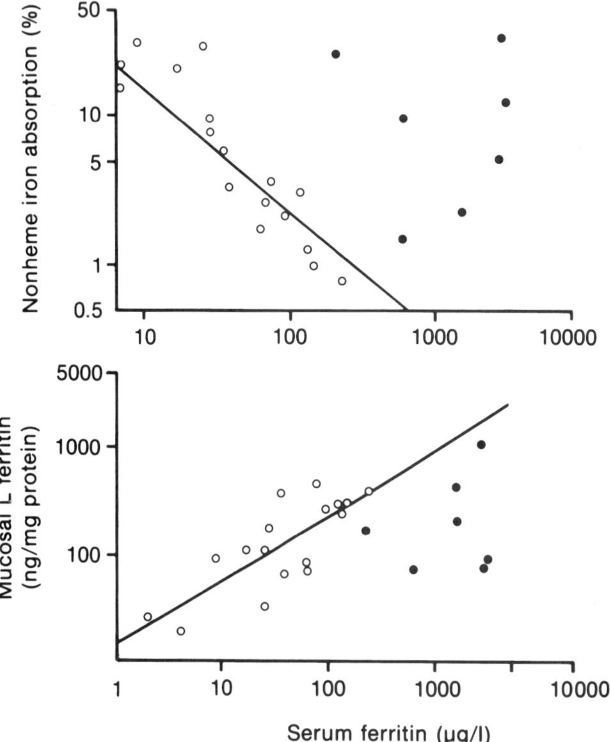

Fig. 127-7 The upper panel shows the relationship between the absorption of nonheme iron and the serum ferritin concentration in 17 normal subjects and in 7 patients with hereditary hemochromatosis. The lower panel shows the relationship between mucosal L ferritin and the serum ferritin concentration. The open symbols represent normal subjects; closed symbols are from patients with hereditary hemochromatosis. (*From Whittaker et al.*[241] *Used by permission.*)

generally deficient in CD4-CD8 T cells.[81,82] The relationship of the T cell changes to the pathogenesis of the disorder is unclear, but it seems likely that they are secondary to the underlying defect and do not play a direct role in pathogenesis.

Role of *HFE* Mutations

Two mutations of *HFE* are clearly associated with hemochromatosis, a major mutation, 845 G → A (C282Y) and a phenotypically weaker mutation, 187 C → G (H63D). The 845A mutation results in the replacement of a cysteine involved in a disulfide bond in the molecule with a tyrosine. This substitution was presumed[79] and subsequently demonstrated[247] to prevent binding of the protein to β_2-microglobulin and hence the transport of the HFE protein to the cell surface. The other *HFE* mutation, 187G, does not affect binding to β_2-microglobulin, and this mutant protein is normally displayed on the surface of the cell. However, it has been suggested that its interaction with the transferrin receptor is impaired.[80]

The actual role of HFE in iron hemostasis remains unclear. Although it is an HLA class I-like molecule, the crystal structure has been interpreted as indicating that the homologue of the peptide-binding cleft of HLA molecules could not bind a peptide. HFE binds to the transferrin receptor.[80,84] Studies on cell-associated transferrin at 37°C suggest that the overexpressed wild-type HFE protein decreases the affinity of the transferrin receptor for transferrin. However, the overexpressed H63D HFE protein made by the 187G mutation does not have this effect, suggesting the functional basis for this mutation. Moreover a soluble complex of HFE and β_2-microglobulin inhibited binding of transferrin to HeLa cell transferrin receptor in a concentration-dependent manner. Scatchard plots of these data indicated that the added heterodimer substantially reduced the affinity of the transferrin receptor for transferrin. Thus it is possible that HFE acts in some way to modulate the binding of transferrin-iron to its receptor.

However, a number of earlier findings are inconsistent with such a model.[227–229,231] Ward et al.[231] reported that: "No differences in the properties of transferrin receptors were found between patients with hereditary hemochromatosis and normal individuals." In another study,[228] the affinity of the transferrin receptor of hemochromatosis monocytes for diferric transferrin was measured and not found to differ significantly from normal. Although there seems to be little doubt that HFE can bind to the transferrin receptor, it is not clear whether, how, or where this plays a role in iron uptake.

Hemochromatosis Without Mutations of *HFE*. In a considerable number of patients with hemochromatosis, including some with a clear-cut genetic pattern, complete sequencing of the coding region of the *HFE* gene failed to reveal any abnormality.[153,248] While promoter and enhancer mutations have not been ruled out in such patients, it seems likely that there are mutations involving other genes that can cause hereditary hemochromatosis.

Many studies were carried out in attempts to identify the defect in hereditary hemochromatosis before cloning of the *HFE* gene and even before linkage of hemochromatosis to the HLA complex on chromosome 6 had been discovered. Therefore, it was not known whether the patients being studied had the *HFE* mutation, although it can be assumed that in most cases they did, as over 80 percent of unselected hemochromatosis patients are homozygous for the 854A mutation of *HFE*. Candidate genes that were discarded, such as those for transferrin, ferritin, and transferrin receptor, may therefore prove to be involved in the smaller subset of patients who do not have this mutation.

Iron overload is quite a constant feature of congenital atransferrinemia, an exceedingly rare disorder; fewer than 10 families have been reported.[249,250] This suggests that abnormalities in transferrin might be responsible for iron overload, a suggestion made in 1961 by Turnbull and Giblett[251] but not pursued actively because the electrophoretic mobility of transferrin is normal in hemochromatosis. However, no evidence of any abnormality in transferrin metabolism has been found. Transferrin from subjects homozygous for the *HFE* takes up and releases iron normally,[252,253] and transferrin polymorphisms in patients who have hemochromatosis without *HFE* mutations showed no deviations from normal gene frequencies[485].

The possibility that ferritin might be abnormal has also been investigated. The hepatic isoferritin pattern is abnormal in patients with hereditary hemochromatosis,[254] but similar changes are found in other varieties of iron overload, and the abnormal pattern disappears with removal of the excess iron.[255]

The transferrin receptor is a particularly interesting candidate for abnormalities in hemochromatosis, because it has been shown that HFE binds to this receptor.[80,84] It is thus possible that in non-*HFE* mutation associated hemochromatosis, transferrin receptor mutations create phenocopies of hemochromatosis due to *HFE* mutations. The transferrin receptor was missing from hepatocytes in biopsies from most of 21 patients with primary hemochromatosis but was present on all of 50 control biopsies.[233] It seemed likely, however, that this change was secondary to iron overload, as the receptor was present in patients who had been treated by phlebotomy. Serum transferrin receptor levels in patients with hemochromatosis are decreased[235,237] but rise during phlebotomy, indicating that the low levels observed in the untreated patients are secondary to iron storage. Direct sequence analysis of transferrin receptors in patients with hemochromatosis has shown no abnormality.[484]

It was suggested that a deficiency of xanthine oxidase might be responsible[256] but this seems unlikely, because it is now known that the enzyme is not involved in the mobilization of iron from ferritin and thus does not affect iron transport.[257]

A relationship between copper and iron metabolism has long been appreciated,[258] but the precise role of copper metabolism in iron metabolism is only recently beginning to be understood. The transport of iron into yeast has been dissected, and a multicopper oxidase, designated FET3 and catalyzing the conversion of Fe^{++} to Fe^{+++}, is required for high affinity transport of iron to take place.[259] Like FET3 in yeast, ceruloplasmin is known to be a ferroxidase. First described in the Japanese literature by Morita et al.[260] in 1992, a mere handful of cases of ceruloplasmin deficiency have been described in the past 5 years (see "Aceruloplasminemia" below).[261] The distribution of iron in these patients is different from that found in hereditary hemochromatosis, in that there is a tendency for accumulation of iron in the brain, but hepatic iron overload is present as well and diabetes mellitus is a part of the syndrome. Hyperceruloplasminemia has been reported to occur in hemochromatosis,[262] but the significance of this finding is unclear.[257]

The possible involvement of β_2-microglobulin in the etiology of hemochromatosis was suggested by the development of iron storage in a β_2-microglobulin "knockout" mouse (see "Animal Models").[81] The coding region of this gene has been sequenced in 14 chromosomes from patients with hemochromatosis who did not have the common mutation without finding any mutations.[248] Calnexin-HLA complexes promote the association of HLA with β_2-microglobulin.[91,263,264] The HLA-β_2-microglobulin complex is then transferred from calnexin to a soluble calcium-binding protein, calreticulin (see below).[91] Although mutations affecting the function of calnexin could impair transport of HFE to the cell surface, to our knowledge this protein has not yet been examined in hemochromatosis.

Mobilferrin (calreticulin) has been implicated as a major component of the intestinal iron transport pathway delineated by Conrad and his colleagues.[108] The coding region of the calreticulin gene of five patients with hemochromatosis who were not homozygous for the 845A mutation of *HFE* has been sequenced without finding any mutations.[248]

Mutations of the IRE or of IRP-1 or IRP-2 are also potential candidates for the cause of hereditary hemochromatosis. The IRP levels were found to be upregulated in monocytes of hemochromatosis patients, but returned to normal when the iron burden was reduced.[265] In the liver IRP levels were reported to be down-regulated in proportion to the amount of iron that had accumulated; intestinal levels of IRP were normal.[266] Mutations of the ferritin light chain IRE have been implicated in the hereditary hyperferritinemia-cataract syndrome,[267–271] but not in hereditary hemochromatosis.

Environmental Factors

Environmental factors play an important part in the expression of the hereditary hemochromatosis genes. It is obvious that surplus iron cannot be accumulated unless the diet permits its absorption. If the average diet contains little bioavailable iron, and iron deficiency is rife, hemochromatosis will be milder. On the other hand, if the diet is effectively fortified with iron, there will not only be a fall in the prevalence of iron deficiency but also an acceleration in the development of hemochromatosis by homozygotes.[272] There has, in fact, been a steady decline in the prevalence of iron deficiency anemia in industrialized countries over recent decades. While the reasons for the improvement in iron nutrition in industrialized countries are not clear, the current trend suggests that hereditary hemochromatosis homozygotes are likely to present with clinical manifestations earlier than in the past and that hemochromatosis may now develop in a portion of the population who would have remained asymptomatic. At the individual level, the use of iron cooking utensils or iron-containing medicinal preparations will accelerate iron accumulation. On the negative side of the iron balance equation, hookworm infestation could cause the elimination through intestinal blood loss of any superfluous iron absorbed, and regular blood donation would have a similar effect.

Alcohol and Iron Overload. In most published series, a significant proportion of subjects with hereditary hemochromatosis have been more than moderate users of alcohol.[11] This was largely responsible for the earlier view that hemochromatosis was not a genetic disorder, but merely alcoholic or nutritional cirrhosis in subjects whose dietary intake of iron was high.[4,5] Certainly, the association of alcoholic cirrhosis with increased quantities of hepatic hemosiderin has been observed frequently. In southern African blacks, the severity of the unique variety of iron overload still commonly encountered there[273] is closely related to the quantity of home-brewed alcohol consumed by the affected individual. There appear to be several reasons for these associations.[273] The most obvious is the iron present in some varieties of alcoholic beverages. The beers indigenous to sub-Saharan Africa are based on millet and maize and are often brewed in pots or drums made of iron. During fermentation the iron content rises as the pH falls. The final mean concentration in one study was 40 mg/liter[274] and in another 15 mg/liter.[275] The alcohol content is low, and large quantities are regularly consumed by many adult males, so that an additional 50 to 100 mg of iron in a highly bioavailable form is ingested each day. This is several times more than the normal total dietary iron intake. The high bioavailability of the iron, equivalent to that of an inorganic ferric salt, is due to the removal by filtration through cloth of most of the grits, which inhibit iron absorption, and probably certain small molecular fermentation products which serve as solubilizing ligands. Iron overload of a degree that is seen in hereditary hemochromatosis develops in many regular drinkers, with prominent hemosiderin deposits in macrophages throughout the body and in the hepatocytes (see "African Iron Overload" below).[11]

Certain wines have also been found to contain significant amounts of iron, but the tannins that are present in red wines inhibit absorption; in one study only 4.4 percent of the iron in red wine was absorbed.[276] Most alcoholic beverages contain little or no iron, and alcohol abuse is certainly not always associated with an increase in the body iron content;[277] in a group of drinkers of distilled liquor, the amounts were actually lower than normal. Only 7 percent of 157 alcoholics with liver disease studied in London had significant hepatic siderosis,[278] while iron stores were only mildly raised in another group of alcoholics with liver disease of varying severity.[279] Alcohol itself does not increase iron absorption,[280,281] although folate deficiency may have this effect.[280] Enhanced iron absorption has been observed in some patients with cirrhosis.[282] Portacaval anastomosis has been associated with the rapid development of iron overload,[283,284] but seems to lead to an increase in liver iron in only some patients.[285] Iron absorption from the gastrointestinal tract is not greater in patients with portacaval shunts than among other cirrhotics.[286]

While it is clear that, with the exception of African iron overload, the consumption of alcohol does not of itself lead to marked iron overload, there is undoubtedly an association between an increased alcohol intake and the onset of symptomatic hereditary hemochromatosis. There is evidence that alcohol contributes to the organ damage (see "Mechanisms of Chronic Iron Toxicity" below).[287] This cannot be the only reason, however, because in one study the iron load of those subjects with hereditary hemochromatosis who had an alcoholic history was only slightly less than that of the nondrinkers,[288] while in another it was actually 50 percent higher.[289] A single copy of either of the two *HFE* mutations influences neither liver iron content nor the risk of fibrotic disease in alcoholics.[290]

Pathologic and Clinical Findings

Individuals with hereditary hemochromatosis are asymptomatic until toxic concentrations of iron have been accumulated, a process that usually takes decades. The clinical manifestations that may present once this phase has been reached are summarized in Fig. 127-8. At this stage the storage iron concentrations in the liver and pancreas may be as much as 50 to 100 times the normal figures, in the thyroid about 25 times, in the heart and adrenal 10 to 15 times, and in the skin, spleen, kidney, and stomach about 5

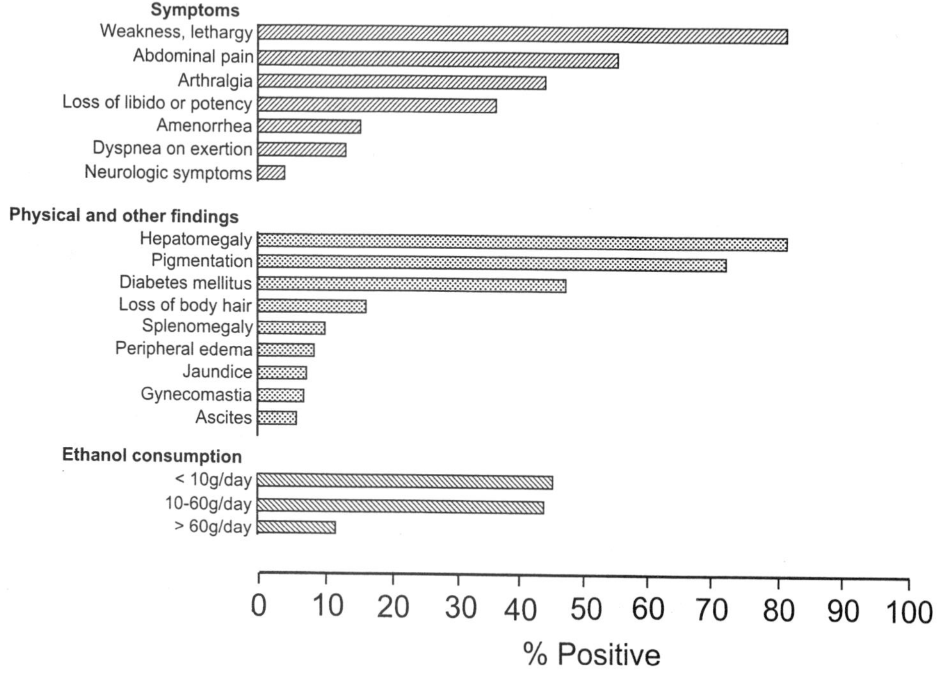

Fig. 127-8 Frequency of clinical features at the time of diagnosis in 251 patients with hereditary hemochromatosis. (*From Niederau et al.*[291] *Reprinted with permission.*)

times normal. The surplus iron is predominantly in the form of hemosiderin and is visible on histologic examination, particularly after staining with potassium ferrocyanide.

Skin. Pigmentation, virtually always present in older series of patients, is less frequently found with earlier diagnosis (30 to 70 percent in recent series[292–294]). It is particularly prominent in exposed areas, the external genitalia, areola of the nipple, flexion creases and old scars, and sometimes the conjunctiva, lid margin, and the oral mucosa.[295] There is increased melanin and hemosiderin, which is most obvious in the sweat glands, but deposits can also be seen in vascular endothelium and in the connective tissue of the corium. The classical bronze skin color is only rarely seen; the shade ranges from brown to slate gray. There is no close correlation with the relative amounts of melanin and iron. The skin is typically fine with soft and scanty facial, pubic, and axillary hair. Xerosis ranging in severity up to generalized ichthyosis has been reported in almost half the patients, together with atrophy of both epidermis and dermis.[295]

Liver. In the early asymptomatic stage discrete granules of hemosiderin can be seen in a proportion of the hepatocytes, typically in the periportal zones.[296,297] At hepatic storage iron concentrations of 0.5 percent dry weight, electron microscopy reveals cytosolic ferritin and some pericanalicular siderosomes in zone 1 hepatocytes with no evidence of organelle damage and no involvement of sinusoidal cells.[298] When the iron concentration is about 1 percent, ferritin can be seen in hepatocytes in all zones and pericanalicular siderosomes are abundant, especially in periportal hepatocytes; some hepatocytes show organelle damage and siderosis is apparent in occasional sinusoidal cells.[298] Once the iron overload is severe (1.5 to 2 percent dry weight) coarse hemosiderin masses are visible in all acinar zones. The bile duct epithelium also frequently contains heavy deposits of hemosiderin,[296] but a striking and diagnostic feature is that there is relatively little iron in the Kupffer cells. There is extensive subcellular pathology and focal necrosis with marked sinusoidal cell siderosis and collagen deposition.[298]

There appears to be a critical hepatic iron concentration beyond which organelle damage occurs and liver cell injury becomes irreversible.[298] This is supported by the observation that the rate of hepatocyte apoptosis is proportional to the iron load,[299] and that hepatic stellate cell activation and collagen deposition are correlated with rising iron concentration.[300] Once the storage iron concentration reaches 2.2 percent dry weight,[297] a slight to moderate increase in portal and periportal fibrosis may be evident. With higher concentrations, cirrhosis may supervene. Typically, the lobules are separated by wide bands of fibrous tissue. Hemosiderin loading may vary from zone to zone and from lobule to lobule, tending to be less in areas of regeneration.[11] A characteristic pattern of fibrosis and lobular disruption has been recognized in subjects who are not alcoholics.[301]

Severe portal hypertension and esophageal varices are seen less frequently than in other forms of cirrhosis. Clinical evidence of ascites is also not common; it is usually associated with cardiac failure.[282] Manifestations of hyperestrogenism such as spider angiomas and gynecomastia, and serious derangement of liver function, usually indicate coexisting alcohol abuse.[289,303–304] Episodes of acute hepatic failure may be provoked by blood loss or surgical procedures.

Hepatoma is an important late complication; its frequency is about 200 times that in the general population.[292,305–307] With rare exceptions[308] it is associated with cirrhosis and may develop years after the successful removal of the iron.[305] Malignant change is suggested by the onset of unexplained weight loss, fever, nodular enlargement of the liver, ascites, jaundice, abdominal pain, anemia, or insulin insensitivity.[302]

Spleen. The average weight of the spleen is about 400 g, somewhat above normal. Hemosiderin deposits are not prominent, and are usually confined to the capsule, blood vessel walls, and trabeculae. The iron concentrations in the spleen and bone marrow are low compared with other varieties of iron overload,[309,310] in keeping with the minimal macrophage involvement in the disease, although lymph nodes, especially those draining markedly siderotic organs, may contain hemosiderin.

Diabetes. Extensive hemosiderin deposits are found in the pancreas and fibrosis is almost invariable. The heaviest iron deposits are seen in the exocrine cells, but no effects on exocrine pancreatic function have been documented. Within the islets, the iron is found only in the beta cells.[311] The islets are of normal size and shape, unlike those found in type 1 diabetes, and do not exhibit the amyloid of type 2 diabetes.[311]

Diabetes is a late manifestation of hemochromatosis. The prevalence in symptomatic subjects is 30 to 60 percent.[292,293,312] However, impaired glucose tolerance may be demonstrable in the absence of diabetes or cirrhosis; it is due to impaired insulin secretion and is reversed by phlebotomy treatment.[313] When diabetes is present it is often associated with cirrhosis.[292,312] In patients with hemochromatosis and cirrhosis who are not diabetic, insulin sensitivity is reduced, and it is not improved by phlebotomy.[313] Diabetes in hemochromatosis is characterized by both impaired insulin secretion[303,313,314] and insulin resistance[303,305,313] and the insulin resistance does not respond to phlebotomy.[313]

Hypogonadism. Diminished sexual function is a frequent finding and is almost invariable in young subjects. Loss of libido, testicular atrophy, impotence, amenorrhea, and sparse body hair are common. The body hair may be scanty for many years before other manifestations of the disease appear. These are typical features of cirrhosis, but in hereditary hemochromatosis they may be present before liver function is significantly impaired.[305] Moreover, although testosterone levels are low in both conditions, the gynecomastia which is characteristic of other varieties of cirrhosis is uncommon in hemochromatosis.[315] Plasma estrogen concentrations are not elevated,[315] and luteinizing hormone and follicle-stimulating hormone levels are low.[316–318] The hypogonadism is due to gonadotropin deficiency, and the low responses to gonadotropin-releasing hormone suggest that the lesion is at the pituitary level[303,316,319] although there is also evidence suggesting hypothalamic dysfunction.[317,318] A decrease in prolactin reserve has also been demonstrated.[317] In contrast, the secretion of other tropic pituitary hormones is not markedly impaired, in keeping with the observation that the hemosiderin in the pituitary is predominantly located within the gonadotropic cells.

Heart. In young subjects cardiac manifestations are not infrequently the presenting feature, and almost always the cause of death, which follows within a year of diagnosis unless the iron is removed.[11] The onset may be acute, with cardiac failure developing over a few days, and the pulmonary congestion and peripheral edema may be very severe. In older individuals the presentation is often more gradual; ischemic heart disease may play a part in some of these. Arrhythmias or cardiac failure eventually develop in more than one-third of untreated cases; the average age of onset is 56 years.[289,292,294]

Clinically, the picture is usually that of a congestive cardiomyopathy with bilateral ventricular dilation, but restrictive features have also been described.[11,320] The presence of an arrhythmia is an adverse prognostic sign. Ventricular ectopic beats are the commonest manifestations, but supraventricular and ventricular tachycardias, ventricular fibrillation, and varying degrees of heart block may also occur.[11] Other rather nonspecific EKG changes such as low voltage, left axis deviation, and flattening or inversion of T waves may be noted.

Before left ventricular function is impaired, thickening of the ventricular wall can be demonstrated by echocardiography,[321] but with the onset of cardiac failure, chamber dilatation and global systolic dysfunction are seen, and ventricular wall thickening is no longer apparent.[322] On radiographic investigation the cardiac profile has a globular appearance, with a decrease in the amplitude of the cardiac pulsations. At necropsy the weight of the heart is often two or three times normal. Hemosiderin is visible in both the interstitial cells and the myocardial fibers; conducting tissue is generally less affected and the sinoatrial node in particular is largely spared. The hemosiderin deposits are particularly prominent in the perinuclear region;[323] in the ventricles deposits are most marked in the subepicardial zone, least in the middle third, and of intermediate density in the subendocardial region and papillary muscles.[322] Degeneration, fragmentation, and necrosis of myocardial cells with fibrosis and interstitial edema have been described.[11,324,325] The atria are less heavily involved.

Joints. Arthropathy was recognized as a manifestation of hemochromatosis only in 1964,[326] but it is actually present in 40 to 85 percent of subjects[294,305,327,328] and is often the presenting feature.[293,294,329] It is not related to the amount of iron or the presence of cirrhosis.[328] The incidence and severity of arthritis increase as the years pass in spite of the removal of the iron by venesection therapy. The classical presentation resembles degenerative joint disease with bony swelling, deformity, and limitation of movement, usually without serious disablement. However, hip arthroplasty may be required[330] and arthritis was rated the clinical finding with the greatest impact on the quality of life by 50 consecutive hemochromatosis patients.[331] Involvement of the second and third metacarpophalangeal and proximal interphalangeal joints together with the radiographic features of narrowing of the joint spaces, loss of cartilage, cysts, and osteopenic metacarpal heads with hooked osteophytes is virtually diagnostic.[329] However, arthralgia with no radiographic changes may also be encountered.[332]

Chondrocalcinosis is present in about half the cases,[329,333] typically asymptomatic, but in some subjects attacks of acute inflammatory synovitis occur (pseudogout). Similar findings in other forms of iron overload[334] suggest that the iron is directly responsible, but the mechanism has not been established. In vitro, ferric ions inhibit pyrophosphatase, increasing the concentration of pyrophosphate and thus the propensity to crystallize. Iron is present in the chondrocytes, but there is no constant relationship with the pyrophosphate crystals.[335] The synovial lining cells are heavily laden with hemosiderin; in contrast to rheumatoid arthritis the type B cells are more affected than the type A.[329]

Osteoporosis. Osteoporosis was demonstrated by radiographic spinal and forearm bone mineral density estimation in 10 of 22 male subjects[336] and 9 of 32 subjects.[328] There was no evidence of osteomalacia. Using dynamic skeletal histomorphometry, diminished bone formation was observed as well as increased resorption.[336] Why osteoporosis should develop in hemochromatosis has not been established. Diamond[336] found the closest correlation to be with hypogonadism, but Sinigaglia et al.[328] related it to the amount of iron. Spinal[337,338] and femoral head[339] osteoporosis have been noted as a complication of African iron overload (see below). In such subjects the mineral density of iliac crest bone correlates inversely with the hepatic storage iron concentration.[338]

Abdominal Pain and Infections. Cirrhotic subjects in particular may experience chronic ache in the epigastrium or right hypochondrium.[305] It may have a variety of causes, including peptic ulceration, hepatoma, variceal bleeding, ascites, cholecystitis, and nephrolithiasis.[289] Rarely, gram-negative bacterial peritonitis may occur, presenting as acute abdominal pain and shock.[340] *Yersinia enterocolitica* has been particularly incriminated.[341–343] Unlike most microorganisms, it does not possess a high affinity iron chelating system, and seldom causes systemic infections because it is unable to obtain sufficient iron from the internal environment of the body. However, the organism is able to proliferate in hereditary hemochromatosis, in which the transferrin is saturated and nontransferrin-bound iron may be present.[344] Septicemias due to other organisms including *Vibrio vulnificus*, other *Yersinia* species, Listeria, and *Escherichia coli*[341,345,346] and zygomycosis[347] have also been described. In addition to making iron more easily available to the parasites, the iron overload may compromise immune cell function.[348] The proliferative response of peripheral blood mononuclear cells is defective in untreated hereditary hemochromatosis patients, and C8p561ck activity is decreased in peripheral blood T-lymphocytes,[246] but the number of CD8-positive T cells is increased.[349] Although monocyte phagocytosis is decreased, no alteration in complement receptors or Fc gamma RIIa polymorphism was found.[350]

MECHANISMS OF CHRONIC IRON TOXICITY

The ability of iron to accept and release electrons is the main basis of its importance to living organisms. The same capacity to undergo reversible oxidation-reduction reactions appears to be the basis of the harm that excessive amounts of iron can inflict. One of the pathways that is considered to be of greatest importance is the Haber-Weiss reaction:

$$Fe^{++} + H_2O_2 \rightarrow Fe^{+++} + OH^- + {}^{\cdot}OH$$

$$O_2^{\cdot-} + Fe^{+++} \rightarrow O_2 + Fe^{++}$$

The sum of these two reactions is the Fenton reaction:

$$O_2^{\cdot-} + H_2O_2 \rightarrow O_2 + OH^- + {}^{\cdot}OH$$

The hydroxyl radical (${}^{\cdot}OH$) is second in reactivity only to atomic oxygen and has been implicated in producing damage to polysaccharides, DNA, and enzymes and in causing lipid peroxidation.[351] Although there is no direct evidence that hydroxyl radical generation is the main pathway of tissue damage in hemochromatosis, this common conjecture seems to be a reasonable one. It has also been suggested that ferryl ions (FeO_2^+) may play a role in mediating tissue damage.[352]

Lipid Peroxidation. In the presence of experimentally induced iron overload, lipid peroxidation can be demonstrated both in vitro[353] and in vivo.[194,354] The rate of peroxidation is a function of the iron concentration, and it is inhibited by the iron chelator deferoxamine, apotransferrin, and antioxidants such as α-tocopherol.[355,356] Evidence of damage to lysosomes, mitochondria, and microsomes has been obtained.[357] In the precirrhotic stage of hereditary hemochromatosis, the first ultrastructural changes have been reported to be in the lysosomes, which are enlarged and iron-laden.[358] Both lipid peroxidation and inhibited oxidative metabolism have been demonstrated in mitochondria from iron-loaded hepatocytes in experimental rats.[359,360] There is evidence that alcohol also induces hepatic lipid peroxidation, perhaps by mobilizing ferritin iron. Alcohol and iron may act synergistically.[361,362]

Fibrosis. Fibrosis is a feature of most organs containing excessive amounts of storage iron, even when there is little or no parenchymal-cell damage. The evidence indicates that collagen synthesis is directly stimulated[363,364] and this is not corrected by vitamin E.[362] In rat experiments the level of pro-a 2(I)-collagen mRNA rises;[364] the activity of a key enzyme in the biosynthetic pathway, prolyl hydroxylase, is increased; the hydroxyproline content rises; and before collagen is visible by light microscopy, electron microscopy reveals collagen fibrils adjacent to the hepatocytes, although no fibroblasts, inflammatory cells, or damage to hepatocyte organelles are visible.[365] Alcohol also stimulates hepatocyte collagen synthesis[287] and this, together with its effect on lipid peroxidation, may explain the development of cirrhosis at lower hepatic iron concentrations in alcoholic subjects.

Ascorbic Acid Depletion. A proportion of the available dietary ascorbic acid is irreversibly oxidized. Administration of large amounts of ascorbic acid to normal subjects soon leads to the excretion of most of the dose unchanged in the urine. But if iron overload is present, there is instead an increase in the excretion of the oxidation product of dehydroascorbate, oxalic acid.[366] With physiological amounts of ascorbic acid, the major oxidation product is carbon dioxide.[367] No adverse effects have been documented in well-nourished subjects, but in siderotic South African blacks, clinical scurvy is seen, mainly in late winter and early spring, when the dietary ascorbic acid content is at its lowest.[337] Ascorbic acid deficiency in turn affects the metabolism of storage iron, reducing the availability of the stored iron for erythropoiesis or chelation by deferoxamine. Of possibly greater significance is the circumstantial evidence that chronic ascorbic acid deficiency can lead to osteoporosis (see "Osteoporosis" above).[11]

Diagnosis

Once toxic concentrations of iron have accumulated, the resultant damage to certain organs is irreversible or only partially reversible (see "Prognosis" below). Every effort must therefore be made to identify homozygous individuals before symptoms appear. A program of phlebotomies can then be instituted and the prospects of morbidity and reduced life expectancy averted. A presymptomatic diagnosis can be made only if clinical or laboratory findings compatible with hereditary hemochromatosis are recognized during investigation of unrelated complaints or through screening of family members or during population screening (see below). The possibility of hereditary hemochromatosis must be considered whenever a raised plasma iron concentration, transferrin saturation, or serum ferritin concentration or evidence of minor liver dysfunction such as a raised serum ALT or unexplained hepatomegaly are encountered. Once diagnosed, those of a new patient's family members who could also be affected should be investigated (see "Identification of Affected Relatives" below).

Even after symptoms have developed, the diagnosis of hereditary hemochromatosis will usually be reached only if an awareness of its protean manifestations is constantly borne in mind. The classical "bronzed diabetes" triad of pigmentation, diabetes, and cirrhosis is actually rare[368] and is seen today only in patients in whom the diagnosis has been missed for many years. Even with the present-day greater awareness of the diversity of presentation, there is an average delay between the development of symptoms and diagnosis of 3.8 years in women and 7.3 years in men.[292] Cases will be missed unless hereditary hemochromatosis is always thought of as a possible cause of skin pigmentation, diabetes, cirrhosis, cardiopathy, arthritis, impotence or sterility, abdominal pain, weakness, tiredness, asymptomatic hepatomegaly, or unexplained elevation of serum transaminases,[296,369] alone or in combination. It is essential to cultivate a high index of clinical suspicion. Observations compatible with hereditary hemochromatosis should trigger further investigation even when the patient's complaints do not appear to be related to iron overload. In a recent review of 195 patients, abnormal blood tests or hepatomegaly found during investigation for an incidental illness had led to the diagnosis in the majority of cases.[292] The commonest presenting symptoms ascribable to hereditary hemochromatosis were weakness, abdominal pain, or joint pains. While impotence was present in most males, it had not caused the patient to consult the physician. Hepatomegaly, skin pigmentation, and diabetes were commonly found on examination. The findings in 251 German[293] and 371 French subjects[294] were similar. Increased awareness of the disease in recent years was reflected by reductions in the average delay in diagnosis after symptoms developed. Of 40 newly diagnosed patients referred to a hepatology clinic from 1990 to 1995, 73 percent were asymptomatic and 78 percent had no abnormal physical signs.[370] In another series[371] only 25 percent of 51 homozygous relatives of the probands were symptomatic, but 3 of them already had hepatic fibrosis and 2 had cirrhosis. While more homozygous individuals are therefore being identified in good time to prevent morbidity, there is no room for complacency; in three recent reports of patients undergoing orthotopic liver transplantation the diagnosis of hereditary hemochromatosis was missed preoperatively in 40 percent, with disastrous consequences.[372]

Once the possibility of hereditary hemochromatosis has come to mind, tests of the patient's iron status must be done. In considering their interpretation, the pathogenesis of the iron overload in hereditary hemochromatosis should be recalled. The earliest manifestations reflect the fact that more iron is being delivered to the plasma than is required by the erythron and other tissues. The plasma iron concentration and the transferrin saturation therefore rise. This occurs before the iron stores are measurably increased. The transferrin saturation is more useful than the plasma iron concentration alone; factors other than hereditary hemochromatosis, such as iron medication, may be responsible for a plasma iron concentration above normal, especially for a single high value.

A persistently high fasting transferrin saturation is highly suggestive of a diagnosis of hereditary hemochromatosis. The College of American Pathologists recommends that individuals with a transferrin saturation persistently above 60 percent should be followed up.[296] Adams and Chakrabarti[373] reported that the transferrin saturation was below 55 percent in only 10 percent of 122 845A (C282Y) homozygotes. A cutoff value of 60 percent identified 90 percent of 107 male Australian homozygotes, but only 74 percent of 35 females; taking 45 percent as the screening level included 100 percent of the males and 91 percent of the females.[374] No normal subjects had fasting transferrin saturations persistently above 45 percent, but significant numbers of heterozygotes did (29 percent of male heterozygotes and 17 percent of females). Seven percent of both male and female heterozygotes had transferrin saturations above 60 percent. The normal circadian variation in the transferrin saturation is not seen in homozygotes.[375] Transferrin saturation may be lowered however by intercurrent infection or a hepatoma.

As the years pass, storage iron accumulates, reaching a peak in the fifth decade.[376] Various studies have confirmed that the values in females tend to be lower than in males of comparable age, the main reason being menstrual iron loss. The most useful test for assessing the degree of storage iron loading is the serum ferritin concentration. In untreated fully developed hereditary hemochromatosis, its value is typically several thousand micrograms per liter, but the complete range from normal values to such high levels may be found. In 122 845A (C282Y) homozygotes, the serum ferritin concentrations were greater than 300 μg/liter in 96 percent of the males and greater than 200 μg/liter in 97 percent of the women; in 4 subjects the serum ferritin was not elevated.[373] It is necessary to take the subject's age and sex into account in evaluating the significance of storage iron measurements. At the same time, it is clear that the combination of the plasma iron concentration, transferrin saturation, and serum ferritin concentration is a valuable screen for homozygosity.[296,377,378]

Useful though the measurement of the serum ferritin concentration has proved to be, it is certainly not infallible, and both false positive and false negative results occur. If necessary, other tests for the presence of iron overload (see below) can be performed. Causes of an elevated serum ferritin concentration other than enlarged iron stores have been considered under "Plasma Ferritin as a Measure of Storage Iron" above. Falsely low concentrations may be due to laboratory error.

Computed tomography can be used to estimate the iron content of the liver, but the sensitivity is low, and moderate iron loading is not detected.[379,380] Magnetic resonance shows more promise:[381] it is accurate in the detection of severe iron overload, but not at lower hepatic iron concentrations[380] unless very short echo times are used.[382] The paramagnetic properties of hemosiderin and ferritin permit the use of a superconducting quantum-interference device to measure the hepatic magnetic susceptibility, which correlates with the hepatic iron concentration,[383] as does the nuclear resonance scattering of gamma rays.[384] The amount of iron in the liver can be calculated from the liver volume as determined by ultrasonography and the storage iron concentration in the biopsy specimen.[385]

The amount of body iron can be measured by invasive or by noninvasive means. The necessity for performing liver biopsy, long regarded as required for the diagnosis of hemochromatosis,[180] has increasingly been questioned.[386] While only liver biopsy provides reliable information regarding the amount of hepatic damage and hence prognosis, the results do not materially alter treatment. Serial phlebotomy measures the amount of body iron and treats the disease at the same time at a lower cost and lower risk than liver biopsy.

In liver biopsies from patients with hemochromatosis, iron is present in the hepatocytes, but the Kupffer cells are spared.[387] The presence or absence of cirrhosis, which has considerable prognostic significance, as discussed in a later section, can also be determined. While semiquantitative estimates of the degree of siderosis can be made visually,[388,296] it is important that it be quantitated using either a chemical technique[389] or atomic absorption spectrophotometry.[390,391] With such measurements it has been possible to differentiate clearly between hereditary hemochromatosis and other forms of liver disease in which hemosiderin may also be visible (see "Differential Diagnosis" below).[392,393] However, among 15 Ohio (U.S.) patients of unstated ethnic origin diagnosed as having hemochromatosis by conventional histopathologic criteria, only 5 were found to be 845A (C282Y) homozygotes by appropriate molecular study of the tissue blocks.[394] It is most likely that such a low frequency of this mutation and absence of the 187G (H63D) mutation was caused by inclusion of several samples from African-American and southern European patients with non-HFE hemochromatosis.

A systematic phlebotomy program is an alternative, noninvasive method for the diagnosis of hemochromatosis. Phlebotomies should be performed until the serum ferritin concentration falls to iron deficiency levels and the hemoglobin concentration to 11 g/dl.[296] The initial iron load can be calculated from the amount of iron removed (500 ml blood contains about 250 mg iron).

The diagnosis of the commonest variety of hereditary hemochromatosis, namely that due to an *HFE* gene mutation, can be established easily using the polymerase chain reaction-based methods as described by Feder et al.[79] or one of the many variations of the technique that have been described. DNA is most conveniently obtained from blood but can be extracted from buccal cells. Large scale screening is better accomplished using an allele-specific oligonucleotide (ASOH)-based technique.[151] Homozygosity for the 845A (C282Y) variant accounts for 69 to 100 percent of cases, with occasional individuals being 845A/187G compound heterozygotes (see "Mode of Inheritance" above). The genetic basis for the other cases remains to be established, and the diagnosis of hemochromatosis is not disproved if the genetic test is negative.

In addition to establishing the presence or absence of fibrosis in the liver, the possibility that other consequences of the iron overload may have developed should be investigated, but a detailed discussion of the special tests used for the assessment of hepatic, cardiac, or endocrine function is beyond the scope of this chapter.

Identification of Affected Relatives. Once a hereditary hemochromatosis homozygote has been identified all first-degree relatives, particularly the sibs, should be screened. If the proband is homozygous for an *HFE* mutation, any other homozygotes, heterozygotes, and unaffected individuals can be easily identified by DNA analysis. If neither *HFE* mutation is present, until the genetic basis of other hereditary hemochromatosis variant(s) is established the iron status of all first-degree relatives should be determined.

If the relevant tests suggest the homozygous state, venesections should be initiated if the serum ferritin level is elevated or there are any clinical stigmata of hemochromatosis. Homozygous sibs who do not show evidence of iron load should be reassessed every 2 to 3 years in order to detect the earliest manifestations of iron overload. In an Australian long-term prospective study of 40 families, the only affected homozygote of either sex who did not develop iron overload had chronic inflammatory bowel disease.[371]

All children of affected homozygotes with the classical mutation are obligate heterozygotes, and may be homozygous if the other parent is a heterozygote; 11 presumable homozygotes were identified among 255 children of homozygous individuals.[213] The interpretation of iron-related tests among family members can be difficult if the hereditary hemochromatosis is not due to an HFE mutation. The use of all appropriate tests in a family setting, such as transferrin saturation and ferritin, is therefore advisable. In some cases, liver biopsy may be considered, but the initiation of a phlebotomy regimen may be a simple way of resolving such a problem if no definite diagnosis can be made, because it will start to deplete a homozygote of potentially noxious iron and among heterozygotes it will soon indicate the lack of increased iron stores.

Differential Diagnosis. The differential diagnosis of homozygosity for hereditary hemochromatosis requires the consideration of iron overload secondary to a chronic anemia and alcoholic liver disease with siderosis. The hyperferritinemia-cataract syndrome is a more remote possibility when an increased serum ferritin level is the only finding.[269,270] Simple heterozygotes for the 845A *HFE* mutation probably develop iron storage only very rarely or not at all. A non-HLA linked syndrome of increased serum ferritin and iron stores with normal plasma iron saturation, usually associated with diabetes and obesity, has been described.[395]

Iron-loading Anemia. Differentiation from iron-loading anemias is usually obvious, although in thalassemia intermedia, congenital dyserythropoietic anemias, and refractory sideroblastic anemias, a near-normal hemoglobin concentration can lead to a diagnostic error.

Alcoholic Hepatic Siderosis. If *HFE* mutations can be demonstrated, most such diagnostic dilemmas will be resolved, but the small fraction of non-*HFE* hereditary hemochromatosis cases may pose a more difficult problem. Until specific tests for the other hereditary hemochromatosis variant or variants become available, the key to distinguishing alcoholic liver disease from non-*HFE* hereditary hemochromatosis plus alcohol abuse is the quantity of hepatic storage iron, and this should be established by chemical analysis rather than by relying on histologic grading. The cellular localization of hemosiderin provides a useful clue, and if there is little Kupffer-cell involvement, hereditary hemochromatosis is probable.[387] But it is the concentration of storage iron that is critical, particularly when it is related to the subject's age.[392] Using this approach, a number of investigators have reported that figures in the hereditary hemochromatosis range are not found in alcoholic cirrhosis (Fig. 127-9).[135,393,396] (The dietary siderosis of sub-Saharan Africa represents a special situation.) In most alcoholic cirrhotic patients without hemochromatosis, the hepatic iron concentration is not more than twice the upper limit of normal.[297,396,397] The calculation of the hepatic tissue iron index,[392] which relates the iron load to the age (mMole iron/g dry weight divided by age in years), helps to identify homozygotes.[296,393] In an analysis of 509 liver biopsy specimens, the hepatic iron index was greater than 1.9 in 51 of the 55 hereditary hemochromatosis samples and in none of the 454 others.[397] However, Adams et al.[398] found hepatic iron indices greater than 1.9 in 12 out of 189 patients who they considered did not have hereditary hemochromatosis. Some investigators have found the hepatic iron index to be unreliable in the presence of cirrhosis.[399,400]

Heterozygotes. Separation of heterozygotes and compound heterozygotes from affected homozygotes poses no problems in *HFE* hemochromatosis with molecular diagnosis, but can be difficult when the *HFE* gene is not mutated, and the subject has a moderately increased transferrin saturation with some increase in iron stores.

Given current gene frequency estimates, about 30 percent of the Caucasian population is heterozygous for one of the two known *HFE* mutations (10 to 12 percent for the classical 845A [C282Y] mutation and 18 to 24 percent for the 187G [H63D] variant) (Table 127-4). Nothing is known of the effect of heterozygosity for the more common 187G (H63D) mutation, but various family studies in the past were performed on 845A (C282Y) heterozygotes who had been identified by HLA haplotyping. We now recognize that such a population of "carriers" is a mixture of simple heterozygotes for the 845A (C282Y) mutation as well as compound heterozygotes for both the 845A (C282Y) and 187G (H63D) mutations. Based on heterozygote population frequencies and appropriate Hardy-Weinberg calculations, approximately 18 percent of the "heterozygotes" may be presumed to be compound heterozygotes. Iron indices of compound heterozygotes are higher on the average than those of simple heterozygotes for the classical 845A (C282Y) mutation. About one third of presumed "heterozygotes" of earlier studies had raised values for one or more of the tests of iron status, including transferrin saturation, serum ferritin, and liver iron,[1,137,181,302,310,319,401–404] but marked iron overload did not occur unless there was a coexisting iron-loading disorder such as hereditary spherocytosis or idiopathic refractory sideroblastic anemia.[405]

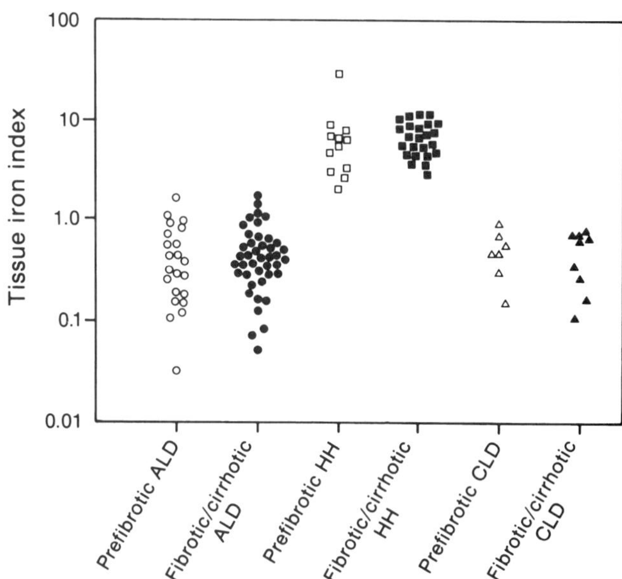

Fig. 127-9 Tissue iron index (iron concentrations divided by age in years) was calculated in patients with alcoholic liver disease (ALD), hereditary hemochromatosis (HH), and other forms of chronic liver disease (CLD). (*From Sallie et al.*[393] *Used by permission.*)

The calculated hepatic storage iron index was somewhat useful in ruling out the heterozygous state before molecular analysis became possible (Fig. 127-10).[134,392] In a prospective study of 40 families, only one of the 98 putative heterozygotes required venesection treatment;[371] this might have been a compound heterozygote 845A/187G. None of the others showed any evidence that their iron stores were increasing during the period of study (up to 24 years). In contrast, only 4 of 51 putative homozygous relatives of the probands did not accumulate iron. Serial observations over a number of years should therefore enable the physician to distinguish between the heterozygous and the homozygous states if it is not initially clear. If the individual in question is the first family member to be encountered, the iron status of the others should be determined, not only to help with the diagnosis of the proband, but also to identify possible homozygotes. An analysis of the number of hemochromatosis patients who are simple heterozygotes, based on mutation analysis, shows no excess over the number of heterozygotes in the general population.[406] This finding is consistent with the older data among heterozygotes, which show abnormal indices of iron metabolism at a frequency approximating that of the prevalence of compound heterozygotes (845A [C282Y]/187G [H63D]) in the population (i.e., about 18 percent).

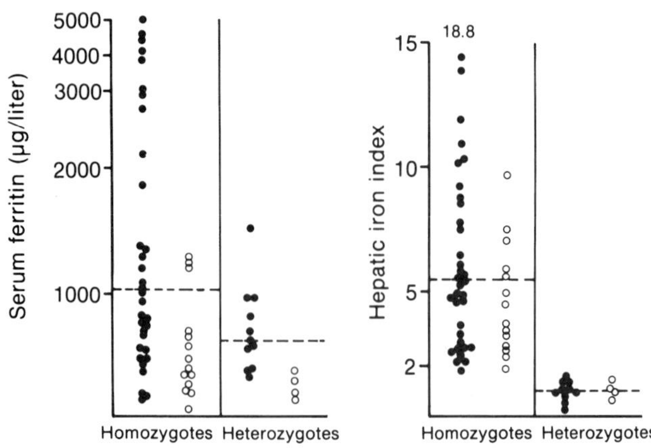

Fig. 127-10 The left panel shows the range of serum ferritin values in 48 individuals homozygous for the HLA-linked iron-loading gene and in 15 heterozygotes. The black circles are males and the open circles females. The right panel shows the hepatic iron index (hepatic iron concentration divided by age) in the same subjects. The broken lines represent median values. (*From Summers et al.*[134] *Used by permission.*)

Heterozygosity for the 845A (C282Y) mutation appears to be associated with a higher frequency of fibrosis and cirrhosis among patients with hepatitis C and is an unfavorable risk factor.[407] Whether venesection might be preventive in such patients is unknown.

Hereditary Hyperferritinemia-Cataract Syndrome. An autosomal dominant syndrome characterized by elevations of serum ferritin (400 to 2250 µg/liter) and congenital nuclear cataracts is described under "Hemochromatosis Without Mutations of *HFE*," above. There is no systemic iron overload and phlebotomy rapidly results in iron deficiency anemia.

HFE Mutations in Other Diseases

Porphyria Cutanea Tarda. The frequency of the 845A (C282Y) hemochromatosis mutation is significantly increased in patients with porphyria cutanea tarda (PCT).[408–410] This condition often is sporadic but can be due to an autosomal dominant deficiency of the enzyme uroporphyrinogen decarboxylase. Phlebotomy treatments are known to be helpful. Homozygosity for the common hemochromatosis mutation 845A (C282Y) was found in 10 to 17 percent of PCT patients. Heterozygotes for this mutation ranged between 26 to 76 percent in different series. In Italy there was no increased frequency of the 845A (C282Y) mutation, but one half of patients had the 187G (H63D) mutation.[411] Abnormal iron indices were also observed in patients without *HFE* mutations. Another frequent etiologic factor among patients with PCT was chronic infection with hepatitis C virus, which was detected in as many as 56 percent of such patients. Hepatitis C virus infections appear to act independently of the *HFE* mutations.[407]

Nonalcoholic Steatohepatitis. Originally described as a disease predominantly of obese middle-aged women, commonly associated with diabetes mellitus and hyperlipidemia, nonalcoholic steatohepatitis has recently been recognized also in males and in individuals of both sexes who are neither obese nor diabetic.[175,412] A proportion of patients have stainable iron in the liver, increased hepatic iron concentrations, and/or raised serum transferrin saturations.[175,412] Bacon et al.[175] suggested that such individuals might be hereditary hemochromatosis heterozygotes. George et al.[412] found four 845A (C282Y) homozygotes and twelve heterozygotes among 51 patients with nonalcoholic steatohepatitis. The presence of the mutation was associated with slightly to moderately increased liver iron stores and a raised transferrin saturation, but not all such subjects had increased stores and one third of the patients with increased liver iron stores did not carry the 845A (C282Y) mutation. Seven men and three women had hepatic storage iron concentrations greater than 40 mM/g dry weight; the highest concentration was 81 mM/g dry weight. Increased hepatic storage iron was associated with hepatic fibrosis, and negatively associated with the degree of steatosis, suggesting that iron may contribute to the development of fibrosis in this condition at concentrations well below the reported fibrogenic threshold of 250 to 400 mM/g dry weight.[392]

X-linked Pyridoxine Responsive Anemia Modified by *HFE* Mutations. Two middle-aged brothers had X-linked pyridoxine responsive sideroblastic anemia with ring sideroblasts.[413] The younger man (59 years) was a compound heterozygote for the 845A/187G (C298Y/H63D) mutations, while the older brother (65 years) had no *HFE* mutations. Ferritin levels were higher in the brother with the *HFE* mutations (3500 versus 1058 µg/liter), as were his body iron stores assessed by phlebotomies (21 g versus 10 g). Presumably, the more severe degree of iron storage was caused by the compound heterozygote status for the *HFE* mutations.

Iron loading may occasionally be found in a variety of other anemias, such as in hereditary spherocytosis,[414,415] and pyruvate kinase deficiency[416] in the absence of blood transfusions or medicinal iron administration. Such cases may sometimes be caused by the simultaneous presence of homozygosity for the major *HFE* 845A (C282Y) mutations.

IRON LOADING DISEASES NOT RELATED TO *HFE* MUTATIONS

Non-*HFE* Hemochromatosis Resembling *HFE* Hemochromatosis

The basic lesion or lesions in hemochromatosis that are not associated with *HFE* mutations are unknown.

Juvenile Hemochromatosis

Juvenile hemochromatosis clearly is a different rare genetic disease of unknown etiology and causes clinical symptoms before 30 years of age and even during childhood. Unlike in hereditary hemochromatosis, both males and females are affected in equal proportions. Inheritance is autosomal recessive and consanguinity has frequently been reported. *HFE* mutations have not usually been detected.[239,417] Whether the heterozygous state for the 845A (C282Y) mutation in two patients with juvenile hemochromatosis[156] was incidental requires further investigation. As in hereditary hemochromatosis with *HFE* mutations, the excess iron distribution in the liver largely affects parenchymal cells. The clinical course is severe. Hypogonadotropic hypogonadism, cardiac arrhythmias, and intractable heart failure are characteristic. Unless treated by periodic venesections, death will occur.

Hemochromatosis in Hereditary Anemias

Clinical and pathologic features similar to those found in hereditary hemochromatosis have been reported in patients suffering from a variety of chronic anemias.[11] These fall into two distinct groups on the basis of the degree of erythropoietic activity. Hemochromatosis tends to develop more slowly in the hypoplastic anemias because of the initial predominantly macrophage localization of the iron from the transfused blood. In a retrospective analysis of 20 such individuals who had heavy iron loads, cirrhosis of the liver had developed in only one, although four had impaired glucose tolerance and five had overt diabetes.[128] As the years pass, however, there is redistribution of iron from macrophages into parenchymal tissues.[418] In the chronic hyperplastic anemias in which erythropoiesis is largely ineffective and there is enhanced absorption of dietary iron as well as multiple transfusions, parenchymal-cell loading takes place in parallel with macrophage loading, and organ damage develops more quickly.[11]

This group is typified by thalassemia major, sometimes thalassemia intermedia,[419] and the various dyserythropoietic and sideroblastic anemias.

By far the commonest of the anemias complicated by hemochromatosis is thalassemia major (see Chap. 181 for details). Thalassemia heterozygotes do not usually accumulate excessive amounts of iron,[420,486] but iron overload is a feature of some patients carrying two different globin gene mutations such as in β-thalassemia-hemoglobin E disease.

The congenital dyserythropoietic anemias are a heterogeneous group of rare nonthalassemic anemias with ineffective erythropoiesis and morphologic alterations of both mature red cells and their precursors (multinuclear erythroblasts).[421,422] Iron overload is common. Three types have been distinguished. Type I and type II are inherited as recessive diseases. Type III is transmitted by autosomal dominant inheritance. Type I is very rare and has megaloblastic features with provisional localization to chromosome 15q15.1 - 15.3. The gene has not been identified. Type II is characterized by hereditary erythroblastic multinuclearity with a positive acidified-serum test (HEMPAS). Provisional gene localization is at chromosome 20q11.2. Type III has grossly disorganized giant erythroblasts. Benign monoclonal gammopathy as well as myelomas are not uncommon. The type III gene has been provisionally mapped to chromosome 15q21. Many cases of dyserythropoietic anemia cannot be clearly categorized.

The sideroblastic anemias are characterized by mitochondrial iron loading and are clinically and hematologically heterogeneous.[423] A definitive X-linked type of sideroblastic anemia that often responds to pyridoxine treatment has been identified. This disease can be of late onset and is caused by missense mutations of the delta amino levulinic synthase gene.[424] Extensive iron loading with heart failure and cirrhosis has been observed and can be cautiously treated with venesections after the anemia is controlled with pyridoxine (see also "*HFE* Mutations In Other Diseases").

African Iron Overload

African iron overload disease has become better defined in recent years and resembles hemochromatosis in some of its aspects. In sub-Saharan African blacks, the severity of the unique variety of iron overload still commonly encountered there[273,425] is closely related to the quantity of home-brewed alcohol consumed by affected individuals (see "Alcohol and Iron Overload" above). Many regular drinkers develop iron overload quantitatively similar to that encountered in hereditary hemochromatosis, but, unlike in hereditary hemochromatosis, macrophages throughout the body as well as hepatocytes contain prominent hemosiderin deposits. Portal fibrosis and micronodular cirrhosis develop, but overt histologic features of alcoholic liver disease are not found.[387] Accelerated ascorbic acid oxidation by the ferric iron deposits has been demonstrated, and together with the usually low dietary ascorbic acid content may lead to scurvy and severe osteoporosis with femoral neck and vertebral fractures.[11,426]

In a small proportion of subjects, usually those with cirrhosis, hemosiderin deposits are also found in the heart, pituitary, thyroid, adrenal, and pancreas. Associated diabetes,[387] cardiomyopathy,[427] and hepatocellular carcinoma[428,429] have been described. The involvement of these tissues has been ascribed to the increased transferrin saturation in such subjects.[11]

A bimodal distribution of transferrin saturations has been demonstrated in beer drinkers of both sexes, but not in nondrinkers.[430] Likelihood analysis of 36 pedigrees to test for dietary iron-gene interaction revealed strong evidence of a genetic effect, with interaction between the ingested amount of dietary iron and a non-HLA-linked gene as shown by mapping studies.[430] A segregation analysis of 351 members of 45 families and a study of 28 spouse pairs with similar heavy beer consumptions supported this conclusion.[102,431] Thus only four of the men and none of the women among the spouses had transferrin saturations greater than 70 percent and high serum ferritin concentrations, although exposure to excessive dietary iron had been comparable. PCR analysis of DNA from 25 individuals identified as probable carriers of the putative African iron-loading gene did not reveal the 845A (C282Y) mutation.[432]

Reports of African-Americans with iron overload have led to the postulation of a non-*HFE* iron-loading gene in this population.[414,433] In one of these reports[414] the iron overload in four male individuals was unexplained, the hepatic iron index was greater than 2, and two had cirrhosis and two cardiopathy. In a review of 326 unselected necropsies on African-Americans, two men and two women, all heavy drinkers, had hepatic iron indices of 1.9 or greater.[428]

Among 808 African-American serum samples (from a Health and Nutrition survey), a suggestive trimodal distribution of transferrin saturation indicative of a mixture of three populations was detected.[434] A small 0.9 percent of the samples clustered around a mean transferrin saturation of 63.4 percent, while 13.6 percent and 85.6 percent had mean saturations of 38 percent and 24.6 percent, respectively. These frequencies are consistent with the hypothesis that 0.9 percent of these samples came from abnormal homozygotes for an undefined non-HLA iron loading gene, while 13 percent were the corresponding heterozygotes and 85 percent were the normal homozygotes for this gene. The isolation of this putative gene should aid in better definition of non-*HFE* hemochromatosis among patients of African origin.

Aceruloplasminemia[435]

A variety of different deletions and nonsense mutations affecting ceruloplasmin (a copper binding glycoprotein) cause complete absence of plasma ceruloplasmin in homozygotes for a mutant gene. A characteristic disorder of iron metabolism caused by loss of the usual ferroxidase activity of ceruloplasmin ensues. Systemic hemosiderosis affecting the pancreas with diabetes mellitus, increased liver iron, pigmentary retinal degeneration, and neurologic findings are observed. In contrast to all other iron storage disorders there is increased iron content in the basal ganglia and in the red and dentate nuclei of the brain. Cerebellar ataxia, extra pyramidal signs, and dementia develop with late adult onset. Treatment with desferrioxamine may prevent progression of neurologic symptoms.

Congenital Atransferrinemia[436,437]

Congenital absence of serum transferrin is a very rare autosomal recessive condition and is caused by mutations of the transferrin gene.[487] Affected individuals have hypochromic anemia refractory to iron therapy and hemosiderosis of the heart and of parenchymal and Kupffer cells in the liver. Heterozygotes have reduced transferrin levels. Therapy with human transferrin and desferrioxamine appears to be effective.

Neonatal Hemochromatosis

Neonatal hemochromatosis (perinatal hemochromatosis) is a rare, almost uniformly rapidly fatal disorder of the newborn, characterized clinically by hepatic insufficiency and often a hemorrhagic diathesis.[438–441] Hemosiderin deposits are very prominent in hepatocytes and other organs, similar to the distribution of hereditary hemochromatosis. In spite of its resemblance to hereditary hemochromatosis, neonatal hemochromatosis seems not to be a neonatal manifestation of it. Neonatal hemochromatosis has only rarely been reported in hereditary hemochromatosis kinships. In the many hereditary hemochromatosis families that have been studied, the young homozygotes show no evidence of having acquired excessive iron *in utero*. In most instances excess iron starts to accumulate only after adulthood is reached, although this occurs during childhood in the juvenile variety of the disease (see "Juvenile Hemochromatosis" section above).

Current evidence suggests that several as yet poorly defined conditions may present as neonatal hemochromatosis. In one the hepatic siderosis is accompanied by defective bile acid synthesis due to delta 4-3 oxosteroid 5 beta-reductase deficiency.[442,443] Two families in which neonatal hemochromatosis was combined with proximal renal tubular dysgenesis have been reported.[444] A third form associated with lactic acidosis and aminoaciduria has been described in a number of Finnish families.[445] Autosomal recessive inheritance was suggested. In other reports sibs have also been affected, and either autosomal recessive or codominant inheritance has been proposed.[439] Autosomal recessive inheritance was highly unlikely in two families in which neonatal hemochromatosis occurred in infants born of different fathers.[446] No *HFE* mutations were detected in 4 cases.[151]

POPULATION SCREENING

The availability of relatively inexpensive diagnostic tests, and the fact that a simple intervention can prevent morbidity and mortality, constitute a strong case for actively searching for hereditary hemochromatosis homozygotes in populations in which the prevalence is high, namely Caucasian populations of European descent.[85,296] While the first task is the prevention of morbidity, finding yet asymptomatic subjects may benefit not only the proband but also asymptomatic homozygotes subsequently identified among relatives. Screening of patients attending diabetic, liver, endocrine, and cardiac clinics for hereditary hemochromatosis may therefore be useful and is currently under study. Conte et al.[447] found 12 persons with hemochromatosis among 894 Italian patients with diabetes, and George et al.[448] found 6 definite and 4 probable homozygotes among 1194 Scottish diabetics. However, Turnbull et al.[449] found only 1 among 727 patients attending a diabetic clinic in northeast England.

There are several reports of more widely based screening studies for hereditary hemochromatosis.[185,319,368,378,450–454] The subjects have typically been blood donors, employees of large corporations, or members of a health maintenance organization, with a raised transferrin saturation being used as the initial screen. The advantages of this approach are that the test is inexpensive, is easy to automate, and can identify affected individuals before iron overload develops. Its disadvantages are that a fasting specimen is required and the test must be repeated to confirm a positive result before proceeding to further investigations.[85] In addition, depending on the cutoff value selected, varying proportions of homozygotes will be missed and heterozygotes included.[374] The serum ferritin concentration has also been used,[319,455] but it is not suitable as the sole initial test as it identifies only those individuals who have already accumulated excess iron. Measurement of the serum ferritin concentration should, of course, form part of the subsequent evaluation of newly identified homozygotes. The unsaturated iron-binding capacity has been proposed as an even cheaper alternative to the transferrin saturation for the screening investigation,[456,457] but its reliability has not yet been established in a large screening program.

In the reports of such programs, the numbers of homozygotes that have been found have usually been lower than the predicted prevalence of about 3 to 5 per 1000. Possible reasons include the diagnostic criteria employed, and age and sex of subjects, their willingness to undergo further investigation, and real differences in prevalence in the populations studied. Olsson et al.[185] in Sweden found three homozygotes among 1311 blood donors using a transferrin saturation of 70 percent as the initial screen and increased stores as the second criterion. In an investigation of 11065 blood donors, Edwards et al.[368] selected a nonfasting transferrin concentration of 50 percent as the initial screen, followed by a fasting transferrin saturation measurement with the decision level for liver biopsy set at 62 percent. Almost one-third of their subjects did not return for collection of the fasting blood sample. Of those who had elevated fasting transferrin saturations, 69 percent were found on biopsy to have marked iron overload. Those who had only moderate increases in liver iron stores were classified as heterozygotes; with hindsight a number of them were probably also homozygotes or compound heterozygotes. Their yield was nevertheless 58 homozygotes, or about 5 per 1000 individuals tested. Bassett et al.[451] found 11 individuals with transferrin saturations greater than 60 percent among 1331 asymptomatic employees. Seven refused further investigation, while the remaining four had hereditary hemochromatosis on liver biopsy. Meyer et al.[319] measured the serum ferritin concentration and unsaturated iron-binding capacity on frozen blood samples collected three years previously from 1783 Afrikaner males over age 40. Of the 192 individuals with a serum ferritin concentration greater than 400 μg/liter or a low unsaturated iron-binding capacity, 150 were available for further study. Homozygosity was defined as a mean serum ferritin concentration above 400 μg/liter plus a mean transferrin saturation greater than 55 percent. There were 17 individuals who met this criterion (0.95 percent of the original 1783 subjects), suggesting a high frequency of hereditary hemochromatosis in this population. Niederau et al.[454] used transferrin saturation combined with serum ferritin concentration as the initial screen, and found hereditary hemochromatosis with gross iron overload in 0.4 percent of males and 0.2 percent of females among 3012 asymptomatic employees. The prevalences were approximately double those figures among 3027 family practitioner outpatients. Smith et al.[458] found five homozygotes among 1875 Caucasian employees of a Massachusetts corporation; most of the grandparents of four of their cases were of Welsh or Irish descent, a finding compatible with the view that the *HFE* gene is of Celtic origin.

Cost-Effectiveness of Population Screening

The question of the cost-effectiveness of screening for hereditary hemochromatosis has been addressed by several groups. Some have constructed models based on various assumptions concerning the percentage of homozygotes identified by the procedure selected, and the costs incurred versus the later costs if iron overload is not prevented,[459–461] while others have reported the actual costs and the number of homozygotes identified.[452,453,458] Estimates of the cost per identified homozygote have ranged widely according to the protocol and assumptions regarding possibilities for minimizing test costs, from 18,041[407] to as little as $4,410.[461] The latter protocol requires all individuals with fasting transferrin saturations greater than 45 percent to be tested for *HFE* mutations rather than to have a liver biopsy as the second step;[461] if more homozygotes found by screening family members of probands are included the figure could be reduced to $2,457.[461] Even at the higher cost levels, opinion is unanimous that screening for hereditary hemochromatosis is cost-effective.

Molecular Testing

The place of molecular testing for abnormal *HFE* genotypes in screening programs has been discussed.[85] The test identifies homozygotes whether or not they have accumulated any excess iron, and eliminates any possible confusion with heterozygotes. Used as the initial screen it has been estimated to be cheaper than transferrin saturation plus serum ferritin concentration.[462] The sample does not have to be drawn in the fasting state and the test does not have to be repeated. However, non-*HFE* hereditary hemochromatosis will be missed. Such individuals may constitute significant percentages of cases. In some recent reports only 59 percent,[159] 87 percent,[463] and 64 percent[153] of hereditary hemochromatosis phenotypes were 845A (C282Y) homozygotes, with a further 7 to 8 percent being compound 845A/187G heterozygotes. The cutoff level for the fasting transferrin saturation should be set at 45 percent so as to include as many homozygotes as possible.[374] (see "Diagnosis" section above). If an abnormal genotype is not present, further tests for the phenotypic abnormality should be pursued. Because of uncertainties regarding testing protocols, the yet unknown clinical penetrance of homozygous hemochromatosis, as well as potential discriminatory misuse of genetic testing in the United States, an expert panel assembled by the Centers for Disease Control and Prevention and the National Human Genome Research Institute recommended deferral of population-wide screening of any sort until more data from various studies became available.[406,464]

TREATMENT

Every patient with hereditary hemochromatosis should undergo repeated phlebotomy until all of the excess of iron has been removed.[11,296] Before initiating the venesection program, it is important to assess the degree of cardiac involvement, both clinically and by special investigations including radiography, electrocardiography, and echocardiography.[465] The quantity of iron removed with each 500 ml of blood is a function of the hemoglobin concentration, averaging about 200 to 250 mg. Guidelines for managing this process have been developed under the auspices of the American College of Pathologists.[296] The erythroid marrow responds to the anemia induced by phlebotomy by increasing the rate of erythropoiesis, and iron to replace that which has been removed is mobilized from the tissues. Most patients tolerate the removal of 500 ml of blood every week for prolonged periods, and even more frequent venesections may be possible.[466] However, it is useful to initiate phlebotomies at intervals of two weeks to give the erythroid marrow an opportunity to approach its maximum rate of proliferation. The hemoglobin should be monitored before each phlebotomy, and the ferritin levels determined every two or three months. As the end of the phlebotomy program is reached, the ferritin level will fall and the MCV will begin to decline as the availability of iron for erythropoiesis decreases. Some clinicians discontinue phlebotomy when the ferritin level falls to below 50 ng/ml; others prefer to induce a mild iron deficiency state. With weekly phlebotomies about 200 mg of iron is removed each week, so that the annual rate of iron removal is 10 g. The length of time phlebotomy needs to be continued depends upon the amount of iron present when treatment is initiated. Typically, the plasma iron concentration remains high until tissue iron stores are almost exhausted, but occasionally a pseudo-iron-deficient state may occur while abundant iron is still present in the tissues. This may be due to the development of a hepatoma or intercurrent infection. Sometimes the plasma iron and ferritin levels will rise rapidly after conclusion of the course of phlebotomies, presumably because some iron pools that are not readily mobilized have gradually equilibrated with other body iron stores. A second short course of phlebotomies may then be required. After the excess iron has been eliminated, reaccumulation can be prevented by periodic venesections, the frequency of which can be tailored to each patient by periodically estimating the serum ferritin level, aiming to maintain it under 50 ng/ml.

Chelating agents, of which the iron-specific deferoxamine is the most effective, can be used to remove excess iron from the body, and indeed this form of treatment is the only one available for the iron overload secondary to refractory anemias. However, the treatment is expensive and cumbersome because nightly subcutaneous infusions are required.[467] Deferoxamine treatment is therefore only rarely recommended in hereditary hemochromatosis, being reserved for the patient who for one reason or another cannot be phlebotomized.

Loss of libido may be treated by the administration of androgens. Diabetes, hepatic failure, and cardiac failure should be managed along conventional lines. In rare cases heart[468,469] and liver[219,221,468,470–473] transplantation has been performed. The outlook for hemochromatosis patients undergoing orthotopic liver transplantation seems to be somewhat less favorable than in patients without hemochromatosis.[219,472]

PROGNOSIS

Removal of iron before cirrhosis or diabetes has occurred prevented all adverse consequences of this inherited condition and was associated with a normal life expectancy.[26,142,474] However, these data were based on small numbers and may have reflected a relatively mild underlying disease[464] with better prognosis. If the tissue iron concentrations do reach critical levels, irreversible morbidity and shortened survival are the results. In an early retrospective analysis of untreated symptomatic hereditary hemochromatosis, the 5-year survival from the time of diagnosis was 18 percent, and the 10-year survival was 6 percent.[475] Removing the iron improves the prognosis dramatically even in symptomatic subjects. In the series described by Niederau et al.,[291] many of the 251 subjects had advanced symptomatic disease (Fig. 127-11). The mean follow-up period was 14 years and some had been observed for as long as 30 years. Survival in those without cirrhosis or diabetes before phlebotomies were initiated was no different from that of age- and sex-matched normal subjects.

Because organ damage correlates with the severity of the iron load, it is not surprising that those who died had significantly more iron that the survivors. Even in those with cirrhosis, the 10-year survival after removing the iron was 70 percent. However, this was significantly reduced compared with age- and sex-matched normal individuals. The findings in a retrospective study of 85 hereditary hemochromatosis subjects were comparable.[476] Markedly disordered liver function and portal hypertension were grave prognostic signs; of 13 such patients, 9 died before all the iron could be removed.[291,477] Cirrhosis is not completely reversed by removing the iron, although there may be some regression of fibrosis and liver function usually improves. In another study some improvement in esophageal varices was noted in 26 percent of patients after six years.[478]

An important late complication of cirrhosis in hereditary hemochromatosis is liver cancer, which may develop years after the removal of the iron. The incidence reported by Niederau et al.[291] was 15 percent of the 142 patients with cirrhosis, and the mean interval between iron depletion and diagnosis of the cancer was 9.4 years. In a retrospective analysis of 649 hemochromatosis subjects with cirrhosis, 18.5 percent developed hepatocellular carcinoma.[479] In an earlier study, as many as 29 percent of treated subjects eventually died of hepatoma.[475] Hepatoma has been reported in a noncirrhotic subject after elimination of the iron overload,[308] but it seems clear that the risk is very small if the patient is treated before cirrhosis develops.

Alcoholism is a further adverse factor; 17 of 18 subjects whose consumption was more than 60 g/day had cirrhosis.[305,480] However, in a later report from these authors, seven out of 20 individuals with this level of consumption were not cirrhotic, possibly a reflection of the significant recent reduction in the interval between the onset of symptoms and the diagnosis.[291] Heavy alcohol consumption has been shown by multivariate analysis to contribute to decreased survival.[304] In another study more alcoholics than nonalcoholics died before the iron could be completely removed.[289]

Arrhythmias or heart failure, especially in young subjects, will prove fatal within a year unless the iron can be removed. Even with careful management, death might not be avoided, but if the iron is successfully eliminated, the cardiopathy usually regresses.[11,481]

Survival in hereditary hemochromatosis patients with diabetes is significantly reduced compared with nondiabetic hemochromatotics, whose survival is similar to that of the normal age- and sex-matched population.[291] In about half the insulin-dependent diabetics, the reduction in insulin resistance following removal of the iron from the hepatocytes means that the dose can be reduced.

The pigmentation regresses in most subjects. Arthropathy improves in about one third, although it may also worsen,[329] but the chance of improved sexual function is slight.[303,305,480,482]

ADDENDUM

Since the preparation of this chapter there has been considerable further progress in the understanding of iron absorption and of hemochromatosis.

The number of proteins that participate in the iron absorption process continues to expand. At least some of these will prove to be important in regulating iron stores. Indeed, in a large study of

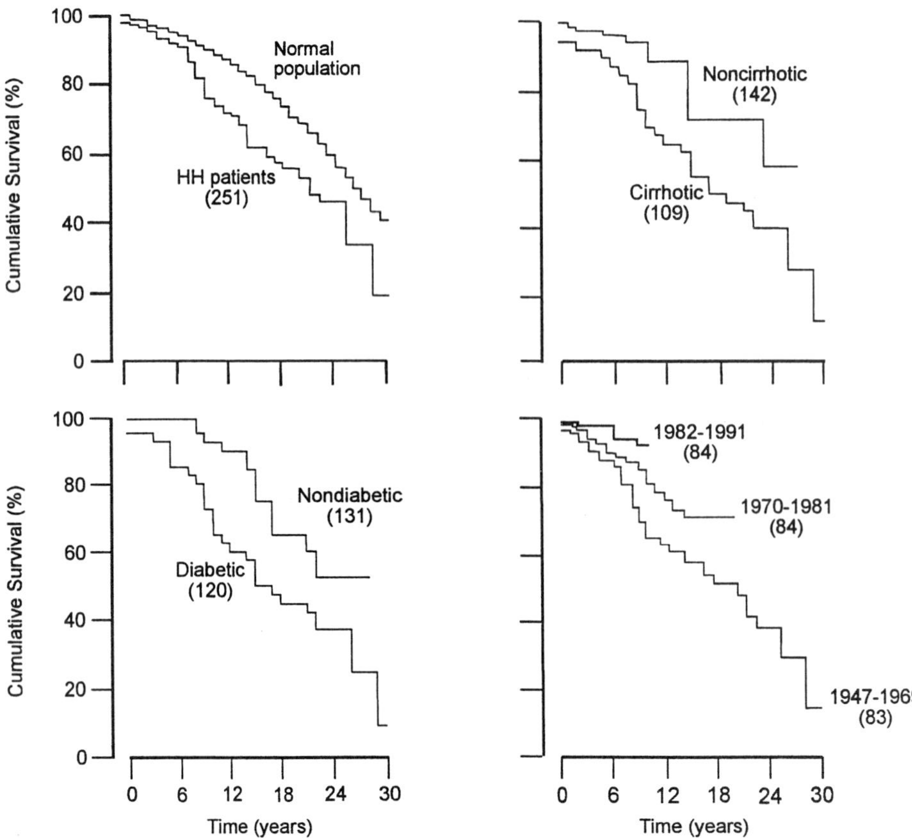

Fig. 127-11 Cumulative survival in 251 patients with hereditary hemochromatosis. Survival was significantly reduced in comparison with expected survival rates for an age- and gender-matched normal population. Results in various subgroups indicated that diabetes and cirrhosis adversely affected prognosis, while cumulative survival has progressively increased in patients initially diagnosed in three periods (1947 to 1968, 1970 to 1981, and 1982 to 1991). (From Niederau et al.[291] Reprinted with permission.)

twins Whitfield et al.[488] showed that there was a strong genetic component in the regulation of transferrin saturation and ferritin levels, but $<5\%$ could be accounted for by *HFE* mutations. A defect in hephaestin, a ceruloplasmin homologue, has been found to be the cause of the sla (sex-linked anemia) mouse.[489] This animal cannot transport iron from the intestinal cell into the blood; presumably hephaestin acts to oxidize Fe^{++} to the Fe^{+++} valence required to bind to plasma transferrin. Conversely, a ferric reductase is required at the luminal side of the mucosal cell, and it has been found that this function is carried out by dihydropteridine reductase as well, probably, as by a cytochrome b-type reductase.[490] A gene encoding a protein quite homologous to the transferrin receptor has been cloned[491] and has been designated the transferrin receptor-2, and been involved in a rare type of genetic hemochromatosis mapping to 7q22.[492] A transport protein has been found to facilitate transport of both ferric and ferrous iron. Designated "stimulator of iron transport" (or SFT), the transcript is iron regulated and it was suggested that it might play a role in iron overload.[493] A homologue of the divalent metal transporter-1 (DCT-1) has been identified and variously designated ferroportin,[494] MTP1,[495] and IREG1. *HFE* knockout mice have been bred with mice deficient in other proteins such as β_2-microglobulin, DMT1, transferrin receptor, and hephaestin to better understand the interaction between these gene products.[496] Another important gene may be located on the long arm of chromosome 1; juvenile hemochromatosis maps to this region.[497]

Although most patients who do not have the mutations at nt 845 or nt 187 do not have any other mutations of *HFE* a few additional mutations have been found,[498,499] and these may cause hemochromatosis in some compound heterozygotes. It has been discovered that polymorphisms exist in both the intron 3[500,501] and intron 4[502] amplimer-binding sites originally recommended by Feder et al. Under some circumstances these can cause misdiagnosis of heterozygotes as homozygotes, because the amplimer would not bind to the normal allele, which would therefore not amplify. In the case of the intron 4 mutation, this does not appear to be a major problem.[503,504] The intron 3 mutation has a very high prevalence among African Americans. Under some conditions this mutation has a profound effect on amplification, and in racially mixed populations in which both the intron 3 mutation and the 845A (C282Y) mutation are present, misdiagnoses have occurred.[500]

One of the major gaps in our knowledge has been in assessing the penetrance of the homozygous state for the 845A (C282Y) mutation. Although the chapter points out the large discrepancy between autopsy data and the assumption of high penetrance that underlies recommendations for screening, the general assumption has been that many or even most homozygotes ultimately develop disease. In retrospect, however, this belief seems to have been based largely on uncontrolled observations of family members of clinically affected patients. Now some population-based surveys based on mutation analysis have been carried out, and the results point to a much lower penetrance of the homozygous state than had previously been believed. Olynyk et al.[505] investigated 3011 white Australian subjects and detected 16 homozygotes for the 845A (C282Y) mutation. Only one had frank cirrhosis, but this patient had mild microvascular steatosis and a history of excessive alcohol intake. Three additional patients had some degree of fibrosis. Several of the patients had clinical symptoms compatible with hemochromatosis, but because there were no controls, the significance of common symptoms such as arthralgia is difficult to evaluate. Our own study of 10,198 patients attending a health appraisal clinic in the United States suggests even lower penetrance of the homozygous state. None of the 43 homozygous subjects that we detected had frank clinical hemochromatosis, and, indeed, responses to questionnaires completed by the patients failed to show any difference between the homozygotes for the 845A (C282Y) mutation and the wild-type controls with respect to any of the stigmata of hemochromatosis.[500] This study has now been expanded to encompass over 23,000 subjects, of whom 100 are homozygous for hemochromatosis. None of the homozygotes have frank clinical stigmata of the disease. Studies by Willis et al.[506] also suggest that the penetrance of the homozygous state is very low; the homozygote frequency was the same in the elderly male population as in the population at large. Clearly any screening strategy must take into account the penetrance of the disease.[507]

Additional studies of the possible effect of the heterozygous state on coronary artery disease have been published. In one study,[508] serum ferritin levels seemed to affect the risk for ischemic heart disease only in the presence of other risk factors. However, in a prospective Finnish study, males who were carriers of the 845A mutation were found to be at 2.3-fold increased risk for myocardial infarction.[509] A review of the literature concluded that there was strong evidence for a relationship between iron levels and cardiovascular disease.[510] However, even though mechanisms involving the generation of active oxygen species are invoked, implying a cause-and-effect relationship, the absence of increased ischemic heart disease in homozygotes for hereditary hemochromatosis makes it likely that the relationship between iron and coronary heart disease may be less direct.

REFERENCES

1. Fairbanks VF, Fahey JL, Beutler E: *Clinical Disorders of Iron Metabolism*, 2d ed. New York, Grune & Stratton, 1971.
2. Mallory FB: Hemochromatosis and chronic poisoning with copper. *Arch Intern Med* **37**:336, 1926.
3. Sheldon JH: *Haemochromatosis*. London, Oxford University Press, 1935.
4. MacDonald RA: Idiopathic hemochromatosis. Genetic or acquired? *Arch Intern Med* **112**:82, 1963.
5. MacDonald RA: Primary hemochromatosis: Inherited or acquired? *Prog Hematol* **5**:324, 1966.
6. Simon M, Pawlotsky Y, Bourel M, Fauchet R, Genetet B: Hémochromatose idiopathique: Maladie associée àl'antigène tissulaire. *Nouv Presse Med* **4**:1432, 1975.
7. Simon M, Bourel R, Fauchet R, Genetet B: Association of HLA-A3 and HLA-B14 antigens with idiopathic hemochromatosis. *Gut* **17**:332, 1976.
8. Kravitz K, Skolnick M, Cannings C, Carmelli D, Baty B, Amos B, Johnson A, Mendell N, Edwards C, Cartwright G: Genetic linkage between hereditary hemochromatosis and HLA. *Am J Hum Genet* **31**:601, 1979.
9. Davis WD, Arrowsmith WR: The effect of repeated phlebotomies in hemochromatosis. *J Lab Clin Med* **39**:526, 1952.
10. Butt EM, Nusbaum RE, Gilmour TC, Didio SL: Trace metal patterns in disease states. I. Hemochromatosis and refractory anemia. *Am J Clin Pathol* **27**:225, 1957.
11. Bothwell TH, Charlton RW, Cook JD, Finch CA: *Iron Metabolism in Man*. Oxford, Blackwell Scientific, 1979.
12. Torrance JD, Charlton RW, Schmaman A, Lynch SR, Bothwell TH: Storage iron in "muscle." *J Clin Pathol* **21**:495, 1968.
13. Finch CA, Deubelbeiss K, Cook JD, Eschbach JW, Harker LA, Funk DD, Marsaglia G, Hillman RS, Slichter S, Adamson JW, Ganzoni A, Giblett ER: Ferrokinetics in man. *Medicine (Baltimore)* **49**:17, 1970.
14. Hershko C, Cook JD, Finch CA: Storage iron kinetics. II. The uptake of hemoglobin iron by hepatic parenchymal cells. *J Lab Clin Med* **80**:624, 1972.
15. Theil EC: Ferritin: structure, gene regulation, and cellular function in animals, plants, and microorganisms. *Annu Rev Biochem* **56**:289, 289, 1987.
16. Harrison PM, Arosio P: The ferritins: Molecular properties, iron storage function and cellular regulation. *Biochim Biophys Acta* **1275**:161, 1996.
17. Weir MP, Gibson JF, Peters TJ: Biochemical studies on the isolation and characterization of human spleen haemosiderin. *Biochem J* **223**:31, 1984.
18. Bell SH, Weir MP, Dickson DP, Gibson JF, Sharp GA, Peters TJ: Mossbauer spectroscopic studies of human haemosiderin and ferritin. *Biochim Biophys Acta* **787**:227, 1984.
19. Crichton RR: Proteins of iron storage and transport. *Adv Protein Chem* **40**:281, 281, 1990.
20. Harrison PM, Clegg JB, May K: Ferritin structure and function, in Jacobs A, Worwood M (eds): *Iron in Biochemistry and Medicine II*. New York, Academic Press, 1980.
21. Ford GC, Harrison PM, Rice DW, Smith JM, Treffry A, White JL, Yariv J: Ferritin: Design and formation of an iron-storage molecule. *Philos Trans R Soc Lond B Biol Sci* **304**:551, 1984.
22. Mann S, Bannister JV, Williams RJ: Structure and composition of ferritin cores isolated from human spleen, limpet (*Patella vulgata*) hemolymph and bacterial (*Pseudomonas aeruginosa*) cells. *J Mol Biol* **188**:225, 1986.
23. Crichton RR: A role for ferritin in the regulation of iron metabolism. *FEBS Lett* **34**:125, 1973.
24. Harrison PM, Treffry A, Lilley TH: Ferritin as an iron-storage protein: Mechanisms of iron uptake. *J Inorg Biochem* **27**:287, 1986.
25. Chasteen ND, Theil EC: Iron binding by horse spleen apoferritin. A vanadyl(IV) EPR spin probe study. *J Biol Chem* **257**:7672, 1982.
26. Grossman MJ, Hinton SM, Minak-Bernero V, Slaughter C, Stiefel EI: Unification of the ferritin family of proteins. *Proc Natl Acad Sci U S A* **89**:2419, 1992.
27. Worwood M: Ferritin. *Blood Rev* **4**:259, 1990.
28. Worwood M, Brook JD, Cragg SJ, Hellkuhl B, Jones BM, Perera P, Roberts SH, Shaw DJ: Assignment of human ferritin genes to chromosomes 11 and 19q13.3 → 19qter. *Hum Genet* **69**:371, 1985.
29. Papadopoulos P, Bhavsar D, Zappone E, David V, Jones C, Worwood M, Drysdale J: A second human ferritin H locus on chromosome 11. *Cytogenet Cell Genet* **61**:107, 1992.
30. Guo W, Adams V, Mason J, McCabe ER: Identification of a ferritin light chain pseudogene near the glycerol kinase locus in Xp21 by cDNA amplification for identification of genomic expressed sequences. *Biochem Mol Med* **60**:169, 1997.
31. Zheng HD, Bhavsar D, Drysdale J: An unusual human ferritin H sequence from chromosome 4. *DNA Seq* **5**:173, 1995.
32. Percy ME, Bauer SJ, Rainey S, McLachlan DR, Dhar MS, Joshi JG: Localization of a new ferritin heavy chain sequence present in human brain mRNA to chromosome 11. *Genome* **38**:450, 1995.
33. Cragg SJ, Drysdale J, Worwood M: Genes for the "H" subunit of human ferritin are present on a number of human chromosomes. *Hum Genet* **71**:108, 1985.
34. Lebo RV, Kan YW, Cheung MC, Jain SK, Drysdale J: Human ferritin light chain gene sequences mapped to several sorted chromosomes. *Hum Genet* **71**:325, 1985.
35. McGill JR, Naylor SL, Sakaguchi AY, Moore CM, Boyd D, Barrett KJ, Shows TB, Drysdale JW: Human ferritin H and L sequences lie on ten different chromosomes. *Hum Genet* **76**:66, 1987.
36. Dugast IJ, Papadopoulos P, Zappone E, Jones C, Theriault K, Handelman GJ, Benarous R, Drysdale JW: Identification of two human ferritin H genes on the short arm of chromosome 6. *Genomics* **6**:204, 1990.
37. Wagstaff M, Worwood M, Jacobs A: Properties of human tissue isoferritins. *Biochem J* **173**:969, 1978.
38. Treffry A, Lee PJ, Harrison PM: Functional studies on rat-liver isoferritins. *Biochim Biophys Acta* **785**:22, 1984.
39. Aziz N, Munro HN: Both subunits of rat liver ferritin are regulated at a translational level by iron induction. *Nucleic Acids Res* **14**:915, 1986.
40. Rogers J, Munro H: Translation of ferritin light and heavy subunit mRNAs is regulated by intracellular chelatable iron levels in rat hepatoma cells. *Proc Natl Acad Sci U S A* **84**:2277, 1987.
41. Cairo G, Bardella L, Schiaffonati L, Arosio P, Levi S, Bernelli-Zazzera A: Multiple mechanisms of iron-induced ferritin synthesis in HeLa cells. *Biochem Biophys Res Commun* **133**:314, 1985.
42. Hentze MW, Caughman SW, Casey JL, Koeller DM, Rouault TA, Harford JB, Klausner RD: A model for the structure and functions of iron-responsive elements. *Gene* **72**:201, 1988.
43. Rouault T, Klausner R: Regulation of iron metabolism in eukaryotes. *Curr Top Cell Regul* **35**:1, 1, 1997.
44. Menotti E, Henderson BR, Kuhn LC: Translational regulation of mRNAs with distinct IRE sequences by iron regulatory proteins 1 and 2. *J Biol Chem* **273**:1821, 1998.
45. Kennedy MC, Mende-Mueller L, Blondin GA, Beinert H: Purification and characterization of cytosolic aconitase from beef liver and its relationship to the iron-responsive element binding protein. *Proc Natl Acad Sci U S A* **89**:11730, 1992.

46. Kaptain S, Downey WE, Tang C, Philpott C, Haile D, Orloff DG, Harford JB, Rouault TA, Klausner RD: A regulated RNA binding protein also possesses aconitase activity. *Proc Natl Acad Sci U S A* **88**:10109, 1991.
47. Rouault TA, Stout CD, Kaptain S, Harford JB, Klausner RD: Structural relationship between an iron-regulated RNA-binding protein (IRE-BP) and aconitase: Functional implications. *Cell* **64**:881, 1991.
48. Butt J, Kim HY, Basilion JP, Cohen S, Iwai K, Philpott CC, Altschul S, Klausner RD, Rouault TA: Differences in the RNA binding sites of iron regulatory proteins and potential target diversity. *Proc Natl Acad Sci U S A* **93**:4345, 1996.
49. Weiss G, Goossen B, Doppler W, Fuchs D, Pantopoulos K, Werner-Felmayer G, Wachter H, Hentze MW: Translational regulation via iron-responsive elements by the nitric oxide/NO-synthase pathway. *EMBO J* **12**:3651, 1993.
50. Hentze MW, Kuhn LC: Molecular control of vertebrate iron metabolism: mRNA-based regulatory circuits operated by iron, nitric oxide, and oxidative stress. *Proc Natl Acad Sci U S A* **93**:8175, 1996.
51. Kim HY, LaVaute T, Iwai K, Klausner RD, Rouault TA: Identification of a conserved and functional iron-responsive element in the 5′-untranslated region of mammalian mitochondrial aconitase. *J Biol Chem* **271**:24226, 1996.
52. Fleming MD, Romano MA, Su MA, Garrick LM, Garrick MD, Andrews NC: Nramp2 is mutated in the anemic Belgrade (b) rat: Evidence of a role for nramp2 in endosomal iron transport. *Proc Natl Acad Sci U S A* **95**:1148, 1998.
53. Gray NK, Hentze MW: Iron regulatory protein prevents binding of the 43S translation pre-initiation complex to ferritin and eALAS mRNAs. *EMBO J* **13**:3882, 1994.
54. Halliday JW, Powell LW: Serum ferritin and isoferritins in clinical medicine. *Prog Hematol* **11**:229, 1979.
55. Siimes MA, Addiego JE Jr, Dallman PR: Ferritin in serum: Diagnosis of iron deficiency and iron overload in infants and children. *Blood* **43**:581, 1974.
56. Ramm GA, Powell LW, Halliday JW: Effect of colchicine on the clearance of ferritin in vivo. *Am J Physiol* **258**:G707, 1990.
57. Jacobs A, Miller F, Worwood M, Beamish MR, Wardrop CA: Ferritin in the serum of normal subjects and patients with iron deficiency and iron overload. *BMJ* **4**:206, 1972.
58. Worwood M, Cragg SJ, Jacobs A, McLaren C, Ricketts C, Economidou J: Binding of serum ferritin to concanavalin A: Patients with homozygous beta thalassaemia and transfusional iron overload. *Br J Haematol* **46**:409, 1980.
59. Bezwoda WR, Bothwell TH, Torrance JD, MacPhail AP, Charlton RW, Kay G, Levin J: The relationship between marrow iron stores, plasma ferritin concentrations and iron absorption. *Scand J Haematol* **22**:113, 1979.
60. Cook JD, Lipschitz DA, Miles LEM, Finch CA: Serum ferritin as a measure of iron stores in normal subjects. *Am J Clin Nutr* **27**:681, 1974.
61. Worwood M: The laboratory assessment of iron status—An update. *Clin Chim Acta* **259**:3, 1997.
62. Dallman PR, Siimes MA, Stekel A: Iron deficiency in infancy and childhood. *Am J Clin Nutr* **33**:86, 1980.
63. Lipschitz DA, Cook JD, Finch CA: A clinical evaluation of serum ferritin as an index of iron stores. *N Engl J Med* **290**:1213, 1974.
64. Elin RJ, Wolff SM, Finch CA: Effect of induced fever on serum iron and ferritin concentrations in man. *Blood* **49**:147, 1977.
65. Baynes RD, Bothwell TH, Bezwoda WR, Gear AJ, Atkinson P: Hematologic and iron-related measurements in rheumatoid arthritis. *Am J Clin Pathol* **87**:196, 1987.
66. Beutler E, Demina A, Laubscher K, Garver P, Gelbart T, Balicki D, Vaughan L: The clinical course of treated and untreated Gaucher disease. A study of 45 patients. *Blood Cells Mol Dis* **21**:86, 1995.
67. Morgan MAM, Hoffbrand AV, Laulicht M, Luck W, Knowles S: Serum ferritin concentration in Gaucher's disease. *BMJ* **286**:1864, 1983.
68. Jacobs A: Serum ferritin and malignant tumours. *Med Oncol Tumor Pharmacother* **1**:149, 1984.
69. Yang F, Lum JB, McGill JR, Moore CM, Naylor SL, van Bragt PH, Baldwin WD, Bowman BH: Human transferrin: cDNA characterization and chromosomal localization. *Proc Natl Acad Sci U S A* **81**:2752, 1984.
70. McKnight GS, Lee DC, Palmiter RD: Transferrin gene expression. Regulation of mRNA transcription in chick liver by steroid hormones and iron deficiency. *J Biol Chem* **255**:148, 1980.
71. Ponka P, Beaumont C, Richardson DR: Function and regulation of transferrin and ferritin. *Semin Hematol* **35**:35, 1998.
72. Lynch SR, Simon M, Bothwell TH, Charlton RW: Circadian variation in plasma iron concentration and reticuloendothelial iron release in the rat. *Clin Sci Mol Med* **45**:331, 1973.
73. Huebers HA, Finch CA: The physiology of transferrin and transferrin receptors. *Physiol Rev* **67**:520, 1987.
74. Evans P, Kemp J: Exon/intron structure of the human transferrin receptor gene. *Gene* **199**:123, 1997.
75. Rabin M, McClelland A, Kuhn L, Ruddle FH: Regional localization of the human transferrin receptor gene to 3q26.2 → qter. *Am J Hum Genet* **37**:1112, 1985.
76. Lebron JA, Bennett MJ, Vaughn DE, Chirino AJ, Snow PM, Mintier GA, Feder JN, Bjorkman PJ: Crystal structure of the hemochromatosis protein HFE and characterization of its interaction with transferrin receptor. *Cell* **93**:111, 1998.
77. Huebers HA, Csiba E, Huebers E, Finch CA: Competitive advantage of diferric transferrin in delivering iron to reticulocytes. *Proc Natl Acad Sci U S A* **80**:300, 1983.
78. Kuhn LC: mRNA-protein interactions regulate critical pathways in cellular iron metabolism. *Br J Haematol* **79**:1, 1991.
79. Feder JN, Gnirke A, Thomas W, Tsuchihashi Z, Ruddy DA, Basava A, Dormishian F, Domingo R, Jr., Ellis MC, Fullan A, Hinton LM, Jones NL, Kimmel BE, Kronmal GS, Lauer P, Lee VK, Loeb DB, Mapa FA, McClelland E, Meyer NC, Mintier GA, Moeller N, Moore T, Morikang E, Prass CE, Quintana L, Starnes SM, Schatzman RC, Brunke KJ, Drayna DT, Risch NJ, Bacon BR, Wolff RK: A novel MHC class I-like gene is mutated in patients with hereditary haemochromatosis. *Nat Genet* **13**:399, 1996.
80. Feder JN, Penny DM, Irrinki A, Lee VK, Lebron JA, Watson N, Tsuchihashi Z, Sigal E, Bjorkman PJ, Schatzman RC: The hemochromatosis gene product complexes with the transferrin receptor and lowers its affinity for ligand binding. *Proc Natl Acad Sci U S A* **95**:1472, 1998.
81. de Sousa M, Reimao R, Lacerda R, Hugo P, Kaufmann SH, Porto G: Iron overload in beta 2-microglobulin-deficient mice. *Immunol Lett* **39**:105, 1994.
82. Rothenberg BE, Voland JR: β_2 Knockout mice develop parenchymal iron overload: A putative role for class I genes of the major histocompatibility complex in iron metabolism. *Proc Natl Acad Sci U S A* **93**:1529, 1996.
83. Parkkila S, Waheed A, Britton RS, Feder JN, Tsuchihashi Z, Schatzman RC, Bacon BR, Sly WS: Immunohistochemistry of HLA-H, the protein defective in patients with hereditary hemochromatosis, reveals unique pattern of expression in gastrointestinal tract. *Proc Natl Acad Sci U S A* **94**:2534, 1997.
84. Parkkila S, Waheed A, Britton RS, Bacon BR, Zhou XY, Tomatsu S, Fleming RE, Sly WS: Association of the transferrin receptor in human placenta with HFE, the protein defective in hereditary hemochromatosis. *Proc Natl Acad Sci U S A* **94**:13198, 1997.
85. Edwards CQ, Griffen LM, Ajioka RS, Kushner JP: Screening for hemochromatosis: Phenotype versus genotype. *Semin Hematol* **35**:72, 1998.
86. Bali PK, Zak O, Aisen P: A new role for the transferrin receptor in the release of iron from transferrin. *Biochemistry* **30**:324, 1991.
87. Gruenheid S, Cellier M, Vidal S, Gros P: Identification and characterization of a second mouse Nramp gene. *Genomics* **25**:514, 1995.
88. Fleming MD, Trenor CC, Su MA, Foernzler D, Beier DR, Dietrich WF, Andrews NC: Microcytic anaemia mice have a mutation in Nramp2, a candidate iron transporter gene. *Nat Genet* **16**:383, 1997.
89. Lee PL, Gelbart T, West C, Halloran C, Beutler E: The human nramp2 gene: Characterization of the gene structure, alternative splicing, promoter region and polymorphisms. *Blood Cells Mol Dis* **24**:199, 1998.
90. Conrad ME, Umbreit JN, Moore EG: Rat duodenal iron-binding protein mobilferrin is a homologue of calreticulin. *Gastroenterology* **104**:1700, 1993.
91. Sadasivan B, Lehner PJ, Ortmann B, Spies T, Cresswell P: Roles for calreticulin and a novel glycoprotein, tapasin, in the interaction of MHC class I molecules with TAP. *Immunity* **5**:103, 1996.
92. Van Leeuwen JEM, Kearse KP: Deglucosylation of N-linked glycans is an important step in the dissociation of calreticulin-class I-TAP complexes. *Proc Natl Acad Sci U S A* **93**:13997, 1996.
93. Umbreit JN, Conrad ME, Moore EG, Latour LF: Iron absorption and cellular transport: The mobilferrin/paraferritin paradigm. *Semin Hematol* **35**:13, 1998.
94. Hallberg L, Hultén L: Iron requirements, iron balance and iron deficiency in menstruating and pregnant women, in Hallberg L, Asp N

(eds): *Iron Nutrition in Health and Disease*. London, John Libby, 1998, p 165.

95. Uzel C, Conrad ME: Absorption of heme iron. *Semin Hematol* **35**:27, 1998.
96. Parmley RT, Barton JC, Conrad ME: Ultrastructural localization of transferrin, transferrin receptor, and iron-binding sites on human placental and duodenal microvilli. *Br J Haematol* **60**:81, 1985.
97. Nathanson MH, Muir A, McLaren GD: Iron absorption in normal and iron-deficient beagle dogs: mucosal iron kinetics. *Am J Physiol* **249**:G439, 1985.
98. Cook JD: Adaptation in iron metabolism. *Am J Clin Nutr* **51**:301, 1990.
99. Conrad ME Jr, Crosby WH: Intestinal mucosal mechanisms controlling iron absorption. *Blood* **22**:406, 1963.
100. Charlton RW, Jacobs P, Torrance JD, Bothwell TH: The role of ferritin in iron absorption. *Lancet* **2**:762, 1963.
101. Hallberg L, Bjorn-Rasmussen E: Measurement of iron absorption from meals contaminated with iron. *Am J Clin Nutr* **34**:2808, 1981.
102. Moyo VM, Gangaidzo IT, Gomo ZA, Khumalo H, Saungweme T, Kiire CF, Rouault T, Gordeuk VR: Traditional beer consumption and the iron status of spouse pairs from a rural community in Zimbabwe. *Blood* **89**:2159, 1997.
103. Benito P, Miller D: Iron absorption and bioavailability: An updated review. *Nutr Res* **18**:581, 1998.
104. Beutler E, Fairbanks VF, Fahey JL: *Clinical Disorders of Iron Metabolism*. New York, Grune & Stratton, 1963.
105. Luke CG, Adel MB, Davis PS, Deller DJ: Gastric iron binding in hemochromatosis, secondary iron overload, cirrhosis, and diabetes. *Lancet* **2**:844, 1968.
106. Multani JS, Cepurneek CP, Davis PS, Saltman P: Biochemical characterization of gastroferrin. *Biochemistry* **9**:3970, 1970.
107. Wynter CV, Williams R: Iron-binding properties of gastric juice in idiopathic haemochromatosis. *Lancet* **2**:534, 1968.
108. Conrad ME, Umbreit JN: Iron absorption—The mucin-mobilferrin-integrin pathway. A competitive pathway for metal absorption. *Am J Hematol* **42**:67, 1993.
109. Conrad ME, Umbreit JN, Peterson RD, Moore EG, Harper KP: Function of integrin in duodenal mucosal uptake of iron. *Blood* **81**:517, 1993.
110. Conrad ME: Introduction: iron overloading disorders and iron regulation. *Semin Hematol* **35**:1, 1998.
111. Raja KB, Pountney D, Bomford A, Przemioslo R, Sherman D, Simpson RJ, Williams R, Peters TJ: A duodenal mucosal abnormality in the reduction of Fe(III) in patients with genetic haemochromatosis. *Gut* **38**:765, 1996.
112. Riedel HD, Remus AJ, Fitscher BA, Stremmel W: Characterization and partial purification of a ferrireductase from human duodenal microvillus membranes. *Biochem J* **309**:745, 1995.
113. Teichmann R, Stremmel W: Iron uptake by human upper small intestine microvillous membrane vesicles. Indication for a facilitated transport mechanism mediated by a membrane iron-binding protein. *J Clin Invest* **86**:2145, 1990.
114. Carpenter CE, Mahoney AW: Contributions of heme and nonheme iron to human nutrition. *Crit Rev Food Sci Nutr* **31**:333, 1992.
115. Wheby MS, Suttle GE, Ford KT: Intestinal absorption of hemoglobin iron. *Gastroenterology* **58**:647, 1970.
116. Hallberg L, Solvell L: Absorption of hemoglobin iron in man. *Acta Med Scand* **181**:335, 1967.
117. Beutler E, Kelly BM, Beutler F: The regulation of iron absorption. II. Relationship between iron dosage and iron absorption. *Am J Clin Nutr* **11**:559, 1962.
118. Hallberg L, Hulten L, Gramatkovski E: Iron absorption from the whole diet in men: how effective is the regulation of iron absorption? *Am J Clin Nutr* **66**:347, 1997.
119. Bezwoda WR, Disler PB, Lynch SR, Charlton RW, Torrance JD, Derman D, Bothwell TH, Walker RB, Mayet F: Patterns of food iron absorption in iron-deficient white and Indian subjects and in venesected haemochromatotic patients. *Br J Haematol* **33**:425, 1976.
120. Lynch SR, Skikne BS, Cook JD: Food iron absorption in idiopathic hemochromatosis. *Blood* **74**:2187, 1989.
121. Gordon DT, Godber JS: The enhancement of nonheme iron bioavailability by beef protein in the rat. *J Nutr* **119**:446, 1989.
122. Grasbeck R, Majuri R, Kouvonen I, Tenhunen R: Spectral and other studies on the intestinal haem receptor of the pig. *Biochim Biophys Acta* **700**:137, 1982.
123. Tenhunen R, Grasbeck R, Kouvonen I, Lundberg M: An intestinal receptor for heme: Its partial characterization. *Int J Biochem* **12**:713, 1980.
124. Young GP, Rose IS, St John DJ: Haem in the gut. I. Fate of haemoproteins and the absorption of haem. *J Gastroenterol Hepatol* **4**:537, 1989.
125. Conrad ME, Benjamin BI, Williams HL, Foy AL: Human absorption of hemoglobin-iron. *Gastroenterology* **53**:5, 1967.
126. Bothwell TH, Pirzio-Biroli G, Finch CA: Iron absorption. I. Factors influencing absorption. *J Lab Clin Med* **51**:24, 1958.
127. Pootrakul P, Kitcharoen K, Yansukon P, Wasi P, Fucharoen S, Charoenlarp P, Brittenham G, Pippard MJ, Finch CA: The effect of erythroid hyperplasia on iron balance. *Blood* **71**:1124, 1988.
128. Bothwell TH, Finch CA: *Iron Metabolism*. Boston, Little, Brown & Co, 1962.
129. Simon M, Alexandre JL, Rauchet R, Genetet B, Bourel M: The genetics of hemochromatosis. *Prog Med Genet* **4**:135, 1980.
130. Powell LW: Iron storage in relatives of patients with haemochromatosis and in relatives of patients with alcoholic cirrhosis and haemosiderosis: A comparative study of 27 families. *QJM* **34**:427, 1965.
131. Saddi R, Feingold J: Idiopathic haemochromatosis: An autosomal recessive disease. *Clinical Genetics* **5**:234, 1974.
132. Scheinberg IH: The genetics of hemochromatosis. *Arch Intern Med* **132**:126, 1973.
133. Simon M, Pawlotsky Y, Bourel M, Fauchet R, Genetet B: Hémochromatose idiopathique: Maladie associée à l'antigène tissulaire HL-A3? *Nouv Presse* **4**:1432, 1975.
134. Summers KM, Halliday JW, Powell LW: Identification of homozygous hemochromatosis subjects by measurement of hepatic iron index. *Hepatology* **12**:20, 1990.
135. Simon M, Bourel M, Genetet B, Fauchet R, Edan G, Brissot P: Idiopathic hemochromatosis and iron overload in alcoholic liver disease: Differentiation by HLA phenotypes. *Gastroenterology* **73**:655, 1977.
136. Lalouel JM, Le Mignon L, Simon M, Fauchet R, Bourel M, Rao DC, Morton NE: Genetic analysis of idiopathic hemochromatosis using both qualitative (disease status) and quantitative (serum iron) information. *Am J Hum Genet* **37**:300, 1985.
137. Beaumont CM, Simon M, Fauchet R, Hespel JP, Brissot P, Benetet B, Bourel M: Serum ferritin as a possible marker of the hemochromatosis allele. *N Engl J Med* **301**:169, 1979.
138. Yaouanq J, Perichon M, Chorney M, Pontarotti P, Le Treut A, El Kahloun A, Mauvieux V, Blayau M, Jouanolle AM, Chauvel B, Moirand R, Nouel O, Le Gall JY, Feingold J, David V: Anonymous marker loci within 400 kb of HLA-A generate haplotypes in linkage disequilibrium with the hemochromatosis gene (HFE). *Am J Hum Genet* **54**:252, 1994.
139. Jazwinska EC, Pyper WR, Burt MJ, Francis JL, Goldwurm S, Webb SI, Lee SC, Halliday JW, Powell LW: Haplotype analysis in Australian hemochromatosis patients: Evidence for a predominant ancestral haplotype exclusively associated with hemochromatosis. *Am J Hum Genet* **56**:428, 1995.
140. Raha-Chowdhury R, Bowen DJ, Stone C, Pointon JJ, Terwilliger JD, Shearman JD, Robson KJH, Bomford A, Worwood M: New polymorphic microsatellite markers place the haemochromatosis gene telomeric to D6S105. *Hum Mol Genet* **4**:1869, 1995.
141. Stone C, Pointon JJ, Jazwinska EC, Halliday JW, Powell LW, Robson KJH, Monaco AP, Weatherall DJ: Isolation of CA dinucleotide repeats close to D6S105 linkage disequilibrium with haemochromatosis. *Hum Mol Genet* **3**:2043, 1994.
142. Dugast IJ, Papadopoulos P, Zappone E, Jones C, Theriault K, Handelman GJ, Benavous R, Drysdale JW: Identification of two human H genes on the short arm of chromosome 6. *Genomics* **6**:204, 1990.
143. Worwood M, Raha-Chowdhury R, Dorak MT, Darke C, Bowen DJ, Burnett AK: Alleles at D6S265 and D6S105 define a haemochromatosis-specific genotype. *Br J Haematol* **86**:863, 1994.
144. Gandon G, Jouanolle AM, Chauvel B, Mauvieux V, Le Treut A, Feingold J, Yves Le Gall J, David V, Yaouanq J: Linkage disequilibrium and extended haplotypes in the HLA-A to D6S105 region: implications for mapping the hemochromatosis gene (HFE). *Hum Genet* **97**:103, 1996.
145. Kerem BT, Rommons JM, Buchanan JA, Markiewicz D, Cox TK, Chakravarti A, Buchwald M, Tsui LC: Identification of the cystic fibrosis gene: Genetic analysis. *Science* **245**:1073, 1989.
146. Hästbacka J, de la Chapelle A, Mahtani MM, Clines G, Reeve-Daly MP, Daly M, Hamilton BA, Kusumi K, Trivedi B, Weaver A, Coloma A, Lovett M, Buckler A, Kaitila I, Lander ES: The diastrophic dysplasia gene encodes a novel sulfate transporter: Positional cloning

by fine-structure linkage disequilibrium mapping. *Cell* **78**:1073, 1994.
147. Henz S, Reichen J, Liechti-Galliati S: HLA-H gene mutations and haemochromatosis. The likely association of H63D with mild phenotype and the detection of S65C, a novel variant in exon 2. *J Hepatol* **26(Suppl 1)**:57, 1997.
148. Beutler E, Felitti VJ, Ho NJ, Gelbart T: Commentary on *HFE* S65C variant is not associated with increased transferrin saturation in voluntary blood donors by Naveen Arya, Subrata Chakrabrati, Robert A. Hegele, Paul C. Adams. *Blood Cells Mol Dis* **25**:358, 1999.
149. Crawford DH, Halliday JW, Summers KM, Bourke MJ, Powell LW: Concordance of iron storage in siblings with genetic hemochromatosis: Evidence for a predominantly genetic effect on iron storage. *Hepatology* **17**:833, 1993.
150. Adams PC: Intrafamilial variation in hereditary hemochromatosis. *Dig Dis Sci* **37**:361, 1992.
151. Beutler E, Gelbart T, West C, Lee P, Adams M, Blackstone R, Pockros P, Kosty M, Venditti CP, Phatak PD, Seese NK, Chorney KA, Ten Elshof AE, Gerhard GS, Chorney M: Mutation analysis in hereditary hemochromatosis. *Blood Cells Mol Dis* **22**:187, 1996.
152. Tay GK, Leelayuwat C, Chorney MJ, Cattley SK, Hollingsworth PN, Witt CS, Daly LN, Hughes A, Dawkins RL: The MHC contains multiple genes potentially relevant to hemochromatosis. *Immunogenetics* **45**:336, 1997.
153. Carella M, D'Ambrosio L, Totaro A, Grifa A, Valentino MA, Piperno A, Girelli D, Roetto A, Franco B, Gasparini P, Camaschella C: Mutation analysis of the HLA-H gene in Italian hemochromatosis patients. *Am J Hum Genet* **60**:828, 1997.
154. Jouanolle AM, Gandon G, Jézéquel P, Blayan M, Campion ML, Yaonang J: Haemochromatosis and HFE. *Nat Genet* **14**:251, 1996.
155. Anonymous (The UK Haemochromatosis Consortium): A simple genetic test identifies 90 percent of UK patients with haemochromatosis. *Gut* **41**:841, 1997.
156. Adams PC, Campion ML, Gardon G, LeGall JY, David V, Jouanolle AM: Clinical and family studies in genetics of hemochromatosis: Microsatellite and HFE studies in five atypical families. *Hepatology* **26**:986, 1997.
157. Borot N, Roth MP, Malfroy L, Demangel C, Vinel JP, Pascal JP, Coppin H: Mutations in the MHC class I-like candidate gene for hemochromatosis in French patients. *Immunogenetics* **45**:320, 1997.
158. Garry PJ, Montoya GD, Baumgartner RN, Liang HC, Williams TM, Brodie SG: Impact of HLA-H mutations on iron stores in healthy elderly men and women. *Blood Cells Mol Dis* **23**:277, 1997.
159. Barton JC, Shih WWH, Sawada-Hirai R, Acton RT, Harmon L, Rivers C, Rothenberg BE: Genetic and clinical description of hemochromatosis probands and heterozygotes: Evidence that multiple genes linked to the major histocompatability complex are responsible for hemochromatosis. *Blood Cells Mol Dis* **23**:135, 1997.
160. Bradley LA, Johnson DD, Palomaki GE, Haddow JE, Robertson NH, Ferrie RM: Hereditary haemochromatosis mutation frequencies in the general population. *J Med Screen* **5**:34, 1998.
161. Willis G, Jennings BA, Goodman E, Fellows I, Wimperis JZ: A high prevalence of HLA-H 845A mutations in hemochromatosis patients and the normal population in Eastern England. *Blood Cells Mol Dis* **23**:288, 1997.
162. Mercier G, Bathelier C, Lucotte G: Frequency of the C282Y mutation of hemochromatosis in five French populations. *Blood Cells Mol Dis* **24**:165, 1998.
163. Jézéquel P, Bargain M, Lellouche F, Geffroy F, Dorval I: Allele frequencies of hereditary hemochromatosis gene mutations in a local population of west Brittany. *Hum Genet* **102**:332, 1998.
164. Mercier G, Bathelier C, Lucotte G: Frequency of the C282Y mutation of hemochromatosis in five French populations. *Blood Cells Mol Dis* **24**:165, 1998.
165. Gottschalk R, Seidl C, Löffler T, Seifried E, Helzer D, Kaltwasser JP: HFE codon 63/282 (H63D/C282Y) dimorphism in German patients with genetic hemochromatosis. *Tissue Antigens* **51**:270, 1998.
166. Bell H, Undlien D, Raha-Chowdhury R, Berg JP, Vartdal F, Raknerud N, Heier HE, Thomassen Y, Haug E, Thorsby E: Prevalence of the hemochromatosis Cys282Tyr mutation among patients with hemochromatosis and blood donors in Norway. *St Malo Symposium* 245, 1997.
167. Cardoso EM, Stal P, Hagen K, Cabeda JM, Esin S, de Sousa M, Hultcrantz R: HFE mutations in patients with hereditary haemochromatosis in Sweden. *J Intern Med* **243**:203, 1998.
168. Merryweather Clarke AT, Pointon JJ, Shearman JD, Robson KJH: Global prevalence of putative haemochromatosis mutations. *J Med Genet* **34**:275, 1997.
169. Cullen LM, Gao X, Easteal S, Jazwinska EC: The hemochromatosis 845 G $\rightarrow$ A and 187 C $\rightarrow$ G mutations: Prevalence in non-Caucasian populations. *Am J Hum Genet* **62**:1403, 1998.
170. Beckman LE, Saha N, Spitsyn V, Van Landeghem G, Beckman L: Ethnic differences in the HFE codon 282 (Cys/Tyr) polymorphism. *Hum Hered* **47**:263, 1997.
171. Beutler E, Gelbart T: HLA-H mutations in the Ashkenazi Jewish population. *Blood Cells Mol Dis* **23**:95, 1997.
172. Merryweather Clarke AT, Liu YT, Shearman JD, Pointon JJ, Robson KJ: A rapid non-invasive method for the detection of the haemochromatosis C282Y mutation. *Br J Haematol* **99**:460, 1997.
173. Roth M, Giraldo P, Hariti G, Poloni ES, Sanchez-Mazas A, Stefano GFD, Dugoujon JM, Coppin H: Absence of the hemochromatosis gene Cys282Tyr mutation in three ethnic groups from Algeria (Mzab), Ethiopia, and Senegal. *Immunogenetics* **46**:222, 1997.
174. Beckman LE, Saha N, Spitsyn V, VanLandeghem G, Beckman L: Ethnic differences in the HFE codon 282 (Cys/Tyr) polymorphism. *Hum Hered* **47**:263, 1997.
175. Barton JC, Edwards CQ, Bertoli LF, Shroyer TW, Hudson SL: Iron overload in African Americans. *Am J Med* **99**:616, 1995.
176. Beutler E, West C: New diallelic markers in the HLA region of chromosome 6. *Blood Cells Mol Dis* **23**:219, 1997.
177. Motulsky AG: Genetics of hemochromatosis. *N Engl J Med* **301**:1291, 1979.
178. Datz C, Haas T, Rinner H, Sandhofer F, Patsch W, Paulweber B: Heterozygosity for the C282Y mutation in the hemochromatosis gene is associated with increased serum iron, transferrin saturation, and hemoglobin in young women: A protective role against iron deficiency? *Clin Chem* **44**:2429, 1998.
179. Finch SC, Finch CA: Idiopathic hemochromatosis, an iron storage disease. A. Iron metabolism in hemochromatosis. *Medicine (Baltimore)* **34**:381, 1955.
180. Olynyk JK, Luxon BA, Britton RS, Bacon BR: Hepatic iron concentration in hereditary hemochromatosis does not saturate or accurately predict phlebotomy requirements. *Am J Gastroenterol* **93**:346, 1998.
181. Cook JD, Finch CA, Smith N: Evaluation of the iron status of a population. *Blood* **48**:449, 1976.
182. MacSween RNM, Scott AR: Hepatic cirrhosis: A clinicopathological review of 520 cases. *J Clin Pathol* **26**:936, 1972.
183. Lindmark B, Eriksson S: Regional differences in the idiopathic hemochromatosis gene frequency in Sweden. *Acta Med Scand* **218**:299, 1985.
184. Valberg LS, Sorbie J, Ludwig J, Pelletier O: Serum ferritin and the iron status of Canadians. *Can Med Assoc J* **114**:471, 1976.
185. Olsson KS, Ritter B, Rosen U, Heedman PA, Staugard F: Prevalence of iron overload in central Sweden. *Acta Med Scand* **213**:145, 1983.
186. Olsson KS, Ritter B, Lundin PM: Liver affection in iron overload studied with serum ferritin and serum aminotransferases. *Acta Med Scand* **217**:79, 1985.
187. Tanner AR, Desai S, Lu W, Wright R: Screening for haemochromatosis in the UK: Preliminary results. *Gut* **26**:1139, 1985.
188. Meyer T, Baynes R, Bothwell T, Jenkins T, Jooste P, Du Toit E, Martell R, Jacobs P: Phenotypic expression of the HLA linked iron-loading gene in males over the age of 40 years: A population study using serial serum ferritin estimations. *J Intern Med* **227**:397, 1990.
189. Meyer TE, Ballot D, Bothwell TH, Green A, Derman DP, Baynes RD, Jenkins T, Jooste PL, du TE, Jacobs PJ: The HLA linked iron loading gene in an Afrikaner population. *J Med Genet* **24**:348, 1987.
190. Jonsson JJ, Johannesson GM, Sigfusson N, Magnusson B, Thjodleifsson B, Magnusson S: Prevalence of iron deficiency and iron overload in the adult Icelandic population. *J Clin Epidemiol* **44**:1289, 1991.
191. Rous P, Oliver J: Experimental hemochromatosis. *J Exp Med* **28**:629, 1918.
192. Brighton CT, Bigley EJ, Smolenski BI: Iron-induced arthritis in immature rabbits. *Arthritis Rheum* **13**:849, 1970.
193. Awai M, Narasaki M, Yamanoi Y, Seno S: Induction of diabetes in animals by parenteral administration of ferric nitrilotriacetate. A model of experimental hemochromatosis. *Am J Pathol* **95**:663, 1979.
194. Bacon BR, Tavill AS, Brittenham GM, Park CH, Recknagel RO: Hepatic lipid peroxidation in vivo in rats with chronic iron overload. *J Clin Invest* **71**:429, 1983.
195. Iancu TC, Ward RJ, Peters TJ: Ultrastructural observations in the carbonyl iron-fed rat, an animal model for hemochromatosis. *Virchows Arch B Cell Pathol Incl Mol Pathol* **53**:208, 1987.
196. Park CH, Bacon BR, Brittenham GM, Tavill AS: Pathology of dietary carbonyl iron overload in rats. *Lab Invest* **57**:555, 1987.

197. Olynyk J, Hall P, Reed W, Williams P, Kerr R, Mackinnon M: A long-term study of the interaction between iron and alcohol in an animal model of iron overload. *J Hepatol* **22**:671, 1995.
198. Lavoie JP, Teuscher E: Massive iron overload and liver fibrosis resembling haemochromatosis in a racing pony. *Equine Vet J* **25**:552, 1993.
199. Pearson EG, Hedstrom OR, Poppenga RH: Hepatic cirrhosis and hemochromatosis in three horses. *J Am Vet Med Assoc* **204**:1053, 1994.
200. House JK, Smith BP, Maas J, Lane VM, Anderson BC, Graham TW, Pino MV: Hemochromatosis in Salers cattle. *J Vet Intern Med* **8**:105, 1994.
201. Gosselin SJ, Kramer LW: Pathophysiology of excessive iron storage in mynah birds. *J Am Vet Med Assoc* **183**:1238, 1983.
202. Randell MG, Patnaik AK, Gould WJ: Hepatopathy associated with excessive iron storage in mynah birds. *J Am Vet Med Assoc* **179**:1214, 1981.
203. Brayton C: Amyloidosis, hemochromatosis, and atherosclerosis in a roseate flamingo (Phoenicopterus ruber). *Ann N Y Acad Sci* **653**:184, 184, 1992.
204. Spalding MG, Kollias GV, Mays MB, Page CD, Brown MG: Hepatic encephalopathy associated with hemochromatosis in a Toco toucan. *J Am Vet Med Assoc* **189**:1122, 1986.
205. Cornelissen H, Ducatelle R, Roels S: Successful treatment of a channel-billed Toucan (*Ramphastos vitellinus*) with iron storage disease by chelation therapy: Sequential monitoring of the iron content of the liver during the treatment period by quantitative chemical and image analyses. *J Avian Med Surg* **9**:131, 1995.
206. Simpson RJ, Konijn AM, Lombard M, Raja KB, Salisbury JR, Peters TJ: Tissue iron loading and histopathological changes in hypotransferrinaemic mice. *J Pathol* **171**:237, 1993.
207. Raja KB, Simpson RJ, Peters TJ: Intestinal iron absorption studies in mouse models of iron-overload. *Br J Haematol* **86**:156, 1994.
208. Santos M, Clevers H, de Sousa M, Marx JJ: Adaptive response of iron absorption to anemia, increased erythropoiesis, iron deficiency, and iron loading in β_2-Microglobulin knockout mice. *Blood* **91**:3059, 1998.
209. Hashimoto K, Hirai M, Kurosawa Y: Identification of a mouse homolog for the human hereditary haemochromatosis candidate gene. *Biochem Biophys Res Commun* **230**:35, 1997.
210. Albig W, Drabent B, Burmester N, Bode C, Doenecke D: The haemochromatosis candidate gene HFE (HLA-H) of man and mouse is located in syntenic regions within the histone gene cluster. *J Cell Biochem* **69**:117, 1998.
211. Zhou XY, Tomatsu S, Fleming RE, Parkkila S, Waheed A, Jiang J, Fei Y, Brunt EM, Ruddy DA, Prass CE, Schatzman RC, O'Neill R, Britton RS, Bacon BR, Sly WS: HFE gene knockout produces mouse model of hereditary hemochromatosis. *Proc Natl Acad Sci U S A* **95**:2492, 1998.
212. Kaikov Y, Wadsworth LD, Hassall E, Dimmick JE, Rogers PCJ: Primary hemochromatosis in children: Report of three newly diagnosed cases and review of the pediatric literature. *Pediatrics* **90**:37, 1992.
213. Adams PC, Kertesz AE, Valberg LS: Screening for hemochromatosis in children of homozygotes: Prevalence and cost-effectiveness. *Hepatology* **22**:1720, 1995.
214. Moirand R, Adams PC, Bicheler V, Brissot P, Deugnier Y: Clinical features of genetic hemochromatosis in women compared with men. *Ann Intern Med* **127**:105, 1997.
215. Adams PC, Kertesz AE, Valberg LS: Clinical presentation of hemochromatosis: A changing scene. *Am J Med* **90**:445, 1991.
216. Walters GO, Jacobs A, Worwood M, Trevett D, Thomson W: Iron absorption in normal subjects and patients with idiopathic haemochromatosis: Relationship with serum ferritin concentration. *Gut* **16**:188, 1975.
217. McLaren GD, Nathanson MH, Jacobs A, Trevett D, Thomson W: Regulation of intestinal iron absorption and mucosal iron kinetics in hereditary hemochromatosis. *J Lab Clin Med* **117**:390, 1991.
218. Sargent T, Saito H, Winchell HS: Iron absorption in hemochromatosis before and after phlebotomy therapy. *J Nucl Med* **12**:660, 1971.
219. Poulos JE, Bacon BR: Liver transplantation for hereditary hemochromatosis. *Dig Dis* **14**:316, 1996.
220. Koskinas J, Portmann B, Lombard M, Smith T, Williams R: Persistent iron overload 4 years after inadvertent transplantation of a haemochromatotic liver in a patient with primary biliary cirrhosis. *J Hepatol* **16**:351, 1992.
221. Farrell FJ, Nguyen M, Woodley S, Imperial JC, Garcia-Kennedy R, Man K, Esquivel CO, Keeffe EB: Outcome of liver transplantation in patients with hemochromatosis. *Hepatology* **20**:404, 1994.
222. Valberg LS, Simon JB, Manley PN, Corbett WE, Ludwig J: Distribution of storage iron as body iron stores expand in patients with hemochromatosis. *J Lab Clin Med* **86**:479, 1975.
223. Cook JD, Barry WE, Hershko C, Fillet G, Finch CA: Iron kinetics with emphasis on iron overload. *Am J Pathol* **72**:337, 1973.
224. Fillet G, Beguin Y, Baldelli L: Model of reticuloendothelial iron metabolism in humans: Abnormal behavior in idiopathic hemochromatosis and in inflammation. *Blood* **74**:844, 1989.
225. Flanagan PR, Lam D, Banerjee D, Valberg LS: Ferritin release by mononuclear cells in hereditary hemochromatosis. *J Lab Clin Med* **113**:145, 1989.
226. Bassett ML, Halliday JW, Powell LW: Ferritin synthesis in peripheral blood monocytes in idiopathic hemochromatosis. *J Lab Clin Med* **100**:137, 1982.
227. Sizemore DJ, Bassett ML: Monocyte transferrin-iron uptake in hereditary hemochromatosis. *Am J Hematol* **16**:347, 1984.
228. Baynes RD, Bukofzer G, Bothwell TH, Meyer TE, Friedman BM, Macfarlane BJ, Lamparelli RD: Iron metabolism in normal and hemochromatotic macrophages. *Am J Hematol* **31**:21, 1989.
229. Beutler E, West C: Ferritin in cultured fibroblasts from patients with idiopathic hemochromatosis. *Haematologia (Budap)* **14**:147, 1981.
230. McLaren GD: Reticuloendothelial iron stores and hereditary hemochromatosis: A paradox. *J Lab Clin Med* **113**:137, 1989.
231. Ward JH, Kushner JP, Ray FA, Kaplan J: Transferrin receptor function in hereditary hemochromatosis. *J Lab Clin Med* **103**:246, 1984.
232. Banerjee D, Flanagan PR, Cluett J, Valberg LS: Transferrin receptors in the human gastrointestinal tract. Relationship to body iron stores. *Gastroenterology* **91**:861, 1986.
233. Sciot R, Paterson AC, Van den Oord JJ, Desmet VJ: Lack of hepatic transferrin receptor expression in hemochromatosis. *Hepatology* **7**:831, 1987.
234. Adams PC, Chau LA, White M, Lazarovits A: Expression of transferrin receptors on monocytes in hemochromatosis. *Am J Hematol* **37**:247, 1991.
235. Thorstensen K, Egeberg K, Romslo I, Dalhoj J, Wiggers P: Variations in serum erythropoietin and transferrin receptor during phlebotomy therapy of hereditary hemochromatosis: A case report. *Eur J Haematol* **47**:219, 1991.
236. Pietrangelo A, Rocchi E, Casalgrandi G, Rigo G, Ferrari A, Perini M, Ventura E, Cairo G: Regulation of transferrin, transferrin receptor, and ferritin genes in human duodenum. *Gastroenterology* **102**:802, 1992.
237. Ledue TB, Craig WY: Serum concentrations of transferrin receptor in hereditary hemochromatosis. *Clin Chem* **41**:1053, 1995.
238. Lombard M, Bomford AB, Polson RJ, Bellingham AJ, Williams R: Differential expression of transferrin receptor in duodenal mucosa in iron overload. Evidence for a site-specific defect in genetic hemochromatosis. *Gastroenterology* **98**:976, 1990.
239. Kaltwasser JP, Gottschalk R, Seidl CH: Severe juvenile haemochromatosis (JH) missing HFE gene variants: Implications for a second gene locus leading to iron overload. *Br J Haematol* **102**:1111, 1998.
240. Moura E, Noordermeer MA, Verhoeven N, Verheul AFM, Marx JJM: Iron release from human monocytes after erythrophagocytosis in vitro: An investigation in normal subjects and hereditary hemochromatosis patients. *Blood* **92**:2511, 1998.
241. Whittaker P, Skikne BS, Covell AM, Flowers C, Cooke A, Lynch SR, Cook JD: Duodenal iron proteins in idiopathic hemochromatosis. *J Clin Invest* **83**:261, 1989.
242. Powell LW, Campbell CB, Wilson E: Intestinal mucosal uptake of iron and iron retention in idiopathic haemochromatosis as evidence for a mucosal abnormality. *Gut* **11**:727, 1970.
243. Boender CA, Verloop MC: Iron absorption, iron loss and iron retention in man: Studies after oral administration of a tracer dose of $^{59}FeSO_4$ and $^{131}BaSO_4$. *Br J Haematol* **17**:45, 1969.
244. Marx JJ: Mucosal uptake, mucosal transfer and retention of iron, measured by whole-body counting. *Scand J Haematol* **23**:293, 1979.
245. Gerhard GS, Ten Elshof AE, Chorney MJ: Hereditary haemochromatosis as an immunological disease. *Br J Haematol* **100**:247, 1998.
246. Arosa F, da Silva AJ, Godinho IM, ter Steege, JC, Porto G, Rudd CE, de Sousa M: Decreased C8p561 ck activity in peripheral blood T-lymphocytes from patients with hereditary hemochromatosis. *Scand J Immunol* **39**:426, 1994.
247. Feder JN, Tsuchihashi Z, Irrinki A, Lee VK, Mapa FA, Morikang E, Prass CE, Starnes SM, Wolff RK, Parkkila S, Sly WS, Schatzman RC: The hemochromatosis founder mutation in HLA-H disrupts β_2-microglobulin interaction and cell surface expression. *J Biol Chem* **272**:14025, 1997.

248. Beutler E, West C, Gelbart T: HLA-H and associated proteins in patients with hemochromatosis. *Mol Med* **3**:397, 1997.
249. Hromec A, Payer J Jr, Killinger Z, Rybar I, Rovensky J: Congenital atransferrinemia. *Dtsch Med Wochenschr* **119**:663, 1994.
250. Hamill RL, Woods JC, Cook BA: Congenital atransferrinemia: A case report and review of the literature. *Am J Clin Pathol* **96**:215, 1991.
251. Turnbull A, Giblett ER: The binding and transport of iron by transferrin variants. *J Lab Clin Med* **57**:450, 1961.
252. Bothwell T, Jacobs P, Torrance JD: Studies on the behaviour of transferrin in idiopathic haemochromatosis. *S Afr J Med Sci* **27**:35, 1962.
253. Wheby MS, Balcerzak SP, Anderson P, Crosby WH: Brief report: Clearance of iron from hemochromatosis and normal transferrin in vivo. *Blood* **24**:765, 1964.
254. Powell LW, Alpert E, Isselbacher KJ, Drysdale JW: Abnormality in tissue isoferritin distribution in idiopathic haemochromatosis. *Nature* **250**:333, 1974.
255. Halliday JW, McKeering LV, Tweedale R, Powell LW: Serum ferritin in haemochromatosis: Changes in the isoferritin composition during venesection therapy. *Br J Haematol* **36**:395, 1977.
256. Mazur A, Sackler M: Haemochromatosis and hepatic xanthine oxidase. *Lancet* **1**:254, 1967.
257. Awai M, Brown EB: Examination of the role of xanthine oxidase in iron absorption by the rat. *J Lab Clin Med* **73**:366, 1969.
258. Kaplan J, O'Halloran TV: Iron metabolism in eukaryocytes: Mars and Venus at it again. *Science* **271**:1510, 1996.
259. Askwith C, Eide D, Van Ho A, Bernard PS, Li L, Davis-Kaplan S, Sipe DM, Kaplan J: The FET3 gene of *S. cerevisiae* encodes a multicopper oxidase required for ferrous iron uptake. *Cell* **76**:403, 1994.
260. Morita H, Inoue A, Yanagisawa N: A case of ceruloplasmin deficiency which showed dementia, ataxia and iron deposition in the brain. *Rinsho Shinkeigaku* **32**:483, 1992.
261. Okamoto N, Wada S, Oga T, Kawabata Y, Baba Y, Habu D, Takeda Z, Wada Y: Hereditary ceruloplasmin deficiency with hemosiderosis. *Hum Genet* **97**:755, 1996.
262. Borda F, Uribarrena R, Miranda MP: Hyperceruloplasminemia in hemochromatosis. *N Engl J Med* **304**:1047, 1981.
263. Nossner E, Parham P: Species-specific differences in chaperone interaction of human and mouse major histocompatibility complex class I molecules. *J Exp Med* **181**:327, 1995.
264. Ortmann B, Androlewicz MJ, Cresswell P: MHC class I/β_2-microglobulin complexes associate with TAP transporters before peptide binding. *Nature* **368**:864, 1994.
265. Cairo G, Recalcati S, Montosi G, Castrusini E, Conte D, Pietrangelo A: Inappropriately high iron regulatory protein activity in monocytes of patients with genetic hemochromatosis. *Blood* **89**:2546, 1997.
266. Flanagan PR, Hajdu A, Adams PC: Iron-responsive element-binding protein in hemochromatosis liver and intestine. *Hepatology* **22**:828, 1995.
267. Mumford AD, Vulliamy T, Lindsay J, Watson A: Hereditary hyperferritinemia-cataract syndrome: Two novel mutations in the L-ferritin iron-responsive element. *Blood* **91**:367, 1998.
268. Arnold JD, Mumford AD, Lindsay JO, Hegde U, Hagan M, Hawkins JR: Hyperferritinaemia in the absence of iron overload. *Gut* **41**:408, 1997.
269. Cazzola M, Bergamaschi G, Tonon L, Arbustini E, Grasso M, Vercesi E, Barosi G, Bianchi PE, Cairo G, Arosio P: Hereditary hyperferritinemia-cataract syndrome: Relationship between phenotypes and specific mutations in the iron-responsive element of ferritin light-chain mRNA. *Blood* **90**:814, 1997.
270. Girelli D, Corrocher R, Bisceglia L, Olivieri O, De Franceschi L, Zelante L, Gasparini P: Molecular basis for the recently described hereditary hyperferritinemia-cataract syndrome: A mutation in the iron-responsive element of ferritin L-subunit gene (the "Verona mutation"). *Blood* **86**:4050, 1995.
271. Aguilar-Martinez P, Biron C, Masmejean C, Jeanjean P, Schved JF: A novel mutation in the iron responsive element of ferritin L-subunit gene as a cause for hereditary hyperferritinemia-cataract syndrome. *Blood* **88**:1895, 1996.
272. Bothwell TH, Derman D, Bezwoda WR, Torrance JD, Charlton RW: Can iron fortification of flour cause damage to genetic susceptibles (idiopathic haemochromatosis and beta-thalassaemia major)? *Hum Genet* **1(Suppl)**:131, 1978.
273. Gordeuk VR, Boyd RD, Brittenham GM: Dietary iron overload persists in rural sub-Saharan Africa. *Lancet* **1**:1310, 1986.
274. Bothwell T, Seftel HC, Jacobs A, Torrance JD, Baumslag N: Iron overload in Bantu subjects. Studies on the availability of iron in Bantu beer. *Am J Clin Nutr* **14**:47, 1998.
275. Derman DP, Bothwell TH, Torrance JD, Bezwoda WR, MacPhail AP, Kew MC, Sayers MH, Disler PB, Charlton RW: Iron absorption from maize (*Zea mays*) and sorghum (*Sorghum vulgare*) beer. *Br J Nutr* **43**:271, 1980.
276. Bezwoda WR, Torrance JD, Bothwell TH, MacPhail AP, Graham B, Mills W: Iron absorption from red and white wines. *Scand J Haematol* **34**:121, 1985.
277. Lundvall O, Weinfeld A, Lundin P: Iron stores in alcohol abusers. I. Liver iron. *Acta Med Scand* **185**:259, 1969.
278. Jakobovits AW, Morgan MY, Sherlock S: Hepatic siderosis in alcoholics. *Dig Dis Sci* **24**:305, 1979.
279. Chapman RW, Morgan MY, Bell R, Sherlock S: Hepatic iron uptake in alcoholic liver disease. *Gastroenterology* **84**:143, 1983.
280. Celada A, Rudolf H, Donath A: Effect of experimental chronic alcohol ingestion and folic acid deficiency on iron absorption. *Blood* **54**:906, 1979.
281. Celada A, Rudolf H, Donath A: Effect of a single ingestion of alcohol on iron absorption. *Am J Hematol* **5**:225, 1978.
282. Callender ST, Malpas JS: Absorption of iron in cirrhosis of liver. *BMJ* **2**:1516, 1963.
283. Plumb V, Ho KJ, Mihas AA: Hemochromatosis associated with side-to-side portacaval shunt. *South Med J* **70**:1369, 1977.
284. Lombard CM, Strauchen JA: Postshunt hemochromatosis with cardiomyopathy. *Hum Pathol* **12**:1149, 1981.
285. Adams PC, Bradley C, Frei JV: Hepatic iron and zinc concentrations after portacaval shunting for nonalcoholic cirrhosis. *Hepatology* **19**:101, 1994.
286. Friedman BI, Schaefer JW, Schiff L: Increased iron-59 absorption in patients with hepatic cirrhosis. *J Nucl Med* **7**:594, 1966.
287. Irving MG, Halliday JW, Powell LW: Association between alcoholism and increased hepatic iron stores. *Alcohol Clin Exp Res* **12**:7, 1988.
288. LeSage GD, Baldus WP, Fairbanks VF, Baggenstoss AH, McCall JT, Moore SB, Taswell HF, Gordon H: Hemochromatosis: Genetic or alcohol-induced? *Gastroenterology* **84**:1471, 1983.
289. Milder MS, Cook JD, Stray S, Finch CA: Idiopathic hemochromatosis, an interim report. *Medicine (Baltimore)* **59**:34, 1980.
290. Grove J, Daly AK, Burt AD, Guzail M, James OFW, Bassendine MF, Day CP: Heterozygotes for HFE mutations have no increased risk of advanced alcoholic liver disease. *Gut* **43**:262, 1998.
291. Niederau C, Fischer R, Purschel A, Stremmel W, Haussinger D, Strohmeyer G: Long-term survival in patients with hereditary hemochromatosis. *Gastroenterology* **110**:1107, 1996.
292. Adams PC, Valberg LS: Evolving expression of hereditary hemochromatosis. *Semin Liver Dis* **16**:47, 1996.
293. Niederau C, Strohmeyer G, Stremmel W: Epidemiology, clinical spectrum and prognosis of hemochromatosis. *Adv Exp Biol Med* **356**:303, 1994.
294. Didelot JM, Epeirier JM, Martinez PA, Morel P, Blanc P, Larrey D, Michel H: First clinical manifestations of hereditary hemochromatosis: About 498 patients. *St Malo Symposium* 1997.
295. Chevrant-Breton J, Simon M, Bourel M, Ferrand B: Cutaneous manifestations of idiopathic hemochromatosis. *Arch Dermatol* **113**:161, 1977.
296. Witte DL, Crosby WH, Edwards CQ, Fairbanks VF, Mitros FA: Hereditary hemochromatosis. *Clin Chim Acta* **245**:139, 1996.
297. Bassett ML, Halliday JW, Powell LW: Genetic hemochromatosis. *Semin Liver Dis* **4**:217, 1984.
298. Iancu TC, Deugnier Y, Halliday JW, Powell LW, Brissot P: Ultrastructural sequences during iron overload in genetic hemochromatosis. *J Hepatol* **27**:628, 1997.
299. Zhao M, Laissue JA, Zimmermann A: Hepatocyte apoptosis in hepatic iron overload diseases. *Histol Histopathol* **12**:367, 1997.
300. Ramm GA, Crawford DH, Powell LW, Walker NI, Fletcher LM, Halliday JW: Hepatic stellate cell activation in genetic hemochromatosis: Lobular distribution, effect of increasing hepatic iron and response to phlebotomy. *J Hepatol* **26**:584, 1997.
301. Powell LW, Kerr JFR: The pathology of the liver in hemochromatosis, in Ioachim HL (ed): *Pathobiology Annual*. New York, Appleton-Century-Crofts, 1975, p 317.
302. Finch SC, Finch CA: Idiopathic hemochromatosis, an iron storage disease. A. Iron metabolism in hemochromatosis. *Medicine (Baltimore)* **34**:381, 1955.
303. Stremmel W, Niederau C, Berger M, Kley HK, Kruskemper HL, Strohmeyer G: Abnormalities in estrogen, androgen, and insulin metabolism in idiopathic hemochromatosis. *Ann N Y Acad Sci* **526**:209, 1988.

304. Adams PC, Agnew S: Alcoholism in hereditary hemochromatosis revisited: Prevalence and clinical consequences among homozygous siblings. *Hepatology* **23**:724, 1996.
305. Niederau C, Fischer R, Sonnenberg A, Stremmel W, Trampisch HJ, Strohmeyer G: Survival and causes of death in cirrhotic and in noncirrhotic patients with primary hemochromatosis. *N Engl J Med* **313**:1256, 1985.
306. Bradbear RA, Bain C, Siskind V, Schofield FD, Webb S, Axelsen EM, Halliday JW, Bassett ML, Powell LW: Cohort study of internal malignancy in genetic hemochromatosis and other chronic nonalcoholic liver diseases. *J Natl Cancer Inst* **75**:81, 1985.
307. Hsing AW, McLaughlin JK, Olsen JH, Mellemkjar L, Wacholder S, Fraumeni JF Jr: Cancer risk following primary hemochromatosis: A population-based cohort study in Denmark. *Int J Cancer* **60**:160, 1995.
308. Fellows IW, Stewart M, Jeffcoate WJ, Smith PG, Toghill PJ: Hepatocellular carcinoma in primary haemochromatosis in the absence of cirrhosis. *Gut* **29**:1603, 1988.
309. Brink B, Disler P, Lynch S, Jacobs P, Charlton R, Bothwell TH: Patterns of iron storage in dietary iron overload and idiopathic hemochromatosis. *J Lab Clin Med* **88**:725, 1977.
310. Charlton RW, Hawkins DM, Mavor MO, Bothwell TH: Hepatic storage iron concentrations in different population groups. *Am J Clin Nutr* **23**:358, 1970.
311. Rahier J, Loozen S, Goebbels RM, Abrahem M: The haemochromatotic pancreas: A quantitative immunohistochemical and ultrastructural study. *Diabetologia* **30**:5, 1987.
312. Buysschaert M, Paris I, Selvais P, Hermans MP: Clinical aspects of diabetes secondary to idiopathic haemochromatosis in French-speaking Belgium. *Diabetes Metab* **23**:308, 1997.
313. Hramiak IM, Finegood DT, Adams PC: Factors affecting glucose tolerance in hereditary hemochromatosis. *Clin Invest Med* **20**:110, 1997.
314. Dymock IW, Cassar J, Pyke DA, Oakley WG, Williams R: Observations on the pathogenesis, complications and treatment of diabetes in 115 cases of haemochromatosis. *Am J Med* **52**:203, 1972.
315. Kley HK, Niederau C, Stremmel W, Lax R, Strohmeyer G, Kruskemper HL: Conversion of androgens to estrogens in idiopathic hemochromatosis: Comparison with alcoholic liver cirrhosis. *J Clin Endocrinol Metab* **61**:1, 1985.
316. Bezwoda WR, Bothwell TH, Van Der Walt LA, Kronhein S, Pimstone BL: An investigation into gonadal dysfunction in patients with idiopathic hemochromatosis. *Clin Endocrinol* **6**:377, 1977.
317. Lufkin EG, Baldus WP, Bergstrahl EJ, Kao PC: Influence of phlebotomy treatment on abnormal hypothalamic-pituitary function in genetic hemochromatosis. *Mayo Clin Proc* **62**:473, 1987.
318. Siminoski K, D'Costa M, Walfish PG: Hypogonadotrophic hypogonadism in idiopathic hemochromatosis: Evidence for combined hypothalamic and pituitary involvement. *J Endocrinol Invest* **13**:849, 1990.
319. Meyer T, Baynes R, Bothwell T, Jenkins T, Jooste P, du Toit E, Jacobs P: Phenotypic expression of the HLA linked iron-loading gene in males over the age of 40 years: A population study using serial ferritin estimations. *J Intern Med* **227**:397, 1990.
320. Cutler DJ, Isner JM, Bracey AW, Hufnagel CA, Conrad PW, Roberts WC, Kerwin DM, Weintraub AM: Hemochromatosis heart disease: An unemphasized cause of potentially reversible restrictive cardiomyopathy. *Am J Med* **69**:923, 1980.
321. Cecchetti G, Binda A, Piperno A, Nador F, Fargion S, Fiorelli G: Cardiac alterations in 36 consecutive patients with idiopathic haemochromatosis: Polygraphic and echocardiographic evaluation. *Eur Heart J* **12**:224, 1991.
322. Olson LJ, Baldus WD, Tajik AJ: Echocardiographic features of idiopathic hemochromatosis. *Am J Cardiol* **60**:885, 1987.
323. Dabestani A, Child JS, Perloff JK, Figueroa WG, Schelbert HR, Engel TR: Cardiac abnormalities in primary hemochromatosis. *Ann N Y Acad Sci* **526**:234, 1988.
324. Buja LM, Roberts WC: Iron in the heart: Etiology and clinical significance. *Am J Med* **51**:209, 1971.
325. Olson LJ, Edwards WD, Holmes DR J: Endomyocardial biopsy in hemochromatosis: Clinicopathologic correlates in six cases. *J Am Coll Cardiol* **13**:116, 1989.
326. Schumacher HR: Hemochromatosis and arthritis. *Arthritis Rheum* **7**:41, 1964.
327. Mathews JL, Williams HJ: Arthritis in hereditary hemochromatosis. *Arthritis Rheum* **30**:1137, 1987.
328. Sinigaglia L, Fargion S, Fracanzani AL, Binelli L, Battafarano N, Varenna M, Piperno A, Fiorelli G: Bone and joint involvement in genetic hemochromatosis: Role of cirrhosis and iron overload. *J Rheumatol* **24**:1809, 1997.
329. Schumacher HR, Straka PC, Krikker MA, Dudley AT: The arthropathy of hemochromatosis: Recent studies. *Ann N Y Acad Sci* **526**:224, 1988.
330. Montgomery KD, Williams JR, Sculco TP, DiCarlo E: Clinical and pathologic findings in hemochromatosis hip arthropathy. *Clin Orthop* **347**:179, 1998.
331. Adams PC, Speechley M: The effect of arthritis on the quality of life in hereditary hemochromatosis. *J Rheumatol* **23**:707, 1996.
332. de Jonge-Bok JM, Macfarlane JD: The articular diversity of early haemochromatosis. *J Bone Joint Surg Br* **69**:41, 1987.
333. Adamson TC, Resnik CS, Guerra J, Vint VC, Weisman MH, Resnick D: Hand and wrist arthropathies of hemochromatosis and calcium pyrophosphate deposition disease: Distinct radiographic features. *Radiology* **147**:377, 1983.
334. Abbott DF, Gresham GA: Arthropathy in transfusional siderosis. *BMJ* **1**:418, 1972.
335. Schumacher HR: Articular cartilage in the degenerative arthropathy of hemochromatosis. *Arthritis Rheum* **25**:1460, 1982.
336. Diamond T, Stiel D, Posen S: Osteoporosis in hemochromatosis: Iron excess, gonadal deficiency, or other factors? *Ann Intern Med* **110**:430, 1989.
337. Seftel HC, Malkin C, Schaman A, Abrahams C, Lynch SR, Charlton RW, Bothwell TH: Osteoporosis, scurvy and siderosis in Johannesburg Bantu. *BMJ* **1**:642, 1966.
338. Lynch SR, Berelowitz I, Seftel HC, Miller GB, Krawitz P, Charlton RW, Bothwell TH: Osteoporosis in Johannesburg Bantu males: Its relationship to siderosis and ascorbic acid deficiency. *Am J Clin Nutr* **20**:799, 1967.
339. Solomon L, Beighton P: Rheumatic disorders in the South African Negro: Part III: Idiopathic necrosis of the femoral head. *S Afr Med J* **49**:1825, 1975.
340. MacSween RNM: Acute abdominal crises, circulatory collapse and sudden death in haemochromatosis. *QJM* **35**:589, 1966.
341. Robins-Brown RM, Rabson AR, Koornhof HJ: Generalized infection with Yersinia enterocolitica and the role of iron. *Contrib Microbiol Immunol* **5**:277, 1979.
342. Olesen LL, Ejlertsen T, Paulsen SM, Knudsen PR: Liver abscesses due to *Yersinia enterocolitica* in patients with haemochromatosis. *J Intern Med* **225**:351, 1989.
343. Conway SP, Dudley N, Sheridan P, Ross H: Haemochromatosis and aldosterone deficiency presenting with *Yersinia pseudotuberculosis* septicaemia. *Postgrad Med J* **65**:174, 1989.
344. Cover TL, Aber RC: *Yersinia enterocolitica. N Engl J Med* **321**:16, 1989.
345. Muench KH: Hemochromatosis and infection: Alcohol and iron, oysters and sepsis. *Am J Med* **87**:40N, 1989.
346. Manso C, Rivas I, Peraire J, Vidal F, Richart C: Fatal Listeria meningitis, endocarditis and pericarditis in a patient with haemochromatosis. *Scand J Infect Dis* **29**:308, 1997.
347. McNab AA, McKelvie P: Iron overload is a risk factor for zygomycosis. *Arch Ophthalmol* **115**:919, 1997.
348. de Sousa M: Immune cell functions in iron overload. *Clin Exp Immunol* **75**:1, 1989.
349. Bryan CF, Leech SH, Kumar P, Gaumer R, Bozelka B, Morgan J: The immune system in hereditary hemochromatosis: A quantitative and functional assessment of the cellular arm. *Am J Med Sci* **301**:55, 1991.
350. Moura E, Verheul AF, Marx JJ: Evaluation of the role of Fc gamma and complement receptors in the decreased phagocytosis of hereditary hemochromatosis patients. *Scand J Immunol* **46**:339, 1997.
351. McCord JM: Iron, free radicals, and oxidative injury. *Semin Hematol* **35**:5, 1998.
352. Gutteridge JM: Iron and oxygen: A biologically damaging mixture. *Acta Paediatr Scand* **361(Suppl)**:78, 1989.
353. O'Connell MJ, Ward RJ, Baum H, Peters TJ: The role of iron in ferritin- and haemosiderin-mediated lipid peroxidation in liposomes. *Biochem J* **229**:135, 1985.
354. Houglum K, Filip M, Witztum JL, Chojkier M: Malondialdehyde and 4-hydroxynonenal protein adducts in plasma and liver of rats with iron overload. *J Clin Invest* **86**:1991, 1990.
355. Sharma BK, Bacon BR, Britton RS, Park CH, Magiera CJ, O'Neill R, Dalton N, Smanik P, Speroff T: Prevention of hepatocyte injury and lipid peroxidation by iron chelators and alpha-tocopherol in isolated iron-loaded rat hepatocytes. *Hepatology* **12**:31, 1990.
356. Pietrangelo A, Gualdi R, Casalgrandi G, Montosi G, Ventura E: Molecular and cellular aspects of iron-induced hepatic cirrhosis in rodents. *J Clin Invest* **95**:1824, 1995.

357. Bacon BR, Britton RS: Hepatic injury in chronic iron overload. Role of lipid peroxidation. *Chem Biol Interact* **70**:183, 1989.
358. Stal P, Glaumann H, Hultcrantz R: Liver cell damage and lysosomal iron storage in patients with idiopathic hemochromatosis. A light and electron microscopic study. *J Hepatol* **11**:172, 1990.
359. Bacon BR, Park CH, Brittenham GM, O'Neill R, Tavill AS: Hepatic mitochondrial oxidative metabolism in rats with chronic dietary iron overload. *Hepatology* **5**:789, 1985.
360. Britton RS: Metal-induced hepatotoxicity. *Semin Liver Dis* **16**:3, 1996.
361. Nordmann R, Ribiere C, Rouach H: Involvement of iron and iron-catalyzed free radical production in ethanol metabolism and toxicity. *Enzyme* **37**:57, 1987.
362. Brown KE, Poulos JE, Li L, Soweid AM, Ramm GA, O'Neill R, Britton RS, Bacon BR: Effect of vitamin E supplementation on hepatic fibrogenesis in chronic dietary iron overload. Am *J Physiol* **272**:G116, 1997.
363. Hunt J, Richards RJ, Harwood R, Jacobs A: The effect of desferrioxamine on fibroblasts and collagen formation in cell cultures. *Br J Haematol* **41**:69, 1979.
364. Rojkind M, Dunn MA: Hepatic fibrosis. *Gastroenterology* **76**:849, 1979.
365. Weintraub LR, Goral A, Grasso J, Franzblau C, Sullivan A, Sullivan S: Pathogenesis of hepatic fibrosis in experimental iron overload. *Br J Haematol* **59**:321, 1985.
366. Lynch SR, Seftel HC, Torrance JD, Charlton RW, Bothwell TH: Accelerated oxidative catabolism of ascorbic acid in siderotic Bantu. *Am J Clin Nutr* **20**:641, 1967.
367. Hankes LV, Jansen CR, Schmaeler M: Ascorbic acid catabolism in Bantu with hemosiderosis (scurvy). *Biochem Med* **9**:244, 1974.
368. Edwards CQ, Griffen LM, Goldgar D, Drummond C, Skolnick MH, Kushner JP: Prevalence of hemochromatosis among 11065 presumably healthy blood donors. *N Engl J Med* **318**:1355, 1988.
369. Olsson KS, Eriksson K, Ritter B, Heedman PA: Screening for iron overload using transferrin saturation. *Acta Med Scand* **215**:105, 1984.
370. Bacon BR, Sadiq SA: Hereditary hemochromatosis: presentation and diagnosis in the 1990s. *Am J Gastroenterol* **92**:784, 1997.
371. Powell LW, Summers KM, Board PG, Axelsen E, Webb S, Halliday JW: Expression of hemochromatosis in homozygous subjects: Implications for early diagnosis and prevention. *Gastroenterology* **98**:1625, 1990.
372. Powell LW: Hemochromatosis: The impact of early diagnosis and therapy. *Gastroenterology* **110**:1304, 1996.
373. Adams PC, Chakrabarti S: Genotypic/phenotypic correlations in genetic hemochromatosis: Evolution of diagnostic criteria. *Gastroenterology* **114**:319, 1998.
374. McLaren CE, McLachlan GJ, Halliday JW, Webb SI, Leggett BA, Jazwinska EC, Crawford DG, Gordeuk VR, McLaren GD, Powell LW: Distribution of transferrin saturation in an Australian population: Relevance to the early diagnosis of hemochromatosis. *Gastroenterology* **114**:543, 1998.
375. Edwards CQ, Griffen LM, Kaplan J, Kushner JP: Twenty-four hour variation of transferrin saturation in treated and untreated haemochromatosis homozygotes. *J Intern Med* **226**:373, 1989.
376. Cartwright GE, Edwards CQ, Kravitz K, Skolnick M, Amos DB, Johnson A, Buskjaer L: Hereditary hemochromatosis: Phenotypic expression of the disease. *N Engl J Med* **301**:175, 1979.
377. Bassett ML, Halliday JW, Powell LW: Value of hepatic iron measurements in early hemochromatosis and determination of the critical iron level associated with fibrosis. *Hepatology* **8**:24, 1988.
378. Wiggers P, Dalhoj J, Kiaer H, Ring-Larsen H, Hyltoft Petersen P, Blaabjerg O, Horder M: Screening for hemochromatosis: Prevalence among Danish blood donors. *J Intern Med* **51**:143, 1991.
379. Guyader D, Gandon Y, Deugnier Y, Jouanolle H, Loreal O, Simon M, Bourel M, Carsin M, Brissot P: Evaluation of computed tomography in the assessment of liver iron overload. *Gastroenterology* **97**:737, 1989.
380. Chezmar JL, Nelson RC, Malko JA, Bernadino ME: Hepatic iron overload: Diagnosis and quantification by noninvasive imaging. *Gastrointest Radiol* **15**:27, 1990.
381. Siegelman ES, Mitchell DG, Rubin R, Hann HWL, Kaplan KR, Steiner RM, Rao VM, Schuster SJ, Burk DL, Rifkin MD: Parenchymal versus reticuloendothelial iron overload in the liver: Distinction with MR imaging. *Radiology* **179**:361, 1991.
382. Kaltwasser JP, Gottschalk R, Schalk KP, Hartl W: Non-invasive quantitation of iron-overload by magnetic resonance imaging. *Br J Haematol* **74**:360, 1990.
383. Brittenham GM, Farrell DE, Harris JW, Feldman ES, Danish EH, Muir WA, Tripp JH, Bellon EM: Magnetic-susceptibility measurement of human iron stores. *N Engl J Med* **3307**:1671, 1982.
384. Wielopolski L, Ancona RC, Mossey RT, Vaswani AN, Cohn SH: Nuclear resonance scattering measurement of human iron stores. *Med Phys* **12**:401, 1985.
385. Peters TJ, Duane P, Raja K: Use of liver volume determination in the assessment of iron overload in patients with haemochromatosis. *Eur J Gastroenterol Hepatol* **3**:137, 1991.
386. Felitti VJ, Beutler E: New developments in hemochromatosis. *Am J Med Sci* **318**:257, 1999.
387. Bothwell TH, Abrahams C, Bradlow BA, Charlton RW: Idiopathic and Bantu hemochromatosis: A comparative histological study. *Arch Pathol* **79**:163, 1965.
388. Edwards CQ, Griffen LM, Kushner JP: Comparison of stainable liver iron between symptomatic and asymptomatic hemochromatosis homozygotes and their homozygous relatives. *Am J Med Sci* **301**:44, 1991.
389. Torrance JD, Bothwell TH: Tissue iron stores, in Cook JD (ed): *Methods in Hematology*. New York, Churchill Livingstone, 1980, p 90.
390. Barry M, Sherlock S: Measurement of liver-iron concentration in needle biopsy specimens. *Lancet* **1**:100, 1971.
391. George PM, Conaghan C, Angus HB, Walmsley TA, Chapman BA: Comparison of histological and biochemical hepatic iron indexes in the diagnosis of genetic hemochromatosis. *J Clin Pathol* **49**:159, 1996.
392. Bassett M, Halliday JW, Powell LW: Value of hepatic iron measurements in early hemochromatosis and determination of the critical iron level associated with fibrosis. *Hepatology* **6**:24, 1986.
393. Sallie RW, Reed WD, Shilkin KB: Confirmation of the efficacy of hepatic tissue iron index in differentiating genetic haemochromatosis from alcoholic liver disease complicated by alcoholic haemosiderosis. *Gut* **32**:207, 1991.
394. Bartolo C, McAndrew PE, Sosolik RC, Cawley KA, Balcerzak SP, Brandt JT, Prior TW: Differential diagnosis of hereditary hemochromatosis from other liver disorders by genetic analysis: Gene mutation analysis of patients previously diagnosed with hemochromatosis by liver biopsy. *Arch Pathol Lab Med* **122**:633, 1998.
395. Moirand R, Mortaji AM, Loreal O, Palliard F, Brissot P, Deugnier Y: A new syndrome of liver iron overload with normal transferrin saturation. *Lancet* **349**:95, 1997.
396. Chapman RW, Morgan MY, Laulicht M, Hoffbrand AV, Sherlock S: Hepatic iron stores and markers of iron overload in alcoholics and patients with idiopathic hemochromatosis. *Dig Dis Sci* **27**:909, 1982.
397. Kowdley KV, Trainer TD, Saltzman JR, Pedrosa M, Krawitt EL, Knox TA, Susskind E, Pratt D, Bonkovsky HL, Grace ND, Kaplan MM: Utility of hepatic iron index in American patients with hereditary hemochromatosis: A multicenter study. *Gastroenterology* **113**:1270, 1997.
398. Adams PC, Bradley C, Henderson AR: Evaluation of the hepatic iron index as a diagnostic criterion for genetic hemochromatosis. *J Lab Clin Med* **130**:509, 1997.
399. Ludwig J, Hashimoto E, Porayko MK, Moyer TP, Baldus WP: Hemosiderosis in cirrhosis: a study of 447 native livers. *Gastroenterology* **112**:882, 1997.
400. Deugnier Y, Turlin B, le Quilleuc D, Moirand R, Loreal O, Messner M, Meunier B, Brissot P, Launoie B: A reappraisal of hepatic siderosis in patients with end-stage cirrhosis: Practical implications for the diagnosis of hemochromatosis. *Am J Clin Path* **21**:669, 1997.
401. David V, Paul P, Simon M, Le Gall JY, Fauchet R, Gicquel I, Dugast IJ, Le Mignon L, Yaouanq J, Cohen D, Bourel M: DNA polymorphism related to the idiopathic hemochromatosis gene: Evidence in a recombinant family. *Hum Genet* **74**:113, 1986.
402. Lord DK, Dunham I, Campbell RD, Bomford A, Strachan T, Cox TM: Molecular analysis of the human MHC Class I region in hereditary haemochromatosis. *Hum Genet* **85**:531, 1990.
403. Youanq J, El Kahloun A, Chorney M, Jouanolle AM, Mauvieux V, Perichon M, Blayau M, Pontarotti P, Le Gall JY, David V: Familial screening for genetic haemochromatosis by means of DNA markers. *J Med Genet* **29**:320, 1992.
404. Sheldon JH: *Haemochromatosis*. London, Oxford University Press, 1935.
405. Powell LW, Jazwinska EC, Halliday JW: Primary iron overload, in Brock JH, Halliday JW, Pippard MJ, Powell LW (eds): *Iron Metabolism in Health and Disease*. London, Saunders, 1994, p 227.
406. Burke W, Thomson E, Khoury MJ, McDonnell SM, Press N, Adams PC, Barton JC, Beutler E, Brittenham G, Buchanan A, Clayton EW, Cogswell ME, Meslin EM, Motulsky AG, Powell LW, Sigal E, Wilfond BS, Collins FS: Hereditary hemochromatosis — Gene discovery and its implications for population-based screening. *JAMA* **280**:172, 1998.

407. Smith BC, Gorve J, Guzail MA, Day CP, Daly AK, Burt AD, Bassendine MF: Heterozygosity for hereditary hemochromatosis is associated with more fibrosis in chronic hepatitis C. *Hepatology* **27**:1695, 1998.
408. Santos M, Clevers HC, Marx JJ: Mutations of the hereditary hemochromatosis candidate gene HLA-H in porphyria cutanea tarda. *N Engl J Med* **336**:1327, 1997.
409. Roberts AG, Whatley SD, Morgan R, Worwood M, Elder GH, Morgan RR: Increased frequency of the haemochromatosis Cys282Tyr mutation in sporadic porphyria cutanea tarda. *Lancet* **349**:321, 1997.
410. Bonkovsky HL, Poh-Fitzpatrick M, Pimstone N, Obando J, Di Bisceglie AM, Tattrie C, Tortorelli K, LeClair P, Mercurio MG, Lambrecht RW: Porphyria cutanea tarda, hepatitis C, and HFE gene mutations in North America. *Hepatology* **27**:1661, 1998.
411. Sampietro M, Piperno A, Lupica L, Arosio C, Vergani A, Corbetta N, Malosio I, Mattioli M, Fracanzani AL, Cappellini MD, Fiorelli G, Fargion S: High prevalence of the His63Asp HFE mutation in Italian patients with porphyria cutanea tarda. *Hepatology* **27**:181, 1998.
412. George KD, Goldwurm S, MacDonald GA, Cowley LL, Walker NI, Ward PJ, Jazwinska EC, Powell LW: Increased hepatic iron concentration in nonalcoholic steatohepatitis is associated with increased fibrosis. *Gastroenterology* **114**:311, 1998.
413. Yaouanq J, Grosbois B, Jouanolle AM, Goasguen J, Leblay R: Haemochromatosis Cys282Tyr mutation in pyridoxine-responsive sideroblastic anaemia. *Lancet* **349**:1475, 1997.
414. Barry M, Scheuer PJ, Sherlock S, Ross CF, Williams R: Hereditary spherocytosis with secondary haemochromatosis. *Lancet* **2**:481, 1968.
415. Edwards CQ, Skolnick MH, Dadone MM, Kushner JP: Iron overload in hereditary spherocytosis: Association with HLA-linked hemochromatosis. *Am J Hematol* **13**:101, 1982.
416. Salem HH, Van der Weyden MB, Firken BG: Iron overload in congenital erythrocyte pyruvate kinase deficiency. *Med J Aust* **1**:531, 1980.
417. Camaschella C, Roetto A, Cicilano M, Pasquero P, Bosio S, Gubetta L, Di Vito F, Girelli D, Totaro A, Carella M, Grifa A, Gasparini P: Juvenile and adult hemochromatosis are distinct genetic disorders. *Eur J Hum Genet* **5**:371, 1997.
418. Schafer AI, Cheron RG, Dluhy R, Cooper B, Gleason RE, Soeldner JS, Bunn HF: Clinical consequences of acquired transfusional iron overload in adults. *N Engl J Med* **304**:319, 1981.
419. Fiorelli G, Fargion S, Piperno A, Battafarano N, Cappellini MD: Iron metabolism in thalassemia intermedia. *Haematologica* **75(Suppl 5)**:89, 1990.
420. Modell B, Berdoukas V: *The Clinical Approach to Thalassemia*. London, Grune & Stratton, 1984.
421. Marks PW, Mitus AJ: Congenital dyserythropoietic anemias. *Am J Hematol* **51**:55, 1996.
422. Beutler E: The congenital dyserythropoietic anemias, in Beutler E, Lichtmann MA, Coller BS, Kipps TJ, Seligson U (eds): *Williams' Hematology*. New York, McGraw-Hill, 2000.
423. Fitzsimmons EJ, May A: The molecular basis of the sideroblastic anemias. *Curr Opin Hematol* **3**:167, 1996.
424. Cotter PD, May A, Fitzsimmons EJ, Houston T, Woodcock BE, Al-Sabah AI, Wong L, Bishop DF: Late-onset X-linked sideroblastic anemia: missense mutations in the erythroid delta-aminolevulinate synthase (ALAS2) gene in two pyridoxine-responsive patients initially diagnosed with acquired refractory anemia and ringed sideroblasts. *J Clin Invest* **96**:2090, 1995.
425. Friedman BM, Baynes RD, Bothwell TH, Gordeuk VR, Macfarlane BJ, Lamparelli RD, Robinson EJ, Sher R, Hamberg S: Dietary iron overload in southern African rural blacks. *S Afr Med J* **78**:301, 1990.
426. Schnitzler CM, MacPhail AP, Shires R, Schnaid E, Mesquita JM, Robson HJ: Osteoporosis in African hemosiderosis: role of alcohol and iron. *J Bone Miner Res* **9**:1865, 1994.
427. MacPhail AP, Simon MO, Bothwell TH, Torrance JD, Isaacson C: Changing patterns of dietary iron overload in black South Africans. *Am J Clin Nutr* **32**:1272, 1979.
428. Gordeuk VR, McLaren CE, MacPhail AP, Deichsel G, Bothwell TH: Associations of iron overload in Africa with hepatocellular carcinoma and tuberculosis: Strachan's 1929 thesis revisited. *Blood* **87**:3470, 1996.
429. Moyo VM, Makinuke R, Gangaidzo IT, Gordeuk VR, McLaren CE, Khumalo H, Saungweme T, Rouault T, Kiire CF: African iron overload and hepatocellular carcinoma. *Eur J Haematol* **60**:28, 1998.
430. Gordeuk V, Mukiibi J, Hasstedt SJ, Samowitz W, Edwards CQ, West G, Ndambire S, Emmanual J, Nkanza N, Chapanduka Z: Iron overload in Africa. Interaction between a gene and dietary iron content. *N Engl J Med* **326**:95, 1992.
431. Moyo VM, Mandishona E, Hasstedt SJ, Gangaidzo IT, Gomo ZA, Khumalo H, Saungweme T, Kiire CF, Paterson AC, Bloom P, MacPhail AP, Rouault T, Gordeuk VR: Evidence of genetic transmission in African iron overload. *Blood* **91**:1076, 1998.
432. McNamara L, MacPhail AP, Gordeuk VR, Hasstedt SJ, Rouault T: Is there a link between African iron overload and the described mutations of the hereditary hemochromatosis gene? *Br J Haematol* **102**:1176, 1998.
433. Barton AL, Banner BF, Cable EE, Bonkovsky HL: Distribution of iron in the liver predicts the response of chronic hepatitis C infection to interferon therapy. *Am J Clin Pathol* **103**:419, 1995.
434. Gordeuk VR, McLaren CE, Looker A, Hasselblad V, Brittenham GM: Distribution of transferrin saturations in the African-American population. *Blood* **91**:2175, 1998.
435. Harris ZL, Klomp LW, Gitlin JD: Aceruloplasminemia: An inherited neurodegenerative disease with impairment of iron homeostasis. *Am J Clin Nutr* **67**:972S, 1998.
436. Hamill RL, Woods JC, Cook BA: Congenital atransferrinemia: A case report and review of the literature. *Am J Clin Pathol* **96**:215, 1991.
437. Hayashi A, Wada Y, Suzuki T, Shimizu A: Studies on familial hypotransferrinemia: unique clinical course and molecular pathology. *Am J Hum Genet* **53**:201, 1993.
438. Goldfischer S, Grotsky HW, Chang CH, Berman EL, Richert RR, Karmarkar SD, Roskamp JO, Morecki R: Idiopathic neonatal iron storage involving the liver, pancreas, heart, and endocrine and exocrine glands. *Hepatology* **1**:58, 1981.
439. Knisely AS, Magid MS, Dische MR, Cutz E: Neonatal hemochromatosis. *Birth Defects* **23**:75, 1987.
440. Silver MM, Beverley DW, Valberg LS, Cutz E, Phillips MJ, Shaheed WA: Perinatal hemochromatosis: Clinical, morphologic and quantitative iron studies. *Am J Pathol* **128**:538, 1987.
441. Sigurdsson L, Reyes J, Kocoshis SA, Hansen TW, Rosh J, Knisely AS: Neonatal hemochromatosis: Outcomes of pharmacologic and surgical therapies. *J Pediatr Gastroenterol Nutr* **28**:85, 1998.
442. Shneider BL, Setchell KD, Whitington PF, Neilson KA, Suchy FJ: Delta 4-3-oxosteroid 5 beta-reductase deficiency causing neonatal liver failure and hemochromatosis. *J Pediatr* **124**:234, 1994.
443. Siafakas CG, Jonas MM, Perez-Atayde AR: Abnormal bile acid metabolism and neonatal hemochromatosis: A subset with poor prognosis. *J Pediatr Gastroenterol Nutr* **25**:321, 1998.
444. Bale PM, Kan AE, Dorney SF: Renal proximal tubular dysgenesis associated with severe neonatal hemosiderotic liver disease. *Pediatr Pathol* **14**:479, 1994.
445. Fellman V, Rapola J, Pihko H, Varilo T, Raivio KO: Iron-overload disease in infants involving fetal growth retardation, lactic acidosis, liver heamosidersosis, and aminoaciduria. *Lancet* **351**:490, 1998.
446. Verloes A, Temple IK, Hubert AF, Hope P, Gould S, Debauche C, Verellen G, Deville JL, Koulischer L, Sokal EM: Recurrance of neonatal haemochromatosis in half sibs born of unaffected mothers. *J Med Genet* **33**:444, 1996.
447. Conte D, Manachino D, Colli A, Guala A, Aimo G, Andreoletti M, Corsetti M, Fraquelli M: Prevalence of genetic hemochromatosis in a cohort of Italian patients with diabetes. *Ann Intern Med* **128**:370, 1998.
448. George DK, Evans RM, Crofton RW, Gunn IR: Testing for haemochromatosis in the diabetes clinic. *Ann Clin Biochem* **32**:521, 1995.
449. Turnbull AJ, Mitchison HC, Peaston RT, Lai LC, Bennett MK, Taylor R, Bassendine MF: The prevalence of hereditary hemochromatosis in a diabetic population. *QJM* **90**:271, 1997.
450. Borwein ST, Ghent CN, Flanagan PR, Chamberlain MJ, Valberg LS: Genetic expression of hemochromatosis in Canadians. *Clin Invest Med* **6**:171, 1983.
451. Bassett ML, Halliday JW, Bryant S, Dent O, Powell LW: Screening for hemochromatosis. *Ann N Y Acad Sci* **526**:274, 1988.
452. Balan V, Baldus W, Fairbanks V, Michels V, Burrit M, Klee G: Screening for hemochromatosis: A cost-effectiveness study based on 12,258 patients. *Gastroenterology* **107**:453, 1994.
453. Baer DM, Simons JL, Staples RL, Rumore GJ, Morton CJ: Hemochromatosis screening in asymptomatic ambulatory men 30 years of age and older. *Am J Med* **98**:464, 1995.
454. Niederau C, Niederau CM, Lange S, Littauer A, Abdel Jalil N, Maurer M, Haussinger D, Strohmeyer D: Screening for hemochromatosis and iron deficiency in employees and primary care patients in western Germany. *Ann Intern Med* **128**:337, 1998.
455. Bell H, Thordal C, Raknerud N, Hansen T, Bosnes V, Halvorsen R, Heier HE, Try K, Leivestad T, Thomassen Y: Prevalence of

hemochromatosis among first-time and repeat blood donors in Norway. *J Hepatol* **26**:272, 1997.
456. Skikne BS, Cook JD: Screening test for iron overload. *Am J Clin Nutr* **46**:840, 1987.
457. Witte DL: Unsaturated iron binding capacity identifies iron overload in ambulatory individuals. *Clin Chem* **41**:S145, 1995.
458. Smith BN, Kantrowitz W, Grace ND, Greenberg MS, Patton TJ, Ookubo R, Sorger K, Semeraro JG, Doyle JR, Cooper AG, Kamat BR, Maregni LM, Rand WM: Prevalence of hereditary hemochromatosis in a Massachusetts corporation: Is Celtic origin a risk factor? *Hepatology* **25**:1439, 1997.
459. Phatak PD, Guzman G, Woll J, Robeson A, Phelps CE: Cost-effectiveness of screening for hemochromatosis. *Arch Intern Med* **154**:769, 1994.
460. Buffone GJ, Beck JR: Cost-effectiveness analysis for evaluation of screening programs: Hereditary hemochromatosis. *Clinical Chemistry* **40**:1631, 1994.
461. Bassett ML, Leggett BA, Halliday JW, Webb S, Powell LW: Analysis of the cost of population screening for haemochromatosis using biochemical and genetic markers. *J Hepatol* **27**:517, 1997.
462. Adams PC, Gregor JC, Kertesz AE, Valberg LS: Screening blood donors for hereditary hemochromatosis: Decision analysis model based on a 30-year database. *Gastroenterology* **109**:177, 1995.
463. Sham RL, Ou CY, Cappuccio J, Braggins C, Dunnigan K, Phatak PD: Correlation between genotype and phenotype in hereditary hemochromatosis: analysis of 61 cases. *Blood Cells Mol Dis* **23**:314, 1997.
464. Burke W, Press N, McDonnell SM: Hemochromatosis: Genetics helps to define a multifactorial disease. *Clin Genet* **54**:1, 1998.
465. Henry WL, Nienhuis AW, Wiener M, Miller DR, Canale VC, Piomelli S: Echocardiographic abnormalities in patients with transfusion-dependent anemia and secondary myocardial iron deposition. *Am J Med* **64**:547, 1978.
466. Crosby WH: Treatment of haemochromatosis by energetic phlebotomy. One patient's response to the letting of 55 litres of blood in 11 months. *Br J Haematol* **4**:82, 1958.
467. Propper RD, Cooper B, Rufo RR, Nienhuis AW, Anderson WF, Bunn HF, Rosenthal A, Nathan DG: Continuous subcutaenous administration of deferoxamine in patients with iron overload. *N Engl J Med* **297**:418, 1977.
468. Surakomol S, Olson LJ, Rastogi A, Steers JL, Sterioff S, Daly RC, McGregor CG: Combined orthotopic heart and liver transplantation for genetic hemochromatosis. *J Heart Lung Transplant* **16**:573, 1997.
469. Koerner MM, Tenderich G, Minami K, zu Knyphausen E, Mannebach H, Kleesiek K, Meyer H, Koerfer R: Heart transplantation for end-stage heart failure caused by iron overload. *Br J Haematol* **97**:293, 1997.
470. Egawa H, Berquist W, Garcia-Kennedy R, Cox K, Knisely AS, Esquivel CO: Rapid development of hepatocellular siderosis after liver transplantation for neonatal hemochromatosis. *Transplantation* **62**:1511, 1996.
471. Kilpe VE, Krakauer H, Wren RE: An analysis of liver transplant experience from 37 transplant centers as reported to Medicare. *Transplantation* **56**:554, 1993.
472. Kowdley KV, Hassanein T, Kaur S, Farrell FJ, Van Thiel DH, Keeffe EB, Sorrell MF, Bacon BR, Weber FLJ, Tavill AS: Primary liver cancer and survival in patients undergoing liver transplantation for hemochromatosis. *Liver Transpl Surg* **1**:237, 1995.
473. Pillay P, Tzoracoleftherakis E, Tzakis AG, Kakizoe S, Van Thiel DH, Starzl TE: Orthotopic liver transplantation for hemochromatosis. *Transplant Proc* **23**:1888, 1991.
474. Gordeuk VR: Hereditary and nutritional iron overload. *Baillieres Clin Haematol* **5**:169, 1992.
475. Bomford A, Williams R: Long term results of venesection therapy in idiopathic haemochromatosis. *QJM* **45**:611, 1976.
476. Adams PC, Speechley M, Kertesz AE: Long-term survival analysis in hereditary hemochromatosis. *Gastroenterology* **101**:368, 1991.
477. Desforges JF, Kalaw E, Gilchrist P: Inhibition of glucose-6-phosphate dehydrogenase by hemolysis inducing drugs. *J Lab Clin Med* **55**:757, 1960.
478. Fracanzani AL, Fargion S, Romano R, Conte D, Piperno A, D'Alba R, Mandelli C, Fraquelli M, Pacchetti S, Braga M: Portal hypertension and iron depletion in patients with genetic hemochromatosis. *Hepatology* **22**:1127, 1995.
479. Adams PC: Hepatocellular carcinoma in hereditary hemochromatosis. *Can J Gastroenterol* **7**:37, 1993.
480. Strohmeyer G, Niederau C, Stremmel W: Survival and causes of death in hemochromatosis: Observations on 163 patients. *Ann N Y Acad Sci* **526**:245, 1988.
481. Conte WJ, Rotter JI: The use of association data to identify family members at high risk for marker-linked diseases. *Am J Hum Genet* **36**:152, 1984.
482. Siemons LJ, Mahler C: Hypogonadotropic hypogonadism in hemochromatosis: Recovery of reproductive function after iron depletion. *J Clin Endocrinol Metab* **65**:585, 1987.
483. Blackwell JM, Barton CH, White JK, Searle S, Baker AM, Williams H, Shaw MA: Genomic organization and sequence of the human NRAMP gene: identification and mapping of a promoter region polymorphism. *Mol Med* **1**:194, 1995.
484. Tsuchihashi Z, Hansen SL, Quintana L, Kronmal GS, Mapa FA, Feder JN, Wolff RK: Transferrin receptor mutation analysis in hereditary hemochromatosis patients. *Blood Cells Mol Dis* **24**:317, 1998.
485. Lee PL, Ho NJ, Olson R, Beutler E: The effect of transferrin polymorphisms on iron metabolism. *Blood Cells Mol Dis* **25**:374, 1999.
486. Edwards CQ, Skolnick MH, Kushner JP: Coincidental nontransfusional iron overload and thalassemia minor: association with HLA-linked hemochromatosis. *Blood* **58**:844, 1981.
487. Beutler E, Gelbart T, Lee P, Trevino R, Fernandez MA, Fairbanks VF: Molecular characterization of a case of atransferrinemia. Submitted. 2000.
488. Whitfield JB, Cullen LM, Jazwinska EC, Powell LW, Heath AC, Zhu G, Duffy DL, et al.: Effects of HFE C282Y and H63D polymorphisms and polygenic background on iron stores in a large community sample of twins. *Am J Hum Genet* **66**:1246, 2000.
489. Vulpe CD, Kuo YM, Murphy TL, Cowley L, Askwith C, Libina N, Gitschier J, et al.: Hephaestin, a ceruloplasmin homologue implicated in intestinal iron transport, is defective in the sla mouse. *Nat Genet* **21**:195, 1999.
490. Lee P, Halloran C, Cross AR, Beutler E: NADH-ferric reductase activity associated with dihydropteridine reductase. *Biochem Biophys Res Commun* **271**:788, 2000.
491. Kawabata H, Yang S, Hirama T, Vuong PT, Kawano S, Gombart AF, Koeffler HP: Molecular cloning of transferrin receptor 2: A new member of the transferrin receptor-like family. *J Biol Chem* **274**:20826, 1999.
492. Camaschella C, Roetto A, Cali A, De Gobbi M, Garozzo G, Carella M, Majorano N, et al.: The gene TFR2 is mutated in a new type of haemochromatosis mapping to 7q22. *Nat Genet* **25**:14, 2000.
493. Yu JM, Yu ZK, Wessling-Resnick M: Expression of SFT (stimulator of Fe transport) is enhanced by iron chelation in HeLa cells and by hemochromatosis in liver. *J Biol Chem* **273**:34675, 1998.
494. Donovan A, Brownlie A, Zhou Y, Shepard J, Pratt SJ, Moynihan J, Paw BH, et al.: Positional cloning of zebrafish ferroportin1 identifies a conserved vertebrate iron exporter. *Nature* **403**:776, 2000.
495. Abboud S, Haile DJ: A novel mammalian iron-regulated protein involved in intracellular iron metabolism. *J Biol Chem* **275**:19906, 2000.
496. Levy JE, Montross LK, Andrews NC: Genes that modify the hemochromatosis phenotype in mice. *J Clin Invest* **105**:1209, 2000.
497. Roetto A, Totaro A, Cazzola M, Cicilano M, Bosio S, D'scola G, Carella M, et al.: Juvenile hemochromatosis locus maps to chromosome 1q. *Am J Hum Genet* **64**:1388, 1999.
498. Barton JC, Sawada-Hirai R, Rothenberg BE, Acton RT: Two novel missense mutations of the HFE gene (I105T and G93R) and identification of the S65C mutation in Alabama hemochromatosis probands. *Blood Cells Mol Dis* **25**:146, 1999.
499. Wallace DF, Dooley JS, Walker AP: A novel mutation of HFE explains the classical phenotype of genetic hemochromatosis in a C282Y heterozygote. *Gastroenterology* **116**:1409, 1999.
500. Beutler E, Felitti V, Gelbart T, Ho N: The effect of *HFE* genotypes on measurements of iron overload in patients attending a health appraisal clinic. *Ann Intern Med*, **133**:329, 2000.
501. Beutler E, Gelbart T: A common intron 3 mutation prevents amplification of the HFE gene. *Blood Cells Mol Dis*, **26**:229, 2000.
502. Jeffrey GP, Chakrabarti S, Hegele RA, Adams PC: Polymorphism in intron 4 of HFE may cause overestimation of C282Y homozygote prevalence in haemochromatosis. *Nat Genet* **22**:325, 1999.
503. Merryweather-Clarke AT, Pointon JJ, Shearman JD, Robson KJH, Jouanolle AM, Mosser A, David V, et al.: Polymorphism in intron 4 of HFE does not compromise haemochromatosis mutation results. *Nat Genet* **23**:271, 1999.
504. Gomez PS, Parks S, Ries R, Tran TC, Gomez PF, Press RD: Polymorphism in intron 4 of HFE does not compromise haemochromatosis mutation results. *Nat Genet* **23**:272, 1999.

505. Olynyk JK, Cullen DJ, Aquilia S, Rossi E, Summerville L, Powell LW: A population-based study of the clinical expression of the hemochromatosis gene. *N Engl J Med* **341**:718, 1999.
506. Willis G, Wimperis JZ, Smith KC, Fellows IW, Jennings BA: Haemochromatosis gene C282Y homozygotes in an elderly male population. *Lancet* **354**:221, 1999.
507. Motulsky AG, Beutler E: Hemochromatosis: The leading genetic disease target for public health intervention. *Ann Rev Public Health* **21**:65, 2000.
508. Klipstein-Grobusch K, Koster JF, Grobbee DE, Lindemans J, Boeing H, Hofman A, Witteman JCM: Serum ferritin and risk of myocardial infarction in the elderly: The Rotterdam Study. *Am J Clin Nutr* **69**:1231, 1999.
509. Tuomainen TP, Kontula K, Nyyssonen K, Lakka TA, Helio T, Salonen JT: Increased risk of acute myocardial infarction in carriers of the hemochromatosis gene Cys282Tyr mutation: A prospective cohort study in men in eastern Finland. *Circulation* **100**:1274, 1999.
510. de Valk B, Marx JJM: Iron, atherosclerosis, and ischemic heart disease. *Arch Intern Med* **159**:1542, 1999.

CHAPTER 128

Molybdenum Cofactor Deficiency and Isolated Sulfite Oxidase Deficiency

Jean L. Johnson ▪ Marinus Duran

1. The molybdenum cofactor is a low-molecular-weight prosthetic group in which the metal is complexed to a unique pterin species termed *molybdopterin*. The cofactor is essential for the function of the human enzymes sulfite oxidase, xanthine dehydrogenase, and aldehyde oxidase. Patients with *molybdenum cofactor deficiency* (OMIM Nos. 252150 and 252160) are deficient in the activity of all three enzymes and exhibit symptoms that include severe neurologic abnormalities, dislocated ocular lenses, and mental retardation. They excrete elevated levels of sulfite, thiosulfate, *S*-sulfocysteine, taurine, xanthine, and hypoxanthine and low amounts of uric acid. Patients with *isolated sulfite oxidase deficiency* (OMIM No. 272300) lack sulfite oxidase activity but are normal with respect to molybdenum cofactor and xanthine dehydrogenase and aldehyde oxidase functions. This form of sulfite oxidase deficiency produces clinical symptoms and neuropathology essentially indistinguishable from those of the combined deficiency disease.
2. More than 100 patients have been diagnosed with molybdenum cofactor deficiency or isolated sulfite oxidase deficiency. Molybdenum cofactor deficiency appears to be more prevalent than the isolated deficiency but is also more likely to be detected in routine screening programs. Patients with milder clinical symptoms and late onset are found more often among those with isolated sulfite oxidase deficiency. Both molybdenum cofactor deficiency and isolated sulfite oxidase deficiency are inherited as autosomal recessive traits, with obligate heterozygotes displaying no symptoms. Patients belong to a variety of ethnic groups and are found among the populations of Europe, North America, Northern Africa, Turkey, and Asia.
3. Although considerable variability in severity of symptoms and age of onset does occur, the key clinical symptom for molybdenum cofactor deficiency and isolated sulfite oxidase deficiency is severe convulsions, presenting early after birth. All patients with this presentation immediately should be subjected to metabolic screening procedures. Many patients display dysmorphic facial features that resemble those in patients with perinatal asphyxia. Patients with this presentation and no apparent hypoxic event at birth should be screened for these disorders.
4. Pathology studies in a number of cases of molybdenum cofactor deficiency and isolated sulfite oxidase deficiency have revealed a severe encephalopathy with marked neuronal loss and demyelination in the white matter accompanied by gliosis and diffuse spongiosis. The observation that neither isolated xanthinuria nor a combined loss of xanthine dehydrogenase and aldehyde oxidase results in encephalopathy supports the conclusion that these effects result from the absence of sulfite oxidase activity. A disturbed development and damage to the brain may occur as a result of accumulation of toxic levels of sulfite in cerebro.
5. Prenatal diagnosis of molybdenum cofactor deficiency and of isolated sulfite oxidase deficiency is accomplished by assay of sulfite oxidase activity in uncultured chorionic villus tissue or in cultured amniotic cells.
6. Molybdenum cofactor deficiency and isolated sulfite oxidase deficiency are serious and often fatal diseases for which no effective therapy is generally available. Some patients, especially those with milder forms of isolated sulfite oxidase deficiency, respond well to the administration of diets low in sulfur-containing amino acids. Some success in seizure control has been achieved with the antiepileptic drug vigabatrin.
7. The genes for sulfite oxidase and for most of the molybdenum cofactor biosynthetic enzymes have been cloned, and the mutations in a number of patients have been characterized at the molecular level. Deletions and insertions, as well as nonsense and missense mutations, have been identified in the sulfite oxidase gene, with one mutation, *R160Q*, identified in more than one patient. Patients with molybdenum cofactor deficiency comprise two complementation classes. Group B patients have mutations in molybdopterin synthase or molybdopterin synthase sulfurylase, whereas group A patients are most likely defective in genes coding for early steps in the biosynthetic pathway, *MOCS1A* or *MOCS1B*.
8. The extreme instability of the isolated molybdenum cofactor precludes its use as effective therapy for correction of molybdenum cofactor deficiency. However, as more is learned of the pathways of biosynthesis and metabolism of this molecule in human tissues, more stable intermediates may be identified with potential efficacy for cofactor replacement therapy in some patients.

The following are gene names, symbols, and GenBank Accession Numbers (where known), respectively, for enzymes and steps in pathways (e.g., Figures 128-2 and 128-4) described in this chapter. Molybdenum cofactor synthesis step 1 (two segments): *MOCS1A* and *MOCS1B*, AJ224328; molybdopterin synthase (two subunits): *MOCS2A* and *MOCS2B*, AF091871; molybdopterin synthase sulfurylase: *MOCS3*, AF102544; sulfite oxidase: *SUOX*, L31573.

A list of standard abbreviations is located immediately preceding the index in each volume.

A combined deficiency of sulfite oxidase and xanthine dehydrogenase was described for the first time in 1978.[1] The patient presented in the neonatal period with feeding difficulties, severe neurologic abnormalities, dislocated ocular lenses, and dysmorphic features of the head. Chemical screening revealed xanthinuria as well as the metabolic characteristics of sulfite oxidase deficiency. The occurrence of two rare inherited defects in a single individual was thought to be highly improbable. However, because molybdenum is an essential component of both xanthine dehydrogenase and sulfite oxidase, a defect in molybdenum metabolism or transport was suspected. Molybdenum deficiency of dietary origin could be excluded, although it was later shown by Abumrad et al.[2] that a dietary deficiency of the metal in a patient receiving total parenteral nutrition led to a similar depressed functioning of both enzymes. The underlying primary defect in the index case of the heritable form of combined deficiency of sulfite oxidase and xanthine dehydrogenase was established[3] as a deficiency of the molybdenum cofactor, the low-molecular-weight prosthetic group of molybdoenzymes in which the metal is complexed to a unique pterin species termed *molybdopterin*. Evidence also was presented indicating that a third molybdenum cofactor-dependent enzyme, aldehyde oxidase, was deficient in this patient.[3] Soon after the description of the first patient, other patents with similar clinical and chemical hallmarks were diagnosed.[4,5] Direct evidence for genetic inheritance was provided by the occurrence of two patients in a single family.[6]

A key to the diagnosis of molybdenum cofactor deficiency was the description, several years earlier, of a patient with an isolated case of sulfite oxidase deficiency.[7,8] This patient subsequently was shown to have normal xanthine dehydrogenase and molybdenum cofactor function.[9] The clinical and biochemical features that were identified in this case laid the groundwork for characterization of the combined-deficiency disease. The number of identified cases of both the isolated and combined deficiency is steadily growing; the combined deficiency appears to be the more common variant of sulfite oxidase deficiency. The emphasis in the sections that follow is on inherited molybdenum cofactor deficiency; however, the isolated deficiency of sulfite oxidase is covered as well and is particularly relevant in view of the clinical similarities of the two variants. The isolated deficiency of xanthine dehydrogenase, known as *xanthinuria*, and the combined deficiency of xanthine dehydrogenase and aldehyde oxidase are covered in Chap. 111.

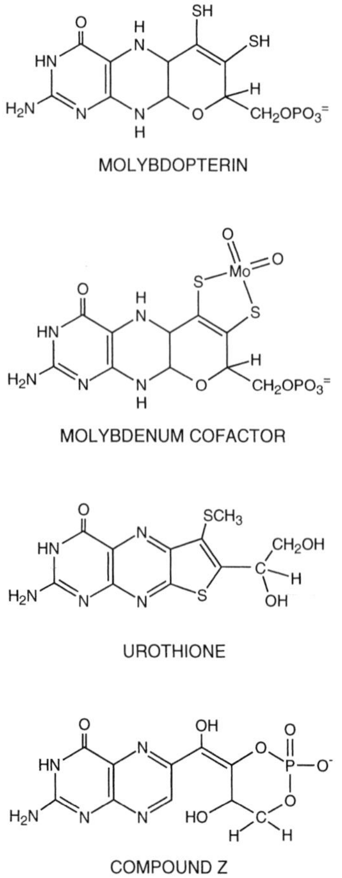

MOLYBDOPTERIN

MOLYBDENUM COFACTOR

UROTHIONE

COMPOUND Z

Fig. 128-1 Chemical structures of molybdopterin, the molybdenum cofactor urothione, and compound Z. Molybdopterin and the molybdenum cofactor are shown in the tricyclic form observed in the crystal structures of several molybdoenzymes. The dioxo ligands of the molybdenum in the molybdenum cofactor structure shown are features of the cofactor in sulfite oxidase. The metal in the cofactor in xanthine dehydrogenase and aldehyde oxidase contains one oxo and one sulfido group as terminal ligands.

THE MOLYBDENUM COFACTOR

Chemistry of the Molybdenum Cofactor

Sulfite oxidase, xanthine dehydrogenase, and aldehyde oxidase, the three known molybdoenzymes present in human tissues, each contain the metal as a part of a molybdenum cofactor in which the metal is complexed to a unique organic moiety termed *molybdopterin*.[10–13] The structures of the molybdenum cofactor and molybdopterin are shown in Fig. 128-1. The molybdenum cofactor within the protective environment of an enzyme is quite stable and very tightly bound to the protein. In some enzymes, the metal is coordinated by ligands provided by the protein as well as those supplied by molybdopterin. The structure of the molybdenum cofactor shown in Fig. 128-1 indicates the presence of two terminal oxo ligands to the metal, as is characteristic of the cofactor in sulfite oxidase and certain other molybdoenzymes of nonanimal origin. The ligand field of the molybdenum in the cofactor of xanthine dehydrogenase and aldehyde oxidase is modified from the structure shown in that one of the oxo ligands is replaced by a terminal sulfide. The sulfo form of the cofactor is essential for the functioning of these two enzymes, as shown by the in vitro inactivation of both by cyanide, which extracts the sulfide as thiocyanate, leaving a nonfunctional dioxo cofactor.[14,15] The incorporation of the terminal sulfide ligand has been established as the function of the *ma-l* locus in *Drosophila melanogaster*,[16] and a deficiency in this sulfuration activity may underlie that class of xanthinuric patients who exhibit a combined deficiency of aldehyde oxidase but normal sulfite oxidase[17] (see Chap. 111).

Extraction of the molybdenum cofactor from a molybdoenzyme requires strong denaturing conditions, disrupts the molybdenum ligand field, and yields an unstable molybdenum-molybdopterin complex. Dissociation of the metal from the free complex, which occurs quite readily, leaves a species with two highly reactive vicinal sulfhydryl groups that can decay into a multitude of products. For these reasons, reversible resolution and reconstitution of the cofactor from molybdoenzymes has not been accomplished. The instability of the side chain and reduced pterin ring in the released complex made chemical characterization of the active species particularly challenging and will have important implications in terms of design of potential therapeutic agents to correct molybdenum cofactor deficiency.

Chemical characterization of the molybdenum cofactor was accomplished by analyzing a number of stable degradation products, two of which are formed in vitro,[12] a third that is produced metabolically and excreted in the urine,[11] and a fourth that was generated by specific chemical modification based on the predicted structure.[13] The structure of urothione, the metabolic degradation product of molybdopterin, is shown in Fig. 128-1. This thienopterin was identified originally in 1940[18] and characterized structurally in 1969[19] as a minor constituent of unknown function present in human urine. The metabolic relationship between the molybdenum cofactor and urothione was established by the discovery that patients with molybdenum cofactor deficiency excrete no detectable urothione.[11,20]

The structure of molybdopterin predicted from the study of stable degradation products has been verified by x-ray crystallographic data obtained on chicken liver sulfite oxidase and several other molybdopterin-containing enzymes.[21–23] In the crystal structure of sulfite oxidase, the pterin was found to exist as part of a tricyclic ring system with a pyran ring fused to the pyrazine ring of the pterin, a feature also observed in the crystalline forms of other molybdopterin-containing enzymes. This three-ringed structure may reflect the state of the cofactor in the native protein; however, the open form is clearly present in the various derivatives of the cofactor, suggesting that ring opening is facile and perhaps even reversible under certain circumstances. The observed three-ringed pterin structure corresponds to an open form wherein the pterin ring is present at a dihydro state of reduction. Gardlik and Rajagopalan[24] have shown that in xanthine oxidase and sulfite oxidase, the molybdenum cofactor is present as a dihydropterin.

Recent discoveries have lent additional complexity to the task of understanding molybdenum cofactor chemistry. Certain molybdoenzymes of bacterial origin have been shown to contain dinucleotide forms of molybdopterin with GMP,[25–29] CMP,[30,31] AMP,[28] and IMP[28] in pyrophosphate linkage to the molybdopterin side chain. Others, including aldehyde ferredoxin oxidoreductase,[22] DMSO reductase,[23,32] and formate dehydrogenase,[33] contain bis(molybdopterin) cofactors wherein the metal is liganded by the dithiolenes of two molybdopterin molecules. The roles of the ribonucleotide and the bis pterin in the cofactor of these enzymes is yet to be understood; however, it has been established that the three molybdoenzymes in humans use exclusively the molybdenum cofactor with one molybdopterin per metal center and no appended ribonucleotide.

Enzymes and Metabolic Pathways Dependent on the Molybdenum Cofactor

Xanthine dehydrogenase (E.C. 1.2.1.37) catalyzes the hydroxylation of hypoxanthine and xanthine to produce uric acid as the final product. The enzyme is also active, to varying degrees, with a variety of other heterocyclic substrates.[34] The reaction mechanism[35] involves abstraction of a hydride ion from the substrate and replacement with a hydroxyl ion ultimately derived from water. Substrate binding and hydroxylation occur at the molybdenum center with concomitant reduction of Mo(VI) to Mo(IV). The molybdenum is reoxidized as electrons are passed on through an enzyme-bound electron transport chain consisting of flavin adenine dinucleotide (FAD) and two 2Fe/2S centers. The physiologic oxidizing substrate for the reaction is NAD^+, although under certain conditions the enzyme is converted to a form that reduces molecular oxygen.[36,37] It is this form of the enzyme that is referred to by the more familiar name, *xanthine oxidase*.

The role of the enzyme in metabolism is in the pathway of purine degradation for excretion. Because hypoxanthine and guanine can be reclaimed to a large extent by the action of hypoxanthine-guanine phosphoribosyl transferase, and because hypoxanthine and xanthine are not highly toxic compounds, deficiencies of xanthine dehydrogenase in humans are largely benign (see Chap. 111). The major clinical symptoms attributed to xanthinuria as the isolated deficiency disease relate to the limited solubility of xanthine at physiologic pH and are manifest as deposits or calculi in kidney and sometimes in muscle.

Xanthine dehydrogenase is a soluble enzyme present in liver and intestine and, at lower levels, in kidney, spleen, and skeletal and heart muscle.[38] It is also a normal constituent of milk, although the function of the enzyme in milk is unknown. Xanthine dehydrogenase activity is not expressed in cultured human cell lines.[39]

Sulfite oxidase (E.C. 1.8.2.1) functions as the terminal enzyme in the pathway of degradation of sulfur amino acids (see Fig. 128-2). Besides functioning to eliminate endogenously produced sulfite, the enzyme fills an important role in detoxifying exogenously derived sulfite and sulfur dioxide.[40] Rats made deficient in sulfite oxidase have been shown to be more sensitive to the deleterious effects of these agents.

Sulfite oxidase exists as a soluble protein compartmentalized in the intermembrane space of the mitochondrion. In this location, it has ready access to its reducing substrate, sulfite, which can diffuse

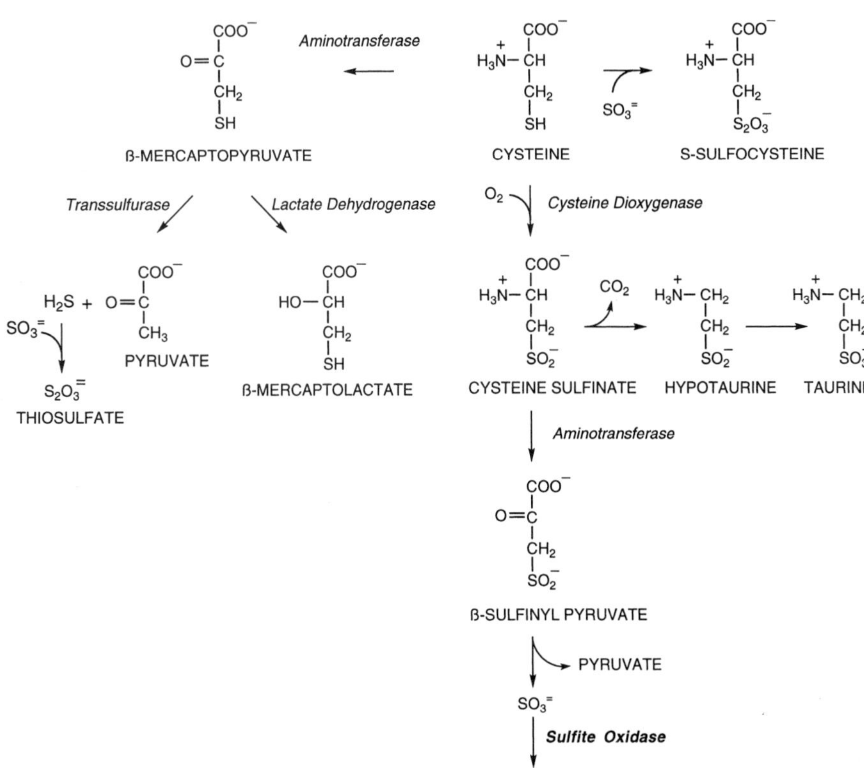

Fig. 128-2 Pathway of cysteine catabolism. The major pathway of degradation, direct oxidation with formation of sulfate, is indicated as the downward branch. The minor pathway of degradation, transamination and transsulfuration, is shown on the left. Pathways of formation of *S*-sulfocysteine, thiosulfate, and taurine, intermediates that accumulate in cases of sulfite oxidase deficiency, are also shown.

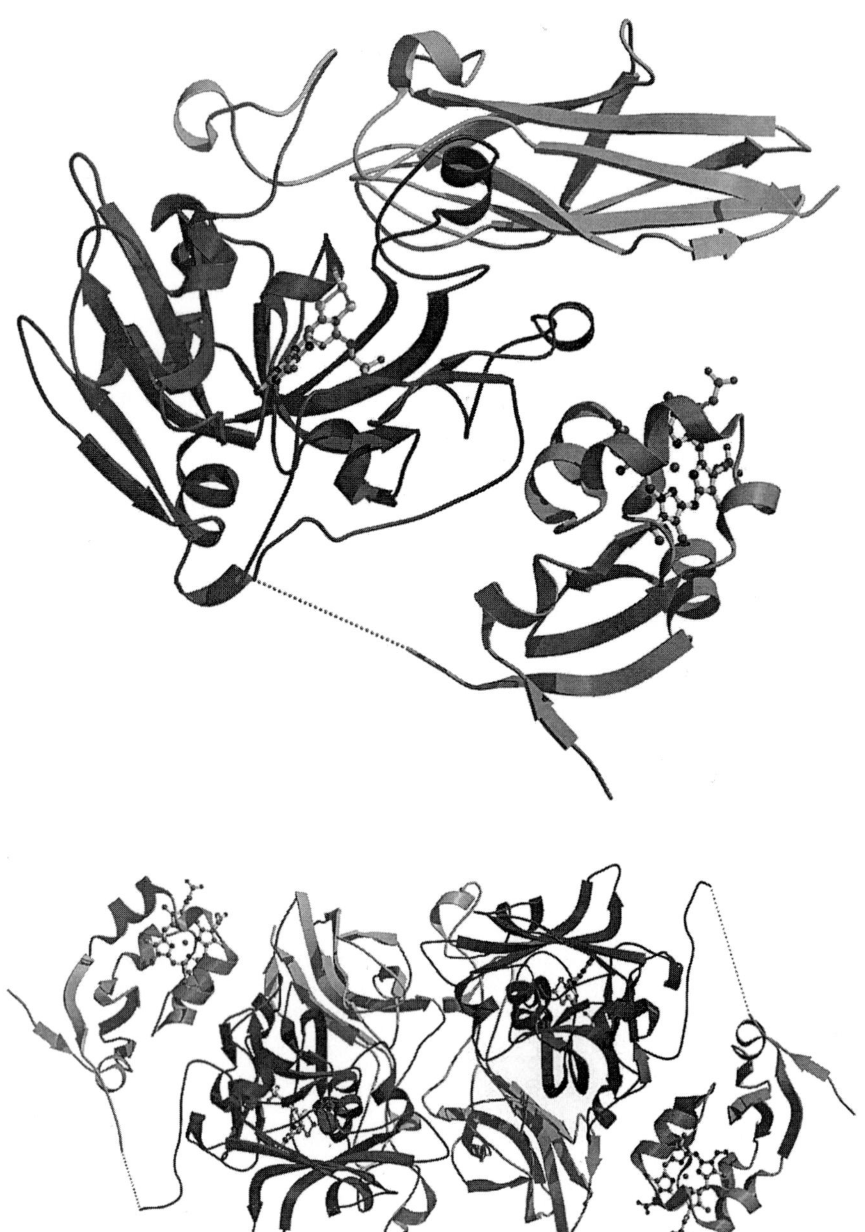

Fig. 128-3 Structure of chicken liver sulfite oxidase monomer (*top*) and dimer (*bottom*). The molybdenum cofactor and the heme are shown in ball-and-stick representation. (*Courtesy of C. Kisker.*)

across the mitochondrial membranes, and to its physiologic electron acceptor, cytochrome c.[41] Oxidation of sulfite occurs at the molybdenum center with reduction of the metal from Mo(VI) to Mo(IV). The electrons are then transferred one at a time through the b_5 heme of the enzyme and from there to cytochrome c. The enzyme exists as a dimer of identical subunits; proteolytic studies revealed that each monomer could be cleaved into a larger molybdenum domain and a smaller heme domain.[42] The three-dimensional structure of chicken liver sulfite oxidase recently has been determined by x-ray crystallography[21] and is illustrated in Fig. 128-3. Each monomer of the dimeric enzyme was found to consist of three domains, a heme, a molybdenum cofactor domain, and a C-terminal domain that contains most of the dimer contact regions. The heme domain possesses a strong antigenic determinant. Polyclonal antibodies generated against the sulfite oxidase protein are directed primarily to this antigenic region and strongly inhibit enzyme activity.[9,43] The enzyme is found in many tissues, with highest levels in liver, kidney, lung, and heart. No detectable activity was found in blood or skeletal muscle.[44] The enzyme is expressed in fibroblasts, cultured amniotic fluid cells, and lymphoblasts.

A deficiency of sulfite oxidase can arise from a specific defect in the enzyme protein or from a lack of functional molybdenum cofactor. The clinical picture is very similar in the two diseases, suggesting that most, if not all, of the devastating sequelae of molybdenum cofactor deficiency stem from the absence of sulfite oxidase, as is considered in more detail below.

Aldehyde oxidase (E.C. 1.2.3.1) shares many physicochemical properties with xanthine dehydrogenase (cofactor composition, molecular weight, and subunit structure) and shows some overlap in substrate specificity as well.[35] Aldehyde oxidase will hydroxylate hypoxanthine to yield xanthine but cannot convert the latter to uric acid.[34] The enzyme works on a wide variety of heterocyclic compounds and xenobiotics and may function as a part of the body's general detoxification system. The enzyme is present in the soluble cell fraction and exists as a constitutive and irreversible oxidase, reducing oxygen to hydrogen peroxide and superoxide. Aldehyde dehydrogenases have been described in various systems, but none of these are molybdoenzymes.

Aldehyde oxidase activity is difficult to assay directly in human tissues in part due to its instability to freezing. Consequently, the absence of aldehyde oxidase activity in patients with molybdenum cofactor deficiency has not been demonstrated directly. In the first case reported, however, an in vivo test of aldehyde oxidase function, measuring the conversion of L-histidine to hydantoin-5-propionic acid, indicated a deficiency of this enzyme as well.[3] An isolated deficiency of aldehyde oxidase in humans has never been reported; however, patients with a combined deficiency of xanthine dehydrogenase and aldehyde oxidase and normal sulfite oxidase have been described.[17] These individuals display the characteristics of xanthinuria and in addition are severely deficient in the ability to convert *N*-methylnicotinamide to its oxidation products in vivo. The combined deficiency of xanthine dehydrogenase and aldehyde oxidase in these individuals is without apparent serious clinical consequences, suggesting that isolated aldehyde oxidase deficiency would be an asymptomatic abnormality and supporting the conclusion that the deficiency of sulfite oxidase is responsible for the severe pathogenesis associated with molybdenum cofactor deficiency.

Molybdenum Cofactor Biosynthesis

The pathway of biosynthesis of the molybdenum cofactor has not yet been fully elucidated. Of the other complex pterins present in human tissues, tetrahydrobiopterin, the cofactor for phenylalanine hydroxylase and related enzymes, is synthesized *de novo* from guanosine triphosphate (GTP), while folic acid is dietarily derived. Studies on the biosynthesis of the molybdenum cofactor in *Escherichia coli* have shown that molybdopterin is synthesized by a unique *de novo* pathway quite unlike that of biopterin synthesis in higher organisms. The requirement for a unique pathway is in fact not unexpected given the requirement for a side chain containing four carbons rather than the three of tetrahydrobiopterin, which are supplied directly by the ribose in the cyclohydrolase I reaction. The cofactor is present in a variety of molybdoenzymes of bacterial, fungal, plant, and animal origin and as such could be supplied in the diet. Recent sequencing of large portions of the human genome, however, has revealed the presence of human homologues of the microbial genes implicated in molybdopterin biosynthesis, strongly suggesting that a *de novo* synthetic pathway related or identical to that in *E. coli* is operative in humans.

A series of molybdopterin mutants (*mol* mutants) of *E. coli* have been identified. In the absence of molybdopterin, the cells are unable to generate functional nitrate reductase and by virtue of this defect are rendered chlorate-resistant.[45] These mutants have been characterized biochemically and the functions of many of the *mol* genes established.

As indicated in Fig. 128-4, molybdopterin is synthesized in *E. coli* from guanosine or a guanosine derivative, as evidenced by the incorporation of label from radioactive guanosine.[46] Two genes in the *moa* locus, *moaA* and *moaC*, are required to convert the guanosine derivative to an intermediate *precursor* Z, a reduced pterin that contains the four-carbon side chain of molybdopterin in the form of a six-membered cyclic phosphate ring.[47,48] The oxidized product of precursor Z, termed *compound* Z, has the structure shown in Fig. 128-1. In the conversion of guanosine to precursor Z, the guanine ring becomes a part of the pterin ring, whereas the carbon atoms of a pentose or pentulose (perhaps the guanosine ribose) are diverted to the C-6 and C-7 of the pterin ring and to the side-chain atoms C-2′, C-3′, and C-4′.[49] Unlike classic pathways, however, in which the C-8 of the guanine ring is eliminated as formate,[50] in molybdopterin biosynthesis, this carbon is fully retained as C-1′ of the molybdopterin side chain, with the remodeling of the ring atoms of the pentose and purine moieties proceeding by intramolecular rearrangement.[46,49] The reactions catalyzed by MoaA and MoaC have not been characterized, and the order in which they function is not known, although the gene sequence of *moaA* predicts a protein of 37.3 kDa with a GTP-binding motif.[51] The protein contains two conserved cysteine clusters essential for activity[52,53] and presumably involved in formation of the Fe/S cluster(s) evident from the absorption (M. M. Wuebbens and K. V. Rajagopalan, unpublished data) and epr spectra of the enzyme.[53] The role of

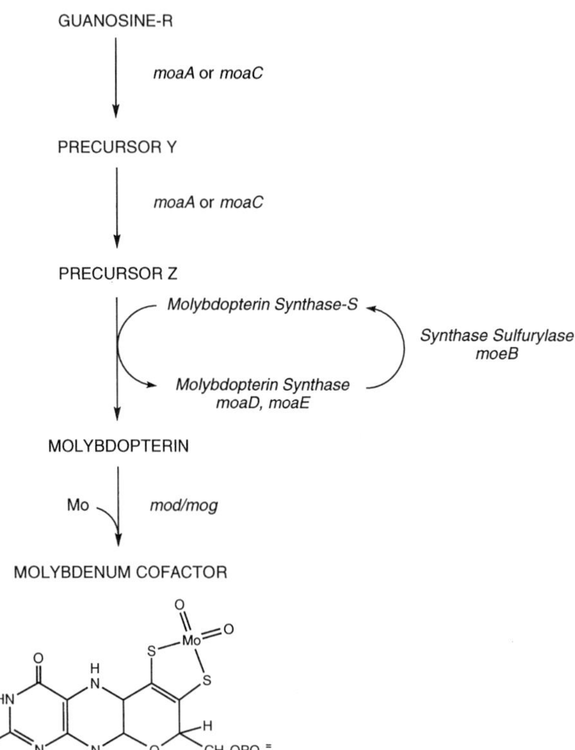

Fig. 128-4 Biosynthesis of the molybdenum cofactor in *E. coli*. Guanosine-R indicates guanosine or one of its phosphorylated derivatives.

an intervening *moaB* gene is undetermined, although its strong homology to *mog* (see below) and the lack of success in generating chlorate-resistant point mutants at the *moaB* locus suggest that it may be redundant.

The conversion of precursor Z to molybdopterin requires decyclization of the side chain concomitant with sulfur incorporation and is effected by a two-subunit protein complex termed *molybdopterin synthase*.[54] Generation of active molybdopterin synthase is itself a multistep process requiring the synthesis of small and large subunits (coded for by genes *D* and *E* at the *moa* locus) and sulfuration of the small subunit, catalyzed by *molybdopterin synthase sulfurylase* (MoeB). The sulfur on the molybdopterin synthase small subunit is apparently transferred to precursor Z as it is converted to molybdopterin, requiring resulfuration of the small subunit before the molybdopterin synthase can function again.[29] The synthase sulfurylase gene has been cloned and sequenced[55]; characterization of the recombinant protein revealed that the enzyme contains stoichiometric zinc that contributes to a strong shoulder at 320 nm in the absorption spectrum (P. Bali and K. V. Rajagopalan, unpublished data). Zinc binding may be accomplished through the cysXXcys motif that occurs twice in the MoeB sequence. The predicted amino acid sequence also shows the presence of a distinct nucleotide-binding motif at the N-terminus and a possible ATP-binding site near the C-terminus.

Clues to the mechanism of action of molybdopterin synthase sulfurylase have come from the identification of significant homologies between MoeB and a number of other proteins, including ubiquitin-activating enzyme and ThiF (in the thiamin biosynthetic pathway). In the ubiquitin-dependent protein degradation system, a cysteine residue of the activating enzyme becomes linked to ubiquitin in an ATP-dependent reaction. A thioester is generated between the ubiquitin-activating enzyme sulfhydryl and the free carboxyl of the C-terminal glycine of ubiquitin. The small subunit of molybdopterin synthase, like ubiquitin, has a C-terminal gly-gly motif, and it has been proposed that a thiocarboxylate is similarly formed on MoaD by the action of MoeB.[56–58] Evidence in support of the presence of a thiocarboxylate on MoaD has been obtained[59] by comparing the molecular masses of the protein purified from a *moeB* mutant with that from *moeB*+ cells. A mass increase of 16 suggests that an oxygen in the *moeB* mutant is replaced by a sulfur in the *moeB*+ cells. The thiocarboxylate hypothesis recently has been corroborated by studies on the ThiS protein in the thiamine biosynthetic pathway. Mass spectrometry showed that the ThiS protein exhibits the same molecular mass increase in the active form.[60] Further characterization of the sulfurylated species using SWIFT (stored waveform inverse Fourier transform) and SORI (sustained off-resonance irradiation) mass spectrometry localized the thiocarboxylate to the terminal glycine residue.[60] A second protein encoded at the *moe* locus, MoeA, is also required for molybdenum cofactor biosynthesis, but very little information is available as to its role.

The molybdopterin that is the product of the molybdopterin synthase reaction remains bound to protein and is converted to molybdenum cofactor by addition of the metal in an appropriate "activated" form. These latter biosynthetic steps require products of the *mod* and *mog* loci. The *modABCD* operon encodes a high-affinity molybdate uptake system, with the *modA* gene encoding a periplasmic binding protein specific for molybdate and tungstate.[61,62] A possible role for Mog as a chelatase responsible for insertion of the metal in molybdenum cofactor formation has been proposed.[63] Both *mod* and *mog* mutants are repaired to some extent by growth on high levels of molybdate, suggesting that molybdate uptake and insertion can occur nonenzymatically, but both Mod and Mog functions are essential for molybdenum cofactor formation under the normally low concentrations of the metal in the culture medium. The final step in cofactor assembly in *E. coli* and many other microorganisms, but not in humans (and not indicated in Fig. 128-4), is ribonucleotide addition catalyzed by MobAB to generate dinucleotide forms of the cofactor.

Molecular Characterization of Molybdenum Cofactor Deficiency

The complex nature of the molybdenum cofactor and the unstable dithiolene group in particular have led to the evolution of elaborate and unique mechanisms for cofactor synthesis. The presence of a multistep pathway for molybdenum cofactor biosynthesis in humans makes it likely that there are multiple sites where genetic lesions could occur, each resulting in the phenotype of molybdenum cofactor deficiency (see footnotes at the beginning of this chapter). Indeed, evidence that this is the case has been presented.[64] When fibroblasts from either of two cofactor-deficient siblings were cocultured with cells from any of seven other unrelated molybdenum cofactor-deficient patients, sulfite oxidase activity was expressed. Complementation occurred without heterokaryon formation and was achieved even when cells from one complementation group (A) were cultured in medium conditioned by prior culture of cells from group B patients, suggesting the presence of a diffusible precursor of molybdopterin in the conditioned medium. The complementation groups were further delineated as representative of defects early (A, OMIM No. 252150) or late (B, OMIM No. 252160) in the biosynthetic pathway based on the presence or absence of precursor Z in the urine.

Patients in the A complementation group are likely to be defective in enzymes equivalent to MoaA or MoaC in *E. coli* and thus unable to synthesize precursor Z. The human homologues of *moaA* and *moaC*, *MOCS1A* and *MOCS1B*, have been identified, and a patient with a single-base deletion in *MOCS1A* and one with a two-base deletion in *MOCS1B* have been reported[65] (see footnotes at the beginning of this chapter). The genes are present as two open reading frames on a single polycistronic nuclear gene, a very unusual occurrence in eukaryotes. As in *E. coli*, however, the specific catalytic function of the two proteins encoded by these genes has not been determined.

Group A patients would be expected to retain a functional molybdopterin synthase. Indeed, the presence of a molybdopterin synthase activity that can activate precursor Z has been demonstrated in fibroblasts and liver tissue from group A cofactor-deficient patients.[64,66] Group B patients, on the other hand, are expected to have defects in this function or in the synthase sulfurylase. The human equivalents of the *E. coli* genes *moaD*, *moaE*, and *moeB* have been identified,[67] and sequencing of the cDNAs from group B patients is underway. The large and small subunits of molybdopterin synthase in humans appear to be coded for by overlapping gene segments, with the reading frames shifted from each other by one base.[67] The predicted human equivalent of the *E. coli* molybdopterin synthase sulfurylase is considerably larger than the *E. coli* protein, with extensions at both the N- and C-terminal ends. The possible role of the extra peptide segments has not been determined.

The final stages of molybdenum cofactor assembly in humans, involving absorption, transport, and incorporation of the metal, are poorly understood at this point, and no patients have been identified who make molybdopterin but fail to generate the functional molybdenum complex. However, one may anticipate that defects in molybdenum uptake, transport, and/or processing could occur and that these would result in molybdenum cofactor deficiency (analogous to *mod* or *mog*). Since these defects potentially could be overcome by administration of higher levels of the metal by appropriate routes, it is important to be alert for those variants of cofactor deficiency which might respond to molybdate administration. A 130-base segment of sequence from the human genome corresponds very closely to a portion of *modA*, suggesting that human homologues of the *mod* operon exist. However, searches of several human cDNA libraries for *mog* homologues[67] detected exclusively the neural portion gephyrin, which has been implicated in the mobilization of glycinergic receptors and has been shown to bind to tubulin.[68] The possible role of gephyrin in molybdenum cofactor biosynthesis is currently being investigated.

Shalata et al.[69] have begun the task of mapping the genetic loci responsible for cofactor biosynthesis in humans using homozygosity mapping and two consanguineous affected kindreds of Israeli-Arab origin including five patients. They have demonstrated the linkage of a molybdenum cofactor synthetic gene to an 8-cM region on chromosome 6p21.3 between the markers *D6S1641* and *D6S1672*. These results provide a conventient method for prenatal diagnosis of molybdenum cofactor deficiency in families affected at this particular locus as well as the first means of identification of heterozygous carriers of the defective gene.

Molecular Analysis of Defects in Isolated Sulfite Oxidase Deficiency

The rat[70] and human[71] sulfite oxidase (symbol *SUOX*) genes have been cloned and sequenced, and molecular defects associated with cases of isolated sulfite oxidase deficiency have been determined, as summarized in Table 128-1. The first mutation identified[72] was a single-base deletion, cytosine 400, leading to a shift in the reading frame with termination of translation following amino acid 145. The last 12 amino acids of the truncated protein are out of frame and unrelated to sulfite oxidase. The heme domain of the sulfite oxidase protein is not affected, but a major portion of the molybdenum domain is absent. Other deletion mutations identified[73] include a 4-base deletion in one patient and a 16-base deletion in another. In the latter case, the deletion is located close to the 3′ end of the sulfite oxidase coding region, suggesting that the C-terminal region of the protein is essential for catalytic function. To date, a single patient with an insertion mutation has been identified. In this individual, an extra cytosine causes a shift in the reading frame and early termination before even the heme domain is completed.

Single-base mutations have been identified in several patients.[73] A nonsense mutation, identified in two sisters, introduces a stop

Table 128-1 Mutations in the Sulfite Oxidase Gene Identified in Patients with Isolated Sulfite Oxidase Deficiency

	Base Change	Predicted Effect	Reference
A. Deletions	400delC	Premature termination	72
	562-565delCTTT	Premature termination	73
	1233-1248del	Premature termination	73
B. Insertions	113-114insC	Premature termination	73
C. Missense	479G > A*	R160Q*	74
	623C > A	A208D	Unpublished†
	634C > T	R212C	Unpublished†
	965A > G	K322R	Unpublished†
	1090C > T	Q364X	73
	1109C > A	S370Y	Unpublished†
	1418G > A	G473D	73

NOTE: Numbering of nucleotides is based on the cDNA sequence, with the A of the ATG of the initiator methionine codon denoted nucleotide +1. Numbering of amino acids is also from the initiator methionine, which is the first amino acid in the 22-residue leader sequence of sulfite oxidase.

*The 479G > A (*R160Q*) mutation has been found in two patients. One is homozygous for the mutation; the other has an *R212C* mutation on the second allele.

†Johnson JL, Garrett RM, Graf TN, Rajagopalan KV, et al.

codon in place of a glutamine (*Q364X*), with truncation of the protein in the molybdenum domain. A glycine-to-aspartate substitution at residue 473 seen in one patient occurs in the third domain of the sulfite oxidase subunit very close to the C-terminus of the protein. Characterization of recombinant protein bearing this mutation has revealed a monomeric protein with little catalytic activity, confirming the significance of the third-domain in maintaining the normal dimeric structure of the enzyme. Another third-domain mutation, *S370Y*, seen in a different patient, also leads to a monomeric, nonfunctional enzyme. Several informative missense mutations occur at the active site of the enzyme and include an arginine-to-glutamine substitution at residue 160.[74] This arginine falls in a region of sequence that is highly conserved between the rat and human sulfite oxidases as well as in related molybdoenzymes from other sources. Kinetic analysis of the purified recombinant mutant protein has shown that it is partially active, but its K_m for sulfite is highly increased, and its K_{cat} is decreased. The apparent in vivo inefficiency of the enzyme results from the significant decrease in K_{cat}/K_m for the mutant protein compared with the wild-type enzyme. The corresponding arginine in the crystallized chicken liver enzyme was positioned within the substrate-binding pocket and has been proposed to attract the negatively charged sulfite ion to the enzyme reactive center.[21] Two other mutations affecting the active site of the enzyme include changes at residues 208 (A to D) and 212 (R to C). Both of these lie within a highly conserved region neighboring cysteine 207, the protein ligand to the molybdenum. A mutation affecting residue 322 (K to R) is of considerable interest because, from the crystal structure, the corresponding lysine in the chicken liver enzyme is predicted to be involved in molybdopterin binding through hydrogen bonding between the lysine main-chain —NH and the pterin N-1, the lysine carbonyl and the 2-amino group of the pterin, and the lysine epsilon amino group and an oxygen of the pterin phosphate. These interactions entail extremely precise alignment such that even conservative replacement of lysine with arginine would likely result in a protein with an altered mode of molybdopterin binding or no incorporation of the pterin.

Of the mutations characterized thus far in patients with isolated sulfite oxidase deficiency, only one, the *R160Q* substitution, has been noted in more than one individual; the allele involves a CpG dinucleotide which is hypermutable and could be recurrent on independent chromosomes. Two patients have been identified with differing mutations on the two alleles, but most are homozygous for a single mutation, consistent with the high degree of consanguinity in the families studied to date. Thus far no extensive correlation has been noted between the specific mutation and the degree of severity of clinical symptoms. However, the residual activity, albeit low, observed in the *R160Q* mutant protein is in accord with the relatively mild clinical course in a patient homozygous for that allele.[74]

CLINICAL ASPECTS OF MOLYBDENUM COFACTOR DEFICIENCY AND ISOLATED SULFITE OXIDASE DEFICIENCY

Clinical Phenotype

Molybdenum cofactor deficiency (OMIM Nos. 252150 and 252160) and isolated sulfite oxidase deficiency (OMIM No. 272300) are not extremely rare inborn errors of metabolism. Thus far more than 100 patients with one of these two defects have been identified. The incidence of molybdenum cofactor deficiency appears to be somewhat higher than that of isolated sulfite oxidase deficiency. However, recognition of the former condition is easier, since severe hypouricemia will be picked up by most clinical laboratories, whereas sulfite oxidase deficiency can only be recognized by the presence of compounds not routinely tested for such as sulfite, thiosulfate, and *S*-sulfocysteine. Data on 52 molybdenum cofactor–deficient patients and 16 sulfite oxidase–deficient patients are shown in Table 128-2. Although the general clinical profiles are similar, the sulfite oxidase–deficient group contains more late-onset patients in whom the disease has a relatively milder course.

Both molybdenum cofactor deficiency and isolated sulfite oxidase deficiency appear in many ethnic groups. Patients have been identified among the populations of Europe, North America, Northern Africa, Turkey, and Asia. Patients identified since the last edition of this work have been heavily concentrated in the Netherlands, Germany, the United Kingdom, France, the United States, and Canada, most probably due to greater recognition of the disease among clinicians in these countries. The patients identified include Caucasian and non-Caucasian individuals, the latter for the most part from Asian and northern African countries now resident in western Europe. The mode of inheritance of both deficiencies is autosomal recessive, with nearly equal numbers of males and females affected. Obligate heterozygotes do not display any symptoms.

Table 128-2 Incidence of Reported Signs and Symptoms in 52 Molybdenum Cofactor–Deficient Patients and 16 Patients with Isolated Sulfite Oxidase Deficiency

	Molybdenum Cofactor Deficiency	Isolated Sulfite Oxidase Deficiency
Seizures	49/52	9/14
Psychomotor retardation	41/43	11/14
Ectopic lenses	22/36	4/7
Dysmorphic signs	20/27	2/2
Hypertonicity	23/26	5/5
Hypotonia	19/26	8/8
Dilated ventricles	20/23	4/5
Brain hypodensity	20/23	5/6
Brain atrophy	16/19	3/4
Spastic tetraplegia	21/23	
Opisthotonus	11/18	
Enophthalmos	7/15	
Hydrocephalus	7/13	
Myoclonus	10/14	
Late onset	5/52	8/13
Feeding difficulties		4/4

Molybdenum cofactor deficiency is a serious and often fatal disease. Many of the known patients died at an early age, and several others were severely affected children cared for in institutions. The onset of symptoms (see Table 128-2) is usually in the first days after birth, although nearly all patients were born after an uneventful pregnancy and delivery with adequate Apgar scores. Feeding difficulties start soon after birth, and severe and characteristic neurologic symptoms develop. The neurologic picture includes tonic/clonic seizures observed in many patients, axial hypotonia, and peripheral hypertonicity. The seizures are difficult to suppress. Progression is variable, although the general level of mental development is extremely poor. Lens dislocation develops in patients who survive the neonatal period. Other ophthamologic abnormalities may include spherophakia, nystagmus, cortical blindness, enophthalmos, and iris coloboma,[75,76] all in varying frequency.

Fewer than 10 percent of the molybdenum cofactor–deficient patients had a late-onset presentation. These patients do present a diagnostic challenge. No clear clinical hallmarks have been defined in these milder cases, but interestingly, one patient had clinical symptoms more typical of classic homocystinuria.[77] In those cofactor-deficient patients who develop symptoms after the neonatal period, some incident such as an infection usually precipitates onset of the disease.

The clinical symptoms of patients with isolated sulfite oxidase deficiency are generally quite similar to those of patients with molybdenum cofactor deficiency (see Table 128-2), even though molybdenum cofactor and xanthine dehydrogenase functions are normal. However, symptoms in the isolated deficiency appear to be somewhat more variable than those of molybdenum cofactor–deficient patients. The first patient described with the isolated deficiency[7,8] was very severely affected with many neurologic abnormalities, including severe mental retardation, seizures, and opisthotonos. Lens dislocation was found at age 2, and the patient died at age $2\frac{1}{2}$. The late-onset patient, especially, may lack the suggestive symptoms, such as seizures or ectopic lenses (see Table 128-2). The onset of change in clinical presentation in these milder cases varied between 6 and 15 months, and in many cases a sudden event such as an infection triggered the onset of symptoms, often dystonia and developmental regression. Increased catabolism associated with the stress may result in an increased availability of cysteine, leading to an acute sulfite intoxication. The harmful potential of excess cysteine was suggested by the death of the first patient with isolated sulfite oxidase deficiency following a cysteine loading test.[7] Ophthamologic abnormalities, including spherophakia, have been described in patients with isolated sulfite oxidase deficiency,[72,75] similar to those reported in molybdenum cofactor deficiency.

Although some variability in severity of symptoms and age of onset does occur, the key clinical symptom for both molybdenum cofactor deficiency and isolated sulfite oxidase deficiency is severe convulsions not responding to therapy appearing soon after birth. All patients with these symptoms immediately should be subjected to the metabolic screening procedures described in this chapter. Even to date the clinical phenotype of sulfite oxidase deficiency is not generally known among pediatricians and neurologists. Diagnostic delay or failure may result in the birth of new patients in families at risk. Patients in whom the primary diagnosis is unrecognized are often described clinically as having *infantile encephalopathy* with reference to anatomic brain anomalies and neurologic symptoms.

As the population of patients identified with molybdenum cofactor deficiency and isolated sulfite oxidase deficiency has increased, it has become possible to carry out more meaningful studies characterizing the dysmorphic facial features associated with these disease states. It has been noted[78] that the majority of patients with molybdenum cofactor deficiency have a remarkably similar appearance, with features that include a long face with puffy cheeks, widely spaced eyes, elongated palpebral fissures, thick lips, a long philtrum, and a small nose. Patients with severe neonatal isolated sulfite oxidase deficiency may display the same dysmorphic features as in molybdenum cofactor deficiency. These features, which resemble those observed in cases of perinatal asphyxia and can be of considerable diagnostic value, are illustrated in a collection of patient photographs presented in Fig. 128-5. Although these patients often have a normal head circumference at birth, progressive microcephaly is common. In contrast, several patients have been described with macrocephaly associated with hydrocephalus. Since virtually all patients with molybdenum cofactor deficiency and with isolated sulfite oxidase deficiency had a normal delivery following an uncomplicated pregnancy, it is advisable to screen for these disorders in every child with the signs and symptoms of perinatal asphyxia but no apparent hypoxic event at birth.

Pathology and Neuroradiologic Evaluation

Results of pathologic investigations are available from several patients with molybdenum cofactor deficiency. The most detailed are from a patient described by Roth et al.[79] Macroscopic study revealed severe cerebral atrophy and extreme microgyria with fine vermiform, tortuous convolutions separated by wide and deep sulci, a feature that was less marked in the gyri hippocampi. No necrosis, softening, hemorrhage, or tumors were noted. There was enlargement of the lateral and fourth ventricles, with multicystic subcortical and juxtacortical focal lesions in the white matter. Microscopic examination revealed lesions in the frontal, temporal, and occipital cortexes characterized by a marked loss of neurons. These were replaced by an astrocytic gliosis and accumulation of microgliocytic granular bodies. In the deeper layers, the cortical lesions were accompanied by microcavitations and spongiosis with an astrocytic granulosis and microgliocytic granular bodies. In the white matter, demyelination was noted, combined with a marked axonal loss. In the cerebellum, granular and Purkinje cells were scarce, but no other noteworthy lesions were seen.

Pathologic studies in a patient described by Barth et al.[80] revealed brain shrinkage and severe loss of neurons, particularly in all layers of the isocortex, thalamus, and basal ganglia. Paucity of myelin in the long tracts was noticed, along with isomorphic gliosis. There was a diffuse spongiosis affecting both the neutrophil and white-matter structures.

In a patient described by Roesel et al.,[20] the right side of the brain was considerably smaller than the left. The left side contained mostly gray matter with only small amounts of white;

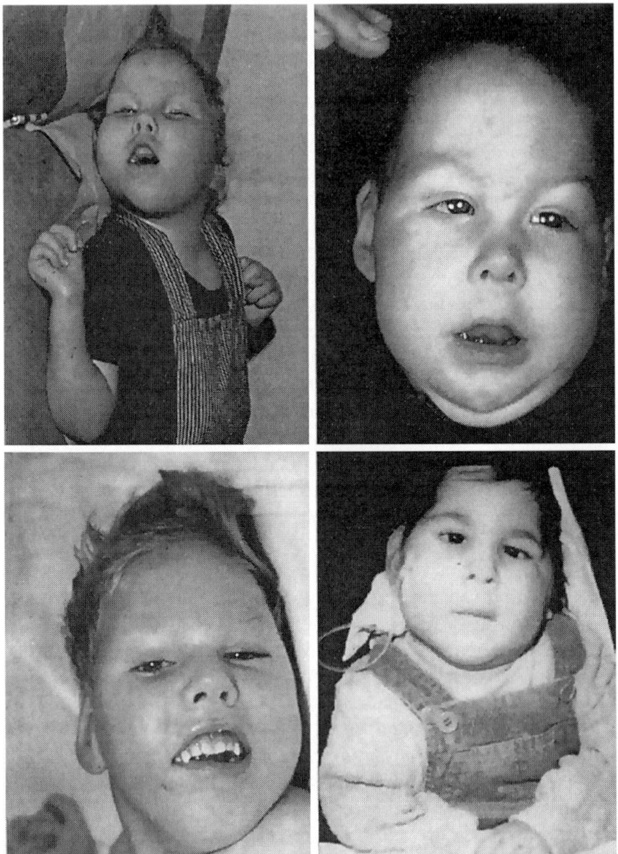

Fig. 128-5 Facial features of patients with molybdenum cofactor deficiency [patient 1, *top left*[4]; *patient 2, top right*[117]; and patient 3, *bottom left*[83]] and isolated sulfite oxidase deficiency [patient 4, *bottom right*[118]]. All had the characteristic puffy cheeks, long philtrum, and small nose. Patient 2 was not microcephalic. All photographs are used with permission. (*In publication of these photographs, we acknowledge the following individuals: patient 1, Dr. F. Beemer; patient 2, Drs. J. B. C. de Klerk and J. G. M. Huijmans; patient 3, Drs. H. D. Bakker and A. H. van Gennip; patient 4, Dr. W. Brussel. The photograph of patient 1 was published originally by Bohn Stafleu Van Loghum Publishers.*)

the right side, more white than gray. There was considerable gliosis on the right side and multiple dark purplish deposits. The right cerebellar hemisphere also was atrophic and showed extensive gliosis. The highly asymmetric effects seen in this patient point to a more complex etiology of disease than simply a uniform exposure to a toxic metabolite. Local tissue destruction may have caused protein breakdown and catabolism of cysteine resulting in excessive sulfite formation.

Cranial computed tomography (CT) on a patient described by Endres et al.[81] revealed decreased density of the white matter at age 4 weeks and at age 3 months a generalized decrease of cerebral substance with hydrocephalus. In a patient described by Aukett et al.,[82] ultrasound examination of the head demonstrated slight dilatation of the ventricles. A CT scan of the head was abnormal, showing marked attenuation of brain tissue, sparing only the most superficial layers of the cortex and the deep central gray matter and subependymal regions.

Neuroradiologic imaging studies have been extended to include additional cases of molybdenum cofactor deficiency. Severe cortical atrophy and thalamic calcifications resembling sequelae of asphyxia were observed by CT in one patient.[83] In a study of two sets of affected siblings,[84] all four showed multicystic leukencephalopathy and a normal newborn pattern of myelination of brain stem. This was followed, however, by a massive, in some cases progressive, destruction of the white matter together with enlargement of the ventricles and cerebrospinal fluid spaces. An abnormal orientation and atypical shape of the frontal horns of the dilated ventricles were noted in all four patients, as well as in several additional patients with CT results published earlier. The distortion was attributed to severe volume loss of the basal ganglia and thinning of the corpus callosum. Magnetic resonance imaging (MRI) was noted to be superior to CT in the demonstration of these lesions. CT studies of two additional patients[85] obtained soon after birth indicated normal brain development in one patient but in the second demonstrated diffuse low attenuation in the cerebral white matter and in the caudate nuclei and thalami. Follow-up MRI studies[85] of these patients demonstrated progressive widening of the sulci, ventricles, and cisterna magna and a loss of brain volume, with cessation of myelination at 31 months and 16 weeks of age, respectively.

The MRI changes of the mildest cases of molybdenum cofactor deficiency[86] showed a bilaterally increased signal intensity in lentiform nuclei extending to involve caudate nuclei and cerebral peduncle. Dilated ventricles were not reported in these patients.

Pathologic studies of a patient with isolated sulfite oxidase deficiency were described by Rosenblum.[87] The brain of this patient also displayed a massive loss of neurons and their axons, with intense demyelination and glial proliferation consisting of multiple discrete cavitary formations in the deep cerebral white matter. Cystic and gliotic lesions also were found in basal ganglia, thalamus, and cerebellum.

Detailed neuroradiologic studies on two patients with isolated sulfite oxidase deficiency have been reported by Brown et al.[88] The first patient showed cerebral edema on CT examination in the neonatal period that progressed to a severe neuropathy by age $3\frac{1}{2}$ years. Gross cerebral and cerebellar atrophy was observed, with a marked increase in the depth of the sulci, an abnormal gyral pattern, and grossly dilated ventricles. There were a number of apparent cystic spaces in the basal ganglia and some areas of focal calcification, particularly in the occipital lobe and parietal cortex. The second patient also showed cerebral edema by CT at 1 week of age. By 1 month, significant cerebral abnormalities were seen, with decreased density throughout the white matter and mild ventricular dilatation, and by 6 months, gross neuropathologic changes comparable with those seen in the first patient at $3\frac{1}{2}$ years were already visible.

Neuropathologic investigations were carried out on the second patient.[88] The brain weight was less than half that of normal. The cerebrum was moderately atrophic and showed severe loss of white matter, with dilatation of the lateral and third ventricles. Numerous subcortical cysts up to 1 cm in diameter were present throughout all lobes. There was complete degeneration of the cerebral cortex in the medial frontal lobes anteriorly and some gyral atrophy in the occipital and parietal lobes. Chalky white areas of calcification were noted in the residual white matter. The thalami, basal ganglia, cerebellar folia, and dentate nucleus were all atrophic. Microscopic examination showed a diffuse loss of myelin in the cerebral white matter with gliosis, cystic spaces, and focal deposits of calcification. In the cerebellum, there was severe loss of Purkinje cells and increased Bergmann layer glia. The dentate nucleus showed virtual total neuron loss and extensive gliosis. The cerebellar white matter had little myelin and marked gliosis.

MRI studies of a fourth patient[72] at 13 months of age revealed marked gyral atrophy, leukomalacia with prominent cystic changes, thinning of the corpus callosum, and ventricular enlargement. The neuropathologic abnormalities in this patient also were noted to resemble changes that might occur as a consequence of severe perinatal asphyxia.

Overall, the similarities between the lesions in the molybdenum cofactor deficiencies and those observed in patients with isolated sulfite oxidase deficiency suggest strongly that the cerebral lesions are due to the consequences of sulfite oxidase deficiency. Xanthine dehydrogenase deficiency does not result in encephalopathy, nor does the combined deficiency of xanthine

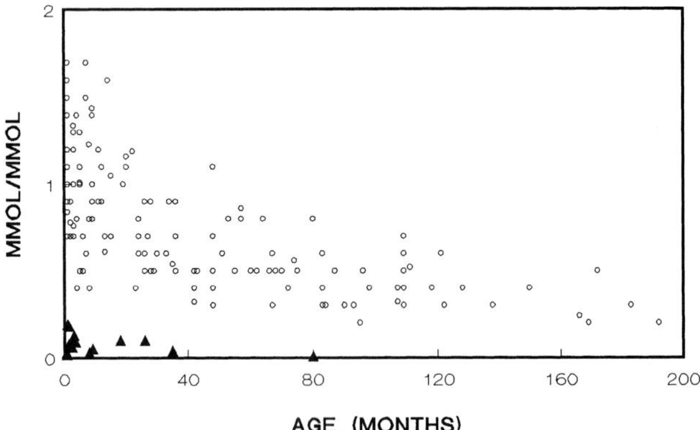

Fig. 128-6 Urinary uric acid excretion expressed as mmol/mmol creatinine in subjects who were referred for selective screening of inborn errors in whom no defect could be found (○) and in patients with molybdenum cofactor deficiency (▲).

dehydrogenase and aldehyde oxidase. Thus the encephalopathy of molybdenum cofactor deficiency can be ascribed to the absence of sulfite oxidase activity.

Biochemical Hallmarks and Clinical Diagnosis

Abnormal Metabolites and Metabolic Screening Procedures. In sulfite oxidase deficiency, sulfite accumulates and sulfate production is decreased. Sulfite overflow is apparently moderated to some extent by an enhanced degradation of cysteine sulfinate to taurine (see Fig. 128-2). Taurine production is invariably increased in this condition. The presence of elevated levels of sulfite leads to accumulation of *S*-sulfocysteine formed by direct reaction of sulfite with cyst(e)ine. Increased levels of thiosulfate are also characteristic of sulfite oxidase deficiency as a consequence of elevated sulfite. Catabolism of cysteine by transamination produces mercaptopyruvate (see Fig. 128-2). Transsulfuration of mercaptopyruvate provides a source of reduced sulfur that combines with sulfite to yield thiosulfate. Urinary sulfate is not a useful parameter because of the lack of a well-defined control range in young children. Molybdenum cofactor–deficient patients still excrete sulfate, which may reflect catabolism of sulfated mucopolysaccharides and glycolipids as well as unused dietary sulfate.

Xanthine dehydrogenase deficiency presents with markedly elevated urinary xanthine and moderately increased hypoxanthine. Uric acid is low, decreased both in urine and in plasma. The evaluation of urinary uric acid expressed as millimoles per millimole of creatinine may be facilitated by comparing the excretion values with those of age-matched controls (see Fig. 128-6). However, since uric acid levels are not always severely depressed, the differential diagnosis of isolated sulfite oxidase deficiency versus molybdenum cofactor deficiency is best made on the basis of the establishment of urinary xanthine and hypoxanthine levels rather than on an analysis of uric acid levels alone. A specific metabolic consequence of molybdenum cofactor deficiency that is useful in diagnosis is the absence of urinary urothione, believed to be the excreted degradation product of molybdopterin.[11] Urothione excretion is normal in patients with an isolated deficiency of sulfite oxidase.

All patients with sulfite oxidase deficiency display a characteristic metabolic profile, although excretory levels of the various metabolites vary substantially due to differences in protein intake, catabolism, and creatinine production. For diagnosis of molybdenum cofactor deficiency or isolated sulfite oxidase deficiency, urinary sulfite is easily detected with a dipstick test (Merkoquant 10013 Sulfit Test or Macherey-Nagel Quantofix $SO_3^{=}$, Gallard Schlesinger, Carle Place, New York), but fresh urine must be used because sulfite is rapidly destroyed by oxidation at room temperature. Not all patients consistently show a positive reaction on the sulfite test strip; in several cases of sulfite oxidase deficiency the initial sulfite test was negative,[82,89,90] whereas in another case the test was only positive on two of three occasions.[72] False-positive reactions are also seen sometimes. The mucolytic drug 2-mercaptoethanesulfonate, for instance, produces a positive test.[91] For these reasons, the dipstick test should be used as a screening procedure only. Quantitative determinations of sulfite, thiosulfate, and sulfate are best performed with anion-column chromatography.[92,93]

S-Sulfocysteine is a stable metabolite and an excellent marker of sulfite oxidase deficiency. It can be identified in urine samples by high-voltage electrophoresis and quantitated by amino acid analysis or derivatized with Dabsyl-Cl and quantitated by HPLC.[94] Electrospray tandem mass spectrometry of dried filter blood spots[95] is also used to quantitate amino acids and can easily detect *S*-sulfocysteine using the 102-Da constant-neutral-loss technique (N. Chamoles, personal communication).

The analysis of other sulfur amino acids can be an additional diagnostic tool. Due to the strong reactivity of sulfite, cyst(e)ine is depleted, and consequently, unusually low plasma cystine levels will be found. Ahomocysteinemia, as measured with the standard HPLC assay for plasma homocysteine, recently has been demonstrated in a patient with molybdenum cofactor deficiency.[96]

To distinguish between molybdenum cofactor deficiency and isolated sulfite oxidase deficiency, numerous procedures are available for quantitation of urinary and plasma oxypurines. The HPLC assay described by Simmonds et al.[97] is very effective. Urothione can be measured by the HPLC assay described by Johnson and Rajagopalan.[11]

Urinary accumulation of *S*-sulfocysteine and thiosulfate, together with sulfothiocysteine, but with normal sulfite, taurine, cystine, and homocysteine, can be found in patients with the so-called ethylmalonic acid syndrome.[98] Affected patients have severe neurologic dysfunction, diarrhea, and petechiae. At least 20 patients are known worldwide. At present, no biochemical defect has been identified, but there is an association with the metabolism of methionine.[99]

Enzyme and Molybdenum Cofactor Assays. When appropriate tissue samples are available, the absence of sulfite oxidase and xanthine dehydrogenase activities can be verified directly. Liver samples from three patients have been tested for the presence of active molybdenum cofactor using a preparation of rat liver demolybdo sulfite oxidase as the acceptor molecule.[100,101] While liver tissue from control individuals contained cofactor that could reconstitute sulfite oxidase activity, samples from the patients failed to do so.[3] Similarly, when liver tissue from these patients was treated to convert molybdopterin to the form A derivative, none was detected.

All molybdenum cofactor–deficient patients tested to date have shown normal levels of plasma molybdenum. However, in the two patients in whom it has been measured, hepatic molybdenum has been found to be severely decreased.[3,20] This finding suggests that virtually all hepatic molybdenum is present in cofactor form and that, in the absence of functional cofactor to bind the metal, any molybdenum taken up by the cells is rapidly exported.

Prenatal Diagnosis. Sulfite oxidase is expressed in amniotic cells, and assay of this activity in cultured amniocytes has been used successfully many times for prenatal diagnosis of molybdenum cofactor deficiency.[102,103] Activities are quite low, however, even in normal cells, so several million cells are required for each assay. Sulfite oxidase is present at high levels in chorionic villi obtained at 10 to 14 weeks' gestation and can be assayed directly in the biopsy sample without cell culture.[104] This assay has been applied successfully to pregnancies at risk for molybdenum cofactor deficiency[104,105] and those at risk for isolated sulfite oxidase deficiency. Measurement of *S*-sulfocysteine in amniotic fluid is of value in prenatal diagnosis and can be accomplished very rapidly.[102] Free sulfite has not been detected in amniotic fluid samples.

Pathogenesis

There is as yet no documented evidence that defines the biochemical basis of the pathology associated with molybdenum cofactor deficiency. We have concluded that the severe neurologic abnormalities are a consequence of the absence of sulfite oxidase activity, but it is not clear whether the brain damage occurs as a result of accumulation of a toxic metabolite or perhaps because of a deficit in the reaction product (sulfate). If the damage arises from a toxic metabolite, a possible candidate is sulfite itself. Exogenous sulfite is classified as a slightly toxic compound that is readily oxidized to sulfate in the intestine, lung, and liver.[40] In patients with sulfite oxidase deficiency, however, there is accumulation of endogenously formed sulfite, sometimes added to by an exogenous burden as well, which overflows into the body fluids. It is not known whether plasma sulfite can pass the blood-brain barrier; however, sulfite oxidase is present in the human brain,[8] suggesting that the sulfinate pathway is operative and cerebral sulfite production occurs. Even before birth, accumulation of sulfite takes place in affected fetuses, as evidenced by the demonstration of *S*-sulfocysteine in amniotic fluid. The toxicity of sulfite at the biochemical level has been discussed extensively.[106] The compound readily attacks disulfide bonds according to the reaction $RSSR' + HSO_3^- \rightarrow RSSO_3^- + R'SH$; reaction with free SH groups can occur as well. Sulfite may destroy thiamine,[107] which could lead to disturbed pyruvate metabolism in cell compartments of the central nervous system. Unsaturated fatty acids are susceptible to attack by sulfite, with possible compromise of membrane integrity.[108] Also, reactions of sulfite with nucleic acids have been considered, but no direct evidence for mutagenic defects in humans have been shown to date.[106]

The mode of interference of sulfite with processes at the molecular level in sulfite oxidase deficiency is completely unknown. The reaction of sulfite with disulfide bonds or with sulfhydryl groups is a general process that would be expected to occur in all organs and not particularly in certain areas of the brain. However, the central nervous system may be especially sensitive to sulfite, with certain parts affected more than others. This could occur either because of local differences in sulfite production or supply of the precursor cysteine or as a result of disturbance of a delicate chemical process such as neurotransmitter function, perhaps unique to specific areas of the brain. Ocular lens subluxation, a common feature of sulfite oxidase deficiency, also might arise as a consequence of disruption of cystine crosslinking by excess sulfite.[7]

Other metabolites that accumulate as a result of sulfite oxidase deficiency appear to be less toxic than sulfite. Thiosulfate and *S*-sulfocysteine might be considered in a sense as detoxification products. However, the severe neurologic abnormalities of the ethylmalonic acid syndrome[98,99] may cast some doubt on this statement. Taurine is a normal metabolite of cysteine oxidation (see Fig. 128-4) and is unlikely to be toxic.

Finally, the possibility that a disturbed development of the brain in sulfite oxidase deficiency occurs as a result of sulfate deficiency must be considered, even though sulfate is a normal dietary constituent and is excreted in the urine by the patients. The extent to which it is made available to brain tissues in the developing fetus and after birth is not clear. Sulfite oxidase may in fact be an important source of the sulfate required for formation of the sulfatides of neural tissue. Percy et al.[109] examined the composition and quantities of sulfate esters in brain and kidney tissue of a patient with isolated sulfite oxidase deficiency and also measured excretion of indoxyl-3-sulfate and tyrosine-*O*-sulfate. Sulfatides were present in normal concentrations and were of normal composition (i.e., substitution of sulfite for sulfate in the esterified products was ruled out). To date, there are no indications of general abnormalities of the sulfation of mucopolysaccharides and glycolipids.

Therapy

Thus far no therapeutic attempts have successfully reversed the clinical symptoms of molybdenum cofactor deficiency. However, certain measures have been implemented that may be of some benefit to individual patients. The first measure is to diminish sulfite production by restriction of the intake of the precursor sulfur-containing amino acids. Considerable success has been achieved with this approach in two patients with mild isolated sulfite oxidase deficiency.[110] Neither patient had seizures under this regimen (during 12 months of therapy), growth was normal, and there were no signs of neurologic deterioration and evident progress in psychomotor development. When selecting diets for this purpose, it is important that the amino acid mixture be low in both methionine and cystine (such as provided by Xmet cys Maxamaid SHS, Liverpool, United Kingdom).

The administration of thiol compounds with the potential to bind sulfite such as penicillamine[81,111] and mercaptoethanesulfonate[81] has been attempted without success. However, it has been noted[112] that these compounds react very poorly with sulfite. In contrast, cysteine, homocysteine, oxidized glutathione, and cysteamine disulfide were readily sulfonated in vitro. Cysteamine in particular may be beneficial in attempts to absorb excess sulfite in patients with sulfite oxidase deficiency. The general problem with this type of approach is to reach sufficiently high intracellular concentrations of the drug, in this case especially in the central nervous system. Extra thiamine may be given to protect against a possible deficiency of this vitamin. In view of the potential ramifications of sulfate deficiency, as have been discussed, it may be beneficial to supplement the diet with inorganic sulfate.

The administration of ammonium molybdate could be useful in patients in whom deficiency of molybdenum cofactor is a consequence of a defect in metal transport or uptake. Thus far, no patients have been identified with such a defect; however, the isolation of bacterial mutants with pleiotropic loss of several molybdoenzymes that is corrected by growth on high molybdate[113] raises the possibility that a similar defect may arise in the human population.

Fujitaka et al.[114] attempted treatment of the combined-deficiency disease in one patient by administration of tetrahydrobiopterin. The absence of clinical or biochemical improvement was consistent with information already available indicating that tetrahydrobiopterin and the molybdenum cofactor are distinct biochemical entities synthesized by nonoverlapping biosynthetic pathways and which serve unique biological functions (see also Chap. 78).

Based on the structural similarities of *S*-sulfocysteine and glutamic acid, it was postulated that molybdenum cofactor deficiency is a model of an *N*-methyl-D-aspartate (NMDA) receptor–related neurodegenerative disease attributed to overstimulation of the NMDA receptor.[115,116] Consequently, Kurlemann et al.[116] treated a 3-year-old patient with dextromethorphan, an NMDA receptor antagonist. With a dose of 12.5 mg/kg of body weight, the seizures stopped, and the EEG showed significant improvement. The drug was well tolerated with minimal side effects.

The seizures associated with molybdenum cofactor deficiency and with isolated sulfite oxidase deficiency have long been considered to be refractive to therapy. With the introduction of novel antiepileptic drugs, this view may change. There are several patients currently being treated with vigabatrin therapy who have become free of convulsions. As the pathways of molybdenum cofactor biosynthesis and metabolism are elucidated in more detail and the defects in human molybdenum cofactor deficiency are further defined at the molecular level, the possibility of effective therapy based on administration of stabilized cofactor derivatives or the appropriate precursors should become possible.

ADDENDUM

Molybdenum Cofactor Biosynthesis

Significant progress has been made in understanding the pathway of molybdenum cofactor biosynthesis, primarily as a result of the purification and crystallization of the various biosynthetic enzymes from *E. coli*. The product of the *moaA* gene has remained refractory to purification due to its extreme insolubility and tendency to aggregate even in the presence of thiol-protecting agents; however, MoaC,[119] the MoaD/MoaE complex (Rudolph, Wuebbens, Rajagopalan and Schindelin, submitted for publication), MoeB (Schindelin et al., unpublished), MogA,[120] and most recently MoeA (Schindelin et al., unpublished) have all yielded diffraction quality crystals, and their structures have been solved at high resolution. MoaC is a tightly packed hexamer with putative active sites located at the interfaces of each monomer pair. MogA is related to the protein gephyrin and has a trimeric structure. The role of gephyrin in molybdenum cofactor biosynthesis in higher organisms has been solidified by the demonstration that gephyrin knockout mice lack molybdoenzyme activity[121] and by the documented ability of gephyrin to reconstitute molybdenum cofactor biosynthesis in a number of mutant cell lines.[122]

Molecular Characterization of Molybdenum Cofactor Deficiency and Isolated Sulfite Oxidase Deficiency

Molecular work characterizing molybdenum cofactor deficiency and isolated sulfite oxidase deficiency has been extended as more patients of both classes have been identified. The genomic structures of *MOCS1A* and *MOCS1B* have been reported along with a number of mutations in each.[123,124] The unusual bicistronic nature suggested that the two genes are transcribed independently generating two distinct proteins. In particular the C-terminal gly-gly motif of MOCS1A, with its parallel in MOCS2A and ubiquitin, implied that MOCS1A is translated exclusively from a monocistronic transcript. However, this conclusion has been called into question by a recent report demonstrating alternative splicing mechanisms that result in fusion of the two open reading frames. These alternative splicings are evolutionarily highly conserved, bypass the normal termination nonsense codon of *MOCS1A*, and produce "no-nonsense" transcripts that encode a single bifunctional protein embodying both MOCS1A and MOCS1B activities, in addition to the MOCS1A translated from monocistronic *MOCS1A*.[125] It is clear that in vivo protein studies will be required to establish with certainty whether the activities in humans exist on independent proteins as in *E. coli* and *Arabidopsis* or whether they are present on a single, bidomain polypeptide.

The structure of the human gene encoding molybdopterin synthase also contains two open reading frames, *MOCS2A* and *MOCS2B*, in this case with overlap and a shift in the reading frame.[126–128] The gene was mapped to chromosome 5[126,128] and comprises seven exons.[128] Mutations were identified in seven patients in whom previous screenings for mutations in *MOCS1A* and *MOCS1B* were negative.[128] Again, although studies reported by Reiss and coworkers suggest that MOCS2A and MOCS2B are made as independent polypeptides, the *MOCS2* locus is also a candidate for "no-nonsense" splicing.[125]

The *MOCS3* cDNA encoding molybdopterin synthase sulfurylase has been sequence,[129] but no patients with mutations in this gene have been identified. This may reflect the essential nature of the sulfurylase in pathways other than molybdopterin biosynthesis or may indicate that other similar activities are adequate substitutes in patients where mutations in *MOCS3* are present, with suppression of identifiable clinical symptoms.

The genomic structure of sulfite oxidase has been determined (Coyne, Johnson and Rajagopalan, unpublished) with the somewhat surprising finding that the gene contains only a single intron which falls within the region encoding the presequence that targets the protein to the mitochondrial intermembrane space. The list of identified mutations *in SUOX* has been extended considerably and includes deletions, insertions, and missense mutations (Johnson et al., unpublished). Many of the latter have been modeled into the three-dimensional structure of the chicken enzyme[130] and characterized biochemically after heterologous expression and purification. A four-basepair deletion that predicts premature termination and results in the complete absence of sulfite oxidase activity has been identified in two families residing in the isolated Lac Brochet community of northern Manitoba. With this information, a PCR-induced mutation restriction analysis method has been developed to allow rapid screening for carriers of the mutation within this inbred population (Johnson et al., unpublished).

Diagnostic and Prenatal Screening Procedures

S-sulfocysteine elevation is the most reliable indication of sulfite oxidase deficiency. It has been routinely quantitated by high voltage electrophoresis, amino acid analysis or HPLC, but each of these methods has serious drawbacks. A more reliable procedure has been developed using tandem mass spectrometry (Stevens, Johnson, Rajagopalan and Millington, unpublished), measuring the molecular ion of the S-sulfocysteine butyl ester at m/z 256 which fragments with specific loss of the S-SO_3 group (113 Da). The values obtained by this new method compare well with those obtained on the same samples by HPLC. Quantitation of *S*-sulfocysteine by mass spectral analysis is available as a service through the Duke University Mass Spectrometry Laboratory (www.duke.edu/~mdfeezor/MSHome/MCDSulfo.html).

With advances in the molecular analysis of the genes encoding the molybdenum cofactor biosynthetic enzymes and sulfite oxidase, prenatal analysis is now routinely carried out by gene sequencing rather than by enzymatic assay. If the mutation(s) in the proband and carrier status of the parents have been established, prenatal analysis is possible using genomic DNA isolated from uncultured CVS material (ref. 131 and Johnson et al., unpublished). Results from this method are rapid, obtainable early in the pregnancy and superior to enzyme assay, in that they allow determination of carrier status as well as distinguishing affected from unaffected fetuses. In those cases where molybdenum cofactor deficiency has been established in large kindreds, prenatal diagnosis and carrier detection can also be carried out using polymorphic DNA markers.[132]

REFERENCES

1. Duran M, Beemer FA, van der Heiden C, Korteland J, de Bree PK, Brink M, Wadman SK, et al.: Combined deficiency of xanthine oxidase and sulphite oxidase: A defect of molybdenum metabolism or transport? *J Inherit Metab Dis* **1**:175, 1978.
2. Abumrad NN, Schneider AJ, Steel D, Rogers LS: Amino acid intolerance during prolonged total parenteral nutrition reversed by molybdate therapy. *Am J Clin Nutr* **34**:2551, 1981.
3. Johnson JL, Waud WR, Rajagopalan KV, Duran M, Beemer FA, Wadman SK: Inborn errors of molybdenum metabolism: Combined deficiencies of sulfite oxidase and xanthine dehydrogenase in a patient lacking the molybdenum cofactor. *Proc Natl Acad Sci USA* **77**:3715, 1980.
4. Wadman SK, Duran M, Beemer FA, Cats BP, Johnson JL, Rajagopalan KV, Saudubray JM, et al.: Absence of hepatic molybdenum cofactor: An inborn error of metabolism leading to a combined deficiency of sulphite oxidase and xanthine dehydrogenase. *J Inherit Metab Dis* **6** (suppl 1):78, 1983.
5. Ogier H, Saudubray JM, Charpentier C, Munnich A, Perignon JL, Kesseler A, Frezal J: Double déficit en sulfite et xanthine oxydase, cause d'encéphalopathie due à une anomalie héréditaire du métabolisme du molybdène. *Ann Méd Interne (Paris)* **133**:594, 1982.
6. Munnich A, Saudubray JM, Charpentier C, Ogier H, Coudé FX, Frézal J, Yacoub L, et al.: Multiple molybdoenzyme deficiencies due to an inborn error of molybdenum cofactor metabolism: Two additional cases in a new family. *J Inherit Metab Dis* **6**(suppl 2):95, 1983.
7. Irreverre F, Mudd SH, Heizer WD, Laster L: Sulfite oxidase deficiency: Studies of a patient with mental retardation, dislocated ocular lenses, and abnormal urinary excretion of *S*-sulfo-L-cysteine, sulfite, and thiosulfate. *Biochem Med* **1**:187, 1967.
8. Mudd SH, Irreverre F, Laster L: Sulfite oxidase deficiency in man: Demonstration of the enzymatic defect. *Science* **156**:1599, 1967.
9. Johnson JL, Rajagopalan KV: Human sulfite oxidase deficiency: Characterization of the molecular defect in a multicomponent system. *J Clin Invest* **58**:551, 1976.

10. Johnson JL, Hainline BE, Rajagopalan KV: Characterization of the molybdenum cofactor of sulfite oxidase, xanthine oxidase and nitrate reductase: Identification of a pteridine as a structural component. *J Biol Chem* **255**:1783, 1980.
11. Johnson JL, Rajagopalan KV: Structural and metabolic relationship between the molybdenum cofactor and urothione. *Proc Natl Acad Sci USA* **79**:6856, 1982.
12. Johnson JL, Hainline BE, Rajagopalan KV, Arison BH: The pterin component of the molybdenum cofactor: Structural characterization of two fluorescent derivatives. *J Biol Chem* **259**:5414, 1984.
13. Kramer SP, Johnson JL, Ribeiro AA, Millington DS, Rajagopalan KV: The structure of the molybdenum cofactor: Characterization of di-(carboxamidomethyl)molybdopterin from sulfite oxidase and xanthine oxidase. *J Biol Chem* **262**:16357, 1987.
14. Massey V, Edmondson D: On the mechanism of inactivation of xanthine oxidase by cyanide. *J Biol Chem* **245**:6595, 1970.
15. Wahl RC, Rajagopalan KV: Evidence for the inorganic nature of the cyanolyzable sulfur of molybdenum hydroxylases. *J Biol Chem* **257**:1354, 1982.
16. Wahl RC, Warner CK, Finnerty V, Rajagopalan KV: *Drosophila melanogaster ma-l* mutants are defective in the sulfuration of desulfo Mo hydroxylases. *J Biol Chem* **257**:3958, 1982.
17. Reiter S, Simmonds HA, Zöllner N, Braun SL, Knedel M: Demonstration of a combined deficiency of xanthine oxidase and aldehyde oxidase in xanthinuric patients not forming oxipurinol. *Clin Chim Acta* **187**:221, 1990.
18. Koschara W: Urothion, ein gelber, schwefelreicher farbstoff aus menschenharn. *Hoppe-Seylers Z Physiol Chem* **263**:78, 1940.
19. Goto M, Sakurai A, Ohta K, Yamakami H: Die struktur des urothions. *J Biochem* **65**:611, 1969.
20. Roesel RA, Bowyer F, Blankenship PR, Hommes FA: Combined xanthine and sulphite oxidase defect due to a deficiency of molybdenum cofactor. *J Inherit Metab Dis* **9**:343, 1986.
21. Kisker C, Schindelin H, Pacheco A, Wehbi WA, Garrett RM, Rajagopalan KV, Enemark JH, et al.: Molecular basis of sulfite oxidase deficiency from the structure of sulfite oxidase. *Cell* **91**:973, 1997.
22. Chan MK, Mukund S, Kletzin A, Adams MWW, Rees DC: Structure of a hyperthermophilic tungstopterin enzyme, aldehyde ferredoxin oxidoreductase. *Science* **267**:1463, 1995.
23. Schindelin H, Kisker C, Hilton J, Rajagopalan KV, Rees DC: Crystal structure of DMSO reductase: Redox-linked changes in molybdopterin coordination. *Science* **272**:1615, 1996.
24. Gardlik S, Rajagopalan KV: The state of reduction of molybdopterin in xanthine oxidase and sulfite oxidase. *J Biol Chem* **265**:13047, 1990.
25. Johnson JL, Bastian NR, Rajagopalan KV: Molybdopterin guanine dinucleotide: A modified form of molybdopterin identified in the molybdenum cofactor of dimethyl sulfoxide reductase from *Rhodobacter sphaeroides* forma specialis *denitrificans*. *Proc Natl Acad Sci USA* **87**:3190, 1990.
26. Johnson JL, Bastian NR, Schauer NL, Ferry JG, Rajagopalan KV: Identification of molybdopterin guanine dinucleotide in formate dehydrogenase from *Methanobacterium formicicum*. *FEMS Microbiol Lett* **77**:213, 1991.
27. Karrasch M, Börner G, Thauer RK: The molybdenum cofactor of formylmethanofuran dehydrogenase from *Methanosarcina barkeri* is a molybdopterin guanine dinucleotide. *FEBS Lett* **274**:48, 1990.
28. Börner G, Karrasch M, Thauer RK: Molybdopterin adenine dinucleotide and molybdopterin hypoxanthine dinucleotide in formylmethanofuran dehydrogenase from *Methanobacterium thermoautotrophicum* (Marburg). *FEBS Lett* **290**:31, 1991.
29. Rajagopalan KV, Johnson JL: The pterin molybdenum cofactors. *J Biol Chem* **267**:10199, 1992.
30. Johnson JL, Rajagopalan KV, Meyer O: Isolation and characterization of a second molybdopterin dinucleotide: Molybdopterin cytosine dinucleotide. *Arch Biochem Biophys* **283**:542, 1990.
31. Hettrich D, Peschke B, Tshisuaka B, Lingens F: Microbial metabolism of quinoline and related compounds: X. The molybdopterin cofactors of quinoline oxidoreductases from *Pseudomonas putida 86* and *Rhodococcus spec. B1* and of xanthine dehydrogenase from *Pseudomonas putida 86*. *Biol Chem Hoppe-Seyler* **372**:513, 1991.
32. Hilton JC, Rajagopalan KV: Identification of the molybdenum cofactor of dimethyl sulfoxide reductase from *Rhodobacter sphaeroides* f. sp. *denitrificans* as bis(molybdopterin guanine dinucleotide)molybdenum. *Arch Biochem Biophys* **325**:139, 1996.
33. Boyington JC, Gladyshev VN, Khangulov SV, Stadtman TC, Sun PD: Crystal structure of formate dehydrogenase H: Catalysis involving Mo, molybdopterin, selenocysteine, and an Fe_4S_4 cluster. *Science* **275**:1305, 1997.
34. Krenitsky TA, Neil SM, Elion GB, Hitchings GH: A comparison of the specificities of xanthine oxidase and aldehyde oxidase. *Arch Biochem Biophys* **150**:585, 1972.
35. Coughlan MP: Aldehyde oxidase, xanthine oxidase and xanthine dehydrogenase: Hydroxylases containing molybdenum, iron-sulphur and flavin, in Coughlan MP (ed): *Molybdenum and Molybdenum-Containing Enzymes*. Oxford, England, Pergamon Press, 1980, p 119.
36. Stirpe F, Della Corte E: The regulation of rat liver xanthine oxidase. Conversion in vitro of the enzyme activity from dehydrogenase (type D) to oxidase (type O). *J Biol Chem* **244**:3855, 1969.
37. Waud WR, Rajagopalan KV: The mechanism of conversion of rat liver xanthine dehydrogenase from an NAD^+-dependent form (type D) to an O_2-dependent form (type O). *Arch Biochem Biophys* **172**:365, 1976.
38. Johnson JL, Rajagopalan KV, Cohen HJ: Molecular basis of the biological function of molybdenum: Effect of tungsten on xanthine oxidase and sulfite oxidase in the rat. *J Biol Chem* **249**:859, 1974.
39. Brunschede H, Krooth RS: Studies on the xanthine oxidase activity of mammalian cells. *Biochem Genet* **8**:341, 1973.
40. Cohen HJ, Drew RT, Johnson JL, Rajagopalan KV: Molecular basis of the biological function of molybdenum. The relationship between sulfite oxidase and the acute toxicity of bisulfite and SO_2. *Proc Natl Acad Sci USA* **70**:3655, 1973.
41. Rajagopalan KV: Sulfite oxidase, in Coughlan MP (ed): *Molybdenum and Molybdenum-Containing Enzymes*. Oxford, England, Pergamon Press, 1980, p 241.
42. Johnson JL, Rajagopalan KV: Tryptic cleavage of rat liver sulfite oxidase: Isolation and characterization of molybdenum and heme domains. *J Biol Chem* **252**:2017, 1977.
43. Johnson JL, Rajagopalan KV: Purification and properties of sulfite oxidase from human liver. *J Clin Invest* **58**:543, 1976.
44. Kessler DL, Johnson JL, Cohen HJ, Rajagopalan KV: Visualization of hepatic sulfite oxidase in crude tissue preparations by electron paramagnetic resonance spectroscopy. *Biochim Biophys Acta* **334**:86, 1974.
45. Stewart V: Nitrate respiration in relation to facultative metabolism in enterobacteria. *Microbiol Rev* **52**:190, 1988.
46. Wuebbens MM, Rajagopalan KV: Investigation of the early steps of molybdopterin biosynthesis in *Escherichia coli* through the use of in vivo labeling studies. *J Biol Chem* **270**:1082, 1995.
47. Johnson JL, Wuebbens MM, Rajagopalan KV: The structure of a molybdopterin precursor: Characterization of a stable, oxidized derivative. *J Biol Chem* **264**:13440, 1989.
48. Wuebbens MM, Rajagopalan KV: Structural characterization of a molybdopterin precursor. *J Biol Chem* **268**:13493, 1993.
49. Rieder C, Eisenreich W, O'Brien J, Richter G, Götze E, Boyle P, Blanchard S, et al.: Rearrangement reactions in the biosynthesis of molybdopterin: An NMR study with multiply $^{13}C/^{15}N$ labelled precursors. *Eur J Biochem* **255**:24, 1998.
50. Brown GM: The biosynthesis of pteridines. *Adv Enzymol* **35**:35, 1971.
51. Rivers SL, McNairn E, Blasco F, Giordano G, Boxer DH: Molecular genetic analysis of the *moa* operon of *Escherichia coli* K-12 required for molybdenum cofactor biosynthesis. *Mol Microbiol* **8**:1071, 1993.
52. Menéndez C, Igloi G, Henninger H, Brandsch R: A pA01-encoded molybdopterin cofactor gene (*moaA*) of *Arthrobacter nicotinovorans*: Characterization and site-directed mutagenesis of the encoded protein. *Arch Microbiol* **164**:142, 1995.
53. Menéndez C, Siebert D, Brandsch R: MoaA of *Arthrobacter nicotinovorans* pA01 involved in Mo-pterin cofactor synthesis is an Fe-S protein. *FEBS Lett* **391**:101, 1996.
54. Pitterle DM, Rajagopalan KV: Two proteins encoded at the *chlA* locus constitute the converting factor of *Escherichia coli chlA1*. *J Bacteriol* **171**:3373, 1989.
55. Nohno T, Kasai Y, Saito T: Cloning and sequencing of the *Escherichia coli chlEN* operon involved in molybdopterin biosynthesis. *J Bacteriol* **170**:4097, 1988.
56. Rajagopalan KV: Biosynthesis of the molybdenum cofactor, in Neidhardt RC (ed): *Escherichia coli and Salmonella: Cellular and Molecular Biology*. New York, ASM Press, 1996, p 674.
57. Rajagopalan KV: Biosynthesis and processing of the molybdenum cofactors. *Biochem Soc Trans* **25**:757, 1997.
58. Johnson JL: Molybdenum, in O'Dell BL, Sunde RA (eds): *Handbook of Nutritionally Essential Mineral Elements*. New York, Marcel Dekker, 1997, p 413.
59. Pitterle DM, Rajagopalan KV: The biosynthesis of molybdopterin in *Escherichia coli*: Purification and characterization of the converting factor. *J Biol Chem* **268**:13499, 1993.

60. Taylor SV, Kelleher NL, Kinsland C, Chiu H-J, Costello CA, Backstrom AD, McLafferty FW, et al.: Thiamin biosynthesis in *Escherichia coli*: Identification of ThiS thiocarboxylate as the immediate sulfur donor in the thiazole formation. *J Biol Chem* **273**:16555, 1998.
61. Rech S, Deppenmeier U, Gunsalus RP: Regulation of the molybdate transport operon, *modABCD*, of *Escherichia coli* in response to molybdate availability. *J Bacteriol* **177**:1023, 1995.
62. Rech S, Wolin C, Gunsalus RP: Properties of the periplasmic ModA molybdate-binding protein of *Escherichia coli*. *J Biol Chem* **271**:2557, 1996.
63. Joshi MS, Johnson JL, Rajagopalan KV: Molybdenum cofactor biosynthesis in *Escherichia coli mod* and *mog* mutants. *J Bacteriol* **178**:4310, 1996.
64. Johnson JL, Wuebbens MM, Mandell R, Shih VE: Molybdenum cofactor biosynthesis in humans: Identification of two complementation groups of cofactor-deficient patients and preliminary characterization of a diffusible molybdopterin precursor. *J Clin Invest* **83**:897, 1989.
65. Reiss J, Cohen N, Dorche C, Mandel H, Mendel RR, Stallmeyer B, Zabot MT, et al.: Mutations in a polycistronic nuclear gene associated with molybdenum cofactor deficiency. *Nature Genet* **20**:51, 1998.
66. Johnson JL, Rajagopalan KV: Molybdopterin biosynthesis in man: Properties of the converting factor in liver tissue from a molybdenum cofactor deficient patient. *Adv Exp Med Biol* **338**:379, 1993.
67. Mendel RR, Bittner F, Bollmann G, Brinkmann H, Eilers T, Greger K, Nerlich A, et al.: Molybdenum cofactor biosynthesis in higher plants, in *Abstracts of Nitrogen Assimilation: Molecular and Genetic Aspects*. Tampa, 1997.
68. Prior P, Schmitt B, Grenningloh G, Pribilla I, Multhaup G, Beyreuther K, Maulet Y, et al.: Primary structure and alternative splice variants of gephyrin, a putative glycine receptor-tubulin linker protein. *Neuron* **8**:1161, 1992.
69. Shalata A, Mandel H, Reiss J, Szargel R, Cohen-Akenine A, Dorche C, Zabot MT, et al.: Localization of a gene for molybdenum cofactor deficiency, on the short arm of chromosome 6, by homozygosity mapping. *Am J Hum Genet* **63**:148, 1998.
70. Garrett RM, Rajagopalan KV: Molecular cloning of rat liver sulfite oxidase: Expression of a eukaryotic Mo-pterin-containing enzyme in *Escherichia coli*. *J Biol Chem* **269**:272, 1994.
71. Garrett RM, Bellissimo DB, Rajagopalan KV: Molecular cloning of human liver sulfite oxidase. *Biochim Biophys Acta* **1262**:147, 1995.
72. Rupar CA, Gillett J, Gordon BA, Ramsay DA, Johnson JL, Garrett RM, Rajagopalan KV, et al.: Isolated sulfite oxidase deficiency. *Neuropediatrics* **27**:299, 1996.
73. Johnson JL, Garrett RM, Rajagopalan KV: The biochemistry of molybdenum cofactor deficiency and isolated sulfite oxidase deficiency. *Int Pediatr* **12**:22, 1997.
74. Garrett RM, Johnson JL, Graf TN, Feigenbaum A, Rajagopalan KV: Human sulfite oxidase *R160Q*: Identification of the mutation in a sulfite oxidase deficient patient and expression and characterization of the mutant enzyme. *Proc Natl Acad Sci USA* **95**:6394, 1998.
75. Lueder GT, Steiner RD: Ophthalmic abnormalities in molybdenum cofactor deficiency and isolated sulfite oxidase deficiency. *J Pediatr Ophthalmol Strabismus* **32**:334, 1995.
76. Parini R, Briscioli V, Caruso U, Dorche C, Fortuna R, Minniti G, Selicorni A, et al.: Spherophakia associated with molybdenum cofactor deficiency. *Am J Med Genet* **73**:272, 1997.
77. Mize CE, Johnson JL, Rajagopalan KV: Defective molybdopterin biosynthesis: Clinical heterogeneity associated with molybdenum cofactor deficiency. *J Inherit Metab Dis* **18**:283, 1995.
78. de Klerk JBC, Bakker HD, Beemer FA, Brussel W, Kohlschütter A, Kurlemann G, Marquard K, et al.: Facial dysmorphism in molybdenum cofactor deficiency/sulfite oxidase deficiency. *Enzyme Protein* **49**:185, 1996.
79. Roth A, Nogues C, Monnet JP, Ogier H, Saudubray JM: Anatomopathological findings in a case of combined deficiency of sulphite oxidase and xanthine oxidase with a defect of molybdenum cofactor. *Virchows Arch [Pathol Anat]* **405**:379, 1985.
80. Barth PG, Beemer FA, Cats BP, Duran M, Wadman SK: Neuropathological findings in a case of combined deficiency of sulphite oxidase and xanthine dehydrogenase. *Virchows Arch [Pathol Anat]* **408**:105, 1985.
81. Endres W, Shin YS, Günther R, Ibel H, Duran M, Wadman SK: Report on a new patient with combined deficiencies of sulphite oxidase and xanthine dehydrogenase due to molybdenum cofactor deficiency. *Eur J Pediatr* **148**:246, 1988.
82. Aukett A, Bennett MJ, Hosking GP: Molybdenum cofactor deficiency: An easily missed inborn error of metabolism. *Dev Med Child Neurol* **30**:531, 1988.
83. Slot HMJ, Overweg-Plandsoen WCG, Bakker HD, Abeling NGGM, Tamminga P, Barth PG, van Gennip AH: Molybdenum-cofactor deficiency: An easily missed cause of neonatal convulsions. *Neuropediatrics* **24**:139, 1993.
84. Schuierer G, Kurlemann G, Bick U, Stephani U: Molybdenum-cofactor deficiency: CT and MR findings. *Neuropediatrics* **26**:51, 1995.
85. Appignani BA, Kaye EM, Wolpert SM: CT and MR appearance of the brain in two children with molybdenum cofactor deficiency. *Am J Neuroradiol* **17**:317, 1996.
86. Hughes EF, Fairbanks L, Simmonds HA, Robinson RO: Molybdenum cofactor deficiency—phenotypic variability in a family with a late-onset variant. *Dev Med Child Neurol* **40**:57, 1998.
87. Rosenblum WI: Neuropathologic changes in a case of sulfite oxidase deficiency. *Neurology* **18**:1187, 1968.
88. Brown GK, Scholem RD, Croll HB, Wraith JE, McGill JJ: Sulfite oxidase deficiency: Clinical, neuroradiologic, and biochemical features in two new patients. *Neurology* **39**:252, 1989.
89. van der Klei-van Moorsel JM, Smit LME, Brockstedt M, Jakobs C, Dorche C, Duran M: Infantile isolated sulphite oxidase deficiency: Report of a case with negative sulphite test and normal sulphate excretion. *Eur J Pediatr* **150**:196, 1991.
90. Barbot C, Martins E, Vilarinho L, Dorche C, Cardoso ML: A mild form of infantile isolated sulphite oxidase deficiency. *Neuropediatrics* **26**:322, 1995.
91. Duran M, Aarsen G, Fokkens RH, Nibbering NMM, Cats BP, de Bree PK, Wadman SK: 2-Mercaptoethanesulfonate-cysteine disulfide excretion following the administration of 2-mercaptoethanesulfonate—a pitfall in the diagnosis of sulfite oxidase deficiency. *Clin Chim Acta* **111**:47, 1981.
92. Wadman SK, Cats BP, de Bree PK: Sulfite oxidase deficiency and the detection of urinary sulfite. *Eur J Pediatr* **141**:62, 1983.
93. Cole DEC, Evrovski J: Screening for sulfite oxidase deficiency with urinary thiosulfate/sulfate ratios determined by anion chromatography. *Clin Chem* **42**:654, 1996.
94. Johnson JL, Rajagopalan KV: An HPLC assay for detection of elevated urinary *S*-sulphocysteine, a metabolic marker of sulphite oxidase deficiency. *J Inherit Metab Dis* **18**:40, 1995.
95. Chace DH, Hillman SL, Millington DS, Kahler SG, Adam BW, Levy HL: Rapid diagnosis of homocystinuria and other hypermethioninemias from newborns' blood spots by tandem mass spectrometry. *Clin Chem* **42**:345, 1996.
96. Graf WD, Oleinik OE, Jack RM, Weiss AH, Johnson JL: Ahomocysteinemia in molybdenum cofactor deficiency. *Neurology* **51**:860, 1998.
97. Simmonds HA, Duley JA, Davies PM: Analysis of purines and pyrimidines in blood, urine, and other physiological fluids, in Hommes FA (ed): *Techniques in Diagnostic Human Biochemical Genetics*. New York, Wiley-Liss, 1991, p 397.
98. Burlina AB, Dionisi-Vici C, Bennett MJ, Gibson KM, Servidel S, Bertini E, Hale DE, et al.: A new syndrome with ethylmalonic aciduria and normal fatty acid oxidation in fibroblasts. *J Pediatr* **124**:79, 1994.
99. Duran M, Dorland L, van den Berg IET, Vredendaal PJCM, de Koning TJ, Poll-The BT, Berger R: The ethylmalonic acid syndrome is associated with deranged sulfur amino acid metabolism leading to urinary excretion of thiosulfate and sulfothiocysteine, in *Abstracts of the 7th International Congress of Inborn Errors of Metabolism, Vienna*. 1997.
100. Johnson JL, Cohen HJ, Rajagopalan KV: Molecular basis of the biological function of molybdenum: Molybdenum-free sulfite oxidase from livers of tungsten-treated rats. *J Biol Chem* **249**:5046, 1974.
101. Johnson JL, Jones HP, Rajagopalan KV: In vitro reconstitution of demolybdosulfite oxidase by a molybdenum cofactor from rat liver and other sources. *J Biol Chem* **252**:4994, 1977.
102. Ogier H, Wadman SK, Johnson JL, Saudubray JM, Duran M, Boue J, Munnich A, et al.: Antenatal diagnosis of combined xanthine and sulphite oxidase deficiencies. *Lancet* **2**:1363, 1983.
103. Desjacques P, Mousson B, Vianey-Liaud C, Boulieu R, Bory C, Baltassat P, Divry P, et al.: Combined deficiency of xanthine oxidase and sulphite oxidase: Diagnosis of a new case followed by an antenatal diagnosis. *J Inherit Metab Dis* **8**(suppl 2):117, 1985.
104. Johnson JL, Rajagopalan KV, Lanman JT, Schutgens RBH, van Gennip AH, Sorensen P, Applegarth DA: Prenatal diagnosis of molybdenum cofactor deficiency by assay of sulphite oxidase activity in chorionic villus samples. *J Inherit Metab Dis* **14**:932, 1991.

105. Gray RGF, Green A, Basu SN, Constantine G, Condie RG, Dorche C, Vianey-Liaud C, et al.: Antenatal diagnosis of molybdenum cofactor deficiency. *Am J Obstet Gynecol* **163**:1203, 1990.
106. Shapiro R: Genetic effects of bisulfite (sulfur dioxide). *Mutat Res* **39**:149, 1977.
107. Til HP, Feron VJ, de Groot AP: The toxicity of sulphite: I. Long-term feeding and multigeneration studies in rats. *Food Cosmet Toxicol* **10**:291, 1972.
108. Southerland WM, Akogyeram CO, Toghrol F, Sloan L, Scherrer R: Interaction of bisulfite with unsaturated fatty acids. *J Toxicol Environ Health* **10**:479, 1982.
109. Percy AK, Mudd SH, Irreverre F, Laster L: Sulfite oxidase deficiency: Sulfate esters in tissues and urine. *Biochem Med* **2**:198, 1968.
110. Rusthoven E, Depondt E, Dorche C, Duran R, Heron B, Rabier D, Russo M, et al.: Attempts at therapy in two patients with a sulfite oxidase deficiency, in *Abstracts of the 7th International Congress of Inborn Errors of Metabolism, Vienna*. 1997.
111. Tardy P, Parvy P, Charpentier C, Bonnefont JP, Saudubray JM, Kamoun P: Attempt at therapy in sulphite oxidase deficiency. *J Inherit Metab Dis* **12**:94, 1989.
112. Kamoun P, Tardy P: Therapeutic attempts in sulphite oxidase deficiency. *Eur J Pediatr* **149**:594, 1990.
113. Johnson JL: The molybdenum cofactor common to nitrate reductase, xanthine dehydrogenase and sulfite oxidase, in Coughlan MP (ed): *Molybdenum and Molybdenum-Containing Enzymes*. Oxford, England, Pergamon Press, 1980, p 345.
114. Fujitaka M, Sakura N, Ueda K, Konishi H, Yoshida S, Yamasaki T: Attempt at treatment with tetrahydrobiopterin in combined deficiency of xanthine oxidase and sulphite oxidase. *J Inherit Metab Dis* **14**:843, 1991.
115. Olney JW, Misra CH, de Gubareff T: Cysteine-*S*-sulfate: Brain damaging metabolite in sulfite oxidase deficiency. *J Neuropathol Exp Neurol* **34**:167, 1975.
116. Kurlemann G, Debus O, Schuierer G: Dextromethorphan in molybdenum cofactor deficiency. *Eur J Pediatr* **155**:422, 1996.
117. Blau N, de Klerk JBC, Thöny B, Heizmann CW, Kierat L, Smeitink JAM, Duran M: Tetrahydrobiopterin loading test in xanthine dehydrogenase and molybdenum cofactor deficiencies. *Biochem Mol Med* **58**:199, 1996.
118. Duran M, de Bree PK, de Klerk JBC, Dorland L, Berger R: Molybdenum cofactor deficiency: Clinical presentation and laboratory diagnosis. *Int Pediatr* **11**:334, 1996.
119. Wuebbens MM, Liu MTW, Rajagopalan KV, Schindelin H: Insights into molybdenum cofactor deficiency provided by the crystal structure of the molybdenum cofactor biosynthetic protein MoaC. *Structure with Folding and Design* **8**:709, 2000.
120. Liu MT, Wuebbens MM, Rajagopalan KV, Schindelin H: Crystal structure of the gephyrin-related molybdenum cofactor biosynthesis protein MogA from *Escherichia coli*. *J Biol Chem* **275**:1814, 2000.
121. Feng G, Tintrup H, Kirsch J, Nichol MC, Kuhse J, Betz H, Sanes JR: Dual requirement for gephyrin in glycine receptor clustering and molybdoenzyme activity. *Science* **282**:1321, 1998.
122. Stallmeyer B, Schwarz G, Schulze J, Nerlich A, Reiss J, Kirsch J, Mendel RR: The neurotransmitter receptor-anchoring protein gephyrin reconstitutes molybdenum cofactor biosynthesis in bacteria, plants, and mammalian cells. *Proc Natl Acad Sci USA* **96**:1333, 1999.
123. Reiss J, Christensen E, Kurlemann G, Zabot M-T, Dorche C: Genomic structure and mutational spectrum of the bicistronic *MOCS1* gene defective in molybdenum cofactor deficiency type A. *Hum Genet* **103**:639, 1998.
124. Reiss J, Cohen N, Dorche C, Mandel H, Mendel RR, Stallmeyer B, Zabot MT, et al.: Mutations in a polycistronic nuclear gene associated with molybdenum cofactor deficiency. *Nat Genet* **20**:51, 1998.
125. Gray TA, Nicholls RD: Diverse splicing mechanisms fuse the evolutionarily conserved bicistronic *MOCS1A* and *MOCS1B* open reading frames. *RNA* **6**:928, 2000.
126. Sloan J, Kinghorn JR, Unkles SE: The two subunits of human molybdopterin synthase: evidence for a bicistronic messenger RNA with overlapping reading frames. *Nucleic Acids Res* **27**:854, 1999.
127. Stallmeyer B, Drugeon G, Reiss J, Haenni AL, Mendel RR: Human molybdopterin synthase gene: identification of a bicistronic transcript with overlapping reading frames. *Am J Hum Genet* **64**:698, 1999.
128. Reiss J, Dorche C, Stallmeyer B, Mendel RR, Cohen N, Zabot MT: Human molybdopterin synthase gene: genomic structure and mutations in molybdenum cofactor deficiency type B. *Am J Hum Genet* **64**:706, 1999.
129. Stallmeyer B, Coyne KE, Wuebbens MM, Johnson JL, Rajagopalan KV, Mendel RR: The cDNA sequence of MOCS3, human molybdopterin synthase sulfurylase. *GenBank accession number AF102544*, 1998.
130. Kisker C, Schindelin H, Pacheco A, Wehbi WA, Garrett RM, Rajagopalan KV, Enemark JH, et al.: Molecular basis of sulfite oxidase deficiency from the structure of sulfite oxidase. *Cell* **91**:973, 1997.
131. Reiss J, Christensen E, Dorche C: Molybdenum cofactor deficiency: first prenatal genetic analysis. *Prenat Diagn* **19**:386, 1999.
132. Shalata A, Mandel H, Dorche C, Zabot MT, Shalev S, Hugeirat Y, Arieh D, et al.: Prenatal diagnosis and carrier detection for molybdenum cofactor deficiency type A in northern Israel using polymorphic DNA markers. *Prenat Diagn* **20**:7, 2000.

PART 15

PEROXISOMES

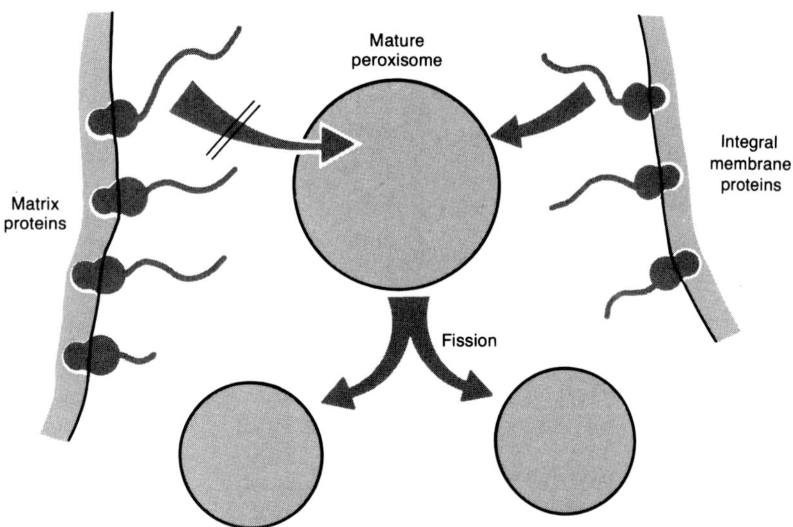

Disorders of peroxisomal function

CHAPTER 129

The Peroxisome Biogenesis Disorders

Stephen J. Gould ■ Gerald V. Raymond ■ David Valle

1. **Peroxisomes are single-membrane lined organelles present in virtually all eukaryotic cells. In most human cells, their abundance ranges from less than a hundred to more than a thousand peroxisomes per cell. The granular matrix of the organelle contains more than 50 matrix enzymes that participate in a wide variety of metabolic pathways including β-oxidation of certain fatty acids and biosynthesis of ether phospholipids, bile acids, and isoprene compounds.**
2. **Peroxisome biogenesis involves synthesis of the matrix proteins on free cytosolic ribosomes followed by receptor-mediated import into the organelle. Most matrix proteins are targeted by a C-terminal peroxisome targeting sequence (PTS1) with a consensus of −S-K-L-COOH that is recognized by a cytosolic receptor, PEX5. A few matrix proteins are targeted by an N-terminal PTS2 with the consensus sequence of −R-L-X_S-H-L−. Peroxisome membrane proteins are specific for the organelle. They are also synthesized on free cytosolic ribosomes and are targeted to the organelle by mechanism(s) that are separate from and less well understood than those used by matrix proteins.**
3. **PEX genes encode peroxins, proteins involved in and necessary for peroxisome biogenesis. These include the PTS1 and 2 receptors, as well as additional cytosolic and integral membrane proteins that are involved in the import of peroxisomal matrix and membrane proteins. To date, 23 PEX genes have been identified, with 15 PEX genes known in humans.**
4. **The peroxisome biogenesis disorders are comprised of at least 12 complementation groups. Defective biogenesis of the organelle leads to complex developmental and metabolic phenotypes that can be organized into two clinical spectra: the Zellweger spectrum with Zellweger syndrome as the most severe example and neonatal adrenoleukodystrophy and infantile Refsum disease as milder variants. The second spectrum is distinctive with classical rhizomelic chondrodysplasia punctata as its exemplar and milder variants described.**
5. **The PEX genes responsible for 11 of the 12 PBD complementation groups are known with multiple mutant alleles identified. Functional analysis of the proteins encoded by these PEX genes together with careful clinical, metabolic, and cellular characterization of the mutant phenotypes has provided insight into the pathophysiology of the peroxisome biogenesis disorders as well as into the normal biology of peroxisome assembly and function.**

In 1964, Dr. Hans Zellweger and colleagues reported the inherited disease that we now know as Zellweger syndrome.[1] Shortly thereafter, Parsage and McAdams reported similarly affected sisters and referred to the disorder as cerebrohepatorenal syndrome.[2] Opitz et al.[3] reviewed these and other reports and suggested the name Zellweger cerebrohepatorenal syndrome (ZS), which we now use to describe this prototypical peroxisome biogenesis disorder. These disorders appear to have an incidence of approximately 1 per 50,000 births.[4,5] The first evidence that peroxisome biogenesis was affected in ZS patients came from Goldfischer et al.,[6] who showed that peroxisomal matrix proteins were not properly compartmentalized in this disease. Over time, the related but milder phenotypes of neonatal adrenoleukodystrophy (NALD)[7] and infantile Refsum disease (IRD)[8] were recognized, although their relationship to ZS was not appreciated until somewhat later.[9–12] These Zellweger spectrum disorders are inherited in an autosomal recessive fashion.[13] Rhizomelic chondrodysplasia punctata (RCDP) was identified later and immediately recognized as a peroxisomal disorder.[14,15]

A series of cell-fusion complementation studies by Brul et al.[16] and others[17] advanced the study of peroxisomal biogenesis disorders (PBD) genetics by demonstrating that ZS, NALD, and IRD appeared to be caused by defects in the same set of genes. These studies also provided strong evidence that PBDs are genetically heterogeneous and that RCDP was genetically homogeneous and distinct from the Zellweger spectrum of disease.[16–18] In general, somatic cell fusion studies are subject to many technical and theoretical caveats and the results are often difficult to interpret. It is therefore notable that the complementation groups of PBD patients reported by Dutch, American, Japanese, and Australian laboratories[16–21] have been a remarkably accurate predictor of gene defect.[22]

Currently, we recognize that ZS, NALD, IRD, and RCDP are complex developmental and metabolic disorders caused by defects in peroxisome biogenesis. The phenotypic variability of these peroxisome biogenesis disorders (PBD) is considerable but can be grouped into two distinct clinical spectra.

The Zellweger spectrum includes ZS at the severe end of the distribution with NALD and IRD as progressively milder segments of the spectrum. ZS patients have severe neurologic deficits, progressive hepatic and renal dysfunction, and skeletal abnormalities. They rarely survive their first year. NALD and IRD patients show similar though less pronounced clinical phenotypes, with many IRD patients surviving into their third and fourth decades. The Zellweger spectrum is generally associated with severe, moderate, or mild defects in virtually all peroxisomal functions. This broad disruption of peroxisomal metabolism is brought about

A list of standard abbreviations is located immediately preceding the index in each volume. Additional abbreviations used in this chapter include: CG = complementation group; DHAPAT = dihydroxyacetone-phosphate acyltransferase; ER = endoplasmic reticulum; IRD = infantile Refsum disease; MRI = magnetic resonance imaging; NALD = neonatal adrenoleukodystrophy; PBD = peroxisome biogenesis disorders; PMP = peroxisomal membrane protein; RCDP = rhizomelic chondrodysplasia punctata; STS = sequence tagged site; TPR = tetratricopeptide repeats; VLCFA = very long chain fatty acids; ZS = Zellweger syndrome.

by severe, moderate, or mild defects in the import of virtually all peroxisomal enzymes, as well as by the inability of many peroxisomal enzymes to function properly when mislocalized to the cytoplasm. Most Zellweger spectrum patients do synthesize peroxisomal membranes and import peroxisomal membrane proteins (PMP) normally and are defective only in the import of peroxisomal matrix enzymes. By contrast, a few ZS patients lack detectable peroxisome membranes, indicating a defect in the synthesis of peroxisome membranes or targeting of integral PMPs, or both with a secondary deficiency of peroxisomal matrix enzymes.

The second phenotypic spectrum, designated the RCDP spectrum, is characterized by a more specific clinical and metabolic phenotype. The typical clinical features include proximal shortening of the limbs (rhizomelia), punctate epiphyseal calcifications, cataracts, and severe developmental delay. At the metabolic level, RCDP patients have defects in just two peroxisomal metabolic functions: plasmalogen biosynthesis and branched chain fatty acid oxidation. The specificity of the RCDP phenotype is partly explained by the cellular phenotype: RCDP cells mislocalize only a small subset of peroxisomal enzymes. As with the Zellweger spectrum of disease, milder variants of RCDP have been identified, leading to an appreciation of the RCDP spectrum of disease.

The PBDs are inherited in an autosomal recessive manner and, in aggregate, occur in approximately 1/50,000 live births. Complementation assays using somatic cell-fusion methods indicate that defects in any of at least 12 complementation groups (CG) or genes produce these phenotypes. Genetic, biochemical, and cellular studies have provided a wealth of information on the probable molecular defects in most PBD patients. In this chapter, we review the current understanding of peroxisome biology, the molecular genetics and cell biology of the PBDs, and the clinical aspects of these complex and challenging disorders.

PEROXISOME MORPHOLOGY AND FUNCTION

Physical and Chemical Properties of Peroxisomes

Human cells typically contain several hundred peroxisomes (Fig. 129-1*A*), though the actual abundance may vary from under a hundred to over a thousand.[5,23] Peroxisomes can vary from 0.1 to 1 μm in diameter and usually appear as simple circular and ovoid vesicles[24–26] (Fig. 129-1*B* and *C*) although their morphology can be more complex. For example, peroxisomes appear to form elongated, tubular structures prior to division[27,28] and convoluted, reticular peroxisomes have been observed in certain cell types.[29] The peroxisome interior is a dense, protein-rich environment. Intraperoxisomal protein concentrations have been estimated at 200 to 300 μg/ml.[30,31] In fact, individual proteins may become so concentrated in the peroxisome lumen that they crystallize.[32,33] In most cells, however, peroxisomes lack protein crystals and these structures cannot be used to identify the organelle.

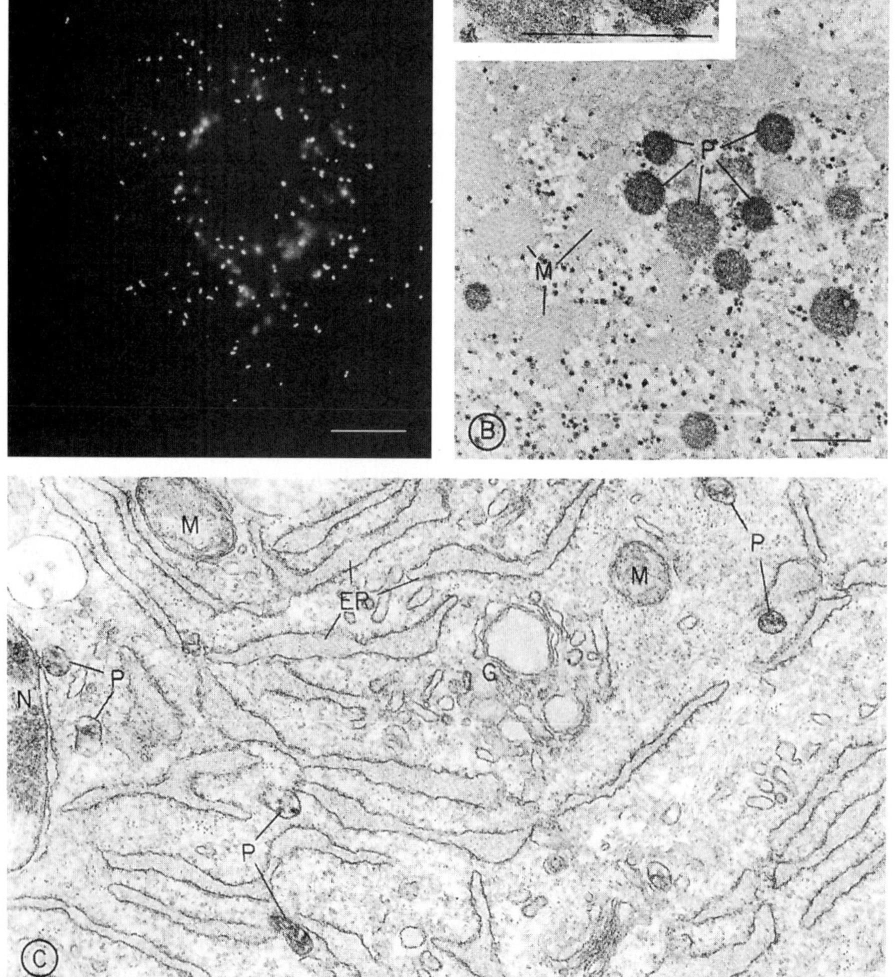

Fig. 129-1 Peroxisome morphology. *A*, Immunofluorescent labeling of a single human hepatoblastoma HepG2 cell with antibodies specific for the integral peroxisomal membrane protein, PMP70. Bar = 20 μM. Note the presence of hundreds of discrete peroxisomes. *B*, Electron microscopy of human liver stained cytochemically for the peroxisomal enzyme, catalase, reveals a cluster of diaminobenzidine-positive peroxisomes in a small region of the cell. Bar = 1 μM. *C*, Electron microscopy of a human amniocyte reveals several peroxisomes distributed throughout the cytoplasm. Bar = 1 μM. P = peroxisome; M = mitochondria; N = nucleus; G = Golgi; ER = endoplasmic reticulum. (*A and* B *from Lazarow et al.*[236] C *from H Shio and PB Lazarow.*)

Recent studies demonstrate that the peroxisome interior is a chemically unique microenvironment. Although prior reports had suggested that the peroxisome membrane was permeable to molecules as large as sucrose,[34–36] this hypothesis was challenged by a series of elegant genetic and biochemical studies in yeast.[37–39] The current view is that the peroxisome membrane is impermeable to a variety of molecules including NAD^+ and acetyl-CoA,[37] $NADP^+$,[38–40] and CoA.[41] The impermeable nature of the peroxisome membrane was confirmed by a recent study of intraperoxisomal pH in human skin fibroblasts, which revealed that the peroxisome matrix is alkaline, with a pH of approximately 8.3.[42] The mechanism by which peroxisomes generate a proton gradient across their membrane is unknown but it may involve a simple metabolic characteristic, such as the presence of proton-consuming enzymes (e.g., decarboxylases[43]) in the peroxisome lumen. Interestingly, most peroxisomal enzymes have a basic pI, which may be an adaptation to the alkaline environment of the peroxisome interior.

Peroxisomal Metabolic Functions

Peroxisomal enzymes participate in a variety of metabolic processes, many of which involve lipids. In humans and other mammals, these include β-oxidation of fatty acids, synthesis of bile acids, α-oxidation of fatty acids and small molecules, such as glyoxylate, and synthesis of ether phospholipids and isoprene compounds.[44,45] These are mediated by an array of intraperoxisomal enzymes but also depend upon metabolite transporters in the peroxisome membrane. Isolated defects in peroxisomal metabolic enzymes and membrane transporters are associated with an array of human diseases. Other chapters describe the deficiencies of peroxisomal fatty acid β-oxidation and etherphospholipid synthesis (Chap. 130), Refsum disease (Chap. 132), primary hyperoxaluria, type 1 (Chap. 133), and X-linked adrenoleukodystrophy (Chap. 131). We refer the reader to these chapters, to several excellent reviews,[44–46] and to the peroxisome Web site (www.peroxisome.org) for detailed discussions of peroxisomal enzymes and their roles in cellular metabolism.

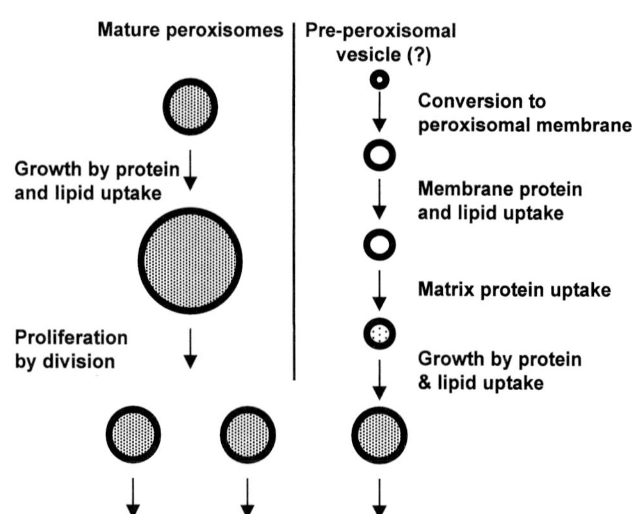

Fig. 129-2 The two pathway model of peroxisome biogenesis. Peroxisomes may arise by growth and division of preexisting peroxisomes as outlined on the left half of the diagram. Post-translation uptake of peroxisomal matrix proteins and peroxisomal membrane proteins delivers protein to the growing organelle. Uptake of lipids occurs through an unknown mechanism. Peroxisomes divide by fission and/or fusion. Peroxisomes can form in the absence of preexisting peroxisomes, indicating that peroxisomes may also form *de novo* by a distinct mechanism. As outlined on the right half of the figure, some other endomembrane of the cell provides a preperoxisomal vesicle, which is then converted into a nascent peroxisome by incorporation of one or more specific factors. These factors then mediate the import of peroxisomal membrane proteins which eventually leads to the formation of a functional matrix protein import apparatus and the ability to divide.

PEROXISOME BIOGENESIS

A General Model of Peroxisome Biogenesis

The peroxisome is one of four distinct organelle systems within mammalian cells. Like the nucleus, the mitochondrion, and the organelles of the secretory/endocytic system (endoplasmic reticulum [ER], Golgi apparatus, lysosomes, endosomes, transport vesicles, secretory vesicles, etc.), the peroxisome appears to use unique mechanisms for its biogenesis. Organelle biogenesis usually follows either of two simple models: growth and division or assembly by vesicle fusion.[47,48] For example, mitochondrial biogenesis involves repeated rounds of mitochondrial growth and division and appears to be relatively independent of other organelle systems.[48] In contrast, the Golgi apparatus depends upon the continuous supply of delivery of protein and lipid by vesicular transport from the endoplasmic reticulum.[47,49,50]

Within this narrow range of options there is surprisingly little agreement on which model best explains peroxisome biogenesis.[22,51–54] A large number of studies provide strong evidence that peroxisomes arise by the growth and division of preexisting peroxisomes.[55] Other equally strong studies demonstrate that peroxisomes can be synthesized in the absence of preexisting peroxisomes.[56–59] Although it is possible to view these results as contradictory we prefer a hypothesis that incorporates both sets of data. Specifically, we propose that peroxisomes may be formed by either of two distinct mechanisms (Fig. 129-2).[56] In this model, the primary route of peroxisome biogenesis involves the growth of preexisting peroxisomes by direct uptake of membrane and matrix proteins, followed by division once a critical threshold is reached. Our model also proposes a second distinct mode of peroxisome biogenesis in which peroxisomes arise from some preperoxisomal vesicle, possibly another endomembrane of the cell. This latter mechanism allows for reappearance of peroxisomes in cells that are completely devoid of the organelle.

As expected for a complex biologic process, the biogenesis of peroxisomes involves a large number of genes and their protein products.[60] As a consequence, genetic disorders of peroxisome biogenesis are heterogeneous. This was first demonstrated by somatic cell-fusion experiments using skin fibroblasts from PBD patients.[16] These early experiments revealed the existence of six distinct CGs of PBD patients and recent studies have expanded the number of PBD CGs to 12.[20] Studies in yeast have identified even more factors that are required for peroxisome biogenesis, with reports of at least 23 distinct fungal peroxisome biogenesis (PEX) genes in the literature.[54,60,61] Humans may have orthologs for all or nearly all of the yeast PEX genes, but only 14 human PEX genes are presently known.[22,62–64]

Distinct Mechanisms for Peroxisomal Matrix and Membrane Protein Import

Any model of peroxisome biogenesis must explain the biogenic route of peroxisomal proteins and the origin of peroxisome membranes. A variety of studies have shown that peroxisomal matrix proteins and PMPs are encoded by nuclear genes, synthesized in the cytoplasm, and imported posttranslationally into peroxisomes.[55] The mechanisms involved in peroxisomal matrix protein import and PMP import appear to be distinct. ZS cells were initially thought to lack peroxisomes entirely,[6] but this hypothesis was revised by studies of PMP fates in PBD cell lines. Santos et al.[65,66] examined cells from two severely affected ZS patients using immunologic reagents directed against PMPs. They found that these cells contained numerous PMP-containing peroxisomes that failed to import peroxisomal matrix proteins.

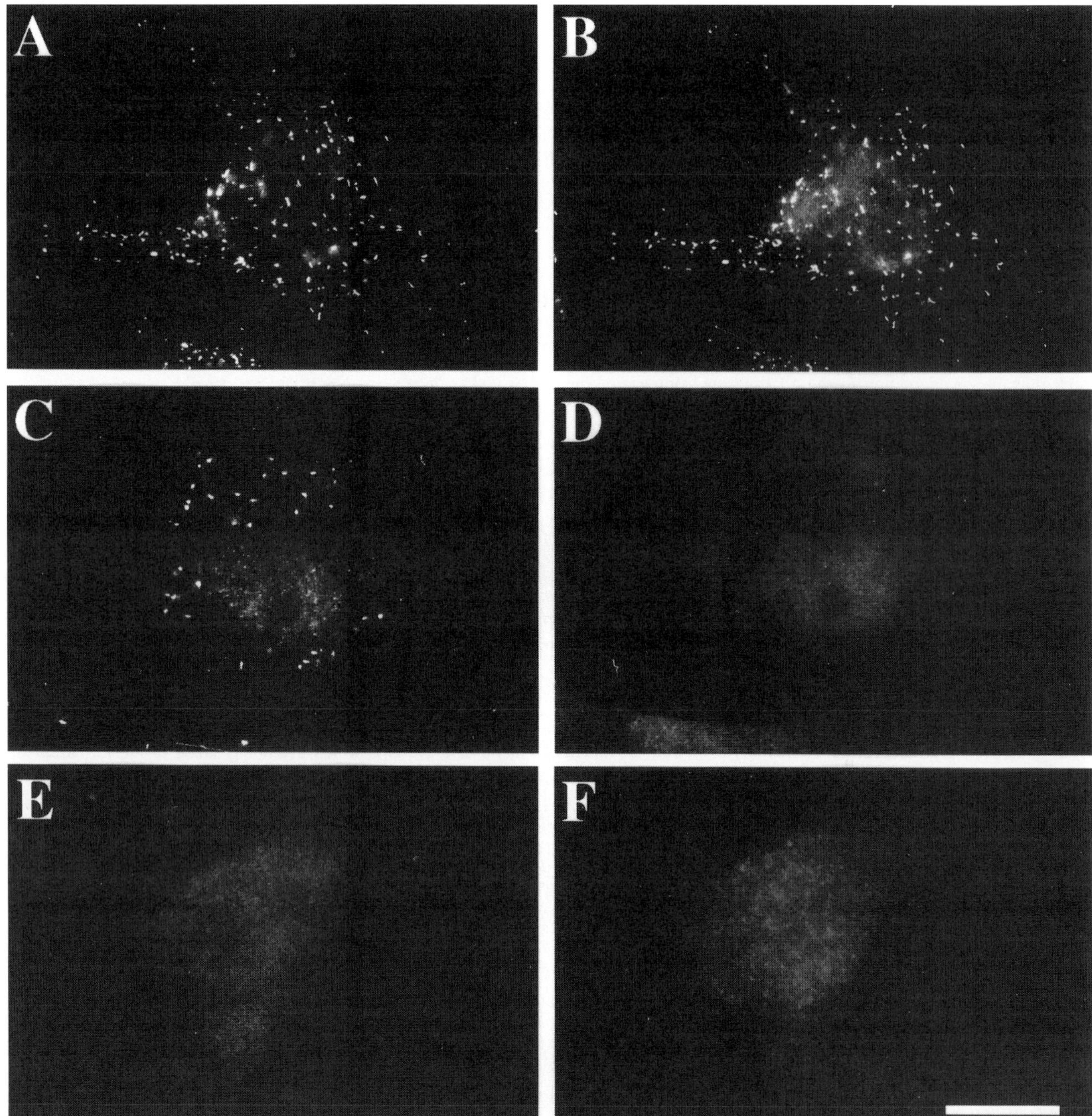

Fig. 129-3 The PBDs can be caused by defects in peroxisomal matrix protein import or peroxisome membrane synthesis. Immunofluorescence microscopy shows that human skin fibroblasts from an unaffected individual (*A, B*) have numerous peroxisomes that contain both integral peroxisomal membrane proteins and peroxisomal matrix proteins, shown here by staining for (*A*) PMP70 and (*B*) the matrix enzyme, catalase. Skin fibroblasts from a PEX10-deficient patient, PBD100[140] have (*C*) numerous PMP70-containing peroxisomes, but (*D*) are unable to import catalase into these peroxisomes, indicating that PEX10 plays a specific role in peroxisomal matrix protein import. In contrast, skin fibroblasts from a PEX3-deficient patient, PBD401,[57] (*E*) lack detectable peroxisomes when stained for PMP70 or (data not shown) any of several other integral peroxisomal membrane proteins. Such cells obviously cannot import peroxisomal matrix proteins (*F*) such as catalase and provide evidence that genes such as PEX3 play important roles in peroxisome membrane biogenesis. Bar = 20 μM. (*Photo courtesy of ST South and SJ Gould.*)

This specific defect in peroxisomal matrix protein import is shown in a series of double indirect immunofluorescence images of normal and PBD fibroblasts (Fig. 129-3). Normal fibroblasts have numerous peroxisomes that contain both integral PMPs and peroxisomal matrix enzymes as shown by the colocalization of the peroxisomal membrane marker, PMP70, and the peroxisomal matrix enzyme catalase in punctate structures distributed throughout the cytoplasm (Fig. 129-3*A* and *B*). In contrast, fibroblasts from a typical Zellweger spectrum patient have numerous PMP-containing peroxisomes but these are unable to import peroxisomal matrix proteins (Fig. 129-3*C* and *D*). This phenotype indicates that the defective genes in these PBD patients encode proteins that play important roles in peroxisomal matrix protein import but that are not required for the import of PMPs or the synthesis of peroxisome membranes.[23,61] The PBD patients that display this cellular phenotype comprise nine of the 12 CG (see Table 129-1). Cells in all of these CGs display the same general phenotype, although differences in allele severity appears to modulate the extent of the matrix protein import defect.[67,68]

A second aspect of the cellular phenotype of these CGs is that the peroxisomes are unusually large and their abundance is roughly 20 percent (approximately 100 per cell) of that in normal

Table 129-1 Summary of PBD Complementation Groups, Numbers of Patients in Each Group and Their Phenotypes, Their Proportion of the PBD Patients, the Associated Gene Defects, Gene Map Position, and Peroxin Characteristics and Presumed Role in Peroxisome Biogenesis

CG	Phenotypes	%	Gene	Location	Peroxin Size, Distribution	Motifs	Function
CG1	75 ZS, 49 NALD, 26 IRD	57%	*PEX1*	7q21-22	143 kDa, n.d.	AAA ATPase	matrix protein import
CG2	1 ZS, 2 NALD, 1 IRD	1%	*PEX5*	12p13	67 kDa, cytosolic/ peroxisomal	TPR domain	matrix protein import, PTS1 receptor
CG3	6 ZS, 2 NALD, 2 IRD	4%	*PEX12*	—	41 kDa, integral PMP	zinc RING	matrix protein import, after docking
CG4	11 ZS, 11 NALD	9%	*PEX6*	6p21.1	104 kDa, n.d.	AAA ATPase	matrix protein import
CG7	4 ZS, 1 NALD	2%	*PEX10*	1p36	37 kDa, integral PMP	zinc RING	matrix protein import, after docking
CG8	4 ZS, 5 NALD, 2 IRD	4%	?		?	?	matrix protein import
CG9	1 ZS	<1%	*PEX16*	—	39 kDa, integral PMP	none known	peroxisome membrane biogenesis
CG10	5 ZS, 2 IRD	3%	*PEX2*	8q21.1	35 kDa, integral PMP	zinc RING	matrix protein import, after docking
CG11	44 RCDP	17%	*PEX7*	6q21-22.2	36 kDa, cytosolic/ peroxisomal	WD-40	matrix protein import, PTS2 receptor
CG12	2 ZS	1%	*PEX3*	6q23-24	42 kDa, integral PMP	none known	peroxisome membrane biogenesis
CG13	1 ZS, 1 NALD	1%	*PEX13*	2p14-16	44 kDa, integral PMP	SH3 domain	matrix protein import, receptor docking
CG14	1 ZS	<1%	*PEX19*	1q22	33 kDa, cytosolic/ peroxisomal	farnesylation	membrane biogenesis, PMP receptor

human fibroblasts (approximately 500 per cell). This numerical reduction may reflect some role for the protein products of the mutant genes in peroxisome membrane biogenesis or it could be a secondary consequence of the metabolic perturbation caused by global peroxisome malfunction. To distinguish between these two possibilities Chang et al.[23] examined peroxisome abundance and morphology in fibroblasts from PBD patients, and in fibroblasts from patients with defects in single peroxisomal enzymes. They found that defects in peroxisomal fatty acid β-oxidation enzymes alone are sufficient to cause the alterations in peroxisome size and abundance seen in most PBD cells.

Recently, a few ZS patients have been identified whose cells lack PMP-containing peroxisomes entirely (Fig. 129-3*E* and *F*). This phenotype is associated with the rapid degradation of some PMPs[20,56,57,59,69] and the mislocalization of other PMPs to the mitochondria,[57,59] indicating that the proteins encoded by the genes defective in these patients are involved in the import of PMPs and/or the synthesis of peroxisomal membranes. This phenotype is characteristic of only three PBD CGs (Table 129-1).[20,56–59]

Peroxisomal Matrix Protein Import

There is a wealth of information on the targeting signals for newly synthesized peroxisomal matrix proteins and their receptors. Studies of these targeting signal receptors have had a profound influence on our models of peroxisomal matrix protein import. Current data indicate that peroxisomal matrix protein import involves cytosolic and peroxisomal processes (Fig. 129-4).

Targeting Signals. Early studies of matrix protein import revealed that the C-terminus of several peroxisomal enzymes was important for their targeting, including firefly luciferase,[70] rat acyl-CoA oxidase,[71] rat L-bifunctional protein,[71] pig D-amino acid oxidase,[71] and human catalase.[71] A detailed analysis of the targeting information in firefly luciferase revealed that its C-terminal three amino acids (–S-K-L-COOH) were both necessary for luciferase import and sufficient to direct other nonperoxisomal proteins into the peroxisome lumen *in vivo*.[72] This first study of the peroxisomal targeting signal (PTS) 1 also revealed that the sequence was variable: alanine or cysteine could substitute for serine at the –3 position, and arginine or histidine could function in place of lysine at the –2 position.

The PTS1 is evolutionarily conserved and functions in species as divergent as protozoans, fungi, plants, insects, and mammals.[73,74] A PTS1 sequence is present at the C-terminus of more

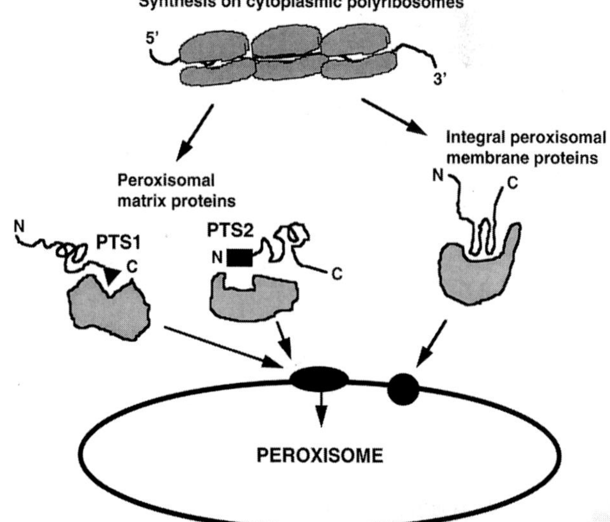

Fig. 129-4 The biogenesis of peroxisomal proteins. Peroxisomal matrix proteins and integral peroxisomal membrane proteins are synthesized on free, cytoplasmic polyribosomes and are imported posttranslationally from the cytoplasm. Peroxisomal proteins contain discrete targeting information. The peroxisomal targeting signals that direct the proteins into the peroxisome matrix are the C-terminal PTS1 and the N-terminal PTS2. The molecular nature of targeting of the integral peroxisomal membrane proteins has yet to be resolved. Newly synthesized peroxisomal matrix proteins and peroxisomal membrane proteins appear to be recognized by distinct, predominately cytoplasmic receptors. The import of matrix and membrane proteins requires additional, distinct sets of peroxisomal membrane proteins.

than 95 percent of the known peroxisomal matrix proteins. While the "consensus PTS1" suggested by Gould et al.[72] ((S/A/C)-(K/R/H)-L-COOH) includes the most commonly used forms of the PTS1,[75,76] many sequence variants have been identified, particularly in lower eukaryotes such as yeast[77,78] and protozoans.[79,80] These include a plethora of single amino acid differences from the consensus (e.g., methionine,[81] isoleucine,[82] or valine[83] in place of the C-terminal leucine and proline,[83a] histidine,[84] or lysine[85] in place of serine at the −3 position). The PTS1 may also vary in the position of the essential basic residue. This is typically found at the −2 position but may also function at the −4 position, extending the length of the PTS1 from a tripeptide to a tetrapeptide.[86,87]

Several peroxisomal matrix enzymes do not contain a functional PTS1, including thiolase,[88,89] acyl-CoA α-hydroxylase,[90,91] and alkyl-dihydroxyacetonephosphate acyltransferase.[92] Instead, these proteins contain an N-terminal PTS2, a signal that was first identified in rat thiolase.[88] The PTS2 consensus is −(R/K)(L/V/I)X_5(Q/H)(L/A) or a conservative variant thereof. Like the PTS1, the PTS2 is both necessary for the import of these proteins and is sufficient to direct soluble proteins into the peroxisome matrix. Unlike the PTS1, which is retained after import, the N-terminal segments of certain PTS2-containing proteins are cleaved following import, although this cleavage event is not essential for PTS2 function.[88]

Factors That Mediate Peroxisomal Matrix Protein Import

All of the known proteins that mediate peroxisomal matrix protein import have been identified through genetic screens, either in yeast or in cultured rodent cells.[93–97] These proteins, known as peroxins, are encoded by PEX genes.[98]

In yeast, fatty acid β-oxidation takes place exclusively in peroxisomes (as opposed to peroxisomes and mitochondria in mammalian cells).[99] This allows design of auxotroph screens that test the ability of yeast to grow on a long-chain fat (oleic acid) as a measure of peroxisome integrity. Thus, it is relatively simple to conduct a mutant screen, and the identification of the corresponding gene is quite straightforward once a mutant is in hand.

Systemic approaches to PEX gene identification have also been pursued in mammalian cells.[100–102] Pex mutants in higher and lower eukaryotes have similar cellular phenotypes (Fig. 129-5). This reflects the general conservation of peroxin function across most species.

The following section represents what is currently known about the various factors that are involved in peroxisomal matrix protein import and is weighted towards data obtained in human and other mammalian cells.

Recognition of PTS1. The PTS1 receptor PEX5 was first identified in the yeast *P. pastoris*. The *P. pastoris pex5* mutant attracted interest because it displayed an isolated defect in the import of PTS1- but not PTS2-containing proteins.[103] This initial study also established that PEX5 bound specifically to PTS1-containing peptides. PEX5 has since been identified in more than 10 species and in all cases consists of an approximately 60 to 70 kDa protein with 6 to 7 tetratricopeptide repeats (TPRs, a 34-amino-acid-long repeat) in its C-terminal half.[103–107] The segment of PEX5 comprised by the TPR repeats appears to define

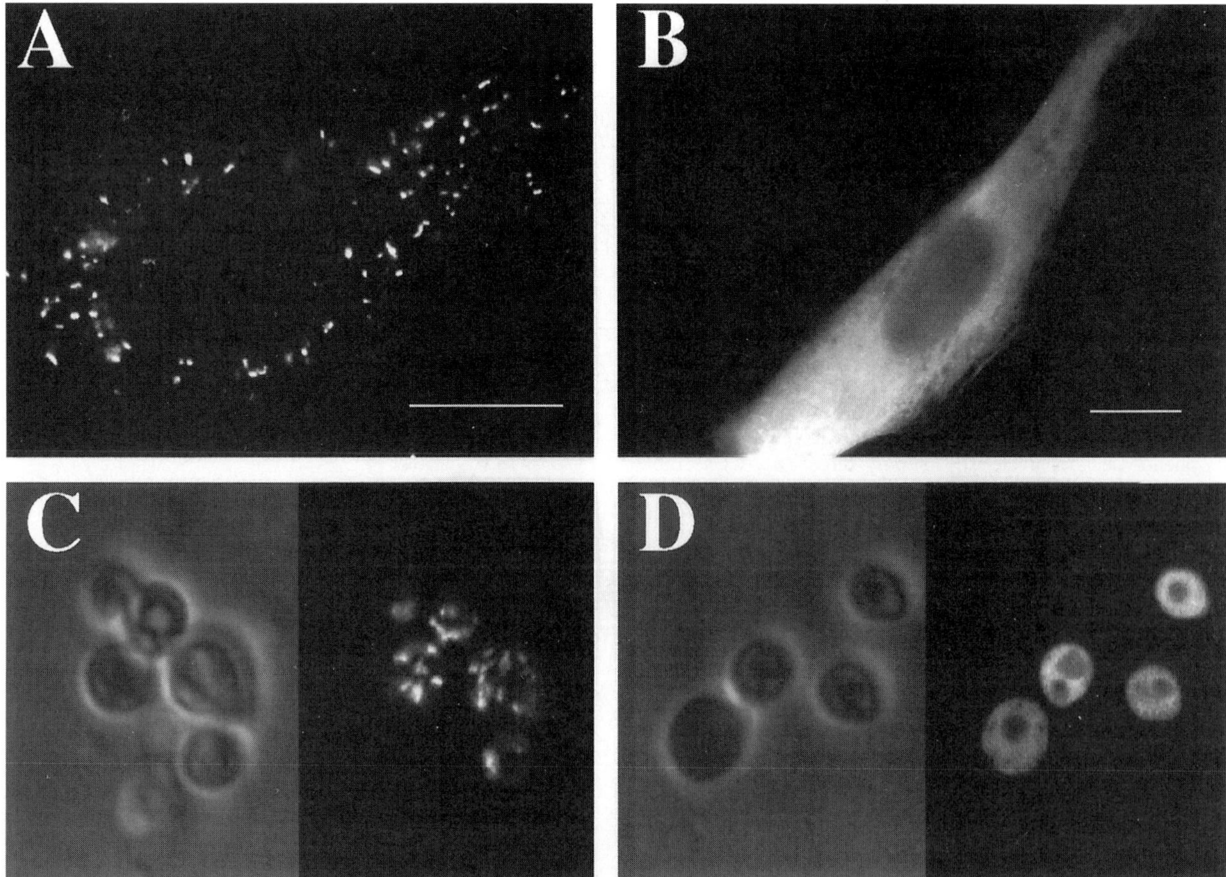

Fig. 129-5 A common cellular phenotype for PBD patients and yeast pex mutants. Immunofluorescence microscopy shows that the peroxisomal matrix enzyme PECI[40] is (*A*) imported into peroxisomes of human skin fibroblasts, but (*B*) accumulates in the cytoplasm of skin fibroblasts from a patient with Zellweger syndrome, PBD100.[140] *C and D*, the inability to import peroxisomal matrix proteins is also observed in yeast pex mutants, as shown here by (*left panels*) phase-contrast and (*right panels*) fluorescence microscopy. A fusion protein between the green fluorescent protein and the PTS1 (*C*) is imported into peroxisomes of wild-type *S. cerevisiae*, but (*D*) accumulates in the cytoplasm of the *S. cerevisiae* pex12 mutant. (*Courtesy of* (A,B) *JM Jones and* (C,D) *CC Chang.*)

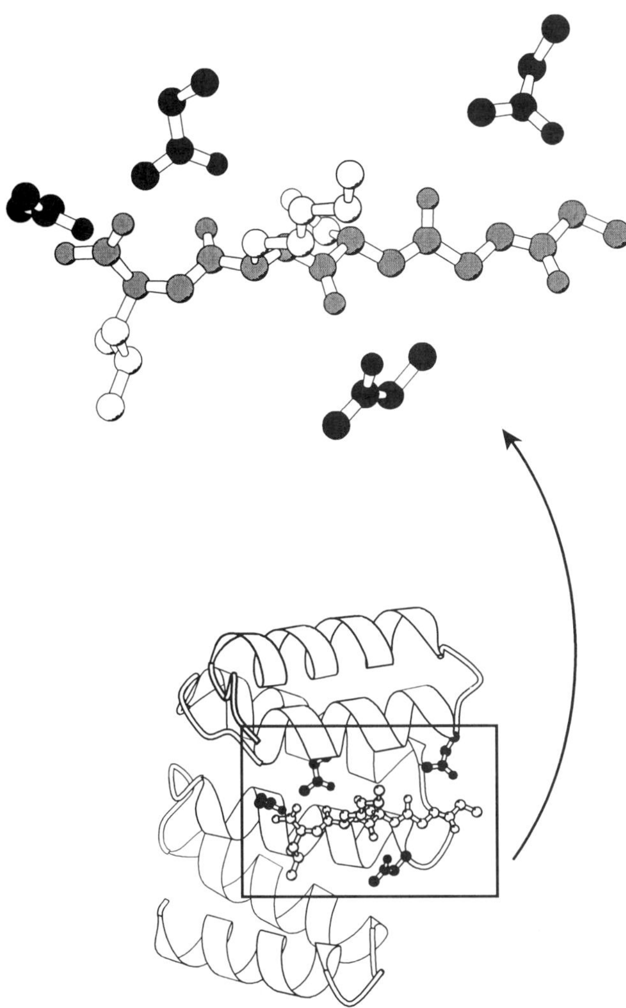

Fig. 129-6 A proposed model for the PEX5-PTS1 complex predicts that conserved asparagine residues bind the PTS1 peptide backbone. The ribbon diagram (*lower image*) shows the receptor ligand complex with the ligand-contacting asparagine residues in black. The upper image shows an expanded view with the ribbon removed, the asparagine side chains in black, the PTS1 peptide backbone in gray, and the PTS1 side chains in white. (*From Gatto et al.*[109] *Used with permission.*)

the PTS1-binding domain because this region retains full PTS1-binding and specificity *in vitro*.[104,108]

A structural model for the PEX5-PTS1 interaction has been proposed.[109] This molecular replacement model is based on the known x-ray crystal structure of three TPRs in protein phosphatase 5.[110] The hypothetical PEX5-PTS1 structure reveals a nearly perfect PTS1-binding pocket formed by TPRs 5, 6, and 7 (Fig. 129-6). The peptide backbone of the PTS1 appears to be bound by three conserved asparagine residues, while a fourth conserved asparagine cooperates with a conserved arginine residue to bind the C-terminal carboxylate of the PTS1. This model also reveals the existence of binding pockets for the side chains at positions −1 and −3 of the PTS1 and proposes that the amino acid side chains at positions −2 and −4 point away from TPRs 5, 6, and 7. Thus, it appears that some other region within the PEX5 TPR domain is responsible for specifying a basic residue at the −2 or −4 positions of the PTS1.

The analysis of PEX5-deficient human fibroblasts has provided an indirect test of this model. Severe mutations in human PEX5 disrupt import of both PTS1- and PTS2-targeted enzymes.[104] This phenotype differs from that of yeast pex5 mutants, which are defective only in PTS1-mediated import, and demonstrates that human PEX5 plays an essential role in both PTS1 and PTS2 protein import. Dodt et al.[104] also identified a more mildly affected PBD patient with a missense mutation in PEX5, N489K. Asparagine 489 is one of the four conserved of the PTS1-binding domain described by Gatto et al.[109] and its alteration is expected to disrupt PTS1 recognition. In accordance with this prediction, the patient with the N489K mutation is defective only in PTS1 protein import and imports PTS2 proteins normally. Furthermore, expression of the N489K mutant of PEX5 restores PTS2 protein import in cells that completely lack PEX5 activity.[111] Thus, the three-dimensional model of the PEX5-PTS1 complex[109] explains the PTS1-specific import defect in cells that are homozygous for the PEX5/N489K mutation.

Studies of human PEX5 have also focused on downstream events that occur following the binding of newly synthesized PTS1-containing proteins. PEX5 is a predominantly cytoplasmic, partly peroxisomal protein[104,112,113] that cycles between the cytoplasm and peroxisome.[114] This dynamic distribution for the PTS1 receptor suggests that peroxisomal matrix protein import involves multiple steps in addition to the translocation of proteins through the peroxisome membrane. These include the recognition of newly synthesized peroxisomal matrix proteins (ligands) in the cytoplasm by the PTS receptor, transport of the receptor-ligand complex to the peroxisome, docking of the complex to the peroxisome membrane, dissociation of receptors from their ligands, ligand import, and receptor recycling (Fig. 129-7). Since its original proposal,[115] a variety of studies have lent indirect support to this model, including the identification of receptor docking factors[112,113,116–118] and receptor recycling factors.[119,120]

Recognition of PTS2. The PEX7 gene was first identified in the yeast *Saccharomyces cerevisiae*.[121] Cells lacking PEX7 are unable to import PTS2-containing proteins but import PTS1 proteins normally. PEX7 contains six WD40 repeats that are preceded by a short N-terminal extension. The WD40 repeat motif is a known mediator of protein-protein interactions.[122] PEX7 has intrinsic PTS2-binding activity,[123,124] but there is no model yet on the regions of PEX7 which contact the PTS2. Studies of *S. cerevisiae* PEX7 distribution indicate that it, like PEX5, may also be a predominantly cytoplasmic, partly peroxisomal protein,[121,123] although there is also some data that suggests it may reside within peroxisomes.[125] An analysis of *Pichia pastoris* PEX7 revealed that it, too, was required only for PTS2 protein import and was a predominantly cytoplasmic, partly peroxisomal protein.[126]

RCDP is associated with a specific defect in PTS2 protein import, suggesting that the gene defective in this disease would encode the PTS2 receptor.[127,128] This hypothesis was confirmed through studies of human PEX7.[129–132] Expression of human PEX7 rescues the cellular phenotype in RCDP cells, and PEX7 mutations have been identified in all RCDP patients examined. The subcellular distribution of endogenously expressed human PEX7 has yet to be elucidated, but an epitope-tagged form of the protein was found to be predominantly cytoplasmic.[129]

Studies in yeast have identified two additional peroxins, PEX18 and PEX21, that appear to physically bind PEX7 and aid in the import of PTS2-containing proteins.[133] PEX18 and PEX21 are homologous to one another and display partial functional redundancy: loss of either has at most a mild effect on PTS2 protein import whereas loss of both peroxins eliminates PTS2 protein import. The pex18, pex21 double-mutant imports PTS1 proteins normally. PEX18 and PEX21 are predominantly cytoplasmic proteins that may aid in the transit of PEX7 between the peroxisome and cytoplasm or facilitate the interaction between PEX7 and PTS2-containing proteins. PEX20 is another protein that appears to play an important role in the import of PTS2-containing proteins, possibly at a step prior to PEX7.[134]

PTS Receptor Docking. Once a newly synthesized peroxisomal matrix protein is recognized by the PTS receptors, receptor-ligand complexes are thought to dock at specific sites in the peroxisomal

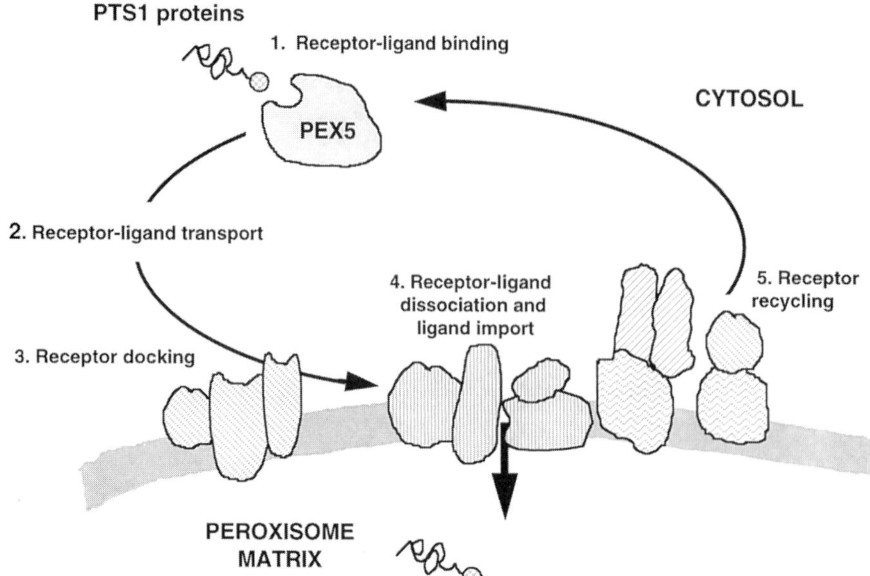

Fig. 129-7 A model of peroxisomal matrix protein import. The predominantly cytoplasmic, partly peroxisomal distribution of PEX5, together with its ability to cycle between peroxisomes and cytoplasm, predicts that matrix protein import involves overlapping cytoplasmic and peroxisomal processes. These are thought to involve (1) binding of newly synthesized peroxisomal matrix proteins (ligands) by the PTS receptor, (2) transport of the receptor ligand complex to the peroxisome, (3) interaction of the complex with specific docking factors, (4) receptor ligand dissociation and matrix protein import, followed by (5) PTS receptor recycling.

membrane. Two peroxisomal membrane proteins, PEX13 and PEX14, have been implicated in this process. PEX13 is an integral peroxisomal membrane that contains a cytoplasmically exposed SH3 domain at its C-terminus.[112,113,116,135,136] Loss of PEX13 results in a defect in import of both PTS1 and PTS2 proteins but does not affect PMP import or peroxisome membrane synthesis. The SH3 domain is a well-known protein-binding domain, and studies in yeast have demonstrated that PEX13 binds to PEX5 via its SH3 domain but also binds to PEX14 via this domain.[112,113,116,117] PEX13 also binds to PEX7 (either directly or indirectly) via an N-terminal, cytoplasmically exposed domain,[117] and is required for the association of PEX5 and PEX7 with peroxisome membranes.

Loss of PEX14 also prevents the PTS receptors from associating with peroxisome membranes.[117,118] In yeast, PEX14 encodes a peripheral peroxisomal membrane protein that is required for both PTS1 and PTS2 protein import but is dispensable for PMP import. In mammals, PEX14 appears to be an integral PMP that also interacts with PEX5 and PEX7.[62–64,137] but there is no evidence on whether mammalian PEX14 is required for PTS receptor docking. PEX14 physically interacts with PEX13 and requires this interaction to associate with peroxisomes, at least in yeast.[117]

Matrix Protein Translocation. Following the docking of PTS receptors to the peroxisome membrane, the newly synthesized matrix proteins must be dissociated from their receptors and then imported into the peroxisome lumen. Peroxisomal matrix protein translocation has yet to be reconstituted biochemically and, thus, there is no unequivocal evidence demonstrating a role for any peroxin in either of these processes. However, likely candidates can be proposed based on expected consequences of translocation defects, the phenotypes of defects in certain PEX mutants, and the biochemical properties of the proteins that are defective in these mutants.

Our model of peroxisomal matrix protein import (Fig. 129-4) predicts two phenotypes for translocation defects. First, the mutant cells should have a severe defect in both PTS1 and PTS2 import, but no defect in peroxisome membrane synthesis or PMP import. Second, docking of the PTS1 receptor should be unaffected and the amount of PTS receptors present on peroxisomes of these mutants should be equal to or greater than the amount of PEX5 detected on peroxisomes of normal cells. Furthermore, the matrix protein translocation factors should interact with the proteins undergoing import. Alternatively, these factors may interact with the PTS receptors themselves, because it is possible that the translocation apparatus will interact with the PTS receptors rather than their ligands.

In both yeast and human cells, loss of either PEX10 or PEX12 results in a severe defect in peroxisomal matrix protein import but no defect in peroxisomal membrane synthesis or PMP import.[23,67,138–142] Furthermore, studies of PEX10- and PEX12-deficient human cells revealed that these peroxins are not required for PEX5 docking on the peroxisome membrane.[114,142] PEX10 and PEX12 are integral peroxisomal membrane proteins and both contain a zinc RING domain at their cytoplasmically exposed C-terminus.[138–141] Zinc RING motifs are thought to mediate protein-protein interactions.[143–145] We found that the zinc RING of PEX12 binds PEX5, the PTS1 receptor, as well as the zing RING domain of PEX10.[142] PEX12, PEX5, and PEX10 appear to associate with one another in vivo, and PEX5 and PEX10 are able to suppress mild mutations in PEX12. Taken together, these results suggest that PEX12 and PEX10 form a complex in the peroxisomal membrane that acts after receptor docking, binds PEX5, and is required for matrix protein translocation.

Loss of PEX2, another integral PMP with a C-terminal zinc RING domain, results in a similar phenotype as PEX10- and PEX12-deficient cells.[23,102,114,146,147] Specifically, PEX2-deficient cells contain numerous peroxisomes, import PMPs normally, and display normal or elevated levels of peroxisome-associated PEX5.[23,114] A recent study in the yeast *S. cerevisiae* also places PEX8 in matrix protein import downstream of receptor docking.[148] PEX8 terminates in the consensus PTS1, serine-lysine-leucine-COOH, but resides in the peroxisome membrane rather than the peroxisome matrix.[148–150] PEX8 interacts with PEX5[148] but does not require its PTS1-like sequence for either transport to peroxisomes or for interaction with PEX5, indicating that its PTS1-like sequence is used for some other process, perhaps in dissociating matrix proteins from PEX5 just prior to or during matrix protein translocation. While circumstantial evidence points to roles for PEX2, PEX8, PEX10, and PEX12 in translocation, *in vitro* translocation studies are required to test this hypothesis directly.

PTS Receptor Recycling. The final step of matrix protein import is thought to occur after translocation and involve the recycling of the PTS receptors to the cytoplasm. The evidence for a recycling event in matrix protein import includes two basic observations. First, the molar ratio of PTS receptors to peroxisomal matrix proteins appears to be on the level of 1:1000 (S. J. Gould, unpublished observation), thus, the receptors must act in a catalytic manner. Second, the PTS receptors appear to be predominantly cytoplasmic proteins and there is evidence that PEX5,[114] and perhaps PEX7 also,[121,123] may cycle between the cytoplasm and peroxisome. Like the matrix protein translocation event, there is as yet, no biochemical system for studying this process. The nomination of particular peroxins to the receptor recycling event is based entirely on expected phenotypes for recycling mutants, observed phenotypes of different PEX mutants, and biochemical properties of the corresponding peroxins.

Based on our model of peroxisomal matrix protein import (Fig. 129-4), we expect that defects in receptor recycling should not affect peroxisome membrane synthesis or PMP import. As for matrix protein import, the absence of any direct defect in receptor docking or matrix protein translocation should allow the peroxisome to import low levels of matrix proteins. Finally, we would expect recycling mutants to display some defect in the return of the receptors to the cytoplasm.

Phenotypes similar to these have been reported for the pex4 mutant of the yeast *Hansenula polymorpha*.[119] PEX4 encodes a peroxisome-associated ubiquitin-conjugating enzyme and its loss affects the import of peroxisomal matrix proteins but has no affect on PMP import.[119,151,152] The *H. polymorpha* pex4 mutant accumulates PEX5 within the peroxisome membrane, and import low to moderate levels of several peroxisomal matrix proteins. Furthermore, matrix protein import in pex4 cells is enhanced by overexpression of PEX5, indicating that loss of PEX4 restricts PEX5 availability, a phenotype expected for a receptor recycling defect.

A recent study[153] established that PEX4, which is only peripherally associated with the outer surface of peroxisome membranes,[119,151,152] physically interacts with PEX22, an integral PMP, and that loss of PEX22 results in the loss of PEX4 from the cell. These results indicate that PEX22 and PEX4 may act together at the same point in peroxisomal matrix protein import. This hypothesis is supported by the fact that cells lacking PEX22 contain peroxisomes and import PMPs. However, there is as yet no data on whether pex22 cells import residual levels of matrix proteins. There is also no data on whether pex22 cells trap PEX5 in the peroxisome membrane. However, loss of either PEX4 or PEX22 results in greatly reduced levels of PEX5, at least in the yeast *P. pastoris*.[120,153] Although we do not yet know the molecular mechanism for reduced PEX5 abundance in pex4 and pex22 cells, it could reflect a mechanism that removes inappropriate protein complexes from protein import sites.

That PEX5 abundance is greatly reduced in cells lacking PEX4 and PEX22, two proteins that appear to act in PTS receptor recycling, also sheds light on the functions of PEX1 and PEX6. Cells lacking PEX1 or PEX6 also display reduced PEX5 abundance and pulse-chase experiments have established that this is due rapid proteolysis of the PTS receptor rather than a reduced rate of PEX5 synthesis.[114,154,155] PEX1 and PEX6 encode a pair of AAA ATPases that physically interact with one another.[156–158] Furthermore, PEX1 and PEX6 genes are able to suppress mild missense mutations in one another, indicating that the physical interactions between their products are likely to have biologic significance.[156,157] That other AAA ATPases such as NSF participate in vesicle trafficking stimulated the hypothesis that PEX1 and PEX6 participate in peroxisome membrane biogenesis.[159] This hypothesis is also supported by observations in the yeast *Yarrowia lipolytica*.[160,161] However, the phenotypes of pex1 and pex6 mutants in human cells,[23,114,154,155] and in the yeasts *P. pastoris*,[162,163] *S. cerevisiae*,[61] and *H. polymorpha*,[164] argue instead that PEX1 and PEX6 act in peroxisomal matrix protein import. In each of these species, loss of PEX1 or PEX6 has no effect on the ability of cells to synthesize peroxisomal membranes or to import PMPs. Peroxisomal matrix protein import is inefficient in pex1 and pex6 mutants but detectable levels of matrix proteins can be found within their peroxisomes, indicating that PEX1 and PEX6 are not required for PTS receptor docking or matrix protein translocation. Furthermore, an epistasis analysis in the yeast *P. pastoris* place PEX1 and PEX6 late in the peroxisomal matrix protein import pathway.[120] Specifically, PEX1 and PEX6 act downstream of peroxisome membrane synthesis, receptor docking and matrix protein translocation but upstream of PEX4 and PEX22. Additional experiments are needed to elucidate the biochemistry of PTS receptor recycling and the role of the PEX1/PEX6 and PEX4/PEX22 complexes in this process.

Other Peroxins Involved in Peroxisomal Matrix Protein Import. It is apparent from the preceding discussion that our knowledge of peroxisomal matrix protein import decreases as we move from the early to later stages of the process. There is still, however, much to be learned about all aspects of peroxisomal matrix protein import. This is particularly apparent when considering PEX9,[165] PEX15,[166] PEX17,[167] and PEX23,[168] all of which appear to play roles in peroxisomal matrix protein import. Current data are insufficient to place any of these peroxins at a particular step of peroxisomal matrix protein import. Furthermore, there appears to be some confusion as to whether PEX17 acts in matrix protein import, as indicated by studies in *S. cerevisiae*,[61,167] or in the import of PMPs, as suggested by one study in the yeast *P. pastoris*.[169]

Based on the studies described above, we may now revisit the model of peroxisomal matrix protein import (Fig. 129-8). This speculative model predicts that most newly synthesized peroxisomal matrix proteins are recognized in the cytosol, followed by transport of the PTS receptor-ligand complex to the peroxisome. Specific docking sites at the peroxisome membrane provide an entry point to the translocation apparatus, which mediates both receptor-ligand dissociation and ligand import. This process is then followed by an ill-defined receptor recycling event that returns the receptors to the cytoplasm.

PMP Import and Peroxisome Membrane Synthesis

Like peroxisomal matrix proteins, integral PMPs are synthesized on free cytosolic ribosomes and are imported posttranslationally into peroxisomes.[55,170,171] However, as we mentioned above, PMP import and peroxisomal matrix protein import are separate processes and require distinct sets of peroxins.[20,22,23,56–59,61,172] The fundamental difference between PMP import and peroxisomal matrix protein import is also revealed by the differences in targeting information used by matrix and membrane proteins of this organelle. PMPs generally lack PTS1- and PTS2-like sequences,[173] PMP import is independent of the PTS1 and PTS2 receptors,[23,61] and the sole PMP targeting signal that has been identified bears no resemblance to either the PTS1 or PTS2.[174,175] In vitro studies also reveal distinctions between PMP import[176,177] and peroxisomal matrix protein import.[178–182] Both processes appear to be time and temperature dependent, but PMP import does not require ATP, whereas ATP depletion strongly inhibits peroxisomal matrix protein import.

Organelle membranes are composed of protein, phospholipids, and a variety of other lipids, such as sterols and fatty acids.[183] Although it is possible to form protein-free lipid bilayers *in vitro*,[184] it is unlikely that organelle membranes could form in the absence of integral membrane proteins. Therefore, the import of integral PMPs may be an essential aspect of peroxisome membrane biogenesis. For a number of years it was thought that all PBD cell lines contained peroxisomal membranes,[185,186] but recent studies identified three different CG Zellweger-spectrum patients who appear to lack detectable peroxisomes.[20,56–59,69,172] The fate of PMPs in these cells is variable, with some being degraded rapidly and others being mislocalized to the mitochondria. Genetic studies revealed that patients from CG9, CG12, and CG14 have inactivating mutations in the PEX3,[57] PEX16,[56,172] and PEX19[58,59] genes, respectively (see Table 129-1).

PEX19

The absence of detectable peroxisomes could be caused by either a defect in the import of PMPs or a defect in the assembly of peroxisome membranes. However, cellular and biochemical

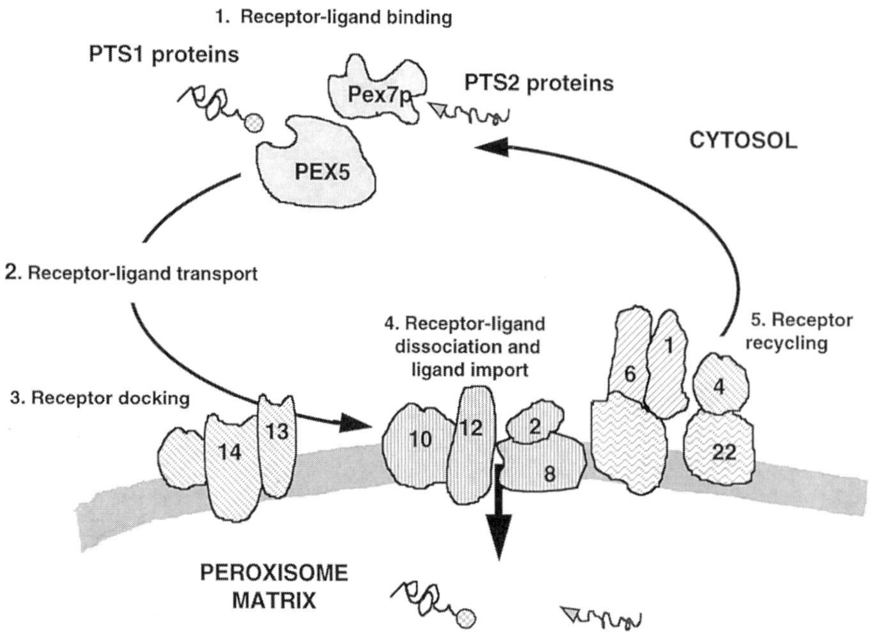

Fig. 129-8 Roles of different peroxins in peroxisomal matrix protein import. PEX5 and PEX7 act as receptors for newly synthesized PTS1- and PTS2-containing peroxisomal matrix proteins, respectively. These receptors require PEX14 and PEX13 for association with peroxisome membranes. The peroxins PEX10, PEX12, PEX2, and PEX8 all appear to be essential for peroxisomal matrix protein translocation but not for receptor docking. These properties, together with the fact that they act upstream of PEX1, PEX4, PEX6, and PEX22, indicate that they may act in matrix protein translocation. PEX1 and PEX6 interact with one another upstream of PEX4 and PEX22 in the terminal steps of matrix protein import.

studies of PEX19 indicate that this protein plays a direct role in PMP import.[59] Human PEX19 was first identified as an abundant farnesylated protein of Chinese hamster ovary cells that was found to be associated with peroxisome membranes.[187] Independent studies in the yeast *S. cerevisiae* and *P. pastoris* identified PEX19 as a small farnesylated protein that was required for peroxisome biogenesis.[188,189] Recently, studies of human and yeast PEX19 converged. Human PEX19 was found to be mutated in a ZS patient who lacked detectable peroxisomes[58] and pex19 was found to be just one of two *S. cerevisiae* pex mutants that lack peroxisome membranes entirely.[61]

Subcellular fractionation experiments revealed that mammalian and yeast PEX19 proteins are predominantly cytoplasmic, partly peroxisomal proteins.[59,188,189] A search for proteins that interact with human PEX19 revealed that this peroxin bound to a wide array of integral PMPs.[59] These included a number of peroxins, including PEX10, PEX11, PEX12, PEX13 and PEX14. It also included a number of metabolite transporters, including PMP34, PMP70, ALDP, and ALDR. The interaction of PEX19 with such a diverse array of integral PMPs indicated that it may participate in their biogenesis rather than their function.

This hypothesis was supported, of course, by the inability of pex19 cells to import PMPs.[58,59] However, it was also supported by several other lines of evidence.[59] First, mislocalization of PEX19 to the nucleus led to an accumulation of newly synthesized integral PMPs in the nucleoplasm, a distribution that is normally never observed for any integral PMP. Second, PEX19 bound to small regions of integral PMPs that were sufficient for peroxisomal localization, indicating that PMP targeting signals contain a PEX19-binding domain. Third, the affinity of PEX19 for integral PMPs is appropriate for a reversible interaction and displays a K_d of approximately 500 nM or less. Taken together, these results demonstrate that PEX19 plays a critical role in PMP import, most likely as a chaperone for newly synthesized PMPs or a PMP targeting signal receptor.

PEX3 and PEX16

While PEX19 appears to play a role in PMP import, the roles of PEX3 and PEX16 in peroxisome membrane biogenesis are less clear.[22] Any cell lacking peroxisome membranes might actually be defective in the genesis of the lipid bilayer rather than PMP import per se and there is no evidence that clearly distinguishes between these two possible roles for PEX3 and PEX16. PEX3 and PEX16 are both integral PMPs and they both interact with PEX19.[59,188–190] While this interaction may simply represent an early step in the biogenesis of these two PMPs, the interaction of PEX19 with PEX3 and/or PEX16 might also reflect some role for these proteins in PMP import more generally. In yeast, PEX3 interacts with a region of PEX3 that is not required for its targeting, raising the possibility that PEX19 may interact with two regions of PEX3 and that PEX3 may participate in PMP import, perhaps as a docking factor for PEX19. There is no evidence as to whether PEX16 interacts with PEX3 or PEX19 other than during its own import into peroxisome membranes.

Peroxisome Synthesis in the Absence of Preexisting Peroxisomes. While there are many questions remaining about what the detailed roles of PEX3, PEX16, and PEX19 are, analysis of these factors has demonstrated one important facet of peroxisome membrane synthesis: peroxisomes can be formed in the absence of preexisting peroxisomes.[56–59,172] Several studies from different laboratories have established that reexpression of PEX3, PEX16, and PEX19 in cells with severe, inactivating mutations in these genes induces the reappearance of peroxisomes.[56–59,172] These restored peroxisomes are morphologically and functionally normal and import PMPs and peroxisomal matrix proteins.

Because PEX3 and PEX16 are integral PMPs there has been much speculation that one or the other of these factors might mediate formation of nascent, preperoxisomal structures from some other endomembrane of the cell, possibly the endoplasmic reticulum.[52–54] Time-course studies of PEX3 and PEX16 targeting failed to support the hypothesis that PEX3 or PEX16 transit through the ER en route to peroxisomes.[56,57] Rather, these studies are most consistent with direct import of these PMPs from the cytoplasm. Furthermore, addition of brefeldin A, a fungal metabolite that blocks the formation of COPI coats on biologic membranes and blocks the transit of membrane beyond the ER, does not inhibit either PEX3- or PEX16-mediated peroxisome synthesis.[56,57] In addition, expression of a dominant negative mutant of SAR1, an ER-associated GTPase required for COPII-mediated vesicle budding from the ER, also fails to inhibit this pathway of peroxisome synthesis.[57]

These results indicate that PEX3- and PEX16-mediated peroxisome membrane synthesis does not involve COPI or COPII, the two coat-protein complexes that mediate most of the known vesicle transport processes that occur early in the secretory pathway. These studies were carried out in human cells and required the indirect inhibition of COPI or COPII by drugs and/or dominant negative mutants. These experiments are therefore subject to experimental caveats that might be avoided if a more facile system such as yeast were used. A systematic side-by-side analysis of 16 known *S. cerevesiae* pex mutants revealed that the pex3 and pex19 mutants also lack detectable peroxisomes but regain peroxisomes after reintroduction of the mutated gene.[61,188,191] The ability to use yeast to study peroxisome synthesis in the absence of preexisting peroxisomes should allow for a more definitive analysis of whether peroxisome biogenesis requires contributions from the endoplasmic reticulum. However, it is notable that *S. cerevisiae* appears to lack a PEX16 gene,[54,56] indicating that the molecular mechanisms of peroxisome membrane synthesis in yeast and humans may display significant differences.

PEX11α and PEX11β

In both yeasts and mammalian cells, the abundance of peroxisomes can vary significantly depending upon the environmental conditions. *S. cerevisiae* utilizes the peroxisomal membrane protein, PEX11, to modulate the abundance of peroxisomes.[192,193] In yeast, the oxidation of fatty acids to acetyl-CoA occurs exclusively in the peroxisome and the presence of fatty acids in the growth medium causes a pronounced increase in peroxisome abundance. This phenomenon requires the transcriptional activation of the PEX11 gene and overexpression of PEX11 under similar conditions leads to hyperproliferation of peroxisomes. Conversely, loss of PEX11 causes an inability to proliferate peroxisomes in response to environmental stimuli, resulting in the accumulation of only a very few, extremely large peroxisomes within the cell.

Humans, like other mammals, contain two forms of PEX11, PEX11α, and PEX11β.[28,194] Expression of either PEX11α or PEX11β alone is sufficient to drive peroxisome proliferation in cultured human fibroblasts.[28] Northern blot experiments revealed that PEX11β is expressed at robust levels in virtually all tissues whereas PEX11α is expressed in a restricted set of tissues,[28] primarily those that respond to peroxisome proliferating agents such as clofibrate.[28,194] The most well-characterized example of peroxisome proliferation in mammals is the response of rodent liver cells to peroxisome proliferating agents. These agents act by stimulating the nuclear hormone receptor PPARα and to a lesser extent PPARγ, which, in turn, alter the transcription of numerous target genes.[195] A 2-week-long exposure to dietary clofibrate results in a tenfold increase in peroxisome abundance[196] and an approximately tenfold increase in the levels of PEX11α.[28,194] Using a tissue culture system, Schrader et al.[28] performed a kinetic study of PEX11β-induced peroxisome proliferation. The first detectable effect of PEX11β overexpression was the elongation of pre-existing peroxisomes, with peroxisome division occurring 12–24 hr later.

Although peroxisome division was not observed directly in these studies, the results suggest that the elongated tubular structures represent an intermediate that forms just prior to peroxisome fission or budding. It has been proposed that PEX11α may act as an assembly factor for ARF and COPI, and that peroxisome proliferation may proceed by COPI-dependent vesicle budding.[194] However, this model cannot explain the mechanism of PEX11β-mediated peroxisome proliferation because it lacks a COPI-binding motif (KXKXX) at its C-terminus. As for why humans and other mammals express two forms of PEX11, it is likely that they perform different functions. Based on the differences in their tissue-specific patterns of expression and their differential regulation by peroxisome proliferating agents, it has been proposed that PEX11β may mediate constitutive peroxisome proliferation, whereas PEX11α may mediate hormone- and diet-induced changes in peroxisome abundance.[28] A direct test of this hypothesis may well require the development of appropriate animal model systems.

A Model for Peroxisome Membrane Synthesis

Any model for peroxisome biogenesis must incorporate the contribution of PEX3, PEX16, and PEX19 to PMP import and peroxisome membrane synthesis, as well as the roles of PEX11 proteins in the division of preexisting peroxisomes. One hypothesis is that peroxisomes can be formed via two distinct pathways (Fig. 129-9).[22,56] This model proposes that peroxisome biogenesis

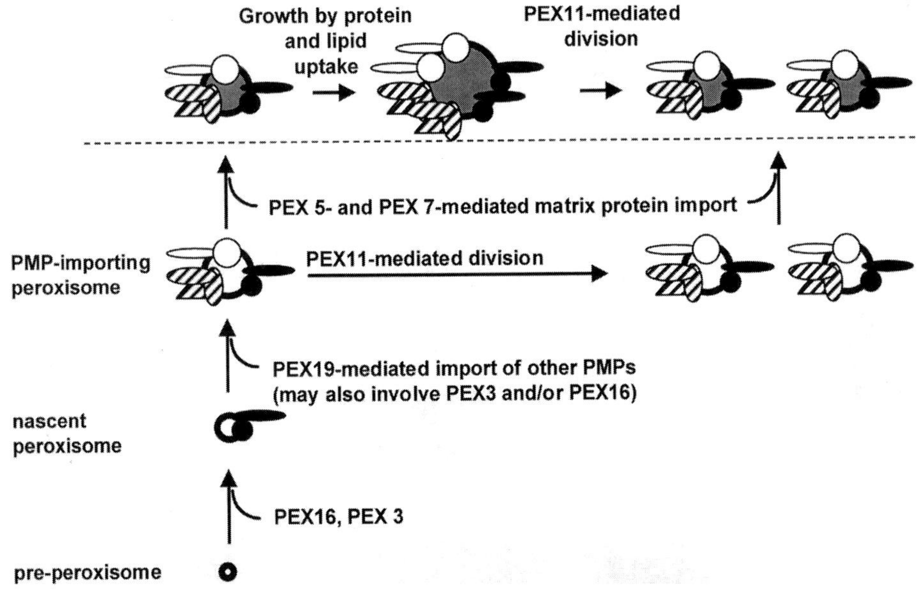

Fig. 129-9 A speculative, two-pathway model for peroxisome biogenesis. The scheme above the dotted line reflects a pathway in which peroxisomes grow by uptake of protein and lipid from the cytoplasm and divide by fission or budding. The scheme below the dotted line reflects a pathway in which peroxisomes are derived from some pre-peroxisomal vesicle. This process appears to first require PEX3 and PEX16, two integral peroxisomal membrane proteins that may normally participate in PMP import. PEX19, the putative PMP receptor, is also required and may facilitate the formation of peroxisomal vesicles that are capable of matrix protein import, PEX11-mediated peroxisome division, or both. These eventually become indistinguishable from mature peroxisomes and become capable of proliferating through the more typical pathway of growth and division of preexisting peroxisomes. The second pathway may occur only in the rescue of peroxisome-deficient mutant cells or may occur at some low frequency in all cells.[56]

typically involves the growth of peroxisomes via uptake of protein and lipids from the cytoplasm, followed by PEX11-mediated peroxisome division. During this mode of peroxisome biogenesis, PEX3, PEX16, and PEX19 would function primarily in PMP import. The two-pathway model also proposes a second route for peroxisome biogenesis in which PEX3 and/or PEX16 mediate the formation of a preperoxisomal vesicle, probably from some other endomembrane of the cell. Once formed, such a vesicle would be competent for PEX19-mediated PMP import, leading to the eventual assembly of a peroxisomal matrix protein import apparatus, matrix protein import, and the genesis of a metabolically active, functional peroxisome. Such a model is attractive because it can explain (a) the ability of PEX11 proteins to drive the proliferation of peroxisomes;[192,193] (b) the presence of only a very few large peroxisomes in cells lacking PEX11;[192,193] (c) the absence of peroxisomes in cells lacking PEX3, PEX16, or PEX19;[56–59,61,172] (d) the ability to synthesize peroxisomes in these cells when the correct gene is introduced; and (e) the extremely slow rate of peroxisome synthesis during rescue of these cells (approximately 1 to 2 days), as compared to the rapid import of PEX3 and PEX16 into preexisting peroxisomes in normal cells (less than 2 h).[56,57]

CLINICAL ASPECTS OF THE PEROXISOMAL BIOGENESIS DISORDERS

Phenotypic Spectra

Two broad phenotypic spectra result from defects in peroxisome biogenesis. The largest of these, the Zellweger spectrum, contains about 80 percent of the PBD patients and includes Zellweger syndrome (MIM 214100),[197,198] neonatal adrenoleukodystrophy (MIM 202370),[199] and infantile Refsum disease (MIM 266510).[8] Each of these clinical syndromes represents a segment of the Zellweger spectrum; ZS is at the severe end of this spectrum, while IRD represents the mildest syndromic phenotype. Patients with even milder problems, isolated, adult onset hearing loss and/or progressive retinal degeneration have been identified and extend the mild end of this phenotypic spectrum.[68,155] A fourth disorder, designated hyperpipecolic acidemia (MIM 239400) and described in only a few children, has the biochemical features that place it in the Zellweger spectrum,[200–202] and should no longer be considered a separate clinical entity.[203,204] The relative frequency of these syndromes among all PBD patients is shown in Table 129-1. Not surprisingly, somatic cell complementation studies[16–19] indicated that the Zellweger spectrum is genetically heterogeneous and we now know that mutations at 11 loci (CG 1 to 4, 7 to 10, 12 to 14) can produce phenotypic features consistent with this spectrum (see Table 129-1). Within this set of 11 genes, there does not appear to be a correlation between phenotypic severity and the responsible gene. Rather, for each of these genes, phenotypic severity seems more correlated with the consequences of the mutation on the function of the protein product (see "Phenotype/Genotype Correlations," below).

The second phenotypic spectrum includes patients with RCDP (MIM 215100). Patients with classical RCDP are distinguished from those in the Zellweger spectrum by more severe skeletal involvement and by specific biochemical parameters. They comprise 15 to 20 percent of all PBD patients. Nearly all are in CG 11 and are due to mutations in *PEX 7* (Table 129-1). Although the phenotypic severity of classical RCDP is relatively uniform, milder variants are known so that, like the Zellweger spectrum, there is a distribution of phenotypic severity.

Zellweger Spectrum

Clinical Presentation and Course. Patients with ZS, also known as the cerebrohepatorenal syndrome, have multiple congenital anomalies as well as ongoing metabolic disturbances as detailed in several reviews.[197,203,205,206] Table 129-2, reproduced from Hugo S.A. Heymans' doctoral dissertation,[13] lists the most common physical findings and their relative frequency in a series of 114 patients he collected from the literature. There are characteristic craniofacial features including large anterior fontanelle, full forehead, hypoplastic supraorbital ridges, epicanthal folds, broad nasal bridge, and small nose with anteverted nares (Fig. 129-10). Ocular abnormalities are common with cataracts, glaucoma, corneal clouding, Brushfield spots, pigmentary retinopathy, and optic nerve dysplasia. Additionally, there is severe hypotonia, weakness, and neonatal seizures. Because of the hypotonia and flattened facies, these infants are sometimes suspected to have Down syndrome.[205] Radiologic examination reveals abnormal punctate calcifications ("calcific stippling") in the patella and epiphyses of the long bones (Fig. 129-11). Renal cysts are common but may be too small to be detected by ultrasound examination (Fig. 129-12).

Affected infants rarely live more than a few months due to the severe hypotonia, feeding difficulty, seizures, liver involvement, and apnea. More than 90 percent show postnatal growth failure. In Wilson's literature survey of 90 patients, 79 had died at an average age of 12.5 weeks.[197] Some apparently classic Zellweger patients live longer. At least two factors may be operative here. Longer-surviving patients may have a somewhat milder disease or they may have survived longer because of the differences in care. While ZS is certainly a severe disorder, the phenotypic overlap with milder syndromes in the Zellweger spectrum dictates caution in making in statements of anticipated life span.

Milder Segments of the Zellweger Spectrum: NALD and IRD

NALD was first described in 1978 by Ulrich et al.[7] and has been reviewed comprehensively.[9,10,199] Ulrich's patient was severely hypotonic at birth, and developed seizures at 4 days and a hypsarrhythmic EEG at 2 months. Seizures continued to be severe and there was no psychomotor development. The boy died at 20 months. Postmortem examination showed widespread demyelination and polymicrogyria involving the cortex and the insula of the temporal operculum. The adrenals were small with atrophic cortices containing ballooned cells with lamellar cytoplasmic inclusions similar to those in X-linked ALD (see Chap. 131). Postmortem studies of brain cholesterol ester fractions showed a marked excess of hexacosanoic acid (25 percent of total fatty acid) (B. Molzer, H. Bernheimer, unpublished results). Based on these findings, Ulrich et al. named this disorder, now known as NALD, *connatal* adrenoleukodystrophy.

Despite the similarity implied by their names, NALD and X-linked ALD must be clearly differentiated. While plasma and tissue accumulation of very long chain fatty acids (VLCFA) is a feature common to both, the mechanism is different. In NALD, there is deficiency of multiple peroxisomal β-oxidation enzymes,[207] while in X-linked ALD the basic defect is limited to the initial step of VLCFA β-oxidation.[208] Additionally, NALD patients have increased plasma levels of pipecolic acid,[209] and elevated levels of bile acid intermediates[210] and their fibroblasts have an impaired capacity to synthesize plasmalogens and oxidize phytanic acid.[211,212] None of these abnormalities are observed in X-linked ALD. Hepatocytes of X-linked ALD patients contain a normal number of morphologiclly normal peroxisomes while in NALD, hepatocyte peroxisomes are present but reduced in number and lack the normal complement of matrix enzymes.[10,23,213,214] Additionally, NALD is inherited as an autosomal recessive trait in contrast to the X-linked pattern of ALD. Finally, recent molecular studies show that the genes responsible for NALD (see Table 129-1) are clearly different from that causing X-ALD (see Chap. 131).

Dysmorphic features are less striking in NALD than in Zellweger syndrome and may even be absent (Fig. 129-13).[199] The clinical course of NALD ranges from that of a severely involved infant who made no psychomotor gains and died at 4 months[215] to patients who are stable but disabled in their midteens.[212,216] These long-surviving patients are severely

Table 129-2 Main Clinical Abnormalities in Zellweger Syndrome

	Cases in which information about the feature was available		Cases in which the feature was present	
Abnormal Feature	Number	Percent	Number	Percent
High forehead	60	53	58	97
Flat occiput	16	14	13	81
Large fontanelle(s), wide sutures	57	50	55	96
Shallow orbital ridges	33	29	33	100
Low/broad nasal bridge	23	20	23	100
Epicanthus	36	32	33	92
High arched palate	37	32	35	95
External ear deformity	40	35	39	97
Micrognathia	18	16	18	100
Redundant skin folds of neck	13	11	13	100
Brushfield spots	6	5	5	83
Cataract/cloudy cornea	35	31	30	86
Glaucoma	12	11	7	58
Abnormal retinal pigmentation	15	13	6	40
Optic disk pallor	23	20	17	74
Severe hypotonia	95	83	94	99
Abnormal Moro response	26	23	26	100
Hyporeflexia or areflexia	57	50	56	98
Poor sucking	77	68	74	96
Gavage feeding	26	23	26	100
Epileptic seizures	61	54	56	92
Psychomotor retardation	45	39	45	100
Impaired hearing	21	18	9	40
Nystagmus	37	32	30	81

SOURCE: From H.S.A. Heymans' survey of 114 patients with Zellweger syndrome reported in the literature.[9]

retarded with sensorineural hearing loss and retinopathy leading to blindness. NALD patients may have an impaired cortisol response to ACTH, but overt adrenal insufficiency is infrequent. While they may achieve the ability to walk and to say a few words, their mental age rarely advances beyond 10 to 12 months. They may also experience regression at 3 to 5 years of age, presumably due to onset and progression of a leukodystrophy. As discussed below, differentiating these patients from IRD is often difficult.

Scotto et al. first recognized IRD in 1982.[8] They described a 5-year-old boy with an enlarged liver, mental retardation, sensorineural deafness, pigmentary degeneration of the retina, anosmia, and dysmorphic features. Ultrastructural study of a liver biopsy specimen revealed lamellar structures resembling those normally found in plant chloroplasts where they contain bound phytol. This microscopic observation led the authors to measure the plasma phytanic acid level, which was found to be 50 to 100 μg/ml (normal less than 3 μg). This important and unexpected observation led to a comparison with "adult" Refsum disease (MIM 266500), an autosomal recessive disorder caused by deficiency of phytanoyl CoA hydroxylase in the peroxisome matrix (see Chap. 132). Elevated phytanic acid levels, pigmentary degeneration of the retina, sensorineural hearing loss and anosmia are observed in both, but dysmorphic features and mental retardation are not part of "adult" Refsum disease. These considerations led to the designation *infantile phytanic acid storage disease*. It was also noted that Kahike et al. had described a similar case in 1974.[217]

The ultrastructural changes in liver led Scotto et al. to focus initially on the phytanic acid abnormality in IRD. Subsequent studies, many of them carried out by the original group of investigators, have demonstrated that IRD is a peroxisome biogenesis disorder. Peroxisomes are absent or severely diminished in number;[11] plasmalogen synthesis is impaired;[12] VLCFA,[218] bile acid intermediates,[219] and pipecolic acid[220] accumulate; and oxidation of phytanic acid is deficient.[218] The phytanic acid oxidation deficiency and phytanic acid accumulation in ZS or NALD patients who survive beyond the fortieth week is equivalent to that in IRD. The emphasis on the phytanic acid abnormality and the name thus reflect a historical sequence rather than a fundamental difference.

IRD patients have moderately dysmorphic features including epicanthal folds, flat bridge of nose, and low set ears (Fig. 129-13).[221] Early hypotonia and enlarged liver with impaired function are common.[8,222] All IRD patients have had sensorineural hearing loss and pigmentary degeneration of the retina. The ERG demonstrates severely subnormal rod- and cone-mediated responses, with greater involvement evident for responses generated by middle and inner retinal neurons compared with responses mediated by photoreceptors.[223] Virtually all IRD patients learn to walk, although their gait may be ataxic and broad-based, and their cognitive function is in the severe retarded range[222] as compared to profound retardation in NALD and ZS.

Chondrodysplasia punctata and renal cortical cysts are not features of IRD. Postmortem study has been reported in only one IRD patient, who died at 12 years of age.[221] This revealed micronodular liver cirrhosis and small, hypoplastic adrenals. The brain showed no malformations except for a severe hypoplasia of the cerebellar granule layer and ectopic locations of the Purkinje cells in the molecular layer. A mild and diffuse reduction of axons and myelin was found in the corpus callosum, the periventricular white matter, corticospinal tracts, and optic nerves. While large numbers of perivascular macrophages were present in the same areas, there was no active demyelination. The retina and cochlea showed severe degenerative changes.

Barth et al.[224] and Bleeker-Wagemaker et al.[225] reported three patients with what they called a mild variant of ZS.

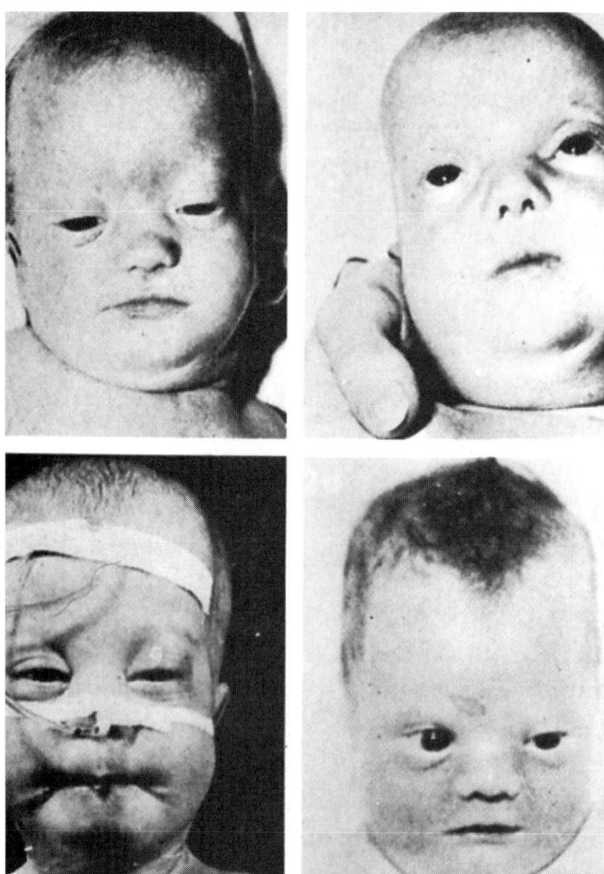

Fig. 129-10 Newborn infants with Zellweger syndrome. Note prominent forehead, hypertelorism, epicanthal folds, hypoplastic supraorbital ridge, and depressed bridge of nose. (*Courtesy of Dr. Hans Zellweger, Iowa.*)

Clinical features and laboratory data (including phytanic acid levels of 34 and 62 μg/ml) resemble those of patients in the IRD category.

Distinguishing Between Phenotypes in the Zellweger Spectrum. The phenotypic boundaries between ZS, NALD, and IRD are imprecise. Plasma VLCFA levels are highest, on average, in ZS, and lowest in IRD, but there is considerable overlap (Fig. 129-14*A*). Plasma phytanic acid levels are low initially but rise with age if the patient ingests chlorophyll-containing foods (Fig. 129-15). Phytanic acid levels are not useful in distinguishing between the phenotypes of the Zellweger patients but are generally lower in this group of patients as compared to RCDP. In the past, phenotypic assignment has been made almost exclusively on age at diagnosis or death. In the Kennedy Krieger series, the mean age at death in ZS is 5.7 ± 6.8 months (n = 50), while that of NALD is 15 ± 31 months (n = 16). The IRD patients are all living at ages 3 to 11 years.

Other clinical distinctions between these phenotypes are less clear. Calcific stippling and renal cysts have only been reported in ZS. Some authors distinguish between NALD and IRD in that the former is often associated with a demyelinating process while this is not a feature of the latter.[226] This delineation is of little clinical value at the present time because it cannot be assigned until the onset of the leukodystrophy and demyelination can apparently occur at any age.

Unusual Presentations. Several unusual PBD presentations have recently come to attention including individuals presenting at an older age with less severe manifestation and a more gradual progression.[18,19] We are aware of two women who are presently blind and deaf, but of low average intelligence and working in sheltered work settings. Both of these women presented in mid- to late childhood with progressive retinitis pigmentosa and sensorineural hearing loss. Biochemically, these individuals have typical abnormalities but less pronounced than those of most ZS patients.

Ek et al.[226] reported a boy who at age 7 months presented with eye findings characteristic of Leber congenital amaurosis. He was hypotonic and retarded and had an enlarged liver, but lacked dysmorphic features and chondrodysplasia punctata. Liver biopsy demonstrated a defect in peroxisomal matrix protein import and biochemical results were characteristic of the disorders of peroxisome biogenesis. The patient's features are most consistent with NALD. This report demonstrates that ocular abnormalities may be a prominent symptom of peroxisome deficiency disorders and should be considered as a possible etiology for Leber congenital amaurosis.

Baumgartner et al. reported an infant with a presentation similar to spinal muscular atrophy.[227,228] Clinical signs included generalized hypotonia, absence of reflexes, muscle wasting, lack of head control, and tongue fasciculations associated with

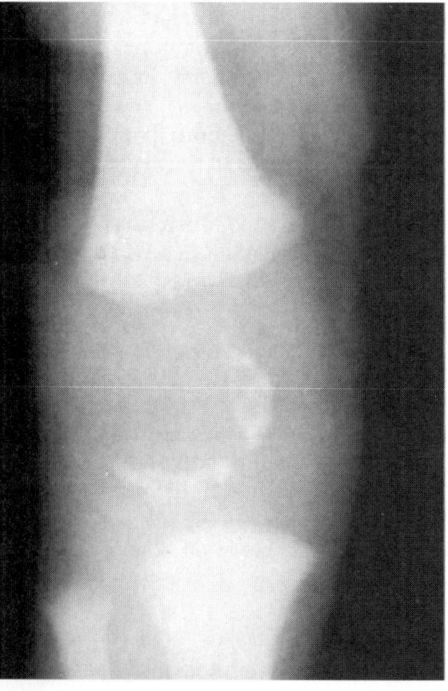

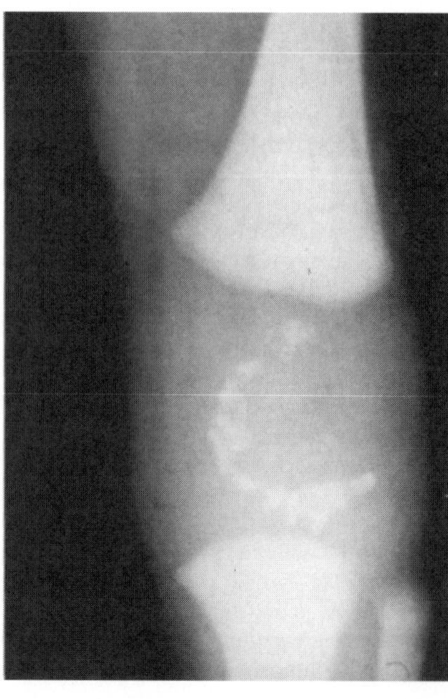

Fig. 129-11 Abnormal calcific stippling of the patella in an infant with Zellweger syndrome. (*Courtesy of Dr. Hans Zellweger.*)

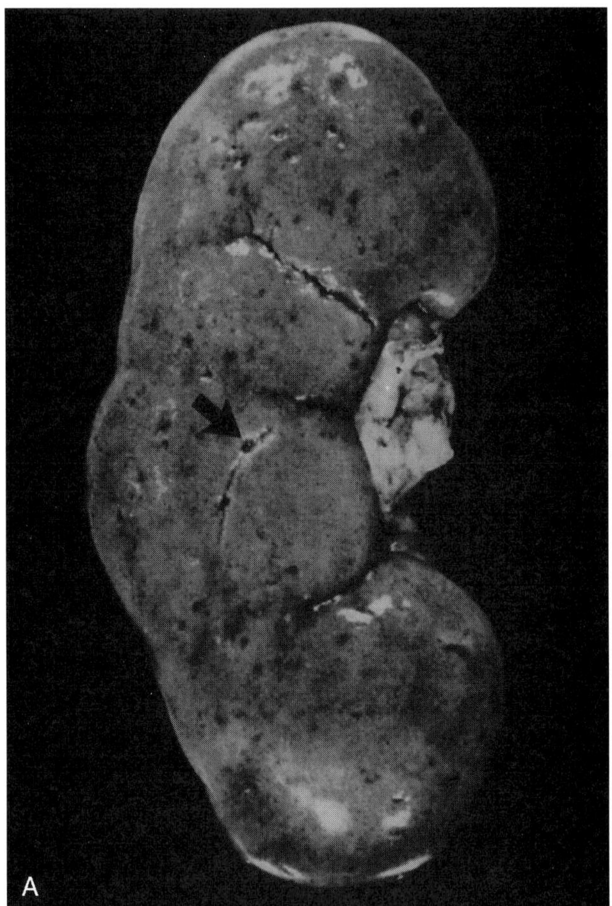

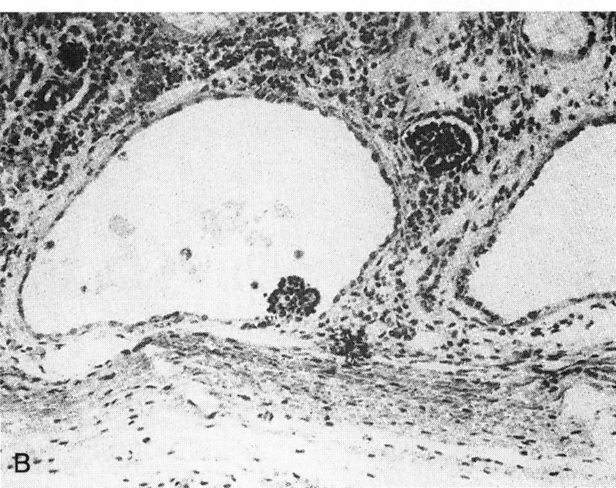

Fig. 129-12 Gross (*A*) and microscopic (*B*) appearance of renal cysts in a patient with Zellweger syndrome. Note that many of the cysts are small (*arrow, A*) and thus may escape detection on ultrasound studies. These cysts are not pathognomic of Zellweger syndrome. They occur also in a number of nonperoxisomal disorders.[198] (*Courtesy of Dr. Hans Zellweger.*)

unaffected facial muscles, and apparently normal intellectual development. Normal muscle histology ruled out infantile spinal muscular atrophy (Werdnig-Hoffmann disease). Elevated plasma concentrations of VLCFA and bile acid intermediates combined with normal plasmalogen levels in erythrocytes suggested defective peroxisomal β-oxidation. This was confirmed by demonstration of deficient pristanic acid and partially deficient C26:0 oxidation in cultured fibroblasts. Severely impaired pipecolic acid oxidation in liver and phytanic acid oxidation in fibroblasts was present. On light and electron microscopy of the liver tissue, abnormal peroxisomes were detected; there were rare peroxisomal membrane ghosts and trilamellar inclusions. Immunoblot analysis revealed absence of peroxisomal β-oxidation enzymes in liver tissue, but normal results in fibroblasts. Remarkably, a peroxisomal defect in fibroblasts was indicated by the observation that catalase was mainly cytosolic, as in the liver of this patient.

MacCollin et al.[229] identified a patient with normal intelligence who presented with ataxia and peripheral neuropathy. This boy showed marked tissue differences in the number of peroxisomes; they were completely absent in fibroblasts but present in the distal renal tubules.

In summary, the range of phenotypes associated with defects in peroxisome biogenesis is wider than previously appreciated, and additional disorders likely to be identified. Because our knowledge of the phenotypic spectrum is still incomplete and the diagnostic tests are relatively simple and reliable, alert clinicians should have a low threshold for pursuing this diagnostic possibility.

Neurophysiological Studies

Neurophysiological studies in ZS have shown profound abnormalities.[230] Govaerts et al. reported 10 of 11 children with ZS with abnormal EEGs consisting mainly of primary vertex sharp waves or spikes during both sleep and wakefulness. No photic driving could be obtained. Takahashi et al.[231] described the EEG and evolution of epilepsy in patients with peroxisomal disorders. In ZS, 5 of 7 patients began having epileptic seizures between 2 days and 1 month. These seizures were partial motor seizures originating in the mouth, arms, or legs. In their series, the patients seizures were controlled by medication and there was no progression to generalized tonic-clonic seizures. The EEG showed infrequent bilateral independent multifocal spikes predominantly in the frontal motor cortex and surrounding regions. Two NALD patients had seizures beginning in infancy; these were tonic in one and infantile spasms in the other. The seizures were intractable. Interictal EEG showed high-voltage slow waves and bilateral independent multifocal spikes evolving in one patient to a flat pattern.

Brain stem auditory-evoked responses are generally not elicitable or, when present, are prolonged. In 6 of 11 patients, there was no recognizable audiometric response to 70 decibels.[230] Somatosensory evoked responses showed a severe propagation defect in ZS, consistent with defects in myelinated pathways. The ERG is extinguished.[232] In the milder phenotypes, the ERG may be present, but is typically diminished.[223]

Neuroradiographic Studies

Magnetic resonance imaging (MRI) studies of children with ZS reveal impaired myelination and diffusely abnormal cortical gyral patterns that consist of regions of microgyria primarily in the frontal and perisylvian cortex, together with regions of thickened pachygyric cortex primarily perirolandic and occipital.

Abnormalities may be appreciated on prenatal ultrasound and include marked dilatation of the lateral ventricles. Germinolytic cysts in the caudothalamic groove, ventricular dilatation, and hypogenesis of the posterior corpus callosum have all been observed (Fig. 129-16).[233–235]

Pathologic Features of the Zellweger Spectrum

Peroxisomes. All PBD patients display some type of defect in peroxisome biogenesis, most of which can be ascertained through microscopic techniques. Early studies suggested that the organelle was typically absent,[6,236,237] or reduced in abundance[236–240] in PBD patients. However, many early claims of "absent peroxisomes" in the Zellweger spectrum of disease were probably incorrect due to an inappropriate assumption that defects in peroxisomal enzyme localization were caused by loss of the entire organelle. This misconception has been laid to rest by a variety of

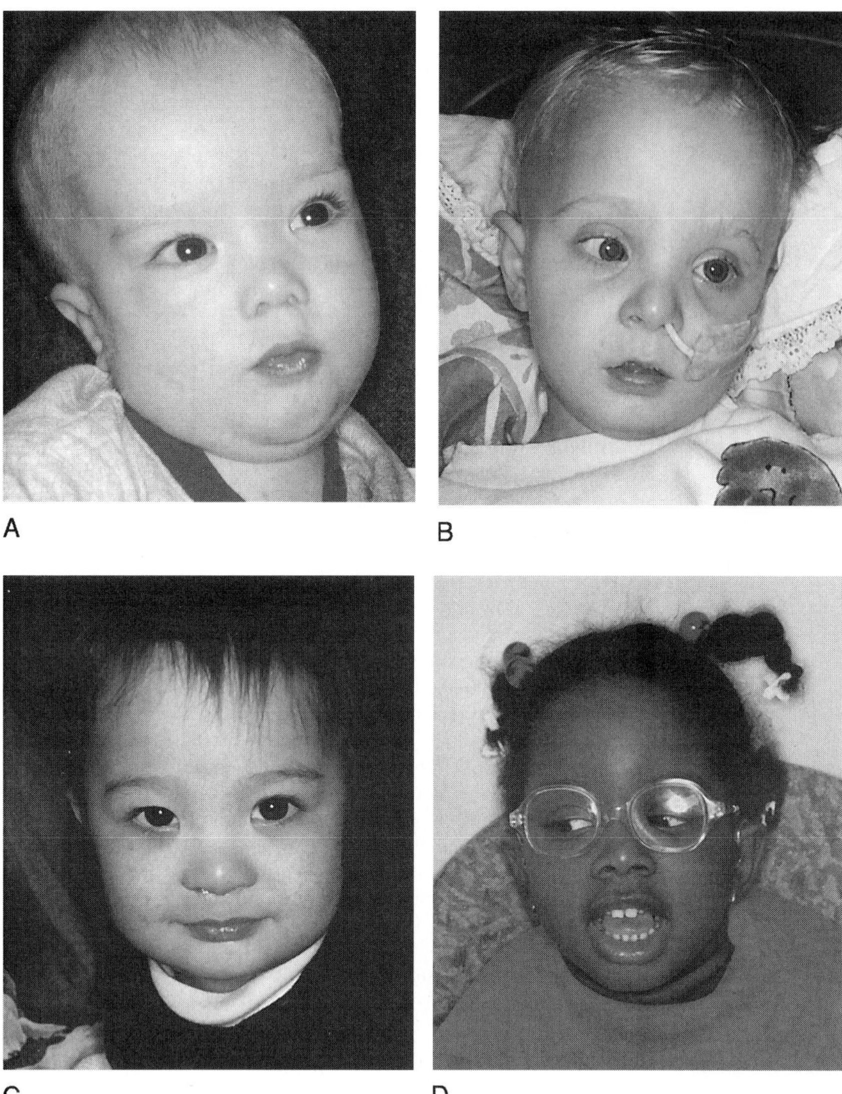

Fig. 129-13 The facial appearance of children with NALD (*A and B*) and IRD (*C and D*).

studies that demonstrate relatively normal import of peroxisomal membrane proteins and peroxisome membrane biogenesis in PBD patients that have no detectable peroxisomal matrix protein import.[23,65,66,186,241] Although the vast majority of PBD patients do contain numerous peroxisomes, recent studies have identified four patients (mutated in PEX3, PEX16, or PEX19) who display a severe defect in import of peroxisomal membrane proteins and appear to lack peroxisome entirely,[20,56–59] the phenotype originally proposed for most PBD patients.[6] A significant proportion of Zellweger spectrum patients (~50%) actually import detectable levels of matrix proteins into their peroxisomes, a finding that has been demonstrated using both immunoelectron microscopic and immunofluorescence techniques.[241–244] The level of matrix protein import observed in these patients appears to correlate with the severity of the mutant alleles in PBD patients, with matrix protein import being greatest in the most mildly affected individuals.[67,68] In addition, there is significant variation in the extent to which different proteins are imported in mildly affected patients. For example, many mildly affected patients import significant amounts of several peroxisomal matrix proteins but display a nearly complete defect in import of catalase.[67,136,244] Such differences are likely to mirror the import kinetics of the various peroxisomal matrix proteins. This hypothesis is supported by the fact that catalase is perhaps the most inefficiently imported peroxisomal matrix protein in mammalian cells[338] and is the most sensitive protein to mild defects in peroxisomal matrix protein import.[139,140] While most Zellweger spectrum patients contain numerous peroxisomes and import membrane proteins normally, peroxisome abundance and morphology in these patients is not normal.[65–67,236–244] To understand the basis for these differences Chang et al.[23] compared peroxisomes of cells from Zellweger spectrum patients, RCDP patients, and patients with single peroxisomal enzyme defects. This study established that there is an 80% reduction in peroxisome abundance in Zellweger spectrum patients who have a severe defect in matrix protein import but no defect in peroxisomal membrane protein import. Interestingly, this study also found an 80% reduction in peroxisome abundance in patients defective in the peroxisomal fatty acid oxidation enzymes acyl-CoA oxidase or D-bifunctional protein. In contrast, no decrease in peroxisome abundance was observed in RCDP patients, X-ALD patients, Refsum disease patients, and patients with defects in plasmalogen biosynthesis enzymes. These and other observations suggest a model in which aberrant peroxisome abundance and morphology is a secondary consequence of matrix protein import defect in Zellweger spectrum patients, which causes a severe defect in peroxisomal fatty acid oxidation. Obviously, this is not intended to explain the absence of peroxisomes in those rare patients with actual defects in peroxisome membrane biogenesis, such as those with mutations in PEX3, PEX16, and PEX19.[56–59]

Brain. There are three typical areas of involvement in the nervous system of individuals with peroxisomal biogenesis disorders: neuronal migration abnormalities, white matter abnormalities,

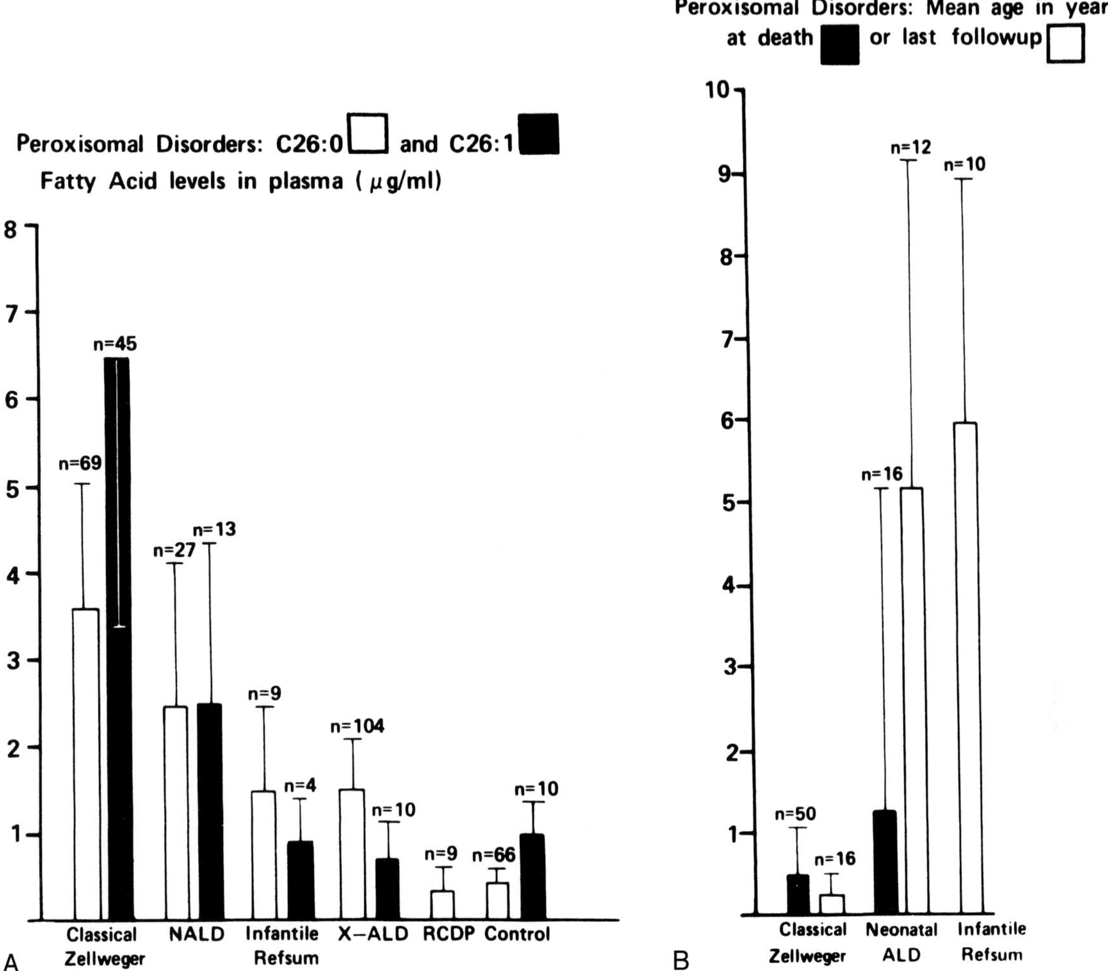

Fig. 129-14 Comparison of plasma VLCFA levels (*A*) and survival (*B*) in patients in the Zellweger spectrum. The values for both *A* and *B* are from patients followed at the Kennedy Krieger Institute.

and selective neuronal involvement.[245] The degree and specific areas of involvement vary with the seriousness of clinical and biochemical involvement and many of the features begin prenatally.

The most striking and intriguing neuropathologic abnormality is a disorder of neuronal migration that has been studied by Volpe and Adams[246] and Evrard et al.[247] (Fig. 129-17). This disordered migration leads to characteristic and unique cytoarchitectonic abnormalities that involve the cerebral hemispheres, the cerebellum, and the inferior olivary complex. In the cerebral hemispheres, neurons that are normally destined for outer cortical layers are distributed within the inner cortical layers and in the underlying white matter. This migration failure causes the cerebral convolutions to be abnormally small (microgyria) or thick (pachygyria). The migration defect involves mainly the perisylvian and medially adjacent frontoparietal convexity, while other areas, such as the anterior frontal and occipital regions, may show a normal convolutional pattern. Evrard et al. concluded that the mechanism of migration was disturbed continuously from the third month of gestation,[247] a conclusion that has been confirmed in subsequent studies of fetuses with ZS.[248] A unique and characteristic feature of the ZS brain malformation is that, despite disturbed migration of multiple neuronal classes throughout the greater duration of the migratory epoch, the defect usually is restricted to certain regions of the cerebral hemispheres. This anatomically restricted disturbance occurs with sufficient consistency that it can be distinguished from all other cerebral malformations. Other characteristic features are migrational defects of the large Purkinje cells in the cerebellum and laminar discontinuities in the principal nucleus of the inferior olivary complex. There is also hypoplasia of the olfactory bulbs[249] and a neuroaxonal dystrophy of the dorsal nucleus of Clarke and the lateral cuneate nucleus.[250,251]

In addition to the neuronal migrational defects, there is also an abnormality of white matter. While the extent and significance of this had been disputed, recent biochemical advances provide insight about its mechanism. Passarge and McAdams noted a severe myelin deficiency and accumulation of sudanophilic lipids and concluded that this finding was consistent with a sudanophilic leukodystrophy.[2] In contrast, brain myelin content was considered to be nearly normal in the Volpe and Adams case.[246] While a destructive myelin process was present, it was restricted to the periventricular region, and its location and restricted distribution suggested to the authors that it was related to hypoxic-ischemic episodes associated with seizures and aspiration.[246] Agamanolis et al.,[249] in consonance with Passarge and McAdams, noted a general deficiency of myelin and an active demyelinative process. They were also the first to note the presence of longitudinal or fiberlike inclusions in both the white and gray matter.[249] Studies by Powers and associates[248,251] demonstrated that these lamellar inclusions are similar to those present in X-linked adrenoleukodystrophy and contain cholesterol esterified with VLCFA. These findings suggest that the white matter abnormality in ZS is related to the defect in VLCFA metabolism, and the mechanism may resemble that in X-linked ALD. Additional defects, particularly the inability to synthesize plasmalogens, a major myelin constituent, probably also contribute to the white matter abnormality.[252]

The neuronal changes in NALD are less consistent and less severe. While some NALD cases showed striking micropolygyria,[7]

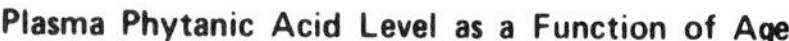

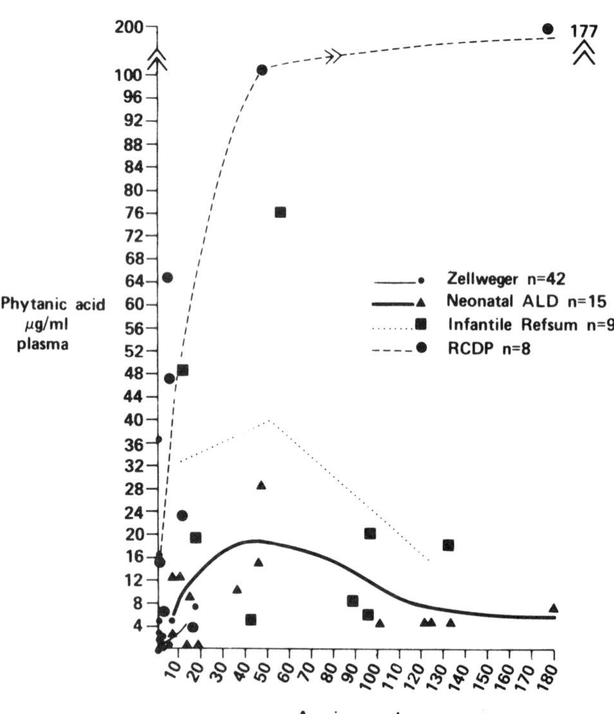

Fig. 129-15 Variation with age of plasma phytanic acid levels in patients with syndromes in the Zellweger and RCDP spectra. These are cross-sectional data from patients followed at the Kennedy Krieger Institute. Because of the scale, only a small proportion of the 42 ZS patients are shown. Twenty-eight of these (ages 0 to 6 months) had normal (<3 μg/ml) plasma phytanic acid levels. While NALD and IRD patients had higher levels, this appears to be related to their longer survival. For unknown reasons, in NALD and IRD patients older than 80 months, the phytanic acids appear to decline. In patients with RCDP, plasma phytanic acid levels become elevated earlier and reach higher levels than the other PBD patients.

other cases showed only mild neuronal migrational defects and heterotopias,[9] and in yet others the cortex and neurons appeared normal.[10,253] The olivary nucleus apparently was normal in all cases. Most NALD cases showed a widespread sudanophilic leukodystrophy, often associated with perivascular accumulation of lymphocytes, as in X-linked ALD, and the white matter involvement actually is more striking than in ZS. This is probably attributable to the longer survival in NALD, because the white matter lesion is known to advance with age.

In a child with IRD who died at 12 years of age, the brain showed no malformations except for a severe hypoplasia of the cerebellar granule layer and ectopic locations of the Purkinje cells in the molecular layer.[221] A mild and diffuse reduction of axons and myelin was found in the corpus callosum, the periventricular white matter, corticospinal tracts, and optic nerves. While large numbers of perivascular macrophages were present in the same areas, there was no active demyelination. The retina and cochlea showed severe degenerative changes.

Eye. In the most severely affected individuals, abnormalities of the anterior segment including corneal clouding, congenital cataract, and congenital glaucoma are present. In patients with ZS or NALD, retinal abnormalities have included photoreceptor degeneration, ganglion cell loss, gliosis of the nerve fiber layer and optic nerve, optic atrophy, and changes resembling those of retinitis pigmentosa in the neural retina and pigment epithelium.[254] The ERG is extinguished[232] in the most severely involved patients, but may be present initially in the less severe.[223]

Ear. Although high frequency of sensorineural hearing loss is frequent in PBD patients, there is little pathologic information. Igarashi et al.[255] found in a child with NALD, the spiral organ of the cochlea was collapsed over the basilar membrane, especially in the basal turns and there was an atrophic tectorial membrane. Mid-modiolus section of the left cochlea showed atrophic views of organ of Corti and severe spiral ganglion cell loss in all turns. Torvik et al. reported that in a child with IRD, the sensory epithelium and the stria vascularis showed severe atrophy.[221]

Liver. Hepatic involvement ranges from normal through severe cirrhosis with organ failure. There is maldevelopment, degeneration with reparative reactions, and storage. In Heymans' review of 114 ZS cases, the liver was enlarged in 78 percent and fibrotic in 76 percent.[13] Thirty-seven percent had micronodular cirrhosis, and cholestasis was present in 59 percent. The changes were more severe in the older infants. In the first 2 months of life, microscopic abnormalities were absent or only mild, while nearly all patients older than 20 weeks showed advanced changes consisting of severe fibrosis and micronodular cirrhosis. Excessive iron deposits in liver were reported in an early study,[256] and were at first thought to be a factor in the pathogenesis of the cirrhosis. This is now considered unlikely, because Gilchrist et al. showed that the liver iron levels diminished with time and were normal in infants living beyond 20 weeks.[257] In Heymans' survey, greater than 85 percent of Zellweger patients had elevated transaminases, and hyperbilirubinemia was present in 13 of 19 cases (60 percent). Hypoprothrombinemia responsive to vitamin K administration

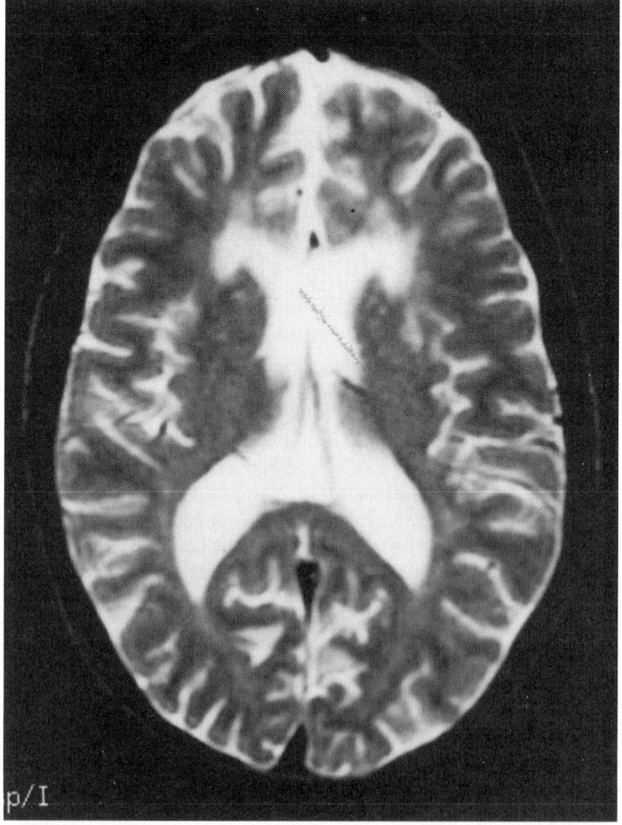

Fig. 129-16 MRI of a 35-year-old patient with a mild variant of peroxisome assembly. The patient had developed hearing loss in childhood and was legally blind by the age of 11. She was diagnosed in her thirties when she was evaluated for sensorineural hearing loss and retinitis pigmentosa. At that time, she was working in a sheltered workshop but had normal intelligence. Her MRI demonstrates bilateral frontal periventricular white matter abnormalities consistent with a leukodystrophy. This highlights both an extremely mild phenotype in some individuals and the difficulty with phenotype assignment based on presence of leukodystrophy.

NEOCORTEX CYTOARCHITECTONIC ANALYSIS

A B C

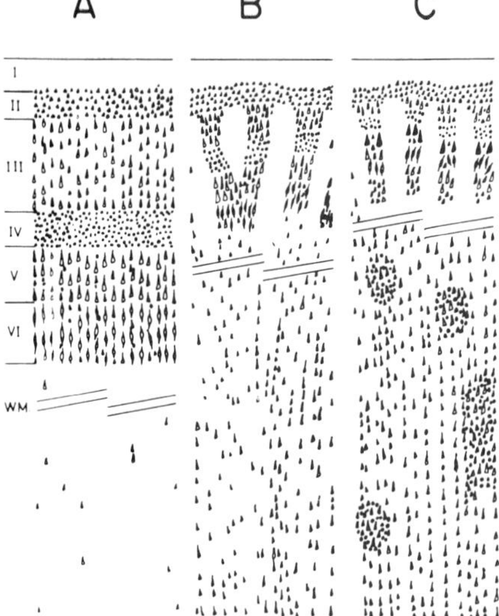

A: normal

B: Zellweger microgyria

C: Zellweger pachygyria

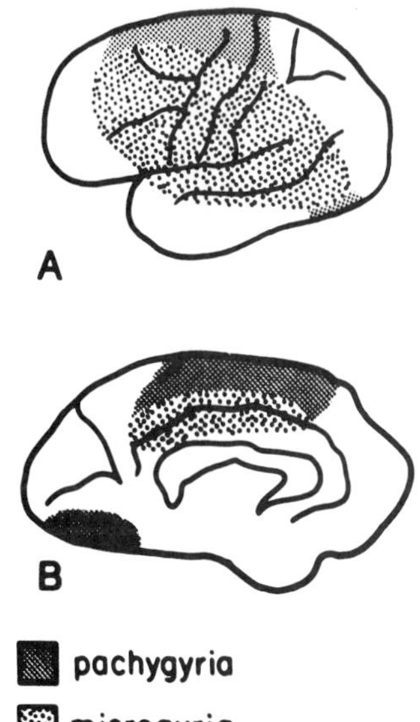

Fig. 129-17 ***A.*** **Schematic representation of cell pattern in normal (A), microgyric (B), and pachygyric (C) neocortical regions. Roman numerals to left correspond to normal cortical layers. White matter and horizontal slashes mark junction of cortex and central white matter. The white matter in B and C contains numerous heterotopic neurons that failed to reach their normal location in the neocortex. In addition, in the abnormal cortex (B and C) the neurons are arranged in fascicles that contain three to six neurons abreast of each other.** ***B.*** **Patterns of pachygyric (fine stippling) and microgyric (coarse stippling) gyral abnormalities on lateral (A) and medial (B) surface of cerebral hemispheres in Zellweger syndrome. The abnormality is restricted, and its pattern is characteristic (see text). The gyri in the unshaded areas are normal. (*Modified from Evrard et al.*[247] *Used by permission.*)**

was reported in 18 patients. This has also been apparent in less affected individuals.[199,222]

Kidney. Renal cysts were observed in 78 of 80 patients with ZS who were studied pathologically (Fig. 129-12).[13] The cysts vary from glomerular microcysts to large cortical cysts of glomerular and tubular origin.[258] The cysts are already present in the fetus.[248] Cysts are not seen in the milder phenotypes.

Adrenal. The adrenal pathology of ZS is similar to that in the more common X-linked ALD and appears to be a function of VLCFA accumulation. The reticularis-inner fasciculata zones contain striated cells, some of which are ballooned. Ultrastructural examination demonstrates the lamellar inclusions identical to those found in X-linked ALD.[259] It has been proposed that VLCFA are toxic to adrenal cortical cells.[260] While overt adrenal insufficiency has not been reported in the ZS, adrenocortical function has been shown to be impaired.[261] Lack of clinically significant disease is probably simply a matter of survival. Similar findings and clinical adrenal insufficiency has been seen in the milder NALD and IRD.

Skeletal Involvement. Calcific stippling of the patella and synchondrosis of the acetabulum occurs in 50 percent of ZS patients.[1,13,262,263] Abnormal mineralization of the patella was already observed at midgestation in two fetuses with ZS.[71] Mineralization of the patella normally begins at 2 to 4 years of age and is completed at about 6 years.[264] Powers et al. suggest that the alteration in ZS represents a premature rather than a dysplastic mineralization.[248] Because of the predominance of involvement in RCDP and in the single disorders of plasmalogen synthesis (see below) there is strong implication of the role of plasmalogens.

Other Organ Involvement. Given the nearly ubiquitous nature of peroxisomes, it is likely that nearly all tissues and organ systems are involved. Congenital cardiovascular malformations occur frequently in ZS patients. In Heymans' review, ventricular septal defects occurred in 32 percent, and 22 percent had various abnormalities of the aorta.[13] Two cases of ZS showed aplasia of the thymus,[265] but postmortem studies of six additional patients[257] and assays of cellular immune responses in peripheral blood lymphocytes[266] have failed to show evidence of cellular immunodeficiency. Study of NALD, has shown lipid inclusions in the thymus.[253,267] While muscle has not been studied in detail in ZS patients, a myopathy has been demonstrated in a patient with NALD,[215] and muscle cells cultured from a patient with ZS showed defective plasmalogen synthesis and cytosolic subcellular localization of catalase.[4] The pancreas may be fibrotic and islet cell hyperplasia has been described in several cases.[4,251,268]

Rhizomelic Chondrodysplasia Punctata (RCDP)

The RCDP phenotype differs significantly from that of ZS. Classical RCDP patients have rhizomelia, striking shortening of their proximal limbs (Fig. 129-18), severely disturbed endochondral bone formation, and coronal clefts of vertebral bodies that are visualized with lateral roentgenograms of the spine. Bilateral cataracts are present in 75 percent of RCDP patients and one quarter develop ichthyosis after birth. There is stippling of the epiphyses especially at the knees, elbows, hips, and shoulders. The facies are abnormal — flattened with frontal bossing, flat nasal bridge, and small nares. RCDP patients have profound psychomotor retardation. The majority of RCDP patients die in the first year or two of life, but several are known to have survived longer, some into their teens.[269]

Heymans et al.[270] demonstrated impaired plasmalogen biosynthesis and phytanic acid accumulation in RCDP patients and assigned this disorder to the peroxisome disease category. Catalase in cultured RCDP fibroblasts is in the particulate fraction.[15] Importantly, Hoefler et al.[15] showed that RCDP is associated with three biochemical abnormalities. The first biochemical abnormality is a defect in plasmalogen biosynthesis that, typically, is more severe than in the ZS. Heymans et al.[14] had previously demonstrated that this defect was due to deficient DHAPAT activity. The second biochemical abnormality is a phytanic acid oxidation

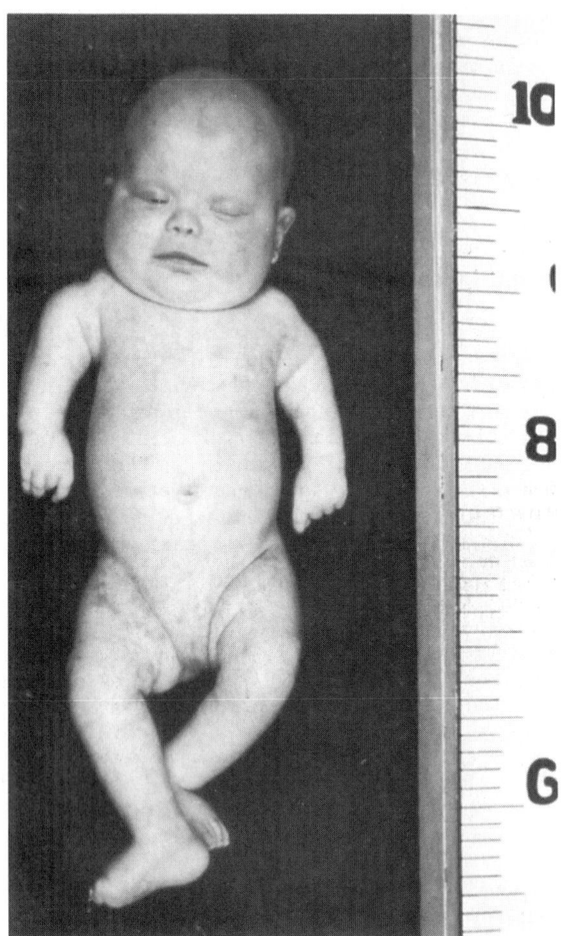

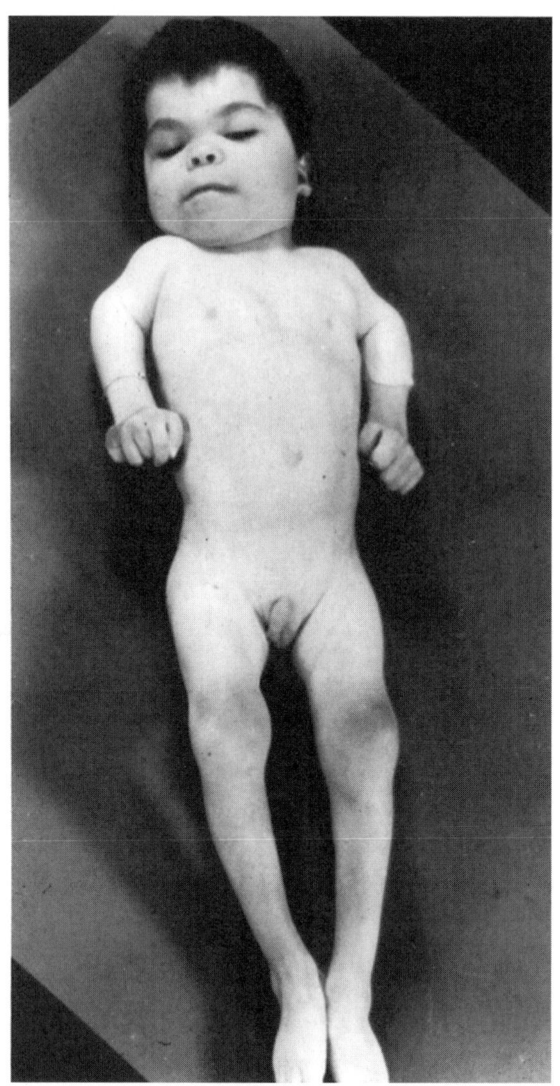

Fig. 129-18 A newborn female (*A*) and a 12-year-old boy (*B*) with RCDP. Note severe shortening of proximal limbs, depressed bridge of nose, hypertelorism, and widespread erythematous and scaling skin lesions in patient *A*. Patient A is case 2 in ref. 15. Patient B is case 7 in ref 297a. Both patients had the biochemical defects characteristic of RCDP (see ref. 15) (*Photo A courtesy of Dr. B. McGillivary, Vancouver, B.C.; photo B courtesy of Dr. R.B.H. Schutgens, Amsterdam, The Netherlands.*)

defect equivalent to that in IRD and ZS. Plasma phytanic acid levels as a function of age are higher in RCDP patients than in patients with other disorders of peroxisome biogenesis (Fig. 129-15). The third defect is the presence of 3-oxoacyl-coenzyme A thiolase in the unprocessed form.[15] This observation suggests failure to import this PTS2 targeted matrix protein. In spite of this last abnormality, VLCFA oxidation and plasma levels are normal. Similarly, levels of bile acid intermediates are not increased.

Studies from several laboratories indicate that the triad of RCDP biochemical abnormalities may be associated with a wider range of phenotypes than had been recognized previously. Poll-The et al.[271] reported a patient with normally proportioned limbs and only moderately impaired psychomotor development. Pike et al.[272] described a patient with a phenotype that resembled the congenital rubella syndrome and Gray[273] described a patient with rhizomelic shortening of limbs but without chondrodysplasia punctata. Moser et al.[18] have reported two sisters with congenital cataracts, the older is not dysmorphic and has normal cognition, the younger has no limb abnormalities, but severe psychomotor retardation.

These results highlight a degree of phenotypic variation and locus heterogeneity in RCDP. The classical biochemical abnormalities may be associated with variable phenotypes and results from mutations in the *PEX7* gene. In contrast, isolated defects in the peroxisomal steps of plasmalogen synthesis, dihydroxyacetone-phosphate acyltransferase (DHAPAT) deficiency[274] and alkyl dihydroxyacetone-phosphate synthase deficiency are clinically indistinguishable from RCDP (see Chap. 130). In these single-enzyme defects, phytanic acid metabolism is normal, thiolase is processed normally, and there is no general defect in import of PTS2-targeted enzymes.

Chondrodysplasia punctata is not specific for RCDP and needs to be differentiated from other conditions with stippling. The chondrodysplasia punctata of RCDP is more widespread and pronounced than in ZS and may involve the vertebral column and some extraskeletal tissues. RCDP must be differentiated from other forms of chondrodysplasia punctata. These include the Conradi-Hünermann form (MIM 118650), which is inherited as an autosomal dominant trait, in contrast to the autosomal recessive inheritance of RCDP. Limb length in Conradi-Hünermann syndrome patients is normal, and they have normal cognition and a longer life span.[275] There are none of the biochemical abnormalities characteristic of RCDP (decreased plasmalogens, increased phytanic acid). There are also X-linked dominant (CDPX2, MIM 302960)[276] and X-linked recessive (CDPX1, MIM 302950)[277] forms of chondrodysplasia punctata, the latter being associated also with defective steroid sulfatase activity. The former has recently been shown to be caused by deficiency of 3β-hydroxysteroid-Δ^8,Δ^7-isomerase an enzyme that catalyzes a step in the post-squalene cholesterol biosynthetic pathway.[278,279] The tattered (Td) mouse is also deficient in this enzyme.[279]

Pathology. All patients in the RCDP spectrum of disease import PTS1-containing peroxisomal proteins normally and contain peroxisomes with a relatively normal morphology and a normal complement of peroxisomal membrane proteins.[23] However, they do display severe to mild defects in import of PTS2-containing proteins such as the PTS2-targeted thiolase, phytanoyl-CoA hydroxylase, and alkyl-dihydroxyacetone phosphate synthase,[88–92] which is consistent with their defects in PEX7, the PTS2 receptor.[129–132] There has been limited information available on pathologic involvement in RCDP and most reports focus on the skeleton and brain. Calcific punctate stippling develops as early as the second trimester and was the sole abnormality in an affected fetus aborted at 20 weeks gestation.[280] On ultrasound, shortening of the humerus and femur with stippling has been seen at 28 weeks gestation.[281,282] The calcific stippling decreases as the patient ages, when osteopenia and delayed skeletal maturation may be evident.[283] The microscopic lesion is characterized by focal degeneration of cartilage cells which become mineralized. Lesions may disrupt the physis and maturation of the cartilage is disturbed. Poor and irregular columnization of chondrocytes and diminished vascularization is seen.[283] Microcephaly is common, but neuropathologic examination has not shown the severe migrational defects characteristic of ZS. Powers et al. described the brain of two children who survived into childhood and noted a postdevelopmental degeneration of the cerebellum with loss of Purkinje cells and granular neurons.[284] They hypothesized that elevated levels of phytanic acid may have toxic effects.[284,285] Abnormalities in other systems have been reported and include cleft palate, cardiac defects, and possible immune abnormalities.[286,287]

DIAGNOSIS OF PEROXISOME BIOGENESIS DISORDERS

The Affected Child

Because the known disorders of peroxisome biogenesis can be diagnosed with accurate and noninvasive tests, it is important to establish guidelines for their application. Such guidelines have been proposed by several groups.[227,288] Theil et al. recommended the performance of these tests in patients who exhibited the combined presence of at least three clinical characteristics that were present in more than 75 percent of the patients (psychomotor retardation, hypotonia, impaired hearing, low/broad nasal bridge, abnormal ERG, hepatomegaly) and one or more characteristics that were present in 50 percent to 75 percent (large fontanelles, shallow orbital ridges, epicanthus, anteverted nostrils, retinitis pigmentosa). Baumgartner and collaborators developed similar age-related clinical indices such as cranial dysmorphism, neurologic dysfunction, hepatomegaly, and failure to thrive in the first 6 months of life; psychomotor retardation, hearing loss, and ophthalmologic manifestations in children between 6 months and 4 years; behavioral changes, dementia, and peripheral neuropathy in individuals older than 4 years of age. As already described, patients with peroxisome biogenesis disorders in the Zellweger spectrum have been misdiagnosed as Down syndrome in the newborn period, Leber congenital amaurosis in infancy, Usher syndrome,[199] Cockayne syndrome,[199] and Werdnig-Hoffman disease.[228] Similarly, RCDP has been misdiagnosed as other chondrodystrophies. We also acknowledge that there are atypical PBD patients who do not meet these criteria.[18,227,228] Because establishment of the diagnosis of a peroxisome disorder has such important implications for genetic counseling and because of the extreme phenotypic variability of the PBDs, we consider it appropriate to apply the screening tests in patients with undiagnosed disorders that are only remotely related phenotypically to patients with classic PBD phenotypes.[289]

Laboratory tests for the diagnosis of disorders of peroxisomes biogenesis have been reviewed[290] and are listed in Table 129-3. The most widely used single assay is the measurement of VLCFA in plasma[291–294] or red blood cell membranes.[295] VLCFA are increased in all of the disorders of Zellweger spectrum and the single-enzyme defects of peroxisomal β oxidation, but they are normal in RCDP.

In the Kennedy Krieger Institute lab, we also perform a series of assays in plasma and red blood cells that permit the detection and preliminary classification of the majority of the known disorders of peroxisome biogenesis.

Blood sample assays include measurement of VLCFA, phytanic acid,[296] pristanic acid,[297] pipecolic acid,[298] bile acid intermediates,[299,300] and the essential fatty acid profile. It must be remembered that abnormalities in phytanic acid[301] and plasmalogens[302] are age dependent. The elevation of phytanic acid may not be demonstrable in young infants or, at times, in older patients (Fig. 129-15). The reduction in red blood cell plasmalogen levels may not be demonstrable in children who are more than 20 weeks old. The above abnormalities in plasma and red blood cells are

Table 129-3 Representative Diagnostic Biochemical Abnormalities in ZS in Blood and Urine

Diagnostic test	Specific value	ZS (Mean ± SD)	Control (Mean ± SD)
VLCFA	C26:0 μg/ml	3.31 ± 1.63	0.22 ± 0.08
	C26:1 μg/ml	1.55 ± 0.55	0.12 ± 0.05
	C24/C22	1.95 ± 0.42	0.84 ± 0.08
	C26/C22	0.52 ± 0.24	0.01 ± 0.01
Phytanic acid	μg/ml plasma	2.35 ± 1.18	0.80 ± 0.40
Pristanic acid	μg/ml plasma	0.42 ± 0.39	0.31 ± 0.41
Pipecolic acid	plasma μM	102.5 ± 88.6	1.9 ± 0.9
	urine μM/g creatinine	79 ± 70	7.0 ± 5.6
Red blood cell plasmalogens	C16:0 DMA/C16:0 fatty acids	0.001–0.025	0.051–0.090
	C18:0 DMA/C18:0 fatty acids	0.001–0.255	0.137–0.255

NOTE: The values for the milder phenotypes, NALD and IRD, are intermediate between those of ZS and controls. In less-affected individuals, one or more studies may approach normal values requiring further analysis with fibroblasts or other tissues. Several of the tests' values are age-dependent. Phytanic acid is normal in the newborn period. The values for pipecolic acid in plasma and urine are for children 7 months to 5 years. Pipecolic acid values are lower in plasma in the first 6 months of life, but the urinary excretion is markedly higher at this time.

most striking in patients with the classical Zellweger phenotype, and may be more subtle in neonatal ALD and infantile Refsum disease patients. In patients with isolated defects in peroxisomal fatty acid oxidation, abnormalities are confined to VLCFA and bile acid intermediates (see Chap. 130).

Studies in cultured skin fibroblasts may be necessary to confirm the diagnosis and suggest a particular CG. These include measurements of VLCFA levels[303] and their β-oxidation;[304,305] acylCoA:dihydroxyacetone phosphate acyltransferase activity[306] or the peroxisomal steps of plasmalogen synthesis;[307] phytanic acid oxidation;[308] and the subcellular localization of catalase.[309] We find the method of Roscher et al.[307] for the assay of the peroxisomal steps of plasmalogen synthesis to be particularly valuable, because it may reveal mild deficiencies in neonatal ALD or infantile Refsum disease that may escape detection by other methods. The disorders of peroxisome biogenesis are distinguished from the single-enzyme defects, by the cytosolic localization of catalase, and by defects in phytanic acid oxidation and plasmalogen synthesis functions that are unimpaired in the single-enzyme defects. In RCDP, plasmalogen synthesis is severely impaired, phytanic acid oxidation is deficient, and thiolase is present in immature form, while VLCFA are normal.[15]

Although metabolic assays for diagnosis of PBD patients have proven to be extremely useful, they are indirect. Rather than measuring the primary defect in peroxisomal protein import, they measure the consequences of the import defect on one or a few peroxisomal metabolic pathways. The metabolism-based assays have the advantage of being relatively non-invasive and have the potential for high-throughput analysis.[300] However, they are not particularly useful for predicting the course of disease in mildly affected PBD patients. While the current inability to predict patient outcomes from biochemical tests may reflect differences in patient care or other environmental factors, it is also possible that more direct measurement of peroxisomal matrix protein import might improve our ability to predict patient outcomes. A number of studies have explored the concept of measuring the primary defect in PBD patients, but these have primarily focused on qualitative measurements of import of just one peroxisomal protein, catalase.[23,185,186,240,244,310–312] As demonstrated by several recent reports, a single defect in peroxisomal matrix protein import can have different effects on the import of different matrix proteins.[136,140,244] In particular, catalase appears to be far more sensitive to mild defects in peroxisomal matrix protein import than other matrix proteins, particularly proteins such as PTE1[41] and PECI[368] that contain good matches to the canonical PTS1.[136] The mechanistic basis for these differences in sensitivity is likely kinetic, with slowly imported proteins being more sensitive to mild defects than efficiently imported proteins. The fact that catalase utilizes an unusual variant of the PTS1[87] and is perhaps the least efficiently imported peroxisomal matrix protein[338] provides at least some support for this hypothesis. It will be interesting to determine whether quantitative measurements of matrix protein import, such as those reported by Liu et al.,[136] can improve our ability to predict disease progression in mildly affected PBD patients.

DNA Diagnosis and Carrier Detection

With elucidation of the molecular defects responsible for many of the peroxisomal disorders, DNA diagnosis, mutational analysis, and carrier determination is presently possible (see below). Complementation analysis remains a mainstay as an initial step in determining the responsible PEX gene.

Prenatal Diagnosis

A variety of techniques are available for the prenatal diagnosis of peroxisomal disorders. They include demonstration of increased VLCFA levels or their impaired oxidation[291,304,313] and deficient plasmalogen synthesis[314,315] in cultured amniocytes, cultured chorionic villus cells, or direct analysis of chorion villus samples; demonstration that peroxisomes are deficient by cytochemical techniques;[316] or by demonstrating the mislocation of catalase to the cell cytosol.[294,309,317] If the molecular basis of the disease segregating in the family is known, DNA diagnosis is possible. When cultured chorion villus samples are used, the possibility of a false negative result due to maternal overgrowth must be kept in mind.[318,319] Other laboratories have combined the use of direct measurement with cultured material confirmation[290] and the use of immunofluorescence staining.[320]

At this time, we continue to recommend use of cultured amniocytes or chorion villus samples for the confirmation of any prenatal diagnosis of the disorders of peroxisome biogenesis. This allows for sampling to be performed elsewhere and for testing to be centralized, it protects against transport accidents, and is not limited by the amount of frozen material, permitting additional testing. Performing two different assays, VLCFA levels and plasmalogen biosynthesis, provides a valuable cross-check.[314]

Results by Rocchiccioli et al.[313] suggest that direct analysis VLCFA in chorion villus samples is feasible. However, in our experience, direct analysis often failed to provide sufficiently reliable differentiation and we have observed one false positive result. We recommend, therefore, that the result be confirmed later by VLCFA and plasmalogen synthesis in cultured chorion villus cells or the immunostaining procedure of Schutgens et al.[290]

Stellaard et al.[300] report promising results with the measurements of bile acid intermediates in amniotic fluid. With the use of a highly sensitive stable-isotope dilution-electron capture-negative ion-mass fragmentography technique, they demonstrated small increases in intermediates in pregnancies with Zellweger fetuses. This potentially rapid approach represents a significant advance for the prenatal diagnosis of those peroxisomal disorders in which the proband had been shown to have elevated levels of bile acid intermediates.

It must be reemphasized that the prenatal diagnosis of RCDP depends upon measurement of plasmalogen synthesis and phytanic acid oxidation activities[15] because VLCFA metabolism is not affected in this condition. Thiolase immunoblotting may be used as a confirmatory test.

The experience of prenatal diagnosis emphasizes the importance of having material from the index case.[290]

MOLECULAR GENETICS OF PEROXISOME BIOGENESIS DISORDERS

Most PBD complementation groups are represented by only a few patients. This is not surprising given their rarity and genetic heterogeneity. Because positional cloning strategies often rely on the availability of large numbers of patients and/or well-studied kindreds with multiple affected individuals, researchers interested in identifying the defective genes in PBD patients have developed alternative approaches to identify the affected genes. Over the past 8 years, these have led to the identification of the genes that are defective in 11 of the 12 known PBD complementation groups and more than 95 percent of PBD patients (Table 129-1).

To date, all of the genes known to be defective in PBD patients have been identified by either or both of two related strategies: homology probing[100] and mammalian cell complementation.[101] The homology-probing approach relies heavily on studies of peroxisome biogenesis in lower eukaryotes and the sequences of peroxisome biogenesis factors from these other organisms. It also relies heavily on the availability of large sequence databases of human expressed sequence tags, which can be searched for genes capable of encoding proteins with significant sequence similarity to the yeast peroxins. Full-length versions of candidate human PEX genes can then be obtained though routine molecular biologic approaches. Expression of the candidate clones in fibroblasts from PBD patients can be used to determine whether the gene can complement the phenotypes of the cell line; if it can, then analysis of the patient's DNA and RNA analysis can reveal whether the gene is mutated in these patients. This general approach was first used to identify PEX5 as the gene responsible for CG2 of the

PBDs[104] and was subsequently used to identify the genes defective in CG1 (PEX1[155,321]), CG3 (PEX12[141]), CG4 (PEX6[154]), CG7 (PEX10[140,322]), CG9 (PEX16[56,172]), CG11 (PEX7[129–131]), CG12 (PEX3[57]), and CG13 (PEX13[135,136]).

The mammalian cell functional complementation approach uses mutant Chinese hamster ovary (CHO) cell lines rather than yeast as the experimental system. Briefly, mutant CHO cells that are unable to import peroxisomal matrix proteins are identified and placed into complementation groups by cell fusion.[94] These CHO pex mutants are then rescued by transfection with mammalian cDNA expression libraries, usually from rat liver.[101] The complementing cDNA can be isolated by a variety of techniques, including the screening of progressively smaller subpools of the cDNA library. The identification of the CHO pex mutants and cloning of the rat PEX genes is generally considered more difficult than the analogous procedures in yeast. However, the identification of human orthologs of rat PEX genes is straightforward, due to the high sequence identity between human and rodent genes, whereas identifying human homologs of yeast PEX genes can be difficult. The CHO pex mutant functional complementation strategy was used to clone the very first PBD gene, PEX2, which is mutated in patients from CG10 of the PBDs.[102] It has since been used to identify the genes defective in CG1 (PEX1[323]), CG3 (PEX12[324,325]), CG4 (PEX6[326]), and CG14 (PEX19[58]).

Defects in Peroxisomal Matrix Protein Import

Eleven distinct PEX gene deficiencies have been identified within the PBDs over the past 8 years (Table 129-1). We discuss those that specifically affect peroxisomal matrix protein import first, in their hypothesized order of action.

PEX5 Deficiency. Human PEX5 cDNA were identified independently by several groups[104,327,328] and the PEX5 gene has been mapped to chromosome 12p13 by a variety of techniques.[327,329] Two forms of the PEX5 mRNA, PEX5S and PEX5L, differ by the presence or absence of 111 bp within the ORF and are generated by alternative splicing of exon 8.[111] PEX5L contains an additional 37 amino acids that are inserted between residues 214 and 215 of PEX5S. PEX5 proteins are predominantly cytoplasmic, partly peroxisomal receptors for newly synthesized peroxisomal matrix proteins. PEX5 binds with high affinity to the type-1 peroxisomal targeting signal (PTS1),[72] the targeting signal that is present on most matrix proteins.[173] A line diagram of PEX5 shows its various functional domains, together with the sites of known PEX5 mutations in PBD patients (Fig. 129-19). A variety of studies have mapped the site of interaction between PEX5 and the PTS1 to the C-terminal TPR domain[103,104,108] and a molecular replacement model of the C-terminal three TPRs predicts that they recognize the PTS1 peptide backbone.[109] PEX5 requires PEX14 for docking to peroxisome membranes.[118] There appear to be multiple PEX14-binding sites within the N-terminal half of PEX5,[137] which may correspond to the repeating tryptophan motif noted by Dodt et al.[104] PEX5 also binds to PEX12, an integral PMP that is required for peroxisomal matrix protein import and that is mutated in patients from complementation group 3 of the PBDs.[145] This interaction, however, is mediated by the C-terminal TPR domain of PEX5.

PEX5 deficiency has been described for just four PBD patients.[104,244,330] PEX5-deficient patients span the phenotypic range of the Zellweger spectrum from ZS to IRD. At the cellular level, all PEX5-deficient patients contain numerous PMP-containing peroxisomes.[23] However, the four PEX5-deficient patients differ in the extent of their peroxisomal matrix protein import defect.

Complete PEX5 deficiency is displayed by PBD005 cells, which were derived from a severely affected ZS patient and are homozygous for a PEX5 nonsense mutation, R390ter.[104] PBD005 cells are unable to import either PTS1- or PTS2-containing peroxisomal matrix proteins but contain numerous PMP-containing peroxisomes.[23,104] The translated product of the PEX5 R390ter allele would be expected to encode the N-terminal half of PEX5. However, PEX5 mRNA levels in PBD005 are below the limit of detection by northern blot, presumably due to nonsense-mediated RNA decay.[331] Expression of PEX5S is sufficient to rescue PTS1 protein import in these cells but restores PTS2 protein import at only 1 percent of the frequency with which it rescues PTS1 protein import.[104,111] In contrast, PEX5L expression rescues both PTS1 and PTS2 protein import in PBD005 cells at equal efficiency.[111] Overexpression of a PEX5L transcript containing the R390ter mutation rescued PTS2 protein import in PBD005 cells, indicating that the severe clinical and cellular phenotypes of PBD005 are due to the combined effects of the PEX5/R390X mutation and nonsense mediated RNA decay.[111]

Two NALD patients, PBD018 and PBD093, are both homozygous for a missense mutation in the PEX5 PTS1-binding domain, N489K.[104,244] These patients import PTS2-containing proteins normally but are unable to import any PTS1-containing proteins. The milder clinical phenotypes of these NALD patients are likely due to the more restricted matrix protein import defect in these cells. Asparagine 489 is though to play a critical role in the binding of PTS1 peptides by PEX5.[109] This residue, together with arginine R520, is predicted to facilitate PTS1-binding by interacting with the C-terminal carboxylate of the PTS1. Biochemical studies reveal that the N489K mutation does not severely affect PEX5 folding but does reduce the affinity of PEX5 for the PTS1 by several orders of magnitude.[332] More recently, an even more mildly affected PEX5-deficient patient was identified, designated 2-03.[330] This IRD patient was homozygous for a missense mutation, S563W, which lies downstream of the last TPR domain of PEX5. This residue is not thought to participate directly in PTS1 recognition. The effects of the S563W mutation appear to be more pronounced for inefficiently imported PTS1-containing

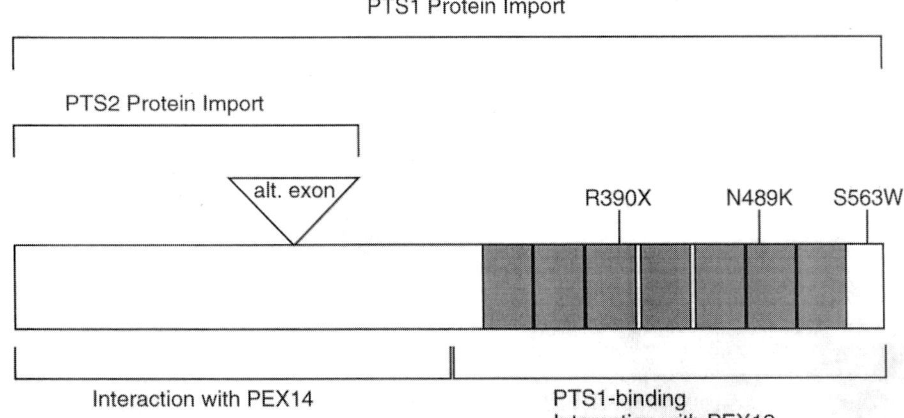

Fig. 129-19 Diagram of the human PTS1 receptor, PEX5 protein. The gray boxes indicate the 7 C-terminal tetratricopeptide repeat (TPR) motifs. The triangle indicates the position of the 37-amino-acid segment encoded by the alternatively spliced exon 8.[111] The brackets indicate regions of the PEX5 protein that interact with other proteins. The positions of three known missense mutations causing clinical phenotypes are indicated; a homozygote for R390K had ZS; a homozygote for N489K had NALD; and a homozygote for S563W had IRD.[104]

proteins such as catalase,[330] whereas the import of efficiently imported PTS1 proteins, such as acyl-CoA oxidase, are barely affected by this mutation. PTS2 protein import is unaffected in this patient.

PEX7 Deficiency. The human PEX7 cDNA was identified independently by three groups, in each instance by homology probing approaches.[129–131] The human PEX7 gene contains 10 exons spanning 102 kb at chromosome 6q21-6q22.2.[132] A number of alternatively spliced forms of PEX7 mRNA have been identified.[132] However, only the cDNAs with the full coding potential are functional in vivo and the shorter transcripts do not interfere with PEX7 function, indicating that they may represent splicing by-products rather than biologically significant transcripts. In yeast, PEX7 encodes the physical receptor for the type-2 peroxisomal targeting signal, PTS2,[123,124] and a similar activity is expected for human PEX7. Human PEX7 appears to be predominantly cytoplasmic,[129] a distribution that has also been observed for the yeast PTS2 receptor,[121,123] but additional studies of PEX7 activity and distribution are necessary. PEX7 appears to interact with PEX5, the PTS1 receptor,[333] an interaction that may explain the essential role of PEX5 in PTS2 protein import.[104] This interaction has not been shown to be direct and may be mediated by other proteins.

RCDP patients represent approximately 20 percent of all PBD cases (Table 129-1) and PEX7 deficiency has been described for more than 40 RCDP patients.[129–131] Although isolated defects in plasmalogen synthesis enzymes cause clinical phenotypes that are indistinguishable from those of RCDP,[274,334] these differ from RCDP in that they have no peroxisome biogenesis defect and are mutated in the two genes that encode peroxisomal enzymes involved in etherphospholipid synthesis.[334,335] All known RCDP patients are mutated in PEX7. RCDP patients all contain numerous PMP-containing peroxisomes, import PTS1 proteins normally, and display severe to mild defects in PTS2 protein import.[23,127]

Complete PEX7 deficiency is displayed by numerous RCDP patients. Braverman et al.[129] reported the identification of a common PEX7 mutation, L292X, that is associated with severe forms of this disease. This mutation is present in approximately two-thirds of RCDP patients and is present on approximately 50 percent of the mutated PEX7 alleles in these individuals. Genotyping studies revealed that the L292X mutation is always found on one particular haplotype, indicating that this mutation arose just once.[132] The high frequency of the L292X allele in RCDP suggests that its prevalence of this allele in populations of European descent may be somewhat elevated.

Braverman et al.[129] also reported the presence of a missense mutation, G217R, in five probands, all of whom were compound heterozygotes for the L292X allele. Three probands contained another missense mutation, A218V, two of whom exhibited relatively mild RCDP phenotypes. Motley et al.[131] reported the identification of the L292X and A218V mutations in RCDP patients and Purdue et al.[130] reported the L292X mutation, as well as an unexplained mutation that results in the PEX7 mRNAs that are 100 bp shorter than normal. More recently, a severely affected RCDP patient with a new mutation, R232X, was reported.[336]

PEX13 Deficiency. During the initial identification and characterization of yeast PEX13, an integral PMP required for peroxisomal matrix protein import, two groups reported human PEX13 cDNAs.[113,116] The PEX13 gene has been localized to chromosome 2p14-16 by both FISH and radiation hybrid mapping, and is contained on at least four exons spanning approximately 11 kb.[337] Human PEX13 is an approximately 44-kDa integral PMP that appears to span the peroxisome membrane twice and extends both its N- and C-termini into the cytoplasm.[113,117] The C-terminal extension of PEX13 contains an SH3 domain, which appears to mediate its interaction with PEX5[113] and with PEX14.[117] The N-terminal extension of PEX13 appears to interact with PEX7, either directly or indirectly.[117] In yeast, loss of PEX13 causes a significant reduction in the levels of peroxisome-associated PEX5 and PEX7, indicating that PEX13 may function as a docking factor for these PTS receptors.

There are only two known cases of PEX13 deficiency, one ZS patient (H-02) and one NALD patient (H-01/PBD222), who together define CG13 of the PBDs.[135,136] H-02 cells have numerous PMP-containing peroxisomes but fail to import peroxisomal matrix proteins.[135] These cells are homozygous for a nonsense mutation in PEX13, W234ter, which truncates PEX13 upstream of its second transmembrane span and removes its SH3 domain. H-01/PBD222 cells display a much milder matrix protein import defect and in fact import detectable levels of both PTS1- and PTS2-containing matrix proteins.[135,136] These cells are homozygous for a missense mutation in the SH3 domain, I326T, and a PEX13/I326T cDNA retains significant PEX13 activity,[136] as one might expect from the mild phenotypes of the H-01/PBD222 patient. The I326T mutation only slightly reduces the import of efficiently import peroxisomal matrix proteins but has a more pronounced effect on the import of inefficiently imported matrix proteins such as catalase[338] and glycolate oxidase, HAOX1.[82]

PEX10 Deficiency. Human PEX10 cDNAs were isolated independently by two different groups,[140,322] in both cases by searching for human homologs of yeast pex10 genes. A sequence tagged site (STS) marks the PEX10 gene, sgc30638, located at the top of the chromosome 1 linkage map. This STS is located 10.26 cR from the top of the chromosome 1 linkage group. The PEX10 coding region is contained on seven exons that are distributed across approximately 8 kb of genomic DNA.[339] Two PEX10 mRNAs, PEX10 and PEX10L, differ by 57 bp and are generated by use of different splice acceptor sites at the 3′ end of intron 3. The shorter form accounts for approximately 95 percent of the PEX10 mRNA in cells.[339] The PEX10L transcript encodes a protein with an additional 19 amino acids inserted following the tyrosine residue at position 200 and appears to be slightly less functional than the shorter, more abundant PEX10 transcript.

PEX10 encodes an integral PMP that spans the membrane twice with its N- and C-termini exposed to the cytosol.[140,322] The C-terminal domain of PEX10 contains a zinc RING motif that is essential for PEX10 function.[339] PEX10 interacts with PEX12 via its C-terminal RING-containing domain.[142] PEX12 is another integral PMP that is required for peroxisomal matrix protein import,[141] and its role in the PBDs is discussed below. Loss of PEX10 results in a severe defect in peroxisomal matrix protein import but no defect in peroxisome synthesis, PMP import, or PTS receptor docking.[23,140,142] Thus, PEX10 appears to participate in an essential step of peroxisomal matrix protein import that occurs after PTS receptor docking. In the yeast *Pichia pastoris*, loss of PEX10 results in the most severe matrix protein import defect yet described.[138]

PEX10 deficiency has been reported in four ZS patients and 1 NALD patient, all of whom were placed in CG7 of the PBDs by cell fusion complementation analysis. The positions of the known *PEX10* mutations are shown relative to the structural domains of the *PEX10* product (Fig. 129-20). The sole NALD patient, PBD052, imports residual levels of both PTS1- and PTS2-containing peroxisomal matrix proteins.[140] PBD052 is a compound heterozygote for a severe nonsense mutation, R125X, and a missense mutation that replaces a zinc-coordinating histidine of the PEX10 zinc RING domain with a glutamine residue, H290Q.[140] This latter mutation only partially reduces PEX10 function.[339] Although the R125X mutation was also reported to retain PEX10 activity, this has since been shown to be an artifact of the cDNA expression system that was used and the R125X mutation actually appears to eliminate PEX10 function.[339]

All four PEX10-deficient ZS patients have mutations that completely eliminate PEX10 activity. PBD100, which is often used as a benchmark PEX10 null cell line,[23] is homozygous for a

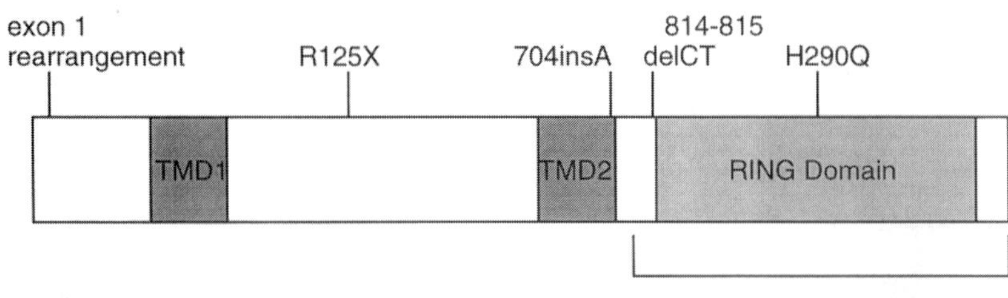

Fig. 129-20 Diagram of the human PEX10 protein. TMD1 and TMD2 indicate transmembrane domains 1 and 2; the large gray rectangle indicates the C-terminal RING domain. The bracket indicates the region of PEX10 that interacts with PEX12. The location of PEX10 mutations in PBD patients is shown above (see Warren et al.[140]). A patient with the NALD phenotype was a compound heterzygote for R125X and H290Q. A patient homozygous for the exon 1 rearrangement had ZS.

splice site mutation at the 5′ boundary of PEX10 intron 3 (GT → AT).[140] This mutation induces aberrant splicing of the PEX10 transcript, leading to the production of a PEX10 mRNA that lacks exon 3 and is 407 bp shorter than normal. A PEX10 cDNA with this mutation lacks activity in vivo. PBD117 is a compound heterozygote for a complicated deletion/insertion/frameshift mutation in exon 1 and a frameshift mutation in exon 4, 704insA, that eliminates the C-terminal zinc RING of PEX10.[339] PBD116 (also known as PBDB-01[322]) and PBD121 are each homozygous for a 2 bp deletion in exon 5 that also precludes expression of the C-terminal zinc RING domain.[339] In fact, all alleles in PEX10-deficient ZS patients preclude the expression of proteins with a zinc RING domain, the region of PEX10 that interacts with PEX12. Three other patients had been placed in complementation group 7 by cell fusion complementation analysis, but these have since been shown to be defective in PEX12, PEX1, and PEX6.[339]

PEX12 Deficiency. Human PEX12 cDNAs were identified both by homology probing[141] and by functional complementation of a CHO pex mutant.[324] The PEX12 gene contains three exons and spans 2.5 kb.[141] There is no evidence for alternative splicing of the PEX12 transcript. The chromosomal location of the PEX12 gene has yet to be determined. PEX12 appears to be an integral PMP that spans the membrane twice and extends its N- and C-termini into the cytoplasm. PEX12 contains an unusual form of the zinc RING motif within its C-terminus. Zinc RING domains typically coordinate two zinc atoms[145,340] but three of the four cysteine residues that normally bind the second zinc atom are missing in the PEX12 RING.[139,141] Nevertheless, the C-terminal RING-containing domain of PEX12 is essential for biological function[139,141,325] and appears to mediate physical interactions between PEX12 and both PEX5, the PTS1 receptor, and PEX10.[142]

PEX12-deficient patients belong to CG 3 of the PBDs. There are currently 10 known PEX12-deficient patients and they display clinical phenotypes that span the range of the Zellweger spectrum (Table 129-1).[18,67,141,142] Peroxisome membrane synthesis and PMP import are unaffected by loss of PEX12, but all patients with mutations in PEX12 display severe-to-mild defects in peroxisomal matrix protein import.[23,67,141] Additional studies have shown that cells lacking PEX12 have normal levels of peroxisome-associated PEX5, the PTS1 receptor.[142] Taken together, the phenotypes of cells lacking PEX12, the localization of PEX12 to the peroxisome membrane, and the physical interaction of PEX12 with both PEX5 and PEX10 suggest that PEX12 acts in peroxisomal matrix protein import downstream of receptor docking, most likely in matrix protein translocation.[145]

Of the 10 known PEX12-deficient patients, 6 display severe ZS phenotypes, 2 display NALD phenotypes, and 2 display IRD phenotypes. The deduced products of all mutant PEX12 alleles in these patients have been identified[67,141,142,324,325] (Fig. 129-21). The five ZS patients carry an array of splice site, frameshift, and nonsense mutations that share one common feature: the inability to express PEX12 proteins that contain their zinc RING domain.[145] In contrast, the NALD and IRD patients all express forms of PEX12 that do include this protein interaction module. The NALD patient PBD095 is homozygous for a mutation that deletes the leucine codon at position 68, L68Δ, and the NALD patient PBD054 is homozygous for a missense mutation in the zinc RING domain.[67] The IRD patient PBD099 initially presented a paradox because this individual is a compound heterozygote for a severe splice-site mutation at the 5′ end of intron 1 and a 2-bp deletion in intron 1.[67] However, translation initiation at an internal ATG codon appears to generate an active, N-terminally truncated form of PEX12 from the second allele, providing an explanation for the relatively mild phenotypes of this patient. The second IRD patient is a sibling of PBD099 and is presumed to have the same alleles and generate PEX12 activity through a similar mechanism.

The PEX12-deficient NALD patient PBD054 was originally placed in CG7 by cell fusion complementation analysis.[142,339] While this could represent an error of the cell fusion technique, we think not. PBD054 cells are phenotypically rescued by overexpression of PEX10, the gene that is normally defective in CG7, and express a missense mutation, S320F, in the PEX12 zinc RING domain, the region of PEX12 that physically interacts with PEX10.[142] Furthermore, this mutation disrupted the ability of PEX12 to bind PEX10, as well as its interaction with PEX5. Thus, we feel that the placement of PBD054 in CG7 might be due to extragenic noncomplementation with the CG7 test cell line PBD052. It is interesting to note that PBD052 cells express a mutant form of PEX10 that has a missense mutation, H290Q, in its zinc RING domain,[140, 339] the region that interacts with zinc RING of PEX12.[145]

The analysis of PEX12-deficient patients provided the first detailed study of phenotype-genotype relationships in the PBDs.[67] This study concluded that there is a relatively straightforward phenotype-genotype relationship in these diseases, with greater loss of gene function causing more severe defects in peroxisomal matrix protein import, which in turn lead to more pronounced metabolic, physiologic, and developmental deficits. Similar trends are apparent in other complementation groups of the PBDs, and are particularly evident from the analysis of PEX1-deficient patients (see below).[68,155]

PEX2 Deficiency. PEX2 was the first PBD gene identified and is defective in patients from CG10 of the PBDs.[101,102] The human PEX2 cDNA was cloned via functional complementation of a CHO pex mutant.[101,341] The PEX2 gene has been mapped to chromosome 8q21.1 by FISH.[342] Although we were unable to delineate the PEX2 gene structure from the literature, the mouse PEX2 gene has been characterized and contains 5 exons with exon 5 containing the entire PEX2 ORF.[343] The product of the human PEX2 gene is a 35-kDa integral PMP.[344] Like PEX10 and PEX12, PEX2 extends its N- and C-termini to the cytoplasm and carries a zinc RING domain within its cytoplasmically exposed C-terminus. Loss of PEX2 is associated with a severe defect in peroxisomal matrix protein import but no defect in peroxisome membrane synthesis or PMP import.[23] Furthermore, cells lacking PEX2 display increased levels of peroxisome-associated PEX5, the PTS1 receptor,[114] indicating that PEX2 functions in peroxisomal matrix protein import downstream of PTS receptor docking.

PEX2 deficiency can manifest with severe or mild phenotypes within the Zellweger spectrum and has been reported for seven patients (Fig. 129-22). The initial PEX2-deficient patient, variously referred to as MM,[102] F-01,[146,147] and PBD062,[23,114,244] is homozygous for a nonsense mutation, R199X, that terminates

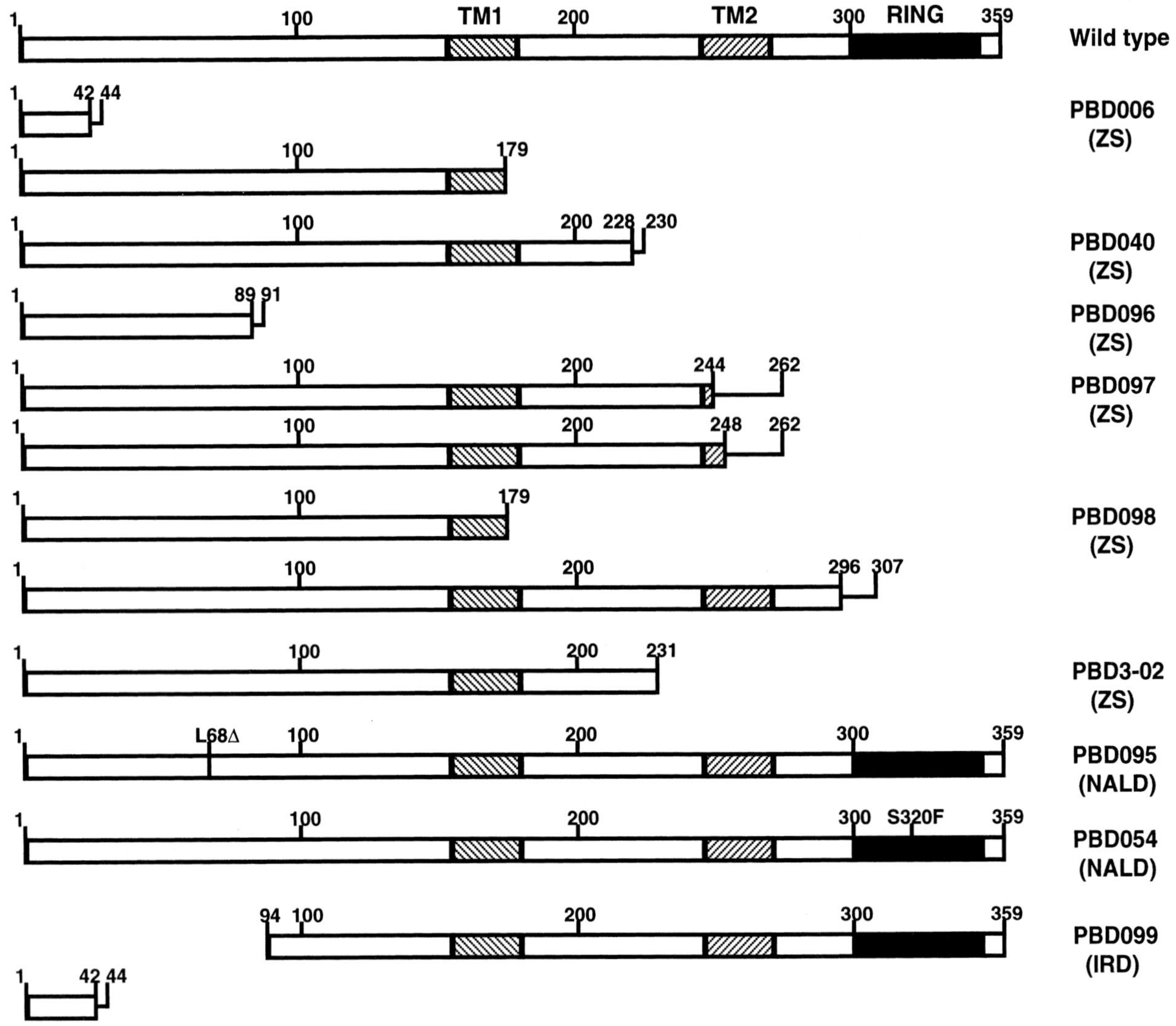

Fig. 129-21 Diagram of the consequences of all currently known *PEX12* mutations on the PEX12 protein. The positions of transmembrane domain 1 (TM1) and the 2 (TM2) and the C-terminal RING domain are indicated. The horizontal rectangles indicate the wild type or mutant PEX12 protein; the thin horizontal black line extending from the C-terminal indicates peptide encoded by an alternative reading frame extending to the indicated premature stop codon (see references 67, 141, and 145 for details). The PBD numbers refer to specific PBD probands and their phenotypes are indicated in the parentheses below.

translation less than half-way through the protein.[102,147] Two other unrelated patients, PBD094 and PBD410, are also homozygous for the same R199X mutation.[345] The ZS patient F-04 is a compound heterozygote for the R119X mutation and a distinct nonsense mutation, R125X.[147] The ZS patient F-08 is homozygous for a frameshift mutation, 550delC, that truncates the PEX2 protein following the isoleucine at position 183, effectively deleting the second transmembrane span and the zinc RING domain.[146]

Peroxisomal matrix protein import was severely affected in all five PEX2-deficient ZS patients, but was only mildly affected in the two PEX2-deficient IRD patients, F-05 and F-06. F-05 is a compound heterozygote for the R119X mutation and a PEX2 missense mutation, E55K.[147] Glutamate 55 is conserved in virtually all PEX2 proteins including those from protozoans, yeast, plants, insects, and mammals. F-06 is homozygous for a frameshift mutation, 642delG, that terminates translation following glutamine 214 and deletes the PEX2 zinc RING domain.[146] Previous mutational studies of PEX2 reported that the zinc RING domain could be removed without affecting PEX2 activity and was therefore dispensable for function.[346] The cellular and clinical phenotypes of F-06 demonstrate that loss of the PEX2 zinc RING domain does, after all, have a significant effect on PEX2 function, though such loss does not abrogate PEX2 activity altogether.

PEX1 Deficiency. The PEX1 gene was first identified in yeast and was in fact the first PEX gene to be identified.[159] The human PEX1 cDNA was identified independently by two groups using homology probing strategies[155,321] and was also identified via functional complementation of a CHO pex mutant.[323] The PEX1 gene resides on chromosome 7 (7q21-q22) and is marked by two

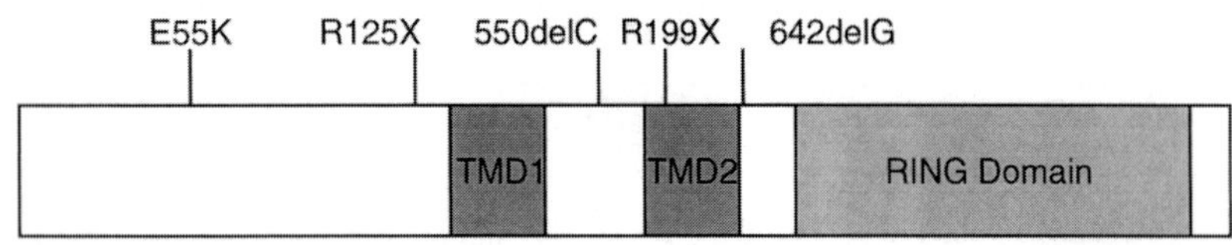

Fig. 129-22 Diagram of the PEX2 protein. The transmembrane domain 1 (TMD1) and 2 (TMD2) and C-terminal RING domain are indicated. The locations of mutations that cause abnormal peroxisome biogenesis are indicated above. See references 102 and 146 for details.

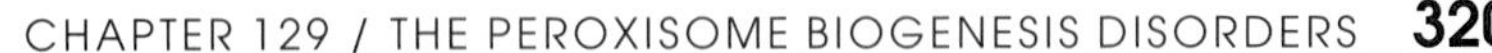

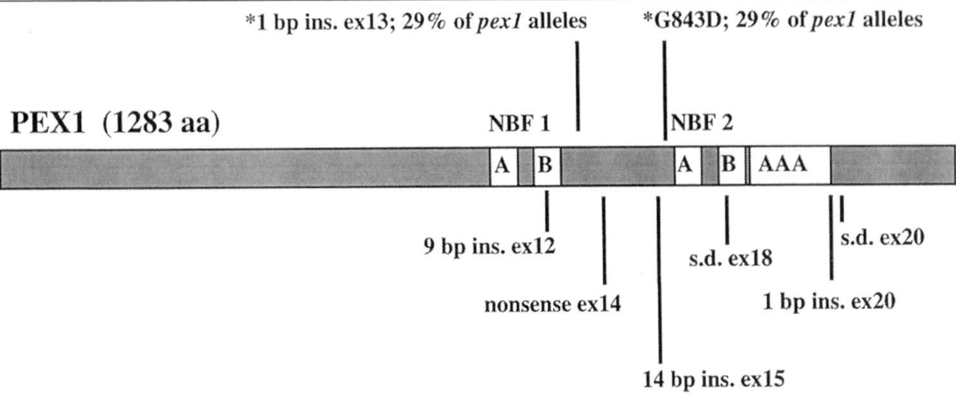

Fig. 129-23 Diagram of the human PEX1 protein. The location of the two nucleotide binding folds (NBF1 and NBF2) are indicated, each comprised of a Walker A and B ATP-binding consensus sequence. The C-terminal AAA motif is indicated. The vertical lines indicate the consequences of the known PEX1 mutation. (See references 68 and 155.)

sequence tagged sites, WI-16251 and sWSS3932.[155,321] The PEX1 gene consists of 24 exons that are distributed over 150 kb of genomic DNA. PEX1 encodes a member of the AAA ATPase protein family and can be found both on the peroxisome and in the cytoplasm.[347] PEX1 physically interacts with PEX6, another AAA ATPase that is required for peroxisomal matrix protein import,[156,158] and overexpression of PEX1 or PEX6 can suppress defects in the other in an allele-specific manner.[156] These two AAA ATPases appear to act late in peroxisomal matrix protein import.[120] Loss of human PEX1 has no effect on peroxisome membrane synthesis or PMP import but reduces the efficiency of both PTS1 and PTS2 matrix protein import.[23,155] PEX5, the PTS1 receptor, is destabilized in PEX1-deficient cells, indicating that PEX1 plays an important role in PEX5 function and matrix protein import.[114]

PEX1 deficiency is responsible for disease in approximately two-thirds of all PBD patients.[18,68,155,348–350] The high frequency of PEX1 deficiency appears to be caused by the presence of two mutated PEX1 alleles in the general population, one that has a PEX1 missense mutation, G843D,[155] and another that carries a PEX1 frameshift mutation, 2097insT.[68] These PEX1 alleles each represent approximately 30 percent of the PEX1 alleles, and one or the other of these alleles are found in roughly 80 percent of PEX1-deficient patients and in 50 percent of all Zellweger spectrum patients. Additional studies have since confirmed the high incidence of the G843D[348,349] and 2097insT[348] mutations in PEX1-deficient patients. The G843D and 2097insT mutations are associated with distinct haplotypes,[68] indicating that they arose once during human evolution and have since expanded in the Caucasian population, the major contributor to our patient population.

The G843D substitution mutation is enriched in IRD and NALD patients.[68,155] In fact, PEX1/G843D homozygotes are among the most mildly affected PBD patients known. One patient who appears to be homozygous for this mutation has survived into her forties and was capable of semi-independent living into her thirties.[18] Using a functional complementation assay, Reuber et al.[155] demonstrated that the G843D mutation does not eliminate PEX1 function and that the PEX1/G843D cDNA retains nearly 15 percent of WT activity. Geisbrecht et al.[156] demonstrated that the G843D mutation reduced the ability of PEX1 and PEX6 to bind to one another *in vitro* and found that overexpression of PEX6 partially suppressed the PEX1/G843D mutation in vivo.

While the frequency of the PEX1/G843D mutation provides an explanation for the large numbers of mildly affected PEX1-deficient patients, the abundance of PEX1-deficient ZS patients is explained by the second common PEX1 mutation, 2097insT. This mutation was first described by Collins and Gould,[68] who detected it in approximately two-thirds of the PEX1-deficient ZS patients and found that it comprised 30 percent of the PEX1 alleles in PEX1-deficent patients. The high frequency of the 2097insT mutation was subsequently confirmed in a group of Australian patients.[348] This exon 13 frameshift mutation results in low steady state PEX1 mRNA levels,[68,348] presumably due to nonsense mediated RNA decay.[331,351] However, the 2097insT mutation does not appear to induce aberrant splicing of the PEX1 transcript.[68] The 2097insT mutation is enriched in severely affected CG1 patients and all 2097insT homozygotes display ZS phenotypes.[68] Using a functional complementation assay, Collins and Gould[68] established that a PEX1/2097insT cDNA lacks detectable PEX1 activity.

In addition to these two common PEX1 mutations, numerous other mutations have been identified in the PEX1 gene, some of which are shown here (Fig. 129-23). These include a missense mutation, L664P,[323] a 9-bp insertion in exon 12,[155,321] a splice donor mutation in intron 18,[155,321] a 14-bp insertion in exon 15,[155] a nonsense mutation in exon 14,[155] a 1-bp insertion in exon 20,[155] and a splice donor mutation in intron 20.[155]

Together, the PEX1 mutation data are consistent with the phenotype-genotype relationship suggested by the recessive nature of the PBDs and prior cell fusion complementation studies.[16–19] Specifically, mutations that are predicted to cause the most severe loss of gene function cause the most severe defects in peroxisomal matrix protein import and are associated with the most severe clinical phenotypes. That one or the other of the two common PEX1 mutations can be found in roughly 80 percent of PEX1-deficient patients and 50 percent of Zellweger spectrum patients indicates that genetic testing technologies may be useful in the PBDs.

PEX6 Deficiency. Human PEX6 cDNAs were identified both by homology probing[154] and by the CHO cell functional complementation assay.[326] The PEX6 gene has been mapped to chromosome 6 both by RFLP analysis[154] and by FISH, which placed it at 6p21.1.[326] This gene contains 17 exons that are dispersed along 14 kb of genomic DNA.[352] PEX6 encodes a 104-kDa member of AAA ATPase protein family[154,326] that physically interacts with PEX1.[156,158] It is therefore not surprising that loss of PEX6 results in phenotypes that are similar to those observed in PEX1 deficiency. PEX6-deficient cells display defects in peroxisomal matrix protein import that vary with allele severity but do not exhibit any detectable defect in peroxisome membrane synthesis or PMP import.[23,154] PEX6 is required for proper stability of PEX5[154] and acts late in peroxisomal matrix protein import.[120]

PEX6 deficiency is the second most common cause of the Zellweger spectrum disorders (Table 129-1).[18,154,326] More than 20 PBD patients have been identified who are defective in PEX6. The peroxisomal matrix protein import defect in these patients varies from severe to mild, but in all cases, it is possible to detect slight import of peroxisomal matrix proteins. For example, Yahraus et al.[154] described a PEX6-deficient ZS patient (PBD106) who lacked detectable levels of PEX6 mRNA and was a compound heterozygote for two frameshift mutations in PEX6, each of which would preclude the synthesis of its essential C-terminal AAA motif. Nevertheless, residual levels of PTS1 protein import could be detected in fibroblasts from this patient.

Additional studies have identified a number of PEX6 mutations in PBD patients, although there is no evidence for any common PEX6 alleles in the CG4 population. Fukuda et al.[326] reported mutations in two ZS patients, one of whom was homozygous for a

1-bp insertion at nucleotide 511 of the PEX6 cDNA sequence (511insT) and another in whom a PEX6 splice site mutation was identified (IVS3 + 1G > A). More recently, Zhang et al.[352] reported an extensive analysis of PEX6 gene structure in 10 PEX6-deficient patients. The mutations described include a variety of splice site, frameshift, nonsense, and missense mutations that are dispersed throughout the gene. Once again, the phenotype-genotype relationships appear to support a straightforward model in which mutations that are expected to create the most significant loss in protein function are associated with the most severe cellular and clinical phenotypes.

CG 8, the Unknown PEX Gene Deficiency. The gene defect in CG 8 of the PBDs has yet to be reported. There are at least 11 known CG 8 patients and these individuals span the phenotypic range of Zellweger spectrum (Table 129-1).[18] Cellular studies of CG 8 cells have found that they all have numerous PMP-containing peroxisomes but display a variable defect in peroxisomal matrix protein import.[23,244] Furthermore, CG 8 cells have reduced levels of PEX5, the PTS receptor, a phenotype that is also observed in PEX1- and PEX6-deficient cells, but not in cells lacking PEX2, PEX7, PEX10, PEX12, or PEX16.[114]

Other Anticipated PEX Gene Deficiencies. Although there is only one complementation group of PBD patients for which the gene is not yet known, it is likely that additional complementation groups will be identified in the future. Human homologs of other yeast PEX genes are likely candidates for being defective in these patients. Currently, PEX14,[62–64] PEX11α,[28] and PEX11β are the only known human PEX genes that are not defective in at least one patient. In yeast, PEX14 participates in peroxisomal matrix protein import, and we would expect a similar role for its human homolog. Loss of yeast PEX11 does not affect peroxisomal protein import, making it unclear whether loss of human PEX11α or PEX11β would result in a disease phenotype.

There are a number of other PEX genes that are required for peroxisomal matrix protein import in yeast but for which the human PEX genes are not known, including the PEX4,[119,151,152] PEX9,[165] PEX15,[166] PEX17,[167] PEX18,[133] PEX20,[134] PEX21,[133] PEX22,[153] and PEX23[168] genes and it is not a certainty that humans have all such genes. However, because these yeast genes all participate in peroxisomal matrix protein import, their human homologs would represent excellent candidates for a PBD gene.

Defects in Peroxisome Membrane Synthesis

Defects in peroxisome membrane synthesis have been observed in just four PBD patients, all of whom display ZS phenotypes. These patients are defective in any of three genes, PEX3, PEX16, and PEX19.

PEX16 Deficiency. The human PEX16 cDNA was identified independently by two groups, in each instance by homology probing approaches.[56,172] The PEX16 gene has yet to be mapped and its organization remains to be determined. The PEX16 product is an integral PMP[56] that extends its N- and C-termini into the cytoplasm. There is only one known PEX16-deficient patient, referred to as either PBD061[56] or PBDD-01.[172] This individual displayed severe ZS phenotypes and was homozygous for the nonsense mutation R176X, which eliminated PEX16 function in vivo. Fibroblasts from this patient lacked detectable peroxisomes, as determined by immunofluorescent staining with antibodies specific for the integral peroxisomal membrane protein, PMP70.[56,172] By immunoblot, these cells lacked detectable levels of PMP70 and of a different integral PMP, P70R, and failed to import a wide variety of integral PMPs.[56]

Reexpression of the PEX16 cDNA restored peroxisome membrane synthesis and PMP import, followed by restoration of peroxisomal matrix protein import.[56] Phenotypic rescue generally required at least 24 h and was not maximal until 72 h after transfection. In contrast, PEX16 targeting to peroxisomes in normal human fibroblasts could be detected as soon as 2 h after transfection.[56] The extreme kinetic difference between PEX16 targeting to peroxisomes and PEX16-mediated peroxisome membrane synthesis suggests that the two processes occur by distinct mechanisms. In addition, the COPI-inhibitor brefeldin A had no effect on either PEX16 targeting to peroxisomes or PEX16-mediated peroxisome membrane synthesis.[56]

PEX19 Deficiency. The human PEX19 cDNA was first identified as HK33, a housekeeping gene expressed in many tissues.[353] The PEX19 gene localizes to chromosome 1q22,[353,354] contains eight exons, and spans approximately 9 kb.[354] Three splice variants of PEX19 have been identified, but their functional significance, if any, remains to be determined. PEX19 encodes a predominantly cytoplasmic, partly peroxisomal protein that binds a wide array of PMPs, including PMPs that are involved in peroxisome biogenesis and PMPs that function in metabolite transport.[59] PEX19 binds PMPs with high affinity, displaying a K_d of 500 nM for the PMP Pex14.

A single PEX19-deficient ZS patient has been identified, PBDJ-01.[58] Cells from this patient are homozygous for a frameshift mutation in PEX19, 764insA, that effectively deletes the C-terminal 45 amino acids from its product.[58] PBDJ-01 cells, which have also been referred to as PBD399 cells,[59] lack detectable peroxisomes, as determined by immunofluorescent staining with antibodies specific for a variety of integral PMPs.[58,59] PMP70, PEX13, and PEX11β simply could not be detected in these PEX19-deficient cells and other PMPs that could be detected, such as PEX14, were mislocalized to their mitochondria. Reexpression of PEX19 restores peroxisome biogenesis in a stepwise fashion with peroxisome membrane synthesis and PMP import preceding peroxisomal matrix protein import.[58]

PEX3 Deficiency. The human PEX3 cDNA was identified independently by two groups, each by homology probing using yeast PEX3 sequences as probes.[190,355] The PEX3 gene is located at chromosome 6q23-24 and contains 12 exons that span approximately 14 kb.[356] PEX3 encodes an integral PMP that physically interacts with PEX19, the putative PMP receptor.[59,190] Two PEX3-deficient patients have been identified, PBD400 and PBD401, both of whom display severe ZS phenotypes.[57] PBD400 fibroblasts are homozygous for a frameshift mutation, 542insT, that would be expected to delete the C-terminal half of PEX3. PBD401 fibroblasts are homozygous for a nonsense mutation, R53X, which would delete the C-terminal 5/6 of PEX3. Both mutations eliminate PEX3 activity.

Reexpression of PEX3 restores peroxisome biogenesis in both PBD400 and PBD401 cells.[57] The earliest time at which rescue could be detected was 24 h after transfection. Complete phenotypic rescue was not maximal until 3 days after transfection. In contrast, PEX3 targeting to peroxisomes could be detected as early as 1 h after transfection, indicating that PEX3 import and PEX3-mediated peroxisome synthesis occur through kinetically distinct mechanisms. PEX3-mediated peroxisome biogenesis occurred in a stepwise fashion, with peroxisome membrane synthesis and PMP import occurring first and peroxisomal matrix protein import detected at later time points. PEX3-medated peroxisome synthesis was unaffected by inhibitors of COPI-mediated and COPII-mediated vesicular transport,[57] raising even more doubts about the origin of the nascent peroxisomes during these instances of de novo peroxisome biogenesis.

Genotype/Phenotype Relationships

Although we are relatively early in our understanding of the pathophysiology of *PEX* gene mutations, some correlations between clinical phenotypic severity, cellular phenotypic severity and genotype are emerging. In CG 1 of the Zellweger spectrum, a frequent *PEX1* missense allele, G843D, has been associated with a mild phenotype.[68,155] Homozygotes for G843D tend to be in the milder region of the Zellweger spectrum (NALD, IRD, and milder still) and, at the cellular level, their peroxisomes appear to import some amount of residual matrix proteins. By contrast, patients homozygous for the common *PEX1* null allele, 2097insT, have typical ZS and their peroxisomes fail to import matrix proteins.[68,348] Similarly, in CG 3, a *PEX12* allele with an early frameshift is apparently rescued by translational initiation at an internal methionine yielding an N-terminal truncated *PEX12* protein with residual activity ($\approx$15 percent).[67] A patient who was a genetic compound for this allele and a *PEX12* null allele had an IRD phenotype and was the least affected of 7 CG 3 probands.

A similar pattern is suggested by early studies in RCDP. Again there is a common allele, *PEX7* L292ter, which produces reduced amounts of a PEX7 protein with no residual function.[129,131] This allele has a high frequency due to a founder effect and accounts for about half of all the *PEX7* genes causing RCDP.[132] Homozygotes for L292ter have a severe cellular defect in the peroxisomal import of PTS2 targeted matrix proteins and have the classical, severe RCDP clinical phenotype.[129,132] By contrast, certain *PEX7* missense alleles (A218V, S25F, H39P, G41V) encode mutant PTS2 receptors that have residual activity and are found in patients with milder phenotypic variants of RCDP.[126,357] The N-terminal location of several of these suggests that this region of the PTS2 receptor may be more tolerant of variation. This prediction is supported by consideration of the structure of proteins homologous to PEX7.

Treatment

The potential of postnatal treatment is limited by the multiple malformations and defects that originate in fetal life. Nevertheless, it may prove of value for patients with milder phenotypes. Wilson et al.[197] and Holmes[358] administered ether lipids orally to mildly affected patients with ZS, and achieved a partial normalization of red blood cell plasmalogen levels. Plasma VLCFA can also be normalized at least in part by a dietary regimen which has been tried in X-linked ALD.[359] This regimen also minimizes phytanic acid intake and has brought about normalization of phytanic acid levels (H.W. Moser, unpublished observation). This dietary approach was used in some patients with the somewhat milder forms of disordered peroxisomes biogenesis.[360] However, given the variability of disease, it has been difficult to evaluate effectiveness.

Two additional approaches were recently proposed, and both have demonstrated positive biochemical effects and anecdotal clinical benefit in studies that have involved single patients. Setchell et al.[361] administered oral cholic and deoxycholic acids in a dosage of 100 mg each per day. They reported improved liver function and an unspecified improvement in neurologic status. Martinez et al.[362] administered oral docosahexaenoic acid in a dosage of 250 mg/day to two patients, one patient died soon after the institution of therapy, the other, a 6-year-old boy with NALD, was reported to show improved alertness, motor performance, vocabulary, and visual-evoked responses. The same group also reported improvement in MRI.[363] In contrast, others have reported that no demonstrable effect. The need for controlled trial of this therapy as well as others has been highlighted.[364]

Administration of clofibrate has failed to induce liver peroxisomes in Zellweger disease patients.[240,365] An interesting observation was that the administration of 4-phenylbutyrate increased the number of peroxisomes in cells of patients with X-ALD.[366]

Often overlooked, symptomatic therapy has been of benefit in children with ZS, NALD, IRD, and RCDP.

ANIMAL MODELS

Two murine models with targeted disruption of PEX genes have been described. In the first of these, the murine PEX5 gene was disrupted by deletion of four exons encoding most of the C-terminal TPR repeats.[367] Affected mice had intrauterine growth retardation but were born alive in the expected Mendelian ratios. All died within the first day or two of life. Histologic examination showed enlarged peroxisomes present in reduced numbers that lacked both PTS1 and PTS2 targeted matrix proteins. This result strongly supports the contention of Braverman et al. that mammalian PEX5 plays a role in both PTS1 and PTS2 import.[111] Interestingly, analysis of the neocortex of these animals showed impaired neuronal migration and maturation with extensive apoptotic neuronal death. This observation is similar to those made on the brains of ZS patients and indicates that the murine model should be a good system for understanding the pathophysiology of the neuronal migration defects.

The second mouse model was produced by disrupting the murine PEX2 gene.[343] Homozygous PEX2-deficient mice were born alive but were hypoactive and hypotonic and died in a few hours. Histologic examination showed the presence of peroxisomes devoid of matrix proteins. Affected mice had elevated VLCFA and decreased erythrocyte plasmalogens. Their central nervous system was abnormal with aberrant neuronal migration. Thus, these animals provide a second model to study the neuronal developmental defects characteristic of human PBD.

REFERENCES

1. Bowen P, Lee CSN, Zellweger H, Lindenberg R: A familial syndrome of multiple congenital anomalies. *Bull Johns Hopkins Hosp* **114**:402, 1964.
2. Passarge E, McAdams AJ: Cerebro-hepato-renal syndrome: A newly recognized hereditary disorder of multiple congenital defects, including sudanophilic leukodystrophy, cirrhosis of the liver and polycystic kidneys. *J Pediatr* **71**:691, 1967.
3. Opitz JM, ZuRhein GM, Vitale L, Shahidi NT, Howe JJ, Chon SM, Shanklin DR, Sybers HD, Dood AR, Gerritsen T: The Zellweger syndrome (cerebrohepatorenal syndrome). *Birth Defects* **5**:144, 1969.
4. Danks DM, Tippett P, Adams C, Campbell P: Cerebro-hepato-renal syndrome of Zellweger: A report of eight cases with comments upon the incidence, the liver lesion and a fault in pipecolic acid metabolism. *J Pediatr* **86**:382, 1975.
5. Lazarow PB, Moser HW: Disorders of peroxisome biogenesis, in Scriver C, Beaudet A, Sly W, Valle D (eds): *The Metabolic and Molecular Bases of Inherited Disease*. New York, McGraw-Hill, 1995, p 2287.
6. Goldfischer S, Moore CL, Johnson AB, Spiro AJ, Valsmis MP, Wisniewski HK, Ritch RH, Norton WT, Rapin I, Gartner LM: Peroxisomal and mitochondrial defects in the cerebro-hepato-renal syndrome. *Science* **182**:62, 1973.
7. Ulrich J, Hershkowitz N, Heits P, Sigrist T, Baelocker P: Adrenoleukodystrophy: Preliminary report of a connatal case, light- and electron microscopical, immunohistochemical and biochemical findings. *Acta Neuropathol (Berl)* **43**:77, 1978.
8. Scotto JM, Hadchouel M, Odievre M, Laudat MH, Saudubray JM, Dulac O, Beucler I, Beaune P: Infantile phytanic acid storage disease, a possible variant of Refsum disease: Three cases including ultrastructural studies of the liver. *J Inherit Metab Dis* **5**:83, 1982.
9. Aubourg P, Scotto J, Rocchiccioli F, Feldmann-Pautrat D, Robain O: Neonatal adrenoleukodystrophy. *J Neurol Neurosurg Psychiatry* **49**:77, 1986.
10. Vamecq J, Draye JP, Van HF, Misson JP, Evrard P, Verellen G, Eyssen HJ, Schutgens RB, Wanders RJ: Multiple peroxisomal enzymatic deficiency disorders: A comparative biochemical and morphologic study of Zellweger cerebrohepatorenal syndrome and neonatal adrenoleukodystrophy. *Am J Pathol* **125**:524, 1986.
11. Roels F, Cornelis A, Poll-The BT, Aubourg P, Ogier H, Scotto J, Saudubray JM: Hepatic peroxisomes are deficient in infantile Refsum disease: A cytochemical study of four cases. *Am J Med Genet* **25**:257, 1986.
12. Wanders RJ, Schutgens RB, Schrakamp G, van den Bosch H, Tager JM, Schram AW, Hashimoto T, Poll-The BT, Saudubray JM: Infantile Refsum disease: Deficiency of catalase-containing particles (peroxisomes), alkyldihydroxyacetone phosphate synthase and peroxisomal beta-oxidation enzyme proteins. *Eur J Pediatr* **145**:172, 1986.
13. Heymans HSA: Cerebro-hepato-renal (Zellweger) syndrome. Clinical and biochemical consequences of peroxisomal dysfunction. University of Amsterdam, 1984.
14. Heymans HS, Oorthuys JW, Nelck G, Wanders RJ, Schutgens RB: Rhizomelic chondrodysplasia punctata: Another peroxisomal disorder. *N Engl J Med* **313**:197, 1985.

15. Hoefler G, Hoefler S, Watkins PA, Chen WW, Moser A, Baldwin V, McGillivary B, Charrow J, Friedman JM, Rutledge L: Biochemical abnormalities in rhizomelic chondrodysplasia punctata. *J Pediatr* **112**:726, 1988.
16. Brul S, Westerveld A, Strijland A, Wanders RJA, Schram AW, Heymans HSA, Schutgens RBH, van den Bosch H, Tager JM: Genetic heterogeneity in the cerebrohepatorenal (Zellweger) syndrome and other inherited disorders with a generalized impairment of peroxisomal functions—A study using complementation analysis. *J Clin Invest* **81**:1710, 1988.
17. Roscher AA, Hoefler S, Hoefler G, Paschke E, Paltauf F, Moser A, Moser H: Genetic and phenotypic heterogeneity in disorders of peroxisome biogenesis. A complementation study involving cell lines from 19 patients. *Pediatr Res* **26**:67, 1989.
18. Moser AB, Rasmussen M, Naidu S, Watkins PA, McGuinness M, Hajra AK, Chen G, Raymond G, Liu A, Gordon D, Garnaas K, Walton DS, Skjeldal OH, Guggenheim MA, Jackson LG, Elias ER, Moser HW: Phenotype of patients with peroxisomal disorders subdivided into sixteen complementation groups. *J Pediatr* **127**:13, 1995.
19. Shimozawa N, Suzuki Y, Orii T, Moser A, Moser HW, Wanders RJA: Standardization of complementation grouping of peroxisome-deficient disorders and the second Zellweger patient with peroxisomal assembly factor-I (PAF-I) defect. *Am J Hum Genet* **52**:843, 1993.
20. Shimozawa N, Suzuki Y, Zhang Z, Imamura A, Kondo N, Kinoshita N, Fujiki Y, Tsukamoto T, Osumi T, Imanaka T, Orii T, Beemer F, Mooijer P, Dekker C, Wanders RJ: Genetic basis of peroxisome-assembly mutants of humans, Chinese hamster ovary cells, and yeast: identification of a new complementation group of peroxisome-biogenesis disorders apparently lacking peroxisomal-membrane ghosts. *Am J Hum Genet* **63**:1898, 1998.
21. Poulos A, Christodoulou J, Chow CW, Goldblatt J, Paton BC, Orii T, Suzuki Y, Shimozawa N: Peroxisomal assembly defects: Clinical, pathologic and biochemical findings in two patients in a newly identified complementation group. *J Pediatr* **127**:596, 1995.
22. Gould SJ, Valle D: The genetics and cell biology of the peroxisome biogenesis disorders. *Trends Genet* **16**:340, 2000.
23. Chang CC, South S, Warren D, Jones J, Moser AB, Moser HW, Gould SJ: Metabolic control of peroxisome abundance. *J Cell Sci* **112**:1579, 1999.
24. Espeel M, Depreter M, Nardacci R, D'Herde K, Kerckaert I, Stefanini S, Roels F: Biogenesis of peroxisomes in fetal liver. *Microsc Res Tech* **39**:453, 1997.
25. Fahimi HD, Reich D, Volkl A, Baumgart E: Contributions of the immunogold technique to investigation of the biology of peroxisomes. *Histochem Cell Biol* **106**:105, 1996.
26. Fahimi HD, Baumgart E: Current cytochemical techniques for the investigation of peroxisomes. A review. *J Histochem Cytochem* **47**:1219, 1999.
27. Schrader M, Burkhardt JK, Baumgart E, Lüers G, Spring H, Völkl A, Fahimi HD: Interaction of microtubules with peroxisomes. Tubular and spherical peroxisomes in HepG2 cells and their alterations induced by microtubule-active drugs. *Eur J Cell Biol* **69**:24, 1996.
28. Schrader M, Reuber BE, Morell JC, Jimenez-Sanchez G, Obie C, Stroh TA, Valle D, Schroer TA, Gould SJ: Expression of *PEX11β* mediates peroxisome proliferation in the absence of extracellular stimuli. *J Biol Chem* **273**:29607, 1998.
29. Gorgas K: Peroxisomes in sebaceous glands. V. Complex peroxisomes in the mouse preputial gland. Serial sectioning and three-dimensional reconstruction studies. *Anat Embryol (Berl)* **169**:261, 1984.
30. Michels PA: The glycosome of trypanosomes: Properties and biogenesis of a microbody. *Exp Parasitol* **69**:310, 1989.
31. Opperdoes FR, Michels PA: The glycosomes of the *Kinetoplastida*. *Biochimie* **75**:231, 1993.
32. Fahimi HD, Baumgart E, Volkl A: Ultrastructural aspects of the biogenesis of peroxisomes in rat liver. *Biochimie* **75**:201, 1993.
33. Veenhuis M, Harder W, van Dijken JP, Mayer F: Substructure of crystalline peroxisomes in methanol-grown *Hansenula polymorpha*: Evidence for an in vivo crystal of alcohol oxidase. *Mol Cell Biol* **1**:949, 1981.
34. Van Veldhoven PP, Just WW, Mannaerts GP: Permeability of the peroxisomal membrane to cofactors of beta-oxidation. Evidence for the presence of a pore-forming protein. *J Biol Chem* **262**:4310, 1987.
35. Verleur N, Wanders RJ: Permeability properties of peroxisomes in digitonin-permeabilized rat hepatocytes. Evidence for free permeability towards a variety of substrates. *Eur J Biochem* **218**:75, 1993.
36. Sulter GJ, Verheyden K, Mannaerts G, Harder W, Veenhuis M: The *in vitro* permeability of yeast peroxisomal membranes is caused by a 31 kDa integral membrane protein. *Yeast* **9**:733, 1993.
37. van Roermund CWT, Elgersma Y, Singh N, Wanders RJA, Tabak HF: The membrane of peroxisomes in *Saccharomyces cerevisiae* is impermeable to NAD(H) and acetyl-CoA under in vivo conditions. *EMBO J* **14**:3480, 1995.
38. van Roermund CW, Hettema EH, Kal AJ, van den Berg M, Tabak HF, Wanders RJ: Peroxisomal beta-oxidation of polyunsaturated fatty acids in *Saccharomyces cerevisiae*: Isocitrate dehydrogenase provides NADPH for reduction of double bonds at even positions. *EMBO J* **17**:677, 1998.
39. Henke B, Girzalsky W, Berteaux-Lecellier V, Erdmann R: IDP3 encodes a peroxisomal NADP-dependent isocitrate dehydrogenase required for the beta-oxidation of unsaturated fatty acids. *J Biol Chem* **273**:3702, 1998.
40. Geisbrecht BV, Gould SJ: The human PICD gene encodes a cytoplasmic and peroxisomal NADP(+)-dependent isocitrate dehydrogenase. *J Biol Chem* **274**:30527, 1999.
41. Jones JM, Nau K, Geraghty MT, Erdmann R, Gould SJ: Identification of peroxisomal acyl-CoA thioesterases in yeast and humans. *J Biol Chem* **274**:9216, 1999.
42. Dansen TB, Wirtz KW, Wanders RJ, Pap EH: Peroxisomes in human fibroblasts have a basic pH. *Nat Cell Biol* **2**:51, 2000.
43. Sacksteder KA, Morrell JC, Wanders RJA, Matalon R, Gould SJ: MCD encodes peroxisomal and cytoplasmic forms of malonyl-CoA decarboxylase and is mutated in malonyl-CoA decarboxylase deficiency. *J Biol Chem* **274**:24461, 1999.
44. Wanders RJA, Tager JM: Lipid metabolism in peroxisomes in relation to human disease. *Mol Aspects Med* **19**:69, 1998.
45. van den Bosch H, Schutgens RBH, Wanders RJA, Tager JM: Biochemistry of peroxisomes. *Annu Rev Biochem* **61**:157, 1992.
46. Wanders RJ, Jansen G, van Roermund CW, Denis S, Schutgens RB, Jakobs BS: Metabolic aspects of peroxisomal disorders. *Ann N Y Acad Sci* **804**:450, 1996.
47. Herrmann JM, Malkus P, Schekman R: Out of the ER—Outfitters, escorts and guides. *Trends Cell Biol* **9**:5, 1999.
48. Neupert W: Protein import into mitochondria. *Annu Rev Biochem* **66**:863, 1997.
49. Nickel W, Wieland FT: Biosynthetic protein transport through the early secretory pathway. *Histochem Cell Biol* **109**:477, 1998.
50. Kuehn MJ, Schekman R: COPII and secretory cargo capture into transport vesicles. *Curr Opin Cell Biol* **9**:477, 1997.
51. Titorenko VI, Rachubinski RA: The endoplasmic reticulum plays an essential role in peroxisome biogenesis. *Trends Biochem Sci* **23**:231, 1998.
52. Kunau W-H, Erdmann R: Peroxisome biogenesis: Back to the endoplasmic reticulum? *Curr Biol* **8**:R299, 1998.
53. Kunau WH: Peroxisome biogenesis: from yeast to man. *Curr Opin Microbiol* **1**:232, 1998.
54. Tabak HF, Braakman I, Distel B: Peroxisomes: Simple function but complex in maintenance. *Trends Cell Biol* **9**:447, 1999.
55. Lazarow PB, Fujiki Y: Biogenesis of peroxisomes. *Annu Rev Cell Biol* **1**:489, 1985.
56. South ST, Gould SJ: Peroxisome synthesis in the absence of preexisting peroxisomes. *J Cell Biol* **144**:255, 1999.
57. South ST, Sacksteder KA, Li X, Liu Y, Santos M, Gould SJ: Inhibitors of COPI and COPII do not block *PEX3*-mediated peroxisome synthesis. *J Cell Biol* **149**:1345, 2000.
58. Matsuzono Y, Kinoshita N, Tamura S, Shimozawa N, Hamasaki M, Ghaedi K, Wanders RJA, Suzuki Y, Kondo N, Fujiki Y: Human *PEX19*:cDNA cloning by functional complementation, mutation analysis in a patient with Zellweger syndrome and potential role in peroxisomal membrane assembly. *Proc Natl Acad Sci U S A* **96**:2116, 1999.
59. Sacksteder KA, Jones JM, South ST, Li X, Liu Y, Gould SJ: *PEX19* binds multiple peroxisomal membrane proteins, is predominantly cytoplasmic, and is required for peroxisome membrane synthesis. *J Cell Biol* **148**:931, 2000.
60. Hettema EH, Distel B, Tabak HF: Import of proteins into peroxisomes. *Biochim Biophys Acta* **1451**:17, 1999.
61. Hettema EH, Girzalsky W, van Den Berg M, Erdmann R, Distel B: *Saccharomyces cerevisiae* pex3p and pex19p are required for proper localization and stability of peroxisomal membrane proteins. *EMBO J* **19**:223, 2000.
62. Will GK, Soukupova M, Hong X, Erdmann KS, Kiel JA, Dodt G, Kunau WH, Erdmann R: Identification and characterization of the human orthologue of yeast Pex14p. *Mol Cell Biol* **19**:2265, 1999.

63. Shimizu N, Itoh R, Hirono Y, Otera H, Ghaedi K, Tateishi K, Tamura S, Okumoto K, Harano T, Mukai S, Fujiki Y: The peroxin Pex14p. cDNA cloning by functional complementation on a Chinese hamster ovary cell mutant, characterization, and functional analysis. *J Biol Chem* **274**:12593, 1999.
64. Fransen M, Terlecky SR, Subramani S: Identification of a human PTS1 receptor docking protein directly required for peroxisomal protein import. *Proc Natl Acad Sci U S A* **95**:8087, 1998.
65. Santos M, Imanaka T, Shio H, Small GM, Lazarow PB: Peroxisomal membrane ghosts in Zellweger syndrome- aberrant organelle assembly. *Science* **239**:1536, 1988.
66. Santos MJ, Imanaka T, Shio H, Lazarow PB: Peroxisomal integral membrane proteins in control and Zellweger fibroblasts. *J Biol Chem* **263**:10502, 1988.
67. Chang C-C, Gould SJ: Phenotype-genotype relationships in complementation group 3 of the peroxisome-biogenesis disorders. *Am J Hum Genet* **63**:1294, 1998.
68. Collins CS, Gould SJ: Identification of a common mutation in severely affected *PEX1*-deficient patients. *Hum Mutat* **14**:45, 1999.
69. Kinoshita N, Ghaedi K, Shimozawa N, Wanders RJA, Matsuzono Y, Imanaka T, Okumoto K, Suzuki Y, Kondo N, Fujiki Y: Newly identified Chinese hamster ovary cell mutants are defective in biogenesis of peroxisomal membrane vesicles (peroxisomal ghosts), representing a novel complementation group in mammals. *J Biol Chem* **273**:24122, 1998.
70. Gould SJ, Keller GA, Subramani S: Identification of a peroxisomal targeting signal at the carboxy terminus of firefly luciferase. *J Cell Biol* **105**:2923, 1987.
71. Gould SJ, Keller G-A, Subramani S: Identification of peroxisomal targeting signals at the carboxy-terminus of four peroxisomal proteins. *J Cell Biol* **107**:897, 1988.
72. Gould SJ, Keller GA, Hosken N, Wilkinson J, Subramani S: A conserved tripeptide sorts proteins to peroxisomes. *J Cell Biol* **108**:1657, 1989.
73. Gould SJ, Keller GA, Schneider M, Howell SH, Garrard LJ, Goodman JM, Distel B, Tabak H, Subramani S: Peroxisomal protein import is conserved between yeast, plants, insects and mammals. *EMBO J* **9**:85, 1990.
74. Gould SJ, Krisans S, Keller GA, Subramani S: Antibodies directed against the peroxisomal targeting signal of firefly luciferase recognize multiple mammalian peroxisomal proteins. *J Cell Biol* **110**:27, 1990.
75. Subramani S: Components involved in peroxisome import, biogenesis, proliferation, turnover and movement. *Physiol Rev* **78**:171, 1998.
76. de Hoop MJ, Ab G: Import of proteins into peroxisomes and other microbodies. *Biochemistry* **286**:657, 1992.
77. Lametschwandtner G, Brocard C, Fransen M, Van Veldhoven P, Berger J, Hartig A: The difference in recognition of terminal tripeptides as peroxisomal targeting signal 1 between yeast and human is due to different affinities of their receptor Pex5p to the cognate signal and to residues adjacent to it. *J Biol Chem* **273**:33635, 1998.
78. Elgersma Y, Vos A, van den Berg M, van Roermund CWT, van der Sluijs P, Distel B, Tabak HF: Analysis of the carboxyl-terminal peroxisomal targeting signal 1 in a homologous context in *Saccharomyces cerevisiae*. *J Biol Chem* **271**:26375, 1996.
79. Blattner J, Swinkels B, Dorsam H, Prospero T, Subramani S, Clayton D: Glycosome assembly in trypanosomes: Variations in the acceptable degeneracy of a COOH-terminal microbody targeting signal. *J Cell Biol* **119**:1129, 1992.
80. Sommer JM, Wang CC: Targeting proteins to the glycosomes of African trypanosomes. *Annu Rev Microbiol* **48**:105, 1994.
81. Swinkels BW, Gould SJ, Subramani S: Targeting efficiencies of various permutations of the consensus C-terminal tripeptide peroxisomal targeting signal. *FEBS Lett* **305**:133, 1992.
82. Jones JM, Morrell JC, Gould SJ: Identification and characterization of HAOX1, HAOX2, and HAOX3, three human peroxisomal 2-hydroxy acid oxidases. *J Biol Chem* **275**:12590, 2000.
83. Jones JM, Gould SJ: Identification and characterization of PTE2, a human peroxisomal long-chain acyl-CoA thioesterase. *J Biol Chem* (in press), 2000.
83a. Geisbrecht BV, Zhang D, Schulz H, Gould SJ: Characterization of PECI, a novel monofunctional Delta(3), Delta(2)-enoyl-CoA isomerase of mammalian peroxisomes. *J Biol Chem* **274**:21797, 1999.
84. Geisbrecht BV, Zhu D, Schulz K, Nau K, Morrell JC, Geraghty MT, Schulz H, Erdmann R, Gould SJ: Molecular characterization of *Saccharomyces cerevisiae* delta3,delta2-enoyl-CoA isomerase. *J Biol Chem* **273**:33184, 1998.
85. Motley A, Lumb MJ, Oatey PB, Jennings PR, De Zoysa PA, Wanders RJA, Tabak HF, Danpure CJ: Mammalian alanine/glyoxylate aminotransferase 1 is imported into peroxisomes via the PTS1 translocation pathway. Increased degeneracy and context specificity of the mammalian PTS1 motif and implications for the peroxisome-to-mitochondrion mistargeting of AGT in primary hyperoxaluria type 1. *J Cell Biol* **131**:95, 1995.
86. Ferdinandusse S, Denis S, Clayton PT, Graham A, Rees JE, Allen JT, McLean BN, Brown AY, Vreken P, Waterham HR, Wanders RJ: Mutations in the gene encoding peroxisomal alpha-methylacyl-CoA racemase cause adult-onset sensory motor neuropathy. *Nat Genet* **24**:188, 2000.
87. Purdue PE, Lazarow PB: Targeting of human catalase to peroxisomes is dependent upon a novel COOH-terminal peroxisomal targeting sequence. *J Cell Biol* **134**:849, 1996.
88. Swinkels BW, Gould SJ, Bodnar AG, Rachubinski RA, Subramani S: A novel, cleavable peroxisomal targeting signal at the amino-terminus of the rat 3-ketoacyl-CoA thiolase. *EMBO J* **10**:3255, 1991.
89. Osumi T, Tsukamoto T, Hata S, Yokota S, Miura S, Fujiki Y, Hijikata M, Miyazawa S, Hashimoto T: Amino-terminal presequence of the precursor of peroxisomal 3-ketoacyl-CoA thiolase is a cleavable signal peptide for peroxisomal targeting. *Biochem Biophys Res Comm* **181**:947, 1991.
90. Jansen GA, Ofman R, Ferdinandusse S, Ijlst L, Muijsers AO, Skjekdal OH, Stokke O, Jakobs C, Besley GT, Wraith JE, Wanders RJ: Refsum disease is caused by mutations in the phytanoyl-CoA hydroxylase gene. *Nat Genet* **17**:190, 1997.
91. Mihalik SJ, Morrell JC, Kim D, Sacksteder K, Watkins PA, Gould SJ: Identification of *PAHX*, a Refsum-disease gene. *Nat Genet* **17**:185, 1997.
92. de Vet EC, van den Broek BT, van den Bosch H: Nucleotide sequence of human alkyl-dihydroxyacetonephosphate synthase cDNA reveals the presence of a peroxisomal targeting signal 2. *Biochim Biophys Acta* **1346**:25, 1997.
93. Erdmann R, Veenhuis D, Mertens D, Kunau WH: Isolation of peroxisome-deficient mutants of *Saccharomyces cerevisiae*. *Proc Natl Acad Sci U S A* **86**:5419, 1989.
94. Tsukamoto T, Yokota S, Fujiki Y: Isolation and characterization of Chinese hamster ovary cell mutants defective in assembly of peroxisomes. *J Cell Biol* **110**:651, 1990.
95. Gould SJ, McCollum D, Spong AP, Heyman JA, Subramani S: Development of the yeast *Pichia pastoris* as a model organism for a genetic and molecular analysis of peroxisome assembly. *Yeast* **8**:613, 1992.
96. Cregg JM, Vankiel IJ, Sulter GJ, Veenhuis M, Harder W: Peroxisome-deficient mutants of *Hansenula polymorpha*. *Yeast* **6**:87, 1990.
97. Nuttley WM, Brade AM, Gaillardin C, Eitzen GA, Glover JR, Aitchinson JD, Rachubinski RA: Rapid identification and characterization of peroxisomal assembly mutants in *Yarrowia lipolytica*. *Yeast* **9**:507, 1993.
98. Distel B, Erdmann R, Gould SJ, Blobel G, Crane DI, Cregg JM, Dodt G, Yujiki Y, Goodman JM, Just WW, Kiel JAKW, Kunau W-H, Lazarow PB, Mannaerts GP, Moser HW, Osumi T, Rachubinski RA, Roscher A, Subramani S, Tabak HF, Tsukamoto T, Valle D, van der Klei I, van Veldhoven PP, Veenhuis M: A unified nomenclature for peroxisome biogenesis factors. *J Cell Biol* **135**:1, 1996.
99. Kunau WH, Beyer A, Franken T, Gotte K, Marzioch M, Saidowsky J, Skaletz-Rorowski A, Wiebel FF: Two complementary approaches to study peroxisome biogenesis in *Saccharomyces cerevisiae*: Forward and reversed genetics. *Biochimie* **75**:209, 1993.
100. Dodt G, Braverman N, Valle D, Gould SJ: From expressed sequence tags to peroxisome biogenesis disorder genes. *Ann N Y Acad Sci* **804**:516, 1996.
101. Tsukamoto T, Miura S, Fujiki Y: Restoration by a 35K membrane protein of peroxisome assembly in a peroxisome-deficient mammalian cell mutant. *Nature* **350**:77, 1991.
102. Shimozawa N, Tsukamoto T, Suzuki Y, Orii T, Shirayoshi Y, Mori T, Fujiki Y: A human gene responsible for Zellweger syndrome that affects peroxisome assembly. *Science* **255**:1132, 1992.
103. McCollum D, Monosov E, Subramani S: The *pas*8 mutant of *Pichia pastoris* exhibits the peroxisomal protein import deficiencies of Zellweger syndrome cells. The PAS8 protein binds to the COOH-terminal tripeptide peroxisomal targeting signal and is a member of the TPR protein family. *J Cell Biol* **121**:761, 1993.
104. Dodt G, Braverman N, Wong C, Moser A, Moser HW, Watkins P, Valle D, Gould SJ: Mutations in the PTS1 receptor gene, PXR1, define

complementation group 2 of the peroxisome biogenesis disorders. *Nat Genet* **9**:115, 1995.

105. Van der Leij I, Franse MM, Elgersma Y, Distel B, Tabak HF: PAS10 is a tetratricopeptide-repeat protein that is essential for the import of most matrix proteins into peroxisomes of *Saccharomyces cerevisiae*. *Proc Natl Acad Sci U S A* **90**:11782, 1993.
106. van der Klei IJ, Hilbrands RE, Swaving GJ, Waterham HR, Vrieling EG, Titorenko VI, Cregg JM, Harder W, Veenhuis M: The *Hansenula polymorpha PER3* gene is essential for the import of PTS1 proteins into the peroxisomal matrix. *J Biol Chem* **270**:17229, 1995.
107. Szilard RK, Titorenko VI, Veenhuis M, Rachubinski RA: Pay32p of the yeast *Yarrowia lipolytica* is an intraperoxisomal component of the matrix protein translocation machinery. *J Cell Biol* **131**:1453, 1995.
108. Terlecky SR, Nuttley WM, McCollum D, Sock E, Subramani S: The *Pichia pastoris* peroxisomal protein PAS8p is the receptor for the C-terminal tripeptide peroxisomal targeting signal. *EMBO J* **14**:3627, 1995.
109. Gatto GJ Jr, Geisbrecht BV, Gould SJ, Berg JM: A proposed model for the PEX5-peroxisomal targeting signal-1 recognition complex. *Proteins* **38**:241, 2000.
110. Das AK, Cohen PW, Barford D: The structure of the tetratricopeptide repeats of protein phosphatase-5: Implications for protein-protein interactions. *EMBO J* **17**:1192, 1998.
111. Braverman N, Dodt G, Gould SJ, Valle D: An isoform of Pex5p, the human PTS1 receptor, is required for the import of PTS2 proteins into peroxisomes. *Hum Mol Genet* **7**:1195, 1998.
112. Elgersma Y, Kwast L, A K, Voorn-Brouwer T, van den Berg M, Metzig B, America T, Tabak HF, Distel B: The SH3 domain of the *Saccharomyces cerevisiae* peroxisomal membrane protein Pex13p functions as a docking site for Pex5p, a mobile receptor for the import of PTS1-containing proteins. *J Cell Biol* **135**:97, 1996.
113. Gould SJ, Kalish JE, Morrell JC, Bjorkman J, Urquhart AJ, Crane DI: Pex13p is an SH3 protein of the peroxisome membrane and a docking factor for the predominantly cytoplasmic PTS1 receptor. *J Cell Biol* **135**:85, 1996.
114. Dodt G, Gould SJ: Multiple PEX genes are required for proper subcellular distribution and stability of Pex5p, the PTS1 receptor: Evidence that PTS1 protein import is mediated by a cycling receptor. *J Cell Biol* **135**:1763, 1996.
115. Braverman N, Dodt G, Gould SJ, Valle D: Disorders of peroxisome biogenesis. *Hum Mol Genet* **4**:1791, 1995.
116. Erdmann R, Blobel G: Identification of Pex13p, a peroxisomal membrane receptor for the PTS1 recognition factor. *J Cell Biol* **135**:111, 1996.
117. Girzalsky W, Rehling P, Stein K, Kipper J, Blank L, Kunau WH, Erdmann R: Involvement of Pex13p in Pex14p localization and peroxisomal targeting signal 2-dependent protein import into peroxisomes. *J Cell Biol* **144**:1151, 1999.
118. Albertini M, Rehling P, Erdmann R, Girzalsky W, Kiel JAKW, Veenhuis M, Kunau W-H: Pex14p, a peroxisomal membrane protein binding both receptors of the two PTS-dependent import pathways. *Cell* **89**:83, 1997.
119. van der Klei IJ, Hibrands RE, Kiel JA, Rasmussen SW, Cregg JM, Veenhuis M: The ubiquitin-conjugating enzyme Pex4p of Hansenula polymorpha is required for efficient functioning of the PTS1 import machinery. *EMBO J* **17**:3608, 1998.
120. Collins CS, Kalish JE, Morrell JC, Gould SJ: The peroxisome biogenesis factors Pex4p, Pex22p, Pex1p, and Pex6p act in the terminal steps of peroxisomal matrix protein import. *Mol Cell Biol* (in press), 2000.
121. Marzioch M, Erdmann R, Veenhuis M, Kunau WH: PAS7 encodes a novel yeast member of the WD-40 protein family essential for import of 3-oxoacyl-CoA thiolase, a PTS2-containing protein, into peroxisomes. *EMBO J* **13**:4908, 1994.
122. van der Voorn L, Ploegh H: The WD-40 repeat. *FEBS Lett* **307**:131, 1992.
123. Rehling P, Marzioch M, Niesen F, Wittke E, Veenhuis M, Kunau WH: The import receptor for the peroxisomal targeting signal 2 (PTS2) in *Saccharomyces cerevisiae* is encoded by the *PAS7* gene. *EMBO J* **15**:2901, 1996.
124. Zhang JW, Lazarow PB: Peb1p (Pas7p) is an intraperoxisomal receptor for the NH_2-terminal, type 2, peroxisomal targeting sequence of thiolase: Peb1p itself is targeted to peroxisomes by an NH_2-terminal peptide. *J Cell Biol* **132**:325, 1996.
125. Zhang JW, Lazarow PB: *PEB1 (PAS7)* in *Saccharomyces cerevisiae* encodes a hydrophilic, intra-peroxisomal protein that is a member of the WD repeat family and is essential for the import of thiolase into peroxisomes. *J Cell Biol* **129**:65, 1995.
126. Elgersma Y, Elgersma-Hooisma M, Wenzel T, McCaffery JM, Farquhar MG, Subramani S: A mobile PTS2 receptor for peroxisomal protein import in *Pichia pastoris*. *J Cell Biol* **140**:807, 1998.
127. Heikoop JC, Van den Berg M, Strijland A, Weijers PJ, Schutgens RBH, Just WW, Wanders RJA, Tager JM: Peroxisomes of normal morphology but deficient in 3-oxoacyl-CoA thiolase in rhizomelic chondrodysplasia punctata fibroblasts. *Biochim Biophys Acta* **1097**:69, 1991.
128. Motley A, Hettema E, Distel B, Tabak H: Differential protein import deficiencies in human peroxisome assembly disorders. *J Cell Biol* **125**:755, 1994.
129. Braverman N, Steel G, Obie C, Moser A, Moser H, Gould SJ, Valle D: Human *PEX7* encodes the peroxisomal PTS2 receptor and is responsible for rhizomelic chondrodysplasia punctata. *Nat Genet* **15**:369, 1997.
130. Purdue PE, Zhang JW, Skoneczny M, Lazarow PB: Rhizomelic chondrodysplasia punctata is caused by deficiency of human PEX7, a homologue of the yeast PTS2 receptor. *Nat Genet* **15**:381, 1997.
131. Motley AM, Hettema EH, Hogenhout EM, Brites P, ten Asbroek ALMA, Wijburg FA, Baas F, Heijmans HS, Tabak HF, Wanders RJA, Distel B: Rhizomelic chondrodysplasia punctata is a peroxisomal protein targeting disease caused by a non-functional PTS2 receptor. *Nat Genet* **15**:377, 1997.
132. Braverman N, Steel G, Lin P, Moser A, Moser H, Valle D: *PEX7* gene structure, alternative transcripts, and evidence for a founder haplotype for the frequent RCDP allele, l292ter. *Genomics* **63**:181, 2000.
133. Purdue PE, Yang X, Lazarow PB: Pex18p and Pex21p, a novel pair of related peroxins essential for peroxisomal targeting by the PTS2 pathway. *J Cell Biol* **143**:1859, 1998.
134. Titorenko VI, Smith JJ, Szilard RK, Rachubinski RA: Pex20p of the yeast *Yarrowia lipolytica* is required for the oligomerization of thiolase in the cytosol and for its targeting to the peroxisome. *J Cell Biol* **142**:403, 1998.
135. Shimozawa N, Suzuki Y, Zhang Z, Imamura A, Toyama R, Mukai S, Fujiki Y, Tsukamoto T, Osumi T, Orii T, Wanders RJA, Kondo N: Nonsense and temperature-sensitive mutations in *PEX13* are the cause of complementation group H of peroxisome biogenesis disorders. *Hum Mol Genet* **8**:1077, 1999.
136. Liu Y, Björkman J, Urquhart A, Wanders RJA, Crane DI, Gould SJ: *PEX13* is mutated in complementation group 13 of peroxisome biogenesis disorders. *Am J Hum Genet* **65**:621, 1999.
137. Schliebs W, Saidowsky J, Agianian B, Dodt G, Herberg FW, Kunau W-H: Recombinant human peroxisomal targeting signal receptor PEX5. *J Biol Chem* **274**:5666, 1999.
138. Kalish JE, Theda C, Morrell JC, Berg JM, Gould SJ: Formation of the peroxisome lumen is abolished by loss of *Pichia pastoris* Pas7p, a zinc binding integral membrane protein of the peroxisome. *Mol Cell Biol* **15**:6406, 1995.
139. Kalish JE, Keller GA, Morrell JC, Mihalik SJ, Smith B, Cregg JM, Gould SJ: Characterization of a novel component of the peroxisomal protein import apparatus using fluorescent peroxisomal proteins. *EMBO J* **15**:3275, 1996.
140. Warren DS, Morrell JC, Moser HW, Valle D, Gould SJ: Identification of *PEX10*, the gene defective in complementation group 7 of the peroxisome biogenesis disorders. *Am J Hum Genet* **63**:347, 1998.
141. Chang C-C, Lee W-H, Moser H, Valle D, Gould SJ: Isolation of the human *PEX12* gene, mutated in group 3 of the peroxisome biogenesis disorders. *Nat Genet* **15**:385, 1997.
142. Chang C-C, Warren DS, Sacksteder KA, Gould SJ: *PEX12* interacts with *PEX5* and *PEX10* and acts downstream of receptor docking in peroxisomal matrix protein import. *J Cell Biol* **147**:761, 1999.
143. Borden KL: RING fingers and B-boxes: Zinc-binding protein-protein interaction domains. *Biochem Cell Biol* **76**:351, 1998.
144. Borden KL: RING domains: Master builders of molecular scaffolds? *J Mol Biol* **295**:1103, 2000.
145. Borden KL, Freemont PS: The RING finger domain: A recent example of a sequence-structure family. *Curr Opin Struct Biol* **6**:395, 1996.
146. Shimozawa N, Zhang Z, Imamura A, Suzuki Y, Fujiki Y, Tsukamoto T, Osumi T, Aubourg P, Wanders RJ, Kondo N: Molecular mechanism of detectable catalase-containing particles, peroxisomes, in fibroblasts from a *PEX2*-defective patient. *Biochem Biophys Res Commun* **268**:31, 2000.
147. Shimozawa N, Imamura A, Zhang Z, Suzuki Y, Orii T, Tsukamoto T, Osumi T, Fujiki Y, Wanders RJ, Besley G, Kondo N: Defective PEX gene products correlate with the protein import, biochemical

abnormalities, and phenotypic heterogeneity in peroxisome biogenesis disorders. *J Med Genet* **36**:779, 1999.

148. Rehling P, Skaletz-Rorowski A, Girzalsky W, Voorn-Brouwer T, Franse MM, Distel B, Veenhuis M, Kunau WH, Erdmann R: Pex8p, an intraperoxisomal peroxin of *Saccharomyces cerevisiae* required for protein transport into peroxisomes binds the PTS1 receptor pex5p. *J Biol Chem* **275**:3593, 2000.
149. Waterham HR, Titorenko VI, Haima P, Cregg JM, Harder W, Veenhuis M: The *Hansenula polymorpha PER1* gene is essential for peroxisomal matrix protein with both carboxy-and amino-terminal targeting signals. *J Cell Biol* **127**:737, 1994.
150. Liu H, Tan X, Russell KA, Veenhuis M, Cregg JM: *PER3*, a gene required for peroxisome biogenesis in *Pichia pastoris*, encodes a peroxisomal membrane protein involved in protein import. *J Biol Chem* **270**:10940, 1995.
151. Wiebel FF, Kunau W-H: The Pas2 protein essential for peroxisome biogenesis is related to ubiquitin-conjugating enzymes. *Nature* **359**:73, 1992.
152. Crane DI, Kalish JE, Gould SJ: The *Pichia pastoris* PAS4 gene encodes an ubiquitin-conjugating enzyme required for peroxisome assembly. *J Biol Chem* **269**:21835, 1994.
153. Koller A, Snyder WB, Faber KN, Wenzel TJ, Rangell L, Keller GA, Subramani S: Pex22p of Pichia pastoris, essential for peroxisomal matrix protein import, anchors the ubiquitin-conjugating enzyme, Pex4p, on the peroxisomal membrane. *J Cell Biol* **146**:99, 1999.
154. Yahraus T, Braverman N, Dodt G, Kalish JE, Morrell JC, Moser HW, Valle D, Gould SJ: The peroxisome biogenesis disorder group 4 gene, *PXAAA1*, encodes a cytoplasmic ATPase required for stability of the PTS1 receptor. *EMBO J* **15**:2914, 1996.
155. Reuber BE, Collins CS, Germain-Lee E, Morrell JC, Ameritunga R, Moser HW, Valle D, Gould SJ: Mutations in *PEX1* are the most common cause of Zellweger syndrome, neonatal adrenoleukodystrophy and infantile Refsum disease. *Nat Genet* **17**:445, 1997.
156. Geisbrecht BV, Collins CS, Reuber BE, Gould SJ: Disruption of a *PEX1-PEX6* interaction is the most common cause of the neurologic disorders Zellweger syndrome, neonatal adrenoleukodystrophy, and infantile Refsum disease. *Proc Natl Acad Sci U S A* **95**:8630, 1998.
157. Faber KN, Heyman JA, Subramani S: Two AAA family peroxins, PpPex1p and PpPex6p, interact with each other in an ATP-dependent manner and are associated with different subcellular membranous structures distinct from peroxisomes. *Mol Cell Biol* **18**:936, 1998.
158. Tamura S, Shimozawa N, Suzuki Y, Tsukamoto T, Osumi T, Fujiki Y: A cytoplasmic AAA family peroxin, Pex1p, interacts with Pex6p. *Biochem Biophys Res Commun* **245**:883, 1998.
159. Erdmann R, Wiebel FF, Flessau A, Rytka J, Beyer A, Frohlich KU, Kunau WH: PAS1, a yeast gene required for peroxisome biogenesis, encodes a member of a novel family of putative ATPases. *Cell* **64**:499, 1991.
160. Titorenko VI, Chan H, Rachubinski RA: Fusion of small peroxisomal vesicles *in vitro* reconstructs an early step in the in vivo multistep peroxisome assembly pathway of *Yarrowia lipolytica*. *J Cell Biol* **148**:29, 2000.
161. Titorenko VI, Ogrydziak DM, Rachubinski RA: Four distinct secretory pathways serve protein secretion, cell surface growth and peroxisome biogenesis in the yeast *Yarrowia lipolytica*. *Mol Cell Biol* **17**:5210, 1997.
162. Spong AP, Subramani S: Cloning and characterization of *PAS5*:A gene required for peroxisome biogenesis in the methylotrophic yeast *Pichia pastoris*. *J Cell Biol* **123**:535, 1993.
163. Heyman JA, Mononsov E, Subramani S: Role of the *PAS1* gene of *Pichia pastoris* in peroxisome biogenesis. *J Cell Biol* **127**:1259, 1994.
164. Kiel JA, Hilbrands RE, van der Klei IJ, Rasmussen SW, Salomons FA, van der Heide M, Faber KN, Cregg JM, Veenhuis M: Hansenula polymorpha Pex1p and Pex6p are peroxisome-associated AAA proteins that functionally and physically interact. *Yeast* **15**:1059, 1999.
165. Eitzen GA, Aitchison JD, Szilard RK, Veenhuis M, Nuttley MW, Rachubinski RA: The *Yarrowia lipolytica* gene *PAY2* encodes a 42-kDa peroxisomal integral membrane protein essential for matrix protein import and peroxisome enlargement but not for peroxisome membrane proliferation. *J Biol Chem* **270**:1429, 1995.
166. Elgersma Y, Kwast L, van den Berg M, Snyder WB, Distel B, Subramani S, Tabak HF: Overexpression of Pex15p, a phosphorylated peroxisomal integral membrane protein required for peroxisome assembly in *S. cerevisiae*, causes proliferation of the endoplasmic reticulum membrane. *EMBO J* **16**:7326, 1997.
167. Huhse B, Rehling P, Albertini M, Blank L, Meller K, Kunau W-H: Pex17p of *Saccharomyces cerevisiae* is a novel peroxin and component of the peroxisomal protein translocation machinery. *J Cell Biol* **140**:49, 1998.
168. Brown TW, Titorenko VI, Rachubinski RA: Mutants of the *Yarrowia lipolytica PEX23* gene encoding an integral peroxisomal membrane peroxin mislocalize matrix proteins and accumulate vesicles containing peroxisomal matrix and membrane proteins. *Mol Biol Cell* **11**:141, 2000.
169. Snyder WB, Koller A, Choy AJ, Johnson MA, Cregg JM, Rangell L, Keller GA, Subramani S: Pex17p is required for import of both peroxisome membrane and luminal proteins and interacts with Pex19p and the peroxisome targeting signal-receptor docking complex in *Pichia pastoris*. *Mol Biol Cell* **10**:4005, 1999.
170. Fujiki Y, Rachubinski RA, Lazarow PB: Synthesis of a major integral membrane polypeptide of rat liver peroxisomes on free polysomes. *Proc Natl Acad Sci U S A* **81**:7127, 1984.
171. Imanaka T, Shiina Y, Takano T, Hashimoto T, Osumi T: Insertion of the 70-kDa peroxisomal membrane protein into peroxisomal membranes in vivo and *in vitro*. *J Biol Chem* **271**:3706, 1996.
172. Honsho M, Tamura S, Shimozawa N, Suzuki Y, Kondo N, Fujiki Y: Mutation in PEX16 is causal in the peroxisome-deficient Zellweger syndrome of complementation group D. *Am J Hum Genet* **63**:1622, 1998.
173. Subramani S: Protein import into peroxisomes and biogenesis of the organelle. *Annu Rev Cell Biol* **9**:445, 1993.
174. Dyer JM, McNew JA, Goodman JM: The sorting sequence of the peroxisomal integral membrane protein PMP47 is contained within a short hydrophilic loop. *J Cell Biol* **133**:269, 1996.
175. McCammon MT, McNew JA, Willy PJ, Goodman JM: An internal region of the peroxisomal membrane protein PMP47 is essential for sorting to peroxisomes. *J Cell Biol* **124**:915, 1994.
176. Pause B, Diestelkotter P, Heid H, Just WW: Cytosolic factors mediate protein insertion into the peroxisomal membrane. *FEBS Lett* **414**:95, 1997.
177. Diestelkotter P, Just WW: In vitro insertion of the 22-kD peroxisomal membrane protein into isolated rat liver peroxisomes. *J Cell Biol* **123**:1717, 1993.
178. Miura S, Kasuya-Arai I, Mori H, Miyazawa S, Osumi T, Hashimoto T, Fujiki Y: Carboxyl-terminal consensus ser-lys-leu-related tripeptide of peroxisomal proteins *in vitro* as a minimal peroxisome-targeting signal. *J Biol Chem* **267**:14405, 1992.
179. Soto U, Pepperkok R, Ansorge W, Just WW: Import of firefly luciferase into mammalian peroxisomes in vivo requires nucleotide triphosphates. *Exp Cell Res* **205**:66, 1993.
180. Miura S, Miyazawa S, Osumi T, Hashimoto T, Fujiki Y: Post-translational import of 3-ketoacyl-CoA thiolase into rat liver peroxisomes *in vitro*. *J Biochem (Tokyo)* **115**:1064, 1994.
181. Fujiki Y, Lazarow PB: Post-translational import of fatty acyl-CoA oxidase and catalase into peroxisomes of rat liver *in vitro*. *J Biol Chem* **260**:5603, 1985.
182. Wendland M, Subramani S: Cytosol-dependent peroxisomal protein import in a permeabilized cell system. *J Cell Biol* **120**:675, 1993.
183. Somerharju P, Virtanen JA, Cheng KH: Lateral organisation of membrane lipids. The superlattice view. *Biochim Biophys Acta* **1440**:32, 1999.
184. Sackmann E, Tanaka M: Supported membranes on soft polymer cushions: Fabrication, characterization and applications. *Trends Biotechnol* **18**:58, 2000.
185. Santos M, Leighton F, Seno S, Okada Y: Subcellular distribution of peroxisomal enzymes in Zellweger syndrome: Activity and subcellular localization in liver. *Intern Cell Biol* **284**, 1984.
186. Santos MJ, Ojeda JM, Garrido J, Leighton F: Peroxisomal organization in normal and cerebrohepatorenal (Zellweger) syndrome fibroblasts. *Proc Natl Acad Sci U S A* **82**:6556, 1985.
187. James GL, Goldstein JL, Pathak RK, W ARG, Brown MS: PxF, a prenylated protein of peroxisomes. *J Biol Chem* **269**:14182, 1994.
188. Gotte K, Girzalsky W, Linkert M, Baumgart E, Kammerer S, Kunau WH, Erdmann R: Pex19p, a farnesylated protein essential for peroxisome biogenesis. *Mol Cell Biol* **18**:616, 1998.
189. Snyder WB, Faber KN, Wenzel TJ, Koller A, Luers GH, Rangell L, Keller GA, Subramani S: Pex19p interacts with pex3p and pex10p and is essential for peroxisome biogenesis in *Pichia pastoris*. *Mol Biol Cell* **10**:1745, 1999.
190. Soukupova M, Sprenger C, Gorgas K, Kunau WH, Dodt G: Identification and characterization of the human peroxin *PEX3*. *Eur J Cell Biol* **78**:357, 1999.

191. Höhfeld J, Veenhuis M, Kunau WH: PAS3, a *Saccharomyces cerevisiae* gene encoding a peroxisomal integral membrane protein essential for peroxisome biogenesis. *J Cell Biol* **114**:1167, 1991.
192. Marshall PA, Krimkevich YI, Lark RH, Dyer JM, Veenhuis M, Goodman JM: Pmp27 promotes peroxisomal proliferation. *J Cell Biol* **129**:345, 1995.
193. Erdmann R, Blobel G: Giant peroxisomes in oleic acid-induced *Saccharomyces cerevisiae* lacking the peroxisomal membrane protein Pmp27p. *J Cell Biol* **128**:509, 1995.
194. Passreiter M, Anton M, Lay D, Frank R, Harter C, Wieland FT, Gorgas K, Just WW: Peroxisome biogenesis: Involvement of ARF and coatomer. *J Cell Biol* **141**:373, 1998.
195. Wahli W, Devchand PR, A IJ, Desvergne B: Fatty acids, eicosanoids, and hypolipidemic agents regulate gene expression through direct binding to peroxisome proliferator-activated receptors. *Adv Exp Med Biol* **447**:199, 1999.
196. Reddy JK, Chu R: Peroxisome proliferator-induced pleiotropic response: Pursuit of a phenomenon. *Ann NY Acad Sci* **804**:176, 1996.
197. Wilson GN, Holmes RG, Custer J, Lipkowitz JL, Stover J, Datta N, Hajra A: Zellweger syndrome: Diagnostic assays, syndrome delineation and potential therapy. *Am J Med Genet* **24**:69, 1986.
198. Zellweger H: The cerebro-hepato-renal (Zellweger) syndrome and other peroxisomal disorders. *Dev Med Child Neurol* **29**:821, 1987.
199. Kelley RI, Datta NS, Dobyns WB, Hajra AK, Moser AB, Noetzel MJ, Zackai EH, Moser HW: Neonatal adrenoleukodystrophy: New cases, biochemical studies and differentiation from Zellweger and related peroxisomal polydystrophy syndromes. *Am J Med Genet* **23**:869, 1986.
200. Gatfield PD, Taller E, Hinton GG, Wallace AC, Abdelnour GM, Haust MD: Hyperpipecolatemia: A new metabolic disorder associated with neuropathy and hepatomegaly: A case study. *Can Med Assoc J* **99**:1215, 1968.
201. Burton BK, Reed SP, Remy WT: Hyperpipecolic acidemia: Clinical and biochemical observations in two male siblings. *J Pediatr* **99**:729, 1981.
202. Thomas GH, Haslam RH, Batshaw ML, Capute AJ, Neidengard L, Ransom JL: Hyperpipecolic acidemia associated with hepatomegaly, mental retardation, optic nerve dysplasia and progressive neurological disease. *Clin Genet* **8**:376, 1975.
203. Schutgens RB, Heymans HS, Wanders RJ, van den Bosch H, Tager JM: Peroxisomal disorders: A newly recognized group of genetic diseases. *Eur J Pediatr* **144**:430, 1986.
204. Wanders RJ, Schutgens RB, Barth PG: Peroxisomal disorders: A review. *J Neuropathol Exp Neurol* **54**:726, 1995.
205. Kelley RI: The cerebrohepatorenal syndrome of Zellweger, morphologic and metabolic aspects. *Am J Med Genet* **16**:503, 1983.
206. Govaerts L, Monnens L, Tegelaers W, Trijbels F, van Raay-Selten A: Cerebro-hepato-renal syndrome of Zellweger: Clinical symptoms and relevant laboratory findings in 16 patients. *Eur J Pediatr* **139**:125, 1982.
207. Chen WW, Watkins PA, Osumi T, Hashimoto T, Moser HW: Peroxisomal beta-oxidation enzyme proteins in adrenoleukodystrophy: Distinction between X-linked adrenoleukodystrophy and neonatal adrenoleukodystrophy. *Proc Natl Acad Sci U S A* **84**:1425, 1987.
208. Mosser J, Lutz Y, Stoeckel ME, Sarde CO, Kretz C, Douar AM, Lopez J, Aubourg P, Mandel JL: The gene responsible for adrenoleukodystrophy encodes a peroxisomal membrane protein. *Hum Mol Genetics* **3**:265, 1994.
209. Kelley RI, Moser HW: Hyperpipecolic acidemia in neonatal adrenoleukodystrophy. *Am J Med Genet* **19**:791, 1984.
210. Manzke HJ, Schuelein M, McCullough DC, Kishimoto Y, Eiben RM: New phenotypic variant of adrenoleukodystrophy. Pathologic, ultrastructural and biochemical study in two brothers. *J Neurol Sci* **45**:245, 1980.
211. Poulos A, Sharp P, Fellenberg AJ, Danks DM: Cerebro-hepato-renal (Zellweger) syndrome, adrenoleukodystrophy and Refsum disease: Plasma changes and skin fibroblast phytanic acid oxidase. *Hum Genet* **70**:172, 1985.
212. Noetzel MJ, Clark HB, Moser HW: Neonatal adrenoleukodystrophy with prolonged survival. *Ann Neurol* **14**:380, 1983.
213. Goldfischer S, Collins J, Rapin I, Coltoff-Schiller B, Chang CH, Nigro M, Black VH, Javitt NB, Moser HW, Lazarow PB: Peroxisomal defects in neonatal onset and X-linked adrenoleukodystrophies. *Science* **227**:67, 1985.
214. Singh I, Moser AE, Goldfischer S, Moser HW: Lignoceric acid is oxidized in the peroxisome: implications for the Zellweger cerebro-hepato-renal syndrome and adrenoleukodystrophy. *Proc Natl Acad Sci U S A* **81**:4203, 1984.
215. Wolff J, Nyhan WL, Powell H, Takahashi D, Hutzler J, Hajra AK, Datta NS, Singh I, Moser HW: Myopathy in an infant with a fatal peroxisomal disorder. *Pediatr Neurol* **2**:141, 1986.
216. Brown RF, McAdams AJ, Cummins JW, Konkol R, Singh I, Moser AB, Moser HW: Cerebro-hepato-renal (Zellweger) syndrome and neonatal adrenoleukodystrophy: Similarities in phenotype and accumulation of very long chain fatty acids. *Johns Hopkins Med J* **151**:344, 1982.
217. Kahlke W, Goerlich R, Feist D: Increased concentration of phytanic acid in plasma and liver of an infant with cerebral damage of unknown etiology. *Klin Wochenschr* **52**:651, 1974.
218. Poulos A, Sharp P, Whiting M: Infantile Refsum's disease (phytanic acid storage disease): A variant of Zellweger syndrome? *Clin Genet* **26**:579, 1984.
219. Poulos A, Whiting MJ: Identification of 3-alpha, 7-alpha, 12-alpha, 12-alpha-trihydroxy-5-beta cholestan-26-oic acid, an intermediate in cholic acid synthesis, in the plasma of patients with infantile Refsum disease. *J Inherit Metab Dis* **8**:13, 1985.
220. Poll-The BT, Saudubray JM, Ogier H, Schutgens RBH, Wanders RJA, Schrakamp G, Van den Bosch H, Trijbels JMF, Poulos A, Moser HW, van Eldere J, Eyssen HJ: Infantile Refsum's disease: Biochemical findings suggesting multiple peroxisomal dysfunction. *J Inherit Metab Dis* **9**:169, 1986.
221. Torvik A, Torp S, Kase BE, Ek J, Skjeldal O, Stokke O: Infantile Refsum's disease: A generalized peroxisomal disorder. Case report with postmortem examination. *J Neurol Sci* **85**:39, 1988.
222. Budden SS, Kennaway NG, Buist NR, Poulos A, Weleber RG: Dysmorphic syndrome with phytanic acid oxidase deficiency, abnormal very long chain fatty acids and pipecolic acidemia: Studies in four children. *J Pediatr* **108**:33, 1986.
223. Weleber RG, Tongue AC, Kennaway NG, Budden SS, Buist NR: Ophthalmic manifestations of infantile phytanic acid storage disease. *Arch Ophthalmol* **102**:1317, 1984.
224. Barth PG, Schutgens RB, Wanders RJ, Heymans HS, Moser AE, Moser HW, Bleeker-Wagemakers EM, Jansonius-Schultheiss K, Derix M, Nelck GF: A sibship with a mild variant of Zellweger syndrome. *J Inherit Metab Dis* **10**:253, 1987.
225. Bleeker-Wagemakers EM, Oorthuys JW, Wanders RJ, Schutgens RB: Long term survival of a patient with the cerebro-hepato-renal (Zellweger) syndrome. *Clin Genet* **29**:160, 1986.
226. Ek J, Kase BF, Reith A, Bjorkhern I, Pedersen JI: Peroxisomal dysfunction in a boy with neurologic symptoms and amaurosis (Leber disease): Clinical and biochemical findings similar to those observed in Zellweger syndrome. *J Pediatr* **108**:19, 1986.
227. Baumgartner MR, Poll-The BT, Verhoeven NM, Jakobs C, Espeel M, Roels F, Rabier D, Levade T, Rolland MO, Martinez M: Clinical approach to inherited peroxisomal disorders: A series of 27 patients. *Ann Neurol* **44**:720, 1998.
228. Baumgartner MR, Verhoeven NM, Jakobs C, Roels F, Espeel M, Martinez M, Rabier D, Wanders RJ, Saudubray JM: Defective peroxisome biogenesis with a neuromuscular disorder resembling Werdnig-Hoffman disease. *Neurology* **51**:1427, 1998.
229. MacCollin M, Moser AB, Beard M: Ataxia and peripheral neuropathy: A benign variant of peroxisome dysgenesis. *Ann Neurol* **28**:833, 1990.
230. Govaerts L, Colon E, Rotteveel J, Monnens L: A neurophysiological study of children with the cerebro-hepato-renal syndrome of Zellweger. *Neuropediatrics* **16**:185, 1985.
231. Takahashi Y, Suzuki Y, Kumazaki K, Tanabe Y, Akaboshi S, Miura K, Shimozawa N, Kondo N, Nishiguchi T, Terada K: Epilepsy in peroxisomal diseases. *Epilepsia* **38**:182, 1997.
232. Hittner HM, Kretzer FL, Mehta RS: Zellweger syndrome. Lenticular opacities indicating carrier status and lens abnormalities characteristic of homozygotes. *Arch Ophthalmol* **99**:1977, 1981.
233. Barkovich AJ, Peck WW: MR of Zellweger syndrome. *Am J Neuroradiol* **18**:1163, 1997.
234. Nakai A, Shigematsu Y, Nishida K, Kikawa Y, Konishi Y: MRI findings of Zellweger syndrome. *Pediatr Neurol* **13**:1995.
235. van der Knaap MS, Valk J: The MR spectrum of peroxisomal disorders. *Neuroradiology* **33**:30, 1991.
236. Takashima S, Chan F, Becker LE, Houdou S, Suzuki Y: Cortical cytoarchitectural and immunohistochemical studies on Zellweger syndrome. *Brain Dev* **13**:158, 1991.
237. Arias JA, Moser AB, Goldfischer SL: Ultrastructural and cytochemical demonstration of peroxisomes in cultured fibroblasts from patients with peroxisomal deficiency disorders. *J Cell Biol* **100**:1789, 1985.
238. Versmold HT, Bremer HJ, Herzog V, Siegel G, Bassewitz DB, Irle U, Voss H, Lombeck I, Brauser B: A metabolic disorder similar to

Zellweger syndrome with hepatic acatalasia and absence of peroxisomes, altered content and redox state of cytochromes and infantile cirrhosis with hemosiderosis. *Eur J Pediatr* **124**:261, 1977.

239. Mooi WJ, Dingemans KP, van den Bergh MA, Jobsis AC, Heymans HS, Barth PG: Ultrastructure of the liver in the cerebrohepatorenal syndrome of Zellweger. *Ultrastruct Pathol* **5**:135, 1983.
240. Lazarow PB, Black V, Shio H, Fujiki Y, Hajra A, Datta N, Bangaru BS, Dancis J: Zellweger syndrome: Biochemical and morphological studies on two patients treated with clofibrate. *Pediatr Res* **19**:1356, 1985.
241. Santos MJ, Hoefler S, Moser AB, Moser HW, Lazarow PB: Peroxisome assembly mutations in humans: Structural heterogeneity in Zellweger syndrome. *J Cell Physiol* **151**:103, 1992.
242. Aikawa J, Chen WW, Kelley RI, Tada K, Moser HW, Chen GL: Low-density particles (W-particles) containing catalase in Zellweger syndrome and normal fibroblasts. *Proc Natl Acad Sci U S A* **88**:10084, 1991.
243. van Roermund CWT, Brul S, Tager JM, Schutgens RBH, Wanders RJA: Acyl-CoA oxidase, peroxisomal thiolase and dihydroxyacetone phosphate acyltransferase: Aberrant subcellular localization in Zellweger syndrome. *J Inherit Metab Dis* **14**:152, 1991.
244. Slawecki M, Dodt G, Steinberg S, Moser AB, Moser HW, Gould SJ: Identification of three distinct peroxisomal protein import defects in patients with peroxisome biogenesis disorders. *J Cell Sci* **108**:1817, 1995.
245. Powers JM, Moser HW: Peroxisomal disorders: Genotype, phenotype, major neuropathologic lesions and pathogenesis. *Brain Pathol* **8**:101, 1998.
246. Volpe JJ, Adams RD: Cerebro-hepato-renal syndrome of Zellweger: An inherited disorder of neuronal migration. *Acta Neuropathol (Berl)* **20**:175, 1972.
247. Evrard P, Caviness VSJ, Prats-Vinas J, Lyon G: The mechanism of arrest of neuronal migration in the Zellweger malformation: A hypothesis bases upon cytoarchitectonic analysis. *Acta Neuropathol (Berl)* **41**:109, 1978.
248. Powers JM, Moser HW, Moser A, Upshur JK, Bradford BF, Pai SG, Kohn PH, Frias J, Tiffany C: Fetal cerebrohepatorenal (Zellweger) syndrome: Dysmorphic, radiologic, biochemical and pathologic findings in four affected fetuses. *Hum Pathol* **16**:610, 1985.
249. Agamanolis DP, Robinson HBJ, Timmons GD: Cerebro-hepato-renal syndrome. Report of a case with histochemical and ultrastructural observations. *J Neuropathol Exp Neurol* **35**:226, 1976.
250. de Leon G, Grover WD, Huff DS, Morinigo-Mestre G, Punnett HH, Kistenmacher ML: Globoid cells, glial nodules, and peculiar fibrillary changes in the cerebro-hepato-renal syndrome of Zellweger. *Ann Neurol* **2**:473, 1977.
251. Powers JM, Tummons RC, Moser AB, Moser HW, Huff DS, Kelley RI: Neuronal lipidosis and neuroaxonal dystrophy in cerebro-hepato-renal (Zellweger) syndrome: Dysmorphic, radiologic, biochemical and pathologic findings in four affected fetuses. *Hum Pathol* **16**:610, 1987.
252. Norton WT: Myelin, in Morrell P (ed): *Isolation and Characterization of Myelin*. New York, Plenum, 1977, p 161.
253. Haas JE, Johnson ES, Farrell DL: Neonatal onset adrenoleukodystrophy in a girl. *Ann Neurol* **12**:449, 1982.
254. Cohen SM, Green WR, de la Cruz ZC, Brown FR, Moser HW, Luckenback WM, Dove DJ, Maumenee IH: Ocular histopathologic and biochemical studies of neonatal and childhood adrenoleukodystrophy. *Am J Ophthalmol* **95**:82, 1983.
255. Igarashi M, Neely JG, Anthony PF, Alford BR: Cochlear nerve degeneration coincident with adrenocerebrokeukodystrophy. *Arch Otolaryngol* **102**:722, 1976.
256. Vitale L, Opitz JM, Shahidi NT: Congenital and familial iron overload. *N Engl J Med* **280**:642, 1969.
257. Gilchrist KW, Gilbert EF, Goldfarb S, Goll U, Spranger JW, Opitz JM: Studies of malformation syndromes of man XIB: The cerebro-hepato-renal syndrome of Zellweger: Comparative pathology. *Eur J Pediatr* **121**:99, 1976.
258. Bernstein J, Brough AJ, McAdams AJ: The renal lesion in syndromes of multiple congenital malformations. Cerebrohepatorenal syndrome, Jeune asphyxiating thoracic dystrophy, tuberous sclerosis, Meckel syndrome. *Birth Defects Orig Art Ser* **10**:35, 1974.
259. Goldfischer S, Powers JM, Johnson AB, Axe S, Brown FR, Moser HW: Striated adrenocortical cells in cerebro-hepato-renal (Zellweger) syndrome. *Virchows Arch* **401**:355, 1983.
260. Schaumburg HH, Powers JM, Raine CS, Suzuki K, Richardson EP Jr: Adrenoleukodystrophy. A clinical and pathological study of 17 cases. *Arch Neurol* **32**:577, 1975.
261. Govaerts L, Monnens L, Melis T, Trijbels F: Disturbed adrenocortical function in cerebro-hepato-renal syndrome of Zellweger. *Eur J Pediatr* **143**:10, 1984.
262. Poznanski AK, Nosanchuk JS, Baublis J, Holt JF: The cerebro-hepato-renal syndrome (CHRS)(Zellweger's syndrome). *AJR Am J Roentgenol* **109**:313, 1970.
263. Williams JP, Secrist L, Fowler GW, Gwinn JL, Dumars KC: Roentgenographic features of the cerebrohepatorenal syndrome of Zellweger. *AJR Am J Roentgenol* **115**:607, 1972.
264. Graham CB: Assessment of bone maturation — methods and pitfalls. *Radiol Clin North Am* **10**:185, 1972.
265. Hong R, Horowitz SD, Borzy MF, Gilbert EF, Arya S, McLeod N, Peterson RD: The cerebro-hepato-renal syndrome of Zellweger: Similarity to and differentiation from the DiGeorge sydrome. *Thymus* **3**:97, 1981.
266. Bakkeren J, Carpay I, Weemaes C, Monnens L: Cellular immunity in cerebrohepatorenal syndrome of Zellweger. *Lancet*: **1029**, 1976.
267. Jaffe R, Crumrine P, Hashida Y, Moser HW: Neonatal adrenoleukodystrophy: Clinical, pathologic and biochemical delineation of a syndrome affecting both males and females. *Am J Pathol* **108**:100, 1982.
268. Patton RG, Christie DL, Smith DW, Beckwith JB: Two patients with islet cell hyperplasia, hypoglycemia and thymic anomalies and comments on iron metabolism. *Am J Dis Child* **124**:840, 1972.
269. Oorthuys JW, Loewer-Sieger DH, Schutgens RB, Wanders RJ, Heymans HS, Bleeker-Wagemakers EM: Peroxisomal dysfunction in chondrodysplasia punctata, rhizomelic type. *Ophthalmic Pediatr Genet* **8**:183, 1987.
270. Heymans HSA, Wanders RJA: Rhizomelic chondrodysplasia punctata, in Moser HW (ed): *Handbook of Clinical Neurology*. New York, Elsevier Science, 1996, p 525.
271. Poll-The BT, Maroteaux P, Narcy C, Quetin P, Guesnu M, Wanders RA, Schutgens RBH, Saudubray JM: A new type of chondrodysplasia punctata associated with peroxisomal dysfunction. *J Inherit Metab Dis* **14**:361, 1991.
272. Pike MG, Applegarth DA, Dunn HG, Bamforth SJ, Tingle AJ, Wood BJ, Dimmick JE, Harris H, Chantler JK, Hall JG: Congenital rubella syndrome associated with calcific epiphyseal stippling and peroxisomal dysfunction. *J Pediatr* **116**:88, 1990.
273. Gray RGF, Green A, Chapman S, McKeown C, Schutgens RBH, Wanders RJA: Rhizomelic chondrodysplasia punctata–A new clinical variant. *J Inherit Metab Dis* **15**:931, 1992.
274. Wanders RJA, Schumacher H, Heikoop J, Schutgens RBH, Tager JM: Human dihydroxyacetonephosphate acyltransferase deficiency: A new peroxisomal disorder. *J Inherit Metab Dis* **15**:389, 1992.
275. Spranger JW, Opitz JM, Bidder U: Heterogeneity of chondrodysplasia punctata. *Hum Genet* **11**:190, 1971.
276. Happle R: X-linked dominant chondrodysplasia punctata. Review of literature and report of a case. *Hum Genet* **53**:65, 1979.
277. Curry CJ, magenis RE, Brown M, Lanman JTJ, Tsai J, O'Lague P, Goodfellow P, Mohandas T, Bergner EA, Shapiro LJ: Inherited chondrodysplasia punctata due to a deletion of the terminal short arm of an X chromosome. *N Engl J Med* **311**:1010, 1984.
278. Braverman N, Lin P, Moebius FF, Obie C, Moser A, Glossmann H, Wilcox WR, Rimoin DL, Smith M, Kratz L, Kelley RI, Valle D: Mutations in the gene encoding 3β-hydroxysteroid-Δ^8, Δ^7-isomerase cause X-linked dominant Conradi-Hünermann syndrome. *Nat Genet* **22**:291, 1999.
279. Derry JMJ, Gormally E, Means GD, Zhao GD, Meindl A, Kelley RI, Boyd Y, Herman GE: Mutations in a Δ^8-Δ^7 sterol isomerase in the tattered mouse and X-linked dominant chondrodysplasia punctata. *Nat Genet* **22**:286, 1999.
280. Gray RG, Green A, Schutgens RB, Wanders RJ, Farndon P, Kennedy CR: Antenatal diagnosis of rhizomelic chondrodysplasia punctata in the second trimester. *J Inherit Metab Dis* **13**:380, 1990.
281. Duff P, Harlass FE, Mililgan DA: Prenatal diagnosis of chondrodysplasia punctata by sonography. *Obstet Gynecol* **76**:497, 1990.
282. Hertzberg BS, Kliewer MA, Decker M, Miller CR, Bowie JD: Antenatal ultrasonographic diagnosis of rhizomelic chondrodysplasia punctata. *J Ultrasound Med* **18**:715, 1999.
283. Gilbert EF, Opitz JM, Spranger JW, Langer LOJ, Wolfson JJ, Viseskul C: Chondrodysplasia punctata — rhizomelic form. Pathologic and radiologic studies of three infants. *Eur J Pediatr* **123**:89, 1976.
284. Powers JM, Kenjarski TP, Moser AB, Moser HW: Cerebellar atrophy in chronic rhizomelic chondrodysplasia punctata: A potential role for phytanic acid and calcium in the death of its Purkinje cells. *Acta Neuropathol (Berl)* **98**:129, 1999.

285. Agamanolis DP, Novak RW: Rhizomelic chondrodysplasia punctata: Report of a case with review of the literature and correlation with other peroxisomal disorders. *Pediatr Pathol Lab Med* **15**:503, 1995.
286. Poulos A, Sheffield L, Sharp P, Sherwood G, Johnson D, Beckman K, Fellenberg AJ, Wraith JE, Chow CW, Usher S: Rhizomelic chondrodysplasia punctata: Clinical, pathologic and biochemical findings in two patients. *J Pediatr* **113**:685, 1988.
287. Wardinsky TD, Pagon RA, Powell BR, McGillivray B, Stephan M, Zonana J, Moser A: Rhizomelic chondrodysplasia punctata and survival beyond one year: A review of the literature and five case reports. *Clin Genet* **38**:84, 1990.
288. Theil AC, Schutgens RB, Wanders RJ, Heymanns HS: Clinical recognition of patients affected by a peroxisomal disorder: A retrospective study in 40 patients. *Eur J Pediatr* **151**:117, 1992.
289. Moser HW, Raymond GV: Genetic peroxisomal disorders: Why, when and how to test. *Ann Neurol* **44**:713, 1998.
290. Schutgens RB, Schrakamp G, Wanders RJ, Heymans HS, Tager JM, van den Bosch H: Prenatal and perinatal diagnosis of peroxisomal disorders. *J Inherit Metab Dis* **12**:118, 1989.
291. Moser AE, Singh I, Brown FRd, Solish GI, Kelley RI, Benke PJ, Moser HW: The cerebrohepatorenal (Zellweger) syndrome. Increased levels and impaired degradation of very-long-chain fatty acids and their use in prenatal diagnosis. *N Engl J Med* **310**:1141, 1984.
292. Moser HW, Moser AB: Measurements of saturated very long chain fatty acids in plasma, in Hommes F (ed): *Techniques in Diagnostic Human Biochemical Genetics*. New York, Wiley-Liss, 1991, p 177.
293. Aubourg P, Bougneres PF, Rocchiccioli F: Capillary gas-liquid chromatographic-mass spectrometric measurement of very long chain (C22 to C26) fatty acids in microliter samples of plasma. *J Lipid Res* **26**:263, 1985.
294. Wanders RJ, Schrakamp G, van den Bosch H, Tager JM, Schutgens RB: A prenatal test for the cerebro-hepato-renal (Zellweger) syndrome by demonstration of the absence of catalase-containing particles (peroxisomes) in cultured amniotic fluid cells. *Eur J Pediatr* **145**:136, 1986.
295. Tsuji S, Suzuki M, Ariga T, Sekine M, Kuriyama M, Miyatake T: Abnormality of long-chain fatty acids in erythrocyte membrane sphingomyelin from patients with adrenoleukodystrophy. *J Neurochem* **36**:1046, 1981.
296. Moser HW, Moser AB: Measurement of phytanic acid levels, in Hommes F (ed): *Techniques in Diagnostic Human Biochemical Genetics*. New York, Wiley-Liss, 1990, p 193.
297. ten Brink H, Wanders RJ, Stellaard F, Schutgens RB, Jakobs C: Pristanic acid and phytanic acid in plasma from patients with a single peroxisomal enzyme deficiency. *J Inherit Metab Dis* **14**:345, 1991.
298. Kelley RI: Quantification of pipecolic acid in plasma and urine by isotope-dilution gas chromatography/mass spectrometry, in Hommes F (ed): *Techniques in Diagnostic Human Biochemical Genetics*. New York, Wiley-Liss, 1991, p 205.
299. Setchell KD, Vestal CH: Thermospray ionization liquid chromatography-mass spectrometry: A new and highly specific technique for the analysis of bile acids. *J Lipid Res* **30**:1459, 1989.
300. Stellaard F, Langelaar SA, Kok RM, Kleijer WJ, Schutgens RB, Jakobs C: Prenatal diagnosis of Zellweger syndrome by determination of trihydroxycoprostanic acid in amniotic fluid. *Eur J Pediatr* **148**:175, 1988.
301. Wanders RJ, Smit W, Heymans HS, Schutgens RB, Barth PG, Schierbeek H, Smit GP, Berger R, Przyrembel H, Eggelte TA: Age-related accumulation of phytanic acid in plasma from a patient with the cerebro-hepato-renal (Zellweger) syndrome. *Clin Chim Acta* **166**:45, 1987.
302. Wanders RJ, Purvis YR, Heymans HS, Bakkeren JA, Parmentier GG, Eyssen H, van den Bosch H, Tager JM, Schutgens RB: Age-related differences in plasmalogen content of erythrocytes from patients with the cerebro-hepato-renal (Zellweger) syndrome: Implications for postnatal detection of the disease. *J Inherit Metab Dis* **9**:335, 1986.
303. Moser HW, Moser AB, Kawamura N, Murphy J, Suzuki K, Schaumburg H, Kishimoto Y, Milunsky A: Elevated C26 fatty acid in cultured skin fibroblasts. *Ann Neurol* **7**:542, 1980.
304. Wanders RJ, van Roermund C, Schutgens RB, van den Bosch H, Tager JM, Nijenhuis A, Tromp A: Prenatal diagnosis of Zellweger syndrome by measurement of very long chain fatty acid (C26:0) beta-oxidation in cultured chorionic villous fibroblasts: Implications for early diagnosis of other peroxisomal disorders. *Clin Chim Acta* **165**:303, 1987.
305. Singh I, Moser AE, Moser HW, Kishimoto Y: Adrenoleukodystrophy: impaired oxidation of very long chain fatty acids in white blood cells, cultured skin fibroblasts, and amniocytes. *Pediatr Res* **18**:286, 1984.
306. Datta NS, Wilson GN, Hajra AK: Deficiency of enzymes catalyzing the biosynthesis of glycerol-ether lipids in Zellweger syndrome: A new category of metabolic disease involving the absence of peroxisomes. *New Engl J Med* **31**:1080, 1984.
307. Roscher A, Molzer B, Bernheimer H, Stockler S, Mutz I, Paltauf F: The cerebrohepatorenal (Zellweger) syndrome: An improved method for the biochemical diagnosis and its potential value for prenatal detection. *Pediatr Res* **19**:930, 1985.
308. Poll-The BT, Skjeldal OH, Stokke O, Poulos A, Demaugre F, Saudubray JM: Phytanic acid alpha-oxidation and complementation analysis of classical Refsum and peroxisomal disorders. *Hum Genet* **81**:175, 1989.
309. Lazarow PB, Small GM, Santos M, Shio H, Moser AB, Moser HW, Esterman A, Black V, Dancis J: Zellweger syndrome amniocytes: Morphological appearance and a simple sedimentation method for prenatal diagnosis. *Pediatr Res* **24**:63, 1988.
310. Roels F, Goldfischer S: The demonstration of hepatic and renal peroxisomes by a high temperature procedure. *J Histochem Cytochem* **27**:1471, 1979.
311. Beard ME, Moser AB, Sapirstein V, Holtzman E: Peroxisomes in infantile phytanic acid storage disease: A cytochemical study of skin fibroblasts. *J Inherit Metab Dis* **9**:321, 1986.
312. Wanders RJA, Kos M, Roest B, Meijer AJ, Schrakamp G, Heymans HSA, Tegelaers WHH, van den Bosch H, Schutgens RBH, Tager JM: Activity of peroxisomal enzymes and intracellular distribution of catalase in Zellweger syndrome. *Biochem Biophys Res Commun* **123**:1054, 1984.
313. Rocchiccioli F, Aubourg P, Choiset A: Immediate prenatal diagnosis of Zellweger syndrome by direct measurement of very long chain fatty acids in chorionic villus cells. *Prenat Diagn* **7**:349, 1987.
314. Hajra AK, Datta NS, Jackson LG, Moser AB, Moser HW, Larsen JW, Powers J: Prenatal diagnosis of Zellweger cerebro-hepato-renal syndrome. *N Engl J Med* **312**:445, 1985.
315. Schutgens RB, Schrakamp G, Wanders RJ, Heymans HS, Moser HW, Moser AE, Tager JM, van den Bosch HV, Aubourg P: The cerebro-hepato-renal (Zellweger) yndrome: Prenatal detection based on impaired biosynthesis of plasmalogens. *Prenat Diagn* **5**:337, 1985.
316. Roels F, Verdonck V, Pauwels M, Lissens W, Liebaers I, Elleder M: Light microscopic visualization of peroxisomes and plasmalogens in first trimester chorionic villi. *Prenat Diagn* **7**:525, 1987.
317. Wanders RJ, Wiemer EA, Brul S, Schutgens RB, van den Bosch H, Tager JM: Prenatal diagnosis of Zellweger syndrome by direct visualization of peroxisomes in chorionic villus fibroblasts by immunofluorescence microscopy. *J Inherit Metab Dis* **12**:301, 1989.
318. Carey WF, Robertson EF, van Bosch CC, Poulos A, Nelson PV, Finikiotis G: Prenatal diagnosis of Zellweger syndrome by chorionic villus sampling—and a caveat. *Prenat Diagn* **6**:227, 1986.
319. Carey WF, Poulos A, Sharp P, Nelson PV, Robertson EF, Hughes JL: Pitfalls in the prenatal diagnosis of peroxisomal beta-oxidation defects by chorionic villus sampling. *Prenat Diagn* **14**:813, 1994.
320. Suzuki Y, Shimozawa N, Kawabata I, Yajima S, Inoue K, Uchida Y, Izai K, Tomatsu S, Kondo N, Orii T: Prenatal diagnosis of peroxisomal disorders. Biochemical and immunocytochemical studies on peroxisomes in human amniocytes. *Brain Dev* **16**:27, 1994.
321. Portsteffen H, Beyer A, Becker E, Epplen C, Pawlak A, Kunau WH, Dodt G: Human PEX1 is mutated in complementation group 1 of the peroxisome biogenesis disorders. *Nat Genet* **17**:449, 1997.
322. Okumoto K, Itoh R, Shimozawa N, Suzuki Y, Tamura S, Kondo N, Fujiki Y: Mutations in *PEX10* is the cause of Zellweger peroxisome deficiency syndrome of complementation group B. *Hum Mol Genet* **7**:1399, 1998.
323. Tamura S, Okumoto K, Toyama R, Shimozawa N, Tsukamoto T, Suzuki Y, Osumi T, Kondo N, Fujiki Y: Human PEX1 cloned by functional complementation on a CHO cell mutant is responsible for peroxisome-deficient Zellweger syndrome of complementation group I. *Proc Natl Acad Sci U S A* **95**:4350, 1998.
324. Okumoto K, Fujiki Y: *PEX12* encodes an integral membrane protein of peroxisomes. *Nat Genet* **17**:265, 1997.
325. Okumoto K, Shimozawa N, Kawai A, Tamura S, Tsukamoto T, Osumi T, Moser H, Wanders RJA, Suzuki Y, Kondo N, Fujiki Y: *PEX12*, the pathogenic gene of group III Zellweger syndrome: cDNA cloning by functional complementation on a CHO cell mutant, patient analysis, and characterization of PEX12p. *Mol Cell Biol* **18**:4324, 1998.

326. Fukuda S, Shimozawa N, Suzuki Y, Zhang Z, Tomatsu S, Tsukamoto T, Hashiguchi N, Osumi T, Masuno M, Imaizumi K, Kuroki Y, Fujiki Y, Orii T, Kondo N: Human peroxisome assembly factor-2 (PAF-2): A gene responsible for Group C peroxisome biogenesis disorder in humans. *Am J Hum Genet* **59**:1210, 1996.
327. Wiemer EAC, Nuttley WM, Bertolaet BL, Li X, Franke U, Wheelock MJ, Anné UK, Johnson KR, Subramani S: Human peroxisomal targeting signal-1 receptor restores peroxisomal protein import in cells from patients with fatal peroxisomal disorders. *J Cell Biol* **130**:51, 1995.
328. Fransen M, Brees C, Baumgart E, Vanhooren JCT, Baes M, Mannaerts GP, Van Veldhoven PP: Identification and characterization of the putative human peroxisomal C-terminal targeting signal import receptor. *J Biol Chem* **270**:7731, 1995.
329. Marynen P, Fransen M, Raeymaekers P, Mannaerts GP, Van Veldhoven PP: The gene for the peroxisomal targeting signal import receptor (PXR1) is located on human chromosome 12p13, flanked by TPI1 and D12S1089. *Genomics* **30**:366, 1995.
330. Shimozawa N, Zhang Z, Suzuki Y, Imamura A, Tsukamoto T, Osumi T, Fujiki Y, Orii T, Barth PG, Wanders RJ, Kondo N: Functional heterogeneity of C-terminal peroxisome targeting signal 1 in PEX5-defective patients. *Biochem Biophys Res Commun* **262**:504, 1999.
331. Maquat LE: When cells stop making sense: Effects of nonsense codons on RNA metabolism in vertebrate cells. *RNA* **1**:453, 1995.
332. Geisbrecht BV: Structural, metabolic, and biotechnological aspects of the PTS1 and its recognition by PEX5. Johns Hopkins University, Baltimore, 2000.
333. Dodt G, Warren DS, Gould SJ: Identification of discrete functional domains of PEX5 that are required for PTS2 protein import and transport of PEX5 to peroxisomes. *J Biol Chem* (in preparation), 2000.
334. de Vet ECJM, IJlst L, Oostheim W, Wanders RJA, van den Bosch H: Alkyl-dihydroxyacetonephosphate synthase: Fate in peroxisome biogenesis disorders and identification of the point mutation underlying a single enzyme deficiency. *J Biol Chem* **273**:10296, 1998.
335. Ofman R, Hettema EH, Hogenhout EM, Caruso U, Muijsers AO, Wanders RJA: Acyl-CoA: Dihydroxyacetonephosphate acyltransferase: Cloning of the human cDNA and resolution of the molecular basis in rhizomelic chondrodysplasia punctata type 2. *Hum Mol Genet* **7**:847, 1998.
336. Shimozawa N, Suzuki Y, Zhang Z, Miura K, Matsumoto A, Nagaya M, Castillo-Taucher S, Kondo N: A novel nonsense mutation of the PEX7 gene in a patient with rhizomelic chondrodysplasia punctata. *J Hum Genet* **44**:123, 1999.
337. Björkman J, Stetten G, Moore CS, Gould SJ, Crane DI: Genomic structure of *PEX13*, a candidate peroxisome biogenesis disorder gene. *Genomics* **54**:521, 1998.
338. Lazarow PB, Robbi M, Fujiki Y, Wong L: Biogenesis of peroxisomal proteins in vivo and *in vitro*. *Ann NY Acad Sci* **386**:285, 1982.
339. Warren DS, Wolfe BD, Gould SJ: Phenotype-genotype relationships in *PEX10*-deficient peroxisome biogenesis disorder patients. *Hum Mutat* **15**:509, 2000.
340. Borden KLB, Boddy MN, Lally J, O'Reilly JO, Martin S, Howe K, Solomon E, Freemont PS: The solution structure of the RING finger domain from the acute promyelocytic leukaemia proto-oncoprotein PML. *EMBO J* **14**:1532, 1995.
341. Shimozawa N, Tsukamoto T, Suzuki Y, Orii T, Fujiki Y: Animal cell mutants represent two complementation groups of peroxisome-defective Zellweger syndrome. *J Clin Invest* **90**:1864, 1992.
342. Masuno M, Shimozawa N, Suzuki Y, Kondo N, Orii T, Tsukamoto T, Osumi T, Fujiki Y, Imaizumi K, Kuroki Y: Assignment of the human peroxisome assembly factor-1 gene (PXMP3) responsible for Zellweger syndrome to chromosome 8q21.1 by fluorescence *in situ* hybridization. *Genomics* **20**:141, 1994.
343. Faust PL, Hatten ME: Targeted deletion of the PEX2 peroxisome assembly gene in mice provides a model for Zellweger syndrome, a human neuronal migration disorder. *J Cell Biol* **139**:1293, 1997.
344. Harano T, Shimizu N, Otera H, Fujiki Y: Transmembrane topology of the peroxin, Pex2p, an essential component for the peroxisome assembly. *J Biochem (Tokyo)* **125**:1168, 1999.
345. Braverman N, Valle D: Unpublished observations, 2000.
346. Tsukamoto T, Shimozawa N, Fujiki Y: Peroxisome assembly factor 1:Nonsense mutation in a peroxisome-deficient Chinese hamster ovary cell mutant and deletion analysis. *Mol Cell Biol* **14**:5458, 1994.
347. Collins CS, Gould SJ: Unpublished observations, 2000.
348. Maxwell MA, Nelson PV, Chin SJ, Paton BC, Carey WF, Crane DI: A common *PEX1* frameshift mutation in patients with disorders of peroxisome biogenesis correlates with the severe Zellweger syndrome phenotype. *Hum Genet* **105**:38, 1999.
349. Gärtner J, Preuss N, Brosius U, Biermanns M: Mutations in *PEX1* in peroxisome biogenesis disorders: G843D and a mild clinical phenotype. *J Inherit Metab Dis* **22**:311, 1999.
350. Wanders RJA, Mooijer PAW, Dekker C, Suzuki Y, Shimozawa N: Disorders of peroxisome biogenesis: Complementation analysis shows genetic heterogeneity with strong overrepresentation of one group (PEX1 deficiency). *J Inherit Metab Dis* **22**:314, 1999.
351. Culbertson MR: RNA surveillance. Unforeseen consequences for gene expression, inherited genetic disorders and cancer. *TIG* **15**:74, 1999.
352. Zhang Z, Suzuki Y, Shimozawa N, Fukuda S, Imamura A, Tsukamoto T, Osumi T, Fujiki Y, Orii T, Wanders RJA, Barth PG, Moser HW, paton BC, Besley GT, Kondo N: Genomic structure and identification of 11 novel mutations of the *PEX6* (peroxisome assembly factor-2) gene in patients with peroxisome biogenesis disorders. *Hum Mutat* **14**:487, 1999.
353. Braun A, Kammerer S, Weissenhorn W, Weiss EH, Cleve H: Sequence of a putative human housekeeping gene (HK33) localized on chromosome 1. *Gene* **146**:291, 1994.
354. Kammerer S, Arnold N, Gutensohn W, Mewes H-W, Kunau W-H, Höfler G, Roscher AA, Braun A: Genomic organization and molecular characterization of a gene encoding HsPXF, a human peroxisomal farnesylated protein. *Genomics* **45**:200, 1997.
355. Kammerer S, Holzinger A, Welsch U, Roscher AA: Cloning and characterization of the gene encoding the human peroxisomal assembly protein Pex3p. *FEBS Lett* **429**:53, 1998.
356. Muntau AC, Holzinger A, Mayerhofer PU, Gartner J, Roscher AA, Kammerer S: The human *PEX3* gene encoding a peroxisomal assembly protein: genomic organization, positional mapping, and mutation analysis in candidate phenotypes. *Biochem Biophys Res Commun* **268**:704, 2000.
357. Braverman N, Lin P, Steel G, Obie C, Moser H, Moser A, Valle D: Mutation analysis of PEX7 in patients with rhizomelic chondrodysplasia punctata. *Am J Hum Genet* **65**:A286, 1999.
358. Holmes RD, Wilson GN, Hajra A: Oral ether lipid therapy in patients with peroxisomal disorders. *J Inherit Metab Dis* **10**:239, 1987.
359. Moser A, Borel J, Odone A, Naidu S, Cornblath D, Sanders DB, Moser HW: A new dietary therapy for adrenoleukodystrophy: Biochemical and preliminary clinical results in 36 patients. *Ann Neurol* **21**:240, 1987.
360. Greenberg CR, Hajra A, Moser A: Triple therapy of a patient with a generalized peroxisomal disorder. *Am J Hum Genet* **41**:A64, 1987.
361. Setchell KD, Bragetti P, Zimmer-Nechemias L, Daugherty C, Pelli MA, Vaccaro R, Gentili G, Distrutti E, Dozzini G, Morelli A: Oral bile acid treatment and the patient with Zellweger syndrome. *Hepatology* **15**:198, 1992.
362. Martinez M, Pineda M, Vidal R, Conill J, Martin B: Docosahexaenoic acid - A new therapeutic approach to peroxisomal-disorder patients: Experience with two cases. *Neurology* **43**:1389, 1993.
363. Martinez M, Vazquez E: MRI evidence that docosahexaenoic acid ethyl ester improves myelination in generalized peroxisomal disorders. *Neurology* **51**:26, 1998.
364. Noetzel MJ: Fish oil and myelin: Cautious optimism for treatment of children with disorders of peroxisome biogenesis. *Neurology* **51**:5, 1998.
365. Bjorkhem I, Blomstrand S, Gaumann H, Strandvik B: Unsuccessful attempts to induce peroxisomes in two cases of Zellweger disease by treatment with clofibrate. *Pediatr Res* **19**:590, 1985.
366. Kemp S, Wei HM, Lu JF, Braiterman LT, McGuinness MC, Moser AB, Watkins PA, Smith KD: Gene redundancy and pharmacologic gene therapy: Implications for X-linked adrenoleukodystrophy. *Nat Med* **4**:1261, 1998.
367. Baes M, Gressens P, Baumgart E, Carmeliet P, Casteels M, Fransen M, Evrand P, Fahimi D, Declercq PE, Collen D, van Veldhoven PP, Mannaerts GP: A mouse model for Zellweger syndrome. *Nat Genet* **17**:49, 1997.

CHAPTER 130

Single Peroxisomal Enzyme Deficiencies

Ronald J. A. Wanders ▪ Peter G. Barth ▪ Hugo S. A. Heymans

1. **Peroxisomes are subcellular organelles present in virtually every eukaryotic cell catalysing a range of essential metabolic functions mainly related to lipid metabolism. These include: (a) fatty acid β-oxidation; (b) etherphospholipid biosynthesis; (c) fatty acid α-oxidation; (d) isoprenoid biosynthesis; (e) L-pipecolate degradation; (f) glutaryl-CoA metabolism; (g) H2O2-metabolism; and (i) glyoxylate detoxification.**
2. **Peroxisomes catalyze the β-oxidation of a variety of fatty acids and fatty acid derivatives which can not be handled by mitochondria. The most important substrates for peroxisomal β-oxidation from a patient's point of view are (a) very long chain fatty acids, (b) pristanic acid as derived predominantly from phytanic acid, and (c) di- and trihydroxycholestanoic acid. The latter two compounds are produced from cholesterol in the liver and undergo β-oxidation in the peroxisome to produce the CoA-esters of chenodeoxycholic and cholic acid, respectively. This implies that "bile acid synthesis" represents in fact a degradative mechanism involving β-oxidation rather than a true biosynthetic process.**
3. **To date, four defined disorders of peroxisomal fatty acid β-oxidation have been identified: (a) acyl-CoA oxidase deficiency (MIM 264470); (b) D-bifunctional protein deficiency (MIM 261515); (c) peroxisomal thiolase deficiency (MIM 261510); and (d) 2-methylacyl-CoA racemase deficiency. Interestingly, the clinical presentation of the first three disorders resembles that of the peroxisome biogenesis disorders (PBDs) in many respects. This is especially true for D-bifunctional protein deficiency since virtually all patients identified sofar (>40) show severe clinical abnormalities including hypotonia, craniofacial dysmorphia, neonatal seizures, hepatomegaly, and developmental delay. Most patients with D-BP deficiency die in the first year of life. A remarkable observation is that patients with D-BP deficiency often show disordered neuronal migration.**
4. **2-Methylacyl-CoA racemase deficiency is a newly identified disorder of peroxisomal β-oxidation in which only the oxidation of the 2-methyl branched-chain fatty acids pristanic acid and di- and trihydroxycholestanoic acid is impaired. In contrast to patients with acyl-CoA oxidase deficiency or any of the other β-oxidation deficiencies, patients with racemase deficiency do not present early in life, but instead develop a late-onset neuropathy.**
5. **Diagnosis of a peroxisomal β-oxidation disorder is based on clinical characteristics combined with a series of tests to assess peroxisomal function. Analysis of very long chain fatty acids is a reliable initial screening method. If abnormal, additional tests should be done in plasma (di- and trihydroxycholestanoic, phytanic, and pristanic acid) and erythrocytes (plasmalogens). Flowcharts may be helpful in reaching the correct diagnosis, which always requires detailed studies in fibroblasts, including enzyme analyses, complementation studies, and molecular analyses.**
6. **Prenatal diagnosis of the various β-oxidation disorders can be done reliably because methods have now been developed that allow analysis in direct chorionic villous material. This obviates the risk associated with culturing chorionic villous cells.**
7. **A second major function of peroxisomes involves the biosynthesis of ether-linked phospholipids, which differ from the regular diacyl phospholipids in one major aspect, which is the ether-bond at the *sn*-1 position of the glycerol backbone. The first two enzymatic steps in etherphospholipid synthesis take place in peroxisomes and are catalyzed by dihydroxyacetonephosphate acyltransferase (DHAPAT) and alkyldihydroxyacetonephosphate synthase (alkyl DHAP synthase) Although many functions for etherphospholipids have been suggested, their true physiological function remains elusive.**
8. **Two isolated defects in etherphospholipid biosynthesis have been described at the level of DHAPAT and alkyl DHAP synthase, respectively. Interestingly, the clinical presentation of patients with DHAPAT- or alkyl DHAP-synthase deficiency resembles that of rhizomelic chondrodysplasia punctata (RCDP) in virtually all aspects, including rhizomelic shortening of the upper extremities, typical facial appearance, congenital contractures, cataract, dwarfism, and severe mental retardation with spasticity.**
9. **If a patient presents with clinical signs and symptoms of RCDP or a variant form, erythrocyte plasmalogen levels should be determined. Measurement of erythrocyte plasmalogens has proven to be extremely reliable because**

A list of standard abbreviations is located immediately preceding the index in each volume. Additional abbreviations used in this chapter include: ACOX1 = acyl-coenzyme A oxidase (straight-chain); ACOX2 = acyl-coenzyme A oxidase (branched-chain); ACOX3 = acyl-coenzyme A oxidase (pristanoyl-CoA); ALD = adrenoleukodystrophy; CAC = carnitine/acylcarnitine carrier; CAT = carnitine acetyltransferase; COT = carnitine octanoyltransferase; CPT = carnitine palmitoyltransferase; D-BP = D-bifunctional protein; DHA = docosahexaenoic acid; DHAP = dihydroxyacetonephosphate; DHAPAT = dihydroxyacetonephosphate acyltransferase; DHCA = dihydroxycholestanoic acid; G3P = glycerol-3-phosphate; G3PAT = glycerol-3-phosphate acyltransferase; IRD = infantile Refsum disease; L-BP = L-bifunctional protein; MTS = mitochondrial targeting signal; NALD = neonatal adrenoleukodystrophy; pTH1 = peroxisomal thiolase (straight-chain specific); pTH2 = SCPx, peroxisomal thiolase (straight- and branched-chain specific); PTS = peroxisomal targeting signal; RCDP = rhizomelic chondrodysplasia punctata; SCP = sterol-carrier-protein; THCA = trihydroxycholestanoic acid; VLCFA = very long chain fatty acids; THC-CoA = 3, 7, 12-trihydroxy-5-cholestanoyl-CoA; ZS = cerebrohepatorenal (Zellweger) syndrome.

all patients identified to date with RCDP type 1, 2, or 3 have shown deficient plasmalogens in erythrocytes. Definitive diagnosis in terms of RCDP type 1, 2, or 3 requires detailed enzymatic studies in fibroblasts followed by molecular analysis of the genes encoding PEX7 (*PEX7*), DHAPAT (*GNPAT*) or alkyl-DHAP synthase (*AGPS*), respectively.

10. **Prenatal diagnosis of RCDP types 1, 2, and 3 can be done reliably in chorionic villous tissue using a combination of enzymatic and immunologic (blotting) methods and, in selected cases, DNA analysis.**
11. **The third major function of peroxisomes concerns their role in isoprenoid biosynthesis. There is growing evidence to suggest that the first part of the isoprenoid biosynthetic pathway from acetyl-CoA to farnesylpyrophosphate is peroxisomal. Consequently, mevalonate kinase deficiency is a peroxisomal disorder. Two types of mevalonate kinase deficiency have been described, a severe form dominated by a series of clinical abnormalities in multiple organs and a milder form associated with periodic fever.**
12. **Peroxisomes also play an indispensable role in glyoxylate detoxification and phytanic acid α-oxidation with hyperoxaluria type 1 and Refsum disease as relevant peroxisomal disorders. These are discussed in other chapters.**
13. **Finally, peroxisomes are also important for the degradation of L-pipecolate, a degradation product of L-lysine, because L-pipecolate oxidase is a peroxisomal enzyme in man. Several cases of hyperpipecolic acidemia have been described in literature, but a specific enzyme deficiency, for instance at the level of L-pipecolate oxidase, has not been described in any of the patients.**

The peroxisomal disorders are relative newcomers in the arena of inherited diseases in man. The reason is that peroxisomes were the last true subcellular organelles to be discovered. In addition, they were long thought to play only a minor role in cellular metabolism. Peroxisomes were first described by Rhodin in the early 1950s as spherical or oval bodies in the cytoplasm of mouse proximal kidney tubules and biochemically characterized by DeDuve and coworkers.[1] The addition of peroxisomes to the group of biochemically defined organelles is closely related to the development of cell fractionation techniques, including density-gradient centrifugation.[1] Indeed, the discovery that several H_2O_2-producing enzymes, such as urate oxidase and D-amino acid oxidase, were truly located in a distinct subcellular particle together with catalase, was based on careful differential and isopycnic gradient centrifugation studies by DeDuve and coworkers.[1] These studies suggested that peroxisomes might play a unique role in H_2O_2 metabolism. The finding, however, that H_2O_2-producing oxidases are also present in other subcellular organelles including mitochondria (monoamine oxidase, sulfite oxidase) indicated that H_2O_2-metabolism is not confined to peroxisomes and questioned the importance of peroxisomes in H_2O_2-metabolism.

In retrospect, it is remarkable that the significance of peroxisomes for mammalian metabolism remained a mystery for so long. Even the seminal observation by Goldfischer et al.[2] that morphologically distinguishable peroxisomes were absent in liver and kidney tubules from patients suffering from the cerebrohepatorenal (Zellweger) syndrome (MIM 214100), attracted little attention. This is, at least partly, due to the fact that the same paper also reported *mitochondrial* abnormalities.[2]

The true significance of peroxisomes became clear only much later because of two key observations. First, Brown et al.[3] reported elevated levels of certain saturated very long chain fatty acids (VLCFA), notably hexacosanoic acid (C26:0) and tetracosanoic acid (C24:0), in plasma from Zellweger patients, whereas the levels of long chain fatty acids such as palmitic, oleic, and linoleic acid were normal. Second, Heymans et al.[4] found strongly decreased levels of a certain type of phospholipids called plasmalogens in erythrocytes and tissues of Zellweger patients. These findings strongly suggested that peroxisomes play an indispensable role in the metabolism of at least two groups of metabolites, that is, VLCFAs and plasmalogens. Subsequent studies confirmed this and it is now clear that peroxisomes catalyze a number of unique metabolic functions.

In this chapter, we describe the major functions of peroxisomes and its constituent enzymes with particular emphasis on fatty acid β-oxidation and etherphospholipid biosynthesis. We then review the clinical, laboratory, pathologic, and molecular findings in patients with a single peroxisomal enzyme deficiency. Table 130-1 lists the single peroxisomal enzyme deficiencies identified so far. Some of these disorders are covered in other chapters. We first discuss peroxisomal fatty acid β-oxidation.

FATTY ACID β-OXIDATION IN PEROXISOMES AND DEFECTS THEREIN

General Characteristics of the Peroxisomal β-Oxidation System

In 1969, Cooper and Beevers[5] reported their remarkable discovery of a fatty acid oxidation system in glyoxysomes of germinating castor bean seedlings. Until then, it was generally believed that fatty acid β-oxidation in eukaryotes was confined to mitochondria. The capacity of the glyoxysomal β-oxidation system was found to increase during germination, together with the activities of the glyoxylate-cycle enzymes, thereby enabling the seedlings to convert lipids into carbohydrates and, thus, to build up cellular constituents from stored lipids.[6] Importantly, the first step in glyoxysomal fatty acid β-oxidation turned out to be catalyzed by an oxidase with direct transfer of reducing equivalents to molecular oxygen to produce H_2O_2. The realization that glyoxysomes and peroxisomes share certain properties and belong to the so-called microbody family, led Lazarow and DeDuve[7] to study fatty acid β-oxidation in rat liver peroxisomes. These studies led to the identification of a complete fatty acid oxidation system in peroxisomes. The activity of this system was stimulated greatly if rats were fed clofibrate, a hypolipidemic drug.[7] Subsequent studies revealed the presence of peroxisomal β-oxidation systems throughout all eukaryotic kingdoms in animals, plants, and a large number of eukaryotic microorganisms (see reference 8 for a review). On the other hand, mitochondrial fatty acid oxidation seems to be limited to animals and some algae indicating that peroxisomal, rather than mitochondrial, oxidation is the dominant fatty acid oxidation pathway in nature.

The mitochondrial and peroxisomal β-oxidation systems have been studied intensively through the years. Although the actual β-oxidation in the two organelles proceeds via the same cyclic process involving four consecutive reactions, the two systems differ markedly.

These differences include:

1. **The peroxisomal and mitochondrial β-oxidation enzymes are different proteins encoded by different genes**. Oxidation of acyl-CoA esters in peroxisomes and mitochondria proceeds via a similar mechanism involving dehydrogenation, hydration, dehydrogenation again, and thiolytic cleavage. Multiple enzymes encoded by different genes catalyze these reactions, as described in detail later. One striking aspect is that in case of peroxisomal fatty acid oxidation the first step is catalyzed by a variety of different FAD-linked acyl-CoA oxidases in which enzyme-bound $FADH_2$ is directly reoxidized by molecular oxygen to produce H_2O_2. In mitochondria, the same reaction is catalyzed by a set of acyl-CoA dehydrogenases, which also carry FAD. The $FADH_2$, which is generated is reoxidized not by O_2, but by electron transfer flavoprotein (ETF), after which the electrons are donated to the respiratory chain via ETF-dehydrogenase (see Chap. 103).

Table 130-1 Overview of the Single Peroxisomal Enzyme Deficiencies Identified To Date

Peroxisomal function involved	Disorder	Phenotype	Deficient enzyme/protein identified	Genetic basis resolved
Fatty acid β-oxidation	X-ALD	X-ALD	ALDP	Yes
	Acyl-CoA oxidase deficiency	NALD-like	Acyl-CoA oxidase	Yes
	D-Bifunctional protein deficiency	ZS/NALD-like	D-Bifunctional protein	Yes
	Thiolase deficiency	ZS-like	Peroxisomal thiolase 1	No
	Branched-chain acyl-CoA oxidase deficiency	No patients identified		
	L-Bifunctional protein deficiency	Not existing any longer*		
	Branched-chain peroxisomal thiolase deficiency	No patients identified		
	Racemase-deficiency	Late-onset neuropathy	Racemase	Yes
Etherphospholipid biosynthesis	DHAPAT-deficiency	(Rhizomelic) chondrodysplasia punctata	Yes	Yes
	Alkyl-DHAP synthase deficiency	(Rhizomelic) chondrodysplasia punctata	Yes	Yes
Fatty acid α-oxidation	Phytanoyl-CoA hydroxylase deficiency	Refsum disease	Yes	Yes
Isoprenoid biosynthesis	Mevalonate kinase (MK) deficiency	1. Classical MK-deficiency 2. Hyper IgD/periodic fever syndrome	Yes	Yes
Pipecolic acid degradation	Isolated hyperpipecolic acidaemia	Variable (see text)	No	No
Glutaryl-CoA metabolism	Glutaryl-CoA oxidase deficiency	Glutaric aciduria type 3	Yes	No
Hydrogen peroxide metabolism	Catalase deficiency	Acatalasaemia	Yes	Yes
Glyoxylate detoxification	Alanine:glyoxylate aminotransferase deficiency	Hyperoxaluria type 1	Yes	Yes

*All patients described with presumed L-bifunctional protein deficiency have now been found to be deficient in D-bifunctional protein due to mutations in the D-bifunctional protein gene (see text).

2. **Mitochondria can oxidize fatty acids to completion whereas peroxisomes cannot**. In plants and fungi in which peroxisomes are the sole site of fatty acid β-oxidation, fatty acids can be degraded into their constituent acetyl-CoA units after which transfer of the acetyl-CoA units occurs to the mitochondria for full oxidation to CO_2 and H_2O. In higher eukaryotes, however, in which both peroxisomes and mitochondria are capable of fatty acid β-oxidation, the general rule for peroxisomes is that fatty acids cannot be fully degraded into acetyl-CoA units. The reason for this is that the peroxisomal acyl-CoA oxidases identified show virtually no activity with shorter-chain acyl-CoA esters like butyryl-CoA and hexanoyl-CoA.[9,10] Hence the peroxisomal β-oxidation system is primarily a *chain-shortening* device tailoring fatty acids for oxidation in mitochondria. For most fatty acids, including C26:0, known to be chain-shortened in peroxisomes, it is not clear at which level chain-shortening stops. An exception is pristanic acid, the α-oxidation product of phytanic acid (3,7,11,15-tetramethylhexadecanoic acid; see Chap. 132), which has been found to undergo three cycles of β-oxidation in peroxisomes followed by transport of the CoA-ester produced (4,8-dimethylnonanoyl-CoA) to mitochondria in the form of a carnitine ester[11] (Fig. 130-1).
3. **Peroxisomal β-oxidation is energetically much less favorable as compared to β-oxidation in mitochondria**. The energy produced in the first step of peroxisomal β-oxidation is not conserved because the hydrogen peroxide produced by the different acyl-CoA oxidases is split into H_2O and O_2 by catalase. This implies that only the energy released in the third step of peroxisomal β-oxidation is conserved whereby the NADH produced is used to synthesize ATP in the mitochondrion.
4. **Different mechanisms are involved in the uptake of fatty acids into peroxisomes and mitochondria**. The mechanism by which fatty acids enter the mitochondria has been resolved in detail. After activation of the fatty acid to its CoA-ester by one of a variety of acyl-CoA synthetases, a three-step mechanism is required to carry the acyl-CoA across the mitochondrial inner membrane. This involves the consecutive action of carnitine palmitoyltransferase 1 (CPT1), the carnitine:acylcarnitine carrier (CAC), and carnitine palmitoyltransferase 2 (CPT2).[12]

   Available evidence suggests that such a mechanism is definitely not operational in peroxisomes, because CoA-esters such as pristanoyl-CoA and trihydroxycholestanoyl-CoA, known to undergo β-oxidation in the peroxisome, cannot be converted into the corresponding carnitine esters.

   At present it is unclear by what mechanism acyl-CoA esters such as C26:0-CoA, pristanoyl-CoA, and trihydroxycholestanoyl-CoA, among others, enter the peroxisome. There is evidence to suggest that this is brought about by the various ABC-transporters known to be present in the peroxisomal membrane. Support for this postulate comes from studies in the yeast *S. cerevisiae* in which two homologues of the human adrenoleukodystrophy (XALD) gene have been identified,[13–15] which physically interact to form a heterodimer in the peroxisomal membrane.[16] Oxidation of oleate was found to be strongly reduced if either of the two genes was deleted. Activation of oleate to oleoyl-CoA occurs outside

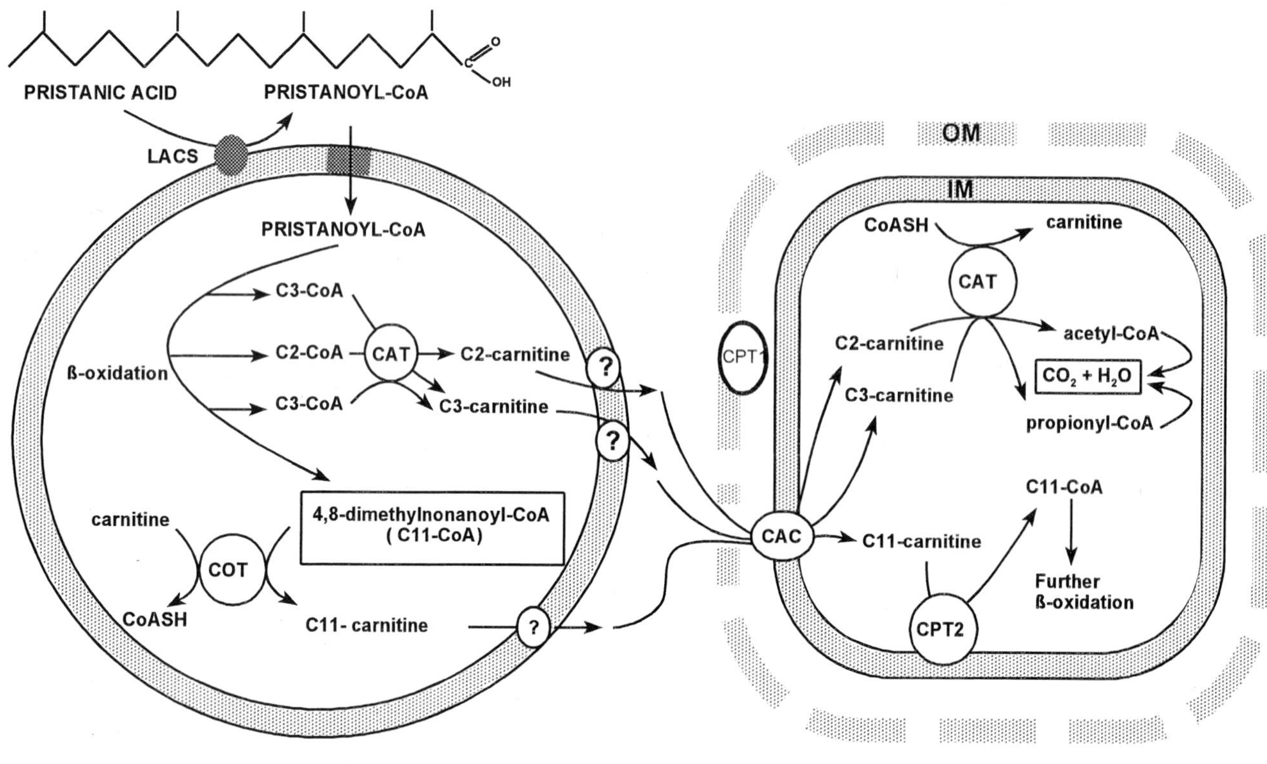

Fig. 130-1 Representation of the functional interaction between peroxisomes and mitochondria in the oxidation of pristanic acid (2,6,10,14-tetramethylpentadecanoic acid). Abbreviations used: CAC = carnitine:acylcarnitine carrier; CAT = carnitine acetyltransferase; COT = carnitine octanoyltransferase; CPT = carnitine palmitoyltransferase; C2 = acetylcarnitine; C3 = propionylcarnitine; IM = inner mitochondrial membrane; LACS = long chain acyl-CoA synthetase; OM = outer mitochondrial membrane. See text for discussion.

peroxisomes,[14] which implies that the dimeric complex formed by the two half-transporters transports oleoyl-CoA. Direct experimental proof for this postulate came from Verleur et al.[17] using selectively permeabilized yeast cells.

In human peroxisomes four half-ABC transporters have been identified to date, including (a) PMP70, the first half-ABC transporter identified,[18,19] (b) ALDP,[20,21] (c) ALDRP,[22,23] and (d) the PMP70-related protein.[24,25] Human ALDRP, PMP70, and PMP70-related protein show 66, 38, and 27 percent amino acid identity with ALDP, suggesting functional similarity. This notion is supported by experimental data showing that overexpression of *PMP70*[26,27] and *ALDR*[27–29] cDNA restored oxidation of VLCFAs in fibroblasts from X-linked adrenoleukodystrophy patients indicating functional similarity among the peroxisomal half-ABC transporters. Because it is likely that half-transporters need to dimerize to exert their function,[30] homo- and heterodimerization of the peroxisomal half-transporters has been studied.[31,32] Using the yeast two-hybrid system, Aubourg and coworkers[32] showed that ALDP, ALDRP, and PMP70 can form homo- as well as heterodimers. These results were verified by coimmunoprecipitation studies that demonstrated homodimerization of ALDP, heterodimerization of ALDP with PMP70 and ALDRP, and heterodimerization of ALDRP and PMP70. If the results obtained in yeast[17] can be extrapolated to human peroxisomes, it may well be that ALDP, either as homodimer or as heterodimer with PMP70 or ALDRP, transports very long chain acyl-CoA esters across the peroxisomal membrane. In this way, each particular heterodimer may transport a specific substrate or set of substrates as shown in *Drosophila* eye pigment cells in which the *white/scarlet/brown* subfamily of half-ABC transporters has been shown to assemble in different heteromeric combinations, each with a different substrate preference.[33]

5. **Mitochondrial and peroxisomal fatty acid oxidation are differentially regulated**. Mitochondrial fatty acid oxidation is strictly regulated at the level of CPT1 as shown in elegant studies by McGarry and Brown.[34] These studies have shown that malonyl-CoA is the central metabolite in the control of fatty acid oxidation in mitochondria by virtue of the fact that malonyl-CoA is a powerful inhibitor of CPT1. A similar type of short-term control of fatty oxidation has not been demonstrated for peroxisomes.
6. **Hypolipidemic drugs affect mitochondrial and peroxisomal fatty acid *β*-oxidation differently**. In rodents, hypolipidemic drugs such as clofibrate exert drastic effects on many enzymes of which most, but not all, are involved in fatty acid metabolism.[35] Administration of hypolipidemic drugs to rodents is associated with strongly increased activities notably of the peroxisomal *β*-oxidation enzymes, whereas the activity of the mitochondrial counterparts is increased to a much more limited extent.[36]
7. **The mitochondrial and peroxisomal *β*-oxidation systems have different substrate specificities**. From a physiological point of view, the most important difference between the mitochondrial and peroxisomal *β*-oxidation systems is that the two systems have different substrate specificities.

Indeed, some substrates, such as C26:0, are exclusively oxidized in peroxisomes. On the other hand, long-chain fatty acids such as palmitate and oleate can be handled by both systems. Current evidence suggests that peroxisomes only play a minor role in long chain fatty acid oxidation, the bulk of long chain fatty acids (>80 percent) being oxidized in mitochondria. Peroxisomes are indispensable, however, for the β-oxidation of a series of fatty acids and fatty acid derivatives as described below.

7.1 β-Oxidation of VLCFAs. Hexacosanoic acid (C26:0) and tetracosanoic acid (C24:0) are exclusively oxidized in peroxisomes. This is immediately clear if it is realized that C26:0 β-oxidation is completely deficient in fibroblasts from patients lacking peroxisomes or in fibroblasts with an isolated deficiency of acyl-CoA oxidase,[37] whereas oxidation is fully normal in cells from a patient with a deficiency at the level of the mitochondrial carnitine acylcarnitine carrier in which oxidation of palmitate is fully deficient (authors' unpublished observations).

There is no information in the literature with respect to the question of how many cycles of β-oxidation actually take place in peroxisomes. In theory, oxidation could proceed until butyryl-CoA is formed, which is no longer a substrate for the two acyl-CoA oxidases identified in human peroxisomes.[9,10] Most likely, butyryl-CoA is then converted into butyrylcarnitine within the peroxisome via carnitine octanoyltransferase (COT) or carnitine acetyltransferase (CAT), followed by export of butyrylcarnitine to the mitochondrion, after which it is taken up by the mitochondria via the mitochondrial carnitine/acylcarnitine carrier (see Fig. 130-2). Once inside, retroconversion to butyryl-CoA occurs followed by β-oxidation into acetyl-CoA units (Fig. 130-1). An alternative possibility is that butyryl-CoA undergoes cleavage inside peroxisomes by one of the acyl-CoA thioesterases (see "Peroxisomal Acxl-CoA Thioesterases"), and that the free butyric acid formed is subsequently exported to the mitochondria, where it is activated in the mitochondrial matrix and undergoes β-oxidation, ultimately giving CO_2 and H_2O.

7.2. β-Oxidation of pristanic acid. Pristanic acid (2,6,10,14-tetramethylpentadecanoic acid) is the α-oxidation product of phytanic (see Chap. 132) but is also directly derived from dietary sources. Before pristanic acid can undergo β-oxidation, activation to its CoA-ester must occur. This is brought about by the long-chain acyl-CoA synthetase (LACS) known to be present at the outer aspect of the peroxisomal membrane as well as in the mitochondrial outer membrane and endoplasmic reticulum membrane.[38] LACS also accepts pristanic acid as substrate.[39]

Recent studies have shed new light on the pathway of pristanic acid β-oxidation, and especially on the involvement of peroxisomes and mitochondria.[11,40] These studies made use of mutant fibroblasts from patients with inherited deficiencies at the level of carnitine palmitoyltransferase 1 (CPT1), the carnitine acylcarnitine carrier (CAC), and carnitine palmitoyltransferase 2 (CPT2). First, it was found that propionyl-CoA leaves the peroxisome as carnitine-ester and enters the mitochondrion via the carnitine:acylcarnitine carrier followed by reconversion of propionylcarnitine into propionyl-CoA via carnitine acetyltransferase (CAT).[40]

Second, Verhoeven et al.[11] found that oxidation of pristanic acid is blocked in fibroblasts with a genetic deficiency of either CAC or CPT2. The identification of 4,8-dimethylnonanoyl-carnitine as accumulating product indicates that pristanic acid undergoes three cycles of β-oxidation within peroxisomes after which the 4,8-dimethylnonanoyl-CoA produced is converted into its carnitine-ester, which leaves the peroxisome via an as yet unidentified transport mechanism (Fig. 130-1).

The carnitine ester enters the mitochondrion via the CAC-carrier and is reconverted into the corresponding CoA-ester

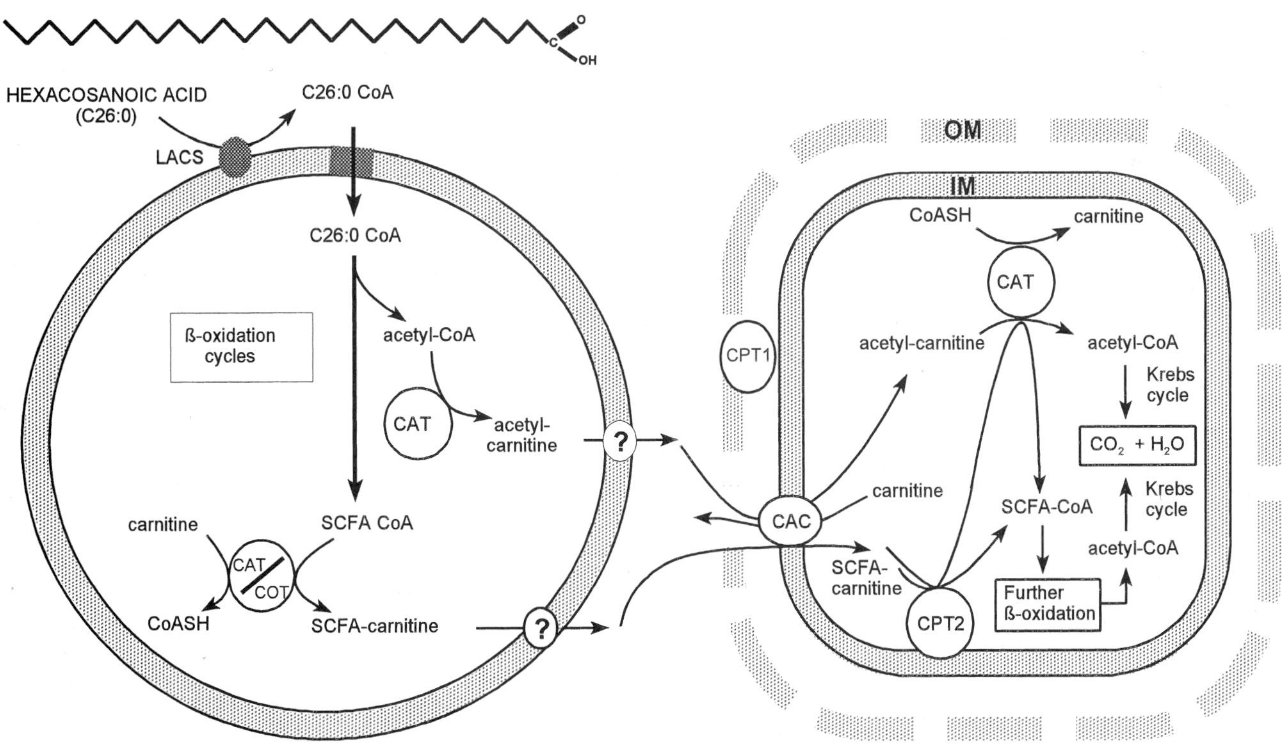

Fig. 130-2 Representation of the intracellular oxidation of C26:0 and the involvement of both peroxisomes and mitochondria. Abbreviations used: CAC = carnitine:acylcarnitine carrier; CAT = carnitine acetyltransferase; COT = carnitine octanoyltransferase; CPT = carnitine palmitoyltransferase; C2 = acetylcarnitine; C3 = propionylcarnitine; IM = inner mitochondrial membrane; LACS = long chain acyl-CoA synthetase; OM = outer mitochondrial membrane; SCFA-CoA = short-chain fatty acyl-CoA; SCFA-carnitine = short-chain fatty acylcarnitine.

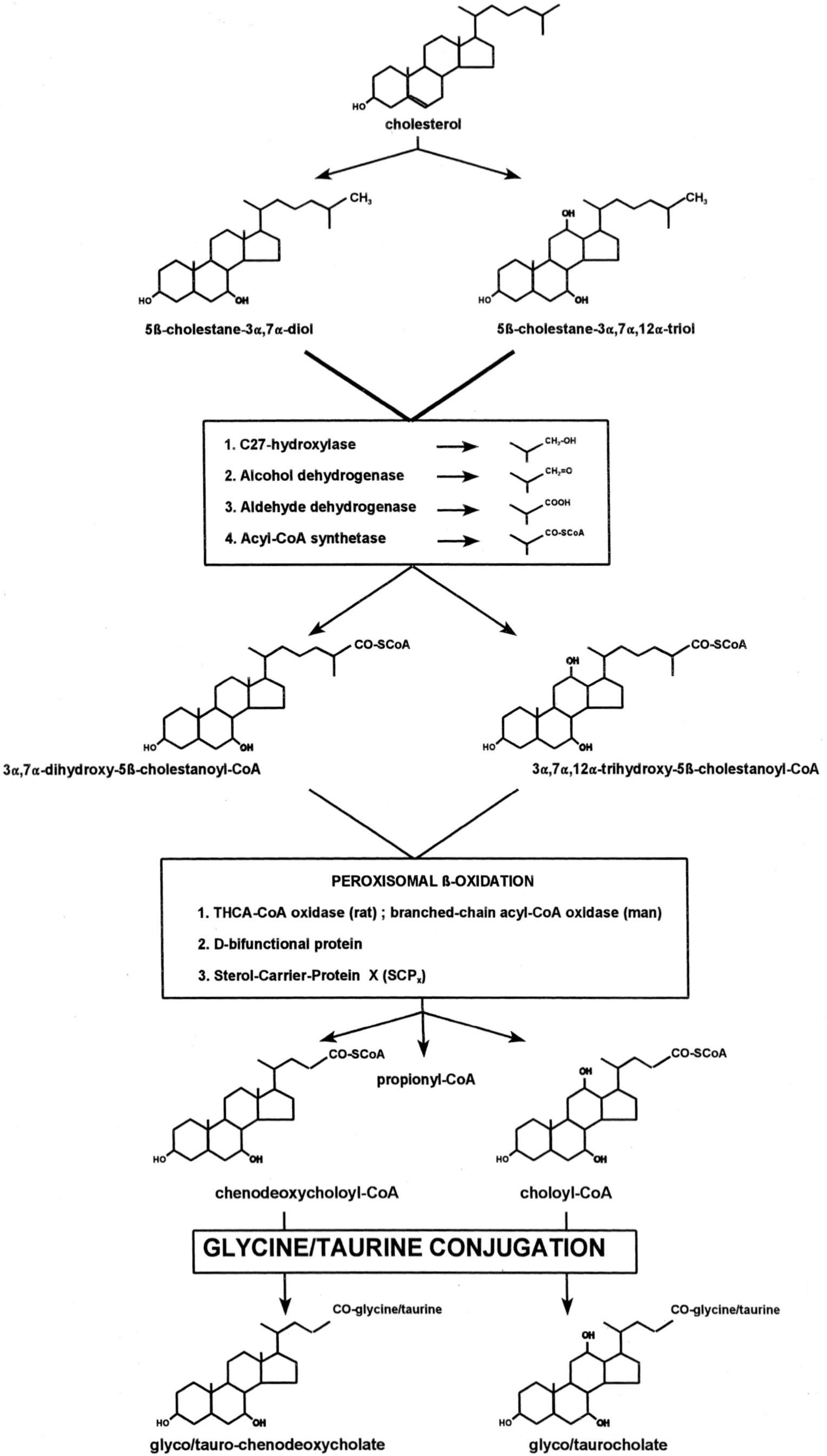

Fig. 130-3 Formation of glyco/taurochenodeoxycholate and glyco/taurocholate from cholesterol. See text for background information.

via CPT2, which is then further degraded by the mitochondrial β-oxidation system (Fig. 130-1).

7.3 β-Oxidation of di- and trihydroxycholestanoic acid (bile acid synthesis). Di- and trihydroxycholestanoic acid are formed in the liver from cholesterol via a complicated set of reactions and are the immediate precursors of chenodeoxycholic acid and cholic acid, respectively. Activation of the two cholestanoic acids occurs at the endoplasmic reticulum membrane.[41] The CoA-esters enter the peroxisome probably via a transport protein possibly made up from two half-ABC transporters as discussed before.

The two cholestanoyl-CoAs are subsequently chain-shortened by one cycle of β-oxidation in the peroxisome, after which the two CoA-esters that are produced, chenodeoxycholoyl-CoA and choloyl-CoA, are transformed into their glycine or taurine conjugates via a specific transferase.[42] This is followed by exit of the conjugates from the peroxisome (Fig. 130-3).

7.4 β-Oxidation of tetracosahexaenoic acid (C24:6 n-3) to docosahexaenoic acid (C22:6 n-3) and the biosynthesis of polyunsaturated fatty acids. Until recently, it was thought that the biosynthesis of docosahexaenoic acid (C22:6 n-3, DHA) from α-linolenic acid occurs by alternating rounds of desaturation and elongation (see Fig. 130-4). However, evidence for the existence of a distinct Δ4-desaturase remained elusive. Elegant studies by Sprecher and coworkers[43] have established the existence of a completely different mechanism in which C22:5 n-3 is converted into C22:6 n-3 via a three-step pathway: (1) microsomal chain elongation of C22:5 to C24:5, followed by (2) desaturation to C24:6 and (3) β-oxidation of C24:6 to C22:6. Subsequent studies[44] showed that β-oxidation of C24:6 to C22:6 is strictly peroxisomal (see reference 45 for a review).

In addition to the compounds listed above which are of direct relevance to human disease, a series of other fatty acids and fatty acid derivatives are known to be β-oxidized in peroxisomes. These include:

7.5 Eicosanoids. Enzymatic oxygenation of polyunsaturated C_{20} fatty acids leads to the formation of a broad range of compounds collectively known as eicosanoids. The three major pathways of eicosanoid formation are (a) the cyclooxygenase pathway leading to prostaglandins and thromboxanes, (b) the lipoxygenase pathway leading to hydroxy fatty acids, leukotrienes and lipoxins, and (c) the cytochrome P450 pathway leading to various epoxy- and hydroxy-metabolites. β-Oxidation is a major mechanism for inactivation of most of these eicosanoids. Many eicosanoids first undergo an initial ω-oxidation followed by β-oxidation as discussed briefly below (see reference 46 for a review):

7.5.1 Prostaglandins.

(a) **Prostaglandins of the F-family** include prostaglandin F2α as the main representative. The main urinary metabolite of prostaglandin F2α is 5α, 7α-dihydroxy-11-ketotetranor-prosta-1,16-dioic acid in rat, monkey, and man, which implies that the molecule has been chain-shortened by two cycles of β-oxidation. Diczfalusy and coworkers[47] reported that this metabolite was *not* present in urine from Zellweger patients, suggesting that β-oxidation of prostaglandin F2α is predominantly, if not exclusively, peroxisomal.

(b) **Prostaglandins of the E-family** include prostaglandin E1 and E2, which both undergo β-oxidation. In vivo loading studies show that 5β,7α-dihydroxy-11-ketotetranorprostanoic acid is the main urinary metabolite, indicating two cycles of β-oxidation. The site of β-oxidation has not been studied.

(c) **Prostaglandins of the D-family** include prostaglandin D2, which produces 9,11-dihydroxy-15-oxo-2,3,18,19-tetranorprost-5-ene-1,20-dioic acid as the main urinary metabolite after intravenous infusion into a male volunteer, indicating two cycles of β-oxidation.

(d) **Prostaglandin I_2 (prostacyclin)** is produced by blood vessels, is a powerful inhibitor of platelet aggregation, and undergoes rapid metabolism in the liver via either β-oxidation or glucuronic acid conjugation. Intravenous administration of radiolabeled prostacyclin revealed a range of metabolites including dinor and tetranor derivatives, implying one or two rounds of β-oxidation. Again, the true site of β-oxidation has not been established.

7.5.2 Thromboxanes such as thromboxane B_2 also undergo β-oxidation. The major metabolite of thromboxane B_2 is 2,3-dinor-thromboxane B_2, which is the product of one cycle of β-oxidation. Diczfalusy et al.[48] reported that 2,3-dinor-thromboxane B_2 was undetectable in urine from Zellweger patients indicating that thromboxane B_2 is predominantly, if not exclusively, β-oxidized in peroxisomes (see also reference 49).

7.5.3 Leukotrienes such as leukotriene B_4, C_4, and E_4 also undergo β-oxidation. Oxidation of LTB_4 appears to take place in both peroxisomes and mitochondria whereas LTE_4 oxidation was strictly peroxisomal as concluded from both in vitro[50] and in vivo[51] studies in Zellweger patients, which revealed strongly increased urinary LTE_4 levels, whereas ω-carboxytetranor-LTE_4, the main urinary product, was completely lacking.[51]

7.5.4 5-, 12-, and 15-Hydroxyeicosatetraenoic acid (HETE) are produced by different lipoxygenases that introduce one molecule of oxygen into polyunsaturated fatty acids containing a 1,4-*cis*, *cis*-pentadiene system. The hydroperoxides are rapidly reduced to the corresponding hydroxy fatty acids in vivo. Studies in a variety of systems show that especially 12- and 15-HETE are readily β-oxidized to shorter-chain products. Studies in Zellweger fibroblasts established that both 12- and 15-HETE are primarily β-oxidized in peroxisomes.[52]

7.6 Long chain dicarboxylic acids. Dicarboxylic acids are formed via ω-oxidation of monocarboxylic acids, especially under conditions of fatty acid overload or in case of an impairment in mitochondrial fatty acid β-oxidation. The first step in the ω-oxidation process involves a cytochrome P450-dependent hydroxylase present in the endoplasmic reticulum followed by oxidation of the ω-hydroxy fatty acid to the corresponding aldehyde and subsequently to the dicarboxylic acid. Activation of long chain dicarboxylic acids occurs at the endoplasmic reticulum membrane[53] followed by β-oxidation, most likely in peroxisomes.[54] It remains to be established at which level β-oxidation of long chain dicarboxylic acids stops.

7.7 Mono- and polyunsaturated fatty acids. There is relatively little information on the precise site of oxidation of mono- and polyunsaturated fatty acids. Based on studies in peroxisome-deficient fibroblasts from Zellweger patients, erucic acid (C22:1 n-9),[55] adrenic acid (C22:4 n-6),[56] and tetracosanoic acid (C24:4 n-6)[57] have been suggested to be oxidized in peroxisomes. The results by Street et al.[57] were questioned by data from the same group[58] showing normal oxidation of C24:4 n-6 in peroxisome-deficient cells. The only difference between the two studies was the use of cells in monolayer[57] or cells in suspension.[58] This obviously needs further study. As discussed above (see 7.4), β-oxidation of tetracosahexanoic acid (C24:6 n-3) to docosahexaenoic acid (C22:6 n-3), the last step in the biosynthesis of this polyunsaturated fatty acid from α-linolenic acid, also occurs in peroxisomes.[44]

Poulos and coworkers[59–61] reported the accumulation of a homologous series of C_{26} to C_{38} polyenoic acids in the brain of Zellweger patients, which suggests that peroxisomes play a major role in the β-oxidation of these fatty acids, too.

7.8 Xenobiotics with aliphatic side chains are often excreted as metabolites possessing a carboxyl side chain shortened by an even number of carbon atoms. This suggests that these

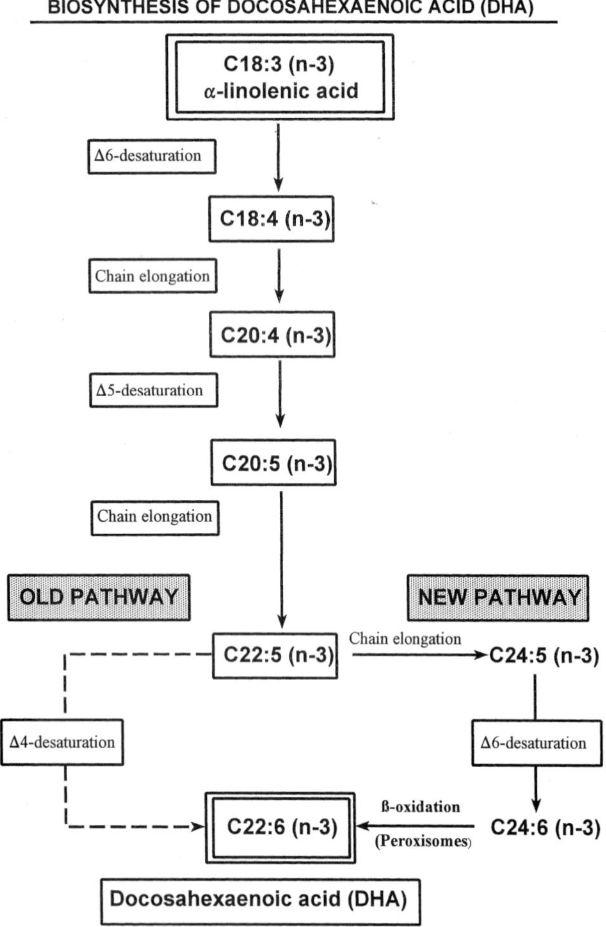

Fig. 130-4 Illustration of the pathway involved in docosahexaenoic acid (DHA) formation. α-Linolenic acid undergoes Δ6-desaturation, chain elongation, Δ5-desaturation, and elongation again, to produce clupanodonic acid (C22:5 n-3). It was long believed that clupanodonic acid undergoes Δ4-desaturation via a Δ4-desaturase. Recent studies, however, show that conversion of C22:5 to C22:6 involves subsequent steps of chain elongation, desaturation, and peroxisomal β-oxidation. See text for more details.

metabolites are formed via ω-oxidation of the terminal methyl-group followed by β-oxidation. Until now, only a few xenobiotics with a carboxyl side chain have been studied.[62–66] In all cases, these compounds were good substrates for peroxisomes, but only poorly handled by mitochondria.

ENZYMOLOGY OF THE PEROXISOMAL β-OXIDATION SYSTEM

Multiple Acyl-CoA Oxidases, Hydratases/3-Hydroxyacyl-CoA Dehydrogenases and Thiolases

In the last few years much has been learned about the enzymes involved in peroxisomal β-oxidation, and it is now clear that the enzymatic organization of the peroxisomal system is much more complicated than originally envisaged. Indeed, until recently it was thought that a single set of β-oxidation enzymes characterized and purified by Hashimoto and coworkers[9,67–69] (see Hashimoto[70] for a review) including acyl-CoA oxidase, bifunctional protein, and peroxisomal thiolase, was involved in the chain-shortening of peroxisomal fatty acids, but this view has dramatically changed now.

Multiple Peroxisomal Acyl-CoA Oxidases. The first peroxisomal acyl-CoA oxidase was purified and characterized by Osumi et al.[9] from rat liver. The substrate specificity of this enzyme was analyzed in detail but did not include pristanoyl-CoA and trihydroxycholestanoyl-CoA as substrates simply because these substrates were discovered as true peroxisomal substrates only much later. The first indication that there had to be another acyl-CoA oxidase came from studies in patients with a deficiency of the classic acyl-CoA oxidase, now called straight-chain acyl-CoA oxidase (LCAX) or acyl-CoA oxidase 1 (ACOX1). Indeed, in such patients, plasma VLCFA levels were greatly increased, whereas the plasma levels of pristanic acid and di- and trihydroxycholestanoic acid were completely normal.[71]

Subsequent studies have clearly established the presence of multiple oxidases. In the rat, two additional peroxisomal acyl-CoA oxidases have been identified. One is pristanoyl-CoA oxidase, which accepts both pristanoyl-CoA and straight-chain acyl-CoAs as substrate.[72,73] Pristanoyl-CoA oxidase is a homohexamer of 70-kDa subunits, is expressed in multiple tissues, and is not induced by hypolipidemic drugs. The third oxidase is expressed in liver only and reacts with di-and trihydroxycholestanoyl-CoA, but not with pristanoyl-CoA.[74,75]

Remarkably, the situation is different in humans in which there are only two oxidases, one straight-chain acyl-CoA oxidase strongly resembling the clofibrate-inducible rat enzyme and the other a branched-chain acyl-CoA oxidase (ACOX2) reacting with *both* pristanoyl-CoA *and* the cholestanoyl-CoA esters (see Fig. 130-5).[10]

The genes encoding the rat[76] and human[77–79] straight-chain acyl-CoA oxidases have all been identified. The same is true for rat pristanoyl-CoA oxidase[80] and rat trihydroxycholestanoyl-CoA oxidase.[81] Finally, the human branched-chain acyl-CoA oxidase has also been characterized at the molecular level.[82]

L- and D-Bifunctional Protein. Early studies by Hashimoto and coworkers have led to the identification of a bifunctional protein with both hydratase and 3-hydroxyacyl-CoA dehydrogenase activities.[67] Interestingly, this protein was also found to harbor

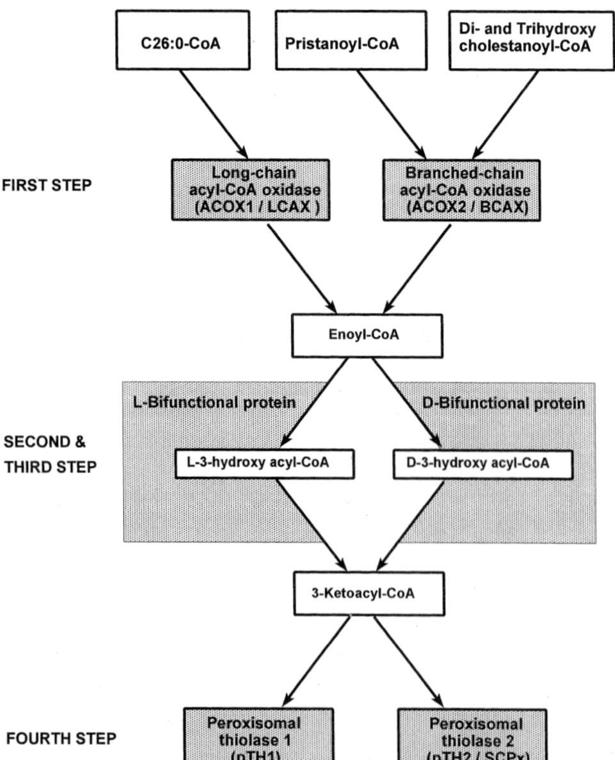

Fig. 130-5 Representation of the peroxisomal enzymes involved in the β-oxidation of C26:0-CoA, pristanoyl-CoA and di- and trihydroxycholestanoyl-CoA.

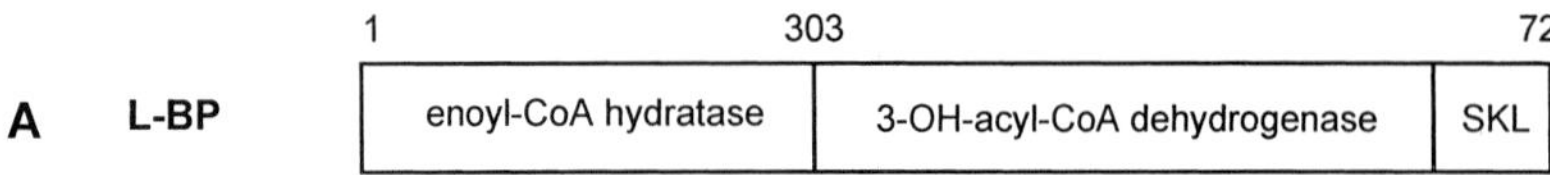

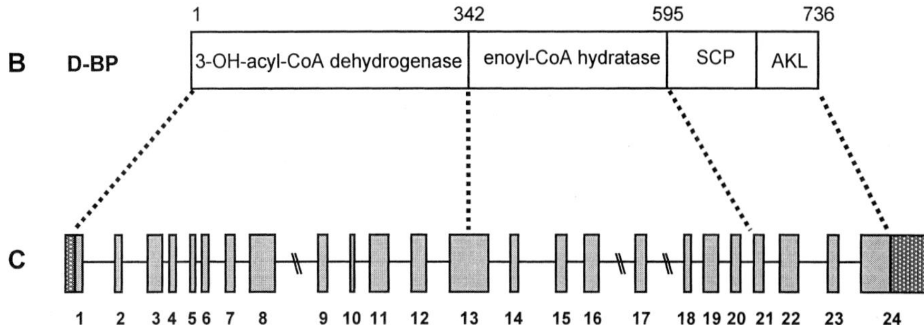

Fig. 130-6 Comparison of the human cDNAs encoding L-BP (A) and D-BP (B). The N-terminal domain of L-BP encodes the enoyl-CoA hydratase and the C-terminal domain encodes the 3-hydroxyacyl-CoA dehydrogenase. In D-BP, the N-terminal domain encodes the 3-hydroxyacyl-CoA dehydrogenase, the middle part encodes the enoyl-CoA hydratase, and the C-terminal domain encodes SCP2. The gene encoding D-BP (C) spans more than 100 kb and consists of 24 exons and 23 introns.[370]

isomerase activity.[83] It is now clearly established that there is also a second bifunctional protein. Several groups identified this protein at about the same time. Using different substrates and peroxisomes from normal-fed rats, Novikov et al.[84] did a systematic study and identified four different 3-hydroxyacyl-CoA dehydrogenases. These studies led to the identification of a new bifunctional protein specifically reacting with the enoyl-CoA esters of di- and trihydroxycholestanoic acid.[85] Coming from a completely different direction Adamski and coworkers reported that the protein they had identified earlier as a 17β-hydroxysteroid dehydrogenase[86] localized in peroxisomes,[87] also exhibited enoyl-CoA hydratase and 3-hydroxyacyl-CoA dehydrogenase activity, whereas the aminoterminal end had strong homology with sterol-carrier-protein 2.[88] Coming from yet another direction, the group of Hiltunen[89] identified the same protein in systematic studies on the presence of enoyl-CoA hydratases in rat liver, elaborating on earlier work from the same group.[90] Finally, this protein was also identified by Hashimoto and coworkers.[91–94] A remarkable aspect of the newly identified bifunctional enzyme is that conversion of *trans*-2-enoyl-CoA esters as produced by the various oxidases, into the corresponding 3-keto compounds does not proceed via a L-3-hydroxyacyl-CoA intermediate, as is the case for the original bifunctional enzyme identified by Hashimoto et al.,[67] but proceeds instead via a D-3-hydroxy intermediate (Fig. 130-5).

Different names have been given to this enzyme including 17β-hydroxysteroid dehydrogenase IV (HSD17B4),[88,95] peroxisomal multifunctional enzyme II (per MFEII),[89] multifunctional protein 2 (MFP2),[85] and peroxisomal multifunctional β-oxidation protein 2 (pMOP2).[96] The name multifunctional protein or enzyme may be confusing especially because a mitochondrial multifunctional enzyme with hydratase, 3-hydroxyacyl-CoA dehydrogenase, and thiolase activity has also been identified (see reference 70 for a review). Hashimoto and coworkers[91–94] coined the name D-bifunctional protein for the newly identified enzyme and renamed the original bifunctional protein as L-bifunctional protein. In the absence of a generally agreed nomenclature, we use L-bifunctional protein (L-BP) and D-bifunctional protein (D-BP) throughout this text.

Importantly, substrate specificity studies revealed clear differences between the two enzyme proteins. First, both enzymes were found to react with straight-chain enoyl-CoAs such as crotonyl-CoA and hexadecenoyl-CoA as substrate.[94] Second, Jiang et al.[94] reported that enoyl-CoA esters with a methyl-group at the 2-position were only handled by D-bifunctional protein and not L-bifunctional protein. One of the substrates tested was (24E)-3α,7α,12α-trihydroxy-5β-cholest-24-enoyl-CoA, the first intermediate in the degradation of 3α,7α,12α-trihydroxy-5β-cholestanoyl-CoA (THC-CoA) to choloyl-CoA. This substrate was handled exclusively by D-BP,[94] indicating that D-BP plays an indispensable role in bile acid synthesis, that is, β-oxidation of THC-CoA. Data from Dieuaide et al.[97] support this conclusion. According to Jiang et al.[94] and Dieuaide et al.,[98] 2-methylhexadecenoyl-CoA is also exclusively handled by D-BP. This is disputed by Qin et al.[89] who reported that pristenoyl-CoA and 2-methyltetradecenoyl-CoA are handled by both D-BP and L-BP. Our finding that pristanic acid β-oxidation is completely deficient in patients lacking D-bifunctional protein,[99] indicates that D-BP is indispensable for both the oxidation of pristanic acid as well as trihydroxycholestanoic acid (THCA).

It should be noted that Xu and Cuebas[100] had already concluded that the classic L-bifunctional enzyme could not be involved in the β-oxidation of di- and trihydroxycholestanoyl-CoA because hydration of the (24E)-7α,12α,15α-trihydroxycholestene-24-enoyl-CoA by L-BP generates 24R,25S-varanoyl-CoA and not 24R,25R-varanoyl-CoA, which is the true in vivo intermediate.[101]

The two bifunctional proteins have been characterized at the molecular level. The cDNA and genomic structure of the gene coding for rat L-bifunctional protein was resolved by Osumi et al.[102] and Ishii et al.,[103] respectively. The cDNA structure of the human L-bifunctional protein is also known.[104] In addition several D-bifunctional proteins from various species have been characterized at the molecular level,[105–109] which includes the cDNA for human D-BP.[110] The complete gene structure of human D-BP was recently resolved.[95] In Fig. 130-6, the cDNAs coding for L-BP and D-BP and the structure of the *D-BP* gene are shown schematically.

Multiple Peroxisomal Thiolases. The first peroxisomal thiolase to be identified and characterized was that discovered by Hashimoto and coworkers.[68,69] The enzyme is synthesized as a 44-kDa precursor and undergoes proteolytic cleavage to the 41-kDa mature protein after import into the peroxisome via the PTS2-route. It is a dimer. Seedorf et al.[111] identified a second peroxisomal thiolase in 1994. The function of this thiolase was initially unclear, but independent studies by Antonenkov et al.[112] and ourselves[96] resolved this problem.

In an effort to establish whether there is a distinct thiolase for the 3-ketoacyl-CoA esters of pristanic acid and di- and trihydroxycholestanoic acid, we measured the 3-ketopristanoyl-CoA thiolase activity in peroxisomes from control and clofibrate-treated rats and found that thiolytic cleavage of 3-ketopristanoyl-CoA was not induced by clofibrate treatment, which argued against a role of the classic thiolase in thiolytic cleavage of 3-ketopristanoyl-CoA.[96] Subsequent studies with purified thiolase 1 (pTH1) and SCPx (peroxisomal thiolase 2; pTH2) showed that 3-ketopristanoyl-CoA and the 3-keto-acylCoA ester of trihydroxycholestanoic acid are handled by SCPx.[96,113] In a systematic study, Antonenkov et al.[111]

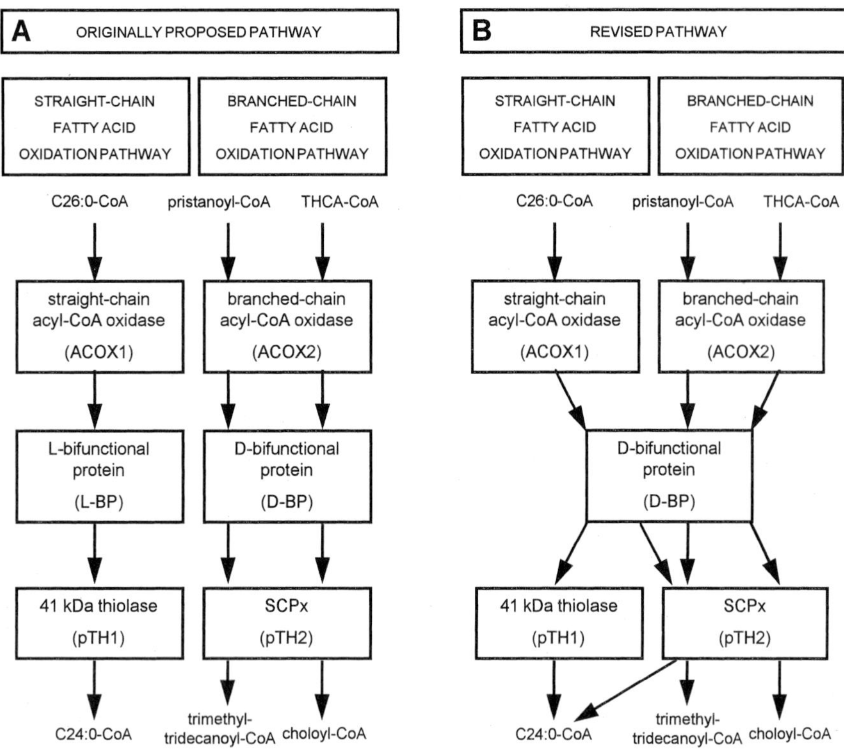

Fig. 130-7 Enzymology of the fatty acid β-oxidation machinery in human peroxisomes involved in the oxidation of straight-chain (C26:0) and 2-methyl branched-chain fatty acids (pristanic acid and trihydroxycholestanoic acid [THCA]). *A* depicts the originally proposed pathway,[127] whereas *B* shows the new, revised pathway described in this chapter. See text for full details.

also found clear evidence for a major role of SCPx in the β-oxidation of 2-methylfatty acids. Very recently, Bunya et al.[114] reached a similar conclusion. The two peroxisomal thiolases have also been characterized at the molecular level.

In the rat, two genes (A and B) for rat peroxisomal 3-ketoacyl-CoA thiolase have been identified.[115,116] Both genes contain 12 exons spanning 8 kb (gene A) and 9.5 kb (gene B). The nucleotide sequences show very high similarity in the exons and in many portions of the introns. Gene A is constitutively expressed at a low level, whereas the transcript of gene B is hardly detectable in normal rat liver but is profoundly induced upon clofibrate feeding.[115,116] The functional significance of these 2 genes is unclear. In humans, there is only a single gene.[117]

Peroxisomal thiolase 2 (SCPx, alternatively called SCP2/3-ketothiolase) has also been characterized at the molecular level.[118] The human gene spans 80 kb and consists of 16 exons. Different transcripts are produced as a result of two different transcription start sites controlled by specific promotors in intron 1 and 12 respectively.[119] The larger transcript codes for the complete 58-kDa protein containing the thiolase domain (amino acids 1 to 404) and the sterol-carrier-protein activity (amino acids 405 to 547).[111,120–122] After import into peroxisomes as mediated by the C-terminal PTS1-signal (AKL) proteolytic cleavage occurs giving rise to a 46-kDa (424 amino acids) thiolase and the 123-amino-acid SCP2 (alternatively called nsL-TP).[123]

When transcription starts at the second site, exons 12 to 16 produce a second transcript coding for a 143-amino-acid containing precursor of sterol-carrier-protein 2, which also undergoes proteolytic cleavage in peroxisomes to produce mature SCP2 (123 amino acids).

Physiological Role of the Various β-Oxidation Enzymes in the Oxidation of Straight-Chain (VLCFA) and 2-Methyl Branched-Chain Fatty Acids (Pristanic Acid and Di- and Trihydroxycholestanoic Acid)

L- and D-Bifunctional Enzyme. The finding that the enoyl-CoA esters of pristanic acid and trihydroxycholestanoic acid are exclusively handled by D-BP and not by L-BP, gives D-BP an indispensable role in 2-methyl branched-chain fatty acid oxidation. This is exemplified by the fact that patients with D-BP deficiency in general show elevated levels of both pristanic acid and trihydroxycholestanoic acid.[99] Remarkably, these patients also have elevated C26:0 levels in plasma, and C26:0 β-oxidation is severely deficient in fibroblasts,[99,124] indicating that D-BP is also the major enzyme in C26:0 β-oxidation.[125]

Peroxisomal Thiolases 1 and 2. Similar considerations apply to the physiological role of peroxisomal thiolases 1 and 2 (SCPx). It is clear that SCPx is the major enzyme involved in pristanic acid and trihydroxycholestanoic acid metabolism. However, SCPx also readily accepts the 3-ketoacyl-CoA esters of straight-chain fatty acids.[96,111,112] It has long been known that patients with RCDP type 1, in which peroxisomal thiolase 1 is lacking from the peroxisomes,[126] have *normal* levels of VLCFAs in plasma and normal C26:0 β-oxidation in fibroblasts. These findings argue against the scheme of Fig. 130-7*A* as proposed by us earlier,[127] and suggest that SCPx may also play a major role in C26:0 β-oxidation. On the other hand, oxidation of C26:0 is completely normal in SCPx-deficient mice,[125,128] suggesting that the two thiolases overlap functionally, at least when C26:0 β-oxidation is concerned. Based on these considerations, we propose the pathway depicted in Fig. 130-7*B*. In this scheme, there is no role for L-bifunctional enzyme. Future studies will show what the true function of L-BP is. The availability of a mouse model lacking L-BP[129] will be important in this respect.

Oxidation of (Poly) Unsaturated Fatty Acids in Peroxisomes: Involvement of Specific Isomerases and Dienoyl-CoA Reductases. Oxidation of unsaturated fatty acids requires the participation of additional, auxiliary enzymes. Fatty acids with a double bond at an odd-numbered position require Δ^3, Δ^2-enoyl-CoA isomerase as auxiliary enzyme, whereas another auxiliary enzyme (2,4-dienoyl-CoA reductase) participates in the β-oxidation of fatty acids with a double bond at an even-numbered position.[130] The differential involvement of Δ^3, Δ^2-enoyl-CoA isomerase and 2,4-dienoyl-CoA reductase in the oxidation of the two C18 monounsaturated fatty acids oleate (C18:1 n-9) and petroselineate

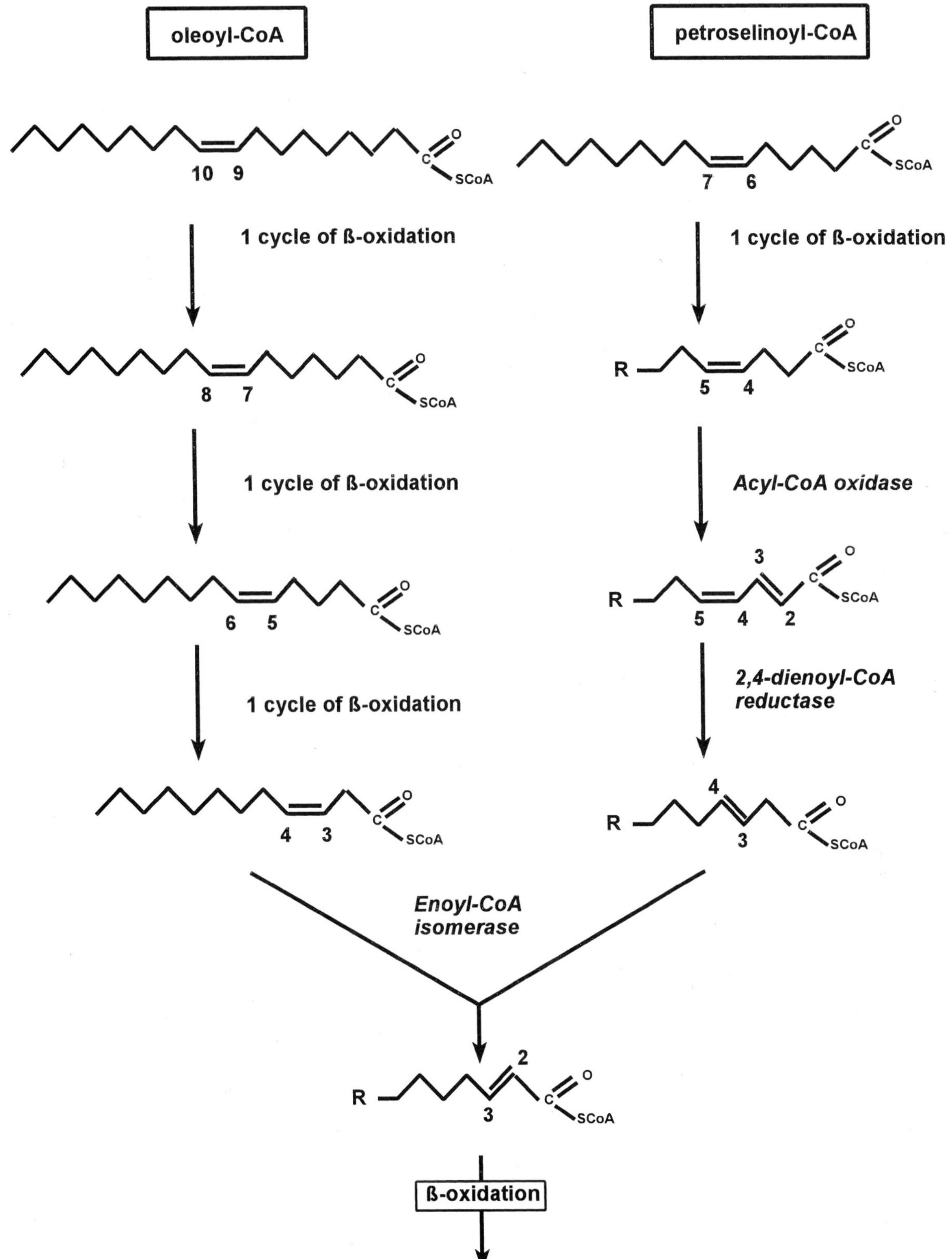

Fig. 130-8 Representation of the enzymes involved in the degradation of unsaturated fatty acids with a double bond at an odd-numbered or even-numbered carbon atom. The differential involvement of Δ^3, Δ^2-enoyl-CoA isomerase and 2,4-dienoyl-CoA reductase in the oxidation of two representative fatty acids, oleate, and petroselineate, is shown. In oleate (C18:1 n-9), the double bond is positioned at an odd-numbered position, whereas in petroselineate, the double bond is at an even-numbered position.

(C18:1 n-6) with a double bond at an odd- or even-numbered position, respectively, is shown in Fig. 130-8.

Δ^3, Δ^2-Enoyl-CoA isomerases catalyze the isomerization of both 3-*cis*- and 3-*trans*-enoyl-CoAs to the corresponding 2-*trans*-enoyl-CoAs. In yeast, isomerization of 3-enoyl-CoAs to 2-enoyl-CoAs is strictly peroxisomal.[131] In higher eukaryotes, however, isomerase activity has been found in both mitochondria and peroxisomes, and the existence of multiple isomerases has been suggested. A short-chain specific isomerase has been purified from various sources, including rat liver, and the corresponding cDNA has been cloned.[132–134] The human cDNA sequence is also known.[135] The active enzyme is a homodimer of two 30-kDa subunits. A second mitochondrial isomerase with specificity for medium and long chain substrates has also been identified and partially purified,[136] but not yet characterized at the molecular level.

Until recently, the situation with respect to peroxisomal isomerases was unclear. Palosaari and Hiltunen[83] have shown that the L-specific bifunctional protein identified by Hashimoto and coworkers[67] also possesses Δ^3, Δ^2-enoyl-CoA isomerase activity as an intrinsic feature of the enzyme making it in fact a trifunctional enzyme. Remarkably, D-specific multifunctional hydratase/3-hydroxyacyl-CoA dehydrogenase β-oxidation enzymes like the *S. cerevisiae* Fox2 protein do not possess isomerase activity,[137] which implies the existence of distinct enoyl-CoA isomerases, at least in yeast. Recent studies by Gurvitz et al.[138] and Geisbrecht et al.[139] have led to the identification of *YLR284C* as the gene coding for the peroxisomal Δ^3, Δ^2-enoyl-CoA isomerase. The corresponding mouse and human cDNAs were rapidly identified making use of the database of expressed sequence tags (dbEST).[140]

2,4-Dienoyl-CoA reductases catalyze the NADPH-dependent reduction of *trans*-2, *cis/trans*-4-dienoyl-CoA into *trans*-3-enoyl-CoA, at least in eukaryotes. Reductases have been purified from various organisms.[141] Mammals possess at least two mitochondrial reductases and a third peroxisomal one.[142,143] The rat[144] and human[145] cDNAs for the 120-kDa mitochondrial isoform have been cloned. The peroxisomal isoform has remained uncharacterized at the molecular level, until very recently. Independent studies by Gurvitz et al.[146] and Van Roermund et al.[147] in the yeast *S. cerevisiae* have led to the cloning of the gene coding for the peroxisomal dienoyl-CoA reductase. A disruption strain was unable to use petroselineate as the sole carbon source, whereas growth on oleate was normal.[146,147] Very recently, both the mouse[148] and human[149] cDNAs coding for peroxisomal 2,4-dienoyl-CoA reductase were identified.

Recent studies have shown that the oxidation of unsaturated fatty acids is more complicated than originally envisaged. The first clue came from studies by Tserng and Jin[150] on the oxidation of 5-enoyl-CoA esters in mitochondria. According to the generally accepted classic pathway, 5-enoyl-CoAs would undergo one cycle of β-oxidation to produce the 3-enoyl-CoA followed by isomerization by the Δ^3, Δ^2-enoyl-CoA isomerase to the 2-enoyl-CoA, which can then undergo further β-oxidation. According to this scheme, no NADPH is required. Tserng and Jin,[150] however, found clear evidence for the obligatory involvement of NADPH and suggested that the 5-enoyl-CoA is directly reduced by a putative NADPH-dependent reductase. Careful studies by Schulz and coworkers[151] failed to identify such an enzyme. Instead, these authors identified a new pathway for the reductive removal of odd-numbered double bonds that involves a new enzyme, $\Delta^{3,5}$, $\Delta^{2,4}$-dienoyl-CoA isomerase. This isomerase, together with 2, 4-dienoyl-CoA reductase and Δ^3, Δ^2-enoyl-CoA isomerase, facilitates the reduction of odd-numbered double bonds (see Fig. 130-9). It remains to be established whether *all* 5-enoyl-CoA esters require the $\Delta^{3,5}$, $\Delta^{2,4}$-dienoyl-CoA isomerase for β-oxidation. Future studies will also have to reveal which unsaturated fatty acids with odd-numbered double bonds are handled by pathway 1 or 2 of Fig. 130-9.

Direct enzyme activity measurements have shown the presence of $\Delta^{3,5}$, $\Delta^{2,4}$-dienoyl-CoA isomerase activity in mitochondria.[152,153] Originally, no $\Delta^{3,5}$, $\Delta^{2,4}$-dienoyl-CoA isomerase activity could be detected in peroxisomes.[153] The observation by Sprecher and coworkers[154] that odd-numbered double bonds are reductively removed during the β-oxidation of arachidonic acid in peroxisomes, suggested the presence of $\Delta^{3,5}$, $\Delta^{2,4}$-dienoyl-CoA isomerase activity in peroxisomes, however. A careful reinvestigation led to the identification of $\Delta^{3,5}$, $\Delta^{2,4}$-dienoyl-CoA isomerase activity in peroxisomes.[155] The mitochondrial $\Delta^{3,5}$, $\Delta^{2,4}$-dienoyl-CoA isomerase was purified by Luo et al.[153] and Chen et al.[152] with conflicting results. Indeed, according to Chen et al.,[152] the enzyme is a tetramer of four identical subunits of 55 kDa each, whereas Luo et al.[153] concluded that the enzyme is a tetramer of four identical 32-kDa subunits.

Recently, Filppula et al.[156] reported the first characterization of a dienoyl-CoA isomerase at the molecular level. These authors showed that the gene identified by FitzPatrick et al.[157] codes for a $\Delta^{3,5}$, $\Delta^{2,4}$-dienoyl-CoA isomerase. Using a subtractive strategy, FitzPatrick et al.[157] identified a peroxisome proliferator-induced rat liver cDNA belonging to the group of hydratases/isomerases. Expression of the cDNA in a bacterial expression system by Filppula et al.[156] showed that the recombinant protein had abundant $\Delta^{3,5}$, $\Delta^{2,4}$-dienoyl-CoA isomerase activity. Interestingly, the 36-kDa isomerase appears to have two targeting signals, a potential mitochondrial targeting signal located at the N-terminus and a true peroxisomal targeting signal type 1 (SKL) at the C-terminal end, which may explain the dual localization of this enzyme. Importantly, transport of the 36-kDa protein into mitochondria is associated with cleavage of the N-terminal sequence, resulting in a mature mitochondrial form of 32 kDa that compares nicely with the data of Luo et al.[153]

Oxidation of 2-Methyl Branched-Chain Fatty Acids: Racemases and the Stereospecificity of Peroxisomal Fatty Acid Oxidation. Naturally occurring phytanic acid is a mixture of two different diastereomers (3S,7R,11R)- and (3R,7R,11R)-phytanic acid.[158] Because α-oxidation does not affect the hydrogen atom in the β-position, pristanic acid is likewise a mixture of diastereomers, (2R,6R,10R)- and (2S,6R,10R)- pristanic acid. The problem is that all mitochondrial acyl-CoA dehydrogenases and peroxisomal acyl-CoA oxidases[159,160] only act on (2S)-2-methylacyl-CoA esters. This implies the indispensable existence of enzymes able to convert (2R)-methyl-branched-chain fatty acids into the corresponding (2S)-fatty acids, otherwise β-oxidation would be blocked. Such enzymes, called racemases, are known to exist. If the pathway of phytanic acid α-oxidation and the subsequent β-oxidation of pristanic acid is considered, racemases in both mitochondria and peroxisomes are required for full oxidation to CO_2 and H_2O. This is a direct consequence of the fact that both mitochondria and peroxisomes participate in the oxidation of pristanic acid. Indeed, pristanic acid undergoes only three cycles of β-oxidation in the peroxisome after which the chain-shortened acyl-CoA, that is, 4,8-dimethylnonanoyl-CoA, is transported to the mitochondrion in the form of a carnitine ester followed by full oxidation to CO_2 and H_2O in the mitochondrion.[11] When the scheme of Fig. 130-10 is inspected, in which all enzymatic steps involved in the oxidation of both (3R,7R,11R)- and (3S,7R,11R)-phytanic acid are depicted, it is clear that in peroxisomes, racemase activity is required twice, whereas in mitochondria, racemase activity is necessary once to convert (2,6R)-dimethylheptanoyl-CoA into (2,6S)-dimethylheptanoyl-CoA. Studies, notably by Conzelmann and coworkers,[161,162] have led to the identification of a 2-methylacyl-CoA racemase, which can rapidly interconvert a variety of (R)- and (S)-2-methyl-branched-chain acyl-CoA esters. A first racemase was purified from rat liver.[161] It is a 45-kDa monomer. The corresponding rat and mouse cDNA species code for proteins of 361 and 360 amino acids, respectively, which both have a KANL-sequence at the extreme C-terminal end, which is a true peroxisomal targeting signal.[163] The rat and mouse racemases lack an apparent mitochondrial targeting signal.

The same racemase as identified by Schmitz et al.[161,163] is probably also involved in the degradation of trihydroxycholestanoic acid to cholic acid. 3α,7α,12α-Trihydroxy-5β-cholestan-27-oic (THCA) (see Fig. 130-3) is produced from 5β-cholestane-3α,7α,12α-triol via a mitochondrial cytochrome P450-dependent 27-hydroxylase. This enzyme is strictly R-specific[164,165] and thus produces the 25R-diastereoisomer of THCA, which is then activated to the (25R)-THC-CoA ester by microsomal THC-CoA synthetase. After transport across the peroxisomal membrane, the

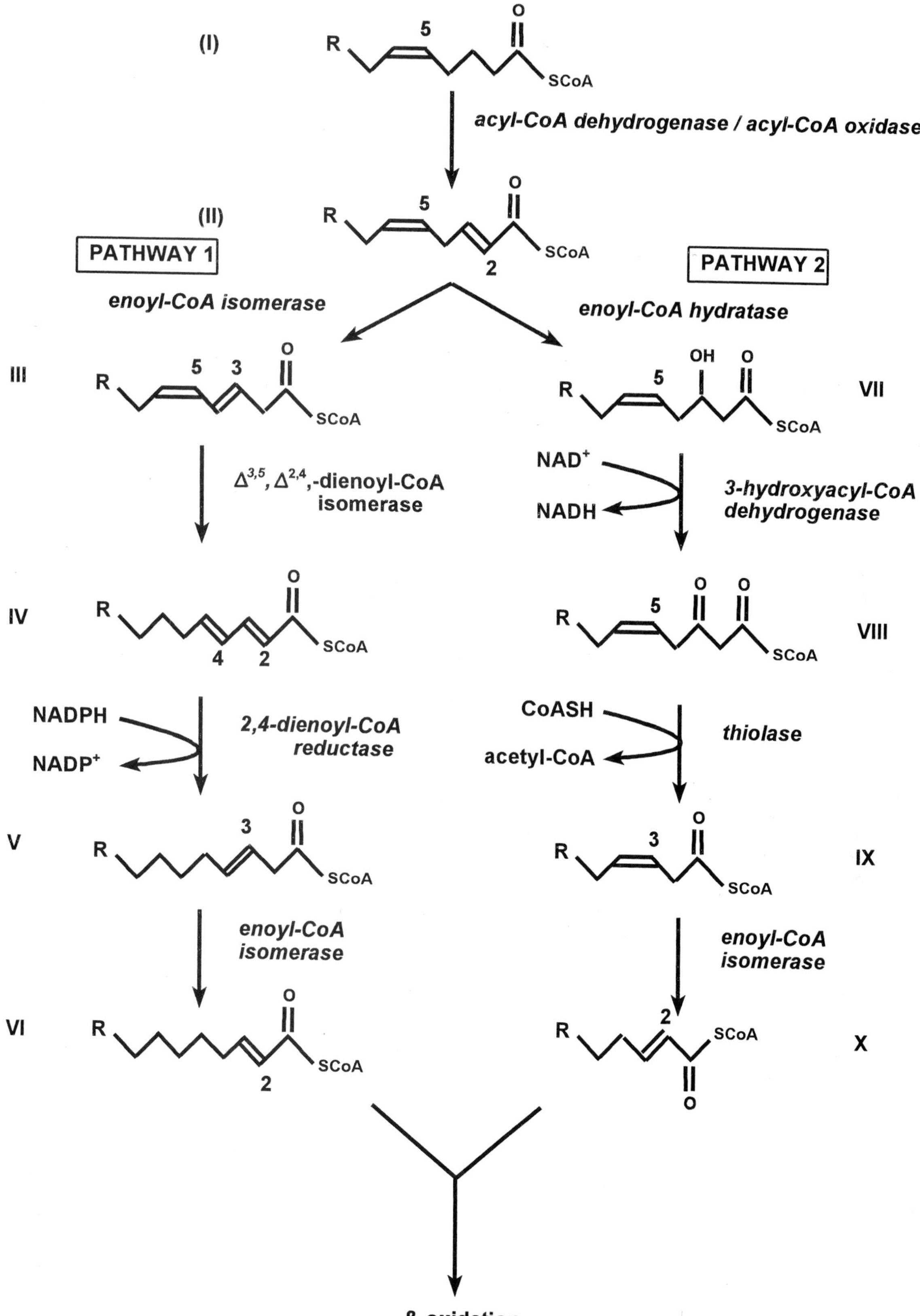

Fig. 130-9 Illustration of the two pathways involved in the oxidation of unsaturated fatty acids with a double bond extending from an odd-numbered carbon atom. *Pathway 1*: The NADPH-dependent reductase pathway. *Pathway 2*: The NADPH-independent isomerase pathway. I = *cis*-5-enoyl-CoA; II = *trans*-2,*cis*-5-dienoyl-CoA; III = *trans*-3,*cis*-5-dienoyl-CoA; IV = *trans*-2,*trans*-4-dienoyl-CoA; V = *trans*-3-enoyl-CoA; VI = *trans*-2-enoyl-CoA; VII = 3-hydroxy-*cis*-5-enoyl-CoA; VIII = 3-keto-*cis*-5-enoyl-CoA; IX = *cis*-3-enoyl-CoA; X = *trans*-2-enoyl-CoA.

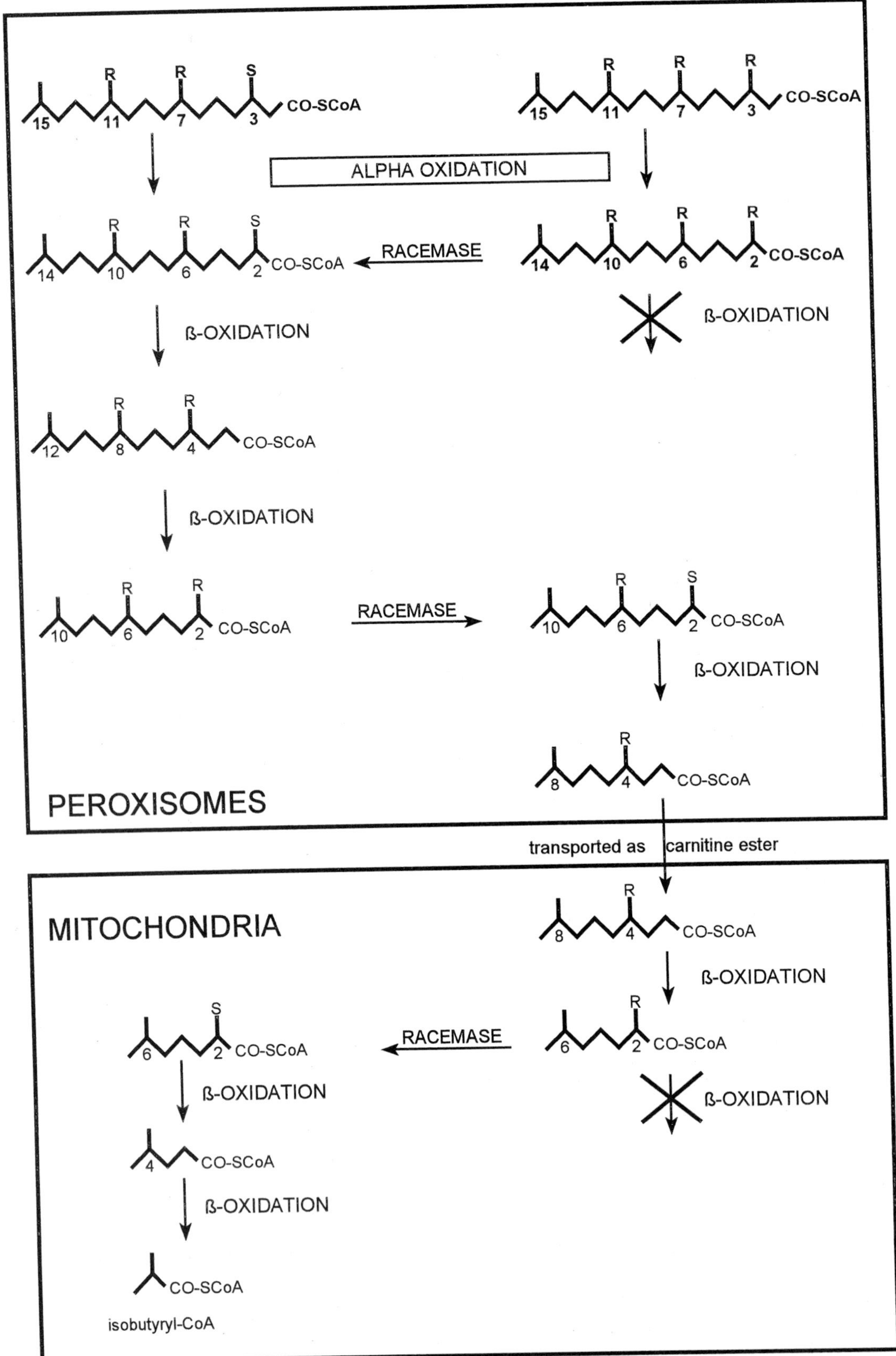

Fig. 130-10 Degradation of phytanic acid and pristanic acid and the involvement of mitochondria and peroxisomes. Naturally occurring phytanic acid is a mixture of both (3S,7R,11R)- and (3R,7R,11R)-phytanic acid. α-Oxidation of the two phytanic acid stereoisomers yields (2S,6R,10R)- and (2R,6R,10R)-pristanic acid, which both undergo β-oxidation as indicated in the figure. Complete oxidation of the two pristanic acid stereoisomers requires the participation of racemase activity in both peroxisomes and mitochondria.

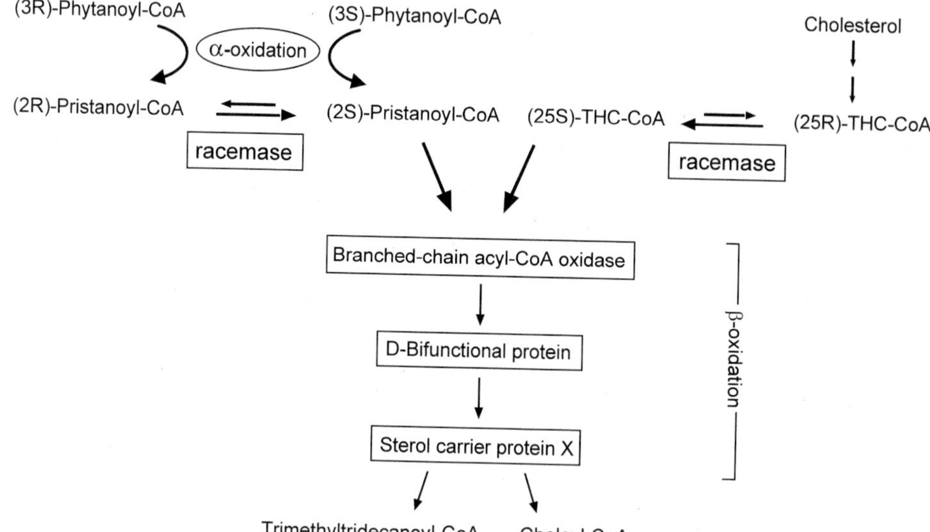

Fig. 130-11 Representation of the steps involved in the oxidation of (3R)- and (3S)-phytanic acid as derived from dietary sources and (25R)-THCA produced from cholesterol in the liver. After the activation of (3R)- and (3S)-phytanic acid to their corresponding CoA esters, they both become substrates for the peroxisomal α-oxidation system, which produces (2R)- and (2S)-pristanoyl-CoA. As branched-chain acyl-CoA oxidase, the first enzyme of the β-oxidation system can only handle the (S)-stereoisomer; (2R)-pristanoyl-CoA needs to be converted by 2-methylacyl-CoA racemase into its (2S)-stereoisomer. The bile-acid intermediates DHCA and THCA are exclusively produced as (25R)-stereoisomers. To be β-oxidized, the CoA esters of the (25R)-stereoisomer also need to be converted by 2-methylacyl-CoA racemase into their (25S)-stereoisomers.

(25R)-THC-CoA must first be converted into the (25S)-THC-CoA ester because this is the true substrate for the acyl-CoA oxidase[159,160] (see Fig. 130-11).

We recently cloned the corresponding human racemase.[166] The human sequence contains an additional 21 amino acids at its N-terminus as compared to the published sequences of the mouse.[163] Translation of the presumed 5′ noncoding regions of the rat and mouse cDNA sequences, however, indicated that the latter two must represent 5′ truncated cDNA species. The human racemase contains a putative type 1 C-terminal peroxisome-targeting signal (−KASL), like the rat (−KANL) and the mouse (−KANL) proteins. In addition, we identified patients with a genetic deficiency of this racemase[166] associated with elevated plasma levels of both pristanic acid and di- and trihydroxycholestanoic acid. These data show that this racemase plays a unique role in the peroxisomal β-oxidation of 2-methyl fatty acids. Interestingly, we recently found that the human racemase is targeted to both mitochondria and peroxisomes by virtue of a double targeting signal in the protein. Furthermore, 2,6-dimethylheptanoyl-CoA turned out to be a good substrate for the recombinant enzyme indicating that a *single* racemase targeted to both mitochondria and peroxisomes catalyzes the three racemization steps required during pristanic acid β-oxidation (Fig. 130-10).

Additional Enzymes Involved in Peroxisomal β-Oxidation

Carnitine Acyltransferases in Peroxisomes. As discussed earlier, it is now clear that during pristanic acid metabolism acetyl-CoA, propionyl-CoA and 4,8-dimethylnonanoyl-CoA leave the peroxisome as carnitine esters,[11,40] which requires the presence of carnitine acyltransferases in peroxisomes (Figs. 130-1 and 130-2). Peroxisomes contain at least three distinct acyltransferases, including carnitine acetyltransferase (CAT),[167,168] carnitine octanoyltransferase (COT),[168,169] and a less-well-characterized medium/long chain acyltransferase.[170] All three enzymes are probably involved in the export of carnitine esters from the peroxisome. Rat carnitine octanoyltransferase was purified by Miyazawa et al.,[169] and the cDNAs for bovine[171] and rat[172] COT have been cloned. We recently cloned the human COT cDNA.[173]

Carnitine acetyltransferase has been purified from different sources including human liver.[174]

Immunoblot analysis in which a monoclonal antibody raised against purified human CAT was used, showed cross-reactive immunologic material in both mitochondria and peroxisomes, although the molecular weight of the two bands differed somewhat.[174] This puzzling observation was resolved by studies from Corti et al.,[175] which revealed that the two forms of human CAT are generated by alternative splicing. In the mRNA encoding the peroxisomal human CAT, the mitochondrial targeting signal (MTS) is disrupted by an intron, so that initiation of translation takes place from a downstream AUG.[175] It appears that the property of one CAT gene coding for two differentially targeted proteins is conserved from yeast to man, although the mechanisms are different. Indeed, the two forms of *S. cerevisiae* CAT are not generated by alternative splicing but by alternative initiation of transcription.[176] The longest mRNA encodes the mitochondrial CAT due to the presence of the MTS, which apparently overrules the peroxisomal targeting signal (AKL). The shorter mRNA initiates downstream of the first AUG. Translation of the shorter mRNA takes place from the second in-frame AUG, resulting in a protein lacking the MTS.[176]

Peroxisomal Acyl-CoA Thioesterases. Acyl-CoA thioesterases, alternatively named acyl-CoA hydrolases, catalyze the hydrolysis of acyl-CoA esters to the free fatty acid plus CoASH. Subcellular fractionation studies have shown the presence of acyl-CoA thioesterase activity in multiple subcellular compartments including mitochondria, microsomes, peroxisomes, and cytosol. Early studies by Osmundsen et al.[177] and Berge et al.[178] revealed the presence of acetyl-CoA, decanoyl-CoA, palmitoyl-CoA, and erucoyl-CoA thioesterase activity in peroxisomes isolated from rat liver. Alexson et al.[179] identified one or more thioesterases in rat brown adipose tissue (BAT) peroxisomes, whereas Bronfman and Leighton[180] demonstrated thioesterase activity in human peroxisomes. Detailed studies by Wilcke and Alexson[181] suggest that peroxisomes contain an inducible short-chain thioesterase active on acetyl-CoA, propionyl-CoA and butyryl-CoA plus one or more medium chain to long chain thioesterases. A long chain acyl-CoA thioesterase was partially purified from isolated peroxisomes and was active only on fatty acyl-CoA species longer than octanoyl-CoA.[181] Until recently, none of the peroxisomal acyl-CoA thioesterases had been resolved at the molecular level. Computer-based screening of the *S. cerevisiae* genome for oleate-induced genes led to the identification of *YJR019C* as the gene coding for a peroxisomal acyl-CoA thioesterase.[182] Disruption of the *YJR019C* gene caused a marked reduction (70 percent) in total cellular thioesterase activity using *n*-decanoyl-CoA as substrate. Importantly, the disruption mutant exhibited a partial growth defect on oleate-containing medium, which stresses the importance of thioesterase activity for fatty acid β-oxidation, although its precise function remains to be established. Jones et al.[182] used the amino acid sequence of YJR019C to scan the EST database. Multiple ESTs were identified, all of which corresponded to a single, previously characterized gene, *hTE*.[183,184] Subsequent studies showed that the product of the *hTE* gene indeed codes for a human peroxisomal thioesterase targeted to peroxisomes via a typical Type 1 peroxisomal targeting signal (−SKL). Recently, Alexson and coworkers[185] cloned four homologous acyl-CoA thioesterases from mouse. Two of these genes were found to code for a cytosolic (CTE-I) and mitochondrial (MTE-I) thioesterase, respectively, whereas the two other genes code for putative peroxisomal thioesterases based on the presence of two presumed type 1 peroxisome-targeting signals (−AKL and −CRL, respectively).[185]

DISORDERS OF PEROXISOMAL β-OXIDATION

Apart from X-linked adrenoleukodystrophy (MIM 300100), only few disorders of peroxisomal β-oxidation have been identified in which the underlying basis has been firmly established. These disorders include (a) acyl-CoA oxidase 1 deficiency, (b) D-bifunctional protein deficiency, (c) peroxisomal thiolase 1 deficiency, and (d) peroxisomal α-methyl-acyl-CoA racemase deficiency.[166]

Acyl-CoA Oxidase Deficiency (Pseudo-Neonatal Adrenoleukodystrophy (NALD)) (MIM 264470)

In 1988, Poll-Thé et al.[37] described two siblings, male and female, from a consanguineous union with neonatal onset hypotonia, delayed motor development, sensory deafness, and retinopathy with extinguished electroretinograms. There was no craniofacial dysmorphia in any of the patients. Although psychomotor development was severely delayed, both patients showed some progress in the first 2 years of life, after which a progressive neurologic regression set in. A cranial CT without contrast enhancement in the neonatal period was minimally abnormal in both patients. At 4 years of age, a repeat cranial CT scan with contrast enhancement was performed in one of the siblings; it revealed bilateral enhancing lesions in the centrum semiovale and a generally hypodense cerebral white matter. Based on these findings, the patients were considered to suffer from neonatal adrenoleukodystrophy (NALD) (MIM 202370). In accordance with this diagnosis, elevated VLCFA levels were found in plasma. However, in contrast to other cases of NALD (see reference 186), normal levels of di- and trihydroxycholestanoic acid, phytanic acid, and pipecolic acid were found. Furthermore, peroxisomes were found to be normally present in liver biopsy specimens from the two patients, although they were enlarged in size and increased in number.[37,187,188]

In fibroblasts from the two patients, C24:0 and C26:0 β-oxidation was found to be strongly deficient, whereas *de novo* plasmalogen synthesis and other peroxisomal parameters were normal, indicating a selective defect in VLCFA β-oxidation. Immunoblot analysis of liver material from one of the patients revealed the absence of the 70-, 50-, and 20-kDa components of acyl-CoA oxidase 1, whereas normal profiles were found for L-bifunctional protein and peroxisomal thiolase 1,[37] thus establishing acyl-CoA oxidase deficiency. The underlying molecular defect was resolved by Fournier et al.[78] who found a large deletion in the acyl-CoA oxidase gene in the two patients.

A second family was reported by Wanders et al.[189] The index patient showed generalized hypotonia, failure to thrive, deafness, hepatomegaly, psychomotor retardation, absent reflexes and frequent convulsions and died at 3 years 11 months. Two additional cases from a single family were described by Suzuki et al.[190] Profound hypotonia, dysmorphic features including hypertelorism, epicanthus, low nasal bridge, low-set ears, and polydactyly were present in both children from the neonatal period. Both siblings showed some development as exemplified by the following milestones in the oldest sibling: head control at 5 months, crawling at 12 months, and walking without assistance at 32 months. Since then, his motor ability regressed and he could not even sit at 41 months. Suzuki et al.[190] used complementation analysis to establish that the defect in the two patients had to be at the level of acyl-CoA oxidase. Using the same strategy, Watkins et al.[191] identified another three patients, which brings the total number of established cases to eight from six families.

Bifunctional Protein Deficiency (MIM 261515)

Bifunctional protein deficiency was first described by Watkins et al.[192] in a male patient with severe hypotonia and neonatal onset seizures. An electroencephalogram revealed multifocal spikes. No developmental progress was observed. There was no dysmorphia and no hepatomegaly. Fontanelles were large with open metopic sutures. Visual-evoked responses and brain stem auditory-evoked responses were grossly abnormal. A brain biopsy at 6 weeks revealed polymicrogyria. The patient died at 5 months of age after a clinical course marked by absent developmental progress and therapy refractory seizures. Visceral autopsy showed minute glomerular cysts in the kidneys, adrenal atrophy with ballooned, lipid-laden cells, and some portal fibrosis in the liver. Neuropathologic studies revealed a polymicrogyric neocortex and focal areas of cortical heterotopia. Based on these clinical features a diagnosis of NALD was considered. Evaluation of peroxisomal metabolites in plasma demonstrated elevated levels of both VLCFA and trihydroxycholestanoic acid with normal values for phytanic acid and pipecolic acid. These findings, plus the observation of abundant peroxisomes in a liver biopsy specimen, clearly distinguished this case from classic NALD.[186] Studies in fibroblasts demonstrated that the defect in this patient was apparently restricted to the peroxisomal β-oxidation pathway. Immunoblot studies of the peroxisomal β-oxidation enzymes revealed the complete absence of L-bifunctional protein in postmortem liver samples, whereas acyl-CoA oxidase and peroxisomal thiolase 1 were present. Immunoblot studies in fibroblasts confirmed this.

Because it is extremely difficult to determine the activity of L-bifunctional protein enzymatically, especially in homogenates, several groups around the world have used complementation analysis to identify new cases of bifunctional protein deficiency.[190,191,193–199] In all these studies, fibroblasts from the patient described by Watkins et al.[192] were used as reference cell line. This strategy has identified more than 40 additional patients. In Table 130-2, data are collected from literature about the clinical features of bifunctional protein deficiency. In general, children with this disorder show severe central nervous system involvement with profound hypotonia (41 of 42), uncontrolled seizures (36 of 38), and failure to acquire any significant developmental milestones. Children are usually full-term and show no evidence of intrauterine growth retardation. Dysmorphic features, including macrocephaly, high forehead, flat nasal bridge, low-set ears, large open fontanelle, and micrognathia, were found in most children. In most cases, neuronal migration is disturbed with areas of polymicrogyria and heterotopic neurons in the cerebrum and cerebellum. A detailed neuropathologic study was done by Kaufmann et al.[200] in a case of bifunctional protein deficiency, which revealed bilateral centrosylvian pachygyria and polymicrogyria, diffuse hemispheric hypomyelination with heterotopic neurons, Purkinje cell heterotopias, and simplified convolutions of the dentate nucleus and inferior olive.

Table 130-2 Clinical Findings in Patients with Established D-Bifunctional Protein Deficiency

	Suzuki et al. (2 patients)	Watkins et al. (15 patients)	Paton et al. (9 patients)	Wanders et al. (18 patients)	Total series
Neonatal hypotonia	2/2 (100%)	15/15 (100%)	7/7 (100%)	17/18 (94%)	41/42 (98%)
Dysmorphic features	2/2 (100%)	11/15 (75%)	5/7 (71%)	12/14 (80%)	30/38 (79%)
Neonatal seizures	2/2 (100%)	14/15 (93%)	9/9 (100%)	11/12 (92%)	36/38 (95%)
Hepatomegaly	1/1 (100%)	ND	4/4 (100%)	3/7 (43%)	8/12 (67%)
Developmental delay	2/2 (100%)	ND	5/5 (100%)	12/12 (100%)	19/19 (100%)
Poor feeding	ND	ND	4/4 (100%)	6/7 (86%)	10/11 (91%)
Neuronal migration defect	ND	7/8 (88%)	1/1 (100%)	7/8 (88%)	15/17 (88%)
Mean age of death	16 months	9 months	7 months	10 months	$10\frac{1}{2}$ months
Consanguinity	1/2 (50%)	ND	5/5 (100%)	10/15 (67%)	16/22 (73%)

The data included in the table were taken from the following papers: Suzuki et al;[190] Watkins et al;[191] Paton et al;[197] and Wanders et al. (in preparation). Data from patients are only included if information about a certain feature is given as being present or absent. ND = not documented.

Bifunctional Protein Deficiency Revisited: Resolution of Its True Enzymatic and Molecular Basis. In 1994, Hoeffler et al.[104] reported the cloning of the cDNA for human L-bifunctional protein, which allowed molecular studies in bifunctional protein-deficient patients. We first concentrated on the patient described by Watkins et al.[192] and found two cDNA species:[124] one cDNA was indistinguishable from the wild-type sequence, whereas in the second cDNA, two nucleotide alterations were found leading to amino acid substitutions of unknown significance in terms of activity. These findings were hard to reconcile with the full deficiency of L-bifunctional protein as found by immunoblot analysis.[192] There was also other evidence suggesting that the defect could not be at the level of L-bifunctional protein. Indeed, as discussed above, studies from a number of groups revealed that the newly identified D-bifunctional protein (and not L-bifunctional protein) is the enzyme involved in di- and trihydroxycholestanoic acid oxidation. Because these two bile-acid intermediates accumulate in virtually all bifunctional protein-deficient patients, including in the case of Watkins et al.,[192] we directed our efforts to D-bifunctional protein and established that the true defect in the patient with presumed L-BP deficiency described by Watkins et al.[192] is at the level of D-bifunctional protein as concluded from enzyme activity measurements and clear-cut mutations in the gene coding for D-bifunctional protein (D-BP).[124] The original observation by Watkins et al.[192] showing the absence of L-BP upon immunoblot analysis, is puzzling and remains unexplained (see reference 124 for discussion).

The finding that D-bifunctional protein is the deficient enzyme in the Watkins case[192] suggested that most patients previously diagnosed as L-bifunctional protein deficient were, in fact, D-BP deficient. This hypothesis was tested in nine patients whose condition was previously diagnosed as L-BP deficiency on the basis of complementation analysis; unambiguous mutations were found in the *D-BP* cDNA from all nine patients.[124] We have now extended these studies to more than 25 patients previously diagnosed as L-BP deficient using a specific enzyme assay for D-bifunctional protein followed by immunoblot/immunofluorescence analysis and 3-DNA analysis. In all cases, the true defect was found in the D-bifunctional protein. So far, no true case of L-bifunctional protein deficiency is known.

D-Bifunctional Protein Deficiency and the Identification of Three Subgroups. Resolution of the true defect in the original patient of Watkins et al.[192] also provided an explanation for another puzzling finding reported by Van Grunsven et al.[199] Using a combined approach based on direct activity measurements of acyl-CoA oxidase 1 and complementation analysis after somatic cell fusion of fibroblasts, these authors classified 13 patients in 4 distinct groups, with 9 of 13 patients in the group of bifunctional protein deficiency.[199] Interestingly, when fusions were carried out with fibroblasts from different patients belonging to this group, clear complementation was found in some of these combinations, leading to the identification of three subgroups within complementation group 2, which represents bifunctional protein deficiency. The authors suggested[199] that this phenomenon may well have to do with the fact that bifunctional protein contains two catalytic activities, including a hydratase and 3-hydroxyacyl-CoA dehydrogenase activity. The recent development of methods to study D-bifunctional protein at the enzyme (activity measurements), protein (immunoblot/immunofluorescence analysis), and molecular levels have allowed confirmation of this hypothesis. In Group 2A, D-bifunctional protein is completely absent, which is associated with the loss of activity of both the hydratase and 3-hydroxyacyl-CoA dehydrogenase components of D-BP. The original patient described by Watkins et al.[192] belongs to this group as shown by Van Grunsven et al.[124] Group 2B in the study of Van Grunsven et al.[199] represents (D-BP)enoyl-CoA hydratase deficiency as described in reference 201, whereas in Group 2C it is the D-3-hydroxyacyl-CoA dehydrogenase component of D-BP that is functionally inactive due to mutations in the part of the *D-BP* gene, which codes for this 3-hydroxyacyl-CoA dehydrogenase part of the D-BP protein. The patient described by Van Grunsven et al.[99] belongs to this group. Enzymatic analysis of D-BP in fibroblasts from the patient revealed normal enoyl-CoA hydratase but deficient 3-hydroxyacyl-CoA dehydrogenase activity (Table 130-3). Subsequent molecular studies identified a G46 → A mutation changing the glycine at position 16 into a serine. The glycine at position 16 is located in an important loop of the Rossman fold forming the NAD-binding site in the dehydrogenase domain of D-BP. This mutation appears to be quite frequent among patients belonging to D-BP subgroup C.[124]

Table 130-3 Biochemical Characteristics of the Peroxisomal β-Oxidation Disorders and Comparison with the Peroxisome Biogenesis Disorders (PBDs)

Parameter measured	Type of peroxisomal disorder						
	Acyl-CoA oxidase deficiency	D-BP deficiency			Thiolase deficiency	Racemase deficiency	PBDs
		IA	IB	IC			
Plasma							
VLCFA	↑	↑	↑	↑	↑	N	↑
THCA	N	↑	N	↑	↑	↑	↑
Pristanic acid (Pris)	N	↑	↑	↑	ND	↑	↑
Phytanic acid (Phyt)	N	↑	↑	↑	ND	N	↑
Pris/Phyt-ratio	N	↑	↑	↑	ND	↑	N
Fibroblasts							
VLCFA	↑	↑	↑	↑	ND	N	↑
Fatty acid oxidation							
C26:0	↓	↓	↓	↓	ND	N	↓
Pristanic acid	N	↓	↓	↓	ND	+/−	↓
Enzyme activities							
Acyl-CoA oxidase 1	↓	N	N	N	ND	N	↓
D-BP activity							
hydratase	N	↓	↓	N	ND	N	↓
3HAD	N	↓	N	↓	ND	N	↓

Abbreviations: ND = not done; +/− means partially deficient

Biochemical Abnormalities in D-Bifunctional Protein Deficiency

Fibroblasts. Studies in fibroblasts from D-BP-deficient patients show that both the oxidation of C26:0 and pristanic acid is deficient. This is not only true for patients with a complete lack of D-BP, such as the patient described by Watkins et al.,[192] but also for patients with a defect in the D-BP at the level of the hydratase (group 2B) or D-3-hydroxyacyl-CoA dehydrogenase component (group 2C) (see Van Grunsven et al.[99,124,201]).

Plasma Metabolites: VLCFAs. In all patients with D-BP deficiency, independent of whether they belong to group 2A, B, or C, VLCFA levels are definitely abnormal, which is important because VLCFA analysis is widely used as an initial screening method for peroxisomal disorders (Table 130-3).

Pristanic and Phytanic Acid. As a consequence of the deficient oxidation of pristanic acid in all types of D-BP deficiency,[99,124,201] pristanic acid is always elevated, provided the patient involved was exposed to phytol-containing foods. If pristanic acid is high, phytanic acid levels are usually also elevated, although to a much lower extent, so that the pristanic acid/phytanic acid ratios are generally much higher as compared to controls. Interestingly, pristanic acid and phytanic acid are usually also elevated in patients affected by a peroxisome biogenesis disorder (PBD), although the pristanic acid/phytanic acid ratio in PBD-patients is usually not elevated.[71] This may help in the initial differential diagnosis of patients as discussed further (see "Postnatal Diagnosis of the Disorders of Peroxisomal β-Oxidation").

Bile Acid Intermediates. Our recent studies clearly show differences between D-BP groups 2A, B, and C with respect to the accumulation of the bile-acid intermediates DHCA and THCA. In case of a complete D-BP deficiency, THCA, DHCA, and the C29-dicarboxylic bile acid accumulate. The same is true for isolated D-3-hydroxyacyl-CoA dehydrogenase deficiency,[99] but not for deficiencies at the level of the hydratase part of D-BP (group 2B). In such patients, we found no THCA, DHCA, and C29.[201] The underlying basis for this peculiar phenomenon is unknown.[201]

Varanic Acid in D-3-Hydroxyacyl-CoA Dehydrogenase Deficiency and the Other Forms of D-Bifunctional Protein Deficiency. Varanoyl-CoA (3α,7α,12α,24-tetrahydroxy-5β-cholestan-26-oyl-CoA) is an intermediate in the β-oxidation of THCA-CoA to choloyl-CoA with a hydroxy group at the β-position. In case of D-3-hydroxyacyl-CoA dehydrogenase deficiency,[99] varanic acid is likely to accumulate. This is also what is observed in vivo: In all patients with a selective defect in the dehydrogenase part of D-BP, varanic acid is very high, which allows easy discrimination between D-BP group C and D-BP groups A and B, respectively, provided that methods used allow resolution of the different varanic acid diastereomers. Vreken et al.[202] have set up a gas chromatography-mass spectrometry method that enables good separation of the four varanic acid diastereomers. A principal feature of this newly developed procedure involves derivatization with 2R-butanol to produce an additional chiral center. Using this technique, the four diastereomers (24S,25S), (24S,25R), (24R,25S) and (24R,25R) resolve as (2R)-butylestertrimethylsilyl-ether derivatives.[202] In patients with an established deficiency of only the D-3-hydroxyacyl-CoA dehydrogenase component of D-bifunctional protein (24R,25R)-varanic acid was most abundant, although there were also significants amounts of the (24R,25S)- and (24S,25S)-diastereomers. The accumulation of (24R,25R)-varanic acid follows logically from the fact that D-bifunctional protein hydrates 24E-3α,7α,12α-trihydroxy-5β-cholest-24-enoyl-CoA (Δ24(E)-THC-CoA) into (24R,25R)-varanoyl-CoA followed by its dehydrogenation to the β-keto compound. Interestingly, in patients with complete D-Bifunctional protein deficiency, no (24R,25R)- and (24R,25S)-varanic acid was found; only (24S,25S)-varanic acid was found.[202]

The accumulation of (24S,25S)-varanic acid results from the reactivity of the enoyl-CoA hydratase part of L-bifunctional protein with Δ24(E)-THC-CoA leading to the specific formation of (24S,25S)-varanoyl-CoA.[100] The accumulation of (24R,25S)-varanic acid in patients with D-3-hydroxyacyl-CoA dehydrogenase deficiency has remained unexplained. That the (24R,25S)-isomer is not observed in complete D-bifunctional protein deficiency suggests that (24R,25S) comes from the (24R,25R)-isomer, possibly catalyzed by the peroxisomal racemase discussed earlier (see "Oxidation of 2-Methyl Branched-Chain Fatty Acids").

Peroxisomal 3-Oxoacyl-CoA Thiolase 1 (PTH1) Deficiency (Pseudo Zellweger Syndrome) (MIM 261510)

In 1986, Goldfischer et al.[203] described a girl, from consanguineous parents, who showed marked facial dysmorphia, muscle weakness, and hypotonia at birth. The patient showed no psychomotor development during her life of 11 months. At autopsy, the patient had renal cysts, atrophic adrenals with striated cells, minimal liver fibrosis, hypomyelination in the cerebral white matter, foci of neuronal heterotopia, and a sudanophilic leukodystrophy. Together, these clinical findings suggested that the patient was affected by Zellweger syndrome. Morphologic analysis of the liver, however, revealed abundant peroxisomes. The subsequent finding that VLCFA in plasma were clearly elevated did suggest a peroxisomal defect possibly restricted to the peroxisomal β-oxidation system. Further proof came when elevated DHCA and THCA-levels were found in a duodenal aspirate. Immunoblot studies revealed the normal presence of the 70-, 50- and 20-kDa components of acyl-CoA oxidase 1 and the 78-kDa L-bifunctional protein, whereas both the 44-kDa precursor form of peroxisomal thiolase 1 and the mature 41-kDa form were completely missing, indicating peroxisomal thiolase deficiency.[204] Unfortunately, cultured skin fibroblasts from the patient are not available, which has severely hampered further studies. It remains to be established whether the primary defect in this patient is, indeed, at the level of peroxisomal thiolase 1 gene or not, especially because there is accumulation of VLCFA in this patient, as well as accumulation of DHCA and THCA. As discussed earlier, β-oxidation of the CoA-esters of DHCA and THCA is catalyzed by branched-chain acyl-CoA oxidase, D-bifunctional protein, and peroxisomal thiolase 2, alternatively called SCPx (see Fig. 130-7*B*). The availability of liver material from the patient allowed us to study the peroxisomal thiolase 1; these studies revealed no mutations in any of the exons (Wanders et al., unpublished). Further studies are underway to resolve the puzzling situation. No additional patients have been described in literature.

Peroxisomal 2-Methylacyl-CoA Racemase Deficiency (MIM 604489): A Newly Identified Peroxisomal Disorder[166]

We recently identified a new defect in the peroxisomal fatty acid β-oxidation pathway in a number of patients suffering from an adult-onset sensory motor neuropathy.[166] Sensory motor neuropathy is associated with inherited disorders including Charcot-Marie-Tooth disease (MIM 118200),[205,206] X-linked adrenoleukodystrophy/adrenomyeloneuropathy,[207] and Refsum disease (MIM 266500) (Chap. 132). In the latter two, the neuropathy is thought to result from the accumulation of VLCFAs and phytanic acid, respectively. We analyzed the plasma of two patients with adult-onset sensory motor neuropathy and additional signs suggesting Refsum disease (patient 1) and X-linked adrenoleukodystrophy (patient 2), and found a similar profile: normal VLCFAs, marginally elevated phytanic acid, and definitely increased levels of the 2-methyl branched-chain fatty acids pristanic acid and di- and trihydroxycholestanoic acid.[166] This suggested a specific defect in the peroxisomal β-oxidation of branched-chain fatty acids, and not in the α-oxidation system, the first enzyme step of which is defective in Refsum disease (Chap. 132). Studies in fibroblasts revealed normal values for all parameters measured except for pristanic acid β-oxidation, which was reduced to 20 to 30 percent of control. We subsequently measured the activities of the enzymes directly involved in the β-oxidation of branched-chain fatty acids, which includes branched-chain acyl-CoA oxidase, D-bifunctional protein, and peroxisomal thiolase 2 (pTH2/SCPx), and found normal values.

We then focused our attention on 2-methylacyl-CoA racemase. As described earlier, (see "Oxidation of 2-Methyl Branched-Chain Fatty Acids"). this enzyme is not directly involved in the β-oxidation process itself, but is important in the β-oxidation of both pristanic acid (Fig. 130-10) and di- and trihydroxycholestanoic acid (Fig. 130-11) because the enzyme catalyzes the interconversion of (2R)- and (2S)-stereoisomers of 2-methyl-branched-chain fatty acyl-CoA esters. The peroxisomal racemase as characterized by Conzelman and coworkers[162,163] accepts pristanoyl-CoA, DHC-CoA, and THC-CoA as substrate. Measurements of racemase activity in fibroblasts from our patients using (25S)-THC-CoA as substrate revealed a complete deficiency of the enzyme.[166] We subsequently cloned the human cDNA that allowed molecular studies in the patients. Clear-cut mutations were found in all patients. Expression studies in *E. coli* showed that the amino acid substitutions resulted in inactive proteins.[166]

The finding of defined abnormalities in patients with late-onset motor neuropathy resulting from a defect in the peroxisomal oxidation of 2-methyl-branched-chain fatty acids at the level of 2-methylacyl-CoA racemase may have major implications for the diagnosis of adult-onset neuropathies of unknown etiology.

UNRESOLVED PEROXISOMAL FATTY ACID β-OXIDATION DISORDERS

In the past, many patients have been described with a defect in peroxisomal β-oxidation of unknown etiology.[208–215] Inspection of the clinical reports of these patients reveals that all patients, except from the case described by Santer et al.,[214] were severely affected with clinical signs and symptoms closely resembling those of established D-bifunctional protein-deficient patients. Preliminary complementation studies (Wanders et al., unpublished) followed by enzymatic and molecular studies of D-BP indicate that in most patients the defect in peroxisomal β-oxidation is caused by a deficient activity of D-bifunctional protein. This is definitely true for the cases described by Clayton et al.,[208] Naidu et al.,[209] Espeel et al.[211] and Van Malderghem et al.[213] (same patient described in both papers), and Van Hole et al.[215]

Di- and Trihydroxycholestanoic Acidemia: Exclusion of Trihydroxycholestanoyl-CoA Oxidase (Branched-Chain Acyl-CoA Oxidase) as the Defective Enzyme. In the past, several patients have been described with di- and trihydroxycholestanoic acidemia.[216–218] Both Christensen et al.[216] and Przyrembel et al.[217] suggested that the defect in their patients had to be at the level of trihydroxycholestanoyl-CoA oxidase. The patient described by Christensen et al.[216] was normal until 18 months of age when her gait became unstable. At age 3 years, severe ataxia of the lower extremities was observed, with dysarthric speech and dry skin. At age 5 years, ataxia had increased, and there was hypotonia and absent reflexes. Hearing was impaired and she was moderately retarded. Originally, only phytanic acid and DHCA, THCA, and the C29 dicarboxylic acid were elevated with normal VLCFA values. Later studies revealed elevated pristanic acid levels, too.[219] The patient was put on a diet low in phytanic acid, which resulted in marked improvement of her condition.

The patient described by Przyrembel et al.[217] showed intrauterine and postnatal growth retardation, complete lack of psychomotor development and hepatic dysfunction progressing to severe liver failure and death at age 6.5 months. THC-CoA oxidase was fully deficient in liver from the patient, but the significance of this finding remained unclear because the specimen was badly preserved.[216] No liver material was available from the patient of Christensen et al.[216] Originally, it was thought that THC-CoA oxidase was expressed in liver only. This is true for the rat but not for humans.[10] Indeed, Vanhove et al.[10] discovered that di- and trihydroxycholestanoyl-CoA are handled by branched-chain acyl-CoA oxidase with ubiquitous expression in many human cells, including fibroblasts. This allowed resolution of the question whether branched-chain acyl-CoA oxidase is the deficient enzyme in these patients or not. We measured the enzyme in fibroblasts from the patients and found completely normal activity. These findings rule out branched-chain acyl-CoA oxidase deficiency in the two patients of Christensen et al.[216] and Przyrembel et al.[217] Two additional patients with di- and trihydroxycholestanoic acidemia have been published;[218] branched-chain acyl-CoA oxidase deficiency was excluded in these patients too (unpublished).

POSTNATAL DIAGNOSIS OF THE DISORDERS OF PEROXISOMAL β-OXIDATION

Acyl-CoA Oxidase, D-Bifunctional Protein and Peroxisomal Thiolase Deficiency

The clinical presentation of patients affected by acyl-CoA oxidase deficiency, D-bifunctional protein deficiency, or peroxisomal thiolase deficiency strongly resembles the clinical presentation of patients affected by a peroxisome biogenesis disorder (PBD) as exemplified by the names pseudo-NALD and pseudo-ZS given to acyl-CoA oxidase deficiency[37] and peroxisomal thiolase deficiency,[203,204] respectively. Table 130-3 lists the biochemical abnormalities observed in patients with either a defect in peroxisome biogenesis or a defect in peroxisomal β-oxidation. In all of the disorders except racemase-deficiency, plasma VLCFA levels are abnormal, which makes VLCFA analysis a good initial screening method to establish whether or not a patient has one of the disorders of peroxisomal β-oxidation or a peroxisome biogenesis disorder. If VLCFA levels are elevated, erythrocyte plasmalogen levels should be measured (see flowchart of Fig. 130-12). If plasmalogens are deficient, a peroxisome biogenesis disorder is established that should be followed up by detailed studies in fibroblasts, including complementation analysis and molecular studies (see Chap. 129). Plasmalogens are strongly deficient in classic Zellweger patients, but may be normal in patients affected by a milder variant, including NALD (MIM 202370) and infantile Refsum disease (IRD; MIM 266510), which implies that the finding of normal plasmalogens does not rule out a PBD. Following the flowchart of Fig. 130-12, phytanic, pristanic, and di- and trihydroxycholestanoic acid should be measured. If all metabolites are normal, acyl-CoA oxidase deficiency is the most probable

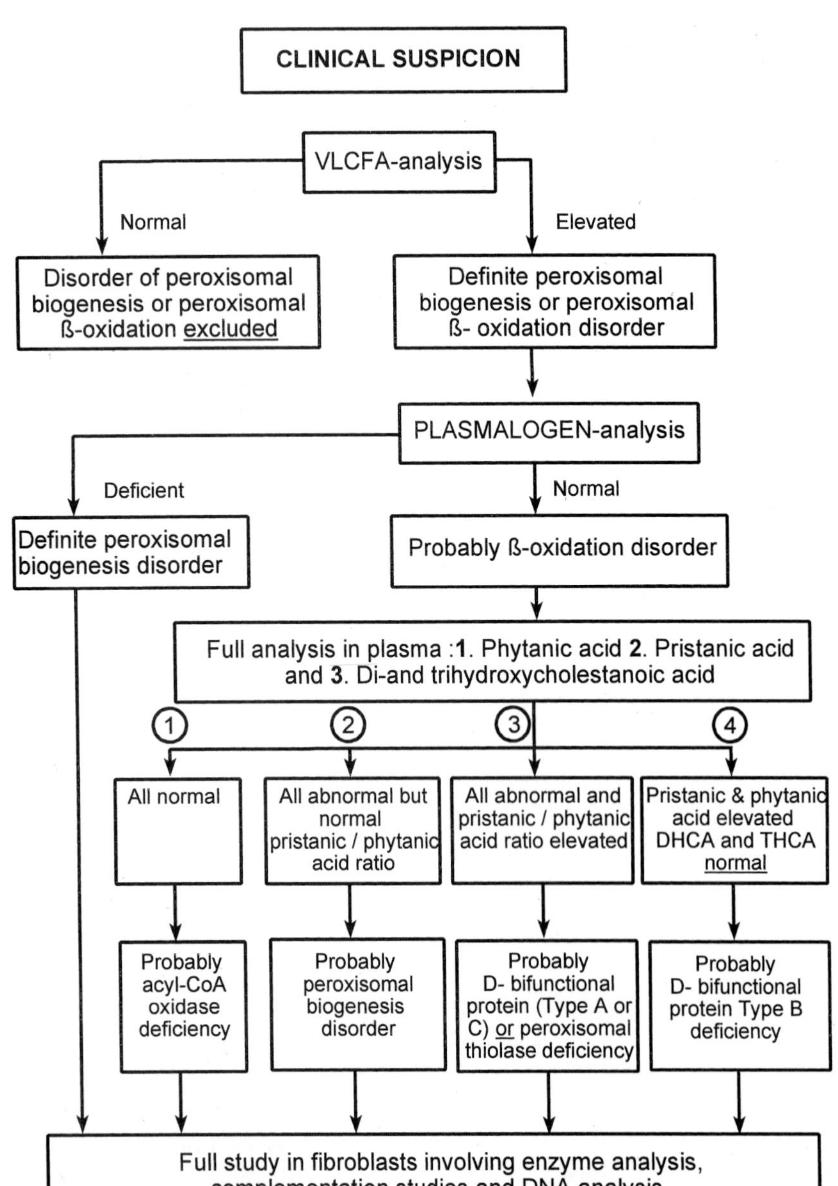

Fig. 130-12 Flowchart for the differential diagnosis of patients clinically suspected to suffer from a peroxisome biogenesis disorder (PBD) or a peroxisomal β-oxidation defect.

diagnosis. If phytanic, pristanic, and di- and trihydroxycholestanoic acid are elevated, two possibilities emerge, dictated by the pristanic acid/phytanic acid ratio. Studies by TenBrink et al.[71] show that pristanic acid/phytanic acid ratios are *normal* in PBD patients, but definitely *abnormal* (four- to twenty-onefold elevated as compared to normal) in β-oxidation-deficient patients. Elevated phytanic and pristanic acid levels in plasma with normal di- and trihydroxycholestanoic acid levels, points to D-bifunctional protein deficiency type B (enoyl-CoA hydratase deficiency).

Although in many cases the correct diagnosis can be made based on the abnormalities in blood following the flowchart of Fig. 130-12, definitive diagnosis requires detailed analyses in fibroblasts including measurements of C26:0 and pristanic acid β-oxidation followed by enzyme activity measurements, complementation studies and molecular analyses.

Acyl-CoA Oxidase. The activity of acyl-CoA oxidase can be measured reliably in fibroblasts homogenates using the method of Souri et al.[220] Furthermore, antibodies have been generated to study the protein by immunoblot and/or immunofluorescence analysis, and the cDNA structure has been resolved.[77–79]

D-Bifunctional Protein. The activity of D-bifunctional protein can be measured in fibroblast homogenates making use of a specific substrate, that is, (24E)-3α,7α,12α-trihydroxy-5β-cholest-24-enoyl-CoA. Van Grunsven et al.[124] showed that formation of the β-ketoacyl-CoA ester of THCA is fully deficient in case of a complete deficiency of D-bifunctional protein, whereas formation of varanoyl-CoA is not completely deficient because of the reactivity of L-bifunctional protein with (24E)-THC-24-enoyl-CoA to produce (24S,25S)-varanoyl-CoA. The availability of antibodies and the identification of the *D-BP* cDNA and gene structure has allowed studies at both the protein and molecular level.[99,124,201,221]

Peroxisomal Thiolase. No methods have been described to date that measure the activity of pTH1 in fibroblast homogenates. Analyses at the protein and cDNA/gene level are possible.

Peroxisomal Racemase Deficiency. The clinical description of the two patients with racemase deficiency reported to date indicates a completely different clinical presentation as compared to the other peroxisomal β-oxidation deficiencies described above. Racemase deficiency should be suspected in all cases of an unexplained sensory motor neuropathy and, in principle, requires analysis of phytanic, pristanic, and di- and trihydroxycholestanoic acid, followed by enzyme analyses in fibroblasts, and, if deficient, DNA analysis (see reference 166).

PRENATAL DIAGNOSIS

Until recently, prenatal diagnosis of acyl-CoA oxidase deficiency and D-bifunctional protein deficiency could only be done in cultured chorionic villous fibroblasts by measuring VLCFA-levels and overall oxidation of C26:0 and/or pristanic acid.[222] The generation of reliable methods for the measurement of acyl-CoA oxidase[220] and D-bifunctional protein[99,124,201] now enables direct analyses in uncultured villi, which eliminates the risks of culturing chorionic villous cells (maternal overgrowth, lack of growth, etc.). If the protein itself is deficient in cells from the index patient, enzyme studies may be backed up by immunoblot analyses. Furthermore, if the molecular defect has been resolved in the index patient, DNA analysis can be done.

ETHER PHOSPHOLIPID BIOSYNTHESIS AND DEFECTS THEREIN

Mammalian glycerophospholipids can be distinguished in two classes with either an ester linkage at the *sn*-1-position of the glycerol backbone (Fig. 130-13*A*) or an ether linkage at that position (Figs. 130-13*B* and *C*). The latter group of phospholipids, called etherphospholipids, can be subdivided into two groups with either an alkyl (Fig. 130-13*A*) or alkenyl (Fig. 130-13*C*) linkage at *sn*-1. The alcohol moiety attached to the phosphate group is almost exclusively confined to ethanolamine or choline, although some exceptions have been found in which inositol or serine is attached. Indeed, the lipid moiety of several mammalian glycosyl phosphatidylinositol (GPI) anchors[223–225] consists of 1-alkyl-2-acylphosphatidylinositol.[226,227] Similarly, a small portion of the free phosphatidylinositol pool is made up of 1-alkyl-2-acyl-phosphatidylinositol.

Ether phospholipids have been found in many organisms including the protozoa *Tetrahymena pyriformis*[228] and *Trypanosoma brucei rhodesiense*,[229] the invertebrates *Meloidogyne javanica*,[230] *Turbatrix aceti*,[231] *Eisenia foetida*,[232] and *Caenorhabditis elegans*,[233] as well as archaebacteria and anaerobic eubacteria.[234] Most yeast species, except *Pullularia pullulans*,[235] lack etherphospholipids. In mammals, ether phospholipids usually occur in their plasmalogen form with plasmenylethanolamine (1-0-alk-1′-enyl-2-acyl-*sn*-glycero-3-phosphoethanolamine) as the primary ether-linked species. Etherphospholipids are present in

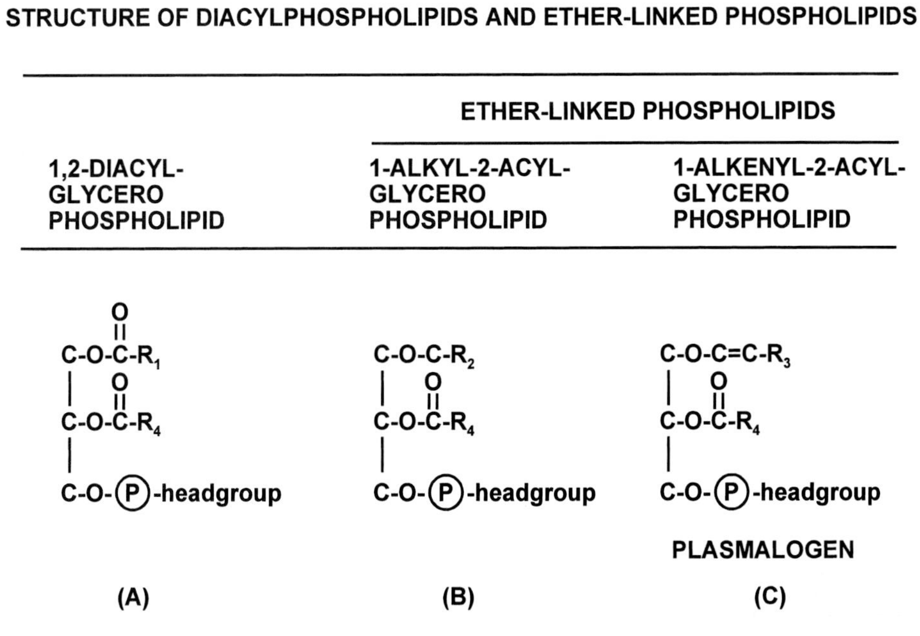

STRUCTURE OF DIACYLPHOSPHOLIPIDS AND ETHER-LINKED PHOSPHOLIPIDS

1,2-DIACYL-GLYCERO PHOSPHOLIPID	ETHER-LINKED PHOSPHOLIPIDS	
	1-ALKYL-2-ACYL-GLYCERO PHOSPHOLIPID	1-ALKENYL-2-ACYL-GLYCERO PHOSPHOLIPID
C-O-C(=O)-R_1 C-O-C(=O)-R_4 C-O-(P)-headgroup	C-O-C-R_2 C-O-C(=O)-R_4 C-O-(P)-headgroup	C-O-C=C-R_3 C-O-C(=O)-R_4 C-O-(P)-headgroup PLASMALOGEN
(A)	(B)	(C)

Fig. 130-13 Structures of glycerophospholipids. R_1, R_2, R_3, and R_4 are aliphatic carbon chains. The head groups in alkyl- and alk-1-enyl-type glycerophospholipids are almost exclusively ethanolamine or choline.

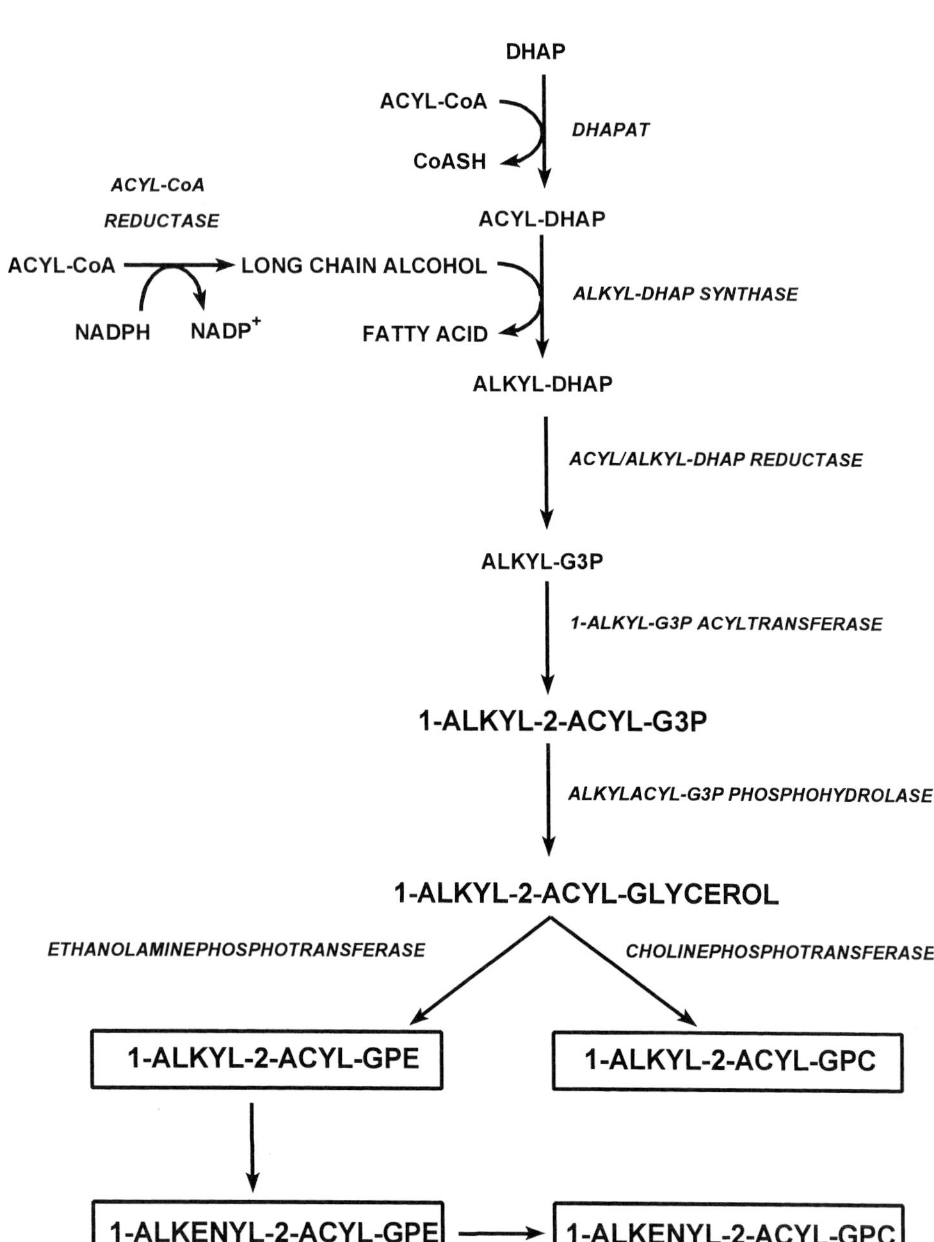

Fig. 130-14 Pathway of ether-phospholipid biosynthesis. DHAP = dihydroxyacetone phosphate; GPC = glycerol-3-phosphocholine; GPE = glycerol-3-phosphoethanolamine; G3P = glycerol-3-phosphate.

virtually all mammalian cells. They account for approximately 15 percent of total phospholipids in humans and are most abundant in heart,[236] brain,[237] neutrophils,[238] and macrophages.[239]

THE DIHYDROXYACETONEPHOSPHATE PATHWAY

In higher organisms, etherphospholipid synthesis starts with the acylation of DHAP with long chain acyl CoAs. Subsequently, the acyl chain in acyl-DHAP is replaced by a long chain alcohol yielding alkyl-DHAP in a reaction catalyzed by alkyl-DHAP synthase. Once synthesized, the alkyl-DHAP then undergoes reduction to alkyl-G3P (1-alkyl-*sn*-glycerol-3-phosphate) via acyl/alkyl-DHAP reductase followed by addition of an acyl-chain at the *sn*-2 position. 1-Alkyl-2-acyl-glycerol-3-phosphate is then converted to 1-alkyl-2-acylglycerol by a phosphohydrolase. This is followed by addition of the polar head groups phosphocholine or phosphoethanolamine from CDP-choline or CDP-ethanolamine, respectively, via the same enzymes as involved in the formation of the diacyl analogs.

1-Alkyl-2-acyl-GPE can be desaturated to yield the plasmalogen form of PE. In contrast, 1-alkyl-2-acyl-GPC *cannot* be desaturated directly in this way, and plasmalogen PC originates from plasmalogen PE via some indirect exchange mechanism (Fig. 130-14).[240,241]

In principle, acylation of DHAP can be brought about by different acyltransferases present in eukaryotic cells, including (a) peroxisomal dihydroxyacetone phosphate acyltransferase (DHAPAT), as well as (b) mitochondrial and (c) microsomal glycerol 3-phosphate (G3P) acyltransferase (G3PAT). The latter two enzymes accept both G3P and DHAP as substrates, whereas peroxisomal DHAPAT is absolutely specific for DHAP. The recent finding that etherphospholipid synthesis is *completely* deficient in patients with an isolated deficiency of peroxisomal DHAPAT[242] due to

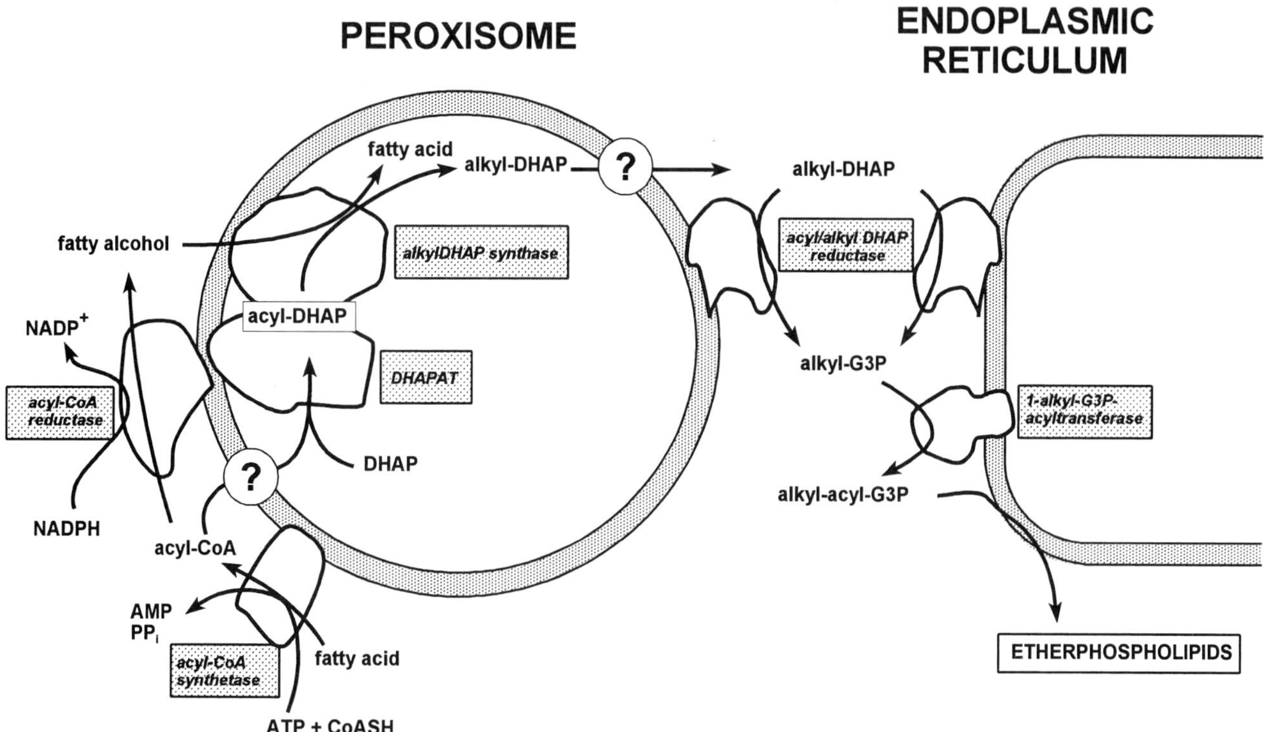

Fig. 130-15 Illustration of the enzymatic organization of etherphospholipid synthesis. See text for details. alkyl-DHAP synthase = alkyldihydroxyacetonephosphate synthase; DHAP = dihydroxyacetonephosphate; DHAPAT = dihydroxyacetonephosphate acyltransferase; G3P = glycerol-3-phosphate.

mutations in the structural gene for DHAPAT[243] indicates that peroxisomal DHAPAT is indispensable for ether-phospholipid synthesis. Apparently, the acyl-DHAP synthesized at the mitochondrial and/or the endoplasmic reticulum membrane is *not* a substrate for alkyl-DHAP synthase. The latter enzyme is exclusively localized in peroxisomes. Because the catalytic site of alkyl-DHAP synthase faces the peroxisomal lumen (see reference 244) these data imply that the peroxisomal membrane is *not* permeable to extraperoxisomal acyl-DHAP.

The next enzyme in the pathway acyl/alkyl-DHAP reductase is predominantly, but not exclusively, peroxisomal because some activity is found in the endoplasmic reticulum.[245] However, DHAPAT, alkyl-DHAP synthase, and acyl/alkyl-DHAP reductase are membrane-bound enzymes with different orientations in the membrane. Indeed, DHAPAT and alkyl-DHAP synthase face the peroxisomal interior,[246,247] whereas the reductase has a cytosolic orientation (see reference 244 for a review).

Interestingly, the enzyme catalyzing the formation of long chain alcohols from acyl-CoA esters, that is, acyl-CoA:NADPH (long chain alcohol-forming) reductase, which was long thought to be a *microsomal* enzyme, has now been found to be a peroxisomal membrane-bound enzyme.[248] Fig. 130-14 is a schematic representation of the enzymatic organization of etherphospholipid synthesis when all available information is taken together. We recently obtained decisive evidence[249] that suggests that DHAPAT is unstable in the absence of alkyl-DHAP synthase, which suggests that they actually form a complex as shown in Fig. 130-15.

SUBCELLULAR LOCALIZATION OF THE ACYL-DHAP PATHWAY ENZYMES

Early studies did not suggest the involvement of peroxisomes in etherphospholipid biosynthesis. Indeed, biosynthesis of acyl-DHAP was first thought to occur in guinea pig liver mitochondria,[250] whereas in rat brain, a microsomal localization was found.[251] However, these studies were done at a time when the existence of peroxisomes had not been well established. Furthermore, subcellular fractionation studies were generally performed using crude subcellular fractions prepared by differential centrifugation. Careful subcellular fractionation of rodent livers by Hajra and coworkers[246,252] using a combination of differential and density-gradient centrifugation methods, revealed that DHAPAT and alkyl-DHAP synthase are predominantly, if not exclusively, peroxisomal (see also reference 253).

This conclusion finds support in the observation that the activity of both DHAPAT and alkyl-DHAP synthase is greatly reduced in cells lacking peroxisomes.[254–256] Both DHAPAT and alkyl-DHAP synthase are strongly bound to the peroxisomal membrane and solubilization of the two enzymes requires detergents.[257,258] However, because both enzymes lack membrane-spanning domains as deduced from the cDNA-derived amino acid sequences, we conclude that they are located at the periphery of the inner face of the peroxisomal membrane (see Fig. 130-15).

PURIFICATION AND MOLECULAR ANALYSIS OF THE ACYL-DHAP PATHWAY ENZYMES

DHAPAT,[258,259] alkyl-DHAP synthase,[257,260,261] and acyl/alkyl-DHAP reductase[262] have all been purified from different sources. N-terminal sequencing of the guinea-pig liver alkyl-DHAP synthase led the way to the identification of the guinea pig cDNA,[263] and this was soon followed by cloning of the human cDNA.[264] Using a similar procedure, we cloned the human DHAPAT cDNA,[243] which was also cloned by Thai et al.[265] using a different approach. Interestingly, the C-terminus of DHAPAT ends in AKL, which is an established type 1 peroxisome-targeting signal (PTS1.) Alkyl-DHAP synthase, however, is a true PTS2-protein.[263,264]

PHYSIOLOGICAL FUNCTIONS OF ETHER-LINKED PHOSPHOLIPIDS

Plasmalogens are major components of cellular membranes and are found in virtually all mammalian cells. Their overall physical-chemical properties are similar to those of the diacylphospholipids, although some differences have been noted.[266] Despite their discovery 75 years ago, little is known about their physiological and cellular functions, although severe possible functions for these phospholipids have been suggested.[267] First, they have been implicated as a major storage depot for arachidonic acid.[268,269] The release of arachidonic acid by plasmalogen-selective phospholipases A_2 has been demonstrated.[266,270,271] Consequently, plasmalogens are a reservoir of prostaglandin and thromboxane precursors.

Furthermore, it has been suggested that plasmalogens facilitate optimal functioning of some receptors, enzymes, and ion pumps,[272–276] and that they are involved in membrane fusion,[277,278] an important process in synaptic transmission, hormone release, and membrane trafficking. In this respect, it was recently postulated that the association of high-density lipoprotein (HDL) with cellular phospholipid is a prerequisite for the process of high-density lipoprotein-mediated cholesterol efflux (HDL-MCE). Plasmalogens have an important function in this HDL-MCE, as was demonstrated by reduced HDL-MCE in plasmalogen-deficient macrophages and skin fibroblasts, and an increase of this efflux upon plasmalogen restoration.[279] Etherphospholipids also play a specific role in glycosylphosphatidylinositol anchors (GPI anchors), which attach several proteins to the cell surface,[227,280–284] and in cellular differentiation, or in maintaining cells in the differentiated state.[285,286]

Another proposed functional role of plasmalogens is protection against certain reactive oxygen species (ROS).[287,288] An etherphospholipid-deficient Chinese hamster ovary (CHO) cell line was shown to be more susceptible to photosensitized killing after incorporation of 12-(1′-pyrene) dodecanoic acid (P12) by exposure to long-wavelength ultraviolet (UV) light, when compared to wild-type CHO cells. Restoration of plasmalogen levels in the etherphospholipid-deficient mutant cells partially normalized resistance to P12/UV treatment.[287] Hoefler et al.[289] and Spinsi et al.[290] reported that plasmalogen-deficient human skin fibroblasts are also hypersensitive to photosensitized killing. Furthermore, they identified products obtained after oxidative breakdown of plasmenyl ethanolamine by singlet oxygen. Plasmalogens have also been suggested to protect the low-density lipoprotein (LDL) particles against oxidation,[291] thereby inhibiting an important early step in the development of atherosclerosis.[292] Further proof for the involvement of plasmalogens in oxidation comes from experiments reporting that plasmalogen levels of ram spermatozoa are selectively reduced by 50 percent upon iron-ascorbate-induced oxidation.[293]

The absence of lipoprotein[a] in the plasma of Zellweger syndrome (ZS) and RCDP patients is probably due to the inability of apolipoprotein[a] to be secreted in these disorders.[294] This inability results from a deficiency in etherphospholipids, because it was only detected in ZS and RCDP patients and not in patients with X-linked adrenoleukodystrophy and the classic form of Refsum disease.

Finally, plasmalogens seem to interact closely with docosahexaenoic acid (DHA), a fatty acid that requires peroxisomes for its production.[295] This was demonstrated by both the beneficial effect of DHA on plasmalogen levels in ZS patients,[296] the preferential acylation of ether lysophospholipids by DHA,[297] and the reduction of DHA levels in plasmalogen-deficient macrophage cell lines.[298] DHA are involved in cholinergic signal transduction,[299] whereas plasmalogens are involved in muscarinic cholinergic signal transduction and secretion of the amyloid precursor protein.[300]

We recently studied the possible role of plasmalogens on the β-adrenergic receptor signaling pathway. In plasmalogen-deficient fibroblasts, formation of cAMP was strongly reduced on stimulation with the β-adrenergic receptor against isoproterenol and epinephrine, whereas cAMP formation was identical on stimulation by forskolin and prostaglandin E1.[301] It remains to be established whether all these different presumed functions of plasmalogens also occur in vivo. Elucidation of this question requires the generation of a mouse model in which the gene for DHAPAT or alkyl DHAP synthase is deleted. Such efforts are underway.

DISORDERS OF ETHERPHOSPHOLIPID SYNTHESIS

Chondrodysplasia punctata (CDP) refers to a genetically heterogeneous group of bone dysplasias, with stippling of the epiphyses in infancy as the common feature. Although several types can be distinguished, there are two major forms, including RCDP with an autosomal recessive mode of inheritance and the Conradi-Hunermann type with autosomal dominant inheritance. RCDP in its classic presentation is clinically characterized by a disproportionally short stature primarily affecting the proximal parts of the extremities, typical facial appearance, congenital contractures, characteristic ocular involvement, dwarfism, spasticity, and severe mental retardation. Radiologic studies reveal shortening, metaphyseal cupping, and disturbed ossification of humeri and/or femora, together with epiphyseal and extra-epiphyseal calcifications.[302] Apart from the severe form of RCDP usually associated with early death, a number of patients have been described with a much milder clinical presentation lacking the classic stigmata such as rhizomelic shortening.[303–307]

The realization that RCDP belongs to the group of peroxisomal disorders came in 1985, when Heymans et al.[308] reported the deficiency of plasmalogens in erythrocytes as well as elevated phytanic acid levels in plasma. More detailed studies in fibroblasts revealed a set of four abnormalities including a deficient activity of DHAPAT, alkyl DHAP synthase, and phytanoyl-CoA hydroxylase. Furthermore, peroxisomal thiolase was present in the 44-kDa precursor form only. The discovery that alkyl DHAP synthase,[263,264] phytanoyl-CoA hydroxylase,[309–311] and peroxisomal thiolase[115,116] are all PTS2-proteins, suggested that the defect in RCDP had to be at the level of the PTS2-receptor, which, indeed, turned out to be true[312–314] (see Chap. 129). Studies in the early 1990s led to the identification of two genetically distinct types of RCDP resulting from mutations in the genes for DHAPAT[243] and alkyl DHAP synthase,[315,316] as described below. We call these various forms RCDP type 1, type 2, and type 3 (see Table 130-4).

Dihydroxyacetone Phosphate Acyltransferase (DHAPAT) Deficiency (RCDP Type 2; MIM 222765)

In 1992, we described the first case of isolated DHAPAT-deficiency in a patient showing all the clinical signs and symptoms of RCDP.[317] In this patient, craniofacial abnormalities were noted at birth, including a high forehead, large fontanels, a low/broad nasal bridge, anteverted nostrils, micrognathia, and a high-arched palate. The patient was extremely hypotonic, had cataracts and pronounced rhizomelic shortening, especially of the upper arms (Fig. 130-16). Furthermore, there were striking radiologic abnormalities consistent with RCDP, although there were no stippled calcifications of patellae and acetabulum. Initial investigations in a blood sample from the patient revealed a full deficiency of erythrocyte plasmalogens consistent with RCDP. A normal phytanic acid level in plasma was found, however. The significance of this finding was not immediately clear because phytanic acid is solely derived from exogenous dietary sources and may be completely normal in young RCDP type 1 patients despite a full block in phytanic acid α-oxidation. Detailed studies in fibroblasts from the patient, however, revealed an isolated DHAPAT-deficiency with normal values for alkyl-DHAP synthase and phytanic acid α-oxidation, and the normal presence of peroxisomal thiolase 1 in its mature 41-kDa form.[317] Barr et al.[318] reported on a second patient with an isolated deficiency of DHAPAT. This patient also had the severe phenotype. In 1994, Clayton et al.[319] reported on a 21-month-old boy and his 3.5-year-old sister, both of whom had isolated DHAPAT deficiency. Both sibs had anteverted nares, normal limbs, hypotonia, growth and

Table 130-4 Overview of the Different Forms of Rhizomelic Chondrodysplasia Punctata and the Biochemical Abnormalities Observed

	(Rhizomelic) Chondrodysplasia Punctata		
Parameter analyzed	Type 1	Type 2	Type 3
Erythrocytes			
Plasmalogens	Deficient	Deficient	Deficient
Plasma			
Very long chain fatty acids	Normal	Normal	Normal
Di- and trihydroxycholestanoic acid	Normal	Normal	Normal
Phytanic acid	Elevated*	Normal	Normal
Pristanic acid	Normal	Normal	Normal
Fibroblasts			
De novo plasmalogen synthesis	Deficient	Deficient	Deficient
DHAPAT-activity	Lowered	Deficient	Deficient/ normal**
Alkyl-DHAP synthase activity	Deficient	Normal	Deficient
Phytanoyl-CoA hydroxylase	Deficient	Normal	Normal
Catalase immunofluorescence (peroxisomes)	Normal	Normal	Normal
Molecular basis			
Affected gene	*PEX7*	*DHAPAT*	*ALKYLDHAP SYNTHASE*

*Because phytanic acid is solely derived from dietary sources, levels may vary from normal to very high depending on the age of the patient and dietary intake.
**See text for explanation.

developmental retardation, and feeding difficulties. Eczema was present in the younger patient. A computed tomographic scan of his head showed mild cerebral atrophy. The older sister had seizures. The same patients plus an additional sibling in the same family were later reported by Sztriha et al.[320] The third patient in the family had a comparable clinical presentation, again without rhizomelia. A similar, mild case of DHAPAT-deficiency was reported by Moser et al.,[195] and later in full detail by Elias et al.,[321] in a 6.5-year-old girl with developmental delay, growth failure, and cataracts, but no rhizomelia and no craniofacial dysmorphism. Table 130-5 lists the clinical findings in the seven cases so far reported.

Molecular Basis of Isolated DHAPAT Deficiency and Phenotype/Genotype Correlation. The identification of the human DHAPAT cDNA by Thai et al.[265] and Ofman et al.[243] enabled studies of DHAPAT-deficient patients at the molecular level, which revealed a variety of different mutations.[243] We performed mutation analysis in five of the seven patients listed in Table 130-5. Interestingly, in cases 1 and 2 we found severe mutations (a 848 TT insertion and a 567del204bp deletion, respectively), causing the complete absence of DHAPAT as reflected in zero activity in fibroblasts (see Table 130-5). On the other hand, in the three mildly affected patients (cases 3, 4, and 5) a homozygous 632G → A mutation was found, changing arginine in position 211 into histidine. Although this mutation is associated with a severe loss of function,[243] some residual activity remains as reflected in the DHAPAT activity measurements in fibroblasts. Taken together, the limited data available indicate a phenotype/genotype correlation.

Alkyl-DHAP Synthase Deficiency (RCDP Type 3) (MIM 600121)

In 1994,[242] we described the first case of isolated alkyl-DHAP synthase deficiency in a patient showing all the clinical characteristics of RCDP. In this patient, erythrocyte plasmalogen levels were completely deficient, whereas plasma phytanic acid levels were normal. Subsequent studies in fibroblasts revealed a complete deficiency of alkyl-DHAP synthase with normal values for DHAPAT and phytanoyl-CoA hydroxylase, and a normally processed peroxisomal thiolase (pTH1).[242] Only a single patient has been described since,[316] although three additional patients have been identified by Dr. H.W. Moser, Baltimore, MD, U.S.A. in which we established isolated alkyl-DHAP synthase deficiency (Wanders and Moser, in preparation). These three patients also show the classic stigmata of RCDP. Two of these patients had early deaths at 25 months and 30 months. The patient described by de Vet et al.[316] is the least affected of the five patients identified so far, and is still alive at 7.5 years of age, with mild to moderate rhizomelia, generalized flexion contractures, inability to sit, roll, or crawl, cataracts, continued seizures, and profound developmental delay.

In the original patient,[242] alkyl-DHAP synthase was fully deficient, whereas DHAPAT, phytanic acid α-oxidation, and peroxisomal thiolase were normal. In the subsequent patient described by de Vet et al.,[316] alkyl-DHAP synthase was deficient

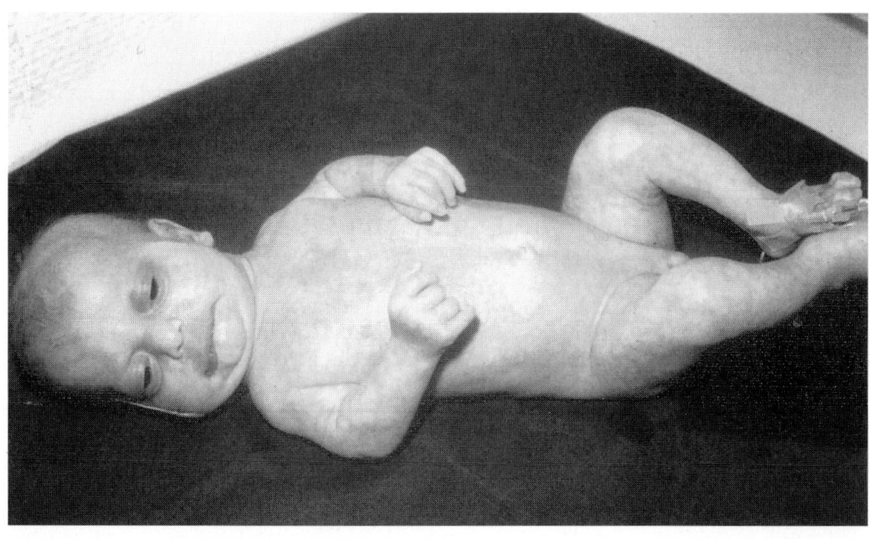

Fig. 130-16 The first patient identified with isolated dihydroxyacetone phosphate acyltransferase (DHAPAT) deficiency. (*Courtesy of Prof. H. Schumacher, Germany.*)

Table 130-5 Summary of the Clinical Findings in the Seven Cases of Isolated DHAPAT Deficiency Reported, To Date

Parameters analyzed	Patients						
	1	2	3	4 ←siblings→	5	6	7
Rhizomelia	+	+	−	−	−	−	+
Facial dysmorphism	+	+	+/−	+/−	−	−	+
Cataract	+	+	−	−	+	+	+
Hypotonia	+	+	+	+	+	+	+
Growth retardation	+	+	+	+	+	+	+
Mental retardation	+	+	+	+	+	+	+
Stippling	+	+	+	+	+	+	+
DHAPAT activity	0.0	0.0	0.1	0.2	0.2	1.6%	0.0
Reference	317	318	319 320	319 320	320	195 321	369

The clinical data in the table are collected from literature as indicated: + = abnormality present; − = abnormality absent. The DHAPAT-activity data are from our own laboratory and, except for case 6 (see ref. 321), reflect activities in fibroblasts (patients 1, 2, 3, 4, and 5; control values [n > 100]: 7.8 ± 2.0 nmol/2 h mg protein) or liver tissue (patient 7; control values [n = 4]: 4.8 ± 0.3 nmol/2 h mg protein).

again, but DHAPAT activity was also deficient with a residual activity of about 15 percent, which closely mimics the findings in RCDP type 1 fibroblasts resulting from a deficiency of the PTS2-receptor. Phytanic acid α-oxidation and peroxisomal thiolase were completely normal in the patient's fibroblasts. To resolve these peculiar findings, we performed complementation studies that revealed that the patient's cell line did belong to RCDP-complementation group 3, which represents alkyl-DHAP synthase deficiency. The solution came when antibodies against the synthase became available[322] and when it became clear that alkyl DHAP synthase and DHAPAT form a complex within the peroxisome.[249] Detailed studies by van den Bosch and co-workers[315,316,322,323] show that the deficient activity of DHAPAT in the second case of alkyl-DHAP synthase deficiency (see Table 2 in de Vet et al:[316] patient 4) is the secondary consequence of the alkyl-DHAP synthase protein being completely absent in this patient due to a homozygous 128-bp deletion that leads to a premature stop. On the other hand, studies in fibroblasts from the first patient with alkyl-DHAP synthase deficiency show that the protein is normally expressed and correctly localized in peroxisomes, but functionally inactive due to a 1256G > A mutation causing the substitution of arginine at position 419 by a histidine. Because DHAPAT is only stable if it forms a complex with alkyl-DHAP synthase within the peroxisome (see Fig. 130-14), these data explain why DHAPAT activity is fully normal in fibroblasts from patient 1 but deficient in patient 2. Furthermore, these data resolve the puzzling situation in RCDP type 1 in which DHAPAT has long been known to be deficient despite its identification as a typical PTS1-protein.[243,265,324]

Postnatal Diagnosis of RCDP and Classification as Type 1, 2, or 3

Table 130-4 lists the biochemical findings in patients in which the diagnosis RCDP type 1 (PTS2-receptor defect), RCDP type 2 (DHAPAT-deficiency), and RCDP type 3 (alkyl-DHAP synthase deficiency) has been established unequivocally by detailed clinical, biochemical, and molecular studies as performed in our center. Our results over the years show that analysis of erythrocyte plasmalogens using the method described by Björhem et al.[325] is an excellent initial screening method if a patient is suspected of suffering from RCDP or a variant thereof. In all cases of RCDP types 1, 2, and 3 that we have analyzed (> 100 cases), erythrocyte plasmalogens have always been clearly abnormal, even in mild cases as described by, for example, Smeitink et al.[305] and Barth et al.[307]. This situation is not observed with the disorders of peroxisome biogenesis because patients suffering from milder variants (NALD, IRD) may have completely normal erythrocyte plasmalogens.[326,327]

If erythrocyte plasmalogen analysis shows a deficiency, we usually proceed by measuring all other peroxisomal metabolites, including VLCFAs, di- and trihydroxycholestanoic acid, pristanic acid, and phytanic acid, although measurement of phytanic acid only may suffice (see flowchart of Fig. 130-17). If phytanic acid is clearly abnormal in the absence of any abnormalities in the other metabolites, RCDP type 1 is virtually established. Definitive diagnosis requires a full study in fibroblasts followed by molecular analysis of the *PEX7* gene.[312–314] If phytanic acid is normal, one is probably dealing with isolated DHAPAT or alkyl-DHAP synthase deficiency, although it should be emphasized that phytanic acid is derived from exogenous sources only and may be normal in young RCDP type 1 patients.[327]

Prenatal Diagnosis of RCDP Types 1, 2, and 3

Prenatal diagnosis of RCDP types 1, 2, and 3 can be done reliably in direct chorionic villous material without the need to culture fibroblasts. In our own center, we prefer to do two (or more) independent tests that include (a) plasmalogens, DHAPAT activity, and immunoblot analysis of peroxisomal thiolase for RCDP type 1; (b) plasmalogen analysis and DHAPAT activity measurements in case of RCDP type 2; and (c) plasmalogen analysis and alkyl-DHAP synthase activity measurements for RCDP type 3 (Table 130-6). These methods are extremely reliable in our hands with no errors made in > 50 prenatal diagnostic procedures. In selected cases, we also perform molecular analysis.

Neuropathologic Findings

Myelogenesis is a highly complex process and abnormalities in myelin formation are seen in a wide range of metabolic diseases. Plasmalogens are major components of myelin. About 80 percent of the ethanolamine phosphoglycerides is of the plasmalogen

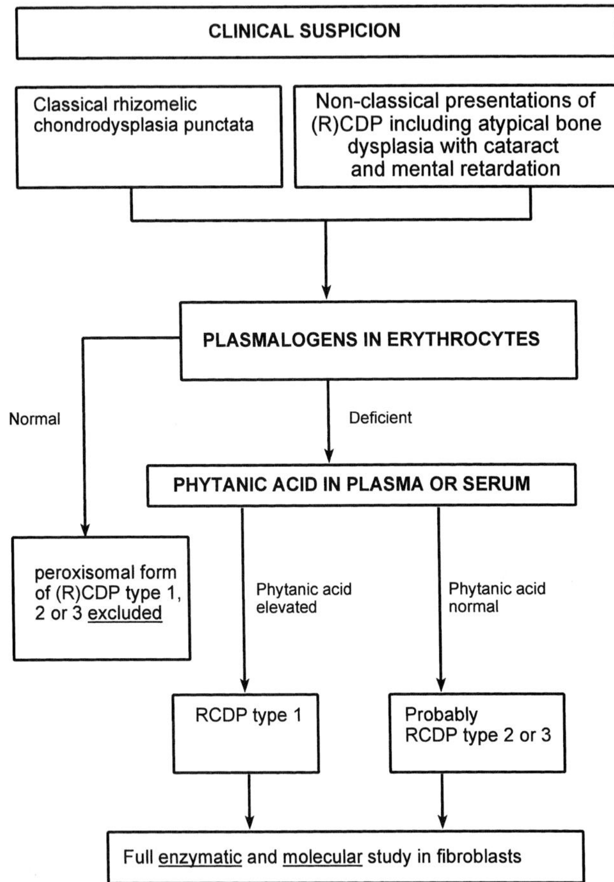

Fig. 130-17 Flowchart for the differential diagnosis of (rhizomelic) chondrodysplasia punctata types 1, 2, and 3.

form. Nevertheless, remarkably little information is available in literature on the neuropathologic lesions of the white matter in RCDP. Even the MRI pathology of the brain in patients with RCDP type 1 has rarely been discussed. Severe delay of myelination and signs of slight demyelination in the occipital white matter were described in a single RCDP type 1 patient,[328] whereas in another case of RCDP type 1, increased signal intensity in the periventricular and subcortical white matter, especially in the occipital regions, were described.[329] Sztriha et al.[320] described delayed myelin formation in two of the three siblings with the nonrhizomelic form of chondrodysplasia punctata type 2 due to isolated DHAPAT deficiency.

Recently, brain MRI findings were reported in another case of isolated DHAPAT deficiency.[330] Brain MRI was performed at the age of 16 months. Sagittal, transverse, and coronal T1-weighted and transverse T2-weighted images were obtained. The subarachnoid spaces and ventricles were enlarged, and there was wide cavum septi pellucidi and Vergae. The T2-weighted images showed high signal intensity in the periventricular white matter and the white matter of the centrum semiovale. The abnormalities were symmetric and extended into the arcuate fibers. The abnormal signal was more accentuated in the frontal and temporal areas than in the parietoccipital regions, and it was less prominent in the perirolandic area. There also was an abnormally high signal in the corticobulbar and corticospinal tracts in the cerebral peduncles. Medial lemniscus and medial longitudinal fasciculus appeared with normal low signal intensity on the T2-weighted images. In contrast with the diffuse abnormality of the peripheral white matter, there was a characteristic sparing of central structures, including corpus callosum, basal ganglia, and thalami. The pons, medulla oblongata, and cerebellum were normal.

Table 130-6 Prenatal Diagnosis of RCDP Types 1, 2, and 3 in Direct Chorionic Villous Material

Type of analysis	RCDP		
	Type 1	Type 2	Type 3
Plasmalogen analysis	+	+	+
DHAPAT activity	(+)	+	−
Immunoblot analysis (thiolase)	+	−	−
Alkyl-DHAP synthase activity	(+)	−	+
Molecular analysis	(+)	(+)	(+)

In our laboratory prenatal diagnosis of RCDP Types 1, 2, and 3 is usually performed using the methods indicated by +, although the other tests indicated by (+) can also be done.

Treatment

To date, there are no reports of treatment of DHAPAT- or alkyl-DHAP-synthase-deficient patients. In principle, treatment with a synthetic ether lipid like 1-*O*-hexadecyl-*sn*-glycerol could be tried, especially in milder affected patients, because 1-*O*-hexadecyl-*sn*-glycerol is an excellent precursor of plasmalogens that enters the biosynthetic pathway for plasmalogens *after* the block at the level of DHAPAT and/or alkyl-DHAP synthase. Indeed, numerous in vitro studies show that hexadecylglycerol is readily taken up by cells, converted into hexadecyl-*sn*-glycerol-3-phosphate, and further metabolized into plasmalogens.

Pathogenesis

The identification of cases with isolated DHAPAT and alkyl-DHAP synthase deficiency clearly shows that etherphospholipids play an indispensable role in the human organism. As described above (see "Physiological Functions of Ether-Linked Phospholipids"), many different functions have been suggested for ether-phospholipids in general, and plasmalogens in particular. Future studies, notably in mutant mice, will tell which of these presumed functions actually predominate in vivo.

PHYTANIC ACID α-OXIDATION AND REFSUM DISEASE

Peroxisomes play a major role in phytanic acid α-oxidation and Refsum disease is the only true disorder of phytanic acid α-oxidation (see Chap. 132).

ISOPRENOID BIOSYNTHESIS AND MEVALONATE KINASE DEFICIENCY

The mevalonate pathway plays a central role in cellular metabolism because it catalyzes the production of a range of isoprenoids that are vital for diverse cellular functions. These isoprenoids include sterols (especially cholesterol), haem A, ubiquinone, dolichol required for glycoprotein synthesis, and isopentenyladenine, which is present in some transfer RNAs. Interest in the mevalonate pathway heightened when it was discovered that growth-regulating $p21^{ras}$ proteins encoded by Ras protooncogenes and oncogenes, as well as other proteins, can undergo protein farnesylation. The covalently linked farnesyl residues anchor these proteins to cell membranes (see reference 331 for a review).

The enzymology of the mevalonate pathway has been studied intensively for many years, and at least the part from acetyl-CoA to farnesylpyrophosphate (FPP) has been well characterized. From previous studies that were almost exclusively based on cell homogenization experiments, the subcellular localization of the cholesterol synthesizing machinery was envisioned to be as follows: (a) condensation of two acetyl-CoA units to aceto-acetyl-CoA followed by condensation of yet another acetyl-CoA to produce 3-hydroxy-3-methylglutaryl-CoA (HMG-CoA) in the cytosol; (b) production of mevalonate from HMG-CoA at the

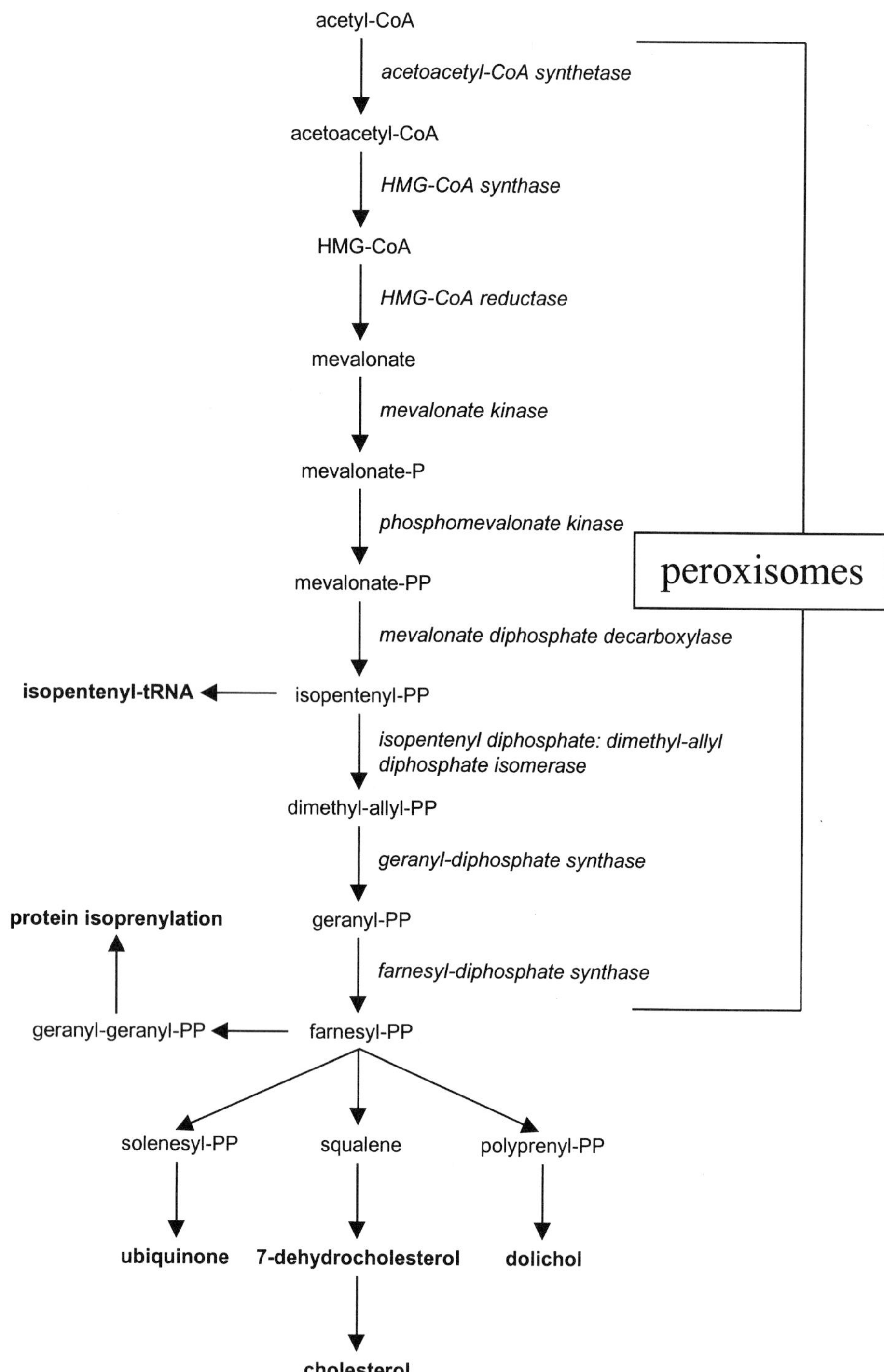

Fig. 130-18 Enzymology of the mevalonate pathway. Synthesis of the various isoprenoids follows a common pathway up to farnesyldiphosphate after which the pathway branches to produce dolichol, ubiquinone, cholesterol, and so on.

endoplasmic reticulum membrane; and (c) conversion of mevalonate to FPP via a series of cytosolic enzymes. At the level of FPP, the pathway branches to produce the different end products shown in Fig. 130-18. Conversion of FPP to cholesterol is generally considered to proceed at the endoplasmic reticulum membrane, although squalene synthase was reported to be present in peroxisomes,[332] a conclusion disproved by Stamellos et al.[333]

The first indication that peroxisomes may play a critical role in the synthesis of isoprenoids came from immunoelectron microscopy studies by Keller et al.[334] that showed the presence of HMG-CoA reductase in the matrix of peroxisomes. In these studies, use was made of antibodies directed against the microsomal HMG-CoA reductase, which is a bona fide transmembrane glycoprotein of two identical 97-kDa subunits. The highly conserved catalytic domain extends into the cytosol and is linked to the membrane portion of the molecule made up of multiple transmembrane elements via a short nonconserved sequence. The puzzling findings by Keller et al.[334] were subsequently confirmed biochemically using quantitative enzyme activity measurements.[335] The relationship between the peroxisomal and microsomal HMG-CoA reductase was recently studied by Aboushadi et al.[336] According to these authors, the peroxisomal reductase is functionally and structurally different from the endoplasmic reticulum HMG-CoA reductase in terms of phosphorylation of the enzyme, rate of degradation in response to mevalonate, and inhibition by statins.

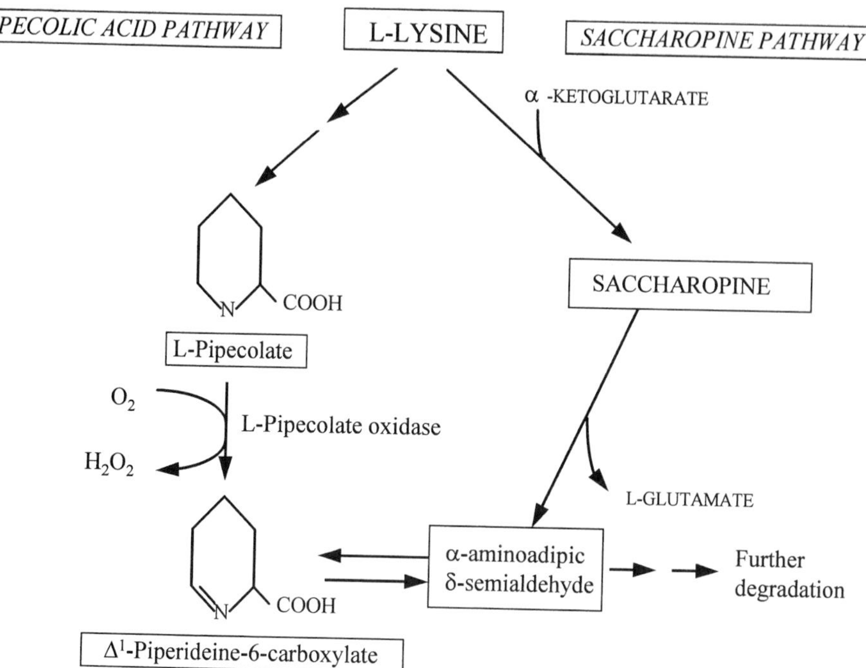

Fig. 130-19 Degradation of L-lysine via the L-pipecolic acid pathway and the saccharopine pathway. The major route of L-lysine degradation is via saccharopine. However, the activity of L-lysine α-ketoglutarate reductase is low in brain, which explains why the L-pipecolic acid pathway is the major route of degradation in brain.

The subsequent enzyme in the pathway, mevalonate kinase,[337,338] is localized in peroxisomes, as well as in farnesyl-diphosphate synthase.[339] Furthermore, phosphomevalonate kinase, mevalonate pyrophosphate decarboxylase, and isopentenyl diphosphate isomerase may also be peroxisomal,[340] suggesting that the whole pathway for the conversion of mevalonate to FPP, or even from acetyl-CoA to FPP, may be present in peroxisomes.[341]

Mevalonate kinase deficiency is the only known disorder involving the peroxisomal part of isoprenoid biosynthesis. Interestingly, apart from the classic form of mevalonate kinase deficiency (MIM 251170), which is associated with severe abnormalities early in life, including profound developmental delay, facial dysmorphia, cataract, hepatosplenomegaly, lymphadenopathy, and early death,[342] mevalonate kinase deficiency has also been observed in hyperimmunoglobulinemia D and periodic fever syndrome (HIDS; MIM 260920).[343,344] This syndrome is an autosomal recessive disorder characterized by recurrent episodes of fever associated with lymphadenopathy, arthralgia, gastrointestinal dismay and skin rash. In HIDS patients, mevalonate kinase is severely reduced (1.2 to 3.4 percent of normal), but not fully deficient as in classic mevalonate kinase deficiency.[343,344]

L-PIPECOLATE METABOLISM IN PEROXISOMES AND ISOLATED HYPERPIPECOLIC ACIDEMIA (MIM 239400)

Pipecolic acid (piperidine-2-carboxylic acid) is an alicyclic imino acid and homologue of proline derived from the metabolism of lysine. The primary route of L-lysine degradation in mammals, including man, is via the saccharopine pathway, which involves the sequential action of L-lysine ketoglutarate reductase and saccharopine dehydrogenase as catalyzed by a single, bifunctional enzyme.[345] In brain, however, the activity of this pathway is negligible[346] and degradation of L-lysine proceeds predominantly via L-pipecolate as intermediate.[347,348] L-Pipecolate is formed from L-lysine via two enzymatic reactions involving formation of 2-keto-6-aminocaproate via L-amino acid oxidase and reduction of Δ^1-piperideine-2-carboxylate, the cyclization product of 2-keto-6-aminocaproate, to L-pipecolate (Fig. 130-19). Subsequently, the enzyme L-pipecolate oxidase converts L-pipecolate to Δ^1-piperideine-6-carboxylate, which opens spontaneously to form L-2-aminoadipic-δ-semialdehyde. This aldehyde is oxidized to 2-aminoadipic acid followed by transamination to 2-ketoadipic acid and oxidative decarboxylation to glutaryl-CoA. L-Pipecolate oxidase is a peroxisomal enzyme in humans.[349,350] In addition, the enzyme is deficient in livers from Zellweger patients,[350–352] which explains the elevated L-pipecolic acid levels in plasma and urine from patients suffering from Zellweger syndrome or one of the other peroxisome biogenesis defects (see Chap. 129). The enzyme has been purified from monkey liver[353] and the corresponding rabbit liver cDNA has been identified.[354]

In literature, several reports have appeared on isolated hyperpipecolic acidemia. The first case was described by Gatfield et al.[355] in a male infant with hepatomegaly, retinopathy, and a progressive neurologic disorder. Three additional patients have been reported in literature, all showing severe clinical abnormalities,[356,357] including hepatomegaly, retinopathy, developmental delay, and several dysmorphic in the two patients of Burton et al.[357] After the recognition that L-pipecolic acid is also elevated in patients suffering from a peroxisome biogenesis disorder, these patients were reevaluated, and in the four patients a deficiency of peroxisomes was found, as concluded from the finding of definite peroxisomal abnormalities in plasma and a generalized loss of peroxisomal functions in fibroblasts (see, for example, reference 358). According to Challa et al.,[359] however, hepatic peroxisomes were normal in the two cases of Burton et al.[357] These results are hard to reconcile with data from several groups, including our own, showing a generalized loss of peroxisomal functions in fibroblasts from the two patients and the absence of punctate immunofluorescence, indicating a true disorder of peroxisome biogenesis. In agreement with these results, Rao et al.[352] reported that both L-pipecolate oxidase and acyl-CoA oxidase were deficient in the first HPA-patient of Burton et al.[357] We recently extended these studies by performing complementation studies. These studies show unambiguously that the defect in HPA-patient 1 of Burton et al.[357] is at the level of the *PEX1* gene (see Chap. 129). Based on these results we conclude that the patients described by Gatfield et al.,[355] Thomas et al.,[356] and Burton et al.[357] were affected by a disorder of peroxisome biogenesis. Since then, additional patients have been described with pipecolic acidemia.

In 1991, Roesel et al.[360] reported increased pipecolic acid levels in plasma and urine of a patient affected by Dyggve-Melchior-Clausen syndrome, which is characterized by mental retardation, dwarfism due to a disturbed spondylometaepiphyseal development, and specific changes of the iliac crest. We have since tested more than 10 patients with this syndrome and have not found elevated pipecolic acid levels, suggesting that the finding of hyperpipecolic acidemia in a single patient with Dyggve-Melchior-Claussen syndrome may have been fortuitous.

In 1996, Vallet et al.[361] reported the fortuitous discovery of major hyperpipecolic acidemia in a 44-year-old man. He is manager of a small commercial firm, his major health problem being recurrent embolism possibly related to a moderate fasting hyperhomocystinemia (20 μM; normal: < 14). Plasma pipecolic acid levels were 250 and 220 μM (normal: < 2.5) at two different occasions in the presence of normal lysine levels. The chirality of the pipecolic acid accumulating in the patient was determined to be L- and not D-. Based on these findings the authors concluded that L-hyperpipecolic acidemia may be a benign trait. On the other hand, Poll-Thé and coworkers[362] recently identified three patients with diverse neurologic abnormalities, all showing isolated hyperpipecolic acidemia.

In two of the three patients, pipecolic acid in CSF was also markedly elevated. Hepatic peroxisomes were normally present.[362] These data indicate that much remains to be learned about this condition.

GLUTARYL-CoA METABOLISM IN PEROXISOMES AND GLUTARYL-CoA OXIDASE DEFICIENCY (MIM 231690)

The classic mechanism for the oxidation of glutaryl-CoA, a catabolite of L-lysine, L-hydroxylysine, and L-tryptophan, involves dehydrogenation to glutaconyl-CoA directly followed by decarboxylation to crotonyl-CoA. Both steps are catalyzed by a single enzyme, glutaryl-CoA dehydrogenase, a mitochondrial FAD-linked acyl-CoA dehydrogenase that donates its electrons via the ETF-system to the respiratory chain.

In 1984, Vamecq et al.[363] identified glutaryl-CoA oxidase activity in rat liver peroxisomes catalyzing the oxidation of glutaryl-CoA to glutaconyl-CoA but not to crotonyl-CoA.[364] Comparative studies suggest that glutaryl-CoA oxidase is a distinct enzyme that is different from acyl-CoA oxidase 1.[363] It could well be that a similar situation is true for human liver because Van Hove et al.[10] reported that both acyl-CoA oxidase 1 and the branched-chain acyl CoA oxidase are not reactive with glutaryl-CoA. On the other hand, data from Horie et al.[365] suggests that the presumed glutaryl-CoA oxidase is identical with acyl-CoA oxidase.

In 1991, Bennett et al.[366] described a patient who was investigated at 11 months of age because of failure to thrive and postprandial vomiting. Two abnormalities were found. First, she was homozygous for β-thalassemia and second, significant glutaric aciduria was found. Studies in fibroblasts revealed *normal* glutaryl-CoA dehydrogenase activity, whereas glutaryl-CoA oxidase activity was not detectable. This study has not been followed up at the enzyme protein and/or DNA level. No additional cases have been identified so far.

HYDROGEN PEROXIDE METABOLISM IN PEROXISOMES AND ACATALASEMIA (MIM 115500)

Catalase is a ubiquitous enzyme present in virtually all aerobic organisms, catalyzing the conversion of H_2O_2 to molecular oxygen and water. Catalase is a tetramer of approximately 240 kDa, with each of the four identical subunits carrying a single ferriprotoporphyrin (heme) group. In normal eukaryotic cells containing peroxisomes, catalase is virtually fully peroxisomal. However, catalase is also active in cells lacking peroxisomes, including erythrocytes and fibroblasts from patients with Zellweger syndrome. Studies have shown that this cytosolic catalase is indistinguishable from peroxisomal catalase in terms of native molecular mass (240 kDa) and kinetic constants.[367]

Acatalasemia is a rare disease that has mainly been described in Japan and Switzerland. In Japan, acatalasemia is associated with ulcerating, often gangrenous, oral lesions, whereas these abnormalities were not seen in Swiss patients. For a detailed account on acatalasemia, see Eaton and Mouchou.[368]

ACKNOWLEDGMENTS

The authors gratefully acknowledge Mrs. Maddy Festen for expert preparation of the manuscript, Mr. Jos Ruiter for preparation of the figures, and the Dutch Organization for Scientific Research (NWO) and the Princess Beatrix Fonds, The Hague, The Netherlands, for financial support.

REFERENCES

1. De Duve C, Baudhuin P: Peroxisomes (microbodies and related particles). *Physiol Rev* **46**:323, 1966.
2. Goldfischer S, Moore CL, Johnson AB, Spiro AJ, Valsamis MP, Wisniewski HK, Ritch RH, et al: Peroxisomal and mitochondrial defects in the cerebro-hepato-renal syndrome. *Science* **182**:62, 1973.
3. Brown FR 3rd, McAdams AJ, Cummins JW, Konkol R, Singh I, Moser AB, Moser HW: Cerebro-hepato-renal (Zellweger) syndrome and neonatal adrenoleukodystrophy: Similarities in phenotype and accumulation of very long chain fatty acids. *Johns Hopkins Med J* **151**:344, 1982.
4. Heymans HSA, Schutgens RBH, Tan R, van den Bosch H, Borst P: Severe plasmalogen deficiency in tissues of infants without peroxisomes (Zellweger syndrome). *Nature* **306**:69, 1983.
5. Cooper TG, Beevers H: Beta oxidation in glyoxysomes from castor bean endosperm. *J Biol Chem* **244**:3514, 1969.
6. Tolbert NE: Metabolic pathways in peroxisomes and glyoxysomes. *Annu Rev Biochem* **50**:133, 1981.
7. Lazarow PB, De Duve C: A fatty acyl-CoA oxidizing system in rat liver peroxisomes; enhancement by clofibrate, a hypolipidemic drug. *Proc Natl Acad Sci U S A* **73**:2043, 1976.
8. Kunau WH, Dommes V, Schulz H: Beta-oxidation of fatty acids in mitochondria, peroxisomes, and bacteria: A century of continued progress. *Prog Lipid Res* **34**:267, 1995.
9. Osumi T, Hashimoto T, Ui N: Purification and properties of acyl-CoA oxidase from rat liver. *J Biochem (Tokyo)* **87**:1735, 1980.
10. Vanhove GF, Van Veldhoven PP, Fransen M, Denis S, Eyssen HJ, Wanders RJA, Mannaerts GP: The CoA esters of 2-methyl-branched chain fatty acids and of the bile acid intermediates di- and trihydroxycoprostanic acids are oxidized by one single peroxisomal branched chain acyl-CoA oxidase in human liver and kidney. *J Biol Chem* **268**:10335, 1993.
11. Verhoeven NM, Roe DS, Kok RM, Wanders RJA, Jakobs C, Roe C: Phytanic acid and pristanic acid are oxidized by sequential peroxisomal and mitochondrial reactions in cultured fibroblasts. *J Lipid Res* **39**:66, 1998.
12. McGarry JD, Brown NF: The mitochondrial carnitine palmitoyltransferase system. From concept to molecular analysis. *Eur J Biochem* **244**:1, 1997.
13. Shani N, Watkins PA, Valle D: PXA1, a possible *Saccharomyces cerevisiae* ortholog of the human adrenoleukodystrophy gene. *Proc Natl Acad Sci U S A* **92**:6012, 1995.
14. Hettema EH, van Roermund CWT, Distel B, van den Berg M, Vilela C, Rodrigues-Pousada C, Wanders RJA, et al: The ABC transporter proteins Pat1 and Pat2 are required for import of long-chain fatty acids into peroxisomes of Saccharomyces cerevisiae. *EMBO J* **15**:3813, 1996.
15. Swartzman EE, Viswanathan MN, Thorner J: The PAL1 gene product is a peroxisomal ATP-binding cassette transporter in the yeast *Saccharomyces cerevisiae*. *J Cell Biol* **132**:549, 1996.
16. Shani N, Valle D: A *Saccharomyces cerevisiae* homolog of the human adrenoleukodystrophy transporter is a heterodimer of two half ATP-binding cassette transporters. *Proc Natl Acad Sci U S A* **93**:11901, 1996.
17. Verleur N, Hettema EH, van Roermund CWT, Tabak HF, Wanders RJA: Transport of activated fatty acids by the peroxisomal ATP-binding-cassette transporter Pxa2 in a semi-intact yeast cell system. *Eur J Biochem* **249**:657, 1997.
18. Kamijo K, Taketani S, Yokota S, Osumi T, Hashimoto T: The 70-kDa peroxisomal membrane protein is a member of the Mdr (P-glycoprotein)-related ATP-binding protein superfamily. *J Biol Chem* **265**:4534, 1990.

19. Kamijo K, Kamijo T, Ueno I, Osumi T, Hashimoto T: Nucleotide sequence of the human 70 kDa peroxisomal membrane protein: A member of ATP-binding cassette transporters. *Biochim Biophys Acta* **1129**:323, 1992.
20. Mosser J, Douar AM, Sarde CO, Kioschis P, Feil R, Moser H, Poustka AM, et al: Putative X-linked adrenoleukodystrophy gene shares unexpected homology with ABC transporters. *Nature* **361**:726, 1993.
21. Mosser J, Lutz Y, Stoeckel ME, Sarde CO, Kretz C, Douar AM, Lopez J, et al: The gene responsible for adrenoleukodystrophy encodes a peroxisomal membrane protein. *Hum Mol Genet* **3**:265, 1994.
22. Lombard-Platet G, Savary S, Sarde CO, Mandel JL, Chimini G: A close relative of the adrenoleukodystrophy (ALD) gene codes for a peroxisomal protein with a specific expression pattern. *Proc Natl Acad Sci U S A* **93**:1265, 1996.
23. Holzinger A, Kammerer S, Berger J, Roscher AA: cDNA cloning and mRNA expression of the human adrenoleukodystrophy related protein (ALDRP), a peroxisomal ABC transporter. *Biochem Biophys Res Commun* **239**:261, 1997.
24. Shani N, Jimenez-Sanchez G, Steel G, Dean M, Valle D: Identification of a fourth half ABC transporter in the human peroxisomal membrane. *Hum Mol Genet* **6**:1925, 1997.
25. Holzinger A, Kammerer S, Roscher AA: Primary structure of human PMP69, a putative peroxisomal ABC-transporter. *Biochem Biophys Res Commun* **237**:152, 1997.
26. Braiterman LT, Zheng S, Watkins PA, Geraghty MT, Johnson G, McGuinness MC, Moser AB, et al: Suppression of peroxisomal membrane protein defects by peroxisomal ATP binding cassette (ABC) proteins. *Hum Mol Genet* **7**:239, 1998.
27. Kemp S, Wei HM, Lu JF, Braiterman LT, McGuinness MC, Moser AB, Watkins PA, et al: Gene redundancy and pharmacological gene therapy: Implications for X-linker adrenoleukodystrophy. *Nat Med* **4**:1261, 1999.
28. Flavigny E, Sanhaj A, Aubourg P, Cartier N: Retroviral-mediated adrenoleukodystrophy-related gene transfer corrects very long chain fatty acid metabolism in adrenoleukodystrophy fibroblasts: Implications for therapy. *FEBS Lett* **448**:261, 1999.
29. Netik A, Forss-Petter S, Holzinger A, Molzer B, Unterrainer G, Berger J: Adrenoleukodystrophy-related protein can compensate functionally for adrenoleukodystrophy protein deficiency (X-ALD): Implications for therapy. *Hum Mol Genet* **8**:907, 1999.
30. Higgins CF: ABC transporters: From microorganisms to man. *Annu Rev Cell Biol* **8**:67, 1992.
31. Smith KD, Kemp S, Braiterman LT, Lu JF, Wei HM, Geraghty M, Stetten G, et al: X-linked adrenoleukodystrophy: Genes, mutations, and phenotypes. *Neurochem Res* **24**:521, 1999.
32. Liu LX, Janvier K, Berteaux-Lecellier V, Cartier N, Benarous R, Aubourg P: Homo- and heterodimerization of peroxisomal ATP-binding cassette half-transporters. *J Biol Chem* **274**:32738, 1999.
33. Ewart GD, Cannell D, Cox GB, Howells AJ: Mutational analysis of the traffic ATPase (ABC) transporters involved in uptake of eye pigment precursors in *Drosophila melanogaster*. Implications for structure-function relationships. *J Biol Chem* **269**:10370, 1994.
34. McGarry JD, Foster DW: Regulation of hepatic fatty acid oxidation and ketone body production. *Annu Rev Biochem* **49**:395, 1980.
35. Lock EA, Mitchell AM, Elcombe CR: Biochemical mechanisms of induction of hepatic peroxisome proliferation. *Annu Rev Pharmacol Toxicol* **29**:145, 1989.
36. Aoyama T, Peters JM, Iritani N, Nakajima T, Furihata K, Hashimoto T, Gonzalez FJ: Altered constitutive expression of fatty acid-metabolizing enzymes in mice lacking the peroxisome proliferator-activated receptor alpha (PPARalpha). *J Biol Chem* **273**:5678, 1998.
37. Poll-Thé BT, Roels F, Ogier H, Scotto J, Vamecq J, Schutgens RBH, Wanders RJA, et al: A new peroxisomal disorder with enlarged peroxisomes and a specific deficiency of acyl-CoA oxidase (pseudo-neonatal adrenoleukodystrophy). *Am J Hum Genet* **42**:422, 1988.
38. Miyazawa S, Hashimoto T, Yokota S: Identity of long-chain acyl-coenzyme A synthetase of microsomes, mitochondria, and peroxisomes in rat liver. *J Biochem (Tokyo)* **98**:723, 1985.
39. Wanders RJA, Denis S, van Roermund CWT, Jakobs C, ten Brink HJ: Characteristics and subcellular localization of pristanoyl-CoA synthetase in rat liver. *Biochim Biophys Acta* **1125**:274, 1992.
40. Jakobs BS, Wanders RJA: Fatty acid beta-oxidation in peroxisomes and mitochondria: The first, unequivocal evidence for the involvement of carnitine in shuttling propionyl-CoA from peroxisomes to mitochondria. *Biochem Biophys Res Commun* **213**:1035, 1995.
41. Schepers L, Casteels M, Verheyden K, Parmentier G, Asselberghs S, Eyssen HJ, Mannaerts GP: Subcellular distribution and characteristics of trihydroxycoprostanoyl-CoA synthetase in rat liver. *Biochem J* **257**:221, 1989.
42. Kase BF, Bjorkhem I: Peroxisomal bile acid-CoA:amino-acid N-acyltransferase in rat liver. *J Biol Chem* **264**:9220, 1989.
43. Voss A, Reinhart M, Sankarappa S, Sprecher H: The metabolism of 7,10,13,16,19-docosapentaenoic acid to 4,7,10, 13,16,19-docosahexaenoic acid in rat liver is independent of a 4-desaturase. *J Biol Chem* **266**:19995, 1991.
44. Moore SA, Hurt E, Yoder E, Sprecher H, Spector AA: Docosahexaenoic acid synthesis in human skin fibroblasts involves peroxisomal retroconversion of tetracosahexaenoic acid. *J Lipid Res* **36**:2433, 1995.
45. Sprecher H, Luthria DL, Mohammed BS, Baykousheva SP: Reevaluation of the pathways for the biosynthesis of polyunsaturated fatty acids. *J Lipid Res* **36**:2471, 1995.
46. Diczfalusy U: Beta-oxidation of eicosanoids. *Prog Lipid Res* **33**:403, 1994.
47. Diczfalusy U, Kase BF, Alexson SE, Bjorkhem I: Metabolism of prostaglandin F2 alpha in Zellweger syndrome. Peroxisomal beta-oxidation is a major importance for in vivo degradation of prostaglandins in humans. *J Clin Invest* **88**:978, 1991.
48. Diczfalusy U, Vesterqvist O, Kase BF, Lund E, Alexson SE: Peroxisomal chain-shortening of thromboxane B2: evidence for impaired degradation of thromboxane B2 in Zellweger syndrome. *J Lipid Res* **34**:1107, 1993.
49. de Waart DR, Koomen GC, Wanders RJA: Studies on the urinary excretion of thromboxane B2 in Zellweger patients and control subjects: evidence for a major role for peroxisomes in the beta-oxidative chain-shortening of thromboxane B2. *Biochim Biophys Acta* **1226**:44, 1994.
50. Jedlitschky G, Huber M, Volkl A, Muller M, Leier I, Muller J, Lehmann WD, et al: Peroxisomal degradation of leukotrienes by beta-oxidation from the omega-end. *J Biol Chem* **266**:24763, 1991.
51. Mayatepek E, Lehmann WD, Fauler J, Tsikas D, Frolich JC, Schutgens RBH, Wanders RJA, et al: Impaired degradation of leukotrienes in patients with peroxisome deficiency disorders. *J Clin Invest* **91**:881, 1993.
52. Gordon JA, Figard PH, Spector AA: Hydroxyeicosatetraenoic acid metabolism in cultured human skin fibroblasts. Evidence for peroxisomal beta-oxidation. *J Clin Invest* **85**:1173, 1990.
53. Vamecq J, de Hoffmann E, Van Hoof F: The microsomal dicarboxylyl-CoA synthetase. *Biochem J* **230**:683, 1985.
54. Suzuki H, Yamada J, Watanabe T, Suga T: Compartmentation of dicarboxylic acid beta-oxidation in rat liver: Importance of peroxisomes in the metabolism of dicarboxylic acids. *Biochim Biophys Acta* **990**:25, 1989.
55. Christensen E, Hagve TA, Christophersen BO: The Zellweger syndrome: Deficient chain-shortening of erucic acid (22:1 (n-9)) and adrenic acid (22:4 (n-6)) in cultured skin fibroblasts. *Biochim Biophys Acta* **959**:134, 1988.
56. Christensen E, Gronn M, Hagve TA, Kase BF, Christophersen BO: Adrenoleukodystrophy. The chain shortening of erucic acid (22:1 (n-9)) and adrenic acid (22:4(n-6)) is deficient in neonatal adrenoleukodystrophy and normal in X-linked adrenoleukodystrophy skin fibroblasts. *Biochim Biophys Acta* **1002**:79, 1989.
57. Street JM, Johnson DW, Singh H, Poulos A: Metabolism of saturated and polyunsaturated fatty acids by normal and Zellweger syndrome skin fibroblasts. *Biochem J* **260**:647, 1989.
58. Poulos A: Very long chain fatty acids in higher animals—A review. *Lipids* **30**:1, 1995.
59. Poulos A, Sharp P, Singh H, Johnson D, Fellenberg A, Pollard A: Detection of a homologous series of C26-C38 polyenoic fatty acids in the brain of patients without peroxisomes (Zellweger's syndrome). *Biochem J* **235**:607, 1986.
60. Sharp P, Poulos A, Fellenberg A, Johnson D: Structure and lipid distribution of polyenoic very-long-chain fatty acids in the brain of peroxisome-deficient patients (Zellweger syndrome). *Biochem J* **248**:61, 1987.
61. Poulos A, Sharp P, Johnson D, Easton C: The occurrence of polyenoic very long chain fatty acids with greater than 32 carbon atoms in molecular species of phosphatidylcholine in normal and peroxisome-deficient (Zellweger's syndrome) brain. *Biochem J* **253**:645, 1988.
62. Gatt S, Bremer J, Osmundsen H: Pyrene dodecanoic acid coenzyme A ester: Peroxisomal oxidation and chain shortening. *Biochim Biophys Acta* **958**:130, 1988.
63. Suzuki H, Mori K, Yamada J, Suga T: Contribution of peroxisomal beta-oxidation system to the chain-shortening of *N*-(alpha-methylbenzol)azelaic acid in rat liver. *Biochem Pharmacol* **39**:1975, 1990.

64. Yamada J, Horie S, Watanabe T, Suga T: Participation of peroxisomal beta-oxidation system in the chain-shortening of a xenobiotic acyl compound. *Biochem Biophys Res Commun* **125**:123, 1984.
65. Yamada J, Ogawa S, Horie S, Watanabe T, Suga T: Participation of peroxisomes in the metabolism of xenobiotic acyl compounds: Comparison between peroxisomal and mitochondrial beta-oxidation of omega-phenyl fatty acids in rat liver. *Biochim Biophys Acta* **921**:292, 1987.
66. Yoshida Y, Yamada J, Watanabe T, Suga T, Takayama H: Participation of the peroxisomal beta-oxidation system in the chain-shortening of PCA16, a metabolite of the cytosine arabinoside prodrug, YNKO1, in rat liver. *Biochem Pharmacol* **39**:1505, 1990.
67. Furuta S, Miyazawa S, Osumi T, Hashimoto T, Ui N: Properties of mitochondrial and peroxisomal enoyl-CoA hydratases from rat liver. *J Biochem (Tokyo)* **88**:1059, 1980.
68. Miyazawa S, Osumi T, Hashimoto T: The presence of a new 3-oxoacyl-CoA thiolase in rat liver peroxisomes. *Eur J Biochem* **103**:589, 1980.
69. Miyazawa S, Furuta S, Osumi T, Hashimoto T, Ui N: Properties of peroxisomal 3-ketoacyl-coA thiolase from rat liver. *J Biochem (Tokyo)* **90**:511, 1981.
70. Hashimoto T: Peroxisomal beta-oxidation: Enzymology and molecular biology. *Ann N Y Acad Sci* **804**:86, 1996.
71. ten Brink HJ, Stellaard F, van den Heuvel CM, Kok RM, Schor DS, Wanders RJA, Jakobs C: Pristanic acid and phytanic acid in plasma from patients with peroxisomal disorders: Stable isotope dilution analysis with electron capture negative ion mass fragmentography. *J Lipid Res* **33**:41, 1992.
72. Van Veldhoven PP, Vanhove G, Vanhoutte F, Dacremont G, Parmentier G, Eyssen HJ, Mannaerts GP: Identification and purification of a peroxisomal branched chain fatty acyl-CoA oxidase. *J Biol Chem* **266**:24676, 1991.
73. Wanders RJA, Denis S, Jakobs C, ten Brink HJ: Identification of pristanoyl-CoA oxidase as a distinct, clofibrate non-inducible enzyme in rat liver peroxisomes. *Biochim Biophys Acta* **1124**:199, 1992.
74. Casteels M, Schepers L, Van Veldhoven PP, Eyssen HJ, Mannaerts GP: Separate peroxisomal oxidases for fatty acyl-CoAs and trihydroxycoprostanoyl-CoA in human liver. *J Lipid Res* **31**:1865, 1990.
75. Van Veldhoven PP, Vanhove G, Assselberghs S, Eyssen HJ, Mannaerts GP: Substrate specificities of rat liver peroxisomal acyl-CoA oxidases: Palmitoyl-CoA oxidase (inducible acyl-CoA oxidase), pristanoyl-CoA oxidase (non-inducible acyl-CoA oxidase), and trihydroxycoprostanoyl-CoA oxidase. *J Biol Chem* **267**:20065, 1992.
76. Osumi T, Ishii N, Miyazawa S, Hashimoto T: Isolation and structural characterization of the rat acyl-CoA oxidase gene. *J Biol Chem* **262**:8138, 1987.
77. Aoyama T, Tsushima K, Souri M, Kamijo T, Suzuki Y, Shimozawa N, Orii T, et al: Molecular cloning and functional expression of a human peroxisomal acyl-coenzyme A oxidase. *Biochem Biophys Res Commun* **198**:1113, 1994.
78. Fournier B, Saudubray JM, Benichou B, Lyonnet S, Munnich A, Clevers H, Poll-Thé BT: Large deletion of the peroxisomal acyl-CoA oxidase gene in pseudoneonatal adrenoleukodystrophy. *J Clin Invest* **94**:526, 1994.
79. Varanasi U, Chu R, Chu S, Espinosa R, LeBeau MM, Reddy JK: Isolation of the human peroxisomal acyl-CoA oxidase gene: Organization, promoter analysis, and chromosomal localization. *Proc Natl Acad Sci U S A* **91**:3107, 1994.
80. Vanhooren JC, Fransen M, de Bethune B, Baumgart E, Baes M, Torrekens S, Van Leuven F, et al: Rat pristanoyl-CoA oxidase. cDNA cloning and recognition of its C-terminal (SQL) by the peroxisomal-targeting signal 1 receptor. *Eur J Biochem* **239**:302, 1996.
81. Baumgart E, Vanhooren JC, Fransen M, Van Leuven F, Fahimi HD, Van Veldhoven PP, Mannaerts GP: Molecular cloning and further characterization of rat peroxisomal trihydroxycoprostanoyl-CoA oxidase. *Biochem J* **320**:115, 1996.
82. Baumgart E, Vanhooren JC, Fransen M, Marynen P, Puype M, Vandekerckhove J, Leunissen JA, et al: Molecular characterization of the human peroxisomal branched-chain acyl-CoA oxidase: cDNA cloning, chromosomal assignment, tissue distribution, and evidence for the absence of the protein in Zellweger syndrome. *Proc Natl Acad Sci U S A* **93**:13748, 1996.
83. Palosaari PM, Hiltunen JK: Peroxisomal bifunctional protein from rat liver is a trifunctional enzyme possessing 2-enoyl-CoA hydratase, 3-hydroxyacyl-CoA dehydrogenase, and delta 3, delta 2-enoyl-CoA isomerase activities. *J Biol Chem* **265**:2446, 1990.
84. Novikov DK, Vanhove GF, Carchon H, Asselberghs S, Eyssen HJ, Van Veldhoven PP, Mannaerts GP: Peroxisomal beta-oxidation. Purification of four novel 3-hydroxyacyl-CoA dehydrogenases from rat liver peroxisomes. *J Biol Chem* **269**:27125, 1994.
85. Dieuaide-Noubhani M, Novikov D, Baumgart E, Vanhooren JC, Fransen M, Goethals M, Vandekerckhove J, et al: Further characterization of the peroxisomal 3-hydroxyacyl-CoA dehydrogenases from rat liver. Relationship between the different dehydrogenases and evidence that fatty acids and the C27 bile acids di- and tri-hydroxycoprostanic acids are metabolized by separate multifunctional proteins. *Eur J Biochem* **240**:660, 1996.
86. Adamski J, Husen B, Marks F, Jungblut PW: The 17 beta-oestradiol dehydrogenase of pig endometrial cells is localized in specialized vesicles. *Biochem J* **290**:777, 1993.
87. Markus M, Husen B, Leenders F, Jungblut PW, Hall PF, Adamski J: The organelles containing porcine 17 beta-estradiol dehydrogenase are peroxisomes. *Eur J Cell Biol* **68**:263, 1995.
88. Leenders F, Tesdorpf JG, Markus M, Engel T, Seedorf U, Adamski J: Porcine 80-kDa protein reveals intrinsic 17 beta-hydroxysteroid dehydrogenase, fatty acyl-CoA-hydratase/dehydrogenase, and sterol transfer activities. *J Biol Chem* **271**:5438, 1996.
89. Qin YM, Poutanen MH, Helander HM, Kvist AP, Siivari KM, Schmitz W, Conzelmann E, et al: Peroxisomal multifunctional enzyme of beta-oxidation metabolizing D-3-hydroxyacyl-CoA esters in rat liver: Molecular cloning, expression and characterization. *Biochem J* **321**:21, 1997.
90. Malila LH, Siivari KM, Makela MJ, Jalonen JE, Latipaa PM, Kunau WH, Hiltunen JK: Enzymes converting D-3-hydroxyacyl-CoA to *trans*-2-enoyl-CoA. Microsomal and peroxisomal isoenzymes in rat liver. *J Biol Chem* **268**:21578, 1993.
91. Jiang LL, Kobayashi A, Matsuura H, Fukushima H, Hashimoto T: Purification and properties of human D-3-hydroxyacyl-CoA dehydratase: Medium-chain enoyl-CoA hydratase is D-3-hydroxyacyl-CoA dehydratase. *J Biochem* (Tokyo) **120**:624, 1996.
92. Jiang LL, Miyazawa S, Hashimoto T: Purification and properties of rat D-3-hydroxyacyl-CoA dehydratase: D-3-Hydroxyacyl-CoA dehydratase/D-3-hydroxyacyl-CoA dehydrogenase bifunctional protein. *J Biochem (Tokyo)* **120**:633, 1996.
93. Jiang LL, Miyazawa S, Souri M, Hashimoto T: Structure of D-3-hydroxyacyl-CoA dehydratase/D-3-hydroxyacyl-CoA dehydrogenase bifunctional protein. *J Biochem (Tokyo)* **121**:364, 1997.
94. Jiang LL, Kurosawa T, Sato M, Suzuki Y, Hashimoto T: Physiological role of D-3-hydroxyacyl-CoA dehydratase/D-3-hydroxyacyl-CoA dehydrogenase bifunctional protein. *J Biochem (Tokyo)* **121**:506, 1997.
95. Moller G, Leenders F, van Grunsven EG, Dolez V, Qualmann B, Kessels MM, Markus M, et al: Characterization of the HSD17B4 gene: D-specific multifunctional protein 2/17beta-hydroxysteroid dehydrogenase IV. *J Steroid Biochem Mol Biol* **69**:441, 1999.
96. Wanders RJA, Denis S, Wouters F, Wirtz KW, Seedorf U: Sterol carrier protein X (SCPx) is a peroxisomal branched-chain beta-ketothiolase specifically reacting with 3-oxo-pristanoyl-CoA: A new, unique role for SCPx in branched-chain fatty acid metabolism in peroxisomes. *Biochem Biophys Res Commun* **236**:565, 1997.
97. Dieuaide-Noubhani M, Novikov D, Vandekerckhove J, Veldhoven PP, Mannaerts GP: Identification and characterization of the 2-enoyl-CoA hydratases involved in peroxisomal beta-oxidation in rat liver. *Biochem J* **321**:253, 1997.
98. Dieuaide-Noubhani M, Asselberghs S, Mannaerts GP, Van Veldhoven PP: Evidence that multifunctional protein 2, and not multifunctional protein 1, is involved in the peroxisomal beta-oxidation of pristanic acid. *Biochem J* **325**:367, 1997.
99. van Grunsven EG, van Berkel E, IJlst L, Vreken P, de Klerk JB, Adamski J, Lemonde H, et al: Peroxisomal D-3-hydroxyacyl-CoA dehydrogenase deficiency: Resolution of the enzyme defect and its molecular basis in bifunctional protein deficiency. *Proc Natl Acad Sci U S A* **95**:2128, 1998.
100. Xu R, Cuebas DA: The reactions catalyzed by the inducible bifunctional enzyme of rat liver peroxisomes cannot lead to the formation of bile acids. *Biochem Biophys Res Commun* **221**:271, 1996.
101. Kinoshita N, Miyata T, Ismail SM, Fujimoto Y, Kakinuma K, Ikekawa N, Morisaki M: Synthesis and determination of stereochemistry of four diastereoisomers at the C-24 and C-25 positions of 3alpha, 7alpha, 12alpha, 24-Tetrahydroxy-5beta-cholestan-26-oic acid. *Chem Pharm Bull* **36**:134, 1988.
102. Osumi T, Ishii N, Hijikata M, Kamijo K, Ozasa H, Furuta S, Miyazawa S, et al: Molecular cloning and nucleotide sequence of the cDNA for

rat peroxisomal enoyl-CoA: Hydratase-3-hydroxyacyl-CoA dehydrogenase bifunctional enzyme. *J Biol Chem* **260**:8905, 1985.

103. Ishii N, Hijikata M, Osumi T, Hashimoto T: Structural organization of the gene for rat enoyl-CoA hydratase: 3-hydroxyacyl-CoA dehydrogenase bifunctional enzyme. *J Biol Chem* **262**:8144, 1987.
104. Hoefler G, Forstner M, McGuinness MC, Hulla W, Hiden M, Krisper P, Kenner L, et al: cDNA cloning of the human peroxisomal enoyl-CoA hydratase: 3-hydroxyacyl-CoA dehydrogenase bifunctional enzyme and localization to chromosome 3q26.3-3q28: A free left Alu Arm is inserted in the 3′ noncoding region. *Genomics* **19**:60, 1994.
105. Leenders F, Adamski J, Husen B, Thole HH, Jungblut PW: Molecular cloning and amino acid sequence of the porcine 17 beta-estradiol dehydrogenase. *Eur J Biochem* **222**:221, 1994.
106. Normand T, Husen B, Leenders F, Pelczar H, Baert JL, Begue A, Flourens AC, et al: Molecular characterization of mouse 17 beta-hydroxysteroid dehydrogenase IV. *J Steroid Biochem Mol Biol* **55**:541, 1995.
107. Corton JC, Bocos C, Moreno ES, Merritt A, Marsman DS, Sausen PJ, Cattley RC, et al: Rat 17 beta-hydroxysteroid dehydrogenase type IV is a novel peroxisome proliferator-inducible gene. *Mol Pharmacol* **50**:1157, 1996.
108. Kobayashi K, Kobayashi H, Ueda M, Honda Y: Expression of 17-beta-hydroxysteroid dehydrogenase type IV in chick retinal pigment epithelium. *Exp Eye Res* **64**:719, 1997.
109. Caira F, Clemencet MC, Cherkaoui-Malki M, Dieuaide-Noubhani M, Pacot C, Van Veldhoven PP, Latruffe N: Differential regulation by a peroxisome proliferator of the different multifunctional proteins in guinea pig: cDNA cloning of the guinea pig D-specific multifunctional protein 2. *Biochem J* **330**:1361, 1998.
110. Adamski J, Normand T, Leenders F, Monte D, Begue A, Stehelin D, Jungblut PW, et al: Molecular cloning of a novel widely expressed human 80 kDa 17 beta-hydroxysteroid dehydrogenase IV. *Biochem J* **311**:437, 1995.
111. Seedorf U, Brysch P, Engel T, Schrage K, Assmann G: Sterol carrier protein X is peroxisomal 3-oxoacyl coenzyme A thiolase with intrinsic sterol carrier and lipid transfer activity. *J Biol Chem* **269**:21277, 1994.
112. Antonenkov VD, Van Veldhoven PP, Waelkens E, Mannaerts GP: Substrate specificities of 3-oxoacyl-CoA thiolase A and sterol carrier protein 2/3-oxoacyl-CoA thiolase purified from normal rat liver peroxisomes. Sterol carrier protein 2/3-oxoacyl-CoA thiolase is involved in the metabolism of 2-methyl-branched fatty acids and bile acid intermediates. *J Biol Chem* **272**:26023, 1997.
113. Wanders RJA, Denis S, van Berkel E, Wouters F, Wirtz KWA, Seedorf U: Identification of the newly discovered 58 kDa peroxisomal thiolase SCPx as the main thiolase involved in both pristanic acid and trihydroxycholestanoic acid oxidation: Implications for peroxisomal beta-oxidation disorders. *J Inherit Metab Dis* **21**:302, 1998.
114. Bunya M, Maebuchi M, Kamiryo T, Kurosawa T, Sato M, Tohma M, Jiang LL, et al: Thiolase involved in bile acid formation. *J Biochem (Tokyo)* **123**:347, 1998.
115. Hijikata M, Ishii N, Kagamiyama H, Osumi T, Hashimoto T: Structural analysis of cDNA for rat peroxisomal 3-ketoacyl-CoA thiolase. *J Biol Chem* **262**:8151, 1987.
116. Hijikata M, Wen JK, Osumi T, Hashimoto T: Rat peroxisomal 3-ketoacyl-CoA thiolase gene. Occurrence of two closely related but differentially regulated genes. *J Biol Chem* **265**:4600, 1990.
117. Bout A, Teunissen Y, Hashimoto T, Benne R, Tager JM: Nucleotide sequence of human peroxisomal 3-oxoacyl-CoA thiolase. *Nucleic Acids Res* **16**:10369, 1988.
118. Ohba T, Rennert H, Pfeifer SM, He Z, Yamamoto R, Holt JA, Billheimer JT, et al: The structure of the human sterol carrier protein X/sterol carrier protein 2 gene (SCP2). *Genomics* **24**:370, 1994.
119. Ohba T, Holt JA, Billheimer JT, Strauss JF 3rd: Human sterol carrier protein x/sterol carrier protein 2 gene has two promoters. *Biochemistry* **34**:10660, 1995.
120. Mori T, Tsukamoto T, Mori H, Tashiro Y, Fujiki Y: Molecular cloning and deduced amino acid sequence of nonspecific lipid transfer protein (sterol carrier protein 2) of rat liver: A higher molecular mass (60 kDa) protein contains the primary sequence of nonspecific lipid transfer protein as its C-terminal part. *Proc Natl Acad Sci U S A* **88**:4338, 1991.
121. Ossendorp BC, Van Heusden GP, De Beer AL, Bos K, Schouten GL, Wirtz KW: Identification of the cDNA clone which encodes the 58-kDa protein containing the amino acid sequence of rat liver non-specific lipid-transfer protein (sterol-carrier protein 2). Homology with rat peroxisomal and mitochondrial 3-oxoacyl-CoA thiolases. *Eur J Biochem* **201**:233, 1991.
122. Seedorf U, Assmann G: Cloning, expression, and nucleotide sequence of rat liver sterol carrier protein 2 cDNAs. *J Biol Chem* **266**:630, 1991.
123. Wirtz KW: Phospholipid transfer proteins revisited. *Biochem J* **324**:353, 1997.
124. van Grunsven EG, van Berkel E, Mooijer PAW, Watkins PA, Moser HW, Suzuki Y, Jiang LL, et al: Peroxisomal bifunctional protein deficiency revisited: Resolution of its true enzymatic and molecular basis. *Am J Hum Genet* **64**:99, 1999.
125. Wanders RJA, van Grunsven EG, Jansen GA: Lipid metabolism in peroxisomes: Enzymology, functions and dysfunctions of the fatty acid alpha- and beta-oxidation systems in humans. *Biochem Soc Trans* **28**:141, 2000.
126. Hoefler G, Hoefler S, Watkins PA, Chen WW, Moser A, Baldwin V, McGillivary B, et al: Biochemical abnormalities in rhizomelic chondrodysplasia punctata. *J Pediatr* **112**:726, 1988.
127. Wanders RJA, Tager JM: Lipid metabolism in peroxisomes in relation to human disease. *Mol Aspects Med* **19**:69, 1998.
128. Seedorf U, Raabe M, Ellinghaus P, Kannenberg F, Fobker M, Engel T, Denis S, et al: Defective peroxisomal catabolism of branched fatty acyl coenzyme A in mice lacking the sterol carrier protein-2/sterol carrier protein-x gene function. *Genes Dev* **12**:1189, 1998.
129. Qi C, Zhu Y, Pan J, Usada N, Maeda N, Yeldandi AV, Rao MS, et al: Absence of spontaneous peroxisome proliferation in enoyl-CoA hydratase/L-3-hydroxyacyl-CoA dehydrogenase-deficient mouse liver. *J Biol Chem* **274**:15775, 1999.
130. Kunau WH, Dommes P: Degradation of unsaturated fatty acids. Identification of intermediates in the degradation of *cis*-4-decenoly-CoA by extracts of beef-liver mitochondria. *Eur J Biochem* **91**:533, 1978.
131. Henke B, Girzalsky W, Berteaux-Lecellier V, Erdmann R: IDP3 encodes a peroxisomal NADP-dependent isocitrate dehydrogenase required for the beta-oxidation of unsaturated fatty acids. *J Biol Chem* **273**:3702, 1998.
132. Muller-Newen G, Stoffel W: Mitochondrial 3-2-*trans*-enoyl-CoA isomerase. Purification, cloning, expression, and mitochondrial import of the key enzyme of unsaturated fatty acid beta-oxidation. *Biol Chem Hoppe Seyler* **372**:613, 1991.
133. Palosaari PM, Kilponen JM, Sormunen RT, Hassinen IE, Hiltunen JK: Delta 3, delta 2-enoyl-CoA isomerases. Characterization of the mitochondrial isoenzyme in the rat. *J Biol Chem* **265**:3347, 1990.
134. Tomioka Y, Hirose A, Moritani H, Hishinuma T, Hashimoto T, Mizugaki M: cDNA cloning of mitochondrial delta 3, delta 2-enoyl-CoA isomerase of rat liver. *Biochim Biophys Acta* **1130**:109, 1992.
135. Kilponen JM, Hayrinen HM, Rehn M, Hiltunen JK: cDNA cloning and amino acid sequence of human mitochondrial delta 3 delta 2-enoyl-CoA isomerase: Comparison of the human enzyme with its rat counterpart, mitochondrial short-chain isomerase. *Biochem J* **300**:1, 1994.
136. Kilponen JM, Palosaari PM, Hiltunen JK: Occurrence of a long-chain delta 3,delta 2-enoyl-CoA isomerase in rat liver. *Biochem J* **269**:223, 1990.
137. Hiltunen JK, Wenzel B, Beyer A, Erdmann R, Fossa A, Kunau WH: Peroxisomal multifunctional beta-oxidation protein of *Saccharomyces cerevisiae*. Molecular analysis of the fox2 gene and gene product. *J Biol Chem* **267**:6646, 1992.
138. Gurvitz A, Mursula AM, Firzinger A, Hamilton B, Kilpelainen SH, Hartig A, Ruis H, et al: Peroxisomal delta 3-*cis*-delta 2-*trans*-enoyl-CoA isomerase encoded by ECI1 is required for growth of the yeast *Saccharomyces cerevisiae* on unsaturated fatty acids. *J Biol Chem* **273**:31366, 1998.
139. Geisbrecht BV, Zhu D, Schulz K, Nau K, Morrell JC, Geraghty M, Schulz H, et al: Molecular characterization of *Saccharomyces cerevisiae* delta3, delta2-enoyl-CoA isomerase. *J Biol Chem* **273**:33184, 1998.
140. Geisbrecht BV, Zhang D, Schulz H, Gould SJ: Characterization of PECI, a novel monofunctional delta(3), delta(2)-enoyl-CoA isomerase of mammalian peroxisomes. *J Biol Chem* **274**:21797, 1999.
141. Hiltunen JK, Filppula SA, Koivuranta KT, Siivari K, Qin YM, Hayrinen HM: Peroxisomal beta-oxidation and polyunsaturated fatty acids. *Ann N Y Acad Sci* **804**:116, 1996.
142. Dommes V, Baumgart C, Kunau WH: Degradation of unsaturated fatty acids in peroxisomes. Existence of a 2,4-dienoyl-CoA reductase pathway. *J Biol Chem* **256**:8259, 1981.
143. Hakkola EH, Hiltunen JK: The existence of two mitochondrial isoforms of 2,4-dienoyl-CoA reductase in the rat. *Eur J Biochem* **215**:199, 1993.

144. Hirose A, Kamijo K, Osumi T, Hashimoto T, Mizugaki M: cDNA cloning of rat liver 2,4-dienoyl-CoA reductase. *Biochim Biophys Acta* **1049**:346, 1990.
145. Koivuranta KT, Hakkola EH, Hiltunen JK: Isolation and characterization of cDNA for human 120 kDa mitochondrial 2,4-dienoyl-coenzyme A reductase. *Biochem J* **304**:787, 1994.
146. Gurvitz A, Rottensteiner H, Kilpelainen SH, Hartig A, Hiltunen JK, Binder M, Dawes IW, et al: The *Saccharomyces cerevisiae* peroxisomal 2,4-dienoyl-CoA reductase is encoded by the oleate-inducible gene SPS19. *J Biol Chem* **272**:22140, 1997.
147. van Roermund CWT, Hettema EH, Kal AJ, van den Berg M, Tabak HF, Wanders RJA: Peroxisomal beta-oxidation of polyunsaturated fatty acids in *Saccharomyces cerevisiae*: Isocitrate dehydrogenase provides NADPH for reduction of double bonds at even positions. *EMBO J* **17**:677, 1998.
148. Geisbrecht BV, Liang X, Morrell JC, Schulz H, Gould SJ: The mouse gene PDCR encodes a peroxisomal delta(2), delta(4)-dienoyl-CoA reductase. *J Biol Chem* **274**:25814, 1999.
149. Fransen M, Van Veldhoven PP, Subramani S: Identification of peroxisomal proteins by using M13 phage protein VI phage display: Molecular evidence that mammalian peroxisomes contain a 2,4-dienoyl-CoA reductase. *Biochem J* **340**:561, 1999.
150. Tserng KY, Jin SJ: NADPH-dependent reductive metabolism of *cis*-5 unsaturated fatty acids. A revised pathway for the beta-oxidation of oleic acid. *J Biol Chem* **266**:11614, 1991.
151. Smeland TE, Nada M, Cuebas D, Schulz H: NADPH-dependent beta-oxidation of unsaturated fatty acids with double bonds extending from odd-numbered carbon atoms. *Proc Natl Acad Sci U S A* **89**:6673, 1992.
152. Chen LS, Jin SJ, Tserng KY: Purification and mechanism of delta 3,delta 5-t-2,t-4-dienoyl-CoA isomerase from rat liver. *Biochemistry* **33**:10527, 1994.
153. Luo MJ, Smeland TE, Shoukry K, Schulz H: Delta 3,5, delta 2,4-dienoyl-CoA isomerase from rat liver mitochondria. Purification and characterization of a new enzyme involved in the beta-oxidation of unsaturated fatty acids. *J Biol Chem* **269**:2384, 1994.
154. Luthria DL, Baykousheva SP, Sprecher H: Double bond removal from odd-numbered carbons during peroxisomal beta-oxidation of arachidonic acid requires both 2,4-dienoyl-CoA reductase and delta 3,5,delta 2,4-dienoyl-CoA isomerase. *J Biol Chem* **270**:13771, 1995.
155. He XY, Shoukry K, Chu C, Yang J, Sprecher H, Schulz H: Peroxisomes contain delta 3,5,delta 2,4-dienoyl-CoA isomerase and thus possess all enzymes required for the beta-oxidation of unsaturated fatty acids by a novel reductase-dependent pathway. *Biochem Biophys Res Commun* **215**:15, 1995.
156. Filppula SA, Yagi AI, Kilpelainen SH, Novikov D, FitzPatrick DR, Vihinen M, Valle D, et al: Delta3,5-delta2,4-dienoyl-CoA isomerase from rat liver. Molecular characterization. *J Biol Chem* **273**:349, 1998.
157. FitzPatrick DR, Germain-Lee E, Valle D: Isolation and characterization of rat and human cDNAs encoding a novel putative peroxisomal enoyl-CoA hydratase. *Genomics* **27**:457, 1995.
158. Ackman RG, Hansen RP: The occurrence of diastereoisomers of phytanic and pristanic acids and their determination by gas-liquid chromatography. *Lipids* **2**:357, 1967.
159. Van Veldhoven PP, Croes K, Asselberghs S, Herdewijn P, Mannaerts GP: Peroxisomal beta-oxidation of 2-methyl-branched acyl-CoA esters: stereospecific recognition of the 2S-methyl compounds by trihydroxycoprostanoyl-CoA oxidase and pristanoyl-CoA oxidase. *FEBS Lett* **388**:80, 1996.
160. Pedersen JI, Veggan T, Bjorkhem I: Substrate stereospecificity in oxidation of (25S)-3 alpha, 7 alpha, 12 alpha-trihydroxy-5 beta-cholestanoyl-CoA by peroxisomal trihydroxy-5 beta-cholestanoyl-CoA oxidase. *Biochem Biophys Res Commun* **224**:37, 1996.
161. Schmitz W, Fingerhut R, Conzelmann E: Purification and properties of an alpha-methylacyl-CoA racemase from rat liver. *Eur J Biochem* **222**:313, 1994.
162. Schmitz W, Albers C, Fingerhut R, Conzelmann E: Purification and characterization of an alpha-methylacyl-CoA racemase from human liver. *Eur J Biochem* **231**:815, 1995.
163. Schmitz W, Helander HM, Hiltunen JK, Conzelmann E: Molecular cloning of cDNA species for rat and mouse liver alpha-methylacyl-CoA racemases. *Biochem J* **326**:883, 1997.
164. Batta AK, Salen G, Shefer S, Dayal B, Tint GS: Configuration at C-25 in 3 alpha, 7 alpha, 12 alpha-trihydroxy-5 beta-cholestan-26-oic acid isolated from human bile. *J Lipid Res* **24**:94, 1983.
165. Shefer S, Cheng FW, Batta AK, Dayal B, Tint GS, Salen G, Mosbach EH: Stereospecific side chain hydroxylations in the biosynthesis of chenodeoxycholic acid. *J Biol Chem* **253**:6386, 1978.
166. Ferdinandusse S, Denis S, Clayton PT, Graham A, Rees JE, Allen JT, Mclean BN, et al: Mutations in the gene encoding peroxisomal-methylacyl-CoA racemase cause adult-onset sensory motor neuropathy. *Nat Genet* **24**:188, 2000.
167. Markwell MA, Tolbert NE, Bieber LL: Comparison of the carnitine acyltransferase activities from rat liver peroxisomes and microsomes. *Arch Biochem Biophys* **176**:497, 1976.
168. Farrell SO, Fiol CJ, Reddy JK, Bieber LL: Properties of purified carnitine acyltransferases of mouse liver peroxisomes. *J Biol Chem* **259**:13089, 1984.
169. Miyazawa S, Ozasa H, Osumi T, Hashimoto T: Purification and properties of carnitine octanoyltransferase and carnitine palmitoyltransferase from rat liver. *J Biochem (Tokyo)* **94**:529, 1983.
170. Singh H, Beckman K, Poulos A: Evidence of two catalytically active carnitine medium/long chain acyltransferases in rat liver peroxisomes. *J Lipid Res* **37**:2616, 1996.
171. Cronin CN: cDNA cloning, recombinant expression, and site-directed mutagenesis of bovine liver carnitine octanoyltransferase—Arg505 binds the carboxylate group of carnitine. *Eur J Biochem* **247**:1029, 1997.
172. Choi SJ, Oh DH, Song CS, Roy AK, Chatterjee B: Molecular cloning and sequence analysis of the rat liver carnitine octanoyltransferase cDNA, its natural gene and the gene promoter. *Biochim Biophys Acta* **1264**:215, 1995.
173. Ferdinandusse S, Mulders J, IJlst L, Denis S, Dacremont G, Waterham HR, Wanders RJA: Molecular cloning and expression of human carnitine octanoyltransferase: Evidence for its role in the peroxisomal beta-oxidation of branched-chain fatty acids. *Biochem Biophys Res Commun* **263**:213, 1999.
174. Bloisi W, Colombo I, Garavaglia B, Giardini R, Finocchiaro G, DiDonato S: Purification and properties of carnitine acetyltransferase from human liver. *Eur J Biochem* **189**:539, 1990.
175. Corti O, DiDonato S, Finocchiaro G: Divergent sequences in the 5′ region of cDNA suggest alternative splicing as a mechanism for the generation of carnitine acetyltransferases with different subcellular localizations. *Biochem J* **303**:37, 1994.
176. Elgersma Y, van Roermund CWT, Wanders RJA, Tabak HF: Peroxisomal and mitochondrial carnitine acetyltransferases of *Saccharomyces cerevisiae* are encoded by a single gene. *EMBO J* **14**:3472, 1995.
177. Osmundsen H, Neat CE, Borrebaek B: Fatty acid products of peroxisomal beta-oxidation. *Int J Biochem* **12**:625, 1980.
178. Berge RK, Flatmark T, Osmundsen H: Enhancement of long-chain acyl-CoA hydrolase activity in peroxisomes and mitochondria of rat liver by peroxisomal proliferators. *Eur J Biochem* **141**:637, 1984.
179. Alexson SE, Osmundsen H, Berge RK: The presence of acyl-CoA hydrolase in rat brown-adipose-tissue peroxisomes. *Biochem J* **262**:41, 1989.
180. Bronfman M, Leighton F: Carnitine acyltransferase and acyl-coenzyme A hydrolase activities in human liver. Quantitative analysis of their subcellular localization. *Biochem J* **224**:721, 1984.
181. Wilcke M, Alexson SE: Characterization of acyl-CoA thioesterase activity in isolated rat liver peroxisomes. Partial purification and characterization of a long-chain acyl-CoA thioesterase. *Eur J Biochem* **222**:803, 1994.
182. Jones JM, Nau K, Geraghty MT, Erdmann R, Gould SJ: Identification of peroxisomal acyl-CoA thioesterases in yeast and humans. *J Biol Chem* **274**:9216, 1999.
183. Liu LX, Margottin F, Le Gall S, Schwartz O, Selig L, Benarous R, Benichou S: Binding of HIV-1 Nef to a novel thioesterase enzyme correlates with Nef-mediated CD4 down-regulation. *J Biol Chem* **272**:13779, 1997.
184. Watanabe H, Shiratori T, Shoji H, Miyatake S, Okazaki Y, Ikuta K, Sato T, et al: A novel acyl-CoA thioesterase enhances its enzymatic activity by direct binding with HIV Nef. *Biochem Biophys Res Commun* **238**:234, 1997.
185. Hunt MC, Nousiainen SE, Huttunen MK, Orii KE, Svensson LT, Alexson SE: Peroxisome proliferator-induced long chain acyl-CoA thioesterases comprise a highly conserved novel multi-gene family involved in lipid metabolism. *J Biol Chem* **274**:34317, 1999.
186. Kelley RI, Datta NS, Dobyns WB, Hajra AK, Moser AB, Noetzel MJ, Zackai EH, et al: Neonatal adrenoleukodystrophy: New cases, biochemical studies, and differentiation from Zellweger and related peroxisomal polydystrophy syndromes. *Am J Med Genet* **23**:869, 1986.
187. Roels F, Cornelis A, Poll-Thé BT, Aubourg P, Ogier H, Scotto J, Saudubray JM: Hepatic peroxisomes are deficient in infantile Refsum disease: A cytochemical study of 4 cases. *Am J Med Genet* **25**:257, 1986.

188. Roels F, Espeel M, De Craemer D: Liver pathology and immunocytochemistry in congenital peroxisomal diseases: A review. *J Inherit Metab Dis* **14**:853, 1991.
189. Wanders RJA, Schelen A, Feller N, Schutgens RB, Stellaard F, Jakobs C, Mitulla B, et al: First prenatal diagnosis of acyl-CoA oxidase deficiency. *J Inherit Metab Dis* **13**:371, 1990.
190. Suzuki Y, Shimozawa N, Yajima S, Tomatsu S, Kondo N, Nakada Y, Akaboshi S, et al: Novel subtype of peroxisomal acyl-CoA oxidase deficiency and bifunctional enzyme deficiency with detectable enzyme protein: Identification by means of complementation analysis. *Am J Hum Genet* **54**:36, 1994.
191. Watkins PA, McGuinness MC, Raymond GV, Hicks BA, Sisk JM, Moser AB, Moser HW: Distinction between peroxisomal bifunctional enzyme and acyl-CoA oxidase deficiencies. *Ann Neurol* **38**:472, 1995.
192. Watkins PA, Chen WW, Harris CJ, Hoefler G, Hoefler S, Blake DC Jr, Balfe A, et al: Peroxisomal bifunctional enzyme deficiency. *J Clin Invest* **83**:771, 1989.
193. Wanders RJA, van Roermund CWT, Brul S, Schutgens RBH, Tager JM: Bifunctional enzyme deficiency: Identification of a new type of peroxisomal disorder in a patient with an impairment in peroxisomal beta-oxidation of unknown aetiology by means of complementation analysis. *J Inherit Metab Dis* **15**:385, 1992.
194. McGuinness MC, Moser AB, Poll-Thé BT, Watkins PA: Complementation analysis of patients with intact peroxisomes and impaired peroxisomal beta-oxidation. *Biochem Med Metab Biol* **49**:228, 1993.
195. Moser AB, Rasmussen M, Naidu S, Watkins PA, McGuinness M, Hajra AK, Chen G, et al: Phenotype of patients with peroxisomal disorders subdivided into sixteen complementation groups. *J Pediatr* **127**:13, 1995.
196. Wanders RJA, Jansen GA, van Roermund CWT, Denis S, Schutgens RBH, Jakobs BS: Metabolic aspects of peroxisomal disorders. *Ann N Y Acad Sci* **804**:450, 1996.
197. Paton BC, Sharp PC, Crane DI, Poulos A: Oxidation of pristanic acid in fibroblasts and its application to the diagnosis of peroxisomal beta-oxidation defects. *J Clin Invest* **97**:681, 1996.
198. van Grunsven EG, Wanders RJA: Genetic heterogeneity in patients with a disorder of peroxisomal beta-oxidation: A complementation study based on pristanic acid beta-oxidation suggesting different enzyme defects. *J Inherit Metab Dis* **20**:437, 1997.
199. van Grunsven EG, van Roermund CWT, Denis S, Wanders RJA: Complementation analysis of fibroblasts from peroxisomal fatty acid oxidation deficient patients shows high frequency of bifunctional enzyme deficiency plus intragenic complementation: Unequivocal evidence for differential defects in the same enzyme protein. *Biochem Biophys Res Commun* **235**:176, 1997.
200. Kaufmann WE, Theda C, Naidu S, Watkins PA, Moser AB, Moser HW: Neuronal migration abnormality in peroxisomal bifunctional enzyme defect. *Ann Neurol* **39**:268, 1996.
201. van Grunsven EG, Mooijer PAW, Aubourg P, Wanders RJA: Enoyl-CoA hydratase deficiency: Identification of an new type of D-bifunctional protein deficiency. *Hum Mol Genet* **8**:1509, 1999.
202. Vreken P, van Rooij A, Denis S, van Grunsven EG, Cuebas DA, Wanders RJA: Sensitive analysis of serum 3alpha, 7alpha, 12alpha, 24-tetrahydroxy-5beta-cholestan-26-oic acid diastereomers using gas chromatography-mass spectrometry and its application in peroxisomal D-bifunctional protein deficiency. *J Lipid Res* **39**:2452, 1998.
203. Goldfischer S, Collins J, Rapin I, Neumann P, Neglia W, Spiro AJ, Ishii T, et al: Pseudo-Zellweger syndrome: Deficiencies in several peroxisomal oxidative activities. *J Pediatr* **108**:25, 1986.
204. Schram AW, Goldfischer S, van Roermund CWT, Brouwer-Kelder EM, Collins J, Hashimoto T, Heymans HS, et al: Human peroxisomal 3-oxoacyl-coenzyme A thiolase deficiency. *Proc Natl Acad Sci U S A* **84**:2494, 1987.
205. Murakami T, Garcia CA, Reiter LT, Lupski JR: Charcot-Marie-Tooth disease and related inherited neuropathies. *Medicine (Baltimore)* **75**:233, 1996.
206. Warner LE, Garcia CA, Lupski JR: Hereditary peripheral neuropathies: clinical forms, genetics, and molecular mechanisms. *Annu Rev Med* **50**:263, 1999.
207. Dubois-Dalcq M, Feigenbaum V, Aubourg P: The neurobiology of X-linked adrenoleukodystrophy, a demyelinating peroxisomal disorder. *Trends Neurosci* **22**:4, 1999.
208. Clayton PT, Lake BD, Hjelm M, Stephenson JB, Besley GT, Wanders RJA, Schram AW, et al: Bile acid analyses in "pseudo-Zellweger" syndrome; clues to the defect in peroxisomal beta-oxidation. *J Inherit Metab Dis* **11(Suppl 2)**:165, 1988.
209. Naidu S, Hoefler G, Watkins PA, Chen WW, Moser AB, Hoefler S, Rance NE, et al: Neonatal seizures and retardation in a girl with biochemical features of X-linked adrenoleukodystrophy: A possible new peroxisomal disease entity. *Neurology* **38**:1100, 1988.
210. Barth PG, Wanders RJA, Schutgens RBH, Bleeker-Wagemakers EM, van Heemstra D: Peroxisomal beta-oxidation defect with detectable peroxisomes: A case with neonatal onset and progressive course. *Eur J Pediatr* **149**:722, 1990.
211. Espeel M, Roels F, Van Maldergem L, De Craemer D, Dacremont G, Wanders RJA, Hashimoto T: Peroxisomal localization of the immunoreactive beta-oxidation enzymes in a neonate with a beta-oxidation defect. Pathological observations in liver, adrenal cortex and kidney. *Virchows Arch A Pathol Anat Histopathol* **419**:301, 1991.
212. Mandel H, Berant M, Aizin A, Gershony R, Hemmli S, Schutgens RBH, Wanders RJA: Zellweger-like phenotype in two siblings: A defect in peroxisomal beta-oxidation with elevated very long-chain fatty acids but normal bile acids. *J Inherit Metab Dis* **15**:381, 1992.
213. Van Maldergem L, Espeel M, Wanders RJA, Roels F, Gerard P, Scalais E, Mannaerts GP, et al: Neonatal seizures and severe hypotonia in a male infant suffering from a defect in peroxisomal beta-oxidation. *Neuromuscul Disord* **2**:217, 1992.
214. Santer R, Claviez A, Oldigs HD, Schaub J, Schutgens RBH, Wanders RJA: Isolated defect of peroxisomal beta-oxidation in a 16-year-old patient. *Eur J Pediatr* **152**:339, 1993.
215. Vanhole C, de Zegher F, Casaer P, Devlieger H, Wanders RJA, Vanhove G, Jaeken J: A new peroxisomal disorder with fetal and neonatal adrenal insufficiency. *Arch Dis Child Fetal Neonatal Ed* **71**:F55, 1994.
216. Christensen E, Van Eldere J, Brandt NJ, Schutgens RBH, Wanders RJA, Eyssen HJ: A new peroxisomal disorder: di- and trihydroxycholestanaemia due to a presumed trihydroxycholestanoyl-CoA oxidase deficiency. *J Inherit Metab Dis* **13**:363, 1990.
217. Przyrembel H, Wanders RJA, van Roermund CWT, Schutgens RBH, Mannaerts GP, Casteels M: Di- and trihydroxycholestanoic acidaemia with hepatic failure. *J Inherit Metab Dis* **13**:367, 1990.
218. Wanders RJA, Casteels M, Mannaerts GP, van Roermund CWT, Schutgens RBH, Kozich V, Zeman J, et al: Accumulation and impaired in vivo metabolism of di- and trihydroxycholestanoic acid in two patients. *Clin Chim Acta* **202**:123, 1991.
219. ten Brink HJ, Wanders RJA, Christensen E, Brandt NJ, Jakobs C: Heterogeneity in di/trihydroxycholestanoic acidaemia. *Ann Clin Biochem* **31**:195, 1994.
220. Souri M, Aoyama T, Hashimoto T: A sensitive assay of acyl-coenzyme A oxidase by coupling with beta-oxidation multienzyme complex. *Anal Biochem* **221**:362, 1994.
221. Suzuki Y, Jiang LL, Souri M, Miyazawa S, Fukuda S, Zhang Z, Une M, et al: D-3-Hydroxyacyl-CoA dehydratase/D-3-hydroxyacyl-CoA dehydrogenase bifunctional protein deficiency: A newly identified peroxisomal disorder. *Am J Hum Genet* **61**:1153, 1997.
222. Wanders RJA, Schutgens RBH, van den Bosch H, Tager JM, Kleijer WJ: Prenatal diagnosis of inborn errors in peroxisomal beta-oxidation. *Prenat Diagn* **11**:253, 1991.
223. Roberts WL, Myher JJ, Kuksis A, Rosenberry TL: Alkylacylglycerol molecular species in the glycosylinositol phospholipid membrane anchor of bovine erythrocyte acetylcholinesterase. *Biochem Biophys Res Commun* **150**:271, 1988.
224. Luhrs CA, Slomiany BL: A human membrane-associated folate binding protein is anchored by a glycosyl-phosphatidylinositol tail. *J Biol Chem* **264**:21446, 1989.
225. Walter EI, Roberts WL, Rosenberry TL, Ratnoff WD, Medof ME: Structural basis for variations in the sensitivity of human decay accelerating factor to phosphatidylinositol-specific phospholipase C cleavage. *J Immunol* **144**:1030, 1990.
226. Butikofer P, Zollinger M, Brodbeck U: Alkylacyl glycerophosphoinositol in human and bovine erythrocytes. Molecular species composition and comparison with glycosyl-inositolphospholipid anchors of erythrocyte acetylcholinesterases. *Eur J Biochem* **208**:677, 1992.
227. Stevens VL, Raetz CR: Class F Thy-1-negative murine lymphoma cells are deficient in ether lipid biosynthesis. *J Biol Chem* **265**:15653, 1990.
228. Fukushima H, Watanabe T, Nozawa Y: Studies on *Tetrahymena* membranes. In vivo manipulating of membrane lipids by 1-O-hexadecyl glycerol-feeding in *Tetrahymena pyriformis*. *Biochim Biophys Acta* **436**:249, 1976.
229. Venkatesan S, Ormerod WE: Lipid content of the slender and stumpy forms of *Trypanosoma brucei rhodesiense*: A comparative study. *Comp Biochem Physiol [B]* **53**:481, 1976.
230. Chitwood DJ, Krusberg LR: Diacyl, alkylacyl, and alkenylacyl phospholipids of meloidogyne javanica females. *J Nematol* **13**:105, 2000.

231. Chitwood DJ, Krusberg LR: Diacyl, alkylacyl and alkenylacyl phospholopids of tre nematode *Turbatrix aceti*. *Comp Biochem Physiol [B]* **69**:115, 1981.
232. Sugiura T, Yamashita A, Kudo N, Fukuda T, Miyamoto T, Cheng NN, Kishimoto S, et al: Platelet-activating factor and its structural analogues in the earthworm *Eisenia foetida*. *Biochim Biophys Acta* **1258**:19, 1995.
233. Satouchi K, Hirano K, Sakaguchi M, Takehara H, Matsuura F: Phospholipids from the free-living nematode *Caenorhabditis elegans*. *Lipids* **28**:837, 1993.
234. Goldfine H, Langworthy TA: A growing interest in bacterial ether lipids. *Trends Biochem Sci* **13**:217, 1988.
235. Goni FM, Dominguez JB, Uruburu F: Plasmalogens in the yeast *Pullularia pullulans*. *Chem Phys Lipids* **22**:79, 1978.
236. Gross RW: High plasmalogen and arachidonic acid content of canine myocardial sarcolemma: A fast atom bombardment mass spectroscopic and gas chromatography-mass spectroscopic characterization. *Biochemistry* **23**:158, 1984.
237. Owens K: A two-dimensional thin-layer chromatographic procedure for the estimation of plasmalogens. *Biochem J* **100**:354, 1966.
238. Mueller HW, O'Flahertry JT, Greene DG, Samuel MP, Wykle RL: 1-*O*-alkyl-linked glycerophospholipids of human neutrophils: Distribution of arachidonate and other acyl residues in the ether-linker and diacyl species. *Lipids* **18**:814, 1983.
239. Sugiura T, Nakajima M, Sekiguchi N, Nakagawa Y, Waku K: Different fatty chain compositions of alkenylacyl, alkylacyl and diacyl phospholipids in rabbit alveolar macrophages: High amounts of arachidonic acid in ether phospholipids. *Lipids* **18**:125, 1983.
240. Blank ML, Fitzgerald V, Lee TC, Snyder F: Evidence for biosynthesis of plasmenylcholine from plasmenylethanolamine in HL-60 cells. *Biochim Biophys Acta* **1166**:309, 1993.
241. Lee TC, Qian CG, Snyder F: Biosynthesis of choline plasmalogens in neonatal rat myocytes. *Arch Biochem Biophys* **286**:498, 1991.
242. Wanders RJA, Dekker C, Horvath VA, Schutgens RBH, Tager JM, Van Laer P, Lecoutere D: Human alkyldihydroxyacetonephosphate synthase deficiency: A new peroxisomal disorder. *J Inherit Metab Dis* **17**:315, 1994.
243. Ofman R, Hettema EH, Hogenhout EM, Caruso U, Muijsers AO, Wanders RJA: Acyl-CoA-dihydroxyacetonephosphate acyltransferase—Cloning of the human cDNA and resolution of the molecular basis in rhizomelic chondrodysplasia punctata type 2. *Hum Mol Genet* **7**:847, 1998.
244. Hajra AK, Das AK: Lipid biosynthesis in peroxisomes. *Ann N Y Acad Sci* **804**:129, 1996.
245. Ghosh MK, Hajra AK: Subcellular distribution and properties of acyl/alkyl dihydroxyacetone phosphate reductase in rodent livers. *Arch Biochem Biophys* **245**:523, 1986.
246. Jones CL, Hajra AK: Properties of guinea pig liver peroxisomal dihydroxyacetone phosphate acyltransferase. *J Biol Chem* **255**:8289, 1980.
247. Hardeman D, van den Bosch H: Rat liver dihydroxyacetone-phosphate acyltransferase: Enzyme characteristics and localization studies. *Biochim Biophys Acta* **963**:1, 1988.
248. Burdett K, Larkins LK, Das AK, Hajra AK: Peroxisomal localization of acyl-coenzyme A reductase (long chain alcohol forming) in guinea pig intestine mucosal cells. *J Biol Chem* **266**:12201, 1991.
249. Biermann J, Just WW, Wanders RJA, van den Bosch H: Alkyl-dihydroxyacetone phosphate synthase and dihydroxyacetone phosphate acyltransferase form a protein complex in peroxisomes. *Eur J Biochem* **261**:492, 1999.
250. Hajra AK: Biosynthesis of acyl dihydroxyacetone phosphate in guinea pig liver mitochondria. *J Biol Chem* **243**:3458, 1968.
251. Hajra AK, Burke C: Biosynthesis of phosphatidic acid in rat brain via acyl dihydroxyacetone phosphate. *J Neurochem* **31**:125, 1978.
252. Hajra AK, Burke CL, Jones CL: Subcellular localization of acyl coenzyme A: Dihydroxyacetone phosphate acyltransferase in rat liver peroxisomes (microbodies). *J Biol Chem* **254**:10896, 1979.
253. Singh H, Beckman K, Poulos A: Exclusive localization in peroxisomes of dihydroxyacetone phosphate acyltransferase and alkyl-dihydroxyacetone phosphate synthase in rat liver. *J Lipid Res* **34**:467, 1993.
254. Datta NS, Wilson GN, Hajra AK: Deficiency of enzymes catalyzing the biosynthesis of glycerol-ether lipids in Zellweger syndrome. A new category of metabolic disease involving the absence of peroxisomes. *N Engl J Med* **311**:1080, 1984.
255. Schutgens RBH, Romeyn GJ, Wanders RJA, van den Bosch H, Schrakamp G, Heymans HSA: Deficiency of acyl-CoA: Dihydroxyacetone phosphate acyltransferase in patients with Zellweger (cerebro-hepato-renal) syndrome. *Biochem Biophys Res Commun* **120**:179, 1984.
256. Schrakamp G, Roosenboom CF, Schutgens RBH, Wanders RJA, Heymans HSA, Tager JM, van den Bosch H: Alkyl dihydroxyacetone phosphate synthase in human fibroblasts and its deficiency in Zellweger syndrome. *J Lipid Res* **26**:867, 1985.
257. Zomer AW, de Weerd WF, Langeveld J, van den Bosch H: Ether lipid synthesis: purification and identification of alkyl dihydroxyacetone phosphate synthase from guinea-pig liver. *Biochim Biophys Acta* **1170**:189, 1993.
258. Ofman R, Wanders RJA: Purification of peroxisomal acyl-CoA: Dihydroxyacetonephosphate acyltransferase from human placenta. *Biochim Biophys Acta* **1206**:27, 1994.
259. Webber KO, Hajra AK: Purification of dihydroxyacetone phosphate acyltransferase from guinea pig liver peroxisomes. *Arch Biochem Biophys* **300**:88, 1993.
260. Brown AJ, Snyder F: The mechanism of alkyldihydroxyacetone-P synthase. Formation of [^{3}H]H_2O from acyl[1-R-^{3}H]dihydroxyacetone-P by purified alkyldihydroxyacetone-P synthase in the absence of acylhydrolase activity. *J Biol Chem* **258**:4184, 1983.
261. Horie S, Das AK, Hajra AK: Alkyldihydroxyacetonephosphate synthase from guinea pig liver peroxisomes. *Methods Enzymol* **209**:385, 1992.
262. Datta SC, Ghosh MK, Hajra AK: Purification and properties of acyl/alkyl dihydroxyacetone-phosphate reductase from guinea pig liver peroxisomes. *J Biol Chem* **265**:8268, 1990.
263. de Vet EC, Zomer AW, Lahaut GJ, van den Bosch H: Polymerase chain reaction-based cloning of alkyl-dihydroxyacetonephosphate synthase complementary DNA from guinea pig liver. *J Biol Chem* **272**:798, 1997.
264. de Vet EC, van den Broek BT, van den Bosch H: Nucleotide sequence of human alkyl-dihydroxyacetonephosphate synthase cDNA reveals the presence of a peroxisomal targeting signal 2. *Biochim Biophys Acta* **1346**:25, 1997.
265. Thai TP, Heid H, Rackwitz HR, Hunziker A, Gorgas K, Just WW: Ether lipid biosynthesis-isolation and molecular characterization of human dihydroxyacetonephosphate acyltransferase. *FEBS Lett* **420**:205, 1997.
266. Paltauf F: Ether lipids in biomembranes. *Chem Phys Lipids* **74**:101, 1994.
267. Lee TC: Biosynthesis and possible biological functions of plasmalogens. *Biochim Biophys Acta* **1394**:129, 1998.
268. Blank ML, Wykle RL, Snyder F: The retention of arachidonic acid in ethanolamine plasmalogens of rat testes during essential fatty acid deficiency. *Biochim Biophys Acta* **316**:28, 1973.
269. Ford DA, Gross RW: Plasmenylethanolamine is the major storage depot for arachidonic acid in rabbit vascular smooth muscle and is rapidly hydrolyzed after angiotensin II stimulation. *Proc Natl Acad Sci U S A* **86**:3479, 1989.
270. Hazen SL, Ford DA, Gross RW: Activation of a membrane-associated phospholipase A2 during rabbit myocardial ischemia which is highly selective for plasmalogen substrate. *J Biol Chem* **266**:5629, 1991.
271. Hirashima Y, Farooqui AA, Mills JS, Horrocks LA: Identification and purification of calcium-independent phospholipase A2 from bovine brain cytosol. *J Neurochem* **59**:708, 1992.
272. Merrill AH Jr, Schroeder JJ: Lipid modulation of cell function. *Annu Rev Nutr* **13**:539, 1993.
273. Turini ME, Holub BJ: The cleavage of plasmenylethanolamine by phospholipase A2 appears to be mediated by the low affinity binding site of the TxA2/PGH2 receptor in U46619-stimulated human platelets. *Biochim Biophys Acta* **1213**:21, 1994.
274. Duhm J, Engelmann B, Schonthier UM, Streich S: Accelerated maximal velocity of the red blood cell Na^+/K^+ pump in hyperlipidemia is related to increase in 1-palmitoyl,2-arachidonoyl-plasmalogen phosphatidylethanolamine. *Biochim Biophys Acta* **1149**:185, 1993.
275. Chen X, Gross RW: Potassium flux through gramicidin ion channels is augmented in vesicles comprised of plasmenylcholine: Correlations between gramicidin conformation and function in chemically distinct host bilayer matrices. *Biochemistry* **34**:7356, 1995.
276. Ford DA, Hale CC: Plasmalogen and anionic phospholipid dependence of the cardiac sarcolemmal sodium-calcium exchanger. *FEBS Lett* **394**:99, 1996.
277. Glaser PE, Gross RW: Plasmenylethanolamine facilitates rapid membrane fusion: a stopped-flow kinetic investigation correlating the propensity of a major plasma membrane constituent to adopt an HII phase with its ability to promote membrane fusion. *Biochemistry* **33**:5805, 1994.
278. Lohner K: Is the high propensity of ethanolamine plasmalogens to form non-lamellar lipid structures manifested in the properties of biomembranes? *Chem Phys Lipids* **81**:167, 1996.

279. Mandel H, Sharf R, Berant M, Wanders RJA, Vreken P, Aviram M: Plasmalogen phospholipids are involved in HDL-mediated cholesterol efflux: Insights from investigations with plasmalogen-deficient cells. *Biochem Biophys Res Commun* **250**:369, 1998.
280. Mato JM, Kelly KL, Abler A, Jarett L: Identification of a novel insulin-sensitive glycophospholipid from H35 hepatoma cells. *J Biol Chem* **262**:2131, 1987.
281. McConville MJ, Bacic A, Mitchell GF, Handman E: Lipophosphoglycan of *Leishmania major* that vaccinates against cutaneous leishmaniasis contains an alkylglycerophosphoinositol lipid anchor. *Proc Natl Acad Sci U S A* **84**:8941, 1987.
282. McConville MJ, Bacic A: A family of glycoinositol phospholipids from *Leishmania major*. Isolation, characterization, and antigenicity. *J Biol Chem* **264**:757, 1989.
283. Ryals PE, Pak Y, Thompson GA Jr: Phosphatidylinositol-linked glycans and phosphatidylinositol-anchored proteins of *Tetrahymena mimbres*. *J Biol Chem* **266**:15048, 1991.
284. de Lederkremer RM, Lima CE, Ramirez MI, Goncalvez MF, Colli W: Hexadecylpalmitoylglycerol or ceramide is linked to similar glycophosphoinositol anchor-like structures in *Trypanosoma cruzi*. *Eur J Biochem* **218**:929, 1993.
285. Chabot MC, Greene DG, Brockschmidt JK, Capizzi RL, Wykle RL: Ether-linked phosphoglyceride content of human leukemia cells. *Cancer Res* **50**:7174, 1990.
286. Naito M, Kudo I, Nakagawa Y, Waku K, Nojiri H, Saito M, Inoue K: Lipids of human promyelocytic leukemia cell HL-60: Increasing levels of ether-linked phospholipids during retinoic acid-induced differentiation. *J Biochem (Tokyo)* **102**:155, 1987.
287. Zoeller RA, Morand OH, Raetz CR: A possible role for plasmalogens in protecting animal cells against photosensitized killing. *J Biol Chem* **263**:11590, 1988.
288. Morand OH, Zoeller RA, Raetz CR: Disappearance of plasmalogens from membranes of animal cells subjected to photosensitized oxidation. *J Biol Chem* **263**:11597, 1988.
289. Hoefler G, Paschke E, Hoefler S, Moser AB, Moser HW: Photosensitized killing of cultured fibroblasts from patients with peroxisomal disorders due to pyrene fatty acid-mediated ultraviolet damage. *J Clin Invest* **88**:1873, 1991.
290. Spisni E, Cavazzoni M, Griffoni C, Calzolari E, Tomasi V: Evidence that photodynamic stress kills Zellweger fibroblasts by a nonapoptotic mechanism. *Biochim Biophys Acta* **1402**:61, 1998.
291. Engelmann B, Brautigam C, Thiery J: Plasmalogen phospholipids as potential protectors against lipid peroxidation of low density lipoproteins. *Biochem Biophys Res Commun* **204**:1235, 1994.
292. Witztum JL, Steinberg D: Role of oxidized low density lipoprotein in atherogenesis. *J Clin Invest* **88**:1785, 1991.
293. Jones R, Mann T: Lipid peroxides in spermatozoa; formation, role of plasmalogen, and physiological significance. *Proc R Soc Lond B Biol Sci* **193**:317, 1976.
294. van der Hoek YY, Wanders RJA, van den Ende AE, Kraft HG, Gabel BR, Kastelein JJ, Koschinsky ML: Lipoprotein[a] is not present in the plasma of patients with some peroxisomal disorders. *J Lipid Res* **38**:1612, 1997.
295. Moore SA, Hurt E, Yoder E, Sprecher H, Spector AA: Docosahexaenoic acid synthesis in human skin fibroblasts involves peroxisomal retroconversion of tetracosahexaenoic acid. *J Lipid Res* **36**:2433, 1995.
296. Martinez M: Docosahexaenoic acid therapy in docosahexaenoic acid-deficient patients with disorders of peroxisomal biogenesis. *Lipids* **31(Suppl)**:S145, 1996.
297. Masuzawa Y, Okano S, Nakagawa Y, Ojima A, Waku K: Selective acylation of alkyllysophospholipids by docosahexaenoic acid in Ehrlich ascites cells. *Biochim Biophys Acta* **876**:80, 1986.
298. Gaposchkin DP, Zoeller RA: Plasmalogen status influences docosahexaenoic acid levels in a macrophage cell line. Insights using ether lipid-deficient variants. *J Lipid Res* **40**:495, 1999.
299. Jones CR, Arai T, Rapoport SI: Evidence for the involvement of docosahexaenoic acid in cholinergic stimulated signal transduction at the synapse. *Neurochem Res* **22**:663, 1997.
300. Perichon R, Moser AB, Wallace WC, Cunningham SC, Roth GS, Moser HW: Peroxisomal disease cell lines with cellular plasmalogen deficiency have impaired muscarinic cholinergic signal transduction activity and amyloid precursor protein secretion. *Biochem Biophys Res Commun* **248**:57, 1998.
301. Biermann J, Wanders RJA, van den Bosch H: Beta-adrenergic receptor-stimulated formation of cAMP is dependent on plasmalogens. *J Clin Invest* (Submitted).
302. Spranger JW, Opitz JM, Bidder U: Heterogeneity of chondrodysplasia punctata. *Humangenetik* **11**:190, 1971.
303. Pike MG, Applegarth DA, Dunn HG, Bamforth SJ, Tingle AJ, Wood BJ, Dimmick JE, et al: Congenital rubella syndrome associated with calcific epiphyseal stippling and peroxisomal dysfunction. *J Pediatr* **116**:88, 1990.
304. Poll-Thé BT, Maroteaux P, Narcy C, Quetin P, Guesnu M, Wanders RJA, Schutgens RBH, et al: A new type of chondrodysplasia punctata associated with peroxisomal dysfunction. *J Inherit Metab Dis* **14**:361, 1991.
305. Smeitink JA, Beemer FA, Espeel M, Donckerwolcke RA, Jakobs C, Wanders RJA, Schutgens RBH, et al: Bone dysplasia associated with phytanic acid accumulation and deficient plasmalogen synthesis: A peroxisomal entity amenable to plasmapheresis. *J Inherit Metab Dis* **15**:377, 1992.
306. Nuoffer JM, Pfammatter JP, Spahr A, Toplak H, Wanders RJA, Schutgens RBH, Wiesmann UN: Chondrodysplasia punctata with a mild clinical course. *J Inherit Metab Dis* **17**:60, 1994.
307. Barth PG, Wanders RJA, Schutgens RBH, Staalman CR: Variant rhizomelic chondrodysplasia punctata (RCDP) with normal plasma phytanic acid: Clinico-biochemical delineation of a subtype and complementation studies. *Am J Med Genet* **62**:164, 1996.
308. Heymans HSA, Oorthuys JW, Nelck G, Wanders RJA, Schutgens RBH: Rhizomelic chondrodysplasia punctata: Another peroxisomal disorder. *N Engl J Med* **313**:187, 1985.
309. Jansen GA, Ofman R, Ferdinandusse S, IJlst L, Muijsers AO, Skjeldal OH, Stokke O, et al: Refsum disease is caused by mutations in the phytanoyl-CoA hydroxylase gene. *Nat Genet* **17**:190, 1997.
310. Mihalik SJ, Morrell JC, Kim D, Sacksteder KA, Watkins PA, Gould SJ: Identification of PAHX, a Refsum disease gene. *Nat Genet* **17**:185, 1997.
311. Jansen GA, Ofman R, Denis S, Ferdinandusse S, Hogenhout EM, Jakobs C, Wanders RJA: Phytanoyl-CoA hydroxylase from a rat liver: Protein purification and cDNA cloning with implications for the subcellular localization of phytanic acid alpha-oxidation. *J Lipid Res* **40**:2244, 1999.
312. Braverman N, Steel G, Obie C, Moser AB, Moser HW, Gould SJ, Valle D: Human PEX7 encodes the peroxisomal PTS2 receptor and is responsible for rhizomelic chondrodysplasia punctata. *Nat Genet* **15**:369, 1997.
313. Motley AM, Hettema EH, Hogenhout EM, Brites P, ten Asbroek AL, Wijburg FA, Baas F, et al: Rhizomelic chondrodysplasia punctata is a peroxisomal protein targeting disease caused by a non-functional PTS2 receptor. *Nat Genet* **15**:377, 1997.
314. Purdue PE, Zhang JW, Skoneczny M, Lazarow PB: Rhizomelic chondrodysplasia punctata is caused by deficiency of human PEX7, a homologue of the yeast PTS2 receptor. *Nat Genet* **15**:381, 1997.
315. de Vet ECJM, IJlst L, Oostheim W, Wanders RJA, van den Bosch H: Alkyl-dihydroxyacetonephosphate synthase: Fate in peroxisome biogenesis disorders and identification of the point mutation underlying a single enzyme deficiency. *J Biol Chem* **273**:10296, 1998.
316. de Vet EC, IJlst L, Oostheim W, Dekker C, Moser HW, van den Bosch H, Wanders RJA: Ether lipid biosynthesis. Alkyl-dihydroxyacetonephosphate synthase protein deficiency leads to reduced dihydroxyacetonephosphate acyltransferase activities. *J Lipid Res* **40**:1998, 1999.
317. Wanders RJA, Schumacher H, Heikoop J, Schutgens RBH, Tager JM: Human dihydroxyacetonephosphate acyltransferase deficiency: A new peroxisomal disorder. *J Inherit Metab Dis* **15**:389, 1992.
318. Barr DG, Kirk JM, al Howasi M, Wanders RJA, Schutgens RBH: Rhizomelic chondrodysplasia punctata with isolated DHAP-AT deficiency. *Arch Dis Child* **68**:415, 1993.
319. Clayton PT, Eckhardt S, Wilson J, Hall CM, Yousuf Y, Wanders RJA, Schutgens RBH: Isolated dihydroxyacetonephosphate acyltransferase deficiency presenting with developmental delay. *J Inherit Metab Dis* **17**:533, 1994.
320. Sztriha LS, Nork MP, Abdulrazzaq YM, al-Gazali LI, Bakalinova DB: Abnormal myelination in peroxisomal isolated dihydroxyacetonephosphate acyltransferase deficiency. *Pediatr Neurol* **16**:232, 1997.
321. Elias ER, Mobassaleh M, Hajra AK, Moser AB: Developmental delay and growth failure caused by a peroxisomal disorder, dihydroxyacetonephosphate acyltransferase (DHAP-AT) deficiency. *Am J Med Genet* **80**:223, 1998.
322. de Vet EC, Biermann J, van den Bosch H: Immunological localization and tissue distribution of alkyldihydroxyacetonephosphate synthase and deficiency of the enzyme in peroxisomal disorders. *Eur J Biochem* **247**:511, 1997.

323. Biermann J, Gootjes J, Humbel BM, Dansen TB, Wanders RJA, van den Bosch H: Immunological analyses of alkyl-dihydroxyacetonephosphate synthase in human peroxisomal disorders. *Eur J Cell Biol* **78**:339, 1999.
324. Ofman R, Hogenhout EM, Wanders RJA: Identification and characterization of the mouse cDNA encoding acyl-CoA: dihydroxyacetone phosphate acyltranferase. *Biochim Biophys Acta* **1439**:89, 1999.
325. Bjorkhem I, Sisfontes L, Bostrom B, Kase BF, Blomstrand R: Simple diagnosis of the Zellweger syndrome by gas-liquid chromatography of dimethylacetals. *J Lipid Res* **27**:786, 1986.
326. Wanders RJA, Purvis YR, Heymans HS, Bakkeren JA, Parmentier GG, Van Eldere J, Eyssen H, et al: Age-related differences in plasmalogen content of erythrocytes from patients with the cerebro-hepato-renal (Zellweger) syndrome: Implications for postnatal detection of the disease. *J Inherit Metab Dis* **9**:335, 1986.
327. Wanders RJA, Schutgens RBH, Barth PG: Peroxisomal disorders: A review. *J Neuropathol Exp Neurol* **54**:726, 1995.
328. van der Knaap MS, Valk J: The MR spectrum of peroxisomal disorders. *Neuroradiology* **33**:30, 1991.
329. Williams DW, Elster AD, Cox TD: Cranial MR imaging in rhizomelic chondrodysplasia punctata. *AJNR Am J Neuroradiol* **12**:363, 1991.
330. Sztriha LS, al-Gazali LI, Wanders RJA, Ofman R, Nork MP, Lestringant GG: Abnormal myelin formation in rhizomelic chondrodysplasia punctata type 2 (DHAPAT-deficiency). *Dev Med Child Neurol*, **42**:492, 2000.
331. Goldstein JL, Brown MS: Regulation of the mevalonate pathway. *Nature* **343**:425, 1990.
332. Ericsson J, Appelkvist EL, Thelin A, Chojnacki T, Dallner G: Isoprenoid biosynthesis in rat liver peroxisomes. Characterization of *cis*-prenyltransferase and squalene synthetase. *J Biol Chem* **267**:18708, 1992.
333. Stamellos KD, Shackelford JE, Shechter I, Jiang G, Conrad D, Keller GA, Krisans SK: Subcellular localization of squalene synthase in rat hepatic cells. Biochemical and immunochemical evidence. *J Biol Chem* **268**:12825, 1993.
334. Keller GA, Barton MC, Shapiro DJ, Singer SJ: 3-Hydroxy-3-methylglutaryl-coenzyme A reductase is present in peroxisomes in normal rat liver cells. *Proc Natl Acad Sci U S A* **82**:770, 1985.
335. Keller GA, Pazirandeh M, Krisans S: 3-Hydroxy-3-methylglutaryl coenzyme A reductase localization in rat liver peroxisomes and microsomes of control and cholestyramine-treated animals: Quantitative biochemical and immunoelectron microscopical analyses. *J Cell Biol* **103**:875, 1986.
336. Aboushadi N, Shackelford JE, Jessani N, Gentile A, Krisans SK: Characterization of peroxisomal 3-hydroxy-3-methylglutaryl coenzyme A reductase in UT2 cells: Sterol biosynthesis, phosphorylation, degradation, and statin inhibition. *Biochemistry* **39**:237, 2000.
337. Stamellos KD, Shackelford JE, Tanaka RD, Krisans SK: Mevalonate kinase is localized in rat liver peroxisomes. *J Biol Chem* **267**:5560, 1992.
338. Biardi L, Sreedhar A, Zokaei A, Vartak NB, Bozeat RL, Shackelford JE, Keller GA, et al: Mevalonate kinase is predominantly localized in peroxisomes and is defective in patients with peroxisome deficiency disorders. *J Biol Chem* **269**:1197, 1994.
339. Krisans SK, Ericsson J, Edwards PA, Keller GA: Farnesyl-diphosphate synthase is localized in peroxisomes. *J Biol Chem* **269**:14165, 1994.
340. Biardi L, Krisans SK: Compartmentalization of cholesterol biosynthesis. Conversion of mevalonate to farnesyl diphosphate occurs in the peroxisomes. *J Biol Chem* **271**:1784, 1996.
341. Krisans SK: Cell compartmentalization of cholesterol biosynthesis. *Ann N Y Acad Sci* **804**:142, 1996.
342. Hoffmann GF, Charpentier C, Mayatepek E, Mancini J, Leichsenring M, Gibson KM, Divry P, et al: Clinical and biochemical phenotype in 11 patients with mevalonic aciduria. *Pediatrics* **91**:915, 1993.
343. Drenth JP, Cuisset L, Grateau G, Vasseur C, van de Velde-Visser SD, de Jong JG, Beckmann JS, et al: Mutations in the gene encoding mevalonate kinase cause hyper-IgD and periodic fever syndrome. International Hyper-IgD Study Group. *Nat Genet* **22**:178, 1999.
344. Houten SM, Kuis W, Duran M, de Koning TJ, van Royen-Kerkhof A, Romeijn GJ, Frenkel J, et al: Mutations in MVK, encoding mevalonate kinase, cause hyperimmunoglobulinaemia D and periodic fever syndrome. *Nat Genet* **22**:175, 1999.
345. Markovitz PJ, Chuang DT, Cox RP: Familial hyperlysinemias. Purification and characterization of the bifunctional aminoadipic semialdehyde synthase with lysine-ketoglutarate reductase and saccharopine dehydrogenase activities. *J Biol Chem* **259**:11643, 1984.
346. Hutzler J, Dancis J: Lysine-ketoglutarate reductase in human tissues. *Biochim Biophys Acta* **377**:42, 1975.
347. Chang YF: Pipecolic acid pathway: the major lysine metabolic route in the rat brain. *Biochem Biophys Res Commun* **69**:174, 1976.
348. Chang YF: Lysine metabolism in the rat brain: Blood-brain barrier transport, formation of pipecolic acid and human hyperpipecolatemia. *J Neurochem* **30**:355, 1978.
349. Wanders RJA, Romeyn GJ, Schutgens RBH, Tager JM: L-pipecolate oxidase: A distinct peroxisomal enzyme in man. *Biochem Biophys Res Commun* **164**:550, 1989.
350. Mihalik SJ, Moser HW, Watkins PA, Danks DM, Poulos A, Rhead WJ: Peroxisomal L-pipecolic acid oxidation is deficient in liver from Zellweger syndrome patients. *Pediatr Res* **25**:548, 1989.
351. Wanders RJA, Romeyn GJ, van Roermund CWT, Schutgens RBH, van den Bosch H, Tager JM: Identification of L-pipecolate oxidase in human liver and its deficiency in the Zellweger syndrome. *Biochem Biophys Res Commun* **154**:33, 1988.
352. Rao VV, Chang YF: Assay for L-pipecolate oxidase activity in human liver: Detection of enzyme deficiency in hyperpipecolic acidaemia. *Biochim Biophys Acta* **1139**:189, 1992.
353. Mihalik SJ, McGuinness M, Watkins PA: Purification and characterization of peroxisomal L-pipecolic acid oxidase from monkey liver. *J Biol Chem* **266**:4822, 1991.
354. Reuber BE, Karl C, Reimann SA, Mihalik SJ, Dodt G: Cloning and functional expression of a mammalian gene for a peroxisomal sarcosine oxidase. *J Biol Chem* **272**:6766, 1997.
355. Gatfield PD, Taller E, Hinton GG, Wallace AC, Abdelnour GM, Haust MD: Hyperpipecolatemia: A new metabolic disorder associated with neuropathy and hepatomegaly: A case study. *Can Med Assoc J* **99**:1215, 1968.
356. Thomas GH, Haslam RH, Batshaw ML, Capute AJ, Neidengard L, Ransom JL: Hyperpipecolic acidemia associated with hepatomegaly, mental retardation, optic nerve dysplasia and progressive neurological disease. *Clin Genet* **8**:376, 1975.
357. Burton BK, Reed SP, Remy WT: Hyperpipecolic acidemia: Clinical and biochemical observations in two male siblings. *J Pediatr* **99**:729, 1981.
358. Wanders RJA, van Roermund CWT, van Wijland MJ, Schutgens RBH, Tager JM, van den Bosch H, Thomas GH: Peroxisomes and peroxisomal functions in hyperpipecolic acidaemia. *J Inherit Metab Dis* **11(Suppl 2)**:161, 1988.
359. Challa VR, Geisinger KR, Burton BK: Pathologic alterations in the brain and liver in hyperpipecolic acidemia. *J Neuropathol Exp Neurol* **42**:627, 1983.
360. Roesel RA, Carroll JE, Rizzo WB, van der Zalm T, Hahn DA: Dyggve-Melchior-Clausen syndrome with increased pipecolic acid in plasma and urine. *J Inherit Metab Dis* **14**:876, 1991.
361. Vallat C, Denis S, Bellet H, Jakobs C, Wanders RJA, Mion H: Major hyperpipecolataemia in a normal adult. *J Inherit Metab Dis* **19**:624, 1996.
362. Kerckaert I, Poll-Thé BT, Espeel M, Duran M, Roeleveld ABC, Wanders RJA, Roels F: Hepatic peroxisomes in isolated hyperpipecolic acidaemia: evidence supporting its classification as a single peroxisomal enzyme deficiency. *Virchows Arch A Pathol Anat Histopathol* (In press).
363. Vamecq J, Van Hoof F: Implication of a peroxisomal enzyme in the catabolism of glutaryl-CoA. *Biochem J* **221**:203, 1984.
364. Vamecq J, de Hoffmann E, Van Hoof F: Mitochondrial and peroxisomal metabolism of glutaryl-CoA. *Eur J Biochem* **146**:663, 1985.
365. Horie S, Ogawa S, Suga T: Identity of acyl-CoA oxidase with glutaryl-CoA oxidase. *Life Sci* **44**:1141, 1989.
366. Bennett MJ, Pollitt RJ, Goodman SI, Hale DE, Vamecq J: Atypical riboflavin-responsive glutaric aciduria, and deficient peroxisomal glutaryl-CoA oxidase activity: A new peroxisomal disorder. *J Inherit Metab Dis* **14**:165, 1991.
367. Wanders RJA, Strijland A, van Roermund CWT, van den Bosch H, Schutgens RBH, Tager JM, Schram AW: Catalase in cultured skin fibroblasts from patients with the cerebro-hepato-renal (Zellweger) syndrome: Normal maturation in peroxisome-deficient cells. *Biochim Biophys Acta* **923**:478, 1987.
368. Eaton JW, Mouchou M: Acatalasemia, in Scriver CR, Beaudet AL, Sly WS, Valle D (eds): *The Metabolic and Molecular Basis of Inherited Disease*, 7th ed. New York, McGraw-Hill, 1995, p 2371.
369. Hebestreit H, Wanders RJA, Schutgens RBH, Espeel M, Kerckaert I, Roels F, Schmausser B, et al: Isolated dihydroxyacetonephosphate-acyl-transferase deficiency in rhizomelic chondrodysplasia punctata: Clinical presentation, metabolic and histological findings. *Eur J Pediatr* **155**:1035, 1996.
370. Leenders F, Dolez V, Begue A, Moller G, Gloeckner JC, de Launoit Y, Adamski J: Structure of the gene for the human 17beta-hydroxysteroid dehydrogenase type IV. *Mamm Genome* **9**:1036, 1998.

CHAPTER 131

X-Linked Adrenoleukodystrophy

Hugo W. Moser ▪ Kirby D. Smith
Paul A. Watkins ▪ James Powers ▪ Ann B. Moser

1. **The term adrenoleukodystrophy (ALD) is used to describe two genetically determined disorders that cause varying degrees of malfunction of the adrenal cortex and nervous system myelin, and are characterized by abnormally high levels of very long chain fatty acids (VLCFA) in tissues and body fluids.**
2. **Two types of ALD must be distinguished. One type is X-linked (MIM 300100), with the biochemical abnormality apparently confined to very long chain fatty acid metabolism, and normal peroxisome structure. The second type has an autosomal recessive mode of inheritance, is referred to as neonatal adrenoleukodystrophy (MIM 202370), and resembles the Zellweger cerebrohepatorenal syndrome (MIM 214100) in that the number and size of peroxisomes are diminished and the function of at least five peroxisomal enzymes is impaired. This chapter is concerned with X-linked ALD (X-ALD). Neonatal ALD is discussed in Chap. 129**
3. **The incidence of males with X-ALD is estimated to lie between 1:20,000 and 1:50,000 of the total population, and appears to be the same in most ethnic groups. There are several distinct phenotypes. Approximately 35 percent of patients have the childhood cerebral form. Affected boys develop normally until 4 to 8 years of age, and then suffer dementia and a progressive neurologic deficit that leads to a vegetative state. More than 90 percent of these have adrenal insufficiency. In approximately 35 to 40 percent of patients, the disorder presents in young adulthood as a slowly progressive paraparesis with sphincter disturbances that involves the long tracts in the spinal cord mainly and is referred to as adrenomyeloneuropathy (AMN). Adrenal insufficiency is present in two-thirds of these patients. Less common phenotypes include adrenal insufficiency without nervous system involvement, progressive cerebral dysfunction in adults, a syndrome that resembles olivopontocerebellar degeneration, and persons who are asymptomatic. The various phenotypes commonly occur within the same kindred. Twenty percent of female heterozygotes develop overt neurologic disturbances that resemble those of adrenomyeloneuropathy. Up to 50 percent of heterozygotes have mild neurologic abnormalities, but overt adrenal insufficiency is rare.**
4. **Tissues and body fluids of patients with X-ALD contain abnormally high levels of unbranched saturated very long chain fatty acids, particularly hexacosanoate (C26:0). This excess is most striking in the cholesterol ester and ganglioside fractions of affected brain white matter and adrenal cortex, but is present to varying degrees in virtually all tissues and body fluids.**
5. **The very long chain fatty acid accumulation is associated with an impaired capacity for their degradation, a reaction that normally takes place in the peroxisome. The defect results in an impaired capacity to form the coenzyme-A derivative of very long chain fatty acids in the peroxisome, a reaction which is catalyzed by very long chain acyl-CoA synthetases (VLCS).**
6. **The gene for X-ALD has been mapped to Xq28. It codes for a peroxisomal membrane protein with homology to the ATP-binding cassette (ABC) transporter superfamily of proteins. The X-ALD protein (ALDP) is closely related to three other peroxisomal membrane ABC proteins. One of these, ALDRP, has 66 percent homology to ALDP and may have some overlapping function. Mutations in this gene have been identified in all X-ALD patients who have been studied in sufficient detail. More than 200 different mutations have been identified (see www.x-ald.nl). There is no correlation between the nature of the mutation and the phenotype. The X-ALD gene has no homology to known VLCS and the mechanisms by which the gene defect leads to VLCFA accumulation and the phenotypic manifestations have not yet been defined.**
7. **The rapidly progressive cerebral forms of X-ALD are associated with an inflammatory response in the brain white matter. A distal axonopathy that involves mainly the long tracts in the spinal cord is the principal abnormality in the more slowly progressive AMN phenotype. Mouse models of X-ALD have been produced by targeted gene disruption. These models have defects of VLCFA metabolism and adrenocortical histological abnormalities that resemble the human disease. They do not have a neurologic phenotype, except for mild changes in advanced age that have some resemblance to AMN.**
8. **Diagnosis of X-ALD can be achieved by demonstration of increased levels of VLCFA in plasma. This diagnosis is accurate in males but normal levels occur in 15 percent of female heterozygotes. Thus, molecular analysis is required to exclude heterozygote status. Prenatal diagnosis is**

A list of standard abbreviations is located immediately preceding the index in each volume. Additional abbreviations used in this chapter include: ABC = ATP-bind cassette; ALD = adrenoleukodystrophy; ALDP = the protein product of the ALD gene; AMS = adrenomyeloneuropathy; BMT = bone marrow transplant; CCER = childhood cerebral ALD; Cho = choline-containing compounds; DHEAS = dehydroepiandrosterone sulphate; DPTA = dimethyl triamine pentaacetic acid; GFAP = glial fibrillary acidic protein; Ins = *myo*-inositol; LCS = long chain acyl-CoA synthetase; MRS = protein magnetic resonance spectroscopy; MS = multiple sclerosis; NAA = *N*-acetyl aspartate; PAS = periodic acid-Schiff; POCA = sodium 2-[5-(4-chlorophenyl)Pentyl]-oxirane-2-carboxylate; TNF = tumor necrosis factor; TOVA = test of variable attention; VLCFA = very long chain fatty acid; VLCS = very long chain acyl-CoA synthetase; X-ALD = X-linked adrenoleukodystrophy.

achieved by measurements of VLCFA levels in cultured amniocytes and by mutation analysis. Brain magnetic resonance imaging (MRI) studies often provide the first clue to the diagnosis, and are of great value in assessing prognosis, and the selection and evaluation of therapeutic approaches.

9. **Adrenal hormone replacement therapy is effective in correcting the adrenal insufficiency associated with adrenoleukodystrophy, but does not alter the neurologic manifestations. Bone marrow transplantation is the most effective therapy in children and adolescents who show early evidence of cerebral involvement. The procedure carries a high risk and selection of candidates requires careful clinical judgment. It is not recommended for patients who do not show evidence of neurologic involvement, patients whose involvement is already advanced, or for adults with adrenomyeloneuropathy. Many patients have received dietary therapy based on the oral administration of a 4:1 mixture of glyceryl trioleate and glyceryl trierucate, also referred to as Lorenzo's Oil. While this therapy reduces or normalizes VLCFA levels in plasma, it does not appear to alter the rate of disease progression in patients who already have neurologic symptoms. An international multicenter study aimed to determine whether administration of the oil to asymptomatic patients can reduce the frequency and severity of later neurologic involvement is in progress.**
10. **Studies in cultured cells and the animal model have suggested two therapeutic approaches based upon lovastatin and 4-phenylbutyrate, which are agents in use for other disease states. Both medications have been reported to increase the capacity of cultured X-ALD cells to metabolize VLCFA. It has been proposed that lovastatin may also reduce the brain inflammatory response. 4-Phenylbutyrate increases the expression of ALDRP and reduces VLCFA levels in the animal model. The clinical efficacy of these agents has not yet been tested. Clinical trials are planned.**
11. **At this time, disease prevention represents the most effective method of diminishing the hardship caused by X-ALD. Disease prevention is facilitated by the fact that less than 5 percent of patients have new mutations, so that most patients can be identified by screening extended families. The combination of plasma VLCFA and mutation analysis can identify all hemizygotes and heterozygotes by noninvasive techniques, and prenatal diagnosis can be established securely. This strategy is complicated by the inability to predict disease severity.**

HISTORY

In retrospect the first case of X-linked adrenoleukodystrophy (X-ALD) (MIM 300100) was reported by Haberfeld and Spieler in 1910.[1] A previously normal boy developed disturbances in eye movement and vision at age of 6 years, became apathetic, and his schoolwork deteriorated. Four months later, his gait became spastic and this progressed to an inability to walk. He was hospitalized at 7 years. Dark skin was noted, but otherwise not commented upon. He died 8 months later. An older brother had died of a similar illness at 8.5 years. Paul Schilder studied the postmortem brain. Because of the severe loss of myelin associated with relative preservation of axons, and the perivascular accumulation of lymphocytes and fat-laden phagocytes and glial cells, he assigned the name "encephalitis periaxialis diffusa." He reported three cases of this type in separate publications.[2–4] These cases later were referred to as Schilder disease. This term was in frequent use until about 20 years ago, when several of the leukodystrophies were defined more precisely, and is still used occasionally. Schilder disease is heterogeneous.[5] In view of the clinical and neuropathologic findings and the presence of melanoderma, the patient referred to here[3] almost certainly had X-ALD. The other two patients reported by Schilder are now thought to have had multiple sclerosis[4] and subacute sclerosing leukoencephalopathy,[2] respectively. Siemerling and Creutzfeldt[6] were the first to describe the combination of adrenocortical atrophy and cerebral demyelination and lymphocytic infiltration in what is now considered the first unequivocal report of X-ALD.

Blaw introduced the name adrenoleukodystrophy in 1970.[7] The key to all subsequent knowledge about the disease was the observation by Powers, Schaumburg, and Johnson[8–11] that adrenal cells of these patients contained characteristic lipid inclusions, followed by the demonstration that these inclusions consisted of cholesterol esters that contained a striking and characteristic excess of very long chain fatty acids (VLCFA).[12] Identification of this biochemical "handle" led to the development of assays capable of demonstrating increases in VLCFA levels in cultured skin fibroblasts,[13] plasma,[14] red blood cells,[15] and amniocytes.[16] These techniques have permitted precise postnatal and prenatal diagnosis, the facilitation of genetic studies and gene mapping,[17–19] and the evaluation of therapeutic approaches.[20,21] Metabolic studies of VLCFA metabolism in patients with X-ALD indicate that they have an impaired capacity to degrade these substances.[22–25] Subcellular localization studies indicate that VLCFA oxidation takes place in the peroxisome,[26] and X-ALD is now assigned to the peroxisomal disease category.[27,28] In 1988, it was shown that the activity of VLCS is diminished.[29,30]

The gene that is defective in X-ALD was mapped to Xq28 in 1981[17] and isolated by positional cloning in 1993.[31] It is a member of the ATP-binding cassette (ABC) transporter family[32] and has no homology to known VLCS. Mouse models of X-ALD by gene targeting were developed in 1997.[33–35]

CLINICAL FEATURES OF X-ALD

Nomenclature

The phenotypic manifestations of X-ALD are more varied than initially realized, and this has caused confusion in nomenclature. Until 1976, the only phenotype that was recognized is what we now refer to as the childhood cerebral form, and Blaw's proposal that it be named adrenoleukodystrophy (ALD) was generally accepted. In 1976, Budka et al.[36] described a more slowly progressive adult form of the disease, and in 1977, Griffin et al.[37] described five additional cases and proposed that this form be named adrenomyeloneuropathy (AMN) because it involved the spinal cord and peripheral nerves.[38] Some authors have used the term adrenoleukodystrophy to designate the childhood cerebral form specifically. Because the various phenotypes frequently occur within the same kindred and the primary defect that underlies the childhood cerebral form and adrenomyeloneuropathy is identical,[31] we propose that the term X-linked adrenoleukodystrophy (X-ALD) be used to embrace all phenotypic variants.

Phenotypes in Male X-ALD Patients

By using as criteria the age at onset, the sites of most severe clinical involvement, and the rate of progression of neurologic symptoms, we have subdivided the clinical spectrum of X-ALD into seven phenotypes in men, and five in the female heterozygotes. These are listed in Table 131-1. Although this subdivision is somewhat arbitrary, it has proved valuable for the study of pathogenetic mechanisms and counseling. Furthermore, quantitative data on the relative frequency of the various phenotypes and of the prognosis of untreated patients in each phenotypic category are essential for the selection and evaluation of various therapies.

Table 131-1 X-ALD Phenotypes

Phenotypes in Males Phenotype	Description	Estimated Relative Frequency
Childhood cerebral (CCER)	Onset at 3–10 years of age. Progressive behavioral, cognitive and neurologic deficit, often leading to total disability within 3 years. Inflammatory brain demyelination.	31–35%
Adolescent	Like childhood cerebral. Onset age 11–21 years. Somewhat slower progression.	4–7%
Adrenomyeloneuropathy (AMN)	Onset 28 ± 9 years, progressive over decades. Involves spinal cord mainly, distal axonopathy inflammatory response mild or absent. Approximately 40% have or develop cerebral involvement with varying degrees of inflammatory response and more rapid progression.	40–46%
Adult cerebral	Dementia, behavioral disturbances. Sometimes focal deficits, without preceding AMN. White matter inflammatory response present. Progression parallels that of childhood cerebral form.	2–5%
Olivo-ponto-cerebellar	Mainly cerebellar and brain stem involvement in adolescence or adulthood.	1–2%
"Addison-only"	Primary adrenal insufficiency without apparent neurologic involvement. Onset common before 7.5 years. Most eventually develop AMN.	Varies with age. Up to 50% in childhood.
Asymptomatic	Biochemical and gene abnormality without demonstrable adrenal or neurologic deficit. Detailed studies often show adrenal hypofunction or subtle signs of AMN.	Diminishes with age. Common < 4 years. Very rare > 40 years.

Phenotypes in Female X-ALD Carriers

Phenotype	Description	Estimated Relative Frequency
Asymptomatic	No evidence of adrenal or neurologic involvement.	Diminishes with age. Most women < 30 years neurologically uninvolved.
Mild myelopathy	Increased deep tendon reflexes and distal sensory changes in lower extremities with absent or mild disability.	Increases with age. Approximately 50% > 40 years.
Moderate to severe myeloneuropathy	Symptoms and pathology resemble AMN, but milder and later onset.	Increases with age. Approximately 15% > 40 years.
Cerebral involvement	Rarely seen in childhood and slightly more common in middle age and later.	Approximately 2%.
Clinically evident adrenal insufficiency	Rare at any age.	Approximately 1%.

CHILDHOOD CEREBRAL ALD (CCER)

The clinical characteristics of CCER have been analyzed in several large series.[39–42] Mean age of onset is 7.2 ± 1.7 years with a range of 2.75 to 10 years (Fig. 131-1). Psychomotor development up to 3 years or later was normal in nearly all reported cases. Neurologic symptoms began before age 3 years in only one case, namely at 2.75 years. In 86 percent of the 167 CCER patients tested at the Kennedy Krieger Institute through 1986, neurologic symptoms preceded signs of adrenal insufficiency, but 85 percent

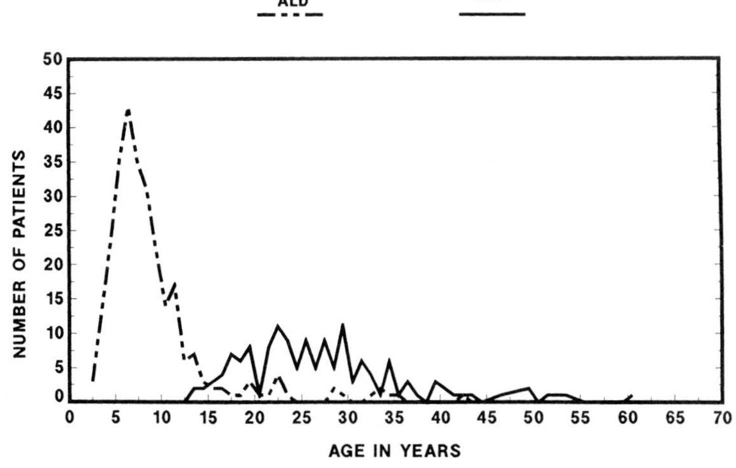

Fig. 131-1 Age at onset of neurologic symptoms of cerebral forms of X-ALD (broken line) and AMN (solid line). While the cerebral forms begin most commonly in childhood, adolescent and adult onset is noted occasionally. The earliest onset of AMN was at age 12 years. These data were assembled in 1992 at a time when AMN was still underdiagnosed. (*From Moser et al.*[256] *Used with permission.*)

Table 131-2 Initial Symptoms in 160 Patients with the Childhood Cerebral Form of Adrenoleukodystrophy

Symptom	Percentage
School difficulty	16
Behavioral disturbances	13
Impaired vision	11
Impaired hearing	8
Poor coordination	8
Dementia	7
Seizure	7
Hyperactivity	6
Squint, double-vision	5
Difficulty walking	4
Speech difficulty	4
Limb weakness	3
Poor handwriting	2
Headaches	2
Loss of athletic ability	1
Urinary incontinence	1
Tics	1
Fecal incontinence	0.3
Increased intracranial pressure	0.3
Difficulty swallowing	0.3
Coma	0.3

of the neurologically involved cases showed diminished cortisol response to ACTH at the time of neurologic diagnosis.[42]

Table 131-2 lists the first overt neurologic symptom in a series of patients with CCER studied at the Kennedy Krieger Institute. Detailed studies of neurologically asymptomatic patients with the X-ALD biochemical defect have also been undertaken. They showed that overt neurologic symptoms may be preceded by a period in which there exist defects of cognitive function that are detected only by detailed neuropsychologic testing.

Early behavioral changes include emotional lability, withdrawn or hyperactive behavior, school failure, or a combination of these symptoms. Difficulty in understanding speech in a noisy room or over the telephone are common early symptoms, and reflect impaired auditory discrimination, often with retention of normal pure tone perception. Diagnosis of an attention deficit disorder and therapy with stimulants are a frequent part of the early history. The attention deficit disorder may evolve rapidly to include clear-cut signs of parietal lobe dysfunction such as constructional and dressing apraxia, higher cortical sensory loss such as astereognosis and graphesthesia, and poor body orientation in space. The resultant behavior from bilateral cerebral hemispheric involvement may be labeled as dementia. Strabismus is common. Visual impairment is an early symptom in approximately one-third of the patients and includes visual field cuts and impaired visual acuity. In the later stages of the disease, vision is lost totally and there is optic atrophy. Nearly all the patients develop focal or generalized seizures at some stage of the illness, and a seizure was the first neurologic manifestation in 7 percent. Once the neurologic symptoms become manifest, progression is rapid. In the 167 patients studied at the Kennedy Krieger Institute, the mean interval between first neurologic symptoms and an apparently vegetative state was 1.9 $\pm$ 2 years (range: 0.5 to 10.5 years).[42] In this state, the child is bedridden, unable to see or speak, and is fed via nasogastric tube or gastrostomy. The child or adolescent may remain in a vegetative state for several years, in some instances more than 5 years. The mean age at death was 9.4 $\pm$ 2.7 years (range: 5.1 to 19 years).

In 85 percent of CCER patients, the MRI shows characteristic symmetric lesions in the parieto-occipital region (Figs. 131-2*A* and *B*).

Recent follow-up studies of X-ALD patients at the Kennedy Krieger Institute indicate that information of prognostic significance can be obtained by subdivision of patients in accordance with age and severity of the brain MRI abnormality. The subdivisions are shown in Table 131-3. Severity of brain involvement was assessed with the brain magnetic resonance imaging (MRI) scoring system developed for X-ALD by Loes et al.[43] This 34-point scale, graded in 0.5-unit intervals, is based on the severity of white matter changes in specific brain regions and on the degree of focal and/or global atrophy. It can be applied to standard MR images. A score of 0 or 0.5 is considered within normal limits. A score of 1 to 3 indicates mild to moderate abnormality, a score greater than 3, moderate to severe involvement. To analyze the data, we constructed Kaplan-Meier survival curves for the groups listed in Table 131-3. The items examined were survival, neurologic, and neuropsychologic function, and MRI. Figures 131-3*A* to *D* are illustrative. Figure 131-3*A* shows the progression in 33 patients, ages 3 to 7 years, whose MRI score was 0 or 0.5 at time of the initial examination. All survived and the neurology score remained normal. By age 10 years, 30 percent developed MRI and neuropsychologic abnormalities. Patients with a normal MRI examination at 7 to 10 years (Fig. 131-3*B*) had a more favorable prognosis. In the 7- to 10-year-old age group, 10 percent developed MRI abnormalities. In the 10- to 13-year-old age group, the MRI remained normal for the duration of the study (data not shown). These findings suggest that patients who reach age 10 years without MRI abnormalities are unlikely to develop cerebral involvement in the next 10 years. Figures 131-3*C* and *D* show disease progression in patients in the same age groups whose MRI score was >3. Irrespective of age, the MRI abnormality progressed in nearly all, and a significant proportion of these patients died. Table 131-4 summarizes the results in the 18 groups.

The prognostic data presented in Fig. 131-3 take into account only age and the Loes MRI score. It is likely that prognostic precision can be increased by inclusion of neurology and neuropsychology scores and by specialized imaging techniques such as magnetic resonance spectroscopy, which are discussed in a later section. Figures 131-4*A* and *B* demonstrate that accumulation of gadolinium, an indicator of the breakdown of the blood-brain barrier, is also of prognostic significance. It should be emphasized that a Loes MRI score greater than 3 does not necessarily indicate that further disease progression will ensue. We have identified 8 patients with abnormal MRI findings who remained stable for periods of up to 10 years. Other such patients have been reported.[44] It is likely that MR spectroscopy[45] or other technical advances[46–48] will permit more precise evaluation of the prognostic significance of neuroimaging abnormalities.

ADOLESCENT CEREBRAL ALD

In one series of 837 patients,[42] there were 42 patients in whom first symptoms occurred between age 11 and 21 years. Symptoms and progression in these patients resemble those in the childhood form.

ADRENOMYELONEUROPATHY (AMN)

Adrenomyeloneuropathy (AMN), characterized by myelopathy and neuropathy, was first described in 1976 in Austria by Budka et al.,[36] and in 1977 by Griffin et al. in the United States.[37] A man in his twenties, who previously had been well, notes stiffness or clumsiness in his legs. Generalized weakness, weight loss, pigmentation, and attacks of nausea and vomiting may have been noted before, after, or concurrent with the neurologic symptoms leading to a diagnosis of Addison disease. The neurologic disability is slowly progressive, so that within the next 5 to 15 years the gait disturbance becomes severe and requires the use of a cane or a wheelchair. Urinary disturbances are noted in the twenties or thirties. Figure 131-1 shows the distribution of age of onset in patients with AMN. Table 131-5 shows that somatosensory and brain stem auditory-evoked responses are

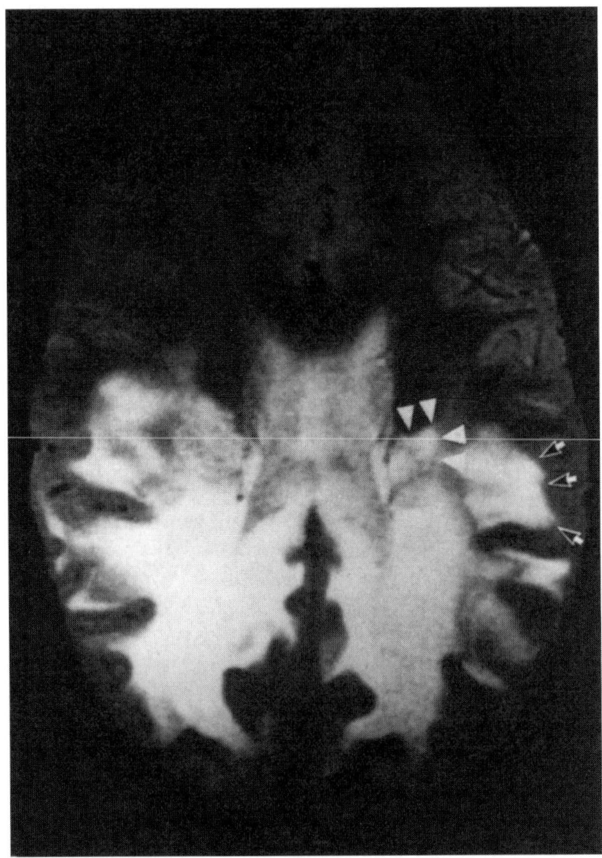

A

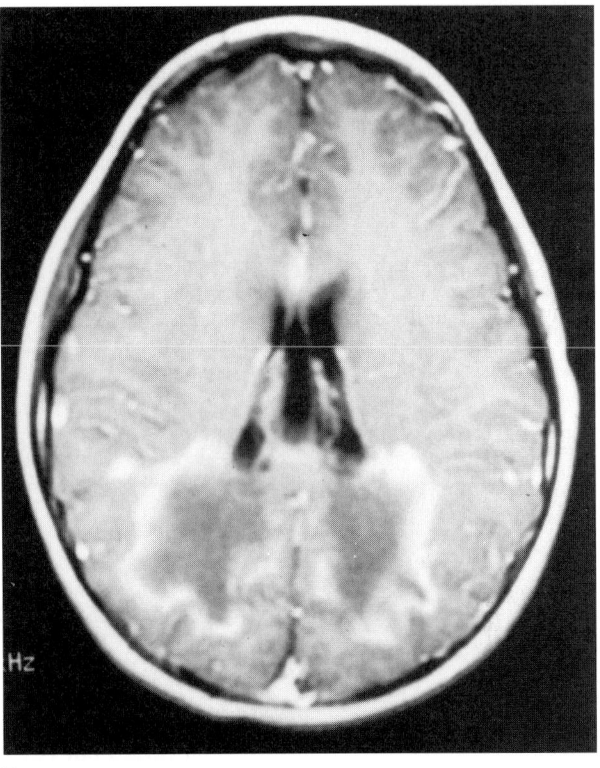

B

Fig. 131-2 T2 (*A*) and T1 (*B*) MRI images in a patient with childhood cerebral form of X-ALD. The T2-weighted image shows the characteristic symmetric areas increased signal in the parieto-occipital region. This pattern is observed in 85 percent of patients with this phenotype. (The T1-weighted image was obtained following the intravenous injection of gadolinium-diethylenetriamine pentaacetic acid. The symmetric regions of decreased signal intensity in the parieto-occipital regions are indicative of loss of myelin and gliosis. The garland of increased signal density that surrounds these regions is the zone in which the gadolinium contrast material has accumulated due to breakdown of the blood-brain barrier associated with the inflammatory response. (*From Kumar et al.*[405] *Used with permission.*).

nearly always abnormal, and that visual-evoked and peripheral nerve abnormalities occur less frequently. Results of neurophys iological studies are described in the section on diagnosis below.

The cerebrum is involved to a variable extent in AMN. Kumar et al.[49] categorized the degree of brain involvement in accordance with the degree and type of MRI abnormality. Brain MRI was

Table 131-3 Stratification of X-ALD Patients by Age and MRI at First Contact with Referral Hospital

Age at First Contact (Years)	MRI (Loes) Score at First Contact (Number of Patients) <1	1–3	>3
<3	25	0	0
3–7	33	6	24
7–10	22	2	35
10–13	19	8	19
13–16	11	2	13
>16	83	25	42
TOTAL	**193**	**43**	**133**

Subdivision of male X-ALD patients by age and severity of MRI abnormality. The study population consisted of 377 patients with X-ALD who have been followed at the Kennedy Krieger Institute for 38 ± 29.5 months (range: 0 to 142 months). The scoring system devised by Loes et al.[43] was used to assess the severity of brain MRI abnormality. A score of <1 is considered within normal limits. A score of 1 to 3 indicates mild or moderate abnormality; and >3 moderate to severe abnormality. BMT in 30 patients; post-BMT data excluded.

normal in 56 percent of the men and 80 percent of the women in a series of 119 men and 45 women with the AMN phenotype. These patients have been referred to as "pure" AMN. Their cognitive functions are intact (Fig. 131-5) except for speed of response, which is probably related to their motor disability. The rate of disease progression in pure AMN patients is more favorable than that in the patients with cerebral involvement. In 16 (13 percent) of the male AMN patients, the brain MRI abnormality was confined to the corticospinal tract fibers in the pons, cerebral peduncles, and internal capsule. Because we have identified patients in whom there was a greater than 25-year interval between onset of neurologic symptoms and tract degeneration demonstrable by MRI, this may represent an axonal "dying back" phenomenon and is not necessarily indicative of primary cerebral involvement, and the prognosis of these patients may be relatively favorable. Forty (34 percent) of the male AMN patients had parenchymal brain MRI abnormalities that resemble those in CCER. These patients, who are sometimes referred to as AMN-cerebral, have a more serious prognosis, and at times neurologic progression is as rapid as in CCER. In addition, follow-up studies now in progress at the Kennedy Krieger Institute indicate that 14 percent of the men who were classified as pure AMN, based upon history and neurologic examination, later developed parenchymal MRI abnormalities that resemble those in CCER (B. van Geel, G.V. Raymond unpublished observation).

Depression or emotional disturbances are common and become more severe as the illness advances. Impotence beginning in the late twenties or thirties is a common occurrence in AMN.[50] In one patient, hypogonadism preceded by 12 years the other manifestations of AMN. In spite of the eventual impairment of sexual function, it is common for AMN patients to have offspring. Seventy-seven percent of male X-ALD patients show subclinical signs of gonadal insufficiency in adulthood.[51]

It was found in retrospect that some men who later developed AMN had been hyperpigmented since early childhood. At the time that AMN is diagnosed, plasma adrenocortical corticotropin hormone (ACTH) levels usually are greatly elevated. Presumably, these men had abnormally high ACTH (and melanocyte stimulating hormone) levels, and in this way, were able to maintain relatively normal adrenocortical function during infancy and childhood. In the Kennedy Krieger Institute series, adrenal insufficiency preceded neurologic deficit in 42 percent of AMN patients. In two patients, Addison disease preceded neurologic dysfunction by 22 and 27 years,[52] and this interval was 32 years in a patient followed at the Kennedy Krieger Institute. Thirty[53] to 50 percent[54] of AMN patients have normal adrenocortical function, and it is in this group that the diagnosis of AMN is most likely to be missed.

ADULT CEREBRAL ALD

The term "adult cerebral ALD" is applied to patients with the biochemical defect of X-ALD who develop cerebral symptoms after 21 years of age, but who do not have signs of spinal cord involvement. This form is relatively rare; 3 percent in the Kennedy Krieger series. Twenty-three cases have been reported in the literature. Age of onset varied from the early twenties to the fifties.[55] Symptoms resembled schizophrenia with dementia or a specific cerebral deficit. One 29-year-old man, who at postmortem examination was found to have bilateral temporal lobe lesions, had symptoms characteristic of the Klüver-Bucy syndrome.[56] Another 34-year-old man presented with dysphasia and a right homonymous hemianopsia.[57] While the presence of Addison disease is a crucial diagnostic clue, adrenal function may be normal in 30 to 50 percent of patients.

The psychiatric manifestations of X-ALD in adults have been reviewed.[58,59] The most common manifestations are signs of mania including disinhibition, impulsivity, increased spending, hypersexuality, loudness, and perseveration. In 10 of 13 cases reported in the English literature, the psychiatric symptoms were the initial symptom. The occurrence of psychotic disturbance in a patient with Addison disease must alert the clinician to the possibility of X-ALD, although psychotic symptoms may occur in other forms of Addison disease also. White matter lesions demonstrated by computer tomography (CT) or MRI often are the first diagnostic clue, with the specific diagnosis being

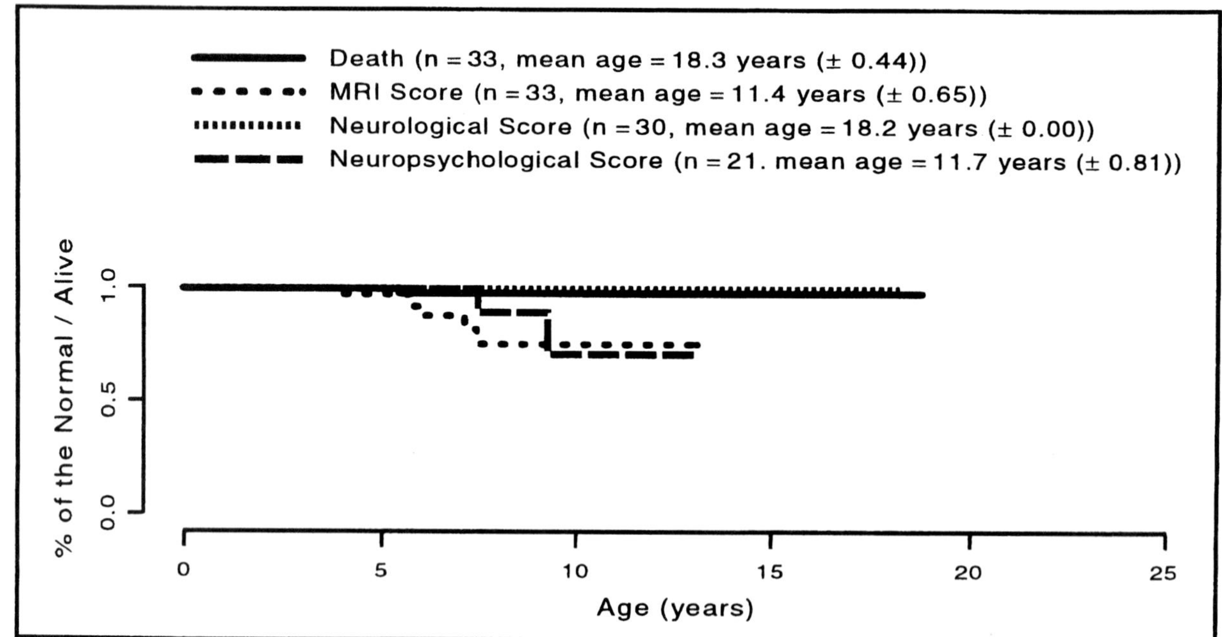

Fig. 131-3 (*A*) Kaplan-Meier plots of survival and disease progression in patients who were between 3 and 7 years old at time of referral and in whom the Loes MRI score (43) was <1 (within normal limits). This group included 33 patients. All patients survived throughout the followup period, and the neurology score remained normal. However, in 30% of patients the neuropsychology score, based upon a 10-point scale devised by Dr. Christine Cox, became >2, and the Loes MRI score increased by more than 1 point. We conclude that 30% of untreated patients in the 3 to 7 year age group whose MRI is normal will develop the CCER phenotype. See reference 409 for a more detailed description of the disease severity scoring system that was used. (*B*) Kaplan-Meier plots of survival and disease progression in patients who were between 3 and 7 years old and in whom the Loes MRI score was >3. Note that 30% of these patients died and that the MRI score increased by more than 2 points in 70%. The neurology and neuropsychology scores were already severely abnormal at baseline. (*C*) Kaplan-Meier plots of survival and disease progression in 22 patients who were 7 to 10 years old and had a Loes MRI score of <1. All survived, and neurology and neuropsychology scores did not increase by more than 1 point. MRI scores increased by more than 2 points in only 5%. These results indicate that patients who retain a Loes MRI score <1 at age 7 to 10 years, are at low risk of developing the rapidly progressive cerebral forms of X-ALD. (*D*) Kaplan-Meier plots of survival and disease progression in 35 7- to 10-year-old patients whose Loes MRI score was >3. Fifty percent of the patients died and MRI score increased by at least 2 points in all of the patients. Neurology and neuropsychology scores were already severely abnormal at baseline.

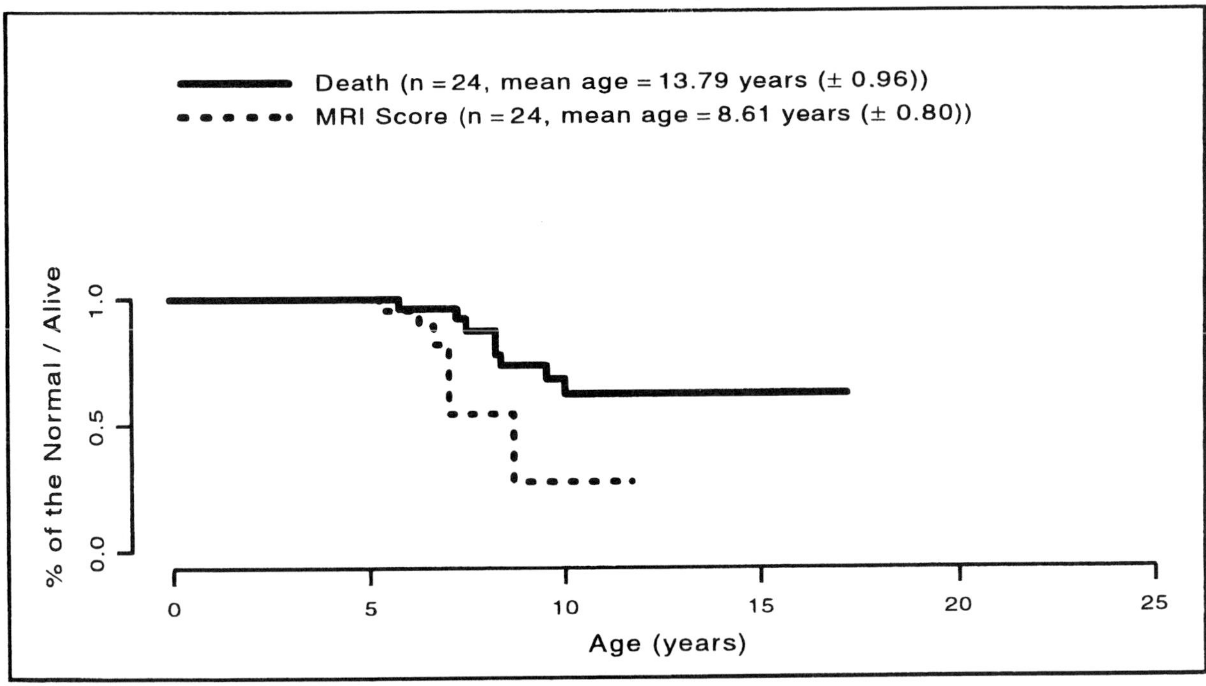

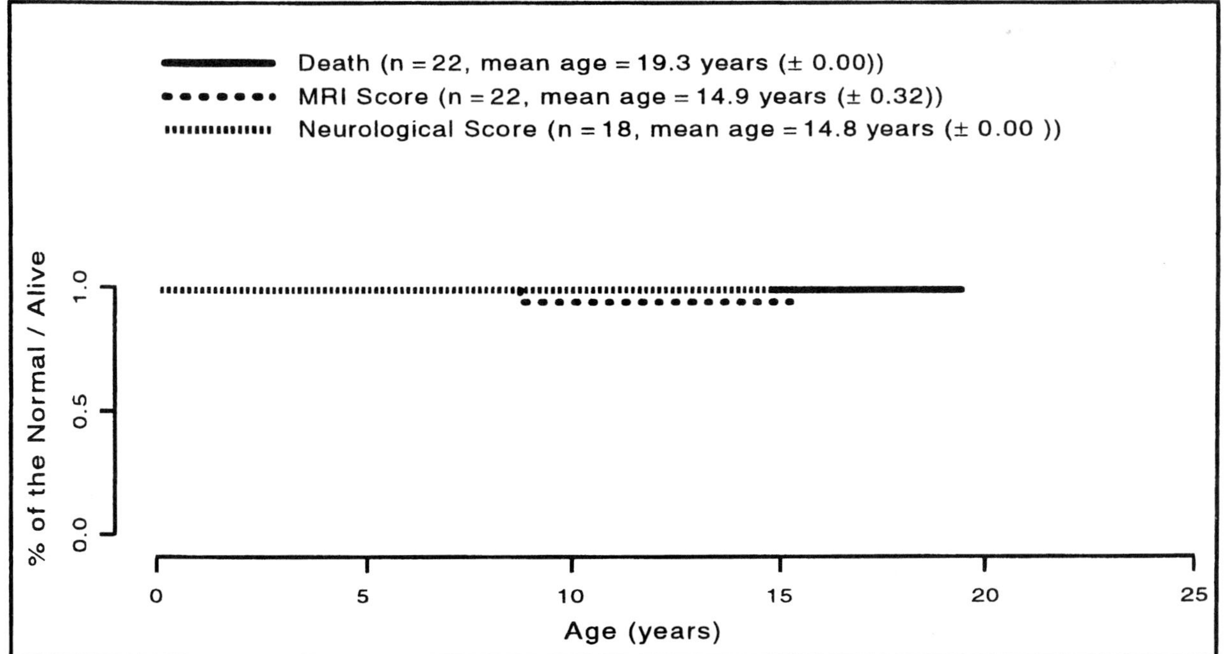

Fig. 131-3 (Continued)

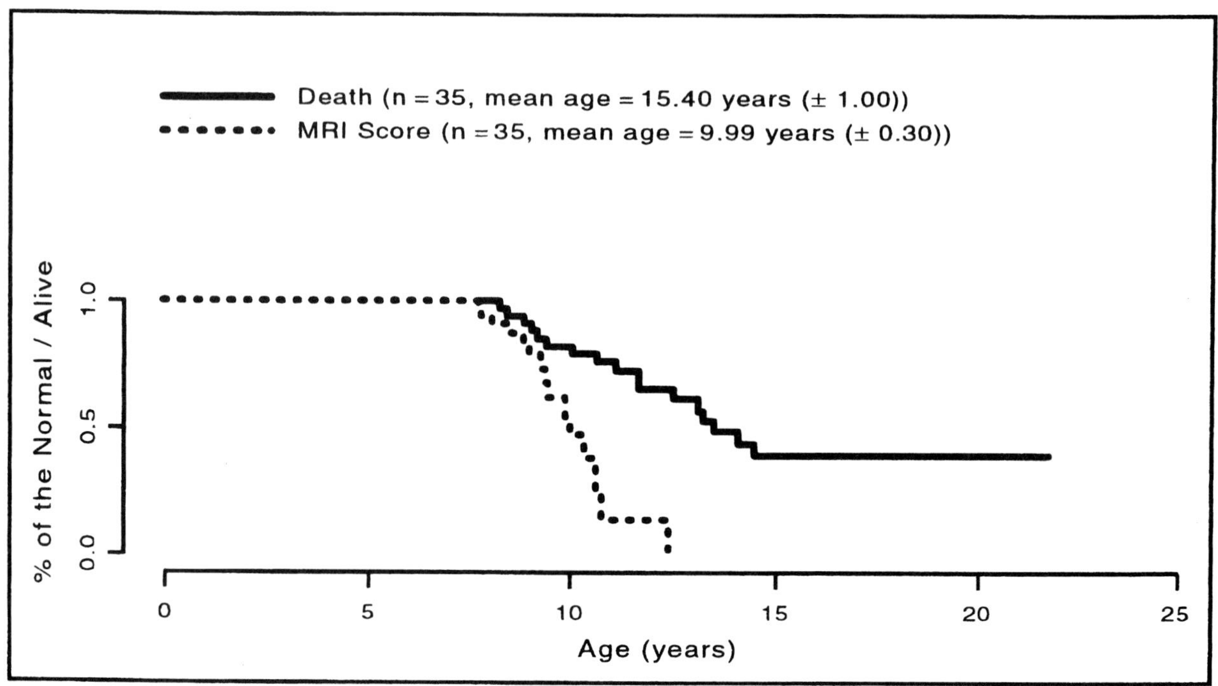

Fig. 131-3 (Continued)

established by biochemical assays. Adult cerebral ALD has a serious prognosis: The interval between first neurologic symptom and an apparently vegetative state or death is 3 to 4 years.

Rapidly progressive cerebral involvement may also supervene in AMN patients who, until then, had exhibited only slowly progressive neurological disability, referred to as "AMN-cerebral." Distinction between the AMN-cerebral and the adult-cerebral classification may be difficult.

ADDISON DISEASE ONLY

X-ALD is one cause of Addison disease in males. In a study at the pediatric endocrine clinic at Tufts University, five of eight males with Addison disease were found to have the biochemical defect of X-ALD.[60] Lauretti et al. identified X-ALD as the cause of adrenal insufficiency in 35 percent of male patients who had previously been diagnosed as having primary idiopathic adrenocortical insufficiency.[61] They noted that none of the X-ALD patients had adrenocortical antibodies. Analogous results were obtained by Jorge et al.,[62] who demonstrated X-ALD as the cause of Addison disease in 5 of 24 patients. Statistical analysis indicated that the likelihood of X-ALD as the cause is age-dependent. It is most likely when Addison disease manifests before the age of 7.5 years. It is important, therefore, that male Addison disease patients be screened for X-ALD. Most of the Addison-only patients will eventually develop neurologic symptoms. In some of the patients this will occur in childhood; in most it will present as AMN in adulthood. In the Kennedy Krieger Institute X-ALD series, we identified 79 Addison-only patients. The interval between the onset of adrenal insufficiency and neurologic disability is variable, but it may be as long as 32 years. Careful neurologic examination often reveals that the Addison-only patients do have slight neurologic involvement, such as hyperreflexia and impaired vibration sense in the legs, or a slight to moderate abnormality on MRI or neuropsychologic testing. In several of these patients, these slight deficits have remained stable for 3 to 4 years. The oldest known adrenal insufficiency-only patient, who died recently of a myocardial infarct at 81 years of age, had a normal neurologic examination and MRI at age 78 (B. van Geel, personal communication). This patient had also been treated for hypothyroidism and had hypogonadism.

We know of two X-ALD pedigrees that each have more than five males with adrenal insufficiency without neurologic involvement. X-linked adrenal insufficiency may also be associated with deficiency of glycerol kinase whose locus is at Xp21 (see Chap. 97).[63] Wakefield and Brown[64] reported another family with X-linked congenital Addison disease studied at a time before the VLCFA assay for the diagnosis of X-ALD was

Table 131-4 Prognosis of X-ALD as a Function of Age and MRI Loes Score

MRI score >3:	70–80% worsen irrespective of age; 8 of 80 remain neurologically stable
MRI score 1–3:	60% worsen irrespective of age; longer survival
MRI score <1:	Ages 3–7: 30% develop cerebral involvement
	Ages 7–10: 10% develop cerebral involvement
	Ages >10: Cerebral involvement rare

Prognosis of X-ALD as a function of age and MRI abnormality. The data presented in this summary table are based on analysis of Kaplan-Meier plots of survival, neurologic and neuropsychologic function, and MRI. These plots were constructed for each of the 18 subgroups shown in Table 131-3. Four of these plots are shown in Figs. 131-3*A* to *D*.

Thirty of the 377 patients had received BMT. Post-BMT data were excluded from analysis. The duration of follow-up is shown in Table 131-3 and in Fig. 131-3.

The conclusions presented in this table are based on follow-up ranging from a few months to 10 years. In spite of this limitation, the data show that consideration of age in combination of degree of MRI abnormality can aid the formulation of prognosis.

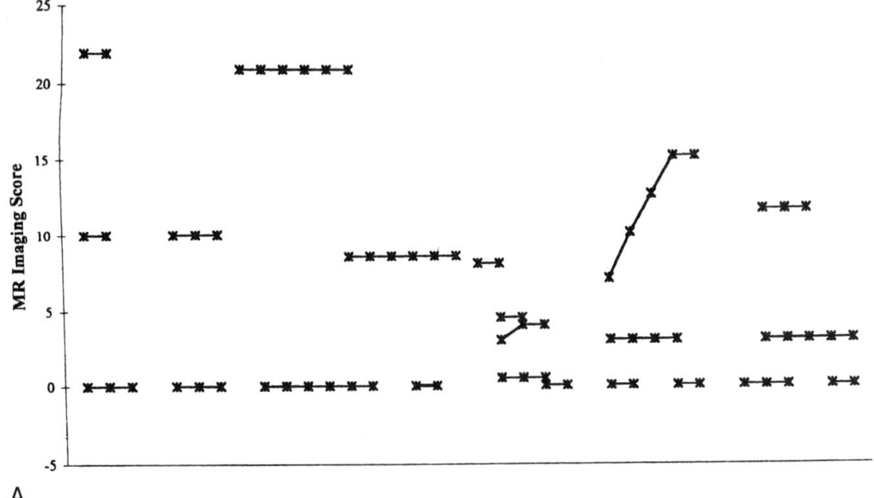

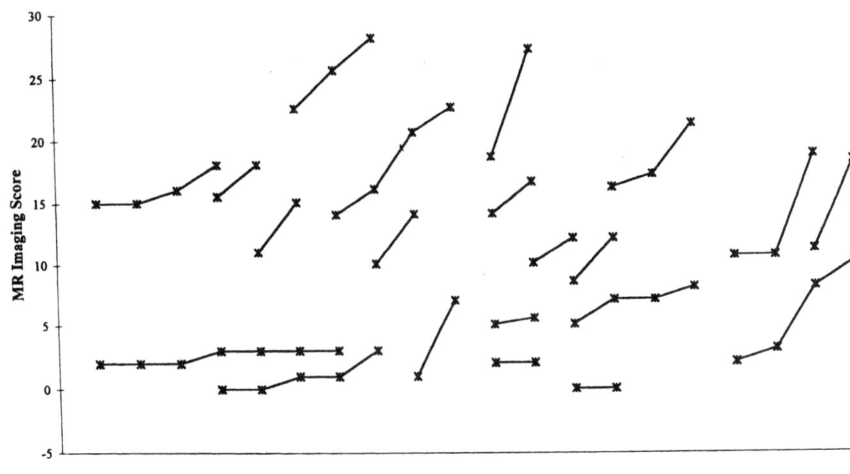

Fig. 131-4 MRI contrast-enhancement and progression of X-ALD. The progression of the brain MRI abnormality was assessed in 43 male X-ALD patients (mean age 12.9 years; range: 3 to 51 years). Severity of brain MRI abnormality was assessed with the scoring system devised by Loes et al.[43] In 22 patients who showed no gadolinium-contrast enhancement on T1-weighted images, the MRI severity score remained constant in 19 (*A*), while the abnormality progressed in 19 out of 21 patients who had shown contrast enhancement (*B*). The results differ statistically with a p value <0.001. (*From Melhem et al.*[406] *Used with permission.*)

Table 131-5 **Survey of 76 Men with Adrenomyeloneuropathy (AMN) and 25 Neurologically Symptomatic Women Heterozygous for Adrenoleukodystrophy**

	Expressed as Percentage with Abnormal Tests	
Test	**AMN***	**Heterozygotes***
Cognitive function	42	39
Brain stem auditory evoked	98	42
Visual evoked	24	5
Somatosensory evoked	100	90
Peroneal nerve velocity	68	29
Median nerve velocity	14	11
Brain MRI	46	16
Cerebral white matter		
Parieto-occipital	28	12
Temporal	43	4
Frontal	11	8
Corpus callosum	17	4
Visual pathways	39	12
Auditory pathways	29	4
Corticospinal tract	41	4
Cerebellar white matter	11	4
Cerebral atrophy	16	4
Overall abnormality	46	16

*Expressed as percentage with abnormal tests.

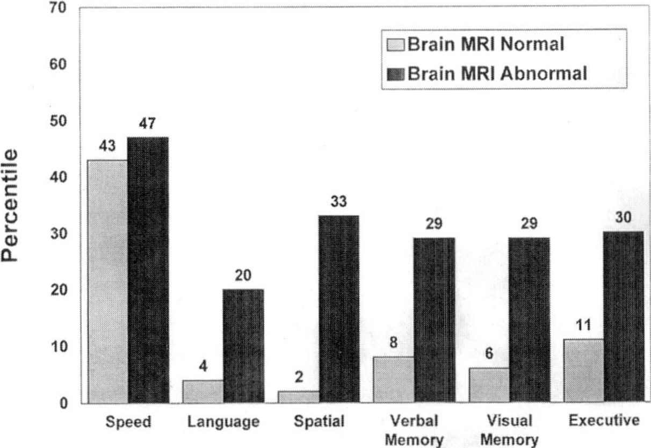

Fig. 131-5 Comparison of impairment of cognitive function in AMN patients with normal MRI, with those whose brain MRI was abnormal. MRI was rated as normal if the Loes score[43] was <1.5, and abnormal if the score was above this number. Well-standardized test instruments were used. Speed of performance, related to motor dysfunction, was impaired equally in both groups, while cognitive function was impaired more severely in all domains when MRI was abnormal. See reference 407 for detail.

available. It is likely that there are a variety of causes of X-linked Addison disease. Investigations to differentiate such cases should include assays of VLCFA and of glycerol kinase activity.

PERSONS WHO HAVE THE BIOCHEMICAL DEFECT OF X-ALD AND ARE FREE OF DEMONSTRABLE NEUROLOGIC OR ENDOCRINE INVOLVEMENT

Among relatives of symptomatic X-ALD patients we have identified 54 males with the biochemical defect of the disease who are said to be free of disability. Twenty-nine of the asymptomatic individuals are less than 10 years old and are at risk of later developing the disability. Twenty-five are 11 years old or older, and most are older than their symptomatic proband relatives. Because AMN and cerebral variants occur frequently within the same kindred, it is likely that these persons will develop AMN when they become adults.

We have identified one man with the biochemical defect of X-ALD, the brother of a patient with adult cerebral ALD, who was neurologically intact and had normal adrenal function at age 62 years. However, 4 years later, he showed mild spastic paraparesis and findings compatible with mild AMN. It is our impression that most adult patients with the biochemical defect of X-ALD who are allegedly asymptomatic will eventually show mild to moderate neurologic abnormalities compatible with AMN.

RARE X-ALD PHENOTYPES

Presentation as Olivopontocerebellar Atrophy

There are eight reports of male patients with documented X-ALD who presented with the clinical manifestations of olivopontocerebellar atrophy.[65–71] Seven of the eight reports were from Japan. In one patient, symptoms presented in childhood at age 5 years 7 months;[69] all others presented in adulthood. Cerebellar ataxia was a presenting symptom. In most instances, it was combined with corticospinal tract involvement. Cerebellar and pontine atrophy were present in all patients in whom imaging studies had been performed and initially may be the only demonstrable abnormality. The illness was progressive, and cerebral white matter abnormalities became evident later in all instances.

Asymmetric Clinical Presentation — Misdiagnosis as Brain Tumor

The initial neurologic and neuroimaging abnormalities of cerebral X-ALD may be asymmetric.[72–74] Figure 131-6 shows the MRI in one of these patients, which differs strikingly from the abnormalities observed in most X-ALD patients (Figs. 131-2*A* and *B*). These patients often are diagnosed as having a brain tumor, and are subjected to brain biopsy. In some instances, the biopsy led to the diagnosis of a leukodystrophy. In other instances, the microscopic findings were interpreted as indicating the presence of a glioma and the patient received radiotherapy. This also occurred in another patient with symmetric frontal lesions.[75] Assay of plasma VLCFA performed after the biopsies showed results characteristic of X-ALD, and this diagnosis was confirmed by additional studies in each instance.

Analysis of Reports of Patients with Spontaneous Remission

The literature includes reports of spontaneous remissions in three patients with X-ALD.[66,76] The first patient was reported by Walsh.[66] In retrospect, he had shown difficulties with schoolwork, behavioral disturbances, and incoordination since 7 years of age. He presented at 9 years of age with drowsiness and apathy, was mute, and his electroencephalogram showed high voltage delta waves without focal or paroxysmal features. He had a favorable response to prednisolone therapy and was able to return to normal activities for 17 days, when drowsiness returned. He then had two additional brief remissions, but after that developed progressive

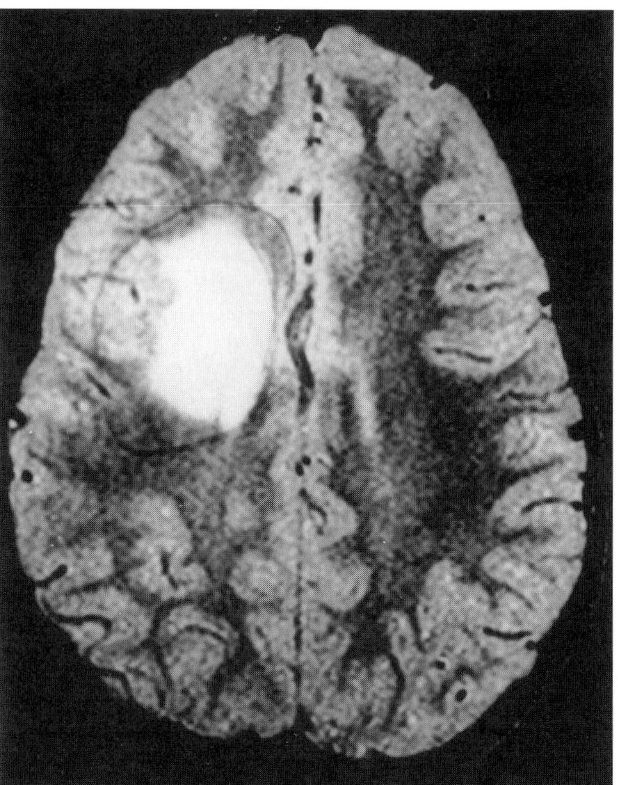

Fig. 131-6 Atypical MRI in a patient with CCER. A 5.8-year-old boy had presented with impaired vision in the right eye, right-sided headache, left-sided weakness, and hyperreflexia. Biopsy of the affected region showed almost complete loss of myelin and gliosis. Plasma VLCFA performed subsequent to the biopsy showed findings characteristic of X-ALD. A bone marrow transplant was performed several months later, and now, 4 years later, his condition appears to have stabilized. (*From Afifi et al.*[72] *Used with permission.*)

and severe neurologic deterioration that led to death at the age of 12 years and 11 months. Autopsy findings were characteristic of X-ALD. Although this patient had brief periods of remission, they appear to have been the result of temporary reductions of brain edema by steroid administration. The two other reported patients had more prolonged remissions, but it is unlikely that they had X-ALD. Subsequent measurements of plasma VLCFA in the second patient reported by Walsh[66] gave normal results and the diagnosis of X-ALD was abandoned (J. Wilson, personal communication, 1991). The diagnosis of X-ALD in the patient reported by Farrell et al.[76] is not confirmed. The diagnosis was based on the demonstration of an elevated C26:0 to C22:0 ratio in plasma and in cultured skin fibroblasts, and on the presence of a color-vision defect. At the time of publication, an association between X-ALD and color-vision defects had been postulated because of the presumed proximity of the genes.[19] More complete studies of VLCFA in cultured skin fibroblasts and plasma of this patient (kindly supplied by Dr. D. Farrell) in the peroxisomal disease laboratory at the Kennedy Krieger Institute failed to reveal abnormalities. Subsequent gene-mapping studies have failed to confirm association between X-ALD and defects in color vision.[31] Analysis of these reports and our own experience with more than 2000 patients fail to document the occurrence of long-term spontaneous remissions in X-ALD.

Relative Frequency and Prognosis of Male Phenotypes

Table 131-6 shows that estimates of the relative incidence of various phenotypes have varied. This variation is attributable to

Table 131-6 X-Linked ALD Phenotype Distributions at Kennedy Krieger Institute (KKI), Baltimore, MD, USA, Academic Medical Center, Amsterdam, The Netherlands, and Hopital De La Salpetriere, Paris, France

Phenotype	KKI Total up to 1995 N = 2088	KKI U.S. & Canada N = 1416	KKI 54 Most Informative U.S. and Canadian Families N = 306	France 1995 N = 303	Netherlands 1994 N = 77
Childhood cerebral	40.5	38.4	34.5	39	31
Adolescent cerebral	4.9	4.8	4.4	—	—
Adult cerebral	2.7	2.8	1.2	2	1
AMN	25.2	26.4	27	39.3	46
Addison only	9.6	9.6	10.3	6	14
Asymptomatic	7.9	8.6	10.3	3.6	8
Insufficient information	9.2	9.4	12.3	Not included	Not included

Estimation of the relative frequency of phenotypes is hampered by ascertainment bias. This bias results from the fact that the milder phenotypes (AMN, Addison-only, and asymptomatic) are often not diagnosed.[77] See text and reference 79 for further discussion.

ascertainment bias and to variance in phenotype designation. Ascertainment bias leads to an underestimate of mildly affected adults[77] and asymptomatic phenotypes. We believe that the most reliable data are those obtained in a comprehensive survey of 30 pedigrees in the Netherlands, in which all pedigree members were traced and examined to the maximum extent possible.[78] As Table 131-6 shows, this survey indicates that 46 percent of the male X-ALD patients had the AMN phenotype, compared to 31 percent for the sum of the CCER plus the adolescent form. Results of an historical survey of the age of onset of X-ALD in patients identified at the Kennedy Krieger Institute are consistent with the conclusion that adult forms are more frequent than CCER. This survey charted the age at onset of neurologic symptoms in 388 male X-ALD patients.[79] Ascertainment bias was eliminated because it included only those patients who belonged to sibships in which the genotype and phenotype of every male member was known (Fig. 131-7 and Table 131-7). Table 131-7 shows that 36 percent of patients developed neurologic symptoms by age 10 and 51 percent by age 20 years. These values resemble the results of the Netherlands and support the conclusion that the later-onset forms of X-ALD are more common than CCER. As Table 131-8 shows, the various phenotypes cooccur frequently within the same kindred or even nuclear family. This finding has implications for genetic counseling because it indicates that the phenotypes of previously identified X-ALD patients in a kindred are not valid predictors of disease expression in future members. Figure 131-1 compares the ages of onset of neurologic symptoms in patients with cerebral involvement and AMN. It is relatively uncommon for phenotypes that present mainly with cerebral involvement, to present after age 15 years. However, approximately half of the AMN patients may develop some degree of cerebral involvement. Figure 131-8 shows the survival analysis of CCER, the adolescent cerebral phenotype, and AMN, and Fig. 131-9 shows the interval between first neurologic symptom and death in these phenotypes.

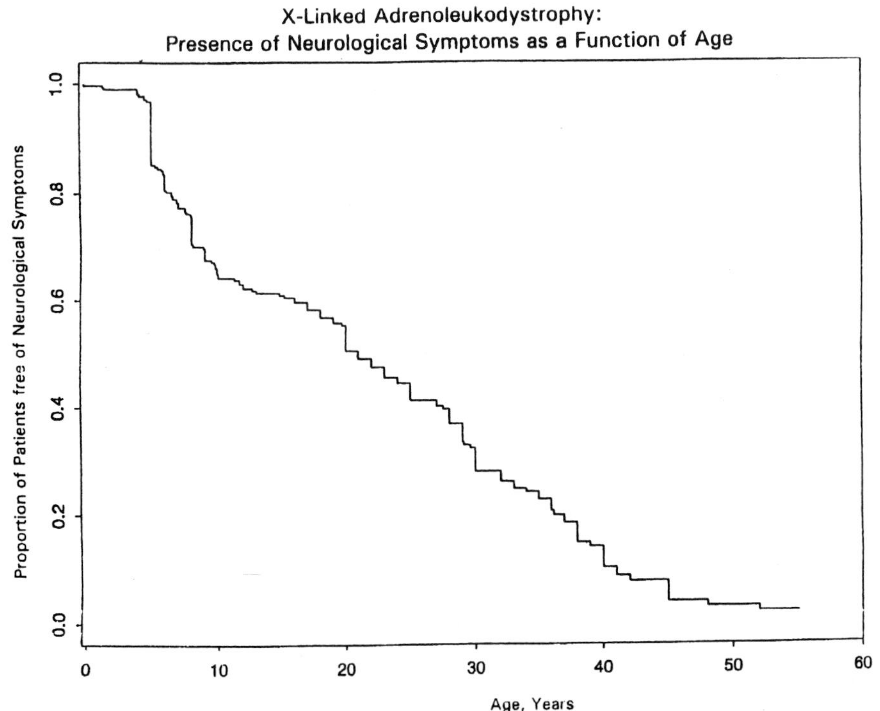

Fig. 131-7 Kaplan-Meier plot of age of first neurologic symptom in 388 X-ALD patients in the U.S. who were members of 253 sibships in which the X-ALD genotype and phenotype of every male member was known. (*From Bezman and Moser.*[79] *Used with permission.*)

Table 131-7 Onset of Neurologic Symptoms of X-ALD as a Function of Age

Age in Years	Fraction of Patients Free of Symptoms	Confidence Limits
4.0	0.9808	0.9800–1.0000
5.0	0.8530	0.8143–0.8936
7.0	0.7718	0.7259–0.8207
8.0	0.7035	0.6532–0.7543
9.0	0.6744	0.6226–0.7303
10.0	0.6413	0.5882–0.6991
14.8	0.6097	0.5554–0.6692
20.0	0.5064	0.4485–0.5717
34.0	0.2423	0.1884–0.3115
52.0	0.0191	0.0050–0.0723

To minimize ascertainment bias, these data are based on an analysis of the clinical course in 388 patients with X-ALD who were members of 253 sibships in which the genotype and phenotype of every male member was known. See text and reference 79 for further discussion.

SYMPTOMATIC X-ALD HETEROZYGOTES

Some degree of neurologic involvement occurs frequently in women who are heterozygous for X-ALD. The largest series is that of Dr. Sakkubai Naidu at the Kennedy Krieger Institute.[55] She examined 104 women who attended the yearly conference of the United Leukodystrophy Foundation (the American leukodystrophy parent organization) because of concern about their affected male relatives rather than their own health, and thus may be a reasonably representative sample of the X-ALD heterozygote population. Their mean age was 32 years (range 15 to 67 years). Sixty-one percent had some neurologic abnormalities that resembled AMN. Disability was severe in 14 percent. Twenty percent had slight to moderately severe symptoms, while another 22 percent had not complained of symptoms but were found to have hyperreflexia and impaired vibration sense in the lower extremities. The mean age at onset of neurologic symptoms was 37.8 ± 14.6 years. Figure 131-10 shows that the frequency and severity of neurologic involvement increases with age. Restuccia et al. studied motor and sensory-evoked responses in 19 heterozygotes.[80] Five of the women had clinical evidence of spinal cord involvement, while 14 were asymptomatic and neurologic examination was normal. As expected, abnormal patterns were observed in all of the symptomatic patients. In addition, mild but unequivocal abnormalities were present in 7 of 14 women who appeared neurologically uninvolved based on history and examination. These studies are consistent with the observation by Naidu et al. that some degree of neurologic involvement develops in more than half of the heterozygotes.

Table 131-8 Phenotype Distribution Among Multiplex Kindreds

	Kindreds	Percent
ALD	54	30.3
ALD/AMN	90	50.7
AMN	34	19.1
Total	178	

Phenotype Distribution Among Multiplex Nuclear Families

	Families	Percent
ALD	66	49.3
ALD/AMN	35	26.1
AMN	33	24.6
Total	134	

Nuclear families include sibships and grandfather-grandson relationship. *Kindreds* include all relatives. CCER indicates that the childhood cerebral form was the only phenotype in the kindred or nuclear family. AMN indicates that this was the only phenotype. ALD/AMN indicates that the childhood cerebral form and AMN were both present. The rarer phenotypes listed in Table 131-1 were not included in this analysis.

A dementing illness beginning in middle age or later has been reported in four heterozygotes.[81–84] Another three had rapidly progressive cerebral symptoms in their late preadolescence or early adolescence similar to what is observed in boys with childhood or adolescent cerebral ALD. Overt adrenocortical insufficiency is rare in X-ALD heterozygotes. It was noted in only 8 of the more than 1600 heterozygotes reported in the literature[83,85,86] or included in the Kennedy Krieger Institute series. Three of the heterozygotes with Addison disease also had severe cerebral involvement. While overt Addison disease is rare, El-Deiry et al. reported that five of eight heterozygous women whose ACTH levels and ACTH stimulation tests were normal showed subclinical decreases of glucocorticoid reserve, as measured by tests with ovine corticosteroid releasing hormone.[87]

In the heterozygotes who had a rapidly progressive dementing illness,[83,84,88] histopathologic studies revealed changes similar to childhood cerebral or adult cerebral ALD. The more mildly affected patients had pathologic changes resembling those in AMN (see "Pathology" below). There was mild involvement of the adrenal cortex, even in a woman with normal adrenal function.[88]

Most X-ALD heterozygotes who presented with paraparesis had previously been diagnosed as having multiple sclerosis.[89] Another was diagnosed as having a dorsolateral cord syndrome of unknown etiology.[90] In all instances, the diagnosis was changed to the manifesting X-ALD heterozygote state only because they had a male child with X-ALD. One previously reported X-ALD heterozygote[89] had noted intermittent paresthesia in her left arm and leg since age 40. At age 44 impaired vibration sense, hyperreflexia in lower extremities, and oligoclonal bands in cerebrospinal fluid led to the diagnosis of multiple sclerosis. When she was 47 years old, the diagnosis of X-ALD was established in her son, and she herself was shown to have unequivocal elevation of VLCFA.[89] A similar sequence was noted in an Australian patient. These histories highlight the phenotypic resemblance between multiple sclerosis and the manifesting heterozygote. The diagnostic difficulty is confounded by the fact that most neurologically impaired heterozygotes have normal adrenocortical function. VLCFA levels in plasma and/or cultured skin fibroblasts are increased in approximately 85 percent of heterozygotes[91,92] but false negative tests with this technique cannot be eliminated. Demonstration of cells that lack immunoreactivity for ALDP is of diagnostic value,[93,94] but this technique is valid only in those families in which lack of this material had been demonstrated in affected male probands. Mutation analysis is the most definitive procedure for the identification of women heterozygous for X-ALD.[95]

Watkiss et al. studied X-inactivation patterns in 12 carriers and found no evidence that skewed patterns were related to clinical manifestations.[96] However, Naidu et al., in studies that included cultured skin fibroblasts of 100 heterozygous women, showed a positive correlation between clinical severity and the proportion of cells that lacked immunoreactivity for ALDP. In three patients with severe neurologic involvement, two of whom also had Addison disease, 98 to 100 percent of cells were immunonegative.[97] In a set of 70-year-old monozygotic twins with elevated VLCFA levels whose clinical manifestations were strikingly different, the severely impaired twin had more than 90 percent immunonegative cells, compared to her unaffected sister who had less than 30 percent of such cells.

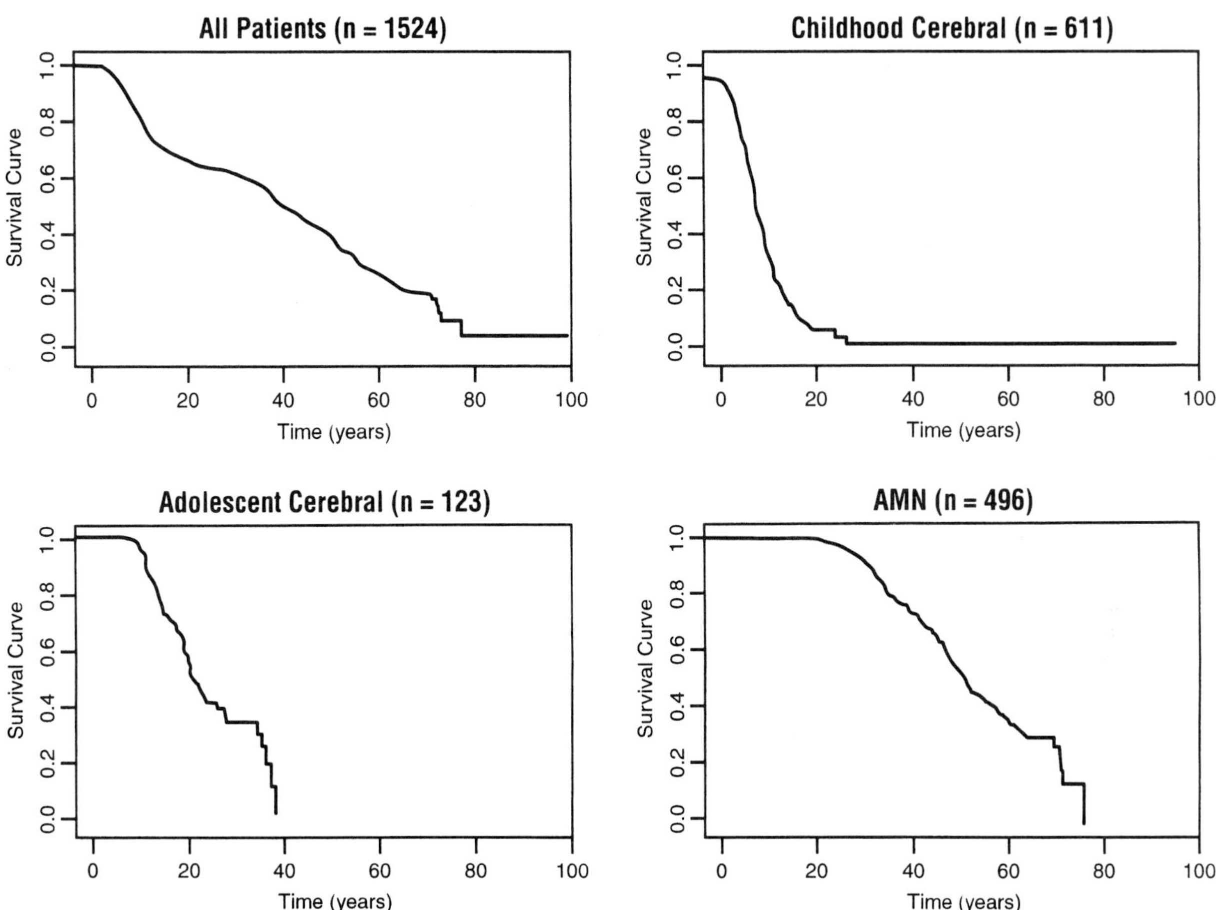

Fig. 131-8 Survival analysis of male patients with X-ALD, based on information in kindreds followed at the Kennedy Krieger Institute. The diagnosis in each patient was based on VLCFA assays and analysis of clinical and pathologic data.

PATHOLOGY OF X-ALD

Nervous System

The pathologic features of the cerebral variants of X-ALD and AMN, except for those in the peripheral nervous system, have been thoroughly studied and reported by several groups and have been reviewed.[38,40,98–100] It is of key importance to note that the pathology of the cerebral forms of X-ALD differs fundamentally from that in pure AMN. The cerebral forms are associated with an inflammatory response in cerebral white matter. Pure AMN is mainly a distal axonopathy,[98] and the inflammatory response is absent or mild.

Nervous System Pathology of Cerebral Forms

Postmortem examination of the brain of cerebrally involved X-ALD patients usually reveals it to be externally normal, except that the optic nerves are often gray and atrophic. Mild to moderate premature atherosclerosis can be seen in the adults. The gray matter is usually intact, but the centrum semiovale is consistently firm (sclerotic) and replaced by large areas of brown to gray translucent tissue. The loss of myelin is confluent, usually symmetric, and most prominent in the parieto-occipital regions. CT and MRI studies have confirmed the caudorostral progression proposed from classical autopsy studies and highlight the contrast-enhancing, advancing edge of the lesion, which is usually frontal. Cavitation and calcification of white matter may be seen in severe cases. Arcuate fibers are relatively spared, but the posterior cingulum, corpus callosum, fornix, hippocampal commissure, posterior limb of the internal capsule, and optic system are typically involved. The cerebellar white matter usually exhibits a similar, but milder, confluent loss of myelin and sclerosis. Secondary corticospinal tract degeneration extending down through the peduncles, basis pontis, medullary pyramids, and spinal cord is characteristic. The brain stem also may display primary demyelinative foci, especially in basis pontis. The spinal cord is spared in the CCER phenotype except for the descending tract degeneration.[40]

Histopathologically, these dynamic white matter lesions of the central nervous system exhibit profound changes in the indigenous elements: marked losses of myelinated axons (myelin > axons) and oligodendrocytes in association with hypertrophic reactive astrocytosis acutely to isomorphic and anisomorphic fibrillary astrogliosis chronically. Apoptotic oligodendrocytes have not been seen with traditional stains, but some appear pyknotic. Random preservation of individual myelinated axons in foci of myelin loss is common, but these myelin sheaths may be thin or irregular. A repertoire of nonresident cells is also recruited. The advancing or active edges of myelin loss are sites of intense perivascular inflammation and lipid-laden macrophage (lipophage) accumulation, in addition to reactive astrocytosis. The composition of the responding cells also varies with the age of the lesion. Diffuse

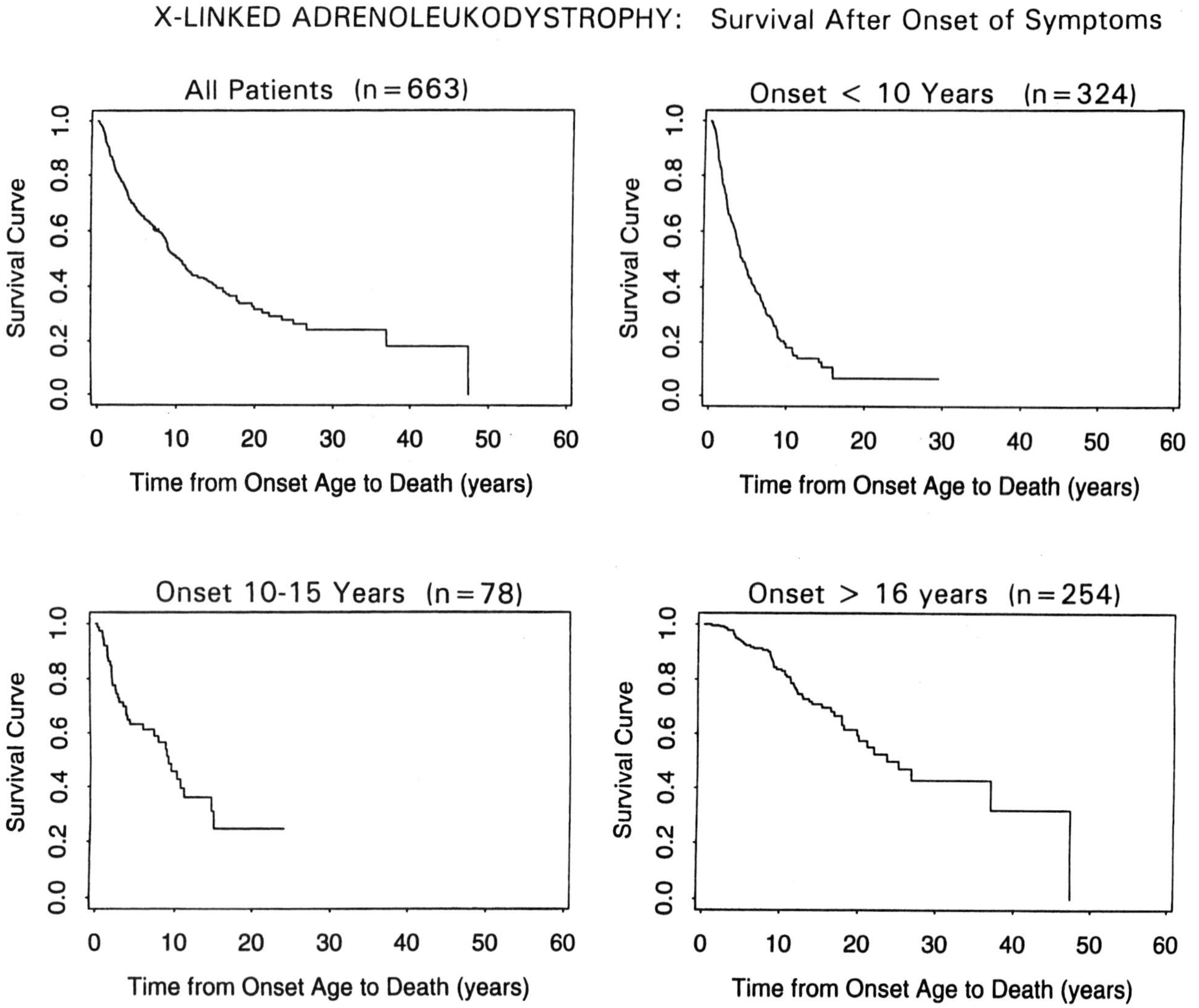

X-LINKED ADRENOLEUKODYSTROPHY: Survival After Onset of Symptoms

All Patients (n=663)

Onset < 10 Years (n=324)

Onset 10-15 Years (n=78)

Onset > 16 years (n=254)

Survival Curve

Time from Onset Age to Death (years)

Fig. 131-9 Survival after onset of symptoms in male patients with X-ALD who were members of kindreds followed at the Kennedy Krieger Institute.

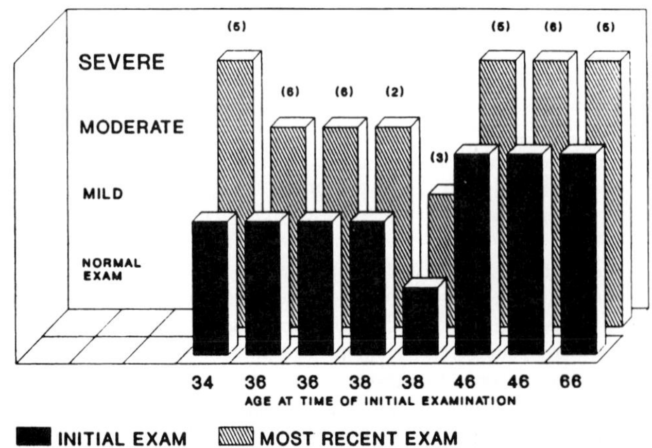

Fig. 131-10 Progression of neurologic disability in women heterozygous for X-ALD. Dr. Sakkubai Naidu obtained the data in study of 104 heterozygous women who attended the annual meetings of the United Leukodystrophy Foundation. Note that disease severity increased in all age groups.

infiltrations of macrophages and large perivascular collections of mononuclear cells (Fig. 131-11), particularly lymphocytes, are highly characteristic of areas of early myelin breakdown, while large perivascular collections of lipophages typify older demyelinative lesions (Fig. 131-12). Small numbers of perivascular lymphocytes, hypertrophic astrocytes, and lipophages are noted even in sclerotic lesions.[98,99] The lymphocytes display both T, including CD4, and B cell phenotypes,[100] with the T cell predominant in our studies.[101] Plasma cells are much less frequent. Lymphocytic perivascular collections are usually most intense immediately within the advancing edge where myelin and oligodendrocytes already have been lost, axons are relatively spared, and many interstitial lipophages are present. Hypertrophy and hyperplasia of glial fibrillary acidic protein (GFAP)-positive astrocytes and macrophage infiltration are seen just outside of the advancing edge, where some splitting of myelin sheaths and edema are observed. Astrocytes and macrophages outside of and at the lesion's edge show both tumor necrosis factor-alpha (TNF-α) and interleukin-1 (IL-1) immunoreactivity; TNF-α is greater in reactive astrocytes and IL-1 greater in macrophages. Adhesion molecule (ICAM) and class I and II molecule up-regulation also are noted.[101]

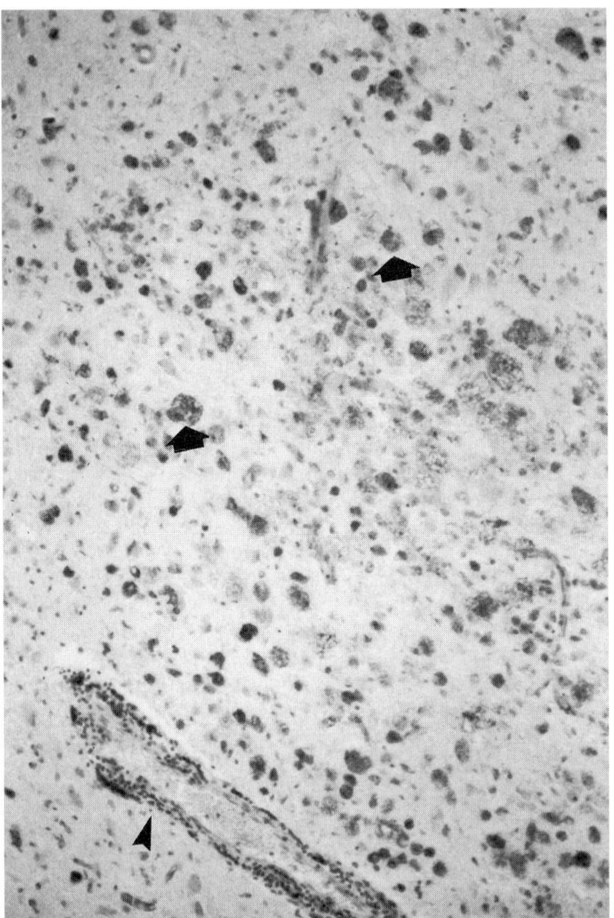

Fig. 131-11 Active edge of white matter demyelinative lesion of CCER showing numerous macrophages ingesting myelin debris (arrows) at outer part of edge and perivascular lymphocytes (arrowhead) inside of the edge. MAC-1 immunoperoxidase stain.

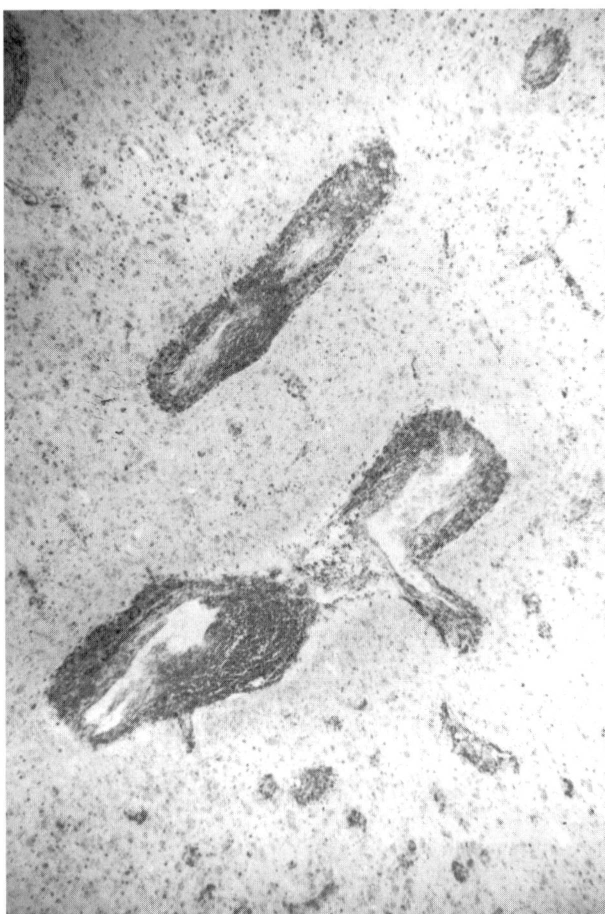

Fig. 131-12 Within the white matter demyelinative lesion of patients with adult cerebral phenotype showing prominent perivascular cuffs of macrophages and fewer lymphocytes. Numerous unstained nuclei in background are reactive astrocytes. MAC-1 immunoperoxidase stain.

Two populations of lipophages are found both perivascularly and diffusely within demyelinated white matter. Both are usually uninucleated; rarely, multinucleated forms are observed. A minor proportion stains less intensely with neutral lipid colorants and the periodic acid-Schiff (PAS) stain, and usually demonstrates striated cytoplasm due to the presence of clear clefts. The number of striations generally correlates inversely with sudanophilia and PAS positivity. These striated macrophages are birefringent and retain their birefringence after acetone extraction.[11] Metachromatic material is inconspicuous.

The corticospinal tracts exhibit equivalent losses of axons and myelin, mild hypertrophy of astrocytes, and a few lipophages. In contrast to secondary tract degeneration in other disorders, X-ALD tract degeneration often contains foci of perivascular lymphocytes and striated lipophages.

Ultrastructural examination of old, sclerotic lesions usually reveals little more than astrocytic processes filled with dense cytofilaments. Active lesions contain demyelinated intact axons, demyelinated degenerated axons, thinly myelinated axons, a variety of inflammatory cells, and two populations of macrophages. The predominant macrophage contains myelin debris and opaque lipid droplets (cholesterol esters), while the other contains lipid droplets, lamellae, lamellar-lipid profiles, and angulate lysosomes containing spicules specificity of ultrastructural changes. Suggestive, but not definitive, evidence of lamellar inclusions in oligodendrocytes has been reported.[102] Beyond the active edge, the extracellular space is enlarged and splitting and fragmentation of myelin sheaths is observed.

Nervous System Lesions in Pure AMN and Heterozygotes

The pathology of AMN was recently reviewed.[103] The central nervous system lesions in "pure" AMN differ from those in CCER, adolescent, and adult cerebral X-ALD.[98–100] The spinal cord bears the brunt of the disease process in AMN, as well as in symptomatic female heterozygotes. Loss of myelinated axons and a milder loss of oligodendrocytes is observed in the long ascending and descending tracts of spinal cord, especially fasciculus gracilis and the lateral corticospinal tracts. The pattern of fiber loss is consistent with a distal axonopathy in that the greatest losses are observed in lumbar corticospinal and cervical gracile tracts. Axonal loss is usually commensurate with the myelin loss. Sudanophilia and inflammation are minimal to absent. Perivascular accumulations of striated lipophages are present, particularly in relatively preserved tracts. Astrogliosis, usually isomorphic, is moderate, and the predominant reactive cells are activated microglia (Powers et al., unpublished observation). Ultrastructurally, the affected tracts may show scant segmental demyelination, myelin corrugation, numerous myelin ovoids, axons with thin myelin sheaths, and probably axonal atrophy. Macrophages with pleomorphic cytoplasmic inclusions, mainly spicules specificity of ultrastructural changes have been visualized under the electron microscope. The medial and lateral lemnisci, brachium conjunctivum, middle cerebellar peduncles, inferior cerebellar peduncles, geniculocalcarine tracts, and optic system also may be involved. The involvement of cerebral and cerebellar white matter in patients with AMN is variable, but is usually minimal compared to cerebral X-ALD. Complete preservation, diffuse or confluent loss of myelin in centrum semiovale without significant inflammation and with arcuate fiber sparing, multifocal loss of myelinated axons and oligodendroglia with indolent astrogliosis, and PAS-positive lipophages (dysmyelination), to localized X-ALD-like inflammatory and demyelinative lesions may be seen. In those AMN patients with a terminal cerebral phase,[101] confluent inflammatory demyelination indistinguishable from CCER is noted, in addition to the expected spinal cord and peripheral nerve lesions.

Peripheral nerve lesions in AMN are variable and mild compared to the myelopathy. Spinal nerve roots and ganglia, sciatic, popliteal, and ulnar nerves have been reported to be unremarkable at autopsy, despite severe myelopathy. Sural and peroneal nerves have displayed a loss of large and small diameter myelinated fibers, endoneurial fibrosis, and thin myelin sheaths.[104,105] Lamellar inclusions in Schwann cells or endoneurial macrophages have been documented at biopsy in peroneal nerve and endomysial nerve twigs.[104,105] Schwann cell lamellar inclusions are usually seen in association with intact myelin sheaths and axons. We have observed segmental demyelination in nerve roots, often in clusters, and atrophy of dorsal root ganglia neurons in AMN; significant ganglion cell loss and Nageotte's nodules have not been seen (Powers et al., unpublished observation). The peripheral nerve in CCER is typically unremarkable at the light microscopic level, but can contain lamellar or lamellar-lipid inclusions in Schwann cells.[9,105]

Adrenal Cortex, Testis, and Pituitary

Adrenocortical cells, particularly those of the inner fasciculata-reticularis, become ballooned and striated due to accumulations of lamellae, lamellar-lipid profiles, and fine lipid clefts (Fig. 131-13).[8,10,106] The striated material, consisting of the same abnormal cholesterol esters as in central nervous system striated lipophages, appears to lead to cell dysfunction, atrophy, and death. Histoenzymatic decreases in mitochondrial alpha glycerophosphate dehydrogenase, 3-β-hydroxysteroid dehydrogenase, and TPNH diaphorase have been reported, and they showed excessive peripheral cytolysis under the electron microscope. Moreover, the striated cells appear to adapt poorly to a tissue culture environment. Ultimately, primary atrophy of the adrenal cortex ensues. Inflammatory cells are rarely observed and are probably an epiphenomenon; antiadrenal antibodies are not detected. The adrenal cortex in AMN displays the same qualitative changes as, but tends to be more atrophic than, in most other X-ALD patients. This probably is related mainly to the longer duration of hypoadrenalism in AMN. The same striated adrenocortical cells have been identified in X-ALD heterozygotes, both symptomatic and asymptomatic; but they are limited to small, multifocal clusters.[88] This finding is in striking contrast to findings in affected males, and even to specimens of affected fetal adrenal cortex,[106] in which this lesion is diffuse.

Testicular lesions in prepubertal X-ALD males are usually present only at the ultrastructural level and consist of lamellae and lamellar-lipid profiles in interstitial cells of Leydig and their precursors. The testis in AMN and adult cerebral X-ALD demonstrates the same Leydig cell alterations as described above in CCER, but there is also some Leydig cell loss. No inflammatory cells have been seen, except in a single case of adult X-ALD. Degenerative changes in seminiferous tubules in AMN appear indistinguishable from those of adult cerebral ALD and vary from maturation arrest to Sertoli cell only. Ultrastructurally, vacuolation of the Sertoli cell's endoplasmic reticulum followed by widened intercellular spaces appears to be the initial lesion of the seminiferous tubules.[50,106,107]

The pituitary may exhibit an increase in basophilic adrenocorticotrophins with varying numbers of stainable granules, depending on the degree and duration of glucocorticoid insufficiency and replacement.

Specificity of Ultrastructural Changes

Electron-dense bi-leaflet structures were first seen in adrenocortical cells lying free in the cytoplasm, fused with each other (multilamellar) or fused with cytoplasmic organelles (Fig. 131-13).[108] These leaflets, referred to as lamellae, have been also demonstrated in Schwann cells, Leydig cells, and macrophages in central nervous system white-matter lesions.[102] The extent to which these lamellae can be classified as truly specific for X-ALD and generalized peroxisomal disorders (see Chap. 129) depends on ultrastructural features that have been described in detail.[10] Ultrastructural demonstration of the characteristic lamellae/lamellar-lipid profiles and biochemical demonstration of an excess of saturated VLCFA are thus a reflection of the same abnormality that is characteristic of X-ALD and other peroxisomal

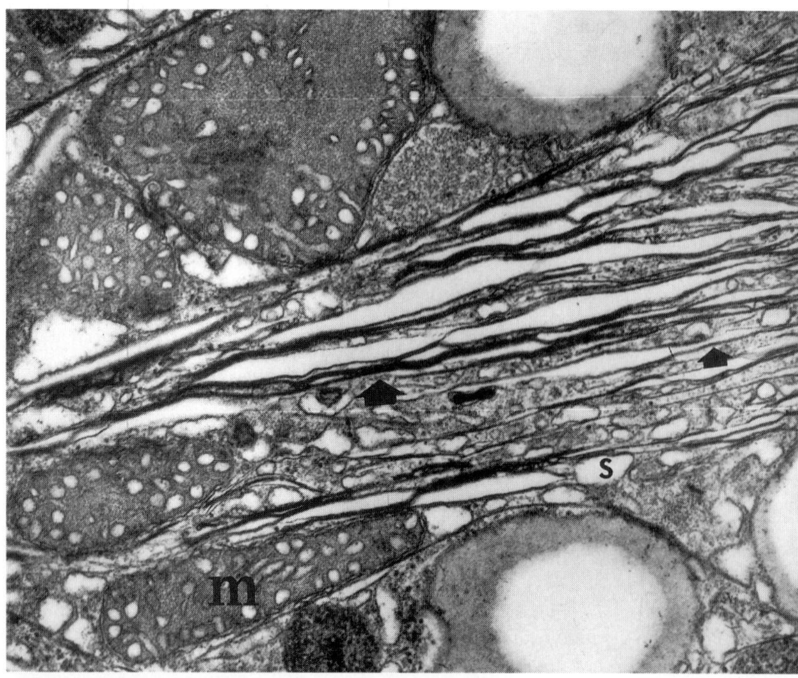

Fig. 131-13 This adrenocortical cell contains both unilamellar and multilamellar inclusions (arrows), which are both free in the cytoplasm and focally contact mitochondria (m) and smooth endoplasmic reticulum (s).

disorders in which VLCFA accumulate. Spicules, usually found within angulate lysosomes of macrophages, are more characteristic of the disorders of peroxisome biogenesis than of X-ALD, but they are less specific for those disorders than are the lamellae and lamellar-lipid profiles.

CHEMICAL PATHOLOGY OF X-ALD

Very Long Chain Fatty Acids (VLCFA): Definition and Normal Tissue Distribution

VLCFA are defined as saturated and unsaturated fatty acids with carbon-chain lengths longer than 22 atoms. Rezanka[109] reviewed the literature about VLCFA, and points out that they are almost omnipresent in the animal and plant kingdoms, varying from 0.1 percent to as much as 10 percent of total fatty acids. Normally saturated VLCFA occur in highest concentration in myelin lipids and red blood cell sphingomyelin. C26:0 accounts for 1 to 5 percent of total fatty acids in brain cerebrosides and sulfatides,[12,110] and in red blood cell sphingomyelin.[15] VLCFA are present in much lower concentration in other tissues. C26:0 constitutes approximately 0.01 percent of total fatty acids in plasma[14] and adipose tissue (Moser HW, unpublished observation) and 0.02 percent in the normal adrenal gland.[16]

Abnormally High Levels of Saturated VLCFA in Tissues and Body Fluids of Patients with X-ALD. Abnormally high levels of saturated VLCFA are the principal biochemical abnormality in the tissues and body fluids of patients with X-ALD. The VLCFA that accumulate in X-ALD are saturated and unbranched, and involve mainly those with a carbon-chain length of 26 (hexacosanoic acid, C26:0) and tetracosanoic acid (C24:0). C26:0 may also be referred to as cerotic acid, and C24:0 as lignoceric acid. Saturated VLCFA with chain lengths up to 32 also accumulate in lesser amounts. This accumulation has a specific pattern. While some degree of excess is present in most tissues, the most striking increases are found in the cholesterol ester fractions of affected brain white matter and in the adrenal cortex.

Sargent and associates have reported that the levels of nervonic acid C24:1 (n-9) is reduced in the brain sphingolipids of X-ALD patients[111] and have hypothesized that a deficit of this fatty acid may contribute to the pathogenesis of the disease.[112]

Cholesterol Ester. Igarashi et al.[12] were the first to report a striking abnormality in the fatty acid composition of cholesterol esters in X-ALD brain and adrenal cortex (Fig. 131-14). Cholesterol esters in control brain contain mostly C16 to C20 fatty acids, whereas cholesterol esters in X-ALD brain contain large amounts of VLCFA (C24 to C30 or more), where they constitute 20 to 67 percent of total fatty acids, compared with 0 to 5 percent in controls.[113] The abnormality of cholesterol ester fatty acids has been confirmed in all subsequent studies.[82,110,114–117]

The cholesterol ester abnormality correlates with histopathology. The greatest excess of cholesterol ester levels and VLCFA enrichment is observed in the actively demyelinating areas.[117–119] In two studies, cholesterol ester levels and fatty acid composition were normal in those regions of X-ALD brain that appeared histologically intact,[117,118] while in another patient, the cholesterol esters in a histologically intact area did contain abnormally high VLCFA levels.[119] "Burned out" gliotic areas of brain contain normal or slightly increased levels of cholesterol esters, with increased VLCFA content.[118]

Phospholipids and Proteolipids. Theda et al.[118] showed that in histologically normal areas of X-ALD white matter, the phosphatidylcholinefraction contained a thirty-ninefold excess of C26:0 in comparison with control, whereas the C26:0 percentage in cholesterol ester, phosphatidylserine, and phosphatidylethanolamine was either normal or increased less than twofold. The phosphatidylcholine fraction in abnormal X-ALD brain tissue

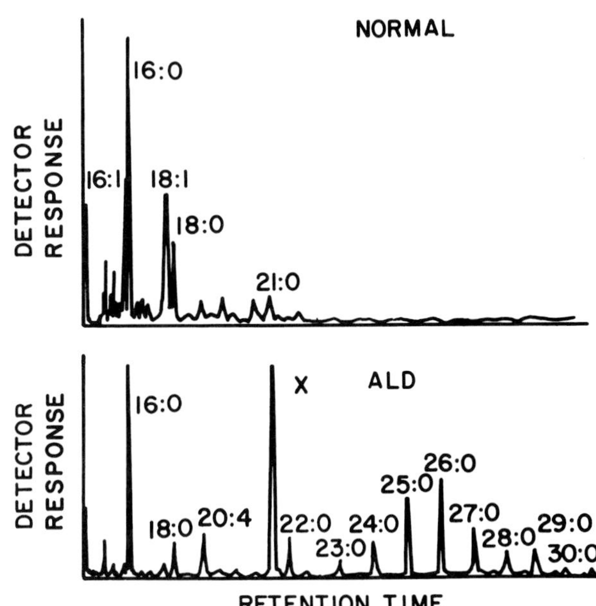

Fig. 131-14 Fatty acid methyl esters of brain cholesterol esters (gas chromatography). ***(From Igarashi et al.[12] Used with permission.)***

contains an excess of C30, C32, and C34 monounsaturated acids,[120] and in myelin, the proportion of saturated and monounsaturated VLCFA bound to proteolipid protein was increased at the expense of oleic acid.[121]

Gangliosides. Fatty acids with a chain length greater than 22 account for 28 to 50 percent of total fatty acids in X-ALD brain gangliosides, compared with 2.5 percent in controls.[113,122] C24:0 and C24:1 (and not C25:0 or C26:0) represent the predominant VLCFA in X-ALD gangliosides, thus differing from the pattern noted in the X-ALD cholesterol ester fraction. All the VLCFAs were attached to the ganglioside by the usual amide linkage. The VLCFA excess was present in all ganglioside species, with those containing multiple sialic acid units showing the greatest excess.

Glycolipids and Triglycerides. Other brain constituents show lesser or no VLCFA excess. Studies of the cerebroside and sulfatide fractions are particularly difficult to interpret because these myelin constituents normally contain VLCFA, and their long chain and VLCFA content is known to be diminished when there is demyelination, as occurs in X-ALD. In two studies, a 1.5- to twofold increase in VLCFA content of cerebrosides and sulfatides was noted,[12,110] while in another study, their levels were unchanged.[117] VLCFA content in the free fatty acid and triglyceride fractions is moderately increased.[110,115,117,118]

Myelin. When X-ALD white matter is fractionated by standard techniques,[123] the myelin content is drastically reduced when compared with normal,[110] while there is a large amount of less dense material, referred to as the floating fraction, that contains large quantities of the abnormal cholesterol esters. Morphologic studies indicate that the abnormal cholesterol esters in X-ALD brain, demonstrable with the electron microscope as lamellar inclusions, are located mainly in invading macrophages.[98] Brown et al.[110] reported that myelin isolated from X-ALD brain contained up to 10 percent of cholesterol esters and that these cholesterol esters were enriched in VLCFA. Normal myelin does not contain cholesterol ester. Such an abnormality in the composition of X-ALD myelin might cause it to be unstable; however, it was not possible to exclude that the X-ALD myelin was contaminated with "floating fraction" material, even though steps were taken to minimize this.[110]

Plasma, Red Blood Cells, Cultured Skin Fibroblasts. As discussed in "Diagnosis of X-ALD" below, a two- to tenfold VLCFA excess was demonstrated in the red blood cells, plasma, and cultured skin fibroblasts of more than 3000 X-ALD hemizygotes and heterozygotes,[92] and the specificity of this finding is confirmed. These studies confirm the significance of the VLCFA abnormality that was first demonstrated in postmortem tissues, and indicate that this biochemical abnormality is an integral part of the disease process.

Occurrence and Metabolism

Source of Saturated VLCFA. VLCFA present in the human body appear to be derived from both the diet and endogenous synthesis. This conclusion is based on studies in two X-ALD patients. In the first study, each day a terminally ill X-ALD patient received 10 mg of (3,3,5,5)-$^2H_4$ hexacosanoic (C26:0) acid by nasogastric tube for a 100-day period. This quantity of C26:0 is equivalent to the C26:0 of the usual American diet. Postmortem study demonstrated that in certain parts of the brain, up to 90 percent of C26:0 contained the label, indicating that in this patient, a substantial portion of brain C26:0 was of dietary origin.[124]

Studies in another X-ALD patient indicate that endogenous synthesis also is a source of VLCFA. This patient received 50 ml of D_2O by mouth each day for a 196-day period. At the end of the study, deuterium enrichment of lignoceric acid (C24:0) and hexacosanoic acid (C26:0) was 72 to 79 percent that of palmitic (C16:0) and stearic (C18:0) acids.[125] This result differs sharply from the findings in respect to phytanic acid in a Refsum disease patient. When this patient received the same amount of oral D_2O over the same time period, plasma phytanic acid was essentially free of label.[126] This result led to the conclusion that phytanic acid in humans is of dietary origin only. The results in the X-ALD patients indicate that C26:0, and presumably other VLCFA, are of both dietary and endogenous origin. The results do not permit conclusions about the relative importance of the two pathways, although the high level of VLCFA label following D_2O administration suggests that the endogenous synthesis may be more important. Dietary studies in X-ALD patients lead to the same conclusion. Dietary restriction of C26:0 failed to lower plasma C26:0 levels,[127] while a reduction was achieved by measures that are presumed to diminish endogenous VLCFA synthesis.[20,21]

Biosynthesis of VLCFA. Synthesis of fatty acids with chain length greater than 16 carbons is carried out by the fatty acid elongation system. This system occurs in both mitochondria and microsomes. The microsomal system appears to be more active and to have greater physiological significance.[128]

The stoichiometry of the elongation reaction in the microsomal system is:

$$\text{Palmitoyl CoA} \pm \text{malonyl CoA} \pm \text{NADPH} \pm \text{H} \pm$$
$$\rightarrow \text{stearoyl CoA} \pm CO_2 \pm \text{NADP}^{\pm} \pm \text{CoA} \pm H_2O$$

With this reaction, a C16 fatty acid (palmitic) is elongated to C18 (stearic acid). VLCFA synthesis is achieved by repeated additions of malonyl CoA, so that two carbon units are added until the desired chain length is achieved. Fatty acid synthesis and elongation are complex and highly regulated processes involving the coordinated action of multiple enzymes and acyl carrier proteins.[129]

The maturational changes in activity of the brain microsomal fatty acid elongation system correlate with the deposition of myelin.[128] This correlation is significant, because myelin lipids contain large amounts of long chain fatty acids. The activity of the microsomal system also is reduced in mouse mutants that are deficient in myelin.[130]

The characteristics of the elongation system vary among tissues.[131] Formation of saturated VLCFA, including C26:0, from [1-^{14}C]C18:0 was first demonstrated in rat sciatic nerve,[132] and was subsequently demonstrated in normal and X-ALD cultured human skin fibroblasts.[133] The factors that control the rate of the elongation are still poorly understood. The chain length of the substrate is an important factor. In a study utilizing swine cerebral microsomes it was found that elongation of C20:0 CoA yielded C22:0 and C24:0 concomitantly, whereas elongation of C22:0 CoA yielded only negligible amounts of C24:0. Kinetic studies in this system suggested that elongation of C20:0 CoA and of C22:0 CoA are carried out through two separate pathways, with that for the C20:0 substrate being more active.[134] Bourre et al. concluded that a single enzyme is responsible for the elongation of behenic acid (C22:0) and its monounsaturated counterpart, erucic acid (C22:1).[130] This finding is relevant to current dietary therapy. It has been shown that administration of monounsaturated fatty acids diminishes synthesis of saturated VLCFA,[135] presumably through competition for the elongating system machinery. On the other hand, the elongation system for polyunsaturated fatty acid is distinct from that for saturated fatty acids.[136]

DEGRADATION OF VLCFA

In 1976, Lazarow and deDuve demonstrated a peroxisomal fatty acid oxidizing system in rat liver,[137] and found that this system was most active toward medium and long chain fatty acids.[138] Three lines of evidence indicate that saturated VLCFA are degraded mainly, and possibly exclusively in the peroxisome: (a) patients who lack peroxisomes invariably have impaired degradation and elevated levels of VLCFA;[28,139] (b) tissue fractionation studies in liver and cultured skin fibroblasts show that C24:0[26] and C26:0[140] are oxidized exclusively in the peroxisomal fractions; and (c) C24:0 oxidation is resistant to inhibitors of mitochondrial function such as cyanide[26] or sodium 2-[5-(4-chlorophenyl)Pentyl]-oxirane-2-carboxylate (POCA).[141] The subcellular localizations of C24:0 degradation in brain is less certain. One group reported that it took place both in mitochondria and peroxisomes,[142] while another group, in an earlier study, found it only in the peroxisomal fraction.[143] Wanders and Tager reexamined this issue.[144] They found that POCA, the inhibitor of carnitine palmitoyl transferase-1, a mitochondrial enzyme, had no effect on the β-oxidation of C26:0 in intact brain cells isolated from adult rats or in cultured glial cells, and they concluded that this reaction in this tissue also took place only in the peroxisome.

In the peroxisomal β-oxidation system, four enzymatic reactions are necessary to shorten fatty acids by two carbons.[145] These reactions are catalyzed by three enzymes: acyl-CoA oxidase, multifunctional protein (containing enoyl-CoA hydratase and hydroxyacyl-CoA dehydrogenase activities), and 3-oxoacyl-CoA thiolase. These enzymes are distinct from their mitochondrial counterparts.[145] This peroxisomal β-oxidation pathway is discussed in more detail in Chap. 130.

Before VLCFA can be degraded by the peroxisomal β-oxidation pathway, however, they must be "activated" by thioesterification to coenzyme A. Enzymes that catalyze this reaction are fatty acid:CoA ligases (AMP-forming), also called acyl-CoA synthetases.[146] The overall reaction is:

$$\rightarrow \text{R-}\overset{\overset{\displaystyle O}{\|}}{\text{C}}\text{-OH} + \text{ATP} + \text{CoA-SH}$$
$$\rightarrow \text{R-}\overset{\overset{\displaystyle O}{\|}}{\text{C}}\text{-S-CoA} + \text{AMP} + PP_i$$

An enzyme-bound acyl-adenylate intermediate is formed during the course of the reaction. Because fatty acids range in size from short (e.g., the 2-carbon-compound acetic acid) to very long (22 or more carbons), no single enzyme is capable of activating all fatty acids. Acyl-CoA synthetases that activate short, medium, long, and very long chain fatty acids have been described, with significant overlap of substrate specificity. For example, lauric acid (C12:0) is activated by both medium chain acyl-CoA synthetase and long chain acyl-CoA synthetase (LCS), and palmitic acid (C16:0) is activated by both LCS and very long chain acyl-CoA synthetase (VLCS).[146] The designation VLCS is used for enzymes that are *capable* of activating VLCFA substrates, and does not imply an inability to activate fatty acid substrates containing less than 22 carbons.

Early evidence for the existence of VLCS enzyme activity is found in a 1971 study of the distribution of acyl-CoA synthetase activity in rat tissues.[147] Peaks of fatty acid chain-length preference were observed in liver, heart, adipose, adrenal, testis, brain, and muscle at 12 carbons and at 16 carbons. The optimal chain-length substrate for LCS purified from several species and tissues is 12 carbons.[148,149] Furthermore, LCS activity with C16 and C18 fatty acids is clearly lower than with C12. Thus, the second peak was suggestive of an enzyme with longer chain-length preference. The first report specifically describing VLCS activity by Singh et al.[150] came a decade later. Most evidence indicates that VLCFA activation takes place in peroxisomes and microsomes, but not in mitochondria. When activation of the C18 fatty acid stearate was compared to that of the C24 VLCFA lignoceric acid, all three organelles produced stearoyl-CoA, but mitochondria were incapable of synthesizing lignoceroyl-CoA.[151] Similar findings of VLCS activity in peroxisomes and microsomes, but not in mitochondria, have been reported for organelles isolated from rat liver, rat brain, human skin fibroblasts, and yeasts.[29,30,152–155]

Biochemical Defect in X-ALD

An impaired capacity to degrade saturated VLCFA has been a consistent finding in various cell preparations from X-ALD patients. The defect was first demonstrated by Singh et al.;[22,156] $[^{14}C]CO_2$ production from $[1\text{-}^{14}C]C24{:}0$ in X-ALD cells was reduced to 17 percent of control. Similar impairments were also demonstrated in the degradation of $[1\text{-}^{14}C]C26{:}0$ in homogenates of white blood cells and cultured amniocytes. $[1\text{-}^{14}C]C16{:}0$ and C18:0 were degraded at normal rates by all these cells. The reduction of peroxisomal VLCFA β-oxidation has been confirmed in several independent laboratories.[23,157,158]

Reports from two laboratories indicate that the defect involves the activity of peroxisomal VLCS. In 1986, Hashmi et al.[159] showed that cultured skin fibroblasts had an impaired capacity to oxidize lignoceric acid, but oxidized lignoceroyl-CoA at a normal rate. This finding focused attention on VLCS. In a total homogenate of X-ALD fibroblasts, activity of this enzyme was normal[160] or reduced slightly to 78 percent of control.[161] However, in the peroxisomal fraction of X-ALD cultured skin fibroblasts, the hexacosanol-CoA synthetase[29] or lignoceroyl-CoA synthetase activity[30] was less than 20 percent of control. Both groups of investigators showed that although VLCS activity is reduced in peroxisomes of X-ALD patients, it is normal in microsomal fractions. Residual VLCS activity in peroxisomal fractions may be due to low-level activation of VLCFA by LCS, because this activity was abolished by addition of an antibody to LCS,[160] although this remains unproven.

Recent findings indicate that more than one enzyme with VLCS activity exists. While this information has greatly expanded our knowledge of these proteins, the task of elucidating the mechanism by which peroxisomal VLCS activity is decreased in cells from X-ALD patients has become more complex. Purification of the first enzyme with VLCS activity was achieved in 1996.[162] Starting with rat liver peroxisomes, classical protein purification techniques were used to isolate a protein that catalyzed the activation of C24:0. The apparent molecular weight of rat VLCS (rVLCS) on sodium dodecyl sulfate-polyacrylamide gels is 70 kDa, distinguishing it from the 78-kDa rat liver LCS. The chain-length specificity of the purified enzyme was not studied in detail, however, the purified VLCS activated the C16:0 at a rate 1.5 times higher than the rate with C24:0. The dual peroxisomal and microsomal subcellular localization of VLCS predicted by activity studies was confirmed by western blots of liver subcellular fractions. Limited proteolysis of purified rVLCS generated peptide fragments that were sequenced and used to clone its cDNA.[152] This, in turn, facilitated cloning and expression studies of mouse VLCS (mVLCS),[163] human VLCS (hVLCS),[164] yeast VLCS (Fat1p),[155,165] and several related proteins (Table 131-9).[166–171]

Rat VLCS cDNA contains an open-reading frame of 1863 nucleotides that encodes a 620-amino-acid protein.[152] The calculated molecular weight of 70,692 was similar to that estimated by electrophoresis of the purified protein. By both western and northern analysis, expression of rVLCS was found only in a limited number of tissues, primarily liver and kidney. Previous studies clearly detected VLCS activity in brain, but neither rVLCS protein nor rVLCS mRNA was detectable in brain, heart, lung, or muscle. These data suggest the existence of other enzymes with VLCS activity. A comparison of the predicted amino acid sequence of rVLCS to the sequences of other known proteins revealed that rVLCS was more homologous to mouse fatty acid transport protein (mFATP)[172] than to other known acyl-CoA synthetases. Subsequently, partial and full-length cDNA clones for additional related proteins have been found. At least six human and five mouse proteins belonging to the VLCS/FATP family have been identified. These proteins can be distinguished from other protein families by the presence of two highly conserved motifs (Fig. 131-15). Motif 1 is an AMP-binding domain that is present in other acyl-CoA synthetases, in CoA ligases, and in luciferases.[173] All of these enzymes' reaction mechanisms involve ATP hydrolysis and formation of an acyl-adenylate or enzyme-adenylate intermediate, suggesting that reactions catalyzed by the VLCS/FATP family also involve the hydrolysis of ATP to AMP and pyrophosphate. The function of motif 2, which is unique to the VLCS/FATP family, is unknown, although the homologous region in the LCS enzyme family has been proposed as an LCS "signature motif."[174]

Table 131-9 Nomenclature and Properties of Mammalian VLCS/FATP Family Proteins

VLCS Designation	FATP Designation	Amino Acids	Tissue Expression	Subcellular Distribution	VLCS Activity	References
VLCS	FATP2	620	Liver, kidney	Peroxisomes, microsomes	Yes	146, 163, 164, 169
VLCS-H1	FATP6	619	Heart	Microsomes	Unknown	146, 169
VLCS-H2	FATP5	689–690	Liver	Microsomes	Yes	146, 167–169
VLCS-H3	FATP3	Unknown	Widespread	Unknown	Unknown	146, 169
FATP1	FATP1	646	Heart, skeletal muscle, adipose	Plasma membrane, ?other intracellular membranes	Yes	146, 169, 170, 172, 178
FATP4	FATP4	641	Small intestine, liver, kidney, brain	Plasma membrane, ?other intracellular membranes	Unknown	169, 171, 180

```
                      Motif 1                Motif 2

hVLCS                 Y T S G T T G L P K    Y F H D R V G D T F R W K - G E N V A T T E V 164
mVLCS (mFATP2)        Y T S G T T G L P K    Y F H D R V G D T F R W K - G E N V A T T E V 163
rVLCS                 Y T S G T T G L P K    Y F H D R V G D T F R W K - G E N V A T T E V 152
hVLCS-H1              F T S G T T G L P K    Y F W D R T G D T F R W K - G E N V A T T E V *
hVLCS-H2              Y T S G T T G L P K    Y F R D R L G D T F R W K - G E N V S T H E V 167
mVLACSR (mFATP5)      F T S G T T G L P K    Y F Q D R L G D T F R W K - G E N V S T G E V 168
hVLCS-H3                                     R F H D R T G D T F R W K - G E N V A T T E V *
mFATP3                F T S G T T G L P K    H F H D R T G D T I R W K - G E N V A T T E V 169
mFATP1                Y T S G T T G L P K    Y F R D R S G D T F R W R - G E N V S T T E V 172
rFATP1                Y T S G T T G L P K    Y F R D R S G D T F R W R - G E N V S T T E V 170
mFATP4                Y T S G T T G L P K    Y F R D R T G D T F R W K - G E N V S T T E V 169
hFATP4                Y T S G T T G L P K    Y F R D R T G D T F R W K - G E N V S T T E V 171
scFAT1p               Y T S G T T G L P K    Y F L D R M G D T F R W K - S E N V S T T E V 155
hLCS                  F T S G T T G N P K    K I I D R K K H I F K L A Q G E Y I A P E K I 408
dmBubblegum           Y T S G T V G M P K    S L T G R S K E I I I T S G G E N I P P V H I 233
```

Fig. 131-15 Highly conserved regions of mammalian VLCS/FATP proteins. Two highly conserved regions of VLCS/FATP proteins were identified. Motif 1 begins at amino acid 224 of hVLCS and motif 2 begins at amino acid 476 of hVLCS. Sequences from all known human, rat, and mouse VLCS/FATP family members are shown. Also included are yeast VLCS (scFat1p), a representative human long-chain acyl-CoA synthetase (hLCS) and the *Drosophila melanogaster* bubblegum protein (dmBubblegum). Vertical bars are used to group proteins thought to be orthologous. Residues identical in all mammalian family members are in bold. Residues in scFat1p, hLCS, and dmBubblegum that are identical to mammalian VLCS/FATP proteins are in *bold italics*. Residues identical in hLCS and dmBubblegum but different from VLCS/FATP proteins are underlined. (*Steinberg SJ and Watkins PA, unpublished.*)

Only limited information is available regarding the specific metabolic roles of VLCS and FATP. Furthermore, there is disagreement among researchers as to the primary function(s) of these proteins. It is generally thought that microsomal VLCS activity produces acyl-CoAs for complex lipid synthesis whereas peroxisomal VLCS activates VLCFA for degradation by β-oxidation. Studies to elucidate specific functions of the homologs of VLCS and FATP are in progress. Investigation of the mouse and human orthologs of rVLCS confirmed both the tissue distribution and subcellular location of this enzyme.[163,164] Antibody to hVLCS was used to show that its C-terminus is oriented in the peroxisomal membrane facing the peroxisomal matrix and not the cytoplasm[175,176] confirming earlier predictions.[177] This orientation is consistent with a role for VLCS in the degradation of potentially toxic VLCFA by peroxisomal β-oxidation. The observation that C24-CoA was a substrate for both peroxisomal and mitochondrial β-oxidation, while nonesterified C24:0 could not be degraded by mitochondria,[159] suggests that activation of VLCFA by either peroxisomes or microsomes yields VLCFA-CoA that is unavailable to mitochondria. Furthermore, this suggests that transport of VLCFA across the peroxisomal membrane and activation to VLCFA-CoA in the matrix may be required for further VLCFA metabolism. When expressed in COS-1 cells, hVLCS activated a wide variety of substrates, including C16:0, C24:0, and branched-chain fatty acids.[164] Activation of branched-chain fatty acids, phytanic acid and pristanic acids, by hVLCS suggests that this enzyme may participate in the degradation of these fatty acids by the sequential action of peroxisomal α-oxidation and β-oxidation pathways. The hVLCS gene is on human chromosome 15q21.2.

A sequence homolog of VLCS has been investigated in man and mouse. Full-length cDNA encoding hVLCS homolog 2 (hVLCS-H2)[167] and the orthologous mouse protein very long chain acyl-CoA synthetase-related (mVLACSR)[168] were cloned. The predicted amino acid sequences of these proteins contain 690 and 689 amino acids, respectively. hVLCS-H2 and mVLACSR are 71 percent identical to each other and both proteins are 45 percent identical to human, rat, or mouse VLCS. By northern analysis, hVLCS-H2 was expressed almost exclusively in liver, and was found in the endoplasmic reticulum in COS-1 cells overexpressing the protein.[167] Although hVLCS-H2 expressed in COS-1 cells activated fatty acids containing 18 to 26 carbons, its specific activity was significantly lower than that of hVLCS expressed in these cells. Recent studies indicate that hVLCS-H2 catalyzes activation of bile acids to their CoA derivatives (PA Watkins and SJ Steinberg, unpublished observations). Thus, it is unlikely that hVLCS-H2 and mVLACSR normally participate in peroxisomal VLCFA metabolism or contribute to the biochemical defect in X-ALD. The hVLCS-H2 gene is found on human chromosome 19.

The protein originally termed mFATP is now designated mFATP1.[172] Initially found in differentiated 3T3-L1 adipocytes, mFATP1 is also expressed in brain, heart, skeletal muscle, and kidney. It localized to the plasma membrane and other intracellular membranes.[172,178] Cellular accretion of fluorescent and radioactive long chain fatty acids was enhanced in 3T3 fibroblasts overexpressing mFATP1.[172] Gargiulo et al.[179] hypothesized that this protein works in concert with a recently identified adipocyte plasma membrane LCS to facilitate the sequential transport of fatty acids across the plasma membrane, followed by their activation to CoA derivatives. Formation of an acyl-CoA, which does not readily traverse biologic membranes, would effectively trap the fatty acid within the cell. Coe et al.[178] recently demonstrated that mFATP1 is also a VLCS capable of activating VLCFA, but not long chain fatty acids. Thus, it is possible that mFATP1 is a multifunctional protein with both transport and acyl-CoA synthetase activity. Direct demonstration of FATP1 in peroxisomes has not been demonstrated, diminishing the likelihood of a role for this protein in X-ALD biochemical pathology. Cloning of human FATP1 has not been reported.

Lodish and coworkers[169,180] studied the mouse VLCS/FATP family. They proposed that all five mouse family members (as well as the six human sequence homologs) are FATP and not VLCS, and named them accordingly. Their hypothesis is based on fatty acid uptake studies with mouse proteins expressed in COS cells. In their nomenclature, mVLCS is mFATP2 and mVLACSR is mFATP5 (Table 131-9). Another of these proteins, termed mFATP4, has been studied in some detail. By northern blot analysis, this protein is endogenously expressed in brain, liver, and kidney.[169] *In situ* hybridization showed that the highest levels of expression are in intestinal mucosal cells.[180] mFATP4 was primarily found in plasma membrane, but it was also found in other cellular membranous structures. Stahl et al.[180] proposed that mFATP4 is vital for the intestinal uptake of dietary fatty acids. By sequence homology, mFATP4 is clearly related to VLCS and mFATP1, and it contains both motifs 1 and 2 (Fig. 131-15). No studies of its ability to activate fatty acids have been reported. The

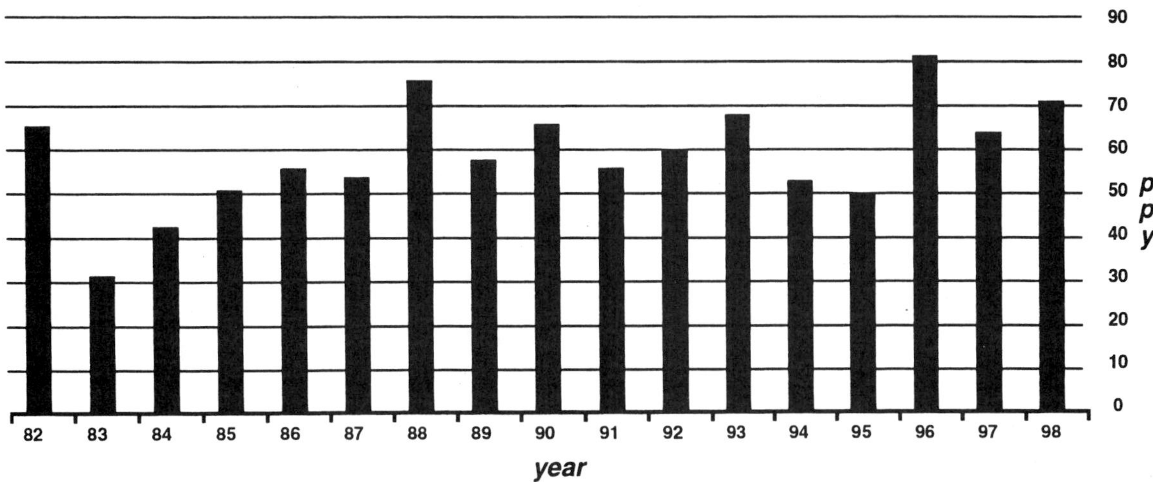

Fig. 131-16 Yearly number of new male X-ALD from the United States diagnosed at the Kennedy Krieger Institute with the plasma VLCFA assay.[92] The diagnosis was confirmed by clinical follow-up in each instance.

two remaining mammalian VLCS/FATP family members are hVLCS homolog 1 (hVLCS-H1) and homolog 3 (hVLCS-H3). In the alternate nomenclature, these are called FATP6 and FATP3, respectively. The sequence of full-length cDNA encoding hVLCS-H1 can be found in public domain databases, but no studies of its biologic function have been reported. Furthermore, there is currently no evidence for a mouse ortholog of hVLCS-H1. The hVLCS-H1 gene is on human chromosome 5. Purification, cloning, and characterization of hVLCS-H3/FATP3 have not been reported.

The *S. cerevisiae FAT1* gene encodes a protein (Fat1p) with significant homology to the VLCS/FATP protein family. The primary role of yeast Fat1p, like mammalian FATP1, was initially thought to facilitate the cellular uptake of long chain fatty acids.[165] Further analysis confirmed that Fat1p is found in both peroxisomal and microsomal subcellular compartments and has VLCS activity.[155] Targeted disruption of the *FAT1* gene resulted in cellular accumulation of VLCFA and decreased VLCS activity. Choi and Martin[181] proposed that Fat1p acts on excess VLCFA produced by the elongation of long chain fatty acids, activating them for subsequent degradation by peroxisomal β-oxidation. Thus, Fat1p appears to influence cellular fatty acid levels by participating in a complex system of regulation of VLCFA homeostasis, not by facilitating uptake.

While there is convincing evidence for impaired degradation of VLCFA in cells from X-ALD patients, Tsuji and associates demonstrated increased rates of C26:0 synthesis from long chain fatty acid precursors in fibroblasts from X-ALD patients.[133,182–184] Thus, the increased levels of VLCFA in X-ALD patients appear to result both from decreased degradation in peroxisomes and increased production in microsomes. The mechanism of VLCFA overproduction is unknown. However, if the hypothesis proposed by Choi and Martin[181] for yeast is applicable to mammalian systems, apparent overproduction may reflect disruption of VLCFA homeostasis primarily at the level of the peroxisome. As is discussed in the section on therapy, monounsaturated fatty acids such as oleic (C18:1) and erucic (C22:1) acids normalize the levels of saturated VLCFA in the plasma of X-ALD patients. Koike et al.[185] have shown that this effect is due to inhibition of the microsomal fatty acid elongating system.

GENETICS

Patterns of Inheritance and Incidence

Pedigree analyses in more than 1000 kindreds have been consistent with an X-linked recessive mode of inheritance in all instances. The availability of noninvasive diagnostic tests, such as the plasma assay for VLCFA,[92] has led to the recognition that X-ALD is more common than had been realized in the past. Since 1981, the peroxisome disease diagnostic laboratory at the Kennedy Krieger Institute has identified 3031 male patients and 1640 women heterozygous for this disorder. They are members of 1038 kindreds. Of the male patients, 1833 came from the United States, 165 from Canada, and the remaining 1033 from all continents and ethnic groups. Figure 131-16 shows the number of new male patients with X-ALD from the United States diagnosed at the Kennedy Krieger Institute between 1981 and 1999. There is a minimum incidence of 1:67,500 based on the number of cases identified each year in this laboratory alone, divided by the number of total births in the U.S. during each of these years. Analogous calculations for Canadian cases identified at the Kennedy Krieger Institute lead to an incidence value of 1:62,000. These are minimum values, because other laboratories also perform the VLCFA assay, and not every patient who has X-ALD is tested. During the last 4 years, the Mayo Clinic Laboratory has performed an increasing number of VLCFA assays. When the cases identified at Mayo Clinic during the last 4 years are added to those diagnosed at Kennedy Krieger Institute, taking care to count only once those who were tested in both laboratories, there is a minimum incidence of 1:42,000. Using an analogous approach in France, P. Aubourg (personal communication) estimated the incidence in France to be 1:22,500. The higher incidence in France may reflect the fact that the X-ALD testing program in that country is more centralized than in the U.S. As already noted, X-ALD has been identified in all ethnic groups. Comparison of incidence in various ethnic groups is limited by the fact that the VLCFA assay is not readily available or utilized in many countries. The minimum incidence in Australasia was estimated at 1:62,500.[186] It should be noted that all these estimates are based on the number of male patients with X-ALD in the total population. The proportion of females heterozygotes for X-ALD can be estimated from calculations of the Hardy Weinberg equilibrium using the faster 2pq where p is the frequency of the normal ALDP gene and q the frequency of the disease gene and of affected hemizygous males (1: 42,000 in the United States based on the data presented above). Since X-ALD can result in death in childhood, for the purpose of this calculation this frequency is reduced to 1−the estimated fraction of X-ALD hemizygotes who die prior to reproductive age. We have set this figure 0.37, thefraction of X-ALD hemizygotes who have the childhood cerebral phenotype.Using this figure we estimate that the combined male and female frequency of X-ALD in the United States is 1:18,000, a value that approaches the frequency of phenylketonuria (1:12,000).

Table 131-10 X-ALD Pedigrees Studied at Kennedy Krieger Institute 1981 to October 1999; Estimated Percentage of New Mutations

	Kindred Category	Number Kindreds	Number Patients
A	Multiple affected males	599	1919
B1	Single case, mother VLCFA normal and lacks mutation	3	3
B2	Single case, mother VLCFA normal	28	28
B3	Single case, pedigree data incomplete	71	71
	Total	701	2021
Estimated maximum percent of new mutations (patients B1 + B2 + B3/total)		5%	

These data are based on analysis of kindreds studied at the Kennedy Krieger Institute. The estimate that 5 percent of patients have new mutations is a maximum value. Category B2 probably includes heterozygotes who had false negative plasma VLCFA assays, and it is likely that category B3 includes relatives with X-ALD who were not identified because of incomplete information.

Table 131-10 demonstrates that at most 5 percent of patients with X-ALD have new mutations.

The X-ALD Gene and Protein

The X-ALD gene was mapped to Xq28 through linkage with the gene G-6-PD[17] and a polymorphic DNA marker DXS52.[18,187,188] A putative gene for X-ALD was identified by positional cloning within Xq28.[31] The X-ALD gene occupies approximately 26 kb of genomic DNA.[31] It is composed of 10 exons and encodes a mRNA of 4.3 kb and a predicted protein (ALDP) of 745 amino acids.[189] Surprisingly, the deduced amino acid sequence of ALDP is related to the superfamily of ABC transmembrane transporter proteins and not VLCS.[152,167,168] The existence of ALDP was unknown and not hypothesized prior to its cloning. Its function in VLCFA β-oxidation and its role in X-ALD pathology have yet to be determined. That mutations in the X-ALD gene are responsible for this disease has been established by the presence of mutations in all patients thoroughly studied[190] (www.x-ald.nl) and by complementation studies showing that expression of X-ALD cDNA restores VLCFA β-oxidation in fibroblasts from X-ALD patients.[191–193]

ABC transporters transport a variety of ligands including ions, fatty acids, and proteins. The typical eukaryotic ABC transporter is a dimer transcribed from a single gene and consists of two hydrophobic transmembrane domains and two hydrophilic domains, each containing a nucleotide-binding fold (Fig. 131-17). In contrast, ALDP has only one hydrophobic and hydrophilic domain and is designated a half-transporter.[31] ALDP has been localized to the peroxisomal membrane with the hydrophilic C-terminal domain oriented toward the cytoplasm.[94,194]

Mutation Analysis, Gene Expression, and Genotype-Phenotype Correlation

Several groups have reported mutational analyses in relatively large series of patients in various ethnic groups.[190,195–200] A mutational database Web site is now available at www.x-ald.nl. More than 300 mutations have been identified. An analysis of 200 mutations reported up to 1998 [190] reveals that 53.5 percent of the mutations are missense, 24 percent are frameshift, 5 percent are in-frame deletions or insertions, and 2.5 percent are splicing defects. The majority of kindreds have private mutations; 68.5 percent were nonrecurrent. As shown in Fig. 131-18, the mutations are spread throughout the entire genome but are not evenly distributed. There is a clustering of mutations in the putative membrane-spanning region (38 percent), the putative nucleotide-binding domain (29 percent), and in a "hot spot" on exon 5 (16 percent). The remaining mutations (17 percent) occur throughout the rest of the coding region. Only 2 mutations have been described in exon 10,[201,202] which encodes the C-terminal 81 amino acids (10.9 percent) of ALDP. The mutational hot spot on exon 5 is a dinucleotide deletion at nucleotide 1801 and 1802.[196,203] This results in a frameshift at amino acid residue E471 and a premature stop codon at position 554. The predicted protein lacks the nucleotide-binding fold and would likely be inactive. This mutation has been identified in 12 percent of all reported kindreds.[190] Haplotype analyses in 12 of these kindreds established that they were unrelated.[196,203] No promoter mutations or complete gene deletions have been reported. Immunofluorescent analyses of fibroblast cell lines from X-ALD patients in several laboratories[93,94,204] have shown that 67 percent of nonrecurrent mutations result in nondetectable ALDP. Because all X-ALD patients have ALDP mRNA, independent of the type or location of mutation, the lack of detectable ALDP is likely due to protein instability.

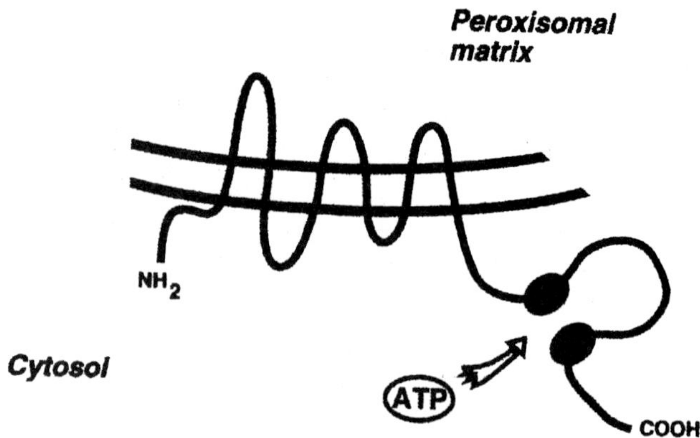

Fig. 131-17 Topologic model of the adrenoleukodystrophy protein. The transmembrane arrangement shown here is predicted by hydropathy analysis of the deduced amino acid sequence. The predicted nucleotide-binding fold is indicated as a loop containing an ATP site. (*From Gartner et al.*[200] *Used with permission.*)

No correlation has been found between disease severity and the presence or absence of immunologically reactive material, or the nature of the mutation. As noted previously and shown in Table 131-8, males in the same family often express different phenotypes. A striking demonstration of this is the presence of five different phenotypes in six male members in a family with a P484R missense mutation.[205] All phenotypes have been observed in patients with the frequent hot spot deletion of nucleotides 1801 and 1802.[196,203] Mild phenotypes have been observed in patients with large deletions[31] and severe phenotypes in patients with missense mutations and presence of immunologically detectable ALDP.[196] Thus, with the data available at this time, mutation analysis does not aid the prediction of phenotype.

ALDP Homologs and Orthologs

Homologs and orthologs of ALDP have been identified in many species from yeast to mammals.[190] All are peroxisomal ABC half-transporters, and include the yeast genes PXA1 and PXA2.[206,207] Three human homologs of ALDP have been identified; PMP70,[208,209] P70R/PMP69,[210,211] and ALDRP.[212–215] Table 131-11 shows their relative sequence identity with ALDP and their chromosomal locations. ALDRP is of particular interest because its amino acid composition[212] and exon organization[214] resemble that of ALDP so closely. Overexpression studies suggest that ALDR can substitute for the function of ALDP, at least in part.[213,216]

The function of these orthologs and homologs has not yet been established. However, the yeast homologs PXA1 and PXA2 have been shown to be necessary for the transport of long chain fatty

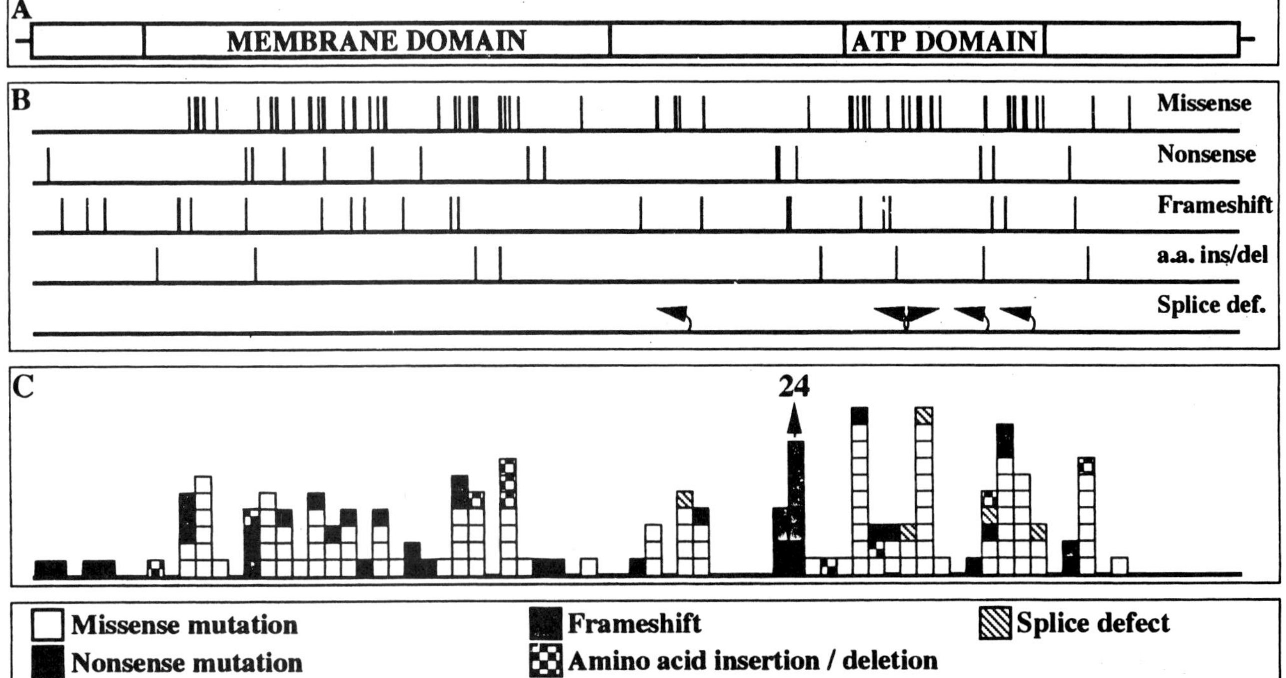

Fig. 131-18 Representation of X-ALD mutations. *A*: Representation of ALDP indicating the putative membrane-spanning and ATP-binding domains. *B*: Depiction of mutation locations grouped by the type of mutation. The vertical lines represent the location of each nonrecurrent mutation. *C*: All known X-ALD mutations are shown except for 13 large deletions that affect two or more exons. Each box represents one patient. (*From Smith et al.*[190] *Used with permission.*)

acids into yeast peroxisomes.[217] Also there is evidence that overexpression of PMP70 cDNA in CHO cells increases uptake of long chain fatty acids into peroxisomes.[218] Because overexpression of ALDRP or PMP70 can partially or completely restore the capacity of cultured cells from X-ALD patients to metabolize VLCFA (Fig. 131-19),[127,213,216,219] it is likely that all are involved in peroxisomal fatty acid transport. By comparison to other ABC half-transporter proteins, it has been suggested that ALDP may function as a homodimer and/or heterodimer with one or more of the other peroxisomal ABC half-transporters.[220,221] The formation of ALDP homodimers and heterodimers with ALDP and PMP70 have been demonstrated by co-immunoprecipitation of *in vitro* synthesized proteins[190] and with the yeast 2 hybrid system.[222]

To date there has been no direct demonstration of endogenous dimers *in vivo*. The patterns of expression of each of the peroxisomal half-transporters differ.[223–226] For example, ALDP and ALDRP, but not PMP70, are expressed in oligodendrocytes, while only ALDRP and PMP70 are found in central nervous system neurons. Thus, it is possible that the peroxisomal half-transporters may transport a variety of fatty acids across the peroxisomal membrane. The various patterns of expression may serve to modulate peroxisomal function in a cell-specific manner resulting in the accumulation of metabolites other than VLCFA possibly contributing to the clinical manifestation of the disease.[223]

Table 131-11 Peroxisomal ABC Half-Transporters

Protein	% Identity to ALDP	Chromosomal Location
ALD	100	Xq28
ALDR	66	12q11
PMP70	38	1p21
P70R (PMP69)	27	14q24

Pathogenesis of Biochemical Defects in X-ALD

There is strong evidence for both mutations in the gene encoding the peroxisomal protein ALDP and impaired VLCFA β-oxidation due to decreased peroxisomal VLCS activity in cells from X-ALD patients. However, the mechanism by which the genetic defect leads to the biochemical defect remains obscure. Several laboratories have now shown that overexpression of ALDP in cells from X-ALD patients or X-ALD mice clearly improves VLCFA β-oxidation rates.[191,213,227–229] Overexpression of hVLCS alone in human X-ALD fibroblasts did not have a significant effect on β-oxidation.[175] In comparable experiments, fibroblasts from the murine X-ALD model transfected with mVLCS showed improvement in one laboratory[190] but not in another.[230] However, a synergistic effect on VLCFA β-oxidation was reported when both VLCS and ALDP were overexpressed in human[175] and mouse fibroblasts.[230] This observation implies that there may be functional interaction between ALDP and peroxisomal VLCS.

Several hypotheses were initially proposed to explain the role of ALDP in VLCFA metabolism. One suggested that ALDP might be required for association of VLCS with the peroxisomal membrane.[31,231] Immunologic studies of fibroblasts from X-ALD patients demonstrated that abundant VLCS was detectable in peroxisomes.[175] This was confirmed by western analysis showing no decrease in VLCS abundance in X-ALD fibroblast peroxisomes.[176] In contrast, in a mouse model of X-ALD, Yamada et al.[230] reported that affected animals had a 33 percent decrease in the liver peroxisomal VLCS/total VLCS ratio by western analysis. Whether this decrease is sufficient to account for the impairment in VLCFA β-oxidation is not certain.

Another hypothesis suggested that ALDP might translocate VLCS into peroxisomes.[31] The observation that VLCS is found on

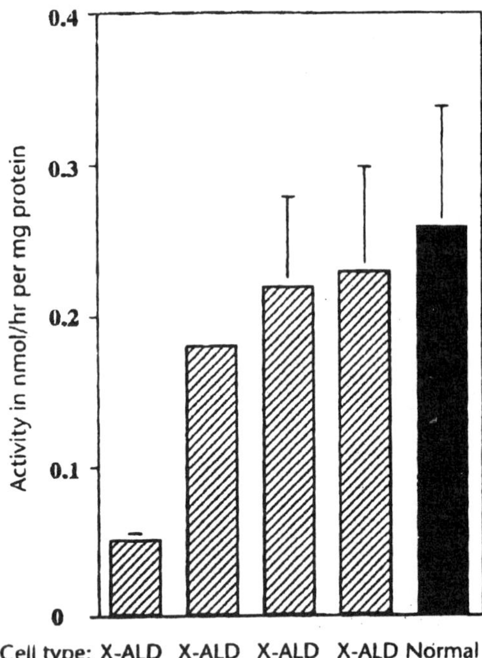

Fig. 131-19 Peroxisomal ABC half-transporter complementation of C24:0 β-oxidation. Human X-ALD fibroblasts transformed with SV40T antigen were transfected with recombinant expression vector (pCDNA3) alone or with vector-containing cDNA for PMP70, ALDP, or ALDRP (hatched bars). The rates of C24:0 β-oxidation in the transfected cells were corrected for the fraction of cells expressing the transgene, as determined by immunofluorescence staining of the transgene. The adjusted rates were compared with the rates of C24:0 β-oxidation determined in transformed fibroblasts from normal individuals (filled bar). The indicated values are the mean and standard deviation for pCDNA3 (n = 6); ALDP (n = 5); ALDRP (n = 4); and normal m (n = 5). PMP70, n = 1. (*From Kemp et al.*[216] *Used with permission.*)

the matrix side of the peroxisomal membrane supported this notion. However, immunologic studies in normal and X-ALD fibroblasts permeabilized with different detergents revealed no differences in the topographic localization of peroxisomal VLCS.[175]

Several hypotheses regarding the relationship between ALDP and VLCS remain to be evaluated. A physical interaction between the two proteins may be required for the optimal expression of peroxisomal VLCS activity. Alternatively, such a physical interaction may be required for coupling of VLCFA import into peroxisomes to the activation of these fatty acids. Aubourg et al.[232] suggested that ALDP could be required for import of a substrate necessary for the activation and/or stabilization of VLCS. Evaluation of these and other mechanisms are in progress in several laboratories.

Studies reported to date that investigated ALDP/VLCS function have focused on hVLCS (or mVLCS). While this protein is the only member of the VLCS/FATP family with a documented peroxisomal subcellular localization, the potential role(s) of other family members in the biochemical pathogenesis of X-ALD remains untested. The observations that (a) the brain is a primary site of pathology in X-ALD, (b) brain has significant VLCS activity, and (c) none of the currently known VLCS/FATP enzymes are expressed to a significant extent in brain, suggest that additional enzymes with VLCS activity exist and may be deficient in X-ALD. Min et al.[233] described one such candidate VLCS in a study the *Drosophila melanogaster* mutant *bubblegum*. Flies with this mutation exhibited neurodegeneration and the males had elevated VLCFA levels that were reduced by feeding monounsaturated fatty acids. The protein encoded by the *bubblegum* gene has sequence homology to both LCSs and VLCSs. Examination of bubblegum protein regions corresponding to motifs 1 and 2 (Fig. 131-15) suggest that it is an acyl-CoA synthetase belonging to a new protein family. The role of the bubblegum ortholog in humans (if there is one) in X-ALD pathology merits investigation.

Effect of VLCFA on Membrane Structure and Function. The greater length of the aliphatic chain causes VLCFA to be insoluble and alters their physiological properties. While albumin has six or more high- and low-affinity binding sites for fatty acids with 12- to 18-carbon chain length,[234,235] it has only a single low-affinity binding site for hexacosanoic acid (C26:0).[236] Desorption of C26:0 from phospholipid membranes is 10,000 times slower than that of fatty acids with a 14- to 18-carbon chain length (Fig. 131-20).[236] Microcalorimetric studies have shown that inclusion of C26:0 in a model membrane disrupts membrane structure (Fig. 131-21). The microviscosity of red cell membranes is increased in patients with X-ALD.[237] The most direct evidence that abnormally high VLCFA levels can alter membrane function is provided by the study of Whitcomb et al.,[238] who assessed ACTH-stimulated cortisol release in cultured human adrenocortical cells. The addition of C26:0 or C24:0 to the culture medium in concentrations equivalent to those in X-ALD plasma increased the microviscosity of adrenocortical cell membranes and decreased ACTH-stimulated cortisol secretion (Fig. 131-22). They concluded that the VLCFA excess altered membrane structure and suppressed the availability of the ACTH receptor. Analogous effects may exist in neural membranes, but while this has not been demonstrated experimentally, it is possible that these alterations in membrane structure contribute to the pathogenesis of the axonopathy in AMN. It should be noted, however, that mice lacking ALDP-targeted disruption of the gene by targeted homologous recombination do not show cerebral, or spinal cord demyelination, or any clinical symptoms up to 2 years of age,[34,35,239] despite a marked increase in brain VLCFA. Thus, an increase in VLCFA accumulation is not necessarily linked to demyelination.

Pathogenesis of Adrenal Dysfunction. Adrenal dysfunction in X-ALD is due to primary adrenocortical insufficiency and elevation of plasma ACTH levels is the initial manifestation.[240] Although the extent of clinically evident adrenal insufficiency is variable, as noted above, a substantial proportion of AMN patients, and most heterozygotes, fail to show clinical or biochemical evidence of adrenal insufficiency. Microscopic study reveals some

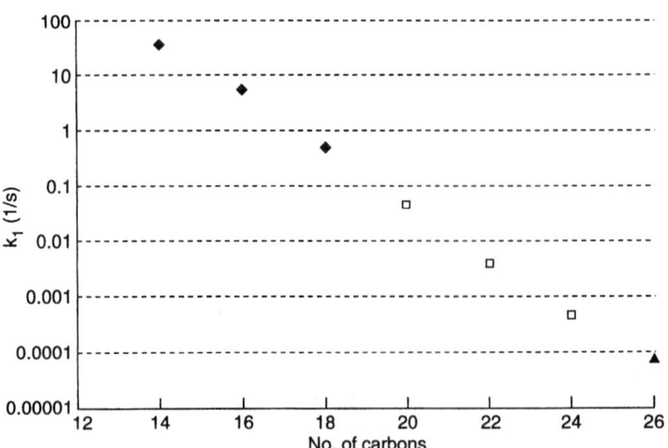

Fig. 131-20 The rate constant for desorption of saturated fatty acids from phospholipid vesicles as a function of chain length. The linear relationship on a semi-log plot of these two variables indicates that the rate of desorption decreases exponentially with increased chain length. (*From Ho et al.*[236] *Used with permission.*)

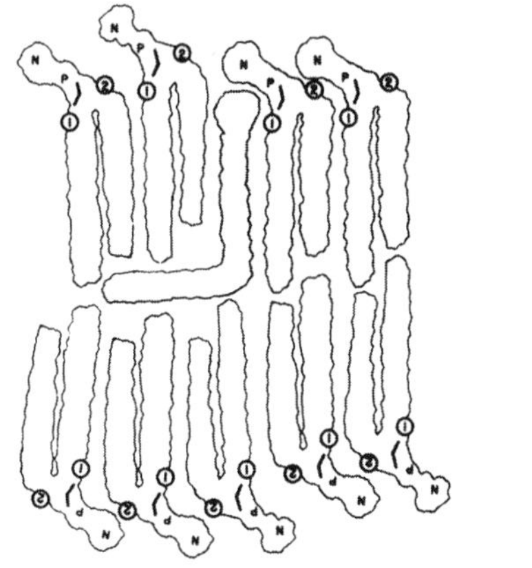
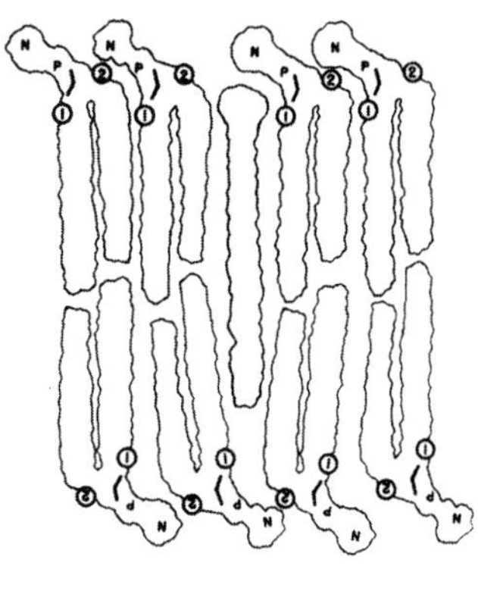

Fig. 131-21 Representation of possible binding modes of C26:0 molecules in phospholipid bilayer. The acyl chains of the phospholipid have 16 (sn-1) and 18 (sn-2) carbons. The molecules could fit linearly and penetrate about halfway through the opposing phospholipid minolayer or could bend in the middle of the bilayer. Calorimetric studies have shown that the C26:0 excess disrupts membrane stability. (*From Ho et al.*[236] *Used with permission.*)

degree of adrenal involvement in nearly all patients. Powers et al.[88] demonstrated characteristic inclusions in a heterozygous woman who had a normal cortisol response to ACTH stimulation.

Powers et al.[241] conducted a correlative morphologic and cytochemical study that provides insight into the pathogenesis of the adrenal dysfunction. They concluded that the adrenal pathology is due to accumulation of abnormal lipids that contain VLCFA. The earliest change is the appearance of birefringent, cytoplasmic striations with lamellae in cortical cells of the inner zonae fasciculata-reticularis. The lamellae represent the formation or precipitation of lipid-protein aggregates or lipid bilayers (Fig. 131-13), which contain cholesterol esterified with VLCFA. Cells that contain these inclusions showed a reduction in mitochondrial and microsomal enzymes. Inflammatory cells were not present. As the disease advances the adrenocortical cells atrophy.

Several factors can contribute to the accumulation of these abnormal cholesterol esters:

1. The impaired capacity to degrade VLCFA. This leads to an increased proportion among the fatty acid precursors of cholesterol esters.
2. Cholesterol esterifying enzyme activity for C26:0 fatty acids is reduced to 16 to 38 percent of that for oleic acid (C18:1). This is, nevertheless, far in excess of the rate of hydrolysis of C26:0-containing cholesterol esters, which is 1/1000 of those that contain C18:1.[242] This imbalance between the formation and degradation of C26:0-containing esters would be expected to lead to their increasing accumulation, and is the most likely cause for the lipid accumulation and the impaired adrenal function. The VLCFA-containing cholesterol esters would not be available as precursors for steroid hormone synthesis.
3. The previously cited studies by Whitcomb et al.[238] indicate that VLCFA excess in the plasma membrane may impair the function of the ACTH receptor (Fig. 131-22).

Pathogenesis of AMN Distal Axonopathy. The nervous system pathology in X-ALD displays two apparently disparate types: (a) the distal axonopathy associated with "pure" AMN,[36,38,98,103] which manifests most commonly in late adolescence or adulthood; and (b) the inflammatory demyelinating lesion associated with the rapidly progressive cerebral forms of the disease,[40,101] which, in

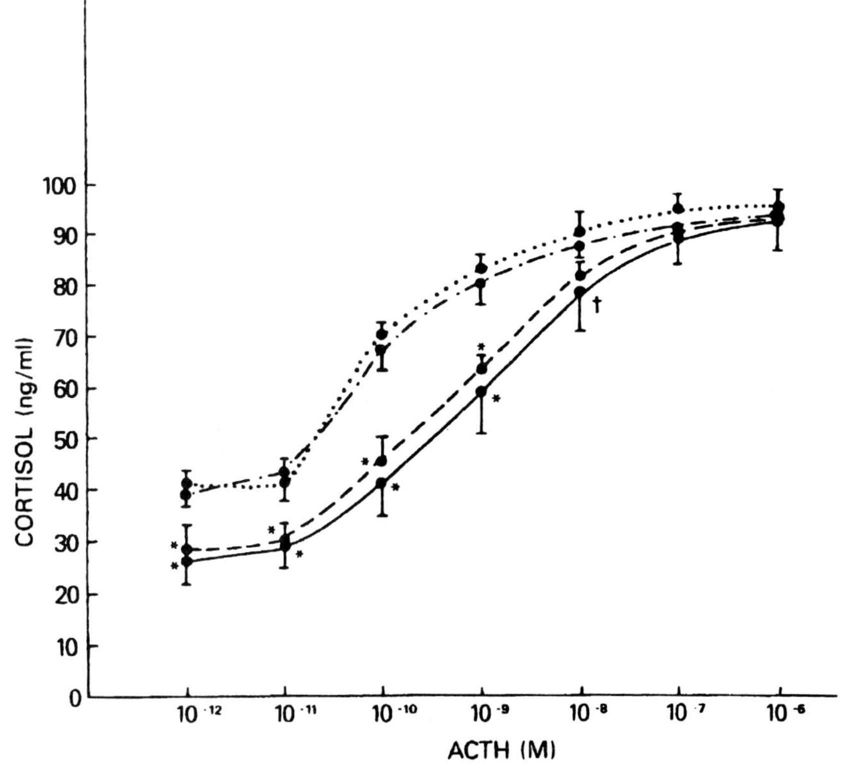

Fig. 131-22 Cortisol response to stimulation with increasing concentrations of ACTH from adrenocortical cells cultured in the presence of the indicated fatty acids or 0.05 percent ethanol (control). Cortisol release after stimulation with 10^{-12} to the 10^{-9} M ACTH was significantly lower ($P < 0.002$) from cells cultured in the presence of 5 μM concentrations of C26:0 (dashed line); C24:0 (continuous); linoleic acid (18:2) (dot-dash); or control (dotted). Note that the saturated VLCFA impaired the ACTH response, whereas the unsaturated fatty did not. The concentration of C26:0 used is equivalent to that in the plasma of X-ALD patients. (*From Whitcomb et al.*[238] *Used with permission.*)

the childhood form, often leads to death prior to the age at which AMN manifests. Analysis of the long-term course of the asymptomatic and Addison-only phenotypes suggests that all X-ALD patients who survive to adulthood will eventually develop the manifestations of AMN. The pathogenesis of the axonopathy is unknown. We speculate that the alterations in membrane structure and function associated with the accumulation of VLCFA may play a pathogenetic role described in the previous section, but at this time, there is no direct evidence for this. Studies in cultured Schwann cells,[243] or oligodendrocytes,[244] or other nervous system cell culture systems may help to clarify the pathogenesis of the axonopathy.

Pathogenesis of the Inflammatory Demyelination Lesion. Correlation of clinical and pathologic findings indicates that the rapid progression in cerebral X-ALD is related to the perivascular infiltration of lymphocytes in the brain white matter. Areas in which these lesions are present show breakdown of the blood-brain barrier and accumulation of contrast material on CT or gadolinium MRI (see below). The inflammatory response is absent or mild in patients with AMN or other noncerebral phenotypes. Both the cause of the inflammatory reaction and why it is present in only about 50% of X-ALD patients lack explanation.

Griffin et al.[100] typed immune cells in autopsy material from four X-ALD patients and found the distribution of immune (T and B) cells to be similar to that found in the central nervous system during a cellular immune response. Bernheimer and coworkers demonstrated increased levels of free IgG and IgA in brain tissue from X-ALD patients comparable to those found in the brain of patients with multiple sclerosis (MS) and 2 to 10 times higher than control levels.[245] The inflammatory demyelination in X-ALD is superficially similar to that seen in MS. In both, inflammatory cells are mostly macrophages and T lymphocytes with infrequent B cells.[101] In MS, these cells are located at the leading edge of the inflammatory lesion, while in X-ALD they are behind the lesion edge. This suggests that in X-ALD cells the inflammatory reaction may be in response to an initial primary demyelinating process.[40] The intracellular accumulation of VLCFA and their altered metabolism could poison cells leading to cell death and the induction of an inflammatory response. The pattern of inflammatory cytokine expression differs in MS and X-ALD. Th2 cytokines, which promote production of B cells, characterize MS lesions, while Th1 cytokines are found in X-ALD lesions.[101,246,247] TNFα is expressed in macrophages and astrocytes in the active lesions of X-ALD patients.[101,247] TNFα is able to activate macrophages, damage myelin sheaths, and/or kill oligodendrocytes *in vitro* and thus may contribute to the initiation of demyelination in X-ALD.[223] Powers et al.[101] have suggested that excess VLCFA stimulates nearby astrocytes, perivascular cells, and macrophages to initiate a TNFα cytokine cascade that leads to demyelination mediated primarily by cytokines, with superimposed destruction of myelin by T cells and to a minimal degree by complement and B cells. Gilg et al.[248] have recently demonstrated an excess of inducible nitric oxide synthetase in postmortem brain tissue of X-ALD patients and propose that this contributes to the pathogenesis of the inflammatory response.

Possible Triggers for the Inflammatory Response. In X-ALD, VLCFA excess is already present in fetal life[16] and precedes the development of brain pathology. We postulate that lipids containing an abnormally high proportion of VLCFA can act as triggers that initiate the cascade of inflammatory demyelination that appears to be cytokine-mediated, perhaps by stimulating TNFα production in a manner analogous to the well-known effect of lipopolysaccharide.[249] Whereas a mild to moderate excess of VLCFA is present in all brain lipid species, the greatest excess occurs in the ganglioside, phosphatidylcholine proteolipid, and cholesterol ester fractions. Even though in active demyelinating lesions the cholesterol ester fraction contains the greatest excess of VLCFA, this appears to be a consequence rather than a cause of demyelination, because the fatty acid composition of this fraction was normal in regions of X-ALD brain in which myelin was still intact.[118] It is thus unlikely that cholesterol esterified with VLCFA acts as a trigger for the inflammatory response. However, each of the three other components could play such a role, with gangliosides a particularly plausible candidate. The gangliosides in X-ALD brain contain 27.8 to 50 percent of fatty acids with a chain length >21.[122] Such fatty acids are virtually absent in normal brain gangliosides.[122] Gangliosides have been implicated in a variety of neuroimmunologic disorders.[250] They have been shown to suppress Theiler's murine encephalomyelitis demyelinating disease.[251] The immunologic properties of gangliosides vary with their fatty acid composition.[252] Gangliosides that contain 22 to 24 fatty acids are 6 to 10 times less effective immunosuppressants than those that contain fatty acids with 16 to 20 carbons.[253] Phosphatidylcholine is another possible trigger. Theda et al.[118] correlated the fatty acid composition of various lipid fractions in X-ALD brain with histopathologic findings, reasoning that abnormalities in trigger molecules should precede histopathologic alterations. They found that in regions in which myelin was intact, the phosphatidylcholine fraction showed the greatest VLCFA excess — its VLCFA content was 16 times that of control. Phosphatidylcholine is a major constituent of the plasma membrane and neurologic disorders with antiphospholipid antibodies have been described.[254] Bizzozero et al.[121] demonstrated an abnormally high VLCFA content in myelin proteolipid isolated from X-ALD brain, a finding that is of interest because antibodies to proteolipid protein have been implicated in the pathogenesis of MS.[255]

Basis of the Intrafamilial Phenotype Variability

The striking intrafamilial phenotypic variability in X-ALD has already been mentioned and is well documented.[256,257] Because of the frequency of phenotypic discordance within families, it was unlikely that there would be a genotype/phenotype correlation in X-ALD. Mutation analysis has confirmed that X-ALD phenotype cannot be predicted based on X-ALD genotype. As noted in the section on mutation analysis, all X-ALD phenotypes are observed in patients with the same mutation, including null mutations, that lack ALDP. As discussed in the section on diagnosis, there is no correlation of disease phenotype and the degree of measurable VLCFA accumulation. Thus, the X-ALD phenotype is not predictable and may be influenced by genetic[256–258] and environmental[259,260] factors. It has been proposed that differences within the immune system account for variable expression of inflammatory demyelination. While this remains a possibility, HLA haplotype association, pattern of cytokine expression, and known TNFα polymorphisms do not correlate with X-ALD phenotype.[246,247]

Animal Models: Potential to Clarify Pathogenesis and Evaluate Therapy

Three laboratories have produced models of X-ALD generated in the mouse by targeted inactivation of the X-ALD gene.[34,35,239] The VLCFA levels in the brain and adrenal gland were comparable to those in the human disease, and the adrenal gland contains lamellar inclusions characteristic of the human disease. The animals have not shown clinical symptoms or evidence of cerebral or spinal cord demyelination up to 2 years of age. Kemp et al.[216] showed that the oral administration of 4-phenylbutyrate to these animals reduced the levels of VLCFA in the brain and adrenal, which has led to the proposal of a new therapeutic approach that is discussed in the section on therapy. The lack of a neurologic phenotype has limited the potential of the animal model to evaluate pathogenesis and therapy. Work is in progress to determine whether a neurologic phenotype is producible by combining knockouts of ALDP with other inactivated genes that have a role in VLCFA metabolism. A "double-knockout" of ALDP and PMP70 has been produced (G Jimenez-Sanchez, J-F Lu, KD Smith, D Valle, personal communication).[261] This

Table 131-12 Differential Diagnosis of X-Linked ALD

Phenotype	Symptom or Sign
Childhood neurologic deficit *without* overt adrenal insufficiency	Hyperactivity, attention deficit, minimal brain damage, emotional disturbance Seizure disorder Brain tumor Metachromatic or globoid leukodystrophy Batten disease Encephalitis Subacute sclerosing panencephalitis Schilder myelinoclastic diffuse sclerosis
Childhood neurologic deficit *with* adrenal insufficiency	Hypoglycemic or anoxic damage associated with Addison disease X-linked glycerol kinase deficiency Central pontine myelinolysis Glucocorticoid deficiency with achalasia and deficient tear production
Adrenal insufficiency only	All other types of adrenal insufficiency
Adrenomyeloneuropathy	Multiple sclerosis Familial spastic paraparesis Spinocerebellar or olivopontocerebral degeneration Cervical spondylosis Spinal cord tumor
Adult cerebral	Schizophrenia Depression Seizure disorders, organic psychosis Alzheimer disease Brain tumor
Symptomatic heterozygote	Multiple sclerosis Chronic nonprogressive spinal cord disease Spinal cord tumor Cervical spondylosis

double-knockout displayed the biochemical characteristics of each of the individual knockouts, but the defects were not synergistic and the animals had not developed neurologic symptoms by 18 months of age. Efforts to produce double-knockouts of ALDP and ALDRP and of ALDP and VLCS are in progress. Cross-breeding of ALDP-deficient mice with mouse strains that are highly susceptible to brain inflammatory disorders such as experimental allergic encephalitis has not produced a neurologic phenotype (P. Aubourg, personal communication).

DIAGNOSIS OF X-ALD

Differential Diagnosis on Basis of Clinical Presentation

The two most common phenotypes of X-ALD (CCER and AMN) are well known and diagnosis is established easily based on clinical findings and biochemical assays described earlier. However, X-ALD continues to be underdiagnosed. This can have serious consequences because it means that there is a loss of opportunity to offer genetic counseling, the provision of adrenal steroid replacement, or the timely provision of therapies such as bone marrow transplantation. Because accurate noninvasive biochemical assays are readily available, the most common reason for diagnostic delay is the failure to include X-ALD in the differential diagnosis.

Table 131-12 lists the conditions that have been mistaken for X-ALD. The most common settings in which diagnosis is delayed or missed are:

1. AMN, that is, progressive paraparesis, distal sensory loss, and sphincter disturbances, when there is no clinical evidence of adrenocortical insufficiency, as may be the case of 30 to 50 percent of men,[54] and nearly all women. In one series, the mean interval between the consultation with a neurologist because of abnormal gait and the establishment of the correct diagnosis was 6.7 years.[77] Multiple sclerosis and progressive spastic paraparesis are the most common misdiagnoses.
2. Primary adrenocortical insufficiency without apparent neurologic involvement. As noted previously, X-ALD is a relatively common cause of primary adrenal insufficiency in males. At present, autoimmune adrenalitis is the most common cause of primary adrenal insufficiency.[262] The two disorders can be distinguished easily because X-ALD patients have increased levels of VLCFA in plasma and they lack adrenocortical antibodies.[61] The converse is observed in patients with autoimmune adrenalitis. We recommend measurement of plasma VLCFA levels in all patients with primary adrenal insufficiency who do not have adrenocortical antibodies in their plasma.
3. Asymptomatic at-risk relatives of X-ALD patients. This requires biochemical or DNA screening of at-risk relatives in the extended, as well as nuclear, families.
4. Patients with atypical brain MRI abnormalities. Approximately 85 percent of patients with childhood cerebral X-ALD (CCER) have the characteristic parieto-occipital lesions shown in Fig. 131-2, and in most instances these findings led the neuroradiologist to suggest the diagnosis of X-ALD. However, in approximately 15 percent of X-ALD patients who have abnormal MRI findings, the lesions are atypical. Initial lesions in the frontal lobes represent the most common variant. Initial lesions may also be found in the cerebellum or pons,[67,70–72] or they may be unilateral.[74] The diagnosis is often delayed in patients with atypical MRI findings. Several patients with asymmetric lesions had been diagnosed to have brain tumors and were treated with radiotherapy.

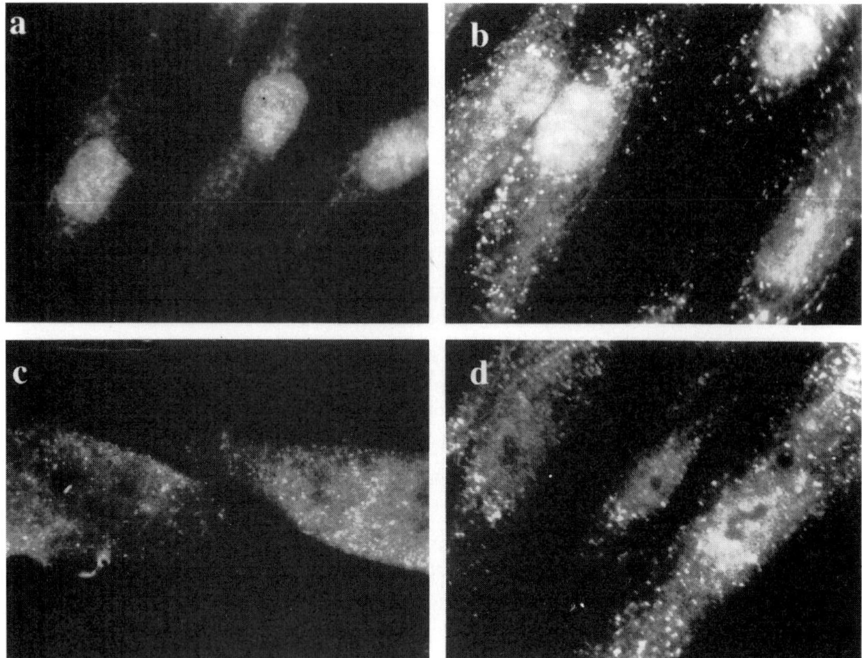

Fig. 131-23 ALP immunofluorescence of fibroblasts from X-ALD patients. Panel *A* shows the absence of punctate immunoreactive material; *C*, weakly positive immunoreactivity, and *D*, normal immunostaining material. Panel *B* shows the immunoreactivity of cells in panel *A* toward peroxisomal 3-oxoacyl-CoA thiolase, which is not deficient in X-ALD, and demonstrates that the lack of immunoreactive material in these cells is ALDP-specific. (*From Watkins et al.*[94] *Used with permission.*)

Table 131-12 also lists conditions other than X-ALD in which primary adrenal insufficiency is combined with neurologic deficits. The most common of these is the "triple A" or Allgrove syndrome (MIM 231550): adrenocortical insufficiency, achalasia, and alacrima,[263] which is often associated with upper and lower motor neuropathy, sensory impairment, and mental retardation. It has been mapped to 12q13.[264] VLCFA levels are normal in patients with this syndrome.[92] Differentiation from X-ALD is important for genetic counseling, because the triple A syndrome has an autosomal recessive mode of inheritance.

Biochemical, Immunocytochemical, and Molecular Assays

Biochemical assays depend upon the demonstration of abnormally high levels of saturated VLCFA in tissues or body fluids, such as plasma,[14,92,265] red blood cells,[15,266] white blood cells,[267,268] "Guthrie" blood spots on filter paper,[269] cultured skin fibroblasts,[13,270,271] cultured amniocytes and chorion villus cells,[16,272] and cultured muscle.[273] Techniques used include gas-liquid chromatography,[274] gas-liquid chromatography-mass spectrometry[265] including stable isotope dilution,[275,276] and high-performance gas-liquid chromatography.[277–279] Gas-liquid chromatography assays and gas-liquid chromatography-mass spectrometry stable isotope dilution assays performed on aliquots of the same samples have given equivalent results (Moser HW, Rinaldo P, Vreken P, unpublished observations).

Indirect immunofluorescence or immunoblotting assays to examine the expression of ALDP have been performed in cultured skin fibroblasts,[93,204] white blood cells,[93] and cultured amniocytes and chorion villus cells.[280] Normal cultured skin fibroblasts or white blood cells show punctate peroxisomal immunofluorescence (Fig. 131-23). This immunoreactivity is lacking in approximately 70 percent of male X-ALD patients.[93,94]

Mutation Analysis. As noted in previous sections, mutations in the X-ALD gene have been demonstrated in all male X-ALD patients in whom the entire gene has been examined.[190] More than 300 different mutations have been identified. Mutational analysis has been complicated by the existence of autosomal paralogs with 92 to 96 percent identity to the X-ALD gene. One strategy that avoids coamplification of autosomal sequences is based on amplification of exons 6 to 10 as a single 4-kb amplicon, using an X-specific primer around exon 6 and a reverse primer in exon 10, followed by a nested PCR of individual exons.[196] An alternative strategy relies on analysis of the entire X-ALD transcript by reverse transcription-PCR and subsequent nested PCR of subfragments.[281] While these techniques have been of great value for research, neither is ideal for clinical application, due to the labile nature of RNA, and the concern that particular mutations may adversely affect expression levels and stability of the mutant transcript, and this may result in underrepresentation of the mutant template in an RT-PCR protocol. This could potentially lead to a false negative diagnosis in carriers. Boehm et al.[95] have developed a procedure that minimizes these pitfalls. It uses a nonnested genomic amplification of the X-ALD gene, followed by fluorescent dye-primer sequencing and analysis. The procedure has been validated for the identification of carriers.

Postnatal Diagnosis of Affected Males

Assay of the levels of saturated VLCFA in plasma is the most frequently used test for the diagnosis of X-ALD. The assay is technically demanding and erroneous results may be obtained in laboratories that have limited experience with the assay. A proficiency-testing program is being developed. The experience with this assay in 3000 patients with peroxisomal disorders and 29,000 controls tested at the Kennedy Krieger Institute was recently analyzed.[92] The test relies on three parameters: the level of hexacosanoic acid (C26:0), the ratio of C26:0 to docosahexanoic acid (C22:0), and the ratio of C26:0 to tetracosanoic acid (C24:0). Figure 131-24 compares the results in 1096 X-ALD patients with those in 17,788 male controls. While there was some overlap between patients and controls for each of the three parameters, this overlap could be eliminated by the application of a computer-derived discriminant function (Fig. 131-24*D*). Figure 131-25 shows that the distribution of VLCFA levels is independent of phenotype, and confirms previous data obtained by Boles et al.[282] VLCFA levels in X-ALD patients do not vary with age.[92] In six affected male neonates, levels were already abnormal in cord blood or plasma obtained on the day of birth. This indicates that neonatal screening may be feasible.

False Positive Tests. Elevations of plasma VLCFA equivalent or greater than those in X-ALD occur in the disorders of peroxisome biogenesis (see Chap. 129) and in other defects of peroxisomal

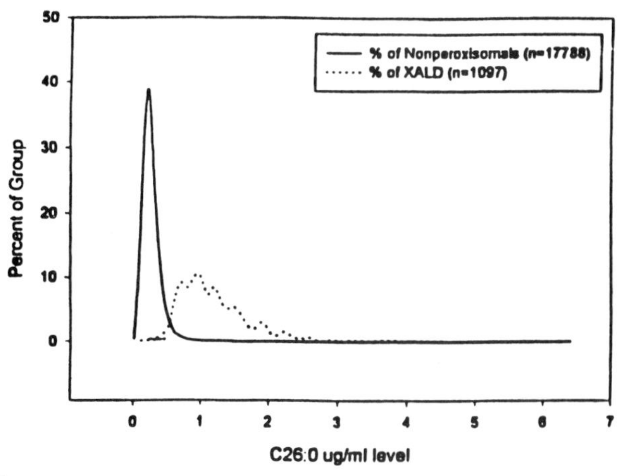

A

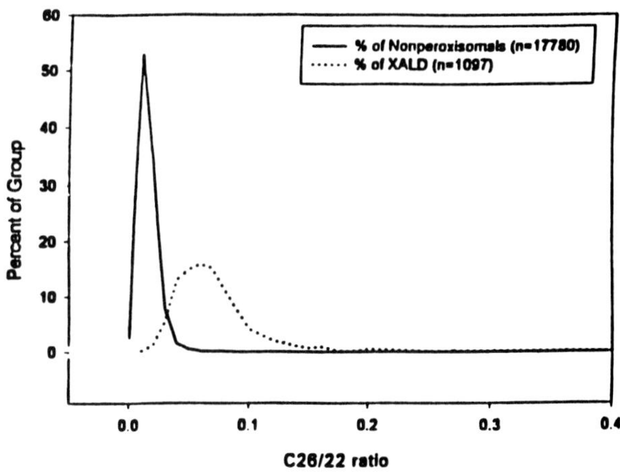

C

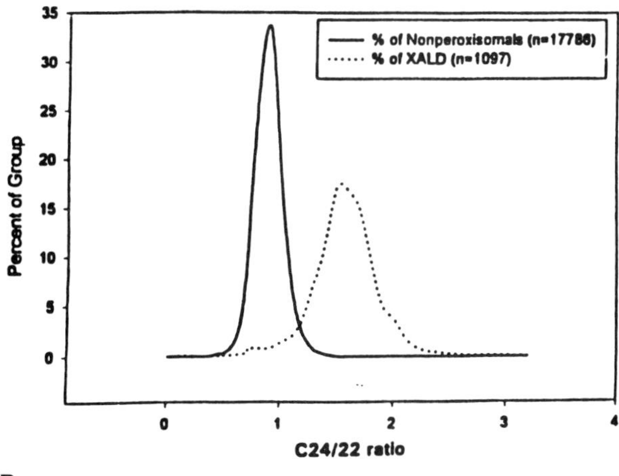

B

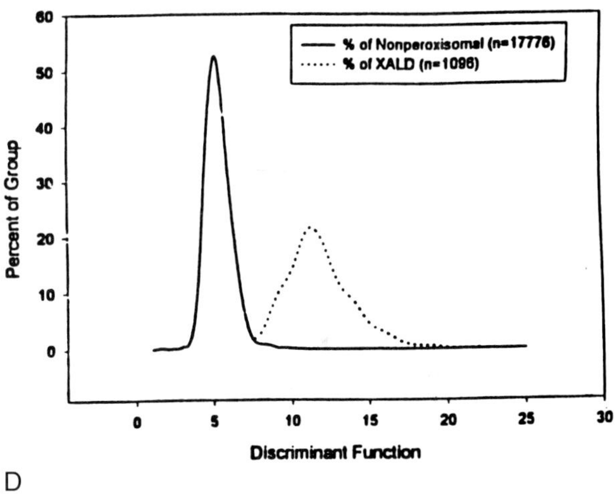

D

Fig. 131-24 Density plots of plasma VLCFA levels in 1097 male patients with X-ALD and 17,788 males who did not have a peroxisomal disorder. The control group included normal individuals and persons with a variety of disorders that did not appear to involve the peroxisome. *A, B,* and *C* show plots for the individual diagnostic parameters. Separately, each demonstrates an overlap between X-ALD and controls, which overlap is eliminated by

β-oxidation (see Chap. 130). However, these disorders can be distinguished because of their strikingly different clinical presentation. They manifest during the neonatal period and usually are associated with hypotonia, dysmorphic features, and multiple malformations. Plasma VLCFA levels may also be increased in children who receive the ketogenic diet to treat seizure disorders.[283] They return to normal when the diet is discontinued and VLCFA levels in cultured skin fibroblasts are normal. Elevated plasma VLCFA levels have been reported in patients with aceruloplasminemia[284] and in patients with crush injuries.[285] In some persons, elevated C26:0 levels and C26:0/C22:0 levels may be present postprandially and are normal in samples obtained before breakfast. These results indicate that false positive results can be identified relatively easily based on clinical presentation in other disorders that affect VLCFA metabolism, or by repeat plasma analysis after an overnight fast.

False Negative Tests in Persons Who Are Consuming Lorenzo's Oil or a Diet with High Erucic Acid Content. As discussed in the section on therapy, "Lorenzo's Oil" reduces or normalizes plasma levels of VLCFA in patients with X-ALD. Erucic acid (C22:1 omega 9), the active component in Lorenzo's Oil, is also a component of mustard and rapeseed oils. These oils may form part of the diet in India and in China.[286] The peroxisome laboratory at the Kennedy Krieger Institute recently tested a 10-year-old boy from India whose plasma VLCFA levels were within normal limits, but whose clinical presentation, brain MRI, and VLCFA levels in cultured skin fibroblasts were characteristic of X-ALD. Erucic acid constituted 0.44 percent of total plasma fatty acids, compared to 0.03 ± 0.03 percent in the U.S. population and a mean of 0.88 percent in X-ALD patients treated with Lorenzo's Oil.[287] He had not taken Lorenzo's Oil. The high erucic acid level was traced to consumption of a mustard oil that contained 40 to 60 percent of erucic acid as part of his customary diet. This experience indicates that the erucic acid level, which is obtained routinely when plasma VLCFA levels are assayed, should be evaluated along with VLCFA levels. Significantly elevated erucic acid levels in plasma indicate that in this sample the VLCFA assay is not a reliable tool for the diagnosis of X-ALD.

Do False Negative Tests Occur in Patients with Normal Erucic Acid Levels? Does a normal plasma VLCFA assay in a male

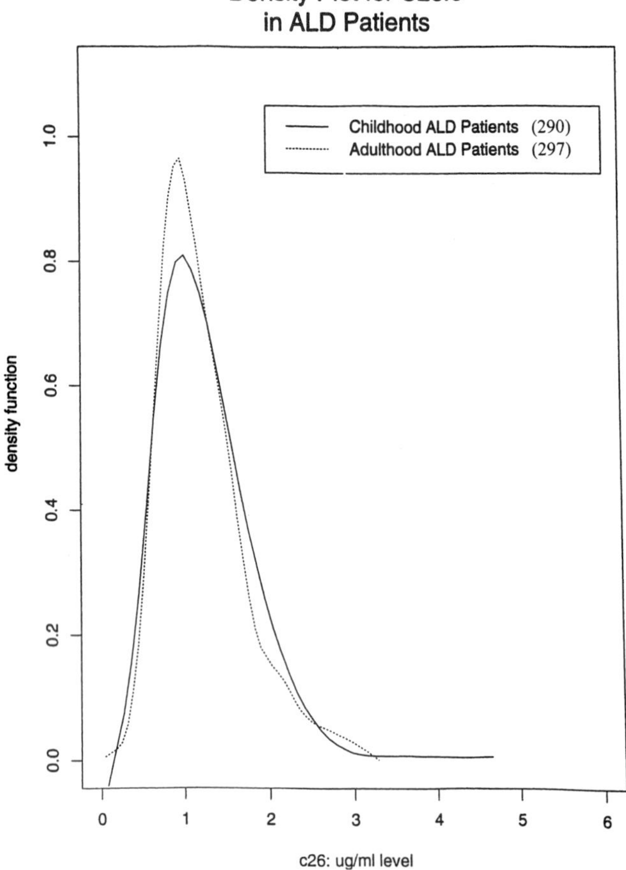

Fig. 131-25 Density plot of plasma VLCFA levels in male patients with the CCER phenotype and those with AMN. The two curves overlap, indicating that plasma VLCFA levels do not correlate with phenotype. The smooth density estimate of the frequency was derived by the density function in S-PLUS and the plot was prepared by using the function plot with the function density. (*From Moser et al.*[92] *Used with permission.*)

whose erucic acid levels are also normal exclude the diagnosis of X-ALD? This is an important question because the plasma VLCFA is the most commonly use diagnostic test, and false negative tests have serious consequences in respect to management and genetic counseling. No false negative results were documented in the series at the Kennedy Krieger Institute, which included samples from more than 30,000 persons. All patients with normal VLCFA levels in whom clinical findings nevertheless suggested X-ALD were shown to have other conditions such as the triple A syndrome.[263,264] However, two false negative plasma VLCFA assays are reported in the literature.[288,289] Assays of VLCFA levels in the cultured skin fibroblasts of these patients were unequivocally abnormal. We conclude that false negative plasma VLCFA assays are rare, but cannot be excluded.

Follow-up Procedures if Results of Plasma VLCFA Assay Are Equivocal. Follow-up procedures include (a) assay of VLCFA levels[13,271] and β-oxidation[290] in cultured skin fibroblasts. False negative results have not been observed. (b) Immunocytochemical analysis of the expression of ALDP[93,94,204] in cultured skin fibroblasts or white blood cells. Seventy percent of X-ALD patients are immunonegative. (c) Mutation analysis.[95] Mutations have been identified in all patients who have been studied in sufficient detail. The test is now available on a service basis.

Heterozygote Identification

VLCFA levels in plasma are increased in approximately 85 percent of women who are obligate heterozygotes for X-ALD.[91,92] Application of the discriminant function does not eliminate overlap between obligate heterozygotes and controls. Two-thirds of the obligate heterozygous women with normal plasma VLCFA levels had increased VLCFA levels in cultured skin fibroblasts.[91] However, even with this combined approach, false negative or equivocal results were obtained in 10 percent of obligate heterozygotes. Mutation analysis[95] provides the most definitive technique. When the nature of the mutation has been identified in the family, a targeted search for this mutation can be conducted conveniently and relatively inexpensively in at-risk family members. Even when affected male relatives are not available for study, the technique developed by Boehm et al[95] permits identification of the mutation in carriers in most instances. Immunocytochemical studies for the expression of ALDP are of great value when affected male relatives are immunonegative. Feigenbaum et al.[93] demonstrated that 15 of 15 obligate heterozygote members of these families had a mixture of immunopositive and immunonegative cells in white blood cells or cultured skin fibroblasts. Under these circumstances, this technique can provide a rapid and convenient method for the identification of heterozygotes.

Prenatal Diagnosis

Prenatal identification of affected male fetuses has been achieved by the demonstration of increased VLCFA levels in cultured amniocytes or chorion villus cells[16] and has been applied at the Kennedy Krieger Institute in a series of 255 pregnancies.[272] There was no overlap between affected and unaffected male fetuses. Sixty-three male affected fetuses were identified. There were no known false negative results, but with the important proviso that follow up was incomplete for 70 of the 180 male fetuses with normal results. There are two reports of normal VLCFA in cultured chorion villus cells of fetuses who were later shown to have X-ALD.[291,292] These results indicate the desirability to additional approaches. Immunocytochemical analysis for the expression of ALDP is of great value when male probands in the family are known to be immunonegative.[280,293,294] When the mutation in the family is known, mutation analysis in fetal cells provides the most definitive diagnostic technique, but it must be emphasized that it is not predictive of phenotype.[294,295]

Neuroimaging Studies

Neuroimaging studies often provide the first clue to the diagnosis of X-ALD. They provide valuable information about prognosis (Figs. 131-3 and 131-4), selection of candidates for bone marrow transplantation, and the evaluation of therapies. CT was shown to be a valuable diagnostic tool in the 1970s and 1980s.[296–300] At this time MRI is the most widely used imaging technique for the diagnosis of X-ALD and other white-matter disorders.[301] It reveals abnormalities that are not detected by CT.[302–305] MRI abnormalities often precede neurologic and neuropsychologic changes.[303] Still greater sensitivity is offered by recently developed techniques such as proton magnetic resonance spectroscopy (MRS) (Fig. 131-26),[45,306–310] magnetization transfer,[46] and three-dimensional diffusion magnetic resonance imaging.[48] These techniques, which are still being refined and are not yet generally available, provide the potential for the detection of brain involvement at still earlier stages and will aid the assessment of the severity of the inflammatory response and of axonal damage.

Eighty percent of CCER patients show cerebral white matter lesions that are characteristic in respect to location and attenuation pattern. In these patients, the lesions are symmetric and involve the periventricular white matter in the posterior parietal and occipital lobes.[305] Noncontrast CT scans show bilateral hypodensities in this location.[311] These regions are hyperintense in proton-density or T2-weighted MRI images.[312] Use of the contrast material gadolinium-diethylenetriamine pentaacetic acid (DPTA) demonstrates a garland of accumulated contrast material adjacent and anterior to the posterior hypodense lesions shown on T1-weighted MRI (Fig. 131-2*B*). The accumulation of contrast material on MRI

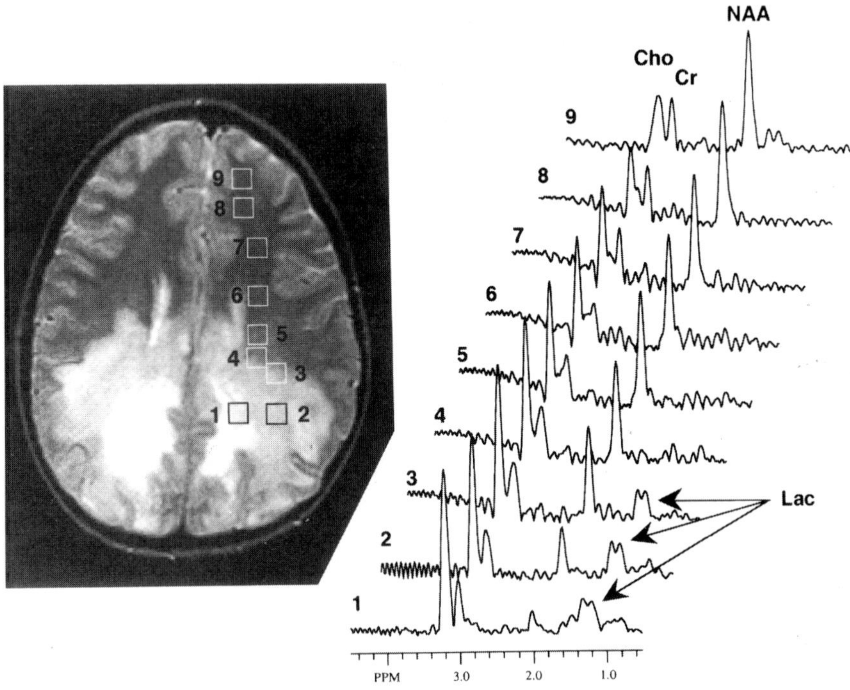

Fig. 131-26 MRI and MS patterns in a patient with CCER. The signal hyperintensities in the occipitoparietal white matter demonstrated in the MR indicate demyelinated areas. The spectra referring to individual voxels are shown on the right. As expected, voxels 1 and 2 show severe reduction of the NAA peak and increased choline peaks. The spectra in the far anterior voxels 8 and 9 are normal. However in voxels 5, 6, and 7 the NAA and choline peaks are abnormal, even though the MRI image in these regions is not altered. This and other studies cited in reference 306 indicate that MS is a more sensitive indicator of brain involvement in X-ALD than MRI.

or CT correlates well with the histopathologic zones described by Schaumburg et al.[40] The outer zone corresponds to the zone of active demyelination with partial loss of myelin and without inflammation. The middle zone enhances with gadolinium-DPTA because of blood-brain barrier breakdown and corresponds to the area of inflammation. In the more posterior hyperintense area on T2-weighted MRI the destructive process is no longer active and myelin is replaced by glial tissues. Although caudorostral progression is most common, initial lesions may be frontal.[75,313–315] Initial lesions were frontal in 5 of 40 patients with childhood and adolescent cerebral X-ALD that were described by Kumar et al.[305] In other patients, who have what is referred to as the Di Chiro type II pattern,[298] there is early involvement of the internal capsule, corpus callosum, corona radiata, forceps major, and cerebral peduncles. The initial lesions may also be in the cerebellum and pons.[65,67,69–71] Occasionally, the initial lesion is asymmetric (Fig. 131-6) and may be mistaken for a brain tumor.

Kumar et al.[49] described the MRI findings in 119 men with AMN and 45 adult heterozygotes. The brain MRI was normal in 54 percent of the men and 80 percent of the women. Diffuse spinal cord atrophy, mainly in the thoracic cord, was present in 18 of 20 men and in 6 of 10 heterozygotes. Thirteen percent of the men had brain MRI abnormalities confined to the corticospinal tract and internal capsule. These changes were interpreted to represent a centripetal extension of the distal axonopathy of AMN. Twenty-seven percent of the AMN patients had diffuse lobar brain involvement resembling that in the childhood cerebral form of X-ALD.

Recently developed techniques of proton magnetic resonance spectroscopy permit the measurement of brain levels of several nervous system metabolites that are of clinical interest. They include *N*-acetyl aspartate (NAA), choline-containing compounds (Cho) *myo*-inositol (Ins) and lactate.[45,306,307–310] NAA is present mainly in neurons.[316] Reduction in this peak is considered to be an index of neuronal or axonal damage, although a recent report indicates that loss of oligodendrocytes may also contribute to this reduction.[317] The Cho peak consists mainly of phosphocholine and glycerophosphocholine. These substances are metabolic products of cell membrane turnover and their elevation is thought to reflect demyelination.[45,318] The Ins peak is a composite peak, due not only to *myo*-inositol but also includes minor contributions of other inositol-containing compounds.[318] An increased Ins peak is interpreted to be a marker of glial proliferation.[45,319] An increase in the lactate peak is thought to arise from the anaerobic metabolism of infiltrating macrophages and lymphocytes and indicative of an inflammatory response.[45]

Several reports indicate that MRS alterations in the cerebral forms of X-ALD precede changes demonstrable by MRI.[45,306–310] Figure 131-26 is illustrative. It shows a comparison of MRI and MRS studies in a patient with CCER. The MRI shows the characteristic abnormalities in the parieto-occipital regions, while the frontal regions appear normal. MRS studies, however, demonstrate diminished NAA and increased Cho peaks in the frontal regions adjacent to the parietal zone, indicating that the disease process has already extended to the posterior frontal region, while the most anterior frontal regions are still unaffected. Pouwels et al.[45] reported quantitative proton magnetic resonance spectra in 39 male X-ALD patients, 23 of whom were asymptomatic. An increase of both Cho and Ins peaks appeared to indicate the onset of demyelination. Markedly increased concentrations of Cho, Ins, and glutamine peaks reflect active demyelination and glial proliferation. A simultaneous reduction in the concentration of NAA and glutamate was considered to indicate neuronal loss or damage. The utilization of these techniques for the selection of patients for bone marrow transplant is discussed in the section on therapy.

Adrenal Function

Previous studies had shown that 35 to 45 percent[40,41] of patients with CCER have overt adrenal insufficiency, but 80 percent show subnormal cortisol increases in response to ACTH stimulation.[53] Eighty percent of patients with the childhood cerebral ALD had overt adrenocortical insufficiency, while 20 percent had a normal cortisol response to ACTH stimulation. Normal adrenocortical function is observed somewhat more frequently in AMN: 30 percent[30] to 50 percent[54] of patients had normal cortisol response to ACTH stimulation. Approximately 1 percent of heterozygotes has Addison disease. Increased plasma ACTH levels are observed frequently in male patients. This was first reported by Rees et al.[320] All of Aubourg's 17 childhood X-ALD patients in whom this measurement was obtained had increased plasma ACTH levels.[41] In summary, adrenocortical function is impaired in the great majority of patients with childhood cerebral X-ALD. However, it is normal in 30 to 50 percent of men with AMN[54] and in 99 percent of women heterozygous for X-ALD.

The need for adrenal function tests to establish the diagnosis of X-ALD has diminished somewhat now that more specific VLCFA assays are available. Nevertheless, it continues to be of importance to assess adrenal function in every case. It is essential to be aware of the extent of impaired adrenal reserve so that replacement therapy can be instituted promptly.

Elevated levels of LH or FSH in plasma have been reported in 40 to 70 percent of AMN patients.[51,53,321] Plasma testosterone levels are low or borderline low in 22 percent of AMN patients.[53] Plasma dehydroepiandrosterone sulphate (DHEAS) levels were below normal in all the 26 X-ALD patients in whom the level of this substance was measured and who included all phenotypes.[322] This included eight AMN patients whose cortisol and ACTH levels were normal. Assies et al. speculated that the abnormally low DHEAS levels may contribute to the pathogenesis of the inflammatory brain disease. They note that the cortisol-DHEAS ratio is reported to mediate the balance between humoral and cellular immunity,[323] and that the secretion of DHEAS normally rises steeply between the ages of 6 to 8 years. This is also the age at which the neurologic symptoms of CCER manifest most frequently (Fig. 131-1).

Neurophysiological Studies

Neurophysiological studies have been performed in large series of AMN patients and women heterozygous for X-ALD. Although hearing and language function are usually intact, brain stem auditory-evoked responses were abnormal in 98 percent of AMN patients and 42 percent of the heterozygotes (Table 131-5). The most common abnormality is a prolongation of the wave I to III interval, pointing to involvement of the medullopontine pathway.[324] The abnormal BAER responses in women heterozygous for X-ALD were first reported by Garg et al.[325] and Moloney et al.[326] BAER responses were abnormal in four of six boys with the childhood cerebral form of X-ALD and in one asymptomatic boy with the biochemical defect.[324]

Visual-evoked responses are less frequently abnormal. Kaplan et al.[327] studied pattern reversal visual-evoked potentials in 82 men with AMN and in 26 heterozygotes with neurologic disability that resembled AMN. Latency was increased in 17 percent of the men and in none of the women. In contrast, VER latencies were increased in 70 percent of boys with early or advanced cerebral involvement.[328]

Several large studies of peripheral nerve function in AMN patients were recently reported. Chaudhry et al.[329] studied 13 variables of peripheral nerve function in 99 men with AMN and 38 heterozygous women. At least one variable was abnormal in 87 percent of the men and 67 percent of the women. Abnormalities were more common in the legs than in the arms. They concluded that the abnormalities represented a mixture of axonal loss and multifocal demyelination. Van Geel et al. demonstrated a polyneuropathy in 65 percent in a study of 23 men with AMN and 5 neurologically symptomatic heterozygotes.[330] They concluded that the patients had a primary axonopathy. Twenty-six percent of the patients partially fulfilled the neurophysiological criteria of a primary demyelination. Kaplan et al. studied somatosensory-evoked responses in 67 men with AMN and 16 women heterozygous for this disorder.[331] Tibial somatosensory-evoked responses were abnormal in all the men and in 14 of 15 women. The men showed abnormalities of both peripheral and central pathways, whereas in the women the abnormality tended to be confined to central pathways. Restuccia et al. demonstrated abnormalities of motor and sensory evoked responses in 12 of 19 heterozygotes. Abnormalities were found in 7 of 14 women who had no other evidence of neurologic involvement.

The electroencephalogram in CCER patients often shows irregular large amplitude slow activity, which is more prominent over the posterior region of the brain.[332,333] The electroretinogram was normal, while the visual-evoked responses were abnormal in 4 of 14 cases.[332]

Neuropsychologic Tests

The importance of performing standardized and quantitative neuropsychologic tests was recently emphasized.[334–336] Neuropsychologic abnormalities usually precede overt neurologic symptoms and the nature and severity of neuropsychologic disturbances affect decisions about therapeutic interventions such as bone marrow transplantation (BMT). The neuropsychologic tests assess five major domains: language, visual perception, visuomotor/constructional function, memory, and executive function-attention. Test batteries that are standardized according to age and cross-culturally include the Wechsler Intelligence Scales for ages ranging from preschool to adult.[337–339] Visual perception of spatial location can be assessed by the Benton Test of Line Orientation.[340] The Rey-Osterrieth Complex Figure is a test of visuospatial perceptual skill.[341] The Bead Memory subtest of the Stanford-Binet Intelligence Scale IV is a test of immediate visual memory,[342] and the Rey Auditory Verbal Learning Test[341,343] tests for verbal memory. The Stroop Color and Word Test[344] and the Test of Variable Attention (TOVA)[345] are examples of tests that are used for the evaluation of executive function and attention. The nature, severity, and rate of progression of neuropsychologic deficits vary with the location of the initial white matter abnormalities as assessed by MRI studies of the brain.[334–336] When lesions begin in the parieto-occipital regions and the splenium of the corpus callosum, as is most commonly the case, deficits involve visuospatial functions and difficulties in auditory processing. Lesions that involve mainly the frontal lobes of patients lead to deficits of executive functions such as impaired flexibility in problem solving strategies and difficulties in anticipatory processing. In contrast with the occipital forms, these deficits have an early impact on school performance. Progression of frontal demyelinating lesions leads to typical frontal lobe syndromes with behavioral disturbances such as hyperactivity, distractibility, apathy, emotional lability, and sexual disinhibition in adolescents.[335]

Biopsy Diagnosis of X-ALD

Electron-microscopic study of nerve twigs contained in conjunctival or skin biopsies[105,346–348] reveals characteristic curved clefts and leaflets in Schwann cells surrounding myelinated axons. Characteristic lamellar inclusions have also been observed in sural nerve biopsy specimens.[104] However, availability of biochemical and genetic assays has eliminated the need for diagnostic biopsy procedures.

THERAPY

Supportive Care

The progressive behavioral and neurologic disturbances associated with the childhood form of X-ALD provide an extreme challenge for the family. Treatment following confirmation of the diagnosis of X-ALD requires the establishment of a comprehensive management program and partnership between the family, physician, visiting nurses, dietitian, school authorities, and counselors.[349] In addition, parental support groups such as the United Leukodystrophy Foundation (2304 Highland Drive, Sycamore, IL 60178) have proven to be of great value. Communication with school authorities is important because under the provision of Public Law 94-142, Education for All Handicapped Children, children with conditions such as X-ALD qualify for special services. Children with leukodystrophies are classified as "other health impaired" or multihandicapped." Depending on the rate of progression of the disease, special needs range from relatively low-level resource services within a regular school program (to correct deficiencies in isolated academic subjects) to self-contained services (for children with attention deficit disorder and multiple academic deficiencies) to home- and hospital-based teaching programs for children who are nonmobile.[349]

Management challenges vary with the stage of the illness. The early stages are characterized by subtle changes in affect, behavior, and attention span. Counseling and communication with school authorities are of prime importance.

Painful muscle spasms often cause severe discomfort. They are treated most commonly with diazepam or baclofen. Diazepam is generally started at 1 to 2 mg every 4 to 6 h, but because it has tachyphylaxis, it often needs to be increased rapidly. Some patients have required as much as 10 mg every 3 to 4 h by mouth or gastrostomy tube. For baclofen, a dosage of 5 mg twice daily may be increased gradually to 25 mg four times daily. While respiratory depression is a concern, in our experience, this is always preceded by loss of alertness. If an awake patient continues to have painful spasms, it is our policy to increase the dosage of muscle relaxant. Other agents, such as dantrolene or tizanidine may also be used, taking care to monitor for the occurrence of side effects and drug interactions.[349]

As the leukodystrophy progresses, bulbar muscular control is lost. Although initially this can be managed by changing to soft and pureed foods, most patients eventually require nasogastric tubes or surgical procedures such as gastrostomy or lateral esophagostomy. Almost all patients have focal or generalized seizures at some stage of the illness. They usually respond readily to standard anticonvulsant medications.

For the child who is ineligible for BMT, parents must consider the level of life-maintaining support that they want for their child as the disease progresses. With the placement of a feeding tube, need for suctioning, and the options of a tracheotomy and mechanical breathing support, the amount of nursing care increases. A number of states have instituted special programs to allow children who would not normally qualify for medical assistance to be eligible for support with actual hours of nursing care and many of the equipment and supply needs in the home provided under a federal and state-funded medicaid waiver program, rather than take on the enormous cost of hospital or institutional care.

Parents also need to use the expertise and help of related organizations. The United Cerebral Palsy programs often have respite care programs or access to special funds to help with therapy and wheelchair costs. The Association for Retarded Citizens has a long history of offering programs to support parents and children in the community. The Epilepsy Foundation may have information and training for school staff and family as well as being able to provide other support.

Supportive care is of great importance for patients with AMN. This includes physiotherapy, urologic consultation for impaired bladder control, erectile dysfunction, and prevention and treatment of urinary infection, avoidance of constipation, vocational and psychological counseling, and the detection and management of adrenal insufficiency. Oral baclofen, dantrolene, or tizanidine may aid management of spasticity and quality of life. The use of an intrathecal baclofen delivery system may help when oral medication is ineffective.[350] Behavioral disturbances are frequent in patients with the AMN-cerebral phenotype[58,59,351] and these patients may require psychiatric consultation.

Supportive care for other family members is also of great importance. The AMN patient may find that he can no longer function in his present employment, which often leads to depression, alcohol dependence, and major problems within the family. A social worker or family counseling is appropriate in many instances to prevent the number of separations that occur.

Many apply for, and eventually receive, disability payments through Social Security, which also makes them eligible for medicare. However, this provides minimal support at best, and without a strong physician advocate, most patients lack the appropriate medical follow up and referrals. Use of a wheelchair to maintain active family participation is often resisted, and switching to hand controls on the family car needs to be done for everyone's safety as the legs become more involved. Referral to vocational rehabilitation may provide the way back to a new career. If not, there needs to be an emphasis on staying involved through one of the many athletic programs that now are available for the handicapped, or volunteering in an organization or school. The organizations that specialize in work with paraplegics are often able to provide excellent information on bowel control, urinary continence, and erectile dysfunction. Time on the telephone or on the computer may bring much needed help.

The AMN-cerebral patient presents a series of problems to the patient's family and friends, and to the community as a whole. Inappropriate behavior may involve the police and require commitment to a psychiatric facility, and as the disease progresses, may require placement in a nursing home. Some states are able to provide home health aides for a certain number of hours, and hospice is available as the disease enters its final state with families faced with making decision about the level of life support. It is almost impossible for the family to organize the appropriate help on their own, and the aid of a social worker may be required as discharge planning takes place from a hospital or other institution.

Adrenal and Gonadal Insufficiency

The importance of evaluating adrenal function and providing appropriate replacement therapy cannot be overemphasized. Steroid replacement therapy does not alter the progression of the neurologic disability, but can increase sense of well being and could be life saving. We are aware of more than 10 patients who died in adrenal crisis, some of whom were free of neurologic involvement. Most X-ALD patients have increased plasma ACTH levels and impairment of cortisol responsiveness to a 0.25-mg intravenous dose of cosyntropin (Cortrosyn) after 60 min. We recommend that at least one of these tests be performed yearly. Isolated measurements of plasma cortisol levels are insufficient and may lead to the false conclusion that adrenal insufficiency has been ruled out. The 8:00 a.m. plasma cortisol level may be normal even when it is unresponsive to ACTH stimulation and the ACTH level is more than 1000 picogram/ml (normal <70).

Glucocorticoid dose requirements are generally the same as those used for other forms of primary adrenal insufficiency.[53] To mimic the diurnal rhythm of physiological cortisol secretion, adult patients receive 25 mg cortisone acetate or 20 mg hydrocortisone administered in the early morning with a smaller second dose of 12.5 mg or 10 mg, respectively, given in the late afternoon. The dosage in children is 5 to 10 mg/24 h. Patients are instructed in a protocol to augment glucocorticoid coverage during physical or mental stress, provided with a parenteral methylprednisolone dose for potential use if vomiting prevents oral dosing, and strongly encouraged to wear Medic-Alert identification declaring their dependency on adrenal steroid therapy. Not all patients require mineralocorticoid replacement. When postural hypotension, hyponatremia, or hyperkalemia does persist despite adequate glucocorticoid therapy, fludrocortisone, 0.05 mg to 0.1 mg per day, is prescribed. Males with clinical manifestations of hypogonadism (e.g., delayed pubertal masculinization, impotence, or diminished libido) that are associated with a low serum testosterone concentration should receive androgens. Impotence, in most instances, is due to spinal cord involvement or neuropathy, rather than testosterone deficiency. Sildenafil, which has been effective in patients with spinal cord injury,[352] has not been tested systematically in patients with AMN, but should be considered. Several AMN patients have reported that it improved erectile function.

Bone Marrow Transplantation

BMT is currently the most effective therapy for cerebral forms of X-ALD in children and adolescents, if the cerebral forms of X-ALD are detected in the early stages of the disease. The mechanism of its favorable effect is not yet understood. Because it carries a high risk, the indications for the procedure must be considered with great care.

Initial Reports. The first BMT was performed in 1981, in a boy with adolescent onset and cerebral demyelination, and reported in 1984.[353] The patient was a 12.5-year-old boy who presented with severe impairment of word discrimination, impaired visual acuity (20/70 left eye and 9/100 in the right eye), a superior temporal quadrantanopia, and slight dysmetria. Verbal IQ was 94, and performance IQ 90. Because of his impaired auditory discrimination, spoken language could not be used to test intelligence. However, when verbal instructions for the intelligence test were written out, the patient read and followed written instructions and answered written questions with well-articulated expressive speech. Plasma VLCFA levels showed the changes characteristic of X-ALD and the capacity of white blood cells to metabolize VLCFA was reduced to 20 percent of control. The preparative regimen for BMT included oral busulfan followed by intravenous cyclophosphamide. The donor was his HLA-identical brother. Intravenous cyclosporine and methylprednisolone were started on the day of the transplant. On day 24, skin biopsy showed a mild (grade 2) histologic graft versus host reaction, but there was no clinically evident graft versus host disease in other organs.

Although biochemical effects were favorable, the clinical outcome was deeply discouraging. On day 18, the patient reported that he could not see and his pupils were unreactive to light. When added to the preexisting defect in auditory discrimination, it was virtually impossible to communicate with him. Plantar responses became extensor and neurologic function deteriorated. He died of an adenovirus infection on day 141. Postmortem examination showed alterations characteristic of cerebral X-ALD. There were no new demyelinative lesions that could be related to the BMT-associated deterioration. Biochemical studies showed that engraftment had occurred, because post-BMT circulating white cells had normal capacity to degrade VLCFA. In addition, the plasma VLCFA levels diminished progressively toward the upper limit of normal. Despite these favorable biochemical effects, the possibly accelerated progression of the neurologic deficit dampened enthusiasm for additional transplants.

In 1985 and 1986 BMT's were performed in two brothers with X-ALD. The older brother, who was 9.4 years old and severely involved neurologically, died 34 days after BMT due to severe neurologic progression. The younger brother, who was neurologically normal, was transplanted at 3.7 years of age. Ten years later, his neurologic exam and brain MRI were normal but he had unexplained behavioral disturbances (S. Winter, personal communication).

The attitude toward BMT was revolutionized by the report of Aubourg et al. in Paris,[354] who, in 1988, transplanted an 8-year-old boy with mild neurologic, neuropsychologic, and MRI abnormalities. An unaffected nonidentical twin was the donor. While at 4 months post-BMT there was slight worsening of the neurologic deficit, this returned to pre-BMT status by 6 months, and at 12 and 18 months, the neurologic, neuropsychologic, and MRI abnormalities had disappeared and the patient's school performance was slightly better than that of his twin.[354] Eleven years later he continues to be normal (P. Aubourg, personal communication). This study suggests that mildly involved patients can withstand the moderate short-term worsening of neurologic status associated with BMT and then may gain long-term benefit. Subsequent experience supports this conclusion.

Current Experience with BMT. A series of reports about BMT in X-ALD have been published.[328,336,355–360] Dr. Charles Peters at the University of Minnesota (personal communication) analyzed the outcome in 124 X-ALD patients who received BMT between July 1981 and January 1999. The procedure was performed in 43 different centers throughout the world. Information was incomplete for some patients. The median age at BMT was 8.6 years (range: 1.9 to 16.1). Preparative therapy included chemotherapy alone in 45 percent and radiation combined with chemotherapy in 55 percent. Median follow-up was 2.8 years (range: 0.4 to 13). The 5-year actuarial probability of survival in 112 patients was 62 percent. The median interval between transplant and death was 4.8 months, range 0.0 to 59 months. The primary causes of death were progression of X-ALD, graft versus host disease, and infection.

While randomized prospective studies have not been performed, several lines of evidence suggest that the procedure can be of long-term benefit. One author (HW Moser, unpublished observation, May 1997) conducted a survey of the neurologic outcome in 59 patients (Fig. 131-27). Forty percent of the survivors remained stable, 9 percent improved slightly, and 13 percent improved unequivocally. Note that improvement persists for at least 4 to 8 years after BMT. This contrasts with the previously cited observation that there is no documented instance of spontaneous long-term remission in X-ALD. Neurologic status may worsen during the first 6 months following BMT, even in those patients who later improve. Additional evidence is provided in the report of Shapiro et al. on long-term effects of BMT in 12 engrafted CCER patients who have been followed for 5 to 10 years.[358] Verbal intelligence remained within normal range for 11 patients and motor function remained normal or improved in 10. Of special significance is the experience at the Hospital Saint Vincent-Paul in Paris during the period 1988 to 1992. During that period, 13 boys with mild to moderate abnormalities on MRI and/or neuropsychologic testing were identified as potential BMT candidates. At that time, it was hospital policy to perform BMT

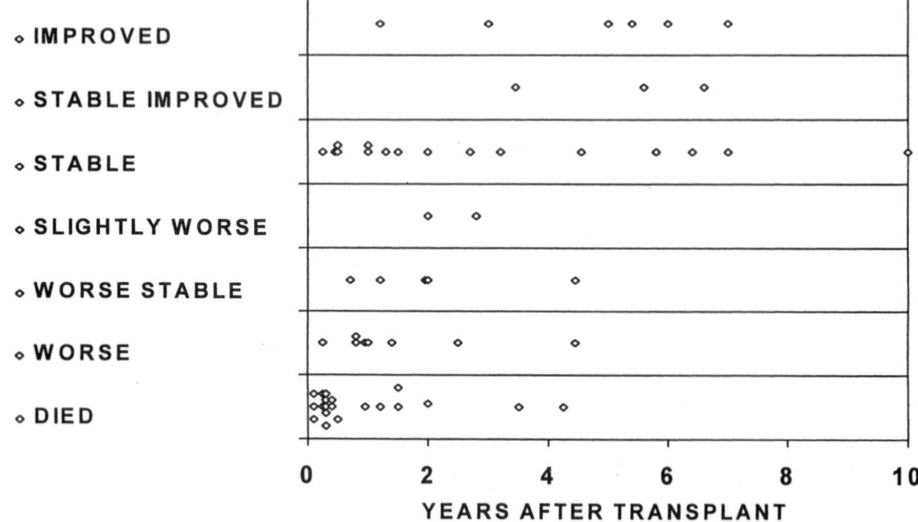

Fig. 131-27 A preliminary appraisal of the result of BMT in X-ALD. Systematic follow-up of X-ALD patients who have received BMT is still in progress. One author (HWM) has made a preliminary appraisal of results by personal contact with physicians and families of 59 patients and these are summarized here. Twenty (34 percent) of the patients died, most often during the first year. Of the 39 survivors, 24 (62 percent) stabilized or improved. Six patients had unequivocal improvement, and in four patients, this persisted more than 5 years after BMT.

only on those patients who had a matched sibling donor. Four of the five patients in that category who were transplanted remained stable or improved. Neurologic deterioration, leading to death in four, was observed in all of the eight patients who were not transplanted because they did not have a matched sibling donor but who were otherwise comparable to the transplant group (P. Aubourg, personal communication).

Mechanism of Beneficial Effect. The mechanism of the beneficial effect of BMT in X-ALD is unknown. It must differ from what occurs in patients with lysosomal disorders where the enzyme that is deficient can be secreted by BMT-derived normal cells and taken up by host cells.[361] This cannot occur in X-ALD because the defect involves a peroxisomal membrane protein. Krivit et al. propose that the effect is mediated by brain microglia.[362] BMT-derived cells do enter the nervous system[363] and brain microglia are bone marrow derived at least in part.[364,365] Donor-derived microglia may have a favorable effect on local brain metabolism. Microglia have a slow turnover rate.[366] This could account for the finding that BMT beneficial effects are not observed until 6 to 12 months after BMT and may continue to increase thereafter.[354]

Beneficial effects of BMT have so far been observed only in patients with CCER or the adolescent cerebral forms of X-ALD. As noted previously, inflammatory and autoimmune mechanisms may play a pathogenetic role in these phenotypes. Preparation for BMT requires immunosuppression. The possibility that the benefit of BMT results from immunosuppression cannot be excluded. It is made less likely by the observation that neurologic disability continued to worsen in all patients who received the immunosuppressive preparative regimen for BMT but who then autoengrafted. One such patient has been reported[359] and progression of the neurologic deficit continued in four others (G. Raymond, unpublished observation). If the presence or absence of the cerebral disease is the result of inherited differences in the inflammatory response, then the success of BMT may be influenced by the genotype of the donor cell.

Indications for BMT. Decisions about the indications for BMT are complicated by the great variability of the natural history of X-ALD and by the risk of the procedure. Assessment of risk-benefit ratio is aided by the data in Figs. 131-3 and 131-4 on the prognosis of nontransplanted patients as a function of age and MRI abnormality. Dr. Charles Peters' analysis of outcome in 124 patients who had received BMT indicates 38 percent mortality in 5 years. Figure 131-27 shows that most of the deaths occurred within the first year. The mean interval between transplant and death was 7.7 months. It is likely that the risk of BMT will be reduced by new techniques that extend the use of partially mismatched donors[367] and the use of cord blood.[368]

There is general agreement that the prime indication for BMT is in boys or adolescents who have mild progressive brain involvement. Because of the risk of the procedure, BMT is not indicated in patients whose brain is uninvolved, because up to half of these patients may escape brain involvement even without therapy. Most patients who are already severely involved at time of BMT continue to deteriorate following transplant. The group at the University of Minnesota noted that all patients whose performance IQ at time of BMT was < 80 remained severely demented or died. They believe that this deterioration may be aggravated by the preparative regimen in current use and are testing a myelin-sparing protocol that eliminates brain irradiation and busulfan and provides for the administration of cyclosporin as a continuous infusion rather than as a bolus (C. Peters, personal communication).

BMT has not been tested systematically in AMN because the risk-benefit ratio is less favorable due to greater risk of graft versus host disease in adults, and the milder disability caused by the disease. It is not known whether BMT will benefit AMN, because the basic pathology in that disorder is a distal axonopathy and the inflammatory response is mild or absent. It is of key importance to determine whether patients who received BMT when they were boys will develop AMN in adulthood.

The selection of candidates for BMT requires careful clinical judgment and periodic monitoring, particularly during the ages of 4 to 12 years when boys are at greatest risk of developing the rapidly progressive disease. It is recommended that they be monitored at least at yearly intervals, but a 6-month interval should be considered. Monitoring should include MRI and neuropsychologic studies. It is important to remember that overt neurologic symptoms develop relatively late, and that when they do occur, the window of opportunity for BMT may already have closed. Neuroimaging and neuropsychologic examinations provide the best opportunity for the identification of patients who can benefit. Abnormal MRI or MRS studies usually provide the first evidence of brain involvement. When these are present, it is particularly important to perform neuropsychologic tests. In 1995, Shapiro et al.[369] recommended that BMT should be considered when neuroimaging abnormalities are associated with mild and progressive neuropsychologic changes, such as a decline of 1 SD in any one of the following scores: (a) IQ (full-scale, verbal, or nonverbal); (b) tests of visual processing or memory, which must be confirmed by other measures or clinical corroboration; or (c) one domain of neuropsychologic function, such as auditory processing, language, nonverbal ability, and motor.

It was recently suggested that the policy to offer BMT only if there is evidence of some impaired neuropsychologic function may delay the procedure excessively and permit the disease to progress to a level that compromises the benefit potential.[357] This suggestion led to the proposal that the procedure should be considered when there are progressive brain MRI abnormalities, even if there is no demonstrable decline in neuropsychologic function. The refinement of imaging techniques adds weight to this recommendation. It must be noted, however, that some patients with unequivocally abnormal MRI remain neurologically stable.[44] The challenge is to determine whether nervous system involvement is progressive. Studies with gadolinium-DPTA contrast material and application of newly developed techniques of MRS[45] and magnetization transfer[46] may be of help, and careful clinical evaluation is a requirement. If the decision is made to proceed with the transplant, we recommend that it be performed in a center experienced in BMT therapy of X-ALD.

Dietary Therapy

The concept of dietary therapy for X-ALD derived from the study of Kishimoto et al.[124] who administered deuterated C26:0 to a terminally ill patient with X-ALD during the last 100 days of his life, and demonstrated that a substantial portion of brain C26:0 contained the label. This led to the development of a diet which restricts C26:0 to less than 15 percent of customary U.S. intake.[370] This diet was administered to six X-ALD patients for 1 to 2 years,[127] but had no effect on clinical course or plasma VLCFA levels. It was later shown that most of the VLCFA that accumulate in X-ALD patients are derived from endogenous synthesis,[125,135,182] and this led to the abandonment of dietary VLCFA restriction as a sole therapy.

Interest in dietary therapy was reawakened by the observation of Rizzo et al. that addition of oleic acid to the medium normalizes the levels of saturated VLCFA in cultured skin fibroblasts,[135] presumably by competing for the microsomal enzyme system that elongates saturated long chain fatty acids.[130] Oral administration of glyceryl trioleate reduced the levels of VLCFA in the plasma of patients with X-ALD[20,21] by 50 percent and was associated with a statistically significant improvement in 1 of 12 parameters of peripheral nerve function (peroneal nerve amplitude).[371] A still more striking effect on plasma VLCFA levels was achieved with the administration of a 4:1 mixture of glyceryl trioleate and glyceryl trierucate,[371–373] which normalizes plasma VLCFA levels within 4 weeks. This mixture is referred to as Lorenzo's Oil. This striking biochemical result, combined with the relentless progression of the disease, and with anecdotal reports of benefit in the literature[372] and the media,[374,375] prompted the utilization of open rather than placebo-controlled randomized therapeutic trials.[376] This decision has hampered the evaluation of clinical efficacy. Experience gained since then indicates that plasma VLCFA levels do not represent valid surrogate markers of therapeutic effectiveness. They are the same in severely and in mildly involved patients (Fig. 131-20) and the degree of normalization of VLCFA levels does not correlate with clinical progression.[327] Erucic acid, the active component of Lorenzo's Oil, does not appear to enter the brain to a significant extent.[377,378]

Eleven years after introduction of Lorenzo's Oil therapy, evaluation of its efficacy is still incomplete, although the results of treatment suggest that benefit is limited at best. In patients who are already symptomatic, most reports indicate that the neurologic disability continues to increase.[379–385] In the absence of controlled studies, it is not possible to determine whether the frequency and rate of deterioration differ from natural history. W. Köhler (personal communication, 1999) presented preliminary data based upon comparison disease progression during therapy with historical information about the rate of progression before the therapy was initiated, which data suggest that strict dietary control may diminish the rate of disease progression in patients with pure AMN. Lorenzo's Oil therapy does not improve endocrine function.[380]

Whether the administration of Lorenzo's Oil can prevent neurologic disability is the subject of an international multicenter study that is still in progress. The study involves 250 boys with X-ALD who started dietary therapy when they were neurologically asymptomatic. Two endpoints will be examined: (a) comparison of the frequency and age at onset of neurologic symptoms in the treated group with that in the historical control group as shown in Fig. 131-7 and Table 131-7; and (b) the degree to which lowering of plasma VLCFA correlates with clinical outcome. The study will be completed at the end of the year 2000. Some patients who started on the diet at 3 years of age have developed CCER while on treatment. Statistical analysis is still incomplete.

Lorenzo's Oil therapy has side effects, most of which can be controlled by careful monitoring. Some reduction of platelet count occurs in more than 30 percent of patients,[380,386–388] but clinically significant abnormal bleeding has not been observed. It is our policy to discontinue Lorenzo's Oil when platelet count falls below 80,000, and the patients are then maintained on glycerol trioleate. This usually results in restoration of platelet count to pretreatment levels, and the Lorenzo's Oil may be resumed at a lower level. Platelets also show decreased membrane anisotropy,[389] and there may be slight lymphocytopenia,[390] elevation of liver enzymes,[380] and a reduction in the levels of polyunsaturated very long chain fatty acids such as docosahexaenoic acid.[287,391] The levels of polyunsaturated fatty acids can be restored to normal by providing dietary supplements of fish oils, safflower oil, or English walnut oil in a dose so that linoleic acid provides approximately 5 percent of total calories.

It is our view that Lorenzo's Oil therapy is not warranted in most patients who already have neurologic symptoms. The clinical benefit of Lorenzo's Oil is limited at best. In addition, moderate side effects are relatively common, and the dietary therapy involves a change in life style and considerable expense. Decision concerning its efficacy as a preventive agent in neurologically asymptomatic patients should be deferred until the multicenter study is completed.

Other Therapeutic Approaches That Have Been Tested

Modification of Inflammatory Response. Because the rapid progression of X-ALD is associated with a brain inflammatory response, reduction of this response could be of therapeutic benefit. So far, efforts to accomplish this have not been successful. Agents tested include cyclophosphamide[392] and interferon-β-1a.[393] Dr. Gerald Raymond at the Kennedy Krieger Institute is conducting a double-masked interferon-β-1b and placebo controlled study of thalidomide. While data analysis is not yet complete, clinical progression continued in all of the patients enrolled in the study at approximately the same rate (G. Raymond, personal communication). Intravenous immunoglobulins were reported to be helpful in one patient with adolescent cerebral ALD.[394] We tested this approach in 12 patients,[256] and found it to be helpful in 1 patient, but without clear benefit in the others.

Plasma exchange[395] and the oral administration of *carnitine* and *clofibrate*[127] did not alter the course of the disease. Carnitine did not alter the levels of VLCFA in plasma.

Potential New Therapies

Lovastatin. Singh and associates have proposed lovastatin as a possible therapeutic agent. They have shown that lovastatin increases the capacity of cultured X-ALD cells to metabolize lignoceric acid (C24:0) and that it normalizes the levels of VLCFA in these cells.[396] They reported that the oral administration of lovastatin in a dosage of 40 mg per day lowered the levels of VLCFA in the plasma of X-ALD patients.[397,398] They also suggested that lovastatin may have a favorable effect on the inflammatory response, which leads to rapid neurologic deterioration in X-ALD patients. They carried out studies in rats with experimental allergic encephalitis, an animal model of multiple sclerosis in which there is an inflammatory response that resembles what is seen in X-ALD. Lovastatin had a favorable effect on mortality and morbidity in these animals.[399] The favorable effect appears to be mediated by the capacity of lovastatin to abolish the cytokine-induced increase of nitric oxide synthase in the affected animals. The clinical efficacy of lovastatin in X-ALD has not yet been tested. It offers an attractive approach, because studies in thousand of patients with hypercholesterolemia have shown that side effects are rare. A multicenter double-masked placebo-controlled clinical trial is planned.

4-Phenylbutyrate. Kemp et al.[216] have presented data that suggest that 4-phenylbutyrate (4-PBA) could benefit patients with X-ALD. In studies with cultured cells from X-ALD patients and a mouse model of X-ALD,[34] they demonstrated that 4-PBA improves the capacity of these cells to oxidize VLCFA and lowered the levels of VLCFA. Most significantly, it also lowered the levels of VLCFA in the brain and adrenal in the X-ALD mouse model. Two possible mechanisms of action were demonstrated. The medication induced peroxisome proliferation, and increased the expression of the peroxisomal protein ALDRP. The latter finding is of particular interest, because ALDRP, which is encoded on Chromosome 12, has 66 percent identity to ALDP, and can substitute for the action of ALDP in cultured skin fibroblasts of X-ALD patients.[34,213] Because of its capacity to increase expression of a redundant gene, the effect of 4-PBA may be viewed as an example of pharmacologic gene therapy.

Based upon the above results and the well-documented observation that this medication increased levels of fetal hemoglobin and ameliorated crises in sickle cell disease,[216,400] we have conducted preliminary studies of the effect of 4-PBA administration in seven men with AMN (G. Raymond, P. Watkins, H. Moser, unpublished observations). They received 20 g per day orally in 3 divided doses. This dose had been used previously in patients with sickle cell anemia.[400] They received the medication consisting of 40 pills a day for 6 weeks, then went 2 weeks without, and then resumed the medication for another 6 weeks. Other than the inconvenience associated with taking such a large number of pills, none experienced side effects, such as gastrointestinal upsets or abnormal odor. Brain magnetic resonance studies performed in one patient 30 min after an oral dose revealed a 4-PBA peak in cerebrospinal fluid and brain white matter.[401] Serial measurements were made of VLCFA levels in plasma, red cells, white blood cells, and platelets, and of VLCFA oxidation in white blood cells. A reduction of C22:0 and C24:0 levels was noted in platelets following 4-PBA administration, but none of the other parameters were altered. Analysis of the expression of the

ALDR gene in the white blood cells of three of these patients showed no differences following 4-PBA administration (P. Aubourg, personal communication). Additional studies with different dosage schedules of 4-PBA and other agents that may lead to increased expression of ALDR are planned.

Gene Replacement Therapy. Retroviral transfer of the X-ALD gene into C34+ cells of X-ALD patients has been achieved,[227] but is not yet sufficiently efficient to warrant clinical trials.

Transplants with Marrow-Derived Mesenchymal Cells. Recent studies have shown that marrow-derived mesenchymal cells can differentiate into various tissues of mesenchymal origin, including adipocytes, chondrocytes, and perhaps astrocytes.[402,403] Transplantation of these cells may make it possible to introduce the normal gene into a larger number and variety of nervous system cells, and thus enhance the effectiveness of BMT. Additional studies of this approach are required, since with current techniques bone marrow-derived mesenchymal stem cells after allogeneic BMT remained host-derived.[404]

PREVENTION OF X-ALD

X-ALD causes severe disability in most persons, and therapy is only partially effective, and it is invasive and expensive. Prevention therefore represents the most effective measure to reduce the hardship caused by this disease. The pattern of heredity and recent technologic advances make prevention feasible for the following reasons:

1. The estimates shown in Table 131-10 indicate that fewer than 5 percent of X-ALD patients have new mutations. Systematic screening of relatives thus could identify the majority of patients and carriers.
2. The combined use of plasma VLCFA assays[92] and DNA analysis[95] can identify all affected males and females by noninvasive techniques.
3. As discussed previously, prenatal diagnosis is feasible and accurate. The potential for preimplantation diagnosis exists. Counseling based on prenatal diagnosis must be balanced with the knowledge that approximately 50 percent of patients with X-ALD have the milder AMN phenotype.

Efforts should be made to screen not only the immediate family but also more distant family members. One-third of the X-ALD patients identified at the Kennedy Krieger Institute were distant relatives, in one instance dispersed in three continents. One hundred seventy-four family members were screened in one kindred, and in many instances screening involved more than 50 members. In our experience, the extended family screens are accomplished most effectively at the time that a symptomatic patient is diagnosed, and are facilitated by enlistment of the aid of one family member who relates well to other members of the kindred and has organizational skills. While this preventive effort is time-consuming, it is strongly justified for humanistic reasons. It can also be justified financially because it is possible to screen 1000 at-risk relatives at the cost of one bone marrow transplant.

REFERENCES

1. Haberfeld W, Spieler F: Zur diffusen Hirn-Rueckenmarksclerose im Kindesalter. *Dtch Z Nervenh* **40**:436, 1910.
2. Schilder P: Die encephalitis periaxilis diffusa. *Arch Psychiatr Nervenkr* **71**:327, 1924.
3. Schilder P: Zur frage der encephalitis periaxialis diffusa (sogenannet diffuse sklerose). *Z Neuro Psych* **15**:359, 1913.
4. Schilder P: Zur Kenntnis der Sogenannten Diffusen Sklerose. *Neur u Pscyh* **10**:1, 1912.
5. Poser CM, van Bogaert L: Natural history and evolution of the concept of Schilder's diffuse sclerosis. *Acta Psych Et Neurol Scand* **31**:(3)285, 1956.
6. Creutzfeldt HG,Siemerling E: Bronzekrankheit und sklerosierende encephalomyelitis. *Arch Psychiatr Nervenkr* **68**:217, 1923.
7. Blaw ME: *Melanodermic type leucodystrophy (adreno-leukodystrophy)* in Neurodystrophies and Neuorolipidoses, Vinken PJ and Bruyn GW (eds) North Holland Publishing Co, 1970, p 128.
8. Powers JM, Schaumberg HH: The adrenal cortex in adrenoleukodystrophy. *Arch Pathol* **96**:305, 1973.
9. Powers JM, Schaumburg HH: Adreno-leukodystrophy: Similar ultrastructural changes in adrenal cortical and Schwann cells. *Arch Neurol* **30**:406, 1974.
10. Powers JM, Schaumburg HH: Adrenoleukodystrophy (sex-linked Schilder's disease). A pathogenetic hypothesis based on ultrastructural lesions in adrenal cortex, peripheral nerve and testis. *Am J Pathol* **76(3)**:481, 1974.
11. Johnson AB, Schaumburg HH, Powers JM: Histochemical characteristics of the striated inclusions of adrenoleukodystrophy. *J Histochem Cytochem* **24**:725, 1976.
12. Igarashi M, Schaumburg HH, Powers J, Kishimoto Y, Kolodny E, Suzuki K: Fatty acid abnormality in adrenoleukodystrophy. *J Neurochem* **26**:851, 1976.
13. Moser HW, Moser AB, Kawamura N, Murphy J, Milunsky A, Suzuki K, Schaumburg H, Kishimoto Y: Adrenoleukodystrophy: Elevated C-26 fatty acid in cultured skin fibroblasts. *Ann Neurol* **7**:542, 1980.
14. Moser HW, Moser AB, Frayer KK, Chen WW, Schulman JD, O'Neill BP, Kishimoto Y: Adrenoleukodystrophy: Increased plasma content of saturated very long chain fatty acids. *Neurology* **31**:1241, 1981.
15. Tsuji S, Suzuki M, Ariga T, Sekine M, Kuriyama M, Miyatake T: Abnormality of long-chain fatty acids in erythrocyte membrane sphingomyelin from patients with adrenoleukodystrophy. *J Neurochem* **36**:1046, 1981.
16. Moser HW, Moser AB, Powers JM, Nitowsky HM, Schaumburg HH, Norum RA, Migeon BR: The prenatal diagnosis of adrenoleukodystrophy. Demonstration of increased hexacosanoic acid in cultured amniocytes and fetal adrenal gland. *Pediatr Res* **16**:172, 1982.
17. Migeon BR, Moser HW, Moser AB, Axelman J, Sillence D, Norum RA: Adrenoleukodystrophy: Evidence for X-linkage, inactivation and selection favoring the mutant allele in heterozygous cells. *Proc Natl Acad Sci U S A* **78**:5066, 1981.
18. Aubourg P, Sack GH, Meyers DA, Lease JJ, Moser HW: Linkage of adrenoleukodystrophy to a polymorphic DNA probe. *Ann Neurol* **21**:349, 1987.
19. Aubourg P, Sack GH, Moser HW: Frequent alteration of visual pigment genes in adrenoleukodystrophy. *Am J Hum Genet* **42**:408, 1988.
20. Moser AB, Borel J, Odone A, Naidu S, Cornblath D, Sanders DB, Moser HW: A new dietary therapy for adrenoleukodystrophy: Biochemical and preliminary clinical results in 36 patients. *Ann Neurol* **21**:240, 1987.
21. Rizzo WB, Phillips MW, Dammann AL, Leshner RY, Jennings SVK: Adrenoleukodystrophy: Dietary oleic acid lowers hexacosanoate levels. *Ann Neurol* **21**:232, 1987.
22. Singh I, Moser AB, Moser HW, Kishimoto Y: Adrenoleukodystrophy: Impaired oxidation of very long chain fatty acids in white blood cells, cultured skin fibroblasts and amniocytes. *Pediatr Res* **18(3)**:286, 1984.
23. Rizzo WB, Avigan J, Chemke J, Schulman JD: Adrenoleukodystrophy: Very long-chain fatty acid metabolism in fibroblasts. *Neurology* **34**:163, 1984.
24. Poulos A, Singh H, Paton B, Sharp P, Derwas N: Accumulation and defective β-oxidation of very long chain fatty acids in Zellweger's syndrome, adrenoleukodystrophy and Refsum's disease variants. *Clin Genet* **29**:397, 1986.
25. Wanders RJA, van Roermond CWT, van Wijland MJA, Nijenhuis AA, Tromp A, Schutgens RBH, Brouwer-Kelder EM, Schram AW, Tager JM, van den Bosch H, Schalkwijk C: X-linked adrenoleukodystrophy: Defective peroxisomal oxidation of very long chain fatty acids but not of very long chain fatty acyl-CoA esters. *Clin Chim Acta* **165**:321, 1987.
26. Singh I, Moser AB, Goldfischer S, Moser HW: Lignoceric acid is oxidized in the peroxisomes: Implications for the Zellweger cerebro-hepato-renal syndrome and adrenoleukodystrophy. *Proc Natl Acad Sci U S A* **81**:4203, 1984.
27. Moser HW: Peroxisomal disorders. *J Pediatr* **108**:89, 1986.
28. Schutgens RBH, Heymans HSA, Wanders RJA, van den Bosch H, Tager JM: Peroxisomal disorders: A newly recognized group of genetic diseases. *Eur J Pediatr* **144**:430, 1986.

29. Wanders RJA, van Roermund CWT, van Wijland MJA, Schutgens RBH, van den Bosch H, Schram AW, Tager JM: Direct evidence that the deficient oxidation of very long chain fatty acids in X-linked adrenoleukodystrophy is due to an impaired ability of peroxisomes to activate very long chain fatty acids. *Biochem Biophys Res Commun* **153**:618, 1988.
30. Lazo O, Contreras M, Hashmi M, Stanley W, Irazu C, Singh I: Peroxisomal lignoceroyl-CoA ligase deficiency in childhood adrenoleukodystrophy and adrenomyeloneuropathy. *Proc Natl Acad Sci U S A* **85**:7647, 1988.
31. Mosser J, Douar A-M, Sarde C-O, Kioschis P, Feil R, Moser H, Poustka A-M, Mandel J-M, Aubourg P: Putative X-linked adrenoleukodystrophy gene shares unexpected homology with ABC transporters. *Nature* **361**:726, 1993.
32. Higgins CF: ABC transporters: From microorganisms to man. *Annu Rev Cell Biol* **8**:67, 1992.
33. Kobayashi T, Shinnoh N, Kondo A, Tamada T: Adrenoleukodystrophy protein-deficient mice represent abnormality of very long chain fatty acid metabolism. *Biochem Biophys Res Commun* **232**:631, 1997.
34. Lu J-F, Lawler AM, Watkins PA, Powers JM, Moser AB, Moser HW, Smith KD: A mouse model for X-linked adrenoleukodystrophy. *Proc Natl Acad Sci U S A* **94**:9366, 1997.
35. Forss-Petter S, Werner H, Berger J, Lassmann H, Molzer B, Schwab MH, Bernheimer H, Zimmermann F, Nave K-A: Targeted inactivation of the X-linked adrenoleukodystrophy gene in mice. *J Neurosci Res* **50**:829, 1997.
36. Budka H, Sluga E, Heiss WD: Spastic paraplegia associated with Addison's disease: Adult variant of adrenoleukodystrophy. *J Neurol* **213**:237, 1976.
37. Griffin JW, Goren E, Schaumburg H, Engel WK, Loriaux L: Adrenomyeloneuropathy: A probable variant of adrenoleukodystrophy. *Neurology* **27(12)**: 1107, 1977.
38. Schaumburg H, Powers JM, Raine CS, Spencer PS, Griffin JW, Prineas JW, Boehme DM: Adrenomyeloneuropathy: A probable variant of adrenoleukodystrophy. II. General pathologic, neuropathologic, and biochemical aspects. *Neurology* **27(12)**:1114, 1977.
39. Blaw ME, Vinken PJ, Bruyn CWE (eds): *Adrenoleukodystrophy*, vol 10. Amsterdam, North Holland, 1970, p 128.
40. Schaumburg HH, Powers JM, Raine CS, Suzuki K, Richardson EP: Adrenoleukodystrophy: A clinical and pathological study of 17 cases. *Arch Neurol* **33**:577, 1975.
41. Aubourg P, Chaussain JL, Dulac O, Arthuis M: Adrenoleukodystrophy in childhood: A review of 20 cases. *Arch Fr Pediatr* **39**:663, 1982.
42. Moser HW, Naidu S, Kumar AJ, Rosenbaum AE: The adrenoleukodystrophies. *CRC Crit Rev Neurobiol* **3**:29, 1987.
43. Loes DJ, Hite S, Moser HW, Stillman AE, Shapiro E, Lockman L, Latchaw RE, Krivit W: Adrenoleukodystrophy: A scoring method for brain MR observation. *Am J Neuroradiol* **15**:1761, 1994.
44. Korenke GC, Pouwels PJW, Frahm J, Hunneman DH, Stoeckler S, Krasemann E, Jost W, Hanefeld F: Arrested cerebral adrenoleukodystrophy: A clinical and proton MRS study in 3 patients. *Pediatr Neurol* **15**:103, 1996.
45. Pouwels PJW, Kruse B, Korenke GC, Mao X, Hanefeld FA, Frahm J: Quantitative proton magnetic resonance spectroscopy of childhood adrenoleukodystrophy. *Neuropediatrics* **29**:254, 1998.
46. Melhem ER, Breiter SN, Ulug AM, Raymond GV, Moser HW: Improved tissue characterization in adrenoleukodystrophy using magnetization transfer imaging. *Am J Radiol* **166**:689, 1996.
47. Pierpaoli C, Jezzard P, Basser PJ, Barnett A, DiChiro G: Diffusion tensor MR imaging of the human brain. *Radiology* **201**:637, 1996.
48. Mori S, Crain BJ, Chacko VP, van Zijl P: Three-dimensional tracking of axonal projections in the brain by magnetic resonance imaging. *Ann Neurol* **45**:265, 1999.
49. Kumar AJ, Koehler W, Kruse B, Naidu S, Bergin A, Edwin D, Moser HW: MR findings in adult-onset adrenoleukodystrophy. *Am J Neuroradiol* **16**:1227, 1995.
50. Powers JM, Schaumburg HH: A fatal cause of sexual inadequacy in men: Adrenoleukodystrophy. *J Urol* **124**:583, 1980.
51. Assies J, van Geel B, Barth P: Signs of testicular insufficiency in adrenomyeloneuropathy and neurologically asymptomatic X-linked adrenoleukodystrophy; a retrospective study. *Int J Androl* **20**:315, 1997.
52. O'Neill BP, Swanson JW, Brown III FR, Griffin JW, Moser HW: Familial spastic paraparesis: An adrenoleukodystrophy phenotype. *Neurology* **35**:1233, 1985.
53. Moser HW, Bergin A, Naidu S, Ladenson PW: Adrenoleukodystrophy: New aspects of adrenal cortical disease, in Nelson DHE (ed): *Endocrinology and Metabolism Clinics of North America: New Aspects of Adrenal Cortical Disease*, vol 20. Philadelphia, WB Saunders, 1991, p 297.
54. Brennemann W, Koehler W, Zierz S, Klingmuller D: Occurrence of adrenocortical insufficiency in adrenomyeloneuropathy. *Neurology* **47**:605, 1996.
55. Moser HW, Moser AB, Naidu S, Bergin A: Clinical aspects of adrenoleukodystrophy and adrenomyeloneuropathy. *Dev Neurosci* **13**:254, 1991.
56. Powers JM, Schaumburg HH, Gaffney CL: Klüver-Bucy syndrome caused by adrenoleukodystrophy. *Neurology* **30**:1131, 1980.
57. DeLong R: Case records of Massachusetts General Hospital. *N Engl J Med* **306**:282, 1982.
58. Kitchin W, Cohen-Cole SA, Mickel SF: Adrenoleukodystrophy: Frequency of presentation as a psychiatric disorder. *Biol Psychiatry* **22**:1375, 1987.
59. Garside S, Rosebush PI, Levinson AJ, Mazurek MF: Late-onset leukodystrophy associated with long-standing psychiatric symptoms. *J Clin Psychiatry* **60**:460, 1999.
60. Sadeghi-Nejad A, Senior B: Adrenomyeloneuropathy presenting as Addison's disease in childhood. *N Engl J Med* **322**:13, 1990.
61. Laureti S, Casucci G, Santeusanio F, Angeletti G, Aubourg P, Brunetti P: X-linked adrenoleukodystrophy is a frequent cause of idiopathic Addison's disease in young adult male patients. *J Clin Endocrinol Metab* **81**:470, 1996.
62. Jorge P, Quelhas D, Oliveira P, Pinto R, Nogueira A: X-linked adrenoleukodystrophy in patients with idiopathic Addison disease. *Eur J Pediatr* **153**:594, 1994.
63. Wise JE, Matalon R, Morgan AM, McCabe ERB: Phenotypic features of patients with congenital adrenal hypoplasia and glycerol kinase deficiency. *Am J Dis Child* **141**:744, 1987.
64. Wakefield MA, Brown RS: X-linked congenital Addison's disease. *Arch Dis Child* **56**:73, 1981.
65. Tateish J, Sato Y, Suetsugu M, Takshiba T: Adrenoleukodystrophy with olivopontocerebellar atrophy-like lesions. *Clin Neuropath* **5(1)**:34, 1986.
66. Walsh PJ: Adrenoleukodystrophy: Report of two cases with relapsing and remitting courses. *Arch Neurol* **37**:448, 1980.
67. Marsden CD, Obeso JA, Lang AE: Adrenoleukomyeloneuropathy presenting as spinocerebellar degeneration. *Neurology* **32**:1031, 1982.
68. Kuroda S, Kirano A, Yuasa S: Adrenoleukodystrophy: Cerebello-brainstem dominant case. *Acta Neuropath* **60**:149, 1983.
69. Kurihara M, Kumagai K, Yagishita S, Imai M, Watanabe M, Suzuki Y, Orii T: Adrenoleukomyeloneuropathy presenting as cerebellar ataxia in a young child: A probable variant of adrenoleukodystrophy. *Brain Dev* **15**:377, 1993.
70. Takada K, Onoda J, Takahashi K, Nakamura H, Taketomi T: An adult case of adrenoleukodystrophy with features of olivo-ponto-cerebellar atrophy. *Jpn J Exp Med* **57(1)**:53, 1987.
71. Ohno T, Tsuchida H, Fukuhara N, Yuasa T, Harayama H, Tsjui S, Miyatake T: Adrenoleukodystrophy: A clinical variant presenting as olivopontocerebellar atrophy. *J Neurol* **231**:167, 1984.
72. Afifi AK, Menenez X, Reed LA, Bell WA: Atypical presentation of X-linked childhood adrenoleukodystrophy with an unusual magnetic resonance imaging pattern. *J Child Neurol* **11**:497, 1996.
73. Young RSK, Ramer JC, Lehman R, Weidner W, Towfighi J, Moser HW: Adrenoleukodystrophy: Unusual CT appearance. *Arch Neurol* **39**:782, 1982.
74. Close PJ, Sinnott SJ, Nolan KT: Adrenoleukodystrophy: A case demonstrating unilateral abnormalities. *Pediatr Radiol* **23**:400, 1993.
75. Sundgren PC, Blennow G, Englund E, Holtas S: Adrenoleukodystrophy — Unusual CT and MR findings in two siblings. *Acta Radiol* **39**:77, 1998.
76. Farrell DF, Hamilton SR, Knauss TA, Sanocki E, Deeb SS: X-linked adrenoleukodystrophy: Adult cerebral variant. *Neurology* **43**:1518, 1993.
77. Van Geel BM, Assies J, Haverkort EB, Barth PG, Wanders RJA, Schutgens RBH, Keyser A, Zwetzloot CP: Delay in diagnosis of X-linked adrenoleukodystrophy. *Clin Neurol Neurosurg* **95**:115, 1993.
78. van Geel BM, Assies J, Weverling GJ, Barth PG: Predominance of the adrenomyeloneuropathy phenotype of X-linked adrenoleukodystrophy in the Netherlands: A survey of 30 kindreds. *Neurology* **44**:2343, 1994.
79. Bezman L, Moser HW: The incidence of X-linked adrenoleukodystrophy and the relative frequency of its phenotypes. *Am J Med Genet* **76**:415, 1998.

80. Restuccia D, Di Lazzaro V, Valeriani M, Oloviero A, Le Pera D, Colosimo C, Burdi N, Call M, Berini E, Di Biase A, Tonali D: Neurophysiological abnormalities in adrenoleukodystrophy carriers. Evidence of different degrees of central nervous system involvement. *Brain* **120**:1139, 1997.
81. Morariu MA, Chasan JL, Norum RA, Moser HW, Migeon BR: Adrenoleukodystrophy variant in a heterozygous female. *Neurology* **32**:A81, 1982.
82. Molzer B, Bernheimer H, Budka H, Pilz P, Toifl K: Accumulation of very long chain fatty acids is common to 3 variants of adrenoleukodystrophy. *J Neurol Sci* **51**:301, 1981.
83. Pilz P, Schiener P: Kombination von Morbus Addison und Morbus Schilder bei einer 43 Jahrigen Frau. *Acta Neuropathol* **26**:357, 1973.
84. Simpson RHW, Rodda J, Reinecke CJ: Adrenoleukodystrophy in a mother and son. *J Neurol Neurosurg Psychiatry* **50**:1165, 1987.
85. Gerhard L, Reinhardt V, Solbach HG: Zu morphologie un atiologie der encephalopathie bei morbus addison. *Verh Dtsch Ges Path* **54**:305, 1970.
86. Dumic M, Gubarev N, Sikic N, Roscher A, Plavsic V, Filipovic-Grcic B: Sparse hair and multiple endocrine disorders in two women heterozygous for adrenoleukodystrophy. *Am J Med Genet* **43**:829, 1992.
87. El-Deiry SS, Naidu S, Blevins LS, Ladenson PW: Assessment of adrenal function in women heterozygous for adrenoleukodystrophy. *J Clin Endocrinol Metabol* **82**:856, 1997.
88. Powers JM, Moser HW, Moser AB, Chan KMA, Elias SB, Norum RA: Pathological findings in adrenoleukodystrophy heterozygotes. *Arch Pathol Lab Med* **111**:151, 1987.
89. Dooley JM, Wright BA: Adrenoleukodystrophy mimicking multiple sclerosis. *Can J Neurol Sci* **12**:73, 1985.
90. Noetzel MJ, Landau WM, Moser HW: Adrenoleukodystrophy carrier state presenting as a chronic nonprogressive spinal cord disorder. *Arch Neurol* **44**:566, 1987.
91. Moser HW, Moser AB, Trojak JE, Supplee SW: The identification of female carriers for adrenoleukodystrophy. *J Pediatr* **103**:54, 1983.
92. Moser AB, Kreiter N, Bezman L, Lu S-E, Raymond GV, Naidu S, Moser HW: Plasma very long chain fatty acids in 3,000 peroxisome disease patients and 29,000 controls. *Ann Neurol* **45**:100, 1999.
93. Feigenbaum V, Lombard-Platet G, Guidoux S, Sarde C, Mandel JL, Aubourg P: Mutational and protein analysis of patients and heterozygous women with X-linked adrenoleukodystrophy. *Am J Hum Genet* **58**:1135, 1996.
94. Watkins PA, Gould SJ, Smith MA, Braiterman LT, Wei HM, Kok F, Moser AB, Moser HW, Smith KD: Altered expression of ALDP in X-linked adrenoleukodystrophy. *Am J Hum Genet* **57**:292, 1995.
95. Boehm CD, Cutting GR, Lachtermacher MB, Moser HW, Chong SS: Accurate DNA-based diagnostic and carrier testing for X-linked adrenoleukodystrophy. *Mol Genet Metab* **66**:128, 1999.
96. Watkiss E, Webb T, Bundey S: Is skewed X inactivation responsible for symptoms in female carriers for adrenoleukodystrophy. *J Med Genet* **30**:651, 1993.
97. Naidu S, Washington C, Thirumalai S, Smith KD, Moser HW, Watkins PA: X-chromosome inactivation in symptomatic heterozygotes of X-linked adrenoleukodystrophy. *Ann Neurol* **42**:498a, 1997.
98. Powers JM: Adrenoleukodystrophy (Adreno-testiculo-leuko-myelo-neuropathic-complex). *Clin Neuropathol* **4(5)**:181, 1985.
99. Powers JM, Moser HW: Peroxisomal disorders: Genotype, phenotype, major neuropathological lesions, and pathogenesis. *Brain Pathol* **8**:101, 1998.
100. Griffin DE, Moser HW, Mendoza Q, Moench T, O'Toole S, Moser AB: Identification of the inflammatory cells in the nervous system of patients with adrenoleukodystrophy. *Ann Neurol* **18**:660, 1985.
101. Powers JM, Liu Y, Moser A, Moser H: The inflammatory myelinopathy of adreno-leukodystrophy: Cells, effector molecules, and pathogenetic implications. *J Neuropathol Exp Neurol* **51(6)**:630, 1992.
102. Schaumburg HH, Powers JM, Suzuki K, Raine CS: Adrenoleukodystrophy (sex-linked Schilder disease): Ultrastructural demonstration of specific cytoplasmic inclusions in the central nervous system. *Arch Neurol* 31:210, 1974.
103. Powers JM, DeCiero DP, Ito M, Moser AB, Moser HW: Adrenomyeloneuropathy: A neuropathologic review featuring its noninflammatory myelopathy. *J Neuropathol Exp Neurol* **59(2)**:89, 2000.
104. Julien J, Vallat JM, Vital C, Lagueny A, Ferrer X, Darriet D: Adrenomyeloneuropathy: Demonstration of inclusions at the level of the peripheral nerve. *Eur Neurol* **20**:367, 1981.
105. Martin J-J, Ceuterick C, Libert J: Skin and conjunctival nerve biopsies in adrenoleukodystrophy and its variants. *Ann Neurol* **8(3)**:291, 1980.
106. Powers JM, Moser HW, Moser AB, Schaumburg HH: Fetal adrenoleukodystrophy: The significance of pathologic lesions in adrenal gland and testis. *Hum Pathol* **13**:1013, 1982.
107. Powers JM, Schaumburg HH: The testis in adrenoleukodystrophy. *Am J Pathol* **102(1)**:90, 1981.
108. Schaumburg H, Richardson EP, Johnson PC, Cohen RB, Powers JM, Raine CS: Schilder's disease: Sex-linked recessive transmission with specific adrenal changes. *Arch Neurol* **27**:458, 1972.
109. Rezanka T: Very long chain fatty acids from the animal and plant kingdoms. *Prog Lipid Res* **28**:147, 1989.
110. Brown III FR, Chen WW, Kirschner DA, Frayer KL, Powers JM, Moser AB, Moser HW: Myelin membrane from adrenoleukodystrophy brain white matter—Isolation and physical/chemical properties. *J Neurochem* **41**:341, 1983.
111. Wilson R, Sargent JR: Lipid and fatty acid composition of brain tissue from adrenoleukodystrophy patients. *J Neurochem* **61**:290, 1993.
112. Sargent JR, Coupland K, Wilson R: Nervonic acid and demyelinating disease. *Med Hypotheses* **42**:237, 1994.
113. Kishimoto Y, Moser HW, Suzuki K: Neurochemistry of adrenoleukodystrophy, in Lajtha AE: *The Handbook of Neurochemistry*, vol 10. New York, Plenum, 1984, p 125.
114. Menkes JH, Corbo LM: Adrenoleukodystrophy: Accumulation of cholesterol esters with very long chain fatty acids. *Neurology* **27**:928, 1977.
115. Ramsey RB, Banik NL, Davison AN: Adrenoleukodystrophy brain cholesteryl esters and other neutral lipids. *J Neurol Sci* **40**:189, 1979.
116. Moller JR, Yanagisawa K, Brady RO, Tourtellotte WW, Quarles RH: Myelin-associated glycoprotein in multiple sclerosis lesions: A quantitative and qualitative analysis. *Ann Neurol* **22(4)**:469, 1987.
117. Taketomi T, Hara A, Kitazawa N, Takada K, Nakamura H: An adult case of adrenoleukodystrophy with features of olivo-ponto-cerebellar atrophy: 2. Lipid abnormalities. *Jpn J Exp Med* **57**:59, 1987.
118. Theda C, Moser AB, Powers JM, Moser HW: Phospholipids in X-linked adrenoleukodystrophy white matter—Fatty acid abnormalities before the onset of demyelination. *J Neurol Sci* **110**:195, 1992.
119. Reinecke CJ, Knoll DP, Pretorius PJ, Steyn HS, Simpson RHW: The correlation between biochemical and histopathological findings in adrenoleukodystrophy. *J Neurol Sci* **70**:21, 1985.
120. Sharp P, Johnson D, Poulos A: Molecular species of phosphatidylcholine containing very long chain fatty acids in human brain: Enrichment in X-linked adrenoleukodystrophy brain and diseases of peroxisome biogenesis brain. *J Neurochem* **56**:30, 1991.
121. Bizzozero OA, Zuniga G, Lees MB: Fatty acid composition of human myelin proteolipid protein in peroxisomal disorders. *J Neurochem* **56**:872, 1991.
122. Igarashi M, Belchis D, Suzuki K: Brain gangliosides in adrenoleukodystrophy. *J Neurochem* **27**:327, 1976.
123. Norton WT, Poduslo ES: Myelination in rat brain: Method of myelin isolation. *J Neurochem* **21**:749, 1973.
124. Kishimoto Y, Moser HW, Kawamura N, Platt M, Pallante B, Fenselau C: Evidence that abnormal very long chain fatty acids of brain cholesterol esters are of exogenous origin. *Biochem Biophys Res Commun* **96**:69, 1980.
125. Moser HW, Pallante SL, Moser AE, Rizzo WB, Schulman JD, Fenselau C: Adrenoleukodystrophy: Origin of very long chain fatty acids and therapy. *Pediatr Res* **17**:293a, 1983.
126. Steinberg D, Mize CE, Avigan J, Fales HM, Eldjarn L, Try K, Stokke O, Refsum S: Studies on the metabolic error in Refsum's disease. *J Clin Invest* **40(3)**:313, 1967.
127. Brown III FR, Van Duyn MA, Moser AB, Schulman JD, Rizzo WB, Snyder RD, Murphy JV, Kamoshita S, Migeon CJ, Moser HW: Adrenoleukodystrophy: Effects of dietary restriction of very long chain fatty acids and of administration of carnitine and clofibrate on clinical status and plasma fatty acids. *Johns Hopkins Med J* **151**:164, 1982.
128. Murad S, Kishimoto Y: Chain elongation of fatty acid in brain: A comparison of mitochondrial and microsomal enzyme activities. *Arch Biochem Biophys* **185(2)**:300, 1978.
129. Volpe JJ, Vagelos RP: Mechanism and regulation of biosynthesis of saturated fatty acids. *Physiol Rev* **56**:339, 1976.
130. Bourre J-M, Daudu O, Baumann N: Nervonic acid biosynthesis by erucyl CoA elongation in normal and quaking mouse brain microsomes. Elongation of other unsaturated fatty acyl-CoAs (mono- and polyunsaturated). *Biochim Biophys Acta* **424**:1, 1976.
131. Christiansen N, Rortveilt T, Norum KR, Thomassen MS: Fatty acid chain elongation in rat small intestine. *Biochem J* **237**:293, 1986.
132. Cassagne C, Darriet D: Biosynthesis of very long chain fatty acids by the sciatic nerve of the rabbit. *FEBS Lett* **90(2)**:336, 1978.

133. Tsuji S, Ohno T, Miyatake T, Suzuki A, Yamakawa T: Fatty acid elongation activity in fibroblasts from patients with adrenoleukodystrophy (ALD). *J Biochem (Tokyo)* **96**:1241, 1984.
134. Yoshida S, Takeshita M: Analysis of the condensation step in elongation of very-long-chain saturated and tetraenoic fatty acyl-CoAs in swine cerebral microsomes. *Arch Biochem Biophys* **254(1)**:170, 1987.
135. Rizzo WB, Watkins PA, Phillips MW, Cranin D, Campbell B, Avigan J: Adrenoleukodystrophy: Oleic acid lowers fibroblast saturated C22-C26 fatty acids. *Neurology* **36**:357, 1986.
136. Ludwig SA, Sprecher H: Substrate specificity on the malonyl-CoA-dependent chain elongation of all-*cis* polyunsaturated fatty acid by rat liver microsomes. *Arch Biochem Biophys* **197**:333, 1979.
137. Lazarow PB, de Duve C: A fatty acyl-CoA oxidizing system in rat liver peroxisomes: Enhancement by clofibrate, a hypolipidemic drug. *Proc Natl Acad Sci U S A* **73(6)**:2043, 1976.
138. Osmundsen H, Thomassen MS, Hiltunen JK, Berge RK: Physiological role of peroxisomal beta-oxidation, in Fahimi HD, Sies HE (eds): *Peroxisomes in Biology and Medicine*. Berlin: Springer, 1987, p 152.
139. Moser AB, Singh I, Brown III FR, Solish GI, Kelly RI, Benke PJ, Moser HW: The cerebro-hepato-renal (Zellweger) syndrome: Increased levels and impaired degradation of very long chain fatty acids, and prenatal diagnosis. *N Engl J Med* **310**:1141, 1984.
140. Singh H, Derwas N, Poulos A: Very long chain fatty acid β-oxidation by rat liver mitochondria and peroxisomes. *Arch Biochem Biophys* **259(2)**:382, 1987.
141. Suzuki Y, Shimozawa N, Yajima S, Yamaguchi S, Orii T, Hashimoto T: Effects of sodium 2-[5-(4-chlorophenyl)pentyl]-oxirane-2-carboxylate (poca) on fatty acid oxidation in fibroblasts from patients with peroxisomal diseases. *Biochem Pharmacol* **41(3)**:453, 1991.
142. Singh H, Usher S, Poulos A: Mitochondrial and peroxisomal beta-oxidation of stearic and lignoceric acids by rat brain. *J Neurochem* **53(6)**:1711, 1989.
143. Singh RP, Singh I: Peroxisomal oxidation of lignoceric acid in rat brain. *Neurochem Res* **11**:281, 1986.
144. Wanders RJA, Tager JM: Peroxisomal fatty acid beta-oxidation in relation to adrenoleukodystrophy. *Dev Neurosci* **13**:262, 1991.
145. Hashimoto T: Individual peroxisomal beta-oxidation enzymes. *Ann N Y Acad Sci* **386**:5, 1982.
146. Watkins PA: Fatty acid activation. *Prog Lipid Res* **36(1)**:55, 1997.
147. Aas M: Organ and subcellular distribution of fatty acid activating enzymes in the rat. *Biochem Biophys Acta* **1(1)**:32, 1971.
148. Kornberg A, Pricer WE Jr: Enzymatic synthesis of the coenzyme A derivatives of long chain fatty acids. *J Biol Chem* **204**:329, 1953.
149. Tanaka T, Hosaka K, Hoshimaru M, Numa S: Purification and properties of long-chain acyl-coenzyme A synthetase from rat liver. *Eur J Biochem* **98**:165, 1979.
150. Singh I, Kang MS, Phillips LA: Lignoceryl CoA ligase activity in rat brain microsomal fraction. *Fed Proc* **41**:1192, 1982.
151. Singh H, Poulos A: Distinct long chain and very long chain fatty acyl CoA synthetases in rat liver peroxisomes and microsomes. *Arch Biochem Biophys* **266**:486, 1988.
152. Uchiyama A, Aoyama T, Kamijo K, Uchida Y, Kondo N, Orii T, Hashimoto T: Molecular cloning of cDNA encoding rat very long chain acyl-CoA synthetase. *J Biol Chem* **271(48)**:30360, 1996.
153. Singh I, Lazo O, Kremser K: Purification of peroxisomes and subcellular distribution of enzyme activities for activation and oxidation of very long chain fatty acids in rat brain. *Biochem Biophys Acta* **1170**:44, 1993.
154. Kalish JE, Chen CI, Gould SJ, Watkins PA: Peroxisomal activation of long and very long chain fatty acids in the yeast Pichia Pastoris. *Biochem Biophys Res Commun* **206**:335, 1995.
155. Watkins PA, Lu J-F, Steinberg SJ, Gould SJ, Smith KD, Braiterman LT: Disruption of the *Saccharomyces cerevisiae* FAT1 gene decreases very long chain fatty acyl-CoA synthetase activity and elevates intracellular very long chain fatty acid concentrations. *J Biol Chem* **273**:18210, 1998.
156. Singh I, Moser HW, Moser ABKY: Adrenoleukodystrophy: Impaired oxidation of long chain fatty acids in cultured skin fibroblasts. *Biochem Biophys Res Commun* **102**:1223, 1981.
157. Singh H, Derwas N, Poulos A: Very long chain fatty acid β-oxidation by subcellular fractions of normal and Zellweger syndrome skin fibroblasts. *Arch Biochem Biophys* **257(2)**:302, 1987.
158. Wanders RJA, van Roermund CWT, van Wijland MJA, Heikoop J, Schutgens RBH, Schram AW, Tager JM, van den Bosch H, Poll-The BT, Saudubray JM, Moser HW, Moser AB: Peroxisomal very long chain fatty acid β-oxidation in human skin fibroblasts: Activity in Zellweger syndrome and other peroxisomal disorders. *Clin Chim Acta* **166**:255, 1987.
159. Hashmi M, Stanley W, Singh I: Lignoceroyl-CoASH ligase: Enzyme defect in fatty acid beta-oxidation system in X-linked childhood adrenoleukodystrophy. *FEBS Lett* **196**:247, 1986.
160. Lazo O, Contreras M, Bhushan A, Stanley W, Singh I: Adrenoleukodystrophy: Impaired oxidation of fatty acids due to peroxisomal lignoceroyl-CoA ligase deficiency. *Arch Biochem Biophys* **270(2)**:722, 1989.
161. Wanders RJA, van Roermund CWT, van Wijland MJA, Schutgens RBH, Heikoops J, van den Bosch H, Schram AW, Tager JM: Peroxisomal fatty acid β-oxidation in relation to the accumulation of very long chain fatty acids in cultured skin fibroblasts from patients with Zellweger syndrome and other peroxisomal disorders. *J Clin Invest* **80**:1778, 1987.
162. Uchida Y, Kondo N, Orii T, Hashimoto T: Purification and properties of rat liver peroxisomal very long chain Acyl-CoA synthetase. *J Biochem* **119**:565, 1996.
163. Berger J, Truppe C, Neumann H, Forss-Petter S: cDNA cloning and mRNA distribution of a mouse very long chain acyl-CoA synthetase. *FEBS Lett* **425**:305, 1998.
164. Steinberg SJ, Wang SJ, Kim DG, Mihalik SJ, Watkins PA: Human very-long-chain acyl-CoA synthetase: Cloning, topography, and relevance to branched-chain fatty acid metabolism. *Biochem Biophys Res Commun* **257**:615, 1999.
165. Faergeman NJ, DiRusso CC, Elberger A, Knudsen J, Black P: Disruption of the *Saccharomyces cerevisiae* homologue to the murine fatty acid transport protein impairs uptake and growth on long-chain fatty acids. *J Biol Chem* **272(13)**:8531, 1997.
166. Watkins PA, Pevsner J, Steinberg SJ: Human very long chain acyl-CoA synthetase and two human homologs: Initial characterization and relationship to fatty acid transport protein. *Prostaglandins Leukot Essent Fatty Acids* **60**:323, 1999.
167. Steinberg SJ, Wang SJ, McGuinness MC, Watkins PA: Human liver-specific very long chain acyl-coenzyme A synthetase: cDNA cloning and characterization of a second enzymatically active protein. *Mol Genet Metab* **618(1)**:32, 1999.
168. Berger J, Truppe C, Neumann H, Forss-Petter S: A novel relative of the very long chain acyl-CoA synthetase and fatty acid transporter protein genes with a distinct expression pattern. *Biochem Biophys Res Commun* **247(2)**:255, 1998.
169. Hirsch D, Stahl A, Lodish HF: A family of fatty acid transporters conserved from mycobacterium to man. *Proc Natl Acad Sci U S A* **95(15)**:8625, 1998.
170. Schaap FG, Hamers L, Von der Vusse GJ, Glatz JFC: Molecular cloning of fatty acid-transport protein cDNA from rat. *Biochim Biophys Acta* **1354**:29, 1997.
171. Fitscher BA, Riedel HD, Young KC, Stremmel W: Tissue distribution and cDNA cloning of a human fatty acid transport protein (hsFATP4). *Biochim Biophys Acta* **1443**:381, 1998.
172. Schaffer JE, Lodish HF: Expression cloning and characterization of a novel adipocyte long chain fatty acid transport protein. *Cell* **79**:427, 1994.
173. Babbitt PC, Kenyon GL, Martin BM, Charest H, Slyvestre M, Scholten JC, Chang KH, Liang PH, Dunaway MD: Ancestry of the 4-chlorobenzoate dehalogenase: Analysis of amino acid sequence identities among families of acyl:adenyl/isomerases, and acyl-CoA thioesterases. *Biochemistry* **31(24)**:5594, 1992.
174. Black PN, Zhang Q, Weimar JD, DiRusso CC: Mutational analysis of a fatty acyl-coenzyme A synthetase signature motif identifies seven amino acid residues that modulate fatty acid substrate specificity. *J Biol Chem* **272**:4896, 1997.
175. Steinberg SJ, Kemp S, Braiterman LT, Watkins PA: Role of very long-chain acyl-CoA synthetase in X-linked adrenoleukodystrophy. *Ann Neurol* **46**:409, 1999.
176. Smith BT, Sengupta TK, Singh I: Intraperoxisomal localization of very long chain fatty acyl-CoA synthetase: Implication in X-adrenoleukodystrophy. *Exp Cell Res* **254**:309, 2000.
177. Lazo O, Contreras M, Singh I: Topographical localization of peroxisomal acyl-CoA ligases—Differential localization of palmitoyl-CoA and lignoceroyl-CoA ligases. *Biochemistry* **29(16)**:3981, 1990.
178. Coe NR, Smith AJ, Frohnert BI, Watkins PA, Bernlohr DR: The fatty acid transport protein (FATP1) is a very long chain acyl-CoA synthetase. *J Biol Chem* **274(51)**:36300, 1999.
179. Gargiulo CE, Stuhlsatz-Krouper SM, Schaffer JE: Localization of adipocyte long chain fatty acyl-CoA synthetase at the plasma membrane. *J Lipid Res* **40(5)**:881, 1999.

180. Stahl A, Hirsch DJ, Gimeno RE, Punreddy S, Ge P, Watson N, Patel S, Kotler M, Raimondi A, Tartaglia LA, Lodish HF: Identification of the major intestinal fatty acid transport protein. *Mol Cell* **4(3)**:299, 1999.
181. Choi JY, Martin CE: The *Saccharomyces cerevisiae* FAT1 gene encodes an acyl-CoA synthetase that is required for maintenance of very long chain fatty acid levels. *J Biol Chem* **274**:4671, 1999.
182. Tsuji S, Sano-Kawamura T, Ariga T, Miyatake T: Metabolism of (17,18-3H2) hexacosanoic acid and (15,16-3h2) lignoceric acid in cultured skin fibroblasts from patients with adrenoleukodystrophy (ALD) and adrenomyeloneuropathy (AMN). *J Neurol Sci* **71**:359, 1985.
183. Tsuji S, Sano T, Ariga T, Miyatake T: Increased synthesis of hexacosanoic acid (C26:0) by cultured skin fibroblasts from patients with adrenoleukodystrophy (ALD) and adrenomyeloneuropathy (AMN). *Biochem J (Tokyo)* **90**:1233, 1981.
184. Tanaka Y, Ando S, Tsuji S, Miyatake T: Enhanced synthesis of hexacosanoic acid in the cultured fibroblasts from patients with adrenoleukodystrophy. *Biomed Res* **9(6)**:451, 1988.
185. Koike R, Tsuji S, Ohno T, Suzuki Y, Orii T, Miyatake T: Physiological significance of fatty acid elongation system in adrenoleukodystrophy. *J Neurol Sci* **103**:188, 1991.
186. Kirk EP, Fletcher JM, Sharp P, Carey B, Poulos A: X-linked adrenoleukodystrophy: The Australasian experience. *Am J Med Genet* **76**:420, 1998.
187. Oberle I, Drayna D, Camerino G, White R, Mandel JL: The telomere of the human X-chromosome long arm: Presence of a highly polymorphic DNA marker and analysis of recombination frequency. *Proc Natl Acad Sci U S A* **82**:2824, 1985.
188. Willems PJ, Vits L, Wanders RJ, Coucke PJ, Van der Auwera BJ, Van Elsen AF, Raeymaekers P, Van Broeckhoven C, Schutgens RB, Dacremont G, et al: Linkage of DNA markers at Xq28 to adrenoleukodystrophy and adrenomyeloneuropathy present within the same family. *Arch Neurol* **47**:665, 1990.
189. Sarde C-O, Mosser J, Kioschis P, Kretz C, Vicaire S, Aubourg P, Poustka A, Mandel JL: Genomic organization of the adrenoleukodystrophy gene. *Genomics* **22**:13, 1994.
190. Smith KD, Kemp S, Braiterman LT, Lu J-F, Wei H-M, Geraghty M, Stetten G, Bergin JS, Pevsner J, Watkins PA: X-linked adrenoleukodystrophy: Genes, mutations, and phenotypes. *Neurochem Res* **24(4)**:521, 1999.
191. Cartier N, Lopez J, Moullier P, Rocchiccioli F, Rolland M-O, Jorge P, Mosser J, Mandel J-M, Bougneres P-F, Danos O, Aubourg P: Retroviral-mediated gene transfer corrects very-long-chain fatty acid metabolism in adrenoleukodystrophy fibroblasts. *Proc Natl Acad Aci U S A* **92**:1674, 1995.
192. Shinnoh N, Yamada T, Yoshimura T, Furuya H, Yoshida Y, Suzuki Y, Shimozawa N, Orii T, Kobayashi T: Adrenoleukodystrophy: The restoration of peroxisomal beta-oxidation by transfection of normal cDNA. *Biochem Biophys Res Commun* **210(3)**:830, 1995.
193. Braiterman LT, Zheng S, Watkins PA, Johnson G, Moser AB, Moser HW, Smith KD: Functional studies of the X-linked adrenoleukodystrophy protein. *Ann N Y Acad Sci* **84**:763, 1996.
194. Mosser J, Lutz Y, Stoeckel ME, Sarde C-O, Kretz C, Douar AM, Lopez J, Aubourg P, Mandel JL: The gene responsible for adrenoleukodystrophy encodes a peroxisomal membrane protein. *Hum Mol Genet* **3(2)**:265, 1994.
195. Takano H, Koika R, Onodera O, Sasaki R, Tsuji S: Mutational analysis and genotype-phenotype correlation of 29 unrelated Japanese patients with X-linked adrenoleukodystrophy (ALD). *Arch Neurol* **56**:295, 1999.
196. Kok F, Neumann S, Sarde C-O, Zheng S, Wu K-H, Wei H-M, Bergin J, Watkins PA, Gould S, Sack G, Moser H, Mandel J-L, Smith KD: Mutational analysis of patients with X-linked adrenoleukodystrophy. *Hum Mutat* **6**:104, 1995.
197. Ligtenberg MJL, Kemp S, Sarde C-O, van Geel BM, Kleijer WJ, Barth PJ, Mandel JL, van Oost A, Bolhuis PA: Spectrum of mutations in the gene encoding the adrenoleukodystrophy protein. *Am J Hum Genet* **56**:44, 1995.
198. Krasemann EW, Meier V, Korenke GC, Hunneman DH, Hanefeld F: Identification of mutations in the ALD-gene of 20 families with adrenoleukodystrophy/adrenomyeloneuropathy. *Hum Genet* **97**:194, 1996.
199. Dodd A, Rowland SA, Hawkes SLJ, Kennedy MA, Love DR: Mutations in the adrenoleukodystrophy gene. *Hum Mutat* **9**:500, 1997.
200. Gartner J, Braun A, Holzinger A, Roerig P, Lenard H-G, Roscher AA: Clinical and genetic aspects of X-linked adrenoleukodystrophy. *Neuropediatrics* **29**:3, 1998.
201. Korenke GC, Krasemann E, Meier V, Beuche W, Hunneman DH, Hanefeld F: First missense mutation (W679R) in exon 10 of the adrenoleukodystrophy gene in siblings with adrenomyeloneuropathy. *Hum Mutat* **1(Suppl)**:S204, 1998.
202. Holzinger A, Maier E, Stockler-Ipsiroglu S, Braun A, Roscher AA: Characterization of a novel mutation in exon 10 of the adrenoleukodystrophy gene. *Clin Genet* **53**:482, 1998.
203. Kemp S, Ligtenberg JL, van Geel BM, Barth PG, Wolterman RA, Schoute F, Sarde C-O, Mandel J-L, van Oost BA, Bolhuis PA: Identification of a two base pair deletion in five unrelated families with adrenoleukodystrophy: A possible hot spot for mutations. *Biochem Biophys Res Commun* **202(2)**:647, 1994.
204. Kemp S, Mooyer PAW, Bolhuis PA, van Geel BM, Mandel JL, Barth PG, Aubourg P, Wanders RJA: ALDP expression in fibroblasts of patients with X-linked adrenoleukodystrophy. *J Inherit Metab Dis* **19**:667, 1996.
205. Berger J, Molzer B, Fae I, Bernheimer H: X-linked adrenoleukodystrophy (ALD): A novel mutation of the ALD gene in 6 members of a family presenting with 5 different phenotypes. *Biochem Biophys Res Commun* **205**:1638, 1994.
206. Shani N, Valle D: A *Saccharomyces cerevisiae* homolog of the human adrenoleukodystrophy transporter is a heterodimer of two half ATP-binding cassette transporters. *Proc Natl Acad Sci U S A* **93**:11901, 1996.
207. Shani N, Sapag A, Valle D: Characterization and analysis of conserved motifs in a peroxisomal ATP-binding cassette transporter. *J Biol Chem* **271**:8725, 1996.
208. Kamijo K, Taketani S, Yokota S, Osumi T, Hashimoto T: The 70-kDa peroxisomal membrane protein is a member of the Mdr (P-glycoprotein)-related ATP-binding protein superfamily. *J Biol Chem* **265(8)**:4534, 1990.
209. Gartner J, Moser H, Valle D: Mutations in the 70K peroxisomal membrane protein gene in Zellweger syndrome. *Nat Genet* **1**:16, 1992.
210. Shani N, Steel G, Dean M, Valle D: Identification of a fourth half ABC transporter in the human peroxisomal membrane. *Hum Mol Genet* **6**:1925, 1997.
211. Holzinger A, Kammerer S, Roscher AA: Primary structure of human PMP69, a putative peroxisomal ABC-transporter. *Biochem Biophys Res Commun* **237(1)**:152, 1997.
212. Lombard-Platet G, Savary S, Sarde C-O, Mandel J-L, Chimini G: A close relative of the adrenoleukodystrophy (ALD) gene codes for a peroxisomal protein with a specific expression pattern. *Proc Natl Acad Sci U S A* **93**:1265, 1996.
213. Netik A, Forss-Petter S, Holzinger A, Molzer B, Unterrainer G, Berger J: Adrenoleukodystrophy-related protein can compensate functionally for adrenoleukodystrophy protein deficiency (X-ALD): Implications for therapy. *Hum Mol Genet* **8(5)**:907, 1999.
214. Broccardo C, Troffer-Charlier N, Savary S, Mandel JL, Chimini G: Exon organization of the mouse gene encoding the adrenoleukodystrophy related protein (ALDR). *Eur J Hum Genet* **6**:638, 1998.
215. Braun A, Kammerer S, Ambach H, Roscher AA: Characterization of a partial pseudogene homologous to the adrenoleukodystrophy gene and application to mutation detection. *Hum Mutat* **7**:105, 1996.
216. Kemp S, Wei H-M, Lu J-F, Braiterman LT, McGuinness MC, Watkins PA, Moser AB, Smith KD: Gene redundancy and pharmacological gene therapy: Potential for X-linked adrenoleukodystrophy. *Nat Med* **4**:1261, 1998.
217. Hettema EH, van Roermund CWT, Distel B, van den Berg M, Vilela C, Rodrigues-Pousada C, Wanders RJA, Tabak HF: The ABC transporter proteins Pat1 and Pat2 are required for import of long chain fatty acids into peroxisomes of *Saccharomyces cerevisiae*. *EMBO J* **15(15)**:3813, 1996.
218. Imanaka T, Aihara K, Takano T, Yamashita A, Sato R, Suzuki Y, Yokota S, Osumi T: Characterization of the 70-kDa peroxisomal membrane protein, an ATP binding cassette transporter. *J Biol Chem* **274(17)**:11968, 1999.
219. Braiterman LT, Zheng S, Watkins PA, Geraghty MT, Johnson G, McGuinness MC, Moser AB, Smith KD: Suppression of peroxisomal membrane protein defects by peroxisomal ATP binding cassette (ABC) proteins. *Hum Mol Genet* **7(2)**:239, 1998.
220. Shani N, Steel G, Dean M, Valle D: Four half ABC transporters may heterodimerize in the peroxisome membrane. *Am J Hum Genet* **59(Suppl 4)**:42A, 1996.
221. Valle D, Gartner J: Penetrating the peroxisome. *Nature* **361**:682, 1993.
222. Liu LX, Janvier K, Berteaux-Lecellier V, Cartier N, Benarous R, Aubourg P: Homo- and heterodimerization of peroxisomal ATP-binding cassette half-transporters. *J Biol Chem* **274(46)**:32738, 1999.

223. Aubourg P, Dubois-Dalcq M: X-linked adrenoleukodystrophy enigma: How does the ALD peroxisomal transporter mutation affect CNS glia? *Glia* **29(2)**:186, 2000.
224. Fouquet F, Zhou JM, Ralston E, Murray K, Troalen F, Magal E, Robain O, Dubois-Dalcq M, Aubourg P: Expression of the adrenoleukodystrophy protein in the human and mouse central nervous system. *Neurobiol Dis* **3**:271, 1997.
225. Pollard H, Moreau J, Aubourg P: Localization of mRNAs for adrenoleukodystrophy and the 70 kDa peroxisomal (PMP70) proteins in the rat brain during post-natal development. *J Neurosci Res* **42**:433, 1995.
226. Troffer-Charlier N, Doerflinger N, Metzger E, Fouquet F, Mandel J-L, Aubourg P: Mirror expression of adrenoleukodystrophy and adrenoleukodystrophy related genes in mouse tissues and human cell lines. *Eur J Cell Biol* **75**:254, 1998.
227. Doerflinger N, Miclea JM, Lopez J, Chommiene C, Bougneres P, Aubourg P, Cartier N: Retroviral transfer and long-term expression of the adrenoleukodystrophy gene in human CD34+ cells. *Hum Gene Ther* **9**:1025, 1998.
228. Braiterman LT, Watkins PA, Moser AB, Smith KD: Peroxisomal very long chain fatty acid beta-oxidation activity is determined by the level of adrenoleukodystrophy protein (ALDP) expression. *Mol Genet Metab* **66**:91, 1999.
229. Flavigny E, Sanhaj A, Aubourg P, Cartier N: Retroviral-mediated adrenoleukodystrophy-related gene transfer corrects very long chain fatty acid metabolism in adrenoleukodystrophy fibroblasts: Implications for therapy. *FEBS Lett* **448**:261, 1999.
230. Yamada T, Taniwaki T, Shinnoh N, Uchiyama A, Shimozawa N, Ohyagi Y, Asahara H, Kira J: Adrenoleukodystrophy protein enhances association of very long chain acyl-coenzyme A synthetase with the peroxisome. *Neurology* **52(3)**:614, 1999.
231. Contreras M, Mosser J, Mandel JL, Aubourg P, Singh I: The protein coded by the X-adrenoleukodystrophy gene is a peroxisomal integral membrane protein. *FEBS Lett* **344(2-3)**:211, 1994.
232. Aubourg P, Dubois-Dalcq M: X-linked adrenoleukodystrophy enigma: How does the ALD peroxisomal transporter mutation effect CNS glia? *Glia* **29**:186, 2000.
233. Min K-T, Benzer S: Preventing neurodegeneration in the *Drosophila* mutant bubblegum. *Science* **284**:1985, 1999.
234. Spector AA: Fatty acid binding to plasma albumin. *J Lipid Res* **16**:165, 1975.
235. Hamilton JA, Era S, Bhamidipati SP, Reed RG: Locations of the three primary binding sites for long-chain fatty acids on bovine serum albumin. *Proc Natl Acad Sci U S A* **88**:2051, 1991.
236. Ho JK, Moser H, Kishimoto Y, Hamilton JA: Interaction of very long chain fatty acid with model membranes and serum albumin: Implications for the pathogenesis of adrenoleukodystrophy. *J Clin Invest* **96**:1455, 1995.
237. Knazek RA, Rizzo WB, Schulman JD, Dave JR: Membrane microviscosity is increased in the erythrocytes of patients with adrenoleukodystrophy and adrenomyeloneuropathy. *J Clin Invest* **72**:245, 1983.
238. Whitcomb RW, Linehan WR, Knazek RA: Effects of long-chain, saturated fatty acids on membrane microviscosity and adrenocorticotropin responsiveness of human adrenocortical cells in vitro. *J Clin Invest* **81**:185, 1988.
239. Kobayashi T, Yamada T, Yasutake T, Shinnoh N, Goto I, Iwaki T: Adrenoleukodystrophy gene encodes an 80-kDa membrane protein. *Biochem Biophys Res Commun* **201**:1029, 1994.
240. Blevins LS, Shankroff J, Moser HW, Ladenson PW: Elevated plasma adrenocorticotropin concentration as evidence of limited adrenocortical reserve in patients with adrenomyeloneuropathy. *J Clin Endocrinol Metab* **78**:261, 1994.
241. Powers JM, Schaumburg HH, Johnson AB, Raine CS: A correlative study of the adrenal cortex in adrenoleukodystrophy: Evidence for a fatal intoxication with very long chain fatty acids. *Invest Cell Pathol* **3**:353, 1980.
242. Ogino T: Biochemical study of adrenoleukodystrophy (ALD). *Folia Psychiatr Neurol Japonica* **34(2)**:117, 1980.
243. Rutkowski JL, Kirk CJ, Lerner MA, Tennekoon GI: Purification and expansion of human Schwann cells in vitro. *Nat Med* **1(1)**:80, 1995.
244. Ishii S, Volpe JJ: Glycoprotein processing is required for completion but not initiation of oligodendroglial differentiation from its bipotential progenitor cell. *Dev Neurosci* **14**:221, 1992.
245. Bernheimer H, Budka H, Muller P: Brain tissue immunoglobulins in adrenoleukodystrophy: A comparison with multiple sclerosis and systemic lupus erythematosus. *Acta Neuropathol (Berl)* **59**:95, 1983.
246. McGuinness MC, Griffin DE, Raymond GV, Washington CA, Moser HW, Smith KD: Tumor necrosis factor-alpha and X-linked adrenoleukodystrophy. *J Neuroimmunol* **61**:161, 1995.
247. McGuinness MC, Powers JM, Bias WB, Schmeckpeper BJ, Segal AH, Gowda VC, Wesselingh SL, Berger J, Griffin DE, Smith KD: Human leukocyte antigens and cytokine expression in cerebral inflammatory demyelinative lesions of X-linked adrenoleukodystrophy and multiple sclerosis. *J Neuroimmunol* **75**:174, 1997.
248. Gilg AG, Pahan K, Singh AK, Singh I: Inducible nitric oxide synthase in the central nervous system of patients with X-linked adrenoleukodystrophy. *J Neuropathol Exp Neurol* (In press), 2000.
249. Beutler B, Cerami A: The history, properties, and biological effects of cachectin [Review]. *Biochemistry* **27**:7575, 1988.
250. Pestronk A: Motor neuropathies, motor neuron disorders, and antiglycolipid antibodies. *Muscle Nerve* **14**:927, 1991.
251. Inoue A, Koh C-S, Yanagisawa N, Taketomi T, Ishihara Y: Suppression of Theiler's murine encephalomyelitis virus induced demyelinating disease by administration of gangliosides. *J Immunol* **64**:45, 1996.
252. Kannagi R, Nudelman E, Hakomori S-I: Possible role of ceramide in defining structure and function of membrane glycolipids. *Proc Natl Acad Sci U S A* **79**:3470, 1982.
253. Ladish S, Li R, Olson E: Ceramide structure predicts tumor ganglioside immunosuppressive activity. *Proc Natl Acad Sci U S A* **91**:1974, 1994.
254. Levine SR, Welch KMA: Antiphospholipid antibodies. *Ann Neurol* **26(3)**:386, 1989.
255. Warren KG, Catz I, Johnson E, Mielke B: Anti-myelin basic protein and anti-proteolipid protein specific forms of multiple sclerosis. *Ann Neurol* **35**:280, 1994.
256. Moser HW, Moser AB, Smith KD, Bergin A, Borel J, Shankroff J, Stine OC, Merette C, Ott J, Krivit W, Shapiro E: Adrenoleukodystrophy: Phenotypic variability: Implications for therapy. *J Inherit Metab Dis* **15**:645, 1992.
257. Smith KD, Sack G, Beaty T, Bergin A, Naidu S, Moser A, Moser HW: A genetic basis for the multiple phenotypes of X-linked adrenoleukodystrophy. *Am J Hum Genet* **49**:165, 1991.
258. Maestri NE, Beaty TH: Predictions of a 2-locus model for disease heterogeneity: Applications to adrenoleukodystrophy. *Am J Hum Genet* **44**:576, 1992.
259. Korenke GC, Fuchs S, Krasemann E, Doerr HG, Wilichowski E, Hunneman DH, Hanefeld F: Cerebral adrenoleukodystrophy (ALD) in only one of monozygotic twins with an identical ALD genotype. *Ann Neurol* **40**:254, 1996.
260. Sobue G, Ueno-Natsukari I, Okamoto H, Connell TA, Aizawa I, Mizoguchi K, Honma M, Ishiwaka G, Mitsuma T, Natsukari N: Phenotypic heterogeneity of an adult form of adrenoleukodystrophy in monozygotic twins. *Ann Neurol* **36**:912, 1994.
261. Jimenez-Sanchez G: Targeted disruption of mammalian peroxisomal ABC transporters. Johns Hopkins University, School of Medicine, Baltimore, MD, PhD 1998.
262. Oelkers W: Adrenal insufficiency. *N Engl J Med* **355**:1206, 1996.
263. Allgrove J, Clayden GS, Grant DB: Familial glucocorticoid deficiency with achalasia of the cardia and deficient tear production. *Lancet* **1**:1284, 1978.
264. Weber A, Wienker TF, Jung M, Easton D, Dean HJ, Heinrichs C, Reis A, Clark AJL: Linkage of the gene for the triple A syndrome to chromosome 12q13 near the type II keratin gene cluster. *Hum Mol Genet* **5**:2061, 1996.
265. Aubourg P, Bougneres PF, Rocchiccioli F: Capillary gas-liquid chromatographic-mass spectrometric measurement of very long chain (C22 to C26) fatty acids in microliter samples of plasma. *J Lipid Res* **26**:263, 1985.
266. Antoku Y, Sakai T, Goto I, Iwashita H, Kuroiwa Y: Adrenoleukodystrophy: Abnormality of very long-chain fatty acids in the erythrocyte membrane phospholipids. *Neurology* **34**:1499, 1984.
267. Molzer B, Bernheimer H, Heller R, Toifl K, Vetterlein M: Detection of adrenoleukodystrophy by increased C26:0 fatty acid levels in leukocytes. *Clin Chim Acta* **125**:299, 1982.
268. Antoku Y, Ohtsuka Y, Nagara H, Sakai T, Tsukamoto K, Iwashita H, Goto I: A comparison of erythrocytes, lymphocytes and blood plasma as samples in fatty acid analysis for the diagnosis of adrenoleukodystrophy. *J Neurol Sci* **94(1-3)**:193, 1989.
269. Nishio H, Kodama S, Yokoyama S, Matsuo T, Mio T, Sumino K: A simple method to diagnose adrenoleukodystrophy using a dried blood spot on filter paper. *Clin Chim Acta* **159**:77, 1986.
270. Kawamura N, Moser AB, Moser HW, Ogino T, Suzuki K, Schaumburg H, Milunsky A, Murphy J, Kishimoto Y: High concentration of

hexacosanoate in cultured skin fibroblast lipids from adrenoleukodystrophy patients. *Biochem Biophys Res Commun* **82**:114, 1978.

271. Sakai T, Antoku Y, Goto I, Ochiai J, Iwashita H, Kuroiwa Y, Katafuchi Y: Very long-chain fatty acids in neutral lipids and glycerophospholipids of adrenoleukodystrophy-cultured skin fibroblasts. *J Neurol Sci* **71**:301, 1985.
272. Moser AB, Moser HW: The prenatal diagnosis of X-linked adrenoleukodystrophy. *Prenat Diag* **19**:46, 1999.
273. Askanas V, McLaughlin J, Engel WK, Adornato BT: Abnormalities in cultured muscle and peripheral nerve of a patient with adrenomyeloneuropathy. *N Engl J Med* **301(11)**:588, 1979.
274. Moser HW, Moser AB: Measurements of saturated very long chain fatty acids in plasma, in Hommes F (ed): *Techniques in Diagnostic Human Biochemical Genetics*, Chap 12. New York, Wiley-Liss, 1991, p 177.
275. Verhoeven NM, Kulik W, Van den Heuvel CMM, Jacobs C: Pre- and post-natal diagnosis of peroxisomal disorders using stable-isotope dilution gas chromatography-mass spectrometry. *J Inherit Metab Dis* **18**:45, 1995.
276. Vreken P: Rapid stable isotype dilution analysis of very long chain fatty acids, pristanic acid, and phytanic acid using gas chromatography-electron impact mass spectrometry. *J Chromatog* **713**:218, 1998.
277. Alberghina M, Fiumara A, Pavone L, Giuffrida AM: Determination of C20-C30 fatty acids by reversed-phase chromatographic techniques: An efficient method to quantitate minor fatty acids in serum of patients with adrenoleukodystrophy. *Neurochem Res* **9(12)**:1719, 1984.
278. Zamir I: Derivatization of saturated long-chain fatty acids with phenacyl bromide in non-ionic micelles. *J Chromatogr* **586**:347, 1991.
279. Kobayashi T, Katayama M, Suzuki S, Tomoda H, Goto I, Kuroiwa Y: Adrenoleukodystrophy: Detection of increased very long chain fatty acids by high-performance liquid chromatography. *J Neurol* **230**:209, 1983.
280. Ruiz M, Coll MJ, Pampols T, Giros M: ALDP expression in fetal cells and its application in prenatal diagnosis of X-linked adrenoleukodystrophy. *Prenat Diag* **17**:651, 1997.
281. Ligtenberg MJL, Kemp S, Sarde CO, van Geel BM, Kleijer WJ, Barth PJ, Mandel JL, van Oost A, Bolhuis PA: Spectrum of mutations in the gene encoding the adrenoleukodystrophy protein. *Am J Hum Genet* **56**:44, 1995.
282. Boles DJ, Craft DA, Padgett DA, Loria RM, Rizzo WB: Clinical variation in X-linked adrenoleukodystrophy—Fatty acid and lipid metabolism in cultured fibroblasts. *Biochem Med Metab Biol* **45(1)**:74, 1991.
283. Theda C, Woody RC, Naidu S, Moser AB, Moser HW: Increased very long chain fatty acids in patients on a ketogenic diet: A cause of diagnostic confusion. *J Pediatr* **122**:724, 1993.
284. Miyajima H, Adachi J, Tatsuno Y, Takahashi Y, Fujimoto M, Kaneko E, Gitlin JD: Increased very long-chain fatty acids in erythrocyte membranes of patients with aceruloplasminemia. *Neurology* **50**:130, 1998.
285. Miwa A, Adachi J, Mizuno K, Tatsuno Y: Very long-chain fatty acid pattern in crush syndrome patients in the Kobe earthquake. *Clin Chim Acta* **258**:125, 1997.
286. Laryea MD, Jiang YF, Xu GL, Lombeck I: Fatty acid composition of blood lipids in Chinese children consuming high erucic acid rapeseed oil. *Ann Nutr Metab* **36**:273, 1992.
287. Moser AB, Jones DS, Raymond GV, Moser HW: Plasma and red blood cell fatty acids in peroxisomal disorders. *Neurochem Res* **24(2)**:187, 1999.
288. Kennedy CR, Allen JT, Fensom AH, Steinberg SJ, Wilson R: X-linked adrenoleukodystrophy with non-diagnostic plasma very long chain fatty acids. *J Neurol Neurosurg Psych* **57**:759, 1994.
289. Wanders RJA, van Roermund CWT, Lageweg W, Jakobs BS, Schutgens RBH, Nijenhuis AA, Tager JM: X-linked adrenoleukodystrophy: Biochemical diagnosis and enzyme defect. *J Inherit Metab Dis* **15**:634, 1992.
290. McGuinness MC, Moser AB, Moser HW, Watkins PA: Peroxisomal disorders: Complementation analysis using beta-oxidation of very long chain fatty acids. *Biochem Biophys Res Commun* **172(1)**:364, 1990.
291. Carey WF, Poulos A, Sharp P, Nelson PV, Robertson EF, Hughes JL, Gill A: Pitfalls in the prenatal diagnosis of peroxisomal beta oxidation defects by chorionic villus sampling. *Prenat Diag* **14**:813, 1994.
292. Gray RGF, Green A, Cole T, Davidson V, Giles M, Schutgens RBH, Wanders RJA: A misdiagnosis of X-linked adrenoleukodystrophy in cultured chorionic villus cells by the measurement of very long chain fatty acids. *Prenat Diag* **15**:486, 1995.
293. Wanders RJA, Mooyer PW, Decker C, Vreken P: X-linked adrenoleukodystrophy: Improved prenatal diagnosis using both biochemical and immunological methods. *J Inherit Metab Dis* **21**:285, 1998.
294. Maier EM, Roscher AA, Kammerer S, Mehnert K, Conzelmann E, Holzinger A: Prenatal diagnosis of X-linked adrenoleukodystrophy combining biochemical, immunocytochemical and DNA analyses. *Prenat Diagn* **19**:364, 1999.
295. Imamura A, Suzuki Y, Song XQ, Fukao T, Shimozawa N, Orii T, Kondo N: Prenatal diagnosis of adrenoleukodystrophy by means of mutation analysis. *Prenat Diagn* **16**:259, 1996.
296. Eiben RM, DiChiro G: Computer assisted tomography in adrenoleukodystrophy. *J Comput Assist Tomogr* **1(3)**:308, 1977.
297. Greenberg HS, Halverson D, Lane B: CT scanning and diagnosis of adrenoleukodystrophy. *Neurology* **27**:884, 1977.
298. DiChiro G, Eiben RM, Manz HJ, Jacobs IB, Schellinger D: A new CT pattern in adrenoleukodystrophy. *Radiology* **137(3)**:687, 1980.
299. Duda EE, Huttenlocher PR: Computed tomography in adrenoleukodystrophy: Correlation of radiological and histological findings. *Radiology* **120**:349, 1976.
300. Aubourg P, Diebler C: Adrenoleukodystrophy—Its diverse CT appearances and an evolutive or phenotypic variant: The leukodystrophy without adrenal insufficiency. *Neuroradiology* **24**:33, 1982.
301. Van der Knaap MS, Valk J: *Magnetic Resonance of Myelin, Myelination, and Myelin Disorders*, 2d ed. Berlin, Springer, 1995, p 216.
302. Bewermeyer H, Bamborschke S, Ebhardt G, Hunermann B, Heiss WD: MR imaging in adrenoleukomyeloneuropathy. *J Comput Assist Tomogr* **9(4)**:793, 1985.
303. Aubourg P, Adamsbaum C, Lavallard-Rosseau MC, Lemaitre A, Boureau F, Mayer M, Kalifa G: Brain MRI and electrophysiologic abnormalities in preclinical and clinical adrenomyeloneuropathy. *Neurology* **42**:85, 1992.
304. Aubourg P, Sellier N, Chaussain JL, Kalifa G: MRI detects cerebral involvement in neurologically asymptomatic patients with adrenoleukodystrophy. *Neurology* **39(12)**:1619, 1989.
305. Kumar GS, Das UN, Kumar KV, Madhavi N, Das NP, Tan BKH: Effect of n-6 and n-3 fatty acids on the proliferation of human lymphocytes and their secretion of the TNF-a and IL-2 in vitro. *Nutr Res* **12**:815, 1992.
306. Kruse B, Barker PD, van Zijl PCM, Duyn JH, Moonen CTW, Moser HW: Multislice proton MR spectroscopic imaging in X-linked adrenoleukodystrophy. *Ann Neurol* **36**:595, 1994.
307. Rajanayagam V, Grad J, Krivit W, Loes DJ, Lockman L, Shapiro E, Baltazor M, Aeppli D, Stillman AE: Proton MR spectroscopy of childhood adrenoleukodystrophy. *Am J Neuroradiol* **17**:1013, 1996.
308. Tourbah A, Stievenart JL, Iba-Zizen MT, Lubetzki C, Baumann N, Eymard B, Moser HW: Localized proton magnetic resonance spectroscopy in patients with adult adrenoleukodystrophy. *Arch Neurol* **54**:586, 1997.
309. Confort-Gouny S, Vion-Dury J, Nicoli E, Cozzone PJ: Localized proton magnetic resonance spectroscopy in X-linked adrenoleukodystrophy. *Paediatr Neuroradiol* **37**:568, 1995.
310. Tzika AA, Ball WS Jr Vigneron DB, Dunn RS, Nelson SJ, Kirks DR: Childhood adrenoleukodystrophy: Assessment with proton MR spectroscopy. *Radiology* **189**:467, 1993.
311. Dubois PJ, Freemark M, Lewis D, Drayer BP, Heinz ER, Osborne D: Atypical findings in adrenoleukodystrophy. *J Comput Assist Tomogr* **5(6)**:888, 1981.
312. Melhem ER, Barker PB, Raymond GV, Moser HW: Review of genetic, clinical, and MR imaging characteristics. *Am J Roentgenol* **173**:1575, 1999.
313. Huckman MS, Wong PWK, Sullivan T, Zeller P, Geremia GK: Magnetic resonance imaging compared with computed tomography in adrenoleukodystrophy. *Am J Dis Child* **140**:1001, 1986.
314. Castellote A, Vera J, Vazques E, Riug M, Belmonte JA, Rovirs A: MR in adrenoleukodystrophy: Atypical presentation as bilateral frontal demyelination. *Am J Neuroradiol* **16**:814, 1993.
315. MacDonald JT, Stauffer AE, Heitoff K: Adrenoleukodystrophy: Early frontal lobe involvement on computed tomography. *J Comput Assist Tomogr* **8(1)**:128, 1984.
316. Birken DJ, Oldendorf WH: N-acetyl-L aspartic: A literature review of a compound prominent in ^{1}H NMR spectroscopic studies of brain. *Neurosci Biobehav Rev* **13**:23, 1989.
317. Bhakoo KK, Pearce JD: In vitro expression of *N*-acetyl aspartate by oligodendrocytes: Implications for proton magnetic resonance spectroscopy signal in vivo. *J Neurochem* **74**:254, 2000.
318. van der Knaap M, Valk J: *Magnetic Resonance of Myelin, Myelination, and Myelin Disease*, 2d ed. Berlin, Springer, 1995.
319. Brand A, Richter-Landsberg C, Leibfritz D: Multinuclear NMR studies on the energy metabolism of glial and neuronal cells. *Dev Neurosci* **15**:289, 1993.

320. Rees LH, Grant DB, Wilson J: Plasma corticotrophin levels in Addison-Schilder's disease. *BMJ* **3**:201, 1975.
321. Brennemann W, Koehler W, Zierz S, Klingmueller D: Testicular dysfunction in adrenomyeloneuropathy. *Eur J Endocrinol* **137**:34, 1997.
322. Assies J, vanGeel B, Barth P: Low dehydroepiandrosterone sulphate (DHEAS) levels in X-linked adrenoleukodystrophy. *Clin Endocrinol* **49(5)**:691, 1998.
323. Rook GA, Hernandez-Pando R, Lightman SL: Hormones, peripherally activated prohormones and the regulation of the Th1/Th2 balance. *Immunol Today* **15**:301, 1994.
324. Shimizu H, Moser HW, Naidu S: Auditory brainstem response and audiologic findings in adrenoleukodystrophy: Its variant and carrier. *Otolaryngol Head Neck Surg* **98(3)**:215, 1988.
325. Garg BP, Markand ON, DeMyer WE, Warren C: Evoked response studies in patients with adrenoleukodystrophy and heterozygous relatives. *Arch Neurol* **40**:356, 1983.
326. Moloney JBM, Masterson JG: Detection of adrenoleukodystrophy carriers by means of evoked potentials. *Lancet* **2**:852, 1982.
327. Kaplan PW, Tusa RJ, Shankroff J, Heller JE, Moser HW: Visual evoked potentials in adrenoleukodystrophy: A trial with Lorenzo Oil. *Ann Neurol* **34(2)**:169, 1993.
328. Krivit W, Shapiro E, Lockman L, Torres F, Stillman A, Moser A, Moser H: Recommendations for treatment of childhood cerebral form of adrenoleukodystrophy, in Hobbs JR, Riches PGE (eds): *Correction of Certain Genetic Diseases by Transplantation*. London: Cogent Trust, 1992, p 38.
329. Chaudhry V, Moser HW, Cornblath DR: Nerve conduction studies in adrenomyeloneuropathy. *J Neurol Neurosurg Psychiatr* **61**:181, 1996.
330. Van Geel BM, Koelman HTM, Barth PG, Ongerboer de Visser BW: Peripheral nerve abnormalities in adrenomyeloneuropathy: A clinical and electrodiagnostic study. *Neurology* **46**:112, 1996.
331. Kaplan PW, Tusa RJ, Rignani E, Moser HW: Somatosensory evoked potentials in adrenomyeloneuropathy. *Neurology* **48**:1662, 1997.
332. Battaglia A, Harden A, Pampiglione G, Walsh P: Adrenoleukodystrophy: Neurophysiological aspects. *J Neurol Neurosurg Psychiatry* **44**:781, 1981.
333. Mamoli B, Graf M, Toifl K: EEG, pattern-evoked potentials and nerve conduction velocity in a family with adrenoleukodystrophy. *Electroencephalogr Clin Neurophysiol* **14**:411, 1979.
334. Shapiro EG, Klein KA: Dementia in childhood: Issues in neuropsychological assessment with application to the natural history and treatment of degenerative storage diseases, in Tramontana MG, Hooer SRE (eds): *Advances in Child Neuropsychology*. New York, Springer-Verlag, 1994, p 119.
335. Aubourg P: X-linked adrenoleu kodystrophy, in Moser H, Vinken OJ, Bruyn GWE (eds) *Handbook of Clinical Neurology*, vol 22. Amsterdam, Elsevier, 1996.
336. Shapiro E, Lockman L, Balthazor M, Loes D, Rajanygam V, Ziegler R, Peters C, Krivit W: Neuropsychological and neurologic function and quality-of-life before and after bone marrow transplantation for adrenoleukodystrophy, in Ringdon O, Hobbs JR, Steward CG (eds): *Correction of Genetic Diseases by Transplantation IV*. London, Cogent Trust, 1997, p 52.
337. Wechsler D: *Wechsler Preschool and Primary Scale of Intelligence (WPPSI-R), revised*. San Antonio, The Psychological Corporation, 1989.
338. Wechsler D: *Wechsler Intelligence Scale for Children (WISC III)*, 3rd ed. San Antonio, The Psychological Corporation, 1991.
339. Wechsler D: *Wechsler Adult Intelligence Scale (WAIS III)*, 3rd ed. San Antonio, The Psychological Corporation, 1997.
340. Benton AL, Hamsher K, Varney N, Spreen O: *Judgment of Line Orientation. Contributions to Neuropsychological Assessment*. New York, Oxford University Press, 1983.
341. Rey A: L'examen psychologique dans les cas d'encephalopatie traumatique. *Arch Psychol* **28**:268, 1941.
342. Thorndike TL, Kagen EP, Sattler JM: *Stanford Binet Intelligence Scale*, 4th ed. Chicago, Riverside Publishing, 1986.
343. Schmidt M: *Rey Auditory and Verbal Learning Test: A Handbook*. Los Angeles, CA, Western Psychological, 1996.
344. Golden CJ: *Stroop Color and Word Test*. Chicago, Stoelting, 1978.
345. Greenberg LM: *Test of Variables of Attention (TOVA)*. Los Alamitos, CA, Universal Attention Disorders, 1989.
346. Martin JJ, Ceuteric C, Martin L: Skin and conjunctival biopsies in adrenoleukodystrophy. *Acta Neuropathol* **38**:247, 1977.
347. Martin JJ, Ceuteric C: Morphological study of skin biopsy specimens: A contribution to the diagnosis of metabolic disorders with involvement of the nervous system. *J Neurol Neurosurg Psychiatry* **41**:232, 1978.
348. Arsenio Nunes ML, Goutieres F, Aicardi J: An ultramicroscopic study of skin and conjunctival biopsies in chronic neurological disorders of childhood. *Ann Neurol* **9**:163, 1981.
349. Brown FRI, Stowens DW, Harris JC Jr, Moser HW: The leukodystrophies, in Johnson RTE (ed): *Current Therapy in Neurologic Disease*. Philadelphia, Decker, 1985, p 313.
350. Middel B, Kuipera-Upmeyer H, Bouma J, Staal M, Oenema D, Postma T, Terpstra S, Stewart R: Effect of intrathecal baclofen delivered by an implanted programmed pump on health related quality of life in patients with severe spasticity. *J Neurol Neurosurg Psychiatry* **63**:204, 1997.
351. Menza MA, Blake J, Goldberg L: Affective symptoms and adrenoleukodystrophy: A report of two cases. *Psychosomatics* **29(4)**:442, 1988.
352. Derry FA, Dinsmore WW, Fraser M, Gardner BP, Glass CA, Maytom MC, Smith MD: Efficacy and safety of oral sildenafil (Viagra) in men with erectile dysfunction caused by spinal cord injury. *Neurology* **51**:1629, 1998.
353. Moser HW, Tutschka PJ, Brown FR III, Moser AB, Yeager AM, Singh I, Mark SA, Kumar AJ, McDonnell JM, White CL, Maumenee IH, Green WR, Powers JM, Santos GW: Bone marrow transplant in adrenoleukodystrophy. *Neurology* **34**:1410, 1984.
354. Aubourg P, Blanche S, Jambaque I, Rocchiccioli F, Kalifa G, Naud-Saudreau C, Rolland M-O, Debre M, Chaussain JL, Griscelli C, Fischer A, Bougneres P-F: Reversal of early neurologic and neuroradiologic manifestations of X-linked adrenoleukodystrophy by bone marrow transplantation. *N Engl J Med* **322**:1860, 1990.
355. Krivit W, Lockman LA, Watkins PA, Hirsch J, Shapiro EG: The future for treatment by bone marrow transplantation for adrenoleukodystrophy, metachromatic leukodystrophy, globoid cell leukodystrophy and Hurler syndrome. *J Inherit Metab Dis* **18**:398, 1995.
356. Loes DJ, Stillman AE, Hite S, Shapiro E, Lockman L, Latchaw RE, Moser HW, Krivit W: Childhood cerebral form of adrenoleukodystrophy: Short-term effect of bone marrow transplantation on brain MR observations. *Am J Neuroradiol* **15**:1767, 1994.
357. Malm G, Ringden O, Anvert M, von Doblen U, Hagenfeeldt L, Isberg B, Knuutila S, Nennesmo I, Winiarski J, Marcus C: Treatment of adrenoleukodystrophy with bone marrow transplantation. *Acta Paed* **86**:484, 1997.
358. Shapiro EKW, Lockman L, Jambaque I, Peters C, Cowan M, Harris R, Bordigoni P, Loes D, Moser H, Fisher A, Aubourg P: Long-term beneficial effect bone marrow transplantation for childhood onset cerebral X-linked adrenoleukodystrophy. *Lancet* **356**:713, 2000.
359. Nowaczyk MJM, Saunders EF, Tein I, Blaser SI, Clarke JTR: Immunoablation does not delay the neurologic progression of X-linked adrenoleukodystrophy. *J Pediatr* **131**:453, 1997.
360. Baker KS, Leslie N, Ris MD, Fogelson MH, Caraway B, Ball W, Farris RE: Matched unrelated bone marrow transplantation for X-linked adrenoleukodystrophy, in Hobbs JR, Riches PG (eds): *Correction of Certain Genetic Diseases by Transplantation*. Ruislip, U.K., Cogent Trust, 1991, p 50.
361. Walkley SU, Thrall MA, Dobrenis K, Hunang M, March PA, Siegel DA, Wurzelman S: Bone marrow transplantation corrects the enzyme defect in neurons in the central nervous system in a lysosomal storage disease. *Proc Natl Acad Sci U S A* **91**:2970, 1994.
362. Krivit W, Peters C, Shapiro EG: Bone marrow transplantation as effective treatment of central nervous system disease in globoid leukodystrophy, metachromatic leukodystrophy, adrenoleukodystrophy, mannosidosis, fucosidosis, aspartylglutaminuria, Hurler Maroteaux-Lamy and Sly syndromes, and Gaucher disease type III. *Curr Opin Neurol* **12**:167, 1999.
363. Unger ER, Sung JH, Manivel JC, Chenggis ML, Blazar BR, Krivit W: Male donor-derived cells in the brains of female sex-mismatched bone marrow transplant receipients: A Y-chromosome specific in situ hybridization study. *J Neuropathol* **52(5)**:460, 1993.
364. Hickey WF, Kimura H: Perivascular microglial cells of the CNS are bone marrow-derived and present antigen in vivo. *Science* **239**:290, 1988.
365. Hickey WF, Vass K, Lassmann H: Bone marrow-derived elements in the central nervous system: An immunohistochemical and ultrastructural survey of rat chimeras. *J Neuropathol Exp Neurol* **51**:246, 1992.
366. Duggan DE, Chen I-W, Bayne WF, Halpin RA, Ducan CA, Schwartz MS, Stubbs RJ, Vickers S: The physiological disposition of lovastatin. *Drug Metabol Dispos* **17(2)**:166, 1989.

367. Aversa F, Tabilio A, Velardi A, Cunningham I, Terenzi A, Falzetti F, Ruggeri L, Barababietola G, Aristei C, Latini P, Reisner Y, Martelli MF: Treatment of high-risk acute leukemia with T-cell depleted stem cells from related donors with one fully mismatched HLA haplotype. *N Engl J Med* **339**:1186, 1998.
368. Rubinstein P, Carrier C, Scaradavou A, Kurtzberg J, Adamson J, Migliaccio AR, Berkowitz RL, Cabbad M, Dobrila NL, Taylor PE, Rosenfield RE, Stevens CE: Outcomes among 562 recipients of placental-blood transplants from unrelated donors. *N Engl J Med* **339**:1565, 1998.
369. Shapiro EG, Lockman LA, Balthazor M, Krivit W: Neuropsychological outcomes of several storage diseases with and without bone marrow transplantation. *J Inherit Metab Dis* **18**:413, 1995.
370. Van Duyn MA, Moser AB, Brown III FR, Sacktor N, Liu A, Moser HW: The design of a diet restricted in saturated very long chain fatty acids: Therapeutic application in adrenoleukodystrophy. *Am J Clin Nutr* **40**:277, 1984.
371. Moser HW, Aubourg P, Cornblath D, Borel J, Wu Y-W, Bergin A, Naidu S, Moser AB: The therapy for X-linked adrenoleukodystrophy, in Desnick RJ (ed): *Treatment of Genetic Diseases*, chap 7. New York, Churchill-Livingstone, 1991, p 111.
372. Odone A, Odone M: Lorenzo's Oil. A new treatment for adrenoleukodystrophy. *J Pediatr Neurosci* **5**:55, 1989.
373. Rizzo WB, Leshner RT, Odone A, Dammann AL, Craft DA, Jensone ME, Jennings SS, Davis S, Jaitly R, Sgro JA: Dietary erucic acid therapy for X-linked adrenoleukodystrophy. *Neurology* **39(11)**:1415, 1989.
374. Moser HW: Lorenzo's Oil. Film review. *Lancet* **341**:544, 1993.
375. Rosen FS: Pernicious treatment. *Nature* **361**:695, 1993.
376. Moser HW: Suspended judgment: Reactions to the motion picture "Lorenzo's Oil." *Control Clin Trials* **15**:161, 1994.
377. Rasmussen M, Moser AB, Borel J, Khangoora S, Moser HW, : Brain, liver and adipose tissue erucic and very long chain fatty acid levels in adrenoleukodystrophy patients treated with glyceryl trierucate and irlolease oils (Lorenzo's Oil). *Neuro Chem Res* **19**:801, 1994.
378. Poulos A, Gibson R, Sharp P, Beckman K, Grattan-Smith P: Very long chain fatty acids in X-linked adrenoleukodystrophy brain after treatment with Lorenzo's Oil. *Ann Neurol* **36**:741, 1994.
379. Aubourg P, Adamsbaum C, Lavallard-Rousseau M-C, Rocchiccioli F, Cartier N, Jambaque I, Jakobezak C, Lemaitre A, Boureau F, Wolf C, Bougneres P-F: A two-year trial of oleic and erucic acids ("Lorenzo's Oil") as treatment for adrenomyeloneuropathy. *N Engl J Med* **329**:745, 1993.
380. van Geel BM, Assies J, Haverkort EB, Koelman JHTM, Verbeeten B, Wanders RJA, Barth PG: Progression of abnormalities in adrenomyeloneuropathy and neurologically asymptomatic X-linked adrenoleukodystrophy despite treatment with "Lorenzo's Oil." *J Neurol Neurosurg Psychiat* **67(3)**:290, 1999.
381. Moser HW: Lorenzo Oil therapy for adrenoleukodystrophy: A prematurely amplified hope. *Ann Neurol* **34(2)**:121, 1993.
382. Rizzo WB, Leshner RT, Odone A, Craft DA, Jennings SS, Jaitly R, Segro JA: X-linked adrenoleukodystrophy: Biochemical and clinical efficacy of dietary erucic acid therapy, in Uziel G, Wanders RJA, Cappa ME (eds): *Adrenoleukodystrophy and Other Peroxisomal Disorders,* International Congress Series 898. Amsterdam, Excerpta Medica, 1990, p 149.
383. Rizzo WB: Lorenzo's Oil — Hope and disappointment. *N Engl J Med* **329(11)**:801, 1993.
384. Uziel G, Bertini E, Rimoldi M, Gambetti M: Italian multicentric dietary therapeutical trial in adrenoleukodystrophy, in Uziel G, Wanders RJA, Cappa ME (eds): *Adrenoleukodystrophy and Other Peroxisomal Disorders: Clinical, Biochemical, Genetic and Therapeutic Aspects,* International Congress Series 898. Amsterdam, Elsevier Science Publishers, 1990, p 163.
385. Poulos A, Robertson EF: Lorenzo's Oil: A reassessment. *Med J Australia* **160**:315, 1994.
386. Stockler S, Molzer B, Plecko B, Zenz W, Muntean W, Soling U, Hunneman DH, Korenki C, Hanefeld F: Giant platelets in erucic acid therapy for adrenoleukodystrophy. *Lancet* **341**:1414, 1993.
387. Zinkham WH, Kickler T, Borel J, Moser HW: Lorenzo's Oil and thrombocytopenia in patients with adrenoleukodystrophy. *N Engl J Med* **328(15)**:1126, 1993.
388. Zierz S, Schroder R, Unkrig CJ: Thrombocytopenia induced by erucic acid therapy in patients with X-linked adrenoleukodystrophy. *Clin Investig* **71**:802, 1993.
389. Stoeckler S, Opper C, Hunneman DH, Korenke GC, Unkrig CJ, Hanefeld F: Decreased platelet membrane anisotropy in patients with adrenoleukodystrophy treated with erucic acid (22:1)-rich triglycerides. *J Inherit Metab Dis* **20**:54, 1997.
390. Unkrig CJ, Schroder R, Scharf RE: Lorenzo's Oil and lymphocytopenia. *N Engl J Med* **330**:577, 1994.
391. Ruiz M, Pampols S, Giros M: Glycerol trioleate/glycerol trierucate therapy in X-linked adrenoleukodystrophy: Saturated and unsaturated fatty acids in blood cells: Implications for follow-up. *J Inherit Metab Dis* **19(2)**:188, 1996.
392. Stumpf DA, Hayward A, Haas R, Schaumburg HH: Adrenoleukodystrophy. Failure of immunosuppression to prevent neurological progression. *Arch Neurol* **38**:48, 1981.
393. Korenke GC, Christen HJ, Hunneman DH, Hanefeld F: Progression of X-linked adrenoleukodystrophy under interferon-beta therapy. *J Inherit Metab Dis* **20**:59, 1997.
394. Miike T, Taku K, Tamura T, Ohta J, Ozaki M, Yamammoto C, Sakai T, Antoku Y, Yadomi C: Clinical improvement of adrenoleukodystrophy following intravenous gammaglobulin therapy. *Brain Dev* **11**:134, 1989.
395. Murphy JV, Marquardt KM, Moser HW, Van Duyn MA: Treatment of adrenoleukodystrophy by diet and plasmapheresis. *Ann Neurol* **12**:220, 1982.
396. Singh I, Pahan K, Khan M: Lovastatin and sodium phenylacetate normalize the levels of very long chain fatty acids in skin fibroblasts of X-adrenoleukodystrophy. *FEBS Lett* **426(3)**:342, 1998.
397. Singh I, Khan M, Key L, Pai S: Lovastatin for X-linked adrenoleukodystrophy. *N Engl J Med* **339(10)**:702, 1998.
398. Pai GS, Khan M, Barbosa E, Key L, Cure JK, Betros R, Singh I: Lovastatin therapy for X-linked adrenoleukodystrophy: Clinical and biochemical observations on twelve patients. *Mol Genet Metab* **69**:312, 2000.
399. Stanislaus R, Pahan K, Singh AK, Singh I: Amelioration of experimental allergic encephalomyelitis in Lewis rats by lovastatin. *Neurosci Lett* **269**:71, 1999.
400. Dover GJ, Brusilow S, Samid D: Increased fetal hemoglobin production in patients receiving 4-phenylbutyrate. *N Engl J Med* **229**:569, 1992.
401. Barker PB, Artemov D, Raymond GV, Horska A, Moser HW: Detection of 4-phenylbutyrate in the human brain by in vivo proton MR spectroscopy. Presentation at 1999 meeting of International Society of Magnetic Resonance in Medicine Denver, Colorado.
402. Azizi SA, Stokes D, Augelli BJ, DiGirolamo C, Prockop DJ: Engraftment and migration of human marrow stroma cells implanted in the brains of albino rats — Similarities to astrocyte grafts. *Proc Natl Acad Sci U S A* **95**:3908, 1998.
403. Eglitis MA, Mezey E: Hematopoietic cells differentiate into both microglia and macroglia in the brains of adult mice. *Proc Natl Acad Sci U S A* **94**:4080, 1997.
404. Koc ON, Peters C, Aubourg P, Raghaven S, Dyhouse S, DeGasperi R, Kolodny EH, BenYoseph Y, Gerson SL, Lazarus HM, Caplan AI: Bone marrow-derived mesenchymal stem cells remain host-derived despite successful hematopoietic engraftment after allogeneic transplantation in patients with lysosomal and peroxisomal storage diseases. *Exp Hematol* **27**:1675, 1999.
405. Kumar AJ, Rosenbaum AE, Naidu S, Wenger L, Citrin CM, Lindenberg R, Kim WS, Ziureich SJ, Molliver ME, Mayber HS, Moser HW: Adrenoleukodystrophy: Correlating MR imaging with CT. *Radiology* **165**:496, 1987.
406. Melhem ER, Loes DJ, Georgiadis C, Raymond GV, Moser HW: X-linked adrenoleukodystrophy: The role of contrast-enhanced weighted spin-echo MR imaging in predicting disease progression. *Am J Neuroradiol* **21**:839, 2000.
407. Edwin D, Speedie LJ, Kohler W, Naidu S, Kruse B, Moser HW: Cognitive and brain magnetic resonance imaging findings in adrenomyeloneuropathy. *Ann Neurol* **40**:675, 1996.
408. Abe T, Fujino T, Fukuyama R, Minoshima S, Shimizu N, Toh H, Suzuki H, Yamamoto T: Human long-chain acyl-CoA synthetase — Structure and chromosomal location. *J Biochem* **111**:123, 1992.
409. Moser HW, Loes DJ, Melhem ER, Raymond GV, Bezman L, Cox CS, Lu S-E: X-linked adrenoleukodystrophy: Overview and Prognosis as a Function of Age and Brain Magnetic Resonance Abnormality. A study involving 372 patients. *Neuropediatrics* (in press).

CHAPTER 132

Refsum Disease

Ronald J. A. Wanders ▪ Cornelis Jakobs ▪ Ola H. Skjeldal

1. Heredopathia atactica polyneuritiformis was first delineated as a distinct disease entity on a clinical basis by Sigvald Refsum in 1946. According to Refsum, the cardinal manifestations of the disease include retinitis pigmentosa, cerebellar ataxia, chronic polyneuropathy, and an elevated protein level in cerebrospinal fluid with a normal cell count. Less constant features are sensorineural hearing loss, anosmia, ichthyosis, skeletal malformations, and cardiac abnormalities. The clinical picture of Refsum disease is often that of a slowly developing, progressive peripheral neuropathy manifested by severe motor weakness and muscular wasting, especially of the lower extremities.

2. As first shown by Klenk and Kahlke in 1963, Refsum disease (MIM 266500) is associated with the accumulation of an unusual 20-carbon, branched-chain fatty acid called phytanic acid (3,7,11,15-tetramethylhexadecanoic acid) in blood and tissues. These findings identified Refsum disease as an inborn error of lipid metabolism inherited as an autosomal recessive trait.

3. Accumulation of phytanic acid reliably distinguishes Refsum disease from the large number of neurologic disorders with which Refsum disease shares some features. The availability of a biochemical marker has clearly established that the classical tetrad of abnormalities is not seen in all patients. Indeed, several patients have been described lacking cerebellar ataxia.

4. Accumulation of phytanic acid is not unique to Refsum disease. Phytanic acid also accumulates in a number of other disorders with a clinical course very different from that of Refsum disease. This includes patients affected by a disorder of peroxisome biogenesis (Zellweger syndrome, neonatal adrenoleukodystrophy, infantile Refsum disease) and rhizomelic chondrodysplasia punctata, type 1. To clearly distinguish between Refsum disease and infantile Refsum disease, in which phytanic acid oxidation is deficient due to the absence of peroxisomes, the term "classical Refsum disease" is used to designate those patients in which phytanic acid is elevated due to a selective defect in phytanic acid α-oxidation with all other peroxisomal functions being normal.

5. Phytanic acid is a 3-methyl fatty acid that cannot be β-oxidized directly. The major mechanism by which phytanic acid is degraded, involves an initial α-oxidation to generate the 19-carbon (n-1) homologue, pristanic acid (2,6,10,14-tetramethylpentadecanoic acid) plus CO_2. Pristanic acid is a 2-methyl fatty acid that can be degraded by β-oxidation.

6. The precise mechanism by which phytanic acid is α-oxidized remained obscure until the recent discovery of the enzyme phytanoyl-CoA hydroxylase (PhyH), that catalyzes the hydroxylation of phytanoyl-CoA to 2-hydroxyphytanoyl-CoA, a reaction requiring 2-oxoglutarate, Fe^{2+} and ascorbate (vitamin C). The subsequent steps in the α-oxidation pathway have also been identified and include the enzyme 2-hydroxyphytanoyl-CoA lyase producing pristanal plus formyl-CoA and an aldehyde dehydrogenase catalyzing the formation of pristanic acid from pristanal. Finally, pristanic acid is activated to its CoA-ester, which can now undergo β-oxidation.

7. *In vivo* and *in vitro* studies have shown that α-oxidation of phytanic acid is grossly deficient in patients with Refsum disease. Recent studies show that in all classical Refsum patients studied so far, the defective enzyme is phytanoyl-CoA hydroxylase due to mutations in the structural gene coding for this enzyme. Phytanoyl-CoA hydroxylase is also deficient in the disorders of peroxisome biogenesis including Zellweger syndrome, neonatal adrenoleukodystrophy, infantile Refsum disease, and rhizomelic chondrodysplasia punctata type 1. In the latter disorders, deficiency of phytanoyl-CoA hydroxylase is the secondary consequence of the disturbance in peroxisome biogenesis due to mutations in one of the genes involved in peroxisome biogenesis.

8. In humans, phytanic acid cannot be synthesized *de novo*, but is exclusively exogenous in origin. Dietary phytanic acid itself is the major source. Dairy products, meat, ruminant fats, and fish are rich sources of phytanic acid. Free phytol, which can readily be converted to phytanic acid in the human body, is also a source of phytanic acid, although the phytol present in chlorophyll, in principle the major dietary source of phytol, is poorly absorbed.

9. Because phytanic acid is solely derived from exogenous sources, treatment with diets low in phytanic acid have been tried. In virtually all patients, a considerable fall in plasma phytanic acid levels was achieved. In some patients, plasma levels even normalized. In most patients, a definite clinical improvement was observed, reflected in a partial, but usually not complete, restoration of peripheral nerve functions along with reduction in the skin abnormalities and electrocardiographic aberrations. Plasmapheresis combined with dietary measures is helpful to bring about a more rapid decrease in phytanic acid levels. Treatment should be instituted as early as possible and continued for life.

The history of Refsum disease (MIM 266500) dates to 1946 when Sigvald Refsum, a Norwegian neurologist, published his seminal monograph in which he described five patients from two inbred Norwegian families suffering from an apparently new, familial neurologic syndrome.[1] The main clinical features found in these

A list of standard abbreviations is located immediately preceding the index in each volume. Additional abbreviations used in this chapter include: DHAPAT = dihydroxyacetonephosphate acyltransferase; ERG = electroretinogram; EST = expressed sequence tags; FALDH = fatty aldehyde dehydrogenase; LCS = long chain acyl CoA synthetase; PBD = peroxisome biogenesis disorders; PhyH = phytanoyl-CoA hydroxylase; PPAR = peroxisome proliferator-activated receptor; PPRE = peroxisome proliferator-response elements; RAR = retinoic acid receptor; RCDP = rhizomelic chondrodysplasia punctata; RXR = retinoid X-receptors; VLCFA = very long chain fatty acids.

patients included hemeralopia, a concentric limitation of the visual fields associated with an atypical retinitis pigmentosa, a polyneuritis-like condition with paresis in a peripheral distribution, and ataxia of cerebellar origin. In addition pupillary abnormalities, a neurogenic impairment of hearing, abnormalities in the electrocardiogram, and elevated cerebrospinal fluid protein concentrations were found.

Refsum's clinical skills allowed him to recognize that all five patients suffered from a specific disease entity (a "Morbus *sui genesis*") distinct from the many clinically related heredoataxic syndromes with an autosomal recessive mode of inheritance. Remarkably, when Refsum discussed the possible nature of "heredopathia atactica polyneuritiformis" in his 1946 paper, he suggested that the disease might well be "an obscure type of lipidosis." To emphasize the important contribution of Sigvald Refsum, Viets[2] suggested the name Refsum disease.

In 1963, Klenk and Kahlke[3] published an exciting paper marking Refsum disease as a disorder of lipid metabolism. They analyzed postmortem tissues from a 7-year-old girl diagnosed as having Refsum disease by Richterich and coworkers[4] in Berne. Following the initial publication by Klenk and Kahlke[3] this patient was described in more detail in 1965, both clinically[4] and biochemically.[5] Analysis of the patient's tissues revealed gross infiltration of lipids, mostly neutral, in liver and kidney, whereas no unusual complex lipids were detected. Gas chromatographic analysis of the fatty acids as their methyl esters revealed the presence of one large, abnormal peak. This component was isolated in pure form and fully characterized as phytanic acid (3,7,11,15-tetramethylhexadecanoic acid), a 20-carbon, branched-chain fatty acid not previously reported in human tissues (Fig. 132-1). It was soon established[5] that the accumulation of phytanic acid is not restricted to tissues, but also occurs in plasma from Refsum disease patients, thus allowing easy, noninvasive diagnosis.

Beginning in 1966, a series of studies, notably by Steinberg and coworkers, established that the accumulation of phytanic acid in Refsum disease patients is due to its defective oxidation.[6–10] Subsequent studies that focused on the way in which phytanic acid is degraded, revealed that phytanic acid undergoes oxidative decarboxylation with CO_2 and pristanic acid as products. Despite intense efforts, the exact mechanism of phytanic acid α-oxidation remained obscure until very recently.[11] In recent years, the structure of the α-oxidation pathway has been resolved completely and the enzymatic and molecular basis of Refsum disease identified. In this chapter, we describe the current state of knowledge with respect to phytanic acid oxidation in relation to Refsum disease.

REFSUM DISEASE: CLINICAL SIGNS AND SYMPTOMS

The age at onset of Refsum disease can vary from early childhood to the third or fourth decade of life. In most of the patients, however, clinical manifestations begin in the second decade. Based on earlier studies, it was concluded that 25 to 40 percent of the patients experience their first symptoms before the age of 10, and 50 to 75 percent before the age of 20.[12,13] An early onset of the disease does not necessarily indicate a particularly poor prognosis as to life span. A few patients have been reported who remained asymptomatic until adulthood.[13]

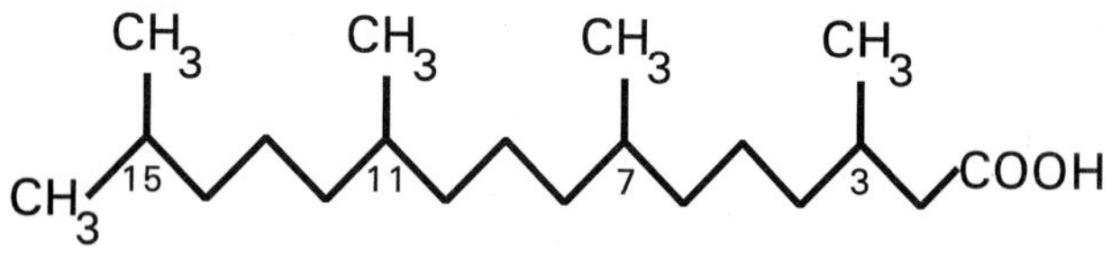

CH_3 CH_3 CH_3 CH_3 — CH_3 15 11 7 3 COOH

Fig. 132-1 Structure of phytanic acid (3,7,11,15-tetramethylhexadecanoic acid), a 20-carbon, fully saturated, fatty acid with methyl-groups at positions 3, 7, 11 and 15 as indicated.

Table 132-1 Clinical and Laboratory Findings in Refsum Disease

Clinical findings:	• Retinitis pigmentosa
	• Peripheral neuropathy (motor and sensory)
	• Cerebellar findings
	• Cardiac abnormalities
	• Symptoms of cranial nerve involvement
	Neurogenic hearing loss
	Anosmia
	Abnormal pupillary reflex
	Miosis
	• Skeletal abnormalities
	• Skin changes—ichthyosis
Laboratory findings:	• Increased CSF protein without pleocytosis (albumino-cytological-dissociation)
	• Elevated plasma phytanic acid concentration

The onset of the disease is insidious, and for many patients, it is difficult to know when the disease started. However, retinitis pigmentosa is, in most cases, a very early clinical feature (see below), and if accurate histories of patients are obtained, many of them will confirm that they suffered from night-blindness in their childhood.

Refsum disease must not be confused with so-called infantile Refsum disease. Both are peroxisomal disorders as discussed in detail later. However, the biochemical and genetic basis is totally different (see below). The name "infantile Refsum disease" dates back to the early 1980s when Scotto and colleagues[14] found elevated levels of phytanic acid in three infants and suggested that this "infantile phytanic storage disease" was a variant of Refsum disease. However, other biochemical abnormalities not found in typical Refsum disease patients were present in these cases, including elevated plasma levels of very long chain fatty acids and pipecolic acid, decreased plasmalogen synthesis, and abnormal subcellular catalase distribution.[15] Because of these additional findings, it is now well established that phytanic acid accumulation in these children is secondary to a disorder of peroxisome assembly (see Chap. 129). This group of patients includes those diagnosed with the Zellweger syndrome and neonatal adrenoleukodystrophy.[15] The term infantile Refsum disease is now generally used to describe a subset of patients with a disorder of peroxisome assembly with the longest survival. The condition described by Refsum[1] is now commonly referred to as classical Refsum disease.

As originally described by Sigvald Refsum, all patients with the disorder bearing his name have a diagnostic tetrad of clinical findings: retinitis pigmentosa, peripheral polyneuropathy, cerebellar ataxia, and a high protein content in the cerebrospinal fluid without an increased number of cells (albuminocytologic dissociation). In most cases additional features, such as cardiac involvement, neurogenic hearing deficit, skin changes, and skeletal malformations are present. Also, anosmia, pupillary abnormalities and cataracts have been described as part of the clinical features (Table 132-1).

Heterozygotes for classical Refsum disease usually do not manifest clinical neurologic signs or symptoms, and generally have normal plasma phytanic acid levels.

Ophthalmologic Signs

Pigmentary retinal degeneration (tapetoretinal degeneration or retinitis pigmentosa) and night-blindness are present in all cases. To our knowledge, there are no convincing reports of classical Refsum disease without any signs of retinitis pigmentosa. Indeed, in a series of 17 patients described by one of us,[13] retinitis pigmentosa was present in all. Usually the retinal degeneration is a very early sign and, in many cases, precedes biochemical diagnosis by several years.[13,16] It is not uncommon that patients with Refsum disease have complained of night blindness many years before additional clinical symptoms appear. Disturbed visual function, often in association with anosmia, is often the first clinical manifestations of the disease. Night blindness, however, is difficult to ascertain, particularly in children. Electroretinography (ERG), which shows a reduction or complete absence of rod and cone responses, can be of great help supporting the diagnosis at early stages. Over the years, a concentric visual field constriction gradually develops until only tubular vision remains.

The appearance of the ocular findings may be of several types and may depend on the stage of development of the disease. Often the typical "bone spicule type"[17] of pigmentary retinal degeneration is lacking, and the pigmentation appears as fine granules or has a "salt and pepper" appearance. In some cases, the retinal disturbance is characterized as "retinitis pigmentosa sine pigmento."[1]

Central vision may be only slightly impaired or normal for a long time. In some cases, however, optic atrophy, cataract, and vitreous opacities may also contribute to visual failure. Refsum did not mention cataract in any of his original patients. Subsequently, it was described in approximately half[13] to one-third of patients.[17] The physician should always consider Refsum disease as a diagnostic possibility in patients with cataract in combination with some neurologic deficit(s).

It has been suggested that as much as 4 to 5 percent of patients with retinitis pigmentosa may have Refsum disease.[18] Because there is an effective treatment, it is important to consider the diagnosis of Refsum disease in all patients who have retinitis pigmentosa. It is this clinical feature, in particular, that can be arrested if dietary treatment is started early enough.[19]

The retinal degeneration seems to be due to the excessive deposition of phytanic acid in ocular tissue.[20] Pathologic examinations reveal an almost complete loss of photoreceptors, thinning of the inner nuclear layer and reduction in the number of ganglion cells of the retina.[21]

Poor vision is due not only to retinitis pigmentosa and cataract, but also to the miosis and poor reaction of the pupils to light, sometimes also to accommodation-convergence. Slow and incomplete dilatation following administration of mydriatics is encountered in less than half of the patients, particularly the older ones, whereas in the children the pupillary responses are mostly normal. In this context, it is interesting to note that Refsum's first patient was described as having an Argyll Robertson syndrome.[1]

Nystagmus, usually of moderate degree, has also been recorded in about one quarter of patients. Remarkably, a patient with retinal arteriovenous communication and Refsum disease has been described.[22]

Polyneuropathy

Chronic or progressive polyneuropathy is well recognized in Refsum disease, although it is not always clinically apparent at the start of the illness. Sometimes it is preceded by visual and auditory dysfunctions for several years. The polyneuropathy of Refsum disease is of the mixed motor and sensory type, is symmetric, and initially affects mainly the distal parts of the lower limbs with muscular atrophy, weakness, and sensory disturbances (Fig. 132-2). It is chronic and progressive if untreated. However, it is not unusual for the symptoms to wax and wane in the early stages. Over the course of years, muscular weakness can become widespread and disabling, involving both the limbs and the truncal musculature.

Almost without exception, patients with Refsum disease have peripheral sensory disturbances.[17] In most cases, it is the deep sensation that is impaired, particularly vibration and position-motion qualities in distal parts of the legs. Some patients also have loss of superficial sensation (cutaneous hypesthesia of the glove and stocking type). Paresthesias, dysesthesias, and spontaneous pains occur in some cases. The peripheral nerves (mostly ulnar, peroneal, and great auricular) may be palpably enlarged and firm.

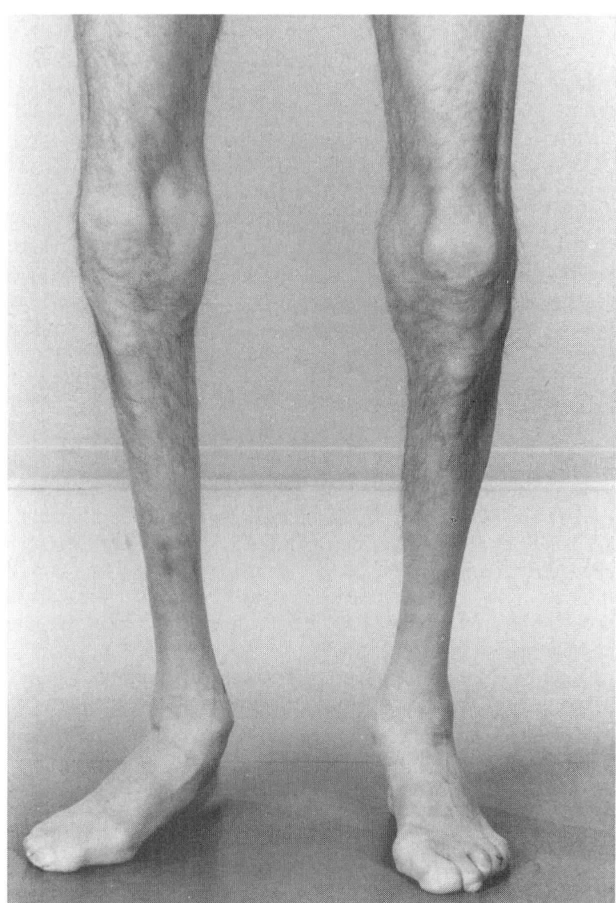

Fig. 132-2 Patient with classical Refsum disease and a long-standing polyneuropathy. Note the marked muscular atrophy.

The clinical neurologic examination in most cases reveals loss of deep reflexes, mostly starting with ankle jerks. Generally, the plantar responses are flexor or absent. Neurophysiological studies show a reduced sensory nerve condition velocity. The reductions are sometimes very marked. However, there does not seem to be a uniform pattern of slowing of the condition velocities as expected in patients with a genetic demyelinative neuropathy.[23] This is in accord with the varying degrees of segmental demyelination that have been reported in studies of nerve biopsies.[17] Kuntzer et al.[24] reported the results of repeated clinical and electrophysiological examinations during a 21-year-period. Their results indicated that patients with Refsum disease have a nonuniform sensorimotor demyelinating neuropathy in which recurrent segmental demyelination with temporal dispersion and possible conduction block of the motor units can occur in parallel with periods of clinical exacerbation. They also found some evidence of chronic reinnervation periods giving a more stable muscle function over time. Interestingly, Gelot and coworkers[25] reported a patient with Refsum disease with primary axonal neuropathy.

Cerebellar Findings

The occurrence of cerebellar dysfunctions in patients with classical Refsum disease has been discussed for many years. Refsum himself regarded cerebellar abnormalities among the main clinical signs of the disease. It should be stressed, however, that cerebellar dysfunction presents relatively late especially when compared with retinopathy and neuropathy. Nevertheless, unsteadiness of gait has been reported in several patients suffering from Refsum disease.[1,17,26] Accordingly, many patients have been misdiagnosed as having Friedreich ataxia (see Chap. 232). The ataxia is characteristically more marked than the degree of muscular weakness and sensory loss would indicate. Nystagmus of cerebellar origin and intention tremor have also been found in several cases. In other descriptions of Refsum disease, cerebellar signs were found to be less constant.[13,17,27] Probably it is a question of the duration of the disease before the clinical signs of cerebellar dysfunction develop.

Additional Clinical Features

Cranial Nerve Changes. Both the olfactory and auditory nerves are most often affected. In fact, anosmia is, in many patients, together with retinitis pigmentosa, a very early clinical manifestation of the disease.[17,26] The loss of hearing is of the cochlear type and may be almost complete.[28] Vestibule function is usually unimpaired. Other cranial nerve involvement is extremely rare.

Cardiac Manifestations. Sudden death among patients with Refsum disease has been striking, and is related to primary cardiac malfunctions.[29–31] Cardiomyopathy with cardiomegaly, heart failure, conduction disturbances and electrocardiographic changes is common.[17] We are aware of one case of classical Refsum disease where the patient underwent a heart transplantation with a good outcome, with respect to both the cardiovascular and the neurologic abnormalities.

Although it has been claimed that cardiac abnormalities only occur in the advanced stages of the disease,[30] Milliaire and coworkers (cited in reference 17) reported two young brothers who both had serious cardiac failure before the clinical stage of the peripheral neuropathy. Both had acute pulmonary edema and dilated hypokinetic cardiomyopathy combined with retinitis pigmentosa, ptosis, and anosmia.

Skeletal Malformations. The first patients reported by Refsum had skeletal malformations in the form of symmetric epiphyseal dysplasia in the knee joints, elbows, and shoulders.[1] A common finding has been bilateral shortening or elongation of the metatarsal bones, particularly the third and fourth metatarsals. Other malformations reported are syndactyly, shortened and widened digits or metacarpals, and hammer toes. These skeletal changes have been recorded in about half of the patients.[13]

Skin Changes. The involvement of the skin is highly variable. Some patients never develop skin changes, while in others, this seems to be one of the presenting manifestations.[32] Cutaneous manifestations, ranging from slightly dry skin, especially on the trunk, to florid ichthyosis, have been reported in several patients.[32] Children have often shown the most marked changes, while the skin involvement in adults is usually less severe. The pathogenesis of the skin changes is uncertain. Dykes et al.[33] found a high epidermal labeling index in patients with Refsum disease. Davies et al.[34] proposed that the accumulation of phytanic acid in the epidermis causes an imbalance in long and short chain fatty acids and suggested that this altered corneocyte adhesiveness.

Other Clinical Signs. Symptoms and signs suggestive of autonomic nerve system involvement, in the gastrointestinal tract and the skin, have been reported in single cases.[35] Renal impairment has been found in a few patients. Dick et al.[36] reported a patient who showed renal dysfunction, possibly at the tubular level, that partially reversed as the serum level of phytanic acid was reduced.

BIOCHEMICAL DIAGNOSIS OF REFSUM DISEASE

The diagnosis of Refsum disease should be established by the demonstration of an isolated phytanic acid accumulation in plasma together with studies in cultured skin fibroblasts to establish defective α-oxidation of phytanic acid and deficient phytanoyl-CoA hydroxylase activity as discussed later.

Plasma Phytanic Acid

Plasma phytanic acid is usually measured by gas chromatography using one of a variety of different methods. Because it is important to demonstrate an isolated accumulation of phytanic acid in the absence of other peroxisomal abnormalities, we prefer methods in which phytanic, pristanic, and very long chain fatty acids (VLCFAs) are measured simultaneously. Although a number of methods have been published for either the analysis of VLCFAs, pristanic or phytanic acid, only very few methods include the simultaneous analysis of these compounds.[37] The latter methods allow easy and reliable quantification of phytanic acid, as well as of VLCFA and pristanic acid. We strongly advocate use of these methods.

Cultured Skin Fibroblasts

Studies in fibroblasts should be performed to pinpoint the precise defect. This first involves studies on the oxidation of [^{14}C] phytanic acid preferably [1-^{14}C] phytanic acid as advocated by Poulos,[38] and not [U-^{14}C] phytanic acid. If deficient, other peroxisomal functions including *de novo* plasmalogen biosynthesis, pristanic acid β-oxidation, and catalase immunofluorescence should also be studied to establish that only phytanic acid α-oxidation is defective. The recent identification of the primary enzyme defect in classical Refsum disease at the level of phytanoyl-CoA hydroxylase[11] now allows direct enzyme activity measurement in fibroblasts followed by mutation analysis as described later.

DISTRIBUTION OF PHYTANIC ACID AMONG VARIOUS LIPIDS

Studies on the distribution of phytanic acid among the various lipid fractions in plasma from Refsum disease patients, revealed that only a small fraction of phytanic acid is in the free form. Virtually all phytanic acid is present in an esterified form with most phytanic acid present in triglycerides and less in the form of phospholipids and cholesterol esters.[39–41] When the triglyceride fraction was studied in more detail, mono- and diphytanoyl-triglycerides were found in addition to the normal nonphytanoyl triglyceride fraction, thus producing a specific pattern characteristic for Refsum disease.[41,42] Indeed, thin-layer chromatography demonstration of this triglyceride pattern has been used for the diagnosis of Refsum disease. Molzer et al.[42] found that the diphytanoyl triglyceride:nonphytanoyl triglyceride ratio is a powerful tool to monitor patients on a phytanic acid free diet.

In plasma of Refsum disease patients phytanic acid principally resides in LDL and HDL, although the contribution of VLDL may be much higher postprandially.[43,44]

PHYTANIC ACID ACCUMULATION IS NOT RESTRICTED TO CLASSICAL REFSUM DISEASE

For many years, it was thought that accumulation of phytanic acid was specific for Refsum disease. It is now clear, however, that accumulation of phytanic acid is observed in a variety of other disorders as discussed below.

Infantile Refsum Disease (MIM 266510) and Other Peroxisome Biogenesis Disorders

The first clue suggesting that phytanic acid accumulation is not unique to Refsum disease came in 1974, when Kahlke et al.[45] described an infant with cerebral damage, arrested development, icterus, and hepatomegaly in whom phytanic acid was clearly elevated in serum and liver. The clinical picture was decidedly not that of classical Refsum disease. This report was unnoticed until the early 1980s when Scotto et al.[14] and Boltshauser et al.[46] described a number of patients suffering from an infantile form of phytanic acid storage disease. The patients showed facial dysmorphia, growth and/or mental retardation, hepatomegaly, failure to thrive, and osteopenia, in addition to retinitis pigmentosa and neurosensory deafness. Because of these two abnormalities, phytanic acid levels were measured and found strongly elevated. Scotto et al.[14] recognized the similarity between their patients and the case described by Kahlke et al.[45] and suggested that the patients either suffered from a severe, early onset form of Refsum disease or a genetically distinct form of phytanic acid storage disease. The latter possibility was considered the most likely[14] for various reasons, including because the infantile and classical forms of Refsum disease were not observed in the same family. The name infantile Refsum disease was subsequently coined. This puzzling situation was resolved when it was found that biochemical abnormalities in infantile Refsum disease patients were not restricted to the accumulation of phytanic acid. Indeed, as first shown by Poulos et al.,[47] the plasma of patients with the infantile but not the adult form of Refsum disease contained elevated levels of VLCFA, di- and trihydroxycholestanoic acid, and pipecolic acid. These abnormalities were earlier described in patients suffering from the cerebrohepatorenal (Zellweger) syndrome, which is characterized by the absence of morphologically distinguishable peroxisomes due to a genetic defect in peroxisome biogenesis. These findings suggested that infantile Refsum disease and Zellweger syndrome are related.[47] As discussed in more detail in Chap. 129, infantile Refsum disease does, indeed, belong to the group of peroxisome biogenesis disorders (PBDs) caused by a genetic defect in one of the many genes involved in peroxisome biogenesis. Other disorders belonging to this group are Zellweger syndrome and neonatal adrenoleukodystrophy. In addition, many patients with a defect in peroxisome biogenesis have been described with intermediate phenotypes that do not allow unequivocal assignment to one of these categories.

Rhizomelic Chondrodysplasia Punctata Type 1 (MIN 215100)

In 1985, Heijmans et al.[48] reported the deficiency of erythrocyte plasmalogens in rhizomelic chondrodysplasia punctata (RCDP) patients, and elevated levels of phytanic acid in serum marking RCDP, as another peroxisomal disorder. Subsequent studies led to the remarkable finding of multiple peroxisomal abnormalities in RCDP patients, including a deficiency of dihydroxyacetonephosphate acyltransferase (DHAPAT) and alkyldihydroxyacetonephosphate synthase (alkyl DHAP synthase), the first two enzymes of ether-phospholipid biosynthesis (see references 49 and 50 for review and Chap. 130). Furthermore, phytanic acid α-oxidation appeared deficient, which explains the accumulation of phytanic acid in plasma from RCDP patients, and finally, peroxisomal thiolase was found to be deficient. As described in more detail in Chap. 129, the underlying basis for this peculiar combination of enzyme deficiencies was recently resolved by three different groups.[51–53] The gene defective in RCDP encodes a receptor protein, Pex7p, which plays an essential role in peroxisome biogenesis by catalyzing the targeting of peroxisomal proteins equipped with a PTS2 signal to the peroxisome. The deficiency of multiple peroxisomal enzymes in RCDP, including phytanoyl-CoA hydroxylase, follows logically from the fact that all PTS2 proteins are not properly targeted to the peroxisome in the absence of a functionally active PTS2 receptor.

Disorders of Peroxisomal Branched-Chain Fatty Oxidation

Many patients have been described with a defect in peroxisomal fatty acid β-oxidation distinct from X-linked adrenoleukodystrophy. In most of these patients, elevated levels of VLCFA are found in plasma in combination with elevated di- and trihydroxycholestanoic acid, pristanic acid and phytanic acid levels (see references 50 and 54 to 56 for review and Chap. 130). The clinical presentation of these patients is usually severe and may be associated with the full spectrum of clinical abnormalities as observed in classical Zellweger syndrome, although milder presentations are also known. In general, the clinical presentation of patients affected by a disorder of peroxisomal β-oxidation resembles that of the disorders of peroxisome biogenesis (see Chap. 129). The accumulation of phytanic acid follows logically from the impaired oxidation of pristanic acid, the product of the phytanic acid α-oxidation pathway. As a consequence, both pristanic and phytanic acid are elevated in these patients with pristanic acid accumulating much more than phytanic acid.[57]

COMBINED PHYTANIC/PIPECOLIC ACIDEMIA

Combined phytanic/pipecolic acidemia has been described as a possibly new entity by Tranchant et al.[58] in a single family with three affected members. One affected patient died at age 17 from a severe, rapidly progressive, neurologic disorder with unusual clinical and neuropathologic abnormalities distinct from classical Refsum disease. Homozygosity mapping studies by Nadal and coworkers[59] localized the mutant locus to chromosome 10p. The same authors suggested several possibilities to explain the peculiar combination of phytanic and pipecolic acidemia. We recently studied this family in some detail and found that phytanoyl-CoA hydroxylase, the enzyme deficient in classical Refsum disease, is also deficient in fibroblasts from the index patient of the family described by Tranchant et al.[58]

Furthermore, molecular analysis revealed clear-cut mutations in the hydroxylase gene (Jansen and coworkers, unpublished). These data are in line with the homozygosity mapping data of Nadal et al.,[59] as we localized the hydroxylase gene to 10p. The apparent defect in pipecolic acid degradation remains unexplained. It should be noted that there is consanguinity within the family, suggesting the possibility of two separate genetic defects.

ORIGIN OF PHYTANIC ACID

Evidence Against Endogenous Synthesis as the Origin of Phytanic Acid

A branched-chain fatty acid was isolated in the butter fat of bovine milk in the early 1950s.[60] Full characterization of this compound with sophisticated analytic techniques such as gas-liquid chromatography and nuclear magnetic resonance spectroscopy was reported 10 years later.[61] These studies revealed that this fatty acid has four methyl groups on a C_{16} backbone and has the systematic name 3,7,11,15-tetramethylhexadecanoic acid. Interestingly, the chemical preparation of this fatty acid from phytol (3,7,11,15-tetramethylhexadec-*trans*-2-ene-1-ol) was already reported in 1911.[62] Based on its polyisoprenoid-like structure Kahlke and Richterich[5] suggested that phytanic acid might be synthesized from four molecules of mevalonic acid analogous to the synthesis of farnesol from mevalonic acid followed by oxidation of farnesol to farnesoic acid. Attempts to demonstrate formation of phytanic acid from [2-^{14}C] mevalonic acid in a Refsum disease patient were negative,[6] however, and neither labeled acetate nor mevalonate was incorporated into phytanate in experimental animals.[63,64]

Origin from Exogenous Sources

After this demonstration that phytanic acid is not synthesized endogenously, it soon became clear that free phytol and phytanic acid, but not chlorophyll-bound phytol, were the true sources of phytanic acid as derived from dietary sources.

Phytol. Dairy products and ruminant fats are probably the most important sources of phytanic acid in the human diet. Ruminants ingest large quantities of chlorophyll, which undergoes effective degradation by resident bacteria in the rumen, releasing phytol from its linkage to the propionic acid side-chain of porphyrin. Free phytol is readily converted to phytanic acid via a mechanism not well-understood (see below). Phytol administered orally is efficiently absorbed both by normal human subjects (61 to 94 percent of tracer dose) as well as by Refsum disease patients.[63]

Phytanic Acid. Like phytol, free phytanic acid is readily absorbed. In the rat, orally administered phytanate is well absorbed, even when fed in large doses.[64] Most absorption occurs by way of the lymph.[65]

In mice fed a diet containing 2 percent (w/w) phytanate, there is profound accumulation of phytanate in liver and serum amounting to 20 to 30 percent of total fatty acids. These levels approach those seen in Refsum patients. Interestingly, when the animals are returned to a normal diet, the stored phytanate disappears within a week or two.

Chlorophyll-Bound Phytol. It was originally thought that chlorophyll with its ubiquitous presence in green vegetables, would be an important dietary precursor because it contains 1 mol of phytol per mol of chlorophyll. Elegant studies by Baxter and Steinberg[66] using [^{14}C] pheophytin, revealed that little, if any, bound phytol is absorbed. A similar conclusion was reached in other studies in which a healthy volunteer ingested 180 g of spinach with only very little effect on the plasma levels of phytanic acid.[67]

PATHOGENESIS OF REFSUM DISEASE

Although much has been learned about the biochemical basis for the accumulation of phytanic acid, less is known about the mechanism by which the accumulation of phytanic acid leads to the clinical manifestations of Refsum disease. Several hypotheses have been proposed as discussed by Steinberg,[68] including the molecular distortion hypothesis, the antimetabolite hypothesis, and the "double-function" hypothesis. Furthermore, it has been proposed that phytanic acid may interfere with the generation of prenylated proteins with consequences for their function. A large and growing body of evidence indicates that covalent modification of proteins by conjugation with farnesyl pyrophosphate or geranylgeranyl pyrophosphate is essential for their function. This covalent modification allows proteins to become associated with membranes and carry out their specific function. Because phytanic acid has a similar structure as compared to the farnesyl and geranylgeranyl groups that are attached covalently to proteins, it has been suggested that phytanic acid might inhibit the enzymes catalyzing the prenylation of target proteins. Although this prenylation hypothesis is attractive, it currently lacks experimental support.

As discussed below, recent studies[69–72] have shed new light on the physiological consequences of elevated phytanic acid levels because phytanic acid turns out to be an effective regulator of gene expression by virtue of its capacity to activate certain nuclear receptors.

PHYTANIC ACID: A LIGAND FOR MEMBERS OF THE NUCLEAR HORMONE RECEPTOR SUPERFAMILY

Kitareewan et al.[69] were the first to report that phytol metabolites are dietary factors that can activate the nuclear retinoid-X receptor (RXR). RXR belongs to an expanding group of nuclear receptors that are transcription factors regulating gene expression in response to lipophilic ligands such as steroid hormones.[73] The family of nuclear receptors include the estrogen receptors, thyroid hormone receptors, retinoic acid receptors, retinoid-X receptor and the more recently identified group of peroxisome proliferator-activated receptors (PPARs). Kitareewan et al.[69] identified a unique RXR effector from organic extracts of bovine serum by following RXR-dependent transcriptional activity. Structural analysis led to phytanic acid as the active compound. Phytanic acid appeared to be a ligand for all three RXRs, including RXRα, β and γ with comparable affinities.

Studies by Seedorf and coworkers[70] provided in vivo evidence indicating that phytanic acid is indeed a potent modulator of gene expression affecting nuclear signal transduction pathways. This was concluded from studies in mutant mice in which the sterol carrier protein X (SCPx) gene was disrupted. As discussed in more detail elsewhere (Chap. 130), SCPx plays a central role in the degradation of phytanic and pristanic acid by catalyzing the last step in the β-oxidation of pristanic acid. As expected, oxidation of pristanic acid is fully deficient in these mice, leading to elevated levels of pristanic and phytanic acid especially when phytol is fed to the animals.

Interestingly, these mutant mice were completely free of symptoms on a normal laboratory diet. However, when phytol was added to the diet, the mice developed severe abnormalities, including lethargy, reduced muscle tone, ataxia, loss of body weight, and a peripheral neuropathy with uncoordinated movements, unsteady gait, and trembling. This was followed by early death, probably due to the extensive neurologic disturbances. Furthermore, profound abnormalities in lipid and glucose homeostasis were found upon phytol feeding. In addition, there was peroxisome proliferation in livers from the mutant mice and gene expression was greatly altered with increased expression of liver fatty acid binding protein (L-FABP), peroxisomal and mitochondrial thiolase, acyl-CoA oxidase, and cholesterol-7α-hydroxylase, and decreased expression of phosphoenolpyruvate carboxykinase.

The results of these studies in mice lacking sterol carrier protein and fed phytol showed striking similarities to the results in rodents fed certain peroxisome proliferators including hypolipidemic agents such as clofibrate.

Studies by Gonzalez and coworkers[74] demonstrated that peroxisome proliferators mediate their effects via activation of the peroxisome proliferator-activated receptor-alpha (PPARα). Activated PPARα dimerizes with the retinoid-X receptor alpha (RXRα) and this heterodimer binds to peroxisome proliferator-response elements (PPREs). PPREs are two direct repeats separated by 1 bp of the sequence TGACCT in the promotor regions of their target genes, including genes involved in lipid metabolism.[73]

For example, the L-FABP gene contains a functional PPRE[73] and it's transcription is up-regulated by peroxisome proliferators. These considerations suggest that phytanic acid might be a transcriptional activator of L-FABP and other genes containing a PPRE by virtue of phytanic acid being a ligand for PPARα. Both predictions proved to be true.[71,72]

The implications of these exciting new findings for Refsum disease remain to be established.

THERAPEUTIC ASPECTS

The view that phytanic acid, which accumulates in Refsum disease, is of exogenous origin, led to an attempt to treat the patients by dietary means. Elimination of phytanic acid and it's precursors from the diet should prevent further accumulation and, because most of the patients retain some capacity to degrade phytanic acid, it also should be possible to reduce the body stores.

Dietary treatment of Refsum disease has been practiced for many years. A test diet was instituted in three patients in 1965,[75] and was subsequently revised and improved.[76] The first patient treated was a man with neurologic symptoms characteristic of Refsum disease starting in childhood. In 1966, he was severely neurologically disabled with a phytanic acid level of 40 mg/dl. On a phytanic acid restricted diet, his phytanic acid fell to 7.5 mg/dl. Furthermore, his polyneuropathy improved markedly and his retinitis pigmentosa stabilized. Now, 34 year later, he is clinically stable with only a mild increase in his plasma phytanic acid (Skjeldal, unpublished).

Many other patients have now been subjected to dietary treatment at various institutions with reduction of plasma phytanic acid levels.[76–95] Severe cases have been described with a dramatic fall in the plasma phytanic acid concentration; for example, from 174 to 13.5 mg/dl in one patient, and in another patient, with plasma exchange in addition to diet, from 145 to 13 mg/dl.[96]

After institution of dietary treatment, the serum phytanic acid level may initially increase.[86,97] A decrease in the plasma phytanic acid level may in fact be delayed for months after starting the diet. This suggests that tissue stores are mobilized when intake is reduced.

In the body, phytanic acid is mainly present in the phospholipids and triglycerides of the various lipoproteins. In liver lipids, it can account for as much as 50 percent of the fatty acids, a concentration higher than that in plasma. If, therefore, liver lipids are mobilized, the level of phytanic acid in plasma will rise, sometimes considerably. The percentage of phytanic acid in adipose tissue is lower (1 to 5 percent of total fatty acids). If adipose tissue lipids are rapidly mobilized, the percentage of phytanic acid in plasma may not increase immediately, and sometimes may even fall while the absolute concentration rises. For this reason, it is recommended to follow responses to diet in terms of *absolute* phytanic acid levels (mg/dl) and *relative* phytanic acid content (percentage of total fatty acids). On the other hand, even though the percentage of phytanic acid in adipose tissue is low, most of the total content of phytanic acid in the body is located there. In one patient, the total amount of phytanic acid was calculated to be 381 g of which 286 g (75 percent) was in adipose tissue. Thus, mobilization of phytanic acid from enormous reservoir in adipose tissue is a potential risk factor in every patient with Refsum disease under dietary treatment. When starting dietary treatment of patients with high levels of phytanic acid in plasma, it is important to avoid an increased flow from the body stores. The diet should provide sufficient calories to keep the body weight nearly constant. If the caloric intake is reduced and the patient starts to lose weight, a paradoxical rise in plasma phytanic acid can occur with an accompanying clinical relapse.[79,80,83,88,90,97] A reduced caloric intake associated with various stress factors such as pregnancy, surgery, infections, or other intercurrent illnesses, are also potential risk factors.

Dietary Prescriptions

In the treatment of patients with Refsum disease, it is necessary to reduce the intake of all sources of phytanic acid drastically. Our knowledge of the occurrence of phytanic acid in different lipids is still limited. It is conceivable that some natural lipids contain no phytanic acid, and that these lipids may be included in the diet. It should also be remembered that in different geographical areas, the same food item may contain different amounts of phytanic acid. Ackman and Hooper demonstrated this many years.[98] The amount of phytanic acid in a sample of cow butter-fat from Canada was 0.008 percent of total fatty acids, from Norway 0.45 percent, from Brazil 0.10 percent, from Argentina and South Africa 0.04 percent, and from Tasmania 0.10 percent. The phytanic acid content of cheese fat also showed great variations from one country to another. These great geographical, and probably also seasonal, variations within the same country, make it difficult to suggest general dietary rules. Of special importance, however, are dairy products of all kinds, ruminant fats, and ruminant meats. These are the major sources of phytanic acid and must be eliminated from the diet. Green vegetables were originally excluded from the diet. The reason for this was the possibility that phytol in chlorophyll might be absorbed and converted to phytanic acid. However, phytol bound to chlorophyll is liberated only to a small extent in the intestines, and is probably of minor importance as a source of phytanic acid in the patients. For this reason, the exclusion of green vegetables is unnecessary, although cooking may release some bound phytol. Some values for phytanic acid content of foods are shown in Table 132-2. More information on dietary management is available in several publications.[77,80,82,83,89,95,98,99] In particular, the papers by Master-Thomas and coworkers[80,99] are very helpful. These publications give information on the phytanic acid content of many ordinary foodstuffs (see Tables 132-2 and 132-3). The authors suggest a practical dietary regimen to maintain phytanic acid intake at less than 10 mg daily.[80]

Table 132-2 Phytanic Acid Content of Foods

Food	Phytanic acid content (mg in 100 g wet weight)
Butter	5–500
Tuna, canned in oil	57
Lamb, cook and minced	49
Cheeses	5–50
Beef, stewed	24
Cod, grilled	4.2
Haddock, steamed	2.6
White bread	1.6
Cornflakes	1.2
White rice, boiled	1.0
Potato, boiled	0.66
Egg white	0.03

The values given represent in many cases analyses of only a single sample and should not be generalized. The wide variations in the phytanic acid contents as for instance observed for butter and cheeses in part reflect seasonal differences in cattle-feeding practices or differences in total fat content (cheeses).

From Masters-Thomas et al.[99] Used with permission.

Very high plasma levels of phytanic acid (above 100 mg/dl) may precipitate toxic and life-threatening symptoms. Several patients have shown such a reaction.[86,97] As an emergency measure, patients with very high levels of phytanic acid may be treated by plasmapheresis, as first suggested by Lundberg et al.[86] Once a week, for a period of several months, 400 ml of plasma was removed from the patient. The decrease of the plasma phytanic acid concentration took place much more rapidly as compared with dietary means alone. Periodic plasmapheresis can also be useful as a supplementation to the ordinary dietary treatment. This combination has been reported to be effective and has helped to keep plasma level low.[83,86,89,91,93,94,100] Repeated plasmapheresis or plasma exchange during early stages of dietary management appears to be a rational way to obtain a good initial response. However, this aggressive treatment strategy is not always succesful,[101] and a lifetime institution of such a treatment may be unreasonably burdensome.

Prognosis

The prognosis of untreated patients of Refsum disease is poor. Ten of 11 patients registered in Norway before the treatment had been introduced were practically blind. Half the untreated patients died before the age of 30 years. Cardiomyopathy has probably been the most frequent cause of sudden death, both in young and middle-aged patients. The dietary treatment has largely changed the natural course of the disease. In patients who respond with a fall in plasma phytanic acid levels, the peripheral neuropathy will stabilize and may even improve. An increase in nerve-conduction velocity has been demonstrated in 10 patients.[81,82,86,87,89,91,95,102] Sural-nerve biopsies have been examined before and after about 2 years of dietary treatment.[94] Demyelination had stopped and there was considerable remyelination and regeneration.

As a result of better neurophysiological parameters, muscle strength and gait will improve and sensory deficits will recede. Other clinical features, such as the retinitis pigmentosa, hearing deficits, cardiomyopathy, and skin manifestations, have been more difficult to improve. However, dietary treatment seems to stop progression of both auditory and visual deficits. To our knowledge, no serious clinical relapses have occurred in patients on dietary treatment associated with significant lowering of the serum phytanic acid level. The well-being and general condition of the patients has been remarkably good. It is reasonable to believe that the efficacy of dietary treatment will be enhanced by its early institution. Once demyelination is extensive, restoration of

Table 132-3 Weights of Food Containing 1, 2, or 5 mg Phytanic Acid (Rounded to Nearest 5 g)

1 mg Phytanic acid portion		2 mg Phytanic acid portion		5 mg Phytanic acid portion	
	wt (g)		wt (g)		wt (g)
White rice, boiled	100	Spaghetti, canned	170	Cottage cheese	270
Spaghetti, canned	85	Cottage cheese	110	Macaroni and cheese, canned	190
White bread	60	Macaroni and cheese, canned	80	Veal, stewed	226
Cornflakes	85	Margarine, Flora	15	Pork, stewed	130
"Rice crispies"	35	Veal, stewed	90	Duckling, roast	65
"Sugar puffs"	95	Pork, stewed	50	Ham, boiled	95
"Weetabix"	65	Ham, boiled	40	Tongue, lamb's (canned)	190
Custard, skim milk	120	Tongue, lamb's (canned)	75	Cod, grilled	120
Margarine, Flora	5	Cod, grilled	50	Smoked haddock	195
Chick peas, canned	50	Smoked haddock	80	Dressed crab, canned	100
Potato (estimate)		Dressed crab, canned	40	Baked beans, canned	170
Boiled	150	Baked beans, canned	70		
Chips	100	Chick peas, canned	100		
Roast	120				
Saute	120				
Chicken soup, dried	50				
Marmite	25				

Data from Masters-Thomas et al.[80] Used with permission.

function is unlikely even if progression is arrested. Every effort should be made to establish the diagnosis and to institute treatment as early as possible.

DEFECTIVE OXIDATION OF PHYTANIC ACID IN REFSUM DISEASE

In Vivo Studies

The discovery by Klenk and Kahlke[3] of the accumulation of phytanic acid in Refsum disease patients was rapidly followed by studies to identify the underlying defect. The first studies done by Stoffel and Kahlke[103] and Steinberg and coworkers[6] used universally labeled phytol ([U-^{14}C] phytol) as precursor. Steinberg and coworkers[6] found that orally administered [U-^{14}C] phytol was rapidly oxidized to $^{14}CO_2$ in a control subject, but not in a patient with Refsum disease. In addition, after administration of [U-^{14}C] phytol, a rapid rise in ^{14}C-phytanic acid was observed in plasma of both the control subject and the patient with Refsum disease. In the control subject, plasma phytanic acid rapidly decreased thereafter, while in the Refsum patient plasma phytanic acid increased to very high levels. Subsequent experiments in which [U-^{14}C] phytanic acid was administered to additional Refsum patients confirmed these observations.[10]

These studies allowed a number of important conclusions. First, that phytol is readily converted into phytanic acid both in normal subjects as well as in Refsum patients. Second, that phytanic acid undergoes rapid oxidation in control but not in Refsum patients.

That phytanic acid is a 3-methyl fatty acid that makes β-oxidation impossible, immediately raised the question of the mechanism by which phytanic acid is oxidized. In principle, several options are possible including: (a) α-oxidation; (b) ω-oxidation; and (c) oxidative carboxylation (Fig. 132-3). In analogy to the situation observed with propionate, which is first activated to its CoA-ester and then undergoes oxidative carboxylation to methylmalonyl-CoA, it was postulated that phytanic acid might also undergo oxidative carboxylation to homophytanic acid (4,8,12,16-tetramethylheptadecanoic acid). Homophytanic acid lacks the methyl group at the 3-position and thus can be β-oxidized normally. Initial experiments by Eldjarn and coworkers[104] provided support for this notion but later results from the same group disproved this idea.[105]

Oxidation from the omega-end (see Fig. 132-3) is another mechanism by which phytanic acid might be oxidized. In vitro studies by Try[106] have shown that phytanic acid can undergo ω-oxidation, but only at a slow rate. Furthermore, in studies by Eldjarn and coworkers[107] using various branched-chain compounds, the capacity for ω-oxidation was found to be normal in Refsum disease patients. These studies suggested that phytanic acid is oxidized via a different mechanism. Subsequent studies showed that the main mechanism of oxidation of phytanic acid is by α-oxidation.

The first clue came from in vivo studies by Mize et al.[108] in which [U-^{14}C]-labeled phytol and phytanic acid were administered to mice. Analysis of fatty acids in the livers of these mice revealed the presence of pristanic acid (2,6,10,14-tetramethylpentadecanoic acid), 4,8,12-trimethyltridecanoic acid, and 4,8-dimethylnonanoic acid. Later, more refined studies led to the identification of additional intermediates including 2-hydroxyphytanic acid.[109] These studies strongly suggested that phytanic acid first undergoes α-oxidation to pristanic acid followed by normal β-oxidation of pristanic acid. Pristanic acid itself is a 2-methyl fatty acid that, like any 2-methyl fatty acid, can readily be β-oxidized.

Eldjarn and coworkers[105,110] had taken a different, very elegant approach based on the use of model compounds. These model compounds (3,6-dimethyloctanoic acid and 3,14,14-trimethylpentadecanoic acid) resemble phytanic acid in having a methyl group at the 3-carbon position that blocks straightforward β-oxidation. After ingestion of 3,6-dimethyl-[8-^{14}C] octanoic acid, healthy control individuals expired $^{14}CO_2$ and in addition excreted the expected product of α-oxidation 2,5-dimethylheptanoic acid in urine. When the same was done in patients with Refsum disease, no $^{14}CO_2$ was produced and no 2,5-dimethylheptanoic acid was found in urine.[110] These data indicated that the oxidative decarboxylation of 3-methyl fatty acids is indeed defective in Refsum disease.

Studies in Cultured Skin Fibroblasts

Virtually all of the studies described above were done by administration of radiolabeled compounds to animals and humans. Subsequent studies[7,8,10] clearly establish that cultured human skin fibroblasts are a perfect model system to study phytanic acid α-oxidation. In agreement with the in vivo studies, phytanic acid oxidation was found to be deficient in Refsum disease fibroblasts, whereas oxidation of 2-hydroxyphytanic acid and pristanic acid

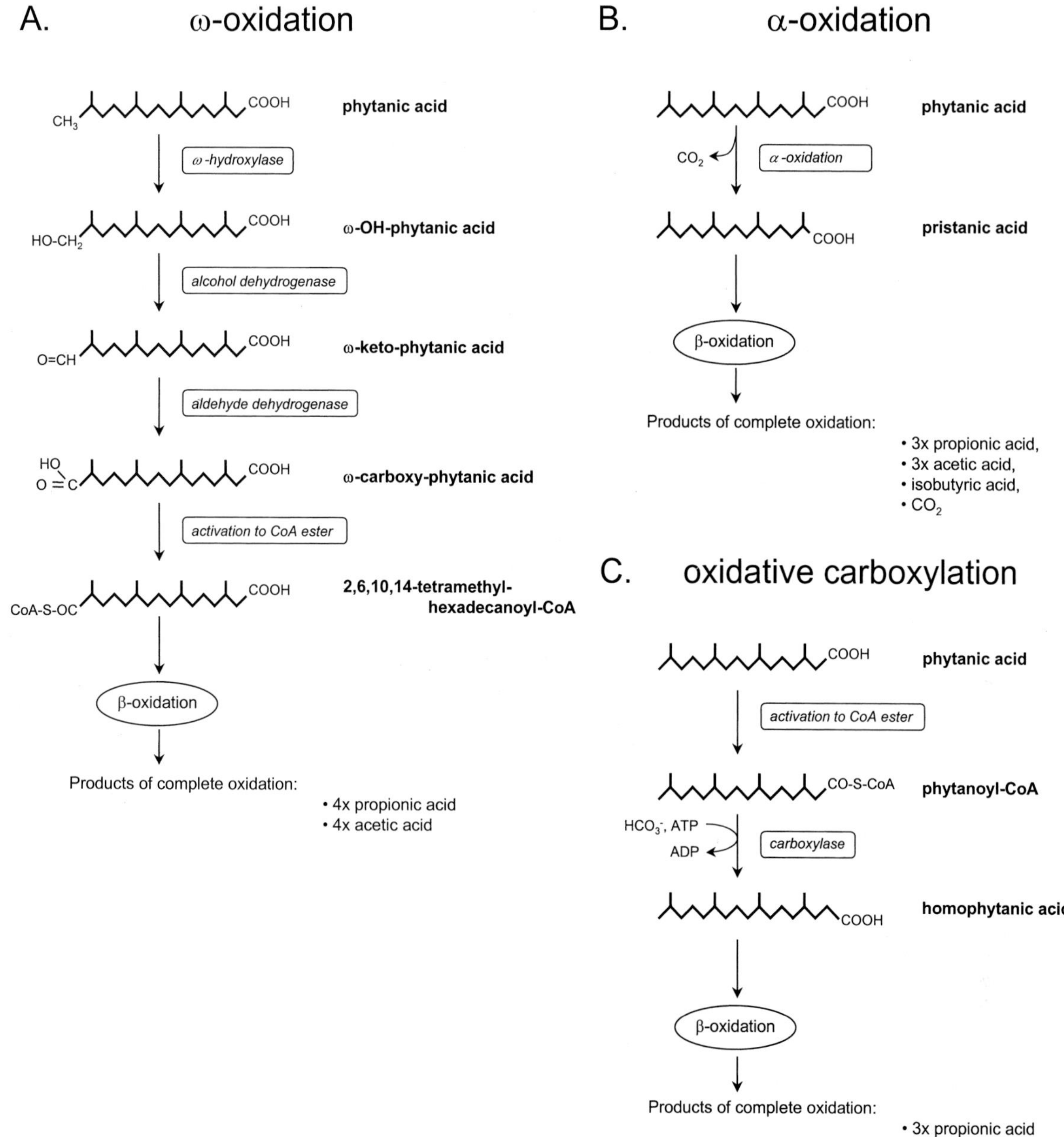

Fig. 132-3 Representation of the theoretically possible initial modes of oxidative attack on the phytanic acid molecule.

was normal, emphasizing that the defect in Refsum disease involved the conversion of phytanic acid to 2-hydroxyphytanic acid.[8,10]

Since then, measurement of phytanic acid α-oxidation in fibroblasts, especially using [1-^{14}C] phytanic acid as substrate,[38] has generally been regarded as an obligatory step in the definite diagnosis of Refsum disease, which is now superseded by direct measurement of the deficient enzyme (phytanoyl-CoA hydroxylase) in fibroblasts as discussed later.

FORMATION OF PHYTANIC ACID FROM PHYTOL

As discussed, phytol is readily oxidized, as shown in vivo in experimental animals, normal human beings, and patients with Refsum disease.[6,10,64,103,108,111–113] Little information is available about the exact mechanism by which phytol is converted into phytanic acid.[114,115] Phytol and phytanic acid differ in two respects including the presence of a double bond between carbon atoms 2 and 3 and the presence of a terminal carboxy group in phytanic acid and an alcohol group in phytol (see Fig. 132-4).

Muralidharan and Muralidharan[114] studied the conversion of phytol to phytanic acid in rat liver homogenates, as well as in mitochondrial fractions. These authors detected phytanic acid but not dihydrophytol, suggesting that the alcohol is first oxidized to a carboxylic acid, which is then followed by removal of the double bond. This system was further characterized by the same authors[115] who reported that formation of phytanic acid from phytol may take place both in mitochondria as well as in microsomes. Clearly, additional work has to be done to resolve the true mechanism.

RESOLUTION OF THE STRUCTURE OF THE PHYTANIC ACID α-OXIDATION PATHWAY

Studies in Broken Cell Preparations

The in vivo studies described above had clearly shown that degradation of phytanic acid occurs primarily by α-oxidation. It was obvious that resolution of the structure of the pathway required studies in cell free systems and whole-cell homogenates

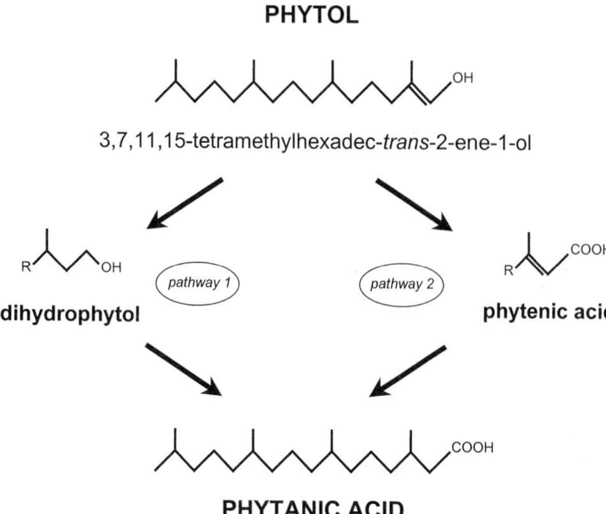

Fig. 132-4 Representation of the two possible mechanisms involved in the formation of phytanic acid from phytol. In humans, pathway 2 is the predominant, if not exclusive, route of formation of phytanic acid from phytol.

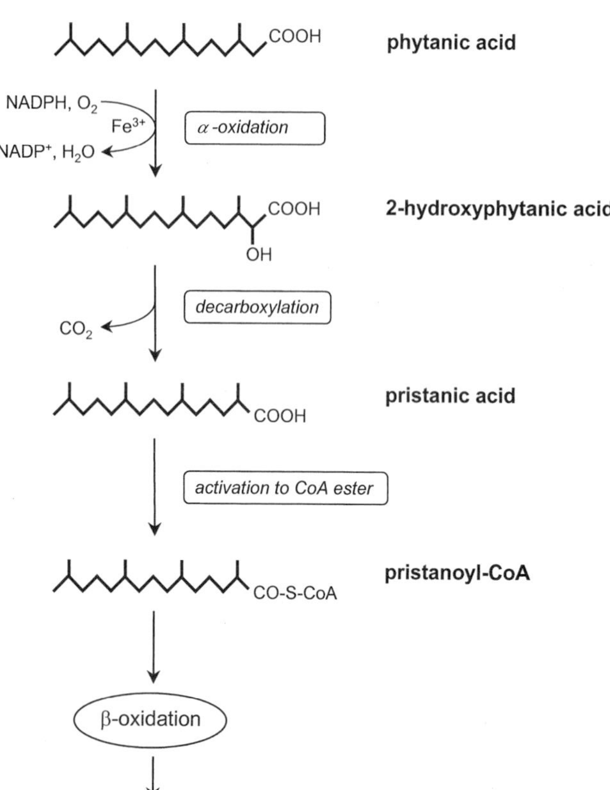

Fig. 132-5 Proposed pathway for the oxidation of phytanic acid as suggested by Tsai et al.[116] Based on studies in rat liver mitochondria, Tsai et al.[116] concluded that the first step in the degradation of phytanic acid is catalyzed by a mitochondrial NADPH- and O_2-dependent ω-hydroxylase converting *free* phytanic acid to *free* 2-hydroxyphytanic acid, followed by its decarboxylation to pristanic acid that, after activation to its CoA-ester, undergoes a series of successive β-oxidations.

fortified with appropriate cofactors. To define these cofactor requirements, Tsai and coworkers[116] performed a systematic study in whole rat liver homogenates and compared the oxidation of phytanic, pristanic and palmitic acid. The conclusions of this important paper can be summarized as follows.

Phytanic acid was found to be readily oxidized in whole liver homogenates fortified with ATP, Mg^{2+}, NAD^+, CoA, $NaHCO_3$, Na-fumarate, and nicotinamide.

Upon oxidation of phytanate, the following products were found: 2-hydroxyphytanic, pristanic, and trimethyltridecanoic acid. Later studies by Steinberg et al.[109] led to the identification of yet other metabolites, including 2,6,10-trimethylundecanoic acid and 4,8-dimethylnonanoic acid.

Systematic studies on the cofactor requirements of phytanate oxidation, measured as the release of $^{14}CO_2$ from [U-^{14}C] phytanate, revealed that oxidation was virtually completely dependent upon ATP and NAD whereas oxidation was blocked upon anaerobiosis. Furthermore, NADPH stimulated oxidation considerably (twofold). The most striking effect was found on addition of ferric (Fe^{3+}) chloride, which stimulated oxidation more than ninefold. Remarkably, oxidation was not dependent upon free CoASH. In fact, omission of CoA led to an *increase* (2.5-fold) rather than a decrease in the rate of phytanate oxidation. The authors interpreted this effect of CoASH as evidence in favor of free phytanic acid as substrate for α-oxidation because diversion of phytanic acid into phytanoyl-CoA apparently inhibited α-oxidation. Based on the results described above Tsai and coworkers proposed the pathway shown in Fig. 132-4 with the following essential elements:

1. Free phytanic acid and *not* phytanoyl-CoA is the true substrate for α-oxidation.
2. α-Hydroxylation is brought about by an NADPH-dependent, oxygen-dependent P450-type of hydroxylase producing 2-hydroxyphytanate.
3. 2-Hydroxyphytanate is converted into pristanic acid via some unknown mechanism.
4. Pristanic acid undergoes β-oxidation to produce 4,8,12-trimethyltridecanoic acid, 2,6,10-trimethylundecanoic acid, 4,8-dimethylnonanoic acid, and its subsequent products of β-oxidation (see Fig. 132-5).
5. The α-oxidation process is primarily if not exclusively mitochondrial as concluded from subcellular distribution studies in which rat livers were homogenized and subjected to successive rounds of centrifugation to prepare a nuclear (700 × *g*, 8 min), mitochondrial (10,000 × *g*, 20 min), microsomal (100,000 × *g*, 45 min) and soluble fraction.

All studies performed by Tsai and coworkers[116] were done with universally labeled [^{14}C] phytanic acid. Muralidharan and Kishimoto[117] pointed out that studies with [U-^{14}C] phytanic acid may give erroneous results because the labeled carbon dioxide produced may stem from the α-oxidation of phytanic acid *per se* but may also derive from the breakdown of pristanic acid, the product of α-oxidation of phytanic acid. For this purpose they synthesized [1-^{14}C] phytanic acid so that release of [1-^{14}C]CO_2 could now be taken as a direct estimate of α-oxidation capacity. Muralidharan and Kishimoto used the same medium as Tsai et al.[116] with the exception that β-cyclodextrin rather than bovine serum albumin was used to solubilize phytanic acid. When these workers studied the effect of each of the constituents in the medium, major differences were found when compared with the data of Tsai et al.[116] Firstly, in accordance with Tsai et al.[116] [1-^{14}C]CO_2-release from [1-^{14}C] phytanic acid was found to be fully dependent on (Mg^2) ATP. Furthermore, nicotinamide stimulated activity considerably (twofold) whereas activity was reduced upon anaerobiosis. Remarkably, no effect of Fe^{3+} and NADPH was found. On the other hand [^{14}C] CO_2 release was inhibited by chelating agents (EDTA but *not* EGTA, α-dipyridyl and *o*-phenanthrolene), respiratory chain inhibitors (KCN, but *not* azide) and uncouplers of oxidative phosphorylation (2,4-dinitrophenol). Furthermore, cytosol was required for optimal activity, which, again, was contrary to the results of Tsai et al.[116]

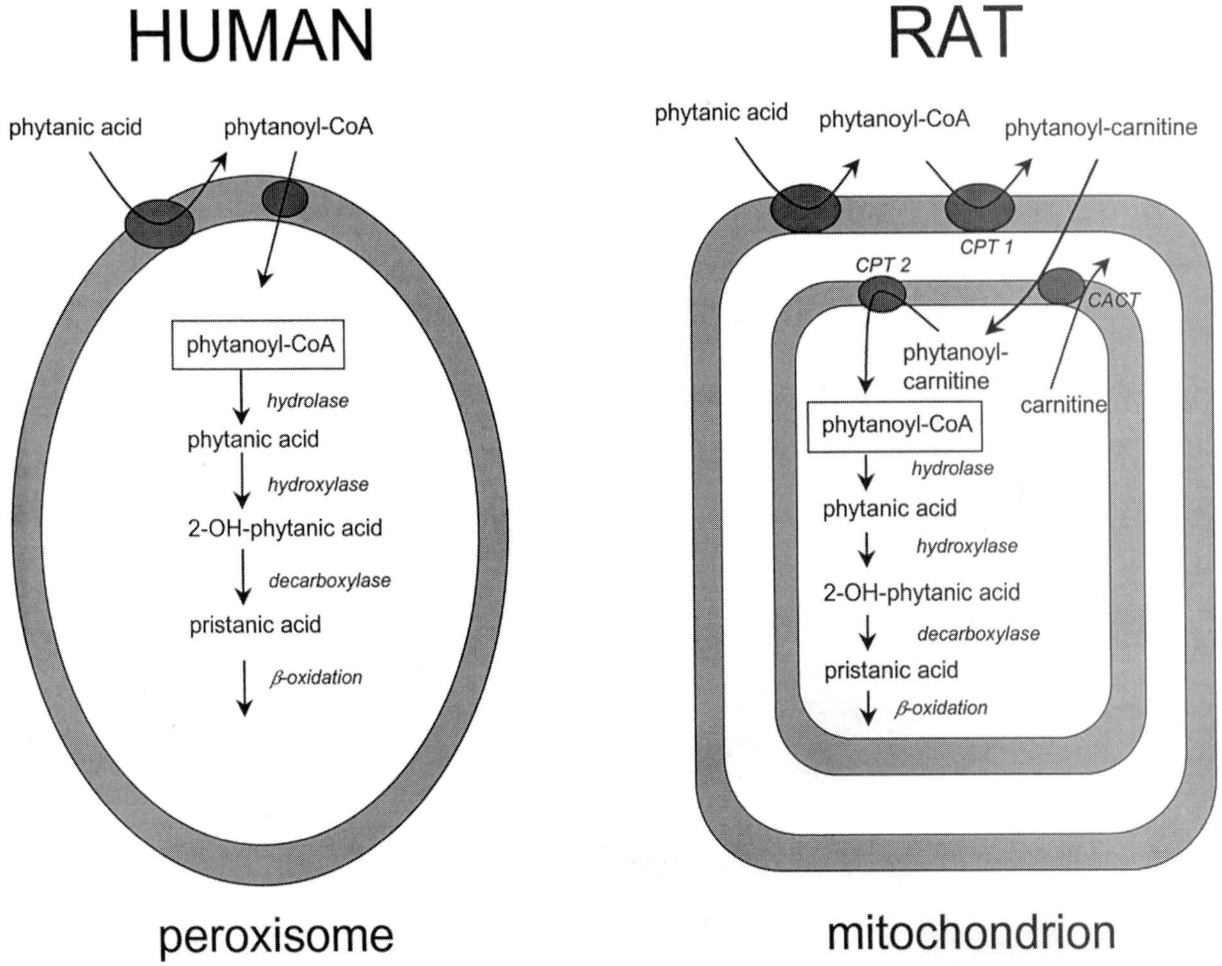

Fig. 132-6 Models proposed by Singh and coworkers for the differential oxidation of phytanic acid in rat and human. See text for details.

Based on these results the authors concluded that: (a) α-oxidation may indeed follow the mechanism suggested by Tsai et al.[116] with free phytanic acid as substrate and 2-hydroxyphytanic acid as product; (b) α-oxidation resides primarily in mitochondria, and (c) a cytosolic, dialyzable factor is required for activity.

In 1987,[118] the question of the subcellular localization of phytanic acid α-oxidation was reconsidered, again based on Poulos and coworkers[47] having shown that phytanic acid α-oxidation is also deficient in fibroblasts from patients suffering from a disorder of peroxisome biogenesis (Zellweger syndrome, infantile Refsum disease), which would suggest a peroxisomal involvement in phytanic acid α-oxidation. The subcellular localization was studied in fractions obtained by differential centrifugation using a protocol allowing preparation of fractions enriched in mitochondria, peroxisomes, and microsomes respectively; all activity was found to be mitochondrial.[118] A similar conclusion was reached by Wanders and Van Roermund[119] who used density-gradient centrifugation techniques based on Nycodenz to prepare peroxisomes and mitochondria of high purity. Activity was again measured as the release of [^{14}C] CO_2 from [1-^{14}C] phytanic acid. All activity was found mitochondrial. Furthermore, activity was drastically reduced by inhibitors of the respiratory chain (antimycin, rotenone) and uncouplers of oxidative phosphorylation (dinitrophenol).[119]

Later studies by Watkins and Mihalik[120] and ourselves[121] revealed that oxidation of phytanic acid measured as release of [^{14}C] CO_2 from [1-^{14}C] phytanic acid was also mitochondrial in human liver. Huang and coworkers[122] also studied the subcellular localization of the α-oxidation process in rat liver and found a *microsomal* localization. These finding were disputed by Singh and coworkers.[123] According to these authors phytanic acid oxidation is mitochondrial in the rat but peroxisomal in man. In their studies α-oxidation was measured as the release of [^{14}C] CO_2 from [1-^{14}C] phytanic acid in a medium containing ATP, $MgCl_2$, CoASH, NAD, FAD, L-carnitine, NADPH, and L-malate. The conclusion that α-oxidation would be peroxisomal in human but mitochondrial in the rat, was based on experiments with (a) POCA, an inhibitor of carnitine palmitoyltransferase 1 that blocks α-oxidation in homogenates of rat liver and rat skin fibroblasts, but not in homogenates of human liver and fibroblasts and (b) subcellular localization studies using Nycodenz.

Based on these[123] and subsequent[124,125] studies, Singh and coworkers proposed the following mechanisms in rat and human, respectively (Fig. 132-6): (a) in both species, the first step involves activation of phytanic acid to phytanoyl-CoA; (b) both in rat and human, phytanic acid α-oxidation follows a similar pathway with *free* phytanic acid as substrate; (c) the enzymes involved in the α-oxidation of phytanic acid to pristanic acid are mitochondrial in the rat and peroxisomal in the human; (d) transport of phytanoyl-CoA across the mitochondrial membrane in the rat involves the concerted action of carnitine palmitoyltransferase 1 (CPT1), the carnitine acylcarnitine carrier, and carnitine palmitoyltransferase 2 (CPT2), whereas in the human situation, phytanoyl-CoA would enter the peroxisome directly; (e) once inside the mitochondrial (rat) and peroxisomal (human) interior, phytanoyl-CoA is converted into free phytanic acid and CoASH via a specific hydrolase; (f) the first step in the α-oxidation of phytanic acid is catalyzed by a peroxisomal (human) and mitochondrial (rat) cytochrome P450 monooxygenase. This was concluded from the finding that ketoconazole and other imidazole derivatives were found to be potent inhibitors of phytanic acid α-oxidation.[126]

The conclusion that phytanic acid α-oxidation is peroxisomal in human but mitochondrial in the rat was hard to reconcile with the discovery of the enzyme 2-hydroxyphytanic acid oxidase with the same (peroxisomal) localization in both rat and human.[127] Early studies by Steinberg and coworkers[116,128,129] had indicated that 2-hydroxyphytanic acid is an obligatory intermediate in the phytanic acid α-oxidation pathway. This was later disputed.[130] The finding that 2-hydroxyphytanic acid accumulates in patients in which pristanic acid β-oxidation is defective, was strong evidence in favor of 2-hydroxyphytanic acid being an intermediate in the pathway formed by hydroxylation of phytanic acid. In analogy to the pathway lactate → pyruvate → acetyl-CoA, we[127] postulated the reaction sequence 2-hydroxyphytanate → 2-ketophytanate → pristanoyl-CoA and, indeed, identified an enzyme capable of converting 2-hydroxyphytanate into 2-ketophytanate.[127]

More compelling evidence against the concept of phytanic acid α-oxidation having a different subcellular localization in rat (mitochondrial) and human (peroxisomal) came when Poulos and coworkers[131,132] reported that branched-chain fatty acids like phytanoyl-CoA are no substrates for CPT1. These and other findings made it clear that there was something fundamentally wrong with all studies performed so far and this indeed turned out to be true as described below.

PHYTANIC ACID α-OXIDATION: RESOLUTION OF THE TRUE STRUCTURE OF THE PATHWAY

Identification of Phytanoyl-CoA Hydroxylase, the Long-Sought Enzyme

When studying phytanic acid α-oxidation in hepatocytes, we[119,127] and others[122] discovered that the rates of phytanic acid α-oxidation in intact hepatocytes were much higher as compared to homogenates of rat liver. Indeed, in our studies rates of phytanic acid α-oxidation in homogenates amounted to only a few percent as compared to the activity in whole cells. Similar low rates have been found in all studies performed in whole homogenates, enriched fractions or isolated organelles. We concluded[127] that all conclusions drawn from studies in homogenates should be viewed with caution.

Another important finding that revolutionized the way of thinking about phytanic acid α-oxidation, was made by Poulos and coworkers.[133] These workers reported that formic acid is the primary product of phytanic acid α-oxidation, and not CO_2. This not only suggested that rates of phytanic acid α-oxidation had long been underestimated but also implied that the concept of a 2-ketoacid (NAD^+) dehydrogenase catalyzing the production of pristanoyl-CoA from 2-ketophytanic as suggested by us could not be true.

The solution came in 1995, when Mihalik and coworkers[134] identified a new enzyme catalyzing the formation of 2-hydroxyphytanoyl-CoA from phytanoyl-CoA. This enzyme appeared to be a dioxygenase requiring 2-ketoglutarate, Fe^{2+} and ascorbate for activity. In the absence of 2-ketoglutarate, *no* activity could be measured. In collaboration with Mihalik and coworkers, we established that phytanoyl-CoA hydroxylase is also present in human liver. Furthermore, the enzyme was localized exclusively in peroxisomes.[135]

Interestingly, in *all* studies performed before 1995 in which phytanic acid oxidation was studied in homogenates, and isolated organelles, *no* 2-ketoglutarate was added, suggesting that the low rates of oxidation measured simply reflect the inadequacy of the assay-medium lacking 2-ketoglutarate.

Studies by Mannaerts and coworkers in rat hepatocytes provided further evidence for the obligatory involvement of a Fe^{2+}- and 2-ketoglutarate-dependent hydroxylase in the α-oxidation process.[136] In these studies, use was made of model compounds including 3-methylhexadecanoate and 3-methylheptadecanoate rather than phytanic acid itself. Although one has to be careful in extrapolating data obtained with model compounds, earlier studies had shown that these model substrates were valid substitutes for phytanic acid.[137] That iron-specific chelators such as desferrioxamine and *o*-phenanthrolene strongly suppressed the α-oxidation of 3-methyl-substituted fatty acids in intact hepatocytes, provided strong evidence for the involvement of iron in the α-oxidation process. This inhibitory effect was specific because the β-oxidation of different substrates was not affected. Furthermore, subsequent studies in permeabilized rat hepatocytes[138] showed very low rates of α-oxidation unless Fe^{2+} and ascorbate were added to the medium in addition to ATP, Mg^{2+}, CoASH, and 2-oxoglutarate. Taking all data together,[134,135,138] it is clear that phytanoyl-CoA hydroxylase is, indeed, the long-sought enzyme that is involved in phytanic acid α-oxidation localized in peroxisomes in both rat and human.

Phytanoyl-CoA Hydroxylase Is Deficient in Classical Refsum Disease

The discovery of phytanoyl-CoA hydroxylase immediately suggested that the deficient α-oxidation of phytanic acid in these patients may result from a deficiency in this enzyme. The work of Jansen et al.[11] showed this to be true. At that time, PhyH activity measurements could only be performed in liver biopsy specimens making use of [^{14}C] phytanoyl-CoA followed by resolution of radiolabeled phytanoyl-CoA and 2-hydroxyphytanoyl-CoA by HPLC. Unfortunately, PhyH activity could not be detected in cultured skin fibroblasts using this assay procedure.

We recently developed a new method that enables PhyH activity to be measured in cultured cells. This method is based on the use of nonradiolabeled phytanoyl-CoA followed by quantification of the 2-hydroxyphytanoyl-CoA produced as the free acid obtained after alkaline hydrolysis using gas chromatography. Table 132-4 summarizes the results obtained in homogenates of human liver and cultured skin fibroblasts, respectively.

Phytanoyl-CoA Hydroxylase Is Also Deficient in the PBDs and in RCDP Type 1

Earlier studies had shown that phytanic acid oxidation is not only deficient in Refsum disease but also in the disorders of peroxi some biogenesis and RCDP type 1, which results from a genetic defect in the PTS2-receptor (Pex7p) encoded by the *HsPEX7* gene.[51–53] Recent studies show that phytanoyl-CoA hydroxylase is also deficient in these disorders.[139] The deficiency of PhyH activity in these peroxisomal disorders probably has to do with the reduced stability of the enzyme in the cytosolic compartment in PBD and RCDP type 1 cells. In these cells, PhyH, being a PTS2-protein (see next section), is not properly targeted to the peroxisome.

Table 132-4 Phytanoyl-CoA Hydroxylase Activity Measurements in Homogenates of Human Liver Specimens and Cultured Skin Fibroblasts from Patients with Refsum Disease and Other Peroxisomal Disorders

	Phytanoyl-CoA hydroxylase activity*			
Patient analyzed	**Liver**		**Fibroblasts**	
Controls	2.45 ± 0.88	(11)	0.30 ± 0.08	(5)
Refsum disease	≤0.05	(1)	N.D.	(8)
Zellweger syndrome	≤0.05	(3)	0.05 ± 0.02	(3)
RCDP Type 1	≤0.05	(3)	0.03≤0.01	(3)
X-linked ALD	2.41; 2.72		0.19 ± 0.05	(3)

*Values represent mean ± SD with the number of control or patient liver samples and cell lines analyzed between parentheses. Activities are in nmol/h · mg protein. Data from Jansen et al.[163] and Jansen et al., unpublished. N.D. = not detectable.

Purification of Phytanoyl-CoA Hydroxylase and Cloning of the Rat, Mouse, and Human cDNAs

We purified the enzyme from rat liver peroxisomes using classic column chromatography procedures to apparent homogeneity.[140] The molecular weight on SDS-PAGE was 35 kDa. The purified enzyme was used for N-terminal protein sequencing and the sequence obtained allowed screening of the database of expressed sequence tags (dbEST). Many human EST-clones were identified, which led to the *in silico* construction of the complete *PHYH* cDNA. This composite human *PHYH* cDNA contained an open-reading frame of 1014 bp encoding a 338-amino-acid protein with a calculated molecular weight of 38.6 kDa, which is much larger than the 35 kDa of the purified protein. Interestingly, at residues 9 to 17 of the deduced amino acid sequence, a typical PTS2 sequence (RLQIVLGHL) was found that directs the PhyH protein to peroxisomes. This targeting depends on the PTS2-receptor (Pex7p). The discovery of PhyH being a PTS2-protein immediately explains the deficiency in RCDP type 1 in which the PTS2-receptor is defective.[51–53]

Expression of the *PHYH* cDNA in *S. cerevisiae* confirmed that this cDNA does code for phytanoyl-CoA hydroxylase. We recently cloned the rat and mouse *PHYH* cDNAs;[141] the deduced amino acid sequences show high homology with clear PTS2-sequences in all three proteins in line with a peroxisomal (and *not* mitochondrial) localization in all three species.

The human *PHYH* cDNA was also identified by Mihalik and coworkers[142] using a different approach based on the concept that PhyH would be a PTS2-protein. Screening of the EST database provided several candidate cDNAs, which allowed construction of a full-length cDNA[142] identical to the cDNA identified by Jansen et al.[140]

Comparison between the cDNA deduced amino acid sequence and the N-terminal amino acid sequence of PhyH as purified from peroxisomes[140] revealed that the purified protein lacks the first 30 amino acids. This implies that after import of the precursor protein into the peroxisome, the N-terminal prepiece containing the PTS2-signal is cleaved off as occurs in certain other PTS2-proteins such as peroxisomal thiolase[143] and alkyldihydroxyacetonephosphate synthase.[144,145]

From 2-Hydroxyphytanoyl-CoA to Pristanic Acid: Resolution of the Complete Structure of the Pathway

Recent studies have shown that 2-hydroxyphytanoyl-CoA is converted into pristanic acid via two enzymatic steps (Fig. 132-7).[146,147] In the first step 2-hydroxyphytanoyl-CoA undergoes cleavage into pristanal and formyl-CoA, which rapidly hydrolyses to formic acid and CoASH.[148] Pristanal is subsequently oxidized to pristanic acid via an aldehyde dehydrogenase. After activation to its CoA-ester, pristanoyl-CoA can be β-oxidized via the peroxisomal β-oxidation system.

The subcellular localization of the enzymes involved in the conversion of 2-hydroxyphytanoyl-CoA to pristanic acid has not been resolved definitively. According to Verhoeven et al.[149] the combined activity of the 2-hydroxyphytanoyl-CoA lyase plus pristanal dehydrogenase measured as the formation of pristanic acid from 2-hydroxyphytanoyl-CoA, is localized in the endoplasmic reticulum, at least in human liver. Recent studies in rat liver by ourselves[150] and others[151] have shown that 2-hydroxyphytanoyl-CoA lyase is a peroxisomal enzyme and *not* a microsomal enzyme. These studies on the subcellular localization of the lyase in the rat showing a strict peroxisomal localization are further supported by data from Foulon et al.,[151] who recently cloned the human 2-hydroxyphytanoyl-CoA lyase cDNA. The C-terminus was found to end in the sequence SNM, which is an atypical PTS1 signal. This was concluded from transfection studies with constructs coding for 2-hydroxyphytanoyl-CoA lyase fused to green-fluorescent-protein (GFP). These studies showed that the construct was targeted to peroxisomes in

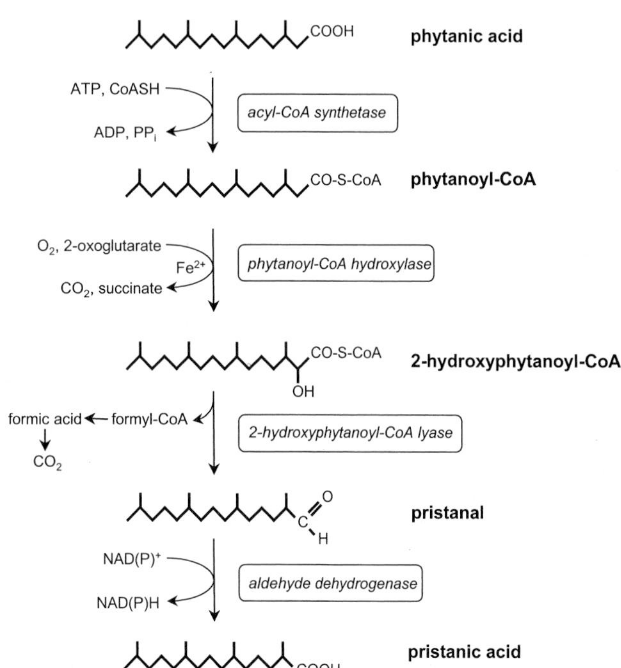

Fig. 132-7 Structure of the phytanic acid α-oxidation pathway as recently elucidated. See text for details.

fibroblasts from PEX5 (+/+) and PEX5 (+/−) mice, whereas in fibroblasts from PEX5 (−/−) mice that lack the PTS1 import receptor (see Chap. 129) a cytosolic localization was found. The finding that a GFP construct, containing only the last five amino acids of the lyase (TRSNM), was also targeted to peroxisomes in a PTS1 import receptor-dependent manner, indicates that the targeting information must be present in this pentapeptide. Apparently, the PTS1 signal found in the 2-hydroxyphytanoyl-CoA lyase protein belongs to the group of nonconsensus PTS1 signals characterized by a C-terminal tripeptide preceded by a positive charge[152] as identified in other peroxisomal proteins like catalase.[153]

The situation with respect to the next step in the pathway, the conversion of pristanal to pristanic acid is less clear. Our own data in human skin fibroblasts[154] have shown that the oxidation of pristanal to pristanic acid is predominantly catalyzed by a microsomal aldehyde dehydrogenase, which is the same enzyme as the one deficient in Sjögren-Larsson syndrome (see Chap. 98). This was concluded from studies with the recombinant Sjögren-Larsson aldehyde dehydrogenase (FALDH) that readily oxidized pristanal to pristanic acid, and from studies on fibroblasts from patients with Sjögren-Larsson syndrome in which oxidation of pristanal to pristanic acid was found to be strongly deficient (13 percent of normal).[154]

On the other hand, studies by Croes et al.,[146] which made use of model compounds rather than the true physiological substrates, showed that isolated rat liver peroxisomes are capable of converting 2-hydroxy-3-methylhexadecanoyl-CoA into both 2-methylpentadecanal and 2-methylpentadecanoic acid. In addition, we recently found that peroxisomes also contain pristanal dehydrogenase activity next to the activity in microsomes and mitochondria (Jansen and Wanders, unpublished data). It is clear that the current data are not conclusive. It may well be that all steps from phytanoyl-CoA to pristanic acid are peroxisomal (Fig. 132-8) including the aldehyde dehydrogenase step. In this respect, it is important to mention that patients suffering from Sjögren-Larsson syndrome do *not* show elevated phytanic acid levels in plasma (authors' unpublished data), which argues against a major role of the Sjörgen-Larsson aldehyde dehydrogenase in phytanic acid α-oxidation. Furthermore, [1-^{14}C] phytanic acid

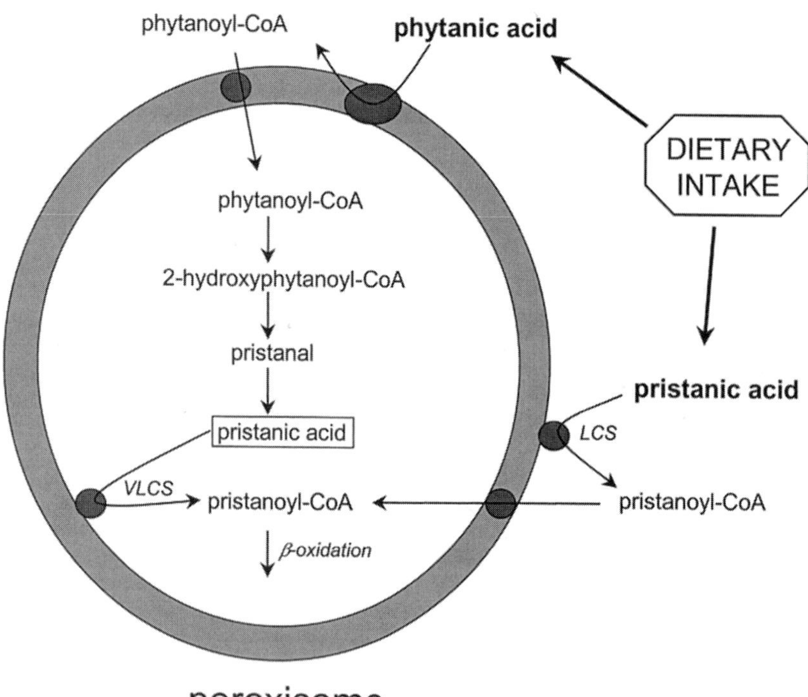

Fig. 132-8 Enzymatic organization of the phytanic and pristanic acid degrading systems in peroxisomes, with particular emphasis on the activation of pristanic acid within the peroxisomal interior or outside peroxisomes. See text for full details.

oxidation iscompletely normal in fibroblasts from Sjögren-Larsson patients.

Activation of Pristanic Acid and Phytanic Acid to Their CoA-Esters

If peroxisomes do contain the complete enzymatic machinery to catalyze the formation of pristanic acid from phytanoyl-CoA, it would make sense if the activation of pristanic acid to pristanoyl-CoA would also take place in peroxisomes. Until recently, it was thought that activation of pristanic acid to pristanoyl-CoA occurs at the cytosolic phase of the peroxisomal membrane, which would imply export of pristanic acid out of the peroxisome. This was concluded from the finding[155] that long-chain acyl-CoA synthetase (LCS), with its catalytic site facing the cytosol,[156] is also able to activate pristanic acid to pristanoyl-CoA. Recent studies, however, suggest that the situation may well be different.

Steinberg et al.[157] recently cloned the human ortholog (HsVLCS) of the gene encoding rat liver very-long-chain acyl-CoA synthetase. The enzyme was localized to both peroxisomes and endoplasmic reticulum and showed high activity with straight- and branched-chain fatty acids including pristanic acid. The authors conclude that HsVLCS is topographically oriented facing the matrix and *not* the cytoplasm, and suggest that the enzyme plays a role in the *intra*peroxisomal activation of pristanic acid to pristanoyl-CoA.

It may well be that the newly identified synthetase and the LCS are both involved in pristanic acid oxidation but play different roles. Because pristanic acid is not only derived from phytanic acid by α-oxidation but also comes directly from dietary sources, it may well be that LCS is involved in the activation of dietary pristanic acid in the cytosol, whereas the VLCS would be involved in the activation of intraperoxisomal pristanic acid generated from phytanic acid (see Fig. 132-8).

Because phytanoyl-CoA is the true substrate for α-oxidation, phytanic acid must also be activated. According to Singh and coworkers,[158] peroxisomes contain a distinct acyl-CoA syn thetase specific for phytanic acid. This view was disputed by Watkins et al.[159] who showed that LCS also reacts with phytanic acid. It remains to be established whether there is a distinct phytanoyl-CoA synthetase. Importantly, both authors agree that phytanoyl-CoA synthetase faces the cytosol which implies that the phytanoyl-CoA ester has to traverse the peroxisomal membrane.

STEREOCHEMISTRY OF THE PHYTANIC ACID α-OXIDATION SYSTEM

As described before, naturally occurring phytanic acid is a racemic mixture of two stereoisomers including (3R,7R,11R,15)-tetramethylhexadecanoic acid and (3S,7R,11R,15)-tetramethylhexadecanoic acid. Studies by Tsai et al.[129] show that both stereoisomers are oxidized at comparable rates. The same authors concluded that the introduction of the hydroxyl group at position 2 is stereospecific and determined by the configuration of the methyl group at position 3. The absolute configuration of the isomers of 2-hydroxyphytanic acid as formed during α-oxidation was not determined, however. This was recently accomplished by Croes et al.[160] making use of model compounds rather than the true phytanic acid stereoisomers. These studies revealed that under physiological conditions only, the (2S,3R) and (2R,3S) isomers are formed demonstrating that the hydroxylation occurs at the opposite side of the methyl-group in position 3, which may have to do with a reduced degree of steric hindrance. Fig. 132-9 shows the metabolism of the two stereoisomers.

MOLECULAR BASIS OF REFSUM DISEASE

The identification of the human *PHYH* cDNA by Jansen et al.[140] and Mihalik et al.[142] and the availability of an expression system[141] made it possible to study the consequences of certain mutations (Jansen et al., unpublished data). The first report on the molecular basis of Refsum disease[140] in five patients describes several mutations, including: (a) a single nucleotide deletion leading to a frameshift and a premature stop codon; (b) an in-frame deletion of 111 nucleotides resulting in a protein product lacking 37 amino acids; and (c) an missense mutation (805A > C) resulting in substitution of a histidine for an asparagine (N269H). Expression studies show that the N269H substitution is associated with loss of PhyH activity (unpublished experiments of Jansen and Wanders).

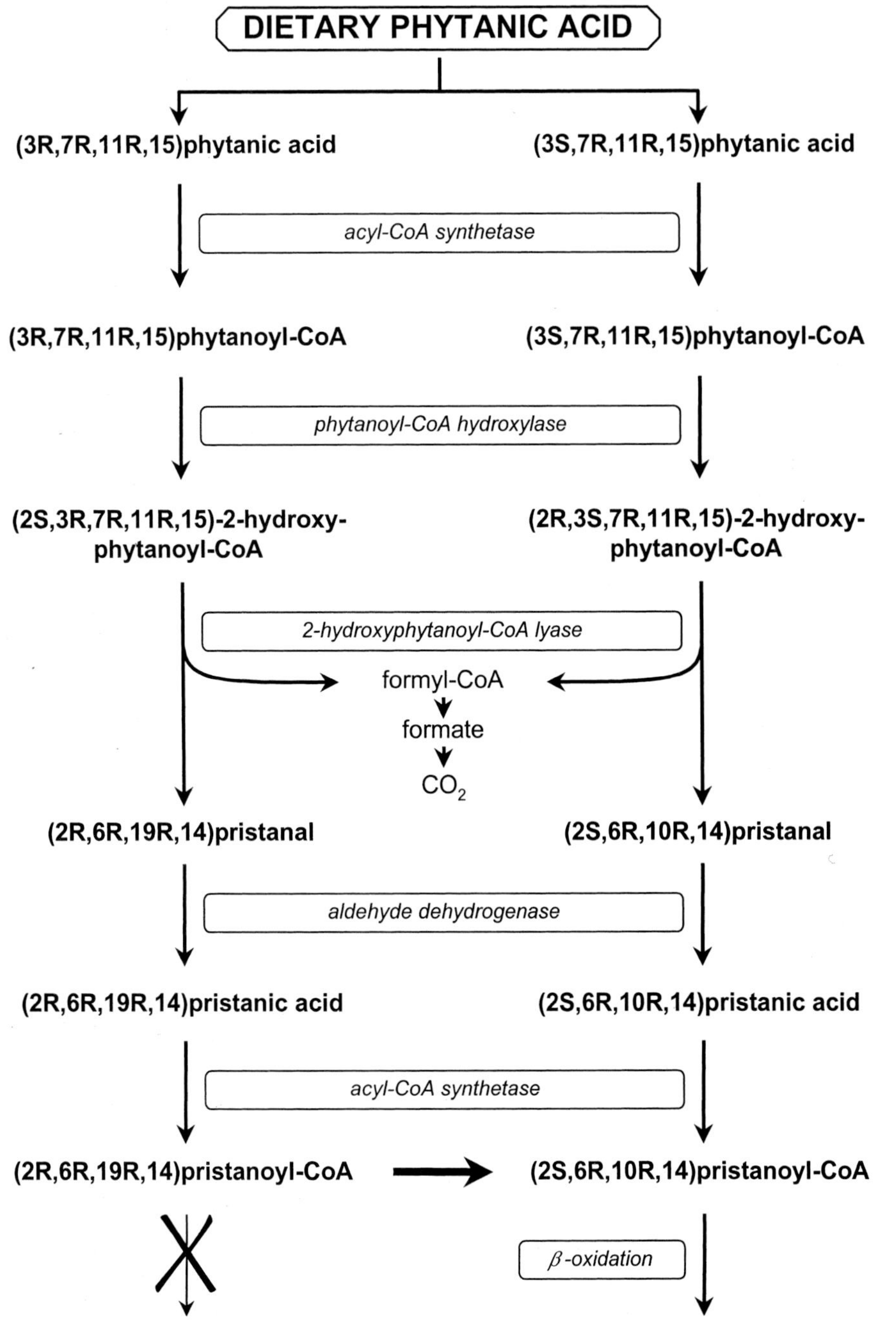

DIETARY PHYTANIC ACID

(3R,7R,11R,15)phytanic acid | (3S,7R,11R,15)phytanic acid

acyl-CoA synthetase

(3R,7R,11R,15)phytanoyl-CoA | (3S,7R,11R,15)phytanoyl-CoA

phytanoyl-CoA hydroxylase

(2S,3R,7R,11R,15)-2-hydroxy-phytanoyl-CoA | (2R,3S,7R,11R,15)-2-hydroxy-phytanoyl-CoA

2-hydroxyphytanoyl-CoA lyase

formyl-CoA → formate → CO_2

(2R,6R,19R,14)pristanal | (2S,6R,10R,14)pristanal

aldehyde dehydrogenase

(2R,6R,19R,14)pristanic acid | (2S,6R,10R,14)pristanic acid

acyl-CoA synthetase

(2R,6R,19R,14)pristanoyl-CoA → (2S,6R,10R,14)pristanoyl-CoA

β-oxidation

Fig. 132-9 Stereochemistry of the phytanic acid α-oxidation system. Naturally occurring phytanic acid is a mixture of two different stereoisomers (3S,7R,11R) and (3R,7R,11R) phytanic acid, both of which can be α-oxidized according to the mechanism shown.

Although the molecular defects have been published for only a few patients,[140,142,161,162] we have identified many different mutations in a series of 35 patients. We recently determined the structure of the *PHYH* gene that spans 21.5 kb on chromosome 10p of the human genome and encodes an mRNA of about 1.6 kb. The 1014 nucleotides of the open-reading frame sequence are separated by 8 introns that range in size from 0.9 to 4.5 kb (Fig. 132-10).

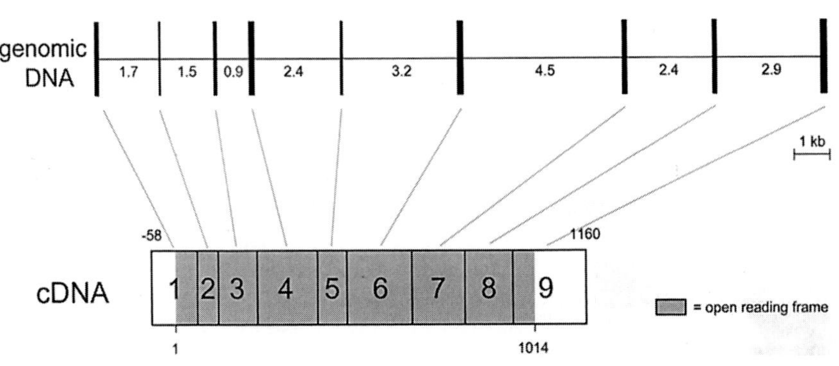

Fig. 132-10 Organization of the human phytanoyl-CoA hydroxylase gene.

ACKNOWLEDGMENTS

The authors gratefully acknowledge the expert help of Mrs. Maddy Festen and Mrs. Iet van der Gracht in preparation of the manuscript. Dr. Gerbert Jansen is gratefully thanked for his many contributions to this chapter. This work was financially supported by grants from the Prinses Beatrix Fonds (The Hague, The Netherlands) and The Netherlands Organization for Scientific Research (NWO, project no. 901-03-133).

REFERENCES

1. Refsum S: Heredopathia atactica polyneuritiformis. *Acta Psychiatr Scand (Suppl)* **38**:1, 1946.
2. Viets HR: Refsum's disease. *N Engl J Med* **236**:996, 1947.
3. Klenk E, Kahlke W: Ueber das Vorkommen der 3,7,11,15-tetramethylhexadecansaure (phytansaure) in den cholesterinestern und anderen lipidfraktionen der organe bei einem krankheitsfall unbekanter genese (Verdacht auf Heredopathia atactica polyneuritiformis, Refsum's syndrome). *Hoppe Seylers Z Physiol Chem* **333**:133, 1963.
4. Richterich R, Van Mechelen P, Rossi E: Refsum's disease (heredopathia atactica polyneuritiformis): An inborn error of lipid metabolism with storage of 3,7,11,15-tetramethylhexadecanoic acid. *Am J Med* **39**:230, 1963.
5. Kahlke W, Richterich R: Refsum's disease (heredopathia atactica polyneuritiformis): an inborn error of lipid metabolism with storage of 3,7,11,15-tetramethylhexadecanoic acid. II. Isolation and identification of the storage product. *Am J Med* **39**:237, 1965.
6. Steinberg D, Avigan J, Mize C, Eldjarn L, Try K, Refsum S: Conversion of U-C14-phytol to phytanic acid and its oxidation in heredopathia atactica polyneuritiformis. *Biochem Biophys Res Commun* **19**:783, 1965.
7. Steinberg D, Herndon JH Jr, Uhlendorf BW, Mize CE, Avigan J, Milne GWA: Refsum's disease: Nature of the enzyme defect. *Science* **156**:1740, 1967.
8. Herndon JH Jr, Steinberg D, Uhlendorf BW, Fales HM: Refsum's disease: characterization of the enzyme defect in cell culture. *J Clin Invest* **48**:1017, 1969.
9. Herndon JH Jr, Steinberg D, Uhlendorf BW: Refsum's disease: Defective oxidation of phytanic acid in tissue cultures derived from homozygotes and heterozygotes. *N Engl J Med* **281**:1034, 1969.
10. Mize CE, Herndon JH Jr, Blass JP, Milne GW, Follansbee C, Laudat P, Steinberg D: Localization of the oxidative defect in phytanic acid degradation in patients with Refsum's disease. *J Clin Invest* **48**:1033, 1969.
11. Jansen GA, Wanders RJA, Watkins PA, Mihalik SJ: Phytanoyl-coenzyme A hydroxylase deficiency—The enzyme defect in Refsum's disease. *N Engl J Med* **337**:133, 1997.
12. Richterich R, Moser H, Rossi E: Refsum's disease (heredopathia atactica polyneuritiformis). An inborn error of lipid metabolism with storage of 3,7,11,15 tetramethyl hexadecanoic acid. A review of the clinical findings. *Humangenetik* **1**:322, 1965.
13. Skjeldal OH, Stokke O, Refsum S, Norseth J, Petit H: Clinical and biochemical heterogeneity in conditions with phytanic acid accumulation. *J Neurol Sci* **77**:87, 1987.
14. Scotto JM, Hadchouel M, Odievre M, Laudat MH, Saudubray JM, Dulac O, Beucler I, et al: Infantile phytanic acid storage disease, a possible variant of Refsum's disease: Three cases, including ultrastructural studies of the liver. *J Inherit Metab Dis* **5**:83, 1982.
15. Poll-The BT, Saudubray JM, Ogier HA, Odievre M, Scotto JM, Monnens L, Govaerts LC, et al: Infantile Refsum disease: An inherited peroxisomal disorder. Comparison with Zellweger syndrome and neonatal adrenoleukodystrophy. *Eur J Pediatr* **146**:477, 1987.
16. Claridge KG, Gibberd FB, Sidey MC: Refsum disease: The presentation and ophthalmic aspects of Refsum disease in a series of 23 patients. *EYE* **6**:371, 1992.
17. Skjeldal OH: Heredopathia atactica polyneuritiformis (Refsum's disease), in Moser HW (ed): *Handbook of Clinical Neurology.* Amsterdam, Elsevier Science BV, 1996, p 485.
18. Goldman JM, Clemens ME, Gibberd FB, Billimoria JD: Screening of patients with retinitis pigmentosa for heredopathia atactica polyneuritiformis (Refsum's disease). *BMJ* **290**:1109, 1985.
19. Hansen E, Bachen NI, Flage T: Refsum's disease. Eye manifestations in a patient treated with low-phytol low-phytanic acid diet. *Acta Ophthalmol (Copenh)* **57**:899, 1979.
20. Levy IS: Refsum's syndrome. *Trans Ophthalmol Soc U K* **90**:181, 1970.
21. Toussaint D, Danis P: An ocular pathologic study of Refsum's syndrome. *Am J Ophthalmol* **72**:342, 1971.
22. Abu el-Asrar AM, Kahtani ES, Tabbara KF: Retinal arteriovenous communication in retinitis pigmentosa with Refsum's disease-like findings. *Doc Ophthalmol* **89**:313, 1995.
23. Lewis RA, Sumner AJ: The electrodiagnostic distinctions between chronic familial and acquired demyelinative neuropathies. *Neurology* **32**:592, 1982.
24. Kuntzer T, Ochsner F, Schmid F, Regli F: Quantitative EMG analysis and longitudinal nerve conduction studies in a Refsum's disease patient. *Muscle Nerve* **16**:857, 1993.
25. Gelot A, Vallat JM, Tabaraud F, Rocchiccioli F: Axonal neuropathy and late detection of Refsum's disease. *Muscle Nerve* **18**:667, 1995.
26. Gibberd FB, Billimoria JD, Goldman JM, Clemens ME, Evans R, Whitelaw MN, Retsas S, et al: Heredopathia atactica polyneuritiformis: Refsum's disease. *Acta Neurol Scand* **72**:1, 1985.
27. Salisachs P: Is the "cerebellar" incoordination of Refsum's disease due to structural lesions in the cerebellum? *J Neurol Neurosurg Psychiatry* **45**:473, 1982.
28. Bergsmark J, Djupesland G: Heredopathia atactica polyneuritiformis (Refsum's diseases). An audiological examination of two patients. *Eur Neurol* **1**:122, 1968.
29. Refsum S: Heredopathia atactica polyneuritiformis. Phytanic acid storage disease (Refsum disease), in Vinken PJ, Bruyn GW, de Jong JMB (eds): *Handbook of Clinical Neurology. System Disorders and Atrophies*. Amsterdam, North-Holland, 1975, p 181.
30. Leys D, Petit H, Bonte-Adnet C, Millaire A, Fourrier F, Dubois F, Rosseaux M, et al: Refsum's disease revealed by cardiac disorders. *Lancet* **1**:621, 1989.
31. Posada Rodriguez IJ, Gutierrez-Rivas E, Cabello A: Cardiac involvement in neuromuscular diseases. *Rev Esp Cardiol* **50**:882, 1997.
32. Refsum S, Stokke O: Refsum's disease (heredopathia atactica polyneuritiformis), in Gomez M (ed.): *Neurocutaneous Disease-A practical approach.* Boston, Butterworths, 1987, p 80.
33. Dykes PJ, Marks R, Davies MG, Reynolds DJ: Epidermal metabolism in heredopathia atactica polyneuritiformis (Refsum's disease). *J Invest Dermatol* **70**:126, 1978.
34. Davies MG, Marks R, Dykes PJ, Reynolds D: Epidermal abnormalities in Refsum's disease. *Br J Dermatol* **97**:401, 1977.
35. Ashenhurst EM, Millar JHD, Milliken TG: Refsum's syndrome affecting a brother and two sisters. *BMJ* **2**:415, 1958.
36. Dick JP, Meeran K, Gibberd FB, Rose FC: Hypokalaemia in acute Refsum's disease. *J R Soc Med* **86**:171, 1993.
37. Vreken P, Van Lint AEM, Bootsma AH, Overmars H, Wanders RJA, Van Gennip AH: Rapid stable isotope dilution analysis of very-long-chain fatty acids, pristanic acid and phytanic acid using gas chromatography-electron impact mass spectrometry. *J Chromatogr* **713**:281, 1998.
38. Poulos A: Diagnosis of Refsum's disease using [1-14C] phytanic acid as substrate. *Clin Genet* **20**:247, 1981.
39. Reynolds DJ, Marks R, Davies MG, Dykes PJ: The fatty acid composition of skin and plasma lipids in Refsum's disease. *Clin Chim Acta* **90**:171, 1978.
40. Dulaney JT, Williams M, Evans JE, Costello CE, Kolodny EH: Occurrence of novel branched-chain fatty acids in Refsum's disease. *Biochim Biophys Acta* **529**:1, 1978.
41. Yao JK, Dyck PJ: Tissue distribution of phytanic acid and its analogues in a kinship with Refsum's disease. *Lipids* **22**:69, 1987.
42. Molzer B, Bernheimer H, Barolin GS, Höfinger E, Lenz H: Di-, mono- and nonphytanyl triglycerides in the serum: A sensitive parameter of the phytanic acid accumulation in Refsum's disease. *Clin Chim Acta* **91**:133, 1979.
43. Laurell S: Separation and characterization of phytanic acid-containing plasmatriglycerides from a patient with Refsum's disease. *Biochim Biophys Acta* **152**:75, 1968.
44. Wierzbicki AS, Hardman TC, Lumb P, Sankaralingam A, Morrish Z, Patel, F, et al: Influence of plasma phytanic acid levels in Refsum's disease on the behaviour of the erythrocyte membrane sodium-lithium countertransporter. *Eur J Clin Invest* **28**:334, 1998.
45. Kahlke W, Goerlich R, Feist D: [Increased concentration of phytanic acid in plasma and liver of an infant with cerebral damage of unknown etiology.] *Klin Wochenschr* **52**:651, 1974.
46. Boltshauser E, Spycher MA, Steinmann B, Briner J, Isler W, Kuster T, Poulos A, et al: Infantile phytanic acid storage disease: A variant of Refsum disease? *Eur J Pediatr* 139:317, 1982.

47. Poulos A, Sharp P, Whiting M: Infantile Refsum's disease (phytanic acid storage disease): A variant of Zellweger's syndrome? *Clin Genet* **26**:579, 1984.
48. Heymans HSA, Oorthuys JW, Nelck G, Wanders RJA, Schutgens RBH: Rhizomelic chondrodysplasia punctata: Another peroxisomal disorder. *N Engl J Med* **313**:187, 1985.
49. van den Bosch H, Schutgens RBH, Wanders RJA, Tager JM: Biochemistry of peroxisomes. *Annu Rev Biochem* **61**:157, 1992.
50. Wanders RJA, Tager JM: Lipid metabolism in peroxisomes in relation to human disease. *Mol Aspects Med* **19**:69, 1998.
51. Braverman N, Steel G, Obie C, Moser AB, Moser HW, Gould SJ, Valle D: Human PEX7 encodes the peroxisomal PTS2 receptor and is responsible for rhizomelic chondrodysplasia punctata. *Nat Genet* **15**:369, 1997.
52. Motley AM, Hettema EH, Hogenhout EM, Brites P, ten Asbroek AL, Wijburg FA, Baas F, et al: Rhizomelic chondrodysplasia punctata is a peroxisomal protein targeting disease caused by a non-functional PTS2 receptor. *Nat Genet* **15**:377, 1997.
53. Purdue PE, Zhang JW, Skoneczny M, Lazarow PB: Rhizomelic chondrodysplasia punctata is caused by deficiency of human PEX7, a homologue of the yeast PTS2 receptor. *Nat Genet* **15**:381, 1997.
54. Wanders RJA, Schutgens RBH, Barth PG, Tager JM, van den Bosch H: Postnatal diagnosis of peroxisomal disorders: a biochemical approach. *Biochimie* **75**:269, 1993.
55. Wanders RJA, Schutgens RBH, Barth PG: Peroxisomal disorders: A review. *J Neuropathol Exp Neurol* **54**:726, 1995.
56. Verhoeven NM, Wanders RJA, Poll-The BT, Saudubray JM, Jacobs C: The metabolism of phytanic acid and pristanic acid in man: A review. *J Inherit Metab Dis* **21**:697, 1998.
57. ten Brink HJ, Stellaard F, van den Heuvel CM, Kok RM, Schor DS, Wanders RJA, Jakobs C: Pristanic acid and phytanic acid in plasma from patients with peroxisomal disorders: Stable isotope dilution analysis with electron capture negative ion mass fragmentography. *J Lipid Res* **33**:41, 1992.
58. Tranchant C, Aubourg P, Mohr M, Rocchiccioli F, Zaenker C, Warter JM: A new peroxisomal disease with impaired phytanic and pipecolic acid oxidation. *Neurology* **43**:2044, 1993.
59. Nadal N, Rolland MO, Tranchant C, Reutenauer L, Gyapay G, Warter JM, Mandel JL, et al: Localization of Refsum disease with increased pipecolic acidaemia to chromosome 10p by homozygosity mapping and carrier testing in a single nuclear family. *Hum Mol Genet* **4**:1963, 1995.
60. Hansen RP, Shorland FB: The branched chain fatty acids of butterfat. II. Isolation of a multibranched, C20 saturated fatty acid fraction. *Biochem J* **50**:358, 1952.
61. Sonneveld W, Haverkamp Begemann P, Van Beers GJ, Keuning R, Schogt JCM: 3,7,11,15-Tetramethylhexadecanoic acid, a constituent of butterfat. *J Lipid Res* **3**:351, 1962.
62. Willstaetter R, Mayer EW, Huni E: Untersuchungen uber Phytol. *Liebigs Ann* **378**:73, 1911.
63. Steinberg D, Mize CE, Avigan J, Fales HM, Eldjarn L, Try K, Stokke O, et al: Studies on the metabolic error in Refsum's disease. *J Clin Invest* **46**:313, 1967.
64. Mize CE, Avigan J, Baxter JH, Fales HM, Steinberg D: Metabolism of phytol-U-14C and phytanic acid-U-14C in the rat. *J Lipid Res* **7**:692, 1966.
65. Baxter JH, Steinberg D, Mize CE, Avigan J: Absorption and metabolism of uniformly 14C-labeled phytol and phytanic acid by the intestine of the rat studied with thoracic duct cannulation. *Biochim Biophys Acta* **132**:277, 1967.
66. Baxter JH, Steinberg D: Absorption of phytol from dietary chlorophyll in the rat. *J Lipid Res* **8**:615, 1967.
67. Baxter JH: Absorption of chlorophyll phytol in normal man and in patients with Refsum's disease. *J Lipid Res* **8**:615, 1967.
68. Steinberg D: Refsum disease, in Scriver CR, Beaudet al, Sly WS, Valle D (eds): *The Metabolic and Molecular Bases of Inherited Disease*, 7th ed. New York, McGraw-Hill, 1995, p 2351.
69. Kitareewan S, Burka LT, Tomer KB, Parker CE, Deterding LJ, Stevens RD, Forman BM, et al: Phytol metabolites are circulating dietary factors that activate the nuclear receptor RXR. *Mol Biol Cell* **7**:1153, 1996.
70. Seedorf U, Raabe M, Ellinghaus P, Kannenberg F, Fobker M, Engel T, Denis S, et al: Defective peroxisomal catabolism of branched fatty acyl coenzyme A in mice lacking the sterol carrier protein-2/sterol carrier protein-x gene function. *Genes Dev* **12**:1189, 1998.
71. Wolfrum C, Ellinghaus P, Fobker M, Seedorf U, Assmann G, Börchers T, Spener F: Phytanic acid is ligand and transcriptional activator of murine liver fatty acid binding protein. *J Lipid Res* **40**:708, 1999.
72. Ellinghaus P, Wolfrum C, Assmann G, Spener F, Seedorf U: Phytanic acid activates the peroxisome proliferator-activated receptor alfa (PPARalfa) in sterol carrier protein 2-/sterol carrier protein x-deficient mice. *J Biol Chem* **274**:2766, 1999.
73. Lemberger T, Desvergne B, Wahli W: Peroxisome proliferator-activated receptors: A nuclear receptor signaling pathway in lipid physiology. *Annu Rev Cell Dev Biol* **12**:335, 1996.
74. Lee SS, Pineau T, Drago J, Lee EJ, Owens JW, Kroetz DL, Fernandez-Salguero PM, et al: Targeted disruption of the alpha isoform of the peroxisome proliferator-activated receptor gene in mice results in abolishment of the pleiotropic effects of peroxisome proliferators. *Mol Cell Biol* **15**:3012, 1995.
75. Eldjarn L, Try K, Stokke O, Munthe-Kaas AW, Refsum S, Steinberg D, Avigan J, et al: Dietary effects on serum-phytanic-acid levels and on clinical manifestations in heredopathia atactica polyneuritiformis. *Lancet* **1**:691, 1966.
76. Stokke O: Dietary treatment of patients with Refsum's disease. Effect of diet on serum phytanic acid levels, in Try K, Stokke O (eds): *Biochemical and Dietary studies in Refsum's Disease (Heredopathia Atactica Polyneuritiformis)*. Oslo, Universitetsforlaget, 1969, p 77.
77. Steinberg D, Vroom FQ, Engel WK, Cammermeyer J, Mize CE, Avigan J: Refsum's disease — A recently characterized lipidosis involving the nervous system. Combined clinical staff conference at the National Institutes of Health. *Ann Intern Med* **66**:365, 1967.
78. Refsum S: Heredopathia atactica polyneuritiformis (Refsum's disease), in Dyck PG, Thomas PK, Lambert EH, Bunge R (eds): *Peripheral Neuropathy*. Philadelphia, WB Saunders, 1984, p 71.
79. Steinberg D, Herndon JH Jr: Refsum's disease: Phytanic acid storage disease, in Goldensohn ES, Appel SH (eds): *Scientific Approaches to Clinical Neurology*. Philadelphia, Lea & Febriger, 1977, p 994.
80. Masters-Thomas A, Bailes J, Billimoria JD, Clemens ME, Gibberd FB, Page NG: Heredopathia atactica polyneuritiformis (Refsum's disease): 1. Clinical features and dietary management. *J Hum Nutr* **34**:245, 1980.
81. Kark RAP, Engel WK, Blass JP, Steinberg D, Walsh GO: Heredopathia atactica polyneuritiformis (Refsum's Disease): A second trial of dietary therapy in two patients. *Birth Defects Orig Artic Ser* **7**:53, 1971.
82. Laudat PH: [Phytol intolerance: Refsum's disease.] *Biochimie* **54**:735, 1972.
83. Gibberd FB, Billimoria JD, Page NG, Retsas S: Heredopathia atactica polyneuritiformis (Refsum's disease) treated by diet and plasma-exchange. *Lancet* **1**:575, 1979.
84. Wolf LM, Laudat PH, Chaumont P, Bonduelle M: [Refsum's disease. Clinical and biochemical evolution under a phytol-free diet. Complementary biochemical studies. Supplement of the 1966 report.] *Rev Neurol (Paris)* **120**:89, 1969.
85. Quinlan CD, Martin EA: Refsum's syndrome: Report of three cases. *J Neurol Neurosurg Psychiatry* **33**:817, 1970.
86. Lundberg A, Lilja LG, Lundberg PO, Try K: Heredopathia atactica polyneuritiformis (Refsum's disease). Experiences of dietary treatment and plasmapheresis. *Eur Neurol* **8**:309, 1972.
87. Sahgal V, Olsen WO: Heredopathia atactica polyneuritiformis (phytanic acid storage disease). A new case with special reference to dietary treatment. *Arch Intern Med* **135**:585, 1975.
88. Dry J, Pradalier A, Delporte MP, Leynadier F: [Two new cases of Refsum's disease. Course during diet.] *Sem Hop* **52**:1675, 1976.
89. Thumler R, Atzpodien W, Kremer GJ, Haferkamp G: [Refsum's syndrome.] *Dtsch Med Wochenschr* **102**:1454, 1977.
90. Penovich PE, Hollander J, Nusbacher JA, Griggs RC, MacPherson J: Note on plasma exchange therapy in Refsum's disease. *Adv Neurol* **21**:151, 1978.
91. Dickson N, Mortimer JG, Faed JM, Pollard AC, Styles M, Peart DA: A child with Refsum's disease: Successful treatment with diet and plasma exchange. *Dev Med Child Neurol* **31**:92, 1989.
92. Moser HW, Batshaw ML, Murray C, Braine H, Brusilow SW: Management of heritable disorders of the urea cycle and of Refsum's and Fabry's diseases. *Prog Clin Biol Res* 34:183, 1979.
93. Hungerbuhler JP, Meier C, Rousselle L, Quadri P, Bogousslavsky J: Refsum's disease: Management by diet and plasmapheresis. *Eur Neurol* **24**:153, 1985.
94. Lenz H, Sluga E, Bernheimer H, Molzer B, Purgyi W: [Course of Refsum's disease under diabetic treatment. Clinical, biochemical and neuropathological data.] *Nervenarzt* **50**:52, 1979.
95. Steinberg D, Mize CE, Herndon JH Jr, Fales HM, Engel WK, Vroom FQ: Phytanic acid in patients with Refsum's syndrome and response to dietary treatment. *Arch Intern Med* **125**:75, 1970.

96. Feldmann H: [Refsum syndrome, heredopathia atactica polyneuritiformis in the view of the otolaryngologist.] *Laryngol Rhinol Otol (Stuttg)* **60**:235, 1981.
97. Fryer DG, Winckleman AC, Ways PO, Swanson AG: Refsum's disease. A clinical and pathological report. *Neurology* **21**:162, 1971.
98. Ackman RG, Hooper SN: Isoprenoid fatty acids in the human diet: Distinctive geographical features in butterfat and importance in margarines based on marine oil. *Can Inst Food Technol J* **6**:159, 1969.
99. Masters-Thomas A, Bailes J, Billimoria JD, Clemens ME, Gibberd FB, Page NG: Heredopathia atactica polyneuritiformis (Refsum's disease): 2. Estimation of phytanic acid in foods. *J Hum Nutr* **34**:251, 1980.
100. Harari D, Gibberd FB, Dick JP, Sidey MC: Plasma exchange in the treatment of Refsum's disease (heredopathia atactica polyneuritiformis). *J Neurol Neurosurg Psychiatry* **54**:614, 1991.
101. Leppert D, Schanz U, Burger J, Gmur J, Blau N, Waespe W: Long-term plasma exchange in a case of Refsum's disease. *Eur Arch Psychiatry Clin Neurosci* **241**:82, 1991.
102. Barolin GS, Hodkewitsch E, Hofinger E, Scholz H, Bernheimer H, Molzer, B: [Clinical and biochemical follow up of Refsum's disease.] *Fortschr Neurol Psychiatr Grenzgeb* **47**:53, 1979.
103. Stoffel W, Kahlke W: The transformation of phytol into 3,7,11,15-tetramethylhexadecanoic (phytanic) acid in heredopathia atactica polyneuritiformis (Refsum's syndrome). *Biochem Biophys Res Commun* **19**:33, 1965.
104. Eldjarn L, Try K, Stokke O: The existence of an alternative pathway for the degradation of branched-chain fatty acids, and its failure in heredopathia atactia polyneuritiformis. *Biochim Biophys Acta* **116**:395, 1966.
105. Eldjarn L, Stokke O, Try K: Alpha-oxidation of branched chain fatty acids in man and its failure in patients with Refsum's disease showing phytanic acid accumulation. *Scand J Clin Lab Invest* **18**:694, 1966.
106. Try K: The in vitro omega-oxidation of phytanic acid and other branched chain fatty acids by mammalian liver. *Scand J Clin Lab Invest* **22**:224, 1968.
107. Eldjarn L, Try K, Stokke O: The ability of patients with heredopathia atactica polyneuritiformis to alpha-oxidize and degrade several isoprenoid branch-chained fatty structures. *Scand J Clin Lab Invest* 18:141, 1966.
108. Mize CE, Steinberg D, Avigan J, Fales HM: A pathway for oxidative degradation of phytanic acid in mammals. *Biochem Biophys Res Commun* **25**:359, 1966.
109. Mize CE, Avigan J, Steinberg D, Pittman RC, Fales HM, Milne GWA: A major pathway for the mammalian oxidative degradation of phytanic acid. *Biochim Biophys Acta* **176**:720, 1969.
110. Stokke O, Try K, Eldjarn L: Alpha-oxidation as an alternative pathway for the degradation of branched-chain fatty acids in man, and its failure in patients with Refsum's disease. *Biochim Biophys Acta* **144**:271, 1967.
111. Steinberg D, Avigan J, Mize C, Baxter JH: Phytanic acid formation and accumulation in phytol-fed rats. *Biochem Biophys Res Commun* **19**:412, 1965.
112. Steinberg D, Avigan J, Mize CE, Baxter JH, Cammermeyer J, Fales HM, Highet PF: Effects of dietary phytol and phytanic acid in animals. *J Lipid Res* **7**:684, 1966.
113. Klenk E, Kremer GJ: Untersuchungen zum Stoffwechsel des Phytols, Dihydrophytols und der Phytansaure. *Hoppe Seylers Z Physiol Chem* **343**:39, 1965.
114. Muralidharan FN, Muralidharan VB: In vitro conversion of phytol to phytanic acid in rat liver: Subcellular distribution of activity and chemical characterization of intermediates using a new bromination technique. *Biochim Biophys Acta* **835**:36, 1985.
115. Muralidharan FN, Muralidharan VB: Characterization of phytol-phytanate conversion activity in rat liver. *Biochim Biophys Acta* **883**:54, 1986.
116. Tsai SC, Avigan J, Steinberg D: Studies on the alpha oxidation of phytanic acid by rat liver mitochondria. *J Biol Chem* **244**:2682, 1969.
117. Muralidharan VB, Kishimoto Y: Phytanic acid alpha-oxidation in rat liver. Requirement of cytosolic factor. *J Biol Chem* **259**:13021, 1984.
118. Skjeldal OH, Stokke O: The subcellular localization of phytanic acid oxidase in rat liver. *Biochim Biophys Acta* **921**:38, 1987.
119. Wanders RJA, van Roermund CW: Studies on phytanic acid alpha-oxidation in rat liver and cultured human skin fibroblasts. *Biochim Biophys Acta* **1167**:345, 1993.
120. Watkins PA, Mihalik SJ: Mitochondrial oxidation of phytanic acid in human and monkey liver: Implication that Refsum's disease is not a peroxisomal disorder. *Biochem Biophys Res Commun* **167**:580, 1990.
121. Wanders RJA, van Roermund CW, Jakobs C, ten Brink HJ: Identification of pristanoyl-CoA oxidase and phytanic acid decarboxylation in peroxisomes and mitochondria from human liver: implications for Zellweger syndrome. *J Inherit Metab Dis* **14**:349, 1991.
122. Huang S, Van Veldhoven PP, Vanhoutte F, Parmentier G, Eyssen HJ, Mannaerts GP: Alpha-oxidation of 3-methyl-substituted fatty acids in rat liver. *Arch Biochem Biophys* **296**:214, 1992.
123. Singh I, Pahan K, Dhaunsi GS, Lazo O, Ozand P: Phytanic acid alpha-oxidation. Differential subcellular localization in rat and human tissues and its inhibition by Nycodenz. *J Biol Chem* 268:9972, 1993.
124. Pahan K, Singh I: Intraorganellar localization of CoASH-independent phytanic acid oxidation in human liver peroxisomes. *FEBS Lett* **333**:154, 1993.
125. Pahan K, Gulati S, Singh I: Phytanic acid alpha-oxidation in rat liver mitochondria. *Biochim Biophys Acta* **1201**:491, 1994.
126. Pahan K, Khan M, Smith BT, Singh I: Ketoconazole and other imidazole derivatives are potent inhibitors of peroxisomal phytanic acid alpha-oxidation. *FEBS Lett* **377**:213, 1995.
127. Wanders RJA, van Roermund CW, Schor DS, ten Brink HJ, Jakobs C: 2-Hydroxyphytanic acid oxidase activity in rat and human liver and its deficiency in the Zellweger syndrome. *Biochim Biophys Acta* **1227**:177, 1994.
128. Tsai SC, Herndon JH Jr, Uhlendorf BW, Fales HM, Mize CE: The formation of alpha-hydroxy phytanic acid from phytanic acid in mammalian tissues. *Biochem Biophys Res Commun* **28**:571, 1967.
129. Tsai SC, Steinberg D, Avigan J, Fales HM: Studies on the stereospecificity of mitochondrial oxidation of phytanic acid and of alpha-hydroxyphytanic acid. *J Biol Chem* **248**:1091, 1973.
130. Skjeldal OH, Stokke O: Evidence against alpha-hydroxyphytanic acid as an intermediate in the metabolism of phytanic acid. *Scand J Clin Lab Invest* **48**:97, 1988.
131. Singh H, Beckman K, Poulos A: Peroxisomal beta-oxidation of branched chain fatty acids in rat liver. Evidence that carnitine palmitoyltransferase I prevents transport of branched chain fatty acids into mitochondria. *J Biol Chem* **269**:9514, 1994.
132. Singh H, Poulos A: Substrate specificity of rat liver mitochondrial carnitine palmitoyl transferase I: Evidence against alpha-oxidation of phytanic acid in rat liver mitochondria. *FEBS Lett* **359**:179, 1995.
133. Poulos A, Sharp P, Singh H, Johnson DW, Carey WF, Easton C: Formic acid is a product of the alpha-oxidation of fatty acids by human skin fibroblasts: Deficiency of formic acid production in peroxisome-deficient fibroblasts. *Biochem J* **292**:457, 1993.
134. Mihalik SJ, Rainville AM, Watkins PA: Phytanic acid alpha-oxidation in rat liver peroxisomes. Production of alpha-hydroxyphytanoyl-CoA and formate is enhanced by dioxygenase cofactors. *Eur J Biochem* **232**:545, 1995.
135. Jansen GA, Mihalik SJ, Watkins PA, Moser HW, Jakobs C, Denis S, Wanders RJA: Phytanoyl-CoA hydroxylase is present in human liver, located in peroxisomes, and deficient in Zellweger syndrome: Direct, unequivocal evidence for the new, revised pathway of phytanic acid alpha-oxidation in humans. *Biochem Biophys Res Commun* **229**:205, 1996.
136. Croes K, Casteels M, Van Veldhoven PP, Mannaerts GP: Evidence for the importance of iron in the alpha-oxidation of 3-methyl-substituted fatty acids in the intact cell. *Biochim Biophys Acta* **1255**:63, 1995.
137. Van Veldhoven PP, Huang S, Eyssen HJ, Mannaerts GP: The deficient degradation of synthetic 2- and 3-methyl-branched fatty acids in fibroblasts from patients with peroxisomal disorders. *J Inherit Metab Dis* **16**:381, 1993.
138. Croes K, Casteels M, de Hoffmann E, Mannaerts GP, Van Veldhoven PP: alpha-Oxidation of 3-methyl-substituted fatty acids in rat liver. Production of formic acid instead of CO_2, cofactor requirements, subcellular localization and formation of a 2-hydroxy-3-methylacyl-CoA intermediate. *Eur J Biochem* **240**:674, 1996.
139. Jansen GA, Mihalik SJ, Watkins PA, Moser HW, Jakobs C, Heijmans HSA, Wanders RJA: Phytanoyl-CoA hydroxylase is not only deficient in classical Refsum disease but also in rhizomelic chondrodysplasia punctata. *J Inherit Metab Dis* **20**:444, 1997.
140. Jansen GA, Ofman R, Ferdinandusse S, IJlst L, Muijsers AO, Skjeldal OH, Stokke O, et al: Refsum disease is caused by mutations in the phytanoyl-CoA hydroxylase gene. *Nat Genet* **17**:190, 1997.
141. Jansen GA, Ofman R, Denis S, Ferdinandusse S, Hogenhout EM, Jakobs C, Wanders RJA: Phytanoyl-CoA hydroxylase from rat liver: Protein purification and cDNA cloning with implications for the subcellular localisation of phytanic acid a-oxidation. *J Lipid Res* **40**:2244, 1999.

142. Mihalik SJ, Morrell JC, Kim D, Sacksteder KA, Watkins PA, Gould SJ: Identification of PAHX, a Refsum disease gene. *Nat Genet* **17**:185, 1997.
143. Swinkels BW, Gould SJ, Bodnar AG, Rachubinski RA, Subramani S: A novel, cleavable peroxisomal targeting signal at the amino-terminus of the rat 3-ketoacyl-CoA thiolase. *EMBO J* **10**:3255, 1991.
144. de Vet EC, Zomer AW, Lahaut GJ, van den Bosch H: Polymerase chain reaction-based cloning of alkyl-dihydroxyacetonephosphate synthase complementary DNA from guinea pig liver. *J Biol Chem* **272**:798, 1997.
145. de Vet EC, van den Broek BT, van den Bosch H: Nucleotide sequence of human alkyl-dihydroxyacetonephosphate synthase cDNA reveals the presence of a peroxisomal targeting signal 2. *Biochim Biophys Acta* **1346**:25, 1997.
146. Croes K, Casteels M, Asselberghs S, Herdewijn P, Mannaerts GP, Van Veldhoven PP: Formation of a 2-methyl-branched fatty aldehyde during peroxisomal alpha-oxidation. *FEBS Lett* **412**:643, 1997.
147. Verhoeven NM, Schor DS, ten Brink HJ, Wanders RJA, Jakobs C: Resolution of the phytanic acid alpha-oxidation pathway: Identification of pristanal as product of the decarboxylation of 2-hydroxyphytanoyl-CoA. *Biochem Biophys Res Commun* **237**:33, 1997.
148. Croes K, Van Veldhoven PP, Mannaerts GP, Casteels M: Production of formyl-CoA during peroxisomal alpha-oxidation of 3-methyl-branched fatty acids. *FEBS Lett* **407**:197, 1997.
149. Verhoeven NM, Wanders RJA, Schor DS, Jansen GA, Jakobs C: Phytanic acid alpha-oxidation: Decarboxylation of 2-hydroxyphytanoyl-CoA to pristanic acid in human liver. *J Lipid Res* **38**:2062, 1997.
150. Jansen GA, Verhoeven NM, Denis S, Romeijn GJ, Jakobs C, ten Brink HJ, Wanders RJA: Phytanic acid alpha-oxidation: Identification of 2-hydroxyphytanoyl-CoA lyase in rat liver and its localisation in peroxisomes. *Biochim Biophys Acta* **1440**:176, 1999.
151. Foulon V, Antonenkov VD, Croes K, Waelkens E, Mannaerts GP, Van Veldhoven PP, Casteels M: Purification, molecular cloning, and expression of 2-hydroxyphytanoyl-CoA lyase, a peroxisomal thiamine pyrophosphate-dependent enzyme that catalyzes the carbon-carbon bond cleavage during alpha-oxidation of 3-methyl-branched fatty acids. *Proc Natl Acad Sci U S A* **96**:10039, 1999.
152. Lametschwandtner G, Brocard C, Fransen M, Van Veldhoven P, Berger J, Hartig A: The difference in recognition of terminal tripeptides as peroxisomal targeting signal 1 between yeast and human is due to different affinities of their receptor Pex5p to the cognate signal and to residues adjacent to it. *J Biol Chem* **273**:33635, 1998.
153. Purdue PE, Lazarow PB: Targeting of human catalase to peroxisomes is dependent upon a novel COOH-terminal peroxisomal targeting sequence. *J Cell Biol* **134**:849, 1996.
154. Verhoeven NM, Jakobs C, Carney G, Somers MP, Wanders RJA, Rizzo WB: Involvement of microsomal fatty aldehyde dehydrogenase in the alpha-oxidation of phytanic acid. *FEBS Lett* **429**:225, 1998.
155. Wanders RJA, Denis S, van Roermund CWT, Jakobs C, ten Brink HJ: Characteristics and subcellular localization of pristanoyl-CoA synthetase in rat liver. *Biochim Biophys Acta* **1125**:274, 1992.
156. Mannaerts GP, Van Veldhoven P, Van Broekhoven A, Vandebroek G, Debeer LJ: Evidence that peroxisomal acyl-CoA synthetase is located at the cytoplasmic side of the peroxisomal membrane. *Biochem J* **204**:17, 1982.
157. Steinberg SJ, Wang SJ, Kim DG, Mihalik SJ, Watkins PA: Human very-long-chain acyl-CoA synthetase: Cloning, topography, and relevance to branched-chain fatty acid metabolism. *Biochem Biophys Res Commun* **257**:615, 1999.
158. Pahan K, Cofer J, Baliga P, Singh I: Identification of phytanoyl-CoA ligase as a distinct acyl-CoA ligase in peroxisomes from cultured human skin fibroblasts. *FEBS Lett* **322**:101, 1993.
159. Watkins PA, Howard AE, Gould SJ, Avigan J, Mihalik SJ: Phytanic acid activation in rat liver peroxisomes is catalyzed by long-chain acyl-CoA synthetase. *J Lipid Res* **37**:2288, 1996.
160. Croes K, Casteels M, Dieuaide-Noubhani M, Mannaerts GP, Van Veldhoven PP: Stereochemistry of a alpha-oxidation of 3-methyl-branched fatty acids in rat liver. *J Lipid Res* **40**:601, 1999.
161. Jansen GA, Ferdinandusse S, Skjeldal OH, Stokke O, de Groot CJ, Jakobs C, Wanders RJA: Molecular basis of Refsum disease: Identification of new mutations in the phytanoyl-CoA hydroxylase cDNA. *J Inherit Metab Dis* **21**:288, 1998.
162. Chahal A, Khan M, Pai SG, Barbosa E, Singh I: Restoration of phytanic acid oxidation in Refsum disease fibroblasts from patients with mutations in the phytanoyl-CoA hydroxylase gene. *FEBS Lett* **429**:119, 1998.
163. Jansen GA, Mihalik SJ, Watkins PA, Jakobs C, Moser HW, Wanders RJA: Characterization of phytanoyl-coenzyme A hydroxylase in human liver and activity measurements in patients with peroxisomal disorders. *Clin Chim Acta* **271**:203, 1998.

CHAPTER 133

Primary Hyperoxaluria

Christopher J. Danpure

1. **The term *primary hyperoxaluria* includes two rare, well-characterized autosomal recessive diseases, primary hyperoxaluria type 1 (PH1, MIM 259900) and type 2 (PH2, MIM 260000). The clinical phenotype of PH1, which is the more common of the two, is one of progressive renal deposition of calcium oxalate (CaOx) as urolithiasis and/or nephrocalcinosis leading to renal failure. Decreasing renal function is accompanied by increasing deposition of CaOx throughout the body as systemic oxalosis. In PH2, which is often considered to be a milder disease than PH1, renal failure is less common. At the biochemical level, PH1 is characterized by concomitant hyperoxaluria and hyperglycolic aciduria and PH2 by hyperoxaluria and hyper-L-glyceric aciduria.**
2. **PH1 is caused by a functional deficiency of the liver-specific peroxisomal enzyme alanine:glyoxylate aminotransferase (AGT) and PH2 by a deficiency of the cytosolic enzyme D-glycerate dehydrogenase/glyoxylate reductase (DGDH/GR). One-third of PH1 patients have significant levels of AGT catalytic activity, which in some cases is similar to the levels found in asymptomatic obligate heterozygotes. These patients have disease due to a unique intracellular protein trafficking defect in which AGT is erroneously localized to the mitochondria instead of the peroxisomes.**
3. **The AGT gene (*AGXT*) has been cloned and sequenced both at the cDNA and the genomic levels. The gene consists of 11 exons spanning about 10 kb and has been localized to chromosome 2q37.3. At least 18 mutations have been identified, many of which are associated with specific enzymic PH1 phenotypes, including the peroxisome-to-mitochondrion targeting defect, intraperoxisomal AGT aggregation, absence of AGT catalytic activity, and absence of both AGT catalytic activity and immunoreactivity.**
4. **AGT is targeted to peroxisomes via the peroxisomal targeting sequence type 1 (PTS1) import pathway, even though its C-terminal tripeptide (Lys-Lys-Leu) does not fit the conservative PTS1 consensus motif. AGT mistargeting to mitochondria is caused by a combination of a common polymorphism that generates a functionally weak mitochondrial targeting sequence (MTS) and a disease-specific mutation that, together with the polymorphism, enhances the efficiency of the MTS by inhibiting AGT dimerization.**
5. **A canine analogue of PH1 and a feline analogue of PH2 have been identified, but their clinical usefulness has yet to be determined.**
6. **Recent years have seen the development of new strategies for diagnosis, prenatal diagnosis, and treatment of PH1. The disease can be diagnosed definitively by AGT assay of percutaneous liver needle biopsies. Such a procedure can diagnose PH1 even in patients who present in renal failure and in whom urinalysis is not available. PH1 also can be diagnosed prenatally by AGT analysis of fetal liver biopsies obtained in the second trimester and DNA analysis of chorionic villus samples or amniocytes in the first trimester. The greatest change in the clinical management of PH1 over the past decade has been the introduction of liver transplantation as a form of enzyme-replacement therapy. Combined hepatorenal transplantation replaces not only the enzymically defective organ (i.e., the liver) but also the pathophysiologically defective organ (i.e., the kidney). Such treatment can correct the clinical and metabolic sequelae of PH1 and lead to resolution of some of the long-term ravages of systemic CaOx deposition.**
7. **The future for PH1 patients is brighter now than it has ever been. Our increasing understanding of the molecular genetics of the *AGXT* gene, the liver-specific localization of the gene product, and the lack of neurologic involvement all go to make PH1 a good candidate for gene therapy. Our increased understanding of the roles of AGT and GR as determinants of endogenous oxalate synthesis may contribute to a wider understanding of the processes involved in more common problems of inappropriate CaOx deposition, such as that which occurs in idiopathic CaOx stone disease.**

OXALATE IN BIOLOGY AND MEDICINE

The relationship between oxalic acid and living systems is ambivalent to say the least. For some forms of life, oxalate is a very useful, or even essential, metabolite, whereas for others, it is a poisonous, nonmetabolizable waste product. In the plant kingdom, oxalate can have both structural and defensive functions, and it can play an important role in calcium homeostasis.[1,2] In some bacteria, such as *Oxalobacter formigenes*, oxalate is an important carbon food source.[3,4] However, for animals in general and mammals in particular, oxalate fulfills no known useful purpose. In fact, as far as mammals are concerned, oxalate is a potentially lethal poison. The life-threatening properties of oxalate, rather than resulting from any biochemical mechanism, are largely due to the physical properties of its calcium salt, which is very insoluble at physiologic pHs.[2] The complex anatomic and physiologic organization of mammals makes them extremely susceptible to the inappropriate deposition of calcium oxalate (CaOx). Crystallization of CaOx can cause pathology simply due to its physical presence, by obstructing tubular lumens, by disrupting intercellular and possibly intracellular interactions and communications, or simply by killing cells within which or next to which crystallization occurs.

Although natural selection has enabled mammals to evolve mechanisms to cope with the presence of oxalate in the external and internal environments, they still appear to be poorly adapted to its presence. Therefore, even in normal circumstances, the relationship between mammals and oxalate is finely balanced

A list of standard abbreviations is located immediately preceding the index in each volume. Nonstandard abbreviations used in this chapter include: PH1 = primary hyperoxaluria type 1; PH2 = primary hyperoxaluria type 2; LDH = lactate dehydrogenase; DAO = D-amino acid oxidase; GO = L-2-hydroxyacid oxidase isoenzyme A (glycolate oxidase); AGT = alanine:glyoxylate aminotransferase isoenzyme 1; GGT = glutamate:glyoxylate aminotransferase; GR = glyoxylate reductase; CL = 2-oxoglutarate:glyoxylate carboligase; DGDH = D-glycerate dehydrogenase; PTS1 = peroxisomal targeting sequence type 1; PTS2 = peroxisomal targeting sequence type 2; MTS = mitochondrial targeting sequence.

with little margin for error. Oxalate frequently is presented with the opportunity to manifest its adverse effects, and relatively minor perturbations in oxalate homeostasis can lead to catastrophe.

OXALOSIS AND HYPEROXALURIA

The complex ionic and macromolecular composition of physiologic fluids means that the concentration of CaOx frequently can exceed its aqueous solubility product.[5] Crystallization of CaOx will occur from an already supersaturated solution when its concentration increases beyond a certain critical level, determined at least in part by pH, ionic composition, the presence of nucleation sites, and the concentration of any crystallization-inhibitory factors.[5] In most cases it is the oxalate rather than the calcium concentration that is the major determinant of CaOx crystallization in the body.[6,7] Because the kidney is the main route by which oxalate is cleared from the body,[8] increased oxalate concentration in the body leads to increased urinary excretion (i.e., hyperoxaluria). The kidney's role in oxalate excretion makes it the prime target for CaOx crystallization. However, under appropriate conditions, CaOx can be deposited at almost any site within the body. CaOx deposition (oxalosis) can be caused by many different conditions that lead to increases in the body's oxalate load.

The causes of hyperoxaluria and oxalosis can be divided into those which are secondary (environmental) and those which are primary (genetic). Secondary hyperoxaluria/oxalosis can be caused by (1) increased ingestion and/or absorption of oxalate due to dietary changes, intestinal disease or surgery, or alterations in intestinal flora, (2) increased endogenous synthesis of oxalate due to the administration of various oxalate precursors, and (3) decreased oxalate clearance from the body due to renal failure. Many of the causes of secondary, or even primary, hyperoxaluria/oxalosis are interactive. For example, renal oxalosis caused by increased oxalate absorption or synthesis can lead to renal failure, a condition itself that can lead to systemic oxalosis.

Infrequently, hyperoxaluria/oxalosis is caused by genetic factors—the so-called primary hyperoxalurias, which are the prime consideration of this chapter. However, although the initiating causes of the primary hyperoxalurias are distinct from those which cause the secondary hyperoxalurias, the pathologic consequences are frequently indistinguishable from each other. This has lead to the cross-fertilization of ideas concerning pathophysiology and etiology from one area to another. Extrapolation is often done between metabolic pathways determined from, for example, ethylene glycol toxicity studies and those operating under normal conditions, and the rationale for the symptomatic treatment of secondary hyperoxaluria or oxalosis and idiopathic CaOx stone disease is often transferred to the primary hyperoxalurias. In some cases these extrapolations are justified, whereas in others they are not.

PRIMARY HYPEROXALURIA

Primary hyperoxaluria is a collective term that encompasses an indeterminate number of inheritable conditions, of which only two, primary hyperoxaluria type 1 (PH1) (MIM 259900) and primary hyperoxaluria type 2 (PH2) (MIM 260000), have been well characterized.* Certain other hyperoxaluric syndromes, such as those involving primary enteric hyperabsorption (the so-called type 3 hyperoxaluria[9,10]) or other familial oxalate transport defects (such as MIM 167030[11–13]), eventually also may be properly considered within this category. This also may be the case for the hyperoxaluria associated with some patients with idiopathic CaOx stone disease.[6,14] However, *because* of the general lack of understanding of the latter hyperoxaluria syndromes and the absence of conclusive evidence concerning their genetic basis, only PH1 and PH2 will be considered in this review.

Many general reviews have been written on the primary hyperoxalurias in recent years.[15–17] In addition, there have been four European Workshops on them since 1990, the proceedings of the last two in 1994 and 1997 having been published.[18,19] Although some of the more general aspects of the primary hyperoxalurias will be included for balance, the present review will concentrate on the metabolic and molecular aspects of these diseases and how our recent understanding of their pathogenesis has influenced their clinical management.

CLINICAL CHARACTERISTICS

Lepoutre is generally credited with having identified the first case of primary hyperoxaluria in 1925.[20] However, it was not until 1950 that the condition was described in detail.[21] The metabolic basis of primary hyperoxaluria was not recognized until 1957,[22] some 30 years after the first description of the disease. In 1968, with the identification of PH2,[23] it was realized that primary hyperoxaluria was more than one disease. Since that time, there have been numerous case reports of primary hyperoxaluria in the literature, as well as many general reviews,[15,17] including four previous contributions on this subject in earlier editions of this book.[16,24–26]

Descriptions of the clinical pathology associated with PH1 and PH2 have been complicated by a tendency of authors not to define a patient's disease beyond primary hyperoxaluria or primary oxalosis, especially in the older literature, or not to describe the criteria used to make such diagnoses. In the vast majority of cases, patients described as having primary hyperoxaluria are assumed to have PH1. The clinical pathology of PH1 has been surveyed in a number of reviews, two of the largest being those by Hockaday et al.,[27] who reviewed over 100 patients in 1964, and Latta and Brodehl,[28] who more recently reviewed 330 published cases.

Clinical Pathology

PH1. At the clinical level, PH1 is characterized by progressive CaOx urolithiasis, nephrocalcinosis, and systemic oxalosis (Fig. 133-1). However, the clinical manifestations are quantitatively and qualitatively heterogeneous with respect to both the timing and the specific contribution made by each of these pathologic sequelae. In most patients, the first symptoms (e.g., renal colic, asymptomatic gross hematuria) occur before the age of 5 years due to the presence of urolithiasis. However, there is an enormous spread in the ages at which the disease first becomes apparent, which can be as early as the first year of life or as late as the seventh decade.[25,27–36] Deposition of CaOx within the kidney parenchyma (nephrocalcinosis) or the renal pelvis/urinary tract (urolithiasis) continues inexorably until eventually renal function is impaired. The further sequelae associated with PH1 (i.e., uremia and systemic oxalosis) are either due to or exacerbated by the renal failure. The inability to clear oxalate from the body leads to its deposition in almost all areas of the body (Table 133-1). The chronic multisystemic pathology following renal failure in PH1, at least, is similar to that found in various secondary hyperoxalurias, but because this pathology is compounded by basic disruptions in oxalate metabolism, it is usually much more severe in PH1.

In PH1 patients, CaOx starts to accumulate even when renal function is only slightly impaired.[37] Following renal failure, systemic CaOx deposition can occur at numerous sites within the body. In many cases, such deposition is associated with pathology appropriate to the tissue concerned (see Table 133-1). For example, deposition in the bone is associated with bone pain, multiple fractures, and osteosclerosis[38–45]; in the myocardium it is associated with heart block, myocarditis, and cardioembolic stroke[46–51]; and in the peripheral vasculature and skin it is associated with livedo reticularis, calcinosis cutis metastatica, and

*In the most recently updated (September 1997) version of McKusick's catalogue OMIM (Online Mendelian Inheritance in Man), PH1 is variously described as oxalosis I, hyperoxaluria I, glycolic aciduria, peroxisomal alanine:glyoxylate aminotransferase deficiency, hepatic AGT deficiency, and serine:pyruvate aminotransferase deficiency, whereas PH2 is described as oxalosis II, hyperoxaluria II, glyceric aciduria, and D-glycerate dehydrogenase-deficiency. Throughout this review the terms *primary hyperoxaluria type 1* (PH1) and *type 2* (PH2) are used.

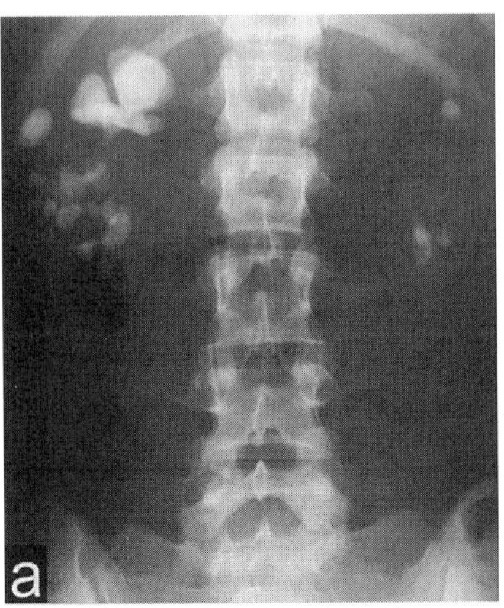

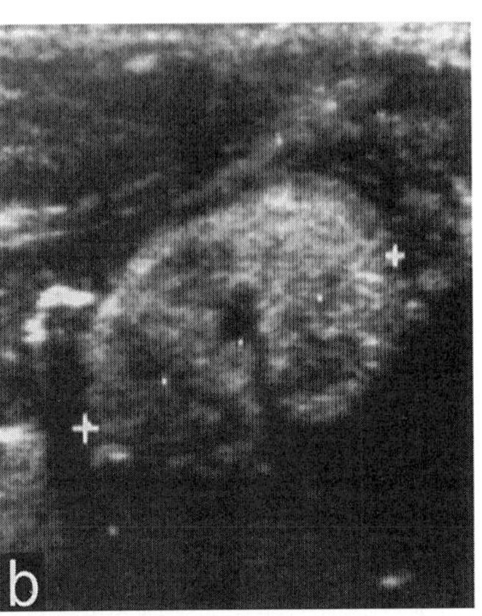

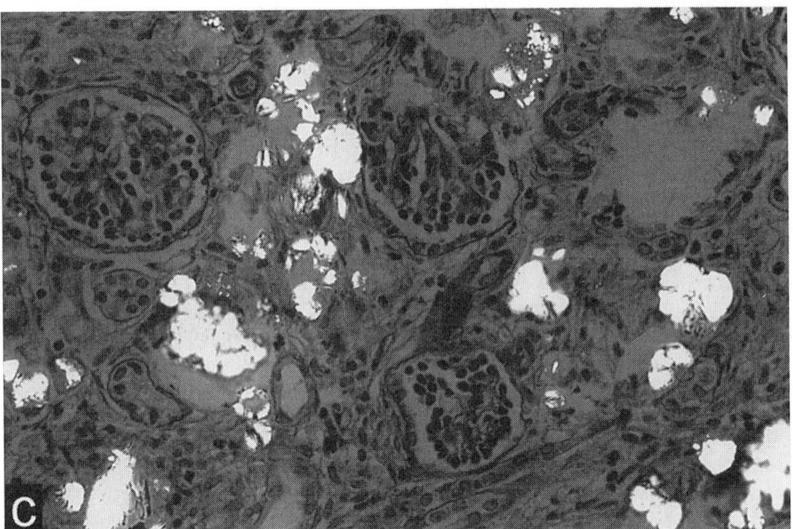

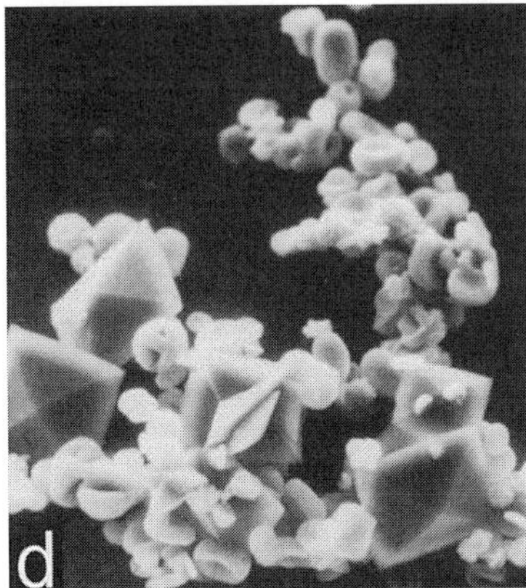

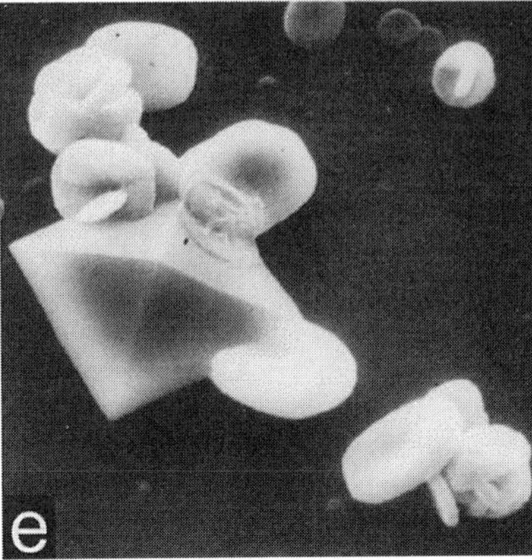

Fig. 133-1 CaOx deposition in PH1. (*A*) X-ray of multiple renal stones including a classic "staghorn" calculus. (*B*) Ultrasound of nephrocalcinosis. (*C*) CaOx crystal deposition in renal cortical tissue. (*D, E*) Scanning electron micrographs of CaOx crystalluria. (*Panels B and C reproduced with permission from Barratt et al.[68]; original photographs kindly provided by Professors R. A. Risdon and T. M. Barratt, Departments of Histopathology and Paediatric Nephrology, The Hospitals for Sick Children, London. Panels D and E reproduced with permission from Danpure and Smith[17]; original photographs kindly provided by Professor L. H. Smith, University of Kansas School of Medicine.*)

peripheral gangrene.[41,43,50,52–57] The pathology of bone oxalosis following renal failure is frequently complicated by renal osteodystrophy and secondary hyperparathyroidism.[41,42,58,59] The histologic aspects of CaOx crystal deposition have been reviewed by Williams and Smith.[25] It is noteworthy, considering the site of the basic enzyme defect in PH1 (see "Enzymic and Metabolic Defects," below), that CaOx deposition has not been observed in the liver parenchyma (see Latta and Brodehl[28]). It has been estimated previously that greater than 80 percent of patients with primary hyperoxaluria (largely PH1) die from renal failure before the age of 20 years[25]. However, with modern treatments (see "Treatment," below), this estimate is almost certainly in need of revision (see Milliner et al.[36]).

A minority of PH1 patients, possibly about 10 percent, have a much more severe, very early onset form of the disease. These patients typically present in the first few months of life with renal failure due to nephrocalcinosis without urolithiasis.[60–67] Presenting symptoms, which result from the renal failure and uremia, include vomiting, severe metabolic acidosis, anorexia, and anemia (for a review, see Leumann[60]). Systemic oxalosis often is apparent at the time of presentation, and the patients frequently die within 1 year from uremic and/or oxalotic complications. Despite

Table 133-1 Some Tissues Involved in Systemic CaOx Deposition in PH1

Tissue	Clinical Symptom and Pathology
Kidney and urinary tract	Urolithiasis, nephrocalcinosis, renal failure, hematuria, pyelonephritis, and hydronephrosis
Bone	Bone pain, multiple fractures, and osteosclerosis
Eye	Retinopathy and optic atrophy
Teeth, mouth, and associated structures	Root resorption, pulp exposure, tooth mobility, and dental pain
Nerves	Peripheral neuropathy (axonal degeneration and segmental demyelination)
Brain and meninges	
Heart	Heart block, myocarditis, and cardioembolic stroke
Deep vasculature	Vasospasm
Peripheral vasculature and skin	Livedo reticularis, peripheral gangrene, and calcinosis cutis metastatica
Bone marrow	Pancytopenia and hepatosplenomegaly
Cartilage, ligaments, and synovial tissue	Arthropathy
Miscellaneous: thymus, adipose tissue, skeletal muscle, and liver blood vessels	

NOTE: See text and Table 75-1 in the previous edition of this chapter[16] for the original references used to compile this table.

suggestions to the contrary (e.g., see Hillman[26]), this fulminant neonatal form of PH1 is not a distinct disease entity but rather the extreme end of a continuous spectrum of clinical severity.[68] As will be seen later (see "Enzymic and Metabolic Defects," below), there are no biochemical or enzymologic distinctions between the two forms of the disease, and examples do occur of patients with intermediate clinical phenotypes, e.g., early-presenting infantile patients with CaOx urolithiasis.[67] The course of the disease in many neonatal patients is so rapid that, unlike the more chronically progressing form, the chronologic order of events cannot be determined with any certainty. For example, it is not known whether systemic oxalosis occurs before, after, or concurrently with the renal failure.

PH2. PH2 appears to be considerably rarer than PH1. At the time of writing this review, only 20 to 30 PH2 patients have been described in the literature.[23,36,69–73] Therefore, the complete range of clinical symptoms has not necessarily been fully explored. It has been thought generally that PH2 is a milder disease than PH1.[36,70,74,75] There does not appear to be an acute neonatal variant of PH2, and patients typically present with urolithiasis in childhood with hematuria, urinary tract infection, and renal colic.[23,69,70] Although in many cases disease appears to progress more slowly than in PH1, there have been several reports recently of PH2 patients presenting with nephrocalcinosis and in whom disease progresses to end-stage renal failure.[72,76–79]

Clinical Biochemistry

PH1. It is the elevated endogenous synthesis of oxalate that leads to the most important biochemical phenotype of PH1 (i.e., hyperoxaluria[27,80] and hyperoxalemia[81–83]). The 24-h urinary oxalate excretion in PH1 patients can reach 2 to 10 times that normally found.[80] While renal function is adequate, the plasma oxalate concentration may be only modestly raised,[84] but in anuric patients, when the effects of the elevated endogenous oxalate synthesis are compounded by the failure to remove oxalate from the body, the concentration increases enormously.[81] The plasma oxalate-creatinine ratio may be elevated by a factor of 4 to 5 relative to normal controls and individuals with chronic renal failure from other causes.[85] Although hyperoxalemia is also found in patients suffering from renal failure due to other causes, the levels found in PH1 are usually much higher.[82,86–90] A number of authors have pointed out that as PH1 patients approach renal failure, the 24-h excretion rate of oxalate appears to normalize (see Williams and Smith[25]), a finding that has considerable diagnostic implications (see "Diagnosis," below).

The increased body fluid levels of oxalate in PH1 are usually, but not always,[34] associated with hyperglycolic aciduria[80] and possibly hyperglycolic acidemia.[91] In fact, the presence of hyperglycolic aciduria frequently is used to distinguish PH1 from secondary hyperoxaluria and other forms of primary hyperoxaluria. However, it is important to note that hyperglycolic aciduria is not uniquely associated with PH1 and, therefore, could lead to misdiagnosis if other factors are not taken into consideration (see "Diagnosis," below). There have been reports in the past of elevated excretion of glyoxylic acid in PH1.[80] However, this is rarely measured owing to the difficulty of obtaining accurate values.

Two variants of PH1 have been defined in biochemical rather than clinical terms. The first of these, *mild metabolic hyperoxaluria,*[92,93] is characterized by hyperglycolic aciduria but only very mild hyperoxaluria. The second is *renal hyperoxaluria,*[1,83] in which the majority of the urinary oxalate appears to be synthesized directly by the kidney rather than being cleared from the bloodstream.

PH2. As in PH1, the prominent biochemical feature of PH2 is hyperoxaluria. Although reports are scarce, it is thought that the level of oxalate excretion in PH2 is somewhat lower than that found in PH1. Hyperglycolic aciduria is not found in PH2. However, concomitant with the hyperoxaluria is hyper-L-glyceric aciduria.[23,94]

Relationship Between Clinical Biochemistry and Clinical Pathology

It is generally, and reasonably, assumed that at least part of the characteristic clinical biochemistry associated with PH1 and PH2 is causally related to the disease pathology. Although dysfunction at the organ level in the primary hyperoxalurias appears to be due to the physical consequences of CaOx oxalate deposition (i.e., tubular obstruction), the cause of damage at the cellular level is not so clear. Understanding the mechanism of cell damage is important because it is thought that hyperoxaluria leads to CaOx kidney stones not only by providing the source material but also by inducing damage to renal epithelial cells, which in turn promotes crystal formation, aggregation, and adherence.[95] Of the metabolites known or predicted to accumulate in primary hyperoxaluria, oxalate and especially glyoxylate are potentially toxic in the biochemical sense. On the other hand, glycolate and L-glycerate are not known to be directly poisonous.

A number of mammalian enzymes are inhibited by oxalate in vitro, e.g., lactate dehydrogenase (LDH),[96–98] pyruvate kinase,[99] and pyruvate carboxylase.[100] Oxalate is taken up by mitochondria, where it appears to bind to the inner membrane.[101,102] It competitively inhibits mitochondrial uptake and oxidation of malate and succinate and may affect membrane integrity or permeability [103].

Using various transformed cell lines derived from renal epithelial cells, it has been found that oxalate is highly toxic, causing increases in DNA synthesis mediated by increased *c-myc* expression,[104,105] vacuolation, nuclear pyknosis, DNA fragmentation, and increased plasma membrane permeability.[106] Oxalate also increases free radical production and lipid peroxidation.[107,108] CaOx crystals also can cause damage. For example, crystal attachment to the outside of the cell can lead to changes in membrane composition and fluidity,[109,110] and crystal endocytosis can lead to the increased expression of numerous genes and cell proliferation.[111–113]

Glyoxylate is a highly reactive molecule and is known to be toxic to animals.[114] In the presence of oxaloacetate, glyoxylate inhibits aconitase and citrate oxidation.[115,116] The 2-oxoglutarate:glyoxylate carboligase (CL) enzyme activity of 2-oxoglutarate dehydrogenase[117–120] may be a manifestation of another potential site of glyoxylate interference with the citric acid cycle. Glyoxylate could inhibit 2-oxoglutarate dehydrogenase by causing a redundant recycling of the first decarboxylating component (see Fig. 75-2 in the previous edition of this chapter[16]). Although glycolate does not appear to be particularly toxic, it has been shown to inhibit human erythrocyte pyruvate kinase at high concentrations.[121]

Incidence, Genetics, and Environment

That the primary hyperoxalurias are uncommon is of no doubt, but their exact incidence has been difficult to determine not least due to the absence, up until a few years ago, of definitive criteria for their diagnosis. According to Barratt et al.,[68] 11 of 165 children with nephrocalcinosis or urolithiasis over a 9-year period were shown to have PH1, which was the same frequency as cystinuria and distal renal tubular acidosis. The proportion of children with end-stage renal disease who have primary hyperoxaluria has been estimated to be 1 percent in one study[122] and between 2 and 2.7 percent in another.[28] An estimate made by Latta and Brodehl[28] was that 1 in 5 to 15 million children between 0 and 15 years of age will present with renal failure due to primary hyperoxaluria. Cochat et al.[35] calculated the average prevalence of PH1 to be 1.05 per 10^6 individuals and the average incidence rate to be 0.12 per 10^6 individuals per year in France. In Switzerland, Kopp and Leumann[123] estimated the prevalence of PH1 to be 2 per 10^6 with a minimal incidence rate of 1 per 10^5 live births. However, bearing in mind the late presentation of some patients and the wide clinical heterogeneity of PH1, the true incidence is likely to be somewhat greater than these estimates. Because of the much lower incidence of PH2, patients with primary hyperoxaluria have been assumed frequently in the past to have PH1, with little or no evidence. However, it is not difficult to appreciate the self-perpetuating nature of such assumptions. In fact, a number of authors have recently suggested that PH2 may be less rare than previously thought.[36,75,124]

Several authors have addressed the issue of the familial or genetic basis of PH1[125–131] and PH2.[23,69] The obvious autosomal recessive pattern of inheritance in the vast majority of families has been confirmed, in the case of PH1 at least, by the cloning and chromosomal localization of the defective gene (see "Molecular Genetics and Cell Biology of PH1," below). Although the rare occurrence of PH1 in more than one generation occasionally has led to the suggestion of dominant inheritance, in at least one family this has been shown to be caused by the presence of more than two mutant alleles (i.e., pseudodominance).[132]

The wide clinical spectra of PH1 and PH2 and the knowledge that other conditions possibly both genetic and environmental can have similar clinical phenotypes suggest that despite clearly being monogenic diseases, severity could be determined significantly by other genetic factors, such as the activities of other enzymes, or environmental factors, such as diet, hydration, gut flora, etc. The relative importance of "nature" and "nurture" is not clear partly because there are very few studies on the variability of primary hyperoxaluria within individual families. Early studies[128] indicated that the severity of disease, at least as determined by the age of onset, was similar in different affected family members. However, recent work[132] has shown that PH1 disease severity can vary enormously within a family. Even individuals with the same level of oxalate excretion and enzyme deficiency (see "Enzymic and Metabolic Defects," below) can have very different clinical phenotypes.[36,132]

METABOLISM OF OXALATE AND ITS PRECURSORS

PH1 and PH2 are clearly metabolic diseases. Therefore, a proper understanding of their molecular etiology and pathogenesis requires, at least in the first instance, a thorough knowledge of the intermediary metabolic pathways likely to be perturbed (i.e., those involved directly and indirectly in the synthesis of oxalate and its precursors).

Oxalate

Synthesis. Several studies have shown that oxalate is only poorly absorbed from the alimentary tract.[133–136] It has been estimated that only about 10 percent of the oxalate excreted in the urine is dietary in origin, the vast majority being endogenously derived.[2,25] However, more recent studies have suggested that this estimate is too low and that dietary oxalate may make a much greater contribution to oxalate excretion than previously thought.[137,138] Oxalate is a nonfunctional, undesirable metabolic end product that is excreted in the urine without further alteration.[2,139–141] It has been proposed that oxalate synthesis, in mammals at least, results from evolutionary limitations on the development of adequate substrate specificities for the various enzymes involved directly or indirectly in its production, all of which have other primary metabolic functions.[139]

Dietary precursors of oxalate are mainly sugars[142,143] and amino acids. About 40 percent of oxalate production appears to be derived from glycine metabolism.[144,145] Ascorbate also appears to be a major precursor of oxalate.[146,147] However, its quantitative importance is not clear, since an increase in dietary absorption of ascorbate leads to only a marginal increase in urinary oxalate excretion.[148,149]

Most oxalate precursors are metabolized via glyoxylate and/or glycolate[139,150–158] (Figs. 133-2 and 133-3), the oxidation of which is the main regulatory step in the metabolism of carbohydrates to oxalate.[159,160] Ascorbate is probably one of the few important precursors of oxalate that is not metabolized

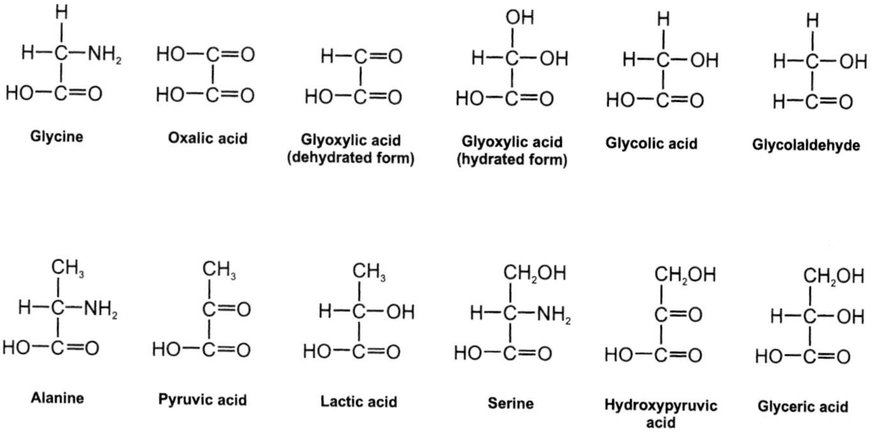

Glycine | Oxalic acid | Glyoxylic acid (dehydrated form) | Glyoxylic acid (hydrated form) | Glycolic acid | Glycolaldehyde

Alanine | Pyruvic acid | Lactic acid | Serine | Hydroxypyruvic acid | Glyceric acid

Fig. 133-2 Structures of some 2/3 carbon compounds important in PH1 and PH2.

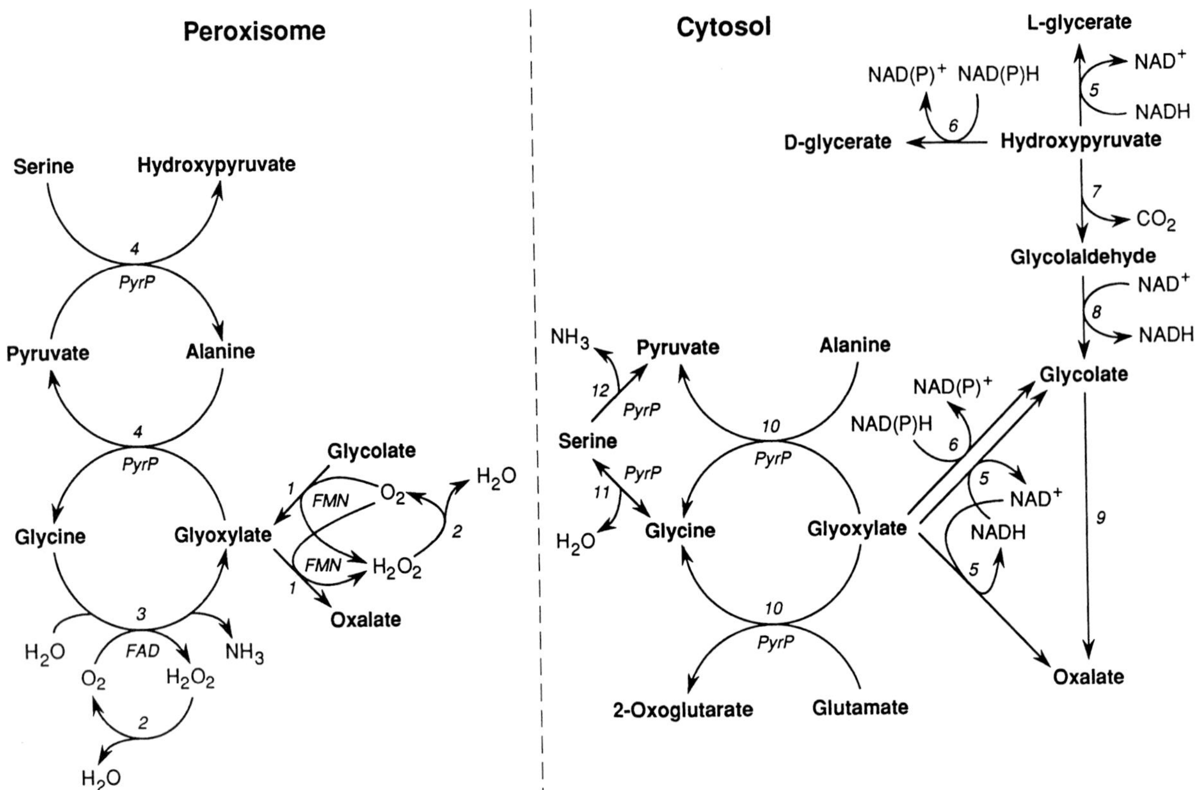

Fig. 133-3 Pathways involved in oxalate, glyoxylate, and glycolate metabolism in the human hepatocyte. *Peroxisomal enzymes*: (1) L-2-hydroxy acid oxidase A/glycolate oxidase (EC 1.1.3.1), (2) catalase (EC 1.11.1.6), (3) D-amino acid oxidase/glycine oxidase (EC 1.4.3.3), and (4) alanine:glyoxylate aminotransferase/serine:pyruvate aminotransferase (EC 2.6.1.44/2.6.1.51). *Cytosolic enzymes*: (5) lactate dehydrogenase (EC 1.1.1.27), (6) D-glycerate dehydrogenase/glyoxylate reductase (EC 1.1.1.29/1.1.1.27/1.1.1.79), (7) hydroxypyruvate decarboxylase (EC 4.1.1.40) (also occurs in the mitochondria[231]), (8) aldehyde dehydrogenase (EC 1.2.1.5) (various isoforms are also found in other intracellular compartments, such as mitochondria, peroxisomes, and microsomes[551]), (9) glycolate dehydrogenase (EC 1.1.99.14), (10) glutamate:glyoxylate aminotransferase/alanine:2-oxoglutarate aminotransferase (EC 2.6.1.4/2.6.1.2), (11) serine hydroxymethyltransferase (EC 2.1.2.1), and (12) serine dehydratase (EC 4.2.1.13). PyrP, pyridoxal phosphate; FAD, flavin-adenine dinucleotide; FMN, flavin mononucleotide; NAD(P)$^+$/NAD(P)H, oxidized and reduced forms of nicotinamide-adenine dinucleotide (phosphate). Note that the relative importance of the various metabolic pathways is not universally agreed on (see text for details).

through this regulatory bottleneck. Most of the conversion of ascorbate to oxalate is probably nonenzymic in nature.[139,147,161]

Renal Excretion. Because oxalate cannot be further metabolized, its elimination from the body can only be by way of physiologic, rather than biochemical, mechanisms. The vast majority of oxalate, whether endogenously or exogenously derived, is excreted in mammals by the kidney, probably by a combination of glomerular filtration and tubular secretion.[141,162–164] However, the net directional flux of oxalate across the tubular epithelium may depend, at least in part, on the luminal/plasma oxalate concentration, since the oxalate-creatinine ratio is indicative of net tubular resorption in normal individuals but net secretion in PH1 patients [85].

Enteric Oxalate Metabolism. There is increasing evidence that oxalate can be degraded within the alimentary tract by anaerobic bacteria such as *O. formigenes*.[165,166] Enteric colonization by this bacterium and the level of oxalate degradation are at least partly dependent on diet and vary from species to species and individual to individual. The extent to which this influences oxalate absorption and renal excretion in humans is, at present, unclear.

Glyoxylate

Synthesis. The most important immediate precursors of glyoxylate are glycine and glycolate (see Fig. 133-3). The oxidative deamination of glycine to glyoxylate can be catalyzed by D-amino acid oxidase (DAO), or glycine oxidase, whereas the oxidation of glycolate to glyoxylate is catalyzed by L-2-hydroxy acid oxidase A, or glycolate oxidase (GO) (for a review, see Masters and Holmes[167]), both reactions yielding hydrogen peroxide as a toxic by-product.

Of the two isozymes of L-2-hydroxy acid oxidase, only the liver-specific isozyme A can use glycolate as a substrate.[168,169] Isozyme B, which is found mainly in nonhepatic tissues, especially the kidney, is inactive toward glycolate.[170,171] DAO is found in many tissues, the activity in the kidney being greater than that in the liver.[172,173] The importance of DAO is demonstrated by the observation that competitive inhibition of DAO in isolated rat liver perfusions leads to a marked inhibition of glycine-to-oxalate metabolism.[154] However, the role of DAO in glyoxylate synthesis has been questioned recently following studies on purified guinea pig peroxisomes.[174] The alkaline pH optimum of DAO and its high K_m for glycine have led some authors to suggest that DAO-catalyzed oxidative deamination of glycine may not be a very efficient reaction.[174,175] Both GO and DAO are peroxisomal enzymes,[170,176,177] an intracellular location that facilitates the rapid removal of the toxic hydrogen peroxide, catalyzed by peroxisomal catalase. In human liver, the activity of DAO is somewhat higher than that of GO.

Transamination. Transamination to glycine has long been recognized as an important route for the metabolism of glyoxylate. Pyridoxal phosphate is an essential cofactor for all aminotransferases, and numerous studies in a variety of species have shown that pyridoxine deficiency leads to an increase in oxalate excretion, whereas pyridoxine supplementation leads to a decrease.[178–182]

Two enzymes in humans are able to catalyze the transamination of glyoxylate, alanine:glyoxylate aminotransferase (AGT)*,[183] and glutamate:glyoxylate aminotransferase (GGT).†,[184] In the human, AGT is liver-specific[185] and normally localized within the peroxisomes.[186–188] However, GGT activity is widely dispersed and localized mainly in the cytosol.[189] The activity of AGT toward glyoxylate in human liver is substantially greater than that of GGT.[184] In fact, AGT is by far the most important enzyme involved in the transamination of glyoxylate in mammals.[190]

Reduction. The reduction of glyoxylate to glycolate can be catalyzed by two enzymes, at least in vitro, namely, glyoxylate reductase (GR)[191] and LDH.[192–198] The former can use either NADH or NADPH as cofactor, whereas LDH can only use NADH. Both enzymes are cytosolic[170] and widely dispersed. There is some disagreement about the relative importance of these two enzymes in glyoxylate reduction (see "Unresolved Metabolic Controversies," below).

Oxidation. Three enzymes are potentially capable of oxidizing glyoxylate to oxalate, namely, GO,[139] xanthine oxidase,[158] and LDH[157,194,196,197,199] (see Fig. 133-3). Xanthine oxidase is probably not a viable candidate in vivo because the inhibitor allopurinol has no effect on urinary oxalate, and xanthinuric patients have normal levels of oxalate excretion.[200,201] However, there is still considerable disagreement about the relative importance of GO and LDH.

Superficially, glyoxylate would not appear to be a suitable substrate for an oxidation reaction catalyzed by either GO or LDH. However, in aqueous solution, glyoxylate is largely hydrated (see Fig. 133-2) and therefore a candidate substrate for both GO[168] and LDH.[193,198] The kinetics of GO-catalyzed glyoxylate oxidation are unfavorable certainly when compared with glycolate oxidation.[202] On the other hand, glyoxylate is as good a substrate for LDH-catalyzed oxidation as is lactate.[194,196] To counter this is the fact that the lactate concentration in liver cell cytosol is orders of magnitude greater than that of glyoxylate.[202,203]

In vitro studies have suggested that LDH is the major enzyme involved with glyoxylate oxidation, certainly in the liver, heart, and blood cells.[25,199,204] However, in such systems, the NAD concentration is a major determinant of LDH activity.[160] The role of LDH in vivo is, however, cast into doubt by the finding that patients deficient in various LDH isozymes have normal urinary oxalate excretion.[202]

Numerous in vitro and in vivo studies have led to the conclusion that GO is more important than LDH in glyoxylate oxidation. The GO inhibitors phenyllactate and *n*-heptanoate completely inhibit glyoxylate-to-oxalate oxidation in isolated perfused rat liver,[205] as does phenyllactate in isolated rat hepatocytes.[206] GO is considered by some authors to be the major enzyme catalyzing glyoxylate oxidation in vivo.[154,155,207] Urinary excretion of oxalate in rats correlates with the levels of GO, not LDH or xanthine oxidase.[208] However, glyoxylate is clearly a much poorer substrate for GO than glycolate,[202] and added to this is the finding that glycolate actually inhibits GO-catalyzed glyoxylate oxidation.[160] In fact, the predicted high intracellular levels of glycolate and lactate have led some authors to suggest that GO is unlikely to contribute significantly to the oxidation of glyoxylate.[174,175,209]

*Alanine:glyoxylate aminotransferase (AGT) is the same enzyme as serine:pyruvate aminotransferase[253,254,263,557] and histidine:pyruvate aminotransferase.[558] Because of the greater relevance of the alanine:glyoxylate reaction to primary hyperoxaluria, the term AGT is used throughout this review.

† Glutamate:glyoxylate aminotransferase (GGT) has been shown to be the same enzyme as alanine:2-oxoglutarate aminotransferase.[189] Because of the greater relevance of the glutamate:glyoxylate reaction to primary hyperoxaluria, the term GGT is used throughout this review.

Other studies have shown that phenyllactate and the LDH inhibitor NAD-pyruvate adduct both inhibit glyoxylate/glycolate oxidation in isolated rat hepatocytes, implicating both GO and LDH in the oxidative processes.[210] It has been suggested that GO and LDH may cooperate in the oxidation of glyoxylate.[156] The steady-state glyoxylate concentration in the peroxisomes is predicted to be low, but if the intraperoxisomal glyoxylate concentration should increase for any reason, e.g., in PH1 (see "Metabolic Consequences of AGT Deficiency," below), then the glyoxylate would leak out into the cytosol to be oxidized by LDH.

Carboligation. Several workers have shown that glyoxylate can be metabolized by isolated rat and human liver mitochondria in the presence of 2-oxoglutarate.[117,120,211] The reaction, which has been described as the "synergistic decarboxylation of glyoxylate and 2-oxoglutarate," leads to the decarboxylation of glyoxylate and the formation of 2-hydroxy-3-oxo-adipate or 2-oxo-3-hydroxy-adipate. The enzyme responsible for this reaction, 2-oxoglutarate:glyoxylate carboligase (CL),[120,211,212], is probably the same enzyme as the citric acid cycle enzyme 2-oxoglutarate dehydrogenase.[118,119,213] Thiamine pyrophosphate is an essential cofactor of CL, and thiamine deficiency in rats has been reported to lead to an increase in glyoxylate in the blood, tissues, and urine.[214,215] In addition, blood glyoxylate has been shown to be increased in thiamine-deficient humans.[216] However, the reactivity of glyoxylate and the technical difficulties associated with its assay cast some doubt on these observations. Therefore, the quantitative significance of the carboligation reaction in vivo remains uncertain.

Glyoxylate Cycle. The glyoxylate cycle, which is characterized by the presence of the two enzymes isocitrate lyase and malate synthase, is found in bacteria, fungi, and germinating seeds of some higher plants.[217–220] Isocitrate lyase catalyzes the cleavage of isocitrate to glyoxylate and succinate, whereas malate synthase catalyzes the condensation of glyoxylate with acetyl CoA to form malate. It has been generally accepted that animals do not possess a glyoxylate cycle,[221,222] although there have been several reports of the existence of both the key enzymes in mammalian tissues,[223–226] including fetal guinea pig liver[227] and rat liver.[228] Counter to this, more recent studies could find no evidence for the presence of isocitrate lyase or malate synthase activity in guinea pig, rat, or embryonic chick liver.[229] Notwithstanding these differences of opinion, there is no evidence that any of the putative components of a glyoxylate cycle have any significant role to play in glyoxylate metabolism and oxalate synthesis in humans.

Glycolate and Hydroxypyruvate

Of the two main glyoxylate precursors, the metabolic pathways leading to the synthesis of glycolate are much more poorly understood than those leading to the production of glycine. In addition to glyoxylate, glycolaldehyde is a recognized precursor of glycolate. Glycolaldehyde is synthesized from hydroxypyruvate (see Figs. 133-2 and 133-3) and possibly ethanolamine.[230]

The metabolism of hydroxypyruvate to oxalate has received considerable attention because it is the main route by which carbohydrates, such as glucose and fructose, are converted to oxalate.[142,143] Evidence for such a pathway has come largely from experiments with intact rats,[150] isolated perfused rat liver,[155] and isolated rat hepatocytes.[142,143,231] The first step in the reaction sequence involves the conversion of hydroxypyruvate to glycolaldehyde catalyzed by hydroxypyruvate decarboxylase (see Fig. 133-3). This enzyme is found in various tissues,[232,233] and in rat liver it is localized in the mitochondria and cytosol.[231] The glycolaldehyde is then presumed to be oxidized to glycolate catalyzed by aldehyde dehydrogenase.

The route from hydroxypyruvate to oxalate may or may not proceed by way of glyoxylate (see Fig. 133-3). There is some evidence that glycolate can be oxidized directly to oxalate. In the rat, hepatectomy leads to an 80 percent reduction in the conversion of glycolate to oxalate but does not affect the metabolism of glyoxylate to oxalate.[153] The remaining 20 percent was attributed to oxidation catalyzed by LDH in extrahepatic tissues. The direct oxidation of glycolate to oxalate[207] is catalyzed by glycolate dehydrogenase,[161] which is concentrated mainly in the liver.[153] The residual glycolate oxidation that occurs in isolated rat hepatocytes in the presence of phenyllactate and NAD-pyruvate adduct has been suggested to be due to glycolate dehydrogenase activity.[210] According to some authors, complete conversion of glycolate to oxalate appears to involve both GO and glycolate dehydrogenase.[161,234]

Despite the preceding evidence, the quantitative role of glycolate dehydrogenase is not clear. Using rat and human liver fractions, it has been shown that most glycolate is indeed oxidized to oxalate via glyoxylate, with no evidence being found for glycolate dehydrogenase activity.[202]

The in vivo relevance in normal circumstances of the hydroxypyruvate-to-oxalate pathway is uncertain because the majority of the cellular hydroxypyruvate would be expected to be reduced to D-glycerate catalyzed by D-glycerate dehydrogenase (DGDH) (see Fig. 133-3).

Tissue Specificities of Metabolic Pathways

The vast majority of research on the metabolic pathways leading to oxalate synthesis have concentrated on the liver. Clearly, the liver is quantitatively the most important organ in the synthesis of oxalate from various sources such as xylitol, glyoxylate, glycolate, glycine, serine, and ethanolamine.[153,154,159] In states of excessive oxalate synthesis, extrahepatic oxalate deposition is presumed to occur due to transport of oxalate out of the liver.[159] Some enzymes involved directly or indirectly in oxalate synthesis are liver-specific, such as AGT and GO. Others, such as LDH, are more widely spread. The distribution of GR is unclear. Recent studies show that whereas DGDH activity is found in several tissues in the human body, GR activity is mainly confined to the liver, with some also in the kidney.[235,236] DAO is much more active in the kidney than in the liver. Since human kidney does not possess AGT activity, glyoxylate detoxification in this organ may depend on GR activity. In addition, the kidney may have to deal with its own synthetic load of oxalate in addition to the bulk of that released from the liver. To counter this suggestion, isolated perfused rat kidney, unlike isolated perfused rat liver, does not appear to synthesize oxalate from a variety of possible metabolic substrates.[154]

Unresolved Metabolic Controversies

Despite many decades of research into the metabolic pathways leading to oxalate synthesis in normal and hyperoxaluric individuals, disagreements still abound in certain areas. For example, differences of opinion can be found concerning the enzymes responsible for glyoxylate oxidation and reduction, the role of glycolate dehydrogenase, and the mechanism of increased oxalate synthesis in PH2 (see "Metabolic Consequences of DGDH/GR Deficiency," below). These arguments can be attributed, at least in part, to two important misunderstandings.

The first is a tendency to ignore the intracellular compartmentation of the enzymes, and therefore the specific metabolic reactions, being investigated. There are at least three compartments involved, namely, cytosol, peroxisomes, and mitochondria. All metabolic experiments, however, introduce substrates (radiolabeled or otherwise) into the cytosol, since this is the first compartment encountered whether a substrate is injected into a whole animal, introduced into an isolated liver perfusion system, or added to the tissue culture medium surrounding cultured hepatocytes. Such approaches may be valid approximations of the endogenous compartmentation of some substrates, but they certainly are not for glyoxylate. Based on the subcellular distribution of DAO and GO, the main site of glyoxylate synthesis is likely to be within the peroxisomes. Peroxisomal glyoxylate would be expected to subjected to quite different metabolic influences than cytosolic glyoxylate. In addition, the various in vitro techniques themselves can give very different results from each other. For example, the metabolic characteristics of isolated liver perfusions can differ widely from those of tissue slices or homogenates.[154]

The second fallacy is the tendency to extrapolate from laboratory animals, especially rats, to humans without allowing for the many differences between these species. The rat and human have very different levels of some key enzymes, the level of AGT being 40 times lower in the former than in the latter, whereas the level of GO is some 10 times higher.[237] The rat has an additional enzyme able to transaminate glyoxylate (i.e., AGT2) not found in humans. AGT2 is a mitochondrial enzyme and, unlike AGT, is not restricted to the liver. On top of these differences is the finding that AGT, which is the major glyoxylate-metabolizing (detoxifying) enzyme in humans, has a different subcellular location in the rat. Only part of it is peroxisomal, with the remainder being mitochondrial. On the basis of these facts, it would be expected that the relative importance of particular metabolic pathways involved in oxalate synthesis would be very different in rats and in humans.

In addition to these problems, it may not always be valid to extrapolate the observations made on normal metabolic processes to those found in states of oxalate overload (e.g., as found in the primary hyperoxalurias). Enzymes that make major contributions to the baseline level of oxalate synthesis may play only minor roles in its elevated synthesis, due to substrate limitation, changes in compartmental fluxes, etc.

The first metabolic studies on primary hyperoxaluria were carried out over 40 years ago. Since then, our understanding of the metabolic routes through to oxalate has improved but is still far from complete, and reappraisal of the established metabolic dogma is urgently needed (e.g., see Holmes et al.[174,175,238]).

ENZYMIC AND METABOLIC DEFECTS

PH1

Attempts to identify the basic enzymic defect in PH1 have been cognizant of the fact that the disease is primarily one of excessive oxalate synthesis and that the main immediate metabolic precursor of oxalate in mammals is glyoxylate (see "Metabolism of Oxalate and Its Precursors," above). In mammals, the three main catalytic reactions involving glyoxylate as substrate are oxidation to oxalate, reduction to glycolate, and transamination to glycine (see Williams and Smith[25] and "Metabolism of Oxalate and Its Precursors," above). A fourth (carboligation) reaction of uncertain metabolic significance also has been identified.[120,211] Because the elevated synthesis of oxalate and glycolate in PH1 precluded the possibility of deficiencies in these redox pathways, attention was directed toward the enzymes responsible for catalyzing the carboligation and transamination reactions.

CL. Although it had been reported previously that the activity of CL in isolated liver mitochondria was unaltered in PH1 patients compared with controls,[120,211] the role of this enzyme was reexamined by Koch et al.[239] These authors showed that there was a deficiency in a soluble (presumably cytosolic) form of the enzyme in liver, kidney, and spleen of PH1 patients even though the activity of the mitochondrial form was normal. Thus soluble CL deficiency became generally accepted as the probable cause of PH1 for 20 years (see Williams and Smith[25] and McKusick[240]). Although there was little direct evidence to the contrary, doubts about the role of CL in PH1 began to accumulate. For example, other workers failed to find a reduction of soluble CL in PH1 patients.[213,241] In addition, doubts were raised about whether soluble CL existed at all in cells or whether it was an artefact of the experimental procedure (i.e., leakage from damaged mitochondria).[118,119,213] The identity of CL also was called into question by the observations that it is probably identical to the mitochondrial citric acid cycle enzyme 2-oxoglutatate dehydrogenase.[118,119] The carboligase reaction possibly could be explained by a redundant recycling of the first decarboxylating component of the 2-oxoglutarate dehydrogenase complex (see Fig. 75-2 in the previous edition of this chapter[16]).

Thiamine pyrophosphate is an essential cofactor of both the CL and 2-oxoglutarate dehydrogenase reactions. Although thiamine deficiency may affect glyoxylate metabolism (see "Metabolism of Oxalate and Its Precursors," above), its effect on oxalate production is more equivocal. Oxalate excretion has been reported to be elevated in thiamine-deficient rats,[242] although this has been disputed by others.[215] Humans with thiamine deficiency do not have hyperoxaluria or CaOx renal stones.[243,244] In fact, some studies have suggested the opposite relationship between thiamine and oxalate synthesis.[179,245]

AGT. Numerous in vivo metabolic studies had pointed to abnormal glyoxylate transamination as a possible cause of PH1[246] (reviewed in Danpure[247] and Williams and Smith[25]), but initial attempts to identify specific enzyme defects were unsuccessful. The transamination of glyoxylate in liver fractions from PH1 patients in vitro was found to be unimpaired.[24,120,211] However, it did appear to be diminished in PH1 kidney homogenates,[248,249] although the significance of the latter observation has been questioned.[250]

The final identification of the enzymic defect in PH1 resulted from the convergence of two independent lines of thought. First, a role for the glyoxylate aminotransferases GGT and AGT in the etiology of primary hyperoxaluria was suggested by Thompson and Richardson.[183,184] Second, because of the localization of the enzymes thought to be involved in glyoxylate synthesis (i.e., DAO and GO) in the peroxisomes,[176] a role for these organelles in the pathogenesis of primary hyperoxaluria also was advanced.[171,221,251] These two ideas converged when it was discovered that various glyoxylate aminotransferases were partly located in the peroxisomes of rat liver[252–255] and especially when it was discovered that AGT, which is the most quantitatively important enzyme for glyoxylate transamination in mammals,[190] was solely peroxisomal in human liver.[186,256] The latter authors speculated that a deficiency of peroxisomal AGT may be the cause of primary hyperoxaluria.

In humans, AGT is a liver-specific enzyme,[185] and the first direct evidence that peroxisomal AGT deficiency was the cause of PH1 was obtained when it was found to be markedly depleted in the livers of two PH1 patients.[257,258] Subsequently, this observation was extended to cover 20 patients[259] and then 59 patients,[34] and now well over 150 PH1 patients have been shown to have hepatic AGT deficiency.[260,261] The specificity of the hepatic AGT deficiency in PH1 was demonstrated by the fact that activities of a number of other peroxisomal enzymes, such as catalase, DAO, and GO, and other aminotransferases, such as GGT, alanine:2-oxoglutarate aminotransferase, and aspartate:2-oxoglutarate aminotransferase, were normal in the livers of PH1 patients.[257,259] The only other enzyme activity shown to be deficient was serine:pyruvate aminotransferase,[259,262] the catalytic activity of which has been shown to be due to the same protein as AGT.[254,263] In addition to decreased AGT enzyme activity, many patients also were shown to be deficient in immunoreactive AGT protein.[34,264] There now can be no doubt that the clinical condition called PH1 is caused by a deficiency of peroxisomal AGT and not cytosolic CL. Because of the heterogeneity and possible ambiguity of the clinical and biochemical descriptions of PH1, it is recommended that PH1 should now be redefined in terms of this AGT deficiency.

Heterogeneity of AGT Expression. PH1 is characterized by marked heterogeneity at the enzymic level[34,259,260] (Fig. 133-4). Although about two-thirds of all patients have undetectable levels of AGT catalytic activity (ENZ$^-$), the remainder have activities that vary from 2 percent to as high as 48 percent of the mean normal activity (ENZ$^+$).[34,259,265] Solely on the basis of enzyme activity, many of the patients in the latter category cannot be distinguished from asymptomatic heterozygotes, who can have activities as low as 25 percent of the mean normal level.[259] About two-thirds of ENZ$^-$ patients also have no immunoreactive AGT protein (CRM$^-$). In the remaining third of ENZ$^-$ patients and all ENZ$^+$ patients, immunoreactive AGT protein can be detected (CRM$^+$).[34,260,261] This can vary from barely detectable levels to normal, or even supranormal, levels. In ENZ+ patients, the level of immunoreactive protein is usually approximately proportional to the level of enzyme activity.

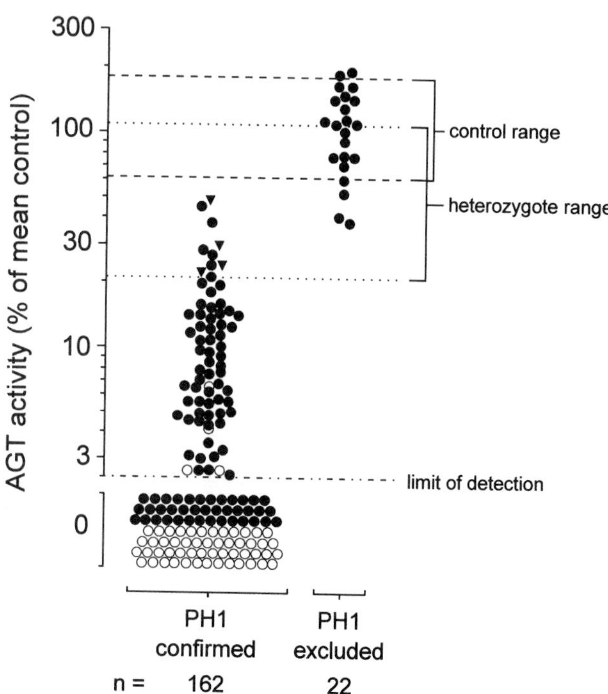

Fig. 133-4 Range of hepatic AGT activities found in PH1 patients. The data show the AGT enzyme activity, expressed as a percentage of the mean control value, in liver biopsies obtained from 184 individuals of whom 162 were diagnosed as having PH1 and 22 were not. Solid symbols = CRM$^+$ individuals; open symbols = CRM$^-$ individuals. Triangles = a diagnosis of PH1 was probable in these patients due to family and other biochemical data but not absolutely certain due to lack of any subcellular data. (*Modified with permission from Danpure and Rumsby.*[261])

Intracellular Mistargeting of AGT. Although the intracellular compartmentation of AGT varies between different vertebrate species (see "Animal Models of Primary Hyperoxaluria," below), in normal human hepatocytes, AGT is exclusively localized within the peroxisomes[186–188,256,266] (Fig. 133-5*A*). In most of the PH1 patients who are ENZ$^-$/CRM$^+$ (~20 percent of the total), the immunoreactive but catalytically defunct AGT protein is also localized totally within the peroxisomes[187,266] (see Fig. 133-5*E*). However, in all ENZ$^+$/CRM$^+$ PH1 patients studied so far, the intracellular distribution of AGT is very different. In these patients, who are predicted to comprise about one-third of the total,[34,260] about 90 percent of the immunoreactive AGT is localized in the mitochondria and only 10 percent in the peroxisomes[267] (see Fig. 133-5*C*). This intracellular protein trafficking defect, which is without precedent in human genetic disease, is specific for AGT, since the subcellular distribution of other peroxisomal enzymes, such as catalase, acyl-CoA oxidase, thiolase, hydratase, DAO, and GO, is unchanged.[267] It would appear that AGT in human liver is unable to perform at least one of its metabolic functions (i.e., glyoxylate transamination/detoxification) properly when located within the mitochondria instead of the peroxisomes.

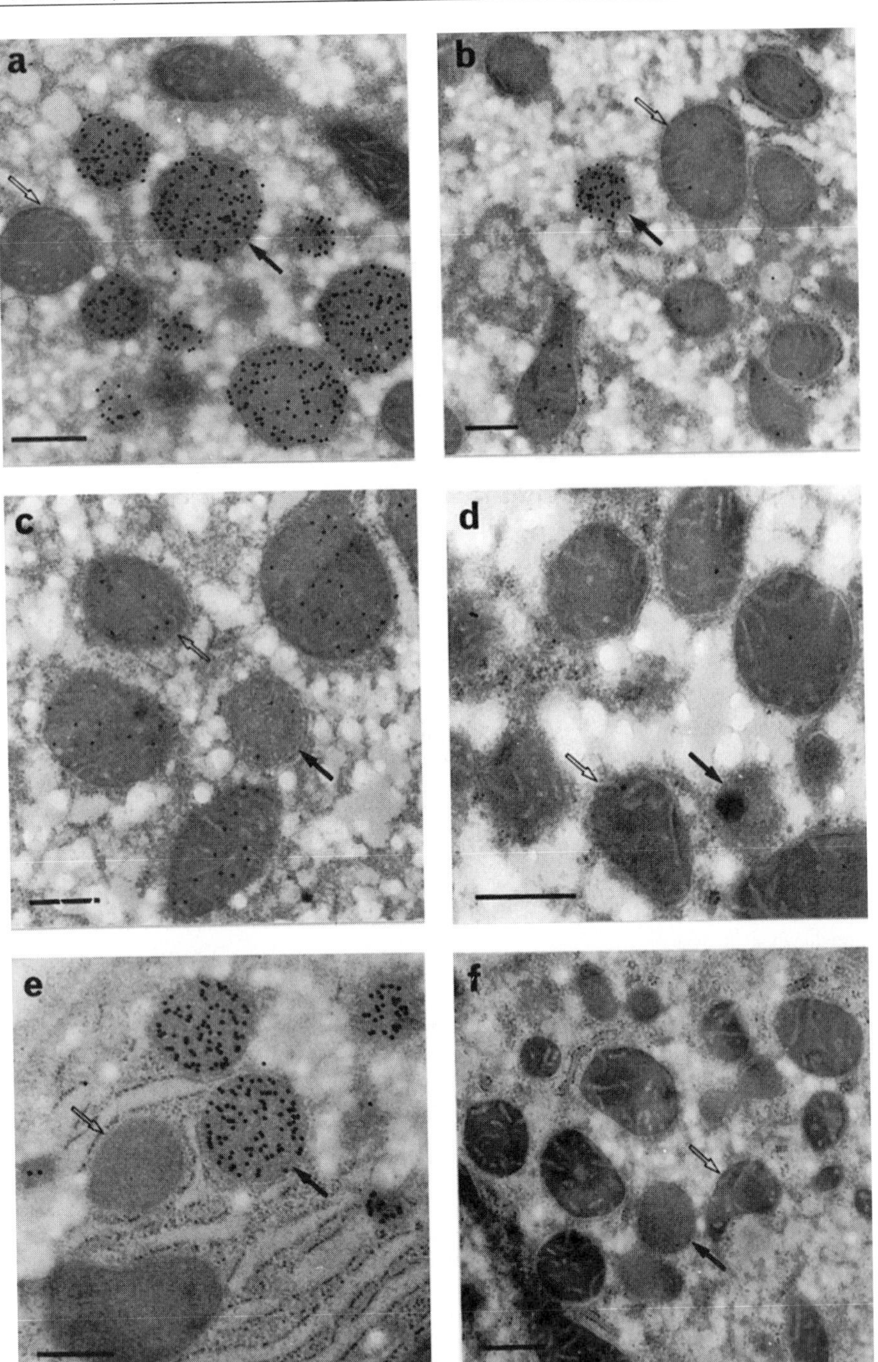

Fig. 133-5 Subcellular distribution of AGT in controls and PH1 patients. Postembedding protein A-gold immunoelectron microscopy of human liver sections using rabbit anti-human liver AGT antiserum. (*A*) Control (homozygous for the major allele) (100 percent peroxisomal AGT). (*B*) Control (homozygous for the minor allele) (90 percent peroxisomal AGT and 10 percent mitochondrial AGT). (*C*) CRM^+/ENZ^+ PH1 patient with the peroxisome-to-mitochondrion trafficking defect (homozygous for the minor allele and the 630G>A mutation) (90 percent mitochondrial AGT and 10 percent peroxisomal AGT). (*D*) $CRM^+/ENZ^\pm$ PH1 patient (compound heterozygote for the 630G>A and 243G>A mutations) (50 percent mitochondrial AGT and 50 percent peroxisomal AGT-the latter is aggregated into cores). (*E*) CRM^+/ENZ^- PH1 patient (homozygous for the 367G>A mutation) (100 percent peroxisomal AGT). (*F*) CRM^- PH1 patient (no labeling). Closed arrows = peroxisomes; open arrows = mitochondria; bars = 0.5 μm. (*Panels A and E reproduced and modified with permission from Purdue et al.*[318]; *photomicrographs courtesy of S. Griffiths.*)

A small number of PH1 patients express a variation of the mistargeting phenotype. These $CRM^+/ENZ^\pm$ patients have low but detectable levels of immunoreactive AGT protein but little or no AGT catalytic activity. AGT immunoreactivity in these individuals is more or less equally divided between peroxisomes and mitochondria. However, that in the peroxisomes appears to be aggregated into matrical corelike structures[268] (see Fig. 133-5*D*). These cores do not stain for other peroxisomal enzymes such as catalase, acyl-CoA oxidase, GO, thiolase, or hydratase.

PH1 as a Peroxisomal Disease. In the light of the preceding findings, PH1 was added to the growing list of peroxisomal diseases, more specifically diseases characterized by deficiencies of single peroxisomal enzymes (see Chap. 130). However, PH1 differs from most other peroxisomal diseases in a number of respects. For example, lipid metabolism remains unperturbed, and there is no evidence of generalized neurologic involvement in PH1. In addition, unlike the generalized diseases of peroxisome biogenesis (see Chap. 129), but like the other single peroxisomal enzyme deficiencies, cells from PH1 patients possess normal numbers of relatively normal-looking peroxisomes, albeit somewhat smaller than usually found[269,270] (Fig. 133-6).

Metabolic Consequences of AGT Deficiency. As with all aminotransferases, AGT is a pyridoxal phosphate-dependent enzyme. It catalyzes an essentially irreversible transamination reaction in which the amino group of alanine is transferred to glyoxylate, yielding pyruvate and glycine, respectively[183] (Table 133-2). The enzyme suffers from substrate inhibition at glyoxylate concentrations greater than 20 mM,[183] a factor that may be predicted to exacerbate the effect of partial AGT deficiency. Unlike GGT, the cofactor is only loosely bound to the apoprotein in AGT and can be removed easily by treatments such as laboratory dialysis.[183] AGT is identical to serine:pyruvate

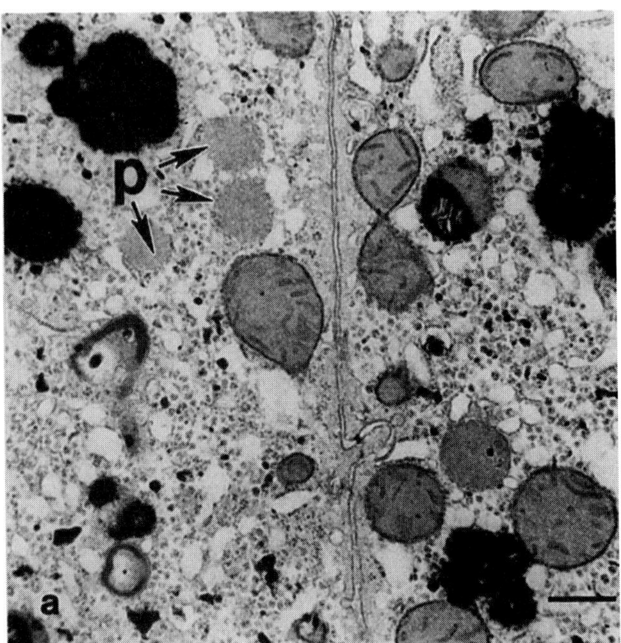

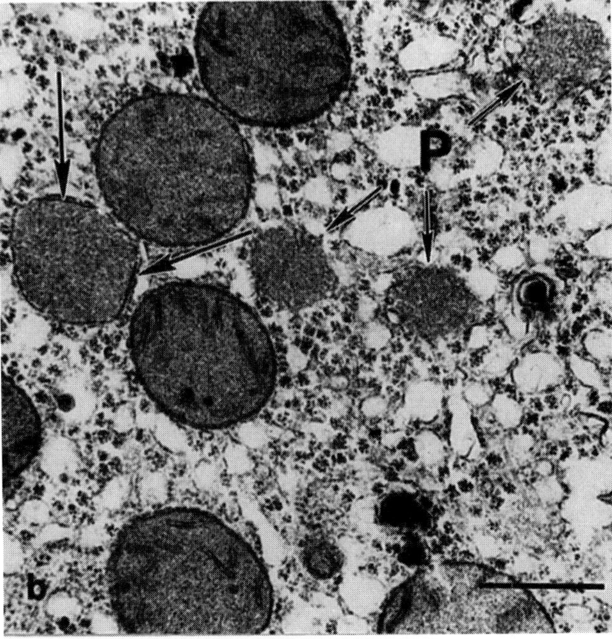

Fig. 133-6 Electron micrograph of a PH1 liver. P, peroxisomes. Note the extensive deposition of lipofuscin in the top panel; unlabeled arrows in the bottom panel indicate marginal plates in a larger than usual peroxisome; bars = 0.5 μm. (*Reproduced and modified with permission from Iancu and Danpure.*[269])

aminotransferase[263] (see Table 133-2), its activity toward serine and pyruvate being about 5 to 10 percent of that toward alanine and glyoxylate in human liver.

AGT plays a major role in glyoxylate transamination and detoxification.[190,271] Failure to detoxify glyoxylate within the peroxisomes, its main site of synthesis, allows one or more of a number of possibilities to occur (see Fig. 133-3). Glyoxylate could be oxidized to oxalate within the peroxisomes, catalyzed by GO. Alternatively, it could diffuse through the peroxisomal membrane into the cytosol, where it could be oxidized to oxalate (catalyzed by LDH), reduced to glycolate (catalyzed by GR or LDH), or transaminated to glycine (catalyzed by GGT).[257,258] The resulting

Table 133-2 Principal Reactions Catalyzed by AGT/SPT and GR/DGDH

AGT (deficient in PH1)
1. Alanine + glyoxylate → pyruvate + glycine
2. Serine + pyruvate → hydroxypyruvate + alanine
GR/DGDH (deficient in PH2)
3. Glyoxylate + NAD(P)H + H^+ → glycolate + $NAD(P)^+$
4. Hydroxypyruvate + NAD(P)H + H^+ → D-glycerate + $NAD(P)^+$

NOTE: Refer to Fig. 133-2 for the structures of the various substrates and products.

excessive synthesis of oxalate and glycolate by the liver is the biochemical hallmark of PH1.

AGT deficiency explains most of the biochemical manifestations of PH1. However, uncertainty still exists about the enzymes responsible for glyoxylate oxidation and reduction (see "Metabolism of Oxalate and Its Precursors," above). It is possible that both GO and LDH contribute to glyoxylate oxidation,[156] with the importance of LDH increasing as the glyoxylate concentration gets higher. The factor likely to determine the relative roles of GO and LDH is the rate of intraperoxisomal oxidation of glyoxylate compared with the rate of its translocation from the peroxisomal matrix into the cytosol. The peroxisomal membrane has been shown to be freely permeable to hydrophilic molecules up to a molecular weight of about 800 Da.[272,273] Therefore, it is unlikely to present any significant barrier to the passage of glyoxylate or any of the other metabolites involved. When in the cytosol, LDH is the only viable candidate for the catalysis of glyoxylate oxidation (see Fig. 133-3).

At least in vitro, LDH can catalyze both the oxidation and the reduction reactions of glyoxylate (see "Metabolism of Oxalate and Its Precursors," above). Disproportionation of two molecules of glyoxylate into one of glycolate and one of oxalate catalyzed by LDH has been suggested to occur in vivo.[204] Anecdotal evidence of equimolar synthesis of oxalate and glycolate in PH1 has been taken as evidence in support of this,[274] the determining factor being the balanced ratio of NAD/NADH maintained by the redox reactions. However, there is no direct evidence that the excessive synthesis of oxalate in PH1 is matched by an equimolar increase in glycolate synthesis (see Hockaday et al.[27]). Certainly there is enormous variation in the urinary oxalate-glycolate ratio in patients with proven AGT deficiency (i.e., PH1 patients). In addition, the urinary oxalate-glycolate ratio appears to vary with age.[68,275] Results obtained in PH2 suggest that GR may be the most important enzyme involved in the reduction of glyoxylate to glycolate (see "Metabolic Consequences of DGDH/GR Deficiency," below).

The biochemical heterogeneity in PH1 with respect to the ratio of oxalate and glycolate excreted in the urine could be explained by differences in the relative contributions made by GO and LDH to the oxidation of glyoxylate and LDH and GR to its reduction. For example, PH1 patients with isolated hyperoxaluria may have most of their glyoxylate metabolized intraperoxisomally by GO, whereas patients with combined hyperoxaluria and hyperglycolic aciduria may have a greater proportion of their glyoxylate diffuse into the cytosol to be oxidized and reduced by the combined actions of LDH and GR. The few PH1 patients with urinary glycolate excretion greatly in excess of the urinary oxalate excretion (e.g., patient 5 in Watts et al.[276]) may have most of their glyoxylate metabolized by GR rather than LDH. Clearly, all these parameters, such as relative enzyme activities and NAD(P)/NAD(P)H ratios, will be genetically influenced.

Once in the cytosol, relatively little glyoxylate would be expected to be transaminated by GGT. Although the activity of GGT is low (when compared with the normal level of peroxisomal AGT), genetic variations in its activity could still be a contributory factor in determining the biochemical and clinical heterogeneity of the disease.[34,247]

PH1 is the most convincing proof of the importance of AGT in the detoxification of glyoxylate. However, not only does it show that the activity of AGT is important, it also shows that its intracellular location is important. Clearly, in humans at least, AGT is unable to fulfill its proper metabolic role when located in the mitochondria. Efficient detoxification of glyoxylate requires transamination at its site of synthesis (i.e., the peroxisome), thus minimizing the chances of it diffusing into the cytosol to be oxidized by LDH. This is not the case, however, with a number of other vertebrates that have their AGT principally within mitochondria (see "Animal Models of Primary Hyperoxaluria," below).

Although under normal circumstances it is assumed that oxalate synthesis occurs throughout the body, in states of excessive oxalate synthesis, extrahepatic oxalate deposition is presumed to occur due to transport out of the liver.[159] This is indeed likely in PH1 because the deficient enzyme is liver-specific. Nevertheless, the baseline oxalate synthesis by other tissues may play a significant role in the overall disease pathology. In some cases of PH1, oxalate synthesis by the kidney may contribute significantly to the level of hyperoxaluria.[1,83]

Relationship Between Enzymic, Biochemical, and Clinical Heterogeneity. Although there is an approximate relationship between residual AGT enzyme activity and clinical severity (as determined by the age of the patient at the time of liver biopsy),[34] it is not clinically useful. There are patients with the acute neonatal form of PH1 who look identical at the enzymic level to mildly affected patients whose first symptoms do not occur until the fifth decade.[34] In addition, there are patients described as having "mild metabolic hyperoxaluria" and "renal hyperoxaluria" who cannot be distinguished enzymically from their counterparts with "normal" PH1 (Jennings and Danpure, unpublished observations). In all these cases, although the underlying disease is undoubtedly caused by AGT deficiency, the specific clinical and biochemical manifestations are likely to be modified by a variety of other factors (Fig. 133-7). For example, disease severity could easily be influenced by other genetic factors, such as the activities of enzymes (other than AGT) involved directly or indirectly in oxalate synthesis. Nongenetic (environmental) factors, such as diet and enteric/renal infection, also could be involved.

The rather poor relationship between enzymic, metabolic, and clinical phenotypes in PH1 has been highlighted in a family containing four patients in two generations recently studied by Hoppe et al.[132] Mother and son with the same degree of AGT enzyme deficiency had very different disease progression, even though they had similarly elevated levels of oxalate excretion. In addition, brother and sister with the same mutations in the gene encoding AGT (see "Molecular Genetics and Cell Biology of PH1," below), and therefore presumed to have similar levels of enzyme deficiency, had markedly different levels of oxalate excretion and clinical phenotypes.[132]

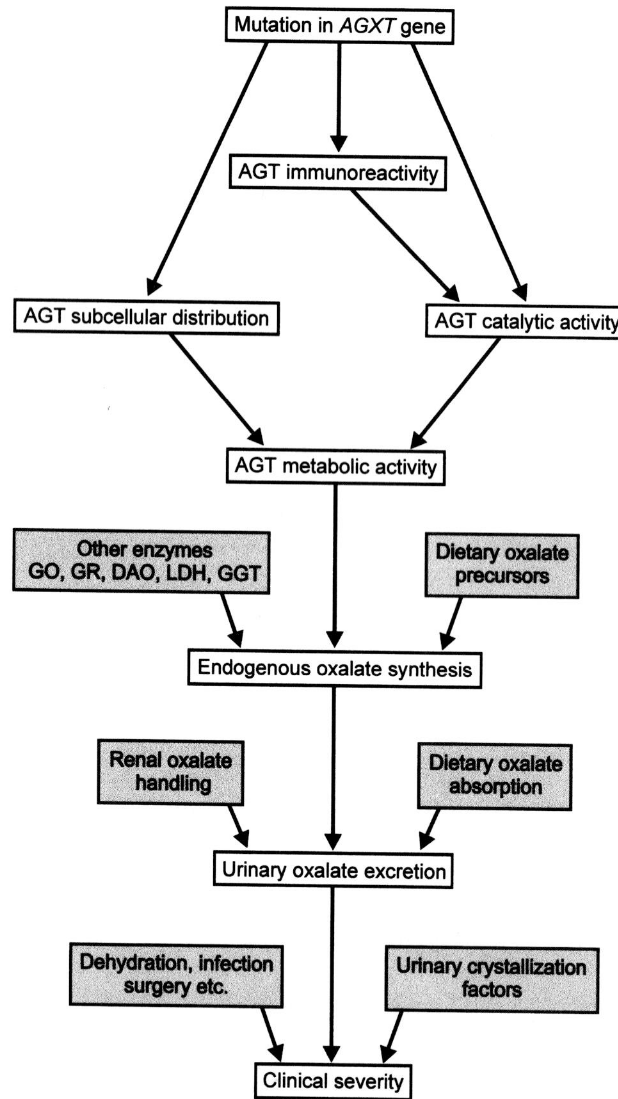

Fig. 133-7 Multifactorial determinants of disease severity in PH1. Unshaded boxes = parameters determining the relationship between the *AGXT* genotype, AGT phenotype, and clinical phenotype; gray-shaded boxes = other genetic and environmental factors likely to perturb the relationship between AGT deficiency and clinical severity.

PH2

DGDH and GR. Considerably less attention has been paid to the elucidation of the basic enzymic defect in PH2, not least because of the greater rarity of this condition compared with PH1. The main distinguishing feature of PH2 is the elevated synthesis of L-glycerate, instead of glycolate, concomitant with elevated synthesis of oxalate.[23] L-Glycerate, which is an abnormal metabolite of hydroxypyruvate, is not normally detectable to any extent in urine, and its increased synthesis in PH2 appears to be due to a failure to metabolize hydroxypyruvate by one of its other metabolic routes (see Williams and Smith[25]). Peripheral blood leukocytes from PH2 patients were found to be deficient in the activity of DGDH, an enzyme that catalyses the reduction of hydroxypyruvate to D-glycerate[23] (see Table 133-2), a finding that was confirmed a long time afterwards by another laboratory.[69] DGDH also possesses GR activity[277,278] (see Table 133-2). GR deficiency in PH2 was first described by Mistry et al.,[279] who showed a marked depletion of GR and DGDH activity in the liver of a PH2 patient. This also has been shown subsequently by another laboratory.[70] Interestingly, recent studies have shown that there are at least two enzymes in human tissues with DGDH activity, only one of which also has GR activity.[236] It is the enzyme with both DGDH *and* GR activities, which is present at high levels in the liver, that appears to be the one deficient in PH2. The activity of the enzyme with only DGDH activity, which is present in leukocytes, is normal in PH2.

Metabolic Consequences of DGDH/GR Deficiency. Notwithstanding the latter comments, there is no doubt that DGDH and GR are simply different catalytic manifestations of the same enzyme. There are two main reactions catalyzed by this protein, namely, the reduction of hydroxypyruvate to D-glycerate and the reduction of glyoxylate to glycolate (see Fig. 133-3 and Table 133-2). Both NAD(H) and NADP(H) can be used as cofactors.

The reaction catalyzed by DGDH is weighted heavily toward the reduction reaction. Therefore, a deficiency of DGDH causes a buildup of hydroxypyruvate that is instead reduced to L-glycerate catalyzed by LDH.[23,94] Although there is no disagreement about this hypothesis, there has been much controversy concerning the mechanisms involved in the cause of the excessive oxalate synthesis in PH2. At least four hypotheses have been advanced.

The first is based on the fact that DGDH is the same enzyme as GR. If GR is an important factor in the metabolism of glyoxylate to glycolate (see "Metabolism of Oxalate and Its Precursors," above), then its deficiency in PH1 could lead to a buildup of glyoxylate in the cytosol, where its oxidation to oxalate, catalyzed by LDH, would increase.[23] The second hypothesis has been developed largely using the experimental model systems of isolated rat liver perfusions and isolated rat liver hepatocytes.[155,161] This hypothesis proposes that the buildup of hydroxypyruvate due to the deficiency of DGDH causes more to be decarboxylated to glycolaldehyde, which is then oxidized to glycolate and then oxidized directly to oxalate, catalyzed by glycolate dehydrogenase, without glyoxylate as an intermediate.[155,161] The third hypothesis suggests that the putative buildup of hydroxypyruvate, due to DGDH deficiency, has a direct effect on LDH, increasing its oxidative role and diminishing its reductive role, due to a shift in NADH/NAD ratios.[280] The fourth hypothesis suggests that hydroxypyruvate could autooxidize to oxalate nonenzymically.[281]

High levels of hydroxypyruvate have never been demonstrated in PH2, and it is likely that the vast majority is reduced to L-glycerate catalyzed by LDH. Therefore, a direct role for hydroxypyruvate in the etiology of the hyperoxaluria in PH2 seems unlikely. In addition, PH2 is not accompanied by hyperglycolic aciduria.[94] This would be difficult to understand if the second hypothesis[155,161] was substantially correct, because glycolate would be an intermediate in the conversion of hydroxypyruvate to oxalate. The third hypothesis[280] is cast into doubt because other workers have found that hydroxypyruvate inhibits both GO and LDH-catalyzed oxidation of glyoxylate,[281] whether using purified LDH[282] or isolated perfused rat livers.[155]

The demonstration of combined DGDH and GR deficiency in both human PH1 liver[279] and in the livers of a feline analogue of PH2[283] (see "Animal Models of Primary Hyperoxaluria," below) is compatible with the first hypothesis of Williams and Smith.[23] This hypothesis has the virtue of being the simplest and, to this author at least, the most plausible.

Relative Importance of AGT and GR in the Metabolism and Detoxification of Glyoxylate

The metabolic and clinical sequelae of PH1 and PH2 demonstrate the important roles played by AGT and GR in the metabolism (detoxification) of glyoxylate, at least in humans (Fig. 133-8). The activities of both enzymes would appear to be major determinants in the level of endogenous oxalate synthesis. The observations that PH1 tends to be a more severe disease than PH2 and that the level of hyperoxaluria also tends to be higher would suggest that AGT has a quantitatively more important role than GR. This is also compatible with the suggestion (see above) that glyoxylate detoxification is more efficient if it occurs in the peroxisomes than in the cytosol.

Nevertheless, AGT and GR are unlikely to be the sole factors. The activities of GO, DAO, LDH, GGT, and possibly the NAD(P)(H) status could all influence the level of oxalate and glycolate synthesis (see Fig. 133-7). Attention to these other possible genetic determinants of oxalate and glycolate synthesis has been increased recently with the observations that isolated hyperglycolic aciduria[284] and concomitant hyperoxaluria and hyperglycolic aciduria[285] can occur for reasons other than AGT deficiency.

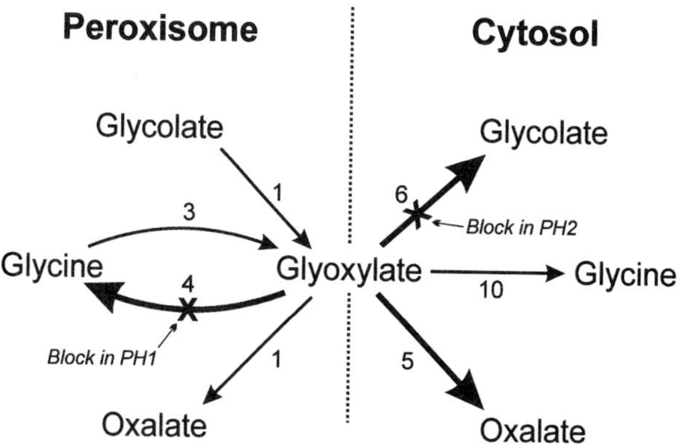

Fig. 133-8 Importance of AGT and GR in the metabolism/detoxification of glyoxylate. Central role of glyoxylate metabolic dysfunction in the excess synthesis of oxalate in PH1 and PH2. Enzymes are numbered as in Fig. 133-3.

MOLECULAR GENETICS AND CELL BIOLOGY OF PH1

Following identification of the causal relationship between AGT deficiency and disease in PH1, there have been significant advances in recent years in our understanding of the molecular genetics and cell biology of this intractable disease. Unfortunately, similar advances have yet to be made in the case of DGDH/GR deficiency and PH2.

The Normal Human AGT Gene

AGT is encoded by a single gene (*AGXT*) that maps to chromosome 2q37.3.[286,287] It consists of 11 exons, ranging from 65 to 407 bp, and spans approximately 10 kb.[286] The longest cDNA clone so far isolated (from a HepG2 library) contains an open reading frame of 1179 nucleotides (including the termination codon), a 5′-UTR of 122 bp, and a 3′-UTR of 299 bp [not including the poly(A) tail].[288] The 10 introns vary in size from 139 bp to approximately 1.65 kb. The deduced amino acid sequence of 392 residues (Fig. 133-9) predicts a polypeptide with a molecular mass of 43,046 kDa,[288,289] a size that is compatible with that observed by SDS-PAGE of AGT purified from human liver.[186,256] Apart from N-terminal acetylation, there is no evidence for any posttranslational modification.[290] The human AGT amino acid sequence is very similar (78-89 percent identical) to those predicted for marmoset, rabbit, rat, guinea pig, and cat.[291-294] As is the case with AGT from these other mammals, the human polypeptide contains a consensus pyridoxal phosphate-binding site at Lys209.[292] As expected for a liver-specific protein, several cis-acting elements thought to be involved in regulation of liver-specific gene expression have been identified in the 1253-bp sequence upstream of the transcription initiation site.[286]

Normal Allelic Variations in the AGT Gene. A number of intragenic polymorphisms have been identified at the *AGXT* locus (Table 133-3). Five point nucleotide substitutions have been found spread across exons 1, 2, 6, 10, and 11. One 1342C > A is in the 3′-UTR,[295] and four are in the coding region. Of these, two, 386C > T and 776G > A, are synonymous changes[286,296] and two, 154C > T and 1142A > G, are nonsynonymous,[296] leading to P11L and I340M amino acid replacements, respectively.

Two intronic polymorphisms of note also have been identified. Intron 1 contains a polymorphic 74-bp duplication[297] that segregates with the 154C > T and 1142A > G point substitutions. These three changes define the "minor" (as opposed to the "major") *AGXT* allele. Recently, it has been shown that the synonymous 386C > T polymorphism segregates more specifically with the 154C > T and intron 1 duplication polymorphisms than does 1142A > G.[298] The minor allele has a frequency of 15 to 20 percent in Caucasian populations but only approximately 2 percent in Japanese.[299]

Intron 4 contains an unusual mildly polymorphic variable number tandem repeat (VNTR) that has some similarities to the

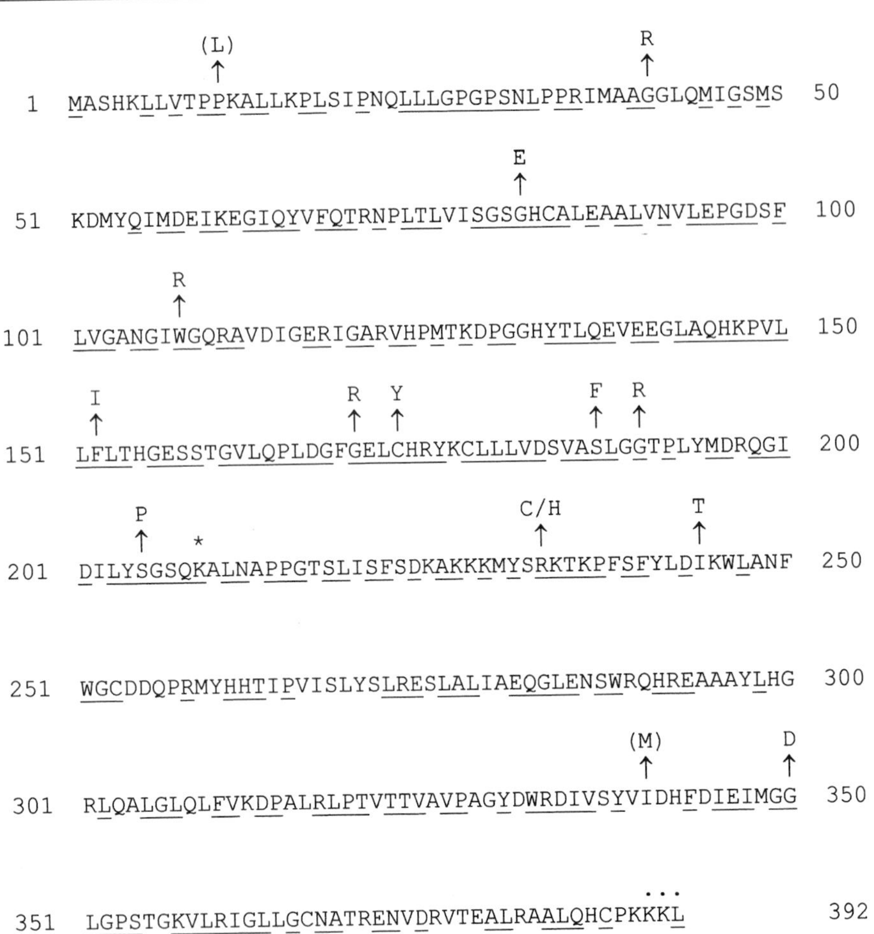

Fig. 133-9 Deduced amino acid sequence of human AGT. The main sequence shows the polypeptide encoded by the more common major *AGXT* allele; underline = amino acids conserved in all six mammals studied so far (i.e., human, marmoset, rabbit, rat, guinea pig, and cat); periods = C-terminal nonstandard PTS1; * = pyridoxal phosphate binding site; ↑ = point amino acid replacements listed in Tables 133-3 and 133-4, those in brackets indicate the polymorphisms associated with the minor *AGXT* allele (see text for details).

Epstein-Barr IR_3 repetitive element and consists of 12, 17, approximately 32 or approximately 38 copies of a 29/32-bp repeating unit.[299] The allelic frequencies of these four polymorphic variations are 33, 7, 0, and 60 percent, respectively, in Caucasians and 31, 45, 5, and 19 percent, respectively, in Japanese[299] (see Table 133-3). The minor *AGXT* allele is always found on the background of the type I (~38 copy number) intron 4 VNTR.

With the exception of the 154C > T (P11L) substitution, none of the preceding polymorphisms are known to have any functional significance (see below). However, many (especially those in introns 1 and 4) have been found to be invaluable in the prenatal diagnosis of PH1 (see "Prenatal Diagnosis of PH1," below). The frequencies of the minor *AGXT* allele and the type I VNTR are much higher in PH1 patients than in the general population (see Table 133-3). This appears to be without functional significance and is simply a reflection of the high frequency of the 630G > A mutation (see below) that cosegregates with these polymorphisms.

Table 133-3 Frequency of Intragenic Polymorphisms at the *AGXT* Locus in Normal Individuals and PH1 Patients

Polymorphism	Location	Amino Acid Replacement	% Allelic Frequency: Normal Population	% Allelic Frequency: PH1 Patients	Detection Method	References
154C > T	Exon 1	P11L	15–20 (~2)	40–50	PCR + *StyI*	296
386C > T*	Exon 2	None			PCR + *AvaII*	296, 298
776G > A	Exon 6	None				286
1142A > G*	Exon 10	I340M	15–20 (~2)	40–50	PCR + *AvaII*	296
1342C > A	Exon 11 (3′UTR)	None				295
74-bp duplication*	Intron 1	None	15–20 (~2)	40–50	PCR	297
Type I VNTR*	Intron 4	None	60 (19)	78	*PstI* + Southern blot	298, 299
Type II VNTR			7 (45)	5		
Type III VNTR			33 (31)	15		
Type IV VNTR			0 (5)	1		

NOTE: Polymorphisms marked with asterisks indicate those which segregate with the minor *AGXT* allele. The values for the % allelic frequency in normal individuals refer to mixed European and North-American populations, but those in brackets refer to Japanese.

Table 133-4 Mutations Identified at the *AGXT* Locus

Mutation	Exon Location	Amino Acid or Other Alteration	Frequency	Polymorphic Allele	Associated Phenotype: CRM	ENZ	Other	Ref.	Method of Identification
243 G > A	1	G41R	3(3) [1%]	Minor	±	±	Perox cores	268	PCR + *Msp*I
320 C > G	2	Y66ter	1(1)		−	−		297	PCR + *Rsa*I
367 G > A	2	G82E	3(6)	Major	+	−		318	PCR + *Ava*I
444 T > C	2	W108R	1(1)					553	
545 G > T	3	Splicing defect or E141D	1(2)					553	
576 T > A	4	F152I	4(4) [1%]	Minor	±	−		268	PCR + *Mbo*I
630 G > A	4	G170R	30% [25%]	Minor	+	+	Perox-to-mito mistargeting	296	PCR + *Msp*I
640 G > A	4	C173Y	1(1)					553	
682 C > T	5	S187F	2(2) [1%]	Major	−	−		554	PCR + *Bsm*I
690 G > A	5	G190R	2(4)					553	PCR + *Fau*I
735 T > C	6	S205P	1(2) [< 1%]		−	−		319	PCR + *Sma*I
819 C > T	7	R233C	1(2) [1%]					295	PCR + *Aca*I
820 G > A	7	R233H	1(1) [< 1%]		−	−		295	PCR + *Aca*I
853 T > C	7	I244T	[9%]	Minor	−/+	−/±		295	PCR + *BstX*I
860 G > A	7	W246ter	1(1) [< 1%]		±	−		295	PCR + *Mae*III
CATCA920-924 → ACAATCTCAG (deletion/insertion)	8	I267 → Q,S,Q,A,C,T,A, ter (frameshift)	2(4)					555	PCR + *Stu*I
GCG1008-1010 → Δ	9	A296Δ	1(1)					553	
1171 G > A	10	G350D	1(2)					553	

NOTE: *Frequency*: This indicates the % allelic frequency in PH1 patients (data not in brackets derived from Table 1 in Danpure[556]; data in square brackets derived from Table 2 in Tarn et al.[298]). Where the % frequency is too low to estimate, the frequency is presented as the number of patients (or alleles in round brackets) found with that particular mutation.

PH1-Specific Mutations in the AGT Gene (*AGXT*)

At the time of writing this review, at least 18 mutations have been identified in *AGXT* (Table 133-4). It has been estimated that these comprise the causal mutations in the expressed alleles of about 40 to 50 percent of the PH1 patients studied so far.[260,298] In a number of cases, particular mutations are consistently associated with particular enzymic phenotypes, such as presence or absence of AGT catalytic activity or immunoreactivity, peroxisome-to-mitochondrion mistargeting, etc. However, in relatively few cases have the mutations been shown actually to cause the enzymic phenotype associated with their presence. More often than not, the causal relationship between a particular mutation and disease is assumed following analysis of the pattern of its segregation with disease within a particular family and its absence in a normal control population. Some of the more interesting examples of proven genotype-enzymic phenotype relationships are discussed below.

Peroxisome-to-Mitochondrion AGT Mistargeting. By far the most remarkable enzymic phenotype associated with PH1 is the mistargeting of AGT from peroxisomes to mitochondria (see Fig. 133-5*c*), a phenomenon that is without parallel in human genetic disease. Such organelle-to-organelle mistargeting is especially surprising because, despite some superficial similarities, the molecular requirements for protein import into mitochondria and peroxisomes are so different. For example, mitochondrial matrix proteins are targeted by cleavable N-terminal presequences of about 10 to 80 residues that are typically positively charged amphiphilic α helices.[300,301] On the other hand, most peroxisomal matrix proteins are targeted by noncleavable C-terminal tripeptides based on the consensus motif Ser-Lys-Leu or conservative variants thereof.[302,303] The latter are called *type 1 peroxisomal targeting sequences* (PTS1s) to distinguish them from type 2 peroxisomal targeting sequences (PTS2s), which are found in a few peroxisomal proteins and are characterized by cleavable N-terminal sequences based on the X_n-Arg-Leu-X_5-His/Gln-Leu-X_n consensus motif.[304,305] In addition to differences in the nature of the topogenic information, mitochondrial proteins can only be imported as unfolded or loosely folded monomers,[306] whereas at least some peroxisomal proteins can be imported as complex folded oligomers.[307,308]

Normal AGT is imported into peroxisomes by way of the PTS1 import receptor Pex5p[309] (see Chap. 129) and, therefore, would be presumed to possess a PTS1. However, the C-terminus of AGT (Lys-Lys-Leu) has only a two out of three match with the consensus PTS1 motif. Although, as expected for a targeting sequence, this tripeptide is necessary for the peroxisomal import of AGT,[309] it is insufficient to target a variety of reporter proteins.[309,310] It is likely that AGT possesses additional (as yet unidentified) topogenic information both adjacent and not adjacent to the C-terminus. The "nonstandard" PTS1 of AGT is remarkable both with respect to its context specificity (i.e., it will target AGT to peroxisomes but not firefly luciferase, bacterial chloramphenicol acetyl transferase, or jellyfish green fluorescent protein) and its allowable degeneracy. For example, the nonconsensus tripeptides Lys-Lys-Leu, Ser-Gln-Leu, Asn-Lys-Leu, His-Arg-Leu, and Ser-Ser-Leu will all target AGT correctly to peroxisomes, as will the consensus tripeptide Ser-Lys-Leu.[309]

All PH1 patients with mistargeted AGT so far studied express at least one minor *AGXT* allele.[260] In addition, in most such patients, this allele contains an additional PH1-specific 630G > A point nucleotide substitution that is predicted to lead to a G170R amino acid replacement.[296] This PH1-specific mutation is the most common so far found, accounting for about 25 to 30 percent of the mutant alleles in European and North American patients.[260,298] Patients who are homozygous for this mutation usually possess significantly more AGT enzyme activity (> 25 percent of normal levels) than those who are heterozygous (< 20 percent).[260] In the latter patients, the other (nonmistargeting)

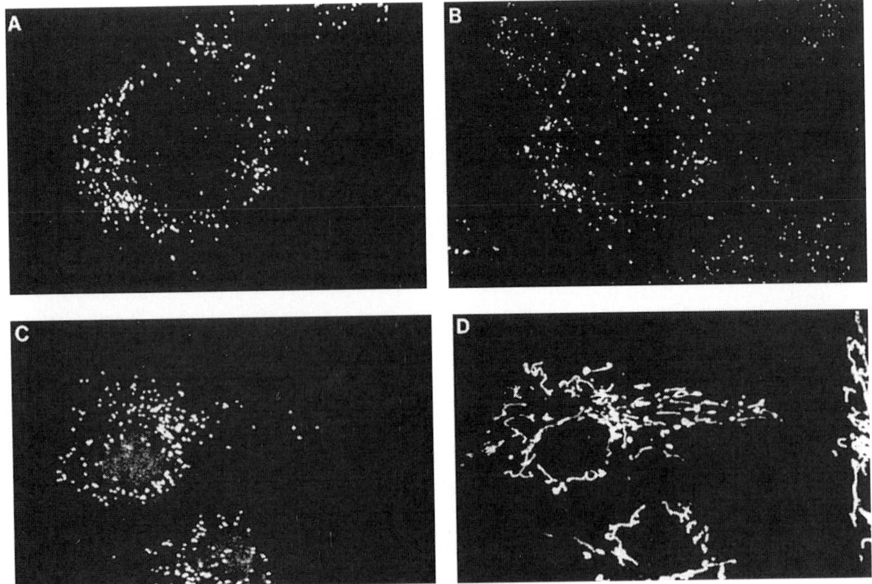

Fig. 133-10 Subcellular distribution of normal AGT encoded by the major *AGXT* allele after transfection of COS-1 cells. Confocal immunofluorescence microscopy of cells either double-labeled for AGT (*A*) and catalase as the peroxisomal marker (*B*) or AGT (*C*) and MitoTracker as the mitochondrial marker (*D*). AGT in these cells is entirely peroxisomal (i.e., it colocalizes with catalase not MitoTracker). (*Reproduced with permission from Danpure et al.*[316])

allele is often not expressed, at least in terms of detectable AGT protein or mRNA.

That this mutant AGT is not just associated with mistargeting but actually causes it can be easily seen in transfected monkey kidney (COS-1) cells or human fibroblasts that do not normally express AGT.[309] Expression in these cells of normal AGT encoded by the major *AGXT* allele leads, as expected, to a peroxisomal localization (Fig. 133-10). On the other hand, expression of the mutant form leads to a distribution resembling that found in the livers of PH1 patients with mistargeted AGT (i.e., mainly mitochondrial but with some peroxisomal) (Fig. 133-11).

P11L Generates a Weak Mitochondrial Targeting Sequence. In order to understand the molecular basis for AGT mistargeting in PH1, it is necessary to consider first the effect of the normal polymorphisms encoded by the minor *AGXT* allele. Normal individuals who are homozygous for the minor *AGXT* allele (~4 percent of the Caucasian population) have relatively normal levels of AGT. However, it is distributed slightly differently from those who are homozygous for the major allele (~64 percent of the population). Whereas AGT is 100 percent peroxisomal in the latter, it is approximately 95 percent peroxisomal and approximately 5 percent mitochondrial in the former[296] (see Fig. 133-5*B*). This partial "rerouting" of AGT to the mitochondria appears to be without any overt clinical consequences. The minor allele contains two nonsynonymous polymorphisms that lead to P11L and I340M amino acid replacements (see Fig. 133-9), and there are a number of pieces of evidence that suggest that the former, but not the latter,

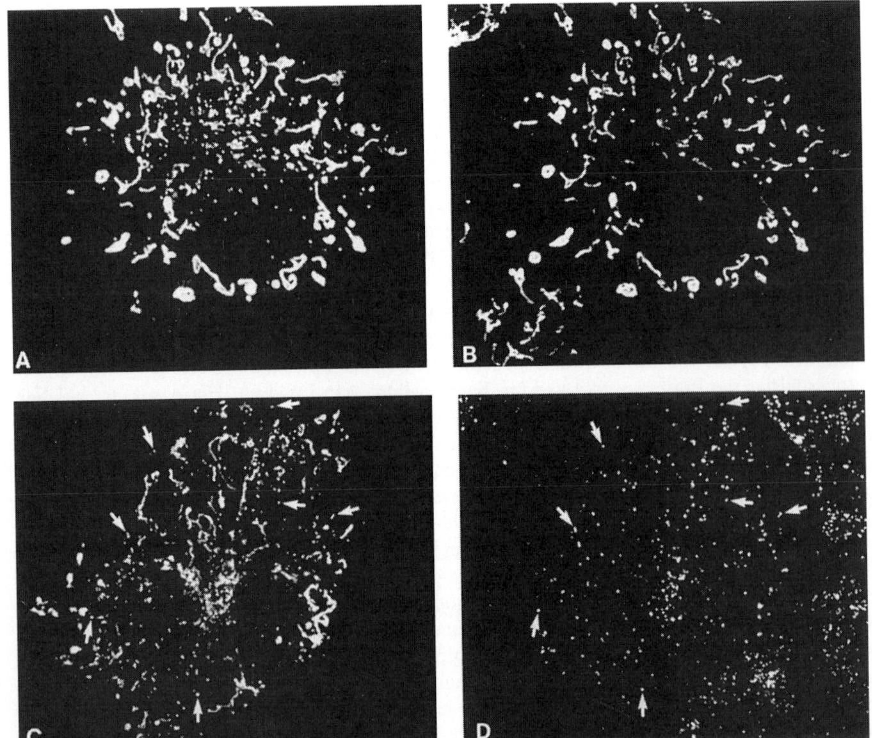

Fig. 133-11 Subcellular distribution of mutant (mistargeting) AGT containing the P11L polymorphism and the G170R mutation after transfection of COS-1 cells. Confocal immunofluorescence microscopy of cells either double-labeled for AGT (*A*) and MitoTracker as the mitochondrial marker (*B*) or AGT (*C*) and catalase as the peroxisomal marker (*D*). The arrows in *C* and *D* help with the alignment of the punctate AGT and catalase. AGT in these cells is mainly mitochondrial (colocalizing with MitoTracker), but some peroxisomal AGT (colocalizing with catalase) is also clearly detectable. (*Reproduced with permission from Danpure et al.*[316])

is likely to have functional consequences. Pro11 is absolutely conserved in all five other mammals so far studied, whereas Ile340 is not. In fact, in three mammals (i.e., cat, rabbit, and guinea pig), residue 340 is actually Met anyway. In addition, using the criteria of Chou and Fasman[311] and Garnier et al.,[312] the P11L replacement is predicted to increase the likelihood of the N-terminus of AGT folding into an α helix, whereas no structural changes are predicted to ensue from the I340M replacement.[296] The extent to which the N-terminus of AGT really does fold into an α helix under physiologic conditions in unclear. Circular dichroism (CD) of synthetic 20-mer peptides based on the N-terminal sequences of AGT with or without the P11L replacement showed that the presence of this polymorphism only marginally increased the proportion that folded into a helical conformation.[559] (Fig. 133-12). Nevertheless, the amino acids at the N-terminus are typical of those found in a mitochondrial targeting sequence (MTS), including the presence of basic, hydroxyl, and hydrophobic but the absence of acidic amino acids. In addition, helical wheel analysis showed that should an α helix actually form, it would be strongly amphiphilic[296] (see Fig. 133-12). In vitro studies with an isolated rat mitochondrial protein import system[313] have shown that the P11L replacement is all that is necessary to target AGT to mitochondria. In such a system, the I340M replacement is not only unable to direct the mitochondrial import of AGT, it also has no effect on the ability of P11L to do so.

Luckily, the P11L-generated MTS appears to be functionally weak, especially under more physiologic conditions. This is best demonstrated by the small proportion (~5 percent) of AGT that is targeted to mitochondria in the liver cells of individuals homozygous for the minor *AGXT* allele (see above). In fact, when this allele is expressed in transfected human fibroblasts or COS-1 cells in culture, mitochondrial localization cannot be seen at all.[309] Presumably, if the P11L-generated MTS had been more efficient, the incidence of PH1 would have been approximately 4 percent in Caucasians instead of approximately 0.0004 percent (see "Incidence, Genetics, and Environment," above).

***G170R* Increases the Efficiency of the *P11L*-Generated MTS.** Efficient mitochondrial targeting of AGT in whole cells only seems to occur when the PH1-specific G170R mutation is present in addition to the P11L polymorphism (see Fig. 133-5*c*). How can G170R increase the functional efficiency of the P11L-generated MTS? Isolated mitochondrial import and cell culture transfection studies have shown that the G170R replacement provides no mitochondrial targeting information itself, and it does not inhibit peroxisomal import.[309,313] In fact, if this mutation had by chance arisen on the major, rather than the minor, *AGXT* allele, then it probably would not have led to any recognizable clinical phenotype, and PH1 would have been 30 percent rares in Caucasian populations than it actually is.

The reason for the remarkable synergism between P11L and G170L with respect to AGT mitochondrial targeting has been established only recently. The explanation highlights one of the most surprising differences between the structural requirements for protein import into peroxisomes and mitochondria. Whereas proteins can be imported into peroxisomes as folded oligomers, they can be imported into mitochondria only as unfolded or partially folded monomers (see above). In vitro translated AGT, encoded by either the major or minor allele, dimerizes rapidly and effectively irreversibly in rabbit reticulocyte lysate[314] (Fig. 133-13) and is likely to do the same in the cytosol of liver cells and transfected tissue culture cells. In the latter system, AGT is imported into peroxisomes as a fully folded catalytically active dimer.[314] However, even when it possesses an MTS (such as that generated by the P11L polymorphism), AGT can only be imported into mitochondria as an unfolded monomer. One of the reasons why the P11L-generated MTS is functionally weak appears to be that it is unable to maintain AGT in a conformation (i.e., unfolded and monomeric) compatible with mitochondrial import. Recent studies suggest that this may be related to its rather weak tendency

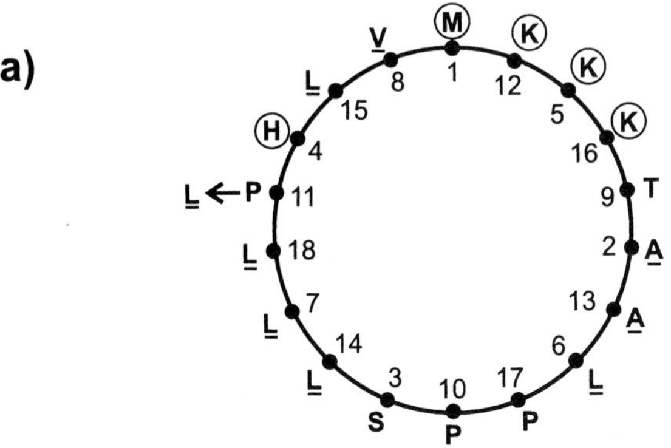

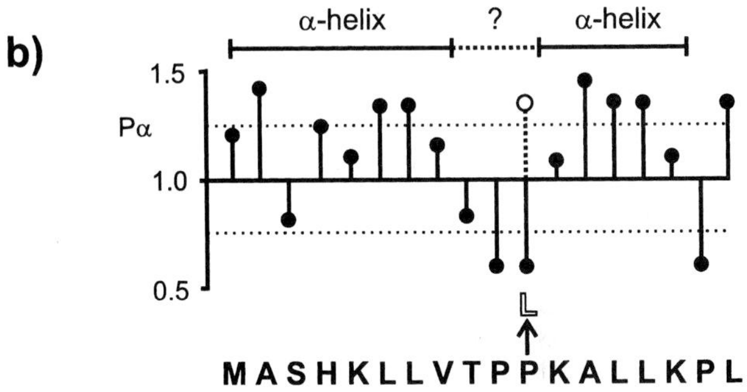

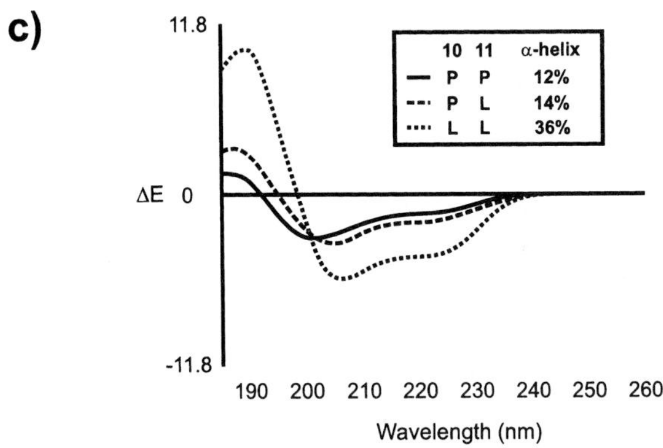

Fig. 133-12 Consequences of the P11L substitution on the structure of the N-terminus of AGT. (*A*) Helical wheel analysis of the N-terminal 18 amino acids of AGT showing its potential amphiphilic nature. Ringed amino acids = positively charged; underlined amino acids = hydrophobic. (*B*) Chou and Fasman plot of the N-terminal 18 amino acids of AGT showing its potential to form an α helix. Pα, the α-helix-forming potential[311] of the individual amino acids. Amino acids with a Pα > 1 favor helix formation, whereas those with Pα < 1 do not. Those above the upper horizontal dotted line (Pα > 1.25) are strong helix formers, whereas those below the bottom horizontal dotted line (Pα < 0.75) are strong helix breakers (note the increased tendency to form an α helix when Pro11 is substituted by Leu). (*C*) Circular dichroism of synthetic peptides in 50 percent trifluoroethanol. PP, 20-mer N-terminal peptide of AGT encoded by the major allele (i.e., with Pro10 + Pro11); PL, 20-mer N-terminal peptide of AGT encoded by the minor allele (i.e., with the P11L substitution); LL, 20-mer N-terminal peptide of AGT with both Pro10 and Pro11 substituted by Leu (not found naturally). As the helix-breaking prolines are substituted by helix-forming leucines, there is increasing tendency for the peptides to fold into α helices. (Peptides made by Mr. P. Purkiss, MRC Clinical Research Centre, Harrow, U.K., and circular dichroism carried out by Dr. A. Drake, Birkbeck College, London, U.K.). (*Panels A and B modified with permission from Purdue et al.*[296])

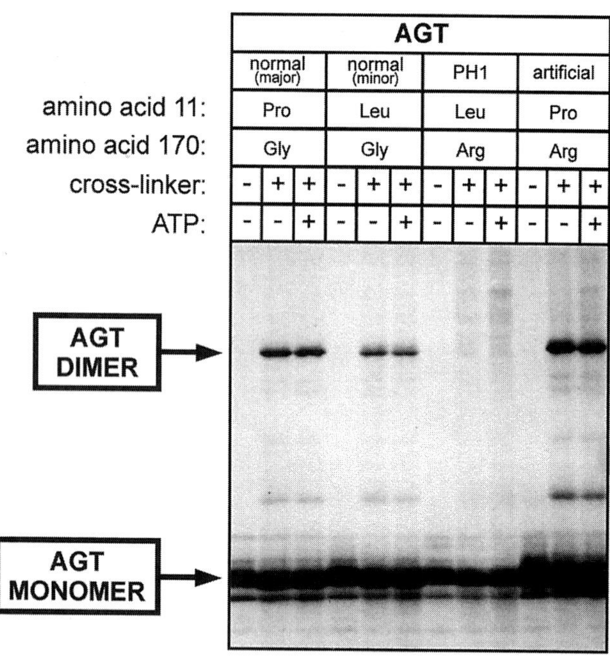

Fig. 133-13 Effect of the P11L polymorphism and G170R mutation on AGT dimerization. SDS-PAGE of normal and mutant forms of in vitro translated AGT before and after chemical crosslinking. Normal AGT encoded by the major allele, normal AGT encoded by the minor allele (containing the P11L polymorphism), and an artificial AGT construct (containing the G170R mutation) all dimerize, but PH1 AGT (containing both polymorphism and mutation) does not. (*Modified with permission from Leiper and Danpure.*[552])

to adopt an α-helical conformation (Lumb and Danpure, unpublished observations[559] (see above).

An artificial AGT construct containing the G170R mutation but not the P11L polymorphism (this construct does not occur naturally) also dimerized rapidly. However, when the P11L and G170R replacements were present together, dimerization was abolished following in vitro translation[314] (see Fig. 133-13). In transfected tissue culture cells, dimerization is retarded rather than halted altogether. Thus, following the double amino acid replacement, AGT can be imported into mitochondria (directed by the P11L-generated MTS) unimpeded by the protein folding and dimerizing. Although it is still unclear how dimerization is inhibited, it is possible that the G170R mutation allows the P11L-generated MTS to fold more readily into an α helix. Circumstantial evidence in support of this comes from recent studies using an artificial AGT construct in which both Pro10 and Pro11 are mutated to Leu. This double replacement of two helix breakers by two helix formers increases markedly the ability of the N-terminal 20 amino acids to fold into an α helix[559] (see Fig. 133-12), as well as inhibiting AGT dimerization and causing peroxisome-to-mitochondrion mistargeting in transfected tissue culture cells. The effect of the artificial P10L replacement appears to have the identical effect on the P11L-generated MTS as does the PH1-specific G170R replacement.

Thus the unparalleled peroxisome-to-mitochondrion mistargeting of AGT in PH1 has an equally unparalleled molecular explanation. The normally occurring P11L polymorphism generates a weak MTS at the N-terminus of AGT. The additional presence of the PH1-specific G170R mutation enhances the efficiency of this MTS, possibly by allowing it to fold more readily into an α helix. This increased helical nature of the MTS delays AGT dimerization so that AGT can be targeted to and imported into mitochondria unimpeded by any structural constraints[315–317] (Fig. 133-14).

Partial Peroxisome-to-Mitochondrial Mislocalization and Intraperoxisomal AGT Aggregation. Three CRM+/ENZ$\pm$ patients have been identified who have a complex enzymic phenotype characterized by the presence of low levels of mitochondrial AGT and intraperoxisomal AGT aggregations or *cores* (see "Enzymic and Metabolic Defects," above, and Fig. 133-5*d*). In at least one of these patients, AGT mRNA of normal size and abundance was present. All three patients were homozygous for the minor *AGXT* allele, two being compound heterozygotes for 243G > A and 576T > A mutations that lead to G41R and F152I amino acid replacements, respectively.[268] The third patient was a compound heterozygote for G41R and G170R.

There are several pieces of evidence that suggest that the F152I and G170R mutations, probably in association with the P11L polymorphism of the minor allele, are responsible for the presence of mitochondrial AGT, albeit at low levels, in these patients. On the other hand, the G41R mutation is likely to be responsible for the presence of peroxisomal AGT aggregates. In two asymptomatic carriers of the F152I mutation (i.e., parents of two different patients), mitochondrial AGT was present, but peroxisomal cores were not. However, in a carrier of the G41R mutation (i.e. a parent of one of the patients), peroxisomal AGT cores were present but very little mitochondrial AGT [268]. The F152I replacement is only 18 residues away from G170R which had already been shown to cause AGT mistargeting in association with P11L (see above). Further support for the role of F152I comes from the finding that two other CRM+/ENZ$\pm$ patients who were heterozygous for this mutation (but not G41R), also on the background of the minor *AGXT* allele, had low levels of immunoreactive AGT protein most of which was in the mitochondria. No peroxisomal cores were present. Attempts to formally prove the roles of these mutations at the mechanistic level have so far not been possible. When expressed in transfected COS-1 cells or human fibroblasts, constructs derived from both types of mutant allele (i.e., P11L + G41R and P11L + F152I) have proven to be unstable and rapidly degraded (Oatey and Danpure, unpublished observations.

Normally Localized but Catalytically Inactive AGT. Several CRM+/ENZ$-$ PH1 patients have been identified who had normal amounts of normally localized (i.e., peroxisomal) immunoreactive AGT protein but zero AGT catalytic activity. In at least one of these, AGT mRNA of normal abundance and size was present.[288] Unlike the patients described earlier, all these CRM+/ENZ$-$ patients were shown to be homozygous for the major *AGXT* allele. In addition, they were homozygous for a 367G > A point mutation predicted to cause a G82E amino acid substitution.[318] Using the criteria of Chou and Fasman[311] and Garnier et al.,[312] the presence of a G82E substitution in the AGT protein is predicted to cause considerable local structural alterations. Although this substitution is at some distance, at least in linear terms, from the putative pyridoxal phosphate-binding site at Lys209,[288,292] it is situated in a well-conserved region of the protein (see Fig. 133-9) and may come into the proximity of the active site in the correctly folded protein. Formal proof of the effect of this mutation has been obtained recently by showing that although recombinant AGT containing G82E can be stably expressed at high levels in *Escherichia coli,* it is almost completely inactive (Lumb and Danpure, unpublished observations.

Absence of AGT Catalytic Activity and Immunoreactivity. A large, rather amorphous group of PH1 patients fits into the CRM$-$/$\pm$ and ENZ$-$/$\pm$ category. The apparent enzymic uniformity of this group is largely illusory, because it is associated with numerous different mutations in *AGXT* (Table 133-4). Although the causal relationship between genotype and phenotype has not been proved in most of these cases, there is one where it has. A single patient was found with almost no AGT catalytic activity and vastly reduced but normally targeted immunoreactivity. This patient was homozygous for the major *AGXT* allele and for a 735T > C mutation that was predicted to cause an S205P

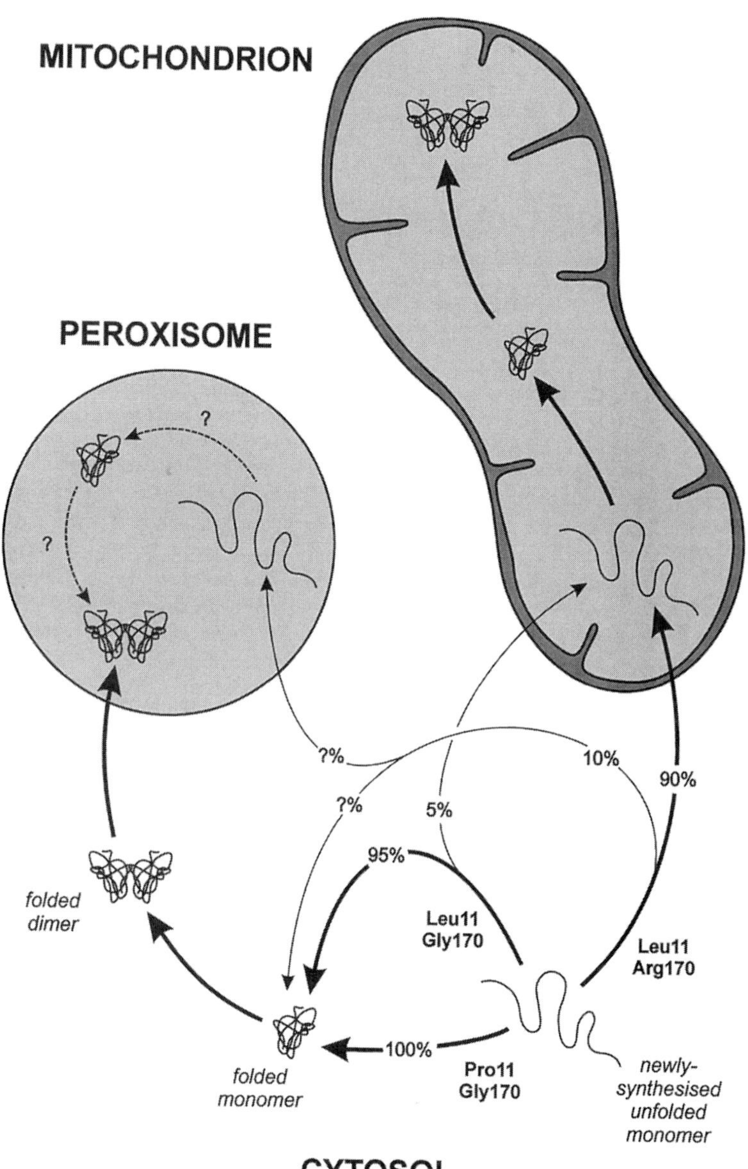

Fig. 133-14 Molecular basis for the peroxisome-to-mitochondrion mistargeting in PH1. ***Pro11Gly170*****: Newly synthesized AGT encoded by the *major AGXT* allele folds and dimerizes rapidly in the cytosol and is then imported into the peroxisomes.** ***Leu11Gly170*****: Most (~95 percent) of the newly synthesized AGT encoded by the *minor AGXT* allele follows the same pattern. However, a small proportion (~5 percent) is imported into the mitochondria due to the presence of an MTS generated by the P11L polymorphism before it has chance to fold and dimerize.** ***Leu11Arg170*****: Newly synthesized mutant PH1 AGT folds only slowly in the cytosol due to the combined presence of both the P11L polymorphism and the G170R mutation. Therefore, the majority (~90 percent) can be imported into the mitochondria due to the presence of the MTS generated by the $P_{11}L$ polymorphism before folding and dimerization have a chance to block the process. It is not certain whether the remaining 10 percent that is imported into peroxisomes folds and dimerizes before import or not. If not, then it is also not known whether any unfolded AGT that may be imported into peroxisomes can subsequently fold and dimerize. It should be noted that the percentage distributions indicated in this figure assume *AGXT* homozygosity. The ability of normal/mutant heterodimers to form normally suggests that carriers of the mutant mistargeting allele would have much more peroxisomal than mitochondrial AGT. The sizes of the arrows represent the relative proportions using each pathway. (*Reproduced with permission from Danpure.*[317])**

amino acid replacement close to the pyridoxal phosphate-binding site.[319] AGT mRNA levels were higher than normal in this patient, indicating a problem with translation or protein stability rather than transcription or RNA stability. In vitro translated mutant AGT containing this mutation was much less stable than normal in rabbit reticulocyte lysate, as it was when expressed in transfected COS-1 cells or transformed *E. coli*.[320,321] At least in the reticulocyte system, its rapid degradation was ATP-dependent.

ANIMAL MODELS OF PRIMARY HYPEROXALURIA

Evolutionary Perspectives

Advances in the understanding of the pathophysiology of human genetic diseases and the development of rational treatment strategies are frequently aided by the identification and characterization of good animal models, either naturally occurring or artificially produced. However, extrapolation from animal to human can be fraught with difficulties due to unexpected genetic or metabolic differences between the species. This is certainly the case with the primary hyperoxalurias, where most of the metabolic studies have been done in the rat. Especially for PH1, the rat is particularly unsuitable because of major differences in the way it metabolizes glyoxylate (see "Metabolism of Oxalate and Its Precursors," above).

AGT and GR are clearly major determinants of the synthesis of oxalate in humans, as shown by the effects of their respective deficiencies in PH1 and PH2 (see Fig. 133-8). The comparative biology of GR has hardly been studied, but the comparative biology of AGT has been the subject of intensive investigation. Within Mammalia, AGT has been shown to vary with respect to overall level of expression, patterns of developmental expression, tissue specificity, and subcellular distribution.

Variable Expression of AGT in Mammals. Some mammals, such as humans, some old-world monkeys (macaque and baboon), new-world monkeys (marmoset), lagomorphs (rabbit), carnivores (cat, dog, and ferret), insectivores (mole, hedgehog, and shrew), and American marsupials (opossum), express high levels of hepatic AGT. Other mammals, most notably rodents and related species (e.g., rat, mouse, hamster, and guinea pig), express lower levels. Yet other mammals, such as the pig, sheep, and ox, express extremely low levels, which in some cases are barely detectable.[322] Although in the human AGT is more or less liver-specific,[185] it is also expressed in other tissues, especially the kidney, in other animals such as the cat, dog, rat, and guinea

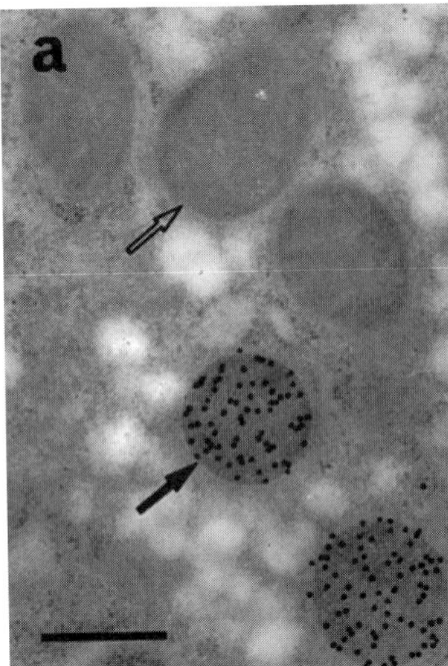

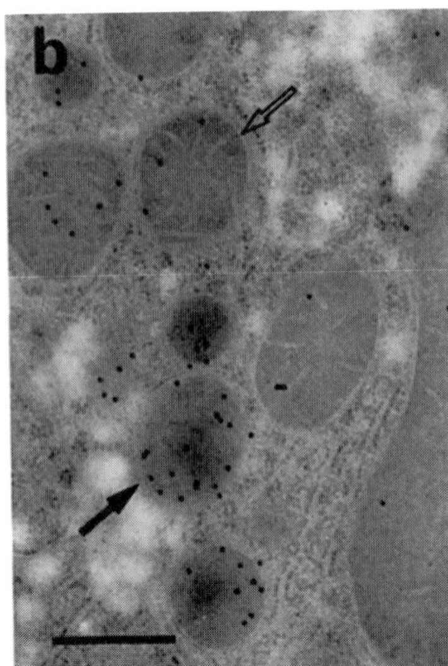

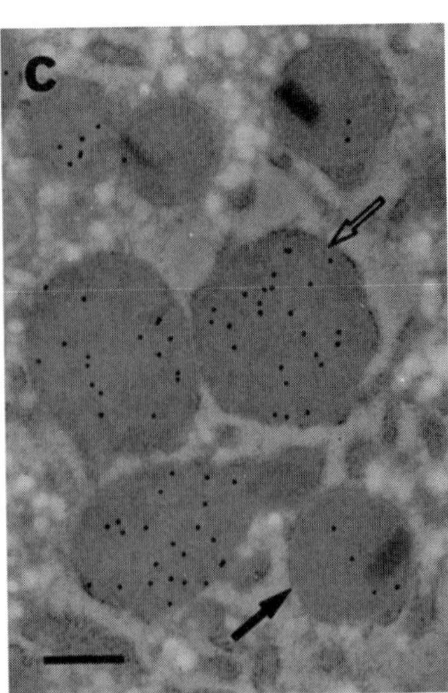

Fig. 133-15 Subcellular distribution of AGT in various mammalian livers. Postembedding protein A-gold immunoelectron microscopy using rabbit anti-human liver AGT antiserum. (*A*) Rabbit (100 percent peroxisomal AGT). (*B*) Opossum (~50 percent peroxisomal AGT + ~50 percent mitochondrial AGT). (*C*) Cat (~5 percent peroxisomal AGT + ~95 percent mitochondrial AGT). Closed arrows = peroxisomes; open arrows = mitochondria; bars = 0.5 μm. (*Photomicrographs courtesy of S. Griffiths.*)

pig.[323–325] The level of AGT in human liver during the neonatal period (i.e., ~2 days postpartum) is little different to that in adulthood (see Fig. 133-18). However, in dog[325] and rat[326,327] liver, the level of AGT immediately after birth is negligible. It increases until weaning, when it reaches its maximum value, after which it plateaus out at the adult level in the dog[325] or decreases substantially to the adult levels in the rat.[326,327]

Variable Subcellular Distribution of AGT in Mammals. By far the most remarkable species difference is the variation in the subcellular distribution of AGT (Fig. 133-15). Notwithstanding the different levels of expression, the intracellular compartmentation of hepatic AGT can be fitted into three main categories.[322] In some species, such as rabbits and most humans, AGT is solely peroxisomal.[186–188,256,328] In others, such as cats and dogs, AGT is mainly (>90 percent) mitochondrial, the remainder being peroxisomal.[328,329] In yet others, such as marmosets, rats, and opossums, AGT is more evenly divided between the peroxisomes and mitochondria.[255,328,330] In addition some animals, such as guinea pigs, have significant proportions of cytosolic AGT (in addition to peroxisomal AGT).[322]

Molecular Evolution of the AGT Gene. The evolution of AGT in mammals has been addressed by Takada and Noguchi.[331] These authors, using immunologic distance of AGT in different species as their yardstick, considered that its subcellular distribution and substrate specificity had evolved during rapid molecular evolution but that the different subcellular forms were not produced by divergent evolution after gene duplication. Subsequent molecular genetic analysis of the AGT gene in different mammalian species is compatible with this view.

In all the animals studied so far (i.e., human, marmoset, rabbit, rat, cat, and guinea pig), AGT is encoded by a single-copy gene.[286,291,293,294,332] The mechanism by which a single AGT gene can produce a protein that is targeted to more than one intracellular location has been studied by a number of workers.[288,292,296,313,332–334] The archetypal AGT gene possesses two in-frame translation start sites 66 bp apart (sites 1 and 2 in Fig. 133-16). The region between these two sites encodes an MTS of 22 amino acids. The "nonstandard" PTS1 is at the C-terminus. If translation initiates from site 1, the polypeptide possesses both an N-terminal MTS and a C-terminal PTS1. Since the former is functionally dominant over the latter,[334] the AGT is targeted to the mitochondria. On the other hand, if translation initiates at site 2, the polypeptide possesses only a PTS1, and the AGT is targeted to the peroxisomes. The situation is complicated by the presence of two transcription start sites (A and B in Fig. 133-16), one being located upstream of both translation start sites and one between sites 1 and 2. In the archetypal situation, transcription from site A leads to translation from site 1, whereas transcription from site B leads to translation from site 2. However, the Kozak translation initiation sequence[335,336] around site 1 is poor, whereas that around site 2 is good. This leads to leaky ribosome scanning of the longer transcript and some translational readthrough to site 2.

The rat and marmoset fit the archetypal situation most closely, the approximately even distribution of AGT between peroxisomes and mitochondria presumably reflecting the similar levels of transcription from sites A and B (see Fig. 133-16). The human, rabbit, and guinea pig have all lost translation start site 1, but on three separate occasions, so the region encoding the MTS is permanently bypassed. The resulting polypeptide therefore is targeted exclusively to the peroxisomes. In addition, the guinea pig also has lost transcription start site A, and the human and rabbit possibly also have lost transcription start site B. However, these are likely to be events secondary to the loss of translation start site 1. The cat, like the marmoset and rat, has kept both translation start sites but has lost transcription start site B. Most translation initiates from site 1, but due to its nonideal Kozak sequence (see above), there is some readthrough to site 2 (see Fig. 133-16). Therefore, in the cat, although most AGT is mitochondrial, a small proportion (5-10 percent) is also peroxisomal.

Dietary Selection Pressure. Within the evolution of mammals, the intracellular targeting of AGT appears to have changed radically on many occasions.[317,322,328] The pathology associated with inappropriate intracellular localization of AGT in some PH1 patients shows that the intracellular distribution of AGT, for some animals at least, is very important. Therefore, the question arises as to what is the nature of the evolutionary selection pressure under which these remarkable fluctuations in compartmentalization have occurred. It has been suggested that this selection pressure could be diet.[328] Certainly, the subcellular localization of AGT in different mammalian species is strongly correlated with diet (natural or ancestral diet, not necessarily current diet) (Fig. 133-17). Herbivores tend to have peroxisomal AGT, carnivores mitochondrial AGT, and omnivores both peroxisomal and mitochondrial AGT.[322] AGT is predicted to have the dual metabolic roles of gluconeogenesis in the mitochondria[190,327,337–341] and glyoxylate

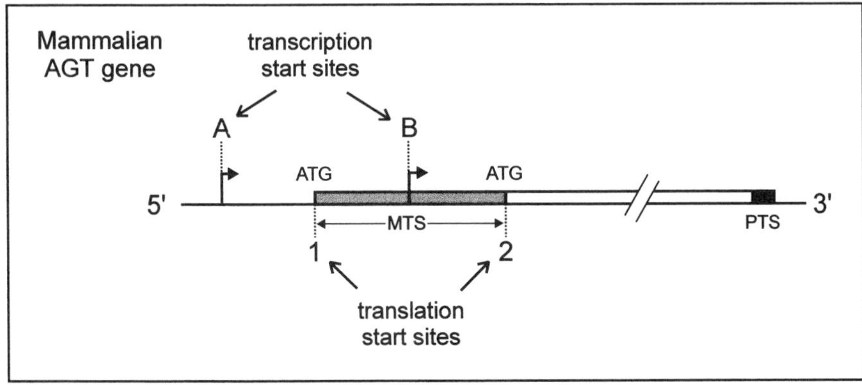

Species	Transcription start	Translation start	Subcellular distribution
Cat	A	1 2	M P → M + P
Marmoset & Rat	A	1 2	M P
	B	2	P → M + P
Human & Rabbit	A	2	P → P
Guinea pig	B	2	P → P

Fig. 133-16 Archetypal mammalian AGT gene and alternative transcription and translation initiation. The archetypal AGT gene contains two potential transcription start sites (A and B) and two in-frame potential translation start sites (1 and 2), the sequence between which (gray-shaded) has the potential to encode the N-terminal mitochondrial targeting sequence (MTS). The C-terminal peroxisomal targeting sequence (PTS) is encoded by the 3' end of the gene (darkly shaded region). The table below shows the different utilization of sites A, B, 1, and 2 in different species and the consequences for AGT subcellular distribution (M, mitochondria; P, peroxisomes). The size of each character represents the relative proportions of each site used and organelle localization. (*Modified with permission from Danpure.*[317])

detoxification in the peroxisomes.[271,342] The differences in subcellular distribution of AGT are presumed to reflect different degrees of importance attached to these roles in different animals, depending on diet. For carnivorous animals, with high-protein, low-carbohydrate, low-oxalate/oxalate precursor diets, a gluconeogenic role for AGT would be favored. On the other hand, for herbivorous animals, on high-carbohydrate, high-oxalate/oxalate precursor diets,[2] a glyoxylate-detoxifying role would be favored [328].

The importance of the glyoxylate-detoxification role for peroxisomal AGT is best demonstrated by the effect of its deficiency or mistargeting to mitochondria in PH1 (see above). On the other hand, the gluconeogenic role of mitochondrial AGT is well shown by the effect of gluconeogenic stimuli. In some rodents (e.g., rat, mouse, hamster, and chipmunk), but not others (e.g., guinea pig), and not members of others orders (e.g., cat, dog, and rabbit), AGT can be induced by glucagon or a high-protein diet.[343,344] In the rat and hamster at least, the increased AGT is confined exclusively to the mitochondria[343–345] due to selective induction of transcription from site A[345,346] (see Fig. 133-16). The metabolic effects of glucagon are mediated by the cAMP signal-transduction pathway, and as might be expected, the upstream region of the rat AGT gene contains cAMP response elements.[347] Such elements have not been identified in the human gene.[286]

Although dietary oxalate or oxalate precursors may very well be determinants of the subcellular distribution of AGT on an evolutionary time scale, the relationship is clearly not simple. The artiodactyls (cattle, sheep, etc.) are typical herbivores predicted to have high oxalate/oxalate precursor diets,[2] yet the level of expression of AGT in these animals is extremely low. However, little, if any, of the dietary oxalate ever gets a chance of being absorbed in these animals because it is likely to be degraded in the rumen by the resident flora.[348–352] In fact, the oxalate-degrading bacterium *O. formigenes* has been found in the intestine of a number of mammals, including rat, guinea pig, and human.[3,4,165,353,354] There appears to be a direct relationship between the level of oxalate-degrading bacteria in the rumen or large bowel of herbivores and the amount of oxalate in the diet.[355,356] Therefore, the presence of oxalate-degrading bacteria in the gut of certain herbivores may modify their evolutionary requirement for AGT.

In addition, in some mammals such as the rat, there is an additional enzyme (AGT2) capable of transaminating glyoxylate, using alanine as the amino donor.[254] When present, AGT2, which is enzymologically, immunologically, and physically distinct from AGT,* is always localized in the mitochondria.[357] The presence of an additional enzyme potentially capable of detoxifying glyoxylate (albeit in an apparently inappropriate organelle) in some mammals also would be likely to modify the evolutionary relationship between AGT expression and diet.

Canine PH1

An analogue of PH1 has been identified in Norwegian Tibetan spaniels.[358] This oxalate nephropathy was found in two litter mates and was characterized by a variety of symptoms, including the deposition of CaOx crystals in the proximal renal tubules.

*Human AGT and the homologous protein in other mammals is often called AGT1 to clearly distinguish it from AGT2.

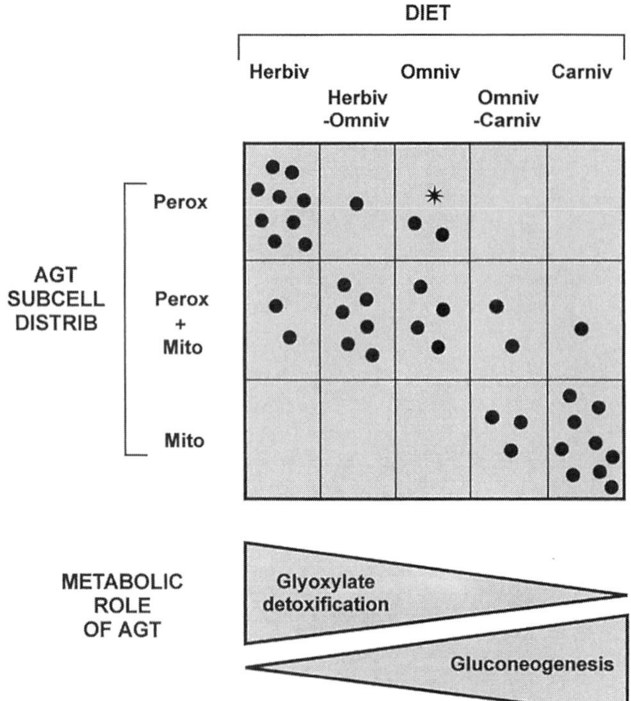

Fig. 133-17 Relationship between diet and AGT subcellular distribution in 40 different vertebrates. *AGT subcellular distribution*: Perox, only peroxisomal; Mito, mainly mitochondrial; Perox + Mito, both peroxisomal and mitochondrial. *Diet*: Herbiv, herbivorous; Omniv, omnivorous; Carniv, carnivorous; Herbiv-Omniv and Omniv-Carniv, self-explanatory intermediates. The star indicates the position of normal humans. It has been suggested (see text) that glyoxylate detoxification is more important in herbivores, whereas gluconeogenesis is more important in carnivores. (*Modified with permission from Danpure et al.*[322])

Analysis of the livers and kidneys of these dogs showed them to be markedly deficient in AGT and serine:pyruvate aminotransferase enzyme activity and immunoreactivity.[325] Immunoreactive AGT was lost from both the mitochondria and peroxisomes (Griffiths, Fryer, and Danpure, unpublished observations). Although urinalysis has not so far been carried out, it would appear that this canine condition is an analogue, at least in enzymic terms, of human PH1. Whether this turns out to be a useful clinical model for the human condition will depend on the results of further analysis. However, bearing in mind the major differences likely to occur in the metabolism of oxalate precursors in the dog due to the radical differences in AGT subcellular distribution, the usefulness of this analogue may be expected to be rather limited.

Feline PH2

The first animal analogue for a primary hyperoxaluria was identified in cats.[359,360] A familial condition was found in a colony of cats that was characterized by acute renal failure due to intratubular deposition of CaOx crystals. The affected cats had massive hyper-L-glyceric aciduria with intermittent hyperoxaluria. Subsequent enzymic analysis of the livers of the affected cats showed them to be markedly deficient in DGDH and GR,[283] which together with the urinary biochemistry data suggested the disease to be analogous to PH2. In the cat colony, the condition was inherited in an autosomal recessive fashion. Heterozygotes could be identified by having levels of DGDH/GR intermediate between the levels found in unrelated normal cats and affected cats.[283] The use of this feline PH2 analogue as a clinical model for the human disease has yet to be evaluated. However, there are a number of reasons for thinking that its usefulness will be somewhat limited. First, the feline disease is much more severe and acute than human PH2. Second, the biochemistry differs significantly. For example, although hyper-L-glyceric aciduria is apparent, hyperoxaluria is much less and intermittent. Third, the pathology is rather different from the human disease. For example, stones or interstitial nephrocalcinosis is not apparent in the cats. In addition, neurologic manifestations are apparent in the cat[360] but not in the human. Whether these differences are due to fundamental differences between feline and human biochemistry and metabolism or to differences in diet or renal physiology are not known. However, it should be borne in mind that the metabolism and dietary handling of oxalate and oxalate precursors may be very different in the cat, the latter being predicted as a consequence of the different subcellular distribution of AGT.

Drug-Induced Rodent Models of Metabolic Hyperoxaluria

Unfortunately, no naturally occurring analogues of primary hyperoxaluria have been discovered so far in rodents. Hepatic AGT activity in rats and mice is considerably less than that found in humans. In fact, some PH1 patients have activities higher than those found in some rodents. Therefore, it is possible that AGT is not required for glyoxylate detoxification in rats to anywhere near the same extent as it is in humans. Even if a natural genetic deficiency of AGT was identified in rats or mice, the resulting pathologic phenotype, if any, might not be relevant to PH1 in humans. Similarly, the generation of artificial AGT knockouts may not yield useful phenotypes.

However, relevant animal models for primary hyperoxaluria, especially PH1, are essential to enable the testing of radical treatment strategies such as enzyme-replacement or gene therapy (see "Treatment," below). Because the main purpose of testing such therapy protocols in animals is to answer very specific questions concerning efficacy, practicality, and safety, the model used does not necessarily have to look like PH1 in its widest sense but only needs to meet certain well-defined criteria. At least some of these may be met in well-characterized model systems in which hyperoxaluria is induced in rats pharmacologically.

Hyperoxaluria can be induced in rats by dietary manipulation, such as increasing the levels of oxalate, glycolate, or ethylene glycol or by decreasing the level of vitamin B_6.[361,362] Although these systems were developed originally to gain insights into the mechanism of stone formation in idiopathic CaOx stone disease, some have potential use in the testing of enzyme-replacement and gene therapy protocols for PH1. The key criterion for usefulness is that the hyperoxaluria results, directly or indirectly, from increased glyoxylate synthesis in the peroxisomes of liver cells. Clearly, this rules out oxalate-induced hyperoxaluria. In addition, hyperoxaluria induced by vitamin B_6 deficiency is ruled out because of the adverse effect it is likely to have on the activity of any newly introduced AGT. However, it is likely that both the glycolate- and ethylene glycol-induced hyperoxalurias do indeed result from increased intraperoxisomal glyoxylate synthesis. Successful targeting of the AGT gene and its expression in hepatocytes, correct subcellular localization of the gene product to the peroxisomes of these cells, and its correct folding, cofactor binding, and acquisition of catalytic activity, leading to increased conversion of intraperoxisomal glyoxylate to glycine, would be manifested in a reduction in oxalate excretion. Therefore, although a naturally occurring rodent analogue for PH1 does not exist, and although the generation of rodent AGT knockouts may not yield such an analogue, the combination of naturally low levels of AGT together with pharmacologically increased oxalate synthesis may provide a workable model to test the potential of enzyme-replacement and gene therapies for PH1 (see "Treatment," below).

DIAGNOSIS

The various methods available for the diagnosis of the primary hyperoxalurias have evolved in parallel with our increased understanding of the diseases at the clinical, biochemical, enzymic, and molecular genetic levels (see "Clinical Characteristics," "Enzymic and Metabolic Defects," and "Molecular Genetics and Cell Biology," above). For a recent more practical guide to the diagnosis of primary hyperoxaluria, readers are referred to Byrd and Latta.[363]

Clinical Diagnosis

Although a combination of renal failure in a child or young adult together with a history of urolithiasis or a family history of urolithiasis or nephrocalcinosis may make the clinician aware of the possibility of primary hyperoxaluria, this is not enough in itself.[28] Unfortunately, none of the clinical symptoms of primary hyperoxaluria are unique, although most are likely to be more severe than those found in renal failure due to other causes. Unexplained nephrocalcinosis (see Fig. 133-1*B*), recurrent urolithiasis (see Fig. 133-1*A*), or even systemic oxalosis in the absence of any obvious secondary causes is frequently taken as being diagnostic of primary hyperoxaluria. Renal CaOx deposition is not specific for primary hyperoxaluria because it also can occur in other conditions such as chronic glomerulonephritis, chronic pyelonephritis, renal tubular acidosis, and acute tubular necrosis.[25] CaOx crystalluria (see Fig. 133-1*D, E*) is not specific enough to be diagnostically useful.[25] Detection of nephrocalcinosis in infants by ultrasound has been used in the diagnosis of PH1[66,364] (see Fig. 133-1*B*). However, the specificity of such a procedure has been called into question.[365,366] Histologic identification of CaOx deposition in kidney or bone biopsies also has been used diagnostically[40,58,367–369] (see Fig. 133-1*C*). As has been pointed out,[25] the results obtained from soft tissue or bone biopsies are difficult to use as diagnostic criteria due to a lack of specificity compared with patients in renal failure for other reasons. However, the characteristic histology of crystal deposition in PH1[40,369] may allow a diagnosis to be made.

Despite the well-recognized clinical heterogeneity, there is no doubt that there is a characteristic clinical pathology associated with primary hyperoxaluria. However, because it is not uniquely so, definitive diagnosis cannot be made without further biochemical and/or enzymic follow-up studies (see below).

Biochemical Diagnosis

By far the most common method of diagnosing the primary hyperoxalurias is by measuring oxalate excretion. Markedly elevated levels of urinary oxalate in the absence of any likely causes of secondary hyperoxaluria is usually taken to indicate the presence of primary hyperoxaluria.[27,80] Determination of the plasma oxalate level[82,83,370] is a more contentious issue, partly due to problems with methodology and partly due to the lack of disease specificity (see "Clinical Characteristics," above). In any case, plasma oxalate levels may not be raised significantly in PH1 until the onset of renal failure.[83,371] Neither urinary nor plasma oxalate determination can distinguish between PH1 and PH2. For such differential diagnosis, urinary glycolate (for PH1)[80,372] and urinary L-glycerate (for PH2)[94] determinations can be used. Therefore, in most cases, a definitive diagnosis of PH1 is based on concomitant hyperoxaluria and hyperglycolic aciduria.[2] However, difficulties can arise with this approach as patients approach end-stage renal failure due to the apparent normalization of 24-hour urinary oxalate excretion.[25,37] This problem can be overcome, at least in part, by codetermination of creatinine excretion and expression of the results as oxalate-creatinine ratios. The plasma glycolate level can be invaluable in distinguishing PH1 from secondary hyperoxaluria in patients with renal failure,[91,373] as can measurement of oxalate[374] and glycolate[373] in the dialysate. The methodology of urine/plasma oxalate/glycolate assays has been reviewed on several occasions.[375–378] Despite much research on the methodology of organic acid analysis in body fluids, the normal ranges quoted for plasma oxalate, for example, in the literature still vary by an order of magnitude (e.g., see Laker[377]).

For several decades, concomitant hyperoxaluria and hyperglycolic aciduria have been used as definitive criteria for distinguishing not only PH1 from PH2 but also "metabolic" from "nonmetabolic" hyperoxaluria.[92] However, recent findings have cast doubt on the universal applicability of this approach. A significant number of PH1 patients (perhaps up to 25 percent) with proven AGT deficiency have hyperoxaluria but little or no increase in glycolate excretion.[34] At the other extreme, some PH1 patients have extreme hyperglycolic aciduria with only mildly elevated oxalate excretion. In addition, isolated hyperglycolic aciduria[284] and concomitant hyperoxaluria and hyperglycolic aciduria[285] have been found in patients with normal AGT levels. Clearly, there must be other genetic defects that cause elevated oxalate and/or glycolate synthesis and excretion, and therefore, these parameters can no longer be considered uniquely pathognomic for PH1.

Enzymic Diagnosis

With the introduction of more "heroic" treatments in recent years for PH1 (see "Treatment," below), it is now essential that a differential diagnosis between PH1 and PH2 be made in patients in whom primary hyperoxaluria is suspected. Some treatments for PH1, such as liver transplantation, may be inappropriate for PH2 or other types of primary hyperoxaluria (but see below). Clinicians should not be satisfied with a diagnosis of primary hyperoxaluria without further subtyping. Because of the problems associated with metabolite analysis (see above), the only way to definitively diagnose PH1, at least, is to measure the activity of the deficient enzyme.

PH1. PH1 is caused by a deficiency of the liver-specific peroxisomal enzyme AGT (see "Enzymic and Metabolic Defects," above) and can be definitively diagnosed[379] and excluded[380] by analysis of AGT in percutaneous liver needle biopsies. Various methods have been developed to enable enzymic diagnosis to be achieved successfully on as little as a few milligrams of material.[259,381–388] Successful diagnoses have now been carried out by AGT assay in several hundred patients, and the method is able to distinguish PH1 from all other forms of hyperoxaluria, even in patients with renal failure.

Unfortunately, AGT is not the only enzyme in human liver able to use alanine and glyoxylate as substrates (see "Metabolism of Oxalate and Its Precursors," above). For example, GGT also can catalyze alanine-glyoxylate transamination[184] and therefore must be corrected for.[259] Because the additional measurement of GTT can lead to extra inaccuracies, a new assay has been devised recently that uses the AGT-specific inhibitor aminooxyacetic acid.[387] AGT enzyme assay in the presence and absence of inhibitor obviates the need to measure GGT at all.

The enzymic phenotypes associated with PH1 are complex, and enzymic assay alone cannot always distinguish between patients and carriers. In such cases (e.g., when the residual level of AGT is greater than ~15 percent), it is also necessary to determine the subcellular distribution of the immunoreactive AGT protein, usually by immunoelectron microscopy.[187] This is also important because other generalized liver diseases, such as cirrhosis, can lead to decreased activities of AGT.[389] AGT immunoreactive protein can be determined by Western blotting as a final diagnostic check.[264] AGT immunoreactivity is considerably more stable than catalytic activity and can be of use in the resolution of ambiguities caused by the biopsy thawing out during transit.

PH2. Because of the lower frequency of PH2 and the lower tendency to relapse into renal failure, there has been less incentive to develop enzymic methods for the diagnosis of PH2, even though urinary L-glycerate is more difficult to measure than glycolate. Leukocyte DGDH assay has been used for such diagnoses.[23,69] Although leukocytes are more easily obtainable than liver biopsies, the differentiation between affected and nonaffected individuals is much more pronounced when liver is used, especially when coupled with the assay of GR.[279] Recently, the GR/DGDH assay procedure has been critically analyzed and improved so that enzymic diagnosis of PH2 is now as straightforward as that for PH1.[236] However, there appears to be more than one enzyme in human tissues with DGDH activity, only one of which also has GR activity. Because the activities of these enzymes depend on the tissue, and because only the enzyme that has both GR and DGDH activity is deficient in PH2,[236] the tissue used for enzymic diagnosis has to be chosen with care.

Diagnosis of PH1 by DNA Analysis

Although the *AGXT* gene has been cloned and sequenced and various mutations identified (see "Molecular Genetics and Cell Biology of PH1," above), "front line" diagnosis of PH1 by mutational analysis has not yet become a practicable proposition. Most patients are predicted to be compound heterozygotes. Therefore, although the causal mutations have been identified in the expressed alleles in 40 to 50 percent of patients (at least in Caucasian populations), it is estimated that on the basis of these mutations alone, in only 5 to 10 percent of cases could patients be distinguished from carriers. Nevertheless, bearing in mind the wide clinical heterogeneity of PH1 even within families, mutational analysis (or even linkage analysis) has considerable potential for the subsequent diagnosis of presymptomatic siblings of patients already diagnosed by other means. A good example of this approach is to be found in a recent study[132] in which 630G > A mutational homozygosity was used to show that an asymptomatic sibling of a severely affected infant did indeed have PH1. Clearly, such presymptomatic diagnosis would allow the introduction of more prophylactic approaches to treatment.

PRENATAL DIAGNOSIS OF PH1

Many peroxisomal diseases can now be diagnosed prenatally,[390,391] but until recently, there has been less incentive to develop procedures for the prenatal diagnosis of the primary hyperoxalurias. This is due at least in part to the fact that primary hyperoxalurias are, in general, much less severe than most peroxisomal diseases. Some authors have even suggested that with the exception of the fulminant neonatal form of PH1, prenatal diagnosis for primary hyperoxaluria is not warranted.[390] No attempts have been made to diagnose PH2 prenatally, and only a few laboratories have attempted to do so in PH1. Just as with postnatal diagnosis, the development of procedures used for the prenatal diagnosis of PH1 has paralleled our increased understanding of its molecular basis.[392] Metabolite analysis of amniotic fluid, which was unsuccessful, led to enzyme analysis of fetal liver, which was successful but complicated, and this in turn led to DNA analysis of chorionic villus or amniocytes, which is both successful and simple.

Glyoxylate Metabolites in Amniotic Fluid

Two laboratories have tried to measure the increased products of abnormal glyoxylate metabolism in amniotic fluid, with varying degrees of success. Rose et al.[393] were unable to detect oxalate in amniotic fluid from normal pregnancies at gestational ages of 15 to 16 weeks but were able detect low levels of oxalate in amniotic fluid from a fetus subsequently found to have PH1. However, Leumann et al.,[67,394] although able to detect oxalate and glycolate in amniotic fluid in normal pregnancies at 15 to 18 weeks, were unable to find any increase when the fetus was affected. It is by no means clear what the metabolic role of AGT is in fetal liver in the second trimester. It is possible that the metabolic manifestations of AGT deficiency, i.e., excessive oxalate and glycolate synthesis, are not expressed in a fetus of this age. Alternatively, any oxalate or glycolate synthesized by the fetus could be cleared much more efficiently by the placenta than by the fetal kidneys.

AGT Assay of Fetal Liver Biopsies

An alternative approach to the prenatal diagnosis of PH1 became available following discovery of the enzymic defect. Unfortunately, unlike most other peroxisomal enzymes, AGT is only expressed in hepatocytes.[185] It is not found to any extent in fibroblasts, leukocytes, chorionic villus, amniocytes, or amniotic fluid.[395,396] Therefore, prenatal diagnosis of PH1 by enzyme analysis requires a fetal liver biopsy.

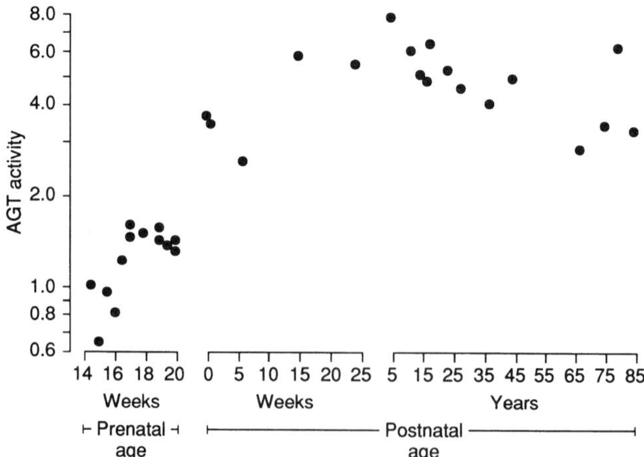

Fig. 133-18 Developmental expression of human hepatic AGT. Changes in AGT catalytic activity (expressed as μmol/h/mg protein) during prenatal and postnatal life. (*Modified with permission from data in Danpure et al.*[397])

The specific activity of AGT in fetal liver in the second trimester is much lower than that found postnatally. AGT catalytic activity is barely detectable earlier than 14 weeks' gestation.[397] Catalytic activity and immunoreactivity increase up to 18 weeks, when the levels plateau until at least 21 to 24 weeks. By this time, the activity is still only about one-third of that found in the immediate postnatal period (Fig. 133-18). The reason for this is not clear but may be a combination of the presence of fewer and smaller peroxisomes and the presence of nonhepatic non-AGT-expressing cells, such as hemopoietic cells, in immature fetal liver.[398–401] However, intraperoxisomal immunoreactive AGT protein can be detected by immunoelectron microscopy as early as 9 weeks' gestation, at which time the peroxisomes are very small and low in number[402] (Fig. 133-19*A*). This gestational age is close to the time of the earliest appearance of easily recognizable peroxisomal structures in human fetal liver.[403]

PH1 has been excluded[404,405] and positively diagnosed[397] prenatally at 20 to 24 weeks' gestation by a combination of AGT enzyme assay, immunoblotting, and immunoelectron microscopy of fetal liver biopsies obtained by ultrasound-guided needle aspiration (see Fig. 133-19*C, D*). The combined use of these three procedures is able to detect all known PH1 phenotypes without any studies on the affected family beforehand.[406] At least eight successful enzymic prenatal diagnoses had been carried by the early 1990s (Jennings and Danpure, unpublished observations), after which time the procedure was supplanted by DNA analysis.

DNA Analysis of Chorionic Villus Samples and Amniocytes

Although it is highly accurate and can be carried out without any prior knowledge of the family concerned, the main disadvantage of prenatal diagnosis by enzymic analysis of a fetal liver biopsy is that the earliest practicable limit for such a procedure is set by the technical difficulties of the sampling procedure rather than the detection method itself. Fetal liver biopsy cannot be performed before 16 weeks' gestation even though AGT can be detected by immunoelectron microscopy as early as 9 weeks.[402]

Cloning of the *AGXT* gene and identification of a number of mutations, intragenic polymorphisms (see Tables 133-3 and 133-4), and closely linked extragenic polymorphisms (mainly microsatellites)[407] mean that DNA analysis of chorionic villus samples or amniocytes obtained in the first trimester (9-10 weeks) is now the prenatal diagnosis method of choice for PH1.[392] The intron 1 duplication and intron 4 VNTR polymorphisms have been

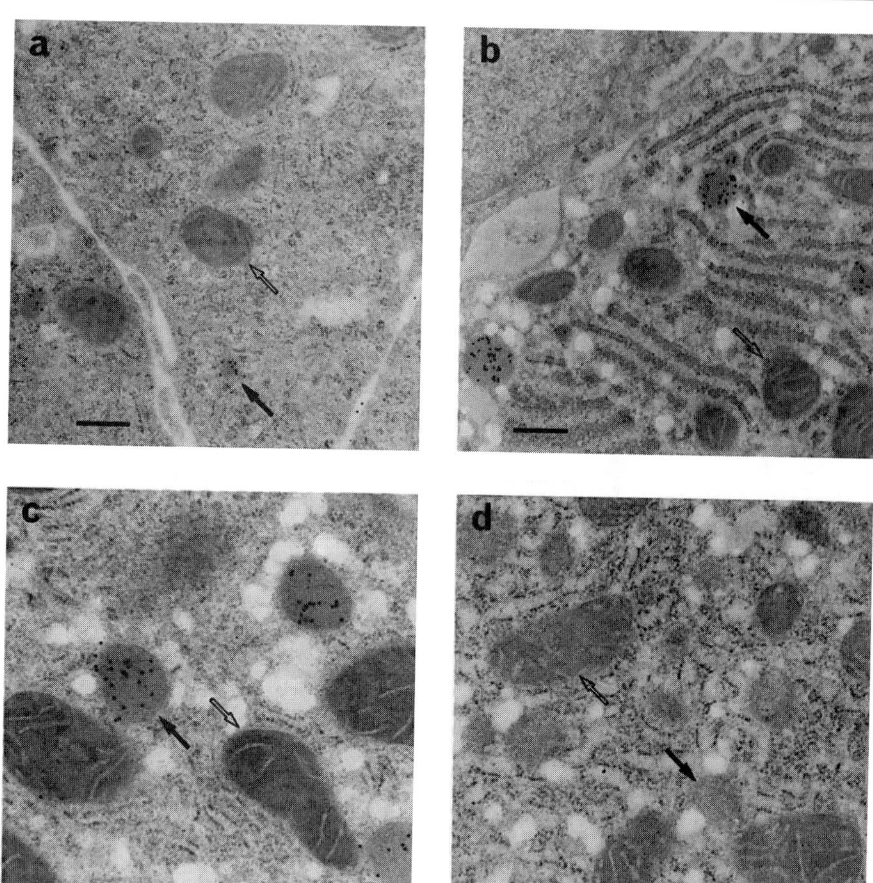

Fig. 133-19 Subcellular distribution of AGT in fetal liver. Postembedding protein A-gold immunoelectron microscopy using rabbit anti-human liver AGT antiserum. (*A, B*) Control fetuses at 9 and 18 weeks, respectively. Note the small, sparsely-labeled peroxisomes at 9 weeks (*A*). (*C, D*) Fetuses at risk for PH1: (*C*) unaffected, 20 weeks; (*D*) affected, 24 weeks. Closed arrows = peroxisomes; open arrows = mitochondria; bars = 0.5 μm. (*Panels B, C, and D reproduced and modified with permission from Danpure et al.*[397]*; photomicrographs courtesy of S. Griffiths.*)

shown to be especially useful.[408,409] These and other intragenic polymorphisms are predicted to be informative in most families. For example, a recent analysis of 22 prenatal diagnostic procedures[407] showed that intragenic polymorphisms alone were informative in 16 cases, extragenic microsatellites alone were informative in 4 cases, and a combination of the two were informative for the remaining 4 cases. Mutational analysis, together with linkage analysis using both intragenic and extragenic polymorphisms, is predicted to be successful in more than 99 percent of prenatal diagnoses of PH1.[392,410]

TREATMENT

General

Approaches to the treatment of the primary hyperoxalurias have been multifarious and, like pre- and postnatal diagnoses, have evolved in parallel with our increased understanding of the disease processes involved. Many of the early attempts to treat the primary hyperoxalurias were in ignorance of the basic molecular defects. As a result, many approaches could only target disease symptoms rather than its causes and were not specific to PH1 or PH2 but shared instead with secondary hyperoxalurias and idiopathic CaOx stone disease (for a review on the treatment of urolithiasis in general, see Smith[411]). Attempts to treat primary hyperoxaluria have been directed toward almost all aspects of the disease process (Fig. 133-20), and although treatment strategies often are categorized at the level of technical procedure (i.e., dietary manipulation, drug therapy, transplantation, etc.), a more rational grouping is based on the specific aspects of primary hyperoxaluria pathogenesis to which the individual treatments are directed. Thus, following the likely order of disease progression (Table 133-5), the first strategy is to decrease the amount of oxalate in the body. This can be achieved either by restricting intake and/or absorption of exogenous dietary oxalate and its precursors or by decreasing endogenous oxalate synthesis. The latter can involve pharmacologic manipulation of the various metabolic pathways leading to oxalate formation or replacement of the deficient enzyme (see Fig. 133-20). The second strategy is to prevent the CaOx from crystallizing out of solution by the use of hydration and crystallization inhibitors or, if it does, to remove the agglomerations by lithotripsy or open surgery. The third strategy, which is the strategy of failure or "last resort," is the treatment of the renal failure and associated uremia by dialysis or kidney transplantation (see Fig. 133-20). Although this is the more "logical" order for the implementation of treatments for primary hyperoxaluria, it is rarely the order that is actually used in practice. This is so because patients present in all stages of disease, so treatments of "last resort," for example, may have to be first. Also, some treatments are complex and not without risk and frequently are not considered until other (possibly less successful) treatments have been tried and failed.

Many papers have been written over the years on various aspects of the clinical treatment of primary hyperoxaluria. The practices advocated by many of the earlier reviews are still relevant and in use today. However, there have been enormous changes in the treatment of PH1 in the last few years as a result of discovery of the basic enzyme defects, and modern approaches to its management, as exemplified by liver transplantation (see below), are much more positive than the mere holding or delaying operations advocated previously (see Williams and Smith[25]).

Corporeal Oxalate Load

Exogenous Oxalate Intake. Although attempts to decrease the total body's load of oxalate by limiting oxalate ingestion and absorption have been shown to be of some use in idiopathic CaOx

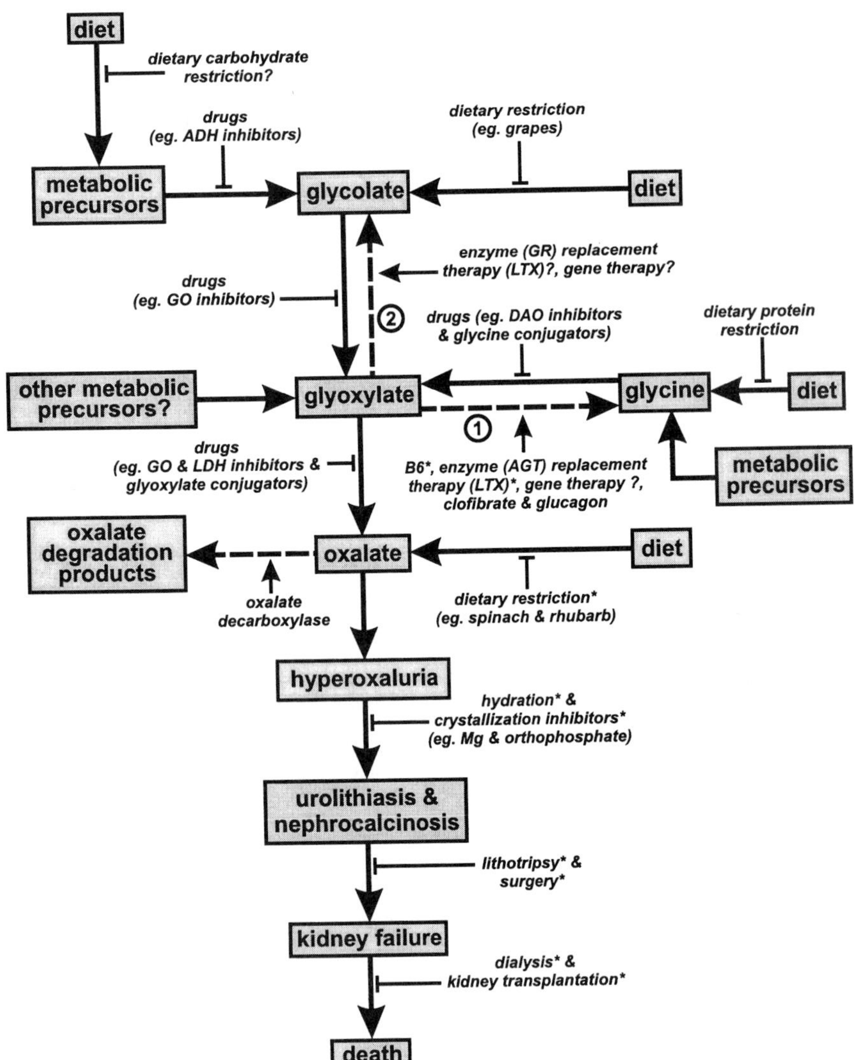

Fig. 133-20 Possible treatment strategies for primary hyperoxaluria. The diagram shows the various possible approaches to treatment discussed in the text together with their metabolic and pathophysiologic targets. Large solid arrows indicate routes toward the terminal consequence of disease (i.e., death). Large dashed arrows indicate routes away from disease. Treatments attempt to inhibit (small T-bars) the former but stimulate (small arrows) the latter. Refer to the text for a discussion of the pros and cons of these procedures. Note that not all the potential treatments included have been shown to work. ? = potential treatments of the future (i.e., not yet tried); * = treatments in current regular use; ADH, aldehyde dehydrogenase; GO, glycolate oxidase; DAO, D-amino acid oxidase; LDH, lactate dehydrogenase; GR, glyoxylate reductase; AGT, alanine:-glyoxylate aminotransferase, B_6, pyridoxine; LTX, liver transplantation. Reaction 2 is that catalyzed by GR (deficient in PH2). Reaction 1 is that catalyzed by AGT (deficient in PH1). Note that the oxalate degradation reaction included in the figure is not normally found in mammals.

stone disease, enteric hyperoxaluria, and possibly some milder cases of primary hyperoxaluria,[412–416] generally they are not regarded as being very helpful. This is so possibly because very little of the oxalate consumed in the diet is absorbed anyway[133–136] (but see Holmes et al.[137,138]). Early attempts to prevent CaOx deposition within the body by restricting dietary calcium were counterproductive. When bound to calcium in the gut, less oxalate is absorbed. Therefore, dietary restriction of calcium, without concomitant restriction of oxalate, can lead to increased urinary oxalate excretion and should be avoided.[417–419]

Endogenous Oxalate Synthesis. As Hillman[26] has pointed out, many early attempts at metabolic intervention in primary hyperoxaluria were done in ignorance of basic enzyme defects and metabolic perturbations. Nevertheless, they have helped shape our understanding of the metabolic processes involved directly and indirectly in the synthesis of oxalate (see "Metabolism of Oxalate and Its Precursors," above). In retrospect, it is now clear why many of the empirically based attempts to pharmacologically manipulate various intermediary metabolic pathways failed to have any effect on the excessive oxalate synthesis in PH1. Even before identification of the enzyme defect in PH1, it was realized that the excessive synthesis of oxalate was caused by a failure to metabolize glyoxylate (the major precursor of oxalate) properly via other routes[420] (for a review of the evidence, see Williams and Smith[25]). Therefore, therapeutic attempts to normalize endogenous oxalate synthesis in PH1 have centered largely around glyoxylate metabolism and can be divided into three main areas, namely, glyoxylate oxidation to oxalate, glyoxylate synthesis, and glyoxylate metabolism to products other than oxalate (see Fig. 133-20).

Glyoxylate and Glycolate Oxidation. Attempts to decrease the rate of oxidation of glyoxylate to oxalate by inhibiting the three enzymes originally thought to be involved, namely, xanthine oxidase, GO, and LDH (see "Metabolism of Oxalate and Its Precursors," above), have proved largely unsuccessful. For example, the xanthine oxidase inhibitor allopurinol has no effect urinary oxalate excretion,[200,201,421] which confirms the lack of involvement of this enzyme in glyoxylate oxidation.

The key role of LDH in intermediary metabolism has precluded any attempt to pharmacologically manipulate its activity as an approach to the treatment of hyperoxaluria. However, GO does not appear to be essential for normal cell function, and many attempts have been made to interfere with its activity, albeit without much success. GO inhibitors, such as hydroxymethanesulfonic acid and hydroxymethanesulfinic acid,[25,420] inhibit the oxidation of glyoxylate to oxalate in human liver supernatant and particulate fractions[422] and that catalyzed by partially purified rat liver and human erythrocyte GO.[423] However, they have no effect on urinary oxalate in laboratory animals.[25] Recent studies using the GO inhibitor DL-2-hydroxy-3-butanoic acid showed that although oxalate excretion was not diminished in normal rats, it was in rats made hyperoxaluric by the administration of glycolate.[424]

Table 133-5 Actual and Potential Treatments of Primary Hyperoxaluria and Their Metabolic and Pathophysiologic Targets

1. Corporeal oxalate load
   - 1.1. Exogenous oxalate intake
     - 1.1.1. *Dietary restriction*
   - 1.2. Endogenous oxalate synthesis
     - 1.2.1. Glyoxylate and glycolate oxidation
       - 1.2.1.1. *GO and LDH inhibitors, glyoxylate trapping*
     - 1.2.2. Glyoxylate and glycolate synthesis
       - 1.2.2.1. *GO, LDH, and ADH inhibitors, glycine trapping*
     - 1.2.3. Glyoxylate transamination
       - 1.2.3.1. *Pyridoxine*
       - 1.2.3.2. *Enzyme replacement therapy by liver transplantation (PH1)*
       - 1.2.3.3. *Gene therapy (PH1)*
       - 1.2.3.4. *Peroxisomal proliferators and gluconeogenic stimuli*
     - 1.2.4. Glyoxylate reduction
       - 1.2.4.1. *Enzyme replacement therapy by liver transplantation (PH2)*
     - 1.2.5. Glyoxylate carboligation
       - 1.2.5.1. *Thiamine*
   - 1.3. Oxalate degradation
     - 1.3.1. *Oxalate oxidase and oxalate decarboxylase*
2. Renal CaOx deposition
   - 2.1. *CaOx solubilization*
   - 2.2. *Lithotripsy and surgery*
3. Renal failure
   - 3.1. *Peritoneal dialysis, hemodialysis, and hemofiltration*
   - 3.2. *Renal transplantation*

NOTE: 1, 2, and 3 are the principal metabolic and pathophysiologic targets for the treatment of primary hyperoxaluria. They are listed in an order determined by the generally accepted causal life history of the disease (i.e., increased corporeal oxalate load → renal CaOx deposition → renal failure). Attempts to treat PH1 rarely occur in this order for two main reasons: (1) patients present in all stages of the disease, so the treatment of "last resort" (i.e., target 3), for example, might have to be the first; (2) some treatments in category 1 are complex and not without risk (e.g., liver transplantation) and are frequently not considered until other treatments (e.g., kidney transplantation) have been tried and failed. The pharmacologic approaches (1.2.1.1, 1.2.2.1, 1.2.3.4, and 1.2.5.1) have not been proven to be successful and are not in current use. Gene therapy for PH1 (1.2.3.3) and liver transplantation for PH2 (1.2.4.1) remain potential treatments for the future. The targets are in normal case and the treatments described in the text are in italics.

DL-α-lipoic acid has been shown to inhibit GO, but not LDH, and to lower oxalate excretion in rats with glyoxylate-induced hyperoxaluria.[425] However, bearing in mind that the reduced form of lipoic acid (i.e., dihydrolipoic acid) contains two thiol groups and could form adducts with glyoxylate (see below), it is not certain that any effect of lipoic acid on oxalate metabolism is necessarily related to its effect on GO. Oxamate, which also inhibits LDH, inhibits the oxidation of glyoxylate in erythrocyte lysates, and oxalatehydrazide and oxamatehydrazide inhibit oxalate synthesis in vivo in the rat.[423] Hydroxybutanesulfonate had no affect on urinary oxalate excretion in monkeys in vivo.[126] Also, tris-hydroxymethylaminomethane, which inhibits glycolate oxidation in vitro,[426] had no effect on urinary oxalate in normal or PH1 humans.[25] However, *n*-heptanoate and phenyllactate, which inhibit glycolate oxidation in vitro, do reduce oxalate synthesis in perfused rat liver, and phenyllactate reduces oxalate synthesis from ethylene glycol in rats in vivo.[205]

The prevention of glyoxylate oxidation by trapping the glyoxylate as a thiol adduct has been suggested as a possible treatment of primary hyperoxaluria or CaOx stone disease in general.[427,428] Thiazolidines can form between glyoxylate and a variety of thiols, including cysteine[427,429] and penicillamine.[428] Cysteine has been shown to inhibit oxalate formation from glyoxylate in rat liver homogenates and hepatocytes and oxalate production in vivo in ethylene glycol-fed and glycolate-fed rats.[427,430] Penicillamine inhibits the synthesis of oxalate from glycolate in isolated rat hepatocytes, but unfortunately, in vivo it has the opposite effect.[429,431] The cysteine precursor L-2-oxathiazolidine-4-carboxylate also has been used to produce glyoxylate adducts. Preliminary evidence suggests that it can decrease oxalate excretion in both rats[432] and humans.[433] Whether glyoxylate trapping has any role to play in the treatment of primary hyperoxaluria has yet to be determined.

Glyoxylate and Glycolate Synthesis. A number of attempts have been made to decrease glyoxylate synthesis. Glyoxylate synthesis from glycolate has effectively been covered by the GO inhibition studies above. Other attempts mainly have been concerned with its synthesis from glycine, catalyzed by DAO.

Attempts have been made to decrease glyoxylate synthesis from glycine by depletion of the available glycine pool, either by conjugating glycine with benzoate or hippurate or by dietary protein restriction.[434,435] In general, these approaches have not been very successful. Although glycine trapping does reduce oxalate production modestly, it is considered not to be useful as a long-term treatment.[436] The very high turnover rate of glycine in vivo and its low fractional conversion to glyoxylate/oxalate have meant that dietary restriction would be unlikely to meet with success. Competitive inhibition of DAO by large oral doses of D-amino acids, such as glutamate and histidine, has no effect on urinary oxalate excretion in PH1 patients.[437]

Various attempts have been made to use aldehyde dehydrogenase inhibitors to lower oxalate synthesis, the rationale being that a decrease in the conversion of glycolaldehyde to glycolate would decrease the synthesis not only of glycolate but also of glyoxylate and oxalate. Calcium carbimide has been used by a number of workers with conflicting results.[438–441] Disulfiram, another aldehyde dehydrogenase inhibitor, had no affect on urinary oxalate excretion in PH1 patients[201,422] or oxalate synthesis in human erythrocytes[442] or human liver supernatant or particulate fractions.[422]

Monoamine oxidase inhibition by isocarboxazide caused a slight reduction in urinary oxalate in a PH1 patient,[241] but this result was not confirmed by others.[126]

Glyoxylate Transamination. Since PH1 is caused by a failure of glyoxylate transamination, it is not surprising that this metabolic reaction has been the target of many attempts at treatment (see Fig. 133-20). Some of these, both pharmacologic (i.e., pyridoxine therapy) and surgical (i.e., enzyme-replacement therapy by liver transplantation), are currently also the most successful.

Pyridoxine. Pyridoxal phosphate is an essential cofactor for all aminotransferases, and numerous studies have been concerned with the affects of pyridoxine (vitamin B_6) administration on urinary oxalate excretion in PH1 patients. Pharmacologic doses of pyridoxine cause varying degrees of reduction in oxalate excretion in some, but not all, PH1 patients.[93,126,129,393,437,440,443–451] Urinary oxalate also can be reduced by pyridoxine in patients with recurrent idiopathic CaOx stones,[452] patients with "mild metabolic hyperoxaluria,"[93] patients suffering from pyridoxine deficiency,[182] and even in nonhyperoxaluric individuals.[179,437]

Although the mechanism of action of pyridoxine is probably related to the activity of AGT, the molecular basis is currently unknown. It has been suggested that large doses of pyridoxine may increase glyoxylate transamination by inducing the synthesis or inhibiting the catabolism of the AGT apoenzyme, similar to the affect of pyridoxine on tyrosine aminotransferase in rat liver.[453] In rat liver, the concentration of peroxisomal AGT apoprotein, as well as holoprotein, appears to be mediated by cofactor

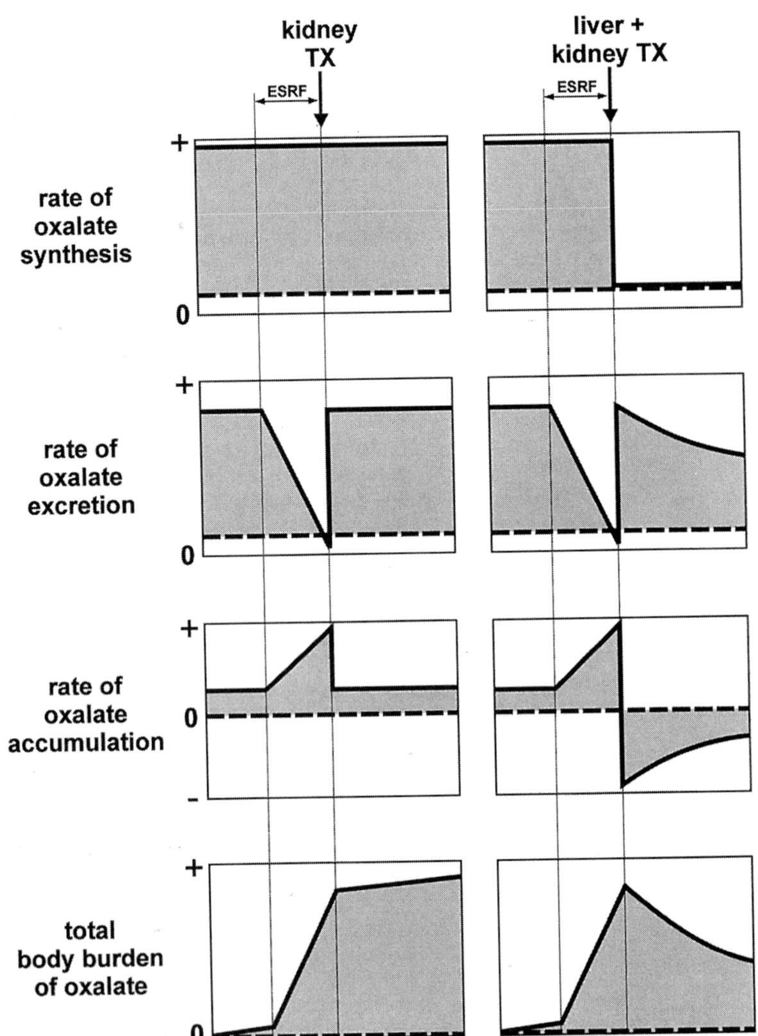

Fig. 133-21 Predicted effects of kidney and liver-kidney transplantation on oxalate dynamics in a PH1 patient with end-stage renal failure (ESRF). Predicted changes to the rates of oxalate synthesis, excretion, and accumulation and total corporeal oxalate burden following isolated kidney transplantation and liver-kidney transplantation in a patient with ESRF. Dotted lines = levels in a normal individual; solid lines = levels in a PH1 patient. The diagram clearly demonstrates the effects of oxalate dynamics on oxalate accumulation and long-term curative value of combined liver-kidney transplantation but not isolated kidney transplantation. Note the decrease in oxalate excretion as kidney function deteriorates. Even though isolated kidney transplantation following ESRF leads to a decrease in the rate of oxalate accumulation to pre-ESRF values, it has no effect on oxalate synthesis, so the total-body burden of oxalate still increases, albeit at a slower rate than immediately before transplantation. On the other hand, combined liver-kidney transplantation leads to normalization of oxalate synthesis and a negative rate of oxalate accumulation, which results in a net decrease in the total-body burden of oxalate. Ordinate = amount; abscissa = time.

concentration.[271] Pharmacologic doses of pyridoxine also could conceivably overcome the effects of mutations in the AGT gene that might interfere with cofactor binding. However, such mutations have yet to be identified. Studies on pyridoxine deficiency in rats indicate that intestinal absorption of oxalate also may be influenced by pyridoxine supplementation,[454–457] but interpretation of these findings in the context of pyridoxine-responsive PH1 is not clear.

Although no proper studies have been carried out on the relationship between pyridoxine responsiveness and AGT activity in PH1 patients, a subjective retrospective analysis of the clinical histories of the patients who have had AGT levels determined in my laboratory indicates that most responsive patients are CRM+/ENZ+. As in most of the latter patients, AGT is mistargeted to the mitochondria (see "Enzymic and Metabolic Defects," above), it follows that pyridoxine responsiveness is related to AGT mistargeting. However, it should be noted that not all patients with mitochondrial AGT are pyridoxine-responsive. A proper understanding of the way pyridoxine works is hampered by the absence of any general agreement on what degree of reduction in urinary oxalate excretion genuinely indicates a meaningful response. In fact, many primary hyperoxaluric patients are given pyridoxine routinely even in the absence of any evidence of responsiveness.

Enzyme-Replacement Therapy by Liver Transplantation in PH1. The discovery of the basic enzyme defect in PH1 has allowed the introduction of a new rational approach to its treatment by enzyme-replacement therapy.[458] In humans, at least, AGT is only found to any significant extent in the liver,[185] where, in most people at least, it is localized exclusively within the peroxisomes of the parenchymal cells.[186–188] Therefore, liver transplantation offers the possibility of not only replacing the total body's requirement for AGT but also providing it in the correct cell and intracellular location.[458] The rationale behind liver transplantation in PH1 is completely different from that behind kidney transplantation (see Fig. 133-20 and Table 133-5). The former attempts to cure the disease, whereas the latter attempts to recover from its consequences (see later). Combined liver-kidney transplantation replaces not only the biochemically defective organ but also the pathophysiologically defective organ at the same time.

The first liver transplantation for PH1 was carried out in 1985.[459] Although there were preliminary indications of biochemical correction before the patient succumbed to a cytomegalovirus infection, the first real success was achieved 2 years later.[460] This patient previously had had two failed kidney transplants and was moribund at the time he received a combined liver-kidney transplantation. At the time of writing this review, he is still well after 11 years (M. Mansell, personal communication), his genetic disease having been corrected clinically, enzymically, and metabolically.

Well over 100 liver transplantations have been carried out for PH1, the vast majority being combined with kidney transplantation.[459–486] The overall European experience has been surveyed on three occasions in the past few years under the auspices of the European PH1 Transplant Registry. The results of 24 patients were reported in 1990,[487] 61 patients in 1994,[488] and 80 patients in 1997.[489]

Normal

Soluble pool
Liver
Glyoxylate
Oxalate
Glycolate
Glycine
Urine
Glycolate Oxalate

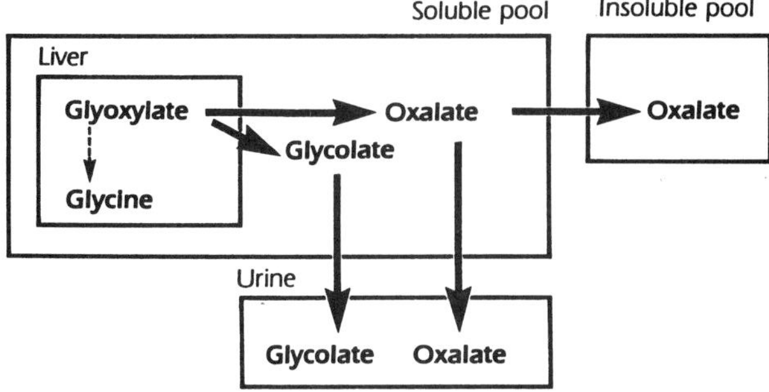

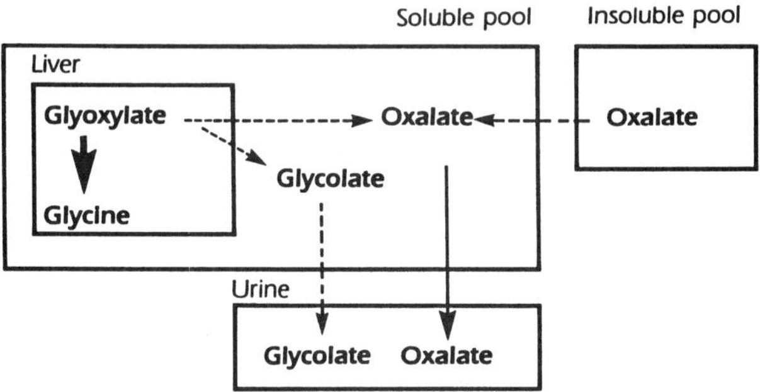

Fig. 133-22 Metabolite fluxes before and after liver transplantation in PH1. Note that oxalate translocation from the soluble pool into the urine is still greater than normal after liver transplantation, while the CaOx deposits in the "insoluble" pool are being mobilized. Since glycolate does not enter the "insoluble pool," urinary glycolate excretion is normalized immediately (see Fig. 133-23*C*). (*Adapted with permission from Danpure.*[247])

Following liver transplantation, the rate of endogenous oxalate and glycolate synthesis would be expected to drop to normal levels immediately, irrespective of whether kidney transplantation is carried out simultaneously or not. However, normalization of the plasma and urinary oxalate concentrations may take very much longer to reflect this decreased synthesis, due to the remobilization of the CaOx stores deposited throughout the body (Figs. 133-21 and 133-22). Calcium glycolate is not insoluble and therefore does not accumulate in the body. Glycolate excretion is normalized very rapidly[247,460,461,469] (Fig. 133-23*C*).

Resolubilization of the systemic oxalotic deposits would be expected to be a slow process, the speed of which will depend on, among other things, the accessibility of the CaOx stores to the blood system. Oxalate deposits in slow-turnover bone, for example, would be expected to be very much more slowly dissolved than those in well-vascularized soft tissues. The rate of normalization of plasma and urinary oxalate levels would be expected to be slowest in PH1 patients with the longest histories of disease and especially in those who have spent the greatest lengths of time with compromized renal function. The oxalate levels in such patients may take several years to return to normal[460,463,464,473,482] (see Fig. 133-23*B*). On the other hand, in young patients with short disease histories and reasonable renal function, oxalate levels can be normalized within 24 hours.[461] The fact that this resolubilization occurs can be seen directly as a decrease in systemic oxalosis and an improvement in the symptoms associated with it following liver transplantation[462,463,468,473,479,480,482,486,490] (Fig. 133-24). In one PH1 patient with severe bone oxalosis, urinary oxalate dropped to near-normal levels by 6 to 8 months but then increased markedly after 12 to 18 months[463] (see Fig. 133-23*B*), presumably due to the remobilization of CaOx deposited in the bone several years earlier.[473]

Because of the morbidity associated with the liver transplantation procedure per se, most PH1 patients have not been transplanted until the disease has progressed to its terminal phases. That is, most patients were in end-stage renal failure, frequently having received one or more kidney transplants previously. Therefore, combined hepatorenal transplantation has been more common than isolated liver transplantation. In some cases the liver was transplanted a few months before the kidney,[469] whereas in others the reverse applied.[462] The relative merits of these various approaches have been discussed previously.[458] The overall outcome of liver transplantation in PH1 depends not only on the normalization of endogenous oxalate synthesis but also on the maintenance of good renal function. In fact, it appears that success depends more on the kidney's function than on that of the liver, the kidney being very sensitive to the accumulated body oxalate load (while the liver is very refractory to it). Isolated liver transplantation in the presence of poor or rapidly declining renal function does not appear to be very successful,[465,483] although sometimes it is unavoidable.[484]

In general, the metabolic outcome of liver transplantation in PH1 is maximized if patients are transplanted before end-stage renal failure so that renal transplantation is unnecessary[461,475,491] (Fig. 133-25). Even after end-stage renal failure, the earlier liver-kidney transplantation is performed, the better, so as to minimize the ravages of systemic oxalosis.[482]

The morbidity and irrevocability of the liver transplantation procedure have encouraged surgeons to think of partial auxiliary procedures. As discussed previously,[458] this is to be discouraged. The patient's defective liver remaining in the body will continue to synthesize excessively nonmetabolizable oxalate independent of the functioning of the new liver (Fig. 133-26).

At the moment, liver transplantation remains the only long-term "cure" for patients with pyridoxine-unresponsive PH1. However, despite the theoretical considerations, the actuarial benefits of such a procedure, especially compared with kidney transplantation, have yet to be determined. Liver transplantation for PH1 was started only 13 years ago, with the longest surviving patient being well and metabolically normal for more than 11 years. On the other hand, kidney transplantation has been used in PH1 for over 30 years, with a few patients surviving for longer than 10 years (see below). The relative merits and long-term outcomes of liver, liver-kidney, and kidney transplantations in PH1 have been debated extensively in recent years.[488,489,492–496]

The Possibility of Gene Therapy for PH1? In many respects, liver transplantation can be considered as a form of gene therapy for PH1 as much as a form of enzyme-replacement therapy.[261,497] The AGT present in the liver graft at the time of transplantation will last only for a few days or weeks at most. It is the properly functioning *AGXT* gene that continues to make more AGT that leads to the long-term success of the procedure. However, as a form of gene therapy, liver transplantation is far from ideal, not least because it involves the replacement of thousands of perfectly normal genes (and indeed enzymes), just to replace the one that is abnormal. A more sensible, and certainly more economical (at least at the genetic level), approach to gene therapy would be to replace only the abnormal gene, leaving all the other normal ones intact.

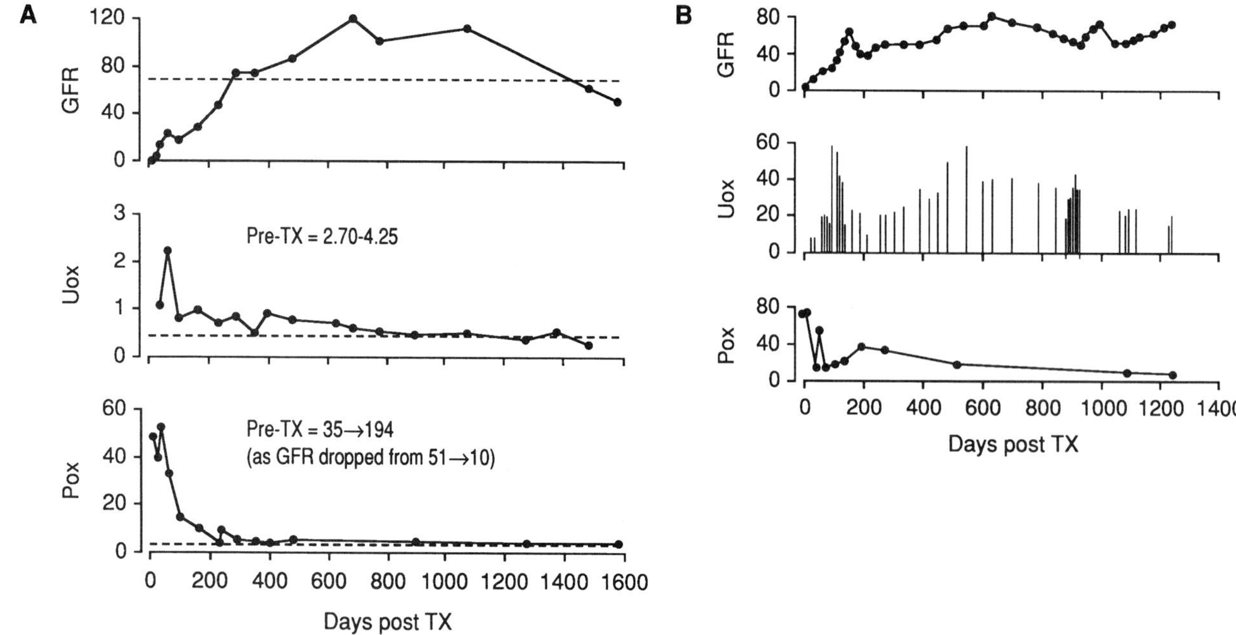

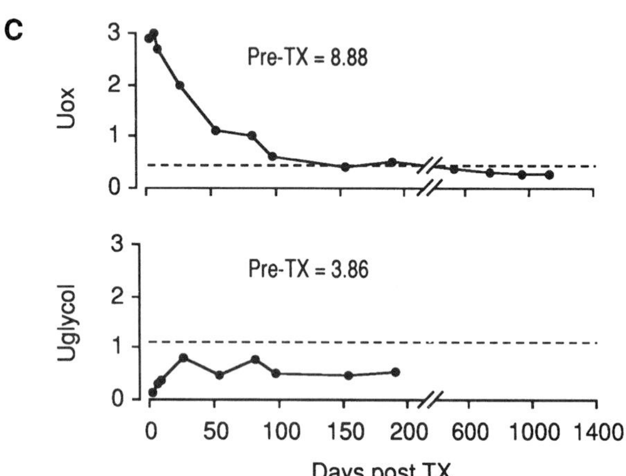

Fig. 133-23 Metabolic normalization following liver-kidney transplantation in PH1. GFR, glomerular filtration rate (ml/min); U_{ox}, urinary oxalate excretion (mmol/24 h in *A* and *C* and μmol/24 h/kg in *B*); P_{ox}, plasma oxalate (μmol/liter); U_{glycol}, urinary glycolate excretion (mmol/24 h); - - - - = lower limit of normal for GFR or upper limit of normal for U_{ox}, P_{ox}, and U_{glycol}; abscissa = days after liver-kidney transplantation; pre-TX = representative values before liver-kidney transplantation. Note the slower normalization of U_{ox} compared with P_{ox} in *A*, the immediate normalization of U_{glycol} compared with U_{ox} in *C* (see Fig. 133-22), and the apparent normalization of U_{ox} after 200 days in *B*, followed by an increase in U_{ox} over the next 300 to 400 days, presumably due to remobilization of bone CaOx deposits (see Fig. 133-24). (*Data for panel A adapted with permission from Watts et al.*[469]*; extra data kindly provided by Dr. G. P. Kasidas, University College & Middlesex School of Medicine, London, and Dr. M. A. Mansell, St. Peter's Hospital, London. Panel B reproduced and modified with permission from Toussaint et al.*[473]*; original figure and data kindly provided by Professor C. Toussaint, Hopital Erasme, Bruxelles. Data for panel C taken with permission from Watts et al.*[469]*; extra data kindly provided by Professor L. H. Smith, Mayo Clinic, Rochester, MN.*)

As outlined previously,[497] there are a number of characteristics of PH1 that make it a suitable candidate for gene therapy. For example, at least at the level of genetic malfunction, if not at the level of clinical pathology, PH1 is a liver-specific disease. The liver represents an excellent target organ for gene therapy, and a considerable amount of current research concerns the development of suitable vectors and clinical protocols aimed at maximizing the expression of transgenes in hepatocytes. Just as liver transplantation is presumed to replace almost all the body's requirement for AGT, so liver-targeted gene therapy at least has the potential to do so.

Even some of the most severe consequences of systemic oxalosis in PH1 appear to be at least partially reversible following liver transplantation (see above). Therefore, there is no reason to believe that the same would not also be the case following gene therapy. Even in advanced stages of systemic oxalosis, the central nervous system seems to be spared. Therefore, the expected resolution of the physical consequences of PH1 following gene therapy would leave no residue of untreatable intellectual or motor impairment.

However, notwithstanding these potential advantages of gene therapy, there are a number of specific difficulties particular to PH1 that will need to be overcome, in addition to those associated with gene therapy in general. These special considerations are due to the enzymic and metabolic peculiarities of PH1, as follows: (1) PH1 is a disease of increased synthesis of storage product (i.e., oxalate), not one of its decreased degradation, (2) the pathologically accumulated material (i.e., oxalate) is not further metabolizable, (3) glyoxylate detoxification catalyzed by AGT can only take place efficiently in hepatocyte peroxisomes, and (4) there is no known mechanism by which peroxisomal enzymes can be taken up from the extracellular environment. This combination of characteristics also has had implications for the enzyme-replacement therapy of PH1 by liver transplantation.[458]

Asymptomatic PH1 heterozygotes can have total liver AGT activities as low as 25 percent of the mean normal level.[260] Therefore, gene therapy should aim at this overall level of expression as a minimum. However, although only the liver needs to be targeted, it is important that the great majority of the hepatocytes (say >75 percent) take up and express the transgene (see Fig. 133-26). If only 10 percent of hepatocytes could be made to take up the transgene, the level of hepatic oxalate synthesis would hardly change, even if each transfected cell expressed 10 times the normal level of AGT (i.e., the total liver activity of AGT would be normal). The 90 percent of hepatocytes that fail to take up or express the AGT transgene will continue to synthesise (excessively) oxalate at the same rate as before. AGT activity in one cell can in no way exert any influence on oxalate production in its AGT-deficient neighbours. Its is exactly for this reason that partial or auxiliary liver transplantation would not be expected

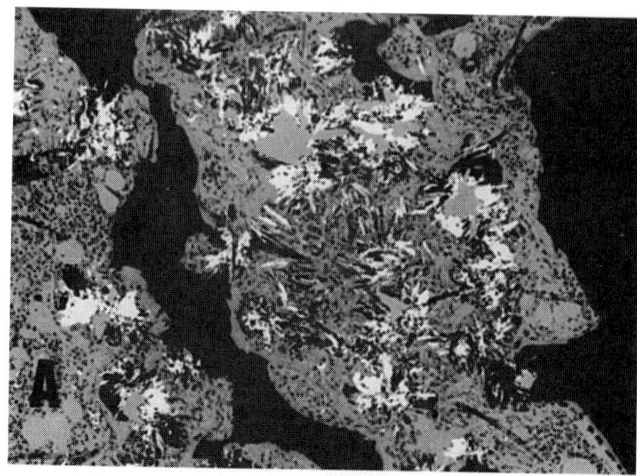

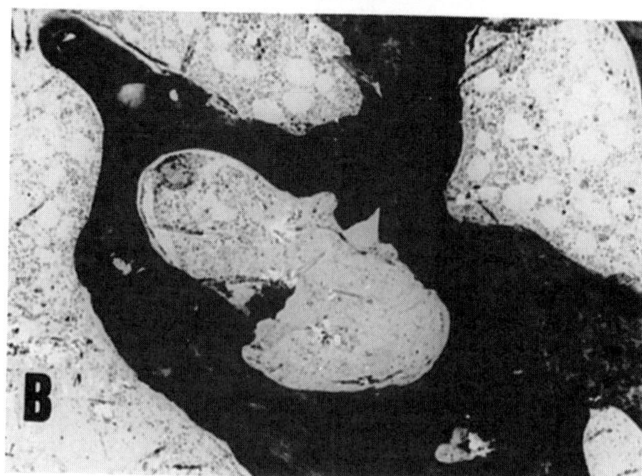

Fig. 133-24 Resolubilization of bone CaOx deposits following combined liver-kidney transplantation in PH1. Iliac crest biopsies of a 15-year-old female PH1 patient 7 months (*A*) and 18 months (*B*) after transplantation (same patient as in Fig. 133-23*B*). Note the decrease in size and number of CaOx crystals and improvement of osteomalacia (toluidine blue, polarized light, bars = 500 μm). (*Reproduced with permission from Watts et al.*[487]*; original photographs kindly provided by Professor C. Toussaint, Hopital Erasme, Bruxelles.*)

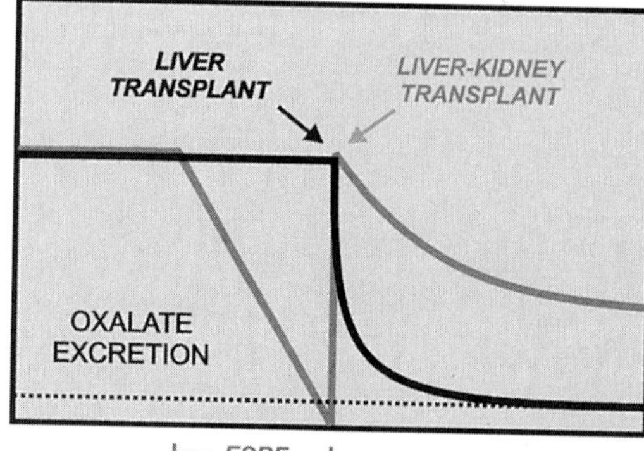

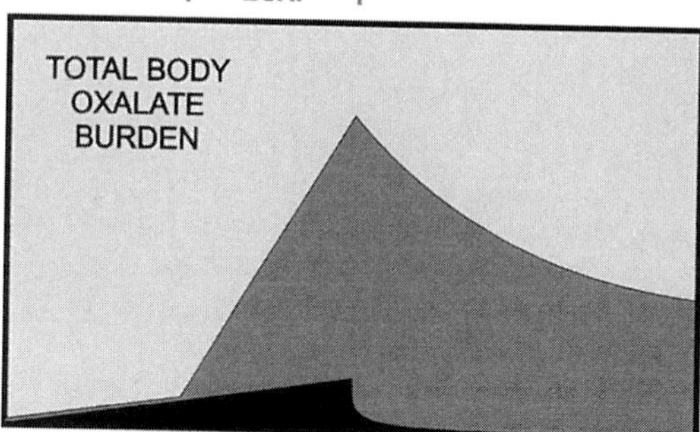

Fig. 133-25 Advantages of isolated liver transplantation before kidney failure over combined liver-kidney transplantation afterwards. *Oxalate excretion*: Black line = theoretical urinary excretion pattern before and after isolated liver transplantation in a patient who did not have compromised renal function; gray line = theoretical excretion pattern before and after combined liver-kidney transplantation in a patient who did have end-stage renal failure (ESRF). *Total oxalate body burden*: Black area = theoretical total accumulation of oxalate in the body in the former case; gray area theoretical total accumulation of oxalate in the body in the latter case. Decreased oxalate excretion, and hence increased oxalate accumulation, during ESRF would be expected to lead much slower normalization of body oxalate levels and excretion following correction of the enzyme defect by liver transplantation than would occur if transplantation had been carried out before ESRF. Ordinate = amount; abscissa = time.

to produce any significant benefit in PH1 (see above and see Fig. 133-26). In the present state of the art, whether in vivo or ex vivo approaches are used for the gene therapy of PH1, using retroviral or adenoviral vectors, treatment would need to be repeated many times in order to achieve the levels of AGT expression necessary to significantly decrease hepatic oxalate synthesis.

It is unfortunate that a suitable naturally occurring animal model for PH1 is not available in which to test the various possible approaches to gene therapy (see "Animal Models of Primary Hyperoxaluria," above). As discussed already, an AGT knockout mouse is unlikely to be an adequate alternative. However, the glycolate/ethylene glycol-fed rat fulfills at least some of the most important requirements of a model and would be a good starting point for testing the potential efficacy of gene therapy.

Despite the anticipated problems, gene therapy for PH1 is a distinct possibility within the next decade. The potential benefits far outweigh the potential difficulties. Just as treatments aimed at the consequences of PH1 (e.g., kidney transplantation) have slowly given way to treatments aimed at its basic cause (i.e., liver transplantation), so liver transplantation itself will give way to treatments aimed more selectively at its cause (i.e., gene therapy).

Peroxisomal Proliferators and Gluconeogenic Stimuli. Clofibrate is a hypolipidemic drug that interferes with various aspects of lipid metabolism.[498] One of its several morphologic effects, which it shares with a number of derivatives and unrelated compounds such as di-(2-ethylhexyl)phthalate, is to cause peroxisomal proliferation.[499,500] Concommitantly with expansion in the peroxisomal compartment size in rat liver is an increase in a variety of peroxisomal enzyme activities, including AGT, serine:pyruvate aminotransferase, and histidine:glyoxylate aminotransferase.[501–503] However, the peroxisome proliferation properties of these agents appears to be remarkably species-specific, with little or no effect on human liver peroxisomes.[504–506] Nevertheless, Streefland et al.[39] treated two PH1 patients with clofibrate without success, in one patient the drug having to be withdrawn due to toxic side effects. Even if the toxicity of clofibrate could be overcome, it seems unlikely to be of any use in the treatment of PH1. In fact, in rats, clofibrate actually increases oxalate synthesis, possibly due to a stimulatory effect on LDH.[507]

In the livers of rats and a number of other rodents, AGT can be induced up to 40 times the baseline level by gluconeogenic stimuli, such as glucagon or a high-protein diet.[337,343–345,502,508] However, glucagon has this effect only on mitochondrial AGT, peroxisomal AGT remaining unaffected. In mammals with only peroxisomal AGT, such as rabbit and guinea pig, AGT is not induced by such treatment.[343] The effect of glucagon on AGT transcription in the rat is mediated by the cAMP signal-transduction pathway.[345,347] However, cAMP response elements have not been found in the human gene.[286] Therefore, it is unlikely that such treatment could be beneficial in PH1, even if only restricted to the third of patients with mitochondrial AGT. In fact, in guinea pigs[209] and transformed

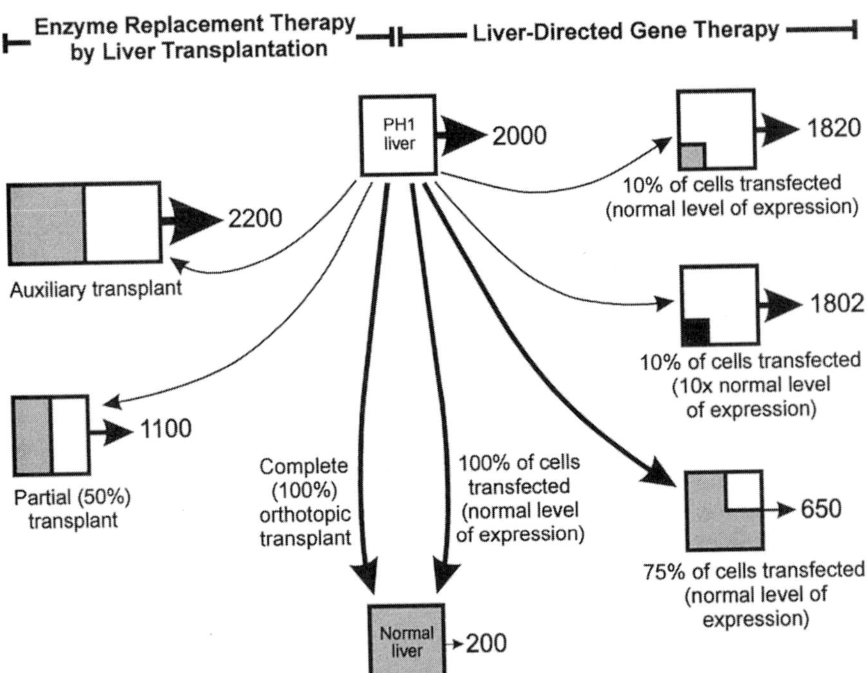

Fig. 133-26 Appropriate and inappropriate strategies for enzyme-replacement and gene therapy of PH1 and their likely metabolic consequences. Numbers indicate an approximation of the daily rate of oxalate synthesis by the liver in micromoles (based on typical daily excretion rates and assuming most of the urinary oxalate is derived from endogenous synthesis by the liver). Open boxes represent uncorrected PH1 liver cells; shaded boxes represent normal or completely corrected liver cells; black box represents liver cells over expressing AGT. Those treatment strategies likely to be successful are denoted by the bold extended arrows. (*Modified with permission from Danpure and Rumsby.*[261])

human liver cells (HepG2),[509] glucagon actually increases, rather than decreases, oxalate synthesis.

Glyoxylate Reduction. Although the activity of GR contributes significantly to the detoxification of glyoxylate and the level of oxalate synthesis (see Fig. 133-8), unlike the other main contributor, AGT, it has received almost no attention as a route by which primary hyperoxaluria may be treated. This is especially surprising because it is a deficiency of GR that leads to the pathologic sequelae of PH2 (see "Enzymic and Metabolic Defects," above). Unlike pyridoxine for PH1, no drugs are known that could be used to stimulate GR activity.

The Possibility of Enzyme-Replacement Therapy by Liver Transplantation for PH2? Although enzyme-replacement therapy by liver transplantation has become an established procedure for the treatment of pyridoxine-resistant PH1, it has not yet been considered for PH2. This has been due in part to the view that PH2 is, in general, a milder disease than PH1 and therefore does not warrant such a "heroic" procedure and in part to an uncertainty about the tissue distribution of GR/DGDH. For liver transplantation to work as a form of enzyme-replacement therapy, this organ must contain a significant proportion of the body's requirement for the enzyme.

However, there is increasing realization that PH2 patients can succumb to renal failure and require kidney transplantation, although there are not enough data available to determine the likely long-term success of the procedure. In addition, recent studies[236] suggest that the liver may very well contain much of the body's GR activity. Therefore, the rationale for liver transplantation in PH2 is much stronger now than it was a few years ago.

Glyoxylate Carboligation. Thiamine pyrophosphate is an essential cofactor for CL. This enzyme, which was shown to be identical to 2-oxoglutarate dehydrogenase, originally was thought to be the cause of PH1 (see "Enzymic and Metabolic Defects," above). Thiamine administration to three PH1 patients failed to have any effect on urinary oxalate,[126] again calling into question the role of this enzyme in glyoxylate/oxalate metabolism.

Oxalate Degradation. Humans and other mammals are unable to degrade oxalate. Therefore, several authors have considered the possibility of treating hyperoxaluric patients by introducing either the gene or gene product of oxalate-degrading enzymes from bacteria or plants, such as oxalate decarboxylase[510] or oxalate oxidase,[511] respectively. Such possibilities have so far remained largely theoretical due to the time and expense of producing enough enzyme and the problem of antigenicity. However, it has been shown that oxalate oxidase implanted within dialysis membrane capsules in the rat peritoneal cavity is able to catalyze the metabolism of peritoneally administered oxalate and glyoxylate.[511] Another approach would be to entrap the oxalate-degrading enzyme within erythrocyte ghosts. Accessibility of such entrapped enzyme to the circulating oxalate does not appear to be a problem, since the transport of organic acids, such as oxalate, glyoxylate, and glycolate, across the erythrocyte ghost membrane appears to be maintained.[512]

Renal CaOx Deposition

CaOx Solubilization. Attempts to prevent CaOx stone formation by increasing its solubility have been widely used.[513] High fluid intake, alkaline citrate,[514–516] trace metal ions,[517] methylene blue,[518] colloids,[519] magnesium oxide,[520] and inorganic phosphates[521] have all been used with varying degrees of success. Magnesium oxalate is some 50 times more soluble than CaOx,[2] and magnesium oxide dietary supplementation has been shown to be beneficial in vitamin B_6-deficient, hyperoxaluric, stone-forming rats[522] and for some patients with recurrent idiopathic CaOx stone disease.[452] The urine from such patients, treated with magnesium, had an increased capacity to keep CaOx in solution. Magnesium oxide therapy also has been shown to be beneficial to some primary hyperoxaluria patients.[520,523] A high phosphate intake has been shown to be beneficial for some patients with recurrent oxalate stone disease in general[513,521] and primary hyperoxaluria patients in particular,[524,525] although the mechanism of action is not understood.

Lithotripsy and Surgery. Failure to prevent CaOx deposition in the kidney and urinary tract may lead to the need for surgical removal or extracorporeal shock-wave lithotripsy if the calculus blocks urine flow or otherwise interferes with renal function.[450,526] Although lithotripsy has revolutionized stone removal, it is not without complications.[527] Lithotripsy for urolithiasis in general has been reviewed previously,[5] but it is generally considered that owing to the progressive nature of PH1, the prognosis following such procedures in this disease is not as good as it is with patients suffering from stones from other causes.

Renal Failure

The various options available for the treatment of renal failure in the primary hyperoxalurias have been reviewed by Watts.[528]

Dialysis. Attempts to treat the uremia associated with the renal failure that follows CaOx deposition are inextricably combined with attempts to diminish the total-body load of oxalate (see above). Hemodialysis, for example, also can remove large quantities of oxalate and its precursors[529] and, together with peritoneal dialysis, has been used extensively in primary hyperoxaluria.[29,529–538] In general, hemodialysis removes oxalate from the body more efficiently than does peritoneal dialysis,[532] but even with hemodialysis, the removal of oxalate is unable to keep up with its excessive synthesis in PH1.[532,534] Therefore, although the uremia can be controlled, the accretion of oxalate continues unabated, leading to CaOx deposition throughout the body.

Renal Transplantation. Dialysis can best be described as a short-term holding operation. A longer-term solution to renal failure is kidney transplantation. Probably more papers have been written about this aspect of the treatment of primary hyperoxaluria than any other. Because the basic defect in PH1 is in the liver rather than in the kidney, renal transplantation itself also can only be regarded as a temporary solution, albeit possibly a longer-term one than is dialysis. Following kidney transplantation, endogenous oxalate synthesis remains elevated, and although the rate of oxalate accumulation in the body may decrease, the total-body oxalate burden is unlikely to decrease significantly (see Fig. 133-21). CaOx deposition can occur rapidly in the transplanted kidney,[39,533,539–546] although in some cases the transplanted kidney can survive for a significant length of time, especially with intensive perioperative management to minimize CaOx reaccumulation in the graft.[494,496,539,543,547–549]

Treatment Summary

The clinician is presented with a plethora of alternatives regarding the treatment of primary hyperoxaluria. The strategy adopted will depend on, among other things, the differential diagnosis and the patient's age, current condition, and clinical history. Some treatments are relatively noninvasive and can be implemented under most circumstances; others are only appropriate if certain strict criteria are met. Not all clinicians agree on the relative merits of different treatment strategies or the order in which they should be used. A flow diagram of the possible decision-making processes regarding the treatment of primary hyperoxaluria in relationship to the differential diagnosis and renal function is shown in Fig. 133-27.

FUTURE

The past 15 years have witnessed enormous advances in our understanding of the pathogenesis and etiology of primary hyperoxaluria, especially PH1. These advances have led to major changes in all aspects of its clinical management. Identification of the basic enzymic and genetic defects in PH1 has enabled a greater appreciation of its wide clinical heterogeneity, further delineation of which could have wider implications for the much more common multifactorial hyperoxaluric syndromes such as idiopathic CaOx stone disease and the metabolic relationship between mammals and oxalate in general. In addition, molecular dissection of the peroxisome-to-mitochondrion AGT trafficking defect has yielded insights beyond the confines of the disease itself and highlighted some of the fundamental structural differences between the peroxisomal and mitochondrial protein import pathways. The next few years promise further advances, especially in the molecular genetics and treatment. Identification of more mutations in the *AGXT* gene may allow definitive diagnosis of PH1

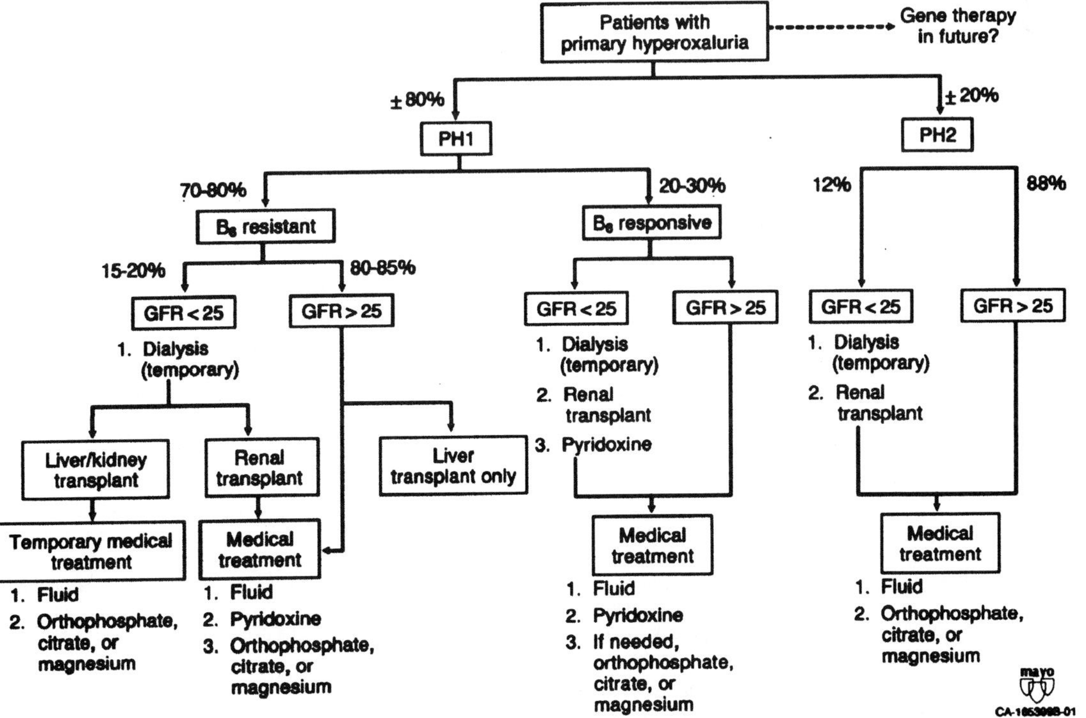

Fig. 133-27 Clinicians' flowchart guide to the treatment of primary hyperoxaluria. A personal view (i.e., that of Professor L. H. Smith, University of Kansas School of Medicine) of the criteria for the implementation of the various commonly used treatment protocols for primary hyperoxaluria depending on the differential diagnosis and disease severity. (*Reproduced with permission from Danpure and Smith[17]; original diagram kindly provided by Professor L. H. Smith, University of Kansas School of Medicine.*)

to be made without the requirement for liver biopsies. Hopefully, in the not too distant future, once the problems associated with gene targeting in general have been overcome, gene therapy will become available for PH1. Gene therapy has greater potential to become the "routine" way to treat PH1 than has enzyme-replacement therapy by liver transplantation. More extensive analysis of the molecular basis for AGT mistargeting has the potential to contribute further to our understanding of the possible relationship between the peroxisomal and mitochondrial import pathways in living cells.

Despite these advances in PH1, there is still an enormous gap in our understanding of the relationship between genotype and clinical/metabolic phenotype. Many controversies about the pathways of oxalate metabolism remain unresolved. The mechanism of pyridoxine responsiveness has still not been determined. More work on the intermediary metabolic pathways leading to and away from oxalate will be required for a proper understanding not only of PH1 but also of CaOx stone disease in general.

Whether equivalent advances will be made with respect to PH2 remains more equivocal. The rate of increase in our understanding and clinical management of PH1 has far outstripped that of PH2 in recent years. This is despite the fact that AGT deficiency in PH1 was identified only 12 years ago, whereas GR/DGDH deficiency in PH2 was identified 30 years ago. The recently renewed interest in the characterization of the pathophysiology of PH2 as a distinct entity from PH1 has stimulated a renaissance of interest in its pathophysiology. The DGDH gene has been cloned recently.[550] Therefore, prenatal diagnosis of PH2 should become available soon. Recent work on the enzymology of PH2 also should allow routine enzymic diagnoses and opens up the possibility of treatment by liver transplantation.

Oxalate in both our external and internal environments remains a threat to our well-being. However, despite our continued ignorance of many aspects of the finely balanced relationship between oxalate and human life, the future of at least one particularly severe example of the perturbation of this balance remains brighter and more positive than it has ever done before.

ACKNOWLEDGMENTS

I would like to acknowledge the invaluable help received from many of my colleagues with the preparation of this chapter. Thanks are due to Professor C. Toussaint (Departement Medico-Chirurgical de Nephrologie, Dialyse et Transplantation, Hopital Erasme, Bruxelles, Belgium), Professor T. M. Barratt (Department of Paediatric Nephrology, The Hospitals for Sick Children, London, U.K.), Dr. G. P. Kasidas (Department of Chemical Pathology, University College & Middlesex School of Medicine, London, U.K.), Dr. M. A. Mansell (St. Peter's Hospital, London, U.K.), Professor L. H. Smith (University of Kansas School of Medicine), and Dr. G. Rumsby and Dr. C. von Schnakenburg (both at the Department of Molecular Pathology, University College London Hospitals, London, U.K.) for allowing the reproduction of previously published figures, providing original photographs, or communicating unpublished extra data for the current and previous editions of this chapter.

I also would like to thank various colleagues, including Professor R. W. E. Watts (Wellington Hospital, London, U.K.), Dr. R. P. Holmes (Wake Forest University, Winston-Salem, NC), Professor C. Toussaint (Hopital Erasme, Bruxelles, Belgium), Dr. G. Rumsby (University College London Hospitals, London, U.K.), Dr. B. Hoppe (University Children's Hospital, Cologne, Germany), Dr. J. I. Scheinman (Medical College of Virginia, Richmond, VA), Professor D. A. Applegarth (British Columbia Children's Hospital, Vancouver, Canada), and Dr. P. Cochat (Hôpital Édouard Herriot, Lyon, France), who have taken the time to read the previous edition of this chapter and given me their suggestions for improvements to the present edition.

I would especially like to express my gratitude and acknowledge the debt owed to my past and present colleagues at the MRC Clinical Research Centre, Harrow, U.K., and the MRC Laboratory for Molecular Cell Biology and Department of Biology, University College London, U.K. (Miss J. Allsop, Dr. G. M. Birdsey, Dr. P. J. Cooper, Dr. P. Fryer, Mr. S. Griffiths, Mr. K. M. Guttridge, Mrs. P. R. Jennings, Dr. J. M. Leiper, Mr. M. J. Lumb, Dr. P. B. Oatey, Dr. P. E. Purdue, and Dr. P. J. Wise,), without whose hard work and dedication over the past 12 years our understanding of primary hyperoxaluria, especially PH1, would be considerably less well advanced than it actually is.

REFERENCES

1. Rose GA: Introduction, in Rose GA (ed): *Oxalate Metabolism in Relation to Urinary Stones*. London, Springer-Verlag, 1988, p 1.
2. Hodgkinson A: *Oxalic Acid in Biology and Medicine*. New York, Academic Press, 1977.
3. Allison MJ, Dawson KA, Mayberry WR, Foss JG: *Oxalobacter formigenes* gen. nov., sp. nov.: oxalate-degrading anaerobes that inhabit the gastrointestinal tract. *Arch Microbiol* **141**:1, 1985.
4. Daniel SL, Hartman PA, Allison MJ: Intestinal colonization of laboratory rats with *Oxalobacter formigenes*. *Appl Environ Microbiol* **53**:2767, 1987.
5. Lingeman JE, Smith LH, Woods JR: *Urinary Calculi: ESWL, Endourology and Medical Therapy.* Philadelphia, Lea and Febiger, 1989.
6. Robertson WG, Peacock M: The cause of idiopathic calcium stone disease: Hypercalciuria or hyperoxaluria? *Nephron* **26**:105, 1980.
7. Larsson L, Tiselius HG: Hyperoxaluria. *Miner Electrolyte Metab* **13**:242, 1987.
8. Osswald H, Hautmann R: Renal elimination kinetics and plasma half-life of oxalate in man. *Urol Int* **34**:440, 1979.
9. Watts RW, Mansell MA: Primary hyperoxaluria, in Rose GA (ed): *Oxalate Metabolism in Relation to Urinary Stones*. London, Springer-Verlag, 1988, p 65.
10. Yendt ER, Cohanim M: Absorptive hyperoxaluria: A new clinical entity-Successful treatment with hydrochlorothiazide. *Clin Invest Med* **9**:44, 1986.
11. Baggio B, Gambaro G, Marchini F, Cicerello E, Borsatti A: Red blood cell transmembrane oxalate flux in calcium-oxalate nephrolithiasis. *Contrib Nephrol* **49**:118, 1985.
12. Baggio B, Gambaro G, Marchini F, Cicerello E, Tenconi R, Clementi M, Borsatti A: An inheritable anomaly of red-cell oxalate transport in "primary" calcium nephrolithiasis correctable with diuretics. *New Engl J Med* **314**:599, 1986.
13. Baggio B, Gambaro G, Marchini F, Cicerello E, Borsatti A: Raised transmembrane oxalate flux in red blood cells in idiopathic calcium oxalate nephrolithiasis. *Lancet* **2**:12, 1984.
14. Yendt ER: Hyperoxaluria in idiopathic calcium oxalate nephrolithiasis. *Md Med J* **37**:857, 1988.
15. Barratt TM, Danpure CJ: Hyperoxaluria, in Holliday MA, Barratt TM, Avner ED (eds): *Pediatric Nephrology.* Baltimore, Williams & Wilkins, 1994, p 557.
16. Danpure CJ, Purdue PE: Primary hyperoxaluria, in Scriver CR, Beaudet AL, Sly WS, Valle D (eds): *The Metabolic and Molecular Bases of Inherited Disease*, 7th ed. New York, McGraw-Hill, 1995, p 2385.
17. Danpure CJ, Smith LH: The primary hyperoxalurias, in Coe FL, Favus MJ, Pak CY, Parks JH, Preminger GM (eds): *Kidney Stones: Medical and Surgical Management*. Philadelphia, Lippincott-Raven, 1996, p 859.
18. Proceedings of the Third Workshop on Primary Hyperoxaluria, Lyon, France, October 21-22, 1994. *Nephrol Dial Transplant* **10**(suppl 8):1, 1995.
19. Proceedings of the Fourth Workshop on Primary Hyperoxaluria, Torino, Italy, March 7-8, 1997. *J Nephrol* **11**(suppl 1):1, 1998.
20. Lepoutre C: Calculs multiples chez un enfant: Infiltration du parenchyme renal par des depots cristallins. *J Urol* **20**:424, 1925.
21. Davis JS, Klingberg WG, Stowell RE: Nephrolithiasis and nephrocalcinosis with calcium oxalate crystals in kidneys and bones. *J Pediatr* **36**:323, 1950.
22. Archer HE, Dormer AE, Scowen EF, Watts RW: Primary hyperoxaluria. *Lancet* **2**:320, 1957.
23. Williams HE, Smith LH Jr. L-Glyceric aciduria: A new genetic variant of primary hyperoxaluria. *New Engl J Med* **278**:233, 1968.
24. Wyngaarden JB, Elder TD: Primary hyperoxaluria and oxalosis, in Stanbury JB, Wyngaarden JB, Fredrickson DS (eds): *The Metabolic Basis of Inherited Disease*. New York, McGraw-Hill, 1966, p 189.

25. Williams HE, Smith LH Jr: Primary hyperoxaluria, in Stanbury JB, Wyngaarden JB, Fredrickson DS, Goldstein JL, Brown MS (eds): *The Metabolic Basis of Inherited Disease*. New York, McGraw-Hill, 1983, p 204.
26. Hillman RE: Primary hyperoxalurias, in Scriver CR, Beaudet AL, Sly WS, Valle D (eds): *The Metabolic Basis of Inherited Disease*. New York, McGraw-Hill, 1989, p 933.
27. Hockaday TDR, Clayton JE, Frederick EW, Smith LH Jr: Primary hyperoxaluria. *Medicine* **43**:315, 1964.
28. Latta K, Brodehl J: Primary hyperoxaluria type I. *Eur J Pediatr* **149**:518, 1990.
29. Boquist L, Lindqvist B, Ostberg Y, Steen L: Primary oxalosis. *Am J Med* **54**:673, 1973.
30. Hall HE, Scowen EF, Watts RW: Clinical manifestations of primary hyperoxaluria. *Arch Dis Child* **35**:108, 1960.
31. Verbruggen LA, Bourgain C, Verbeelen D: Late presentation and microcrystalline arthropathy in primary hyperoxaluria. *Clin Exp Rheumatol* **7**:631, 1989.
32. Cochran M, Hodgkinson A, Zarembski PM, Anderson CK: Hyperoxaluria in adults. *Br J Surg* **55**:121, 1968.
33. Helin I: Primary hyperoxaluria: An analysis of 17 Scandinavian patients. *Scand J Urol Nephrol* **14**:61, 1980.
34. Danpure CJ: Molecular and clinical heterogeneity in primary hyperoxaluria type 1. *Am J Kidney Dis* **17**:366, 1991.
35. Cochat P, Deloraine A, Rotily M, Olive F, Liponski I, Deries N: Epidemiology of primary hyperoxaluria type 1: Societe de Nephrologie and the Societe de Nephrologie Pediatrique. *Nephrol Dial Transplant* **10**(suppl 8):3, 1995.
36. Milliner DS, Wilson DM, Smith LH: Clinical expression and long-term outcomes of primary hyperoxaluria types 1 and 2. *J Nephrol* **11**(suppl 1): 56, 1998.
37. Morgan SH, Purkiss P, Watts RW, Mansell MA: Oxalate dynamics in chronic renal failure: Comparison with normal subjects and patients with primary hyperoxaluria. *Nephron* **46**:253, 1987.
38. Schnitzler CM, Kok JA, Jacobs DW, Thomson PD, Milne FJ, Mesquita JM, King PC, et al: Skeletal manifestations of primary oxalosis. *Pediatr Nephrol* **5**:193, 1991.
39. Streefland M, Donckerwolcke RA: Vitamin B_6-resistant primary hyperoxaluria type I: Report of 5 cases. *Helv Paediatr Acta* **43**:313, 1989.
40. Mathews M, Stauffer M, Cameron EC, Maloney N, Sherrard DJ: Bone biopsy to diagnose hyperoxaluria in patients with renal failure. *Ann Intern Med* **90**:777, 1979.
41. Day DL, Scheinman JI, Mahan J: Radiological aspects of primary hyperoxaluria. *AJR* **146**:395, 1986.
42. Benhamou CL, Pierre D, Geslin N, Viala JF, Maitre F, Chavassieux P, Edouard C, et al: Primary bone oxalosis: The roles of oxalate deposits and renal osteodystrophy. *Bone* **8**:59, 1987.
43. Martijn A, Thijn CJ: Radiologic findings in primary hyperoxaluria. *Skeletal Radiol* **8**:21, 1982.
44. Marangella M, Vitale C, Petrarulo M, Tricerri A, Cerelli E, Cadario A, Barbos MP, et al: Bony content of oxalate in patients with primary hyperoxaluria or oxalosis-unrelated renal failure. *Kidney Int* **48**:182, 1995.
45. Vichi GF, Bongini U, Seracini D, Lavoratti GC: Progression of bone lesions in a child with primary hyperoxaluria type 1: Evaluation by roentgenology and MRI. *Pediatr Radiol* **25**(suppl 1):S102, 1995.
46. Haqqani MT: Crystals in brain and meninges in primary hyperoxaluria and oxalosis. *J Clin Pathol* **30**:16, 1977.
47. Di Pasquale G, Ribani M, Andreoli A, Zampa GA, Pinelli G: Cardioembolic stroke in primary oxalosis with cardiac involvement. *Stroke* **20**:1403, 1989.
48. Tonkin AM, Mond HG, Mathew TH, Sloman JG: Primary oxalosis with myocardial involvement and heart block. *Med J Aust* **1**:873, 1976.
49. Coltart DJ, Hudson RE: Primary oxalosis of the heart: A cause of heart block. *Br Heart J* **33**:315, 1971.
50. Spiers EM, Sanders DY, Omura EF: Clinical and histologic features of primary oxalosis. *J Am Acad Dermatol* **22**:952, 1990.
51. Saatci U, Ozdemir S, Besbas N, Ozen S, Erbay A, Bakkaloglu A, Kotiloglu E, et al: Late cardiac and vascular complications of primary hyperoxaluria in childhood (letter). *Pediatr Nephrol* **10**:677, 1996.
52. Greer KE, Cooper PH, Campbell F, Westervelt FB Jr: Primary oxalosis with livedo reticularis. *Arch Dermatol* **116**:213, 1980.
53. Smeenk G, Vink R: Calcinosis cutis metastatica in a patient with primary hyperoxaluria. *Dermatologica* **134**:356, 1967.
54. Freiberg AA, Fish DN, Louis DS: Hand manifestations of oxalosis. *J Hand Surg Am* **18**:140, 1993.
55. Somach SC, Davis BR, Paras FĄ, Petrelli M, Behmer ME: Fatal cutaneous necrosis mimicking calciphylaxis in a patient with type 1 primary hyperoxaluria. *Arch Dermatol* **131**:821, 1995.
56. Plorer A, Zelger B: Acute livedo racemosa in a patient with type 1 primary hyperoxaluria (letter). *Arch Dermatol* **132**:349, 1996.
57. Farreli J, Shoemaker JD, Otti T, Jordan W, Schoch L, Neu LT, Bastani B: Primary hyperoxaluria in an adult with renal failure, livedo reticularis, retinopathy, and peripheral neuropathy. *Am J Kidney Dis* **29**:947, 1997.
58. Canavese C, Salomone M, Massara C, Portigliatti Barbos M, Cadario A, Pavan I, Marangella M, et al: Primary oxalosis mimicking hyperparathyroidism diagnosed after long-term hemodialysis. *Am J Nephrol* **10**:344, 1990.
59. Stull MA, Glass Royal M: Musculoskeletal case of the day: Primary oxalosis with renal osteodystrophy. *AJR* **154**:1334, 1990.
60. Leumann EP: Primary hyperoxaluria: An important cause of renal failure in infancy. *Int J Pediatr Nephrol* **6**:13, 1985.
61. de Zegher FE, Wolff ED, van den Heijden J, Sukhai RN: Oxalosis in infancy. *Clin Nephrol* **22**:114, 1984.
62. Morris MC, Chambers TL, Evans PW, Malleson PN, Pincott JR, Rose GA: Oxalosis in infancy. *Arch Dis Child* **57**:224, 1982.
63. Srinivas HN, Ramkumar C: Primary hyperoxaluria in infancy. *Australas Radiol* **30**:332, 1986.
64. Giugliani R, Jardim L, Edelweiss MI, Rosa A: Early and unusual presentation of type I primary hyperoxaluria. *Child Nephrol Urol* **10**:107, 1990.
65. Rinaldi S, Rizzoni G: Clinical quiz: Primary hyperoxaluria (PH) type 1. *Pediatr Nephrol* **5**:365, 1991.
66. Brennan JN, Diwan RV, Makker SP, Cromer BA, Bellon EM: Ultrasonic diagnosis of primary hyperoxaluria in infancy. *Radiology* **145**:147, 1982.
67. Leumann EP, Niederwieser A, Fanconi A: New aspects of infantile oxalosis. *Pediatr Nephrol* **1**:531, 1987.
68. Barratt TM, von Sperling V, Dillon MJ, Rose GA, Trompeter RS: Primary hyperoxaluria in children, in Rose GA (ed): *Oxalate Metabolism in Relation to Urinary Stones*. London, Springer-Verlag, 1988, p 83.
69. Chalmers RA, Tracey BM, Mistry J, Griffiths KD, Green A, Winterborn MH: l-Glyceric aciduria (primary hyperoxaluria type 2) in siblings in two unrelated families. *J Inherited Metab Dis* **7**(suppl 2):133, 1984.
70. Seargeant LE, deGroot GW, Dilling LA, Mallory CJ, Haworth JC: Primary oxaluria type 2 (L-glyceric aciduria): A rare cause of nephrolithiasis in children. *J Pediatr* **118**:912, 1991.
71. Mateos Anton F, Garcia Puig J, Jimenez Ortiz A, Perez Castro E, Gomez Mantilla JM: Type 2 primary hyperoxaluria: Description of 2 cases and therapeutic results. *Med Clin Barc* **88**:810, 1987 (in Spanish).
72. Kemper MJ, Conrad S, Muller Wiefel DE: Primary hyperoxaluria type 2. *Eur J Pediatr* **156**:509, 1997.
73. Vilarinho L, Araujo R, Vilarinho A, Pereira E, Abdo K, Bardet J, Parvy P, et al: A new case of hyperoxaluria type II. *J Inherit Metab Dis* **16**:896, 1993.
74. Hicks NR, Cranston DW, Charlton CA: Fifteen-year follow-up of hyperoxaluria type II (letter). *New Engl J Med* **309**:796, 1983.
75. Chlebeck PT, Milliner DS, Smith LH: Long-term prognosis in primary hyperoxaluria type II (l-glyceric aciduria). *Am J Kidney Dis* **23**:255, 1994.
76. Sonmez F, Mir S, Cura A: Nephrocalcinosis in a patient with primary hyperoxaluria type 2 (letter). *Pediatr Nephrol* **11**:265, 1997.
77. Kemper MJ, Muller Wiefel DE: Nephrocalcinosis in a patient with primary hyperoxaluria type 2. *Pediatr Nephrol* **10**:442, 1996.
78. Marangella M, Petrarulo M, Cosseddu D: End-stage renal failure in primary hyperoxaluria type 2 (letter). *New Engl J Med* **330**:1690, 1994.
79. Mansell MA: Primary hyperoxaluria type 2. *Nephrol Dial Transplant* **10**(suppl 8):58, 1995.
80. Hockaday TDR, Frederick EW, Clayton JE, Smith LH Jr: Studies on primary hyperoxaluria: II. Urinary oxalate, glycolate, and glyoxylate measurement by isotope dilution method. *J Lab Clin Med* **65**:677, 1965.
81. Crawhall JC, Watts RW: The oxalate content of human plasma. *Clin Sci* **20**:357, 1961.
82. Constable AR, Joekes AM, Kasidas GP, O Regan P, Rose GA: Plasma level and renal clearance of oxalate in normal subjects and in patients with primary hyperoxaluria or chronic renal failure or both. *Clin Sci* **56**:299, 1979.

83. Kasidas GP, Nemat S, Rose GA: Plasma oxalate and creatinine and oxalate/creatinine clearance ratios in normal subjects and in primary hyperoxaluria: Evidence for renal hyperoxaluria. *Clin Chim Acta* **191**:67, 1990.
84. Zarembski PM, Hodgkinson A: The renal clearance of oxalic acid in normal subjects and in patients with primary hyperoxaluria. *Invest Urol* **1**:87, 1963.
85. Boer P, Prenen JA, Koomans HA, Dorhout Mees EJ: Fractional oxalate clearance in subjects with normal and impaired renal function. *Nephron* **41**:78, 1985.
86. Tomson CR, Channon SM, Ward MK, Laker MF: Plasma oxalate concentration, oxalate clearance and cardiac function in patients receiving haemodialysis. *Nephrol Dial Transplant* **4**:792, 1989.
87. Borland WW, Payton CD, Simpson K, Macdougall AI: Serum oxalate in chronic renal failure. *Nephron* **45**:119, 1987.
88. Kasidas GP, Rose GA: Measurement of plasma oxalate in healthy subjects and in patients with chronic renal failure using immobilised oxalate oxidase. *Clin Chim Acta* **154**:49, 1986.
89. Tomson CR, Channon SM, Parkinson IS, Morley AR, Lennard TW, Parrott NR, Laker MF: Plasma oxalate concentration and secondary oxalosis in patients with chronic renal failure. *J Clin Pathol* **41**:1107, 1988.
90. Mitwalli A, Oreopoulos DG: Hyperoxaluria and hyperoxalemia: One more concern for the nephrologist. *Int J Artif Organs* **8**:71, 1985.
91. Petrarulo M, Marangella M, Linari F: High-performance liquid chromatographic determination of plasma glycolic acid in healthy subjects and in cases of hyperoxaluria syndromes. *Clin Chim Acta* **196**:17, 1991.
92. Rose GA: Mild metabolic hyperoxaluria: A new syndrome, in Rose GA (ed): *Oxalate Metabolism in Relation to Urinary Stones*. London, Springer-Verlag, 1988, p 121.
93. Gill HS, Rose GA: Mild metabolic hyperoxaluria and its response to pyridoxine. *Urol Int* **41**:393, 1986.
94. Williams HE, Smith LH Jr: The identification and determination of glyceric acid in human urine. *J Lab Clin Med* **71**:495, 1968.
95. Scheid CR, Koul HK, Kennington L, Hill WA, Luber Narod J, Jonassen J, Honeyman T, et al: Oxalate-induced damage to renal tubular cells. *Scanning Microsc* **9**:1097, 1995.
96. Nisselbaum JS, Packer DE, Bodansky O: Comparison of the actions of human brain, liver and heart lactic dehydrogenase variants on nucleotide analogues and on substrate analogues in the absence and the presence of oxalate and oxamate. *J Biol Chem* **239**:2830, 1964.
97. Novoa WB, Winer AD, Glaid AJ, Schwert GW: Lactic dehydrogenase: V. Inhibition by oxalate and oxamate. *J Biol Chem* **234**:1143, 1959.
98. Ottolenghi P, Denstedt OF: Mechanism of action of the lactic dehydrogenase of the mammalian erythrocyte: I. Influence of inhibitors. *Can J Biochem Physiol* **36**:1075, 1958.
99. Reed GH, Morgan SD: Kinetic and magnetic resonance studies of the interaction of oxalate with pyruvate kinase. *Biochemistry* **13**:3537, 1974.
100. Seubert W, Huth W: On the mechanism of gluconeogenesis and its regulation: II. The mechanism of gluconeogenesis from pyruvate and fumarate. *Biochem Z* **343**:176, 1965.
101. Laxmanan S, Selvam R, Mahle CJ, Menon M: Binding of oxalate to mitochondrial inner membranes of rat and human kidney. *J Urol* **135**:862, 1986.
102. Strzelecki T, Menon M: The uptake of oxalate by rat liver and kidney mitochondria. *J Biol Chem* **261**:12197, 1986.
103. Strzelecki T, McGraw BR, Scheid CR, Menon M: Effect of oxalate on function of kidney mitochondria. *J Urol* **141**:423, 1989.
104. Koul H, Kennington L, Nair G, Honeyman T, Menon M, Scheid C: Oxalate-induced initiation of DNA synthesis in LLC-PK1 cells, a line of renal epithelial cells. *Biochem Biophys Res Commun* **205**:1632, 1994.
105. Koul H, Kennington L, Honeyman T, Jonassen J, Menon M, Scheid C: Activation of *c-myc* gene mediates the mitogenic effects of oxalate in LLC-PK1 cells, a line of renal epithelial cells. *Kidney Int* **50**:1525, 1996.
106. Scheid C, Koul H, Hill WA, Luber Narod J, Jonassen J, Honeyman T, Kennington L, et al: Oxalate toxicity in LLC-PK1 cells, a line of renal epithelial cells. *J Urol* **155**:1112, 1996.
107. Scheid C, Koul H, Hill WA, Luber Narod J, Kennington L, Honeyman T, Jonassen J, et al: Oxalate toxicity in LLC-PK1 cells: Role of free radicals. *Kidney Int* **49**:413, 1996.
108. Thamilselvan S, Khan SR: Oxalate and calcium oxalate crystals are injurious to renal epithelial cells: Results of in vivo and in vitro studies. *J Nephrol* **11**(suppl 1):66, 1998.
109. Bigelow MW, Wiessner JH, Kleinman JG, Mandel NS: The dependence on membrane fluidity of calcium oxalate crystal attachment to IMCD membranes. *Calcif Tissue Int* **60**:375, 1997.
110. Bigelow MW, Wiessner JH, Kleinman JG, Mandel NS: Surface exposure of phosphatidylserine increases calcium oxalate crystal attachment to IMCD cells. *Am J Physiol* **272**:F55, 1997.
111. Hackett RL, Shevock PN, Khan SR: Madin-Darby canine kidney cells are injured by exposure to oxalate and to calcium oxalate crystals (editorial). *Urol Res* **22**:197, 1994.
112. Hammes MS, Lieske JC, Pawar S, Spargo BH, Toback FG: Calcium oxalate monohydrate crystals stimulate gene expression in renal epithelial cells. *Kidney Int* **48**:501, 1995.
113. Kohjimoto Y, Ebisuno S, Tamura M, Ohkawa T: Interactions between calcium oxalate monohydrate crystals and Madin-Darby canine kidney cells: endocytosis and cell proliferation. *Urol Res* **24**:193, 1996.
114. Barnes RH, Lerner A: Metabolism of glycolic and glyoxylic acids. *Proc Soc Exp Biol* **52**:216, 1943.
115. Ruffo A, Romano M, Adinolfi A: Inhibition of aconitase by glyoxylate plus oxaloacetate. *Biochem J* **72**:613, 1959.
116. D'Abramo F, Romano M, Ruffo A: Inhibition of citrate oxidation by glyoxylate in rat liver homogenates. *Biochem J* **68**:270, 1958.
117. Kawasaki H, Okuyama M, Kikuchi G: Alpha-ketoglutarate-dependent oxidation of glyoxylic acid in rat-liver mitochondria. *J Biochem (Tokyo)* **59**:419, 1966.
118. O'Fallon JV, Brosemer RW: Cellular localization of alpha-ketoglutarate: Glyoxylate carboligase in rat tissues. *Biochim Biophys Acta* **499**:321, 1977.
119. Schlossberg MA, Bloom RJ, Richert DA, Westerfield WW: Carboligase activity of alpha-ketoglutarate dehydrogenase. *Biochemistry* **9**:1148, 1970.
120. Crawhall JC, Watts RW: The metabolism of glyoxylate by human and rat liver mitochondria. *Biochem J* **85**:163, 1962.
121. Fujii S, Sato Y, Kaneko T: The inhibition of human erythrocyte pyruvate kinase by a high concentration of glycolate. *Blood* **72**:1097, 1988.
122. Rizzoni G, Broyer M, Brunner FP, Brynger H, Challah S, Kramer P, Oules R, Selwood NH, Wing AJ, Balas EA: Combined report on regular dialysis and transplantation of children in Europe, XIII, 1983. *Proc Eur Dial Transplant Assoc Eur Ren Assoc* **21**:69, 1984.
123. Kopp N, Leumann E: Changing pattern of primary hyperoxaluria in Switzerland. *Nephrol Dial Transplant* **10**:2224, 1995.
124. Marangella M, Petrarulo M, Cosseddu D, Vitale C, Cadario A, Barbos MP, Gurioli L, Linari F: Detection of primary hyperoxaluria type 2 (L-glyceric aciduria) in patients with maintained renal function or end-stage renal failure. *Nephrol Dial Transplant* **10**:1381, 1995.
125. Holmgren G, Hornstrom T, Johansson S, Samuelson G: Primary hyperoxaluria (glycolic acid variant): A clinical and genetical investigation of eight cases. *Ups J Med Sci* **83**:65, 1978.
126. Watts RW, Chalmers RA, Gibbs DA, Lawson AM, Purkiss P, Spellacy E: Studies on some possible biochemical treatments of primary hyperoxaluria. *Q J Med* **48**:259, 1979.
127. Archer HE, Dormer AE, Scowen EF, Watts RW: Observations on the possible genetic basis of primary hyperoxaluria. *Ann Hum Genet* **22**:373, 1958.
128. Shepard TH, Lou-sein W, Lee MS, Krebs EG: Primary hyperoxaluria: II. Genetics studies in a family. *Pediatrics* **25**:25, 1960.
129. Yano S, Yoshino M, Nishiyori A, Nakao M, Matsumoto T, Ito Y, Yamashita F, Shimada A, Inokuchi T: Hyperoxaluria type I: Therapeutic effects of pyridoxine hydrochloride and inheritance patterns of the disease in a family. *Kurume Med J* **35**:127, 1988.
130. Scowen EF, Watts RW, Hall EG: Further observations on the genetic basis of primary hyperoxaluria. *Ann Hum Genet* **23**:367, 1959.
131. Witzleben CL, Elliott JS: Hereditary hyperoxaluria: Study of a family. *Am J Dis Child* **111**:56, 1966.
132. Hoppe B, Danpure CJ, Rumsby G, Fryer P, Jennings PR, Blau N, Schubiger G, Neuhaus T, Leumann E: A vertical (pseudodominant) pattern of inheritance in the autosomal recessive disease primary hyperoxaluria type 1: Lack of relationship between genotype, enzymic phenotype and disease severity. *Am J Kidney Dis* **29**:36, 1997.
133. Archer HE, Dormer AE, Scowen EF, Watts RW: Studies on the urinary excretion of oxalate by normal subjects. *Clin Sci* **16**:405, 1957.
134. Zarembski PM, Hodgkinson A: Some factors influencing the urinary excretion of oxalic acid in man. *Clin Chim Acta* **25**:1, 1969.
135. Marshall RW, Cochran M, Hodgkinson A: Relationships between calcium and oxalic acid intake in the diet and their excretion in the urine of normal and renal-stone-forming subjects. *Clin Sci* **43**:91, 1972.

136. Chadwick VS, Modha K, Dowling RH: Mechanism for hyperoxaluria in patients with ileal dysfunction. *New Engl J Med* **289**:172, 1973.
137. Holmes RP, Goodman HO, Assimos DG: Dietary oxalate and its intestinal absorption. *Scanning Microsc* **9**:1109, 1995.
138. Holmes RP, Goodman HO, Assimos DG: Metabolic effects of an oxalate-free formula diet, in Pak CY, Resnick MI, Preminger GM (eds): *Urolithiasis 1996 (Proceedings of the 8th International Symposium on Urolithiasis)*. Dallas, Millet the Printer, 1996, p 167.
139. Richardson KE, Tolbert NE: Oxidation of glyoxylic acid to oxalic acid by glycolic acid oxidase. *J Biol Chem* **236**:1280, 1961.
140. Elder TD, Wyngaarden JB: The biosynthesis and turnover of oxalate in normal and hyperoxaluric subjects. *J Clin Invest* **39**:1337, 1960.
141. Hodgkinson A, Wilkinson R: Plasma oxalate concentration and renal excretion of oxalate in man. *Clin Sci Mol Med* **46**:61, 1974.
142. James HM, Bais R, Edwards JB, Rofe AM, Conyers AJ: Models for the metabolic production of oxalate from xylitol in humans: a role for fructokinase and aldolase. *Aust J Exp Biol Med Sci* **60**:117, 1982.
143. Rofe AM, James HM, Bais R, Edwards JB, Conyers RA: The production of [^{14}C]oxalate during the metabolism of [^{14}C]carbohydrates in isolated rat hepatocytes. *Aust J Exp Biol Med Sci* **58**:103, 1980.
144. Atkins GL, Dean BM, Griffin WJ, Scowen EF, Watts RW: Primary hyperoxaluria: The relation between ascorbic acid and the increased urinary excretion of oxalate. *Lancet* **2**:1096, 1963.
145. Crawhall JC, de Mowbray RR, Scowen EF, Watts RW: Conversion of glycine to oxalate in a normal subject. *Lancet* **2**:810, 1959.
146. Atkins GL, Dean BM, Griffin WJ, Scowen EF, Watts RW: Quantitative aspects of ascorbic acid metabolism in patients with primary hyperoxaluria. *Clin Sci* **29**:305, 1965.
147. Baker EM, Saari JC, Tolbert BM: Ascorbic acid metabolism in man. *Am J Clin Nutr* **19**:371, 1966.
148. Lamden MP, Chrystowski GA: Urinary oxalate excretion by man following ascorbic acid ingestion. *Proc Soc Exp Biol Med* **85**:190, 1954.
149. Takiguchi H, Furuyama S, Shimazono N: Urinary oxalic acid excretion by man following ingestion of large amounts of ascorbic acid. *J Vitaminol (Kyoto)* **12**:307, 1966.
150. Gambardella RL, Richardson KE: The formation of oxalate from hydroxypyruvate, serine, glycolate and glyoxylate in the rat. *Biochim Biophys Acta* **544**:315, 1978.
151. Hauschildt S, Chalmers RA, Lawson AM, Schultis K, Watts RW: Metabolic investigations after xylitol infusion in human subjects. *Am J Clin Nutr* **29**:258, 1976.
152. Hauschildt S, Watts RW: Studies on the effect of xylitol on oxalate formation. *Biochem Pharmacol* **25**:27, 1976.
153. Farinelli MP, Richardson KE: Oxalate synthesis from [^{14}C1]glycollate and [^{14}C1]glyoxylate in the hepatectomized rat. *Biochim Biophys Acta* **757**:8, 1983.
154. Liao LL, Richardson KE: The metabolism of oxalate precursors in isolated perfused rat livers. *Arch Biochem Biophys* **153**:438, 1972.
155. Liao LL, Richardson KE: The synthesis of oxalate from hydroxypyruvate by isolated perfused rat liver: The mechanism of hyperoxaluria in L-glyceric aciduria. *Biochim Biophys Acta* **538**:76, 1978.
156. Asker H, Davies D: Purification of rat liver enzymes involved in the oxidation of glyoxylate. *Biochim Biophys Acta* **761**:103, 1983.
157. Weinhouse S, Friedmann B: Metabolism of labelled 2-carbon acids in the intact rat. *J Biol Chem* **191**:707, 1951.
158. Ratner S, Nocito V, Green DE: Glycine oxidase. *J Biol Chem* **152**:119, 1944.
159. James HM, Williams SG, Bais R, Rofe AM, Edwards JB, Conyers RA: The metabolic production of oxalate from xylitol: activities of transketolase, transaldolase, fructokinase and aldolase in liver, kidney, brain, heart and muscle in the rat, mouse, guinea pig, rabbit and human. *Int J Vitam Nutr Res Suppl* **28**:29, 1985.
160. Bais R, Nairn JM, Rofe AM, Conyers RA: Enzymology of endogenous oxalate formation. *Adv Clin Enzymol* **5**:43, 1987.
161. Fry DW, Richardson KE: Isolation and characterization of glycolic acid dehydrogenase from human liver. *Biochim Biophys Acta* **567**:482, 1979.
162. Williams HE, Johnson GA, Smith LH Jr: The renal clearance of oxalate in normal subjects and patients with primary hyperoxaluria. *Clin Sci* **41**:213, 1971.
163. Cattell WR, Spencer AG, Taylor GW, Watts RW: The mechanism of the renal excretion of oxalate in the dog. *Clin Sci* **22**:43, 1962.
164. McIntosh GH, Belling GB: An isotopic study of oxalate excretion in sheep. *Aust J Exp Biol Med Sci* **53**:479, 1975.
165. Allison MJ, Cook HM, Milne DB, Gallagher S, Clayman RV: Oxalate degradation by gastrointestinal bacteria from humans. *J Nutr* **116**:455, 1986.
166. Marangella M, Petrarulo M, Vitale C: Biochemical diagnosis of primary hyperoxalurias, in Jungers P, Daudon M (eds): *Renal Stone Disease: Crystallization Process, Pathophysiology, Metabolic Disorders and Prevention*. Amsterdam, Elsevier, 1997, p 41.
167. Masters C, Holmes R: Peroxisomes: New aspects of cell physiology and biochemistry. *Physiol Rev* **57**:816, 1977.
168. Schuman M, Massey V: Purification and characterization of glycolic acid oxidase from pig liver. *Biochim Biophys Acta* **227**:500, 1971.
169. Nakano M, Ushijima Y, Saga M, Tsutsumi Y, Asami H: Aliphatic L-alpha-hydroxyacid oxidase from rat livers: Purification and properties. *Biochim Biophys Acta* **167**:9, 1968.
170. McGroarty E, Hsieh B, Wied DM, Gee R, Tolbert NE: Alpha hydroxy acid oxidation by peroxisomes. *Arch Biochem Biophys* **161**:194, 1974.
171. Tolbert NE: Peroxisomal redox enzymes. *Methods Enzymol* **52**:493, 1978.
172. Neims AH, Hellerman L: Specificity of the D-amino acid oxidase in relation to glycine oxidase activity. *J Biol Chem* **237**:976, 1962.
173. Dixon M, Kleppe K: D-Amino acid oxidase: II. Specificity, competitive inhibition and reaction sequence. *Biochim Biophys Acta* **96**:368, 1965.
174. Poore RE, Hurst CH, Assimos DG, Holmes RP: Pathways of hepatic oxalate synthesis and their regulation. *Am J Physiol* **272**:C289, 1997.
175. Holmes RP: Pharmacological approaches in the treatment of primary hyperoxaluria. *J Nephrol* **11**(suppl 1):32, 1998.
176. De Duve C, Baudhuin P: Peroxisomes (microbodies and related particles). *Physiol Rev* **46**:323, 1966.
177. Hayashi H, Taya K, Suga T, Niinobe S: Studies on peroxisomes: VI. Relationship between the peroxisomal core and urate oxidase. *J Biochem (Tokyo)* **79**:1029, 1976.
178. Gershoff SN, Faragalla FF, Nelson DA, Andrus SB: Vitamin B_6 deficiency and oxalate nephrocalcinosis in the cat. *Am J Med* **27**:72, 1959.
179. Gershoff SN: Vitamin B_6 and oxalate metabolism. *Vitamins Hormone* **22**:581, 1964.
180. Gershoff SN, Mayer AL, Kulczycki LL: Effect of pyridoxine administration on the urinary excretion of oxalic acid, pyridoxine, and related compounds in mongoloids and nonmongoloids. *Am J Clin Nutr* **7**:76, 1959.
181. Gershoff SN, Faragalla FF: Endogenous oxalate synthesis and glycine, serine, deoxypyridoxine interrelationships in vitamin B_6-deficient rats. *J Biol Chem* **234**:2391, 1959.
182. Faber SR, Feitler WW, Bleiler RE, Ohlson MA, Hodges RE: The effects of an induced pyridoxine and pantothenic acid deficiency on excretion of oxalic and xanthurenic acids in the urine. *Am J Clin Nutr* **12**:406, 1963.
183. Thompson JS, Richardson KE: Isolation and characterization of an L-alanine: Glyoxylate aminotransferase from human liver. *J Biol Chem* **242**:3614, 1967.
184. Thompson JS, Richardson KE: Isolation and characterization of glutamate: Glycine transaminase from human liver. *Arch Biochem Biophys* **117**:599, 1966.
185. Kamoda N, Minatogawa Y, Nakamura M, Nakanishi J, Okuno E, Kido R: The organ distribution of human alanine-2-oxoglutarate aminotransferase and alanine-glyoxylate aminotransferase. *Biochem Med* **23**:25, 1980.
186. Noguchi T, Takada Y: Peroxisomal localization of alanine:glyoxylate aminotransferase in human liver. *Arch Biochem Biophys* **196**:645, 1979.
187. Cooper PJ, Danpure CJ, Wise PJ, Guttridge KM: Immunocytochemical localization of human hepatic alanine:glyoxylate aminotransferase in control subjects and patients with primary hyperoxaluria type 1. *J Histochem Cytochem* **36**:1285, 1988.
188. Yokota S, Oda T, Ichiyama A: Immunocytochemical localization of serine:pyruvate aminotransferase in peroxisomes of the human liver parenchymal cells. *Histochemistry* **87**:601, 1987.
189. Noguchi T, Takada Y, Kido R: Glutamate-glyoxylate aminotransferase in rat liver cytosol: Purification, properties and identity with alanine-2-oxoglutarate aminotransferase. *Hoppe Seylers Z Physiol Chem* **358**:1533, 1977.
190. Rowsell EV, Snell K, Carnie JA, Rowsell KV: The subcellular distribution of rat liver l-alanine-glyoxylate aminotransferase in relation to a pathway for glucose formation involving glyoxylate. *Biochem J* **127**:155, 1972.

191. Suzuki S, Suga T, Niinobe S: Studies on peroxisomes: 4. Intracellular localization of $NADH_2$-glyoxylate reductase in rat liver. *J Biochem* **73**:1033, 1973.
192. Sawaki S, Yamada K: Glyoxylate reductase activity of lactate dehydrogenase. *J Vitaminol (Kyoto)* **11**:294, 1965.
193. Sawaki S, Hattori H, Yamada K: Glyoxylate dehydrogenase activity of lactate dehydrogenase. *J Biochem (Tokyo)* **62**:263, 1967.
194. Sawaki S, Hattori N, Morikawa N, Yamada K: Oxidation and reduction of glyoxylate by lactate dehydrogenase. *J Vitaminol (Kyoto)* **13**:93, 1967.
195. Duncan RJ: The disproportionation of glyoxylate by lactate dehydrogenase. *Arch Biochem Biophys* **201**:128, 1980.
196. Duncan RJ, Tipton KF: The oxidation and reduction of glyoxylate by lactate dehydrogenase. *Eur J Biochem* **11**:58, 1969.
197. Romano M, Cerra A: The action of crystalline lactate dehydrogenase from rabbit muscle on glyoxylate. *Biochim Biophys Acta* **177**:421, 1969.
198. Warren WA: Catalysis of both oxidation and reduction of glyoxylate by pig heart lactate dehydrogenase isozyme 1. *J Biol Chem* **245**:1675, 1970.
199. Gibbs DA, Watts RW: The identification of the enzymes that catalyse the oxidation of glyoxylate to oxalate in the 100,000 g supernatant fraction of human hyperoxaluric and control liver and heart tissue. *Clin Sci* **44**:227, 1973.
200. Gibbs DA, Watts RW: An investigation of the possible role of xanthine oxidase in the oxidation of glyoxylate to oxalate. *Clin Sci* **31**:285, 1966.
201. Gibbs DA, Watts RW: Biochemical studies on the treatment of primary hyperoxaluria. *Arch Dis Child* **42**:505, 1967.
202. Yanagawa M, Maeda Nakai E, Yamakawa K, Yamamoto I, Kawamura J, Tada S, Ichiyama A: The formation of oxalate from glycolate in rat and human liver. *Biochim Biophys Acta* **1036**:24, 1990.
203. Funai T, Ichiyama A: High-performance liquid chromatographic determination of glyoxylate in rat liver. *J Biochem (Tokyo)* **99**:579, 1986.
204. Smith LH, Bauer RL, Williams HE: Oxalate and glycolate synthesis by hemic cells. *J Lab Clin Med* **78**:245, 1971.
205. Liao LL, Richardson KE: The inhibition of oxalate biosynthesis in isolated perfused rat liver by dl-phenyllactate and *N*-heptanoate. *Arch Biochem Biophys* **154**:68, 1973.
206. Rofe AM, Chalmers AH, Edwards JB: [^{14}C]oxalate synthesis from [U-^{14}C]glyoxylate and [1-^{14}C]glycollate in isolated rat hepatocytes. *Biochem Med* **16**:277, 1976.
207. Richardson KE, Farinelli MP, Smith LH, Robertson WG, Finlayson B (eds): *Urolithiasis: Clinical and Basic Research.* New York, Plenum Press, 1981, p 855.
208. Richardson KE: Effect of testosterone on the glycolic acid oxidase levels in male and female rat liver. *Endocrinology* **74**:128, 1964.
209. Holmes RP, Hurst CH, Assimos DG, Goodman HO: Glucagon increases urinary oxalate excretion in the guinea pig. *Am J Physiol* **269**:E568, 1995.
210. Bais R, Rofe AM, Conyers RA: Inhibition of endogenous oxalate production: Biochemical considerations of the roles of glycollate oxidase and lactate dehydrogenase. *Clin Sci* **76**:303, 1989.
211. Crawhall JC, Watts RW: The metabolism of [1-^{14}C]glyoxylate by the liver mitochondria of patients with primary hyperoxaluria and non-hyperoxaluric subjects. *Clin Sci* **23**:163, 1962.
212. Koch J, Stokstad EL: Partial purification of a 2-oxoglutarate:glyoxylate carboligase from rat liver mitochondria. *Biochem Biophys Res Commun* **23**:585, 1966.
213. Danpure CJ, Purkiss P, Jennings PR, Watts RW: Mitochondrial damage and the subcellular distribution of 2-oxoglutarate:glyoxylate carboligase in normal human and rat liver and in the liver of a patient with primary hyperoxaluria type I. *Clin Sci* **70**:417, 1986.
214. Liang CC: Studies on experimental thiamine deficiency: Trends of keto acid formation and detection of glyoxylic acid. *Biochem J* **82**:429, 1962.
215. Hauschildt S, Rudolph R, Feldheim W: Oxalatstoffwechsel und Thiamin-Pyridoxin-Versorgung bei der Ratte. *Int J Vitam Nutr Res* **42**:457, 1972.
216. Buckle RM: The glyoxylic acid content of human blood and its relationship to thiamine deficiency. *Clin Sci* **257**:207, 1963.
217. Kornberg HL, Elsden SR: The metabolism of 2-carbon compounds by micro-organisms. *Adv Enzymol* **23**:401, 1961.
218. Kornberg HL: Anaplerotic sequences and their role in metabolism, in Campbell PN, Greville GD (eds): *Essays in Biochemistry.* London, Academic Press, 1966, p 1.
219. Kornberg HL: Travelling to, and along, the glyoxylate bypass: A commentary on "Synthesis of C4-dicarboxylic acids from acetate by a 'glyoxylate bypass' of the tricarboxylic acid cycle." *Biochim Biophys Acta* **1000**:271, 1989.
220. Kornberg HL, Madsen NB: Synthesis of C4-dicarboxylic acids from acetate by a "glyoxylate bypass" of the tricarboxylic acid cycle, 1957. *Biochim Biophys Acta* **1000**:275, 1989.
221. Tolbert NE: Metabolic pathways in peroxisomes and glyoxysomes. *Annu Rev Biochem* **50**:133, 1981.
222. Madsen NB: Test for isocitrase and malate synthetase in animal tissues. *Biochim Biophys Acta* **27**:199, 1958.
223. Brown VK, Box VL: Occurrence of the glyoxylate-shunt in the epidermis of rats. *Br J Dermatol* **80**:740, 1968.
224. Davis WL, Goodman DB, Crawford LA, Cooper OJ, Matthews JL: Hibernation activates glyoxylate cycle and gluconeogenesis in black bear brown adipose tissue. *Biochim Biophys Acta* **1051**:276, 1990.
225. Davis WL, Jones RG, Farmer GR, Cortinas E, Matthews JL, Goodman DB: The glyoxylate cycle in rat epiphyseal cartilage: The effect of vitamin D_3 on the activity of the enzymes isocitrate lyase and malate synthase. *Bone* **10**:201, 1989.
226. Davis WL, Jones RG, Farmer GR, Matthews JL, Goodman DB: Glyoxylate cycle in the epiphyseal growth plate: isocitrate lyase and malate synthase identified in mammalian cartilage. *Anat Rec* **223**:357, 1989.
227. Jones CT: Is there a glyoxylate cycle in the liver of the fetal guinea pig? *Biochem Biophys Res Commun* **95**:849, 1980.
228. Davis WL, Matthews JL, Goodman DB: Glyoxylate cycle in the rat liver: Effect of vitamin D_3 treatment. *FASEB J* **3**:1651, 1989.
229. Holmes RP: The absence of glyoxylate cycle enzymes in rodent and embryonic chick liver. *Biochim Biophys Acta* **1158**:47, 1993.
230. Dean BM, Watts RW, Westwick WJ: The conversion of (1-^{13}C)glycine and (2-^{13}C)glycine to (^{13}C)oxalate in primary hyperoxaluria: Evidence for the existence of more than one metabolic pathway from glycine to oxalate in man. *Clin Sci* **35**:325, 1968.
231. Rofe AM, James HM, Bais R, Conyers RA: Hepatic oxalate production: The role of hydroxypyruvate. *Biochem Med Metab Biol* **36**:141, 1986.
232. Dickens F, Williamson DH: Studies on the metabolism of hydroxypyruvate in animal tissues. *Biochem J* **72**:496, 1959.
233. Hedrick JL, Sallach HJ: The metabolism of hydroxypyruvate: II. The enzymatic oxidation and decarboxylation of hydroxypyruvate. *J Biol Chem* **236**:1872, 1961.
234. Fry DW, Richardson KE: Isolation and characterization of glycolic acid oxidase from human liver. *Biochim Biophys Acta* **568**:135, 1979.
235. Giafi CF, Rumsby G: Primary hyperoxaluria type 2: Enzymology. *J Nephrol* **11**(suppl 1):29, 1998.
236. Giafi CF, Rumsby G: Kinetic analysis and tissue distribution of human D-glycerate dehydrogenase/glyoxylare reductase and its relevance to the diagnosis of primary hyperoxaluria type 2. *Ann Clin Biochem* **35**:104, 1998.
237. Vamecq J, Draye JP: Pathophysiology of peroxisomal beta-oxidation. *Essays Biochem* **24**:115, 1989.
238. Holmes RP, Assimos DG: Glyoxylate synthesis, its modulation, and its influence on oxalate synthesis. *J Urol.* **160**:1617, 1998.
239. Koch J, Stokstad EL, Williams HE, Smith LH Jr: Deficiency of 2-oxo-glutarate:glyoxylate carboligase activity in primary hyperoxaluria. *Proc Natl Acad Sci USA* **57**:1123, 1967.
240. McKusick VA: *Mendelian Inheritance in Man: Catalogs of Autosomal Dominant, Autosomal Recessive and X-Linked Phenotypes.* Baltimore, John Hopkins University Press, 1986.
241. Bourke E, Frindt G, Flynn P, Schreiner GE: Primary hyperoxaluria with normal alpha-ketoglutarate: glyoxylate carboligase activity: Treatment with isocarboxazid. *Ann Intern Med* **76**:279, 1972.
242. Takasaki E: The urinary excretion of oxalic acid in vitamin B_1 deficient rats. *Invest Urol* **7**:150, 1969.
243. Williams HE, Smith LH Jr: Disorders of oxalate metabolism. *Am J Med* **45**:715, 1968.
244. Salyer WR, Salyer DC: Thiamine deficiency and oxalosis. *J Clin Pathol* **27**:558, 1974.
245. King JS, Lehner DM: Effects of some compounds on urinary oxalate excretion by the human and the squirrel monkey. *Invest Urol* **8**:391, 1971.
246. Smith LH Jr, Hockaday TD, Efron ML, Clayton JE: The metabolic defect of primary hyperoxaluria. *Trans Assoc Am Physicians* **77**:317, 1964.

247. Danpure CJ: Recent advances in the understanding, diagnosis and treatment of primary hyperoxaluria type 1. *J Inherit Metab Dis* **12**:210, 1989.
248. Dean BM, Watts RW, Westwick WJ: Metabolism of 1-^{14}C glyoxylate, 1-^{14}C glycollate, 1-^{14}C glycine and 2-^{14}C glycine by homogenates of kidney and liver tissue from hyperoxaluric and control subjects. *Biochem J* **105**:701, 1967.
249. Dean BM, Griffin WJ, Watts RW: Primary hyperoxaluria: The demonstration of a metabolic abnormality in kidney tissue. *Lancet* **1**:406, 1966.
250. Williams HE, Wilson M, Smith LH Jr: Studies on primary hyperoxaluria: 3. Transamination reactions of glyoxylate in human tissue preparations. *J Lab Clin Med* **70**:494, 1967.
251. Vandor SL, Tolbert NE: Glyoxylate metabolism by isolated rat liver peroxisomes. *Biochim Biophys Acta* **215**:449, 1970.
252. Hsieh B, Tolbert NE: Glyoxylate aminotransferase in peroxisomes from rat liver and kidney. *J Biol Chem* **251**:4408, 1976.
253. Noguchi T, Minatogawa Y, Takada Y, Okuno E, Kido R: Subcellular distribution of pyruvate (glyoxylate) aminotransferases in rat liver. *Biochem J* **170**:173, 1978.
254. Noguchi T, Okuno E, Takada Y, Minatogawa Y, Okai K, Kido R: Characteristics of hepatic alanine-glyoxylate aminotransferase in different mammalian species. *Biochem J* **169**:113, 1978.
255. Noguchi T, Takada Y, Oota Y: Intraperoxisomal and intramitochondrial localization, and assay of pyruvate (glyoxylate) aminotransferase from rat liver. *Hoppe Seylers Z Physiol Chem* **360**:919, 1979.
256. Noguchi T, Takada Y: Peroxisomal localization of serine:pyruvate aminotransferase in human liver. *J Biol Chem* **253**:7598, 1978.
257. Danpure CJ, Jennings PR: Peroxisomal alanine:glyoxylate aminotransferase deficiency in primary hyperoxaluria type I. *FEBS Lett* **201**:20, 1986.
258. Danpure CJ, Jennings PR: Deficiency of peroxisomal alanine:glyoxylate aminotransferase in primary hyperoxaluria type I, in Fahimi HD, Sies H (eds): *Peroxisomes in Biology and Medicine*. Berlin, Springer-Verlag, 1987, p 374.
259. Danpure CJ, Jennings PR: Further studies on the activity and subcellular distribution of alanine:glyoxylate aminotransferase in the livers of patients with primary hyperoxaluria type 1. *Clin Sci* **75**:315, 1988.
260. Danpure CJ, Jennings PR, Fryer P, Purdue PE, Allsop J: Primary hyperoxaluria type 1: Genotypic and phenotypic heterogeneity. *J Inherit Metab Dis* **17**:487, 1994.
261. Danpure CJ, Rumsby G: Enzymology and molecular genetics of primary hyperoxaluria type 1: Consequences for clinical management, in Khan SR (ed): *Calcium Oxalate in Biological Systems*. Boca Raton, FL, CRC Press, 1995, p 189.
262. Danpure CJ, Jennings PR: Alanine:glyoxylate and serine:pyruvate aminotransferases in primary hyperoxaluria type I. *Biochem Soc Trans* **14**:1059, 1986.
263. Noguchi T, Takada Y: Purification and properties of peroxisomal pyruvate (glyoxylate) aminotransferase from rat liver. *Biochem J* **175**:765, 1978.
264. Wise PJ, Danpure CJ, Jennings PR: Immunological heterogeneity of hepatic alanine:glyoxylate aminotransferase in primary hyperoxaluria type 1. *FEBS Lett* **222**:17, 1987.
265. Danpure CJ, Jennings PR: Enzymatic heterogeneity in primary hyperoxaluria type 1 (hepatic peroxisomal alanine:glyoxylate aminotransferase deficiency). *J Inherit Metab Dis* 11(suppl 2):205, 1988.
266. Cooper PJ, Danpure CJ, Wise PJ, Guttridge KM: Immunoelectron-microscopic localisation of alanine:glyoxylate aminotransferase in normal human liver and type 1 hyperoxaluric livers. *Biochem Soc Trans* **16**:627, 1988.
267. Danpure CJ, Cooper PJ, Wise PJ, Jennings PR: An enzyme trafficking defect in two patients with primary hyperoxaluria type 1: Peroxisomal alanine/glyoxylate aminotransferase rerouted to mitochondria. *J Cell Biol* **108**:1345, 1989.
268. Danpure CJ, Purdue PE, Fryer P, Griffiths S, Allsop J, Lumb MJ, Guttridge KM, Jennings PR, Scheinmann JL, Mauer SM, Davidson NO: Enzymological and mutational analysis of a complex primary hyperoxaluria type 1 phenotype involving alanine:glyoxylate aminotransferase peroxisome-to-mitochondrion mistargeting and intraperoxisomal aggregation. *Am J Hum Genet* **53**:417, 1993.
269. Iancu TC, Danpure CJ: Primary hyperoxaluria type I: Ultrastructural observations in liver biopsies. *J Inherit Metab Dis* **10**:330, 1987.
270. De Craemer D, Rickaert F, Wanders RJ, Roels F: Hepatic peroxisomes are smaller in primary hyperoxaluria type 1 (PH1): Cytochemistry and morphometry. *Micron Microsc Acta* **20**:125, 1989.
271. Takada Y, Mori T, Noguchi T: The effect of vitamin B6 deficiency on alanine:glyoxylate aminotransferase isoenzymes in rat liver. *Arch Biochem Biophys* **229**:1, 1984.
272. Van Veldhoven P, Debeer LJ, Mannaerts GP: Water- and solute-accessible spaces of purified peroxisomes: Evidence that peroxisomes are permeable to NAD^+. *Biochem J* **210**:685, 1983.
273. Van Veldhoven PP, Just WW, Mannaerts GP: Permeability of the peroxisomal membrane to cofactors of beta-oxidation: Evidence for the presence of a pore-forming protein. *J Biol Chem* **262**:4310, 1987.
274. Watts RW: Oxaluria. *J R Coll Phys Lond* **7**:161, 1973.
275. Barratt TM, Kasidas GP, Murdoch I, Rose GA: Urinary oxalate and glycolate excretion and plasma oxalate concentration. *Arch Dis Child* **66**:501, 1991.
276. Watts RW, Veall N, Purkiss P: Sequential studies of oxalate dynamics in primary hyperoxaluria. *Clin Sci* **65**:627, 1983.
277. Willis JE, Sallach HJ: Evidence for a mammalian D-glyceric dehydrogenase. *J Biol Chem* **237**:910, 1962.
278. Dawkins PD, Dickens F: The oxidation of D- and L-glycerate by rat liver. *Biochem J* **94**:353, 1965.
279. Mistry J, Danpure CJ, Chalmers RA: Hepatic D-glycerate dehydrogenase and glyoxylate reductase deficiency in primary hyperoxaluria type 2. *Biochem Soc Trans* **16**:626, 1988.
280. Williams HE, Smith LH Jr: Hyperoxaluria in l-glyceric aciduria: Possible pathogenic mechanism. *Science* **171**:390, 1971.
281. Raghavan KG, Richardson KE: Hyperoxaluria in l-glyceric aciduria: Possible nonenzymic mechanism. *Biochem Med* **29**:114, 1983.
282. Raghavan KG, Richardson KE: Hydroxypyruvate-mediated regulation of oxalate synthesis by lactate dehydrogenase and its relevance to primary hyperoxaluria type II. *Biochem Med* **29**:101, 1983.
283. Danpure CJ, Jennings PR, Mistry J, Chalmers RA, McKerrell RE, Blakemore WF, Heath MF: Enzymological characterization of a feline analogue of primary hyperoxaluria type 2: A model for the human disease. *J Inherit Metab Dis* **12**:403, 1989.
284. Craigen WJ: Persistent glycolic aciduria in a healthy child with normal alanine-glyoxylate aminotransferase activity. *J Inherit Metab Dis* **19**:793, 1996.
285. Van Acker KJ, Eyskens FJ, Espeel MF, Wanders RJ, Dekker C, Kerckaert IO, Roels F: Hyperoxaluria with hyperglycoluria not due to alanine:glyoxylate aminotransferase defect: A novel type of primary hyperoxaluria. *Kidney Int* **50**:1747, 1996.
286. Purdue PE, Lumb MJ, Fox M, Griffo G, Hamon Benais C, Povey S, Danpure CJ: Characterization and chromosomal mapping of a genomic clone encoding human alanine:glyoxylate aminotransferase. *Genomics* **10**:34, 1991.
287. Lu-Kuo J, Ward DC, Spritz RA: Fluorescence in situ hybridization mapping of 25 markers on distal human chromosome 2q surrounding the human Waardenburg syndrome, type1 (*WS1*) locus (*PAX3* gene). *Genomics* **16**:173, 1993.
288. Takada Y, Kaneko N, Esumi H, Purdue PE, Danpure CJ: Human peroxisomal L-alanine: glyoxylate aminotransferase: Evolutionary loss of a mitochondrial targeting signal by point mutation of the initiation codon. *Biochem J* **268**:517, 1990.
289. Nishiyama K, Berstein G, Oda T, Ichiyama A: Cloning and nucleotide sequence of cDNA encoding human liver serine-pyruvate aminotransferase. *Eur J Biochem* **194**:9, 1990.
290. Lee IS, Takio K, Kido R, Titani K: Purification and amino- and carboxyl-terminal amino acid sequences of alanine-glyoxylate transaminase 1 from human liver. *J Biochem (Tokyo)* **116**:12, 1994.
291. Purdue PE, Lumb MJ, Danpure CJ: Molecular evolution of alanine:glyoxylate aminotransferase 1 intracellular targeting: Analysis of the marmoset and rabbit genes. *Eur J Biochem* **207**:757, 1992.
292. Oda T, Miyajima H, Suzuki Y, Ichiyama A: Nucleotide sequence of the cDNA encoding the precursor for mitochondrial serine:pyruvate aminotransferase of rat liver. *Eur J Biochem* **168**:537, 1987.
293. Birdsey GM, Danpure CJ: Evolution of alanine:glyoxylate aminotransferase intracellular targeting: Structural and functional analysis of the guinea pig gene. *Biochem J* **331**:49, 1998.
294. Lumb MJ, Purdue PE, Danpure CJ: Molecular evolution of alanine/glyoxylate aminotransferase 1 intracellular targeting: Analysis of the feline gene. *Eur J Biochem* **221**:53, 1994.
295. von Schnakenburg C, Rumsby G: Primary hyperoxaluria type 1: A cluster of new mutations in exon 7 of the *AGXT* gene. *J Med Genet* **34**:489, 1997.
296. Purdue PE, Takada Y, Danpure CJ: Identification of mutations associated with peroxisome-to-mitochondrion mistargeting of alanine/glyoxylate aminotransferase in primary hyperoxaluria type 1. *J Cell Biol* **111**:2341, 1990.

297. Purdue PE, Lumb MJ, Allsop J, Danpure CJ: An intronic duplication in the alanine:glyoxylate aminotransferase gene facilitates identification of mutations in compound heterozygote patients with primary hyperoxaluria type 1. *Hum Genet* **87**:394, 1991.
298. Tarn AC, von Schnakenburg C, Rumsby G: Primary hyperoxaluria type 1: Diagnostic relevance of mutations and polymorphisms in the alanine:glyoxylate aminotransferase gene (*AGXT*). *J Inherit Metab Dis* **20**:689, 1997.
299. Danpure CJ, Birdsey GM, Rumsby G, Lumb MJ, Purdue PE, Allsop J: Molecular characterization and clinical use of a polymorphic tandem repeat in an intron of the human alanine:glyoxylate aminotransferase gene. *Hum Genet* **94**:55, 1994.
300. Attardi G, Schatz G: Biogenesis of mitochondria. *Annu Rev Cell Biol* **4**:289, 1988.
301. von Heijne G: Mitochondrial targeting sequences may form amphiphilic helices. *EMBO J* **5**:1335, 1986.
302. Gould SJ, Keller GA, Hosken N, Wilkinson J, Subramani S: A conserved tripeptide sorts proteins to peroxisomes. *J Cell Biol* **108**:1657, 1989.
303. Swinkels BW, Gould SJ, Subramani S: Targeting efficiencies of various permutations of the consensus C-terminal tripeptide peroxisomal targeting signal. *FEBS Lett* **305**:133, 1992.
304. Swinkels BW, Gould SJ, Bodnar AG, Rachubinski RA, Subramani S: A novel, cleavable peroxisomal targeting signal at the amino-terminus of the rat 3-ketoacyl-CoA thiolase. *EMBO J* **10**:3255, 1991.
305. Osumi T, Tsukamoto T, Hata S, Yokota S, Miura S, Fujiki Y, Hijikata M, Miyazawa S, Hashimoto T: Amino-terminal presequence of the precursor of peroxisomal 3-ketoacyl-CoA thiolase is a cleavable signal peptide for peroxisomal targeting. *Biochem Biophys Res Commun* **181**:947, 1991.
306. Eilers M, Schatz G: Protein unfolding and the energetics of protein translocation across biological membranes. *Cell* **52**:481, 1988.
307. McNew JA, Goodman JM: An oligomeric protein is imported into peroxisomes in vivo. *J Cell Biol* **127**:1245, 1994.
308. Glover JR, Andrews DW, Rachubinski RA: *Saccharomyces cerevisiae* peroxisomal thiolase is imported as a dimer. *Proc Natl Acad Sci USA* **91**:10541, 1994.
309. Motley A, Lumb MJ, Oatey PB, Jennings PR, De Zoysa PA, Wanders RJ, Tabak HF, Danpure CJ: Mammalian alanine:glyoxylate aminotransferase 1 is imported into peroxisomes via the PTS1 translocation pathway: Increased degeneracy and context specificity of the mammalian PTS1 motif and implications for the peroxisome-to-mitochondrion mistargeting of *AGT* in primary hyperoxaluria type 1. *J Cell Biol* **131**:95, 1995.
310. Oatey PB, Lumb MJ, Jennings PR, Danpure CJ: Context dependency of the PTS1 motif in human alanine:glyoxylate aminotransferase 1. *Ann NY Acad Sci* **804**:652, 1996.
311. Chou PY, Fasman GD: Prediction of protein structure. *Biochemistry* **13**:222, 1974.
312. Garnier J, Ogusthorpe DJ, Robson B: Analysis of the accuracy and implications of simple methods for predicting the secondary structure of globular proteins. *J Mol Biol* **120**:97, 1978.
313. Purdue PE, Allsop J, Isaya G, Rosenberg LE, Danpure CJ: Mistargeting of peroxisomal L-alanine:glyoxylate aminotransferase to mitochondria in primary hyperoxaluria patients depends upon activation of a cryptic mitochondrial targeting sequence by a point mutation. *Proc Natl Acad Sci USA* **88**:10900, 1991.
314. Leiper JM, Oatey PB, Danpure CJ: Inhibition of alanine:glyoxylate aminotransferase dimerization is a pre-requisite for its peroxisome-to-mitochondrion mistargeting in primary hyperoxaluria type 1. *J Cell Biol* **135**:939, 1996.
315. Leiper JM, Danpure CJ: A unique molecular basis for enzyme mistargeting in primary hyperoxaluria type 1. *Clin Chim Acta* **266**:39, 1997.
316. Danpure CJ, Jennings PR, Leiper JM, Lumb MJ, Oatey PB: Targeting of alanine:glyoxylate aminotransferase in normal individuals and its mistargeting in patients with primary hyperoxaluria type 1. *Ann NY Acad Sci* **804**:477, 1996.
317. Danpure CJ: Variable peroxisomal and mitochondrial targeting of alanine:glyoxylate aminotransferase in mammalian evolution and disease. *Bioessays* **19**:317, 1997.
318. Purdue PE, Lumb MJ, Allsop J, Minatogawa Y, Danpure CJ: A glycine-to-glutamate substitution abolishes alanine:glyoxylate aminotransferase catalytic activity in a subset of patients with primary hyperoxaluria type 1. *Genomics* **13**:215, 1992.
319. Nishiyama K, Funai T, Katafuchi R, Hattori F, Onoyama K, Ichiyama A: Primary hyperoxaluria type I due to a point mutation of T to C in the coding region of the serine:pyruvate aminotransferase gene. *Biochem Biophys Res Commun* **176**:1093, 1991.
320. Nishiyama K, Funai T, Yokota S, Ichiyama A: ATP-dependent degradation of a mutant serine: pyruvate/alanine:glyoxylate aminotransferase in a primary hyperoxaluria type 1 case. *J Cell Biol* **123**:1237, 1993.
321. Suzuki T, Nishiyama K, Funai T, Tanaka K, Ichihara A, Ichiyama A: Energy-dependent degradation of a mutant serine:pyruvate/alanin:-glyoxylate aminotransferase in a primary hyperoxaluria type 1 case. *Adv Exp Med Biol* **389**:137, 1996.
322. Danpure CJ, Fryer P, Jennings PR, Allsop J, Griffiths S, Cunningham A: Evolution of alanine:glyoxylate aminotransferase 1 peroxisomal and mitochondrial targeting: A survey of its subcellular distribution in the livers of various representatives of the classes Mammalia, Aves and Amphibia. *Eur J Cell Biol* **64**:295, 1994.
323. Yokota S, Oda T: Immunocytochemical demonstration of serine:pyruvate amino-transferase in peroxisomes and mitochondria of rat kidney. *Histochemistry* **83**:81, 1985.
324. Hayashi S, Noguchi T: Alanine: glyoxylate aminotransferase 1 is present in the peroxisomes of guinea pig kidney. *Biochem Biophys Res Commun* **166**:1467, 1990.
325. Danpure CJ, Jennings PR, Jansen JH: Enzymological characterization of a putative canine analogue of primary hyperoxaluria type 1. *Biochim Biophys Acta* **1096**:134, 1991.
326. Snell K, Walker DG: Regulation of hepatic L-serine dehydratase and L-serine-pyruvate aminotransferase in the developing neonatal rat. *Biochem J* **144**:519, 1974.
327. Rowsell EV, Al Tai AH, Carnie JA: Increased liver L-serine-pyruvate aminotransferase activity under gluconeogenic conditions. *Biochem J* **134**:349, 1973.
328. Danpure CJ, Guttridge KM, Fryer P, Jennings PR, Allsop J, Purdue PE: Subcellular distribution of hepatic alanine:glyoxylate aminotransferase in various mammalian species. *J Cell Sci* **97**:669, 1990.
329. Okuno E, Minatogawa Y, Nakanishi J, Nakamura M, Kamoda N, Makino M, Kido R: The subcellular distribution of alanine-glyoxylate aminotransferase and serine-pyruvate aminotransferase in dog liver. *Biochem J* **182**:877, 1979.
330. Yokota S, Oda T: Fine localization of serine:pyruvate aminotransferase in rat hepatocytes revealed by a post-embedding immunocytochemical technique. *Histochemistry* **80**:591, 1984.
331. Takada Y, Noguchi T: The evolution of peroxisomal and mitochondrial alanine:glyoxylate aminotransferase 1 in mammalian liver. *Biochem Biophys Res Commun* **108**:153, 1982.
332. Oda T, Funai T, Ichiyama A: Generation from a single gene of two mRNAs that encode the mitochondrial and peroxisomal serine: pyruvate aminotransferase of rat liver. *J Biol Chem* **265**:7513, 1990.
333. Yokota S, Funai T, Ichiyama A: Organelle localization of rat liver serine:pyruvate aminotransferase expressed in transfected COS-1 cells. *Biomed Res* **12**:53, 1991.
334. Oatey PB, Lumb MJ, Danpure CJ: Molecular basis of the variable mitochondrial and peroxisomal localisation of alanine:glyoxylate aminotransferase. *Eur J Biochem* **241**:374, 1996.
335. Kozak M: The scanning model for translation: an update. *J Cell Biol* **108**:229, 1989.
336. Kozak M: Structural features in eukaryotic mRNAs that modulate the initiation of translation. *J Biol Chem* **266**:19867, 1991.
337. Snell K: The regulation of rat liver l-alanine-glyoxylate aminotransferase by glucagon in vivo. *Biochem J* **123**:657, 1971.
338. Snell K: Mitochondrial-cytosolic interrelationships involved in gluconeogenesis from serine in rat liver. *FEBS Lett* **55**:202, 1975.
339. Snell K, Walker DG: The adaptive behaviour of isoenzyme forms of rat liver alanine aminotransferases during development. *Biochem J* **128**:403, 1972.
340. Rowsell EV, Snell K, Carnie JA, Al Tai AH: Liver L-alanine-glyoxylate and L-serine-pyruvate aminotransferase activities: an apparent association with gluconeogenesis. *Biochem J* **115**:1071, 1969.
341. Rowsell EV, Carnie JA, Wahbi SD, Al Tai AH, Rowsell KV: L-Serine dehydratase and L-serine-pyruvate aminotransferase activities in different animal species. *Comp Biochem Physiol [B]* **63**:543, 1979.
342. Noguchi T: Amino acid metabolism in animal peroxisomes, in Fahimi HD, Sies H (eds): *Peroxisomes in Biology and Medicine*. Berlin, Springer-Verlag, 1987, p 234.
343. Hayashi S, Sakuraba H, Noguchi T: Response of hepatic alanine:-glyoxylate aminotransferase 1 to hormone differs among mammalia. *Biochem Biophys Res Commun* **165**:372, 1989.

344. Oda T, Yanagisawa M, Ichiyama A: Induction of serine:pyruvate aminotransferase in rat liver organelles by glucagon and a high-protein diet. *J Biochem (Tokyo)* **91**:219, 1982.
345. Miyajima H, Oda T, Ichiyama A: Induction of mitochondrial serine:pyruvate aminotransferase of rat liver by glucagon and insulin through different mechanisms. *J Biochem (Tokyo)* **105**:500, 1989.
346. Oda T, Ichiyama A, Miura S, Mori M, Tatibana M: In vitro synthesis of a putative precursor of serine: pyruvate aminotransferase of rat liver mitochondria. *Biochem Biophys Res Commun* **102**:568, 1981.
347. Oda T, Nishiyama K, Ichiyama A: Characterization and sequence analysis of rat serine:pyruvate/alanine:glyoxylate aminotransferase gene. *Genomics* **17**:59, 1993.
348. Morris MP, Garcia-Rivera J: The destruction of oxalates by the rumen contents of cows. *J Dairy Sci* **38**:1169, 1955.
349. Dodson ME: Oxalate ingestion studies in the sheep. *Aust Vet J* **35**:225, 1959.
350. Watts PS: Decomposition of oxalic acid in vitro by rumen contents. *Aust J Agric Res* **8**:266, 1957.
351. Dawson KA, Allison MJ, Hartman PA: Isolation and some characteristics of anaerobic oxalate-degrading bacteria from the rumen. *Appl Environ Microbiol* **40**:833, 1980.
352. Dawson KA, Allison MJ, Hartman PA: Characteristics of anaerobic oxalate-degrading enrichment cultures from the rumen. *Appl Environ Microbiol* **40**:840, 1980.
353. Argenzio RA, Liacos JA, Allison MJ: Intestinal oxalate-degrading bacteria reduce oxalate absorption and toxicity in guinea pigs. *J Nutr* **118**:787, 1988.
354. Daniel SL, Hartman PA, Allison MJ: Microbial degradation of oxalate in the gastrointestinal tracts of rats. *Appl Environ Microbiol* **53**:1793, 1987.
355. Allison MJ, Littledike ET, James LF: Changes in ruminal oxalate degradation rates associated with adaptation to oxalate ingestion. *J Anim Sci* **45**:1173, 1977.
356. Allison MJ, Cook HM: Oxalate degradation by microbes of the large bowel of herbivores: The effect of dietary oxalate. *Science* **212**:675, 1981.
357. Takada Y, Noguchi T: Subcellular distribution, and physical and immunological properties of hepatic alanine:glyoxylate aminotransferase isoenzymes in different mammalian species. *Comp Biochem Physiol [B]* **72**:597, 1982.
358. Jansen JH, Arnesen K: Oxalate nephropathy in a Tibetan spaniel litter: A probable case of primary hyperoxaluria. *J Comp Pathol* **103**:79, 1990.
359. Blakemore WF, Heath MF, Bennett MJ, Cromby CH, Pollitt RJ: Primary hyperoxaluria and L-glyceric aciduria in the cat. *J Inherit Metab Dis* **11**(suppl 2):215, 1988.
360. McKerrell RE, Blakemore WF, Heath MF, Plumb J, Bennett MJ, Pollitt RJ, Danpure CJ: Primary hyperoxaluria (L-glyceric aciduria) in the cat: A newly recognised inherited disease. *Vet Rec* **125**:31, 1989.
361. Khan SR, Hackett RL: Calcium oxalate urolithiasis in the rat: Is it a model for human stone disease? A review of recent literature. *Scan Electron Microsc* **II**:759, 1985.
362. Khan SR: Experimental calcium oxalate nephrolithiasis and the formation of human urinary stones. *Scanning Microsc* **9**:89, 1995.
363. Byrd DJ, Latta K: Hyperoxaluria, in Blau N, Duran M, Blaskovics M (eds): *Physicians Guide to the Laboratory Diagnosis of Metabolic Diseases*. London, Chapman and Hall, 1996, p 375.
364. Wilson DA, Wenzl JE, Altshuler GP: Ultrasound demonstration of diffuse cortical nephrocalcinosis in a case of primary hyperoxaluria. *AJR* **132**:659, 1979.
365. Dietrich RB, Kangarloo H, Boechat MI, Fine RN: The significance of increased echogenicity in the detection and differentiation of pediatric disease. *Int J Pediatr Nephrol* **6**:215, 1985.
366. Rosenfield AT: Ultrasonic diagnosis of primary hyperoxaluria in infancy (letter). *Radiology* **148**:578, 1983.
367. Lindholm J: Intra-vitam diagnosis of oxalosis. *Acta Med Scand* **178**:155, 1965.
368. Gilboa N, Largent JA, Urizar RE: Primary oxalosis presenting as anuric renal failure in infancy: Diagnosis by x-ray diffraction of kidney tissue. *J Pediatr* **103**:88, 1983.
369. Murty ML, Garg I, Date A, Jacob CK, Kirubakaran MG, Shastry JC: Renal histology for the diagnosis of primary hyperoxaluria in patients with end-stage renal disease. *Nephron* **53**:81, 1989.
370. Petrarulo M, Bianco O, Marangella M, Pellegrino S, Linari F, Mentasti E: Ion chromatographic determination of plasma oxalate in healthy subjects, in patients with chronic renal failure and in cases of hyperoxaluric syndromes. *J Chromatogr* **511**:223, 1990.
371. Benhamou CL, Bardin T, Tourliere D, Voisin L, Audran M, Edouard C, Lafage MH, Sebert JL, de Vernejoul MC, Wendling D: Bone involvement in primary oxalosis: Study of 20 cases. *Rev Rhum Mal Osteoartic* **58**:763, 1991.
372. Niederwieser A, Matasovic A, Leumann EP: Glycolic acid in urine: A colorimetric method with values in normal adult controls and in patients with primary hyperoxaluria. *Clin Chim Acta* **89**:13, 1978.
373. Marangella M, Petrarulo M, Bianco O, Vitale C, Finocchiaro P, Linari F: Glycolate determination detects type I primary hyperoxaluria in dialysis patients. *Kidney Int* **39**:149, 1991.
374. Wolthers BG, Meijer S, Tepper T, Hayer M, Elzinga H: The determination of oxalate in haemodialysate and plasma: A means to detect and study "hyperoxaluria" in haemodialysed patients. *Clin Sci* **71**:41, 1986.
375. Kasidas GP: Assay of oxalate and glycollate in urine, in Rose GA (ed): *Oxalate Metabolism in Relation to Urinary Stone*. London, Springer-Verlag, 1988, p 7.
376. Kasidas GP: Assaying of oxalate in plasma, in Rose GA (ed): *Oxalate Metabolism in Relation to Urinary Stone*. London, Springer-Verlag, 1988, p 45.
377. Laker MF: The clinical chemistry of oxalate metabolism. *Adv Clin Chem* **23**:259, 1983.
378. Kasidas GP: Plasma and urine measurements for monitoring of treatment in the primary hyperoxaluric patient. *Nephrol Dial Transplant* **10**(suppl 8):8, 1995.
379. Danpure CJ, Jennings PR, Watts RW: Enzymological diagnosis of primary hyperoxaluria type 1 by measurement of hepatic alanine:-glyoxylate aminotransferase activity. *Lancet* **1**:289, 1987.
380. Morgan SH, Danpure CJ, Bending MR, Eisinger AJ: Exclusion of primary hyperoxaluria type I (PHI) in end-stage renal failure by enzymatic analysis of a percutaneous hepatic biopsy. *Nephron* **55**:336, 1990.
381. Allsop J, Jennings PR, Danpure CJ: A new micro-assay for human liver alanine:glyoxylate aminotransferase. *Clin Chim Acta* **170**:187, 1987.
382. Wanders RJ, Ruiter J, van Roermund CW, Schutgens RB, Ofman R, Jurriaans S, Tager JM: Human liver L-alanine-glyoxylate aminotransferase: characteristics and activity in controls and hyperoxaluria type I patients using a simple spectrophotometric method. *Clin Chim Acta* **189**:139, 1990.
383. Toone JR, Applegarth DA: Micromethod for the assay of glutamate:glyoxylate aminotransferase and modifications of a micromethod for the assay of alanine:glyoxylate aminotransferase: Implications for the prenatal diagnosis of type I hyperoxaluria by fetal liver biopsy. *Clin Chim Acta* **203**:105, 1991.
384. Petrarulo M, Pellegrino S, Marangella M, Cosseddu D, Linari F: High-performance liquid chromatographic microassay for L-alanine: glyoxylate aminotransferase activity in human liver. *Clin Chim Acta* **208**:183, 1992.
385. Horvath VA, Wanders RJ: Rapid identification of primary hyperoxaluria type I patients using a novel, fully automated method for measurement of hepatic alanine:glyoxylate aminotransferase. *J Inherit Metab Dis* **17**:336, 1994.
386. Horvath VA, Wanders RJ: Re-evaluation of conditions required for measurement of true alanine:glyoxylate aminotransferase activity in human liver: implications for the diagnosis of hyperoxaluria type I. *Ann Clin Biochem* **31**:361, 1994.
387. Andy V, Horvath P, Wanders RJ: Aminooxyacetic acid: A selective inhibitor of alanine: glyoxylate aminotransferase and its use in the diagnosis of primary hyperoxaluria type I. *Clin Chim Acta* **243**:105, 1995.
388. Rumsby G, Weir T, Samuell CT: A semiautomated alanine:glyoxylate aminotransferase assay for the tissue diagnosis of primary hyperoxaluria type 1. *Ann Clin Biochem* **34**:400, 1997.
389. Nakatani T, Kawasaki Y, Minatogawa Y, Okuno E, Kido R: Peroxisome localized human hepatic alanine-glyoxylate aminotransferase and its application to clinical diagnosis. *Clin Biochem* **18**:311, 1985.
390. Schutgens RB, Schrakamp G, Wanders RJ, Heymans HS, Tager JM, van den Bosch H: Prenatal and perinatal diagnosis of peroxisomal disorders. *J Inherit Metab Dis* **12**(suppl 1):118, 1989.
391. Wanders RJ, Schutgens RB, van den Bosch H, Tager JM, Kleijer WJ: Prenatal diagnosis of inborn errors in peroxisomal beta-oxidation. *Prenat Diagn* **11**:253, 1991.
392. Danpure CJ, Rumsby G: Strategies for the prenatal diagnosis of primary hyperoxaluria type 1. *Prenat Diagn* **16**:587, 1996.

393. Rose GA, Arthur LJ, Chambers TL, Kasidas GP, Scott IV: Successful treatment of primary hyperoxaluria in neonate (letter). *Lancet* **1**:1298, 1982.
394. Leumann E, Matasovic A, Niederwieser A: Primary hyperoxaluria type I: Oxalate and glycolate unsuitable for prenatal diagnosis. *Lancet* **2**:340, 1986.
395. Danpure CJ: Peroxisomal alanine:glyoxylate aminotransferase and prenatal diagnosis of primary hyperoxaluria type 1. *Lancet* **2**:1168, 1986.
396. Wanders RJ, van Roermund CW, Jurriaans S, Schutgens RB, Tager JM, van den Bosch H, Wolff ED, Przyrembel H, Berger R, Schaaphok FG: Diversity in residual alanine glyoxylate aminotransferase activity in hyperoxaluria type I: Correlation with pyridoxine responsiveness. *J Inherit Metab Dis* **11**(suppl 2):208, 1988.
397. Danpure CJ, Jennings PR, Penketh RJ, Wise PJ, Cooper PJ, Rodeck CH: Fetal liver alanine:glyoxylate aminotransferase and the prenatal diagnosis of primary hyperoxaluria type 1. *Prenat Diagn* **9**:271, 1989.
398. Zamboni L: Electron microscopic studies of blood embryogenesis in humans: I. The ultrastructure of the fetal liver. *J Ultrastruct Res* **12**:509, 1965.
399. Peschle C, Migliaccio G, Lazzaro D, Petti S, Mancini G, Care A, Russo G, Mastroberardino G, Migliaccio AR, Testa U: Hemopoietic development in human embryos. *Blood Cells* **10**:427, 1984.
400. Hoyes AD, Riches DJ, Martin BG: The fine structure of haemopoiesis in the human fetal liver: I. The haemopoietic precursor cells. *J Anat* **115**:99, 1973.
401. Grasso JA, Swift H, Ackerman GA: Observations on the development of erythrocytes in mammalian fetal liver. *J Cell Biol* **14**:235, 1962.
402. Cooper PJ, Danpure CJ, Penketh RJ: Prenatal differentiation of primary hyperoxaluria type 1 phenotypes in the first trimester using immuno-electron microscopy. *Clin Sci* **76**(suppl 20):13, 1989.
403. Espeel M, Jauniaux E, Hashimoto T, Roels F: Immunocytochemical localization of peroxisomal beta-oxidation enzymes in human fetal liver. *Prenat Diagn* **10**:349, 1990.
404. Danpure CJ, Jennings PR, Penketh RJ, Wise PJ, Rodeck CH: Prenatal exclusion of primary hyperoxaluria type 1. *Lancet* **1**:367, 1988.
405. Illum N, Lavard L, Danpure CJ, Horn T, Aerenlund Jensen H, Skovby F: Primary hyperoxaluria type 1: Clinical manifestations in infancy and prenatal diagnosis. *Child Nephrol Urol* **12**:225, 1992.
406. Danpure CJ, Cooper PJ, Jennings PR, Wise PJ, Penketh RJ, Rodeck CH: Enzymatic prenatal diagnosis of primary hyperoxaluria type 1: Potential and limitations. *J Inherit Metab Dis* **12**(suppl 2):286, 1989.
407. von Schnakenburg C, Weir T, Rumsby G: Linkage of microsatellites to the *AGXT* gene on chromosome 2q37.3 and their role in prenatal diagnosis of primary hyperoxaluria type 1. *Ann Hum Genet* **61**:365, 1997.
408. Rumsby G, Uttley WS, Kirk JM: First trimester diagnosis of primary hyperoxaluria type I (letter). *Lancet* **344**:1018, 1994.
409. Rumsby G, Mandel H, Avey C, Geraerts A: Polymorphisms in the alanine:glyoxylate aminotransferase gene and their application to the prenatal diagnosis of primary hyperoxaluria type 1. *Nephrol Dial Transplant* **10**(suppl 8):30, 1995.
410. Rumsby G: Experience in prenatal diagnosis of primary hyperoxaluria typ1. *J Nephrol* **11**(suppl 1):13, 1998.
411. Smith LH: The pathophysiology and medical treatment of urolithiasis. *Semin Nephrol* **10**:31, 1990.
412. Yendt ER, Cohanim M, Peters L: Reduction of urinary oxalate excretion in primary hyperoxaluria by diet. *Trans Am Clin Climatol Assoc* **91**:191, 1979.
413. Trinchieri A, Mandressi A, Luongo P, Longo G, Pisani E: The influence of diet on urinary risk factors for stones in healthy subjects and idiopathic renal calcium stone formers. *Br J Urol* **67**:230, 1991.
414. Smith LH: Diet and hyperoxaluria in the syndrome of idiopathic calcium oxalate urolithiasis. *Am J Kidney Dis* **17**:370, 1991.
415. Marangella M, Bianco O, Martini C, Petrarulo M, Vitale C, Linari F: Effect of animal and vegetable protein intake on oxalate excretion in idiopathic calcium stone disease. *Br J Urol* **63**:348, 1989.
416. Jaeger P, Portmann L, Jacquet AF, Burckhardt P: Influence of the calcium content of the diet on the incidence of mild hyperoxaluria in idiopathic renal stone formers. *Am J Nephrol* **5**:40, 1985.
417. Hodgkinson A, Pyrah LN: The urinary excretion of calcium and inorganic phosphate in 344 patients with calcium stone of renal origin. *Br J Surg* **46**:10, 1958.
418. Nordin BEC, Barry H, Bulusu L, Speed R: Dietary treatment of recurrent calcium stone disease, in Cifuentes Delatte L, Rapado A, Hodgkinson A (eds): *Urinary Calculi: Recent Advances in Aetiology, Stone Structure and Treatment*. Basel, Karger, 1973, p 170.
419. Peacock M, Knowles F, Nordin BEC: Effect of calcium administration and deprivation on serum and urine calcium in stone-forming and control subjects. *Br Med J* **2**:729, 1968.
420. Frederick EW, Rabkin MT, Smith LH, Jr. Primary hyperoxaluria: a defect in glyoxylate metabolism. *J Clin Invest* **41**:1358, 1962.
421. King JS, Wainer A: Glyoxylate metabolism in normal and stone-forming humans and the effect of allopurinol therapy. *Proc Soc Exp Biol Med* **128**:1162, 1968.
422. Gibbs DA, Watts RW: Oxalate formation from glyoxylate in primary hyperoxaluria: Studies on liver tissue. *Clin Sci* **32**:351, 1967.
423. Smith LH, Bauer RL, Craig JC, Williams HE: Inhibition of oxalate synthesis: In vitro studies using analogues of oxalate and glycolate. *Biochem Med* **6**:317, 1972.
424. Kameda K, Yanagawa M, Ichiyama A, Kawamura J: The role of glycolate oxidase in oxalogenesis: An effect of DL-2-hydroxy-3-butanoic acid as an inhibitor of glycolate oxidase. in Pak CY, Resnick MI, Preminger GM (eds): *Urolithiasis 1996 (Proceedings of the 8th International Symposium on Urolithiasis)*. Dallas, Millet the Printer, 1996, p 66.
425. Jayanthi S, Saravanan N, Varalakshmi P: Effect of DL-alpha-lipoic acid in glyoxylate-induced acute lithiasis. *Pharmacol Res* **30**:281, 1994.
426. Baker AL, Tolbert NE: Glycolate oxidase (ferredoxin-containing form). *Methods Enzymol* **9**:338, 1966.
427. Bais R, Rofe AM, Conyers RA: The inhibition of metabolic oxalate production by sulfhydryl compounds. *J Urol* **145**:1302, 1991.
428. Bringmann G, Feineis D, Hesselmann C, Schneider S, Koob M, Henschler D: A "chemical" concept for the therapy of glyoxylate-induced oxalurias. *Life Sci* **50**:1597, 1992.
429. Baker PW, Bais R, Rofe AM: Formation of the L-cysteine-glyoxylate adduct is the mechanism by which L-cysteine decreases oxalate production from glycollate in rat hepatocytes. *Biochem J* **302**:753, 1994.
430. Saravanan N, Senthil D, Varalakshmi P: Effect of L-cysteine on some urinary risk factors in experimental hyperoxaluric rats. *Br J Urol* **78**:22, 1996.
431. Baker PW, Bais R, Rofe AM: (*D*)-Penicillamine increases hepatic oxalate production resulting in hyperoxaluria. *J Urol* **157**:1130, 1997.
432. Baker PW, Bais R, Rofe AM: The efficacy of (*L*)-2-oxothiazolidine-4-carboxylate (OTC) and (*L*)-cysteine in reducing urinary oxalate excretion. *J Urol* **152**:2139, 1994.
433. Holmes RP, Assimos DG, Leaf CD, Whalen JJ: The effects of (*L*)-2-oxothiazolidine-4-carboxylate on urinary oxalate excretion. *J Urol* **158**:34, 1997.
434. Daniels RA, Michels R, Aisen P, Goldstein G: Familial hyperoxaluria. *Am J Med* **29**:820, 1960.
435. Archer HE, Dormer AE, Scowen EF, Watts RW: The aetiology of primary hyperoxaluria. *Br Med J* **1**:175, 1958.
436. Swartz D, Israels S: Primary hyperoxaluria. *J Urol* **90**:94, 1963.
437. Smith LH Jr, Williams HE: Treatment of primary hyperoxaluria. *Mod Treat* **4**:522, 1967.
438. Zarembski PM, Hodgkinson A, Cochran M: Treatment of primary hyperoxaluria with calcium carbimide. *New Engl J Med* **277**:1000, 1967.
439. Gibbs DA, Watts RW: Investigation of possible effect of calcium carbimide on urinary oxalate excretion in primary hyperoxaluria. *Arch Dis Child* **43**:313, 1968.
440. Solomons CC, Goodman SI, Riley CM: Treatment of hyperoxaluria. *New Engl J Med* **277**:1425, 1967.
441. Solomons CC, Goodman SI, Riley CM: Calcium carbimide in the treatment of primary hyperoxaluria. *New Engl J Med* **276**:207, 1967.
442. Fisher V, Watts RW: The metabolism of glyoxylate in blood from normal subjects and patients with primary hyperoxaluria. *Clin Sci* **34**:97, 1968.
443. Gibbs DA, Watts RW: The action of pyridoxine in primary hyperoxaluria. *Clin Sci* **38**:277, 1970.
444. Gibbs DA, Watts RW: The action of pyridoxine in primary hyperoxaluria. *Clin Sci* **37**:565, 1969.
445. Alinei P, Guignard JP, Jaeger P: Pyridoxine treatment of type 1 hyperoxaluria (letter). *New Engl J Med* **311**:798, 1984.
446. Watts RW, Veall N, Purkiss P, Mansell MA, Haywood EF: The effect of pyridoxine on oxalate dynamics in three cases of primary hyperoxaluria (with glycollic aciduria). *Clin Sci* **69**:87, 1985.
447. Yendt ER, Cohanim M: Response to a physiologic dose of pyridoxine in type I primary hyperoxaluria. *New Engl J Med* **312**:953, 1985.
448. Leumann E, Matasovic A, Niederwieser A: Pyridoxine in primary hyperoxaluria type I. *Lancet* **2**:699, 1986.

449. Ludwig GD: Renal calculi associated with hyperoxaluria. *Ann NY Acad Sci* **104**:621, 1963.
450. Amato M, Donzelli S, Lombardi M, Salvadori M, Carini M, Selli C, Caudarella R: Primary hyperoxaluria: Effect of treatment with vitamin B_6 and shock waves. *Contrib Nephrol* **58**:190, 1987.
451. de Zegher F, Przyrembel H, Chalmers RA, Wolff ED, Huijmans JG: Successful treatment of infantile type I primary hyperoxaluria complicated by pyridoxine toxicity. *Lancet* **2**:392, 1985.
452. Gershoff SN, Prien EL: Effect of daily MgO and vitamin B_6 administration to patients with recurring calcium oxalate kidney stones. *Am J Clin Nutr* **20**:393, 1967.
453. Greengard O, Gordon M: The cofactor-mediated regulation of apoenzyme levels in animal tissues: I. The pyridoxine-induced rise of rat liver tyrosine transaminase level in vivo. *J Biol Chem* **238**:3708, 1963.
454. Koul HK, Thind SK, Nath R: Oxalate binding to rat intestinal brush-border membrane in pyridoxine deficiency: A kinetic study. *Biochim Biophys Acta* **1064**:184, 1991.
455. Sidhu H, Gupta R, Farooqui S, Thind SK, Nath R: Absorption of glyoxylate and oxalate in thiamine and pyridoxine deficient rat intestine. *Biochem Int* **12**:71, 1986.
456. Gupta R, Sidhu H, Rattan V, Thind SK, Nath R: Oxalate uptake in intestinal and renal brush-border membrane vesicles (BBMV) in vitamin B_6-deficient rats. *Biochem Med Metab Biol* **39**:190, 1988.
457. Farooqui S, Nath R, Thind SK, Mahmood A: Effect of pyridoxine deficiency on intestinal absorption of calcium and oxalate: Chemical composition of brush border membranes in rats. *Biochem Med* **32**:34, 1984.
458. Danpure CJ: Scientific rationale for hepatorenal transplantation in primary hyperoxaluria type 1, in Touraine JL (ed): *Transplantation and Clinical Immunology, Vol 22*. Amsterdam, Excerpta Medica. 1991, p 91.
459. Watts RW, Calne RY, Williams R, Mansell MA, Veall N, Purkiss P, Rolles K: Primary hyperoxaluria (type I): Attempted treatment by combined hepatic and renal transplantation. *Q J Med* **57**:697, 1985.
460. Watts RW, Calne RY, Rolles K, Danpure CJ, Morgan SH, Mansell MA, Williams R, Purkiss P: Successful treatment of primary hyperoxaluria type I by combined hepatic and renal transplantation. *Lancet* **2**:474, 1987.
461. Cochat P, Faure JL, Divry P, Danpure CJ, Descos B, Wright C, Takvorian P, Floret D: Liver transplantation in primary hyperoxaluria type 1. *Lancet* **1**:1142, 1989.
462. McDonald JC, Landreneau MD, Rohr MS, DeVault GAJ: Reversal by liver transplantation of the complications of primary hyperoxaluria as well as the metabolic defect. *New Engl J Med* **321**:1100, 1989.
463. de Pauw L, Gelin M, Danpure CJ, Vereerstraeten P, Adler M, Abramowicz D, Toussaint C: Combined liver-kidney transplantation in primary hyperoxaluria type 1. *Transplantation* **50**:886, 1990.
464. Ruder H, Otto G, Schutgens RB, Querfeld U, Wanders RJ, Herzog KH, Wolfel P, Pomer S, Scharer K, Rose GA: Excessive urinary oxalate excretion after combined renal and hepatic transplantation for correction of hyperoxaluria type 1. *Eur J Pediatr* **150**:56, 1990.
465. Schurmann G, Scharer K, Wingen AM, Otto G, Herfarth C: Early liver transplantation for primary hyperoxaluria type 1 in an infant with chronic renal failure. *Nephrol Dial Transplant* **5**:825, 1990.
466. Jamieson NV, Watts RW, Evans DB, Williams R, Calne R: Liver and kidney transplantation in the treatment of primary hyperoxaluria. *Transplant Proc* **23**:1557, 1991.
467. Polinsky MS, Dunn S, Kaiser BA, Schulman SL, Wolfson BJ, Elfenbein IB, Baluarte HJ: Combined liver-kidney transplantation in a child with primary hyperoxaluria. *Pediatr Nephrol* **5**:332, 1991.
468. Rodby RA, Tyszka TS, Williams JW: Reversal of cardiac dysfunction secondary to type 1 primary hyperoxaluria after combined liver-kidney transplantation. *Am J Med* **90**:498, 1991.
469. Watts RW, Morgan SH, Danpure CJ, Purkiss P, Calne RY, Rolles K, Baker LR, Mansell MA, Smith LH, Merion RM, Lucey MR: Combined hepatic and renal transplantation in primary hyperoxaluria type I: Clinical report of nine cases. *Am J Med* **90**:179, 1991.
470. de Pauw L, Watts RW, Danpure CJ, Toussaint C: Which transplantation strategies in primary hyperoxaluria type 1? *Nephrologie* **12**:147, 1991.
471. Lloveras JJ, Dupre Goudable C, Rey JP, Sporer P, Durand D, Ton That H, Suc JM: The European experience of liver-kidney transplantation for primary hyperoxaluria type I: Prevention of recurrent intrarenal oxalate deposits. *Presse Med* **20**:2016, 1991.
472. Jouvet P, Hubert P, Jan D, Niaudet P, Beringer A, Narcy C, Daudon M, Broyer M, Revillon Y: Hepatic and renal transplantation in the treatment of type I hyperoxaluria. *Arch Fr Pediatr* **48**:637, 1991.
473. Toussaint C, de Pauw L, Vienne A, Gevenois PA, Quintin J, Gelin M, Pasteels JL: Radiological and histological improvement of oxalate osteopathy after combined liver-kidney transplantation in primary hyperoxaluria type 1. *Am J Kidney Dis* **21**:54, 1993.
474. Janssen F, Hall M, Schurmans T, de Pauw L, Hooghe L, Gelin M, Goyens P, Kinnaert P: Combined liver and kidney transplantation in primary hyperoxaluria type 1 in children. *Transplant Proc* **26**:110, 1994.
475. Coulthard MG, Lodge JP: Liver transplantation before advanced renal failure in primary hyperoxaluria type 1 (letter). *Pediatr Nephrol* **7**:774, 1993.
476. Uribarri J, Miller C, Burrows L: Combined liver-kidney transplantation: For the genetic disorder primary hyperoxaluria type I. *Mt Sinai J Med* **61**:32, 1994.
477. Fauchald P, Flatmark A, Jellum E, Sodal G, Jorstad S: Combined hepatic and renal transplantation in primary hyperoxaluria type 1 (PH1): Long-term results. *Transplant Proc* **26**:1799, 1994.
478. Bufi M, Rossi A, Costa MG, Riccini T, Picarazzi A, Calzecchi E, Antonelli M, Conti G: Primary hyperoxaluria: a case report of combined liver-kidney transplantation. *Transplant Proc* **26**:3645, 1994.
479. Solmos GR, Ali A, Rodby RA, Fordham EW: Rapid reversal of bone scan abnormalities in a patient with type 1 primary hyperoxaluria and oxalosis. *Clin Nucl Med* **19**:769, 1994.
480. Fyfe BS, Israel DH, Quish A, Squire A, Burrows L, Miller C, Sharma SK, Murthy S, Machac J: Reversal of primary hyperoxaluria cardiomyopathy after combined liver and renal transplantation. *Am J Cardiol* **75**:210, 1995.
481. Garnier JL, Boillot O, Gille D, Delafosse B, Colon S, Boujet C, Dubernard JM, Touraine JL: Combined liver-kidney transplantation for primary hyperoxaluria: A report of two cases. *Transplant Proc* **27**:1731, 1995.
482. Toussaint C, Vienne A, de Pauw L, Gelin M, Janssen F, Hall M, Schurmans T, Pasteels JL: Combined liver-kidney transplantation in primary hyperoxaluria type 1: Bone histopathology and oxalate body content. *Transplantation* **59**:1700, 1995.
483. Haffner D, Cochat P, Otto G, Steffen H, Scharer K: When should isolated liver transplantation be performed in primary hyperoxaluria type 1? Follow-up report of two children. *Nephrol Dial Transplant* **10**(suppl 8):47, 1995.
484. Latta A, Muller Wiefel DE, Sturm E, Kemper M, Burdelski M, Broelsch CE: Transplantation procedures in primary hyperoxaluria type 1. *Clin Nephrol* **46**:21, 1996.
485. Bunchman TE, Majors H, Majors G, Gardner JJ, DeVee J, Dennerll EM, Hesford JL, Mitchell CL, Punch JD: The infant with primary hyperoxaluria and oxalosis: from diagnosis to multiorgan transplantation. *Adv Ren Replace Ther* **3**:315, 1996.
486. Broyer M, Jouvet P, Niaudet P, Daudon M, Revillon Y: Management of oxalosis. *Kidney Int Suppl* **53**:S93, 1996.
487. Watts RW, Danpure CJ, de Pauw L, Toussaint C: Combined liver-kidney and isolated liver transplantations for primary hyperoxaluria type 1: The European experience. *Nephrol Dial Transpl* **6**:502, 1991.
488. Jamieson NV: The European Primary Hyperoxaluria Type 1 Transplant Registry report on the results of combined liver/kidney transplantation for primary hyperoxaluria 1984-1994. European PH1 Transplantation Study Group. *Nephrol Dial Transplant* **10**(suppl 8):33, 1995.
489. Jamieson NV: The results of combined liver/kidney transplantation for primary hyperoxaluria (PH1) 1984-1997. The European PH1 transplant registry report. *J Nephrol* **11**(suppl 1):36, 1998.
490. de Pauw L, Vienne A, Toussaint C: Crippling bone disease in a 15-year-old girl treated by haemodialysis. *Nephrol Dial Transplant* **11**:550, 1996.
491. Cochat P, Scharer K: Should liver transplantation be performed before advanced renal insufficiency in primary hyperoxaluria type 1? *Pediatr Nephrol* **7**:212, 1993.
492. Latta K, Jamieson NV, Scheinman JI, Scharer K, Bensman A, Cochat P, Legendre C, Ruder H, de Pauw L, Toussaint C: Selection of transplantation procedures and perioperative management in primary hyperoxaluria type 1. *Nephrol Dial Transplant* **10**(suppl 8):53, 1995.
493. Cochat P, Mahmoud A: Transplantation in primary hyperoxaluria type 1 (editorial). *Nephrol Dial Transplant* **10**:1293, 1995.
494. Scheinman JI, Alexander M, Campbell ED, Chan JC, Latta K, Cochat P: Transplantation for primary hyperoxaluria in the USA. *Nephrol Dial Transplant* **10**(suppl 8):42, 1995.
495. Jamieson NV: European PH1 transplant registry report on the results of combined liver/kidney transplantation for primary hyperoxaluria 1984 to 1992. European PHI Transplantation Study Group. *Transplant Proc* **27**:1234, 1995.

496. Scheinman JI: Recent data on results of isolated kidney or combined kidney/liver transplantation in the USA for primary hyperoxaluria. *J Nephrol* **11**(suppl 1):42, 1998.
497. Danpure CJ: Advances in the enzymology and molecular genetics of primary hyperoxaluria type 1: Prospects for gene therapy. *Nephrol Dial Transpl* **10**(suppl 8):24, 1995.
498. Lazarow PB, De Duve C: A fatty acyl-CoA oxidizing system in rat liver peroxisomes: Enhancement by clofibrate, a hypolipidemic drug. *Proc Natl Acad Sci USA* **73**:2043, 1976.
499. Hess R, Staubli W, Riess W: Nature of the hepatomegalic effect produced by ethyl-chlorophenoxy-isobutyrate in the rat. *Nature* **208**:856, 1965.
500. Svoboda DJ, Azarnoff DL: Response of hepatic microbodies to a hypolipidemic agent, ethyl chlorophenoxy isobutyrate (CPIB). *J Cell Biol* **30**:442, 1966.
501. Takada Y, Noguchi T: Increase in hepatic pyruvate (glyoxylate) aminotransferase activity on administration of clofibrate to the rat. *Biochem Pharmacol* **30**:393, 1981.
502. Yokota S: Quantitative immunocytochemical studies on differential induction of serine:pyruvate aminotransferase in mitochondria and peroxisomes of rat liver cells by administration of glucagon or di-(2-ethylhexyl)phthalate. *Histochemistry* **85**:145, 1986.
503. Panchenko LF, Popova SV, Antonenkov VD: Inducing effect of clofibrate on alkaline phosphatase and histidine-glyoxylate aminotransferase in rat liver. *Experientia* **38**:433, 1982.
504. Gariot P, Barrat E, Drouin P, Genton P, Pointel JP, Foliguet B, Kolopp M, Debry G: Morphometric study of human hepatic cell modifications induced by fenofibrate. *Metabolism* **36**:203, 1987.
505. Gariot P, Barrat E, Mejean L, Pointel JP, Drouin P, Debry G: Fenofibrate and human liver. Lack of proliferation of peroxisomes. *Arch Toxicol* **53**:151, 1983.
506. Blaauboer BJ, van Holsteijn CW, Bleumink R, Mennes WC, van Pelt FN, Yap SH, van Pelt JF, van Iersel AA, Timmerman A, Schmid BP: The effect of beclobric acid and clofibric acid on peroxisomal beta-oxidation and peroxisome proliferation in primary cultures of rat, monkey and human hepatocytes. *Biochem Pharmacol* **40**:521, 1990.
507. Sharma V, Schwille PO: Clofibrate feeding to Sprague-Dawley rats increases endogenous biosynthesis of oxalate and causes hyperoxaluria. *Metabolism* **46**:135, 1997.
508. Fukushima M, Aihara Y, Ichiyama A: Immunochemical studies on induction of rat liver mitochondrial serine:pyruvate aminotransferase by glucagon. *J Biol Chem* **253**:1187, 1978.
509. Holmes RP, Nataluk E, Poore RE, Assimos DG: Oxalate synthesis by Hep G2 cells, in Pak CY, Resnick MI, Preminger GM (eds): *Urolithiasis 1996 (Proceedings of the 8th International Symposium on Urolithiasis)*. Dallas, Millet the Printer, 1996, p 42.
510. Lung HY, Cornelius JG, Peck AB: Cloning and expression of the oxalyl-CoA decarboxylase gene from the bacterium, *Oxalobacter formigenes*: Prospects for gene therapy to control Ca-oxalate kidney stone formation. *Am J Kidney Dis* **17**:381, 1991.
511. Raghavan KG, Tarachand U: Degradation of oxalate in rats implanted with immobilized oxalate oxidase. *FEBS Lett* **195**:101, 1986.
512. Hubbard AR, Sprandel U, Chalmers RA: Organic-acid transport in resealed haemoglobin-containing human erythrocyte "ghosts." *Biochem J* **190**:653, 1980.
513. Howard JE, Thomas WC: Control of crystallization in urine. *Am J Med* **45**:693, 1968.
514. Butz M, Klan R, Karadzic G: First long-term results of oxalate stone prevention by alkali citrate. *Urol Res* **14**:95, 1986.
515. Leumann E, Hoppe B, Neuhaus T: Management of primary hyperoxaluria: Efficacy of oral citrate administration. *Pediatr Nephrol* **7**:207, 1993.
516. Leumann E, Hoppe B, Neuhaus T, Blau N: Efficacy of oral citrate administration in primary hyperoxaluria. *Nephrol Dial Transplant* **10**(suppl 8):14, 1995.
517. Elliot JS, Eusebio E: Calcium oxalate solubility: The effect of trace metals. *Invest Urol* **4**:428, 1967.
518. Sutor DJ: The possible use of methylene blue in the treatment of primary hyperoxaluria. *Br J Urol* **42**:389, 1970.
519. Maclagan NF, Anderson AJ: Some observations on urinary colloids in relation to renal calculi. *Br J Urol* **30**:269, 1958.
520. Silver L, Brendler H: Use of magnesium oxide in management of familial hyperoxaluria. *J Urol* **106**:274, 1971.
521. Thomas WC, Miller GH: Inorganic phosphates in the treatment of renal calculi. *Mod Treat* **4**:494, 1967.
522. Lyon ES, Borden TA, Ellis JE, Vermeulen CW: Calcium oxalate lithiasis produced by pyridoxine deficiency and inhibition with high magnesium diets. *Invest Urol* **4**:133, 1966.
523. Dent CE, Stamp TC: Treatment of primary hyperoxaluria. *Arch Dis Child* **45**:735, 1970.
524. Smith LH, Thomas WC, Arnaud CD: Orthophosphate therapy in calcium renal lithiasis, in Cifuentes Delatte L, Rapado A, Hodgkinson A (eds): *Urinary Calculi: Recent Advances in Aetiology, Stone Structure and Treatment*. Basel, Karger, 1973, p 188.
525. Milliner DS, Eickholt JT, Bergstralh E, Wilson DM, Smith LH: Results of long-term treatment with orthophosphate and pyridoxine in patients with primary hyperoxaluria. *New Engl J Med* **331**:1553, 1994.
526. Boddy SA, Duffy PG, Barratt TM, Whitfield HN: Hyperoxaluria and renal calculi in children: The role of extracorporeal shock wave lithotripsy. *J R Soc Med* **81**:604, 1988.
527. Grateau G, Grunfeld JP, Beurton D, Hannedouche T, Crosnier J: Post-surgical deterioration of renal function in primary hyperoxaluria. *Nephrol Dial Transplant* **1**:261, 1987.
528. Watts RW: Treatment of renal failure in the primary hyperoxalurias. *Nephron* **56**:1, 1990.
529. Saxon A: Hemodialysis for oxaluric renal failure. *New Engl J Med* **288**:526, 1973.
530. Walls J, Morley AR, Kerr DN: Primary hyperoxaluria in adult siblings: With some observations on the role of regular haemodialysis therapy. *Br J Urol* **41**:546, 1969.
531. Blackburn WE, McRoberts JW, Bhathena D, Vazquez M, Luke RG: Severe vascular complications in oxalosis after bilateral nephrectomy. *Ann Intern Med* **82**:44, 1975.
532. Zarembski PM, Rosen SM, Hodgkinson A: Dialysis in the treatment of primary hyperoxaluria. *Br J Urol* **41**:530, 1969.
533. Jacobsen E, Mosbaek N: Primary hyperoxaluria, treated with haemodialysis and kidney transplantation. *Dan Med Bull* **21**:72, 1974.
534. Watts RW, Veall N, Purkiss P: Oxalate dynamics and removal rates during haemodialysis and peritoneal dialysis in patients with primary hyperoxaluria and severe renal failure. *Clin Sci* **66**:591, 1984.
535. Ahmad S, Hatch M: Hyperoxalemia in renal failure and the role of hemoperfusion and hemodialysis in primary oxalosis. *Nephron* **41**:235, 1985.
536. Skinner R, Tomson CR, Tapson JS: Long term survival on haemodialysis in primary hyperoxaluria. *Int J Artif Organs* **13**:412, 1990.
537. Calzavara P, Vianello A, Calconi G, Maresca MC, Da Porto A, Bertolone G: Long survival in hemodialysed patients with oxalosis. *Int J Artif Organs* **14**:380, 1991.
538. Bunchman TE, Swartz RD: Oxalate removal in type I hyperoxaluria or acquired oxalosis using HD and equilibration PD. *Perit Dial Int* **14**:81, 1994.
539. Morgan JM, Hartley MW, Miller AC Jr, Diethelm AG: Successful renal transplantation in hyperoxaluria. *Arch Surg* **109**:430, 1974.
540. Halverstadt DB, Wenzl JE: Primary hyperoxaluria and renal transplantation. *J Urol* **111**:398, 1974.
541. Saxon A, Busch GJ, Merrill JP, Franco V, Wilson RE: Renal transplantation in primary hyperoxaluria. *Arch Intern Med* **133**:464, 1974.
542. Koch B, Irvine AH, Barr JR, Poznanski WJ: Three kidney transplantations in a patient with primary hereditary hyperoxaluria. *Can Med Assoc J* **106**:1323, 1972.
543. Leumann EP, Wegmann W, Largiader F: Prolonged survival after renal transplantation in primary hyperoxaluria of childhood. *Clin Nephrol* **9**:29, 1978.
544. Klauwers J, Wolf PL, Cohn R: Failure of renal transplantation in primary oxalosis. *JAMA* **209**:551, 1969.
545. Deodhar SD, Tung KS, Zuhlke V, Nakamoto S: Renal homotransplantation in a patient with primary familial oxalosis. *Arch Pathol* **87**:118, 1969.
546. Knols G, Leunissen KM, Spaapen LJ, Bosman FT, van der Wiel TW, Kootstra G, van Hooff JP: Recurrence of nephrocalcinosis after renal transplantation in an adult patient with primary hyperoxaluria type I. *Nephrol Dial Transplant* **4**:137, 1989.
547. Scheinman JI, Najarian JS, Mauer SM: Successful strategies for renal transplantation in primary oxalosis. *Kidney Int* **25**:804, 1984.
548. Katz A, Kim Y, Scheinman J, Najarian JS, Mauer SM: Long-term outcome of kidney transplantation in children with oxalosis. *Transplant Proc* **21**:2033, 1989.

549. Thervet E, Legendre C, Daudon M, Chretien Y, Mejean A, Jungers P, Mamzer Bruneel MF, Chauveau D, Kreis H, Is there a place for isolated renal transplantation in the treatment of primary hyperoxaluria type 1? Experience from Paris. *Nephrol Dial Transplant* **10**(suppl 8):38, 1995.
550. Cramer SD, Lin K, Holmes RP: Towards identification of the gene responsible for primary hyperoxaluria type 2: A cDNA encoding human D-glycerate dehydrogenase (abstract). *J Urol* **159**(suppl):173, 1998.
551. Antonenkov VD, Pirozhkov SV, Panchenko LF: Aldehyde dehydrogenase in mammalian peroxisomes, in Fahimi HD, Sies H (eds): *Peroxisomes in Biology and Medicine*. Berlin, Springer-Verlag, 1987, p 244.
552. Leiper JM, Danpure CJ: The role of dimerization of alanine:glyoxylate aminotransferase 1 in its peroxisomal and mitochondrial import. *Ann NY Acad Sci* **804**:765, 1996.
553. von Schnakenburg C: *Molecular analysis of the AGXT* gene and linkage studies in primary hyperoxaluria type 1. PhD thesis, University of London, 1998.
554. Minatogawa Y, Tone S, Allsop J, Purdue PE, Takada Y, Danpure CJ, Kido R: A serine-to-phenylalanine substitution leads to loss of alanine:glyoxylate aminotransferase catalytic activity and immunoreactivity in a patient with primary hyperoxaluria type 1. *Hum Mol Genet* **1**:643, 1992.
555. von Schnakenburg C, Hulton SA, Milford DV, Roper HP, Rumsby G: Variable presentation of primary hyperoxaluria type 1 in 2 patients homozygous for a novel combined deletion and insertion mutation in exon 8 of the *AGXT* gene. *Nephron* **78**:485, 1998.
556. Danpure CJ: Advances in the molecular biology of primary hyperoxaluria type 1 and their consequences for clinical management, in Jungers P, Daudon M (eds): *Renal Stone Disease: Crystallization Processes, Pathophysiology, Metabolic Disorders and Prevention.* Amsterdam, Elsevier, 1997, p 35.
557. Okuno E, Minatogawa Y, Nakamura M, Kamoda N, Nakanishi J, Makino M, Kido R: Crystallization and characterization of human liver kynurenine-glyoxylate aminotransferase: Identity with alanine-glyoxylate aminotransferase and serine-pyruvate aminotransferase. *Biochem J* **189**:581, 1980.
558. Hayashi H, Fukui K, Yamasaki F: Association of the liver peroxisomal fatty acyl-CoA beta-oxidation system with the synthesis of bile acids. *J Biochem (Tokyo)* **96**:1713, 1984.
559. Lumb MJ, Drake AF, Danpure CJ: Effect of N-terminal α-helix formation on the dimerization and intracellular targeting of alanine:-glyoxylate aminotransferase. *J Biol Chem* **274**:20587, 1999.

STANDARD ABBREVIATIONS

Abbreviation	Name
ACTH	corticotropin (adrenocorticotropin, adrenocorticotropic hormone)
ADA	adenosine deaminase
AdoMet	s-adenosylmethionine
Ag	antigen
AIDS	acquired immunodeficiency syndrome
ALT	alanine aminotransferase
AMP, ADP, and ATP*	adenosine 5′-mono-, di-, and triphosphates
AP1, AP2	activator protein 1, 2; transcription factors
apo A-I	apolipoprotein A-I
apo A-II	apolipoprotein A-II
apo A-III	apolipoprotein A-III
apo B	apolipoprotein B
apo C-I	apolipoprotein C-I
apo C-II	apolipoprotein C-II
apo C-III	apolipoprotein C-III
apo D	apolipoprotein D
apo E	apolipoprotein E
APRT	adenine phosphoribosyltransferase
ASO	allele-specific oligonucleotide
AST	aspartate aminotransferase
ATPase	adenosine triphosphate
α_1AT	α_1-antitrypsin
B cell	B lymphocyte
BAC	bacterial artificial chromosome
cAMP, cGMP, etc.	cyclic AMP (adenosine 3′: 5′-monophosphate), etc.
CAT	chloramphenicol acetyltransferase
CD	cluster of differentiation or cluster determinant (e.g., CD34)
cDNA	complementary DNA
CHO cells	Chinese hamster ovary cells
CoA (or CoASH)	coenzyme A
CoASAc	acetyl coenzyme A
cM	centimorgan
Cm-cellulose	O-(carboxymethyl)cellulose
CMP, CDP, and CTP*	cytidine 5′-mono-, di-, and triphosphates
CNS	central nervous system
COS cells	CV-I origin, SV40; cells widely used for transfection studies
CPK	creatine phosphokinase
CRM, CRM$^+$, CRM$^-$	cross-reacting material, CRM positive, CRM negative
CT	computerized tomography
CVS	chorionic villus sampling
DEAE-cellulose	O-(diethylaminoethyl)cellulose
DNA	deoxyribonucleic acid
DNase	deoxyribonuclease
DOPA	3,4-dihydroxyphenylalanine
DPN, DPN$^+$, DPNH$^+$	diphosphopyridine nucleotide and its oxidized and reduced forms
DPT	diphtheria, pertussis, tetanus vaccine
dTMP, dTDP, and dTTP*	thymidine 5′-mono-, di-, and triphosphates
DTT	dithiothreitol
EBV	Epstein-Barr virus
EDTA	ethylenediaminetetraacetate
EEG	electroencephalogram
EGF	epidermal growth factor
EGTA	[ethylenebis(oxyethylenenitrilo)] tetraacetic acid
EKG	electrocardiogram
ELISA	enzyme-linked immunosorbent assay
EM	electron microscopy or microscopic
ER	endoplasmic reticulum
ES cells	embryonic stem cells
FAD and FADH$_2$	flavin-adenine dinucleotide and its fully reduced form
FISH	fluorescence *in situ* hybridization
FITC	fluorescein isothiocyanate
FMN	riboflavin 5′-phosphate
G, G$_i$, G$_s$	guanine nucleotide binding protein, inhibitory form, stimulatory form
G-6-PD	glucose 6-phosphate dehydrogenase
GABA	γ-aminobutyric acid
GC	gas chromatography
GC/MS	gas chromatography/mass spectroscopy
GERL	Golgi endoplasmic reticulum-like
GFR	glomerular filtration rate
GMP, GDP, and GTP*	guanosine 5′-mono-, di-, and triphosphates
GSH and GSSG	glutathione and its oxidized form
Hb, HbCO, HbO$_2$	hemoglobin, carbon monoxide hemoglobin, oxyhemoglobin
HDL	high density lipoprotein
HEPES	4-(2-hydroxyethyl)-1-piperazine ethanesulfonic acid
Hep G2	hepatocellular carcinoma human cell line
HIV	human immunodeficiency virus
HLA	human leukocyte antigens
HMG-CoA	3-hydroxy-3-methylglutaryl-coenzyme A
HPLC	high performance (or pressure) liquid chromotography
HPRT	hypoxanthine-guanine phosphoribosyltransferase
IDDM	insulin-dependent diabetes mellitus
IFN	interferon
Ig	immunoglobulin
IgA	gamma A immunoglobulin
IgG	gamma G immunoglobulin
IgM	gamma M immunoglobulin
IL	interleukin, including IL-1, IL-2, etc.
IM or i.m.	intramuscular
IMP, IDP, and ITP*	inosine 5′-mono-, di, and triphosphates
LDH	lactate dehydrogenase
LDL	low density lipoproteins
LINE	long interspersed repeat element
lod	logarithm of the odds
MCH	erythrocyte mean corpuscular hemoglobin
MCHC	erythrocyte mean corpuscular hemoglobin concentration
MCV	erythrocyte mean corpuscular volume
MHC	histocompatibility complex
MPS	mucopolysaccharide or mucopolysaccharidosis
MRI	magnetic resonance imaging
mRNA	messenger RNA
MS	mass spectrometry
mtDNA, mtRNA	mitochondrial DNA, RNA
Myc	oncogene homologous to avian myelocytomatosis virus including *c-myc*, N-*myc*, and L-*myc*
NAD, NAD$^+$, and NADH†	nicotinamide adenine dinucleotide and its oxidized and reduced forms
NADP, NADP$^+$, and NADPH†	nicotinamide adenine dinucleotide phosphate and its oxidized and reduced forms
NIDDM	non-insulin-dependent diabetes mellitus

(Continues)

STANDARD ABBREVIATIONS (*Cont.*)

Abbreviation	Name	Abbreviation	Name
NK cells	natural killer cells	SE	standard error
NMN	nicotinamide mononucleotide	SEM	standard error of mean
NMR	nuclear magnetic resonance	SER	smooth endoplasmic reticulum
p	probability	SH1, SH2, SH3	Src homology domains 1, 2, 3
P_i	inorganic phosphate		
PAC	P1-derived artificial chromosome	SNP	single nucleotide polymorphism
PAS	periodic acid Schiff	*src*	oncogene homologous to Rous sarcoma virus
PCR	polymerase chain reaction	SSCP	single strand conformational polymorphism
PEG	polyethylene glycol	STR	short tandem repeat
PFGE	pulsed-field gel electrophoresis	SV40	Simian virus 40
PKA	protein kinase A	T_3	triiodothyronine
PKC	protein kinase C	T_4	thyroxine
PKU	phenylketonuria	T cell	T lymphocyte
PP_i	inorganic pyrophosphate	TMP, TDP, and TTP*	ribosylthymine 5′-mono-, di-, and triphosphates
PP-ribose-P	phosphoribosylpyrophosphate		
ras	oncogenes homologous to sarcoma retroviruses including HRAS, KRAS, and NRAS, H-*ras*, K-*ras*, and N-*ras*	TNF	tumor necrosis factor (e.g. TNF-1)
		TPN, TPN^+, TPNH†	triphosphopyridine nucleotide and its oxidized and reduced forms
RER	rough endoplasmic reticulum	Tris	tris(hydroxymethyl)aminomethane
RFLP	restriction fragment length polymorphism	tRNA	transfer RNA
RIA	radioimmunoassay	UDP-Gal	uridine diphosphogalactose
rRNA	ribosomal RNA	UDP-Glc	uridine diphosphoglucose
RNase	ribonuclease	UMP, UDP, and UTP*	uridine 5′-mono-, di-, and triphosphates
RT-PCR	reverse transcription-polymerase chain reaction		
		UV	ultraviolet light
SD	standard deviation	VLDL	very low density lipoprotein
SDS	sodium dodecyl sulfate	VNTR	variable number tandem repeat
SDS-PAGE	sodium dodecyl sulfate polyacrylamide gel electrophoresis	YAC	yeast artificial chromosome

*The d prefix may be used to represent the corresponding deoxyribonucleoside phosphates, e.g., dADP.
†Note that DPN = NAD and TPN = NADP.

AMINO ACID SYMBOLS

Name	Symbols		Name	Symbols	
alanine	Ala	A	leucine	Leu	L
arginine	Arg	R	lysine	Lys	K
asparagine	Asn	N	methionine	Met	M
aspartic acid	Asp	D	phenylalanine	Phe	F
cysteine	Cys	C	proline	Pro	P
glutamic acid	Glu	E	serine	Ser	S
glutamine	Gln	Q	threonine	Thr	T
glycine	Gly	G	tryptophan	Trp	W
histidine	His	H	tyrosine	Tyr	Y
isoleucine	Ile	I	valine	Val	V

CARBOHYDRATE SYMBOLS

Name	Symbols	Name	Symbols
fructose	Fru	N-acetylgalactosamine	GalNAc
fucose	Fuc	N-acetylglucosamine	GlcNAc
galactose	Gal	N-acetylneuraminic acid	NeuAc
glucosamine	GlcN	ribose	Rib
glucose	Glc	sialic acid	Sia
glucuronic acid	GlcA	xylose	Xyl
mannose	Man		

INDEX

Page numbers followed by an "f" indicate figures; numbers followed by a "t" indicate tables.

ISBN 0-07-913035-6

90000

9 780079 130358

SCRIVER/MMBID, 8E SET

ISBN 0-07-136320-3

90000

9 780071 363204

SCRIVER/MMBID, 8E VOLII

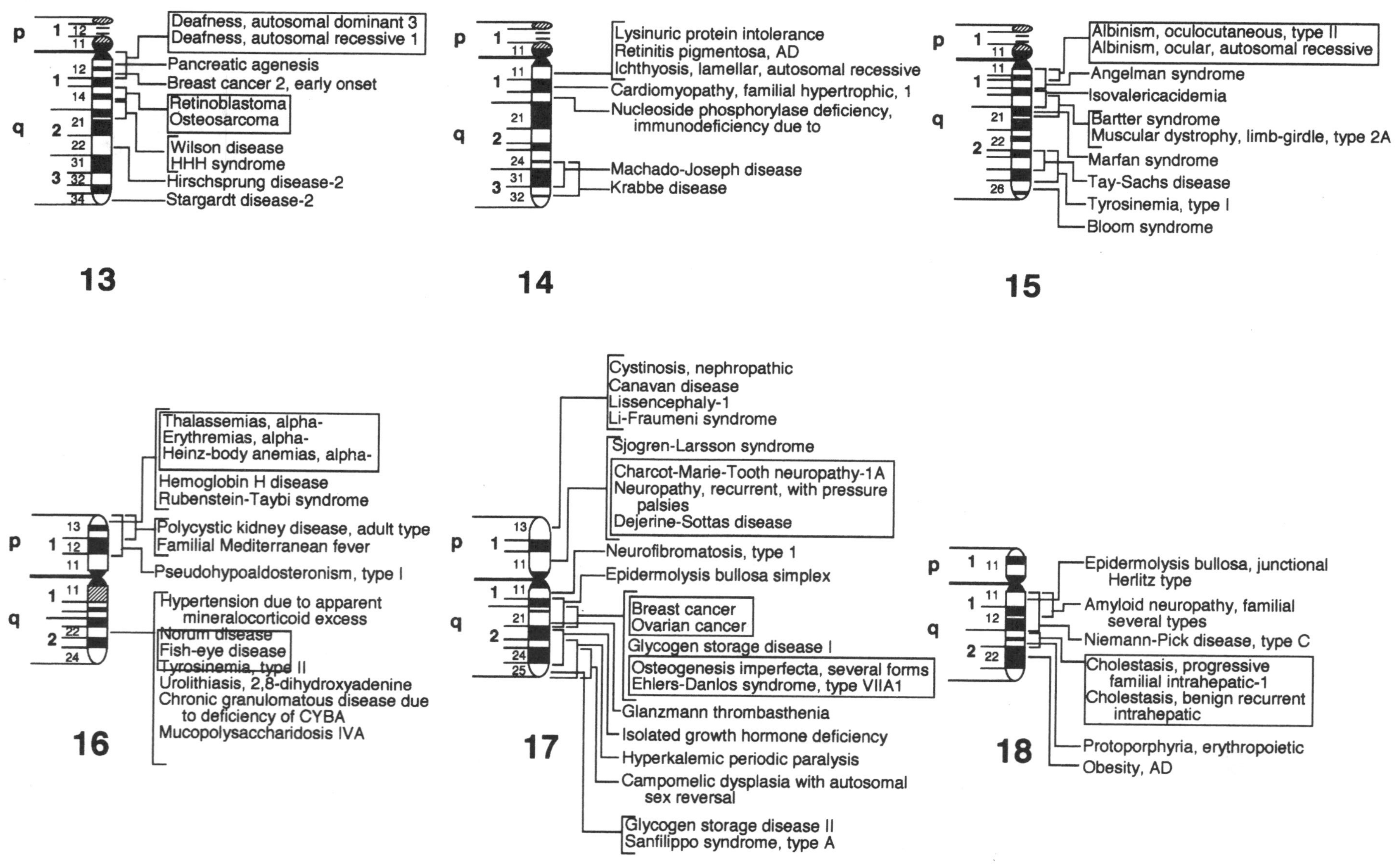

Deafness, autosomal dominant 3
Deafness, autosomal recessive 1
Pancreatic agenesis
Breast cancer 2, early onset
Retinoblastoma
Osteosarcoma
Wilson disease
HHH syndrome
Hirschsprung disease-2
Stargardt disease-2
13
Lysinuric protein intolerance
Retinitis pigmentosa, AD
Ichthyosis, lamellar, autosomal recessive
Cardiomyopathy, familial hypertrophic, 1
Nucleoside phosphorylase deficiency, immunodeficiency due to
Machado-Joseph disease
Krabbe disease
14
Albinism, oculocutaneous, type II
Albinism, ocular, autosomal recessive
Angelman syndrome
Isovalericacidemia
Bartter syndrome
Muscular dystrophy, limb-girdle, type 2A
Marfan syndrome
Tay-Sachs disease
Tyrosinemia, type I
Bloom syndrome
15
Thalassemias, alpha-
Erythremias, alpha-
Heinz-body anemias, alpha-
Hemoglobin H disease
Rubenstein-Taybi syndrome
Polycystic kidney disease, adult type
Familial Mediterranean fever
Pseudohypoaldosteronism, type I
Hypertension due to apparent mineralocorticoid excess
Norum disease
Fish-eye disease
Tyrosinemia, type II
Urolithiasis, 2,8-dihydroxyadenine
Chronic granulomatous disease due to deficiency of CYBA
Mucopolysaccharidosis IVA
16
Cystinosis, nephropathic
Canavan disease
Lissencephaly-1
Li-Fraumeni syndrome
Sjogren-Larsson syndrome
Charcot-Marie-Tooth neuropathy-1A
Neuropathy, recurrent, with pressure palsies
Dejerine-Sottas disease
Neurofibromatosis, type 1
Epidermolysis bullosa simplex
Breast cancer
Ovarian cancer
Glycogen storage disease I
Osteogenesis imperfecta, several forms
Ehlers-Danlos syndrome, type VIIA1
Glanzmann thrombasthenia
Isolated growth hormone deficiency
Hyperkalemic periodic paralysis
Campomelic dysplasia with autosomal sex reversal
Glycogen storage disease II
Sanfilippo syndrome, type A
17
Epidermolysis bullosa, junctional Herlitz type
Amyloid neuropathy, familial several types
Niemann-Pick disease, type C
Cholestasis, progressive familial intrahepatic-1
Cholestasis, benign recurrent intrahepatic
Protoporphyria, erythropoietic
Obesity, AD
18